Essential Surgical Practice

Higher Surgical Training in General Surgery

Fourth edition

Edited by

Sir Alfred Cuschieri MD(Malta) MD(Liverpool) ChM(Liverpool) FRSE FRCS(Ed) FRCS(Eng) FRCS(Glas) FRCSI FMedSci FIBiol

Professor of Surgery and Honorary Consultant Surgeon
Department of Surgery and Molecular Oncology, University of Dundee
Honorary Consultant Surgeon, Tayside University Hospitals NHS Trust

Robert J. C. Steele MD FRCS(Ed) FRCS(Eng) FCS(Hong Kong)

Professor and Head of Surgical Oncology and Honorary Consultant Surgeon
Department of Surgery and Molecular Oncology, University of Dundee
Honorary Consultant Surgeon, Tayside University Hospitals NHS Trust

Abdool Rahim Moossa MD FRCS(Eng) FACS

Professor and Chairman, Surgeon-in-Chief, Department of Surgery
University of California, San Diego Medical Center

ARNOLD

A member of the Hodder Headline Group
LONDON • NEW YORK • NEW DELHI

First published in 1982 by Butterworth Heinemann
Second edition in 1988 by Butterworth Heinemann
Third edition in 1995 by Butterworth Heinemann
Fourth edition published in 2002
by Arnold, a member of the Hodder Headline Group,
338 Euston Road, London NW1 3BH

http://www.arnoldpublishers.com

Distributed in the United States of America by
Oxford University Press Inc.,
198 Madison Avenue, New York, NY 10016
Oxford is a registered trademark of Oxford University Press

British Library Cataloguing in Publication Data
A catalogue record for this book is available from the British Library

Library of Congress Cataloging-in-Publication Data
A catalog record for this book is available from the Library of Congress

ISBN 0 340 80638 9

1 2 3 4 5 6 7 8 9 10

Publisher: Georgina Bentliff
Production Controller: Bryan Eccleshall
Cover Design: Mouse Mat Design

Produced and typeset by Gray Publishing, Tunbridge Wells, Kent
Printed and bound in India by Ajanta Offset, New Delhi

Contents

Section 2: Vascular surgery
Editors: Peter Stonebridge and Gareth D. Griffiths

Section 3: Neurosurgery
Editor: Douglas Gentleman

Section 4: Head and neck surgery
Editor: Robin L. Blair

Section 5: Thoracic surgery
Editor: Alan J. Mearns

List of contributors

Donald J. Adam MB ChB FRCS(Ed)
Specialist Registrar in Surgery
Vascular Surgery Unit
University Department of Clinical and Surgical Sciences
Royal Infirmary
Edinburgh, UK

Meena Agarwal PhD MB MS FRCS(Urol)
Specialist Registrar in Urology
Stirling Royal Infirmary
Stirling, UK

Bankole Akomolafe MB BS BSc FWACS FRCS
Specialist Registrar in Vascular Surgery
Freeman Hospital
Newcastle upon Tyne, UK

Mohamed S. Baguneid MB ChB FRCS(Ed)
Specialist Registrar
Department of Vascular Surgery
Manchester Royal Infirmary
Manchester, UK

Eric Ballantyne BSc(Hons) MD FRCS(Ed) FRCS(SN)
Consultant Neurosurgeon
Ninewells Hospital
Dundee, UK

Richard Barnes MB ChB FCS(Urol)
Consultant Urological Surgeon
Groote Schuur Hospital
Capetown, Republic of South Africa

Keith Baxby BSc MB BS FRCS
Consultant Urological Surgeon
Ninewells Hospital
Dundee, UK

Adrian Bianchi MOM(Malta) MD FRCS(Eng) FRCS(Ed)
Consultant Specialist Paediatric and Neonatal Surgeon
The Neonatal Surgical Unit, St Mary's Hospital;
The Royal Manchester Children's Hospital
Manchester, UK

Jill F. Belch MD FRCP
Professor of Vascular Medicine and Consultant Physician
University of Dundee
Ninewells Hospital and Medical School
Dundee, UK

David C. Berridge DM FRCS(Ed) FRCS(Eng)
Consultant Vascular Surgeon
Department of Vascular and Endovascular Surgery
St James' and Seacroft University Hospitals
Leeds, UK

Robin L. Blair FRCS(Ed) FRCS(C) FACS
Head, Department of Otolaryngology
University of Dundee
Consultant Otorhinolaryngologist – Head and Neck Surgeon
Tayside University Hospitals NHS Trust
Dundee, UK

Michael Bouvet MD
Assistant Professor of Surgery in Residence at UCSD
Department of Surgery
University of California, San Diego Medical Center
San Diego, California, USA

Andrew W. Bradbury BSc MB ChB(Hons) MD FRCS(Ed)
Professor of Vascular Surgery
University Department of Vascular Surgery
Heartlands and Solihull NHS Trust (Teaching)
Bordesley Green East, Birmingham, UK

Paul F. Bradley MD BDS FRCS FDSRCS(Eng) FDSRCS(Edin)
Head of Department
Department of Oral and Maxillofacial Surgery
St Bartholomew's and the Royal London School of Medicine and Dentistry
London, UK

Michael J. Callam MB ChB FRCS E ChM
Consultant Surgeon
Bedford Hospital
Bedford, UK

Kenneth L. Campbell MB ChB MD FRCS(Ed)
Consultant Colorectal Surgeon
Tayside University Hospitals NHS Trust
Honorary Senior Lecturer
University of Dundee
Dundee, UK

Roderick T. A. Chalmers MB ChB MD FRCSEd(Gen)
Consultant Surgeon and Honorary Senior Lecturer
Royal Infirmary of Edinburgh
Edinburgh, UK

Nicholas J. W. Cheshire MD FRCS
Consultant Vascular Surgeon
Regional Vascular Unit
St Mary's Hospital
London, UK

Ian C. Chetter MB ChB MD FRCS
Specialist Registrar and Honorary Clinical Lecturer
Hull Royal Infirmary
Hull, UK

Raul Coimbra MD
Associate Professor in Residence
Department of Surgery, University of California
San Diego Medical Center
San Diego, California, USA

John Connolly FRCSI
Consultant Surgeon
Belfast City Hospital
Belfast, UK

Garth Cruickshank BSc PhD MD FRCS FRCS(Ed)
Professor of Neurosurgery
Queen Elizabeth Hospital
Edgbaston, Birmingham, UK

Sir Alfred Cuschieri MD(Malta) MD(Liverpool) ChM(Liverpool) FRSE FRCS(Ed) FRCS(Eng) FRCS(Glas) FRCSI FMedSci FIBiol
Professor of Surgery and Honorary Consultant Surgeon
Department of Surgery and Molecular Oncology
University of Dundee
Honorary Consultant Surgeon
Tayside University Hospitals NHS Trust, UK

John A. Dewar MA FRCR(London) FRCP(Ed)
Consultant Radiotherapist and Oncologist
Department of Radiotherapy and Oncology
Ninewells Hospital and Medical School
Dundee, UK

Lesley A. Duncan MB ChB FRCA
Consultant Anaesthetist
Department of Anaesthesia
Ninewells Hospital and Medical School
Dundee, UK

John F. Dunn MD
Associate Clinical Professor
Director, Kidney and Kidney-Pancreas Transplantation
Department of Surgery
University of California at San Diego Medical Center
San Diego, California, USA

Sandra Engelhardt MD
Clinical Instructor of Surgery
University of California at San Diego Medical Center
San Diego, California, USA

Y. C. Gan MB ChB FRCS
Specialist Registrar in Neurosurgery
Queen Elizabeth Hospital
Edgbaston, Birmingham, UK

Reza A. Gamagami MD FACS
Assistant Clinical Professor
Kewanee Hospital
Kewanee, Illinois, USA

Douglas Gentleman BSc(Hons) MB ChB(Hons) FRCS(Glasgow) FRCS(England)
Honorary Consultant Neurosurgeon
Ninewells Hospital, Tayside University Hospitals NHS Trust; Consultant,
Centre for Brain Injury Rehabilitation
Royal Victoria Hospital
Dundee, UK

Gareth D. Griffiths MB ChB MD FRCS
Consultant Vascular Surgeon
Vascular Surgical Services Medicine and Cardiovascular Group
Tayside University Hospitals NHS Trust
Ninewells Hospital and Medical School
Dundee, UK

John F. Hansbrough MD
Director, Regional Burn Center
Professor of Surgery
University of California at San Diego Medical Center
San Diego, California, USA

Barney J. Harrison MS FRCS
Consultant Surgeon
Northern Hospital
Sheffield, UK

Marquis E. Hart MD
Associate Professor
Director, Abdominal Transplant Program
Department of Surgery
University of California at San Diego Medical Center
San Diego, California, USA

Michael Hehir MB BCh BAO FRCS(Urol)
Consultant Urological Surgeon
Stirling Royal Infirmary
Stirling, UK

J. Graeme Houston MD FRCP FRCR
Consultant Radiologist, Ninewells Hospital
Tayside University Hospitals NHS Trust
Dundee, UK

David B. Hoyt MD
Chief, Division of Trauma
The Monroe E. Trout Professor of Surgery
University of California at San Diego Medical Center
San Diego, California, USA

Badie K. Jacob MB ChB MD FRCP(London) FCCP
Consultant Chest Physician
Senior Lecturer (Leeds University)
Head of Thoracic Medicine
Bradford Royal Infirmary
Bradford, UK

Francis X. Keeley Jr MD FRCS(Urol)
Consultant Urological Surgeon
Southmead Hospital
Bristol, UK

Ajai Khanna MD
Assistant Professor
Director, Pediatric Abdominal Transplantation and Transplantation Research
Department of Surgery
University of California at San Diego Medical Center
San Diego, California, USA

P. V. Sunil Kumar MB MS FRCS
Specialist Registrar in Urology
Southmead Hospital
Bristol, UK

Rosemary A. Levison BSc MSc
Head of Vascular Laboratory
Ninewells Hospital
Dundee, UK

Rhoda MacKenzie MB ChB FRCSEd
Research Fellow
University Department of Vascular Surgery
Heartlands and Solihull NHS Trust (Teaching)
Bordesley Green East, Birmingham, UK

Paul R. Maddox MCh FRCS(Ed) FRCS(Eng)
Consultant Surgeon
Royal United Hospital
Bath, UK

Khalid R. Makhdoomi FRCSI FRCS(Gen. Surg.)
Honorary Consultant Vascular Surgeon
Regional Vascular Unit
St Mary's Hospital
London, UK

Peter T. McCollum MBBCh MCh FRCSI FRCSEd
Professor of Vascular Surgery
Hull Royal Infirmary
Hull, UK

Alan J. Mearns MB ChB FRCS(Eng) FRCS(Ed)
Consultant Cardiothoracic Surgeon
Bradford Royal Infirmary
Bradford, UK

Andrew Mikulaschek MD
Clinical Instructor of Surgery
University of California at San Diego Medical Center
San Diego, California, USA

Alan A. Milne MB ChB MD FRCS(Glasg)
Consultant Surgeon
Queen Margaret Hospital
Dunfermline, UK

Abdool Rahim Moossa MD FRCS(Eng) FACS
Professor and Chairman, Surgeon-in-Chief
Department of Surgery
University of California at San Diego Medical Center
San Diego, California, USA

Rodney E. Mountain MB ChB FRCS(ORL) Ed
Consultant Otolaryngologist
Tayside University Hospitals NHS Trust
Honorary Senior Lecturer in Otolaryngology
University of Dundee
Dundee, UK

Janos Nagy MD FRCS
Specialist Registrar in Vascular Surgery
Department of Vascular Surgery
Ninewells Hospital and Medical School
Dundee, UK

A. Ross Naylor MD FRCS
Consultant Vascular Surgeon and Honorary Senior Lecturer
Department of Surgery
Leicester Royal Infirmary
Leicester, UK

Graham R. Ogden BDS FDS MDSc PhD
Professor of Oral and Maxillofacial Surgery
Head of Unit of Oral Surgery and Medicine
University of Dundee, Dental Hospital and School
Dundee, UK

Robert Pickard MD FRCS(Urol)
Consultant Urological Surgeon
Freeman Hospital
Newcastle upon Tyne, UK

Peter W. H. Rae MB ChB(Edin)
Consultant in Biochemistry
Department of Clinical Biochemistry
Western General Hospital
Edinburgh, UK

Alasdair W. S. Ritchie BSc MD ChB FRCS
Consultant Urological Surgeon
Gloucestershire Royal Hospital
Gloucester, UK

Ilan Rubinfeld MD
Clinical Instructor of Surgery
University of California at San Diego Medical Center
San Diego, California, USA

C. Vaughan Ruckley MB ChB ChM FRCSE
Emeritus Professor of Vascular Surgery
Vascular Surgery Unit
University Department of Clinical and Surgical Sciences
Royal Infirmary
Edinburgh, UK

Gregory P. Sadler MD FRCS(Ed) FRCS Gen Surg(Eng)
Consultant Surgeon
Department of Surgery
John Radcliffe Hospital
Oxford, UK

Declan Sheppard MB BCh BAO MRCPI FRCR
Consultant Radiologist
Ninewells Hospital
Dundee, UK

Sami M. Shimi MD BSc FRCS
Senior Lecturer
Department of Surgery and Molecular Oncology
University of Dundee
Honorary Consultant Surgeon
Tayside University Hospitals NHS Trust
Dundee, UK

David M. Smith MD FRCS(Ed)
Consultant Surgeon and Hon Senior Lecturer
Ninewells Hospital and Medical School
Tayside University Hospitals NHS Trust
Dundee, UK

Owen Sparrow MB BCh Mmed(Neurosurgery) FRCS(Ed) FRCS FCS(SA)(Neurological Surgery)
Consultant Neurosurgeon
Wessex Neurological Centre
Southampton General Hospital
Southampton, UK

Robert J. C. Steele MD FRCS(Ed) FRCS(Eng) FCS(Hong Kong)
Professor and Head of Surgical Oncology and Honorary Consultant Surgeon
Department of Surgery and Molecular Oncology
University of Dundee
Honorary Consultant Surgeon
Tayside University Hospitals NHS Trust
Dundee, UK

J. Howard Stevenson MD FRCS(Ed)
Consultant Plastic Surgeon
Tayside University Hospitals Trust, Honorary Senior Lecturer, Department of Surgery, Faculty of Medicine
University of Dundee
Dundee, UK

Peter Arno Stonebridge ChM MD ChB FRCS(Ed)
Consultant Vascular Surgeon, Vascular Surgical Services, Medicine and Cardiovascular Group
Tayside University Hospital, NHS Trust
Ninewells Hospital and Medical School
Dundee, UK

Mark A. Stott MD ChB FRCS
Consultant Urological Surgeon
The Royal Devon and Exeter Hospital
Exeter, UK

Ahmed Taha MD FRCS
Specialist Registrar in Neurosurgery
Queen Elizabeth Hospital
Edgbaston, Birmingham, UK

Mayer Tenenhaus MD
Associate Clinical Professor
Department of Surgery
University of California at San Diego Medical Center
San Diego, California, USA

Alastair M. Thompson MD FRCSEd(Gen)
Senior Lecturer and Honorary Consultant Surgeon
Department of Surgery and Molecular Oncology
University of Dundee
Honorary Consultant Surgeon
Tayside University Hospitals NHS Trust
Dundee, UK

Nicholas Todd MD FRCS
Consultant Neurosurgeon and Spinal Surgeon
Newcastle General Hospital
Newcastle upon Tyne, UK

Isobel D. Walker MD FRCP FRCPath
Consultant Haematologist
Department of Haematology
Glasgow Royal Infirmary
Glasgow, UK

Michael G. Walker MB ChB ChN FRCS(Ed) FRCS
Consultant Vascular Surgeon
Department of Vascular Surgery
Manchester Royal Infirmary
Manchester, UK

William S. Walker MA MB BChir FRCS FRCSE
Consultant Cardiothoracic Surgeon
Department of Thoracic Surgery
Edinburgh Royal Infirmary
Edinburgh, UK

Jonathan Wasserberg BSc(Hons) FRCS(SN)
Senior Lecturer in Neurosurgery
Queen Elizabeth Hospital
Edgbaston, Birmingham, UK

Robert J. Winchell MD
Associate Professor of Clinical Surgery
University of California at San Diego Medical Center
San Diego, California, USA

Malcolm H. Wheeler MD FRCS
Professor of Surgery, Consultant Endocrine Surgeon
Department of Surgery
University Hospital of Wales
Cardiff, UK

Michael G. Wyatt MB BS MSc MD FRCS
Consultant Vascular Surgeon
Northern Vascular Centre
Freeman Hospital
Newcastle upon Tyne, UK

Preface

For the editors, as well as the authors, a new edition of *Essential Surgical Practice* (*ESP*) is always a major undertaking, but, nonetheless, a rich and rewarding experience. The production of the fourth edition has been no exception. Indeed, it represents a milestone in the life of this surgical textbook for three reasons: the recruitment of Professor Robert Steele as one of the editors, new publishers for the book, and most importantly, the decision to produce a total re-write rather than a revision as was the case with the previous editions. In so doing we decided on a completely new approach necessitated by the changing needs of surgical practice and training world-wide.

ESP is now in two volumes. The first (already published) deals with the *Generality of Surgical Practice* and is overtly topic oriented with the emphasis on basic pathophysiology of surgical illness and management of patients in the various clinical settings. The second (the present volume) is addressed to higher surgical trainees (specialist registrars and residents) and young consultants in *General Surgery* and in *Vascular Surgery*. These two main sections have been written to provide detailed information of the disease processes and their management expected of higher surgical trainees and chief residents completing their specialist surgical training and embarking on professional careers as independent consultant/attending surgeons. Furthermore, these sections should serve as reference sources for established surgeons requiring information on management of particular topics within these two surgical specialties.

The other surgical specialties (Head and Neck, Burns, Trauma, Chest, Neurosurgery and Urology) are covered in separate *Other Specialty Sections* at a level that provides the general and vascular surgeon with a professional working knowledge of current surgical practice in these areas. In this respect, we are most grateful and indebted to our section editors: Mr K. Baxby (Urology), Mr R. Blair (Head and Neck Surgery), Mr D. Gentleman (Neurosurgery), Dr D. Hoyt (Trauma), Mr A. J. Mearns (Thoracic Surgery), Mr P. Stonebridge and Mr G. Griffiths (Vascular Surgery) for their very significant efforts and contributions. The section editors were responsible for outlining content, recruiting the authors, collating and proofreading the material in their sections. As in previous editions, however, the editors have proofread all the material covered in this volume. Thus, we hope that typographical mistakes in the present edition will be few and far between. In addition we have included separate modules on Transplantation (Dr E. Hart *et al.*) and Neonatal/Paediatric Surgery (Mr A. Bianchi) and Plastic and Reconstructive Surgery (Dr M. Tenehaus).

We are delighted with our new publishers, especially for the commitment they have shown to *ESP*, and the support they have provided since they took over from the previous publishers. Finally, we are grateful to our PAs, Anna Pilley, Edna Finney and Rachel Ramiro, who have, by their assistance, greatly facilitated progress and completion of the work. We hope that this second volume of the fourth edition of *ESP* will prove to be useful and beneficial to all surgical trainees world-wide. This has always been our objective and is the only measure of success that we cherish as surgical authors and educators. Indeed, we dedicate this fourth edition of *ESP* to *all the young surgeons* who will take the baton from us to practise, develop and lead this demanding but rewarding profession.

A. Cuschieri, R. J. C. Steele and A. R. Moossa

MODULE 1

Trauma – specific injuries

1 • Soft tissue injuries of the neck

2 • Chest trauma

3 • Abdominal and pelvis injuries

4 • Vascular trauma

Section 1.1 • Soft tissue injuries of the neck

The neck is an anatomically complex region that acts as a conduit for multiple structures, including vital components of the vascular, neurological, respiratory, endocrine and digestive systems. Of particular importance, the neck is enveloped by the platysma and the superficial fascia just beneath the skin and subcutaneous tissue, and by the deep cervical fascia, which includes the pre-tracheal and the pre-vertebral planes. The space between the pre-tracheal layer and the pre-vertebral layer is called the visceral compartment, where all the vital structures are located. The density and relative vulnerability of these structures dictates that injuries to this region be given a high priority in the management of multiply injured patients. The frequency of serious injury and the diagnostic challenge that neck trauma presents has generated considerable controversy regarding the 'best' diagnostic approach. The policy of mandatory operative exploration of all penetrating injuries was developed as a result of wartime experience that demonstrated reduced mortality with this approach. However, more recent civilian experience has shown similar results with a policy of selective operative management. Developments in pre-hospital care, rapid transport to designated facilities and improvements in non-invasive diagnostic methods have further acted to reduce the morbidity and mortality in patients with neck injuries.

Initial resuscitation

The propensity of respiratory compromise in patients with vascular or tracheal injuries makes the early establishment of a secure airway a priority.

- Approximately 10% of patients with neck injuries will have some degree of airway compromise.

Haematoma, laryngeal fractures, soft tissue swelling or intraluminal bleeding may cause upper airway obstruction. Many patients with blunt injuries will have major associated craniofacial trauma, requiring intubation for both airway management and control of intracranial hypertension. Endotracheal intubation is mandatory in patients with significant obstructive signs and should be considered as a prophylactic measure with injuries capable of producing obstruction. The establishment of a surgical airway via cricothyroidotomy is necessary in patients who cannot be intubated easily by the oral or nasal route.

Hypovolaemic shock is treated by the establishment of large bore i.v. cannulas and the infusion of Ringer lactate or type-specific blood. Obvious external haemorrhage from cervical wounds often can be controlled by direct external pressure. Massive external haemorrhage from major vascular wounds requires more direct digital control by the insertion of a gloved finger through the wound. Blind clamping in an effort to control haemorrhage is dangerous and should not be attempted.

Overlooked occult haemorrhage from seemingly innocuous penetrating neck wounds is a dangerous pitfall. Wounds at the base of the neck may produce sudden, unexpected and massive internal bleeding into the mediastinum, pleural space, or into an adjacent tracheal wound. Massive haemorrhage from these injuries can be controlled occasionally by direct pressure, but more often requires immediate transport to the operating room. Anterolateral thoracotomy or sternotomy for proximal vascular control may be necessary in some of these patients.

Following initial resuscitation, patients who are haemodynamically stable must be assessed for the need of operative intervention. The details of this assessment will be discussed, but during this period, any manoeuvre that may act to exacerbate or produce recurrent haemorrhage should be avoided. Probing of the injury beneath the platysma muscle may disrupt haemostasis. Similarly, gagging or coughing also increases the risk of recurrent haemorrhage, and nasogastric tube placement therefore should be deferred. Patients with suspected or known vascular injuries requiring operative exploration should undergo skin cleansing and be draped prior to anaesthetic induction in the event that straining during induction disrupts local haemostasis. There is, in addition, a risk of venous air embolism during induction. Suspected venous injuries should be managed with gentle pressure on the cervical wound with the patient in the supine position.

All patients with neck injuries should undergo a careful neurological evaluation including cranial nerves, particularly VII and IX–XII, and motor and sensory examination and the pre-operative findings should be documented.

Methods of evaluation

The need for operative intervention is the central issue that must be addressed by any method of evaluation. Operative treatment may be deemed necessary on the basis of clinical findings shown in Table 1.1. While this list is not universally accepted the presence of any of these findings is associated with a high incidence of clinically significant injuries. A small percentage of patients will present with active bleeding, shock or an expanding haematoma and require immediate operative intervention. Other patients with superficial wounds to the platysma or with complete absence of any clinical signs may require no further evaluation. For clinically stable patients, invasive and non-invasive studies (plain and contrast radiography, arteriography, computed tomography (CT), endoscopy) may be necessary. They may be used for localization of a known or suspected lesion and aid in planning the operative approach. They are often necessary to exclude (with varying degrees of reliability) potential injuries. In the case of arteriographic embolization, the procedure also may be therapeutic.

Chest and simple anteroposterior and lateral films are routinely obtained in all patients with penetrating injuries. Occult haemorrhage into the chest, associated pneumothorax and cervical soft tissue air are reliable indicators of serious injury. Neck films may be useful for detecting foreign bodies (e.g. glass) and in the assessment of approximate gunshot trajectories.

Arteriography is perhaps the most widely used invasive method. In high cervical injuries, arteriography is very accurate. The reliability of arteriography in excluding mediastinal vascular injuries has been questioned, however, due to the size and orientation of the aorta and great vessels. Arteriographic definition of venous injuries is not particularly reliable.

The use of contrast oesophagography in the evaluation of cervical oesophageal injuries is controversial. Because of the fascial investments of the cervical oesophagus, the sensitivity of contrast extravasation in defining injury is not as high as it is for the intrathoracic oesophagus, where leakage of contrast from a laceration or perforation tends to be less contained. While oesophagography is used in some centres, several investigators have found the incidence of missed injuries associated with this method to be as high as 50%. Sensitivity can be increased by distending the oesophagus with water-soluble contrast, under slight pressure, through a proximal nasogastric tube. Similarly, oesophagoscopy has not proven to be a reliable means of excluding injury, with a reported sensitivity of only 40–50% in several studies. The sensitivity of oesophagoscopy may be improved by the use of a rigid scope, but this entails the administration of a general anaesthetic and a small risk of perforation.

Table 1.1 Indications for operative intervention in the management of neck injuries

- *Vascular injuries*
  - Hypotension/shock
  - Active external bleeding
  - Large or expanding haematoma
  - Distal pulse deficit
  - Bruit
  - Hemispherical deficit or hypoperfusion
  - Significant haemothorax or haemomediastinum
  - Peripheral nerve lesion adjacent to major vascular structures
- *Aerodigestive injuries*
  - Subcutaneous air/crepitus
  - Air emanating from wound
  - Unexplained blood in aerodigestive tract
  - Respiratory stridor
  - Dysphagia/hoarseness
- *Neurological injuries*
  - Cranial nerves: VII, IX, X, XI, XII
  - Impaired diaphragmatic motion – phrenic nerve
  - Brachial plexus deficits

Penetrating neck injuries

For purposes of diagnostic strategy and operative approach, the neck has been divided into three zones (Figure 1.1).

Injuries that occur above the angle of the mandible (zone 3) may involve the petrous or cavernous portions of the internal carotid artery, the vertebral artery or deep branches of the external carotid artery. Wide exposure of this area and distal vascular control may be difficult to obtain. Routine exploration as a diagnostic manoeuvre may be both hazardous and inaccurate. Gunshot wounds account for the majority of these

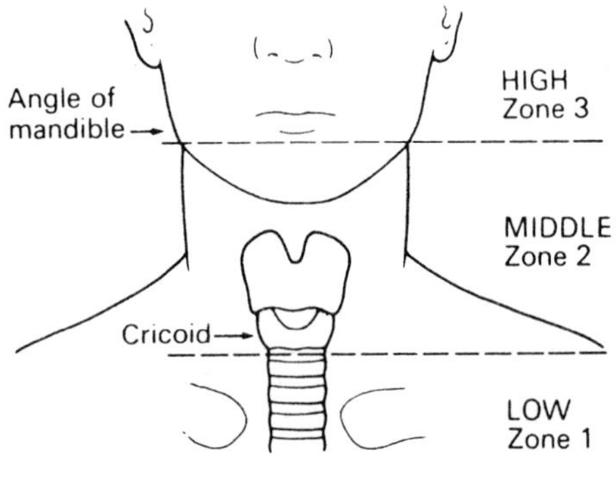

Figure 1.1 Classification of neck injuries.

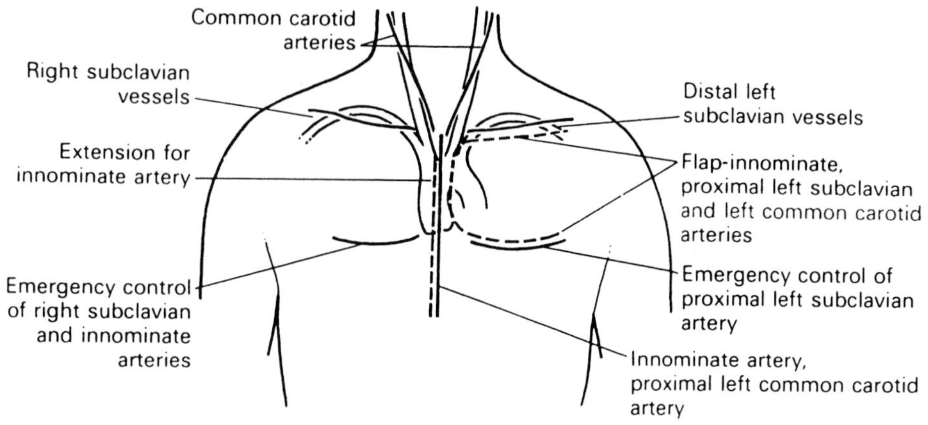

Figure 1.2 Operative approaches for zone 1 injuries to the neck.

injuries, and patients may present with haematoma or haemorrhage from the mouth, nose, throat or the wound. There are often associated neurological injuries.

Arteriography is the diagnostic method of choice for zone 3 injuries. It has proven to be both highly sensitive and specific, and a negative study generally eliminates the need for further evaluation or treatment. The intracranial circulation also can be assessed by arteriography in patients with dense neurological deficits. Therapeutic embolization may be performed for injuries to inaccessible branches of the external carotid artery.

Zone 1 injuries occur at the base of the neck and, like zone 3 injuries, do not allow easy accessibility from an operative standpoint. Injuries in zone 1 may involve proximal carotid, subclavian or innominate vessels, and patients are at risk for exsanguinating haemorrhage, which may be occult if the blood tracks into the chest or mediastinum. As many as 39% of patients with zone 1 vascular injuries presented with unexplained shock in some series. It is of note that 32% of patients in one series had no clinical signs suggesting a major vascular injury.

Management strategy for zone 1 injuries consists of early operative exploration for patients with obvious clinical signs of major vascular injury, i.e. shock, major external or intrathoracic or mediastinal bleeding, or pulse deficit. Asymptomatic patients sustaining zone 1 injuries are evaluated by angiography. Asymptomatic zone 1 patients with negative arteriograms may be safely managed non-operatively.

A variety of incisions have been used to gain exposure and vascular control for thoracic inlet injuries (Figure 1.2). The operative approach will be determined by the specificity of localizing signs, pre-operative arteriography or associated intrathoracic injuries. Transverse clavicular incisions are used for access to distal subclavian injuries. Injuries to the mid portion of the subclavian vessels usually will require either a clavicular osteotomy or elevation/resection of a portion of the clavicle to obtain vascular access. Proximal access to right subclavian or innominate vessels is best obtained through a median sternotomy with supraclavicular lateral extension for additional exposure. Left proximal subclavian injuries will generally require a posterolateral thoracotomy for control. 'Trapdoor' or 'book' incisions simply combine an anterior thoracotomy with a median sternotomy and supraclavicular extension for wide exposure to left-sided and aortic arch injuries. More distal carotid injuries can be best approached via an anterior sternocleidomastoid incision.

It is injuries to zone 2 that have generated the greatest controversy regarding management. The experience gained with these injuries during military conflicts demonstrated the value of routine exploration in reducing morbidity and mortality, and was subsequently applied to civilian trauma. Recently, the policy of mandatory exploration in asymptomatic patients was re-examined because of the high incidence of negative explorations. Some centres now follow a policy of selective exploration of zone 2 injuries. There is a lower threshold, however, to explore gunshot wounds to the neck due to a significant number of injuries caused directly by the missile or indirectly by cavitation.

The controversy regarding mandatory versus selective neck exploration remains unsolved. The principal arguments for each approach are summarized in Table 1.2. The debate is one of diagnostic methods, not therapy. There is no role for non-operative management of patients with clinically suspected vascular or aerodigestive injuries.

A summary of the results for selective and mandatory exploration policies in several series is presented in Table 1.3. This experience suggests that there is little difference in clinical outcome between these policies. It is possible to use ancillary investigations to evaluate zone 2 injuries and avoid a non-therapeutic surgical exploration. However, if a complete and adequate evaluation cannot be performed, surgical exploration remains a safe and appropriate diagnostic modality.

Table 1.2 Mandatory versus selective neck exploration

• Mandatory exploration	
For	*Against*
Risk of injury is high	Many negative explorations
Diagnosis established with certainty	Significant morbidity with negative exploration
No delay in diagnosis/treatment	More costly than selective management
No serious morbidity with negative exploration	Injuries may still be missed
• Selective exploration	
For	*Against*
Avoids unnecessary exploration	Incurs potentially dangerous delay
No significant mortality with delayed treatment	Serious injuries may be missed by non-invasive studies
Cost and hospital stay less or equal to mandatory exploration	Requires more hospital resources
Non-invasive tests are very accurate in defining major injuries	

Table 1.3 Cumulative results: mandatory versus selective management

	Total patients	*Patients explored*	*Negative exploration*	*Total deaths*	*Deaths explored*	*Deaths observed*
Mandatory	477	408 (85%)	231 (56%)	16 (3.3%)	16 (3.3%)	0
Selective	316	148 (47%)	29 (19.6%)	12 (3.8%)	10 (3.2%)	2 (0.6%)

Patients with isolated neck wounds not found to have significant injuries can be managed in the ward post-operatively and discharged within 24–48 hours, minimizing hospital time and expense, and maximizing diagnostic efficiency. The choice between mandatory and selective policies will depend to a large extent on institutional resources, personnel and available expertise.

Specific injuries

The repair of most arterial injuries can be accomplished by lateral arteriorrhaphy, primary re-anastomosis or graft interposition. Ligation is rarely indicated for major vessels except in cases of certain carotid lesions, or when a patient's condition demands a short operative time. Vertebral artery ligation is generally tolerated without sequelae. Injury to major veins should be repaired if possible, although ligation does not lead to significant morbidity.

Lacerations of the larynx and trachea are repaired primarily. Mucosal approximation should be performed carefully with fine absorbable sutures to avoid intraluminal granulation tissue. Tracheal rings and cartilage can be reapproximated using non-absorbable extramucosal sutures.

Oesophageal and pharyngeal injuries

Cervical injuries to the oesophagus and pharynx are repaired in one or two layers and drained using soft Penrose or closed suction drains. More distal oesophageal injuries may be repaired primarily if diagnosed early. Late repair of intrathoracic oesophageal injuries should not be attempted. These injuries are best treated by wide drainage and oesophageal diversion and exclusion.

Blunt neck injuries

Blunt neck injuries are caused frequently by a direct blow to the thyroid or cricoid cartilage as the result of motor vehicle or 'clothes-line' accidents. Severe injuries may also follow acceleration–deceleration forces, significant flexion–extension of the cervical spine or inadequate use of seat belts. Injuries to the larynx, trachea or oesophagus may result. Severe injuries may not be obvious on initial examination. Patients may present with airway obstruction, hoarseness, dysphagia, subcutaneous air, laryngeal deformities, blood in the aerodigestive tracts, haematoma or simply soft tissue swelling. Airway obstruction usually requires placement of a surgical airway. In the presence of severe laryngotracheal trauma, a cricothyroidotomy often is not feasible, and tracheostomy will be required.

Signs of major vascular injury may be more subtle than those associated with penetrating trauma. Carotid dissections are frequently missed, and may present in a delayed manner with a developing neurological deficit. In fact, blunt injuries to the carotid artery account for 3–5% of all carotid injuries.

Carotid duplex scanning is a reliable method of screening for dissections, with arteriography reserved for positive scans or patients with clinical indications. Non-invasive diagnostic methods are used initially in clinically stable patients, and include contrast radiography and CT. The cervical spine also must be carefully evaluated in the initial assessment. Arteriography, bronchoscopy and oesophagoscopy may be indicated.

Vascular injuries are given highest priority and neck exploration is performed on the basis of arteriographic findings. Oesophageal and pharyngeal lacerations are repaired and drained. Laryngeal fractures are generally repaired with the use of a stent.

Complications of cervical trauma

- Massive haemorrhage leading to hypovolaemic cardiac arrest and complications arising from spinal cord injuries are the leading causes of mortality in patients with cervical trauma. Missed injuries involving the oesophagus may lead to fistula formation, abscess and occasionally to mediastinitis. Undiagnosed vascular injuries have produced late sequelae including arteriovenous fistula and false aneurysms. Glottic or subglottic stenosis may complicate laryngeal and tracheal injuries.

Section 1.2 • Chest trauma

Surgeons have been involved in the treatment of chest injuries throughout recorded history. The Smith Papyrus (*c.* 3000 BC) describes treatment of penetrating chest wounds by application of fresh meat. Though therapeutic techniques have improved considerably, chest injuries from both penetrating and blunt mechanisms remain a significant problem. It has been estimated that approximately 20–25% of all trauma-related deaths are due to chest injury. In most areas, blunt chest injuries are by far the most common but the incidence of penetrating trauma in many urban hospitals in the USA is much higher, reflecting a high level of urban violence. The majority of penetrating injuries are still produced by stab wounds, though the relative frequency of gunshot wounds is increasing. Overall mortality for stab wounds to the chest is in the range of 2–3% in contrast to the 15–20% mortality seen with gunshot wounds. Many chest injuries, including tension pneumothorax, myocardial tamponade and massive haemothorax, present with imminent threat to life. These injuries require rapid diagnosis and immediate treatment. In addition, chest injury can result in significant late morbidity and mortality. An understanding of the anatomy and pathophysiology of chest injuries is essential for the optimal management of the trauma patient.

Anatomical considerations

The chest and its contents can be divided into four anatomical zones: the chest wall, the pleural space, the lung parenchyma and the mediastinum. The chest wall consists of the bony thorax and the associated musculature. Injuries to the chest wall consist primarily of fractures of the ribs and sternum, as well as soft tissue injuries. The pleural space is a virtual space between the lung and the chest wall. Though it is normally empty, the pleural space can become filled with air (pneumothorax) or blood (haemothorax) as a result of injury to other organs in the chest. In addition, alteration of the normally negative intrapleural pressure will cause collapse of the lung and ventilatory compromise. The lung parenchyma includes the lung tissue itself, along with associated airways. Injuries to the lung parenchyma include laceration, contusion, haematoma and pneumatocele. The mediastinum contains a number of major structures, including the heart, aorta and great vessels, trachea, proximal bronchi and oesophagus. Injuries within the mediastinum have the potential to involve many critical structures, and require an aggressive diagnostic and therapeutic approach.

Initial management

The initial management of patients with suspected chest injury follows the same general outline used for all other injured patients. An initial primary survey should be done, evaluating the patency of the airway, the efficacy of breathing and the adequacy of circulation. This rapid head to toe examination is aimed at identifying immediate life-threatening problems and treatment should be instituted as soon as such injuries are found. This concept is especially important in the patient with chest injuries, as many immediately life-threatening situations are a result of chest trauma, e.g.:

- airway obstruction
- massive open pneumothorax
- tension pneumothorax
- massive haemothorax
- pericardial tamponade.

For example, tachypnoea, dyspnoea and hypotension associated with decreased breath sounds and deviation of the trachea away from the site of injuries suggest the presence of a tension pneumothorax. If suspected, the pneumothorax should be immediately decompressed by placement of a large bore needle thoracostomy followed by expeditious placement of a chest tube. The site for needle placement should be chosen to allow the most rapid decompression of the chest with the least risk of injury to other intrathoracic structures. Common teaching has suggested the use of the second intercostal space in the midclavicular line. Placement of the needle in the fifth or sixth intercostal space at the anterior axillary line, corresponding to the level of the inframammary crease, is frequently easier and further removed from vital mediastinal structures.

Similarly, profound hypotension, distended neck veins and a parasternal stab wound strongly suggest pericardial tamponade. Rapid thoracotomy and release of tamponade can be life-saving, and should be undertaken immediately.

Once all immediately life-threatening problems have been addressed, and two large bore intravenous lines placed, a second more detailed head-to-toe examination is done. The first step in thorough assessment of the chest is a careful visual inspection for overt signs of injury including deformities, contusions, lacerations and penetrating wounds. Radio-opaque markers should be placed at all entrance and exit wounds. The location and direction of penetrating injuries can aid in the determination of structures at risk for injury.

- It is important to be aware that structures within the chest may be damaged by penetrating wounds with entrance sites well outside the boundaries of the thorax. The rate and pattern of the patient's breathing should be evaluated. Direct observation can detect paradoxical chest wall motion, splinting and retractions associated with inadequate ventilation.

Palpation of the chest can reveal point tenderness, deformity and crepitance. Tenderness and deformity may be diagnostic of fractures of the ribs or sternum. Marked crepitance is indicative of subcutaneous emphysema, which can result from major bronchial injuries, pulmonary parenchymal injuries or injuries of the oesophagus. Probing of chest wounds is rarely indicated and risks converting a simple soft tissue injury into a pneumothorax.

Auscultation of the chest allows assessment of breath sounds, primarily for quality and symmetry. Decreased breath sounds are suggestive of pneumothorax, haemothorax or possible right mainstem intubation. Depth of breathing and adequacy of ventilation can also be assessed. The presence of other adventitial lung sounds should be noted, though detailed examination may be difficult in the resuscitation room setting. The physical examination should suggest likely injuries within the chest, and then necessary diagnostic studies should be obtained as expeditiously as possible.

The plain radiograph of the chest can yield a wealth of useful diagnostic information, and should be obtained as early as possible in the resuscitation of the injured patient. The chest radiograph must be carefully examined in its entirety and allows evaluation of the bony thorax, the soft tissues of the chest wall and mediastinum, as well as the lung parenchyma. The presence of rib fractures, pneumothorax or haemothorax can provide information necessary to direct the ongoing course of the resuscitation.

Serial radiographs of the chest are useful in order to follow the progress of identified pathological processes and should also be obtained after all invasive procedures. The repeat film allows verification that the endotracheal tube, central venous catheter or chest tube is in the correct position and that the desired therapeutic effect has been achieved.

In addition to drawing a blood sample for an initial haematocrit and blood typing, nearly all patients with suspected chest injury should have an arterial blood gas analysis. The blood gas results are invaluable in identifying the patients who are at risk to progress to ventilatory failure. Significant hypoxaemia or hypercarbia may precede overt clinical evidence of impending respiratory failure. In addition, the evaluation of the patient's acid base status offers an important assessment of the degree of metabolic acidosis and therefore the extent of peripheral hypoperfusion due to hypovolemic shock. The resolution of metabolic acidosis is a good guide to the effectiveness of fluid and blood resuscitation.

Other more involved diagnostic studies of the chest are required in special circumstances. Angiography is important in blunt injuries in which aortic injury is likely as well as in penetrating injury with the probability of arterial injury. The role of CT in the assessment of acute chest injuries continues to evolve. CT is certainly a useful modality in the long-term follow-up of many chest injuries. The utility of CT in the acute diagnosis of thoracic injuries has been controversial, but improvements in CT technology have led to more widespread use. Centres with an interest in CT of the chest have reported very good results. In some circumstances, ultrasound may be of use in detecting the presence or absence of pericardial tamponade or determining the presence or absence of aortic injury. Endoscopy and various contrast techniques may be important in identifying potential injuries to the oesophagus.

Injuries by anatomical zone

Specific organ system injuries within the chest can be organized by the anatomical zones outlined above. Though the pleural space contains no structures of its own, many other intrathoracic injuries present with haemothorax or pneumothorax, and this zone will be addressed first, followed by the chest wall, pulmonary parenchyma and the mediastinum.

Manifestations of chest injury in the pleural space

Despite the diverse nature of potential injuries in the chest, many patients present initially with either haemothorax or pneumothorax. Prior to the advent of thoracic surgery, chest wounds were treated expectantly, and the external wounds addressed several days later, if the patient survived. Drainage of haemothorax remained controversial through the middle of the 20th century. The use of tube thoracostomy in the management of haemothorax and pneumothorax did not become standard until the 1970s. Treatment of haemothorax or pneumothorax is often the sole intervention required in patients with chest trauma, and aggressive early intervention is critical in achieving the optimal outcome.

Pneumothorax

A simple pneumothorax occurs when air escapes from the injured lung, or enters through a penetrating wound, and collects in the pleural cavity. Pneumothorax is common after either penetrating or blunt trauma. Approximately 90% of patients with pneumothorax due to blunt trauma have an associated rib fracture. Physical findings suggestive of pneumothorax include diminished breath sounds, hyperresonance of the chest to percussion, decreased respiratory expansion on the side of the injury, and subcutaneous emphysema. The diagnosis is readily confirmed on chest radiograph (Figure 1.3).

Traumatic pneumothorax should be treated by tube thoracostomy. The presence of air in the pleural space results in a loss of the normally negative intrapleural pressure and a variable degree of collapse of the lung. The degree of respiratory embarrassment is dependent upon the degree to which normal ventilatory mechanics are disturbed. The most extreme example is the *open pneumothorax,* or so-called *sucking* chest wound. If the wound is sufficiently large, intrapleural pressure remains equal to atmospheric pressure. Attempts at spontaneous

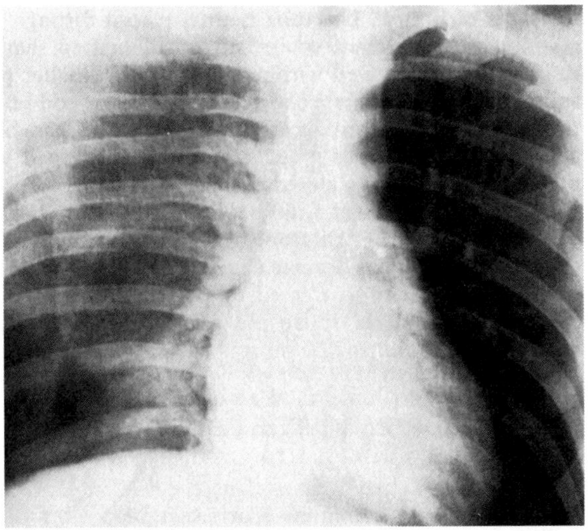

Figure 1.3 Right haemopneumothorax. Note the collapsed lung. The diffuse haziness in the right hemithorax is caused by blood layering out posteriorly.

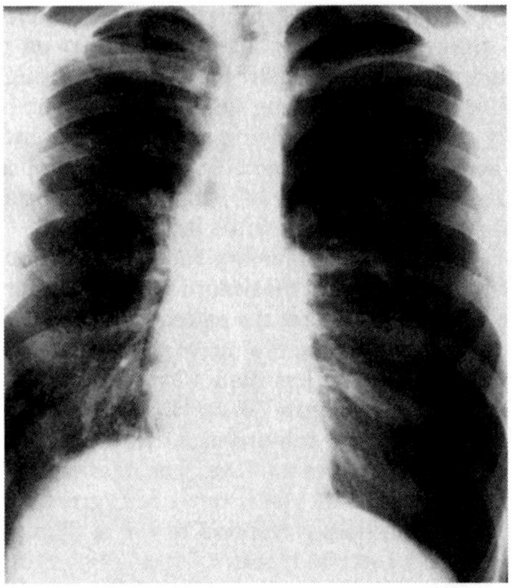

Figure 1.4 Left tension pneumothorax. Note collapsed lung and hyperlucent left hemithorax. Tension pneumothorax is evidenced by shift of mediastinum to the right, depression of the left hemidiaphragm and widened intercostal spaces.

ventilation will result only in movement of air in and out of the body wall defect. No significant ventilation of the lung is possible and respiratory compromise is severe. Such a patient may improve dramatically with simple occlusion of the defect, creating a closed pneumothorax, which subsequently can be treated by tube thoracostomy.

Another special case is the *tension pneumothorax,* which is created if air continues to accumulate in the pleural space, creating pressures above atmospheric.

- This can result in a shift of the mediastinum away from the site of the injury, causing a significant decrease in venous return to the heart and resultant hypotension, as well as severely compromised ventilation of the opposite lung (Figure 1.4).

Tension pneumothorax may be produced as a result of repeated Valsalva manoeuvres in a patient with a laceration of the lung that acts as a one-way valve allowing air to enter but not to leave the pleural space.

- A much more common cause of tension pneumothorax is the use of positive pressure ventilation in a patient with pulmonary parenchymal injury.

In either circumstance, air is forced into the pleural cavity under positive pressure, creating the tension pneumothorax. The patient with chest injury who will be on positive pressure ventilation, either in the operating room or the intensive care unit (ICU), must be monitored closely. Consideration should be given to performing a prophylactic tube thoracostomy prior to the development of symptomatic pneumothorax if the patient has significant rib fractures or penetrating injuries likely to result in pneumothorax.

The diagnosis of tension pneumothorax is often readily apparent from physical examination. The patient is usually dyspnoeic and haemodynamically unstable. The affected hemithorax is hyperexpanded and breath sounds are decreased. There may also be distension of the neck veins and shift of the trachea away from the site of the injury. Treatment consists of immediate decompression with a large bore needle followed by expeditious tube thoracostomy. As previously discussed, the needle should be placed at a site that allows the most rapid and safe decompression of the chest.

Regardless of the underlying cause, most pneumothoraces will resolve with tube thoracostomy alone. The chest tube allows restoration of normal intrapleural pressure and re-expansion of the lung. With re-expansion and reapproximation of the pleural surfaces, all but the largest parenchymal defects will seal in a period of a few days. Positive pressure ventilation can greatly prolong the time required for parenchymal air leaks to seal, especially if mean airway pressures are high.

Haemothorax

The accumulation of blood in the pleural space is also a frequent result of either blunt or penetrating trauma. The bleeding may range from minimal to massive, life-threatening haemorrhage depending on the nature of the injury. The presenting symptoms may also vary widely depending on the degree of haemorrhage. Breath sounds generally will be decreased on the side of the injury and a supine chest radiograph will show a diffuse haziness as blood layers posteriorly (Figures 1.5 and 1.6). Initial treatment of haemothorax requires placement of a chest tube that is large enough to ensure evacuation of the accumulated blood. In general, this requires a 36 Fr or larger tube. The majority of lacerations to the pulmonary parenchyma involve low-pressure vessels of the pulmonary circulation. Such bleeding can be expected to stop after placement of the chest tube and re-expansion of the lung. Injuries to systemic arteries, including the intercostal arteries and the internal mammary arteries, can lead to massive haemorrhage, especially if the vessels are only partially transected.

Most cases of haemothorax can be treated by tube thoracostomy alone. In situations of truly massive initial haemorrhage or significant ongoing haemorrhage, thoracotomy is required for control of the bleeding. The decision for thoracotomy must be individualized to the case at hand. In general, an initial return of 1000–1500 ml or significant continued bleeding in excess of 200–300 ml/h over a period of time should alert one to the possible need for thoracotomy and surgical control of the bleeding.

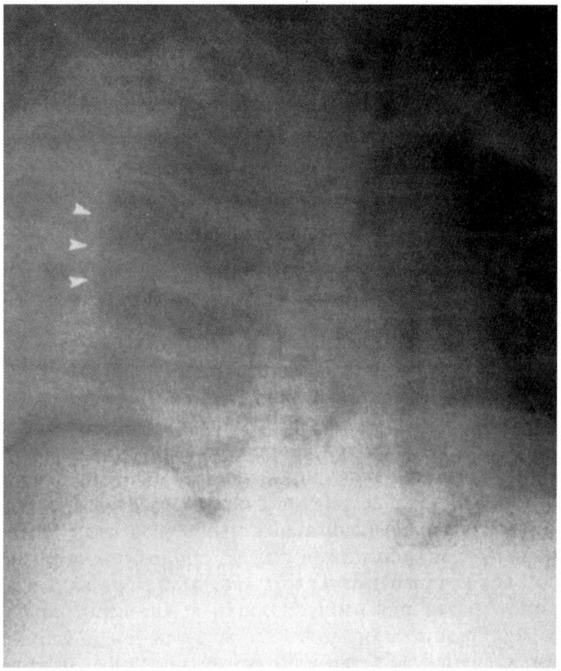

Figure 1.5 Massive haemothorax. Note near complete opacification of left hemithorax.

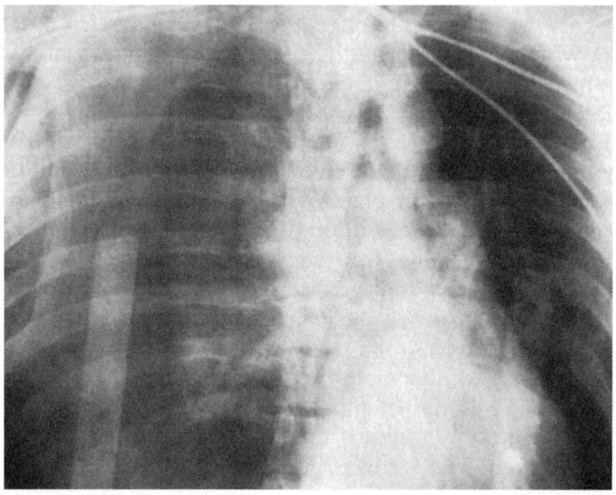

Figure 1.6 Tension haemopneumothorax. Note collapse of right lung, with collection of blood in right hemithorax and marked shift of mediastinum to the left.

Technique of tube thoracostomy

The initial therapy in most patients with either haemothorax or pneumothorax is tube thoracostomy regardless of mechanism of injury. The tube often must be placed rapidly, during the course of resuscitation. Under these circumstances, the site of entry is generally chosen to be the fourth or fifth intercostal space in the anterior axillary line. This site is chosen to avoid inadvertent injury to the diaphragm and to allow easy access to the chest without going through major muscle mass. The proposed site should be thoroughly prepped, draped and infiltrated with a liberal amount of local anaesthetic if time allows. The chest tube should be 36 Fr or larger to allow for adequate evacuation of the haemothorax.

An incision is made approximately one interspace below the intended site of entry into the chest and a short subcutaneous tunnel is made extending over the upper border of the rib. The pleural space is entered over the superior aspect of the rib to avoid injury to the intercostal neurovascular bundle. The chest should be entered carefully with a blunt clamp to avoid potential injury to the underlying structures. Once the pleural cavity is entered, the surgeon's gloved finger should be inserted into the chest to confirm entry into the pleural space and to assess the presence or absence of adhesions to the pulmonary parenchyma. This 'digital thoracotomy' also affords the opportunity for the surgeon to palpate the pericardium, lung and diaphragm to assess for signs of injury. The tube is then placed through the opening in the pleural space and positioned so that all draining holes are well within the chest. In small persons this may necessitate shortening the distal end of the tube by several centimetres. Once the tube has been adequately placed, it is securely sutured and taped in place and attached to a closed drainage system.

Post-procedure chest radiography is mandatory both to confirm placement of the tube and to ensure the desired therapeutic effect has been achieved. Persistent haemothorax or pneumothorax may be treated by the placement of a second tube, but should also raise the question of the need for a thoracotomy to control the injury.

Injuries to the chest wall

Rib fractures

By far the most common injury sustained after blunt chest trauma is rib fracture. In older patients, rib fractures can occur after relatively minor injuries, due to decreased bone density and loss of chest wall compliance. The primary manifestation of rib fractures is pain and this can lead to significant complications if inadequately treated. The pain of rib fractures is often intense and causes splinting and poor inspiratory effort on the affected side. This can result in an ineffective cough and progressive atelectasis leading to pneumonia.

- The elderly, especially those with underlying pulmonary parenchymal disease, are particularly vulnerable to these complications. Thus, adequate analgesia is of paramount importance in the management of the patient with rib fractures.

The use of bedside pulmonary function tests, including forced vital capacity and maximum inspiratory force, can give an objective estimate of the patient's degree of ventilatory compromise. Tidal volume of <5 ml/kg, forced vital capacity of <10 ml/kg, or maximum inspiratory force of <30 cm of water are indicators of significant ventilatory compromise. Initial attempts at pain control using oral or parenteral analgesics are appropriate, but additional measures must be aggressively pursued in those who do not respond to initial therapy. The use of intercostal nerve blocks with long-acting local anaesthetic is effective, but requires relatively frequent re-administration. In addition, it is impractical for large numbers of broken ribs. The use of epidural narcotics or epidural narcotic and local anaesthetic combinations can be of great benefit, especially in the elderly or in those with associated abdominal operations.

- Rib fractures may serve as a marker for more serious associated injuries. Historically, fracture of the first rib has been taken as a hallmark of very high-energy transfer and has been associated with major chest, abdominal and vascular injuries. Certainly, the presence of a first rib fracture must alert one to the possibility of associated major injuries in the chest or abdomen. Fractures of the lower ribs are associated with either liver or splenic injury. A 20% incidence of splenic injury has been associated with fracture of the tenth to twelfth ribs on the left side.

Flail chest

The flail chest is caused by multiple contiguous comminuted or segmented rib fractures resulting in a free-floating section of the chest wall. It can also occur without radiographically apparent fractures by disruption of the cartilaginous or ligamentous attachments of the ribs. This injury results in a segment of the chest wall moving in response to changes in intrapleural pressure, rather than in co-ordination with the muscular action of the chest wall. Thus, the flail segment moves *paradoxically* inwards with inspiration and outwards with expiration.

Older theories on the pathophysiology of flail chest were based on the belief that this paradoxical chest wall movement caused ineffective air movement between the lungs. Historical attempts at treating flail chest were aimed at stabilizing the chest wall to prevent this paradoxical movement. Despite significant advances in the technology of chest wall stabilization, this therapeutic approach did not significantly change the overall mortality rate associated with flail chest. It is now felt that the underlying injury to the lung rather than the paradoxical movement of the flail segment *per se* is responsible for the morbidity associated with flail chest.

The current therapy of flail chest is focused on treating the underlying pulmonary contusion and achieving adequate analgesia to allow the patient to make effective spontaneous ventilatory efforts. The need for intubation and mechanical ventilatory support is determined by:

- the patient's clinical appearance
- the ability to ventilate adequately, and
- the degree of pulmonary dysfunction.

The patient without evidence of respiratory distress and with good pulmonary function can be managed without intubation if pain relief is adequate. Patients with significant arterial hypoxaemia or ventilatory insufficiency should be intubated and mechanical ventilation initiated. The patient should be supported in this fashion until there is evidence of resolution of the pulmonary parenchymal damage and until the pain is sufficiently controlled to allow adequate ventilatory mechanics.

Some patients with large flail segments have very severe chest wall deformity, and subsequent loss of volume in the affected hemithorax. Chest wall reconstruction and mechanical stabilization of the flail segment is advocated by some for highly selected cases. A significant percentage of these patients will suffer long-term disability due to the chest wall deformity.

Sternal fracture

In the past, sternal fractures (Figure 1.7) were most commonly the result of severe blunt trauma to the anterior chest. In older series, sternal fractures were associated with a significant incidence of severe chest injuries, including traumatic rupture of the aorta, rupture of the oesophagus, rupture of major bronchi and myocardial contusion. These injuries resulted from crashes in which the sternum was fractured by impact

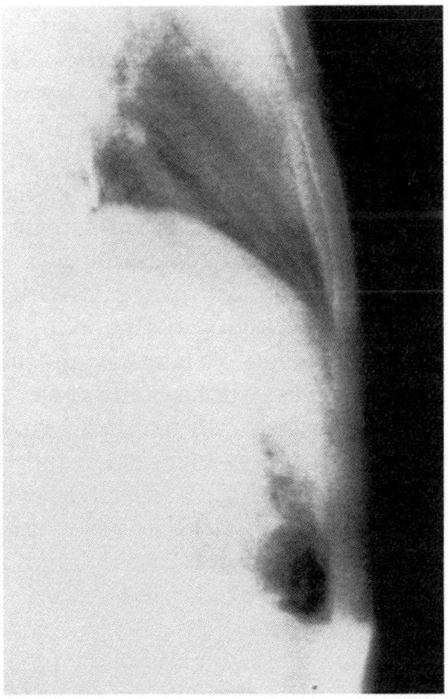

Figure 1.7 Sternal fracture. Lateral chest film showing non-displaced sternal fracture.

with the rigid steering column or dashboard. The presence of a sternal fracture would often mandate additional diagnostic studies such as arch angiography to rule out associated injuries.

- The aetiology of sternal fracture, and therefore its association with severe thoracic injury, has changed with changes in automobile design, as well as changes in the average age of drivers.

In more recent experience, the majority of sternal fractures are sustained as a result of the use of shoulder restraints, especially in older patients with decreased bone density. Under these circumstances, the sternal fracture is often an isolated injury and is much less commonly associated with significant intrathoracic injury. The need for additional evaluation in patients with sternal fracture should be based on the overall circumstance, not the mere existence of the sternal fracture.

Treatment of the sternal fracture itself is generally conservative with an emphasis on pain relief. Fewer than 25% of patients with a complete fracture of the sternum will require operative fixation. Indications for operative fixation include significant posterior displacement of the fracture or persistent chest wall instability.

Pulmonary parenchymal injuries

Pulmonary laceration

Simple lacerations of the pulmonary parenchyma are common after penetrating trauma but are relatively rare after blunt trauma. The patient with a pulmonary laceration usually presents with pneumothorax and a variable degree of haemothorax. Initial treatment consists of placement of a tube thoracostomy to drain the haemothorax and re-expand the lung. The majority of bleeding and air leak from pulmonary lacerations will stop after the lung has been re-expanded. Tube thoracostomy is definitive therapy in most cases.

Some patients may develop a large persistent air leak. This situation can be exacerbated by the need for continued positive pressure ventilation. Massive air leak should alert one to the possibility of significant bronchial injury. If the leakage rate is high enough, effective alveolar ventilation is lost, greatly complicating ventilatory management. Under these circumstances, a number of methods can be used to try to control the leakage rate, including lowering driving pressures, selective bronchial intubation, or the use of endoscopic techniques to occlude the bronchial orifice leading to the damaged lobe. In extreme cases, the patient can be managed with split lung ventilation. In split lung ventilation, a double lumen tube and two separate ventilators are used to allow independent ventilation of each lung. Fortunately, development of such large bronchopleural fistulas is uncommon.

Pulmonary contusion

Blunt injury is more likely to lead to the production of pulmonary contusion. Contusion is a result of haemorrhage and oedema formation in the lung parenchyma without associated tissue disruption. Some degree of contusion occurs in up to 70% of patients with severe blunt chest trauma and the mortality rate is highly variable depending on age, underlying lung disease and associated injuries. Significant pulmonary contusions can cause major local changes in pulmonary compliance and alveolar function, leading to significant ventilation perfusion mismatch. The resulting arterial hypoxaemia can be severe, depending on the amount of lung involved. The decrease in compliance can also significantly increase the patient's work of breathing. The situation is complicated by pain from associated chest wall injuries, which decreases the patient's ventilatory effort and cough. This combination of factors can lead to a rapidly progressive ventilatory failure, necessitating intubation and mechanical ventilatory support.

The diagnosis of pulmonary contusion is generally made on the basis of mechanism of injury, arterial hypoxaemia and chest radiograph showing a poorly defined infiltrate in the area of the injury (Figure 1.8). The radiographic changes are usually apparent in the early phase, within 1 or 2 hours after injury. The treatment of pulmonary contusion is dependent on the severity of the parenchymal injury, as well as the nature and severity of associated injuries.

Minor pulmonary contusions can be managed with general supportive measures. Patients who manifest signs of early respiratory failure should be intubated and given mechanical ventilatory support. The period of time needed for return of adequate ventilatory function and gas exchange may vary from 1 day to several weeks. No efficacy has been shown for either prophylactic antibiotics or steroids in changing the course of pulmonary contusion.

- Since fluid overload is likely to be detrimental in the patient with pulmonary contusion, resuscitation should be done judiciously and should be titrated to physiological endpoints. Invasive monitors such as pulmonary artery catheters and arterial lines should be used frequently in the severely injured. Measurement of filling pressures, cardiac output and mixed venous blood gases can provide invaluable information needed to adjust therapy.

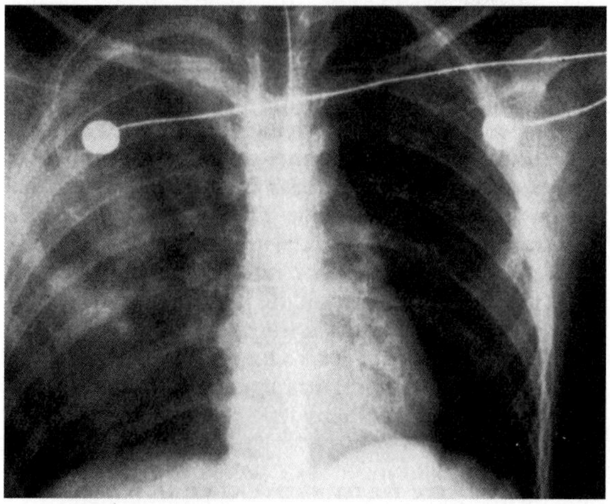

Figure 1.8 Pulmonary contusion. Note poorly defined infiltrate in right mid-lung field and multiple posterior rib fractures.

Pulmonary haematoma

An intraparenchymal haematoma is produced by bleeding into the lung substance that is contained by the parenchyma or the pleura. The mechanism of injury and presenting symptoms are similar to those of pulmonary contusion. In a pure pulmonary haematoma, alveolar dysfunction may be minimal, and the clinical manifestations less severe than the chest radiograph might suggest. The radiographic findings are also similar, but haematomas tend to have a sharper margin and a more spherical shape (Figure 1.9). Resolution of a pulmonary haematoma is generally slower than that of contusion, and occurs over a period of 2–3 weeks. Treatment is conservative for those patients not showing evidence of respiratory compromise.

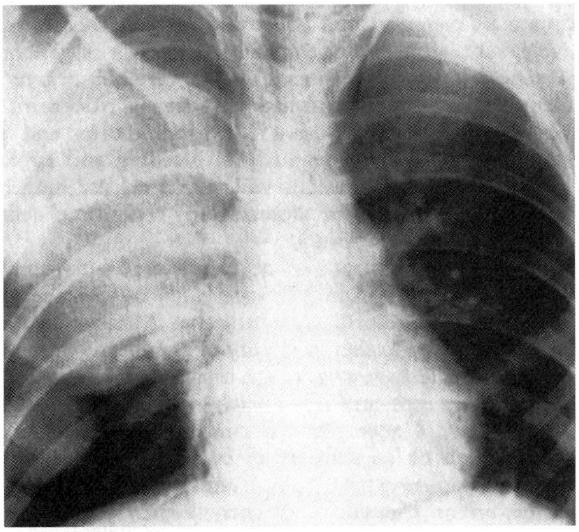

Figure 1.9 Pulmonary haematoma. Note well-defined margins of this lesion compared to the pulmonary contusion.

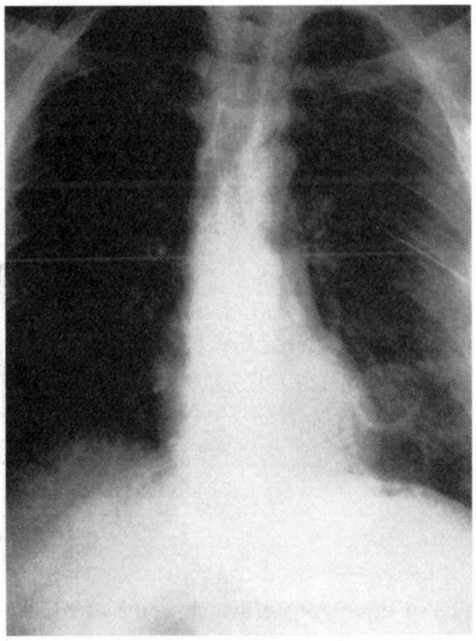

Figure 1.10 Pulmonary pneumatocele. Note well-defined cavities in the left lower lung field.

Traumatic pneumatocele

A pulmonary pneumatocele can develop from the resolving stages of a pulmonary haematoma or after injury to a small bronchus without significant haemorrhage. Either mechanism results in the formation of a cavity in the pulmonary substance. As an isolated injury, pneumatocele is well tolerated and the patient may be relatively asymptomatic. The chest film will show an air-filled cavity and possibly an air fluid level (Figure 1.10). The major potential complication is infection but this is fairly rare. Resolution is generally slow, over a period of many weeks. Specific intervention is rarely required.

Injury to the large airways

The incidence of major tracheobronchial injury in most trauma centres is low. This is due to a combination of high scene mortality from associated injuries and a tendency for some injuries to remain relatively asymptomatic, presenting in delayed fashion. In most cases, tracheobronchial injury due to blunt trauma occurs within 2.5 cm of the carina and wounds are generally circumferential. Penetrating injuries may occur at any level.

Patients generally present in one of two ways, depending on the location of the bronchial rupture. Patients in whom the bronchus ruptures into the pleural cavity will present with pneumothorax and massive air leak after placement of a chest tube. Symptoms may include haemoptysis and massive subcutaneous or mediastinal emphysema. If the bronchial rupture occurs within the mediastinum, the presentation can be much less acute. Respiratory distress in this group is uncommon, though most patients have some degree of haemoptysis. In addition, there may be subcutaneous emphysema in the neck or discernible to auscultation of the chest. Mediastinal emphysema is the most common radiographic finding (Figure 1.11). The primary injury frequently heals, though the patient may present with later complications due to stricture at the site of injury.

Patients with suspected tracheobronchial injury should be evaluated by bronchoscopy. In patients with acute respiratory distress, this evaluation may need to be done in the operating room or after endotracheal intubation. Treatment depends on the extent of the injury and patient's clinical course. In general, injuries involving less than one-third of the circumference of the trachea or major bronchus can be observed. Injuries greater than one-third of the circumference are usually repaired primarily in order to prevent or minimize stricture formation.

Injuries to mediastinal structures

Blunt injury to the thoracic aorta

Traumatic rupture of the aorta is a common cause of automobile crash fatalities, resulting in 10–15% of such deaths. Older experience suggests that approximately 80% of these victims died at the scene or *en route* to the hospital. Of the remaining patients reaching the

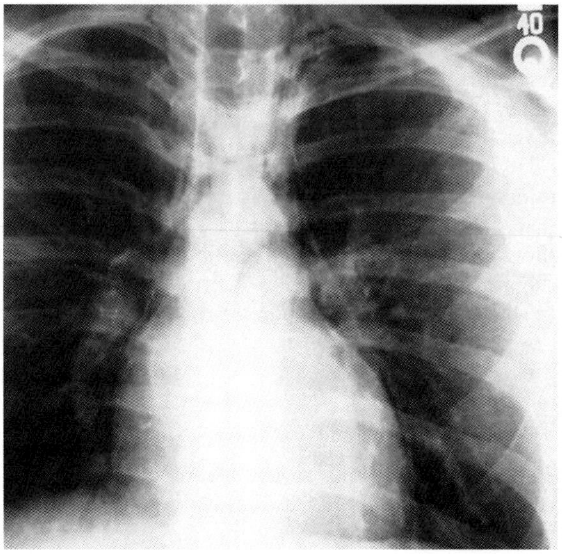

Figure 1.11 Mediastinal emphysema. Pneumomediastinum can be seen along the left edge of the cardiac silhouette. In addition, there is a small left apical pneumothorax, and subcutaneous emphysema in the soft tissue of the left neck.

hospital, 30% died within 6 hours and 50% within 24 hours if no surgical treatment was undertaken. The estimated mortality at 10 weeks was 90% without surgical treatment. More recent data suggest that patients with blunt aortic injury fall into two broad categories. Those patients with haemodynamic instability and evidence of leak from the aortic injury are at extreme risk of rupture and death, necessitating immediate surgical intervention. A second group of patients may present with a small and very stable pseudoaneurysm, and are at relatively low risk of acute rupture. Overall, the incidence of blunt aortic injury remains low in patients presenting alive to the hospital, resulting in only one to four such injuries per year in a busy trauma centre.

The two most common sites of blunt aortic injury are in the descending aorta just distal to the origin of the left subclavian artery and in the ascending aorta proximal to the innominate artery. Injury may occasionally occur at the diaphragmatic hiatus. Injuries to the ascending aorta are frequently associated with severe cardiac damage, tamponade and death. Almost all patients surviving long enough to reach the hospital will have injuries located just distal to the origin of the left subclavian artery, at the level of the ligamentum arteriosum.

Aortic injury is commonly associated with a mechanism of rapid deceleration causing horizontal shear at the relatively fixed portions of the aorta. In addition, significant anteroposterior compression of the chest or significant lateral impact may result in traumatic disruption of the aorta. Whatever the mechanism, these forces result in complete disruption of the vessel wall over all or part of its circumference. Survivors are those in whom the haemorrhage is contained by the tissues of the mediastinum with the formation of a pseudoaneurysm.

Clinical presentation can be extremely variable. Patients may appear to have no external signs of significant trauma or may present *in extremis* with massive haemothorax and significant respiratory distress. The presence of other significant thoracic injuries must raise suspicion of blunt aortic injury. In addition, there may be abnormal pulses in the extremities. The patient may present with a pseudo-coarctation syndrome manifested by upper extremity hypertension and diminished pulses in the lower extremities. Conversely, pulses in the upper extremities may be decreased due to occlusion of the origin of the vessels of the aortic arch. It is also important to do a thorough neurological evaluation, as patients may present with neurological compromise due to spinal cord ischaemia. Additionally, spinal cord ischaemia is one of the major complications of surgical management and it is vital to document the neurological status prior to surgery.

The diagnosis of blunt aortic injury requires a high degree of suspicion based on mechanism and associated injuries. Findings in the chest radiograph suggestive of blunt aortic injury include:

- widening of superior mediastinum to more than 8 cm
- loss of the aortic knob or blurring of the aortic contour
- left apical cap
- massive left haemothorax, especially in the absence of rib fractures
- depression of the left mainstem bronchus
- deviation of nasogastric or endotracheal tube to the right
- widening or loss of the paravertebral stripe.

Widening of the superior mediastinum is the most commonly described finding, but loss of the normal contour of the aortic knob may be more sensitive (Figure 1.12). It is important to remember that all of the above findings can be very subtle or may be entirely absent. The plain film of the chest can offer information that may heighten suspicion, but cannot be relied upon to exclude the injury.

Patients with chest radiograph findings suggestive of thoracic aortic injury or with highly suspicious mechanism and clinical findings should undergo a definitive study to exclude the possibility of aortic injury. Historically, arch aortography has been the accepted standard. The aortogram will usually indicate the location and extent of injury, though biplanar films may be required to demonstrate subtle injuries. Digital subtraction studies may lack sufficient sensitivity to exclude the diagnosis. The role of CT of the chest in the diagnosis of blunt aortic injury is in evolution. Improvements in CT technology, including helical scanning and dynamic CT, have greatly improved the utility of this modality as a primary screening tool. Centres with a dedicated interest in the use of CT have reported results comparable to those obtained with arch aortography. In centres without the requisite expertise in CT interpretation, arch aortography is still the most appropriate definitive examination.

Trans-oesophageal echocardiography has also been used with good success in some centres. This study can

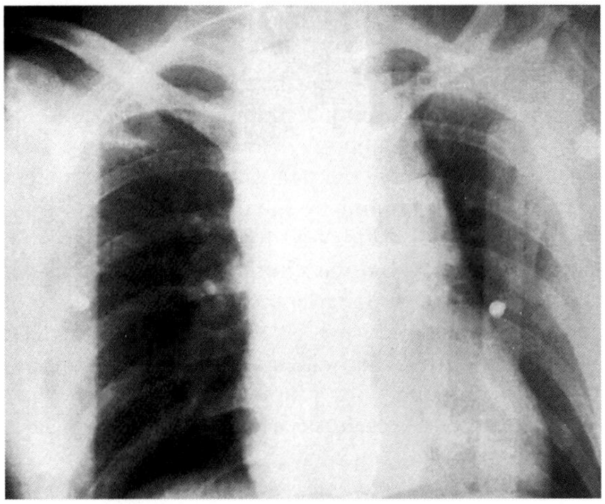

Figure 1.12 Traumatic aortic rupture. Note widening of the superior mediastinum, with loss of the aortic contour.

be done at the patient's bedside, and offers very good visualization of the aortic arch. The primary barrier to extended use of trans-oesophageal echo is the considerable expertise required for its performance and interpretation. Trans-oesophageal echo should be considered in patients at high risk for aortic injury who cannot be transported for CT or angiography.

The treatment of traumatic disruption of the thoracic aorta is surgical, requiring resection of the damaged segment and primary repair. In older series, primary repair of the injury without adjunctive bypass techniques was felt to be sufficient but current experience suggests that perfusion of the distal aorta via partial cardiopulmonary bypass should be done in the majority of cases to minimize the likelihood of spinal ischaemic injury. It is critical that the diagnosis is made and surgical repair initiated rapidly, as operative mortality rises dramatically if the pseudoaneurysm ruptures prior to surgical control.

In the pre-operative period it is important to avoid hypertension, which may cause untimely rupture of the containing pseudoaneurysm. The patient should have appropriate monitoring lines placed but the subclavian route for central venous catheterization should probably be avoided to prevent violation of the mediastinal haematoma. Judicious use of beta-blockers to lower overall blood pressure as well as the rate of rise of blood pressure is important, in addition to ensuring that the patient is not subjected to situations that might cause undue pain and anxiety.

Penetrating injuries to the thoracic aorta

Injuries to the thoracic aorta and great vessels are more commonly due to penetrating injuries. In these circumstances the diagnostic problems are considerably more clear cut. Those patients presenting with initial haemodynamic instability and a penetrating wound to the chest require urgent thoracotomy. In the haemodynamically stable patient with a penetrating wound in proximity to the great vessels, angiography should be considered. This study can be of paramount importance in determining the best surgical approach, especially if more than one major vessel may be involved. It must be remembered that angiography for penetrating trauma has a finite incidence of false negativity and a highly suspicious injury should be explored despite negative angiograms.

The approach to major vascular injuries in the thorax may involve significant blood loss and preparations for large-scale fluid and blood replacement should be made. Proximal and distal control may require cross-clamping of the descending aorta with associated risk of spinal injury. Partial bypass techniques have greatly improved over the past several years and should be used within the trauma setting whenever practical. Under most circumstances, systemic heparinization is not required. Primary repair of injury should be attempted when feasible but intercostal vessels must not be sacrificed to obtain mobility, due to the increased risk of spinal cord ischaemia. Short interposition grafts should be used for defects too large for primary repair.

Blunt myocardial injury

Significant blunt trauma to the chest can result in injury to the heart. The most severe injuries can cause cardiac rupture, which is almost uniformly fatal. Patients succumb from exsanguination if the pericardium is also ruptured or from tamponade if the pericardium remains intact. It is uncommon for a patient with this diagnosis to survive to reach the hospital, but those who do are almost certain to have suffered an atrial rupture. Atrial rupture must be suspected in a patient with severe blunt chest trauma who develops signs and symptoms of cardiac tamponade, or otherwise unexplained hypotension. The patient should be supported by volume infusion as rapid preparations are made for surgical decompression and attempt at repair. If time allows, two-dimensional echocardiography is useful to confirm or exclude the diagnosis in the patient with suspicious findings. Needle pericardiocentesis occasionally may be useful as a temporizing measure awaiting surgical availability.

Less severe blunt injuries to the heart can result in myocardial contusion. There is very little agreement in the definition of significant myocardial contusion, its diagnosis or its treatment. The incidence of significant myocardial contusion is difficult to estimate but is probably less than 10% of patients with severe chest trauma. Patients with clinically significant myocardial contusion are those who suffer potentially life-threatening complications, such as dysrhythmia or pump failure, or those who die with contusion demonstrated at autopsy. More subtle forms of myocardial contusion also may be important but are more difficult to characterize.

Blunt injury to the myocardium can produce wall motion abnormalities as well as render the heart prone to dysrhythmias. These factors are rarely dangerous in patients under observation in an ICU setting but can cause significant problems during surgery for associated injuries. Unfortunately, there are no classic signs or symptoms suggestive of myocardial contusion. There are no universally accepted diagnostic criteria and the utility of various modalities is highly variable and institution dependent. The electrocardiogram (ECG) is generally accepted as the first diagnostic test. Most frequent ECG abnormalities are alterations in T wave and ST segments, as well as sinus tachycardia. Supraventricular and ventricular dysrhythmias as well as sinus and AV nodal dysfunction are occasionally reported. The specificity of ECG in the diagnosis of myocardial contusion is low.

In analogy to myocardial infarction, the measurement of the cardiac enzymes creatinine phosphokinase and, more recently, troponin has been suggested to be helpful in the diagnosis of myocardial contusion. Recent experience suggests that abnormalities in cardiac enzymes are not useful in predicting which patients will develop significant complications. The specificity is low and the diagnostic threshold is not well established. Studies aimed at directly visualizing the function of the heart have some utility. Most common is two-dimensional echocardiography. A general global picture of cardiac function as well as individual wall motion abnormalities can be detected fairly accurately. Other pathology including intramural haematoma, intracavitary thrombus, pericardial effusion and valvular dysfunction also can be identified. The procedure is non-invasive and can be performed easily at the bedside. However, the significance of echocardiographic abnormalities in the otherwise asymptomatic patient is unclear. Subtle motion abnormalities are commonly seen, but do not correlate with likelihood of complications, especially dysrhythmia. Radionuclide imaging has been suggested, but it is impractical and unlikely to provide information that is clinically relevant.

Once the diagnosis of myocardial contusion has been reached, there is no consensus as to appropriate management, but the trend is towards a short period of monitoring and treatment of dysrhythmia and pump dysfunction as they arise. There are no data to support the use of prophylactic anti-dysrhythmics. Those patients with probable myocardial contusion who require surgery for associated injuries should be aggressively monitored, including a pulmonary arterial catheter and arterial line. The use of trans-oesophageal echocardiography may also provide useful information in the intra-operative assessment of myocardial function.

As a general rule, patients with a normal admission ECG and normal haemodynamic parameters do not require ECG monitoring. The length of time that patients with evidence of myocardial contusion should be monitored is also not well established. Clinical judgement must be used in determining when the patient is stable for discharge. A period of 24 hours is probably sufficient in the absence of significant dysrhythmias.

Penetrating myocardial injuries

Penetrating injuries to the heart are encountered in approximately 2–4% of penetrating chest and abdominal injuries. These injuries were once felt to be uniformly fatal but since the first successful repair of right ventricular stab wound by Rehn in 1896, significant progress has been made. Most patients with penetrating cardiac injuries who reach a hospital alive are victims of stab wounds. Survival may approach 80% in the case of single chamber injury with a small pericardial defect, resulting in tamponade rather than rapid exsanguination. Most patients with gunshot wounds to the heart do not survive to reach the hospital and among those who do, mortality is very high due to extensive tissue damage and more frequent exsanguination. The keys to maximizing survival are recognition, fluid resuscitation and rapid operative intervention.

The outcome of potentially survivable injuries to the heart is in large part determined by the size of the associated pericardial defect. Wounds producing large defects in the pericardium lead to rapid exsanguinating haemorrhage and death. Smaller pericardial defects may lead to the development of tamponade rather than exsanguination. While this too can cause circulatory collapse and death, the chances of successful resuscitation are much higher. In a sense, a tamponade can be a life-saving situation.

Pericardial tamponade must be suspected in all patients with penetrating injuries in proximity to the heart, especially those with wounds in the parasternal region. Patients with tamponade are often relatively stable as pressure within the pericardium rises. Once a critical level is reached, cardiac output falls precipitously. Profound shock and death ensue if aggressive therapy is not instituted immediately. The patient with tamponade is frequently anxious and muffled heart tones with pulsus paradoxus may be present. Marked elevation of central venous pressure is a useful associated clinical finding. Patients with tamponade often have distended neck and upper extremity veins in contrast to a hypovolaemic patient with collapsed veins. However, a patient with both tamponade and significant hypovolaemia may not exhibit abnormally elevated central venous pressure.

A thorough search for potential injury must be conducted in a haemodynamically stable patient with penetrating injuries in proximity to the heart. Measurement of central venous pressure has been advocated as a screening test. Unfortunately, this test lacks both sensitivity and specificity, so findings must be interpreted with great caution. Ultrasonic imaging of the heart can be useful if available in a timely fashion. Two-dimensional echocardiography can be useful both in the detection of fluid within the pericardium and in determination of overall pump function. If a high degree of suspicion persists, the diagnosis should be aggressively pursued by direct visualization of the pericardium. This can be done easily through a subxiphoid pericardial window.

Definitive management of penetrating injury to the heart consists of thoracotomy and opening the pericardial sac. After tamponade is relieved, bleeding usually can be controlled by digital pressure while preparations for definitive repair are made. Small lacerations can be repaired using pledgetted sutures on the beating heart, while large or complex wounds should be repaired on cardiopulmonary bypass. Almost all patients with tamponade can be supported temporarily with aggressive volume resuscitation while preparations for surgery are made. Pericardiocentesis is rarely indicated, except as a temporizing measure if facilities for thoracotomy are unavailable.

Injuries to the oesophagus

Because of its protected location in the posterior mediastinum, blunt injury to the thoracic oesophagus is exceedingly rare in patients presenting to the hospital alive. When it occurs, blunt rupture of the oesophagus is usually seen in the distal third just above the gastro-oesophageal junction similar to Boerhaave's syndrome. The injury is probably produced by sudden increases in intra-oesophageal pressure due to blunt upper abdominal trauma in the presence of a full stomach.

Penetrating injuries to the oesophagus are more common and may occur at any level. One must conduct a thorough search for injury to the oesophagus if a penetrating wound has a trajectory that is in proximity to the thoracic oesophagus. There is a high incidence of major associated injury with either blunt or penetrating mechanism.

Specific signs and symptoms due to perforation of the oesophagus are few and generally the patient's complaints are related to associated injuries. As noted, early diagnosis is the single most important factor in determining ultimate outcome. Findings on chest radiography of pneumomediastinum, widened mediastinum, air in the prevertebral space or left pleural effusion, as well as penetrating injury with proximity to the oesophagus must seriously suggest the diagnosis. Suspicious cases must be aggressively pursued.

The best initial study is probably contrast oesophagography though this test does have a significant false-negative rate. Adjunctive flexible oesophagoscopy can add to the sensitivity. Early operative repair is the key to successful therapy for thoracic oesophageal perforations. Mediastinal contamination and eventual sepsis lead to prohibitively high mortality rates in patients whose operative repair is delayed beyond approximately 12–24 hours.

The upper two-thirds of the thoracic oesophagus are best approached through right thoracotomy while injuries confined to the lower third may be more easily accessible from the left. The general operative principles are to attempt surgical closure of the injury when possible and establish wide mediastinal drainage. Extensive tissue destruction or massive mediastinal contamination may preclude primary repair and constitute indications for an exclusion technique.

Section 1.3 • Abdominal and pelvis injuries

In civilian life, the majority of abdominal injuries are due to blunt trauma secondary to high-speed automobile accidents. Penetrating injuries, although often associated with wartime combat, are seen with increasing frequency in hospital emergency departments, particularly in urban areas. The failure to manage abdominal injuries successfully accounts for the majority of preventable deaths following multiple injuries. Failure to recognize occult abdominal haemorrhage and to successfully control bleeding from intra-abdominal organs leads to significant morbidity, and such injuries account for approximately 10% of traumatic deaths that occur annually in the USA. Even today, with the development of trauma systems, failure to manage abdominal injuries continually accounts for significant morbidity.

There are many mechanisms that account for abdominal injuries. The recognition of two major groups, penetrating and non-penetrating, is of greatest importance for treatment and has direct implications for the diagnostic work-up and therapy. The abdomen encompasses a large area of the body, from the diaphragm superiorly to the infragluteal fold inferiorly, including the entire circumference of this region. Penetrating or blunt injury to the back also may result in significant intra-abdominal injury. Multiple system injuries, particularly those involving the central nervous system, chest and musculoskeletal system, are often associated and may obscure injury to the abdominal contents and symptoms from this area. The importance of repeated assessment of a patient suspected of having intra-abdominal injury cannot be overemphasized.

- In patients with multiple system trauma in whom speciality consultation is needed, the overall responsibility for treatment must reside with one physician, preferably the general surgeon, to provide consistent serial examinations.

Experience shows that accurate categorization of injuries allows the development of treatment protocols that minimize wasted time and improve efforts in pre-operative and intra-operative management of abdominal injuries.

Anatomical considerations

A practical knowledge of the contents of the abdomen is important. Assessment of the abdomen is influenced by its differing anatomical features. For evaluation purposes, the abdomen is divided into four areas: intrathoracic abdomen, true abdomen, pelvic abdomen and retroperitoneal abdomen (Figure 1.13). All the other areas are difficult to assess on physical examination, with the exception of the true abdomen.

The intrathoracic abdomen is that portion of the upper abdomen that lies beneath the rib cage. The contents include the diaphragm, liver, spleen and stomach, but bony and cartilaginous structures make this portion essentially inaccessible to palpation. Each structure may

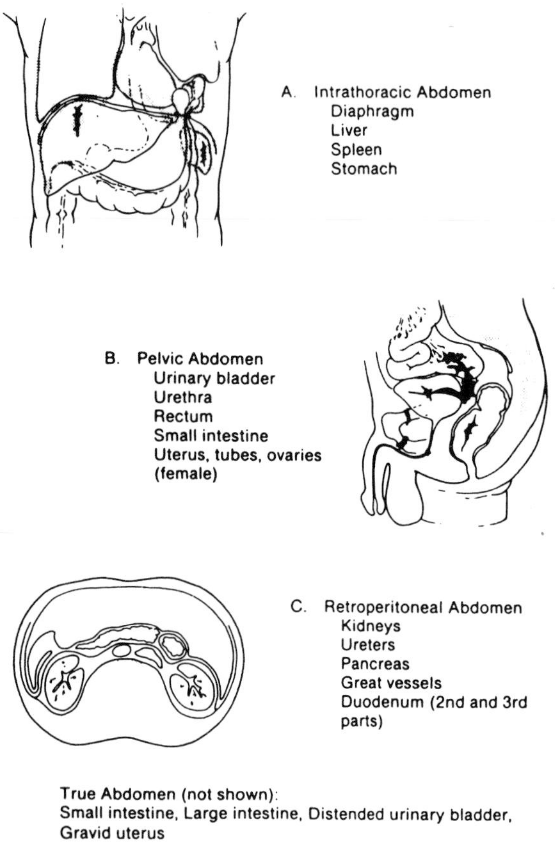

Figure 1.13 Contents of the abdomen. (After Hardy, J. D. ed. (1977). *Rhoad's Textbook of Surgery*, 5th edn. Philadelphia, PA: Lippincott.)

be injured when blunt or penetrating injury is delivered to the rib cage and peritoneal lavage becomes useful in evaluating this area of anatomy.

The pelvic abdomen lies in the hollow of the pelvis. It is surrounded on all sides by the bony pelvis and its contents include the rectum, bladder, urethra, small bowel, and in females, the uterus, fallopian tubes and ovaries. Trauma to the pelvis, particularly pelvic fractures, may damage the organs within, and penetrating injuries of the buttocks may injure any or all of the pelvic organs. Injury to these structures may lack physical findings and be difficult to diagnose. As such, suspected injuries to this area of the abdomen must be investigated using adjunctive procedures such as bladder catheterization, urethrocystography and sigmoidoscopy.

The retroperitoneal abdomen contains the kidneys, ureter, pancreas, second and third portion of the duodenum, the ascending and descending colon, and the great vessels, the aorta and vena cava. Injury to these structures may occur secondary to penetrating or blunt trauma as well. The kidneys may be damaged by injury to the lower ribs posteriorly, and crushing injuries to the front or sides of the trunk may damage any of these structures. As with the thoracic and pelvic abdomen, injury to these structures may result in few physical findings, and physical examination and peritoneal lavage may be of little or no help. Evaluation of the retroperitoneal abdomen requires utilization of radiographic procedures including intravenous pyelography, angiography and CT. In addition, serum amylase determinations may be helpful. The true abdomen contains the small and large intestines, the bladder when distended, and uterus when gravid. Injuries to any of these organs are usually manifested by pain from peritonitis and are associated with abdominal findings. Peritoneal lavage is a useful adjunct when an injury is suspected and a plain abdominal film may be helpful when free air is present.

In summary, the abdomen consists of four distinct anatomical areas. Each of these must be suspected of sustaining injury and must be investigated systematically with knowledge of the limitations of physical examination, and the appropriate radiographic or diagnostic procedures that may reveal the diagnosis.

Classification of injuries

The classification of abdominal injuries based upon aetiology is extensive (Table 1.4). Classifications involving the amount of injury or the number of organs injured are not practical from the standpoint of diagnosis or treatment of abdominal injuries. It is most useful to categorize injuries into penetrating and nonpenetrating, as this correlates best with the likelihood of significant intra-abdominal injury, the speed with which diagnosis and treatment must be accomplished, and the associated mortality and morbidity.

Penetrating wounds

The handgun has replaced the knife as the most common cause of significant penetrating injury to the abdomen. Significant intra-abdominal injury occurs about 80% of the time following a gunshot wound, whereas significant injury occurs approximately 20–30% of the time following stab wounds. The frequency of injury following penetrating abdominal trauma is shown in Table 1.5.

Injuries to both thoracic and abdominal cavities occur in 25% of patients with penetrating wounds of the abdomen, and conversely, patients with penetrating wounds of the thorax often have significant intra-abdominal injury since the wound may traverse the diaphragm and result in abdominal injury. Whether

Table 1.4 Aetiology of abdominal injuries

Penetrating	*Blunt*	*Iatrogenic*
Stab wounds	Crush injury	Endoscopic
Gunshot wounds	Blast injury	External cardiac massage
Shotgun wounds	Seatbelt syndrome	Peritoneal dialysis
		Paracentesis
		Percutaneous transhepatic cannulation
		Liver biopsy
		Barium enema

Table 1.5 Frequency of injury in penetrating abdominal trauma

Organ	*Percentage*
Liver	37
Small bowel	26
Stomach	19
Colon	17
Major vascular	13
Retroperitoneal	10
Mesentery and omentum	10
Spleen	7
Diaphragm	5
Kidney	5
Pancreas	4
Duodenum	2
Biliary system	1
Other	1

selective management or mandatory laparotomy is the best method for treating stab wounds is debated and discussed further below. Most agree that gunshot wounds to the abdomen should be explored, as the probability of significant intra-abdominal injury is high. The difference in injury potential is a function of the increased kinetic energy associated with a gunshot wound.

Blunt trauma

Incidence of blunt abdominal trauma is increasing because of the increased automobile and motorcycle accident rate. The car remains the cause of non-penetrating trauma in at least 70% of patients with this injury. The incidence of specific organ injuries is listed in Table 1.6.

The sudden application of pressure to the abdomen is more likely to rupture a solid organ than a hollow viscus, and this accounts for the greater incidence of solid organ injury. More elastic tissues of the young tolerate trauma better than the less resilient or fixed tissue of older people and this accounts for the difference in significant intra-abdominal injury following blunt trauma in children and adults.

Iatrogenic injuries

Significant intra-abdominal injury can follow iatrogenic causes, listed in Table 1.4, and these represent a variety of commonly performed diagnostic and therapeutic procedures that can lead to significant intra-abdominal injury. The principles of diagnosis and treatment are no different from other traumatic injuries.

Table 1.6 Frequency of injury in blunt abdominal trauma

Organ	*Percentage*
Spleen	25
Kidney	12
Intestine	15
Liver	15
Retroperitoneal haematoma	13
Mesentery	5
Pancreas	3
Diaphragm	2
Urinary bladder	6
Urethra	2
Vascular	2

Pre-hospital care

Little can be done for patients with abdominal injuries in the field. General features of stabilization and evaluation include ensuring an adequately functioning airway, inserting intravenous lines, preferably in the upper extremity, and the beginning of fluid resuscitation. For penetrating wounds, sterile dressings should be applied and the patient carefully monitored. Any foreign bodies embedded in the trunk should not be removed as major bleeding might follow removal. Evisceration is best left undisturbed, except to apply a sterile dressing and protect the patient from further injury.

Hospital care and diagnosis

In the patient with suspected abdominal injury, the history of injury as well as the physical examination remain important factors in the surgeon's decision-making process. Diagnosis and treatment should proceed concurrently following established protocols, many of which have been reviewed previously.

Diagnosis: history

History that exists should be transferred at the time of the field report by the paramedics. Penetrating injuries present few diagnostic challenges, other than whether or not to explore the abdomen. An attempt should be made to establish details of the weapon involved. Blunt trauma assessment can be greatly aided by accurate history. Obtaining a history from the paramedical team that the patient was involved in an automobile accident in which the steering wheel was impacted strongly suggests the possibility of duodenal or pancreatic trauma.

- If the patient has sustained rib fractures on the lower left chest, there is a 20% chance of associated splenic injury, and with rib fractures on the right there is a 10% chance of liver injury.

Back pain associated with a compression fracture of the upper limb or spinal region carries an associated 20% chance of significant renal injury. This, in combination with the aspects of physical diagnosis and adjuncts to physical diagnosis as discussed below, assists in the initial assessment of abdominal injury.

Resuscitation

The ABC of emergency resuscitation - airway, breathing and circulation – should be initiated. A patent functioning airway must be established, particularly in the comatose patient, prior to evaluation of the abdomen. If necessary, an endotracheal tube is placed and assisted ventilation begun. Upper extremity, large-bore i.v. cannulae are started and resuscitation is begun with Ringer lactate. Blood samples are drawn for basic studies, including haemoglobin (Hb), electrolytes, and blood for type and cross-match. Arterial blood gases are determined and repeated to assess ventilatory status and acidosis. An early rapid assessment of the abdomen is performed.

The key objective of the physical diagnosis of abdominal injury is to identify the need for operation. The precise determination of organ injury is unnecessary. Physical examination becomes the determination of intra-abdominal bleeding or peritoneal irritation. Unfortunately, because of anatomical constraints, evaluation of bleeding or peritoneal irritation may not be able to be determined by examining the abdominal wall. Associated injuries often cause tenderness and spasm in the abdominal wall and make this diagnosis complex. Lower rib fractures, pelvic fractures or abdominal wall contusion may mimic the signs of peritoneal irritation and it may be impossible to determine whether there is significant intra-abdominal bleeding or peritoneal irritation from a ruptured viscus.

Since the primary manifestation of solid organ injury is haemorrhage, particularly following blunt trauma, the patient should be monitored closely during the initial assessment and resuscitation for evidence of continuing or refractory haemorrhagic shock, and further evaluation should occur in the operating room. A patient who remains haemodynamically stable allows for an objective and complete evaluation, including diagnostic peritoneal lavage (DPL) or image studies and laboratory tests.

Physical examination

Physical assessment should proceed in an orderly fashion. The patient should be evaluated for signs of blunt trauma and for penetrating wounds. Small abrasions or areas of ecchymosis may represent warnings of significant intra-abdominal injury.

- All the penetrating wounds should be marked with radio-opaque clips and a subsequent radiograph taken to delineate the trajectory of the bullet or path of the knife and allow for an intelligent assessment of the likelihood of associated injury.

The abdominal wall and back should be carefully inspected and posterior ecchymosis should raise the possibility of retroperitoneal injury. Determining the absence of bowel sounds may be helpful to assess significant peritoneal irritation from blood or intestinal contents, but is difficult to hear in a noisy emergency department and likely to take significant time to develop. This is more often likely to be a late finding following injury.

The patient's respiratory pattern should be evaluated. It may be a clue to significant abdominal trauma. Halted, laboured breathing may be from diaphragmatic irritation or accompany upper abdominal injury. Pain in the shoulder with inspiration (Kehr's sign) on the left side corresponds with irritation of the diaphragm from bleeding. Palpation may reveal localized tenderness, spasm or rigidity of the abdominal wall. This finding or direct rebound tenderness should make the clinician very suspicious of significant intra-abdominal injury. In the conscious patient, suprapubic tenderness and pelvic lateral wall tenderness are assessed for a pelvic fracture. Inspection of the perineum and urethral meatus for blood may raise the possibility of pelvic fracture as well.

- The passage of a Foley catheter should be delayed until radiographic evaluation of the pelvis can be obtained and signs of urethral injury are absent.

As assessment continues, an indwelling urinary catheter is placed and a sample of urine is sent to the laboratory to evaluate for microscopic haematuria. If injury to the lower urinary tract, bladder or urethra is suspected because of an associated pelvic fracture, catheterization should be delayed until urethrography is performed to rule out injury to the urethra. Rectal examination is performed and sphincter tone is evaluated. The integrity of the rectal wall, the position and mobility of the prostate are evaluated, and the examining finger should be tested for the presence of gross or occult blood. A nasogastric tube is passed, aspirated and tested for blood. The presence of blood becomes an indication for operation in penetrating trauma.

Interpretation of physical findings

Intraperitoneal injuries can occur in vascular, solid and hollow organs. Interpretation of the physical findings associated with these different structures is often a function of the amount of time that each of these types of organ requires to create peritoneal irritation.

The spectrum of injury can vary from a patient with rapid intra-abdominal bleeding, secondary to a mesenteric artery laceration, with no physical findings except hypovolaemic shock, to a patient with immediate peritoneal irritation from inflammation following injury to the stomach or colon. Small intestinal injury may not produce significant intra-abdominal findings for 24 hours. Because of the spectrum the interpretation of physical findings may represent, frequent re-evaluation becomes an essential component of any management protocol that is short of definitive diagnosis.

Adjunctive studies for assessment of abdominal trauma

Several laboratory tests, radiological studies and ancillary diagnostic procedures are useful in evaluating a patient suspected of having abdominal injury.

Radiological studies and ancillary diagnostic procedures

Laboratory tests of value in the evaluation of a patient with abdominal trauma include haematocrit, urinalysis and serum amylase. White count, serum creatinine, glucose and electrolyte determinations are often obtained for baseline values but make little contribution to early management. The diagnosis of massive haemorrhage is usually obvious and haematocrit merely confirms it.

Urinalysis will indicate the presence of microscopic haematuria. In blunt trauma, greater than 30–50 red blood cells (RBCs) should lead to radiographic evaluation of the kidneys and urinary bladder. Serum amylase can be normal in the face of major pancreatic injury or enteric injury, but elevated values should raise suspicion of significant intra-abdominal injury. Serum amylase can be elevated in patients without significant visceral injury. Any suspicion of pancreatic or duodenal injury ultimately should be ruled out in the patient with a history of epigastric trauma with a contrast enhanced CT scan. Persistently elevated amylase always should be investigated. Radiological studies of potential value in the evaluation of abdominal trauma include abdominal plain films, urethrography and cystography, intravenous urography (IVU), CT scan, radionuclide scans, ultrasound and angiography.

All injuries from penetrating trauma should be evaluated with a plain radiograph with radio-opaque markers to allow evaluation of the injuring trajectory. In blunt trauma, plain radiographs may delineate fractures with associated visceral injury potential, show free intraperitoneal air, retroperitoneal 'stippling,' associated duodenal injury, or loss of the psoas shadow indicating retroperitoneal bleeding.

Abdominal CT is the best method available to identify and grade solid organ injury, helping in the decision whether to treat some of these injuries non-operatively. Furthermore, CT is also superior compared to DPL and ultrasound to diagnose retroperitoneal injuries. The advantage of using CT relies on the fact that it is non-invasive and repeatable; however, it is expensive and time consuming, requiring transfer of the patient to the radiology department. Another important drawback of CT is its low sensitivity to identify bowel and diaphragmatic rupture.

- CT should **not** be used in the haemodynamically unstable trauma patient.

Sensitivity, specificity, positive predictive value, negative predictive value and accuracy vary greatly depending on the quality of the equipment (helical vs conventional) and the experience of those interpreting it. Although solid organ injuries can be graded by CT, several reports have emphasized that CT grading does not correlate with operative findings, and the decision whether to operate or not is based on the haemodynamic status, transfusion requirements, metabolic derangement and physical examination.

Most of the experience with the utilization of ultrasound in the trauma setting was accumulated in Europe and Japan. Recently, American trauma centres have started using ultrasound to evaluate the presence of haemoperitoneum in the blunt trauma patient. Ultrasound in this scenario is not intended to diagnose specific injuries, but rather to provide information about free fluid in the peritoneal cavity and in the pericardial sac. This focused utilization of ultrasound in the emergency department or in the resuscitation room is known as FAST.

Obesity, gas interposition, subcutaneous emphysema and injuries that do not cause changes in tissue interface are limiting factors for FAST evaluation. In the trauma victim, a significant drawback of FAST is that small amounts of free fluid are difficult to identify. Other limitations of FAST include its dependency on the operator and on the interpreter. As with CT, sensitivity, specificity and accuracy are variable, but as experience increases, the results also improve.

The advantages of FAST are that it is rapid, cheap, non-invasive, does not require radiation, can be repeated over time, and can be performed in parallel to the initial assessment in the resuscitation room. In the unstable trauma patient, a positive FAST eliminates the need for further tests and indicates the necessity for abdominal exploration. A negative FAST indicates that the bleeding source is other than the abdomen.

- In the haemodynamically stable patient, a positive FAST does **not**, *per se*, indicate the need for surgical exploration.

In such instances, an abdominal CT scan is obtained to evaluate the bleeding source, and as described above, to help in the determination of the appropriate therapy (operative vs non-operative). Diagnostic laparoscopy may be the most reliable method to determine peritoneal violation in anterior or flank stab wounds. However, drawbacks of laparoscopy include, but are not limited to, the necessity for general anaesthesia, high cost and equipment availability. These disadvantages are overcome if laparoscopy is performed in the operating room immediately prior to a diagnostic laparotomy whenever this is considered necessary.

As a general rule, the use of diagnostic laparoscopy in the blunt trauma patient is very limited and this method does not seem to be superior to any other method commonly used in the decision-making process. Reported missed injury rates in blunt trauma cases vary from 10 to 35%. Diagnostic laparoscopy has been considered the most appropriate method to evaluate penetrating abdominal injuries (confirms intact peritoneal lining) and diaphragmatic injuries, and several reports also have described the potential of repairing the diaphragm using laparoscopy in the absence of other intraperitoneal injuries, avoiding an exploratory laparotomy. There is a risk of tension pneumothorax in the presence of diaphragmatic injuries and thus a low pressure pneumoperitoneum (10 mmHg or lower) or a gas-less technique is advisable.

Patients with major hepatic injuries (central liver haematomas) treated non-operatively who have a persistent drop in the haematocrit and increased volume of the haematoma shown on CT scan may benefit from angiography and selective embolization. Arteriography is also indicated in patients with suspected renal artery thrombosis.

Peritoneal lavage

Peritoneal lavage is the standard technique used to detect significant intra-abdominal haemorrhage following blunt trauma and can be used to evaluate significant intra-abdominal injury following stab wounds. Its applicability following low-velocity gunshot wounds is limited, and it has no place in the management of high-velocity gunshot wounds. Abdominal paracentesis can be used rarely instead of peritoneal lavage when intra-abdominal haemorrhage is suspected, and paracentesis will expedite going to the operating room. It should be emphasized that a negative abdominal paracentesis is of no diagnostic significance, and it is best to practise peritoneal lavage.

Peritoneal lavage, like paracentesis, is of greatest value in those patients whose physical findings are difficult to evaluate. The specific indications for peritoneal lavage include:

- unconscious trauma patients with signs of abdominal injury
- patients with high energy transfer, suspected intra-abdominal injury and equivocal physical findings
- patients with multiple injuries and unexplained shock
- patients with spinal cord injury
- intoxicated patients in whom abdominal injury is suspected.

An additional indication includes patients who are candidates for intra-abdominal injury who have equivocal diagnostic findings, and will be undergoing prolonged general anaesthesia for other injuries and thus are unavailable for continued re-evaluation.

Contraindications include:

- patients with previous abdominal operations
- pregnancy
- morbid obesity
- patients with an obvious surgical abdomen.

A pelvic radiograph should be taken before performing peritoneal lavage when pelvic fractures are suspected so that, if necessary, the incision can be made in the supra-umbilical position. This avoids a false-positive test from passing the catheter through the pelvic haematoma that has dissected onto the anterior abdominal wall below the umbilicus.

Lavage is rarely used with a gunshot wound. Essentially all gunshot wounds are explored by laparotomy. When local exploration of stab wounds is positive for peritoneal penetration or suspected because the anterior fascia is penetrated, peritoneal lavage can be performed as a screening tool. In blunt trauma, peritoneal lavage is considered positive when 5–10 ml of grossly bloody aspirate is obtained or when the lavage fluid has greater than 100 000 RBC/mm^3. Evaluation of lavage fluid in stab wounds should be based upon a protocol. In general, greater than 1000 RBC/mm^3 is considered a positive lavage and laparotomy should follow.

Technique of peritoneal lavage

Prior to initiation of peritoneal lavage, the bladder should be emptied by drainage with a catheter. The abdomen is prepared with povidone iodine and draped with sterile towels. The midline of the lower abdomen is infiltrated with lidocaine and epinephrine, and a small incision is made and carried down to the linea alba. This is incised, a peritoneal dialysis catheter is placed and seated against the peritoneum, and the peritoneum is penetrated. This is known as the 'semi-open' technique. Once the peritoneum is entered, the stylet is withdrawn and the catheter directed at a 45° angle into the pelvis. The catheter is aspirated, and if the aspirate returns with 10 ml of non-clotting blood, the study is positive. If little or no blood is aspirated, a 1000 ml bag of normal saline or Ringer lactate is infused into the peritoneal cavity. Once infused, the empty i.v. bottle is placed on the floor, allowing the intraperitoneal fluid to siphon back into the bottle. Grossly bloody fluid indicates a positive lavage and pink fluid is sent for a cell count, with greater than 100 000/mm^3 red cells being considered positive.

Generally accepted criteria for a positive peritoneal lavage in blunt trauma include grossly bloody fluid, red blood cell count greater than 100 000/mm^3, white blood cell count greater than 500/mm^3, amylase greater than 200 units, and the presence of bile, faeces or bacteria. A rough index of cloudiness in the lavage fluid is the ability to read newsprint through the fluid in the i.v. tubing. If the words can be read, the lavage is considered to have less than 100 000 RBC/mm^3 and a formal count should be obtained.

Establishing priorities and indications for surgery

Indications for laparotomy include signs of peritoneal injury, unexplained shock, evisceration of a viscus, a positive diagnostic peritoneal lavage and deterioration of findings during routine follow-up.

It is the job of the general surgeon caring for the trauma patient to integrate various specialties that may be called upon to participate in the care of the multiply injured patient. This often may require a two-team approach, for instance, with the simultaneous management of a major intracranial injury and intra-abdominal injury.

In preparation for laparotomy, certain aspects must be considered to protect the patient from severe hypotension during the early stages of surgical exploration. Vascular access must be secure. If the patient has suffered major blood loss, central venous catheterization should be performed. An arterial cannula should be placed to allow peri-operative recording of the blood pressure. Broad spectrum antibiotics should be given as soon as the decision to perform laparotomy is made, and these should be continued into the post-operative period, determined by the operative findings and the presence of associated injuries. Hypothermia is often a problem in patients who have prolonged intra-abdominal operations for multiple injuries and have large volumes of transfusion. Anticipating the need for warming is important.

Operative approach

The operative approach for abdominal trauma is straightforward. A midline incision is preferred, and there are few reasons to deviate from this. It allows extension into a median sternotomy in the event that more proximal control of the vena cava or aorta is needed. The patient should be routinely cleaned from the sternal notch to the mid thigh to allow harvesting of the saphenous vein for any encountered vascular injury.

Once the abdomen is opened, obvious blood and clot is removed by packing all four quadrants of the abdomen. These are sequentially removed from the lower abdomen first and next from the upper abdomen. Any area that is found to be the source of haemorrhage can be repacked. Additional inflow occlusion can be accomplished by clamping the aorta at the diaphragmatic hiatus. Obvious leaking hollow viscus wounds are rapidly sutured and contamination is thereby minimized during the course of the operation. Retroperitoneal haematomas may be the source of exsanguinating haemorrhage if rupture into the free peritoneal cavity has occurred. If not, these can be left for investigation at a later time, depending on the location. Haematomas of the pelvis associated with pelvic fractures should not be disturbed. Stable haematomas in the perinephric space lateral to the midline that are not expanding are best left undisturbed. Central haematomas that may involve injury to the major vascular structures, pancreas or duodenum are noted and exploration of these is carried out after control of injuries within the peritoneal cavity is accomplished.

Once haemorrhage has been controlled by packing and ongoing contamination stopped, time must be taken to allow re-establishment of the patient's circulating blood volume and cardiac output. Prolonged periods of hypotension should be avoided at all costs and this generally can be done with packing. Once the intra-abdominal injuries have been repaired, a thorough completion exploratory laparotomy methodically investigating the entire abdominal contents is performed.

Specific injuries

Diaphragmatic injuries

Following blunt trauma, the diaphragm is involved in about 3% of injuries, most commonly involving the left hemidiaphragm. The right hemidiaphragm can be involved and massive visceral herniation is possible. All should be repaired to avoid the long-term consequence of herniation that may be fatal to the patient. The diagnosis is suspected when respiratory distress and radiological evidence of pleural effusion are not relieved by intercostal catheter decompression or when an upright radiograph demonstrates visceral herniation. Herniation is inevitable due to the pressure differential that exists between the thoracic and abdominal cavity.

Penetrating injuries below the nipples and below the costal margins should be assumed to have penetrated the diaphragm. These should be evaluated with peritoneal lavage, thoracoscopy in patients with haemothorax or pneumothorax, or laparoscopy in those with a normal chest film. At the time of exploratory laparotomy in blunt or penetrating trauma, the entire diaphragmatic surface should be explored to rule out injury. Simple holes may be repaired with interrupted horizontal mattress sutures and larger lacerations or actual defects may have to be repaired with prosthetic material.

Repair of acute traumatic diaphragmatic rupture is accomplished through the abdomen because of the potential for associated intraperitoneal injuries. Defects discovered at a later time are satisfactorily repaired by a transthoracic, an abdominal or a combined approach. The complications of diaphragmatic rupture result primarily from missing the injury and delayed presentation with incarceration and possible strangulation of intestinal viscera.

Spleen

The spleen is the intra-abdominal organ most frequently injured in blunt trauma. The history is helpful in the patient who can describe a blow, fall or sports injury to the left chest, flank or left upper abdomen. Often, it is accompanied by rib fractures on the left side. The spleen lies in the left upper quadrant of the abdomen and in the intrathoracic abdomen. It lies to the left and slightly behind the stomach. During increased intra-abdominal pressure accompanying blunt trauma, compression of the spleen may occur between the anterior wall and the posterior rib cage. Likewise, in penetrating trauma, a wound of entry or exit in this area should arouse suspicion. Clinical signs may be surprisingly few and a thorough search must be undertaken based on injury mechanism. The clinical picture of splenic injury includes left upper quadrant abdominal pain, signs of blood loss and pain in the left shoulder (Kehr's sign).

The management of splenic trauma has been the subject of major re-examination since the early 1990s, and an increased appreciation is emerging of the danger of intra-abdominal abscess and post-splenectomy sepsis following routine splenectomy. The recognition of fatal pneumococcal septicaemia in patients undergoing splenectomy has led to an interest in splenic salvage. The spectrum of injury may vary from a simple laceration or contusion without capsular disruption to total fragmentation of the spleen.

Adjunctive laboratory studies in general are not helpful. Leucocytosis and decreased haematocrit will occur, but these are not specific for splenic injury. Plain abdominal films may show enlargement of the splenic shadow, medial displacement of the splenic shadow, or medial displacement of the stomach. Stable patients with suspected abdominal trauma now undergo ultrasound examination as stated above. If free fluid is found and the patient remains stable, an abdominal CT scan is obtained to identify the source of bleeding, to rule out contrast extravasation and other intra-abdominal injuries that would require an operation, and to grade the severity of the splenic injury.

- Fifty to 70% of all splenic injuries in stable patients are currently treated by means of a non-operative approach.

During the course of laparotomy, the spleen is evaluated for haemorrhage. If haemorrhage from the spleen is present, one must make a decision regarding splenic salvage. Adequate mobilization of the spleen from its attachments is essential to the success of splenic salvage. Care must be taken during the course of mobilization to prevent further injury. Once mobilized, the tail of the pancreas is freed from the posterior retroperitoneum and the spleen is delivered into the abdominal incision. Ongoing bleeding can be controlled from the spleen during mobilization by digital compression. Capsular tears of the spleen can be controlled by topical haemostatic agents. Lacerations into the splenic substance can be controlled with interlocking absorbable sutures. Major lacerations of the splenic substance involving less than 50% of the splenic tissue can be treated with segmental splenic resection. Splenic salvage should not be pursued if:

- the patient has protracted hypotension
- undue delay is anticipated in attempting to repair the spleen
- the patient has other severe injuries.

With penetrating injury, damage to adjacent structures such as stomach, pancreas, colon and diaphragm must be considered and investigated.

Complications following splenectomy include early transient thrombocytosis, which resolves spontaneously over 1–3 months. Anticoagulation should not be utilized. Delayed haemorrhage, pancreatitis and subphrenic abscess also occur. The incidence of subphrenic abscess probably is increased by post-operative drainage and most would advise against it.

Post-splenectomy sepsis

The incidence of life-threatening sepsis in adult patients seems to be increasing. It is clear that fatal pneumococcal septicaemia in children under the age of 4 is a real risk. The significance of the clinical incidence is less easy to define. When splenectomy is indicated or required, post-operative follow-up and management are essential. Immunization with the polyvalent pneumococcal vaccine and booster immunization every 3 years should be done. These patients should be advised of their increased potential risk for post-splenectomy sepsis and should carry an identification card to alert health care workers of this possibility whenever they have an infection. All infections should be considered as emergencies and treated with antibiotics. Prophylactic antibiotics should be used whenever the patient is to undergo instrumentation, such as during dental repair or surgery.

Liver injuries

The liver is the largest organ in the abdominal cavity and is commonly damaged in blunt and penetrating abdominal trauma and in thoraco-abdominal injuries.

- Because of its size, injuries sufficient to lacerate the liver are associated with injuries to other organs in about 80% of cases.

Spontaneous haemostatic mechanisms that characterize liver tissue may contribute to the pervasive observation that 85% of liver injuries do not bleed at the time of laparotomy, and patients tolerate these injuries very well.

- Most liver injuries will in fact require only documentation and no drainage.

Thus, only a minority of liver injuries require definitive surgical care. These, however, present as complex a problem to the surgeon as any other injury.

The history is helpful in that there is usually an indication of blunt energy transfer, particularly to the right rib cage or upper abdomen. Physical findings may be minimal in that early bleeding may not cause peritoneal irritation. The abdomen may or may not be distended.

- A patient who has a history of being in shock at the scene following blunt trauma should be suspected of having a major liver injury and any patient who is hypotensive after blunt abdominal trauma must be suspected of having a severe liver injury. Haemodynamically unstable patients, those with altered mental status, or those who will undergo general anaesthesia for extra-abdominal procedures should be evaluated with DPL. However, stable patients without peritoneal signs are better evaluated by CT scan due to the possibility of non-operative treatment.

Injuries vary from capsular tears and non-bleeding lacerations to large fractures and lobar destruction, with extensive parenchymal disruption and hepatic artery and venous injuries. The type of injury dictates the amount of surgical therapy required. The principles of surgical management of liver injury are the same regardless of the severity of injury. They involve:

- control of bleeding
- removal of devitalized tissue
- establishment of adequate drainage.

Simple lacerations that have stopped bleeding at the time of surgery do not require drainage unless they are deep into the parenchyma with the high possibility of post-operative biliary leakage. Subcapsular haematomas can be simply evacuated if there is no associated parenchymal injury (Figure 1.14). Lacerations that continue to bleed despite attempts at local control will require opening the liver wound – a tractotomy. The depths of the liver wound are explored and specific vessels and biliary radicals individually ligated. In the event that bleeding continues despite segmental ligation of parenchymal vessels, the porta hepatis should be compressed (Pringle manoeuvre). If the bleeding stops, it can be assumed to be from the portal veins or hepatic artery. If the bleeding continues, it is assumed to be coming from the hepatic veins or the retrohepatic vena cava. The portal triad also can be intermittently clamped to allow visualization during placement of sutures as parenchymal vessels are ligated.

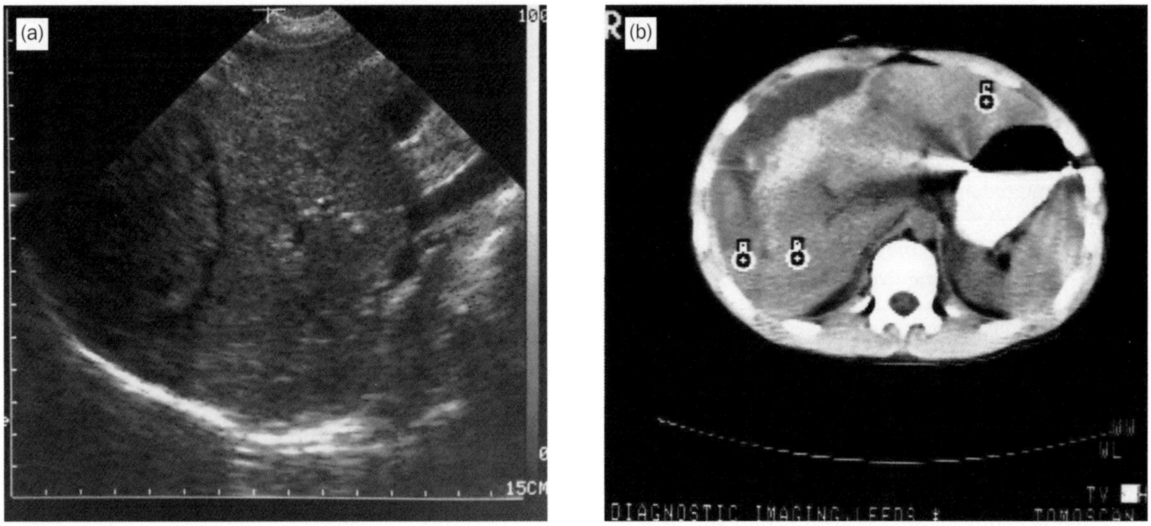

Figure 1.14 (a) Ultrasound of liver, showing large haematoma. (b) CT scan of liver in the same patient showing encapsulated haematoma and underlying liver damage.

When selective ligation fails, ligation of the hepatic artery is an alternative. It may produce dramatic haemostasis without subsequent liver failure, but this should be done as close to the liver as possible and only as a last resort. Packing the liver is an alternative to ligation of the hepatic artery, as discussed below.

An alternative for deep lacerations with persistent bleeding is resectional debridement of the segment of the liver. This is accomplished with finger fracture, removing devitalized liver or a portion of the segment, whole segment or lobe to allow access and control of bleeding. This will be required in approximately 3% of all liver injuries. Subsegmental resection may be adequate; if segmentectomy or lobectomy is required, knowledge of the anatomy is imperative in order not to compromise inflow or outflow to the remaining segments. If this course is to be followed, a decision should be made early, the blood bank notified, and adequate help and exposure obtained. Exposure is best accomplished by complete division of the capsular attachments. Finger fracture through the parenchyma with individual ligation of vessels and biliary radicals as they are encountered after adequate control of the porta hepatis is the best technique.

Inability to control bleeding by clamping the porta hepatis implies significant retrohepatic vena caval bleeding or bleeding from the hepatic veins. If this is unilobular, then debridement and resection should be sufficient. With bilobar involvement or uncontrollable haemorrhage from a single lobe, early consideration should be given to the placement of the intracaval shunt (Figure 1.15). To accomplish this, the sternum is split and a chest tube is placed through the right atrium. Proximal and distal control are obtained above and below the liver, above the renal veins. This will allow better visualization of hepatic vein and vena caval lacerations, which can be directly suture ligated.

In the event that parenchymal or hepatic vein bleeding cannot be controlled and the patient remains difficult to resuscitate, packing of the injury and resuscitation is most appropriate. Subsequent removal of the packs 24–72 hours post-operatively can be followed with resection and suture ligation in a resuscitated patient. Often, bleeding will have stopped and nothing further is needed. If packing is to be used, a blanket of disposable plastic draping material between the liver and the pack will prevent bleeding when the packs are removed. Packing can be accomplished as long as intra-abdominal pressure does not exceed 40 mmHg. If packing cannot be accomplished without excessive

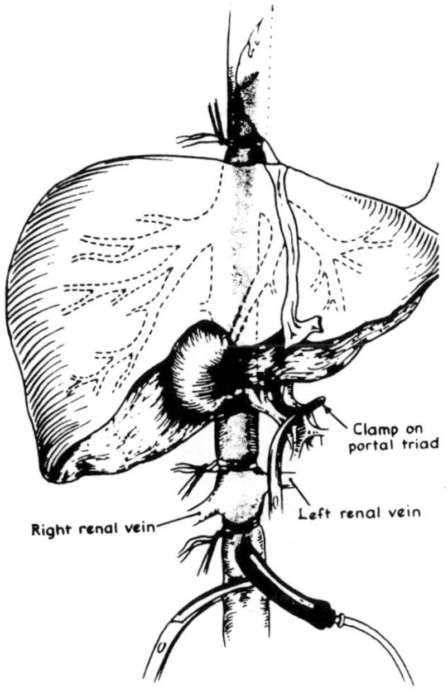

Figure 1.15 The placement of a caval catheter may be achieved by introducing the catheter into the abdominal vena cava as shown or by a route through the atrial appendage if the chest has been opened.

increases in intra-abdominal pressure, towel clamp closure can be used as a temporary measure and the fascia closed when the packs are removed.

When haemostasis is achieved, non-viable tissue should be debrided and the area drained. When extensive parenchymal damage or central penetrating injuries are encountered, active drainage with sump tubes is indicated. T tubes in the common duct have no place unless the extrahepatic biliary tree is injured. Significant complications following liver injury include:

- pulmonary complications
- coagulopathy
- hypoglycaemia
- jaundice
- biliary fistulas
- haemobilia
- subdiaphragmatic and intraparenchymal abscess formation.

Disseminated intravascular coagulation and impaired liver synthesis can be implicated in the aetiology of the coagulopathy following liver resection, but the most important factor is usually hypothermia and inadequate blood component replacement. Patients undergoing major hepatic resection following trauma need continuous glucose infusion during the early post-operative period, but hypoalbuminaemia, though present, does not require specific albumin administration. Aggressive nutritional support should be used. Hyperbilirubinaemia is transient, will peak in 2–3 weeks, and usually does not go above 10 mg/dl. Intra-abdominal abscesses (intrahepatic and subphrenic) can develop, particularly when large amounts of debridement have been necessary, and are diagnosed with clinical signs of sepsis and imaging with ultrasound or CT. Biliary fistulas usually close spontaneously.

Haemobilia is a rare complication, which presents with intrahepatic bleeding into the bile ducts and can be diagnosed with endoscopy and treated with angiographic embolization.

Stomach injuries

Injuries of the stomach are very rare in blunt trauma and common in penetrating trauma. The stomach is intrathoracic, partially protected by the rib cage, and gastric injuries are relatively difficult to diagnose. Any penetrating wound in this area should be suspected of causing injury to the stomach and requires investigation of the anterior and posterior surface at the time of laparotomy.

A nasogastric tube should be inserted during initial evaluation, and aspirate positive for blood may point to a gastric injury and should raise suspicion. The intra-operative evaluation of stomach injury includes good visualization of the oesophageal hiatus, evaluation of the anterior portion of the stomach, division of the gastrocolic ligament, and complete visualization of the posterior aspect of the stomach. If there is any question regarding injury, the stomach should be distended with saline and vital dye to evaluate for leaking. Penetrating wounds are debrided and primary closure is performed. Maceration of the stomach from significant penetrating or blunt injury may require gastric resection. Postoperative complications include intra-abdominal abscess, particularly in the lesser sac, but are rare. The other complication of gastric injury is gastric fistula. The treatment is immediate re-operation and repair using healthy tissue. Due to its proximity to the diaphragm, the stomach is frequently injured following thoracoabdominal wounds. Depending on the severity of contamination due to spillage of gastric contents, empyema is another complication.

Injuries to the duodenum

Isolated injury to the duodenum usually does not cause significant hypotension and signs of peritonitis may be delayed if the retroperitoneal duodenum is injured. Failure to recognize this injury is associated with high morbidity and mortality caused by abscess formation in the lesser sac and the development of sepsis. Entry wounds between the xiphoid and umbilicus suggest possible injury to the duodenum, and non-penetrating duodenal injury may be caused by crushing injuries where intraperitoneal and extraperitoneal duodenum is macerated or contused against the spine. A closed loop compression of an air-filled loop following a seatbelt injury can account for maceration injury often seen in the duodenum. History of trunk injury or localized blow to the epigastrium with handle bars, steering wheel or fist should suggest these types of injury.

Adjunctive diagnostic tests might include hyperamylasaemia. This occurs in about half of the patients with blunt injury to the duodenum as a result of extravasation of intra-abdominal pancreatic amylase. Elevated serum amylase following blunt trauma is not diagnostic of an injury but raises suspicion and necessitates further diagnostic study. Abdominal radiographs may suggest duodenal injury showing obliteration of the psoas shadow, absence of air in the duodenal bulb, or air in the retroperitoneum outlining the kidney. Psoas muscle and lumbar spine abnormalities, such as spastic lordosis in association with transverse process fractures, indicate major injury in this area.

Definitive diagnosis requires contrast duodenography or CT scan with oral contrast. Extravasation of contrast material is an absolute indication for laparotomy. Distortion of the duodenum indicates significant injury and is a relative indication for laparotomy. The radiographic picture of an intramural duodenal haematoma is not an indication to operate immediately. If this causes obstruction that fails to resolve, then operative management is indicated.

Intra-operative evaluation of the duodenum requires complete mobilization of the duodenum (Kocher manoeuvre). The hepatic flexure of the colon is taken down to expose the anterior aspect of the second portion of the duodenum, and inspection of the third and fourth portions of the duodenum at the base of the transverse colon should be done. Retroperitoneal haematomas in the area of the duodenum must be explored and the lesser sac should be entered to exclude associated pancreatic injuries.

Limited perforations or simple lacerations of the duodenum within 6 hours of injury are treated with primary closure. After 6 hours, the risk of duodenal leak increases. Suction decompression of the duodenum with a transpyloric nasogastric tube, tube jejunostomy or tube duodenostomy is advisable if repair is in any way compromised.

If the laceration of the first and second portion of the duodenum is extensive and primary closure would be associated with obstruction, Roux-en-Y jejunoduodenostomy is indicated. Multiple or extensive lacerations that narrow the lumen and jeopardize the vascularity of the duodenum are best managed by pyloric exclusion. The proximal duodenum is defunctionalized by closing the pylorus and establishing gastric drainage with a gastrojejunostomy. Wounds of the first and second portion of the duodenum are closed primarily and the duodenum is drained with a tube duodenostomy. The area around the duodenum is also drained.

Pancreaticoduodenectomy is occasionally indicated for massive injury in the right upper quadrant in which the proximal duodenum cannot be repaired, usually due to devascularization. This is usually accompanied by maceration of the head of the pancreas, and thereby becomes the indication for pancreaticoduodenectomy. This is rarely needed, however.

The distal duodenum (third and fourth portions) can be primarily closed as with the proximal duodenum if the injury is treated within 6 hours of insult. More than 6 hours after injury, or when there is maceration of the distal duodenum, resection of the third and fourth portions of the duodenum and duodenal jejunostomy should be performed.

Duodenal haematomas confirmed by radio contrast study can be expected to resolve, and management consists of nasogastric suction until peristalsis returns and slow introduction of solid food. Persistent duodenal obstruction will require operative treatment.

Other than post-operative bleeding, the most significant complication following duodenal injury is the development of a duodenal fistula, which occurs in 5–10% of patients following anastomosis. Unlike a gastric fistula, it is generally managed non-operatively with nasogastric suction, nutritional support and aggressive stoma care. In addition, antibiotics are indicated if infection occurs. Uncomplicated fistulas will close in 6 weeks and should be treated operatively if they persist beyond 6 weeks.

Pancreatic injuries

Blunt trauma to the abdomen from a direct kick, blow or seatbelt injury may crush the pancreas over the vertebral column. Epigastric and posterior penetrating wounds likewise can penetrate the pancreas and are often associated with significant injuries involving the kidney, vena cava and colon. This is of particular concern in that enzymatically active pancreatic juice increases the possibility of anastomotic leak following these injuries if they are not recognized and treated appropriately. The shared blood supply between the pancreas and duodenum makes the likelihood of these two injuries occurring in combination very high. Diagnosis is by history and associated clinical findings, although these may be non-existent. Suspicion must be raised and serial re-evaluation undertaken if there is any doubt. Elevation of serum and urinary amylase following blunt injury is not diagnostic, but a persistent elevation suggests pancreatic injury, and this must be ruled out. Contrast duodenography may reveal widening of the C-loop. A loss of the psoas shadow, anterior displacement of the stomach and duodenum from a pancreatic phlegmon, and left pleural effusion are all suggestive of a pancreatic injury but not specifically diagnostic. CT scan is of potential value but its role is still unclear.

Patients seldom undergo laparotomy because of pancreatic injury alone. Instead, they are generally operated on because of intraperitoneal blood loss or peritonitis. At the time of laparotomy, the pancreas should be examined and any evidence of adjacent injury excluded (i.e. duodenal haematoma, haematoma in the transverse mesocolon, or trauma to the anterior wall of the stomach or spleen). Any retroperitoneal haematoma around the pancreas should be explored, and retroperitoneal bile staining indicating a concurrent duodenal or biliary tract injury must be investigated. If there is any evidence that the pancreas has been contused, it should be drained. Injury to the body and tail, which is refractory to simple debridement, should be treated with partial pancreatic resection splenectomy and distal pancreatectomy. Injuries to the mid-portion of the pancreas can theoretically be treated with pancreaticojejunostomy, but little is to be gained over splenectomy and distal pancreatectomy in this circumstance.

Penetrating wounds to the right of the superior mesenteric vein should be treated with debridement and direct suture ligation of areas of bleeding. Debridement must be conservative in that bile ducts may be injured and blood supply compromised.

Significant injury to the head of the pancreas or to the right of the superior mesenteric vessels will be associated with a 30–60% probability of temporary pancreatic fistula, and this should be accepted. Severe trauma to the head of the pancreas in association with duodenal injuries should be treated with debridement of the pancreas, closure of the duodenal wound, and pyloric exclusion as described above. Extensive damage to the head of the pancreas and duodenum may require total pancreatoduodenectomy. Wide drainage is the rule and should be anticipated even when the pancreas is only locally debrided. This should be accomplished with sump drains brought out to the flank and left in place until drainage has stopped. The most common complication of pancreatic injury is a persistent pancreatic fistula; if well controlled it should close spontaneously unless there is obstruction to the pancreatic duct. Somatostatin has been used to expedite healing of pancreatic fistulas, but results remain controversial.

Small intestine injuries

Injuries to the small intestine occur in approximately 15–20% of patients who require laparotomy after blunt trauma. The postulated mechanisms are:

- Crushing injury of the bowel between the spine and the blunt object, such as a steering wheel or handlebars.
- Deceleration shearing of the small bowel at fixed points such as the ileocaecal valve and around the superior mesenteric artery.
- Closed loop rupture caused by increased intra-abdominal pressure.

Injuries to the small intestine are present in approximately 25–30% of patients who require laparotomy after penetrating trauma. Diagnosis is often either directly apparent secondary to peritoneal injury, or indirectly due to bleeding from the raw surface of the enterotomy. Antibiotics should be started pre-operatively.

At operation, significant bleeding will be the first priority. After application of packs and vascular control of exsanguinating haemorrhage, non-crushing clamps should be applied to prevent further leakage of small bowel contents. The small bowel should be carefully examined from the ligament of Treitz all the way to the ileocaecal valve. Contusion of the antimesenteric wall of the bowel may result in delayed perforation, and seromuscular sutures can be used to imbricate the contusion into the lumen. Mesenteric haematomas that extend up to the bowel should be incised and evacuated such that the underlying bowel can be adequately examined.

Single holes from stab wounds or shotgun pellets can be closed without debridement. Since penetrating injuries in general occur in pairs, careful examination of the bowel wall on the opposite side must be done to avoid missing any small perforations. If two adjacent holes are found, they can be connected across the bridge of bowel and a transverse closure effected so as not to narrow the lumen. Large lacerations are debrided and closed. Transection of the small bowel is debrided and closed in routine fashion and the mesenteric defect should be closed to prevent herniation. Any large segments of bowel that are devascularized or have multiple defects should be resected and re-anastomosed. Patients are maintained on post-operative decompression with a nasogastric tube until peristalsis returns and feeding is then begun.

Major complications include intra-abdominal abscess anastomotic leakage and enterocutaneous fistulas, as well as intestinal obstruction. Intra-abdominal abscess must be drained. If obstruction occurs early, it can generally be treated conservatively with a nasogastric tube, but may require re-operation. Enterocutaneous fistulas can be treated conservatively if the output is low and should be expected to close spontaneously with parenteral nutrition.

Injuries to the colon and rectum

The greatest number of injuries to the colon and rectum are the result of penetrating or perforating trauma. The amount of force required to damage the colon is considerable and, thus, the colon is relatively refractory to blunt injury. Blunt trauma accounts for only 5% of colonic injuries. Rectal injuries can occur in association with pelvic fracture and any patient with a significant pelvic fracture must have the possibility of rectal injury considered in addition to evaluation of other pelvic viscera, such as the bladder, distal ureters and vagina.

Signs and symptoms are not specific for injury to the colon and rectum. Indirectly, they will create peritoneal irritation and tenderness, which occur relatively early following injury. Laboratory studies are not helpful; radiological studies may show free air in the peritoneal cavity. Peritoneal lavage is of value if intraperitoneal colonic injury is present and may return fluid with blood or bacteria. If the injury is confined to the extraperitoneal colon and rectum, lavage is of no value. Extraperitoneal colonic or rectal injury is extremely difficult to diagnose.

- The possibility of rectal injury must be considered in any patient with penetrating trauma to the lower abdomen or buttocks.

Digital examination is essential. The presence of blood on examination is strong evidence for colon or rectal injury, and proctoscopic and sigmoidoscopic examinations should be performed. About 95% of colon injuries are caused by gunshot, shotgun or stab wounds, and whenever the possibility of colonic injury is entertained, prophylactic antibiotics should be started intravenously immediately. The number of doses continued post-operatively is determined by the degree of colon injury and local contamination.

- The central debate in the operative management of colonic injury is between primary repair of low-risk colonic injuries versus repair and proximal colostomy or resection and colostomy.

Primary repair can be selected when known associated complicating factors have been excluded. Complications increase in primary repair when there is pre-operative hypotension, intraperitoneal haemorrhage exceeding 1 litre, more than two associated organs injured (hepatic, pancreatic and splenic injuries are the most dangerous) or significant faecal spillage, or more than 6 hours have elapsed since injury. Many patients with low-risk penetrating colon injuries can be treated with primary closure or resection and primary anastomosis following these guidelines. All high-risk colon injuries or those associated with severe injuries as indicated above should be treated with resection and colostomy. An alternative or compromise between colostomy and primary repair has been advocated with exteriorization of the repaired segment. The success of this technique varies and it has no benefit over colostomy. Post-operative complications include abscess formation, anastomotic leak, parastomal hernia, and the morbidity and mortality associated with colostomy closure.

Rectal injuries cause morbidity and mortality primarily due to inadequate initial therapy and the complications associated with delayed sepsis. Rectal injury must be suspected when there is any penetrating injury or a sacral fracture that produces a pelvic ring disruption. Sigmoidoscopic examination is essential.

The principles of operative management include:

- Placement of the patient in the lithotomy position, which allows simultaneous exposure of both the perineum and abdomen.
- Wide debridement of all dead and devitalized tissue.
- A totally defunctioning colostomy (simple loop colostomy is inadequate).
- Rectal wall closure, if possible.
- Retrorectal drainage with coccygectomy, when necessary, to attain adequate rectal drainage.
- Antibiotics, nutritional support and repeat debridement.

Complete rectal destruction is an indication for a primary abdominal perineal resection, with packing that should be removed in approximately 48 hours. Complications following rectal injuries include pelvic abscesses, urinary or rectal fistulas, rectal incontinence and stricture, loss of sexual function, and urinary incontinence.

Retroperitoneal haematomas

The optimum management of retroperitoneal haematoma depends on a number of factors including aetiology, location and other associated injuries. Management of the retroperitoneal haematoma in patients with multisystem trauma has been a source of confusion and controversy for years.

The retroperitoneum can be divided into anatomical zones for purposes of decision making (Figure 1.16). Central retroperitoneal haematomas (zone 1) are associated with pancreaticoduodenal injuries or major abdominal vascular (aorta and vena cava) injury. Flank or perinephric haematomas (zone 2) may be associated with injuries to the genitourinary tract, or in the case of penetrating trauma, with injuries to the colon. Zone 3 injuries, which are confined to or originate from the pelvis, are most often associated with pelvic fractures. Retroperitoneal haematomas in zone 1 are explored regardless of aetiology or size because of the high incidence of associated major vascular, pancreatic or duodenal injuries, and the high morbidity and mortality if these are overlooked.

Retroperitoneal haematomas caused by a penetrating mechanism should be routinely explored. The only exception would be those located in zone 2, which should be explored only if:

- They are adjacent to the colon and may be concealing an occult colonic injury.
- They are expanding.
- Pre-operative evaluation with either nephrotomography or computed tomography has demonstrated a major renal injury that is felt to need repair.

Increased non-operative management of renal injury, even with urine extravasation, has been advocated. If the complication of urinoma develops, this can be managed with percutaneous drainage as long as there is neither significant bleeding nor sepsis. Proximal control of the renal pedicle should be gained in any exploration of the perinephric haematoma. Zone 2 haematomas caused by blunt trauma can be left alone if they are not expanding or if the IVU or CT scan is normal, or a non-operative management course is to be followed.

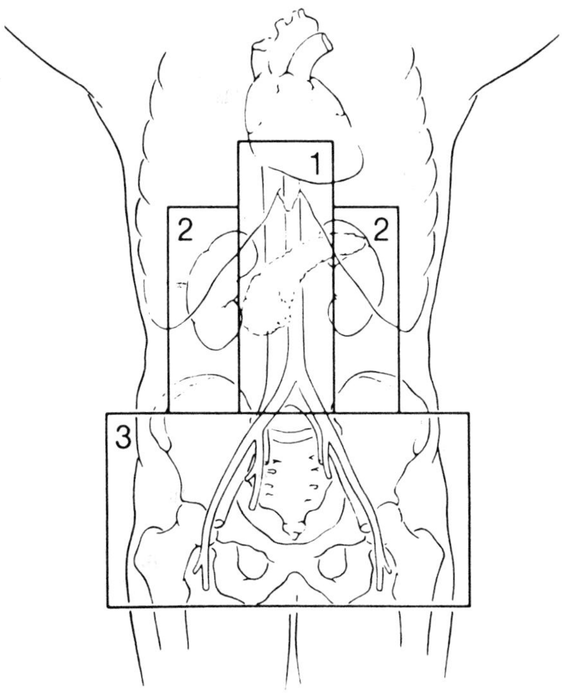

Figure 1.16 Zones of the retroperitoneum (see text).

Zone 3 retroperitoneal haematomas generally are explored in patients with penetrating injuries in order to exclude major vascular or ureteral injuries. Local bleeding encountered at exploration under these circumstances is generally easy to control and the associated injuries can be identified. Patients with zone 3 haematomas secondary to blunt trauma usually have associated pelvic fractures, and exploration of the haematoma can be hazardous. There is often extensive injury to the rich presacral venous and arterial circulation. Incision to the peritoneum destroys the tamponade effect, and dissection in the haematoma may produce catastrophic bleeding. Exploration of these haematomas is associated with an increased transfusion requirement and a high mortality, as discrete bleeding points can rarely be identified.

Management of pelvic fractures

Pelvic fractures continue to be a major cause of morbidity and mortality in patients with blunt abdominal injury. Pedestrian and motor vehicle accidents account for the majority of these injuries, with an associated mortality between 10 and 25%. Massive haemorrhage and coagulopathy continue to account for 40–60% of the mortality in this group of patients.

Pelvic fractures have been classified by a number of different schemes.

- The most useful classification is that by Trunkey (Figure 1.17).

Type I injuries represent comminuted or crush fracture of the pelvis and involve three or more elements of the pelvic rings. These fractures have the highest morbidity and mortality, and are accompanied by massive haemorrhage and severe soft tissue injury. Type II fractures are unstable injuries and involve at least two breaks in the pelvic ring. These include diametric fractures with cephalad displacement of the hemipelvis (Malgaigne), and 'open book' fractures. Type III pelvic fractures are stable fractures generally involving a single element in the pelvic ring or fractures of the pubic rami.

The initial management of the patient with pelvic fractures will depend on associated injuries. In patients with severe pelvic fractures who are haemodynamically unstable, intracavitary haemorrhage must be excluded using conventional means, including radiological studies and diagnostic peritoneal lavage. The incidence of false-positive peritoneal lavage is high in this group of patients due to free dissection of blood from the pelvis into the abdominal cavity and passage of the lavage catheter into an expanded preperitoneal space filled with haematoma. The latter can be minimized by performing diagnostic peritoneal lavage through a supra-umbilical midline incision. Laparotomy is performed immediately for patients with positive lavage. Intra-abdominal visceral injuries are treated, and the pelvic haematoma is not explored.

Control of ongoing pelvic retroperitoneal bleeding represents the greatest challenge in these patients and is the main cause of mortality. Both arterial and venous bleeding may be present and patients may lose in excess of 20 units of blood in a major pelvic injury. Methods of haemorrhage control that have been developed in recent years include:

- Application of the military anti-shock trousers (MAST).
- Pelvic arteriography and arterial embolization.
- Early reduction of the pelvic fracture using external pelvic fixation.

The use of the MAST for early control of haemorrhage has resulted in increased survival and appears to decrease transfusion requirements. MAST suits have been used most often for 'field resuscitation'. Recently they have been used for extended time in the hospital for non-operative control of venous retroperitoneal pelvic bleeding.

Pelvic arteriography and embolization plays an essential role in the early management of massive or persistent pelvic retroperitoneal haemorrhage. The selection of patients for arteriography depends on the magnitude of pelvic haemorrhage, and should be performed when transfusion requirements exceed approximately 4–6 units. Embolization is a safe and effective means of non-operative control and has resulted in reduced morbidity and mortality. Ligation of the hypogastric artery for control of pelvic haemorrhage has been advocated in the past. Because of the rich arterial supply, this is an ineffective manoeuvre for control of arterial haemorrhage and arteriography is preferable. No effect on venous bleeding is achieved by hypogastric ligation.

The best algorithm for management of haemorrhage from pelvic fractures utilizes early arteriography. Indications are:

- recurrent hypotension following initial resuscitation (attributed to the pelvic fracture) or
- if the transfusion requirements exceed 4–6 units within the first 2 hours following injury.

Patients should be maintained in the MAST suit until arteriography can be performed. Following arteriography, patients remain in the MAST suit while any hypothermia and coagulopathy is corrected.

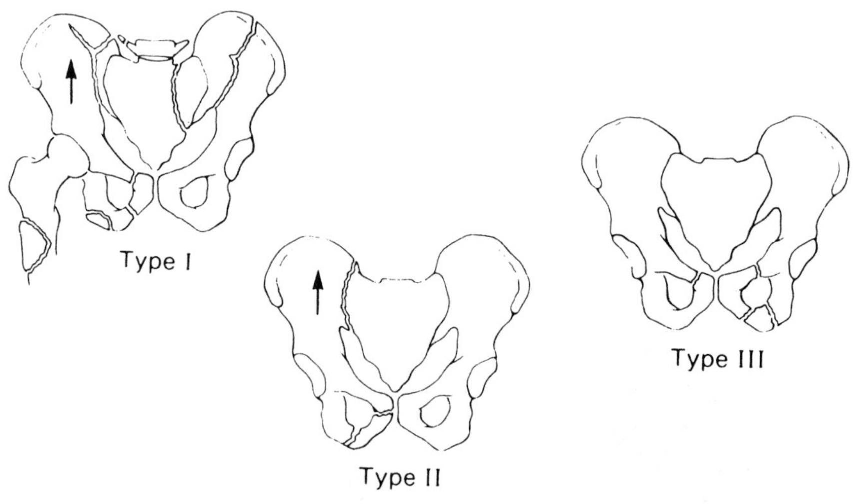

Figure 1.17 Pelvic fracture classification (see text).

Pelvic external fixation is performed in selected cases where there is wide fracture displacement, particularly in anterior or 'open-book' fractures. Decreasing pelvic volume may decrease venous bleeding; however, arterial bleeding, which occurs most frequently in fractures of the posterior elements of the pelvic ring, may not improve with external fixation.

Pelvic fractures associated with deep perineal lacerations, or rectal or vaginal lacerations, are classified as compound pelvic fractures.

- These injuries are associated with a high incidence of septic complications and carry a mortality of approximately 50%.

The primary source of contamination is the faecal stream, and complete diversion is necessary to reduce septic complications. A double-barrelled colostomy should be performed after adequate control of the retroperitoneal haemorrhage has been obtained. A loop colostomy does not provide complete diversion and should not be used under these circumstances.

Urinary tract injuries

General

Because of its location, injuries to the genitourinary tract often are clinically silent and frequently overlooked in the face of more obvious abdominal or thoracic injuries. An awareness of the subtle manifestations of genitourinary injuries is necessary to avoid missing injuries. The physical examination is unreliable in diagnosing urinary tract injuries, but these injuries are amenable to radiological diagnosis. Systematic, orderly evaluation of the urinary tract reduces the chance of missing injury and limits the number of unnecessary retroperitoneal explorations for minor trauma.

Different criteria should exist for initial evaluation of the urinary tract in blunt as opposed to penetrating trauma. In blunt trauma, fractures of the lower portion of the rib cage or spinous processes fractures have been associated with an incidence of renal injuries as high as 20%. Findings of a flank haematoma or ecchymosis on physical examination or associated solid viscus injuries found at laparotomy are also associated with increased incidence of significant renal trauma.

Penetrating trunk trauma, particularly to the back or the flank, has the potential of significant renal injury without any obvious clinical manifestations. A suspicion of renal injury should exist with any penetrating trauma in the vicinity of the renal tract despite outwardly negative clinical signs. Bladder catheterization allows evaluation of the presence and degree of haematuria. The presence of haematuria, either microscopic or gross, is indicative of urinary tract injury, but the absence of haematuria does not exclude the presence of a urinary tract injury. Of patients with penetrating injuries to the renal tract, 15–20% will not present initially with haematuria, and renal artery occlusion may occur in blunt trauma without associated haematuria. Nevertheless urinalysis remains the most sensitive screening test. Intravenous pyelography (IVP) is usually the next step in the radiological evaluation of renal injuries. The degree of haematuria necessary to prompt further evaluation by IVP has not been clearly defined. Penetrating injuries in the vicinity of the urinary tract should be evaluated by IVP regardless of the presence of haematuria. Patients who have sustained major axial or anteroposterior deceleration injuries should undergo evaluation using IVP regardless of the findings of urinalysis. The majority of patients with blunt trauma and haematuria are found to have a normal IVP.

- Current data suggest that 50 RBCs per high-powered field distinguishes between patients with minor and potentially major urinary tract trauma.

This results in a decreased number of intravenous pyelograms performed without any apparent increase in missed urinary tract injuries.

Retrograde cystography is used to diagnose rupture of the bladder. Rupture of the bladder should be suspected in a patient with haematuria and lower pelvic or abdominal trauma. Patients with pelvic fractures involving the anterior arch are particularly prone to have an associated bladder injury. Cystography is performed by the infusion of 50 ml of contrast under gravity flow and if no injury is apparent initially, an additional 250 ml is used to delineate my injury. Intra- and extraperitoneal bladder rupture usually can be differentiated using these methods, but a post-void filling must be obtained to evaluate carefully for extraperitoneal injury.

Retrograde urethrography (RUG) is used to define suspected urethral tears, which occur predominantly in males. Absolute indications for performing retrograde urethrogram include blood at the urethral meatus and a free-floating prostate. Suspicion for urethral injuries also should exist in male patients who present with large perineal haematomas or other perineal injuries. Patients who are suspected of having urethral rupture should not be catheterized. RUG is performed by slow infusion of undiluted contrast material through a small Foley catheter with a balloon inflated in the meatal fossa. Extravasation is seen with injury.

CT is being used increasingly to evaluate patients with a variety of abdominal and retroperitoneal injuries, and has been found to be useful in the preoperative staging of renal injuries. Patients in whom the results of IVP are either indefinite or abnormal should be followed up with a CT scan.

Renal injuries

The kidney is the most commonly injured part of the urinary tract. Classification of renal injury is divided into minor and major injuries, with minor injuries comprising approximately 85% of the cases. Renal contusions comprise the vast majority of minor renal trauma and almost invariably can be treated without operation. Major renal trauma includes deep cortical medullary lacerations with extravasation and large perinephric haematomas, and vascular injuries of the renal pedicle. Microscopic or gross haematuria is usually present, but the degree of haematuria in most seriously injured patients is a poor predictor of the degree of renal injury.

With penetrating injuries, approximately 80% will require laparotomy for associated intra-abdominal injuries. The problem at laparotomy is the decision of whether or not to explore a perinephric haematoma. If the patient's condition has not allowed adequate pre-operative evaluation with IVP, it is best to explore all perinephric haematomas produced by penetrating injuries. Perinephric haematomas associated with blunt injuries are not explored unless they are pulsatile or expanding. The incidence of nephrectomy under these circumstances has been shown to be greatly reduced with a transabdominal approach. Vascular control of the renal pedicle prior to mobilization of the kidney is worthwhile but probably does not lessen the incidence of nephrectomy *per se*.

In patients suspected of having renal injury because of an abnormal or indefinite IVP, evaluation using CT provides a more precise definition of the degree of renal injury. The use of CT under these circumstances allows some patients with isolated renal injuries to be managed non-operatively. Patients with suspected major renal vascular trauma are further evaluated using arteriography.

Indications for operative exploration in patients with penetrating trauma include:

- a suspected renal injury found at laparotomy with incomplete pre-operative staging
- patients with IVP or CT scans demonstrating renal pedicle injury, urinary extravasation
- parenchymal laceration with significant perinephric haematoma.

Indication for operative intervention in patients with blunt trauma is more controversial, but in general includes:

- patients with large renal lacerations and extravasation
- renal pedicle injuries
- patients with a large or expanding perinephric haematoma.

The increasing use of CT scan has allowed more patients with both blunt and penetrating renal injuries to be managed non-operatively. The precise definition of non-operative injury has not been determined, but stable haematomas and minimal extravasation can be safely managed non-operatively. Options at the time of exploration for renal trauma include nephrectomy, partial nephrectomy, and repair of transcapsular lacerations using omental and/or peritoneal patch grafts.

Ureteral injuries

Injury to the ureter is uncommon and occurs mostly with penetrating trauma. The presence of haematuria in ureteral injury is not a consistent finding. Ureteral injury is generally suspected pre-operatively by the location of the penetrating injury, or in the case of blunt injury, by the presence of concomitant intra-abdominal or other genitourinary tract injuries. In 80–85% of cases of ureteral injury, IVP will confirm the diagnosis; 15–20% of ureteral injuries are not demonstrated on IVP and require demonstration by retrograde ureterography.

- Many ureteral injuries are missed at initial evaluation and present late as urinomas with associated fever, flank mass and pain, or as a urinary fistula, often presenting as urine extravasation through the cutaneous site of the penetrating injury.

In those patients whose clinical condition does not allow for pre-operative IVP, the diagnosis of ureteral injury may be made at the time of laparotomy by chromo-ureterography. This is accomplished by the intravenous injection of 5 ml of methylene blue or indigo carmine dye. Extravasation of the blue-tinged urine into the operative field usually serves to confirm the presence of ureteral injury and to locate its site. Surgical options for repair of injured ureters include uretero-ureterostomy, or ureteral reimplantation into the bladder. In cases of extensive ureteral loss, auto-transplantation of the kidney into the iliac fossa may be necessary for injuries to the upper third of the ureter. Middle third injuries may require reimplantation of the damaged ureter into the normal ureter across the midline, or renal and bladder mobilization to allow for a tension-free anastomosis. Long segment ureteral losses in the lower third may be managed by the creation of an anterior bladder flap tube into which a shortened ureter may be reimplanted.

Bladder injuries

The majority of bladder injuries occur as a result of blunt external trauma, and should be strongly suspected in patients with haematuria and pelvic fractures. Bladder rupture may be extraperitoneal or intraperitoneal. The former is usually a result of perforations by adjacent bony fragments from the site of the pelvic fracture, and the latter the result of rupture of the dome that occurs when a full bladder sustains a direct blow. Diagnosis is made by cystography. Intravenous pyelography is often necessary to evaluate the upper urinary tract. The possibility of ureteral injury also should be considered in any patient with a bladder injury. Repair of intraperitoneal rupture of the bladder is accomplished via a transabdominal approach, and includes a suprapubic cystostomy with drainage.

The management of extraperitoneal rupture of the bladder is primarily non-operative. The non-operative management of extraperitoneal rupture by the use of prolonged Foley catheter drainage requires that the patient has no intra-abdominal injuries, no significant local haemorrhage and no urinary tract infection. A 20–25% complication rate has been reported with non-operative management of extraperitoneal bladder rupture, but this is probably excessive. Patients with severe pelvic fractures and massive retroperitoneal bleeding are always managed non-operatively. A delayed repair of their extraperitoneal rupture can be done if required once the retroperitoneal bleeding is controlled and their condition stabilized. These patients are at very high risk for haemorrhagic complications associated with dissection into the retroperitoneal pelvic haematoma.

Injuries to the urethra

Disruption of the urethra is an injury found mostly in men, and associated with either pelvic fractures or so-called straddle injury.

- Posterior urethral tears are present in approximately 10% of pelvic fractures.

Ruptures of the anterior urethra are generally associated with straddle injuries and are often isolated lesions. Urethral injuries are suspected on the basis of mechanism, associated pelvic fracture, perineal haematoma or perineal injury, blood at the urethral meatus, and displacement of the prostate gland. Diagnosis is made by a retrograde urethrogram. Intravenous pyelography generally is performed in patients with associated injuries. The majority of patients with rupture of the posterior urethra will have a complete tear. About half of the patients with anterior urethral injuries will have complete tears.

The initial management of urethral injuries has undergone significant change in the past several years. Conventional early urethral realignment has given way to initial bladder decompression by suprapubic cystostomy and a delayed urethroplasty. Delayed repair has served to markedly diminish the incidence of stricture, impotence and incontinence associated with urethral repair at the time of injury.

Complications of genitourinary trauma

Stepwise systematic evaluation of suspected genitourinary injuries will result in a low incidence of delayed diagnosis, and the associated haemorrhagic and infectious complications. Early complications of genitourinary injury include:

- haemorrhage
- urinary extravasation
- infection.

Haemorrhage may be massive with severe renal injuries and can result in exsanguination. Urinary extravasation from renal fracture, ureteral lacerations and bladder rupture may result in retroperitoneal urinomas. These collections are prone to infection and may lead to abscess formation. Large retroperitoneal haematomas, associated urinary extravasation and urinary tract infection can result in seeding of the haematoma and, eventually, abscess formation and sepsis.

Late complications of genitourinary trauma include:

- hypertension, arteriovenous fistula and pyelonephritis with renal injuries
- stricture formation and hydronephrosis with ureteral transections
- stricture, incontinence and impotence with disruptions of the urethra.

Table 1.7 Consequences of increased intra-abdominal pressure

- *Increase*
  - Cardiac rate
  - Pulmonary capillary wedge pressure
  - Peak inspiratory pressure
  - Central venous pressure
  - Intrapleural pressure
  - Systemic vascular resistance
- *Reduction*
  - Cardiac output
  - Central venous return
  - Visceral blood flow
  - Renal blood flow
  - Glomerular filtration

Abdominal compartment syndrome following trauma

Trauma patients with severe intra-abdominal injuries, presenting in profound shock and requiring large amounts of intravenous fluids are those most susceptible to the development of sudden increase in intra-abdominal pressure. This syndrome is characterized by abdominal distension, oliguria, hypoxia and increased pulmonary inspiratory pressure. The diagnosis is confirmed by measuring the intra-abdominal pressure directly or the intravesical pressure. In the presence of these signs, an early and immediate decompression, by means of leaving the abdominal wall open, is indicated. The physiological derangements determined by a significant increase in intra-abdominal pressure are listed in Table 1.7.

Section 1.4 • Vascular trauma

Penetrating or blunt injuries to arteries and veins are a major cause of morbidity and mortality in the trauma patient. Vascular injuries to the extremities can be life or limb-threatening. Rapid diagnosis and repair is crucial to the successful management of these injuries. Many of the current principles of management of serious vascular injuries and their complications have been developed through the cumulative military experience since World War II. The modern experience in urban trauma centres with injuries due to low-velocity missiles and motor vehicle accidents has led to further refinements in the management of vascular trauma. During World War II when extremity arterial injuries were treated primarily by ligation, DeBakey reported a 48% amputation rate. Increasing use of arterial repair in the Korean conflict resulted in a reduction of the amputation rate to 13%, and the lessons of the Vietnam War further contributed to the capability to treat vascular trauma with good success. This improvement can be attributed to the shortened evacuation time, which minimizes ischaemia, the repair of accompanying venous injuries and the widespread availability of experienced surgeons. Subsequent technological advancements in angiography, non-invasive imaging, Doppler examination, and improved prosthetic grafts and suture materials have facilitated successful treatment of these difficult problems.

Aetiology

Direct penetrating injury (primarily stab and gunshot wounds) or blunt trauma is responsible for the majority of vascular injuries encountered in civilian practice. Although advances in motor vehicle safety may improve the outlook for blunt vascular injury, the current epidemic of urban violence is likely to result in an even greater increase in the number of penetrating injuries. The rapidly increasing use of intravascular diagnostic and interventional techniques in the medical community has also significantly raised the number of iatrogenic injuries that are encountered.

The trauma produced by a bullet is proportional to its kinetic energy, which is primarily determined by the velocity of the projectile ($= 1/2 \text{ mass} \times \text{velocity}^2$). A high-velocity missile not only results in significant direct injury but also produces a cavitational and suction effect (blast injury) that can cause a more extensive intimal injury than is initially expected or apparent. As a consequence, major complications may present in a delayed fashion. While low-velocity projectile and stab wounds are not associated with a 'blast injury' of this nature, they nevertheless can produce major vascular disruption with attendant ischaemia, haemorrhage or arteriovenous fistulas.

Pathophysiology

The spectrum of blood vessel injury consists of laceration, transection, contusion and spasm. Arterial or venous laceration is the most common type of vascular injury due to penetrating trauma. Any arterial injury can result in thrombosis, haematoma, pseudoaneurysm or communication with a venous channel forming an arteriovenous fistula. Complete transection of an artery often induces retraction of the intima and media, which prevents exsanguinating haemorrhage. Partial transection precludes this mechanism and often results in more significant blood loss. Since the intima is the weakest layer of the artery, its disruption can lead to thrombosis in the absence of external signs of blood loss or significant haematoma suggestive of a vascular injury. Traumatic arterial spasm is a rare entity that is difficult to diagnose with certainty, but represents a myogenic reaction independent of the autonomic nervous system in medium sized muscular arteries. If not recognized early, these injuries can lead to significant morbidity from ischaemia. Arterial spasm is an angiographic rather than a clinical diagnosis. It must be emphasized that other types of arterial injury must be ruled out before it is assumed that spasm is responsible for poor limb perfusion.

Diagnosis and initial management

Rapid evaluation and institution of effective treatment are critical factors in the successful management of traumatic vascular injuries. This includes airway management, vigorous resuscitation with crystalloid infusion, administration of blood products and appropriate prioritization of any other accompanying life-threatening injuries. Although most vascular injuries are diagnosed promptly, others may be more insidious and their detection requires a thorough search. It is clear that the surgeon is the key individual responsible for ensuring that an occult injury is not overlooked. A history of persistent arterial bleeding, a large or expanding haematoma, major haemorrhage with hypotension, diminished or absent distal pulse, an injury to anatomically related nerves, or a bruit at or distal to a suspected injury, alone or in combination, are useful clinical signs of vascular injury. The classical signs of severe distal extremity ischaemia: pain, pallor, pulselessness, paralysis and paraesthesia, are helpful in determining the urgency of repair.

In the setting of severe extremity ischaemia, time is of critical importance. Whereas brain tissue dies within minutes in the face of acute ischaemia, muscle and peripheral nerve tissue may tolerate anoxia for 4–6 hours. Despite this window of opportunity, delay in diagnosis and failure to act promptly will lead to a low flow state with intravascular stasis, activation of intravascular coagulation and thrombosis. The eventual outcome is irreversible damage to skeletal muscle, peripheral nerves and visceral organ function.

- It is paramount to recognize that the presence of pulses does not exclude major vascular injury.

Distal pulses are present in over 35% of cases of proximal arterial injury. This is a consequence of pulse wave propagation through soft clot or an intimal flap, or by way of collateral blood flow around a thrombosed vessel. In this setting there are usually no clinical signs of ischaemia.

Biplanar angiography can confirm and localize injuries, and aid in determining surgical planning. As a consequence, angiography has obviated the need for many surgical explorations by excluding the presence of injury. The accuracy of angiography is between 92% and 98%, with the majority of errors being false-positive interpretations. Several studies have shown that angiography accurately confirms the absence of significant vascular injury even when an injury is clinically suspected. More importantly, angiography discloses a 20% incidence of clinically unsuspected vascular injuries. Thus, exclusion arteriography is useful in the management of vascular trauma to eliminate the need for exploration in a stable patient with equivocal signs of arterial injury.

Despite its accuracy, several recent studies have critically questioned the indications for exclusion arteriography, particularly for 'proximity' wounds. Data from these indicate that arteriography for proximity of a penetrating wound alone, in the absence of other clinical findings, results in a very high incidence of negative arteriograms. Digital subtraction angiography (DSA) also has been demonstrated to be useful in the evaluation of the trauma patient. The advantages of intra-arterial DSA as compared to conventional angiography include the use of less contrast material, a shorter time for the procedure and cost-effectiveness.

As a general rule, patients with a single penetrating injury to the extremity presenting with absent or diminished distal pulses, massive external bleeding, signs of distal ischaemia, pulsatile or expanding haematoma, or palpable thrill (hard signs) should be explored. Patients with multiple penetrating wounds in one extremity or victims of blunt trauma with associated orthopaedic injuries presenting with hard signs of arterial injury should undergo angiography (in the radiology suite or in the operating room) prior to surgical exploration. Angiography in these circumstances helps to determine the surgical approach.

The expense, morbidity and time delay associated with conventional arteriography has prompted the use of non-invasive technology to evaluate the vascular system, particularly in the extremities. B-mode ultrasound has been found to have a specificity of nearly 100; however, its sensitivity, approximately 80%, limits its usefulness as a screening tool. Johansen has utilized the 'arterial pressure index' (arterial pressure in the injured limb divided by the pressure in an uninvolved arm), with a ratio of less than 0.90 being considered significant as a predictor of arterial injury. This modality has been found to have a negative predictive value of 99% and can be easily and rapidly performed at the bedside. Duplex scanning also has been evaluated in a number of centres and has been found to have a sensitivity, specificity and accuracy of 95% or greater, approximately that of the 'gold standard', arteriography. Furthermore, experience may not only confirm its utility as a screening device but also allow exploration and repair of arterial injuries without the necessity for arteriography. While these non-invasive techniques have been evaluated predominantly in penetrating trauma, early experience indicates applicability for blunt injury as well.

The Brink's classification can be used to simplify initial management of vascular injuries:

- Category I – patients in shock from ongoing haemorrhage.
- Category II – vascular injuries occurring in haemodynamically stable patients but having potential for significant morbidity.
- Category III – a clinically suspected injury in a stable patient.

According to Brink, category I patients require immediate operative intervention. Although the source of haemorrhage usually will be obvious following penetrating trauma, localization in major blunt trauma can be particularly perplexing. This point is typified by the classic dilemma of managing combined thoracic and abdominal trauma in the unstable hypotensive patient. In this setting, laparotomy is performed prior to angiography when no obvious source of bleeding is discovered by chest radiography or intercostal intubation. Category II and III patients merit thorough and rapid evaluation, often including angiography as part of the initial evaluation.

During the initial management of the trauma patient, obvious sources of external bleeding can be controlled in most cases with manual compression or packing. Blind clamping or the use of tourniquets is condemned. Blind probing of a stable wound should not be attempted unless one is certain of the ability to control any suspected vascular injury that might be disrupted. Since shock and associated injuries contribute to overall morbidity and mortality, these problems may demand priority in saving the patient's life. Co-ordination of the overall effort by an experienced trauma surgeon leads to optimal establishment of priorities.

The refinement of interventional radiology techniques has provided the trauma surgeon with a new tool in the armamentarium to manage arterial injuries that would otherwise be explored on a regular basis. The use of vascular stents in intimal injuries and graft covered stents in full thickness injuries with minor extravasation is now possible, and may replace mandatory surgical exploration in the future.

General operative principles

Operative procedures are almost invariably performed under general anaesthesia. Endotracheal intubation must be carefully performed and can be hazardous, particularly when a patient has vascular injuries of the neck and great vessels. The patient should undergo skin preparation and be draped widely with consideration given to potential sources of autogenous vein and artery for subsequent repair. Broad-spectrum antibiotics are routinely administered prior to surgery and in the immediate post-operative period. A complete selection of vascular instruments, clamps and sutures must be available, as well as embolectomy catheters. Use of intraluminal shunts in extremity injuries has permitted long delays in definitive repair of the vascular injury while other life-threatening or stabilizing orthopaedic procedures are completed.

Incisions generally should be made parallel to the injured vessel with transverse extensions at joint creases. It is useful to excise previous scars when possible, as they can be a source of wound complication. Attempts should be made to preserve arterial and venous collaterals to optimize extremity perfusion. The contralateral saphenous vein is preferentially used when a venous conduit is required for major lower extremity arterial and venous injuries. The time-honoured principle of gaining proximal and distal control prior to evacuation of haematomas remains critical in operative management of vascular injuries. In situations where proximal or distal access is difficult, the use of balloon catheters for occlusion has been found to be invaluable. Systemic heparin at a dose of 50–75 units/kg is generally administered prior to clamping unless other injuries contraindicate its use. Regional heparinization is appropriate for cases that prohibit systemic anticoagulation. Careful use of balloon catheter thrombectomy is essential prior to vascular repair to remove proximal and distal thrombi, minimizing post-operative thromboembolic complications.

Arterial repair often can be performed by simple lateral arteriorrhaphy or resection of a short segment (<2 cm) of artery with primary anastomosis. It is important to adequately debride damaged arterial tissue. More extensive injuries require replacement with either autogenous saphenous vein or prosthetic material. Experimental and clinical data suggest polytetrafluoroethylene (PTFE) is the most infection-resistant of available prostetic grafts. Vascular injuries in the presence of massive contamination may be treated by placing an extra-anatomic bypass to provide flow continuity; however, recent reports have not confirmed an increased incidence of graft infection when placed *in situ* in a grossly contaminated wound.

Accompanying venous injuries, particularly to the deep femoral and popliteal veins, should be repaired to maximize the chances of success when the artery is repaired. Adjunctive use of intermittent venous compression stockings or arteriovenous fistulas may improve patency of venous repairs.

Management of specific injuries

Vascular injuries of the intrathoracic aorta and great vessels

Injuries to the aortic arch and great vessels are usually caused by penetrating rather than blunt trauma. The morbidity and mortality rates of these injuries are among the highest in vascular trauma. Most of these patients expire prior to arrival at the hospital from profound shock secondary to massive haemorrhage. Successful management of these injuries depends upon aggressive resuscitation, often utilizing lower extremity intravenous lines, early intubation, prompt diagnosis and rapid surgical control of haemorrhage. The diagnostic signs suggestive of great vessel trauma are described in Table 1.8.

About one-third of these injuries will have no obvious clinical signs of vascular trauma, except for a penetrating cutaneous wound. High-grade arteriography is useful, but should not delay surgery in the haemodynamically unstable patient.

Table 1.8 Signs suggestive of major thoracic vascular injuries

- Cardiac arrest
- Persistent shock
- Cardiac tamponade
- A mediastinum widened to > 8 cm
- Recurring haemothorax
- Blunting of the aortic knob
- Pleural capping
- Deviation of the left main stem bronchus
- Displacement of the nasogastric tube
- Neurological deficits
- Pulse deficits
- Bruits

Wide preparation of the neck and chest is essential. Access to injuries of deep mediastinal vessels may require median sternotomy. When necessary, this incision easily can be extended into the supraclavicular fossa or obliquely anterior to the sternocleidomastoid muscle in the neck, to approach the more distal innominate or carotid arteries. The proximal left subclavian artery is difficult to repair through a median sternotomy. Although a high, left lateral thoracotomy is preferred, a 'trapdoor' thoracotomy extension may be made into the left third or fourth intercostal space if anterior mediastinal exposure is also required (Figure 1.18).

During repair of the innominate artery, one must consider the need for adequate cerebral blood flow and utilization of an intraluminal shunt. Poor distal back bleeding, stump pressures in the carotid artery <60 mmHg or electroencephalographic (EEG) changes during intra-operative monitoring suggest the need for shunt placement to maintain cerebral perfusion while repairing the innominate artery.

The majority of thoracic aortic pseudoaneurysms produced by blunt trauma occur at the aortic isthmus, just distal to the origin of the left subclavian artery. If not recognized and repaired, the pseudoaneurysm has an unpredictable course, and can rupture hours or even months later. Aortography is the definitive test to identify this problem although CT scans and trans-oesophageal echocardiography have been used recently. This injury is best approached through a fourth or fifth intercostal space posterolateral thoracotomy. The incidence of paraplegia following thoracic aortic repair has been reported as varying from 1 to 20%. Recent studies suggest that the incidence of paraplegia may be reduced by short clamp times or by the use of active or passive bypass when long cross-clamp times are anticipated.

Innominate vascular injury

Innominate vascular injuries are most frequently caused by penetrating trauma. Although minor arterial

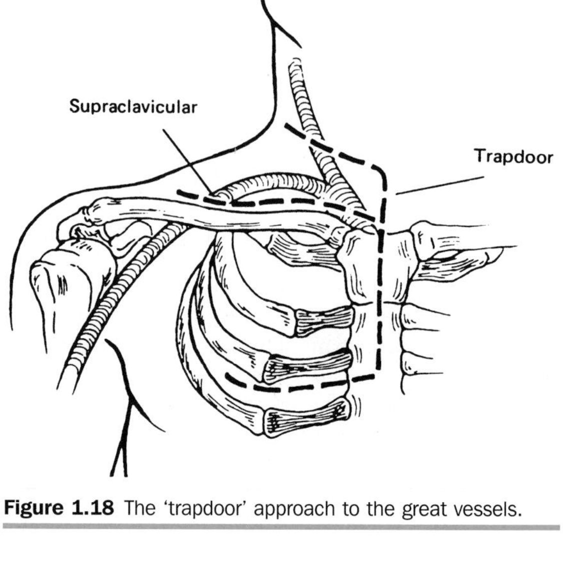

Figure 1.18 The 'trapdoor' approach to the great vessels.

injuries can be repaired primarily or with a patch graft, major injuries require bypass grafting, usually originating from the proximal aorta. Prosthetic grafts are usually used, although the saphenous vein is an acceptable alternative. If there is significant contamination, ligation and extrathoracic bypass (carotid–carotid, subclavian–subclavian, axillary–axillary, subclavian–carotid) through uncontaminated tissue planes has been used successfully to eliminate the need for prosthetic graft material.

Accompanying injuries to the superior vena cava (SVC) and innominate vein are common. The SVC always should be repaired and may require temporary shunting to allow venous return. Although repair of innominate venous injuries is desirable, unilateral ligation is tolerated in most cases. Bilateral ligation results in a SVC-like syndrome.

Both SVC and innominate vein injuries may be a source for air embolization. In the event of this complication, immediate direct aspiration of air from the pulmonary artery, right ventricle, atrium and SVC is required.

Subclavian vascular injuries

Penetrating trauma continues to be responsible for the majority of subclavian vascular injuries. Mortality from these injuries has declined to 5%. The majority may be repaired by primary anastomosis or an interposition graft. Right subclavian injuries usually can be managed through a right supraclavicular incision with clavicular resection if necessary. Proximal left subclavian injuries require lateral thoracotomy or a 'trapdoor' approach for repair. Subclavian venous injuries can be ligated with relative impunity.

Blunt trauma resulting in fracture of the clavicle and the underlying first rib can produce significant injury to the subclavian vessels lying between these bony elements. The incidence of subclavian injuries with first rib and clavicular fractures is reported to be 14%. Subclavian vascular injuries often have accompanying spinal cord or brachial plexus injuries that are responsible for significant and sometimes devastating disability.

Carotid artery injuries

Diagnosis and management of carotid artery injuries is a critical aspect in the treatment of neck trauma. Significant carotid trauma is often accompanied by injury to other arterial or venous structures as well as to the larynx, pharynx, trachea, oesophagus, salivary glands, thoracic duct, and adjacent cranial and cervical nerves. Carotid artery injuries as a consequence of penetrating trauma often present with haemorrhage, haematoma, a threatened airway or shock. The common carotid artery is injured most frequently. The patient's neurological status is the most crucial factor that determines therapeutic options for management. It is controversial whether restoration of cerebral blood flow in the presence of a neurological deficit can convert a region of ischaemic infarction to haemorrhagic infarction. A 40% operative mortality rate has been noted in patients with pre-operative coma. However, recent studies indicate that an aggressive approach to revascularization of the carotid artery even in the setting of a significant neurological deficit is safe and may result in improvement of the patient's neurological deficit. Reversal of neurological deficits also has been reported in patients who have undergone extracranial-to-intracranial (EC-IC) bypasses for high cervical or intracranial internal carotid injuries. Most authors now favour carotid reconstruction in patients with mild to moderate deficits when antegrade flow has been preserved. Major carotid artery injuries also should be repaired in the setting of profound neurological deficit or coma of short duration, but results are unpredictable. Repair in this setting may increase function and appears to do no harm though reports are limited.

Carotid injuries are most often approached through a vertical incision along the anterior border of the sternocleidomastoid muscle (Figure 1.19). Adequate debridement with resection/primary anastomosis or interposition grafting is utilized. Shunts should be used liberally when there is concern regarding the adequacy of collateral perfusion.

Blunt trauma to the carotid artery is more difficult to detect and evaluate since patients often have accompanying closed head injuries or other complications of blunt trauma. Diagnosis is delayed in approximately 50% of patients. The neurological sequelae of blunt carotid trauma may manifest themselves in a delayed fashion since they are usually due to intimal disruption or mural contusion with subsequent thrombosis or embolization. These deficits may occur hours to days after a reported injury. Limb paralysis in an alert patient, a lucid interval, transient ischaemic attacks, Horner's syndrome, or a history of hyperextension, forceful trauma to the neck or extensive maxillofacial injury should alert the surgeon to the possibility of blunt carotid injury. Resection of the damaged artery and an interposition graft with autogenous tissue

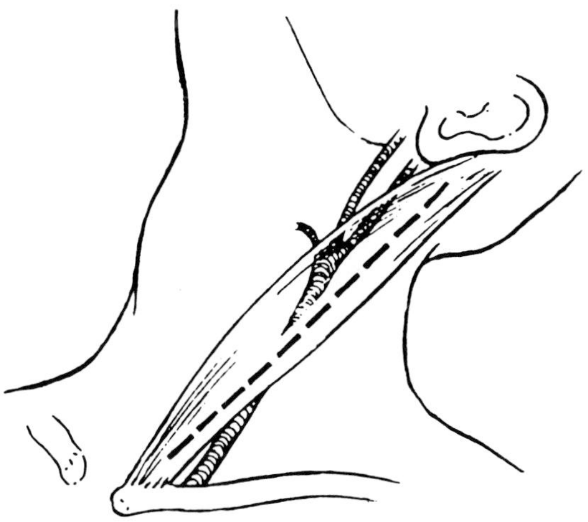

Figure 1.19 Incision and approach to the carotid vessels.

or primary anastomosis is recommended for injuries in accessible anatomical locations. Dissection of the internal carotid artery without complete occlusion may be treated with anticoagulants. The patient with a dense stroke and occlusion is unlikely to benefit from operation.

Vertebral artery injuries

Traumatic injury of the vertebral artery is rare because of the protection afforded by its anatomical course through the cervical vertebrae. Penetrating trauma accounts for the majority of injuries, although blunt trauma with fracture of the cervical spine also can produce vertebral artery injury. Suspicion of an injury to the vertebral artery necessitates immediate angiography. These injuries can result in significant haemorrhage, thrombosis, or development of a pseudoaneurysm or arteriovenous fistula. Because of the confluence of the vertebral arteries to form the basilar artery, ligation alone is inadequate treatment for most injuries. Percutaneous occlusion with detachable balloons is useful adjunct in treating these injuries.

Intra-abdominal vascular injuries

Injuries to major intra-abdominal vascular structures are associated with both significant haemorrhage and risk of visceral ischaemia. Patients are most often victims of penetrating trauma and may present with shock, necessitating emergency laparotomy. Although optimal treatment is repair and restoration of normal vascular pathways, knowledge of the anatomy and collateral circulation allows ligation of many injuries when necessary. Proximal arterial control, most frequently of the aorta, is usually necessary prior to exposure and repair of the injury. This can be achieved through a left thoracotomy or by clamping the supracoeliac aorta below the diaphragm through a midline laparotomy incision unless the patient also requires chest exploration or open cardiac message (Figure 1.20).

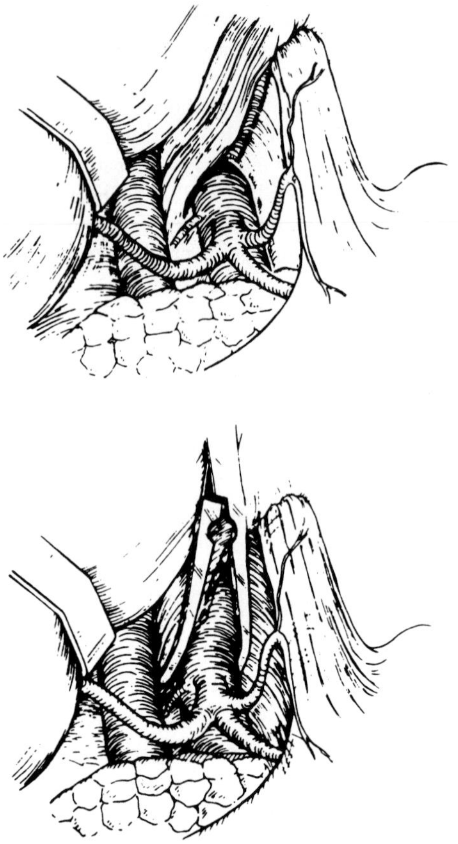

Figure 1.20 To gain access to the supracoeliac aorta, the liver is retracted upwards, the stomach downwards and the posterior peritoneum incised. The muscular crus of the diaphragm is incised.

Intra-abdominal venous injuries are associated with mortality as high as 50% and pose complicated technical and decision-making problems for the surgeon. The aetiology of the injury, associated injuries and condition of the patient on arrival to the hospital a re important determinants of survival. The present authors recently have found retroperitoneal tamponade to be the most important factor related to survival following abdominal aortic and inferior vena cava (IVC) injuries. Difficulty in exposure and control of venous injuries, as well as problems in suturing the venous wall without tension or tearing, are factors contributing to the challenge of venous repair. Because of low flow rates, venous repairs are more prone to thrombosis, particularly when prosthetic materials are used.

When venous ligation is required, fluid sequestration occurs in the affected vascular bed and patients require additional fluid administration to maintain intravascular volume until collateral flow improves. When collateral flow is inadequate, infarction secondary to venous obstruction can occur. Classification of injuries according to regions of the abdomen (central zone, lateral peri-renal and lateral pelvic zones) aids in guiding optimal exposure. The central zone is divided into supramesocolic and inframesocolic regions. Cephalad to the transverse mesocolon, injuries may occur to the supracoeliac aorta, coeliac axis, superior mesenteric artery or vein, portal vein, and renal arteries or veins. Exposure, control and repair are facilitated by right medial rotation of the left colon, left kidney, spleen, pancreas and stomach (Figure 1.21). Aortic injuries often are reparable by direct suture or patch aortoplasty. Grafts are rarely required and should be avoided in the setting of significant enteral contamination.

Although repair is desirable, coeliac axis injuries can be ligated without consequence in almost all patients because of the rich collateral circulation in the foregut. Common hepatic artery ligation distal to the origin of the gastroduodenal artery can result in hepatic ischaemia, particularly if the portal vein is also compromised. Splenic artery ligation is well tolerated.

Injuries to the superior mesenteric artery proximal to the inferior border of the pancreas can similarly be ligated although simple or isolated injuries should be repaired. Injury distal to the pancreas demands repair

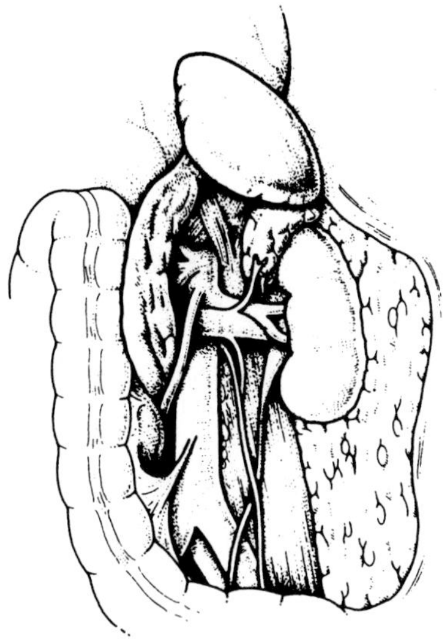

Figure 1.21 Exposure of the infra- and suprarenal cava as well as portal vein by reflecting the left colon, spleen and pancreas. (After Blaisdell, F. W. and Trunkey, D. D. eds. *Abdominal Trauma*, Vol. 1. New York: Thieme-Stratton.)

with lateral arteriorrhaphy or bypass graft because of the high likelihood of ischaemia. Superior mesenteric venous injuries distal to the pancreas should be repaired with lateral venorrhaphy or saphenous vein bypass whenever possible, although in the multiply injured patient ligation is an acceptable alternative. 'Second look' laparotomy 24–48 hours after repair is appropriate for mesenteric vascular injuries whenever concern exists regarding bowel viability.

The exposure for access to the suprarenal aorta allows easy assessment of the posterior left renal artery and the anterior artery can be evaluated by leaving the kidney *in situ*. Renovascular repair is discussed later. The primary concern with wounds in the inframesocolic central zone is aortic or vena caval injury. Access is obtained by opening the midline retroperitoneum after eviscerating the small bowel to the right. The aorta is controlled at the level of the left renal vein, inspected, and appropriate repair is then performed. Infrarenal vena caval injuries can be approached in the same fashion and controlled with either partial occluding clamps or sponge sticks. Exposure of the entire subhepatic vena cava can be obtained by an extended Kocher manoeuvre deflecting the duodenum and colon to the left (Figure 1.22). Primary repair or patch cavaplasty should be performed, although extensive injuries may require ligation. Rapid diagnosis and repair of injury to renal vessels is essential for preservation of renal function. The stable patient with haematuria should undergo intravenous pyelography followed by arteriography if there is non-visualization of one or both kidneys. Although injury secondary to penetrating trauma is more common, renal artery thrombosis is seen more often with blunt trauma.

Renovascular injuries may be evidenced by either central retroperitoneal haematomas or lateral perirenal haematomas. Exposure should be obtained through the mid-line retroperitoneum with dissection of the aorta and control of the renal arteries and veins. Approach to the injury itself usually requires lateral exposure by deflection of the colon and other viscera on the appropriate side.

Although renal artery repair should be attempted in most cases, renal salvage beyond 6 hours post-injury is rare. Saphenous vein is the optimal conduit when a graft is required. Nephrectomy should be performed in the unstable patient or the patient with a complex renal injury in whom the contralateral kidney is uninjured. Autotransplantation or *ex vivo* renal artery repair may be contemplated in the haemodynamically stable patient with bilateral renal injuries to avoid chronic renal failure.

Despite an aggressive approach to renal artery repair, it is successful in < 30% of cases. Injury to the left renal vein can be treated safely with ligation near the IVC provided that adrenal and gonadal collaterals have been preserved. Inability to repair the right renal vein necessitates nephrectomy due to the limited collateral drainage.

Vascular injuries in the region of the portohepatic and retrohepatic area are rare but associated with very high mortality. These challenging injuries lead to exsanguination in a short period of time, and surgical approach is difficult due to the proximity of other vital structures and important organs, that may be injured as well. Proximal control of injuries in the hepatoduodenal ligament can be obtained by compression with fingers or a vascular clamp, the Pringle manoeuvre. The mortality from portal venous injury ranges from 40% to 70%. The portal vein is exposed by medial retraction

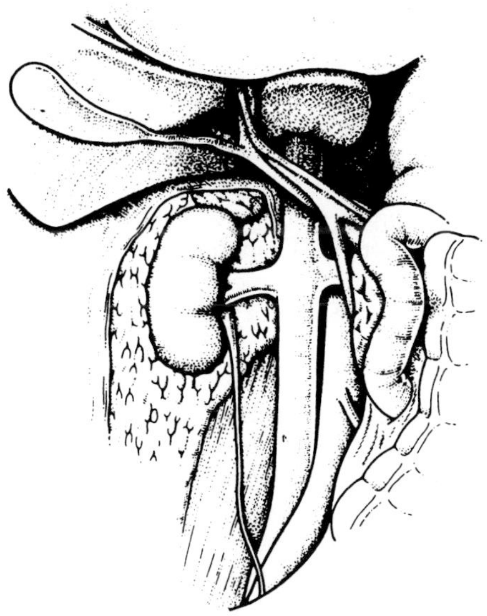

Figure 1.22 Exposure of the upper abdominal aorta and visceral vasculature by reflection of the right colon and head of pancreas and duodenum. (After Blaisdell, F. W. and Trunkey, D. D. eds. *Abdominal Trauma*, Vol. 1. New York: Thieme-Stratton.)

of the common bile duct and repair with lateral venorrhaphy or primary anastomosis should be performed if at all possible. Approach to the more proximal portal vein requires deflection of the pancreas and duodenum via a Kocher manoeuvre. Extensive injury may require ligation, which is tolerated in 90% of cases if hepatic artery flow is uninterrupted. Concomitant hepatic artery injury mandates portal vein repair. Following ligation, fluid sequestration in the gut will occur and patients may develop portal hypertension. Injury to the retropancreatic portal vein requires mobilization and division of the overlying pancreas to achieve repair. Injury to the suprarenal, retrohepatic vena cava is a particularly difficult injury to treat. Bleeding is usually massive and the diagnosis should be suspected when major hepatic parenchymal bleeding persists despite the Pringle manoeuvre. Mobilization and division of the hepatic ligaments are required and vascular control by isolation and clamping of the portal vein, supracoeliac aorta, infrarenal and suprahepatic vena cavae may be necessary. Occlusion of these veins is poorly tolerated due to the abrupt decrease in venous return to the heart. Extension of the laparotomy incision into a median sternotomy with insertion of an atriocaval shunt isolates the injury and permits venous return during repair, but mortality still exceeds 50%.

Hepatic venous injury usually can be treated with lateral repair after mobilization and division of the hepatic ligaments, but ligation of a single hepatic vein is well tolerated. Iliac arterial and venous injuries most often are due to penetrating trauma and are associated with haematomas in the lateral pelvic zones. Haemorrhage usually can be managed with direct pressure while proximal arterial control is obtained at the aortic bifurcation and distal control at the inguinal ligament. Lateral repair, resection, and primary anastomosis or interposition grafting with saphenous vein or PTFE is performed. Extensive injuries or grossly contaminated wounds may be managed by ligation if the ankle pressure by Doppler is >60 mmHg or by extra-anatomical bypass if reconstruction is required. Iliac venous injuries can be difficult to expose due to the overlying arteries. Compression is utilized for control to avoid injury to these thin walled veins and lateral repair is preferred. Ligation is reasonably well tolerated.

Injuries to the extremities

Extremity vascular injuries are common sequelae of both blunt and penetrating trauma. Although tolerance to ischaemia is greater than that of the viscera or brain, rapid diagnosis and treatment is essential. Accompanying nerve and soft tissue injuries often limit the success of vascular reconstruction. The femoral artery is the most commonly injured vessel in the lower extremity. Although such injuries are most often due to penetrating trauma fractures, dislocations and iatrogenic injuries from percutaneous catheterization or placement of intra-aortic balloon pumps are also important causes. Femoral artery injuries are often associated with injury to accompanying veins and nerves. In addition to arterial repair, extensive attempts at deep vein reconstruction are warranted to minimize early and late morbidity. In general, injuries to the profunda femoris artery also should be repaired because of the significant incidence of subsequent atherosclerotic vascular disease involving the superficial femoral artery. Injuries to the superficial femoral artery are repaired by resection and primary anastomosis or interposition graft with the contralateral saphenous vein.

The popliteal vessels are particularly susceptible to blunt traumatic injury from fractures and dislocations. The amputation rate for unreconstructed injuries in this area reaches as high as 61%. Concomitant popliteal vein injury decreases the likelihood of success of arterial reconstruction. Therefore, expeditious repair of both the vein and artery is essential.

Although the ideal sequence of repair in patients with combined orthopaedic and popliteal vascular injuries has been debated for many years, most surgeons feel that vascular repair should precede repair of skeletal injuries when there is threatened limb loss from ischaemia. If not contraindicated, heparinization and the use of mannitol to minimize muscle compartment swelling are valuable adjuncts. Intraluminal shunts have been utilized to maintain distal blood flow to the extremities while other life-threatening injuries are being repaired. Others have advocated use of shunts to perfuse the extremity while orthopaedic stabilization is performed, allowing subsequent vascular repair in a stabilized limb. Heparin should be continued if possible in the post-operative period to enhance vein patency.

Injury to the small vessels below the popliteal trifurcation can pose difficult management problems. When both tibial arteries are injured, the amputation rate may reach 65%, whereas with injury to only one vessel the rate is much lower. Arteriography in this area is important in defining the sites and extent of all the injuries. This is particularly true with multiple pellet wounds from a shotgun blast. If arteriography demonstrates only a single isolated arterial injury below the knee without active bleeding, pseudoaneurysm or arteriovenous fistula, and the patient does not have an ischaemic limb, then observation without surgical intervention is justified. On the other hand, any patient who demonstrates ischaemia, bleeding or a vascular complication of the injury should undergo immediate exploration and repair of the artery. If a vein graft is required for repair, it should be harvested from the contralateral extremity. Fasciotomy is often required when prolonged ischaemia or soft tissue injury is present. Salvage of a useful limb is often more dependent on the extent of neuromuscular injury than vascular injury.

Vascular injuries of the upper extremity are extremely common. These injuries are seen not only with penetrating trauma, but also after use of the brachial artery for arteriographic and cardiac catheterization,

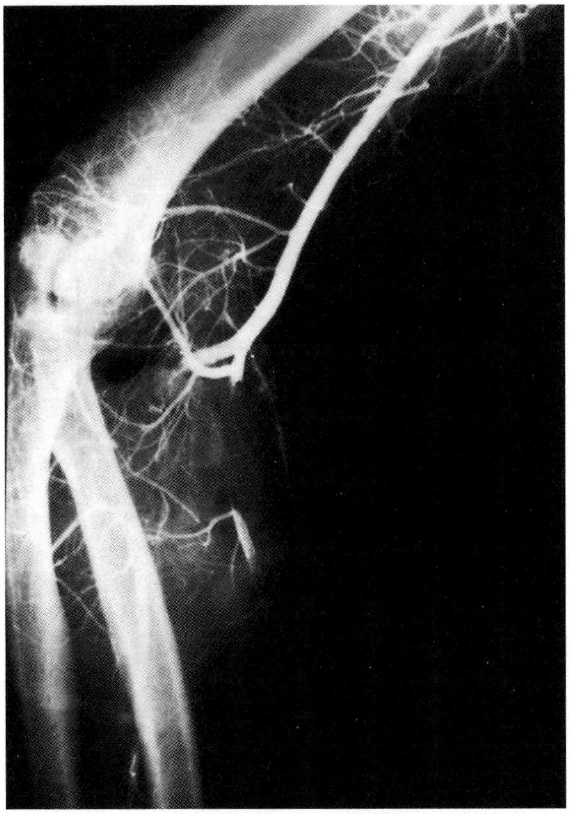

Figure 1.23 The patient sustained a severe crush injury to an elbow resulting in a massive haematoma, complete transection of the proximal ulnar artery and contusion/thrombosis of the proximal radial artery. Circulation was restored using a reversed autogenous saphenous vein graft between the brachial and radial arteries.

Table 1.9 Orthopaedic injuries associated with vascular trauma

- Posterior knee dislocation
- Distal femur
- Proximal tibia
- Supracondylar fracture of the humerus
- Clavicular fracture
- Shoulder dislocation
- First rib fracture

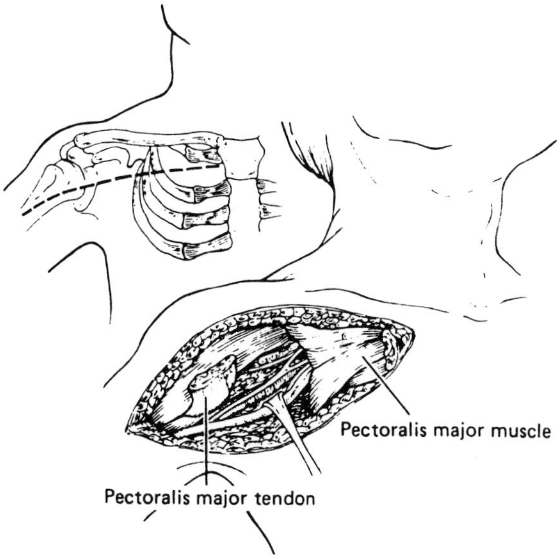

Figure 1.24 Approach to the axillary artery.

and following cannulation for arterial blood gas monitoring. Long bone fractures with or without joint dislocation are another potential source of vascular trauma (Figure 1.23). In children the brachial artery is particularly vulnerable to injury from supracondylar fractures of the humerus. Table 1.9 presents frequent orthopaedic injuries associated with extremity vascular trauma.

Most upper extremity vascular injuries do not result in limb-threatening ischaemia, and physical examination or angiography can establish the diagnosis. Injuries to the axillary and brachial arteries require urgent exploration and usually can be managed by thrombectomy and primary repair with or without a vein patch (Figure 1.24). Injuries to the radial and ulnar arteries often are easily repaired but can be ligated if an intact palmar arch is present. Fasciotomy of the forearm may be needed if ischaemia or soft tissue injury causes a compartment syndrome.

Major vascular injuries in pelvic trauma

The high mortality (30–60%) of major pelvic fractures is secondary to unrelenting haemorrhage. Bleeding occurs from lacerations of both small and medium-sized arteries and veins, as well as fractured bone. Most arterial bleeding is from branches of the internal iliac artery. Success in managing these patients requires rapid assessment, vigorous resuscitation, and reversal of systemic effects of prolonged shock.

Haemorrhage can be controlled to some extent by compression of the pelvic area with the use of a MAST suit. Similarly, early external fixation of the pelvis provides compression, immobilization, and amelioration of the bleeding caused by movement of unstable large bony fragments. Patients who require transfusion in excess of 4–6 units of blood attributable to the pelvic injury are candidates for therapeutic embolization of pelvic arterial bleeding in the angiography suite. Whether this is performed before or after external fixation depends on the relative speed and efficiency with which each procedure can be performed in an individual circumstance. In general, angiography should occur first. Hypogastric artery ligation has few advocates, as it has been shown to be almost totally ineffective. However, it remains an alternative in conjunction with packing the pelvis and re-exploring the patient at a later time.

Acute and chronic sequelae of vascular injury

Haemorrhage

Bleeding subsequent to arterial repair is uncommon, occurring in less than 5% of cases. It may present as frank haemorrhage from the operative incision or as a rapidly expanding haematoma. In virtually all cases, the cause is a technical error, resulting from inadequate haemostasis in the wound or from the suture line of the vascular repair. Rarely, bleeding may be due to a missed arterial or major venous injury. Patients who develop this complication should be returned to the operating room immediately for evacuation of any surrounding haematoma, identification and correction of the problem.

Thrombosis

Occlusion of a vascular repair is the most frequently encountered acute complication of vascular surgery. Depending on the vessel involved and the type of repair (i.e. lateral arteriorrhaphy, interposition grafting, etc.) thrombosis occurs after arterial repair for trauma in approximately 10% of cases. If late thromboses are included, the incidence rises to about 20%.

- Early thrombosis is due to a technical problem, most commonly stenosis of the repair or inadequate thrombectomy.

Other causes include intimal dissection with prolapse and missed injury. Because these technical problems are easily corrected if discovered early, it is prudent to perform completion arteriography at the initial operation. Thrombosis presents with a loss of distal pulses associated with signs of ischaemia (i.e. pallor, poikilothermia, pain, paralysis and paraesthesia). If pulses that were initially present disappear, the diagnosis is thrombosis and there is no need for confirmatory arteriography. These patients should be returned as soon as possible to the operating room for thrombectomy, repair and completion arteriography. On the other hand, if pulses were never palpable after the repair and the patient is hypothermic, vasospasm may be present. In such cases, every effort should be made to rewarm the patient and improve perfusion to the extremity. If pulses do not return, either arteriography or exploration should be considered.

Arteriovenous fistula

Arteriovenous fistula after arterial trauma occurs in 2–7% of cases. The most common causes are fragment, shrapnel or shotgun wounds. Numerous physiological changes occur as flow increases through the fistula, going from the high-pressure arterial system to the low-resistance venous system. Among these changes are increases in cardiac output, heart rate, central venous pressure and blood volume. Local changes in the region of the fistula include dilatation of the proximal artery and the distal vein, distal varicosities and extremity oedema. Most of these changes are reversible with correction of the fistula. Patients may present with signs of venous stasis disease, arterial insufficiency or frank congestive heart failure. The physical findings are often suggestive of the diagnosis and include a palpable thrill and an audible bruit or a continuous machinery type murmur. Occlusion of the fistula may cause a decrease in the elevated pulse rate (Nicolandani-Branham's sign). Arteriography always should be performed to confirm the diagnosis, localize the lesion anatomically and determine the presence of any associated pathology. Less than 2% of fistulas will close spontaneously, so treatment is required. Although percutaneous techniques have been used in some cases, surgery remains the mainstay of therapy.

Pseudoaneurysm

The incidence of pseudoaneurysm following trauma is difficult to ascertain since it is often reported in association with arteriovenous fistulas. A pseudoaneurysm may cause symptoms by encroachment on local structures as it expands or it may present acutely with rupture, distal embolization or thrombosis. Small pseudoaneurysms (< 3 cm) will often thrombose spontaneously, particularly when due to iatrogenic injury. In stable patients without local complications, a period of observation is reasonable. If the pseudoaneurysm is large or persistent, arteriography should be obtained pre-operatively to define the anatomy and associated pathology. Surgical resection with end-to-end anastomosis or interposition grafting is usually necessary, although some injuries can be repaired primarily.

Infection

- Infection of an arterial suture line is a disastrous complication often leading to haemorrhage, thrombosis, distal ischaemia and eventual amputation.

Factors predisposing to infection include:

- closure of a contaminated wound
- inadequate soft tissue coverage of an arterial repair
- inadequate debridement of a traumatized, contaminated vessel.

This complication is best avoided by vigorous cleansing of contaminated wounds, use of appropriate antibiotics, aggressive debridement of devitalized tissues, and coverage of arterial repairs with well-vascularized soft tissue.

Compartment syndrome

- A compartment syndrome is the result of trauma or reperfusion following severe prolonged ischaemia, which leads to swelling within a closed fascial space.

This contained swelling results in a rise in tissue hydrostatic pressure to the point that blood flow is compromised. If untreated, a compartment syndrome will result in myonecrosis and limb dysfunction. The most commonly involved areas are the anterior compartment in the lower leg and the volar compartment in the forearm. Since nerve tissue is more susceptible to ischaemia than is muscle tissue, initial symptoms include paraesthesia and pain in the involved extremity. The muscle is usually tense and pain may be severe, especially with passive movement of the involved compartment. Pulses are usually palpable, even in advanced stages, and are not a reliable indicator of the severity of the syndrome. If one suspects development of a compartment syndrome, compartmental pressure should be measured. This can be done by insertion of a plastic cannula or a wick catheter directly into the involved muscle or muscle group. Fasciotomy is indicated in those patients with a compartmental pressure greater than 40 mmHg initially or a pressure of 30 mmHg that is sustained for more than 4 hours. If compartmental pressures cannot be obtained, one must proceed based upon the clinical impression. For example, if a patient with a popliteal artery injury undergoes revascularization of the lower extremity approximately 8–10 hours after injury and develops a tense anterior compartment associated with a peroneal nerve palsy and loss of sensation in the distribution of the peroneal nerve (first web space), fasciotomy is indicated. The treatment of a compartment syndrome should not be delayed, since irreversible myonecrosis with resultant contracture will occur within 12 hours.

MODULE 2

Disorders of the skin and soft tissues

The diseases of the skin and soft tissues which have important surgical implications are largely although not exclusively neoplastic. In this module, a section on anatomy and function of the skin is followed by sections on benign and malignant conditions of skin, fibrous tissue, muscle, adipose tissue and the lymphatic system. There is also a section on vascular tumours.

2.1 • Anatomy and function of skin

The skin is divided into two main layers: the surface epithelium or epidermis and the underlying dermis (Figure 2.1). The epidermis is a keratinized stratified squamous epithelium and for descriptive purposes it can be divided into five layers, the stratum basale, the stratum spinosum, the stratum granulosum, the stratum lucidum and the stratum corneum (Figure 2.2).

The stratum basale is the deepest layer and consists of a single layer of cylindrical cells with deeply basophilic cytoplasm and centrally placed nuclei. Interspersed between the basal cells are melanocytes, a specialized group of dendritic cells which synthesize the pigment melanin. Above the stratum basale is the stratum spinosum which consists of two to six rows of cuboidal cells which become flattened as they approach the surface. Mitotic activity in the resting epidermis occurs mainly in the stratum basale although in regeneration following injury this extends to the stratum spinosum.

The next layer is the stratum granulosum which is made up of one to three layers of diamond-shaped cells with darkly staining pyknotic nuclei. This layer is most

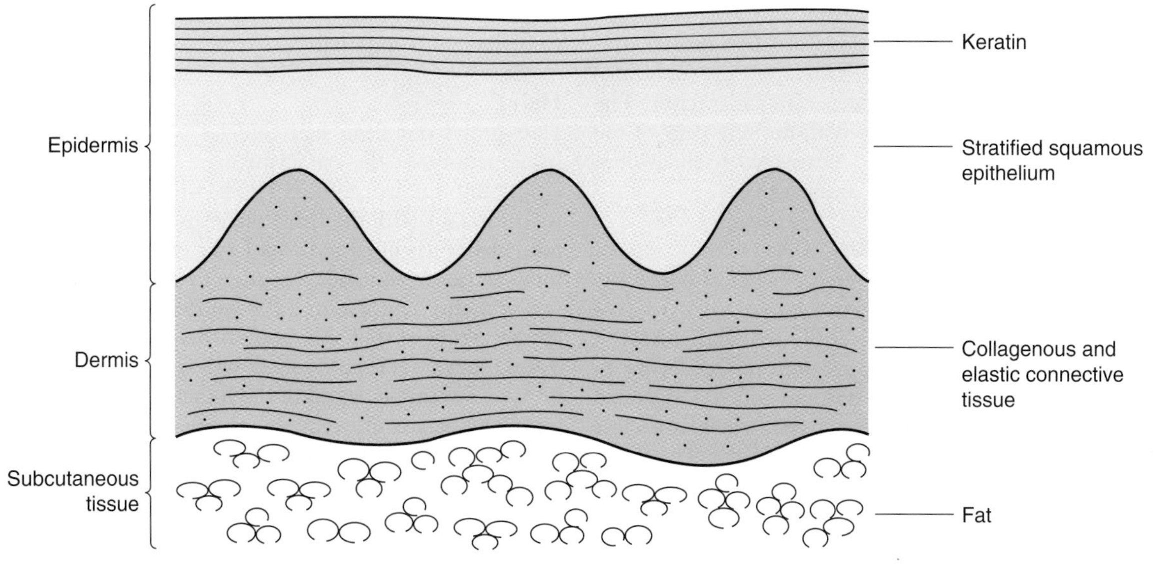

Figure 2.1 Anatomy of the skin.

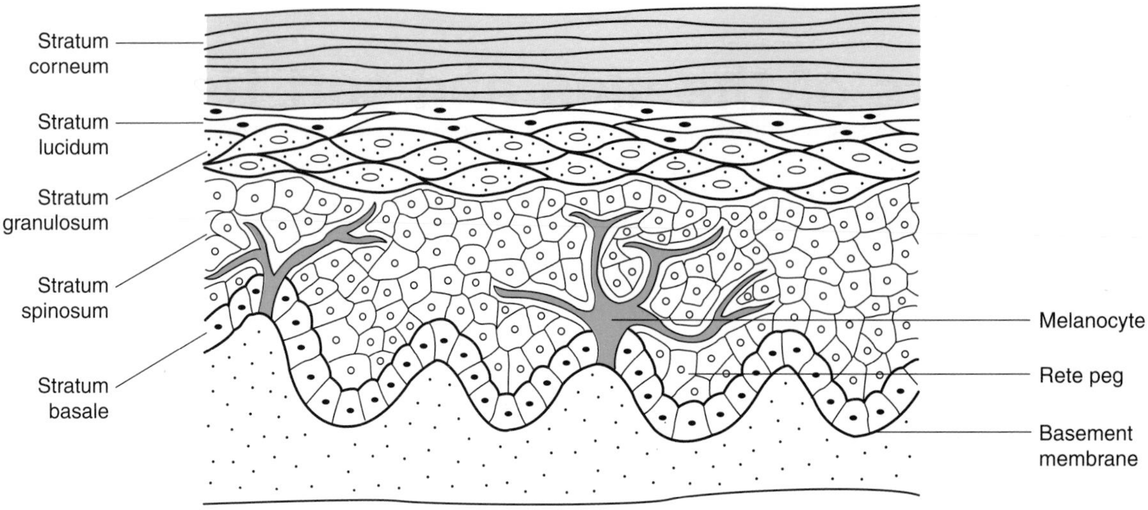

Figure 2.2 Layers of the epidermis.

obvious in the thick skin of the palms and soles of the feet and it is in this layer that the fibrous protein keratin is produced. In thick skin immediately above the stratum granulosum is a single layer of hyaline anucleate cells called the stratum lucidum. This layer is absent in most parts of the skin other than the palms of the hands and the soles of the feet. The outer layer of the skin is the stratum corneum consisting of a variable number of flattened anucleate dead cells containing keratin. Over pressure areas such as the hands and the feet the keratin layer is dense and compact whereas over the rest of the body surface it forms a loose covering.

The undersurface of the epidermis consists of downward epithelial projections into the dermis called rete or interpapillary pegs. The dermis itself is a fibroelastic bed which supports the epidermis and its appendages. This layer becomes continuous with the subcutaneous fascia. In the dermis there are two layers, the superficial papillary bodies and the deeper reticular layer. The papillary bodies interdigitate with the rete pegs of the epidermis. The dermis is relatively acellular but contains tissue macrophages and mast cells.

The epidermal appendages

Sweat glands

Sweat glands are found all over the skin and consist of simple tubular glands extending from the epidermis to the mid-dermis where they become coiled. The coiled portion of the gland produces sweat which is a clear fluid, hypotonic in relationship to plasma. The main solute is sodium chloride but it also contains potassium, lactic acid and urea. Sweating is a mechanism for regulating body temperatures and is controlled by the hypothalamus via the cholinergic fibres of the sympathetic nervous system. It is stimulated by a rise in body temperature brought about by an increase in environmental temperature or exercise. It is also induced by hypotension, anxiety or fear.

Apocrine glands

These glands are found in the axilla, anogenital region, the mammary areola and the canal of the external ear. Similar to the sweat gland, this is a coiled tubule but much larger and is situated in the lower dermis and upper part of the subcutaneous fat. Unlike the sweat gland, however, which penetrates the epidermis, it opens into a hair follicle above the ducts of the sebaceous glands. The secretion from the apocrine glands has a milky appearance and its production is stimulated by adrenergic stimuli such as fear or pain. Apocrine glands become active only after puberty but their function is not clear. Blockage of the apocrine glands leads to hydradenitis suppurativa.

Hair

Hair grows out from hair follicles which are tubular invaginations of the epidermis, and sebaceous glands empty into the hair follicle. The fact that the epidermis is continuous with the hair follicles is of importance as follicular epithelium and to a lesser extent the epithelium of the sweat glands can grow upwards to resurface the skin after epithelium has been denuded by trauma or the taking of split skin graft. A hair itself is basically a long, dead keratinized shaft which starts as a small growth area in the depths of the follicle known as a hair bulb. This area is situated in the upper part of the subcutaneous fat and is invaginated on the underside by vascular connective tissue known as the hair papilla. Above the hair bulb the cells become elongated and undergo keratinization and from this point the hair shaft is a dead structure made up of an outer cortex and a looser inner medulla. Inserted into the walls of the follicles are small strips of smooth muscle, the erectores pilorum. These are supplied by adrenergic nerve fibres and lead to the erection of hair that occurs during cold and emotional stress.

Sebaceous glands

These glands are absent from the palms of the hands and the soles of the feet but are otherwise found all over the skin surface. They are holocrine glands which produce their secretion by disintegration of the contents of the cells which are then discharged directly into the sebaceous duct which enters into the hair follicle (Figure 2.3). The function of the secretion (sebum) is to lubricate the skin and act as a physical protective barrier. It consists of a mixture of fatty acids, glycerides, cholesterol and other substances. Sebaceous gland activity rapidly increases after puberty.

Nails

Nails are made up of semi-transparent keratin and are surrounded proximally and laterally by folds of skin. They arise from the nail bed which is a modified epidermis lacking a stratum granulosum. It is associated with a highly vascular dermis which is continuous on deep aspect with the periosteum of the distal phalanx.

Pigmentation

In man the main function of pigmentation of the skin appears to be protection against the harmful effects of sunlight, and dark skin appears to be the result of selective adaptation to intense prolonged sunlight. The cells responsible for pigmentation are the melanocytes found between the cells of the stratum basale at the junction of the epidermis and the dermis. These synthesize the black pigment melanin from the amino acid tyrosine by means of the copper-dependent oxidase tyrosinase. Melanin is transferred to the surrounding basal cells by the dendritic processes of the melanocytes. Pigmentation by melanin is controlled by the melanocyte stimulating hormone (MSH) produced by the anterior lobe of the pituitary gland. Excess MSH secretion results in increased melanin pigmentation. Interestingly, the number of melanocytes per unit area of skin is the same in all races and increased pigmentation must therefore reflect an increased melanin synthesis.

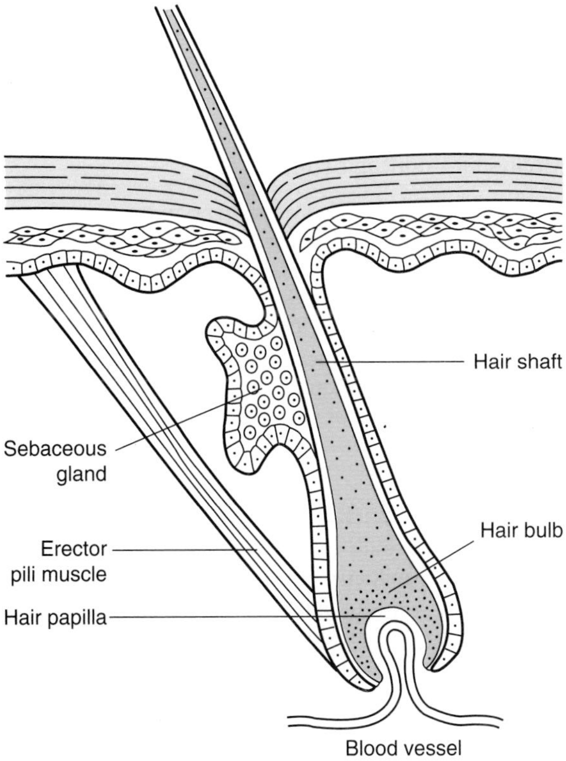

Figure 2.3 Anatomy of the hair follicle.

Blood supply of skin

The blood supply to the skin not only supplies oxygen and nutrients but also plays an important role in temperature regulation. Skin requires a minimum flow of 0.8 ml of blood per minute per 100 ml of tissue to supply its oxygen requirements but there is an abundant blood supply which allows considerable variation in blood flow. Small arterial branches penetrate the subcutaneous fat and form a plexus just above it and loops of vessels go up to supply the individual papillae. Branches from these plexuses supply glands and hair roots. The blood is returned via venous plexuses which are situated below the arterial ones and arteriovenous shunts known as glomus bodies are found in certain regions, particularly the palms, the soles, the ears and the central part of the face. These allow the capillary circulation to be short circuited and are concerned with temperature regulation. The very smallest cutaneous arterioles contain muscle fibres which are again important for thermoregulation. The epidermis itself is avascular and receives nourishment from the vessels in the tip of the papillae via the intercellular spaces. The dermis also has a rich network of lymphatics which start in the papillae eventually joining the larger subcutaneous blood vessels.

Nerve supply of skin

Sensations appreciated by the skin are touch, pressure, pain and temperature and these are detected by a network of myelinated and non-myelinated fibres from which terminals arise in the dermis. The receptors for these sensations are complex and the two which are probably responsible for light touch are Merkel's disks and Meissner's corpuscles. The Pacinian corpuscle is sensitive to pressure. Pruritus (itch) is a common symptom and may be produced by a variety of physical stimuli and disease processes. It seems to be closely related to pain as it travels in the C fibres of sensory nerves and ascends in the spinothalamic tracts of the spinal cord in association with the pain fibres.

Section 2.2 • Benign surgical conditions of skin

Epidermoid cysts

Often called sebaceous cysts these lesions are derived from the epidermis lining the hair follicle and the sebaceous gland. They may occur anywhere on the skin but particularly on the head, face, neck and the trunk. They are unilocular dermal cysts giving rise to visible and palpable cystic swellings which are fixed to the skin (Figure 2.4). There is usually a visible central punctum at the site of the follicle. Histologically, the cyst is made up of layers of epidermal cells interspersed with keratin layers. An epidermoid cyst may become inflamed and present as a tender indurated swelling.

Treatment involves excision usually along with an ellipse of overlying skin and it is important to excise the whole cyst to prevent recurrence. In the infected state an epidermoid cyst should be incised to allow drainage and the remnant can be excised at a later date.

True sebaceous cysts occur in a rare condition known as steatocystoma multiplex which is characterized by the presence of multiple cysts containing oily sebum. Another type of cyst which may be mistaken for an epidermoid cyst arises from the epidermis of the external root sheath of the hair follicle. These are known as pilar cysts or trichilemmal cysts. These tend to occur in women and appear to be familial. Occasionally the walls may rupture and the proliferative reaction may mimic a squamous cell carcinoma.

Keratoacanthoma

This is self-limiting lesion which typically appears as a rapidly growing nodule with a central crater containing a keratin plug (Figure 2.5). Over 6 weeks the lesion grows to its maximum size and then it begins to shrink over a period of about 6 weeks leaving a depressed scar at the site of the lesion. The nodule rarely exceeds 2.5 cm in maximum diameter. Histological differentiation from a squamous cell carcinoma can be difficult but the clinical course is typical. The aetiology is not clear but keratoacanthomas are thought to be derived from hair follicles and to be associated with exposed and ageing skin. If the diagnosis is made confidently then treatment can be expectant. If however, there is any doubt an incisional biopsy should be taken of the specimen. If a lesion which is thought to be a keratoacanthoma does not regress within 6 weeks then excisional biopsy should be carried out.

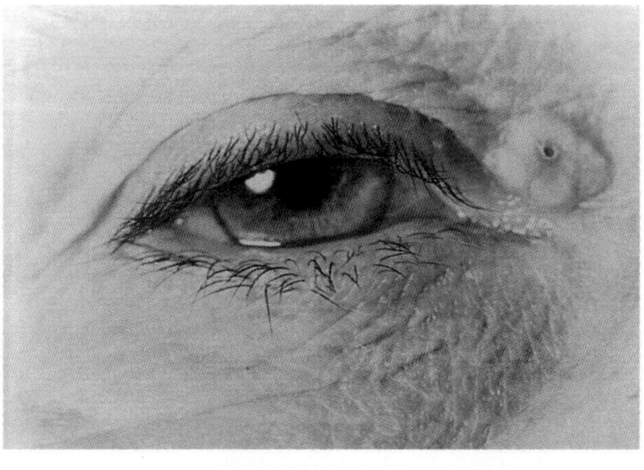

Figure 2.4 Typical epidermoid (commonly known as sebaceous) cyst, this example being situated at the inner canthus of the right eye. (Courtesy of Dr Sally Ibbotson, Senior Lecturer in Dermatology, University of Dundee, Dundee, Scotland.)

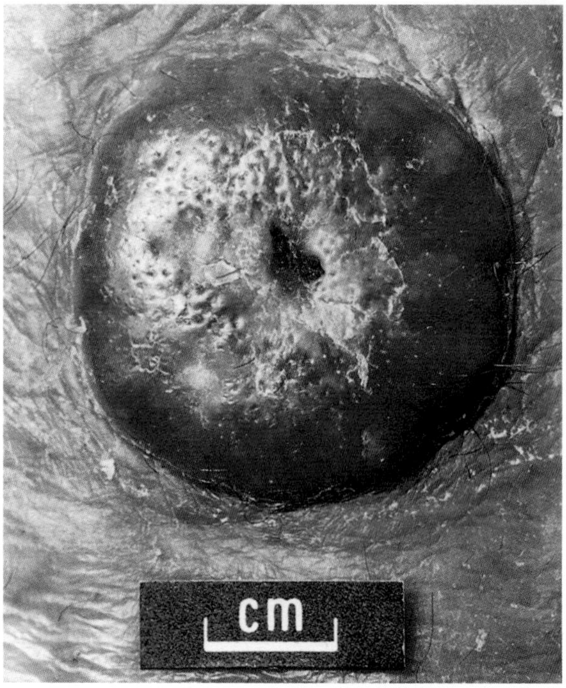

Figure 2.5 Keratoacanthoma. (Courtesy of Dr Sally Ibbotson, Senior Lecturer in Dermatology, University of Dundee, Dundee, Scotland.)

Molluscum contagiosum

This lesion is caused by a pox virus and is contagious but with a low virulence. It tends to occur in children and young adults. The virus multiplies in the deep layers of the epidermis and destroys the low-lying tissue producing a central pore. The most typical clinical presentation is a crop of smooth umbilicated lesions up to 1 cm in diameter. The usual form of treatment is curettage but cryotherapy or topical trichloroacetic acid can be effective.

Warts

Warts arise as a result of epithelial hyperplasia triggered by a human papilloma virus (HPV). They commonly occur on the hands of children and may regress spontaneously. If they fail to do so they may be treated with cryotherapy, coagulation, desiccation or surgical excision.

Keloid

The term keloid is used to describe proliferation of fibrous tissue following trauma. This is commonly the

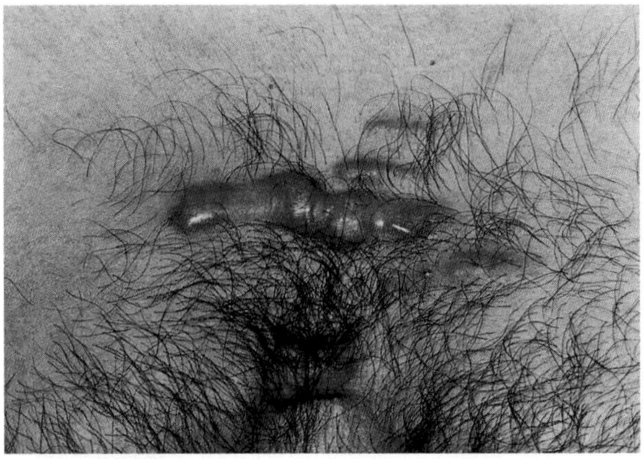

Figure 2.6 Keloid scarring. (Courtesy of Dr Sally Ibbotson, Senior Lecturer in Dermatology, University of Dundee, Dundee, Scotland.)

result of a surgical incision or a burn and appears as a raised red sensitive area which transgresses the original margins of the injury. It gradually stabilizes into a prominent unsightly overgrowth of scar tissue (Figure 2.6). Keloid scarring is extremely rare in white skin races being much more common in black skin by a ratio of about 12:1. It occurs particularly in young people with a peak incidence between 10 and 25 years. It may occur anywhere on the body but the back, the neck, the earlobes, the pre-sternal and deltoid regions seem to be at particular risk. Histological examination shows an overgrowth of collagenous tissue with disorganized fibrillar structure. There is little elastic tissue and there are few blood cells. It is important to distinguish keloid from hypertrophic scarring which gives rise to a similar red raised lesion but does not transgress the boundaries of the injury.

The treatment of keloid scarring is extremely difficult. Surgical excision is usually contraindicated as this will merely result in further keloid scarring, although in very large areas, intralesional excision may be of value. Spontaneous regression may occur but this cannot be guaranteed. Intralesional injection of steroids may be of value and specially designed tight fitting elastic garments providing continuous firm pressure have been used with some success.

Section 2.3 • Malignant and pre-malignant conditions of skin

Cancer of the skin taken as an overall entity is by far the commonest malignant tumour to affect humans. The three main types are squamous cells carcinoma, basal cell carcinoma and malignant melanoma. These will be dealt with in turn but first the general aetiology and pathology of skin cancer will be considered followed by an examination of pre-malignant lesions.

Aetiology

There are two major aetiological factors, the human papilloma virus and solar radiation. For some reason it is usually only the skin of the perineum which is affected by malignant change unequivocally associated with HPV (see section on anal intraepithelial neoplasia). However, papilloma virus particles have been found in squamous cell carcinomas from other parts of the body and it may have a more widespread role.

Table 2.1 Classification of ultraviolet light

Class	*Wavelength (nm)*	*Source*	*Effect*
UVA	320–400	Sunlight	Darkening of melanin; phototoxicity
UVB	280–320	Sunlight	Sunburn; carcinogenesis; melanin production
UVC	>280	Arc welders; sterlizing lamps	Carcinogenesis

Both pre-malignant and malignant lesions of the skin occur more frequently in those areas which are exposed to the sun. The causative agent is ultraviolet (UV) light which may be classified according to its wavelength (Table 2.1). UVA (wavelength 320–420 nm) is probably the least damaging to skin but may have an additive effect to that of UVB (wavelength 290–320 nm). UVB is more damaging and UVC (200–290 nm) is the most damaging. Relatively little UVC reaches the earth's surface as it is filtered by the ozone layer but it can be produced by arc welders and sterilizing lamps. It should be noted that although sunbeds generally emit UVA radiation they are still potentially dangerous.

Ultraviolet light causes dimerization of adjacent pyrimidines in the epidermal DNA. This decreases the efficiency of cellular repair mechanisms and thereby may lead to malignant transformation. Malignant and pre-malignant skin lesions are rare in negroid populations and common in Australia, New Zealand and South Africa where the skins of migrant North Europeans are exposed to high levels of sunlight. The absorptive effect of the atmospheric ozone layer is least at the Equator but increases with increasing longitude as the suns rays strike the ozone layer more obliquely and have a longer passage through it.

Pathology of solar damage

Solar radiation creates changes in skin known as actinic change which involves degeneration of collagen in the dermis and an increase in the amount of elastin. As a consequence there is failure of the supportive dermal structure and the skin becomes wrinkled. In the epidermal layer actinic change affects all the cells. The epidermis becomes thin and atrophic, melanocytes become irregularly distributed and atypical and there is an increase in the number of suppressor T-lymphocytes.

The epidermal keratinocytes undergo hyperkeratinization and parakeratinization. In the early stages of dysplastic change, excessive amounts of keratin are produced and the keratin fails to separate from the skin resulting in hyperkeratosis. Clinically, this forms scales. With further accumulation of damage the pattern changes to the more severe dysplastic form, parakeratosis. Here the cells fail to mature and as they pass to the surface they retain their nuclei. In addition, cellular atypia of individual epithelial cells is seen with pleomorphism, hyperchromatism, irregular nuclei and an increase in the ratio of nuclear area to cytoplasmic area. Extreme dysplastic changes are described as carcinoma *in situ* and when the basement membrane is breached the lesion becomes an invasive tumour.

Actinic keratosis

Actinic keratosis is also known as senile keratosis or solar keratosis. It is most commonly seen in Caucasians and it presents clinically as a red scaly patch on the exposed skin of elderly individuals. The clinical course is slow with regression of some lesions and progression of others to malignancy. Histologically the skin exhibits a variable degree of solar damage as described above. Although the most effective treatment for actinic keratosis is excision this may be difficult in large and awkward areas. It may therefore be appropriate to treat this conservatively and only advise excision when there are suspicious clinical indications of malignancy, i.e. the beginnings of ulceration or bleeding.

Carcinoma *in situ*

Carcinoma *in situ*, sometimes known as Bowen's disease, can be difficult to distinguish from actinic keratosis and indeed represents the more severe end of the spectrum of this condition. Histologically the picture is identical to that of squamous cell carcinoma without penetration of the basement membrane. Clinically it presents as a rough reddened patch of skin, which persists over many months or years. Owing to the risk of malignant change, it should be excised unless there is a compelling reason to treat it expectantly for reasons of size or anatomical position.

Squamous cell carcinoma of the skin

As with carcinoma *in situ*, squamous cell carcinoma of the skin tends to occur in the exposed areas of white-skinned elderly individuals, particularly those who have spent a lot of time in the open.

Pathology

Squamous cell carcinomas arise from the epidermal keratinocytes. Histologically, abnormal squamous cells are seen growing downwards from the epidermis into the dermis and subcutaneous tissues in strands or sheets. The tumour may be classified as well differentiated, moderately differentiated or poorly differentiated. Typically the well-differentiated type of tumour will show keratinization and formation of keratin pearls composed of concentric layers of cells with increasing keratinization towards the centre. The cells are large and polygonal with eosinophilic cytoplasm, mitotic figures and nucleoli are few. By contrast, the poorly differentiated tumours are made up of anaplastic cells with multiple mitoses and nucleoli and no keratinization. There is a four-part classification of squamous cell carcinoma based on differentiation described by Broder but this is not widely used.

Squamous cell carcinomas spread locally via lymphatics and via the blood. Local invasion is horizontal and vertical and in neglected tumours can give rise to widespread destruction of skin and underlying structures. Erosion of large blood vessels can be a terminal event. Lymphatic spread is to the lymph nodes that are draining the affected part of the skin and the blood-borne spread tends to manifest itself in lungs, bone and brain. However, the tendency to metastasize in squamous cell carcinoma is relatively low and only about 3% will have metastasized at the time of diagnosis. For some reason, squamous cell carcinomas that arise in chronic scars tend to behave more aggressively but it is not clear whether this is a biological feature of the disease or whether tumours arising in scars tend to be neglected.

Aetiology

As outlined above the most important aetiological factor is the ultraviolet component of sunlight but others include exposure to ionizing radiation, chronic heat, tobacco, chronic scarring and ulceration (Marjolin's ulcer) and immunosuppression. The role of the human papilloma virus is not clear but papilloma virus particles have been isolated in squamous cell carcinomas.

Clinical features

Clinically there are two patterns of growth which are recognized although these can overlap to a certain extent. The infiltrative type begins as a warty nodule which breaks down to form an ulcer with a rolled edge overlying the surrounding indurated skin (Figure 2.7).

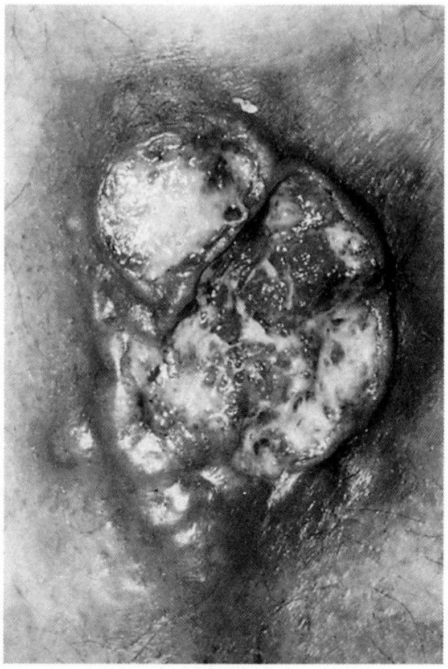

Figure 2.7 Infiltrative squamous carcinoma.

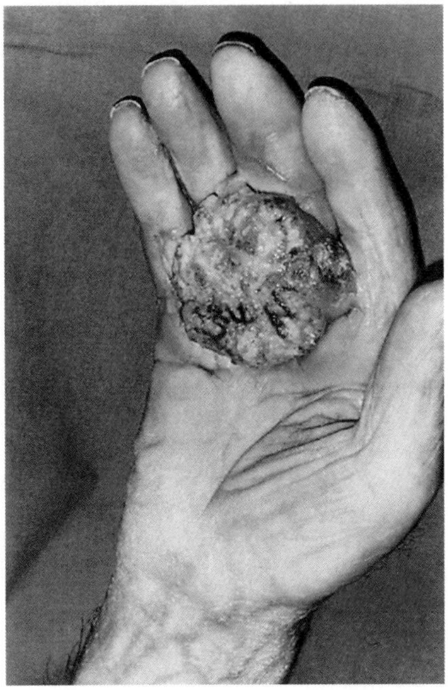

Figure 2.8 Protuberant squamous carcinoma.

The protuberant type produces a raised cauliflower-like lesion (Figure 2.8). The degree of induration felt clinically gives an indication of the depth of invasion of the tumour as does the extent of ulceration.

Diagnosis

The diagnosis tends to be evident clinically but must be confirmed by either an incisional or where possible an excisional biopsy.

Prognosis

The best predictor of tumour behaviour in terms of metastatic disease is the vertical tumour thickness but the surface area of the tumour also has implications for local recurrence. Tumours arising in apparently normal skin have a poorer prognosis in terms of recurrence and distance spread than those arising in skin showing solar damage. Histological differentiation is also a factor in prognosis as the poorly differentiated tumours have an increased tendency to metastasize. The anatomical site of the tumours is also important. Tumours of the trunk and limbs have a worse prognosis than those of the head and neck.

Treatment

As mentioned above, diagnosis should be made by excisional biopsy wherever possible and this will also serve as treatment if the tumour is completely excised. Small lesions may be excised under local anaesthetic but the incision should be planned prior to introduction of the anaesthetic to avoid mistakes created by distortion of the skin. When deciding on the extent of excision the lesion should be inspected under a good light and by palpation as induration indicating tumour extension may be felt more easily than it is seen. The incision should be marked in ink after measuring a margin of clearance. In the head and neck area a margin of 5 mm is considered an adequate compromise between tumour clearance and the cosmetic and functional result. On the trunk and limbs however, a wider margin is taken.

When removing the lesion it is important to remember that a deep clearance is as important as lateral clearance and it is important to palpate and inspect the deep margin during excision. In the limbs the possibility of extension along fascial planes must be considered and perineural spread must also be taken into account. A history of pain or unusual sensations associated with the tumour may suggest perineural spread. Whatever the site of the tumour it is essential that a margin of normal tissue is excised on all aspects of the tumour and if the tumour is adherent to tendon or bone this tissue must also be excised. Problems of reconstruction must not compromise the tumour clearance otherwise the surgery will fail. After excision it is important to mark the affected piece of skin in order to allow the histopathologist to orientate the specimen. With this in mind the specimen should always be accompanied by a diagram showing its site and orientation.

Although surgery is the treatment of choice for the majority of squamous cell carcinomas this tumour is radiosensitive and radiotherapy has an important part to play in its management. In practice, radiotherapy is reserved for tumours which are inoperable by virtue of involvement of vital structures and for post-operative treatment of tumours which have been inadequately excised because of anatomical considerations. Having said this, radiotherapy may be used as the primary treatment modality for all squamous cell carcinomas with the following reservations:

- Pre-treatment biopsy is essential.
- Radiation of exposed skin in young people may increase the risk of future carcinoma.
- Areas of chronic friction or poor vascularity, e.g. the shoulders and pretibial area, should not be irradiated as this will lead to chronic skin damage.
- Treatment of skin around the eye may lead to radiation keratitis.

Recurrent disease

If histological examination of an excised squamous cell carcinoma reveals resection margin involvement the risk of recurrence is in the region of 50%. A second procedure should therefore be undertaken immediately unless this is contraindicated by the involvement of vital structures. In this case radiotherapy is indicated. If recurrence occurs after a lesion has been excised with adequate histological margins this indicates deep infiltration along tissue planes. This tends to occur in lesions of the ear and requires either wide excision or radiotherapy. When wide excision is performed, intra-operative frozen section will help to define the extent of excision.

Treatment of metastatic disease

When metastatic deposits in the regional lymph nodes are detected, *en bloc* resection of the local lymph node group is indicated and post-operative radiotherapy should be considered for poorly differentiated tumours. Metastatic lesion of the bone and brain may be treated by radiotherapy to reduce local symptoms but widespread disease will require chemotherapy. Overall, the 5 year survival in patients with metastatic disease at presentation is 25%. The 10 year survival is 13% and the 15 year survival is 8%.

Basal cell carcinoma

Basal cell carcinoma (BCC) is the commonest skin malignancy in white-skinned races.

Pathology

BCC arises from epithelial cells and it is thought that the cell of origin is from the follicular adnexal basal lining the hair follicle rather than cells from the basal layer of the epidermis. Histologically the tumour consists of clumps of basophilic cells surrounded by a stroma of connective tissue. At the periphery of the tumour, columnar cells form a palisade, which is a hallmark of the tumour. Mucin is found in the stroma but not elastin in contradistinction to squamous cell carcinomas. The ratio of cells to stroma varies according to the five types of BCC: noduloulcerative, superficial spreading, morphoeic, pigmented and fibroepithelioma of Pinkus.

Noduloulcerative BCC

This is a well-circumscribed tumour with islands of basal cells embedded in a fibroblastic stroma. Centrally the cells are arranged randomly but peripherally the cells form palisades. The basal cells may show differentiation towards the adnexal structures of the skin or may demonstrate squamous metaplasia.

Superficial spreading BCC

In this variant there are nests of basaloid cells with peripheral palisading lying in the level of the basal layer of the epidermis with atrophy of the epidermis above this.

Morphoeic BCC

Here there is a dense fibrous dermal stroma with scanty strands and groups of cells embedded within it. The tumour cell strands may stream from the undersurface of the tumour into the deeper tissues. Proliferation of the stroma may also occur in the horizontal plane beneath apparently normal epidermis. This makes for difficulty in judging the margin of the tumour with the naked eye and is responsible for the high incidence of recurrence of this type of BCC.

Pigmented BCC

This type of BCC is similar to the noduloulcerative type but contains melanocytes.

Fibroepithelioma of Pinkus

In this variant strands of basaloid cells extend into the deeper fibrous stroma and there is no palisading.

Although BCCs behave like malignant tumours locally with both horizontal and vertical invasion patterns, metastases are extremely rare occurring in less than 0.1% of cases.

Aetiology

Exposure to sunlight appears to be the most important aetiological factor in BCC. However, the risk is increased by ionizing radiation burns or chemical damage to the skin. Ingestion of arsenic and general immunosuppression also appear to be important. There may also be a familial component, and the Gorlin-Goltz syndrome, which is inherited as an autosomal dominant trait, predisposes to the development of multiple BCCs as well as craniofacial abnormalities, abnormal development of the costal cartilages and palmoplantar pits.

Clinical features

The clinical features of BCCs can be subdivided according to type.

Noduloulcerative BCC

Also known as cystic BCC, ulcerative BCC or a rodent ulcer, this is by far the commonest form of the tumour accounting for approximately 50% of all BCCs. Clinically it presents as a slowly growing nodule with a waxy or pearly appearance associated with telangiectasia. Later in the course of the disease the skin ulcerates to form a typical rodent ulcer (Figure 2.9).

Superficial spreading BCC

This type of BCC is also described as superficial cicatrizing or 'field fire' BCC. It presents as a scaling erythematous lesion, usually on the trunk. It does not become indurated and it does not ulcerate. Instead it spreads radially while appearing to heal in the centre. The central scar area contains sweat glands but the hair follicles are destroyed producing characteristic alopecia. The tumour is frequently multi-focal and is commonly advanced at presentation owing to the insidious nature of its development.

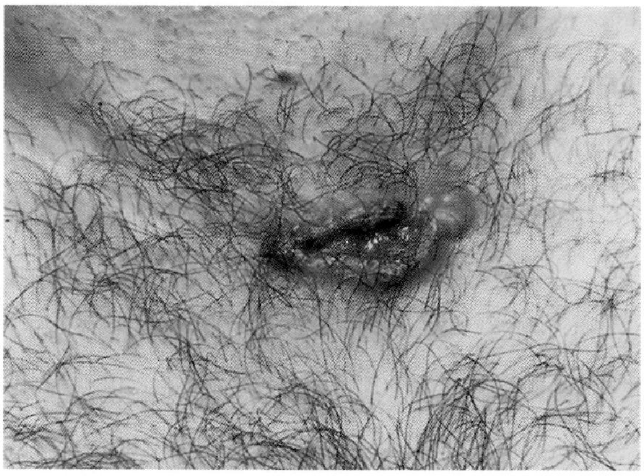

Figure 2.9 Rodent ulcer.

Morphoeic BCC

This presents as a dense greyish yellow plaque which increases in size gradually. Around the eyelids contraction of the fibrous stroma may result in distortion. Ulceration may also occur.

Pigmented BCC

Clinically this type of BCC is similar to the noduloulcerative type but with a pearly black sheen.

Fibroepithelioma of Pinkus

This presents as a papilloma without scaling or ulceration.

Diagnosis

The diagnosis of BCC is clinical but must be confirmed by histology. Wherever possible this should be an excisional biopsy.

Treatment

BCCs may be treated by surgical excision, curettage, cryotherapy, laser treatment or radiotherapy.

Surgical excision

As mentioned above the most satisfactory approach is excisional biopsy which allows examination of the entire specimen and evaluation of the resection margins. A simple excision is usually carried out as an ellipse around the tumour with a margin of 2–3 mm for nodulocystic lesions. In morphoeic or recurrent lesions the clearance should be 1 cm. As with squamous cell carcinoma the excised specimen should be marked to allow the pathologist to orientate the specimen. After excision in most cases primary closure is possible but it may be necessary to use partial thickness or full thickness grafting. On the face large lesions may require flap reconstruction after excision.

Curettage

Noduloulcerative BCCs can sometimes be excised with a curette and the wound allowed to heal by secondary intention. The rationale behind this method is that the soft tumour is scraped out while the firmer more resistant normal skin is spared. However, this method is not suitable for lesions greater than 1 cm in diameter or for morphoeic lesions as the risk of persistent tumour is too great. In general, formal general surgical excision is to be preferred.

Cryotherapy and laser

BCCs can be treated by cryotherapy using a liquid nitrogen probe at minus 50°C for between 30 and 120 s. Similarly the CO_2 laser can be used to treat BCCs. Neither allows histological examination of the specimen and both produce cicatrization. Again surgical excision is to be preferred but these methods may be useful for multiple small BCCs.

Radiotherapy

The overall cure rate of BCCs using radiotherapy is about 90% which is in the same order as all the other methods used. This option may seem attractive as operation is avoided but it does require multiple visits to hospital as the exposure required is 4000–6000 Gy over several fractions to obtain the best results. Despite this, radiotherapy often causes skin atrophy and alopecia. Previous radiotherapy is a contraindication to further similar treatment in the same area.

The choice of treatment depends on the site and size of the tumour, its histological nature, the condition of the patient and, in recurrent tumour, the methods previously used.

Benign pigmented naevi

Naevi are extremely common and have little clinical significance in themselves. However, they may mimic malignant melanoma or they may be cosmetically unacceptable to the patient. A small proportion of naevi may also have malignant potential.

Aetiology and pathology

Melanocytes, which are responsible for skin pigmentation, arise from the neural crest and in the first weeks of embryonic development they migrate to the skin as well as to the meninges, uveal tract and ectodermal mucosa. In the skin, melanocytes are distributed through the dermis and epidermis. At birth, most cutaneous melanocytes are present in the basal layer of the epidermis but over the first three decades of life some will migrate into the dermis. In the dermis melanocytes lose their ability to undergo mitosis and therefore have no malignant potential.

Melanocytes may clump together in the basal layer of the epidermis to form a simple lentigo or mole, which is commonly seen in infants. This may be regarded as the first stage in the progression towards a mature intradermal naevus. As the child grows, the melanocytes aggregate at the dermo-epidermal junction. These are called junctional naevi. The melanocytes gradually become incorporated into the dermis by fibroblast migration. When this has taken place naevi consist of a combination of junctional aggregates and intradermal aggregates of melanocytes and are termed compound naevi. Finally as the naevus matures all the melanocytes aggregate into the dermis and an intradermal naevus is formed. Thus junctional naevi are common in children and have virtually no malignant potential. In adults, they are rare but do carry a risk of malignant transformation and tend to be found on the palms of the hands and the soles of the feet.

Clinical features

The junctional naevus is either a macule or papule and is brown, smooth and hairless. It may occur anywhere but when these lesions are seen on the palms or the soles in adults they may be pre-malignant. The intradermal type of naevis is a papule often hairy and well defined. It may be brown or flesh coloured. It is most commonly seen on the face and on the neck.

Diagnosis

The diagnosis is usually self-evident but excision biopsy and histological examination are necessary for definitive diagnosis.

Treatment

The only treatment for a naevus is excision but this should only be done when the lesion is inconvenient or where there is a possibility of malignancy. The latter is suggested by rapid growth, a deepening of the pigmentation or bleeding (see next section).

Malignant melanoma

Malignant melanoma predominantly affects white-skinned races, particularly Caucasians who are exposed to intense sunlight. The highest incidence in the world is in Queensland in Australia (33 per 100 000). The disease is extremely rare in black-skinned races and when it does occur it is found almost exclusively on the sole of the foot, the subungual region or on the mucus membranes. Women are more commonly affected than men by a ratio of 2:1 and it is very rare in children.

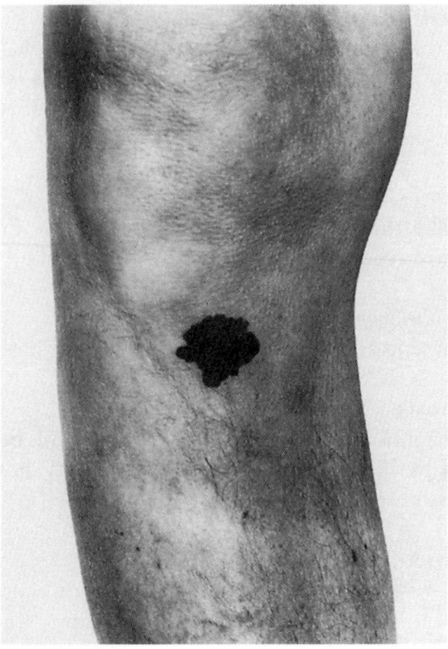

Figure 2.10 Superficial spreading melanoma.

Pathology

Malignant melanomas are classified into four groups according to their clinical presentation. These are: (1) lentigo maligna, (2) superficial spreading, (3) nodular and (4) acral lentiginous. Each of these categories has a characteristic macroscopic and microscopic appearance although in terms of prognosis the histological depth of penetration is the most important feature.

Lentigo maligna melanoma

This is a slow growing, flat, pigmented lesion, sometimes known as Hutchinson's melanotic freckle and it tends to exist for a long time in a pre-malignant state. It is relatively non-aggressive and rarely metastasizes. It typically develops in some damaged skin, usually on the face in elderly individuals.

Superficial spreading melanoma (Figure 2.10)

This is the commonest type of melanoma and typically presents as an alteration in a pre-existing naevus on the trunk or limbs of an individual aged between 40 and 50. It appears as a flat pigmented lesion with an irregular edge and non-homogeneous pigmentation. Histologically the tumour cells often excite a local lymphocytic response which appears to result in regression of parts of the tumour.

Nodular melanoma (Figure 2.11)

Again usually arising in a pre-existing naevus this has appearance of a nodule growing from a pigmented area of skin usually on the head, neck or trunk of an individual aged between 50 and 70 years. Histologically the tumour has a strong vertical growth component with relatively little radial growth.

Acral lentiginous

This term is used to describe melanomas arising in the nail beds or on the palmar or plantar skin. They grow slowly and seldom metastasize.

Spread

The main route of spread is metastasis to the regional lymph nodes but a tumour may also metastasize to local skin giving rise to satellite lesions. These may occur in an excision scar and often occur between the excision site and the regional lymph nodes. Distant blood-borne metastases tend to occur in the liver, lung or brain. The majority of patients who develop distant metastases do so within 3 years of the diagnosis of the primary lesion although later metastases have been reported.

Aetiology

The aetiological factors in malignant melanoma are: (1) sun exposure, (2) racial predisposition, (3) pre-malignant states and (4) recurrent trauma. The most important pre-malignant state is the junctional or compound naevus as it appears that melanocytes that remain in the epidermis have malignant potential. The reason for this is unclear. A minority of malignant melanomas are associated with congenital giant naevi or the dysplastic naevus syndrome. Congenital giant naevi are defined as naevi occupying more than 1% of the body surface area. These may be very large and may sometimes cover the trunk, upper arms and upper thighs (bathing trunk naevus). The risk of malignant change in such lesions varies from 2 to 28% according to the series. Of melanomas which occur in giant congenital naevi, 50% develop in the first 5 years of life. The dysplastic naevus syndrome is a familial condition inherited as an autosomal dominant with variable penetrance. It is characterized by multiple pale, non-homogeneous naevi with an irregular edge. Most commonly they occur on the back and start to develop around puberty. The risk of developing malignant melanoma in these individuals is several hundred times that of the normal population.

Clinical features

The clinical features of a malignant melanoma vary according to the classifications which are described in the pathology section. The most important principle to appreciate however, is that melanomas may develop either as pre-existing naevi or as a development of pigmentation and normal skin. The changes in a naevus which suggest malignancy include an increase in size, loss of homogeneity with areas of darker or lighter pigmentation, irregularity of outline, nodularity, bleeding and ulceration. Itching may also be a feature and occasionally a patient may notice satellite lesions.

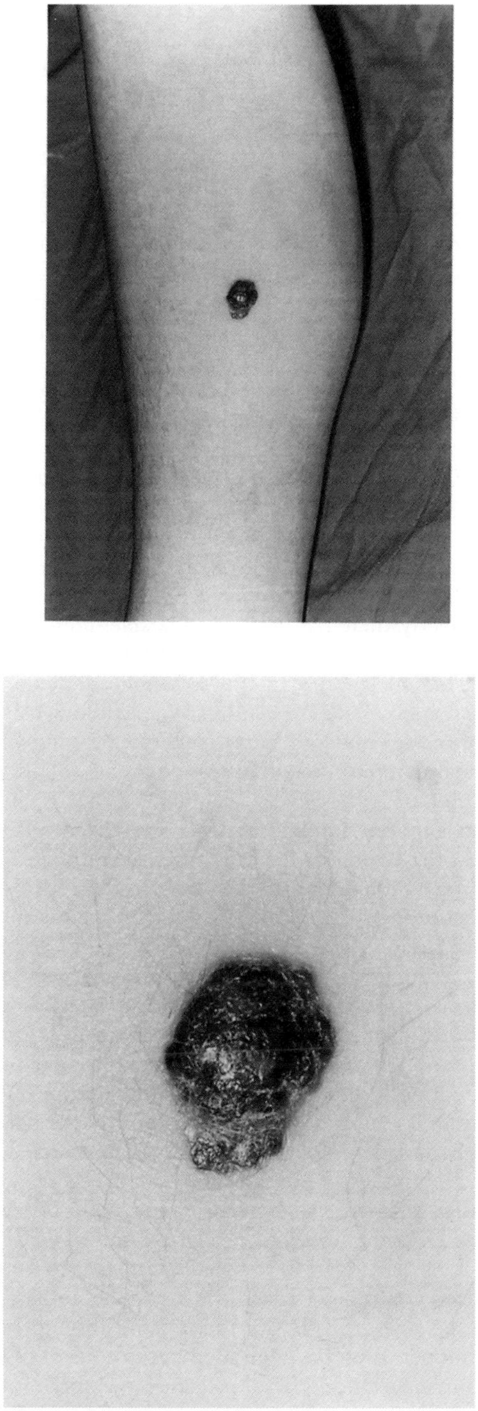

Figure 2.11 Nodular melanoma.

Diagnosis

Suspicious lesions must be dealt with urgently by excisional biopsy. Incisional biopsy should be avoided as malignancy may be missed and some clinicians feel that incisional biopsy may encourage metastatic spread, although the evidence for this is lacking. Complete excision of the lesion is also necessary for proper staging of the tumour. Another important feature is the presence of lymph node metastases and careful palpation of the regional lymph nodes should always be carried out when a malignant melanoma is suspected.

Prognosis

The prognosis of a malignant melanoma is most accurately estimated by the histological depth of the tumour. This can be estimated either by measuring the depth of penetration (the Breslow thickness) or by using the Clarke classification.

Breslow thickness

The Breslow thickness is measured from the granular layer of the epidermis to the deepest melanoma cell of the lesion in a fixed specimen. Breslow separated melanomas into three bands according to the prognostic significance of the depth of penetration. Tumours less than 0.76 mm in depth were associated with a 100% long-term survival. Tumours between 0.76 and 1.5 mm have a poor prognosis and those greater than 1.5 mm have an extremely poor prognosis. This classification was merely developed for convenience, however, and in reality prognosis deteriorates progressively with increasing thickness. In thin tumours, which have stimulated an immune response resulting in the regression of tumour cells (superficial spreading melanoma) measurement of the thickness may be unreliable. In these cases survival will be less than predicted for the apparent thickness.

Clarke levels

Clarke classified levels of invasion of malignant melanoma in terms of the histological layers of the skin (Table 2.2). This system requires accurate histological assessment of the penetration of the tumour through defined layers of the dermis and is subject to considerable inter-observer variability. It has been shown to be less accurate than Breslow thickness in determining prognosis and Breslow thickness has become the standard system for histological classification.

Table 2.2 Clarke's levels of invasion of the skin by melanoma cells

Level 1	Tumour cells confined to epidermis above basement membrane
Level 2	Tumour cells present in papillary dermis
Level 3	Tunour cells penetrating through the full depth of the papillary dermis to the level of the reticular dermis
Level 4	Tumour cells in the reticular dermis
Level 5	Tumour cells in the subcutaneous fat

Staging

In addition to Breslow thickness and Clarke level staging systems have to take into account metastatic spread. The simplest staging system is the McNeer and Dasgupta system (Table 2.3) but the more complex system of the American Joint Committee on Cancer is more widely used (Table 2.4).

Treatment

The treatment of malignant melanoma is essentially surgical. The initial excisional biopsy should be carried out with a sufficient margin to ensure local clearance. Following histological confirmation of the diagnosis and measurement of the Breslow thickness, further treatment may be planned. The basic principle is wide excision to prevent local recurrences caused by micrometastasis present in the skin at the time of primary excision but there is still some controversy surrounding the margin required to achieve adequate clearance.

For many years, a 5 cm margin in all directions and including deep fascia was recommended but there is no evidence that this approach improves the survival rate and little evidence that it affects the rate of local recurrence. Recent studies indicate that for lesion of 0.76 mm or less in thickness a 1 cm excision margin is adequate and curative. Thicker lesions require a wider excision margin of at least 2 cm but extending the margin beyond 3 cm even for the thickest lesions does not appear to affect prognosis.

There is also controversy surrounding the treatment of regional lymph nodes in patients with stage 1 disease, i.e. those with localized disease and no clinically involved nodes. Elective regional lymph node dissection in such patients has shown that tumour may be present in the regional lymph nodes in 5–25%. For this reason some surgeons will perform an elective regional lymph node clearance in those patients with tumours thicker than 1.5 mm in diameter, even when the lymph nodes are impalpable. For patients with clinical lymph node involvement but no distant metastases it is generally agreed that regional lymph node excision should be performed. Following this, the 5 year survival is related to the original Breslow thickness with 80% survival in patients with melanoma less than 3.5 mm and 27% survival in those with tumours greater than 3.5 mm.

Recently, there has been considerable interest in the concept of probe-directed sentinel node dissection in malignant melanoma. In this technique, patients with clinical stage 1 and 2 melanomas (i.e. without palpable lymph node) undergo intra-operative mapping of the regional lymph node. This is done by intradermal injection of ^{99m}Tc-labelled sulphur colloid or human serum albumin administered pre-operatively into the skin in the region of the tumour or excision area. The draining lymph nodes are then detected by a hand-held gamma probe (Figure 2.12). If the lymph node nearest to the tumour detected in this way is histologically positive for tumour, then a complete inguinal lymph node dissection is carried out. This approach holds out the hope of a rational surgical approach to patients with lymph nodes which are not clinically involved.

In patients with palpable lymph nodes, fine needle aspiration cytology can be used to confirm the diagnosis of metastatic disease before dissection is carried out. In the groin there is considerable controversy regarding whether a superficial inguinal lymph node dissection should be combined with a pelvic lymph node dissection. This has not been resolved and there are no randomized controlled trials in this area. Chemotherapy is of little value in malignant melanoma although isolated limb perfusion has been used in the control of local tumour recurrence. Useful palliation may be obtained but there is no evidence that regional or systemic chemotherapy has an effect on survival.

Table 2.3 Staging of malignant melanoma

Stage 1:	Primary tumour only, with no evidence of metastases
Stage 2:	Primary lesion with metastatic spread to the regional lymph nodes detectable on clinical examination
Stage 3:	Primary lesion with metastasis to more than one lymph node group or to another area

Table 2.4 American Joint Committee on Cancer staging system for malignant melanoma

Stage IA:	Localized disease less than 0.76 mm or Clarke level 2
Stage IB:	Localized disease 0.76–1.5 mm or Clarke level 3
Stage IIA:	Localized disease 1.5–4 mm or Clarke level 4
Stage IIB:	Localized disease 4.1 mm or more or Clarke level 5
Stage III:	Melanoma with involvement of regional lymph node group
Stage IV:	Melanoma with advanced regional lymph node involvement, multiple regional lymph node group involvement or distant metastases

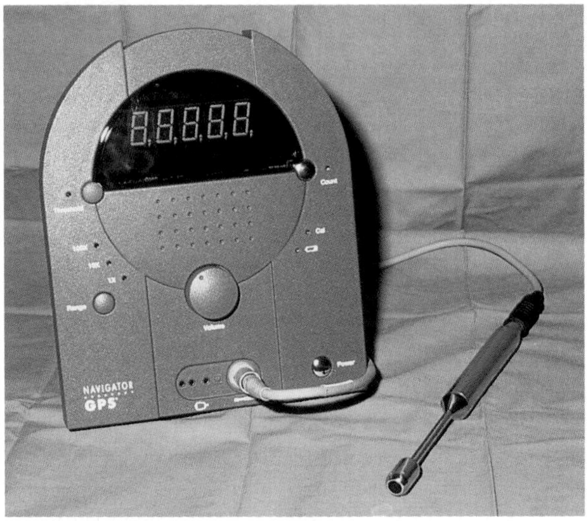

Figure 2.12 Hand-held gamma probe for sentinal node biopsy.

Section 2.4 • Tumours of fibrous tissue

Tumours of fibrous tissue are derived from fibroblasts and may demonstrate abnormal ground substance or collagen fibre formation. Myofibroblasts may also be present and these probably arise from fibroblasts.

Fibroma

This is a benign encapsulated fibrous nodule which may be a soft subcutaneous nodule (fibroma mole) or a pedunculated lesion of the oral mucosa (fibroma durum). Fibromas may be treated by enucleation.

Fibrous histiocytoma

This condition is also called sclerosing haemangioma or dermatofibroma. They are benign and occur on the arms and legs in adults. They are seldom more than 1 cm in diameter and histologically they are made up of thin walled capillary vessels surrounded by fibroblasts and histiocytes. Treatment is by excision.

Desmoid

The term desmoid is derived from the Greek word *desmos* which means a band or a tendon and desmoid tumours arise from fascial sheaths or musculoaponeurotic structures. Desmoids may arise as a result of familial adenomatous polyposis (FAP) and this is generally known as Gardner's syndrome (see module on colorectal disease). Desmoids may however present without associated polyposis and abdominal desmoid tumours tend to occur in post-partum women. These may be related to changes in the abdominal wall during pregnancy. Extra-abdominal desmoids are commonest in the third and fourth decades but may present at any age. They are commoner in males and affect the back, chest wall and head and neck, particularly at the site of previous scars.

Histological examination reveals well-differentiated collagenous fibroblasts with a low mitotic rate. The treatment is by wide local excision although this can sometimes be difficult and hazardous. Desmoids have a particularly rich blood supply and considerable blood loss during surgery can be anticipated. Although these lesions are technically benign they do have a tendency to recur locally and this happens in about 50% of cases after excision. Desmoids are also sensitive to irradiation and radiotherapy may be appropriate in some situations **[see Module 6: Disorders of the abdominal wall and peritoneal cavity]**.

Fibrosarcoma

Fibrosarcoma is a malignant tumour which tends to occur in adults between the ages of 35 and 55. It is commoner in males than females and it may occur any where in the body although the incidence appears to be highest in the thigh and arm. It may be related to trauma and has been reported to arise from burn scars, injection sites, ulcers and areas of previous irradiation. On histology the tumour may be classified as low or high grade. Low-grade fibrosarcomas have abundant collagenous stroma, few cells and few mitotic figures or giant cells. These are the better differentiated tumours and have a relatively good prognosis. High-grade fibrosarcomas have abnormal fibroblasts arranged in a herringbone pattern with giant cells and mitotic figures. These have a poorer prognosis.

Clinically, a fibrosarcoma presents as a firm rubbery mass, usually with a long history of slow painless enlargement (Figure 2.13). The incidence of metastatic disease in high-grade fibrosarcoma is high although regional lymph nodes are rarely involved. The commonest sites for secondary deposits are the lungs, bones and liver. Treatment is by surgical excision with clear margins and to ensure a good result resection should extend to one tissue plane beyond the involved tissue. This may involve removing muscle and some patients require complex plastic reconstruction.

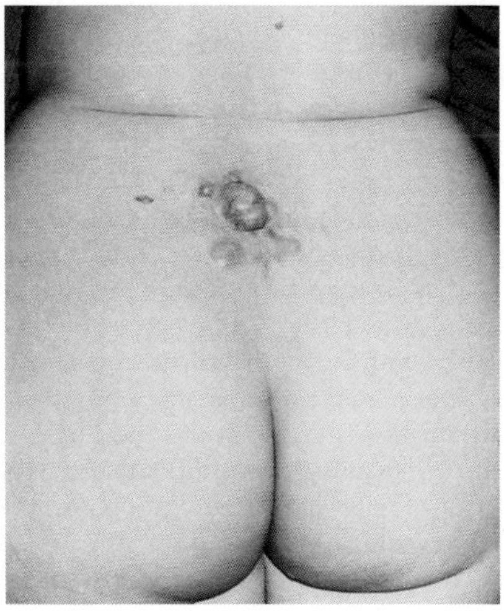

Figure 2.13 Fibrosarcoma.

Dermatofibrosarcoma protuberans is a rare form of fibrosarcoma which presents clinically as one or more red or bluish dermal nodules usually on the trunk or shoulders. They tend to occur in young adults and although they grow slowly they may suddenly start to enlarge and ulcerate. They are extremely locally aggressive but metastatic disease is relatively rare. On histology there are non-collagenous fibroblasts arranged in bundles around a central acellular area to produce a characteristic cartwheel appearance. Treatment is by wide local excision.

Section 2.5 • Tumours of muscle

Rhabdomyoma

These rare benign tumours arise from striated muscle and are probably related to fetal tissue. They affect adult males and are predominantly tumours of head and neck although they have been found in the heart and in limb muscles. They are treated by excision.

Leiomyoma

These are benign tumours of smooth muscle and usually occur in the uterus (fibroids) and in the gastrointestinal tract. They tend to occur in middle-aged females and there may be a familial tendency. Complete excision is usually curative.

Rhabdomyosarcoma

Rhabdomyosarcoma is a malignant tumour of skeletal muscle and although rare, the so-called embryonal rhabdomyosarcoma of children accounts for about 10% of all malignant tumours in children under the age of 15 years. The site of the tumour varies with the age at presentation and in children there are two peaks in age distribution. Head and neck and genitourinary tumours are commonest in children soon after birth whereas during adolescence the tumours are typically paratesticular. Histologically the tumours consist of undifferentiated mesenchymal cells.

In adults, rhabdomyosarcoma is a deep-seated lesion that often only presents when it projects into the skin as a reddish brown tumour. It is most commonly seen in the thigh, shoulder and upper arm. On histology, pleomorphic cells are seen and it can be difficult to differentiate from other types of sarcoma. The diagnosis has to be made on histology but magnetic resonance imaging (MRI) may be helpful in planning treatment as it will demonstrate the tumour in relation to the surrounding tissue planes.

In children with embryonal rhabdomyosarcoma treatment involves a multi-disciplinary approach involving surgery, irradiation and chemotherapy. The 5-year survival is greater than 50% and tumours of the orbit and genitourinary region have a better prognosis than other tumours. In adults, rhabdomyosarcoma is a highly aggressive form of sarcoma which metastasizes readily. The treatment of local disease is surgical and chemotherapy and radiotherapy have little to contribute.

Leiomyosarcomas

These are malignant tumours of smooth muscle and are most commonly seen in the uterus and gastrointestinal tract. However, they may also originate from the smooth muscle of major blood vessels, the oral and nasal cavities and the gallbladder. Treatment is surgical but local recurrence is common and the overall prognosis is poor.

Section 2.6 • Tumours of adipose tissue

Lipoma

Lipomas are benign tumours of adipose tissue and they are among the commonest of all benign neoplasms. They may occur in any organ as fat is present throughout the body but they are most often found in the subcutaneous tissue of the neck and shoulders, chest and thigh. The incidence of lipomas increases over the age of 40 and they are more commonly found in females than in males.

Histologically, lipomas are usually simple but there are several other types which are defined by their histological appearance. Fibroblastic or spindle cell lipomas are made up of fat cells and fibroblasts in a myxomatous stroma. These are benign but may be difficult to distinguish from liposarcomas on histology. Angiolipomas are characterized by a dense vascular plexus.

Clinically, a lipoma presents as a slow growing asymptomatic mass in the subcutaneous tissue. Occasionally deeper lipomas may cause nerve compression and are then associated with paraesthesia, pain and other functional problems. On examination, they are typically circumscribed, non-tender and are characteristically mobile, as they are not attached to skin. Small lipomas may be difficult to palpate as they slip from under the examining fingers. Angiolipomas are characterized by pain and Dercum's disease or adiposis dolorosa is a syndrome in which diffuse adipose tissue is deposited around the ankles, knees and elbows in menopausal women. This is often associated with pain.

Although most lipomas are subcutaneous, they may infiltrate fascia, muscle, periosteum or bone. They may recur after excision, but do not behave like malignant tumours. The treatment of a single lesion is excision in order to obtain histological diagnosis. Patients who have multiple lipomas should only have those lesions excised which are causing problems. If these are confirmed histologically as lipomas, it is safe to assume that the other lesions are similar.

Liposarcoma

These malignant tumours of adipose tissue are rare but must always be considered in the differential diagnosis when a lipoma is suspected. Unlike lipomas, liposarcomas usually arise from deeper tissues. They occur most frequently in older patients and are commoner in males than in females. The commonest sites are the limbs and the retroperitoneum. Histologically, liposarcomas are classified according to their malignant potential and there are five subtypes: (1) well differentiated, (2) myxoid, (3) fibroblastic, (4) lipoblastic and (5) pleomorphic.

The *well-differentiated* subtype is made up of mature adipocytes which show some pleomorphism and occasional mitotic figures. These tumours have a good prognosis. They do not metastasize but are invasive and tend to recur locally. The second subtype, *myxoid liposarcomas*, consist of pleomorphic adipocytes and pre-adipocytes and fibroblast-like cells or prolipoblasts. This subtype is commonly found in the groin, thigh, trunk, popliteal fossa and the retroperitoneum. It is most commonly seen in the fifth and sixth decades of life. These tumours may metastasize and have a 50% risk of local recurrence after excision. The *fibroblastic* subtype is made up largely of prolipoblasts with a few pre-adipocytes. It presents clinically very much as the myxoid liposarcoma but has a poor prognosis with a 62% recurrence rate after surgical excision. *Lipoblastic liposarcoma* is made up of round cells with pre-adipocytes and lipoblasts in a myxoid stroma. This tumour shows a similar malignant potential to the fibroblastic type. The *pleomorphic liposarcoma* is made up of undifferentiated cells with a high mitotic rate. The tissue of origin is demonstrated by the presence of occasional pre-adipocytes, lipoblasts or intracytoplasmic hyalin globules. This tumour has a strong tendency to metastasize and is associated with very poor prognosis.

Treatment of liposarcoma is by wide excision and for the less differentiated types radiotherapy should be considered either as adjuvant treatment or as an alternative where surgical excision is impossible or incomplete.

Section 2.7 • Tumours of the lymphatic system

Cystic hygroma

This lesion occurs in babies and consists of a diffuse soft swelling usually found in the neck. It may also occur in the lymphatic tissue of the axilla or groin. It is a hamartomatous overgrowth of lymphatics leading to a multiloculated cystic lesion which may reach large dimensions. Infection of or haemorrhage into the cyst may result in rapid painful enlargement. The only effective method of treatment is surgical excision.

Lymphangioma

Lymphangioma is a cystic lesion of lymphatic tissue. Lymphangioma simplex rises in the skin or mucosa and is common on the tongue. Several cystic lesions may occur together and this is called lymphangioma circumscripta. Treatment is usually by excision although recurrence is relatively common. Electrocoagulation and argon laser therapy have also been used to good effect. The cavernous lymphangioma is more extensive than lymphangioma simplex. They occur at any time between birth and about 20 months of age. They resemble cavernous haemangiomata but lack the blue colour seen with this lesion. Initially they are soft but after repeated infections they become fibrotic. Some may resolve spontaneously and if this occurs it happens usually before the age of 8 years. If they persist after this age then treatment should be by wide surgical excision if this is possible.

Lymphangiosarcoma

Lymphangiosarcoma is a malignant tumour of the lymphatic system which arises in areas of chronic lymphoedema particularly in the limb. It was most commonly seen in lymphoedema following mastectomy for carcinoma of the breast but may also be seen in congenital lymphoedema. Clinically, it appears as macules which may coalesce and ulcerate. The disease spreads rapidly and may spread to the lungs. Radiotherapy is the usual first line treatment but surgery may also be necessary.

Section 2.8 • Vascular tumours

The majority of vascular tumours are benign and previous classifications been based on their clinical appearance, the architecture of the vascular channels and the embryology. However, Mullikan has introduced a classification based on cellular activity, which has been generally accepted because of its clinical implications. Vascular abnormalities can be divided into true haemangiomas and vascular malformations.

The term *haemangioma* should be restricted to those lesions which grow by proliferation of endothelial cells. Clinically they are absent at birth and tend to grow rapidly in a proliferative phase for the first year of life. During this time its growth is disproportionately high to the child's growth. It then enters an involutional phase during which it regresses spontaneously. Pyogenic granulomas are included under this category. *Vascular malformations* on the other hand are structural abnormalities that result from embryonic defects in morphogenesis. These grow in parallel with the patient's growth and do not regress. Many lesions which were formally termed cavernous haemangiomas fall into this group.

Haemangiomas

The haemangioma is the commonest tumour of childhood and affects 10–12% of Caucasian children at 1 year of age. They occur predominantly in the head and neck but are also found on the trunk and limbs (Figure 2.14). The diagnosis is based on clinical grounds and relies on a history of a lesion arising soon after birth and growing at a rate parallel to the child's growth.

A superficial haemangioma or strawberry naevus is bright red and raised with a characteristic appearance. As it begins to involute, generally in the second year of life, it develops a pitted appearance. Deeper lesions may appear blue through the overlying skin. Because of rapid enlargement haemangiomas may give rise to a

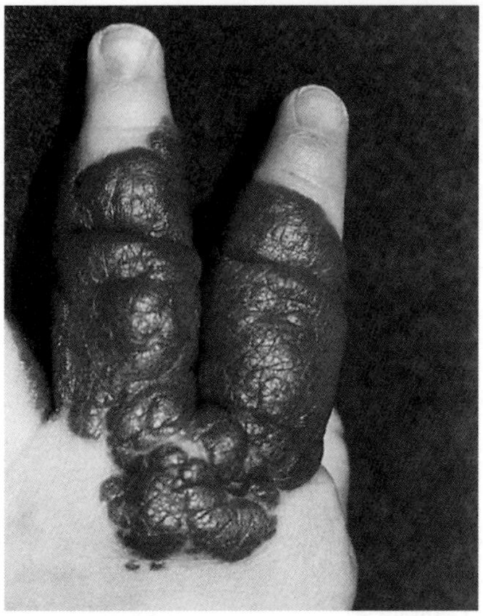

Figure 2.14 Haemangioma.

number of complications. About 5% ulcerate and a small proportion develop infection. The resulting tissue destruction can be severe and these have been called wildfire haemangiomas.

Occasionally the anatomical position of a haemangioma may cause problems, e.g. haemangiomas of the respiratory or alimentary tracts may give rise to obstruction and haemangiomas on the eyelid may result in amblyopia and failure to develop binocular vision. Bleeding may occur locally or rarely the patient may develop platelet thrombi within the haemangioma leading to a consumptive thrombocytopenia (Kasabach-Merit syndrome). These patients should be treated by steroid therapy. In general the treatment of haemangioma should be expectant although occasionally when there is severe bleeding or infection, excision may be required.

Pyogenic granuloma

Pyogenic granuloma is a proliferative vascular lesion common in children and young adults, typically found on the face or limbs. There may be history of trauma but it frequently arises spontaneously. It is a pedunculated lesion which often ulcerates and may become infected or bleed. As with other types of haemangioma it may involute if treated expectantly, but if bleeding or infection occurs, the lesion may be treated by silver nitrate cautery, electrocoagulation or surgical excision.

Vascular malformations

As indicated above, vascular malformations are structural abnormalities which are determined during embryological development. This may result in a capillary, venous, lymphatic or combined abnormality. Any of these can produce a low flow malformation. In some cases however, an arteriovenous fistula may develop leading to a high flow malformation.

Port wine stain

The port wine stain is a low flow capillary malformation, sometimes called a capillary haemangioma or naevus flammeus. It presents at or soon after birth as a flat area of discoloration. Initially it is pink or scarlet but with age it deepens to purple. It grows in parallel with the patient's growth but with increasing age it may become macular, giving a cobblestone type of appearance. On histological examination, it is made up of mature vascular endothelium. Port wine stains on the trunk and limbs may be associated with lymphatic or venous abnormalities (Klippel-Trenauney syndrome). Port wine stains of the face may be associated with underlying abnormalities of the meningeal and choroid plexus vasculature resulting in focal seizures (Sturge-Weber syndrome). Port wine stains are best treated using photocoagulation with a tuneable dye laser. This lightens the colour of the lesion and reduces the cobblestone effect in older lesions. Very rarely, excision and skin grafting may be necessary.

Capillary lymphatic malformations

These lesions, also known as lymphangioma circumscriptum or verrucous haemangioms, are commonly found on the limbs and trunk. They present at birth as clearly demarcated raised red areas. With age they become hyperkeratotic giving them a warty appearance. On histology they are made up of dermal and subcutaneous vessels and lymphatics. Treatment, where necessary, is by surgical excision and it is important to remove any deep extensions of the lesion to prevent recurrence.

Angiokeratoma

Angiokeratomata are abnormalities of the microvasculature presenting as dark red papules up to 1 cm in diameter. There are two main patterns of distribution. Angiokeratomata of Mibelli are found on the hands and feet, whereas angiokeratomata of Fordyce are found in linear groups on the abdomen and thigh. In Fabry's disease, angiokeratomata are found on the bathing trunk area. The appearance of angiokeratoma is the result of a sex-linked recessive disorder of glycolipid metabolism. Patients may also develop renal failure and hypertensive cardiovascular disease.

Telangiectasia

The telangiectasia lesion is known as a spider naevus and consists of a dilated vessel with radiating branches. It is commonly found on the face, arms and chest and because of its vascular nature it blanches on pressure over the feeding vessel. Spider naevi are found in pregnancy and in liver cirrhosis where they are thought to be related to oestrogen levels. Hereditary haemorrhagic telangiectasia (Osler-Weber-Rendu disease) is characterized by multiple telangiectasia and is complicated by widespread bleeding and the late development of arteriovenous pulmonary malformations. Individual spider naevi rarely require treatment but if removal is required for cosmetic reason, thermocoagulation may be used.

Venous malformations

Venous malformations are also known as cavernous haemangiomas. Clinically they are soft, compressible and non-pulsatile and may present in any site. They are often dark blue but in deep tissue when they are covered by skin they may have a normal colour. If combined with a capillary malformation they may be dark red. The adjacent bone may become distorted or hypertrophied in response to the blood flow through the lesion. Phlebothrombosis may develop within the abnormality giving rise to pain and induration of the lesion. Minor injury may lead to rapid enlargement of the vessels or the formation of the arteriovenous fistula. Treatment of venous malformations must be planned by delineating the extent of the abnormal vessels. Angiography can confirm the venous nature of the lesion and define feeding vessels, and MRI may be useful to define the extent of the lesion which is not seen on angiography. Treatment depends on the size of the lesion and its anatomical site but may consist of intravascular coagulation, selective arterial embolization of feeding vessels or surgical resection.

Arteriovascular malformations

Compared with low flow abnormalities (above) high flow vascular malformations are rare. They tend to occur on the head and neck and limbs and may arise from an innocent low flow capillary vascular malformation. Trauma or the hormonal changes of puberty and pregnancy may precipitate the formation of arteriovenous communications in such a lesion. Clinically they present as a raised, warm lesion with a palpable thrill and a bruit on auscultation. The overlying skin may become ischaemic and the lesion may haemorrhage spontaneously or as a result of relatively minor trauma. The high flow may cause gigantism of the limb or the digit and the pulsatile flow may erode bony structures. There may also be a systemic effect as the shunt effect of the fistula may give rise to cardiac failure. Treatment of an arteriovascular malformation generally involves surgical excision although pre-operative embolization may help to reduce intra-operative blood loss.

Malignant vascular tumours

Haemangiopericytoma

Haemangiopericytoma is a rare tumour of the blood vessel wall arising from pleuripotential cells. It is highly malignant and metastasizes in about 50% of cases. Treatment is by surgical excision.

Haemangiosarcoma

This again is a rare tumour and occurs in adult males. It arises from the vascular endothelial cells and presents as a deep soft tissue mass. It may be multi-focal and grows rapidly with local invasion. Treatment involves wide surgical excision.

Kaposi's sarcoma

Kaposi's sarcoma is a tumour of endothelial cells which is becoming increasingly recognized for its prevalence in immunosuppressed patients, particularly those with human immunodeficiency virus (HIV) infection. Four types of Kaposi sarcoma are recognized. The first is a rare tumour of East European Jews which develops as indolent nodules particularly in the lower limbs. Treatment is by excision of the individual lesions or radiotherapy. The second clinical type is described amongst Bantu males in Africa. Again nodules occur in the lower extremity but the tumour behaves much more aggressively. The third clinical type affects renal transplant patients who are immunosuppressed. The fourth type is so-called epidemic Kaposi's sarcoma. This arises in patients carrying HIV and presents with single or multiple nodules, usually in the head and neck. It may occur in many different anatomical sites, however, including the intestine. The prognosis of this type of tumour is difficult to determine as outcome is probably related to the progress of the HIV infection rather than the sarcoma itself. Depending on the site, treatment may be surgical but chemotherapy has been used although this has the disadvantage of causing increased immunosuppression and simple regimens using vincristine and bleomycin tend to be used. This can produce a response rate of up to 75% with a low risk of bone marrow suppression. Alpha interferon may also be used to induce remission but high doses are needed and side-effects including fatigue, fever and alopecia are common.

Further reading

Hughes, T. M. D., Thomas, J. M. (1999). Combined inguinal and pelvic lymph node dissection of stage III melanoma. *Br J Surg* **86**: 1493–8.

Jansen, L., Nieweg, O. E., Peterse, J. L. *et al.* (2000). Reliability of sentinel lymph node biopsy for staging melanoma. *Br J Surg* **87**: 484–9.

Safai, B. (1993). Cancers of the skin. In: DeVita, V. T. Jr, Hellman, S., Rosenberg, S. A., eds. *Cancer Principles and Practice of Oncology*. Vol. 2, 4th edn. Philadelphia, PA: Lippincott, pp. 1567–611.

MODULE 3

Disorders of the breast

Many women develop breast symptoms during their lifetime, most of which are self limiting and resolve in time. Some symptoms should be referred to a breast specialist (Table 3.1a) whilst others can be managed in the community (Table 3.1b).

Breast conditions can be subdivided into benign and malignant diseases. Whatever the underlying pathological process, a concise history and examination followed by appropriate radiological imaging and cytological/pathological investigation is required.

Section 3.1 • Organization of services

Ideally, breast clinics should be established and served by staff trained in breast disease: surgeons, breast physicians, radiologists, diagnostic radiographers and breast care nurses, with specialist pathology/cytology, oncology and plastic surgery back-up.

Patients attending for diagnostic purposes should be seen by a clinician with special training in breast diseases. Based on evidence that patients with breast cancer managed in a breast unit/centre have a better outcome, patients with breast cancer should be managed by a multidisciplinary team within a designated breast unit.

While delay in being seen at a breast clinic is associated with marked anxiety, delays of onset of treatment of less than 3 months are unlikely to be associated with a measurable difference in survival. Hence, in the UK, it has been suggested that more than 80% of urgent referrals are seen within 5 working days and the remainder within 10 working days (after receipt of referral).

History

The history for a patient with breast symptoms can be subdivided into:

- History of the presenting problem.
- Hormonal history.
- Gynaecological history.
- Family history.
- Other medical/surgical history.

History of the presenting problem

Having established the age and the sex of the patient, answers to the following questions should be recorded (Table 3.2).

Hormonal and gynaecological history

This should include age at menarche and (where appropriate) menopause, number and timing of pregnancies, use of oral contraception and hormone replacement therapy (and whether oestrogen and/or progesterone containing, duration and timing of usage).

Family history

This should include any cancers diagnosed in the wider family and the age and type of cancer in each family member. Breast, ovarian, prostate and colon cancers are of particular relevance in familial predisposition to breast cancer.

Other medical/surgical history

Here your aim is to assess your patient's general medical, mental and social health especially as regards fitness for surgery, possible radiotherapy or chemotherapy and breast reconstruction. In particular you need to know about medications, if the patient smokes and any history of venous thrombosis.

The patient's age (Figure 3.1) and the history will direct you towards the likely diagnosis but a systematic breast examination is necessary to pick up additional features.

Table 3.1a Patient referral

Conditions that require referral to a breast specialist include:

Lump
- Any new discrete lump
- New lump in pre-existing nodularity
- Asymmetrical nodularity that persists at review after menstruation
- Abscess or breast inflammation which does not settle after one course of antibiotics
- Cyst persistently refilling or recurrent cyst (if the patient has recurrent multiple cysts and the general practitioner (GP) has the necessary skills, then aspiration is acceptable)

Pain
- If associated with a lump
- Intractable pain that interferes with a patient's lifestyle or sleep and which has failed to respond to reassurance, simple measures such as wearing a well-supporting bra, and common drugs
- Unilateral persistent pain in postmenopausal women

Nipple discharge
- All women aged 50 and over
- Women under 50 with:
  - Blood-stained discharge; or
  - Bilateral discharge sufficient to stain clothes; or
  - Persistent single duct discharge

Nipple retraction or distortion, nipple eczema
- Change in skin contour

Table 3.1b Patient referral

Conditions that can be initially managed in general practice:

- Young women (<35 years) with tender, lumpy breasts and older women with symmetrical nodularity, provided that they have no localized abnormality
- Women with minor and moderate degrees of breast pain who do not have a discrete palpable lesion
- Women aged under 50 years who have nipple discharge that is from more than one duct or is intermittent and is neither bloodstained nor troublesome

Examination

Examination includes the key steps outlined below.

The patient (naked to the waist) is examined in the presence of a chaperone.

With the patient sitting, the breast should be inspected for changes in contour due to skin or nipple tethering which may be emphasized by asking the patient to raise her arms above her head and lean slightly forward. Tethering of a lesion to the chest wall can be assessed by asking the patient to put her hands on her hips and press onto both hips thus contracting the pectoral muscles.

Next, with the patient lying comfortably with her hands behind her head, explain you will examine the normal breast first. Examine each breast, including the axillary tail, with the flattened fingers of your hand.

Table 3.2 History for breast conditions

- Is there a lump?
- Where is the lump?
- How big is it?
- When was it first noted?
- Is it a single/are they multiple lump(s)?
- Have there been any previous lumps?
- Does it change with menses?
- Is it tender/mobile/hard/soft?
- Are there any lumps elsewhere?
- Are there any associated features?
- Skin changes
- Nipple indrawing
- Nipple discharge – single or multiple ducts; blood stained or not
- Are there any problems in the other breast, axilla, supraclavicular fossae or neck?

Any lump should be assessed for size (measured with calipers), shape, consistency, tenderness, mobility and fixity to the overlying skin/underlying chest wall.

Both axillae should be examined thoroughly for palpable nodes ensuring the anterior, medial, posterior and apical node groups are palpated. The size, number and fixity should be recorded. Although clinical assessment of axillary nodes may not reflect their pathology status, for patients with breast cancer the clinical TNM system requires an assessment of node involvement.

The supraclavicular and infraclavicular fossae and cervical region should also be examined for palpable lymph nodes.

Any other symptomatic regions should be examined as required for signs (in a patient with breast cancer) of metastatic disease.

Your examination findings must be recorded in sketch or written form, as part of good clinical practice and for medicolegal reasons.

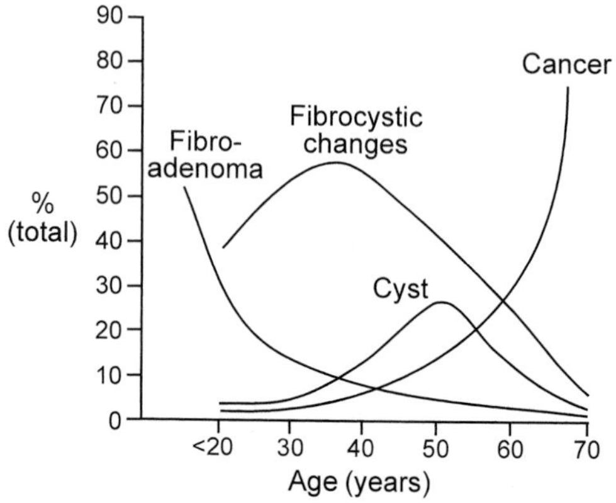

Figure 3.1 Incidence of breast lesions presenting to a breast clinic: fibroadenoma, fibrocystic changes, cyst and cancer as percentage of breast lumps in patients presenting to a breast clinic compared with patient age.

Initial assessment, investigation and staging of breast symptoms

Methods of assessment of a breast abnormality include clinical history and examination, imaging and sampling the lesion with a needle for cytological/histological assessment (fine needle aspiration cytology (FNAC) or core biopsy). These three investigations collectively comprise **triple assessment**. There is strong evidence that triple assessment provides more accurate diagnosis than a smaller number of tests. Clinical examination, mammography, ultrasound, FNA and core biopsy range in sensitivity from 85 to 95%.

All patients should have a full clinical examination. Where a localized abnormality is present, patients should have imaging usually followed by FNA or core biopsy. A lesion considered malignant on either clinical examination, imaging or cytology alone should have histopathological confirmation of malignancy before any definitive surgical procedure, e.g. mastectomy or axillary clearance. Clearly there are medicolegal implications if triple assessment is not performed prior to mastectomy if the subsequent definitive pathology turns out to be non-malignant.

Section 3.2 • Benign breast conditions

Aberrations of normal development and involution (ANDI)

The cyclical variations in oestrogen and progesterone result in increased mitosis around days 22–24 of the menstrual cycle but apoptosis restores the balance across the cycle.

Benign proliferations in the breast are often considered as aberrations of normal development and involution (ANDI).

Localized benign nodularity

Localized benign nodularity, previously termed fibroadenosis or fibrocystic disease, occurs commonly in young women, often with bilateral nodularity which is usually accentuated premenstrually. Any focal nodularity should disperse after two menses (approximately 6 weeks). Lumpy, normal breast tissue is usually managed by general practitioners following repeat examination, with reassurance, but any persistent localized abnormality requires referral for triple assessment.

Fibroadenoma (Figure 3.2)

There is a spectrum of ANDI that ranges from a single fibroadenoma (termed a juvenile fibroadenoma in teenage girls) through giant fibroadenoma to phyllodes tumour (formally known as cystosarcoma phyllodes). A fibroadenoma forms from a breast lobule, a smooth, non-tender, mobile lump, usually in a young woman. It may be single, lobulated or multiple and does not show any changes in size with menstruation. Following diagnostic triple assessment the fibroadenoma can be excised if >4 cm or at the patient's request or monitored using ultrasound and if it fails to change in size over 6–12 months may be left *in situ*; indeed one-third may disappear completely. Rarely, cytological assessment alone of a fibroadenoma in a young woman may be reported as C5 (malignant). This is where the principle of triple assessment becomes extremely important; radiology and diagnostic biopsy will confirm the diagnosis. A giant fibroadenoma should be excised as its increasing size may distort the shape of the breast. Phyllodes tumours progressively increase in size, and range between a benign histological appearance and more sarcoma-like appearance with an increasing number of mitotic figures. Local recurrence is common if excision is incomplete and therefore a phyllodes tumour should be excised with a margin of normal tissue to prevent local recurrence; even then further recurrence may require mastectomy; metastasis is very rare.

Cyst (Figure 3.3)

Rare before the age of 30 years, the incidence of cysts declines after the menopause. However, 7% of women develop a symptomatic cyst at some point during their life. Cysts may be single, multiple, unilateral or bilateral and range in size from 2 mm to several centimetres. Whereas ultrasound may be particularly useful in demonstrating the site and number of cysts, aspiration yields clear or turbid fluid ranging in colour from white to dark green; a cyst may disperse spontaneously; approximately 10% of cysts recur and require re-aspiration. Clinically worrisome cysts are those which contain fresh blood, those where there is a residual mass after aspiration (the residual mass should then be aspirated for cytology), or cysts which recur more than twice, any of which may signify a carcinoma in the wall of the cyst. While routine cytology of a cyst aspirate is not useful in clinical diagnosis, recurrent or suspicious cysts should be excised and sent for histology. Endocrine agents such as danazol have been used to reduce the formation of further cysts in those prone to multiple cyst formation.

Duct papilloma

A duct papilloma classically presents as a blood-stained nipple discharge from a single duct; pressure on the areolar margin overlying the duct papilloma results in expression of a blood-stained discharge. The discharge can be tested for blood using a urinary testing stick. Under general anaesthetic a lachrymal probe should be inserted into the duct and the single duct excised through a circumareolar incision and sent to pathology. Rarely, the symptoms of a blood-stained nipple discharge may be due to an intraduct carcinoma.

Epithelial hyperplasia

Epithelial hyperplasia (previously termed epitheliosis or papillomatosis) is usually an incidental finding on

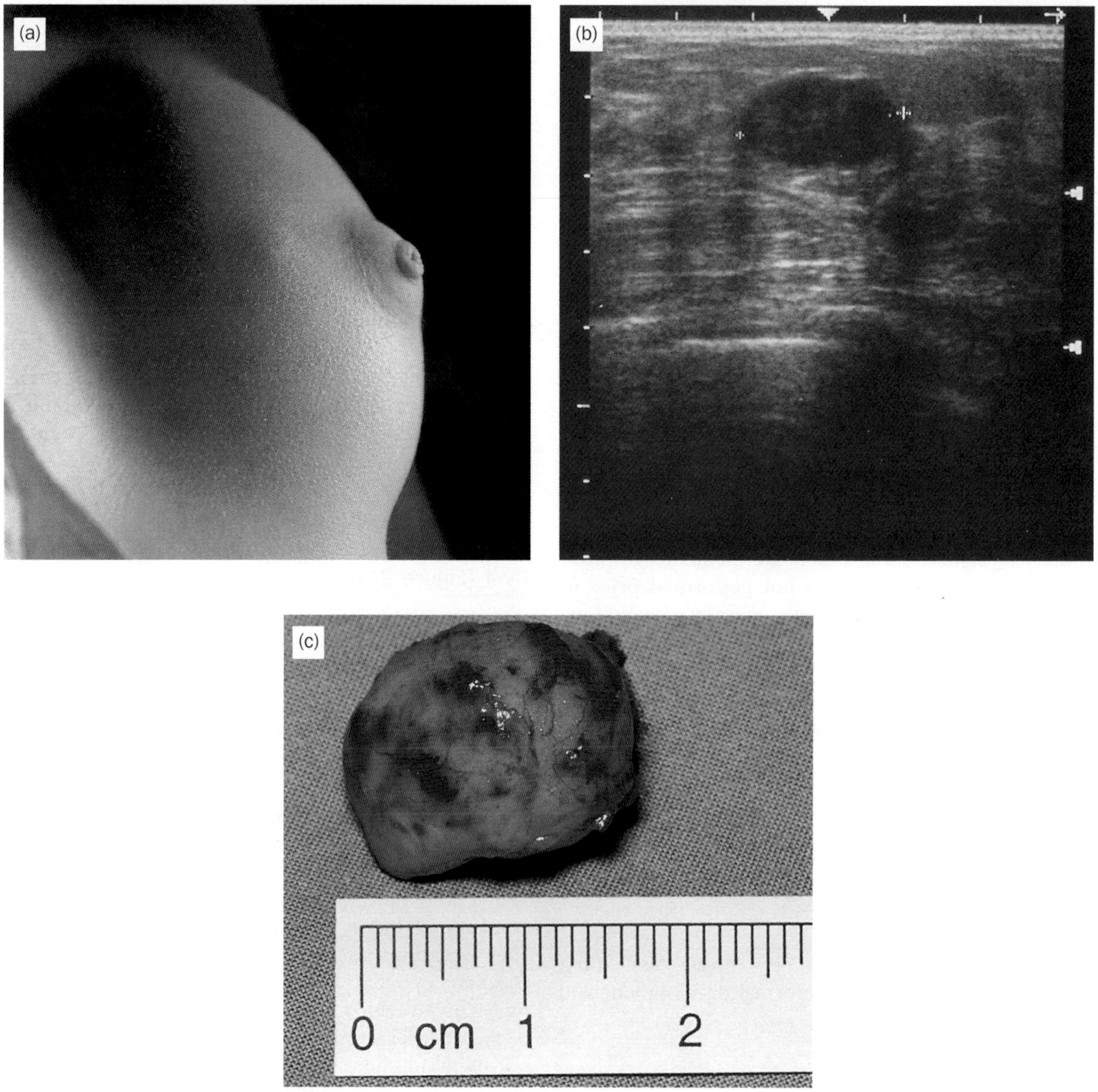

Figure 3.2 Fibroadenoma: (a) clinical appearance; (b) ultrasound appearance; (c) surgical specimen.

biopsy and can be graded as mild, moderate or florid. Cellular atypia (atypical hyperplasia) increases the risk of breast cancer two- to four-fold.

Sclerosing lesions

Usually detected on mammography, radial scars also known as complex sclerosing lesions (localized areas of fibrosis) may require biopsy to exclude cancer.

Inflammatory/infectious processes

Abscess (Figure 3.4)

Abscess formation may occur on the breast tissues or in the skin underlying the breast (in a sebaceous cyst) or in the inframammary fold. The typical symptoms of pain, redness and swelling are present.

A breast abscess may be lactational, occurring in a young breast-feeding woman, and usually staphylococcal in origin. Non-lactational abscesses tend to occur in middle aged females who smoke and are secondary to streptococci and anaerobic bacteria. Periareolar infection, occurring in women in their 30s, results from active periductal inflammation (periductal mastitis). Periareolar abscess formation may proceed to a fistula (see below). Peripheral non-lactating breast abscess may be associated with diabetes, steroid therapy or rheumatoid arthritis. There may be multiple peripheral abscesses requiring drainage and antibiotics. At an early stage, abscess formation may be aborted by the use of appropriate antibiotics (such as amoxycillin, safe in breast-feeding mothers, with its anti-anaerobic and anti-staphylococcal action). Once an abscess is established, antibiotics are required for the surrounding

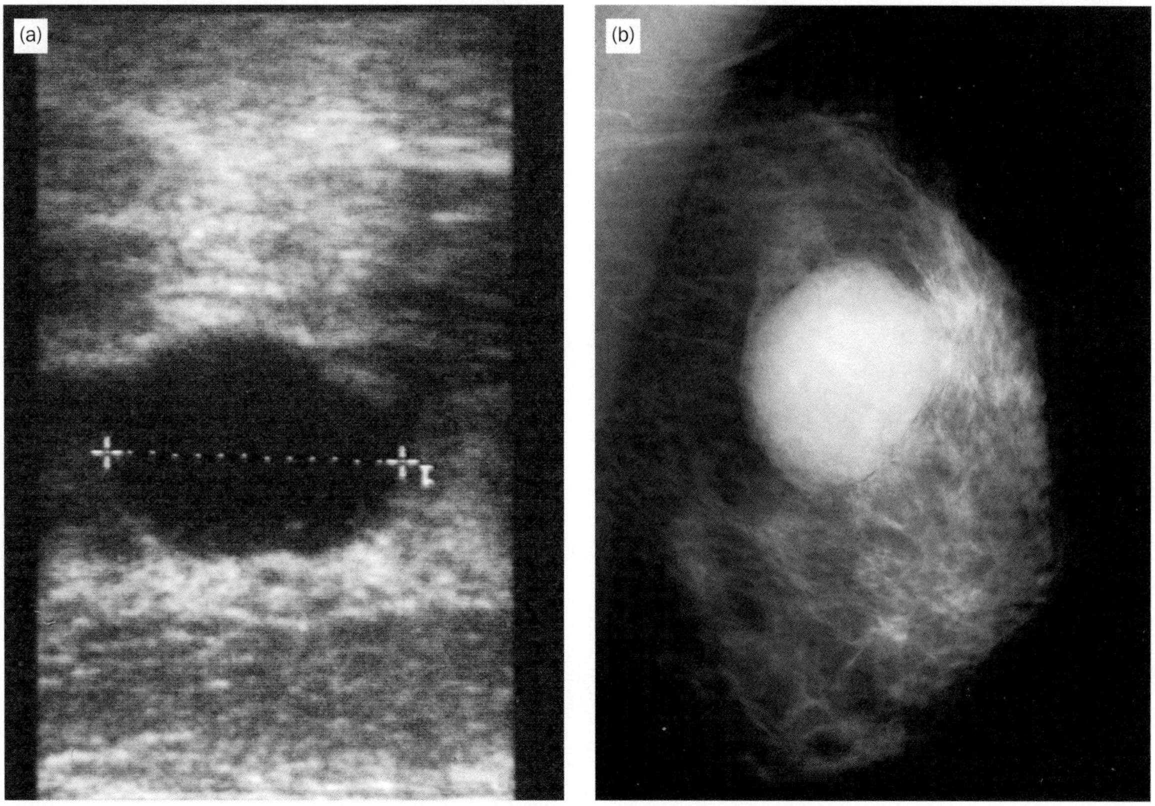

Figure 3.3 Cyst: radiological appearances using (a) ultrasound; (b) mammogram of a breast cyst.

cellulitis plus drainage either under local anaesthetic using a 19 g needle or by formal incision and drainage under local or general anaesthesia. Inserting a drain, as described in older surgical texts, is ***not*** required. A breast abscess may require more than one drainage procedure (particularly if needle aspiration is used) and may be complicated by fistula formation. Tuberculosis and actinomycosis are rarer but recognized causes of breast abscess.

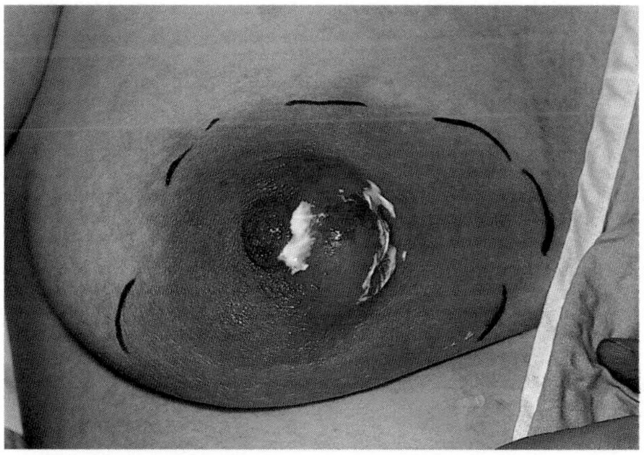

Figure 3.4 Breast abscess in breast-feeding mother demonstrating erythema marked to determine whether it is spreading, pointing abscess adjacent to the areola with local anaesthetic cream in place prior to needle aspiration.

Inflammatory breast cancer should be excluded in patients with a solid inflammatory lesion or an abscess which does not respond to appropriate treatment.

Fistula (Figure 3.5)

A fistula between the epithelium of a breast duct and the skin may follow on as a consequence of an abscess with the discharge site/fistula usually opening at the areolar margin. Excision of the fistula through a circumareolar incision including the duct up to the back of the nipple under antibiotic cover is the treatment of choice, rather than laying open the length of the fistula with the resultant scarring and deformity.

Duct ectasia (periductal mastitis)

These represent a spectrum of inflammatory process where the subareolar ectatic, enlarged, ducts are surrounded by a mild inflammatory infiltrate. The ectatic duct may result in a retracted slit shaped nipple (in contrast to the nipple retraction seen with an underlying cancer). Creamy discharge from multiple bilateral ducts is a feature of duct ectasia and is distinct from the single blood-stained discharge of a duct papilloma/intraduct carcinoma.

Fat necrosis

Fat necrosis in the breast usually appears in postmenopausal women following trauma to the breast (such as a seatbelt injury) as a localized inflammatory

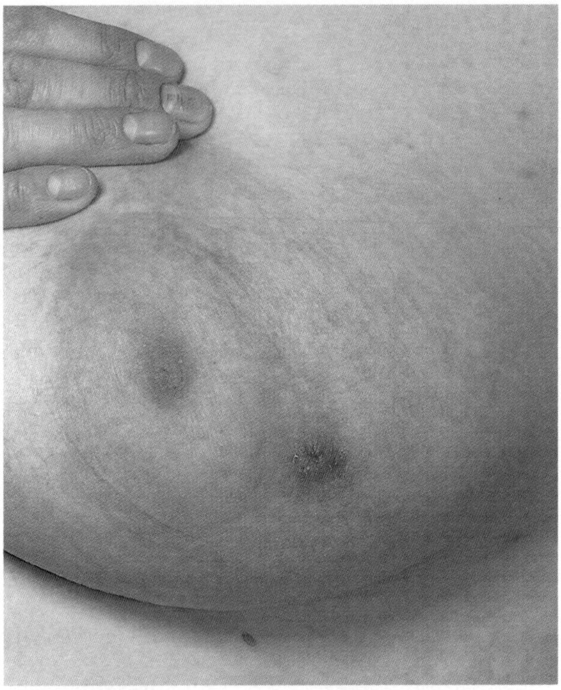

Figure 3.5 Fistula as a consequence of a breast abscess; note the classical position at the areolar margin.

response. Fat necrosis may be suggested from the history but should be diagnosed using triple assessment as a small cancer may clinically and radiologically mimic fat necrosis. Treatment is by reassurance or, if suspicion remains or the patient requests, excisional biopsy.

Hormonal changes

Nipple discharge

Single or multiple duct discharge producing a clear, creamy, green or black fluid is a common physiological finding but also occurs from ectatic ducts. Physiological nipple discharge from multiple ducts, usually bilateral, is not uncommon in premenopausal women. Following triple assessment to exclude concomitant disease, a careful drug history (particularly for psychotrophic drugs which may cause hyperprolactinaemia) and measurement of serum prolactin to exclude a (rare) pituitary prolactin secreting tumour, surgical intervention (duct excision or disconnection) is only required if blood can be detected on stick testing raising the suspicion of an underlying papilloma or rarely a carcinoma, or if there is a profuse discharge causing patient distress.

Breast pain (mastalgia)

While some breast discomfort or pain is reported in two-thirds of women, mastalgia can be defined as breast pain of sufficient severity for a woman to seek medical advice. While breast pain is a symptom of breast cancer in <10% of women, appropriate reassurance is required.

Mastalgia may be unilateral, bilateral, unifocal or multifocal, cyclical (worse pre-menses) or acyclical. It is important to exclude concomitant pathology. Cyclical mastalgia is worst in the days pre-menses, usually affects the outer half of the breast, occurs in women often in their thirties and may persist for months or years. Cyclical mastalgia ceases with the menopause. Acyclical mastalgia may be continuous or have a random pattern and is more common in women in their forties. Hormone replacement therapy may exacerbate mastalgia, at least initially. Following triple assessment of any focal abnormalities to exclude malignancy, conservative measures include reassurance and explanation, simple analgesia (e.g. paracetamol), dietary modification (avoiding caffeine in tea, coffee and soft drinks; avoiding fatty foods), wearing a supportive bra especially at night, stopping smoking and regular exercise. Keeping a breast pain chart (Figure 3.6) can be helpful for the patient to record the timing and severity of the pain and for the clinician to establish any pattern of pain.

Although mastalgia is self limiting, it may persist for months or years. For cyclical mastalgia, medication such as gammalinoleic acid (oil of evening primrose) given for a minimum of 3 months' duration in an adequate dose (80 mg tid) shows a response in 40–60% of patients. If the pain is persistent and severe, medical therapy such as 100–200 mg danozol or bromocriptine have similar response rates, but one-third of women experience side-effects. Tamoxifen 10 mg/day (although not licensed for breast pain) or

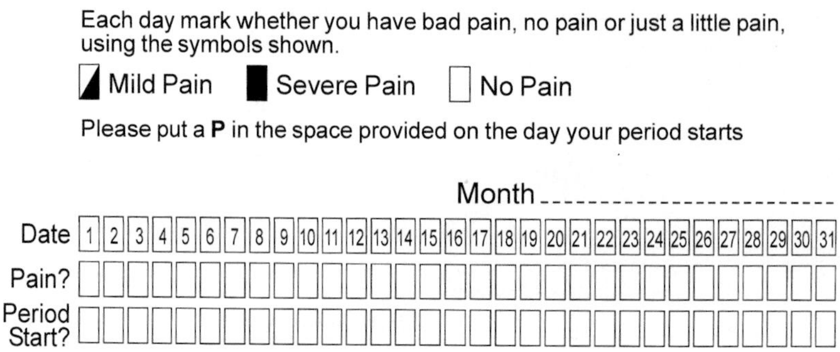
Each day mark whether you have bad pain, no pain or just a little pain, using the symbols shown.
Mild Pain
Severe Pain
No Pain
Please put a P in the space provided on the day your period starts
Month
Date
1 2 3 4 5 6 7 8 9 10 11 12 13 14 15 16 17 18 19 20 21 22 23 24 25 26 27 28 29 30 31
Pain?
Period Start?

Figure 3.6 Breast pain chart for a patient to complete indicating the severity of pain and timing in relation to menses; the first month's chart (usually completed for 3 months).

ovarian suppression (by a luteinizing hormone-releasing hormone analogue) is increasingly used for refractory mastalgia; psychological referral for the management of the pain may be required. Rarely, mastectomy is needed to remove the painful breast, but should be performed only when chest wall disease has been excluded, other measures have been exhausted and following patient counselling, as surgery tends to make mastalgia worse not better.

Acyclical mastalgia may respond to the conservative measures used for cyclical pain. A persistent localized painful area may respond to local anaesthesia/steroid injection.

Chest wall pain, musculoskeletal pain (e.g. Bornholm myalgia), costochondritis (particularly of the second rib/cartilage joint – Tietze's syndrome), thrombophlebitis of the chest wall veins (Mondor's condition, Figure 3.7) intra-abdominal (gall stones) or intrathoracic (cardiac, pleural) pain may all present as breast pain to a breast clinic. Exclusion of significant breast pathology, reassurance and non-steroidal drugs can provide symptomatic relief.

Other conditions

An accessory nipple, accessory breast tissue (which occur along the milk lines) or, conversely, breast hypoplasia (which may be associated with pectoral/upper limb abnormalities – Poland's syndrome) are developmental abnormalities of variations in the site and the volume of breast tissue. Surgical treatment is only required when swollen accessory breast tissue is symptomatic. Rarely, hamartoma, angioma or neurofibroma may occur in the breast.

Lipoma

Lipomata are not uncommon in the breast and can mimic other breast lumps including carcinoma. They require triple assessment followed by excision if the patient wishes.

Sebaceous cyst

This lies within the skin of the breast usually adjacent to the sternum or an inframammary fold. The classic punctum is often visible and the cyst may become inflamed/infected. This lesion may be left or if the patient requests excised.

Surgery for benign breast conditions

Many benign breast conditions are self limiting and following triple assessment the patient may require simple reassurance, conservative measures or a course of medication. Follow-up of patients with benign breast conditions is not usually required in the hospital setting. A benign lump may be excised (under local or general anaesthetic) at the request of the patient. In women over 40 years, even with benign findings on triple assessment, many surgeons advocate excisional biopsy of a new, focal lump to exclude the small false negative risk (i.e. missing a cancer) on triple assessment. Surgical scars should be placed circumferentially, in the line of skin tension (Figure 3.7) or at the areolar margin, or in the skin lines of the axilla.

Gynaecomastia (Figure 3.8)

Gynaecomastia, the growth of breast tissue in males, is a benign, reversible condition affecting 3% of the male population at any one time. Teenage boys undergoing puberty (pubertal gynaecomastia) and elderly men (senescent gynaecomastia) are most commonly affected and between them account for half of the patients with gynaecomastia. Gynaecomastia secondary to drug therapy, liver disease, primary hypogonadism (e.g. Klinefelter's syndrome), testicular tumours, hyperthyroidism or renal disease should be excluded. Withdrawal of the drug (cimetidine, digoxin, spironolactone, anabolic steroids, oestrogen) should result in symptom resolution.

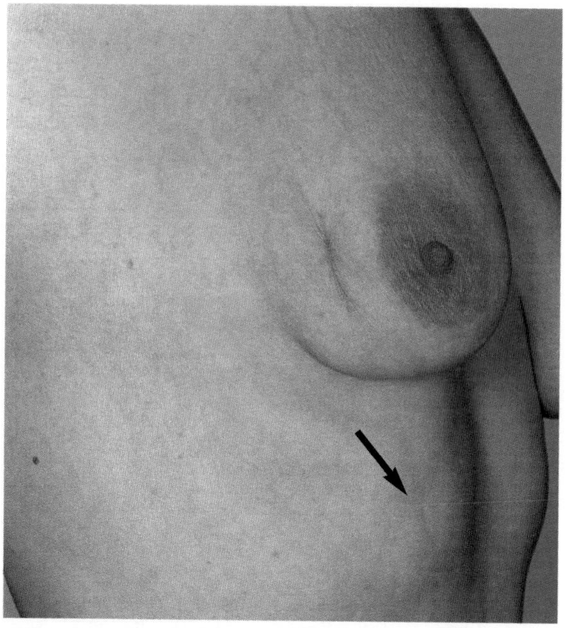

Figure 3.7 Mondor's disease (thrombophlebitis) (arrow) and a benign breast biopsy scar in the skin lines.

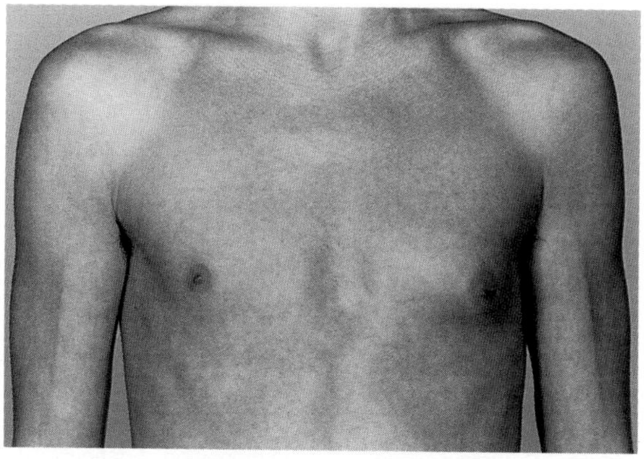

Figure 3.8 Unilateral (left) gynaecomastia in a teenage boy.

Clinical examination, revealing a tender, palpable lump deep to the areolar and often, surprisingly, unilateral, may be supplemented by mammography and FNA if male breast cancer is suspected. In young men, the testes should be examined to exclude testicular tumours and human chorionic gonadotropin and oestrogen levels measured. Surgical excision (through a circumareolar incision), danazol or tamoxifen have all been used for the treatment of gynaecomastia.

Section 3.3 • Female breast cancer

Natural history of breast cancer

The therapeutic strategy for any disease presupposes an understanding of its natural history. Figure 3.9 shows the relationship between tumour size, as measured clinically at presentation, and the development of distant metastases. Since patients with distant metastases are incurable, the latter is ultimately equivalent to death from breast cancer. This series comprises 2648 patients, first seen at the Institut Gustave Roussy, Paris, between 1954 and 1972, before systemic adjuvant therapy was used and for those with operable tumours, mastectomy was generally performed. Four observations can be made on the basis of these curves:

- The risk of developing distant metastases increases with tumour size.
- The larger the tumour, the shorter the average time to the development of distant metastases.
- The risk of having metastases at presentation is only significant for those patients presenting with large (approximately >5 cm) tumours.
- Nevertheless, the majority of patients will develop distant metastases at some time (usually within the first 10 years) after initial presentation. Even for patients with the smallest tumours (<2.5 cm), a significant proportion will die of breast cancer.

This leads to the concept of a threshold size for the tumour before distant dissemination occurs. While there will be considerable individual variation, the threshold size will on average be smaller for those

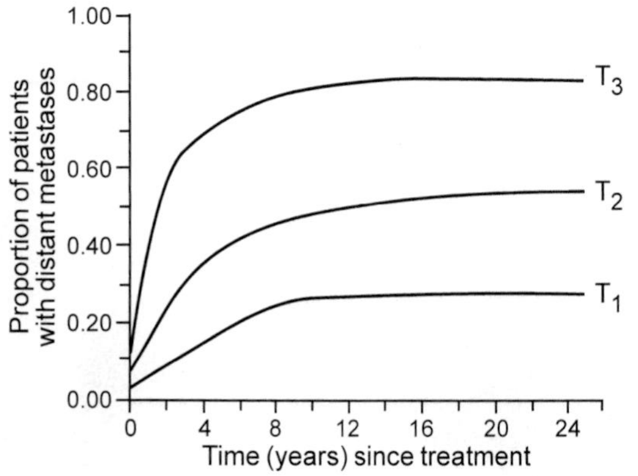

Figure 3.9 Tumour size in relation to proportion of patients with metastases following initial treatment for breast cancer.

patients with histologically high grade (grades 2 or 3) tumours, compared with grade 1 and for those patients with axillary or internal mammary lymph node involvement, compared to those without. Two further observations can be drawn from these data:

- If patients can be diagnosed when the tumour is very small, then the prognosis should be better. This is the rationale of the breast screening programme using mammography as a means of 'early' detection of breast cancers.
- Many patients, even though they have no clinical evidence of distant metastases at presentation, have occult distant metastases that will become clinically apparent in future years. Local therapies (such as surgery and radiotherapy) for the primary tumour will not affect these occult metastases, and hence such patients need systemic therapy. This is the rationale of systemic adjuvant therapy (see later).

Epidemiology of breast cancer

It is estimated that the world burden of breast cancer is some 1 million women newly diagnosed each year. The extent of the breast cancer problem can be illustrated based on the data from Scotland. Breast cancer is the most common incident cancer among women in Scotland with 3168 new registrations from a total (male and female) population of 5.5 million in 1995 and accounts for 25% of the female cancer burden excluding non-melanoma skin cancer. For women the risk of developing breast cancer up to the age of 74 years is approximately 8%; it is the commonest cause of death in women aged 40–50 years.

Breast cancer is the second most common cause of death from cancer in women (after lung cancer), with 1244 deaths recorded in Scotland in 1995. Survival has improved over the past 20 years in Scotland, with 56% 5 year relative survival having been reported for those diagnosed between 1968 and 1972, compared to 70% for those diagnosed between 1988 and 1992. However, even allowing for pathological stage there is evidence of variation between different patient groups.

The rising incidence of breast cancer may be due to the increasingly aged population together with earlier detection (including DCIS which may never develop into invasive cancer) through screening programmes in addition to the factors listed below. This increasing incidence may be offset by the improved survival secondary to the effect of early detection of small cancers prior to metastasis, use of adjuvant tamoxifen, radiotherapy and chemotherapy.

Aetiological factors in breast cancer

While the aetiology of breast cancer is multifactorial and may differ between individual women and racial groups, it is clear that breast cancer has a genetic basis upon which internal hormonal influences, diet and external environmental factors act.

Endocrine influences on breast epithelium result in stimulation then involution of breast tissue. The number of cycles of stimulation/involution together with the stimulatory effect of exogenous steroid hormones (oestrogen, progesterone) may additively increase the risk of breast cancer.

Age

The risk of breast cancer increases with age, although there is a flattening of the age/incidence curve after the menopause. The median age for breast cancer is 60 years.

Hormonal influences

- Age at menarche (younger age increases the risk).
- Age at menopause (menopause at age 55 doubles the risk compared to menopause at age 45).
- Number of pregnancies (higher number is protective).
- Age at first pregnancy (if over 30 double the risk compared to <20 years at first pregnancy).
- Breast feeding history (breast feeding is protective).
- Oral contraceptive use (high oestrogen pills increase risk, low oestrogen/progesterone pills are safer; use before age of 20 increases risk; note that oral contraceptive use decreases the risk of ovarian cancer). Risk is elevated during and for 10 years after use.
- Hormone replacement therapy (HRT). A recent analysis of pooled published data on HRT and risk of breast cancer has shown that the relative risk for each year of use is 1.023 and for 5 years or more of use the relative risk is 1.350. For women under the age of 50 this risk is equivalent to having normal menses and therefore women under 50 are at no increased risk. Five years after cessation of HRT, the risk returns to normal levels. A baseline mammogram prior to commencement of HRT is not recommended. Cancers diagnosed in women on HRT tend to be at an earlier stage and hence HRT is not associated with increased breast cancer mortality. Breast cancer risk from HRT should be balanced against the benefits of HRT including those on the cardiovascular system and bony skeleton.
- Oophorectomy in premenopausal women greatly reduces the risk of breast cancer, the benefit being greatest when oophorectomy is conducted at a young age, presumably by reducing the cyclical oestrogenic stimulation of breast tissue.

Family history

A family history of breast, ovarian, colon, prostate or other cancers is associated with increased risk of breast cancer (see also section on breast cancer genetics).

Where a family member has had breast or ovarian cancer one should record age at onset, whether unilateral/bilateral, the menopausal status of the individual and the relationship to the individual consulting – first degree relative (mother, sister or daughter), second degree relative, maternal or paternal side. There are now guidelines (Table 3.3) for patients to attend risk assessment clinics for screening which, when conducted at centres with expertise and interest in the field, can detect cancers with similar success to breast screening programmes conducted in postmenopausal women.

Diet

Dietary influences on breast cancer risk are most startling when noting the increased risk of breast cancer in Japanese women moving to the USA. Some evidence suggests that soya and phytoestrogens are protective but eating saturated fat and red meat, drinking alcohol and obesity in postmenopausal women increase the risks of breast cancer.

Table 3.3 Familial breast cancer: criteria for identifying women at substantial increased risk

The following categories identify women who have three times (or more) the population risk of developing breast cancer:

A woman who has:

- One first degree relative with bilateral breast cancer or breast and ovarian cancer or
- One first degree relative with breast cancer diagnosed under the age of 40 or one first degree male relative with breast cancer diagnosed at any age or
- Two first or second degree relatives with breast cancer diagnosed under the age of 60 or ovarian cancer at any age on the same side of the family or
- Three first or second degree relatives with breast or ovarian cancer on the same side of the family
- In this context a first degree female relative is mother, sister or daughter. A second degree female relative is grandmother, granddaughter, aunt or niece.

Socioeconomic factors

In the Western world, breast cancer has an increased incidence in higher social class women, possibly related to different hormonal profiles (age at menarche, age at first pregnancy, etc.) in different social classes. Women from the lowest social classes present with later stage disease and appear to have a poorer outcome, despite receiving similar therapies. The reasons for this are unclear.

Other influences

Atypical epithelial hyperplasia holds a four-fold increased risk of developing breast cancer compared with women who have no proliferative changes. Radiation (as in those exposed to the atomic bomb) doubles the risk in later life.

Breast cancer genetics

Familial predisposition

About 5–10% of breast cancer in the West is attributed to a genetic predisposition – there are probably several genes of limited penetrance, inherited in an autosomal dominant fashion.

BRCA1 (17q) and BRCA2 (13q) account for many of the larger families with multiple (four or more) breast and other cancers in close relatives. Within certain populations, the particular mutation identified (e.g. BRCA2 deletion at position 999 in half of familial cancers in Iceland) demonstrates the genetic lines of inheritance. However, population screening for mutations in BRCA1 and BRCA2 is not, at present, realistic given the large size of these genes and the scatter of mutational sites. Inheritance of mutant p53 (Li-Fraumeni syndrome) or PTEN (Cowden's syndrome) is even less common. These four genes have comparatively high penetrance resulting in multiple cancer sites within each family and sometimes within each individual. The breast cancers usually occur before the age of 65 years and may be bilateral. Based on a detailed family history, risk estimates can be computed using established tables to help inform women whether their risk is sufficient to warrant intervention. Other genes such as ataxia telangiectasia (ATM), and some as yet unknown, probably account for many of the smaller families (two or three cases) where BRCA1 and BRCA2 have been excluded.

There appears to be a wide range of molecular abnormalities in breast cancer which probably interact with the cellular environment and play a role in the aetiology, development, invasion and metastasis of breast cancer. Using whole genome scanning techniques, such as comparative genomic hybridization (CGH) or genetic profiling (with microarray or chip-based technology for gene expression and gene deletion), it is clear that individual cancers vary markedly from each other. Few genes are of genuine widespread clinical utility but include the oestrogen receptor gene protein product (ER) and a cell surface receptor HER2 (erbB2, NEU). Some can provide useful information for clinical decision making (PgR, pS2/PNR2, p53) while others (Ki67 or PCNA as a proliferation marker, percentage of cells in S phase, DNA content of tumour) relate to the biological aggressiveness of the cancer.

ER

Oestrogen receptor (ER), originally measured by radioimmunoassay or the dextran coated charcoal method, on cell lysates, is now assessed by immunohistochemistry on tissue sections (Figure 3.10), for which a variety of scoring systems exist. Two forms of ER exist: ER alpha (detected and measured clinically in breast cancer samples) and ER beta (recently detected and of uncertain significance in breast cancer). Tumours with moderate or high ER are much more likely to respond to endocrine therapy than those with no or low ER. In addition, ER expression correlates with survival, at least in the first 5 years following diagnosis. However, only two-thirds of patients with ER expression appear to have intact, functioning downstream effector pathways so some centres also measure progesterone receptor (PgR) and/or the insulin-like growth factor peptide pS2 in immunohistochemical sections. Expression of PgR and/or pS2 along with ER suggests the cancer is more likely to respond to endocrine therapy.

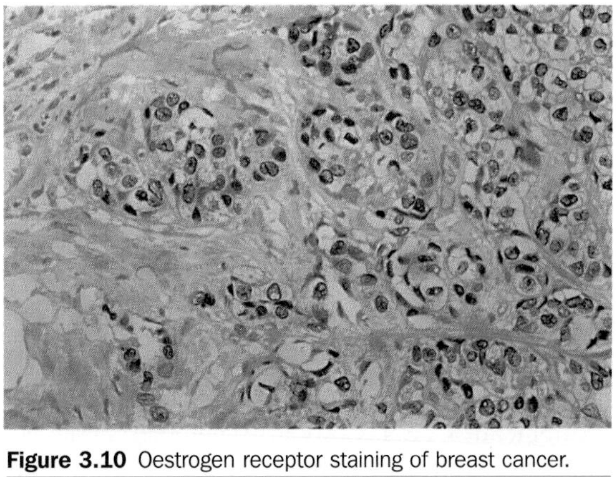

Figure 3.10 Oestrogen receptor staining of breast cancer.

HER2

HER2 (erbB2, neu) is a transmembrane growth factor receptor, expressed in 15–30% of invasive breast cancer (and, for reasons which are unclear, up to 80% of DCIS) associated with poor prognosis in invasive breast cancer. It is one of a family of growth factor receptors (including epidermal growth factor receptor, erbB3, erbB4) but unlike most other molecular markers now forms a target for 'biological therapy'. For patients in whom amplified HER2 can be detected (i.e. multiple copies for the gene best detected by fluorescence *in situ* hybridization, FISH) and is overexpressed (on immunohistochemistry), humanized mouse antibody, trastuzumab (herceptin) is the first new 'biological' therapy to enter clinical use. What is perhaps of greatest clinical significance is that this therapy may be most effective in node positive patients with invasive breast cancer whose disease is relatively insensitive to chemotherapy or endocrine therapy.

p53

p53 has acquired the nickname 'guardian of the genome' due to its essential role in the cellular response to injury with subsequent cell cycle arrest or apoptosis. In breast cancer mutant p53 has been associated with poor prognosis and resistance to treatment by chemotherapy. Thus, detection of p53 mutation may be important in clinical therapeutic decision making and is the subject of clinical trials. Unfortunately immunohistochemistry for p53 in breast cancer is less reliable than other methods of detecting p53 mutation and this has held back the application of p53 research in the clinical arena.

Other genes

Several other genes (multiple drug resistance mdr glycoprotein), oncogenes (c-myc), apoptotic pathway genes (bcl2, bax), tumour suppressor genes (Rb), growth factors (transforming growth factors alpha and beta families, insulin-like growth factors), growth factor receptors (epidermal growth factor receptor), proteases (cathepsin D) and cell cycle related genes (p21, cyclin D) have been among the many studied in breast cancer. Each has its enthusiasts, but to date they have added little to clinical practice.

Early detection and prevention of breast cancer

Based on the concept that detecting and treating precancerous lesions and small cancers (before they have metastasized to the regional nodes and/or further afield) could save lives, breast screening and, more recently, chemoprevention of breast cancer in high risk groups have been implemented.

Breast screening

There is currently no evidence to support the view that clinical breast examination by doctor, nurse or patient should be considered as a primary screening technique. However, since the majority of breast cancers are found by women themselves, women should be encouraged to become aware of the feel and shape of their breasts, so that they are familiar with what is normal for them and to report any change from normal to a medical practitioner.

Breast screening in the UK, performed by mammography, aims to reach 70% of the target population and requires considerable organization with a built-in quality assurance programme. Two-view mammography (craniocaudal + oblique), with double reading of films performed every 2–3 years should maximize the detection of small (<15 mm) breast cancers.

The UK breast screening programme aims to detect 36 invasive and four DCIS lesions per 10 000 women at the initial (prevalent) screen age 50–52 years and at least 40 invasive and five DCIS per 10 000 women at subsequent (incident) rounds. The current detection rate in the UK NHSBSP runs at five per 1000. More than 50% of the cancers detected should be <15 mm pathological size.

Some two-thirds of screen detected abnormalities prove to be insignificant on further mammographic/ultrasound review. For the remainder, triple assessment is required, and since two-thirds are impalpable, ultrasound or mammographic guided biopsy with fine needle, core or very wide bore core biopsy should establish the diagnosis. Stellate lesions and the minority where the diagnosis is in doubt require excision. For malignant lesions a pre-operative diagnosis may be achieved in up to 95% of patients.

Screen detected cancers are, in general, smaller, better differentiated, more likely to be of special type and node negative when compared with symptomatic cancers; these features agree with the concept of detecting 'early' cancers, where the chances of metastasis are less and mortality is lower. Thus, screening by mammography can reduce mortality from breast cancer by up to 40% in those who attend.

In the UK, women in the 50–64 year age range are invited every 3 years for screening through the National Health Service (NHS) breast screening programme (NHSBSP) with extension up to 70 years likely to achieve a 29% reduction in mortality. Meta-analyses of the international screening mammography trials also show statistically significant mortality reduction, of 18–29%, in the 40–49 year age group. The efficacy of screening in the UK is being evaluated in the 40–41 years trial. Thus, with evidence that screening can be effective in the 40–70 years age group, there is the potential for reducing the mortality of breast cancer by using population-based screening. Unfortunately, this approach cannot be adopted throughout the world, due to constraints on resources or the pattern of clinical care in some countries.

Radiation risk and mammography

It is thought that ionizing radiation increases the risk of breast cancer development after a latent period of 10 years, that the risk is cumulative, and that the risk is greatest for adolescent exposure and decreases with increasing age at exposure. In those aged over 50 years, the risk of cancer induction is, very approximately, 1:100 000 per single-view examination. The average dose per examination (single-view per breast) is approximately 1–2 mGy, the dose being dependent on breast thickness and exposure factors used.

Women at increased risk of breast cancer

It is estimated that some 5% of all cases of breast cancer are attributable to inheritance of a gene conferring a high lifetime risk of breast cancer. A characteristic of many cases of genetically determined breast cancer is early age of onset. Several genes predisposing to breast cancer have been identified including BRCA1, BRCA2, ATM and p53.

Some women with histologically identifiable lesions, e.g. lobular carcinoma *in situ* (LCIS) or severe atypical hyperplasia, are at a higher relative risk (of about four) of breast cancer. The risk is further increased when there is a positive family history. Thus, women with LCIS or severe atypical hyperplasia should have annual or biennial mammography. Ductal carcinoma *in situ* (DCIS) is considered below.

Only those women judged to be at substantially increased risk (see Table 3.3) should be considered at present for detailed genetic assessment and follow-up in specialist clinics. In families with four or more relatives affected with either breast or ovarian cancer in three generations and one living affected individual, direct gene testing might be appropriate.

Management of women at high risk of breast cancer

For some families, the risk decreases with age and this should be reflected in their management. Women at high risk of breast cancer have three options: increased frequency of screening, chemoprevention with tamoxifen or prophylactic surgery.

Increased frequency of screening

Regular clinical and mammographic examination has been offered to young women at high risk of breast cancer without controlled trials. The efficacy of screening of young, high-risk women is at present uncertain, but a recent review by the UK Familial Breast Cancer Group suggested targeted screening may be as efficacious in this age group as in the NHSBSP.

In the UK, it is suggested that mammography (initial two-view then at least single oblique) should start at the age of 35 years, or 5 years younger than the youngest affected family member, whichever is younger. For women at high risk of breast cancer:

- <40 years: biennial mammography and annual clinical examination
- 40–50 years: annual mammography and clinical examination
- 50+ years: depending on the risk, either discharge to NHSBSP or continue more frequent screening.

In the UK, known gene carriers (or women at equivalent risk) who do not opt for prophylactic surgery are eligible to take part in a MRC study examining magnetic resonance imaging (MRI) and breast screening in women at high risk of breast cancer.

Chemoprevention

In the adjuvant setting, tamoxifen was noted to reduce the incidence of contralateral breast cancers; hence chemoprevention with tamoxifen is of major interest. The effect of tamoxifen on women at increased risk of breast cancer should gain a definitive answer from a double blind randomized trial (International Breast Cancer Interventional Study, IBIS) involving some 8000 women randomized to tamoxifen 20 mg daily or placebo for 5 years. The NSABP trial was stopped when an interim analysis showed a 50% reduction in the rate of DCIS and 47% reduction in invasive breast cancers. The additional benefits (reduced osteoporotic fractures) and detrimental effects (increased risk of endometrial cancer, DVT, PE, stroke in >50 years age group) were noted. Two European trials made public at the same time failed to confirm the benefit. Raloxifene, given for osteoporosis, has also been evaluated and early results show a reduction in breast cancers comparable to tamoxifen; direct comparisons of tamoxifen and raloxifene have yet to be reported.

Prophylactic surgery

Some women at very high risk (>35% lifetime risk) of breast cancer may wish to consider prophylactic bilateral mastectomy, usually with reconstruction. If subcutaneous mastectomy is considered, the risk from residual ductal tissue deep to the nipple or in the tail of the breast must be recognized as any familial genetic defect would theoretically be carried by all remaining cells. The reduction in the incidence of breast cancer by 90% is considered worthwhile by some women.

Management of women who develop breast cancer with autosomal dominant inheritance

At present causal mutations can be identified in some 20% of high-risk breast cancer families. Genetic testing must involve formal pre- and post-testing counselling in person by a clinical geneticist. Predictive tests should only be undertaken in diagnostic laboratories with appropriate quality control.

Women who carry a mutant BRCA1 or BRCA2 gene and develop early breast cancer have a risk of developing cancer in the contralateral breast of up to 64%. In such patients presenting with good prognosis tumours, bilateral mastectomy should be discussed with the patient by her surgeon.

The risk of ovarian cancer is dependent on the family history. Both high-risk (63% lifetime risk at 70 years) and low-risk (<40%) families exist. Preliminary data suggest that prophylactic oophorectomy does reduce the risk of ovarian cancer. Prophylactic bilateral oophorectomy may be considered but may also be appropriate systemic adjuvant therapy for premenopausal patients with ER positive breast cancer (see page 84).

Section 3.4 • Assessment, investigation and staging of breast cancer

Methods of assessing breast conditions, including breast cancer, are based on triple assessment: clinical assessment, radiological assessment and cytological/histological assessment.

Imaging of symptomatic breast disease

Mammography on its own does not exclude breast cancer and must be performed as part of triple assessment. In patients with symptomatic disease two view mammography should be performed: craniocaudal and oblique views (Figure 3.11) supplemented by compression/paddle or magnification views. The radiological classification of breast appearances is listed in Table 3.4. Mammography is not recommended under the age of 35 years unless there is a strong clinical suspicion of carcinoma. Ultrasound examination may provide additional information to mammography (Figure 3.3), and can be useful to visualize focal breast disease in women under 35 years where the breast is radiologically dense and lesions may be more difficult to detect.

Stereotactic (mammographic) or ultrasound guided FNA or core biopsy should be performed on impalpable lesions that are suspicious or equivocal on radiological review. This may provide sufficient information to allow a benign lesion to be left *in situ*, but if clinical doubt persists or the patient requests, needle localiza-

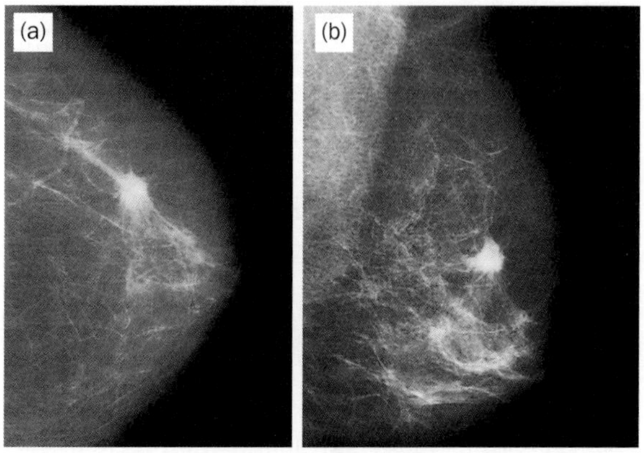

Figure 3.11 Two-view mammograms of a screen-detected breast cancer.

Table 3.4 Classification of radiological appearances

Mammograms		*Breast type*		*Ultrasound*	
R1	Normal	N1	Good visualization; no masses/calcification/ deformities	U1	Normal/diffuse benign
R2	Benign	P1		U2	Single cyst
R3	Indeterminate	P2		U3	Solid benign
R4	Probably malignant	PDY	Dense; cannot rule out masses.	U4	Suspicious of malignancy
R5	Malignant	DY		U5	Malignant
				U6	Multiple cysts

tion biopsy of the impalpable lesion with specimen radiographs is necessary to allow histological examination of the appropriate portion of the biopsy specimen.

Other imaging modalities

The role of MRI in the primary investigation of breast symptoms is not yet defined. MRI has been shown to be helpful in patients with implants who have developed symptoms where ultrasound has not been diagnostic. Patients with suspected recurrent disease in the conserved breast may benefit from MRI if mammography, ultrasound and cytology have been unhelpful. Positron emission tomography (PET) scanning remains, at present, an experimental tool for examining breast cancers and lymph node metastases.

Cytology/pathology in diagnosis of breast cancer

Fine needle aspiration cytology of a focal breast abnormality using a 21 G or (less painfully) 23 G needle can yield representative material for cytological examination (Figure 3.12). Appropriately dried/fixed and stained, expert cytological review based on cytological appearances can grade needle aspiration smeared on a slide as C_1 (insufficient for diagnosis), C_2 (benign), C_3 (atypia), C_4 (suspicious of cancer) or C_5 (malignant). After an equivocal result, or insufficient material (C_1) the FNAC can be repeated or supplemented by core biopsy (under local anaesthesia) or surgical excision biopsy. Markers such as oestrogen receptors may be performed on the aspiration and provide useful clinical information in elderly unfit patients in whom primary tamoxifen is likely to be of therapeutic benefit if the tumour cytology is oestrogen receptor positive.

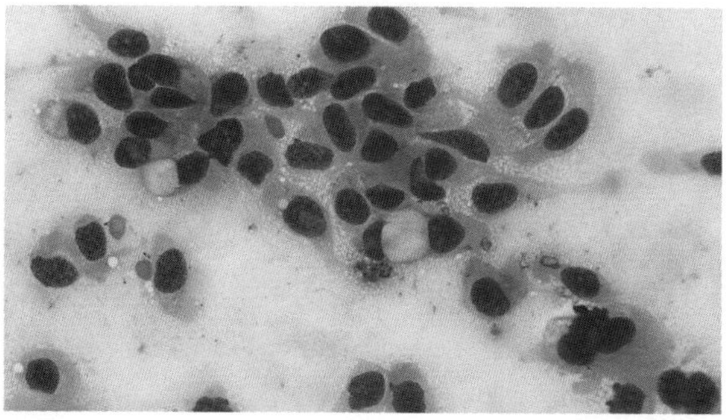

Figure 3.12 Cytology (C5) of a fine needle aspirate of a breast cancer.

Staging of breast cancer

Patients are staged clinically according to the UICC TNM classification (see Table 3.5). Although clinical assessment of tumour size is not completely accurate, and radiological imaging can be more accurate, there is reasonable correlation between clinical tumour size and final pathological assessment. All patients with a breast mass should have a careful clinical examination and the mass should be measured with callipers. The presence or absence of any signs of local advancement (inflammation, peau d'orange, ulceration, satellite nodules, direct chest wall involvement, fixed axillary nodes) should be noted and recorded. Clinical examination is an unreliable guide as to whether there is involvement of the axillary nodes by metastatic breast cancer.

In early operable breast cancer (T1–2, N0–1), there is no current evidence to support routine screening for metastatic disease in asymptomatic women. Such patients should normally only have minimal staging investigations, which may include a chest X-ray, full blood count and liver function tests. Patients with symptoms suggestive of metastases at a particular site do require appropriate investigation. The incidence of asymptomatic metastases increases as the T and N stage of the locoregional cancer increases. If it will affect treatment, patients with more advanced but operable disease (T3, N1–2) may require staging to exclude distant metastases. The staging tests required include isotope bone scan (Figure 3.13) (with additional supplementary radiographs to determine whether abnormalities are likely to be due to metastatic disease), liver ultrasound or abdominal CT scan. If metastases are detected, the tumour markers CEA and CA15-3 may be elevated and are useful for monitoring disease progression.

Pathology

The nature of specimens submitted to the pathologist varies widely, depending on surgical practice and protocols of management. FNA cannot distinguish DCIS from invasive cancer and a minimum of four core biopsies targeted on a focal lesion are needed to provide histological material to demonstrate and classify invasive malignancy.

Histology of breast cancer

Breast cancers originate from the epithelium of the terminal duct lobular unit. Those remaining within the basement membrane are classified as *in situ*, and have

Table 3.5 TNM staging

T Primary tumour		
TX	Primary tumour cannot be assessed	
T0	No evidence of primary tumour	
Tis	Carcinoma *in situ*: intraductal carcinoma, or lobular carcinoma *in situ*, or Paget's disease[a] of the nipple with no tumour	
T1	Tumour 2 cm or less in greatest dimension	
	T1mic	Microinvasion[b] 0.1 cm or less in greatest dimension
	T1a	More than 0.1 cm but not more than 0.5 in greatest dimension
	T1b	More than 0.5 cm but not more than 1 cm in greatest dimension
	T1c	More than 1 cm but not more than 2 cm in greatest dimension
T2	Tumour more than 2 cm but not more than 5 cm in greatest dimension	
T3	Tumour more than 5 cm in greatest dimension	
T4	Tumour of any size with direct extension to chest wall[c] or skin	
	T4a	Extension to chest wall
	T4b	Oedema (including peau d'orange), or ulceration of the skin of the breast, or satellite skin nodules confined to the same breast
	T4c	Both 4a and 4b, above
	T4d	Inflammatory carcinoma[d]
N Regional lymph nodes		
NX	Regional lymph nodes cannot be assessed (e.g. previously removed)	
N0	No regional lymph node metastasis	
N1	Metastasis to movable ipsilateral node(s)	
N2	Metastasis to ipsilateral axillary node(s) fixed to one another or to other structures	
N3	Metastasis to ipsilateral internal mammary lymph node(s)	
M Distant metastasis		
MX	Distant metastasis cannot be assessed	
M0	No distant metastasis	
M1	Distant metastasis	

Notes:
[a]Paget's disease associated with a tumour is classified according to the size of the tumour.
[b]Microinvasion is the extension of cancer cells beyond the basement membrane into the adjacent tissues with no focus more than 0.1 cm in greatest dimension. When there are multiple foci of microinvasion, the size of only the largest focus is used to classify the microinvasion. (Do not use the sum of all the individual foci.) The presence of multiple foci of microinvasion should be noted, as it is with multiple larger invasive carcinomas.
[c]Chest wall includes ribs, intercostal muscles and serratus anterior muscle but not pectoral muscle.
[d]Inflammatory carcinoma of the breast is characterized by diffuse, brawny induration of the skin with an erysipeloid edge, usually with no underlying mass. If the skin biopsy is negative and there is not localized measurable primary cancer, the T category is pTX when pathologically staging a clinical inflammatory carcinoma (T4d). Dimpling of the skin, nipple retraction or other skin changes, except those in T4b and T4d, may occur in T1, T2 or T3 without affecting the classification.

characteristic patterns as do invasive cancers which disseminate beyond the basement membrane.

Invasive cancers are now classified as no special type (NST, or not otherwise specified) (Figure 3.14) or special types: lobular, tubular, medullary, mucoid, papillary, which may have characteristic histopathological features and some of which have a better prognosis. For cancers of NST, prognosis is related to tumour grade I, II, III based on gland formation, nuclear pleomorphism, and frequency of mitoses originally described by Scarff, Bloom and Richardson. For invasive cancer some 80% is NST, 10% lobular and the remainder

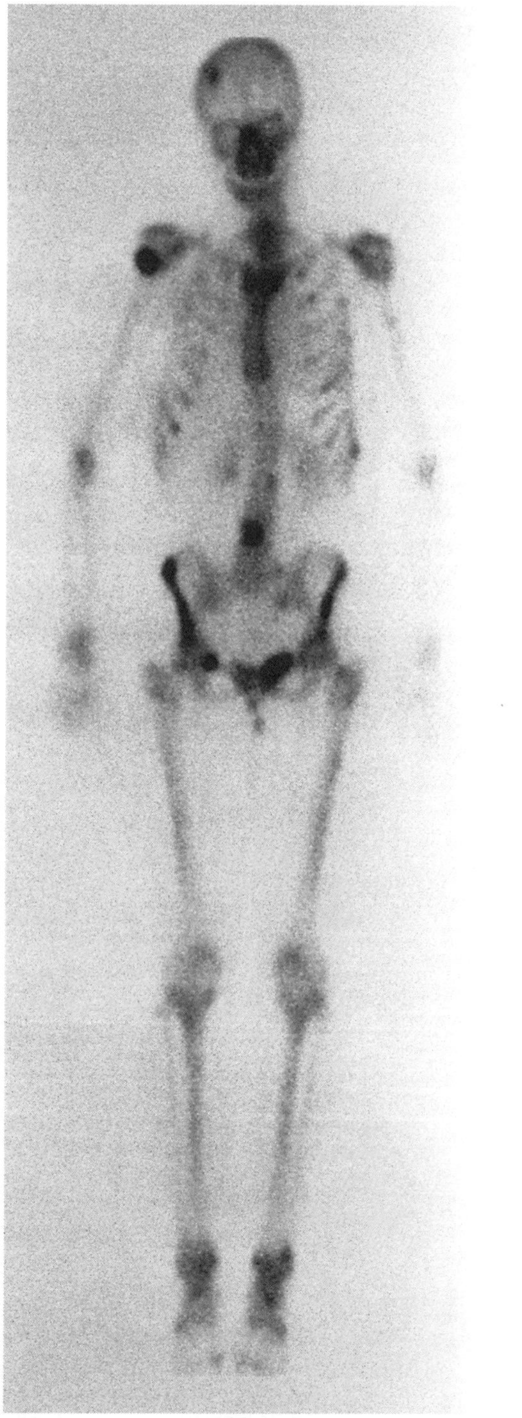

Figure 3.13 Staging bone scan demonstrating bone metastases of the right humerus, thoracic and lumbar spine, pelvic bones and skull.

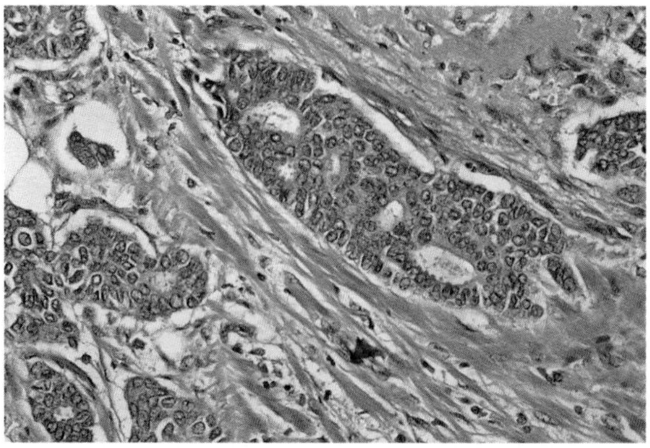

Figure 3.14 Haematoxylin and eosin stained section of invasive breast cancer.

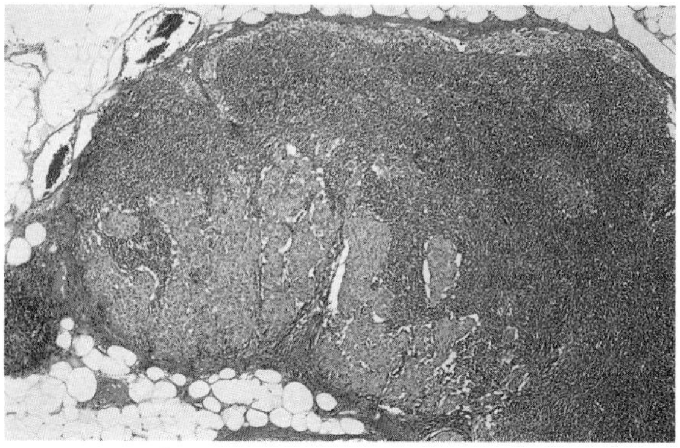

Figure 3.15 Haematoxylin and eosin stained section of an axillary lymph node showing extensive node involvement with invasive breast cancer.

(10%) tubular, medullary, mucoid, papillary or other even rarer types. Lymphatic or vascular invasion on histological assessment is also a marker for both local and systemic recurrence. Patients with perineural invasion or extensive (>25%) *in situ* cancer within the tumour mass are more likely to develop local recurrence.

Paget's disease is an eczematous infiltration of large breast cancer cells into the nipple/areolar skin which occurs in approximately 2% of presenting cancers. It is symptomatic of an underlying usually invasive cancer or less commonly *in situ* disease. Diagnosis is from incisional biopsy after triple assessment which may reveal an underlying cancer.

Metastatic spread from breast carcinoma is via lymphatic channels to regional lymph nodes (Figure 3.15), predominantly in the axilla. Even in the absence of detectable lymph node metastasis, lymphatic or vascular invasion in the breast tissue is suggestive of the propensity of the cancer to spread to distant metastatic sites.

Synoptic reporting is proving increasingly acceptable to standardize and optimize communication, with the format determined locally for macroscopic and microscopic details. An illustrative example is provided in Table 3.6.

Table 3.6 Synoptic pathology report

- Invasive cancer: Invasive carcinoma, no special type
- Grade: III (Glands 3, Nuclei 3, Mitosis 2)
- Size: 27 mm
- *In situ* cancer. Present: comedo type
- Grade: High
- Extent: Extensive, within main lesion
- Calcification: Yes; associated with *in situ* cancer
- Margins: Nearest is medial at 5 mm, all others >10 mm
- Multifocal: No
- Vascular/lymphatic invasion: Yes, at the edge of the cancer in two blocks
- Lymph nodes: Number confirmed 5; number positive 1 (microscopic)
- Oestrogen receptor (specify scoring system): Histoscore = 120, heterogeneity present

Summary: Right breast wide local excision – invasive carcinoma grade 3 with one lymph node metastasis.

Carcinoma *in situ*

A spectrum of pre-invasive neoplastic change in the breast includes DCIS (4% of symptomatic, 25% of screen detected 'cancers'), lobular carcinoma *in situ* (LCIS; <1% symptomatic and 1% of screen detected lesions) and hyperplastic appearances (ductal or lobular atypia) which can cause diagnostic difficulties.

DCIS (Figure 3.16) covers a heterogeneous group of lesions and is classified by histological type, grade and the presence of necrosis. However, no internationally agreed classification system exists. High-quality mammography is required to determine the extent of disease, although DCIS can be present without mammographic signs. The majority of cases are now detected in screening programmes, although the natural history of the disease is not fully understood.

DCIS characterized by ducts expanded by large irregular cells with large irregular nuclei may be classified in a variety of ways: comedo DCIS has high-grade cytology, extensive necrosis and branched calcifications. Non-comedo DCIS (cribriform, solid or micropapillary) has low-grade cytology, lacks necrosis and calcification is inconsistent. As one might expect, there are patients with intermediate histology. DCIS is increasing in the frequency of detection, largely due to screening techniques. The risk of developing invasive cancer at the site of DCIS is about 40% over a 30 year period (usually during the first 10 years). The average age of diagnosis is 55 and most women are postmenopausal. The biology remains poorly understood (for example 80% of DCIS is HER-2 expressing but unlike invasive cancer (see page 70) this is not a poor prognostic sign).

Atypical ductal hyperplasia (ADH)

ADH forms part of a spectrum with DCIS – membrane bound spaces of 2–3 mm with cellular atypia. ADH holds a four-fold risk of developing breast cancer which is additive with any family history of breast cancer.

Lobular carcinoma *in situ* (LCIS)

LCIS, usually an incidental histological finding, is an expansion of the breast lobule by smaller, regular cells with regular row/oval nuclei. The risk of developing

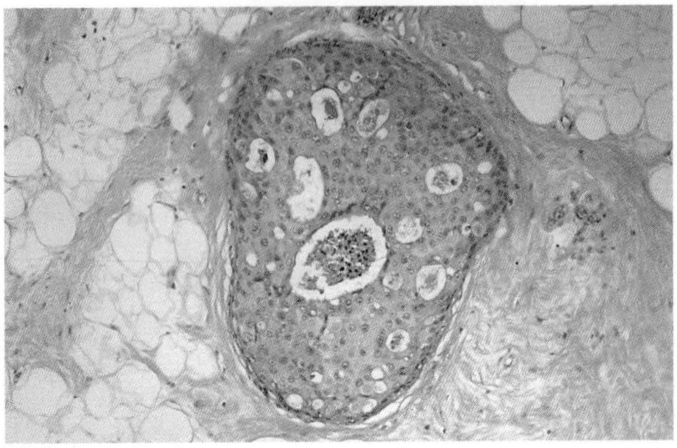

Figure 3.16 Haematoxylin and eosin stained section demonstrating DCIS (of cribriform type).

invasive breast cancer is about 25% (and contralateral breast cancer about 10%) at 20 years; since most women (70%) with LCIS are premenopausal (mean age 45 years) this may be significant.

Other malignancies in the breast

Primary lymphoma affecting nodes within the breast or in the axilla is perhaps the most common non-breast malignancy and is treated, following staging with or without local excision/tumour biopsy, by conventional anti-lymphoma regimens. Sarcoma is treated by excision with the widest possible margin at mastectomy followed by post-operative radiotherapy.

While primary breast cancer is by far the most common breast malignancy, secondary spread from other organs such as bronchogenic carcinoma or from the gynaecological organs is recognized. Usually, the cellular morphology of the lesion gives clues as to its origin (which may be suggested from a past history of e.g. leiomyosarcoma of the uterus) and the use of special stains suggesting the lesion is not breast cancer (e.g. oestrogen receptor negative) or positive molecular markers (e.g. for lymphoma) give clues to the primary.

Prognostic factors

In the management of breast cancer, prognostic factors aid the selection of treatment for individual patients. Age (patients <35 years have a poorer prognosis), tumour size (histological measured size and larger means worse prognosis), axillary node metastasis (Figure 3.17) (on pathology, not clinical, grounds; survival is directly correlated with the number of lymph nodes involved – women with over 10 nodes do particularly badly) and distant metastasis.

Combined with tumour grade, histological tumour size and pathological node status have been used to construct the Nottingham Prognostic Index, where NPI = (tumour size in cm $\times$ 0.2) + lymph node stage (1 = no nodes, 2 = 1 to 3 nodes positive, 3 = 4 or more nodes involved) + grade (1, 2 or 3). Originally forming three prognostic groups (good, moderate, poor) the NPI is now used to place patients in one of five prognostic groups (Blamey, 1996).

Prognostic group	*NPI*	*10 year survival (%)*
Excellent	≤2.4	94
Good	≤3.4	83
Moderate I	≤4.4	70
Moderate II	<5.4	51
Poor	>5.4	19

Section 3.5 • Overview of breast cancer management

It is well established that breast cancer is a spectrum of diseases associated with different clinical behaviours and treatment should be tailored appropriately. Therefore management of patients with breast cancer may involve surgery, radiotherapy, systemic therapy (hormonal and/or chemotherapy), or a combination of these. Since there remain uncertainties in the management of breast cancer, consenting patients should be entered into appropriate clinical trials where possible. Many patients want and benefit from being fully informed of the possible treatment options, and being involved in the decisions about their treatment. The availability of a breast care nurse and discussion within a multidisciplinary team is helpful in this respect.

Management options by stage

- All patients with T1–3, N0 or 1, M0 should be considered for primary surgery.
- Some patients with larger T2 (>3 cm) or T3, N0 or 1, M0 may be considered for primary systemic therapy (neoadjuvant endocrine or chemotherapy) prior to surgery.
- Most T4 tumours are initially inoperable but may become operable after a course of primary systemic therapy or radiotherapy.
- Very small numbers of patients (usually elderly) with potentially operable breast cancer are not medically fit for any surgical procedure.
- Patients with established distant metastatic disease should be managed palliatively but actively. FNA and/or core biopsy are used to confirm the diagnosis, and through the use of these samples for oestrogen receptor, progesterone receptor and HER-2, the likely sensitivity to systemic therapy may be assessed.

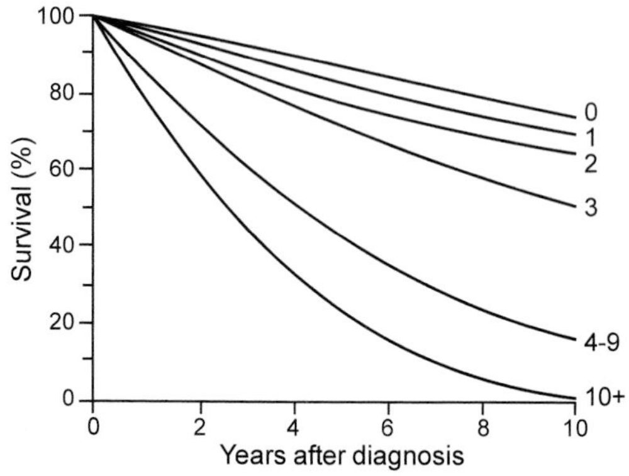

Figure 3.17 Axillary node involvement (number of nodes on pathology review) compared with survival following the diagnosis of breast cancer.

Most patients will complete their initial treatment and then be followed up.

Operable breast cancer

Surgery to the breast

There are three established surgical procedures for invasive breast cancers:

- Wide local excision.
- Quadrantectomy or segmentectomy.
- Mastectomy.

Both wide local excision and segmentectomy would normally be followed by radiotherapy. The combination of wide local excision or segmentectomy and radiotherapy is often called breast conservation. Randomized controlled clinical trials have shown that in tumours up to 4 cm in size treatment by mastectomy or breast conservation (surgery and radiotherapy) results in no significant difference in overall survival. Local recurrence rates are similar with a non-significant relative reduction in favour of mastectomy. Patients undergoing conservation have similar psychological morbidity to those undergoing mastectomy, but have greater freedom of dress and better body image than women who have had mastectomy.

Conservation surgery

Wide local excision is excision of a tumour with a margin of clearance of both invasive and *in situ* disease. Wide local excision (sometimes referred to a lumpectomy) should be performed with due respect to the skin lines of the breast and the likely cosmetic result (Figure 3.18); for invasive disease, an axillary procedure (see below) may be conducted under the same anaesthetic (Figure 3.18). Lateral margins (histopathological) should be 1 mm or more clear of disease. There are no direct comparisons between wide local excision (1 cm macroscopic clearance) and segmental excision (1 cm macroscopic clearance but the excision incorporating tissue from the nipple right out to the periphery of the breast) or quadrantectomy (similar excision to segmental excision but with 2–3 cm macroscopic margin clearance). The most important factor related to cosmetic outcome is the volume of tissue excised and therefore quadrantectomies if not followed by reconstruction (e.g. a latissimus dorsi miniflap) produce less good cosmetic results than wide local excision or segmental excision.

A central tumour is not a contraindication to conservation although it may necessitate removal of the nipple and areola, which may compromise cosmesis for some patients.

The decision whether to recommend mastectomy or breast conservation will depend on factors listed in Table 3.7.

Mastectomy

Mastectomy is indicated for operable breast cancer which is either large or at multiple sites, when radiotherapy is to be avoided, or by patient preference. A modified radical mastectomy removes the skin overlying the cancer, nipple areolar complex and all breast tissue including the axillary tail, but leaves the pectoral muscle intact (removed in a radical mastectomy) and may avoid the need for radiotherapy in many cases. Patients with high-grade tumours, pathology size ≥4 cm, lymphatic permeation or multiple axillary node involvement have a significantly higher risk of locoregional recurrence which can be reduced by supplementing mastectomy with radiotherapy. When mastectomy is carried out axillary clearance is usually performed.

Mastectomy may be complicated postoperatively by haematoma or seroma formation beneath the skin flaps (and hence most surgeons leave in a vacuum drain beneath the skin flaps), wound infection (which should complicate <2% of operations) or, rarely, flap necrosis.

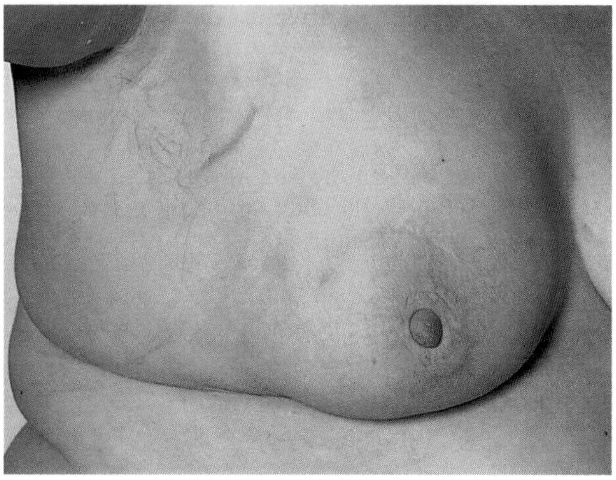

Figure 3.18 Breast conservation: surgical scars following wide local excision of a breast cancer from the 12 o'clock position and axillary node sampling.

Table 3.7 Factors influencing choice of breast surgery

The ratio of the size of the tumour to the size of the breast:
- smaller tumours in larger breasts are more suitable for breast conservation than larger tumours in smaller breasts: a cut off of 4 cm is often quoted.

The pathological features of the tumour (if known)
- extensive *in situ* component
- histological grade II or III
- lymphatic/vascular invasion.

There is an increased risk of local recurrence if disease (invasive or DCIS) is <1 mm from the margins of excision or present at multiple sites.

Age of patient
- Patients aged <35 years are at increased risk of local recurrence.

The patient's own preference.

Fitness for surgery and/or radiotherapy.

Breast reconstruction after mastectomy

Many women are distressed at the prospect of a mastectomy. For these women, discussion of some form of breast reconstruction may help.

Breast reconstruction does not appear to be associated with an increase in the rate of local cancer recurrence, nor to impede the ability to detect recurrence if it develops and can yield psychological benefit. Breast reconstruction may be performed either at the time of mastectomy or as a delayed procedure. Immediate reconstruction has been reported to produce better cosmetic results. The psychosocial effects of breast reconstruction, and the relative merits of immediate and delayed surgery, have not been adequately studied.

The choice of operation for an individual patient depends on several factors including breast size, the adequacy of skin flaps and whether radiotherapy is planned or has been previously used.

Methods comprise:

- An implant filled with silicone or saline which can be placed subcutaneously or subpectorally. Silicone implants are still licensed in most countries for breast reconstruction. Despite some adverse publicity there is no evidence that silicone prostheses are associated with significant systemic problems. Soya-bean implants have now been withdrawn worldwide leaving saline filled implants as the only alternative.
- Use of a tissue expander, placed in either the subpectoral or subcutaneous plane, which can be expanded to provide a matched size with a contralateral side and then partially deflated to allow ptosis or replaced with a silicone or saline implant with repositioning as necessary (Figure 3.19). Tissue expansion is not recommended following radiotherapy due to the fibrotic process induced by radiation.
- Myocutaneous flaps: (a) latissimus dorsi (LD) flap together with overlying skin based on the neurovascular supply to LD may be used to replace a defect postmastectomy but often requires a prosthesis deep to the muscle to ensure adequate bulk and ptosis on the reconstructed side (Figure 3.20). Latissimus dorsi mini flaps where skin is not taken can be used to replace bulk following quadrantectomy and may be harvested using laparoscopic equipment and techniques. (b) Transverse rectus abdominus mycutaneous flap (TRAM flap) may be performed either as a pedicle flap based on the superior epigastric artery or as a free flap based on the inferior epigastric artery with a microvascular anastomosis between the inferior epigastric and the subscapular vessels or vascular bundle to latissimus dorsi. This provides a good bulk of tissue of similar consistency to normal breast and together with contralateral surgery and nipple reconstruction or tattooing can give outstanding results (Figure 3.21).

Surgery to the opposite breast, mastopexy or reduction mammoplasty, may be required to achieve symmetry. Techniques for reconstruction of the nipple/areola complex have been described. Alternatively acceptable nipple prostheses may be made by taking a mould from the existing nipple or nipple tattooing.

Complications of breast reconstruction include infection of the prosthesis, necrosis of skin or flap tissue (ranging from minor fat necrosis to necrosis of the whole flap in <5% of patients), puncture or leakage of implants (10% at 10 years); fibrotic capsule formation around the implant (requiring capsulotomy or capsulectomy) is now less common (<10% at 1 year) due to the use of textured implants, but cosmetically unsatisfactory results can still occur.

Who should perform breast reconstruction? Should it be the same surgeon who performs the mastectomy? There are advantages and disadvantages to the same surgeon performing both operations. Certainly, the surgeon performing the reconstruction should be fully trained in all the appropriate techniques and, in most units, will be a plastic surgeon. Patients who are being prepared for a mastectomy should be informed of the option of reconstruction and, if appropriate, should discuss the options with a surgeon trained in reconstructive techniques, prior to their surgery.

Impalpable tumours

Mammographic screening is increasingly detecting lesions which are radiologically suspicious of malignancy but impalpable. While stereotactic FNAC or core biopsy may provide satisfactory diagnostic material, excision of an impalpable lesion may be required for diagnosis and excision of histologically proven cancer for therapeutic breast conservation requires localization of the radiologically detected lesion. Excision of a needle localized radiological abnormality (Figure 3.22a) may thus be considered diagnostic (if lesser procedures have failed to establish the diagnosis) where the procedure will simply excise the area targeted or a therapeutic procedure to excise the radiologically abnormal area with a 10 mm rim of normal tissue while at the same time axillary surgery may be performed. The diagnostic biopsy of a benign lesion should weigh less than 30 g, the intention being to minimize breast disruption by the diagnostic procedure.

Localization can be performed either under ultrasound guidance or by fixing the breast in a mammographic grid and then guiding one or more fine wires to the localized lesion. A check film is taken to allow

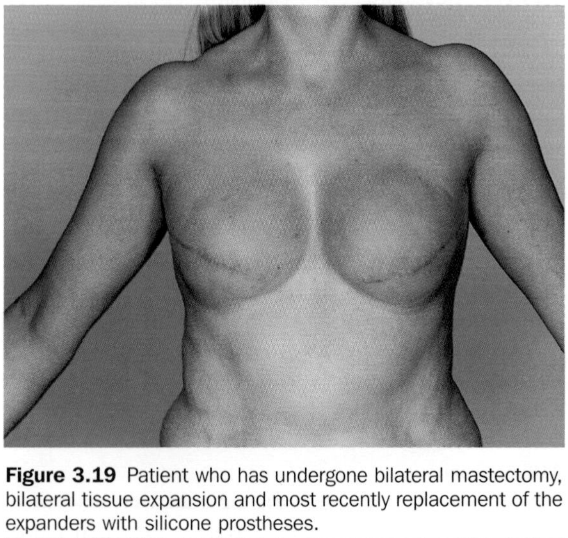

Figure 3.19 Patient who has undergone bilateral mastectomy, bilateral tissue expansion and most recently replacement of the expanders with silicone prostheses.

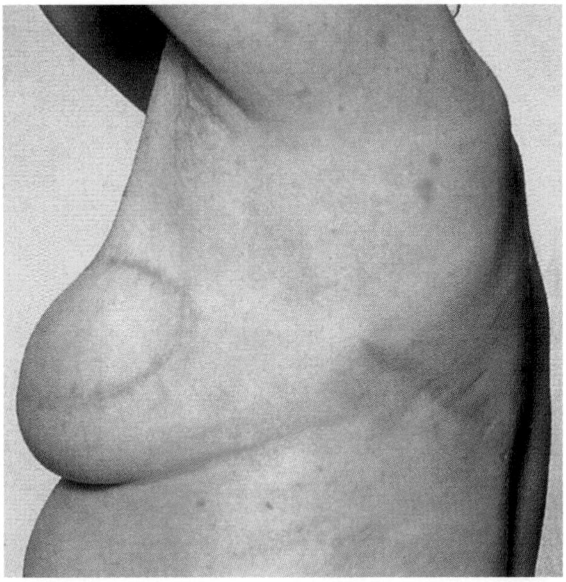

Figure 3.20 Lateral view of latissimus dorsi reconstruction showing the posterior scar, skin/muscle reconstruction (with silicone implant) demonstrating good ptosis.

the surgeon to place an appropriate incision and excise the abnormal area (Figure 3.22b).

Specimen radiology of the excised lesion while the patient remains anaesthetized (local anaesthesia or general anaesthesia may be used for this procedure) ensures the correct area of tissue has been removed by comparison with pre-operative mammography and subsequent histological examination is required to confirm the adequacy of the excision. Excised specimens should be marked for orientation so that the pathologist can indicate whether any margins of excision are inadequate.

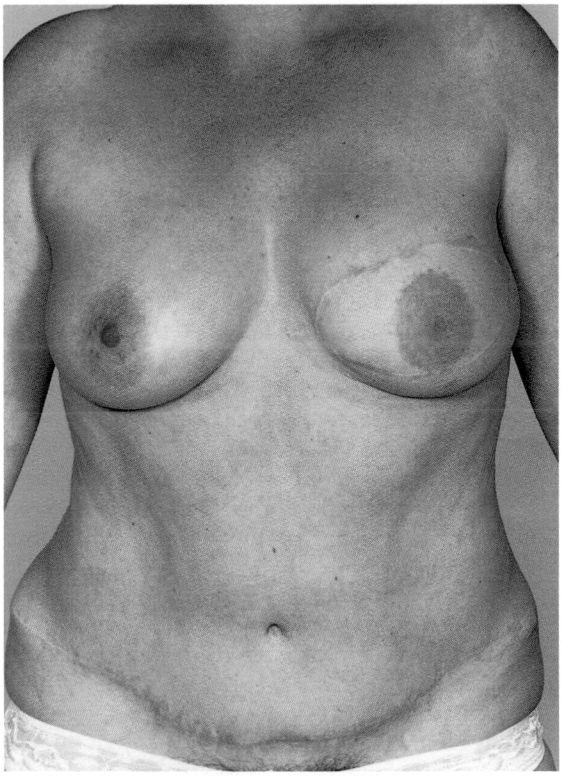

Figure 3.21 Left TRAM flap free flap reconstruction plus nipple tattooing. Note abdominal scars.

Paget's disease

Depending on the site of any underlying primary, wide local excision (+ radiotherapy) or mastectomy (if the lesion is distinct from the centre) is satisfactory.

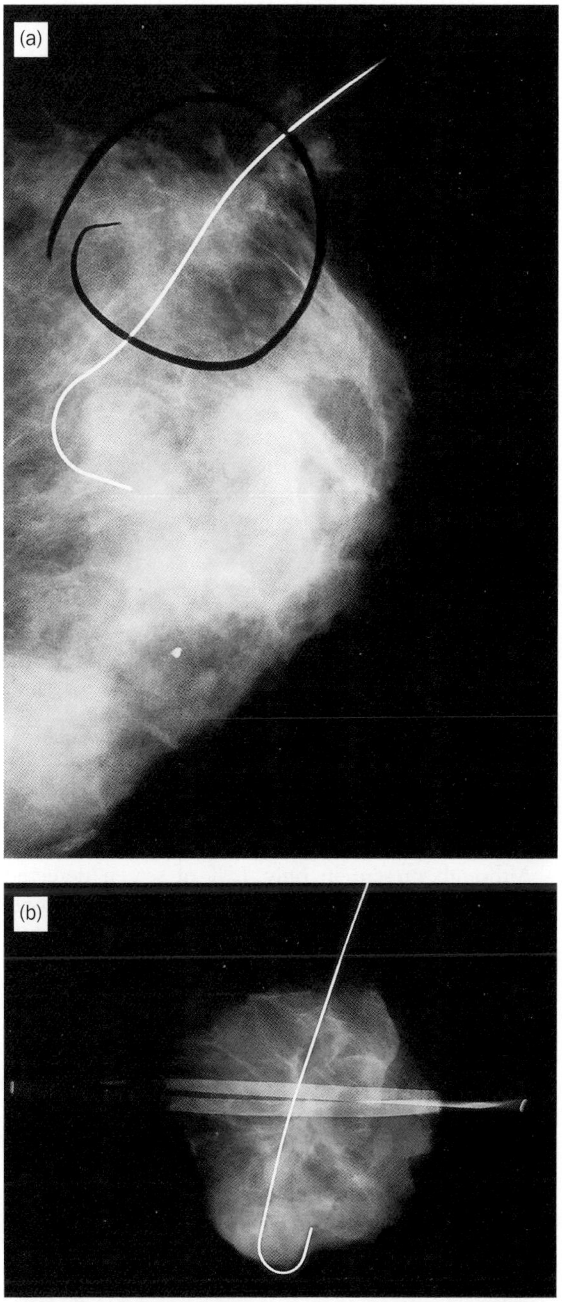

Figure 3.22 Needle localization for impalpable screen detected cancer: (a) mammogram with localizing wire in place; (b) excision biopsy confirmatory film.

Ductal carcinoma *in situ* (DCIS)

Localized areas of DCIS should be completely excised with a wide margin on pathology review.

In patients with extensive DCIS (over 4 cm) (Figure 3.23) or disease affecting more than one quadrant a mastectomy should be performed and results in 98% 5 year survival. Surgical staging of the axilla is not required.

Following adequate local excision of DCIS, patients should be considered for radiotherapy to the breast. While a 1 cm margin of normal tissue around DCIS may be sufficient to gain local control, there is a reduction of recurrence or the development of invasive cancer in those given radiotherapy following wide local excision of high-grade DCIS. The role of systemic hormonal treatment is not established but may reduce recurrence in the breast.

Axillary surgery is not recommended in patients with DCIS alone, although 1-2% of patients with large, high-grade DCIS may have axillary metastasis.

LCIS

While observation, tamoxifen treatment or local excision may have their advocates, mastectomy (or bilateral mastectomy) with reconstruction is the treatment of choice.

Surgery to the axilla

Lymphatic drainage from the breast is predominantly to the axilla, although metastatic breast cancer may spread via internal mammary, intercostal or interpectoral nodes.

One of the most important prognostic indicators is whether there has been spread of cancer to the axillary lymph nodes (Figure 3.17), and hence it is used as one of the major determinants of appropriate systemic adjuvant therapy. Axillary surgery should be performed in all patients with invasive operable breast cancer. Axillary nodes lie inferior to the axillary vein and are classified in relation to the pectoralis minor muscle – level I lateral, II posterior to and III medial to pectoralis minor.

Although present in only 15% of screen detected cancers, some 50% of symptomatic cancers have axillary metastases.

For larger tumours (T2 and above) a complete level III axillary clearance is the treatment of choice.

Since only 5% of node metastases are 'skip metastases', missing the lower level I nodes but involving level II or III, for small cancers there is no consensus as to the best way to manage the axilla (Table 3.8).

The following procedures are practised.

Table 3.8 Recommended management of axillary nodes for operable breast cancer

Impalpable cancer or less than 2 cm	Node sample, or sentinel node biopsy (in trial) or level I, II and III clearance
All other operable cancer	Level I, II and III clearance

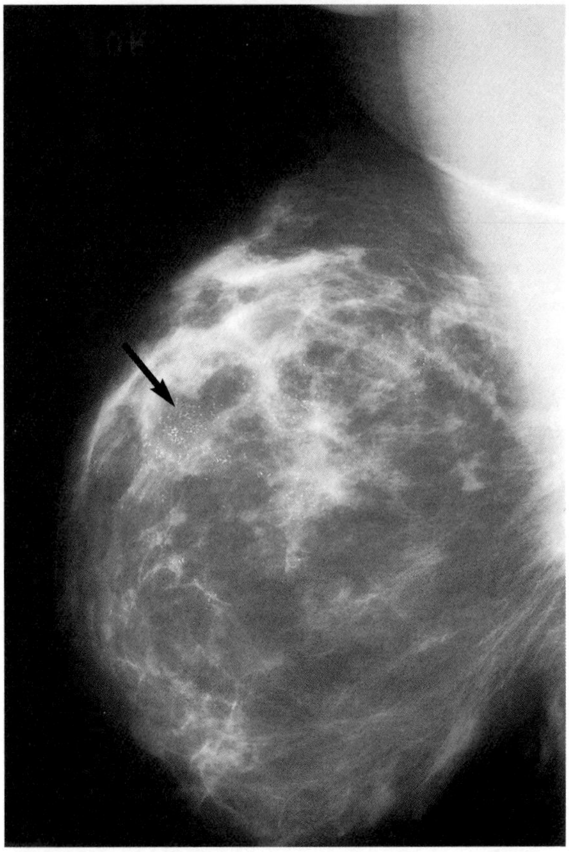

Figure 3.23 DCIS on breast screening mammogram.

To stage the axilla

Sentinel node biopsy. Based on the concept that there is a first or sentinel axillary node draining breast cancer, radiolabelled albumin is injected adjacent to the cancer 4–18 hours prior to surgery; breast scintigraphy may be performed to confirm the label has travelled and highlighted an axillary node. Combined with injecting patent blue dye around the cancer at the time of surgery, lymphatic channels and the sentinel node containing the blue dye can be visually identified (Figure 3.24) and a gamma probe used to confirm the hottest (sentinel) node. A second node may also be identified by this means. The combination of gamma and visual detection is superior to either alone but still has a false negative rate of 5%. The concept is that immediate histological examination of the sentinel node, if negative, will prevent the need for further axillary surgery, while if positive, the surgeon will proceed to axillary clearance. While an established technique for melanoma, the role of sentinel node biopsy in breast cancer, particularly for small cancers (which are likely to be node negative) has yet to be established in multicentre clinical trials.

Axillary node sampling. Picking out at least four individual lymph nodes from the lower axillary fat through a small axillary skin crease incision (Figure 3.18) stages the axilla, but is not a form of treatment. However, for small cancers (less than 2 cm) which are axillary sam-

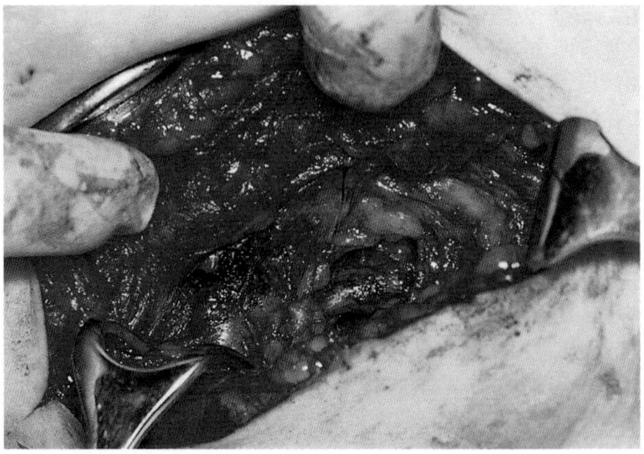

Figure 3.24 Sentinel node biopsy: blue dye staining a lymphatic and two sentinel nodes. The lower node contained a high radiolabel signal and had a small focus of metastatic breast cancer.

ple negative it may prevent the need for a full axillary clearance with less morbidity than axillary clearance. A positive node sample should be followed by axillary irradiation or axillary clearance.

To stage and treat the axilla

Axillary node clearance – a block dissection of the axillary contents comprises the tissue bounded by the axillary vein (superiorly), latissimus dorsi, serratus anterior and pectoralis major, and the apex is situated at the point where the axillary vein passes over the first rib.

Level I is up to the lateral border of pectoralis minor, level II is up to the medial border of pectoralis minor and level III is up to the apex of the axilla. Care is taken to preserve the neurovascular supply to serratus, latissimus and pectoralis major and cutaneous nerves and not to dissect superior to the axillary vein.

Complications of axillary clearance include seroma formation (50%), infection (5%), cutaneous nerve damage, shoulder stiffness (5%) and pain. Long-term complications include upper limb lymphoedema (up to 15%), neural damage or restricted shoulder movement (10%).

There is no advantage of level III clearance over axillary radiation in terms of survival at 10 years, nor does either have an advantage in terms of regional control of disease.

Only level III dissection fully stages the axilla and treats nodal disease. Further treatment of the axilla (radiotherapy or surgical re-excision) may be required for patients who have had a level I or II dissection to achieve local disease control if involved nodes are identified histologically, but risks lymphoedema. Further treatment after level III dissection is only considered if the nodes cannot be adequately cleared or if there is extranodal spread of the tumour. Clearance and radiotherapy increases the risk of lymphoedema of the upper limb to some 40%.

Only 5% of women with breast cancer have internal mammary node metastases, usually from medially placed cancers, but 90% of these women also have axillary metastases so most surgeons do not perform internal mammary node biopsy.

Rarely, breast cancer may present with axillary nodes but no clinically evident breast primary. While mammography and MRI may identify an occult lesion in two-thirds of these patients, in the remainder level III axillary clearance with observation (clinical and radiological) of the breast may be the treatment of choice.

Section 3.6 • Adjuvant radiotherapy

Radiotherapy has been used after surgery for breast cancer for decades. Indeed the move from radical mastectomy was facilitated by trials showing that simple mastectomy and radiotherapy produced results equivalent to radical mastectomy, without the loss of function. A generation later, trials showed that for patients with small operable tumours, local surgery (wide local excision) and post-operative radiotherapy were equivalent in terms of survival and local control to conventional mastectomy. Post-operative radiotherapy is now used following mastectomy or breast conservation for operable breast cancer.

Post-mastectomy radiotherapy

Radiotherapy and local control

Radiotherapy given after mastectomy will reduce the risk of isolated local recurrence by approximately two-thirds. The absolute benefit will depend on the risk of recurrence: thus if the risk of recurrence without radiotherapy is 39%, this will be reduced to 13% with radiotherapy, an absolute benefit of 39 − 13 = 26%. Conversely, a risk of recurrence of 3% would be reduced to 1%, an absolute benefit of 2%. The former would certainly be clinically useful, whereas for the latter patient, the disadvantages of radiotherapy would probably outweigh the (modest) benefit.

Radiotherapy after mastectomy is thus generally recommended only for those patients judged to be at a particular risk of recurrence, i.e. large tumour size (>5 cm), involved nodes, high histological grade, lymphatic and/or vascular invasion and involved (usually deep) margins. Risk of local recurrence is a summation of these factors, although there is no convenient formula to quantify them.

Systemic adjuvant therapy (see page 83) does reduce the risk of local recurrence, but radiotherapy confers additional benefit and the relative reduction in local recurrence is independent of any systemic therapy. Thus the decision as to whether to recommend post-mastectomy radiotherapy depends on the perceived risk of recurrence, bearing in mind the pathological factors considered above and the systemic therapy to be offered.

Extent of radiotherapy

For the reasons mentioned above, radiotherapy will normally certainly include the chest wall. Whether the axilla is included depends on the type and results of axillary surgery. If the axilla has been formally sampled and at least four nodes show no evidence of tumour involvement, then axillary radiotherapy will not improve local control within the axilla. If the validity of sentinel node biopsy is confirmed, it is likely that it will be equivalent to a sample. Conversely, a positive (or inadequate) sample should be followed by either level III axillary clearance or axillary radiotherapy. A surgical clearance of the axilla should both stage and treat the axilla. Radiotherapy following axillary clearance will substantially increase the risk of morbidity without any increase in local control. The only exceptions are where a clearance is known to have left residual disease and/or there is extensive extracapsular spread – these patients are at high risk of local recurrence with its associated morbidity which must be balanced against the morbidity of treatment.

The supraclavicular fossa and internal mammary chain of nodes (IMC) have been irradiated as part of standard therapy in some centres, but without clear evidence of benefit. Isolated IMC recurrence is rare and supraclavicular recurrence is an early manifestation of metastatic relapse. At present the results of a large EORTC trial of IMC irradiation are awaited and the role of nodal radiotherapy in terms of survival benefit is discussed below.

Effect on survival

Whilst the importance of local treatment (surgery, radiotherapy) on local control has long been recognized, the concept of breast cancer as a systemic disease at presentation used to discount the importance of local therapy in terms of survival. Recent studies examined post-mastectomy radiotherapy (chest wall and nodes) in patients who were also receiving systemic adjuvant therapy, showed that the addition of radiotherapy to the chest wall and nodal areas was associated with a highly significant improvement in overall survival, at 10 years, of about 9%. An overview of all trials of post-operative radiotherapy (including post-mastectomy and breast conservation trials) showed a reduction in breast cancer mortality of 3.0% at 10 years and 4.8% at 20 years. This benefit was offset by an excess of non-breast cancer deaths (mostly vascular) in the irradiated patients, so the absolute benefit of radiotherapy was only 2.1% at 10 years and 1.2% at 20 years. The long-term results are inevitably dominated by studies initiated 30–40 years ago, when systemic therapy was less used and radiotherapy techniques were less sophisticated (less care was taken to minimize the dose received by the heart, probably accounting for the excess vascular deaths). There is however good evidence that local control can affect survival, presumably by the recurrence acting as the focus for metastatic reseeding. The practical implications are that local control is important and needs meticulous technique by both surgeon and radiotherapist to minimize morbidity, maximize local control and hence to improve survival.

Radiotherapy after breast conservation

All studies have shown that radiotherapy to the breast following limited breast surgery reduces the risk of local recurrence. Table 3.9 shows the recurrence rate for three trials in which different surgical procedures were used. Whilst these are not direct comparisons, the data suggest that when more extensive surgery (quandrantectomy or sector resection) is used, the local recurrence rate without radiotherapy is less (albeit at the cost of an impaired cosmetic result). Nevertheless, even with more extensive surgery, radiotherapy significantly reduces the local recurrence rate.

If the patient has systemic adjuvant therapy, as well as surgery, radiotherapy further reduces the risk of local recurrence; the magnitude of the effect is very similar to that seen after mastectomy. For the small group of patients with small, adequately excised, grade 1 tumours (or of special type such as tubular cancer), and node negative, a trial (BASO II) is examining whether radiotherapy confers an advantage for this group of patients with a low risk of recurrence. All other studies have demonstrated that radiotherapy reduces the risk of recurrence. Thus radiotherapy is of potential benefit to all patients undergoing breast conservation and should only be omitted if the clinician feels, after discussion with the patient, that the morbidity of radiotherapy does not justify the excess recurrence risk for that patient.

Dosage and complications

Radiotherapy doses of 40–50 Gy delivered in 15–25 fractions over 3–5 weeks (+ tumour bed boost of 10–20 Gy) are standard radiotherapy regimens. There

Table 3.9 Comparison of effect of radiotherapy and the extent of breast surgery on recurrence rate

Type of surgery	*Wide local excision*	*Sector resection*	*Quadrantectomy*
Name of trial	NSABP	Uppsala-Orebro	Milan
No. of patients	1450	381	579
No radiotherapy	39%	7.6%	10%
Radiotherapy	10%	2.9%	0%
Duration	8 years	3 years	3 years

are ongoing trials examining the optimal dosage regimen and the need for a boost.

Historically, patients were treated with orthovoltage machines that resulted in skin reactions, telangiectasia, cardiac arterial damage, brachial plexopathy and, rarely, haemangiosarcoma. Current megavoltage treatment with tangential fields means that reactions are much less, with skin erythema and fatigue most common. Supraclavicular radiotherapy may cause a transient oesophagitis. In the long term, a small number of patients develop breast oedema and/or fibrosis.

Section 3.7 • Adjuvant systemic therapy

For many patients, breast cancer is a systemic disease at presentation, albeit the metastases are not detectable and only become apparent during the ensuing years. The rationale of systemic adjuvant therapy given after surgery is to treat and hopefully eradicate the occult distant metastases and hence improve survival. There have been numerous trials of adjuvant therapy and the results of these have contributed to the overviews of the Early Breast Cancer Trialists' Collaborative Group. These confirm that adjuvant endocrine and/or cytotoxic therapy can improve both recurrence free and overall survival.

Choice of adjuvant therapy

The choice of appropriate therapy from polychemotherapy, oophorectomy and tamoxifen will be determined by:

- the woman's risk of recurrence (based mainly on nodal status, tumour size and tumour grade)
- the hormone receptor status of the patient's tumour (mainly oestrogen receptor, but progesterone receptor may be important)
- the patient's menopausal status.

Clearly this requires individual discussion of pathology findings which may be helped by using the Nottingham Prognostic Index as an aid to decision making (see page 76).

The magnitude of the benefits of adjuvant therapy can be illustrated by considering the results of trials of ovarian ablation. For premenopausal women not receiving chemotherapy, ovarian ablation reduces the odds of death by 24%, but Figure 3.25 shows firstly that there is a slightly greater effect on recurrence free survival than overall survival, and secondly that the absolute reduction varies according to the risk of relapse. In other words, node positive women have a higher absolute benefit because they are at a higher risk of relapse.

In effect there are three groups of women, as summarized in Table 3.10 (percentage defined at 10 years).

Group A have significant occult metastatic disease which is either resistant to or not eradicated by the systemic therapy. They may gain some prolongation of disease free survival but they will not gain any survival advantage.

Group B have occult distant metastases that are eradicated by systemic therapy and hence achieve a personal cure; they are thus the true beneficiaries of systemic adjuvant therapy (and represent the difference between the curves in Figure 3.25).

Group C had no metastases at presentation and do not benefit from systemic therapy since they would have survived anyway.

Table 3.10 also summarizes the relative size of the groups for both node positive and negative patients. Adjuvant systemic therapy can significantly improve the outlook for patients with breast cancer and has probably contributed to the recent improvement in survival. Nevertheless, most patients will not derive personal benefit from it and it is important to balance the morbidity of treatment (for all) against the benefit (for a minority).

Endocrine therapy

Tamoxifen

Tamoxifen is a steroidal drug which acts predominantly as as antioestrogen blocking oestrogen receptor alpha receptors and is the most widely used adjuvant systemic therapy. The EBCTCG (1998a) overview confirms that it reduces the odds of recurrence by about 25% and of death by about 17%, which translates to an absolute survival benefit of about 6% at 10 years (but more for node positive and less for node negative patients). This effect is largely confined to patients with oestrogen receptor positive tumours (or possibly oestrogen receptor and/or progesterone receptor positive tumours) and

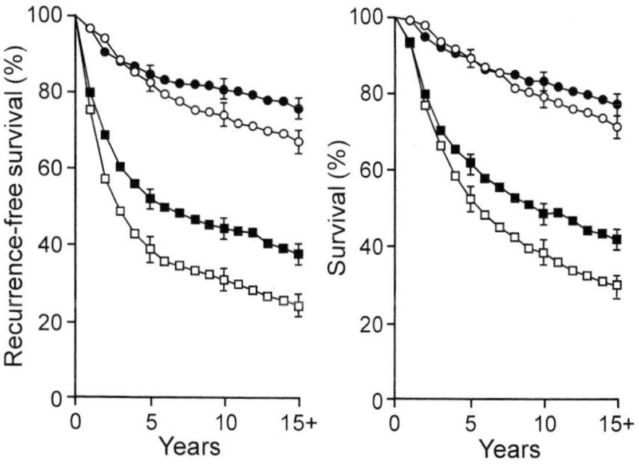

Figure 3.25 Effects of ovarian ablation alone in breast cancer. Left-hand figure: recurrence free survival for node negative women <50 years (upper pair of curves) demonstrating improved survival for women who had ovarian ablation (top line) versus controls (second line); for node positive women <50 years (lower pair of curves) better survival for patients who received ovarian ablation (third line down) versus control (bottom line). Right-hand figure: overall survival for node positive women <50 years (upper pair of curves) demonstrating improved survival for women who had ovarian ablation (top line) versus controls (second line); for node positive women <50 years (lower pair of curves) better survival for patients who received ovarian ablation (third line down) versus control (bottom line).

Table 3.10 Relative benefit of ovarian ablation on survival (see text)

Group	*A*	*B*	*C*	*Total*
Node negative	24%	6%	70%	100%
Node positive	58%	13%	29%	100%
Occult metastases	Resistant	Sensitive	None	

is seen in all age groups, both premenopausal and postmenopausal patients, independent of node status and chemotherapy. In addition, tamoxifen reduces the risk of contralateral breast cancer by up to 50%. Studies have shown a clear benefit in taking tamoxifen 20 mg/day for at least 2 years and preferably up to 5 years, but any longer is the subject of ongoing evaluation. Tamoxifen is generally well tolerated, but 40% of women complain of symptomatic side-effects including hot flushes, weight gain, gastrointestinal upset, loss of libido and vaginal dryness or discharge. Hot flushes may be relieved using clonidine, megestrol acetate (20 mg bd) or fluoxetine; the role of HRT in women who have had breast cancer is currently the basis of clinical trials. For postmenopausal women, tamoxifen also functions as an oestrogen agonist on non-breast tissue, gives some protection against osteoporosis and reduces blood cholesterol. It is, however, associated with a small increased risk of venous thrombotic disease; long-term use is associated with endometrial hyperplasia (occasionally progressing to endometrial cancer, hence vaginal bleeding should be investigated) and retinal changes have been reported. Despite these potential hazards (which are of particular importance to the chemoprevention of breast cancer using tamoxifen), it is important to remember that tamoxifen is associated with a reduction in overall mortality for patients with breast cancer.

Treatment of elderly women

Elderly fit patients (>70 years) who comprise 40% of women with potentially operable tumours have in the past been managed with tamoxifen alone. Although there is no adverse effect on survival, two randomized controlled trials have shown that tamoxifen alone is associated with a higher rate of local recurrence than surgery and adjuvant tamoxifen. Thus, elderly patients with potentially operable tumours able to undergo surgery should be managed in the same way as younger women, rather than by giving tamoxifen as sole therapy. Some elderly women with larger cancers or inoperable disease which express oestrogen receptor may respond to neoadjuvant tamoxifen to render the tumour operable with the response rate of 75% in oestrogen receptor positive patients similar to that of neoadjuvant chemotherapy.

Ovarian ablation

Ovarian ablation reduces the odds of recurrence by 25% and of death by 24% (a similar order of improvement to that achieved by polychemotherapy; EBCTCG, 1998b) but is only of benefit to premenopausal women. Many of the trials of ovarian ablation were carried out before hormone receptor status was measured, but more recent studies suggest that the benefit is largely confined to women with hormone receptor positive tumours. Ovarian ablation can be performed either surgically (and increasingly laparoscopically), by a short course (usually four fractions) of low-dose radiotherapy to the pelvis ('radiation menopause') or medically using a gonadotrophin analogue (usually given as a monthly subcutaneous injection into the abdominal wall). The optimal duration of 'medical oophorectomy' has not been established but has generally been 2–5 years. All methods seem to work, though there are few comparative data on them. The main side-effects of all of them are those of a menopause – flushes, sweats, mood changes, etc., often worse than a physiological menopause, because the artificial menopause is precipitate.

Other hormonal agents

No other hormonal agents are of established benefit when used in the adjuvant setting, although some of the newer aromatase inhibitors (letrozole, anastrozole, exemestane) are the subject of ongoing trials.

Cytotoxic chemotherapy

The EBCTCG overview (1998b), confirms that chemotherapy can reduce the odds of recurrence by 28% and of death by 17%, translating to an absolute survival benefit of about 6% at 10 years. As for endocrine therapy, the proportional benefit was seen for both node positive and negative disease, but the absolute benefit was greater for women with positive nodes. The benefit of chemotherapy, however, declines with age. The reduction in the odds of death is 27% for patients aged <50 years, 14% for those aged 50–59 years, 8% for those aged 60–69 years and there are inadequate data for women aged >70 years. Thus, the absolute survival benefit at 10 years for node positive women aged <50 years is 11%, but for node positive women aged 50–59 years it is only 3%. Chemotherapy seems to be of benefit to patients with both oestrogen receptor positive and negative tumours.

Historically, since a combination of drugs is more effective than one alone and a prolonged course more effective than a single dose, the standard regimen was a combination of cyclophosphamide, methotrexate and 5-fluorouracil (CMF) giving a total of six cycles. More recent studies have incorporated an anthracycline (usually adriamycin or epirubicin), and the overview shows that these drugs can produce a further reduction in the odds of recurrence or death (compared with CMF) of about 11–12%, which translates to an absolute survival gain of about 2–3%. These studies were mostly on patients aged <50 years, so caution should be exercised in applying these findings to older patients. However, they suggest an anthracycline-based regimen should be considered for women at high risk of disease relapse where four cycles of doxorubicin and cyclophosphamide may be as effective as six cycles of CMF. The addition of newer agents, such as taxanes and vinorelbine, may confer additional survival benefit in patients with node positive disease and these are the subject of clinical trials.

The side-effects of chemotherapy are acute and chronic. The main acute ones are fatigue/lethargy, nausea and vomiting (usually well controlled with 5-HT_3 antagonist anti-emetics), alopecia (uncommon with CMF, nearly invariable with anthracyclines but may be reduced by scalp cooling) and neutropenia. The latter is the main acute medical hazard since neutropenic sepsis can supervene rapidly and patients should always be warned to seek prompt medical assistance (intravenous antibiotics and fluids) for what may initially appear as a minor 'flu-like illness. Chemotherapy can induce cessation of menses, which especially for women over 40 years may be permanent; thus premenopausal patients should always be warned of the risk of an early menopause and loss of fertility with chemotherapy. Conversely, premenopausal patients should be warned to avoid conception, since all chemotherapy drugs are damaging to the fetus. Anthracyclines can cause a cardiomyopathy, though not usually in the doses used in adjuvant regimens; there is the possibility of interaction with radiation and this underlines the need for minimizing the radiation dose to the heart.

Combined adjuvant therapies

For patients with oestrogen receptor/progesterone receptor negative tumours, adding endocrine therapy to chemotherapy will not confer any additional benefit. For patients with oestrogen receptor and/or progesterone receptor positive tumours, however, the evidence is that chemotherapy can add to the benefit of tamoxifen and tamoxifen. Trials are ongoing to quantify this benefit. For ovarian ablation and chemotherapy, there are fewer data; from the trials that there are, ovarian ablation seems to add to the benefit of chemotherapy although by less than the benefit of ovarian ablation alone, possibly because chemotherapy itself may induce ovarian ablation.

Standard treatments

Standard treatments (Table 3.11) are based on risk of disease recurrence which may be calculated using the NPI. In general, low-risk disease = mostly T1/T2, node negative; intermediate/high risk = node positive or node negative; but grade 3 or T3 cancers. Where doubt exists, women should be offered entry into clinical trials.

Neoadjuvant chemotherapy

Neoadjuvant chemotherapy involves giving chemotherapy before surgery to patients with non-metastatic primary breast cancer which is potentially operable. In these cases, the diagnosis should be confirmed by a core biopsy, since a positive FNA does not discriminate between invasive and *in situ* disease. Neo-adjuvant therapy has two potential advantages over adjuvant (postoperative) chemotherapy. Firstly, since the tumour is still in the breast, it is possible to assess whether the tumour (and by implication any occult metastases) is sensitive to the particular regimen used. Secondly, if there is a satisfactory response to chemotherapy, there may be sufficient reduction in the size of the tumour that the surgical approach can be changed (i.e. a mastectomy avoided). A significant clinical response is usually observed in about 70–90% of patients, but a complete pathological response is seen in <15% of patients; tumour progression during treatment is rare. A large NSABP study showed that there was no survival advantage in neoadjuvant over adjuvant chemotherapy, but a higher proportion of the neoadjuvant patients were able to have breast conservation. Neoadjuvant chemotherapy has generally been used in patients with relatively larger tumours – clinical size >3 cm – and should normally be followed by surgery, even when complete clinical response is obtained.

High-dose chemotherapy

High-dose chemotherapy (which may require stem cell rescue) has not yet demonstrated an improvement in survival rate, and indeed carries a mortality of ~1%. It should only be used within the context of clinical trials.

Locally advanced breast tumours

These are defined as primary tumours greater than 5 cm in size (or fixed) or, less often, patients with bulky or fixed axillary lymph nodes. These patients would thus be staged as T3–4, N0–2, M0. As previously mentioned, there is a significant risk of these patients having detectable metastatic disease, and they should be formally staged including bone and liver scans even

Table 3.11 Standard treatments for breast cancer

Premenopausal or perimenopausal women
- Women with low-risk disease should be considered for tamoxifen if ER positive.
- Women with intermediate or high-risk disease who are ER positive should be offered chemotherapy and/or ovarian ablation.
- Women with intermediate or high-risk disease who are ER negative should be offered adjuvant chemotherapy including an anthracycline. Tamoxifen or ovarian ablation is likely to hold no benefit.

Postmenopausal women
- Women with low-risk disease should be considered for tamoxifen if ER positive.
- Women with intermediate or high-risk disease and ER positive tumours should be considered for tamoxifen and/or CMF.
- Women with intermediate or high-risk disease and ER negative tumours should, if fit, be considered for chemotherapy.

if asymptomatic, to confirm the absence of overt metastases.

Some of these patients ('small' T3 tumours, 'localized' T4 tumours) will be operable but for most patients, their initial management will be non-surgical. The diagnosis should be confirmed by core biopsy and the receptor status measured.

Induction therapy

The aim of treatment is to obtain and then maintain local control of the tumour. This is usually best achieved by initial systemic therapy ('induction therapy') and then local surgery or radiotherapy. For patients with hormone sensitive tumours, especially if elderly, initial therapy should be hormonal and tamoxifen is the most widely used. Chemotherapy can also be effective initial management. The response rate is about 70%, although a complete pathological response is only seen in 10–15%, with little evidence that different regimens improve efficacy.

If induction therapy has been effective the patient should proceed to surgery (usually a mastectomy with level III axillary clearance) and then post-operative radiotherapy since they will usually be at high risk of local recurrence. If the tumour remains inoperable after induction therapy, then radiotherapy may be used to try to obtain local control. High-dose local radiotherapy alone has been used in the treatment of locally advanced breast cancer (Figure 3.26), but the local control rate at 5 years is only 20–50% (depending on case selection). Thus induction systemic therapy is recommended first.

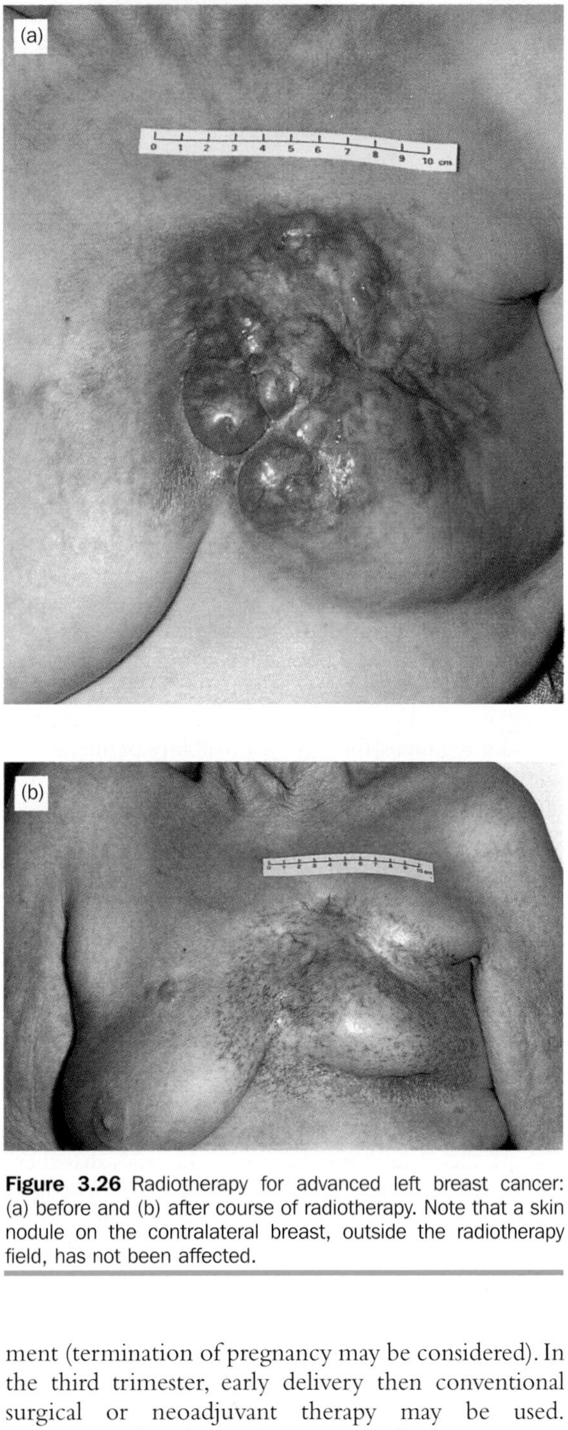

Figure 3.26 Radiotherapy for advanced left breast cancer: (a) before and (b) after course of radiotherapy. Note that a skin nodule on the contralateral breast, outside the radiotherapy field, has not been affected.

Inflammatory breast cancer

This is an aggressive type of locally advanced breast cancer. Clinically, the breast is inflamed and tender; the patient may well have been initially treated with antibiotics. The diagnosis should be confirmed by core biopsy, although this may need more than one attempt, since the inflammatory reaction within the breast may make it difficult to obtain a positive sample. Inflammatory breast cancer is associated with high morbidity and mortality, a 5 year survival of 50% and only 30% disease free at 10 years.

These tumours do not respond well to hormonal management and because of their rapid growth, should be treated with initial chemotherapy and then subsequent surgery/radiotherapy to achieve the best local control, disease free survival and overall survival.

Intra-arterial chemotherapy has had reported successes in non-trial settings, but carries a risk of mortality and has not been widely taken up.

Breast cancer in pregnancy

About 1% of breast cancers occur during pregnancy or lactation, and are thus diagnosed in 1:10 000 pregnancies. The difficulties of detecting a lump in the enlarging breast result in later detection (two-thirds have nodal metastasis). In the first 6 months of pregnancy, mastectomy and clearance form the mainstay of treatment (termination of pregnancy may be considered). In the third trimester, early delivery then conventional surgical or neoadjuvant therapy may be used. Pregnancy after diagnosis/treatment for breast cancer does not appear to reduce survival.

Patients who are unfit for surgery

These will generally be elderly patients and because of their co-morbidity, the principles of their management will be closer to those applicable to metastatic disease than operable breast cancer. In general, the aim of treatment is to control the primary tumour with the least morbidity, maintaining quality of life, so tamoxifen is usually the most appropriate therapy.

Radiotherapy alone is not recommended for local control of advanced tumours, although local control rates of 20–40% at 5 years may be obtained in selected cases after using at least 60 Gy conventionally fractionated.

Section 3.8 • Local recurrence

Local recurrence is defined as recurrence in the treated breast or chest wall, axilla and previously the ipsilateral supraclavicular fossa, although the latter is now regarded as a distant relapse.

Relapse in the chest wall, axilla or supraclavicular fossa (Figure 3.27) is usually found clinically, 80% occur within 2 years and most occur within 5 years of initial surgery; it is frequently a harbinger of distant spread. Distant metastases will be found at the time of local relapse in about 20% of patients and about a further 70% will develop distant metastases within 5–10 years. Local relapse should be confirmed histologically, by either FNAC or biopsy. Patients with local relapse should be restaged (full blood count, plasma viscosity, blood biochemistry, chest X-ray, bone and liver scans), and those with distant metastases managed appropriately (page 88).

For patients with apparently isolated local recurrence, the best predictor of prognosis is the disease-free interval (time from initial treatment to local relapse) – the longer the interval the better the prognosis.

Management of local recurrence

Local recurrence may be classified as single spot relapse, multiple spot relapse or a field change.

The aim of treatment is to regain local control – uncontrolled local disease is miserable for the patient and difficult to manage. The management strategy will be determined by the previous treatment, the site of recurrence, its operability and hormone receptor status. The patient should be assessed jointly by the surgeon and oncologist and treatment individualized. In general, recurrence in the chest wall or axilla should be removed surgically if feasible, as it usually is for single spot or sometimes multiple spot recurrence. This may be easier if it is first reduced in extent by systemic therapy (hormone therapy or chemotherapy) and, if not previously used, radiotherapy which should be employed for field change recurrence. Systemic therapy should be reviewed and may be changed depending on the patient's condition, previous systemic adjuvant therapy and the hormone receptor status of the tumour. Intra-arterial chemotherapy, infusional 5-fluorouracil or photodynamic therapy have all been used to try to achieve local control. Tissue necrosis with infection may become a significant problem requiring topical metronidazole gel, charcoal dressings or oral antibiotics. Confirmed progression of local disease recurrence often causes troublesome bleeding and may progress to carcinoma 'en cuirasse' encircling and constricting the chest wall.

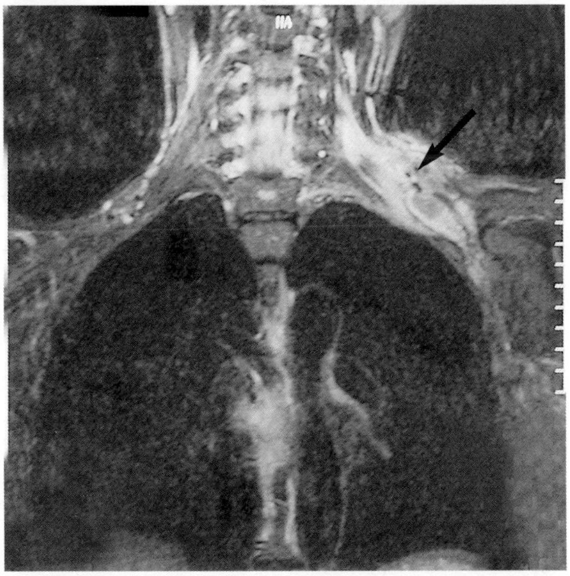

Figure 3.27 Supraclavicular fossa disease on MRI surrounding and infiltrating the left brachial plexus.

Local recurrence in the treated breast

Unlike recurrence after mastectomy, recurrence in the conserved breast occurs at a more constant rate (approximately 1%/annum), and is much less commonly associated with distant relapse. It is usually detected clinically and/or mammographically. Further surgery (most commonly mastectomy) is recommended and after this, the patient may have no further recurrence.

Section 3.9 • Metastatic disease

About 8% of patients have distant metastases at first presentation, but most patients with distant metastases will have been previously treated for breast cancer that was apparently localized to the breast and the axillary lymph nodes some time previously.

Patients with metastatic breast cancer are incurable. Treatment is therefore palliative, the aim being to relieve symptoms and maintain the best quality of life. Median survival after the diagnosis of metastatic breast cancer is about 2 years, but there is a 'tail' of patients who survive for 5–10 years. Thus, management varies from the treatment of a patient with a rapidly fatal cancer to the management of what is a chronic, albeit serious, disease.

For the patient with metastatic disease, proper working of the multidisciplinary team is crucial. Her needs will vary over time and she will need access to a wide variety of disciplines. Most patients will be primarily under the care of their family doctor and the practice team, and the secondary sector should aim to support the GP so the patient has prompt access to surgeon, oncologist, orthopaedic specialist and palliative care team at the appropriate times.

The presentation of the patient with metastases are legion, but among the commonest sites are bone (Figure 3.13) with pain or fracture, pleura (effusion causing dyspnoea; Figure 3.28), liver (lethargy, nausea, anorexia), peritoneal cavity (ascites causing abdominal distension) (Figure 3.29), lung (dyspnoea, dry cough) supraclavicular fossa/cervical nodes (Figure 3.27), spine (Figure 3.30), brain (headaches, imbalance, fits) and marrow (lethargy, infections, anaemia). Whatever the site of initial metastasis, patients should be staged to assess the extent of metastatic spread, by at least a full blood count, biochemistry (including bone and liver chemistry), isotope bone scan, X-ray of chest and a liver scan (CT or ultrasound); tumour markers (CEA, CA15-3) can be used to monitor the disease.

In general, the patient presenting with visceral metastases (e.g. liver, lymphangitis carcinomatosis of lung) will have aggressive, usually hormone insensitive, disease with a poor prognosis, whereas relapse in soft tissue, pleura and/or bone is associated with a survival measured in many months or years (and often hormone sensitive disease).

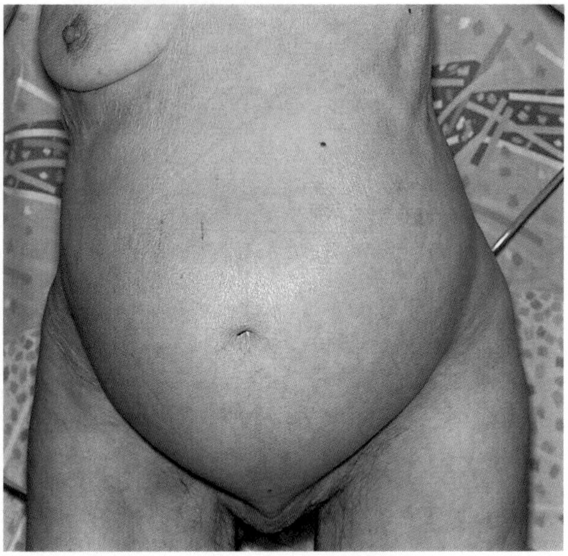

Figure 3.29 Gross ascites from metastatic breast cancer; previous left mastectomy.

Principles of treatment

Since there is no evidence that treating asymptomatic metastases alters survival, treatment is aimed at symptom control and can be considered as:

- Control of specific symptoms.
- Systemic therapy to control the disease.
- Local therapies for local symptoms.

Symptom control

Symptom control should be used in combination and comprise analgesic regimens including non-steroidal

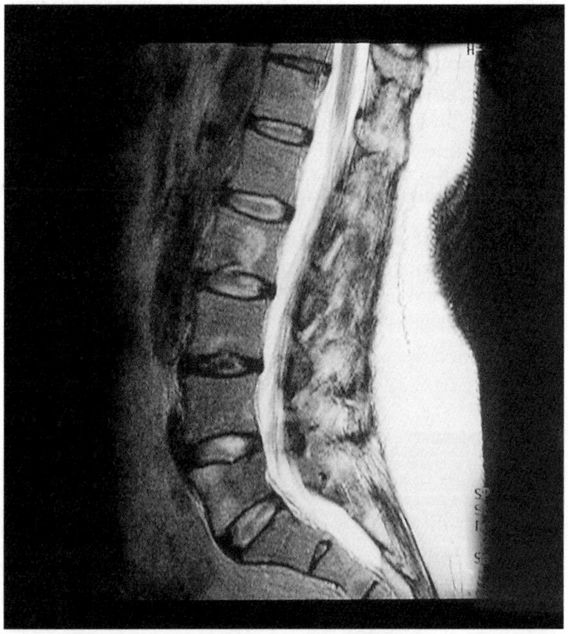

Figure 3.30 Spinal metastases of L2 and L5 on MRI scan.

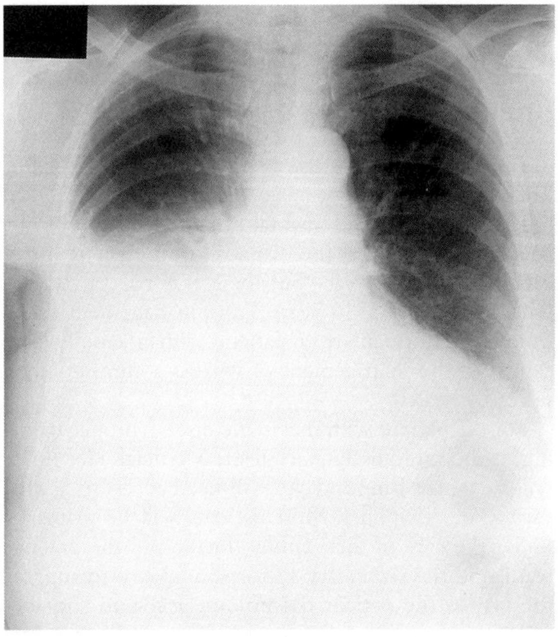

Figure 3.28 Pleural effusion from secondary breast cancer.

anti-inflammatory drugs, opioid drugs, amitriptyline/carbamazepine/gabapentin, transcutaneous electrical nerve stimulation and psychological control techniques.

Hypercalcaemia often presents as non-specific deterioration of health, confusion, abdominal symptoms, dehydration and ultimately renal failure and coma. Rehydration (oral, IVI), bisphosphonates and therapy against the underlying cancer is required.

Systemic therapy

Since metastatic breast cancer is a systemic disease, the best way to control it is with effective systemic therapy.

In general, hormone therapy is considered as first line therapy, since it is less toxic than cytotoxic chemotherapy. The best predictor of response to hormone therapy is the hormone receptor status of the primary tumour. A positive oestrogen receptor status is associated with response in about 60% of patients, whereas a negative status is associated with response in <10%; response to second line endocrine treatment is half that seen to first line treatment. Thus patients with oestrogen receptor positive tumours will normally be treated hormonally in the first instance, unless they have advanced visceral metastases (e.g. liver), when the response to hormonal therapy is low and the delay in waiting for a hormonal response may compromise the patient's survival. Such patients should normally be considered for chemotherapy. Patients with oestrogen receptor negative tumours should be considered for chemotherapy only since hormonal therapy is unlikely to help them; a balance must be struck between achieving response and limiting side-effects. Response in ~50% patients (again with response to second line treatments half of this) may achieve control for 6–10 months.

Choice of hormonal therapy

The hormonal measures available are:

- ovarian ablation (medical or surgical) (for premenopausal patients)
- anti-oestrogens, of which the most established is tamoxifen
- aromatase inhibitors (for post-menopausal women). Examples are the non-steroidal such as anastrozole and letrozole and steroidal such as formestane and exemestane. Non-selective drugs such as aminoglutethamide are no longer prescribed
- progestagens, e.g. megesterol acetate and medroxypregesterone acetate
- surgical adrenalectomy and surgical pituitary ablation (using a yttrium screw) are no longer practised as they have been surpassed by pharmaceutical developments.

The choice of hormonal agent will be determined by menopausal status and any previous adjuvant hormonal therapy. Response to hormone therapy may take some time to become apparent, and should not be assessed before about 6-8 weeks. A good response to first time hormone therapy predicts that about half of such patients will respond to second line hormonal therapy, so therapies can be used in sequence. There is no evidence that combining hormone and chemotherapy is better than the same agents used sequentially. Progesterone or, increasingly, aromatase inhibitors (which may be superior in terms of morbidity and survival to progesterones) are used as second line therapy.

Choice of chemotherapy

Chemotherapy will normally be used for patients with hormone receptor negative disease, advanced visceral disease or on failure of hormone therapy. Generally, chemotherapy drugs are more effective used in combinations (e.g. CMF) than as single agents, and the highest response rates are seen with combinations containing an anthracycline (e.g. adriamycin or epirubicin), though increased response does not seem to translate into a survival advantage. The choice of drugs will be determined by any previous adjuvant chemotherapy, the sites of disease and the acceptable toxicities for that patient. Chemotherapy should always be given under the supervision of an experienced oncologist and by a specialist team.

Newer agents

Taxanes may be effective against anthracycline resistant disease with a response rate of ~30%; vinorelbine has some activity as a second line drug. Immunotherapy with trastuzumab antibody to erbB-2 oncogene (expressed in up to 25% of invasive cancers) may become increasingly used but can have cardiotoxicity.

Bisphosphonates

These are drugs that are of established value in the treatment (and prevention) of malignant hypercalcaemia, but there are also good data from trials that given regularly, they can reduce the morbidity of bony metastatic disease (Figure 3.13) (less pain, fewer pathological fractures). They can be given either as a monthly intravenous injection or as a single daily oral dose. Their role in the prophylaxis of bone metastasis is currently under study.

Local therapies

Patients need careful assessment of their symptoms and many may be helped by appropriate local therapies. Examples would include:

- Drainage of pleural effusions (Figure 3.28) ± instillation of bleomycin as a tumoricidal and pleuradhesis agent.
- Drainage of ascites (Figure 3.29).
- Surgical stabilization of sites of bony weakness due to metastases – most commonly in the long bones. Prophylactic fixation is preferred, but some patients will need fixation following pathological fracture.
- Palliative radiotherapy, most commonly for painful bony metastases (Figure 3.30). A single fraction of 7–8 Gy will give substantial pain relief in 80% of patients but will not be effective if there is mechanical pain. NSAIDs may confer additional benefit.
- Spinal cord compression. This is an oncological emergency and patients require rapid neurosurgical/radiotherapy assessment, usually following an urgent MRI scan to show the nature and level of the block(s) within the spinal canal.
- Brain metastases. High-dose cortisteroids (4 mg qid dexamethasone) to reduce oedema followed by radiotherapy are usually employed. Local excision + radiotherapy can be effective for single metastases depending on the site.
- Photodynamic therapy for extensive chest wall disease previously treated by conventional modalities.

Section 3.10 • Male breast cancer

The incidence of male breast cancer increases with age but still accounts for less than 1% of breast cancers. For example, in Scotland it accounted for only 18 of 3168 registrations in 1995 and in the USA the death of only one in a million men.

Risk factors include Klinefelter's syndrome (testicular atrophy and insufficiency, gynaecomastia) where the ratio of oestrogen to androgen is elevated and increases the risk of breast cancer some 20 times. BRCA2 mutation in breast cancer families is associated with breast cancer in male members of the families and hence screening male relatives in such families may be justified. p53 gene mutations have been identified in 40% of male breast cancers.

Presentation is as a palpable, painless, firm lump which is often eccentric to the nipple and fixed to the chest wall and skin (Figure 3.31).There may be erythema progressing to ulceration through the skin, nipple retraction or a bloody nipple discharge.

Diagnosis

As for female breast cancer diagnosis is by triple assessment: clinical examination, mammography and FNAC allow the distinction between gynaecomastia and male breast cancer. Staging should include full blood count, blood biochemistry, chest radiograph, liver ultrasound and bone scan.

Histologically, most male breast cancer is ductal; DCIS accounts for 10%; lobular cancer and special types are comparatively rare.

Treatment

Modified radical mastectomy, or radical mastectomy if the pectoralis major muscle is directly infiltrated by breast cancer, accompanied by axillary node clearance is the standard treatment even for advanced disease (T4) involving the skin or underlying chest wall muscle. Radiotherapy is based on data from female breast cancer, and used to assist local disease control together with surgery.

While the use of adjuvant endocrine or chemotherapy has not been the subject of the major clinical trials undertaken for female breast cancer, 65–85% of male breast cancer is oestrogen receptor positive and 67% progesterone receptor positive. Not surprisingly, endocrine therapy can be effective: orchidectomy (medical or surgical), tamoxifen (with a 70% response rate) and as second line therapy cyproterone acetate or LHRH analogues have largely replaced oestrogens as therapy. CMF or anthracycline-based chemotherapy as for female breast cancer is used both adjuvantly and palliatively.

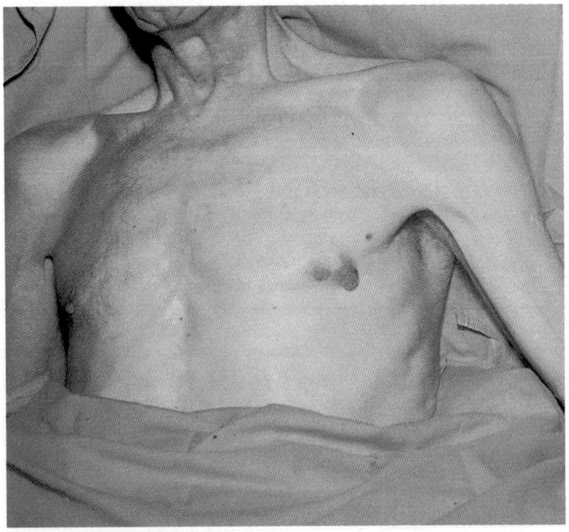

Figure 3.31 Male breast cancer (T4 disease).

Section 3.11 • Follow-up

Most patients with breast cancer will complete their primary treatment (surgery, radiotherapy, chemotherapy, etc.) and return to the community. Traditionally, they have then been followed up in the hospital outpatient department. The aim of follow-up is to detect local recurrence (when treatable) or contralateral disease. For those patients with established metastatic disease and/or uncontrolled local disease, continued follow-up is appropriate since they are likely to need ongoing care tailored to the pace of the disease and the patient's needs. For those patients who are apparently disease free, the purpose of follow-up is less clear but includes detection of local disease recurrence or detection of a second, contralateral cancer or metastatic disease, assessment of treatment morbidity or may simply provide reassurance.

Some patients find regular follow-up reassuring but others find it stressful. The optimal frequency and length of follow-up is not defined. It is, however, important that there is a strategy of care agreed between the patient, the GP and the hospital, so that the appropriate care can be offered to the patient should any problems develop.

Detection of distant metastases

Metastatic relapse will present unpredictably and usually between clinic visits. Routine screening for metastases by regular scans, X-rays, etc., in patients who are asymptomatic does not improve survival. Thus, investigations for metastases should be restricted to patients with symptoms suggestive of metastatic relapse.

Detection of local recurrence

Relapse in the chest wall after mastectomy or in the axilla or supraclavicular fossa is usually detected clinically. Local recurrence after conservation occurs at a constant rate each year, hence follow-up should be continued to 10 years. Following mastectomy the risk of local recurrence is greatest in the first 2 years and decreases thereafter. Follow-up may be discontinued, if disease free, at 5 years. Whilst these relapses may be found at a routine hospital visit, they may also be found by the patient between visits. It is important that the patient can be referred back promptly to the clinic.

Relapse in the treated breast (following conservation treatment) may be found clinically or on follow-up mammography. The latter is therefore recommended every 1–2 years.

Relapse in the contralateral breast
Breast cancer in one breast is associated with a ~1% per annum increased risk of developing cancer in the contralateral breast. The other breast should therefore be examined at each visit and a mammogram performed every 1–2 years.

Morbidity of therapy

Follow-up is also the opportunity to assess the morbidity of treatment, especially complications such as lymphoedema and breast oedema.

Other considerations

Arm mobility
Women with breast cancer may develop arm stiffness directly related to their surgery and radiotherapy. Women undergoing breast and/or axillary surgery need shoulder exercises to enable them to recover a full range of arm and shoulder mobility.

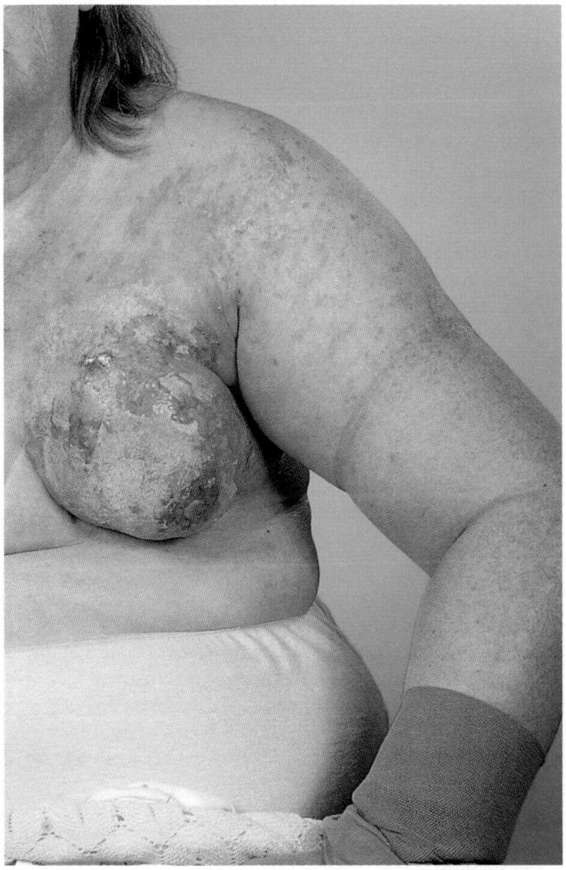

Figure 3.32 Lymphoedema of the left upper limb secondary to advanced breast cancer with chest wall disease and infiltration of the axilla. Note the armlet to symptomatically treat the lymphoedema.

Lymphoedema
Lymphoedema of the arm may occur in women with breast cancer due to lymphatic damage caused by surgery and/or radiotherapy, or because of obstruction caused by local tumour (Figure 3.32). Thus, all patients undergoing surgery and/or radiotherapy treatment to the axilla should receive pre-treatment information on lymphoedema. The incidence of lymphoedema has been cited at between 5 and 38%, depending on treatment combinations. Although there is currently no cure for lymphoedema, it is possible to reduce the size of the arm. The most effective management and maintenance comprises multimodal physical therapy (skin care, external support, exercise, massage) and education. Diuretics or pneumatic compression pumps should not be relied upon. Lymphoedema should be treated at the first sign of swelling when management will be more effective. The lymphoedematous arm is prone to streptococcal infection after minor injury (e.g. gardening); patients should be instructed to seek medical attention, including antibiotics, at the first signs of infection (tenderness, redness, increased swelling, pain on movement of the limb).

Menopausal symptoms
Menopausal symptoms are beginning to be recognized as an issue for women with breast cancer.

Many women who receive treatment for breast cancer subsequently experience menopausal symptoms, either as a result of their adjuvant treatment, or as a natural process. The average age at menopause is 50 years, but in 25% of women who develop breast cancer premenopausally and undergo adjuvant treatment, it is 10 years earlier. Although HRT is widely advocated for the treatment of menopausal symptoms, its use in women with a personal or family history of breast cancer remains controversial, and alternative methods of coping with menopause have not yet been fully explored. Some studies show progestogens such as megestrol acetate and soya protein are useful in all eviating menopausal symptoms. (See also section on tamoxifen, page 83.)

Women should be informed regarding the potential effect of cancer treatment on their menopausal status, and advised regarding non-oestrogen alternatives and self-care strategies which might alleviate their symptoms.

Prostheses
External breast prostheses are the most common method of restoring breast symmetry following surgery, and a wide variety of shapes and sizes are available. A soft temporary breast prosthesis should be fitted before hospital discharge, and a permanent prosthesis should be fitted either 6–8 weeks post-operatively (or when the wound is fully healed), or following completion of radiotherapy once any skin reaction has resolved. Women should also be given advice on bras, swimwear and replacement prostheses.

Psychological considerations
Women (and men) with breast symptoms may suffer considerable emotional distress, even once a benign diagnosis is made.

Breast cancer is a high-profile disease the progression and treatment of which results in substantial physical and psychological morbidity.

To participate effectively in decision making, women and their families need to receive adequate information and sufficient time to discuss treatment options. Breast care nurses and voluntary sector organizations can provide verbal, written and multimedia information. Studies of the physical impact of screening and genetic counselling appear to be reassuring. There is no clear evidence that mastectomy and breast conservation differ in terms of clinically significant anxiety or depression; some studies have found that breast conservation is associated with fewer problems related to body image, although conservation may carry an increased risk of worrying about recurrence. Hence some women choose mastectomy although not all women wish to share in the decision making. Significant numbers of women develop psychological problems after anti-cancer therapy treatment and some require formal treatment. Psychological factors may influence the course of malignant disease but can certainly be harnessed to combat the side-effects of treatment, particularly chemotherapy. Disease recurrence is associated with increased psychological morbidity; formal psychological interventions can be used successfully should it occur.

Acknowledgements
The authors thank Mr J. H. Stevenson (Figures 3.19, 3.20, 3.21), Dr C. Purdie (Figure 3.2b, 3.12, 3.14, 3.15, 3.16), Mr D. C. Brown (Figures 3.24) and Dr D. McLean (Figures 3.3, 3.11, 3.22) for permission to use clinical slides.

Further reading

Bates, T. *et al.* (1991). Breast cancer in elderly women: a Cancer Research Campaign trial comparing treatment with tamoxifen and optimal surgery with tamoxifen alone. *Br J Surg* **78**: 591–4.

Blamey, R. W. (1996). The design and clinical use of Nottingham Prognostic Index in breast cancer. *Breast* **5**: 156–7.

Breast Specialty Group of the British Association of Surgical Oncology (1999). The management of metastatic bone disease in the United Kingdom. A BASO guideline. *Eur J Surg Oncol* **25**: 3–23.

Collaborative Group on Hormonal Factors in Breast Cancer (1997). Breast cancer and hormone replacement therapy: collaborative reanalysis of data from 51 epidemiological studies of 52705 women with breast cancer and 108411 women without breast cancer. *Lancet* **350**: 1047–59.

Dixon, J. M. and Thompson, A. M. (1991). Effective surgical treatment for mammary duct fistula. *Br J Surg* **78**: 1185–6.

Dixon, J. M. *et al.* (1984). Fine needle aspiration cytology in relationship to clinical examination and mammography in the diagnosis of a solid breast mass. *Br J Surg* **71**: 593–6.

Early Breast Cancer Trialists' Collaborative Group (1996). Ovarian ablation in early breast cancer: overview of the randomised trials. *Lancet* **348**: 1189–96.

Early Breast Cancer Trialists' Collaborative Group (1998a). Tamoxifen for early breast cancer: an overview of the randomised trials. *Lancet* **351**: 1461–7.

Early Breast Cancer Trialists' Collaborative Group (1998b). Polychemotherapy for early breast cancer: an overview of the randomised trials. *Lancet* **352**: 930–42.

Early Breast Cancer Trialists' Collaborative Group (2000). Favourable and unfavourable effects on long-term survival of radiotherapy for early breast cancer: an overview of the randomised trials. *Lancet* **355**: 1757–70.

Fisher, B. *et al.* (1995). Reanalysis and results after 12 years of follow-up in a randomised clinical trial comparing total mastectomy with lumpectomy with or without irradiation in the treatment of breast cancer. *N Engl J Med* **333**: 1456–61.

Fisher, B. *et al.* (1997). Effect of preoperative chemotherapy on local-regional disease in women with operable breast cancer: findings from the National Surgical Adjuvant Breast and Bowel Project B-18. *J Clin Oncol* **15**: 2483–93.

Fisher, B. *et al.* (1998). Tamoxifen for the prevention of breast cancer: report of the National Surgical Adjuvant Breast and Bowel Project P-1 study. *J Natl Cancer Inst* **90**: 1371.

Gillis, C. R. and Hole, D. J. (1996). Survival outcome of care by specialist surgeons in the west of Scotland: a study of 3786 patients in the west of Scotland. *BMJ* **312**: 145–8.

GIVIO Investigators (1994). Impact of follow-up testing on survival and health-related quality of life in breast cancer patients: a multi-centre randomized controlled trial. *JAMA* **271**: 1587–92.

Hendrick, R. E. *et al.* (1997) Benefit of screening mammography in women aged 40–49: a new meta-analysis of randomised controlled trials. *Monogr Natl Cancer Inst* **22**: 87–92.

Hermansen, C. *et al.* (1987). Diagnostic reliability of combined physical examination, mammography and fine-needle puncture ('triple-test') in breast tumours. A prospective study. *Cancer* **60**: 1866–71.

Information and Statistics Division. Scottish Health Statistics (1997). Edinburgh ISD NHS in Scotland 1998.

Koscielny, S. *et al.* (1984). Breast cancer: relationship between the size of the primary tumour and the probability of metastatic dissemination. *Br J Cancer* **49**: 709–15.

McIntosh, S. A. and Purushotham, A. D. (1998). Lymphatic mapping and sentinel node biopsy in breast cancer. *Br J Surg* **85**: 1347–56.

Macmillan, R. D. (2000). Screening women with a family history of breast cancer – results from the British Familial Breast Cancer Group. *Eur J Surg Oncol* **26**: 149–52.

Overgaard, M. *et al.* (1997). Postoperative radiotherapy in high-risk premenopausal women with breast cancer who receive adjuvant chemotherapy. *N Engl J Med* **337**: 949–55.

Overgaard, M. *et al.* (1999) Postoperative radiotherapy in high-risk post-menopausal breast cancer patients given adjuvant tamoxifen. *Lancet* **353**: 1641–8.

Pain, S. J. and Purushotham, A. D. (2000). Lymphoedema following surgery for breast cancer. *Br J Surg* **87**: 1128–41.

Robertson, J. F. R. *et al.* (1999). The objective measurement of remission and progression in metastatic breast cancer by the use of serum tumour markers. *Eur J Cancer* **35**: 47–53.

Rosselli Del Turco M. *et al.* (1994). Intensive diagnostic follow-up after treatment of primary breast cancer: a randomized trial. National Research Council Project on Breast Cancer follow up. *JAMA* **271**: 1593–7.

Silverstein, M. J. (1998). Ductal carcinoma in situ of the breast. *BMJ* **317**: 734–9.

Slamon, D. J. and Clarke, G. M. (1988). Amplification of c-erbB-2 and aggressive human breast tumours. *Science* **240**: 1795–8.

Steele, R. J. C. *et al.* (1985). The efficacy of lower axillary sampling in obtaining lymph node status in breast cancer: a controlled randomised trial. *Br J Surg* **72**: 368–9.

Thompson, A. M. (1999). Axillary node clearance for breast cancer. *J R Coll Surg Edin* **44**: 111–17.

Veronesi, U. *et al.* (1993). Prognostic significance of number and level of axillary node metastases in breast cancer. *Breast* **2**: 224–8.

Ziyaie, D. *et al.* (2000). p53 and breast cancer. *Breast* **9**: 239–46.

MODULE 4a

Disorders of the thyroid gland

Section 4a.1 • Thyroid embryology, anatomy and physiology

Thyroid embryology

The thyroid is principally of **endodermal** origin, and is derived from the floor of the pharynx between the tuberculum impar (the medial swelling of the tongue) and the cupola. The thyroid migrates down the neck in front of the hyoid bone and thyroid cartilage, and remains connected to the tongue (at a point called the foramen caecum, located at the junction of the anterior and posterior tongue) by the thyroglossal duct. The duct normally closes at around the fifth week, and the only remnant is the foramen caecum. A portion of the duct may, however, persist (a thyroglossal cyst) or occasionally, a portion of the thyroid may become detached and arrest at any point along the thyroglossal duct (ectopic thyroid). Papillary carcinoma of the thyroid may develop in an ectopic thyroid gland. Complete failure of descent may result in a lingual thyroid, at the back of the tongue. The thyroid is in its normal position just inferior to the cricoid cartilage by the seventh week. Follicles appear and the thyroid begins to secrete hormones by the twelfth week, one of the first organs to do so. The thyroid also has a **neural** crest origin from the ultimobranchial body, which is derived from the fifth pharyngeal pouch (which in turn is usually considered to be a part of the fourth pharyngeal pouch). The ultimobranchial body becomes incorporated into the lateral portion of the thyroid, which can persist as a small nodule on the lateral aspect of the thyroid lobe (the tubercle of Zuckerkandl). The ultimobranchial body gives rise to the parafollicular cells, which secrete calcitonin. Hence, the thyroid gland is derived from both the primitive pharynx (the follicular cells) and the neural crest (the parafollicular cells).

Surgical anatomy of the thyroid gland

The thyroid is a highly vascular gland, weighing about 15 g, and consists of two lobes, united in the midline by the isthmus, which overlies the second and third tracheal rings. There may also be a pyramidal lobe present, superior to the isthmus and often to the left of the median plane. This is present in 50% of cases and is the remnant of the thyroglossal tract. A fibrous capsule, which septates into the gland, surrounds the thyroid. This capsule is enveloped by the visceral layer of the pre-tracheal cervical fascia. Posteriorly, the gland is attached to the cricoid cartilage and the superior tracheal rings by dense connective tissue (Berry's ligament). This attachment of the thyroid to the trachea causes the thyroid to move on swallowing, which helps distinguish thyroid nodules from other causes of lumps in the neck.

The arterial supply is from the superior and inferior thyroid arteries, which lie in the plane between the thyroid capsule and the pre-tracheal fascia. The superior thyroid artery originates from the external carotid artery and divides into an anterior and posterior branch at the superior pole of the thyroid. The external branch of the superior laryngeal nerve has an intimate relationship with the superior thyroid artery as it overlies the cricothyroid in 20% of cases (in a further 20% of cases the nerve passes deep to cricothyroid and is therefore not routinely seen at operation). Care must be taken to ligate the superior thyroid artery on the capsule of the thyroid at operation and to avoid damage to the nerve when applying diathermy to the small branches of the superior thyroid artery to the posterior constrictor and cricothyroid. Damage to the superior laryngeal nerve results in paralysis of the cricothyroid muscle. The inferior thyroid artery originates from the thyrocervical trunk, which in turn is from the first part of the subclavian artery. It enters the thyroid on its lateral aspect and has an intimate relationship with the recurrent laryngeal nerve. On the left, the recurrent laryngeal nerve runs deeper in the tracheo-oesophageal groove and is usually medial to the inferior thyroid artery. On the right, the recurrent laryngeal nerve runs more lateral and has a more intimate relationship to the branches of the inferior thyroid artery. Superiorly, the nerve passes through the posterior portion of Berry's ligament (an area where it is prone to damage) before entering the larynx, usually adjacent to the inferior cornu of the thyroid cartilage. The recurrent laryngeal nerve is the motor supply to the intrinsic muscles of the larynx, with an injury to the nerve causing ipsilateral vocal cord palsy. In about 1% of cases there is a non-recurrent right laryngeal nerve, due to a vascular anomaly in the development of the aortic arches. In 10% of patients there is a thyroidea ima artery, which arises from the brachiocephalic trunk, and passes into the inferior portion of the isthmus.

The venous drainage of the thyroid is by the superior and middle thyroid veins, which drain into the internal jugular and the inferior thyroid veins, which drain into the brachiocephalic vein. The lymphatic drainage of the thyroid is by the pre-laryngeal, pretracheal and paratracheal lymph nodes medially and then to the inferior deep cervical lymph nodes laterally in the carotid sheath.

Thyroid physiology

The thyroid gland consists of two main types of cells – the follicular and parafollicular cells. The follicle is the basic functional unit of the thyroid and consists of a single layer of cuboidal (follicular) cells around a store of colloid. The follicular cells synthesize thyroid hormone in four stages, which include:

- Iodide trapping – iodide is actively transported (ATP dependent) into the thyroid gland. The average daily requirement of iodine is 150 μg, with the normal daily Western dietary intake containing approximately 500 μg.
- Organification – the iodide is oxidized by the enzyme thyroid peroxidase and then combined with tyrosine to form the inactive iodotyrosines: 3-monoiodotyrosine (MIT) and 3,5-diidotyrosine (DIT). The iodotyrosines are incorporated into the soluble protein, thyroglobulin, and are then stored as colloid in the follicular lumen of the thyroid.
- Coupling – the iodotyrosines in the thyroglobulin are then coupled – MIT and DIT to form tri-iodothyronine (T3) and the coupling of DIT and DIT to form thyroxine (T4).
- Release – colloid is taken up by the thyroid cell by endocytosis to form endosomes. The thyroglobulin is then hydrolysed to liberate T4, T3, MIT and DIT. The MIT and DIT are deiodinated and the released iodide is reused by the thyroid cell. The active hormones, T4 and T3, are secreted into the blood.

The vast majority of the released thyroid hormone is in the form of T4 (90%). Most of the T3 (80–90%) is produced by the peripheral conversion of T4, and is much more potent than T4. The metabolic activity of thyroid hormone is determined by the amount of free T3 and free T4. Thyroxine is very highly protein bound in plasma (99.95% bound to thyroid-binding globulin [TBG], transthyretin [TTR] and albumin, with about 0.05% free). When bound, T4 is not physiologically active but provides a storage pool of thyroid hormone, which can last 2–3 months (mean half-life of T4 is 6.5 days). Reverse T3 (rT3) is also produced by the deiodination of T4 – it is not physiologically active and increased levels of rT3 are produced in hyperthyroidism, and periods of excess catabolism (e.g. burns, sepsis).

Peripheral action of thyroid hormone

Thyroid hormones act predominantly via a nuclear thyroid receptor (TR), which modulates gene synthesis of the cell, which can, in turn, increase protein synthesis. T4 is relatively inactive in the periphery, due to a low affinity for TR, whereas there is a high affinity between T3 and TR.

Thyroid hormone regulation

Thyroid stimulating hormone (TSH) is the major regulator of thyroid activity, with increased levels causing hypertrophy of the thyroid. TSH is secreted by the anterior pituitary, and is a glycoprotein with an alpha and beta subunit (the alpha subunit being common to follicle-stimulating hormone (FSH), luteinizing hormone (LH) and human chorionic gonadotropin (hCG)). TSH acts by binding to the TSH receptor on the follicular cell, leading to increased thyroid hormone synthesis, via cAMP. Thyroid releasing hormone (TRH) is the most important positive stimulus to the production of TSH. TRH is produced in the paraventricular nucleus of the hypothalamus and passes through the median eminence to the anterior pituitary via the hypophyseal portal system. T3 has a negative feedback on both the anterior pituitary and the hypothalamus.

Parafollicular cells

The parafollicular, or C cells, secrete calcitonin. Calcitonin is a 32-amino acid peptide that lowers calcium largely by the inhibition of osteoclasts. It is of little physiological importance as there is no disturbance of calcium regulation following thyroidectomy, provided that the parathyroids are preserved. It is a sensitive tumour cell marker for medullary thyroid carcinoma (see differentiated thyroid carcinoma section). Calcitonin also has a role in the treatment of Paget's disease of the bone.

Section 4a.2 • Hypothyroidism

Causes

Hypothyroidism is one of the most common endocrine disorders, with approximately 5% of the female population developing hypothyroidism at some stage in their lives. The vast majority are caused by primary hypothyroidism, with secondary (anterior pituitary gland disorders) and tertiary hypothyroidism (hypothalamic disorders) being rare. Primary hypothyroidism is usually caused by autoimmune thyroiditis (Hashimoto's thyroiditis) (85% of all cases), or by treatment for thyrotoxicosis – by either surgery or radioactive iodine. About 50–70% of patients with thyrotoxicosis treated by subtotal thyroidectomy are hypothyroid at 10 years, related to the remnant size and the degree of lymphocytic infiltration of the thyroid. The use of radioactive iodine in the management of thyrotoxicosis results in 50% of patients developing hypothyroidism in the first year, with 3% per annum subsequent to that. Lifelong follow-up of these patients with TSH assessments is therefore required. External beam radiotherapy to the neck can cause up to 50% of patients to become hypothyroid (usually 2–7 years after treatment). In addition, certain drugs can cause hypothyroidism, including amiodarone and lithium.

Symptoms

Symptoms of hypothyroidism include dry skin (90%), tiredness (70%), cold intolerance, coarse hair, weight gain, hoarseness (unrelated to recurrent laryngeal nerve palsy) and constipation.

Hashimoto's (chronic lymphocytic) thyroiditis

Hashimoto's thyroiditis is an autoimmune disorder with a familial predisposition. Females are more affected (9:1), with the usual age of onset being 40–50 years, although it can occur at any age. The usual clinical presentation is with a painless thyroid enlargement (a firm, rubbery gland); occasionally, the patient may present with pain or pressure in the neck. The gland enlarges due to the lymphocytic infiltrate and areas of focal hyperplasia, caused by TSH stimulation. In the early stages the free T4 and T3 may be normal, with an elevated TSH (so-called compensated hypothyroidism). The patient may also present with thyrotoxicosis (4%), caused by release of thyroxine in the early stage of the disease, before becoming hypothyroid in the long term.

Tests/investigations

These are:

- TSH (with free T4 and T3 if the TSH is suppressed).
- Thyroid antibodies – antimicrosomal antibodies (antithyroid peroxidase) are found in 90% of patients with Hashimoto's thyroiditis, but are not specific as they are also found in 70% of patients with Graves' disease. Antithyroglobulin antibodies are found in 60% of patients and are more specific to Hashimoto's thyroiditis.

The use of thyroid ultrasound or isotope scans is usually not required in the diagnosis of Hashimoto's thyroiditis.

Treatment

The aim of treatment is to normalize the TSH level by giving thyroxine – usually in a dose of 100–150 μg for an adult. Care must be taken when instituting therapy in the elderly or patients with coronary artery disease, when a lower dose should be initially administrated (starting at 25 μg and increasing by 25 μg increments every fortnight). Around 5% of the female population is on thyroxine and follow-up of all patients is usually by automated computer follow-up, to check the TSH level on an annual basis.

Complications

Complications of Hashimoto's thyroiditis include hypothyroidism, increased predilection for other autoimmune disorders (such as pernicious anaemia) and thyroid lymphoma. Eighty per cent of all B-cell thyroid lymphomas develop on a background of Hashimoto's thyroiditis (Figure 4a.1).

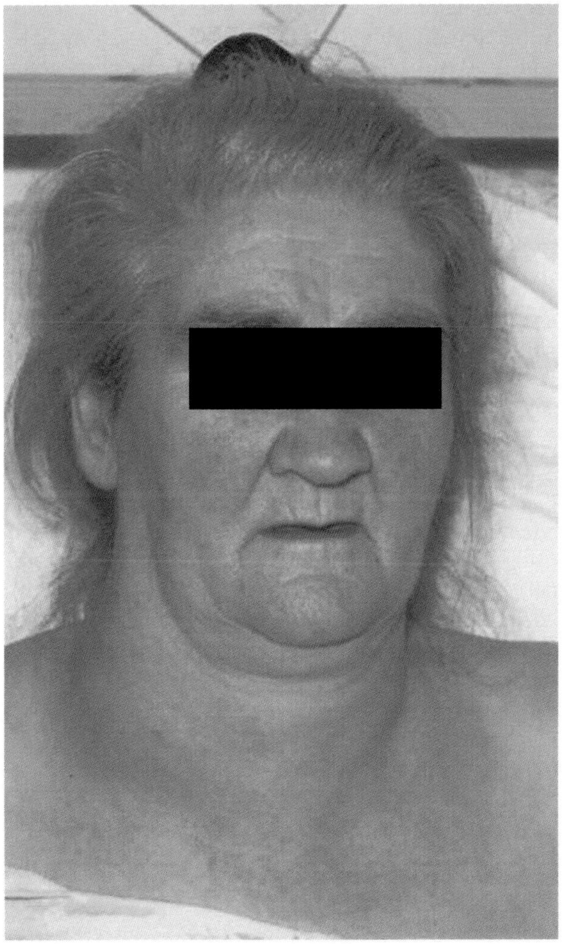

Figure 4a.1 Patient who developed lymphoma on a background of Hashimoto's thyroiditis

Section 4a.3 • Hyperthyroidism

Causes

Thyrotoxicosis is defined as an excess production of thyroid hormones – the vast majority of which is caused by primary thyrotoxicosis (including Graves' disease, toxic multinodular goitre and solitary toxic adenoma). Secondary thyrotoxicosis is rare and may be caused by exogenous administration of thyroxine, struma ovarii (ectopic hormone) and choriocarcinoma. An unusual cause of thyrotoxicosis is the Jod–Basedow phenomenon, which is caused by the excessive release of thyroxine in an iodine-deficient patient on resumption of dietary iodine intake, or administration of intravenous contrast. The phenomenon is most commonly observed in patients over 50 years with a long-standing multinodular goitre.

Graves' disease

Diffuse toxic goitre

Graves' disease (also called Basedow's disease) is an autoimmune disorder, characterized, in 90% of cases, by the presence of an IgG antibody which reacts with the TSH receptor. The antibody is termed thyroid stimulating immunoglobulin (TSI) or TSH receptor antibody (TRAb) and stimulates the follicular cells, leading to excess production of thyroxine, hyperplasia and hypertrophy of the gland. Graves' disease is commoner in females (7:1) and is not pre-malignant, though there is a natural incidence of differentiated thyroid carcinoma, and indeed a malignant nodule associated with Graves' disease is usually an aggressive tumour.

Symptoms and signs

Classically, symptoms include weight loss, heat intolerance, palpitations, irritability, tiredness and tremor. On examination there may be a goitre (although the gland may be normal sized), tachycardia (or atrial fibrillation in the elderly), sweaty palms and hyperactive reflexes. Eye signs include periorbital oedema, chemosis, lid retraction (upper lid retraction may occur due to stimulation of the sympathetic portion of the oculomotor nerve and is not necessarily indicative of proptosis), lid lag and exopthalmos. Other peripheral signs of thyrotoxicosis include proximal upper limb myopathy (Figure 4a.2) and an infiltrative dermopathy (pretibial myxoedema).

Investigations

These are:

- TSH – the TSH is suppressed in thyrotoxicosis. If TSH is suppressed, measure T_3/T_4.
- Antibodies – antimicrosomal (thyroid peroxidase antibody) and antithyroglobulin antibodies are raised in 70% of patients, while the TRAb antibody is raised in 90% of patients.

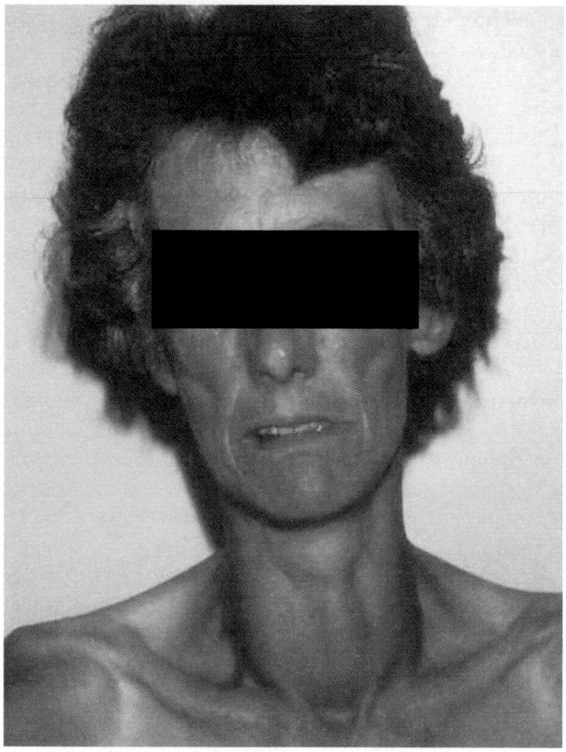

Figure 4a.2 Proximal upper limb myopathy in patient with thyrotoxicosis.

- Scanning – Ultrasound or isotope scans are generally unhelpful in the investigation of Graves' disease, except in post-partum thyrotoxicosis, when isotope scanning maybe helpful to differentiate from self-limiting post-partum thyroiditis.
- Fine needle aspiration (FNA) – FNA is not required, unless there is a palpable nodule within the gland, in which case a potentially aggressive carcinoma needs to be excluded.

Other causes of primary thyrotoxicosis

Plummer's disease (originally described in 1913) is the term given to a hyperfunctioning thyroid, which may be either multinodular or a solitary nodule. A **toxic multinodular goitre** usually develops in a large, long-standing multinodular goitre, of at least 10 years' duration. Isotope scanning will usually show multiple hot areas, and will help determine whether the gland is retrosternal. The preferred treatment for toxic multinodular goitre is by total thyroidectomy, following initial medical therapy to render the patient euthyroid. A **solitary toxic adenoma** (STA) is an autonomous nodule that produces enough thyroid hormone to cause hyperthyroidism. Investigations will reveal a suppressed TSH and negative antibodies. A thyroid isotope scan will reveal the hot nodule with the extranodular thyroid tissue suppressed, and will also help differentiate a solitary toxic adenoma from a toxic multinodular goitre. The treatment of choice for a solitary toxic adenoma is a total lobectomy of the affected side, although radioactive iodine may be considered in the elderly patient.

Treatment of Graves' disease

Antithyroid drugs

The thionamides, carbimazole and propylthiouracil, block the organification (iodination) of the tyrosine residues on the thyroglobulin molecule, by interacting with the enzyme thyroid peroxidase, and inhibiting thyroxine formation. Carbimazole is converted to its active constituent methimazole (primarily used in USA). A recent study in Japan suggested the use of carbimazole and 100 μg of thyroxine with a markedly reduced relapse rate following cessation of therapy, although the findings of this study have failed to be replicated in Europe. Side-effects of carbimazole include fever, rash and neutropenia; rarer side-effects include arthritis, vasculitis, hepatitis and agranulocytosis. Treatment with recombinant granulocyte colony-stimulating factor (rh G-CSF) has been reported to shorten recovery time in patients with thionamide-induced agranulocytosis. If the patient develops a reaction to carbimazole, then they can be switched to propylthiouracil, as there is only a 1:10 000 cross-reaction between the two drugs.

Surgery

The original standard of surgery in Graves' disease was to render the patient euthyroid and to perform a subtotal thyroidectomy, leaving around 5 cm^3 of thyroid tissue. However, following subtotal thyroidectomy there may be a 10% recurrence rate of thyrotoxicosis, and in addition, 70% of the patients may develop hypothyroidism at 10 years. The current trend is to perform a near total or total thyroidectomy, which eliminates the disease with negligible recurrence rates and the patient can be immediately commenced on thyroxine, as they will become inevitably hypothyroid.

Radioactive iodine (RAI)

This modality uses the high-energy beta particles, emitted by 131-iodine, to ablate the follicular cells. It is the treatment of choice in elderly patients, patients with small glands or those unfit for surgery.

Contraindications to RAI

These are:

- Pregnancy – RAI crosses the placenta freely, and activity in the maternal bladder causes fetal irradiation
- Breast feeding – both iodine and pertechnetate are excreted in breast milk
- Severe toxicity – patients may develop thyroid storm if markedly toxic and should be pretreated with beta blockers.

Carbimazole is stopped 48 hours before and restarted 3–5 days after RAI. The usual dose of ^{131}I given is between 500–750 mBq and the maximum effects of treatment occur 3–4 months after the dose of RAI. Hypothyroidism is an almost inevitable consequence of treatment (see hypothyroidism section). RAI may exacerbate clinically evident ophthalmopathy and the use of systemic corticosteroids may be indicated.

The risk of thyroid carcinoma is reduced with the use of RAI, while the risk of leukaemia or other malignancies is the same as the general population. The risk to the fetus is about 1 in 10 000 of developing severe abnormalities and women are advised to refrain from becoming pregnant for at least 6-12 months following treatment.

Section 4a.4 • Management of thyroid nodules

Nodular thyroid disease is common and the incidence increases with age. The prevalence of palpable nodules in the general population is 4–7%, but autopsy studies and ultrasonography have shown that the true incidence to be much greater with around 50% of adults having nodules. Thyroid cancer, however, is rare, affecting around 4 in 100 000 individuals per year and constituting 1% of all malignancies.

The diagnostic dilemma for the clinician therefore revolves around the anxiety induced by the fear of malignancy within the solitary or dominant thyroid nodule, against a background of common benign nodular disease (Figures 4a.3 and 4a.4). The approach to thyroid nodule management must therefore be a selective one, utilizing continually improving diagnostic techniques to reliably identify those patients with malignancy who require surgery, whilst avoiding thyroidectomy in the majority of patients with benign pathology.

Clinical features

There are certain clinical risk factors, which may help differentiate benign from malignant nodules (Table 4a.1), but the majority of thyroid nodules are asymptomatic being found fortuitously on routine clinical examination. Malignancy usually presents as a painless lump, but may occasionally cause discomfort in the

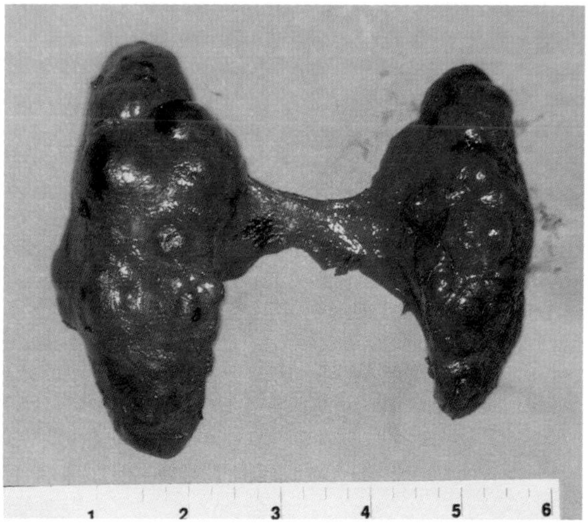

Figure 4a.3 Dominant nodule in the right upper thyroid lobe of a multinodular goitre.

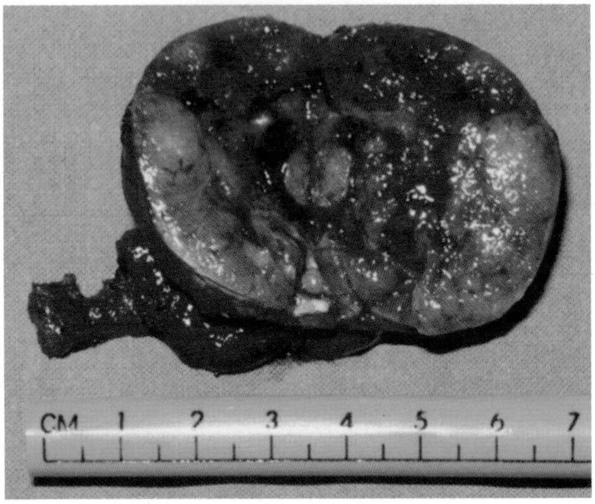

Figure 4a.4 Solitary nodule – benign.

Table 4a.1 Risk factors for thyroid malignancy

- Age – a new thyroid nodule in patients less than 20 or older than 50 years
- Male sex
- Clinical features – consistency, fixation, size – solitary vs multiple nodules
- A history of head and neck irradiation
- Familial history of thyroid malignancy or multiple endocrine neoplasia type 2 (MEN 2)
- Recurrent laryngeal nerve palsy
- Cervical lymphadenopathy

neck. In contrast, the sudden presentation of a painful swelling is almost pathognomonic of haemorrhage into a simple colloid nodule. Development of a new solitary nodule or rapid growth of an existing dominant nodule may suggest malignancy, but a malignant tumour can also be extremely slow growing, present for many years before being discovered. The very young and elderly are at increased risk for malignancy, possibly related to exposure to ionizing radiation. There is an increased incidence of follicular cancer in iodine-deficient endemic goitrous areas, which is counterbalanced by an increase in papillary cancer in iodine-rich regions. Solitary nodules convey a greater risk of malignancy in males and a family history of endocrine disease points towards the diagnosis of medullary thyroid carcinoma. Papillary carcinoma may also be familial and has been described with familial adenomatous polyposis (Gardner's syndrome) and also ataxia-telangiectasia. Palpation can be misleading and although a hard fixed nodule is likely to be malignant, a benign colloid nodule can also be hard with dystrophic calcification. Associated cervical lymphadenopathy and recurrent laryngeal nerve palsy is highly suggestive of malignancy with direct nerve invasion.

Diagnostic investigations

The majority of patients with a thyroid nodule are euthyroid, but the presence of thyroid dysfunction may aid in diagnosis. For example, a hyperthyroid patient with a solitary nodule suggests a benign toxic autonomous nodule, whereas hypothyroidism may indicate nodular Hashimoto's disease possibly with lymphomatous change. With a positive family history, serum calcitonin should be measured to aid diagnosis (and subsequent monitoring) of medullary thyroid cancer with MEN 2 syndrome. Chest X-ray, computed tomography (CT) and magnetic resonance imaging (MRI) have little role in the differentiation of malignancy, but do help in the assessment of goitre size and retrosternal extension and extent of tracheal deviation or narrowing.

Isotope scanning is extremely poor in differentiating between malignant and benign lesions and its role is now limited to the identification of an autonomously functioning nodule (solitary toxic adenoma).

High-resolution ultrasonography is operator dependent but is sensitive in identifying impalpable nodules as small as 0.3 mm in diameter. It differentiates cystic from solid lesions but has a low specificity for detecting malignancy and therefore has limited routine practical value in the assessment of thyroid nodules.

Fine needle aspiration cytology (FNAC) has now become the dominant investigation for the diagnosis of thyroid malignancy. Cytological assessment may be performed using a wet-fixed or air-dried preparation or alternatively utilizing a cell block method in which the thyroid architecture is preserved. The author performs at least 10 passes of the needle in each case and finds good patient compliance with few complications for the procedure, which can easily be repeated (see Figures 4a.5–4a.8). A confident diagnosis of colloid nodule, thyroiditis, papillary, medullary and anaplastic carcinoma, lymphoma and even metastatic deposits can be made. One major limitation for the technique is the evaluation of follicular lesions where histology is

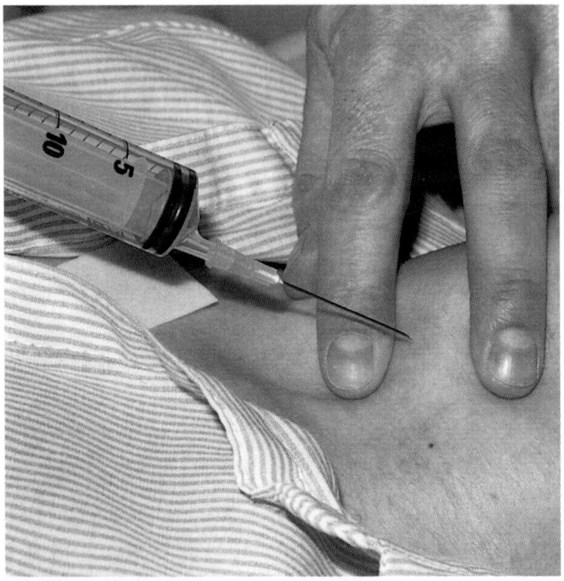

Figure 4a.5 Fine needle aspiration – fixation of nodule with index and middle finger prior to aspiration.

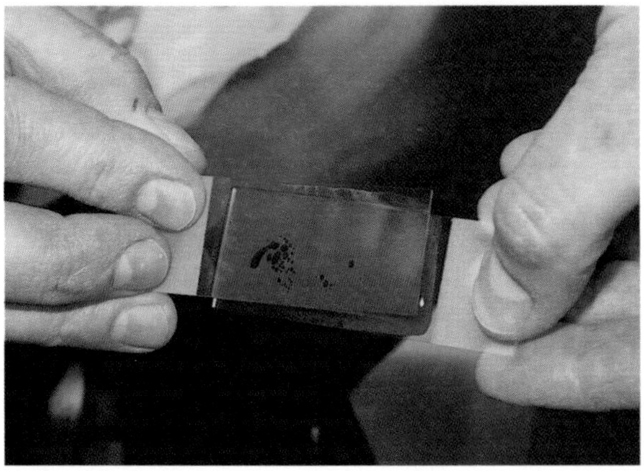

Figure 4a.6 Fine needle aspiration – aspirate spread evenly between two slides.

required to differentiate benign follicular adenoma from carcinoma, a diagnosis which is dependent upon the presence of capsular and vascular invasion. Core biopsy for these follicular lesions may be helpful if the lesion is big enough but any follicular neoplasm should be regarded as potentially malignant and selected for surgical excision. To rely on FNAC for overall assessment and selection for surgery there must be a low false-negative and false-positive rate, which has been well demonstrated in a number of studies. False-positive rates vary from 0 to 1.1% and false-negative rates from 0.7 to 6%. Inadequate specimens should lead to repeat aspiration. The suspicious FNAC is a difficult grey area, which may be improved with immunocytochemical techniques. However, if there is any doubt (clinical or cytological suspicion or two inadequate FNACs), then surgery is indicated and one study demonstrated that 23% of suspicious lesions are malignant, which has been echoed by other reports.

The widespread use of FNAC in diagnostic assessment has led to an increased incidence of malignancy in patients selected for surgery from 10–50%, with a concomitant reduction in cases requiring thyroid surgery producing a favourable cost-reduction. FNAC is therefore a highly accurate and cost-effective diagnostic technique of low morbidity providing a valuable

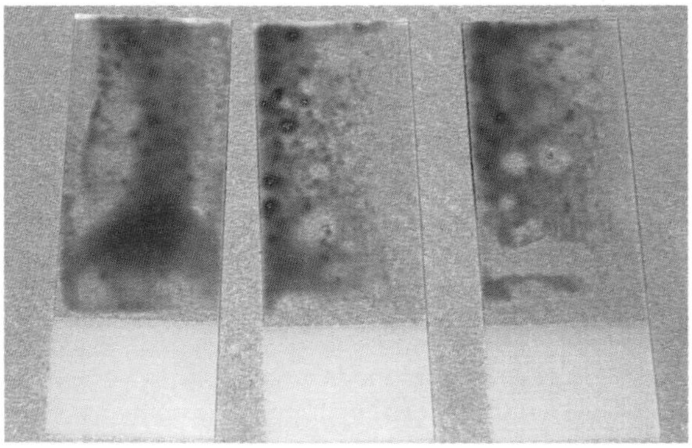

Figure 4a.7 Fine needle aspiration – specimen to be air-dried before sending to laboratory.

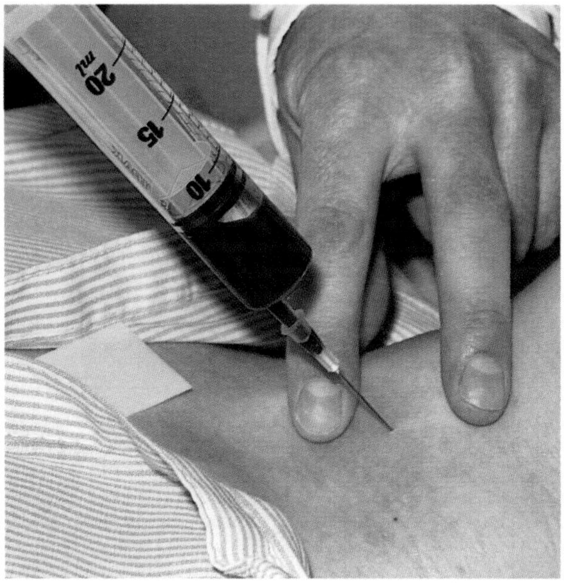

Figure 4a.8 Fine needle aspiration cytology – a diagnostic and also sometimes a therapeutic procedure (as seen here with aspiration of a thyroid cyst).

adjunct to the clinical assessment in the overall selection of patients with thyroid nodules for surgery (Figure 4a.9).

Conservative management

FNAC may be both a diagnostic and therapeutic tool for the management of simple thyroid cysts. However, surgical excision may still be required in a small number of patients where there is persistent cyst formation or a suspicious residual nodule. Where this is the case after cyst aspiration, FNAC of the nodular area should be carried out in all cases. The sudden painful presentation of an acute haemorrhagic colloid nodule produces the typical blood-stained aspirate from the lesion which usually resolves spontaneously.

A long-term follow-up study of putatively benign thyroid nodules has demonstrated that just over a third of nodules disappear and most nodules reduce in size over a 10–30 year period (Kuma *et al.*, 1992). However, 26% of enlarging nodules were found to be malignant. The overall number studied was large and a further study by the same group (Kuma *et al.*, 1994) utilizing clinical re-examination, FNAC and ultrasound-guided FNAC to assess nodules over 9–11 years has clearly demonstrated that 99% of benign nodules remain benign, with the majority decreasing in size or disappearing during the follow-up period. The worrying clinical feature remains an increase in nodule size, which in this series amounted to a malignancy rate of 4.5%. Clearly there should be a high index of suspicion for enlarging lesions during follow-up, which should be long term.

Medical treatment with exogenous thyroxine for suppressive therapy may be useful in diffuse colloid goitre but once nodule formation has developed, patients are unlikely to benefit.

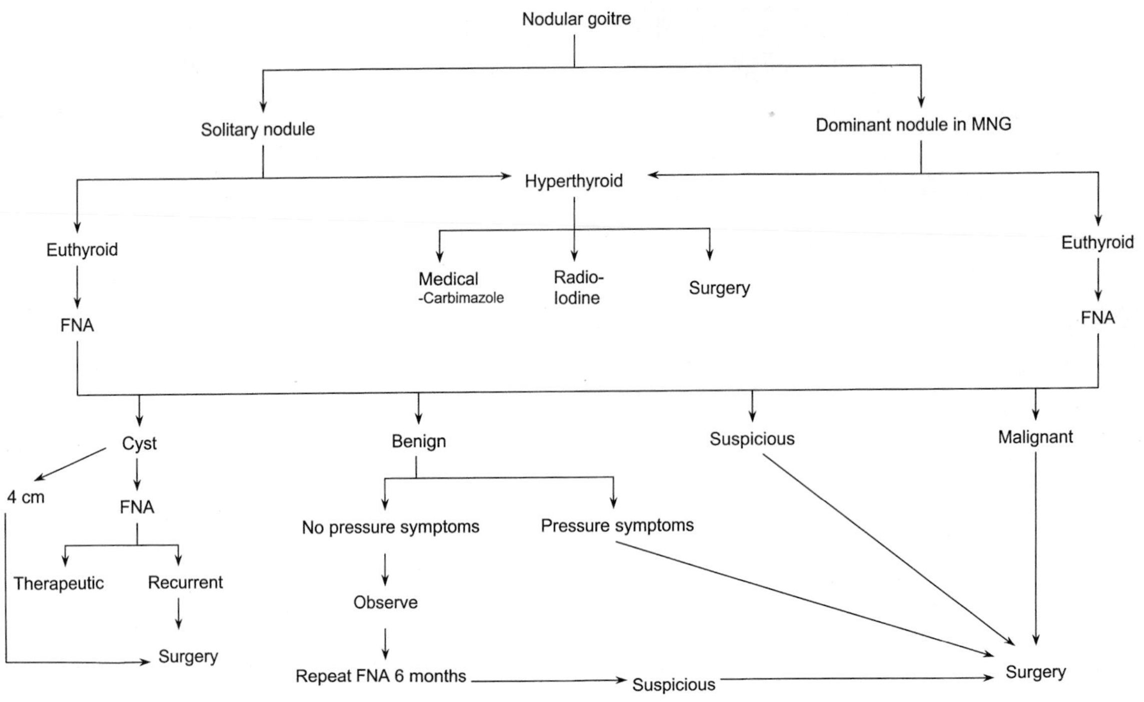

Figure 4a.9 Algorithm for management of patients with thyroid nodules.

Surgical management

The indications for surgery stem from the overall assessment of clinical risk factors coupled with the findings of FNAC that may suggest suspicious or frankly malignant lesions. Large nodules may also cause pressure symptoms, especially in patients from endemic goitrous areas (for example, dyspnoea, dysphagia or choking sensation) which may be an indication irrespective of a benign work-up. A multidisciplinary approach should now be well established in most centres bringing together the endocrinologist, anaesthetist and surgeon who should all be skilled in this particular field.

At operation the nodule is examined and any lymphadenopathy noted along with palpation of the contralateral lobe through the strap muscles. If the nodule is truly unilateral a total thyroid lobectomy removing isthmus and pyramidal lobe *en bloc* is performed preserving parathyroid glands, external branch of superior laryngeal and recurrent laryngeal nerves. This enables a full histological examination of the lesion without any risk of tumour spillage and is a safe procedure with low morbidity when performed in experienced hands. The details will not be discussed further as this is described elsewhere in the module. Frozen section may be useful in confirming malignancy leading to total thyroidectomy and avoiding a second operation. If there is any doubt (particularly with follicular lesions) then the neck is closed and formal paraffin histology is awaited.

Summary

Thyroid nodular disease is a common entity whereas malignancy is rare. Differentiation of a malignant from a benign nodule may be reliably determined in the majority of cases utilizing clinical assessment coupled with FNAC. This is a safe, reliable and cost-effective method to select patients with potential malignancy for thyroidectomy and avoid unnecessary surgery in those with benign disease who do not have any cosmetic or pressure symptoms.

Section 4a.5 • Multinodular goitre

Incidence/pathophysiology

Benign enlargement of the thyroid (goitre) is a common endocrine problem, with an incidence of 5–12% in females and 2–5% in males in areas of adequate iodine intake, whereas in areas of severe iodine deficiency, the incidence can be as high as 90%. Enlargement of the thyroid tends to start as diffuse hyperplasia of the gland, with subsequent areas of focal hyperplasia (which may be dependent on TSH stimulation) and areas of regression and colloid degeneration, leading to a multinodular goitre (MNG) (Figure 4a.10); a multinodular goitre may be non-toxic (euthyroid) or toxic (Plummer's disease).

Causes

The aetiology of a multinodular goitre is poorly understood, but is multifactorial in origin; environmental causes are important with iodine deficiency causing the vast majority of (endemic) goitres world-wide. In areas of adequate iodine intake, drugs (notably amiodarone and

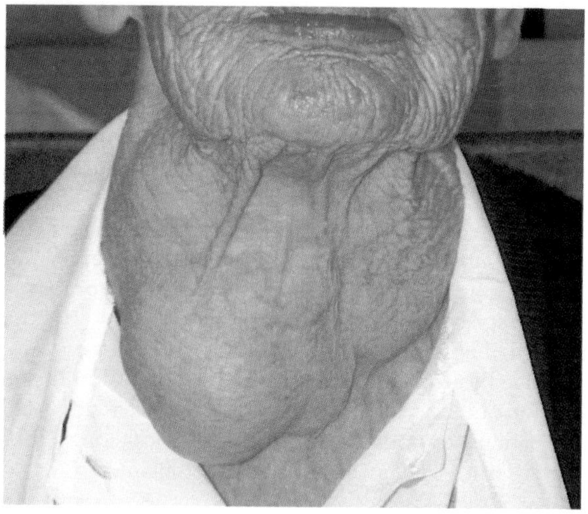

Figure 4a.10 Patient with long-standing multinodular goitre.

lithium), ingestion of brassica vegetables and genetic causes of dyshormonogenesis all have a role to play, but the most common cause of a goitre in the Western world is autoimmune thyroiditis (Hashimoto's thyroiditis).

History and examination

History

The vast majority of multinodular goitres are asymptomatic, and are discovered incidentally at a routine medical examination; 80% are euthyroid at presentation. It is important to check for symptoms that may point to the goitre being malignant, e.g. the rate of increase in size of the swelling, previous neck irradiation or whether there is a family history of thyroid carcinoma. Hoarseness is usually an ominous sign of involvement of the recurrent laryngeal nerve by tumour, although rarely a recurrent nerve neuropraxia caused by compression can be found in patients with a long-standing multinodular goitre. Patients with significant goitres may complain of dysphagia (due to extrinsic pressure on the oesophagus), dyspnoea (pressure on the trachea) or a sensation of choking when lying down. Compressive or obstructive symptoms are more common when the goitre grows posteriorly or in a retrosternal direction; around 10% of multinodular goitres will have a retrosternal extension.

Examination

The examination should ascertain whether the swelling is a solitary thyroid nodule (STN) or a dominant swelling in a multinodular goitre. In practice, a clinical diagnosis of a STN is in fact a dominant nodule in a MNG in 50% of the cases as shown on subsequent investigations. Examination for tracheal deviation and regional lymphadenopathy is done. Raising the arms above the head may induce obstructive symptoms in patients with a retrosternal goitre (Pemberton's sign). The presence of stridor should be sought, as this is a significant symptom, caused by tracheal compression. Venous compression by the goitre, particularly in the antero-superior mediastinum, can cause distended and engorged veins to appear in the neck and anterior chest wall. The consistency of the goitre is usually soft, although areas of calcification may occur in long-standing goitres.

Investigation

All patients with a multinodular goitre should have their TSH level checked to establish their thyroid status, with estimation of the free T4 and T3 if the TSH is abnormal. Any dominant nodule within a multinodular goitre should be essentially treated as a solitary thyroid nodule, as they have an incidence of malignancy of around 10%; they should all have FNAC performed. A chest X-ray or X-ray of the thoracic inlet is required if clinical examination demonstrates tracheal deviation. Further examination by CT scan or MRI will be helpful in delineating the extent of tracheal deviation or compression (Figure 4a.11), the extent of any retrosternal component and the relationship to the major vessels. Thyroid isotope scanning is useful to confirm that the gland is multinodular and the retrosternal extension of the gland, but gives little information as regards the trachea and oesophagus. Thyroid ultrasound is of little benefit in the investigation of a multinodular goitre.

Management and treatment of multinodular goitres

The majority of multinodular goitres can be treated conservatively, but there are some indications for surgery.

The indications for the treatment of patients with multinodular goitre are as follows:

- Suspected or proven malignancy on fine needle aspiration (FNA).
- Compression of the trachea or oesophagus.
- Most patients with a retrosternal component of the goitre.
- Significant recent growth of a dominant nodule (suggestive of malignancy).
- Local neck discomfort.
- Cosmetic reasons.

The treatment modalities of multinodular goitres include suppressive thyroxine therapy, radioactive iodine or surgery.

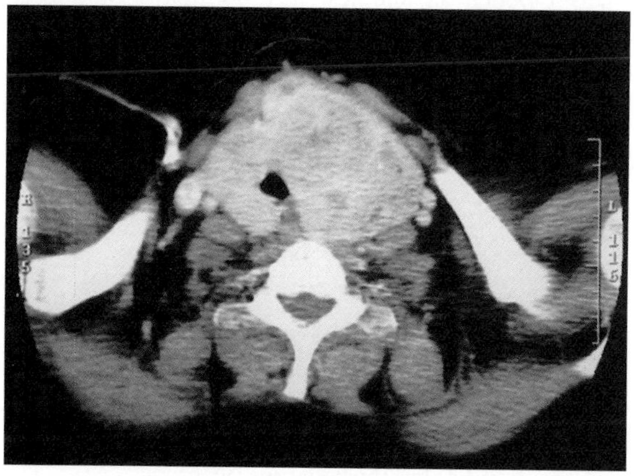

Figure 4a.11 CT scan of neck demonstrating tracheal deviation and compression.

Suppressive thyroxine therapy

The use of suppressive thyroxine therapy remains controversial; protagonists say that suppression of the TSH to <0.1 mU/l for at least a period of 6 months will shrink the size of a multinodular goitre by 20–30% in about 30% of all patients. Recent studies have refuted this and shown no difference between patients receiving suppressive doses or replacement doses of thyroxine. Some concerns have been raised as regards the development of osteoporosis in postmenopausal patients with suppressed TSH levels. It is not the author's current practice to use thyroxine therapy.

Radioactive iodine

Recent evidence suggests that the size of multinodular goitres may be reduced by up to 40% by RAI, with a 30% incidence of hypothyroidism. While RAI does not clear the problem of the multinodular goitre, it may be useful in patients who are unfit or refuse surgery, and in recurrent multinodular goitres following surgery.

Surgery

Surgery remains the mainstay in the treatment of multinodular goitres, particularly if there is a suspicion of malignancy or tracheal compression. If only one lobe of the thyroid is multinodular and the other lobe is normal, then a unilateral total lobectomy will suffice. Suppressive thyroxine therapy following surgery has no benefit in reducing the incidence of progression of the contralateral lobe to becoming multinodular. If both lobes are affected, then a total thyroidectomy is usually required, with subsequent thyroxine replacement therapy.

Section 4a.6 • Differentiated thyroid cancer (DTC)

Diagnosis

The diagnosis of thyroid cancer may be made on clinical grounds, by thyroid cytology, or after a previous thyroid operation. Clinical features that should raise suspicion of malignancy in a patient with a thyroid nodule are shown in Table 4.a1 (thyroid nodule section).

Clinical examination and pre-operative assessment

This should ascertain the extent and nature of the palpable thyroid/lymph node abnormalities. A chest X-ray is required to exclude metastases. Ultrasound may be of use in detecting gross nodal disease in the central neck or posterior triangles. Cross-sectional imaging with CT/MRI may be of value in some patients with locally advanced disease to identify gross nodal disease and/or identify extrathyroidal spread.

Ultrasound and/or isotope scanning are not routinely required in the diagnosis of patients with suspected or proven thyroid cancer. These tests are neither specific nor sensitive for the diagnosis of malignancy.

A pre-operative diagnosis will allow a planned therapeutic intervention specific to the subtype of cancer identified, i.e. total lobectomy versus total thyroidectomy ± lymph node surgery (sampling, central neck clearance, modified neck dissection).

Informed consent must be obtained from all patients prior to surgery. The nature of the proposed operation and its potential risks to the recurrent/superior laryngeal nerves, parathyroid insufficiency including the possible need for calcium/vitamin D replacement, and the need for thyroxine replacement/suppression therapy must be discussed. Prior to operation it is advisable for patients to undergo assessment of vocal cord status, and a serum calcium level should be obtained.

Treatment of DTC

Once thyroid cancer is diagnosed the patient should ideally be cared for by an experienced multidisciplinary team that allows ready access to a surgeon, pathologist, biochemist, clinical and molecular geneticist, endocrinologist and oncologist.

Surgery

Surgery is the primary treatment for most patients with DTC. Although **the minimum operation required for DTC is total thyroid lobectomy and isthmectomy** there remains controversy about the extent of surgery required for patients with DTC. Most surgeons recommend total or near total thyroidectomy for DTC but there is a substantial body of opinion that argues the case for lobectomy and isthmectomy alone for unifocal tumours less than 5 cm in diameter without extrathyroidal spread. For **low-risk** patients with DTC (see below) unilateral lobectomy and isthmectomy may be appropriate.

Three factors are relevant in consideration of the choice of surgery for DTC:

- Potential surgical morbidity.
- The risk of local recurrence.
- The impact on prognosis.

The arguments for total thyroidectomy as opposed to near total (leaving *less than 2 g of tissue on the contralateral side*) include: lower local recurrence rates, increased survival for tumours greater than 1.5 cm in diameter, opportunity to use serum thyroglobulin as a marker for persistent/recurrent disease and the low morbidity of this procedure, if performed by an experienced surgeon. In all cases, care should be taken to preserve parathyroid tissue and function of the external branch of the superior laryngeal nerve and recurrent laryngeal nerves.

In the following scenarios there is consensus as to the 'correct' treatment

- Papillary microcarcinoma (less than 1 cm diameter) – lobectomy and isthmectomy.
- Minimally invasive follicular cancer with capsular invasion only – lobectomy and isthmectomy.

- DTC with extrathyroidal spread – near/total thyroidectomy.
- Bilateral/multifocal DTC – near/total thyroidectomy.
- DTC with distant metastases – near/total thyroidectomy.
- DTC with extensive nodal involvement – near/total thyroidectomy.

In some patients a diagnosis of thyroid cancer is only made following previous thyroid surgery. Completion thyroidectomy should be performed within 3–4 days or after 3 months have elapsed from primary surgery to minimize risks of morbidity associated with post-operative scarring.

Lymph node surgery

Thyroid cancer is unusual in that although lymph node involvement in some studies is not associated with an adverse prognosis, other studies have shown node surgery may have a beneficial effect on long-term survival

Lymph node involvement appears to be dependent upon the histological subtype (papillary 35–65% involvement, follicular less than 20%), the local extent of the tumour, the surgical procedure performed (sampling bias) and the thoroughness of pathological examination of excised tissue.

Although DTC most frequently involves lymph nodes from the central compartment (paratracheal/oesophagotracheal), posterior triangle node involvement is also commonly seen. In patients with papillary thyroid cancer, routine unilateral lymph node surgery in the absence of macroscopic node involvement will identify node involvement in at least 35% of cases, but the long-term benefit on prognosis of such routine procedures is unclear. Lymph node dissection is an efficient procedure for the 'treatment' of nodal metastases, but is associated with a higher risk of complications (parathyroid insufficiency, recurrent laryngeal nerve injury). The 'absolute' indication for lymph node dissection in patients with DTC is macroscopic cervical node involvement identified pre-operatively or at the time of operation. The extent of lymph node surgery in patients with DTC is also controversial – current practice ranges from node 'picking' procedures to functional neck dissection conserving non-lymphatic structures.

Non-surgical treatment of DTC

Normal thyroid cell differentiation and proliferation is TSH dependent. TSH receptors are present in most differentiated thyroid cancer cells and on that basis patients with DTC should receive lifelong thyroxine, with the smallest dose of thyroxine necessary to suppress TSH to undetectable levels (TSH < 0.1 μg/l). Triiodothyronine (T3) may be used if follow-up RAI scans are required, as it has a shorter half-life than thyroxine, and only requires to be stopped 1 week prior to scanning (see Follow-up of patients with DTC).

In many patients, an ablative dose of radioiodine is given post-operatively to destroy any residual thyroid tissue. This facilitates the use of thyroglobulin as a marker of residual or recurrent disease and the use of whole body isotope scanning as a diagnostic/therapeutic technique. External beam radiotherapy to the neck is used only in patients with extensive extrathyroidal disease and those whose tumour does not take up radioiodine as neoadjuvant therapy.

While near/total thyroidectomy, post-operative RAI ablation and TSH suppression with thyroxine may be advocated in all patients with DTC there is insufficient evidence to justify this. A selective approach to treatment is indicated. Ideally the extent of surgical intervention should be guided by the risk grouping of the patient at presentation (see prognosis section).

Follow-up of patients with DTC

Recurrent thyroid cancer may occur soon after initial therapy or years later. Patients with thyroid cancer should be followed up in a multidisciplinary thyroid cancer clinic.

Serum thyroglobulin should not be detectable in patients who have undergone thyroid ablation. High/rising titres of thyroglobulin in the blood indicate persistent or recurrent disease. Thyroglobulin levels will increase on thyroxine withdrawal, as its production is TSH dependent. Clinical trials in the use of recombinant human TSH suggest recombinant TSH to be an effective alternative to thyroxine withdrawal during follow-up of patients with differentiated thyroid cancer. ^{131}I whole-body scanning has to some extent been superseded. Once residual thyroid tissue has been ablated after surgery, metastases from DTC may take up radioactive iodine in the presence of high serum TSH concentration. Whole body scanning can be used to identify metastases in patients with DTC in whom thyroglobulin levels are increasing.

Recurrent DTC

Recurrence may be local or regional (in the neck) or systemic. Treatment will depend to some extent on the original nature of the disease and its treatment. Surgery is the mainstay of treatment of local/regional recurrence. Surgery is followed by radioactive iodine scanning ± ablation or external beam radiotherapy. Distant metastases will usually occur in the lungs or skeletal system. Although distant metastases cause cancer death in 10–15% of patients with DTC, they are compatible with long-term survival. They may present as a result of local symptoms, neurological complications or rising thyroglobulin levels. Palliative surgical procedures may be appropriate if there are orthopaedic/spinal complications. It should be remembered that metastases may be solitary. Remission will occur in 50% of patients with distant metastases that take up radio-iodine (10 year survival 25–40%).

Prognosis

In general terms, the prognosis from DTC is worse in men, patients less than 16 or greater than 45 years of age at presentation, when there is incomplete resection of primary disease, extrathyroidal spread or distant metastases. Specific histological subtypes of papillary cancer (tall cell/columnar cell), and follicular cancer (insular/Hurthle cell) are also associated with a worse prognosis. Various scoring systems allow risk stratification of patients with DTC. These include:

- AMES – **A**ge, **M**etastases, **E**xtent of primary tumour, **S**ize at presentation.
- AGES – **A**ge, **G**rade, **E**xtent of primary tumour, **S**ize of tumour.
- MACIS – **M**etastases, **A**ge, **C**ompleteness of resection, **I**nvasion of extrathyroidal tissues, **S**ize of tumour.
- TNM – T1 < 1 cm, T2 >1 to 4 cm, T3 > 4 cm, T4 extends beyond the thyroid.

In general terms, 80–90% of patients will fall within the 'best' prognostic group in whom disease-specific death will occur in no more than 2% of patients. In the worst prognosis groups the 20 year mortality rate will be 75–95%.

Summary

To date there have been no controlled, prospective studies of long-term outcome in patients with DTC treated by conservative versus more radical surgery. Post-operative radioiodine ablation of thyroid remnants has been shown to decrease local recurrence rates and facilitate serum thyroglobulin estimation and iodine-131 scanning to identify metastatic spread. Evidence to support a benefit from RAI ablation in terms of decreased local recurrence and increased survival in all patients is controversial, particularly in patients whose tumours are completely excised.

Medullary thyroid cancer (MTC)

Five to ten per cent of thyroid cancer cases arise from C cells of the thyroid. The disease may occur in one of four clinical settings:

- sporadic
- familial – MEN 2A
- familial – MEN 2B
- familial non-MEN associated MTC.

Diagnosis and pre-operative assessment

Sporadic MTC will usually present as a thyroid nodule and/or lymph node enlargement. Symptoms include those secondary to airway/oesophageal compression, pain, diarrhoea and rarely Cushing's syndrome due to gut peptide or adrenocorticotropic hormone (ACTH) release by the tumour. The diagnosis may be confirmed on thyroid cytology or as a result of a previous operation. The absence of a family history does **not** preclude an apparently sporadic MTC being the index case of genetically determined disease. In all cases a family history of thyroid cancer/phaeochromocytoma should be excluded.

If the diagnosis of MTC is made prior to operation pre-operative investigation should include basal calcitonin and CEA, ultrasound of neck to identify multiple thyroid lesions (a marker of familial disease) and lymph node enlargement. CT/MRI may identify mediastinal node involvement. **Phaeochromocytoma must be excluded prior to operation in all cases by a normal 24 hour urine collection for catecholamines/metanephrines.** Germ-line analysis (venous blood sample) for a Ret proto-oncogene mutation is required in all patients to exclude familial disease.

In families affected or, likely to be affected by genetically determined MTC, screening for Ret mutations in individuals at risk (ante- and post-cedent) should be performed. Prophylactic thyroidectomy is indicated in kindred members without clinically apparent disease but who are carriers of the germ-line Ret mutation. Provocative biochemical testing is not required in Ret positive individuals, but baseline calcitonin concentrations should be taken, though they may be normal in the presence of MTC. There is no evidence on which to base a firm recommendation for the age at which prophylactic surgery should be performed but, on current knowledge, it should be between 5 and 7 years of age.

Surgical treatment

Irrespective of gene status the current standard operation for this disease is total thyroidectomy and central neck node clearance from the hyoid bone superiorly to the innominate vein inferiorly. Biopsy of the jugulo-carotid lymph nodes from both sides of the neck and frozen section should be performed. If these nodes are positive they should be removed and frozen section examination of posterior triangle nodes should be performed. If these biopsied nodes are positive, the respective nodal group should be formally cleared. In the absence of soft tissue involvement, muscle, vessel and nerve resection procedures are inappropriate. If there is evidence of involvement of anterior/superior mediastinal node involvement at presentation, these nodes should be cleared (sternotomy would be required).

In all cases the parathyroid gland should be identified and preserved. In MEN 2 patients only enlarged parathyroid glands should be excised (see Section 6.3).

After surgery replacement doses of thyroxine are given. There is no indication in MTC for TSH suppression.

Follow-up of patients with MTC

Long-term follow-up of these patients is required. At review, basal calcitonin and CEA levels should be measured. Patients with MEN 2 require exclusion of the adrenal and parathyroid manifestations of disease at least annually.

Basal levels of calcitonin/CEA may be:

- Undetectable – if a subsequent pentagastrin stimulation test is negative, cure is possible.
- Detectable/raised – indicating residual disease. The multidisciplinary team should carefully consider the management of each patient but options include a search for residual disease or close observation. Factors that affect the decision to 'chase' the biochemical abnormality will include the age of the patient and disease burden at presentation.

Identification of residual MTC will require the use of high-resolution CT of the neck/chest/liver, and/or one or more of the isotope scans with pentavalant DMSA, ^{123}I MIBG or radiolabelled octreotide. Laparoscopy may be the most sensitive test to identify liver metastases that are typically small and 'miliary'. Selective venous catheterization for calcitonin gradients may be useful. Surgical intervention to remove 'occult' disease may reduce calcitonin levels but there are no long-term follow-up data to confirm that this approach affects the long-term prognosis.

Treatment of recurrent/metastatic disease

Surgery is the treatment of choice for local/regional recurrence. MTC is resistant to chemotherapy. The response to radiotherapy is generally poor, but may be useful in patients with inoperable disease or symptomatic bone metastases. Diarrhoea may be severe and intractable in recurrent disease and should be controlled by the use of anti-diarrhoeal agents including codeine phosphate or loperamide.

Prognosis

The mortality rate for MTC exceeds that of differentiated thyroid cancer; in patients who present with symptomatic MTC the 10 year survival rate is in excess of 60%. Factors that indicate a poor prognosis include age more than 40 years at presentation, male sex, extrathyroidal spread, nodal involvement, metastases, tumour aneuploidy, negative amyloid staining and familial disease. Long-term survival of patients with metastatic disease is common in MTC.

Lymphoma (less than 5% of thyroid cancers)

This is more common in women (3:1), with the incidence increasing with age (most patients are aged greater than 60 years). The diagnosis will be made clinically often by the history of long-standing goitre/hypothyroidism (Figure 4a.1) and a rapidly enlarging neck mass with a minority complaining of compressive symptoms. Thyroid lymphoma is often associated with a history of autoimmune thyroid disease (80% of patients). FNA and core biopsy will often confirm the diagnosis and allow immunohistochemical subtyping of the lymphoma. Most thyroid lymphomas are mucosa-associated lymphoid tissue (MALT)-L lymphomas. CT scanning will often show homogeneous thyroid enlargement without evidence of invasion of adjacent structures.

Treatment of lymphoma

Some patients will present with acute airway obstruction. Intravenous steroids can achieve rapid resolution of symptoms after a tissue diagnosis has been obtained. External beam radiotherapy is used subsequently. There is no evidence that surgery offers any benefit to patients with lymphoma. Following diagnosis and treatment of upper airway symptoms the patient should be referred to an oncologist. Staging with CT scanning, liver function tests and full blood count is appropriate. Treatment for this disease may include radiotherapy and/or chemotherapy (CHOP).

Section 4a.7 • Undifferentiated thyroid carcinoma

Undifferentiated or anaplastic thyroid carcinoma (1.5% of thyroid cancers), in contrast to well-differentiated thyroid carcinoma, is a highly aggressive tumour, with 70% of patients having metastases at the time of presentation. Patients generally present with a large, hard, ill-defined cervical mass, usually invading adjacent structures, which is often associated with a long-standing goitre. The sex incidence is similar and most patients present aged 60–70 years. Occasionally, undifferentiated thyroid carcinoma may develop as a transformation of a previously treated well-differentiated thyroid carcinoma, which may have been in remission for a considerable time. Diagnosis can usually be confirmed by a core biopsy under local anaesthetic, as fine needle aspiration for cytology may not be diagnostic.

Undifferentiated thyroid carcinoma may be classified as small cell, large cell or spindle cell, which may resemble sarcomas. Small cell carcinomas must be distinguished pathologically from lymphoma, which has a far more favourable prognosis.

Treatment

Treatment of these patients is by total thyroidectomy, if no extrathyroidal spread, when possible, although this is rarely achieved in undifferentiated thyroid carcinoma. Palliative surgery may be necessary to relieve symptoms. Surgical debulking may be attempted, and often a tracheostomy is required. Tracheal/oesophageal stenting should be considered. External beam radiotherapy is usually given to these patients in an attempt to slow tumour progression. Undifferentiated thyroid carcinoma is not responsive to ^{131}I therapy, but chemotherapy, particularly with doxyrubicin, can give partial remission in up to 30% of patients. However, no current treatment protocol exists as a standard treatment for these patients and evidence of significant therapeutic benefit after radiotherapy and/or chemotherapy is lacking. The prognosis remains appalling, with the majority of patients dead within a year of diagnosis.

Section 4a.8 • Thyroidectomy

Introduction

It was not until the early twentieth century that thyroidectomy became a safe and acceptable operation with the advent of general anaesthesia, antisepsis and haemostatic techniques. Theodore Kocher of Berne was the chief protagonist of these methods and for his lifetime devotion to the development of safe thyroid surgery was awarded the Nobel Prize in 1909, by which time the previous high mortality had fallen to less than 1%. Further advances by William Halsted, Charles Mayo and George Crile were subsequently developed by Frank Lahey and remain the basis of safe thyroid surgery that is continued to be practised today by trained endocrine surgeons.

Surgical principles

Successful thyroid surgery depends upon an intimate knowledge of the surgical anatomy of the neck with the provision of good operative exposure and skilful dissection to identify and preserve the laryngeal nerves and parathyroid glands. A bloodless field should be maintained throughout with minimum usage of bipolar diathermy and suction.

Pre-operative preparation

This should include indirect laryngoscopy to exclude a pre-existing unilateral nerve palsy, especially if the patient has undergone previous thyroid surgery. General anaesthesia with endotracheal intubation and muscle relaxation is deployed and the patient is placed supine on an operating table 15° head up with the neck in near full extension and a sandbag in the interscapular position.

Access to the gland

A collar incision is used two finger-breadths above the sternal notch extending to both sternomastoid muscles. The incision is extended through subcutaneous fat and platysma down to the deep fascia and by a process of blunt and sharp dissection this plane (anterior to the anterior jugular vessels) is extended superiorly to the level of the thyroid notch and inferiorly to the sternal notch and the skin flaps are then held apart using a self-retaining retractor (Jolls or two wishbone retractors). The strap muscles are then separated with a midline incision through the deep fascia and retracted laterally. This should be as long as possible to enable full access to the operative field. Transverse division of the strap muscles is not routinely required but may be occasionally used for safe access to a large or vascular goitre.

The deeper sternothyroid muscle is usual slightly adherent to the capsule and is separated from it with careful blunt and sharp dissection, dividing middle thyroid veins when present with 3/0 vicryl or surgiclips.

The thyroid lobe is then delivered using traction from the index finger on a small swab over the lobe with the strap muscles retracted laterally by use of two small Langenbeck retractors to expose the superior thyroid artery and laryngeal nerve. The forefinger is passed upwards in the plane behind the superior pole breaking down areola tissue and then gently retracting the superior pole betwixt finger and thumb inferolaterally to expose the space between the superior thyroid vessels and the cricothyroid muscle (Figure 4a.12). Skeletalization of the superior thyroid artery is then achieved and the vessel or its branches ligated with absorbable suture material (0 vicryl × 2 proximally) and divided well away from the external branch of superior laryngeal nerve which usually runs along the surface

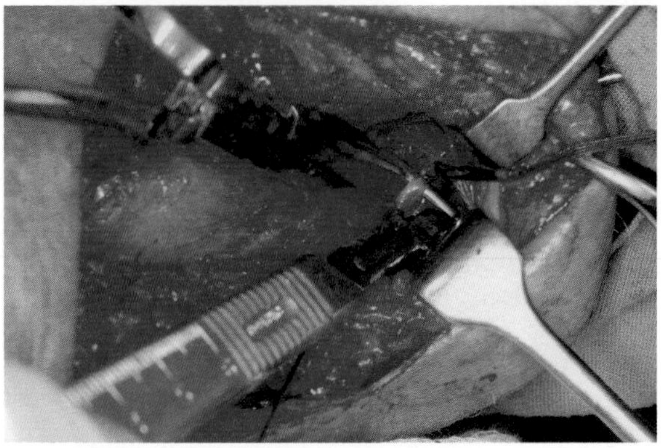

Figure 4a.12 Division of left superior thyroid artery.

of (or within) the cricothyroid but may also pass between the branches of the vessels, where it is in great danger if mass ligation is carried out.

The recurrent laryngeal nerve and parathyroid glands

The superior pole of the lobe may now be delivered partially into the mid-line joined by the lower lobe when inferior thyroid veins are ligated (with 3/0 vicryl or clips) close to the capsule being careful to avoid injury to the inferior parathyroid gland. Further finger retraction on the lobe will now bring into view the deeper aspect of the middle third of the thyroid lobe and the adjacent junction between the inferior thyroid artery and recurrent laryngeal nerve (see Figure 4a.13). This should be carefully identified by gentle dissection of the overlying fascial layers with a small artery clip and is recognized as a white cord with an overlying vasa-nervosum usually coursing latero-medially deep to the inferior thyroid artery. However, there is enormous variability of its course, especially on the right side where in 1% of cases the nerve may even be non-recurrent arising from the vagus and passing medially close to the inferior thyroid artery before turning to ascend to enter the larynx. It also may divide into several branches before entering the larynx where the inferior cornu of the thyroid cartilage is a fairly constant landmark for its point of entry. The parathyroid glands are most commonly located either side of the neurovascular intersection and are then dissected carefully downwards preserving individual branches of the inferior thyroid artery supplying them wherever possible. If they are rendered ischaemic at operation the individual gland is minced into 1 mm cubes and autotransplanted into a pocket in the sternomastoid muscle. The individual branches of the inferior thyroid artery are then ligated close to the thyroid capsule with clips or 3/0 vicryl. The main inferior thyroid artery trunk is not ligated to preserve the blood supply to the parathyroid glands.

The nerve is perhaps most in danger at its point of entry into the larynx as it passes through the suspensory ligament of Berry, where it often adopts a curving

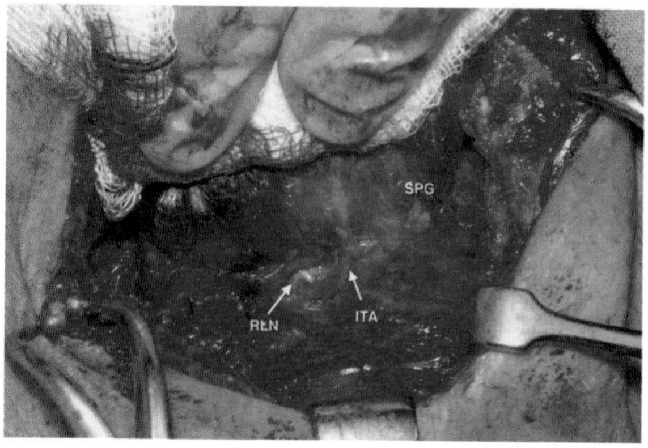

Figure 4a.13 Exposure of the neurovascular intersection of the inferior thyroid artery (ITA) and recurrent laryngeal nerve (RLN). The superior parathyroid gland (SPG) can be found within a 2 cm radius cranial to the intersection, usually posterior to the RLN and thyroid gland. Note the looping of the RLN within Berry's ligament close to its insertion beneath the cricothyroid.

loop (see Figure 4a.13) and the nerve must be carefully identified in this region before dividing the suspensory fascia by staying close to the thyroid capsule at all times.

Resection of the lobe

Dissection is continued further medially by dividing the vascular fascia binding the thyroid lobe to the trachea and larynx with particular attention to careful clipping and ligation near Berry's ligament where troublesome bleeding may obscure the entry point of the recurrent laryngeal nerve to the larynx. The mobilization is now complete and resection is continued to include the isthmus and pyramidal lobe where present. The cut surface of the contralateral thyroid lobe is usually sutured with 3/0 vicryl absorbable sutures to the tracheal fascia to obtain haemostasis.

Wound closure

The sandbag is now removed from under the patient's spine and the neck space is re-examined for bleeding with a Valsalva manoeuvre by the anaesthetist. With haemostasis secured, a suction drain is placed deep to the strap muscles and brought out laterally leaving one or two holes in the subcutaneous plane to drain any haemorrhage which may collect superficially. The strap muscles are closed with continuous 3/0 vicryl and the wound closed with subcutaneous 3/0 vicryl to platysma and clips to skin.

Total and subtotal thyroidectomy

With total thyroidectomy for cancer, gross multinodular disease or Graves' disease, the opposite lobe will be mobilized in a similar manner to that described above with or without an appropriate lymph node clearance for malignancy.

Subtotal thyroidectomy is carried out as above except a small remnant (usually 4–5 g of tissue) is left on each side of the trachea sutured to it with 3/0 vicryl absorbable sutures to secure haemostasis. Some surgeons perform a unilateral total lobectomy leaving a single large remnant on the contralateral side, which is an acceptable alternative strategy.

Retrosternal goitre

Ligation and division of the superior vessels is essential before any attempt is made to deliver a retrosternal goitre. This is achieved by introducing a finger down into the mediastinum behind the sternum and using gentle traction, which may be aided by the use of a bent dessert spoon when dealing with a very large multinodular gland. A mediastinal split is seldom necessary.

Complications of thyroid surgery

General surgical complications are those of anyone undergoing a general anaesthetic such as cardiac or pulmonary, with a current mortality rate in several large series approaching zero. The morbidity of thyroidectomy from its specific complications, however, continues to be a matter of concern (Table 4a.2). Clearly meticulous attention to operative technique is required and this is now an area for the trained endocrine surgeon rather than a general surgeon. Litigation for thyroidectomy complications amount to approximately 5% of general surgical claims, most of which involve recurrent laryngeal nerve injury.

To avoid damage to the recurrent laryngeal nerve (RLN) a detailed knowledge of the variable anatomy of its course is required and identification is fundamental to avoiding trauma. This has been controversial in the past but many workers, including large series of total thyroidectomies, have reported no permanent laryngeal nerve damage. Clearly it is important to have pre- and post-operative assessment of vocal cord function by an ENT surgeon, which has important medicolegal implications. Bilateral palsy is exceedingly rare, but may lead to temporary or permanent tracheostomy. This is most likely to be a problem where re-operation is performed when one recurrent laryngeal nerve has already been permanently damaged. The frequency of the RLN injury following thyroid surgery should be below 1% although this will clearly reflect case-mix and operative experience. The external branch of superior laryngeal nerve is also at risk during thyroidectomy and permanent voice damage following its injury is surprisingly common although difficult to detect on indirect laryngoscopy. Such injury may be

Table 4a.2 Specific complications of thyroidectomy

- Recurrent laryngeal nerve palsy
- Injury to external branch of superior laryngeal nerve
- Hypoparathyroidism
- Acute laryngeal oedema
- Reactionary haemorrhage
- Persistent hyperthyroidism
- Residual hypothyroidism
- Wound problems

minimized if the nerve is identified and preserved during superior thyroid artery ligation.

Patients should be informed of this and other complications before surgery, emphasizing a greater risk when re-exploration or cancer surgery is performed. A specific consent form is a useful documentation of good pre-operative counselling.

Parathyroid damage producing hypocalcaemia is the second largest category of thyroid related medicolegal claims and although usually temporary, a permanent hypocalcaemic state has been shown to occur in 1–3% of cases. Most cases occur due to disruption of the parathyroid blood supply and the inferior thyroid artery vessel branches should be handled gently and ligated near to the thyroid as discussed above.

Hypothyroidism is inevitable after total thyroidectomy where thyroxine replacement is given and also increases with time after subtotal resection. Although hypothyroidism is easily treated with thyroxine replacement recurrent hyperthyroidism presents more of a problem with re-operation carrying a significant increase in complications and in this scenario, radioiodine ablation is probably a safer option.

Post-operative reactionary haemorrhage is potentially catastrophic, but can be avoided with meticulous haemostasis. However, the most serious and life-threatening complication is post-operative airway obstruction due to acute laryngeal oedema which may or may not be associated with haematoma and has a curious aetiology most likely to be related to impaired lymphatic drainage of the larynx causing this internal oedema. It is an extremely rare complication which can be minimized by meticulous attention to haemostasis and avoidance of unnecessary manipulation of the larynx during surgery.

Wound complications still stimulate complaints but a well-positioned collar incision within the skin creases can give adequate exposure and an excellent cosmetic result. Suture granuloma can be minimized by the use of absorbable suture material or clips (preferred by the author). Wound infection is rare but hypertrophic scarring may occur particularly if the patient has a propensity to keloid formation.

Thyroidectomy is a routine and safe surgical procedure with a low morbidity and negligible mortality when performed by trained endocrine surgeons and most of the complications of thyroidectomy may be avoided by careful surgical technique.

Further reading

Clark, O. H. *et al.* (1982). *Ann Surg* **196**: 361–70.
Grant, C. S. *et al.* (1989). *Surgery* **106**: 980–6.
Hysmans, D. A. *et al.* (1994). *Ann Intern Med* **15**; **121**: 757–62.
Kuma, K. *et al.* (1992). *World J Surg* **16**: 583–8.
Kuma, K. *et al.* (1994). *World J Surg* **18**: 495–9.
Paggi, A. *et al.* (1999). *Endocr Res* **25**: 229–38.

Further recommended reading (for thyroid and parathyroid modules)

Clark, O. H. and Quan-Yang Duh. (1997). *Textbook of Endocrine Surgery*. Philadelphia, PA: W. B. Saunders.
Clark, O. H., Quan-Yang Duh and Siperstein, A. E. *The Surgical Clinics of North America. Endocrine Surgery*. Philadelphia, PA: W. B. Saunders.
Frieser, S. R. and Thompson, N. W. (1997). *Surgical Endocrinology: Clinical Syndromes*. Philadelphia, PA: Lippincott.
Lynn, J. and Bloom, S. R. *Surgical Endocrinology*. Oxford: Butterworth-Heinemann.
Wheeler, M. H. and Richards, S. H. The laryngeal nerves. *Curr Surg Pract* **5**: 237–50.

MODULE 4b

Disorders of the parathyroid glands

Section 4b.1 • Parathyroid embryology, anatomy and physiology

Embryology

The superior parathyroid glands originate from the dorsal tips of the fourth pharyngeal pouch, which is incorporated into the lateral aspect of the thyroid along with the ultimo-branchial body; this common origin occasionally leads to an intra-thyroidal location for the superior parathyroid gland, although this is rare.

The inferior parathyroid glands arise from the dorsal aspect of the third pharyngeal pouch, with the thymus originating from the ventral aspect. Together, they descend as a complex in a plane ventral to the fourth pharyngeal pouch, and the lower parathyroids are therefore found in a more anterior position than the upper parathyroids, usually dissociating from the thymus near the lower pole of the thyroid, but this migration can vary widely. With an absence of migration, the inferior parathyroid gland may be found superior to the upper pole of the thyroid mimicking a superior gland, but surrounding thymic tissue clarifies the true origin. If the inferior parathyroid remains attached to the thymus, it will migrate to the anterior mediastinum.

Surgical anatomy

Awareness of the common pathways of migration is invaluable in parathyroid surgery (see Figure 4b.1). Eighty per cent of the upper parathyroid glands lie within a localized area of a 2 cm radius, cranial to the intersection of the recurrent laryngeal nerve (RLN) and the inferior thyroid artery (ITA). This is a very common symmetrical position for the superior glands, which are usually tucked away posterior to the upper pole of the thyroid. If the glands are sited more anteriorly they are located on the surface of the thyroid frequently beneath its capsule, where there is typically freedom of movement as opposed to prominent thyroid nodules which are fixed. Approximately 1% of superior glands are found in the para-oesophageal or retro-oesophageal space, from where they may descend to the posterior mediastinum due to the effect of negative intra-thoracic pressure of respiration.

More than half of the inferior parathyroid glands are located around the lower pole of the thyroid, with a quarter being found within the thyro-thymic ligament or within the thymus itself. As the inferior gland becomes enlarged, it tends to migrate into the thymus

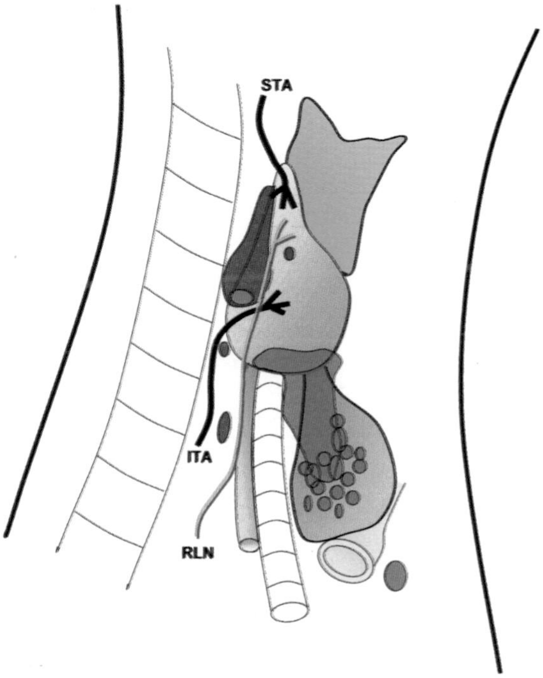

Figure 4b.1 Sites of migration rest for superior (shaded red) and inferior (shaded blue) parathyroid glands. (STA/ITA, superior and inferior thyroid artery; RLN, recurrent laryngeal nerve).

within the anterior mediastinum, where up to one-third of all missed parathyroid tumours can be found.

Parathyroid physiology

The parathyroid glands secrete parathormone (PTH). PTH is a polypeptide with 84 amino acid residues and a molecular weight of 9500. It is formed from preproPTH (115 amino acids), which is cleaved in the endoplasmic reticulum to form proPTH (90 amino acids). Six further amino acids are cleaved in the Golgi apparatus and the PTH is then stored in secretory granules in the chief cells of the parathyroid glands. The N-terminal portion is felt to be the biologically active portion of PTH. The half-life of PTH is only 10–15 min, as it is rapidly cleaved by the Kupffer cells in the liver. The main mechanism for the regulation of PTH is a negative feedback with plasma ionized calcium. Accurate measurement of circulating intact PTH is now obtained using two site radioimmunoassay, with an assay against both the C-terminal and the N-terminal. This enables it to be differentiated from parathyroid hormone-related protein (PTHrP), which has PTH like activity. PTHrP has a similar N-terminal, but has 140 amino acids, and is found in breast milk, the renal tubules and the brain. PTHrP is also responsible for 80% of the hypercalcaemia associated with malignancy – the humoral hypercalcaemia of malignancy.

PTH has effects on the bone, kidney and the gastrointestinal tract. In the bone, it promotes bone reabsorption, by the activation of osteoblasts, to mobilize calcium. In the kidney, PTH increases the excretion of phosphate, by decreasing proximal tubular reabsorption. In normal circumstances, PTH increases calcium reabsorption at the distal tubules. However, this effect is overwhelmed in patients with hyperparathyroidism by the raised levels of calcium being filtered, leading to hypercalciuria. This effect helps distinguish primary hyperparathyroidism from rarer causes of hypercalcaemia, such as benign familial hypocalciuric hypercalcaemia (FHH). PTH also converts 25-hydroxycholecalciferol to the active 1,25-hydroxycholecalciferol, which aids the mobilization of calcium from the bone and promotes the absorption of calcium from the gastrointestinal tract.

Section 4b.2 • Hyperparathyroidism

Primary hyperparathyroidism (HPT) is the inappropriate secretion of PTH associated with excessive growth and abnormal function of one or more parathyroid glands. These abnormalities cause hypercalcaemia in most but not all patients ('normocalcaemic' HPT). The prevalence of HPT is 0.1–2%, being highest in post-menopausal women. HPT occurs most commonly in its sporadic form, familial cases accounting for less than 5% of cases.

Diagnosis

Although patients with HPT may present with severe 'classic' symptoms and signs, these are relatively uncommon today in the UK. The most common complaints are non-specific and are vague (Table 4b.1). The symptoms of HPT do not correlate with the severity of the hypercalcaemia and many patients (at least 30%) are diagnosed consequent on the incidental detection of a raised serum calcium. Although these patients are often described as having 'asymptomatic' HPT, the term 'mild' HPT is more appropriate because truly asymptomatic disease is uncommon. The prevalence of neuropsychiatric symptoms and cardiovascular risk factors in such individuals is frequently ignored.

The diagnosis of HPT is confirmed by the finding of an inappropriately high level of 'intact' PTH, the biologically active hormone, in a patient with hypercalcaemia. If the PTH level is low, normal or suppressed the hypercalcaemia is not caused by HPT. The differential diagnosis of HPT (Table 4b.2) includes hypercalcaemia of malignancy mediated by PTH-related peptide (PTHrP) and other growth factors secreted by the primary tumour which stimulate osteoclastic bone resorption and the presence of multiple bone metastases. Patients with FHH should be excluded by the absence of symptoms, a family history of the disorder and/or failed neck exploration, low urinary calcium and a calcium creatinine clearance ratio less than 0.01.

Pathology

At least 80% of patients with HPT will have single gland disease, a parathyroid adenoma. Most abnormal glands will weigh 200–1000 mg (normal glands weighing up to 50 mg). They are usually reddish brown in colour and have a low fat content, in contrast to a 'suppressed' normal gland. A remnant of normal compressed tissue may be visible to the pathologist; this 'rim' of parathyroid may be used as a criterion to distinguish parathyroid adenoma from hyperplasia. Multiple gland disease in HPT may be due to multiple adenomas (more frequent in older patients) in up to 10% of

Table 4b.1 Symptoms and signs of hyperparathyroidism

- Renal
  - Urinary frequency/polyuria and thirst
- Urinary tract calculi
  - Nephrocalcinosis
  - Renal failure
- Bone
  - Bone and joint pains
  - Chondrocalcinosis
  - Reduced bone mineral density
  - Fracture
- Gastrointestinal
  - Poor appetite
  - Nausea and vomiting
  - Constipation
  - Abdominal pain
  - Peptic ulcer
  - Pancreatitis
- Cardiovascular
  - Hypertension
  - Various myocardial changes
- Neuropsychiatric
  - Depression, psychosis
  - Fatigue, weakness, poor memory

Table 4b.2 Causes of hypercalcaemia

- Primary hyperparathyroidism
  - Primary hyperparathyroidism
  - Familial hyperparathyroidism
- Malignancy
- Sarcoidosis
- Vitamin D excess
- Thyrotoxicosis
- Drugs – thiazide diuretics, lithium
- Familial hypocalciuric hypercalcaemia
- Prolonged immobilization

patients or parathyroid hyperplasia (sporadic or associated with familial disease). In an individual patient with parathyroid hyperplasia the glands may be of varied size. Two histological subtypes are recognized – chief cell hyperplasia and water clear-cell hyperplasia.

Pre-operative localization studies

An experienced parathyroid surgeon will cure at least 95% of patients at initial bilateral neck exploration without the need for pre-operative localization. On that basis the routine use of localization studies is not recommended. The use of unilateral neck exploration and the arrival of minimally invasive parathyroid surgery has, particularly in European and US institutions, led to renewed interest in 'scan-directed' first-time surgery, to date without clear evidence of outcome/cost benefit.

The most frequently used non-invasive localization studies are:

- **Ultrasound.** Published series report that 50–80% of enlarged parathyroid glands can be identified prior to surgery. The skill of the user, the size and position of the abnormal gland and the presence of co-existing thyroid nodules will affect the sensitivity, specificity and accuracy of this technique.
- **Technetium-99m sestamibi (MIBI).** Up to 85% of parathyroid adenomas and 50% of abnormal glands in patients with multiglandular disease can be localized. The use of SPECT (single photon emission computed tomography) allows sagittal and transverse scans and better localization particularly of ectopic parathyroid tissue.

The use of CT, MRI, selective angiography, selective venous catheterization for PTH gradients and positron emission tomography (PET) scans is well described, but are best reserved for localization of abnormal parathyroid glands when initial surgery has failed.

Natural history of primary hyperparathyroidism

There is no doubt that patients with significant hypercalcaemia and/or 'symptomatic' hyperparathyroidism should undergo neck exploration and excision of abnormal parathyroid glands. There is long-standing dispute as to what is appropriate management for patients with minimally elevated serum calcium levels and/or 'minimal' symptoms. In this group, surgery results in a reduction in the HPT associated risk of death from cardiovascular disease, an increase in cancellous bone density, reversal of neuromuscular deficit and improvement in quality of life. Non-surgical 'treatment' of HPT consists of observation and long-term follow-up. Hormone replacement therapy for postmenopausal women with HPT at risk of osteoporosis does reduce the serum calcium. Although long-term observational follow-up studies show that as many as 25% of untreated patients have progression of their disease, there are no prospective randomized controlled trials on which to base guidelines for treatment. On that basis, a liberal approach to surgery is recommended.

Section 4b.3 • Familial hyperparathyroidism

Multiple endocrine neoplasia type 1 (MEN 1)

This autosomal dominant disorder, in which the causative gene is located on chromosome 11q13, and is characterized by hyperparathyroidism (90%), multiple neuroendocrine tumours of the pancreas (75%) – usually gastrinoma, and pituitary tumours (>30%) – usually prolactinoma. The hyperparathyroidism is multiglandular, and surgical intervention less than subtotal parathyroidectomy is associated with recurrence rates of up to 40%. Supernumerary parathyroid glands are common in this disease (up to 20%), most frequently sited in the thymus. The surgical approach should therefore include *at least* subtotal parathyroidectomy and transcervical thymectomy.

Multiple endocrine neoplasia type 2 (MEN 2A and MEN 2B)

This autosomal dominant disorder, in which the gene is localized to chromosome 10q, and is characterized by medullary thyroid cancer (invariable), phaeochromocytoma (50%) and hyperparathyroidism (25%). Patients with MEN 2B have a Marfanoid phenotype and multiple mucosal ganglioneuromata. The hyperparathyroidism of MEN 2 is less severe, single gland disease is more frequent, and only enlarged parathyroid glands should be removed at operation.

Familial non-MEN hyperparathyroidism is very rare and frequently associated with multiglandular disease, supernumary glands and parathyroid carcinoma. In some families the disorder is associated with mandibular tumours.

It is recommended that patients and families with genetically determined disease should be treated in specialist centres, as the treatment and screening strategies required for both MEN 1 and MEN 2 require a multidisciplinary approach that includes endocrine surgeons and physicians, clinical and molecular geneticists, interventional radiologists, histopathologists, biochemists and pathologists.

Section 4b.4 • Hypercalcaemic crises in HPT

Acute severe hypercalcaemia (corrected calcium >3.5 mm/l) may occur in patients with HPT, often precipitated by intercurrent illness (associated with vomiting/diarrhoea) or diuretic therapy. The clinical presentation may include fatigue, weakness, polyuria, confusion, coma, pancreatitis and cardiovascular instability. Hypotension, pancreatitis and cardiac failure predict a poor outcome.

Treatment

The treatment of hypercalcaemic crises in HPT involves:

- Aggressive rehydration with normal saline – up to 200 ml per hour – to promote a good urine output. This may require monitoring of CVP in elderly or unfit patients. Diuretic therapy is best avoided.
- Bisphosphonates act by inhibiting bone resorption. Treatment is usually by giving Pamidronate 60–90 mg intravenously over 4–24 hours. Multiple doses may be required.

Surgery should be delayed until the corrected serum calcium is below 3 mmol/l.

Section 4b.5 • Parathyroid carcinoma

Parathyroid carcinoma is found in approximately 1% of primary/HPT cases. Patients will typically have a long history, calcium levels >3.5 mm/l (70%), a palpable neck mass (50%) and severe bone disease (60%). At operation, the diagnosis is made on the basis of a firm, adherent grey–white gland (sometimes an atypical 'old' benign adenoma) or local invasion.

- Biopsy is contra-indicated.
- *En-bloc* resection of the parathyroid gland, thyroid lobe and isthmus and other involved tissue should be performed.

Completion surgery should be performed if the diagnosis is made by the pathologist (a thick fibrous capsule with trabeculated fibrous bands traversing the tumour). Half the patients will have a favourable prognosis, although recurrent disease (local/regional and/or metastases with hypercalcaemia) usually occurs within 3 years.

Section 4b.6 • Surgical approaches to hyperparathyroidism

The definitive treatment for patients with primary HPT is surgery, which should ensure a high rate of cure with a low complication rate. Doppman noted that 'the only localizing study indicated in a patient with untreated primary hyperparathyroidism is to localize an experienced parathyroid surgeon'. It is therefore axiomatic that the surgeon should have a good understanding of embryology and surgical anatomy of the parathyroid glands, to ensure a successful outcome (see section on parathyroid embryology and anatomy).

Pathology

The normal shape of a parathyroid gland depends on its location. In loose tissue it classically appears as a light-brown ovoid or sphere floating within surrounding yellow fat, but under a capsule the shape is flat with sharp edges. When enlarged, however, it assumes a spherical shape indicating hyperactivity of the parathyroid gland. The greatest diameter of a normal parathyroid gland is usually no more than 5 mm with an upper limit of normal weight of 50 mg.

Surgical technique

Pre-operative preparation is as previously described for thyroidectomy except for the use of methylene blue (5 mg per kg body weight methylene blue in 500 ml of dextrose/saline infused intravenously over an hour before surgery), which selectively stains parathyroid tissue and is a valuable aid to the difficult case. It is fundamental for the endocrine surgeon to identify all four (or possibly more) parathyroid glands in the neck. The parathyroid exploration is usually started by searching for the upper parathyroid gland just above the neurovascular intersection of the RLN/ITA on the dorsum of the thyroid gland, retracting the thyroid with a finger on a gauze swab. Careful dissection of the fat and fibrous attachments to the thyroid at this point usually reveals the majority of upper glands. The dissection should be under direct vision at all times to prevent injury to the RLN, which usually runs antero-medially to the upper gland. When it cannot be found in its usual site exploration of the para/retro-oesophageal space is undertaken with digital exploration of the posterior mediastinum and capsulotomy of the upper thyroid pole to inspect for a subcapsular intrathyroidal gland.

The search for the inferior parathyroid gland begins with a thorough inspection of the lower thyroid pole, the thyrothymic ligament and the thymus itself. Usually the lower parathyroid lies in the fat between inferior thyroid veins but rarely it may be found in the anterior surface of the thyroid gland.

Bilateral exploration should be undertaken and in 85% of patients there will be a solitary parathyroid adenoma. The adenoma is gently dissected using a gauze pledget (to push the gland forward) and fine clips (taking care not to break the capsule) to release it from its fascial coverings. The pedicle is defined, clipped and divided, and the adenoma removed (Figures 4b.2 and 4b.3). If three normal parathyroid glands are found the adenoma should be removed and examined by frozen section. It is controversial whether a biopsy of one of the normal glands is undertaken but the author does not routinely biopsy unless the appearances at operation are suspicious. If two enlarged glands are found they should be removed and the two normal glands should be biopsied and marked with clips. Microscopic distinction between adenomas and hyperplasia can be difficult and the role of the pathologist intra-operatively is therefore limited to the identification of parathyroid tissue. If all parathyroid glands are enlarged three parathyroid glands should be removed along with a half of the fourth and a thymectomy should be performed, as supernumerary parathyroid glands are frequently located in the thymus. The parathyroid remnant should be approximately 50 mg of tissue and an easily accessible gland with a reliable vascular stalk should be chosen and biopsied first before the others

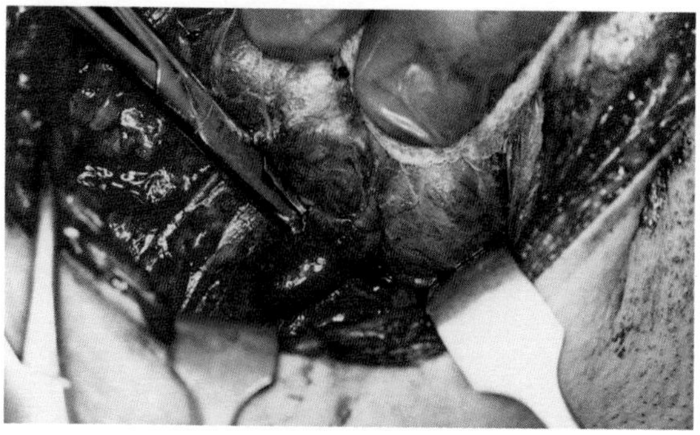

Figure 4b.2 Cervical exploration – left superior parathyroid adenoma (stained with methylene blue) being gently 'teased out' from surrounding fascia.

are removed to ensure that it remains viable. An alternative surgical strategy is to remove all four glands and re-implant half of one as an autotransplant into a pocket of the sternomastoid muscle.

Secondary hyperparathyroidism

In patients with secondary HPT, familial HPT or MEN 1 syndrome all parathyroid glands are involved and the rate of recurrent HPT in these patients ranges from 10–15%. A subtotal parathyroidectomy should therefore be performed leaving behind a remnant of a lower parathyroid (with a clip marker) or autotransplantation is performed as described above. Cryopreservation of some parathyroid tissue may also be considered.

Mediastinotomy

Following a thorough exploration of the neck when an abnormal gland is not found normal glands should never be removed and the cervical wound should be closed and full investigation carried out, including high-resolution ultrasound scanning, CT, MRI, Sestamibi subtraction scan and selective venous sampling to confirm the location of the ectopic adenoma which is usually to be found within the chest (see Figure 4b.4) in either the anterior mediastinum (for an inferior gland) or posterior mediastinum (for a superior gland). Surgery can then be planned accordingly for either a

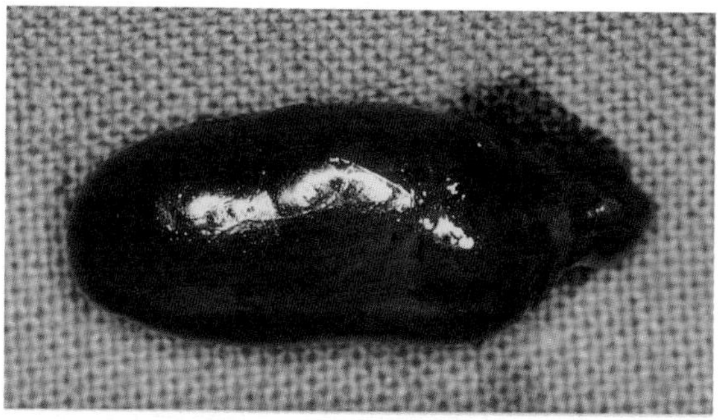

Figure 4b.3 Left superior parathyroid adenoma weighing 630 mg – note intact glistening capsule.

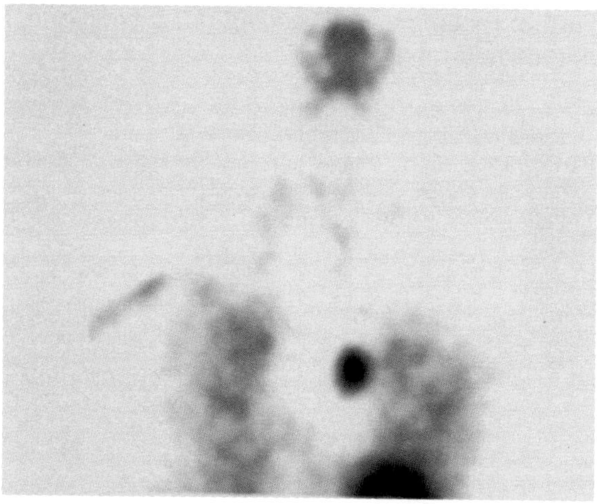

Figure 4b.4 Sestamibi scan demonstrating ectopic adenoma of fifth parathyroid gland in aorto-pulmonary window of middle mediastinum.

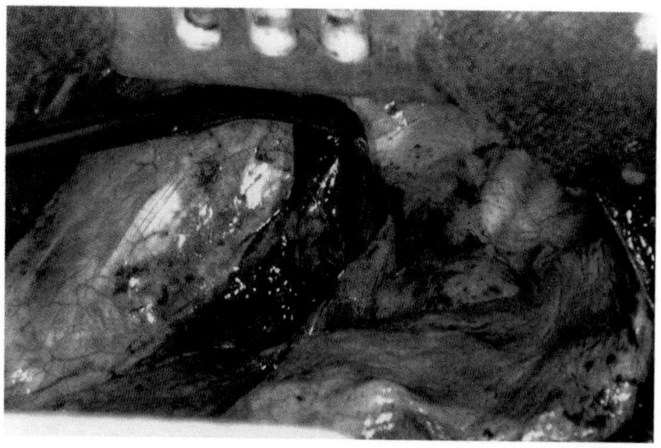

Figure 4b.5 Removal of ectopic fifth parathyroid adenoma (7 g) from aorto-pulmonary window through a left fourth rib thoracotomy (courtesy of Mr C. Forrester-Wood, BRI).

mediastinotomy or lateral thoracotomy, respectively (see Figure 4b.5). More recently thoracoscopy or mediastinoscopy has been reported to be a successful minimally invasive technique to remove mediastinal adenomas.

Unilateral or bilateral exploration

Unilateral neck exploration for primary HPT is controversial because of the concern about missing multiglandular disease and the inaccuracy of pre-operative localization tests. Protagonists claim decreased complications and cost-effectiveness for the technique but drawbacks are obviously missing double adenomas or hyperplasia. Retrospective data analysis reveals no differences between two techniques and to date no prospective studies have compared unilateral versus bilateral exploration. Bilateral neck exploration is therefore the standard approach because it is safe, avoids missing a second adenoma and avoids unnecessary expensive pre-operative localization studies as over 95% of patients can be cured when treated by an experienced endocrine surgeon using a bilateral neck exploration.

Further recommended reading (for thyroid and parathyroid modules)

Clark, O. H. and Quan-Yang Duh. (1997). *Textbook of Endocrine Surgery*. Philadelphia, PA: W. B. Saunders.

Clark, O. H., Quan-Yang Duh and Siperstein A. E. *The Surgical Clinics of North America. Endocrine Surgery*. Philadelphia, PA: W. B. Saunders.

Frieser, S. R. and Thompson, N. W. (1997). *Surgical Endocrinology: Clinical Syndromes*. Philadelphia, PA: Lippincott.

Lynn, J. and Bloom, S. R. *Surgical Endocrinology*. Oxford: Butterworth-Heinemann.

Wheeler, M. H. and Richards, S. H. The laryngeal nerves. *Curr Surg Pract* **5**: 237–50.

MODULE 5

Disorders of the adrenal glands

The Roman anatomist Bartholomaeus Eustachius first described the adrenal glands in 1552 in his *Opuscula Anatomica* referring to them as 'glandulae renibus incumbentes' (glands lying on the kidneys). The function of the adrenal glands, however, remained a mystery to workers for 300 years, until in 1856 the French physiologist Charles Brown-Séquard demonstrated these glands were essential to life in a series of experiments on dogs and rats. Brown-Séquard had been inspired by a report the previous year by Thomas Addison of London, describing the clinical findings of 11 patients in whom the adrenal glands had been found at post-mortem to be destroyed, through either tuberculosis or cancer (a condition later termed Addison's disease).

General consensus held that the adrenals secreted a substance essential to life, though what this substance was remained an enigma and Addison's disease remained untreatable. Whilst working on a cure for Addison's disease in 1893 the physiologists George Oliver of Harrogate and Edward Sharpey-Schäfer of London prepared an extract from the adrenal medulla (the anatomical distinction between cortex and medulla had been made in the 1805 by Baron Georges Cuvier and the terms coined by Emil Huschke in 1845). The extract failed to cure Addison's but produced a marked constriction of blood vessels. This preparation was later purified and termed adrenaline (1897) or epinephrine (1901). It was not until the late 1920s when American workers prepared an adrenal cortical extract termed 'cortin' that Addison's disease was treated successfully.

The adrenal glands are now known to secrete a wide variety of hormones that regulate many essential physiological functions including blood pressure, carbohydrate, fat and protein metabolism. It is not surprising, therefore, that development of hyperplastic or neoplastic conditions may lead to overproduction of various hormones, resulting in a wide variety of clinical syndromes.

The current day endocrine surgeon with an ever-increasing diversity of biochemical tests, pharmaceutical agents, localizing modalities and operative techniques, has a unique opportunity to correct profound physiological and often life threatening disturbances and restore the patient to complete normality.

Section 5.1 • Anatomy

The adrenals are retroperitoneal structures, each weighing approximately 2–6 g and located on either side of the vertebral column within Gerota's fascia, in close proximity to the crura of the diaphragm and the superior poles of the kidneys. The right adrenal gland is triangular or pyramidal in shape with the apex superiorly and the base towards the right kidney. It lies on the right crux of the diaphragm posteriorly, the bare area of the liver anteriorly, the inferior vena cava antero-medially and the superior pole of the right kidney infero-laterally. The left gland is crescenteric in shape, related anteriorly to the stomach and pancreas and posteriorly to the diaphragm. Anteriorly the gland is covered by the peritoneum of the lesser sac.

Arterial supply is drawn from the aorta, renal artery and inferior phrenic artery, though some tumours (particularly phaeochromocytoma) may demonstrate marked vascular neogenesis. Main venous drainage on the right side is via a short adrenal vein (5 mm) directly to the inferior vena cava, usually entering posteriorly. On the left side drainage is directly to the left renal vein. Frequently venous drainage is supplemented by additional veins running directly to the vena cava or hepatic veins on the right and the phrenic vein on the left.

Macroscopically the adrenal glands are a golden yellow colour, which contrasts with the surrounding perinephric fat. When sectioned the outer cortical layer (which makes up 80% of the normal gland in volume) is lipid rich and golden or yellow, in contrast to the well-vascularized medulla which tends to be reddish-brown in colour. The cortex consists of three layers. From outer to inner these are: the zona glomerulosa (aldosterone production), zona fasciculata (cortisol production) and zona reticularis (androgen production).

The adrenals have a rich sympathetic nerve supply from the coeliac plexus but pre-ganglionic fibres from the splanchnic nerves pass through the coeliac plexus to supply the adrenal medulla.

Section 5.2 • Physiology

The principal hormone secretions of the adrenal gland, aldosterone, cortisol and the androgens (mainly testosterone) are synthesized via intermediates such as pregnenolone and progesterone, from cholesterol by a series of metabolic steps, each requiring a specific enzyme.

Aldosterone is a mineralocorticoid with the principal action of stimulating sodium reabsorption in exchange for potassium and hydrogen ions. This occurs in the distal renal tubule, ascending loop of Henle and collecting ducts. Plasma oncotic pressure is increased thus expanding plasma volume. Synthesis and secretion of aldosterone is regulated by angiotensin II and by plasma levels of sodium and potassium. Aldosterone is produced in the zona glomerulosa in response to a fall in blood volume, registered in the juxtaglomerular apparatus of the afferent tubules of the kidney. These cells release renin which splits angiotensinogen to angiotensin I, which is then converted to angiotensin II by angiotensin-converting enzyme (ACE). Sodium retention is directly linked to potassium exchange, the rate being dependent on the rate at which sodium is presented to the tubule.

Glucocorticoid production, mainly cortisol and small amounts of corticosterone are produced in the zona fasciculata. The rate of production is directly dependent on adrenocorticotrophic hormone (ACTH) from the pituitary, which in turn is suppressed directly by cortisol, via a direct negative feedback mechanism of cortisol on the pituitary. ACTH secretion is stimulated by corticotrophin releasing hormone (CRH), produced by the hypothalamus (CRH production is also suppressed by cortisol). Cortisol has a wide range of physiological actions involving fat, carbohydrate and protein metabolism and is subject to a specific diurnal variation in synthesis and production, with highest levels being achieved early in the morning and lowest levels at night.

Androgen production is from the zona reticularis and is also stimulated by ACTH. In the adult, however, the main site of sex hormone production is the gonads. Sex hormones produced from the adrenals play a role in growth and sexual differentiation.

Section 5.3 • Addison's disease and adrenal insufficiency

Adrenal insufficiency was first recognized and described by Thomas Addison in a presentation in 1849. His classic 1855 publication documented the symptoms and physical findings in 11 patients with adrenal destruction noted at post-mortem. The major causative factor was tuberculosis, although metastatic carcinoma and atrophy were also documented. The term Addison's disease was first used by Armand Trousseau of Paris the following year. Trosseau had read Addison's monograph '*On the Constitutional and Local Effects of Disease of the Supra-renal Capsules*' and noted the same symptoms, clinical and post-mortem findings in a patient with tuberculosis of the adrenal glands.

Addison's disease has always been a rare condition and until recently reduction in the numbers of patients with tuberculosis decreased the incidence even further but the incidence of tuberculosis has risen and this, coupled with acquired autoimmune deficiency syndrome (AIDS) and autoimmune adrenalitis has meant that the incidence of Addison's disease has increased. In 1974 the recorded incidence in Denmark was six cases per 100 000 population.

A number of conditions have now been described that can destroy or interfere with the adrenal cortex, resulting in Addison's disease. The most common cause is autoimmune disease, which is responsible for 65% of all cases of primary adrenal insufficiency and association with other autoimmune conditions such as autoimmune thyroiditis and insulin-dependent diabetes is common. Other causes include tuberculosis, AIDS, sarcoidosis, amyloidosis, haemochromatosis, histoplasmosis, metastatic carcinoma, congenital adrenal hyperplasia, adrenocortical haemorrhage (particularly in anticoagulated patients), adrenal venography or meningococcal septicaemia (Waterhouse–Friderichsen syndrome).

AIDS is increasingly responsible for patients with Addison's disease by a number of mechanisms. Adrenal destruction and insufficiency can be caused by infection with *Mycobacterium tuberculosis*, *M. avium-intracellulare*, toxoplasmosis, histoplasmosis and *Pneumocystis carinii*. Neoplastic destruction by Kaposi's sarcoma or lymphoma has also been described. Ketocanozole, rifampicin, phenytoin and corticosteroids, drugs used in the treatment of AIDS-related illness may all cause adrenal impairment. As patients with AIDS frequently present with similar symptoms to those with Addison's disease, a high index of suspicion is required.

Bilateral surgical removal is an obvious cause of adrenal insufficiency. By definition, however, adrenal insufficiency following bilateral adrenalectomy is not Addison's disease. Acute adrenal failure may also result following the sudden withdrawal of long-term steroid treatment precipitating cardiovascular collapse or even death.

Adrenal insufficiency is characterized by lassitude, weakness, anorexia and amenorrhea. Physical findings include hypotension, pigmentation of the buccal mucosa (particularly on pressure areas), vitiligo and loss of body hair. In acute and extreme cases drowsiness, confusion, coma and death occur. In the collapsed patient, stigmata of disease for which steroids may be prescribed or bilateral adrenalectomy scars may provide important clues to the diagnosis. Features of adrenal, hypothalamic or pituitary disease may also be present.

The diagnosis of Addison's disease may be confirmed by intramuscular injection of 250 μg of tetracosactrin and the plasma cortisol response at 0, 30 and 60 min recorded (short-term Synacthen test). In normal patients the plasma cortisol level should rise. The response is absent or impaired in patients Addison's disease. A long-term Synacthen test (depot test) helps to distinguish primary adrenal insufficiency from secondary adrenal dysfunction, usually from pituitary disease. Subsequent investigations including chest and abdominal X-ray and auto-antibody screening are directed at establishing the cause of adrenal insufficiency.

Treatment of acute adrenal insufficiency

The signs and symptoms of acute adrenal insufficiency listed above progress rapidly. In patients with meningococcal septicaemia (often children) characteristic petechial skin haemorrhages may be noted in addition to hyperpyrexia, rigors and vomiting. The onset of profound shock with tachycardia and hypotension may occur suddenly. If appropriate therapy is not immediately instituted, coma and death ensue. The most common finding on routine laboratory testing is hyponatraemia, although this is not always present.

Once the diagnosis is suspected patients should be given 100 mg of hydrocortisone intravenously and rapidly resuscitated with intravenous normal saline. Intravenous antibiotics are given immediately if septicaemia is suspected as the underlying cause. Recovery is usually prompt but hydrocortisone (100 mg i.v.) should be continued every 6 hours until the patient is stabilized. Subsequently, patients can be changed to oral hydrocortisone or dexamethasone. Mineralocorticoids are not necessary when the dose of cortisol exceeds 60 mg/day. Chronic adrenal insufficiency will require maintenance therapy with hydrocortisone, usually 20 mg in the morning and 10 mg in the evening. Additional mineralocorticoid may be necessary in patients with impaired salt-retaining ability (0.05–0.1 mg fludrocortisone). Hypertension, oedema and hypokalaemia are signs of overtreatment. Fatigue, hypotension and hyperkalaemia are signs of undertreatment. The relative potency of various steroid preparations are shown in Figure 5.1.

Surgery and steroid replacement therapy

- **Bilateral adrenalectomy**: Hydrocortisone sodium succinate is given i.m. (or i.v.) with the premedication and a further 100 mg given at the time of gland removal. In the post-operative period hydrocortisone 100 mg 6 hourly i.v. is continued for between 48 and 72 hours, reducing to 50 mg 6 hourly before the introduction of 20 mg of oral hydrocortisone in the morning and 10 mg at night. Mineralocorticoid is given as oral 0.05–0.1 mg fludrocortisone acetate daily.
- **Unilateral adrenalectomy** normally does not require steroid cover but if performed for Cushing's syndrome due to an adrenal adenoma, hydrocortisone sodium succinate 100 mg i.m./i.v. is given with the premedication and a further 100 mg given during the operation and continued 6 hourly, reducing with the introduction of 20 mg of oral hydrocortisone in the morning and 10 mg at night. Gradual reduction of steroid replacement is made on a monthly basis with complete weaning often taking up to 12–18 months, as the remaining adrenal gland recovers normal function.
- **Surgery in the hypoadrenal patient**, e.g. after bilateral adrenalectomy and in patients with adrenal suppression from steroid therapy. If these patients are having major surgery, additional steroids are required: hydrocortisone sodium succinate 100 mg i.m./i.v. is given with the premedication and a further 100 mg i.v. given during the operation and continued 6 hourly until the patient is able to return to the usual oral replacement steroid dose. If the post-operative period is prolonged, e.g. after a gastrointestinal operation, the parenteral hydrocortisone is reduced to 50 mg and then 25 mg 8 hourly until the patient is able to take oral medication.

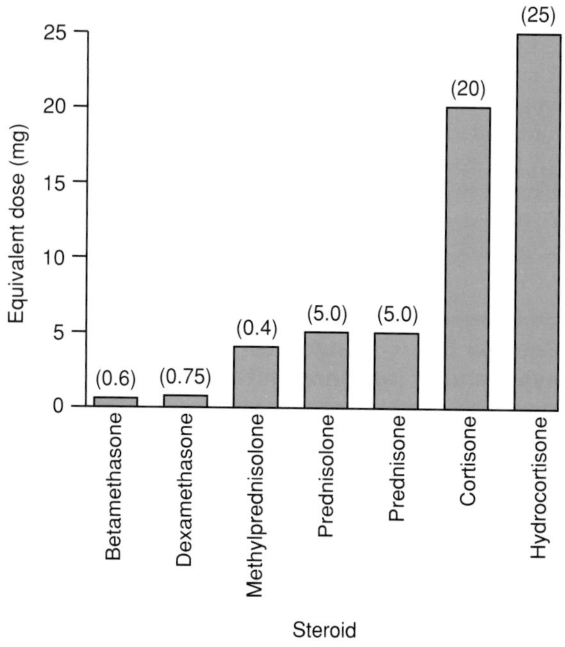

Figure 5.1 Relative potency of steroid compounds.

For most minor surgery, where oral intake is not restricted, intramuscular hydrocortisone is only required for 24 hours post-operatively and for minimal surgical procedures such as endoscopy, a single dose of hydrocortisone 100 mg is all that is required.

Patients who are on steroid therapy, who have undergone bilateral adrenalectomy or who suffer from primary hypoadrenalism must be fully advised by the medical staff on the nature of their condition and the symptoms to be expected with inadequate steroid replacement. They are instructed to double the usual dose of steroid immediately and seek medical assistance in the event of illness or severe stress. The crucial importance of this treatment must be emphasized. All patients should carry a steroid warning card and the wearing of a Medic Alert® bracelet is to be encouraged. Patients who have had total adrenalectomy in some hospitals in the USA are given a steroid-containing syringe for emergency self-administration.

Section 5.4 • Congenital adrenal hyperplasia (adrenogenital syndrome)

The principal hormone secretions of the adrenal gland, aldosterone, cortisol and the androgens (mainly testosterone) are synthesized via intermediates such as pregnenolone and progesterone, from cholesterol by a series of metabolic steps, each requiring a specific enzyme. A deficiency in one of the enzymes (inherited in an autosomal recessive manner) leads to a deficiency in cortisol and/or aldosterone production. The lack of negative feedback to the pituitary results in excessive ACTH production. The growth stimulating effect of ACTH leads to the development of bilateral adrenal hyperplasia.

The most common cause of adrenal hyperplasia is a deficiency of the enzyme 21-hydroxylase (90% of cases). This enzyme catalyses progesterone to deoxycorticosterone and 17-OH progesterone to 11-deoxycortisol. Deficiency leads directly to lack of production of aldosterone and cortisol. The backlog of metabolites are subsequently diverted into production of the androgens dehydroepiandrosterone, androstenedione and testosterone. Other enzyme deficiencies reported include 11β-hydroxylase, 3β-hydroxy steroid dehydrogenase and 17α-hydroxylase. Impaired production of aldosterone leads to *salt wasting* from excessive urinary salt loss. This is characterized in the newborn by vomiting, and failure to feed and thrive.

The condition termed *congenital adrenal hyperplasia* is fortunately rare, with a reported incidence of 1 in 5000 to 1 in 15 000. Excessive androgen production in the female fetus leads to virilization, pseudohermaphroditism with ambiguous external genitalia, clitoral enlargement and fusion of the genital folds. In the male fetus the effects of androgen excess are not so obvious but penile enlargement occurs during childhood and pseudoprecocious puberty may ensue (infant Hercules). Early epiphyseal closure leads to short stature in adult life.

Diagnosis of congenital adrenal hyperplasia

Lack of the enzyme 21-hydroxylase leads to excess of the precursors progesterone and 17-OH progesterone. Measurement of the plasma level of 17-OH progesterone by radioimmunoassay is the most reliable method of confirming the diagnosis.

Treatment

Hydrocortisone (5 mg/day in divided doses) is administered to replace the glucocorticoid deficiency and totally suppress ACTH drive. Adequate suppression can be monitored by assessing 17-OH progesterone levels in urine and plasma. *Salt wasting* is treated by intravenous normal saline and mineralocorticoid replacement. Early diagnosis, adequate medical therapy and careful follow-up should ensure growth development, fertility and life expectancy are all normal.

Section 5.5 • Cushing's syndrome

The physiological and clinical features of Cushing's syndrome are due to excessive levels of circulating glucocorticoids. The predominant clinical features of the disease include moon type facies, centripedal obesity with prominent interscapular fat pad formation, abdominal striae, diabetes and hypertension. The causes of Cushing's syndrome are divided into two main groups, ACTH dependent and non-ACTH dependent.

ACTH-dependent Cushing's syndrome

Cushing's disease

Harvey Cushing (a Boston neurosurgeon) described the classical clinical features of the syndrome in 1932. He termed the condition 'pituitary basophilism', indicating that the condition was caused specifically by a pituitary basophil adenoma. Pituitary (ACTH)-dependent Cushing's syndrome (referred to as Cushing's disease) accounts for 70% of all cases of the syndrome. An ACTH-producing pituitary adenoma or microadenoma is responsible in approximately 75% of patients. Tumours are small (usually <1 cm) and malignancy is rare. The primary defect is probably located in the hypothalamus with overproduction of CRH. Chronically raised ACTH levels result in adrenal cortical hyperplasia and cortisol excess. ACTH secretion is still subject to negative feedback but at a higher set point than normal. Women are affected eight times more commonly than men and the disease is most common between 35 and 50 years of age.

Ectopic ACTH syndrome

Ectopic ACTH production accounts for 10% of cases of Cushing's syndrome and is caused by a spectrum of tumours originating from neuro-endocrine cells. The commonest cause is a small cell carcinoma of the lung (previously referred to as oat cell tumours). Other causes include thymoma, medullary thyroid cancer, phaeochromocytoma, pancreatic islet cell tumours, certain ovarian cancers, pancreas, stomach and bronchial carcinoids.

The first case of ectopic ACTH syndrome was described by Brown in 1928, although the term 'ectopic ACTH syndrome' was originally coined by Liddle and colleagues in 1962. Cases caused by benign carcinoids may be difficult to diagnose as the onset of

Cushing's syndrome may be insidious over several years. The tumours may also be small and therefore difficult to locate.

In patients with small cell carcinoma of the lung, the onset of symptoms is usually rapid, making the diagnosis easier. Tumours are aggressive and the primary malignancy frequently kills the patient before significant or severe effects of glucocorticoid excess supervene. The peak incidence of ACTH syndrome is in the fourth and fifth decades and the condition is twice as common in men as in women.

Non-ACTH-dependent Cushing's syndrome

The commonest cause of the syndrome is the administration of steroids for the treatment of other conditions. This iatrogenic group will not be considered further.

Adrenal tumours

Approximately 20% of cases of Cushing's syndrome are caused by either benign adrenal adenoma (10%) or frankly invasive adrenocortical carcinoma (10%). Benign adenoma is more common in adults and malignancy more common in the young. Excessive glucocorticoid secretion suppresses ACTH production from the pituitary, resulting in atrophy of the contralateral adrenal gland.

Macronodular adrenal cortical hyperplasia

This unusual condition, in which ACTH-independent cortisol secretion results from bilateral adrenal nodular hyperplasia, is sometimes seen in the young and may be associated with severe osteopenic bone disease. The cause is unknown.

Primary pigmented nodular adrenal cortical disease

Primary pigmented nodular adrenal cortical disease (PPND) producing autonomous adrenal hyperfunction occurs in conjunction with cardiac, breast and cutaneous myxomas. The adrenal nodules in this rare condition are normally small and the adrenal glands may even appear to be normal on imaging. Lentigines are found on the face, lips and conjunctivae. Pituitary adenomas and neuroectodermal tumours also occur.

Clinical features of Cushing's syndrome

The most common features of Cushing's syndrome are truncal obesity, weight gain, facial plethora, hirsutism, mild or moderate hypertension, menstrual irregularities, bruising and abdominal striae (Figure 5.2).

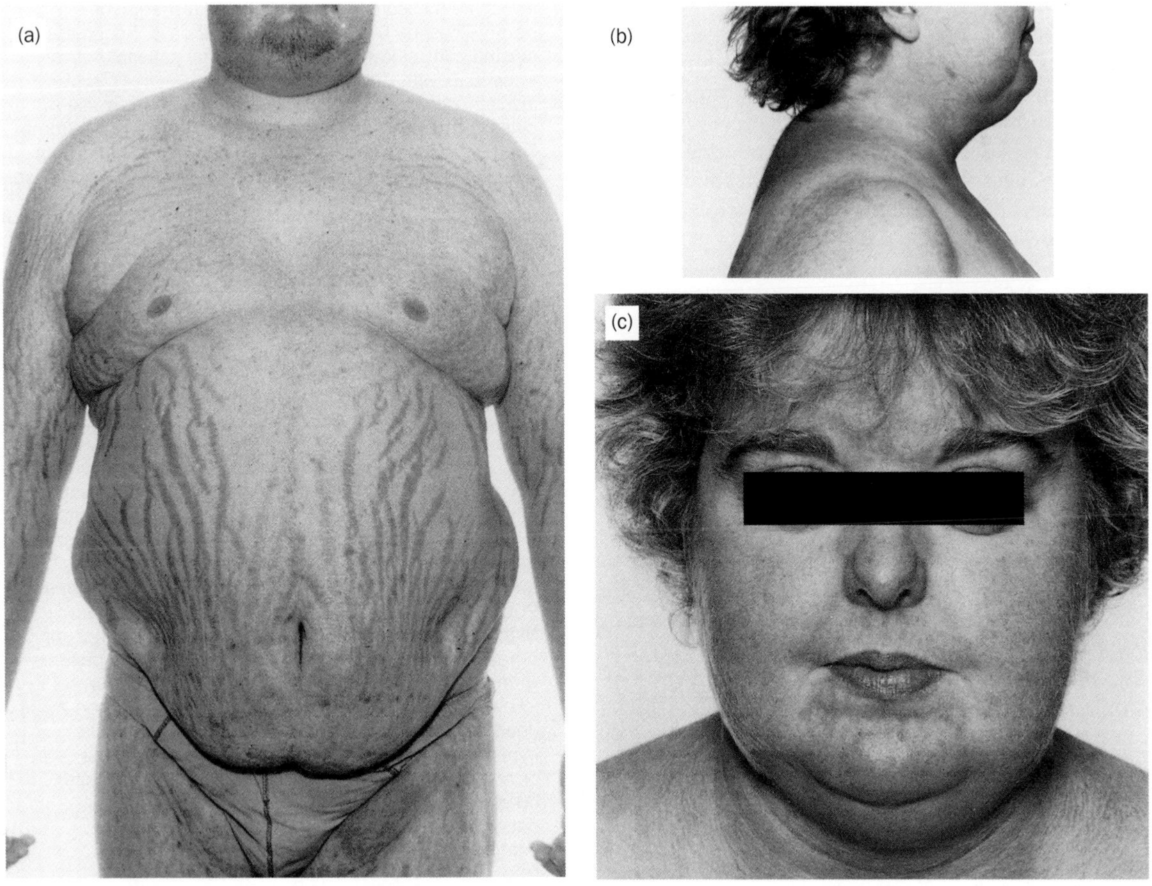

Figure 5.2 Cushing's syndrome. (a) Marked truncal obesity, abdominal striae and wasted limbs. (b) Interscapular fat pad. (c) Plethoric moon face.

Obesity is caused by excessive cortisol stimulating appetite and promoting gluconeogenesis which releases glucose for fat synthesis. Patients develop plethoric, rounded 'moon-like' facies, whereas truncal fat distribution results in interscapular fat pad formation. In contrast, the toxic effect of cortisol on muscles leads to muscle wasting and weakness. The proximal limb muscles are affected most and patients may develop a 'lemon on a stick' appearance.

Skin changes result from excessive cortisol depleting skin collagen. Thinning of the skin, striae and excessive bruising (either spontaneously or with minor trauma) are all features. In ACTH-dependent Cushing's syndrome, high levels of ACTH melanocyte stimulating hormone cause skin pigmentation. This is more commonly encountered in ectopic ACTH syndrome due to malignancy and Nelson's syndrome (high ACTH levels following bilateral adrenalectomy for pituitary disease).

Hirsutism and acne from excessive androgen secretion are often distressing features for the patient. Adrenocortical carcinoma should be suspected, particularly if virilisim is marked.

Poor wound healing is a direct outcome of decreased collagen synthesis and increased protein catabolism. This is an important consideration in all patients in whom surgery is contemplated, particularly when an anterior abdominal approach is employed.

Hypertension and oedema are a consequence of the glucocorticoid effects of cortisol resulting in salt and water retention. Congestive cardiac failure is present in 20% of patients. Untreated this is a major cause of mortality in Cushing's syndrome.

Diabetes mellitus, approximately 15% of patients develop diabetes because of the action of cortisol on carbohydrate metabolism. An abnormal glucose tolerance test (GTT), however, may be present in 70% of patients.

Osteoporosis is common (70%) and may lead to pathological fractures particularly in the ribs and also vertebral collapse. Urinary calcium excretion is raised (hypercalciuria) leading to renal stone formation and hypocalcaemic alkalosis.

Menstrual disturbance, male impotence, psychiatric illness and growth retardation (particularly in children) are also associated features of Cushing's syndrome.

Differential diagnosis

The clinical features of Cushing's syndrome may be mistakenly confused with those of the obese diabetic, particularly when there is a plethoric face or hirsutism. Polycystic ovary syndrome, with sterility and hirsutism also poses diagnostic difficulties but Cushing's syndrome rarely causes hirsutism alone. Alcoholic patients can present with pseudo-Cushing's syndrome, the signs and symptoms of which resolve following cessation of excessive alcohol intake.

Biochemical investigation of Cushing's syndrome

Cushing's syndrome will be initially suspected on the basis of the above clinical features. It is then necessary to confirm the presence of hypercortisolism and subsequently identify the cause of excessive cortisol production.

Tests to confirm hypercortisolism

These are:

- *Plasma cortisol levels* (under ACTH control) in normal individuals exhibit a diurnal variation. The highest levels are recorded at 9.00 am (<140–800 nmol/l) and lowest at midnight (<190 nmol/l). Loss of this diurnal variation is frequently exhibited in Cushing's syndrome. Plasma cortisol levels recorded at 9.00 am and particularly at midnight are elevated above normal limits. False positive and false negative observations may be caused by acute illness or depression. Even the relatively minor trauma of venupuncture can falsely elevate midnight levels.
- *Urinary free cortisol* in 24 hour urine collection is invariably raised in Cushing's syndrome. Normal values are <360 nmol/day for men and <280 nmol/day for women.
- *Dexamethasone suppression tests*. In normal individuals ACTH secretion and cortisol production may be suppressed by the administration of an exogenous corticosteroid (dexamethasone). Although patients with Cushing's syndrome may also exhibit ACTH suppression, it is far less marked than in normal individuals. *Overnight dexamethasone test:* 2 mg of dexamethasone (a powerful corticosteroid) is administered orally at midnight and plasma cortisol levels are measured at 9.00 am. When results of the overnight test are equivocal a *low-dose dexamethasone test* may be performed: plasma cortisol levels are measured prior to oral administration of dexamethasone 0.5 mg 6 hourly for 2 days. Suppression of plasma cortisol levels is seen in normal patients but rarely in patients with Cushing's syndrome.
- *Insulin-induced hypoglycaemia* fails to produce a rise in plasma cortisol levels in patients with Cushing's syndrome. The test is useful in differentiating between patients with the syndrome from patients with depression who may have elevated basal cortisol levels.

Identification of the cause of cortisol excess

Having confirmed a diagnosis of Cushing's syndrome the following tests are used to establish whether the disease is ACTH or non-ACTH dependent (i.e. pituitary or non-pituitary in origin):

- *Plasma ACTH measurement by radioimmuno-assay.* Patients with adrenal tumours have low or undetectable levels of plasma ACTH (<10 pg/ml), compared to patients with pituitary disease who tend to have elevated levels, although in some patients with pituitary disease ACTH levels may be in the normal range. In patients with ectopic ACTH syndrome, levels may be very high, sometimes in excess of 200 pg/ml.
- *High-dose dexamethasone test.* Patients are given 2 mg of dexamethasone 6 hourly for 2 days. In nearly all patients with pituitary disease (ACTH dependent) serum cortisol levels are suppressed. In contrast, patients with non-ACTH dependent disease (adrenal tumour, adrenal nodular hyperplasia and ectopic ACTH syndrome) show little or no suppression. False positive and negative results do occur and are more likely to be encountered in patients with adrenal nodular hyperplasia and ectopic ACTH syndrome than patients with adrenal tumours.
- *Metapyrone test.* This test is now rarely performed. Metapyrone is an 11μ-hydoxylase inhibitor which blocks the final step in cortisol synthesis, reducing plasma cortisol

levels, stimulating ACTH secretion and increasing production of the cortisol precursors (compound S). The test is performed by giving patients metapyrone 750 mg (125 mg/4 hourly). A 24 hour urine collection is performed on the day before, the day of and the day after metapyrone administration and 17 OHCS levels are measured. In normal patients and patients with pituitary disease (ACTH dependent) urinary excretion of 17 OHCS is increased. In contrast, the majority of patients with adrenal tumours exhibit a decrease in 17 OHCS urinary excretion. Patients with nodular hyperplasia or ectopic ACTH syndrome usually demonstrate an impaired or absent response to metapyrone.

Choice of test in Cushing's syndrome

When Cushing's syndrome is suspected clinically, diagnosis is usually confirmed by:

- measuring plasma cortisol (9.00 am and midnight)
- measuring urinary free cortisol and
- performing a low-dose dexamethasone test.

Confirming the cause of Cushing's syndrome is best achieved by:

- measuring basal plasma ACTH
- performing a high-dose dexamethasone test and
- in cases of diagnostic difficulty, performing a metapyrone test.

Localizing procedures in Cushing's syndrome

Pituitary tumour (Cushing's disease)

Magnetic resonance imaging (MRI) is considered the investigation of choice in localizing pituitary tumours and approximately 85% of pituitary adenomas are detectable by this technique. MRI, however, may fail to identify microadenomas of 5–10 mm in size. In these patients, bilateral selective catheterization of the petrosal sinus and ACTH measurement after CRH stimulation is the most sensitive test in confirming the presence of a microadenoma. Plain skull X-ray is not helpful in identifying pituitary tumours even with thin section tomography.

Computed tomography (CT) scanning, although formally popular, will only identify approximately 50% of tumours and has now largely been replaced by MRI. A routine chest X-ray should be performed and may show a lung or bronchial tumour responsible for ectopic ACTH secretion.

Adrenal tumour

CT scanning is very effective in localizing adrenal tumours even as small as 1 cm in diameter. When an adrenal tumour is suspected as the cause of Cushing's syndrome, early CT scanning may prove useful to focus other investigations. Adrenal tumours larger than 6 cm on CT scanning are more likely to be malignant.

Benign adrenal tumours demonstrate increased uptake of ^{131}I-6β-iodomethylnorcholesterol (NP59) or selenium-75 cholesterol, with a corresponding decrease in contralateral adrenal gland uptake (Figure 5.3). This is a useful adjunct to CT scanning and contrasts with

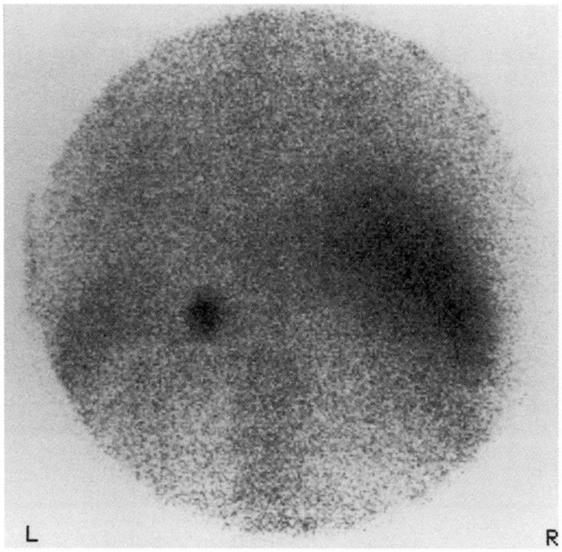

Figure 5.3 Seleno-cholesterol scan of a patient with Cushing's syndrome due to an adenoma in the left adrenal gland.

adrenocortical carcinoma which rarely takes up NP59 but because contralateral adrenal gland suppression is still present with adrenocortical carcinomas, neither gland demonstrates significant uptake. A bilateral scintigram image is seen in Cushing's disease where there is bilateral adrenal gland hyperplasia.

MRI is also capable of demonstrating adrenal tumours (Figure 5.4).

Ectopic ACTH

Ectopic ACTH-producing tumours are often small and may be difficult to locate. Chest X-ray may identify benign or malignant bronchial tumours. CT or MRI scanning may aid in locating bronchial,

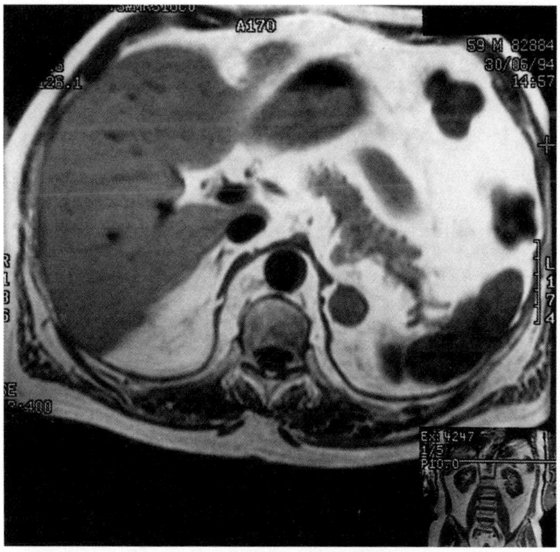

Figure 5.4 MRI scan of patient with Cushing's syndrome due to an adenoma in the left adrenal gland.

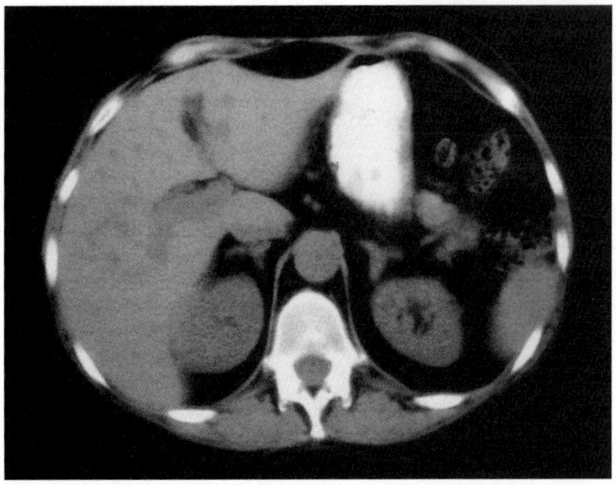

Figure 5.5 CT scan of abdomen showing bilateral enlarged hyperplastic adrenal glands in the ectopic ACTH syndrome.

pulmonary, thymic or pancreatic tumours which may be the source of ACTH production. The adrenal glands are enlarged and usually demonstrable on CT scan (Figure 5.5).

Treatment of Cushing's syndrome

Medical treatment

Patients with Cushing's syndrome (either pituitary or adrenal in origin) in whom surgery is contraindicated may be treated by long-term metapyrone therapy. This 11β-hydroxylase inhibitor reduces circulating levels of cortisol by inhibiting its synthesis from 11-deoxycortisol. Metapyrone is also useful in the preparation of patients with Cushing's syndrome for definitive treatment such as adrenalectomy, transsphenoidal microsurgery or pituitary irradiation. Initial dosage is 250 mg eight hourly, increasing over a week to 500 mg 6 hourly. In full dosage complete adrenal blockade is achieved, necessitating replacement therapy with 0.25 mg dexamethasone twice daily. Side-effects of metapyrone are often unpleasant and include nausea, vomiting, hirsutism and acne.

Other drugs have also been used in the medical management of Cushing's syndrome, including ketoconazole, which reduces cortisol levels by inhibiting cytochrome P-450 enzymes, aminoglutethamide, which inhibits the conversion of cholesterol to pregnenolone, bromocryptine, a dopamine agonist and mitotane (discussed in the section on adrenocortical carcinoma).

Pituitary disease

Transsphenoidal microsurgery

Selective removal of the pituitary basophil microadenoma by transsphenoidal microsurgery is currently the treatment of choice for patients with Cushing's disease. When tumours have been localized pre-operatively and removed completely at operation by an experienced surgeon, cure rates are high (80–90%). These patients rarely require pituitary replacement therapy. When tumours are not localized pre-operatively and not readily identified at operation, partial hypophysectomy (removing two-thirds of the gland) is usually performed. Cure rates in these patients fall in comparison to the former group.

Pituitary surgery will be complicated by pituitary insufficiency when complete hypophysectomy is performed. Patients may require replacement therapy with one or more of the following agents: corticosteroid, thyroxine, testosterone, oestrogen and anti-diuretic hormone (diabetes insipidus). Complications such as infection, meningitis or anosmia occur rarely.

Pituitary irradiation

Radiotherapy using either an external proton beam, linear accelerator or interstitial irradiation using ^{198}gold or ^{90}yttrium is also effective. Resolution of the clinical syndrome however, is more protracted and may take 6–18 months. Pituitary insufficiency occurs in about 50% of patients but less frequently in children, making pituitary irradiation treatment an appropriate and acceptable therapy.

Bilateral adrenalectomy

Formerly the treatment of choice in Cushing's disease, improved techniques in pituitary surgery have meant that bilateral adrenalectomy is reserved for the following situations:

- When pituitary surgery has failed or is technically not feasible.
- Palliative treatment of patients with ectopic ACTH syndrome.
- Patients with primary adrenal hyperplasia.
- Patients with rapidly progressive or severe hypercortisolism.

Prior to surgery, treatment with metapyrone is necessary to reduce cortisol production and correct metabolic defects. When present diabetes mellitus and hypertension should be controlled. Appropriate venous thrombosis prophylaxis and support stockings are employed. Adequate steroid replacement therapy is essential in this procedure, the details of which are outlined earlier in this module. Adrenalectomized patients are dependent on lifelong glucocorticoid and mineralocorticoid replacement therapy.

A rare, late complication of bilateral adrenalectomy in patients with Cushing's syndrome was first described by Nelson and colleagues in 1960. This condition is characterized by the development of an ACTH-producing pituitary tumour following bilateral adrenalectomy, accompanied by skin hyperpigmentation, headache, visual field defects and hypopituitarism. The condition may be controlled by hypophysectomy or pituitary irradiation. Prophylactic pituitary irradiation in patients undergoing bilateral adrenalectomy will reduce the incidence of Nelson's syndrome.

Overall, results for bilateral adrenalectomy in the treatment of Cushing's disease are good. Montgomery and Welbourn (1978) reported 65% of patients in remission at 5–15 years following surgery with 50% alive at 20 years.

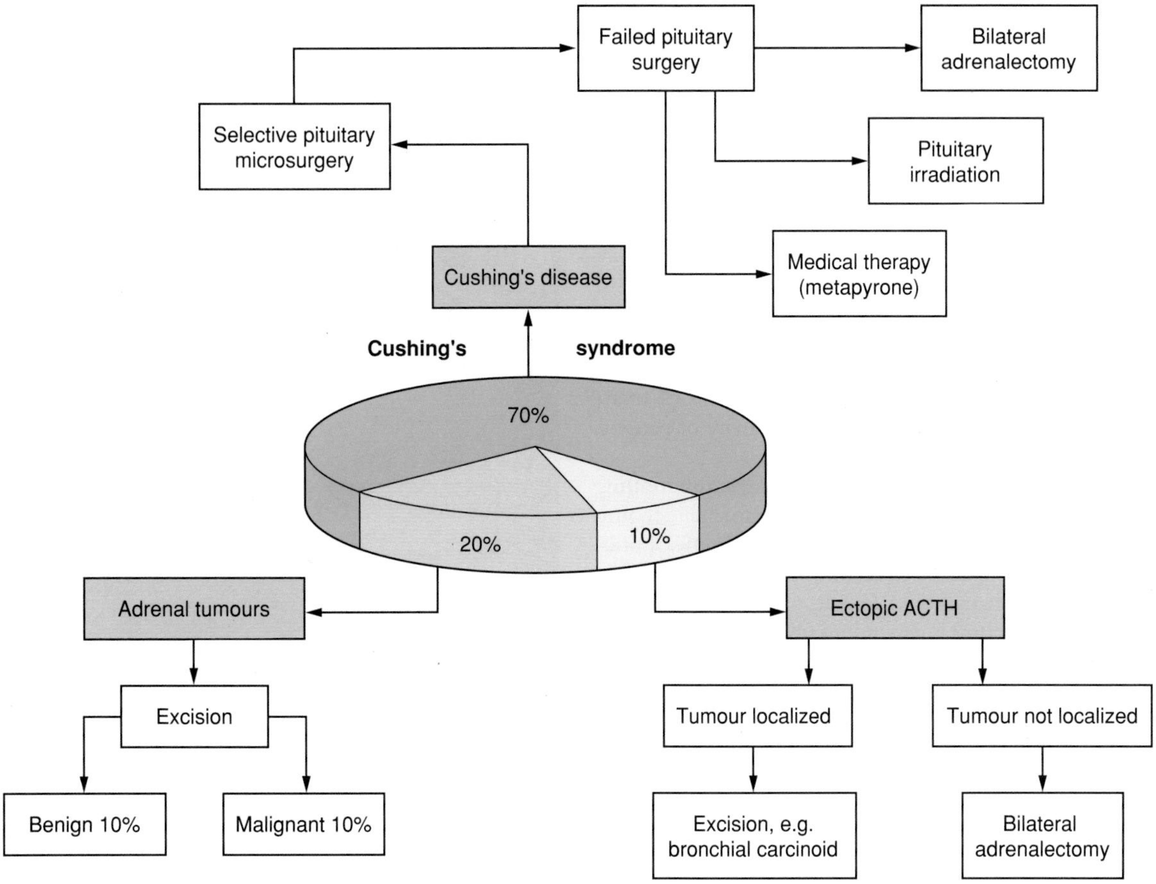

Figure 5.6 Causes and treatment of Cushing's syndrome.

Adrenal adenoma

When Cushing's syndrome is caused by an adrenal adenoma the treatment of choice is unilateral adrenalectomy, with most endocrine surgeons currently favouring a laparoscopic approach. The contralateral adrenal gland is suppressed in this condition and patients require steroid support both per-operatively (at tumour removal) and post-operatively. Complete weaning off steroid replacement may take more than a year. Cure rate and long-term survival are excellent.

Summary

The causes and treatment of Cushing's syndrome are summarized in Figure 5.6.

Section 5.6 • Adrenocortical carcinoma

Pathology

Adrenocortical carcinoma is a rare tumour responsible for 10% of all cases of Cushing's disease with a peak incidence in the fourth and fifth decades. Tumours are usually >5 cm in diameter and may be palpable. Macroscopically, they have a lobulated appearance, are

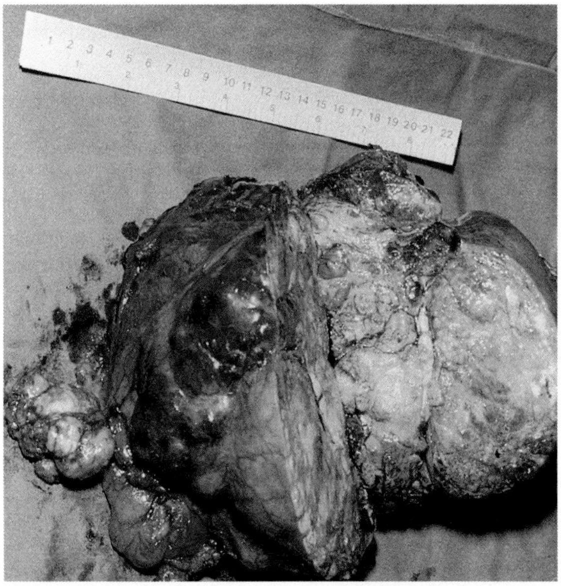

Figure 5.7 Gross specimen of adrenocortical carcinoma: haemorrhagic cut surface of a partly necrotic tumour.

greyish pink in colour and exhibit areas of haemorrhage and necrosis (Figure 5.7). They may invade local structures such as pancreas, kidney, diaphragm and bowel. Venous invasion is also common and may be gross to involve the inferior vena cava. Microscopically tumours display numerous mitosis, nuclear pleomorphism and vascular invasion. Sometimes the true malignant potential may not be apparent on conventional histological appraisal.

Adrenocortical carcinomas are aggressive malignancies with a high recurrence rate after surgery and a poor response to radiotherapy. Distant metastases to liver, lungs, bone and skin are common and often present at the time of presentation. Most forms of treatment are disappointing and only a minority of patients survive beyond 2–3 years.

Tumours are divided into two groups, functioning (60%) and non-functioning (40%). The former account for 10% of all cases of Cushing's syndrome. Functioning tumours are more common in younger patients (<40 years) and exhibit a female to male ratio of 4:1. The clinical picture is dependent upon the hormone or hormones secreted. In contrast, non-functioning tumours are more common in older patients (>40 years) and exhibit a female to male ratio of 2:1 but may produce steroid precursors such as pregnenolone.

Surgical staging

Adrenocortical carcinomas may be staged into the following groups:

Stage I	Tumour <5 cm in diameter, with no local invasion, nodal or distant metastases.
Stage II	Tumour >5 cm in diameter, with no local invasion, nodal or distant metastases.
Stage III	Tumour with local invasion *or* local lymph node metastases but no distant metastases.
Stage IV	Tumour with local invasion *and* local lymph node *or* distant metastases.

At presentation approximately 70% of patients have either stage III or stage IV disease.

Clinical presentation

Non-functioning or minimally functioning tumours may grow to a massive size (>20 cm) before they become clinically apparent. Despite the term 'non-functioning' these tumours do produce steroid precursors and measurement of dehydroepiandrosterone may be of value in the diagnosis of malignant disease. Patients usually present with weight loss, fatigue, abdominal pain or in rare incidences with haemorrhagic necrosis of the tumour leading to acute pain, fever and/or shock. A palpable abdominal mass may be present. Functioning tumours secrete excessive steroids which may cause Cushing's syndrome, hyperaldosteronism, virilization, feminization or a mixed clinical picture. Indeed a mixed hormonal secretion is highly suspicious of malignancy.

The development of Cushing's syndrome in a child is likely to be due to an adrenocortical carcinoma. It occurs in association with virilization, acne and amenorrhoea in the young female, virilization in a prepubital female and feminization in the male. In contrast to benign secreting tumours the onset of symptoms is likely to be rapid. Functioning tumours may also be large at presentation. Adrenocortical cancers are not

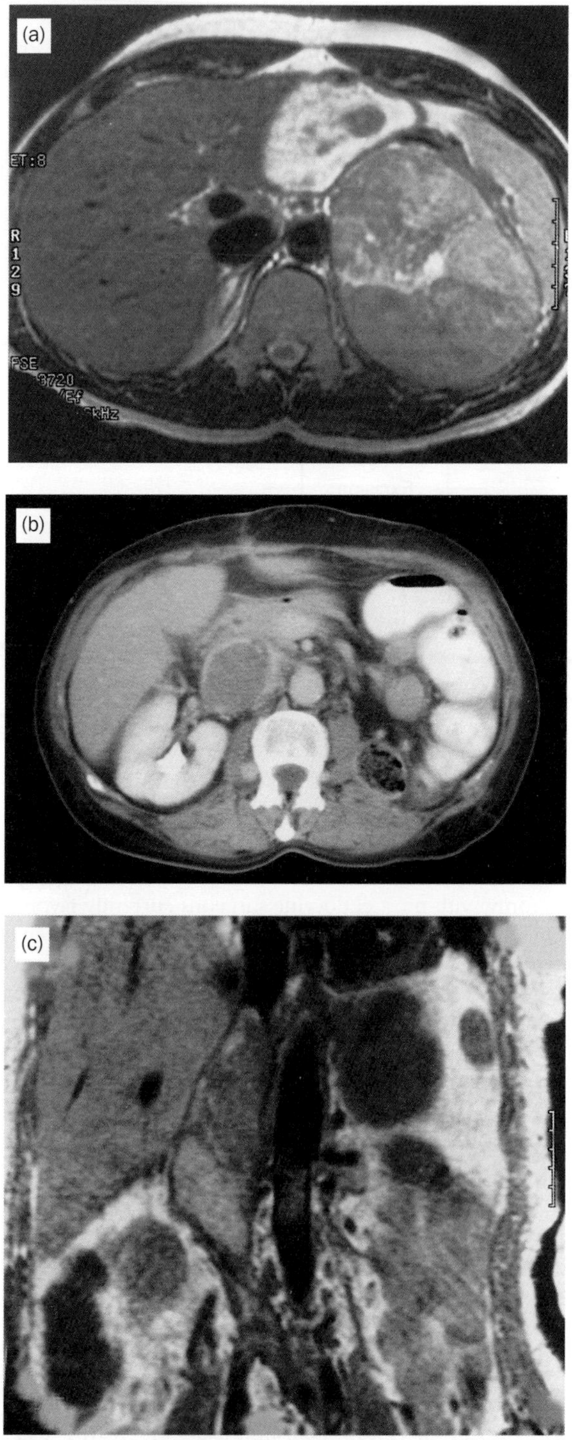

Figure 5.8 (a) MRI scan of patient with massive left adrenocortical carcinoma. (b) CT scan showing tumour within lumen of IVC. (c) MRI scan showing tumour invasion of IVC.

ACTH dependent and like benign adrenocortical tumours fail to suppress with high doses of dexamethasone.

Pre-operative imaging with CT or MRI will provide valuable information regarding tumour size, local invasion and distant metastases (Figure 5.8a, b). The presence of inferior caval invasion can also be determined by MRI, rendering caval venography unnecessary (Figure 5.8c). NP59 or seleno-cholesterol scintigraphy will show absent or low uptake bilaterally.

Treatment

Surgical resection offers the only prospect of cure. Unfortunately most patients at presentation have advanced incurable disease and only palliation is possible. In patients with stage I or II disease, aggressive surgical resection in the form of an *en-bloc* resection, sacrificing adjacent organs such as the spleen, kidney and distal pancreas is necessary to achieve adequate clearance. Occasionally large tumours require a thoraco-abdominal approach and clearance of an involved inferior vena cava may be best achieved using cardiopulmonary bypass. Should local recurrence occur, further surgical resection has been shown to lead to prolonged survival. Steroid replacement should be given at the time of adrenalectomy for functioning tumours and maintained post-operatively.

These tumours demonstrate little radiosensitivity and radiotherapy has proved disappointing. Chemotherapy with mitotane (o,p' DDD) has been of value particularly when used in patients prior to the development of metastatic disease following surgical resection for stage I and II disease and in an individual subsequently undergoing repeated surgical resection for recurrent disease. It is unlikely however that this agent significantly improves overall survival. Mitotane induces selective necrosis of the zona fasiculata and zona reticularis and results in destruction of the contralateral adrenal gland. Replacement steroid therapy is therefore essential. Metapyrone is useful in controlling the symptoms of cortisol excess in patients who are unfit or unsuitable for surgery.

Survival rates for adrenocortical carcinoma are poor and are dependent on disease stage at presentation. The overall 5 year survival is as low as 16% but stage I and II disease may have a survival of more than 50% compared with 0% for those with stage IV tumours.

Section 5.7 • Aldosteronism

Primary aldosteronism

Primary hyperaldosteronism is a rare syndrome characterized by hypertension, hypokalaemia, hypernatraemia and suppressed plasma renin activity (PRA). It is caused by excessive aldosterone secretion from the zona glomerulosa of the adrenal cortex. This potentially curable condition accounts for less than 1% of all patients with hypertension and was first described by Dr Jerome Conn in 1955, 3 years after the hormone aldosterone had been identified.

Excessive aldosterone production causes expansion of plasma volume and elevation of the blood pressure (see physiology section). The rise in blood volume and sodium ion concentration is detected by the juxtaglomerular apparatus and renin secretion falls in response. Loss of potassium and hydrogen ions in the urine leads to hypokalaemia and metabolic alkalosis.

Adrenocortical adenoma (Conn's tumour) is by far the most common cause of primary hyperaldosteronism, accounting for approximately 85% of cases. Other less common causes are bilateral adrenocortical hyperplasia (idiopathic hyperaldosteronism), aldosterone-producing adrenocortical carcinoma, glucocorticoid-suppressible hyperaldosteronism (familial type 1), non-glucocorticoid-suppressible hyperaldosteronism (familial type 2, which may be adenoma or hyperplasia) and aldosterone-producing ovarian carcinoma.

Pathology of primary hyperaldosteronism

Conn's tumours are classically unilateral, less than 2 cm in size, project from the adrenal gland and have a characteristic golden or canary yellow appearance (Figure 5.9). Tumours are composed of lipid-laden clear cells and occur more frequently on the left side. Bilateral tumours are in found in 10% of patients. The remainder of the adrenal cortex in patients with Conn's tumours is not always normal. Microscopic and/or macroscopic nodular hyperplasia is a frequently

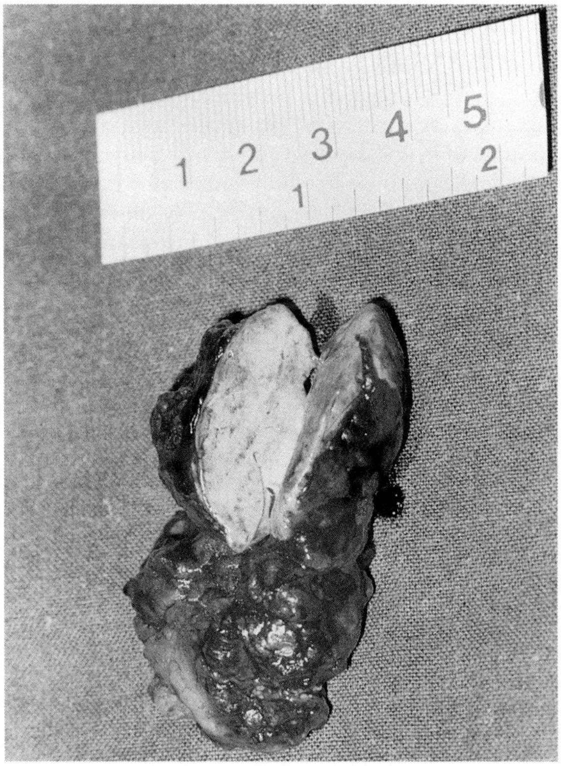

Figure 5.9 Conn's adrenal adenoma – gross specimen.

associated feature, present in approximately 40–50% of patients.

Idiopathic hyperaldosteronism is found in 10–15% of patients with primary hyperaldosteronism. The disease is bilateral and composed of both diffuse and focal areas of microscopic and macroscopic hyperplasia. Nodule formation is frequently present, probably caused by hypertensive vascular changes. The nodules are capable of producing cortisol but not aldosterone. The dividing line between solitary adenoma, adenoma in a background of zona glomerulosa hyperplasia and hyperplasia with no dominant nodule is somewhat blurred. Indeed variations may represent a spectrum of disease. Identifying the cause of primary hyperaldosteronism is crucial and has a direct bearing on appropriate management.

Clinical presentation

The syndrome of primary hyperaldosteronism is characterized by continuous hypertension which is often severe but rarely malignant. Patients may present at any age but more commonly between the third and fifth decades. Conn's tumours occur twice as commonly in women, though idiopathic hyperplasia is equally distributed between sexes and tends to occur at a later age.

The duration of hypertension prior to diagnosis is reported to be around 7 years and may be resistant to usual antihypertensive medication. Where hypokalaemia is marked, patients may experience muscle weakness, cramps, headaches, polydipsia, polyuria and nocturia. In rare cases where hypokalaemia is particularly severe, patients may experience episodes of intermittent flaccid paralysis or even tetany. Symptoms of hypokalaemia may be brought on by the administration antihypertensive diuretics, particularly the thiazides. On rare occasions excessive salt intake may also cause episodes of hypokalaemia. Patients may be symptomless and the diagnosis is often only suspected when routine biochemical analysis characteristically reveals hypokalaemia associated with mild hypernatraemia.

Biochemical investigation and diagnosis

When hyperaldosteronism is suspected clinically, confirmation of the diagnosis is obtained by demonstrating elevated plasma aldosterone concentration (PAC) with suppressed PRA. This contrasts with secondary hyperaldosteronism, where both PAC and PRA are raised. Prior to carrying out biochemical studies potassium stores should be replenished (hypokalaemia inhibits aldosterone secretion) and drugs affecting renin–aldosterone regulation should be discontinued for 4–6 weeks. This includes spironolactone, ACE inhibitors and all diuretics. In patients in whom hypertension is marked, antihypertensive medication may be continued with agents such as prazosin and guanethidine, although calcium channel blockers and β-blockers probably do not significantly affect results.

Primary hyperaldosteronism is confirmed if in a hypertensive patient PAC is increased (normal 2.2–15 ng/dl) in association with PRA being suppressed below normal (0.2–0.5 ng/dl). It has been suggested that a PAC:PRA ratio of >50 is diagnostic. Urinary potassium excretion should be in excess of 40 mmol/day.

Aldosterone suppression test

Where results are equivocal further evaluation is deemed necessary. Diagnosis of primary hyperaldosteronism in this situation may be confirmed by failure to demonstrate suppression of urinary aldosterone secretion in response to a sodium load. Caution is necessary in performing these tests as biochemical disturbances can be severe and marked hypokalaemia may ensue. Patients should therefore be normokalaemic prior to testing and have potassium supplementation throughout the test. Oral sodium loading takes place over 3 days at a dose of 9 g/day, on the third day a 24 hour urine collection is made and urinary aldosterone, potassium and sodium levels are measured. The 24 hour urinary sodium excretion should exceed 200 mEq (documenting adequate sodium loading) and the diagnosis of hyperaldosteronism is confirmed if aldosterone levels exceeds 12 μg.

Differentiation between adenoma and idiopathic hyperplasia

Following diagnosis of primary hyperaldosteronism it is necessary to distinguish between an aldosterone-producing adenoma and idiopathic hyperplasia. This distinction has important therapeutic implications, as only cortical adenomas are likely to benefit from surgery.

Aldosterone-producing cortical adenomas remain relatively unresponsive to angiotensin but still respond to ACTH and follow the corticotrophin circadian rhythm. In idiopathic hyperplasia there is a hypersensitivity to angiotensin II. These mechanisms can be used as the basis for a test to distinguish between the two conditions.

PAC is measured after overnight recumbancy and after the patient has been ambulatory for 4 hours. In those with adenomas, PAC falls, whereas in patients with idiopathic hyperplasia, PAC rises. Although this test is not absolutely reliable Young reported an overall accuracy of 85% in 246 patients in a collective review of the literature.

Reports of subtypes of primary hyperaldosteronism termed primary adrenal hyperplasia (PAH) and aldosterone-producing renin-responsive adenoma (both responding to unilateral adrenalectomy) further confuse the issue.

Localization

CT scanning has proven to be reliable in localizing Conn's tumours greater than 1 cm in size in more than 90% of patients. Identification of an obvious adrenal cortical adenoma increases confidence of the diagnosis of Conn's tumour versus idiopathic hyperplasia in patients with primary hyperaldosteronism. Tumours are usually homogeneous with decreased attenuation both

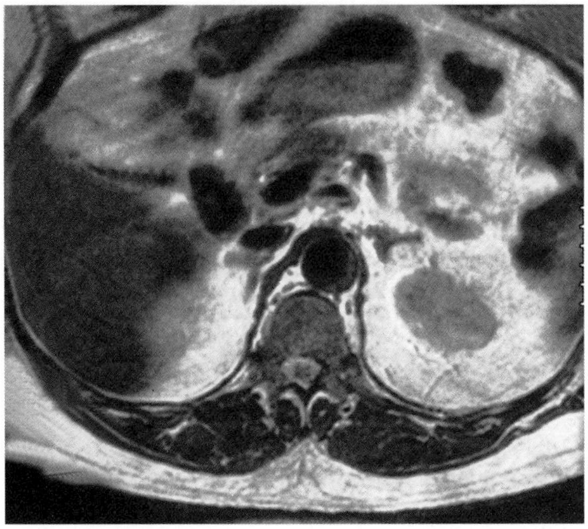

Figure 5.10 MRI scan of the abdomen in a patient with Conn's syndrome due to microadenoma in the left adrenal gland.

before and after contrast enhancement because of their low lipid content. Most tumours measure less than 2 cm but those smaller than 1 cm may be missed, particularly in thin patients with little perinephric fat. MRI has also proved useful in identifying tumours and may well become the method of choice (Figures 5.10 and 5.11).

Adrenal scanning with ^{131}I-6β-iodomethylnorcholesterol (NP59) or selenocholesterol following dexamethasone suppression for 5 days (to decrease activity in surrounding adrenal tissue) provides excellent localization (90%), although it has limitations with smaller tumours. It also has the disadvantage of administering a significant dose of radiation. It has particular value in cases where it has proved difficult to localize an adenoma or to distinguish adenoma from bilateral adrenal hyperplasia by CT and/or MRI.

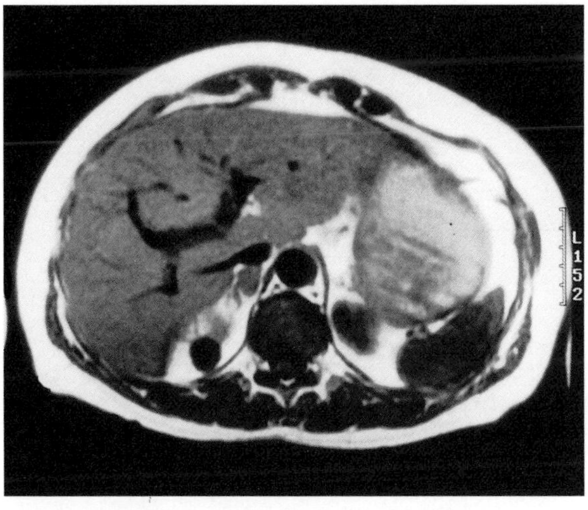

Figure 5.11 MRI of the abdomen in a patient with Conn's syndrome due to right adrenal cortical adenoma.

Table 5.1 Selective venous sampling results in the patient with microadenoma shown in Figure 5.10

Results of bilateral adrenal vein sampling

Vein	*Aldosterone (pmol/l)*	*Cortisol (nmol/l)*	*A/C ratio*
Right adrenal	2910	5300	0.5
Left adrenal	17 000	1810	9.4
Peripheral	660	320	2.1

The most accurate functional method of localizing Conn's tumours remains selective venous catheterization (Table 5.1). The technique, however, is invasive and potentially hazardous, with reported extravasation of contrast, intra-adrenal haemorrhage and adrenal necrosis. Use is most appropriate in patients where CT, MRI and NP59 have failed to precisely localize the tumour, when an abnormal nodule demonstrated by CT is non-functioning and when bilateral nodules are present and may be interpreted as hyperplasia. Difficulty in placing the catheter into the right adrenal vein (which is short and at 90° to the cava) may lead to sampling errors. These errors can be minimized by simultaneously measuring cortisol and employing the aldosterone:cortisol ratio as an indicator of any true increase in hormone concentration.

Treatment

Once an aldosterone-secreting cortical adenoma is confirmed biochemically and localized by CT or radioisotope scan the treatment of choice in patients deemed medically fit for surgery is unilateral adrenalectomy. Traditionally an open posterior approach has been used but this is a tumour which lends itself to laparoscopic adrenalectomy very well and is now currently the preferred technique for most endocrine surgeons. Patients are prepared for surgery by correction of hypokalaemia and hypertension, usually with spironolactone 100 mg/day. Those in whom hypertension responds well to spironolactone pre-operatively tend to have a more favourable outcome from surgery.

Patients with idiopathic hyperplasia, those where hypertension persists following adenoma excision and those who are unfit for surgery because of medical reasons should be treated with spironolactone. Potassium sparing diuretics also have a significant effect in controlling blood pressure and restoring potassium balance.

Post-operative follow-up

Unilateral adrenalectomy for adenomas has been reported to improve hypertension in the majority and to achieve normotension in 44–98% of patients, although the average cure rate appears to be about 70% at 1 year. Some patients may have persistent hypertension immediately post-operatively and others develop further hypertension over a period of time.

Sex and age have been demonstrated to be the only two significant prognostic factors in determining operative success. The older the patient, the less likely adrenalectomy is to restore normotension. This is probably because long-term hypertension causes irreversible pathological changes in blood vessel walls and co-existing causes of hypertension are also present. Hypertension is also more likely to be labelled 'essential' in elderly patients compared to younger ones, which may lead further to a delay in diagnosis and thus long-term vessel damage. Women also have a more favourable response to adrenalectomy than men, possibly because female hormones confer a protective effect on blood vessels.

Summary

The investigation and treatment of primary aldosteronism is summarized in Figure 5.12.

Secondary hyperaldosteronism

Severe hypertension from cardiovascular or renal disease may be associated with excessive secretion of aldosterone termed secondary hyperaldosteronism. Hypertensive stimulation of the juxtaglomerular apparatus produces renin, which in turn leads to aldosterone secretion via the renin–angiotensin mechanism. Raised

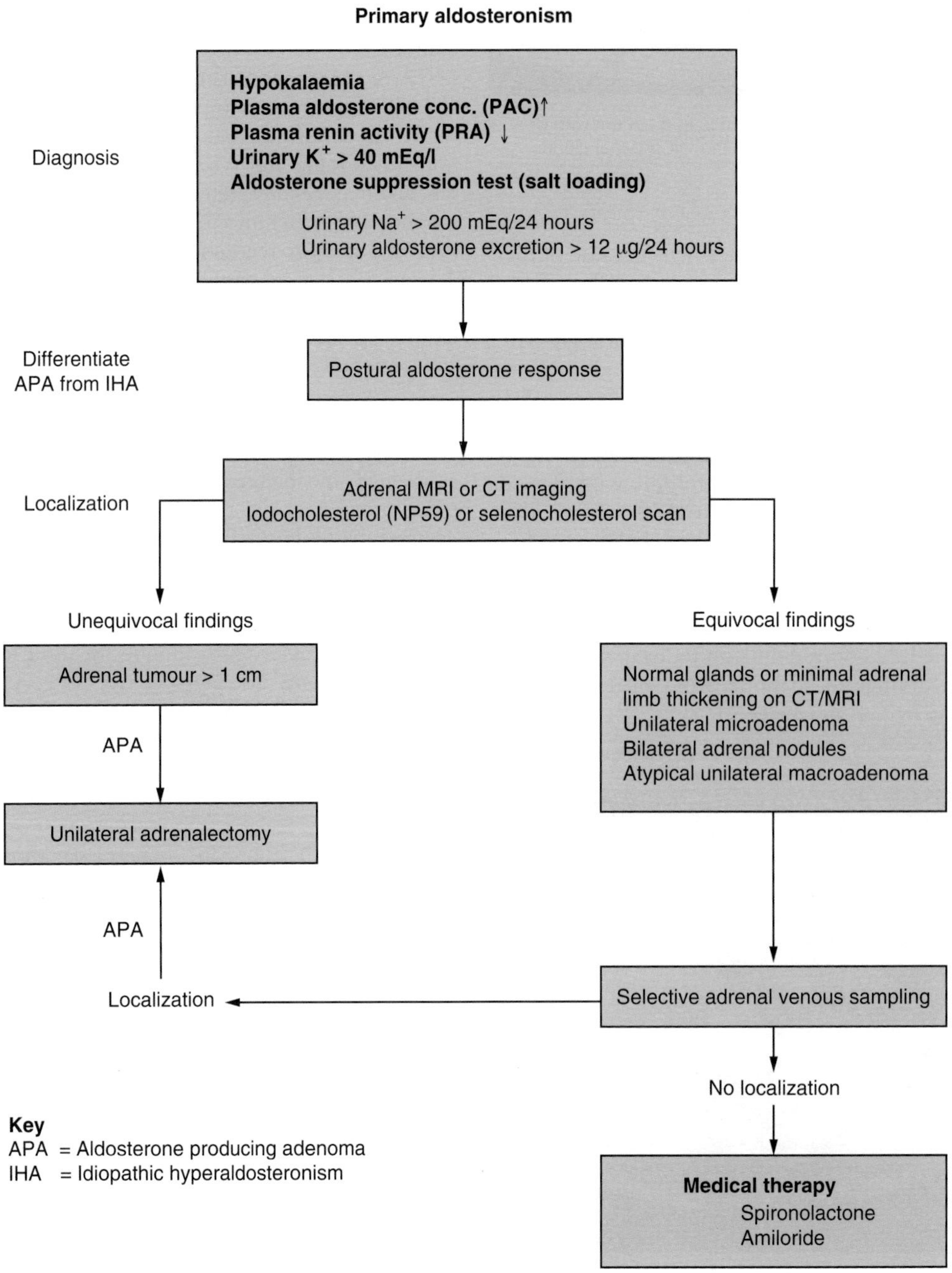

Figure 5.12 Investigation and treatment of primary aldosteronism.

PRA therefore distinguishes secondary hyperaldosteronism from primary hyperaldosteronism (where PRA is suppressed), this being an important clinical distinction.

Section 5.8 • Phaeochromocytoma

Phaeochromocytoma is a functioning tumour of the catecholamine-producing chromaffin cells. Derived from the Greek *phaeo* meaning dusky and *chroma* meaning colour, the tumour is characterized by a syndrome resulting from excess catecholamine production. The condition was first described in 1886 by Frankel, following a post-mortem that had demonstrated bilateral adrenal tumours in an 18-year-old patient who had presented with hypertension, sudden collapse and death. The term phaeochromocytoma was first used by Pick in 1912 but it was not until 1926 that the first successful surgical removal of such a tumour was performed by Roux in Lausanne, a feat repeated by C. H. Mayo in the USA during the following year.

In recent years, advances in biochemical diagnosis, accurate pre-operative localization, preparation with α- and β-adrenergic receptor blocking agents and enhanced surgical skills have meant that patients with phaeochromocytoma can expect a favourable outcome from appropriate treatment.

Pathology

Most tumours are unilateral, more common on the right side and range considerably in size from 1 cm to more than 15 cm. Weight varies accordingly but usually tumours are between 50 and 200 g. Sporadic tumours are usually unilateral and unifocal. In contrast, familial tumours are more likely to be bilateral (50–70%) and multifocal.

Macroscopically, tumours are well-encapsulated, frequently cystic-containing areas of haemorrhage and necrosis. When sectioned the cut surface is pinkish grey in colour and highly vascular.

Chromaffin cells are of neuroectodermal origin and although located primarily in the adrenal medulla they may also be found in small numbers in the sympathetic ganglia. Tumours developing in these extra-adrenal sites are termed *catecholamine-secreting paragangliomas*. These tumours are more common in children and may be located along the course of the sympathetic chain but predominate at the aortic bifurcation (the organ of Zuckerkandl). Approximately 40% of paragangliomas are malignant.

Phaeochromocytoma has been termed the '10%' tumour. Approximately 10% are extra-adrenal, 10% bilateral, 10% malignant, 10% are in children and 10% are familial, associated with other genetically determined conditions such as multiple endocrine neoplasia (MEN) types 2A and 2B, von Hippel–Lindau disease or von Recklinghausen's neurofibromatosis.

Histologically, diagnosis of malignancy in these tumours is rarely possible as many lesions, both benign and malignant, exhibit evidence of capsular and vascular invasion. The only reliable indicator of malignancy is demonstration of local invasion into adjacent structures such as the renal or inferior vena caval veins, or localization of tumour in sites other than the sympathetic chain such as bone, lung and liver.

Incidence

Phaeochromocytoma may be found at post-mortem in approximately 0.1% of hypertensive patients. The incidence in the population is of the order of one to two cases per 100 000 and approximately 800 deaths per year occur in the USA from phaeochromocytoma. The condition remains undiagnosed in 35% of sufferers during their lifetime. In patients in whom phaeochromocytoma is not diagnosed, death may ensue from myocardial infarction or cerebrovascular accident during or immediately after even a minor surgical operation. A high index of suspicion is therefore necessary to make the diagnosis and avoid this potential catastrophe.

Clinical presentation

Hypertension is by far the most common manifestation, mimicking 'essential' hypertension by being continuous in 50% of patients but paroxysmal in the remaining 50%. Excess noradrenaline, adrenaline or dopamine secretion predisposes to hypertension usually associated with palpitations, sweating and headache. So commonly are these symptoms associated with phaeochromocytoma, that the absence of all three has been said to rule out the diagnosis in patients with hypertension.

Events which raise intra-abdominal pressure such as bladder emptying, sexual activity, defecation or exercise may trigger attacks which may last from several minutes to several hours. Other less common causative factors are alcohol, drugs (notably tricyclic antidepressants) and foods containing high levels of tyramine.

In undiagnosed patients, labour or invasive procedures such as angiography may precipitate particularly severe hypertensive episodes resulting in peripheral circulatory failure and even cardiac arrest.

The incidences of myocardial infarction, hypertensive encephalopathy, cerebrovascular accident and catecholamine cardiomyopathy are all raised in these patients. Other manifestations of phaeochromocytoma, resulting from increased levels of catecholamines, are flushing, pallor, pupillary dilation, Raynaud's phenomenon, fever, tremors, nausea, weakness, nausea, vertigo, anxiety and an impending sense of doom. Gastrointestinal manifestations may be generalized abdominal pain, pseudo-obstruction, ileus, ischaemic enterocolitis and acute megacolon. Malignant tumours may also be responsible for glucose intolerance and severe hyperglycaemia.

Physical examination frequently reveals a thin, pale, anxious patient. Hypertension may be severe and in contrast to essential hypertension, 70% of patients exhibit a postural drop in blood pressure usually associated with concomitant tachycardia. An abdominal mass may be present in up to 15% of patients, palpation of which may precipitate paroxysmal symptoms and should be conducted with care in patients where there is a high index of suspicion. Clinical features such as a thyroid nodule, Marfinoid habitus or neurofibromatosis may be suggestive of familial disease such as MEN 2A, 2B or von Recklinghausen's disease.

The differential diagnosis includes, 'essential' and 'labile' hypertension, anxiety neurosis and other psychiatric disorders, hyperthyroidism, diabetes mellitus and functional bowel disorder. It is not surprising therefore that phaeochromocytoma has been labelled the great 'mimic' with all the attendant diagnostic difficulties.

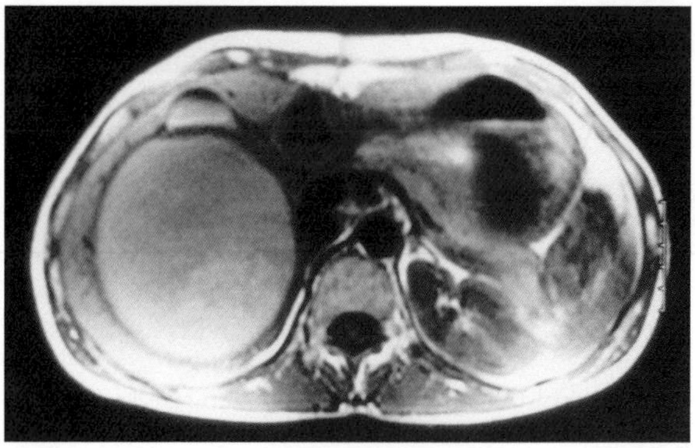

Figure 5.14 MRI scan (T2 weighted) of large right adrenal phaeochromocytoma. This lesion was originally referred as a possible hepatic cyst.

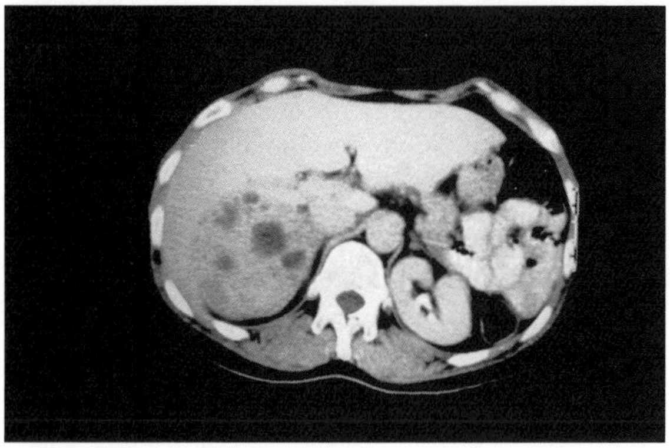

Figure 5.15 CT scan of malignant phaeochromocytoma in the right adrenal gland. Typical heterogeneous appearance with areas of haemorrhage.

Investigation and diagnosis

Diagnosis of phaeochromocytoma is provided by establishing catecholamine excess, followed by localization of the tumour. Armstrong and colleagues described the metabolic pathways of catecholamine production and excretion, which provide the basis for biochemical investigation of phaeochromocytoma. Dopamine, noradrenaline and adrenaline are formed in the chromaffin cells of adrenal medulla from phenylalanine and tyrosine. Noradrenaline and adrenaline are converted to normetadrenaline and metadrenaline prior to excretion in the urine. These metanephrines are then further converted to vanillyl mandelic acid (VMA), also excreted in the urine.

Diagnosis is thus established by 24 hour urine collection in an acidified container and measurement of the metanephrine and VMA content of the urine. Adrenaline, noradrenaline and dopamine are also assayed by high pressure liquid chromatography (HPLC), reducing the possibility of drug interactions producing spurious results. In borderline cases, measurement of plasma free catecholamine levels may be helpful during acute hypertensive attacks but is otherwise unnecessary. Pharmacological provocation tests are potentially dangerous and are only of historic interest.

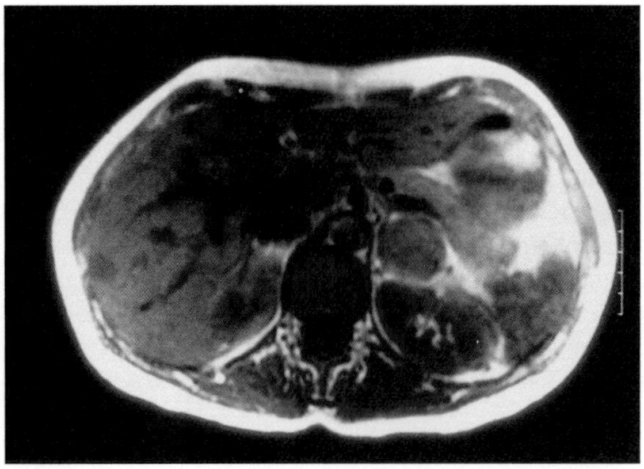

Figure 5.13 MRI scan of left adrenal phaeochromocytoma.

Localization

Once the diagnosis of phaeochromocytoma has been confirmed the exact site of the tumour or tumours must be identified. MRI is now established as the localizing procedure of choice, in preference to CT (Figures 5.13–5.15). Tumours are displayed as low-signal intensity T1-weighted images with a characteristic, almost unique, hyperintense signal on T2-weighted images. This contrasts with non-functioning adrenal adenomas which have the same signal characteristics as normal adrenal tissue. MRI is of particular value in locating extra-adrenal paragangliomas, especially those located in the urinary bladder and paracardiac regions (Figure 5.16). MRI negates the need for contrast enhancement of tumours necessary with CT imaging, thus avoiding the potential hypertensive crises which contrast material can precipitate, although a recent report suggest that use of non-ionic contrast material is probably safe.

When MRI or CT has failed to accurately localize the tumour ^{123}I-metaiodobenzylguanidine (MIBG) or indium-111 pentetreotide may be useful (Figures 5.17 and 5.19). MIBG has been reported to have a sensitivity of 90% and a specificity of 100% in tumour localization, although to achieve this it may be necessary to

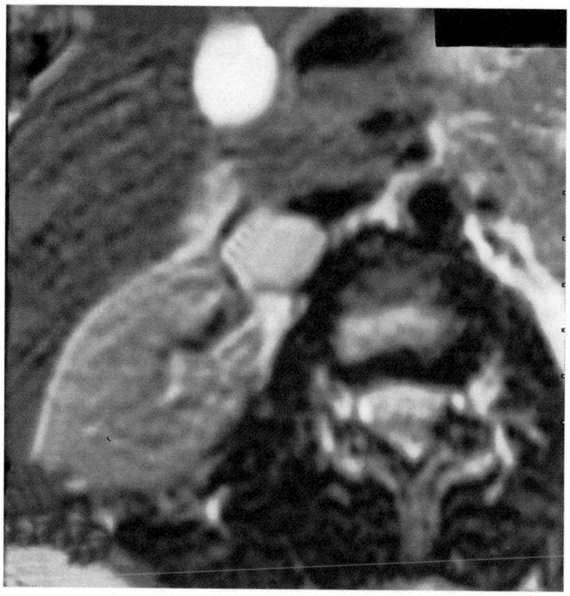

Figure 5.16 MRI scan (T2 weighted) of extra-adrenal phaeochromocytoma situated close to the right renal hilum.

repeat the scan several times in the 72 hour period after administration of the tracer. Invasive procedure such as selective venous catheterization and selective adrenal angiography are no longer deemed necessary in tumour localization.

Treatment

Catecholamine secreting tumours are treatable causes of hypertension and surgical resection of the tumour following pharmaceutical control of hypertension is the recommended management. Patients who have medical contraindications to surgery or patients have

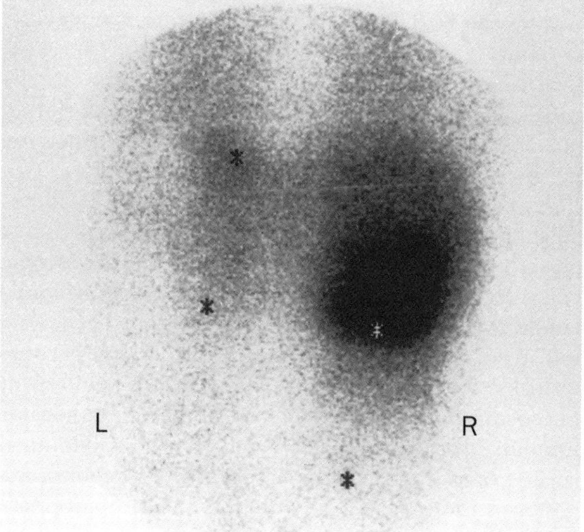

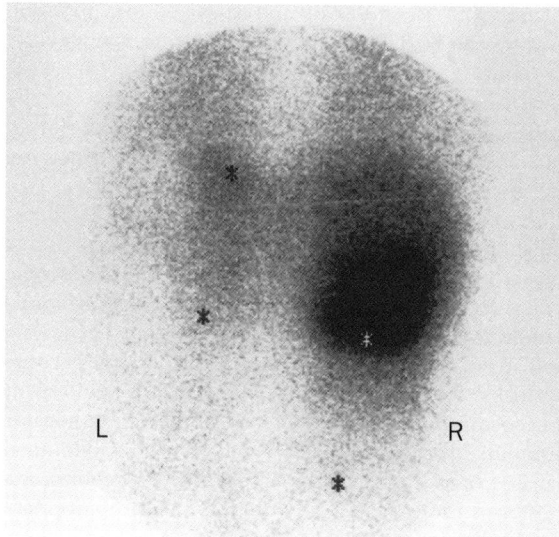

Figure 5.17 MIBG (metaiodobenzylguanadine) scan of malignant right phaeochromocytoma.

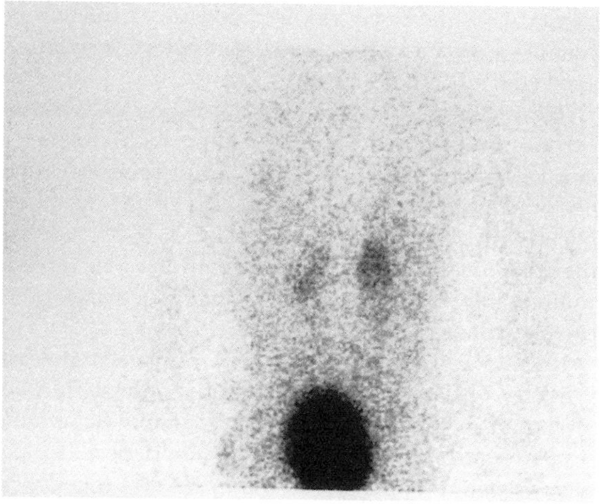

Figure 5.18 MIBG scan of a 5-year-old boy with bilateral phaeochromocytoma (right tumour within the adrenal gland, left tumour extra-adrenal).

widespread metastatic disease from malignant phaeochromocytoma (in whom there is little hope of obtaining a surgical cure) will not be considered candidates for surgery. These patients in this group may benefit from treatment with α-methyl-ρ-tyrosine, an inhibitor of catecholamine synthesis which can reduce circulating levels by as much as 50%, offering some symptomatic control.

Pre-operative control of hypertension

Anaesthetic induction or even minimal manipulation of adrenal or extra-adrenal phaeochromocytomas may cause dramatic and dangerous fluctuations in blood pressure. It is therefore vital to control blood pressure pre-operatively. The agent of choice in the routine patient is the long acting α-adrenergic blocker phenoxybenzamine. Medical control of hypertension in a patient thought to have a phaeochromocytoma should be commenced once the tumour is suspected, prior to any localizing procedures. Untreated patients are at

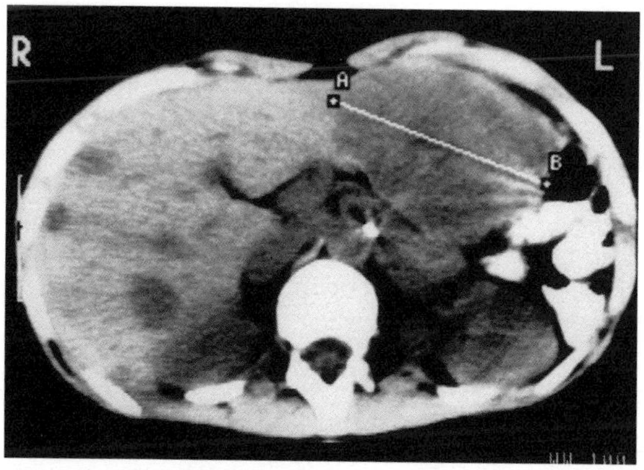

Figure 5.19 CT scan of recurrent malignant phaeochromocytoma in the left adrenal tumour bed. Multiple metastases are seen in the right lobe of the liver.

significantly increased risk of myocardial infarction, cerebrovascular accident, acute heart failure, arrythmias and sudden death.

Treatment with non-competitive α-blockade allows expansion of the intravascular volume, with concomitant fall in blood pressure, leading to the essential benefit of reduced frequency and intensity of per-operative hypertensive episodes. A disadvantage of α-blockade is the risk of hypotension following removal of the tumour and withdrawal of the α-agonist activity of the catecholamines.

Phenoxybenzamine should be commenced at least 7–10 days prior to surgery. The initial dose should be 10 mg bd, increasing by 10–20 mg/day, until hypertension is controlled and the patient experiences orthostatic hypotension. Often a dose up to 160 mg/day is required to achieve this effect. Patients should be encouraged to take liberal fluids and salt to help replace the expanded intravascular volume. Side-effects of phenoxybenzamine include sedation, weakness, lassitude, nausea, nasal congestion and pedal oedema.

Three to four days prior to surgery, gentle β-blockade with propranolol 40 mg/day is instituted. The use of pre-operative β-blockade had been somewhat controversial though it is of particular use in patients with pure adrenaline-secreting tumours and those experiencing tachycardia and arrythmias. Asthma and cardiac failure are absolute contraindications to the use of β-blockers and β-adrenergic blockade should not be used without prior α-blockade, as unopposed vasoconstriction can lead to potentially catastrophic hypertension.

The use of selective α1-blockers such as prazosin hydrochloride and the newer α1-blockers, such as terazosin and doxazosin (which selectively block postsynaptic α1-receptors and have a shorter duration of action) may allow reduction in blood pressure without the reflex tachycardia associated with non-competitive α blockade. Labetalol which has α- and β-adrenergic blocking properties has a much shorter action than phenoxybenzamine and may employed by anaesthetists per-operatively in controlling blood pressure. Other drugs reported to control blood pressure in phaeochromocytoma are calcium channel blockers such as nifedipine. Use is somewhat controversial but a claimed advantage of nifedipine is that patients are unlikely to experience unpleasant orthostatic hypotension.

Anaesthesia for phaeochromocytoma

Close co-operation among endocrinologist, anaesthetist and surgeon should ensure that the patient arrives in theatre in the optimal condition for surgery. Subsequently a co-ordinated team approach between surgeon and anaesthetist should ensure a safe outcome.

Patients are prepared for surgery by insertion of central venous and arterial lines. Electrocardiograph monitoring and intravenous access are essential and urinary catheterization is helpful. Swan–Ganz catheterization to monitor pulmonary wedge pressure has been advocated but its use is probably best restricted to patients in whom cardiac function is known to be seriously compromised, especially those with catecholamine cardiomyopathy.

Anaesthesia is best maintained by isoflurane rather than halothane which has the potential for unwanted cardiac arrythmias. A range of pressure-regulating agents (phentolamine, sodium nitroprusside, noradrenaline and dopamine) should be available in order to maintain and control blood pressure on a minute to minute basis throughout the procedure. Intravenous lignocaine (50–100 mg) is of value in controlling arrythmias. Propranolol (1 mg) may also be of benefit. Cardioversion equipment must be readily available.

Danger periods during surgery for phaeochromocytoma include induction, intubation and per-operative handling of the tumour. Another crucial period may be immediately after tumour resection when hypotension can ensue. This situation is best managed by co-ordinated effort by surgeon and anaesthetist. Volume expansion with blood or colloids is usually sufficient but in refractory cases it may be necessary to give an adrenaline or a dopamine infusion. Failure of the blood pressure to fall following tumour removal may suggest a second tumour or undiagnosed metastatic disease. When bilateral adrenalectomy is performed the procedure must be covered with hydrocortisone 100 mg pre-operatively on induction and further hydrocortisone at the time of gland removal. Intravenous hydrocortisone (100 mg 6 hourly) is continued post-operatively, reducing as full oral steroid replacement therapy is instituted.

Surgery for phaeochromocytoma

Surgical approaches for phaeochromocytoma have changed over recent years. Formerly an anterior transabdominal approach was advocated, through either a midline or bilateral subcostal incision. This approach enabled a laparotomy to be performed to accurately identify the site of disease and to ensure that no lesion was overlooked. Transabdominal access is especially necessary in large tumours, particularly on the right side where the disease may extend posterior to the vena cava and lead to problems of vascular control. In rare instances a thoracoabdominal procedure may be necessary.

As localizing techniques improved a unilateral focused approach was advocated, usually via the posterior or postero-lateral route. The advent of laparoscopic adrenalectomy and the increasing refinement of localizing procedures such as MRI has meant that now a unilateral, focused, endoscopic approach has become virtually the routine surgical method for removal of phaeochromocytomas. This may be accomplished for tumours up to 6 cm in diameter via a transabdominal laparoscopic approach (favoured by most surgeons) or a posterior route (technically more difficult), appropriate for smaller tumours.

Technical aspects are covered in the section on adrenal surgery in this module but special considerations in surgery for phaeochromocytoma include minimal handling of the tumour (made easier by a laparoscopic approach), complete haemostasis (venous ooze is a potential hazard in the α-blocked patient) and close communication with the anaesthetist.

Extra-adrenal phaeochromocytomas are managed by a variety of surgical approaches depending on their location. In the case of bladder tumours, partial, segmental or even total cystectomy may be necessary, particularly when tumours are suspected to be malignant.

Post-operative management

Post-operatively intensive care monitoring of arterial blood pressure, central venous pressure and urinary output is vital. Requirements for intravenous fluid replacement of blood and plasma expanders will be largely determined by the above measurements. Often large amounts of fluid will be necessary because of the relative disproportion between vascular capacitance and circulating blood volume following the removal of the chronic catecholamine vasoconstrictor drive. Residual phenoxybenzamine can also causes fluid loss into the retroperitoneal space.

When hypotension persists, haemorrhage rather than refractory vasodilation should be considered. Care should be taken to avoid overtransfusion leading to pulmonary oedema. Blood glucose levels should also be closely monitored, particularly in the first 6 hours post-operatively as dangerous, even life-threatening hypoglycaemia may ensue, requiring glucose infusion. Where hypertension persists this may be due to residual tumour, metastatic disease or chronic renal damage secondary to long-standing severe hypertension.

All patients should have urinary catecholamine and VMA measurements repeated post-resection and annually thereafter. In patients with malignant disease the true nature of the condition may not become apparent for many years, thus long-term follow-up is advised and even benign tumours may occasionally reoccur. Overall however prognosis in well-prepared patients undergoing careful elective surgery is excellent, with low morbidity and mortality.

Phaeochromocytoma in special circumstances

Unsuspected phaeochromocytoma encountered during surgery

This potentially fatal condition presents a considerable challenge to both surgeon and anaesthetist. Warning signs include unexplained tachycardia, arrythmias or hypertension during anaesthetic induction, at attempted tumour removal or for surgery for a completely unrelated condition in an unprepared patient. Should these warning signs go unheeded patients may develop cardiac failure, pulmonary oedema and fatal cardiac arrest. In this situation α-blockade should be instituted immediately and the procedure terminated. The patient should then undergo full investigation, preparation and localization prior to excision of the tumour at a later date.

Malignant phaeochromocytoma

Malignancy occurs in about 10% of phaeochromocytomas but this rises to 40–50% in extra-adrenal tumours. The difficulties of diagnosing malignancy histologically have already been referred to. Surgical resection remains the principal therapeutic measure.

Localization of metastatic disease may be aided by an MIBG scan, though this has a false negative rate of approximately 10%. In some instances ^{131}I-MIBG may have a therapeutic as well as a diagnostic role. Where possible recurrent disease should be resected, debulked or ablated (Figure 5.19). Chemotherapy has not proved very effective but radiotherapy has been reported to occasionally provide useful palliation, particularly in bony metastases. Symptoms of catecholamine excess may to some extent be alleviated by α-methyl-ρ-tyrosine.

Survival rates in malignant phaeochromocytoma are between 35 and 40% at 5 years, although on rare occasions patients with distant metastases have been reported to survive longer. Extra-adrenal tumours, however, carry a less favourable prognosis.

Phaeochromocytoma in pregnancy

Phaeochromocytoma in pregnancy is a potentially lethal condition: maternal mortality of 40% and fetal mortality of 40–56% have been reported. Hypertension is common in pregnancy and phaeochromocytoma may be mistaken for pre-eclampsia. Therefore, catecholamine excess should be excluded in all hypertensive pregnant women. A high index of suspicion should be maintained in pregnant women who present with unexplained cardiovascular collapse, or exhibit severe or labile hypertension in early pregnancy, or in patients who have a positive family history. Maternal and fetal mortality rates are greatly reduced if the diagnosis is made prior to the onset of labour as hypertensive paroxysms will be precipitated by uterine contractions, anaesthesia or caesarean section.

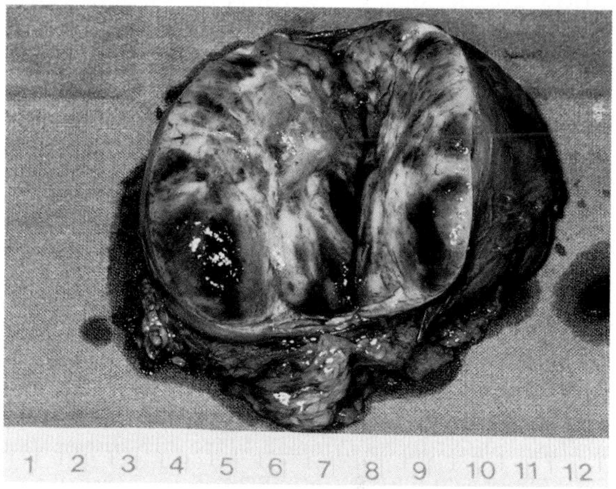

Figure 5.20 Gross specimen of phaeochromocytoma diagnosed during pregnancy and excised at 36 weeks synchronously with caesarean section delivery. The tumour shows typical haemorrhagic appearances on the cut surface.

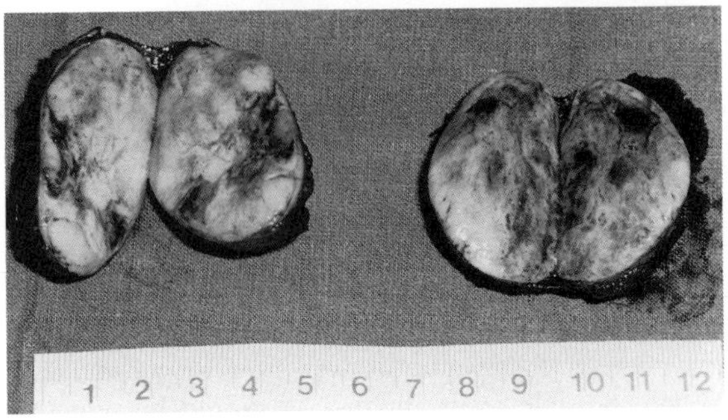

Figure 5.21 Gross specimen of bilateral phaeochromocytomas excised from a 5-year-old boy.

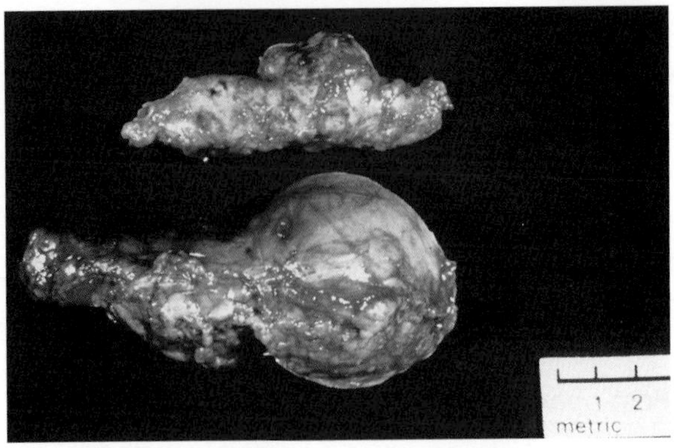

Figure 5.22 Gross specimen of bilateral phaeochromocytomas excised from a patient who had previously undergone total thyroidectomy for medullary thyroid carcinoma as part of the MEN 2B syndrome.

Following diagnosis, tumours may be localized with MRI, avoiding excessive use of X-rays.

After instigating the usual α-blockade and β-blockade 2–3 days pre-operatively in the first and second trimesters surgical excision of tumours may be performed. Some patients may elect for termination of the pregnancy. In the third trimester caesarean section followed by removal of the phaeochromocytoma under the same anaesthetic is appropriate (Figure 5.20). Vaginal delivery should be avoided at all costs.

Phaeochromocytoma in children

When phaeochromocytoma occurs in children there is an increased incidence of bilateral, multiple and extra-adrenal tumours because of the association with MEN 2 syndromes (Figure 5.21). In contrast to adults the tumours are less commonly malignant and the hypertension more often sustained. Hypertension in children always demands the fullest investigation and surgical resection of a phaeochromocytoma is usually followed by an excellent clinical result.

Phaeochromocytoma and MEN 2A and 2B

Multiple endocrine neoplasia (MEN) is a syndrome characterized by medullary thyroid carcinoma and phaeochromocytoma. In the MEN 2A variant, primary hyperparathyroidism is also associated, whilst in MEN 2B, patients have characteristic facies, Marfinoid habitus, skeletal abnormalities and mucocutaneous ganglioneuromas. Hyperparathyroidism does not occur in MEN 2B.

Germ-line mutations in the RET proto-oncogene are responsible for MEN 2A and 2B. The gene is inherited in an autosomal dominant fashion with high penetrance and variable expression. All patients with MEN 2 will develop medullary thyroid cancer but development of phaeochromocytoma is variable.

When present adrenal disease in MEN 2 is bilateral, passing through a phase of hyperplasia to nodularity and multiple phaeochromocytomas. Once the disease has been confirmed through measurement of urinary catecholamines and their metabolites, bilateral adrenalectomy should be performed. Some advocate unilateral adrenalectomy when the disease appears localized to one side but this approach remains controversial as the natural history of the disease clearly indicates that bilateral disease eventually develops in all affected individuals (Figure 5.22). After adrenalectomy careful follow-up is mandatory in all patients but after unilateral adrenalectomy this is especially pertinent in order to monitor the development of disease in the contralateral gland.

Summary

The investigation and treatment of phaeochromocytoma is summarized in Figure 5.24.

Section 5.9 • Other adrenal tumours

Adrenal incidentaloma

Increasing use of sophisticated imaging modalities such as ultrasound, CT and MRI and the ever increasing resolution that both software and hardware are achieving, has meant that the number of incidentally discovered adrenal masses has increased over the past 10 years. Silent adrenal masses are now identified in 0.5–4.5% of patients undergoing CT for reasons other than suspected adrenal pathology, a figure approaching the incidence of incidentalomas identified at postmortem (1.5–5.7%). Adrenal incidentalomas present the clinician with a diagnostic problem, particularly in excluding malignancy tumour but also with respect to functioning potential.

The essential step in the investigation of an incidentally discovered adrenal tumour is to establish whether the lesion is functioning. Biochemical screening should include measurement of electrolytes, 24 hour urinary VMA and metanephrine levels, 9.00 am and midnight serum cortisol and aldosterone. The 1 mg overnight dexamethasone suppression test should exclude Cushing's syndrome.

The majority of incidentalomas (35–95%) are benign, non-functioning adrenal adenomas. They are more prevalent in older women and in obese, diabetic patients. Tumours are classically smooth, round and less

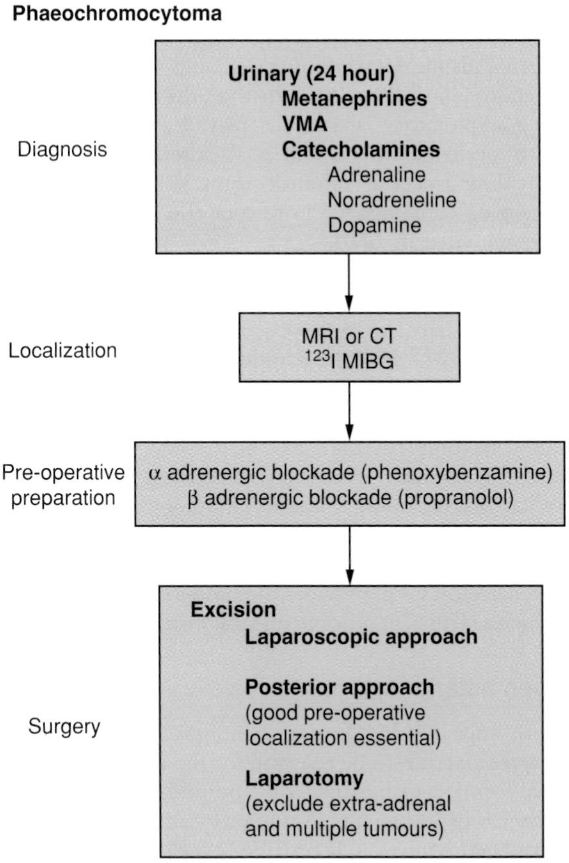

Figure 5.23 Investigation and treatment of phaeochromocytoma.

than 3 cm in size. They are homogeneous and enhance only minimally after contrast injection on CT. With MRI, signal intensity is the same as normal adrenal tissue; this is helpful in distinguishing secondary metastatic lesions in the adrenal which tend to have intense T2 weighted images (Figure 5.23). Calcification, haemorrhage and necrosis are uncommon.

Where diagnosis is in doubt NP59 or selenocholesterol scintigraphy may identify functioning adenomas causing subclinical Cushing's (5%) or aid in the diagnosis of malignancy. Following the exclusion of a phaeochromocytoma, fine needle aspiration cytology can be selectively and carefully employed if a secondary adrenal malignant deposit is suspected.

Adrenal cysts also cause diagnostic confusion. These are usually small and symptomless but when large may present as a tumour mass displacing the kidney. Drainage under ultrasound or CT guidance is recommended and the fluid sent for cytological analysis. Adenomyelolipomas are benign, non-functioning tumours which have a characteristic appearence on MRI and only require excision if there are significant symptoms.

The incidence of malignancy in adrenal tumours increases with size of lesion and for this reason surgical resection is recommended for all lesions greater than 4 cm. MRI or CT scans demonstrating non-homogeneity may also influence the decision to perform surgery.

Smaller lesions can be monitored by interval CT, MRI or ultrasound scans and excision considered when there is an increase in size. Surgical excision should also be performed in patients under 50 years of age because of the increased malignancy risk for adrenal lesions in the younger subject.

Secondary adrenal tumours

Many malignant neoplasms metastasize to the adrenal glands. Among the more common tumours are breast, bronchus and melanoma. Adrenocortical hormone production may be reduced where large metastases cause significant adrenal destruction resulting in an acute Addisonian crisis.

Neuroblastoma

Presentation

These tumours of neural crest origin occur mainly in children, over 60% presenting in the first year of life. They occur in the adrenal medulla, adjacent retroperitoneal tissue and along the sympathetic ganglia. The majority of the tumours occur in the abdomen (75%), the remainder occurring in the thorax (20%) and neck (5%). Aggressive malignancies, they invade adjacent local structures such as kidney, spleen, liver and pancreas. Metastatic spread occurs early via the blood stream and lymphatics and is frequently present at initial presentation. Two distinct patterns of metastatic spread are recognized, *Hutchinson's type* (tumour on the left side producing metastases to the orbit, skull and long bones) and *Pepper's type* (tumour on the right side with metastatic spread to the liver).

Approximately 50% of children with this tumour present with a large, symptomless abdominal mass. The other 50% present with symptoms including anorexia, nausea, vomiting and diarrhoea (tumours producing vasoactive intestinal peptide). Over 90% of neuroblastomas produce catecholamines and hypertension and/or flushing may be a feature. A 24 hour urine collection for VMA, metanephrine's and catecholamines is therefore mandatory in these patients. Dumb-bell tumours (tumours extending into the spinal canal) may produce neurological symptoms. The main differential diagnosis of neuroblastoma is nephroblastoma (Wilms' tumour).

Tumour staging

Tumours are staged with a combination of chest X-ray, CT/MRI scanning and skeletal survey. MIBG scintography may be useful in identifying primary tumours as well as residual or recurrent tumour:

- Stage I: tumours are confined to the adrenal gland and are totally excised.
- Stage II: tumours extend beyond the organ of origin but do not cross the midline; ipsilateral lymph nodes may be involved.
- Stage III: tumours cross the midline.
- Stage IV: distant metastatic spread present.

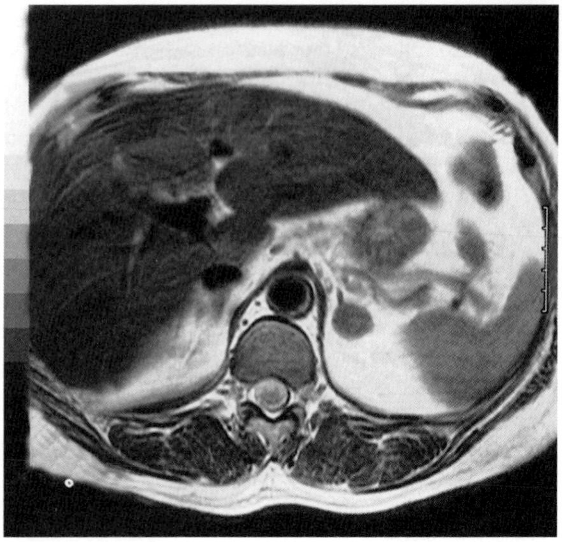

Figure 5.24 MRI scan of a non-functioning left adrenal incidentaloma.

Treatment

Surgical excision remains the mainstay of treatment. When complete excision is not possible, tumour debulking followed by either radiotherapy and/or combination chemotherapy with vincristine and cyclophosphamide may be of benefit. Radiotherapy is of particular benefit in painful metastatic deposits.

Prognosis

Prognosis is dependent on age and tumour stage. Children aged less than 2 years have a better 2 year survival rate compared to their older counterparts (77% compared to 38%). The 2 year survival rate worsens with stage: stage I (100%), stage 2 (82%), stage III (42%) and stage IV (30%). Factors improving stage-specific prognosis include a high urinary VMA to homovanillic acid ratio and low serum neurone-specific enolase level.

Section 5.10 • Adrenalectomy

Background

The first description of an adrenalectomy was provided by Thornton in 1890. He employed an approach to the right adrenal gland using an incision for cholecystectomy, previously described by Carl von Langenbüch of Berlin in 1882. For many years the adrenal glands were approached via incisions described for renal surgery. Unfortunately these incisions were frequently too low to gain adequate exposure and surgeons began to site incisions progressively higher. In 1932 Lennox Broster of London (a pioneer of adrenal surgery) described a posterior, intercostal, transpleural adrenalectomy. He had performed a laparotomy a few weeks previously in the same patient to inspect the adrenals and look for any extra-adrenal tissue. In 1936 Hugh Young of Baltimore devised a simultaneous, bilateral, posterior approach, enabling him to inspect both adrenal glands, a technique associated with little post-operative morbidity. Prior to the advent of CT scanning, exploratory laparotomy played a pivotal role in both localizing adrenal and extra-adrenal tumours and providing access for adrenalectomy. With modern-day localizing techniques, however, this approach has become virtually obsolete.

The main approaches to the adrenal glands are anterior and posterior or postero-lateral. The description by Gagner in 1992 of an endoscopic technique has provided surgeons with the additional option of performing adrenalectomy as either an 'open' or a 'minimally invasive' (endoscopic) procedure. Each method of adrenalectomy has both advantages and disadvantages and the approach of choice is dependent on a number of factors including tumour pathology, tumour size, patient physique, previous surgery and the personal preference of the surgeon. Despite the various options, adrenalectomy still provides the modern-day endocrine surgeon with a significant surgical challenge.

Open anterior approach

With improved localization techniques the *open anterior approach* tends to be reserved for the removal of large (<6–8 cm), malignant or potentially malignant tumours or in patients in whom localizing procedures have been equivocal. It provides excellent exposure of one or both adrenal glands and enables examination of the abdominal viscera and sympathetic chain to search for extra-adrenal tissue. The patient is placed supine on the operating table and a transverse, subcostal incision made. This may either be unilateral or be extended across the midline when exposure of both adrenal glands is required. Alternatively a vertical midline incision made be preferred.

The major disadvantages of this approach are:

- in patients with Cushing's syndrome, when wound complications including infection and dehiscence contribute significantly to morbidity
- it necessitates entering the peritoneal cavity producing a post-operative ileus and
- there is an increased incidence of atelectasis, pulmonary collapse and chest infection.

Laparoscopic 'anterior' approach

Laparoscopic adrenalectomy can be performed effectively and safely. This approach was quickly popularized and subsequent reports confirmed its feasibility. Most surgeons currently use a lateral flank approach with the patient lying with the side to be operated on uppermost. A pneumoperitoneum is created and three, or when needed, four laparoscopic ports are inserted below the costal margin. All the ports should be 10 mm in size which enables the camera to be moved from port to port to improve visualization. A significant advantage of the flank approach is that once the spleen is mobilized on the left side it acts as a retractor under its own weight. Similarly the liver on the right requires minimal retraction.

The anterior laparoscopic approach allows excellent visualization of the adrenal glands and the vascular pedicles both sides, particularly the adrenal veins. It is an ideal approach for Conn's tumours and smaller phaeochromocytomas (<6 cm) as the adrenal vein can be divided early in the procedure. Operative times have dramatically improved with experience and new instrumentation to an extent that bilateral laparoscopic adrenalectomy is now readily performed.

Post-operatively patients can be mobilized quickly and inpatient stay is significantly reduced compared to open adrenalectomy. Perhaps the major advantage of laparoscopic adrenalectomy is seen in patients with Cushing's syndrome. Wound size is markedly reduced in these patients and consequently the wound-associated morbidity has dramatically improved.

Anterior laparoscopic adrenalectomy is unsuitable for adrenal tumours >8 cm, malignant and potentially malignant tumours. A relative contraindication is previous abdominal surgery. Identification of smaller left-sided tumours may prove difficult.

Open posterior approach

The posterior approach to the adrenal gland was originally described by Hugh Young in 1936. Most endocrine surgeons, however, favour the Turner–Warwick modification of the posterior approach, where the eleventh or twelfth ribs are removed extrapleurally. This incision may also be slightly modified by making a 'hockey-stick'-shaped incision that initially runs parallel to the spinal column. The approach is suitable for smaller adrenal tumours including Conn's, adenomas and Cushing's syndrome due to bilateral adrenal hyperplasia. Recent improvements in adrenal imaging techniques have enabled surgeons to employ this approach for selected patients with phaeochromocytoma. The incision is associated with a low morbidity and mortality and hospital inpatient time is reduced compared to the open anterior approach. As peritoneum is not entered post-operative ileus is a rare complication.

The main disadvantages of this approach are restricted visualization and access, particularly on the right side where the right adrenal vein is short and may be difficult to secure.

Posterior endoscopic approach

Some authors have described a posterior endoscopic approach to the adrenal glands. Patients are positioned as for an open posterior approach and a balloon is inserted and inflated in the retroperitoneal space below the twelfth rib. Ports are inserted into the artificial space and the adrenal gland is visualized. The approach is most appropriate for small adrenal tumours (<3 cm), particularly Conn's tumours and also in patients with bilateral adrenal hyperplasia. Post-operative recovery is quicker and hospital inpatient stay even shorter than anterior laparoscopic adrenalectomy.

The major drawbacks with this approach are:

- difficult anatomical orientation compared to the anterior laparoscopic approach
- very limited operating space
- normal endoscopic instruments may be too long and
- even minor bleeding may cause significant visualization problems.

Because of these problems the approach has not proved popular with most surgeons. The approach, however, does offer an alternative technique in patients with suitable adrenal tumours in whom an anterior laparoscopic approach is not feasible because of previous extensive abdominal surgery.

Further reading

Abel, J. J. and Crawford, A. C. (1897). On the blood pressure raising constituents of the supra renal capsule. *Johns Hopkins Hosp Bull* **8**: 151.

Addison, T. (1855). *On the Constitutional and Local Effects of Disease of the Supra Renal Capsules*. London: Samuel Highley.

Amador, E. (1965). Adrenal hemorrhage during anticoagulant therapy. A clinical and pathological study of ten cases. *Ann Intern Med* **63**: 559–71.

Armstrong, M. D., McMillan, A. and Shaw, K. N. F. (1957). 3-Metoxy-4-hydroxy-D-mandellic acid, a urinary metabolite of norepinephrine. *Biochim Biophys Acta* **25**: 422–8.

Auda, S. P., Brennan, M. F. and Gill, J. R. Jr (1980). Evolution of the surgical management of primary aldosteronism. *Ann Surg* **191**: 1–7.

Azzopardi, J. G. and Williams, E. D. (1968). Pathology of 'nonendocrine' tumors associated with Cushing's syndrome. *Cancer* **22**: 274–86.

Biglieri, E. G., Irony, I. and Kater, C. E. (1989). Identification and implications of new types of mineralocorticoid hypertension. *J Steroid Biochem* **32**(1B): 199–204.

Boggan, J. E., Tyrrell, J. B. and Wilson, C. B. (1983). Transsphenoidal microsurgical management of Cushing's disease. Report of 100 cases. *J Neurosurg* **59**: 195–200.

Boutros, A. R., Bravo, E. L., Zanettin, G. and Straffon, R. A. (1990). Perioperative management of 63 patients with pheochromocytoma. *Cleveland Clin J Med* **57**: 613–17.

Bravo, E. L. (1989). Physiology of the adrenal cortex. *Urol Clin North Am* **16**: 433–7.

Bravo, E. L. (1994). Evolving concepts in the pathophysiology, diagnosis, and treatment of pheochromocytoma. *Endocr Rev* **15**: 356–68.

Broster, L. R., Hill, H. G. and Greenfield, J. G. (1932). Adrenogenital syndrome and unilateral adrenalectomy. *Am J Surg* **19**: 557–70.

Brown, W. H. (1928). A case of pleuriglandular syndrome: diabetes of bearded woman. *Lancet* **ii**, 1022–7.

Brown-Séquard, C. (1856). Recherches experimentales sur la physiologie et la pathologie des capsules suurenales C: *Arch Gen Med (Paris)* **8**, 385.

Burke, C. W. and Beardwell, C. G. (1973). Cushing's syndrome. An evaluation of the clinical usefulness of urinary free cortisol and other urinary steroid measurements in diagnosis. *Q J Med* **42**: 175–204.

Burke, C. W., Adams, C. B., Esiri, M. M. *et al.* (1990). Transsphenoidal surgery for Cushing's disease: does what is removed determine the endocrine outcome? *Clin Endocrinol* **33**: 525–37.

Carney, J. A., Sizemore, G. W. and Tyce, G. M. (1975). Bilateral adrenal medullary hyperplasia in multiple endocrine neoplasia, type 2: the precursor of bilateral pheochromocytoma. *Mayo Clin Proc* **50**: 3–10.

Chang, A., Glazer, H. S., Lee, J. K., Ling, D. and Heiken, J. P. (1987). Adrenal gland: MR imaging. *Radiology*. **163**: 123–8.

Cirillo, R. L. Jr., Bennett, W. F., Vitellas, K. M. *et al.* (1998). Pathology of the adrenal gland: imaging features. *Am J Roentgenol* **170**: 429–35.

Conn, J. W. (1955) Part I. Painting background. Part II. Primary aldosteronism, a new clinical syndrome. *Lab Clin Med* **45**: 3.

Crapo, L. (1979). Cushing's syndrome: a review of diagnostic tests. *Metab Clin Exp* **28**: 955–77.

Cushing, H. (1932). The pituitary body and its disorders. *Johns Hopkins Hosp Bull* **50**: 137.

Cutroneo, K. R., Rokowski, R. and Counts, D. F. (1981). Glucocorticoids and collagen synthesis: comparison of *in vivo* and cell culture studies. *Collagen Relate Res* **1**: 557–68.

Daly, P. A. and Landsberg, L. (1992). Phaeochromocytoma: diagnosis and management. *Baillières Clin Endocrinol Metab* **6**: 143–66.

Doppman, J. L., Oldfield, E., Krudy, A. G. *et al.* (1984). Petrosal sinus sampling for Cushing syndrome: anatomical and technical considerations. *Radiology* **150**: 99–103.

Duh, Q. Y., Siperstein, A. E., Clark, O. H. *et al.* (1996). Laparoscopic adrenalectomy. Comparison of the lateral and posterior approaches. *Arch Surg* **131**: 870–5; discussion 875–6.

Dunnick, N.R., Heaston, D., Halvorsen, R. *et al.* (1982). CT appearance of adrenal cortical carcinoma. *J Comput Assist Tomogr* **6**: 978–82.

Dwyer, A. J., Frank, J. A., Doppman, J. L. *et al.* (1987). Pituitary adenomas in patients with Cushing's disease: initial experience with Gd-DTPA-enhanced MRI imaging. *Radiology* **163**: 421.

Edis, A. J., Grant, C. S. and Egdahal, R. H. (eds) (1984). *Manual of Endocrine Surgery*, 2nd edn. New York: Springer.

Edwards, C. R. and Besser, G. M. (1974). Diseases of the hypothalamus and pituitary gland. *Clin Endocrinol Metab* **3**: 475–505.

Evans, A. E., D'Angio, G. J. and Randolph, J. (1971). A proposed staging for children with neuroblastoma. Children's Cancer Study Group A. *Cancer* **27**: 374–8.

Farwell, A. P., Devlin, J. T. and Stewart, J. A. (1988). Total suppression of cortisol excretion by ketoconazole in the therapy of the ectopic adrenocorticotropic hormone syndrome. *Am J Med* **84**: 1063–6.

Favio, G. and Lumachi, F. N. (1997). Cushing's syndrome. In: Clark, O. H. and Duh, Q. Y. eds. *Textbook of Endocrine Surgery*. Philadelphia, PA: W. B. Saunders.

Ferriss, J. B., Brown, J. J., Fraser, R. *et al.* (1975). Results of adrenal surgery in patients with hypertension, aldosterone excess, and low plasma renin concentration. *BMJ* **1**(5950): 135–8.

Finkelstein, M. and Shaefer J. M. (1979). Inborn errors of steroid biosynthesis. *Physiol Rev* **59**: 353–406.

Fishman, L. N., Liddle, G. W., Island, D. P. *et al.* (1987). Effects of aminogluthamide on adrenalfunction in man. *J Clin Endocrinol Metab* **27**: 481–8.

Frankel, F. (1886). Ein Fall von doppelseitigem, vollig latent verlaufen Nebennierentumor und zleichzeitizer Nephritis. *Vichows Arch Pathol Anat Klin Med* **103**: 244–63.

Friesen, S. R. and Thompson, N. W. eds (1990). *Surgical Endocrinology*. Philadelphia, PA: Lippincott.

Fudge, T. L., McKinnon, W. M. and Geary, W. L. (1980). Current surgical management of pheochromocytoma during pregnancy. *Arch Surg* **115**: 1224–5.

Gagner, M., Lacroix, A. and Bolte, E. (1992). Laparoscopic adrenalectomy in Cushing's syndrome and pheochromocytoma [letter]. *N Engl J Med* **327**: 1033.

Granberg, P. O., Adamson, U., Cohn, K. H. *et al.* (1982). The management of patients with primary aldosteronism. *World J Surg* **6**: 757–64.

Grant, C. S., Carney, J. A., Carpenter, P. C. and van Heerden, J. A. (1986). Primary pigmented nodular adrenocortical disease: diagnosis and management. *Surgery* **100**: 1178–84.

Grant, C. S., Carpenter, P., van Heerden, J. A. and Hamberger, B. (1984). Primary aldosteronism. Clinical management. *Arch Surg* **119**: 585–90.

Gross, M. D., Wilton, G. P., Shapiro, B. *et al.* (1987). Functional and scintigraphic evaluation of the silent adrenal mass. *J Nucl Med* **28**: 1401–7.

Hall, R. (1981). Addison's disease. *Med Int* **6**: 276–8.

Henley, D. J., van Heerden, J. A., Grant, C. S. *et al.* (1983). Adrenal cortical carcinoma – a continuing challenge. *Surgery* **94**: 926–31.

Herrera, M. F., Grant, C. S., van Heerden, J. A. *et al.* (1991). Incidentally discovered adrenal tumors: an institutional perspective. *Surgery* **110**: 1014–21.

Horgan, S., Sinanan, M., Helton, W. S. and Pellegrini, C. A. (1997). Use of laparoscopic techniques improves outcome from adrenalectomy. *Am J Surg* **173**: 371–4.

Hughes, I. A. (1982). Congenital and acquired disorders of the adrenal cortex. *Clin Endocrinol Metab* **11**: 125–31.

Hughes, I. A. and Read, G. F. (1982). Simultaneous plasma and saliva steroid measurements as an index of control in congenital adrenal hyperplasia (CAH). A longitudinal study. *Horm Res* **16**: 142–50.

Hughes, I. A. and Winter, J. S. (1978). The relationships between serum concentrations of 17OH-progesterone and other serum and urinary steroids in patients with congenital adrenal hyperplasia. *J Clin Endocrinol Metab* **46**: 98–104.

Hughes, I. A., Riad-Fahmy, D. and Griffiths, K. (1979). Plasma 17OH-progesterone concentrations in newborn infants. *Arch Dis Child* **54**: 347–9.

Hunt, T. K., Schambelan, M. and Biglieri, E. G. (1975). Selection of patients and operative approach in primary aldosteronism. *Ann Surg* **182**: 353–61.

Javadpour, N., Woltering, E. A. and Brennan, M. F. (1980). Adrenal neoplasms. *Curr Prob Surg* **17**: 1–52.

Jeffcoate, W. J., Rees, L. H., Tomlin, S. *et al.* (1977). Metyrapone in long-term management of Cushing's disease. *BMJ* **ii**: 215–17.

Johnston, R. R., Eger, E. I., II. and Wilson, C. (1979). A comparative interaction of epinephrine with enflurane, isoflurane, and halothane in man. *Anesth Analg* **55**: 709–12.

Landsberg, L. and Young, J. B. (1980). In: Bondy, P. K. and Rosenburg, L. E. eds. *Metabolic Control and Disease*. Philadelphia, PA: W. B. Saunders.

Liddle, G. W. (1960). Test of pituitary-adrenal suppressibility in the diagnosis of Cushing's syndrome. *J Clin Endocrinol Metab* **20**: 1539.

Liddle, G. W., Island, D. and Meador, C. K. (1962). Normal and abnormal regulation of corticotrophin secretion. *Recent Prog in Horm Res* **15**: 125–66.

Manger, W. M. and Gifford, R. W. Jr (1977). *Pheochromocytoma*. New York: Springer.

Marescaux, J., Mutter, D. and Wheeler, M. H. (1996). Laparoscopic right and left adrenalectomies. *Surg Endosc* **10**: 912–15.

Mayo, C. H. (1927). Paroxysmal hypertension with tumour of retroperitoneal nerve. *JAMA* **89**: 1047.

Minno, A. M., Bennett, W. A. and Kvale, W. F. (1954). Phaeochromocytoma. *N Engl J Med* **251**: 959–65.

Montgomery, D. A. D. and Welbourn, R. B. (1978). Cushing's syndrome: 20 years after adrenalectomy. *Br J Surg* **65**: 210–20.

Mukherjee, J. J., Peppercorn, P. D., Reznek, R. H. *et al.* (1997). Pheochromocytoma: effect of nonionic contrast medium in CT on circulating catecholamine levels. *Radiology* **202**: 227–31.

Mulligan, L. M., Kwok, J. B., Healey, C. S. *et al.* (1993). Germ-line mutations of the RET proto-oncogene in multiple endocrine neoplasia type 2A. *Nature* **363**: 458–60.

Navaratnarajah, M. and White, D. C. (1984). Labetalol and phaeochromocytoma [letter]. *Br J Anaesth* **56**: 1179.

Nelson, D. H., Meakin, J. W. and Thorn, G. W. (1960). ACTH producing pituitary tumours following adrenalectomy for Cushing's syndrome. *Ann Intern Med* **52**: 560.

Nerup, J. (1974). Addison's disease – clinical studies. A report of 108 cases. *Acta Endocrinol* **76**: 127–41.

Neumann, P. J. (1997): Addison's disease and acute adrenal haemorrhage. In: Clark, O. H. and Duh, Q. Y. eds. *Textbook of Endocrine Surgery*. Philadelphia, PA: W. B. Saunders.

Nicholson, J. P. Jr, Vaughn, E. D. Jr, Pickering, T. G. *et al.* (1983). Pheochromocytoma and prazosin. *Ann Intern Med* **99**: 477–9.

Obara, T., Ito, Y., Okamoto, T. *et al.* (1992). Risk factors associated with postoperative persistent hypertension in patients with primary aldosteronism. *Surgery* **112**: 987–93.

Oldfield, E. H., Chrousos, G. P., Schulte, H. M. *et al.* (1985). Preoperative lateralization of ACTH-secreting pituitary microadenomas by bilateral and simultaneous inferior petrosal venous sinus sampling. *N Engl J Med* **312**: 100–3.

Oliver, G. and Sharpey-Shafer, E. A. (1895). The physiological effects of extracts of the supra renal capsule. *J Physiol (Lond)* **18**, 230.

Orth, D. N. (1978). Metyrapone is useful only as adjunctive therapy in Cushing's disease. *Ann Intern Med* **89**: 128–30.

Padberg, B. C., Holl, K. and Schroder, S. (1992). Pathology of multiple endocrine neoplasias 2A and 2B: a review. *Horm Res* **38**(Suppl 2): 24–30.

Pavlatos, F. C., Smilo, R. P. and Fordham, P. H. (1965). A rapid screening test for Cushing's syndrome. *JAMA* **193**: 720.

Peppercorn, P. D., Grossman, A. B. and Reznek, R. H. (1998). Imaging of incidentally discovered adrenal masses. *Clin Endocrinol* **48**: 379–88.

Pick, L. (1912). Das Ganglioma embryonale sympathicum. *Berlin Klin Wochenschr* **19**: 16–22.

Plumpton, F. S., Besser, G. M. and Cole, P. V. (1969). Corticosteroid treatment and surgery. 2. The management of steroid cover. *Anaesthesia* **24**: 12–18.

Pommier, R. F. and Brennan, M. F. (1992). An eleven-year experience with adrenocortical carcinoma. *Surgery* **112**: 963–70; discussion 970–1.

Pont, A., Williams, P. L., Loose, D. S. *et al.* (1982). Ketoconazole blocks adrenal steroid synthesis. *Ann Intern Med* **97**: 370–2.

Proye, C. A., Huart, J. Y., Cuvillier, X. D. *et al.* (1993). Safety of the posterior approach in adrenal surgery: experience in 105 cases. *Surgery* **114**: 1126–31.

Quinn, S. J. and Williams, G. H. (1988). Regulation of aldosterone secretion. *Ann Rev Physiol* **50**: 409–26.

Remine, W. H., Chong, G. C., Van Heerden, J. A. *et al.* (1974). Current management of pheochromocytoma. *Ann Surg* **179**: 740–8.

Rolleston, H. D. (1936). *The Endocrine Organs in Health and Disease*. Oxford: Oxford University Press.

Roux: Thesis Lausanne. Cited by Barbeau, A., Marc-Aurele, J., Brouillet, J. *et al.* (1958). Le pheochromocytome bilateral: presentation d'un cas et revue de la litterature. *J Union Med Can* **87**: 165–72.

Rovit, R. L. and Duane, T. D. (1969). Cushing's syndrome and pituitary tumors. Pathophysiology and ocular manifestations of ACTH-secreting pituitary adenomas. *Am J Med* **46**: 416–27.

Ruder, H. J., Loriaux, D. L. and Lipsett, M. B. (1974). Severe osteopenia in young adults associated with Cushing's syndrome due to micronodular adrenal disease. *J Clin Endocrinol Metab* **39**: 1138–47.

Savage, M. O. (1985). Congenital adrenal hyperplasia. *Clin Endocrinol Metab* **14**: 893–909.

Schenker, J. G. and Chowers, I. (1971). Pheochromocytoma and pregnancy. Review of 89 cases. *Obstet Gynecol Surv* **26**: 739–47.

Schenker, J. G. and Granat, M. (1982). Phaeochromocytoma and pregnancy – an updated appraisal. *Aust NZ J Obstet Gynaecol* **22**: 1–11.

Schteingart, D. E., Motazedi, A., Noonan, R. A. and Thompson, N. W. (1982). Treatment of adrenal carcinomas. *Arch Surg* **117**: 1142–6.

Schteingart, D. E., Seabold, J. E., Gross, M. D. and Swanson, D. P. (1981). Iodocholesterol adrenal tissue uptake and imaging adrenal neoplasms. *J Clinical Endocrinol Metab* **52**: 1156–61.

Scott, H. W. Jr, Dean, R. H., Lea, J. W. *et al.* (1982). Surgical experience with retrogastric and retropancreatic pheochromocytomas. *Surgery* **92**: 853–65.

Serfas, D., Shoback, D. M. and Lorell, B. H. (1983). Phaeochromocytoma and hypertrophic cardiomyopathy: apparent suppression of symptoms and noradrenaline secretion by calcium-channel blockade. *Lancet* **ii**: 711–13.

Soreide, J. A., Brabrand, K. and Thoresen, S. O. (1992). Adrenal cortical carcinoma in Norway, 1970–84. *World J Surg* **16**: 663–7.

Staren, E. D. and Prinz, R. A. (1996). Adrenalectomy in the era of laparoscopy. *Surgery* **120**: 706–11.

Tam, P. K. (1994). Paediatric solid tumours. In: Morris, P. J. and Malt, R. A. eds. *Oxford Textbook of Surgery*. New York: Oxford University Press.

Thompson, G. B., Grant, C. S., van Heerden, J. A. *et al.* (1997). Laparoscopic versus open posterior adrenalectomy: a case control study of 100 patients. *Surgery* **122**: 1136.

Thompson, N. W. and Cheung, P. S. (1987). Diagnosis and treatment of functioning and nonfunctioning adrenocortical neoplasms including incidentalomas. *Surg Clin North Am* **67**: 423–36.

Thornton, J. K. (1890). Abdominal nephrectomy for large sarcoma of the left suprarenal capsule. *Clinical Society Transactions (London)* **23**: 150–3.

Tibblin, S., Dymling, J. F., Ingemansson, S. and Telenius-Berg, M. (1983). Unilateral versus bilateral adrenalectomy in multiple endocrine neoplasia IIA. *World J Surg* **7**: 201–8.

Troncone, L., Rufini, V., Montemaggi, P. *et al.* (1990). The diagnostic and therapeutic utility of radioiodinated metaiodobenzylguanidine (MIBG). 5 years of experience. *Eur J Nucl Med* **16**: 325–35.

Turner-Warwick, R. T. (1965). The supra costal approach to the renal area. *Br J Urol* **37**: 671–6.

van Heerden, J. A., Grant, C. S. and Weaver, A. C. (1993). *Acta Chir Austrica* **25**: 216.

van Heerden, J. A., Sheps, S. G., Hamberger, B. *et al.* (1982). Pheochromocytoma: current status and changing trends. *Surgery* **91**: 367–73.

Veldhuis, J. D., Iranmanesh, A., Lizarralde, G. and Johnson, M. L. (1989). Amplitude modulation of a burstlike mode of cortisol secretion subserves the circadian glucocorticoid rhythm. *Am J Physiol* **257**(1 Pt 1): E6–14.

Verner, J. V. and Morrison, A. B. (1974). Endocrine pancreatic islet disease with diarrhea. Report of a case due to diffuse hyperplasia of nonbeta islet tissue with a review of 54 additional cases. *Arch Intern Med* **133**: 492–9.

von Langenbuch, C. (1882). Ein Fall von Exstirpation der Gallenblase. *Berlin Klin Wochenschr* **19**: 725–7.

Walz, M. K., Peitgen, K., Hoermann, R. *et al.* (1996). Posterior retroperitoneoscopy as a new minimally invasive approach for adrenalectomy: results of 30 adrenalectomies in 27 patients. *World J Surg* **20**: 769–74.

Welbourn, R. B. ed. (1990). *The History of Endocrine Surgery*. New York: Praeger.

Welbourn, R. B. and Manolas, K. J. (1983). *Endocrine Surgery*. London: Butterworth.

Werbel, S. S. and Ober, K. P. (1993). Acute adrenal insufficiency. *Endocrinol Metab Clin North Am* **22**: 303–28.

White, F. E., White, M. C., Drury, P. L. *et al.* (1982). Value of computed tomography of the abdomen and chest in investigation of Cushing's syndrome. *BMJ Clin Res Ed.* **284**: 771–4.

Young, A. E. and Smellie, W. J. B. (1997). The adrenal glands. In: Fardon, J. R. ed. *Breast and Endocrine Surgery*. London: W. B. Saunders.

Young, H. G. (1936). A technique for simultaneous exposure and operation on the adrenals. *Surg Gynecol Obstet* **54**: 179.

Young, W. F. Jr (1997). Pheochromocytoma and primary aldosteronism: diagnostic approaches. *Endocrinol Metab Clin North Am* **26**: 801–27.

Young, W. F. Jr and Klee, G. G. (1988). Primary aldosteronism. Diagnostic evaluation. *Endocrinol Metab Clin North Am* **17**: 367-95.

MODULE 6

Disorders of the abdominal wall and peritoneal cavity

Section 6.1 • Surgical anatomy

The two terms abdomen (or abdominal cavity) and peritoneal cavity are not strictly synonymous. The abdomen (or abdominal cavity) refers to the musculo-aponeurotic and bony walls that enclose a region lined on the inside by the peritoneum. By contrast, the peritoneal cavity denotes the space enclosed by the peritoneal lining and contains some but not all of the abdominal viscera. The retroperitoneal space lies behind the posterior wall of the peritoneal cavity and contains adipose and areolar 'packing tissue' in which lie the retroperitoneal organs. This is continuous with the rest of the extraperitoneal space filled with the same packing tissue separating the musculo-aponeurotic anterolateral walls from the peritoneal membrane. Underneath the packing tissue is a fascial layer (endo-abdominal fascia) that covers the muscles of the back and this is continuous with the transversalis fascia anterolaterally on both sides.

The abdominal cavity is subdivisible into the abdomen proper and the pelvis. When viewed from one side of the sagittal plane, the pelvis lies below and behind the abdominal cavity as a basin-shaped extension with a centrally sloping muscular floor (pelvic diaphragm) part of which (the puboccygeus) is continuous with the muscular coat of the rectum. The upper boundary of the abdominal cavity is made up of the diaphragm and because of this, a substantial part of the abdominal cavity (almost equal to the thoracic cavity) lies under the lower rib cage. The anterolateral walls of the abdomen are made up of the musculo-aponeurotic layer: the recti muscles on either side of the midline anteriorly separated by a median raphe (linea alba) and three pairs of flat wide muscles (external oblique, internal oblique and transversus abdominis).

The peritoneal cavity itself consists of the greater sac (or general peritoneal cavity) and the lesser sac (also known as the omental bursa) which lies behind the stomach, lesser omentum and transverse colon/mesocolon, and below the inferior surface of the liver. The two sacs communicate on the right side via a small slit (foramen of Winslow), the anterior fold of which, sometimes referred to as the hepatoduodenal ligament, contains the bile duct, common hepatic artery and the portal vein. It provides a readily accessible site for temporary occlusion of the hepatic inflow vessels during hepatic resections and in the event of bleeding from the hepatic vascular parenchyma or the hepatic arteries (Pringle's manoeuvre).

Anterolateral abdominal wall

The subcutaneous fat becomes divisible into two layers in the lower part of the abdomen: superficial fatty Camper's fascia and the deep membranous Scarpa's fascia that inserts into the fascia of the thigh below and parallel to the inguinal ligament. The deep fascia of the anterolateral wall is thin and covers the superficial abdominal muscles. The two musculo-aponeurotic halves of the anterior abdominal wall are joined by the mid-line linea alba, which essentially consists of interwoven fibres of the rectus sheath forming a distinctive pattern. At the umbilical pit the skin is adherent to the linea alba and this marks the narrowest point of the abdominal wall (consisting of skin, linea alba and attachment of the ligamentum teres).

Thinning and stretching of the linea alba especially in females after multiple pregnancy results in separation (divarication) of the two rectus muscles with an intervening bulge. In the upper half of the anterior abdominal wall, the rectus muscles have both an anterior and a posterior sheath. This arrangement changes at the level of the anterior superior iliac spines where the posterior sheath is absent with its lower margin forming a crescentic outline referred to as the arcuate line (linea semicircularis). Hence, below this point, the abdominal wall is weaker. Internally the anterior abdominal wall is covered by the transversalis fascia, which is separated from the parietal pneumoperitoneum by intervening areolar-fatty tissue. The fat of this layer tends to become more abundant and the connection between the peritoneal membrane and the abdominal wall looser in the lower abdomen and pelvis.

Just above the umbilicus, the parietal peritoneum is carried backwards as a two layered membrane (falciform ligament) which is attached to the anterosuperior surface of the liver and the diaphragm. It contains a variable amount of fat (excessive and pendulant in the obese) and along its lower margin the round ligament or ligamentum teres which is attached to the recessus of Rex at the bottom of the umbilical fissure of the liver. It represents the obliterated left umbilical vein, which connects with the left portal vein in the fetus. The muscles and skin of the anterolateral abdominal wall are supplied by the following nerves, which run in the neurovascular plane between the internal oblique and transversus abdominis muscles:

- thoraco-abdominal (inferior intercostal) nerves (T7–T11)
- subcostal nerves (T12)
- ilioinguinal and iliohypogastric nerves (L1).

Below the umbilicus five structures lying between the peritoneum and the parieties form ridges or folds separating shallow fossae. In the midline, there is the median umbilical ligament (urachus, remains of the allantois) which forms a slender fibrous band between the apex of the urinary bladder and the umbilicus. The medial umbilical ligaments (obliterated portions of the umbilical arteries) run upwards and medially one on either side of the median umbilical ligament with which they merge at the umbilicus. The inferior epigastric vessels arising from the external iliac arteries run upwards and medially lateral to the medial umbilical ligaments to supply the rectus muscles and eventually enter the rectus sheath beneath the arcuate line. They form the lateral umbilical folds. Inadvertent damage to these vessels especially during laparoscopic surgery can lead to substantial haematoma formation. The named peritoneal fossae on either side are:

- supravesical – between median and medial umbilical folds
- medial inguinal – between the lateral and medial umbilical folds (site of direct inguinal hernia)
- lateral inguinal – lateral to the lateral umbilical folds (inferior epigastric arteries), includes the deep inguinal ring (site of indirect inguinal hernia).

The iliopubic tract is a condensation of the transversus abdominis fascia overlying the inner surface of the inguinal ligament when viewed from the peritoneal side (laparoscopic surgery) and separates the inferior edge of the deep inguinal ring from the femoral canal and vein below. In the early days of laparoscopic hernia surgery, this region was referred to as the triangle of doom in view of iatrogenic damage to the femoral vessels and nerve when the surgeon dissected or clipped below the iliopubic tract.

Inguinal and femoral canals

Inguinal canal

This is an oblique channel above and parallel to the medial half of the inguinal ligament and averages 4 cm in length. It contains the spermatic cord in the male and the much more tenuous round ligament of the uterus in the female – hence the inguinal canal is intrinsically weaker in the male accounting for the much higher incidence of inguinal hernia. The canal starts at the internal (deep) inguinal ring situated just lateral to the inferior epigastric artery at the midpoint of the inguinal ligament, where the transversalis fascia extends as a cone inside the internal ring and actually forms the internal spermatic fascia (innermost lining of the spermatic cord).

The vas deferens (round ligament in the female) and the testicular vessels enter the inguinal canal at the deep ring and these together with the artery to the vas deferens (derived from the inferior vesical artery), cremasteric artery (from inferior epigastric), genital branch of the genitofemoral nerve, pampiniform plexus, sympathetic fibres and lymphatic vessels form the contents of the spermatic cord. This acquires two further sheaths in its passage down the inguinal canal on its way to the scrotum – the cremasteric fascia (from the internal oblique) and the external spermatic fascia (from the external oblique aponeurosis).

The other important structure in the inguinal canal in both sexes is the ilioinguinal nerve, which lies external to the spermatic cord in the male.

The external or superficial inguinal ring is a slit-like opening in the external oblique aponeurosis situated just above and lateral to the pubic tubercle. Its margins are known as the crura (medial and lateral) and are held together by means of the intercrural fibres. Normally the spermatic cord exits the inguinal canal beneath these intercrural fibres, which are supposed to prevent stretching of the superficial inguinal ring. The anterior wall of the inguinal canal is made up of the aponeurosis of the external oblique; the posterior wall by the transversalis fascia throughout reinforced medially by the fibres of the conjoint tendon.

There is considerable controversy regarding the importance of the transversalis fascia in contributing to the strength of the posterior wall of the inguinal canal, and hence, to the pathogenesis of inguinal hernia, with some regarding it as a crucial factor that must be taken into consideration during fascial repair. Others consid-

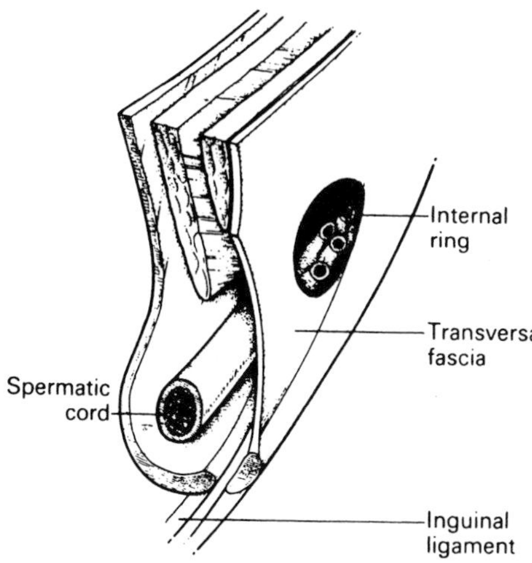

Figure 6.1 The internal view of the deep inguinal ring and cord contents. (Derived from Nyhus, L. M. and London, R. E. eds (1978). *Hernia*, 2nd edn. Philadelphia, PA: Lippincott.)

er that the strength of the posterior wall of the canal is largely dependent on the conjoint tendon. The arching fibres of the internal oblique and transversus abdominis form the roof of the inguinal canal, whereas the floor is made of the grooved inguinal ligament (Figure 6.1). This expands medially to form the lacunar ligament – a crescentic extension from the inguinal ligament to the pectineal line of the pubis that forms the medial margin of the femoral ring/canal.

Femoral canal

The cone-shaped femoral fascial sheath (derived from the endoabdominal fascia) extends into the thigh below the inguinal ligament and has three components from lateral to medial – lateral compartment (femoral artery), intermediate compartment (femoral vein) and medial compartment (femoral canal). The femoral canal itself is funnel shaped with an average length of 1.25 cm and with its oval base (the femoral ring) upwards (facing the abdominal cavity). Below it tapers to the

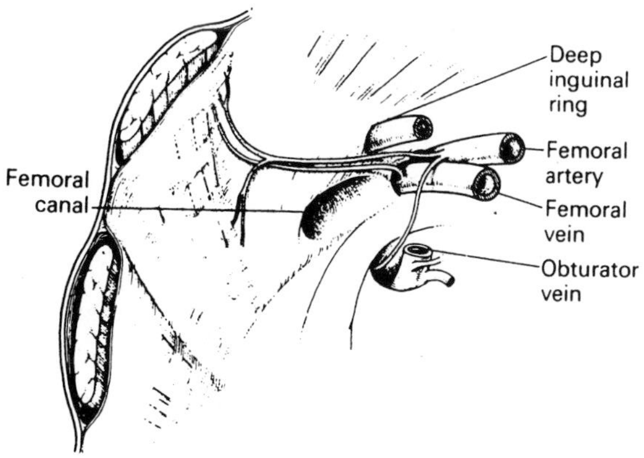

Figure 6.2 The inner aspect of the inguinal region which demonstrates the position of the femoral canal in relation to the femoral vessels and obturator forament. (Derived from Nyhus and London, 1978.)

junction of the long saphenous with femoral vein. The femoral canal normally contains loose connective tissue and a few lymphatics, and sometimes one of the deep inguinal nodes (Figure 6.2).

The boundaries of the femoral ring are the sheath covering the femoral vein laterally, the edge of the lacunar ligament medially, the inguinal ligament anteriorly and the superior pubic ramus and pectineus posteriorly. Normally it is sealed by a condensation of extraperitoneal fatty tissue known as the femoral septum, which is covered superiorly by peritoneum.

Posterior abdominal wall and retroperitoneum

From both anatomical and functional aspects, this is best considered from its ventral aspect. In the midline are the bodies, transverse processes and the intervertebral discs of the five lumbar vertebrae. Laterally the musculo-aponeurotic wall (external and internal oblique and transversus abdominis muscles) extends from the twelfth rib to the pelvic brim. The psoas muscles take origin from the bodies and transverse processes of the upper four lumbar vertebrae and are joined by the iliacus muscles on their lateral aspect. Posteriorly and laterally, the quadratus lumborum muscles form the remaining support for the lumbar nerves and vessels (Figure 6.3). The lower part of the posterior abdominal wall is made up of the iliacus muscles covering the iliac bones of the bony pelvis. The complex anatomy of the posterior abdominal wall is of great importance during surgery on retroperitoneal organs and retroperitoneal tumours. In this respect, the muscles of the posterior abdominal wall are covered by the endoabdominal fascia that is given various names depending on the underlying muscles:

- Psoas fascia or sheath covering the psoas major muscles – attached medially to the lumbar vertebrae and below to the pelvic brim.
- Quadratus lumborum fascia – attached to the transverse processes of the lumbar vertebrae and continuous laterally with the anterior layer of the thoracolumbar fascia.
- Thoracolumbar fascia – splits to enclose the deep muscles of the back and is thick and strong in the lumbar region where it extends from the costal margin to iliac crests and is attached laterally to the internal oblique and transversus abdominis muscles (Figure 6.4).

The retroperitoneal space is bounded above by the diaphragm and below by the pelvic brim but is of course continuous with the retroperitoneal space of the pelvis. The space contains the aorta, vena cava, cysterna chylii, para-aortic glands and vessels, the kidneys and ureters, the adrenal glands, the second and third parts of the duodenum, the lower end of the bile duct, pancreas, the various nerve plexuses and the lumbar sympathetic chain.

The somatic nerves of the posterior abdominal wall are:

- subcostal nerves
- lumbar nerves
- lumbar plexus – located in the posterior part of the psoas major (L1–L4).

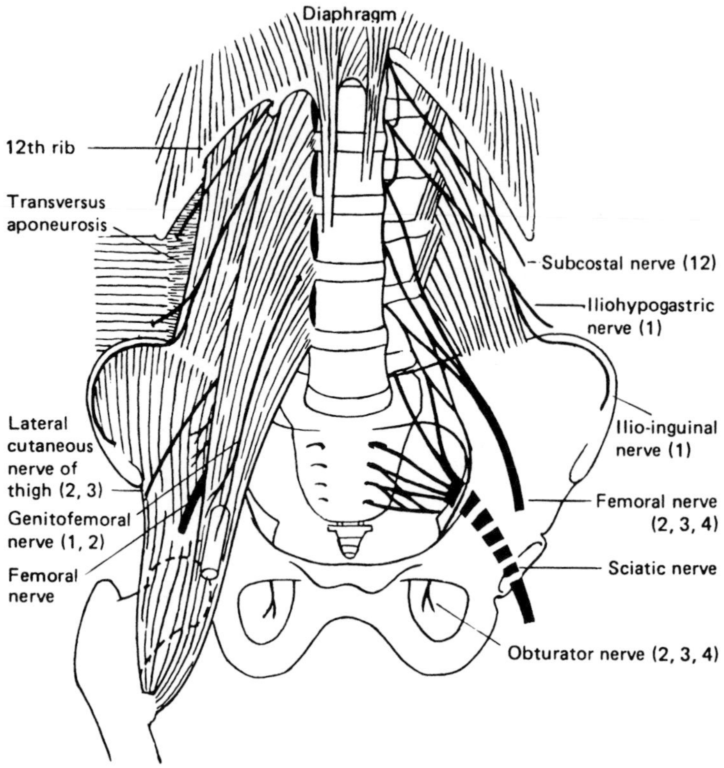

Figure 6.3 The anatomical freatures of the posterior abdominal wall.

In turn, the lumbar plexus gives rise to the following nerves (on either side):

- *Obturator* nerve (L2–L4) exits from the medial border of the psoas and descends medially through the pelvis to reach the thigh where it supplies the adductor muscles
- *Femoral* nerve (L2–L4) – exits from the lateral border of the psoas major, supplies the iliacus and then exits the abdomen deep to the inguinal ligament lateral to the femoral artery. Supplies hip flexor muscles and knee extensors
- *Lumbosacral trunk* – crosses the sacral wing to enter the pelvis to form the sacral plexus together with S1–S4 nerves
- *Genitofemoral* nerve (L1, L2) – exits from the anterior surface of the psoas major but stays deep to the psoas fascia and lower down (lateral to common iliac arteries) it divides into its femoral and genital branches
- *Ilioinguinal* and *iliohypogastric* nerves (both from L1) – descend in front of the quadratus lumborum, penetrate the transversus abdominis near the anterior superior iliac spine and then travel through the internal and external oblique muscles (to which they give branches) to the skin of the groin and pubic region. Only the ilioinguinal nerve courses through the inguinal canal on its way to the skin.
- *Lateral femoral cutaneous* nerve (L2, L3) – runs downwards and laterally across the iliacus muscle and exits the abdomen below the inguinal ligament and close to the anterior superior iliac spine. It supplies skin of the anterolateral aspect of the thigh.

The autonomic nerves consist of:

- vagal branches
- abdominopelvic splanchnic nerves – thoracic (T5–T12) and lumbar (L1–L3)
- pre-vertebral sympathetic ganglia
- abdominal autonomic plexuses.

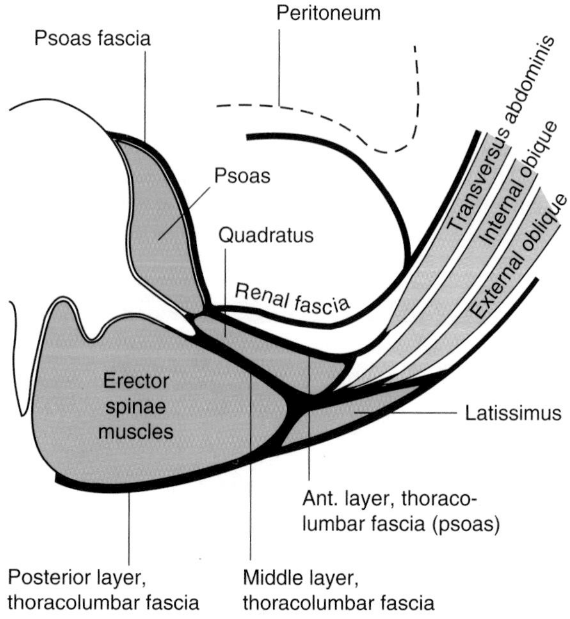

Figure 6.4 Thoracolumbar fascia. This splits to enclose the deep muscles of the back and is thick and strong in the lumbar region where it extends from the costal margin to iliac crests and is attached laterally to the internal oblique and transversus abdominis muscles.

The lumbar splanchnic nerves (thee to four in number) enter three nerve plexuses (intermesenteric, inferior mesenteric and superior hypogastric) which supply pre-synaptic fibres to the pre-vertebral ganglia and plexuses, situated close to the major branches of the aorta (coeliac, superior mesenteric, aortorenal and inferior mesenteric). The post-synaptic fibres from these pre-vertebral ganglia form peri-arterial plexuses that supply the various organs.

The parasympathetic supply to the various plexuses is derived from the vagi and the pelvic splanchnic nerves, which originate directly from the ventral rami of S2–S4. The location of the abdominal nerve plexuses is as follows:

- *Coeliac* (solar) – surrounds the coeliac trunk.
- *Superior mesenteric* – around the origin of the superior mesenteric artery.
- *Inferior mesenteric* – surrounds the corresponding artery as it arises from lower aorta.
- *Intermesenteric* – plexus on the anterior surface of the aorta between the superior and inferior mesenteric arteries.
- *Superior hypogastric* – continuous with the intermesenteric and inferior mesenteric plexi and located over the bifurcation of the aorta. It gives rise to the *hypogastric nerves/plexi,* which continue towards the pelvic floor lateral to the rectum, urinary bladder and uterine cervix. These nerves/plexuses must be preserved in males during rectal and prostatic pelvic surgery because they are responsible through their parasympathetic fibres (S2–S4) for erection and ejaculation.

Trauma to the space from blunt or penetrating injury is common, particularly in high-speed vehicle accidents. Damage to the contained structures leads to haemorrhage and haematoma formation **[Trauma module, Vols I and II]**. Haemorrhage into the retroperitoneal space may also occur spontaneously from leaking abdominal aneurysm, and in patients with bleeding disorders and those taking anticoagulants.

Pelvic floor

This is largely made of the levator ani muscle which slopes downwards from the lateral pelvic walls, pubic bones, ischial spines and coccygeus towards the centre of the pelvis. Together with the coccygeus muscles posteriorly, the levator ani muscle forms the pelvic diaphragm through the centre of which pass the rectum and urethra in both sexes, separated by the vagina in the female. The levator ani which has a separate nerve supply (S3, S4) has three components – the pubococcygeus (stretching from the pubis to the coccyx, the puborectalis which forms a sling around the anorectal junction and the ileococcygeus which forms the posterior part. Aside from forming the floor of the pelvis and providing support for the rectum, bladder and uterus, the levator ani plays an important part in the voluntary control of micturition and defecation.

The pelvic diaphragm is covered by fascia on both its upper and lower surfaces. The ischiorectal fossa is the space between the sloping inferior surface of the pelvic diaphragm and the ischial tuberosity. It is normally packed by fatty tissue and is traversed by the inferior rectal vessels (Figure 6.5). The important nerves associated with the pelvic floor are the pelvic splanchnic (S2–S4), nerves to the levator ani and coccygeus muscles and the pudendal nerve. The pudendal nerve (S2–S4) exits the pelvis through the greater sciatic foramen to enter the pudendal canal on the medial side of the ischial tuberosity. Although it is the chief sensory nerve to the external genitalia in both sexes, it supplies muscular branches to the external anal and urethral sphincters and to the perineal muscles.

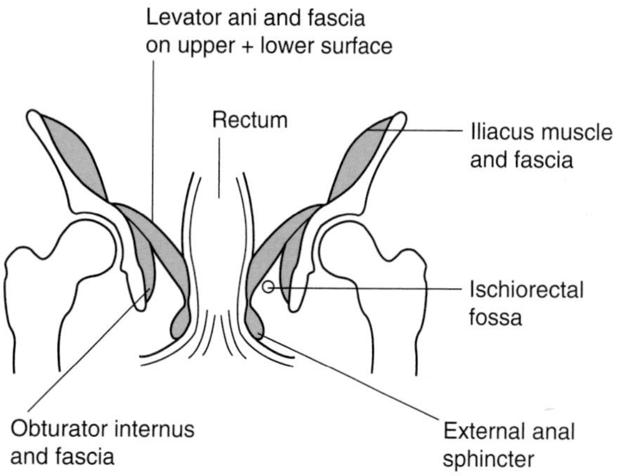

Figure 6.5 The pelvic diaphragm is covered by fascia on both its upper and lower surfaces. The ischiorectal fossa is the space between the sloping inferior surface of the pelvic diaphragm and the ischial tuberosity. It is normally packed by fatty tissue and is traversed by the inferior rectal vessels.

Section 6.2 • The umbilicus

The umbilicus normally lies in the plane of the disc between the third and fourth lumbar vertebrae although clearly this varies with sex, age and degree of obesity. When examined from the deep surface, four fibrous cords are seen radiating from it, and these represent structures which in fetal life traverse the umbilical cord: the umbilical vein, right and left umbilical arteries and the urachus. The additional structure to pass through the cord in embryonic development is the vitello-intestinal duct with the accompanying vitelline veins. Not surprisingly, subclinical defects in the umbilical cicatrix are common and these give rise to paraumbilical hernias usually in obese females.

Omphalitis

Infection of the umbilicus is fortunately a rare complication of the neonate. Faulty technique in dealing with the umbilical cord at birth leads to infection by *Staphylococcus aureus* or haemolytic streptococcal organisms with local suppuration and cellulitis of the adjacent abdominal wall. Treatment with appropriate antibiotics and local drainage is essential for bacteraemia is common. There is an association between umbilical sepsis and portal vein thrombosis with the development of portal hypertension in these children.

In the adult, infection of the umbilicus is a more chronic condition with a seropurulent, often foul smelling, discharge and the development of granulation tissue. In the majority of patients, the fault lies in a lack of hygiene but occasionally small foreign bodies are present and these include 'umbilical stone', a concretion due to desquamated dead superficial epidermal cells. Pilonidal cysts can also occur, albeit rarely in the umbilical pit.

Congenital abnormalities

Patent urachal remnant

A persistent discharge of urine from the umbilicus results from a completely patent urachus. This complication may be delayed into childhood or early adult life, but in these circumstances, there is almost always an underlying urinary obstruction that has forced open the near-obliterated urachal remnant. It is important that prior to excision of the urachal remnant, the bladder should be shown to be free from any form of obstruction, e.g. posterior urethral valves.

Two other urachal abnormalities may be delayed into adult life: urachal sinus and urachal cysts. In the former, an intermittent umbilical discharge is the prominent symptom, and in the latter, the development of a very tender infected swelling in an infra-umbilical position leads to exploration and demonstration of an infected urachal cyst. In both instances excision is indicated but repair of the bladder is not usually required.

Vitello-intestinal duct remnant

The persistence of this remnant may show as a faecal fistula at the umbilicus, a bud or polyp of intestinal mucosa at the umbilicus, a cyst lying deep to the umbilicus between the abdominal wall and the ileum, a deep umbilical sinus, or a Meckel's diverticulum with or without a fibrous band attached to the posterior aspect of the umbilicus and responsible for intestinal obstruction by volvulus or band obstruction (Figure 6.6).

The umbilical sinus, polyp or cyst requires excision. The completely patent vitello-intestinal duct may be complicated by partial or complete prolapse of the ileum through the umbilicus and requires early correction before this complication occurs. Meckel's diverticulum is discussed elsewhere [**Disorders of the Small Intestine, Vol. II**].

Abdominal wall defects

A failure of the umbilical defect to close leads to the development of omphalocele or an umbilical hernia. Major defects in the development of the abdominal wall are associated with exstrophy of the bladder and other forms of developmental abnormality including intestinal malrotation. The 'prune belly' baby has a gross deficiency of muscular development, and the abdominal contents are covered only with skin, peritoneum and an intervening hypoplastic muscular layer.

Rectus sheath haematoma

This presents acutely usually following surgery but may arise spontaneously when it can be misdiagnosed for a vascular tumour. It is invariably located on one side below the umbilicus. The haematoma develops from rupture of the inferior epigastric vessels (usually artery). In the spontaneous variety, there is usually a history of sudden strain or paroxysm of coughing followed by severe abdominal pain and the development of nausea, anorexia and vomiting. A tender swelling can be felt in the abdominal wall, about 5.0 cm in diameter, though much larger haematomas may be encountered. A mild pyrexia and leucocytosis may occur. The condition is easily confirmed by an ultrasound scan of the abdominal wall (Figure 6.7). Surgical treatment is advisable with evacuation of clot and ligature of the inferior epigastric vessels. There has been a significant increase in the incidence of post-operative rectus sheath haematomas since the advent of laparoscopic surgery. The trauma to the inferior epigastric vessels is caused by blind insertion of ports and is entirely preventable.

Section 6.3 • Disorders of the peritoneum

Primary peritonitis

In surgical practice, peritonitis is usually *secondary* to gastrointestinal perforation/injury/anastomotic dehiscence or a gangrenous/infected hollow visceral organ [**Patients Undergoing Emergency Operations, Vol. I**]. Bacterial peritonitis can however be primary, i.e. develops in the absence of surgery/trauma or any primary intra-abdominal focus of infection. This is usually encountered in patients with chronic disease in whom the term *spontaneous bacterial peritonitis* is used as opposed to the rarer *primary bacterial peritonitis* which is reserved for the disease occurring in previously normal individuals (usually females and children).

A fourth category of peritonitis is recognized – *tertiary peritonitis* (TP). This occurs in intensive care patients and is defined as the persistence or recurrence of intra-abdominal infection following apparently adequate therapy of primary or secondary peritonitis. In one reported series tertiary peritonitis developed in 74% of patients admitted with intra-abdominal infection to a surgical intensive care unit (ICU). Patients who develop TP have a significantly longer ICU stay and more advanced organ dysfunction reflected in higher ICU mortality (64% vs 33%) than patients with uncomplicated secondary peritonitis. The most common infecting organisms in patients with TP are *Enterococcus, Candida, Staphylococcus epidermidis* and *Enterobacter*. The infectious foci are rarely amenable to percutaneous drainage and these patients do not benefit from laparotomy as the infection is diffuse and poorly localized. In common with nosocomial pneumonia in the critically ill patients, TP appears to be more a reflection than a cause of an adverse outcome.

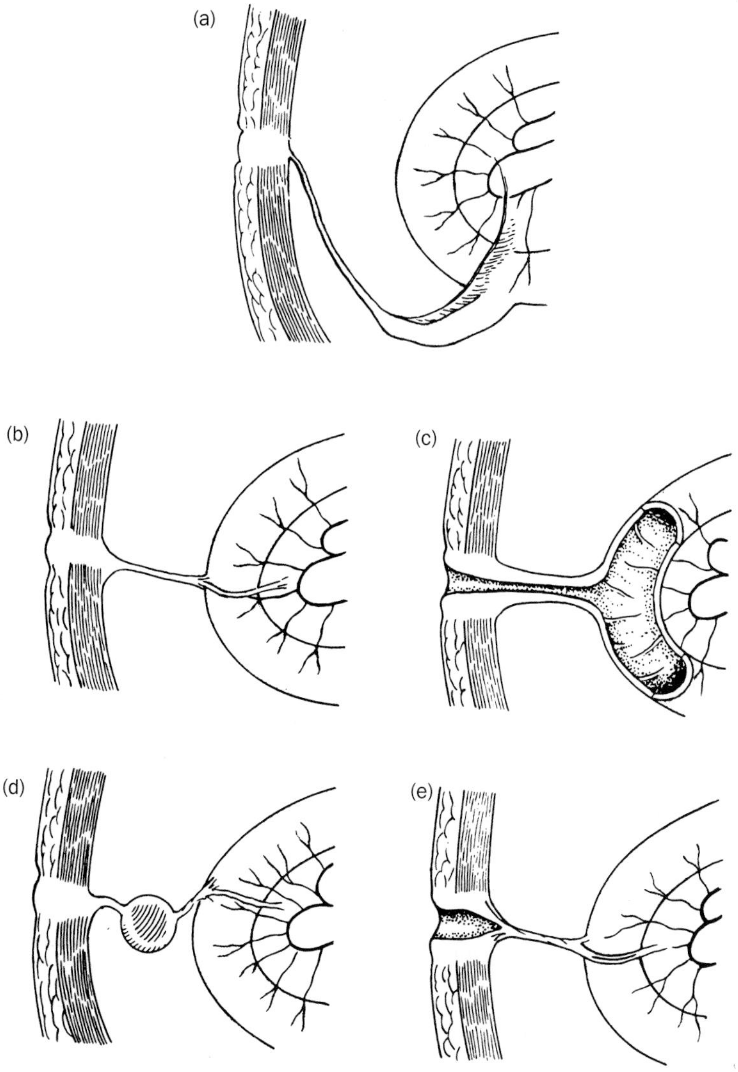

Figure 6.6 The vitello-intestinal duct may connect with the umbilicus as: (a) a fibrous cord extending from a Meckel's diverticulum; (b) a simple fibrous cord to a loop of ileum; (c) an umbilical intestinal fistula; (d) a fibrous cord with cyst; (e) an umbilical sinus.

Primary bacterial peritonitis

By definition, primary bacterial peritonitis occurs in healthy individuals and the infecting organism is of the Gram-positive type, most commonly *Streptococcus pneumoniae* and group A streptococci. The disease is encountered in children, adolescents and adult females in whom it may follow childbirth, chest and urinary tract infection. In most instances, the infection is haematogenous.

Infants and children who develop primary pneumococcal peritonitis usually present with acute abdominal pain, vomiting and fever, and abdominal signs indicative of peritoneal inflammation. Diagnosis is made on clinical grounds helped by abdominal X-rays and ultrasound examination. The blood cultures may be positive in these patients. Treatment is with intravenous antibiotics in the first instance. Awareness of the condition is important as primary peritonitis is a rare condition in children, and thus it will be overlooked unless it is con-

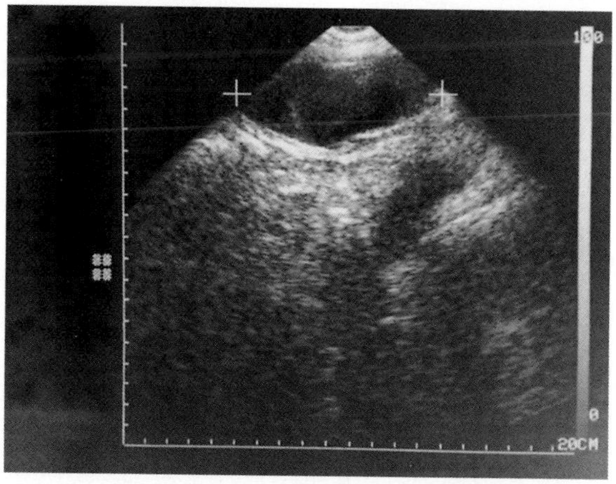

Figure 6.7 Ultrasound of lower abdominal wall of a patient on dicoumarin therapy, who developed severe abdominal pain after a coughing spasm. The area next to the '+' shows a haematoma confined by rectus sheath.

sidered in the differential diagnosis of children presenting with an acute abdomen.

The disease in adults is confined to females, and although the infection is commonly pneumococcal, instances of gonococcal peritonitis have been reported. The typical patients are usually young adolescent girls or women of childbearing age. Some cases are reported in association with acute (non-perforated) appendicitis. Primary peritonitis caused by *S. pneumoniae* may follow childbirth. The patients become pyrexial and develop abdominal pain, diarrhoea and clinical signs of peritonitis. In addition to antibiotic therapy, laparotomy is usually necessary to remove pus and for abdominal lavage. Culture of vaginal swabs is usually positive for pneumococcus in patients who develop the condition after childbirth. The prognosis of primary peritonitis with early diagnosis and treatment (antibiotics and abdominal lavage) is good with recovery of the vast majority of patients.

Management

In many of these patients, the differentiation between primary and secondary bacterial peritonitis is difficult, if not impossible. In practice all are explored surgically and the condition is diagnosed because of the absence of a primary focus, although the surgeon must be aware of the mild (non-perforated) appendicitis associated with a seropurulent peritonitis usually in young females. These are now considered as instances of 'primary peritonitis'. At operation, adequate samples of the peritoneal fluid are taken for culture, the appendix is removed if it appears mildly inflamed and abdominal lavage is undertaken before closure. As the infection is most commonly due to *S. pneumoniae*, the initial antibiotic should consist of augmentin (amoxycillin + clavulanic acid).

Spontaneous bacterial peritonitis

This carries a worse prognosis and has a definite mortality from septic shock and multi-organ system failure. It is an infection of intraperitoneal fluid (ascites or peritoneal dialysate). In general patients with a low ascitic protein concentration (<1.0 g/dl) irrespective of the nature of the underlying disease (liver or renal) are prone to spontaneous bacterial peritonitis (SBP). The groups of patients who are prone to develop SBP include:

- cirrhotic patients with ascites, Wilson's disease, chronic active hepatitis
- renal failure patients on chronic peritoneal dialysis
- patients with the nephrotic syndrome
- immunocompromised patients.

The common factor in these patients is reduced resistance to bacterial infection. The infecting organisms are often Gram-negative.

Clinical features of SBP due to liver and renal disease

About 30% of patients with SBP have no symptoms or signs directly referable to the abdomen, and therefore, a high index of suspicion must be kept especially in susceptible groups. Early diagnosis is imperative, as otherwise the mortality is high, ranging from 50 to 80%. In other patients, the disease develops insidiously and localizing signs of peritonitis are present but often minimal. The most common manifestations include abdominal pain, fever, rebound-tenderness and diminished or absent bowel sounds. The full-blown picture is accompanied by septic shock and is invariably fatal. Once suspected, a 100 ml specimen of ascitic fluid is taken for culture and Gram-staining of the deposit after centrifugation. The fluid is also examined for polymorphonuclear count (PMN) and pH. A PMN count >250 ml and a pH < 7.37 are diagnostic and indicate the need for antibiotic therapy, even if the culture of the ascitic fluid is negative. A blood culture should also be taken and is positive in 70% of cases.

SBP in cirrhotic patients with ascites

In this instance there is bacterial infection of ascitic fluid in the absence of any intra-abdominal, surgically treatable source of infection. The reported incidence of SBP in cirrhotics with ascites varies from 18 to 25%. Most of the infections are aerobic and 50–60% of the reported cases have been caused by *Escherichia coli*. The aetiology is thought to involve:

- bacterial translocation from the gut to mesenteric lymph nodes
- depressed activity of the reticuloendothelial phagocytic system
- decreased antimicrobial capacity of ascitic fluid – low levels of C3, opsonins and fibronectin.

Diagnosis is based on clinical suspicion and analysis of ascitic fluid (white cell count and culture in blood culture bottles). Treatment is with a third-generation cephalosporin. This achieves a cure rate higher than 80%. Cytological cure is obtained in 65% of patients who are culture positive and sensitive to ceftriaxone after 48 hours of treatment and 95% are cured of their infection after 5 days of treatment. Even so many patients (up to 30%) die during the hospitalization despite documented cure of their spontaneous bacterial peritonitis from complications related to their end-stage liver disease (renal failure, gastrointestinal bleed, cerebral oedema). Infection-related mortality does occur, and is related to the onset of bacteraemia (often from *Pseudomonas* spp.).

Prophylactic selective intestinal decontamination with oral norfloxacin is recommended for the prevention of SBP in cirrhotic patients who are at high risk for developing SBP. These include:

- hospitalized cirrhotic patients with gastrointestinal haemorrhage
- patients with low ascitic fluid total protein (≤1 g /dl)
- patients with high bilirubin level and/or low platelet count.

The long-term prognosis of SBP patients is poor, and these patients should be considered for liver transplantation.

SPB in patients on CAPD

As in cirrhotic patients, SPB in patients on chronic peritoneal dialysis (CAPD) can be culture positive or negative. The infection may be caused by either Gram-positive cocci or Gram-negative bacilli. SPB in this patient group can also arise as a consequence of catheter-related infections (subcutaneous tunnel or catheter exit site). The risk factors for catheter exit-site infection documented in a prospective randomized trial by univariate analysis and multiple logistic regression analysis are:

- younger age (<50 years)
- low serum albumin level (<35 g/l)
- number of previously placed PD catheters
- short cuff-exit distance (<2 cm)
- *Staphylococcus aureus* nasal carriage.

The standard primary treatment of CAPD spontaneous bacterial peritonitis is with intraperitoneal netromycin combined with intermittent intraperitoneal vancomycin.

However, in a larger randomized clinical trial, oral levofloxacin in combination with intermittent intraperitoneal vancomycin was found to be equally effective. This regimen is simpler to administer and less costly. It is currently recommended as the primary therapy in centres with relatively low exposure and, thus low background resistance to fluoroquinolones.

The primary cure rate of CAPD spontaneous bacterial peritonitis averages 75% but varies considerably from centre to centre. Higher cure rates are obtained in patients with culture-negative and Gram-positive infections (75–80%) than Gram-negative infections (55%).

SPB in patients with the nephrotic syndrome

Spontaneous bacterial peritonitis associated with the nephrotic syndrome is largely encountered in children, and is rare in adults. The patients usually have active nephrosis and present with diffuse abdominal pain, ascites, fever and rigors. The infection is caused by either Gram-positive or negative pathogens but culture-negative cases have been reported. When it is severe and unresponsive to antibiotic therapy, the patients die of septic shock.

Granulomatous peritonitis

The formation of multiple peritoneal granulomas with the development of ascites may rarely occur as a manifestation of sarcoidosis when differentiation from tuberculous peritonitis can be difficult and is based on a positive Kveim test, negative tuberculosis (TB) cultures and a lack of response to anti-tuberculous therapy.

Starch peritonitis (starch granuloma syndrome) used to be a more common cause of granulomatous peritonitis in surgical practice and caused substantial morbidity. Talc (magnesium silicate) was the initial lubricant for surgical gloves and its implantation during surgery caused severe granuloma formation, chemical peritonitis and adhesion formation. It was replaced by Bio-Sorb in 1949. This is the epichlorohydrinated polymer of cornstarch mixed with 2% magnesium oxide and small amounts of sodium sulfate and sodium chloride. When introduced, it was claimed to be completely absorbed by the peritoneal membrane and was thus free of the disadvantages encountered with talc. Subsequent experience has shown that reactions to Bio-Sorb do occur and include a syndrome of starch peritonitis (starch granuloma syndrome) which has a characteristic and well-recognized clinical picture. The disease starts 2–6 weeks after abdominal surgery with a low-grade fever, anorexia, nausea, vomiting, abdominal distension, cramp-like pain and tenderness. The abdominal distension is due to ileus and to the accumulation of ascitic fluid. Multiple granulomas develop on both the visceral and parietal pneumoperitoneum. The ascitic fluid is usually amber but may be serosanguinous and contains many leucocytes made up largely of lymphocytes and monocytes. The granulomatous nodules consist of collections of lymphocytes, macrophages, polymorphs and eosinophils around starch granules which have a characteristic Maltese-cross appearance on microscopy (Figure 6.8). There is debate concerning the nature of the reaction. Some ascribe its development to a state of hypersensitivity to cornstarch, which can be

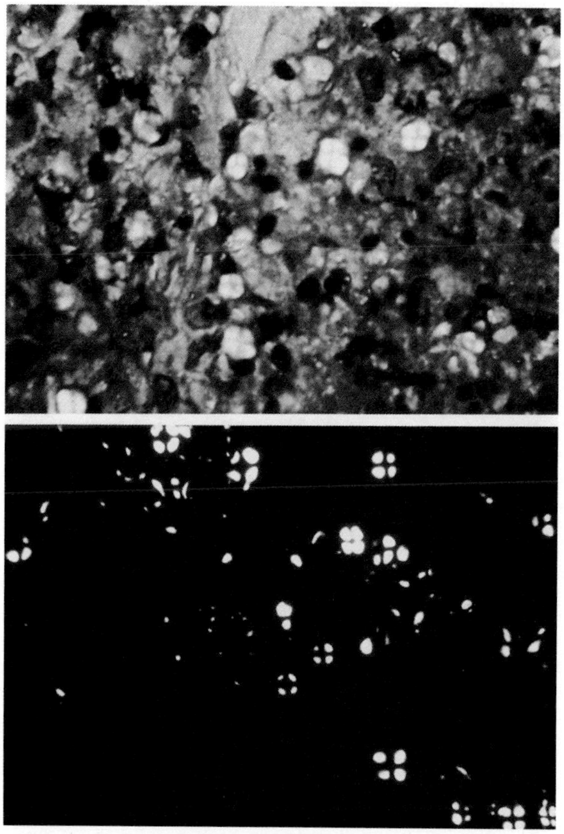

Figure 6.8 Maltese-cross appearance of corn-starch granules visualized with polarized light. (Courtesy of I. Capperauld, Ethicon Laboratories, Edinburgh.)

demonstrated by skin patch testing in patients who develop the condition. Others argue that it represents a foreign body reaction. This is unlikely in view of the rare occurrence. The diagnosis is made on the clinical picture together with the demonstration of starch granules in the ascitic fluid obtained by an abdominal tap (iodine staining and polarized light microscopy). Surgery is avoided if the diagnosis is certain and treatment is conservative. Rapid resolution is seen with systemic corticosteroid therapy. The complications of starch peritonitis include sinus and fistula formation, adhesion formation and intestinal obstruction.

Bio-Sorb is seldom used in gloves nowadays, but if it is, the following measure is advisable. After the gloves have been put on by the surgeon, 10 ml of povidone iodine (Betadine) is applied and smeared on the surface of the gloves. The black starch-iodine granules are then washed off by pouring 500 ml of sterile water from a container. In most instances, hydrogel polymers are used nowadays as lubricants for surgical gloves.

Meconium peritonitis

Meconium peritonitis is an unusual and not uncommonly fatal form of neonatal peritonitis. It is caused by antenatal extravasation of meconium into the peritoneal cavity and this results in a serious illness characterized by intraperitoneal calcification, dense inflammatory fibrosis with or without giant pseudocyst formation. In the majority of cases, no obvious cause can be found for the meconium peritonitis. In neonates and infants in whom a cause is found at laparotomy, this is either jejunal or ileal atresia and less commonly perforation of the appendix. The most striking and common findings during surgery are gross inflammatory adhesion bands with matted intestinal loops. Giant pseudocysts or intestinal perforation are present in 50–60% of cases. The surgical treatment depends on the exact operative findings in the individual neonate/infant. Some need adhesiolysis alone. Pseudocysts are partially resected and temporary enterostomy should be done for perforated bowel or when resection is needed with no attempt at primary anastomosis.

Non-surgical pneumoperitoneum

The introduction of as little as 10 ml of air into the peritoneal cavity may be demonstrated by erect films of the abdomen and chest in the right subdiaphragmatic region. Intraperitoneal air introduced during laparotomy is rapidly absorbed in infants (within 12 h), often takes longer in older children and adults (38–48 h) but may persist for 3–4 weeks in adults. Studies on operating room air have indicated the presence of deleterious substances including endotoxin. The absorption of this through the serosal surfaces of the exposed bowel and peritoneal membrane has been incriminated, in part, for the post-operative 'stress response' after open surgery.

In surgical practice, pneumoperitoneum detected by an erect abdominal or chest X-ray usually indicates perforation of a hollow viscus and is accompanied by clinical signs of peritoneal irritation indicative of serious intra-abdominal disease necessitating urgent surgical intervention. However, 10% of all cases of pneumoperitoneum are not accompanied by physical abdominal signs or evidence of significant underlying disease. The common causes of this non-surgical pneumoperitoneum are:

- Escape of air from the tracheobronchial tree in patients with chronic obstructive airways disease and in patients on intermittent positive pressure ventilation.
- Free air after laparotomy, abdominal paracentesis and peritoneal dialysis. About 25% of patients still have demonstrable air under the diaphragm after an abdominal operation.
- Sealed subclinical perforation. This may be spontaneous or after gastrointestinal endoscopy including colonoscopy (iatrogenic subclinical perforation).
- Gynaecological causes – tubal insufflation, pelvic examination, douching, etc.
- Pneumatoides cystoides intestinalis.
- Idiopathic – no ascertainable cause.

Pneumoperitoneum can occur after laparoscopic surgery undertaken with CO_2 insufflation but usually clears rapidly within 12 hours due to the rapid absorption of this gas. Complete aspiration of CO_2 after a laparoscopic operation is important for two reasons – less severe immediate post-operative CO_2 narcosis and reduction of shoulder pain the day after surgery.

In all cases, pneumoperitoneum is of significance only in the presence of symptoms and signs of peritoneal irritation. Otherwise a conservative approach is indicated. An overdistended viscus (e.g. hepatic flexure), adventitial gas shadows, subdiaphragmatic extraperitoneal fat and basal pulmonary collapse may produce radiological appearance simulating free air in the peritoneal cavity – *pseudopneumoperitoneum*.

Haemoperitoneum

The presence of blood in the peritoneal cavity is a major feature of trauma to the intraperitoneal and retroperitoneal organs **[Trauma modules, Vols I and II]**. Other causes of haemoperitoneum include bleeding from the puncture site following percutaneous liver biopsy or other related interventions, and after hepatic resections. In both cases, there is the added problem of abnormal coagulation that often precludes spontaneous arrest. Thus active intervention without any delay is needed in these patients.

The bleeding from puncture site(s) following percutaneous interventions may be substantial if a major intrahepatic vessel is damaged. The initial step during the operation is the application of a vascular clamp across the foramen of Winslow (Pringle's manoeuvre). This is left for 10–20 min, after which the clamp is removed and if the bleeding does not recur, the puncture hole is injected with fibrin glue. Recurrence of the bleeding after release of the vascular clamp indicates damage to a major intrahepatic vessel. There are the two options. The traditional one is to expose the damaged vessel by extending the puncture wound after re-application of the vascular clamp to the inflow vessels. This is then suture ligated and the clamp released.

A simpler technique (if equipment and expertise are available) is localized thermal ablation using a radiofrequency (RF) probe. There is a risk in patients with these iatrogenic puncture injuries of the development of an intrahepatic arterio-portal fistula, and for this reason, they should be followed by high-dose computed tomography (CT)-based angiography.

Bleeding after hepatic resection necessitates identification of the bleeding points usually in the cut hepatic parenchyma with individual suture ligation. If there are no obvious bleeding points but generalized ooze, argon beam spray coagulation is the best option. If this does not control the oozing, peri-hepatic gauze packing is indicated. The packs are removed 24–48 hours later.

Haemoperitoneum may arise spontaneously from:

- rupture of hepatic neoplasms
- rupture of splenic and hepatic aneurysms
- severe necrotizing pancreatitis
- peritoneal carcinomatosis.

In clinical practice, haemoperitoneum is seldom a feature of patients with leaking abdominal aneurysm who are admitted alive to hospital as intraperitoneal rupture of the aorta is immediately fatal. The clinical picture of spontaneous haemoperitoneum varies with the underlying cause. When the blood loss is substantive, e.g. rupture of liver tumour or splenic artery aneurysm, the clinical picture is that of severe hypovolaemia and abdominal distension. The hypovolaemia is resistant to volume replacement and the only hope of survival of these patients is immediate surgery with subdiaphragmatic aortic cross-clamping.

In the absence of significant hypovolaemia, the presence of blood in the peritoneal cavity causes some irritation of the peritoneal lining with the development of abdominal signs which, however, vary in intensity and can be marked especially if the haemorrhagic exudate is due to an inflamed organ, e.g. severe pancreatitis, or contains irritant secretions, e.g. bile. Adynamic ileus is invariably present in these cases. The clinical features of bleeding peritoneal carcinomatosis include increase in the ascites and abdominal girth and a hypochromic microcytic anaemia. The diagnosis is confirmed by an abdominal tap. Treatment in these terminally ill patients is entirely supportive.

Tumours of the peritoneum

By far the commonest is secondary peritoneal carcinomatosis usually encountered in patients above the age of 40 years. The most common sites of the primary are stomach, breast, pancreas, colon and ovary. As far as tumours of the pancreas, stomach, colon and ovary are concerned, there is now evidence for a stage when viable tumour cells are shed into the peritoneal cavity, before any visible macroscopic appearance of deposits. This stage is identified by lavage cytology with use of specific immunohistochemical stains. In general, exfoliation of tumour cells occurs when the tumour reaches the serosa. In cancer of the colon, 30% of patients have positive lavage cytology at the time of the resection of the primary. In most instances, positive lavage cytology is accompanied by an unfavourable prognosis.

The only reliable method for detection of peritoneal tumour deposits is by laparoscopy and this is far superior to the standard radiological imaging for establishing the diagnosis. However, the development of a special magnetic resonance imaging (MRI) technique has yielded promising results. This technique involves fat-suppression during gadolinium-enhanced MRI after the administration of dilute oral barium solution. This double-contrast MRI enables the detection of carcinomatosis, and tumours <1 cm in diameter in 75–80% of cases. Established peritoneal deposits lead to the formation a turbid or blood-stained ascites.

There is no curative treatment at this stage and most surgeons would manage these patients entirely palliatively. However because of the favourable results obtained in patients with pseudomyxoma peritonei following cytoreduction surgery (peritonectomy and omentectomy) and intraperitoneal chemotherapy (*vide infra*), this form of therapy has been extended to selected patients with peritoneal metastases secondary to colorectal cancer. The preliminary results have been promising in patients:

- with low-volume, low-grade peritoneal metastases
- with perforated cancers
- in whom definitive surgical cytoreduction is complete.

In these patients hyperthermic intraperitoneal chemotherapy with mitomycin C (35 mg/m^2) results in an actuarial 2 year survival of 59%. Obviously further studies are needed before this treatment is advocated routinely.

Pseudomyxoma peritonei

The term pseudomyxoma peritonei (PMP) is used to describe rare conditions characterized by the intraperitoneal accumulation of mucoid ascites/mucinous plaques involving the peritoneal surfaces that may or may not contain epithelial and other cells. There has been considerable confusion regarding both the pathology and aetiology of PMP in the past but this is now largely resolved. There are two main clinicopathological types of PMP:

- *Disseminated peritoneal adenomucinosis* (DPAM) – benign peritoneal lesions that consist mainly of extracellular mucin containing few benign mucinous epithelial cells without cytological atypia or mitotic activity. An appendiceal mucinous adenoma (cystadenoma) is present in 50–55%. The condition may also complicate mucocele of the appendix.
- *Peritoneal mucinous carcinomatosis* (PMCA) – malignant peritoneal lesions composed of abundant mucinous epithelium with cytological features of carcinoma.

PMCAs are further classified into:

- PMCA consistent with origin from an appendiceal or intestinal mucinous adenocarcinoma, or
- PMCA with features intermediate between DPAM and PMCA or with discordant features despite the presence of at least focal areas of carcinoma in the peritoneal lesions, whether or not the primary site demonstrates an unequivocal carcinoma.

This classification of PMP is important because of its prognostic significance. Thus with treatment, the age-adjusted 5 year survival rate for patients with DPAM exceeds 80%, as opposed to 38% for patients with PMCA with intermediate or discordant features, and 7% for patients with PMCA.

Pathology

There is some debate on the exact aetiology, as PMP has been reported in association with a variety of neoplasms: appendix and ovary, and rarely pancreas, colon and urachus. The immunophenotype (cytokeratin-7 negative; cytokeratin-20 and CEA positive) of the lesions of PMP is indicative of a gastrointestinal origin at least in the vast majority of cases. On very rare occasions, the disease involves the retroperitoneal space either alone or in association with intraperitoneal disease (retroperitoneal PMP). The possibility that some cases of PMP arise from primary transformation of the peritoneal mesothelium into neoplastic mucin-secreting tissue (mucinous metaplasia) has been raised although chromosomal analysis of these tumours does not support this hypothesis. Nonetheless, PMP has to be regarded as a heterogeneous lesion and usually develops from appendiceal (benign or malignant) or ovarian lesions (benign).

PMCA is best considered as a diffuse carcinoma derived from gastrointestinal (usually appendiceal) mucinous cystadenocarcinomas. The cancer cells/mucinous plaques are found at pre-determined sites within the abdomen and pelvis and the primary tumour may be small and inconspicuous. The subdiaphragmatic space on both sides, the greater omentum and the pelvis are the sites of maximum disease. Involvement of the intestine is late. Women often have concomitant ovarian mucinous tumours that suggest primary ovarian neoplasia. However, morphological, immunohistochemical and molecular studies in these cases usually indicate that the ovarian tumours are secondary and the PMCA is of intestinal origin. These observations question the existence of a borderline group of mucinous ovarian tumours as a cause for this condition. Thus ovarian tumours exhibiting borderline features should be included in the benign group and designated as atypical proliferative mucinous tumours. Pulmonary parenchymal metastases although rare have been reported in patients with PMCA.

In contrast, DPAM represents the benign form of the disease. In these patients the peritoneal implants are usually derived from the extrusion of epithelial cells from an adenoma of the appendix. It is thought that the mucin deposition occurs in accordance with fluid flow and gravitational forces within the peritoneal cavity. The small bowel is not usually involved. Instances of DPAM have been reported in association with mucocele of the appendix (obstructive dilatation of the appendiceal lumen due to abnormal accumulation of mucus). Mucocele of the appendix has a characteristic CT appearance consisting of spherical or elongated cystic lesions, attached to the wall of the caecum, and may exhibit mural calcification.

Contrary to early reports, cytological examination of the mucin pool/plaques always reveals cells but these vary in count and type (epithelial cells, mesothelial or mesothelial-like cells, histiocytes and fibroblast-like or spindle cells). The epithelial cells may be columnar with mucinous features and may have benign or malignant cytological features. In general, high epithelial cell counts and cytologically malignant cell types are associated with a poor prognosis.

Clinical features

PMP is a rare condition, being reported in approximately two per 10 000 laparotomies. The majority of patients are middle-aged or older patients. Often the primary tumour is slow growing and rarely metastasizes or invades adjacent viscera. In addition to progressive abdominal distension, the condition may present as an acute abdomen with intestinal obstruction. Instances of presentation with spontaneous external fistula in patients with PMP arising from a mucinous carcinoma of the appendix are recorded.

PMP has also been reported in association with splenic mucinous epithelial cyst. These may present with splenomegaly before the development of the disease, i.e. presenting feature of pseudomyxoma peritonei, or be detected after the diagnosis or with recurrence of PMP.

When suspected, confirmation of the disease is obtained by fat-suppressed, gadolinium-enhanced, breath-hold MRI after administration of dilute oral barium solution. This carries a higher diagnostic yield that non-enhanced MR imaging or CT scanning. The characteristic MRI features include thick wall cysts and septa. Laparoscopy carries the highest diagnostic yield and provides an assessment of the extent of the disease and its pathological type (on biopsy).

Treatment

The treatment is multimodal and consists of:

- aggressive surgical debulking and
- intra-operative or post-operative intraperitoneal chemotherapy or systemic combination chemotherapy.

Surgical treatment (usually by laparotomy) entails aggressive surgical evacuation, and resection of the primary and diseased peritoneum. Removal of the appendix is advocated in all cases even if it does not appear to the site of the primary disease.

Currently most centres favour intraperitoneal chemotherapy with alkylating agents, or 5-fluorouracil (5-FU) and mitomycin C or cisplatin. One report has indicated that hyperthermic (40–42°C) intraperitoneal chemotherapy improves the response rates. Others rely on systemic combination chemotherapy including cisplatin. Radiotherapy is generally regarded as being ineffective in PMP. Long-term survival without recurrence of the disease is well documented in patients with DPAM. By contrast, patients with a high-grade malignant process (PCAM) usually die of the disease inside 8 years, but the generally held view is that treatment (if the condition of the patient permits) is the same. In these malignant cases the debulking can be a difficult and time-consuming operation. Others avoid aggressive therapy in view of the high morbidity rates without prospects for significant improvement in survival. This seems to be an unduly pessimistic view. Good results especially for intermediate PCMAs can be obtained. They depend on early diagnosis and treatment before large volumes of disease and multiple surgical procedures lead to small bowel entrapment by tumour.

There have been reports of the laparoscopic management of pseudomyxoma peritonei secondary to adenocarcinoma of the appendix. This approach permits thorough exploration of the abdomen, irrigation and aspiration of the thick mucinous material and the instillation of mucolytic agents (5% dextrose solution). Appendicectomy or right hemicolectomy is performed with minimal disturbance of the anterior abdominal wall. The intraperitoneal catheters for chemotherapy are placed through the port sites.

Peritoneal mesothelioma

Mesothelioma is a relatively rare malignant neoplasm arising from the serosal lining of the pleural, peritoneal and pericardial cavities. In many countries there has been a rising incidence of the disease since 1950 due to exposure to asbestos predominantly in males. Age-specific incidence rates are highest for the older age groups. There is a long latency period between exposure to diagnosis and this averages 20–30 years. Several studies have shown that these asbestos-related tumours are characterized by balanced chromosomal rearrangements. Asbestos-related mesotheliomas occur most commonly in the pleura, but instances of peritoneal mesotheliomas due to asbestos exposure are well documented and asbestos bodies (mainly amosite) have been documented in the peritoneal cavity, the most common sites being the mesentery and omentum usually in patients with heavy-fibre burdens in lung tissue.

Peritoneal mesotheliomas can develop, albeit rarely, in the absence of exposure to asbestos. Perhaps the most important is malignant mesothelioma after radiation therapy for Hodgkin's disease. In these patients, the mesothelioma arises in the field of prior radiotherapy. There is a rare primary variant that occurs in young females, and instances of mesotheliomas have been reported in patients with familial Mediterranean peritonitis.

Pathology

Malignant mesotheliomas (MMs) are pleural, pericardial or peritoneal neoplasms usually associated with asbestos exposure. Since mesothelial cells are biphasic, they may give rise to epithelial and sarcomatous MMs. In addition, benign 'atypical proliferations of mesothelial cells' may occur. The separation of mesothelial hyperplasia from early malignant mesothelioma can be very difficult on histological examination. These lesions are termed 'atypical mesothelial hyperplasia'. Immunostaining for epithelial membrane antigen (EMA) and the quantitation of silver-stained nucleolar organizer regions (AgNORs) can be useful in differentiating benign from malignant histological sections of pleural and peritoneal biopsies. There have been recent reports of simian virus 40 (SV40) DNA large T antigen (Tag) sequences in both pleural and peritoneal epithelial MMs but not in sarcomatous lesions. MM tends to be a diffuse lesion and when associated with asbestos exposure is classified as an industrial disease. Pathological confirmation of asbestos aetiology is necessary for these patients to obtain compensation.

Benign mesotheliomas (BMs) comprise two macroscopic types: fibrous and multicystic. The fibrous type forms well-encapsulated solid tumours composed of spindle-shaped cells. The multicystic variety has a marked tendency for local recurrence after resection. Both types are associated with long survival after surgical resection.

In females, the histological distinction between epithelial peritoneal mesothelioma and ovarian papillary serous carcinoma diffusely involving the peritoneum may be difficult even with immunohistochemistry and usually requires examination of the ultrastructural features by electron microscopy. To compound a difficult problem further, rare instances of primary mesothelioma in young women have been documented and some of these are associated with highly elevated serum levels of CA-125. This makes the differentiation even more difficult since this is the typical marker for epithelial serous tumours from the ovary.

Clinical features

Currently only 2.2 cases of MMs per million population per year are diagnosed. The incidence of the disease continues to increase because of the long latency period, despite the fact that exposure to asbestos in industry has virtually ceased since 1970. Malignant mesotheliomas are encountered mainly in men. The mean age at first diagnosis of malignant mesotheliomas is about 59 years; females on average are 4 years younger at presentation. The most frequent initial symptoms of MMs include fatigue, abdominal pain, anorexia, marked weight loss and abdominal distension caused by intractable ascites. Clinical presentation as fever of unknown origin is exceptional, but when it occurs, it signifies a very aggressive tumour with a bad prognosis. Both benign and malignant disease may present with an abdominal mass or intestinal obstruction or gastric outlet obstruction. More uncommon presentations include dysphagia secondary to pseudo-achalasia, chronic pancreatitis and regional lymphadenopathy. Overall, the mean survival time ranges from about 3 months to 8 years. Prolonged survival is only encountered with benign mesotheliomas.

The current standard non-invasive imaging modality for staging of malignant mesothelioma is CT. However, CT does not determine resectability. Laparoscopy using a multiport technique with diaphragmatic, peritoneal and abdominal wall biopsies provides more accurate staging. The ascitic fluid is examined for malignant cells.

Treatment
This entails surgical exploration with excision (benign lesions) or tumour debulking followed by intraperitoneal chemotherapy. Details of the intraperitoneal chemotherapy vary. Good results have been reported with continuous hyperthermic peritoneal perfusion (CHPP) with cisplatin-based regimens (CDDP). In phase II studies, this combination results in a median progression-free survival of 26 months, and an overall 2 year survival of 80% (for all mesotheliomas including the multicystic variants). The morbidity is acceptable (24%). Re-treatment after initial response can result in a second long-term response.

Some advocate two-stage peritoneal chemotherapy for patients with primary peritoneal mesothelioma. In stage I, patients undergo cytoreductive surgery and placement of an intraperitoneal infusion catheter, through which intraperitoneal chemotherapy is administered for 4 months. In stage II, a second laparotomy with debulking of residual disease and placement of perfusion intraperitoneal catheters is carried out. High-dose intraperitoneal hyperthermic (40–42°C) chemotherapy using a disposable perfusion circuit is then administered. The reported experience with this two-stage treatment is limited and currently there is no evidence that it gives superior results.

MMs are generally regarded as being unresponsive to systemic chemotherapy. However, dramatic regression of the disease has been reported following systemic chemotherapy with gemcitabine. The activity of gemcitabine in malignant mesothelioma has been confirmed by phase II studies. There is also evidence suggesting better response rates when gemcitabine is combined with cisplatin. Other regimens that have shown activity are based on doxorubicin and cisplatin.

Section 6.4 • Special forms of intestinal obstruction

Post-operative intestinal obstruction

It is often incorrectly assumed that a persistent intestinal obstruction (beyond 3–4 days) after abdominal surgery is due to a protracted adynamic ileus. Whilst there are some specific operations in which this is the case, e.g. intestinal intubation with a Baker's tube or complex remedial reconstructive surgery on the gastrointestinal tract, in the majority of cases in whom the obstruction is delayed a mechanical cause is likely to be present. Early obstruction (during the first 5 days) is usually due to non-strangulating causes, e.g. anastomotic oedema, adhesive fibrinous matting with distension and kinking of the intestinal loops. As the obstruction is often incomplete, active surgical intervention is rarely necessary and the majority settle with conservative management. By contrast later post-operative obstructions (occurring or persisting beyond 7 days of surgery) are usually caused by organized bands or abscesses and may be strangulating in nature. Laparotomy is therefore necessary for these late or prolonged post-operative intestinal obstructions.

Bolus obstruction

Intraluminal bolus obstruction, usually of the small intestine, may be caused by tricho- and phytobezoars, gallstones or a mass of worms (*Ascaris lumbricodes*). The latter is usually encountered in children and is often precipitated by antihelminthic therapy.

Phytobezoars
These are firm masses of undigested fruit or vegetable fibres that can cause gastric or small bowel obstruction. The predisposing factors include:

- the ingestion of large amounts of high-fibre foods
- inadequate mastication
- previous gastric surgery producing hypo- or anacidity and loss of the antral pump mechanism.

Often the phytobezoars that form after gastric surgery consist of orange pith.

Patients with gastric bezoars present with epigastric pain, loss of appetite and weight, and episodes of distension and vomiting. The condition is usually diagnosed at endoscopy. Intestinal bezoars present with mechanical small bowel obstruction. Gastric bezoars are multiple in 17% of cases and intestinal bezoars in 4%.

Gastric bezoars may be treated conservatively by cellulase enzymatic digestion (300 ml of 0.5% cellulase solution instilled 4 hourly via a nasogastric tube for 2 days). Alternatively piecemeal removal may be carried out endoscopically but this may be difficult. Laparotomy is needed for patients presenting with small bowel obstruction. Sometimes it is possible to knead the bolus into the caecum. When this is not successful, the phytobezoar is removed by an enterotomy. Gallstone ileus is discussed elsewhere **[Disorders of the Biliary Tract, Vol. II]**.

Intestinal pseudo-obstruction

The tem 'pseudo-obstruction' is used to describe obstruction of the small or large intestine in the absence of a mechanical cause or acute intra-abdominal disease. The term covers a variety of syndromes which result from damage to the myenteric plexus (neuropathy) or smooth muscle abnormality (myopathy) or both. Small intestinal and colonic pseudo-obstruction are best discussed separately.

Small intestinal pseudo-obstruction
This condition may be primary (idiopathic) or secondary. Familial *hollow visceral myopathy*, which is included in the primary category, is a particularly severe disorder which involves the smooth musculature of the oesophagus, entire gastrointestinal tract including the colon and often the urinary bladder. The secondary variety results from a neuropathy/myopathy induced by certain systemic disorders or drug misuse (excess

phenothiazine administration, laxative abuse). The disorders most commonly associated with the development of secondary small intestinal pseudo-obstruction are:

- diabetes mellitus
- scleroderma
- progressive systemic sclerosis
- acute intermittent porphyria
- hypothyroidism
- Chagas' disease.

It has also been reported as a complication of sclerotherapy for oesophageal varices. When the underlying abnormality is a neuropathy (e.g. diabetes mellitus), the pattern of intestinal motor activity is abnormal with derangements of the myoelectrical migratory complexes (MMCs), absence of any normal activity or disorganized non-propulsive hypermotility. By contrast in myopathic conditions (e.g. hypothyroidism), the pattern or motor activity is normal but the intensity of the contractile activity is reduced.

The clinical picture is that of recurrent episodes of subacute intestinal obstruction with colicky abdominal pain, vomiting and distension. The treatment entails correction of any underlying disorder whenever this is possible (e.g. hypothyroidism). Intestinal prokinetics, e.g. metoclopramide and domperidone or cisapride are sometimes beneficial, especially the last. Cisapride acts by increasing the local concentration of acetylcholine in the intestinal smooth musculature. The synthetic peptide ceruletide which has to be administered intravenously or intramuscularly is also beneficial particularly during acute episodes. Intravenous erythromycin may be effective in some patients. Replacement therapy is necessary in patients with hypothyroidism.

Colonic pseudo-obstruction

Two types are recognized: acute and chronic. The acute condition was first described by Ogilvie in 1948 and is sometimes referred to as Ogilvie's syndrome. It consists of a selective dilatation of the caecum and proximal colon with a sharp cut-off usually at the splenic flexure, and less frequently the hepatic flexure and sigmoid, suggestive of mechanical obstruction. It is best considered as a localized form of adynamic ileus, which usually develops in patients with major pre-existing, non-intestinal conditions requiring hospitalization, e.g. major surgery, severe trauma, sepsis, myocardial infarction, severe renal and respiratory disease. The aetiology remains unknown although administration of drugs that impair colonic motility and air swallowing are thought to be contributory factors. The defect appears to be in the smooth muscle or in one of the intestinal control mechanisms, and slow wave activity (electrical control activity) has been reported to be absent in these patients.

The clinical picture is dominated by abdominal distension often without vomiting. The patient complains of increasing discomfort and may develop cramp-like abdominal pain. Radiography shows features of colonic obstruction with caecal distension (7.5–22.0 cm). Caecal perforation is a well-recognized complication and is likely to occur if the radiological size of the caecum exceeds 12 cm.

The standard treatment is by colonoscopic decompression which is successful in the majority of patients. Recurrence of the condition is encountered in 20% of patients. These are treated by further colonoscopy when a Baker's intestinal tube is inserted transanally into the caecum, or the colonoscope left *in situ* for 2 hours, thereby maintaining decompression. Surgical intervention with tube caecostomy is undertaken when colonoscopic treatment fails.

Chronic colonic pseudo-obstruction may be primary or secondary. They latter may result from a motility disorder, diabetes mellitus, hypothyroidism, malignancy, psychosis or drug and laxative abuse. This is covered elsewhere **[Disorders of the Colon and Rectum, Vol. II]**.

Intussusception

Intussusception is a telescoping of a segment of intestine into an adjacent one (Figure 6.9). The condition is encountered most commonly in childhood with a peak incidence at 4 months. Intussusception may, however, be encountered in the adult, in which case a precipitating lesion that initiates the intussusception (the lead point) is usually present, e.g. intestinal polyp or submucous lipoma. By contrast, in infants and children some 70–95% are classed as idiopathic (no lead point) and an associated illness, such as urinary tract infection or gastroenteritis, is encountered in 30%. It is often assumed that hyperplasia of the lymphoid patches in the terminal ileum secondary to common disease in infancy may be involved in the initiation of idiopathic intussusception in this age group. A definite seasonal incidence is observed in infants and children with clear peaks in the spring and summer. This is suggestive of viral infections being the cause of the intestinal lymphoid hyperplasia.

Intussusception is anatomically defined as ileo-ileal, ileo-caecal and ileo-colic depending on the site and extent of the telescoping observed by the time of diagnosis. The condition is a strangulating type of intestinal obstruction and if treatment is delayed, ischaemic necrosis of the involved bowel segments and peritonitis are inevitable.

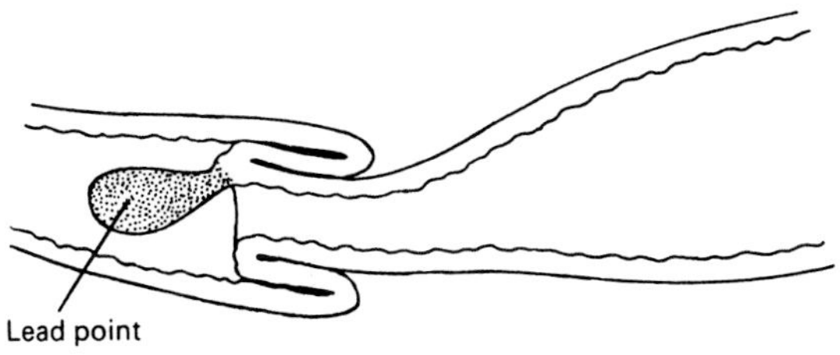

Figure 6.9 Components of an intussusception.

The clinical features include the sudden onset of vomiting, cramp-like abdominal pain and rectal bleeding. An abdominal mass is palpable in 55–60% of cases. Children with intussusception associated with a lead point (Meckel's diverticulum, polyp, duplication, Henoch–Schönlein purpura, suture line, appendix, tumour) are usually older than the idiopathic cases.

In the absence of peritonitis and intestinal obstruction, the initial treatment is by hydrostatic barium enema, which is successful in 50% and is followed by a recurrence rate of 6%. Intussusception caused by a lead point is not likely to reduce with a hydrostatic barium enema and usually requires surgical intervention. Operative treatment is necessary when the hydrostatic reduction is incomplete, uncertain or contraindicated (peritonitis, intestinal obstruction). Operative reduction is usually possible, although the viability of the bowel may be compromised after reduction and resection therefore necessary. In adults, it has to be assumed that a lead point is present and its nature determined by subsequent investigations after recovery, unless of course the lesion is palpable through the bowel wall after reduction.

Volvulus

Volvulus is a twist or rotation of a loop of intestine about its mesenteric attachments. It is therefore a sudden obstruction of the closed loop variety if the rotation is complete (360°) and ischaemia or total vascular occlusion may be present by the time of diagnosis.

The condition may involve the stomach **[Disorders of the Stomach, Vol. II]**, small and large intestine. Two intestinal varieties are described: primary and secondary. Primary volvulus results from malrotation of the gut or congenital excessive mobility from loose fixation or long mesenteric attachments (volvulus of the midgut in the neonate). The more common secondary volvulus is due to rotation of a loop of small intestine around an adhesions/band, an ileostomy or colostomy. Caecal and sigmoid volvulus are considered elsewhere **[Disorders of the Colon and Rectum, Vol. II]**.

Section 6.5 • Intraperitoneal adhesions

Adhesions following abdominal and pelvic surgery are important in view of their morbidity and frequent hospital re-admissions. They occur after elective surgery and following peritonitis from any cause. The morbidity spectrum of intraperitoneal adhesions includes:

- chronic pain
- acute and subacute intestinal obstruction
- secondary female infertility
- increased operating time for subsequent operations
- risk (20%) of iatrogenic bowel injuries during subsequent operations.

Pathology of adhesions

The causes of intraperitoneal adhesions are:

- open abdominal or pelvic surgery
- individual susceptibility
- ischaemic areas – anastomotic sites, reperitonealization of raw areas
- foreign bodies – talc, starch granules, gauze lint, cellulose, etc.
- peritonitis from any cause
- inflammatory bowel disease – Crohn's disease
- radiation enteritis
- sclerosing peritonitis – usually drug induced, e.g. certain beta-blockers.

The most common category is post-operative adhesions. There is undoubtedly an individual susceptibility as some patients are prone to adhesions and others not, even after major operations but the genetics and molecular biological basis for this predisposition to adhesion formation are not known. Talc is no longer a problem. Surgical gloves either incorporate a hydrogel polymer or are powdered with epichlorohydrinated cornstarch. Gauze lint is still important and there is evidence that it is responsible for 25% of cases of intraperitoneal granuloma formation caused by implanted foreign bodies. There is some evidence that some post-operative adhesions develop on a background of ischaemia in the region of surgically constructed anastomoses and following attempts at reperitonealization of raw areas. These should be left unsutured when they are rapidly filled with an inflammatory exudate and thereafter covered by a new serosa derived from free-floating peritoneal macrophages.

The exact pathogenesis of intra-abdominal adhesions is not fully understood but trauma and exposure of the peritoneum and the subsequent biochemical and cellular response to repair this injury are involved. Fibrin deposition is the initiating step as this is essential for mesothelial repair. Normally there is a fine balance between resurfacing of denuded areas by mesothelial cells and fibrinolysis that removes the initial fibrin structural framework. Disturbance of this fine balance between mesothelial repair and fibrinolysis by ischaemia and other factors is thought to be responsible for adhesion formation after abdominal surgery. As the fibrinolytic activity is compromised, the fibrin matrix persists, becomes invaded by fibroblasts and gradually matures into fibrous bands usually within 5–7 days. Adhesions may be parietal (between viscera and abdominal walls and diaphragm) or visceral (between bowel loops and solid organs). Usually both are present in the individual case.

Another factor that is thought to be important in the development of adhesions is disruption of the naturally occurring surface active phospholipid (SAPL) barrier, which normally keeps the peritoneal membrane lubricated and separates the visceral from the parietal peritoneum. The component lipids of this SAPL barrier, which protects other surfaces such as the alveolar membrane, are dipalmitoylphosphatidylcholine (DPPC) and unsaturated phosphatidylglycerol (PG). Three-dimensional studies of the molecular configuration have shown that SAPL barrier is composed of multiple layers (lamellar bodies). The efficacy of SAPL lamellar bodies is due to their ability to bind to the mesothelial epithelium within the microvilli to form molecular structures that keep the surface well lubricated and de-wetted. The protective and lubricating properties of SAPL barrier are compromised during surgery and may account for the development of adhesions.

There is no established classification of adhesions. They can be filmy, dense or string-like, and of variable spread within the peritoneal cavity but are usually centered on the operative site and the parietal access wound. From the symptomatic and pathological viewpoint, parietal adhesions (those binding the intra-abdominal contents) to the parieties are more important than inter-loop/visceral adhesions.

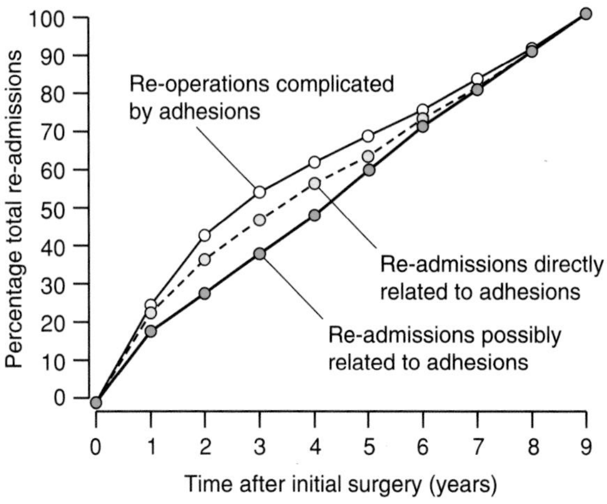

Figure 6.10 Adhesion-related hospital re-admissions after abdominal and pelvic surgery: a retrospective cohort study. (Reproduced by kind permission from Ellis, H. *et al.* (1999). Adhesion-related hospital readmissions after abdominal and pelvic surgery: a retrospective cohort study, *Lancet* **353**: 1476–800.)

Adhesions after elective surgery

Although estimates of the incidence of adhesions vary (40–97%), all the reports indicate that the problem is substantial and results in both a significant morbidity and major added health care costs. In the USA over 400 000 operations were performed for lysis of adhesions in 1993 and the total costs for treating patients with complications and symptoms caused by adhesions has been estimated at $1.2 billion annually. In one retrospective cohort study based on validated data of patients undergoing open abdominal or pelvic surgery (29 760) from the Scottish National Health Service database in 1986, followed up for 10 years, 34.6% were re-admitted a mean of 2.1 times during the study period 'for a disorder directly or possibly related to adhesions, or for abdominal or pelvic surgery that could be potentially complicated by adhesions'. Six per cent of all re-admission during the study period were directly due to adhesions and the majority of these (97%) required an operation during the re-admission. Most of the adhesion-related events are encountered during the first year after surgery (22% of all operative adhesiolysis performed in the first 12 months) but the incidence of adhesion-related morbidity and re-admissions did not decline during the 10 year period (Figure 6.10).

Complications of adhesions requiring re-admission to hospital are much more frequent after surgery on the small bowel and colon than after pelvic gynaecological surgery involving the female reproductive organs. Small bowel obstruction developed in 25% of patients after total colectomy with ileo-anal pouch reconstruction in one large reported series of 1005 patients. Approximately 70% of all hospital admission for small bowel obstruction are due to adhesions.

Clinical features

Patients with intraperitoneal adhesions may develop chronic symptoms or present acutely with intestinal obstruction.

Chronic adhesion syndromes

The most common is abdominal pain with or without nausea in the absence of abdominal signs, except perhaps minimal tenderness. The pain distribution is variable and is not necessarily beneath the abdominal wall scar. These are the most difficult patients to evaluate and usually undergo a series of investigations, often repeated before coming either to laparotomy or laparoscopy. The outcome in terms of pain relief after adhesiolysis is uncertain; some patients obtain pain relief (possibly a placebo effect) but usually the pain recurs. In other patients the pain is episodic and colicky in nature, accompanied by nausea, audible excessive bowel sounds and abdominal distension lasting for variable periods. These attacks terminate in diarrhoea, which relieves both the pain and the abdominal distension. In these patients the symptoms are due to recurrent attacks of subacute small bowel obstruction and indeed, these patients may develop acute obstruction at any time. These patients often lose weight from malabsorption due to bacterial overgrowth. This group undoubtedly benefits from surgery (*vide infra*).

Acute adhesive intestinal obstruction

This is the most common reason for emergency admission/re-admission to hospital. The obstruction is almost always in the small bowel although the level of obstruction varies. Colonic obstruction due to adhesions is rare and other causes should be considered. The severity of vomiting and the extent of abdominal distention vary with the level of the obstruction. The condition is readily diagnosed by the clinical symptoms and signs and abdominal plain films (erect and supine). The possibility of strangulation should be suspected if the pain is constant, there is obvious tenderness on palpation and a marked leucocytosis. Early recourse to surgical intervention may prevent infarction of the intestine.

Treatment of adhesion-related complications

Prophylactic

In the first instance good surgical technique is important. In this context, the specific points include:

- delicate handling of tissues and organs
- avoidance of spillage of visceral contents during surgery
- minimizing operative blood loss
- protection of exposed viscera from drying
- avoidance of closure of parietal peritoneal defects – this induces ischaemia at the suture line
- washing the operative region and peritoneal cavity with isotonic saline at the end of the operation.

There is good evidence that laparoscopic surgery is followed by a significantly reduced incidence of postoperative adhesions and this effect is probably related to maintenance of the 'milieu interier' of the coelomic cavity during the operation, although other factors may be involved.

Even with the best operative techniques, elective surgery on the small intestine and colon and emergency surgery for acute peritonitis is a significant risk factor and there is an increasing argument for specific prophylaxis after these operations. A variety of drugs (anticoagulants, dextrans of various molecular sizes, antihistamines, non-steroidal anti-inflammatory drugs (NSAIDs), povidone, streptokinase etc.) have been investigated as anti-adhesion agents but none have been shown to be effective as chemoprophylactic agents against adhesion formation.

There is to date only one proven prophylactic treatment that should be considered in these patients. This consists of a bio-resorbable membrane based on sodium hyaluronate (Seprafilm) which is placed on the front of the intestinal loops/greater omentum separating them from the parietal wound. The use of this membrane has been shown to be entirely safe (no detectable adverse effects) and in a prospective randomized trial of patients undergoing colectomy and ileal pouch anal anastomosis significantly reduced the incidence of adhesions (15 vs 58%).

Based on the role of SAPL barrier in peritoneal lubrication and its disruption by open surgery, a synthetic mixture of surface-active phospholipids (DPPC and PG – proprietary name ALEC) has been used in experimental studies and shown to reduce adhesions by 70%. The product is available in powder form (identical to surfactant used in neonatal respiratory problems) and is jet sprinkled into the peritoneal cavity at the end of the procedure. Clinical studies are ongoing in patients undergoing emergency colonic operations with ALEC but to date there are no published results.

Another anti-adhesion agent of interest is a 4% icodextrin solution (ADEPT) used extensively in peritoneal dialysis. As these patients do not form peritoneal adhesions, icodextrin has been studied experimentally and in one clinical trial against Ringer's solution in gynaecological laparoscopic surgery. In both instances it reduced the incidence, severity and extent of adhesions. However, its efficacy in general surgical practice remains unproven. It has several advantages. These include proven non-toxicity, low cost and ease of administration, i.e. one litre of the solution is instilled in the peritoneal cavity at the end of the operation. Icodextrin solution is contraindicated in patients with known allergy to starch-based polymers and in patients with maltose or isomaltose intolerance.

Treatment of patients with symptomatic/complicated adhesions

Patients with chronic symptoms

The patients with a clinical picture of subacute small bowel obstruction should undergo surgical adhesiolysis. This may be undertaken by the open approach or laparoscopically depending on local expertise. Following adhesiolysis, insertion of Seprafilm between the contents and the parieties is advocated. The insertion of Seprafilm may prove difficult if the operation is conducted by the laparoscopic approach. The decision for adhesiolysis is difficult in patients with chronic symptoms in the absence of definitive abdominal signs. If the surgeon decides to intervene, the laparoscopic approach is preferable to the open approach in these patients, as the likelihood is that the symptoms will recur after a variable period and the patient will then be insistent on further surgery. The author had a patient referred for remedial surgery to reconstruct the abdominal wall who by the age of 49 years had had 38 operations. The alternative to Seprafilm is ADEPT solution, particularly if the operation is conducted laparoscopically.

Patient with acute small bowel obstruction

In the absence of signs and symptoms of strangulation, these patients are managed conservatively with nasogastric decompression and fluid and electrolyte replacement in the first instance. This conservative management is usually successful but if there is no improvement within 12–24 hours of admission, emergency laparotomy and adhesiolysis is undertaken. These operations should be performed under prophylactic antibiotic cover, and if for any reason the bowel is injured during the operation or resection of an intestinal segment is performed, a full 5 day antibiotic course to cover Gram-negative organisms (anaerobes and aerobes) is necessary. The laparoscopic approach is used by some surgeons in these patients but is technically difficult in view of the distended oedematous intestinal loops and may carry a higher risk of iatrogenic bowel injury than the open conventional approach. In some instances, because of dense adhesions, the bowel may be injured during the mobilization. Inadvertent enterotomy during adhesiolysis occurs in 15–20% and increases the post-operative morbidity and urgent re-laparotomy rate. These patients are also more likely to require intensive care support and parenteral nutrition and have significantly longer post-operative stay in hospital. The risk factors for inadvertent enterotomy during adhesiolysis are:

- obesity
- three or more previous laparotomies
- adhesiolysis in lower abdomen and pelvis
- old age.

If the inadvertent enterotomy is ragged and extensive, it is better to resect this injured segment, otherwise it is oversewn. The insertion of Seprafilm between the intestinal loops/omentum and the parietal wound is advisable in all patients undergoing adhesiolysis for intestinal obstruction (irrespective of iatrogenic bowel injury). Patients with features of strangulating obstruction at or soon after admission (especially those with constant pain and marked leucocytosis) require immediate surgery following resuscitation.

Patients with recurrent episodes of small bowel obstruction

The patients pose real problems in surgical management, as the relative efficacy of the various surgical operations used for this condition has never been adequately assessed by prospective randomized studies. The operations available include:

- adhesiolysis alone
- adhesiolysis with Seprafilm
- Noble intestinal plication
- Child–Phillips plication
- Baker intestinal intubation.

To date there is no evidence of any clear superiority of one procedure and there are no data on the efficacy of Seprafilm in reducing the obstructive episodes after adhesiolysis but this seems a sensible addition to adhesiolysis especially as its use does not incur any adverse effects.

The Noble intestinal plication (Figure 6.11) involves suturing the small intestinal loops with serosal sutures so that the small bowel coils become fixed in gentle curves when adhesions re-form. The procedure is rarely performed nowadays because it is time consuming and carries an appreciable morbidity (perforation, fistula, peritonitis). Furthermore patients complain of chronic abdominal pain and remain subject to recurrent attacks of intestinal obstruction.

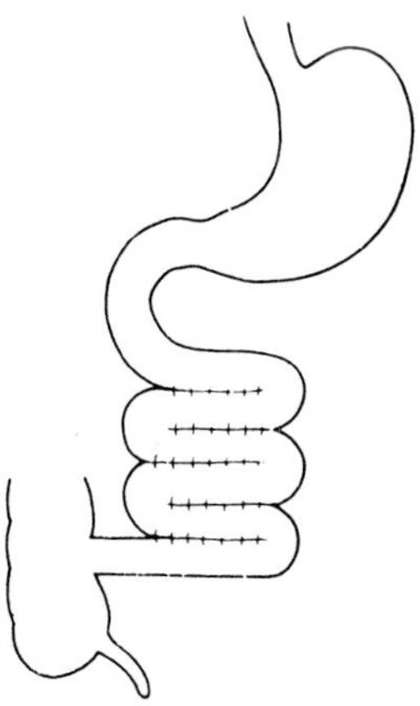

Figure 6.11 Diagrammatic representation of Noble's plication operation. The small intestinal loops are sutured together in smooth curves by means of seromuscular sutures.

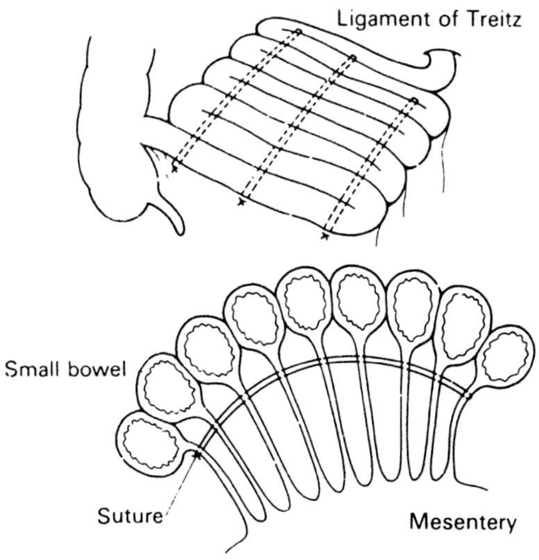

Figure 6.12 Diagrammatic representation of the Child–Phillips operation of transmesenteric plication for recurrent small intestinal obstruction due to adhesions.

In the Child–Phillips operation of transmesenteric plication (Figure 6.12) after adhesiolysis, the small intestine and mesentery are placed in an orderly fashion. Thereafter, the intestinal coils are fixed in position by means of transmesenteric sutures on some 3–5 mm away from the mesenteric border of the intestine, avoiding the terminal branches of the mesenteric arcade. The results of a number of retrospective reports with this procedure for recurrent small bowel obstruction due to adhesions have been good in terms of relative freedom from further episodes of intestinal obstruction.

The intraluminal tube or long intestinal 'stent' tube was first proposed by White as a simple method of achieving gentle curves rather than allowing the bowel to develop acute angulations when adhesions re-form. Baker introduced the jejunostomy tube and advocated its insertion through either a purse-string suture in the

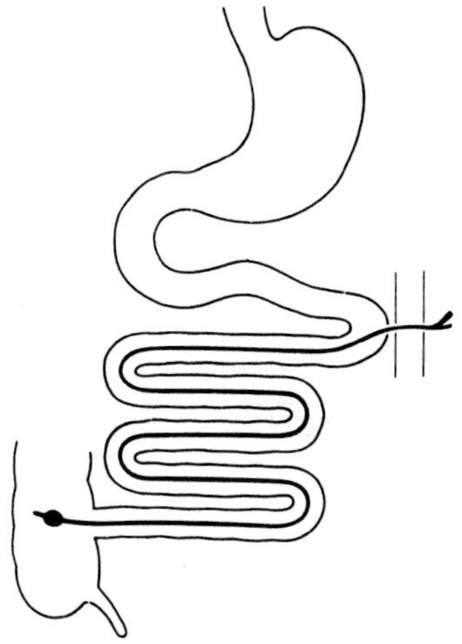

Figure 6.13 Intestinal intubation for recurrent small bowel obstruction usinng a Baker's tube inserted via a Witzel jejunostomy.

upper jejunum or a Witzel jejunostomy (Figure 6.13). The tube has an inflatable balloon near its tip, which facilitates passage down the small intestine into the caecum. Modifications of the technique include gastrostomy stent plication with and without tube exit-caecostomy (Figure 6.14). The latter is unnecessary and increases the risk of infection. One disadvantage of the intestinal intubation method is the long period of ileus after the operation. Reports on the efficacy of intestinal intubation in preventing recurrent intestinal obstruction have been conflicting. Some have found the procedure beneficial and have extended its use as a prophylactic measure in the treatment of patients with generalized peritonitis and following major abdominal surgical procedures. Other reports indicate that intestinal intubation is inferior to adhesiolysis alone.

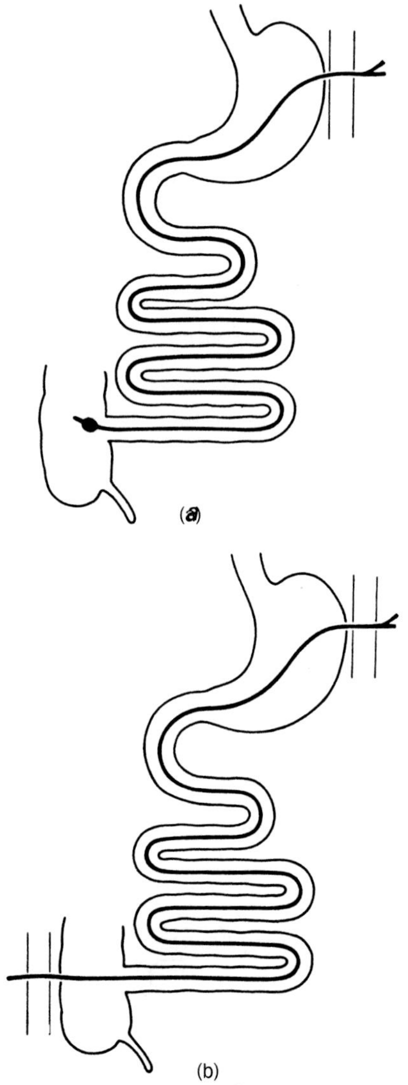

Figure 6.14 (a) Gastrostomy with long intestinal tube plication for recurrent small bowel obstruction. (b) Modification of the technique with gastrotomy and tube exit-caecostomy. This technique is not generally recommended as the exit-caecostomy is considered unnecessary and increases the risk of infection.

Section 6.6 • Desmoid tumours (aggressive fibromatosis)

The pathological disorder underlying the development of these lesions is *aggressive fibromatosis*. Desmoid tumours are considered as locally aggressive but non-metastasizing tumours. This is not strictly true as instances of peritoneal dissemination are documented but are uncommon. These tumours exhibit a marked tendency to recur after surgical excision, lead to considerable morbidity and not uncommonly contribute to death of the patients. Aggressive neurofibromatosis may arise sporadically or in association with familial adenomatous polyposis (FAP) and Gardner's syndrome.

Pathology

Aggressive fibromatosis (myo-fibromatosis in children) is a fibroproliferative disorder of fascial and musculo-aponeurotic structures that most commonly affects the trunk and extremities but variants can affect the intra-abdominal mesenteries and the parietal pleura. The pathological process consists of a monoclonal proliferation of spindle (fibrocyte-like) cells that is locally invasive with a tendency to recurrence but very rarely metastasizes, although instances of peritoneal dissemination have been reported in patients with mesenteric desmoids. Some tumours arise sporadically but a subgroup is associated with FAP. Beta-catenin mutations and beta-catenin dysregulation have been documented in both sporadic aggressive fibromatosis and that occurring in association with FAP, itself caused by germ-line mutations in the adenomatous polyposis coli (APC) gene. It is known that the APC gene is involved in the regulation of the cellular level of beta-catenin which has a cell membrane function (member of the adherens junctions) and binds transcription factors in the nucleus, thereby activating transcription (mediator in Wingless signalling). Cellular beta-catenin protein level is elevated in all desmoid tumours (sporadic and those associated with FAP). The demonstration of mutations in two mediators in the Wnt-APC-beta-catenin pathway implicates beta-catenin stabilization as the key factor in the pathogenesis of aggressive fibromatosis. It appears that truncating APC gene mutations (337 bp insertion of an Alu I sequence into codon 1526 of the APC gene) give aggressive fibromatosis cells a proliferative advantage through elevated cellular levels of beta-catenin protein. What is interesting is the observation that the higher level of beta-catenin protein compared to surrounding normal tissues is associated with normal levels of beta-catenin mRNA. This suggests that the elevated beta-catenin is due to degradation at a lower rate than normal tissues.

Desmoid tumours are oestrogen receptor and progesterone receptor negative. Despite this, antiestrogens (tamoxifen and toremifine) and NSAIDS (sulindac and diclofenac) have been shown to induce objective response rates in both adult patients and children with unresectable or recurrent desmoid tumours and the effect of the combination is synergistic, i.e. increased efficacy compared to either agent alone. Most desmoid tumours express the proliferating cell nuclear antigen (PCNA) although this has not been shown to influence outcome.

Clinical features

Desmoid tumours are rare with a reported incidence of 2–4 per million population. They can occur at any age from childhood to old age but there is an established female preponderance and the majority of sporadic cases occur in women of childbearing age when they usually appear during or after pregnancy. Infantile/juvenile tumours tend to be very aggressive and involve proliferation of fibrous and muscle layers (myo-fibromatosis). The mesenteric variant constitutes about 10% of all desmoid tumours and accounts for 50–70% of lesions developing in patients with FAP. Although the trunk and extremities are the most common sites of external desmoids, lesions can occur anywhere – neck, chest, hands, etc.

The majority of tumours developing in patients with FAP do so after surgery and 50–70% are intra-abdominal (mesenteric variant) and 30–50% external in the abdominal wall. Mesenteric desmoids have a significantly worse prognosis than abdominal wall tumours and cause recurrent intestinal or ureteric obstruction which often contribute to the death of the patient. By contrast abdominal wall desmoids do not cause death or significant morbidity although recurrence is common after excision.

Treatment

In view of rarity of the condition the treatment is not standardized. There are four treatment modalities:

- surgical excision
- radiotherapy
- combined anti-oestrogen and anti-inflammatory drug therapy
- chemotherapy
- newer modalities: isolated limb perfusion and immunotherapy with interferon.

Surgical excision

This remains the most effective, although recurrence rates are high (average 30% at 5 years), recurrence-free survival is good (80–75%) at 5 years for primary extremity and trunk desmoid tumours. Local recurrence after surgical excision is not related to any specific prognostic factors (age, sex, depth and size of tumour, and positive resection margins). Thus attempts at wide excision resulting in unnecessary morbidity may not prevent local recurrence. Surgical excision of these lesions should remove macroscopic disease with preservation of function and structure when possible, as residual microscopic disease does not significantly compromise the 5 year disease-free or overall survival. Conservative surgery is especially indicated in children where it should be accompanied by adjuvant therapy (*vide infra*). In limb lesions, amputation should be reserved only for patients in whom the disease or repeated resections have resulted in a non-functional or chronically painful extremity.

Radiotherapy

Radiation is an effective modality for desmoid tumors, either alone or as an adjuvant to resection. The main indication for radiotherapy is unresectable disease. Post-operative radiation is not recommended for patients with negative resection margins. Patients with positive margins should receive 50 Gy of post-operative radiation. Unresectable tumours are irradiated with a dose of approximately 56 Gy with a 75% expectation of local control. The radiation dose correlates with the incidence of complications. Thus doses of 56 Gy or less produce a 5% complication rate at 15 years as compared to 30% with higher doses.

In 30% of juvenile patients suffering from aggressive fibromatosis primary complete resection is not feasible. In this age group, radiotherapy as primary treatment is indicated only if complete tumour resection is not feasible without mutilation. In general, radiotherapy should be used as a last resort in children with skeletal immaturity because of the risk of growth disturbance, contracture and secondary malignancy.

Combined antioestrogen and anti-inflammatory drug therapy

This can be used at any age but is indicated in patients with unresectable disease/recurrence after radiotherapy, especially children in whom it is recommended prior to resort to chemotherapy. Reasonable response rates (up to 30%) and disease control are well documented.

Chemotherapy

Chemotherapy is indicated in young patients and children:

- with gross residual tumour
- with disease progression
- after failed surgery and radiotherapy.

The most effective regimen is vinblastine and methotrexate, which is accompanied by acceptable toxicity. The treatment should be continued for at least 20 weeks.

Newer modalities

Isolated limb perfusion (ILP) with tumour necrosis factor (TNF) and melphalan has been used with some success as a limb preservation treatment in patients with recurrent desmoids and significant symptoms who would otherwise require mutilating surgery for control of the disease. However, the reported experience, though promising (40% regression rate), is limited. Also interferon-induced remission in aggressive fibromatosis of the lower extremity has been reported.

Section 6.7 • Disorders of the retroperitoneum

Retroperitoneal fibrotic disorders

There is a group of fibrotic disorders of the pneumoperitoneum that are closely related and considered to be distinct from aggressive fibromatosis (desmoids). They include:

- secondary retroperitoneal fibrosis – drug-induced, extravasation of urine, desmoplastic response to a variety of tumours
- idiopathic retroperitoneal fibrosis (Ormond's disease)
- inflammatory aortic aneurysm
- sclerosing mesenteritis
- multifocal retroperitoneal fibrosclerosis.

All are rare. The secondary type accounts for about 30% of cases. The drug-induced type is associated with the administration of methysergide for migraine but other drugs (methyl dopa, phenacetin, etc.) have been implicated.

Idiopathic retroperitoneal fibrosis (IRF, Ormond's disease)

The condition accounts for 70% of cases and results in the development of a flat, grey–white plaque of tissue which is found in the lower lumbar region and then spreads laterally and upwards to encase the common iliac vessels, vena cava and the aorta. Rarely, it may extend upwards above the renal arteries and become contiguous with a similar process in the mediastinum, or forwards into the small bowel mesentery or mesocolon. It may very rarely also involve the bile duct, duodenum and pancreas. The histological picture varies from an active one which shows inflammatory cells and small blood vessels surrounding bundles of collagen fibres, to a more mature process that is relatively avascular and acellular with patches of calcification.

The aetiology of idiopathic retroperitoneal fibrosis is unknown. It has been attributed in the past to lymphatic and venous obstruction and lymphangitis. Leakage of blood or urine from trauma into the retroperitoneal space causing fibrosis is classed as secondary retroperitoneal fibrosis. The majority of idiopathic cases are regarded as part of an obscure collagen disorder. A possible genetic predisposition for IRF is suggested by the presence of the human leucocyte antigen (HLA)-B27 immunophenotype in 44% of cases. The association in some patients with inflammatory aortic aneurysm is now established (*vide infra*). In these patients it appears that the fibrosis is caused by a chronic inflammatory or autoimmune response to antigens leaking into retroperitoneum from atheromatous plaques in the aorta or common iliac arteries.

The average age at presentation is 50–55 years but the disease is documented in young individuals and elderly patients (aged 44–71 years). There is a male predominance in reported cases. Clinical presentation may be insidious with a variable picture but the most common presentation is with hypertension, obstructive uropathy (single or bilateral) and renal failure. A nagging ill-defined low back pain is common and there may be evidence of venous obstruction as shown by swelling of the scrotum and legs. Uncommonly, the patient may present with claudication. Examination reveals anaemia, leucocytosis and an increased sedimentation rate. Biochemical investigation may show a degree of renal failure. The intravenous urogram reveals a characteristic picture consisting of hydronephrosis and medial displacement of the ureters with gross irregularity.

Patients in renal failure will require cystoscopy and ureteric stenting to relieve the obstructive uropathy and permit recovery of the renal function. If stenting is unsuccessful, percutaneous nephrostomy is necessary to improve renal function before definitive treatment. This consists of surgical ureterolysis. The operation is carried out by a transabdominal approach, and the freed ureter(s) are separated from the fibrous tissue by vascularized omental interposition and placed intra- or extraperitoneally. This operation gives the best results (even without subsequent corticosteroid therapy) with complete resolution of the symptoms and long-term successful alleviation of ureteric obstruction in 100% of patients.

Many drugs have been shown to effective in idiopathic retroperitoneal fibrosis. These include corticosteroid, azathioprin, cyclophosphamide, methotrexate, tamoxifen and mycophenolate mofetil. Tamoxifen and corticosteroids seem to be the most effective combination and are indicated in patients with continuous activity of the disease and to prevent recurrence after surgery.

Inflammatory aneurysm

Inflammatory aneurysm (aortitis) accounts for 4% of abdominal aneurysms and has an established association with retroperitoneal fibrosis. Following surgical treatment of the aneurysm, the inflammatory fibrosis resolves completely in only 23%, improves in 35% but remains static in the remainder and can then lead to involvement of the ureter(s) or intestine. The characteristic perivascular distribution of IRF is in support of the hypothesis that the disease is an immune-mediated response to leaking antigens from severe atherosclerosis. It is recommended that patients with inflammatory aneurysms should be followed up and receive medical therapy with corticosteroids and tamoxifen if the fibrosis does not resolve, or progresses.

Sclerosing mesenteritis

This is a very rare idiopathic benign mesenteric lesion and only a few cases have been reported. It is characterized by fat necrosis, fibrosis and chronic inflammation and has been recently reported in human immunodeficiency virus (HIV)-positive patients. It presents with recurrent abdominal pain and weight loss and tends to form masses that involve the pancreas and the small bowel mesentery. The condition responds to tamoxifen and corticosteroids.

Multifocal idiopathic fibrosclerosis

Multifocal idiopathic fibrosclerosis (MIF) is a rare syndrome characterized by exuberant fibrosis involving many organs/systems – mediastinal fibrosis, retroperitoneal fibrosis, orbital pseudotumour, Riedel's thyroiditis and sclerosing cholangitis. Patients may also have Dupuytren's contractures, lymphoid hyperplasia, Peyronie's disease, vasculitis, testicular fibrosis and pachymeningitis.

Retroperitoneal swellings

The term retroperitoneal tumour is usually confined to lesions arising from tissues (muscles, fat, fibrous tissue, lymph nodes, nerves and developmental remnants) of this compartment but excluding origin from the retroperitoneal organs (pancreas, kidneys and ureters and adrenal glands). Retroperitoneal swellings may be cystic or solid, benign or malignant.

Benign cystic lesions

The cystic swellings are usually benign and the majority are discovered accidentally. They include:

- cystic lesions arising from developmental (Wolffian) remnants of the urogenital tract. These are situated near one or other kidney
- mesenteric cysts (intra- and retroperitoneal)
- teratomatous and dermoid cysts
- abdominal cystic lymphangiomas (lymphogeneous cysts)
- parasitic cysts.

Abdominal cystic lymphangiomas are rare and usually present in infants and children, mean age 5 years (range 3 months–8 years) and indeed some are diagnosed on the pre-natal ultrasound examination. They may, however present in adult patients. The majority (90%) of childhood lesions are intraperitoneal (mesentery and gastrointestinal tract) but some (10%) are located in the retroperitoneal space. The symptomatology varies but the most common presentation is with abdominal pain. A palpable tumour is found in 30% of patients. In children, abdominal lymphangiomas may present with complications such as intestinal obstruction (including volvulus), infection and sudden increased pain and swelling caused by intracystic haemorrhage. The diagnosis is established by abdominal ultrasonography. Treatment is with surgical excision, which has to be complete to prevent recurrence.

In adults, symptoms of abdominal cystic lymphangiomas have usually been present for several months to years, and the documented sites include the pancreas, spleen and retroperitoneum. Thus compared to children, a significantly higher proportion involve retroperitoneal structures and acute presentation is rare.

Solid tumours

The majority of solid retroperitoneal tumours are malignant. The benign tumours, which comprise 20%, include:

- lipomas
- neurofibromas, neurilemmomas
- leiomyomas
- extra-adrenal chromaffinomas (phaechromocytomas) – may be malignant
- retroperitoneal mucinous cystadenomas
- haemangiopericytoma.

The Costello syndrome is characterized by mental retardation and the occurrence of benign tumours (usually papillomata) but instances of children with the Costello syndrome who develop retroperitoneal embryonal rhabdomyosarcoma are documented. Adult retroperitoneal tumours of nervous origin account for 20% of the retroperitoneal tumours in this age group. The majority are males (sex ratio 10:3). The main symptom is the abdominal pain (84.6% of all cases) and all the tumours usually reach a large size by the time of presentation. Benign solid lesions such as retroperitoneal neurilemmomas show up as well-demarcated round or oval masses on CT. They may exhibit heterogeneous contrast enhancement, no-enhancement indicative of cyst formation and tumour calcification.

Paraganglioma are tumours of embryological origin from the neural crest and can be found in any location along the aorta and/or in association to the sympathetic chain. These tumours can be non-functioning or secreting (catecholamines – usually norepinephrine) and the secretory state influences the clinical presentation. These secreting neuroendocrine tumours are responsible for 0.1–0.5% cases of hypertension. Only 20% of paragangliomas are catecholamine secreting, and cause a syndrome similar to that of phaeochromocytoma. Paraganglionomas may be multiple and malignant. The malignant types recur locally after excision and spread by the blood stream predominantly to bones and lungs. Immunohistochemical staining of paraganglionomas may exhibit type I cells (chromogranin A and neurone-specific enolase) which have no prognostic significance, or type II cells (S100 protein), the presence of which is associated with a good prognosis. Some paraganglionomas are familial (hereditary paraganglioma) and are associated with germline mutations in the von Hippel–Lindau disease (VHL) tumour suppressor gene and the ret proto-oncogene.

Both benign (mucinous cystadenomas) and malignant (mucinous cystadenocarcinomas) can occur as primary tumours of the retroperitoneum. The immunological staining characteristics of malignant lesions indicate that these tumours have patterns similar to ovarian mucinous tumours. This genotypic similarity with ovarian mucinous tumours may indicate similar mechanisms in their histogenesis.

Hemangiopericytomas are rare vascular benign tumours derived from pericytes and can develop in the retroperitoneal space where they usually present as very bulky but otherwise clinically silent tumours. Tumours as large as 30 cm have been documented. Treatment is by surgical excision.

Although not strictly a primary retroperitoneal tumour as angiomyolipoma (a mesenchymal tumour) usually originates from the kidney, it is considered here for a number of reasons. In the first instance, its pleomorphic appearance and involvement of regional lymph nodes may simulate malignancy, although the lesion is benign. Secondly, angiomyolipomas are very common (approximately 40%) in patients suffering from tuberous sclerosis and are then usually small, bilateral and asymptomatic.

The important clinical feature of angiomyolipomas is spontaneous rupture and retroperitoneal haemorrhage and this usually occurs with larger tumours. Although the tumour has specific ultrasonographic and CT appearances, histological examination is necessary for establishing the diagnosis. The management varies with size. Thus small asymptomatic lesions should be followed up with sequential CT scans and removed by enucleation or partial nephrectomy only if they reach a size >4.0 cm. Emergency surgery is needed for patients with massive bleeding, when it is usually very difficult to preserve the kidney.

Overtly malignant retroperitoneal tumours are of diverse origin:

- lymphomas
- congenital neuroblastoma
- soft tissue sarcomas – fibrosarcoma, liposarcoma, rhabdomyosarcoma, neurofibrosarcoma and other malignant nerve cell tumours
- neoplasms arising from the urogenital ridge.

Congenital neuroblastoma is the most frequent solid neoplasm in infancy. It presents as a retroperitoneal cystic or solid mass and is readily diagnosed by ultrasonography. It is now possible to diagnose these tumours pre-natally usually in the third trimester of pregnancy by means of B-mode ultrasonography as cystic suprarenal masses. The pre-natal detection necessitates delivery in a perinatal centre so that neo-natal surgery can be performed. In general these are highly aggressive tumours but significant cure rates are recorded.

Retroperitoneal sarcomas

Fortunately retroperitoneal sarcomas (fibro-, lipo, leio-, myxo-, rhabdomyosarcomas) are rare with a reported incidence rate of one to two cases per million per year. They can be well-differentiated (low-grade) or undifferentiated (high-grade) tumours when the primary cell origin may be difficult to establish even on histochemistry. Despite advances in molecular oncology, the aetiology in most soft tissue sarcomas remains elusive. At the time of presentation, these tumours are usually large due to their slow relatively asymptomatic growth over a period of many months (Figure 6.15). Local recurrence is very common (33–86%) after surgical resection and local failure is usually the cause of death as distant metastases are rare (up to 30%) in reported series.

Some liposarcomas exhibit on histology peculiar meningothelial-like whorls and metaplastic bone in the whorls or immediate vicinity The meningothelial-like whorls represent a mesenchymal proliferation that may undergo myofibroblastic, or osteoblastic differentiation in liposarcoma. The meningothelial whorls are thought to represent an early sign of dedifferentiation of liposarcomas. In general, the prognosis of liposarcomas is poor.

Clinical features

The age range is varied and some (neuroblastomas) are congenital tumours. Most patients present initially with

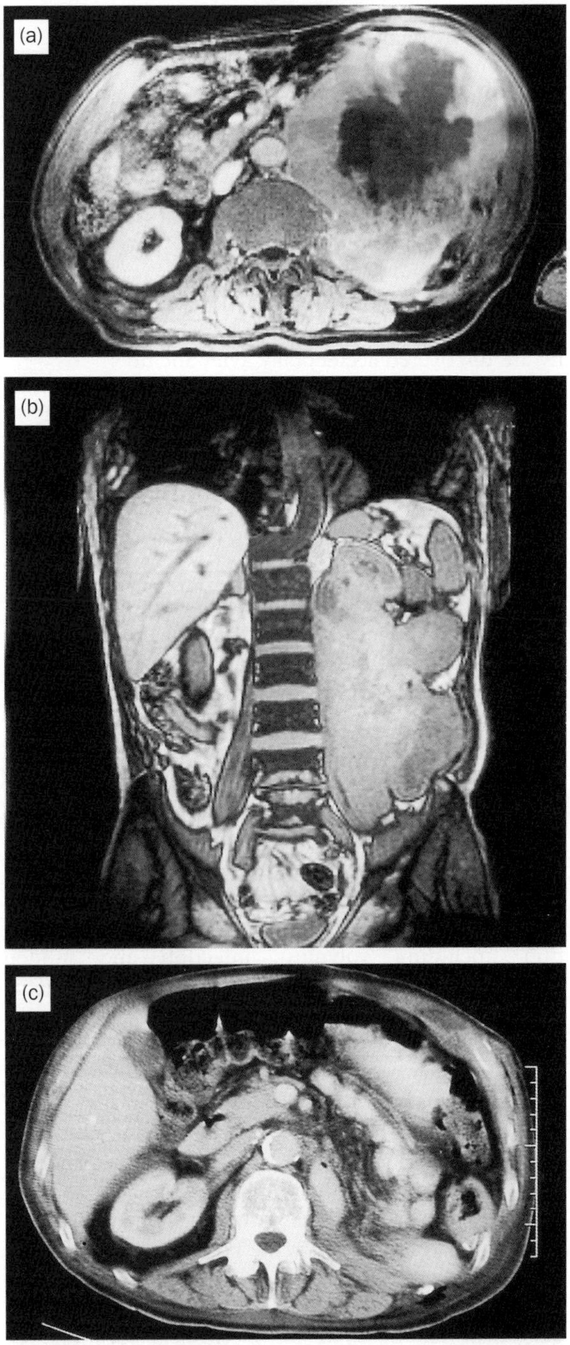

Figure 6.15 Left retroperitoneal high-grade sarcoma: (a) transverse MRI view, (b) axial MRI view, (c) MRI after resection which involved *en-bloc* removal of left kidney and spleen. The tumour did not involve the paraspinal muscles and the abdominal wall muscles.

vague symptoms including fever, abdominal discomfort, back pain, anorexia, vomiting, fatigue and weight loss. In the majority the mass is palpable at the time of presentation. If the mass is pelvic and the patient female, there is a real risk of misdiagnosis of gynaecological (usually) ovarian malignancy. This leads to laparotomy and inappropriate transperitoneal biopsy instead of referral to a soft tissue sarcoma centre. The most common reasons for this error are misinterpretation of clinical signs and over-reliance on ultrasound findings by the gynaecologists. The more frequent utilization of CT is recommended in all patients with pelvic tumours.

In advanced cases, there may be evidence of caval compression with lower limb oedema, varicocele, ascites and dilated abdominal wall veins. The most useful investigations in these patients are MRI or helical CT with contrast enhancement, and if available, positron emission tomography (PET) scan. A retroperitoneal core needle biopsy is performed under CT/ultrasound guidance. These tests have largely replaced other investigations, although an intravenous urogram is advisable as part of the work-up to exclude ureteric involvement and to assess the function of both kidneys (in case one needs to be removed with the tumour). A chest X-ray is performed in all malignant cases.

Retroperitoneoscopy has been used to diagnose infiltrating retroperitoneal lymphadenopathy or masses when retroperitoneal biopsy under CT guidance fails to establish a definite diagnosis but the technique is not in established routine usage. Reported results are, however, good and in one series, a precise diagnosis was obtained in 108 of the 118 patients. The sensitivity of retroperitoneoscopy is 84% for malignant lymphoma, 94% for Hodgkin's lymphoma, 95% for metastatic lymph nodes of carcinomas and 100% for primary retroperitoneal tumours. If these findings are confirmed by other studies, retroperitoneoscopy with visually guided biopsy will replace CT- guided biopsy.

Treatment

The treatment of retroperitoneal tumours depends on their pathological nature and is essentially surgical. Patients with malignant retroperitoneal tumours are best managed in tertiary referral centres that have the necessary surgical expertise in dealing with soft tissue sarcomas. Surgical treatment planning is based on adequate imaging with CT with intravenous and oral contrast. Alternatively MRI imaging provides equivalent information. Distant metastases and infiltration of non-resectable vascular or neural structures preclude resection. Complete *en bloc* surgical excision at the first laparotomy is the treatment of choice in virtually all primary retroperitoneal tumours. Radical *en bloc* resection including adjacent organs is technically demanding and it often proves difficult even in experienced hands to obtain adequate tumour-free margins. Invasion of the retroperitoneal muscles can pose major problems even in experienced hands. Thus complete radical resection is only possible in 30% of cases. The resectability rate in published series ranges from 38 to 100% but the radical (complete) resection rates are lower. Prognosis is influenced by two factors – histological grade and completeness of the surgical excision (R0 = no residual disease). The reported 5 year survival rate after radical resection for cure varies from 62 to 92% in well-differentiated tumours, as distinct from 16–48% in undifferentiated sarcomas.

There is no firm evidence that adjuvant chemotherapy and radiotherapy impart significant benefit in patients with retroperitoneal soft tissue sarcomas, in contrast to soft tissue sarcomas of the extremities where adjuvant radiation is effective in decreasing local recurrence in tumours >5.0 cm. A recent meta-analysis of randomized trials on adjuvant chemotherapy for soft tissue sarcomas has found a small reduction in local and distant relapse and a trend for improved overall survival. New adjuvant and neo-adjuvant treatments are currently being conducted by the EORTC for patients with non-resectable retroperitoneal tumours.

Section 6.8 • Hernias

Internal hernias

Internal hernias are a rare but important cause of intestinal obstruction (0.2–0.9% of all cases) because they are often undiagnosed before emergency laparotomy; and not uncommonly, they lead to infarction necessitating bowel resection (of varying extent), and this contributes to the high morbidity and mortality rates. Internal hernias are often classified as developmental (congenital) or acquired. In the congenital types, except in instances of gross mid-gut malrotation, the presentation occurs over a wide age range, but the majority of patients are in the fifth decade. By definition, developmental internal hernias cause obstructive symptoms in the absence of any previous surgical intervention.

Acquired internal hernias occur in patients who have undergone abdominal surgery, most commonly of the upper gastrointestinal tract, e.g. after gastric bypass surgery for morbid obesity or following Roux-en-Y diversion (especially if this is antecolic). They are well documented after right hemicolectomy (both open and laparoscopic), after laparoscopic extraperitoneal hernia repair (through unrecognized defects in the peritoneum), vascular operations, e.g. intraperitoneal femoro-femoral bypass grafting and after pelvic lymphadenectomy when loops of small intestinal become trapped beneath one or other iliac arteries. A particular group of acquired internal hernia occurs, albeit rarely, in relation to transplantation of the kidneys and liver. There are sometimes referred to as para-transplantation internal hernias and can have serious consequences. Following renal transplantation the internal hernia is caused by entrapment of bowel or omentum through a defect in the peritoneum covering the transplanted kidney. Internal herniation with volvulus of the small intestine is a potentially fatal complication after liver transplantation. The herniation occurs around the Roux-en-Y loop used for the biliary reconstruction. The mortality of this condition (from graft or bowel necrosis) is 50%. In view of the high mortality of peritonitis in transplant patients, early surgical treatment is indicated in all these patients who develop intestinal obstruction after surgery.

Pathological anatomy

This provides a more useful classification and better understanding of the underlying pathology. Thus internal hernias fall into two groups: *true hernias* and *internal prolapses*

True hernias

These have a hernial sac. The orifice involved may be:

- normal, e.g. Winslow's foramen
- paranormal, i.e. peritoneal fossae – paraduodenal, ileocaecal, inter- and mesosigmoidal, paracolic, supravesical.

Internal prolapse

These do not have a sac. The prolapse may occur through:

- an abnormal orifice in a mesentery or an omentum (trans-mesenteric, trans-mesocolonic, trans-omental
- an anomalous orifice – congenital defects in ligament (falciform, gastrosplenic, broad ligaments) or a mesentery (mesentery of Meckel's diverticulum)
- surgical defects or entrapment by surgically altered internal anatomy, e.g. anastomoses, stomas.

Paraduodenal hernias (right and left in close relation to the fourth part) constitute the commonest true internal hernias and account for 30–53% of cases. They are caused by incomplete rotation of the mid-gut such that the small intestine becomes entrapped behind the colon and mesocolon. The most valuable investigation for PDH is a small bowel enema, which usually shows clumping of the small intestine with incomplete rotation of the caecum and ascending colon. Other true internal hernias worthy of specific mention are hernia through the foramen of Winslow (epiploic foramen) and paracaecal hernia. Herniation through the epiploic foramen accounts for 8% of internal hernias. Most commonly the caecum and ascending colon are involved, and in some cases, re-enter the main peritoneal cavity through an additional congenital defect of the lesser omentum. In patients with chronic symptoms, a barium enema may be diagnostic because it shows the caecum lying posterior and medial to the stomach. Paracaecal hernia presents with both subacute and acute low small bowel obstruction.

Internal hernia (prolapse) arises as a complication of gastrointestinal surgery in 0.3–1% of cases. The majority occur after upper gastrointestinal surgery (Billroth II gastrectomy with antecolic gastrojejunostomy and enteroanastomosis, Roux-en-Y reconstruction or diversion, etc.) and less commonly after colon surgery (right hemicolectomy, colostomy). Presentation with intestinal obstruction may occur early or several years after (up to 25) the intervention.

Malrotation of the mid-gut usually presents acutely in the neonatal period but affected individuals may not develop symptoms until much later (2–23 years). The most common symptoms include vomiting (68%), colicky abdominal pain (55%) and diarrhoea (9%). The diagnosis is made by barium meal and follow-through, or preferably, a small bowel enema. A significant number of these late presenting patients (40%) are found to have either a volvulus or internal hernia at operation.

Clinical features

The reported incidence of all internal hernias varies between 0.2 and 0.9% of autopsies, 0.3–2% of parietal hernias, and 0.01% of laparotomies. Overall the condition is more common in males (3:2). The age distribution varies widely but peak symptomatic incidence is in the fifth decade (mean age of 45–50 years). Some (10–15%) are discovered as an incidental finding during laparotomy for another condition. Most commonly, these are paraduodenal hernias.

The symptoms of internal hernia irrespective of type are entirely non-specific and very few cases are diagnosed in the elective situation, with the vast majority (90%) presenting with acute intestinal obstruction, which is often strangulating with evidence of established peritonitis caused by infarcted bowel (30–60%). In a minority of patients recurrent attacks of colicky pain and abdominal distension are followed by imaging tests (contrast radiology, CT scanning, abdominal ultrasound), and these may provide a pre-operative diagnosis. More rarely still, a mass is found on physical examination of the abdomen in a patient with subacute obstructive symptoms. Acute intestinal obstruction with strangulation occurring in a patient without an external hernia or previous abdominal surgical intervention should suggest the possibility of a congenital internal hernia, especially if the patient gives a history of chronic intermittent abdominal pain and a palpable abdominal mass is found on examination.

Treatment

The essence of good management is early intervention (laparotomy) as this is the only means of preventing necrosis of the bowel. The surgical treatment consists of reduction of the hernial contents, resection of necrosed bowel, usually with primary anastomosis and correction of the anatomical defect that caused the herniation in the first instance. The operative reduction of the hernia and the surgical repair must be conducted with extreme care to avoid injury to the major mesenteric vessels juxtaposed to or surrounding the hernial orifice. The hospital stay, morbidity and mortality (up to 30% in large series) depend on the presence/absence of bowel infarction. In the rare instances when an internal hernia is discovered after investigation of chronic symptoms, elective surgery is needed because of the pathogenic potential of this condition.

Diaphragmatic hernias

Strictly speaking diaphragmatic hernias should include hiatal hernias but by convention, these are included with gastroesophageal reflux disease **[Disorders of the oesophagus, Vol. II]**. Diaphragmatic hernias excluding this category fall into three groups:

- congenital diaphragmatic hernia
- traumatic diaphragmatic hernia – secondary to undiagnosed rupture of the diaphragm
- herniations through congenital small defects – through foramina of Morgagni (anterior) and foramina of Bochdalek (posterior).

Congenital diaphragmatic hernia (CDH)

This is a serious congenital anomaly, which is always associated with pulmonary hypoplasia and other abnormalities (35%) particularly of the central nervous system and the skeleton. The condition is diagnosed in the majority (80%) by pre-natal ultrasound when the question of termination arises. With emergency neonatal surgery (reconstruction of the diaphragm with prosthetic mesh) and extracorporeal membrane oxygenation (ECMO) for cases with severe pulmonary impairment, the survival of infants born alive with CDH only averages 60% and more than half (60%) of these have persistent disorders that include respiratory problems, developmental delay, poor growth and gastro-oesophageal reflux. Despite advances in neonatology there is still a high mortality and morbidity associated with CDH.

Rupture of the diaphragm and traumatic diaphragmatic hernia

The primary event is rupture of the diaphragm due to severe blunt trauma, most commonly from motor vehicle accidents. The rupture, which is twice as common on the left side and is rarely bilateral (5%) may be diagnosed immediately or missed when a traumatic hernia is diagnosed because of symptoms or complications. Rupture of the diaphragm is more common in males (4:1) and occurs over a wide age range. Associated injuries are present in the majority of patients (90%) with rupture of the diaphragm. These include rib fractures, splenic, hepatic, pulmonary and bowel injuries. Helical CT with sagittal and coronal reformatted images is the best imaging test for the diagnosis of diaphragmatic rupture after blunt trauma. Findings consistent with diaphragmatic injury include waist-like constriction of abdominal viscera (collar sign), intrathoracic herniation of abdominal contents, and diaphragmatic discontinuity. Helical CT reformatted images detect 78% of left-sided and 50% of right-sided diaphragmatic injuries.

The injury is always a major one with a reported mean Injury Severity Score (ISS) of 30–35. The immediate mortality ranges from 15 to 20%. Predictors of death include old age, high ISS, severe hypovolaemic shock and bilateral injuries. Emergency repair of a ruptured diaphragm can be carried out through a laparotomy, thoracotomy or the thoraco-abdominal approach, depending on the nature of the associated injuries.

Traumatic diaphragmatic hernia (TDH) is usually diagnosed months to several years (average 5 years) after the injury. The patient may have non-specific symptoms (vague chest pain, shortness of breath, palpitations) or presents acutely with clinical signs of intestinal obstruction/strangulation of a hollow organ. In line with its aetiology TDH is more common on the left. The chest X-ray is often suggestive and diagnosis is usually confirmed by barium studies of the gastrointestinal tract. The most common herniated abdominal organs in TDHs are the stomach and colon. The repair involves closure of the defect by a prosthetic mesh and this can be performed through a thoracotomy or laparotomy or laparoscopically.

Iatrogenic diaphragmatic hernia

This is due to damage to the diaphragm during surgery, particularly laparoscopic anti-reflux surgery. The injury is often caused by HF electro-surgery and the resulting defect, which is small, leads to herniation usually of the stomach over the succeeding months. The most common complaint is pain in the left upper quadrant and left shoulder. The condition is diagnosed by a barium meal and is often missed by flexible endoscopy.

Morgagni and Bochdalek hernias

Hernias through the foramina of Morgagni (right and left) are rare congenital hernias that may present in infancy, childhood and adult life. They are situated anteriorly in the immediate retrosternal position. In children Morgagni hernias are usually asymptomatic but they may be associated with mild respiratory distress or cause gastrointestinal symptoms and rarely incarceration of bowel which may be of the partial Richter type. In adults they may present with vague symptoms or intestinal obstruction or gastric volvulus. The foramina of Bochdalek are congenital posterior diaphragmatic defects resulting from persistence of the pleuroperitoneal canal on one or both sides. Bochdalek's hernias are rare and present in adult and elderly patients with digestive symptoms and less frequently with obstruction. Both hernias do not have a sac are thus instances of internal prolapses.

Incisional hernias

Incisional hernias after abdominal surgery are common but with a varied reported incidence depending on case mix (2–20%). Strictly speaking, the term ventral hernia should be restricted to incisional hernia arising in abdominal mid-line operative wounds. There are several factors that contribute to the aetiology of incisional hernias, the most important being adequacy of abdominal wound closure in the first instance and the occurrence of wound infection and subclinical wound dehiscence in the post-operative period. There is no evidence that abdominal wound closure with synthetic monofilament biodegradable sutures carries a higher incidence of incisional hernia than closure with non-absorbable sutures. There are however a number of recognized risk factors, which include:

- obesity, especially morbid obesity – very strong risk factor
- chronic obstructive airways disease (COAD)
- type of incision, i.e. more frequent after vertical than transverse
- steroid dependence – less important than morbid obesity
- creation of a stoma (colostomy, ileostomy, urinary conduit) – parastomal hernias
- age > 70 years
- no prophylactic antibiotic cover during primary operation – increased incidence.

There is some evidence that apart from technical faults and risk factors, incisional hernia may arise in patients with an underlying collagen metabolic disorder, known to play an important role in the development of inguinal hernia. Studies have shown a decreased ratio of collagen I/III due to a concomitant increase in collagen III in patients with incisional and recurrent incisional hernias. This appears to reduce the mechanical strength of connective tissues and may explain the high incidence of recurrence in patients undergoing fascial repair procedures.

Aside from the obvious disfigurement, they cause pain and discomfort and may strangulate although the risk of this complication is low. The diagnosis is obvious and is made on clinical examination, when tensing of the muscles of the anterior abdominal wall (elevation of head from pillow or lower limbs from bed) accentuates the bulge. The vast majority of incisional hernias are reducible when the patient lies down in the supine position.

Treatment

This has to be individualized. Thus if the patient has minimal symptoms and especially if elderly, conservative management with an abdominal support is advisable. Many patients, however, have symptoms and dislike the bulge, and for this reason insist on repair. There are three techniques of surgical repair of incisional hernias:

- primary fascial repair
- tension-free repair by synthetic mesh prosthesis
- autogenous repair by vascularized innervated muscle flaps – reserved for large defects/recurrent hernias (*vide infra*).

There is now sufficient reported evidence that primary fascial repair techniques have an unacceptably high incidence of recurrence (up to 50%) and these operations have largely been abandoned in most centres. By contrast, tension-free repair by a synthetic mesh is accompanied by a much lower recurrence rate (2–10%) and is the technique that is in general use. The most popular prosthetic material used is polypropylene mesh that is available in either mono- or double filament forms. An alternative material is fluorinated polyester mesh that can be gel impregnated for antibiotic bonding immediately before use. There is experimental evidence that adherence of bowel to fluorinated polyester mesh is minimal and this material exhibits minimal contraction and hardening with time. Whatever material is used, it is important that the mesh overlaps the size of the defect by a significant margin, and it should lie loosely rather than be stretched over the defect. Tension-free mesh repair can be undertaken laparoscopically apparently with good results in the short term. The risks of tension-free repair of incisional hernias include:

- wound infection
- infection of the mesh
- seroma formation
- wound sinus
- enterocutaneous fistula formation
- recurrence.

Although wound infection is common (4–17%), actual incidence rates of mesh infection are not known but most such instances resolve with antibiotic treatment, although persistent serious infections necessitating removal of the mesh are well documented. This is a major problem. The management is staged with temporary skin cover until infection is eradicated, followed by abdominal wall reconstruction by muscle transfer flaps (*vide infra*). Seroma formation is also common but its incidence varies (0–22%) with the size of the defect and hence the mesh. Most surgeons insert tunnelled Redivac suction drains to the site to prevent this complication. There is no evidence that these tunnelled small-calibre suction drains increase the incidence of post-operative wound/mesh infection. However, the efficacy of these suction drains in reducing the incidence of seroma formation remains unproven. Wound sinus is reported in 4–18% of cases. It usually heals with conservative management or minor intervention to remove the offending suture. Enterocutaneous fistula has been reported but appears to be a rare complication. Its exact aetiology is not known but adherence of the bowel to the mesh appears to initiate the process. In a recent large retrospective report on 136 cases, the patient-related factors considered important on statistical evaluation in relation to recurrence following tension-free mesh repair with polypropylene were:

- age > 70 years
- hernia > 6 cm
- no prophylactic antibiotic cover
- recurrent hernia
- wound infection.

It is important to stress that the recurrent hernia is usually larger that the initial one and hernial defects larger than 10 cm may require autogenous reconstruction of the abdominal wall by muscle flaps.

Massive midline wall defects

These include large central incisional hernias (usually recurrent) and pose major problems in management. In one reported series of 22 patients, the defects varied in size from 6 by 14 cm to 10–24 cm and the causes included:

- removal of infected synthetic mesh material (32%)
- recurrent incisional hernia (18%)
- removal of split-thickness skin graft and dense abdominal wall cicatrix (18%)
- parastomal hernia (9%)
- primary incisional hernia (9%)
- trauma/enteric/abdominal wall sepsis (9%)
- abdominal wall tumour resection (4.5%).

In view of size of the defect, conservative management with an abdominal support is unsatisfactory, and if the patient is fit, surgical treatment is indicated. Reconstruction of these large central abdominal wall defects is a major surgical undertaking that requires specialist plastic surgical expertise. Modern surgical treatment is based on autogenous tissue reconstruction introduced by Ramirez *et al.* The technique utilizes bilateral, innervated, bi-pedicle, rectus abdominis–transversus abdominis–internal oblique muscle flaps that are transposed medially to reconstruct the central defect.

The results of the Ramirez autogenous tissue reconstruction are good with satisfactory healing and no recurrence in 90%. The morbidity considering the magnitude of the operation is reported to be minimal and confined to superficial infection and wound seroma formation. The post-operative mortality averages 4–5%. Although the Ramirez operation is usually used to treat complicated (trauma, surgical excision) or recurrent central abdominal wall defects, it is also used as a primary repair of large central incisional hernias.

Port site wound (incisional) hernias after laparoscopic surgery

The overall reported incidence of incisional hernias through port side wound is 2–3%. The risk factors include

- size of port > 10 mm
- obesity
- inadequate fascial closure.

The vast majority occur in port wounds greater than 10 mm but instances of herniation have been reported in smaller port wounds (5 mm) especially in the lower abdomen. It has to be remembered that below the arcuate line, there is no posterior rectus sheath and thus the abdominal wall is intrinsically weaker. The commonest reported site is the umbilical region probably because this is usually a large port (used to insert the laparoscope and extract specimen). Patients can present with localized pain and a subcutaneous lump, which is tender and has a cough impulse; or acutely with acute intestinal obstruction. This usually involves the small bowel and is of the Richter's type. In obese patients, the small hernia can be easily overlooked as a cause of the small bowel obstruction (*vide infra*).

Parastomal hernias

A parastomal hernia is an incisional hernia that occurs at the site of surgically constructed intestinal stoma on the abdominal wall. The basic underlying cause for the development of a parastomal hernia is progressive enlargement of the trephine opening in the abdominal wall, due to tangential abdominal forces working on the circumference of the opening through which the bowel emerges. This physical consideration accounts for the unsatisfactory results of surgical repair irrespective of its nature.

Parastomal hernias are common and their management is both difficult and controversial. They continue to pose management problems. In one large series of 316 patients with 322 stomas, an overall incidence of 67% of stoma-related complications was reported. This included a 31% parastomal herniation rate, stenosis of the stoma in 10% and prolapse in 7% at 10 years after surgery. Parastomal hernias include:

- paracolostomy hernia
- ileostomy hernia
- urinary conduit hernia.

After sigmoid colostomies the crude and actuarial risk of complications are 50 and 58% respectively at 13 years with paracolostomy hernia being the highest, 35–40% at 10 years. Paracolostomy hernias are more likely in the elderly and in patients with other abdominal wall hernias. From the published data, the extraperitoneal technique appears to reduce the incidence of paracolostomy hernia. Other technical factors, e.g. mesenteric fixation and siting the stoma through the belly of the rectus abdominis, do not appear to influence the rate of this complication, although there are strong proponents for both measures.

In general, complications are detected much later in patients with a urological stoma than in those with a colostomy. The high incidence of stomal complications requires long-term follow-up of these patients.

Paracolostomy hernia most commonly presents with a bulge, ill-fitting bag and leakage problems, but they may present acutely with intestinal obstruction (usually small bowel), and indeed strangulation. Instances of incarcerated stomach in the hernial sac have been reported. The presumed reduction in the risk of intestinal obstruction with closure of the lateral space has not been confirmed by long-term studies. However, there is a slight reduction in the risk of intestinal obstruction with the extraperitoneal technique.

The stomal complications of ileostomy may occur many years after construction and at 20 years the incidence of stomal complications exceeds 70% in patients operated on for ulcerative colitis, but is lower though still high (50–60%) in patients following colectomy for Crohn's disease. The complications in order of frequency are:

- skin problems (34%)
- intestinal (23%)
- retraction (17%)
- parastomal herniation (16%)
- prolapse.

Thus stomal herniation is distinctly less common after terminal ileostomy than terminal colostomy. Again closure of the lateral space does not diminish the risk of intestinal obstruction and fixation of the mesentery does not reduce the probability of prolapse of the ileostomy. The incidence of parastomal herniation is unaffected by siting the ileostomy through the rectus abdominis as distinct from the oblique muscles.

The incidence of parastomal hernia in patients with ileal conduit diversion is lower than ileostomy after proctocolectomy (4–5%). The most common presentation is with a poorly fitting appliance causing leakage of urine. However, acute presentation with obstruction, anuria and parastomal ileal conduit fistula are well documented.

Treatment of parastomal hernias

The surgical treatment of parastomal hernias presents a continuing challenge and there is no universally effective operation. There are four techniques used in the surgical treatment of parastomal hernias:

- re-location of ostomy with repair of the defect (fascial or with mesh)
- mesh repair of the defect around the ostomy exit site. In this method, the hernia sac (laparocele) is replaced without being opened and the mesh positioned in the properitoneal space
- reduction and mesh repair with two strips of polypropylene mesh through a midline incision
- special prosthesis consisting of a polypropylene ring mounted in the centre of a polypropylene mesh.

Irrespective of technique, repair of parastomal hernia repair is often unsuccessful (average recurrence rate of 30% at 5 years) and rarely without complication. The general consensus for first-time repair is to re-locate the stoma and repair the defect with a tension-free mesh. This, of course, may transfer the problem to the other side. For recurrent parastomal hernias, local repair with prosthetic material (without re-location) is advocated, as it appears to be the best of a bunch of poor alternatives. In either case, fascial repair alone should not be performed owing to an unacceptably high recurrence rate.

There have been other techniques reported but the reported data on their efficacy are limited. As the basic problem is progressive enlargement with time of the hole by the tangential abdominal forces, a ringed prosthesis technique has been reported which appears to give good results in the short term. The prosthesis consists of a polypropylene ring of varying internal diameter (20, 25 or 30 mm), mounted in the centre of a polypropylene mesh. Following mobilization the exteriorized bowel is inserted through the ring and the mesh sutured to the parieties. In a series of 14 patients treated with this technique there was only one recurrence during a follow-up period of 5–35 months. Another procedure uses the mid-line laparotomy approach and after reduction, two trips of polypropylene are sutured on either side of the bowel to prevent enlargement of the orifice.

Non-incisional abdominal wall hernias

These hernias occupy a good deal of surgical time and account for 10–15% of all surgical operations. The majority of operations (80%) are performed for inguinal hernias though this figure is even higher in the male population. The remainder are in the region of the umbilicus (8%), incisional (7%) and femoral hernias (5%). Rarer forms of hernias, though very interesting, form only a tiny proportion of the surgical problem.

Diagnosis of abdominal wall hernias

In the vast majority of patients, the diagnosis is made on history and physical examination (location of the bulge and cough impulse) and no other confirmatory tests are needed. However, diagnostic problems may be encountered especially in obese patients and those presenting with acute intestinal obstruction. Water-soluble contrast herniography is an accurate means of identifying inguinal and femoral hernias in cases presenting diagnostic problems. For other hernias ultrasound and cross-sectional imaging CT or MRI is preferred. These are especially useful in the detection of the rare hernias, e.g. Spigelian, obturator (pelvic floor) hernias.

Epigastric, umbilical and para-umbilical hernias

These hernias are grouped together because herniation occurs through a defect in the linea alba between the xiphisternum and the umbilicus. The paraumbilical hernia is an epigastric hernia situated just above the umbilicus.

Epigastric hernia

This hernia is usually encountered in males above the age of 40 years. About one-quarter of cases are multiple. The defect in the linea alba allows a small pad of extraperitoneal fat to protrude, and as a result of the increased intra-abdominal pressure, the defect enlarges and then permits a sac of peritoneum and eventually the sac may admit omentum or even small bowel. Most epigastric hernias are symptomless and are diagnosed incidentally by the patient or doctor. A small nodule, which is more prominent on standing, is palpable in the mid-line but it is rare for a cough impulse to be elicited. A small number of patients present with vague upper abdominal symptoms, which do not fit a dyspeptic pattern and in whom repair of the hernia gives relief. It may be that in these patients a degree of tension on the peritoneal sac has produced the symptoms.

Small epigastric hernias do not require treatment. Those larger than 2.0 cm have the potential of strangulation because of the narrow neck through the linea alba and are best treated surgically. The procedure consists of excision of the sac and repair of the defect by either a simple longitudinal fascial repair or a transverse overlapping of the Mayo type. The results except in the very obese are generally very good.

Adult paraumbilical hernia

These hernias are more common in females (3:1) and are largely confined to obese patients. The defect lies just above the umbilicus, though deformity of the umbilical button is the earliest manifestation. In adults these are common with an overwhelming female preponderance. In one study of 2100 patients undergoing laparoscopy, paraumbilical fascial defects were found in 18% of patients and only 56% of these had symptomatic or overt umbilical hernias. The hernia may enlarge to the size of an orange but the neck of the sac remains dangerously small so that the risk of strangulation is ever present. The chronicity of the condition leads to firm adhesions forming between the peritoneal sac and its contents so that almost all large hernias are irreducible and should never be treated by the use of abdominal support or truss. Surgical treatment is best carried out effectively in all patients. The majority of patients however present acutely with obstruction/strangulation. The procedure of choice for repair of paraumbilical hernia is that described by W.J. Mayo in 1893. After excision of the sac, the defect is closed by suture, the upper crescent being fixed over the front of the lower half of the defect. The Mayo operation has reported recurrence rates of 2–3%. For large hernias in the elective situation, some now use a prosthetic mesh repair.

Infantile umbilical hernia

The worst defect is exomphalos which fortunately is a rare condition, occurring in about 1: 5000 births and is nowadays diagnosed pre-natally. It is frequently associated with other congenital defects and not surprisingly about one-quarter of the babies have malrotation of the intestine.

Simple umbilical hernia (UH) is common in infants and young children with the highest reported incidence in African-Caribbean babies. In the vast majority of infantile umbilical hernia spontaneous closure occurs (reduction in size by approximately 18% each month) before the age of 4 years and thus management is conservative especially as complications during this age period are rare. However, large infantile umbilical hernias (neck of the sac > 2 cm) are unlikely to close spontaneously and surgical repair is therefore advisable. Irrespective of size, an umbilical hernia that persists beyond 4 years requires surgical repair, as closure then becomes unlikely. It is generally considered important to preserve the umbilical cicatrix after excising the sac and repairing the defect so that the child will not appear different from its fellows.

The most common complication in these children is incarceration with the development of small bowel obstruction. The reported risk of this complication is approximately 1:1500 umbilical hernias. Another very rare complication reported in Nigerian children is spontaneous rupture. This usually occurs in the first year of life and is probably precipitated by raised intra-abdominal pressure from excessive crying. The condition results in partial evisceration and needs urgent intervention.

Adult umbilical hernia

The umbilical hernia that develops in patients with refractory ascites due to chronic liver disease is often overlooked but can assume clinical significance. In the first instance incarceration is well documented as a complication of effective relief of the ascites following diuresis, paracentesis, peritoneovenous shunting and transjugular intrahepatic portasystemic shunt (TIPS). Secondly, these patients have marked atrophy of the abdominal muscles and some have, in addition, large high-pressure veins following recanalization of the umbilical vein (caput medusae). Thus repair can be difficult and should always be conducted using prosthetic mesh, preferably of the double stranded closely knitted variety. In addition, subcutaneous suction drains should be avoided because of the increased risk of infection of the ascitic fluid. The use of prophylactic antibiotics against Gram-negative bacteria is mandatory.

Groin hernias

Because of the erect posture, the inguinofemoral area is subjected to maximum strain from the intra-abdominal pressure especially during exertion. This together with the intrinsic weakness that is caused by the inguinal canal in males accounts for the predominance of these hernias especially in males. The hernia starts as a small pressure-induced diverticulum (hernial sac) that emerges through the deep inguinal and less commonly the femoral ring to enter the respective canal and exit as a lump in the groin that has a cough impulse. The term groin hernia covers inguinal and femoral hernias which are discussed separately.

Complications of groin hernia

The complications of groin hernias are:

- irreducibility
- obstruction
- strangulation.

The majority of patients who are admitted as emergencies with complicated groin hernias have not previously sought medical attention or been diagnosed with the condition in the outpatient department. This observation implies that most hernias that develop complications do so within a relatively short time in the natural history of the disease. Mortality of obstructed hernias is high in patients with co-existing cardiorespiratory disease, whereas morbidity rate is influenced by the viability of contents of the hernial sac. In turn, this is directly related to the duration of irreducibility/incarceration or delay in presentation.

The risk factors for complications of groin hernias are:

- **Adults**
  old age
  duration of hernia – short duration < 1 year
  type of hernia – femoral more than inguinal
  co-existing medical illness especially COAD
- **Children**
  very young (infants)
  gender (male)
  short duration of hernia
  side (right)

Inguinal hernia

By far and away, inguinal hernia is the most common external abdominal hernia, accounting for over 90%. Normally two mechanisms act to prevent herniation through the inguinal canal. With increased intra-abdominal pressure, contraction of the internal oblique and transversus muscles act upon the section of the transversus aponeurosis that arches convexly upwards over the medial half of the canal. The arch is pulled down and flattened and thus reinforces the posterior inguinal wall. The second mechanism, which may in fact be more important, depends upon the attachment of the strong fascial layer forming the deep inguinal ring. This fascial ring is normally firmly adherent to the posterior surface of the transversus muscle so that contraction of this muscle pulls the ring upwards and laterally.

In essence, an inguinal hernia is the consequence of weakness of the posterior abdominal wall. In the past, stretching of the transversalis fascia was considered to be the most important factor and some fascial repair procedures (Shouldice operation) were based on suture plication of this layer. Some however consider the transversalis (endoabdominal) fascia to be the thinnest and least important layer in the prevention of inguinal hernia formation and consider that the strength of the posterior wall of the inguinal canal is due to the muscle fibres and aponeuroses of the internal oblique and transversus abdominis. There is evidence for an increased risk of right inguinal hernia after appendicectomy. This is related to the denervation of the right transversus abdominis muscle fibres. These fibres are responsible for the support of the deep inguinal ring of fascia. Weak fascial support due to an abnormal accumulation of type III collagen has been demonstrated in some patients with direct but not indirect inguinal hernia.

Inguinal hernia exhibits a marked male predominance (20:1) and from the anatomical standpoint is of two types, indirect (or lateral) and direct (or medial). The sac of an indirect sac arises from the processus vaginalis. The hernia travels down the inguinal canal from the internal ring and exits as a subcutaneous lump exhibiting a cough impulse at the external inguinal ring above and medial to the pubic tubercle. The herniation lies inside the spermatic cord (covered by all the three spermatic fascial layers). In view of its indirect course, it does not often reduce itself spontaneously when the patient lies down and is more prone to irreducibility than the direct inguinal variety. Indirect inguinal hernia enters the scrotum as it enlarges whence it qualifies as inguino-scrotal hernia (Figure 6.16). The same pathology occurs in the female. Persistence of the processus vaginalis forms a peritoneal diverticulum (canal of Nuck). This enters the inguinal canal to form the hernia, which after exiting from the superficial inguinal ring, enters the labium majus as it enlarges. The direct hernia results from a weakness of the posterior wall of the inguinal canal medial to the internal ring and hence the inferior epigastric vessels; the sac is thus in close proximity to the external ring. Occasionally, the medial wall of the sac of a direct inguinal hernia is composed of the bladder wall. As the hernia enlarges it exits through the superficial inguinal ring behind or above the spermatic cord. Because of the direct path and wide neck, the vast majority of direct hernias are spontaneously reducible when the patient lies down and rarely strangulate. Moreover, even when large, direct hernias do not enter the scrotum, they tend to enlarge in the groin beneath Scarpa's fascia, which obstructs their entry into the scrotum. Patients with major weakness of the posterior inguinal wall may develop combined direct and indirect hernias with the two hernial sacs straddling the inferior epigastric vessels – this is sometimes referred to as pantaloon hernia.

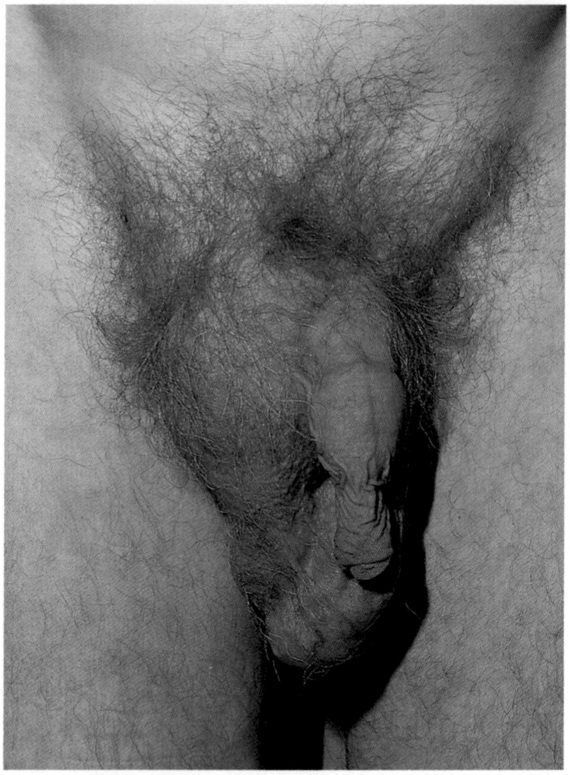

Figure 6.16 Inguino-scrotal hernia.

Clinical features

The complaint common to nearly all patients is the appearance of a lump in the groin. Some patients complain of a dragging sensation or pain in the groin, particularly during the early stages, but many hernias are asymptomatic. There may be a history of a major physical strain or of heavy physical work prior to the development of the hernia. Presumably, increased abdominal pressure can stretch the fascial margins of the deep inguinal ring and open up a pre-formed peritoneal sac.

The hernia may be best shown with the patient standing or precipitated by coughing and straining. The bulge should be above and medial to the pubic tubercle. In patients with large inguinoscrotal hernias the diagnosis is obvious though a cough impulse may be difficult to elicit. The differential diagnosis of inguinal hernia includes femoral hernia, inguinal lymphadenopathy, ectopic testis, hydrocele of the cord, saphena varix and lipoma of the cord. Endometriosis in a hernial sac may be mistaken for an incarcerated hernia, as may malignant tumours in the groin. Patients with chronic groin pain constitute a difficult diagnostic problem. Most cases of chronic pain in athletes are due to soft tissue injuries but in a small number, an undeclared hernia is the cause.

In the vast majority of cases, the diagnosis of an inguinal hernia is made clinically and a good physical examination can distinguish between the two types of hernia. The old practice of inserting a finger into the inguinal canal to detect the exact position of the cough impulse (tip of the finger in indirect and volar aspect of the finger in direct hernia) is no longer practised because it causes considerable patient discomfort. The best technique is to reduce the hernia with the patient in the supine position, and then apply pressure over the internal ring. This should control the hernia only if it is of the indirect variety. When difficulty arises in establishing the diagnosis because the hernia is small, especially if the patient is obese, water-soluble contrast herniography (50–80 ml injected intraperitoneally) may be used.

Sliding inguinal hernia

Essentially, in a sliding inguinal hernia, part of the sac wall is formed by prolapsed viscus and for this reason these hernias are always large (Figure 6.17). The condition can be suspected but not confirmed pre-operatively on clinical examination. Usually the diagnosis is established during surgery, although ultrasound and cross-sectional imaging may identify sliding components pre-operatively. The most common organ associated with a sliding inguinal hernia is the sigmoid colon but other organs can be involved. These include the vermiform appendix, urinary bladder, etc. In neonates large sliding hernias containing Fallopian tubes, ovaries and uterus are well documented and such instances have been reported in middle-aged females.

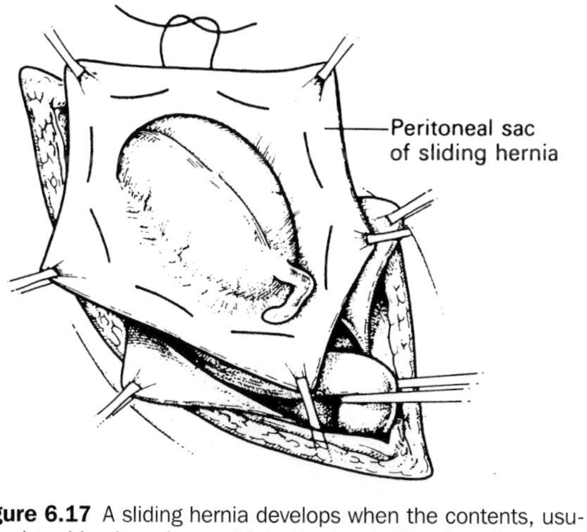

Figure 6.17 A sliding hernia develops when the contents, usually sigmoid colon, descend into the inguinal region. The colon does not lie within the sac but the sac is applied to its surface. The bowel is liable to damage if the sac is fully dissected from the surface and is best managed by a plicating suture after which the bowel can be returned to the abdominal cavity. (Derived from Nuhus and London, 1978.)

The more usual sliding hernia involving the colon forms a large inguinal mass and is often irreducible by the time of diagnosis. Sliding inguinal hernia may present acutely with strangulation involving omentum, small bowel, bladder or colon itself.

Inguinal hernias in children

At this age group, 90% of inguinal hernias occur in males and these often present at about 1 year when the child starts to walk with the vast majority being of the indirect type (patent processus vaginalis). Ten to 20% of children will develop a hernia on the other side; in about 50%, this peritoneal sac will be present at the time of operation on the presenting side. Attempts to detect these occult hernias have included contrast herniography and laparoscopy. There is no indication for routine exploration of the contralateral side. Direct inguinal hernia is extremely rare in children.

The history of a lump appearing in the groin is usually obtained from the mother who notices the hernia after a period of straining or coughing by the child. Quite frequently the hernia cannot be demonstrated by the medical examiner and all that can be felt is a silky sensation on palpation of the spermatic cord as the layers of the processus vaginalis move under the examining fingers. Unfortunately as many of the signs are ignored, there is a tendency for the hernia to become obstructed and strangulated by the time of presentation. This being the case, all children with a strong history should have elective exploration of the affected side. The operation consists of transection and high ligation of the processus vaginalis (herniotomy). Repair of the inguinal canal is not necessary. Differential diagnosis at this age includes undescended testis, hydrocele of the cord and torsion of the testis.

Repair of inguinal hernias

In general, if the patient is fit, an inguinal hernia should be repaired surgically. There are however situations when non-operative management is sensible. This conservative management should only be considered if the hernia is easily reducible and the patient has significant comorbid disease. Small indirect inguinal hernias are controlled by a spring truss, but large indirect and direct hernias require a large pad and firm belt. In all other patients surgical repair should be recommended.

The various repair procedures fall into two categories: fascial repairs (Bassini, Bassini with Tanner's slide, McVay, Ferguson, Shouldice) and tension-free prosthetic (polypropylene or polyester) repairs (Table 6.1) and these may be performed by the anterior open approach or laparoscopically/endoscopically. The fascial repairs are the oldest. Their only advantage is the avoidance of prosthetic material, which may become infected, but they carry the highest incidence of recurrence, particularly the Bassini operation since the repair cannot be

Table 6.1 Inguinal hernia repair procedures

Fascial repairs
Bassini
Bassini with Tanner's slide
Shouldice
Ferguson
McVay
Open tension-free prosthetic repairs
Stoppa
Lichtenstein
Plug repair
Laparoscopic
Transabdominal preperitoneal (TAP)
Total extraperitoneal approach (TEP)
Percutaneous endoscopic external ring repair (PEER)
Lichtenstein
Plug

effected without tension. In practice, infection of the prosthetic mesh, requiring removal has proved to be a rare occurrence, and this category of hernia repair operations is much more favoured nowadays in view of the uniformly reported good results and low recurrence rates. Open tension-free mesh repairs can be carried out under local anaesthesia as day cases and this reduces the costs considerably.

The laparoscopic approach has a number of advantages that include less post-operative pain, earlier return to full activity and work, and reduced incidence of persistent groin pain at 1 year. The initial higher morbidity (including major vascular, bowel, bladder and nerve injuries) and high recurrence rates reflected inexperience with the technique as surgeons were not familiar with the anatomy of the posterior abdominal wall as visualized from the peritoneal side. The morbidity and recurrence rates of the laparoscopic vs open tension-free repairs are now equivalent. The residual disadvantages are increased hospital (but not total) costs and the need for general or epidural anaesthesia. There is now good evidence that the laparoscopic TEP operation gives the best results in patients with large bilateral and recurrent hernias. The recurrence rate after primary laparoscopic TEP repairs at 3 years is under 1%.

Uniformly excellent results have been reported consistently with the open Lichtenstein repair using polypropylene (Marlex) mesh under local anaesthesia. At 5 years, this procedure in hernia centres has a recurrence rate of 0.1%. Most of the recurrences occur at the pubic tubercle usually because the mesh used was too small. The tension-free mesh plug repair was introduced in the late 1980s. A preformed mesh plug is used to fill and expand extraperitoneally occluding the defect. In large hernias, the plug is overlaid with an appropriately sized sheet of mesh. The technique is simple and entails minimal dissection especially in direct hernias. The reported recurrence rates vary from 1 to 3%. In a prospective randomized study comparing open mesh plug repair with laparoscopic TEP, the overall recurrence rate was similar (2.5% for the TEP vs 3% for the mesh-plug hernioplasty). However, patients undergoing the laparoscopic repair required less narcotic analgesic medication and returned to full activity 1 week sooner than the open-surgery group. There were no major post-operative complications in either arm in this study but minor morbidity was lower (13%) after laparoscopic TEP than in the open mesh plug group (23%).

PEER hernioplasty using a special inguinal canal retractor (Figure 6.18) is still in its early evaluation stage but initial results look promising. The actual repair is performed using either Lichtenstein mesh or hernia plug techniques. Irrespective of repair, only one incision (2.5 cm) is necessary. This is placed over the external inguinal ring and following division of the external spermatic fascia from the margins of the external ring, the inguinal canal is entered initially with the index finger. This is then replaced by the endoscopic inguinal canal retractor which houses a 30°, 5 mm telescope. The advantages of PEER repair include minimal pain and avoidance of general or epidural anaesthesia.

The complications of inguinal hernia repair are:

- urinary retention especially in males
- wound infection and haematomas
- scrotal swelling
- orchitis and testicular atrophy
- recurrence
- iatrogenic bladder, bowel, nerve and vascular injuries
- chronic groin pain.

Recurrent inguinal hernias

The recurrence rates vary widely but irrespective of approach, the lowest recurrence rates are encountered

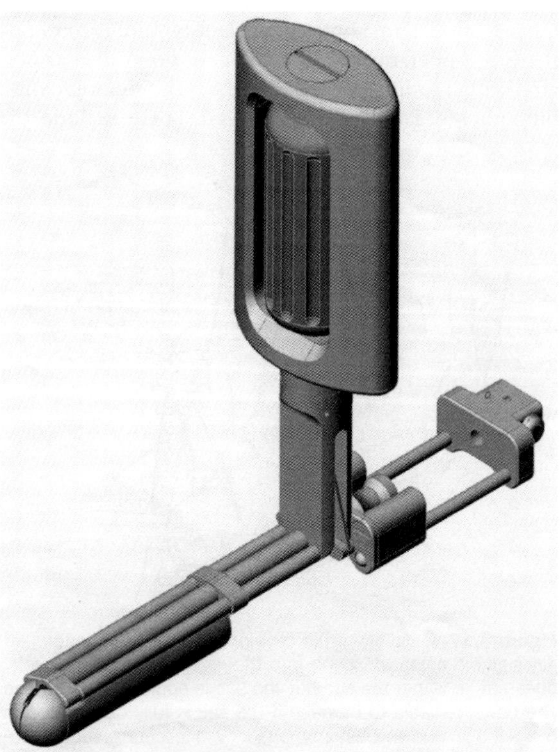

Figure 6.18 Inguinal canal retractor for PEER hernia repair.

after tension-free prosthetic mesh or plug repairs. The majority of recurrence rates occur within the first 2–3 years of the repair. Acceptable recurrence rates should be below 3% at 5 years. A Swedish study on a large cohort (n = 1232) of patients aged 15–80 years operated upon for inguinal or femoral hernia involving several surgeons/hospitals demonstrated the positive effect of audit (closing the loop) over a 10 year period. The recurrence rate decreased from 18% in 1984–6 to 3% in 1993–4. During this interval, there was a corresponding decline in the re-operation rate for recurrence at 3 years from 10.8% to 2.2%.

The surgical treatment of recurrent inguinal hernias is less effective and the risk of further recurrence is higher than after first time repair. It is now generally agreed that all recurrent inguinal hernias require some form of tension-free prosthetic mesh repair (open or laparoscopic). It is essential that the size of the mesh used is large enough to overlap the defect by a significant margin. The risk of further recurrence depends on the technique and the number of previous repairs. Thus in a large reported series patients with a first-time recurrence had recurrence rates of 2% as opposed to 9% in patients who had undergone two or more prior repairs. The morbidity of recurrent hernia repair is higher and includes wound haematoma, scrotal oedema, temporary pain at the wound site, paraesthesiae, injury of the ilioinguinal nerve and femoral hernia, although the overall morbidity can be low with good surgical technique.

Femoral hernias

The pathogenesis of femoral hernias is now thought to be related to the mode of insertion of the fibres of the transversus abdominis and its investing sheath into the superior pubic ramus and develops in two stages. If the insertion of the transversus abdominis fibres on the superior pubic ramus is through a narrow band, a cone-shaped defect overlying the femoral ring (the femoral cone) results. Initially, preperitoneal fat with or without a sac enters this femoral cone as a result of increased abdominal pressure. This is the asymptomatic stage I (internal) femoral hernia that can only be detected if the preperitoneal space is explored during inguinal herniorrhaphy. In time the fatty contents of the femoral cone exit from the narrow distal orifice when a stage II (external) symptomatic hernia results. As the hernia extends downwards, the sac is turned forwards through the cribriform fascia and may then turn upwards to overlie the inguinal ligament, when it may be mistaken for an inguinal hernia. The hernia may however remain quite small and be invisible or scarcely palpable in obese patients. Femoral hernia is particularly prone to incarceration and strangulation. By the time of diagnosis 16% of stage II femoral hernias are irreducible and 25–40% present with incarceration/strangulation. Of the emergency group up to 40% will have strangulation of the hernial sac contents (omentum, small bowel, vermiform appendix) requiring excision.

Femoral hernias can occur at any age with peak incidence in the fifth and sixth decades and are significantly commoner in females especially if multiparous (4:1). The higher incidence on the right side is inexplicable unless the right leg being in use more often than the left in severe exercise is the reason. Femoral hernias are exceedingly rare in children. A small stage II femoral hernia may be difficult to diagnose especially in obese women. The lump may not be easily palpable and the cough impulse difficult to elicit. On other occasions, the nodule, typically below and lateral to the pubic tubercle, may be difficult to differentiate from a lymph node. In such cases, contrast herniography or cross-sectional imaging with CT or MRI can be extremely useful.

Treatment of femoral hernias

All require surgical repair because of risk of obstruction/strangulation. The surgical approach varies with the presentation. In the elective situation, the surgical approach may be from below the inguinal ligament or through the inguinal canal.

Infra-inguinal operations

In the classical low approach, the hernial sac is isolated through an incision below the inguinal ligament. The sac is opened and emptied, with care taken to avoid injury to the bladder wall, which may be close to the medial side of the sac. The peritoneum is closed above the neck of the sac and the stump returned to the abdomen. The femoral canal is repair by interrupted non-absorbable sutures passing from the undersurface of the inguinal ligament to Cooper's ligament behind, or by the insertion of a rolled-up mesh plug. The repair with this cylindrical mesh prosthesis inserted into the femoral canal gives better results that the classical low fascial repair and is favoured nowadays. Alternatively a mesh repair can be effected laparoscopically using the total extraperitoneal approach.

Trans-inguinal approach

The inguinal canal is opened anteriorly and then the neck of the femoral hernia exposed by incising the posterior inguinal canal wall. The sac is open and the contents are reduced after which the peritoneum is closed and a tension-free mesh repair is effected of the posterior wall of the inguinal canal, ensuring this is of adequate size and thus overlaps the pubic tubercle.

Obstructed/strangulated femoral hernia

Although both the above can be used in patients with obstructed femoral hernias, the preperitoneal approach of McEvedy is recommended especially in the presence of strangulation of the contents of the hernial sac because this gives immediate access to the peritoneal cavity. The skin incision may be longitudinal or transverse over the lower abdomen but above the inguinal canal. The musculo-aponeurotic layer is divided lateral to the rectus abdominis, and the extraperitoneal space of the lower abdomen is entered. The hernia is usually easily reducible from above but it may not be. In this case the incision is enlarged and the peritoneal cavity entered above the sac.

Other hernias

Richter's or Richter–Littre's hernia

In 1700, the French surgeon Alexandre de Littre described a hernia in which only the antimesenteric part of the bowel was inside the hernial sac. Subsequently in 1777, Richter described 'the intestinal wall hernia', in which the antimesenteric border of the bowel was incarcerated within the hernial sac. For this reason Richter's hernia is sometimes referred as Richter–Littre hernia. Richter's hernia can complicate any small hernia but the most commonly involved is femoral hernia in which a knuckle of the small intestine becomes incarcerated. The patient presents acutely with symptoms and signs of intestinal obstruction. The diagnosis is often delayed as the obstruction may be incomplete or the small hernia may be overlooked particularly in obese patients. There are now well-documented cases of Richter's hernia complicating small unrecognized port site wound hernias after laparoscopic surgery. The diagnosis should be considered in all patients who develop acute intestinal obstruction after laparoscopic surgery and is established by cross-sectional CT imaging.

All patients irrespective of nature of Richter's hernia require urgent intervention after resuscitation, and if the partial incarceration of the bowel is necrotic, the affected segment of the small intestine is resected.

Littre's hernia

This is defined as any hernial sac that contains a Meckel's diverticulum and may involve inguinal, umbilical, femoral, ventral and lumbar hernias. Littre's hernia is rare, particularly in children, in whom the umbilical variety is the commonest. It may present with evidence of gastrointestinal bleeding, as an incompletely reducible hernia, or acutely with intestinal obstruction and faecal-hernial fistulas. Obstructed/strangulated Littre's hernia usually presents in adult patients with intestinal obstruction. Pre-operative diagnosis is rare with the vast majority being recognized during emergency surgery. The recommended treatment is resection of the Meckel's diverticulum from within the opened hernial sac but extension of the wound is needed when the adjacent loop of small intestine is infarcted usually as the result of a volvulus.

Obturator (pelvic floor) hernia

Herniation through the obturator foramen is a rare clinical entity occurring most commonly in elderly thin (average body weight 35–40 kg) multiparous females and presenting with acute small bowel obstruction. In one report of a large series one-third of the patients were admitted from homes for elderly people and were either bed-ridden or wheelchair-bound. The vast majority of patients with obstructed obturator hernia are high-risk patients and this together with the delayed diagnosis and intervention accounts for the high morbidity and mortality (15–25%) because of the frequent presence of infarcted bowel (60–75%). The pre-operative diagnosis of obturator hernia is difficult since there are no specific clinical features although the Howship-Romberg sign may be positive, but a groin mass is rarely found on physical examination. Recently, pelvic CT has been shown to provide the diagnosis in suspect cases, and may be indicated in elderly patients with mechanical intestinal obstruction of uncertain origin. However, the correct pre-operative diagnosis does not appear to influence the outcome, with survival being determined by early surgical intervention.

Repair of the hernial defect is difficult because adjacent tissues are not easily mobilized and thus requires a polypropylene mesh placed in the preperitoneal space and sutured to Cooper's ligament. Recently there have been a few reports on the laparoscopic repair of obturator hernia but the experience is limited. This approach is inadvisable in the presence of infarcted bowel.

Spigelian hernia

This is an interesting hernia that is probably more common than the number of reported cases suggests. The herniation occurs close to the linea semilunaris (Spigelian line). This marks the transition between the muscular and aponeurotic part of the transversus abdominis muscle (Spigelian aponeurosis) at the edge of the rectus abdominis on either side, and extends from the costal margin to the pubic tubercle. The herniation occurs through a defect in the Spigelian aponeurosis between the linea semilunaris and the lateral edge of the rectus (Figure 6.19). As the hernia is covered by the external oblique aponeurosis, it is initially intramural and may not be palpable externally, i.e. the sac lies between the internal and external oblique muscles (85%) but may penetrate through the external oblique layer as it enlarges (15%). The hernial sac may be empty or contain small bowel, omentum, and more rarely, caecum or sigmoid colon. Although very rare, congenital Spigelian hernia has been reported in children and these cases may be associated with an undescended

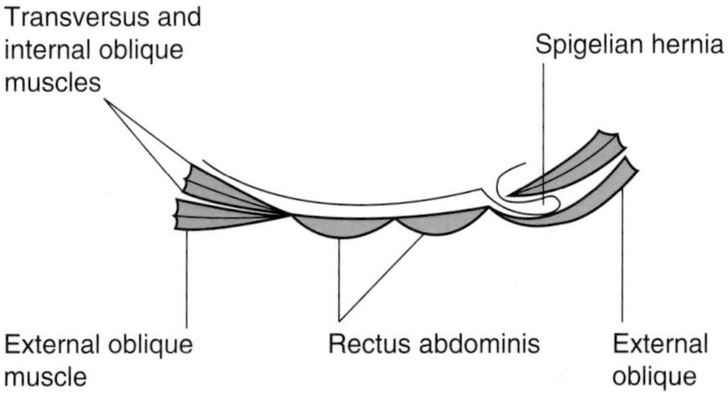

Figure 6.19 Diagrammatic representation of Spigelian hernia. The herniation occurs through a defect in the Spigelian aponeurosis between the linea semilunaris and the lateral edge of the rectus.

testis or an ipsilateral mediastinal neuroblastoma where muscle atrophy caused by the neuropathy of the ninth to twelfth intercostal nerves is thought to be responsible for the hernia.

The mean age at diagnosis is 60 years and the hernia can occur on either side with equal frequency. The clinical presentation varies depending on the contents of the hernia sac and the size/type of herniation. Pain is the most common symptom but varies in intensity and nature. On physical examination, the commonest findings are a palpable hernia and a palpable hernial defect. Some patients (20–25%) present acutely with a tender irreducible mass or intestinal obstruction caused by incarceration of a loop of intestine.

Although large easily palpable Spigelian hernias do not pose diagnostic problems, small hernias are often overlooked. Persistent point tenderness along the Spigelian aponeurosis with associated spasm of the abdominal wall should suggest the diagnosis in these cases. Ultrasound scanning or CT will identify these small impalpable hernias.

The treatment of Spigelian hernia is surgical. A gridiron incision is favoured by many surgeons in patients with palpable hernias. In patients with non-palpable hernias the preperitoneal dissection is carried out through a vertical incision which permits good exposure. The vertical approach is also recommended in patients requiring emergency surgery because of intestinal obstruction as it enables an exploratory laparotomy. Repair can be either fascial or by prosthetic mesh sheet or plug, although as with other hernias tension-free prosthetic repair is favoured nowadays. The repair of uncomplicated Spigelian hernias can be performed laparoscopically. Irrespective of approach, the reported recurrence rates after surgical repair are low.

Further reading

Pseudomyxoma peritonei

Cintron, J. R. and Pearl, R. K. (1996). Colorectal cancer and peritoneal carcinomatosis. *Semin Surg Oncol* **12**: 267–78.

Du Plessis, D. G., Louw, J. A. B. and Wranz, P. A. (1999). Mucinous epithelial cysts of the spleen associated with pseudomyxoma peritonei. *Histopathology* **35**: 551–7.

Guerrieri, C., Franlund, B., Fristedt, S. *et al.* (1997). Mucinous tumors of the vermiform appendix and ovary, and pseudomyxoma peritonei: histogenetic implications of cytokeratin 7 expression. *Hum Pathol* **28**: 1039–45.

Hinson, F. L. and Ambrose, N. S. (1998). Pseudomyxoma peritonei. *Br J Surg* **85**: 1332–9.

Low, R. N., Barone, R. M., Lacey, C. *et al.* (1997). Peritoneal tumor: MR imaging with dilute oral barium and intravenous gadolinium-containing contrast agents compared with unenhanced MR imaging and CT. *Radiology* **204**: 513–20.

Raj, J., Urban, L. M., ReMine, S. G. and Raj, P. K. (1999). Laparoscopic management of pseudomyxoma peritonei secondary to adenocarcinoma of the appendix. *J Laparoendosc Adv Surg Tech A* **9**: 299–303.

Ronnett, B. M., Shmookler, B. M., Sugarbaker, P. H. and Kurman, R. J. (1997). Pseudomyxoma peritonei: new concepts in diagnosis, origin, nomenclature, and relationship to mucinous borderline (low malignant potential) tumors of the ovary. *Anat Pathol* **2**: 197–226.

Ronnett, B. M., Zahn, C. M., Kurman, R. J. *et al.* (1995). Disseminated peritoneal adenomucinosis and peritoneal mucinous carcinomatosis. A clinicopathologic analysis of 109 cases with emphasis on distinguishing pathologic features, site of origin, prognosis, and relationship to 'pseudomyxoma peritonei'. *Am J Surg Pathol* **19**: 1390–408.

Shin, H. J. and Sneige, N. (2000). Epithelial cells and other cytologic features of pseudomyxoma peritonei in patients with ovarian and/or appendiceal mucinous neoplasms: a study of 12 patients including 5 men. *Cancer* **90**: 17–23.

Sugarbaker, P. H. (1996). Pseudomyxoma peritonei. *Cancer Treat Res* **81**: 105–19.

Teixeira, M. R., Qvist, H., Giercksky, K. E. *et al.* (1997). Cytogenetic analysis of several pseudomyxoma peritonei lesions originating from a mucinous cystadenoma of the appendix. *Cancer Genet Cytogenet* **93**: 157–9.

Tsai, C. J. and Lee, H. H. (1998). Disseminated peritoneal adenomucinosis – a diagnostic approach by peritoneoscopy. *Gastrointest Endosc* **48**: 312–14.

Ubhi, S. S., McCulloch, P. and Veitch, P. S. (1997). Preliminary results of the use of intraperitoneal carbon-adsorbed mitomycin C in intra-abdominal malignancy. *Br J Cancer* **76**: 1667–9.

Wirtzfeld, D. A., Rodriguez-Bigas, M., Weber, T. and Petrelli, N. J. (1999). Disseminated peritoneal adenomucinosis: a critical review. *Ann Surg Oncol* **6**: 797–801.

Mesothelioma

Attanoos, R. L. and Gibbs, A. R. (1997). Pathology of malignant mesothelioma. *Histopathology* **30**: 403–18.

Cocco, P. and Dosemeci, M. (1999). Peritoneal cancer and occupational exposure to asbestos: results from the application of a job-exposure matrix. *Am J Ind Med* **35**: 9–14.

Conlon, K. C., Rusch, V. W. and Gillern, S. (1996). Laparoscopy: an important tool in the staging of malignant pleural mesothelioma. *Ann Surg Oncol* **3**: 489–94.

Dodson, R. F., O'Sullivan, M. F., Huang, J. *et al.* (2000). Asbestos in extrapulmonary sites: omentum and mesentery. *Chest* **117**: 486-93.

Janssen-Heijnen, M. L., Damhuis, R. A., Klinkhamer, P. J. *et al.* (1999). Increased but low incidence and poor survival of malignant mesothelioma in the southeastern part of The Netherlands since 1970: a population-based study. *Eur J Cancer Prev* **8**: 311–14.

Mongero, L. B., Beck, J. R., Kroslowitz, R. M. *et al.* (1999). Treatment of primary peritoneal mesothelioma by hyperthemic intraperitoneal chemotherapy. *Perfusion* **14**: 141–5.

Ordonez, N. G. (1998). Role of immunohistochemistry in distinguishing epithelial peritoneal mesotheliomas from peritoneal and ovarian serous carcinomas. *Am J Surg Pathol* **22**: 1203–14.

Park, B. J., Alexander, H. R., Libutti, S. K. *et al.* (1999). Treatment of primary peritoneal mesothelioma by continuous hyperthermic peritoneal perfusion (CHPP). *Ann Surg Oncol* **6**: 582–90.

Pass, H. and Gazdar, A. F. (1999). Presence of simian virus 40 sequences in malignant mesotheliomas and mesothelial cell proliferations. *J Cell Biochem* **76**: 181–8.

Scurry, J. and Duggan, M. A. (1999). Malignant mesothelioma eight years after a diagnosis of atypical mesothelial hyperplasia. *J Clin Pathol* **52**: 535–7.

Stamat, J. C., Chekan, E. G., Ali, A. *et al.* (1999). Laparoscopy and mesothelioma. *J Laparoendosc Adv Surg Tech A* **9**: 433–7.

Sugarbaker, P. H. (1999). Management of peritoneal-surface malignancy: the surgeon's role. *Langenbecks Arch Surg* **384**: 576–87.

Tejido Garcia, R., Anta Fernandez, M., Hernandez Hernandez, J. L. *et al.* (1997). Fever of unknown origin as the clinical presentation of malignant peritoneal mesothelioma. *Ann Med Int* **14**: 573–5.

Weissmann, L. B., Corson, J. M., Neugut, A. I. and Antman, K. H. (1996). Malignant mesothelioma following treatment for Hodgkin's disease. *J Clin Oncol* **14**: 2098–100.

Wolanski, K. D., Whitaker, D., Shilkin, K. B. and Henderson, D. W. (1998). The use of epithelial membrane antigen and silver-stained nucleolar organizer regions testing in the differential diagnosis of mesothelioma from benign reactive mesothelioses. *Cancer* **1**(82): 583–90.

Primary peritonitis

Block, S. L., Adams, G. and Anderson, M. (1998). Primary pneumococcal peritonitis complicated by exudative pleural effusion in an adolescent girl. *J Pediatr Surg* **33**: 1416–17.

Cheng, I. K., Fang, G. X., Chau, P.Y. *et al.* (1998). A randomized prospective comparison of oral levofloxacin plus intraperitoneal (IP) vancomycin and IP netromycin plus IP vancomycin as primary treatment of peritonitis complicating CAPD. *Perit Dial Int* **18**: 371–5.

Guarner, C., Sola, R., Soriano, G. *et al.* (1999). Risk of a first community-acquired spontaneous bacterial peritonitis in cirrhotics with low ascitic fluid protein levels. *Gastroenterology* **117**: 414–19.

Guarner, C. and Soriano, G. (1997). Spontaneous bacterial peritonitis. *Semin Liver Dis* **17**: 203–17.

Hemsley, C. and Eykyn, S. J. (1998). Pneumococcal peritonitis in previously healthy adults: case report and review. *Clin Infect Dis* **27**: 376–9.

Javid, G., Khan, B. A., Shah, A. H. *et al.* (1998). Short-course ceftriaxone therapy in spontaneous bacterial peritonitis. *Postgrad Med J* **74**: 592–5.

Nathens, A. B., Rotstein, O. D. and Marshall, J. C. (1998). Tertiary peritonitis: clinical features of a complex nosocomial infection. *World J Surg* **22**: 158–63.

Pommer, W., Brauner, M., Westphale, H. J. *et al.* (1998). Effect of a silver device in preventing catheter-related infections in peritoneal dialysis patients: silver ring prophylaxis at the catheter exit study. *Am J Kidney Dis* **32**: 752–60.

Adhesions

Becker, J. M., Dayton, M. T., Fazio, V. W. *et al.* (1996). Prevention of postoperative abdominal adhesions by a sodium hyaluronate-based bioresorbable membrane: a prospective randomized double-blind multicentre study. *J Am Coll Surg* **183**: 297–306.

Ellis, H., Moran, B. J., Thompson, J. N. *et al.* (1999). Adhesion-related hospital readmissions after abdominal and pelvic surgery: a retrospective cohort study. *Lancet* **353**: 1476–80.

Peritoneal adhesiolysis (1994). National Inpatient Profile 1993. Baltimore: HCIA Inc., **427**: 653–5.

Van der Kabben, A. A., Dijkstra, M., Nieuwenhuizen, M. M. *et al.* (2000). Morbidity and mortality of inadvertent enterotomy during adhesiotomy. *Br J Surg* **87**: 467–471.

Desmoid tumours-aggressive fibromatosis

Adam, U., Mack, D., Forstner, R. *et al.* (1999). Conservative treatment of acute Ormond's disease. *Tech Urol* **5**: 54–6.

Ballo, M. T., Zagars, G. K. and Pollack, A. (1998). Radiation therapy in the management of desmoid tumors. *Int J Radiat Oncol Biol Phys* **42**: 1007–14.

Ballo, M. T., Zagars, G. K., Pollack, A. *et al.* (1999). Desmoid tumor: prognostic factors and outcome after surgery, radiation therapy, or combined surgery and radiation therapy. *J Clin Oncol* **17**: 158–67.

Barbalias, G. A. and Liatsikos, E. N. (1999). Idiopathic retroperitoneal fibrosis revisited. *Int Urol Nephrol* **31**: 423–9.

Bus, P. J., Verspaget, H. W., van Krieken, J. H. *et al.* (1999). Treatment of mesenteric desmoid tumours with the anti-oestrogenic agent toremifene: case histories and an overview of the literature. *Eur J Gastroenterol Hepatol* **11**: 1179–83.

Clark, S. K., Neale, K. F., Landgrebe, J. C. and Phillips, R. K. (1999). Desmoid tumours complicating familial adenomatous polyposis. *Br J Surg* **86**: 1185–9.

Clark, S. K., Smith, T. G., Katz, D. E. *et al.* (1998). Identification and progression of a desmoid precursor lesion in patients with familial adenomatous polyposis. *Br J Surg* **85**: 970–3.

Fibrotic disorders

Gilkeson, G. S. and Allen, N. B. (1996). Retroperitoneal fibrosis. A true connective tissue disease. *Rheum Dis Clin North Am* **22**: 23–38.

Goy, B. W., Lee, S. P., Eilber, F. *et al.* (1997). The role of adjuvant radiotherapy in the treatment of resectable desmoid tumors. *Int J Radiat Oncol Biol Phys* **39**: 659–65.

Halling, K. C., Lazzaro, C. R., Honchel, R. *et al.* (1999). Hereditary desmoid disease in a family with a germline Alu I repeat mutation of the APC gene. *Hum Hered* **49**: 97–102.

Kottra, J. J. and Dunnick, N. R. (1996). Retroperitoneal fibrosis. *Radiol Clin North Am* **34**: 1259–75.

Lackner, H., Urban, C., Kerbl, R. *et al.* (1997). Noncytotoxic drug therapy in children with unresectable desmoid tumors. *Cancer* **80**: 334–40.

Lev-Chelouche, D., Abu-Abeid, S., Nakache, R. *et al.* (1999). Limb desmoid tumors: a possible role for isolated limb perfusion with tumor necrosis factor-alpha and melphalan. *Surgery* **126**: 963–7.

Lewis, J. J., Boland, P. J., Leung, D. H. *et al.* (1999). The enigma of desmoid tumors. *Ann Surg* **229**: 866–72.

Li, C., Bapat, B. and Alman, B. A. (1998). Adenomatous polyposis coli gene mutation alters proliferation through its beta-catenin-regulatory function in aggressive fibromatosis (desmoid tumor). *Am J Pathol* **153**: 709–14.

Merchant, N. B., Lewis, J. J., Woodruff, J. M. *et al.* (1999). Extremity and trunk desmoid tumors: a multifactorial analysis of outcome. *Cancer* **86**: 2045–52.

Ozener, C., Kiris, S., Lawrence, R. *et al.* (1997). Potential beneficial effect of tamoxifen in retroperitoneal fibrosis. *Nephrol Dial Transplant* **12**: 2166–8.

Serpell, J. W., Tang, H. S. and Donnovan, M. (1999). Factors predicting local recurrence of desmoid tumours including proliferating cell nuclear antigen. *Aust NZ J Surg* **69**: 782–9.

Skapek, S. X., Hawk, B. J., Hoffer, F. A. *et al.* (1998). Combination chemotherapy using vinblastine and methotrexate for the treatment of progressive desmoid tumor in children. *J Clin Oncol* **16**: 3021–7.

Tejpar, S., Nollet, F., Li, C. *et al.* (1999). Predominance of beta-catenin mutations and beta-catenin dysregulation in sporadic aggressive fibromatosis (desmoid tumor). *Oncogene* **18**: 6615–20.

von Fritschen, U., Malzfeld, E., Clasen, A. and Kortmann, H. (1999). Inflammatory abdominal aortic aneurysm: a postoperative course of retroperitoneal fibrosis. *J Vasc Surg* **30**: 1090–8.

Retroperitoneal tumours

Besznyak, I. and Ronay, P. (1993). Surgery of primary retroperitoneal tumours. *Eur J Surg Oncol* **19**: 637–40.

de Perrot, M., Rostan, O., Morel, P. and Le Coultre, C. (1998). Abdominal lymphangioma in adults and children. *Br J Surg* **85**: 395–7.

Fanburg-Smith, J. C. and Miettinen, M. (1998). Liposarcoma with meningothelial-like whorls: a study of 17 cases of a distinctive histological pattern associated with dedifferentiated liposarcoma. *Histopathology* **33**: 414–24.

Hauser, H., Mischinger, H. J., Beham, A. *et al.* (1997). Cystic retroperitoneal lymphangiomas in adults. *Eur J Surg Oncol* **23**: 322–6.

Heling, K. S., Chaoui, R., Hartung, J. *et al.* (1999). Prenatal diagnosis of congenital neuroblastoma. Analysis of 4 cases and review of the literature. *Fetal Diagn Ther* **14**: 47–52.

Herman, K. and Kusy, T. (1998). Retroperitoneal sarcoma – the continued challenge for surgery and oncology. *Surg Oncol* **7**: 77–81.

Karakousis, C. P., Kontzoglou, K. and Driscoll, D. L. (1995). Resectability of retroperitoneal sarcomas: a matter of surgical technique? *Eur J Surg Oncol* **21**: 617–22.

Mann, G. B., Lewis, J. J. and Brennan, M. F. (1999). Adult soft tissue sarcoma. *Aust NZ J Surg* **69**: 336–43.

Merrot, T., Chaumoitre, K., Simeoni-Alias, J. *et al.* (1999). Abdominal cystic lymphangiomas in children. Clinical, diagnostic and therapeutic aspects: apropos of 21 cases. *Ann Chir* **53**: 494–9.

Montresor, E., Iacono, C., Nifosi, F. *et al.* (1994). Retroperitoneal paragangliomas: role of immunohistochemistry in the diagnosis of malignancy and in assessment of prognosis. *Eur J Surg* **160**: 547–52.

Porte, H., Copin, M. C., Eraldi, L. *et al.* (1997). Retroperitoneoscopy for the diagnosis of infiltrating retroperitoneal lymphadenopathy and masses. *Br J Surg* **84**: 1433–6.

Spillane, A. J. and Thomas, J. M. (2000). Gynaecological presentation of retroperitoneal tumours. *Br J Obstet Gynaecol* **107**: 170–3.

Tenti, P., Romagnoli, S., Pellegata, N. S. *et al.* (1994). Primary retroperitoneal mucinous cystoadenocarcinomas: an immunohistochemical and molecular study. *Virchows Arch* **424**: 53–7.

Hernias

Ahmad, A., Gangitano, E., Odell, R. M *et al.* Survival, intracranial lesions, and neurodevelopmental outcome in infants with congenital diaphragmatic hernia treated with extracorporeal membrane oxygenation. *J Perinatol* **19**: 436–40.

Athanassiadi, K., Kalavrouziotis, G., Athanassiou, M. *et al.* (1999). Blunt diaphragmatic rupture. *Eur J Cardiothorac Surg* **15**: 469–74.

Byers, J. M., Steinberg, J. B. and Postier, R. G. (1992). Repair of parastomal hernias using polypropylene mesh. *Arch Surg* **127**: 1246–7.

Cheung, M.T. (1995). Complications of an abdominal stoma: an analysis of 322 stomas. *Aust NZ J Surg* **65**: 808–11.

de Ruiter, P. and Bijnen, A. B. (1992). Successful local repair of paracolostomy hernia with a newly developed prosthetic device. *Int J Colorectal Dis* **7**: 132–4.

Elio, A., Veronese, E., Frigo, F. *et al.* Ileal volvulus on internal hernia following left laparoscopic-assisted hemicolectomy. *Surg Laparosc Endosc* **8**: 477–8.

Gagic, N. M. (1982). Right paraduodenal hernia. *Can J Surg* **25**: 71–2.

Hampel, N. and Zabbo, A. (1985). Parastomal ileal conduit-enteric fistula. *J Urol* **134**: 956–7.

Huddy, C. L., Boyd, P. A., Wilkinson, A. R. and Chamberlain, P. (1999). Congenital diaphragmatic hernia: prenatal diagnosis, outcome and continuing morbidity in survivors. *Br J Obstet Gynaecol* **106**: 1192–6.

Khan, M. A., Lo, A. Y. and Vande Maele, D. M. (1998). Paraduodenal hernia. *Am Surg* **64**: 1218–22.

Khanna, A., Newman, B., Reyes, J. *et al.* (1997). Internal hernia and volvulus of the small bowel following liver transplantation. *Transpl Int* **10**: 133–6.

Khoury, N. (1998). A randomized prospective controlled trial of laparoscopic extraperitoneal hernia repair and mesh-plug hernioplasty: a study of 315 cases. *J Laparoendosc Adv Surg Tech A* **8**: 367–72.

Killeen, K. L., Mirvis, S. E. and Shanmuganathan, K. (1999). Helical CT of diaphragmatic rupture caused by blunt trauma. *Am J Roentgenol* **173**: 1611–16.

Kyriakides, G. K., Simmons, R. L., Buls, J. *et al.* 'Paratransplant' hernia. Three patients with a new variant of internal hernia. *Am J Surg* **136**: 629–30.

Leber, G. E., Grab, J. L., Alexander, A. I. *et al.* (1998). Long-term complications associated with prosthetic repair of incisional hernias. *Arch Surg* **133**: 378–82.

Leong, A. P., Londono-Schimmer, E. E. and Phillips, R. K. (1994). Life-table analysis of stomal complications following ileostomy. *Br J Surg* **81**: 727–9.

Lodha, K., Deans, A., Bhattacharya, P. and Underwood, J.W. (1998). Obstructing internal hernia complicating totally extraperitoneal inguinal hernia repair. *J Laparoendosc Adv Surg Tech A* **8**: 167–8.

Londono-Schimmer, E. E., Leong, A. P. and Phillips, R. K. (1994). Life table analysis of stomal complications following colostomy. *Dis Colon Rectum* **37**: 916–20.

Lynne, C. M., Politano, V. A. and Cohen, R. L. (1974). Parastomal hernia causing anuria; unusual complication of ileal conduit diversion. *Urology* **4**: 603–4.

Marshall, F. F., Leadbetter, W. F. and Dretler, S. P. (1975). Ileal conduit parastomal hernias. *J Urol* **114**: 40–2.

Martin, L. and Foster, G. (1996). Parastomal hernia. *Ann R Coll Surg Engl* **78**: 81–4.

Maxson, R. T., Franklin, P. A. and Wagner, C. W. (1995). Malrotation in the older child: surgical management, treatment, and outcome. *Am Surg* **61**: 135–8.

Molloy, R. G., Moran, K. T., Waldron, R. P. *et al.* (1991). Massive incisional hernia: abdominal wall replacement with Marlex mesh. *Br J Surg 1991* **78**: 242–4.

Morris-Stiff, G. and Hughes, L. E. (1996). The continuing challenge of parastomal hernia: failure of a novel polypropylene mesh repair. *Ann R Coll Surg Engl* **80**: 184–7.

Newsom, B. D. and Kukora, J. S. (1986). Congenital and acquired internal hernias: unusual causes of small bowel obstruction. *Am J Surg* **152**: 279–85.

Ortiz, H., Sara, M. J., Armendariz, P. *et al.* (1994). Does the frequency of paracolostomy hernias depend on the position of the colostomy in the abdominal wall? *Int J Colorectal Dis* **9**: 65–7.

Ozenc, A., Ozdemir, A. and Coskun, T. (1998). Internal hernia in adults. *Int Surg* **83**: 167–70.

Rai, S., Chandra, S. S. and Smile, S. R. (1998). A study of the risk of strangulation and obstruction in groin hernias. *Aust NZ J Surg* **68**: 650–4.

Renvall, S. and Niinikoski, J. (1991). Internal hernias after gastric operations. *Eur J Surg* **157**: 575–7.

Rivkind, A. I., Shiloni, E., Muggia-Sullam, M. *et al.* (1986). Paracecal hernia: a cause of intestinal obstruction. *Dis Colon Rectum* **29**: 752–4.

Robbins, A. W. and Rutkow, I. M. (1998). Mesh plug repair and groin hernia surgery. *Surg Clin North Am* **78**: 1007–23.

Rubin, M. S., Schoetz, D. J. Jr and Matthews, J. B. (1994). Parastomal hernia. Is stoma relocation superior to fascial repair? *Arch Surg* **129**: 413–18.

Sandblom, G., Gruber, G., Kald, A. and Nilsson, E. (2000). Audit and recurrence rates after hernia surgery. *Eur J Surg* **166**: 154–8.

Schumpelick, V., Steinau, G., Schluper, I. and Prescher, A. (2000). Surgical embryology and anatomy of the diaphragm with surgical applications. *Surg Clin North Am* **80**: 213–39.

Shestak, K. C., Edington, H. J. and Johnson, R. R. (2000). The separation of anatomic components technique for the reconstruction of massive midline abdominal wall defects: anatomy, surgical technique, applications, and limitations revisited. *Plast Reconstr Surg* **105**: 731–8.

Toms, A. P., Dixon, A. K., Murphy, J. M. *et al.* (1999). Illustrated review of new imaging techniques in the diagnosis of abdominal wall hernias. *Br J Surg* **86**: 1243–9.

Vrijland, W., Jeekel, J., Steyerberg, E. W. *et al.* (2000). Intraperitoneal polypropylene mesh repair of incisional hernia is not associated with enterocutaneous fistula. *Br J Surg* **87**: 348–52.

White, T. J., Santos, M. C. and Thompson, J. S. (1998). Factors affecting wound complications in repair of ventral hernias. *Am Surg* **64**: 276–80.

Complications that develop in groin hernias (term covers inguinal and femoral)

Berliner, S. D. (1990). The femoral cone and its clinical implications. *Surg Gynecol Obstet* **171**: 111–14.

Harrison, L. A., Keesling, C. A., Martin, N. L. *et al.* (1995). Abdominal wall hernias: review of herniography and correlation with cross-sectional imaging. *Radiographics* **15**: 315–32.

Papagrigoriadis, S., Browse, D. J. and Howard, E. R. (1998). Incarceration of umbilical hernias in children: a rare but important complication. *Pediatr Surg Int* **14**: 231–2.

Ramachandran, C. S. (1998). Umbilical hernial defects encountered before and after abdominal laparoscopic procedures. *Int Surg* **83**: 171–3.

Sanchez-Bustos, F., Ramia, J. M. and Fernandez Ferrero, F. (1998). Prosthetic repair of femoral hernia: audit of long term follow-up. *Eur J Surg* **164**: 191–3.

Skandalakis, L. J., Androulakis, J., Colborn, G. L. and Skandalakis, J. E. (2000). Obturator hernia. Embryology, anatomy, and surgical applications. *Surg Clin North Am* **80**: 71–84.

Trotter, J. F. and Suhocki, P. V. (1999). Incarceration of umbilical hernia following transjugular intrahepatic portosystemic shunt for the treatment of ascites. *Liver Transpl Surg* **5**: 209–10.

MODULE 7

Disorders of the oesophagus

Section 7.1 • Anatomy and physiology of the oesophagus

Embryology of the oesophagus

The oesophagus starts to develop in the fourth week of embryonic development from the foregut immediately caudal to the primordial pharynx and extends to the fusiform dilatation in the foregut, this time to become the stomach. The oesophagus is short initially but it elongates rapidly due to the growth and descent of the heart and lungs, reaching its final relative length by the seventh week. As the laryngo-tracheal groove grows from the ventral wall of the primordial pharynx, longitudinal tracheo-oesophageal folds grow and approach each other to fuse and form a septum between the developing trachea and oesophagus. Incomplete fusion of the tracheo-oesophageal folds results in a defective tracheo-oesophageal septum and fistula formation. By the fifth week of development the oesophageal epithelium is two cells thick and is composed of columnar cells, which develop cilia by 10 weeks. The epithelium lining proliferates and partly or completely obliterates the lumen by the eighth week of development and large vacuoles appear in the centre. In succeeding weeks the vacuoles coalesce and the oesophageal lumen re-canalizes but with a multi-layered ciliated epithelium. During the fourth month this epithelium finally becomes replaced with the stratified squamous epithelium that characterizes the mature oesophagus. Failure of re-canalization of the oesophagus in this period results in oesophageal atresia and possibly oesophageal stenosis. Surrounding the oesophageal epithelium, layers of muscle begin to differentiate from the mesoderm. The inner circle of muscular layer is recognizable by 5 weeks of gestation and the outer longitudinal layer of muscle begins to take shape by 8 weeks of gestation. The striated muscle in the superior third of the oesophagus is derived from mesenchyme in the caudal pharyngeal arches, whereas the smooth muscle in the inferior third of the oesophagus develops from the surrounding splanchnic mesenchyme. Both types of muscle are innervated by branches of the vagus nerve, which supply the caudal pharyngeal arches. A dorsal mesentery more developed inferiorly connects the oesophagus to the developing aorta and may, on occasion, have smooth muscle remnants in adult life. Vagal trunks run alongside the oesophagus, but as the stomach rotates to the right, the right vagus assumes a posterior position and the left trunk crosses the lower oesophagus to lie anterior to the oesophagogastric junction. The oesophagus attains its final length at the seventh week of gestation, having a length at birth of 8–10 cm.

Anatomy of the oesophagus

The oesophagus is a hollow muscular tube, which is about 25 cm long, and connects the pharynx to the stomach. It commences in the neck, level with the lower border of the cricoid cartilage (sixth cervical vertebra), and descends mainly anterior to the vertebral column traversing the diaphragm at the level of the tenth thoracic vertebra, ending in the abdomen at the cardiac orifice of the stomach, at the level of the eleventh thoracic vertebra. Topographically, the oesophagus is generally vertical but has two shallow curves. Immediately below the pharynx it is a midline structure but inclines to the left as far as the root of the neck, gradually returning to the midline near the fifth thoracic vertebra, and deviates to the left again at the seventh thoracic vertebra, finally turning anteriorly as it traverses the diaphragm. The oesophagus also curves in a coronal plane, to follow the cervical and thoracic curvatures of the vertebral column. The surgical relevance of these deviations is that the cervical oesophagus is best approached from the left side of the neck, and the thoracic portion through the right side of the thorax, except the lower third (below the thoracic arch) which is more accessible from the left thorax.

The oesophagus is arbitrarily divided into three segments.

The cervical part (5 cm long) is behind the trachea and attached to it by loose areolar tissue. It lies in front of the pre-vertebral fascia, separated from it by loose areolar tissue. The recurrent laryngeal nerves ascend on each side in the groove between the trachea and the oesophagus. The left recurrent laryngeal nerve is positioned closer to the oesophagus than the right one as it ascends along the oesophagus for a larger distance. The cervical oesophagus commences with cricopharyngeus muscle at the inferior portion of the inferior pharyngeal constrictor, clearly identified by its transverse fibres. Just above the cricopharyngeus, the transition between the oblique fibres of the inferior constrictor muscle and the transverse fibres of cricopharyngeus creates a point of potential weakness termed Killian's dehiscence, which is the site of origin of a pharyngo-oesophageal (Zenker's) diverticulum (Figure 7.1). Cricopharyngeus muscle fibres blend into the longitudinal and circular muscles of the cervical oesophagus.

The thoracic oesophagus runs in the superior mediastinum between the trachea and the vertebral column, passing behind and to the right of the aortic arch to descend in the posterior mediastinum along the right side of the descending thoracic aorta as it proceeds behind the pericardium overlying the left atrium. The oesophagus then deviates further to the left and anteriorly entering the oesophageal diaphragmatic hiatus at the level of the tenth thoracic vertebra. On either side the thoracic oesophagus is bound by the parietal pleura. Clinically, the thoracic oesophagus is divided into three parts. The upper thoracic oesophagus extends from the cricopharyngeus to the level of the carina. The middle thoracic oesophagus extends from the level of the carina to halfway between the carina and the oesophago-gastric junction and the lower thoracic oesophagus from halfway between the carina and the oesophago-gastric junction to include the lower third of the oesophagus. Oncologically, the thoracic oesophagus is divided into the supra-carinal oesophagus (upper oesophagus) and the infra-carinal oesophagus (middle and lower oesophagus).

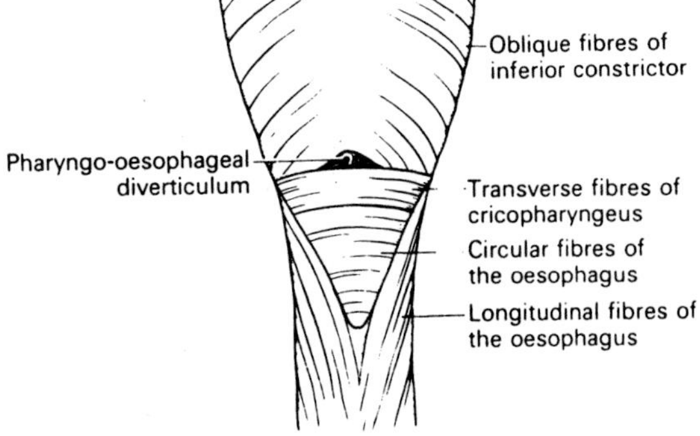

Figure 7.1 Diagrammatic representation of the posterior aspect of the upper oesophagus and pharynx showing Killian's dehiscence as the longitudinal fibres of the oesophagus sweep anteriorly. The pharyngo-oesophageal diverticulum emerges between the oblique fibres of the inferior constrictor and the transverse fibres of the cricopharyngeus.

The abdominal oesophagus emerges from the right diaphragmatic crus slightly to the left of the midline at the level of the tenth thoracic vertebra. It forms an inverted cone (1–2 cm in length) which curves sharply to the left and its base continuous with the gastric cardiac orifice. It is covered by peritoneum on its front and left side, and the peritoneum reflected from its posterior surface to the diaphragm is part of the gastrophrenic ligament. Behind it is the left crus of the diaphragm.

Oesophageal attachments

The oesophagus is loosely bound to adjacent structures by fibro-areolar tissue throughout its course except at the upper and lower ends. Superiorly, the longitudinal muscle fibres of the oesophagus are inserted into the cricoid cartilage. The lower attachments consist of serous reflections and the phreno-oesophageal membrane. The subdiaphragmatic pleural reflection is continuous with the mediastinal pleura and is separated from the lower segment of the oesophagus by a condensation of the endothoracic fascia which constitutes the phreno-oesophageal membrane. This important fibro-elastic membrane fixes the lower gullet but permits its continuous vertical displacement as occurs with respiration. The phreno-oesophageal membrane consists of a superior and an inferior limb. The latter is inserted into the cardia and the superior limb into the lower 3 cm of the thoracic oesophagus. The fibres of the membrane are disposed in bundles and lamelli and are inserted deeply into the oesophageal walls, some reaching the submucous layer. Approximately 40–60% of the fibres are made of elastin. The membrane has both strength and resilience, which are necessary to cope with the continuous movement of the hiatus during life. The phreno-oesophageal membrane is easily identified during mobilization of the oesophagus.

Structure of the oesophagus

The oesophagus consists of four layers. The fibrous adventitia is irregular, and consists of loose, areolar connective tissue containing elastin fibres. The looseness permits considerable movement of the oesophagus during swallowing. The fibres penetrate and surround the fasciculae of muscle in the deeper layers. The muscular layer is composed of an outer thicker longitudinal and inner circular layer. The longitudinal fibres surround the whole length of the oesophagus with a continuous coat except postero-superiorly where the longitudinal fibres separate and sweep round to the anterior aspect of the oesophagus before their insertion into the posterior aspect of the cricoid cartilage. The V-shaped interval between these fasciculae is filled by cricopharyngeus above and circular muscle fibres below. The potential weak area posteriorly may become the site of acquired pulsion diverticulae (Zenker's above and Laimer's below). A natural constriction occurs at this point due to the presence of the hypopharyngeal fold and the cricopharyngeus muscle. Accessory slips of non-striated muscle sometimes pass between the oesophagus and left pleura or the root of the left principal bronchus, trachea, pericardium or aorta. The circular fibres are continuous with those of the cricopharyngeus superiorly and with the oblique gastric muscle fibres inferiorly. The two muscle layers of the upper quarter of the oesophagus are striated. Below this there is a gradual replacement with smooth muscle. Although similar in appearance to striated skeletal muscle it is not under voluntary control but rather under autonomic nervous control. At the lower end of the oesophagus, the circular muscle layer is thickened but a definite anatomical sphincter is not present. The external longitudinal muscle of the oesophagus continues longitudinally along the gastric greater and lesser curvatures. These muscle bundles turn upwards towards the fundus, interlacing with fibres of the internal muscle layer. The circular muscle layer of the lowermost portion of the oesophagus becomes semi-circular (clasps) and continues down the lesser curvature aspect of the cardia to insert in the submucosal connective tissue on the opposite side. Gastric sling fibres are also semi-circular in the opposite direction and at an oblique angle to the posterior attachments of the oesophageal semi-circular muscles.

The submucosa is very loose in order to permit dilatation of the oesophagus during swallowing. It loosely connects mucosal and muscular layers and contains large blood vessels, nerves and mucous glands. The mucosa is made of non-keratinized squamous epithelium, which is arranged in longitudinal folds especially at the lower end where the oesophageal mucosal folds form a rosette. The mucosal layer consists of the lining epithelium, connective tissue with papilli (lamina propria) and non-striated muscularis mucosa. At the upper oesophagus the muscularis mucosa is absent or sparse and becomes a considerable stratum below this. At intermediate levels its fascicles are mainly longitudinal but become more plexiform towards the gastro-oesophageal junction. There are small oesophageal glands of compound racimose mucous type in the submucosa deep to the muscularis mucosas each with a long duct traversing it and the other layers of the mucosa. Glands of the abdominal portion of the oesophagus resemble gastric cardia glands and lie superficial to the muscularis mucosa.

The cardio-oesophageal junction

This consists of the supra-diaphragmatic portion, the inferior oesophageal constriction, the vestibule and the cardia (Figure 7.2). Radiologically the supra-diaphrag-

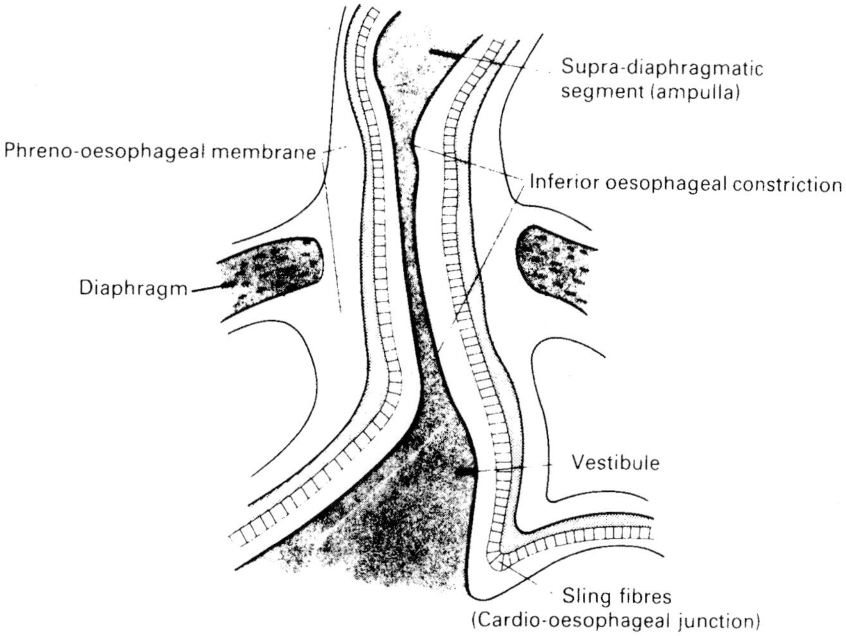

Figure 7.2 Diagrammatic representation of the anatomy of the lower oesophagus. (Reproduced from Hennessy and Cuschieri, 1992, *Surgery of the Oesophagus*, 2nd edn, Butterworth Heineman, Oxford, by permission.)

matic portion consists of an ampulla and the empty segment just distal to it. The ampulla is not an anatomical dilatation and is caused by the primary peristaltic wave (during a contrast examination) acting in conjunction with the negative intra-thoracic pressure, which momentarily expand the segment just before the lower oesophageal sphincter (LOS) relaxes. (Note: in the USA, lower esophageal sphincter would be abbreviated as LES.) The inferior oesophageal constriction consists of a concentric narrowing of the oesophageal lumen at the level of the diaphragmatic hiatus. On average, it is situated some 2 cm from the cardio-oesophageal junction. It is not synonymous with the LES although the sphincter region extends to include this area. The longitudinal oesophageal mucosal folds are very prominent inside the inferior constriction but disappear readily when the oesophagus is distended. The intra-abdominal segment of the oesophagus is also known as the vestibule. It is often described as an inverted funnel or cone which inclines to the left before joining the stomach at an angle (cardiac angle or angle of His). When viewed endoscopically from within the stomach it forms a well-marked ridge at the left margin of the gastro-oesophageal junction, which is occasionally referred to as the incisura. The cardia denotes the junction between the oesophagus and stomach. The only reliable and constant anatomical landmark of this is made by the slim or oblique muscle fibres of the stomach but these cannot be identified endoscopically. Clinically the term cardia is used to describe the junction between the oesophagus and stomach. It contains the squamo-columnar junction, which forms the serrated Z-line marking an abrupt change from the tough smooth pale squamous epithelium of oesophagus to the epithelium of the stomach. A zone of junctional epithelium is interposed between the squamous lining of the oesophagus and the gastric mucosa. It is lined by columnar cells which contain simple tubular mucosal glands which are superficial to the muscularis mucosa and hence resistant to acid and peptic digestion.

Vascular supply, venous and lymphatic drainage

The oesophagus receives a segmental arterial supply from several small arterioles throughout its course. These come from the inferior thyroid, common carotid, costocervical and vertebral arteries in the neck, bronchial and direct aortic branches in the thorax, and branches of the left gastric and left inferior phrenic artery at the lower end including the abdominal portion. The arterioles terminate in a fine capillary network before penetrating the oesophageal muscle layer. After penetrating and supplying the oesophageal muscle layer, the arterioles join a capillary plexus in the submucosa. These capillary networks run longitudinally in the submucosa allowing mobilization of segments of the oesophagus without compromise to the blood supply. The venous drainage is to the inferior thyroid and hypopharyngeal veins in the neck, the azygos, hemi-

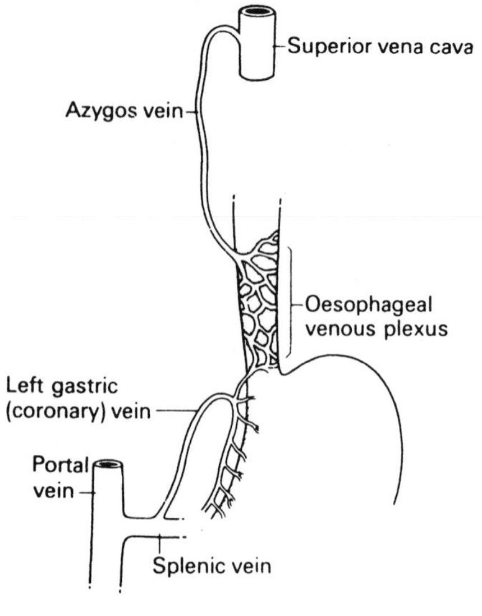

Figure 7.3 Venous drainage of the lower oesophagus.

azygos and intercostal veins in the chest, except at the lower end which drains into the left gastric vein (Figure 7.3). The lower oesophagus is clinically the most important site of communication between the portal and systemic venous radicles, being the site of occurrence of varices in the majority of patients with portal hypertension. In the lower oesophagus the veins are mainly situated within the lamina propria whereas in the more proximal oesophagus and stomach they reside in the submucous plane. This is held responsible for the propensity of the lower oesophagus to bleed in variceal portal hypertension. The lymphatics form extensive mucosal (lamina propria), submucosal, muscularis and adventitial plexuses which communicate freely, and lymph flows long distances in the large submucosal plexus before passing through the muscular coat to reach the adventitial plexus and draining lymph nodes. These are grouped into three main tiers: the first is composed of nodes alongside the oesophagus (para-oesophageal), the second or intermediate group is made up of mediastinal lymph nodes, and the third are the deep cervical, supraclavicular, tracheo-bronchial and coeliac nodes from above downwards. In general, lymph drainage from the upper two-thirds of the oesophagus proceeds in a proximal direction towards the cervical region whereas the lower third drains distally to the subdiaphragmatic region and coeliac lymph nodes. In view of the anatomical distribution and communication of oesophageal lymphatics, oncological resection should include 10 cm above and below the tumour. Lymphatic drainage of the gastro-oesophageal junction mainly follows the arteries supplying the junction.

The thoracic duct arises from the cysterna chyli, which lies in the abdomen to the right of the aorta, approximately at the level of the second lumbar vertebra. The duct enters the chest through the aortic hiatus coursing in the posterior mediastinum to the right of the midline between the aorta and the azygos vein behind the oesophagus. At the level of the fifth thoracic vertebra, it crosses behind the oesophagus to the left under the aortic arch and continues along the left side of the oesophagus, ascending behind the left subclavian artery to the base of the neck. There, it curves to the right and caudally to drain into the internal jugular vein near its junction with the left subclavian vein. The majority of people have a single thoracic duct and the remainder have two or more ducts.

Nerve supply of the oesophagus

Two plexuses of nerves in the oesophageal wall (Meissner's plexus in the submucosa and Auerbach's plexus in the muscularis) form networks of multipolar ganglion cells, the processes of which are in contact with one another and receive axons from the vagus. Post-ganglionic fibres of these plexuses innervate the smooth muscle cells. Post-ganglionic sympathetic fibres from the prevertebral ganglia enter the plexuses without synapsing to reach the muscles of the blood vessels of the oesophageal wall.

Swallowing and oesophageal motility are co-ordinated by the swallowing centre in the brain stem. This is an area in the medulla oblongata and lower portion of the pons, which is closely associated with the tractus solitarius. It receives and co-ordinates sensory inputs from peripheral mechanoreceptors in the pharynx and oesophagus. Motor impulses that initiate the swallowing reflex are transmitted from the swallowing centre to the pharynx and upper oesophagus via the trigeminal, glossopharyngeal, vagus and hypoglossal nerves.

The nerve supply of the oesophagus is parasympathetic (vagal) and sympathetic. The parasympathetic fibres, which are predominantly motor, are derived from neurones of the vagal motor nuclei and travel in the glossopharyngeal, vagus and recurrent laryngeal nerves terminating in the myenteric plexus. The sensory component is formed by axons of the nodose ganglion, the cells of which are unipolar with their peripheral axons transmitted via the sensory portion of the trigeminal and glossopharyngeal nerves, which terminate in receptors situated in the pharynx and oesophagus. The central axons of the cells of the nodose ganglion communicate with the swallowing centre in the brain stem.

The sympathetic nerve supply consists of preganglionic fibres derived from neurones situated in the intermediolateral columns of spinal cord segments T5 and T6 and terminate in the cervical, thoracic and coeliac ganglia. The post-ganglionic sympathetic fibres then reach the oesophagus as a periarterial plexus.

The rami reaching the oesophagus communicate with a plexus containing groups of ganglion cells between the two layers of the muscular coat, the myenteric plexus. The submucous plexus of the oesophagus is rather sparse and consists mainly of nerve fibres.

Endoscopic appearance of the oesophagus

The oesophagus proper starts just distal to the cricopharyngeus muscle at around 15 cm from the incisor teeth. The mucosa is pale and lacks lustre. The lumen is collapsed until insufflated with air and then the wall is smooth. There are a number of naturally occurring anatomical narrowings in the oesophagus. The cervical constriction occurs at the level of the cricopharyngeus muscle at approximately 15 cm from the incisor teeth. The next constriction is expected where the oesophagus is crossed by the aortic arch at 22 cm, by the left main bronchus at 27 cm, and where it passes through the diaphragmatic hiatus at the cardio-oesophageal junction at 37–40 cm from the incisors, depending on the sex and build of the patient. Although the left atrium is in front of the lower part of the oesophagus below the left main bronchus, it is only when the atrium is enlarged that it indents the oesophagus. At the cardio-oesophageal junction the stratified squamous epithelium is abruptly succeeded by gastric columnar epithelium, the junction is visible as a serrated line with the greyish pink smooth oesophageal mucosa contrasting with the red mamillated gastric mucosa.

Physiology of the oesophagus

The basic function of the oesophagus is to transport swallowed material from the pharynx into the stomach. It has little secretory function and no absorptive function. The pharynx is central to the swallowing complex. Besides other functions, the pharynx facilitates the propulsion of food for a few seconds at a time.

Conventionally, swallowing has been divided into three stages. The *voluntary stage* initiates the swallowing process. A food bolus is rolled (squeezed) posteriorly into the pharynx by pressure of the tongue upwards and backwards against the palate. Subsequently, the process of swallowing becomes automatic and involuntary. The *pharyngeal stage* constitutes the passage of food through the pharynx into the oesophagus. As food enters the pharynx it stimulates mechanoreceptors around the opening of the pharynx and on the tonsillar pillars. This stimulates a series of automatic pharyngeal muscular contractions. The soft palate is pulled upwards to close the posterior layers preventing reflux of food into the nasal cavities. The palato-pharyngeal folds on either side approximate each other to form a sagittal slit allowing properly masticated food to pass with ease and yet impeding the passage of large objects. The vocal chords are strongly approximated and the larynx is pulled upwards and posteriorly against the epiglottis, which swings backwards over the opening of the larynx. This prevents passage of food into the trachea. The upward movement of the larynx enlarges the opening of the oesophagus and stimulates relaxation of the tonically active upper oesophageal sphincter (crico-pharyngeus). As the larynx is raised and the upper oesophageal sphincter is relaxed the entire muscular wall of the pharynx contracts, beginning in the superior constrictor and spreading downwards as a rapid peristaltic wave over the middle and inferior constrictors and thence into the oesophagus. This peristaltic wave propels the food into the oesophagus. This stage of swallowing is principally a reflex act. It is almost always initiated by voluntary movement of food into the back of the mouth, which in turn elicits the swallowing reflex. The *oesophageal stage* is also involuntary and promotes passage of food from the pharynx to the stomach. Food is propelled down the oesophagus by peristaltic waves. Primary peristalsis is simply a continuation of the peristaltic wave that commenced in the pharynx and spreads into the oesophagus during the pharyngeal phase of swallowing. This wave passes all the way from the pharynx to the stomach in approximately 8 s. However, food swallowed in the upright position is usually transmitted down the oesophagus in about 5–8 s because of the additional effect of gravity. If the primary peristaltic wave fails to move all the food that has entered the oesophagus into the stomach secondary peristaltic waves result from the distension of the oesophagus by the retained food and these continue until all the food has emptied into the stomach. The secondary peristaltic waves are initiated partly by intrinsic neuronal circuits in the myenteric plexus and partly by reflexes that are transmitted through vagal fibres from the brain stem. It is important to note that a denervated oesophagus will continue to generate these secondary peristaltic waves in response to distension. The other type of contraction exhibited by the oesophagus is tertiary contractions which occur spontaneously and are non-propulsive. They are usually encountered in various oesophageal motility disorders but are also observed in apparently healthy individuals especially in older age. These tertiary contractions may be generalized involving the whole of the oesophageal body or localized. They are usually seen on a double contrast barium meal examination.

In between swallows the body of the oesophagus is flaccid and the lumen largely collapsed. However, both the upper and lower oesophageal sphincters are tonically contracted. The upper oesophageal sphincter (UOS, cricopharyngeus) is closed by tonic contraction induced through constant discharge from neurones originating in the cranial nuclei. (Note: in the USA, upper esophageal sphincter would be abbreviated UES.) The sphincter remains in tonic contraction with a resting pressure of about 100 mmHg. The physiological function of the sphincter is to prevent passage of air from the pharynx into the oesophagus and reflux of oesophageal contents into the pharynx. This reflex action is essentially protective and is aimed at preventing aspiration. In the resting state the oesophageal body has no motor activity. When stimulated by passage of food or saliva a contraction is initiated in the upper oesophagus, which progresses distally towards the stomach. Oesophageal peristaltic waves travel at 3–4 cm/s, last between 3 and 4.5 s, and reach a peak amplitude of 30 mmHg in the upper oesophagus which progressively gets larger as it travels down the oesophagus to around 120 mmHg in the lower oesophagus. In the resting state the pressure within the body of the oesophagus is similar to the intra-thoracic pressure, being negative during inspiration and reaching 5 mmHg during expiration. At the lower 2–4 cm of the oesophagus, a high-pressure zone (HPZ) is encountered. This is due to tonic contraction of the lower oesophageal sphincter (intrinsic component) and to mechanical factors (extrinsic component).

The intrinsic part of the HPZ constitutes the 2–4 cm tonically contracted segment just proximal to the gastro-oesophageal junction. Its normal resting tone ranges from 15 to 25 mmHg relative to intra-gastric pressure. Three-dimensional mapping of this region shows asymmetry of the pressure profile (Figure 7.4). The segment has a spontaneous tendency to relax periodically at times unrelated to swallowing. These periodic relaxations have been termed 'transient lower

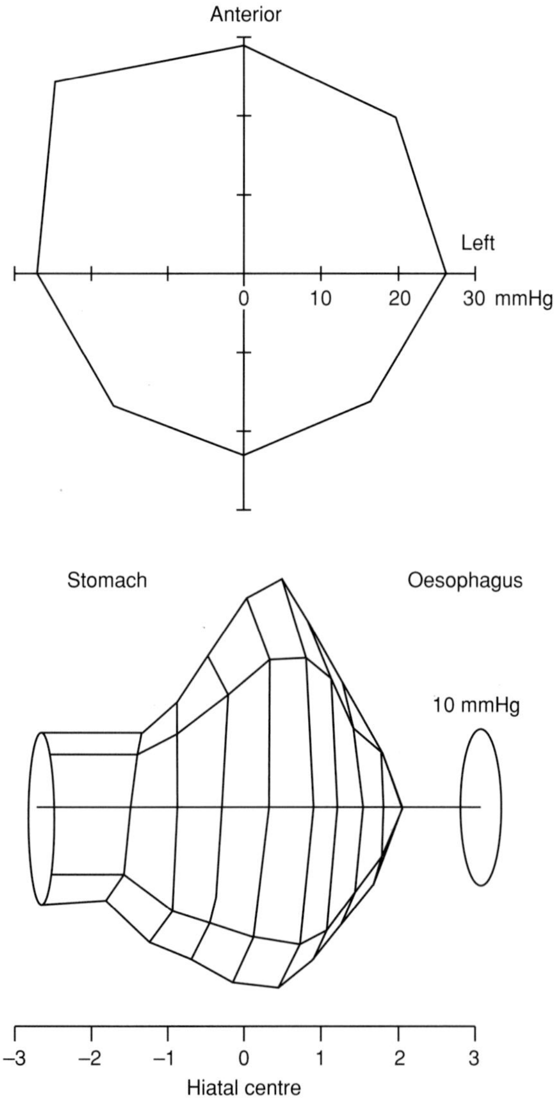

Figure 7.4 Radial (top) and axial (bottom) pressure profile of the gastro-oesophageal junction in an asymptomatic subject obtained using the technique of vector manometry. Position zero on the axial scale is the mid-point of the diaphragmatic hiatus.

oesophageal sphincter relaxations' (TLOSRs) to distinguish them from relaxations triggered by swallows. They account for the small amount of physiological reflux found in normal subjects. To allow a food bolus to enter the stomach, the LOS relaxes for 5–10 s and then tonic contraction returns. Relaxation is probably due to non-adrenergic non-cholinergic neurotransmitters such as vasoactive intestinal polypeptide (VIP) and nitric oxide. The resting tone is largely dependent on the intrinsic muscular activity because it persists after neural input is abolished by treatment with neurotoxins. During fasting the LOS has cyclic phasic contractile activity synchronous with phases 2 and 3 of the interdigestive motor complex. This is probably regulated by motilin, which acts on the LOS, by preganglionic stimulation of cholinergic nerves.

The extrinsic component is largely determined by contractions of the diaphragmatic crura. The increase in LOS pressure is mainly during inspiration and can be as much as 100 mmHg with maximum diaphragmatic contraction. This pinchcock action of the diaphragm is a protective mechanism against reflux induced by sudden increases in intra-abdominal pressure. This mechanism is obviated when a hiatal hernia is present.

Section 7.2 • Assessment of oesophageal disease

This includes a careful history, physical examination and appropriate investigations to establish the nature of the underlying pathology.

Symptoms

The presentation of oesophageal disease is often typical with one or more of the well-known classic symptoms. Atypical presentation is not, however, infrequent and oesophageal disease may be mistaken for cardiac and pulmonary disorders. In these patients differentiation is only possible after specialized investigations are carried out. A small cohort of patients with oesophageal symptoms have no abnormality on physical examination and intensive investigations. In some, but not all of these patients, the symptoms reflect a psycho-neurotic state. The typical symptoms of oesophageal disease are: dysphagia, regurgitation, odynophagia, chest pain and water brash.

Dysphagia

Difficulty in swallowing or a sensation of food bolus arrest or delay during swallowing may be due to mechanical obstruction or functional disorder. The patient feels the food sticking and often points to a particular site on the sternum although this does not correlate well with the exact anatomical location of the obstruction. Dysphagia for solids implies significant disease which may be mechanical or functional, whereas dysphagia for liquids only is more likely to be functional (oesophageal motility disorder). In the latter, difficulty with swallowing may be intermittent or its severity variable with exacerbations and periods of relative remission. Some patients with dysphagia find that food transit through the oesophagus can be facilitated by sipping fluid after each solid bolus or by repeated swallows and various postural manoeuvres such as expiration against a closed glottis (Valsalva). On the other hand, persistent and progressive dysphagia indicates mechanical narrowing of the oesophageal lumen. This is usually associated with regurgitation and is not relieved by sipping fluids or repeated swallowing. Eventually, with progression to total dysphagia, the patient is unable to swallow saliva and exhibits constant drooling. In obstructive dysphagia, the symptom begins when 20–30% of the oesophageal lumen is lost and patients usually present when 50% of the oesophageal lumen is compromised.

The sensation of a substernal lump (globus)

When this is present a short period after eating or when fasting it is termed 'globus hystericus'. It is a neurotic symptom in patients with emotional instability but requires thorough examination to exclude organic disease. Dysphagia is never an expression of a purely psychiatric disorder. However, some patients with well-established oesophageal disease may report that their dysphagia is worse during severe emotional periods.

Regurgitation

This symptom results from regurgitation of gastric or oesophageal fluid into the throat accompanied by a sour taste in the mouth. It is often postural and occurs predominantly in the supine position especially at night, with the regurgitated material often staining the pillow. Postural regurgitation, which is a very common symptom of reflux disease, is precipitated by meals and activities associated with a rise in the intra-abdominal pressure, i.e. bending and straining. Regurgitation may also occur as an overflow phenomenon due to the accumulation of food in the oesophagus proximal to a stenosing lesion. This spillback into the pharynx and mouth at night may lead to aspiration pneumonitis. In oesophageal motility disorders both overflow and postural regurgitation may occur, although the former is more commonly encountered in these conditions.

Odynophagia

This complaint consists of localized pain, usually in the lower sternal region, which occurs immediately on swallowing certain foods or liquids. It always indicates organic disease, most commonly oesophagitis. Hot drinks, acid citrus beverages, coffee and heavily spiced foods are among the most frequent dietary items which induce this symptom. It can be severe enough to condition patients not to eat or drink the offending item, or food in general. Odynophagia can be seen after involvement of the mucosa by reflux, radiation, viral or fungal infections. Less commonly odynophagia can be a manifestation of ulceration or cancer of the oesophagus.

Heartburn

This is the most common manifestation of oesophageal disease and may occur in up to 50% of the population. It is due to reflux of gastric juice, which is injurious to the oesophageal mucosa. The chemical injury is accentuated by a defective clearing of the refluxate by the oesophagus consequent on an impaired motility. This increases the contact time of the acid and any other injurious substance (e.g. bile salts) with the oesophageal mucosa. Some patients complain of severe heartburn, yet on endoscopy there is little or no evidence of inflammation. These individuals may still have reflux with an abnormal oesophageal mucosal sensitivity. Heartburn is often worsened by recumbency and increase in intra-abdominal pressure, and may follow fatty meals or alcoholic beverages. Heartburn is usually relieved, even temporarily, by taking antacids. This symptom can increase in intensity until it is perceived as chest pain.

Chest pain

Oesophageal anterior chest pain is often described as a tightening or gripping pain, which closely simulates angina pectoris. Thus it may radiate to the back, jaw, arm and ear and may even be relieved by sublingual nitrates. This type of pain is commonly found in patients with reflux oesophagitis or oesophageal motility disorders. It may occur in association with meals when it persists for about an hour after eating, but is also experienced in the fasting state and is frequently precipitated by emotion and exercise.

Water brash

This symptom is uncommon and is restricted to patients with reflux disease. It is due to excessive salivation, the mouth becoming full of fluid, which has a salty taste, clear and frothy.

Atypical presentation of oesophageal disease

Patients with oesophageal disease may present with anaemia due to chronic blood loss and, less commonly, with acute upper gastrointestinal bleeding (haematemesis, melena). Chronic blood loss is usually due to erosive oesophagitis and active bleeding results from the Mallory–Weiss syndrome or peptic ulceration in a hiatus hernia. Incarceration and strangulation of a para-oesophageal hiatus hernia and spontaneous perforation of the oesophagus (Boerhaave syndrome) present acutely with a severe life-threatening illness.

Reference has already been made to the frequently encountered difficulty in distinguishing oesophageal from cardiac pain. Often, patients are treated for angina for a while until persistence/aggravation of symptoms indicates the need for coronary angiography. Approximately 20–40% of patients with chest pain and normal coronary angiography are subsequently found to have oesophageal disease.

Presentation with pulmonary symptoms is common. These include attacks of coughing, choking and repeated chest infections due to aspiration pneumonitis in patients with overflow or postural regurgitation. The chest radiograph shows areas of consolidation, abscess formation and pleural effusion. Furthermore, intrinsic asthma is often exacerbated by gastro-oesophageal reflux with aspiration particularly in infants and children. Effective treatment of the reflux disease is often followed by a considerable improvement in the asthmatic condition of these patients.

Physical signs

The oesophagus is a mediastinal structure and is inaccessible to physical examination. However, patients presenting with oesophageal diseases may have physical signs, which should be sought during the examination. These include evidence of weight loss; pallor due to anaemia; swelling in the neck due to pharyngeal pouch; enlarged lymph nodes in the left supra-clavicular or cervical regions; chest signs on auscultation and percussion of the lung fields; epigastric mass due to carcinoma of the cardia enlarging downwards, hepatomegaly with or without clinical jaundice; tylosis of the hands and/or feet.

Investigations for oesophageal diseases

These are outlined in Table 7.1. Some of the physiological tests require special expertise in their execution and interpretation and are therefore only available in major or specialist centres. In addition to these investigations, tests to exclude cardiac disease, e.g. electrocardiogram at rest and after exercise and coronary angiography, may be necessary in a subset of patients who present with episodes of anterior chest pain.

Radiology

Chest radiography

This time-honoured investigation continues to be necessary in all patients admitted acutely with oesophageal symptoms to detect or exclude aspiration pneumonitis, mediastinal widening which may suggest nodal involvement in patients with oesophageal and other malignancies and, in addition, to outline any soft tissue shadows and fluid gas levels (intra-thoracic stomach, achalasia). In patients with suspected oesophageal perforations or suture line dehiscence after an oesophagectomy, a chest radiograph to detect mediastinal emphysema and pleural effusion is an essential investigation which should be performed before contrast studies. A plain chest radiograph should serve as a background study against which contrast radiographs can be compared.

Contrast radiology

The standard contrast investigation is the barium swallow, which is particularly useful in the following categories of patients:

- Patients with dysphagia from any cause.
- Patients with gastro-oesophageal reflux should have this investigation to determine the presence or absence of a hiatus hernia and to exclude oesophageal shortening.
- Patients with previous surgery to the oesophagus or oesophagogastric junction.
- Patients with known benign or malignant strictures about to undergo surgery or endoscopic therapeutic manoeuvres.

Table 7.1 Investigations for oesophageal disease

Category	*Test*	*Indications*
Radiological	Chest radiograph	Aspiration pneumonitis, oesophageal perforation
	Contrast swallow	Dysphagia, perforation, motility disorders
	Cine-radiology	Motility disorders, reflux disease
	CT scanning	Staging of malignant disease
Ultrasound scanning	External	Motility disorders, reflux disease
	Endoscopic	Staging of malignant disease
Radio-isotope studies	Labelled liquid or solid bolus studies	Oesophageal transit, reflux disease
Endoscopy	Fibreoptic, rigid + biopsy, cytology	All patients with oesophageal symptoms, especially dysphagia
Physiological	Stationary manometry	Pre-pH metry, reflux disease
	Ambulatory manometry	Oesophageal motility disorders, non-cardiac chest pain
	Acid perfusion test (Bernstein's test)	Oesophageal sensitivity to acid
	24 hour pH monitoring	Reflux disease
	Bilitec	Alkaline reflux disease

In the standard barium meal test, reflux of barium into the oesophagus may be observed in the upright position and is always significant. Screening with the patient in the Trendelenberg supine position is conventionally used to enhance and therefore better detect this reflux. However, radiological demonstration of reflux in this way is present in 20% of individuals without oesophagitis and radiological reflux is absent in 40% of patients with moderate to severe oesophagitis. The use of the barium swallow in the detection of gastro-oesophageal reflux is therefore inadequate. Its main value lies in the demonstration of an associated hiatus hernia, which is present in some patients, and in detecting the extent and severity of stricture formation. Although oesophagitis can be detected with special radiological contrast techniques designed to obtain details of the mucosa, barium swallow is distinctly inferior to endoscopy in establishing this diagnosis. A contrast swallow is an essential investigation in patients suspected of oesophageal perforation or leaking oesophageal anastomosis. Because extravasated barium can cause granuloma formation and because once extravasated into tissues, it remains for the rest of the patient's life, most radiologists prefer a water-soluble contrast medium in the first instance and proceed to diluted barium only if the diagnosis is still in doubt. Water-soluble contrast media are iodine-containing contrast media with the iodine being radio-opaque. In the event of a perforation, the contrast medium finds its way into either the mediastinal or peritoneal cavity and is absorbed and finally excreted via the kidneys. Evidence suggests the absence of irritant effects on the peritoneal membranes, nor do they exacerbate established inflammation. They are, however, hypertonic and may lead to serious complications, which include electrolyte imbalance and significant fluid shifts. In addition, the iodine base may be allergenic and merits particular careful consideration in the case of latent hyperthyroid disease. However, they are fully absorbed from the gastrointestinal tract and because of their high osmolality may occasionally cause diarrhoea, which ceases as soon as the intestine has been emptied. Gastrografin (meglumine diatrozoate) is the conventional water-soluble contrast medium for examination of the upper gastrointestinal tract. It is an ionic contrast medium with high osmolality and aspiration of gastrografin into the lungs may cause pulmonary oedema. Caution is needed with tracheo-oesophageal fistulae to avoid passage of the medium into the lungs. Gastromyro (iopamidol, flavoured niopam) is a contrast medium belonging to the new generation of non-ionic compounds whose solubility is due to the presence of hydrophilic substituents in the molecule. This results in a solution of low osmolality when compared with ionic media. Due to this property it has a good margin of safety for examinations in which there is the risk of accidental aspiration of the diagnostic medium or its introduction into the lung via a fistula.

Barium meal is an essential investigation in the evaluation of patients with dysphagia. The barium meal examination may provide evidence for a mechanical obstructive lesion (Figure 7.5). However, importantly it provides a record of the extent and length of the stricture and any angulation or tortuosity. This becomes useful in evaluating the length of a tumour and when dilating a benign stricture. In motility disorders, barium meal examination excludes a mechanical obstruction and may show characteristic features of a motility disorder such as achalasia. A barium-marshmallow swallow or bread and barium swallow is also useful in delineating peristaltic progress in the oesophagus.

Fluoroscopy/video-radiology

The use of cine-fluoroscopy/video recording is largely restricted to the investigation of patients with cricopharyngeal dysfunction and oesophageal motility disorders. The three phases of swallowing can be identified with remarkable accuracy and any deviations from the normal pattern are illustrated, evaluated and compared after treatment. Fluoroscopy plays but a minor role in the evaluation of oesophageal motility disorders. Its

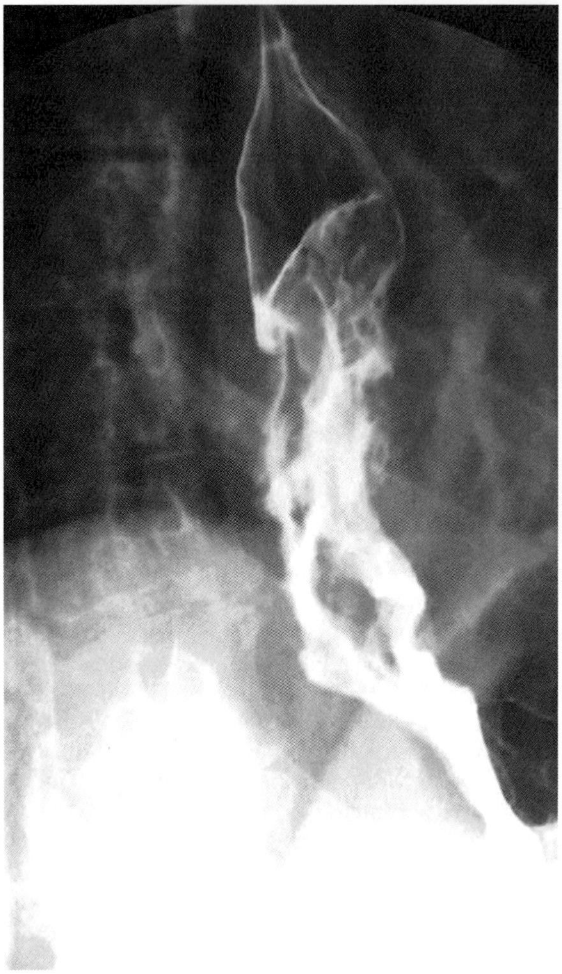

Figure 7.5 Barium swallow showing a large exophytic tumour in the lower oesophagus in a patient presenting with dysphagia.

value is limited to the exclusion of mechanical obstruction in the oesophagus and oesophagogastric junction.

CT scanning

Reports on the use of CT scanning have confirmed its general usefulness in the pre-operative assessment of oesophageal malignancy (Figure 7.6). The extent of mural invasion and the size of the lesion are sufficiently accurate. The accuracy of CT scanning in determination of the involvement of adjacent structures has been controversial. Signs of adjacent structure-tumour invasion include budding, deformation or growth extension beyond the structure. Aortic invasion can be predicted with accuracy if there is an excess of 90° contact between the circumference of the aorta and the tumour. Loss of the paravertebral fat space in the triangle formed by the aorta, oesophagus and vertebral body is another accurate sign of invasion of the aorta. CT is inaccurate in predicting diaphragmatic invasion. In addition, CT is not reliable in detecting lymphadenopathy and it is impossible to differentiate nodal deposits from reactive lymphadenopathy. This applies to both mediastinal, subdiaphragmatic and cervical lymph nodes. CT is however useful in the detection of distant metastases (Figure 7.7). The overall accuracy in detecting metastases is more than 80%. CT is also sufficiently accurate for the detection of pulmonary metastases but small peritoneal deposits are not usually recognized by CT.

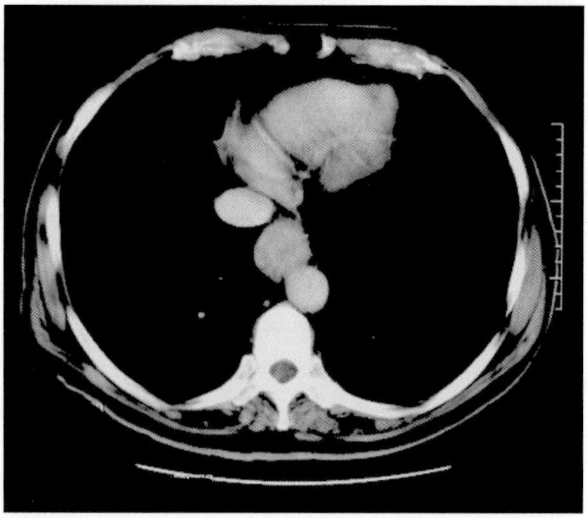

Figure 7.6 A CT scan of the lower chest showing a large tumour in the lower oesophagus which is adherent to the thoracic aorta making the tumour unresectable.

Ultrasound scanning

Screening for diaphragmatic respiratory movement by real time ultrasound has largely replaced X-ray fluoroscopy for this purpose. Paralysis of one hemidiaphragm with paradoxical movement results from phrenic nerve paralysis and indicates advanced inoperable intramediastinal malignancy (oesophageal and bronchial carcinoma). Endoscopic ultrasonography (EUS) has rapidly been established as a very accurate technique for the assessment of the extent of intramural involvement and enlargement of adjacent lymph nodes. Ultrasound probes between 7.5 and 12 MHz frequency forming an integral part of the endoscope are used for this purpose. The wall of the oesophagus is seen as a five-layer structure. The first two layers correspond to the superficial and deep mucosa, the third layer to the submucosa, the fourth layer to the muscularis propria and the fifth layer to the adventitia. Endoscopic ultrasound provides sufficient information on lymph nodes so that rounded sharply demarcated homogeneous hypoechoic lymph nodes are most likely malignant. The overall accuracy in the detection of malignant lymph nodes is in excess of 80%. If the tumour is sufficiently stenotic to preclude the passage of the endosonography probe then the tumour can be dilated to enable this. Endosonographic imaging of the proximal end of the tumour without dilatation is not sufficiently accurate. New small diameter (2–3 mm) endosonographic probes are currently marketed and

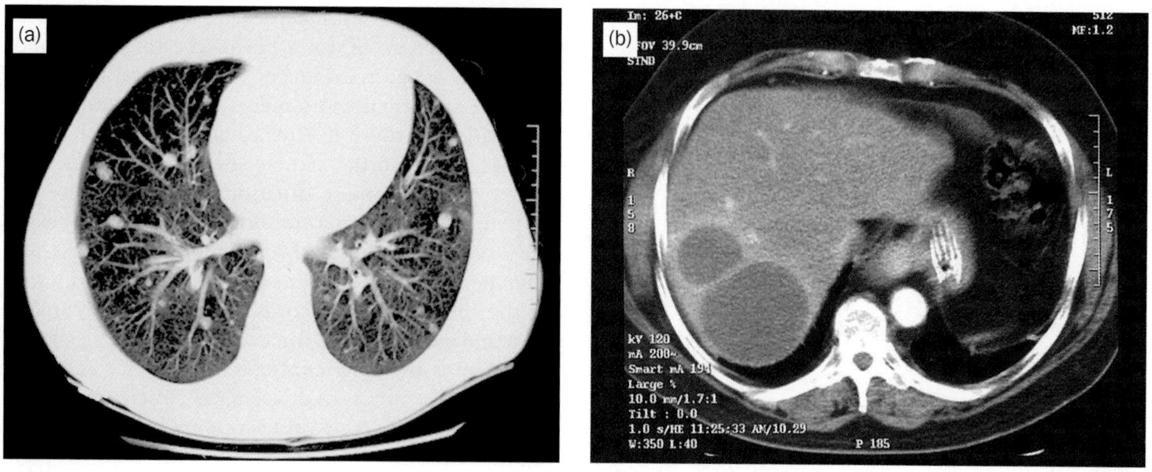

Figure 7.7 (a) CT scan of the thorax showing bilateral pulmonary metastases from primary oesophageal cancer; (b) CT scan of the upper abdomen showing large hepatic metastases from primary oesophageal cancer.

may overcome this difficulty. Tumour stenosis however is by itself a sign associated with advanced tumour stage.

Radio-isotope studies

These are used to evaluate oesophageal transit of liquid and solid boluses in individuals with motility disorders. When a labelled liquid bolus is used, the patient is placed in the supine position and swallows on demand the labelled liquid previously held in the mouth. Normal individuals clear 90% of the liquid from the oesophagus into the stomach in 4–15 s. A more physiological modification employs the use of a standardized solid bolus, which is swallowed by the patient in the erect position. The bolus consists of 10 ml poached egg-white labelled with ^{99m}Tc pertechnitate. External scintiscanning is started as the patient swallows the chewed bolus. The normal transit time for this test is 10 s. Special software can generate time versus radioactivity curves, which outline transit in the upper, middle and lower thirds separately in addition to the total oesophageal transit. Using row summation, a condensed image can also be generated. This outlines graphically the spatial arrangement of the labelled egg-white bolus (vertical axis) with respect to time on the horizontal axis (Figure 7.8). Prolonged transit times are encountered in oesophageal motility disorders with an oscillatory pattern encountered in achalasia (Figure 7.9). The condensed image shows a striking sinuous outline resulting from the up and down oscillations of the bolus in patients with achalasia and diffuse oesophageal spasm.

Endoscopy

Flexible endoscopy has largely replaced rigid oesophogoscopy because it provides better visualization, is safer and permits concomitant examination of the stomach. With the endoscope in the stomach and the use of the J-manoeuvre, the cardiac orifice can be inspected which is not possible with the rigid endoscope (Figure 7.10). Fibre-optic endoscopy is essential in all patients with dysphagia. It provides direct visual information on the presence or absence of pathology. Both biopsy and brush cytology are used in the diagnosis of oesophageal malignancy and their combined accuracy rate is 96% which is better than the accuracy of either test alone. Cytology appears to be more reliable in stenosing lesions whereas endoscopic biopsy carries a higher positive yield in exophytic tumours. Endoscopic biopsies are also necessary in the diagnosis and histological grading of reflux oesophagitis and in the detection of Barrett's epithelium and its surveillance in patients with long-standing reflux disease. Rigid

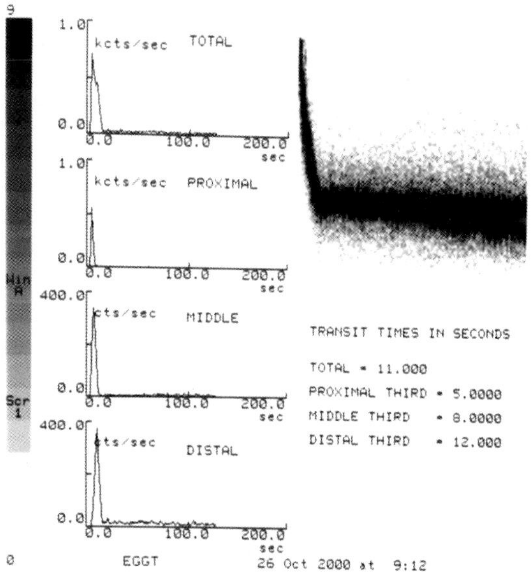

Figure 7.8 Oesophageal isotope-labelled egg transit study. Time activity curves in a normal subject in the whole oesophagus and in different segments of the oesophagus. The condensed image shows normal transit through the oesophagus into the stomach.

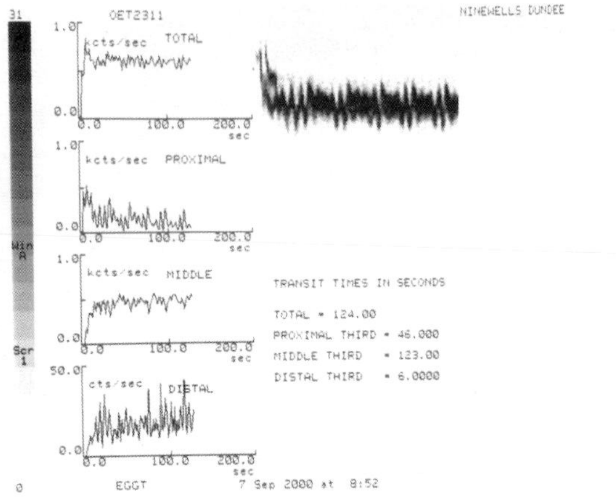

Figure 7.9 Oesophageal isotope-labelled egg transit study in a patient with achalasia. The time activity curves show step delay of transit throughout the different segments of the oesophagus. The condensed image shows an oscillatory pattern of radioactivity as it oscillates backwards and forwards in the oesophagus.

oesophagoscopy is still infrequently used for the removal of foreign bodies and when it is necessary to obtain larger biopsies than is possible by the fibre-optic technique.

Physiological tests

These include manometry, pH-metry and tests to assess bile reflux. The Bernstein test continues to be used when a correlation between symptoms and acid reflux is required. The standard acid reflux test (SART) and the acid clearance test have largely been replaced by pH-metry in the assessment of patients with reflux symptoms.

Oesophageal manometry

This technique measures the mechanical function of the oesophageal musculature and its sphincters by recording intra-luminal pressure profiles caused by the contractions. Intra-luminal pressure recording is carried out using a system of water-perfused catheters or solid-state strain-gauge transducers built into catheters. For sphincter pressure measurements there is a potential for the position of the sphincter to alter in relation to the pressure sensor on the catheter especially in prolonged measurements. In these situations the Dent sleeve can be used. This is a thin, 6 cm long, open-ended, silastic sleeve which surrounds the pressure sensor ports of a water-perfused catheter. The sleeve operates by traversing the sphincter and records the averaged circumferential and axial pressure forces acting on the sleeve. An alternative is the sphinctometer. This device is usually sited distally in a multi-channel micro-transducer catheter and consists of a side-mounted transducer surrounded by a silicone, oil-filled silastic tube of 6 cm length and of the same diameter as the catheter. The water-perfused catheter is connected to a low compliance hydraulic pump, which in turn is connected to a system of strain gauges and a system of readout, most

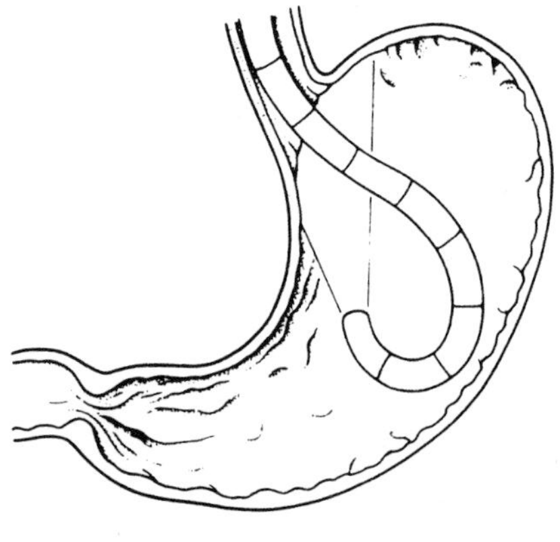

Figure 7.10 With the endoscope in the stomach and the use of the J-manoeuvre the cardiac orifice can be inspected, which is not possible with the rigid endoscope.

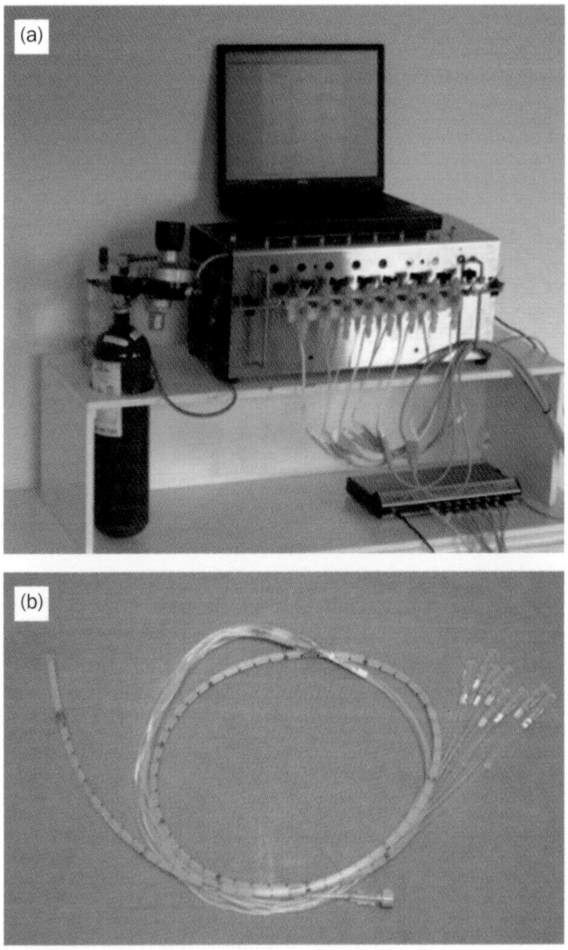

Figure 7.11 (a) Stationary manometry is performed using a low compliance gas-driven hydraulic pump infusing water through a multi-channel catheter connected to a system of strain gauges which feed the back pressure signal into a digital converter and it is displayed on the computer screen. (b) A multi-channel silicone catheter.

commonly a computer (Figure 7.11). The solid-state strain-gauge micro-transducers can be connected directly to the readout system. The study commences by determination of the position of the lower oesophageal sphincter/high-pressure zone. This is done by inserting the catheter into the stomach and withdrawing it either rapidly (rapid pull-through) or slowly (stationary pull-through), taking pressure recordings at each of the stations from both the sphincter and oesophageal body. The rapid pull-through technique provides information on the position and length of the sphincter. The manometry catheter can then be positioned with one pressure sensor in the middle of the sphincteric area and three pressure sensors separated by 5 cm intervals on the catheter lying within the oesophageal body. In stationary manometry pressure recordings are taken from the sensors in response to a number of water swallows separated by 30 s. This method provides sufficient information on the position, length and pressure of the lower oesophageal sphincter in addition to pressure, peristalsis and propagation of contractions within the oesophageal body (Figure 7.12). The information obtained from manometric studies is analysed according to set criteria (Table 7.2) to diagnose oesophageal motility disorders. This method is indicated for the accurate placement of pH electrodes prior to 24 hour ambulatory pH monitoring in patients suspected of having gastro-oesophageal reflux disease. This method can also be diagnostic in patients with classical motility disorders of the oesophagus. In patients where the stationary manometry reveals a motility disorder of the oesophagus and in those patients suspected of having an oesophageal motility disorder, prolonged ambulatory manometry is preferred. This method employs solid-state pressure transducer catheters attached to a portable recording system with event markers triggered by the patient when symptoms occur (Figure 7.13). They are particularly useful for patients with non-cardiac chest pain who may have transient motility disturbances in the oesophagus and for patients with non-specific motility disorders. Because of the diverse aetiology of these disorders, a combined recording of manometry and pH metry is indicated. Analysis of both manometry and pH metry may reveal the disorder (Figure 7.14). More recently, vector manometry of the lower oesophageal sphincter has been obtained using a water-perfused catheter with eight radial channels. Although this technique has provided illustrative three-dimensional representation of the lower oesophageal sphincter, the technique suffers from poor reproducibility.

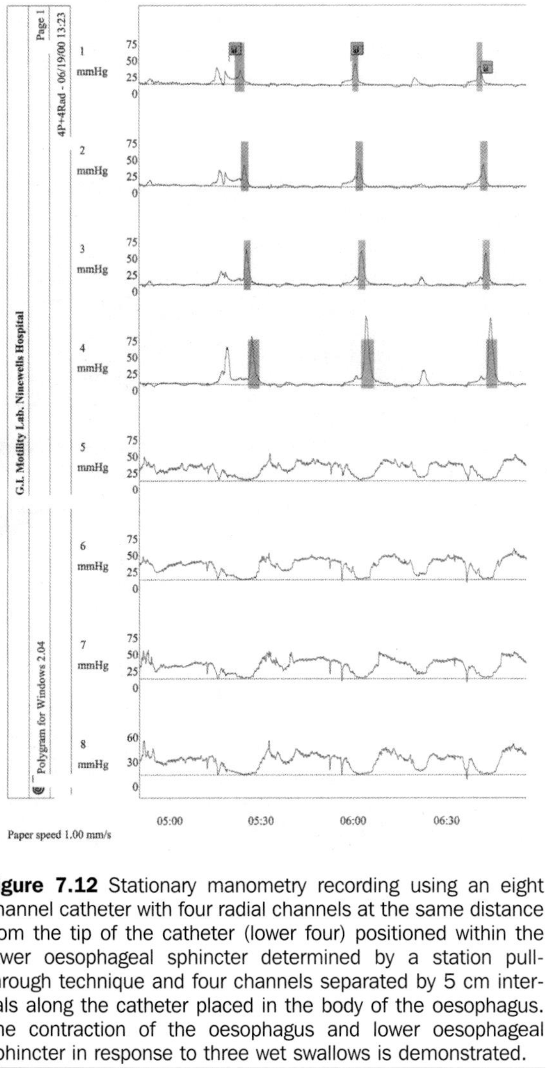

Figure 7.12 Stationary manometry recording using an eight channel catheter with four radial channels at the same distance from the tip of the catheter (lower four) positioned within the lower oesophageal sphincter determined by a station pull-through technique and four channels separated by 5 cm intervals along the catheter placed in the body of the oesophagus. The contraction of the oesophagus and lower oesophageal sphincter in response to three wet swallows is demonstrated.

24 Hour pH monitoring

This technique involves the transnasal placement of a pH measuring electrode sited 5 cm above the manometrically identified lower oesophageal sphincter. The pH electrode monitors the changes in intra-oesophageal pH over a circadian cycle (24 hours) with the information stored in a portable recording device (Figure 7.15). A 24 hour pH profile is subsequently obtained from the recording device. This includes the frequency, duration and pattern of reflux episodes together with temporal correlation with symptoms (Figure 7.16). Conventionally, a reflux episode is defined as a pH drop to below pH 4. Specially designed software analyses the data in two ways. In reflux event analysis, all individual reflux episodes are identified and characterized: their number, mean duration, number of long reflux events more than 5 min and the duration of the longest reflux episodes. Cumulative oesophageal exposure analysis depicts the frequency distribution of the oesophageal pH data for the erect and supine parts of the study as well as for the whole period of study. The generated data for any one patient are then compared with those which pertain to a 'normal' population. Indications for 24 hour ambulatory pH monitoring include the definitive diagnosis of gastro-oesophageal reflux in patients who are sufficiently symptomatic to have warranted endoscopy, but in whom endoscopy is normal. In addition, it is used to investigate patients suspected of having gastro-

Table 7.2 Oesophageal manometry indices and criteria

Index	*Normal*	*Abnormal*
HPZ (sphincter) pressure	10–26 mmHg	<10.0 mmHg, >26.0 mmHg
HPZ relaxation	Relaxes when reached by primary wave	No relaxation with swallowing
Oesophageal body contractions	Primary peristaltic waves generated by wet/dry swallows	>10% aperistaltic waves, retrograde or segmental contractions
Amplitude	30–140 mmHg	< 0 mmHg, >140 mmHg
Duration	2–10 s	>15 s
Wave form	Mostly single or double peaked wave forms	Abnormal and multi-peak wave forms
Additional contractions	Secondary peristaltic waves	Repetitive (tertiary, non-propulsive) contractions

oesophageal reflux as a cause of atypical symptoms such as non-cardiac chest pain, respiratory and laryngeal symptoms, in whom the relevant investigations have been normal and to correlate such symptoms with reflux episodes. Further, it is used when established gastro-oesophageal reflux responds poorly to optimal medical therapy and particularly when surgical treatment is contemplated. It may also be used in the assessment of patients with complex oesophageal disorders prior to surgery.

24 Hour oesophageal bile monitoring (by spectrophotometry) In the last decade, an optical fibre sensor has been developed which can spectrophotometrically detect bilirubin in the oesophagus as a marker of entero-gastro-oesophageal reflux. A fibre-optic probe inserted transnasally into the oesophagus and positioned 5 cm above the manometrically determined HPZ is connected to an ambulatory spectrophotometer. The system is marketed under the name 'Bilitec 2000' (Figure 7.17). This device registers the presence of bilirubin when it

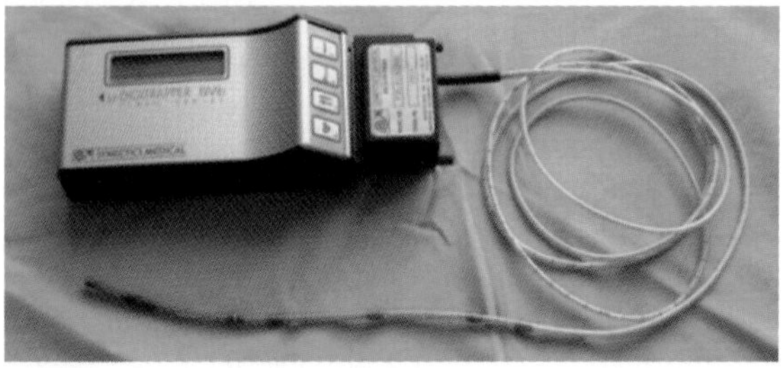

Figure 7.13 A portable recording device connected to a catheter on which three pressure transducers measure pressure and a pH electrode measures the hydrogen ion concentration.

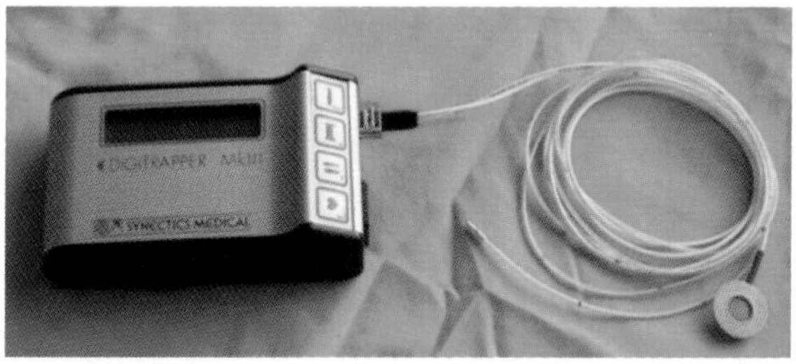

Figure 7.15 Portable recording device connected to a pH catheter with a surface electrode used for 24 hour pH monitoring.

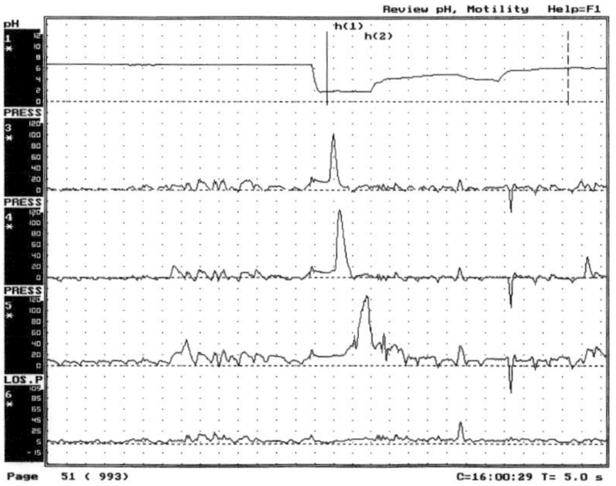

Figure 7.14 Part of a recording of 24 hour combined pressure and pH study showing a drop in pH in the lower oesophagus stimulating a peristaltic contraction to clear the oesophagus.

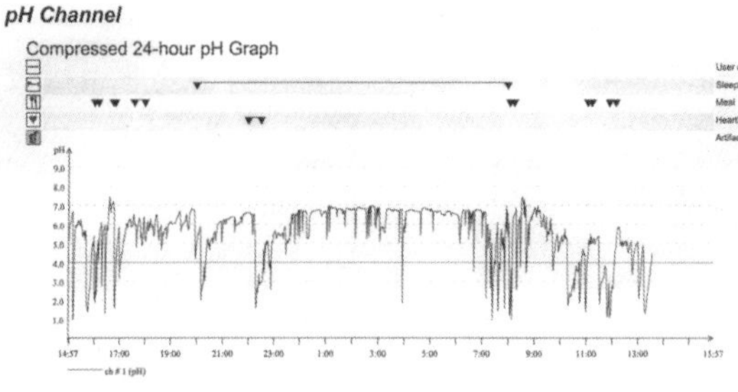

Item	Total	Upright	Supine	Meal	PostP	HrtBrn
Duration of period (HH:MM)	21:20	10:35	12:00	01:15	07:22	00:30
Number of acid refluxes (#)	33	26	12	8	14	3
Number of long acid refluxes (#)	9	6	3	1	4	2
Longest acid reflux (min)	26	26	8	8	16	8
Total time pH below 4.00 (min)	144	124	36	16	58	14
Fraction time pH below 4.00 (%)	11.2	19.6	5.0	21.6	13.0	45.2
Symptom Index (%)	n/a	n/a	n/a	n/a	n/a	100.0

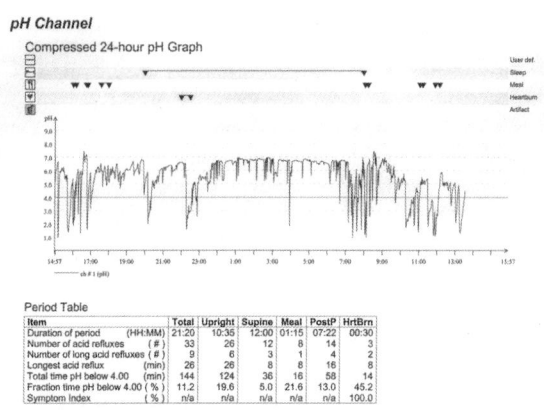

Figure 7.16 A compressed recording of 24 hour pH metry showing episodes of acid reflux in the lower oesophagus and analysis of the reflux episodes.

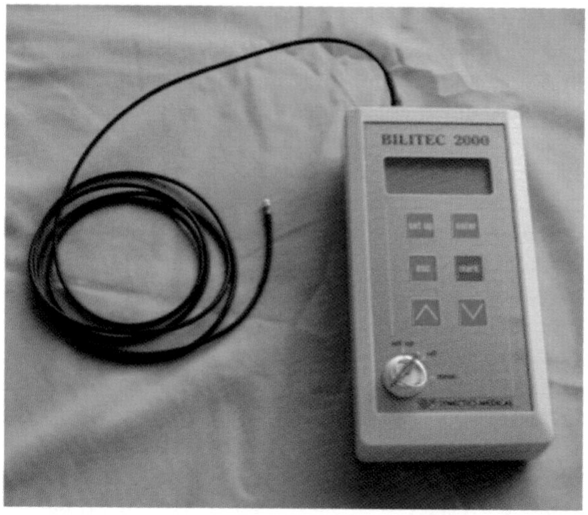

Figure 7.17 An ambulatory spectrophotometer connected to a fibre-optic probe used for prolonged ambulatory bile reflux monitoring.

detects an absorption peak around 453 nm. This peak is said to be easily detectable both in the bile spectrum and in the spectrum of gastric juice combined with other substances (e.g. bile, food, drinks and blood). The presence of bilirubin is, for practical purposes, equivalent to the presence of bile and the detection of an absorption peak around 453 nm implies the presence of bile. The ambulatory spectrophotometer transfers the signals to a data logger and a 24 hour profile can be recorded. The data can then be off-loaded to a computer and an absorbance curve (for 453 nm) is produced for the recording period (24 hours). An episode of bile reflux is defined as an increase in absorbance over 0.14 absorbance units. This threshold has been set arbitrarily to avoid false positive results, which can be caused by the absorbance at 453 nm of dietary substances consumed during the test. It is important to use a standard diet avoiding coloured food substances and beverages during the test. In addition, bile reflux in an acidic medium ($pH < 3.5$) may be underestimated as a result of dimer isomerization of bilirubin and a shift in absorption wavelength in this environment. Further, in a few medical conditions (Gilbert's and Dubin–Johnson syndromes), there is a disproportionate secretion of bilirubin compared to bile acids. This test is indicated in patients with symptomatic gastro-oesophageal reflux with poor response to an adequate dose of proton pump inhibitors. It is also indicated in patients with complications of gastro-oesophageal reflux disease such as Barrett's metaplasia, strictures and ulcers and in patients with reflux symptoms after gastrectomy. Normal values for this test have been published. Validation tests suggest that the overall accuracy of the system is sufficient for clinical use but not reliable enough to study disease mechanisms caused by duodeno-gastro-oesophageal reflux.

Bernstein's acid perfusion test

This detects oesophageal mucosal sensitivity to acid and is very useful in the determination of the oesophageal origin of chest pain. The patient is studied in the fasting upright position. A nasogastric tube is positioned in the middle of the oesophagus. Infusion is initially started with isotonic saline and then switched to 0.1 M HCl without informing the patient. Acid perfusion will reproduce the pain in patients with a sensitive oesophageal mucosa. After stopping the infusion the pain should subside within 20 min.

Section 7.3 • Gastro-oesophageal reflux disease and non-reflux oesophagitis

Gastro-oesophageal reflux disease is the commonest upper digestive disorder with approximately 45% of the population having reflux symptoms. Peptic oesophagitis is the commonest endoscopic diagnosis being found in 25% of patients having an upper gastrointestinal endoscopy. The prevalence of the disease is relatively constant over the age of 30 years and does not seem to increase with age. It is best to think of this disease as a syndrome of excessive gastro-oesophageal reflux. Gastro-oesophageal reflux *per se* is a physiological phenomenon, which usually occurs during the post-prandial period in most people. Up to 50 reflux episodes may occur in a 24 hour period, but most of these episodes are short-lived. Exposure of the lower oesophageal mucosa to acid pH less than 4 should not exceed 5% of a 24 hour period. Gastro-oesophageal reflux in excess of this amount is considered pathological and leads to oesophageal mucosal sensitization. This in turn contributes to the appearance of symptoms of the disease. In many patients the symptoms are mild and intermittent with no macroscopic mucosal damage (non-erosive reflux disease). In 10% of patients, however, oesophagitis develops. In these patients further major complications of ulceration, stricture and columnar metaplasia occur at the rate of 10% for each complication. Approximately 10% of patients with columnar metaplasia can go on to develop dysplasia in the metaplastic segment of the oesophagus.

Gastro-oesophageal reflux disease is predominantly a condition of the Western world. This general pattern of distribution suggests that dietary factors are important in the aetiology of this disease.

Pathophysiology of gastro-oesophageal reflux disease

Pathological gastro-oesophageal reflux occurs when the balance between those factors, which promote reflux, exceeds the effect of those factors that resist reflux and its damaging effects.

Factors resisting reflux and damage

The anti-reflux mechanism that constitutes the basic defence mechanism against gastro-oesophageal reflux is due to several components acting in concert. These include competence of the lower oesophageal sphincter 'complex', oesophageal clearance of refluxed material and mucosal resistance to the damaging effects of the refluxate.

Competence of the cardio-oesophageal junction

There is now general agreement that competence of the cardio-oesophageal segment is due to the combined action of the lower oesophageal sphincter in addition to mechanical factors which interact and function in concert, which together form the 'lower oesophageal sphincter complex' otherwise known as the high pressure zone.

The lower oesophageal sphincter is the single most important factor accounting for the competence of the gastro-oesophageal junction. Anatomically, the lower oesophageal sphincter and cardia represent a two-compartment arrangement of clasp-like bands of muscle above and a sling-like muscle below. The clasps are clustered on the gastric lesser curve aspect of the oesophagus extending for several centimetres above and below the squamo-columnar junction. The sling is a condensation of the oblique muscle layer of the stomach, located on the greater curvature of the stomach at the angle of His. The muscles of the lower oesophageal sphincter and proximal cardia have unique and characteristic physiological function, which are largely myogenic but with neuro-endocrine influences. Several drugs, hormones and food substances are known to influence the contractile activity of the lower oesophageal sphincter (Table 7.3). The resting tone of the lower oesophageal sphincter increases following the administration of gastrin, cholinergic and alpha-adrenergic agents, and decreases after secretin, cholecystokinin and glucagon. Dietary agents such as coffee, foods containing fat, and nicotine reduce the lower oesophageal sphincter pressure, as do some drugs including calcium channel blockers and theophylene. Pro-kinetic agents such as cisapride and metoclopromide produce an increase in the resting tone of the lower oesophageal sphincter. In general, the effects of hormones on the lower oesophageal sphincter have been achieved by pharmacological doses and it is not possible to ascribe with certainty a physiological role to these peptides or hormones. The normal resting tone of the lower oesophageal sphincter pressure is 10–25 mmHg and is radially asymmetrical. Temporary inhibition of the lower oesophageal sphincter occurs just prior to the arrival of a primary peristaltic wave induced by swallowing, to allow entry of food into the stomach. The sphincter relaxes to equal the gastric baseline pressure of 1–3 mmHg and subsequently resumes its contracted state. Precise measurement of the sphincteric function of the lower oesophageal sphincter has shown that the tonically contracted lower oesophageal sphincter relaxes to equal gastric pressure just prior to the arrival of a peristaltic wave down the oesophagus induced by swallowing. However, the lower oesophageal sphincter, essential as it may be, is one component of a complex and multi-factorial anti-reflux mechanism.

The length of the intra-abdominal segment of oesophagus is another important factor in the competence of the lower oesophageal sphincter. Any increase in intra-abdominal pressure would be equally applied to the intra-abdominal segment of oesophagus maintaining its walls in apposition (Figure 7.18). Approximately 2 cm of intra-abdominal oesophagus seems

Table 7.3 Effect on lower oesophageal sphincter pressure (high pressure zone) by hormones, drugs and foodstuffs

	Decrease HPZ activity	*Increase HPZ activity*
Hormones/peptides	Glucagon Secretin Cholecystokinin VIP GIP Progesterone Oestrogens Serotonin (N-receptors) Histamine (H_2-receptors) Enkephalins	Gastrin Motilin Bombesin Histamine (H_1-receptors) Serotonin (M-receptors)
Prostaglandins	E_1, E_2, A_2	F_2
Drugs	Atropine Antihistamines Ca^{2+}-blockers Ganglion-blockers Tricyclic antidepressants	Metoclopramide Domperidone Cisapride Cholinergic drugs Anticholinesterases
Foodstuffs	Caffeine Fats Chocolate Alcohol	Protein meal
Others	Smoking	

sufficient for competence of the lower oesophageal sphincter in most people.

The diaphragmatic crural mechanism also seems important. This component seems to exert its effect mainly during deep inspiration or during periods of sudden increases in intra-abdominal pressure such as during coughing or sneezing. It is the diaphragmatic crural mechanism which is responsible for the radial asymmetry of the high-pressure zone as measured by vector manometry.

The acute angle of His is also thought to be important by providing an abrupt insertion of the oesophagus into the stomach. As such, it also maintains a small diameter aperture of the distal oesophagus as it joins the stomach. This component seems to be mainly important during gastric distension.

Although the phreno-oesophageal membrane has no direct effect on closure of the lower oesophagus, it plays an important role by fixing the lower oesophagus and maintaining a sufficient intra-abdominal segment within the abdomen. As such, this component seems secondary and supportive in nature.

The mucosal rosette in the lower oesophagus seems to provide the substance for the valve to maintain its closure when the lower oesophageal sphincter is contracted. As such, it also provides support to the primary function of competence of the gastro-oesophageal junction.

Oesophageal clearance

- Clearance of the refluxate from the oesophagus is by volume clearance due to normal peristalsis of all but 1 ml of the refluxate and by chemical clearance due to neutralization in a step-wise fashion by swallowed saliva.

Volume clearance is achieved by primary and secondary peristalsis of the oesophageal body. Primary peristalsis occurs in response to swallowing and secondary peristalsis in response to oesophageal distension by the refluxate. Although it is established that 25–50% of patients with gastro-oesophageal reflux disease have impairment of peristaltic function, it is controversial as

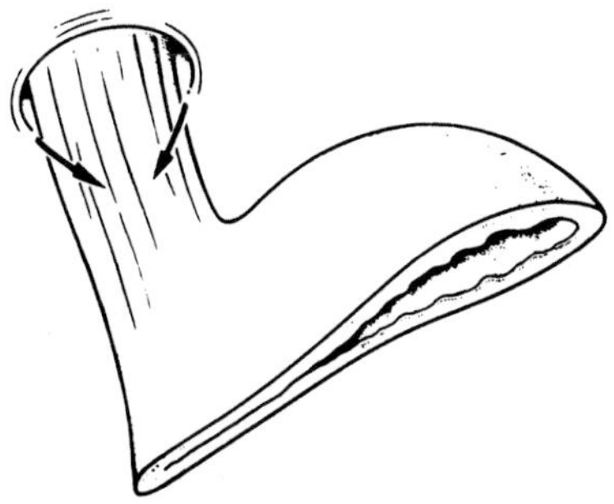

Figure 7.18 Competence is the result of a flutter valve, the abdominal segment being flattened anteroposteriorly against the aorta by the intra-abdominal pressure. The mechanism is similar to a Heimlich valve used for chest drains instead of an underwater-seal drain.

to whether this is a primary pathology contributing to reflux or whether it is resultant from it. However, once the abnormality is established, it is non-reversible even after reflux control either medically or surgically.

In chemical clearance saliva assumes an important role. The bicarbonate content of saliva is capable of neutralizing small acid volumes but in practice this seems to have a minor effect. It is important to emphasize that oesophageal clearance only shortens the contact time between the injurious refluxate and the oesophageal mucosa.

Mucosal resistance

This term is less well understood. However, four mechanisms are thought to be responsible for the integrity of the oesophageal mucosa:

- The submucosal glands producing bicarbonates are probably important for neutralization of acid reflux during sleep when salivary secretion is decreased.
- A hydrophobic mucosal surface due to phospholipids in mucus.
- Resistance to transmucosal ion diffusion is due to tight luminal cell layers and to an intercellular lipid matrix.
- Cellular mechanisms include the Na^+/H^+ antiport, which maintains intracellular pH by inhibition of free-radical production and by increasing cellular turnover when damage has occurred.

It is, however, clear that once the mucosal barrier is breached there is the potential for the injurious refluxate to manifest its damage. Once damaged, it is not clear what contribution components of the mucosal barrier have, and it is less clear at this stage whether it is amenable to pharmacological manipulation.

Factors promoting reflux and damage

Dysfunctional gastro-oesophageal sphincter

The primary event in gastro-oesophageal reflux disease is failure of the anti-reflux barrier (the lower oesophageal sphincter complex). This failure consists of a combination of the following components:

- Primary weakness of the smooth muscle of the lower oesophageal sphincter. It is not clear whether this is genetic or dietary in origin.
- Short length of the intra-abdominal segment of oesophagus. Both sphincter length and resting pressure influence the sphincter vector volume, which is thought to be the key factor of mechanical sphincter competence. The acute component of a shortened sphincter occurs during gastric distension and the chronic component is in the presence of a hiatus hernia.
- Defective hormonal and neural control of the sphincter. This is most commonly diet induced and transient.
- Abnormally high number of transient lower oesophageal sphincter relaxations. Approximately 65% of reflux episodes in GORD patients and 90% of reflux episodes in normal subjects occur during transient lower oesophageal sphincter relaxations. These occur in the absence of swallows and last 5–30 s in comparison with less than 5 s for swallow-induced relaxations. They are thought to be associated with gastric distension. It has been suggested that mechanoreceptors in the gastric cardia initiate vagal reflexes, which lead to sphincter relaxations.
- The presence of a hiatal hernia. This results in a change of the pressure environment, shortening of the lower oesophageal sphincter, changes in the anatomy and

reflexes of the gastric cardia. Approximately 50% of patients symptomatic of GORD have a hiatal hernia and 90% of patients with reflux oesophagitis have a hiatus hernia. However, many patients with a hiatus hernia are asymptomatic and 40–50% have no oesophagitis.

The majority of patients with gastro-oesophageal reflux disease can be categorized into one of three mechanisms with a disordered gastro-oesophageal sphincter.

- Patients with a hypotensive resting lower oesophageal sphincter pressure of less than 6 mmHg have free reflux of gastric contents into the lower oesophagus.
- Patients with a borderline lower oesophageal sphincter pressure and intermittent increases in the intra-gastric pressure have what is termed 'stress reflux'.
- Patients with an increased frequency and duration of transient lower oesophageal sphincter relaxations are termed to have 'reflex reflux'. They account for approximately 40% of patients with gastro-oesophageal reflux disease and 65% of patients with reflux oesophagitis.

Gastric distension

Physiological gastric distension occurs in the post-prandial period. Gastric emptying, however, may be impaired by organic outlet obstruction or by functional gastric dysmotility either due to disease processes or as a result of the ingestion of food which slows the rate of gastric emptying such as fat. Approximately 40% of patients with gastro-oesophageal reflux disease have impaired gastric emptying. Gastric distension exerts pressure against the physiological anti-reflux barrier, shortening the sphincter and impairing its function. In addition, gastric distension stimulates an increased rate of transient lower oesophageal sphincter relaxations. The combination contributes to an ineffective anti-reflux barrier.

The refluxate

The principal physiological components of gastric juice are acid and pepsin. Acid alone is injurious to the oesophageal mucosa at pH less than 2. At pH 2–4.5 pepsin is activated and is capable of permeating the mucosal cell membrane. Approximately a quarter of patients with reflux oesophagitis have gastric hypersecretion. Bile salts in the pH range 2–7 are capable of producing severe mucosal damage. This damage is amplified in the presence of acid and pepsin. Clinically, pure acid and pepsin reflux occurs in 42% of patients and mixed reflux of gastric and duodenal juices occurs in 58% of patients. Pure alkaline reflux is uncommon and occurs in the setting of post-gastric surgery or with conditions causing achlorhydria.

Pathology of gastro-oesophageal reflux disease

The histological appearances of the early stages of gastro-oesophageal reflux disease are best appreciated from examination of deep biopsies. The normal oesophageal mucosa consists of three layers; the basal (germinal) layer, the prickle cell layer (polygonal cells with numerous bridges) and the superficial or functional layer (flattened cells with pyknotic nuclei). In the normal mucosa inflammatory cells are few and scanty

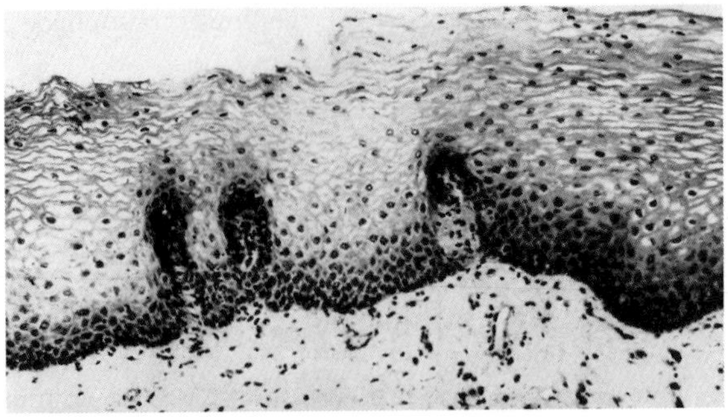

Figure 7.19 Suction biopsy of the lower oesophageal mucosa. Normal histology: the basal layer is less than 15% of the total epithelial thickness. The papillae of the lamina propria extend less than two-thirds of the way to the luminal surface. No polymorphonuclear leucocytes are present in either lamina propria or epithelium. Mononuclear cells, normal constituents of the lamina propria, are present.

and the vascular dermal papillae project from the lamina propria to no more than half the thickness of the epithelium (Figure 7.19). The histological changes of early damage include widening of the basal layer so as to constitute more than 15% of the total epithelial thickness. In addition, the dermal papillae extend to more than two-thirds of the way through the epithelium to the luminal surface (Figure 7.20). These changes are indicative of an increased rate of epithelial turnover.

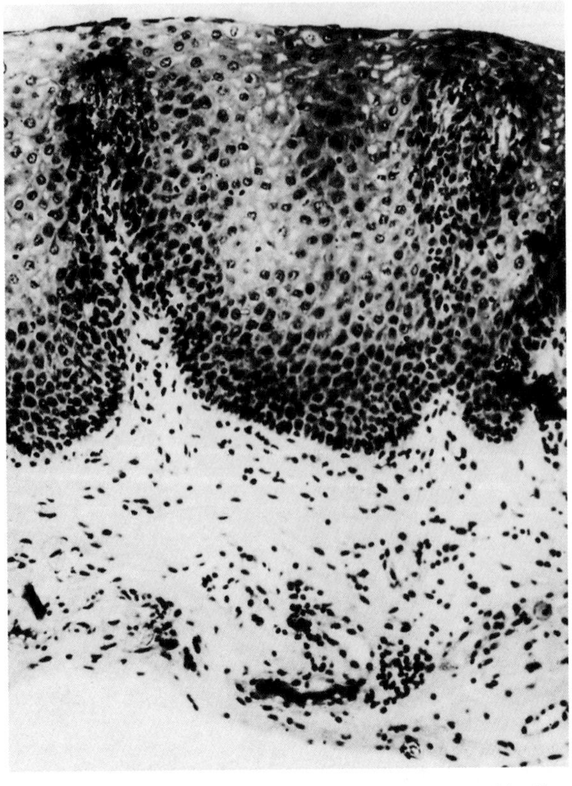

Figure 7.20 Mild to moderate oesophagitis due to acid reflux. The basal layer occupies about 30% of the total epithelial thickness and the papillae extend nearly to the surface. No polymorphonuclear leucocytes are present.

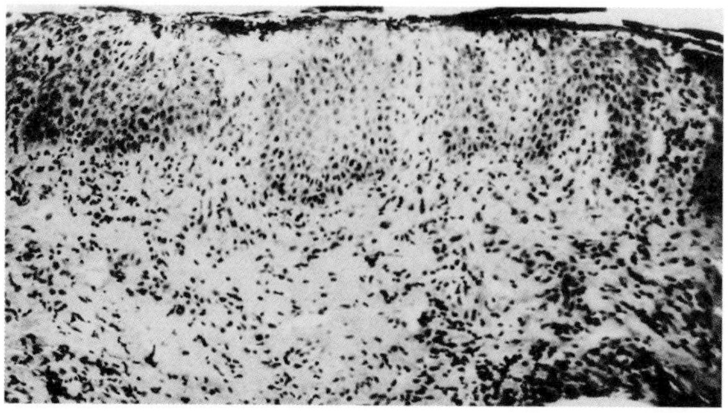

Figure 7.21 Severe gastro-oesophageal reflux with gross erosion and exudate visible endoscopically. The total epithelial thickness is less than normal and is composed entirely of basal cells. The papillae are widened and extend all the way to the luminal surface where superficial necrosis is present. Many polymorphonuclear leucocytes are present in the lamina propria and within the epithelium.

With more severe damage there is an accumulation of inflammatory cells (mainly polymorphs). The total epithelial thickness is reduced and becomes entirely composed of basal cells. The papillae become widened and extend to the surface when superficial necrosis and ulceration supervene (Figure 7.21). These acute ulcers are situated superficial to the muscularis mucosa. Their base consists of granulation tissue surrounded by an inflammatory infiltrate, which is accompanied by submucosal oedema. Healing of these superficial ulcers does not result in fibrosis and the regenerated epithelium is of the squamous variety. However, if the ulceration and inflammation reaches the submucous layer or beyond, some fibrosis is inevitable and the regenerated mucosa may eventually consist, entirely or in part, of columnar epithelium.

Helicobacter pylori and gastro-oesophageal reflux disease

Epidemiological, pathophysiological and clinical studies have demonstrated that *Helicobacter pylori* infection, particularly the cagA-positive strain, is protective against the development of gastro-oesophageal reflux disease and its complications. This protective effect is dependent on the extent of *Helicobacter*-induced corpus gastritis, with severe corpus gastritis causing profound reduction of acid secretion. In addition, development of reflux oesophagitis after *H. pylori* eradication therapy has been reported suggesting that the disappearance of *H. pylori* increases the risk for the development of reflux oesophagitis. Although the mechanism of reflux oesophagitis development after eradication therapy is unknown, the severity of corpus gastritis before eradication has been shown to be an important factor in predicting the occurrence of reflux oesophagitis. The severity of corpus gastritis is known to be negatively associated with gastric acid secretion. Several studies have shown that gastric acid secretion increases to normal or near normal levels in patients with hypochlorhydria after successful *H. pylori* eradication therapy. It is presumed that healing of gastritis (parietal cell dysfunction) and increased acid secretion after successful *H. pylori* eradication therapy contributes to the development of reflux oesophagitis. The available evidence suggests that this phenomenon has no clinical relevance for the treatment of gastro-oesophageal reflux disease. During treatment with proton pump inhibitors, the 24 hour oesophageal pH does not depend on the *H. pylori* status, nor does the medication dose required for maintenance therapy.

Clinical features of gastro-oesophageal reflux

The typical symptoms of gastro-oesophageal reflux are heartburn, regurgitation and dysphagia. Symptoms are aggravated by posture and can be especially severe at night, after large meals and activities which increase the intra-abdominal pressure, e.g. bending, stooping, gardening, etc. Other symptoms which may occur include pain on swallowing hot or spicy foods (odynophagia) and water brash. Dysphagia may be due to spasm or oedema of the inflamed lower oesophagus in which case it remits with improvement of the oesophagitis consequent on treatment. In some patients dysphagia arises as a result of a secondary motility disorder in the lower oesophagus due to chronic reflux induced fibrosis. Resistant dysphagia indicates stricture formation. A scoring system introduced by DeMeester is very useful for assessing the extent of symptomatic severity (Table 7.4). A typical presentation with chest pain which can closely mimic coronary artery disease and with pulmonary symptoms including asthma is common. Some patients present with laryngeal symptoms manifesting as a persistent dry cough, changes in the voice or choking episodes. Others have palatal and dental erosions associated with gastro-oesophageal reflux. Rarely, patients present with anaemia or haematemesis and are found to have florid oesophagitis at endoscopy.

Table 7.4 DeMeester's scoring system for symptoms of gastro-oesophageal reflux

Symptoms	*Grade*	*Description*
Heartburn		
None	0	No heartburn
Minimal	1	Occasional episodes
Moderate	2	Reason for medical visit
Severe	3	Interference with daily activities
Regurgitation		
None	0	No regurgitation
Minimal	1	Occasional episodes
Moderate	2	Predictable on position or straining
Severe	3	Episodes of pulmonary aspiration with chronic nocturnal cough or recurrent pneumonitis
Dysphagia		
None	0	No dysphagia
Minimal	1	Occasional episodes
Moderate	2	Requires fluids to clear
Severe	3	Episode of meat impaction requiring medical treatment

Table 7.5 Savary–Miller classification of reflux oesophagitis

Grade	*Description*
1	Single or isolated erosive lesion(s), oval or linear but affecting only one longitudinal fold
2	Multiple erosive lesions, non-circumferential, affecting more than one longitudinal fold, with or without confluence
3	Circumferential erosive lesions
4	Chronic lesions: ulcer(s), stricture(s) and/or short oesophagus. Alone or in association with lesions of grades 1–3
5	Columnar epithelium in continuity with the Z line, non-circular, star-shaped or circumferential. Alone or associated with lesions of grades 1–4

The important and clinically useful tests in establishing a diagnosis are flexible endoscopy with biopsy followed by pH metry. Oesophageal manometry is used to locate the high-pressure zone prior to insertion of the pH probe but in itself is of limited use for the diagnosis of gastro-oesophageal reflux. In patients with dysphagia without a stricture oesophageal manometry may be valuable in assessing the motility of the oesophageal body. Prior to surgical treatment a barium swallow is essential to demonstrate the presence, type and size of any associated hiatal hernia. In addition it may provide information on a shortened oesophagus.

Complications of gastro-oesophageal reflux disease

The complications of gastro-oesophageal reflux disease are reflux oesophagitis, ulcerative oesophagitis, formation of strictures and webs and columnar metaplasia.

Reflux oesophagitis

The development of a spectrum of changes in the oesophageal mucosa which are discernible by endoscopy represents a complication of gastro-oesophageal reflux disease. A variety of grading systems have been suggested to reflect the severity of the oesophagitis and to provide a useful basis for comparison before and after treatment and using different treatments either in the same centre or across literature. The most popular grading system is that advocated by Savary and Miller and modified subsequently (Table 7.5). This system, however, suffers from significant inter-observer variability and has not been submitted to a validation programme. An alternative system, which clinically and functionally correlates to the severity of reflux and its treatment and which has been submitted to validation with success, is the 'Los Angeles classification' system (Table 7.6).

Table 7.6 The Los Angeles classification of oesophagitis

Grade	*Description*
Grade A	One (or more) mucosal break no longer than 5 mm, that does not extend between the tops of two mucosal folds
Grade B	One (or more) mucosal break more than 5 mm long that does not extend between the tops of two mucosal folds
Grade C	One (or more) mucosal break that is continuous betweeen the tops of two or more mucosal folds but which involves less than 75% of the circumference
Grade D	One (or more) mucosal break which involves at least 75% of the oesophageal circumference

Oesophagitis is present in 30–40% of patients referred for investigation. Not all patients with oesophagitis are symptomatic. Further, oesophagitis can decrease in severity or resolve completely, or can persist or progress to a more severe grade without treatment.

Deep ulceration with peri-oesophagitis

This complication is usually found in long-standing symptomatic disease. These patients usually have more severe symptoms and tend to have more severe reflux. The ulcers involve the oesophagus beyond the submucous layer and cause a peri-oesophagitis and extensive mural fibrosis, which may eventually lead to stricture formation and oesophageal shortening. Full thickness penetration may involve the peri-oesophageal arterial plexus and cause massive haemorrhage. However, this complication and overt perforation are rare. Chronic blood loss, however, is a recognized sequel.

Strictures and webs

Oesophageal webs which may form at sites of ulcerative oesophagitis are the result of submucous fibrosis in a localized area of the oesophagus and are most commonly found at the lower end or at the level of the aortic arch. They may cause dysphagia with intermittent solid bolus obstruction but are easily treated by endoscopic dilatation and seldom recur thereafter. The exact nature of the distinctive circular mucosal ridge situated at the oesophago-gastric junction and known as Shatski's ring is still debatable. Shatski's rings tend to occur in association with hiatus hernia and are not usually associated with any evidence of oesophagitis (Figure 7.22). The majority are asymptomatic but those with a ring aperture less than 13 mm cause mild intermittent dysphagia with sudden episodes of total obstruction, sometimes referred to as the 'steakhouse syndrome'. In the majority of symptomatic patients, an underlying motility disorder is present in addition to the ring.

Stricture formation is the result of repeated oesophageal damage with fibrosis replacing the muscular coat of a segment of the oesophagus. The majority occur in elderly patients over 60 years of age with long-standing symptoms. Oesophageal stricturing occurs in approximately 10% of patients with gastro-oesophageal reflux disease. Peptic strictures with a lumen of less than 3 mm in diameter and a length greater than 3 cm are classified as severe (Figure 7.23). They account for 10% of strictures in most series and are both difficult and dangerous to dilate. In addition, there is evidence that the initial severity of the stricture

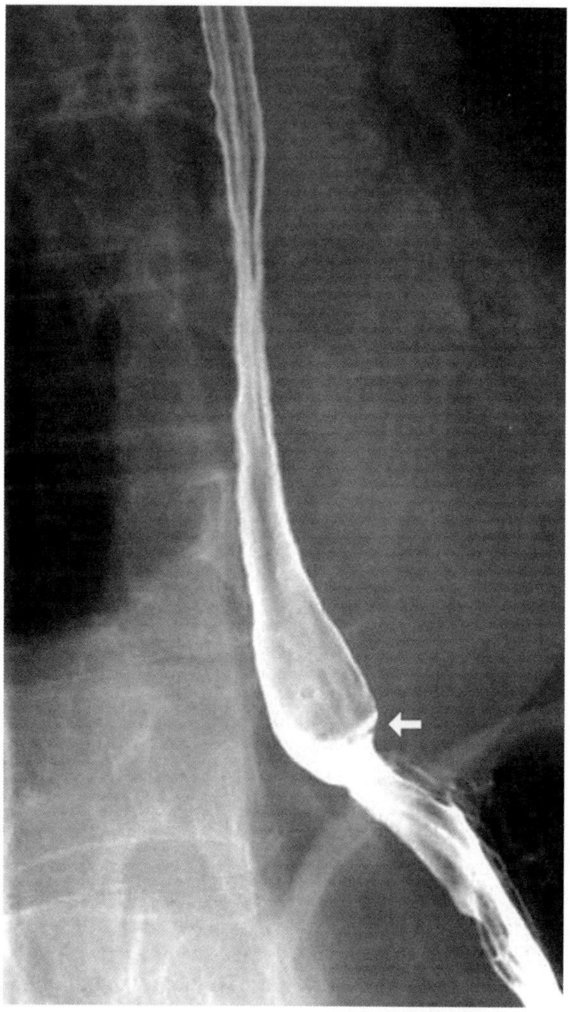

Figure 7.22 Barium swallow showing a Shatski's ring just above the oesophago gastric junction causing hold-up to the flow of barium in a patient presenting with dysphagia.

is an indicator of the propensity for recurrence after dilatation. The incidence of oesophageal peptic strictures has been noted to decrease with the advent of proton pump inhibitors.

Columnar metaplasia of the oesophagus (Barrett's oesophagus)

The development of intestinal metaplasia in the lower oesophagus is a recognized complication of severe gastro-oesophageal reflux. Continued reflux trauma leads to the accumulation of genetic instability in areas of intestinal metaplasia and the development of dysplasia and cancer in a proportion of these patients. This condition will be discussed separately.

Treatment of gastro-oesophageal reflux

Treatment of gastro-oesophageal reflux disease is dependent on the severity and persistence of symptoms and onset of complications. Management is conservative in the first instance and is designed to minimize reflux episodes, reduce chemical damage and improve

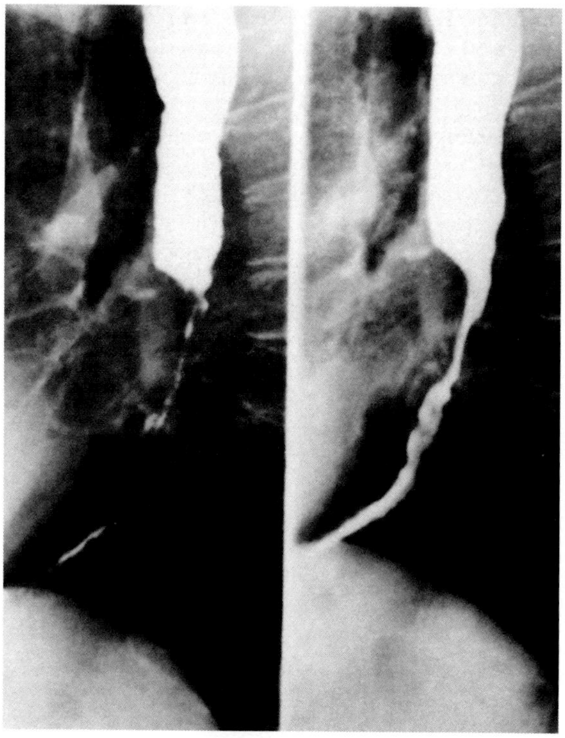

Figure 7.23 Barium swallow showing severe reflux stricture. It exceeds 3.0 cm in length.

oesophageal clearance by specific medication. The patient's co-operation is essential in achieving weight reduction and abstinence from smoking. Dietary advice includes the avoidance of large meals especially within three hours of recumbency and replacing these with frequent small dry snacks with fluids in between meals, and avoidance of fatty, spicy and acidic foods, fruit juices and spirits, and substances which impair the lower oesophageal sphincter tone such as chocolate and coffee. Posture advice includes sleeping propped up as near to 45° as possible by using several pillows or raising the head of the bed (Figure 7.24). In addition patients should avoid bending and stooping.

Medical treatment

Specific medical treatment is indicated when symptoms persist. The medical treatment can be approached in two different fashions. The correction of mecha-

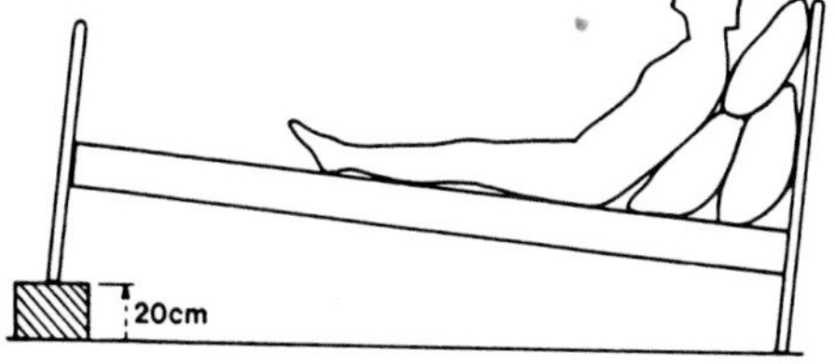

Figure 7.24 The patient is advised to sleep propped up as near to 45° as possible by using several pillows. To avoid sliding down the bed, 20 cm blocks are placed under the foot of the bed.

nisms involved in the pathogenesis of reflux includes a decrease in the frequency of transient lower oesophageal sphincter relaxations and improvement of oesophageal clearance of the refluxate to minimize the oesophageal exposure time. The more popular approach employs neutralization or suppression of intragastric acidity to render the refluxate less harmful to the oesophageal mucosa. This approach provides symptomatic relief and prevents mucosal injury in the majority of patients. The various drugs which are used alone or in combination in the medical treatment of gastro-oesophageal reflux disease are shown in Table 7.7.

In practice, most patients would have already used over the counter antacids prior to seeking advice. Although antacids provide some symptomatic relief in mild cases, this is relatively short lived. Antacid–alginate mixtures, e.g. Gaviscon, form a viscous solution which appears to float on the surface of gastric contents, theoretically providing a barrier between the oesophageal mucosa and the refluxate. There is no evidence that any of the above agents heal oesophagitis. For more severe and persistent symptoms H_2-receptor blockers (e.g. cimetidine, ranitidine) are given commonly as a single bedtime ulcer-healing dose. Many patients with mild disease can achieve symptomatic control and endoscopic healing of oesophagitis on an appropriate course of H_2-receptor antagonists. A full course of treatment for 3 months should be followed by maintenance therapy indefinitely, otherwise the symptoms inevitably recur. If symptoms persist despite H_2 receptor antagonists, and for more reliable healing of oesophagitis a 'step-up' approach to proton pump inhibitors (e.g. omeprazole, lansoprazole, pantoprazole) is indicated. They are potent inhibitors of gastric acid secretion, which act specifically by inhibiting the enzyme H^+/K^+-ATPase, the final step in the formation of hydrochloric acid in the parietal cell. Using these agents, healing of endoscopic oesophagitis occurs in 80–90% of patients using high-dose treatment for 8 weeks. Recurrence of oesophagitis is universal unless maintenance therapy is administered indefinitely. Maintenance therapy is best used regularly on a daily basis rather than on demand when symptoms occur. There is evidence that the addition of ranitidine to maintenance therapy using proton pump inhibitors can establish total acid release suppression and prevent the development of metaplasia. The additional use of prokinetic agents is advocated in the management of reflux in an effort to reduce oesophageal exposure time. In addition many patients have impaired peristaltic function and lower oesophageal sphincter function and would benefit from augmentation of these. Agents such as metoclopromide and domperidone produce brief improvements of symptoms but no healing of oesophagitis. In comparison, cisapride which acts directly to enhance the release of acetylcholine in the myenteric plexus has a sustained effect and leads to healing of oesophagitis when combined with antisecretory agents but this drug has withdrawn because of serious side-effects. For control of transient lower oesophageal sphincter relaxations, the $GABA_B$ agonist baclofen is proving a useful agent. Mucosal protection agents such as sucralfate, misoprostol and carbenoxolone are most useful in combination treatment with antisecretory agents and increase the healing rate of oesophagitis.

It is important to emphasize that some patients with gastro-oesophageal reflux disease have troublesome symptoms, which interfere with their work, sleep or leisure activities but are found not to have oesophagitis at endoscopy. These patients have what is termed 'non-erosive reflux disease'. These symptomatic patients may be found to have microscopic evidence of oesophagitis. Provided they are proven to have excessive acid reflux on pH metry, then every attempt should be made to treat their symptoms either medically or surgically.

The conservative management of neutral/alkaline reflux after gastric surgery is difficult and seldom effective. The administration of bile salt-binding agents such as cholestyramine or mucosal protective agents such as sucralfate may help temporarily. However, medical treatment is usually unsuccessful in the long term and surgical intervention is required in these patients.

Surgical treatment of gastro-oesophageal reflux

The majority of patients with gastro-oesophageal reflux will have limited periods plagued with episodes of reflux controlled by lifestyle adjustments and

Table 7.7 Drug therapy in gastro-oesophageal reflux disease

Drug class	*Examples*	*Mode of action*
Antacids with silicone	Dimethylpolysiloxane	Defoaming agents
Antacids with alginate	Anti-reflux floating alginate	Antacid platform on top of gastric juice
Prokinetic drugs	Bethanecol, metoclopramide, domperidone	Motility enhancing (improve clearance)
Antisecretory drugs	Cimetidine, ranitidine, famotidine	H_2-receptor blockers
	Omeprazole, lansoprazole, pantoprazole	Proton pump inhibitors
Mucosal protectors	Carbenoxolone with alginate, sucralfate, misoprostil	Various actions

pharmacological agents with or without maintenance therapy. Approximately 10–15% of patients will be referred for consideration to have anti-reflux surgery. The indications for surgical treatment are as follows:

- Failure of medical therapy. This should be considered when the patient has received the appropriate medications at the appropriate dosage with development of side-effects of the medication, persistence of symptoms, or inability to comply with the medication or lifestyle adjustments. Disease progression despite appropriate medical therapy also falls under this category. The persistence of vomiting or regurgitation in patients with an incompetent gastro-oesophageal sphincter and usually with a hiatus hernia is a strong indication for surgical intervention.
- Development of complications. These include ulcers, strictures, columnar metaplasia of the lower oesophagus and secondary motility disorders of the oesophagus. Many of these patients may be elderly and frail with comorbid disease and surgical intervention in this group is inappropriate. Young and fit patients who develop these complications should be considered for surgery. Patients with high-grade oesophagitis should be included in this category from the outset although this is controversial.
- Persistence of reflux in children beyond the age of 2 years.
- Reflux after previous upper abdominal surgery, particularly alkaline reflux.
- Atypical symptoms of gastro-oesophageal reflux including respiratory, pharyngeal and dental problems.
- Individualized assessment. This includes young patients who can only be maintained in remission by the administration of continuous and life-long medication. While the consequences of this approach may have been overstated, the prospects of life-long medication in the young patient should not be underrated. Within this category, socioeconomic considerations are also important for both the state and the individual. It is estimated that the cost of maintenance therapy for 10 years using proton pump inhibitors far exceeds the costs of an anti-reflux procedure.

The primary goal in the management of gastro-oesophageal reflux is to improve the quality of life in these patients by complete symptom resolution and maintenance of symptom control. Additional therapeutic end points include the healing of damage already incurred and prevention of long-term complications of reflux.

The aim of the technical procedure in anti-reflux surgery is to restore and anchor the oesophagogastric junction below the diaphragm to achieve an adequate length of intra-abdominal oesophagus. In addition a mechanism must be created at the oesophagogastric junction to restore competency of the gastro-oesophageal/lower oesophageal sphincter mechanism. In this respect closure of the hiatus is not always needed but hiatal repair and crural approximation is indicated if there is an associated hiatus hernia. The most commonly performed anti-reflux operation is the Nissen total fundoplication or one of its modifications (Rosetti-Hell, partial anterior or posterior wraps). The Belsey mark IV repair is a carefully constructed partial fundoplication through thoracic access. Other operations include the Hill posterior gastropexy and placement of the Angelchick prosthesis.

It is not entirely clear how fundoplications exert their action. Numerous studies have shown an increase in lower oesophageal sphincter tone after a variety of fundoplication procedures and that the pressure was substantially higher after a total fundoplication than after a partial fundoplication. In addition, recent studies have shown that a total fundic wrap reduces post-prandial reflux by reducing the frequency of transient lower oesophageal sphincter relaxations and rendering swallowing-induced relaxations incomplete. After a partial wrap patients maintain their ability to vent air from the stomach without jeopardizing the anti-reflux mechanism. In addition, the total fundoplication has been shown to prevent shortening of the lower oesophageal sphincter during gastric distension. In addition to fundoplication, anti-reflux surgery entails reduction of the hiatal hernia with crural approximation. This anatomical restoration has the potential to prevent reflux by reducing the hiatal hernia, and by improving oesophageal clearance and crural and diaphragmatic function by enhancing the lower oesophageal sphincter pressure.

All anti-reflux surgical procedures can be done using minimal access surgery. The introduction of minimal access surgery in this field offered a more acceptable surgical option for patients with gastro-oesophageal reflux disease. This is due to a reduction in post-operative pain, rapid recovery and early discharge from hospital, minimum morbidity and next to zero mortality.

Floppy Nissen fundoplication

This procedure is designed to create a circumferential 2–3 cm loose wrap of gastric fundus around the mobilized abdominal oesophagus. The vagal trunks are preserved and so are the vagal branches to the liver that run through the pars flaccida. Adequate mobilization of the fundus may entail division of the upper short gastric vessels and adhesions between the posterior surface of the upper stomach and the pancreas. Crural repair is performed posteriorly with interrupted sutures. The fundoplication is fixed using seromuscular sutures and include the oesophageal wall. The uppermost suture also approximates the anterior margin of the diaphragmatic hiatus (Figure 7.25). This prevents slipping of the wrap, which is a serious complication as it causes constriction of the stomach. The wrap must be loose (floppy Nissen) to avoid post-operative dysphagia and dehiscence of the wrap. In order to ensure this, a variety of prostheses can be introduced perorally into the oesophagus prior to ligation of the sutures. The operation is performed through the abdomen and has the advantage of access to other upper intra-abdominal pathology which might require surgical attention at the same time, e.g. gall stones. The operation can also be done laparoscopically conferring all the benefits of minimal access surgery. The main disadvantage of the classic Nissen fundoplication is that it results in a supercompetent sphincter with the development of the gas bloat syndrome in 20% of patients. This is due to gaseous distension of the stomach following the inability to belch and vomit. With a properly constructed loose Nissen, post-operative dysphagia is rare and is usually transient.

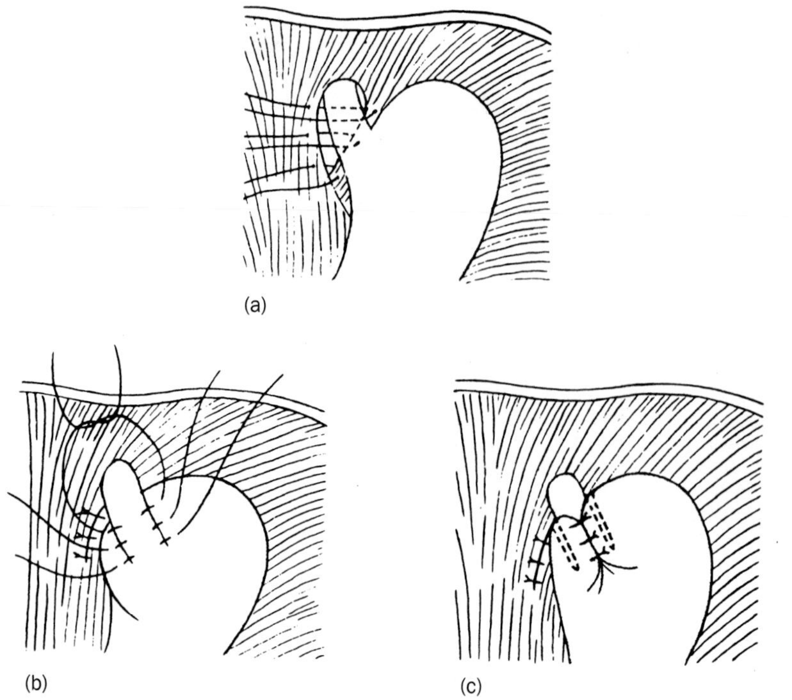

Figure 7.25 Steps in the performance of the Nissen fundoplication. (a) The distal oesophagus has been mobilized to restore its intra-abdominal segment and the diaphragmatic hiatus is being narrowed posteriorly. (b) Placement of the sutures between the stomach and the oesophagus to create the 360° wrap. (c) Fundoplication completed.

Modifications of the classic Nissen are the Rosetti-Hell procedure (Figure 7.26) which was advocated for obese and difficult patients. This creates a smaller wrap from the anterior wall of the fundus. The oesophageal mobilization is as extensive as in classical Nissen. It is important that the posterior wall of the fundus is mobilized fully from the left crus. The division of the upper short gastric vessels is rarely required. The anterior fundus is brought around the oesophagus and sutured to the stomach just to the left edge of the abdominal oesophagus. The sutures do not include the oesophageal wall. Fixation of the wrap to prevent slippage is achieved by 2–3 sutures, which anchor the lower edge of the wrap to the adjacent lesser curvature of the stomach. Crural repair is necessary.

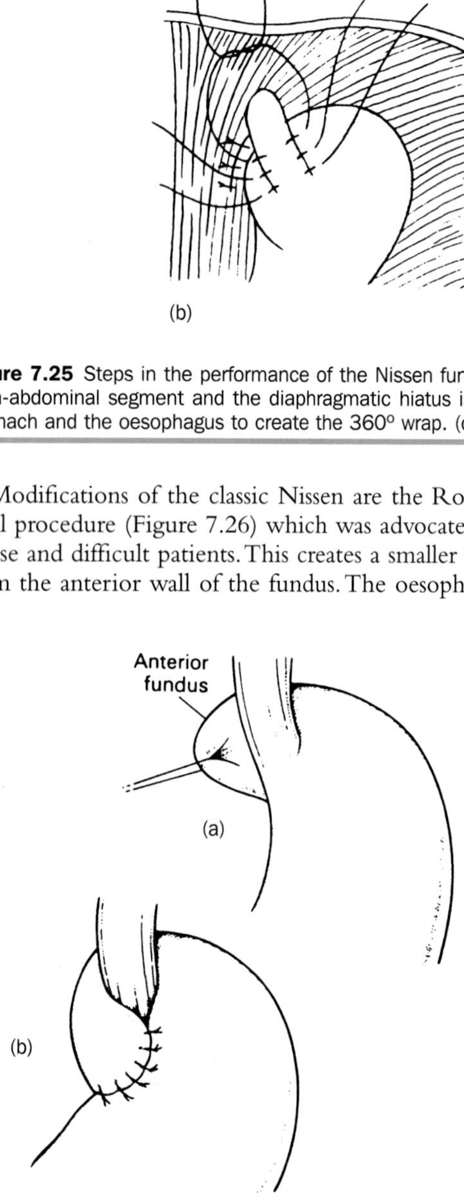

Figure 7.26 Rosetti-Hell modification of the Nissen fundoplication. This creates a smaller wrap and consists of complete mobilization of the oesophagus and gastric fundus. The latter is then brought behind and around the right edge of the oesophagus by means of a stay suture (a); it is then sutured to the adjacent anterior wall of the stomach and the lower edge of the wrap is anchored to the lesser curvature (b).

Partial fundoplication (incomplete wraps)

These procedures have become popular in order to minimize the problem of the gas bloat syndrome frequently encountered after a complete wrap. The two procedures that provide good reflux control comparable to that achieved by total loose fundoplication are the modified Toupet partial fundoplication (posterior) and the Dor (Watson) fundoplication (anterior). In addition the Belsey mark IV repair is a thoracic partial fundoplication.

Modified Toupet partial posterior fundoplication

This entails full mobilization of the abdominal oesophagus and oesophagogastric junction. After the right (posterior) vagus is freed from the oesophagus, the fundus and the upper part of the posterior wall of the stomach are first anchored to the right and left crura by interrupted sutures before the partial (270°) fundoplication is fashioned by suturing the stomach to the

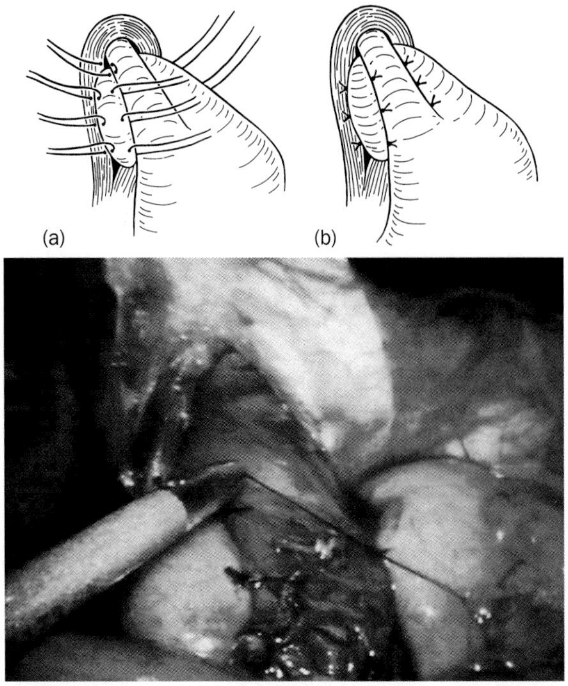

Figure 7.27 (a, b) Diagrammatic representation of the posterior Toupet partial fundoplication. (Reproduced from *Reflux Oesophagitis*.) (c) Laparoscopic Toupet partial fundoplication.

anterior wall of the oesophagus on either side of the anterior vagus nerve. The fixation of the partial wrap to the crura is important and serves two objectives (Figure 7.27). It prevents herniation through the hiatus and abolishes any drag on the oesophageal sutures. Lind described a similar procedure with a 300° posterior fundoplication. Two rows of sutures are placed between the posterior wrap and the oesophagus on either side. A third row of sutures is placed anteriorly leaving a 60° bare area of oesophagus anteriorly. Crural approximation is necessary if there is a hiatal defect.

Anterior partial fundoplication (180°)

This was first described by Dor and has been modified by Watson. The hiatus is repaired behind the oesophagus which is anchored to the right crus. Thereafter the mobilized fundus is brought in front of the oesophagus and sutured to it and to the adjacent oesophagogastric junction and to the right crus, in effect achieving a 180° wrap around the front of the oesophagus. The overall effect is to accentuate the angle of His and anchor 3–5 cm of oesophagus in the abdomen.

Belsey mark IV repair

The operation is performed through a left posterolateral thoracotomy through the bed of the sixth rib. The stomach is rolled around the lower 3–5 cm of the anterior two-thirds (270°) of the mobilized oesophagus by two wraps, the second burying the first and including the diaphragm. When the sutures of the second wrap are tied the intra-abdominal segment of the oesophagus is restored (Figure 7.28). With experience this

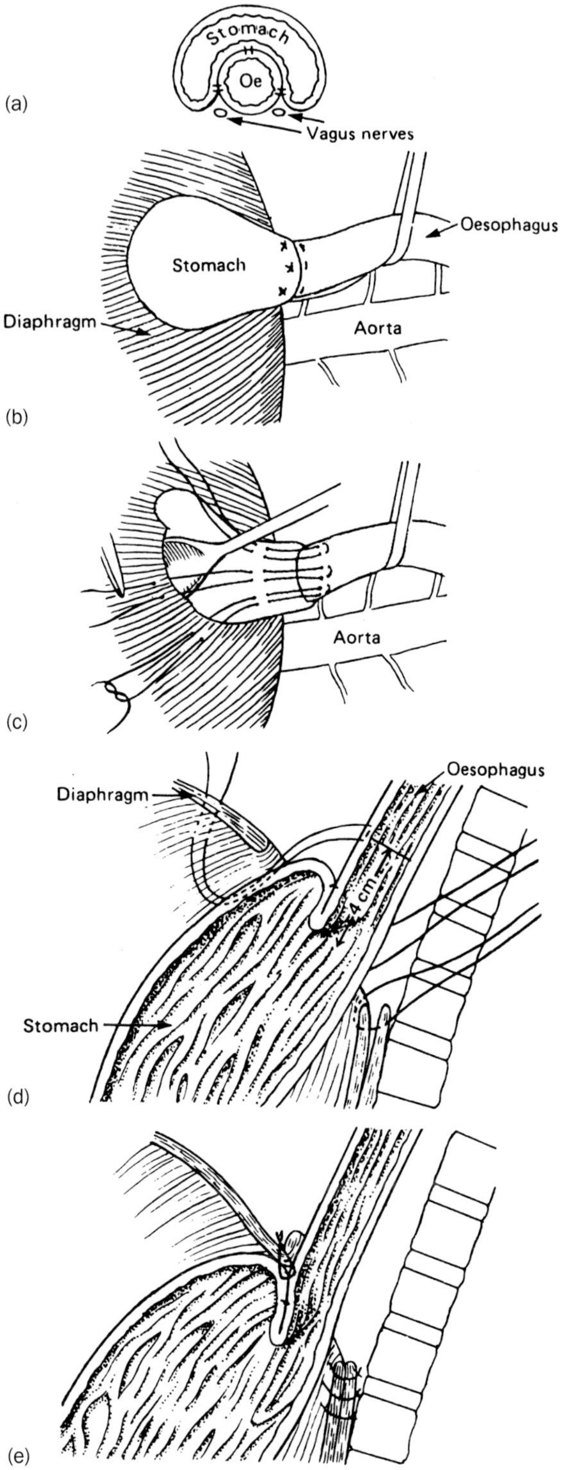

Figure 7.28 The Belsey mark IV repair (transthoracic). (a) The completed 270° gastric wrap around the oesophagus (Oe). (b) The first row of mattress sutures between the oesophagus and the stomach has been completed. (c) Placement of the second row of mattress sutures through the diaphragm as well as stomach and oesophagus. Vertical cross-section of the repair: (d) at time of placement of the second row of mattress sutures; (e) at completion of the repair.

operation gives good results. Since the wrap is not circumferential, the gas bloat syndrome is rarely encountered. A crural repair is considered an essential component of the operation.

Hill posterior gastropexy

This procedure is performed transabdominally. After mobilization of the lower oesophagus, the coeliac axis is identified and the median arcuate ligament overlying the aorta is dissected. Crural repair is performed with non-absorbable sutures so that the hiatus is narrowed to an orifice, which admits one finger along the oesophagus. The gastropexy is achieved by 2–3 cm plicating sutures, which pick up the cardio-oesophageal junction in front and behind the oesophagus on the medial side, in addition to the median arcuate ligament or the pre-aortic fascia. When these sutures are tied, approximately 180° of the distal oesophagus is included in a partial gastric wrap which is fixed firmly to the arcuate ligament and pre-aortic fascia (Figure 7.29). Hill employs an oesophageal manometry catheter and advocates the intra-operative monitoring of pressures during the repair to ascertain that a satisfactory narrowing of the cardia has been achieved.

Insertion of Angelchick prosthesis

The prosthesis consists of an incomplete annular silicone gel filled implant with a tape at either end. These are tied together after insertion and constitute the only anchorage mechanism (Figure 7.30). It requires mobilization of the oesophagus, just enough to enable insertion of the implant. Indeed, excessive mobilization favours migration of the prosthesis, which weighs some 45 g. The most common displacement is distal which results in gastric obstruction. The operation is easy and

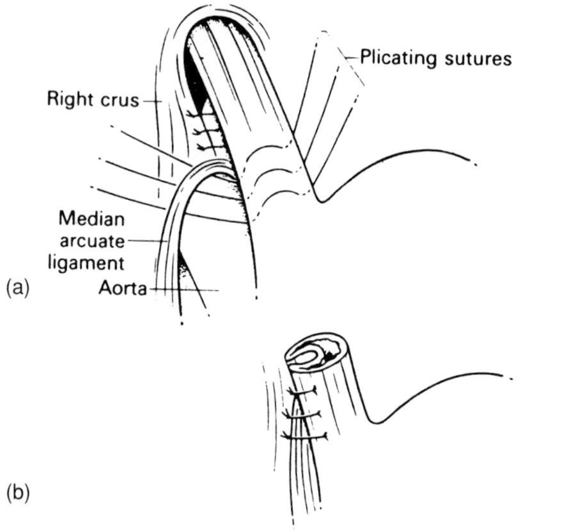

Figure 7.29 The Hill posterior gastropexy. (a) Crural repair has been completed. The plicating sutures in the gastro-oesophageal junction and median arcuate ligament have been inserted. (b) The plicating sutures have been tied resulting in a 180° wrap on the medial side of the gastro-oesophageal junction which is also fixed to the median arcuate ligament.

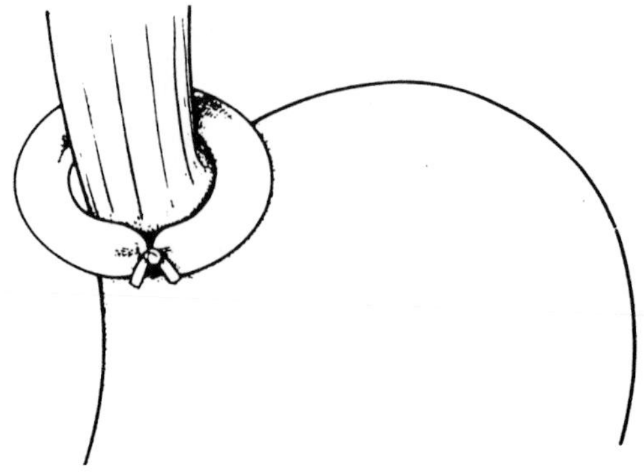

Figure 7.30 The silicone gel Angelchik split-ring prosthesis is inserted around the gastro-oesophageal junction and the tapes are tied anteriorly. Only a very limited mobilization of the oesophagus is performed. This operation has been largely abandoned.

quick to perform. Follow-up studies, however, have shown a high initial dysphagia rate with persistence of this distressing symptom in 8–10% of patients. This requires removal of the prosthesis as the dysphagia is unresponsive to dilatation. Erosion through the wall of the gastro-oesophageal junction is another serious complication but is fortunately rare. The risk of this eventuality is enhanced if the implant is inserted near a suture line. At present the Angelchick prosthesis cannot be recommended for routine use in anti-reflux surgery and is contraindicated after previous subdiaphragmatic surgery.

Collis gastroplasty

In some patients with chronic reflux, the oesophagus is found to be shortened to the extent that despite adequate mediastinal mobilization, there is insufficient length to allow construction of a tension free fundoplication. The oesophagus in these patients can be lengthened by means of a gastroplasty as described by Collis. A tube of lesser curvature is fashioned as a substitute for the intra-abdominal segment of oesophagus (Figure 7.31). The success of the operation was initially thought to be dependent on the restoration of the cardiac angle of His. This is now known to be incorrect and experimental studies have shown that competence is due to the construction of an intra-abdominal muscular tube, which is continuous with the intra-thoracic oesophagus. A partial or complete gastric wrap may be added around the neo-oesophagus. The Collis gastroplasty can be performed through the thoracic access as an adjunct to the Belsey repair or more commonly transabdominally. The procedure can be performed by the hand-assisted laparoscopic approach.

In addition to the above, a number of antireflux procedures such as the ligamentum teres cardiopexy were described by enthusiasts but are only practised by a limited number of surgeons today.

Choice of anti-reflux operation

Aside from individual preference and experience, most general surgeons prefer the abdominal route and use

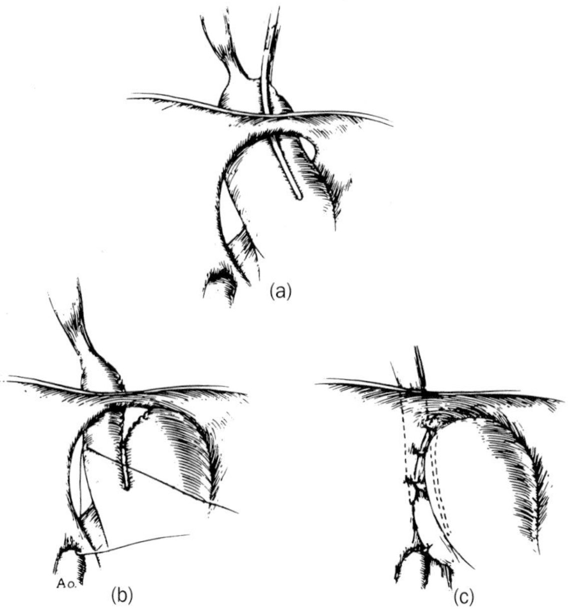

Figure 7.31 The Collis gastroplasty. The oesophageal stricture is dilated intraoperatively. A tube is cut from the lesser curve side of the stomach. This intra-abdominal gastric tube acts as the lower oesophageal segment. It demonstrates a high-pressure zone on manometry and reflux is corrected.

the Nissen procedure or one of its modifications. Fundoplication may, however, be difficult in obese patients, in those with dense adhesions due to previous upper abdominal surgery and those with a narrow subcostal angle and barrel-shaped chest with a deep subdiaphragmatic region. In these patients, a thoracic approach using the Belsey mark IV procedure is a better and safer alternative.

Laparoscopic anti-reflux and hiatal hernia surgery
Minimal access anti-reflux and hiatal hernia surgery has become increasingly established throughout the world. The minimal access route confers the benefits of reduced post-operative pain, early recovery and discharge from hospital, and minimum morbidity. All the minimal access procedures reproduce the essential steps of the equivalent open operation. Short-term results have largely mirrored the experience with the open operations. If the long-term results of efficacy are confirmed this will result in a significant change in the management of patients with gastro-oesophageal reflux disease.

Results and complications of anti-reflux surgery
Success in anti-reflux surgery describes improvement or abolition of reflux symptoms with healing of oesophagitis and reduction of lower oesophageal acid exposure to within physiological levels, in the largest proportion of operated patients, for a long period, with minimum adverse technical and post-operative consequences. Symptomatic improvement after anti-reflux surgery has been reported between 65% and 96% whereas symptom abolition was in the range of 32–82%. Healing of oesophagitis after anti-reflux surgery is reported between 63% and 91% whereas restoration of lower oesophageal acid exposure to normal was in the range of 67–85%.

Mortality after anti-reflux surgery is less than 1% and is mainly related to comorbid factors. Intra-operative complications depend on the experience of the surgeon, and the procedure performed and can be as high as 10%. Post-operative complications include persistent troublesome dysphagia 6 months after surgery (5.5%), early satiety (49%), abdominal bloating (36%), inability to belch or vomit (31%), diarrhoea (20%), nausea (8%) and recurrent reflux symptoms (8%) of which 3–6% will require revisional surgery. At revisional surgery the fundoplication may be found to be too tight, too loose, too long, incorrectly positioned, disrupted or slipped either up above the diaphragm or down around the stomach. Disruption of the crural approximation can facilitate wrap migration and para-oesophageal herniation.

Laparoscopic anti-reflux surgery appears equivalent to the open approach in terms of symptomatic and objective reflux control. However, the incidence of complications appears to be slightly higher than following the open approach, especially troublesome dysphagia and proximal migration of the wrap. The exact reasons for these complications are not clear. Prior to revisional surgery medical therapy a comprehensive re-evaluation should be attempted. At surgery the reason for failure of the anti-reflux procedure should be identified and corrected for each individual patient. The size of the hiatus and crural approximation should be evaluated, the length and diameter of the wrap should be explored and fixation of the wrap to the gastro-oesophageal junction and a length of intra-abdominal oesophagus should be ascertained.

Management of benign oesophageal strictures

The general principles for the management of patients with benign oesophageal strictures are:

- Establishing an accurate diagnosis on the nature of the stricture and its cause.
- Dilatation of the stricture to obviate dysphagia.
- To establish a long-term treatment strategy for the individual patient. This may be by medical therapy using proton pump inhibitors with a chronic dilatation regimen, demand dilatation, specific anti-reflux therapy or surgery, stricturoplasty, or oesophageal intubation, replacement or bypass.

An accurate diagnosis is essential as it affects the treatment options for the oesophageal stricture itself and any underlying disease. The initial assessment is with a clinical history, which includes an evaluation of the patient's perception of and response to the complaint of dysphagia. The history should also seek symptoms of coughing, aspiration and symptoms of neuromuscular disorders in addition to previous symptoms of reflux. History of odynophagia and weight loss should also be established. Drug therapy should also be enquired

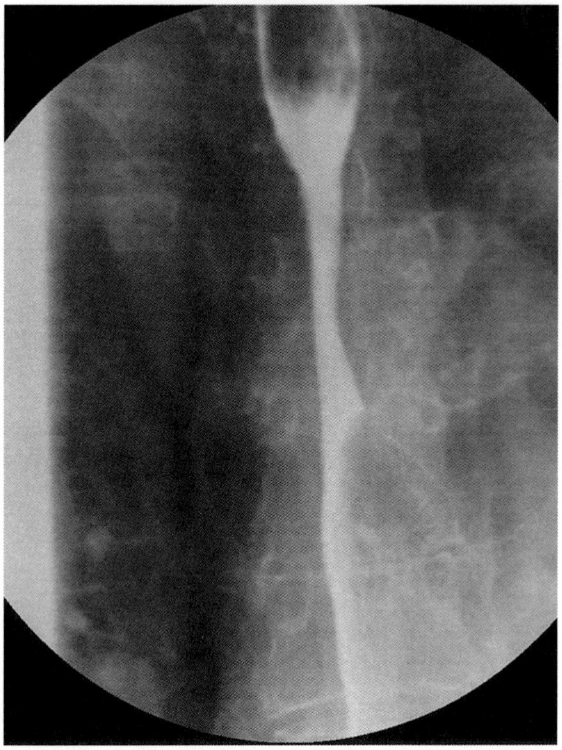

Figure 7.32 Barium swallow showing a benign oesophageal stricture with smooth tapering ends causing hold-up to the flow of barium.

about. A barium swallow is probably the best initial diagnostic test. This should establish the length and width of the stricture and will provide additional mucosal detail (Figure 7.32). In addition it provides useful information for planning the endoscopy and dilatation. The presence of a hiatus hernia and evidence of reflux may also be ascertained from the barium swallow. Endoscopic visualization with biopsy and brush cytology should establish the nature of the stricture. The flexible endoscope can also be used for dilatation of the stricture in order to obtain more representative biopsies. A normal barium swallow and endoscopy should rule out a stricture and in these circumstances a motility disorder of the oesophagus should be considered.

Gastro-oesophageal reflux is the most common cause of benign oesophageal strictures with 10% of reflux patients developing strictures. The stricture is caused by chronic fibrosis and scarring in response to chronic reflux injury in the lower oesophagus. Reflux and Barrett's strictures usually occur at the gastro-oesophageal junction. Medication induced strictures are associated with the use of tetracycline, doxycycline, potassium chloride, quinidine and non-steroidal anti-inflammatory agents. These strictures frequently occur in the mid-oesophagus at the level of the aortic arch but can occur anywhere in the oesophagus. Oesophageal rings and webs should not be confused with oesophageal strictures. Although webs and strictures can be caused by reflux oesophageal strictures are usually longer than 3 mm, are fibrotic and frequently require multiple gradual dilatations. Another cause of benign strictures is ingestion of caustic agents. Caustic stricture formation occurs in up to 30% of patients within 8 weeks and persists. These strictures are often long and may involve the whole length of the oesophagus. They usually require multiple dilatations. Benign strictures of the oesophagus occur following oesophageal variceal sclerotherapy in up to 30% of patients and less commonly following oesophageal variceal ligation. Benign oesophageal strictures also arise following radiation therapy. Radiation induced strictures are usually difficult to treat by oesophageal dilatation. Rarely connective tissue disorders such as scleroderma are associated with benign oesophageal strictures. Prolonged nasogastric intubation may also result in long oesophageal strictures.

The principal aim of dilatation is to stretch the fibrous component of the stricture gradually to achieve an oesophageal lumen of 10–15 mm in diameter. The end point of dilatation depends on the initial size of the stricture, the general condition of the patient and the predisposing factors. Most strictures can be dilated but severe long and tortuous strictures are difficult, carry an increased risk of perforation and can recur quickly following dilatation.

Various types of dilating systems are currently available (Table 7.8).

Mercury-filled rubber bougies are useful for mild strictures. The Maloney dilators have a tapered tip and the Hurst dilators have a blunt tip. Both are easy to use and are well tolerated. However, they impose a burden on the patient who has to be instructed on their repeated use and many patients experience difficulty in swallowing them. Sizes less than 36 Fr are very difficult to use because they are too pliable and tend to bend or coil if the oesophagus is too tortuous or the stricture is narrow.

Wire-guided dilators such as the Savery/Gillard dilators, Puestow, Celestin and Gruntzig are useful in all types of strictures. They are more rigid and are less likely to bend or coil. They have a central core so that they can be passed over a pre-inserted guidewire. Some consist of metal olives (Eder/Puestow) and some are more substantial graduated polyvinyl dilators (Savery/Gillard, Celestin). The guidewire should have a flexible tip and can be inserted either endoscopically or using fluoroscopy. Hydrophilic guidewires tend to be less rigid, more expensive but easier to pass through long and tortuous strictures. When the guidewire is inserted endoscopically it is safer to check the position of the wire by fluoroscopy. When the guidewire is in position the endoscope can be withdrawn and the dilators passed over the guidewire across the strictured part of the oesophagus. Advancement of the dilator should be coupled with rotation of the dilator around the guidewire. When undue resistance is encountered dilatation should be halted. For severe strictures the dilatation needs to be gradual and the procedure may necessitate two or more sessions with rest intervals of 1–2 weeks between sessions. During each session,

Table 7.8 Dilating systems

Procedure	*Comment*
Rigid oesophagoscopy with rigid dilators without guidewire	Requires general anaesthesia, higher risk of perforation
Flexible endoscopy with guidewire-guided dilators: Puestow, Clestin,Gruntzig, TTS and OTW hydrostatic balloons	Can be performed under sedation, lower risk of perforation
Fluoroscopy (without endoscopy) and guidewire-guided dilators: OTW hydrostatic balloons	Performed under sedation, low risk of perforation
Non-rigid dilators: mercury-weighted rubber (e.g. Maloney)	Self-administered, lower risk of perforation. Ineffective for severe strictures, poor patient compliance

dilatation should not exceed 6–8 mm increase in diameter. If available, routine fluoroscopy should be used for all wire-guided dilatations.

Hydrostatic polyurethane balloon dilators are of two types. Through the scope type (TTS) are used endoscopically whereas over the wire type (OTW) are mainly wire guided and less popular. The balloons are hydrostatically pressurized to inflate to a maximum diameter (Figure 7.33). Some versions produce a variable balloon maximum diameter dependent on the hydrostatic pressure. The balloon catheter tip is flexible and atraumatic and can negotiate tortuous or narrow strictures. Hydrostatic balloons are largely safe and can be used progressively to dilate long strictures, but are expensive.

The complications of dilatation include haemorrhage, perforation and septicaemia.

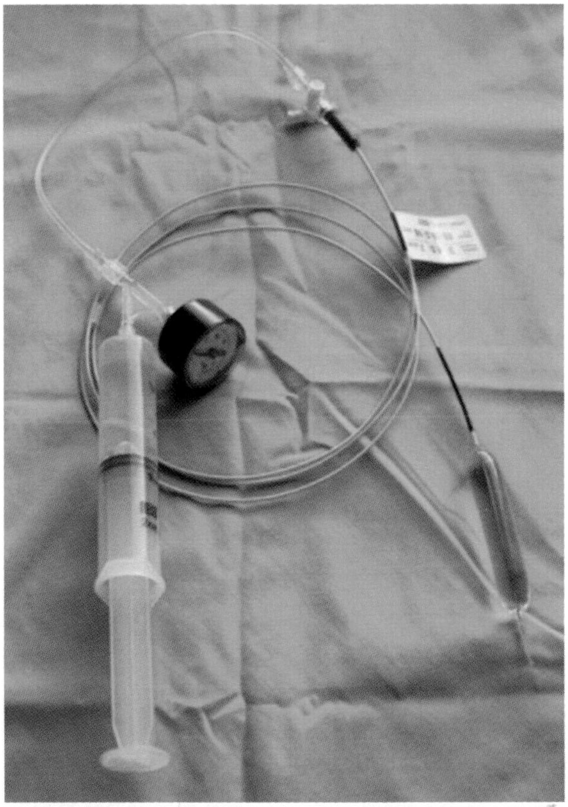

Figure 7.33 Hydrostatic polyurethane balloon dilator.

Although there is universal agreement that dilatation is the first line treatment in patients with dysphagia due to a benign oesophageal stricture, there is considerable controversy regarding the subsequent treatment.

Once adequate dilatation is achieved patients should be advised on lifestyle adjustment and should be prescribed proton pump inhibitors. Up to 50% of patients will achieve a satisfactory freedom from dysphagia using this approach. The rest will require frequent dilatations. Of those who will require repeated dilatations 50% will be elderly and unsuitable for anti-reflux surgery. These patients should be on a chronic dilatation regimen at predetermined intervals with demand dilatations carried out as required. The rest of the patients should have anti-reflux surgery with or without a stricturoplasty (Thal fundic patch). A small cohort of young patients will have severe strictures, which require frequent dilatations. These can be managed by either intubation or resection with oesophageal replacement. Intubation should be reserved for elderly unfit patients and should be combined with lifelong proton pump inhibitors. Younger and fit patients should be considered for resection and replacement. If the stricture is short it can be replaced by an interposed isoperistaltic jejunum or colon and if the stricture is long oesophagectomy should be considered with replacement using a gastric pull through or a colonic segment. This operation is clearly reserved for fit patients.

A single dilatation usually obviates all oesophageal rings and webs, however, medication and caustic induced strictures, radiation strictures and those strictures sustained after prolonged nasogastric intubation may require repeat dilatations. If the strictures are resistant to dilatation and the patients are fit oesophagectomy and replacement should be considered.

Surgical treatment of strictures

Indications for surgery include:

- Young patients with reflux strictures.
- Frequent and especially increasingly difficult dilatations.
- Intractable/impassable strictures or strictures associated with Barrett's oesophagus.

All young patients with peptic strictures that respond to dilatation and proton pump inhibitors should be considered for *anti-reflux surgery*. If the stricture is impassable pre-operatively this can be facilitated intra-operatively. Access through a left posterolateral or left

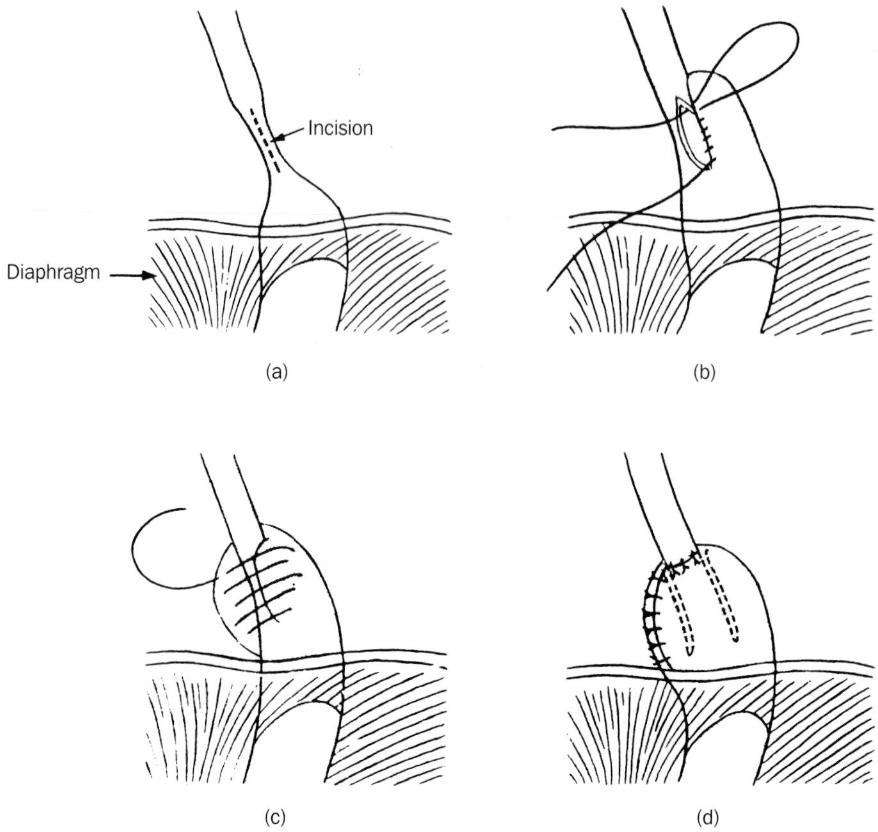

Figure 7.34 The Thal fundic patch operation for distal oesophageal stricture. (a) Incision and dilatation of stricture. (b) Oesophageal defect covered by gastric serosa. (c) Full fundoplication to prevent further reflux. (d) Completed procedure.

thoracoabdominal approach facilitates exposure and mobilization of the lower oesophagus. The negotiation of the stricture can be guided by the surgeon's hand. Once the stricture is dilated attempts should be made to reduce the gastro-oesophageal junction below the diaphragm. A standard anti-reflux procedure such as Belsey mark IV or the Nissen fundoplication is then performed. If there is significant oesophageal shortening a Collis gastroplasty is indicated to create a neo-oesophagus around which a wrap is formed.

If the stricture is severely fibrotic and cannot be dilated then the *Thal fundic patch* should be considered. The stricture is incised longitudinally and the lumen of the oesophagus allowed to gape open. The mobilized fundus of the stomach is applied as a serosal patch to the margins of the opening in the distal oesophagus. A full fundoplication around the rest of the oesophagus completes the procedure (Figure 7.34). Resection of these severe impassable strictures with replacement by interposed isoperistaltic jejunum or colon is nowadays considered preferable to the Thal fundic patch as it gives better long-term results.

Subtotal oesophagectomy with replacement by stomach or colon is reserved for long strictures. The best long-term results are probably achieved by a vagus sparing oesophagectomy with an interposed isoperistaltic jejunum (Figure 7.35) or left colon placed in

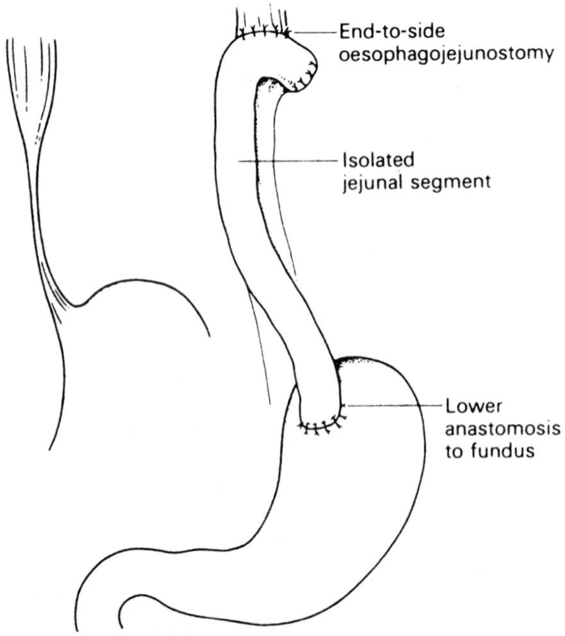

Figure 7.35 Replacement of a severe intractable stricture with a loop of isoperistaltic jejunum isolated on a vascular pedicle. Following resection, the jejunal segment is interposed between the oesophagus and the stomach. Alternatively, a loop of colon can be used to restore continuity.

the posterior mediastinum. The use of a gastric pull through would necessarily incur division of the vagus but would make the operation technically easier and less demanding for the surgeon. Transhiatal dissection of the oesophagus (Orringer) would also obviate a thoracotomy.

Columnar metaplasia of the oesophagus (Barrett's oesophagus)

Columnar cell lined oesophagus was first described by Barrett as ectopic islands of gastric epithelium associated with deep ulceration and stricture formation. This description has undergone several modifications in light of new knowledge but the condition continues to be referred to as Barrett's oesophagus. The condition is usually diagnosed when a segment of salmon pink columnar epithelium is seen endoscopically to extend well above the gastro-oesophageal junction. The diagnosis must be confirmed histologically. The gastro-oesophageal junction in normal individuals is the point at which the tubular oesophagus joins the saccular stomach. However, the squamocolumnar mucosal junction does not always coincide with the gastro-oesophageal junction and can be above it. Thus gastric columnar epithelium in the lower oesophagus (<3 cm) is not abnormal, nor is junctional epithelium with mucus secreting cells abnormal. However, metaplastic columnar epithelium with goblet cells is abnormal anywhere in the oesophagus. This metaplastic epithelium is histologically identical to intestinal metaplasia of the incomplete type found in the stomach and has been termed 'specialized' intestinal metaplasia. This specialized columnar epithelium is often flat but occasionally has a villiform surface and always with mucus secreting columnar cells and goblet cells. The goblet cells contain acidic mucin. The columnar cells may resemble normal gastric foveolar cells or intestinal absorptive cells, but they do not have all the typical features of either. Goblet cells are the key cells that distinguish ordinary columnar epithelium from specialized epithelium.

The terms 'long segment Barrett's oesophagus' (LSBE) and 'short segment Barrett's oesophagus' (SSBE) describe the extent of intestinal metaplasia in the oesophagus to be more than or less than 3 cm respectively. The distinction has clinical significance since SSBE is 3.5 times more prevalent than LSBE but the prevalence of dysplasia in LSBE is three times that in SSBE. Demographically patients with LSBE and SSBE tend to be white male smokers.

The term 'oesophagogastric junction specialized intestinal metaplasia' (OGJ-SIM) has been coined to describe the presence of specialized intestinal metaplasia in biopsies obtained from the area just distal to the oesophagogastric junction. This condition is as prevalent as SSBE and can progress to dysplasia and cancer but is more likely related to *H. pylori* gastritis. There may however be a subset of patients in this entity who represent a continuation of the spectrum of Barrett's oesophagus.

Barrett's oesophagus is an acquired condition, which seems to have a particular predilection for white males in the Western world. Autopsy studies suggest that the majority of cases of Barrett's oesophagus in the general population are unrecognized. The clinical prevalence of the condition is around 22.6 cases per 100 000 of population. Up to 4% of all patients referred for endoscopy, up to 20% of patients with reflux symptoms, 44% of patients with a reflux stricture, 37% of patients with scleroderma and up to 26% of institutionalized, handicapped patients have Barrett's oesophagus. It is controversial as to how quickly the condition develops but there are suggestions that Barrett's oesophagus can develop within 3 years and once formed, the surface area of the oesophagus covered by intestinal metaplasia remains constant in most individuals. Up to 10% of patients can progress with continued reflux and up to 2% may regress.

Columnar metaplasia of the lower oesophagus develops in up to 20% of patients with reflux symptoms. Patients with Barrett's oesophagus have more severe symptoms of reflux for a longer duration. However, community prevalence figures suggest that the majority of patients with Barrett's oesophagus are asymptomatic. This has prompted a search for a serum marker for the condition, but no sensitive serum marker has thus far been found. The majority of patients with Barrett's oesophagus are found to have a hiatus hernia. Oesophageal motility profiles in these patients show a particularly low pressure of the lower oesophageal sphincter and relatively weak oesophageal body contractions. In addition, these patients are found to have a significantly higher prevalence of abnormal oesophageal bilirubin exposure than those patients without Barrett's with or without oesophagitis.

It is generally accepted that columnar replacement at the gastro-oesophageal junction is a response to reflux trauma at that site but the reasons for intestinal specialization remain unclear. There is evidence that the basal cells in the squamous oesophageal epithelium give rise to the development of intestinal metaplasia rather than cephalad creeping substitution of the denuded squamous epithelium in the lower oesophagus. One model of the possible pathophysiology of Barrett's oesophagus stipulates that the adaptive response to the increased cell loss caused by reflux oesophagitis is an increase in the proliferative zone height and length. The functional stem cells in the basal zone become more accessible and susceptible to refluxed material and ingested carcinogens and mutagens. For some reason, the rapidly proliferating multi-potential cells in the basal layer assume a metaplastic phenotype, which survives natural selection in the reflux milieu.

This condition has stimulated substantial interest recently in view of the escalating incidence of adenocarcinoma of the lower oesophagus and gastrooesophageal junction in the Western world. Neoplastic progression in Barrett's oesophagus develops within the metaplastic columnar epithelium when genetic changes occur that lead to the development of dysplasia. The accumulation of additional genetic changes within the dysplastic epithelium may lead to the development of adenocarcinoma. Dysplasia in Barrett's oesophagus is recognized histologically by a combination of architectural and cytological abnormalities. Dysplastic glands may retain their normal configuration, but more often have irregular or even grossly distorted architecture. In low-grade dysplasia, the glands are limited by cells with crowded, stratified, hyperchromatic nuclei. In high-grade dysplasia, the nuclei are larger and more hyperchromatic, have irregular nuclear membranes and have lost their polarity. Because the epithelial abnormalities in dysplasia form a continuous spectrum from relatively mild atypia to overt dysplasia the boundaries separating negative, indefinite, low and high-grade dysplasia cannot be sharply defined. Thus, significant inter-observer variation in the diagnosis and grading of dysplasia exists. Indeed, when severe dysplasia has been confirmed, approximately 40% of patients will harbour adenocarcinoma of the oesophagus as found at resection. The other problems in the diagnosis of dysplasia include sampling error and differentiation from reactive change. It is suggested that four quadrant biopsies using 'jumbo' forceps at intervals of 2 cm or less throughout the length of the Barrett's segment should overcome the majority of sampling errors. Reactive or regenerative hyperplasia due to inflammation or ulceration may be difficult to differentiate from dysplasia. This situation is termed indefinite for dysplasia and warrants further biopsies after intensive medical therapy.

The molecular alterations that underlie the process of malignant transformation in Barrett's oesophagus include aneuploidy, microsatellite instability, and mutations or deletions in several loci. One of the earliest events in the malignant transformation is the selection and propagation of the metaplastic clones with specialized intestinal metaplasia. Subsequently, altered expression of growth factors, such as epidermal growth factor (EGF) and transforming growth factor-alpha (TGFα) and genomic alterations of cell cycle-associated genes are noted. Cell cycle gene abnormalities include increased cyclin D1 expression (chromosome 11q13), hypermethylated or mutated p16 (chromosome 9p21), mobilization of cells from G0 to G1, loss of control of the G1/S phase transition and accumulation of cells in G2. Over-expression of p53 protein is frequently observed with an increasing rate from metaplasia to dysplasia and cancer. The increase in p53 expression is accompanied by an increase in Ki67 labelling indicating proliferative activity and an upward shift of the proliferative compartment. The prevalence of DNA aneuploidy increases with increasing histological grade of abnormality from metaplasia to cancer. Neoplastic progression occurs when genomic instability produces multiple aneuploid subclones and one or more develop the capacity for invasion. Inhibition of apoptosis is a late event and probably occurs in a subpopulation of cells. Alteration of cell adhesion and increased cell migration precede cancer invasion. The expression of CD44H and its variants increases progressively in dysplasia and infiltrating cancer.

Surveillance for Barrett's oesophagus is aimed to detect dysplasia, the first step in the neoplastic transformation. The surveillance interval is based on the grade of dysplasia. The recommended frequency of surveillance endoscopy in patients with Barrett's oesophagus is shown in Table 7.9. Representative four quadrant biopsies should be taken from every 2 cm level of intestinal metaplasia. In addition, biopsies should be obtained from areas of nodularity, ulcers or strictures. The biopsies should be stained with specialized stains (periodic acid–Schiff, high iron diamine) in addition to the standard stains (haemoxylin and eosin). The majority of pathologists have agreed to adhere to reporting in accordance with the Vienna classification of gastrointestinal epithelial neoplasia (Table 7.10). Algorithms of surveillance and management have developed for the different categories.

Medical treatment of Barrett's oesophagus without dysplasia using proton pump inhibitors reduces the acid exposure to the oesophagus, and by inhibiting acid production reduces the volume of refluxed material that includes bile. However, both acid and bile reflux

Table 7.9 Recommended surveillance programme for patients with intestinal metaplasia and dysplasia

No dysplasia	After two negative biopsies every 3 years
Indefinite dysplasia	Repeat biopsy after a course of PPIs
Low-grade dysplasia	Every 6 months for 1 year and then every year
High-grade dysplasia	Expert confirmation and resection for surgical candidates

Four large biopsy specimens should be taken from every 2 cm level of the Barrett's oesophagus.

Table 7.10 Vienna classification of gastrointestinal epithelial neoplasia

Category 1	Negative for neoplasia/dysplasia
Category 2	Indefinite for neoplasia/dysplasia
Category 3	Non-invasive low-grade neoplasia (low-grade adenoma/dysplasia)
Category 4	Non-invasive high-grade neoplasia
	4.1 High-grade adenoma/dysplasia
	4.2 Non-invasive carcinoma (carcinoma *in situ*)[a]
	4.3 Suspicion of invasive carcinoma
Category 5	Invasive neoplasia
	5.1 Intramucosal carcinoma[b]
	5.2 Submucosal carcinoma or beyond

[a]Non-invasive indicates absence of evident invasion.
[b]Intramucosal indicates invasion into the lamina propria or muscularis mucosae.

(Table reproduced from Schlemper *et al.*, The Vienna classification of gastrointestinal epithelial neoplasia. *Gut* 2000; **47**: 251–5.)

into the oesophagus while patients are on maintenance therapy, and in some patients the degree of oesophageal exposure to gastric juice remains abnormal. There is also concern that raising the pH of the gastric environment allows bile acids to remain in solution in a non-polar form that is noxious to the oesophageal mucosa. Surgical treatment of these patients by fundoplication will correct pathological oesophageal reflux of both acid and duodenal content. There is evidence that surgically treated patients are protected from the development of dysplasia and oesophageal cancer. There is also evidence that an anti-reflux procedure in patients with Barrett's oesophagus may induce partial or even complete regression of Barrett's epithelium but the impact of this regression on the subsequent development of adenocarcinoma is not clear. There is further evidence that *de novo* development of Barrett's oesophagus is exceedingly rare in patients who have had effective anti-reflux surgery. This is in marked contrast to reports of long-term medical treatment where up to 34% of patients on long-term acid suppression developed Barrett's oesophagus while on therapy.

The concern over the premalignant nature of Barrett's oesophagus has stimulated efforts to reverse the metaplastic process. Medical therapy, even with high-dose proton pump inhibitors or anti-reflux surgery has claimed only partial and unpredictable regression of the columnar epithelium. Further, there is uncertainty whether surgery or high-dose medical therapy can hold the progression to dysplasia and carcinoma. Consequently, efforts have been turned to ablating the Barrett's mucosa by thermal, chemical or mechanical means. Laser therapy, electrosurgery (monopolar, bipolar) and argon-enhanced electrosurgery are thermal. These have been used with variable success. Ablated areas heal with squamous cells but require multiple treatments and strictures may form during the healing process. There are also reports of squamous regeneration overlying Barrett's epithelium. Photodynamic therapy is chemical. A photoactive drug is administered that is preferentially absorbed in highly proliferating cells and subsequently activated by light of a specific wavelength. When the drug is activated, singlet oxygen and superoxide radicals are created which destroy cellular organelles thereby killing the tissue. The depth of treatment is limited to the penetration of light and is therefore controllable. The technique is limited by systemic photosensitization, which requires patients to stay out of direct sunlight for varying periods; it is also limited by the incomplete and unreliable nature of the columnar ablation and the high incidence of stricture formation. Surgical ultrasound is a primarily mechanical means of ablation. With this method the mucosal cells are mechanically removed or destroyed by scrubbing, abrading or separating layers. The cavitron ultrasonic surgical aspirator is a surgical ultrasound system that was designed for this purpose. The system can be set to optimal energy frequencies to ablate only the epithelium superficial to the muscularis mucosa. Early results of this technique are promising.

The optimum management of patients with high-grade dysplasia detected on biopsy consists of oesophagectomy. When high-grade dysplasia is confirmed to be present, approximately 40% of these patients may harbour an occult cancer not detected on surveillance biopsies. In addition the surrogate changes of high-grade dysplasia and intramucosal cancer are not reliably differentiated. Further, the rate of progression from high-grade dysplasia to invasive cancer can be as fast as 10–14 months. For all these reasons it is prudent to recommend early oesophagectomy for these patients provided expert confirmation of the severity of dysplasia is obtained.

Since intramucosal cancer is different in biological behaviour from invasive cancer, it has been suggested that it may be amenable to endoscopic mucosal resection (EMR). This type of approach would require that intramucosal tumours be distinguished from those that are more deeply invasive. Despite endoscopic ultrasound, it is questionable whether this is possible. Further, up to 18% of patients with intramucosal lesions have positive lymph nodes. This type of approach may be more suitable for patients with comorbid disease or in combined modality treatment schedules.

Non-reflux oesophagitis

The classification of non-reflux induced oesophageal damage is outlined in Table 7.11. Some are the result of accidental or deliberate ingestion of corrosive agents. The commonest infective oesophagitis seen nowadays is due to monilia infestation. Iatrogenic oesophageal damage may be drug induced or follow radiotherapy or instrumentation of the oesophagus including insertion of a nasogastric tube. There are well-documented cases of the development of severe strictures after nasogastric intubation but considering the frequency of usage of this procedure in general surgery, this complication is very rare although transient oesophagitis is very common.

Corrosive oesophagitis

The ingestion of solid or liquid caustic agents is accidental in children, but in adults it usually represents attempted suicide. The most common chemicals which are swallowed are alkaline caustics, acids and household bleaches. The alkaline caustics consist of sodium hydroxide (the active ingredient in household lye and drain cleaners), sodium carbonate (washing soda), sodium metasalicylate (dishwashing detergent) and ammonia water (household cleaners). Oesophageal burns have also been reported following the ingestion of clinitest tablets which contain a significant amount of anhydrous sodium hydroxide. Severe damage also results in children who swallow small alkaline batteries, which consist of 45% potassium hydroxide of approximately 8 M.

These corrosive substances cause an initial burn with necrosis of the mucosa and underlying tissue, the extent of which is proportional to the concentration, amount and duration of tissue contact. In general, acid ingestion

Table 7.11 Types of non-reflux oesophagitis

Type	*Causative agent*	*Clinical features*
Corrosive	Lye, acid, sodium hypochlorite, etc.	Burns, stricture, motility disorders, reflux disease
Infective	Candidosis	Occurs in chronic illnesses, immunosuppressive or antibiotic therapy, secondary to other oesophagitis, AIDS
	Herpes virus	Occurs in debilitated, immunosuppressed patients particularly with lymphoproliferative disorders
Drug-induced	Tetracycline, NSAIDs, doxycycline, etc.	Higher incidence in patients with motility disorders and reflux disease
Radiation	Doses greater than 20–40 Gy to the mediastinum if combined with adriamycin or actinomycin D	Ulceration and stricture formation, may simulate recurrence of neoplasm
Specific disorders		Bullous dermatoses, Behçet's syndrome, Crohn's disease, aphthous oesophagitis, etc.

results in a higher incidence of stricturing and mortality, which is reported to be 18% as opposed to 2% following ingestion of lye. The speed of lye injury is so great that attempts to neutralize the caustic are usually futile. The severity of the burn is classified as follows:

- First degree: mucosal hyperaemia
- Second degree: transmucosal ulceration
- Third degree: deep ulceration, mediastinal, plural or peritoneal perforation.

All ingested corrosives commonly affect other sites in addition to the oesophagus. These include the oropharynx, larynx, stomach, duodenum and jejunum (rare). The oesophageal/gastric involvement may be total or segmental. In severe injuries, necrosis of the tracheal wall leads to the early development of a tracheo-oesophageal fistula, which unless recognized early and treated promptly by surgical intervention, carries a prohibitive mortality.

The burned wound progresses through acute, subacute and chronic cicatrical stages. The acute inflammatory phase occurs in the first few days following injury and is characterized by tissue coagulation, inflammatory reaction, vascular thrombosis and secondary bacterial infection. During the subacute phase, which may last up to 2 weeks (depending on the severity of the injury), all necrotic tissue is lysed and replaced by granulation tissue. The injured oesophagus is potentially weakest during this intermediate phase (7–14 days post-injury). Symptoms of pain and dysphagia may well improve or disappear during this period. The process of epithelialization is usually complete by the third to the sixth week following injury. Maturation and contraction of the fibrous tissue results in the formation of strictures which may be multiple, short or long (tubular). At times, the fibrosis is not circumferential, and on contraction, leads to a shelf stricture. Other long-term consequences of severe corrosive oesophagitis are the development of carcinoma of the oesophagus, motility disorders of the oesophagus, hiatus hernia and gastro-oesophageal reflux. The latter is held responsible for strictures which develop years after the injury. Although there is evidence for the association between corrosive strictures and the development of oesophageal carcinoma, the risk appears small and does not justify prophylactic oesophagectomy. Careful long-term follow-up of all patients with regular endoscopy is, however, necessary.

Management

After early resuscitation the goals of therapy are to prevent perforation and to avoid progressive fibrosis of the oesophagus. The early management consists of assessment of the extent and severity of the injuries, supportive therapy, antibiotics and steroid administration. On admission, the whole of the oropharynx is carefully inspected. Substernal and back pain or abdominal signs may suggest mediastinal or intra-abdominal perforation. Hoarseness, stridor and dyspnoea suggest laryngeal oedema. The initial radiological investigations consist of chest radiography and abdominal films. Monitoring by pulse oximetry and intermittent arterial blood gas analysis should be carried out and tracheostomy should be performed if airway obstruction or respiratory distress is severe or progressive. Systemic antibiotic therapy is commenced with broad-spectrum antibiotics. In addition, some favour the oral administration of an anti-fungal agent in severe injuries to prevent candida infestation. Shock is treated with intravenous fluids as necessary. Sedatives and analgesics are administered to relieve anxiety and pain. Fibre-optic endoscopy should be performed within the first 24 hours to assess severity of the oesophageal injury. Antacids are administered for first degree burns. Although controversial, corticosteroids are recommended at an initial dose of 80 mg per day tapering to 20 mg per day until the oesophagus heals. These patients are kept without oral intake until they can swallow their saliva. Patients with third degree burns, especially after liquid lye, require further investigation with water-soluble contrast agents swallow and on confirmation of necrosis/perforation are subjected to emergency oesophago-gastrectomy. In less severely injured patients, a contrast swallow investigation is rarely necessary in the early stages and is usually performed together with repeat endoscopy 3 weeks after the injury. Regular dilatation should commence for all patients with strictures. The optimal time for commencement of dilatation varies with the severity of the injury and is best delayed until re-epithelialization is complete. This can take from 10 days to several weeks depending on the severity of the burn.

The indications for surgical reconstruction of the oesophagus after corrosive injury are:

- Extensive persistent strictures.
- The need for frequent dilatations.
- Presence of high strictures or late fistula between the oesophagus and the tracheobronchial tree.
- Physical and psychological trauma to a child which may impair normal growth and development.
- Late oesophageal shortening with reflux oesophagitis.
- Severe dysplasia, carcinoma *in situ* or invasive carcinoma during follow-up.

The surgical alternatives for patients with extensive oesophageal scarring are total oesophagectomy and its replacement with colon, isoperistaltic jejunum or stomach. When the mediastinum is frozen, which is a common occurrence, the scarred oesophagus is left *in situ* and a bypass procedure is used. Colon bypass is generally preferred. The mobilized left colon, based on the ascending branch of the left colic artery and the inferior mesenteric vein, is placed in an isoperistaltic fashion and tunnelled through the anterior mediastinum (retro-sternal) space into the neck, to be anastomosed end to end with the transected oesophagus above, and to the anterior wall of the stomach as an end to side anastomosis below. Using the right colon, the procedure is technically easier and the terminal ileum is anastomosed to the proximal oesophagus. Long-term results suggest that an isoperistaltic left colon is superior to the right colon. A reversed gastric tube based proximally on the greater curvature of the stomach and receiving its blood supply from the left gastro-epiploic artery, is used when the colon proves unsuitable for oesophageal reconstruction, provided that the stomach has not sustained severe injury. The reversed gastric tube is also tunnelled retrosternally to the neck for anastomosis with the cervical oesophagus.

Oesophagitis in AIDS patients

Candida oesophagitis is frequently present in patients infected with the human immunodeficiency virus (HIV) and is one of the recognized indicator diseases for the acquired immunodeficiency syndrome (AIDS). In addition, candida oesophagitis may cause acute dysphagia soon after the primary infection before sero-conversion has occurred. When established, candida oesophagitis in AIDS patients responds to long-term systemic anti-fungal therapy with fluconazole.

AIDS patients are also prone to severe ulcerative viral oesophagitis caused by cytomegalovirus and herpes simplex virus. The symptoms caused by either infection include dysphagia or odynophagia. In some patients, deep ulcers develop which may indeed progress to broncho-oesophageal fistulae. Infection by microbacteria and tuberculosis has been documented at least in some of these AIDS patients and the lesions may heal with anti-tuberculous chemotherapy (isoniazid, rifampicin and pyrazinamide). Other bacterial oesophageal infections in AIDS patients may be caused by streptococci, staphylococci and klebsiella organisms.

Medication induced oesophagitis

Medication induced injury is a common but often unrecognized cause of oesophageal strictures. The injury is often extensive and related to direct mucosal damage, but this is commonly localized. Tetracycline, doxycycline, potassium tablets, ascorbic acid, quinidine and non-steroidal anti-inflammatory agents are the principal agents that cause damage but other drugs have been implicated. Patients usually experience heartburn or chest pain accompanied by odynophagia occurring 4–6 hours after ingestion of the medication. At endoscopy a localized mucosal ulcer is found and this may heal without a scar or lead to stricture formation. Patients should be instructed to take their medication in the upright position with fluids and to remain upright for 30–60 min after ingestion. Medication induced ulcers and strictures are frequently found in the mid oesophagus at the level of the aortic arch (site of normal oesophageal constriction), but they can occur anywhere in the oesophagus. Patients with pre-existing strictures are at a greater risk of medication induced injury.

Radiation oesophagitis

The incidence of ulcerative oesophagitis following radiation therapy alone or combined modality therapy ranges from 5% to 53%. Treatment with chemotherapy or radiotherapy, which includes the oesophagus within its contours, destroys rapidly dividing cells including those in the basal epithelial layer. Cell death decreases the renewal rate of the basal epithelium, causing mucosal atrophy, ulceration and initiation of the inflammatory response. Synergy between chemotherapy and radiotherapy may increase the severity and extent of oesophagitis observed in combined modality treatment.

There is no effective prophylactic measure for radiation oesophagitis. Management is for established oesophagitis. Nutrition must be ensured and symptomatic relief of sequelae, especially dysphagia is important. The latter can be improved by topical or systemic analgesia. If oesophageal spasm occurs, calcium antagonists may provide some relief. Gastro-oesophageal reflux symptoms can be helped by proton pump inhibitors. Nutrition can be ensured by endoscopic dilatation, stent implantation or endoscopic percutaneous gastrostomy (PEG). Late significant side-effects are rare. Local injections of steroids may be useful to prevent recurrent stenosis.

Section 7.4 • Diaphragm

The diaphragm (Figure 7.36) is a dome shaped musculotendinous structure, which separates the thoracic from the abdominal cavity. It is attached anteriorly to the lower sternum, laterally to the costal margins and posteriorly (crura) to the first three lumbar vertebrae. The aortic hiatus (median arcuate ligament) is situated posteriorly in front of the twelfth thoracic vertebra and through it pass the aorta, the thoracic duct and the azygos vein. To the left and anteriorly is situated the oesophageal hiatus at the level of the tenth thoracic vertebra (seventh left costal cartilage). In the majority of individuals, the oesophageal hiatus is formed entirely by the fibres of the right crus, which is more substantial than the left and arises from the bodies of the first three lumbar vertebrae and intervertebral discs. It is connected to the left crus by the median arcuate ligament after it arches over the aorta. The most common arrangement which is found in up to 60% of individuals is for the right crus to split into a large right (anterior) and a smaller left (posterior) limb. The splitting is in the ventrodorsal rather than the sagittal plain, which results in a waistcoat effect and the creation of an obliquely disposed oval diaphragmatic canal rather than an orifice. The vagus nerves, oesophageal branches of the left gastric artery, veins and lymphatics accompany the oesophagus through the hiatus. Slightly to the right of the midline, at the level of the ninth thoracic vertebra (sixth right costal cartilage), is the vena caval foramen in the central tendon. This allows the passage of the inferior vena cava and small branches of the right phrenic nerve.

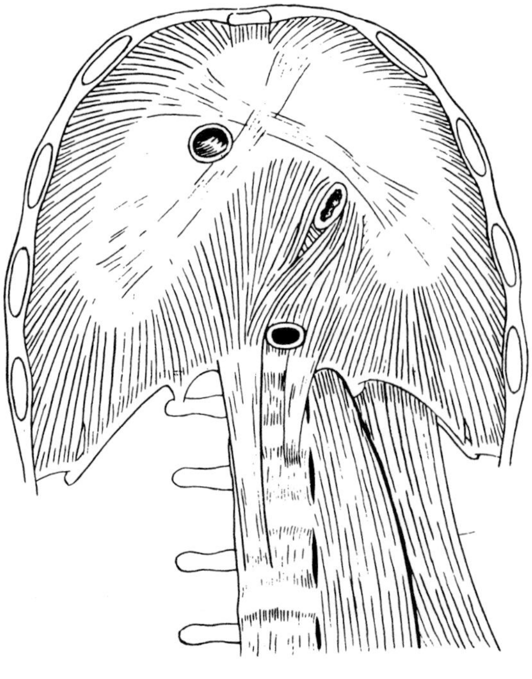

Figure 7.36 Inferior surface of the diaphragm viewed from the abdomen.

The arterial blood supply to the diaphragm comes from the phrenic arteries and the lower intercostal arteries, which arise directly from the aorta and the terminal branches of the internal mammary arteries.

Several other structures pass through the diaphragm. The splanchnic nerves pierce each crus, the sympathetic trunks pass behind the medial arcuate ligament, and the subcostal nerves and vessels pass behind the lateral arcuate ligament, while the left phrenic nerve pierces the left dome of the diaphragm to supply its abdominal surface. There is a rich communication between the lymphatic vessels of the posterior mediastinum and the upper abdominal lymph channels.

Congenital diaphragmatic herniae

The development of the diaphragm is usually complete by the eighth to tenth week of intrauterine life. Complete absence of the diaphragm occurs rarely. Congenital hernias are the result of maldevelopment of the septum transversum. The prevalence of the condition can be up to 1 in 2100 births and the male to female ratio is 2:1. Approximately 80% of fetuses with congenital diaphragmatic herniae also have polyhydramnios and most cases can now be diagnosed by ultrasonography before the 25th week of gestation. Attempts at intrauterine diaphragm repair have had limited success. Attempts to temporarily occlude the main bronchus of the hypoplastic lung have also had limited success. The sites of congenital herniation are shown in Figure 7.37. In general terms 30% of fetuses with congenital diaphragmatic herniae are stillborn. Fifty percent of those born alive with a congenital diaphragmatic hernia also have other congenital malformations, most frequently of the nervous system. The associations with trisomy 18, 20 and 21 and with Pierre Robin syndrome are also documented. The majority of

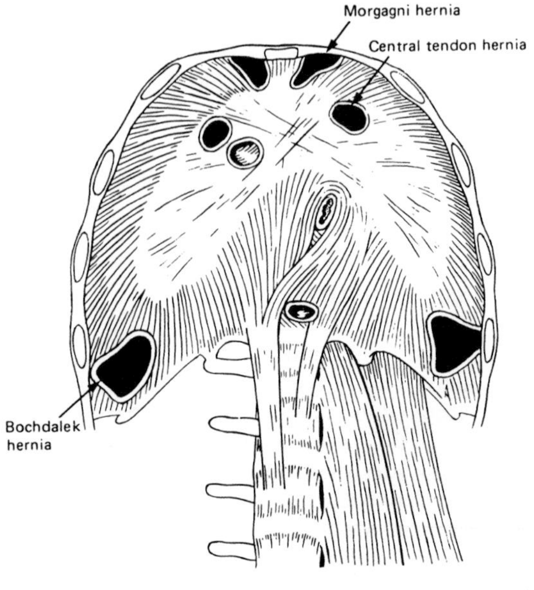

Figure 7.37 Site of congenital diaphragmatic herniae.

diaphragmatic herniae are left-sided (75%), some are right-sided (22%) and few are bilateral defects (3%). The commonest type of diaphragmatic defect is a posterolateral hernia (90%), followed in frequency by eventration of the diaphragm (5%), and the least common defect being a retrosternal hernia (2%).

Posterolateral hernia (through foramen of Bochdalek)

These herniae are posteriorly situated and are due to persistence of the pleuro-peritoneal canals, which are the last part of the diaphragm to close. The hernia, which is usually left-sided, presents acutely with respiratory distress in the neonatal period. In adults most of them are asymptomatic. Symptomatic patients present with digestive symptoms due to herniation of the colon, stomach or small bowel.

Parasternal hernia (through foramen of Morgagni or Magendie)

The diaphragmatic hernia described by Morgagni in 1761 is a rare diaphragmatic anomaly that is nearly always congenital. This hernia is more common on the right and occurs through a triangular anterior defect lateral to the sternum between the sternal and costal attachments of the diaphragm where the superior epigastric artery, veins and lymphatics pass from the chest into the abdomen. It is usually asymptomatic in the first years of life; it may be discovered by chance on a routine radiograph or cause problems in adult life with episodes of pain and tenderness in the right subcostal region and intermittent obstructive symptoms. Complete intestinal obstruction may supervene. The posteroanterior chest film in these patients shows a rounded gas-containing shadow to the right of the cardiac outline. This shadow is seen to lie behind the sternum on lateral chest films. In doubtful cases, a radiological contrast study is needed to confirm the diagnosis. Surgical treatment is recommended in all cases because of the risk of intestinal obstruction and strangulation. The best approach is through a midline upper abdominal incision. After reduction of the contents into the abdomen, the sack, which is usually present, is excised and repair is performed by approximating the two diaphragmatic edges with non-absorbable interrupted sutures. Closure with a Marlex or propylene mesh is necessary for large defects. Repair of these hernias can also be performed laparoscopically. This hernia can be associated with cardiac anomalies as in the pentalogy of Cantrell.

Herniation through the central tendon

The deficiency in the central tendon may be situated at the apex of the right or left cupola or involve the central part in relation to the pericardium. On the right side, a hernia through the central tendon contains a mushroom shaped portion of liver parenchyma, which grows through the opening and enlarges on the thoracic surface of the diaphragm. The condition is usually diagnosed accidentally by a routine chest radiograph. It can be easily differentiated from a primary tumour of the diaphragm by ultrasound scanning or three-dimensional imaging. In left-sided hernias the fundus of the stomach usually protrudes as an air-containing cyst on the top of the diaphragm. A central hernia is usually associated with a defect in the pericardium, and small intestine can herniate into the pericardial cavity.

A small defect in the central tendon on the right side does not require any treatment. However, surgical repair of the other two defects is usually recommended because of the risk of mechanical gastric or intestinal complications.

Congenital hiatal hernia

This is usually of the sliding type and is associated with gastro-oesophageal reflux. More rarely the hernia is of the para-oesophageal variety. Both can present in infancy and childhood.

Congenital short oesophagus

In the absence of congenital defects, gastro-oesophageal incompetence is often present in the neonate. The condition corrects itself spontaneously during the first few months of life, probably by further development of the intra-abdominal oesophagus. True congenital shortening of the oesophagus in infancy and childhood is very rare. In this condition, the cardia and a large portion of the fundus of the stomach are situated in the mediastinum without any obvious hernial sack or sliding.

Most instances of congenital shortening of the oesophagus are acquired and result from prolonged pathological reflux with fibrosis, ulceration and stricture formation. The fibrosis draws the stomach further into the chest and in extreme cases, the oesophageal stricture may be situated at the level of the aortic arch.

Regardless of the aetiology, the most common symptoms are those of spontaneous regurgitation when the infant or child is in the reclining position and recurrent attacks of chest infection or asthma. Aspiration may also result in the development of a lung abscess. The condition requires treatment with an anti reflux procedure. Most authorities favour a Collis type gastroplasty with a partial fundal wrap. Others recommend an intra-thoracic Nissen fundoplication.

Eventration of the diaphragm

Anomalous congenital development of the diaphragm or its innervation may result in unilateral elevation of the diaphragm. Alternatively, phrenic nerve injury at birth or later, or injury to the diaphragm, may result in the same problem. Differentiation between eventration of the diaphragm and a large congenital hernia, especially of the Bochdalek type, may be difficult or impossible until surgical exploration.

Eventration of the diaphragm has clinical significance only if it is associated with symptoms or when it cannot be differentiated from other serious conditions. The symptoms of eventration which are identical to those of large congenital diaphragmatic herniae may

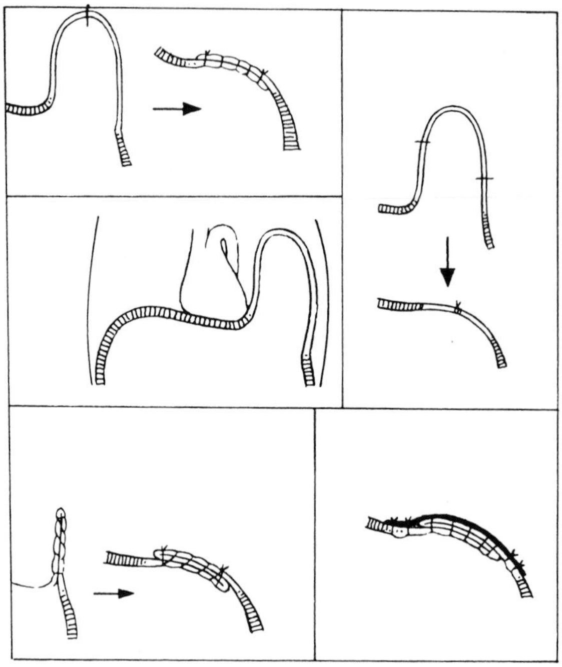

Figure 7.38 Techniques for correction of eventration of the diaphragm.

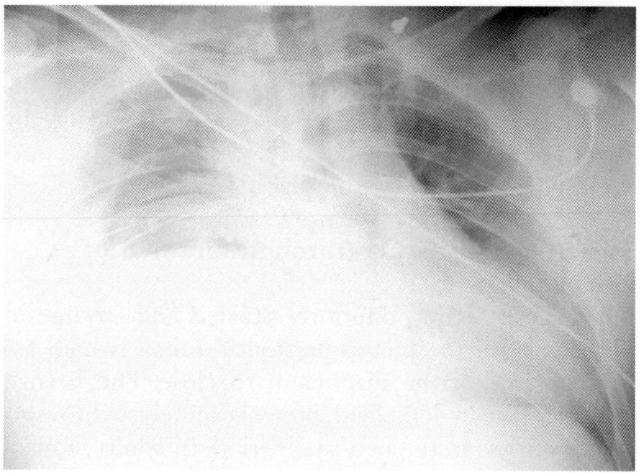

Figure 7.39 Plain chest X-ray showing liver herniation through the ruptured right hemidiaphragm after a road traffic accident.

occur in the neonatal period and include respiratory distress and tachycardia with impaired cardiac function. In older children, digestive and respiratory symptoms are aggravated by obesity.

In adult patients, the symptoms may be minimal and management is then conservative. Surgical treatment is necessary if symptoms are severe or disabling. Approach is through a left thoracotomy. The procedures which can be used to restore the diaphragm to its normal position are illustrated in Figure 7.38. They include incision or partial excision with plication of the diaphragm. In severe cases, prosthetic replacement of a very attenuated diaphragm with a synthetic mesh is required.

Traumatic diaphragmatic hernia

Traumatic rupture of the diaphragm may result from penetrating (25%) or blunt (75%) trauma to the abdomen and chest. The tendinous portion, especially on the left side, is the usual side of rupture (68%) as the liver protects the right side of the diaphragm from most injuries except the penetrating type. The rupture is associated with herniation of abdominal contents and may present acutely following the injury or escape detection until several months to years later. The herniation of abdominal viscera may occur acutely at the time of the injury or be delayed until some time later. The symptoms are related to the size of the herniated contents and to the onset of mechanical complications such as intestinal obstruction, strangulation, haemorrhage or progressive cardiorespiratory insufficiency.

The diagnosis is usually established on plain chest and abdominal films in when a space occupying lesion or bowel gas shadow is seen in the chest. If the omentum spleen or liver is the main herniated structure, the shadow appears solid (Figure 7.39). The herniated spleen is usually ruptured and accompanied by severe haemorrhage. This may result in total opacification of the left chest. Otherwise, air fluid levels may be observed indicative of herniation of hollow viscera (colon, small bowel). Passage of a nasogastric tube identifies a herniated stomach above the diaphragm. Contrast radiological studies may be needed to confirm the diagnosis. A significant proportion (40%) of traumatic diaphragmatic herniae do not produce any visible effects on plain chest radiography or three dimensional imaging using computed tomography (CT), magnetic resonance imaging (MRI) or ultrasonography, making diagnosis elusive in the acute setting. The rupture may be discovered by laparoscopy (gas-free, using abdominal wall lift), thoracoscopy or at laparotomy for associated injuries or subsequently on repeat investigations or as a result of bowel obstruction or strangulation.

In acute rupture, there are often associated injuries, which take precedence over the diaphragmatic injury. However, repair of the acute tear should be performed at the same sitting whenever possible. Elective repair of a traumatic diaphragmatic hernia may be performed through either a left thoracotomy or an upper abdominal approach. In delayed cases, the operation may be difficult due to the presence of adhesions and/or atrophy of the damaged diaphragm. Primary repair is usually possible using interrupted non-absorbable sutures. Otherwise closure with prosthetic mesh is performed.

Hiatal hernia

The oesophageal hiatus is an elliptical opening in the muscular part of the diaphragm. The crura arise from the anterior surface of the first four lumbar vertebrae on the right and from L2 and L3 vertebrae on the left to insert anteriorly into the transverse ligament of the central tendon of the diaphragm. There is some reported variability in the configuration of the oesophageal hiatus. The diaphragmatic crura are thick, musculo-tendinous bundles that become more tendinous and more muscular near their vertebral origins. The lowermost portions of the oesophagus and the gastro-oesophageal junction are held in place through the hiatus by the phreno-oesophageal membrane. With age, the phreno-oesophageal membrane becomes less definite and more fatty. It is also virtually non-existent in patients with long-standing hiatal hernia. This condition is commonly encountered from the fifth decade onwards in the Western world and there is a strong aetiological association with obesity. Excessive body weight is a significant independent risk factor for hiatal hernia. Hiatal hernia, however, is not synonymous with gastro-oesophageal reflux. A hiatus hernia can exist without any symptoms. Further, gastro-oesophageal reflux and reflux oesophagitis can occur in the absence of a hiatus hernia. However, in the presence of hiatus hernia there is probably a higher chance of developing oesophagitis. It is possible that in the presence of sphincter dysfunction, a hiatus hernia exacerbates reflux disease and its symptoms are worse than in the absence of such a hernia. There are rare instances of post-traumatic herniation of the stomach through the hiatus and these must be differentiated from traumatic rupture of the diaphragm. In the vast majority of cases, however, the development of hiatus hernia is spontaneous. Gall stones and colonic diverticular disease are commonly present in patients with a hiatus hernia (Saint's triad) and difficulty may be encountered in establishing which of the three disorders accounts for the patient's symptoms.

Pathology

Conventionally, three types of hiatal hernia are recognized: type 1: axial, sliding; type 2: para-oesophageal; and type 3: mixed.

Axial hernia

This accounts for the majority (70–80%) of cases. The gastro-oesophageal junction and a variable portion of the adjacent stomach slide upwards into the mediastinum carrying with them a peritoneal sac (Figure 7.40). This results in loss of the cardiac angle of His and, commonly, incompetence of the cardio-oesophageal junction. There is no uniform definition of what constitutes a sliding hiatus hernia. Surgeons, anatomists, radiologists and endoscopists all differ slightly in their views and this must be taken into account when evaluating a symptomatic patient. The symptoms and complications of this type of hernia are those which are consequent on gastro-oesophageal reflux and reflux oesophagitis (chronic blood loss, stricture formation, Barrett's epithelium, etc.).

Para-oesophageal hernia

In this type, the fundus of the stomach rotates in front of the oesophagus and herniates through the hiatus into the mediastinum (Figure 7.41). As the cardio-

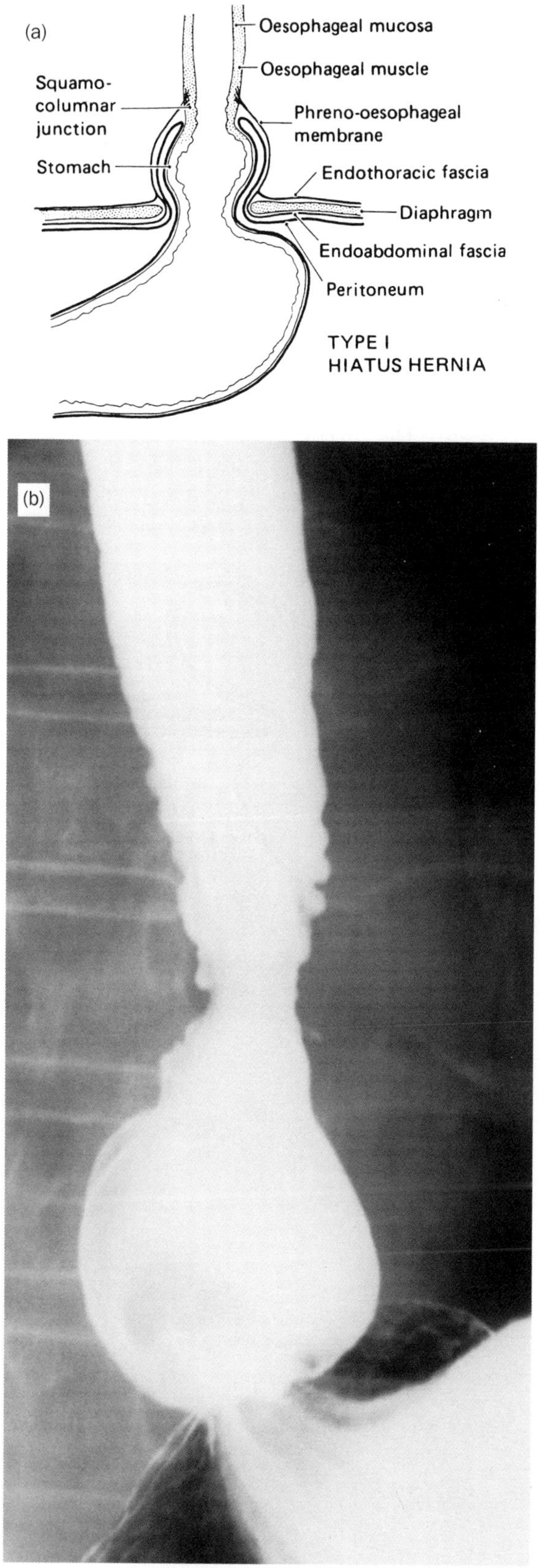

Figure 7.40 (a) Diagrammatic representation of type 1 (axial, sliding) hiatal hernia. (b) Barium swallow showing type 1 (axial, sliding) hiatal hernia. Note displacement of the cardio-oesophageal junction into the chest.

oesophageal junction remains *in situ* within the abdomen (except in large herniae) cardiac incompetence and reflux are not usually encountered. This type of hernia accounts for 8–10% of cases and is found predominantly in the elderly. In large herniae the entire stomach and pylorus may be found within the chest inside a large hernial sac which may also contain the spleen and hepatic flexure of the colon. These large herniae are prone to incarceration and strangulation with infarction and perforation of the stomach. Large herniae can also progress to complete volvulus, which results in pyloric or duodenal obstruction. When a para-oesophageal hernia bleeds, this is due either to chronic gastric ulceration in the intra-thoracic stomach or to an erosive gastritis in a congested and strangulated organ. The majority of uncomplicated para-oesophageal herniae can be easily reduced through the abdomen.

(a)

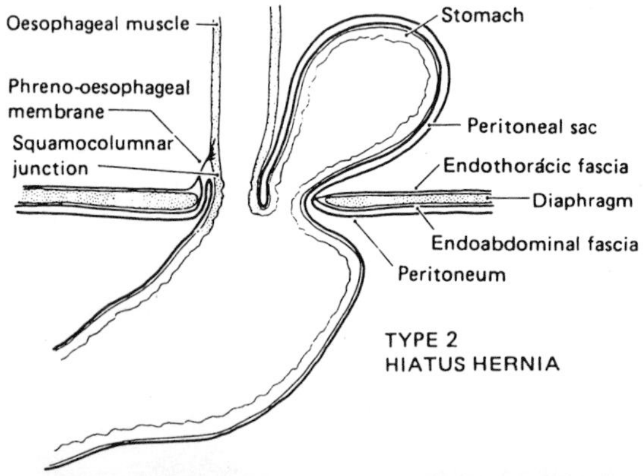

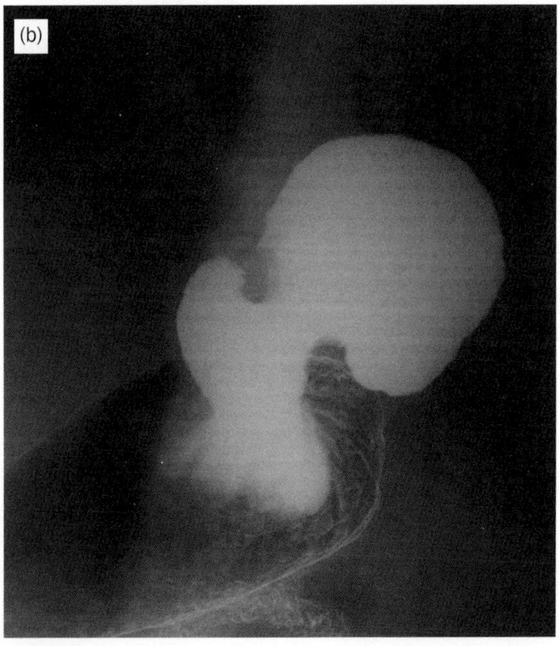

Figure 7.41 (a) Diagrammatic representation of type 2 (para-oesophageal) hiatal hernia. (b) Barium swallow showing large type 2 (para-oesophageal) hiatal hernia. Note rotation of the fundus as it rolls up in front of the cardio-oesophageal junction.

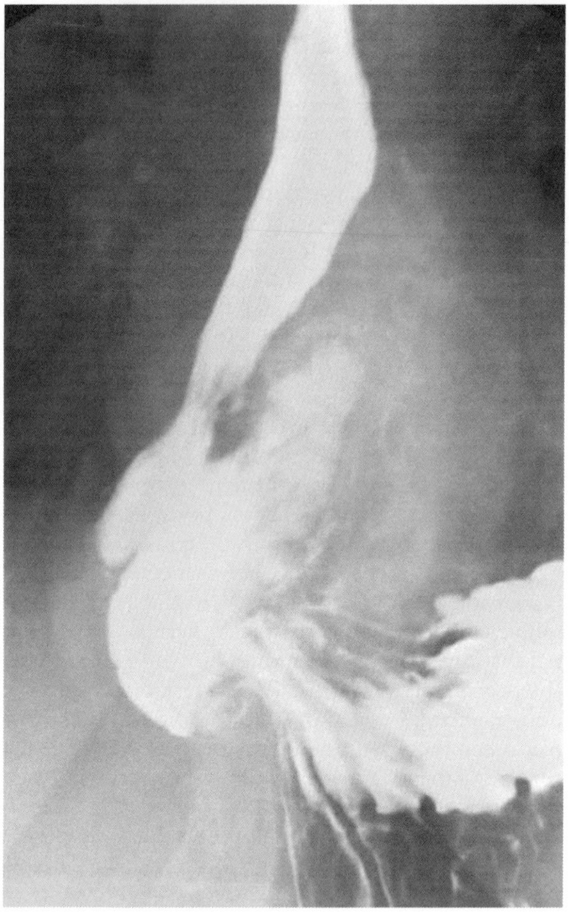

Figure 7.42 Barium swallow showing herniation of the fundus and gastro-oesophageal junction into the chest.

Mixed hernia

This resembles a large para-oesophageal hernia but the gastro-oesophageal junction is also herniated above the diaphragm (Figure 7.42). It has features and complications of both types 1 and 2 herniae. It is found in 10–15% of patients. This type of hernia is generally considered to be a late stage of the para-oesophageal variety.

Clinical features

These depend on the type of hernia and the onset of acute life-threatening complications, which can occur with the para-oesophageal and mixed varieties.

Axial herniae

The condition may be asymptomatic, particularly in elderly patients with limited activity and a sedentary lifestyle. When symptoms occur, they are largely due to gastro-oesophageal reflux and reflux oesophagitis. Chronic blood loss resulting in iron deficiency anaemia is common but active haemorrhage is rare. Some patients may present with dysphagia due to stricture formation without a preceding symptomatic history. Others present with dysphagia secondary to obstruction by diaphragmatic impingement on the herniated stomach.

Para-oesophageal and mixed herniae

The symptoms of para-oesophageal herniae are due to the pressure effects of the herniated stomach especially when it becomes distended with food or gas. Reflux is rare, occurring in only 3% of individuals unless the hernia is or becomes mixed. Common symptoms include pain, dyspnoea, feeling of distension and tiredness, which are precipitated by meals, bending and stooping. The pain is sharp, situated beneath the lower sternum and radiating to the back. It is often accompanied by a bloated sensation, anxiety, palpitation and dyspnoea. The attacks may simulate angina pectoris very closely and even cardiac arrythmias may be present during an episode. The pain, however, is often relieved by belching or vomiting. Dysphagia is found in 20% of patients with para-oesophageal hernia.

Acute presentation

Approximately 20% of patients with large para-oesophageal/mixed herniae may present acutely with severe upper gastrointestinal haemorrhage or strangulation/infarction/perforation of the intra-thoracic stomach. In the latter instance the patient develops severe retrosternal pain and shock which are often mistaken for myocardial infarction. A chest radiograph shows a large gastric gas/fluid shadow overlying the heart. With gastric infarction and perforation, mediastinal widening and emphysema, left basal collapse and pleural effusion may be outlined by this investigation. Gastric infarction and perforation carry a high mortality rate from septic mediastinitis and bacteraemia.

Treatment

Clinical assessment and appropriate investigations must establish that the symptoms are due to the hiatal hernia. In elderly patients and in individuals with comorbid disease, case selection for surgery requires astute clinical judgement based on the severity of the symptoms and cardiorespiratory reserve. Middle-aged patients with significant coronary artery disease may require myocardial revascularization before surgical treatment of the hiatal hernia.

Type 1, axial herniae are treated by reduction with an anti-reflux procedure. This is best achieved by a laparoscopic procedure in the majority of patients. The majority of uncomplicated para-oesophageal herniae can also be approached similarly and are easily reducible via this approach. Following reduction of the hernia, a small and moderate sized hiatus is repaired with interrupted non-absorbable sutures and the gastro-oesophageal junction fixed beneath the diaphragm after restoring the oesophagogastric angle (Allison's repair). Some surgeons advocate a Nissen fundoplication in addition to reduction and crural repair of these herniae. If the hiatal defect is large, a synthetic mesh can be fashioned around the oesophagus and sutured to the edge of the large defect. In addition to the above, some surgeons advocate a gastropexy in the form of a tube, gastrostomy or otherwise to prevent recurrence. These patients can be managed by the laparoscopic approach by experienced surgeons. They are, however, challenging cases in time and effort.

Patients presenting with persistent bleeding from a chronic gastric ulcer in an intra-thoracic stomach require emergency partial gastrectomy and repair of the hernia. Strangulated/infarcted para-oesophageal and mixed herniae require an emergency thoracotomy. If the stomach is viable it is unrotated and reduced into the abdomen and crural repair is performed. A Belsey anti-reflux procedure is unwise in this situation as it may lead to gastric/oesophageal perforation. Resection of the infarcted stomach with mediastinal and pleural toilet is necessary for those patients presenting with this serious complication.

Section 7.5 • Motility disorders of the oesophagus

Oesophageal motility disorders may be primary where the oesophagus is the major site of involvement or secondary where the oesophageal abnormalities are due to more generalized neural, muscular or systemic diseases, to metabolic disturbances or to inflammatory or neoplastic lesions of the oesophageal wall. The accepted classification of the primary oesophageal motility disorders is shown in Table 7.12. It is important to emphasize that this section deals with clinical motility disorders of the oesophagus, in contrast to manometric or contraction abnormalities identified manometrically with an unclear symptomatology. It is best to think of the various motility disorders as syndromes since controversy exists regarding the aetiology of the various primary motility disorders. The classification is also fraught with difficulty since the boundary between them is vague and progression from one disorder to another has been documented. The differentiation of the main primary varieties is based largely on the symptoms and manometric profile (Table 7.13) (Figure 7.43) and on radiological appearances. There is little doubt that primary oesophageal disorders, apart from causing distressing symptoms, which affect the nutritional state and social life of the individual, carry a significant morbidity from early and late complications. The management of these patients can be difficult and surgical intervention, which should not be undertaken lightly, requires careful case selection and accurate diagnosis.

Table 7.12 Classification of primary oesophageal motility disorders

Specific	Achalasia Vigorous achalasia Diffuse oesophageal spasm Nutcracker oesophagus (symptomatic high-amplitude oesophageal peristalsis)
Non-specific	Hypertensive HPZ Hypo-/aperistalsis Abnormalities of peristaltic sequence

Table 7.13 Manometric criteria for oesophageal motility disorders

Motility disorder	*Manometric criteria*
Achalasia	Simultaneous contractions (aperistalsis) High LOS pressure Incomplete LOS relaxation
Diffuse oesophageal spasm	Simultaneous contractions (>10% of swallows) Intermittent normal peristalsis
Nutcracker oesophagus	High-amplitude (>140 mmHg) peristaltic contractions
Hypertensive LOS	High resting LOS pressure (>45 mmHg) Normal LOS relaxation Normal peristalsis
Non-specific motility disorders	Non-propagated contractions Retrograde contractions Low-amplitude (<30 mmHg) contractions Prolonged duration (>6 s) contractions Multi-peaked and disordered contractions Aperistalsis in oesophageal body with normal LOS Abnormal LOS function

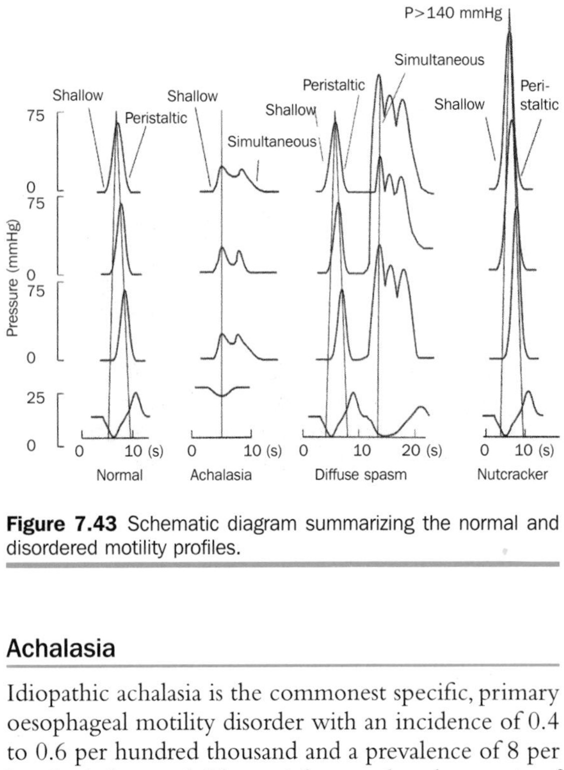

Figure 7.43 Schematic diagram summarizing the normal and disordered motility profiles.

Achalasia

Idiopathic achalasia is the commonest specific, primary oesophageal motility disorder with an incidence of 0.4 to 0.6 per hundred thousand and a prevalence of 8 per hundred thousand. The aetiology and pathogenesis of this disease remains unknown. However, primary achalasia has been shown to be a result of one or more neuromuscular defects. The commonest neuro-anatomical change seen in the oesophagus of achalasia patients is a decrease or loss of myenteric ganglion cells with some neural fibrosis and variable degrees of chronic inflammation within the myenteric plexus. It is thought that achalasia results from a primary inflammatory process with secondary ganglion cell and nerve damage. Vagus nerve and dorsal motor nuclei abnormalities have also been reported but in a smaller number of patients with achalasia. Histologically there is a paucity of nerve fibres within the distal smooth muscle segment of the oesophagus. Recent studies show selective destruction of non-cholinergic, non-adrenergic inhibitory neurones. It is thought that the cholinergic system remains intact in patients with achalasia. The manometric profile that characterizes achalasia includes absence of peristaltic contractions within the oesophageal body and incomplete relaxation of the high-pressure zone in response to swallowing. In addition the high-pressure zone pressure is usually elevated (more than 25 mmHg) and some patients exhibit an increased intra-oesophageal resting pressure relative to the gastric base line. Loss of propulsive peristaltic contractions and in particular the defective sphincter relaxations result in stasis of food in the oesophagus which progressively dilates and lengthens and thereby assumes a sigmoid shape in advanced cases. The mucosa of the oesophagus often shows oesophagitis with mucosal ulceration. This is largely due to stasis and bacterial proliferation and fermentation consequent on retention of food debris. Monilial infestation may occur spontaneously or be induced by antibiotic therapy. Leucoplakia is commonly encountered in long-standing cases of achalasia and oesophageal carcinoma is reported to develop in 3–5% of patients at an average of 20 years after diagnosis. It seems unlikely that this risk is influenced by effective treatment of the condition. An association between achalasia and other neurological diseases has been reported. These include Parkinson's disease and hereditary cerebellar ataxia.

Clinical features

The main symptoms are dysphagia, regurgitation and chest pain. The dysphagia is mainly for solid food with variable degrees of liquid dysphagia. Initially it is intermittent, of variable severity and may be aggravated by emotional stress and cold liquids. A gradual onset and eventual plateau are typically seen, with an average duration of dysphagia of around 2 years prior to presentation. Often patients find that swallowing is improved by drinking liquids, by repeated swallowing or by the adoption of certain manoeuvres such as Valsalva, eating upright and breath holding. These manoeuvres increase the intra-oesophageal pressure and thereby help to overcome the functional resistance at the cardio-oesophageal junction.

When oesophageal dilatation is minimal, odynophagia as well as spontaneous episodes of chest pain, which may be severe and simulate angina pectoris, accompany the dysphagia. With the onset of moderate dilatation of the oesophagus, both the chest pain and the dysphagia become less severe but spontaneous and postural regurgitation of foamy mucoid saliva becomes a frequent complaint in 60–90% of patients. Often, patients maintain their weight and the condition may be discovered accidentally by a chest radiograph taken for some other purpose. Other patients may seek medical advice largely because of halitosis and persistent eructations of foul smell. Heartburn may accompany symptoms in long-standing disease as a result of bacterial fermentation of food retained in the flaccid oesophageal body. Advanced achalasia with massive dilatation of the gullet is usually accompanied by severe dysphagia, frequent regurgitation, weight loss, anaemia and prominent symptoms of respiratory complications (pneumonia, bronchiectasis, lung abscess, fibrosis and tuberculosis) with fever, sweating, cough, breathlessness and expectoration of muco-purulent material. The anaemia is nutritional in origin and may be accompanied by avitaminosis.

It is crucial in the investigation of patients with idiopathic achalasia to exclude secondary achalasia syndromes that may be seen with gastro-oesophageal malignancies or as part of a para-neoplastic syndrome

The essential investigations are chest radiography, contrast radiology, endoscopy and manometry. Plain chest radiography may reveal a soft tissue shadow with or without a fluid level due to the dilated oesophagus. Contrast radiology is usually diagnostic. The classic radiological features include dilatation of the oesophageal body, a beak like tapering of the oesophagus at the gastro-oesophageal junction and in 50% of patients absence of the gastric air bubble (Figure 7.44). Endoscopy is mandatory to exclude peptic stricture and carcinoma of the lower end of the oesophagus and cardia. The unhindered passage of the endoscope through the gastro-oesophageal junction should be possible in patients with idiopathic achalasia and provides further reassurance that an organic stenosis is not present. The oesophagus is usually found to be dilated and may have extensive mucosal friability and ulceration due to stasis of food and secretions. The lower oesophageal sphincter often appears puckered and fails to open with air insufflation but should be easily traversed with minimal pressure.

Manometry is the gold standard for confirming the diagnosis of achalasia and may establish the severity of the disease. The classic picture is that of aperistalsis in the oesophageal body with failure of a hypertonic lower oesophageal sphincter to relax completely in response to swallowing (Figure 7.45). As the oesophagus dilates the pressure peaks tend to become broader and of lower amplitude. Some patients may exhibit high-amplitude simultaneous and repetitive contractions not induced by swallowing. These are sometimes associated with cramp-like pain across the chest. The solid radio-nucleotide oesophageal transit study usually shows an oscillatory pattern with retention of the radio-isotope bolus in the oesophagus.

Treatment

Some benefit may be derived from the administration of long-acting nitrates. Nitrates decrease lower oesophageal sphincter pressure by 66% for up to 90 min. Although initial response in achalasia patients range from 50% to 70%, there is a tachyphylaxis such that less than 50% of patients have a sustained response. Calcium channel blockers interfere with calcium uptake by smooth muscle cells, which are dependent on intracellular calcium for contractions. Controlled trials in patients with achalasia have not shown consistent clinical benefit when these agents are compared with placebo. With such poor response to pharmacotherapy the current treatment of achalasia is by botulinum toxin injection, pneumatic dilatation or surgical myotomy. Botulinum toxin binds to presynaptic receptors and irreversibly inhibits axonal acetylcholine release. When injected into the lower oesophageal sphincter, the toxin theoretically removes the influence of the excitatory myenteric plexus neurones, thereby reducing lower oesophageal sphincter pressure. An immediate response has been reported in 90% of patients, with symptomatic improvement and a reduction in lower oesophageal sphincter pressure of 33–45%. There is, however, no significant improvement in oesophageal emptying. Furthermore, the symptomatic benefit is not permanent, and there is diminution of response with repeat injections. Nevertheless, the therapy is safe and can be used effectively as a temporizing measure in elderly patients or in individuals with atypical features that cast uncertainty on the diagnosis. However, in classical achalasia, botulinum toxin injection is inferior to the more definitive therapies of pneumatic dilatation or surgical myotomy.

Pneumatic dilatation using polyethylene balloons 30–40 mm in diameter has become a standard form of oesophageal dilatation for treating achalasia. Long-term benefit can only be achieved with dilatation to a diameter of at least 3 cm. Low-compliance balloon dilators, which have a maximal designated diameter, are probably safer than high-compliance balloon systems, which adapt to the surrounding oesophagus with resultant increase in oesophageal wall tension. To date, the influence of the balloon diameter, rate of inflation, dilatation pressure, duration of dilatation and the number of dilatations per session remain controversial. For effective dilatation the balloon should be placed to straddle the gastro-oesophageal junction and inflated to its maximum diameter. Simultaneous fluoroscopy

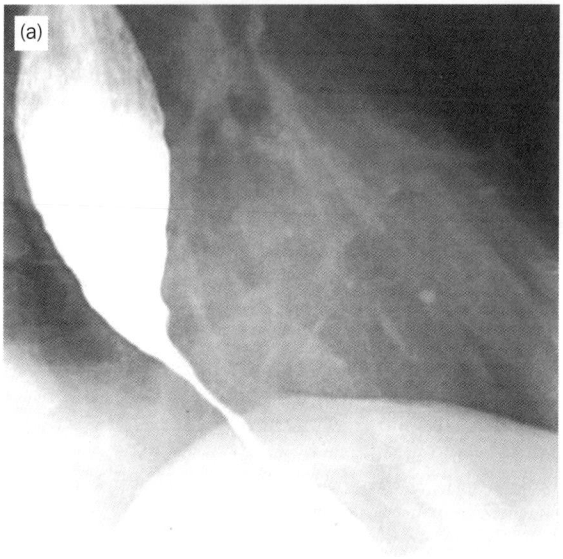

should demonstrate waist obliteration by the end of the procedure. No more than two dilatations are recommended in a single session. Immediate complications occur in up to 16% of cases with oesophageal perforation rates of up to 13%. Presence of a hiatal hernia or an epiphrenic diverticulum increases the perforation risk and is considered a relative contraindication to pneumatic dilatation. Response to pneumatic dilatation is variable, with 60–80% of patients receiving benefit. This however is short term and more than 50% of patients have recurrence of their symptoms within 5 years. These patients can be treated by repeat dilatation or surgical myotomy. However, oesophageal dissection and myotomy may be technically more difficult owing to scarring and have a higher risk of mucosal perforation. Manometric studies show return of intermittent peristaltic waves in the distal oesophagus in up to 20% of patients and although lower oesophageal sphincter relaxation does not return to normal it improves significantly. Gastro-oesophageal reflux as a complication of dilatation occurs in only 2% of patients and typically responds to standard anti-reflux therapy.

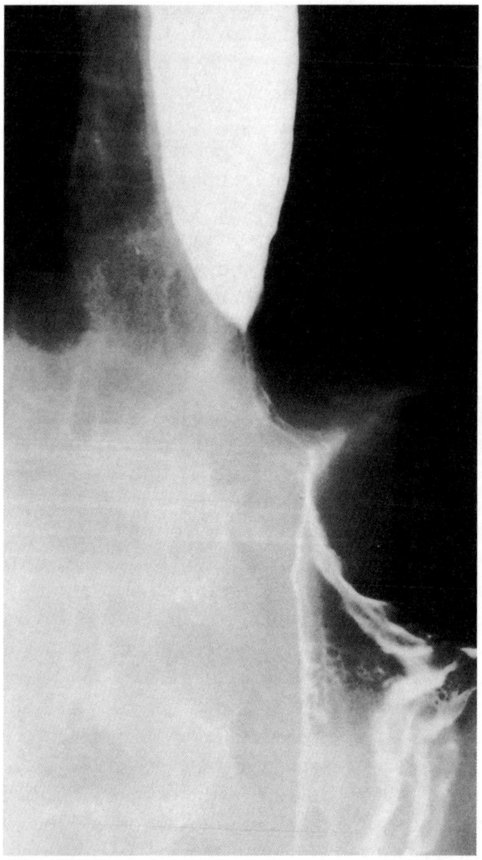

(b)

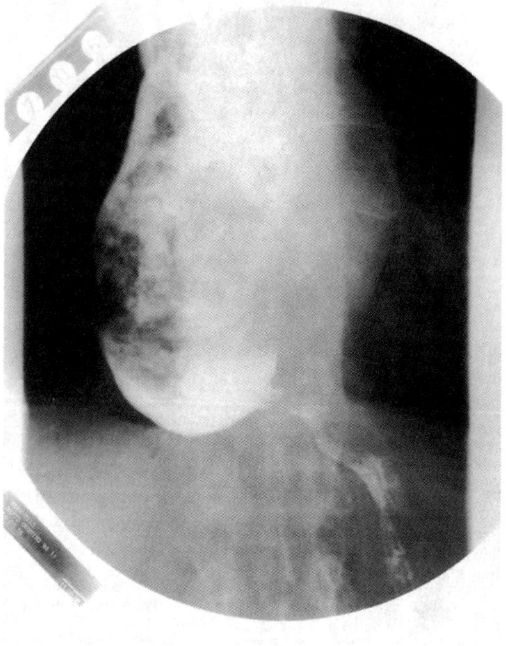

Figure 7.44 (a) Barium swallows in a patient with achalasia. The oesophagus is grossly dilated above an apparent narrowing of the cardia. The tapering of the oesophagus to the cardia has been likened to a 'bird's beak'. (b) Barium swallow showing grossly dilated sigmoid oesophagus in a patient with longstanding achalasia.

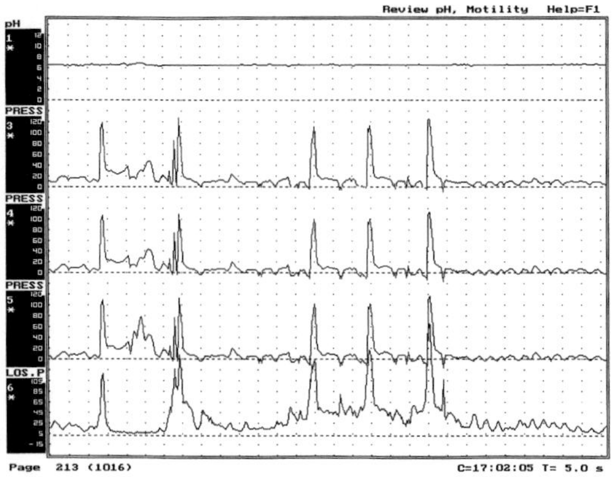

Figure 7.45 Manometric tracing obtained from a 24 hour combined pH and manometry study on a patient with achalasia. The top channel shows the pH in the lower oesophagus. Channels 3, 4 and 5 (5 cm apart in the body of the oesophagus) show aperistaltic contractions in the oesophagus and channel 6 (in the lower oesophageal sphincter) shows failure of relaxation.

Surgical treatment of achalasia is indicated in the following groups of patients:

- In children and young adults in whom repeated treatments will incur procedure related morbidity.
- After failure of pneumatic dilatation or botulinum toxin injection therapy. Failure in this regard indicates recurrent symptoms after a short period of treatment. It is controversial as to how many repeated treatments patients should be subjected to before they should be considered for surgical cardiomyotomy.
- Patients with co-existent pathology requiring surgical intervention or making non-surgical treatment excessively risky, e.g. hiatal hernia, epiphrenic diverticulum, tortuous distal oesophagus.
- Informed patient's choice.

Although referred to as Heller's cardiomyotomy, the modern operation consists of an anteriorly placed division of the musculature of the lower end of the oesophagus down to the mucosa, which bulges out once the contracted muscle is divided (Figure 7.46). Some surgeons prefer to excise a muscle strip. The modern anterior cardiomyotomy is performed through a left thoracoscopic or laparoscopic approach with the latter being more popular. The muscle coat of the distal oesophagus is divided longitudinally which traverses behind the anterior vagus nerve, which must be elevated to prevent damage or division. Experts differ on the distal extent and limit of the myotomy. Some prefer to carry the incision on to the stomach only far enough to ensure complete division of the lower oesophageal musculature. Others insist on continuing the myotomy on to the cardia. There is also controversy regarding the necessity to suture the divided muscle edges to the corresponding diaphragmatic crus. Further, there is controversy regarding the need and type of fundoplication following the myotomy. Some surgeons believe that the myotomy invariably destroys the lower oesophageal sphincter mechanism with inevitable reflux in up to 14% of patients and oesophagitis in up to 3% of patients, unless an anti-reflux procedure is added. Others prefer to carry the myotomy without incurring any damage to the phreno-oesophageal membrane and without the excessive dissection of the diaphragmatic hiatus. The incidence of gastro-oesophageal reflux with this technique is thought to be very low. The most popular fundoplications performed after a Heller's cardiomyotomy are a posterior 180° fundoplication (Toupet) and an anterior 180° fundoplication (Dor). The results of surgical myotomy are excellent in over 90% of patients. Poor results are usually attributed to an incomplete myotomy and gastro-oesophageal reflux with its complications. Morbidity is due to recognized or missed perforations with their sequelae which occur at a rate of 0.1%.

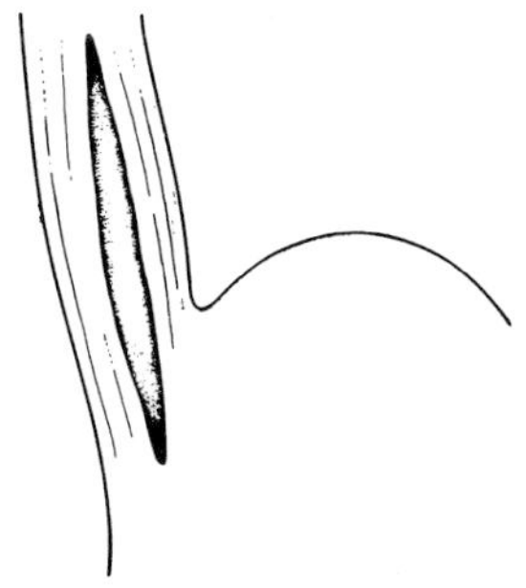

Figure 7.46 Anterior cardiomyotomy for achalasia. The myotomy is made on the anterior surface of the lower end of the oesophagus and extends to the cardio-oesophageal junction. Some advocate the performance of a loose fundal wrap to prevent post-operative reflux.

Infrequently patients are encountered with longstanding untreated achalasia with a huge tortuous mega-oesophagus (Figure 7.47) which may even form a bulge in the lower neck. In this group of patients where the gullet is totally immotile and tortuous from the redundant length, cardiomyotomy is ineffective. These patients require a subtotal oesophagectomy with gastric pull through and cervical anastomosis. Due to the chronicity of the condition and the neovascularization of the dilated oesophagus this procedure can represent a surgical challenge and requires careful assessment preoperatively.

Vigorous achalasia

This condition is a variant of achalasia. It has features of both classic achalasia and diffuse oesophageal spasm. Manometrically, it is characterized by repetitive high-amplitude aperistaltic contractions and failure of relaxation of the lower oesophageal sphincter. There is often minimal oesophageal dilatation and prominent tertiary contractions on radiographs. Chest pain is a more prominent feature than in typical achalasia. In addition, the clinical manifestations include dysphagia and regurgitation.

Medical management with long-acting nitrates or calcium channel blockers may give some symptomatic relief although the long-term results of this medication

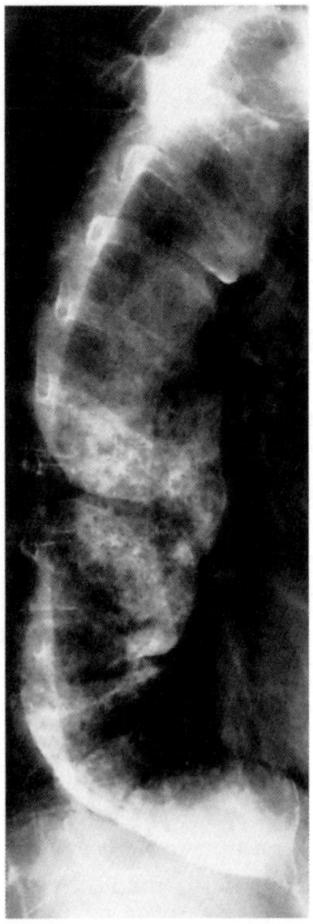

Figure 7.47 Barium swallow in long-standing achalasia. The patient presented with dysphagia and a neck lump which disappeared after insertion of nasogastric tube. These patients do not benefit from a cardiomyotomy and, if fit, are best treated by oesophagectomy with gastric replacement.

are poor. Pneumatic dilatation and botulinum toxin injection also produce temporary relief of dysphagia. Current surgical management consists of a long myotomy from the level of the aortic arch to the gastro-oesophageal junction. This procedure which gives good results can now be performed through a left thoracoscopic approach thus obviating the need for an extensive left posterolateral thoracotomy.

Chagas' disease

This disorder, the oesophageal component of which is known as Chagas' mega-oesophagus, is the result of an infestation with *Trypanosoma cruzi*. The disease is endemic in rural parts of Latin America. The parasite invades the reticulo-endothelial system, muscles and the nervous system. Destruction of the myenteric plexus of the oesophagus leads to a condition which simulates achalasia both radiologically and manometrically. Furthermore, the symptoms of the oesophageal disorder which occur in up to 25% of patients with Chagas' disease are similar to those of classic achalasia. Laparoscopic cardiomyotomy is the treatment of choice for these patients and good or excellent results are achieved in 95% of patients long term. Patients with a poor general condition due to the chronic infestation should preferably be treated by pneumatic dilatation or botulinum toxin injection.

Diffuse oesophageal spasm

Diffuse oesophageal spasm is characterized by multiple spontaneous contractions and by swallow-induced repetitive contractions of simultaneous onset, large amplitude and long duration which alternate with periods of normal peristalsis. The high-pressure zone is of normal resting pressure with normal relaxation in response to swallowing. The aetiology of diffuse oesophageal spasm is still unknown. Physiological studies suggest that in this disorder the oesophagus is sensitive to cholinergic stimuli, emotional states and olfactory stimuli and there are case reports suggesting a reversal through inhalation of the anti-cholinergic agent apratropium bromide. The clinical and manometric patterns of diffuse oesophageal spasm may overlap with achalasia. There are also reports that patients may progress from diffuse oesophageal spasm to achalasia and from other non-specific oesophageal motility disorders to oesophageal spasm, suggesting that these oesophageal motility disorders overlap clinically and pathophysiologically.

The major clinical symptoms of diffuse oesophageal spasm are substernal midline chest pain, odynophagia and dysphagia. The typical sufferers tend to have an emotional personality. Pain is most commonly described as sharp, burning or constricting and is often misdiagnosed as ischaemic heart disease. Radiation of the pain to the back, neck and jaws is common. Not infrequently, the diagnosis of diffuse oesophageal spasm is considered after normal coronary angiography. Although at times the pain seems to be precipitated by the ingestion of gassy beverages and hot or cold substances, it is more often spontaneous and unrelated to swallowing or other events. Dysphagia is also common. It is of variable severity, often intermittent and may be precipitated by emotional upsets. Typically, the dysphagia is as severe for liquids as it is for solids. However, weight loss is not usually encountered and episodes of complete obstruction do not occur.

Multiple mechanisms have been proposed for the pain associated with diffuse oesophageal spasm, including occult gastro-oesophageal acid reflux, myoischaemia, luminal distension and visceral hypersensitivity. Some cases of diffuse oesophageal spasm are undoubtedly associated with gastro-oesophageal reflux disease and the spasm may improve after treatment with anti-reflux measures. In up to 50% of patients with diffuse oesophageal spasm, a constellation of symptoms suggestive of irritable bowel syndrome is present. The term irritable oesophagus has been applied to this group of patients. In addition, the psychological profile of patients with diffuse oesophageal spasm shows a higher incidence of emotional disturbances.

Diagnosis of diffuse oesophageal spasm requires confirmation by manometry. Other useful investigations are barium swallow, radionucleotide oesophageal transit studies and rarely provocation tests. The barium swallow may demonstrate repetitive tertiary contractions which result in the typical corkscrew appearance

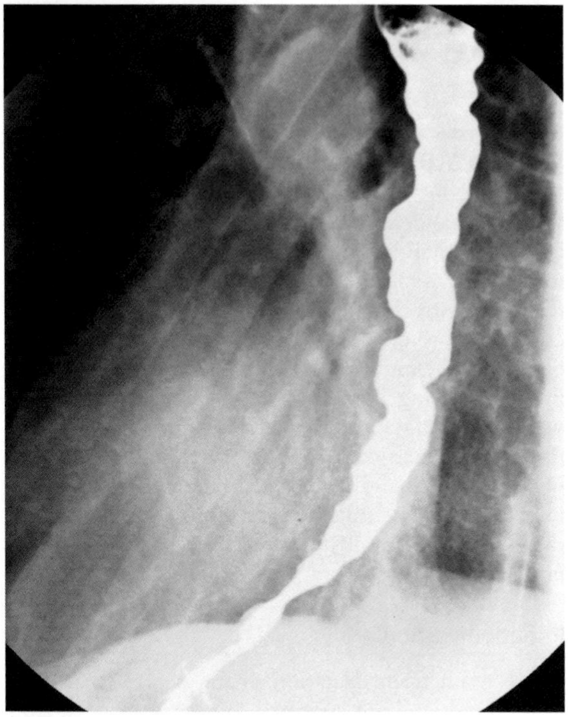

Figure 7.48 Barium swallow in a patient with diffuse oesophageal spasm showing typical 'corkscrew' appearance.

(Figure 7.48). The oesophageal radionucleotide transit tests shows an oscillatory or non-clearance pattern from the oesophagus. Provocative tests with cholinergic compounds and edrophonium chloride demonstrate the hypersensitivity of the oesophageal musculature to these agents but these tests rarely differentiate between diffuse oesophageal spasm and achalasia. An endoscopic examination is mandatory in all cases to exclude organic disease causing partial obstruction at the cardio-oesophageal junction. Infrequently 24 hour pH monitoring may detect occult acid reflux.

Treatment should only be considered after excluding a cardiac cause for the chest pain and ruling out gastro-oesophageal acid reflux as a mechanism. Treatment is aimed at symptom amelioration but achieving therapeutic benefit remains a challenge. Long-acting nitrates can provide temporary relief of symptoms and calcium channel blockers are of limited efficacy. Anti-cholinergics have produced variable results. Benzodiazepines and psychotropic drugs have recently received remarkable attention and the results of their use are pending. Pneumatic dilatation is beneficial although the results are not as consistent and dramatic as in achalasia and the benefit may be related to a placebo effect in the psychologically dependent patients. Surgical intervention is considered only after the above measures have failed and consists of a long oesophageal myotomy tailored to the extent of the manometric abnormality. At times this involves the entire extent of the thoracic oesophagus but more commonly extends from the aortic arch to the oesophagogastric junction. The myotomy can be done thoracoscopically obviating the need for a thoracotomy. Post-myotomy reflux can be treated by anti-secretory therapy or by a loose partial fundoplication.

Nutcracker oesophagus

This condition is characterized by high-amplitude (more than 140 mmHg) peristaltic contractions. These hypercontractile waves of contraction can be limited to the distal oesophagus or can be found throughout the whole oesophagus. The nutcracker oesophagus is more often associated with non-cardiac chest pain than with dysphagia. The pathophysiology of the nutcracker oesophagus is unclear. Together with the changes in motility, there is a muscular hypertrophy, which can be seen on endoscopic ultrasound investigation.

Diagnosis by manometry should establish normal peristaltic waves on swallowing which are of high amplitude (more than 140 mmHg) and with increased duration (more than 5.5 s). There should be a normal peristaltic sequence and a normal high-pressure zone pressure and relaxation. Gastro-oesophageal reflux may be a phenomenon in a minority of patients and prolonged pH monitoring should establish this. Endoscopy should be performed to establish the presence or absence of oesophagitis. Treatment should be considered after exclusion of a cardiac cause for the pain. Patients found to have gastro-oesophageal reflux should be treated with anti-secretory agents. Treatment with long-acting nitrates or calcium channel blocking agents has produced unsatisfactory results. Most patients continue to experience recurrent non-cardiac chest pain despite the medication. Weak sedatives, antidepressants and behavioural therapy with biofeedback have also been reported to provide symptomatic improvement. Intermittent dilatation has also been reported to relieve the symptoms of chest pain and dysphagia temporarily but there is evidence that this effect can also be achieved by a sham dilatation. Surgery in the form of a long oesophageal myotomy has also produced variable results.

Non-specific oesophageal motility disorders

In non-specific oesophageal motility disorders, a variety of symptoms such as dysphagia, non-cardiac chest pain, regurgitation, heartburn and globus sensation in the absence of an organic disease are reported. The understanding of these motility disorders is still limited, the patients present with a variety of abnormal manometric patterns, but they do not meet the strict criteria of the classical primary oesophageal motility disorders. Therefore, these motor abnormalities have been grouped in a broad category termed non-specific oesophageal motility disorders. The main findings within this group are ineffective (non-propagated) and low-amplitude contractions, associated with delayed oesophageal transit of radioisotopes. Some patients with gastro-oesophageal reflux exhibit these findings, pointing to an association between the two disorders. Whether the motility disorder is the cause or the effect of increased oesophageal acid exposure remains to be determined.

This is a difficult group of patients to diagnose and treat. Although the motility disorder may be apparent on manometry, there is difficulty in associating the motility disorder with symptoms. Prolonged pH monitoring may isolate a subset of patients who might respond to anti-secretory agents. Treatment should be aimed at ameliorating symptoms with medication, which may include sedatives and psychotropic agents.

Motility disorders secondary to systemic disorders

The most common condition which may lead to severe oesophageal motor dysfunction is progressive systemic sclerosis. Less commonly, patients with dermatomyositis, lupus erythematosus, rheumatoid arthritis and diabetes mellitus may be similarly affected. The oesophageal motor disorder in patients with systemic sclerosis is characterized by incompetence of the lower oesophageal sphincter and weakness to the point of complete loss of peristaltic activity of the distal two-thirds of the oesophagus. The myopathy is confined to the smooth muscle portion of the oesophagus and the function of the upper striated segment and the pharynx remains normal. Histologically, marked atrophy of the smooth muscle is present together with fibrosis in the submucosa and muscularis propria. Barium swallow shows a flaccid hypotonic, slightly dilated organ with gross radiological reflux.

Nearly all patients with scleroderma and oesophageal involvement have symptoms of gastro-oesophageal reflux and these are often severe. Gross peptic oesophagitis and stricture formation are common since oesophageal clearance is grossly impaired due to the hypo–aperistalsis. The other manifestations of the disorder such as Raynaud's phenomenon, calcinosis and tight skin are present and should point to the diagnosis in patients who present with dysphagia and severe reflux symptoms.

The management of these patients is extremely difficult. There is no specific medical therapy although prokinetic agents such as domperidone, metoclopromide and cisapride are often used with variable and inconsistent results. Gastro-oesophageal reflux must be treated vigorously by standard medical regimens and any peptic strictures are dilated. Some advocate anti-reflux operations but these are less often successful than in ordinary gastro-oesophageal reflux because the atrophied oesophageal musculature holds sutures poorly. Furthermore the incidence of persistent post-operative dysphagia is high because of the absence of effective peristalsis such that even a loose fundal wrap may lead to a hold up at the lower end of the oesophagus. The other surgical alternative is resection of the oesophagus with replacement using colon or an isoperistaltic jejunal segment. However, the reports with these procedures for this condition are few and the collective experience reported in the literature is limited such that it is not possible to comment on their overall benefit.

Section 7.6 • Oesophageal diverticula

Oesophageal diverticula may be congenital or acquired. Congenital diverticula are very rare and are due to incomplete duplication of the oesophagus. Acquired diverticula are classified into pulsion and traction varieties. Pulsion diverticula arise as a consequence of pathological elevation of the intra-luminal oesophageal pressure causing herniation of the mucosa through a weak area in the muscular wall. Traction diverticula are the consequence of inflammatory adhesions between the oesophagus and mediastinal structures, particularly lymph nodes. The subsequent fibrous contracture pulls the oesophageal wall (mucosa and muscle) to form a pouch.

Pseudodiverticula

These result from dilatation of the oesophageal racemose glands and are confined to the submucosal layer of the oesophagus. They are rare, usually multiple and are often associated with extensive strictures or motility disorders. Candidosis frequently complicates the clinical picture. The disorder is most commonly encountered in late middle age and a higher incidence has been reported in individuals with chronic alcoholism, immune deficiency and tuberculosis. The aetiology of oesophageal pseudodiverticulosis is obscure. The most consistent symptom of the disorder is dysphagia, which becomes very painful when monilial infestation supervenes.

The clinically important oesophageal diverticula are:

- Pharyngo–oesophageal diverticulum (Zenker's diverticulum) (65%).
- Mid–thoracic diverticulum (15%).
- Epiphrenic diverticulum (20%).

Pharyngo-oesophageal (Zenker's) diverticulum

This diverticulum is of the pulsion variety and is usually secondary to cricopharyngeal dysfunction and less commonly to an oesophageal motility disorder. It develops as a midline mucosal out-pouching on the posterior aspect of the pharyngo-oesophageal junction between the fibres of the inferior pharyngeal constrictor and the transverse fibres of the cricopharyngeus and is usually manifest on the left side. The anatomical defect in this area, first described by Killian, is triangular in shape and is further accentuated by the absence of the longitudinal fibres of the oesophagus as they sweep anteriorly prior to their insertion into the posterior surface of the cricoid cartilage. As posterior extension is limited by the spine, the enlarging diverticulum comes to lie to the side (usually left) as well as

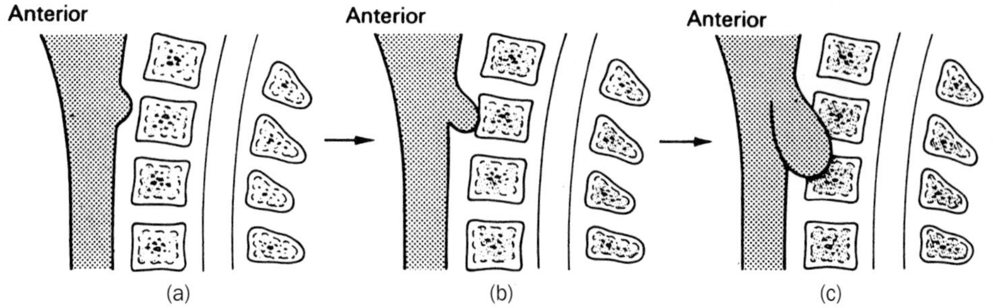

Figure 7.49 Diagrammatic representation of the development and progress of a pharyngo-oesophageal diverticulum. The cricopharyngeal dysfunction and resultant high intraluminal pressure cause a mucosal herniation between the oblique fibres of the inferior constrictor and the transverse fibres of the cricopharyngeus. Enlargement of the pouch is limited posteriorly by the spine (b). It therefore becomes dependent and bulges lateral to the oesophagus usually on the left side (c). As it becomes dependent, food tends to enter the sac rather than the oesophageal lumen which may also be compressed by the pouch.

behind the oesophagus. There is evidence that more than one type of motility disturbance may be responsible for the development of a pharyngo-oesophageal diverticulum. Most commonly, cricopharyngeal dysfunction is the cause although controversy exists as to its exact nature. Some ascribe it to failure of relaxation of the cricopharyngeus with swallowing (cricopharyngeal achalasia), others to premature contraction of this upper oesophageal sphincter before the pharyngeal contraction is complete and another theory postulates a hypertonic sphincter secondary to excessive gastro-oesophageal reflux. In some patients, the diverticulum is secondary to oesophageal motility disorders such as achalasia or diffuse oesophageal spasm and some reports have documented an association between the development of a pharyngo-oesophageal diverticulum and gross gastro-oesophageal reflux with or without hiatal hernia.

The diverticulum consists mainly of mucosa and submucosa with a sparse and incomplete muscular coat. As it enlarges, the pouch tends to assume a vertical lie and compresses and displaces the oesophagus such that its axis becomes in line with the pharynx (Figure 7.49). Ingested food then enters the pouch more readily than the oesophagus. Symptoms such as coughing and spluttering with meals become more marked and the risks of aspiration are increased. In addition, there is a great danger of iatrogenic perforation of the diverticulum at endoscopy as the endoscope tends to enter the diverticulum rather than the oesophagus. The complications of pharyngo-oesophageal diverticulum are:

- Pneumonitis, lung abscesses, pulmonary collapse.
- Bleeding from the diverticulum (rare).
- Perforation (usually iatrogenic).
- Development of carcinoma (0.3%).

Clinical features

Pharyngo-oesophageal diverticulum is three times more common in males than females and usually occurs in late middle age and in the elderly. Occasionally the development of the diverticulum is preceded by a period of high dysphagia characterized by difficulty in the transfer of food from the pharynx to the oesophagus. As the condition progresses, the patients complain of regurgitation, constant throat irritation, gurgling noises during swallowing, chronic cough and recurrent chest infections due to aspiration. With compression of the oesophagus, dysphagia becomes more severe and attacks of coughing and spluttering are experienced with each meal. Other symptoms include halitosis, hoarseness and anorexia. These patients typically require a long period to eat even a small meal. The regurgitated material is non-acid. Rarely, the pouch enlarges sufficiently to become clinically palpable. More usually, a gurgling sound can be elicited on palpation/massage of the left side of the neck at the level of the cricoid performed after the patient is asked to swallow several gulps of air.

The diagnosis is best confirmed by a barium swallow. The lateral films demonstrate the diverticulum better and outline its neck and any oesophageal compression (Figure 7.50). It is important that a full barium swallow investigation is performed to exclude gross oesophageal motility disorders and a hiatal hernia. Endoscopy is not necessary for the diagnosis and carries a risk of iatrogenic perforation, especially if the pouch is dependent and in line with the pharynx. If endoscopy is considered necessary, it should be done by an experienced surgeon and the introduction of the endoscope from the level of the cricopharyngeus onwards should be performed under vision. Oesophageal manometry, including pressure profiles of the cricopharyngeus should be done to exclude an oesophageal motility disorder. Prolonged pH monitoring is advisable in patients with hiatal hernia and those with reflux symptoms or endoscopic evidence of oesophagitis.

Treatment

The management of pharyngo-oesophageal diverticulum is usually by surgical intervention either through an open approach along the anterior margin of the left sternomastoid from the level of the hyoid bone to the anterior end of the clavicle or endoscopically. The surgical options are (Figure 7.51):

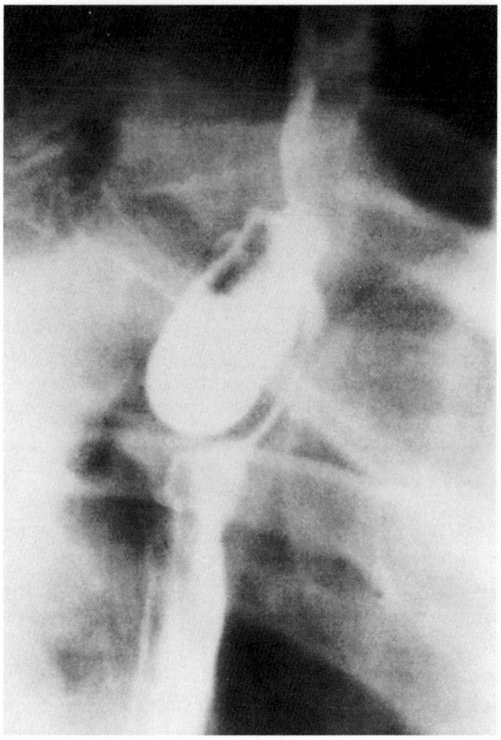

Figure 7.50 Barium swallow demonstrating a large pharyngeal pouch. The patient had marked dysphagia and aspiration lung abscess.

- Cricopharyngeal myotomy: this is suitable for small non-dependent diverticula.
- Diverticulectomy: this is necessary for large dependent pouches and should be combined with a cricopharyngeal myotomy.
- Diverticulopexy: this consists of invagination and plication of the pouch. It is suitable for moderate sized pouches which are not grossly infected or adherent to adjacent structures and is often combined with cricopharyngeal myotomy.
- Endoscopic division of the septum: in elderly poor-risk patients with large dependent diverticula, endoscopic electrocautery, laser and stapled division of the septum formed by the opposed walls of the diverticulum and the oesophagus is increasingly popular and can be done under regional anaesthesia.

Mid-thoracic diverticula

These are of three kinds: congenital, traction and pulsion. The congenital and traction varieties have a similar radiological appearance (tented triangular shape with a wide neck) and possess a muscular coat. The congenital ones are thought to represent foregut duplications and the traction types are secondary to fibrous adhesions to healed tuberculous lymph nodes. Both the congenital and traction mid-oesophageal diverticula are rare, and the vast majority of pouches in this region of the oesophagus are secondary to specific (diffuse oesophageal spasm, high-amplitude peristaltic contractions) or non-specific oesophageal motility disorders which cause a persistent elevation of the oesophageal

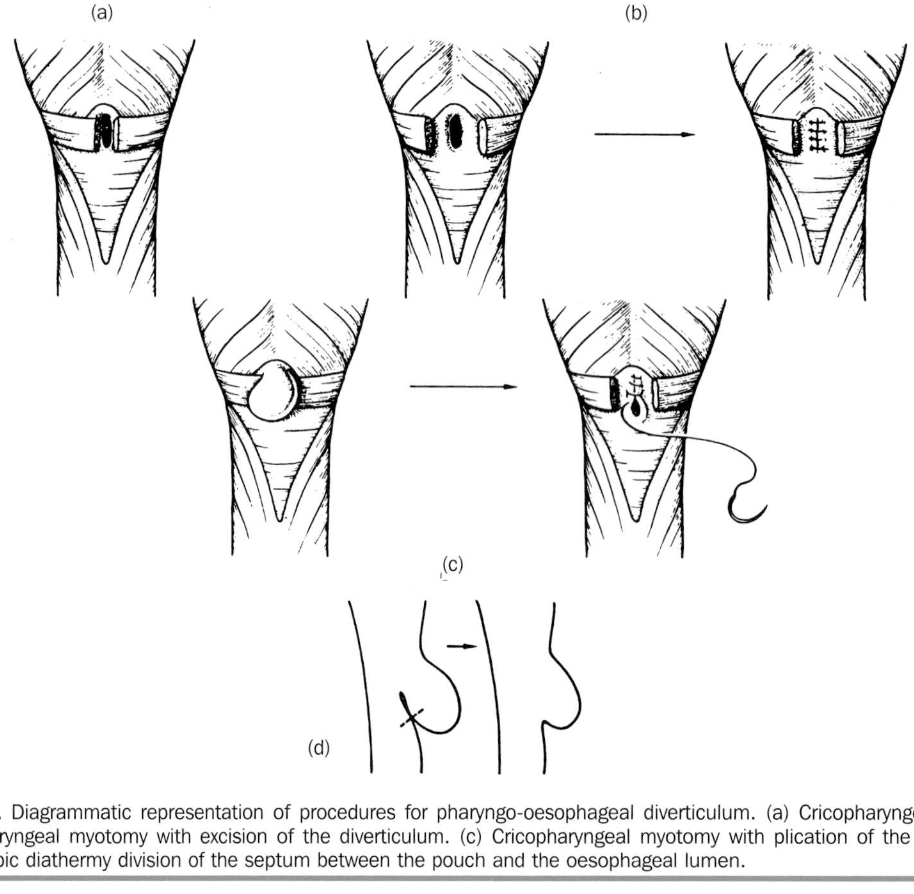

Figure 7.51 Diagrammatic representation of procedures for pharyngo-oesophageal diverticulum. (a) Cricopharyngeal myotomy. (b) Cricopharyngeal myotomy with excision of the diverticulum. (c) Cricopharyngeal myotomy with plication of the diverticulum. (d) Endoscopic diathermy division of the septum between the pouch and the oesophageal lumen.

intra-luminal pressure with subsequent mucosal herniation through a weak defect. These pulsion diverticula are usually narrow-necked and globular in shape and do not possess a muscular coat. The complications of mid-oesophageal diverticula are inflammation and perforation, usually by a swallowed fish bone, foreign body leading to abscess formation and tracheo/broncho-oesophageal fistula. The surgical approach to symptomatic or complicated mid-thoracic diverticula is through a right thoracotomy. Excision of the sack is followed by layered closure of the oesophagus. Asymptomatic mid-thoracic diverticula do not require any active treatment. Repair of these diverticula can now be performed through a right thoracoscopic approach.

Epiphrenic diverticula

Although a few are congenital, the vast majority of epiphrenic diverticula are acquired and of the pulsion variety. The raised intra-luminal pressure is secondary either to a specific motility disorder, usually diffuse oesophageal spasm or achalasia, or to a hiatal hernia and gastro-oesophageal reflux. The symptoms are largely due to the underlying disorder although ulceration is known to occur in the diverticulum and to be a rare cause of haematemesis, which may be severe. Halitosis, anorexia and obscure chest pain are reported to be specific features of epiphrenic diverticula. Although carcinoma has been reported in these pouches, it appears to be rare and a causal relationship remains unproven. The treatment of symptomatic patients is that of the underlying disorder. If the pouch is small, it usually resolves after successful therapy of the motility disorder or reflux disease. Excision of the diverticulum in addition to surgical correction of the underlying disorder is indicated if the pouch is dependent and has a narrow neck such that it cannot drain adequately, or if the sack is inflamed or is compressing the oesophagus by virtue of its size.

Sideropenic dysphagia (Patterson–Kelly, Plummer–Vinson syndrome)

This syndrome is usually associated with iron-deficiency anaemia but may persist for long periods after adequate replacement therapy. It affects predominantly postmenopausal females and consists of dysphagia, microcytic, hypochromic anaemia, glossitis, atrophic inflammation of the mucosa of the pharynx and upper oesophagus with areas of hyperkeratosis, ulceration and the formation of high, usually anteriorly placed, oesophageal webs. Other features include dry skin and eyes, koilonychia, splenomegaly and angular stomatitis. Cases associated with reflux oesophagitis have been described, as have rare instances of the condition after gastric surgery. The oesophageal webs are flimsy and best demonstrated by barium swallow (Figure 7.52). They are easily missed and are readily ruptured at endoscopy. The dysphagia is thought to result more from oesophageal spasm associated with the inflamed atrophic mucosa than partial obstruction due to the oesophageal webs. The anaemia is usually accompanied by a low serum iron concentration. Patients with this condition require long-term follow-up because of the substantial risk of the development of upper oesophageal cancer, usually in the post-cricoid region. The incidence of oesophageal cancer in these patients is variously reported at 10–30%.

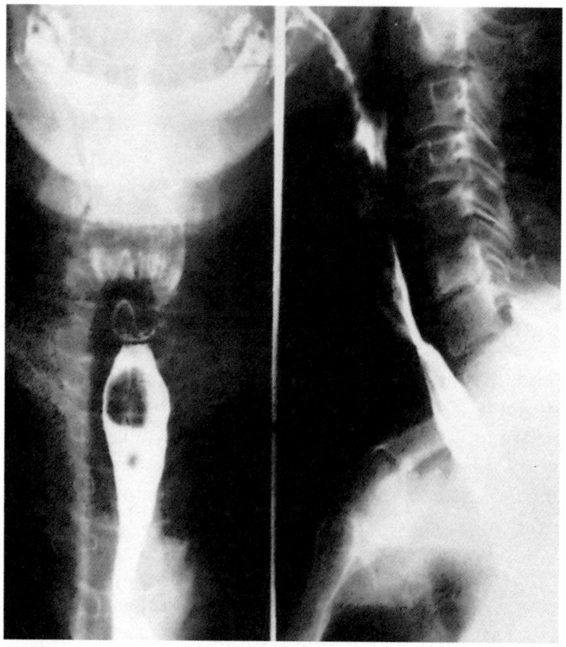

Figure 7.52 Barium swallow showing oesophageal web in a patient with sideropenic dysphagia.

Oesophageal cysts and duplications

Oesophageal cysts are very rare and may be acquired or congenital. The acquired variety are retention cysts of the submucous racemose glands and usually occur at the lower end of the oesophagus. They are rarely symptomatic but if large, may cause dysphagia. Removal is achieved through an oesophageal myotomy over the lesion, which shells out easily and without incurring a breach of the oesophageal mucosa.

Congenital (enterogenous) cysts and re-duplications share the same developmental origin and represent embryonal rests within or attached to the oesophageal walls. The cysts are most commonly lined with ciliated columnar epithelium. They usually present in infancy and childhood with pressure effects, i.e. dysphagia, and bronchial obstruction with respiratory distress as they expand within the confined space of the mediastinum. Whenever possible, enucleation of the cyst is performed without resection of the oesophagus but this is not always possible as the cyst may be densely adherent to the oesophageal mucosa as a result of previous inflammatory episodes. Re-duplications are elongated structures, which possess a muscular coat and are lined with squamous epithelium.

Section 7.7 • Oesophageal perforations

Perforation of the oesophagus constitutes a serious life-threatening condition, which is accompanied by a high morbidity, prolonged hospital stay and an appreciable mortality. Survival depends on prompt recognition and early surgical intervention for the majority of cases, although there is a place for non-operative management in selected patients.

Pathology

The categories of oesophageal perforations are outlined in Table 7.14. The commonest cause of oesophageal perforations is endoscopy especially when associated with dilatation and/or intubation of strictures. The incidence of oesophageal perforation following insertion of a rigid endoscope is 0.5% as opposed to 0.05% after flexible endoscopy. Dilatation considerably increases the risk, the incidence of perforation varying from 0.1% with the Maloney dilators, 0.3% with the Eder–Puestow metal olives to 1–5% after pneumatic dilatation for achalasia using 3.5–4 cm balloons. The pathology of oesophageal perforations caused by dilatation is shown in Figure 7.53. Post-operative perforations refer to oesophageal damage sustained during para-oesophageal surgery, e.g. Nissen fundoplication, repair of hiatus hernia, bariatric surgery and vagotomy. The risk factors for oesophageal iatrogenic perforation during upper abdominal surgery are oesophagitis and poor surgical exposure.

Penetrating gunshot wounds of the oesophagus are common in the USA. The cervical oesophagus is the segment most commonly involved. Most cervical oesophageal injuries due to external trauma are associated with the injuries to adjacent structures: spinal cord, thyroid gland, jugular vein, carotid arteries, larynx, etc.

Overall, the thoracic oesophagus (lower end) is the most commonly affected segment (55%) and the left side is more commonly affected than the right. Thoracic injuries also carry the worst prognosis. From the clinical standpoint, oesophageal perforation is classified into early (acute) and late (chronic). An acute perforation is one which is recognized immediately or within a few hours of its occurrence. It carries a good prognosis with a reported mortality of 10% as sepsis is not established and repair is feasible since oedema of the oesophageal wall is minimal. Late perforations

Table 7.14 Categories of oesophageal perforations

Category	*Example/comment*
Iatrogenic	Instrumental Post-operative
Swallowed foreign bodies	
External trauma	Usually penetrating
Corrosive ingestion	
Spontaneous	Neonatal Intramural haematoma (incomplete perforation) Mallory–Weiss syndrome
Progressive disease	Peptic ulceration Hiatus hernia Tumours

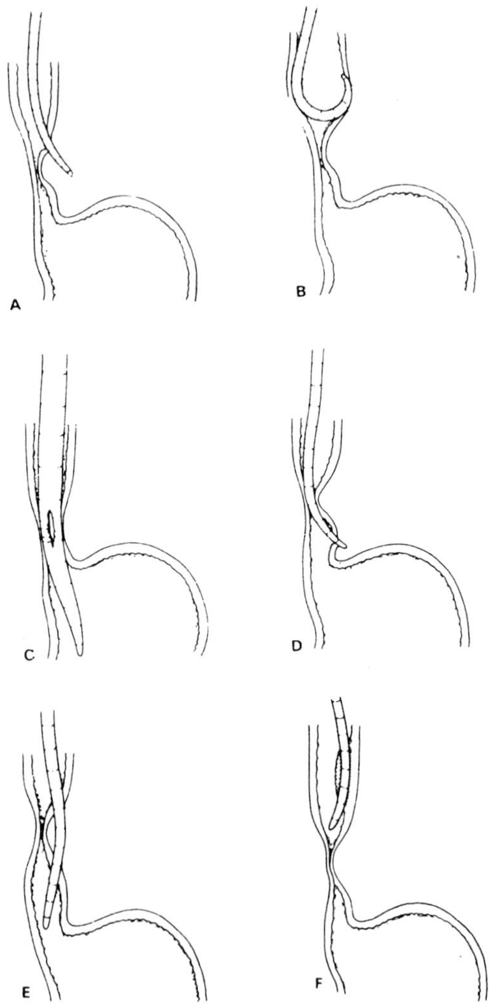

Figure 7.53 Pathology of oesophageal injuries caused by dilatation. Injuries A and B are more prone to occur in the presence of ulceration or pseudodiverticula above the stricture or hiatal hernia. Injury C is especially likely to complicate pneumatic dilatation for achalasia and stenting of malignant strictures. Injury D occurs as a result of a sudden give, the tip of the dilator perforating the oesophagus or stomach distal to the stricture. This type of injury can also result from the use of the Eder-Puestow guidewire when an excess length of wire is introduced and curls in the distal oesophagus and stomach. Perforation occurs as the dilator is pushed down coaxially along the curved guidewire. Injury E has a re-entry hold in the distal oesophagus and occurs in relation to strictures affecting the midoesophagus or higher, particularly malignant lesions. Injury F is an incomplete one (intramural haematoma, dissection) and usually occurs in the cervical oesophagus at, or just distal to, the cricopharyngeus; it is often caused by the endoscope, especially the rigid variety. There may or may not be a re-entry hole lower down. (Reproduced from Hennessy and Cuschieri, 1992, by permission.)

denote missed injuries, which are diagnosed beyond 24 hours of onset. By then, there is considerable transmural oedema of the oesophagus and this precludes safe primary suture of the tear. In addition, sepsis within the mediastinum and pleural cavity is well established and the patient's cardiovascular state is unstable from sepsis. The reported mortality of late perforations ranges from 40 to 60%.

Clinical features

The early manifestations of an oesophageal perforation are pain, tachycardia and fever. The site of the pain and its radiation vary with the oesophageal segment involved. The pain is, however, always severe. Patients with cervical injuries often develop a nasal voice and may have dysphagia. Haematemesis may also be found in cervical perforations. This is also a feature of incomplete injuries of the thoracoabdominal segment. Supraclavicular swelling and crepitus (subcutaneous emphysema) are observed in 60% of cervical and 30% of mid-oesophageal injuries. In thoracic injuries, respiratory distress is common and is accompanied by dullness on percussion and diminished air entry and breath sounds on the affected side (effusion). Upper abdominal tenderness with rebound and infrequent or absent bowel sounds indicates perforation of the abdominal segment of the oesophagus. However, these abdominal signs may be absent with small perforations (e.g. guidewire-induced, small unrecognized tears during para-oesophageal surgery) and the first intimation of this complication may be the development of a subphrenic abscess.

In late perforations, clinical evidence of established sepsis is present with fever, cardiovascular instability or fully developed septic shock. The infection is polymicrobial with aerobic, anaerobic and fungal organisms. The diagnosis is confirmed by plain and contrast radiology. Plain radiographs (neck, posteroanterior and lateral chest) are frequently diagnostic but may not accurately localize the perforation. The radiological features include presence of surgical emphysema in the mediastinum or neck (Figure 7.54), widening of the mediastinum and an increased distance between the trachea and the vertebral column. Irregularity of the mediastinal air interface is a radiological sign of mediastinitis. Free air beneath the diaphragm may be detected in patients with injuries to the abdominal oesophagus.

A contrast swallow is always required in patients with suspected oesophageal perforation. This is to confirm the perforation and to localize it (Figure 7.55). In addition it will indicate to which side of the chest the perforation has occurred although that may be evident from plain radiography. Endoscopy is not required for complete injuries but is indicated when clinical suspicion persists despite negative contrast studies, e.g. blood-stained nasogastric aspirate or frank haematemesis. Its main indications are:

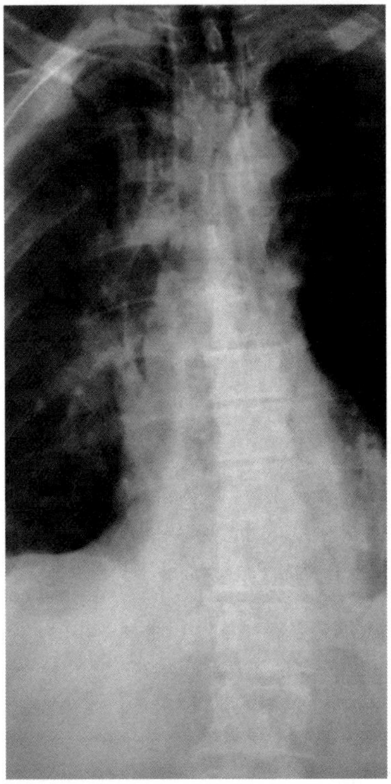

Figure 7.54 Plain radiograph of the chest showing surgical emphysema in the mediastinum following oesophageal perforation.

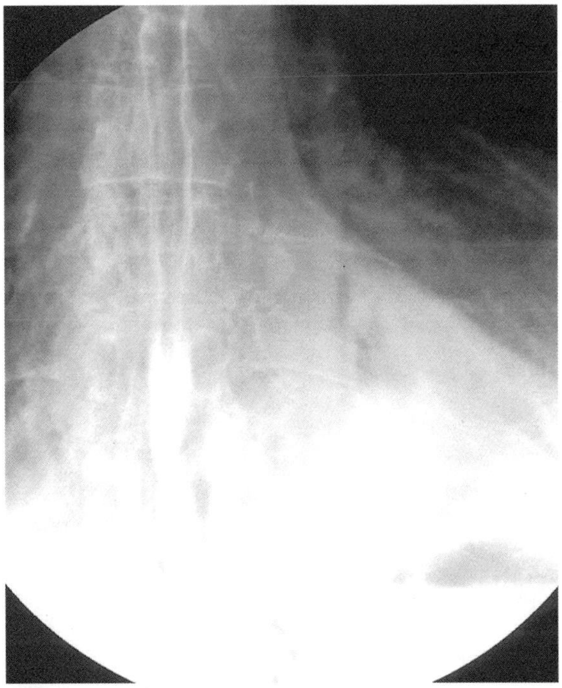

Figure 7.55 Water-soluble contrast swallow confirming and outlining the site of perforation in the lower oesophagus.

- Diagnosis of incomplete (intramural) perforation and Mallory–Weiss syndrome.
- Retrieval of foreign bodies and endoscopic control of bleeding.
- Assessment of the burn severity after ingestion of corrosive agents.

Neonatal and paediatric oesophageal perforations

Neonatal perforations are rare and may be traumatic or spontaneous. Both occur more commonly in premature babies and are attended with a substantial mortality, 19% for the traumatic variety and 33% for spontaneous perforation. The main distinguishing features of the two conditions are shown in Table 7.15.

Oesophageal injuries in children are either iatrogenic following dilatation or result from ingestion of foreign bodies and corrosive agents. The range of foreign bodies swallowed is extreme and includes coins, pins, aluminium can tops, alkaline pencil batteries, etc. Unless corrosive in nature, the symptoms following ingestion of foreign bodies may be delayed for several weeks to months. The swallowed object gradually burrows through the oesophageal walls and adjacent tissue often leading to the development of a tracheo-oesophageal fistula and respiratory infection. Pyrexia and persistent cough are common presenting features and paradoxically, dysphagia is rare. Endoscopy often fails to reveal the foreign body but may show an area of granulation tissue. Confirmation of the diagnosis is best achieved by radiology.

Spontaneous oesophageal injuries in the adult

Traditionally, three conditions come under this category:

- Intramural haematoma (incomplete perforation).
- Mucosal laceration (Mallory–Weiss syndrome).
- Complete spontaneous perforation (Boerhaave syndrome).

Intramural haematoma

This lesion, which is extremely rare, arises as an oesophageal mucosal tear associated with submucosal bleeding with dissection of this plane by the expanding intramural haematoma. The clinical picture is said to be distinctive with a history of gagging or choking while eating, followed by sharp mid-epigastric/lower retrosternal pain radiating to the back and associated with haematemesis. A contrast radiological swallow demonstrates a double barrel oesophagogram. The condition is self-limiting in the majority of cases and there have been no reported incidences of progression to a complete perforation. Rarely, endoscopic incision of the septum between the true and false lumens of the oesophagus is required.

Mallory–Weiss syndrome

This syndrome consists of painless haematemesis after vomiting, retching and straining usually induced by excess alcohol intake. However, there are notable and frequent exceptions to this definition. In particular, there is a high incidence of associated gastro-oesophageal disease. The Mallory–Weiss syndrome is common and accounts for 5–10% of patients undergoing endoscopy for haematemesis.

The lesion consists of a longitudinal mucosal tear involving the mucosa alone or the mucosa and submucosa on the gastric side of the oesophago-gastric junction. The tear, which may be single or multiple, is located on the lesser curve side in the majority of cases (85%). Associated lesions are found in 75% of patients and include hiatal hernia, oesophagitis, oesophageal varices and duodenitis/peptic ulceration. Although the bleeding stops spontaneously in the majority of patients, it may be severe and recurrent.

The condition is more often found in males (70%) and a history of alcoholism is frequently present (40–70%) but not invariable. Hypovolaemia requiring blood transfusion is found in one-third of patients. The diagnosis is confirmed by upper gastrointestinal endoscopy, which is delayed until resuscitation with blood transfusion is achieved in all shocked patients. The treatment is conservative with gastric acid suppression and antacids. Endoscopic photo- or electro-coagulation is reserved for patients with actively bleeding tears at the time of endoscopy. Surgical treatment is only indicated for those patients who continue to bleed or in whom the haemorrhage recurs after the above measures. It consists of suture ligation of the bleeding mucosal tears through a generous gastrotomy. Percutaneous embolization of the left gastric artery is used in poor-risk patients such as cirrhotic individuals.

Table 7.15 Distinguishing features of traumatic and spontaneous oesophageal perforations in the neonate

	Traumatic	*Spontaneous*
Site	Hypopharynx and cervical oesophagus	Distal oesophagus
Prematurity	30–35%	20%
Sex	Female preponderance	Equal
Aetiology	Trauma: intubation, oral suction	Unknown, ?oesophagitis
Clinical features	Difficulty in passing gastric catheter, increased oral secretions/drooling	Respiratory distress
Radiographic findings	Non-specific changes on chest radiograph, posterior tract on contrast studies	Right-sided pneumothorax or hydropneumothorax
Mortality	19%	33%

Boerhaave syndrome

The fatal condition of acute gastric distress, forceful vomiting, severe chest pain and collapse due to a complete tear of the lower thoracic oesophagus, just above the cardia, was first described by Herman Boerhaave in a Dutch admiral. This aristocratic gentleman succumbed in this way following a bout of over-indulgence of food and drink. However, only a minority of complete spontaneous perforations of the lower thoracic oesophagus fit the classical description of Boerhaave. The condition is uncommon and occurs usually between the ages of 40 and 60 years with a male-to-female ratio of 2:1. There is frequently a long history of indigestion and chronic gastrointestinal disease such as duodenal ulcer, reflux oesophagitis and hiatal hernia. Apart from overeating, other pre-disposing factors include neurological disorders, tumours and gastrointestinal obstruction. Boerhaave syndrome has also been reported during childbirth, severe convulsions and even straining during defecation.

The manifestations consist of sudden severe epigastric pain radiating to the left chest and shoulder and upper abdomen, which develops after a violent retching episode or straining. Dyspnoea and shock rapidly supervene. The correlation between retching/vomiting and the onset of pain is only encountered in 40% of patients. Aside from shock, physical findings include surgical emphysema in the neck, dullness and diminished air entry over the base of the left lung, tenderness and guarding in the upper abdomen and absent or infrequent bowel sounds. The condition may simulate very closely myocardial infarction, perforated peptic ulcer, pulmonary embolism, dissecting aortic aneurysm and severe acute pancreatitis, with any of which it is often misdiagnosed. The chest radiograph shows a left-sided plural effusion and the contrast swallow establishes the diagnosis.

Management of oesophageal perforations

The management of oesophageal perforations consists of simultaneous diagnosis and resuscitation for these severely ill patients at presentation. Antibiotic therapy with broad-spectrum antibiotics, which includes anaerobic cover, is commenced as soon as a diagnosis is made. Monitoring of vital signs, which include central venous pressure, must accompany intravenous fluid resuscitation. Inotropic support may be necessary at the outset in a proportion of patients. After a period of optimization, the vast majority of patients require surgical intervention. There are however certain specific indications for adopting non-operative management:

- Incomplete injuries: traumatic perforation of the neonate, intramural haematoma and the Mallory–Weiss syndrome.
- Complete injuries: these include minor guidewire-induced subdiaphragmatic perforations and certain thoracic perforations. The accepted criteria for a conservative approach in thoracic injuries are a localized perforation contained within the mediastinum or between the mediastinum and the visceral pleura, the cavity drains easily into the oesophageal lumen, minimal symptoms are present and clinical sepsis is minimal.

If non-operative management is contemplated this entails cessation of oral intake, antibiotic therapy, nasogastric aspiration, parenteral nutrition and underwater seal pleural drainage if the radiograph shows a pleural effusion. The condition of the patient is monitored closely and frequently and surgical intervention is undertaken if there is lack of progress or deterioration on the development of clinical sepsis.

Surgical management of oesophageal perforations

Several options for the treatment of oesophageal perforations are available. Once the diagnosis is confirmed, treatment should be tailored to the individual patient and factors such as delay in presentation, underlying oesophageal disease, location of the perforation and cause of the perforation all influence the results of therapy. Overall the aim of treatment is to seal the leak while maintaining gastrointestinal continuity, drain the infected area and the oesophageal contents and aggressively treat sepsis.

Endoscopic treatment of oesophageal perforations

This is indicated in elderly, frail or compromised patients especially those with comorbid disease. Sealing the leak can be achieved by the endoscopic application of fibrin glue sealant or cyanoacrylate. This however is limited to small perforations. Oesophageal intubation with covered self-expanding metallic stents is gaining popularity as the preferred method for sealing oesophageal perforations in the above category of patients. They can be used for early and late diagnosed perforations and for small or large tears. They are however limited to perforations in the thoracic oesophagus. Temporary drainage of gastric contents can be achieved by a percutaneous endoscopic gastrostomy, which can be performed at the same sitting, and through this aperture a jejunal feeding tube can be introduced and directed through the pylorus for nutritional support. The additional measures of antibiotics and chest drainage when there is an infusion are mandatory in all cases.

Surgical treatment of oesophageal perforations

The best results are obtained with early perforations, the mortality rising four- to five-fold if the perforation is treated surgically beyond 24 hours of onset. The approach depends on the segment of oesophagus involved: cervical injuries are approached through an incision along the anterior border of the left sternomastoid muscle, thoracic injuries through a right or left thoracotomy (depending on the exact level) and lower end/abdominal injuries through a left thoracoabdominal approach.

Early perforations. The surgical treatment depends on whether the perforation has occurred through an otherwise normal oesophagus or it is associated with significant oesophageal disease, e.g. carcinoma, stricture. In the absence of significant oesophageal disease, the perforation is closed in layers with non-absorbable sutures and drainage established. This is sufficient for early cervical injuries but for thoracic perforations most surgeons recommend additional buttressing with pleural or intercostal flaps for high lesions and a diaphragm flap (Figure 7.56), pericardial patch or omental patch for low lesions. Alternatively, the latter may be reinforced by a Thal fundal patch or a Nissen fundoplication, which is particularly useful in posterior injuries of the abdominal segment.

If the perforation is associated with significant oesophageal disease then resection (usually oesophagogastrectomy) with primary reconstruction is performed. If the condition of the patient is unstable, the reconstruction is delayed, in which case a totally diverting cervical oesophagostomy is carried out (see below) and the stomach end is closed.

Late perforations. If the diagnosis of the injury is delayed, direct suture of the oesophageal tear is not possible due to the severe transmural oedema. The options available are the following:

- Closure of the defect with a suitable flap of gastric fundus.
- Oesophageal diversion with or without exclusion.
- Endoscopic management.

Closure of the defect should be attempted in lower thoracic and abdominal perforations by the use of diaphragm flap, omental patch or gastric fundus. In either event, no attempt is made to suture the perforation; the gap is either covered with a diaphragmatic flap which is sutured to healthy oesophageal wall beyond the tear (Figure 7.57) or plugged with a Thal fundal patch over which a fundoplication is fashioned (Figure 7.58).

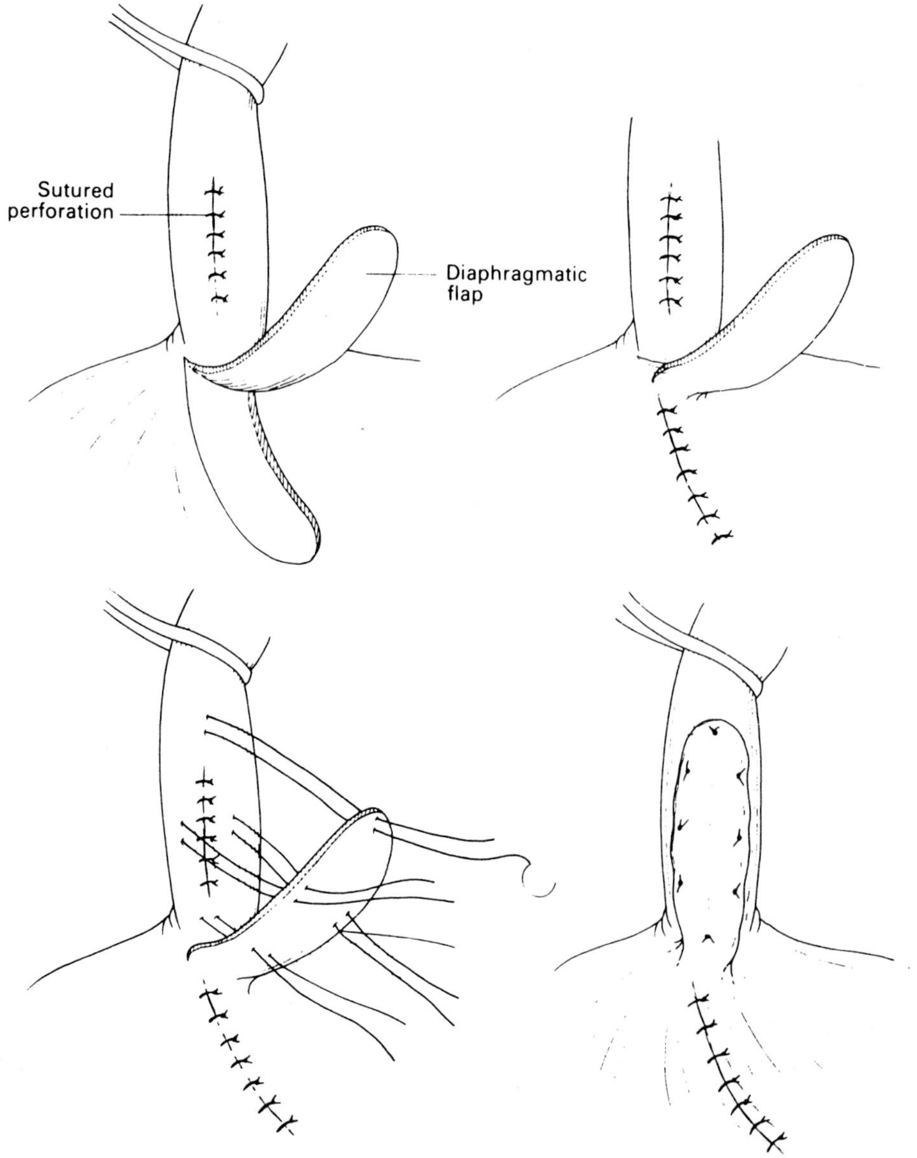

Figure 7.56 Technique of diaphragmatic flap reinforcement of sutured oesophageal perforation. (Reproduced from Hennessy and Cuschieri, 1992, by permission.)

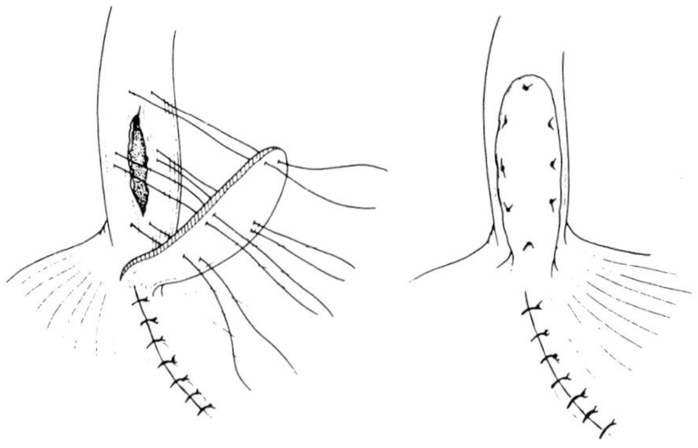

Figure 7.57 In late perforations, the flap is used to plug the tear by sutures which are inserted from within the oesophageal lumen. (Reproduced from Hennessy and Cuschieri, 1992, by permission.)

Diversion is appropriate for high thoracic injuries. After pleural toilet and insertion of drains down to the perforation and in the pleural cavity, the chest is closed and a cervical oesophagostomy is performed by the technique described by Ergin (Figure 7.59). Some advocate diversion with exclusion for late perforations. A cervical oesophagostomy is performed and, through a thoracotomy, the oesophagus is banded with Teflon distal to the perforation. Definitive treatment is carried out at a later stage if the patient survives. The disadvantage of exclusion is that a second thoracotomy is always necessary to remove the band even if the patient does not require oesophageal resection.

Oesophageal intubation is another option, which is indicated in late diagnosed perforations in poor-risk patients. It entails a thoracotomy or a thoracoscopy, pleural drainage and the insertion of a large T tube (preferably silicone, size 22–24 Fr) into the oesophageal lumen through the perforation. Drains are also left to the mediastinum and the pleural cavity. Some surgeons advocate the repeated endoscopic application of cotton wool pledgets soaked in 20% sodium hydroxide followed by 30% acetic acid to the edges of the perforation.

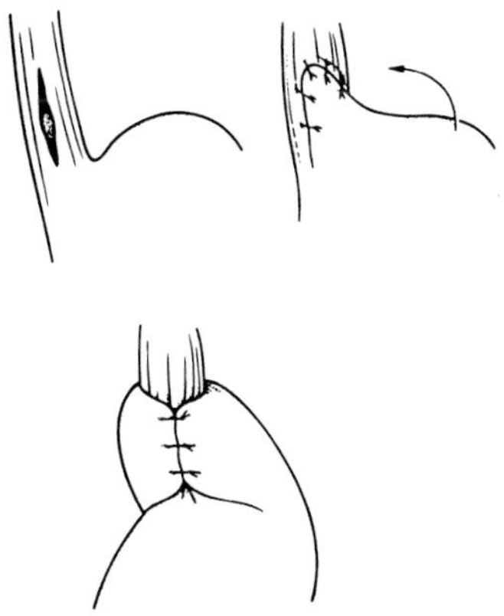

Figure 7.58 Closure of late perforation of the lower oesophagus by a Thal fundic patch which is reinforced by a fundoplication.

Section 7.8 • Neoplasms of the oesophagus

Tumours of the oesophagus are predominantly malignant. Symptomatic benign tumours are rarely encountered in clinical practice and account for less than 1% of all oesophageal neoplasms.

Benign tumours

The commonest benign tumour of the oesophagus is leiomyoma (smooth muscle tumour). They occur most commonly in the lower oesophagus (Figure 7.60) and may be multiple. The majority are small and asymptomatic but larger ones can be seen as uniform oval swellings which project into the lumen of the oesophagus and are covered by an intact mucosa. Some lesions

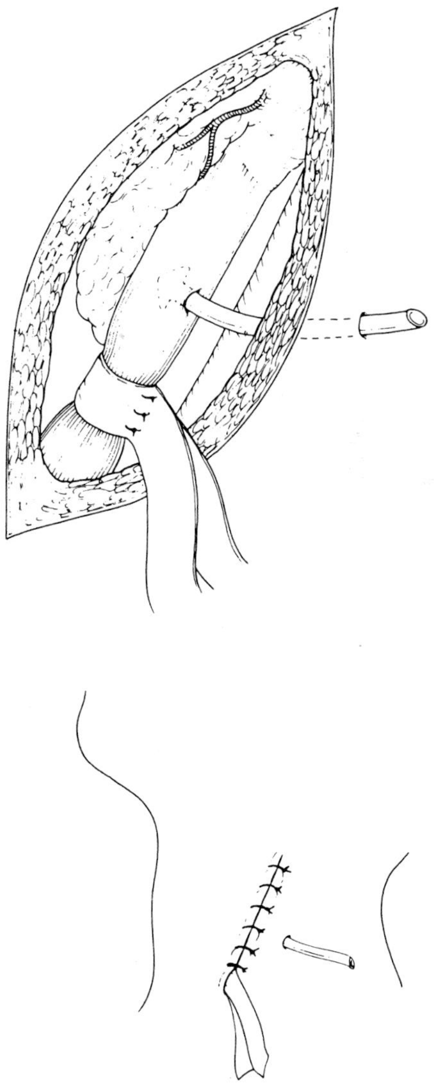

Figure 7.59 Technique of temporary totally diverting cervical oesophagostomy. The long limbs of the band are brought out through the lower end of the incision. (Reproduced from Hennessy and Cuschieri, 1992, by permission.)

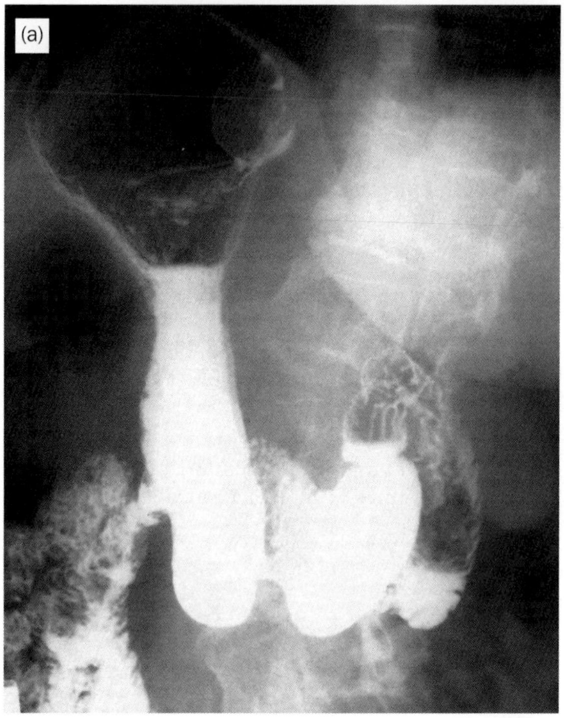

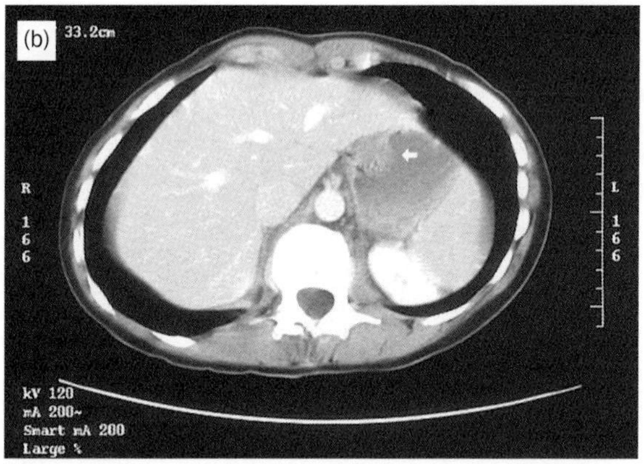

Figure 7.60 (a) Barium swallow showing a smooth ovoid tumour at the gastro-oesophageal junction. The lesion was a benign smooth muscle tumour (leiomyoma). (b) CT scan showing an ovoid leiomyoma at the oesophago-gastric junction.

may calcify. The most common presentation is with dysphagia. Bleeding due to ulceration is less common than with gastric leiomyomas although it is well documented. Malignant transformation can occur but is rare. As the tumours are well encapsulated, they can be removed by enucleation without oesophageal resection. Endoscopic removal is suitable for small pedunculated lesions. Localized resection is indicated if the lesion is large, adherent to the mucosa or at the gastro-oesophageal junction.

The next most common benign tumours in the oesophagus are fibrous or fibrovascular polyps. They occur commonly in the upper third of the oesophagus and are covered by squamous epithelial lining, which may be ulcerated. Inflammatory polyps, also called oesophagogastric polyps, are encountered at the gastro-oesophageal junction, are covered by both gastric and oesophageal epithelium and are associated with chronic oesophagitis. Adenomatous polyps are usually encountered at the lower end of the oesophagus and may be sessile or pedunculated. Most adenomatous oesophageal polyps arise as a consequence of reflux oesophagitis or columnar metaplasia.

Squamous cell papillomas (caused by the human papilloma virus) may occur anywhere in the oesophagus. They are usually single and multi-lobulated with a granular or warty surface and can vary in size. Granular cell tumours, which are rare, arise from Schwann cells. They affect middle-aged women and are usually found in the distal oesophagus. Haemangiomas are rare in the oesophagus and are usually discovered incidentally. Neurofibromas are also rare and occur as a manifestation of neurofibromatosis.

Malignant oesophageal neoplasms

Malignant oesophageal neoplasms are mostly carcinomas and carry a poor prognosis with an overall 5 year survival of 5%. In the West, cancer of the oesophagus is predominantly a disease of elderly (more than 60 years) men with an overall incidence of 10–20 per hundred thousand of population per annum. The highest incidence in the Western hemisphere is found in France, followed by Scotland where the frequency of the disease has more than doubled in the past 30 years. Carcinoma of the oesophagus is some 20–30 times more common in China, Iran and the Transkei region of South Africa than in the West. The endemic cancers in these high-incidence countries occur at a younger age and the male predominance of the disease is not as marked as in Western countries. Throughout the world, the incidence of cancer of the oesophagus is increasing in both sexes with a trend towards a greater increase in women. In contrast, there is a clear declining trend in Finland, with a decrease in incidence and mortality of about 10% every 5 years for both sexes.

Aetiology

The aetiology of oesophageal cancer remains unknown but is currently thought to be multi-factorial. The biology and aetiology of squamous cell cancer of the oesophagus and adenocarcinoma of the oesophagus are different. The important factors for squamous cell cancer of the oesophagus include the following:

- Excess alcohol intake.
- Smoking.
- Absence of protective substances in fruits and green vegetables.
- Ingestion of exogenous carcinogens and promoting factors.

Various epidemiological surveys have shown a good correlation between excess alcohol intake and smoking and the incidence of oesophageal cancer. Alcohol is thought to act as a promoter rather than a direct carcinogen. Tobacco however is considered a direct carcinogen. Certain vitamins (A, B_{12}, C, E, folic acid and riboflavin) and trace elements (iron, zinc, selenium and molybdenum) are thought to be protective. Deficiency of these substances either from inadequate ingestion of green vegetables and fruits or as a consequence of soil depletion (in the case of trace elements) is associated with a high incidence of oesophageal cancer. The carcinogenic compounds and promoters which have been implicated in endemic areas are nitrosamines, tannins (polyhydrophenyls), alcohol and phorbol esters (present in herbal/medicinal teas).

In addition, there are certain disorders which are known to predispose to the development of cancer of the oesophagus. These are outlined in Table 7.16.

Tylosis palmaris et plantaris is a hereditary autosomal dominant disorder transmitted by a single autosomal gene. It is characterized by the development of hyperkeratosis of the skin of the palms and feet during the first and second decades and the subsequent development of cancer of the oesophagus in virtually all affected individuals by the seventh decade.

The risk of oesophageal cancer in patients with *achalasia* is not reduced by myotomy. When carcinoma develops in this condition and in patients with long-standing strictures, it is usually diagnosed late and therefore carries a poor prognosis. The slightly increased risk in patients with *scleroderma* is secondary to gastro-oesophageal reflux rather than the condition itself. There is controversy as to whether infection with the human papilloma virus predisposes to squamous cell cancer of the oesophagus. Other high-risk diseases include *Plummer–Vinson syndrome* and strictures associated with lye ingestion.

For adenocarcinoma of the oesophagus, case control studies indicate that smoking, obesity and a history of chronic gastro-oesophageal reflux are significant factors. There is a clear racial, gender and site predilection for oesophageal adenocarcinoma. Approximately 95% of patients are white, men outnumber women 5:1 and approximately 80% of patients have tumours in the distal third of the oesophagus or gastro-oesophageal junction.

Table 7.16 Conditions which predispose to the development of oesophageal cancer

High risk	
	Tylosis type A
	Plummer–Vinson syndrome
Intermediate risk	
	Reflux disease and Barrett's oesophagus
	Achalasia
	Ectopic gastric mucosa
	Radiotherapy for Hodgkin's and non-Hodgkin's lymphomas
	Previous squamous cell carcinoma of the head/neck
Low risk	
	Oesophageal diverticula
	Corrosive strictures
	Coeliac disease
	Scleroderma

Pathology

The vast majority of malignant neoplasms of the oesophagus are carcinomas. Typical squamous cell carcinoma (SCC) and adenocarcinoma (AC) account for 95% of oesophageal cancers. The remaining cases include unusual histological variants of squamous cell carcinoma such as verrucose carcinoma, basaloid squamous carcinoma (adenoid cystic carcinoma), pseudosarcomatous squamous cell carcinoma (carcinosarcoma), variants of adenocarcinoma such as adenosquamous carcinoma and mucoepidermoid carcinoma, and a variety of other tumour types including choriocarcinoma, gastrointestinal stromal tumours (leiomyosarcoma), liposarcoma, malignant fibrous histiocytoma, synovial sarcoma, rhabdomyosarcoma, small cell carcinoma and melanoma. In addition, the oesophagus can be involved in metastatic cancer primarily from the lung and breast (Table 7.17).

The predominant histological type throughout the world is squamous but adenocarcinomas, especially of the lower oesophagus and gastro-oesophageal junction are increasing, particularly in the West. Adenocarcinoma of the gastric cardia can behave biologically similar to adenocarcinoma of the oesophagus. These are however classified separately into three types (Table 7.18) and should be considered separately from oesophageal and gastric neoplasms. In the West, the peak incidence of the disease is found over the age of 60 years and predominantly in males although in the past decade there has been an increased incidence in the younger age group (30–50 years), and the male-to-female sex predominance is narrowing.

Macroscopically the disease assumes one of three forms:

- Polyploid (fungating, protruded) (60%) (Figure 7.61).
- Stenosing (scirrhous, flat, diffuse, infiltrative) (15%) (Figure 7.62).
- Ulcerative (excavated) (25%) (Figure 7.63).

Growth of oesophageal cancer (SCC or AC) occurs by intra-oesophageal spread, direct extension and

Table 7.17 Histology of malignant oesophageal neoplasms

Carcinoma	
Squamous (95%)	
Adenocarcinoma (1–2%)	
Squamous cell variants:	
	Verrucous carcinoma
	Basiloid squamous carcinoma (adenoid cystic carcinoma)
	Pseudosarcomatous squamous cell carcinoma (carcinosarcoma)
Adenocarcinoma variants:	
	Mucoepidermoid carcinoma
	Adenosquamous carcinoma
Oat cell	
Melanoma	
Sarcoma	
	Leiomyosarcoma
	Rhabdomyosarcoma
	Fibrosarcoma
	Lymphoma

Table 7.18 Classification of oesophagogastric junctional tumours

Type 1	Adenocarcinoma of the distal oesophagus that usually arises from an area with specialized intestinal metaplasia of the oesophagus, and may infiltrate the oesophagogastric junction from above
Type 2	Cancer of the true cardia arising from the cardiac epithelium or short segments with intestinal metaplasia at the oesophagogastric junction
Type 3	Subcardia gastric cancer which infiltrates the oesophago-gastric junction and distal oesophagus from below

Extract from Consensus Conference of the International Gastric Cancer Association (IGCA) and the International Society for Diseases of the Esophagus (ISDE).

lymphatic or haematogenous metastasis. SCC more typically invades adjacent structures than AC. Distant metastasis may be present in 25–30% of patients at the time of diagnosis and in up to 50% of patients at autopsy. The liver (32%), lungs (21%) and bones are the most frequent sites.

Early cancer of the oesophagus (confined to mucosa/submucosa) is rarely encountered in the West because of the absence of screening programmes. The transition between severe dysplasia to carcinoma *in situ* and invasive adenocarcinoma of the oesophagus is well documented. The results of surgical treatment for early oesophageal cancer are extremely favourable with a very low operative mortality and a 5 year survival of 80–85%. There is an increasingly stronger argument for screening programmes, particularly in areas of high incidence and in patients with known predisposing

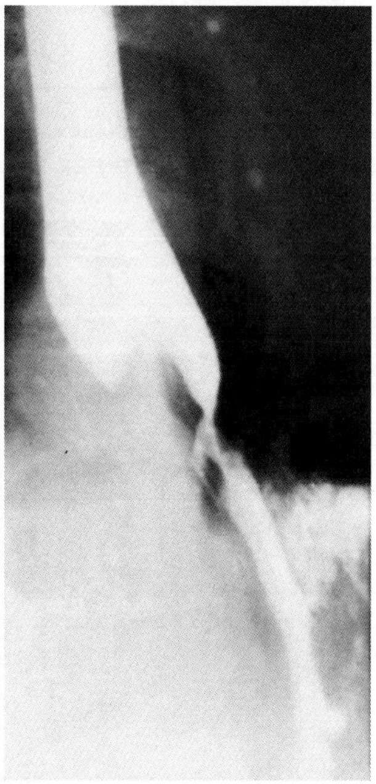

Figure 7.61 Barium swallow showing a polypoid malignant tumour at the lower end of the oesophagus.

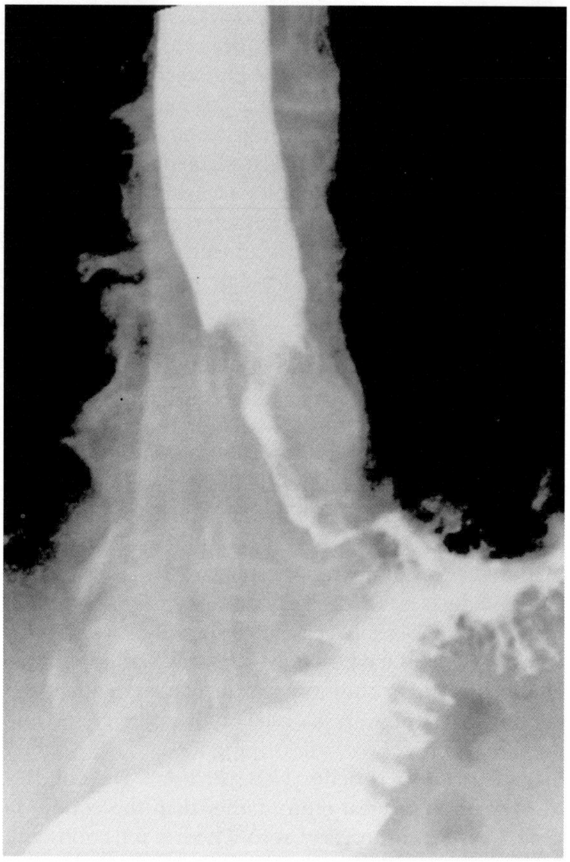

Figure 7.62 Barium swallow demonstrating a long irregular stenosing lesion of the distal oesophagus. This neoplasm has a tendency to spread along the longitudinal axis in the submucosal layer.

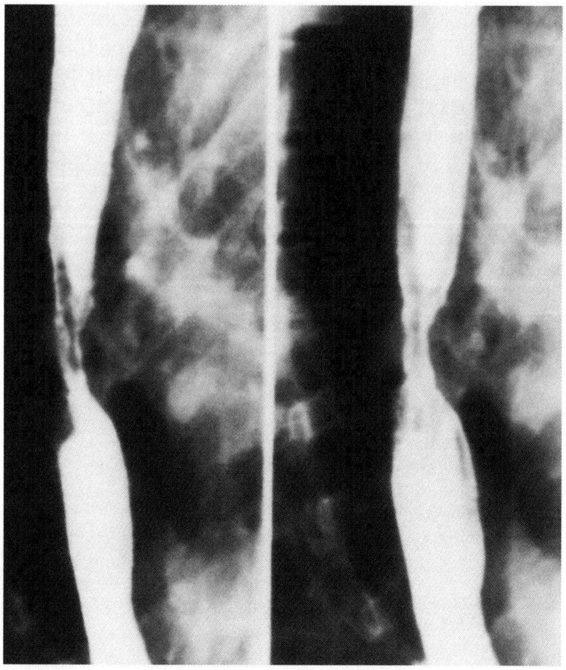

Figure 7.63 Ulcerating type of oesophageal carcinoma situated at the lower third of the gullet.

conditions. The increased incidence of adenocarcinoma in the West and its relationship to columnar metaplasia has prompted structured surveillance programmes for patients with metaplasia and dysplasia.

Histology

The histological types of oesophageal cancer are outlined in Table 7.17.

Squamous cell carcinoma

This accounts for 90% of oesophageal cancers (excluding gastric cardia cancers). Squamous cell cancers occur throughout the length of the oesophagus and are equally common in the middle and lower thirds but are less frequent in the upper third. Early lesions appear as small, grey–white, plaque-like thickenings or elevations of the mucosa. Depending on the degree of keratinization and cytological atypia, the histological appearance can be well-, moderately or poly-differentiated. The degree of differentiation does not seem to correlate with the extent of the disease, the presence of metastases or the prognosis. Two histological variants are occasionally seen. These are the verrucose carcinoma and the carcinosarcoma, which has a mixture of squamous and spindle cells and is less aggressive. The carcinoma invades the muscle walls of the oesophagus and the adjacent mediastinal structures, particularly nerves (recurrent laryngeal, phrenic) and/or the major bronchi and trachea and pericardium. Lymph node spread from tumours of the upper third is predominantly to the supraclavicular, cervical and upper mediastinal nodes; from the middle third neoplasms may involve all the mediastinal nodes and those along the left gastric and coeliac vessels, whereas neoplasms in the lower third usually spread preferentially to the lower mediastinal and subdiaphragmatic nodes. Metastatic spread is preferentially to the liver, lungs and bones. Most symptomatic tumours are quite large by the time they are diagnosed and have already invaded mediastinal structures and metastasized. Squamous cell carcinoma of the oesophagus is sensitive to radiotherapy.

Adenocarcinoma

The majority of adenocarcinomas of the oesophagus usually originate from Barrett's epithelium following long-standing gastro-oesophageal reflux. Consequently, they are usually located in the distal oesophagus and may invade the adjacent gastric cardia. A few adenocarcinomas may arise from ectopic gastric epithelium or from the oesophageal submucous glands.

The sequence of progression from intestinal metaplasia through dysplasia to carcinoma *in situ* and invasive carcinoma is well documented. The time interval between each of the phases, however, is unknown. The lesion initially appears as a flat or raised patch of an otherwise intact mucosa. It can then assume one of the three macroscopic features. Microscopically most tumours are mucin-producing glandular tumours. The tumours may exhibit intestinal-type features or less often are made up of diffusely infiltrative signet-ring cells of a gastric type. Occasionally squamous cells, adenosquamous cells and adenocarcinoid cells can be found within the tumour. The mode of spread of adenocarcinoma is similar to that of squamous tumours. The prognosis of oesophageal adenocarcinoma is poor and these tumours are relatively insensitive to radiotherapy.

Squamous cell variants

These include verrucose carcinoma, basiloid squamous carcinoma (adenoid cystic carcinoma) and pseudosarcomatous squamous cell carcinoma (carcinosarcoma). Verrucose carcinoma is a tumour with a low-grade malignancy; however, prognosis can be fairly poor. Oesophageal resection is the treatment of choice. Carcinosarcoma is a polypoid tumour with squamous cells as well as spindle cell components. The tumour behaves biologically like squamous cell carcinoma and the treatment is similar. Adenoid cystic carcinomas are histologically and biologically identical to adenoids cystic carcinoma of the salivary gland. They are intramural tumours and are believed to arise from oesophageal submucosal glands. The tumours are slow growing indolent lesions. Basiloid squamous carcinoma is a locally aggressive malignant lesion which generally metastasizes late in its course. Oesophageal resection is indicated for these tumours.

Adenocarcinoma variants

Mucoepidermoid carcinoma and adenosquamous carcinoma have oesophageal squamous cell cancer with a mucin-secreting component. They are uncommon and are thought to arise from oesophageal submucosal glands. The tumours behave biologically similarly to primary oesophageal squamous cell carcinoma. Oesophageal resection is the treatment of choice.

Other tumours

Leiomyosarcoma of the oesophagus arises from the muscularis propria or more rarely from the muscularis mucosa. They consist of irregular whorls of neomorphic spindle cells. They appear more frequently in the lower third of the oesophagus, with the remainder equally distributed in the middle and upper thirds. These tumours are slow growing, of a low grade and uncommonly metastasize. The treatment of choice is wide surgical resection. Although these tumours are considered radio resistant, radiotherapy can be considered for some patients with comorbid disease.

Liposarcoma, malignant fibrous histiocytoma, synovial sarcoma and rabdomyosarcoma are rare in the oesophagus and should be treated by radical resection when possible. Primary lymphomas are very uncommon and most of the reported cases have been of the non-Hodgkin's type.

Peptide-secreting malignant oesophageal tumours

Although rare, these are well documented. Most, but not all, have been instances of oat cell type tumour with secretory granules but others are histologically squamous cell carcinomas. Inappropriate secretion of adrenocorticotropic hormone, calcitonin, parathormone and, more recently, VIP has been reported.

Oncogenes and tumour biochemistry

To date, there has been no useful tumour marker for oesophageal cancer. Tumour antigen 4 (first isolated from cervical squamous carcinoma) is present in the majority of squamous cell oesophageal carcinomas and its concentration correlates with the degree of differentiation of the tumour. The antigen is shed in the circulation and early reports suggested that the serum levels reflect the size of the tumour burden. Further studies however did not establish the usefulness of this tumour marker in squamous cell cancer of the oesophagus. Tumour marker CA 19-9 has been used to monitor response to therapy and tumour recurrence, but its low sensitivity (34%) and modest specificity (84%) preclude its use for screening and diagnosis. EGF DNA is amplified in squamous cell cancer of the oesophagus. There is also amplification and overexpression of the epidermal growth factor receptor (EGFR) gene (ERB-B). Overexpression of this oncogene correlates with an increased frequency of lymph node metastasis. TGFα is often co-expressed with EGF and EGF receptor gene. The overexpression of the protein products correlates with a decrease in survival. The hst-1 and int-2 oncogenes code for proteins that are homologous to EGF. They are often co-amplified but are not overexpressed. Their co-amplification correlates with advancing clinical stage and worse prognosis of squamous cancer of the oesophagus. Cell cycle check-point regulator cyclin D1 is overamplified and has been observed to be co-amplified with hst-1 oncogene in squamous cancer of the oesophagus. Gene inactivation on chromosome 17p and loss of heterozygosity are detected in at least half of oesophageal cancers. In addition p53 mutations are detected in one-third of oesophageal cancers. Homozygous deletion and denovo methylation of the CDKN2 tumour suppressor gene may lead to its inactivation. This is more commonly observed with the more advanced stage of oesophageal squamous cancer. Overexpression of protein p21 encoded for by the Ras oncogene has been observed in some oesophageal squamous cancers. Overexpression of the cell surface glycoproteins encoded for by the CD44 gene correlates with increased dysplasia in oesophageal squamous cancer. Further molecular biological research will continue to shed light on the molecular events in oesophageal cancer.

Diagnosis

The majority of patients in the West present with advanced stages of the disease. Dysphagia may not become apparent until two-thirds of the oesophageal lumen has been obliterated. Oesophageal obstruction will result in malnutrition, weight loss, regurgitation and occasionally aspiration. Some patients may have palpable cervical lymph nodes and hepatic or cutaneous metastases at presentation.

The key investigations for establishing the diagnosis in patients with progressive dysphagia with or without weight loss are barium swallow and endoscopy with biopsy and cytology. Contrast radiology gives a good assessment of the length of the lesion. Resectability and cure rates decline sharply for lesions longer than 5 cm. Endoscopy gives precise information on the site and extent of circumferential involvement of the oesophagus by the tumour. As such both endoscopy and contrast radiology are essential and complementary. One or other technique is sufficient for screening in high-risk areas and in individuals with known predisposing conditions.

The advanced stages of this disease are associated with non-resectability and poor survival even after resection. Detecting the disease at an early stage is proven to increase the resectability and survival rates. The most sensitive and cost-effective screening method is endoscopy. Screening can only be justified however in areas of high prevalence and in individuals with predisposing conditions. Serum markers have not been shown to be useful in the detection of oesophageal tumours.

Staging

Once a diagnosis of oesophageal cancer is made, staging of the disease is essential to choose the best therapeutic option for the patient, and for assessing tumour resectability. In addition, the stage of the disease at the time of diagnosis is the single most important prognostic factor. The most common clinical staging system used is the TNM classification, which is based on independent measures of the depth of oesophageal wall penetration, regional lymph node involvement and the presence or absence of distant metastatic disease (Table 7.19). This staging system offers a reasonable correlation to prognosis but underestimates the importance of the number and location of lymph node metastases, and the length of the tumour. In a large retrospective review of Japanese patients with surgically treated oesophageal cancer, tumour invasion was shown to have a substantial impact on 5 year survival (T1: 46.1%, T2: 29%, T3: 21.7%, and T4: 7.0%).

For the assessment of oesophageal wall depth of invasion, CT and EUS are the standard investigations. The accuracy of CT is poor with medium sensitivity and good specificity. This is due to limitations in determining the primary tumour stage (T) and regional lymph node stage (N). In contrast, CT scanning is highly sensitive and specific for detecting metastatic disease to the lung, liver and adrenal glands. MRI has shown similar limitations in sensitivity and specificity as CT and currently offers no additional advantage in the pre-operative staging of patients with oesophageal cancer. The early experience with positron emission tomography (PET) has provided encouraging results for the detection of distant and regional lymph node metastasis as well as organ metastasis. The role of this modality is currently being evaluated. EUS, using a radial scanning echoendoscope, provides detailed

Table 7.19 The TNM staging system for oesophageal cancer

Primary tumour (T)			
TX	Primary tumour cannot be assessed		
T0	No evidence of primary tumour		
Tis	Carcinoma *in situ*		
T1a	Tumour invades lamina propria		
T1b	Tumour invades submucosa		
T2	Tumour invades muscularis propria		
T3	Tumour invades adventitia		
T4	Tumour invades adjacent structures		
Regional lymph nodes (N)			
NX	Regional lymph nodes cannot be assessed		
N0	No regional lymph node metastasis		
N1	Regional lymph node metastasis		
Distant metastasis			
MX	Presence of distant metastasis cannot be assessed		
M0	No distant metastasis		
M1	Distant metastasis		
Stage grouping			
Stage 0	Tis	N0	M0
Stage I	T1	N0	M0
Stage IIA	T2	N0	M0
	T3	N0	M0
Stage IIB	T1	N1	M0
	T2	N1	M0
Stage III	T3	N1	M0
	T4	Any N	M0
Stage IV	Any T	Any N	M1

Source: American Joint Committee on Cancer. Esophagus. In Fleming, I.D., Cooper, J.S., Henson, D.E. *et al.* eds. *AJCC Cancer Staging Handbook*, 5th edn. Philadelphia, PA: Lippincott, 1998.

examination of five ultrasonic layers in the wall of the oesophagus. Local structures around the oesophagus can also be identified and the regional lymph nodes are seen. The T staging of the primary tumour with EUS has an accuracy of 80–90%. EUS is also reported to be 80–90% accurate in detecting mediastinal lymph node metastasis. Interventional EUS using a curved linear echoendoscope can provide aspirates of suspect lesions around the oesophagus for cytological confirmation. The main difficulty with EUS is the slow acquisition of experience to confidently analyse the images. The introduction of higher frequency probes with better imaging may overcome the initial difficulties. The other main difficulty is in assessment of stenotic tumours. Slim echoprobes, which pass over a guidewire introduced endoscopically, have been developed to overcome this difficulty. Oesophageal ultrasound is limited to evaluation of the oesophagus and peri-oesophageal structures but has no utility in the detection of visceral metastasis. EUS and CT are complementary in providing the TNM stage of the disease.

Bronchoscopy should be performed for proximal oesophageal tumours to determine bronchial involvement, which is considered a contraindication to surgical resection. Vocal cord paralysis determined by ENT examination and phrenic nerve paralysis (diaphragmatic screening by fluoroscopy or ultrasound) are indications of inoperability as is distant organ metastasis.

Treatment

The treatment of patients with oesophageal cancer depends on the stage of the disease and the condition of the patient. Some patients with resectable lesions are unfit for surgery by virtue of significant comorbid disease. The nutritional state of the patient must also be considered and assessed. Anthropomorphic measurements (e.g. skin fold thickness, triceps girth) and biochemical and haematological tests (albumin, transferrin, haemoglobin, serum iron, prothrombin time, etc.) taken together would give a valuable estimation of the nutritional state of the patient. In malnourished patients, a period of parenteral or preferably enteral nutrition for a few weeks before surgery should be undertaken.

Treatment strategy

Surgery is the 'gold standard' primary treatment for local and regional tumours of the oesophagus in resectable disease and in patients fit for major surgery. The aim of surgery in these patients should be an R0 resection (complete macroscopic and microscopic removal of tumour) for cure, although palliation of dysphagia is an important secondary objective. In general, some 30–40% of oesophageal tumours are resectable (20% for T4, 50% for T3, and 80–90% for T1–T2). At operation, a few are found to be inoperable and in some there is residual tumour after the resection. Mortality rate of oesophagectomy is 5–10% in specialized centres. This rate is largely dependent on surgical expertise, caseload and patient selection. Higher mortality rates are reported from occasional oesophagectomists. The most frequent complications are anastomotic leakage and bronchopulmonary complications. Recent favourable reports suggest that the 5 year survival of all resected patients is 24% and of those patients resected with a curative intent (R0) is approximately 40% independent of the histology. These favourable results are thought to be due to lower operative mortality, increased surgical radicality, better staging and selection of patients and multi-modality treatment.

For tumours localized in the oesophageal segment below the tracheal bifurcation (T1–T3), without evidence of nodal disease or with only limited nodal disease, oesophagectomy with local lymphadenectomy should be considered and may be regarded as potentially curative. In patients with early cancer (T1a, N0) oesophagectomy is the best treatment. Lymphadenectomy is not necessary for this subset of patients. The oesophageal resection can be in the form of a vagal preserving oesophagectomy. Endoscopic mucosal resection, laser therapy or photodynamic therapy may be considered for individual patients. The choice of pre-operative or post-operative radiochemotherapy for these patients is dictated by staging tests, operative findings and post-operative histopathological assessment. For patients with more advanced but potentially curable cancer (T1b, NX; T2, NX) treatment is by oesophagectomy or oesophago-gastrectomy with local lymphadenectomy. Distal tumours can be removed by a transhiatal subtotal oesophagectomy or oesophagogastrectomy with a one-field lymphadenectomy. More proximal tumours require a transthoracic oesophagectomy with or without a two-field lymphadenectomy. Pre-operative chemoradiotherapy may incur a survival benefit and post-operative chemoradiation is recommended for the more advanced lesions with residual disease or involved lymph nodes.

For locally advanced resectable patients (T3NX), the treatment options include surgery in the form of transthoracic oesophagectomy with or without a two- or three-field lymphadenectomy, neoadjuvant chemoradiation followed by surgery and definitive chemoradiation. There is little evidence to suggest that the second approach is superior to the others. For locally advanced unresectable patients (T4NX) or unfit patients, chemoradiation should be offered followed by restaging tests. In those patients in whom the disease was down-staged surgery should be considered.

The management of patients with locally advanced or metastatic oesophageal cancer and patients with poor general medical condition must be individualized based on stage, characteristics of the tumour, patient's medical condition and patient preference. The aim of palliative treatment is rapid and sustained relief of dysphagia. Chemotherapy alone or in combination with radiotherapy should be considered with other palliative measures.

For squamous cell carcinoma with its multi-focal potential, subtotal oesophagectomy with a cervical anastomosis should be the treatment of choice. For adenocarcinoma, curative resection should include 10 cm proximal and distal margins and must include the part of the oesophagus lined with columnar metaplasia.

For tumours in the upper oesophagus (cervical oesophagus and proximal part of the thoracic oesophagus above the tracheal bifurcation) virtually all of these are squamous cell cancers. Pharyngolaryngectomy is the treatment of choice for T1 and T2 tumours of the cervical oesophagus and radiotherapy is advocated for more advanced lesions. A combined chemoirradiation approach followed by salvage or curative surgery may be appropriate in some individuals. Due to the reconstruction procedure, post-operative radiotherapy is seldom undertaken. For resectable tumours (T1–T3) of the thoracic oesophagus above the tracheal bifurcation, the therapeutic options include oesophagectomy with or without lymphadenectomy, pre-operative chemoradiotherapy followed by surgery or chemoradiotherapy alone. There is little evidence in favour of the second option. More advanced tumours should necessarily have pre-operative chemoradiation followed by staging to assess resectability.

Resection

Tumours of the cervical oesophagus. The majority of proximal tumours arise from the hypopharyngeal area (pyriform fossa, posterior wall of the pharynx and postcricoid region) and tumours of the cervical oesophagus are rare. They carry a poor prognosis and survival beyond 1 year after treatment is uncommon. Radiotherapy is the treatment of choice for these tumours since the majority of them are large at presentation. Pharyngolaryngectomy is indicated for early lesions or for lesions which have recurred after radiotherapy. These patients have a permanent tracheostomy. Until recently, reconstruction was achieved with colon (brought up retrosternally or subcutaneously), stomach or myocutaneous flaps. Viscus transposition increases the operative mortality in this group of patients while myocutaneous flap repairs have a high incidence of complications, mainly strictures and fistulae. However, the best results in terms of swallowing, voice production and early hospital discharge are achieved with free revascularized jejunal or greater curve gastric grafts which are interposed between the proximal pharynx and the distal oesophagus after the blood supply has been restored to the graft by anastomosis of the artery and vein to the superior thyroid artery and facial vein (Figure 7.64).

Tumours of the thoracic oesophagus. Surgical approach to the oesophagus can be transthoracic or through the mediastinum. In general, transthoracic operations have a higher degree of operative mortality and morbidity.

The procedure may consist of a subtotal oesophagectomy with a cervical anastomosis or a partial oesophagectomy with a midthoracic anastomosis. Because of the multi-focal potential of squamous cell carcinoma, subtotal oesophagectomy is carried out, the anastomosis for reconstruction being carried out in the neck. For adenocarcinoma, curative resection should include 10 cm proximal and distal margins as part of the *en-bloc* resection, and all of the columnar lined oesophagus.

Some surgeons prefer partial oesophagectomy (Lewis–Tanner operation) as the routine procedure for tumours of the lower two-thirds of the oesophagus and

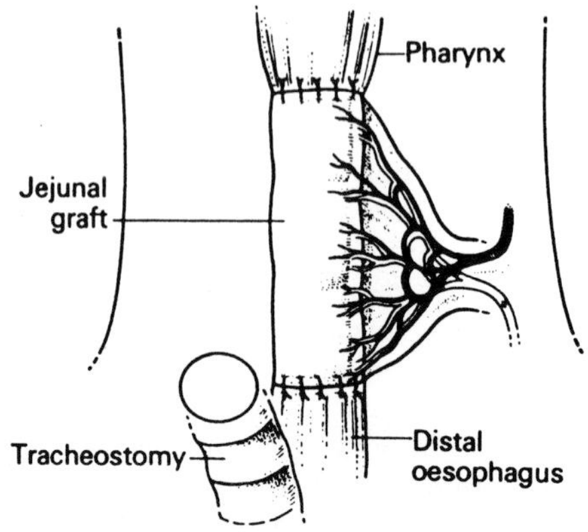

Figure 7.64 Free revascularized jejunal graft for reconstruction after pharyngolaryngectomy. This microvascular technique gives the best results and is replacing other methods of reconstruction.

reserve subtotal oesophagectomy for high thoracic oesophagus tumours. The advantages of subtotal oesophagectomy are better tumour clearance and an easier anastomosis in the neck, dehiscence of which is rare and less life threatening in this situation. The important complication of intra-thoracic oesophageal anastomosis is leakage with the development of empyema. This complication is the major cause of post-operative mortality after oesophageal resection. Careful attention in the performance of this anastomosis to ensure mucosa to mucosa coaptation, experience good vascularity and avoidance of any tension are the most important factors in the prevention of anastomotic dehiscence.

Partial oesophagectomy. The two-stage Lewis–Tanner procedure (Figure 7.65) was the standard operation for resection of tumours of the lower two-thirds of the oesophagus (excluding carcinoma of the cardia). It achieves better clearance than the left thoracotomy approach, which is seldom used nowadays. The abdominal or first stage of the Lewis-Tanner operation is usually performed through a mid-line epigastric incision. The entire stomach is mobilized and its vascular supply maintained through the right gastro-epiploic and right gastric vessels. The short gastric vessels are ligated individually and then the left gastric artery is ligated at its origin through the coeliac axis. The duodenum and head of pancreas are mobilized sufficiently to expose a long segment of the vena cava and to enable their reflection to the midline or beyond. Proximally, the peritoneum over the gastro-oesophageal junction and the phreno-oesophageal membrane are divided. The abdominal oesophagus is mobilized, the vagal trunks are sectioned and blunt dissection of the lower posterior mediastinum around the oesophagus is performed. In lower third lesions, the tumour should become palpable at this stage. Gastric pyloromyotomy or pyloroplasty is unnecessary unless there is duodenal scarring or deformity.

The thoracic or second stage is performed through a right posterolateral thoracotomy carried out through the bed of the fifth rib. The oesophagus is eminently accessible through this approach and the only overlying structure is the azygos vein. A minimum of 5 cm proximal clearance from the upper margin of the tumour is necessary because of the submucosal spread of oesophageal cancer. The stomach is pulled into the chest after the oesophagus and the tumour have been mobilized. The distal resection margin is at the cardio-oesophageal junction or upper third of the stomach depending on the lower extent of the disease. The gastric end is closed and the stomach then anastomosed to the intrathoracic oesophagus either manually or using a stapler. In transecting the oesophagus, the muscle coat should be divided all the way around to expose the mucosal tube which is then transected 1.0 cm further distally (Figure 7.66). This prevents retraction of the oesophageal mucosa inside the muscular layers and therefore facilitates and ensures the safety of the anastomosis. A tension free anastomosis can be carried out with a single layer technique using interrupted sutures or preferably using a mechanical stapler.

Subtotal oesophagectomy. For squamous cell cancer and for proximal lesions and for surgeon's preference subtotal oesophagectomy with anastomosis of the mobilized stomach or colon to the cervical oesophagus can be carried out. This is achieved either by means of a three-stage operation (McKeown's oesophagectomy) or by the technique of transhiatal oesophagectomy without thoracotomy, popularized by Orringer. Endoscopic oesophagectomy also achieves subtotal oesophagectomy without thoracotomy.

The first stage of the McKeown's procedure is identical to that of the Lewis–Tanner oesophagectomy.

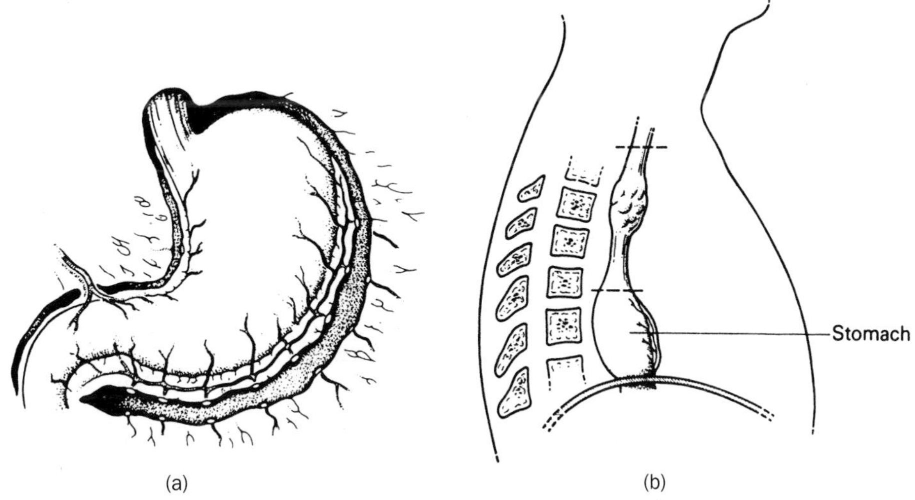

Figure 7.65 The Lewis–Tanner two-stage oesophagectomy. (a) Abdominal stage – the stomach and duodenum have been completely skeletonized with preservation of the right gastric and gastro-epiploic vessels. (b) The oesophagus and tumour are mobilized through a right thoracotomy, and the previously mobilized stomach is then drawn into the chest.

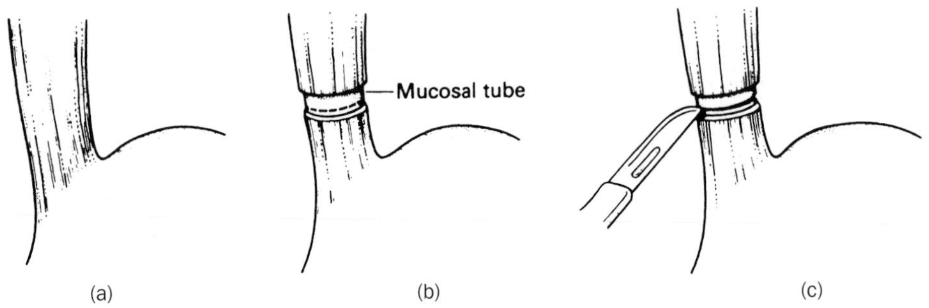

Figure 7.66 The oesophageal muscular coat is divided all the way round down to the mucosal tube which is then transected 1.0 cm lower down. This prevents retraction of the mucosa inside the muscular layers.

The second stage differs in that it entails total mobilization of the thoracic oesophagus up to and including the thoracic inlet, after which the chest is closed and the patient is re-positioned in the supine posture. A variant of the described McKeown's procedure is '*en-bloc* oesophagectomy'. This aims to remove an envelope of tissue surrounding the tumour bearing oesophagus, including adjacent pleura and pericardium and the posterior mediastinal tissues anterior to the vertebral bodies, including the azygos vein and the thoracic duct.

The cervical or third stage is conducted through an oblique or transverse incision on the left side of the neck 2.0 cm above the clavicle. After mobilization of the cervical oesophagus, the distal gullet with tumour is pulled up into the neck until the cardia appears. The gastro-oesophageal junction and the lesser curvature, together with associated lymph nodes are then clamped, divided and closed, and the oesophagus is then resected. The anastomosis is performed in the neck between the proximal cervical oesophagus and the fundus of the stomach tube.

Endoscopic oesophagectomy

Transhiatal oesophagectomy. In oesophagectomy without thoracotomy, the stomach is skeletonized as described previously. The thoracic oesophagus is mobilized by manual dissection through the hiatus, which may be divided to facilitate the procedure. The cervical and upper thoracic oesophagus are mobilized through an approach along the anterior border of the left sternomastoid. The cervical oesophagus is then transected and a long rubber tube is attached to the distal end. The thoracic oesophagus with the tumour is then withdrawn into the abdomen, and the gastro-oesophageal junction is transected and closed. The oesophagus is then detached from the rubber tube and removed. The tube is anchored to the fundus of the stomach. Traction at the cervical end of the rubber tube is used to pull up the stomach through the posterior mediastinum into the neck for anastomosis to the cervical oesophagus (Figure 7.67). The advantage of this procedure is the avoidance of a thoracotomy, especially in elderly patients and patients with significant bronchopulmonary disease.

A variant of the transhiatal oesophagectomy is the vagal-sparing oesophagectomy. This operation is described for proven severe dysplasia in patients with intestinal metaplasia of the oesophagus. A vein stripper is advanced through a limited gastrotomy into the cervical oesophagus. The cervical oesophagus is then divided after securing the vein stripper in the distal segment. The stripper is then pulled through the gastrotomy to strip the oesophagus from surrounding structures preserving the vagi in the process. The stripped oesophagus is then divided from the stomach and the gastrotomy wound closed. An isoperistaltic colon segment is then passed retrosternally or in the posterior mediastinum. The colon is anastomosed proximally to the oesophagus and distally to the stomach. The advantages of this procedure include those of the transhiatal oesophagectomy in addition to excellent functional results.

Endoscopic oesophagectomy is a recent advance on blunt transhiatal oesophagectomy. The principal benefit of both approaches is the avoidance of a thoracotomy, which is particularly relevant in oesophageal cancer as the majority of patients suffering from this disease are above the age of 60 years. The advantages of the endoscopic procedure over the blunt transhiatal resection include a precise visually guided dissection, with minimum blood loss and less risk of injury to the azygos vein, left bronchus and recurrent laryngeal nerves.

There are two techniques of endoscopic oesophagectomy; the mediastinascopic approach of Buess and the right thoracoscopic technique first introduced by Cuschieri. The mediastinascopic dissection is performed using a special operating rigid mediastinascope, which is introduced through a left cervical incision along the anterior margin of the sternomastoid. It allows perivisceral mobilization of the intra-thoracic oesophagus up to the abdominal hiatus. After the oesophagus is resected and removed through the abdomen by the abdominal operator (operating synchronously), the mobilized stomach or gastric tube is brought up through the mediastinum for anastomosis to the proximal cervical oesophagus. The main disadvantage of the mediastinascopic approach is the difficulty of dissection and removal of the para-oesophageal

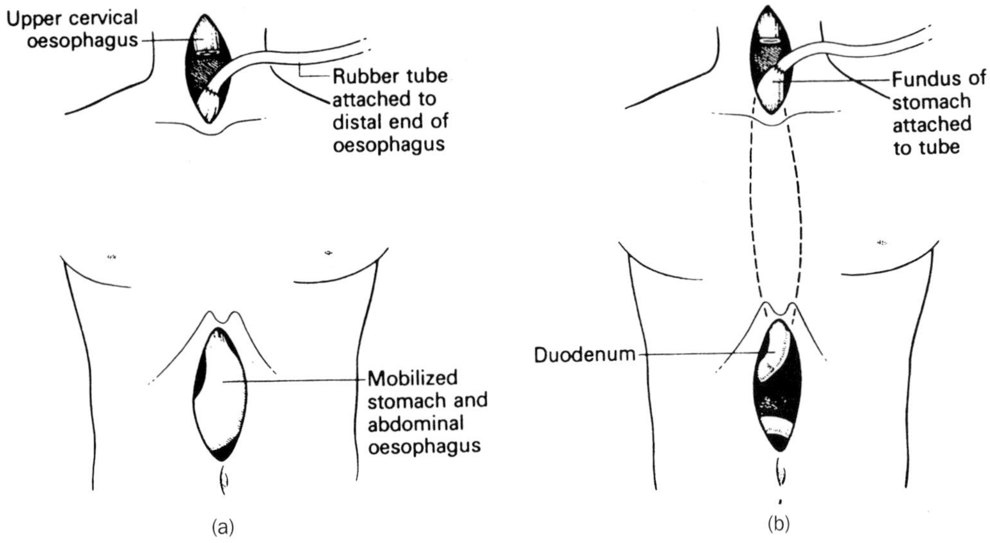

Figure 7.67 Subtotal oesophagectomy without thoracotomy. (a) The stomach and duodenum have been mobilized with preservation of the right gastric and epiploic vessels. The thoracic oesophagus is mobilized by hand dissection through the hiatus. The cervical and upper thoracic oesophagus are mobilized through an incision along the anterior border of the left sternomastoid muscle. The cervical oesophagus is then transected and a rubber tube attached to the distal end. The oesophagus with tumour is then withdrawn into the abdomen until the attached end of the rubber tube is encountered. The oesophagus is then resected, and the cardio-oesophageal junction closed and attached to the rubber tube. (b) The stomach is brought to the neck for anastomosis to the cervical oesophagus by means of traction on a rubber tube from its cervical end.

lymph nodes, which are often left behind. In this respect, the resection is usually non-curative but in view of the advanced nature of most oesophageal cancers this is acceptable in most instances. The dissection of the lower thoracic oesophagus is also difficult with this technique due to the bulge and pulsation of the aorta on which the operating mediastinascope tends to impinge.

The right thoracoscopic operation (Figure 7.68) is conducted using a double lumen endobronchial tube for isolating the left lung in order to achieve collapse of the right lung. The procedure is identical to the thoracic stage of the McKeown operation and permits precise visually guided dissection of the oesophagus and the regional para-oesophageal and tracheo-bronchial lymph nodes with little blood loss. In tumours of the lower third, the azygos vein is simply mobilized from the oesophagus but in middle third lesions, the vein is ligated and divided. Another advantage of the procedure is the ability to perform the dissection of the lower cervical oesophagus through the right chest by extending the mobilization beyond the thoracic inlet. After the endoscopic mobilization is completed, the patient is turned in the supine position for the second stage. The neck is opened through an oblique or transverse incision. The mobilized cervical oesophagus is then transected. At the same time, the abdominal surgeon performs the standard gastric mobilization and after resection of the oesophagus, the stomach tube is pulled up to the neck for proximal anastomosis to the cervical oesophagus. The results of right thoracoscopic oesophagectomy for cancer to date have been excellent in a few centres with appropriately selected patients. The procedure entails single lung anaesthesia for 90–120 min. Patients with inadequate respiratory reserve cannot tolerate this intra-operatively and tend to develop more respiratory problems post-operatively. The haemodynamic upset caused by single lung ventilation may be misinterpreted as overinfusion. In addition, shunting tends to occur with subsequent lung damage, which becomes apparent 48 hours post-operatively. The main advantages of this procedure are: minimizing blood loss, abolition of post-thoracotomy pain, reduction in post-operative ventilatory difficulty and early discharge from hospital.

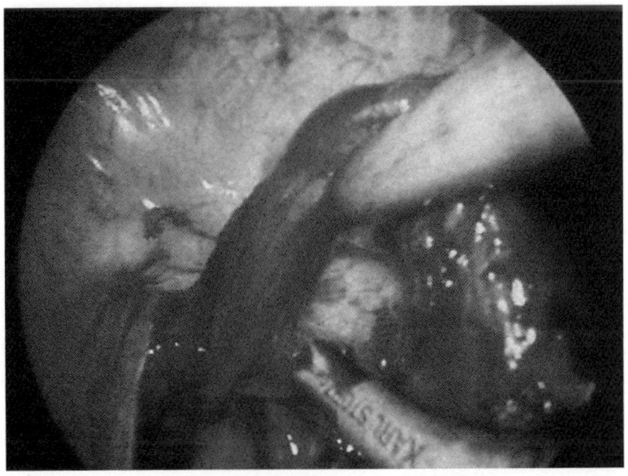

Figure 7.68 Right thoracoscopic dissection of the oesophagus with level 2 lymphadenectomy for a carcinoma of the middle third.

Tumours of the oesophagogastric junction. Resection of the tumour with a limited lymphadenectomy of the field surrounding the tumour is the goal of surgical resection. This can be achieved by oesophago-gastrectomy or partial oesophagectomy with resection of the proximal margin of the stomach. Oesophago-gastrectomy is carried out through the abdominal route, removing an oncologically safe margin of the oesophagus with the upper third of the stomach. The lower oesophageal dissection can be carried out through the transhiatal route or transthoracically. Partial oesophagectomy is more appropriate for type 1 oesophagogastric junction tumours with an oesophagogastrectomy being more appropriate for type 2 and 3 tumours.

Lymphadenectomy. The goal of extensive lymphadenectomy is to remove all regional lymph node groups with potential metastatic deposits (Table 7.20) in order to improve the pathological staging of the disease. Whether this translates into improved survival or disease free interval remains unproven. A *one-field* lymphadenectomy only involves the dissection of the diaphragmatic, right and left paracardiac, lesser curvature, left gastric, coeliac and common hepatic nodes. A *two-field* lymphadenectomy includes the para-aortic (mediastinal) nodes together with the thoracic duct, the right and left pulmonary hilar nodes, the para-oesophageal nodes and the para-tracheal bronchial nodes. *Three-field* lymphadenectomy additionally includes the brachio-cephalic, deep lateral and external cervical nodes including the right and left recurrent nerve lymphatic chains (deep anterior cervical nodes). Approximately 75% of patients with lower third cancers have involved lymph nodes in the coeliac trunk, left gastric and common hepatic territories. These will be removed in a single field (abdominal) lymphadenectomy. Approximately, 60% of patients with middle and lower oesophageal tumours have mediastinal and sub-diaphragmatic lymph node involvement. This would be covered by a two-field lymphadenectomy. Due to the lower incidence of cervical node metastases in patients with cancer of the sub-carinal oesophagus and due to the little difference in 5 year survival between patients undergoing a three- or a two-field dissection, dissection of cervical nodes in these patients is questionable. A three-field lymphadenectomy incurs an additional morbidity and mortality even in experienced centres. For patients with upper third tumours, three-field lymphadenectomy should be considered in clinical trial protocols. In addition, a subset of patients in which lymph node metastases are detectable only by cervical ultrasound, three-field lymphadenectomy should be considered, especially for low-risk patients. This may necessitate referral to a specialist centre which practises this type of surgery in the context of clinical trials. To date, there is very little evidence to suggest that extensive lymphadenectomy carries a survival benefit or improves locoregional control in Western oesophageal surgical practice.

Table 7.20 Regional lymph nodes around the oesophagus

Group	*Site of lymph nodes*
A	Superficial cervical nodes Cervical para-oesophageal nodes Deep cervical nodes Supraclavicular nodes
B	Bilateral recurrent laryngeal nodes Infra-aortic arch nodes
C	Tracheal bifurcation nodes Paratracheal nodes Pulmonary hilar nodes
D	Upper thoracic para-oesophageal nodes Middle thoracic para-oesophageal nodes Lower thoracic para-oesophageal nodes Posterior mediastinal nodes Diaphragmatic nodes
E	Right cardiac nodes Left cardiac nodes Lesser curvature nodes
F	Left gastric artery nodes Common hepatic artery nodes Coeliac axis nodes

Reconstruction. The standard reconstruction of the alimentary tract after oesophagectomy is performed using the gastric pull-up (Figure 7.69). This guarantees good functional results with a safe and quick operation. If the stomach is unsuitable due to previous surgery or concurrent disease, an isoperistaltic colonic segment on a vascular pedicle should be considered with the left colon being preferred to the right colon. This is claimed to reduce post-operative reflux oesophagitis, which occurs in 30% of patients after a partial oesophagectomy and in 15% of patients after a subtotal oesophagectomy. After a lower third oesophagectomy or oesophago-gastrectomy a pedicled isoperistaltic jejunal loop would suffice. The transposition path of choice is the posterior mediastinum as it is the most direct, and guarantees less morbidity and better post-operative functional results. The alternative retrosternal transposition route is preferred for bypass purposes and in patients in whom residual disease is left behind. The retrosternal route would avoid involvement of the transposed viscus either by local recurrence or by post-operative irradiation.

Non-surgical treatment

Radiotherapy. Treatment by supervoltage external beam radiotherapy may be curative (radical) or palliative to relieve dysphagia and metastatic bone pain in patients with advanced disease. It can also be given as an adjunct to surgical treatment either in the form of multi-modality treatment or after oesophagectomy to improve locoregional control. In many institutions, complete surgical resection has been the 'gold standard' against which other therapies are compared. It is difficult to make a meaningful comparison between surgery and radical radiation therapy for the primary treatment of resectable oesophageal cancer in the absence of comparative clinical trials between these two modalities in otherwise fit patients with early (resectable) oesophageal cancer. An analysis of retrospective series indicates that patients selected for radical treatment with radiotherapy have similar overall results to surgery except that the mortality of radical radiotherapy is small and its morbidity is significantly lower than that accrued by surgery. In general, radiotherapy achieved relief of dysphagia and local control of the disease but remote failure was common. There are, however, certain definite contraindications to radical radiotherapy. These include large tumours (more than 9.0 cm) and the presence of a tracheal broncho-oesophageal fistula. The main disadvantages of radical radiotherapy are the development of a fibrous stricture in half the patients treated. A variety of radiation therapy regimens have been described (40–70 Gy in 20–30 fractions), but no survival benefit was detected between them. Accelerated fractionation regimens that decrease the overall time of treatment may enhance local control at the expense of increased stricture rate.

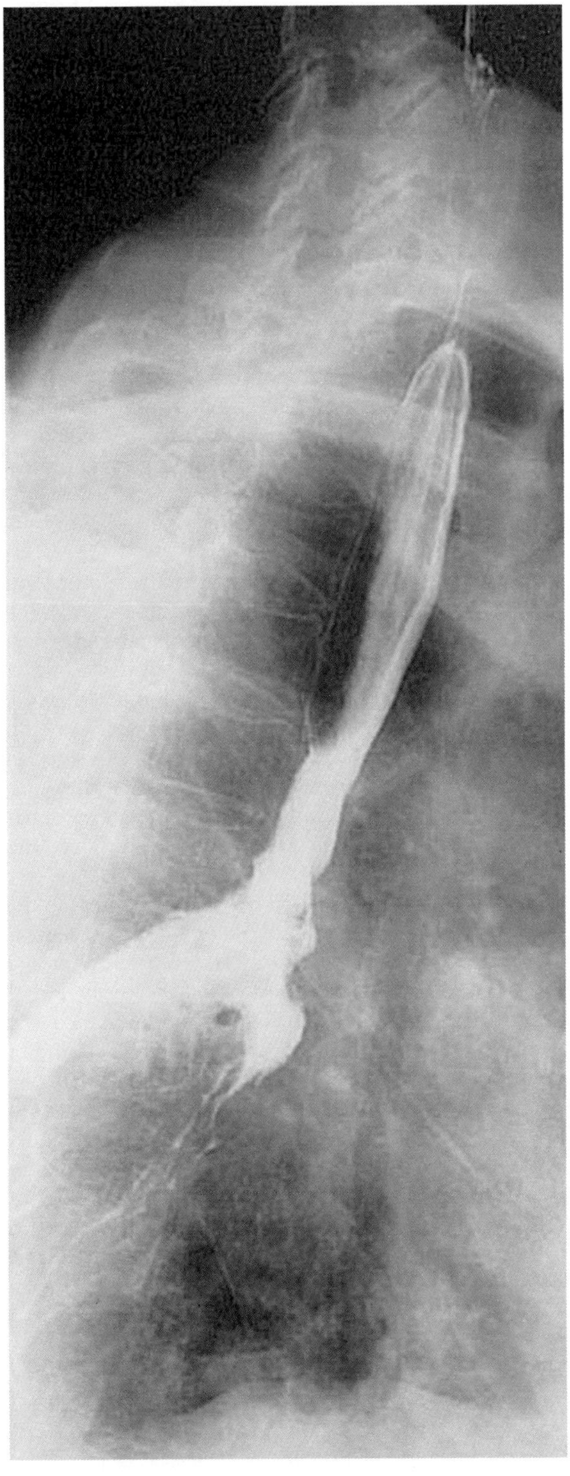

Figure 7.69 Barium swallow showing a gastric pull-up reconstruction after a partial oesophagectomy.

Brachytherapy (intracavity irradiation) with caesium or iridium pellets loaded into an applicator and placed in the lumen of the oesophagus is another technique for delivering radiotherapy locally. The main limitation of this technique is the effective treatment distance, which in the case of iridium is 1 cm. Larger tumours would be irradiated in the centre but not peripherally. As such this technique is useful for palliation of dysphagia but not for radical treatment unless combined with external-beam super-voltage radiotherapy.

Radiotherapy is the treatment of choice for patients with cervical oesophageal cancer and for some patients with upper thoracic oesophageal cancer. Squamous carcinomas are considered radio-sensitive and adenocarcinomas are considered relatively radio-resistant. For patients considered healthy enough to receive radical radiation therapy, concomitant chemotherapy is the preferred option.

Palliative treatment to relieve dysphagia is usually administered by external-beam super-voltage radiotherapy using a dose of 45–50 Gy. Dysphagia may temporarily worsen during the course of treatment and it may take up to 2 months before effective palliation of dysphagia is realized. In addition, the duration of palliation after radiation therapy is variable but is generally poor and can be accompanied by the development of fibrotic strictures in 30% of patients. Combined chemo/irradiation produces better palliation of dysphagia at the expense of a higher rate of toxicity. Brachytherapy as a palliative measure is reported to give excellent results with relief of dysphagia in 65%.

Chemotherapy. In view of the metastatic rate of oesophageal cancer the disease should be regarded as systemic in the majority of patients, regardless of the stage of the disease at presentation. Systemic chemotherapy is advocated to address this problem. Several agents have been identified which can be used in combination treatment regimens for oesophageal cancer. These include 5-fluorouracil (5-FU), cisplatin, vindesin, mitomycin C, paclitaxel and etoposide. Paclitaxel is one of the new group of taxanes with a high response rate in metastatic oesophageal cancer, which also acts as a radiation sensitizer and as such a useful adjunct to radiotherapy. Combination regimens are preferred to single agent use to increase the response rate using agents with different mechanisms of action and different toxicity profiles. Most combination regimens have the antimetabolite 5-FU in bolus injections or low-dose continuous infusions with or without leucovorin. The second most common agent used in combination regimens is cisplatin. The combination of cisplatin and 5-FU has consistently produced a complete pathological response rate of around 10% and a partial response rate (regression) of 50–60% but with significant toxicity, which can be up to 60%. Adding a third agent, such as bleomycin, has only fractionally improved the response rate at the expense of universally worse toxicity.

Multi-modality treatment. The majority of patients with oesophageal cancer present with advanced stages of the disease, which jeopardizes the chances of a curative resection. This has led to the use of various multi-modality treatment schedules with or without surgery. The combined use of chemotherapy and radiotherapy is based on the rationale that different tumour cell subpopulations may be resistant to one modality but sensitive to another. In addition, apart from activity against micrometastases, some chemotherapeutic agents have radio-sensitizing properties. In early resectable disease, it seems that survival rate is not significantly influenced by multi-modality regimens compared to surgery alone. However, in locally advanced disease, the potential benefit of the regimens becomes more evident with substantial numbers of patients having the stage of their disease lowered and becoming eligible for resection.

The combined use of chemotherapy and radiation therapy for the primary treatment of oesophageal cancer has produced better response rates, in terms of tumour and metastatic disease response with improved survival, than either modality alone. One popular regimen which is used in the treatment of patients with metastatic disease is the Herskovic regimen. This consists of 50 Gy of radiation delivered over 6 weeks (25 fractions) with cisplatin and 5-FU given on weeks 1, 5, 8 and 11 (two courses of chemotherapy during and two after radiation).

Since residual disease after standard oesophagectomy is between 35 and 67%, radiotherapy has been commonly used with surgical resection for locoregional control. Theoretically, pre-operative radiotherapy is potentially advantageous from the radiobiology viewpoint. The dissected post-operative field is ischaemic and likely to be hypoxic. Tumour cell hypoxia is one mechanism of radio-resistance. In practice, however, pre-operative radiotherapy does not appear to have a significant effect on locoregional control or on survival. However, post-operative radiotherapy seems to improve locoregional control (disease-free interval) in node negative patients but has no impact on overall survival.

Pre-operative chemotherapy (neoadjuvant) followed by surgery is used to downstage advanced tumours in order to increase the resectability rate and to improve survival. Giving the treatment pre-operatively should result in better drug delivery to the tumour, as the local blood supply has not been disturbed by operative dissection. Distant control should also be enhanced as micrometastases are treated early without having to wait for post-surgical recovery. In addition, pre-operative treatment allows for the identification of responders who may benefit from additional post-operative therapy. Results from the UK MRC trial using 5-FU and cisplatin in two courses pre-operatively vs surgery alone suggest a 9% 2 year survival benefit in patients who received pre-operative chemotherapy. The response seems to be similar for adenocarcinoma and squamous cell cancer.

The additional use of radiotherapy to chemotherapy pre-operatively has many theoretical advantages. However, there are only limited data which suggest the safety of pre-operative chemoirradiation with marginal survival benefit. There are too few data on post-operative chemoirradiation to reach any meaningful conclusion.

Despite the early enthusiasm, immunotherapy with biological response modifiers (interferons, interleukin-2 and lymphokine activated killer cells) has not been successful in oesophageal and other gastrointestinal tumours.

Palliation of advanced oesophageal cancer

Surgical bypass. These are less popular than intubation procedures because they carry a high mortality, which averages around 30%, and are major operations, which do not seem justified in patients with advanced disease or poor general condition with very limited survival. When successful, however, relief of dysphagia is better than that obtained by intubation and the patient can swallow ordinary meals. Surgical bypass is the most effective method of dealing with a malignant oesophago-tracheal fistula in selected patients. The procedures are outlined in Table 7.21.

The most commonly used bypass procedures are the reversed gastric tube and colon bypass. Gastro-oesophageal anastomosis warrants a thoracotomy and for this reason is seldom performed electively. However, it is the best option when a tumour which was deemed resectable on pre-operative staging is found to be inoperable at thoracotomy. The reversed gastric tube is fashioned along the greater curvature using staplers and is based on the left gastro-epiploic vessels (Figure 7.70). It is brought up to the neck for anastomosis to the cervical oesophagus via either the subcutaneous or retrosternal route. Necrosis of the transposed colon is the main disadvantage of colon bypass for inoperable oesophageal malignancy (Figure 7.71).

Table 7.21 Palliative bypass procedures

Reversed gastric tube
Gastro-oesophagostomy proximal to the tumour
Colon bypass, right or left, retrosternal or subcutaneous
Jejunal bypass

Laser canalization. Laser photocoagulation is an effective method of oesophageal canalization in patients with obstructive, advanced oesophageal cancer. In most instances the Nd:YAG laser is used as it produces good destruction of malignant tissue and its energy is not absorbed by blood.

Two techniques are employed: the sequential and the dilatation – single treatment methods. With the sequential technique, a channel is established by laser photocoagulation at the proximal end of the tumour and the burrowing is progressively continued over the entire length of the tumour in several sessions. With the single treatment method, the tumour is first dilated to allow the passage of the flexible endoscope and photocoagulation of the entire tumour is applied as the endoscope is withdrawn gradually. Laser photocoagulation is only effective in the destruction of mucosal tumour and is difficult in lesions of the upper third and of the oesophagogastric junction. Complications of laser canalization include perforation and the development of a fibrous stricture. In addition, the treatment has to be repeated frequently to obtain sustained relief from dysphagia. Laser canalization using the Nd:YAG laser provides similar relief of dysphagia to endoscopic intubation. However, more complications occur in intubated patients with a higher incidence of recurrent dysphagia.

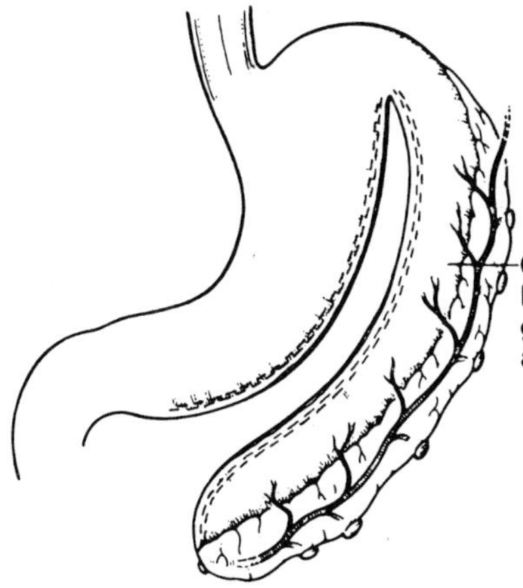

Figure 7.70 Reversed gastric tube based on the left gastro-epiploic vessels used for bypass of inoperable oesophageal malignancy.

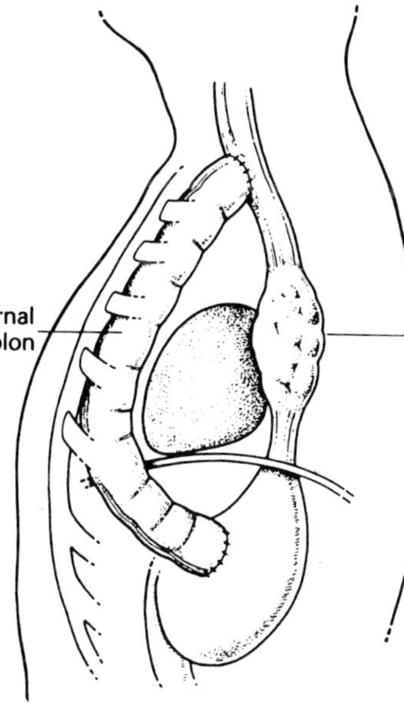

Figure 7.71 Retrosternal colon bypass. The disadvantage of this technique is the risk of impaired venous drainage of the transposed colon with the development of necrosis which is usually fatal.

Photodynamic therapy is another form of palliative re-canalization of the oesophagus using laser light energy for advanced oesophageal neoplasms. The principle entails a prior intravenous administration of a photosensitizer, usually a haematoporphyrin derivative (HpD) or oral administration of 5-amino-laevulanic acid (5-ALA). These photosensitizers are taken up and retained by the tumour. After 6–24 hours the tumour is irradiated by light (wavelength of 630 nm). This type of light energy excites the photosensitizer in the tumour to the triplet state with the production of highly reactive species such as singlet oxygen, which induce necrosis of the tumour (largely by occlusion of the tumour circulation). Although undoubtedly effective and safe, photodynamic therapy is not used frequently because of the difficulty in generating the laser light using either argon-pump dye laser or gold metal vapour lasers. Both machines are difficult to operate. The other disadvantage of photodynamic therapy is the retention of the photosensitizer in the tissues for several weeks. This results in cutaneous hypersensitivity to sunlight from which the patient has to be protected during this period to avoid severe sunburn. The results with intravenous photosensitizers are better than with the oral ones. Each treatment achieves necrosis of a proportion of the luminal tumour and the treatment has to be repeated frequently for sustained relief of dysphagia.

Electrocoagulation – BICAP probe. Endoscopic guided fulguration of advanced oesophageal neoplasm is possible with the BICAP probe (Figure 7.72). This is passed over a guidewire to the proximal margin of the tumour, which is coagulated under endoscopic control. The procedure continues with antegrade coagulation of the tumour until the lower end of the lesion is reached, when the probe is rotated 180° and retrograde coagulation applied creating a sizeable channel through the neoplastic mass. Comparative studies have shown similar palliative efficacy to laser photocoagulation for circumferential tumours. The advantages of the BICAP electrocoagulation technique include portability, low cost and ability to treat submucosal lesions, long or high oesophageal cancers, in one session. However, the BICAP probe is less safe then the Nd:YAG photocoagulation for exophytic non-circumferential cancers. Like laser photocoagulation, multiple treatment sessions are

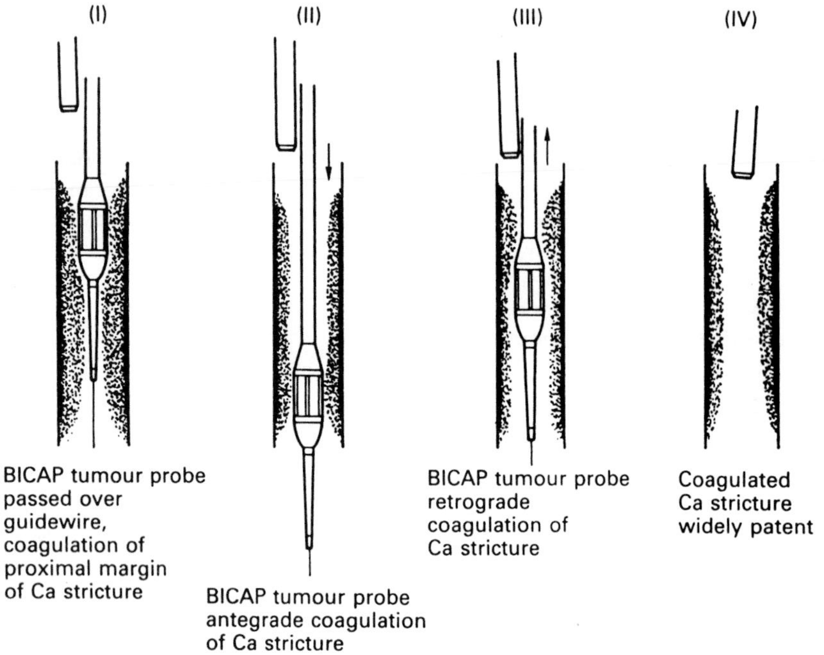

Figure 7.72 Technique of electrocoagulation of obstructing advanced oesophageal cancer using the BICAP tumour probe (tumour shown shaded).

required for a sustained improvement in dysphagia. The complication rate varies from 5 to 20% and includes perforation, fistula formation and haemorrhage.

Ethanol injection. Absolute alcohol can be injected under endoscopic control via a variceal injection needle into the obstructing tumour tissue to induce necrosis. This method, though cheap, quick and painless, has had limited application. The technique can be applied for lesions anywhere in the oesophagus and may be useful when the oesophageal lumen is completely obstructed by tumour. It is generally used as an adjunct to other methods such as stenting when it can be used to manage tumour overgrowth and tumour ingrowth through the stents.

Intubation. This is still the most popular method of palliation of dysphagia for inoperable oesophageal cancer. Traction intubation entails surgical intervention to railroad the tube in position and anchor it to the stomach. The most common types of traction tube used are the Mousseau–Barbin and Celestin tubes (Figure 7.73). Increasingly, pulsion is preferred since this avoids a laparotomy. Pulsion tubes which can be placed through the lesion by means of a flexible introducer inserted over a guidewire are commonly used nowadays (Atkinson's pulsion tubes) (Figure 7.74). A preliminary dilatation is usually necessary before insertion of pulsion tubes. Intubation is more effective for distal than proximal lesions. The main advantage of intubation is that the treatment is performed in a single session with dramatic restoration of swallowing. However, plastic tubes have several disadvantages in that they are rigid, with a large external diameter and small internal diameter lumen of 12 mm. As a result, most patients are only able to swallow liquidized food. Care of the tube is important and these patients are advised to take aerated drinks in between meals to prevent blockage, which is a common complication. Perforation of the oesophagus is a real risk at the time of insertion of the tube (5–19%). Later complications include the erosion of the tube through the tumour (13%) and dislodgement (11–15%) with upper airway obstruction. The hospital mortality of oesophageal intubation for advanced oesophageal cancer can be up to 20%.

More recently, self-expanding metallic stents have been used for the palliation of advanced oesophageal cancer. They provide excellent palliation of dysphagia. They are relatively easy to insert by practising endoscopists and interventional radiologists. The stents are introduced with the deployment device over a guidewire and positioned across the marked malignant stricture in the oesophagus. The guidewire can be introduced endoscopically or radiologically. Fluoroscopy is necessary to mark the limits of the stricture. Preliminary dilatation of the stricture up to 12 mm (depending on the type of stent) is required. This reduced extent of dilatation has reduced the risk of perforation markedly with consequent reduction in hospital mortality. Once the stent is expanded, the large lumen achieved (16–20 mm) and the flexibility of the stent allow for restoration of swallowing with little dietary modification (Figure 7.75). The stents can be used for proximal and distal oesophageal obstruction but have had limited success in oesophagogastric junction tumours due to angulation and migration. Several types are available (Figure 7.76)

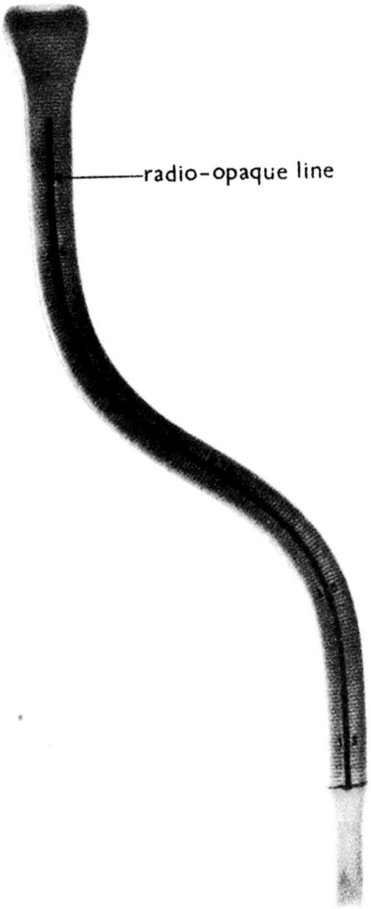

Figure 7.73 Celestin traction tube.

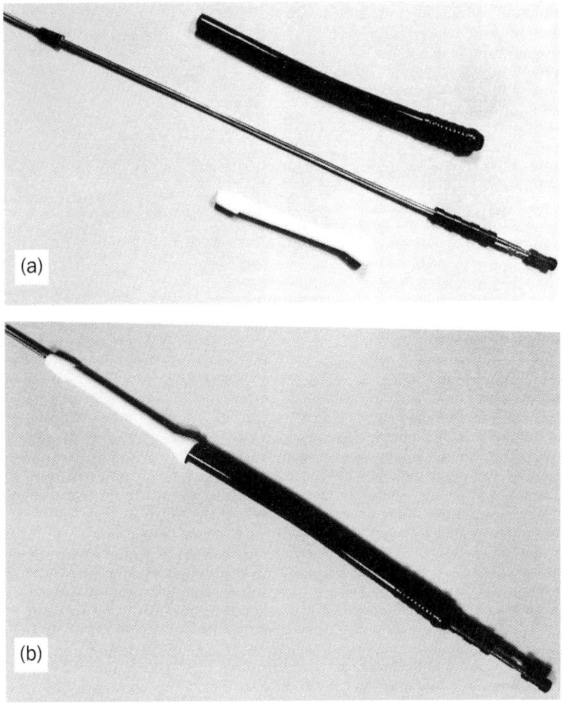

Figure 7.74 (a) Atkinson pulsion oesophageal tube (white) and the Nottingham introducer. The tube is made of silicone rubber and has distal shoulders to prevent upward displacement. (b) Atkinson's tube and Nottingham oesophageal tube introducer assembled for insertion. The stricture is first dilated and then the tube-introducer assembly is guided in place over a guidewire. The introducer has a mechanism to release the tube and allow the removal of the introducer and guidewire.

with varying diameters and lengths. Some have a polyethylene coating over the mesh of the stent (covered stents) and some have distal anti-reflux valves. Delayed stent failure however can occur in a number of patients due to migration of the stent in up to 29% of patients, tumour ingrowth through the mesh of uncovered stents in up to 36% of patients, tumour overgrowth above or below the stent (15%), symptomatic gastro-oesophageal reflux after stenting across the oesophagogastric junction, stent related haemorrhage (6–9%) and post-stenting chest pain requiring opiate analgesia in up to 10% of patients. The major limitation of self-expanding metallic stents is their cost.

The most difficult patients to palliate are those who develop a malignant tracheo-oesophageal fistula either spontaneously (5%) or as a result of radiotherapy. Some fistulae arise as a result of pressure necrosis caused by a plastic prosthesis or a stent or as a result of a canalization procedure. Supportive care provides a median life expectancy of about 3 weeks and death usually results from pulmonary complications. The aim of palliation therapy is to seal the fistula rapidly in order to improve the quality of life for this group of patients. The conservative method of management, with cessation of oral intake and providing nutritional support is indicated for

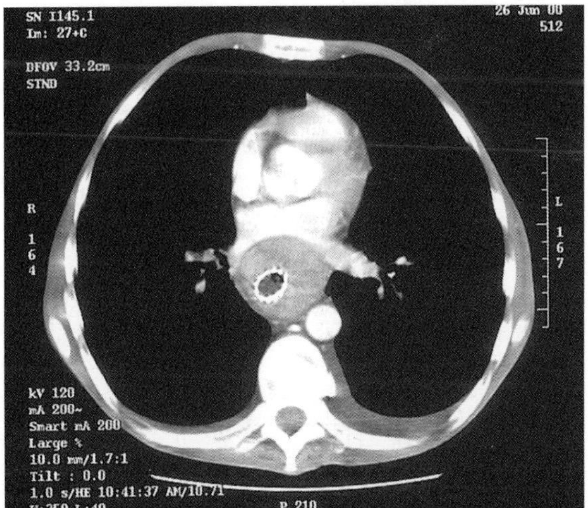

Figure 7.75 CT scan showing a large mid-oesophageal tumour which has been stented with an ultraflex stent maintaining patency of the oesophagus.

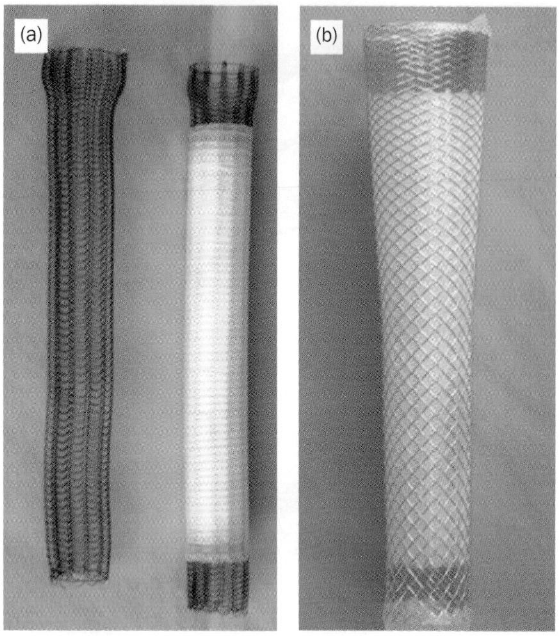

Figure 7.76 (a) Ultraflex stents (covered and uncovered). (b) Flamingo stent which is covered.

a short period as a temporary measure to improve the patient's condition. Surgical closure or bypass surgery is associated with high morbidity and mortality. Closure by means of cyanoacrylates and fibrin has had varying degrees of success. Placement of plastic balloon endoprostheses is associated with considerable morbidity and mortality without consistent closure of the fistula. Covered self-expanding metallic stents are reported to have a success rate of sealing tracheo/broncho-oesophageal fistulae in 67–100%. Despite their cost, covered stents are the most reliable and cost-effective method in the management of these patients.

Further reading

Anatomy and physiology of the oesophagus

Bombeck, C. T., Dillard, D. H. and Nyhus, L. M. (1966). Muscular anatomy of the gastro-oesophageal junction and the role of phrenoesophageal ligament. *Ann Surg* **164**: 643.

Chevallier, J. M., Vitte, E., Derosier, C. *et al.* (1991). The thoracic oesophagus: sectional anatomy and radiosurgical applications. *Surg Radiol Anat* **13**: 313.

Davies, M. R. Q. (1996). Anatomy of the extrinsic motor nerve supply to mobilised segments of the oesophagus disrupted by dissection during repair of oesophageal atresia with distal fistula. *Br J Surg* **83**: 1268.

Delattre, J.-F., Avisse, C., Marcus, C. and Flament, J.-B. (2000). Functional anatomy of the gastroesophageal junction. *Surg Clin North Am* **80**: 241–60.

Gahagan T. (1962). The function of the musculature of the oesophagus and stomach in the oesophagogastric sphincter mechanism. *Surg Gynecol Obstet* **114**: 293.

Gray, S. W., Rowe, J. S. Jr and Skadalakis, J. E. (1979). Surgical anatomy of the gastroesophageal junction. *Am Surg* **45**: 575.

Hayward, J. (1961). The lower end of the oesophagus. *Thorax* **16**: 36.

Hermann J. D. and Murugasu, J. J. (1966). The blood supply of the esophagus in relation to esophageal surgery. *Aust NZ Surg* **35**: 195.

Jordan, P. H. Jr and Kinner, B. M. (1999). New look at epiphrenic diverticula. *World J Surg* **23**: 147.

Kuwano, H., Ikebe, M., Baba, K. *et al.* (1993). Operative procedures of reconstruction after resection of esophageal cancer and the postoperative quality of life. *World J Surg* **17**: 773.

Liebermann-Meffert, D. (1993). Anatomical aspects in surgery of esophagus and cardia. *Postgrad Gen Surg* **5**: 122.

Libermann-Meffert, D., Allgower, M., Schmid, P. *et al.* (1979). Muscular equivalent of the lower esophageal sphincter. *Gastroenterology* **76**: 31.

Liebermann-Meffert, D. and Siwert, J. R. (1992). Arterial anatomy of the esophagus: a review of literature with brief comments on clinical aspects. *Gullet* **2**: 3.

Marshall, R. E., Anggiansah, A., Anggiansah, C. L. *et al.* (1999). Esophageal body length, lower esophageal sphincter length, position and pressure in health and disease. *Dis Esophagus* **12**: 297–302.

Patti, M. G., Gantert, W. and Way, L. W. (1997). Surgery of the esophagus: anatomy and physiology. *Surg Clin North Am* **77**: 959.

Skandalakis, J. E. and Ellis, H. (2000). Embryology and anatomic basis of esophageal surgery. *Surg Clin North Am* **80**: 85–155.

Assessment of oesophageal disease

Barrett, M. W., Myers, J. C., Watson, D. I. and Jamieson, G. G. (2000). Detection of bile reflux: in vivo validation of the Bilitec fibreoptic system. *Dis Esophagus* **13**: 44–50.

Buecker, A., Wein, B. B., Neuerburg, J. M. and Guenther, R. W. (1997). Esophageal perforation: comparison of use of aqueous and barium-containing contrast media. *Radiology* **202**: 683–6.

Flamen, P., Lerut, A., Van Cutsem, E. *et al.* (2000). Utility of positron emission tomography for the staging of patients with potentially operable esophageal carcinoma. *J Clin Oncol* **18**: 3202–10.

Galmiche, J. P., Lehur, P. A., Bruley des Varannes, S. and Denis, P. (1986). Twenty-four hour intraesophageal pH monitoring. *Gastroenterology* **91**: 1581–3.

Griffith, J. F., Chan, A. C., Chow, L. T. *et al.* (1999). Assessing chemotherapy response of squamous cell oesophageal carcinoma with spiral CT. *Br J Radiol* **72**: 678–84.

Griffith, J. F., Kew, J., Chan, A. C. and Metreweli, C. (1999). 3D CT imaging of oesophageal carcinoma. *Eur J Radiol* **32**: 216–20.

Hampton, F. J. and MacFadyen, U. M. (1990). Reproducibility of oesophageal pH monitoring. *Gut* **31**: 1420–1.

Helmberger, H. (1999). CT for local staging of esophageal cancer. *Dis Esophagus* **12**: 202–4.

Katzka, D. A. and Castell, D. O. (1998) Esophageal manometry and modern medicine. *Dig Dis* **16**: 189–91.

McCray, W. H. Jr, Chung, C., Parkman, H. P. and Miller, L. S. (2000). Use of simultaneous high-resolution endoluminal sonography (HRES) and manometry to characterize high pressure zone of distal esophagus. *Dig Dis Sci* **45**: 1660–6.

Nakazawa, S. (2000). Recent advances in endoscopic ultrasonography. *J Gastroenterol* **35**: 257–60.

Nellemann, H., Aksglaede, K., Funch-Jensen, P. and Tommesen, P. (2000). Bread and barium. Diagnostic value in patients with suspected primary oesophageal motility disorders. *Acta Radiol* **41**: 145–50.

Okholm, M., Sorensen, H., Wallin, L. and Boesby, S. (2000). Bile reflux into the esophagus. Bilitec 2000 measurements in normal subjects and in patients after Nissen fundoplication. *Scand J Gastroenterol* **34**: 653–7.

Rice, T. W. (2000). Clinical staging of esophageal carcinoma. CT, EUS, and PET. *Chest Surg Clin North Am* **10**: 471–85.

Sawczenko, A., Gray, G. and Sandhu, B. K. (2000). Reproducibility of 24-hour intraesophageal pH monitoring. *Pediatrics* **105**: 1371–2.

Tanomkiat, W. and Galassi, W. (2000). Barium sulfate as contrast medium for evaluation of postoperative anastomotic leaks. *Acta Radiol* **41**: 482–5.

Wallace, K. L., Middleton, S. and Cook, I. J. (2000). Development and validation of a self-report symptom inventory to assess the severity of oral-pharyngeal dysphagia. *Gastroenterology* **118**: 678–87.

Wetcher, G. J., Hinder, R. A., Perdikis, G. *et al.* (1996). Three-dimensional imaging of the lower esophageal sphincter in healthy subjects and gastroesophageal reflux. *Dig Dis Sci* **41**: 2377–82.

Gastro-oesophageal reflux disease and non-reflux oesophagitis

Armstrong, D., Monnier, P., Nicolet, M. *et al.* (1991). Endoscopic assessment of oesophagitis. *Gullet* **1**: 63–7.

Banerjee, S. and LaMont, J. T. (2000). Treatment of gastrointestinal infections. *Gastroenterology* **118**: S48–67.

Barbezat, G. O. (2000). New treatment for Barrett's oesophagus. *Biomed Pharmacother* **54**: 362–7.

Bremner, C. G. and Demeester, T. R. (1998). Proceedings from an international conference on ablation therapy for Barrett's mucosa. *Dis Esophagus* **11**: 1–27.

Cadiot, G., Bruhat, A., Rigaud, D. *et al.* (1997). Multivariate analysis of pathophysiological factors in reflux oesophagitis. *Gut* **40**: 167–74.

Cuschieri, A., Shimi, S. M. and Nathanson, L. K. (1992). Laparoscopic reduction, crural repair, and fundoplication of large hiatal hernia. *Am J Surg* **163**: 425–30.

DeGroen, P. C., Lubbe, D. F., Hirsch, L. J. *et al.* (1996). Esophagitis associated with the use of alendronate. *N Engl J Med* **335**: 1016–21.

Drabek, J., Keil, R. and Namesny, I. (1999). The endoscopic treatment of benign esophageal strictures by balloon dilatation. *Dis Esophagus* **12**: 28–9.

Ell, C., May, A., Gossner, L. *et al.* (2000). Endoscopic mucosal resection of early cancer and high-grade dysplasia in Barrett's esophagus. *Gastroenterology* **118**: 670–7.

Hamada, H., Haruma, K., Mihara, M. *et al.* (2000). High incidence of reflux oesophagitis after eradication therapy for *Helicobacter pylori*: impacts of hiatal hernia and corpus gastritis. *Aliment Pharmacol Ther* **14**: 729–35.

Hirota, W. K., Loughney, T. M., Lazas, D. J. *et al.* (1999). Specialized intestinal metaplasia, dysplasia, and cancer of the esophagus and esophagogastric junction: prevalence and clinical data. *Gastroenterology* **116**: 227–85.

Geboes, K. and Van Eyken, P. (2000). The diagnosis of dysplasia and malignancy in Barrett's oesophagus. *Histopathology* **37**: 99–107.

Galamiiche, J. P. and Bruleu des Varannes, S. (1994). Symptoms and disease severity in gastro-oesophageal reflux disease. *Scand J Gastroenterol* **29**: 62–8.

Jankowski, J. A., Wright, N. A., Metzer, S. J. *et al.* (1999). Molecular evolution of the metaplasia-dysplasia-adenocarcinoma sequence in the esophagus. *Am J Pathol* **154**: 965–73.

Kahrilas, P. J. (1999). The role of hiatus hernia in GERD. *Yale J Biol Med* **72**: 101–11.

Kahrilas, P. J., Shi, G., Manka, M. and Joehl, R. J. (2000). Increased frequency of transient lower esophageal sphincter relaxation induced by gastric distention in reflux patients with hiatal hernia. *Gastroenterology* **118**: 688–95.

Kahrilas, P. J., Lin, S., Chen, J. and Manka, M. (1999). The effect of hiatus hernia on gastro-oesophageal junction pressure. *Gut* **44**: 476–82.

Klauser, A. G., Schindlbeck, N. E. and Muller-Lissner, S. A. (1990). Symptoms in gastro-oesophageal reflux disease. *Lancet* **335**: 205–8.

Klinkenberg-Knol, E. C., Nellis, F., Dent, J. *et al.* (2000). Long-term omeprazole treatment in resistant gastro-esophageal reflux disease: efficacy, safety, and influence on gastric mucosa. *Gastroenterology* **118**: 661–9.

Lidums, I., Lehmann, A., Checklin, H. *et al.* (2000). Control of transient lower esophageal sphincter relaxations and reflux by the GABAB agonist baclofen in normal subjects. *Gastroenterology* **118**: 7–13.

Lundell, L. R., Dent, J., Bennett, J. R. *et al.* (1999). Endoscopic assessment of oesophagitis: clinical and functional correlates and further validation of the Los Angeles classification. *Gut* **45**: 172–80.

McClave, S. A., Brady, P. G., Wright, R. A. *et al.* Does fluoroscopic guidance for Maloney oesophageal dilation impact on the clinical endpoint of therapy: relief of dysphagia and achievement of luminal patency. *Gastrointest Endosc* **43**: 93-7

McDougall, N. I., Johnston, B. T., Kee, F. *et al.* (1996). Natural history of reflux oesophagitis: 10 year follow up of its effect on patient symptomatology and quality of life. *Gut* **38**: 481–6.

Maguire, P. D., Sibley, G. S., Zhou, S. M. *et al.* (1999). Clinical and dosimetric predictors of radiation-induced esophageal toxicity. *J Radiat Oncol Biol Phys* **45**: 97–103.

Miller, L. S., Jackson, W., McCray, W. and Chung, C. Y. (1998). Benign non-peptic esophageal strictures. Diagnosis and treatment. *Gastrointest Endosc Clin North Am* **8**: 329–55.

Saeed, Z. A., Winchester, C. B., Ferro, P. S. *et al.* (1995). Prospective randomised comparison of polyvinyl bougies and through the scope balloons for dilation of peptic strictures of the oesophagus. *Gastrointest Endosc* **41**: 189–95.

Sagar, P. M., Ackroyd, R., Hosie, K. B. *et al.* (1995). Regression and progression of Barrett's oesophagus after antireflux surgery. *Br J Surg* 1995 **82**: 806–10.

Sampliner, R. E. (1998). Practice guidelines on the diagnosis, surveillance, and therapy of Barrett's oesophagus. The Practice Parameters Committee of the American College of Gastroenterology. *Am J Gastroenterol* **93**: 1028–32.

Schlemper, R. J., Riddell, R. H., Kato, Y. *et al.* (2000). The Vienna classification of gastrointestinal neoplasia. *Gut* **47**: 251–5.

Sontag, S. J. (1999). Defining GERD. *Yale J Biol Med* **72**: 69–80.

Watson, A. (2000). Barrett's oesophagus – 50 years on. *Br J Surg* **87**: 529–31.

Weston, A. P., Sharma, P., Topalovski, M. *et al.* (2000). Long term follow-up of Barrett's high grade dysplasia. *Am J Gastroenterol* **95**: 1888–93.

Wolfe, M. M. and Sachs, G. (2000). Acid suppression: optimizing therapy for gastroduodenal ulcer healing, gastroesophageal reflux disease, and stress-related erosive syndrome. *Gastroenterology* **118**: S20–4.

Zaninotto, G., Parenti, A. R., Ruol, A. *et al.* (2000). Oesophageal resection for high-grade dysplasia in Barrett's oesophagus. *Br J Surg* **87**: 1102–5.

Diaphragm

Andrade-Alegre, R. (1999). Chronic diaphragmatic hernia. *Chest* **116**: 1838–9.

Cairns, A. M. and Ewig, J. M. (1996). Diaphragmatic hernia. *Paediatr Rev* **17**: 102.

Carre, I. J., Johnston, B. T., Thomas, P. S. and Morrison, P. J. (1999). Familial hiatal hernia in a large five generation family confirming true autosomal dominant inheritance. *Gut* **45**: 649–52.

Clark, R. H., Hardin, W. D., Hirschl, R. B. *et al.* (1998). Urgent surgical management of congenital diaphragmatic hernia: a report from the congenital diaphragmatic hernia study group. *J Pediatr Surg* **33**: 1004.

David, T. J. and Illingworth, C. A. (1976). Diaphragmatic hernia in the south-west of England. *J Med Genet* **13**: 253–62.

Delattre, J. F., Avisse, C., Marcus, C. and Flament, J. B. (2000). Functional anatomy of the gastroesophageal junction. *Surg Clin North Am* **80**: 241–60.

Harrison, M. R., Adzik, M. S., Bullard, K. M. *et al.* (1997). Correction of congenital diaphragmatic hernia in utero VII: a prospective trial. *J Pediatr Surg* **32**: 1637.

Hubbard, A. M., Crombleholme, T. M., Azdick, N. S. *et al.* (1999). Prenatal MRI evaluation of congenital diaphragmatic hernia. *Am J Perinatol* **16**: 407–13.

Katranci, A. O., Gork, A. S., Rizalar, R. *et al.* (1998). Pentalogy of Cantrell. *Ind J Paediatr* **65**: 149–53.

Lang-Lazdunski, L., Mouroux, J., Pons, F. *et al.* (1997). Role of videothoracoscopy in chest trauma. *Ann Thorac Surg* **63**: 327.

Moore, E. E., Malngoni, M. A., Cogvill, T. H. *et al.* (1994). Organ injury scaling, IV: thoracic vascular, lung, cardiac and diaphragm. *J Trauma* **36**: 299.

Naunheim, K. S. (1998). Adult presentation of unusual diaphragmatic hernias. *Chest Surg Clin North Am* **8**: 359–69.

Oddsdottir, M. (1996). Paraesophageal hernia. *Surg Clin North Am* **80**: 1243–52.

Ortega, A. E., Tang, E., Froes, E. T. *et al.* (1996). Laparoscopic evaluation of penetrating thoracoabdominal traumatic injuries. *Surg Endosc* **10**: 19.

Pettiaux, N., Cassart, M., Pavia, M. *et al.* (1997). Three-dimensional reconstruction of human diaphragm with the use of spiral computed tomography. *J Appl Physiol* **82**: 998.

Reys, C., Chang, L. K., Waffaran, F. *et al.* (1998). Delayed repair of congenital diaphragmatic hernia with early high-frequency oscillatory ventilation during postoperative stabilisation. *J Pediatr Surg* **33**: 1010.

Shapiro, M. J., Heiberg, E., Durham, R. M. *et al.* (1996). The unreliability of CT scans and initial chest radiographs in evaluating blunt trauma induced diaphragmatic rupture. *Clin Radiol* **51**: 27.

Schumpelick, V., Steinau, G., Schluper, I. and Prescher, A. (2000). Surgical embryology and anatomy of the diaphragm with surgical applications. *Surg Clin North Am* **80**: 213–39.

Weissberg, D. and Refaely, Y. (1995). Symptomatic diaphragmatic hernia: surgical treament. *Scand J Thorac Cardiovasc Surg* **29**: 201–6.

Wilson, J. M., Lund, D. P., Lillechei, C. W. *et al.* (1997). Congenital diaphragmatic hernia: a tale of two cities: the Boston experience. *J Pediatr Surg* **32**: 401.

Motility disorders of the oesophagus

Bowery, D. J., Blom, D. and Lord, R. V. (2000). Surgical treatment of achalasia: thoracoscopic or laparoscopic? *Am J Gastroentrol* **95**: 1087–8.

Champion, J. K., Delisle, N. and Hunt, T. (2000). Laparoscopic esophagomyotomy with posterior partial fundoplication for primary esophageal motility disorders. *Surg Endosc* **14**: 746–9.

Chelimsky, G., Hupertz, V. and Blanchard, T. (2000). Manometric progression of achalasia. *J Pediatr Gastroenterol Nutr* **31**: 303–6.

Goldenberg, S. P., Burrell, M., Fette, G. G. *et al.* (1991). Classic and vigorous achalasia: a comparison of manometric, radiographic and clinical findings. *Gastroenterology* **101**: 743–8.

Gideon, R. M., Castell, D. O. and Yarze, J. (1999). Prospective randomized comparison of pneumatic dilation technique in patients with idiopathic achalasia. *Dig Dis Sci* **44**: 1853–7.

Harris, A. M., Dresner, S. M. and Griffin, S. M. (2000). Achalasia: management, outcome and surveillance in a specialist unit. *Br J Surg* **87**: 362–73.

Kahrilas, P. J. (2000). Esophageal motility disorders: current concepts of pathogenesis and treatment. *Can J Gastroenterol* **14**: 221–31.

Kelly, J. H. (2000). Management of upper esophageal sphincter disorders: indications and complications of myotomy. *Am J Med* **6**(108 Suppl) S43–6.

Kumar, V., Shimi, S. M. and Cuschieri, A. (1998). Does laparoscopic cardiomyotomy require an antireflux procedure? *Endoscopy* **30**: 8–11.

Mearin, F., Fonollosa, V., Vilardell, M. and Malagelada, J. R. (2000). Mechanical properties of the gastro-esophageal junction in health, achalasia, and scleroderma. *Scand J Gastroenterol* **35**: 705–10.

Moreto, M. and Ojembarrena, E. (2000). Treatment of achalasia by injection of botulinum toxin or sclerosants? *Endoscopy* **32**: 361–2.

Morino, M. and Rebecchi, F. (2000). Pneumatic dilatation and laparoscopic cardiomyotomy in the management of achalasia. *Surg Endosc* **14**: 870.

Pandolfino, J. E., Howden, C. W. and Kahrilas, P. J. (2000). Motility-modifying agents and management of disorders of gastrointestinal motility. *Gastroenterology* **118**: S32–47.

Patti, M. G. and Pelligrini, C. A. (1996). Endoscopic surgical treatment of primary oesophageal motility disorders. *J R Coll Surg Edinb* **41**: 137.

Shimi, S., Nathanson, L. K. and Cuschieri, A. (1991). Laparoscopic cardiomyotomy for achalasia. *J R Coll Surg Edinb* **36**: 152–4.

Shimi, S. M., Nathanson, L. K. and Cuschieri, A. (1992). Thorascopic long oesophageal myotomy for nutcracker oesophagus: initial experience of a new surgical approach. *Br J Surg* **79**: 533–6.

Storr, M. and Allescher, H. D. (1999). Esophageal pharmacology and treatment of primary motility disorders. *Dis Esophagus* **12**: 241–57.

Vaezi, M. F. (1999). Achalasia: diagnosis and management. *Semin Gastrointest Dis* **10**: 103–12.

Oesophageal diverticula

Allen, M. S. (1999). Treatment of epiphrenic diverticula. *Semin Thorac Cardiovasc Surg* **11**: 358–62.

Baker, M. E., Zuccaro, G. Jr, Achkar, E. and Rice, T. W. (1999). Esophageal diverticula: patient assessment. *Semin Thorac Cardiovasc Surg* **11**: 326–36.

Chami, Z., Fabre, J. M., Navarro, F. and Domergue, J. (1999). Abdominal laparoscopic approach for thoracic epiphrenic diverticulum. *Surg Endosc* **13**: 164–5.

Jordan, P. H. Jr and Kinner, B. M. (1999). New look at epiphrenic diverticula. *World J Surg* **23**: 147–52.

Rice, T. W. and Baker, M. E. (1999). Midthoracic esophageal diverticula. *Semin Thorac Cardiovasc Surg* **11**: 352–7.

Rocco, G., Deschamps, C., Martel, E. *et al.* (1999). Results of reoperation on the upper oesophageal sphincter. *J Thorac Cardiovasc Surg* **117**: 28–30.

Oesophageal perforations

Antonacci, R., Perkins, A. B., Hillstrom, M. and Tung, G. A. (1996). General case of the day. Perforated Barrett ulcer of the distal esophagus. *Radiographics* **16**: 197–9.

Bak-Romaniszyn, L., Malecka-Panas, E., Czkwianianc, E. and Planeta-Malecka, I. (1999). Mallory–Weiss syndrome in children. *Dis Esophagus* **12**: 65-7.

Drabek, J., Keil, R. and Namesny, I. (1999). The endoscopic treatment of benign esophageal strictures by balloon dilatation. *Dis Esophagus* **12**: 28–9.

Fernandez, F. F., Richter, A., Freudenberg, S., Wendl, K. and Manegold, B. C. (1999). Treatment of endoscopic esophageal perforation. *Surg Endosc* **13**: 962–6.

Guillem, P. G., Porte, H. L., Saudemont, A., Quandalle, P. A. and Wurtz, A. J. (2000). Perforation of Barrett's ulcer: a challenge in esophageal surgery. *Ann Thorac Surg* **69**: 1707–10.

Lawrence, D. R., Ohri, S. K., Moxon, R. E. *et al.* (1999). Primary esophageal repair for Boerhaave's syndrome. *Ann Thorac Surg* **67**: 818–20.

Liu, K., Wang, Y.-J., Cheng, Q.-S. and Ma, Q.-F. (1998). Surgical treatment of Boerhaave's syndrome: when, how and why? *Dis Esophagus* **11**: 248–53.

Soll, A. H. and McCarthy, D. (1999). NSAID-related gastrointestinal complications. *Clin Cornerstone* **1**: 42–56.

Urbani, M. and Mathisen, D. J. (2000). Repair of esophageal perforation after treatment for achalasia. *Ann Thorac Surg* **69**: 1609–11.

Valji, A. M., Maziak, D. E., Allen, M. W. and Shamji, F. M. (2000). The stomach as a microvascularly augmented flap for esophageal replacement. *Ann Thorac Surg* **69**: 1593–4.

Younis, Z. and Johnson, D. A. (1999). The spectrum of spontaneous and iatrogenic esophageal injury: perforations, Mallory–Weiss tears, and haematomas. *J Clin Gastroenterol* **29**: 306–17.

Neoplasms of the oesophagus

Akiyama, H., Tsurumaru, M., Ono, Y. *et al.* (1994). Esophagectomy without thoracotomy with vagal preservation. *J Am Coll* 1994; **178**: 83–5.

Akiyama, H., Tasurumaru, M., Vdagawa, Y. *et al.* (1994). System lymph node dissection for esophageal cancer – effective or not? *Dis Esophagus* **7**: 1–12.

Ando, N., Iizuka, T., Kakegawa, T. *et al.* (1997). A randomized trial of surgery with and without chemotherapy for localized squamous carcinoma of the thoracic esophagus. *J Thorac Cardiovasc Surg* **114**: 205–9.

Bartels, H., Stein, H. J. and Siewert, J. R. (1998). Pre-operative risk analysis and postoperative mortality of oesophagectomy for resectable oesophageal cancer. *Br J Surg* **85**: 840–4.

Belsey, R. (1983). Reconstruction of the oesophagus. *Ann R Coll Surg Engl* **65**: 360–4.

Beuzen, F., Dubois, S. and Flejou, J. F. (2000). Chromosomal numerical aberrations are frequent in oesophageal and gastric adenocarcinomas: a study using in-situ hybridization. *Histopathology* **37**: 241–9.

Bosset, J. F., Gignoux, M., Triboulet, J. P. *et al.* (1997). Chemotherapy followed by surgery compared with surgery alone in squamous-cell cancer of the oesophagus. *N Engl J Med* **337**: 161–7.

Chandawarker, R. Y., Kakegawa, T., Fujita, H. *et al.* (1996). Comparative analysis of imaging modalities in preoperative assessment of nodal metastasis in esophageal cancer. *J Surg Oncol* **61**: 214–17.

Cuschieri, A., Shimi, S. M. and Banting, S. (1992). Endoscopic oesophagectomy through a right thoracoscopic approach. *J R Coll Surg Edinb* **37**: 7–11.

DeCamp, M. M., Swanson, S. J. and Jaklitsch, M. T. (1999). Esophagectomy after induction chemoradiation. *Chest* **116**(Suppl.): 466–9S.

Devesa, S. S., Blot, W. J. and Fraumeni, J. F. Jr (1998). Changing pattern in the incidence of esophageal and gastric carcinoma in the United States. *Cancer* **83**: 2049–53.

Ell, C., May, A., Gossner, L. *et al.* (2000). Endoscopic mucosal resection of early cancer and high-grade dysplasia in Barrett's esophagus. *Gastroenterology* **118**: 670–7.

Fumagalli, U. and Panel of Experts (1996). Resective surgery for cancer of the thoracic esophagus: results of a consensus conference. *Dis Esophagus* **9**: 3–19.

Kuwano, H., Ikebe, M., Baba, K. *et al.* (1993). Operative procedures of reconstruction after resection of esophageal cancer and the postoperative quality of life. *World J Surg* **17**: 773.

Lehnert, T. (1999). Multimodal therapy for squamous carcinoma of the esophagus. *Br J Surg* **86**: 727–39.

Natsugoe, S., Mueller, J., Stein, H. J. *et al.* (1998). Micrometastasis and tumour cell microenvolvement of lymph nodes from esophageal squamous cell cancer: frequency, associated tumour characteristics and impact on prognosis. *Cancer* **83**: 858–66.

Orringer, M. B. and Sloan, H. (1978). Esophagectomy without thoracotomy. *J Thorac Cardiovasc Surg* **76**: 643–54.

Poplin, E. A., Jacobson, J., Herskovic, A. *et al.* (1996). Evaluation of multimodality treatment of locoregional esophageal carcinoma by Southwest Oncology Group 9060. *Cancer* **78**: 1851.

Ruol, A. and Panel of Experts (1996). Multimodality treatment for non-metastatic cancer of the thoracic oesophagus: results of a consensus conference. *Dis Esophagus* **9**: 39–54.

Shimi, S. (1999). Self-expanding metallic stents in the management of advanced oesophageal cancer: a review. *Semin Laparosc Surg* **7**: 9–21.

Siewert, J. R. and Stein, H. J. (1996). Adenocarcinoma of the gastroesophageal junction: classification, pathology and extent of resection. *Dis Esophagus* **9**: 173–82.

Siewert, J. R. and Stein, H. J. (1998). Classification of carcinoma of the esophagogastric junction. *Br J Surg* **85**: 1457–9.

Spechler, S. J. (2000). Barrett's esophagus: an overrated cancer risk factor. *Gastroenterology* **119**: 587–9.

Van Dekken, H., Geelen, E., Dinjens, W. N. M. *et al.* (1999). Comparative genomic hybridization of cancer of the gastroesophageal junction: deletion of 14q31–32.1 discriminates between esophageal (Barrett's) and gastric cardia adenocarcinoma. *Cancer Res* **59**: 748–52.

Vaughn, T. L., Davis, S., Kristal, A. *et al.* (1995). Obesity, alcohol and tobacco as risk factors for cancers of the esophagus and gastric cardia: adenocarcinoma versus squamous cell carcinoma. *Cancer Epidemiol Biomarkers Prev* **4**: 85.

Walsh, T. N., Noonan, N., Hollywood, D. *et al.* (1996). A comparison of multimodal therapy and surgery for esophageal adenocarcinoma. *N Engl J Med* **335**: 462.

Wu, T. T., Watanabe, T., Heitmiller, R. *et al.* (1998). Genetic alterations in Barret esophagus and adenocarcinomas of the esophagus and esophagogastric junction. *Am J Pathol* **153**: 287–94.

MODULE 8

Disorders of the stomach and duodenum

Section 8.1 • Surgical anatomy

Stomach

The stomach has an irregular pyriform shape tapering towards the duodenum and curved anteriorly so that its proximal (cardiac) orifice at the junction with the oesophagus and the distal part (pyloric sphincter) are at a more posterior plane near the retroperioneum than the middle part (body) of the organ. It is anatomically divisible into three parts: fundus, body and pyloric region (antrum and pyloric canal). The fundus is the globular proximal portion to the left of the oesophagus separated from it by the cardiac notch and attached by fascia to the left crus and adjacent diaphragm and the gastro-phrenic peritoneal fold. The pyloric region extends from the angular notch on the lesser curvature to the pyloric sphincter and consists of the antrum (proximal tapering section) and pyloric canal (tubular distal part just proximal to the pyloric sphincter) which is made up of a thickening of the circular muscle coat discontinuous with the equivalent muscle layer of the duodenum. The site of the pylorus is marked by a shallow superficial serosal notch and by the two veins of Mayo (superior and inferior) that cross its anterior surface. The anterior wall of the stomach is more voluminous than the posterior wall and this is important in anti-reflux surgery. The stomach is lined by two types of mucosa:

- Parietal or oxyntic lining the fundus and stomach – contains parietal (acid secreting) and chief cells (secrete pepsins). Surface of mucosa has rugae and is acid
- Antropyloric mucosa – contains mucus secreting and G cells that secrete gastrin. Surface of mucosa is smooth and neutral or slightly alkaline.

There are no surface markings to mark the antro-parietal junction and the extent of the antral mucosa varies but on average is approximately 5.0 from the pyloric orifice.

The stomach rests on the stomach bed consisting of retroperitoneal structures and organs: spleen, diaphragm, left kidney and adrenal, pancreas, splenic artery, transverse colon and mesocolon – hence the complexity of its vascular supply and lymph node drainage. It is almost completely lined by peritoneum anteriorly from the greater sac and posteriorly from the omental bursa (lesser sac). Above the lesser curvature of the stomach these meet to form the lesser omentum which is attached to the liver. This is usually thin, encloses the bile duct, hepatic artery and portal vein at the right extremity and has a clear segment on the extreme left (pars flaccida) that overlies the caudate lobe of the liver near the right crus of the diaphragm. The branches of the left gastric and right gastric arteries run along the lesser curvature between the two layers of the lesser omentum. The two peritoneal layers meet along the greater curvature of the stomach to form a much larger and fattier fold which has different names in its various sections, but which from the surgical standpoint should be considered as one structure sweeping from the entire margin of the greater curvature and fundus:

- Greater omentum – attached to transverse colon and mesocolon (from which it can be separated through the embryonic vascular plane)
- Gastrosplenic ligament – contains the short gastric vessels to the spleen
- Gastrophrenic ligament – small peritoneal fold that joins the stomach to the diaphragm to the left of the oesophagus.

Duodenum

Although anatomically part of the small intestine, the duodenum is closely related to surgery of the stomach and pancreas. It is almost entirely retroperitoneal and is fixed by fascia to the posterior abdominal wall. It forms an eccentric curve 28 cm long opening to the left and joining the stomach at the pylorus with the rest of the small intestine at the duodeno-jejunal junction marked by a peritoneal fold known as the ligament of Treitz. It is divided into four parts: first (duodenal bulb) second (descending part – contains the duodenal papilla), third (transverse) and fourth (ascending). The duodenal bulb passes backwards from the pylorus before turning down to form the second part and the fourth part bends forwards at the duodeno-jejunal junction. The superior relation on the outside of the curve is the gallbladder. On the right side and posteriorly are the inferior vena cava, the right renal vessels and pelvis/upper ureter of the right kidney and the aorta. Anteriorly the second part is crossed by the transverse colon to which it is attached by loose areolar tissue and the third part is crossed by the superior mesenteric vessels and the root of the small bowel mesentery. The head of the pancreas nestles inside the duodenal curve. In the groove between the duodenum and the pancreas runs the gastroduodenal artery which arises from the common hepatic and descends behind the duodenal bulb to reach the groove.

The duodenal mucosa contains Brunner's glands, which secrete a highly alkaline mucus which acts as a protective mechanism to the mucosa from the acid chyme delivered into the duodenum by the stomach. Usually the Brunner epithelium stops just beyond the duodenal papilla and never reaches the duodeno-jejunal junction.

Blood supply of the stomach and duodenum

Stomach

The stomach is supplied by the left gastric, right gastric, right gastroepiploic and left gastroepiploic arteries and thus directly or indirectly its blood supply is from the coeliac axis. The left gastric (origin from the coeliac axis or aorta) gives off an ascending oesophageal branch and then runs down between the two layers of the lesser omentum close to the lesser curvature to form an anastomotic arcade with the right gastric artery (origin from the hepatic artery). This arcade gives off delicate branches to the lesser curve but most of its bigger branches pierce the seromuscular coat anteriorly and posteriorly to join the submucous vascular plexus of the stomach. Likewise the right gastroepiploic (origin from the gastroduodenal artery) forms an arcade along the greater curvature and joins up with the left gastroepiploic (origin from splenic artery). All the branches from the gastroepiploic arcade pierce the seromucular layer to join the submucous vascular plexus of the stomach (no direct branches to the greater curvature). Extensive arterio-arterial and arterio-venous connections are present within the gastric submucosal vascular plexus. The nutritional blood supply to the stomach (with the exception of the lesser curvature) is derived from this plexus and this accounts for the viability of the stomach when only one artery (right gastroepiploic) is retained during gastric reconstruction after oesophagectomy. It also underlies the increased safety of tubulization of the stomach (which entails removal of the lesser curve) over intact stomach reconstruction. The other benefit of tubulization is increased length. The venous drainage of the stomach parallels roughly the arterial supply.

Duodenum

The duodenal blood supply is through the duodeno-pancreatic arcades, which supply both the duodenum and pancreas and form an important collateral route between the coeliac and superior mesenteric arterial territories. The duodenopancreatic aracades are formed by the gastroduodenal artery (origin hepatic artery) and the anterior and posterior inferior pancreatic arteries (originating from the superior mesenteric). The gastroduodenal artery soon after its origin behind the duodenal bulb gives off the posterosuperior pancreaticoduodenal (or retroduodenal) artery which curves round the lower common bile duct in its descent to the posterior aspect of the head of the pancreas and the duodenum. The gastroduodenal artery then continues in the groove between the duodenum and the pancreas and divides into the right gastroepiploic and the anterior superior pancreaticoduodenal artery. The latter together with the retroduodenal artery anastomose with the anterior and posterior inferior pancreaticoduodenal arteries derived from the superior mesenteric artery. Hence the difficulty in devascularizing the duodenum in bleeding duodenal ulcer. The collateral circulation between the coeliac and superior mesenteric artery through the duodeno-pancreatic arcades also explains the unpredictable results of ligation of the common hepatic artery.

Nerve supply

The sympathetic supply is through the splanchnic nerves (T5/6–T9/10) with the preganglionic efferent fibres ending in the coeliac plexus and then the postganglionic fibres travel in the periarterial plexuses along the arteries to the stomach. The sympathetic fibres subserve visceral sensation and pain. The parasympathetic supply is from the vagi. There is considerable variation in the anatomical distribution of the vagal branches to the stomach, which is not helped by confusing eponymous nomenculature and lack of precise knowledge regarding the origin of some of the branches. Classically the anterior vagus has the following branches:

- Hepatic branches – constant – travel up towards the liver in the pars flaccida of the lesser omentum
- The pyloric nerve of McCrae – inconstant nerve to the pyloric region
- Anterior gastric division or nerve of Latarget – constant antral branches of which are preserved in highly selective vagotomy.

The posterior vagus gives off:

- The posterior gastric division – posterior nerve of Latarget, smaller but essentially mirror image of the anterior nerve
- The coelic division to the coeliac plexus.

The proximal gastric branches to the fundus have a variable origin from the nerves of Latarget, from the main vagal trunks at or above the hiatus and even from the oesophageal nerve plexus in the mediastinum. One of the these nerves arising from the anterior trunk close to the oesophagogastric junction is known as the nerve of Grassi and is held responsible for some of the recurrences after vagotomy, although other proximal gastric branches are equally important in this respect.

In addition there are gastroepiploic nerves which travel along the related vessels in the greater omentum and are said to innervate the parietal mass alongside the greater curve. There is no doubt regarding the existence of these nerves as they can be demonstrated in thin patients, but their origin and function has not been established although some regard them as important in ulcer recurrence after highly selective vagotomy and for this reason advocate their section (extended highly selective vagotomy – Donahue operation).

Lymph node drainage

This is exceedingly complex and has been mapped out by the Japanese Society for Gastric Cancer into numbered stations that form the basis of the various types of gastric resection for cancer in terms of the level of regional lymphadenectomy performed (Table 8.1).

Gastric physiology

The most important physiological function of the stomach is to act as a receptacle for ingested food which is partially digested and hydrolysed by acid and pepsin, milled into semifluid chyme in the antropyloric region and then delivered into the small intestine. To enable ingestion of an adequate amount of food, the stomach possesses the property of adaptive relaxation or accommodation, which enables it to enlarge its capacity without a significant rise in intraluminal pressure. The adaptive relaxation is mediated by stretch reflexes and vagal afferents and is therefore greatly impaired after vagotomy. It is also reduced to varying extents after partial gastrectomy and fundoplication. Loss of adaptive relaxation is manifested clinically as early satiety and can be caused by disease (usually malignant) that infiltrates the wall of the stomach.

The mucosa lining the proximal stomach contains the parietal and chief cells whereas the mucosa lining the more muscular antropyloric segment secretes predominantly an alkaline mucus but contains specialized

Table 8.1

Lymph node station number	*Constituent lymph nodes*
1	Right cardial nodes – right side of the abdominal oesophagus and O-G junction
2	Left cardial nodes – left side of the abdominal oesophagus and O-G junction
3	Nodes along the lesser curvature
4	Nodes along the greater curvature, sa: Nodes along the short gastric vessels; sb: Nodes along the left gastroepiploic vessels; d: Nodes along the right gastroepiploic vessels
5	Suprapyloric nodes
6	Infrapyloric nodes
7	Nodes along the left gastric artery
8	Nodes along the common hepatic artery, a: Anterosuperior group; p: Posterior group
9	Nodes around the coeliac axis
10	Nodes at the splenic hilum
11	Nodes along the splenic artery
12	Nodes in the hepatoduodenal ligament
13	Nodes on the posterior surface of the pancreatic head
14	Lymph nodes at the root of the mesentery, A: Nodes along the superior mesenteric artery; V: Nodes along the superior mesenteric vein
15	Nodes along the middle colic vessels
16	Nodes around the abdominal aorta, a1: Nodes in the aortic hiatus; a2: Nodes around the abdominal aorta from coeliac to lower margin of the left renal vein; b1: Nodes around abdominal aorta from lower margin of left renal vein to upper margin of the inferior mesenteric; b2: Nodes around the aorta from lower margin of inferior mesenteric artery to the aortic bifurcation
17	Nodes on the anterior surface of the pancreatic head
18	Nodes along the inferior margin of the pancreas
19	Infradiaphragmatic nodes
20	Nodes in the oesophageal hiatus

endocrine (G) cells that release gastrin in a co-ordinated fashion under the influence of gastrin releasing peptide (GRP). The parietal cells secrete hydrochloric acid and intrinsic factor (necessary for the absorption of vitamin B_{12} in the terminal ileum), whereas the chief cells are responsible for the production and secretion of pepsinogens that are then converted to active pepsins by the HCl.

The motility of the stomach is a highly organized event controlled by the enteric nervous system. The initial adaptive relaxation after eating is followed by an increased activity of the antropyloric segment (antral mill), the contractions of which together with the acid/pepsin digestion convert the food into semifluid chyme before onward controlled passage into the intestinal tract via the pyloric sphincter. Normal gastric secretion consists of three interconnected phases:

- cephalic
- gastric
- intestinal.

The cephalic phase follows stimulation of the vagal centres in the hypothalamus from the psychosensory input: expectation, sight, smell and chewing of food. The effect is mediated by direct cholinergic stimulation of the parietal cell mass and by cholinergic potentiation of other stimuli including histamine release. The gastric phase has two components. The first is consequent on intragastric stimulation via stretch and chemoreceptors in the body that activate local and vagovagal reflexes evoking acid secretion. The second is the release of gastrin from the antrum by stimulation of stretch receptors and activation of antral chemoreceptors by peptides and amino acids released from the food acting via GRP. The intestinal phase is initiated by the entry of chyme into the duodenum when bile, pancreatic juice and various hormones are released. A delicate feedback inhibition occurs whereby acid and fat in the duodenum inhibit further gastric acid secretion by the release of secretin and cholecystokinin.

Peripheral mechanisms of gastric acid secretion

Gastric acid secretion is stimulated by acetylcholine, gastrin and histamine. Special receptors for these substances are present on the surface of the gastric mucosal cells. The H_2 receptor (for histamine) is the most efficacious receptor in stimulating acid secretion and has been cloned and shown to belong to the same family as the beta-adrenergic receptors. Its blockage by H_2 receptor antagonists (cimetidine, ranitidine, etc.) forms the basis of one type of acid reducing medical therapy for duodenal ulcer disease and reflux oesophagitis. Acetylcholine is released from the post-ganglionic neurones of the vagal parasympathetic system and this is referred to as the neurocrine secretion. Gastrin is released from the specialized antral G cells into the blood stream and exerts a hormonal action. Histamine is released from three sites (mast cells, enterochromaffin-like cells and nerves) into the interstitial fluid and thus acts by a paracrine action.

The main inhibitor of gastric secretion is somatostatin which is released from the D cells and exerts a continuous inhibitory paracrine effect on the parietal cells of the fundus and on the G cells of the antrum. Various hormones such as secretin, cholecystokinin, vasoactive intestinal polypeptide (VIP), etc., inhibit gastric secretion through release of somatostatin. More recent studies on the role of somatostatin have identified a further mechanism for stimulation of gastric secretion. This involves the inhibition of somatostatin secretion. Thus increased vagal cholinergic activity results in both direct stimulation of acid secretion and indirect stimulation by suppression of somatostatin restraint. The latter process is referred to as disinhibition. Other substances that inhibit gastric secretion include neurotensin, substance P and high concentrations of alcohol.

The acid pump

Irrespective of the chemical messenger (histamine, acetylcholine, gastrin), the ability of the parietal cells to secrete acid is dependent on the integrity of the enzyme H^+,K^+ adenosine triphosphatase (ATPase) which is also referred to as the acid pump. The system exchanges the H^+ from the intracellular water for extracellular K^+ present in the lumen of the canaliculus. Reversible inhibition of the ATPase pump can be achieved by proton pump inhibitors (PPIs), e.g omeprazole. PPIs are inactive when administered but in the highly acid environment of the acid secretory canaliculus of the parietal cell, omeprazole is converted to cationic sulfenamide which reacts covalently with groups on the outside of the pump producing long-lasting total but reversible inhibition of acid secretion. PPIs have largely replaced H_2 blockers in the treatment of peptic ulcer disease and reflux oesophagitis. They, however, cause a significant hypergastrinaemia at a much higher level than that encountered with H_2 blockers which do not achieve total suppression of acid secretion. In experimental animals prolonged administration of PPIs results in the development of benign tumours of the enterochromaffin cells.

Gastric secretion of pepsinogens

Pepsins are aspartic proteinases and are synthesized and secreted by the chief cells as prozymogens. The three important pepsins are: pepsin I, pepsin II (gastricsin) and pepsin III (chymosin or rennin). Their main physiological role is acid-dependent digestion of dietary proteins within the stomach. The released peptides and amino acids then mediate gastrin release and, through this mechanism, the food-dependent gastric secretion of both acid and pepsins. Although pepsins are involved in the pathophysiology of gastritis, peptic ulceration and reflux oesophagitis, the precise mechanisms are still poorly defined, although digestion of the collagen IV component of the basement membrane, with delayed healing of any mucosal injury, may be important.

Gastroduodenal mucosal defence mechanisms

The important defence mechanisms that protect the gastroduodenal mucosa agains a variety of insults, including drugs such as ethanol and non-steroidal anti-inflammatory drugs (NSAIDs), are:

- surface mucous gel
- bicarbonate secretion
- reactive hyperaemia
- epidermal growth factor
- polyamines and ornithine carboxylase.

The outer surface of the gastric mucosa is covered by a mucous gel, which is hydrophobic. This property is dependent on phosopholipid-containing vesicles, myelinated structures and a phospholipid band in the deeper layers of the mucous gel covering the luminal surface of the mucosa. The gastric mucosal cells extract bicarbonate from the mucosal blood and secrete it into the gastric lumen across the apical plasma membrane. Bicarbonate also reaches the gastric lumen by tracking between the gastric cells (paracellularly). This constant bicarbonate flux is reduced by smoking, certain drugs (e.g. cyclooxygenase inhibitors) and somatostatin. Enhanced secretion of bicarbonate is induced by prostaglandins and theophylline. When acid or other noxious agents enter the gastric mucosal cells, sensory neurones are stimulated, which the cause the release of vasodilatory neuropeptides (calcitonin gene-related peptide), nitric acid and prostaglandins with a resultant reactive hyperaemia. This increased blood flow permits the neutralization of the back-diffusing acid before significant tissue damage occurs. If the surface of the epithelium is damaged, the increased bicarbonate load brought to the mucosa by the reactive hyperaemia spills out and is trapped within the surface mucus, cellular debris and fibrin forming a mucoid cap that covers the injured area, thereby providing a protective microenvironment with a stable pH of 5–6 despite the high luminal acidity within the stomach.

Epidermal growth factor (EGF) which is produced by the salivary and Brunner's glands under physiological conditions is concerned both with mucosal defence against injury and in the repair of established mucosal damage. Deficient secretion of EGF in patients with rheumatoid arthritis and the sicca syndrome is thought to be responsible for the enhanced susceptibility to NSAID-induced erosive disease exhibited by these patients. When ulceration develops anywhere in the gastrointestinal tract, special cells derived from the crypts adjacent to the ulceration site appear and secrete abundant amounts of EGF. This together with the synthesis of polyamines (required for cell growth and differentiation) by the enzyme ornithine carboxylase and other growth peptides is responsible for the reparative process.

Physiological consequences of gastrectomy

Loss of weight or failure to regain pre-operative or ideal weight is very common after gastrectomy and may be particularly marked in patients who experience significant post-cibal symptoms. The resulting diminished dietary intake is the major factor and far outweighs others such as malabsorption and decreased transit times. Mild steatorrhoea occurs in 70% of patients but severe steatorrhoea is rare and is then usually encountered in patients who develop bacterial overgrowth. Anaemia is a frequent adverse consequence of both gastrectomy and vagotomy and drainage, and its incidence increases with duration of follow-up. Iron-deficiency anaemia accounts for the majority with an incidence of 60% and 75% in males and females, respectively, 10–20 years after gastric surgery. The pathogenesis of the iron-deficiency anaemia remains unclear. Malabsorption of iron may play a role but several other factors have been incriminated: shift to trivalent ferric iron at high pH, loss of gastric juice factor facilitating iron absorption, increased binding of iron to proteins, diminished hydrolysis of iron–protein complexes and chronic blood loss from gastritis and erosions. Whatever the exact cause(s), sufficient oral iron can be absorbed even after total gastrectomy to restore the serum iron level to normal, and if prophylactic iron supplementation is administered (300 mg qid), the development of post-gastrectomy iron-deficiency anaemia is prevented.

Vitamin B_{12} malabsorption is invariable after total gastrectomy and unless replacement therapy is initiated, megaloblastic anaemia develops within 3–4 years when the body stores of the vitamin become depleted. Although malabsorption of B_{12} is well documented after partial gastrectomy, frank megaloblastic anaemia is rare. The main factor responsible in these patients is the lack of a sufficiently acid environment that is normally required to release vitamin B_{12} bound to food. Although intrinsic factor secretion is reduced after partial gastrectomy (and vagotomy and drainage), it is not known whether the residual secretion is inadequate in physiological terms.

Post-gastrectomy bone disease is less frequently encountered nowadays. Although osteomalacia accounts for the majority, cases with features of both osteoporosis and osteomalacia are well documented. The aetiology is multifactorial. Diminished dietary intake of calcium and vitamin D is important and malabsorption follows bypass of the duodenum, which is the major site of calcium absorption. Most commonly, the disease is encountered after total or Polya-gastrectomy in elderly patients. There is latent period of several years and a female preponderance. The biochemical features (raised alkaline phosphatase and serum calcium) and radiological changes (rarefaction) pre-date the onset of symptoms which include generalized bone pain, weakness from associated myopathy and stress fractures.

Section 8.2 • Symptomatology

Dyspepsia

The functions of the stomach and duodenum are concerned with the initiation of the process of digestion. This is achieved by a combination of mechanical fragmentation and acid/peptic digestion of foodstuffs together with an orderly delivery of the resulting acid chyme into the duodenum where further chemical digestion in an alkaline medium ensues. In health we are unaware of these activities, which are the result of co-ordinated secretory and motor functions by neural and humoral mechanisms. Gastroduodenal disease disturbs many of these physiological mechanisms and produces varied symptoms described clinically under the collective term 'dyspepsia'. Dyspeptic symptoms are extremely common in the general population with reported prevalence rates of 14–41% but show marked regional differences. It has been estimated that only 25% of patients with dyspepsia seek medical attention and in these endoscopy is normal in a substantial but varying extent (25–76%). One of the several reasons for this problem has been defining what constitutes dyspepsia in the general population. Several international Working Parties and Consensus Conferences have addressed this issue with some measure of but not total agreement on the constituent symptoms, severity grades and the appropriateness of endoscopy.

An agreed recent international definition of dyspepsia is 'episodic or persistent abdominal symptoms, often related to the intake of food, which patients or physicians believe to be due to disorders of the proximal portion of the digestive tract'. The symptoms included in the generic definition of dyspepsia agreed at the Maastricht consensus conference are:

- pain or discomfort in the upper abdomen
- nausea and vomiting
- early satiety
- epigastric fullness and regurgitation.

Maastricht consensus conference 1997

Heartburn and dysphagia are not considered dyspeptic symptoms by the Maastricht consensus statement and this is now agreed internationally.

There are two broad categories of dyspepsia: organic and non-organic. Organic dyspepsia is produced by organic disease, e.g. peptic ulceration, oesophagitis, gastric carcinoma, whereas non-organic dyspepsia is restricted to symptoms occurring in patients without any demonstrable focal lesion in the upper gastrointestinal tract. The prevalence of organic dyspepsia (symptoms and abnormal endoscopic changes) increases with age with a distinct threshold around 40–45 years. In particular, gastric cancer is rare below the age of 40 years.

Four subgroups of dyspeptic patients have been recognized. These are based on the predominant symptoms and generally reflect the most likely aetiology of the symptoms:

- ulcer-like
- reflux-like
- dysmotility-like
- non-specific.

While this subgrouping is clinically useful, the results of several prospective studies have demonstrated quite unequivocally that symptoms alone are not able to differentiate between organic and non-organic causes of disease. In essence, conventional history taking is not always reliably predictive of the underlying cause of dyspepsia. The important practical issue in the management of patients with dyspepsia relates to which patients should be investigated by upper gastrointestinal endoscopy before treatment. In practice, there are a number of clinical variables that influence this decision although practice varies between centres. Thus patients with the following generally have non-organic disease and are thus likely to be endoscopy negative:

- age < 45 years
- patients who are *H. pylori* negative
- patients without a history of NSAID usage
- patients without alarm/sinister symptoms – loss of appetite, weight loss, bleeding.

Specific symptoms of surgical importance

Altered motility (primary or following gastric surgery) can result in rapid emptying of the stomach (dumping), delayed emptying (from gastroparesis) or abnormal reflux of duodenal contents into the stomach and oesophagus (enterogastric reflux). The symptom complex produced is varied but is determined by the functional abnormality. In some cases, the functional abnormality may in turn may cause organic disease, e.g. gastritis from enterogastric reflux.

Loss of appetite, weight loss, recent onset dyspepsia, constant upper abdominal pain and evidence of bleeding (overt or occult) have to be regarded as *alarm* or *sinister symptoms* and thus require urgent investigation by endoscopy particularly if the patient is over 40 years of age. Weight loss is common, if not universal, in patients with post-gastric surgery symptoms and is largely the result of a reduced oral dietary intake as in many of these patients, the symptoms are precipitated by food or the patient is only able to eat small meals because of early satiety due to either a reduced gastric reservoir or loss of adaptive gastric relaxation after meals. Loss of appetite associated with early satiety/abdominal discomfort in a patient without previous gastric surgery is suspicious of a gastric neoplasm and pre-dates obstructive symptoms (vomiting). In most Western countries pyloric obstruction with vomiting of ingested food not mixed with bile is very rarely caused by benign disease. In young female patients loss of appetite and weight is commonly caused by psychological disorders including anorexia nervosa.

Acute severe constant epigastric pain accompanied by abdominal signs of peritoneal irritation implies a breach in the integrity of the gastric/duodenal wall most commonly by peptic ulceration. Constant chronic back pain is indicative of a posterior ulcerating lesion penetrating the pancreas. When this involves the head/neck of the pancreas, erosion of the gastroduodenal artery as it runs down in the groove between the two organs can result in severe upper gastrointestinal haemorrhage.

Section 8.3 • Investigation of patients with gastric disorders

Endoscopy

The development of the modern flexible fibre-optic endoscopes has allowed accurate diagnosis of both acute and chronic gastroduodenal disease, and in many instances altered its management. Undoubtedly the experienced endoscopist has an accuracy rate superior to that of the radiologist. Its value in the bleeding patient has already been mentioned and nowadays it is axiomatic that all patients admitted with acute upper gastrointestinal bleeding require an upper gastrointestinal endoscopy within 24 hours of admission and when indicated, therapeutic control of the bleeding is achieved by this approach in the first instance.

The management of gastroduodenal disorders has changed radically with the recognition of the important pathogenetic role of infection with *Helicobacter pylori* and related organisms. This is reflected in the recommendation that testing for *H. pylori* should constitute the initial step in the management of patients below 45 years with dyspepsia and if positive, eradication therapy commenced – *the test and treat strategy* according to which, endoscopy is avoided in patients who are rendered symptom free by this treatment. This approach has the potential for considerable savings of endoscopy-related costs. This strategy has some advantages. It lowers the *H. pylori* prevalence and hence the risk of *H. pylori*-related disease including gastric carcinoma, and significantly reduces of the endoscopic workload with substantial cost savings. However, this strategy has a number of risks. In the first instance, none of the tests for *H. pylori* are sufficiently sensitive (10–20% false negative rates). The test-and-treat policy results in overtreatment of patients who do not require eradication (e.g. patients with reflux oesophagitis whose symptoms can be worsened by eradication) and may miss significant disease, e.g. Barrett's columnar cell change, gastric ulcer or gastric neoplasia. In addition it incurs a morbidity related to the side-effects of antibiotics and the emergence of resistant strains.

The *test and scope strategy* establishes the diagnosis before treatment, permits biopsy of organic disease and excludes gastric neoplasia. Furthermore it reduces anxiety of the patients and avoids overtreatment. It is cost effective in Europe where the endoscopy costs (under $500) are significantly lower than in the USA. The morbidity of upper gastrointestinal endoscopy is low but it is considered an unpleasant experience by most patients. In the current state of knowledge, the *test and scope strategy* is preferable certainly in European countries. To a large extent the validity of the test-and-treat strategy relates to the prevalence of *H. pylori* in the community. In most Western countries this has declined substantially during the past decade and now is of the order of 10%, whereas high prevalence rates (40–70%) are still encountered in underprivileged countries. If *the test-and-treat policy* is adopted on the basis of high community prevalence, endoscopy should be done in dyspeptic patients who either are *H. pylori* negative or have alarm symptoms irrespective of their *H. pylori* status.

In light of the rather confusing situation the European Panel on the Appropriateness of Gastrointestinal Endoscopy (EPAGE) considers upper gastrointestinal endoscopy to be *necessary* in the following:

- In individuals >45 years testing positive for *H. pylori*, with persistent symptoms despite eradication treatment.
- In individuals > 45 years, never investigated, *H. pylori*-negative and no NSAID intake, with persistent symptoms despite acid lowering treatment.
- In individuals > 45 years with a previous history of gastric ulcer, no *H. pylori* testing or *H. pylori* test negative, with persistent symptoms despite acid-lowering drugs.

Upper gastrointestinal endoscopy is a safe technique. Full facilities for resuscitation should always be available and pulse oximetry is nowadays considered essential during the procedure. Sedation should always be kept to the minimum, particularly in any patient who may have hypovolaemia or hypoxaemia. Diazepam or midazolam in small incremental doses is usually adequate. Fortral should not be used as with any opiate it may depress respiration significantly, and it also delays gastric emptying, thus making subsequent regurgitation and aspiration more likely. In addition, Fortral can cause pulmonary hypertension, which can be significant in a patient recovering from haemorrhagic shock. Spasmolytic agents, such as Buscopan, are sometimes useful to allow visualization of the antrum, passage of the endoscope through into the duodenum and duodenoscopy.

Radiology

Barium meal examination is commonly used in investigating the stomach and duodenum. Although gross lesions are usually seen, the technique does have its limitations. Subtle mucosal changes of gastritis and of early mucosal cancer can only be detected if a meticulous double contrast technique is used in which the stomach is filled with air and the lining coated with a thin film of barium. Even with these precautions, endoscopy usually gives superior results. A barium meal examination is notoriously unreliable in the assessment of a patient with acute upper gastrointestinal bleeding. The presence of clot within the stomach produces a variety of bizarre appearances. Even when a lesion can be identified, contrast radiology cannot demonstrate whether this has been responsible for the bleeding. For these reasons, endoscopy is the preferred investigation for the bleeding patient. Despite these criticisms, barium meal remains an extremely valuable investigation. A normal radiological appearance should not be accepted, however, in a patient with continuing dyspepsia, and supplementary endoscopy should be performed. Barium swallow/meal is invaluable in outlining the exact topography of upper gastrointestinal cancer.

Endoscopic ultrasonography

Ultrasound examination of the stomach can be performed with either external or endoluminal probes. It is used to measure gastric wall thickness, to assess the extent of intramural involvement of the stomach wall by tumour, and to establish enlargement of the perigastric lymph nodes. The normal stomach wall thickness measured by ultrasound (internal or external) is 5–6 mm. An endoscopy and biopsy is indicated when the ultrasound gastric wall thickness exceeds 5 mm.

Over the past few years, there have been significant advances in the technology of flexible endoscopic ultrasonography (EUS) with high-frequency (20 MHz) mini-probes capable with the appropriate software of distinguishing the layers of the oesophagus and stomach. Although considerable experience is needed for valid interpretation of EUS findings, there is no doubt the EUS provides the most sensitive modality for the staging of oesophageal and gastric tumours. In both organs EUS is superior to all other imaging tests in the staging of infiltrative mural lesions. In the stomach EUS is particularly useful in:

- the pre-treatment staging of early gastric cancer in detecting absence, superficial and deep involvement of the submucosa
- the staging and follow-up of gastric mucosa-associated lymphoid tissue (MALT) lymphomas
- the diagnosis of stromal (mesenchymal) tumours.

Deep involvement of the submucosa in early gastric cancer (EGC) is associated with a significantly increased risk of lymph node spread. Thus whereas EGCs limited to the mucosa have a 3% incidence of regional node involvement, this increases to 20% with deep invasion of the submucosa, thereby precluding any form of 'local' endoscopic treatment. EUS is also capable of identifying advanced gastric cancer (involvement of the muscularis propria) and infiltration of adjacent organs but is unreliable in detecting lymph node involvement (as opposed to enlargement) and peritoneal deposits.

EUS has an overall diagnostic accuracy for gastric non-Hodgkin's lymphoma approximating 95%. It is also reliable in assessing depth of invasion (85% accuracy) and to a lesser extent (60%) in detecting metastatic spread to the perigastric lymph nodes. The characteristic echo pattern consists of an extended hypoechoic thickening of the second and third layers with preservation of identity of all the layers. A similar picture is obtained in linitis plastica except that the hypoechoic thickening is more longitudinally extensive and involves the entire circumference of the stomach. In patients with MALT lymphomas associated with *H. pylori* infection, if the lesion is confined to second or third layer on EUS staging (mucosa or submucosa), eradication of the infection results in remission in 85% of cases. By contrast if the EUS staging shows deeper infiltration, eradication of the *H. pylori* infection has no effect on the tumour and indicates the need for chemotherapy or surgery.

Mesenchymal (stromal) tumours appear as hypoechoic masses continuous with the fourth ultrasound layer (muscularis propria). The EUS features suggestive of malignancy are tumour size >4 cm, irregular extraluminal border, echogenic foci and cystic spaces. If all these features are absent, the stromal tumour can be confidently predicted as benign. However, a confident diagnosis of malignancy cannot be made on the basis of EUS findings.

Helical computed tomography

Computed tomography (CT) is useful in the staging and assessment of operability of patients with gastric cancer. The technique involves ingestion of water (hydro-CT) or dilute contrast by the patient followed by helical CT scanning with the patient in the prone position (Figure 8.1). This technique allows documentation of extent of mural involvement, extragastric extension and involvement of retrogastric organs such as the pancreas. Helical CT also enables detection of lymph node enlargement especially of the coeliac/para-aortic lymph nodes. By contrast CT is unreliable in the staging of primary gastric lymphomas both in terms of the extent of mural invasion and in regional node involvement.

Other investigations

In most cases the morphological assessment of the stomach and duodenum by contrast radiology and endoscopy gives sufficient information for further management decisions to be made. In selected cases it may be necessary to obtain a functional evaluation of the gastroduodenal region. This can be achieved by gastric secretory testing, measurement of gastric emptying and enterogastric reflux, and determination of the plasma concentration of the antral hormone gastrin.

Gastric secretory tests

Because of the association of duodenal ulceration with hypersecretion of acid, measurement of gastric acid output has held a fascination for many surgeons. In practice, however, measurement of acid secretion has little

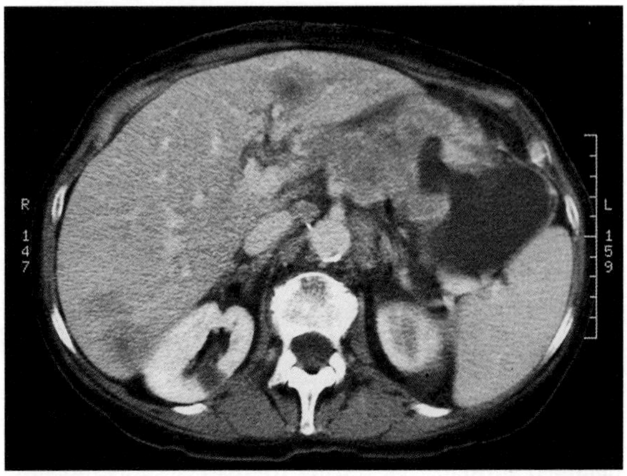

Figure 8.1 Hydro-helical CT in a patient with advanced gastric cancer.

clinical relevance in the management of patients with upper gastrointestinal disorders unless the Zollinger–Ellison syndrome is suspected. Thus acid secretory studies are now carried out largely for research purposes.

Basal and maximal acid output

Basal secretion is usually measured over 1 hour. Maximal secretion is best stimulated with the synthetic gastrin analogue 'pentagastrin', which is given by intramuscular injection in a dose of 6 μg/kg (10 pg/kg in the post-vagotomy patient). Secretion is then followed for 1 hour and the maximal response (peak 15 min × 4) calculated. There are many pitfalls in acid secretory tests. The overlap between normal and disease is considerable, and the results obtained vary with body weight and sex. Typical values in pre-operative and post-operative patients are shown in Table 8.2. The only clinical reason for acid secretory studies nowadays is in the diagnosis of pernicious anaemia and the Zollinger–Ellison syndrome. In the post-operative patient, maximal acid output is reduced by 70% or more after gastrectomy and 50–70% by vagotomy. A post-operative maximal acid response of 20 mmol/hour greater is a fairly reliable indication of a persisting hypersecretory state (incomplete vagotomy).

The measurement of basal acid output after gastric surgery has particular relevance to the question of ulcer recurrence caused by a pancreatic gastrin-producing tumour (Zollinger–Ellison syndrome). If hypergastrinaemia exists, 'basal' secretion is already being stimulated and the characteristic findings will be of a high basal secretion, which does not increase much further, when a maximal stimulus is given. If basal secretion is greater than 10 mmol/hour, and this represents more than 60% of the maximal response, a gastrinoma should be suspected. Proof of this requires measurement of plasma gastrin concentration.

The insulin test

After complete denervation of the parietal cell mass, acid output is reduced by 50% or more. Incomplete denervation will not achieve this, and the chance of a recurrent ulcer is increased. Nowadays, an assessment of the adequacy of vagotomy is indicated only in *H. pylori*-negative patients who develop recurrent ulceration after this procedure. The insulin test, originally described by Hollander, depends upon the fact that insulin-induced hypoglycaemia stimulates hypothalamic nuclei which induce a parasympathetic response. If vagal innervation of the parietal cell mass persists, acid will be secreted in response to the hypoglycaemia. The test is performed by giving an intravenous injection of soluble insulin (0.2 U/kg) after basal secretion has been collected in four 15 min aliquots. Secretion is then followed for a further 2 hours. If the acid concentration in any 15 min sample after insulin is 20 mmol/l greater than in the basal period, the test is regarded as positive. If no free acid is secreted basally, then a post-insulin concentration of more than 10 mmol/l is taken as positive. Subsequent to Hollander's original description, the interpretation of the test has been modified in many ways. The modification most commonly used is to divide a positive response into 'early' (during the first hour) or 'late' (second hour).

A positive insulin test indicates residual vagal innervation of the parietal cell mass. An 'early' positive response usually implies a fairly generous residual innervation and the actual amount of acid secreted (i.e. volume as well as concentration) is quite large. If a patient with a recurrent ulcer has an early positive response to insulin, and a maximal acid output of 20 mmol/hour or more, then incomplete vagotomy is the likely cause. A 'late' positive response may not be so significant, particularly if the acid outputs to insulin and pentagastrin are small. Cephalic stimulation can also be produced by sham feeding ('chew and spit'). The gastric secretory response to sham feeding is used in some centres instead of the insulin test, as it is safer and just as reliable. One of the problems with the insulin test is that many asymptomatic patients can show a positive response. Furthermore, when serial tests have been performed after vagotomy it has been shown that negative responses in the first few months after operation can revert later. Thus, the insulin test must be interpreted with caution, and considered only in the context of all other clinical, endoscopic and secretory information. The deliberate production of hypoglycaemia is not without problems, and the test should not be carried out in patients with significant cardiac disease, cerebrovascular disease or epilepsy.

Table 8.2 Typical values for basal and maximally stimulated acid secretion

	Acid output (mmol/hour)*	
	Basal secretion	*Maximal secretion*
Normal	2	20–30
Per-operative duodenal ulcer	>5	>35
Post-vagotomy	<2	10–20
Post-gastrectomy	1	<10

*These values are approximations only. Secretion increases with increasing body weight and decreases progressively with age. Females secrete about two-thirds the amount of acid secreted by males.

Gastric emptying

Measurement of gastric emptying is indicated in patients with symptomatology indicative of dysmotility type dyspepsia. The symptoms fall into two groups:

- gastroparesis – early satiety, fullness and gastric retention with vomiting
- rapid emptying with early vasomotor dumping.

In surgical practice, the majority of these patients have post-gastric surgery symptoms and are investigated with a view to possible remedial surgery. Delayed gastric emptying can however be encountered in diabetic patients and those with dysmotility disorders including hollow visceral myopathy which affects the entire gastrointestinal tract. A variety of radionuclide 'meals' are used. The patient drinks or ingests the meal and the radioactivity in the stomach is then monitored with an external gamma camera, thus obtaining radioactivity–time curves. The most useful index is the T1/2, which is the half-emptying time, i.e. the time taken for half of the ingested meal to leave the stomach. Assessment of both liquid and gastric emptying (on separate occasions) is necessary to document the pattern of abnormal gastric emptying. Thus in many post-gastrectomy patients, the liquid emptying is fast but the solid emptying is delayed (Figure 8.2). Rapid gastric emptying of liquids is often associated with a much shorter small bowel transit time. Useful qualitative information can be obtained using a 'physiological' food and barium meal if the more sophisticated isotope techniques are not available.

Tests for enterogastric reflux

Measurement of gastroduodenal reflux can assist in assessing patients with bile vomiting and bile gastritis. In

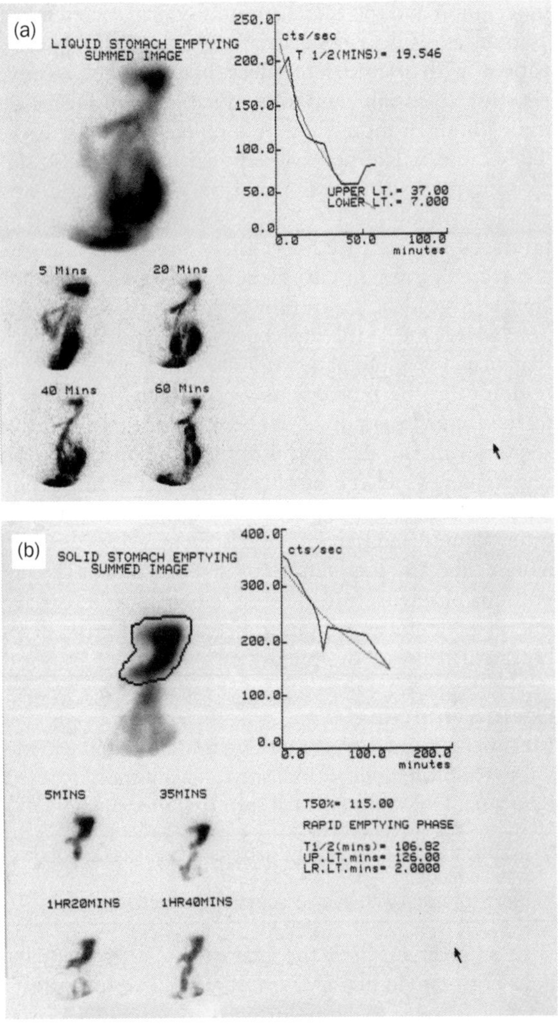

Figure 8.2 Isotope gastric emptying in a patients with vasomotor dumping after truncal vagotomy and drainage: (a) liquid meal showing fast emptying, (b) solid meal demonstrating slow emptying.

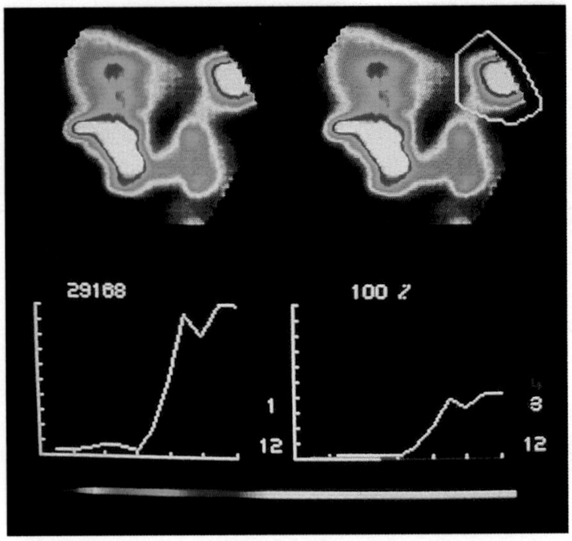

Figure 8.3 Extensive reflux of bile into the gastric remnant in a patient with bile gastritis and vomiting after Polya-gastrectomy.

the latter case, demonstration of increased quantities of bile in the stomach may suggest that re-operation for bile diversion may be profitable. Enterogastric bile reflux is best quantitated by combining biliary excretion scintigraphy (Hida scan) with cholecystokinin or preferably a milk meal (the milk-Hida test – see Figure 8.3).

Plasma gastrin concentration

The peptide hormone gastrin is elaborated in specific endocrine cells in the gastric antrum and, to a lesser extent, the duodenum. Gastrin secretion occurs in response to distension of the antrum and the presence of food, particularly protein. When the pH in the antrum falls, gastrin release is inhibited, so that a negative feedback control exists. The concentration of gastrin in the plasma can be measured by specific radioimmunoassay. This is indicated if clinical or gastric secretory features suggest the possibility of the Zollinger–Ellison syndrome. The reported levels of plasma gastrin vary between laboratories, but values greater than 200 pg/ml are regarded as abnormally high. Values in excess of 1000 pg/ml are virtually diagnostic of a gastrinoma, provided that the patient is secreting acid. The reason for this proviso is that in an achlorhydric patient, e.g. one with pernicious anaemia, there is no fall in antral pH to shut off gastrin secretion. Not uncommonly the plasma gastrin concentration will be found to be elevated, but not sufficiently so for the diagnosis of the Zollinger–Ellison syndrome to be made confidently. There are a number of causes of hypergastrinaemia (Table 8.3). Many of these can be excluded simply, but difficulty will be experienced in distinguishing a gastrinoma from antral hyperplasia, retained antrum or merely an exaggeration of the usual rise in gastrin that follows acid reduction by vagotomy. Three stimulatory tests are useful (Figure 8.4):

Table 8.3 Causes of hypergastrinaemia

Primary autonomous increased secretion
Tumour – Zollinger–Ellison syndrome
Antral G-cell hyperplasia
Increased stimulation
Hypercalcaemia
Decreased inhibition
Hypo- or achlorhydria, e.g. pernicious anaemia, post-vagotomy
Retained, excluded gastric antrum
Small bowel resection
Decreased removal
Renal failure
Small bowel resection

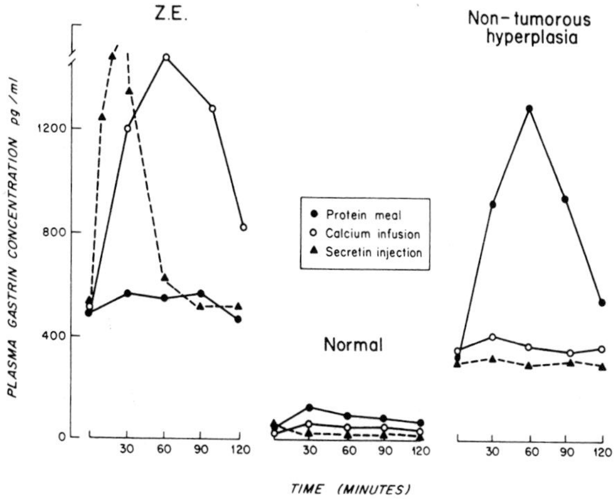

Figure 8.4 The use of provocative gastrin stimulation tests to differentiate between the hypergastrinaemia of the Zollinger–Ellison syndrome (Z.E.) and that due to antral G-cell hyperplasia.

- *Protein meal* – gastrin of antral origin is stimulated by protein. Provided that the antrum is present, and in continuity, gastrin levels will rise after such a meal. An exaggerated response is found in G-cell hyperplasia. Gastrin secretion from a tumour is autonomous and not affected by a meal.
- *Calcium stimulation* – calcium is involved in the release of many peptide hormones. Under normal circumstances an infusion of calcium causes a slight rise in gastrin concentration. If a gastrin-producing tumour is present there is a very marked release of gastrin by calcium. The usual procedure is to infuse 5 mg/kg/hour for 3 hours.
- *Secretin challenge* – an intravenous injection of secretin, 4 U/kg, does not affect antral gastrin, or may actually cause a slight fall in concentration. For reasons not understood, secretin causes an immediate and large release of gastrin from tumours. If this stimulus is employed it is important to use pure secretin, since many preparations of secretin contain some contaminating gastrin, or cross-reacting cholecystokinin.

Section 8.4 • *Helicobacter pylori* infection

Gastroduodenal disease

Helicobacter pylori, previously known as *Campylobacter pylori*, is a spiral-shaped organism (Figure 8.5) which has assumed increasing importance in certain gastroduodenal disorders. The infection is acquired by oral ingestion. Transmission by inadequately cleaned and disinfected endoscopes is now well documented. There is also evidence of transmission between cohabiting parties as spouses of duodenal ulcer patients have a higher seroprevalence of *H. pylori* infection than controls. The organism is often identified in children complaining of abdominal pain. Indeed population studies indicate that the infection is acquired in childhood and thereafter the acquisition rate slows down exponentially with age. A high rate of infection is documented amongst endoscopy staff (endoscopists and endoscopic nurses) with prevalence rates as high as 75–80% compared to 20–65% background infectivity rate (varies in different countries). Indeed in most Western countries *H. pylori* infection is disappearing spontaneously at a fast rate.

Pathology

Within the stomach, *H. pylori* localizes on to the epithelial surface beneath the viscid mucous layer where it exerts its pathological effects via the elaboration of various enzymes and toxins. The gastric mucous barrier is disturbed by the production of an endopeptidase, which has a powerful mucolytic action and by the generation of large amounts of ammonia with an increase in the epithelial surface pH. The latter alters the mucosal charge gradient, cellular permeability and epithelial Na^+,K^+-ATPase activity leading to back-diffusion of H^+. The adhesion of the organism to the surface of the gastric epithelial cells is mediated by a specific substance, adhesin, which also causes haemagglutination of erythrocytes (*in vitro*). In addition to surface attachment, the organism can invade the gastric epithelial cells. *Helicobacter pylori* produces two cytotoxins. One of these induces vacuolization of the affected cells. This vacuolizing cytotoxin is much more commonly encountered in isolates from patients with duodenal ulceration than those with gastritis and no ulceration. The clinical relevance of the other toxin which is a weak haemolysin remains unknown. The other adverse effects of *H. pylori* infection include

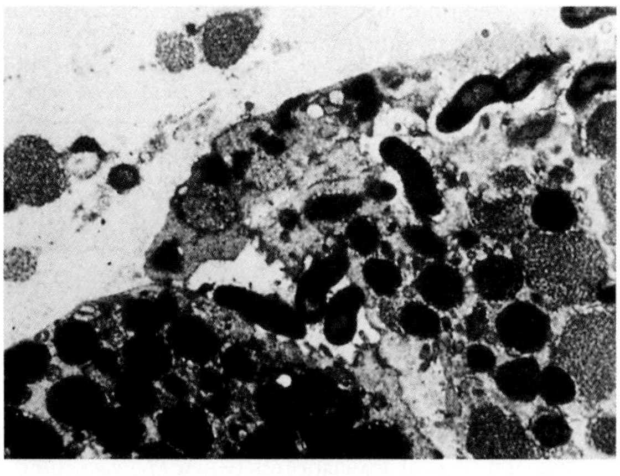

Figure 8.5 *Helicobacter pylori* in gastric mucosa.

reduced epithelial cell turnover (impaired healing), reduction of surface hydrophobicity and increased lipolytic activity, release of chemotactic factors for neutrophils and monocytes and degranulation of eosinophils (with release of cytotoxic cationic proteins), activation of the classical complement pathway with the release of potent inflammatory mediators and stimulation of the G cells with increased release of gastrin as a result of the high surface pH consequent on the locally produced NH_3.

Not all patients with *H. pylori* infections develop gastroduodenal disease, which has to be regarded as a complication of the infection. Aside from host factors, the virulence and genetic type of the organism, age of the host and environmental factors (smoking, diet especially the protective effect of dietary fruit and vegetables) are important and determine the development of specific gastroduodenal disease and its incidence. *Helicobacter pylori* exhibits marked genetic variation and hence the presence of virulent and less virulent strains. Virulence is associated with the 'cag pathogenicity island' (segment of DNA) which has 40 genes, one of which is the *cytotoxin associated gene A* (*cagA*) that codes for the protein CagA that is highly antigenic and hence can be detected by antibody tests. The pathogenicity island (PAI) is associated with the vacuolating toxin and hence mucosal damage and inflammation. Long-standing inflammation then leads to atrophy and intestinal metaplasia. The *H. pylori* antigens also induce the appearance of MALT follicles in the gastric submucosa. Hence the entire spectrum of gastroduodenal disease caused by *H. pylori* – gastroduodenitis, duodenal and gastric ulcers, atrophic gastritis, carcinoma of the body and antrum of the stomach and MALT-associated gastric lymphoma.

What is interesting is that the PAI including its cagA gene does not produce the vacuolating toxin. This is coded by another gene (vacA) that is located in the genome of *H. pylori* outside the PAI. However, only organisms that possess the PAI can secrete the vacuolating toxin. Whilst infections with virulent CagA-positive organisms cause serious gastroduodenal disease, paradoxically they may protect the host from the development of reflux oesophagitis and possibly Barrett's columnar metaplasia and carcinoma of the gastrooesophageal junction.

Extradigestive disease

There are several mechanisms whereby gastric infection with *H. pylori* could contribute to the development of extradigestive disease:

- immunological responses to the *H. pylori* antigens
- constant production of proinflammatory substances: cytokines, eicosanoids, acute phase proteins
- mimicry between bacterial and host antigens
- reduced folate and iron absorption.

There has been considerable research interest into the possible aetiological association between *H. pylori* infections and a variety of extradigestive disorders (Table 8.4). The reported studies in patients with ischaemic heart disease (IHD) have tended to confirm this association but with extremely wide variation on the estimates of the degree of risk of infected patients. A recent review indicated that at best infected patients carry a low (10–20%) excess risk. The association between *H. pylori* infection and carotid artery stenosis is based on reports that show significantly more severe stenosis in infected compared to non-infected patients with this condition. The hypothesis suggested for the role of *H. pylori* infection in atherosclerosis, aside from the long-standing inflammatory cascade, is folate malabsorption by the infected stomach. Low serum folate is a well-documented risk factor for ischaemic vascular disease.

Table 8.4 Extradigestive disorders with possible association with *H. pylori* infection

- Ischaemic heart disease
- Ischaemic cerebrovascular disorders including carotid artery stenosis
- Functional vascular disorders – Raynaud's phenomenon and idiopathic migraine
- Immunological disease: Henoch–Schönlein purpura, Sjögren's syndrome, autoimmune thrombocytopenia
- Extra-gastric MALT-lymphomas
- Sideropenic anaemia – possible iron malabsorption
- Skin disorders – idiopathic chronic urticaria, acne rosacea and alopecia aerata
- Hepatobiliary disease – cirrhosis, cholesterol stones, chronic cholecystitis (other Helicobacter species, e.g. *H. bilis*, *H. pullorum*)

Helicobacter heilmannii infections

This organism, previously known as *Gastrospirillum hominis*, can also infect the stomach although it is much less commonly encountered in clinical practice and is reported to be present in 0.08–1% of endoscopies. Infection produces a gastritis that differs from that caused by *H. pylori* in several respects. In the first instance, the mononuclear infiltrate is mild, the inflammation is unusually inactive, the bacterial mucosal load is low and the degenerative/regenerative lesions in the surface gastric epithelium are focal and mild. Contrary to *H. pylori*, the bacteria do not adhere to the surface epithelium. Nonetheless, infection with *H. heilmannii* can cause peptic ulcer disease, gastric cancer and gastric MALT lymphomas. Thus when present the condition requires eradication therapy.

Tests for *Helicobacter pylori* infection

The most commonly performed are the *rapid urease tests*. These are carried out on endoscopic biopsies and use test kits such as the CLO, Hpfast and Pyloritec, etc., and provide a result within 3 hours of the endoscopy. The sensitivity and specificity of these tests at the final reading are similar at 90 and 100% respectively. Therapy with PPIs at the time of endoscopy significantly reduces the sensitivity of antral and corpus biopsies for detection of infection by both rapid urease tests and

Table 8.5 Comparative sensitivity and specificity of the various tests used for diagnosis of *Helicobacter pylori* infections

Test	*Sensitivity (%)*	*Specificity (%)*
Rapid urease tests	90	100
Culture	98	100
Polymerase chain reaction	97	100
Histology of antrum and corpus	98	99
^{13}C breath test	100	100
Serology	98	88

histology. Thus if PPI therapy cannot be discontinued, the urease test should not be read before 24 hours after biopsy and in addition a serological test should be performed.

Other tests include culture in a microaerobic environment, the polymerase chain reaction, histology of the antrum and corpus (Giemsa or the Warthin-Starry silver stain), the ^{13}C urea breath test and serology for the detection of *H. pylori* specific antibodies (IgG). The modern immunological test kits are based on purified antigen preparations and use the enzyme-linked immunosorbent assay (ELISA).

There is little to choose between these various tests in terms of sensitivity and specificity (Table 8.5) and in practice, the choice of test used depends on the clinical situation. In symptomatic patients undergoing endoscopy, a biopsy-based test is the appropriate one (rapid urease, histology, culture) and the accuracy is increased if more than one test is performed. In asymptomatic patients a serological test is first performed and if this is positive, confirmation is achieved by the ^{13}C breath test. This test is also indicated in patients with recurrent symptoms after previous eradication even if the endoscopy is normal. Serological tests within 6–12 months of eradication are unreliable. It is now recommended that the outcome of any eradication treatment needs to be confirmed by a non-invasive test 4–8 weeks after the end of the treatment, and the best test for this purpose is the ^{13}C breath test.

Section 8.5 • Acute gastroduodenal disorders

The various surgical disorders of the stomach and duodenum are discussed later in this chapter. Many of these diseases present with varying degrees of urgency, as either perforation, bleeding or stenosis. The general management of these situations is discussed here.

Perforation

Clinical features

Free perforation into the general peritoneal cavity is a catastrophic event the signs and symptoms of which do not usually cause diagnostic problems. When perforation of a chronic ulcer occurs there will often have been an increase in the severity of the dyspepsia for a few days prior to the perforation. When an acute ulcer perforates there may be no premonitory symptoms, particularly in younger patients. The pathology of steroid-induced perforations is not fully understood. For instance, perforation is much more common in patients with rheumatoid arthritis on steroids than in patients with ulcerative colitis. This may be a reflection of the primary disease process or, alternatively, may be a feature of the concomitant use of other drugs. The use of NSAIDs has been shown to be associated with an increased incidence of peptic ulceration and with an increased risk of the complications of both perforation and bleeding.

Acute perforations also accompany situations of stress, such as burns, multiple injuries and sepsis, and can occur in patients receiving intensive chemotherapy and radiotherapy. Such perforations may be duodenal, pyloric or gastric. Perforation of malignant gastric ulcers is common and although most perforated gastric ulcers will be benign, biopsy is important if the ulcer is not removed. The moment of perforation is often identified by the patient as an excruciating epigastric pain. The subsequent symptoms depend in part on the degree of peritoneal soiling and whether or not the perforation becomes sealed. The pain usually becomes generalized. In addition, it may be felt over the shoulder if diaphragmatic irritation ensues. Sometimes the spread of gastroduodenal content is maximal along the right paracolic gutter so that pain may localize to the right iliac fossa and simulate appendicitis. Significant vomiting is uncommon unless the diagnosis is delayed and an ileus becomes established. Occasionally in the elderly or seriously ill patient, the perforation does not occur as a dramatic episode and there is a slower development of generalized peritonitis with its accompanying and symptoms.

The physical signs accompanying perforation will again depend upon the degree and rate of soiling. Tenderness, with guarding, may vary from being localized to the upper abdomen to being generalized. If contamination of the general peritoneal cavity has occurred there will usually be rigidity and a silent abdomen. Abdominal distension is a late feature and is due to paralytic ileus in the absence of significant spasm of the abdominal musculature. In the elderly and ill patient this may be the only significant finding. A variable degree of peripheral circulatory failure may be present with tachycardia, hypotension, a cold periphery and a decreased urinary output. Respiration will often be shallow and grunting.

Diagnosis

The key to the diagnosis, suspected from the signs and symptoms, is the plain abdominal or chest radiograph taken in the erect position (the lateral decubitus position may need to be used instead of the erect in an ill patient). Although free peritoneal gas may come from any of the alimentary hollow organs, in practice the finding of subdiaphragmatic air usually on the right side is virtually pathognomonic of gastroduodenal perforation. Radiological features of an ileus may be present in more advanced cases. If a pneumoperitoneum is not seen radiologically, the diagnostic problem is to differentiate between a sealed perforation with minimal localized soiling and an acute pancreatitis. In some cases of the former, identification may not be too important if the clinical state of the patient is improving. When it is important to differentiate between the two, contrast radiology with a water-soluble contrast medium may be very useful. Such studies are also helpful if a diagnosis of perforation of a gastric ulcer into the lesser sac is suspected.

In the absence of a pneumoperitoneum, serum amylase estimation should be performed. Moderate elevation of amylase concentration may be present in 10–20% of perforated ulcers, but it is uncommon to find concentrations in excess of 700 Somogyi units unless renal function is impaired as a result of hypovolaemia. If doubt persists, a diagnostic peritoneal tap or lavage may help. The amylase content will usually be very high in either condition, but it should be possible to differentiate between gastroduodenal content and the brown-coloured fluid of pancreatitis.

Management

Initial treatment should be directed towards correction of hypovolaemia and any electrolyte imbalance. Oliguria and poor peripheral perfusion are contraindications to immediate operative treatment, and their correction should take precedence even over radiological studies. If necessary, resuscitation should be monitored with measurement of central venous pressure and urine output from a urinary catheter. Colloids can be used for resuscitation, but crystalloid in the form of a balanced salt solution is equally effective. Any patient needing such aggressive therapy should also be given oxygen by mask. Pain relief should be given as soon as the physical signs have been assessed. Pethidine is usually very effective, and a small dose can be given intravenously if absorption from a poorly perfused periphery is likely to be a problem. Nasogastric aspiration should be instituted. Antibiotics are not recommended routinely since the initial peritonitis is chemical. However, if operative cleansing of the peritoneal cavity is to be delayed much beyond 8 hours from perforation, or if the patient has chronic respiratory problems, the use of a broad-spectrum antibiotic such as cefuroxime is justified.

Operative or conservative management

There is no doubt that some patients with perforated ulcers can be managed non-operatively with a successful outcome. A policy of nasogastric suction, intravenous fluids, antibiotics and analgesics will allow many perforations to seal spontaneously and the ileus to resolve. An H_2-blocker administered parenterally is usually added to reduce both acid secretion and gastric juice volume. The problem with this approach, which is usually reserved for poor-risk elderly patients, is a high incidence of residual abscess formation, particularly in the subphrenic region which will subsequently require drainage. An operative approach (closure of the perforation and peritoneal lavage) is therefore strongly recommended in the vast majority of patients. This can be performed laparoscopically or through a midline laparotomy. Irrespective of the approach (open surgical or laparoscopic), adequate peritoneal toilet with thorough debridement of the peritoneal gutters and warm saline irrigation (3–4 litres) is as important as closure of the perforation. Insertion of drains is of doubtful value and is not generally recommended. There is controversy regarding the additional definitive surgical treatment in these patients at the time of the surgery for the perforation. This consideration arises only in those patients with a long history of peptic ulceration and in whom the perforation is early (within 6–8 hours) and whose *H. pylori* status is not known. This constitutes a rare group nowadays. If a definitive surgical treatment is considered necessary, this should consist of a highly selective vagotomy rather than truncal vagotomy and drainage.

Following suture closure of a perforated duodenal ulcer, two important factors determine future management:

- the *H. pylori* status
- the requirement of the patient for NSAIDs.

All these patients require testing for *H. pylori* and if positive eradication therapy is instituted. Some advocate eradication therapy in all patients who have sustained a perforated duodenal ulcer but this management policy is not recommended in regions of low *H. pylori* infection prevalence. If the patient has been and requires to continue to take NSAIDs, consideration should be given to changing to a selective cyclo-oxygenase-2 inhibitor. If this proves ineffective, then the addition of an H_2 blocker or PPI may reduce the future risk of recurrent ulceration.

In patients undergoing emergency surgery for perforated gastric ulcer, biopsy is essential if suture closure is contemplated. This is best achieved by local excision of the ulcer. As 10% of perforated gastric ulcers are due to malignant disease (lymphoma or carcinoma), there is a case for partial gastrectomy with wide margins beyond the perforated area. If this is not feasible, usually because of the poor general condition or frailty of the patient, then excision of the ulcer is followed by closure of the perforation. Some would perform vagotomy, either truncal with drainage or highly selective vagotomy (HSV). Review of the ulcer histology is essential to exclude malignancy in these patients.

Pyloric stenosis (gastric outlet obstruction)

Pyloric stenosis is, in fact, rarely due to stenosis at the pylorus. More commonly, the site of the obstruction is on one side or the other of the pylorus – either the first part of the duodenum at the site of chronic scarring from ulceration or the antrum where a benign ulcer or a cancer is the problem. True pyloric stenosis can arise from a pyloric channel ulcer or very rarely from a congenital web or adult hypertrophic pyloric stenosis. Other stenotic complications of peptic ulcer disease include hourglass deformity and teapot deformity (gastric ulcer). All complications result in outlet obstruction. The stenotic complications arise from repeated cycles of ulceration and healing resulting in dense fibrosis with narrowing and deformity. Some instances of pyloric stenosis are, however, caused by inflammatory oedema surrounding an active ulcer and these often resolve with medical and conservative treatment. Considerable hypertrophy occurs in response to the outlet obstruction. Sometimes, difficulty is encountered in distinguishing between benign gastric outlet obstruction and obstructing antral gastric cancer. This may require repeated endoscopy with biopsy and brush cytology before the true nature of the disease is established. In practical terms this distinction is pedantic since the problems are the same. The common causes of gastric outlet obstruction are:

- chronic duodenal ulceration/fibrosis
- antral gastric carcinoma
- carcinoma of the head of the pancreas.

Rare causes of gastric outlet obstruction

Rare causes of delayed gastric emptying include a variety of benign tumours, lymphomas, Crohn's disease, duodenal haematoma, adult pyloric hypertrophy, annular pancreas, mucosal diaphragm and Wilkie's disease.

Adult pyloric hypertrophy

Thickening of the circular muscle of the pylorus to produce outlet obstruction can occur in adults. The relationship to congenital pyloric stenosis is unclear, although about 25% of such adults give a history dating back to childhood. At operation a focal or generalized thickening of the pylorus is found. There is nearly always a degree of fibrosis so that pyloroplasty rather than pyloromyotomy is the usual operation of choice.

Mucosal diaphragm

Symptoms due to an incomplete diaphragm are often not apparent until middle age. Presumably muscular hypertrophy in the stomach is capable of overcoming the obstruction until this time. The diaphragm, consisting of mucosa and submucosa and being found in the antrum, pylorus or duodenum, represents a failure of recanalization of the embryonic gut. Gastric ulcers are sometimes found in association with this lesion. Excision of the diaphragm, with or without pyloroplasty, is all that is needed.

Megaduodenum

Rarely, a dilated stomach is found without an organic obstruction. The dilatation may extend into the duodenum for a variable extent. Some such cases have been well documented as being associated with degeneration of the myenteric nerve plexus. This may be as part of Chagas' disease, but in the UK the cause of the degeneration is usually unknown. Gastrojejunostomy is usually beneficial in the short term, although progression of the degeneration to other parts of the gastrointestinal tract may occur may occur.

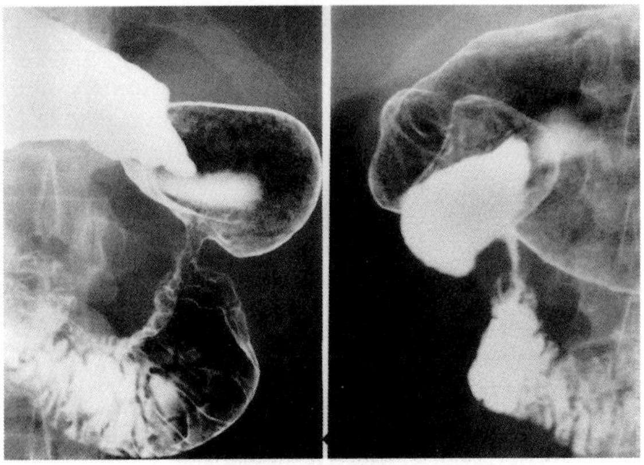

Figure 8.6 Barium meal in a patient with annular pancreas who presented with intermittent episodes of vomiting after meals.

Annular pancreas

Rare instances of annular pancreas presenting in adult life as pyloric stenosis have been described. The precipitating cause is usually an attack of pancreatitis. If symptoms persist, a gastrojejunostomy is advised (Figure 8.6).

Arteriomesenteric compression (Wilkie's disease)

The fourth part of the duodenum is potentially compressible between the vertebral column and the superior mesenteric vessels. Acute weight loss and immobilization in a plaster cast are cited as predisposing factors to this very rare problem. In many patients diagnosed as Wilkie's syndrome the obstruction is caused by other disease, the most important being tumours (lymphoma or carcinoma) at the duodenojejunal junction.

Clinical features of gastric outlet obstruction

Pyloric stenosis due to a duodenal ulcer usually occurs in a patient with long-standing symptoms of ulceration. A short preceding history with little in the way of characteristic ulcer pain suggests that the obstruction may be malignant. In most Western countries the majority of cases of gastric outlet obstruction are caused by distal gastric cancer. In the typical case of benign pyloric stenosis, the patient experiences yet another exacerbation of his ulcer symptoms. As obstruction develops, however, the character of the pain may change to become more of a generalized upper abdominal discomfort. Vomiting and anorexia supervene. As vomiting increases, pain may become less of a feature. The typical vomiting of pyloric stenosis is effortless and projectile and the vomitus is characterized by an absence of bile and the presence of partially digested food eaten hours or even days previously. With repeated vomiting and failure to eat, the patient often becomes constipated, although in some cases diarrhoea may develop.

Examination will usually show an underweight patient who is dehydrated and often with a degree of iron-deficiency anaemia. In such a relatively advanced cases there will nearly always be evidence of gastric stasis in the form of a succussion splash. Visible peristalsis may be apparent passing across the upper abdomen from left to right, and the dilated stomach may actually be palpable.

Metabolic features

Prolonged vomiting of gastric contents results in a characteristic series of electrolyte disturbances. Initially the major loss is fluid rich in hydrogen and chloride ions so that a minor degree of dehydration may accompany a hypochloraemic alkalosis. At this stage the serum sodium is usually normal and hypokalaemia may not be obvious. The more marked metabolic changes which accompany unrelieved gastric outlet obstruction result from a combination of continued losses with secondary changes in renal function. In the early stages the urine is characterized by a low chloride content and is appropriately alkaline because of enhanced bicarbonate excretion. This tends to compensate for the metabolic alkalosis, but it does so at the expense of losing sodium. If the gastric losses continue the patient thus becomes progressively more dehydrated and hyponatraemic. In an attempt to conserve circulating volume, sodium is retained by the kidneys and hydrogen ions and potassium are excreted preferentially. At this late stage, therefore, the patient with a metabolic alkalosis will have paradoxically acid urine. Hence the alkalosis becomes more severe and hypokalaemia is more marked. As a secondary effect of the alkalosis, the concentration of plasma-ionized calcium may fall so that disturbances of conscious level and tetany may be apparent.

Management

Gastric outlet obstruction due to chronic duodenal ulcer is treated by truncal vagotomy and gastroenterostomy. Other benign causes not associated with acid hypersecretion are managed with gastroenterostomy alone. Hourglass deformity and the teapot stenosis which are complications of gastric ulcer disease are best managed by gastrectomy if the patient's condition permits.

The priority in management of the advanced case of pyloric stenosis is correction of the fluid and electrolyte disturbances. Blood transfusion may be needed. This will often become apparent as dehydration is corrected and the spuriously high haemoglobin value falls to its actual level. Rehydration should be achieved by saline infusions with potassium supplements as indicated by electrolyte determinations. Provision of adequate sodium allows excretion of alkaline urine so that the alkalosis becomes correctable. Success is indicated by clinical improvement in the state of hydration, by an increase in urine output, a fall in blood urea and haematocrit, and restoration to normal of electrolyte concentrations.

Gastric lavage should be performed with a wide-bore tube using saline for irrigation. This should be performed twice daily initially and until the returning fluid is quite clear of particulate matter. The patient should not be allowed to eat, but fluids may be given, and milky drinks or elemental diets should be encouraged. One benefit of bed rest, rehydration, lavage and milk drinks is that an ulcer will begin to heal and with subsidence of the inflammatory changes the obstruction will begin to remit. Such improvement is often apparent even when the cause of the obstruction is a malignancy. There must be no undue rush over this stage of management which will often take a week or more. The objective is to get the patient into the best possible state for surgery, and it is a mistake to accept less than this ideal. During this time the patient will often benefit from chest physiotherapy. In nutritionally compromised patients, provision of adequate nutrition may require intravenous feeding. It may be difficult to make a firm clinical diagnosis of the cause of the pyloric stenosis. Even when the stomach has been well prepared, radiological studies may merely confirm outlet obstruction and fail to reveal the cause. Flexible endoscopy with biopsy is appropriate once the stomach is cleansed.

Sometimes pyloric stenosis first manifests itself when active ulcer disease within the duodenum has 'burnt itself out'. A non-operative approach to the problem may then be justifiable, particularly in the elderly or medically unfit patient. Balloon dilatation of the stenosed area, via an endoscope, can sometimes relieve the obstruction. Although this may need to be repeated at intervals of a few weeks for a period, on occasions this approach can obviate the need for surgery. The surgical treatment of benign pyloric stenosis caused by duodenal ulceration/fibrosis is by truncal vagotomy and posterior gastroenterostomy.

Gastric volvulus

Malrotation is associated with abnormal or incomplete fixation of the intestinal mesenteries so that acute twisting may occur. As commonly as volvulus, abnormal peritoneal bands associated with the intestinal malrotation (Ladd's bands) can cause duodenal obstruction.

The stomach is normally well anchored, particularly at the hiatus and pylorus. For volvulus to take place the points of tethering must be stretched and weakened. This can occur in patients with connective tissue disorders (e.g. Ehlers–Danlos syndrome), when there is extra space for the stomach to be pulled into (e.g. diaphragmatic or hiatal hernias, or anterior abdominal wall defects) or when a large tumour has caused lengthening of the connective attachments of the stomach. Volvulus can occur around two axes – mesenterico-axial or organo-axial (Figures 8.7 and 8.8). In either type the presentation may be with chronic symptoms of epigastric distress and vomiting. Acute volvulus, more common with the organo-axial variety, presents as severe pain and ineffectual retching.

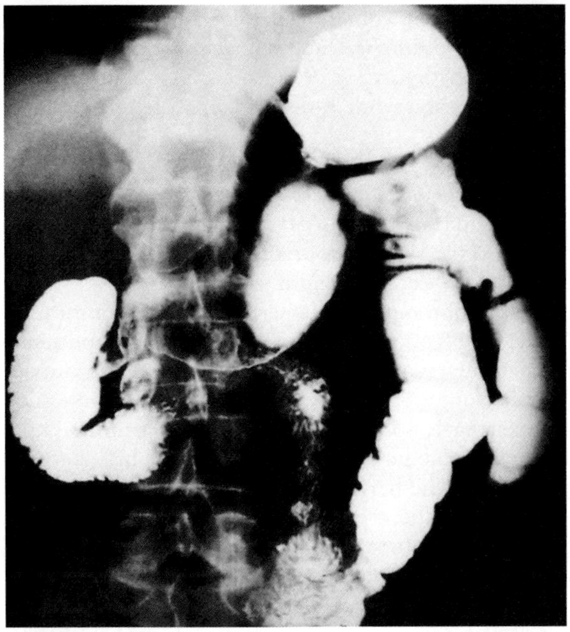

Figure 8.7 Gastric volvulus.

Distension, tenderness and signs of shock follow rapidly, and urgent surgery is indicated if strangulation and perforation are to be avoided. At operation the anatomy should be returned to normal and the stomach fixed with non-absorbable sutures. The predisposing cause should be dealt with if the patient's condition permits.

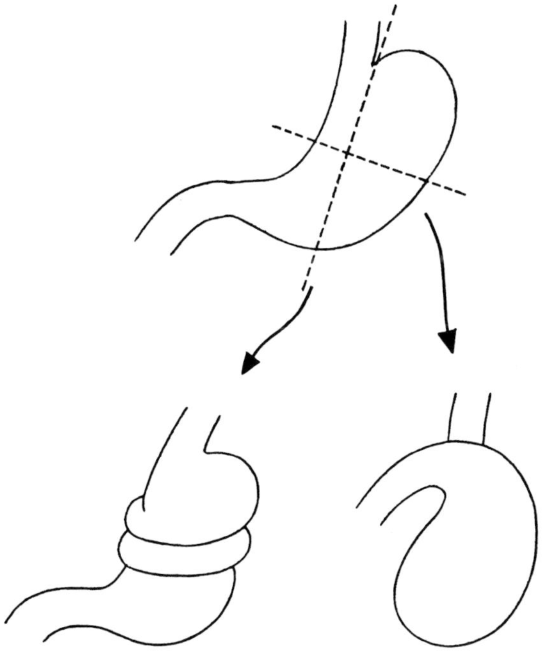

Figure 8.8 The two types of gastric volvulus: (a) organo-axial; (b) mesenterico-axial.

Haematemesis and melaena

Patients presenting with acute upper gastrointestinal haemorrhage still pose management problems and despite the advances in medical treatment, including diagnostic and interventional endoscopy, the overall mortality from acute upper gastrointestinal bleeding has not changed appreciably during the past decade and probably averages 20%, although there is sufficient evidence from good prospective and retrospective reports that with the appropriate management strategy, the hospital mortality of these patients can be reduced to 5%.

Aetiology

The causes of upper gastrointestinal haemorrhage are discussed in **Module 6, Vol. I**. The vast majority (> 90%) are caused by chronic peptic ulceration, NSAID-induced bleeding and oesophagogastric varices. On occasions the source of an acute upper gastrointestinal bleed may remain unknown. If the presenting problem is melaena alone and no blood is found in the stomach or duodenum on repeat endoscopy, then attention should turn to the lower small bowel and colon. Sometimes, however, there will be clear evidence of upper alimentary tract bleeding without apparent cause. In these patients the urge to intervene by laparotomy should be resisted until all efforts to establish the diagnosis have been exhausted. In these problematic cases, good emergency mesenteric angiography and small bowel enteroscopy often locate the source of the bleeding, allowing effective focused surgical intervention and obviating the totally unsatisfactory situation when a surgeon finds the gastrointestinal tract full of blood at operation with no palpable or macroscopic pathology being evident.

Chronic peptic ulcers

Despite the current more effective medical treatment, bleeding from duodenal and gastric ulcers still remains one of the common causes of life-threatening upper gastrointestinal haemorrhage. Some attribute the bleeding caused by NSAIDs to be largely due to the exacerbation of chronic ulcer disease, especially gastric ulcers in the elderly females. The problem inherent to bleeding peptic ulcers is their tendency to rebleed after spontaneous or therapeutic arrest. This propensity to recurrent haemorrhage has been attributed to the acid environment of the stomach and the proximal duodenum that impairs platelet aggregation and blood coagulation, and to the digestion of the clots by pepsin. In an interesting study on human volunteers, intraduodenal infusion of blood resulted in decreased pentagastrin-stimulated acid and pepsin secretion, suggesting a natural protective mechanism.

NSAID-induced bleeding

Aspirin and non-aspirin NSAID usage in the elderly is widespread in the general population and a recent population based study documented annual prevalence rates of 60% and 26% respectively. A meta-analysis of 16 studies has shown that NSAID users have a three-fold risk of gastrointestinal hemorrhage, surgery and death compared to non-users. The risk from bleeding is greatest:

- in the first few months of treatment
- in the elderly (>65 years)
- in patients with concomitant steroid use
- in patients with a previous history of gastrointestinal events.

The incidence of bleeding and perforation according to the Nottingham study is 1:6000 and 1:33 000 prescriptions respectively. Of all the NSAIDs known to cause bleeding or perforation (indomethacin, naproxen, etc.), aspirin produces the most damage. There is some evidence that the newer NSAIDs, e.g. nabumetone, that inhibit selectively cyclooxygenase-2 are less damaging to the gastroduodenal mucosa and hence significantly less ulcerogenic but they appear to be less effective clinically in relieving pain. The other problem with NSAIDs concerns the development of non-specific ulceration of the upper small intestinal mucosa in 8–9% of users. These can bleed and perforate.

Dieulafoy's lesion (exulceration simplex)
This was first described in 1978 and consists of a nodule containing a visible vessel covered with apparently normal mucosa. Some of the lesions have an overlying clot at the time of endoscopy. The diagnosis is difficult and is usually made after repeated endoscopic examinations. Treatment is by endoscopic electrocoagulation or sclerotherapy.

Portal hypertensive gastropathy
Although macroscopic abnormalities of the gastric mucosa are frequent in patients with cirrhosis and portal hypertension, clinically significant mucosal vascular changes causing bleeding and anaemia occur in a minority of these patients. This gastropathy occurs in patients with progressive liver damage and affects predominantly the fundus, although no region is exempt and the condition may be generalized (Figure 8.9). The histological appearances of portal congestive gastropathy consist of mucosal and submucosal vascular dilatation with little evidence of inflammatory changes.

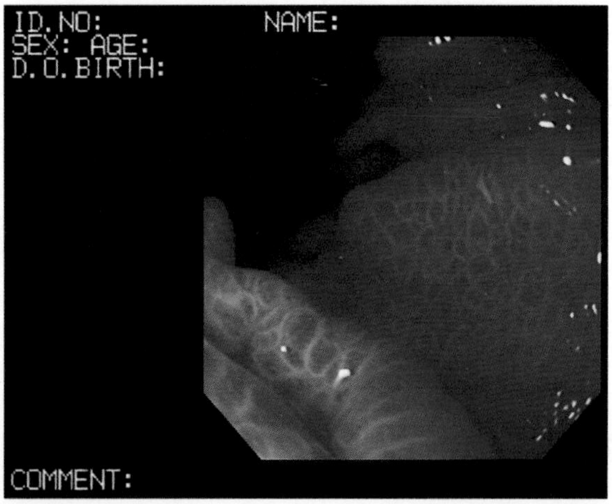

Figure 8.9 Endoscopic appearance of portal hypertensive gastropathy. (Courtesy of Dr John F Dillon, consultant gastroenterologist, Ninewells Hospital, Dundee, Scotland.)

Diffuse vascular ectasia (watermelon stomach)
This condition consists of ectatic mucosal sacculated vessels in the lamina propria traversing the antrum and sometimes the duodenum. Histology shows fibrin thrombi, fibromuscular hyperplasia and a significantly increased blood vessel area. The endoscopic appearance bears some resemblance to the stripes of a watermelon. The disorder presents with upper gastrointestinal haemorrhage. Some of the patients are cirrhotic but it is unclear whether all subjects have portal hypertension or indeed whether the underlying pathology is common to all patients who develop diffuse vascular ectasia which is usually associated with reduced acid secretion. The bleeding is often recurrent requiring multiple transfusions. The localized nature of the lesion renders it amenable to endoscopic electrocoagulation or sclerotherapy. The relationship between gastric vascular ectasia and portal hypertensive gastropathy remains unclear at the moment.

Tumours
Gastrointestinal haemorrhage may be caused by both benign and malignant tumours. Acute haemorrhage is, however, more commonly associated with benign lesions such as neurofibromatosis and mesenchymal (smooth muscle) tumours. Malignant tumours (carcinoma and lymphomas) more usually cause chronic blood loss with the development of iron-deficiency anaemia, although massive bleeding may be precipitated by combination chemotherapy (see below).

Chemotherapy
Life-threatening bleeding or perforation from necrosis of the tumour may complicate chemotherapy for gastrointestinal tumours especially lymphomas. The bleeding is aggravated by the frequent thrombocytopenia induced by the treatment. In addition to haematological support, surgical intervention with resection of the tumour (if possible) is indicated.

Stress ulceration
There has been a substantial decrease in the incidence of stress ulceration in intensive care units and this has been attributed to better methods of supportive care. Stress ulceration causing bleeding in intensive care patients is treated by ranitidine or sucralfate. The latter was shown to be marginally better in one clinical trial in that fewer transfusions were needed. In another study of patients with severe bleeding from stress ulceration, which had failed to respond to ranitidine, sucralfate administered via a nasogastric tube after gastric aspiration (to remove intragastric blood) in aliquots of 60 ml repeated every 2–4 hours resulted in cessation of the bleeding in all cases.

Aorto-enteric fistula

This usually complicates aortic replacement with prosthetic grafts but may arise spontaneously. The aetiology is thought to be graft infection. Small repeated warning haemorrhages usually precede catastrophic gastrointestinal bleeding. The acute episode often leads to fatal exsanguination although prompt aggressive surgical intervention with ligature of the aorta, removal of the graft and axillofemoral bypass may save some of these patients.

Duodenal diverticulum

Although fairly common (Figure 8.10), and usually located in the periampullary region, bleeding from a duodenal diverticulum is rare. Acute haemorrhage may be caused by erosion of a major vessel, bleeding ectopic gastric mucosa, an intradiverticular polyp or local inflammatory process. Duodenal diverticula are managed conservatively unless complications (bleeding or perforation) arise. A solitary duodenal diverticulum is a frequent occurrence. It does not usually cause bleeding but may pose difficulties with cannulation of the bile/pancreatic duct during ERCP. It also increases the risk of duodenal perforation in patients undergoing endoscopic sphincterotomy.

Management

The successful treatment of acute upper gastrointestinal haemorrhage demands aggressive treatment and a policy that is flexible enough to deal with the problems peculiar to the individual patient. There is good evidence that the best outcome is achieved by combined management between gastroenterologists and surgeons working as a team and in close co-operation from the time of admission of the patient. There are three phases in the management of the bleeding patient: resuscitation, diagnosis and definitive treatment [**see Module 6, Vol. I**].

Acute dilatation of the stomach

Acute dilatation of the stomach is a serious condition, which may cause death by aspiration. Although it is encountered most commonly as a complication of upper abdominal surgery (especially splenectomy) and pelvic surgery, it occurs in other situations including orthopaedic patients immobilized in plaster casts. It is more common in malnourished and debilitated patients. Other predisposing factors include aerophagy (apprehensive patients), excessive inadvertent distension of the stomach during endotracheal intubation and ventilation, administration of oxygen by nasal catheter, endoscopy with vigorous insufflation of gas and the use of opiate analgesia. Contrary to expectations, acute dilatation of the stomach is rarely encountered after surgery for gastric outlet obstruction. The exact aetiology is unknown. The stomach becomes atonic and this has been attributed to reflex inhibition of the myenteric neurones supplying the gastric musculature or failure of the gastric pacemaker.

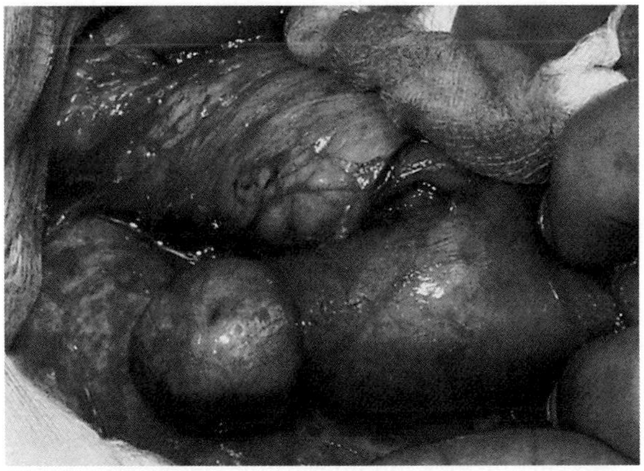

Figure 8.10 Duodenal diverticulum which caused upper gastrointestinal bleeding.

Acute dilatation of the stomach is well documented in patients (usually young females) suffering from anorexia nervosa or bulimia (compulsive eating followed by self-induced vomiting) and instances of gastric necrosis and rupture of the stomach have been reported in these patients. The suggested mechanisms for acute gastric dilatation in anorexia nervosa include muscular atrophy from starvation and neurogenic paralysis. In both conditions gastric necrosis supervenes when the intragastric pressure exceeds the gastric venous pressure.

The hugely dilated stomach, which may occupy the whole of the abdomen, is filled with dark blood-stained fluid. Evidence of hypovolaemia due to fluid and electrolyte sequestration is often present and the patient is frequently hypokalaemic. Premonitory symptoms include hiccups, vague feelings of unease in the epigastric region and small vomits that may contain altered blood. A gastric succussion splash is diagnostic. The more dramatic presentation which usually follows these symptoms but may occur *de novo* is either severe pain mimicking myocardial infarction or severe collapse from hypovolaemia (simulating pulmonary embolism) or sudden marked vomiting of litres of foul-smelling fluid with inevitable aspiration and the development of acute respiratory distress syndrome (ARDS; Mendelson's syndrome).

The treatment of this emergency situation is prompt decompression of the stomach by a large-bore nasogastric tube, preferably of the Salem sump suction variety, and replacement of the hypovolaemia and electrolyte deficit by crystalloid solutions. Pulmonary aspiration is treated by bronchoscopic suction and lavage, antibiotics and steroids together with endotracheal intubation and ventilatory support in the intensive care unit. The mortality of acute gastric dilatation accompanied by pulmonary aspiration remains high. Early detection of the condition with appropriate intervention will prevent the vast majority of these deaths.

Nasogastric suction

Routine nasogastric suction by a Ryle's tube was introduced as a precaution against complications such as acute gastric dilatation in all patients undergoing abdominal surgery. This practice is now considered unnecessary and indeed counterproductive as a number of prospective controlled clinical trials have demonstrated that the routine use of nasogastric suction is accompanied by a higher incidence of post-operative complications, delays recovery and induces considerable patient discomfort. In an effort to reduce gastric secretion, H_2-receptor antagonists (H_2RAs) have been administered but these agents do not impart any benefit and may indeed result in an increased incidence of infection as the suppression of acid secretion in the stomach is accompanied by bacterial proliferation.

Although routine prophylactic nasogastric decompression is not favoured, early therapeutic nasogastric suction is mandatory and is recommended in all patients in whom the ileus persists for more than 24 hours after the operation. Therapeutic nasogastric decompression is best achieved by the use of the Salem sump suction tube rather than the more popular single lumen Ryle's tube. If a nasogastric tube is considered necessary, then continuous drainage with intermittent aspiration to establish continuous patency is essential. There is never an indication to plug the tube and this amounts to bad practice since aside sfrom causing patient discomfort, the tube is not contributing any possible benefit to the patient under these circumstances.

Section 8.6 • Peptic ulcer disease

Although there are differences in the clinical picture, it is customary to consider duodenal and gastric ulcers together.

Epidemiology

In the Western world, the incidence and prevalence of duodenal ulcer disease and its complications increased from the beginning of the twentieth century to reach a peak in the period 1960–1970 and thereafter declined. During this same period the incidence of duodenal ulcer disease started to increase in other parts of the world such as Kenya and South Africa, suggesting an increased exposure to environmental ulcerogens. World-wide, duodenal ulcers are more common than gastric ulcers and there is a significantly higher incidence of duodenal ulceration in males at all age groups. In Africa and India almost all ulcers are duodenal and stenosis with obstruction is a frequent complication. In Europe duodenal ulcers are two to four times as common as gastric ulcers but there are some regional variations, e.g. duodenal ulcers are twice as frequent in Scotland than in England. Duodenal ulceration is fairly common in North America and gastric ulcer is probably less common than in Europe. Although duodenal ulcers are prevalent in Australia, a relatively high incidence of gastric ulcers is encountered in younger females.

Aetiology

Aside from genetic factors (increased prevalence of duodenal ulcers in patients with blood group O-non-secretors and in individuals with hyperpepsinogenaemia I), dietary factors, drug ingestion (NSAIDs) and smoking are important. The latter is associated both with an increased incidence of gastric and duodenal ulceration and with a higher relapse rate following successful healing by medication or surgical therapy.

The aetiology of peptic ulceration is varied and not completely understood. The most common causes are environmental ulcerogens (chemical or infective) acting in concert with factors that impair the gastric mucosal resistance to injury and the healing of mucosal lesions thereby leading to chronicity. This in turn is influenced by diet (vegetables and fruit) and social habits (smoking and alcohol).

Ulcerogens

These are environmental rather than endogenous and may be infective or chemical in nature. The most important infective agent that is responsible for peptic ulceration (duodenal and gastric) is *H. pylori*. Not all patients who are infected with this organism develop ulcers. The risk of peptic ulceration is determined by the severity of the *H. pylori* associated gastritis and not the titre of the *H. pylori* antibodies. The vacuolizing toxin of this organism appears to be involved in duodenal ulcer disease and undoubtedly the infection, by impairing the mucus-bicarbonate protective layer, plays an important role in the chronicity of the lesion, and the tendency to relapse as evidenced by the enhanced healing rates and reduced recurrence when the infection is eradicated by appropriate antibiotic therapy. Strains of *H. pylori* with vacA signal-sequence type S1A are associated with severe gastritis and duodenal ulcers, whereas vacA S2 strains cause mild gastric mucosal inflammation without ulceration. There is also evidence that strains of *H. pylori* that produce cytotoxin and induce a neutrophil oxidative burst are associated with peptic ulcer disease.

Patients with acute exacerbations of duodenal ulceration have higher levels of circulating antibodies to herpes simplex type I than controls and express greater than normal titres of antibodies to this virus in their duodenal contents. This has been implicated as a possible cause for some recurrent ulcers although treatment of duodenal ulcer subjects with acyclovir does not reduced the relapse rate.

The chemical ulcerogens include substances in food and drugs. Information on dietary ulcerogens is scanty apart from the association with excessive alcohol, coffee and cola consumption in the West. Although chronic ingestion of hot spicy foods is often incriminated, there has not been any good epidemiological evidence to support this hypothesis. By contrast, there is growing interest and information on dietary protective factors. These include a high-fibre diet, increased consumption of essential fatty acids (gamma-linolenic acid which is a prostaglandin precursor) and fresh green vegetables (particularly raw cabbage and lentils). However, the importance and influence of these anti-ulcerogens in the incidence of peptic ulcer disease remain to be established although it is likely that they protect against gastroduodenal disease in *H. pylori* infected individuals.

The most important group of chemical ulcerogens is constituted by aspirin and other NSAIDs. These are the commonest cause of peptic ulceration in *H. pylori* negative individuals. However, these drugs cannot be regarded as specific gastroduodenal ulcerogens since they also induce damage and ulceration of the small and large intestine. There are some differences between ulcers cause by *H. pylori* and those caused by NSAIDs. These include:

- NSAID-associated ulcers are more likely to cause gastrointestinal haemorrhage. Thus overall 75% of patients with upper gastrointestinal bleeding from peptic ulcers are on NSAID medication.
- Gastric ulcers caused by *H. pylori* are rarely encountered on the greater curve (5%), being most commonly situated on the lesser curve (85%), whereas NSAIDs ulcers (in the absence of *H. pylori infection*) occur along the lesser and greater curvatures in 35% and 45% respectively.

The exact relation between NSAID usage and *H. pylori* infection in the pathogenesis of peptic ulcer disease has not been resolved. *Helicobader pylori* infection and NSAID usage is encountered in 20% of patients. Eradication of the infection does not appear to influence the healing and recurrence of gastric and duodenal ulcers associated with chronic NSAID medication. Other drugs that can cause both gastric and duodenal ulcers include cocaine and amphetamines.

Role of acid and pepsin

The maxim 'no acid, no ulcer' is no longer tenable. Although some 30–40% of duodenal ulcer patients exhibit acid hypersecretion and there are well-established syndromes of persistent gastric hypersecretion associated with intractable ulceration, the overlap between the acid secretory status of duodenal ulcer patients and controls is considerable and there are many 'normal individuals' who hypersecrete acid and do not develop ulcers. Furthermore, duodenal ulcers can develop in individuals with normal or even reduced gastric acid output and almost all patients with gastric ulcers have normal or reduced acid secretion. None the less, gastric acid is an important factor in the chronicity of the disease and undoubtedly suppression of acid secretion by medical or surgical treatment permits healing in the majority of patients. The secretory characteristics of the usual duodenal ulcer patients (the norm as distinct from all patients) include an increased acid secretory capacity (enlarged parietal cell mass and enhanced maximal acid output in response to pentagastrin), increased gastrin response to food and insulin, increased sensitivity to gastrin and defective inhibition of acid secretion (normally elicited by antral acidification, antral distension and intraduodenal fat). There is an increased concentration of pepsins in the gastric juice of patients with duodenal ulceration, especially pepsin I which is the most mucolytic. The disruption of the mucus-bicarbonate layer by pepsin I exposes the underlying mucosa to injury by ulcerogens and impairs healing by removal of the protective mucous cap (blister effect).

Impaired healing and chronicity

The chronic nature of peptic ulcers implies impaired healing of a mucosal injury. This important aspect of the pathogenesis of ulcer disease has been previously overlooked but has received considerable attention in recent years in view of its crucial importance in treatment of the ulcer diathesis. The exact mechanisms involved in the impaired healing process are still poorly understood but are likely to be multifactorial and involve defective cellular migration and proliferation, inadequate supply or degradation of important growth factors such as salivary EGF, down-regulation of EGF receptors, persistent *H. pylori* infection with destruction of the protective mucous gel cap under which re-epithelization of a mucosal defect proceeds without further injury by acid and pepsin, low tissue pO_2, changes in the ulcer base and intraluminal factors (in the gastric juice). A recent interesting observation is the slower healing of gastric ulcers arising in normal gastric mucosa when compared to those that develop in areas of atrophic gastritis. It seems likely that the increased proliferation of the gastric mucosal cells that characterizes atrophic gastritis is responsible for the rapid healing of ulcers in gastritic mucosa.

Other factors

Enterogastric reflux of bile salts and lysolecithin with destruction of the mucus-bicarbonate layer and mucosal injury was first suggested by Capper as the cause of gastric ulceration. Although bile salts in particular can lead to back-diffusion of acid following disruption of the mucous gel, this theory has never been conclusively proven. Similarly antral stasis with delayed gastric emptying resulting in antral distension and increased gastrin release has been implicated in the development of pyloric channel and pre-pyloric ulcers. As a group, these 'gastric' ulcers behave like duodenal ulcers and tend to be associated with hyperacidity as distinct from the more usual proximal gastric ulcers, which originate on a background of normal or hypoacidity and are often accompanied by atrophic gastritis. Despite the extensive literature on the potential vascular cause of ulcers as exemplified by instances of gastric ulceration after highly selective vagotomy and in association with mesenteric ischaemia or experimental restriction of the blood supply to the stomach in animals, there has been no confirmation that focal vascular insufficiency is important in the pathogenesis of peptic ulcer disease.

Peptic ulcers occur at specific local sites: duodenal ulcers in the bulb, gastric ulcers at the antropyloric junction on the lesser curve, etc. This has been interpreted as indicative of trauma resulting from the action of ulcerogens being specifically directed to these sites. Frequently quoted examples illustrative of this effect include the lesser curve location of gastric ulcers following reflux of duodenal contents and the occurrence of 'sump ulcers' following ingestion of ulcerogenic tablets which gravitate to the most dependent part of the stomach. The same mechanism has been proposed by Kirk for explaining the location of duodenal ulcers, i.e. the 'jets' of gastric contents repeatedly hit the duodenal bulb in the same region causing focal ulceration. There are other explanations, which have been proposed to explain the localized nature of peptic ulcers. These include the concepts of mucosal boundaries, adverse strain-inducing relationships between the mucosa and the underlying musculature and the distribution of the mucosal and submucosal blood vessels. Undoubtedly some junctional mucosal ulcers, typified by pre-pyloric ulcers are notoriously resistant to healing. The kinetic strain imposed by the circular muscle on the fundopyloric mucosal boundary in the case of lesser curve gastric ulcers; and where the pyloric musculature ends (in duodenal ulcers), is an attractive though unconfirmed hypothesis.

Stress induces gastric hypersecretion and can lead to acute (stress) ulceration in seriously ill patients. In the more common situation, stress is regarded as an aggravating factor rather than primary cause and in this respect there is an important individual predisposition determined by personality traits and environmental factors, which may arise early in life. However, there is no evidence that patients with ulcer disease are psychologically or psychiatrically different from normal before the onset of the disease. Uncommonly, duodenal ulceration may be associated with other disorders, which include liver disease (particularly after shunt surgery), persistent hypercalcaemia, renal failure and after massive small bowel resection.

Clinical features

Chronic duodenal ulceration

This occurs at all age groups but the peak incidence is between 25 and 50 years. Whereas mortality caused by duodenal ulceration is low to negligible in this age range, the age-specific death rate (from complications of the disease) rises to 24/100 000 and 7/100 000 above 65 years in males and females respectively. This difference in mortality is due to the significantly higher incidence of duodenal ulceration in males with a sex ratio of 2–4:1. Duodenal ulceration is a remitting disease characterized by periods of activity and quiescence. Exacerbations may be associated with periods of stress, dietary or alcoholic indiscretions and smoking. It tends to have a seasonal variation. Early in the history of the disease, remissions may be associated with complete healing of the ulcer, but as the disease progresses, there is a tendency towards fibrous scarring so that evidence of past disease may be found on investigation even when the patient is free from symptoms. Typically, the epigastric pain is experienced during fasting (hunger pain) when the stomach is empty and there is nothing to buffer the acid secretions. Relief usually follows eating, ingestion of milk or alkalis. Failure to produce relief, particularly if the pain radiates to the back, is suggestive of posterior ulcer penetration into the pancreas. The post-prandial pain relief lasts for varying periods but usually averages several hours before it recurs and often occurs at night waking the patient up. Vomiting is not usually a feature of uncomplicated disease but may develop in severe exacerbation of an inflamed ulcer with surrounding gross oedema of the duodenal bulb or result from fibrosis causing organic outlet obstruction (pyloric/duodenal stenosis).

As the patients are constantly nibbling food to ward off painful indigestion, they are usually overweight. Other than this, physical signs may amount to no more than diffuse epigastric tenderness, although this is sometimes well localized. Occult bleeding may produce marked iron-deficiency anaemia. The presence of a succussion splash indicates delayed gastric emptying.

Chronic gastric ulcer

Chronic ulceration of the stomach is less common than that in the duodenum in most countries, the ratio of gastric to duodenal ulcers varying from 1:4 to 1:20. There are two quite distinct types of gastric ulcer: type I, which occurs in the body of the stomach along the lesser curve, and type II, which is referred to as the pyloric channel ulcer and includes pre-pyloric ulcers. The natural history, acid secretory profile and therapeutic response of type II ulcers are akin to those of duodenal ulceration. Type I chronic gastric ulcer may arise in a normal mucosa or on a mucosal background of atrophic gastritis. The disease is not associated with hyperacidity and indeed hypoacidity is frequently encountered, particularly in patients with atrophic gastritis. There is a male preponderance but this is not as marked as in duodenal ulceration and the peak incidence is encountered after middle age. The age-specific mortality from complicated gastric ulcer disease in patients above the age of 65 years is 57/100 000 and 42/100 000 in males and females respectively.

Gastric ulceration is most commonly encountered in late middle-aged and elderly patients. In Australia an association with chronic ingestion of NSAIDs and the relatively high prevalence in younger females has been documented. The association with chronic ill health and lower socioeconomic class is not as obvious as it was early in the twentieth century. The main clinical feature is pain, or perhaps more commonly a feeling of acute discomfort and fullness in the epigastrium. Unlike duodenal ulcer, the pain of gastric ulceration is not experienced during fasting when the stomach is empty. Indeed, the converse is true, as eating produces or exacerbates the pain. For this reason, patients suffering from the disease are afraid of eating and because of the reduced dietary intake, they are usually underweight. It is important to stress that this symptom complex of indigestion immediately after meals and weight loss is indistinguishable from that produced by gastric cancer and clinically it is impossible to differentiate between the two disorders unless the cancer is advanced and incurable. Nausea and vomiting are more common symptoms than in duodenal ulcer, even in the absence of outlet obstruction. Although periodicity with remissions and relapses of symptoms is encountered, this is not as obvious as in duodenal ulceration.

Aside from weight loss, physical examination is not usually rewarding, with epigastric tenderness being the only fairly consistent finding. Gastric ulcers may obstruct, perforate or bleed. Occasionally, a large inflammatory mass around an ulcer may be palpable, particularly if the patient has lost weight, but for all practical purposes, a palpable epigastric mass in a patient with this dyspeptic background indicates advanced gastric cancer.

Investigations

In most centres upper gastrointestinal endoscopy has replaced double contrast barium meals because of the greater diagnostic accuracy. In patients with duodenal ulcer the findings vary from a definite crater in the first part of the duodenum to severe duodenitis. Endoscopic biopsy of the antrum is necessary for establishing the *H. pylori* status but the ulcer itself should not be biopsied as it is always benign and the biopsy may precipitate bleeding. Although double contrast barium meal carries a high diagnostic yield and, if performed expertly, will differentiate benign gastric ulcer disease from early ulcerating cancer, endoscopy and multiple biopsies with brush cytology are mandatory in all patients with gastric ulceration. The *H. pylori* status is best determined on the endoscopic biopsies (histology). Furthermore, the endoscopy should be repeated after 2–3 months and if the ulcer healing is not documented, further biopsies are taken and surgical treatment is indicated even if the second biopsies are reported as benign.

Medical treatment of ulcer disease

Until the recognition of the importance of *H. pylori* in the pathogenesis of peptic ulcer disease medical therapy was based on acid suppression. Whereas there is little doubt concerning the efficacy of ulcer healing by inhibitors of gastric acid secretion, there are several problems with this therapy, the most important of which is ulcer recurrence. For this reason, the mortality from complications of ulcer disease did not decline with the introduction of effective acid reducing drugs. The most commonly used anti-secretory agents for peptic ulcer disease are the H_2RAs. There is little to choose between the various agents currently available except that information confirming long-term safety is available for cimetidine and ranitidine only. A therapeutic course should last 2–3 months and heals 90% of ulcers with symptom relief being achieved within 2–3 days of initiation of therapy. PPI, e.g. omeprazole, lanzoprazole, and are more effective because they achieve complete (but reversible) acid inhibition and virtually heal all ulcers including ulcers resistant to H_2RAs.

The main problem with the H_2RAs and PPIs concerns recurrence, which is universal unless maintenance therapy is continued indefinitely. Even so, a proportion of patients 'break through' maintenance treatment. The cumulative rate of symptomatic relapse (which underestimates the true relapse rate) during 5 years' maintenance treatment is 16% and 26% for ranitidine and cimetidine respectively. The groups which are likely to recur despite maintenance therapy include patients whose ulcers were slow to heal in the first instance, those with pre-pyloric ulcers, smokers and patients with high gastric secretory capacity. Other problems that arise as a result of the need for long-term indefinite maintenance therapy include decreasing compliance and increasing costs. Undoubtedly, the most effective anti-secretory agents for healing both duodenal and gastric ulcers are the PPIs. Again maintenance therapy is required to prevent relapse. There are, however, justifiable fears relating to the long-term use of these PPIs, which induce total achlorhydria, sustained hypergastrinaemia and proliferation of the gastric fundic endocrine cells and G cells in the rats with the development of carcinoid tumours. Although initial reports showed no effect on the endocrine cell population of the gastric fundic mucosa in patients with the Zollinger-Ellison syndrome on long-term therapy with omeprazole, instances of carcinoid tumours developing in such patients have now been documented. Another worry concerning protracted use of omeprazole is the overgrowth of nitrosating bacteria, which inevitably follows the achlorhydria induced by this drug, leading to excess formation of N-nitroso compounds. Sucralfate appears useful in maintenance therapy for gastric ulcers. Bismuth is accompanied by a low recurrence rate, presumably because it eradicates *H. pylori*. The synthetic prostaglandin analogues have been disappointing and yield inferior ulcer healing rates to the H_2RAs.

In patients who are *H. pylori* positive, acid suppression has been replaced with eradication therapy which now constitutes the first line treatment. Initially this was referred to as triple therapy because of the original three-drug regimen (bismuth, metronidazole or tinidazole and amoxycillin) which was administered for 4 weeks. There are now several eradication regimens administered over a 1–2 week period:

- dual therapy – combination of an antibiotic with omeprazole
- bismuth-based triple therapy
- triple therapy with PPI and two antibiotics (clarithromycin + amoxycillin or metronidazole
- quadruple therapy (PPI, bismuth, metronidazole and tetracycline)
- ranitidine bismuth citrate (RBC) and two antibiotics.

Current eradication therapy results in average permanent healing rates without recurrence in 90% (range 81–100%). Eradication therapy has however some limitations:

- The incidence of *H. pylori* ulcers is declining rapidly in many countries and in some *H. pylori* infection prevalence rates are as low as 10%.
- Eradication therapy fails in 10–19% of patients due to several factors: non-compliance, bacterial resistance.
- Treatment related issues – the eradication regimen used and its duration.
- Re-infection.

There is a high incidence of failure when the infection is caused by cagA-strains. Rescue treatment is indicated in patients in whom eradication therapy fails. This should always include three drugs (triple therapy) and the course should be given for at least 2 weeks. If bacterial resistance is documented by culture (usually resistance to metronidazole or clarithromycin), these antibiotics are replaced and an RBC based triple therapy used.

Indications for surgical treatment of ulcer disease

Elective surgery for duodenal ulcer disease has declined substantially during the past 20 years and is now largely restricted to the treatment of complicated disease. The situation may however change as the prevalence of *H. pylori* infection declines. Even in *H. pylori* positive patients, gastroenterologists now acknowledge the real problem with failures of re-eradication therapy since long-term acid suppression therapy is costly and attended by poor compliance. Laparoscopic elective ulcer surgery may well provide the answer to these resistant ulcers.

Operations for duodenal ulcer

The aim of all operations for uncomplicated duodenal ulceration is to reduce acid secretion to such levels that the ulcer will heal permanently. The only exception to this is the operation of gastroenterostomy, which aims at directing acid away from the area of ulceration. Although effective, this procedure is attended by a high incidence of anastomotic or jejunal ulceration, amounting perhaps to 50% in the long term. Thus this operation is seldom used except in some elderly patients with pyloric stenosis. In the majority of patients, the surgeon is faced with the choice of gastric resection (to reduce the size of the parietal cell mass and remove the antrum – the source of the gastric phase of secretion), vagal denervation (to abolish the cephalic phase of secretion and reduce the sensitivity of the parietal cells to secretory stimuli), or a combination of the two. Although the purpose of the operation is to achieve permanent cure of the ulcer diathesis, this is not the only consideration, and a comparison of the various procedures demands that operative morbidity and mortality, and the incidence of side-effects need to be weighed carefully against success rate in terms of recurrent ulcer risk.

The relative advantages and disadvantages of gastrectomy, vagotomy and drainage, and highly selective vagotomy, are summarized in Figure 8.11. Subtotal gastrectomy with gastrojejunal anastomosis is an excellent anti-ulcer operation, but its merits are seriously marred by the increased morbidity and mortality which would be expected to follow a return to the widespread use of this operation, as well as the incidence of troublesome side-effects and nutritional sequelae. The initial hope that the operation of truncal vagotomy and drainage would avoid the problems of alimentary side-effects and maintain good nutrition has not materialized, and many surgeons feel dissatisfied with this approach. Truncal vagotomy and antrectomy possesses the advantages of a dual attack on acid secretory mechanisms, and as a result carries the lowest recurrent ulcer risk. Unfortunately, it incurs the disadvantages of both resection and vagotomy. Truncal vagotomy and antrectomy is probably the operation of choice for resistant ulcers, including pyloric channel and pre-pyloric ulcers, as these are attended by high recurrence rates.

Vagotomy procedures

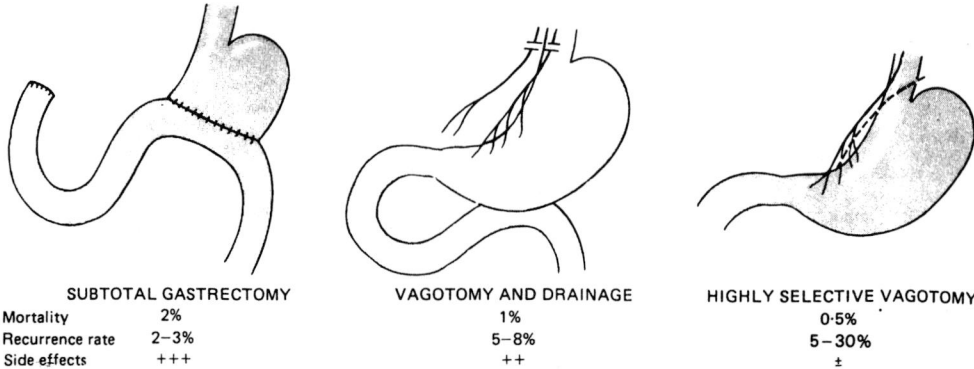

The alternatives to truncal vagotomy and drainage are bilateral selective vagotomy with drainage, highly selective vagotomy (parietal cell, proximal gastric, selective proximal gastric), posterior truncal vagotomy and ante-

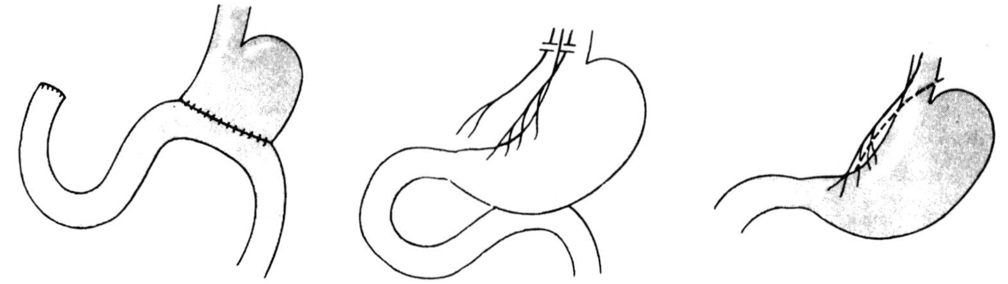

	SUBTOTAL GASTRECTOMY	VAGOTOMY AND DRAINAGE	HIGHLY SELECTIVE VAGOTOMY
Mortality	2%	1%	0·5%
Recurrence rate	2–3%	5–8%	5–30%
Side effects	+++	++	±

Figure 8.11 The relative advantages and disadvantages of various operative procedures used for chronic duodenal ulceration. The figures given for mortality and recurrence rates are average values only. Choice of the 'best' operation involves a careful balance of these three factors.

rior seromyotomy, posterior truncal vagotomy and anterior highly selective vagotomy.

Bilateral selective vagotomy confines the denervation to the stomach and preserves the vagal branches to the liver (hepatic plexus). The operation requires additional gastric drainage as the antrum is denervated. Gastric stasis and ulceration have been documented in patients in whom drainage was omitted. Although bilateral selective vagotomy does reduce the incidence of diarrhoea and achieves adequate gastric denervation, the overall clinical results obtained by this procedure have been no better than those of truncal vagotomy with drainage, and for this reason, the operation has been largely abandoned.

Undoubtedly, HSV is the most physiological procedure since it denervates the parietal cell mass but leaves the antral mill (antropyloric segment) innervated and therefore obviates the need for a drainage procedure. Herein lies the distinct advantage of this operation as the avoidance of drainage leads to a virtual abolition of the alimentary side-effects, although diarrhoea can still occur, albeit extremely rarely. The drawback of HSV is the higher incidence of recurrent ulceration documented by some long-term reports (20–30%). These reports have, however, included cases for which HSV is unsuitable. Thus the operation should not be performed in patients with pyloric channel ulcers (including pre-pyloric), in patients with stenosis (previously these were managed with HSV and pyloric dilatation) and in patients with bleeding ulcers. There is some controversy regarding the efficacy of HSV in patients with ulcers resistant to H_2RAs. In the author's experience these patients are best managed by truncal vagotomy and antrectomy.

Alternatives to HSV include the Taylor procedure (posterior truncal vagotomy and anterior seromyotomy) and the Hill procedure (posterior truncal vagotomy and anterior highly selective vagotomy). Several reports and one clinical trial have demonstrated that the Taylor procedure gives equivalent results to the classical HSV. There have been no large series or clinical trials with the Hill procedure, although on a priori grounds it should achieve equivalent results to these two procedures.

Drainage procedures

Truncal vagotomy and bilateral selective vagotomy necessitate a drainage procedure. This can be achieved by posterior gastrojejunostomy or pyloroplasty. Controlled clinical trials have not indicated any obvious superiority of one procedure over the other, but there are some important practical considerations. Bile vomiting is slightly commoner after gastroenterostomy but this is offset by a slightly higher incidence of dumping after pyloroplasty. Gastroenterostomy is a safer alternative when the ulcer area is the seat of an inflammatory mass or when there is significant fibrous scarring. If a post-vagotomy patient develops bile vomiting or dumping, it is easy to close the gastroenterostomy. By contrast, reconstruction of the pylorus is more demanding and the results are less certain.

Operations for gastric ulcer

The objectives of gastric ulcer surgery are the removal of the ulcer, thus dealing with the problem of possible malignancy, and prevention of further ulcer recurrence. Ideally the ulcer should be removed as part of a gastrectomy procedure but on occasion local excision of the ulcer is combined with vagotomy. The standard treatment is the Billroth I gastrectomy. This resection includes the ulcer, the lesser curve and the antrum. Restoration of continuity by gastroduodenal anastomosis is seldom a problem as the duodenum is normal. Both the mortality and the ulcer recurrence rate following this procedure are low (2%) and it is now acknowledged as the standard treatment for gastric ulcer disease. Post-operative alimentary side-effects can follow this operation but their frequency and severity are less than those encountered after Polya-gastrectomy and truncal vagotomy with drainage. Likewise, long-term nutritional problems are not usually marked or frequent after Billroth I gastrectomy.

The main alternative to gastrectomy in the treatment of gastric ulcer is vagotomy and drainage, which carries a lower operative mortality (1%). If this operation is used, it is ideally combined with local excision of the ulcer. If this is not possible because of the ulcer location, then a full-thickness biopsy of the lesion is mandatory. The recurrence rate after truncal vagotomy and drainage with excision of the gastric ulcer is high and averages 10–20% in the long term. Furthermore, the symptomatic results, in terms of alimentary problems, are no better than those achieved by gastrectomy. There is therefore little justification in using this operation as the routine surgical procedure for uncomplicated type I gastric ulcer. It is, however, indicated in the poor-risk elderly patient. The reported experience of HSV with ulcer excision is limited but the results appear to approximate to those achieved by truncal vagotomy and drainage, although one report documented an unacceptably high recurrence rate.

A special problem is posed by the high lesser curve ulcer situated at the cardio-oesophageal junction. The options here include a resection distal to the ulcer, leaving it *in situ* (Kelling-Madlener procedure) or, preferably, to excise all the lesser curve using the Pauchet type of gastrectomy where the new lesser curve is reconstituted without the use of clamps. Unfortunately, very high lesser curve ulcers are often encountered in the elderly where the questions of malignancy and operative mortality are especially pertinent. Proximal or total gastrectomy are inadvisable in these patients and whenever possible medical therapy should be persisted with. An HSV with local excision of the ulcer is considered for patients who prove refractory to medical treatment.

Some 30% of patients with lesser curve ulceration are said to have evidence of past or present duodenal ulceration. Such ulcers have been designated as type III. It is usually assumed that the duodenal ulcer precedes the gastric, but the precise relationship is not always clear. In theory, both delayed gastric emptying from pyloric stenosis or bile reflux through an incompetent diseased duodenal bulb could be responsible for the gastric ulcer. In practice, the evidence for both these theories is not impressive.

Gastric ulcers coexisting with duodenal ulcer disease tend to be situated fairly distally in the stomach, usually at or beyond the incisura. Levels of gastric acid secretion are normal or high, but below levels found in patients with duodenal ulcer disease alone. Surgical treatment of combined ulcer disease is by the operation normally favoured by the surgeon for duodenal ulcer. The risk of the gastric ulcer being malignant when it is associated with a duodenal ulcer is small but, none the less, present. In one large series, gastric carcinoma was present in 8% of patients with gastric ulcer alone and 1.2% of patients with coexisting duodenal ulceration. All forms of gastric ulcer must be biopsied.

Laparoscopic elective ulcer surgery

All these elective operations for peptic ulcer disease can be performed laparoscopically. The laparoscopically assisted approach is particularly suited to partial gastrectomy as the small midline incision enables a more functionally effective reconstruction after the resection. Hand access devices are now available that permit the insertion/withdrawal of the surgeon's hand without loss of pneumoperitoneum (Figure 8.12a, b). They expedite complex operations such as partial gastrectomy and permit the conduct of these operations even in the presence of obesity. Hand assisted laparoscopic surgery (HALS) is likely to replace the laparoscopically assisted approach as the assisting hand of the surgeon is used throughout the operation for exposure and controlled traction. The laparoscopic operations have been shown to achieve the same acid reduction and ulcer healing rates as the equivalent open operations in the short term. The advantage of these laparoscopic operations over the conventional open procedures is the short hospital stay and the accelerated recovery to full activity. It seems likely that laparoscopic ulcer surgery may play a role in the management of intractable ulcer disease following failure of eradication therapy.

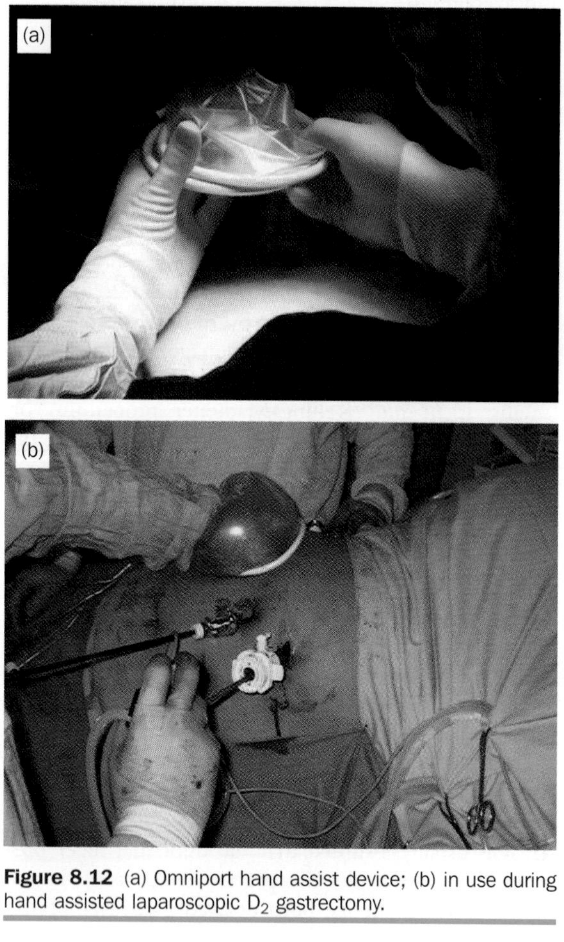

Figure 8.12 (a) Omniport hand assist device; (b) in use during hand assisted laparoscopic D_2 gastrectomy.

Section 8.7 • Failures of gastric surgery

Unsatisfactory results follow ulcer surgery in 10–20% of patients. The reported incidence varies considerably and no doubt depends, to some extent, on the thoroughness and length of follow-up. Poor results may be due to recurrent ulceration, alimentary side-effects or adverse nutritional consequences. Thus the failures of gastrectomy are largely nutritional or due to post-cibal or alimentary sequelae and rarely caused by recurrent ulceration, with the opposite being the case after HSV. The poor results of truncal vagotomy and drainage may be due to either recurrent ulceration or functional alimentary side-effects.

Recurrent ulcer

Recurrence of type I gastric ulcer after an appropriate gastrectomy is rare, so the problem concerns mainly duodenal and pyloric channel ulcers (type II). Recurrent ulceration may appear in the stomach, the duodenum, or at the site of the gastrointestinal stoma. The overall rate depends on the procedure performed, the ulcer type and smoking. Thus the highest recurrent ulcer rates are reported after HSV and the lowest after truncal vagotomy and antrectomy. Pre-pyloric ulcers exhibit a higher recurrence rate than duodenal ulcers. A Swedish study has demonstrated that continued smoking is an important factor and resulted in a recurrence rate of 24% as opposed to 7% in non-smokers after HSV. Several studies over the years have confirmed that the two most important factors are inadequate vagotomy and incomplete drainage (gastric hold-up) and these probably account for 80% of recurrences. It should be stressed, however, that these data on recurrent ulceration after surgical treatment pre-date the *H. pylori* era.

The laboratory tests associated with recurrent ulcer after surgical treatment are shown in Table 8.6. In patients with recurrent ulcer after vagotomy with drainage or antrectomy, the basal serum pepsinogen I (PG I) levels are significantly higher than in patients without recurrence. Furthermore, following injection of beta-

Table 8.6 Laboratory findings associated with recurrent ulcer after surgery

Test	
Basal acid output	>4 mmol/hour
Post-op % reduction of basal acid output	>70%
Maximal acid output	>25 mmol/hour
Post-op % reduction of maximal acid output	<50%
Insulin test	Positive
Sham feeding test	Positive
Basal serum group I pepsinogen	>100 ng/ml
Betazole stimulated group I pepsinogen	>100% of basal

zole, patients with recurrent ulcer exhibit a rise in the serum PG I level whereas those without (or with a complete vagotomy) demonstrate a paradoxical decrease in the serum level of this pepsinogen. Rare causes include inadequate gastric resection, retained antrum, Zollinger–Ellison syndrome and hypercalcaemia.

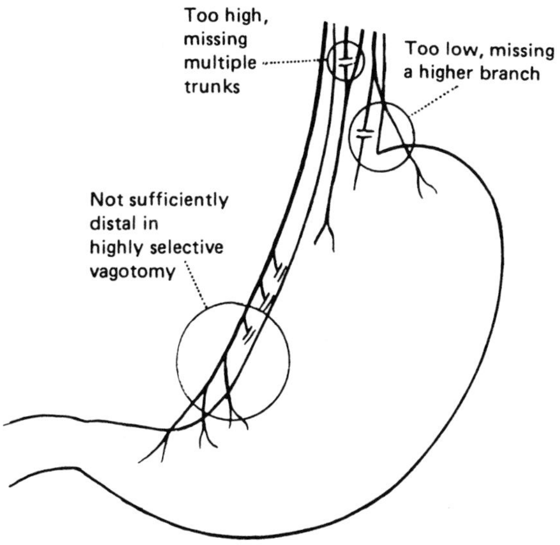

Figure 8.13 The causes of incomplete vagotomy.

Inadequate vagotomy

Failure to achieve complete denervation of the parietal cell mass is the commonest cause of recurrent ulceration. The incidence of incomplete vagotomy may be as high as 20% after truncal vagotomy, as judged by the results of the early post-operative insulin tests. It is true that some of these positive tests are only technically positive and may be the result of very small fibres only, but some are due to a major vagal trunk, which is missed, and under these circumstances recurrence is inevitable. Peroperative tests have been described which are reputed to improve visualization of the nerve fibres (leucomethylene blue) or permit a check on the completeness of the vagotomy by observing a failure of peristalsis or absence of acid secretion after electrical stimulation after pentagastrin or histamine infusion (as shown by an intragastric dye, Congo red, or pH probe). In practice, these techniques are all time-consuming, give variable results and have not become established in routine practice. The most important prerequisites for successful vagotomy are appreciation of the variable anatomy of the vagus, patience and meticulous technique.

Truncal vagotomy can be carried out at two levels: the hiatus or above (as advocated by Dragstedt), or at the cardia. At either level, it is possible to miss vagal fibres (Figure 8.13), although there is less liability to overlook a significant trunk if the vagotomy is carried low down on the oesophagus. The solution to the problem is to divide the anterior and the posterior trunks at the hiatus initially. This will enable the oesophagus to be pulled down and the region of the cardia then becomes more accessible. The lower oesophagus is then cleared methodically all the way round of all nerve fibres down to the longitudinal muscular fibres. With this length of abdominal oesophagus cleared, it is quite easy to inspect the region of the fundus and thus ensure against missing nerve fibres (Grassi) to this region.

If complete parietal cell denervation is to be achieved by HSV, three aspects of the technique need special attention. Clearance of at least 5 cm of the distal oesophagus is mandatory. In addition, the lesser curve denervation must be carried out distally far enough to ensure that the parietal cell mass is completely denervated. In practice, this means leaving only one recognizable antral branch of the nerve of Latarget. Finally, the innervation of the fundus by the nerves of Grassi must be disrupted.

Antral stasis

This arises when there is duodenal fibrosis. Previously these cases were treated by pyloric dilatation during HSV. Undoubtedly this has been one of the factors involved in ulcer recurrence after this procedure. Nowadays it is recognized that these patients require a drainage operation. The nature of the vagotomy (HSV or truncal) then becomes a matter of individual choice. Another unsatisfactory practice is the performance of bilateral truncal vagotomy without drainage. The ulcer recurrence (usually pyloric channel) in these patients with time is unacceptably high. This operation is bad whether performed transthoracically, thoracoscopically, abdominally or laparoscopically.

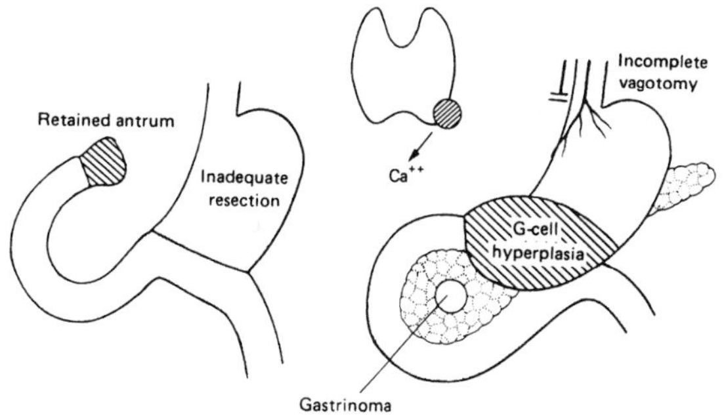

Figure 8.14 The causes of recurrent duodenal or stomal ulceration after previous ulcer surgery.

Rare causes of ulcer recurrence

These include inadequate gastric resection, retained gastric antrum, the Zollinger–Ellison syndrome and hypercalcaemia (Figure 8.14).

Inadequate gastric resection

If gastrectomy is the method used for reducing acid secretion, a 75% resection is needed. A related consideration is the method of restoring continuity after resection. In terms of ulcer recurrence, it is generally believed that a gastrojejunal anastomosis (Billroth II, Polya) is better than gastroduodenostomy although it is difficult to substantiate this claim with certainty from the published literature. The difference in ulcer recurrence rates may be related more to the extent of gastric resection since more stomach is likely to be retained in Billroth I operations to achieve a gastroduodenal anastomosis without tension.

Retained gastric antrum

If retained antral tissue (after gastric resection) is left in continuity with the duodenal stump, the antral G cells, now in a permanent alkaline environment, will secrete gastrin continuously. Under this constant stimulus, the remaining parietal cells will produce sufficient acid for stomal ulceration to develop. Whenever hypergastrinaemia is found after partial gastrectomy, the retained antrum syndrome must be considered. Differentiation of this condition from autonomous tumour production of gastrin is usually possible from the results of the secretin and calcium tests, but direct confirmation of retained antral tissue may be more difficult. Radioisotope scanning with pertechnetate may help. Treatment entails excision of the retained antral tissue.

Zollinger–Ellison syndrome

The most dramatic ulcer recurrences are those associated with occult gastrin-producing tumours (gastrinomas), usually of the pancreas, less often of the duodenum, and which constitute the Zollinger–Ellison syndrome (ZES). The usual picture is that of a severe ulcer diathesis causing stomal and multiple jejunal ulcers associated with extreme gastric acid hypersecretion. Because the parietal cell mass is under constant stimulation by the persistent autonomous gastrin release, the basal acid secretion amounts to more than 60% of the response to pentagastrin or histamine. The diagnosis is confirmed by assay of the serum gastrin level. Although gastrinomas are rare and probably account for no more than 2% of recurrent ulcers, the diagnosis should be entertained in all cases since the vast majority of gastrinomas (70%) present in this fashion. Gastrinomas may occur in association with multiple endocrine neoplasia type 1 (MEN 1, Werner's syndrome). In this situation, the presence of multiple endocrine neoplasia has neither a favourable nor a deleterious effect on the prognosis of the ZES.

The treatment of ZES is not standardized and to some extent depends on the pathological stage of the disease. Undoubtedly, omeprazole is highly effective and in one large review of 80 patients, this drug in doses of 60–120 mg daily (dose has to be individualized) provided satisfactory control in 90% of cases. These results are much better than those previously achieved by H_2RAs. It seems sensible therefore to start every patient on omeprazole. Following investigation and imaging tests (computed tomography (CT), magnetic resonance imaging, positron emission spectroscopy scanning), patients with lesions that are deemed to be operable probably deserve a laparotomy with excision of the tumour (pancreas or duodenum) and this may be curative in the absence of lymph node or hepatic deposits. Total gastrectomy is now reserved for patients in whom control of acid hypersecretion cannot be achieved by omeprazole.

Antral G cell hyperplasia

This is a rare cause of recurrent ulcer. In this condition, the hypergastrinaemia results either from an increased number of antral gastrin secreting cells or from an exaggerated response to feeding (post-prandial hypergastrinaemia without hyperplasia). The syndrome is therefore better referred to as antral G-cell hyperactivity or hyperfunction. All patients with this condition are cured by antrectomy.

Hypercalcaemia

Primary hyperparathyroidism can on rare occasions cause peptic ulceration in the absence of a gastrinoma. These patients do not usually have hypergastrinaemia or gross acid hypersecretion. In addition, hyperparathyroidism can coexist with gastrinoma and other endocrine neoplasia (MEN 1). In practice, if hypercalcaemia is found in a patient with peptic ulcer, recurrent or otherwise, both parathormone and gastrin levels should be measured. If primary hyperparathyroidism only is established and corrected surgically, the ulcer should heal. There is some evidence that this is more likely to occur if the patient has a parathyroid adenoma than hyperplasia. If MEN 1 syndrome is established (20% of ZES), both parathyroid surgery and treatment of the gastrinoma are required.

Management of patients with recurrent dyspepsia

The persistence of indigestion, or its return after a period of freedom from symptoms, suggests the possibility of recurrent ulceration. Other possibilities should not, however, be overlooked. These include unrelated pathology such as reflux disease, gallstones and pancreatitis. On other occasions, the dyspepsia is caused by complications of the ulcer surgery, e.g. enterogastric reflux or gastric stasis. It is not always easy to diagnose recurrent ulceration. Sometimes, the character of the pain is similar to that experienced by the patient before operation but on other occasions it is different in type, site or both. If vomiting is a feature, the presence of bile or food may suggest gastritis or stasis as the underlying cause of the problem. Recurrent ulcers may present with bleeding or, less commonly, perforation with no accompanying dyspepsia. The rapid return of symptoms, haemorrhage or perforation, particularly in a younger patient should suggest the possibility of the ZES. Coexisting diarrhoea may be indicative of this condition or gastrojejunocolic fistula, although simple post-vagotomy diarrhoea is much more common than either of these two conditions. Gastrojejunocolic fistula is an extremely rare complication of benign ulcer disease nowadays and the vast majority of these cases are neoplastic in origin.

Following gastric surgery, radiological contrast studies of the stomach and duodenum, though occasionally useful, are often difficult to interpret. Scarring of the duodenum will persist even if the ulcer has healed and the presence of a pyloroplasty makes radiological identification of a recurrent ulcer in this region virtually impossible. Endoscopy with assessment of the *H. pylori* status is the best method for the investigation of patients with recurrent dyspepsia and for the detection of ulcer recurrence. It may also provide additional information relating to adverse consequences of gastric surgery, particularly enterogastric bile reflux and gastritis. The diagnosis of recurrent ulceration may (rarely nowadays) be followed by further investigation to assess the post-operative secretory status (see Table 8.6). These tests will provide information on the completeness or otherwise of the vagotomy and the persistence of acid hypersecretion which, if excessive, should raise the possibility of ZES.

Estimation of serum gastrin is wise in all patients with recurrent ulcer. If hypergastrinaemia is encountered, further investigations are required to exclude gastrinoma and differentiate it from antral G-cell hyperplasia or retained antrum. Not all recurrent ulcers require surgical treatment. Indeed those that are associated with *H. pylori* should heal with eradication therapy. Most *H. pylori* negative cases are best managed with H_2RAs or proton pump inhibitors. Particular indications for surgical intervention include antral stasis associated with pyloric channel ulcers or incomplete vagotomy (following truncal vagotomy) in patients who are *H. pylori* negative, failure of eradication therapy in *H. pylori* positive patients, and the retained antrum (following gastrectomy). The most common cause is incomplete vagotomy. This can be treated by re-vagotomy and antrectomy if the patient is *H. pylori* negative.

Section 8.8 • Sequelae of gastric surgery

Minor post-prandial complaints are commonly experienced by patients after gastric operations. These usually improve with time and dietary adjustments. In a cohort of patients, however, variously estimated at 5–20%, the symptoms are severe, persistent and cause considerable disability and malnutrition. The various post-gastric surgery syndromes arise on a background of altered anatomy and physiology of the upper gastrointestinal tract although the exact mechanisms responsible for some of the severe symptoms remain unclear. A useful classification of the sequelae of gastric surgery is shown in Table 8.7.

Table 8.7 Sequelae of gastric surgery

Recurrence of the disease
Recurrent ulcer, recurrence of gastric carcinoma
Nutritional consequences
Weight loss, anaemia – iron deficiency, B_{12} deficiency
Milk intolerance
Bone disease
Dumping symptoms
Reactive hypoglycaemia
Bile vomiting
Diarrhoea
Small stomach syndrome
Mechanical complications
Afferent/efferent loop obstruction, jejunogastric intussusception, gastroesophageal reflux
Others
Cholelithiasis, bezoar formation, gastric carcinoma

Disabling symptoms after gastric surgery are more often encountered in the following:

- female sex
- operations for peptic ulceration in the young (below 30 years of age)
- extensive gastrectomy with duodenal diversion (Polya).

Severe and persistent symptoms are rarely encountered after highly selective vagotomy but occur with the same frequency as that reported after gastrectomy in patients who undergo truncal vagotomy with drainage or truncal vagotomy and antrectomy. The type of drainage procedure (pyloroplasty or gastrojejunostomy) does not affect the incidence of the post-prandial symptoms and other sequelae.

Nutritional consequences of gastric surgery

These consist of weight loss, anaemia and bone disease.

Weight loss

Loss of or failure to gain weight is very common after gastric surgery and tends to be more marked after extensive gastrectomy, particularly of the Polya type. Significant weight loss is usually encountered in patients who obtain a bad result and experience severe post-cibal symptoms. The resulting diminished calorie intake is the major factor although malabsorption of fat and nitrogen and decreased small bowel transit time may be operative at least in some patients. Although mild steatorrhoea is common, severe fat malabsorption is rare unless there is a coexisting subclinical small intestinal disease (e.g. gluten enteropathy) or gross bacterial overgrowth.

Anaemia

Iron-deficiency anaemia

Microcytic hypochromic anaemia is very common after vagotomy and drainage and gastric resections, especially in females. The incidence of this complication increases with time and approximates to 60 and 80% at 10–20 years in males and females respectively. The exact pathogenesis of the iron-deficiency anaemia is unclear but is probably multifactorial. The mechanisms thought to be important include:

- shift to trivalent ferric iron at high pH followed by polymerization
- loss of a gastric juice factor which normally facilitates the absorption of iron
- diminished splitting of iron–protein complexes by the reduced peptic activity of the gastric juice
- enhanced binding of dietary iron to specific proteins (e.g. gastroferrin).

In view of the high incidence of iron-deficiency anaemia after gastric surgery, prophylactic treatment with oral iron (300 mg qds) is nowadays recommended in all patients after gastrectomy and truncal vagotomy and drainage. This amount of daily iron supplementation allows sufficient absorption to restore serum iron levels to normal.

Macrocytic anaemia

This is the result of vitamin B_{12} deficiency. Malabsorption of this vitamin is invariable after total gastrectomy due to the loss of intrinsic factor. However, megaloblastic anaemia takes several years to develop due to the large body stores of vitamin B_{12}. These patients have an abnormal Schilling test and require 3-monthly injections of cyanocobalamin indefinitely. Subclinical deficiency of this vitamin is also encountered in some patients after partial gastrectomy or truncal vagotomy and drainage, although frank megaloblastic anaemia is rare in these groups. The main factor responsible for the impaired absorption of dietary vitamin B_{12} in patients after partial gastrectomy and truncal vagotomy is the lack of acid environment which normally facilitates the release of vitamin B_{12} bound to the ingested food. The reduced secretion of intrinsic factor reported in some of these patients is considered to be less important in this group of patients in whom the Schilling test is normal. Treatment is with oral crystalline vitamin B_{12}, which is administered between meals. Malabsorption of vitamin B_{12} may also be the consequence of bacterial overgrowth and steatorrhoea. Folate deficiency is rare and is only encountered in patients after extensive or total gastrectomy. It results from an inadequate dietary intake.

Bone disease

This complication develops several years after gastric resection with duodenal exclusion (Polya) as the duodenum is the major site of calcium absorption. The majority of patients are females who develop osteomalacia 10–20 years after gastrectomy. However, cases with features of both osteomalacia (bone demineralization) and osteoporosis (loss of bone substance) are well documented. The biochemical features (raised alkaline phosphatase and serum calcium) and radiological changes (rarefaction) usually pre-date the clinical symptoms by several months to years. The clinical features of post-gastrectomy bone disease include generalized bone pains, weakness due to an associated myopathy and the development of stress fractures. Treatment is with oral calcium and vitamin D supplements or with bis-phosphonates.

Dumping

Considerable confusion has been generated by the inclusion of patients with reactive hypoglycaemia in this group under the heading 'late dumping' to differentiate them from patients with vasomotor symptoms which occur soon after eating and in this terminology are referred to as 'early dumpers'. There is now general agreement that patients with symptoms due to reactive hypoglycaemia which occur 2–3 hours after a meal should be considered outside the dumping category.

Although the term 'dumping' was introduced by Mix in 1922, the first description of the dumping syndrome was reported by Hertz in 1913. The syndrome, which is one of the commonest sequelae of gastric surgery, consists of post-prandial vasomotor (systemic) and gastrointestinal symptoms (Table 8.8). The dumping syndrome is associated with rapid gastric emptying (Figure 8.15) although some have postulated that enterogastric reflux of bile is responsible for some of the symptoms. The vasomotor symptoms (palpitation, vasodilatation, hypotension and fainting/having to lie down, etc.) occur within minutes of eating and are due to hypovolaemia, which is accompanied by diminished cardiac output and peripheral resistance. The attacks are typically precipitated by high carbohydrate meals. The hypovolaemia is secondary to a massive outpouring of fluid from the vascular compartment into the bowel lumen as a consequence of the hyperosmolar nature of the intestinal contents resulting from the precipitous gastric emptying. Several vasoactive peptides have been held responsible for the vascular and gastrointestinal manifestations of the dumping syndrome. These include kinins, substance P, enteroglucagon, gastric inhibitory polypeptide (GIP) and neurotensin. The gastrointestinal symptoms, which include diarrhoea, occur later during the course of a dumping attack and may be absent.

Patients with mild to moderate dumping symptoms are managed satisfactorily with dietary manipulations.

Table 8.8 Manifestations of the dumping syndrome

Vasomotor (systemic)	*Gastrointestinal*
Weakness	Fullness
Tiredness	Epigastric discomfort/heaviness
Dizziness	Nausea
Headache	Vomiting
Fainting/wanting to lie down	Distension
Warmth	Excessive borborygmi/distension
Palpitations	Diarrhoea
Dyspnoea	
Sweating	

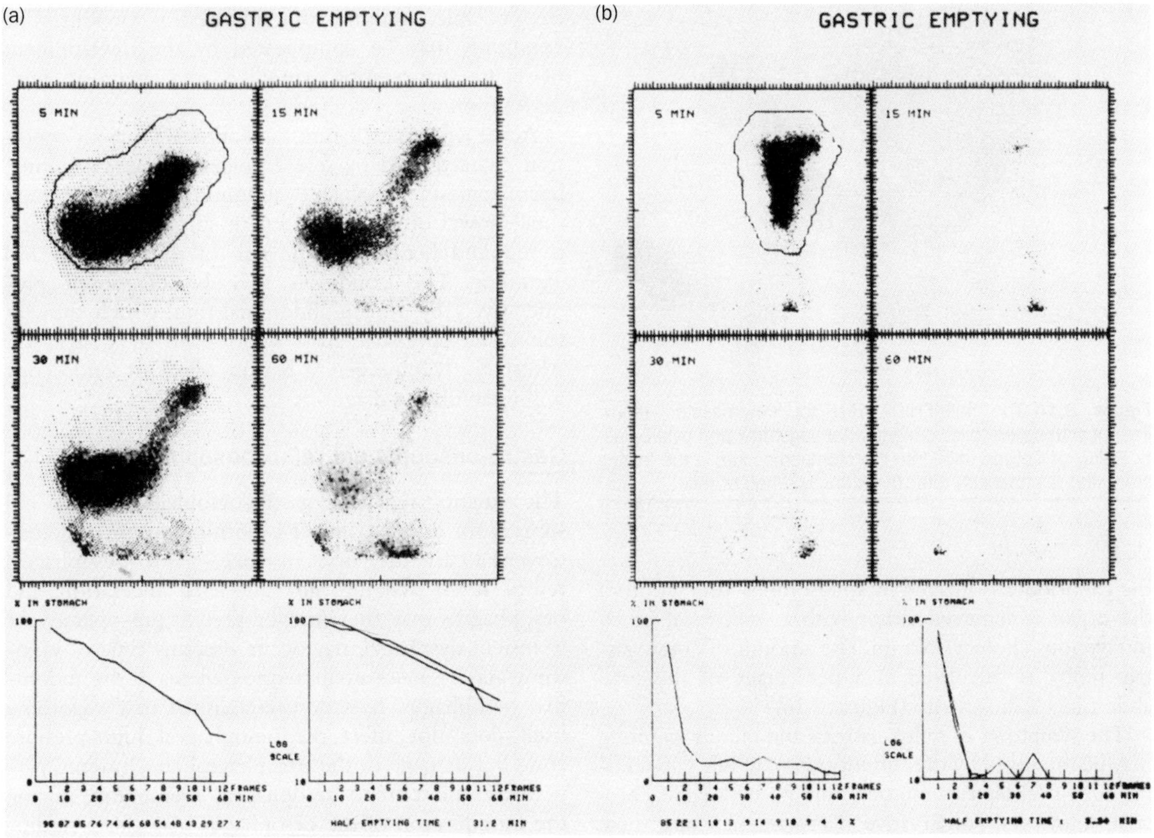

Figure 8.15 Gastric emptying of an isotope-labelled meal: (a) normal single exponential emptying; (b) rapid initial gastric emptying in a patient with severe dumping symptoms.

These patients are advised to eat small, dry meals rich in protein and fat but low in carbohydrate. Additives that slow gastric emptying, such as methoxy-pectin or bran, are beneficial. However, remedial gastric surgery is required for patients with severe and persistent dumping symptoms (see below).

Reactive hypoglycaemia

This complication is relatively uncommon and has a reported incidence of 1-6% of patients after gastric surgery. Reactive hypoglycaemia often coexists with other symptoms, including vasomotor dumping and diarrhoea. The symptoms which occur 2–3 hours after a meal are due to hypoglycaemia and include sweating, tremor, difficulty in concentration and, rarely, fainting. The diagnosis is best confirmed by an extended oral glucose tolerance test, which demonstrates an initial hyperglycaemia. This is accompanied by an exaggerated insulin release with elevated plasma insulin and enteroglucagon that are followed by the hypoglycaemia. Reactive hypoglycaemia usually responds to dietary measures including low-carbohydrate, high-protein meals.

Bile vomiting

Vomiting of bile or bile-stained fluid before or after meals is a common complaint after gastric surgery. It may be a manifestation of the following disorders:

- recurrent ulceration
- enterogastric reflux
- intermittent obstruction of the afferent or efferent loop of a gastroenterostomy
- cardio-oesophageal incompetence.

Enterogastric reflux/reflux gastritis

Reflux of upper intestinal secretions (bile/pancreatic juice/succus entericus) into the stomach causes a reflux erosive gastritis and bile vomiting. The symptoms include epigastric pain, nausea and vomiting in the early post-prandial period. The pain is usually of a burning nature, is aggravated by food and is not relieved by antacids. The attack usually culminates in the vomiting of bile-stained fluid 1–2 hours after a meal. Less commonly, the vomiting occurs in the early morning and is preceded by nocturnal burning pain. The erosive gastritis leads to chronic blood loss with the development of an iron-deficiency anaemia and, occasionally, to severe acute gastric haemorrhage. The diagnosis is established by upper gastrointestinal endoscopy, which shows a diffuse gastritis with an oedematous friable mucosa and superficial gastritis, in addition to pooling of bile-stained fluid. Quantitation of the enterogastric reflux is obtained by the modified EHIDA test. In this investigation, EHIDA is injected intravenously and is followed by external scintiscanning of the upper abdomen with a gamma camera. When

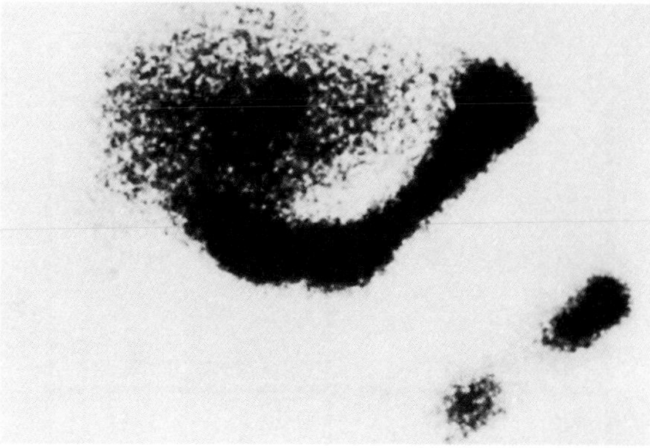

Figure 8.16 The milk-EHIDA test for enterogastric reflux. Patient with severe bile vomiting after vagotomy and pyloroplasty. Reflux of isotope (bile) into the stomach occurs in the fasting state and is enhanced after the administration of milk.

the gallbladder is imaged by the isotope, contraction of the organ is achieved either with a milk meal or by intravenous cholecystokinin. The amount of enterogastric reflux is calculated as a percentage of the total abdominal radioactivity (Figure 8.16).

The symptoms of reflux gastritis and bilious vomiting may be improved by the administration of bile salt-binding agents (cholestyramine, aluminium hydroxide, charcoal). However, conservative management along these lines often fails, when remedial surgical intervention becomes necessary. Prolonged enterogastric reflux can result in atrophic gastritis and intestinal metaplasia. It has been incriminated as a factor in the development of carcinoma of the stomach after gastric surgery although evidence for this hypothesis remains lacking.

Extrinsic loop obstruction

This rare complication occurs after truncal vagotomy and gastroenterostomy and usually affects the afferent loop. The predisposing factors to the development of afferent loop obstruction include an antecolic anastomosis and long loops (exceeding 20 cm). The causes of extrinsic loop obstruction are:

- internal herniation
- kinking of the anastomosis
- adhesions
- volvulus
- stenosis
- jejunogastric intussusception
- development of carcinoma of the gastric remnant.

Obstruction of afferent or efferent loops is usually chronic and intermittent but may be acute. The symptoms of chronic afferent loop obstruction include fullness, cramp-like pain and nausea within 1 hour of eating. The attack culminates in vomiting of copious amounts of bile-stained fluid that relieves the symptoms. The presentation of acute afferent loop obstruction is with severe colicky abdominal pain, nausea and vomiting which is characteristically free of bile. Abdominal tenderness is present. The condition may be complicated by the development of acute pancreatitis, jaundice and necrosis with perforation.

Acute jejunogastric intussusception is a serious condition characterized by severe epigastric pain, vomiting, haematemesis, a palpable abdominal mass and high small bowel obstruction. Urgent surgical intervention is required because of the risk of strangulation and gangrene. The condition may be diagnosed pre-operatively by a plain abdominal film, which shows a soft-tissue epigastric mass surrounded by gastric air. Alternatively, emergency barium meal or endoscopy will establish the diagnosis.

Gastro-oesophageal reflux/oesophagitis

The situation regarding gastro-oesophageal reflux and surgery for duodenal ulcer is both confusing and controversial. In the first instance, gastro-oesophageal reflux often accompanies duodenal ulceration and oesophagitis may, therefore, be present pre-operatively. Transient dysphagia may occur after any type of vagotomy and has been attributed to oedema of the abdominal oesophagus. It is now established that vagotomy itself does not affect the oesophageal high-pressure zone but damage to the oesophageal attachments, particularly the phreno-oesophageal membrane, during the mobilization of the oesophagus may cause cardio-oesophageal incompetence. If this is associated with enterogastric reflux, a severe form of oesophagitis due to reflux of bile and pancreatic juice (neutral or alkaline) may ensue and lead to stricture formation of the lower oesophagus.

Diarrhoea

The reported incidence of this complication varies widely, largely due to varying definitions. Three patterns of diarrhoea are encountered after gastric surgery:

- frequent loose motions
- intermittent episodes of short-lived diarrhoea and
- severe intractable explosive diarrhoea.

Severe, explosive diarrhoea is a serious, but rare, disability, being encountered in 2% of patients after truncal vagotomy. It is often accompanied by dumping symptoms and is precipitated by food. Severe intractable diarrhoea is characterized by extreme urgency and often causes incontinence during an acute attack. Although often associated with rapid gastric emptying, the exact mechanism of intractable explosive diarrhoea is unknown. Malabsorption of bile salts and/or fatty acids consequent on the intestinal denervation has been implicated. The small bowel transit is markedly accelerated.

A full malabsorption survey is necessary in all patients with severe diarrhoea as in a few patients this disability is secondary to a previously undiagnosed gastrointestinal disease (e.g. adult coeliac) or bacterial overgrowth consequent on a blind loop. Medical management is with a low animal fat diet, intestinal sedatives (codeine phosphate, lomotil) and bile-salt binding agents such as cholestyramine. Although temporary improvement can be obtained in this way, long-term benefit is rarely obtained with conservative management, particularly in severe cases.

Small stomach syndrome

This term is sometimes used for the early satiety complained of by some patients after vagotomy which causes loss of receptive relaxation of the stomach during eating. It is best reserved, however, for the inability to eat experienced by some unfortunate patients, usually females, after extensive gastrectomy. The patients usually complain of a multiplicity of symptoms that preclude an adequate oral intake. The condition leads to gross malnutrition and is refractory to conservative management. Some patients can be managed by elemental diets administered via a clinifeed tube and an IVAC pump or via a feeding jejunostomy. Although many can be trained to use this in their homes and maintain an adequate nutritional state in his way, the quality of life is poor. Thus, if the patient's age and general condition are satisfactory, surgical intervention designed to reconstruct a gastric reservoir and restore duodenal continuity is indicated.

Other complications

These include the formation of gallstones and bezoars and the development of gastric carcinoma. Vagotomy causes dilatation of the gallbladder. However, although there are a number of reports indicating an increased risk of gallstone formation after both vagotomy and partial gastrectomy, there is no firm evidence that gastric surgery predisposes to cholelithiasis.

The factors implicated in the formation of bezoars after gastric surgery include hypoacidity, impaired proteolytic activity, inadequate mastication and loss of the antral pump. The majority of bezoars, which develop after gastric surgery, consist of undigested vegetable/fruit matter (notably orange pith). Bezoars can cause chronic symptoms such as nausea, vomiting, abdominal discomfort, halitosis and early satiety. They can also lead to serious complications, e.g. small bowel obstruction, severe gastritis and ulceration, bleeding, perforation and malnutrition. Treatment is initially conservative by enzymic (cellulase) digestion or endoscopic fragmentation/removal. Surgical intervention is undertaken if medical/endoscopic therapy fails or because of the development of a complication.

There is good evidence that previous gastric surgery (partial gastrectomy, gastro-enterostomy) predisposes to the development of gastric carcinoma in the stomach remnant. Vagotomy does not appear to be implicated in this condition. Although reflux gastritis with the development of intestinal metaplasia, particularly of the type III variety, and bacterial overgrowth with formation of nitrosamines in the hypochlorhydric gastric stump have been implicated, the exact mechanism for the development of invasive carcinoma remains unknown. Also it seems likely that many of these patients had *H. pylori* gastritis that was not recognized at the time. This may well have contributed to the development of gastric carcinoma. There is a long latent period of 15–20 years and the risk, though definite, is small.

Remedial surgical treatment for post-gastric surgery syndromes

General considerations

As the majority of symptoms improve with time, initial management is always conservative and surgical treatment should not be undertaken before 18 months have elapsed since the gastric operation. Only patients with severe symptoms, which persist beyond this time despite conservative management, should be considered as candidates for remedial surgery. All these patients ought to be investigated and assessed thoroughly to establish the dominant symptom and the underlying altered gastric physiology. Although remedial surgery may impart considerable benefit to these patients, a totally symptom-free outcome is rarely obtained.

Despite the classical descriptions of separate syndromes, most patients have a mixture of symptoms but a careful history always determines the *dominant symptom/disability*, i.e. that which is most disruptive of the patient's life style. Remedial surgery is directed in the first instance to correction/improvement of this symptom/disability.

Dumping

The easiest patients to manage are those who experience severe dumping after truncal vagotomy and drainage. In these patients, the remedial surgery consists of either take down of the gastroenterostomy or pyloric reconstruction (Figure 8.17) depending on the type of drainage used. Surprisingly, gastric retention is rarely encountered, although post-prandial fullness is common after these remedial operations. For dumping after partial gastrectomy, an isoperistaltic jejunal interposition (10–15 cm) between the gastric remnant and the duodenum acts as an effective brake to slow down the gastric emptying (Figure 8.18).

Bile vomiting

The commonest cause of this is enterogastric reflux. Excellent results are obtained in patients with vagotomy and gastroenterostomy by take down of the latter. Pyloric reconstruction for bilious vomiting due to enterogastric reflux in patients after vagotomy and pyloroplasty does not give satisfactory results. Severe enterogastric reflux after partial gastrectomy is usually treated by Roux-en-Y diversion. Although very effective in abolishing the bile vomiting, this procedure may lead to bacterial overgrowth. An alternative approach is the construction of an isoperistaltic jejunal segment between the gastric remnant and the duodenum.

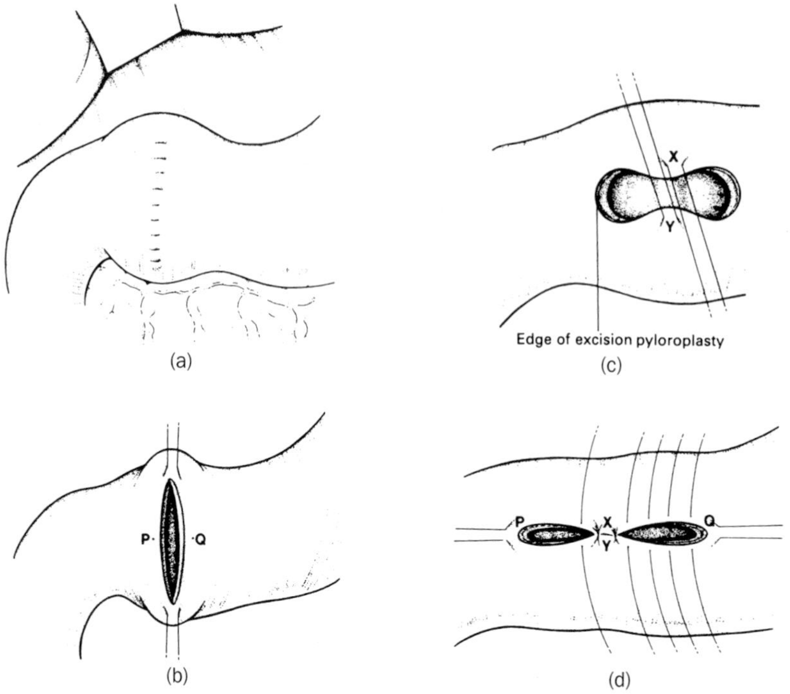

Figure 8.17 Pyloric reconstruction for dumping after Heinicke-Mikulicz pyloroplasty: (a) exposure of the pyloroplasty; (b) insertion of stay sutures beyond both ends of the pyloroplasty scar which is incised; (c) restoration of the alignment of the pyloric muscular ring; (d) the realigned antropyloric segment is closed with fine interrupted non-absorbable sutures.

Small stomach syndrome

This is the most difficult condition to treat. The patients are usually grossly malnourished and require a period of parenteral nutrition before surgical treatment. The best procedure consists of completion gastrectomy and the creation of a jejunal reservoir with an isoperistaltic conduit between the oesophagus and the duodenum (see Figure 8.19). In many of these patients, the gastric stump is inflamed and immotile. An improved outcome following this type of remedial surgery reflected in the ability to sustain weight by an oral diet is encountered in 50–60% of these patients. The problem has been the prediction of patients who are likely to benefit from such extensive remedial surgery. Obviously psychological factors are important in this respect although abnormal psychological states may be the result of the disability. Pre-operative weight

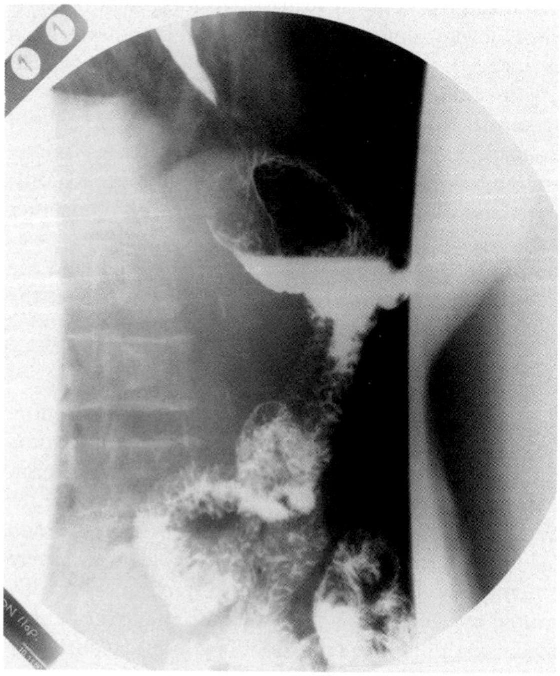

Figure 8.18 Isoperistaltic jejunal interposition between gastric remnant and the duodenum.

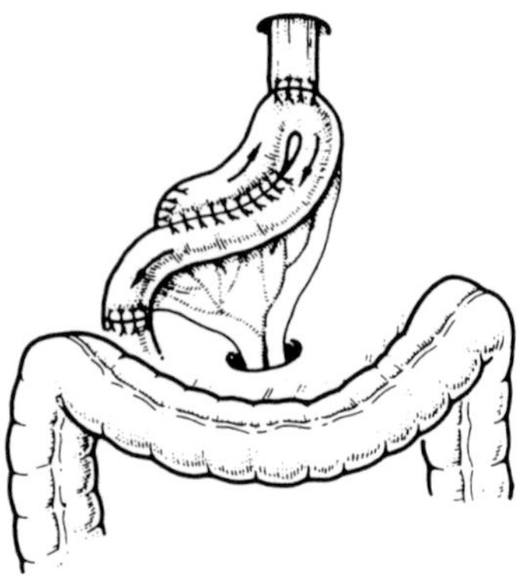

Figure 8.19 Jejunal pouch interposition with isoperistaltic conduit.

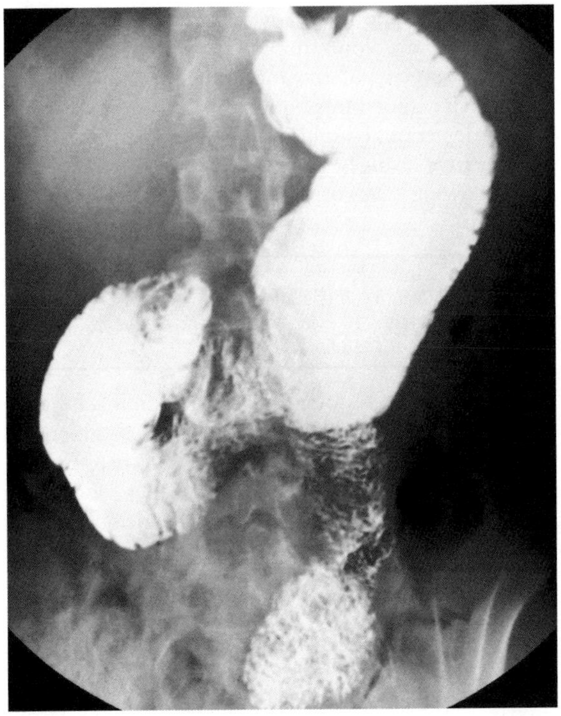

Figure 8.20 Barium series in a patient with completion gastrectomy and reconstruction with jejunal reservoir with isoperistaltic conduit. The operation was performed for severe symptoms (small stomach syndrome and vasomotor dumping) with good symptomatic result and weight gain.

gain on enteral feeding is reported to be a good indicator of a positive outcome after remedial surgery for the small stomach syndrome (Figure 8.20). In patients who do not improve after completion gastrectomy and creation of a reservoir, or in those who decline this remedial operation, nutrition can be maintained by a surgically constructed feeding jejunostomy. This is preferable to intravenous nutrition.

Severe explosive diarrhoea

Although the use of reversed jejunal segments has been advocated, the outcome of these operations is poor due to the development of episodes of post-prandial colic, intestinal obstruction, distension and bacterial overgrowth. The best results are obtained by the distal onlay ileal graft procedure which is designed to create a passive non-propulsive segment of the small intestine some 30–60 cm proximal to the ileocaecal junction (Figure 8.21). Some 50% of patients obtain significant benefit following this procedure if they avoid fat/dairy products. Some patients complain of post-prandial colic after this operation with some abdominal distension. Revision (reduction of the length of the reversed distal onlay graft) may be necessary if these symptoms are severe. Remedial surgery fails in half the patients, and in these, a temporary loop ileostomy should be offered. If the patient finds this acceptable after a trial period of 3 months, the ileostomy is made permanent, otherwise it is reversed.

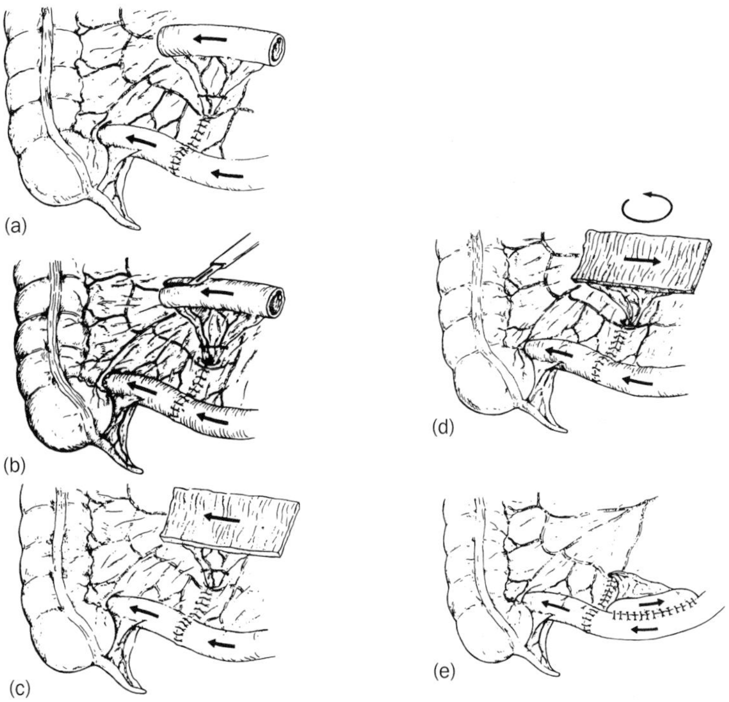

Figure 8.21 Reversed ileal onlay graft for severe explosive diarrhoea: (a) a 10 cm segment of ileum is isolated on an intact pedicle some 30 cm proximal to the caecum; (b) continuity of the small bowel is restored by an entero-enteric anastomosis; (c) the isolated segment is split longitudinally along its antimesenteric border; (d) reversal of the flap; (e) suture of the reversed graft as an onlay to the adjacent ileum, thereby creating a passive non-propulsive segment. (From Cuschieri, A. (1986) *British Journal of Surgery* **73**, 981–4, by permission).

Table 8.9 Classification of gastritis

Common
Non-atrophic gastritis (*H. pylori*)
Atrophic gastritis type A (autoimmune)
Atrophic gastritis type B (associated by *H. pylori* infection)
Reflux gastritis (enterogastric reflux)
Stress gastritis (seriously ill patients)
Erosive gastritis (drugs and alcohol)
Rare
Lymphocytic gastritis
Granulomatous gastritis (TB, Crohn's disease)
Gastritis cystica polyposa
AIDS gastritis (cryptosporidiosis)
Eosinophilic gastritis
Suppurative gastritis
Emphysematous gastritis

Section 8.9 • Gastritis

There is considerable confusion regarding the nomenclature of inflammatory conditions of the gastric mucosa (gastritis). Clinical designations do not always conform with specific histological patterns and in some instances vascular changes are noted with minimal cellular inflammatory response (Table 8.9). The term gastropathy as opposed to gastritis is more appropriate to the latter conditions, typified by alcoholic gastritis.

In the past, there have been several clinical and histological classifications of gastritis producing a rather confusing picture to the clinician. In 1990, the Sydney system was introduced as a basis for the classification and this has now become widely accepted and updated at the international workshop in Houston in 1996; hence it is referred to as the Sydney–Houston classification. The system is based on the histological examination of at least four biopsies, two from the middle body and two from the antrum at least 2 cm proximal to the pylorus (anterior and posterior walls). The Houston update also recommends that additional biopsies from the lesser curvature and the angular notch are necessary especially for the early diagnosis of atrophic gastritis and intestinal metaplasia. The main change in the classification of gastritis outlined by the Houston update is in the designation of two broad categories: *atrophic* and *non-atrophic*, although there is some disagreement on the validity of this subdivision as a mixed picture may be encountered (gland atrophy and metaplasia).

The new classification is based on five histological parameters that are graded separately by the histopathologist as mild, moderate or severe:

- chronic inflammation – mononuclear infiltrates
- activity – acute polymorphonuclear infiltrates
- atrophy – loss of normal glands
- intestinal metaplasia
- extent of colonization of biopsies by *H. pylori* in non-metaplastic epithelium.

Extensive lymphoid follicle formation is indicative of *H. pylori* infection and may lead to the development of MALT lymphomas. In general the grade (mild to severe) of the colonization with *H. pylori* correlates with the severity of the mononuclear inflammation, the activity (polymorphonuclear inflammation), the mucus depletion, lymphoid follicle formation and the degenerative changes. In practice, this system results in the following categorization of the mucosa of the stomach:

- normal
- non-atrophic *H. pylori* gastritis
- atrophic gastritis – *H. pylori* positive or negative
- special forms of gastritis.

Patients with a histologically normal stomach by the Sydney–Houston criteria have a normal functional mucosa with respect to output of acid, pepsinogens, intrinsic factor and peptide hormones and these individuals have a low risk of peptic ulcer and gastric carcinoma. Ulcers when they occur are due to drug ingestion such as NSAIDs or steroids and rarely to Crohn's disease or the Zollinger–Ellison syndrome.

Non-atrophic gastritis is caused by *H. pylori* or much less commonly by *H. heilmannii* (*vide infra*). It involves mainly the antrum and the duodenal bulb (bulbitis) and is strongly associated with the development of peptic ulcers with a cumulative risk of symptomatic peptic ulceration of 30% over a period of 10 years. The acid output is not impaired (parietal cell mass not significantly diseased). Indeed the inflammation tends to increase the gastric acid secretion and the output of some of the peptide hormones. There is nonetheless an increased risk of gastric carcinoma of the diffuse type in patient with non-atrophic gastritis without intestinal metaplasia.

Atrophic gastritis can occur in the absence of *H. pylori* infection (type A) or be caused by infection with this organism (type B). In both types of atrophic gastritis the risk of peptic ulceration, particularly duodenal, is low. The secretory function of the gastric mucosa becomes progressively impaired and if the antral mucosa is severely involved, there is reduction/loss of the gastrin-secreting G cells and the somatostatin-secreting D cells.

Type A atrophic gastritis affects mainly the corpus and appears to be of autoimmune aetiology with the presence of circulating parietal cell antibodies. It typically develops in patients with pernicious anaemia where it is associated with achlorhydria and absent secretion of intrinsic factor and thus malabsorption of vitamin B_{12}. As the antrum is relatively spared, the serum gastrin level is grossly elevated. This chronic hypergastrinaemia may lead to the development of endocrine tumours. There is an increased risk of gastric carcinoma, which is usually of the diffuse type.

Type B atrophic gastritis is the result of infection of the antral mucosa by *H. pylori* and eradication of the infection is followed by documented histological improvement although relapse may occur. Type B gastritis is much more common than the type A variety.

The changes always begin distally in the pyloric region and subsequently spread to the antrum and body of the stomach to a variable extent. This multifocal atrophic gastritis is accompanied by intestinal metaplasia. The atrophy and intestinal metaplasia are marked in both antrum and body and in the lesser curvature and angular notch in particular. There is a significant risk of gastric cancer, of the intestinal type, the risk being dependent on the severity and extent of the atrophy and intestinal metaplasia in the antrum and body of the stomach.

From a clinical standpoint, it is useful to consider gastritis as either acute when the condition is likely to be associated with acute pain and bleeding, or chronic when vague non-specific symptoms predominate and the risk to the patient lies in progression of the condition to peptic ulceration or to dysplasia and the development of gastric cancer.

Special forms of gastritis

Lymphocytic gastritis

This rare form of gastritis account for some 5% of cases of patients presenting with dyspepsia but is more commonly encountered amongst patients with coeliac disease in whom it is present in 15–45%. It is thought to be the result of an abnormal immunological reaction to unidentified luminal antigens. The condition may be intermittent. Histologically it is characterized by infiltration of the gastric epithelium by T-lymphocytes similar to that encountered in coeliac disease (intra-epithelial lymphocytes greater than 25/100 epithelial cells compared to the normal of 3–5/100 epithelial cells). Some cases are associated with infection by *H. pylori*. Although some patients do not exhibit any specific endoscopic features, in the majority a distinctive appearance consisting of nodularity, erosions and enlarged mucosal folds (referred to as varioliform gastritis) is observed.

Reactive/erosive gastritis

This is the result of gastric mucosal damage by exogenous and endogenous irritants. Histologically there is foveolar hyperplasia, severe congestion, oedema and fibrosis of the lamina propria with a paucity of inflammatory cells. Reactive gastritis is commonly caused by drugs, e.g. NSAIDs (present in 25–45% of NSAID users) and alcohol. The usual locations of drug-induced damage are the antral and pre-pyloric regions. The lesions are produced by blockade of the cyclooxygenase pathway with reduction of the cytoprotective gastric prostaglandins. Thus NSAIDs that are prostaglandin sparing (non-acetylated salicylates such as carprofen nabumetone, etc.) and low-dose steroids are less likely to cause erosive gastritis. The alcohol-induced mucosal damage affects in addition the mucosal microvessels, which undergo necrosis with resulting haemorrhage and thrombus formation. The role of leukotrienes in this pathological process is debatable. Other causes of haemorrhagic erosions include cor pulmonale, severe infections such as pneumonia, cirrhosis and blood disorders. Reflux gastritis due to enterogastric reflux of bile (see below) is a form of reactive gastritis with a distinctive pathological change consisting of subnuclear vacuolization of the foveolar epithelium.

Gastritis cystica polyposa

This is a rare late complication of gastric surgery (1–25 years), although instances without a history of previous gastric operations have been reported. The patients present with abdominal pain, nausea, vomiting or gastrointestinal bleeding. Endoscopically a hypertrophic nodular gastritis is present and this may be mistaken for carcinoma.

AIDS gastritis

In patients with the acquired immunodeficiency syndrome (AIDS), vomiting due to gastric outlet obstruction from gross inflammatory oedema of the pyloric ring is caused by infection with cryptosporidiosis. In these patients cryptosporidial oocysts can be recovered from the stools. An interesting confirmed observation is the low prevalence of *H. pylori* infection in human immunodeficiency virus (HIV) positive patients with low CD4 counts (<200) compared to HIV negative patients. This low prevalence is also accompanied by a reduced incidence of peptic ulcers. Gastric toxoplasmosis due to infection with *Toxoplasma gondii* is rare in AIDS patients but when it occurs it causes abdominal pain. Diffuse thickening of the gastric folds is seen at endoscopy. Gastric mucosal biopsy confirms necrosis and intracellular trophozoites in gastric epithelial, smooth muscle and endothelial cells.

Eosinophilic gastritis

This occurs as part of eosinophilic gastroenteropathy in infants and children and has an allergic basis. The pyloric region and adjacent duodenum become diffusely thickened due to oedema of the submucosal and the muscle layers, which are also infiltrated with eosinophils and occasional giant cells. The antrum is the area of the stomach most severely affected. Histological examination of biopsies show extensive eosinophilic infiltrates with oedema and lymphangiectasia. The elevation of the serum IgE correlates with the severity of the disease. In the majority of patients there is a peripheral eosinophilia. Some cases arise as a complication of polyarteritis nodosa, when they tend to be severe and life threatening. The clinical features of eosinophilic gastritis include symptoms of delayed gastric emptying, e.g. early satiety, nausea and vomiting, and gastrointestinal bleeding. The treatment is with sodium cromoglycate and/or prednisolone.

Suppurative (phlegmonous) gastritis

This is a rare and often fatal bacterial infection producing a cellulitis of the stomach wall. Haemolytic streptococci are the commonest infecting organisms. The condition usually complicates a pre-existing gastric lesion and is more commonly encountered in the elderly and alcoholic patients. The presentation is usually one of severe progressive peritonitis. Treatment is with gastric resection and systemic antibiotics. At operation, the stomach exhibits a dusky discoloration and its serosal surface is covered with a fibrinous exudate. Necrotizing gastritis is an especially severe variant, which results in overt infective gangrene. It is caused by a mixed infection with fusiform and spirochaete bacteria from the mouth.

Granulomatous and Crohn's gastritis

Granulomatous gastritis, most commonly of the antrum is encountered in less than 1% of patients undergoing endoscopy. The largest subgroup (50% of cases) is due to Crohn's disease. The reported estimates of Crohn's gastritis in patients with established intestinal Crohn's disease vary from 6 to 24% of cases. Crohn's gastritis may occasionally be the presenting form of the disease. The microscopic features are similar to those of intestinal Crohn's and non-caseating granulomas are present in one-third of cases. In addition there is focal chronic active ulceration with erosions of the epithelium in the absence of *H. pylori* infection, which should always suggest the diagnosis. Involvement of the duodenum is common.

Granulomatous gastritis also includes tuberculous gastritis. The tuberculous infection of the stomach is almost always secondary to active pulmonary disease. It produces multiple ragged ulcers and discrete tubercles may be visualized at endoscopy. Serosal inflammation is common and there is marked loco-regional lymphadenopathy. Treatment is with antituberculous chemotherapy.

Emphysematous gastritis

Air-filled cysts in the gastric wall are rare and are usually accompanied by pneumatoides cystoides intestinalis. Gas cysts in the wall of the stomach can also occur in association with pyloric obstruction and chronic obstructive airway disease with emphysema. Gas can also be introduced in the wall of the stomach following incomplete injuries during endoscopy.

Clinical management of gastritis

It is important to stress that, irrespective of symptoms and presentation, specific diagnosis depends on endoscopy and biopsy which is mandatory in all gastric lesions with the exception of overtly vascular conditions. The management then depends on the effect of the gastritis (e.g. bleeding, chronic symptoms), the removal of the underlying cause when applicable, or specific therapy when indicated. When the chronic gastritis is accompanied by dysplasia, surveillance by endoscopy is indicated and if the dysplasia becomes severe, then gastric resection is indicated.

Section 8.10 • Gastric tumours

Gastric tumours may be benign or malignant. The benign group includes non-neoplastic gastric polyps which are usually of the regenerative (hyperplastic) type. Carcinoma is the predominant malignant gastric tumour, lymphoma being much less common and may occur as a primary lesion or as secondary involvement from lymphomas arising elsewhere. The most common connective-tissue (mesenchymal) neoplasms are the smooth muscle tumours. Although most of these are benign (leiomyoma), some are malignant (leiomyosarcoma). The differentiation between benign and malignant smooth muscle tumours may be difficult to determine even by histological assessment in the individual case.

Adenomas and other benign tumours

True adenomas of the stomach are rare and account for only 5% of benign gastric polyps. Thus although progression to a carcinoma is possible as in cancer of the colon, this sequence is a rare event in the development of invasive gastric carcinomas. The majority of gastric adenomas are found in the antrum and may be single or multiple (Figure 8.22). They may form sessile, villous, pedunculated or lobulated growths. Treatment is advisable and may be achieved endoscopically but if the tumour is large or multiple, surgical local excision or partial gastrectomy is necessary. Other benign tumours include lipomas, neurofibromas, neurilemmomas and glomus tumours.

Non-neoplastic gastric polyps

The commonest site of non-neoplastic polyps of the stomach is the antropyloric region. Various types of gastric polyps are recognized, the commonest being the *regenerative (hyperplastic)* variety. These are also known as types I and II in Japan, account for 75% of gastric polyps and can occur anywhere in the stomach. Regenerative polyps have an inflammatory origin. They often occur in association with gastritis and peptic ulceration, form smooth nodules of variable size and consist of proliferating glands with no cellular atypia. All regenerative polyps should be removed endoscopically and be subjected to histological examination, as a detailed pathological study of 477 lesions

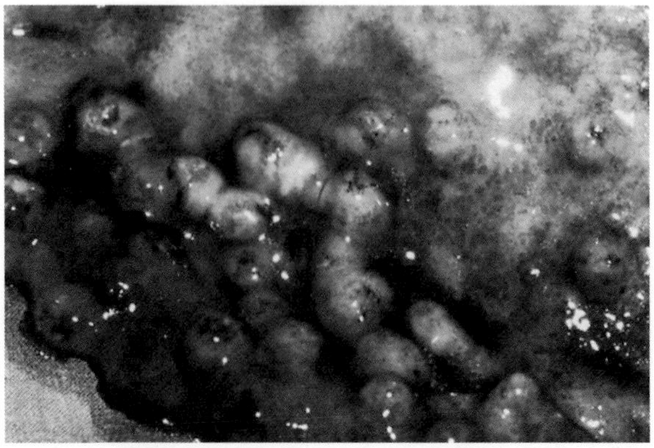

Figure 8.22 Multiple adenomatous polyps treated by partial gastrectomy.

identified focal carcinoma in 2.1% and dysplastic foci in 4%.

The *inflammatory fibroid polyp* (eosinophilic granuloma, haemangiopericytoma) is a rare lesion, which is most commonly found in the gastric antrum and can be sessile or pedunculated. It is usually associated with hypochlorhydria. Histologically, it is composed of a vascular stroma containing numerous capillaries and arterioles, fibroblasts and an inflammatory cell infiltrate with an abundance of eosinophils. However, the lesion is not associated with a systemic eosinophilia or allergic conditions. In this respect it contrasts with eosinophilic gastroenteritis which affects the pyloric antrum and the first part of the duodenum and arises on a background of gastrointestinal allergy.

Myoepithelial hamartomas are composed of glands surrounded by smooth muscle and arise from the submucosal layer of the antrum and pylorus where they form smooth sessile masses. The *hamartomatous polyps* of Peutz-Jeghers syndrome may occur in the stomach. They very rarely become malignant. Heterotopic pancreatic tissue is again most commonly found in the antropyloric region.

Fundic gland polyps are usually small and multiple and situated in the fundus or body of the stomach. Microscopy shows microcysts lined by fundic epithelium including oxyntic cells.

Neoplastic polyps

These are adenomas and constitute types III and IV in Japan. They occur predominantly in the antrum and may be either sessile or pedunculated. They are analogous to colonic adenomas and histologically they consist of atypical glands with pseudostratified epithelium showing nuclear abnormalities and high mitotic figures. They also contain endocrine cells positive for serotonin and other peptide hormones. Like the colonic counterparts they are categorized as *adenomatous* (tubular adenoma), *tubovillous* and *villous*. All have a malignant potential, which is however low (5% invasive malignancy in 5–7 years) and size dependent. Endoscopic removal and surveillance are recommended.

Polyposis syndromes

Multiple gastric polyps of varying types can be found in:

- Familial colonic polyposis and the related Gardner's syndrome – gastric polyps occur in 50% of patients
- Peutz-Jeghers syndrome – occur in 20% of patients
- Generalized juvenile polyposis and related Cronkhite-Canada syndrome
- Cowden's syndrome (multiple hamartomas syndrome).

Giant gastric folds and Menétrier's disease (hypertrophic gastropathy)

Giant gastric folds (or large gastric folds) are found in both benign and malignant diseases, and their differentiation with either upper gastrointestinal X-ray or endoscopy is difficult. Sometimes, even endoscopic biopsy cannot establish a definitive diagnosis. Recently, EUS has been used to investigate patients with giant gastric folds. The causes of giant gastric folds are:

- gastric varices
- gastric lymphangiectasis
- gastritis
- gastric carcinoma (scirrhous type)
- gastric lymphomas
- Menétrier's disease.

EUS is useful in the differential diagnosis of giant gastric folds and avoids the risk associated with biopsy of gastric varices. All patients with gastric varices have anechoic tortuous varicose veins in the submucosal layer. EUS images of gastric lymphangiectasis are similar to those of gastric varices. EUS reveals regular gastric wall thickening of the second (mucosa) and third (submucosa) layers in non-atrophic gastritis. The fourth (muscularis propria) layer is intact in mucosa-associated lymphoid tissue lymphoma (MALToma), but not in the other types of gastric lymphoma. The second and third layers of MALTomas are irregular in thickness and of heterogeneous echogenicity, different from the characteristic EUS findings in gastritis. The fourth layer is markedly thickened only in malignant conditions. Differentiation of gastric cancer from lymphoma with EUS is difficult because of overlapping EUS findings.

Menétrier's disease (polyadenomes en nappe, hypertrophic gastropathy) which can occur in both children and adults, consists of giant hypertrophy of the mucosal folds of the stomach and is associated with a marked protein-losing enteropathy. The giant folds are usually centred along the greater curvature with sharp demarcation between the abnormal and normal gastric mucosa. The histology shows marked foveolar hyperplasia with inflamed and oedematous stroma. There is gastric hypersecretion in terms of volume but the acid content is low. Often polyps form in this condition. The patient may develop acute or, more commonly, chronic blood loss leading to anaemia. The protein-losing enteropathy can result in severe hypoproteinaemia correctable only by gastrectomy. There have been some reports indicating that the condition predisposes to gastric malignancy. A recent study in children has revealed an association between hypertrophic gastropathy and cytomegalovirus infection. A similar morphological change with prominent gastric folds may be encountered in Zollinger–Ellison syndrome, except the histology shows hyperplasia of the parietal cells.

Carcinoma of the stomach

This disease continues to carry a poor prognosis, especially in Western countries where the overall 5 year survival averages 10%. A better outcome is obtained in Japan, which has the highest age-standardized incidence in the world (100/100 000 for males). The improved survival in Japan is due to an active screening programme resulting in earlier diagnosis and an aggressive surgical approach designed to reduce loco-regional recurrence in the gastric bed.

Epidemiology

There has been a decline in the incidence of gastric cancer during the past 30 years throughout the world. The exact reason for this is unknown but the increased consumption of refrigerated in preference to spiced and pickled foods has been postulated as a possible factor. There has been considerable epidemiological research on food intake and risk of cancer of the stomach. A decreased incidence has been observed with increased consumption of fresh vegetables and fruit. The protective vegetables include dark green, cruciferous and allium vegetables (onions, garlic and leeks). Increased dietary carotene, vitamin C and calcium are also protective. By contrast, increased consumption of retinol does not reduce the risk. The sharpest decline has been observed in Finland where the incidence of gastric cancer is now one-third of the rate that prevailed in the early 1950s. Within the UK, the disease is commoner in Scotland and Wales. In Scotland, the current age-standardized rate for gastric cancer is 20 and 10/100 000 for males and females respectively. In contrast to the overall decline in the incidence of gastric cancer, tumours of the upper third of the stomach including the oesophagogastric junction have increased and now account for approximately 40% of gastric cancers. The most marked reduction has been observed in tumours of the middle third of the stomach. The male preponderance (2:1) is encountered world-wide. The disease is rarely seen before 40 years of age and the incidence rises sharply with age to reach a maximum between 70 and 80 years. Cancer of the stomach is three times more common in social classes IV and V (semi-skilled and unskilled labourers) than in social classes I and II (professional, executive and higher management).

Aetiology

It is now believed that gastric carcinogenesis is a multistep process based on the model initially proposed by Pelayo Correa and often referred to the Correa cascade: *chronic gastritis* leads to *atrophy* and *intestinal metaplasia* which then changes to *dysplasia* (nowadays regarded as pre-invasive neoplasia). The underlying mechanisms for this stepwise carcinogenesis (manifested by these histological changes) consists of a series of genetic changes (mostly unknown) that ultimately result in a clone of neoplastic cells which escapes the normal growth control checks and is thus able to proliferate and disseminate. Different gene mutations and growth factors are involved in this cascade. In this context, abnormal p53 tumour suppressor gene (normal gene is responsible for chromosomal repair or apoptosis, i.e. self-destruction without inflammation if the damage is irreparable) is known to be operative late in this sequence probably at the severe dysplasia stage. Over-expression of the p21 product of the RAS oncogene has been detected in some gastric cancers. The p62 product of the C-myc oncogene is also over-expressed in some gastric tumours but this gene is amplified in various tissues associated with cell proliferation, neoplastic or otherwise. It is thus a cell cycle enhancing agent and is unlikely to be specifically involved in the development of gastric cancer. Amplification of the HER2/neu gene has also been documented in some gastric cancers. This gene is related to but is distinct from the HERI gene, which encodes for the epidermal growth factor receptor (EGFr). Although co-amplification of these two oncogenes has not been documented, the EGFr binding of gastric carcinomas is about twice that found in normal tissues. Furthermore, this activity increases from about 4% in early gastric carcinomas to 35% in advanced tumours irrespective of histological type. The hypothesis generated from these findings is that some gastric cancers exhibit autocrine secretion, which is intended for self-stimulation, i.e. the tumour cells secrete EGF for which they have excess receptors. There is evidence that the hormone gastrin is trophic to both neoplastic and normal gastrointestinal cells and this effect appears to be mediated via a high-affinity gastrin receptor. However, there is no direct evidence that gastrin is involved in the development and progression of gastric cancer, and phase I clinical studies on the use of agents which block gastrin binding have not demonstrated any benefit in patients with advanced disease.

As with other neoplasms the presence and degree of aneuploidy appears to be associated with a poor prognosis in gastric cancer. In one study the DNA distribution patterns were grouped as low (diploid) and high ploidies. The more invasive tumours with widespread nodal involvement were largely confined to the high ploidy group. Furthermore, patients with tumours exhibiting high ploidy had a much lower 5 year survival (24%) compared to patients with low ploidy tumours (91%). It is important to stress, however, that the tumour stage and size were not equivalent between the two groups of patients. Other studies have failed to find any association between DNA ploidy, histological grade and tumour type. Thus tumour aggressiveness *per se* may not be directly related to DNA aneuploidy and other factors are certainly involved.

In practice, two major problems have slowed progress and account for different reported outcomes from different centres: different definitions of pre-neoplastic changes between East and West and inter-observer variations in histopathological diagnosis of these changes. During the past 5 years, various international working groups (Padova, Houston) have addressed these issues, and although some issues remain unresolved certain agreements have been reached.

Gastric atrophy is now defined as loss of appropriate or native cells, i.e. glands that are normally present in the gastric mucosa in a given area, viz. loss of mucous glands in antrum/pre-pyloric region and cardia, and loss of oxyntic cells in the body (corpus) of the stomach. The loss of native glands may be accompanied by replacement fibrosis or the appearance of inappropriate glands (not native to the region). The term *metaplasia* is reserved to identify the presence of non-native glands, with two main types:

- *intestinal metaplasia* – epithelium contains goblet cells, absorptive cells with or without a brush border and Paneth cells
- *pyloric or pseudo-pyloric metaplasia* – replacement of oxyntic cells by mucous (pyloric) glands.

The term dysplasia is regarded unequivocally as pre-invasive neoplasia. In the West the neoplastic proliferation categorized by dysplasia is confined to the lamina propria of the original glandular structure. In Japan, the term 'borderline lesions' is used to categorize histological and cytological changes irrespective of whether the lamina propria is involved or not. The Padova conference established the following consensus between Eastern and Western pathologists on five categories:

- negative for dysplasia
- indefinite for dysplasia
- non-invasive neoplasia
- suspicion of invasive cancer
- gastric cancer.

Although the results of several epidemiological studies have failed to demonstrate specific causative factors, the following have been implicated:

- *H. pylori* gastritis
- highly spiced, salted or pickled foods
- polycyclic hydrocarbons, especially those generated by high-temperature pyrolysis of animal fat and aromatic amino acids in grilled and barbecued meats
- inorganic dusts (miners and potters)
- high consumption of animal fat
- high salt consumption (osmotic damage to gastric mucosa)
- protein malnutrition (may lead to achlorhydria)
- viral infections (which may damage the gastric mucosa and cause temporary achlorhydria)
- excess alcohol consumption
- tobacco smoking
- dietary nitrates (drinking water and vegetables)
- refluxed bile acids (as tumour promoters).

Nitrates are thought to be important as they can be converted to N-nitroso compounds in the stomach. However, although these compounds are extremely potent carcinogens in animals there is no definite evidence that they are carcinogenic to humans. Both the reduction of nitrates to nitrites and the nitrosination of the nitrites with amines (with the formation of N-nitrosamines) are known to be catalysed by bacteria such as *Escherichia coli*. Other than *H. pylori* gastritis, bacterial overgrowth which is commonly encountered in the human stomach in conditions of hypo- or anacidity is associated with a high concentration of nitrites and N-nitrosamines. Although plausible, the hypothesis postulating the sequence: increased dietary nitrates → bacterial proliferation in an achlorhydric stomach → excess N-nitrosamine production → cancer of the stomach, has not been confirmed in the human. By contrast, the carcinogenic potential of *H. pylori* induced gastritis is beyond dispute.

The recognized risk factors in the development of gastric carcinoma are:

- persistent infection with *H. pylori*
- atrophic gastritis and pernicious anaemia
- previous partial gastrectomy
- adenomatous and regenerative (hyperplastic) gastric polyps
- familial polyposis
- hypogammaglobulinaemia
- blood group A
- type III intestinal metaplasia.

The most researched risk factor has been atrophic gastritis (*H. pylori* positive or negative) in view of the high incidence of carcinoma (three- to six-fold increase). The incidence of gastric atrophy increases with age and is frequently encountered in patients above the age of 60 years in Western countries. In addition to *H. pylori*, other factors can cause primary damage of the gastric mucosa with the development of atrophic gastritis. There is now established evidence for the progression of gastric atrophy to intestinal metaplasia, dysplasia and carcinoma *in situ*.

Although there is a higher incidence of intestinal metaplasia in gastric carcinoma than in benign conditions, the lesion is too common to be useful for screening purposes. However, the recognition of the various types of intestinal metaplasia by detailed histology and mucin histochemistry has clarified the picture considerably. There are three types of intestinal metaplasia depending on the degree of cell differentiation and abnormal mucus production (Table 8.10). Various studies have now shown a strong association between type III intestinal metaplasia and gastric carcinoma of the intestinal type (see below). This type of intestinal metaplasia (Figure 8.23) is also found in gastric adenomas but not in regenerative polyps. Furthermore, a high incidence of type III intestinal metaplasia has been reported in relatives of patients with gastric carcinoma and in patients with pernicious anaemia.

The most important histological marker of gastric cancer is dysplasia. The subject has attracted considerable research interest and the previous controversial issues have now been largely resolved. The remaining problem is a practical one and concerns the pathological differentiation of the grades of dysplasia, which can pose difficulties even among experienced histopathologists. There are two types of dysplasia. Type A affects metaplastic gastric epithelium and can lead to the

Table 8.10 Types of intestinal metaplasia

- Type I (complete) – Mature absorptive and goblet cells. The latter secrete sialomucin (normal)
- Type II (incomplete) – Absorptive cells are few or absent. Columnar 'intermediate' cells in various stages of de-differentiation are present and secrete sialomucin. The goblet cells secrete sialomucins and occasionally sulphomucins (abnormal mucins)
- Type III (incomplete) – The cell de-differentiation is more marked than in type II. The 'intermediate' cells secrete predominantly sulphomucins (abnormal mucins). The goblet cells secrete both sialo- and sulphomucins. A variable degree of disorganized glandular architecture is present.

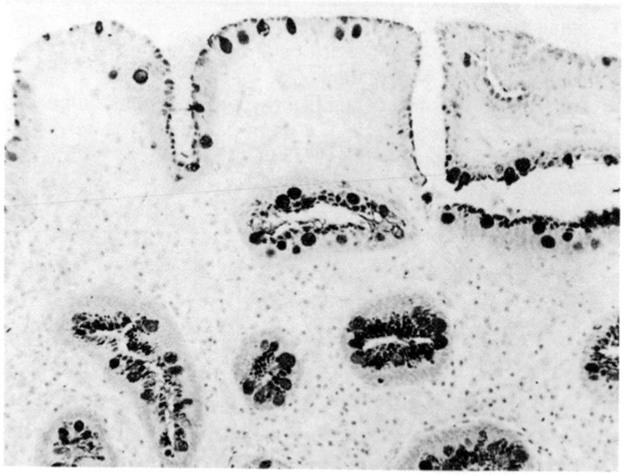

Figure 8.23 Histochemical appearance of type IIB incomplete intestinal metaplasia using high iron diamine alcian blue stain (HID-AB) for mucins. The normal absorptive cells are scanty and have been replaced by de-differentiated 'intermediate' cells which secrete sulphomucin (black). The goblet cells secrete a mixture of sialo- (grey) and sulphomucin. The glandular architecture is disorganized. (Courtesy of MP Holley, Ninewells Hospital, Dundee, Scotland.)

development of intestinal type of gastric cancer. Type B arises in non-metaplastic gastric epithelium and predisposes to diffuse or intermediate gastric cancers. The cell population of the glands in type B dysplasia is largely made up of undifferentiated round cells with a clear or amphophilic cytoplasm lacking a brush border. Dysplasia is graded histologically (by either subjective or morphometric quantitative methods) into mild, moderate and severe. The morphometric grading is based on architectural parameters such as volume and surface densities of glands and epithelium, which describe the arrangement and shape of nuclei and nucleolar size.

Severe dysplasia (Figure 8.24) is now regarded as *in situ* gastric cancer. Several longitudinal studies have demonstrated that whereas mild and moderate dysplasia progress slowly and in some instances remain stable

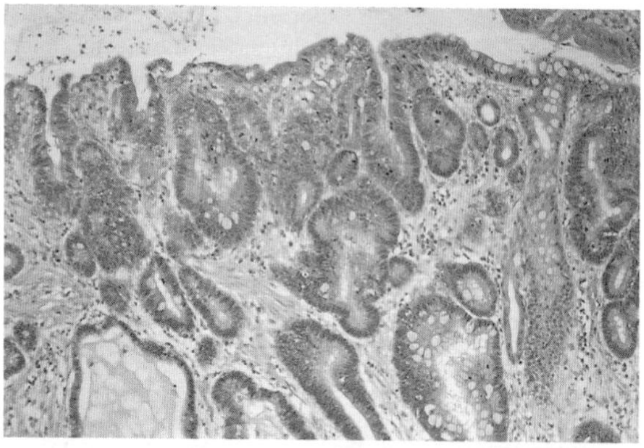

Figure 8.24 Gastric mucosa showing superficial glanular crowding and irregularity with celular atypia amounting to high-grade dysplasia. There is associated intestinal metaplasia. (Courtesy of Dr FA Carey, consultant pathologist, Ninewells Hospital, Dundee, Scotland.)

or even regress, severe dysplasia progresses to invasive cancer in the vast majority of patients. Thus while mild to moderate dysplasia merits endoscopic surveillance only, when severe dysplasia is diagnosed, a second biopsy is mandatory within a few weeks. If severe dysplasia is confirmed in this way, gastrectomy should be performed. In 40–50% of these cases, invasive early gastric cancer will be found on pathological examination of the resected stomach. Whereas genetic factors are important in relation to diffuse carcinoma, there is no evidence for familial predisposition in the development of the intestinal type of gastric cancer. Diffuse gastric carcinoma is significantly more common in patients with blood group A, in relatives of patients with diffuse gastric cancer and in familial hypogammaglobulinaemia. This is a genetically determined disorder, which is characterized by the defective production of IgG antibodies and is usually accompanied by pernicious anaemia. Patients with familial hypo-gammaglobulinaemia have a 50-fold excess risk of developing gastric carcinoma.

Pathology

There are several classifications of gastric carcinoma. The most useful to the clinician and epidemiologist is the Lauren (or Finnish or DIO) classification. This recognizes two main groups with different histogenesis and (probably) aetiology. The first group is known as the *intestinal gastric cancer* (I) as the gastric carcinoma cells exhibit a striated (brush) border and generally resemble intestinal cells. They tend to form localized expanding or ulcerated lesions and are frequently surrounded by intestinal metaplasia especially of the type III variety. The second group is known as the *diffuse gastric cancer* as the lesion infiltrates the gastric wall without forming large discrete masses. The diffuse cancer carries a worse prognosis than the intestinal variety and often arises from apparently normal gastric mucosa usually over a wide field. These cancers are not usually associated with intestinal metaplasia or other precancerous conditions except pernicious anaemia and familial hypo-gammaglobulinaemia.

The intestinal and diffuse cancers account for 90% of all gastric carcinomas. The remainder have a mixed morphology and are referred to as other (0), hence the alternative name, DIO classification. However, the majority of the tumours in the 'other' category behave like the intestinal gastric cancers. Within each category (intestinal or diffuse), the tumours are graded pathologically into well differentiated, poorly differentiated and undifferentiated. The intestinal type of gastric cancer is made up of cohesive neoplastic cells (which stick together) and when the tumour is well differentiated, these neoplastic cells form glandular tubules with a central lumen (Figure 8.25). The various subtypes of the well-differentiated intestinal gastric cancer are: large gland carcinoma, small gland carcinoma and a type of colloid carcinoma and in which mucous lakes are found surrounded by well-differentiated glands. The growth of intestinal cancer is mainly by expansion

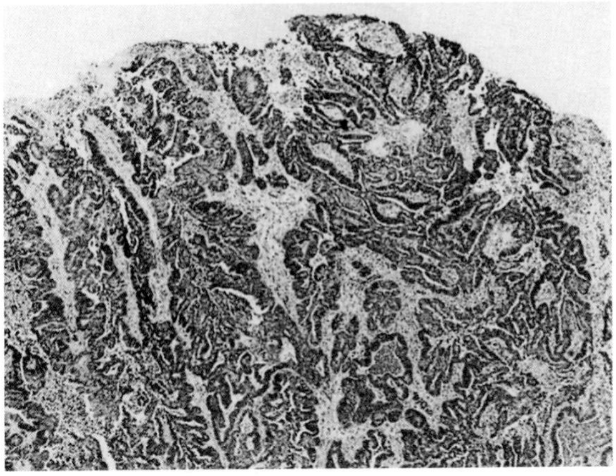

Figure 8.25 Photomicrograph of a well-differentiated gastric cancer of the intestinal type. The cells form well-defined glandular acini.

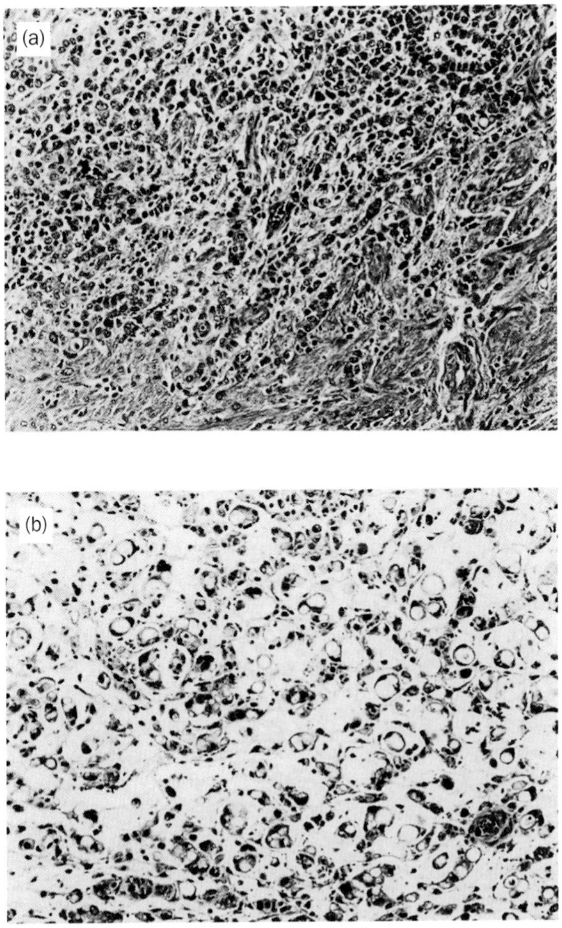

Figure 8.26 (a) Low-power view of the histological appearance of a diffuse type of gastric cancer. The cells have lost all cohesion and stream out into the surrounding stroma; (b) high-power field showing the streaming of the malignant cells which are loaded with mucus resulting in eccentric position of the nucleus, i.e. signet cell appearance. (Courtesy of MP Holley, Ninewells Hospital, Dundee, Scotland.)

and macroscopically they form polypoid or fungating masses, which may ulcerate centrally.

The diffuse gastric carcinomas are made of neoplastic cells which lack cohesion and therefore tend to stream out in single-file fashion and invade the stomach wall with no tendency to organization into tubular or glandular structures (Figure 8.26). They are therefore highly invasive tumours and carry a worse prognosis than the intestinal variety. The well-known linitis plastica (leather-bottle stomach) is a classic example of the diffuse type of gastric cancer. Some diffuse gastric cancers show little tendency to mucin production. Others consist of mucin-laden signet ring cells (signet cell carcinoma) or large lakes of mucus surrounding isolated clusters of signet cells (diffuse colloid carcinoma). The clinicopathological differences between the intestinal and diffuse gastric carcinomas are outlined in Table 8.11.

Serological markers

Various antibodies have been used for the detection of shed surface tumour associated antigens in the peripheral blood of patients with gastric carcinoma (CEA, CAl9 9, CASO, CAl25, CA72 4). These tumour markers are used to detect presence of a given tumour, its recurrence after surgical treatment and progression of the disease. The only reliable marker in patients with gastric cancer is CA72 4. The activity of this antigen correlates well with tumour burden and lymph node involvement. The serum level returns to normal after curative resection and any subsequent elevation indicates loco-regional or distant recurrence of the disease.

Table 8.11 Contrasting features of intestinal and diffuse gastric cancers

	Intestinal	*Diffuse*
Histogenesis	Areas of intestinal metaplasia, type II/III	Normal gastric mucosa
Early cancer	Protruding type	Flat, depressed or excavated
Infiltration	Localized	Diffuse
Peritoneal dissemination	Infrequent	Frequent
Hepatic metastases	Nodular	Diffuse
Sex incidence	More common in males	More frequent in females
Age incidence	More common in the elderly	More common in the young
Association with blood group A	No	Yes
Association with pernicious anaemia	No	Yes
Genetic predisposition	No	Yes
Association with *H. pylori*	Yes	Yes
Prognosis	Survival better than the diffuse	Dismal

Early gastric cancer

This is defined as cancer limited to the mucosa and submucosa and accounts for up to 30–40% of newly diagnosed tumours in Japan as a result of screening for the disease. It is becoming increasingly relevant in Western countries as with early access endoscopy, early gastric cancer is diagnosed much more frequently. The macroscopic type of early gastric cancer seen endoscopically and the extent of submucosal invasion (superficial or deep, sm_{1-2}) determined by endosonography appear to determine the incidence of spread to the level 1 regional lymph nodes (N_1). Overall some 15% of early gastric cancers have lymph node deposits. In the past these were referred to as early-simulating advanced gastric cancer. The prognosis with adequate resection is excellent with 5 year survival rates exceeding 80%. Early gastric cancer assumes different endoscopic appearances which have been classified as follows (Figure 8.27):

- protruding
- superficial: this may be elevated, flat or depressed
- excavated.

In the revised classification of gastric cancer of the Japanese Gastric Cancer Association (JGCA), the recognized macroscopic types are:

- type 1 (polypoid well demarcated)
- type 2 (ulcerated with sharply demarcated margins)
- type 3 (ulcerated without definite limits infiltrating the surrounding walls)
- type 4 (diffusely infiltrating without significant ulceration)
- type 5 (non-classifiable)

Superficial tumours are designated as T0 and five categories are recognized on endoscopic appearances:

- type 0I *protruding type* – lesion has a thickness greater than twice that of the normal mucosa
- type 0IIa *superficial elevated type* – lesion has a thickness of up to twice that of the normal mucosa
- type 0IIb *flat type*
- type 0IIc *superficial depressed type*
- type 0III excavated *type*.

In combined types, the largest component is designated first, e.g. type 0IIc + 0III.

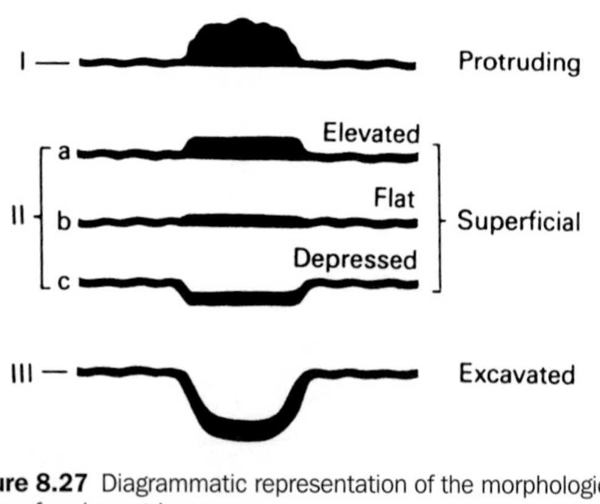

Figure 8.27 Diagrammatic representation of the morphological types of early gastric cancer.

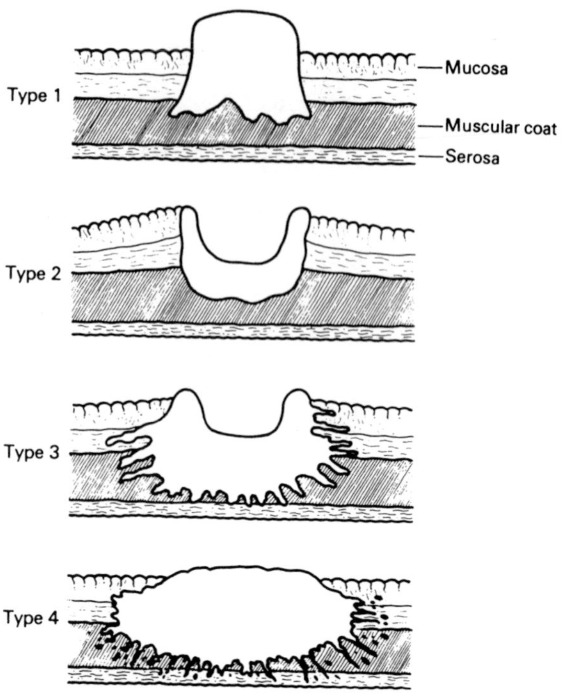

Figure 8.28 Diagrammatic representation of the Borrmann classification of advanced gastric cancer.

Advanced gastric carcinoma

This is defined as a tumour that has involved the muscularis propria of the stomach wall and accounts for >90% of gastric carcinomas diagnosed in the UK. In the vast majority of cases, spread to the regional lymph nodes is present alone or in association with peritoneal and hepatic deposits. Advanced gastric carcinoma is further classified into macroscopic types first described by Borrmann (Figure 8.28). Types 1 and 2 carry a better prognosis than types 3 and 4, which are always incurable despite attempts at radical resection.

Staging of gastric cancer

In the past, there were several staging systems for gastric carcinoma. An international staging system has now been agreed. The new TNM categories are shown in Table 8.12. The important prognostic factors in patients without detectable distant metastases are depth of invasion of the stomach wall by the tumour and lymph node spread. Other significant (by univariate analysis) but lesser prognostic variables are the type of cancer (intestinal or diffuse), location of the tumour (growths of the cardia having a poorer prognosis than lesions of the middle and lower third) and the histological type (degree of differentiation) although multivariate analysis indicates that only clinical stage, extent of involvement of the gastric wall by tumour and lymph node involvement are independent prognostic markers. The MRC study (ST01 trial) has shown that eosinophilic infiltration of the tumour is an independent prognostic marker with marked eosinophilic infiltration being associated with long-term survival after resection.

Table 8.12 Staging of gastric cancer
Surgical stage grouping is based on T, N, P, H and M with each of these components being defined as follows:

T – Primary tumour
T_1 Tumour limited to the mucosa and submucosa
T_2 Tumour involves the muscularis propria or subserosa
T_3 Tumour penetrates the serosa
T_4 Tumour involves contiguous structures

N – Regional lymph nodes
N_0 No metastases to the regional lymph nodes
N_1 Involvement of the perigastric lymph nodes within 3 cm of the primary tumour
N_2 Involvement of the regional lymph nodes more than 3 cm from the primary including those located along the left gastric, common hepatic, splenic and coeliac arteries

P – Peritoneal metastases
P_0 No peritoneal metastases
P_1 Peritoneal metastases to adjacent but not distal peritoneum
P_2 A few metastases to the distant peritoneum
P_3 Numerous metastases to distant pneumoperitoneum

H – Hepatic deposits
H_0 No hepatic deposits
H_1 Metastases limited to one lobe
H_2 A few metastases in both lobes
H_3 Numerous metastases to both lobes

M – Distant metastases
M_0 No evidence of distant metastases
M_1 Evidence of distant metastases

Note. Involvement of lymph nodes beyond level N_2, i.e. N_3, N_4 is regarded as distant metastases according to the new classification.

On the basis of the above, the surgical stage grouping is:

		P_0, H_0, M_0				P_0, H_1
		N_0	N_1	N_2	N_3	$N_{0,1,2}$
P_0	T_1	Ia	Ib	II	IIIa	
H_0	T_2	Ib	II	IIIa	IIIb	IVa
M_0	T_3	II	IIIa	IIIb	IVa	
	T_4	IIIa	IIIb	IVa		
P_1 H_0	$T_{1,2,3}$			IVa		

Spread of gastric carcinoma

The diffuse type of gastric cancer spreads rapidly through the submucosal and subserosal lymphatic plexuses and penetrates the gastric wall at an early stage. The intestinal variety remains localized for a while and has less tendency to disseminate. With both cancers, spread to the lymph nodes along the greater and lesser curvatures tends to occur once the muscular coat of the stomach is invaded by the neoplasm. Thereafter, spread occurs to the nodes along the coeliac axis and its trifurcation (left gastric, splenic and common hepatic arteries), to the nodes in the splenic hilum, the root of the mesentery, the retropancreatic nodes and the hepatoduodenal nodes. Involvement of the para-aortic nodes above and below the transverse colon then ensues. The exact nodal groups which are involved depend on the anatomical site of the primary tumour (upper, middle, lower third). Contrary to general belief, involvement of the duodenum by an antral carcinoma is not unusual, as is extension to the abdominal oesophagus by lesions originating in the upper third of the stomach. Metastatic spread is usually to the peritoneal cavity and the liver. The most common organs involved by direct extension are the omentum, the transverse colon and mesocolon and the left lobe of the liver.

Clinical features

Early gastric cancer of the intestinal type is asymptomatic but early diffuse cancer may present with dyspepsia simulating peptic ulceration. The symptoms may respond to treatment with antacids and H_2-receptor blockers/PPIs and the ulcer may show evidence of healing at follow-up endoscopy. In any event, the early symptoms are often vague and include indigestion, malaise, early satiety, post-prandial fullness and loss of appetite. Weight loss is a significant feature of the disease but usually signifies an advanced lesion that has involved the muscular coat of the stomach or beyond. Lesions of the cardia may present with dysphagia and circumferential growths of the middle third and the pyloric antrum cause obstructive symptoms with vomiting after meals. Acute presentation with haematemesis or melaena is encountered more often with advanced than early lesions.

The most common presentation is that of recent dyspepsia in a patient above the age of 45 years. There are no specific features to the cancer dyspepsia. Thus, all patients who present with indigestion require full investigation including endoscopy to establish the diagnosis before treatment is started. The most frequent reason for the delay in the diagnosis of cancer of the stomach is a period of symptomatic therapy with antacids or H_2-receptor blockers/PPI often lasting several months before referral for endoscopy is undertaken. Irrespective of sex and age, the exact diagnosis of the underlying gastroduodenal disease must be established in all patients above the age of 45 years with indigestion before treatment of any sort is initiated. Anaemia, which is often present at the time of diagnosis, is usually of the iron-deficiency type due to chronic blood loss. Evidence of weight loss is usually present on examination and hypoalbuminaemia is frequent. Although often stressed, enlarged left supraclavicular lymph nodes are a rare physical finding in gastric cancer. A palpable epigastric mass usually signifies incurable, though not necessarily a non-resectable, tumour. Jaundice, hepatomegaly or ascites indicate advanced incurable disease and limited survival. Evidence of spread beyond the peritoneal cavity is unusual at the time of diagnosis of gastric carcinoma.

The key investigations are upper gastrointestinal endoscopy with multiple biopsy and brush cytology and air-contrast barium meal (Figure 8.29). Other tests are used to detect extragastric disease and help in the staging of the lesion. These include chest radiography, liver function tests, hydro-helical CT with the patient in the prone position and gastric endosonography (Figure

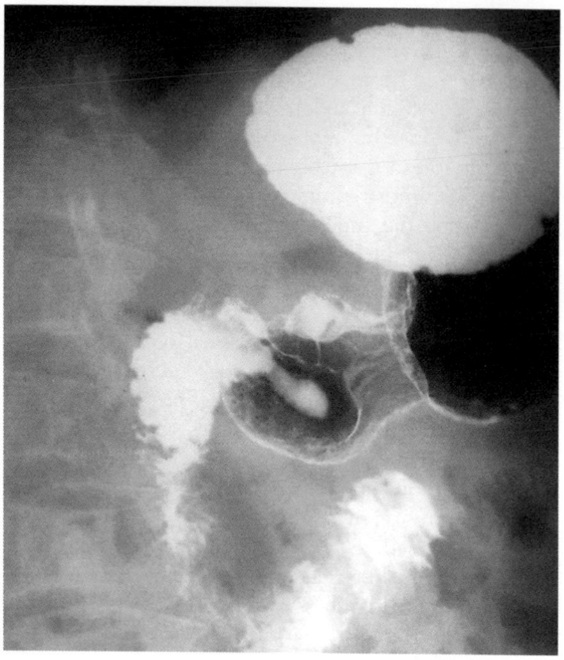

Figure 8.29 Air-contrast (barium) meal showing an antral carcinoma.

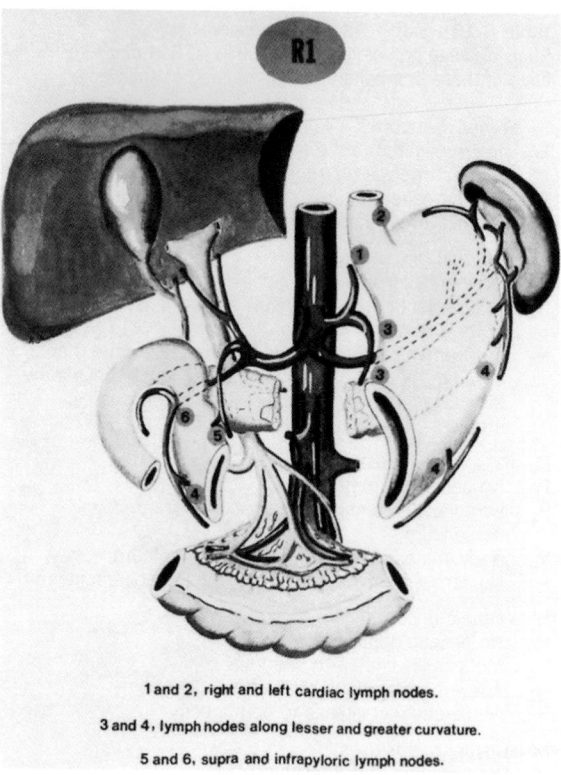

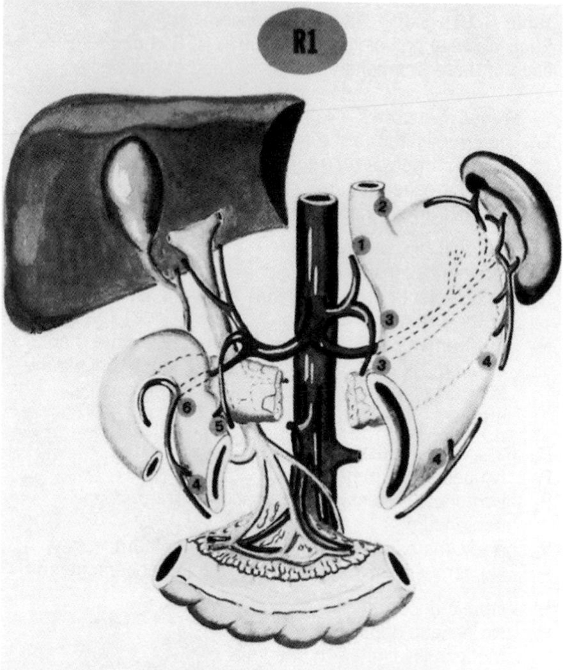

Figure 8.31 Extent of lymph node clearance in D_1 resection.

8.30). Hydro CT scanning with the patient in the prone position is very used for assessing the extent of involvement of the stomach wall by the tumour and posterior fixation (usually to the pancreas). More accurate information of the T staging is obtained by endoscopic gastric ultrasound scanning. Enlarged para-aortic nodes can be detected by CT. Laparoscopy is extremely valuable in assessing resectability and curability. It is the only reliable method of detection of peritoneal seedlings and is nowadays carried out routinely in most centres.

Treatment of advanced gastric carcinoma

An adequate surgical resection remains the only effective treatment which offers a chance of cure or long-term survival. Furthermore, a palliative resection whenever feasible is more effective in relieving symptoms than bypass or intubation procedures. Radiotherapy is largely ineffective.

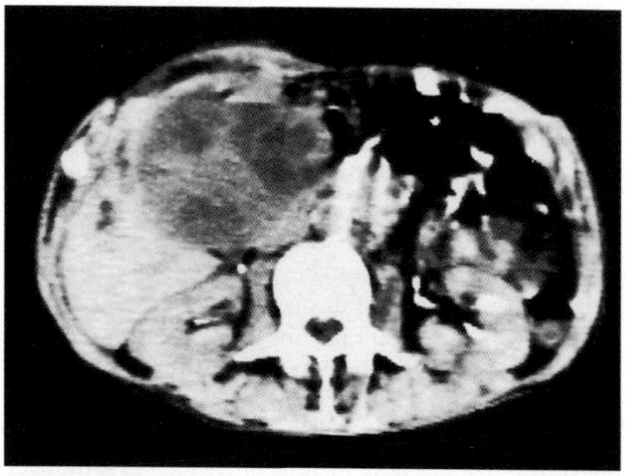

Figure 8.30 CT scan of the liver in a patient with gastric carcinoma of the diffuse type showing multiple hepatic deposits.

The principles underlying a potentially curative resection of a gastric carcinoma are:

- an appropriate resection with adequate tumour-free margins
- a regional lymph node clearance corresponding to the location of the primary tumour in the stomach
- safe and well-functioning reconstruction.

The Japanese Research Society for Gastric Cancer has issued a classification of gastric resections for cancer based on the radicality (D) of the procedure: D_1, D_2 and D_3. In D_1 resections, the lymph node clearance is confined to the primary group of nodes, i.e. those around the cardia, along the greater and lesser curvatures and the juxtapyloric ones (Figure 8.31). In practice, this is achieved by removal of the greater and lesser omenta with the excised stomach. This is the type of resection most frequently carried out in the West and is thought by the Japanese not to achieve adequate control of the disease, resulting in a high incidence of local recurrence in the gastric bed. The D_2 resection (Figures 8.32 and 8.33) necessitates an additional clearance of the lymph nodes around the main arteries: the left gastric, coeliac, common hepatic and splenic arteries, besides the retropancreatic and splenic hilar lymph nodes. In addition to lymph node clearance of the named arteries, a splenectomy and resection of the body and tail of the pancreas may be necessary to

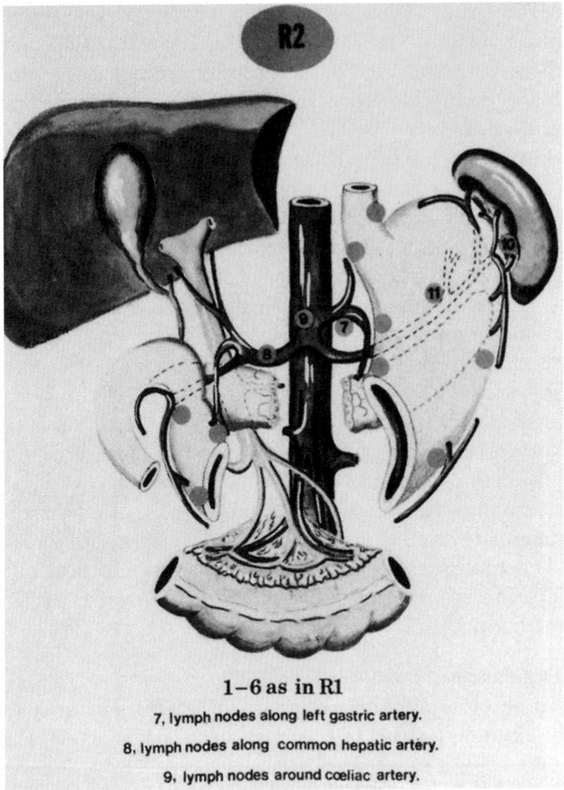

R2
1–6 as in R1
7, lymph nodes along left gastric artery.
8, lymph nodes along common hepatic artery.
9, lymph nodes around cœliac artery.

Figure 8.32 Extent of lymph node clearance in D_2 resection.

achieve this. The D_3 resection extends the lymph node clearance even further to include the nodes present in the porta hepatis, behind the head of the pancreas, in the root of the mesentery, around the middle colic vessels and the para-aortic lymph nodes (Figure 8.34). In some tumours, this will involve partial colectomy, hepatic lobectomy, subtotal pancreatectomy and even pancreaticoduodenectomy.

Extent of gastric resection

A gastrectomy does not need to be total to be curative. Resection which provides a 2.0 cm margin for early or

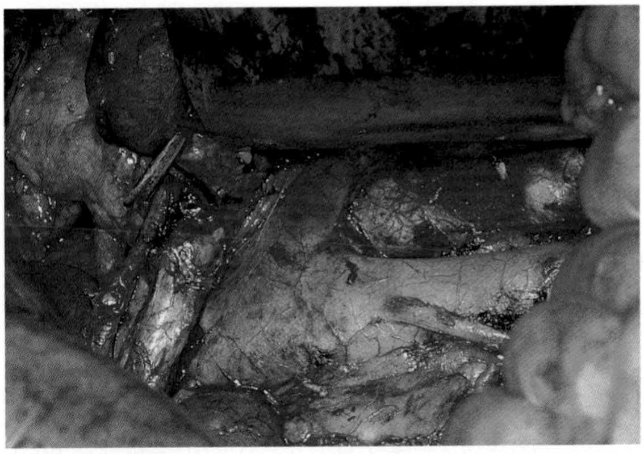

Figure 8.33 Operative photograph of lymph node clearance in a D_2 resection for antral carcinoma.

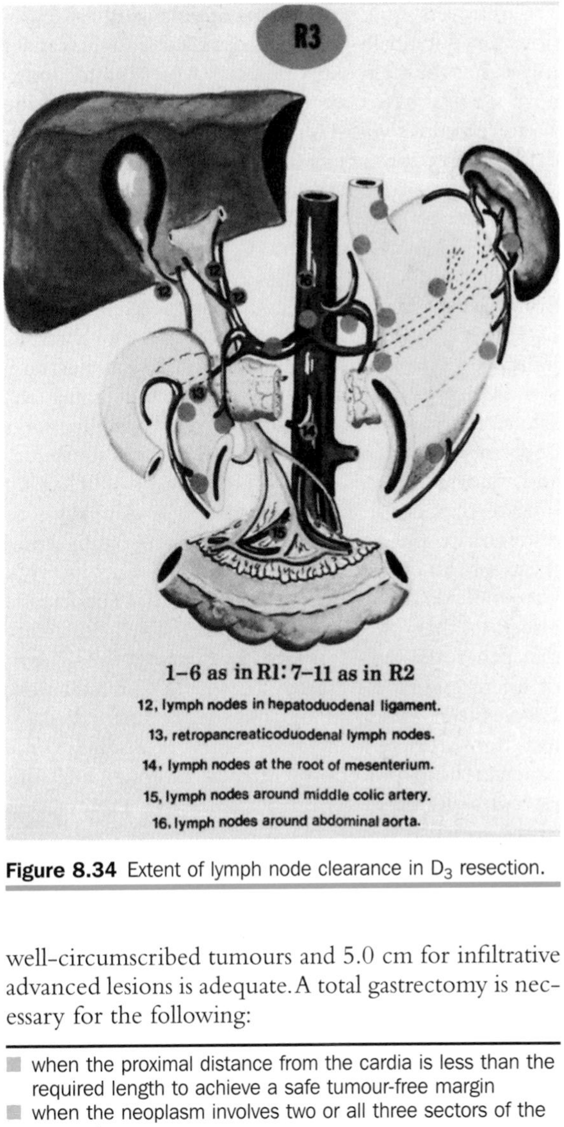

Figure 8.34 Extent of lymph node clearance in D_3 resection.

well-circumscribed tumours and 5.0 cm for infiltrative advanced lesions is adequate. A total gastrectomy is necessary for the following:

- when the proximal distance from the cardia is less than the required length to achieve a safe tumour-free margin
- when the neoplasm involves two or all three sectors of the stomach
- diffuse carcinoma (Borrmann 4) irrespective of size.

Omentectomy

The lesser omentum should be detached from the liver. The removal of the greater omentum must include the anterior leaf of the transverse mesocolon (bursectomy) to bare the colic arteries and veins and ensure the removal of the lymph nodes accompanying these vessels.

Lymph node clearance

This must be adequate and appropriate to the site of the primary neoplasm. Some advocate intra-operative lymph node mapping which is achieved by the peritumoral injection of dyes such as Evans Blue to outline the draining lymph nodes but this is rarely practised outside Japan. The principle of an adequate node clearance is that this should encompass the tier of lymph nodes beyond those that are macroscopically involved. Thus for a tumour which is accompanied by involvement of N_1 nodes, a D_2 type of resection is necessary.

Controversy still exists on the optimal surgical resection for potentially curable advanced gastric cancer (involving the muscularis propria). Much better long-term survival have been reported from Japan and some Western centres with D_2 resections than with the standard D_1 resections but all of these has been either retrospective or non-randomized prospective studies. None of the randomized studies has detected a survival advantage, including the MRC trial. This showed no difference in long-term survival, overall and with death from gastric cancer as the end-point, between D_1 and D_2 surgery. Both the MRC and the Dutch trial results indicate quite clearly that pancreatico-splenectomy should not form part of D_2 resections. Pancreatico-splenectomy appears to disadvantage these patients both in terms of increased post-operative morbidity and mortality and, very probably, by reducing long-term survival. In both studies it is impossible to differentiate the adverse effects of splenectomy from those of pancreatectomy on the long-term survival but multivariate analysis indicates that pancreatic resection has the stronger effect. The possibility that pancreatic resection actually enhances the growth of microresidual disease requires further investigation. Pancreatic resection should only be performed in D_2 resections if there is direct extension of disease to the pancreas from posteriorly situated tumours, and this resection should be regarded as palliative. Preservation of the pancreas is now being recommended and practised by Japanese surgeons in D_2 resections for gastric cancer.

Others have also stressed the importance of spleen preservation during D_2 resections for proximal gastric cancer. Two centres have reported impressive results with low post-operative morbidity and mortality and improved survival with spleen preserving D_2 resections. The argument against splenic preservation is the incidence of lymph node metastases along the distal splenic artery and splenic hilum in patients with proximal tumours. Reported estimates for deposits in these nodes vary from 15 to 27%. In the MRC trial, 25% of patients with proximal (C, CM) tumours had involved splenic nodes. Some, possibly all, of the splenic artery nodes can be removed with preservation of the pancreas and spleen but the splenic hilar nodes cannot be removed safely without a splenectomy. What needs to be addressed is which patients with proximal and cardiac tumours are suitable for splenic preservation. The lymph nodes concerned constitute group 10 in the Japanese classification (nodes in splenic hilum) and are considered N_2 nodes for proximal tumours. If one adheres to the Japanese criteria, the tumours that could be considered for splenic preservation are antral and middle third tumours. In practice, spleen preserving D_2 resection is often undertaken when the tumour is well clear of the fundus and short gastric vessels.

It is difficult to reach any definite conclusions on the influence of the extent of lymphadenectomy on long-term survival. The comparison of the patients in the MRC study who actually underwent radical lymphadenectomy (as defined by the Japanese rules) and those with nodal harvest of 25 or fewer regional nodes indicated no difference. In the German prospective but non-randomized study where the surgeons were allowed to perform their preferred resection, radical lymphadenectomy (26 or more nodes in the specimen) significantly improved survival only in stage II and stage IIIa disease. This effect was, however, restricted to patients with pN_0 and pN_1.

A sensible middle of the road policy is recommended in the midst of this controversy. The resection has to be radical – sufficient resection margins, omentectomy and *adequate lymphadenectomy*. The extent of the lymphadenectomy should, however, be based on the known incidence of N_1 and N_2 deposits in relation not just to the site of the tumour but also to the extent of transmural involvement by tumour (pT). On a purely pragmatic level, all advanced gastric cancers with serosal encroachment/involvement require D_2 resection, but T_1 cancers involving the submucosa are treated by D_1 resection.

Definition of a curative resection

An absolute curative resection for gastric cancer may be deemed to have been performed when:

- there is no peritoneal or hepatic disease
- the serosa is not involved by the tumour
- the resection margins are free of tumour by histological examination
- the D (resection) level exceeds the level of nodal involvement (N).

When the D level equals the N value, the resection is classified as relatively curative.

Reconstruction

There is still considerable controversy regarding the optimum method of reconstruction after gastric resection and the various procedures may be grouped into duodenal bypass procedures and reconstructions which restore duodenal continuity. The important consideration in reconstruction after resection of gastric cancer is whether the surgeon considers that the excision performed is likely to be curative or not. In patients who are considered to have had complete excision (curative resection), the reconstruction should attempt to restore duodenal continuity since these procedures result in the best nutritional outcome in the long term. Thus for patients who have had a curative distal gastrectomy, a Billroth I procedure is the preferred method. A jejunal interposition reservoir type reconstruction (Figures 8.35 and 8.36) is the ideal for patients who have undergone curative subtotal/total gastrectomy.

Duodenal bypass procedures (Polya for distal gastrectomy and Roux-en-Y or loop jejunostomy with entero-enteric anastomosis for more extensive resections) are performed in patients in whom the resection is considered to be non-curative (Figure 8.37) as these reconstructions are less likely to be obstructed by recurrent disease.

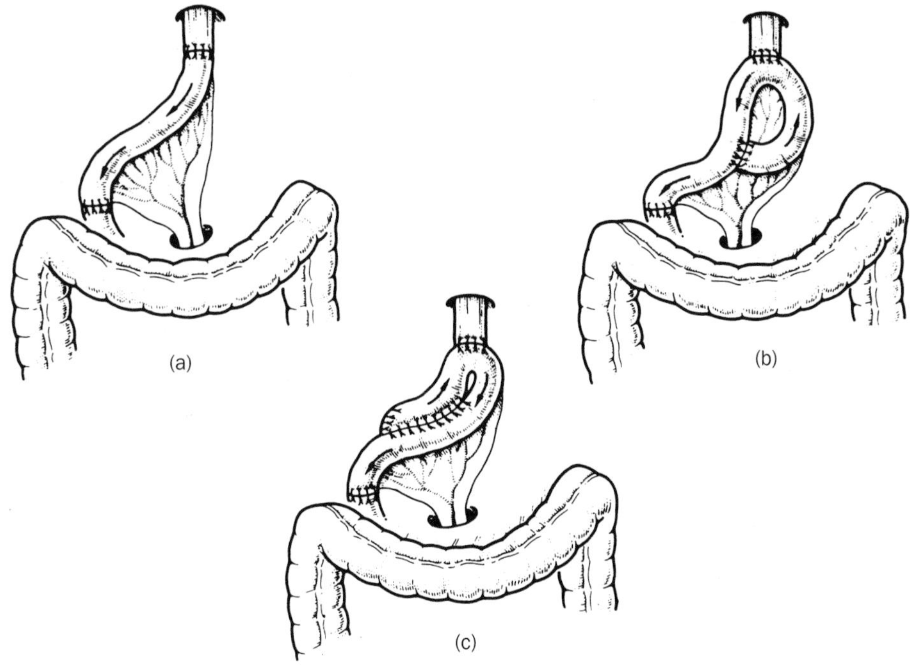

Figure 8.35 Types of jejunal interpositions between the gastric remnant or oesophagus and the duodenum: (a) single isoperistaltic loop; (b) omega loop interposition; (c) reservoir jejunal interposition with isoperistaltic conduit.

Treatment of early gastric cancer

The dilemma in the management of patients with early gastric cancer (local endogastric ablation/removal or wedge resection versus D_1 or D_2 gastrectomy) centres on the selection of tumours that are unlikely to be accompanied by spread to the regional lymph nodes. Data are now available even from Western series to indicate that the incidence of regional node spread increases when early gastric cancer invades the submucosa deeply. The endoscopic macroscopic type of lesion, and level of submucosal involvement by gastric cancer endosonography (sm_1 = superficial invasion, sm_2 = deep invasion) are used in the selection of the appropriate treatment in the individual case as they are reliable indicators of regional node involvement. In a recent study from Japan on the incidence of regional node deposits in patients with early gastric cancer with submucosal invasion, no lymph node metastases were found on pathological examination in any cancer measuring less than 2.0 cm irrespective of the endoscopic macroscopic type. None of the simple type 0IIa lesions was associated with vascular involvement or regional node deposits and only 3% of type 0IIc cancers measuring 3 cm or less had nodal involvement. In contrast, macroscopic type 0I (protruded type) or combined types (0IIA+IIC, 0IIC+III) were more likely to infiltrate deeply with a high incidence (18–25%) of lymph node metastases. The conclusion from this report is that lymphadenectomy is unnecessary in tumours measuring 3.0 cm or less provided they are either simple macroscopic type 0IIa or simple type 0IIc sm_1 cancers.

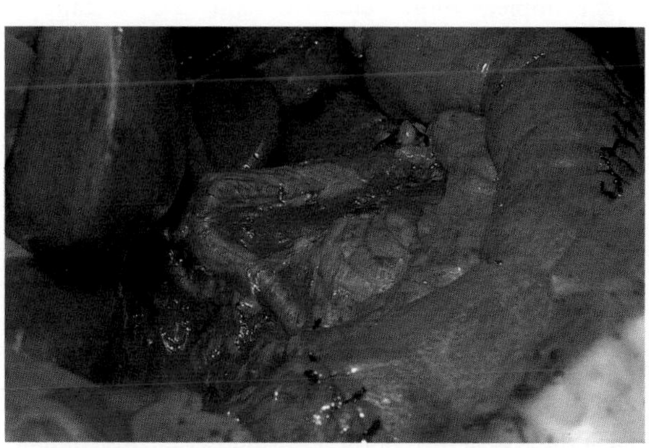

Figure 8.36 Operative photograph of reconstruction with a jejunal reservoir after curative D_2 total gastrectomy for advanced gastric cancer.

Alternative treatment in patients with early gastric cancer

Although adequate gastrectomy with removal of the level 1 lymph nodes (limited extended lymphadenectomy) is the standard treatment for these patients, alternative methods can be employed and provided adequate selection of cases is undertaken, the survival is not compromised.

In early superficial gastric cancer there are four alternative options:

- interventional flexible endoscopic treatment – submucosal resection, photodynamic ablation
- laparo-endoluminal resection
- transgastrostomal endoscopic surgery
- laparoscopic gastric resections (totally laparoscopic, laparoscopically assisted and hand assisted).

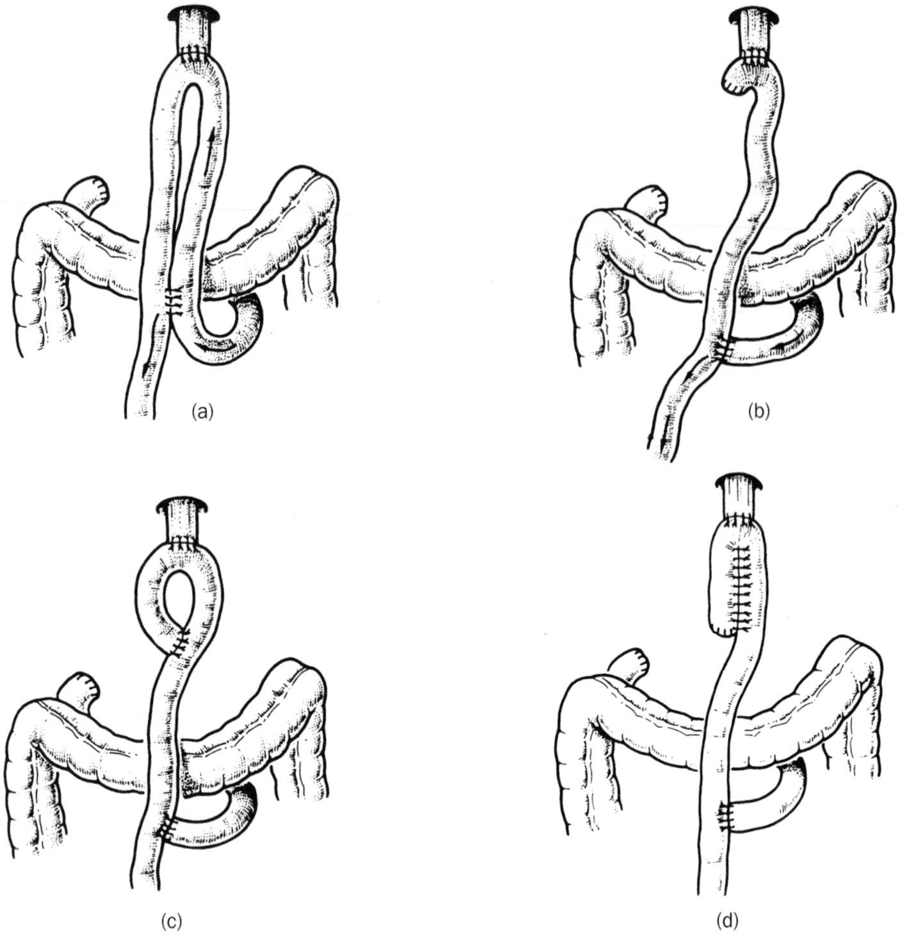

Figure 8.37 Types of reconstruction with closure (bypass) of the duodenum: (a) loop oesophagojejunostomy with distal (40–60 cm) entero-enteric anastomosis; (b) simple Roux-en-Y reconstruction; (c) omega Roux-en-Y; (d) Hunt Lawrence Roux-en-Y pouch.

The interventional flexible endoscopic approach appears to be suitable for superficial early gastric cancer not involving the submucosa and the techniques include mucosectomy (submucosal resection) after adrenaline/saline injection in the submucosal layer and laser ablation. The vast majority of reports of early gastric cancers treated by interventional endoscopic techniques are from Japan. The laparo-endoluminal mucosectomy is an alternative to the above for the same lesions. This technique is particularly suited for lesions on the posterior wall of the stomach and fundus. An experienced laparoscopic surgeon and a skilled endoscopist work together. The procedure starts with a laparoscopic inspection and placement of a detachable clamp just distal to the duodeno-jeunal junction. Following passage of a flexible endoscope and insufflation of the stomach, this is entered from the serosal side between the lesser and greater curvatures with a stretchable (Innerdyne) cannula. This is then expanded to 10 mm for insertion of the laparoscope and insufflation of the stomach with CO_2. Two Innerdyne cannulae are inserted as instrument channels and stretched to 5.0 mm once in place. The third assisting instrument is brought down via the operating channel of the flexible endoscope, which for this reason must have a large instrument channel (3–4 mm). The technique is safe provided it is limited to the right categories of superficial gastric cancer described previously. Since it necessitates CO_2 insufflation of the stomach, the laparo-endoluminal approach is unsuitable for lesions requiring full thickness resection.

A simpler, more effective and less technically demanding technique was first described by Yamashita *et al.* and is referred to as transgastrostomal endoscopic surgery. It is particularly useful for post-wall lesions and since it avoids the need for CO_2 insufflation, it is suitable for both mucosectomies and full thickness excisions. The technique involves a small midline incision. The anterior wall of the stomach is grasped and a limited anterior gastrotomy performed. The edges of the gastrostomy are then sutured to the skin with interrupted sutures. An operating short proctoscope is then inserted into the stomach (Buess operating proctoscope is ideal). A 30° endoscope is then inserted in the channel at the top of the endoscope. Endoscopic instruments are used for the mucosectomy or full thickness excision.

Laparoscopic wedge resection without lymphadenectomy is adequate for small superficial lesions without significant submucosal involvement situated on the anterior wall close to the lesser curvature. Accurate location of the lesion with intra-operative flexible endoscopy is integral to this technique. Laparoscopic D_1 gastrectomy is ideal for early gastric cancer >3.0 cm with submucosal invasion (sm_2) detected by gastric endosonography. However, the reported data are limited and the follow-up period is too short to permit any conclusions on efficacy and safety. A total D_1 gastrectomy is advisable for middle and upper third lesions but a distal D_1 gastrectomy is sufficient for antral lesions. All D_1 gastrectomies include an omentectomy but the spleen is preserved even in upper third lesions. D_2 gastrectomies are best performed with the HALS approach.

Chemotherapy for gastric cancer

The situation regarding the chemotherapy of gastric cancer has changed during the past 5 years. Previously no single agent or combination of agents imparted any significant advantage and all the clinical prospective randomized trials on adjuvant therapy (treatment after potentially curative resection) with various regimens, including FAM (5-fluorouracil (5-FU), adriamycin and mitomycin C) which was considered the most active, showed no evidence of improved survival over resection alone. Furthermore, the chemotherapy incurred a considerable morbidity and was responsible for some deaths. However, a number of newer combinations, usually incorporating cisplatin, have been shown to result in a significant response rate (40%) in patients with advanced gastric cancer with complete objective response in some 15–20%. One of the first effective regimens was the EAP (etoposide, adriamycin (doxorubicin) and cisplatin). This resulted in substantial downgrading of tumours after neoadjuvant therapy (before surgery) so that at subsequent laparotomy some patients became operable and indeed examination of the resected specimens showed minimal and in some instances no histological evidence of residual disease. Other regimens reported to give similar response rates include 5-FU + doxorubicin or epirubicin (less toxic isomer) + cisplatin (FDP) and 5-FU + doxorubicin + triazinate (FDT). The disadvantage of all these combinations is the high toxicity rate, which precludes treatment or necessitates drastic dose reduction in a significant percentage of patients. Currently the most widely used effective regimen, in view of its acceptable toxicity, is the one developed by Cunningham at the Royal Marsden Hospital. This consists of epirubicin (50 mg/m^2 in 3-weekly intravenous boluses), cisplatin (60 mg/m^2 in 3-weekly infusions) and 5-FU 200 mg/m^2 administered daily by continuous infusion through a central Hickman line for 3 weeks. The full treatment consists of six cycles. In one ongoing UK Medical Research Council neoadjuvant study (MAGIC trial), three cycles are administered pre-operatively and three cycles post-operatively in the surgery + chemotherapy arm. In advanced or recurrent disease, the Cunningham–Marsden regimen exhibits a higher response rate than other regimens, averaging 40% overall with 15–20 complete response rates.

Radiotherapy

Adjuvant radiotherapy (pre-, intra- and post-operatively) has been used in some centres on the observation that loco-regional recurrence in the gastric bed is common after surgical excision. However, there have been no clinical trials which have documented any survival improvement following adjuvant radiotherapy for gastric cancer. Intra-operative radiotherapy is used in some Japanese centres for resectable stage II and III disease. Although survival benefit has been reported in one retrospective series, intra-operative radiotherapy is not used elsewhere and has never been validated prospectively.

Palliative surgical treatment

The symptoms which require palliation are pain, vomiting, dysphagia, bleeding and malaise. The best results are obtained by a palliative gastrectomy, which may have to be total if the patient's general condition permits. An antecolic gastrojejunostomy is performed for non-resectable antral neoplasms. The jejunum is anastomosed to the greater curvature after ligature and division of the lower short gastric vessels (Figure 8.38). The posterior short loop gastroenterostomy favoured for benign disease is inappropriate as a palliative procedure for gastric carcinoma. The Devine's exclusion-bypass operation (Figure 8.39), previously popular for inoperable antral neoplasms, is seldom performed nowadays in view of the poor results. Dysphagia due to inoperable lesions of the cardia is best treated by intubation (e.g. plastic or metallic expanding stents) which is preferable to the more difficult and major procedure of jejuno-oesophageal bypass. Alternatively, dysphagia can be relieved by photodynamic therapy using Photofrin II and red laser light (620 nm).

Other malignant epithelial tumours of the stomach

These include adenosquamous, squamous and anaplastic tumours. Adenosquamous carcinomas are rare tumours, which are usually found at the cardia. They

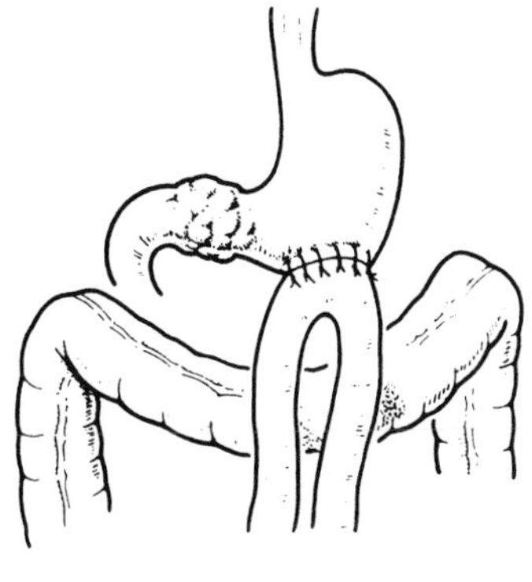

Figure 8.38 An antecolic gastroenterostomy to the greater curvature of the stomach is an effective palliative procedure for inoperable carcinoma of the stomach.

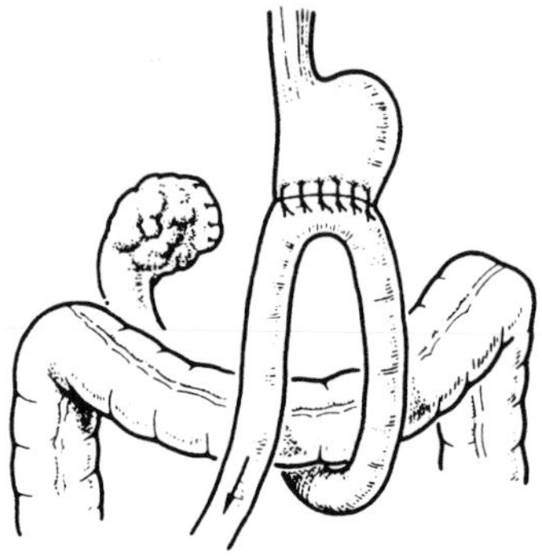

Figure 8.39 Diagrammatic representation of Devine's antral exclusion bypass operation for inoperable carcinoma of the antrum. This operation is seldom performed nowadays. It is difficult to perform in the presence of large antral tumours and the results have been poor. It has largely been replaced by the Tanner's antecolic anastomosis to the greater curvature.

are mixed tumours and both components (squamous and glandular) are histologically and biologically malignant. Until recently, anaplastic malignant tumours caused considerable difficulties with the histological diagnosis and especially the differentiation between an anaplastic carcinoma and a high-grade undifferentiated malignant lymphoma. This problem has been overcome with the advent of specific monoclonal antisera to the common leucocyte antigen (CLA) which is specific for lymphomas. Monoclonal antibodies to the epithelial membrane antigen (EMA) and cytokeratin (CAM 5.2) are used to identify the epithelial origin of anaplastic carcinomas.

Mesenchymal tumours

These include smooth muscle tumours, neurogenic tumours (Schwannomas) and neoplasms of uncommitted mesenchymal cells, often considered as a less differentiated variant of leiomyomas. More recently, the last group has been classified as gastrointestinal stromal tumours (GISTs) separate from leiomyomas and leiomyosarcomas on the basis of their immunohistochemical staining characteristics. All are positive for c-kit (CD117) and CD34 and although some GISTs show positive staining for muscle actin, all are negative for desmin and S100-protein. A Finnish study has confirmed the distinct genetic identity of GISTs with DNA copy number losses in 14q not present in leiomyomas and leiomyosarcomas. The distinction between benign and malignant lesions is difficult. Mitotic activity on histological examination is important in this respect although lesions with little or no mitotic activity have been known to recur or metastasize after excision.

The term *gastrointestinal sarcoma* covers smooth muscle, GIST and neurogenic tumours with malignant potential. These sarcomas are rare and constitute 1% of gastric malignancies. The commonest site is the stomach (50%), followed by small bowel and duodenum (30%). The usual clinical presentation irrespective of site is with pain or bleeding (acute or chronic). Some 20% are asymptomatic and may be found accidentally during operation, and 10–20% of gastrointestinal sarcomas present acutely with tumour perforation. Large tumours may cause massive intraperitoneal bleeding. Carney's syndrome, which usually affects young females, consists of gastric sarcoma in association with pulmonary chrondromas and extra-adrenal paragalionomas that may be secreting causing hypertension.

The stomach is one of the common sites of smooth muscle tumours. Although they are often classified into benign (leiomyoma) and malignant (leiomyosarcoma), the histological differentiation between the two may be difficult. However, the majority of gastric smooth muscle tumours are benign. They are encountered in the upper and middle thirds and rarely in the antrum of the stomach. Malignant tumours tend to be larger, show necrotic and haemorrhagic change and have a mitotic rate, which exceeds 10 per 50 high power fields. All gastric smooth tumours are submucosal but their growth pattern differs. Some grow preferentially towards the serosal side (*predominantly subserosal*), others predominantly into the lumen (*intraluminal*). Large tumours can grow in both directions resulting in *dumb-bell lesions*. The differentiation between benign and malignant may be difficult even by histology and mitotic index but tumours <5.0 cm are usually benign with a reported incidence of nodal deposits of 2%.

Gastric sarcomas occur predominantly in the proximal stomach. In one of the largest published series, the 10 year survival after curative resection was 93% overall (87.5% after gastrectomy and 95% after wedge resection). The survival was not influenced by the type of resection (local resection versus gastrectomy) but was adversely affected by ulceration of tumour, and size >5.0 cm. Metastatic or recurrent disease was observed in 9/103 (8.7%) patients. The site of the recurrence was in the liver or peritoneal cavity.

Some smooth muscle tumours show areas of epithelioid differentiation and are referred to as epithelioid smooth muscle tumours, epithelioid myomas or leiomyoblastomas. Other non-epithelial tumours encountered in the stomach include haemangiopericytoma and Kaposi's sarcomas. Even in the absence of von Recklinghausen's disease, neurogenic tumours occur in the stomach and they usually originate from the autonomic nerve elements. They are macroscopically indistinguishable from smooth muscle tumours but on specific staining with neurogenic markers (neuron-specific enolase), their neurogenic origin is confirmed. The management is identical to that of smooth muscle tumours and indeed the vast majority are clinically diagnosed as such and the true nature of the tumour is only identified if detailed histochemical staining is performed on the resected specimen.

Treatment

For most tumours, local resection without lymphadenectomy is nowadays regarded as the correct surgical treatment. Local resection with a surrounding cuff of 1.0–2.0 cm is a safer option than local enucleation as this encourages spillage and implantation leading to recurrence. For lesions >5.0 cm a formal gastrectomy with lymphadenectomy is necessary. The extent of lymphadenectomy (D_1 vs D_2) remains a matter of individual practice, although the published evidence indicates that the D_1 resection should suffice, as the incidence of lymph node deposits is very low. There is now an extensive reported experience of laparoscopic treatment of gastric mesenchymal tumours and the results have been entirely favourable with low morbidity and short hospital stay. The technique and nature of treatment depend on several factors:

- size of lesion
- its location and
- growth morphology (subserosal or exophytic, intraluminal or endophytic, dumbbell).

Anterior wall subserosal tumours are the easiest tumours to resect by the laparoscopic approach. The lesion is removed with a surrounding cuff of normal stomach. This can be achieved by excision with a linear cutting endostapler or by electrosurgical excision followed by single-layer continuous suture closure of the defect. If the stapling technique is used, the lesion is pulled up and the stapler jaws are applied to normal stomach wall on either side of the lesion in a vertical direction to prevent narrowing of the stomach at the site of excision. The advantage of the stapler technique is ease of execution but the excision-suture technique ensures a more complete circumferential clearance. Posterior wall subserosal tumours are best approached through the lesser sac. The greater curvature is then grasped and pulled up to expose the posterior wall of the stomach and the lesion, which is then excised and the defect closed by continuous suture. Alternatively linear cutting stapler excision can be used. Others use the transgastric approach for posterior lesions.

Intra-operative endoscopy is essential for locating the exact site of gastric intraluminal smooth muscle tumours. For large endophytic lesions some recommend a two step approach, i.e. endoscopic debulking followed by laparoscopic resection. For anterior intraluminal tumours, following endoscopic location, a suture is applied on the gastric wall overlying the tumour and used to tent the anterior wall of the stomach during excision. Excision by high-frequency electrosurgery is preferable to linear cutting stapler excision in this location. There are two options for posterior endophytic lesions: (i) transgastric through a gastrotomy of the anterior wall of the stomach or (ii) by the transgastrostomal endoscopic approach. The laparo-endogastric approach is inadvisable as the full thickness excision that is required for these lesions results in deflation of the gastric lumen rendering the procedure very difficult. The anterior gastrotomy is fashioned opposite the site of the lesion located by flexible endoscopy. It is bad practice to grasp the tumour. Instead a suture is placed on the stomach wall close to the lesion and by traction; this enables prolapse of the tumour and adjacent posterior wall of the stomach through the gastrotomy. The lesion is then excised either by high-frequency electrosurgery or by application of the linear cutting endostapler. The anterior gastrotomy is then closed with continuous single layer suturing. The hand-assist laparoscopic approach can also be used for these tumours.

Gastric smooth muscle tumours within 1.0 cm of the oesophagogastric junction or close to the pyloric ring are difficult to resect laparoscopically and some consider these as contraindications to the laparoscopic approach. Aside from technical difficulties during surgery, the functional outcome may be jeopardized by disruption of the anti-reflux mechanism or emptying of the stomach. In the author's experience, lesions close to the pylorus can be effectively treated by laparoscopic antrectomy with Billroth I or II reconstruction.

Tumours greater than 5.0 cm are best treated with gastrectomy either open or by the laparoscopic hand-assisted laparoscopic approach.

Gastric lymphomas

Primary Hodgkin's disease is extremely rare in the gastrointestinal tract and in practice all gastrointestinal lymphomas are of the non-Hodgkin's type (NHL) arising from either B or T-cells. Non-Hodgkin's lymphoma of the gastrointestinal tract accounts for 4–20% of all NHLs and is the most common extranodal site of presentation. The stomach is the major organ involved by gastrointestinal lymphoma. A significant proportion of gastric lymphomas are of low-grade histology and arise from MALT. Such MALT lymphomas may be associated with *H. pylori* infection and may undergo complete regression following eradication of *H. pylori*.

Pathology of primary gastric lymphomas

Primary gastric lymphomas (PGLs) tend to infiltrate the wall of the stomach in a diffuse fashion causing mucosal thickening with a tendency to ulceration and indeed perforation. The pyloric antrum is the commonest site followed by the body and the cardia. Histologically a PGL consists of follicle centres (non-neoplastic component) that are surrounded and invaded by a malignant cellular infiltrate consisting of centrocyte-like cells and a variable proportion of plasma cells (some reactive, some neoplastic). This malignant infiltrate extends into the surrounding mucosa where it forms characteristic lymphoepithelial lesions and to the submucosa where it induces dense sclerosis. Lymph node spread from B-cell MALT lymphoma is usually limited to the gastric regional lymph nodes. A more aggressive type of PGL is the malignant centrocytic variety. Histologically, this consists of neoplastic centrocytes which form a mantle zone around the reactive follicles which they invade and ultimately replace (mantle cell lymphoma). This tumour has a tendency to form multiple polypoid masses and for this reason, it is often referred to as multiple lymphomatous polyposis.

The lymphoma that arises in response to stimulation by the gluten antigen in patients with coeliac disease is a T-cell lymphoma. It is the most common primary gastrointestinal T-cell lymphoma, arising from the intra-epithelial T-cells, and is always clinically aggressive.

MALT lymphomas

MALT lymphomas arise from sites normally devoid of lymphoid tissue and are preceded by chronic inflammatory, usually immune, disorders that induce the accumulation of lymphoid tissue in the first instance. The stomach is the most common site of MALT lymphoma. In the vast majority of cases (90%) gastric lymphoma arises on a background of *H. pylori* infection/gastritis and much less commonly *H. heilmannii.* MALT and other lymphomas (B or T-cell) can develop in patients with:

- dyspepsia
- coeliac disease – gluten autoimmunity
- virally induced immunodeficiency (HIV)
- immunosuppression after solid-organ transplantation
- inflammatory bowel disease
- other viruses – Epstein–Barr virus (EBV).

The development of primary gastric MALT lymphoma is a multi-stage process. The initial stage is that of *recruitment*: aggregates of normal MALT appear in response to infection/gastritis by these organisms. BCA-1, which functions as a homing chemokine in normal lymphoid tissue, is induced in chronic *H. pylori* gastritis and may be involved in the formation of these gastric lymphoid follicles. The transition chronic *H. pylori*-associated gastritis → low-grade lymphoma → high-grade lymphoma involves both physiological T-cell mediated immune responses and the acquisition of genetic abnormalities. The tumour is thought to originate from an autoreactive MALT marginal zone B-cell as a consequence of a genotoxic insult induced by *H. pylori* infection. This autoreactive progenitor tumour cell proliferates and develops early genetic abnormalities and instability, e.g. t(11;18) translocation, trisomy three, c-myc and p53 mutations resulting in *partial neoplastic transformation*. This abnormal B-cell clone is then stimulated to expand and form a *low-grade lymphoma* by *H. pylori*-specific intratumoral T-cells. The dependence of growth on continued immunological stimulation by the *H. pylori* antigens is demonstrated by *in vitro* experiments confirming growth stimulation of lymphoma cells (harvested from low-grade lymphomas) on contact with T-cells sensitized to heat-killed *H. pylori.* It also explains the regression of early tumours (stage IE) following eradication of *H. pylori.* By contrast large, deeply invasive tumors and those that have undergone high-grade transformation typically do not respond to eradication therapy. This is the consequence of additional genetic abnormalities (complete inactivation of the tumour suppressor genes p53 and p16, activation of c-myc oncogene and overexpression of Bcl-6) that enable this abnormal B-cell clone to become T-cell independent. At this stage *transformation from low-grade to high-grade* lymphoma has occurred. High-grade MALT lymphomas are composed of large-sized lymphoma cells that are morphologically indistinguishable from nodal large B-cell lymphomas. The *H. pylori* strain appears to be important in the development of high-grade lymphoma. Thus the frequency of $CagA^+$ strain infection is significantly higher (77% versus 38%) in high-grade than in low-grade MALT lymphomas indicating that high-grade gastric MALT lymphoma transformation is more likely to occur following infection by $CagA^+$ strains.

High-grade B-cell lymphomas are classified in three groups based on the presence or absence of a low-grade MALT component and lymphoepithelial lesions (LELs):

- high-grade MALT lymphomas appearing in low-grade MALT lymphomas (LG/HG MALT lymphoma)
- large cell lymphoma with LELs composed of large cells (high-grade LELs) but without a low-grade component (HG MALT lymphoma)
- diffuse large B-cell lymphoma without a low-grade MALT lymphoma component or LELs (DLBCL).

EBV may contribute to the pathogenesis of a small proportion of high-grade MALT lymphoma, where virtually all tumor cells harbour EBV. These tumours can be identified because the component cells express the oncogenic viral protein LMP1.

Clinical features

PGL is the most common extranodal lymphoid tumour in the Western world and accounts for 60% of gastrointestinal lymphomas. By contrast, in the Middle East, where small bowel disease predominates, PGL accounts for only 38% of all gut lymphomas. Seen in perspective, PGL is a rare disease and accounts for 2–5% of all gastric malignancies and is less common than secondary involvement of the stomach by primary nodal disease. There is evidence that the incidence has been rising over the past 20 years. The clinical course varies with the grade of the lesion, being slow and indolent in low-grade MALT tumours.

PGL affects both sexes with only a marginal male predominance. The age distribution is wide, with the mean around 55–60 years. The early symptoms of the disease are indistinguishable from those of gastric carcinoma and always include upper abdominal discomfort and dyspepsia, although nausea, vomiting and weight loss are less common. Some patients develop diarrhoea, which is often persistent. Ulceration of the tumour may lead to bleeding and perforation and indeed some 10–15% of patients with high-grade aggressive tumours present as an emergency with acute bleeding or perforation. The risk of both complications is enhanced by chemotherapy. The prognosis is influenced by the grade (low, low-intermediate, high-intermediate), irrespective of age. Within each grade the adverse prognostic factors in patients with non-Hodgkin's lymphoma are:

- age >60 years
- elevated lactate dehydrogenase (× 1 normal)
- performance status
- stage of the disease.

Patients with Hodgkin's disease and nodal non-Hodgkin's lymphomas are known to have an excess risk for other cancers. A high incidence of other cancers has also been suggested in patients with gastric MALT lymphomas. In one large reported series other tumours were detected in 12% of patients either prior to MALT gastric lymphoma or concomitantly or after diagnosis of the lymphoma. The most frequent other tumours are lymphoid neoplasms and gastric carcinoma. This study did not confirm an excess incidence of other tumours on statistical grounds, except perhaps in patients under 50 years. The most important association is with gastric cancer arising concomitantly or after gastric lymphoma.

A palpable mass is present in at least 20% of patients but its detection does not signify inoperability. Occult blood is found on testing in 50% of patients. The erythrocyte sedimentation rate (ESR) is grossly elevated. The diagnosis is confirmed by endoscopy with multiple biopsy. The criteria for establishing a PGL include absence of superficial lymphadenopathy and splenomegaly, normal chest X-ray, no hepatic involvement and appropriate histology.

The endoscopic findings which favour a diagnosis of gastric lymphoma include mucosal oedema with a cobblestone appearance, rugal hypertrophy, multiple tumour nodules and multiple superficial ulcerations overlying a large tumour mass. The endoscopic appearances of low-grade disease most commonly consist of superficial spreading lesions without ulceration (60%). However, both ulcerofungating and ulceroinfiltrating lesions are encountered. Overall, invasion of muscularis propria is encountered in 28% of patients of patients with low-grade disease. Likewise lymph node involvement is common even in low-grade disease confined to mucosa and submucosa. High-grade MALT lymphomas tend to form large solitary tumours. The higher the grade of tumor, the larger the tumor size. Endoscopic ultrasonography is very useful in the assessment of the depth of tumoral infiltration of the gastric wall by PGL. This is reflected by an increased gastric wall thickness, the extent of which (up to 5 mm, 6 mm or greater) differentiates superficial from infiltrative tumours. The mucosal thickness should return to normal following successful treatment (*vide infra*). Persistence of gastric wall thickness indicates evolving disease or relapse even if endoscopic histology is negative. Staging of gastric low-grade MALT lymphomas by endoscopic ultrasonography allows prediction of the response to therapy by eradication of *H. pylori*. Thus complete remission is only encountered in patients with disease limited to mucosa and submucosa.

Table 8.13 Ann Arbor staging of lymphomas

- Stage I: Involvement of a single lymph node region (I) or single extralymphatic organ or site (IE)
- Stage II: Involvement of two or more lymph node regions on the same side of the diaphragm (II) or localized involvement of an extralymphatic organ or site (IIE)
- Stage III: Involvement of lymph node regions on both sides of the diaphragm (III) or localized involvement of an extralymphatic organ or site (IIIE), the spleen (IIIS) or both (IIISE)
- Stage IV: Diffuse or disseminated involvement of one or more extralymphatic organs with or without associated lymph node involvement

Asymptomatic patients are designated as distinct from those with symptoms (B) which include fever, sweats or weight loss <10% body weight.

Treatment

Once a diagnosis of PGL is made, the tumour is staged, most commonly using the Ann Arbor system (Table 8.13), although the modified TNM system used for gastric carcinoma is adopted by some (Table 8.11). Staging is important because multivariate statistical analysis of reported data has demonstrated that clinical stage is the only significant factor in relapse-free and disease-specific survival. Although often performed, CT has low sensitivity in detecting perigastric lymphadenopathy in PGL and understages the disease in 33% of patients. Much more accurate staging is obtained by gastric endoscopic ultrasound scanning and by positron emission tomography after the injection of $[^{18}F]$fluorodeoxyglucose (^{18}FDG PET). This provides the most accurate measure of the extension of PGL in the gastric wall but is available only in a few centres.

The optimal management of PGL has never been determined by prospective randomized clinical trials. Thus management varies from centre to centre. It is best to consider management in accordance with stage of the disease.

Stage I disease

The majority of these patients are *H. pylori/H. heilmannii* positive. In these patients eradication of the infection is followed by complete regression of MALT lymphoma in 50–55%, partial regression in 23–30% and no response in 23–35%. Tumours in the distal stomach appear more likely to respond than tumours in the proximal stomach. The probability of complete regression of lymphoma is 60% at 6 months, 79% at 12 months and 100% at 14 months, respectively. The factors predictive of complete and/or near complete MALT lymphoma regression are:

- *H. pylori* cure
- grade of tumour – complete response limited to low-grade lymphomas
- stage – tumours limited to mucosa/submucosa, up to 5 mm thickness on endoscopic ultrasound.

As histological regression occurs at variable rates following cure of *H. pylori*, long-term follow-up is necessary as small areas of high-grade tumour may lead to recurrence of a lesion that is intrinsically more malignant with totally autonomous growth.

The recommended eradication regimens used vary considerably and are constantly changing in terms of the drug combination used, the duration of each course and the number of courses administered. The most common first line treatment (except in patients with known allergy or intolerance) is full dose PPIs bid, clarithromycin 500 mg bid and amoxycillin 1000 mg bid for 10 days. Others recommend two of three oral antibiotic regimens along with a PPI and bismuth subsalicylate administered sequentially for 21 days and at 8 weeks:

- amoxicillin, 750 mg three times daily, and clarithromycin, 500 mg three times daily
- tetracycline, 500 mg four times daily, and clarithromycin, 500 mg three times daily
- tetracycline, 500 mg four times daily, and metronidazole, 500 mg three times daily.

Eradication has to be confirmed preferably by culture. Overall, eradication therapies are safe and neither the decreased efficacy of acid-lowering drugs, nor the possible increased risk of peptic oesophagitis is considered as a contraindication. It has to be stressed that there are as yet insufficient data with regard to the duration of the remissions induced by eradication of *H. pylori* and thus long-term surveillance is essential. Second tumors/relapses have been reported in 15–20% of patients. Even more worrying are well-documented reports of patients with histological disappearance of the lymphoma following eradication who subsequently developed an aggressive nodal type B-cell non-Hodgkin's lymphoma usually of the diffuse large cell type. In many of these patients the second high-grade lymphoma proved fatal despite intensive chemotherapy. Thus although complete remissions of low-grade gastric MALT lymphomas after the cure of *H. pylori* infection appear to be stable, at present there are insufficient data to conclude that these patients are truly cured of their disease.

Eradication therapy is not indicated in patients who are *H. pylori* negative. The best treatment for these tumours has yet to be defined. The options are chemotherapy versus local treatment, i.e. surgery or radiotherapy. The reported data indicate a similar high 5 year survival (>90%) with all three modalities. On the basis of these data, it would appear that for *H. pylori* negative stage I tumours, the first line treatment rests between radiotherapy and chemotherapy. As radiotherapy is well tolerated and has fewer side-effects than chemotherapy, it has to be regarded as the optimal treatment for these patients with localized *H. pylori* negative gastric MALT lymphoma. Surgery is reserved for treatment failures or complications.

Stage II disease

The optimal management of stage II has not been established despite the use of various treatment modalities. The most widely used management entails surgery (total/partial gastrectomy) followed by chemotherapy initially with m-VEPA (vincristine, cyclophosphamide, prednisolone and doxorubicin). This is followed by consolidation chemotherapy with VEMP (vindesine, cyclophosphamide, methotrexate and prednisolone) or VQEP (vindesine, carbazilquinone, cyclophosphamide and prednisolone). The reported post-operative overall and disease-free survival rates at 10 years with this management are 82% and 92.0%, respectively. Thus stage II PGL appears to be curable when treated with gastrectomy and adjuvant chemotherapy.

Stages III/IV disease

The prognosis is poor especially in patients with stage IV disease. Initially treatment is with chemotherapy or chemo-irradiation. Emergency surgery (gastrectomy) is needed in patients with perforation/bleeding who may arise *de novo* or complicate chemotherapy/radiotherapy. Elective surgical resection is indicated for patients who respond to chemotherapy but have residual disease. Although primary surgical resection was practised widely for stage III disease and resulted in 5 year survival of 20%, this practice has been largely replaced by chemotherapy. If primary gastric resection is undertaken for stage III disease, post-operative chemotherapy should be administered.

Gastric pseudolymphoma (benign lymphoid hyperplasia)

The term pseudolymphoma was used until recently to describe certain lesions found in some patients with active or healed peptic ulcers. The endoscopic appearance of these antral lesions, which can be single or multiple, varies from ulcers with overhanging margins to areas of nodularity and flat plaques with an infiltrative appearance. Histologically, they consist of an infiltrate of small lymphocytes containing germinal cells, e.g. plasma cells, eosinophils and polymorphs, and fibrosis in the submucosal layer. The term 'pseudolymphoma' was used because of the frequent inability to identify the true nature of the lesion: reactive or neoplastic. This problem has now been resolved because with modern immunohistochemical staining and DNA analysis it is always possible to differentiate monotypic (neoplastic lymphocytes) with light-chain restriction from proliferation of polytypic (reactive) non-neoplastic cells. The term pseudolymphoma should therefore be abandoned and replaced by benign or reactive lymphoid hyperplasia, which accurately describes these lesions.

Carcinoid and other endocrine tumours

Gastric carcinoids are rare and account for only 2% of the reported gastrointestinal carcinoids. There is an established association between the atrophic gastritis (type A) and chronic hypergastrinaemia of pernicious anaemia and the development of gastric carcinoids. Initially these patients develop hyperplasia of the gastrin-producing G cells of the antral mucosa and of the argyrophil endocrine cells (enterochromaffin) of the fundic mucosa. This is followed in time by the development of a spectrum of neoplastic change varying from diffuse hyperplasia of the argyrophil cells to multiple focal tumourlets (microcarcinoidosis) to obvious, often multiple, discrete carcinoid tumours. The prevalence of gastric carcinoids in patients with pernicious anaemia is variously reported at 2–9%. More recently, fundal enterochromaffin tumours have been reported in patients with the Zollinger–Ellison syndrome after prolonged therapy with omeprazole.

The gastric carcinoids developing in patients with pernicious anaemia often contain gastrin, somatostatin, serotonin and vasoactive intestinal peptide. By contrast gastric carcinoids arising in a previously normal mucosa do not produce serotonin but may contain histamine. Recently, patients with gastric carcinoids and hyperparathyroidism due to adenoma formation or hyperplasia have been reported. Gastric carcinoids, though generally slow growing and indolent, can metastasize especially if they exhibit atypical histology and are larger than 2.0 cm. They are rarely symptomatic and the majority are discovered during endoscopy or contrast examination of the stomach. They do not have a distinctive macroscopic appearance and can form smooth elevations covered by intact mucosa, polypoid projections or ulcerative lesions, which can cause chronic blood loss and microcytic hypochromic anaemia. Overt haematemesis is, however, rare. The carcinoid syndrome caused by a primary gastric carcinoid has never been reported.

Gastric carcinoids are best treated by local resection, although some advocate and practise endoscopic resection (especially for small tumours) followed by endoscopic surveillance. The use of antrectomy (to abolish the source of gastrin) in patients with diffuse hyperplasia and micro-carcinoidosis is being evaluated in some centres. The prognosis following resection is good even in the presence of regional node deposits and hepatic metastases.

The other endocrine tumours of the stomach arise either from normally resident endocrine cells within the gastric mucosa or from islands of ectopic pancreatic tissue (e.g. insulinoma). They may be single or multiple. Although rare, gastrinomas are well documented in the stomach although they are usually sited in the duodenum and may then be accompanied by neurofibromatosis and phaeochromocytoma.

Primary duodenal carcinoma

Primary duodenal carcinoma is a distinct entity and should be differentiated from ampullary and periampullary tumours. It is closely linked with villous adenoma, which is present in 50% of cases. In addition, adjacent duodenal dysplasia is encountered in 60%. The most common site of origin of primary duodenal carcinoma is the descending (second part) of the duodenum (80%) but tumours can originate in the third and fourth parts. There is an equal sex incidence and the median age at diagnosis is 60 years although the age range of reported cases is wide (21–82 years). Half of the patients present with jaundice. Other common presenting symptoms include pain, iron-deficiency anaemia due to occult blood loss and vomiting from duodenal obstruction. Treatment of operable disease is with pancreatoduodenectomy. The 5 year survival after curative resection averages 40%.

Further reading

General

Caletti, G. and Fusasroli, P. (1999). Endoscopic ultrasonography. *Endoscopy* **31**: 95–102.

Froehlich, F., Bochud, M., Gonvers, J.-J. *et al.* (1999). Appropriatness of gastroscopy: dyspepsia. *Endoscopy* 31: 579–95.

Gabriel, S. E., Jaakkimainen, L. and Bombardier, C. (1991). Risk of serious gastrointestinal complications related to use of nonsteroidal anti-inflammatory drugs. A meta-analysis. *Ann Intern Med* **115**: 787–96.

Misiewicz, J. J. (1991). The Sydney System: a new classification of gastritis. *J Gastroenterol Hepatol* **6**: 207–8.

Price, A. B. (1991). The Sydney System: Histologicaldivision. *J Gastroenterol Hepatol* **6**: 209–22.

Sipponen, P and Stolte, M. (1997). Clinical impact of routine biopsies of the gastric antrum and body. *Endoscopy* **29**: 671–8.

Talley, N. J., Evans, J. M., Fleming, K. C. *et al.* (1995). Nonsteroidal antinflammatory drugs and dyspepsia in the elderly. *Dig Dis Sci* **40**: 1345–50.

Gastric cancer

Bonenkamp, J. J., Songun. J., Hermans, J. *et al.* (1995). Randomised comparison of morbidity after D_1 and D_2 dissection for gastric cancer in 996 Dutch patients. *Lancet* **345**: 745–8.

Cuschieri, A., Weeden, S., Fielding, J. *et al.* (1999). Patient survival after D_1 and D_2 resections for gastric cancer: long-term results of the MRC randomized surgical trial. *Br J Cancer* **79**: 1522–30.

Griffith, J. P. (1995). Preservation of the spleen improves survival after radical surgery for gastric cancer. *Gut* **36**: 684–90.

Japanese Classification of Gastric Carcinoma – 2nd English Edition (1998). *Gastric Cancer* **1**: 10–24.

Lisborg, P. H., Jatzko, G. R., Denk, H. *et al.* (1997). Long-term survival analysis of gastric cancer limited to the submucosa. *J Gastroenterol* **35**: 663–8.

Ohashi, S. (1995). Laparoscopic intraluminal (intragastric) surgery for early gastric cancer. *Surg Endosc* **9**: 161–71.

Siewert, J. R., Bottcher, K., Roder, J. D. *et al.* (1993). Prognostic relevance of systematic node dissection in gastric carcinoma. *Br J Surg* **80**: 1015–18.

Siu, W. T., Leong, H. T. and Li, M. K. (1997). Laparoscopic resection of bleeding gastric polyps. *Surg Endosc* **11**: 283–4.

Smith, J. W., Shiu, M. H., Kelsey, L. and Brennan, M. F. (1991). Morbidity of radical lymphadenectomy in the curative resection of gastric carcinoma. *Arch Surg* **126**: 1469–73.

Spinelli, P., Cerrai, F. G., Cambareri, A. R. *et al.* (1993). Two-step endoscopic resection of gastric leiomyoma. *Surg Edosc* **7**: 90–2.

Sue-Ling, H. M. (1998). Detection and treatment of early cancer in the West. *Gastric Cancer* **1**: 8–9.

Sue-Ling, H. M. and Johnston, D. (1993). Gastric cancer: a curable disease in Britain. *BMJ* **307**: 591–6.

Takeshita, K., Saeki, I., Tani, M. *et al.* (1998). Rational lymphadenectomy for early gastric cancer with submucosal invasion: a clinicopathological study. *Jpn J Surg* **28**: 580–6.

Mesenchymal tumours

Aogi, K., Hirai, T., Mukaida, H. *et al.* (1999). Laparoscopic resection of submucosal gastric tumours. *Surgery Today Jpn J Surg* **29**: 102–6.

Azagra, J. S., Goergen, M., De Simone, P. and Ibanez-Aguirre, J. (1999). Minimally invasive surgery for gastric cancer. *Surg Endosc* **13**: 351–7.

El-Rifai, W., Sarlomo-Rikala, M., Andersson, L. C. *et al.* (1998). DNA copy number changes in gastrointestinal stromal tumours – a distinct genetic entity. *Ann Chir Gynaec* **87**: 287–90.

Katai, H., Sasako, M., Sano, T. and Maruyama, K. (1998). Surgical treatment of gastric leiomyosarcoma. *Ann Chir Gynaec* **87**: 293–6.

Morgan, B. K., Compton, C., Talbert, M. *et al.* (1990). Benign smooth tumours of the gastrointestinal tract. *Ann Surg* **211**: 63–6.

Motson, R. W., Fisher, P. W. and Dawson, J. W. (1995). Laparoscopic resection of a benign intragastric stromal tumour. *Br J Surg* **82**: 1670.

Otani, Y., Ohgami, M., Kubota, T *et al.* (1997). Surgical management of gastric leiomyosarcoma: evaluation of the propriety of laparoscopic wedge resection. *World J Surg* **21**: 440–3.

Sasako, M., Kinoshita, T., Maruyama, K. *et al.* (1989). Surgical management of gastric leiomyosarcoma – a clinicopathological study of 51 resected cases. *Jpn J Gastroenterol Surgery* **22**: 2212–16.

Watson, D. I., Game, P. A. and Devitt, P. G. (1996). Laparoscopic resection of benign tumours of the posterior gastric wall. *Surg Endosc* **10**: 540–1.

Welch, J. P. (1975). Smooth muscle tumours of the stomach. *Am J Surg* **130**: 279–85.

Yamashita, Y., Maekawa, T., Sakai, T. and Shirakusa, T. (1999). Transgastrostomal endoscopic surgery for early gastric carcinoma and submucosal tumour. *Surg Endosc* **13**: 361–4.

Lymphomas

Chang, D. K., Chin, Y. J., Kim, J. S. *et al.* (1999). Lymph node involvement rate in low-grade gastric mucosa-associated lymphoid tissue lymphoma-too high to be neglected. *Hepatogastroenterology* **46**: 2694–700.

Chen, T. K., Wu, C. H., Lee, C. L. *et al.* (1999). Endoscopic ultrasonography in the differential diagnosis of giant gastric folds. *J Formos Med Assoc* **98**: 261–4.

Crump, M., Gospodarowicz, M. and Shepherd, F. A. (1999). Lymphoma of the gastrointestinal tract. *Semin Oncol* **26**: 324–37.

Ferreri, A. J., Ponzoni, M., Cordio, S. *et al.* (1998). Low sensitivity of computed tomography in the staging of gastric lymphomas of mucosa-associated lymphoid tissue: impact on prospective trials and ordinary clinical practice. *Am J Clin Oncol* **21**: 614–16.

Fung, C. Y., Grossbard, M. L., Linggood, R. M. *et al.* (1999). Mucosa-associated lymphoid tissue lymphoma of the stomach: long term outcome after local treatment. *Cancer* **85**: 9–17.

Hsi, E. D., Eisbruch, A., Greenson, J. K. *et al.* (1998). Classification of primary gastric lymphomas according to histologic features. *Am J Surg Pathol* **22**: 17–27.

Ioachim, H. L., Hajdu, C., Giancotti, F. R. and Dorsett, B. (1999). Lymphoid proliferations and lymphomas associated with gastric metaplasia, dysplasia, and carcinoma. *Hum Pathol* **30**: 833–42.

Isaacson, P. G. (1999). Gastrointestinal lymphomas of T- and B-cell types. *Mod Pathol* **12**: 151–8.

Isaacson, P. G. (1999). Mucosa-associated lymphoid tissue lymphoma. *Semin Hematol* **36**: 139–47.

Kodera, Y., Yamamura, Y., Nakamura, S. *et al.* (1998). The role of radical gastrectomy with systematic lymphadenectomy for the diagnosis and treatment of primary gastric lymphoma. *Ann Surg* **227**: 45–50.

Levy, M., Hammel, P., Lamarque, D. *et al.* (1997). Endoscopic ultrasonography for the initial staging and follow-up in patients with low-grade gastric lymphoma of mucosa-associated lymphoid tissue treated medically. *Gastrointest Endosc* **46**: 328–33.

Makela, J., Karttunen, T., Kiviniemi, H. and Laitinen, S. (1999). Clinicopathological features of primary gastric lymphoma. *J Surg Oncol* **70**: 78–82.

Montalban, C., Castrillo, J. M., Lopez-Abente, G. *et al.* (1999). Other cancers in patients with gastric MALT lymphoma. *Leuk Lymphoma* **33**: 161–8.

Neubauer, A., Thiede, C., Morgner, A. *et al.* (1997). Cure of *Helicobacter pylori* infection and duration of remission of low-grade gastric mucosa-associated lymphoid tissue lymphoma. *J Natl Cancer Inst* **89**: 1350–5.

Peng, H., Ranaldi, R., Diss, T. C. *et al.* (1998). High frequency of CagA^{+} *Helicobacter pylori* infection in high-grade gastric MALT B-cell lymphomas. *J Pathol* **185**: 409–12.

Regimbeau, C., Karsenti, D., Durand, V. *et al.* (1998). Low-grade gastric MALT lymphoma and *Helicobacter heilmannii* (Gastrospirillum Hominis). *Gastroenterol Clin Biol* **22**: 720–3.

Rodriguez, M. (1998). Computed tomography, magnetic resonance imaging and positron emission tomography in non-Hodgkin's lymphoma. *Acta Radiol Suppl* **417**: 1–36.

Sackmann, M., Morgner, A., Rudolph, B. *et al.* (1997). Regression of gastric MALT lymphoma after eradication of *Helicobacter pylori* is predicted by endosonographic staging. MALT Lymphoma Study Group. *Gastroenterology* **113**: 1087–90.

Steinbach, G., Ford, R., Glober, G. *et al.* (1999). Antibiotic treatment of gastric lymphoma of mucosa-associated lymphoid tissue. An uncontrolled trial. *Ann Intern Med* **131**: 88–95.

Takenaka, T., Maruyama, K., Kinoshita, T. *et al.* (1997). A prospective study of surgery and adjuvant chemotherapy for primary gastric lymphoma stage II. *Br J Cancer* **76**: 1484–8.

Tursi, A. and Gasbarrini, G. (1999). Acquired gastric mucosa-associated lymphoid tissue (MALT): a review with special emphasis on association with extragastric diseases and management problems of gastric MALT. *J Clin Gastroenterol* **29**: 133–7.

Weston, A. P., Banerjee, S. K., Horvat, R. T. *et al.* (1999). Prospective long-term endoscopic and histologic follow-up of gastric lymphoproliferative disease of early stage IE low-grade B-cell mucosa-associated lymphoid tissue type following *Helicobacter pylori* eradication treatment. *Int J Oncol* **15**: 899–907.

Xu, W. S., Chan, A. C., Lee, J. M. *et al.* (1998). Epstein-Barr virus infection and its gene expression in gastric lymphoma of mucosa-associated lymphoid tissue. *J Med Virol* **56**: 342–50.

Yoshino, T. and Akagi, T. (1998). Gastric low-grade mucosa-associated lymphoid tissue lymphomas: their histogenesis and high-grade transformation. *Pathol Int* **48**: 323–31.

MODULE 9

Disorders of the liver

Section 9.1 • Anatomy of the liver

The liver is the largest organ in the body, with a weight varying from 1200 to 1600 g. It arises from the foregut endoderm as a diverticulum which extends into the septum transversum and connects with the vitelline veins of the yolk sac. The caudal section of the hepatic anlage ultimately forms the biliary tract and gallbladder while the cephalic section forms the hepatic parenchyma. The vitelline veins form the portal and hepatic veins. The left umbilical vein persists as the ductus venosum and diverts oxygenated blood from the placenta around the liver directly into the inferior vena cava. After birth the vestigial ligamentum venosum runs in the free edge of the falciform ligament (round ligament, ligamentum teres). It may recanalize in patients with portal venous hypertension or can be used after dilatation for exchange blood transfusion or to permit radiological investigation of the portal venous system.

Morphology and topographical anatomy of the liver surfaces

The liver can be regarded as a wedge with rounded edges tapering to the left. It has three surfaces: antero-superior, inferior and posterior. The antero-superior surface is marked by the umbilical fissure in the depths of which (recessus of Rex) is inserted the round ligament (obliterated umbilical vein) attached to the cornu of the left portal vein. The umbilical fissure and the falciform ligament divide the antero-superior surface into right and left lobes. The posterior surface of the liver is largely formed of the bare area of the right lobe of the liver attached loosely to the diaphragm and retroperitoneum, and the caval canal that accommodates the retrohepatic vena cava and hepatic veins. The inferior surface of the liver is more complicated. The gallbladder is attached anteriorly some distance to the right of the umbilical fissure. The area between the gallbladder and the umbilical fissure is known as the quadrate lobe. Behind this and the neck of the gallbladder is the transverse hilar fissure that contains the main divisions of the portal vein, hepatic artery and common hepatic duct and forms the posterior limit of the right lobe. The hepatic parenchyma separating the hilar fissure and the inferior surface of the left lobe from the vena cava forms the caudate lobe (Figure 9.1).

Relations

In terms of anatomical relations, the antero-superior surface of the liver is in contact with the diaphragm and its upper margin reaches the level of the fourth interspace on the right and crosses the junction of the xiphisternum and sternum. Inferiorly the tip of the right liver reaches the costal margin, though Riedel's extension commonly extends below the costal margin and can reach the iliac crest. The gallbladder lies in the cystic fossa on the undersurface of the liver. There is a

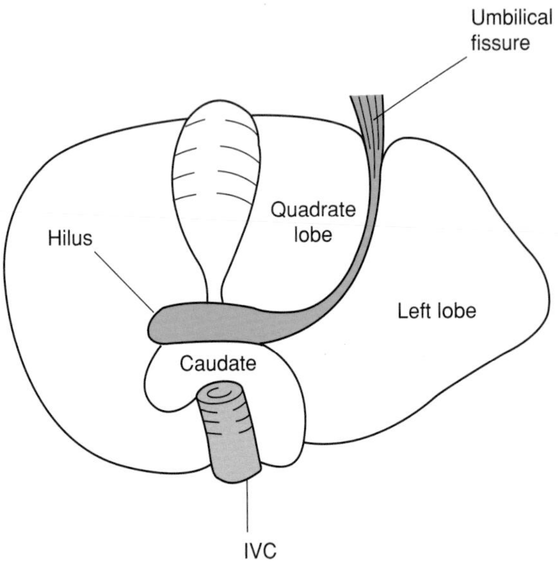

Figure 9.1 Inferior morphological surface of the liver. Note the quadrate lobe (segment IV) lies between the umbilical fissure and the gallbladder. Posteriorly the caudate lobe (segment I) separates the inferior vena cava (IVC) from the hilar fissure and the left lobe. The hepatic veins of the caudate lobe drain directly into the IVC.

layer of fascia between the liver and the gallbladder (which must not be transgressed during cholecystectomy). Inferior relations of the right lobe include the upper pole of the right kidney and the right adrenal vein and more anteriorly the first part of the duodenum as it is overlapped by the gallbladder. The much thinner left lobe overlies the gastro-oesophageal junction. The lesser sac lies below the liver and behind the lesser omentum. It usually communicates with the rest of the peritoneal cavity through the foramen of Winslow lying behind the portal vein, hepatic artery and common bile duct. Occlusion of these structures (by finger, sling or vascular clamp) stops the arterial and portal venous inflow and this manoeuvre first described by Pringle is used to control bleeding during liver surgery and liver trauma.

Ligaments

The right coronary and left triangular ligaments suspend the liver from the diaphragm. The left triangular ligament is a thin peritoneal fold that is relatively avascular. Its two layers separate medially as the caval canal is reached; one sweeps back to the lesser sac and the other forms the left leaf of the falciform ligament. The coronary ligament is composed of two separate peritoneal folds (superior and inferior) between which lies the 'bare area' of the liver that is connected to the diaphragm by loose relatively avascular areolar tissue. The two leaves of the coronary ligaments join laterally, thus forming a V-shaped attachment to the diaphragm and retroperitoneum. The superior layer is an extension of the right leaf of the falciform ligament and attaches the superior surface to the diaphragm. The inferior leaf of the coronary ligament is a reflection of the peritoneum covering the right peri-nephric and adrenal region on to the inferior surface of the liver to the right of the infrahepatic vena cava.

Caval canal

This important region is often ignored in accounts of surgical anatomy. It is essentially a gutter in which lies the retrohepatic vena cava and the hepatic veins, all of which are enveloped in a loose fibrous meshwork rather than membranes. The caudate lobe separates the caval canal from the hilar fissure anteriorly and from the left lobe. The caval canal is best exposed during hepatectomy by a combined superior and inferior approach. Superiorly, the caval canal is covered by the diverging layers of the falciform ligament. When these are divided, a loose fibrous packing tissue envelops the vena cava and the right and left hepatic veins. Below, the caval canal is opened by division of the inferior leaf of the coronary ligament. The fibrous tissue covering the vena cava is loose in this region. A variable number of unnamed hepatic veins are encountered and these include veins to the caudate lobe. The retrohepatic vena cava also receives the phrenic veins and below these, it is loosely attached to the retroperitoneum and thus, provided the correct plane is identified, a sling can be passed around it and including the right and left hepatic veins in the immediate suprahepatic region.

Functional or segmental anatomy of the liver

The details of the segmental anatomy of the liver on which modern hepatic surgery is based come from the anatomical dissections performed by Rex (1888) and Cantlie (1898) more than 100 years ago and subsequently elaborated by Goldsmith and Woodburne (1957), Couinaud (1957), Healy and and Schroy (1953) and Elias and Petty (1952).

In essence the liver should be regarded as a paired organ (right and left livers) that are fused along a line extending from the middle of the gallbladder fossa anteriorly to the left edge of the suprahepatic inferior vena cava posteriorly. Within the liver this corresponds to a vertical plane (the main portal scissura or Cantlie's line) in which lies the middle hepatic vein. The right liver receives the right portal vein, hepatic artery and bile duct and the left liver the corresponding left portal vein, hepatic artery and bile duct.

The right liver

The right liver is further subdivided into two sectors by the vertical right portal scissura in which lies the right hepatic vein. This scissura has no surface makings but is a plane that subtends an angle of 40° with the horizontal and corresponds to a line extending from the anterior edge of the liver (midway between its right corner and the right edge of the gallbladder) to the confluence of the right hepatic vein with the vena cava. The medial sector is composed of segments IV (antero-inferior) and VIII (postero-superior) and the lateral sector of segment VI (antero-inferior) and VII (postero-superior). Thus in the supine patient segments V and VI partially overlap segments VIII and VII, respectively (Figure 9.2). Each segment receives a portal pedicle and is drained by a separate bile duct.

The left liver

This is divided by the left portal scissura, in which lies the left hepatic vein, into a medial sector that forms segment IV and a lateral sector that is further divided into an anterior segment III and a posterior segment II (Figure 9.3).

Caudate (dorsal, Spigel) lobe

Although this is customarily labelled as segment I, it is really a separate 'liver' because it has its own hepatic veins and bile ducts although it receives portal and arterial branches from both right and left sides. The caudate lobe is situated behind the hilar fissure and embraces the vena cava from the left forming an L-shaped structure with the horizonal limb separating the hilar fissure from the vena cava and the vertical limb the left liver from the vena cava.

Because of this segmental liver anatomy, it is possible to resect a single or several segments even in the liver that has been distorted by chronic disease. A careful identification of the vessels and ducts supplying each segment can be achieved by dissection above the portal hilum and each set may be ligated separately prior to resection of the segment.

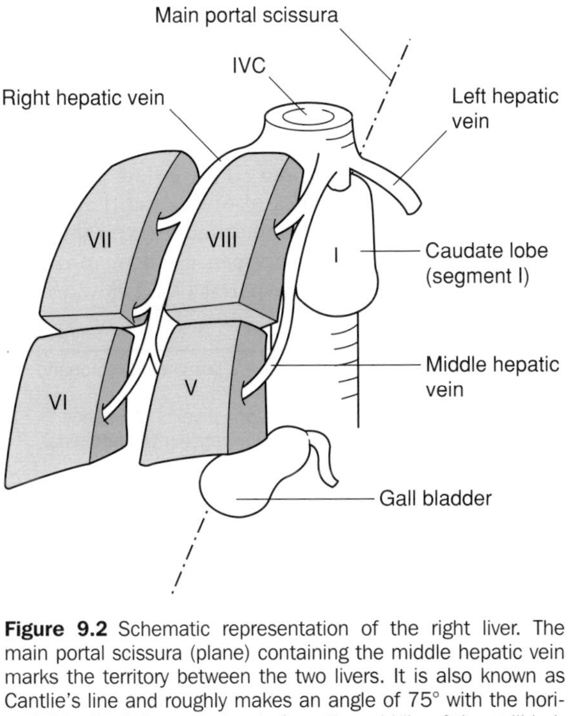

Figure 9.2 Schematic representation of the right liver. The main portal scissura (plane) containing the middle hepatic vein marks the territory between the two livers. It is also known as Cantlie's line and roughly makes an angle of 75° with the horizontal to the left, and extends from the middle of the gallbladder fossa to left side of the vena cava. The right liver is divided into two sectors by the vertical right portal scissura containing the main trunk of the right hepatic vein. These two sectors are split by the plane of the right portal vein into two antero-inferior (V and VI) and two postero-superior (VII, VIII) segments. Thus the right liver is smaller than the right lobe. Unfortunately, the vertical scissurae (planes) are undulating and not straight as shown in the drawing. This precludes a good correlation between radiological and anatomical segmentation (see text).

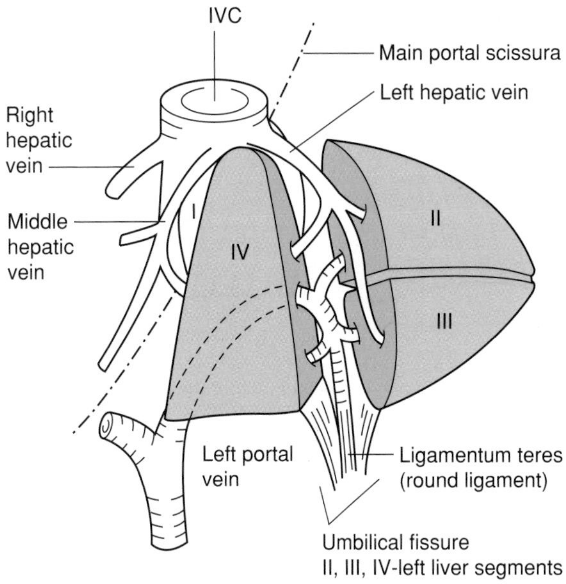

Figure 9.3 Schematic representation of the left liver that is split by the left portal scissura containing the left hepatic vein into segment IV medially and segments II and III laterally. Thus the left liver is larger than the left lobe.

Main hepatic veins

Each numbered segment contributes hepatic veins that coalesce to form the main venous drainage of the livers and lie between the segments. There are three veins of surgical importance: the right hepatic vein drains segments V–VIII by a short vessel directly into the suprahepatic vena cava; the middle hepatic vein drains from both livers (segments IV and V) and empties either directly into the vena cava or into the left hepatic vein. The latter vein drains segments II–IV. Segment I, the caudate lobe, drains by one or more small hepatic veins directly into the retrohepatic vena cava.

In the majority of patients both the right hepatic and the left hepatic veins can be identified and secured extrahepatically within the caval canal but not the middle hepatic vein. The left hepatic vein is exposed by complete division of the left triangular ligament. It slopes down from the vena cava to the liver so that its posterior wall is in contact with the vena cava and separated from it by loose fibrous tissue (Figure 9.4). The right hepatic vein is exposed only after the right lobe is dislocated to the left. It runs directly posteriorly from the liver in intimate contact with the vena cava before entering it more posteriorly (Figure 9.5). Again only a loose layer of fibrous tissue separates the medial wall of the right hepatic vein from the vena cava but the fibrous tissue on its outer surface is usually firm and thickened. Many liver surgeons advise against extrahepatic ligature of the right or left hepatic veins and

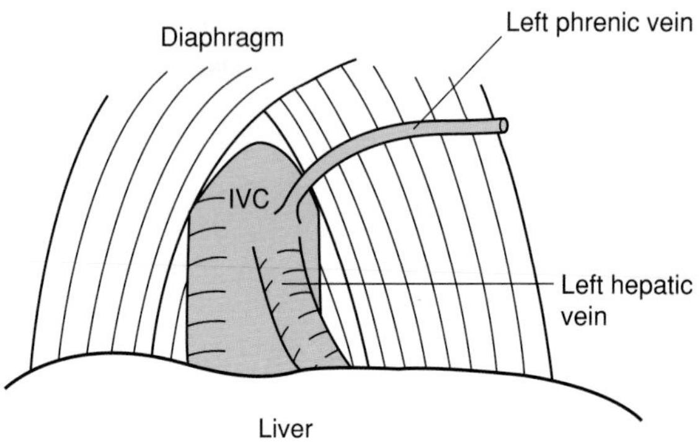

Figure 9.4 Schematic representation of the left hepatic vein.

secure either of these (depending on the resection) intrahepatically during the hepatic resection after temporary occlusion of the inflow vessels (Bismuth modification of the Ton That Tung technique). The author disagrees with this, as in many but not all cases, with careful dissection, there is sufficient length for securing either of these veins extrahepatically by transfixation. Initial control of the relevant hepatic vein at the start of the hepatectomy certainly reduces the operative blood loss.

Portal hilum

In the portal hilum, the portal vein which has formed behind the head of the pancreas by the junction of splenic and superior mesenteric veins, passes along the edge of the lesser omentum for 7.5 cm. It receives branches from the pylorus and the important left coronary vein from the cardio-oesophageal region (Figure 9.6). The portal vein provides the final conduit for the venous return from the gastrointestinal tract and its usual distribution to the various functional segments is shown in Figure 9.7. In the axial plane, the two main branches of the portal vein lie in the same plane (sometimes referred to as the transverse scissura). From right to left, segments VI, V, IV and III are below this plane, whereas segments VII, VIII, I (caudate) and II above it.

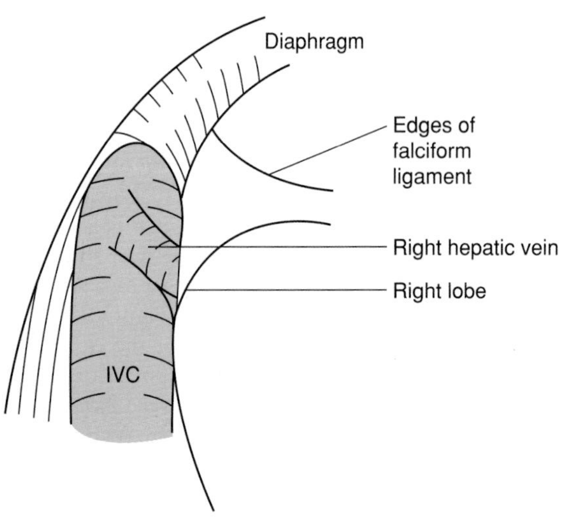

Figure 9.5 Schematic representation of the right hepatic vein after dislocation of the right lobe of the liver.

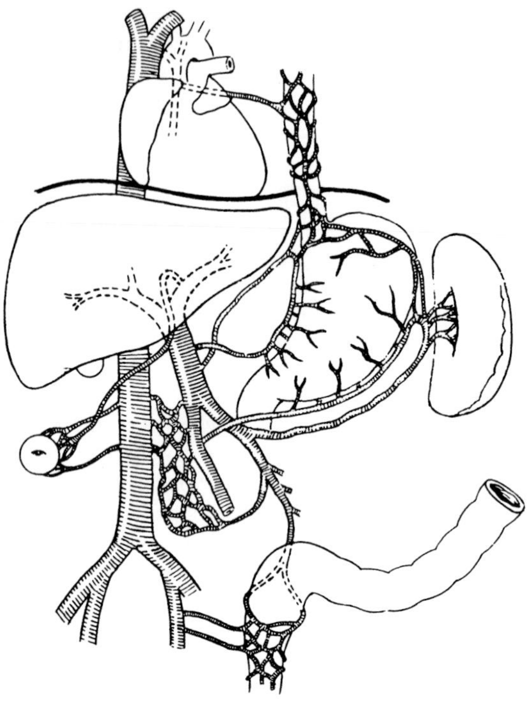

Figure 9.6 This shows the portal venous drainage from the gastrointestinal tract and demonstrates the major anastomotic sites between the portal and systemic systems: the cardio-oesophageal junction leading up to the azygos system, the retroperitoneum, the umbilicus and the inferior rectal plexus.

There are major anastomotic sites between the portal and systemic systems that open up in the presence of occlusion/obstruction to portal blood flow to the liver:

- The cardio-oesophageal junction – left gastric (coronary) vein to the azygos system.
- Communications with retroperitoneal veins of Sappey.
- Umbilicus – recanalized left umbilical vein to abdominal parietal veins – caput medusae.
- Communications with the inferior rectal plexus (see Figure 9.6).

The common hepatic duct draining both livers passes in front of and to the right of the portal vein and receives the cystic duct at a variable point of its course to form the common bile duct. The common hepatic artery runs to the left of the common bile duct giving off the main cystic artery and branches to the common bile duct prior to division into right and left branches.

An understanding of the point of the division of the structures in the portal hilum is essential for the surgeon. The main vessels and ducts, particularly the left branches, are surrounded by the vasculobiliary sheath described originally by Walaeus in 1640 and sometimes referred to as the Glissonian sheath. While the portal vein is loosely enclosed, the bile duct and hepatic artery

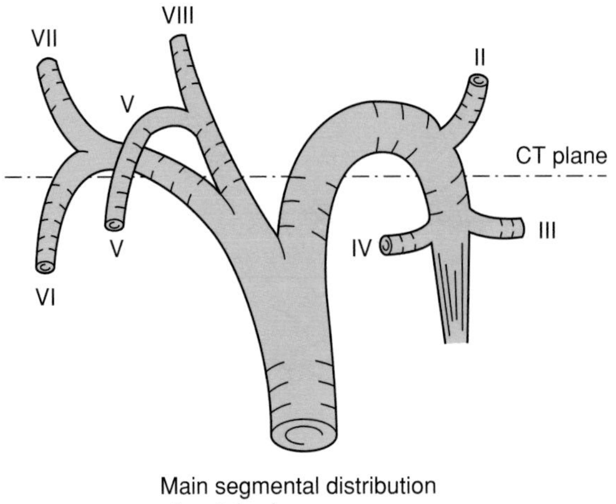

Figure 9.7 Schematic representation of the usual distribution of the portal vein. Above the transverse line (representing the transverse scissura marking the plane of the right and left portal veins) the upper branches supply segments VII, VIII, I, III and the lower branches VI, V, IV, III. The distribution of the portal vein branches varies from patient to patient.

are firmly adherent to the sheath. The upper surface of the sheath which is in contact with the liver parenchyma thickens to become the hilar plate. This structure can be released from the liver surface because there are no branches along it and permits the surgeon to isolate the vessels to the left lobe and proceed to liver resection more safely (Figure 9.8). The right-sided vessels are shorter and not so conveniently enclosed in a hilar plate, thus great care is required in handling.

Radiological anatomy of the liver

The advent of helical computed tomography (CT) and magnetic resonance imaging (MRI) scanning of the liver has identified limitations of the anatomical segmental anatomy used by hepatic surgeons. Initially it was thought that the volumetric data sets obtained with these imaging techniques could be segmented using the three hepatic veins and the plane of the main portal vein branches (in similar fashion to the anatomical segmentation). These recent radiological studies (based on corrosion casts of cadaveric livers) have shown a poor correlation between the radiological and anatomical segments due to the large anatomical variation of the portal venous territories that, in effect, alter the shape, size and number of segments. In addition, the vertical scissurae in which lie the hepatic veins are undulating planes rather than straight as assumed by the anatomical segmentation. The discrepancies between the radiological and anatomical segmentation vary with the axial cuts of the liver on spiral CT but can measure up to 4.0 cm.

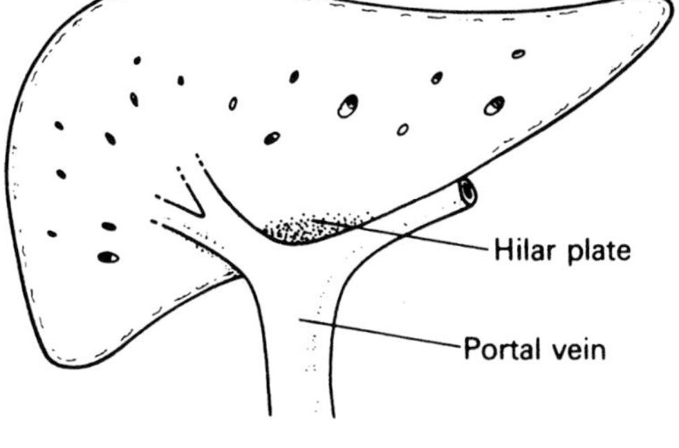

Figure 9.8 To the undersurface of the liver, the bifurcation of the major hilar structures is secured by a dense fibrous sheath termed the hilar plate. After incising this structure the vessels to the left liver segments run for 1.5 cm before dividing into segmental branches.

- In other words, a tumour of this size can be radiologically ascribed to an incorrect segment.

Thus radiological segmentation to provide precise location of the lesion in the liver is not possible and can indeed be misleading. True segmentation will only be possible with the development of techniques that outline the anatomy of the portal vein including its small peripheral branches in the individual case.

Hepatic architecture

Conventional morphology considers that the liver is composed of pyramidal lobules based on a central vein and surrounded on the periphery by portal trunks with terminal radicles of bile duct, portal vein and hepatic artery (Figure 9.9). The two vascular systems of central vein and portal tract lie on planes at right angles to one another and never interdigitate. Thus the sinusoids are arranged perpendicular to the planes of the central veins and portal blood passes to the central vein along a pressure gradient. The walls of the sinusoids are composed of endothelial and phagocytic cells termed Kupffer cells. Between the hepatocytes and Kupffer cells is the space of Disse. Bile canaliculi are shown to be channels or grooves in the hepatocyte surface, lined by microvilli. The network of canaliculi drains the liver lobules into the terminal bile ducts.

It may help in the understanding of liver injury and its consequences to view the liver morphology somewhat differently. The concept of Rappaport is to regard the liver as a series of acini supplied by a portal triad of structures (Figure 9.10). Three zones of sinusoids are envisaged in which the peripheral zone of the acini (zone 3) is damaged more severely in any form of injury. Adjacent forms of injury may coalesce to form areas of bridging necrosis and later to fibrosis, producing the common pattern of post-sinusoidal block. zones 1 and 2 may form the nidus of surviving cells which then regenerate in nodular form.

Section 9.2 • Serum protein changes in liver disease

Acute phase reactant proteins (alpha$_2$-macroglobulin, C-reactive protein, etc.) are often elevated in acute liver

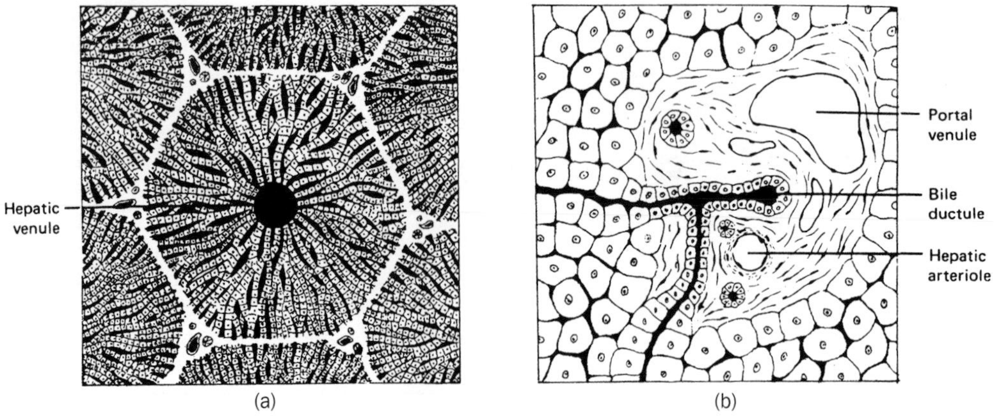

Figure 9.9 (a) This demonstrates the normal liver architecture in which a hepatic plate apparently surrounds a hepatic vein through which blood from the hepatic sinusoids drains. (b) In fact it is more appropriate to centre the hepatic plate on the portal tract which contains the elements of the bile ducts into which bile can directly drain from the hepatocytes and branches of the portal vein and hepatic artery together with connective tissue stroma. Zones closest to this portal tract (zone 1) are protected in most circumstances from liver damage. Liver cells surrounding the hepatic vein (zone 3) are more susceptible to all forms of hepatic damage. Regenerative nodules are normally centred on a portal tract.

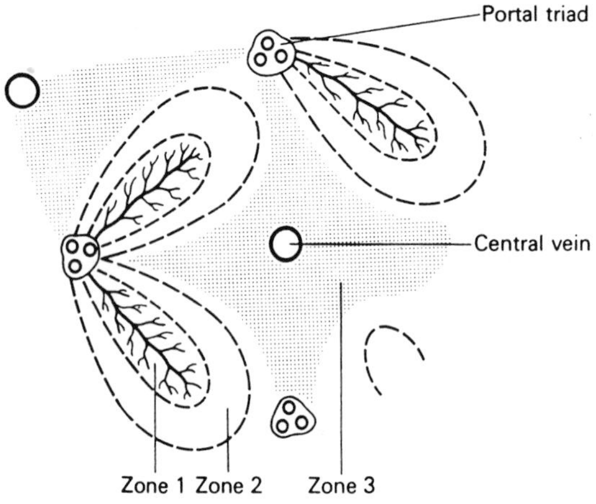

Figure 9.10 According to Rappaport, there are three zones of liver parenchyma. Zone 1 adjacent to the portal triad is the best vascularized and least susceptible to injury. Zone 3 is adjacent to the central vein and most susceptible to injury.

disease. Other changes include lowering of the serum albumin, release of integral proteins, raised immunoglobulins and the appearance of abnormal protein antigens.

Albumin

The serum albumin is often low in patients with chronic liver disease and the hypoalbuminaemia is associated with a complementary rise in the other serum proteins, particularly globulins (altered albumin: globulin ratio). The fall in the serum albumin is often used in the grading of the severity of hepatic decompensation, e.g. Pugh and Child's classifications. When severe, the hypoalbuminaemia is usually accompanied by fluid and salt retention but reduced plasma oncotic pressure is only one of several interrelated factors responsible for ascites in patients with chronic liver disease. The exact mechanism (defects in transcription, mRNA processing or translation, defective export) for the depressed albumin synthesis in patients with hepatic fibrosis or cirrhosis is not known. Paradoxically, in some patients with cirrhosis, albumin synthesis by the liver is actually increased.

Immunoglobulins

Marked elevation of the serum IgG is encountered in patients with cirrhosis and chronic active (aggressive) hepatitis. Serum IgA, which is normally secreted in the bile, is also elevated in these conditions but to a lesser extent. Primary biliary cirrhosis is associated with elevation of the serum IgM and the presence of antimitochondrial antibodies.

Release of integral cellular membrane enzymes

In hepatocellular injury, integral cellular enzymes are released into the circulation. These include aspartate transaminase (AST) and alanine amino transaminase (ALT). The levels of both transaminases in the serum reflect the severity of the ongoing liver cell damage and necrosis. Minor elevations are encountered in cholestasis and chronic liver disease, whereas substantial serum levels (>400 units) are encountered in acute hepatitis with liver cell necrosis from any cause.

The group of isoenzymes responsible for the hydrolysis of phosphate esters in an alkaline medium are termed alkaline phosphatases. These enzymes are found in the liver, biliary tract, bone, intestine, kidney and placenta. The various isoenzymes can now be differentiated by special immunoassays establishing the exact tissue origin of the circulating enzyme. In cholestasis and obstructive jaundice the conjugated hyperbilirubinaemia is accompanied by significant elevation of the serum alkaline phosphatase activity due to impaired excretion of the enzyme in the bile and hepatic induction (over-production). Other (alkaline phosphatase type) enzymes associated with the biliary tract such as

5-nucleotidase and gamma-glutamyl transpeptidase (γ-GT) exhibit a parallel elevation. Gamma-GT is also elevated in alcoholic liver disease.

The biochemical picture in patients with secondary deposits consists of marked elevation of the bile ductular enzymes (alkaline phosphatase, 5-nucleotidase, γ-GT) out of proportion to the small rise in the serum bilirubin.

Marker export proteins

The most important is α-fetoprotein (AFP) which is expressed in the cytoplasm of the majority of cases of hepatocellular carcinoma (HCC) and secreted in the plasma. Thus a raised serum AFP is a very useful marker of HCC. A level of 500 ng/dl is diagnostic of HCC, and a level between 20 and 500 ng/dl may be indicative of a small HCC (<5.0 cm) but is also encountered in benign liver disease associated with necrosis and regeneration, e.g. cirrhosis and chronic active hepatitis, and other tumours. A rising level of AFP even if below the diagnostic range is indicative of a small (occult) HCC. Persistent elevation after resection of HCC indicates residual disease and re-elevation after initial normalization is suggestive of recurrence. A correlation between serum level of AFP, tumour size and survival has been established by a number of studies. Thus patients with marked pre-operative elevation have a poor survival after surgery. The well-differentiated variant of HCC, fibrolamellar carcinoma, does not cause an elevation of AFP and this oncofetal antigen is not expressed by cholangiocarcinoma.

Other export proteins produced by a minority of HCC include ferritin and α_1-antitrypsin but aside from detection in the cytoplasm of the tumour cells by immunohistochemistry these are not of clinical diagnostic value.

Section 9.3 • Hepatic functional reserve

In clinical practice use is made predominantly of standard 'liver function tests' and indeed these together with nutritional state, muscle wasting, water and salt retention with ascites form the basis for assessment of the hepatic reserve. The most commonly used are the Child-Pugh score/grading (modified from the initial Child-Turcotte) and the Paul Brousse hospital classification system (Tables 9.1 and 9.2)

There are in addition tests that give an assessment of the functional capacity (reserve) of the liver. These are not often used clinically except in specialist hepatobiliary centres and in clinical research studies. Some are tests of microsomal function (e.g. antipyrine clearance, caffeine clearance), others of cytosolic function (e.g. galactose elimination capacity) or hepatic perfusion and excretion (e.g. indocyanine green clearance) or synthesis (albumin, urea and prothrombin). In practice, the most commonly used are the indocyanine green (ICG) clearance and the prothrombin activity after administration of vitamin K.

Table 9.1 Child–Pugh classification of disease severity in cirrhotic patients

Parameter	*A*	*B*	*C*
Albumin, g/dl	>3.5	3.0–3.5	<3.0
Bilirubin, µmol/l	<25	25–40	>40
Prothrombin, s >normal	<4	4–6	>6*
Prothrombin, %	>64	40–65	<40
Ascites	None	Controlled	Refractory
Encephalopathy	None	Minimal	Advanced

*In the original Child–Turcotte classification, nutrition was used but this has been substituted with prothrombin activity. The bilirubin has to be adjusted for patients with primary biliary cirrhosis (A = 5–7, B = 8–10, C = 11 or more).

Indocyanine green clearance

This is presently considered to be the best test of hepatic functional reserve. Most commonly, it is used to select patients for hepatic resection. More recently ICG clearance has been reported to be beneficial in liver transplantation – selection of patients and prediction of graft viability. Hepatic clearance of ICG is dependent on many factors, the most important of which are hepatic blood flow, binding to plasma proteins, transport across the sinusoidal-hepatocyte membrane, intracellular transport, export across the canalicular membrane and bile flow. In clinical practice, hepatic clearance is derived from the plasma ICG clearance curve. The test is carried out after an overnight fast when ICG (0.5 g/kg body weight) is injected intravenously usually in the antecubital vein. Blood samples are taken from the contralateral antecubital vein before administration (plasma blank) and at 5, 10, 15 and 20 min after injection of ICG.

- Most consider that a retention of greater than 14% at 15 min precludes major resection as it indicates a significant reduction in the hepatic reserve.

However, good survival has been reported in patients having an ICG retention greater than 14% provided the resection is carried out expertly and is not accompanied by significant blood loss.

Bromsulfthalein clearance

Sodium phenoltetrabromophthalein disulfonate (BSP) is a synthetic dye that is removed from the blood by the liver (similar pharmacokinetics to ICG). After

Table 9.2 Paul Brousse hospital classification system

A = none of the criteria
B = 1–2 criteria
C = 3 or more criteria

Parameter	*Number of criteria*
Albuminaemia <3.0 g/100 ml	1
Hyperbilirubinaemia >30 µmol/l	1
Encephalopathy	1
Clinical ascites	1
Coagulation factors II and V 40–60%	1
Coagulation factors II and V <40%	2

intravenous injection it is bound to albumin and lipoprotein and taken up by the hepatic parenchymal cells where it is conjugated and excreted into the bile. As a test of hepatic function it is given at a dose of 5 mg/kg and less than 6% should be left by 45 mm. It is a sensitive test of hepatic dysfunction but not often used nowadays. The BSP test is not useful in patients with moderate jaundice, fever, severe obesity or following the recent use of radio-opaque drugs. A modification of the test involves administering the BSP by continuous infusion to achieve a steady state. This provides a more accurate estimate of hepatic reserve in patients with cirrhosis and yields information on liver blood flow based on the Fick principle.

Prothrombin activity

This is a sensitive test of hepatic synthesis of vitamin K dependent factors that is impaired in jaundice and hepatocellular disease. In addition to the level of prothrombin activity, the response to a parenteral dose of vitamin K analogue is a most useful test of hepatocyte function. Thus restoration to normal within 24–48 hours is expected in patients with obstructive jaundice without significant impairment of hepatocyte function.

Section 9.4 • Imaging of the liver

The normal liver parenchyma is sufficiently homogeneous for most pathological processes to be demonstrable in contrast.

Plain radiography

A plain abdominal film may give helpful information in terms of liver size and the position of the overlying diaphragm. Rarely a small gas/fluid level may be seen within an abscess. Hydatid cysts are well shown by virtue of calcification within the cyst wall.

Ultrasonography

This is the investigation of choice in patients with suspected biliary tract pain, cholestasis and vague upper abdominal pain of a non-dyspeptic nature. The liver is shown as a large transonic structure in which the portal vein, hepatic veins and inferior vena cave are well shown. In patients with cholestasis, dilated intrahepatic bile ducts clearly pinpoint the presence of large duct obstruction and occasionally the cause for this obstruction may be seen distally in the biliary tree. The demonstration of gallbladder disease is particularly good and gallstones are diagnosed with an accuracy of 95%. Visualization of the portal venous system is also possible and ultrasound is the first investigation required to demonstrate patency of the portal venous system. The patency of the portal vein and other major vascular channels including surgical shunts is much more readily established with duplex ultrasound scanning, and with the colour Doppler facility, the direction of flow in relation to the transducer can also be ascertained.

It is in the screening of the liver parenchyma for focal lesions that ultrasound comes into its own and in ideal circumstances lesions as small as 1 cm can be demonstrated. Particularly well shown are liver cysts and abscesses, but also primary liver tumours and dense multifocal metastases are readily seen. Used as a screening test in patients with hepatitis B antigen it has proved possible to identify patients with small operable hepatocellular cancers in whom prolonged survival has been reported.

Intra-operative ultrasound screening of the liver can demonstrate precisely the anatomy of vascular structures, the boundaries of palpable liver tumours and the presence of impalpable foci enabling a more appropriate resection line or preventing the performance of resection which is destined to fail. Intrahepatic gallstones are also well shown. Intra-operative probes (for open or laparoscopic surgery) are of the linear array configuration with a frequency in the 7.5–10 MHz range. They thus provide high definition in the near field (2.0–3.0 cm depth). Intra-operative contact ultrasonography is invaluable during liver surgery as the precise anatomy and patency of hepatic veins can be established.

Ultrasonography is of considerable help in the guidance of needles and catheters into intrahepatic collections. Solitary echogenic areas may be haemangiomas or localized fatty infiltration and once firmly diagnosed by alternative means, e.g. CT scanning, ultrasound may be used to monitor stability of size. Liver cirrhosis is suggested by areas of increased and irregular attenuation. In steatosis (fatty liver) the parenchyma is diffusely hyperechoic.

CT scanning

This investigation is commonplace in the diagnosis and treatment planning of hepatic disease. With conventional CT thin horizontal slices (about 10) of the liver are performed in order to demonstrate fully the anatomical details. The procedure is often combined with oral contrast to define the stomach and duodenum and intravenous contrast to outline the vessels and focal lesions within the liver. CT scanning is particularly valuable in the diagnosis of focal disease: tumours, cysts or abscesses. Liver injuries including subcapsular haematomas are particularly well demonstrated by conventional CT scanning.

In many centres spiral (helical) CT scanning has replaced the conventional CT for several reasons: much better definition, fast scanning and the acquisition of volumetric data sets from which three-dimensional (3-D) reconstruction of the pathological anatomy can be obtained.

Helical (spiral) computed tomography of the liver

In helical or spiral CT the planar movement of the patient is combined with continuous rotation of the X-ray tube and detector system resulting in a spiral or helical movement of the system relative to the patient.

This enables the acquisition of a volume of data from a block of tissue (volumetric data set). Thus images can be constructed at any position within the scanned volume of tissue. Often intravenous contrast is administered during the investigation when the following imaging can be performed:

Intravenous contrast enhanced helical CT:

- abdominal survey helical CT
- dual helical hepatic CT
- high-dose helical hepatic CT
- delayed iodine CT (DICT)
- helical 3-D CT hepatic angiography.

Intra-arterial contrast enhanced helical hepatic CT can also be used to obtain CT angiography (CT-A, CT-AP).

Abdominal survey helical CT

This is undertaken using powered intravenous contrast injection (150 ml at 3.0 ml/s) with hepatic attenuation threshold set at 50 Hounsfield units (HU) which provides a consistent and uniform hepatic enhancement. All the images of the upper abdomen (liver, pancreas, spleen, etc.) are acquired during a single breath-hold. As far as the liver is concerned, it should detect the size of the liver lobes and the presence of focal lesions within the hepatic parenchyma.

Dual helical hepatic CT

This is used for the detection of hypervascular hepatic lesions, e.g. carcinoid tumour deposits, hepatocellular carcinoma, etc. The technique is based on obtaining scans slices during the hepatic arterial (12–25 s post-injection) and the subsequent arterio-portal venous phase (50–60 s post-injection) following intravenous power contrast injection, 200–180 ml at 5.0 ml/s. During the arterial phase, the hypervascularized lesions 'light up' because of greater enhancement with respect to the normal hepatic parenchyma. During the arterio-portal venous phase these lesions become isodense or hypodense with respect to the hepatic parenchyma.

High-dose helical CT

With this technique, large doses of contrast (200 ml) are injected at a rate of 5 ml/s to produce hepatic contrast enhancement that is almost equivalent to that obtained by arterial injection. With refinements in dosage and technique, the high helical CT technique gives similar detection rates for metastatic disease and is less invasive than direct high-dose arterial injection, such as CT-AP (*vide infra*).

CT-angiography and CT-portography

CT-angiography (CT-A) involves direct injection of contrast in the hepatic artery, whereas in CT-portography (CT-AP) the contrast is delivered to the liver after selective catheterization of the splenic or superior mesenteric arteries. Until recently, CT-AP was regarded as the gold standard for the detection of secondary tumour deposits, e.g. colorectal cancer, because the lesions derive their blood supply exclusively from the hepatic artery. Thus in CT-AP, secondary deposits are seen as defects within the normal enhanced liver parenchyma. By contrast, CT-A produces direct contrast enhancement of tumour deposits against a background of non-enhanced liver parenchyma.

Delayed iodine CT (DICT)

This consists of CT scanning some 4–6 hours after the intravenous administration of iodine-contrast agents, since 10–15% of this is excreted by the liver and thus produces delayed enhancement of the normal hepatic parenchyma but not of tumours. Aside from lesion detection, it is used to sort out perfusion abnormalities during CT-AP that may be misinterpreted as tumours.

MRI of the liver

Until recently MRI has taken second place to helical CT in the diagnosis of liver disease especially in the detection and location of primary and secondary hepatic tumours. The situation is, however, changing with newer techniques of MRI and the introduction of better MRI contrast agents.

In essence the MRI system creates a strong magnetic field (measured in tesla, most imaging machines are in the 1.0–1.5 tesla range) by a resistive or superconducting magnet in which the patient is housed during imaging. This magnetic field causes alignment of the spinning protons (hydrogen nuclei) of the patient's tissues in the north–south position. These protons are then displaced from this magnetic field-induced alignment by the application radiofrequency pulses, but return (relax) to the north–south position thereafter. During this relaxation, the spinning protons emit radiofrequency electromagnetic signals of their own that are picked by receiver coils. Different tissues relax at different rates and thus produce signals of different strength – this forms the basis of the imaging. The contrast between the various tissues can be altered by varying the repetition time between the radiofrequency cycles (to deviate the protons) and the time of sampling the signals emitted from the protons – this is known as 'weighting the image'. In practice, two types of 'weighting' are commonly used – T1- and T2-weighting. T1-weighting provides anatomical detail whereas T2-weighting give high signals for tissues and structures that contain a high free water content: inflammation, ducts containing secretions, etc.

The recent developments in MRI techniques have stemmed from the shortening of the acquisition time by various techniques (fast and ultra-fast spin echo, gradient echo sequences, etc.) designed to reduce the motion artifacts and to enable complete acquisition of the imaging data set in one single breath-hold (15–30 s). The other significant change has been the introduction of new MRI contrast agents.

The contrast agents used in MRI of the liver are:

- *Gadolinium (Gd) chelates with extracellular distribution (e.g. Gd-DTPA)* – following intravenous injection, these leave the intravascular compartment rapidly to equilibrate in the interstitial space. This limits their usefulness in the detection of focal hepatic lesions, but the technique is valuable in characterizing the nature of identified lesions by the different patterns of enhancement and washout, e.g. persistence of enhancement on delayed images in haemangiomas, strong initial transitory enhancement followed by delayed enhancement in focal nodular hyperplasia.
- *Hepatobiliary contrast agents (e.g. Gd-EOB-DTPA)* – these are hepatocyte specific and thus provide prolonged enhancement of normal liver parenchyma and lesions that contain hepatocytes. Thus hepatocellular carcinoma, focal nodular hyperplasia and the regenerative nodules of cirrhosis enhance with these agents, whereas secondary deposits, lymphomas and cholangiocarcinomas do not.
- Macrophage–monocyte–phagocyte system (MMPS) target agents – these consist of superparamagnetic iron oxide (SPIO) particles coated with dextran that are cleared from the blood by the macrophage–monocyte system following intravenous injection. In the liver, they are taken up by the Kupffer cells abolishing the signal on heavily weighted T2-imaging. As focal lesions (tumours in particular) do not contain Kupffer cells, these lesions appear as bright white lesions against the black (negatively enhanced) normal hepatic parenchyma. This contrast imaging provides one of the best techniques currently available for the detection and precise location of hepatic secondary deposit (Figure 9.11) particularly with 3-D reconstruction from the volumetric data set.
- *Intravascular (blood pool) contrast agents* – ultra small superparamagnetic dextran coated particles (USPIO) are used as intravascular contrast agents in view of their long-half life in the blood (200 min). They are useful in the detection of hypervascular lesions (hepatocellular carcinoma, deposits from carcinoid tumours, haemangiomas, etc.) using dynamic MRI in much the same fashion as dual helical CT.

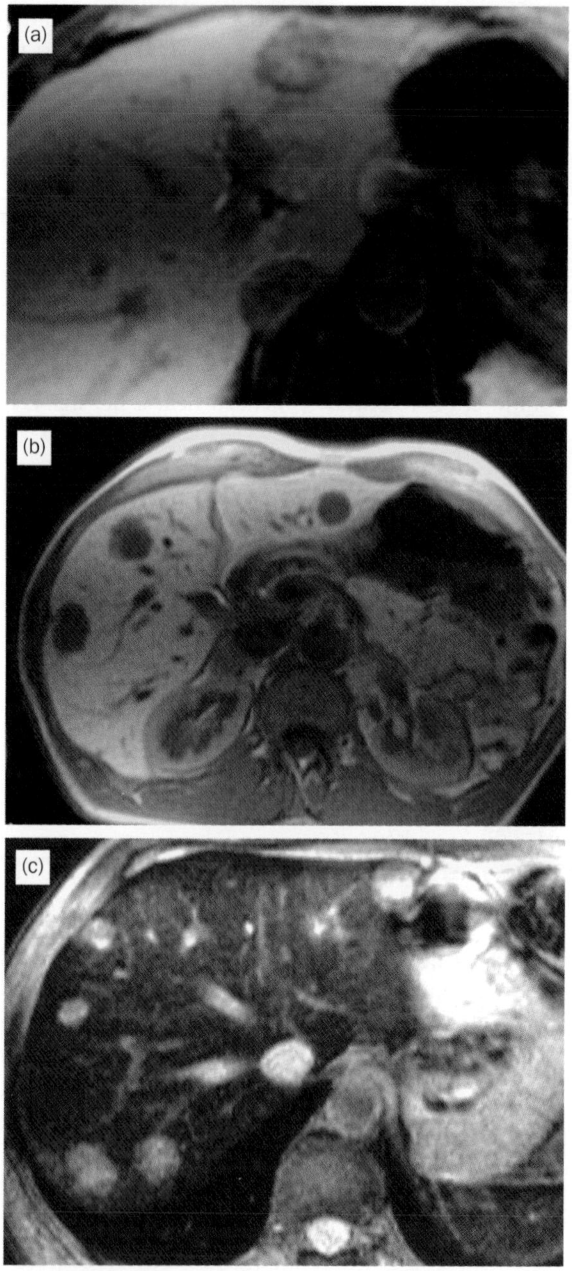

Figure 9.11 MRI scanning for secondary tumour deposits: (a) delayed T1-weighted image following Gd-BOTA, (b) delayed T1-weighted image following Mn-DPDP, (c) T2-weighted imaged following superparamagnetic iron oxide (SPIO) – as the tumour deposits do not contain Kupffer cells, they appear as bright white lesions against the black (negatively enhanced) normal hepatic parenchyma.

Helical CT versus MRI for liver imaging

CT is widely available and remains the first-choice method for imaging the liver in many institutions and high-dose helical CT (CT-AP) is recognized as the gold standard method of pre-operative staging of patients with liver metastases. Advanced MRI techniques are less readily available. MRI is thus used selectively in:

- Differentiating haemangiomas from metastases.
- Distinguishing focal liver fat from tumour deposit (fat suppression technique).
- Screening for deposits in patients with fatty liver.
- Equivocal helical CT.
- Characterization of certain primary liver lesions – hepatocellular carcinoma, focal nodular hyperplasia, hepatocellular adenoma, regenerative nodules in cirrhosis.
- Characterization of fluid collections.

Scintiscanning of the liver parenchyma

This investigation is performed much less commonly nowadays as ultrasound, CT and MRI provide much better definition. ^{99m}Technetium (^{99m}Tc) is taken up by the reticuloendothelial system and may detect focal lesions greater than 2 cm in diameter in about two-thirds of cases. Lesions in the anterior half of the liver are preferentially shown. Generalized liver disease is demonstrated as reduced or patchy uptake with increased uptake of the spleen and bone marrow. In the Budd–Chiari syndrome, reduced uptake of the liver is noted in some patients except in the caudate lobe.

An alternative isotope, ^{67}gallium citrate, is concentrated in neoplastic foci and abscesses, and haemangiomas concentrate the isotope ^{113}indium. In the last decade, isotope-labelled antibodies specific to tumour surface specific antigens have been introduced both for the detection of small tumour deposits and also as a means of guiding specific procedures (radio-guided surgery/ interventions). In so far as the detection of secondary deposits in the liver these labelled antibody techniques have one advantage over both spiral CT scanning and MRI, they outline living tumour deposits, and for this reason have the potential to provide useful information on the presence or absence of viable tumour after *in situ* ablation (*vide infra*, positron emission tomography).

Examples of radio-guided surgery include abdominal interventions following the administration of the appropriate isotope and with the use of a sterile Geiger counter during surgery to detect tumour deposits in nodes, etc., and sentinel lymph node biopsy for cancer of the breast that is now in widespread usage.

Positron emission tomography

Until fairly recently positron emission tomography (PET) has been used to investigate single organs, particularly the heart (myocardial perfusion, oxygen extraction, etc.) and the brain (metabolism, neurotransmitter function, etc.). With the advent of whole body PET scanning, the technique is being introduced in oncology where it has a significant potential and advantages over other imaging modalities:

- In principle, whole body PET can identify a tumour and indicate the presence of spread anywhere in the body at an early stage (micrometastases).
- It can differentiate between benign and malignant tumours (metabolic activity of the lesion).
- It differentiates viable from non-viable tumour – increasingly important for *in situ* ablation of tumours, e.g. liver, prostate.

PET is based on the use of unstable short-lived (minutes to hours) positron-emitting radioisotopes produced by a cyclotron. Positrons (β^+) are positively charged electrons. Positron emission stabilizes the element by removing its excessive protons and positive charge (when the atomic number of the element is reduced by one). The positrons emitted from the nucleus of these decaying radioisotopes travel a short distance and collide with electrons of nearby (host tissue) atoms with annihilation that is accompanied by the generation of gamma rays (photons). Each collision/annihilation between a positron and an electron produces two 511 keV gamma rays that are emitted at 180° to each other (referred to as coincidence lines). These photonic coincidence lines are picked by a circular array of external detectors and used to generate the PET image. The positron emitting isotopes used in PET scanning become stable elements after emission of the positrons, i.e. they are no longer radioactive.

The positron-emitting radioisotopes can be administered to patients as elements, e.g. $^{18}F^-$ for bone scanning or incorporated into tracer substances, e.g. ^{18}F-labelled 2-deoxyglucose (FDG). FDG measures glucose metabolism, and aside from tumour localization, it can differentiate benign from malignant tissue because of the different metabolic rates. The oxygen positron-emitting isotope [$^{15}O{=}O$] can be used to measure tumour necrosis. Whole body PET scanning has been used in breast, colorectal, liver and prostatic cancer.

Examination of the vascular tree

In the past, the demonstration of the vascular tree was dependent on use of invasive techniques of contrast radiology. Increasingly, however with duplex ultrasound scanning, the helical CT techniques and MRI these are used in preference to invasive angiology in the first instance.

Hepatic wedge pressure and hepatic venography

The wedge pressure can be measured by passing a catheter via the brachial vein, through the right atrium and directly into the hepatic veins as far as possible. It represents the sinusoidal pressure and corresponds to some degree with portal vein pressure. This correlation is absent in pre-sinusoidal blocks, e.g. schistosomiasis. The technique is less commonly employed than formerly unless there is a need to demonstrate coincidentally the anatomy of hepatic veins. In patients with suspected Budd–Chiari syndrome, the hepatic venography demonstrates the underlying pathology (acute or chronic) of the obstruction of the vena cava/ hepatic veins responsible for the hepatic congestion and ascites, e.g. thrombus, congenital caval diaphragms, veno-occlusive disease. By careful selective injection of contrast media, it is possible to show individual veins, the presence of thrombus and a degree of completeness of the obstruction. A similar technique is used for trans-internal jugular portosystemic shunt (TIPSS) which is employed in patients with portal hypertension and poor functional reserve (Child–Pugh C) and in some patients with Budd–Chiari syndrome.

Arteriography and splenoportography

The portal venous system may be demonstrated by splenic puncture using an intercostal route. The splenic pulp pressure is readily measured and this equates to the portal venous pressure. Injection of medium outlines the splenic and portal veins and often demonstrates major collaterals. Portography can also be performed via the percutaneous transhepatic route. This technique also allows selective cannulation of the left gastric vein and its embolization in poor-risk patients with bleeding varices. Some centres use the left umbilical vein, after this is dilated and re-canalized, to inject contrast for visualization of the portal venous system.

More commonly, however, the portal system is imaged by arteriography. The superior mesenteric artery or coeliac axis is cannulated by the Seldinger technique. The arterial supply of the liver is first demonstrated and the venous phase of the injection outlines the superior mesenteric, portal veins and the splenic vein, according to the site of injection and amount of contrast injected. The distinctive corkscrew intrahepatic arteries are characteristic of cirrhosis and a good estimate of liver size is made (Figure 9.12).

Needle biopsy of the liver

This valuable investigation is indicated in patients with undiagnosed liver disease and selectively in some with

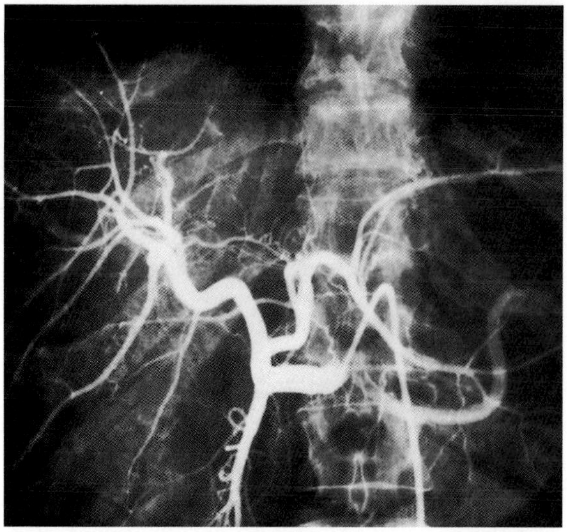

Figure 9.12 Following selective catheterization of the common hepatic artery through the coeliac axis the hepatic arteries are well shown. In this case the terminal branches of the left hepatic artery are stretched around a large metastatic deposit within the left lateral lobe and similar metastases may be detected in the right lobe also. In certain patients the left hepatic artery will arise from the left gastric artery and the right hepatic artery may arise, at least in part, from the superior mesenteric artery (20%).

focal abnormalities of the liver. The mortality rate should be low (less than 0.1%) provided certain precautions are taken. It requires an inpatient stay and should only be performed once the prothrombin time is shown to be not more than 3 s greater than the control and the platelet count greater than 60 000. The Menghini needle has largely been replaced by the Tru-cut needle for both diffuse and local disease.

For diffuse liver disease, e.g. cirrhosis, the procedure may be carried out by the blind percutaneous technique through a right lateral intercostal approach. Because of increased safety, some have abandoned the blind percutaneous approach even for diffuse disease and undertake the liver biopsy under ultrasound guidance. Needle biopsies from cirrhotic livers tend to fragment. Focal lesions require a targeted biopsy with either ultrasound or laparoscopic visual control (*vide infra*).

The important indications for liver biopsy are:

- Chronic liver disease.
- Cholestatic jaundice without dilatation of the biliary tract on ultrasonography.
- Unexplained hepatomegaly.
- Drug-induced liver disease.
- Solid space occupying lesions of the liver.

There is some controversy regarding the biopsy of suspected malignant hepatic tumours (primary and secondary). The consensus view nowadays is that if the suspect malignant lesion is considered operable and resectable, then target biopsy should not be undertaken as this may cause spillage and peritoneal implantation. On the other hand if the lesion is judged to be inoperable biopsy for histological confirmation is mandatory. Vascular lesions, especially haemangiomas should not be biopsied because of the risk of severe intraperitoneal haemorrhage.

The complications of liver needle biopsy include:

- Pleural effusion.
- Haemorrhage from the liver and thoracic wall.
- Intrahepatic haematoma.
- Hepatic arteriovenous fistulas.
- Haemobilia.
- Accidental puncture of the gallbladder and large bile ducts leading to bile peritonitis.
- Tumour cell implantation.

After the procedure the patient is confined to bed for 24 hours with regular and frequent pulse and blood pressure measurement.

Laparoscopy with contact ultrasonography of the liver

This is an invaluable investigation that provides direct information on the state of the liver and the peritoneal cavity. It is particularly useful in the investigation of patients with jaundice, chronic liver disease, ascites of unknown origin, and in the diagnosis and staging of both primary and secondary hepatic tumours. The advent of laparoscopic contact ultrasonography using high-resolution linear array probes has added considerably to the diagnostic yield of laparoscopy for the detection and staging of hepatic tumours. In addition to detecting hepatic secondary deposits in the liver and peritoneal cavity that are too small to be detected by CT scanning and MRI, laparoscopic contact ultrasonography permits the visualization of the hepatic vasculature (portal vein, hepatic artery, hepatic veins and retrohepatic vena cava) and examination of the entire biliary tract. This accurate assessment of the extent of involvement of the liver by tumour and relation to hepatic veins enables surgical planning of the resection necessary in the individual case.

Laparoscopy with contact ultrasonography and colour Doppler readily identifies haemangiomas. Visually guided biopsies or fine needle aspiration cytology of both the hepatic parenchyma (in cirrhosis) and focal lesions (tumours) for histological confirmation carries a higher diagnostic yield than percutaneous liver biopsy, and should bleeding occur from the biopsy site, this can be controlled by compression or electrocoagulation. Laparoscopic cholangiography can be performed during the same sitting in jaundiced patients, either through the gallbladder or transhepatically. Indeed, there is a growing view that laparoscopy with targeted biopsy and cholangiography (when indicated) provides all the information required for the management of these patients and obviates the routine need for expensive imaging tests in patients with jaundice and chronic liver disease. It is the best method of diagnosis and staging of pancreatic cancer and aside from providing histological or cytological confirmation, it allows the performance of bilio-enteric bypass and gastrojejunostomy for inoperable disease (Figure 9.13).

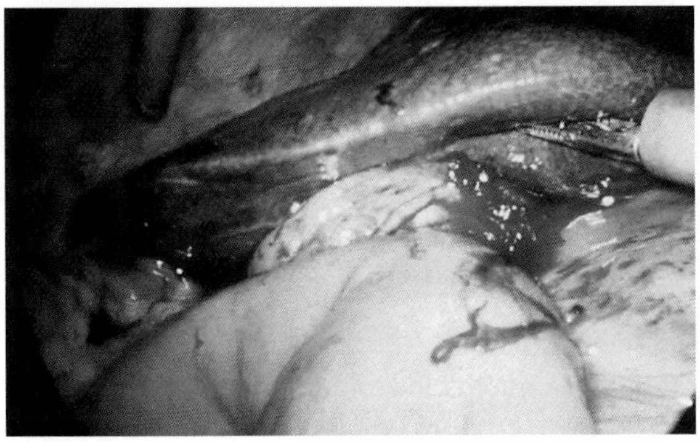

Figure 9.13 Endophotograph of laparoscopic cholecystojejunostomy in a patient with inoperable pancreatic cancer.

Section 9.5 • Clinical features of liver disease

Many of the symptoms which can ultimately be attributed to liver disorders are non-specific, e.g. fatigue, malaise, headache, myalgia, arthralgia and fever are commonly found in hepatitis. Confusion, forgetfulness, poor concentration and personality change are central nervous symptoms of advanced hepatic cirrhosis whereas ascites, weight loss and malnutrition and dependent oedema reflect other functional deficiencies of the same condition.

Anorexia and nausea are common in all forms of hepatic and biliary disease and it is common for pain in the right hypochondrium to be present. It is usually possible to distinguish between biliary tract colic and the dull boring pain of focal hepatic disease. Clearly jaundice is the most obvious symptom and constitutes the greatest diagnostic problem. In many instances jaundice will be accompanied by dark urine, pale stools and pruritus. General examination may reveal early jaundice in the sclerae and palate. Pruritus may lead to scratch marks and may be present earlier than other manifestations of liver disease, especially in primary biliary cirrhosis.

Chronic liver disease may show stigmata in the form of palmar erythema, finger clubbing, leuconychia, spider naevi, particularly over the upper half of the body, central nervous effects with a liver flap, peripheral neuritis and loss of consciousness ranging from confusion to full hepatic coma. In advanced disease with encephalopathy, a sweet musky odour may be apparent on the breath: foetor hepaticus.

On abdominal examination, there may be evidence of collateral veins in the abdominal wall, distension of the abdomen and eversion of the umbilicus from ascites, dependent oedema, gynaecomastia, testicular atrophy and loss of axillary and pubic hair. On palpation, hepatomegaly should be searched for and a decision made whether this is real or apparent, whether it is diffuse, focal or multifocal. Liver tenderness may be elicited either abdominally or by palpation or through the rib cage by percussion. Auscultation may rarely elicit a friction rub over an expanding tumour or abscess and a systolic bruit is sometimes heard. Splenomegaly may accompany hepatomegaly in patients with portal hypertension.

Section 9.6 • Non-surgical disorders of the liver

A full description of all liver disease is beyond the scope of this module. However, certain conditions must be borne in mind in deciding whether a liver disorder has a surgical basis or whether it is best handled by a physician. Many disorders require joint management between hepatologist, hepatic surgeon and in some cases, interventional radiologist.

Drug-related jaundice and hepatotoxicity

Since one of the main functions of the liver is to detoxify or to metabolize many pharmaceutical agents, it is perhaps not surprising that an overdose or abnormal response to the agent may lead to problems. It is not usually the drug but a metabolite that causes the liver cell damage with overt jaundice and in some cases, acute hepatic insufficiency (fulminant liver failure). There are many drugs that cause liver damage to varying extents. Theses may be classified as:

- Directly hepatotoxic agents, e.g. carbon tetrachloride, tetracyclines, paracetamol, DDT and benzene derivatives
- Drugs that interference with bilirubin metabolism/transport:
  - haemolysis, e.g. para-aminosalicylic acid and phenacetin
  - impaired bilirubin excretion, e.g. methyl testosterone and norethandrone
  - interference with uptake and transport of bilirubin, e.g. rifampicin, radiological contrast agents
  - interference with bilirubin conjugation, e.g. novobiocin
  - interference with bilirubin binding, e.g. salicylates and sulfonamides.
- Intrahepatic cholestasis, e.g. phenothiazine derivatives, chlorpromazine.
- Hepatitis-like disease, e.g. iproniazid, halothane, trichloroethylene, oxyphenisin (in laxatives) and many other drugs.
- Hepatic fibrosis (sclerosis) may complicate long-term use of cytotoxic agents especially in regional intra-arterial chemotherapy.

Damage is maximal in zone 3 where metabolizing enzymes are in the highest concentration and oxygen tension is the lowest. The histological picture may resemble acute hepatitis, and if so, has a poor prognosis. In other cases the light microscopy shows only scattered fatty change and no inflammation. A careful history of both prescribed and self-medication is required for all jaundiced patients or those who have abnormal liver function tests.

Drug-induced liver disorders

From a clinical standpoint, there is a wide spectrum of drug-induced liver disorders (DILD):

- cholestatic jaundice
- acute hepatitis
- chronic active hepatitis
- pseudoalcoholic liver disease
- hepatic sclerosis (due to vascular damage)
- hepatic neoplasia
- fulminant liver failure
- hepatic veno-occlusive disease
- vanishing bile duct syndrome.

DILD accounts for 40% of hospitalized cases of 'acute hepatitis'. Over 20% of cases of fulminant hepatic failure are caused by drugs such as halothane, acetaminophen (paracetamol), phenytoin and α-methyl dopa. In surgical practice hepatic injury induced by antimicrobial drugs is not uncommon. Augmentin (amoxicillin conjugated to clavulanate) can cause hepatocellular and mixed hepatocellular cholestatic injury. The mechanism appears to be drug hypersensitivity to the clavulanic acid or a metabolite derived from it. Chronic cholestatic injury can be caused by ketoconazole, and nitrofurantoin can result in chronic hepatitis, whereas erythromycin estolate has been reported to induce hepatic pseudo-tumours.

Rare instances of mild reversible cholestatic or mixed cholestatic hepatocellular injury have been reported following therapy with the commonly used H_2-receptor antagonists (cimetidine, ranitidine, famotidine and nizatidine).

Halogenated anaesthetic agent induced hepatitis

Although rare, halothane hepatitis continues to afflict patients from time to time. Hepatic injury caused by this halogenated anaesthetic agent has been reported in an anaesthetist. Although usually recoverable, severe hepatocellular damage progressing to fulminant liver failure is well documented. The injury appears to be due to hypersensitivity and the impaired liver function is associated with pyrexia, skin rashes and eosinophilia. Moreover the condition develops in patients after previous exposure to halothane. An antibody to a hapten metabolite of the anaesthetic agent (trifluoroacetate) is found in 30% of suspected cases of halothane hepatitis. Biochemically, there is elevation of the serum glutathione 5-transferase activity and this appears to be a more specific and sensitive measure of anaesthetic-induced hepatic injury than the serum aminotransferases. Although there has been only one single case report implicating isoflurane and the hepatotoxic potential of this agent remains debatable, covalently bound antigens which are recognized by antibodies from patients with previous halothane hepatitis have been reported, indicating the distinct possibility of cross-sensitization with halothane or a common immune mediated mechanism. Thus the practice of changing halogenated anaesthetics in patients requiring multiple anaesthetics does not guarantee a reduced risk.

Hepatotoxic herbal remedies

Some of the increasingly popular herbal remedies are hepatotoxic and the spectrum of the disorders range from mild hepatitis to extensive necrosis, prolonged cholestasis, occlusion of the small hepatic veins (veno-occlusive disease), chronic hepatitis and cirrhosis. Chinese herbal teas (popular in the treatment of dermatitis) derived from the plants *Dictamnus dasycarpus* and *Paeonia* sp. have been confirmed to have hepatotoxic substances and cases of severe jaundice and hepatitis have been reported after drinking these teas.

Acute and chronic viral hepatitis

From the surgical standpoint the important infections are hepatitis B, C and to a lesser extent A. Hepatitis A continues to give rise to epidemics. Although the disease is usually benign, complications including prolonged cholestasis and macropapular skin reactions are common. A vaccine developed from killed virus A propagated in fibroblast culture is available. It appears to be particularly effective when combined with recombinant hepatitis B vaccine.

The hepatitis B virus (HBV), which was first isolated in 1966, has infected in excess of 350 million individuals world-wide. It is a leading cause of chronic hepatitis, cirrhosis and hepatocellular carcinoma. Hepatitis B-liver disease is one of the common indications for liver transplantation.

The hepatitis B vaccination programme appears to be altering the epidemiology of hepatitis B. Thus infection in heath care workers and homosexuals (who have accepted the vaccination programme) has fallen, whereas the incidence in drug abusers has increased. It should be stressed that the infectivity of HBV is much greater (eight times) than that of human immunodeficiency virus (HIV).

Specific therapy of chronic hepatitis B disease is now possible with α-interferon which inhibits the replication of HBV and treatment can lead to remission of the disease with clearance of the hepatitis B e antigen and hepatitis B surface antigen [Module 5, Vol. I]. α-Interferon is administered subcutaneously in a dose of 10 MU three times weekly for up to 12 months. Unfortunately interferon is only effective in 30–40% within the first year of treatment. Criteria have now been proposed that predict a good response to α-interferon. These include:

- a raised aminotransferase concentration >100 IU/ml
- low values for hepatitis B virus DNA < 200 ng/l
- liver biopsy showing moderate to severe inflammatory activity
- age <65 years.

One of the most promising antiviral agents is the nucleoside analogue lamivudine (3-thiacytidine). The drug is administered alone or together with hepatitis B virus immunoglobulin. In a recent control trial combined therapy with lamivudine and α-interferon resulted in a higher HbeAg seroconversion rate than either agent alone and this synergistic effect was marked in patients with moderately elevated baseline aminotransferase levels. Lamivudine therapy is now administered before and after liver transplanation to prevent infection of the graft by the hepatitis B virus.

Hepatitis C accounts for 50% of sporadic non-A, non-B hepatitis and for 90% of hepatitis due to transfusion of blood and blood products. It can cause chronic liver disease. Hepato-cellular cancer has also been associated with previous hepatitis C infection in Italy, Spain, the USA and Japan. The vast majority of haemophiliac patients who received blood products prior to screening of donors and blood products (1987) became infected and some of these have progressed to end-stage liver disease requiring transplantation. Currently the only approved treatment is α-interferon (3 MU subcutaneously three times per week for 12 months). Although some 50% of patients respond initially to this treatment, a sustained response is only encountered in 25%. Although patients with cirrhosis do not respond to α-interferon, there is recent evidence that this treatment may reduce the risk of hepatocellular carcinoma in these patients. Following transplantation, nearly all patients become re-infected and 20% develop cirrhosis in the transplanation liver within 5 years. Studies to date indicate that neither Ribavirin nor interferon when given singly has been significantly successful, but combination treatment has yielded promising results when used both prophylactically and therapeutically. The results of clinical trials on this combination are ongoing. If efficacy of combination therapy is confirmed it is likely that antiviral therapy would have to be indefinite in these patients in an effort at prevention of re-infection and progression to chronic liver disease.

Cirrhosis of the liver

Liver cirrhosis is the end result of hepatocyte death and needs to be distinguished from hepatic fibrosis which can occur in the portal regions from chronic bile duct obstruction or congenitally, or around the central veins in chronic cardiac failure. Confluent necrosis of zones 1 and 3 leads to fibrotic bridges and the regeneration of surviving hepatocytes results in a further distortion of hepatic architecture. Three morphological types of cirrhosis can be recognized:

- *Micronodular* has small regenerating nodules throughout the liver separated by thick fibrous septa; it is characteristically associated with alcoholism and malnutrition.
- *Macronodular* has nodules of variable size with normal histological appearances within the larger nodules.
- *Mixed* picture results from regeneration in a micronodular cirrhosis.

Clinical presentation

Not uncommonly the condition will be unsuspected and comes to light because of a routine estimation of liver function tests or found incidentally at laparotomy. Clinical suspicion is aroused by finding palmar erythema, spider naevi, otherwise unexplained peripheral oedema or epistaxis. Alternatively, the patient may present in a later state of disease with muscle wasting and ascites, with gastrointestinal haemorrhage from varices, jaundice or hepatic encephalopathy.

In most patients, liver cirrhosis has a poor prognosis. However, it is now known that certain types, e.g. haemochromatosis and Wilson's disease can be reversed by appropriate treatment. Other diagnoses are less likely to regress but in some the prognosis may be improved with appropriate management. It is of considerable importance that the risks of surgical procedures be assessed. Certain clinical criteria are worth recording:

- Size of liver – large livers have better prognosis than small shrunken organs.
- Jaundice – poor prognostic sign unless diagnosis is primary biliary cirrhosis.
- Ascites – poor prognostic sign.
- Albumin – <25 g/l is a poor prognostic sign.
- Hypoprothrombinaemia – if persistent, is a poor prognostic sign.
- Portosystemic encephalopathy – poor prognostic sign.
- Alcoholic history – if abstains, prognosis is better than cirrhosis of unknown origin (cryptogenic)

These prognostic factors can be combined in various mathematical models and also form the basis of the grading systems previously described.

Ascites in chronic liver disease

Ascites is the most common consequence of cirrhosis and 10% of patients die as a result of secondary morbidity associated with therapy of this complication. Furthermore these patients tend to have more advanced liver disease, are more prone to die from variceal haemorrhage or hepatorenal syndrome and are subject to the development of spontaneous bacterial peritonitis.

In the final analysis, the ascites is the end result of avid sodium and water retention that is invariable in chronic liver disease. However, the exact mechanism for the ascitic fluid formation and its sequestration in the intraperitoneal compartment is unknown. Three suggestions have been put forward: *underfilling*, *overflow* and the *peripheral arterial vasodilatation hypotheses*.

According to the traditional underfilling theory, the ascitic fluid formation develops as a direct result of the portal hypertension. The effective circulating blood volume and the renal blood flow are reduced by the sequestration of fluid in the peritoneal cavity. The fall in the effective blood flow that is detected by volume baroreceptors triggers the compensatory release of hormones which then act on the kidneys to retain sodium and water. However, as the renal sodium and water retention precede the formation of ascites, the underfilling hypothesis seems unlikely.

According to the overflow theory, the primary event is expansion of the plasma volume which then leads to overflow into the peritoneal compartment and increased lymph formation. This theory does not explain the mechanism of the primary event (water and salt retention causing the expansion of the plasma volume), nor does it account for the well-documented secondary humoral and sympathetic nervous responses that are present in patients with cirrhosis.

The currently favoured hypothesis is known as the peripheral arterial vasodilatation theory of renal sodium and water retention. The initial event is loss of arteriolar tone with peripheral arteriolar dilatation and a decreased effective arterial blood flow. This triggers the usual humoral and sympathetic response with release of renin, aldosterone, noradrenaline and vasopressin, leading to water and salt retention and renal vasoconstriction. As the plasma volume expands, the concentrations of these hormones return to normal. Given the progressive increase in the plasma volume and increased lymph formation (caused by the increased hydrostatic pressure), the presence of portal hypertension helps to localize a substantial part of the retained fluid in the peritoneal cavity.

Whatever the mechanism, the blood volume is increased in cirrhotics with ascites and there is an abnormally high urinary excretion of prostaglandins (especially E_2) and immunoglobulin M. There is increasing evidence for abnormal metabolism or impaired action of atrial natriuretic factor (ANF), synthesized and released by the atrial myocardium in ascitic patients, particularly in the presence of renal functional impairment. The plasma ANF is elevated in patients with ascites. This is due to increased cardiac release rather than decreased splanchnic extraction and degradation. The cause of the elevated ANF may be increased stretch of the atrial muscle fibres by the expanded blood volume or it may be secondary to elevated levels of angiotensin II, noradrenaline and vasopressin. Recombinant synthetic ANF induces a marked diuresis when administered to cirrhotic patients without sodium retention, but this effect is absent or diminished in patients with this complication.

Clinically, the ascites is often accompanied with peripheral oedema and pleural effusions. More recently, it has been recognized that pericardial effusion is present in many patients (60%) with ascites secondary to alcoholic cirrhosis. When tense, the ascites may be tender, limits mobility and causes dyspnoea by tenting of the diaphragm. All patients with ascites exhibit marked muscle wasting. A diagnostic sample of peritoneal fluid obtained by aspiration is essential. The serum-ascitic fluid albumin ratio is very important (and correlates with the portal venous pressure). A gradient which is <11 g/litre is present in patients without portal hypertension. Higher values are associated with portal hypertension. This ratio helps to distinguish high protein transudates in patients with portal hypertension from true exudates (e.g. tuberculosis and peritoneal carcinomatosis).

The standard initial medical treatment consists of dietary sodium restriction and diuretics. Initially spironolactone is used and when necessary loop diuretics (e.g. frusemide) are added. Unfortunately, the use of potent loop diuretics, while undoubtedly effective, increases the risk of encephalopathy. This complication is especially prone to occur in patients with renal impairment. The kidney malfunction may be subclinical and undetected by both blood urea and serum creatinine, but if measured, the glomerular filtration rate (GFR) is found to be reduced. It is important that patients with low GFR are identified, as aside from responding unfavourably to loop diuretics, these patients are particularly susceptible to renal compromise by both anti-inflammatory drugs and aminoglycosides which are therefore contraindicated.

When the above medical management fails (refractory ascites) the options are:

- therapeutic paracentesis with intravenous albumin;
- recirculation therapy; or
- peritoneovenous shunting
- saphenoperitoneal shunting.

Large volume paracentesis is an effective and safe method of treatment provided it is accompanied by intravenous infusion of salt-poor albumin solution. Albumin replaced in a dose of 6 g for every litre of ascitic fluid removed is used to achieve volume replacement and prevent renal impairment and hyponatraemia. The disadvantage of therapeutic high volume paracentesis is the rapid recurrence of the ascites.

Recirculation therapy is carried out by devices such as the Rhodiascit machine, which permit the re-infusion of the ascitic fluid into the venous system. This technique avoids the need for albumin infusions and appears to be equally effective and safe. There has been considerable debate regarding the role of peritoneovenous shunting in the management of ascites in patients with cirrhosis. The results of clinical trials comparing this surgical approach with other forms of treatment have now clarified the picture.

Peritoneovenous shunting is an effective form of treatment which reduces hospitalization, increases muscle mass and leads to adequate long-term control of ascites (with diminished diuretic dosage) in patients with ascites and good liver function (child A and B). It is, however, ineffective and accompanied by a significant mortality in patients with advanced disease and is, therefore, contraindicated in these patients. Recurrence of ascites is due to blockage usually of the venous segment of the system. The other complications of peritoneovenous shunting are coagulopathy (DIC) and infection.

More recently, saphenoperitoneal shunt has been introduced for the treatment of intractable ascites due to chronic liver disease. Essentially, this consists of exposure of the long saphenous vein with ligature and division of all its tributaries. The long saphenous vein is then divided at mid thigh level with ligature of the distal end. The proximal end is observed for a few minutes to ensure that there is no back bleeding, i.e. the sapheno-femoral valve is competent. If this is confirmed, the proximal end is turned up and anastomosed to the peritoneum near the internal ring with a continuous suture. Early results with saphenoperitoneal shunting have confirmed its safety and efficacy. It retains the efficacy of peritoneovenous shunting without the need for insertion of prosthetic valve. This operation is, however, not yet in established usage.

Congenital hepatic fibrosis (fibropolycystic disease)

This is a congenital disorder that is inherited as an autosomal recessive trait, the importance of which lies in the development of portal hypertension with variceal bleeding in afflicted individuals. In view of its association with other disorders that are characterized by ectatic ducts or cysts, the more generic name 'fibropolycystic disease' may be more appropriate.

In congenital hepatic fibrosis, there is enlargement of the portal spaces by pronounced fibrosis and bile ductule proliferation. The ductules are dilated (ectatic) to varying degrees but still communicate with the main intrahepatic biliary tree. It is generally thought that the bile duct proliferation is the primary abnormality. Some of the bile ductules may become so dilated as to form communicating microcysts. The disease though diffuse is patchy with areas of unaffected liver and essentially the overall architecture of the liver remains normal, although the portal fibrosis results in a block to the sinusoidal circulation within the liver and hence the development of portal hypertension.

Both sexes are affected and the disease is uncommon with a prevalence of 1:100 000. In most patients the condition is first recognized by the onset of severe gastrointestinal bleeding which on endoscopy is found to be due to ruptured oesophageal or gastric varices usually between the age of 5 and 20 years. Less commonly the condition presents with abdominal discomfort caused by an enlarged spleen or because of hypersplenism. In a small minority of patients, the presentation is with bacterial cholangitis. The clinical findings include hepatosplenomegaly with normal liver function tests except for a slight elevation of the alkaline phosphatase or γ-GT in some patients. The liver is hyperechoic on ultrasound examination. The diagnosis is established by liver biopsy.

In 50% of cases congenital hepatic fibrosis is associated with Caroli's syndrome (ectatic dilatation of the segmental bile ducts causing recurrent bacterial cholangitis). Other associated malformations that may occur include ectatic renal collecting tubules (similar to but distinct from medullary sponge kidney), duplication of the portal vein, cystic dysplasia of the pancreas, pulmonary emphysema, intestinal lymphangiectasia, cerebellar haemangioma, cleft palate and aneurysms of the renal and hepatic arteries.

The clinical course of congenital hepatic fibrosis is that of repeated episodes of variceal haemorrhage and as the liver function remains normal in these patients, the best treatment is by selective decompression by Warren shunt after the acute episode has been controlled by endoscopic banding (*vide infra*).

- Sclerotherapy should be avoided in these patients because of the risk of portal vein thrombosis.

Patients who develop bacterial cholangitis require antibiotic therapy.

Alcoholic liver disease

Alcoholic liver disease is a major problem, especially in the affluent Western countries. The spectrum of liver damage varies from fatty infiltration to alcoholic hepatitis, hepatic fibrosis and cirrhosis. The latter is the commonest chronic liver disease in some Western countries. Despite intensive research, the exact mechanism responsible for the hepatic damage remains unknown. Females develop alcoholic liver disease after exposure to a smaller quantity of alcohol than males. This may partly be explained by the significantly lower gastric alcohol dehydrogenase (ADH) activity in women, resulting in a larger quantity of ingested alcohol reaching the liver. The gastric ADH is significantly reduced in chronic alcoholics of both sexes. Alcoholics have a higher incidence of HBV (44%) and HCV (50%) disease and these viruses may play a part in the development of cirrhosis at least in some patients. The nutritional intake of alcohol abusers is another factor that contributes to the development of liver disease. The majority of alcoholics tend to ingest food that is low in protein and high in fat. There is some evidence that hepatocyte necrosis may be secondary to the reactive oxygen radicals, which are generated during ethanol metabolism. Serum endotoxin levels are known to be increased in patients with alcoholic liver disease and stimulation of the phagocytes by endotoxin with excess production of tumour necrosis factor has been suggested as a possible mechanism for the hepatocyte damage. Alcohol reduces the cellular regeneration by an antiproliferative effect, so that cell damage is less likely to be replaced by functioning parenchyma. Acetaldehyde derived by oxidation from ethanol in the liver is involved in the increased synthesis of type I collagen in the liver and hence the fibrosis. Another factor which has been implicated in the fibrosis is the cytokine transforming growth factor (TGF-β) which is produced in excessive amounts by the Kupffer cells in response to alcohol. The excess TGF-β stimulates the transformation of lipocytes (special forms of Kupffer cells) into active fibroblasts. There is some epidemiological evidence that these lipocytes are more prone to activation when sensitized by a high-fat diet.

The commonest and earliest sign of liver damage is hepatomegaly, which may progress to a tender liver from fatty infiltration of the parenchyma. At this stage the liver biopsy shows the hepatocytes to be distended with fat and sometimes there are hyaline deposits (Mallory's hyaline). In alcoholic hepatitis in addition to tender hepatomegaly, there is jaundice, leucocytosis and elevation of the transaminases. The liver biopsy in alcoholic hepatitis shows a cellular infiltrate, liver cell necrosis, cholestasis, variable degree of fatty change and, sometimes, Mallory's hyaline. The final stage is the development of cirrhosis, which is of the micronodular variety. There are no specific laboratory markers of alcoholic liver disease although the following are highly suggestive: raised levels of γ-glutamyl transpeptidase, presence of carbohydrate-depleted (sialic acid-depleted) transferrin and a specific isoenzyme of alanine aminotransferase (F-AAT). The latter is strongly associated with hepatocyte necrosis.

The most important factor in the treatment of alcoholic liver disease is abstinence from alcohol, and considerable improvement both in the liver function tests and on repeat biopsy can be obtained by this means if the disease has not reached the cirrhotic stage. Corticosteroids are indicated in alcoholic hepatitis. Parenteral nutrition imparts significant benefit in patients with alcoholic hepatitis and may improve survival although this is debatable. Transplantation is now performed for advanced alcohol related chronic liver disease provided a minimum period of 6 months' abstinence can be documented. The results to date have been better than predicted and only about 15% of patients have resumed drinking after the transplantation.

Cholestatic liver disease

Cholestasis, impaired bile secretion/excretion, with the development of conjugated hyperbilirubinaemia and raised bile ductular enzymes can be caused by drugs including alcohol, viral hepatitis, obstructive lesions of the biliary tract and primary hepatic cholestatic liver disorders. These are primary biliary cirrhosis, vanishing bile duct syndrome and sclerosing cholangitis [**Disorders of the biliary tract, Vol. II**].

Primary biliary cirrhosis

This is a disease of unknown aetiology in which the intrahepatic bile ducts are progressively destroyed by an immunological process. It runs a variable course but ultimately ends in primary biliary cirrhosis (as distinct from secondary biliary cirrhosis due to chronic obstruction of the extrahepatic biliary tract, e.g. strictures). Circulating antibodies against mitochondrial constituents (antimitochondrial antibodies) are found in all the patients. These antibodies are non-organ and non-species specific and their relationship to the aetiology of the disease remains speculative but they are useful in the diagnosis of the condition. The most widely held immunological hypothesis for the development of the disease is aberrant expression of class II histocompatibility antigens on the epithelium of the bile ducts which induces a T-cell related progressive immune destruction. There is some evidence that the mitochondrial antigens responsible for the production of antimitochondrial antibodies (e.g. E_2 antigen which is also present in Gram-negative bacteria) may cross-react with the bile duct antigens. Antimitochondrial antibodies specific to primary biliary cirrhosis can be induced by immunizing rabbits by R mutant Enterobacteriaecae organisms. Thus the possibility of an immunological disorder secondary to release of the E_2 antigens by intestinal R-form Gram-negative organisms has been raised.

The disease is often asymptomatic for long periods. Some cases are discovered accidentally because of abnormal liver function tests obtained before blood donation. There is a female preponderance and the mean age at symptomatic presentation is 40 years. The symptoms include itching, weight loss, malaise and icterus. The liver becomes enlarged and with progression of the disease, portal hypertension with splenomegaly develops. There is deposition of cholesterol in the tissues especially around the orbits and on the extensor surface of the large joints. In advanced disease, intrapulmonary shunting is associated with finger clubbing. The malabsorption secondary to the diminished bile salt pool leads to deficiency of fat-soluble vitamins (A, D, E, K) with the development of osteoporosis. In addition to biochemical features of cholestasis and presence of antimitochondrial antibodies, the serum IgM is elevated. Smooth muscle antibodies are also present in many patients.

There is no effective medical therapy but symptomatic relief is obtained by a variety of drugs. Cholestyramine is used for itching and ursodeoxycholate improves symptoms and the liver function tests by replacing the toxic hydrophobic bile acids. Prednisolone seems to reduce fatigue and itching and may improve liver function. Monthly injections of fat-soluble vitamins are administered to counteract the deficiencies caused by the malabsorption. However, the disease process is not influenced by medical treatment and the only effective therapy that imparts a long-term cure is hepatic transplantation. Primary biliary cirrhosis is the second most frequent indication for liver transplantation. Nowadays, this operation is undertaken before the development of end-stage disease and the onset of hyponatraemia or significant bone disease. It is considered in patients whose quality of life has deteriorated or in whom the bilirubin exceeds 100 mmol/l, and in those who develop portal hypertension.

Vanishing bile duct syndrome

This is a condition that results in the progressive destruction of segments of the intrahepatic ductules with the development of persistent jaundice caused by drugs. The disease is usually irreversible, i.e. cessation of the drug does not relieve the cholestasis as shown by persistent jaundice, elevated alkaline phosphatase and γ-glutamyl transpeptidase. Many drugs are responsible for the development of this syndrome but the most important are:

- Co-amoxyclav
- Carbamzepine
- Chlorpromazine
- Co-trimoxazole
- Fluvloxacillin
- Methyltestosterone
- Phenytoin
- Prochlorperazine.

Metabolic liver disease

By definition, this includes a variety of disorders (Table 9.3) of hepatic synthesis, degradation or regulation of endogenous compounds. In practice they fall into two

Table 9.3 Metabolic liver disease

- **Genetic haemochromatosis:** defect of iron metabolism
- **Neonatal haemochromatosis:** defect of iron metabolism
- **Wilson's disease:** defect of copper metabolism
- **Cystic fibrosis**
- **α_1-Antitrypsin deficiency:** sequestration of α_1-antitrypsin granules in endoplasmic reticulum
- **Hereditary tyrosinaemia type 1:** absence/deficiency of fumarylacetoacetate hydrolase
- **Crigler-Najiar syndrome:** absence/deficiency of uridine diphosphate-glucuronosyl transferase

broad categories: disorders associated with defective enzyme production or release (e.g. α_1-antitrypsin deficiency) and disorders of mineral deposition (e.g. haemochromatosis).

Haemochromatosis

This includes genetic haemochromatosis and neonatal haemochromatosis. Both represent a disorder of iron metabolism that is inherited as an autosomal recessive trait. They are thus distinct from secondary (acquired) haemochromatosis, which develops in patients with polycythaemia and those requiring multiple repeated blood transfusions (chronic haemolytic anaemias).

Genetic haemochromatosis is common. The gene carrier rate in the North European population is 10% and the disorder may affect up to 1 in 300 heterozygotes. The precise location of the candidate gene (HFE) has been recently identified. The abnormality consists of a single point mutation, i.e. the HFE encodes a single amino acid substitution from cysteine to tyrosine (C282Y). The discovery of the candidate gene has led to a simple effective screening method for the disorder.

If unrecognized, genetic haemochromatosis results in progressive iron deposition in the liver, heart, pancreas, joints and endocrine glands with sparing of the spleen, lymph nodes and bone marrow. Genetic haemochromatosis is associated with the human leucocyte antigen (HLA) allo-antigens A3, B7 or B14 and is more common in males. However, the precise metabolic defect remains obscure. An abnormally enhanced transport of dietary iron through the intestinal cell is likely and this is caused by failure of the normal mechanism of down-regulation of the villous enterocyte transferrin receptors in response to excess iron stores. The hepatic accumulation of iron leads to cirrhosis with an increased risk of hepatocellular carcinoma, which is one of the commonest causes of death in untreated patients.

The classical clinical picture of the full blown disease is that of a diabetic patient (75%) in whom there is a dusky brown pigmentation of the skin, buccal mucosa and conjunctiva (bronze diabetes) and cirrhosis. About half the patients have a polyarthropathy starting in the small joints and many exhibit other endocrine dysfunctions including hypopituitarism and hypogonadism. The liver biopsy shows excessive iron deposition in the hepatocytes and the Kupffer cells with fibrosis or macronodular cirrhosis. The deposited iron is thought to induce hepatic injury by peroxidation of the intracellular phospholipid membranes. In addition, these patients are subject to cardiomyopathy.

Early diagnosis is essential to prevent the development of multi-organ disease. Characteristically, the serum ferritin is elevated and the transferrin saturation exceeds 55%, in the presence of which a liver biopsy is essential for establishing the diagnosis. Treatment of the disease entails phlebotomy and reduced dietary intake of iron with long-term follow-up of all patients.

Neonatal haemochromatosis has similar features but is genetically different. The condition develops *in utero* and the affected infants exhibit intrauterine growth retardation, are often premature and develop early liver failure and death.

Wilson's disease

This is a rare autosomal recessive inherited disorder of copper metabolism leading to copper overload of various organs: liver, cornea, kidneys and the central nervous system (basal ganglia). The gene for Wilson's disease (ATP7B) is located on the long arm of chromosome 13. Wilson's disease is characterized by a low serum caeruloplasmin level. The basic cellular defect underlying the disease is unknown but there is a markedly decreased biliary excretion of copper, which is largely responsible for the progressive copper overload. The hepatic injury results in fibrosis and cirrhosis at a relatively young age and portal hypertension is common. Neurological features are more common in adult patients. The classical clinical feature is that of the Kayser-Fleischer ring of pigment in the cornea. Aminoaciduria and phosphaturia are the result of renal damage following copper deposition in the proximal tubules. Copper studies (serum copper, serum caeruloplasmin and urinary copper levels) should be undertaken in all young patients presenting with chronic liver disease and slit-lamp examination of the cornea is also carried out. Although there may be difficulty in distinguishing Wilson's disease from other chronic forms of liver disorders as these are often accompanied by increased hepatic copper, the finding of a low plasma caeruloplasmin resolves this diagnostic difficulty.

The treatment of Wilson's disease consists of chelation therapy with penicillamine or tientine together with avoidance of food high in copper content. Zinc supplementation is useful because it protects to some extent against the copper-induced hepatocyte injury and reduces the absorption of copper by the enterocytes. Ammonium tetrathiomolybdate is particularly effective for patients with neurological or psychiatric manifestations of the disease.

Cystic fibrosis

As more patients with cystic fibrosis are surviving to adulthood, the incidence of hepatic disease associated with this congenital disorder is increasing. Some 25% of patients with cystic fibrosis have clinical and biochemical evidence of liver disease. Many of these patients have intrahepatic and extrahepatic biliary strictures. Improvement in the liver function tests may be obtained by therapy with ursodeoxycholic acid which increases the bile flow and alters the composition of bile such that the proportion of the less toxic hydrophilic bile acids in the bile acid pool is enhanced.

Alpha$_1$-antitrypsin deficiency

This inherited disorder affects Caucasians of European descent. The deficiency of the α_1-antitrypsin (which acts as an antiprotease) results in pulmonary damage due to lack of inhibition of neutrophil elastase and to liver disease. The latter appears to be secondary to the sequestration of α_1-antitrypsin granules in the endoplasmic reticulum of the hepatocyte. There is no effective medical therapy and progressive disease is treated with hepatic transplantation.

Hereditary tyrosinaemia type I

This metabolic disorder is characterized by a deficiency of the enzyme fumarylacetoacetate hydrolase (FAH) which is the last enzyme involved in the degradation pathway of tyrosine. The accumulated products of the amino acid together with various catalytic proteins result in renal, hepatic and neurological involvement. There are two clinical forms of this disorder. The acute type (total absence of FAH) is dominated by failure to thrive and progressive liver failure with death in infancy. The chronic variety (reduced levels of FAH) is characterized by renal tubular dysfunction, rickets, progressive liver disease and the development of hepatocellular carcinoma. The best treatment of this condition is hepatic transplantation which abolishes the risk of hepatocellular carcinoma.

Crigler–Najiar syndrome

This congenital disorder which results in hyperbilirubinaemia is covered elsewhere [Disorders of the Biliary Tract, Vol. II].

Section 9.7 • Hepatic encephalopathy

Hepatic encephalopathy (HE) is a term that covers a spectrum of neuropsychiatric disorders which afflict patients suffering from liver disease and/or portosystemic shunting. It remains uncertain whether the same morbid process underlies the various clinical states associated with the development of encephalopathy or whether separate mechanisms are involved, i.e. different types of HE exist. Hepatic coma is encountered in acute liver failure: *acute fulminant encephalopathy*. In chronic liver disease, the hallmarks of HE are intellectual impairment, reduced level of consciousness and abnormalities on psychometric testing. The encephalopathy in chronic liver disease may be subclinical (mild) or overt either as recurrent reversible episodes (often precipitated by bleeding), or as an overt and persistent condition when the HE may be accompanied by permanent structural central nervous system (CNS) changes, predominantly cortical atrophy of the brain.

There is increasing evidence that the encephalopathy of acute liver failure is different from that encountered in chronic liver disease and portosystemic shunting. Aside from the fact that it is not linked to any of the factors known to precipitate encephalopathy in chronic liver disease, it does not respond to standard measures which are effective in chronic HE. More importantly, cerebral oedema, which is frequently present in acute liver failure, is very rarely encountered in chronic liver disease.

Subclinical encephalopathy is detected by psychometric testing and is found in patients with normal or mildly abnormal liver function tests (schistosomiasis, well-compensated inactive Child A cirrhosis, congenital hepatic fibrosis and splenic or portal vein thrombosis). It is probably equivalent to the shunt encephalopathy (after surgical portosystemic shunting) and may be present for several years before overt encephalopathy develops.

Despite considerable research, the exact mechanisms involved (possibly multifactorial) in the production of the encephalopathy remain uncertain. Five hypotheses have been advanced over the years:

- Ammonia toxicity.
- Multiple synergistic neurotoxins.
- False neurotransmitters secondary to an abnormal plasma amino acid profile.
- Overactivity of GABA neurotransmission.
- Depressant cerebral effects of benzodiazepine-like substances.

Ammonia toxicity cannot be overlooked as there is considerable evidence that the raised blood ammonia (found in all cases of HE) plays a pathogenetic role either directly or indirectly via a metabolic consequence. Ammonia induces changes in the brain astrocytes, which are present in patients who die of HE. Furthermore, measures designed to reduce the intestinal absorption of ammonia constitute the most effective means of reversing the encephalopathy of chronic liver disease. The ammonia toxicity is enhanced by hypokalaemic alkalosis as the change from the NH_4^- ion to gaseous NH_3 allows easy passage through the blood-brain barrier.

The accumulation of multiple neurotoxins including various mercaptans remains questionable and recent studies have been non-confirmatory. In many patients with HE, the plasma amino acid profile is distinctly abnormal with a preponderance of aromatic neutral amino acids (phenylalanine, tryptophan and tyrosine) over branched chain aliphatic amino acids (valine, leucine and isoleucine). This observation led to the hypothesis that excessive blood levels of the aromatic amino acids induce the formation of false neurotransmitters (phenyl-ethanolamine and octopamine) by intestinal organisms which are then absorbed and replace or deplete the normal brain neurotransmitters, dopamine and noradrenaline. This hypothesis generated considerable interest and led to the use of specific solutions and diets enriched with high levels of branched chain amino acids in an effort to reverse the process. In fact this hypothesis is now known to be invalid, as studies on human brains in patients dying of HE have not confirmed the depletion of normal neurotransmitters. Branched chain amino acid therapy does not significantly affect the outcome of patients with acute encephalopathy but may be minimally beneficial in patients with chronic encephalopathy.

The GABA hypothesis implicates overactivity of the gamma-aminobutyric acid (GABA) neurotransmission in the development of HE. The excess GABA is synthesized by the enteric flora and reaches the systemic circulation (and hence the brain) via the portosystemic shunts. The evidence in favour of the GABA hypothesis includes high blood levels in patients with HE, increased blood-brain permeability to GABA (in animal models), increased or hypersensitive GABA receptors and improvement of the encephalopathy (in animal models) by GABA antagonists.

The benzodiazepine hypothesis is interesting and is related to the GABA neurotransmission as the receptors for both compounds are linked (GABA-benzodiazepine receptor-chloride inophore complex). Benzodiazepine compounds (diazepam, desmethyldiazepam, etc.) have been detected in the CNS of humans suffering from HE. It is not known whether these are produced locally in the brain, or represent occult ingestion or are synthesized by the gut microflora. In hepatic encephalopathy, the blood level of benzodiazepine is elevated and the level correlates with the severity. The most convincing evidence to date for this hypothesis is the improvement of HE that results from therapy with benzodiazepine antagonists such as flumazenil.

The most common precipitating cause of acute encephalopathy in patients with chronic liver disease is gastrointestinal haemorrhage, usually due to ruptured varices. When severe, the patient becomes deeply comatose. Other precipitating factors include hypokalaemic alkalosis, diuretic therapy, sedation, sepsis and portosystemic surgical shunting. To a large extent the incidence and severity of post-shunt encephalopathy is dependent on the size of the shunt, and for this reason, it is most severe after a portacaval shunt. The clinical features of patients with overt chronic persistent encephalopathy include lack of concentration, incoordination, altered sleep rhythm, deterioration of intellectual function and level of consciousness and neurological signs (apraxia, hyperactive stretch reflexes). Cortical atrophy which occurs in 10% is associated with marked psychometric impairment and chronic disability.

The principles of management of patients with hepatic pre-coma or coma include the search for and correction of any precipitating cause, e.g. withdrawal of sedatives and administration of suitable antagonists, correction of fluid and electrolyte disturbances, arrest of haemorrhage and treatment of sepsis (including primary peritonitis in ascitic patients). In the presence of a gastrointestinal bleed, drastic purgation with oral magnesium sulfate and the use of enemas is needed to reduce the intestinal protein load (and thus the formation of ammonia by the intestinal organisms). This is accompanied by the administration of neomycin (2 g tds) or metronidazole (0.2 g tds) and lactulose (30 ml tds) to reduce the absorption of ammonia (by ionization) and enhance the purgation.

Contrary to widespread belief patients with chronic liver disease should not be subjected to dietary protein restriction. In the first instance, patients with stable cirrhosis have a higher protein requirement than normal, i.e. 1.2–1.5 g/kg body weight to remain in positive balance. It is true that some are intolerant of this amount because of the encephalopathy and protein intake has to be individualized. The European Society for Parenteral and Enteral Nutrition recommends a daily protein intake of 1.0–1.5 g/kg depending on the degree of hepatic decompensation. In patients who are intolerant, the amount is reduced to 0.5 g/kg and the remainder of their requirements achieved by administration of branched chain amino acids. In practice, the most effective way of achieving a sufficient protein intake in patients with liver disease is by frequent small meals and a late evening meal. This has been shown to improve nitrogen balance without exacerbating encephalopathy. Lactilol is used in preference to lactulose as it is equally effective and more palatable. Some benefit may be obtained by therapy with L-dopa or bromocriptine. The use of the benzodiazepine antagonist flumazenil is currently being evaluated in clinical trials. Patients with severe encephalopathy after surgical shunts unresponsive to medical treatment are treated by blocking of the shunts using radiological embolization techniques.

Fulminant liver failure

Acute fulminant liver failure is defined as severe encephalopathy occurring within 6 to 8 weeks of the onset of the illness. Essentially, this consists of acute massive hepatocellular damage in a previously normal liver caused by poisoning such as acetaminophen and ecstasy, viral infections (A, B, C), halothane anaesthesia and mushroom poisoning (*Amanita phylloides*). The disease still carries a high mortality despite newer methods of hepatic support and liver transplantation. Patients with acetaminophen hepatotoxicity, hepatitis A and hepatitis B are more likely to recover than patients with non-A, non-B hepatitis or other drug-induced liver failure.

Biochemical evidence of massive liver cell necrosis in these patients includes marked elevations of the transaminases and deepening jaundice. The coma is accompanied by gross cerebral oedema with raised intracranial pressure. There is multi-system involvement with clotting failure, renal impairment, fall in the peripheral resistance, pulmonary insufficiency and an increased susceptibility to serious infections.

The treatment of fulminant liver failure is supportive and carried out within the setting of an intensive care unit. This and the recognition for the need to treat these desperately ill patients in specialized liver units (with transplant facilities) has led to an overall reduction in the mortality. The useful therapeutic measures that have contributed to the improved survival include:

- early ventilatory support for encephalopathy
- prophylactic antibiotics and antifungal agents
- inotropic support
- renal support with haemofiltration/dialysis [Module 12, Vol. I]
- extraction of poisons
- intracranial pressure monitoring and reduction of cerebral oedema by 20% mannitol infused intravenously
- *N*-acetylcysteine infusion.

N-acetylcysteine infusion is now well established in the treatment of liver failure caused by paracetamol and survival in these patients has improved from 40 to 83%. *N*-acetylcysteine infusion is being used selectively to treat other forms of acute liver failure.

Liver transplantation is used in patients who do not respond to supportive therapy. The problem concerns the availability of a suitable donor within the limited time frame available before the patient dies or the condition becomes irretrievable. For this reason newer forms of artificial hepatic support are currently being evaluated. These include the extracorporeal liver assist (using a pig's liver) and the bioartificial liver device that uses isolated hepatocytes.

Fulminant liver failure due to ecstasy

One of the documented drugs that can cause fulminant liver failure is 3,4-methylenedioxymetamphetamine (ecstasy) taken orally as a stimulant during parties and raves. In addition to the usual clinical manifestations of fulminant liver failure, persistent hyperthermia and rhabdomyolysis are specific features that suggest the diagnosis. The disease is very severe and often requires transplantation for survival.

Renal disease and hepatorenal failure

Renal disease is very common in patients with chronic liver disease and may, for a while, be subclinical and detected only by determination of the GFR. As previously described, the kidneys play a crucial role in the development of ascites. Despite obvious impairment, there are often no histological changes on renal biopsy and the condition is then referred to as functional renal failure. This hepatorenal syndrome is seen as a manifestation of end-stage liver disease but may also complicate the post-operative period after variceal surgery. The urine output may not be significantly reduced but, despite this, sodium, potassium and water retention are pronounced and the blood urea and creatinine rise sharply. The serum biochemistry of the condition is also characterized by a profound hyponatraemia. Functional renal failure may also be precipitated by loop diuretics and often complicates infection of the ascitic fluid (primary bacterial peritonitis). Endotoxin may be involved in the pathogenesis. Hepatorenal failure does not usually recover with renal dialysis and the best chance of reversal is improvement of the liver function.

Structural renal failure (tubular necrosis) can occur following hypotension due to variceal haemorrhage. Chronic liver disease associated with HBV disease and hepatitis B surface antigen (HBsAg) antigenaemia is often accompanied by glomerulonephritis due to mesangial IgA deposits. This presents most commonly as the nephrotic syndrome and may respond to corticosteroid therapy [Module 12, Vol. I].

Section 9.8 • Hepatic abscesses

Abscesses of the liver are less common in temperate than in tropical regions. There are also differences in the underlying aetiology between the two regions. There are two types: pyogenic and amoebic.

Pyogenic abscesses

Pathogenesis

The main aetiological factor is bile duct infection with ascending cholangitis commonly due to *Escherichia coli* and anaerobic Gram-negative organisms. The suppurative process may affect both lobes of the liver and be multiple. Other sources of infection include:

- Ascending pylephlebitis. While any inflammatory process within the abdomen may initiate pylephlebitis, it is most commonly the result of complicated diverticulitis.
- Some hepatic abscesses of staphylococcal and streptococcal origin arise as a complication of bacteraemia (haematogenous).
- Direct extension from intra-abdominal suppuration, e.g. gangrenous cholecystitis, penetrating peptic ulcer disease and subphrenic collections.
- Trauma to the liver, both penetrating and non-penetrating, may devitalize liver tissue and subsequent infection produces an abscess.
- A significant group of patients are found in the geriatric population. No obvious cause is found in many of these patients (cryptogenic). These often have an insidious onset and non-specific specific symptoms such that at the time of diagnosis, the abscess is usually very large. In some cases, the chronic abscess erodes through the diaphragm and bursts into the bronchial tree presenting with chest symptoms (Figure 9.14). The infecting organisms for these abscesses are commonly the *Peptostreptococcus* and *Streptococcus milleri* but other microbes including *Bacteroides fragilis* may be involved.
- Parasitic infestations – *Ascaris lumbricoides*
- Tuberculous liver abscesses
- HIV infection – cholangitis/cholangiopathy

There has been a change in the epidemiology and clinical features of pyogenic hepatic abscesses during the past 15 years. The patients tend to be older (mean age 65 years), identification of the source of the infection is more common and the diagnosis is made earlier with modern imaging techniques. In addition HIV infection is now one of the risk factors and abscesses due to methicillin resistant *Staphylococcus aureus* appear to be on the increase. The infection is polymicrobial in

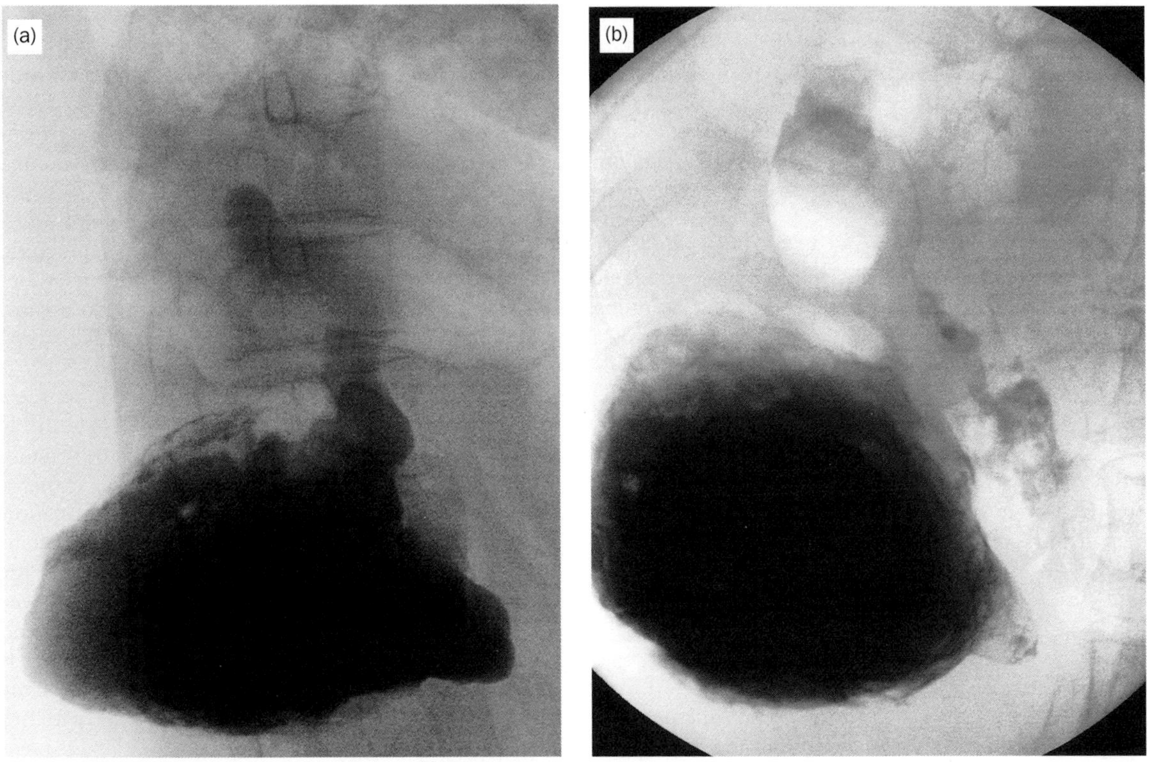

Figure 9.14 Contrast study showing a fistula between the right hepatic abscess and right basal bronchial tree in an elderly patient initially treated with percutaneous drainage.

45%. *Escherichia coli* and *Streptococcus milleri* are the most frequently isolated organisms. In endemic areas of *Ascaris lumbrocoides* infestations, e.g. Kashmir, India, up to 15% of pyogenic hepatic abscesses are associated with this infestation.

Cholangitis/cholangiopathy associated with HIV infection is characterized by chronic abdominal pain, low-grade fever, cholestasis, and sometimes areas of focal or diffuse dilatation of the bile ducts. The disease appears to be the result of immunosuppression and/or secondary opportunistic infections rather than a direct cytopathic effect of the virus itself. Various opportunistic pathogens, including cytomegalovirus, *Cryptosporidium*, *Campylobacter fetus* and *Candida albicans*, have been implicated in the aetiology of HIV-associated cholangitis.

Pylephlebitis usually occurs secondary to infection in the region drained by the portal venous system, the most common being diverticulitis and appendicitis. Infection is caused by *E. coli* in 54%, followed by *Proteus mirabilis* (23%). The pylephlebitis induces a septic thrombosis of the portal vein and its branches, with multiple micro-abscess formation in the liver (honeycomb liver). Early recognition of the disease and timely antibiotic therapy are essential for survival. The overall reported mortality is 32%.

Irrespective of aetiology, liver abscesses are found much more commonly in the right lobe. All abscesses contain areas of liver parenchymal cell necrosis surrounded by polymorphonuclear leucocytes and lymphocyte infiltration with relatively damaged parenchyma and viable bacteria on the periphery. Ultimately a fibrous reaction is initiated which may produce a fibrous capsule containing pus.

Clinical features of hepatic abscesses

Untreated pyogenic liver abscesses carry a high mortality and 10% are diagnosed only at post-mortem. The important determinants of mortality are multiple abscesses, hyperbilirubinaemia and comorbid disease. Since most pyogenic abscesses are secondary to other infective processes, the clinical features may be dominated by the primary disorder. Characteristically there is a high fever, rigors, profuse sweating, anorexia and vomiting, with pain as a relatively late symptom. In the elderly pyogenic liver abscess is commoner in females and the symptoms may be vague. Thus the patients may have minimal abdominal tenderness on physical examination. The clinical features are also less striking in hepatic amoebiasis where the fever is usually low grade. However, pain is a more common feature with amoebic abscess and is aggravated by movement and coughing. An amoebic abscess may reach a very large size before causing pain if situated posteriorly and points to the bare area of the liver. About half the patients with amoebic abscesses will have diarrhoea.

Hepatomegaly is common, particularly with amoebiasis. Occasionally with right lobe abscesses there is bulging and pitting oedema of the intercostal spaces. An abscess in the left lobe may present as a painful epigastric swelling. On investigation, anaemia and leucocytosis may be found, and the erythrocyte sedimentation rate (ESR) is markedly elevated. Disturbances of the liver function tests are not diagnostic, particularly when complicated by cholangitis, and may be absent in amoebiasis.

Blood cultures are usually positive in patients with pyogenic abscesses when taken during the height of pyrexia. Both aerobic and anaerobic cultures are needed. Clinical suspicion of hepatic abscess must be confirmed by ultrasonography or CT scanning (Figure 9.15). The highest diagnostic yield for both pyogenic and amoebic liver abscess is obtained by CT scanning with contrast enhancement. Diagnostic aspiration is a safe and reliable procedure and provides means of identification of the organisms responsible and thus the appropriate antibiotic therapy. Chest radiography is necessary in all cases to outline basal lung changes (consolidation and effusion) and may show direct lung involvement in complicated cases. An elevated immobile diaphragm (radiological screening or ultrasonography) is often encountered, particularly in large abscesses. A plain film of the abdomen may demonstrate gas in the abscess cavity.

Complications

Recurrent bacteraemia is the most common complication of pyogenic abscesses. Extension and rupture of the abscess may occur in any direction. Peritoneal rupture results in widespread peritonitis or in the formation of a subphrenic collection. Extension through the diaphragm may lead to thoracic empyema or to a rupture into the bronchus with expectoration of large volumes of 'anchovy paste' pus from amoebic abscesses and bile-stained pus from cholangitic abscesses. Rarely, the abscess ruptures into the pericardium with high mortality.

Treatment

The initial management of a hepatic abscess is usually non-surgical with administration of antibiotics according to bacterial sensitivity. Precise microbiological identification may result from blood cultures or from aspiration of the abscess cavity under ultrasound control. In the event of a failure to isolate organisms, the choice of antibiotic should be based on the most likely aetiological factor, i.e. cholangitic and pylephlebitic abscesses are usually infected with *E. coli* and anaerobes and may be appropriately treated with cephalosporins, gentamicin and metronidazole. Microaerophilic streptococcus infections are sensitive to penicillin.

Closed percutaneous transhepatic abscess drainage (PTAD) performed under ultrasound or CT control is as effective as open surgical drainage if the pyogenic abscess is single and unilocular. Percutaneous catheter drainage is monitored by serial ultrasound examination to assess degree of resolution. The reported success rate of PTAD averages 85%. The success rate for PTAD for patients with multiple or multilocular abscesses is lower although good results have been reported from some centres in these groups. Thus in some centres, PTAD is used as the primary treatment for liver abscesses irrespective of the number of abscesses and the patient's condition.

As the most frequent cause of hepatic abscess is biliary disease, flexible endoscopic treatment of these hepatic abscesses is practised in some centres. This includes sphincerotomy and insertion of a nasobiliary catheter for continuous antibiotic lavage for 8 to 10 days.

The factors indicating failure of initial non-operative management including PTAD and endoscopic treatment are:

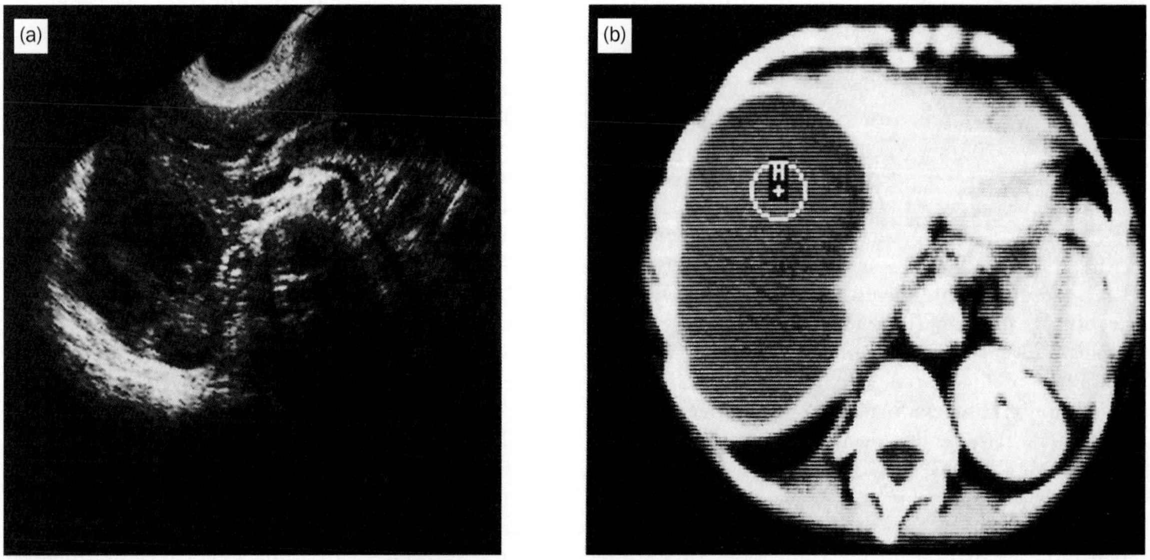

Figure 9.15 (a) An ultrasound of the liver on coronal section shows a cavity within the liver substance. (b) CT scan demonstrates that the abscess cavity occupies most of the right lobe of the liver. Subsequent drainage of the cavity resulted in complete resolution.

- unresolving jaundice
- renal impairment secondary to clinical deterioration
- multiloculation of the abscess
- rupture on presentation
- biliary communication (Figure 9.16).

Deterioration in the general condition of the patient, repeated episodes of septicaemia or a failure of the abscess to decrease in size are indications for open surgical drainage. Posteriorly placed abscesses may be approached by the retroperitoneal route through the bed of the twelfth rib. Larger abscesses require abdominal drainage with wide-bore sump drains and special care being taken to avoid contamination of the peritoneal cavity. Where a pyogenic abscess is secondary to cholangitis, concomitant drainage of the common bile duct with a T-tube and removal of ductal stones may be necessary.

Hepatic amoebiasis

This results from intestinal amoebiasis. The infection spreads to the liver via the portal vein from an ulcer in the bowel wall. Most amoebae lodge in the interlobular veins and degenerate. Some act by cytolysis to invade the portal tracts and lead to cell necrosis and a coalescence of infected triads to form a larger abscess cavity. Hepatic abscess is the most common extra-intestinal manifestation of *Entamoeba histolytica*. There is a male preponderance and the mean age is 40 years. The presenting features include fever (77%), right upper quadrant abdominal pain (72%), cough (16%), chest pain (19%) and chest radiographic abnormalities (57%). The liver function tests are often normal. The diagnosis is usually made by ultrasonography followed by confirmatory serum antibody titre. Early abscesses are solid but pus appears later, characteristically resembling anchovy paste, though in one-third of patients the pus has the usual creamy appearance. Occasionally, amoebic abscesses become secondarily infected with pyogenic bacteria.

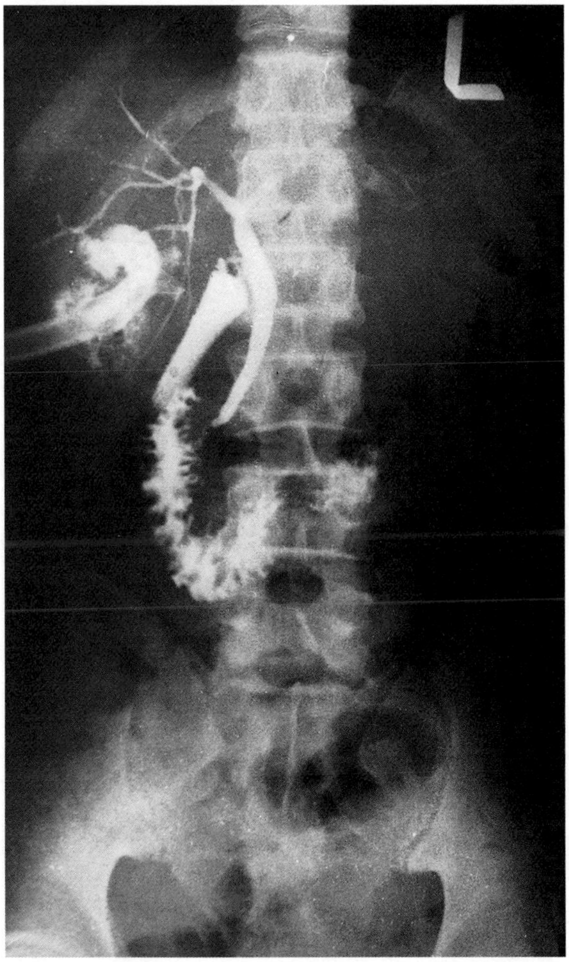

Figure 9.16 Right hepatic abscess communicating with the intrahepatic biliary tree.

In one large series from the USA, patients were divided into groups based on the presumed manner in which they had acquired amoebic liver abscess (ALA): (a) those born or raised in the USA, with a history of travel to an endemic area (Tr-ALA); (b) those from an endemic area, but living in the USA for less than 1 year (En-ALA); and (c) those neither from nor having travelled to an endemic area (N-ALA). In this series, there was a distinctive clinical pattern in patients from different epidemiological groups. Thus patients with Tr-ALA were a decade older than those from endemic areas and were more likely to be male, and to have an insidious onset. In addition patients in the Tr-ALA group were more likely to have hepatomegaly and large abscesses. Thirty per cent of patients had no associated travel history or endemic origin as risk factors (N-ALA). The majority of these had severe immunosuppression, such as infection with HIV, malnutrition or chronic infection.

The diagnosis of amoebic hepatic abscess requires confirmation by positive serological tests, demonstration of amoebic trophozoites in abscess fluid and a rapid response to anti-amoebicides. Amoebic abscesses tend to occur in younger patients than in those with pyogenic liver abscess. In addition, they are much more likely to have abdominal pain and present with a history of symptoms of shorter duration. Both types, however, have the same high incidence of right lower lung abnormalities (50%). Amoebic abscesses are treated with metronidazole with or without chloroquin. Metronidazole therapy is invariably successful and has lowered the mortality of amoebic abscess which is now negligible although recurrence after treatment can occur, albeit rarely. Aspiration of the amoebic abscess is not required routinely and is usually reserved for patients when there is no response within 2 days. Rupture of an amoebic abscess into the lung and bronchus can usually be treated successfully by antibiotics and postural drainage. When the intrapulmonary rupture is associated with cholangitis, bile duct drainage is essential. A persistent bronchopleural fistula may require formal thoracotomy, decortication of the lung and diaphragm with resection of severely damaged pulmonary tissue and diaphragmatic repair. Rupture into the pericardium requires early aspiration of the exudate and occasionally transpleural drainage [Module 5, Vol. I].

Subphrenic extrahepatic abscess

The distribution of intra-abdominal abscesses is directly related to the precipitating lesion and to the potential peritoneal spaces. Abscesses are most common in the right and left lower quadrants as a consequence of appendicitis, diverticulitis and pelvic sepsis. Abscesses around the liver comprise the next most common group of intra-abdominal septic collections. Six spaces around the liver are described. Superiorly, the falciform ligament divides the left and right subphrenic spaces, the latter being divided into anterior and posterior spaces by the triangular ligament. In the infrahepatic region, there are also three spaces – the two on the left side including the lesser sac of the peritoneal cavity and the space immediately below the lateral lobe of the left hepatic lobe (Figure 9.17).

Subphrenic collections may contain a mixture of pus and gastrointestinal secretions and may be large. While any intra-abdominal sepsis may precipitate these collections, most abscesses follow operative intervention with post-operative leaks, spontaneous perforation of hollow organs or accidental abdominal trauma. In the latter situation, extrahepatic collections of blood or serous fluid become encysted and infected (Figure 9.18). Primary causes include pancreatitis, cholecystitis, perforated peptic ulcer, perforated diverticular disease and perforated acute appendicitis.

Clinically, suspicion of an extrahepatic collection is aroused by fever with occasional episodes of septicaemia. Non-specific abdominal symptoms and general ill-health are common, though in some patients attention is drawn to respiratory symptoms resulting from inflammatory changes induced in the lung by a subdiaphragmatic collection. When an abscess is subhepatic, tenderness is elicited and a mass may be palpated or percussed.

The confirmation of an abscess may be difficult and probably many minor collections ultimately resolve and remain unproven. In right posterior subphrenic space collections there is typically elevation of diaphragm on chest radiography with decreased mobility of the diaphragm on screening (Figure 9.19). Inflammation of the diaphragm leads to pneumonic changes in the overlying lung and a pleural effusion. However, diagnosis and location of subphrenic abscesses is nowadays made by ultrasound and CT scanning.

Management

Minor collections may resolve with antibiotics and the frequency of dense adhesions between the liver and diaphragm at elective second laparotomies suggests this is a relatively common event. However, once pus is identified in the subphrenic region, drainage of the abscess is mandatory. With accurate localization using ultrasound or CT scanning, many collections can be aspirated and a catheter left in place. In most instances percutaneous drainage suffices but some require open

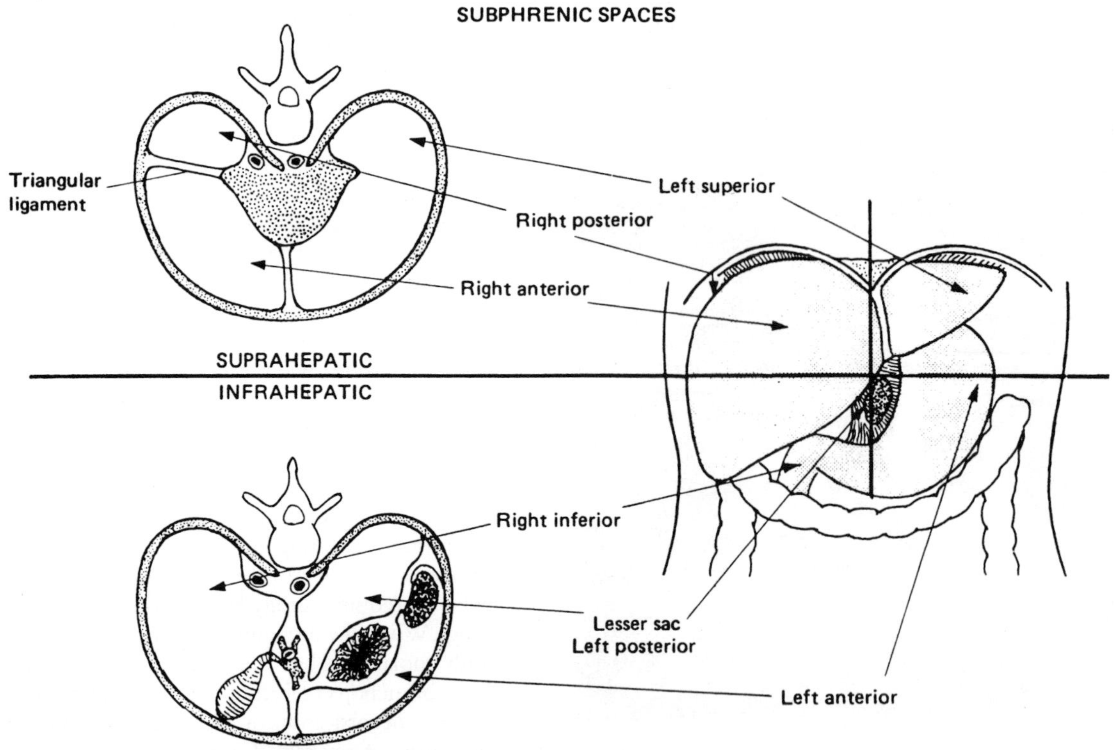

Figure 9.17 The subphrenic spaces may be considered to be supra- and infrahepatic.

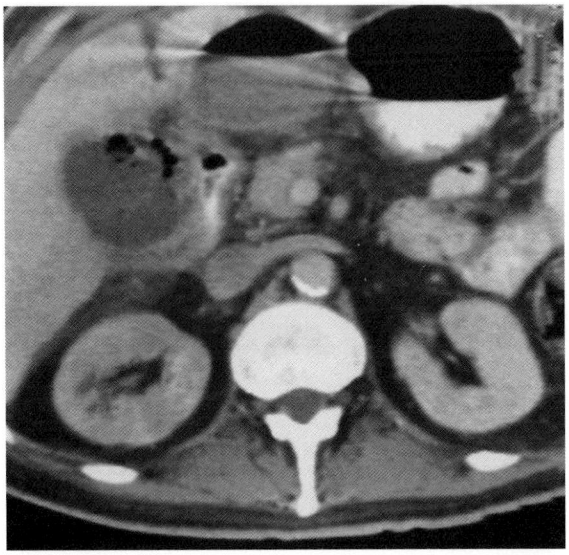

Figure 9.18 CT scan of an infrahepatic abscess with fluid level lying between the gallbladder and gastric antrum. The abscess resulted from the infected gallbladder which contains stones seen on other sections of the CT examination.

surgical drainage. These include multilocular collections, and the presence of thick pus with necrotic slough. Most subhepatic abscesses may be drained surgically by an anterior approach, as may the right anterior subphrenic collection. Occasionally it is possible to enter the abscess without contamination of the peritoneal cavity. Posterior subphrenic collections are most appropriately drained by the classic extraserous approach through the bed of the twelfth rib. In either approach, the abscess cavity is thoroughly explored and all loculi are broken down. Wide calibre drains are inserted to the furthermost point of the cavity. Gradual withdrawal of the drains is indicated, with daily saline irrigation. Repeated sinograms will show loculation beyond the tip of the drain. Culture of the infected fluid is taken at the time of drainage. Further cultures (from drain effluent) are often needed especially if resolution is delayed.

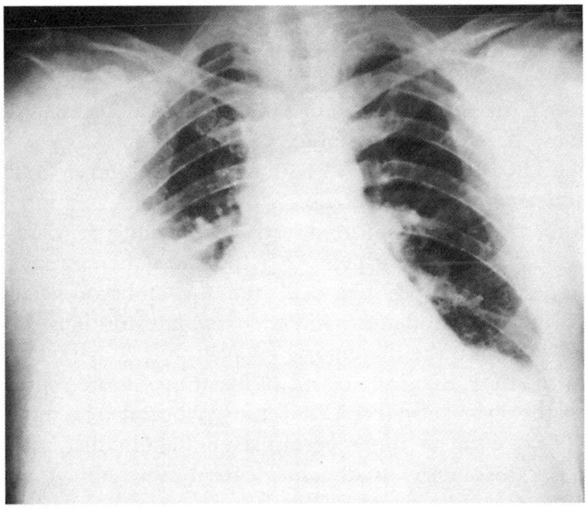

Figure 9.19 Following cholecystectomy the patient developed a high swinging fever, together with signs at the right base and tenderness in the right hypochondrium. A chest radiograph taken at the time shows evidence of a marked pleural effusion on the right side with an underlying subphrenic collection. Drainage of the subphrenic collection led to subsequent resolution of the pleural effusion.

Abscesses occurring as a complication of surgical operations are largely preventable. Prior to abdominal closure, a saline lavage of the peritoneal cavity with special attention to the subphrenic spaces and pelvis will reduce the incidence of post-operative abscesses to a minimum.

Section 9.9 • Liver cysts

These include simple hepatic cysts, choledochal cysts, cystadenoma of the liver, Caroli's disease and parasitic cysts. Choledochal cysts are covered elsewhere [Module on Disorders of the biliary tract, Vol. II]

Non-parasitic hepatic cysts

Within the non-parasitic group there are a variety of clinical conditions that reflect underlying developmental defects of the liver parenchyma or bile ducts. Some cystic lesions follow trauma in which a central rupture has resulted in a collection of bile and serum and these cysts have no epithelial lining. Others are clearly similar to dermoid cysts found in other sites. Most of the remainder are lined by cuboidal or columnar epithelium, contain serous fluid and do not communicate with the biliary tract. These are nowadays referred to as simple cysts and are multiple in 50% of cases. The cysts can grow to a large size and in so doing cause pressure atrophy of the surround hepatic parenchyma. They are generally regarded as developmental abnormalities from aberrant bile ducts. The ultrasound incidence of asymptomatic cysts is 1%, but symptomatic cysts are much rarer. Symptomatic cysts are much commoner in females (9:1) and huge cysts are almost exclusively found in women above the age of 50 years (Figure 9.20).

The ciliated hepatic foregut cyst (CHFC) is a rare small to medium size solitary cystic lesion of the liver that is commoner in males (as distinct from the solitary hepatic cysts) and occurs over a wide age range (35–75 years). CHFC is most commonly located in the medial segment of the left hepatic lobe as distinct from the more common solitary hepatic cysts. CHFC is usually found incidentally on radiological imaging or during surgical exploration, although some may present with abdominal pain, and in a collective review of 52 cases, one patient presented with portal vein compression. Histologically, the lining of the columnar epithelium is composed of ciliated cells, mucin secreting goblet cells and endocrine cells positive for chromogranin, synaptophysin, bombesin and calcitonin (similar to respiratory epithelium). The lesion is thought to be a developmental ventral foregut abnormality arising from a bronchiolar bud of the tracheobronchial diverticulum.

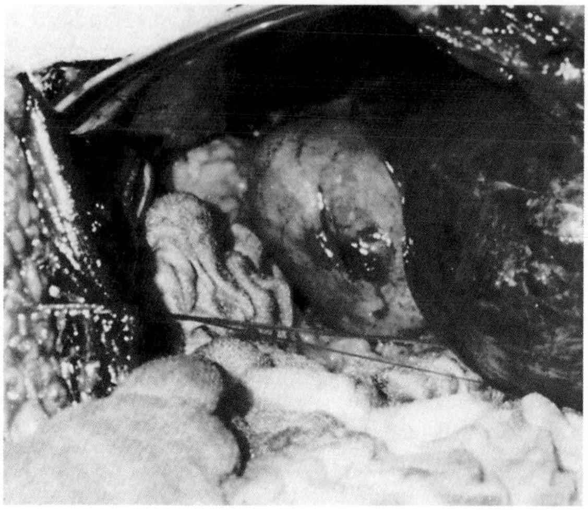

Figure 9.20 This operative photograph shows the undersurface of the liver in which the gallbladder is seen as a whiter structure and lies adjacent to a large lymphogenous cyst of the liver.

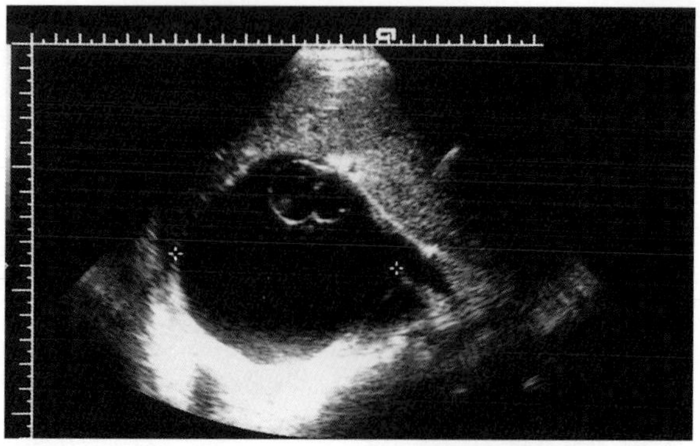

Figure 9.21 Ultrasound scan of hepatic cystadenoma. The lesion recurred three times following de-roofing and needed a right hepatectomy.

Clinical features and treatment

Most simple hepatic cysts are asymptomatic and only become apparent when the cysts reach sufficient size to exert pressure on adjacent viscera, producing non-specific symptoms of vomiting, upper abdominal pain and occasionally diarrhoea. Clinical examination reveals a non-tender smooth mass in the liver. Jaundice is very unusual and liver function tests are usually normal. Plain film of the abdomen may show displacement of the colon or stomach but the diagnosis is best confirmed by ultrasonography. Other investigations including CT are not usually necessary. Complications are uncommon and include intracystic bleeding that causes sudden severe pain and increase in size, fistulation with the intrahepatic biliary tract or duodenum, bacterial infection, compression of the bile duct with obstructive jaundice and compression of the vena cava or portal vein. Differentiation is from parasitic cysts and from adult polycystic disease of the kidney where multiple serous hepatic cysts are often present and may indeed replace a substantial part of the hepatic parenchyma.

Only symptomatic cysts require treatment. This consists of fenestration (deroofing) which is nowadays carried out laparoscopically. Percutaneous aspiration of large cysts with introduction of sclerosing agents is followed by a high recurrence rate. In patients with adult polycystic disease of the kidney and liver cysts causing discomfort, multiple fenestration or hepatic resection is followed by improvement but recurrence is inevitable although symptomatic improvement may last for up to 2 years.

Hepatic cystadenoma

This is rare and affects predominantly females. It forms a large multiloculated cyst filled with mucinous fluid and lined by cuboidal epithelium on a basement membrane and thick compact cellular stroma containing foamy macrophages. In places the lining epithelium forms polypoid projections. Although benign, the lesion is liable to complications, notably cholestasis due to compression of the bile duct, intracystic bleeding, infection, rupture and malignant degeneration to cystadenocarcinoma. Hepatic cystadenoma must be excised completely even when asymptomatic. Fenestration/partial resection is inevitably followed by recurrence and increases the risk of cystadenocarcinoma (Figure 9.21).

Caroli's syndrome

This is not a single entity and covers a spectrum of disorders characterized by congenital multifocal dilatations of the segmental bile ducts. In 50% of cases Caroli's syndrome is associated with congenital hepatic fibrosis, itself an inherited malformation (autosomal recessive). The clinical picture of Caroli's syndrome is dominated by recurrent episodes of bacterial cholangitis [Disorders of the biliary tract, Vol. II].

Hydatid cysts of the liver

This infestation is endemic in certain countries, particularly the southern half of South America, Australasia, New Zealand, France and certain areas of the USA and the UK [Module 5, Vol. I]. Man is a secondary host and becomes infected by ingesting vegetables and water fouled by dogs or more directly by handling the parasite-infested dogs as pets. After ingestion, the egg shell is destroyed by gastric acid and the embryos hatch within the duodenum and then migrate through the gut wall into the mesenteric circulation to lodge within the liver. Eighty per cent of hydatid cysts are found in the liver substance. The embryo becomes a small vesicle with an inner germinal epithelium that produces secondary or daughter brood cysts containing scolices and hooklets. Some cysts never produce brood capsules or become sterilized by secondary infection or calcification. Hydatid cysts caused by *Echinococcus granulosus* are unilocular as distinct from the multilocular alveolar type due to *Echinococcus multilocularis*. This forms a spongy collection of cysts and carries a poor prognosis.

Clinical features

Since the growth of the parasite is slow, many years elapse before the cyst reaches significant size (Figure 9.22). Palpable cysts are therefore rare in children. At all ages, pain, jaundice and ascites are uncommon and, in most patients, general health is good. On physical examination an anteriorly located cyst presents as a smooth rounded tense mass. Secondary infection results in tender hepatomegaly, rigors and pyrexia associated with a deep-seated continuous pain. Further clinical features are the result of cyst complications. Intrabiliary rupture may give biliary colic and usually causes jaundice and fever. Intraperitoneal rupture produces severe pain and shock classically associated with pruritus and urticaria. Some of the implanted brood cysts induce a profound fibrous reaction that sterilizes the infection but other cysts reappear in various parts of the peritoneal cavity years later. Intrathoracic rupture may be preceded by symptoms of diaphragmatic irritation, and rupture into bronchus leads to a partly blood-stained sputum which frequently becomes bile-stained. Hydatid allergy is manifested by urticaria or, very rarely, anaphylactic shock.

Investigations

An unruptured cyst may show on plain radiograph as a calcified reticulated shadow or by displacement of the diaphragm and stomach if not calcified. Following intrabiliary rupture, gas may enter the cyst leading to partial collapse of the cyst wall (Camellotte sign). Ultrasonography reveals an echogenic cyst.

Although the cyst is isolated from the liver by an adventitial layer, there is an absorption of parasitic products which acts as an antigenic stimulus. This is reflected in an eosinophilia in 25% of patients, a complement fixation test which is accurate in 93% of patients. The Casoni test has been largely abandoned. Some cysts never leak and tests are never positive in these patients.

Treatment

The treatment of hydatid cysts of the liver is surgical or radiological. There is no guaranteed response to drug treatment with mebendazole/albendazole and the cyst is a potential source for serious complications. Surgical treatment involves removing the cyst without contaminating the patient. Where there are multiple cysts, several procedures may be necessary. Large cysts found on the antero-inferior and postero-inferior aspects of the liver are approached abdominally. Cysts in the dome may be reached by the posterior extraserous approach or transpleurally through the bed of the ninth rib.

The initial stage involves protection of the operative field against live cysts using multiple coloured towels soaked in hypertonic saline which isolate the main cyst from the exposed serous cavity. Since hydatid fluid is under high pressure, the cyst is decompressed by aspiration as completely as possible, though daughter cysts tend to block the needle frequently. The main cyst is injected through the same needle with 20% hypertonic saline and left for 5 min, after which the main cyst is opened and all daughter cysts are removed. In large cysts it is not feasible to remove the cyst wall and the cavity is drained for a few days and partially occluded by an omental plug which is sutured to the rim of the cyst.

Marsupialization of large cysts may be indicated when secondary infection has occurred but prolonged purulent drainage results and a secondary omentoplasty may be necessary. Cysts with extensive calcification are usually sterile and best left alone. Jaundice after intrabiliary rupture requires choledochotomy and

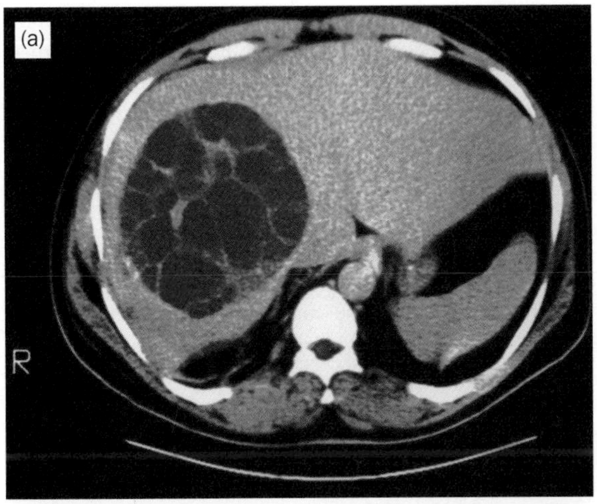

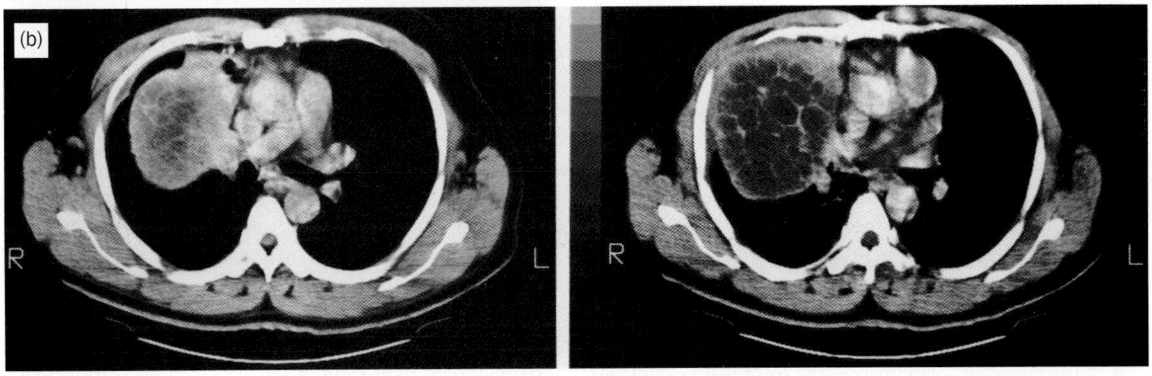

Figure 9.22 CT scan showing multi-septate hydatid cyst (a) in the right lobe and (b) projecting above the right liver surface in the subphrenic space.

clearance of cysts followed by T-tube drainage. Peritoneal rupture is managed by laparotomy and careful toilet followed by lavage. Providing that rupture has not occurred and careful surgical techniques are applied, the prognosis is excellent.

There have been good reported results of percutaneous ultrasound-guided treatment of hepatic hydatid cysts. The treatment involves puncture, aspiration, injection (of scolicidal agents), and re-aspiration (PAIR). In patients with cysts larger than 6 cm in diameter, PAIR is followed by percutaneous drainage (PAIR-PD). In one recent large reported series no recurrence of hydatid disease after PAIR or PAIR-PD was observed during a follow-up period of 72 months (mean, 26 ± 27 months).

Medical treatment with mebendazole and albendazole is unreliable as penetration of the drug into the cysts cavity is uncertain. Thus although many cysts decrease in size, not all scolices are killed. Nowadays medical treatment with these drugs is started before surgery or radiological intervention (PAIR).

Section 9.10 • Liver tumours

Benign solid tumours

Benign tumours of the liver are commonly asymptomatic and discovered accidentally during investigation usually by ultrasound, and during laparotomy for other conditions. More rarely, they reach sufficient size as to cause symptoms or complications that can be quite dramatic. Though the classification of these tumours is not sharply defined several types are identified:

- haemangioma
- infantile haemangioendothelioma
- neoplastic angioendotheliomatosis
- hamartoma
- focal nodular hyperplasia
- adenoma
- cholangioma
- biliary cystadenoma.

Haemangiomas

Haemangiomas are the commonest benign tumour of the liver most commonly found in adults between the ages of 30 and 70 years, but only rarely produce symptoms. They are frequently situated just beneath the liver capsule and are normally of the cavernous type. Histologically the lesion is composed of blood-filled endothelial lined spaces separated by a variable degree of fibrous tissue and inflammatory changes, both of which result from episodes of spontaneous thrombosis.

Infantile haemangioendothelioma is the most common mesenchymal tumour in this age group and the majority present in the first few months of life. The lesion may be solitary or multicentric and often extends over a wide area. Histologically it consists of numerous arteriovenous channels, endothelial lined vascular lakes in a fibrous stroma containing bile ducts. The tumour is locally aggressive and presents with hepatomegaly, coagulopathy (due to thrombosis in the tumour), extramedullary haemopoiesis, cardiac failure(commonest presentation), bleeding and liver failure. Most deaths are due to cardiac failure. A related but histologically different condition is *neoplastic angioendotheliomatosis*. Although essentially benign these diffuse subcapsular haemorrhagic lesions in children have a variable course. They may mature to a cavernous haemangioma or regress spontaneously but rarely they may undergo sarcomatous change. In children the condition may present as high output cardiac failure and is often associated with cutaneous haemangiomas (85%). Other complications are attributed to recurrent thrombotic episodes in the tumour. These include microangiopathic anaemia, thrombocytopenia and hypofibrinogenaemia.

In adults, some of these cavernous haemangiomas, having grown to significant size (> 4.0 cm), will eventually produce pain or dyspepsia and may develop a palpable abdominal mass. A bruit is heard in about 15% of patients. The pain is usually dull but acute posterior pleuritic pain lasting a few weeks may develop and has been attributed to episodes of intratumoral thrombosis and inflammation. In general symptomatic cavernous haemangiomas are more common in females and have been documented to enlarge during pregnancy. Intratumoral thrombosis may be precipitated by oral contraception.

Rupture of cavernous haemangioma is rare. The reported incidence of this complication varies from 0 to 10%. Nonetheless, it is a serious complication in view of the major intra-abdominal haemorrhage with shock and collapse. Cavernous haemangiomas have characteristic appearances on the various imaging modalities:

- hyperechoic lesion on ultrasound
- hypodense on CT without contrast, halo edge enhancement on high-dose contrast helical CT which then fills the centre of the lesion
- dark on T1 and intensely white on T2-weighted MRI images.

The need for arterioportography (Figure 9.23) seldom arises nowadays. A biopsy is not indicated.

The majority of these tumours do not require any treatment except for follow-up liver ultrasound examination. The preferred treatment for clinically significant/symptomatic haemangiomas is segmental/wedge excision where possible, with lobectomy being reserved for large/muliple lesions confined to one lobe. In such cases the residual liver may contain further haemangiomas. Supervoltage radiotherapy is used for symptomatic lesions in adults who are unfit for surgery.

Children presenting in the first year of life have a poorer prognosis. Hepatic angiography in this age group may demonstrate a major feeding vessel from the hepatic artery, when ligation of this vessel or the main hepatic artery may reduce the blood flow through the lesion. With more diffuse lesions, radiotherapy and steroids result in significant shrinkage and a reduction

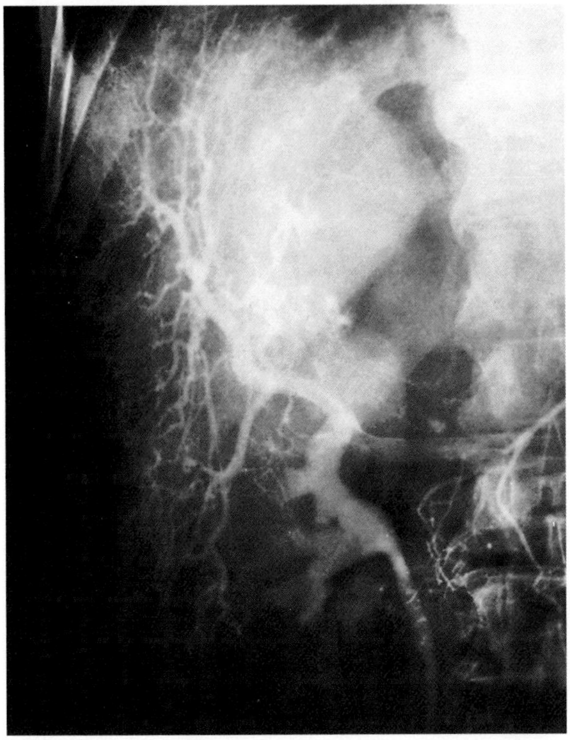

Figure 9.23 This selective arteriogram shows an apparent tumour circulation arising from the left hepatic artery. Subsequent resection of a tumour in the left lobe showed this to be a benign cavernous haemangioma.

in the volume of arteriovenous shunting. It is nowadays the preferred management in this age group. After the first year, the angioendotheliomatosis may regress, as do the cutaneous lesions. Resection of vascular tumours is no longer advocated in children but liver transplantation is the correct treatment for infantile haemangioendothelioma that fails to respond to radiotherapy.

Mesenchymal hamartomas

Hamartomas are tumour-like malformations of congenital origin and consist of normal tissues in a disorderly arrangement. The lesions vary from minute nodules to large solid tumours and may be single or multiple. The tumours are not encapsulated, the fibrous periphery is a pseudocapsule of compressed parenchyma (Figure 9.24) and the histological picture demonstrates irregular distorted hepatic plates, vascular channels, bile ducts, cysts and extensive fibrosis. Children are commonly affected and present with an expanding abdomen and a large palpable mass. Large tumours may displace the stomach and produce vomiting and elevate the diaphragm compressing the right lung. As the tumour expands, inferior vena caval compression occurs.

Mature hepatic teratomas have been reported. All have mesodermal, endodermal and ectodermal components (tridermal). They may be associated with chromosomal abnormalities, e.g. trisomy 13.

Hamartomas show as filling defects in angioCT or scintiscans as they are relatively avascular tumours. Large tumours should be removed, usually by formal lobectomy. Occasionally, large tumours may show evidence of sarcomatous change and have a poor prognosis. Benign lesions have an excellent prognosis and where small and multiple should be kept under observation.

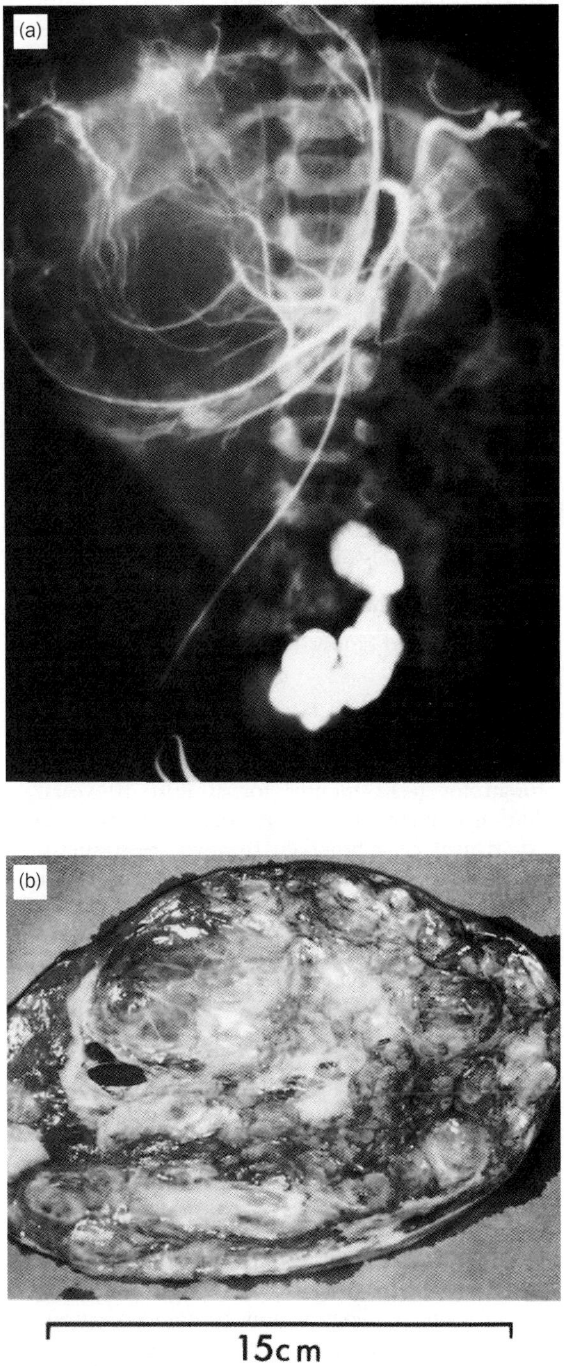

Figure 9.24 (a) A 3-year-old child presented with an expanding liver tumour. Selective arteriogram showed the hepatic vessels to be stretched around the tumour and there is little evidence of tumour circulation. (b) The excised lesion proved to have a distinct capsule and to be multilocular. Histology showed this to be a hamartoma of the liver.

Liver cell adenomas

Adenomas are variable in size (4–30 cm). They are rare and occur in children, postmenopausal women or males. There is an established increased incidence related to use of the contraceptive pill. The risk rises after 4 years of pill usage, particularly in women over 30 years on pills of high oestrogen content. Liver cell adenoma can also occur in patients with type I glycogen storage disease and galactosaemia. Up to 30% of adenomas are multiple.

Macroscopically liver cell adenoma forms a pale soft smooth lesion without a fibrous capsule. Histologically the tumour consists of sheets of hepatocytes containing glycogen, venous lakes and necrotic ghosts cells. The differentiation between liver cell adenoma and well-differentiated hepatocellular (lamellar) carcinoma may be difficult and the two may co-exist. Furthermore hepatocellular carcinoma may develop in patients with biopsy confirmed liver cell adenoma.

The symptoms of liver cell adenoma include upper abdominal pain and mass. The lesion carries an ever-present risk of rupture and haemorrhage, a complication that occurs in 30% of cases (Figure 9.25). A specific diagnosis of liver cell adenoma cannot be made by CT, ultrasound or MRI. Although they have a distinctive arteriographic appearance (enlarged tortuous vessels, peripheral and central feeding), this is also encountered in hepatocellular carcinoma. Nowadays diagnosis is established by ultrasound or laparoscopically guided biopsy.

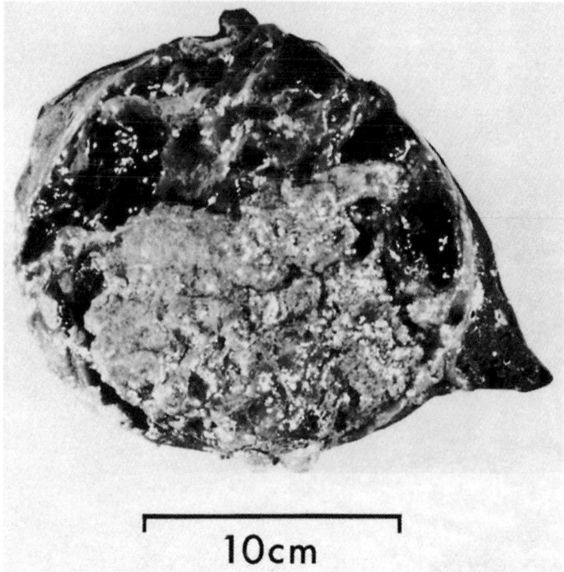

Figure 9.25 This operative specimen of the right lobe of the liver has been cut to show the necrotic contents of a hepatic adenoma into which a major haemorrhage has occurred. The patient presented with severe upper abdominal pain and evidence of massive blood loss.

Treatment

If the diagnosis is certain and the lesion is asymptomatic, it may be monitored by ultrasound and α-fetoprotein for 6–12 months for at least 10 years. In addition, oral contraception is stopped and in this context, it may be appropriate to advocate sterilization. Adenomas that diminish in size should be managed expectantly whereas those that do not regress on follow-up should be excised. If the patient becomes pregnant, the risk of rupture is greater.

Ruptured and bleeding tumours are excised as emergency procedures and since many of these tumours are near the surface, local excision with a thin rim of parenchyma is sufficient, although whenever possible the resection should be anatomical. Intracapsular haemorrhage may produce an extremely large tumour necessitating formal lobectomy.

Focal nodular hyperplasia

Focal nodular hyperplasia (FNH) (Figure 9.26) is nowadays regarded as a separate entity from liver cell adenoma on aetiological and pathological grounds. FNH is best considered as a response to parenchymal injury or to an anomalous arterial supply to a local area of liver tissue. The lesion is usually small and may be multiple (20%), although large lesions presenting as an abdominal mass may occur especially in pregnant females and in children of both sexes. There is no aetiological association with oral contraception and the incidence of FNH has not increased since the introduction of the contraceptive pill. Macroscopically FNH consists of a firm mass, the cut surface of which reveals a central scar with radiating fibrous septa. The microscopic findings are akin to cirrhosis with regenerating nodules and fibrosis. The vast majority of FNH cases are discovered accidentally during surgery or investigation. FNH is not pre-malignant and the natural history is such that it may be observed without serious risk.

Adenomatous hyperplasia

This ill-defined pathological entity refers to sizeable nodules that develop in chronic liver disease. In cirrho-

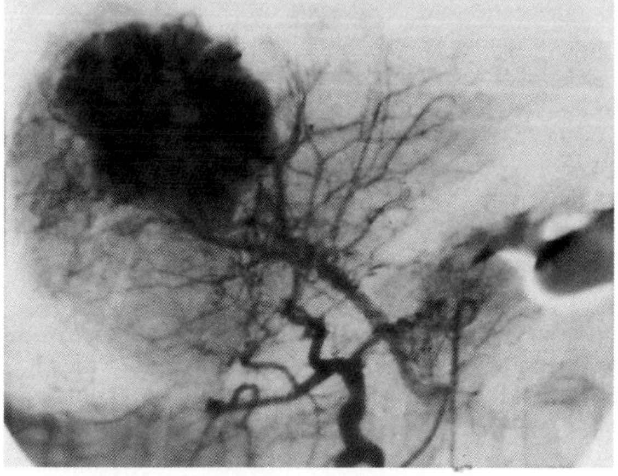

Figure 9.26 Hepatic arteriogram demonstrating the marked nodular appearance of focal nodular hyperplasia seen during both arterial and venous phases of the study.

sis, adenomatous hyperplasia forms part of the spectrum of morbid pathological change which includes small benign regenerative nodules, large size regenerative nodules (adenomatous hyperplasia), atypical adenomatous hyperplasia (dysplastic borderline lesions, considered as low-grade hepatocellular carcinomas by some pathologists) and frank hepatocellular carcinoma. There is some debate as to the malignant potential of adenomatous hyperplasia as some reports have indicated that cancer can develop from the intervening hepatic parenchyma, whereas others consider the transition from regenerative nodules to adenomatous hyperplasia, dysplasia and carcinoma to be the norm.

Cholangioma (Von Meyenburg complexes)

These are derived from bile duct epithelium and form small greyish white nodules consisting of mature bile ducts and fibrous tissue with a cystic component. The condition is entirely asymptomatic and requires no treatment. Most are diagnosed on biopsy for nodules found accidentally during surgery. Von-Meyenburg complexes (VMCs) do carry a small risk of malignant transformation (only 11 cases of neoplastic transformation of VMCs have been reported). The malignant tumour that may develop from VMCs is cholangiocarcinoma usually in patients over 60 years of age.

Primary malignant tumours of the liver

The primary malignant tumours of the liver are dominated by hepatocellular carcinoma (HCC). By comparison, other primary tumours are rare or very rare. They include hepatic cholangiocarcinoma, angiosarcoma and epitheloid haemangioendothelioma.

Hepatocellular carcinoma, hepatoma

Primary HCC is the commonest malignant tumour world-wide and its geographical distribution parallels closely the incidence of hepatitis B and C viral infection. Although the highest prevalence is encountered in the Far East and sub-Saharan Africa, it is also common in selected populations within the USA and Europe. The disease usually develops on a background of cirrhosis (cirrhomimetic) but can originate in normal or non-cirrhotic hepatic parenchyma (non-cirrhomimetic). In the South African black population, where the incidence is high (HCC accounts for 80% of all cancers in the Bantu), 37% of primary hepatic carcinoma occurs in patients without cirrhosis. This is a much higher incidence of non-cirrhomimetic disease than anywhere else in the world, including Japan (11%). In general, there are no marked differences between patients with and without cirrhosis in the symptomology, size of tumours at presentation, serum markers and the HBV status, although a lower incidence of HBsAg is reported in some countries in non-cirrhomimetic cases. It is important to stress that a significant cohort of non-cirrhotic patients have histological evidence in the portal tracts of ongoing chronic liver disease.

The disease is more common in males and, although slow-growing, it is associated with a poor prognosis and a frequently fatal outcome with a median survival of 4 months in patients with symptomatic disease. The outcome is not influenced by racial origin or the presence of chronic liver disease and is largely determined by the stage of the disease.

Aetiological factors

The exact pathogenesis remains unknown but the development of the disease seems to occur in stages with initiation by a genotoxic event followed by transformation due to the action of co-carcinogens. There is no evidence for a genetic predisposition and the high incidence in certain ethnic groups and regions is explained by the correspondingly high prevalence of chronic viral liver disease in these populations.

There is undoubtedly an association between the development of HCC and the presence of chronic (necro-inflammatory) liver disease with or without a background of HBV/HCV disease. One hypothesis, suggested by Dunsford *et al.*, is that irrespective of the aetiology, chronic liver cell injury induces a series of events (cell death, regeneration, cellular metabolic dysfunction and release of inflammatory mediators) which collectively increase the risk of transforming mutations. Chronic liver disorders which are particularly prone to the development of HCC are haemochromatosis, alcoholic liver disease and hereditary tyrosinaemia.

The importance of HBV infection in the development of HCC is undoubted. The risk is increased 94-fold in HBsAg-positive males. In the Far East, 90% of patients who develop HCC are HBsAg positive, although the corresponding figure in the West is substantially lower (10–30%). It is now known that the hepatitis B viral DNA and RNA are present in tissue extracts of the tumour and the viral DNA is commonly integrated in the host genome. However, since the non-neoplastic parenchyma adjacent to the tumour also contains viral DNA, integration alone does not account for the carcinogenesis and the molecular mechanisms by which the hepatitis B viral DNA induces mutation remain obscure. It has been suggested that subsequent to integration, promoting co-factors are important and these include specific carcinogens and the known risk factors, i.e. male sex, alcohol, iron overload and cigarette smoking. Again the molecular mechanisms involved in the action of these co-factors are not known. The other hypothesis concerning the development of HCC in HBV disease implicates the insertion of the viral DNA close to a cellular proto-oncogene, which is then stimulated to produce cellular transformation. Alternatively, the integration of the viral DNA is followed by chromosomal rearrangement leading to carcinogenesis.

Since the identification of hepatitis C, there have been several reports, particularly from southern Europe (Italy and Spain) and the USA that have shown a significantly high incidence of antibodies to HCV in patients with hepatocellular carcinoma. The mechanism is obscure since HCV is not a retrovirus. It is assumed that its oncogenic action is the result of a chronic necro-inflammatory state along the Dunsford hypothesis. Many, but not all these patients, have had alcoholic or HBsAg chronic liver disease. It is now generally accepted that hepatitis C disease predisposes to the development of HCC.

Co-infection with HBV and HCV is not uncommon and results in more severe liver disease and with a significant increased risk for the development of HCC. In one recent study from Japan, 59% of patients with HCV disease and who developed HCC had evidence of past HBV infection and were anti-HBc positive. The mechanism for this synergy between co-infection with HBV and HCV is not known but it has been suggested that the HBV encoded X protein that regulates both cell proliferation and apoptosis on a background of increased hepatocyte turnover present in patients with chronic HCV infection, may be involved.

Of the mycotoxins, the most important is aflatoxin B, produced by a fungus that contaminates grain and nuts, particularly in West Africa. Recently, aflatoxin B has been detected histochemically in patients with HCC. The aetiological role of hepatic helminthosis remains obscure and the only firm association is between infestation with *Clonorchis sinensis* and the development of cholangiocarcinoma as distinct from HCC.

Pathological features of HCC

From a macroscopic viewpoint HCCs are described as:

- *Expanding* – sharp demarcation between tumour mass and the compressed (sometimes atrophied) surrounding parenchyma. Some have a definite capsule. Further classified into single nodular or multinodular
- *Pedunculated* – predominantly extrahepatic growth. This has two subtypes: type I intrahepatic origin, or type II extrahepatic tumour mass that becomes nourished by a branch of the right hepatic artery (not true HCC)
- *Spreading* – lack of demarcation between tumour and surrounding hepatic parenchyma. May involve the whole liver as nodules (usually in cirrhotic livers) or be diffusely infiltrating (non-cirrhotic livers), sometimes referred to as Engel's massive form
- *Multifocal* – several unconnected small tumours of similar size that appear to have arisen synchronously rather than as metastatic foci from an initial single tumour
- *Indeterminate* – no distinct pattern, different features in different parts.

Another perhaps more important distinction is *small HCC*. According to the *Japanese General Rules for Clinical and Pathological Study of Primary Liver Cancer*, this is an HCC of a diameter that is less than 2.0 cm. However during the last 10 years, this limit has been extended by surgeons to tumours smaller than 3.0–5.0 cm. In any event small HCC are nodular and well differentiated. A capsule is not identified when the lesion is smaller than 2.0 cm but larger tumours possess a definite capsule. Histologically, small HCCs are difficult to diagnose and in particular to differentiate from large regenerative nodules. A suggestive histological picture with a rising α-fetoprotein is the basis for establishing the diagnosis. Small HCCs are slow growing and have an excellent prognosis with resection or *in situ* ablation. Recurrence and prognosis are influenced by size, extracapsular growth and involvement of the portal venules.

Some large tumours may have necrotic centres. On cut section there may be a pale appearance with satellite projections into the surrounding liver tissue but some tumours have a homogeneous appearance and merge with the normal cut appearance of the parenchyma. Histologically the tumour cells resemble the normal polygonal hepatocytes and often contain inspissated bile between cells especially when well differentiated. The most commonly used classification of HCC is that of Gibson and Sobin employed by the World Health Organization:

- *Trabecular or sinusoidal* – tumour cells grow in cords or lamellae of variable thickness and are separated by sinusoids
- *Pseudoglandular or acinar* – in addition to the basic trabecular pattern, areas of the tumour exhibit glandular pattern and canaliculi with or without bile plugs
- *Compact* – tumour cells grow in solid masses compressing the sinusoids, which thus become indistinct.
- *Scirrhous* – cords of tumour cells are separated by fibrous septa.

All HCC (and secondary tumours) lack a Kupffer cell population. This is important because some imaging tests, e.g. MRI using superparamagnetic ferric oxide contrast agents, are based on this characteristic. Various histological subtypes are recognized the most common is the clear cell variant which accounts for up to 10%. The tumour cells appear 'clear' because they are laden with glycogen or lipid in the foamy cytoplasm and are sometimes associated with hypoglycaemia or hypercholesterolaemia respectively. The strong male prevalence seen with other HCC is not shared by this histological subtype which has a male/female ratio of 1.6:1.0. Histological grades (I–IV) are used as an index of differentiation by some,

- but is has to be stressed that in general, there is poor correlation between the histology and the prognosis of hepatocellular carcinoma.

α-Fetoprotein secreting tumours may show periodic acid–Schiff (PAS)-positive staining.

HCC may spread to other segments of the liver. In this situation there is usually a large tumour mass with smaller separate satellite nodules. This is different from multifocal cancer where the nodules are of similar size. Spread through the liver is along the lumina of the hepatic and portal veins with the formation of tumour thrombus, which then embolizes to other parts of the liver. HCC is a highly vascular tumour as the neoplastic cells promote angiogenesis. Even tumour thrombus within the portal veins becomes vacularized by arterial tumour vessels and this mechanism is held responsible for the development of arteriovenous shunts that characterize this tumour. HCC can grow into and obstruct the biliary tract causing jaundice (icteric hepatoma).

Fibrolamellar HCC is a distinct variant with specific histological, histochemical and clinical features that occurs in young adults. This tumour has a better prognosis with cures rates of 50% after resection. The histology shows large polygonal cells in a dense fibrous stroma that forms bands or lamellar structures. The histology is similar to that of focal nodular hyperplasia and differentiation by imaging between the two may be difficult. The current consensus is that the two are not related aetiologically and that the FNH represents a hyperplastic response to the HCC. The α-fetoprotein is not elevated in fibrolamellar carcinoma but the serum vitamin B_{12} binding is usually elevated and this has been suggested as a tumour marker for fibrolamellar HCC. Also some patients have elevated plasma neurotensin.

The pattern of recurrent disease after apparently successful resection suggests that direct infiltration along the hepatic veins and suprahepatic vena cava is common. Lymphatic spread to the portal tract is also common and distal lymphatic metastases are seen later in the natural history. Blood-borne metastases in the lungs are common.

Rarer malignant hepatic tumours

Hepatocellular cholangiocarcinoma combines histological features of both types of tumour and probably represents a coincidental occurrence. *Cystadenocarcinoma* occurs as a large lesion usually in adults. Microscopically, cystic spaces are lined in part with cuboidal epithelium with papillary projections.

Angiosarcoma (malignant haemangioendothelioma) consists of proliferating endothelial cells with fibrotic and haemorrhagic areas and large cavernous sinuses lined with dedifferentiated endothelium. The tumour cells may express factor VIII-related antigen. The tumour usually forms multiple nodules throughout the liver rather than a single mass. There is an established association with vinyl chloride production (as soluble monomer and solid PVC) or exposure to arsenic, thorotrast or anabolic steroids. Angiosarcoma can occur in both children and adults. It usually metastasizes within the peritoneal cavity and carries a very poor prognosis. Presentation with life threatening intraperitoneal haemorrhage is common. The related *epithelioid haemangioendothelioma* also expresses factor VIII-related antigen and although it has a somewhat more favourable prognosis, it too can bleed intraperitoneally and develop extrahepatic metastases.

Adult hepatoblastoma is now referred to as malignant hepatic mixed tumour. Although composed of both epithelial and mesenchymal elements, these tumours are different from teratomas. They can form very large tumours.

Hepatic tumours in childhood

Primary liver tumours account for about 15% of abdominal tumours in childhood.

They include:

- Hepatoblastoma
- HCC
- Infantile haemangioendothelioma
- Undifferentiated embryonic sarcoma (embryonal rhabdomyosarcoma)
- Mesenchymal hamartoma
- Malignant rhabdoid tumour
- Mature teratomas.

Hepatoblastoma is the most common liver tumour in children and usually occurs below the age of 5 years with a male predominance. This is an aggressive, rapidly enlarging tumour. Metastases are present in 50% of patients at the time of presentation. The right lobe of the liver is involved in 70%. Various histological types are recognized: HB epithelial, HB mixed epithelial and mesenchymal and HB NOS (not otherwise specified). The HB mixed type includes the teratoid hepatoblastoma which contains elements of the three germ layers. Irrespective of type, the α-fetoprotein is elevated in the majority of cases. Large tumours may rupture with massive intraperitoneal haemorrhage that is often fatal.

Infantile HCC has similar morphological features to the adult type except for the absence of chronic liver disease/cirrhosis. It may occur in infants. Fibrolamellar HCC is encountered in older children

Undifferentiated embryonal sarcoma is usually diagnosed in children between the ages of 6 and 10 years and shows no male preponderance. Histologically the tumour consists of undifferentiated spindle cells and multinucleated giant cells in loose connective tissue. Differentiated components (cartilage, osteoid, striated muscle, etc.) are infrequent. Where possible, liver resection is indicated and about one-third of patients survive long term.

Mesenchymal hamartoma – this may form a lobulated mulitcystic or solid, at times pedunculated mass usually in the right lobe of the liver. It presents in infants (usually about 10 months) but may develop in older children, as a progressively enlarging mass. The tumour consists of epithelial line structures resembling bile ducts in a fibrous/myxoid stroma. The lesion is benign and cure is achieved by resection.

The rare *malignant rhabdoid tumour* is a very aggressive tumour consisting of sheets of cells containing eosinophilic intermediate cytoskeletal filaments. It is almost invariably fatal.

Clinical features of hepatic tumours

The incidence of HCC shows wide geographical variation with high prevalence regions (Mozambique, South Africa, Far Eastern countries) and low prevalence countries (1–2/100 000) such as the USA and UK. Some races seem to be at a higher risk, e.g. black population of South Africa and Chinese. HCC exhibits a male dominance with an average sex ratio of 3:1. In the early stages of the disease, HCC is asymptomatic and is only discovered by screening (by ultrasound and α-fetoprotein) in individuals at risk of the disease.

The predominant symptom results from an abdominal mass, which produces a dragging sensation on exercise. Other symptoms include anorexia, weight loss, abdominal or chest pain, vomiting, fever and, more rarely, changes in bowel habit and weakness. Jaundice and peripheral stigma of chronic liver disease may be present in patients with HCC in a cirrhotic liver or arising in childhood biliary atresia. Also jaundice may supervene from the growth of HCC into the bile ducts (icteric hepatoma). Some liver tumours at all ages present acutely with rupture and massive intraperitoneal bleeding.

Physical findings include obvious abdominal distension due to hepatomegaly or the presence of a hepatic mass. A bruit is heard in about 10% of patients. Ascites is common and is sometimes bloodstained. Additional infrequent clinical features include hypoglycaemia, hypercalcaemia, hyperlipidaemia and hyperthyroidism. Laboratory studies frequently show abnormalities of liver function tests but these may reflect underlying chronic liver disease. Haematological abnormalities may include anaemia due to intratumoral haemorrhage or polycythaemia due to anomalous erythropoietin release. Serum α-fetoprotein levels are elevated in about one-third and are a useful cancer marker after resection. However it is more commonly elevated in the USA, China and African populations. Serum α-fetoprotein is more likely to be elevated in undifferentiated cancers and is a valuable marker for screening the cirrhotic population for HCC development. The reported sensitivity of serum α-fetoprotein in the detection of HCC in patients with cirrhosis varies from 29 to 87%. Despite this, a rising level of AFP or a level greater than 500 ng/ml in patients with chronic active hepatitis or cirrhosis should be followed by real time ultrasonographic examination of the liver and other imaging techniques to exclude HCC.

Hepatitis B and C should be looked for in all patients. For patients undergoing surgery a study of the coagulation parameters is necessary as these may be abnormal and certainly will be affected by a major hepatic resection. Rarely there is hyperlipidaemia or hypercalcaemia with demineralization of the skeleton and spontaneous fractures.

Tumour localization and evaluation

Most patients are initially evaluated by ultrasound scanning to demonstrate size and position of lesions. More detailed information is obtained by helical high-dose CT or MRI which reveals lesions greater than 1.0 cm in size. A chest radiograph may suggest direct diaphragmatic involvement or show pulmonary metastases. Both ultrasound and CT guided biopsy are practised to obtain histological confirmation, but this practice is ill-advised in patients with resectable tumours, as it encourages local implantation and may thus jeopardize cure. Occasionally all imaging modalities (ultrasound, spiral CT, MRI) fail to demonstrate a lesion in a cirrhotic patient who has other indications of the presence of an HCC, e.g. raised α-fetoprotein. In these cases, laparoscopy with laparoscopic contact ultrasonography may be helpful. For large posteriorly placed tumours, cavography is essential to exclude invasion of the inferior vena cava but simple compression or deviation of the inferior vena cava does not preclude a successful resection. There is probably no place for a trial dissection of a hepatocellular carcinoma and the surgeon should have fully assessed the probability of a successful resection before embarking upon it.

With the advent of monoclonal antibodies, newer immunoscintigraphic methods are being developed. These include labelled antibodies against α-fetoprotein and antibodies to surface antigens of human HCC (XF-8, AF-20). Preliminary results look promising.

Surgical treatment

Pre-operative preparation

Disturbance of liver function tests, particularly with regard to serum levels of bilirubin and albumin, may indicate the seriousness of liver damage in patients with chronic liver disease and tumour. Child's classification is used to judge the operative risk prior to resection. Patients classified as grade B or C have effectively lost 50–60% of their liver parenchyma. ICG clearance is used in many centres to evaluate the hepatic reserve and thus the ability to withstand major resection. The arterial ketone body ratio (KBR) of acetoacetate/β-hydroxybutarate is a good indicator of the hepatic mitochondrial redox potential and for this reason is used in some centres in the pre-operative evaluation. Resection is poorly tolerated in patients with a KBR < 0.4.

In some patients with large tumours of the right liver, requiring an extended right hepatectomy (segments 4–8), the residual left lobe (segments 2 and 3) may be too small and in these patients resection will be followed by acute liver failure even if the liver parenchyma is healthy. In these patients pre-operative right portal vein embolization (POPE, *vide infra*) is used to achieve substantial hypertrophy of the left lobe before the resection is undertaken 4 weeks later. Patients with normal liver parenchyma will regenerate the liver bulk but patients with cirrhosis are not able to regenerate further liver tissue. Hence major resections are contraindicated in cirrhotic B and C patients.

Fluid and electrolyte disturbances should be corrected prior to surgery and vitamin K is given routinely. Nutritional supplementation with the maximum protein load tolerable by the patient may elevate the serum albumin though albumin infusions are usually required post-operatively. Patients should receive an intravenous glucose load (1 litre 10% dextrose) prior to surgery in order to ensure that hepatic glycogen is maximal.

Resection

Surgical resection remains the first line treatment of HCC even in patients with cirrhosis provided their hepatic reserve is good. The best results are obtained in patients with lesions less than 2.0 cm and in those with encapsulated well-differentiated tumours. The 5 year survival rate after resection averages 35–38%. Recurrence after resection is common and reaches 55% at 5 years. The risk of intrahepatic recurrent disease after curative resection is enhanced by the presence of a macroscopic portal thrombus at the time of surgery, indicating possible spread of cancer cells from the thrombus during the surgical intervention. Thus only

21% of intrahepatic recurrences are situated near the hepatic resection line and the majority (79%) are located away from the hepatic stump. For this reason, some surgeons advocate intra-operative embolization (with starch microspheres) of the portal branch supplying the tumour at the time of the resection.

The predictors of survival by univariate analysis are vascular invasion, advanced age, multiple tumours and lack of capsule but only vascular invasion remains significantly predictive on multivariate analysis.

The objective of surgical resection is to excise the lesion safely with a margin of healthy liver tissue of 2 cm or more (Figure 9.27). This can be achieved by careful operative assessment. Even so, intra-operative ultrasound is used to locate the lesion in relation to major structures (hepatic veins) and to ensure that no other satellite foci are present. Small liver tumours are amenable to segmental resection providing a tumour free margin of at least 1.5 cm (Figure 9.28). This approach, i.e. segmentectomy, is most suited to patients with chronic liver disease where tumours have been detected relatively early by screening.

Large tumours require a formal dissection along major planes. Where the tumour is localized to segments 5–8, a right hepatectomy is required. If it encroaches on segment 4, an extended right hepatectomy (including segment 4 of the left liver) is necessary. Lesion in segments 2 and 3 are excised by left lobectomy but where, as is often the case, the tumour approaches the falciform ligament and segment 4, then a left hepatectomy (segments 2–4) is necessary. Some cancers extend across the plane between the two livers particularly from the right into segment 4. In some patients requiring major resection for both primary

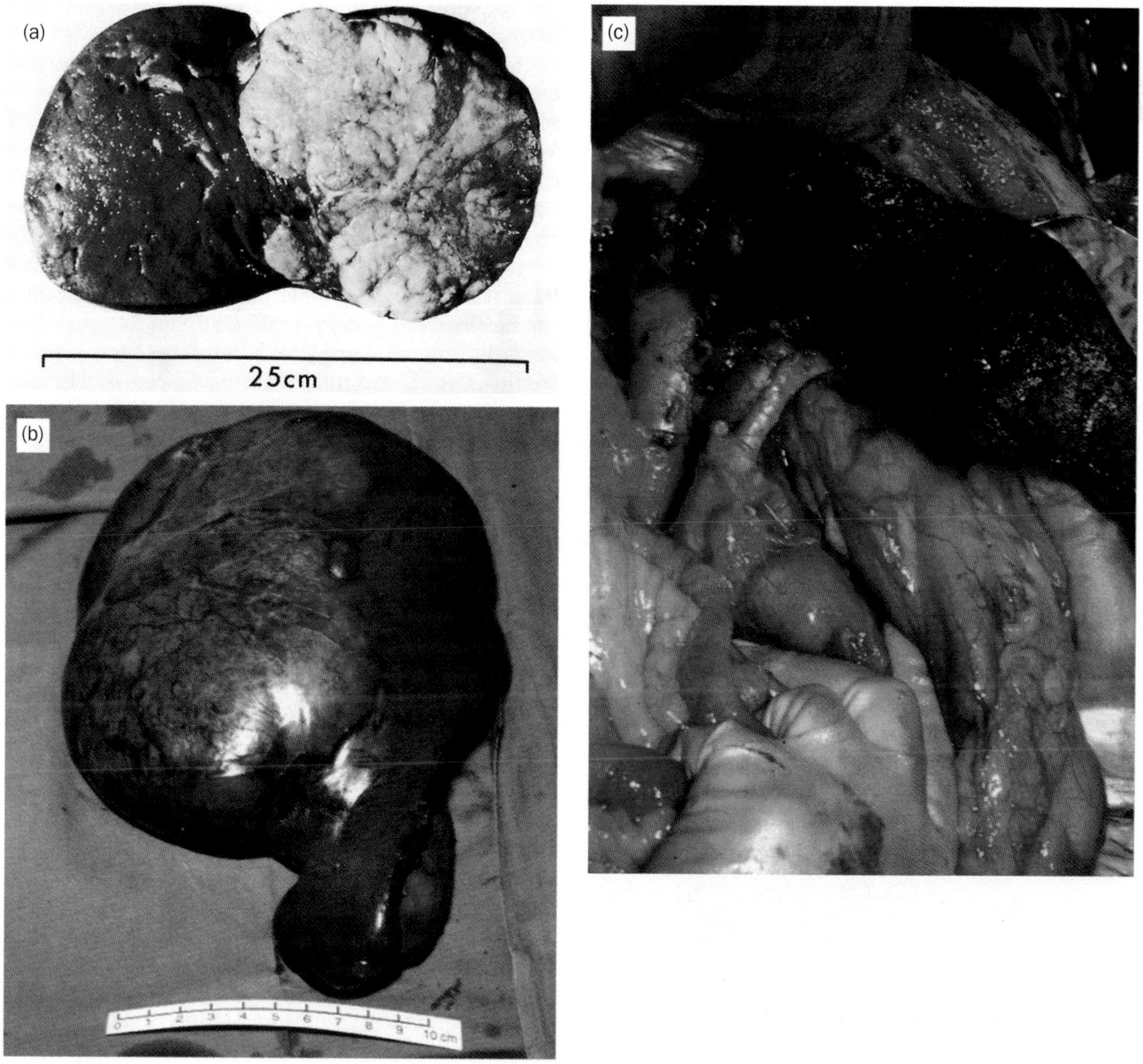

Figure 9.27 (a) This shows the cut surface of a right lobectomy specimen removed for a hepatoma. The large bulky tumour can be seen to be lobulated and to have necrotic areas but there is evidence of a satellite formation apart from the main tumour. (b) Extended right hepatectomy (right hepatectomy together with caudate lobe and segment 4 of the left liver – for massive hepatocellular carcinoma. (c) Residual liver, i.e. segments 2 and 3.

and secondary hepatic tumours, e.g. especially extended right hepatectomy, the residual liver parenchyma (segments 1–3) is too small. Avoidance of major blood loss during major hepatic resections underlies a good post-operative outcome. Bleeding is considerably reduced during the hepatectomy if the CVP is reduced to around zero by head-up tilt and vasodilator therapy.

Hepatic transplantation

The results of hepatic transplantation for HCC have improved with recurrence rates of 20% and survival rates of 45% at 5 years. The best results have been in cirrhotic patients with small tumours where partial resection could have been considered as an alternative. Thus, aside from occult small lesions (<2.0 cm) in patients requiring transplantation for chronic liver disease and cirrhosis, the indication for this surgical treatment is limited to a selected group of patients with fibrolamellar carcinoma. Even in this group, some consider that if the tumour is too large to resect, the outcome following transplantation is not good.

Post-operative care after liver resection

Patients after liver resection require major parenteral support with diminishing daily requirements as liver regeneration takes place. Following hepatectomy/lobectomy there is transient portal hypertension and a sizeable sequestration of blood in the portal venous system.

Jaundice is minimal and lasts about 1 week. More profound and persistent hyperbilirubinaemia may indicate bile duct obstruction and the need for further surgery. Hypoglycaemia can occur in the early post-operative course. Regular monitoring of blood glucose levels is thus necessary. Usually this complication can be avoided by infusing 5–10% glucose during and after operation. Intra- or post-operative coagulation defects can also be countered by the prophylactic use of fresh frozen plasma (at least two units daily during the first 4 days) and vitamin K injections. Since the half-life of albumin is 8–24 hours, hypoalbuminaemia is universal after a major hepatic resection and only partly correctable by plasma infusion. Repeated plasma or albumin infusion may be necessary for at least 1 week post-operatively until hepatic regeneration is sufficient to maintain plasma levels. Regeneration of liver documented by imaging occurs by 3 months if the parenchyma is normal.

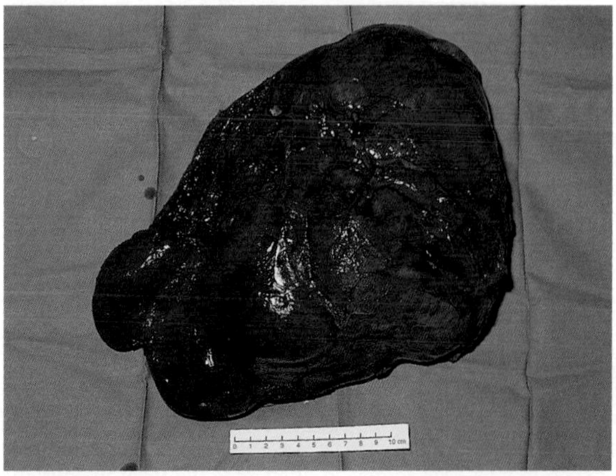

Figure 9.28 Segmentectomy 5 and 6 for metastatic carcinoid tumour.

Non-surgical management of primary hepatic cancer

Chemotherapy

Chemotherapy is used in some patients with unresectable lesions although the results are generally poor. The chemotherapy may be administered systemically or regionally with hepatic arterial infusion using either external or implantable pumps. Only one report has demonstrated that hepatic arterial infusion with floxuridine, doxorubicin and mitomycin C is associated with increased survival compared with systemic intravenous therapy, with the vast majority showing no difference. In general, a higher objective response is obtained by regional chemotherapy but this is offset by a higher rate of post-treatment complications (chemical hepatitis, biliary sclerosis, peptic ulceration and gastritis/duodenitis). A recent retrospective large series of chemotherapy for hepatic malignancy documented an overall response rate of 13% in patients with HCC. Thus it is doubtful whether this poor response justifies the morbidity and costs of this treatment. The results of adjuvant immunotherapy with cytokines such as interleukin-2 (IL-2) and interferons have been equally disappointing to date. Some response to α-interferon can occur in patients with HCC arising on a background of cirrhosis due to hepatitis B or C.

Chemoembolization

Transarterial chemoembolization (TACE) with gelatin sponge and/or ethiodized oil (with or without added chemotherapeutic agents such as cisplatin or doxorubicin) imparts some objective response and symptomatic improvement in patients with unresectable disease. TACE has also been used in the pre-operative setting before surgical resection but there is no evidence that this combined approach improves the survival or reduces the recurrence rates.

Radiotherapy

Supervoltage radiotherapy has been used in unresectable disease but the treatment is limited by the dose-related radiation-induced hepatitis. Thus dosages greater than 30 Gy are not tolerated. Nonetheless, symptomatic relief of pain can be obtained by this therapy. A more recent approach is interstitial radiation using ^{131}I-labelled antibodies to ferritin and α-fetoprotein with the aim of targeting the radiation dose to the tumour. The early results with this targeted interstitial radiotherapy seem promising, with 50% partial response rates.

Metastatic disease of the liver

Direct invasion of the liver may result from locally advanced cancers of the stomach, pancreas and hepatic flexure of the colon. More commonly, hepatic metastases are the result of vascular spread from the primary tumour via either the portal vein or hepatic artery. The liver is by far and away the commonest site of metastatic disease from gastrointestinal, bronchial and breast cancers. In part this is due to its dual blood supply. Though many of the secondary deposits appear necrotic on cut section, there is sufficient blood supply to allow multiple deposits to expand and livers weighing in excess of 10 kg at autopsy have been recorded. Although the histological picture normally reflects the primary tumour, there is a general tendency towards dedifferentiation.

Many hepatic secondaries are asymptomatic but patients with widespread involvement and expansion of the liver suffer pain in the abdomen and back. Some patients experience severe flatulence and nausea, which reduces their nutritional intake. Though many patients appear physically well when liver metastases are first detectable, as the disease progresses, malnutrition, jaundice, ascites and cachexia are inevitable.

By the time liver metastases become symptomatic, there is usually massive involvement. Thus the objective of modern management is the detection of early asymptomatic disease in patients at risk of secondary hepatic deposits, especially with colorectal cancer. Many patients (as much as 35%) with apparently curable primary tumours have overt or occult hepatic metastases at the time of surgery. Routine pre-operative CT scanning downstages about 25% of patients with colorectal cancer due to the presence of hepatic deposits. Intra-operative contact ultrasonography will detect an additional 10%.

Additional information may be obtained from routine liver function tests though these are not likely to show abnormalities until tumour involvement is marked. Serial monitoring of carcinoembryonic (CEA) will detect one-third of metastatic livers with normal liver scans, though the rise in CEA may be due to deposits elsewhere.

Laparoscopy with contact ultrasonography is the best method for the detection of hepatic metastatic disease and peritoneal deposits. In addition, laparoscopic evaluation permits assessment of the disease (site, multiple lesions) and in this respect provides invaluable information concerning the possibility of surgical resection, which in selected cases can be undertaken laparoscopically. On the macroscopic appearance as seen at laparoscopy, metastatic liver disease can be classified as:

- Discretely nodular – single or multiple, unilateral or bilateral
- Miliary – widespread small seeding deposits
- Diffusely confluent disease – involving multiple segments or lobes.

Only the discretely nodular disease is potentially treatable, and cure is rarely obtained if the involvement is greater than 30% of the hepatic substance. The prognosis of patients with miliary or diffusely confluent disease is so poor that no treatment other than symptomatic relief is indicated.

Embolization of the right portal vein prior to right hepatectomy in patients with primary and secondary hepatic tumours

Removal of more than 65% of the liver parenchyma in adults carries a significant risk of post-operative liver failure. Thus the volume of the residual liver or the future remnant liver (FRL) is crucial to survival. This problem is encountered in patients requiring a right hepatectomy and especially extended right hepatectomy, when the remnant liver is judged too small on the pre-operative helical CT scan. Portal venous blood flow promotes hepatic cell regeneration. The responsible hepatotrophic factors are now known to be insulin and glucagon. The principle of pre-operative right portal vein embolization (POPE) is to redistribute the portal flow and thus the hepatotrophic factors to the left liver. The portal vein is accessed via the subxyphoid route under ultrasound control and a catheter is placed for occlusion of the right portal vein by cyanoacrylate-gelatin sponges, gelfoam, etc. Hypertrophy after POPE of the FRL ranges from 50 to 90% after 35 days depending on the embolization agent used. This practice which is now established entails postponing surgery for 4 weeks after the embolization. POPE is reasonably well tolerated although patients may develop ascites and the post-embolization syndrome (*vide infra*) from which the vast majority of patients recover with supportive management.

Treatment of liver metastases

Metastatic hepatic disease is a major problem and in Western countries 90% of liver tumours are metastatic, notably from primaries in the gastrointestinal tract, pancreas, lung and breast. Only a selected group of patients with discretely nodular disease are amenable to treatment. The options available are surgical resection, chemotherapy, chemoembolization and *in situ* ablation.

Surgical resection

Overall, less than 5% of patients with hepatic metastases are suitable for liver resection. The best results are obtained in patients with colorectal metastatic disease. Resection is indicated if the deposits are fewer than four in number, and there is no extrahepatic tumour including hepatic hilar lymph node deposits or comorbid disease, i.e. around 10% of patients with deposits from colorectal cancer. A collective series of resections for hepatic deposits due to colorectal cancer from 24 institutions has shown a 5 year disease-free survival of 25–30%. The resections may be anatomical (resection of recognized anatomical segments or lobes or livers) or non-anatomical. Irrespective of type, a 1.0 cm tumour-free margin is essential. The use of intra-operative ultrasonography (with 7.5 MHz flat probe) is of immense value both in the detection of secondary deposits and in guiding the extent of resection to ensure adequate tumour-free margins. In recent years, re-resection of hepatic secondary deposits has been practised in some centres although the number of reported cases is too small to permit any definite conclusions on the benefit resulting from this aggressive approach. Also resection can be combined with some form of *in situ* ablation (*vide infra*).

Chemotherapy

Despite anecdotal reports, there is no evidence that regional hepatic intra-arterial chemotherapy is followed by a better survival than systemic chemotherapy and randomized clinical studies have shown no difference in survival at 2 years between the two approaches. As in chemotherapy for HCC, regional hepatic arterial infusion chemotherapy for hepatic metastatic disease is accompanied by a higher objective response rate but is attended by a significantly greater hepatic morbidity. Infusion chemotherapy is best administered through implantable ports rather than external Hickman type catheters (lower complication rate). Infusion of 5-fluorouracil (5-FU) in combination with albumin microspheres through the hepatic artery or with pharmacological redistribution of flow to the tumours by the use of noradrenaline and propranolol has not yielded better response rates when compared with equivalent chemotherapy administered through the intravenous route. Currently, intraperitoneal therapy with agents that undergo first pass metabolism in the liver (5-FU, doxorubicin, epirubicin) is being evaluated in a number of centres. This is equivalent to portal vein infusion as the major absorption pathway of these drugs from the peritoneal lining is via the portal venous system. The practical benefit of this approach is the simplicity of the therapy which entails the insertion of an implantable peritoneal access port. The development of chemical irritation of the peritoneal lining with fibrosis may, however, limit the long-term efficacy of intraperitoneal chemotherapy.

The most common systemic chemotherapy regimen used for treating colorectal hepatic deposits is with high-dose infusion 5-FU through a Hickman line with folinic acid (Gramont regimen). Significant responses (objective regression or static disease) are obtained in 30% but the duration of the response is measured in months. Newer agents, e.g. Raltidrex, have been introduced during the past 5 years that are marginally more effective than the Gramont regimen. Early phase II studies have shown good response rates (without prolongation of survival) in patients treated with high-dose 5-FU and recombinant IL-2.

Chemoembolization

TACE is beneficial in secondary ocular melanoma, advanced carcinoid syndrome and deposits from islet cell tumours. The details of the emboli used vary from gelatin sponges to lipiodol, starch granules, etc. The cytotoxic agents most commonly used are 5-FU, doxorubicin and cisplatin. A frequent complication of TACE is the development of the post-embolization syndrome which consists of nausea, vomiting, fever, abdominal pain, paralytic ileus and elevation of the serum transaminases. Other complications include infarction of the gallbladder, pancreatitis, gastroduodenal bleeding and rupture of the tumour. Following chemoembolization of carcinoid hepatic disease, cardiovascular reactions may supervene which require specific pharmacological treatment with somatostatin analogue.

In situ ablation

In essence, *in situ* ablation consists of local destruction of the tumour. This is achieved by thermal methods aimed at heating the tumour to a temperature above 42.5°C for several minutes or by rapid freezing to –40°C or by chemical denaturation. The various ablating technologies include:

- Rapid freezing – cryotherapy.
- Radiofrequency heating probes.
- Microwave heating.
- Interstitial laser hyperthermia.
- Heating by high-intensity focused ultrasound.
- Chemical ablation by alcohol injection.
- Biochemical ablation by p53 induced apoptosis (developmental).

Currently *in situ* ablation of liver tumours is used:

- When the disease is inoperable either because of multiple deposits in both lobes, or in the case of HCC because the functional reserve of the liver precludes safe resection (Child B, C).
- In conjunction with resection for bilateral disease.

In situ ablation can be carried out at open surgery, percutaneously or via the laparoscopic approach. The major advantage of the percutaneous and laparoscopic routes is that the procedure can be repeated several times. This is an important consideration in patients with metastatic liver disease as the majority of these patients develop fresh lesions in time. The laparoscopic approach carries advantages over the percutaneous technique – more accurate ablation and reduced risk of collateral damage to adjacent organs. The actual ablation is monitored by laparoscopic contact ultrasonography. It is likely that the maximal benefit to patients with hepatic deposits is obtained by repeated *in situ* ablation (as necessary) alternating with cycles of systemic chemotherapy. The results of phase II studies with this combined management have to date been promising but the experience is limited.

Cryoablation

Cryotherapy is the oldest *in situ* ablation modality and has been used in the treatment of inoperable liver tumours for more than 25 years. The principle is very rapid freezing followed by a slow thaw. The tumour must be frozen to –40°C for complete destruction. Modern cryo-units use high-efficiency liquid nitrogen (boiling temperature = –190°C) re-circulating implantable probes (2–4 mm) that are impaled in the lesion under ultrasound control. The objective is to achieve an iceball that totally encompasses the tumour and extends into the surrounding normal parenchyma for at least 1.0 cm (Figure 9.29).

Radiofrequency (RF) thermal ablation

With this modality, a high-frequency alternating current (100 000–500 000 Hz) is passed through the tissue to cause intense ionic agitation resulting in frictional heating. Normal and neoplastic tissue is destroyed if heated to above 43°C for 5 min. Multi-electrode probe systems increase the ablative power of RF generators. Even so the ablative zone rarely exceeds 3.5 cm. This is because of charring around the electrodes which increases the impedance and thus limits current flow in the tissue. This problem has been overcome by the introduction of 'cool-tip' electrodes. These are hollow and are kept cool (around 30°C) by closed cold water circulation. Because of the absence of charring around the electrode during use, the ablative capacity is considerably enhanced (Figure 9.30). RF thermal ablation has been used in patients with inoperable primary and secondary hepatic tumours. Most of the reported experience has been on the use of RF ablation by the percutaneous route under radiological or external ultrasound guidance. The laparoscopic/contact ultrasound approach carries a number of potential distinct advantages over the percutaneous route. In the first instance the positive pressure pneumoperitoneum by reducing liver blood flow decreases the heat sink, resulting in a larger ablative zone. Secondly, the approach permits precise visual and contact ultrasound guided insertion of the electrode in the hepatic lesion; and thirdly, the risk of collateral damage is minimized.

Microwave thermal ablation

This is similar in principle to the above but uses microwave energy instead. It seems to be accompanied by a higher morbidity rate, especially of biliary fistula, than RF ablation. It is popular in Japan where it is also used during open surgery for inoperable liver tumours.

High-intensity ultrasound thermal ablation

The technology has now been developed to produce hyperthermia by high-intensity focused ultrasound (HIFU) which can be focused with extreme precision to destroy localized tumour. This technological advance has been described as trackless surgery. The device uses a special transducer that images the lesion and then destroys it by focusing high-intensity ultrasonic energy at a selected point some distance away from the transducer. This point is referred to as the focal point and is the site of heating (up to 90°C) and coagulation necrosis. The profile of the ultrasonic beam is such that heating between the tip of the transducer and the focal point is insufficient to cause any significant thermal damage to the skin, parieties and other intervening tissue. Experience with HIFU is limited but the technique has been used in breast, cerebral and prostate cancer. There are, as yet, no reports on the use of HIFU in the treatment of hepatic metastases.

Interstitial laser hyperthermia (laser thermotherapy)

The underlying principle here is the generation of heat by Nd:YAG laser in the contact mode using quartz fibres that are impaled in the lesion. The problem with

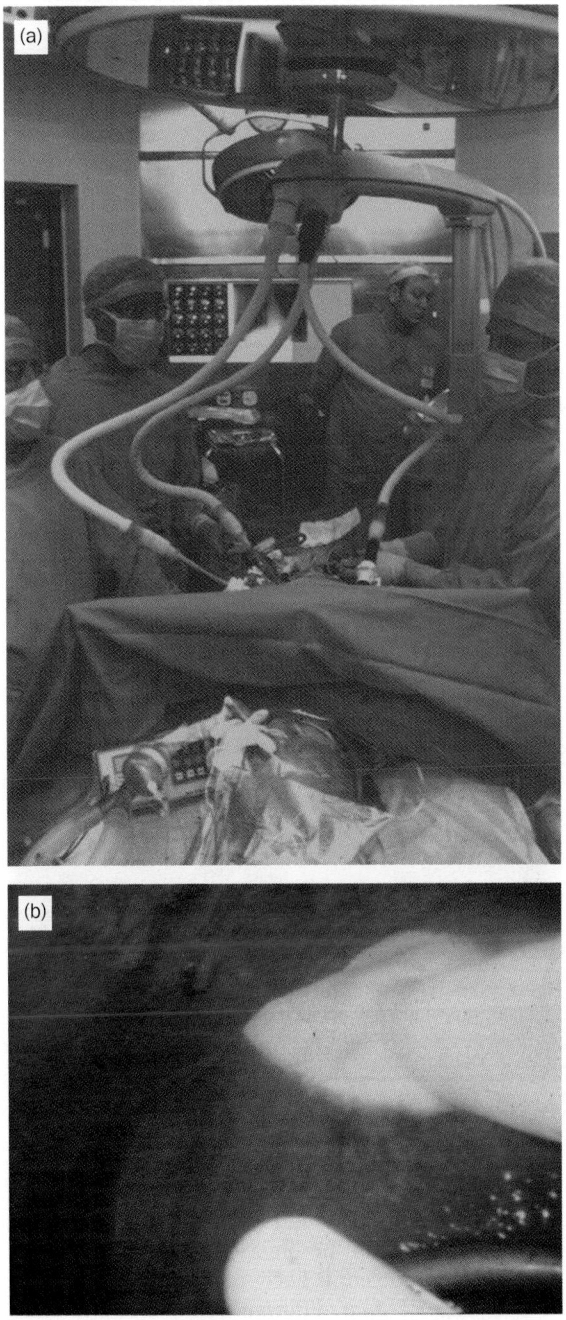

Figure 9.29 (a) Laparoscopic cryoablation of metastatic liver disease. (b) The ablation is monitored by laparoscopic contact ultrasonography – the expanding iceball has a hyperechoic margin that surrounds an acoustic shadow.

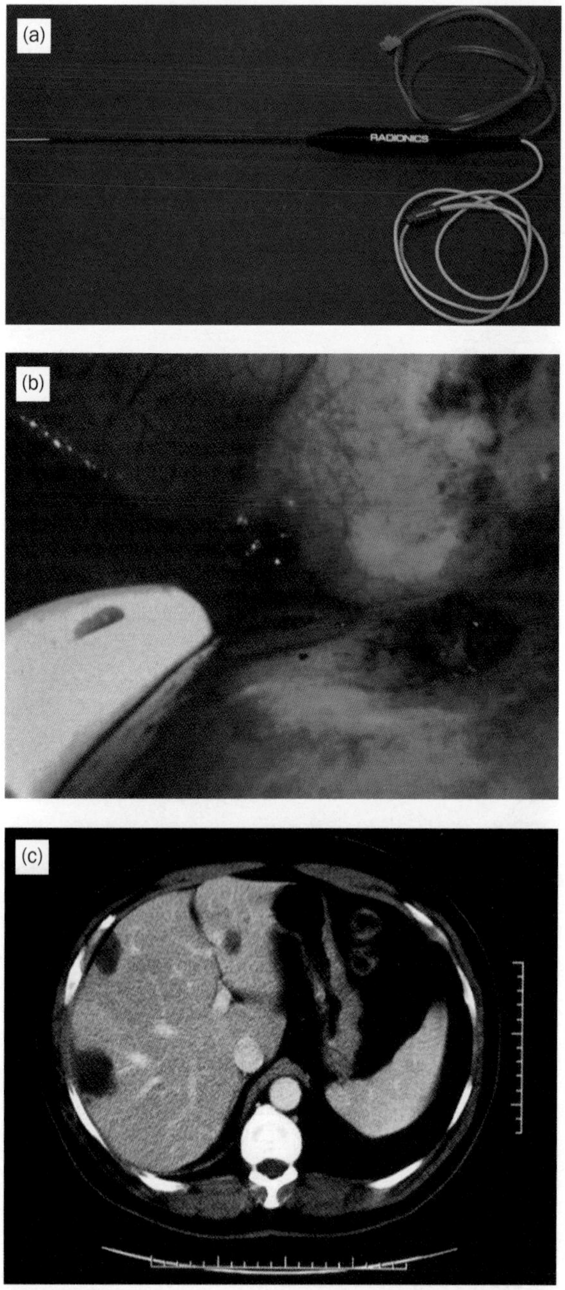

Figure 9.30 (a) Cool-tip electrode for R-F ablation (Radionics); (b) laparoscopic thermal ablation of secondary hepatic deposits; (c) post-operative angio-CT showing ablated tumours (dark holes in liver parenchyma).

interstitial laser hyperthermia has been the limited thermal ablation thermal zone that can be achieved due to carbonization around the bare fibre. Thus multiple fibres have to be inserted into the tumour, although this problem is likely to be overcome by the development of light diffusing tip applicators. Laser thermotherapy is conducted percutaneously or laparoscopically. The disadvantages of laser thermotherapy include laser hazards to personnel, costs, complexity and maintenance of the equipment.

Alcohol injection

This is the simplest and is largely used by the interventional radiologists. Absolute alcohol is used to destroy the tumour. The results are unpredictable as the flow through a single needle may not perfuse the entire lesion even with several passes. Alcohol injection is used only for small lesions (1–2 cm), usually HCC. It is more difficult in the harder secondary deposits. The development of multi-point injection systems may enhance the scope of chemical ablation.

p53-induced apoptosis

This is still in the early phases of clinical evaluation. Wild type p53 carried by a harmless virus (incomplete adenovirus) is injected into the tumour, a process known as transfection. If the tumour cells are infected with the combination, the p53 induces programmed cell death (apoptosis) of the neoplastic cells. Other forms of gene therapy include genes that activate precursor cytotoxic agents.

Section 9.11 • Hepatic trauma

Liver injuries are encountered in civilian practice with regular frequency. Most are caused by blunt trauma from falls or motor vehicle accidents. More rarely in the UK, injuries are due to penetrating stab wounds and still more rarely from high-velocity missiles. Many hepatic injuries are accompanied by other intra-abdominal injury and by injuries to the head and thorax and the clinical features of these injuries may predominate. Fortunately, most liver injuries require only documentation and only a minority of liver injuries require definitive surgical care. These, however, present major surgical and management problems.

When the injury of the liver is penetrating in nature the diagnosis is not difficult and the initial problem is to determine whether the injury extends through the diaphragm into the thoracic cavity. This requires full radiological examination of the chest and upper abdomen. Knife wounds produce a clear incised track into the liver that only rarely devitalizes liver segments and haemorrhage is easily controlled unless a major vascular structure is severed. Gunshot wounds produce much more damage and the external wounds in the body wall and liver surface may not reflect the internal damage to the liver substance where the severity of the tissue damage is directly related to the size and velocity of the missile. Similarly, the bursting type of injury may have a small laceration on the liver surface but wide cracks extend deeply into the liver parenchyma and may lead to devitalization of large segments.

The clinical picture of significant hepatic trauma is dominated by bleeding which can be massive and difficult to control in major injuries. The classification and management of hepatic injuries are considered elsewhere [**Trauma Module, Vol. II**]

- What is important to stress to the general surgeon is that in the event that parenchymal or hepatic vein bleeding cannot be controlled by standard operative measures and the patient remains unstable, packing is the most appropriate option.

Subsequent removal of the packs 24–72 hours later can be followed by definitive surgical treatment of the injury. Often, bleeding will have stopped and nothing further is needed.

Section 9.12 • Disorders of the hepatic vasculature

The unique nature of liver blood supply leads to a series of clinical problems that may be described by considering each system (portal vein, hepatic artery, hepatic veins) separately. However, there are end-points which are common to all three systems, e.g. portal hypertension effects can follow obstruction to portal or hepatic venous systems and pathological changes in these two systems can co-exist. It is advisable when evaluating a patient as hepatic vascular disorder, to demonstrate the anatomy or physiological status of all three systems.

Portal hypertension

Obstruction to portal venous flow leads to a rise in the pressure of the splanchnic venous circulation. While no value is absolute, portal hypertension may be assumed when the portal vein pressure exceeds 20 cm of saline. Obstruction may result from extrahepatic compression or thrombosis of the portal, mesenteric or splenic veins, from compression of portal venous radicles within the liver from a wide variety of liver diseases or from obstruction to the outflow from the liver (Table 9.4). Rarely, anomalous arterio-portal fistulas result in a massive rise in portal venous flow and pressure (*vide infra*).

Most commonly, portal hypertension is post-sinusoidal and results from cirrhosis of the liver. While a precise diagnosis may not be relevant to the immediate management of a patient with variceal bleeding, it may ultimately indicate prognosis and further treatment. Chronic active hepatitis may improve with medical treatment, whereas the histological features of alcoholic hepatitis indicate recent liver injury which will be associated with a poor surgical risk. There is a wide spectrum of metabolic disorders of the liver (Wilson's disease, haemochromatosis) and granulomatous liver disease (toxoplasmosis, schistosomiasis), all of which can be improved by specific treatment with improvement/maintenance of liver function if the gastrointestinal haemorrhage can be controlled.

The portal hypertension in patients with cirrhosis is the result of a combination of increased portal venous resistance and an increased splanchnic blood flow. The latter is secondary to elevated circulating levels of vasodilator substances (including glucagon) and decreased sensitivity of the splanchnic vasculature to endogenous vasoconstrictors. Portal hypertension sometimes develops in patients with liver disease prior to the onset of cirrhosis. This has been attributed to intrahepatic arterioportal anastomoses, hyperdynamic circulation and the accumulation of vasoactive humoral factors which alter the resistance to flow.

Table 9.4 Pathogenesis of portal hypertension

- **Increased blood flow into portal venous system (no obstruction)**
  Hepatic and splenic arterioportal fistulas (rare)
- **Extrahepatic outflow obstruction**
  Hepatic vein thrombosis; Budd–Chiari syndrome, veno-occlusive disease
  tricuspid incompetence, right heart failure
- **Extrahepatic inflow obstruction**
  Congenital malformation of portal vein
  Portal vein thrombosis
  Splenic vein thrombosis (sectorial portal hypertension)
  Portal vein compression, e.g. nodes
- **Intrahepatic obstruction**
  Presinusoidal: periportal fibrosis and schistosomiasis
  Postsinusoidal: cirrhosis (alcoholic, nutritional, postnecrotic, biliary), veno-occlusive diseases, haemochromatosis, Wilson's disease, congenital hepatic fibrosis.

About 25% of patients will have an extrahepatic block and a proportion of these patients will have underlying liver disease or polycythaemia. Chronic pancreaticobiliary disease or pancreatic neoplasms may be precipitating factors for portal or splenic vein thrombosis but only rarely does neonatal umbilical sepsis seem to be an aetiological factor. Extrahepatic outflow block may result from thrombosis or occlusion of the hepatic veins (Budd–Chiari syndrome). Aetiological factors may be protein C deficiency, the contraceptive pill and ingested toxins that include senecio or bush tea poisoning (veno-occlusive disease). Other patients have congenital diaphragms in the suprahepatic vena cava or chronic congestive right heart failure. Such patients rarely present with bleeding varices but suffer with intractable ascites, painful hepatomegaly and rapidly deteriorating liver function. Portal hypertension may also follow thrombosis of the splenic vein from pancreatitis or tumour. In this instance the portal hypertension is left sided (sectorial) and the varices affect the short gastric and gastroepiploic veins.

Obstruction to portal venous flow is followed by enlargement of natural portosystemic communications (see Figure 9.6) and by the development of new collateral channels at surgically constructed mucocutaneous junctions (colostomy, ileostomy). Rarely, portal venous blood is shunted away from the liver by an enlargement of the umbilical vein (Cruveilhier–Baumgarten syndrome) and may be detected by a venous bruit in the midline. Though there is a risk of variceal bleeding from the ileum, colon and haemorrhoidal areas, the major risk of haemorrhage is from the oesophagus and stomach. In the oesophagus the varices are large, tortuous and thin-walled with a tendency to rupture. However, in the stomach there is venous engorgement of the gastric mucosa with a tendency to erosive gastritis and a widespread diffuse haemorrhage (portal hypertensive gastropathy). Most patients suffering this complication will have portal venous pressures in excess of 30 cm of saline. The predilection of the gastric cardia to develop varices is probably due to the drainage of the left coronary vein after portal hypertension has developed. Instead of draining towards the liver, blood passes along paraoesophageal veins and then via 'perforator' veins to the submucosa of the oesophagus. Three columns tend to develop and run upwards for a variable length, usually communicating with the azygos system. Blood flow from the spleen may course through the short gastric vessels to the gastric fundus and link with enlarged collaterals at the cardia. Fundal varices are well seen only after retroflexion of the flexible endoscope once this is in the stomach. Colonic varices may occasionally be seen on sigmoidoscopy though not as commonly as may be expected. Nor is the caput medusa or periumbilical plexus of veins at all common. It is most prominent in patients who develop a small paraumbilical hernia into which an omental plug provides the portal flow.

It has to be recognized that not all patients develop portal hypertension as a result of their chronic liver disease; estimates vary from 15% to 40%. Furthermore only about one-half of the patients with gastro-oesophageal varices ever suffer from gastrointestinal bleeding.

Three clinical syndromes can be attributed to portal hypertension, namely:

- Hypersplenism
- Ascites
- Gastrointestinal bleeding.

Hypersplenism

Splenomegaly is frequently associated with portal hypertension and there may be sufficient sequestration of formed blood elements in the spleen to cause haemolytic anaemia, leucopenia and thrombocytopenia. Only rarely are these features sufficient to produce major symptoms but they do lead to general debility. After portal vein decompression, hypersplenism improves in approximately 50% of patients. Thus pancytopenia in patients requiring portal venous decompression may be an indication for a splenectomy and lienorenal shunt.

Ascites

The development of fluid retention and ascites is extremely common in chronic liver disease and portal hypertension and its incidence correlates with the degree of advancement (stage) of the disease. The pathophysiology of ascites and its management have been outlined earlier.

Gastrointestinal haemorrhage

About 30% of patients with varices suffer gastrointestinal haemorrhage within 2 years of diagnosis and thereafter only a smaller fraction bleed each year. Larger varices appear more likely to bleed than smaller varices and varices that are observed to increase in size over a period of 1 year will almost certainly bleed at some point. The pressure within the veins reaches systemic arterial pressure during coughing and straining and additional factors must initiate the haemorrhage. Aside from size (grades II, III), the risk factors which predispose to variceal haemorrhage are portal pressure and the following endoscopic findings:

- cherry-red spots;
- overlying varices;
- red whale markings; and
- blue varices (as opposed to white).

Once they develop, oesophageal varices do not resolve spontaneously except small (grade I) varices associated with reversible portal hypertension which may develop in patients with intense fatty infiltration due to alcoholism. Improvement in the hepatic condition following medical therapy and abstinence from alcohol can be followed by resolution of the varices in these patients. Children with extrahepatic portal hypertension commonly bleed when suffering from upper respiratory tract infection.

Clinical features

Variceal bleeding may present in the usual fashion of haematemesis of coffee-ground material and repeated melaena. However, there is commonly a minor warning bleed of a mouthful of bright red blood followed some hours later by a major haemorrhage of fresh blood produced without retching. Such patients may be known to have or to show the peripheral stigmata of chronic liver disease. Unless bleeding is massive and continuing, every attempt is made to localize the source of bleeding by fibre-optic endoscopy.

Oesophagogastroscopy should be performed as soon as the patient has been resuscitated and is haemodynamically stable. This is usually possible within 8–12 hours of admission. Flexible endoscopy has largely replaced other methods of diagnosis of bleeding varices such as splenoportography and is often used in the therapeutic control of variceal bleeding. In patients with massive haemorrhage, a clinical diagnosis may have to suffice and resuscitation commenced together with measures to obtain control of the bleeding before the patient exsanguinates. In addition to blood volume replacement and correction of electrolyte and acid-base imbalance, methods to prevent the development of encephalopathy or minimize its severity are instituted.

Control of active variceal haemorrhage

The mainstays of modern management are balloon tamponade followed by sclerotherapy or banding of the varices or primary control with sclerotherapy/banding. Drug therapy remains controversial although there have been some recent advances in this area. Endoscopic band ligation is now well established and is used in preference to sclerotherapy in many centres.

Balloon tamponade

The major standby in the immediate control of variceal haemorrhage remains balloon tamponade. Problems arise with this technique when it is used as the only means of control over a long period and results in a mortality rate greater than if it were not used at all. However, provided the tamponade is to be applied for a limited period of 12–24 hours, followed by alternative action if it fails, the balloon system can be life-saving.

Two balloon systems are commonly used:

- *Sengstaken tube* – with a gastric balloon of about 60–100 ml capacity, which is meant to anchor the tube at the cardia and an oesophageal balloon which is inflated to 30–40 mmHg and compresses the submucosal veins of the oesophagus
- *Linton tube* – with a large gastric balloon of 300–700 ml capacity which is pulled against the diaphragmatic hiatus with traction and disconnects the high-pressure portal venous system from the thoracic azygous veins.

Both systems have disadvantages, the major one being that during use, pharyngeal and oesophageal secretions accumulate and can be aspirated into the bronchial tree. Both balloons are capable of oesophageal rupture if they are inflated when incorrectly placed. The Sengstaken gastric balloon may not anchor the tube at the cardia so that the oesophageal balloon moves headwards to obstruct the airway. It may do this anyway in a short person or in the presence of kyphosis. Prolonged traction with the Linton tube leads to linear ulcers in the oesophagus which bleed profusely and are almost impossible to deal with.

Once the tube is placed, regular half-hourly or hourly aspirations of the oesophagus and stomach are performed to remove blood and secretions and determine whether variceal control has been obtained. Specimens are retained in test tubes and should show a progression from bright red blood to altered blood to clearer gastric secretions. Once control is obtained, time is spent in full resuscitation with blood transfusion, plasma and electrolyte replacement as indicated by clinical parameters and laboratory studies.

Balloon tamponade is discontinued after 12–24 hours but the tube retained initially so that gastric and oesophageal aspiration may continue. By this time, a plan of action should have been evolved to proceed further either immediately or in the event of further haemorrhage (Figure 9.31). This may involve sclerotherapy/banding or a radiological/surgical procedure on the varices or portal venous system and the decision will largely depend upon the experience and views of the attending clinicians.

Endoscopic sclerotherapy

Many clinicians now proceed to variceal injection at the time of diagnostic endoscopy obviating the need for balloon tamponade in the majority of patients. As the bleeding episodes overwhelmingly occur from variceal rupture at the lower end of the oesophagus and cardia, an attempt is made to inject the varices in this region by several punctures in a circumferential fashion. Three techniques are available:

- Techique 1 performed under GA – using the rigid endoscope, the varices can be injected by a long needle usually mounted in tandem with a forward-viewing telescope. After injection, the instrument is passed forward to compress the injection site for a few minutes (rarely used nowadays).
- Technique 2 preferably performed under GA – uses the flexible endoscope with an outer compression over-tube – the objective of the outer tube is to isolate the varices which prolapse into the lumen of the sheath through a small window at the distal end of the outer tube.
- Technique 3 performed under sedation – uses the flexible endoscope without an outer sheath.

A flexible needle passed through the endoscope is used for injection after which the sheath is rotated to cover the injection site (Figure 9.32). There is some debate on the relative efficacy of sclerosant injection around (paravariceal) or in the lumen (intravariceal) of the varices. In practice this is largely irrelevant as both are likely to happen (intentionally or otherwise) during the course of repeated sclerotherapy management of these patients.

There is no doubt about the efficacy of sclerotherapy in achieving arrest of bleeding in patients with variceal haemorrhage and in reducing the incidence of subsequent bleeding episodes. Sclerotherapy is repeated at 3 weekly sessions until all the varices are obliterated (over 3–6 months). In a comparative study on the efficacy and safety of various sclerosants (ethanolamine oleate, 3%, tetradecyl sulfate and absolute alcohol), although all agents had the same success rate, the alcohol treatment required fewer sessions with lesser amounts of sclerosant and was the cheapest.

Sclerotherapy has a number of disadvantages. In the first place, it requires special expertise which is not always available. In addition, there are a number of complications. These include oesophageal ulceration, perforation or stricture, adult respiratory distress syndrome, mediastinitis, bacteraemia (10%) with subsequent endocarditis (especially in patients with prosthetic valves), anaphylactic reactions (ethanolamine oleate), pneumatosis intestinalis, pneumoperitoneum and portal/mesenteric vein thrombosis. A recent report of patients requiring surgical management after previous sclerotherapy showed an incidence of portal vein thrombosis of 36%. Thus sclerotherapy should be used cautiously, especially in good-risk patients (Child A) who may later require a shunt operation. Sclerotherapy also aggravates portal gastropathy, is difficult to apply and is less effective in the control of gastric varices. Recurrence of oesophageal varices after initial obliteration by sclerotherapy occurs in about 60% of patients. There do not appear to be any significant effects on survival following successful sclerotherapy except perhaps in patients with extrahepatic portal hypertension.

The results of endoscopic sclerotherapy are more dependent on operator skill and experience than

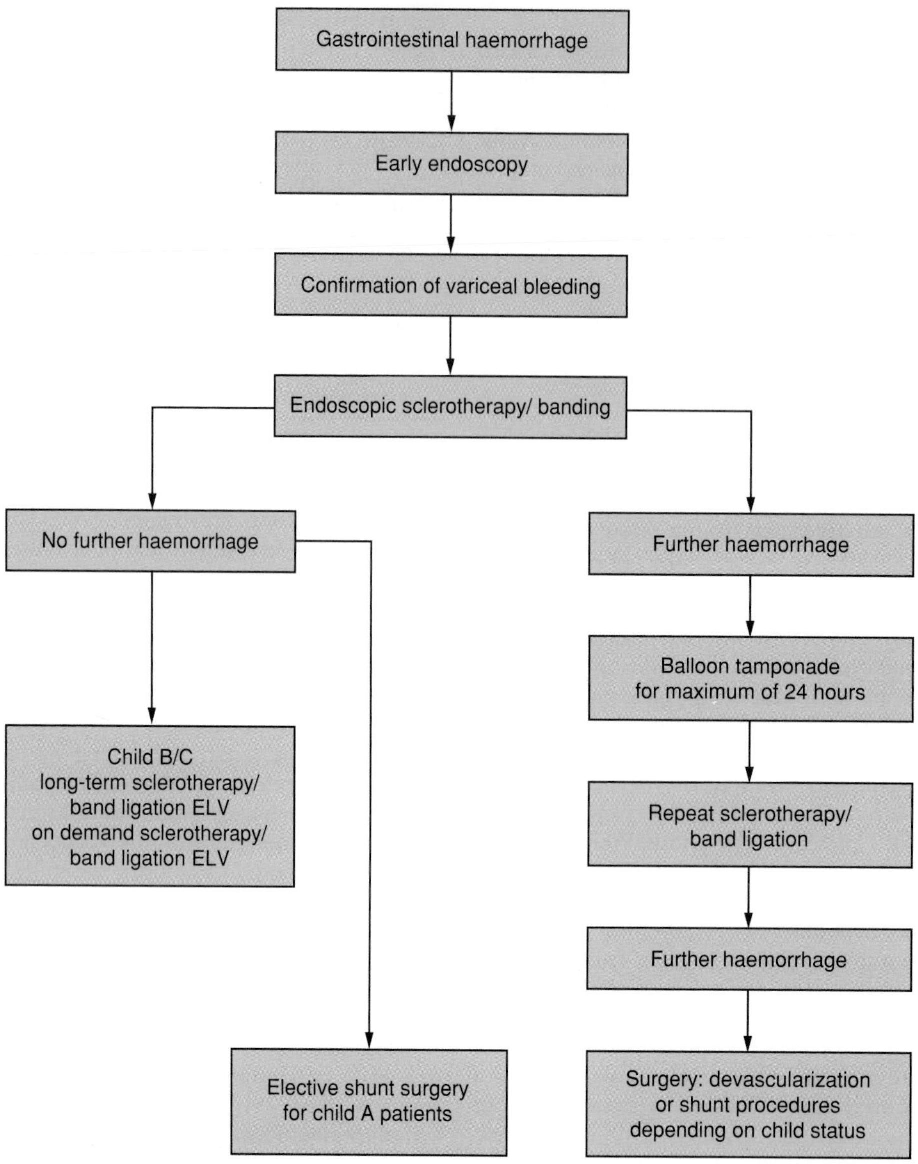

Figure 9.31 Algorithm for the management of patients with variceal haemorrhage.

the choice of technique, schedule or sclerosant used. Schedule refers to the long-term management after effective initial control of variceal haemorrhage with two options:

- Long-term sclerotherapy at regular intervals
- On-demand sclerotherapy, i.e. after bleeds only.

Three clinical trials have shown that patients managed with the 'on-demand' policy continue to experience bleeding for a longer period and have a higher re-bleed rate than long-term sclerotherapy patients but there is no difference in survival and the need for shunt surgery.

Failed sclerotherapy is managed by either an oesophageal transection with or without devascularization or shunt procedure depending on the condition of the patient and the extent of hepatic decompensation.

Endoscopic ligation of varices

Endoscopic ligation of varices (ELV) is achieved by a simple and ingenious device that consists of a circular attachment, which fits on the end of a forward-viewing or oblique-viewing flexible endoscope. A rubber 0 band, mounted on the tubular attachment, is dislodged around the base of the varix after this is sucked inside the ring by activation of the suction of the endoscope. Multiple-fire ELV devices are now available and these have eliminated the previous shortcoming of EVL that entailed removal of the endoscope for reloading. Several randomized trials have now confirmed that ELV is as or more effective than endoscopic sclerotherapy in controlling active variceal bleeding and eradicating varices, and furthermore it is accompanied by a significantly lower morbidity (bacteraemia and infection complications, treatment-induced ulcers and stric-

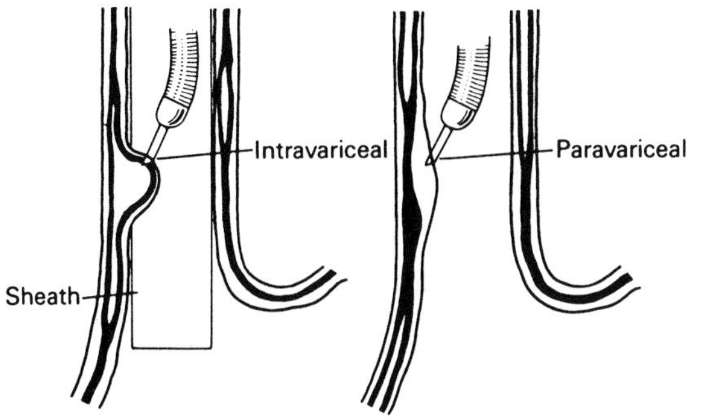

Figure 9.32 Injection sclerotherapy can be achieved by injecting directly into the varix (intervariceal), which may be best, or immediately adjacent (paravariceal).

ture formation). Serious complications following ELV are rare and the majority of these are caused by the overtube that is used by some to facilitate the repeated passage of the band-loaded endoscope. Bleeding and perforation can occur in this situation if the mucosa is pinched between the endocope and the edge of the overtube especially during withdrawal.

ELV is thus rapidly displacing endoscopic sclerotherapy in most centres except for: (a) small or previously treated varices, (b) varices that cannot be aspirated into the cylinder attachment, and (c) very large oesophageal varices and gastric varices.

Percutaneous transhepatic embolization

Varices can be thrombosed by retrograde passage of catheters with embolization (Gelfoam, coils, etc.) following injection of contrast to outline the anatomy and the exact location of the catheter tip (Figure 9.33). The method has been largely abandoned nowadays as it is no more effective than endoscopic sclerotherapy.

Gastric varices

These are difficult to control by ES and EVL and are generally considered as indications for TIPSS or surgical shunting. However, newer endoscopic techniques have shown promising results. These are:

- Cyanoacrylate injection – undergoes instant polymerization when injected in the varix, plugging its lumen within seconds.
- Intravarix bovine thrombin injection.
- Application of detachable snare (Endoloop, Olympus, Japan).

Drug therapy

This remains controversial and there is no standard practice which is generally adopted. Drug therapy is used both in the initial control of bleeding and in the prophylaxis against bleeding subsequent to arrest by established techniques. The efficacy of continuous intravenous infusion of vasopressin (or its analogues, glypressin or terlipressin) in the control of variceal haemorrhage remains unconfirmed although recent reports with high-dose infusions combined with intravenous sodium nitroprusside or nitroglycerin (to minimize the systemic and myocardial adverse effects) have provided evidence of control of bleeding in a significant percentage of patients.

Arrest of bleeding can be obtained by somatostatin and, more recently, by its synthetic long-acting analogue (Octreotide). A randomized trial showed it to be at least as effective as sclerotherapy. Its effects are largely attributed to a lowering of the transhepatic venous gradient. Pentagastrin is reported to reduce the variceal haemorrhage by inducing contraction of the lower oesophageal sphincter. In one clinical report its use followed by the intravenous administration of metoclopramide (a longer acting agent with similar effects on the sphincter) was reported to result in arrest of bleed-

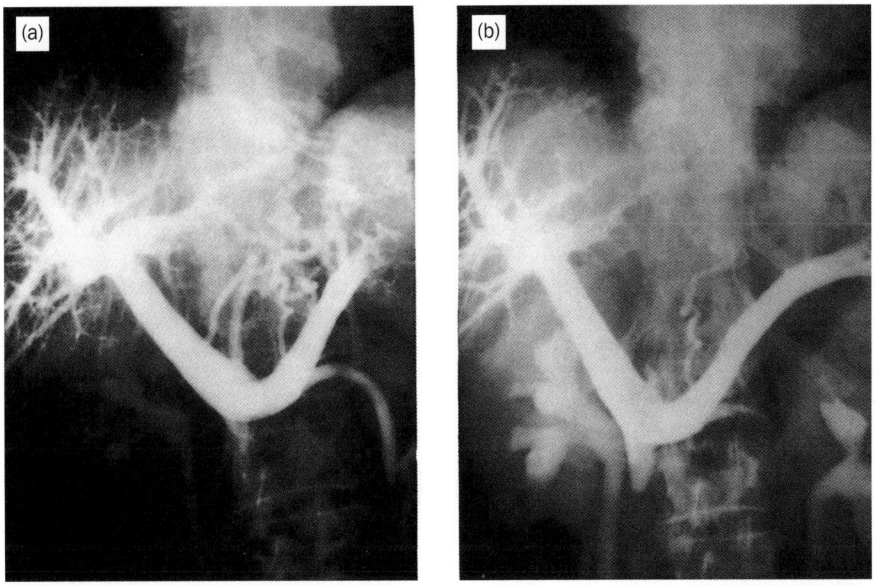

Figure 9.33 Occasionally transhepatic embolization of bleeding varices can be attempted and can give good control of the vessels feeding the cardia, but control is only temporary.

ing in the majority of patients. Further clinical studies are needed to confirm these encouraging results.

Pharmacological lowering of the portal venous pressure by beta-blockers (propranolol and nadolol) has been employed to prevent bleeding after initial control by sclerotherapy. The various reports suggest a reduction of subsequent bleeds by 30%. However, there are concerns about the adverse effects of these agents on hepatic function. One report has demonstrated a significant reduction in the hepatointestinal oxygen uptake in cirrhotic patients with obvious clinical deterioration when assessed by psychometric testing. In addition, propranolol therapy results in an elevation of the blood ammonia and it increases the incidence of encephalopathic episodes.

Surgical treatment

Some 85% of patients with bleeding varices can be controlled by non-surgical measures. The biggest problem group are those patients who continue to bleed or in whom bleeding recurs soon after standard non-operative management. The majority of these patients are high-risk candidates whose liver function is poor from end-stage liver disease or has been downstaged from A/B to C as a consequence of the recurrent hypovolaemic episodes. Unless prior information is available on the patients, it is difficult to distinguish between these two categories at the time of emergency surgical intervention. Portosystemic shunting in this group carries a prohibitive mortality and is contraindicated. The correct surgical management which is likely to prevent death from exsanguination is oesophageal transection.

Two other groups of patients are considered for surgical treatment of portal hypertension in an elective setting. The first consists of patients in whom bleeding has been arrested and who have good liver function (Child A/good B). Since there is no effective safe measure for prevention of further bleeding episodes and since these patients' expected survival is good, elective surgical therapy by portosystemic shunting or oesophageal transection with devascularization (Siguira procedure) is a sensible, cost-effective and safe management approach. The other group concerns patients with end-stage liver disease (Child C) who have been controlled by sclerotherapy. These patients should be considered for hepatic transplantation. For this reason, surgery should be avoided as it increases the morbidity and mortality of the procedure. TIPSS introduced by radiological intervention techniques is employed in these patients to achieve portal decompression and thus avoid further bleeding episodes prior to hepatic transplantation. TIPSS has been used in good-risk patients but follow-up has demonstrated an unacceptably high thrombosis rate beyond 6 months and because of this, a trial comparing TIPSS vs. sclerotherapy has concluded that radiological shunting is not advisable in good-risk patients.

Preparation for surgery

Careful cardiovascular and respiratory assessment prior to surgery is essential and it may be possible to detect an abnormal haemodynamic state, which may determine whether patients should be subjected to emergency surgery, the time of elective surgery and post-operative care. Careful cardiovascular investigation will also indicate the patients with the highest risk from variceal haemorrhage and operation. Three states are recognized:

- a hyperdynamic state characterized by an increased cardiac output without evidence of peripheral vascular or pulmonary dysfunction
- a balanced hyperdynamic response to stress in which a further increase in cardiac output is usually compensated for by an adequate increase in myocardial contractility and oxygen consumption
- an unbalanced hyperdynamic state in which there is evidence of severe peripheral vascular abnormality, impaired oxygen extraction and a tendency to cardiac failure.

High-risk patients may require the use of inotropic drugs and prolonged ventilatory support. Hypokalaemia needs appropriate replacement either orally or intravenously, in patients with a prolonged prothrombin time. Vitamin K (10–30 mg) should be given intramuscularly or intravenously. Prolonged partial thromboplastin time indicates more serious liver dysfunction though it may be present if large amounts of stored blood have been given. Fresh frozen plasma is indicated prior to and during surgery. Patients are also prepared by intestinal sterilization with 6 g of neomycin mixture orally.

If the surgical approach which is favoured is a direct attack on the varices, then there is no particular reason to visualize the portal venous system. However, if this can be done with confidence using duplex ultrasound, then it should be done so that if circumstances change, particularly during operation, the surgeon is aware of other possibilities. Unfortunately ultrasound is often quite difficult in these critically ill patients and the vessels may be obscured by bowel gas from recent endoscopy. If necessary, CT angiography can be performed, provided that adequate care can be given to variceal control in the radiology department.

Direct surgical obliteration

This procedure is now standard in many hospitals. The original transthoracic approach, which had a 50% mortality, has been abandoned in favour of a circular stapling gun introduced via a gastrotomy. The device should transect and remove the segment of oesophagus immediately adjacent to the cardia (Figure 9.34). Care is taken to avoid injury to the vagus nerves and to perform an adequate ligation of the peri-oesophageal veins. In practice, if the surgeon effectively devascularizes the upper half of the gastric lesser curvature as in proximal gastric vagotomy, this achieves the effect of preparing the oesophagus for transection.

If it is suspected that the major source of bleeding is from gastric varices, the oesophageal stapling instrument is not effective. A gastrotomy with double separate straight non-cutting linear stapling across the anterior and posterior walls gives the same effect as the por-

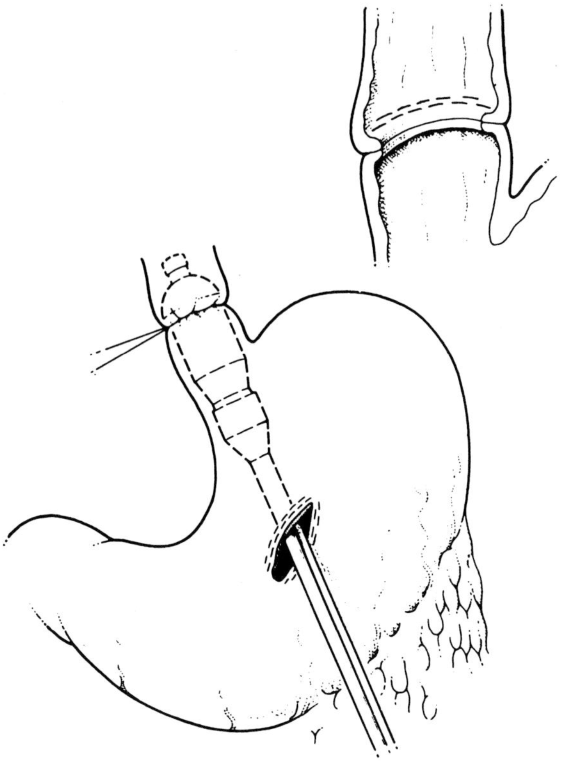

Figure 9.34 Stapled transection of the lower oesophagus is achieved by introducing the circular stapler (28–31 mm) through a gastrotomy and by tying the oesophagus to the central axle with a strong suture before closing the gun and firing.

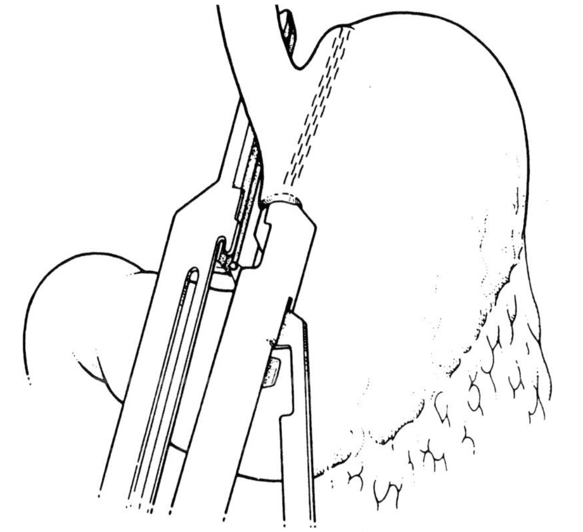

Figure 9.35 Gastric stapling below the cardia is performed by using two applications of linear non-cutting stapler on the anterior and posterior walls through a gastrotomy near the lesser curvature.

toazygos procedure described many years ago by Tanner (Figure 9.35). The procedure may be extended by adding to it a splenectomy and this is indicated if significant hypersplenism is present. Splenectomy is not without its problems, for collaterals in the lienorenal ligament are very difficult to control and the splenic vein is lost should a decompression procedure become advisable at a future date. A staged second procedure in which the peri-oesophageal veins are ligated via a transthoracic approach constitutes the complete Sigiura procedure.

Stapling of the varices and devascularization of the oesophagogastric junction is effective in the control of haemorrhage in a large majority of patients. The operating time is short and intra-operative blood losses are minimal. However, the immediate hospital mortality is still high (35%), particularly in patients who are actively bleeding. Late rebleeding from varices also occurs fairly commonly and it is logical to carry out endoscopic examination at 3 months in survivors and if possible deal with residual varices by sclerotherapy or band ligation.

Portosystemic shunts

Whipple introduced the operation of portacaval shunt in 1945 in which the portal vein was anastomosed to the side of the vena cava. The decompression of the portal venous system reduces the incidence of variceal bleeding and enables ascites to be more easily controlled. The portal pressure falls as does the hepatic venous pressure and the hepatic artery flow increases as compensation. Since these early experiences, other types of portal decompression operations have been devised but relatively few are performed in current practice because of a high incidence of post-shunt encephalopathy. This complication is higher if the patient is older than 50 years, has previous evidence of encephalopathy or has poor liver function (grade C). The procedures are best performed under scheduled urgent or elective conditions, i.e. where other methods have failed to prevent recurrent variceal haemorrhage but the patient can be maintained in a stable condition for some days. Patients with primary biliary cirrhosis, congenital hepatic fibrosis or high portal obstruction are most suited. Alcoholic patients, particularly if still drinking, or those who have evidence of hepatitis and patients with progressive chronic active hepatitis are least suited.

The most effective shunt for portal decompression remains the end-to-side portacaval shunt and it is the easiest to perform. The side-to-side shunt is thought to be nearly as effective in reducing portal pressure and appears more effective in dealing with chronic ascites possibly because decompression of the liver reduces hepatic lymph. Lienorenal or mesentericocaval shunts are also side-to-side shunts and are indicated when ascites appears to be a major complication of the portal hypertension. Significant hypersplenism suggests the need for a lienorenal shunt. These three standard shunts decompress the portal venous system and direct portal blood with its hepatotrophic factors away from the diseased liver. This fact may be responsible for the higher incidence of portosystemic encephalopathy and for the high mortality from hepatic failure in poor-risk patients. Encephalopathy seems less of a problem with lienorenal and mesenterico-caval shunts.

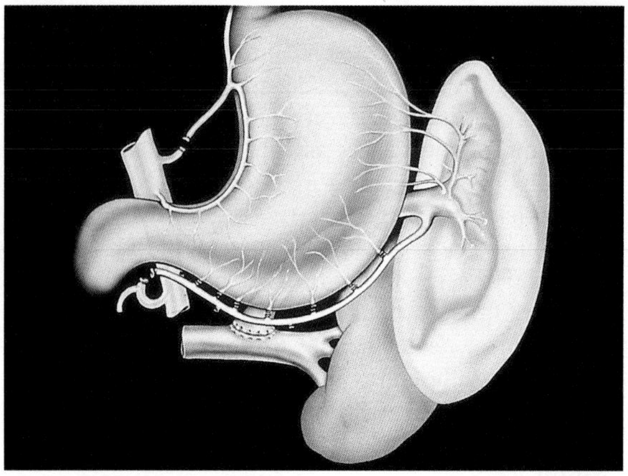

Figure 9.36 Warren distal spleno-renal shunt which results in transplenic decompression.

Selective decompression of the oesophagogastric junction is achieved by the Warren distal splenorenal shunt (Figure 9.36). In this operation, diversion of blood from the cardia is via the short gastric veins into the splenic which is anastomosed to the left renal vein in an end-to-end fashion. The objective is to preserve portal venous flow to the liver and while this is achieved in the post-operative period, it does not seem that it is maintained in the long term.

There is no indication for prophylactic portacaval shunt, for although bleeding is controlled, other complications ensue and there is no improvement in survival.

The operative mortality of shunt surgery performed for the emergency control of variceal bleeding varies from 20 to 70%. However, most results for emergency surgery are reported after prolonged attempts at conservative control and after massive blood transfusion. There is some evidence that if emergency shunts are performed as soon as resuscitation permits, the operative mortality is considerably lessened. Failure of conservative management should be followed by an alternative approach without delay.

Elective shunts can be performed with an operative mortality of about 5%. Shunt patency can be confirmed by ultrasound examination and thrombosis seems to occur in 10–15% of patients with lienorenal or distal splenorenal shunts. The figure may be higher in mesentericocaval shunts (40%) but is very low after portacaval decompression. Late rebleeding rates reflect the incidence of shunt obstruction. The results of the Atlanta trial comparing sclerotherapy with distal splenorenal shunt in the prevention of recurrent variceal haemorrhage have shown that initial sclerotherapy with resort to selective shunt in rebleeders is the optimal approach.

Prophylactic therapy

This refers to treatment of patients with portal hypertension who have never sustained variceal bleeding, the aim of the prophylactic therapy being to prevent the occurrence of haemorrhage. In this context prophylactic portosystemic shunting is contraindicated as it does not impart any benefit, and aside from the mortality, it substitutes the risks of haemorrhage with deterioration of liver function and encephalopathy. Prophylactic pharmacological therapy with beta-blockers (propranolol or nadolol) is used to prevent bleeding episodes. The dose of the beta-blocker is titrated to achieve adequate control of the wedge hepatic vein pressure. Several studies have confirmed that if the pressure is reduced by this therapy to less than 12 mmHg, the incidence of bleeding is significantly reduced. However, as previously described this medical therapy can result in significant deterioration of liver function. For this reason case selection seems sensible and it would seem appropriate to limit this prophylactic treatment to those patients with high risk factors for bleeding and in whom the liver function is good (Child A). Despite several reports, the benefit of prophylactic sclerotherapy remains unproven. The therapeutic value of calcium blocking agents in the prophylactic management of patients with portal hypertension remains uncertain.

Management of portal hypertensive gastropathy

This is a significant problem as it has a great tendency to bleed. The haemorrhage may be acute and life-threatening, or chronic, leading to iron-deficiency anaemia. Portal hypertensive gastropathy is aggravated by sclerotherapy. There is no effective medical or endoscopic management. Standard measures include correction of the coagulopathy, judicious transfusion, administration of vasopressin with nitroglycerin or somatostatin and avoidance of non-steroidal anti-flammatory drugs (NSAIDs). There is some evidence that propranolol therapy may be effective in some patients. Other agents used include sucralfate and prostaglandin analogues although the efficacy of these remains unproved. When bleeding is massive, the only possibility of salvage is total or subtotal gastrectomy but this procedure carries a high mortality in these patients.

Extrahepatic portal block

Infants and children with this condition will generally stop bleeding and require only blood transfusion. Recurrent haemorrhage in the early years is the rule but appears with lessened frequency in teenage and young adult life. Ideally, these patients may be managed with repeated sclerotherapy. With the failure of this approach, mesenteric angiography is performed and the larger venous tributaries can be used to construct 'make do' shunts to the vena cava or renal vein.

Adult patients should be amenable to stapling procedure and it is important that the site of bleeding between staples is accurately localized. If the spleen appears to be draining across the gastric fundus, it should be removed. Careful follow-up with endoscopy and sclerotherapy for residual varices is appropriate. Since most patients do not have liver disease, prognosis may be reasonably good and ascites and encephalopathy are rarely problems.

Rarer hepatic disorders

Variceal haemorrhage from patients suffering with hepatic schistosomiasis appears to have a reasonable prognosis once the condition is recognized and treated. Both devascularization procedures and full portal decompression are reported to control variceal bleeding long term. Similarly, patients with hepatic fibrosis appear to have a favourable prognosis following portal decompression for variceal bleeding. Certain types of storage disorders, e.g. type 6B glycogen storage disease and familial hypercholesterolaemia, may improve following portal venous diversion.

Disorders of the hepatic artery

The anatomy of the hepatic artery is variable and in about 20% of patients additional branches to a single common hepatic trunk arising from the coeliac axis are found. The most common variants are a supply of the left lateral lobe from the left gastric artery and there is often a major trunk running from the superior mesenteric artery alongside the common bile duct, which supplies the right lobe.

Hepatic artery occlusion

This condition may develop spontaneously in an acute fashion in patients with polyarteritis nodosa, or from an embolism or chronically from atheroma. More commonly, the occlusion is from trauma – external, surgical or radiological. Although theoretically there is a risk of hepatic infarction, this does not usually occur provided the portal vein stays patent. Common hepatic artery ligation as a deliberate step has been practised for some years to devascularize tumours and appears quite safe if the hepatic artery parenchyma is normal. Hepatic artery branch embolization by radiological means does not appear to be associated with segmental infarction. This suggests that the collateral circulation is usually quite sufficient to maintain flow via vessels in the subcapsular region, portal triad and phrenic regions. Where hepatic artery occlusion does occur, it is conventional to prescribe broad-spectrum antibiotics for 7 days.

Hepatic artery aneurysm

This interesting condition is rare but may present a diagnostic and technical challenge. Hepatic artery aneurysms account for 20% of all splanchnic artery aneurysms. The aneurysm may occur:

- In the common hepatic artery proximal to the gastroduodenal artery
- In the hepatic artery proper (distal to the gastroduodenal) or in the right or left hepatic arteries
- Within the hepatic parenchyma.

The most common aetiology is atheroma (60%) but some are of mycotic origin (infection complicating bacterial endocarditis) and a few (10%) are caused by trauma including penetrating injuries of the liver, radiological interventions and needle biopsy, cholecystectomy, etc. There is an increased incidence in patients with collagen disorders, particularly systemic lupus erythematosis (SLE).

The risk of rupture is high. Rupture may occur into the peritoneal cavity (usually fatal), the bile duct (haemobilia), the portal vein with the development of an A-V fistula or the duodenum with massive upper gastrointestinal haemorrhage.

Most hepatic artery aneurysms are encountered at middle age (4th and 5th decades) and are commoner in males (2:1). Some aneurysms are asymptomatic and discovered on imaging tests during investigation for other disorders. Two clinical syndromes are seen in symptomatic cases. The patient may present with increasing non-specific pain in the right upper quadrant, which may defy diagnosis. The aneurysm is then usually diagnosed by ultrasound examination and the lesion confirmed by CT-angiography or arteriography. The alternative presentation is similar with pain that resembles biliary colic. Jaundice develops and the patient

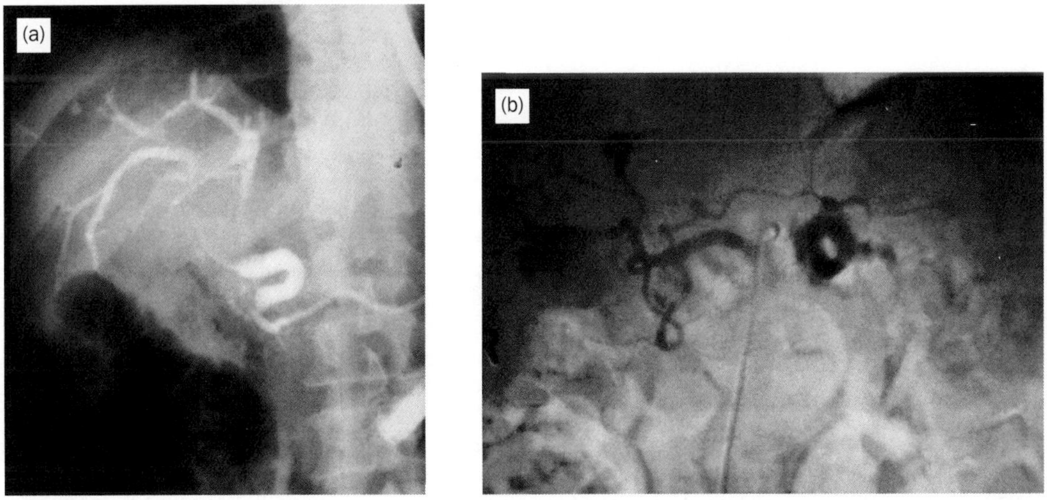

Figure 9.37 (a) An ERCP cholangiogram showing the distortion of the extrahepatic biliary tree of a patient with haemobilia. (b) A hepatic arteriogram revealed a large hepatic aneurysm arising from the right hepatic artery and rupturing into the biliary tree.

shows evidence of upper gastrointestinal haemorrhage. Acute presentation with sudden collapse and peritoneal signs indicates free rupture into the peritoneal cavity (Figure 9.37).

Management

Even asymptomatic hepatic aneurysms should be treated because of the risk of rupture.

Ideally, intrahepatic aneurysms should be managed by percutaneous embolization. The advantage of this approach is that all vessels feeding the aneurysm are identified. Nevertheless, because of the tortuosity produced by atherosclerosis, it may prove impossible to position an arterial catheter. Open operation is then required, at which time the hepatic lobar artery is isolated and filled with Gelfoam. Aneurysms in segment 2, 3 or 4 may be with by local hepatic resection (Figure 9.38).

Extrahepatic artery aneurysms require surgical treatment although transcatheter embolization has been used in some centres. If the aneurysm arises from the common hepatic artery (proximal to the gastroduodenal artery) isolation with exclusion or excision and ligation is safe if the liver function is normal, otherwise an aorto-hepatic bypass (saphenous vein or PTFE graft) is needed in addition to the excision/exclusion. Aneurysms of the hepatic artery proper or of the right/left hepatic arteries are excised with insertion of a saphenous vein graft.

Patients presenting with free intraperitoneal rupture have a dismal prognosis with an immediate or late mortality approaching 100%. Most patients presenting with aneurysm rupture into the biliary tract are salvageable. After achieving control, the aneurysm is treated as outlined above and the defect in the biliary tract closed with insertion of a T-tube.

Hepatic-arteriovenous fistulas

A-V fistulas between hepatic arteries and hepatic veins are very rare and occur as a congenital anomaly. The presentation is in infancy with intractable heart failure. Transplantation is needed for survival.

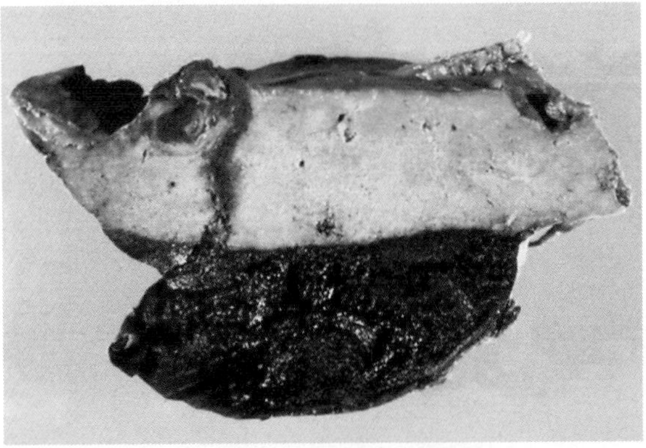

Figure 9.38 Operative specimen of left liver lobe removed from a patient with haemoperitoneum having ruptured an intrahepatic arterial aneurysm which tracked through the liver parenchyma.

A-V fistulas between the hepatic arteries and the portal vein or its branches (arterio-portal fistulas) are much commoner. These lesions are always acquired. The condition may follow the rupture of a hepatic artery aneurysm into the portal venous system (30%). Blunt and penetrating injuries (including percutaneous trans-hepatic interventional procedures) account for one-third of cases. The remainder result from mass ligation/stapling of vessels during splenectomy, pancreatic and small bowel resections. The topographical distribution of these surgical iatrogenic arterio-portal fistulas may thus be splenic, superior mesenteric, gastroduodenal and inferior mesenteric. The pathological anatomy of these iatrogenic arterio-portal fistulas is always complex with the frequent presence of a false aneurysm and multiple feeder vessels. Arterio-portal fistulas may develop spontaneously in hereditary telangliectasia.

Irrespective of origin, all arterio-portal fistulas cause portal hypertension. Initially this is sectorial and accompanied by venous congestion of the related gut mucosa (stomach, duodenum, small intestine, colon) which may cause obscure recurrent gastrointestinal haemorrhage with negative upper and lower gastrointestinal endoscopy. As collaterals develop over a period of years, the venous mucosal congestion (and bleeding) subside but portal hypertension of the entire splenic bed eventually develops with variceal bleeding most commonly from oesophageal varices.

Diagnosis is based on arteriography. In the case of iatrogenic lesions diagnosed by arteriography before the development of total hypertension, therapeutic embolization is the treatment of choice. However, this is ineffective in established cases with false aneurysm and multiple feeder vessels, when a direct surgical approach is needed. This consists of excision of the fistula after ligation of all the feeder vessels identified by pre-operative arteriography. Portal decompression by shunting is universally unsuccessful in these cases.

Budd–Chiari syndrome

The syndrome of abdominal pain with intractable ascites is diagnosed not infrequently and has considerable surgical implications. The problem arises from an obstruction to the hepatic venous system at any point from lobule to right heart. Strictly speaking, the term Budd–Chiari should be restricted to those patients with occlusion (usually thrombosis) in the major hepatic veins and/or adjacent suprahepatic vena cava, and the term veno-occlusive disease to obliteration (usually by sclerosis) of the smaller intrahepatic veins that may develop following ingestion of certain alkaloids, after chemotherapy, bone marrow transplantation and irradiation of the liver.

Budd–Chiari syndrome is more common in women and some cases have been attributed to oestrogen–progesterone oral contraceptives. Others are caused by haematological disorders, e.g. polycythaemia, paroxysmal nocturnal haemoglobinaemia, antithrombin III deficiency and haemolytic anaemias. Collagen disorders such as lupus erythematosus, sarcoidosis and rheumatoid arthritis also predispose the affected individuals to the disorder. As the same effects are produced by suprahepatic vena caval obstruction, about one-third of cases are associated with obstruction of this organ. The aetiology may be fibrosis from previous trauma, primary or secondary tumours of the liver, adrenal, kidney or vena cava itself and a well-established condition in which a web of presumed congenital origin is found across the lumen of the vena cava. This condition is well described in Japanese patients. In veno-occlusive disease, hepatic vein thrombosis may be widespread in the various radicles of the liver or distinctly patchy.

In chronic cases of Budd–Chiari, the veins are replaced by a fibrous band but the caudate lobe which has a hepatic venous drainage survives and even enlarges enough to produce a separate caval obstruction. On histological examination the predominant feature is of centrizonal venous congestion with necrosis of the surrounding cells and areas of haemorrhage.

The condition may present fairly acutely with severe abdominal pain and vomiting and a large tender liver with ascites. Where the problem is secondary to an underlying malignancy, clearly those features may predominate. The condition may progress rapidly over a few weeks to hepatic failure, coma and death. The more chronic form presents in similar fashion but at a reduced tempo and with less evidence of hepatic failure. There is usually peripheral oedema, which extends on to the thighs if the vena cava becomes progressively obstructed. Serum liver function tests show disturbance but are not diagnostic. Provided that the clotting parameters will permit it, an early recourse to liver biopsy is essential. However, given the patchy nature of the condition, other diagnostic tests may be required. Ultrasound can be very effective in the sense that hepatic veins, which are normally demonstrable, are absent and a hepatic scintiscan may be grossly abnormal with poor general uptake except by the caudate lobe, which may show normal or greater than normal uptake. These two tests indicate the need for hepatic venography and inferior vena cavography to demonstrate the site of venous blockade. Other conditions such as cirrhosis, malignant ascites, heart failure and constrictive pericarditis clearly require to be excluded.

Treatment and prognosis

As might be expected the prognosis is variable and dependent upon the extent of venous thrombosis. For patients with a rapid deterioration, hepatic transplantation is needed for survival. Mild cases can be managed with low sodium diet and diuretics and spontaneous improvement appears to occur in some patients, presumably as the veins recanalize, and prolonged survival is recorded. The moderately severe patients present more of a problem as the time course may be relatively short (3–4 years). As anticoagulants and fibrinolysins appear of no benefit, the ascites has to be managed by portal and hepatic decompression. A side-to-side portacaval shunt can accomplish this provided the inferior vena cava is not obstructed. A prosthetic meso-atrial shunt constructed between the superior mesenteric vein and the right atrium with special precautions to avoid constriction at the diaphragm is used in the presence of caval occlusion, although some favour a combined side to side portacaval shunt and a caval atrial shunt in these cases. Inferior vena caval webs or diaphragms can be dealt with by balloon angioplasty but more commonly require surgical finger or dilator 'membranotomy' through the right atrial appendage. Hepatic transplantation is indicated in patients with chronic Budd–Chiari and deteriorating hepatic function or after failed shunt surgery.

Further reading

Alvarez, O. A., Vanegas, F., Maze, G. L. *et al.* (2000). Polymicrobial cholangitis and liver abscess in a patient with the acquired immunodeficiency syndrome. *South Med J* **93**: 232–4.

Barakate, M. S., Stephen, M. S., Waugh, R. C. *et al.* (1999). Pyogenic liver abscess: a review of 10 years' experience in management. *Aust N Z J Surg* **69**: 205–9.

Berenguer, M. and Wright, T. L. (1999). Hepatitis C and liver transplantation. *Gut* **45**: 159–63.

Bismuth, H., Houssin, D., Ornowski, J. and Meriggi, F. (1986). Liver resections in cirrhotic patients: a western experience. *World J Surg* **10**: 311–17.

Chatelain, D., Chailley-Heu, B., Terris, B. *et al.* (2000). The ciliated hepatic foregut cyst, an unusual bronchiolar foregut malformation: a histological, histochemical, and immunohistochemical study of 7 cases. *Hum Pathol* **31**: 241–6.

Cuschieri, A., Bracken, J. and Boni, L. (1999). Initial experience with laparoscopic ultrasound-guided radiofrequency thermal ablation of hepatic tumours. *Endoscopy* **31**: 318–21.

De Baere, T., Roche, A., Elais, D. *et al.* (1996). Preoperative portal vein embolisation for extension of hepatectomy indications. *Hepatology* **24**: 1386–91.

De Baere, T., Roche, A., Vavavasseur, D. *et al.* (1993). Portal vein embolisation: utility for inducing left hepatic lobe hypertrophy befor surgery. *Cardiovascular Radiology* **183**: 73–7.

Dharmarajan, T. S., Tankala, H., Ahmed, S. *et al.* (2000). Pyogenic liver abscess: a geriatric problem. *J Am Geriatr Soc* **48**: 1022–3.

DiChiro, G. and Fulham, M. (1993). Virchow's shackles: can PET-FDG challenge tumour histology? *AJNR* **14**: 524–7.

Dull, J. S., Topa, L., Balgha, V. and Pap, A. (2000). Non-surgical treatment of biliary liver abscesses: efficacy of endoscopic drainage and local antibiotic lavage with nasobiliary catheter. *Gastrointest Endosc* **51**: 55–9.

Fasel, J. H. D., Selle, D., Evertsz, C. J. G. *et al.* (1998). Segmental anatomy of the liver: poor correlation with CT. *Radiology* **206**: 151–6.

Filice, C., Brunetti, E., Bruno, R. and Crippa, F. G. (2000). Clinical management of hepatic abscesses in HIV patients. *Am J Gastroenterol* **95**: 1092–3.

Freeny, P. C. (1997). Helical computed tomography of the liver: techniques, applications and pitfalls. *Endoscopy* **29**: 515–23.

Germer, C. T., Albrecht, D., Roggan, A. and Buhr, H. J. (1998). Technology for *in situ* ablation by laparoscopic and image-guided interstitial laser hyperthermia. *Semin Laparosc Surg* **5**: 195–203.

Hoffner, R. J., Kilaghbian, T., Esekogwu, V. I. and Henderson, S. O. (1999). Common presentations of amebic liver abscess. *Ann Emerg Med* **34**: 351–5.

Ibrarullah, M. D., Sreenivasa, D., Sriram, P *et al.* Padhy, B. P. (1999). Giant non-parasitic hepatic cyst with biliary communication. *Trop Gastroenterol* **20**: 142–3.

Jain, D., Sarode, V. R., Abdul-Karim, F. W. *et al.* (2000). Evidence for the neoplastic transformation ofVon-Meyenburg complexes. *Am J Surg Pathol* **24**: 1131–9.

Jalan, R. and Hayes, P. C. (2000). For British Society of Gastroenterology. UK guidelines on the management of variceal haemorrhage in cirrhotic patients. *Gut* **46**(Suppl): 1–15.

Javid, G., Wani, N. A., Gulzar, G. M. *et al.* (1999). Ascaris-induced liver abscess. *World J Surg* **23**: 1191–4.

Lam, Y. H., Wong, S. K., Lee, D. W. *et al.* (1999). ERCP and pyogenic liver abscess. *Gastrointest Endosc* **50**: 340–4.

Lau, H., Man, K., Fan, S. T. *et al.* (1997). Evaluation of preoperative hepatic function in patients with hepatocellular carcinoma undergoing hepatectomy. *Br J Surg* **84**: 1255–9.

Lim, H. E., Cheong, H. J., Woo, H. J. *et al.* (1999). Pylephlebitis associated with appendicitis. *Korean J Intern Med* **14**: 73–6.

Mahfouz, A.-E., Hamm, B. and Taupiz, M. (1997). Hepatic magnetic resonance imaging: new techniques and contrast agents. *Endoscopy* **29**: 504–14.

Marusawa, H., Osaki, Y., Kimura, T. *et al.* (1999). High prevalence of anti-hepatis B virus serological markers in patients with hepatic C virus related chronic liver disease in Japan. *Gut* **45**: 284–8.

Misra, A., Loyalka, P. and Alva, F. (1999). Portal hypertension due to extensive hepatic cysts in autosomal dominant polycystic kidney disease. *South Med J* **92**: 626–7.

Odev, K., Paksoy, Y., Arslan, A. *et al.* (2000). Sonographically guided percutaneous treatment of hepatic hydatid cysts: long-term results. *J Clin Ultrasound* **28**: 469–78.

Ogata, H., Tsuji, H., Hizawa, K. *et al.* (2000). Multilocular pyogenic hepatic abscess complicating *Ascaris lumbricoides* infestation. *Intern Med* **39**: 228–30.

Ogawa, T., Shimizu, S., Morisaki, T. *et al.* (1999). The role of percutaneous transhepatic abscess drainage for liver abscess. *J Hepatobiliary Pancreat Surg* **6**: 263–6.

Patanakar, T., Prasad, S., Armao, D. and Mukherji, S. K. (2000). Tuberculous abscesses of the liver. *Am J Roentgenol* **174**: 1166–7.

Philosophe, B., Grieg, P. D., Hemming, A. W. *et al.* (1998). Surgical management of hepatocellular carcinoma: resection or transplantation? *J Gastroinest Surg* **2**: 21–7.

Plauth, M., Merli, M., Kindrup, J. *et al.* (1997). ESPEN guidelines for nutrition in liver disease and transplantation. *Clin Nutr* **16**: 43–55.

Schalm, S. W., Heathcote, J., Cianciara, J. *et al.* (2000). Lamivudine and alpha interferon combination treatment of patients with chronic hepatitis B infection: a randomised trial. *Gut* **46**: 562–8.

Seeto, R. K. and Rockey, D. C. (1999). Amebic liver abscess: epidemiology, clinical features, and outcome. *West J Med* **170**: 104–9.

Vadejar, H. J., Doran, J. D., Charnley, R. and Ryder, D. (1999). Saphenoperitoneal shunts for patients with intractable ascites associated with chronic liver disease. *Br J Surg* **86**: 882–5.

Vick, D. J., Goodman, Z. D., Deavers, M. T. *et al.* (1999). Ciliated hepatic foregut cyst: a study of six cases and review of the literature. *Am J Surg Pathol* **23**: 671–7.

Zimmerman, H. and Reichen, J. (1998). Hepatectomy: preoperative analysis of hepatic function and postoperative liver failure. *Dig Surg* **15**: 1–11.

MODULE 10

Disorders of the biliary tract

Section 10.1 • Surgical anatomy

Biliary tract

The right hepatic duct is formed by the intrahepatic union of the dorsocaudal and ventrocranial branches draining the two sectors of the right liver (segments V–VIII) (Figure 10.1). The ventrocranial duct is in direct line with the right hepatic duct and crosses in front of the dorsocaudal branch as this arches downwards before reaching the confluence of the two ducts. The left hepatic duct, which is formed by medial and lateral branches draining segments II–IV, is longer than the right hepatic duct. It follows a partial extrahepatic course (of variable length depending on the width of the quadrate lobe) and, therefore, dilates readily in the presence of distal obstructive disease. The extrahepatic portion of the left duct and its segment III branch can be accessed surgically at the hilum by following the insertion of the round ligament (ligamentum teres) in the depths of the recessus of Rex (Figure 10.2). This 'round ligament' approach is an effective method of bilio-enteric bypass for inoperable cholangiocarcinoma of the extrahepatic ducts.

The union of the right and left hepatic ducts is usually extrahepatic (90% within 1.0 cm of liver parenchyma), high up in the porta hepatis. The resulting common hepatic duct receives the cystic duct lower down, whereupon it becomes the common bile duct. It is customary, however, in surgical anatomy to use the term 'common bile duct' or simply 'bile duct' for the entire extrahepatic conduit as it obviates difficulties in nomenclature, especially when there is a low insertion of the cystic duct. The junction of the right and left hepatic ducts is also referred to as the *hilar bifurcation*. Together with the hepatic artery to its left and the portal vein behind, the common bile duct is surrounded by fibrous tissue known as the Glissonian sheath. At the hilum this is thickened and forms a condensation that

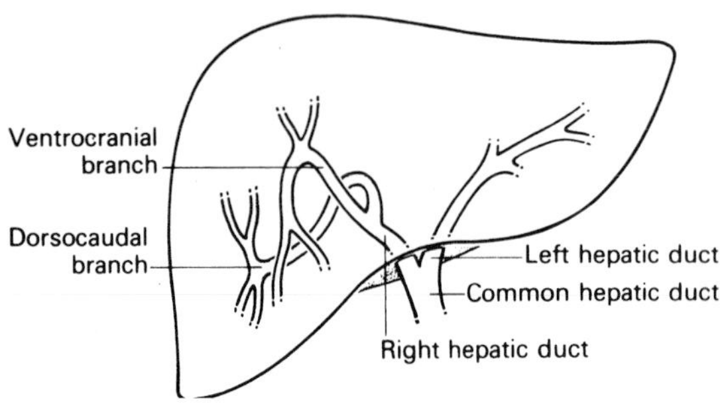

Figure 10.1 Frontal schematic view of the liver illustrating the intrahepatic biliary tree and the ductal arrangement at the hilus. Note the left duct has a longer extrahepatic course. Within the liver, the dorsocaudal branch of the right hepatic duct curves acutely posterior to the ventrocranial branch.

is often referred to as the *hilar plate*. If the liver is incised anteriorly and posteriorly (between the hilum and the caudate lobe) to the hilar plate, finger dissection enables the mobilization of the main divisions of the hepatic duct, hepatic artery and portal vein (Figure 10.3). This manoeuvre allows inferior displacement and thus access in case of high bile duct strictures. It is also used for segmental resections of the liver.

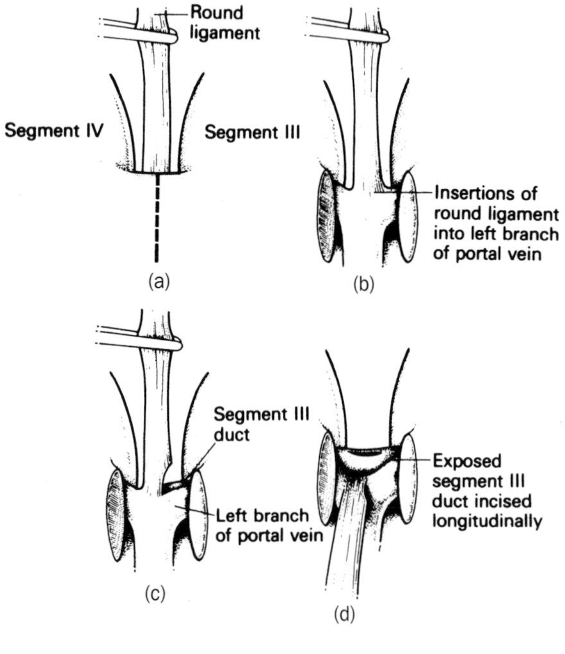

Figure 10.2 Diagrammatic representation of the round ligament approach to segment III duct: (a) the round ligament leads to the umbilical fissure between segment IV and segment III which are often joined by a bridge of liver tissue that overlaps the terminal insertions of the round ligament into the left branch of the portal vein; (b) the bridge of liver tissue has been divided to expose the vascular terminations of the round ligament to the left branch of the portal vein; (c) the terminations of the round ligament have been suture ligated and divided to expose the left branch of the portal vein; (d) downward traction displaces the left branch of the portal vein with exposure of segment III duct which is divided longitudinally for anastomosis to a loop of jejunum.

Ductal anomalies

The intrahepatic arrangement outlined above applies in 75% of cases. A different arrangement is encountered in the remainder when either the right dorsocaudal or ventro-cranial ducts join the left hepatic duct, or the common hepatic duct forms a trifurcation (Figure 10.4a–d). The majority (75–80%) of intrahepatic calculi are located in the left hepatic duct and right-sided calculi, which are far less common, are usually found in the ventrocranial branch of the right hepatic duct.

Important extrahepatic anomalies sometimes referred to as 'aberrant ducts' are encountered in 15–19% of patients. In fact, these 'anomalous/aberrant ducts' represent an extrahepatic confluence of a segmental duct and in the vast majority (95%) affect the right system, when the aberrant duct joins the right hepatic duct (extrahepatically), or common hepatic duct or cystic duct, and very rarely, the gallbladder.

Gallbladder and cystic duct

The gallbladder is a pear-shaped sac about 10 cm in length and is situated on the inferior surface of segment V of the right liver. It is covered with a layer of peritoneum that contains many small veins that require coag-

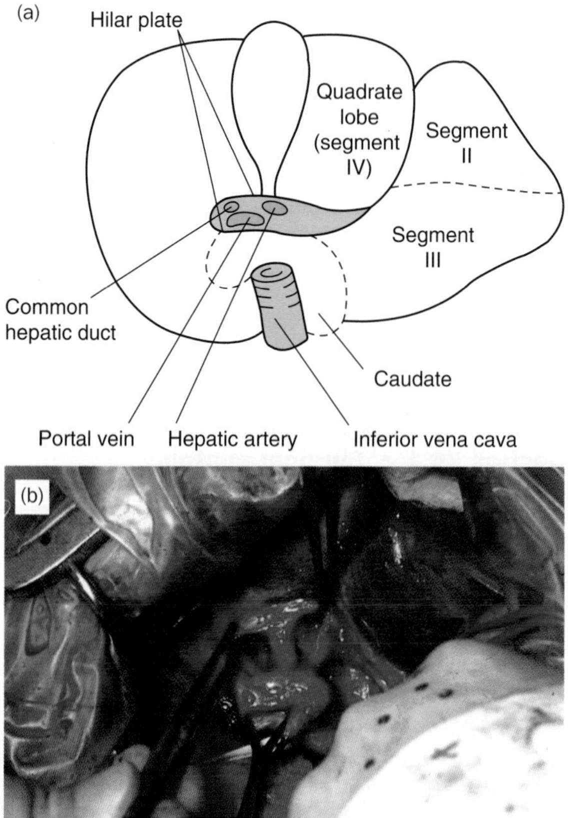

Figure 10.3 (a) Schematic representation of the hilar plate on the inferior surface of the liver. The intrahepatic hilar structures can be displaced downwards by division of the hilar plate anteriorly and behind the portal vein between it and the caudate lobe; (b) operative exposure by this technique during remedial surgery for a high bile duct stricture.

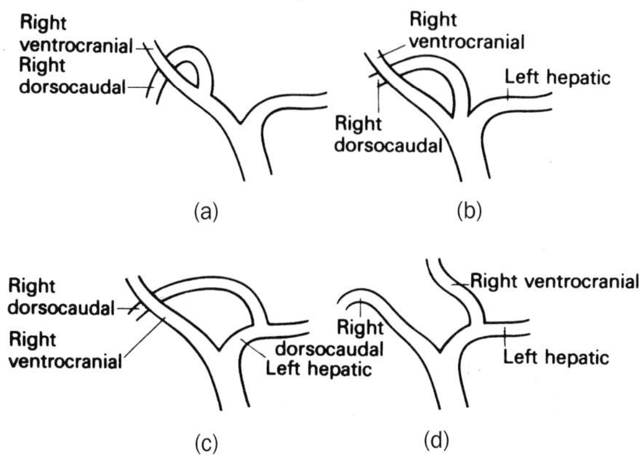

Figure 10.4 Variations in the confluence of the major intrahepatic ducts: (a) normal arrangement which is found in 75% of cases; (b) trifurcation where the right ventrocranial, right dorsocaudal and the left hepatic ducts arise simultaneously from the common hepatic duct, there being no right hepatic duct; (c) termination of the right dorsocaudal branch into the left hepatic duct; (d) termination of the right ventrocranial duct into the left hepatic duct.

ulation during cholecystectomy. It is customarily divided into the fundus, which has the poorest blood supply, especially when the organ is distended, the body and the neck or infundibulum which leads to the cystic duct. Not infrequently, the neck has an abnormal sacculation, which is referred to as Hartmann's pouch. This may become adherent to the surrounding structures of the porta hepatis, particularly the common bile duct, seriously obscuring anatomical relationships during dissection of this region.

The cystic duct runs a variable course from the neck of the gallbladder to join the common hepatic duct. Its mucosa is arranged in a spiral fold or valve (valve of Heister), which often causes difficulties in cannulation during operative transcystic cholangiography. Although most anatomical textbooks indicate that the cystic duct joins the bile duct along its right margin, several large series of surgical dissections and analyses of operative cholangiograms demonstrate clearly that this arrangement is rare and is only encountered in 15–20% of cases. Much more commonly, the cystic duct enters the bile duct either posteriorly or anteriorly (40%). It may also pursue a spiral or a parallel course with the bile duct, with the two structures being enclosed in a common fibrous sheath that tends to obscure the exact location of the entry of the cystic duct into the bile duct (Figure 10.5). The spiral cystic duct runs down and behind the common hepatic duct to enter on its medial aspect (35%). The parallel cystic duct runs parallel to the bile duct for a variable distance before entering it. This is the rarest arrangement and is encountered in 5–7% of patients. Rarely, the cystic duct joins the right hepatic duct and very infrequently the left duct.

Anomalies of the gallbladder

The most common anomaly of the gallbladder encountered during surgery is the Phyrgian cap where the fundus is constricted and turned back on itself. The fully intrahepatic gallbladder is rare. The so-called floating gallbladder, which has a complete serosal covering and a dorsal mesentery, is relatively uncommon, as is malposition of the gallbladder and double gallbladder.

The floating gallbladder predisposes to torsion, which simulates acute cholecystitis. An elongated sausage-shaped gallbladder frequently accompanies congenital cystic disease of the bile ducts. Agenesis (congenital absence) of the gallbladder is very rare and the condition can only be diagnosed at laparotomy in a patient who has not undergone previous biliary tract surgery. Another rare anomaly is the trabeculated gallbladder, but this usually causes symptoms similar to chronic cholecystitis and is associated with abnormal gallbladder emptying.

A left-sided gallbladder is an integral component of *situs inversus*. In the absence of this condition, malposition is generally regarded as a very rare anomaly. Thus a collective review of the Western literature yielded only 24 cases of left-sided gallbladder. Two types of gallbladder malposition have been described – *medioposition* of the gallbladder and *sinistroposition* (transposition). In medioposition, the gallbladder is displaced medially to lie on the under surface of the quadrate lobe (segment IV) but still on the right side of the round ligament. In sinistroposition, the gallbladder lies under the left lobe (segment III) to the left of the round ligament (Figure 10.6). Despite its alleged rare incidence the authors have encountered five cases of sinistroposition in a consecutive series of 1764 patients undergoing laparoscopic cholecystectomy, a prevalence of 0.28%. The resulting pathological anatomy has implications for the safe conduct of laparoscopic cholecystectomy. Despite the left-sided location of the gallbladder, the biliary pain experienced by these

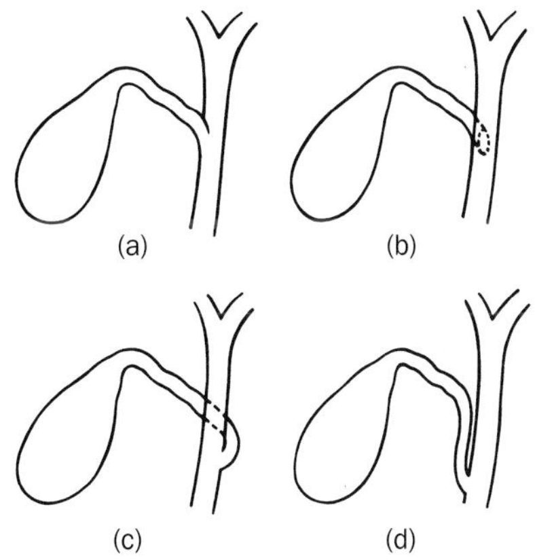

Figure 10.5 Schematic representation of the termination of the cystic duct: (a) lateral insertion often depicted as the usual arrangement but which is only encountered in 15–20% of patients; (b) anterior or posterior termination – this is the most common type and accounts for 40% of cases; (c) spiral cystic duct which courses behind the bile duct to open on its medial aspect – this is fairly common and is found in 35% of patients; (d) parallel cystic duct – this is the rarest arrangement and is encountered in 5–7% of patients.

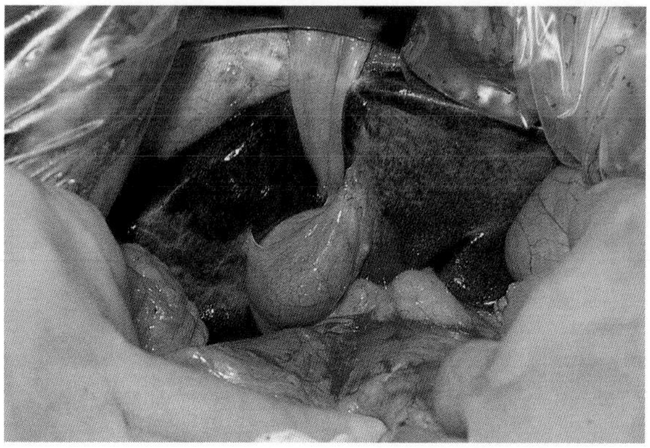

Figure 10.6 Operative photograph of sinistroposition of the gallbladder which lies under the left lobe (segment III) to the left of the round ligament. Despite the left-sided location of the gallbladder, the biliary pain experienced by these patients is always on the right side.

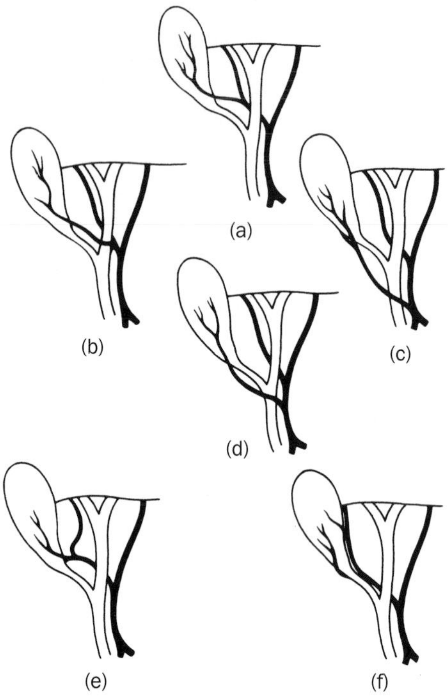

Figure 10.7 Anomalies of the cystic artery: (a) normal arrangement where the cystic artery arises from the right hepatic artery soon after this emerges from behind the common hepatic duct; (b) origin of the cystic artery from the right hepatic to the left of the bile duct, the cystic artery then crossing in front of the common hepatic duct; (c) low origin of the cystic artery from the common hepatic or gastroduodenal arteries; (d) accessory cystic artery arising from the hepatic artery – this second artery can also arise from the left hepatic, right hepatic and gastroduodenal arteries; (e) looped right hepatic artery with a short cystic artery arising from the summit of the right hepatic arterial arch; (f) the right hepatic runs close to the cystic duct and the neck of the gallbladder before giving anterior and posterior cystic branches – this anomaly is the most dangerous since the right hepatic is easily mistaken for a large cystic artery.

patients is always on the right side. The pre-operative diagnosis of this anomaly is made only rarely despite routine preoperative external ultrasonography and selective recourse to endoscopic retrograde cholangiopancreatography (ERCP). In sinistroposition, the cystic artery always crosses in front of the common bile duct from right to left. The cystic duct may open on the left or right side of the common hepatic duct. The anomaly does not preclude safe laparoscopic cholecystectomy but modifications of the port sites and the use of the falciform lift facilitate the procedure in these cases.

The arterial supply of the gallbladder is by means of the cystic artery, which usually arises from the right hepatic artery. The cystic artery is an end-artery and its occlusion is followed by gangrene of the gallbladder. There are several congenital anomalies of the arterial supply of the gallbladder (Figure 10.7), the most important of which is a short cystic artery arising from a looped right hepatic artery. All these arterial anomalies are however important and must be recognized during cholecystectomy before ligature of the 'cystic artery'. Careful display and verification of the anatomy is the single most important factor in the prevention of arterial bleeding and iatrogenic injuries during cholecystectomy and biliary tract surgery.

Common bile duct

The bile duct (choledochus) is formed by the union of the right and left hepatic ducts each draining the respective hemi-liver. It is joined at a variable distance along its course by the cystic duct. In strict anatomical terms, the segment between the hilar bifurcation and the cystic duct is referred to as the common hepatic duct and the term common bile duct is reserved for the portion distal to this junction. From the surgical standpoint, however, it is best to consider it as one structure, which is divisible into the *supraduodenal*, *retroduodenal*, *intrapancreatic* and *intraduodenal* segments. It serves as a conduit of bile from the liver and gallbladder to the duodenal papilla, and in the adult measures 11–12 cm in length with an average diameter of 7 mm, range 4–10 mm.

The supraduodenal segment is important surgically because it is the area that is most commonly explored. It lies in the free edge of the hepatoduodenal ligament to the right of the hepatic artery and anterolateral to the portal vein. The retroduodenal segment curves to the right away from the portal vein behind the first part of the duodenum before entering the head of the pancreas – intrapancreatic segment. However, in 20% of patients the duct has a partial or complete extrapancreatic course. The transduodenal segment (also known as the infundibulum) which traverses obliquely the duodenal wall and usually joins the pancreatic duct, opens into the duodenal lumen at the summit of the major duodenal papilla. The lower end of the common bile duct, therefore, deviates to the right before entering the lumen of the duodenum almost at right angles. This is an important practical consideration since forcible probing through this area may perforate the bile duct

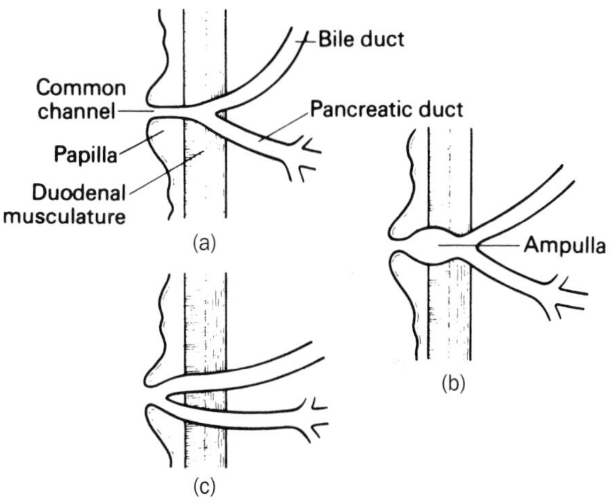

Figure 10.8 Configuration of the lower end of the common bile and pancreatic ducts: (a) the two ducts join to form a common channel, which opens at the summit of the duodenal papilla – this is the most common arrangement; (b) there is a localized dilatation of the common channel to form the ampulla of Vater; (c) the two ducts open separately into the duodenum.

and result in a haematoma, post-operative pancreatitis, choledochoduodenal fistula or stricture of the lower end of the bile duct.

The main pancreatic duct (Wirsung) joins the posteromedial wall of the transduodenal segment of the bile duct to form a common channel in 90% of cases. A localized dilatation of the common channel to form an ampulla of Vater is uncommon (10–20%) and in 10% of patients the two ducts open separately into the duodenum (Figure 10.8).

The Vaterian segment includes the lower 2.5–3.0 cm of the common bile duct, the distal part of the pancreatic duct, the ampulla or common channel and the major duodenal papilla. These structures are surrounded by a condensation of circular and longitudinal smooth muscle fibres often referred to as the sphincter of Oddi, although it was Boyden who described the detailed anatomy of the various components of this sphincteric complex. The inferior sphincter is the strongest component and is also known as the papillary muscular ball (Figure 10.9). It surrounds the terminations of the bile and pancreatic ducts and the common channel. The middle sphincter is the longest and the thinnest of the components and surrounds the transduodenal and a variable portion of the transpancreatic segments of the bile duct and the duct of Wirsung. The superior sphincters consist of localized thickenings of the middle sphincters around the bile and pancreatic ducts at the proximal end of the sphincter complex.

An important variation of the anatomy of the Vaterian segment is the condition known as *pancreas divisum*, which results from failure of fusion of the ventral and dorsal pancreas during embryological development. The duct of the ventral pancreas, which normally forms the main pancreatic duct, remains rudimentary and drains the lower portion of the pancreatic head and the uncinate process. The rest of the pancreas is drained through the duct of the dorsal anlage (duct of Santorini) which opens through the small accessory papilla above the major duodenal ampulla. The incidence of pancreas divisum in the general population is 5–8% but the condition is much commoner in patients with idiopathic recurrent pancreatitis (approximately 25%) and an aetiological relationship has been suggested.

The rest of the common bile duct contains few muscle fibres. Its epithelial lining rests on a loose stroma containing elastic fibres, which disappear with age or disease. Thus, stone impaction, prolonged distension or cholangitis may lead to rigidity of the common bile duct. The narrowest portion of the common bile duct occurs at its point of entrance into the duodenal wall and this area is often indicated by a notch on the cholangiogram. The diameter of the transduodenal segment is normally 5 mm and that of the major duodenal papilla varies from 0.5 to 1.5 mm. The commonest site for calculus arrest or impaction is just proximal to the transduodenal segment. The major duodenal papilla is situated on the posteromedial aspect of the second part of the duodenum about 7.0–10.0 cm from the pylorus. Its appearance may vary from the usual well-defined papilla with varying degrees of projection to a flattened depression between the mucosal folds. Irrespective of its exact configuration, the major duodenal papilla frequently has a dorsal mucosal fold. The papilla is more easily located by ERCP than by direct inspection during surgical intervention. The minor (accessory) papilla is more proximally situated and assumes clinical importance only in patients with pancreas divisum.

The activity of the choledochal sphincteric complex is independent of the duodenal musculature but may be influenced by it. Thus, the effect of certain drugs on the choledochal sphincter differs from their action on the duodenal wall, and duodenal muscular peristaltic activity has no significant effect on the common bile duct pressure. The choledochal sphincter is an active structure and measures up to 2.5 cm in length. It

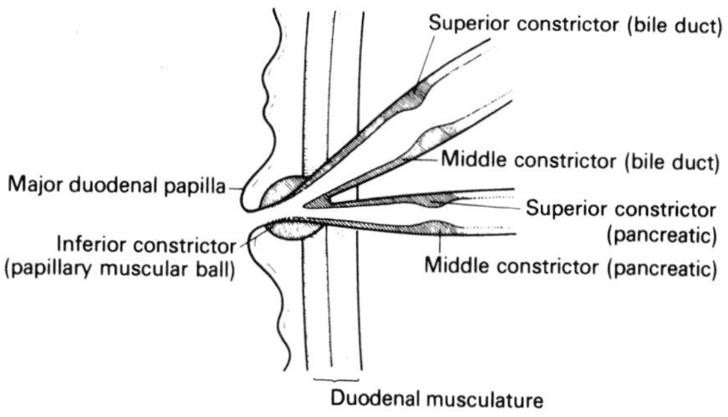

Figure 10.9 Diagrammatic representation of the components of the sphincter complex (sphincter of Oddi) surrounding the Vaterian segment. The bile and pancreatic ducts are illustrated splayed apart to facilitate the demonstration. Normally the terminal portions of both ducts are contiguous.

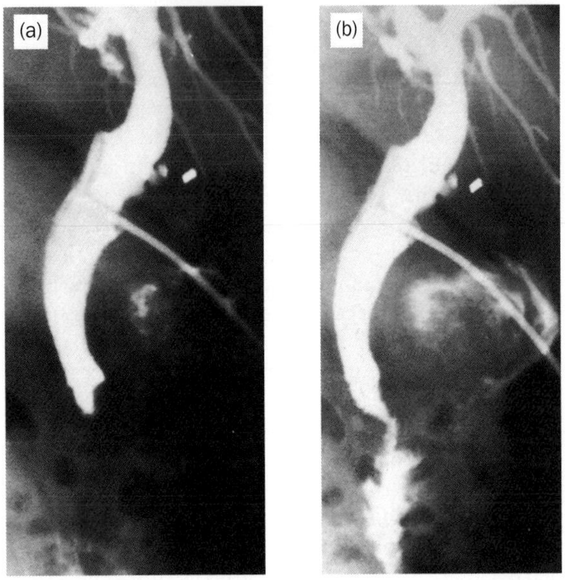

Figure 10.10 The pseudocalculus phenomenon: (a) during the systolic phase of choledochal sphincter action, there is an apparent detachment of the lower end of the common bile duct outline from the duodenal contrast shadow with an inverted meniscus effect, the appearance simulating a stone impacted at this site; (b) this 'filling defect' disappears when the same bile duct is visualized during diastole (relaxation) of the sphincter.

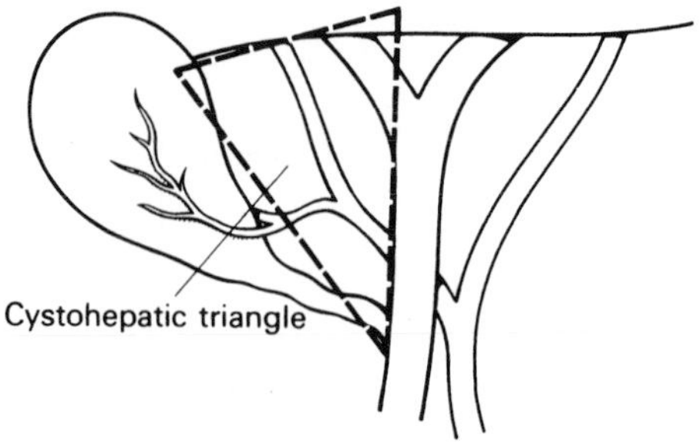

Figure 10.11 Cystohepatic triangle of Calot formed by the cystic duct and neck of the gallbladder inferiorly, the liver edge superiorly and the common hepatic duct medially. It contains the cystic artery and lymph node and the right hepatic artery as it emerges from behind the common hepatic duct. The vast majority of aberrant/anomalous bile ducts arise from the right ductal system (especially the dorsocaudal branch of the right hepatic) and 80% are located in the cystohepatic triangle of Calot.

consists of well-developed longitudinal and circular smooth muscle. Contraction of the longitudinal muscle tends to open the duct lumen, whereas the circular muscle has the opposite effect. These contracted (systolic) and relaxed (diastolic) states of the choledochal sphincter lead to quite distinct appearances of the lower end of the common bile duct at cholangiography. During contraction, contrast often forms a meniscus with the concavity facing downwards simulating a stone (the pseudocalculus phenomenon) (Figure 10.10).

Cystohepatic triangle of Calot

The cystohepatic triangle is important in biliary surgery especially in the performance of cholecystectomy. It is a triangular fold of peritoneum containing the cystic duct, cystic artery, cystic node and a variable amount of fat. It also often contains the right hepatic artery which usually enters the triangle behind the common hepatic duct and before it gives off the cystic artery, after which it curves upwards along the right hepatic duct to the liver. The cystic lymph node is most commonly situated at the junction of the cystic with the common hepatic artery. The vast majority of aberrant/anomalous bile ducts arise from the right ductal system (especially the dorsocaudal branch of the right hepatic) and 80% are located in the cystohepatic triangle of Calot (Figure 10.11). The cystohepatic triangle is virtually obliterated in the presence of Mirizzi's syndrome (*vide infra*).

Lymphatic drainage of the gallbladder

Proximally, the lymphatic channels of the gallbladder communicate with those of the Glisson's capsule of the liver. The hepatic capsular lymphatics drain into the thoracic duct except those on the superior surface of the liver, flow from which reaches the retrosternal lymph nodes via several channels. Distally, the gallbladder lymphatics and those of the extrahepatic bile ducts drain into the cystic lymph node which is situated near the cystic artery close to its origin from the right hepatic artery, and to other nodes lateral to the lower end of the bile duct, particularly the retroduodenal segment.

Hepatic artery

The adult hepatic artery is derived from the middle of the three primordial arteries that supply the fetal liver. The usual arrangement is for the common hepatic artery to arise from the coeliac axis. After giving off the right gastric and gastroduodenal arteries behind the antroduodenal region, it arches upwards along the left side of the bile duct and in front of the portal vein. It then bifurcates into the right and left hepatic arteries usually quite close to the liver. The right hepatic artery usually crosses behind (rarely in front of) the common hepatic duct before giving rise to the cystic artery. Low division of the hepatic artery is encountered in 15% of patients when the right hepatic artery courses behind the portal vein.

The important anomalies are the result of persistence of the left or right primordial hepatic arteries. The most common (20%) is persistence of the left primordial artery. This anomalous vessel then arises from the left gastric artery or directly from the aorta and traverses the lesser omentum to enter the liver in the umbilical fissure. It is very rare for a persistent left primordial hepatic artery to be the main or only arterial supply to the liver; usually it is present in addition to the normal hepatic artery. Persistence of the right primordial artery results in an anomalous right hepatic artery originating from the superior mesenteric. It ascends to the liver behind the pancreas and duodenum to reach the free edge of the hepatoduodenal ligament. Again it is very rare for a persistent right primordial hepatic artery to provide the sole arterial blood supply to the liver.

Section 10.2 • Surgical biliary physiology

Hepatic cholesterol and bile acid physiology

The liver plays a key role in the metabolism of cholesterol. It regulates the uptake of dietary cholesterol, its *de novo* synthesis and the excretion of this lipid in bile either as free cholesterol or as bile acids. There is increasing evidence for metabolic compartmentalization of cholesterol within the hepatocyte, i.e. cholesterol derived from extrahepatic sources is metabolized differently from that synthesized in the liver, the latter being destined for bile acid synthesis via the 7-alpha hydroxylation step, after which it is no longer available for esterification.

Under normal conditions, sufficient bile acids are synthesized to make up for the enteric losses, and to this extent the synthesis of bile acids by the liver is generally believed to be controlled by the circulating bile salt concentration, although there is some debate on the importance of this feedback control mechanism [See Module 11, Vol. 1]. The primary bile acids are conjugated within the hepatocyte with the amino acids glycine and taurine, before being secreted into the bile canaliculi. Toxic relatively insoluble secondary bile salts (reabsorbed from the small intestinal pool) such as lithocholic acid are sulphated prior to excretion. Cholesterol is transported into the bile canaliculi as phospholipid-cholesterol vesicles. The formation of phospholipid-cholesterol-bile acid micelles is a post-canalicular event induced by the high concentrations of bile acids in the hepatic bile. There is evidence that high concentrations of deoxycholic acid may promote the hepatic secretion of cholesterol saturated bile and thereby induce the nucleation of cholesterol crystals.

Bile secretion

The secretion of bile by the liver is largely dependent on the influx of bile acids, which consists of a large component made up of bile salts that have been reabsorbed from the small intestine into the portal venous blood, and a smaller component of newly synthesized bile acids. There is a small bile acid-independent fraction of bile secretion, which is reduced in experimental cholestasis, whereas the bile acid-dependent fraction increases under these conditions.

Somatostatin decreases both the bile acid flow and bile ductular secretion indicating a suppression of *de novo* bile acid synthesis by the hepatocytes. By contrast, vasoactive intestinal polypeptide (VIP) increases the bile flow in man by a mechanism which is similar to that of secretin. The basal or resting (interdigestive) common bile duct pressure that averages 6.0 mmHg ensures the continued patency of the lumen of the choledochus but is insufficient to overcome the resistance of the choledochal sphincter. The hepatic bile is stored and partitioned in the gallbladder, although the patterns of gallbladder filling and emptying are incompletely understood. Eating results in the cholecystokinetic response consisting of contraction of the gallbladder and relaxation of the sphincter of Oddi that results in the timely delivery of bile salts into the intestinal tract. This response is mediated by known hormonal mechanisms (cholecystokinin) and poorly understood neural reflexes. Studies have shown that gallbladder emptying occurs before the onset of gastric emptying of a meal, suggesting a cephalic neural reflex. Gallbladder contractions also occur during the interdigestive period and, in the human, these are coincident with phase II duodenal activity of the intestinal migratory motor complexes.

Biliary motility

The existence of an independent choledochal sphincter is now recognized by electrophysiological criteria. It results in a high-pressure zone just within the papilla. Apart from being responsive to various hormonal influences, the choledochal sphincter has a rich nerve supply via the hepatic vagal plexus, which consists predominantly of motor fibres derived from the left abdominal vagus. The sympathetic component is derived from the spinal segments T8 and 9 via the coeliac and periarterial plexuses. In addition, the lower end of the common bile duct exhibits phasic peristaltic activity with opening (diastolic) and closing (systolic) movements that correlate with pressure waves demonstrated in man. In the fasting state these phasic contractions are cyclical and parallel the duodenal migratory motor complexes. They are considered to regulate the flow of bile and pancreatic juice into the duodenum. The sphincter is in a contracted state and offers a significant resistance to bile flow in between these phasic contractions.

Effect of hormones

Cholecystokinin (CCK) is the main stimulus to gallbladder contraction in response to a meal and CCK administration increases gallbladder pressure, decreases the resistance through the sphincter of Oddi and enhances the bile flow in man. CCK-induced gallbladder contraction is largely inhibited by atropine. In the human, the gallbladder is less sensitive to CCK than the exocrine pancreas since the dose of exogenous CCK required to induce trypsin secretion is lower than that necessary for gallbladder contraction. CCK action on the extraheptic biliary tract is not mediated by the nervous system although the atropine effect in reducing CCK-mediated contraction suggests that its action may be mediated by the release of acetylcholine from intrinsic cholinergic nerves. CCK administration results in the activation in cyclic AMP. CCK induces a relaxation of the sphincter of Oddi, which is concomitant with contraction of the gallbladder, the response resulting in an efficient delivery of bile into the duodenum in response to a meal. CCK and motilin may be involved with the phasic activity of the choledochal sphincter, which is associated with duodenal migratory myoelectrical complexes during the interdigestive stage.

The activity of CCK depends on the COOH-terminal heptapeptide, a sequence found in gastrin which has a cholecystokinetic activity 1/15 that of CCK. Thus, this effect of gastrin is a pharmacological phenomenon in both dog and man, and gastrin has no effect on the biliary pressure of cholecystectomized patients. The synthetic hepta-, octa- and decapeptides of CCK are more potent than the various molecular forms of the naturally occurring CCK. In the human, 20 mg/kg of the COOH-terminal octapeptide of CCK (OP-CCK) reduces the gallbladder size by 40%. Caerulein, a peptide of similar composition to CCK extracted from amphibian skin, has a marked cholecystokinetic effect about three times that induced by CCK in the dog. Both the gallbladder contraction and the relaxation of the sphincter of Oddi are produced by a direct action on the smooth muscle. The synthetic derivative, ceruletide, has been used in the relief of biliary colic and to promote passage of retained ductal stones during saline infusion of the common bile duct through the T-tube.

Secretin does not appear to have a significant cholecystokinetic response in the human. Its effects on the gallbladder muscle vary with the species studied. Glucagon relaxes both the gallbladder musculature and the choledochal sphincter in man and the dog, probably by a direct action. VIP, which has been demonstrated in nerve fibres and neurons within the gallbladder wall, induces relaxation of the gallbladder and inhibits gallbladder contraction induced by CCK. These findings suggest that VIP may act as a local neurotransmitter in the physiological neural regulation of gallbladder function. Somatostatin-containing cells have been demonstrated in the human extrahepatic biliary tract. Somatostatin interferes with the gallbladder emptying and reduces bile flow in man. The mammalian tachykinin substance P (SP) has been detected in the biliary tract. It is a potent stimulator of gallbladder contraction both by a direct action and indirectly by inducing the release of a cholinergic transmitter.

Impaired gallbladder emptying

Impaired gallbladder contraction with poor emptying leads to biliary sludge formation, increases the risk of stone formation and in certain susceptible patient groups may lead to acute acalculous cholecystitis. Emptying of the gallbladder is disturbed:

- in patients after vagotomy
- the morbidly obese
- in patients with chronic pancreatitis and exocrine insufficiency
- in patients on long-term parenteral nutrition, and
- in the critically ill.

In the morbidly obese, both the fasting gallbladder volume and emptying rates are lower than normal and are associated with precipitation of cholesterol crystals. The cause–effect relationship between these two abnormalities (which precedes which) remains debatable.

A recent study has shed some light on the mechanism underlying the poor contractile activity of the gallbladder in vagotomized patients. These patients exhibit an abnormally elevated CCK release after a triglyceride meal when compared to normal subjects. This has been interpreted as a compensatory response to a reduced sensitivity of the gallbladder to CCK following vagal denervation. In patients with chronic pancreatitis, impaired contractility of the gallbladder is encountered in those patients who develop malabsorption. The impaired gallbladder emptying is thus attributed to reduced fat digestion and inadequate triglyceride absorption leading to defective secretion of CCK. Lack of oral alimentation and abrogation of the post-prandial CCK response is involved in the impaired motility of the gallbladder encountered in patients on parenteral nutrition.

Delivery of bile into the duodenum

Studies in the human have demonstrated that the bile salt output through an intact choledochal sphincter is significantly lower than that obtained from the T-tube in patients after common bile duct exploration. Whereas peak bile salt output is significantly increased after cholecystectomy, the total bile salt output is unaffected by this operation when compared to normal. The exogenous administration of CCK results in the production of a more stable bile secretion than the endogenous release of this hormone induced by the intraduodenal infusion of essential amino acids, the rhythmic release of bile following which is related to the concentration of bile salts in the duodenal lumen. The delivery of bile into the duodenum is predominantly influenced by the choledochal sphincter, the activity of which is controlled by complex neurohormonal mechanisms that are as yet poorly understood. Alcohol ingestion induces spasm of the choledochal sphincter and intraduodenal instillation of 0.1 N HCl produces the same effect in the dog.

Neural influences on biliary motility

In man the results of vagal stimulation by insulin-provoked hypoglycaemia suggest that the parasympathetic nervous system is involved in the maintenance of the gallbladder tone. Vagotomy causes dilatation and some delay in the gallbladder emptying when studied by cholescintigraphic techniques. Vagotomy also results in a decrease in the nerve fibres within the gallbladder wall. However, the increased prevalence of gallstones after vagotomy suggested by some retrospective reports remains controversial. Vagal activity appears to influence the tone of the choledochal sphincter. Electrical stimulation of the vagus nerve in the dog has been reported to result in no change or in a decreased bile flow through the sphincter and an increase in its electromyographic activity. In the human, hepatic plexus vagectomy has been reported to lower the passage pressure (the pressure head which opens the sphincter and permits bile to flow into the duodenum), indicating a lowering of the sphincteric muscular activity/contractility.

The role of the sympathetic system remains undefined. An increased threshold for pain induced by biliary distension has been reported in the human following sympathetic blockade. Stimulation of the right splanchnic nerve induces a contraction of the sphincter, which is abolished by alpha-blockade, and gallbladder dilatation that is inhibited by beta-blockade.

Effect of cholecystectomy and sphincterotomy/sphincteroplasty

On *a priori* grounds, removal of the gallbladder would be expected to alter the delivery of bile into the duodenum as this would then depend on the hepatic secretory pressure (maximum 25–30 cmH_2O) and the resistance of the choledochal sphincter which is expressed by the passage (yield) pressure. In practice, cholecystectomy in the human does not lead to any alterations in the total bile salt output compared to the normal situation but there is a redistribution of the pool of bile salts between the gut and the portal venous system. The effect of cholecystectomy on the cholesterol saturation of bile is uncertain, with some reports indicating a reduction and others showing no effect on the bile composition.

Although no changes in the biliary cholesterol content, gallbladder filling and response to CCK are observed after division of the sphincter (endoscopic or surgical), the concentration of lecithin and bile salts in the gallbladder is decreased, as is the concentrating ability of the gallbladder. In addition, the results of animal experiments have shown an increase in the monohydroxy and dihydroxy bile salts in the gallbladder, which becomes colonized by bacteria and develops histological changes of chronic inflammation. In the human, cholecystitis develops in 6% of patients with an *in situ* gallbladder within 6 months of an endoscopic sphincterotomy. A further 30% will develop cholecystitis and biliary symptoms during subsequent years.

Section 10.3 • Investigation of patients with biliary tract disorders

Plain abdominal radiology

The plain abdominal film is rarely used in the diagnosis of gallstones in the elective situation as only 10% of gallstones are radio-opaque. However, a plain film of the abdomen can provide useful diagnostic information in the acute situation. It may demonstrate gas in the biliary tract in patients with bilio-enteric fistulas. The demonstration of this gas together with dilatation of the small intestine provides good evidence of gallstone ileus (intraluminal small distal small bowel obstruction by a large gallstone) although the stone itself is rarely visualized on the film. The plain film also provides valuable diagnostic information in patients with emphysematous cholecystitis. Finally, calcification within the gallbladder wall, which is an established risk factor for carcinoma of the gallbladder, is best detected by a plain abdominal film.

Oral cholecystography and intravenous cholangiography

Both techniques can provide adequate visualization of the gallbladder if the serum bilirubin is below 40–50 μmol/l. Oral cholecystography can also demonstrate gallbladder contractility after a fatty meal or after the injection of cholecystokinin/ceruletide. Failure of the gallbladder to opacify is followed by repeated investigation using a double-dose cholecystogram. Non-visualization by this method is indicative of a diseased gallbladder if ingestion and absorption of the oral contrast agents (Telepaque) can be reasonably assumed (probability exceeds 90%). The sensitivity of a technically satisfactory oral cholecystogram for the detection of radiolucent stones exceeds 90%. However, visualization of the ducts is poor and is obtained in only 20% of patients after a fatty meal, although CCK- or ceruletide-cholecystography enhances the visualization of the ducts considerably (80% of patients). Oral cholecystography is unpredictable in the ill patient who is nauseous and may vomit (e.g. acute cholecystitis). The technique is, however, useful after the acute episode has subsided and in patients with mild attacks. In most centres, however, oral cholecystography has been superseded by ultrasound scanning for the diagnosis of gallstones. Oral cholecystography is still used in the diagnosis of polypoid lesions of the gallbladder.

The gallbladder is less well defined by the intravenous cholangiogram (IVC) but the extrahepatic biliary system can be better visualized by this procedure, especially with an infusion technique used in association with tomography. Infusion cholangiography is an accurate technique for the diagnosis of cystic duct obstruction (acute cholecystitis, where the gallbladder is not opacified but the ducts are outlined). However, the technique has been largely replaced by biliary scintigraphy, which is more accurate. With the advent of laparoscopic cholecystectomy, there was an initial resurgence in the use of intravenous cholangiography to detect ductal calculi in patients with symptomatic gallstone disease prior to operation. A water-soluble contrast agent (iotroxate meglumine) is administered as an intravenous infusion and a tomographic X-ray technique is used to visualize the biliary tract. However, subsequent studies have shown that despite this tomographic infusion technique which undoubtedly enhances the quality of the opacification of the biliary tract, IVC is insufficiently reliable. It cannot, therefore, be regarded as a good substitute for operative cholangiography. In addition, there is a small but definite incidence of severe hypersensitivity reactions. In practice, pre-operative IVC has been abandoned in most centres.

Real-time ultrasonography

This is now the first-line investigation for biliary tract and pancreatic disease in most hospitals. Aside from its non-invasive nature and lack of any radiation exposure, ultrasound scanning can provide simultaneous information on the following:

- presence of gallstones
- presence of gallbladder disease
- dilatation of the biliary tract and hepatic parenchymal disease, e.g. tumour deposits
- lesions in the pancreas.

Real-time ultrasound in experienced hands can detect gallstones in over 90% of cases (Figure 10.12). However, its sensitivity for ductal calculi is much less and varies considerably from centre to centre (10–80%). Gallbladder ultrasound scanning also detects gallbladder enlargement, thickening of the walls and tumours but is less sensitive in the diagnosis of adenomyomatosis than oral cholecystography. Ultrasound examination of the gallbladder is used as the initial diagnostic procedure for acute cholecystitis since it enables the determination of tenderness over the sonographically identified gallbladder and is able to detect pericholecystic fluid collections and gallbladder wall oedema/thickening (ultrasonographic signs of cholecystitis), in addition to sludge and stones. However, the sensitivity and specificity of ultrasound in the diagnosis of acute cholecystitis is lower than that for gallbladder scintiscanning.

The ultrasonographic detection of a dilated biliary tract is the first step in the investigation of patients with biochemical evidence of cholestatic jaundice. In icteric patients, its accuracy in the diagnosis of extrahepatic bile duct obstruction exceeds 90% (Figure 10.13). Its diagnostic yield is lower, however, in mildly jaundiced patients since it may miss minimal dilatation of the intrahepatic biliary tree. As ultrasound examination does not give accurate information on the exact site and extent of the lesion causing the extrahepatic obstruction, further investigation with computed tomography (CT) and magnetic resonance cholangiopancreatography (MRCP) or ERCP is required in most patients. Percutaneous fine needle cytological aspiration of mass lesions in the liver, extrahepatic bile ducts, gallbladder and pancreas is now routinely performed in some centres under ultrasonographic guidance and may establish the definitive diagnosis regarding the benign or malignant nature of the lesion. There are no known biological hazards of ultrasound investigation (at the energy level used for diagnostic purposes).

Ultrasound examination may prove unsatisfactory for technical reasons in the following:

- obese
- following previous surgery
- ascites
- gaseous distension of the upper abdominal viscera.

In these instances, CT scanning provides more reliable information.

CT scanning and magnetic resonance imaging

Helical or spiral CT scanning can provide similar information on the biliary tree as ultrasonography, but in view of cost and radiation exposure it is usually held in reserve when ultrasound examination has failed (usually for technical reasons). Contrast enhancement (vascular or biliary) increases the diagnostic yield. High-dose contrast helical CT scanning provides much better detection of solid lesions in the extrahepatic bile ducts (e.g. cholangiocarcinoma), pancreas and liver.

Magnetic resonance imaging (MRI), also known as nuclear magnetic resonance, is being increasingly used for the detection of hepatobiliary and pancreatic disease at the expense of CT. The technique is based on the behaviour of protons (e.g. hydrogen) of the nuclei of molecules, which act as spinning magnets and align themselves in a specific direction when exposed to an external electromagnetic field. If radiofrequency (magnetic) pulses corresponding to the spinning frequency of the protons are then applied, the alignment is disturbed with each pulse and then returns or 'relaxes' to the original position. The time taken for the nuclear motion to get out of step is known as T2 and that required for the return to the original position is known as T1. Both these time constants vary with the proton density of the tissue and the local atomic and molecular environment of the protons (i.e. chemical state of the tissue). The movement of the nuclei resulting from the externally applied radiofrequency pulses is known as 'resonant absorption' and is accompanied by the re-emission of radio waves that are picked up by a receiver coil placed round the patient. Different techniques of radiofrequency pulses are used to generate

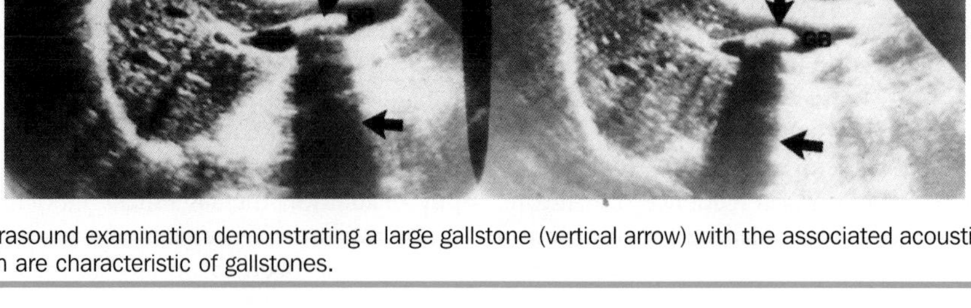

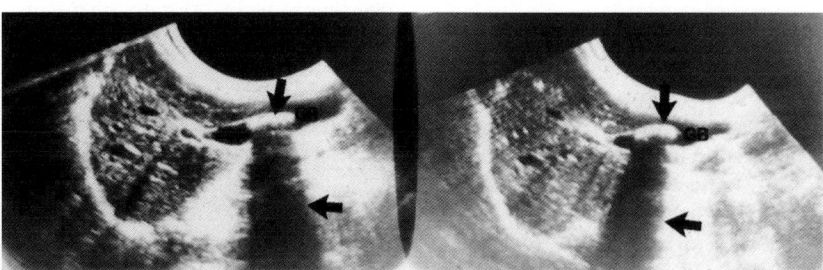

Figure 10.12 Ultrasound examination demonstrating a large gallstone (vertical arrow) with the associated acoustic shadows (transverse arrow) which are characteristic of gallstones.

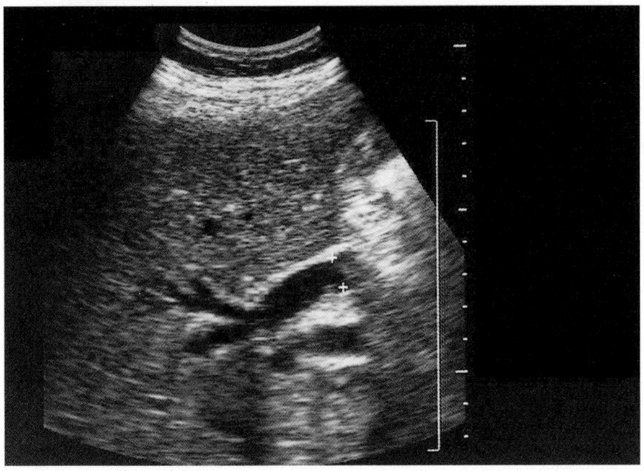

Figure 10.13 Ultrasound examination of the liver showing dilated intrahepatic and common bile ducts in a patient with carcinoma of the pancreas.

images of different slice thickness and in various planes. The advantages of MRI are:

- excellent soft tissue definition, particularly of the central nervous system because of the lipid/water content
- it can image in any plane (coronal, sagittal, transverse) without movement of the patient
- it avoids radiation exposure
- it carries no known biological hazard.

It is likely that magnetic resonance spectroscopy (MRS) will be able to provide the best test of liver function in the not too distant future. Already, it has been used successfully to identify specific inborn errors of metabolism due to specific enzyme deficiencies.

The production of multiplanar images of the pathological anatomy by MRI accounts for its usefulness in the detection of the site and cause of obstruction in patients with cholestatic jaundice. MRI (if available) should be used in preference to CT in patients with suspected hilar cholangiocarcinoma and primary carcinoma of the gallbladder where it is superior to CT in assessing the presence and extent of extramural invasion.

Magnetic resonance cholangiopancreatography (MRCP)

The principle of MRCP is based on heavily weighted T2 pulse sequences (obtained by fast spin echo sequences) since these ensure a very high signal from stationary liquids such as bile and pancreatic juice because of their long T2 relaxation time, in marked contrast to the surrounding vascular liver parenchyma with its high blood flow that generates virtually no signal because of its much shorter T2. Hence the bile column stands out as a hyperintense signal against the background hypo-intense liver tissue. As a result, detailed imaging of the entire biliary tree (intra and extrahepatic) and pancreatic ductal system is possible without the administration of contrast in the vast majority (>90%) of patients.

Studies have shown that MRCP provides useful clinical information that influences management in the following:

- **Biliary calculi** – MRCP detects stones as small as 2 mm in the bile duct even when this is not dilated. With the right sequences it has a sensitivity of 90–95% and specificity of 90–100% (overall diagnostic accuracy of 95%) for the detection of choledocholithiasis. This has been shown in randomized studies to approximate to the diagnostic accuracy of ERCP (Figure 10.14). Pitfalls for stone detection by MRCP include surgical clips, pneumobilia, haemobilia/clots and flow artifacts. In particular, surgical clips used to secure the medial end of the cystic duct after cholecystectomy create signal void artifacts that obscure the related segment of the common bile duct. MRCP should displace ERCP for the detection of ductal calculi in patients with gallstone associated acute pancreatitis, and hence the need when these are obstructing the papilla for endoscopic sphincterotomy. MRCP is the best technique for demonstrating the presence and exact location of intrahepatic stones. MRCP is also very useful in differentiating common hepatic duct obstruction by Mirizzi syndrome from obstruction by gallbladder cancer or enlarged lymph nodes.
- **Choledochal cysts** – MRCP displays all types of choledochal cysts.
- **Bile duct injury** – MRCP outlines both the ducts and the perihepatic bile collection but is unable to establish whether the bile leak is active or not. Thus in this situation both MRCP and ERCP are needed.
- **Bile duct tumours** – MRCP has distinct advantages over ERCP and transhepatic cholangiography in the diagnosis of high bile duct tumours because it provides anatomical information of the entire biliary tract on both sides of the stricture. In addition it detects extension of tumour along intrahepatic ducts and enables complete tumour staging of the disease, i.e. assesses involvement of liver, portal nodes and portal vein (with additional MR pulse sequences, e.g. contrast-enhanced T1 weighted spin echo). MRCP is also valuable in assessing the patency of hepaticojejunostomy following surgery for high bile duct strictures or hilar cholangiocarcionoma (Figure 10.15).

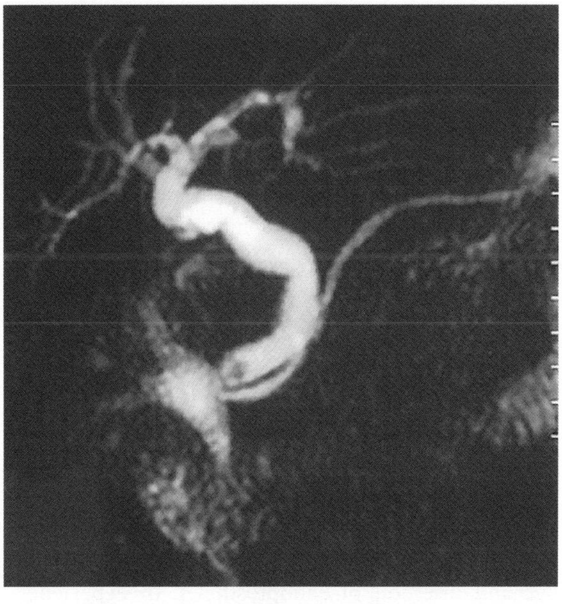

Figure 10.14 MRCP outlining the entire biliary tree and demonstrating a stone at the lower end of the bile duct. Note also that the pelvi-calyceal system of the right kidney is visualized and this obscures the duodenum in this patient who was admitted with acute pancreatitis. The entire pacreatic duct is clearly visible.

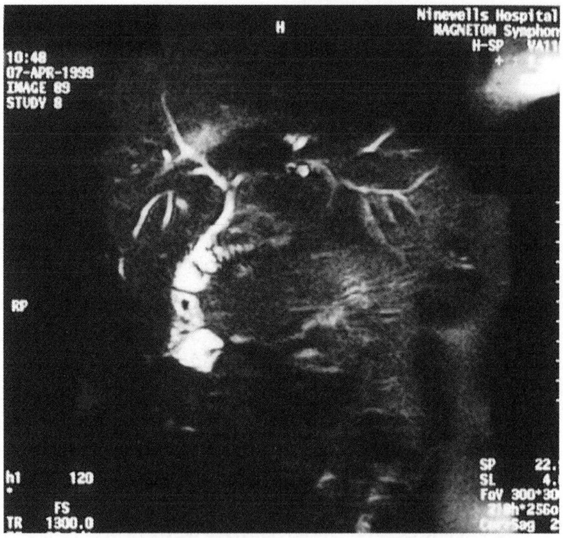

Figure 10.15 MRCP outlining a hepaticojejunostomy after repair of a iatrogenic high bile duct stricture.

- **Pancreatic disease** – The main pancreatic duct is visualized in over 95% of cases. It is highly accurate in the diagnosis of pancreas divisum. In established chronic pancreatitis, MRCP has the same diagnostic accuracy as ERCP but not in early disease with minimal changes in the side branches. MRCP is very useful for ampullary tumours – it detects a dilated bile duct abutting on an irregular ampullary mass indenting the duodenum. Although it can detect proximal and body cancer of the pancreas, it offers no advantages over CT/ultrasound in this respect, except in cystic tumours in view of its ability to detect static fluid collections.

MRCP versus ERCP

MRCP gives the same diagnostic information as ERCP except for the detection of minimal disease chronic pancreatitis. Its distinct advantage is its entirely non-invasive nature. In comparative studies, the failure rate of MRCP (contraindications to MRI, claustrophobia and inadequate examination) is lower than ERCP. MRCP is applicable irrespective of altered or pathological anatomy that precludes ERCP, e.g. duodenal stensosis, hepaticojejunostomy. Thus the trend is to replace diagnostic ERCP with MRCP and restrict ERCP to those patients who require endoscopic intervention, i.e. endoscopic sphincterotomy and stone extraction, stenting, etc.

Percutaneous transhepatic cholangiography (PTC)

This is a commonly used technique for the visualization of the biliary tract in the jaundiced patient and can be modified to allow percutaneous transhepatic drainage and insertion of endoprostheses. In experienced hands, the success rate with PTC approximates to 100% in patients with dilated biliary tracts and exceeds 70% in the absence of bile duct dilatation. The reported accuracy of PTC in detecting the level and cause of the biliary obstruction averages 90% (Figure 10.16). Nowadays, the procedure is carried out under sedation using the Chiba (also known as 'skinny') 22-gauge needle which has an external diameter of 0.7 mm. The use of the Chiba needle has largely replaced the thicker Longdwell-trocar-cannula because of the higher success rate and a lower incidence of complications. The procedure must be covered with systemic antibiotic therapy (usually an aminoglycoside or cephalosporin or pipericillin) and any clotting abnormality must be corrected with vitamin K and/or the administration of fresh frozen plasma prior to its performance.

In practice, PTC is used when ERCP fails or does not provide sufficient information on the proximal intrahepatic biliary tree because of an obstructing lesion of the extrahepatic bile ducts. However, MRCP can provide this information, and if available should be used in preference to PTC.

Pre-operative percutaneous external transhepatic biliary drainage (Figure 10.17) is seldom performed nowadays since several clinical trials have shown no benefit from the procedure in terms of reduced operative morbidity and mortality in severely jaundiced patients and the technique predisposes to infection of the obstructed biliary tract unless a closed collecting system which incorporates bacterial filters is used. However, the percutaneous or endoscopic insertion of endoprostheses (in-dwelling stents introduced over guidewires and positioned through the obstruction by means of pusher tubes) is a valuable method of palliation of patients with large bile duct obstruction due to inoperable/incurable malignancy (Figure 10.18).

The complications of PTC include:

- bacteraemia
- bile leakage
- haemorrhage: free bleeding into the peritoneal cavity and haemobilia
- bile embolization
- intrahepatic arterioportal fistula
- pneumothorax
- contrast reactions.

The reported incidence of major complications with the Chiba needle varies from 3 to 10% with a mortality of 0.1–0.3%.

Endoscopy and endoscopic retrograde cholangiopancreatography (ERCP)

Upper gastrointestinal endoscopy with a forward or oblique-viewing panendoscope should be performed in jaundiced patients as significant gastrointestinal pathology is encountered in 25% of jaundiced patients.

ERCP, which is performed through a side-viewing endoscope, provides useful information in patients with cholestatic jaundice irrespective of whether the ductal system is dilated or not. In experienced hands, successful cholangiography is achieved by ERCP in over 90% of cases. ERCP permits concomitant endoscopic examination and biopsy of lesions encountered during the endoscopic examination although the examination of the stomach and duodenum is more difficult and

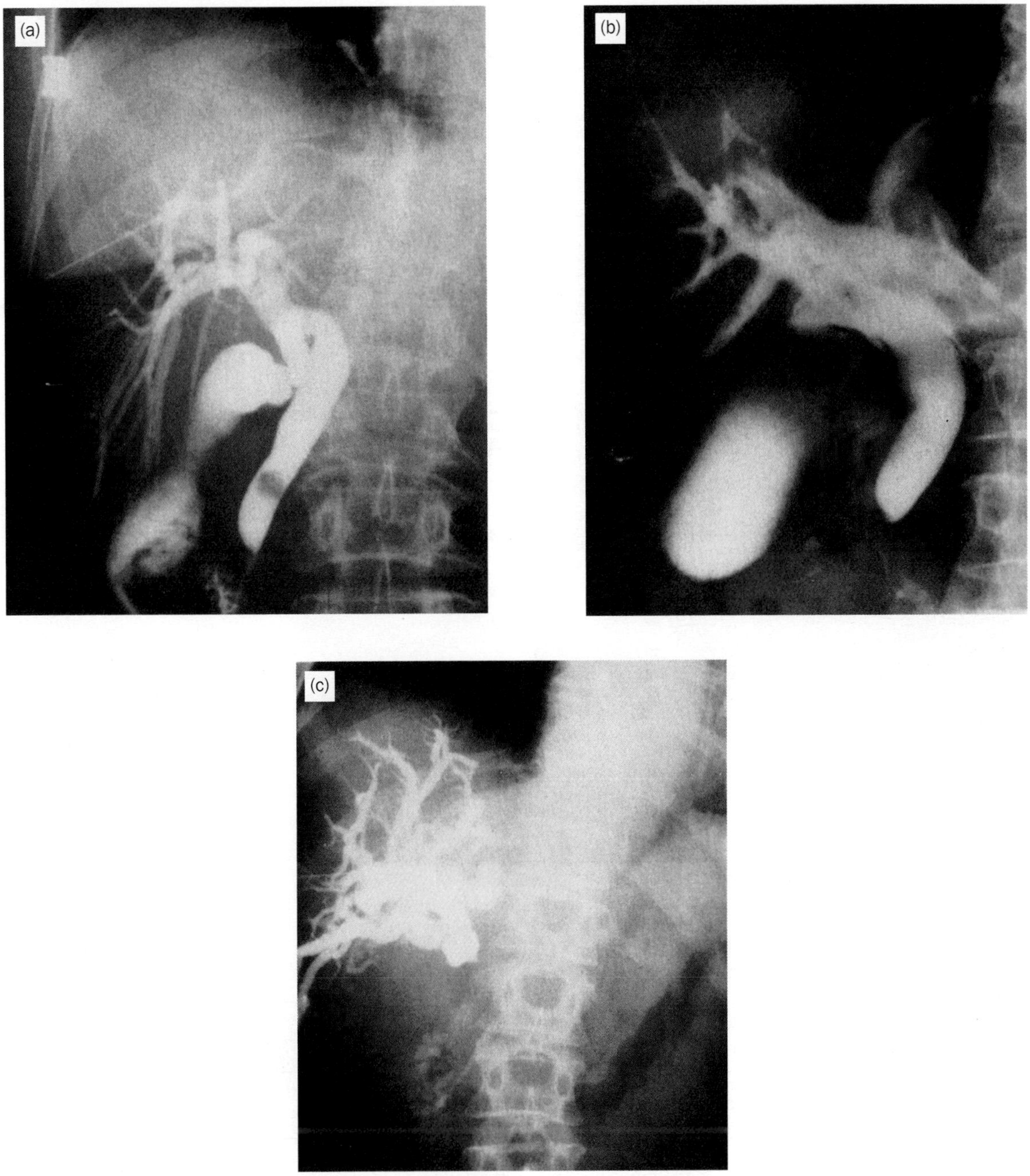

Figure 10.16 Percutaneous transhepatic cholangiograms: (a) ductal calculus proximal to a benign stricture; (b) carcinoma of the pancreas; (c) cholangiocarcinoma.

less optimal than with a forward- or oblique-viewing endoscope. A pancreatogram can be obtained during the same investigation. Certain lesions can be treated or palliated during the procedure, e.g. endoscopic stone removal, endoscopic nasobiliary drainage and stent insertion for inoperable malignant large bile duct obstruction.

Diagnostic ERCP has a very low morbidity largely due to pancreatitis (1.0%) and mortality (0.1%). The morbidity of interventional (therapeutic) ERCP, especially sphincterotomy, is, however, higher (6–10%). The immediate mortality of endoscopic sphincterotomy averages 1.0%, although the 30 day mortality is 3%. The complications which may follow endoscopic sphincterotomy are:

- haemorrhage
- acute pancreatitis
- cholangitis
- retroperitoneal duodenal perforation
- impacted Dormia basket
- acute cholecystitis
- gallstone ileus – following extraction of large stones.

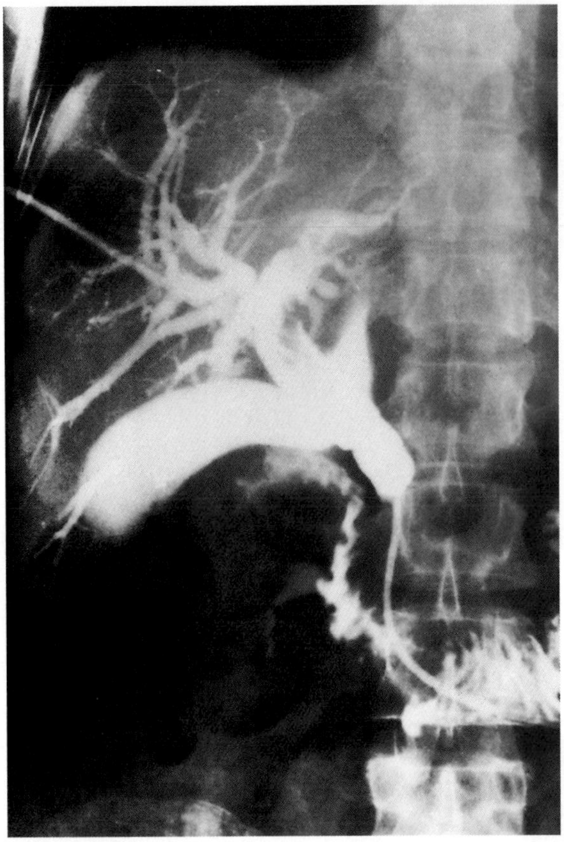

Figure 10.17 Pre-operative external biliary decompression for complete obstruction due to carcinoma of the pancreas. This technique is seldom used nowadays except as a prelude to insertion of an endoprosthesis for palliation of complete obstruction caused by inoperable pancreaticobiliary malignancy.

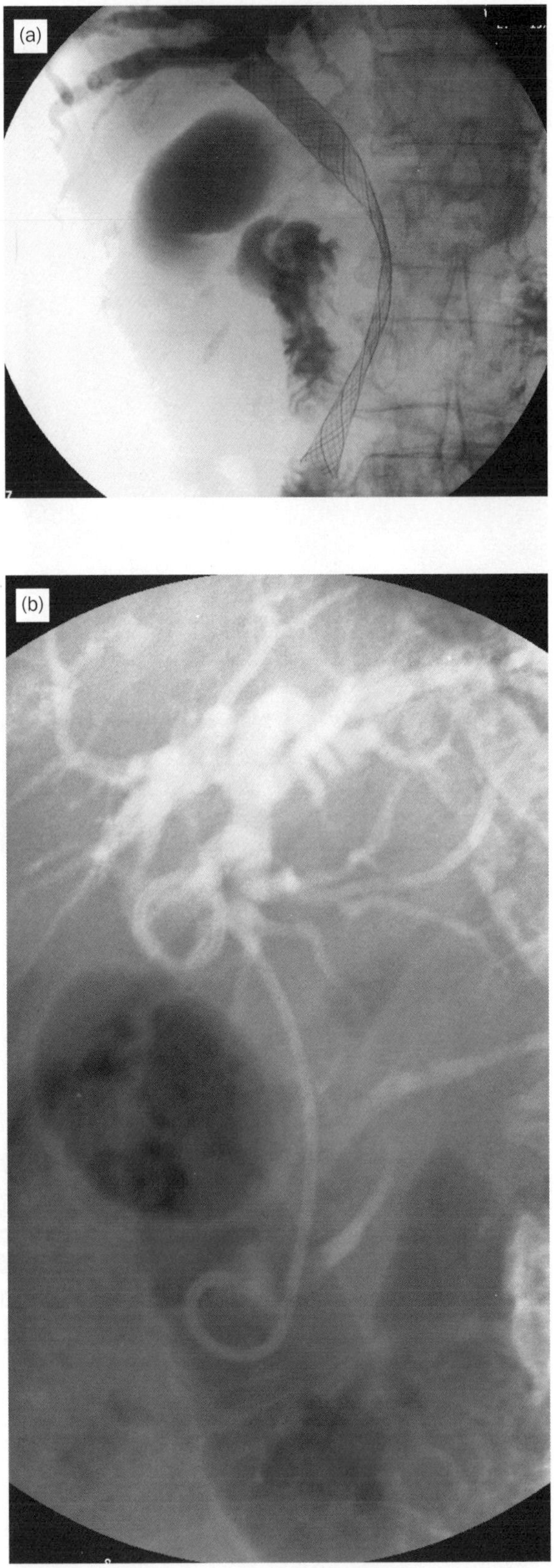

Figure 10.18 Stenting for inoperable disease: (a) expandable metallic endoprosthesis inserted transhepatically under radiological control for palliation of an inoperable hilar cholangiocarcinoma; (b) endoscopic plastic stent for palliation of inoperable carcinoma of the head of the pancreas.

ERCP is very accurate in the diagnosis of ductal calculi (Figure 10.19), tumours of the bile ducts (Figure 10.20) and pancreas (Figures 10.21 and 10.22) and sclerosing cholangitis. In patients with complete biliary obstructive lesions, the proximal biliary tree is not visualized. These patients require further investigation with MRCP or PTC. ERCP is less accurate than ultrasound and oral cholecystography in the diagnosis of gallbladder disease and gallstones.

Technical failure of an attempted ERCP examination may be due to:

- duodenal or pyloric stenosis
- previous Billroth II gastrectomy
- duodenal diverticulum
- uncooperative patient
- inexperience with the procedure.

Biliary scintiscanning

The most widely used radiopharmaceutical compounds are ^{99m}Tc-labelled compounds of IDA (iminodiacetic acid) and EHIDA (diethylacetanilido-iminodiacetic acid). These agents, which are powerful gamma emitters, are administered intravenously, whereupon they are selectively taken up by the hepatocytes and secret-

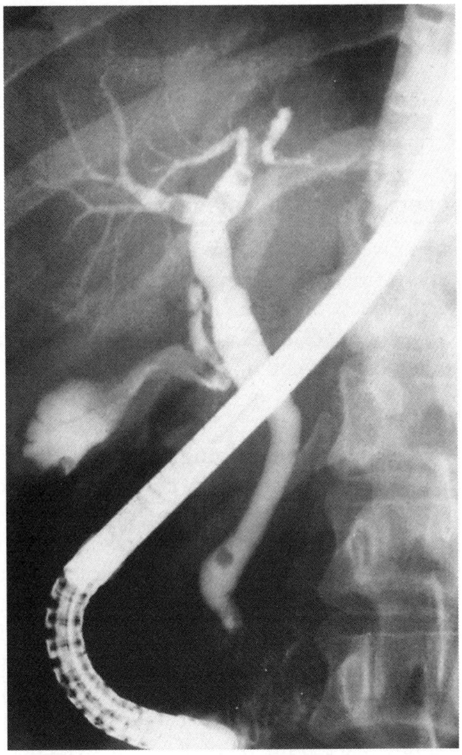

Figure 10.19 ERCP outlining ductal calculi.

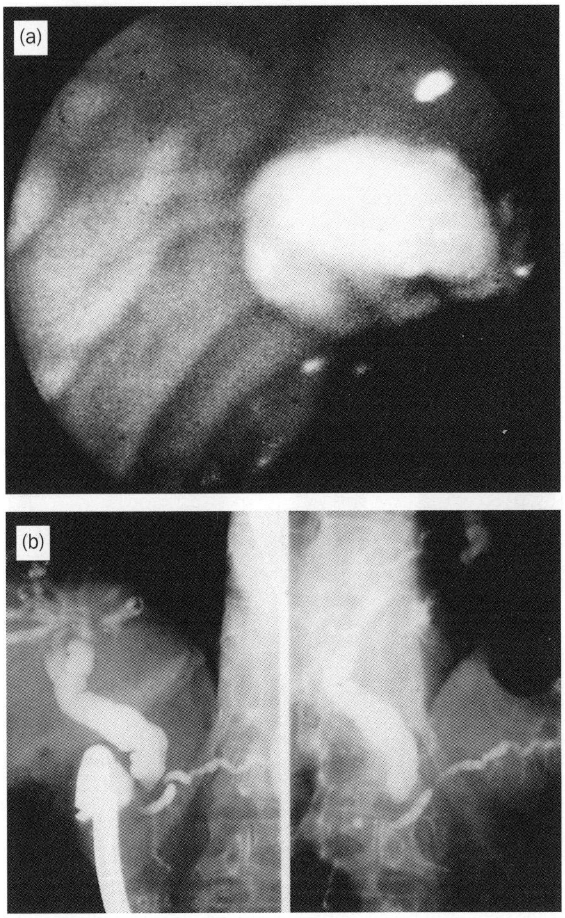

Figure 10.21 (a) Endoscopic view of a periampullary lesion of the pancreas; (b) cholangiopancreatogram of the same patient.

ed into the bile. They are therefore ideal for the imaging of the biliary tree by a gamma camera, especially since their uptake by the liver and excretion into the biliary tract is not influenced by the presence of cholestasis.

EHIDA-cholescintiscanning is the most accurate test of acute cholecystitis irrespective of its nature (acute calculus obstructive, acalculous cholecystitis) and establishes the diagnosis within 1 hour of the intravenous administration of the radiopharmaceutical agent. A diagnosis of acute cholecystitis can be confidently made if the scintigram shows prompt excretion and a normal common bile duct with entry of isotope into the duodenum, but the gallbladder is not imaged (Figure 10.23). The information is stored on magnetic tape/disk for more detailed computer analysis at a later stage. Cholescintiscanning has a sensitivity of 91–97% and a specificity of 87% for the diagnosis of acute cholecystitis. A normal gallbladder scintiscan is virtually 100% accurate in excluding cholecystitis. False-positives are encountered in:

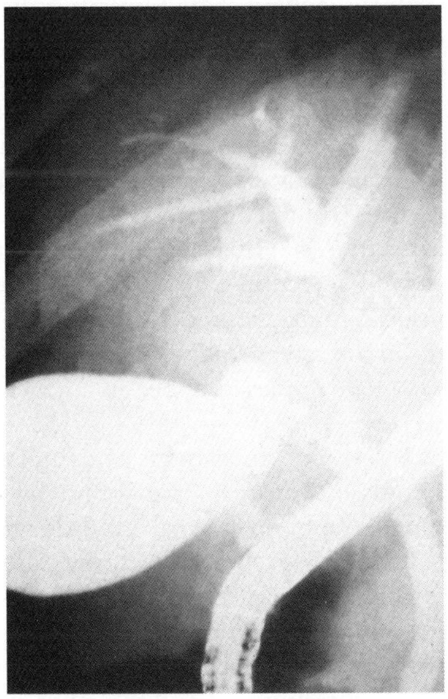

Figure 10.20 ERCP showing a hilar cholangiocarcinoma.

- chronic cholecystitis
- gallstone pancreatitis
- patients with alcoholic liver disease
- patients receiving parenteral nutrition.

The number of false-positive results obtained by cholescintigraphy in the diagnosis of acute cholecystitis can be drastically reduced by the administration of intravenous morphine before the procedure. This opiate causes spasm of the sphincter of Oddi and thereby induces reflux of bile (and radionuclide) in the gallbladder if the cystic duct is patent. The morphine-

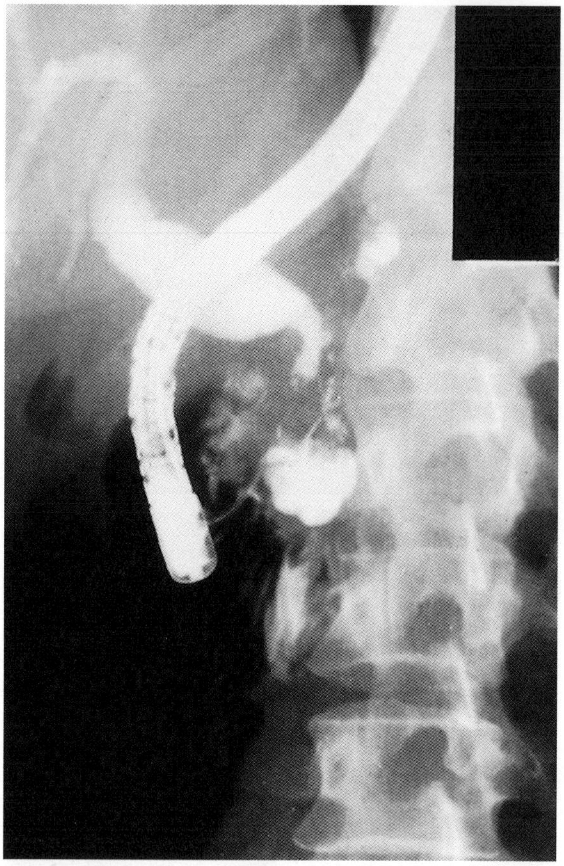

Figure 10.22 ERCP showing a carcinoma of the head of the pancreas.

radionuclide test appears to be very useful in the evaluation of critically ill patients with suspected acute acalculous cholecystitis, in patients who are fasting or receiving parenteral nutrition and as a repeat procedure in those patients in whom the gallbladder was not visualized.

Biliary scintiscanning has also been used to evaluate the jaundiced patient with a bilirubin greater than 50 μmol/l. Hepatocellular disease is diagnosed when poor liver excretion and intestinal activity are demonstrated after 18 hours of injection. Complete biliary obstruction is denoted by the absence of any intestinal activity after 18 hours, and partial obstruction by normal liver excretion, dilated ducts and delayed intestinal activity. However, biliary scintigraphy is not used routinely for the investigation of the jaundiced patient since other techniques (e.g. ultrasound and cholangiography) give more precise information of the underlying pathology. The exception to the above is provided by jaundice in the neonate where biliary scintigraphy and estimation of faecal radioactivity following the intravenous injection of the isotope is one of the routine tests used for the diagnosis of biliary atresia.

EHIDA scintigraphy is also very useful for the functional evaluation of surgically constructed bilio-enteric anastomoses (Figure 10.24). EHIDA scintiscanning after gallbladder contraction induced by a milk meal or intravenous CCK is used to quantitate enterogastric reflux. Normal individuals reflux less than 5–10% of the administered dose of the radionuclide. EHIDA scintigraphy is also useful in documenting the presence and location of biliary leaks after cholecystectomy.

Intra-operative fluorocholangiography

Intra-operative fluorocholangiography (IOFC) is commonly performed via the cystic duct (transcystic) but other techniques (direct puncture of the common bile duct, cholecystocholangiography, intra-operative transhepatic cholangiography) are available and used in certain situations.

Transcystic fluorocholangiography

Although there are many who practise and advocate the selective use of IOFC during cholecystectomy, in the best interest of the patient this investigation must be regarded as an integral part of cholecystectomy whether this is performed by the open or laparoscopic approach. It provides the best road map of the biliary tree and indicates the need, or otherwise, for exploration of the common bile duct. Although it may not reduce the incidence of bile duct injury during laparoscopic cholecystectomy, there is good evidence that routine IOFC results in the detection of bile duct damage during the operation. This is important as the majority of reported bile duct injuries (60%) are missed and discovered in the post-operative period or subsequent to discharge. The arguments for a selective policy for IOFC include increased operating time, unsatisfactory exposures and the safe prediction of a 'normal' common bile duct in the absence of a history of jaundice, normal pre-operative liver function test (LFTs) and a normal sized duct at operation. Intra-operative cholangiography incurs considerable delays and is often unsatisfactory only when performed by a mobile X-ray machine with three blind static films after the sequential injections of contrast medium. The modern procedure entails the employment of portable high-definition C-arm image intensifiers (Figure 10.25). These have digital facilities and an expanded software that enables image storage and advanced image processing: zoom facility, real-time subtraction, road mapping, etc. The entire biliary tree is visualized by screening (fluoroscopy) during injection of contrast medium in all patients inside 5 min. Desired images are selected as they appear on the screen and stored on hard disk from which permanent copies can be obtained on X-ray film cassettes.

Unsuspected stones (in patients with normal LFTs and ultrasound examination) are found by digitized fluorocholangiography in normal sized ducts in 4–7% of patients undergoing cholecystectomy. These stones would all be missed if a selective policy for IOFC were adopted and although some may pass spontaneously without any adverse effects, others will cause acute pancreatitis or cholangitis. Thus the contention that missed stones during cholecystectomy do not matter as

(a)

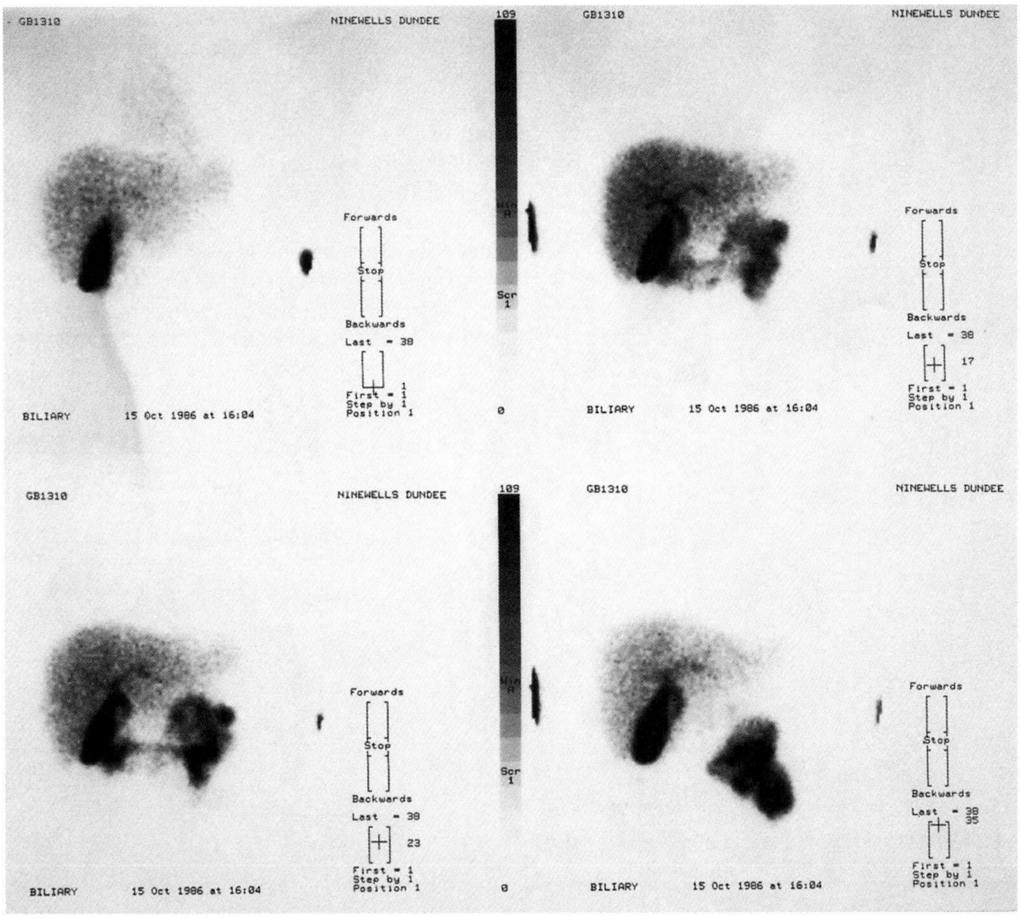

(b)

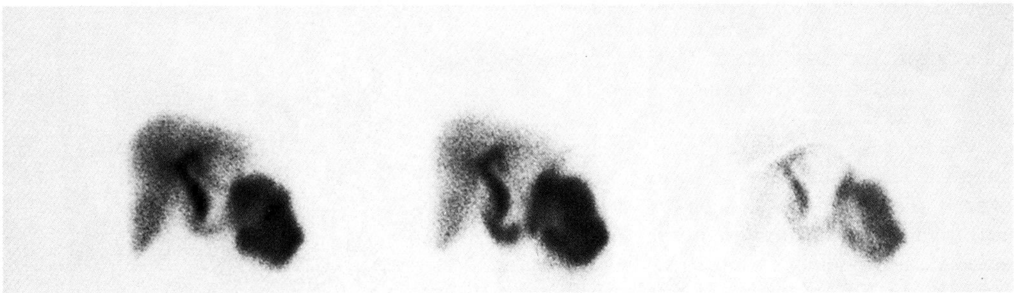

Figure 10.23 Biliary scintigraphy with EHIDA: (a) normal cholescintigram – both the gallbladder and the bile duct are imaged; (b) acute cholecystitis – a normal bile duct with prompt excretion into the duodenum is observed but the gallbladder is not outlined.

they can be treated by endoscopic sphincterotomy when they become symptomatic or cause complications incurs an avoidable morbidity and a small but definite mortality. Anomalies of the biliary tract are encountered in some 19% of patients undergoing routine IOFC during cholecystectomy. Perhaps the most important of these is an abnormal short cystic duct which terminates in either the common hepatic or the right hepatic duct. This anomaly if detected will reduce the risk of bile duct damage, especially during laparoscopic cholecystectomy where tenting of the extrahepatic conduit is produced as a result of the lateral and upward displacement of the gallbladder. If unrecognized, this will result in partial or total compromise of the common hepatic or common duct by the clip used to secure the medial end of the cystic duct. Finally, a selective policy for IOFC will not impart the experience needed to carry out the investigation expeditiously and the familiarity to interpret accurately the cholangiographic findings.

During laparoscopic cholecystectomy, the most commonly used technique involves cannulation of the cystic duct after this is opened by fine curved microscissors. Although a variety of disposable purpose-designed catheter systems are available, the best and most cost-effective is the Cook ureteric catheter (5 Fr)

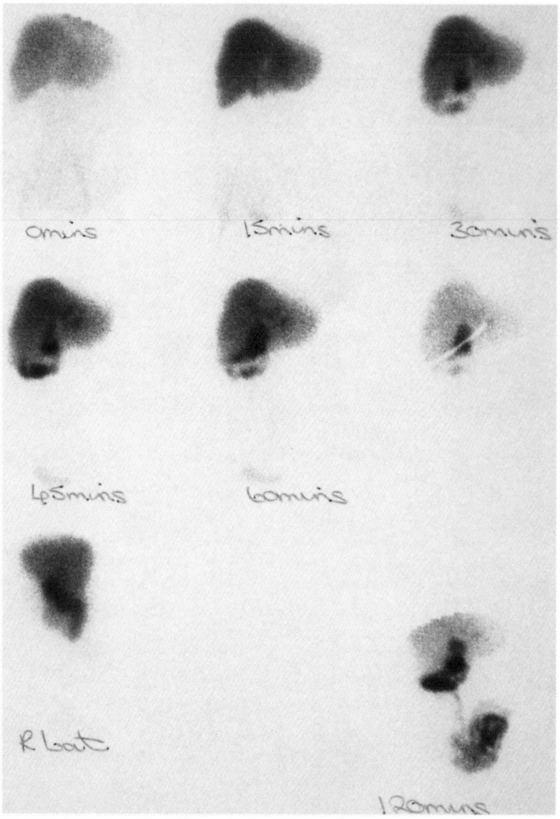

Figure 10.24 EHIDA scintigram showing a functioning hepaticojejunostomy performed for a high bile duct stricture.

inserted inside a cholangiograsper (Figure 10.26). This instrument not only guides the catheter to the cystic duct lumen but its jaws allow the cystic duct walls to be grasped on the catheter once this is safely in the lumen of the cystic duct.

Before screening is commenced, the operating table should be tilted 15° to the right (to obviate an intervening spinal column) and in a slight Trendelenburg position to facilitate proximal filling of the ductal system. Nowadays, water-soluble contrast media, such as sodium diatrizoate (25–50%), are used. The volume required depends on dilatation or otherwise of the biliary tract. If during screening a hold-up is encountered at the lower end of the bile duct which does not appear to be organic, intravenous injection of secretin, ceruletide or glucagon is administered when pharmacological relief of spasm of the choledochal sphincter is followed by entry of dye into the duodenum. Contrast injection should be stopped when pancreatic duct filling is observed because of the risk of pancreatitis.

With experience, use of digitized fluoroscopic screening and meticulous technique, both false-negative and -positive rates of IOFC are very low. Avoidance of metal clips, whenever possible, is desirable as they may obscure small filling defects. The most common artifact leading to unnecessary exploration of the common bile duct remains the air bubble. This can be prevented by ensuring that the delivery system is air-free. If 'bubbles' are observed during screening, aspiration should be avoided as this introduces air into the bile duct from the duodenum. In this situation, the syringe should be disconnected from the cannula or catheter, the external end of which is held low, by the side of the drapings, such that the hydrostatic pressure of bile will cause retrograde flow along the cannula and the 'bubble shadow' disappears. Small blood clots, the tips of the transverse processes of the second lumbar vertebra, calcified costal cartilage and a contracted choledochal sphincter with its meniscus effect can also be misinterpreted as ductal calculi when the X-ray machine and static films are used. These sources of error are dismissed easily when fluoroscopic screening is used.

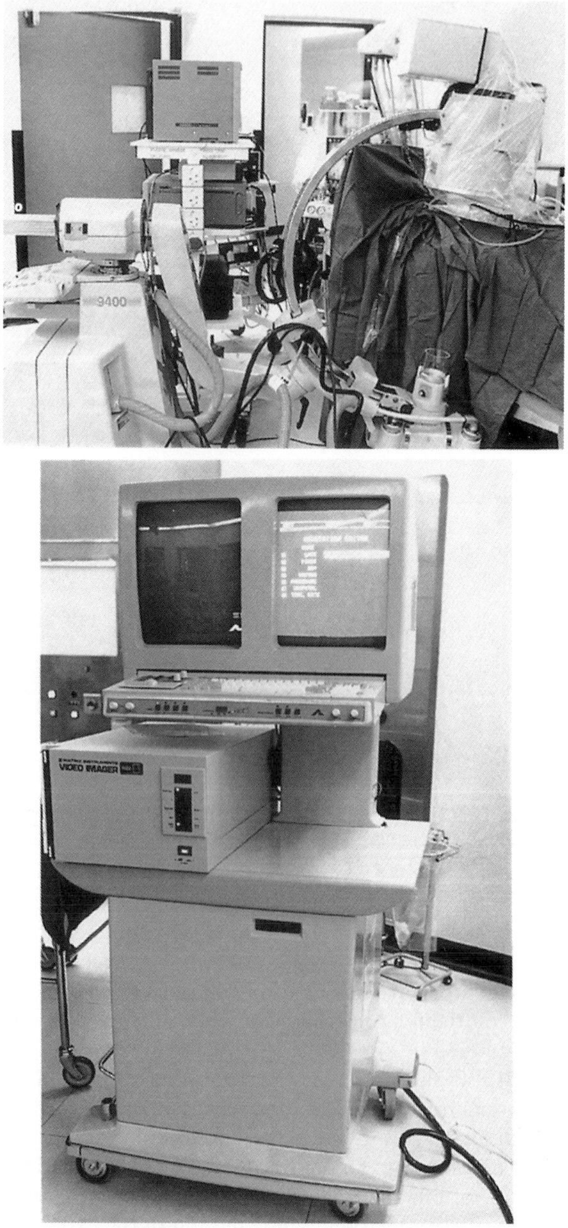

Figure 10.25 Modern C-arm fluoroscopy unit for intra-operative cholangiography.

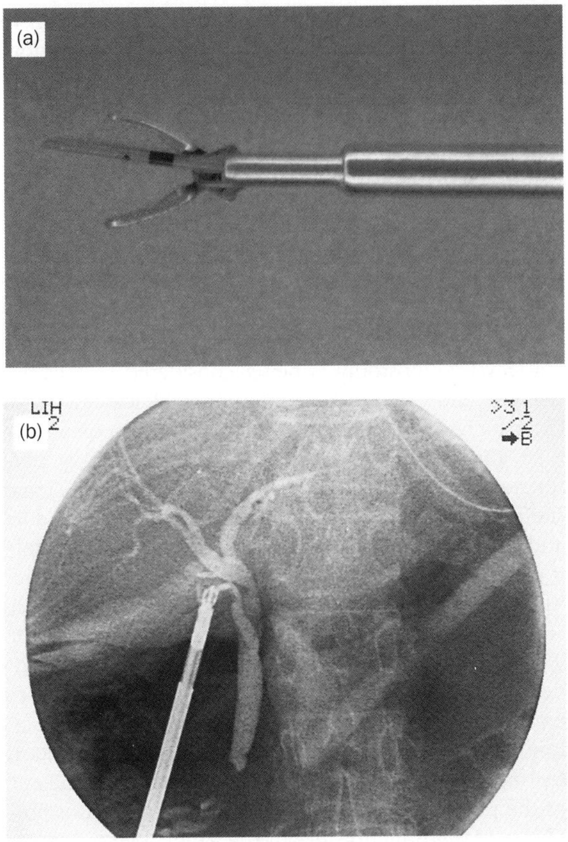

Figure 10.26 Laparoscopic transcystic cholangiography: (a) ureteric catheter inside a cholangiograsper is used for intra-operative transcystic cholangiography during laparoscopic cholecystectomy; (b) intra-operative transcystic cholangiogram during laparoscopic cholecystectomy using a 4 Fr ureteric catheter and cholangiograsper.

The important rules governing the performance and interpretation of IOFC are:

- Rapid and over-filling of the ductal system must be avoided as aside from obscuring small ductal calculi, the resulting raised pressure may cause cholangio-venous reflux.
- Unequivocal flow into the duodenum must be demonstrated in all cases.
- Both intra- and extrahepatic bile ducts must be visualized. Non-filling of the intrahepatic biliary tract, or part of it, is always pathological and cannot be ignored. Aside from technical errors, the most common cause for failure of proximal duct filling is a hilar cholangiocarcinoma. During laparoscopic cholecystectomy, it may be indicative of common duct injury.
- Contrast injection is stopped with the onset of pancreatic duct filling.
- If doubt exists regarding the interpretation of any abnormalities, expert radiological advice should be sought (Figure 10.27). Ideally, a radiologist should see and comment on the films or the fluoroscopic examination (on hard disk or videotape) routinely.

A completion T-tube cholangiogram is performed after common bile duct exploration although this is replaced by completion choledochoscopy in some centres. Before injecting contrast, the T-tube and the extrahepatic bile duct is filled with about 60 ml of saline to remove air bubbles. Spasm of the choledochal sphincter is common after biliary manipulations during common bile duct exploration (e.g. passage of balloon catheters, etc.). This may result in a hold-up of contrast in the lower end of the bile duct. It is easily differentiated from missed organic obstruction by the intravenous administration of spasmolytic agents such as glucagon or ceruletide. (Figure 10.28).

Complications of IOFC are rarely encountered and are usually due to either hypersensitivity to the contrast

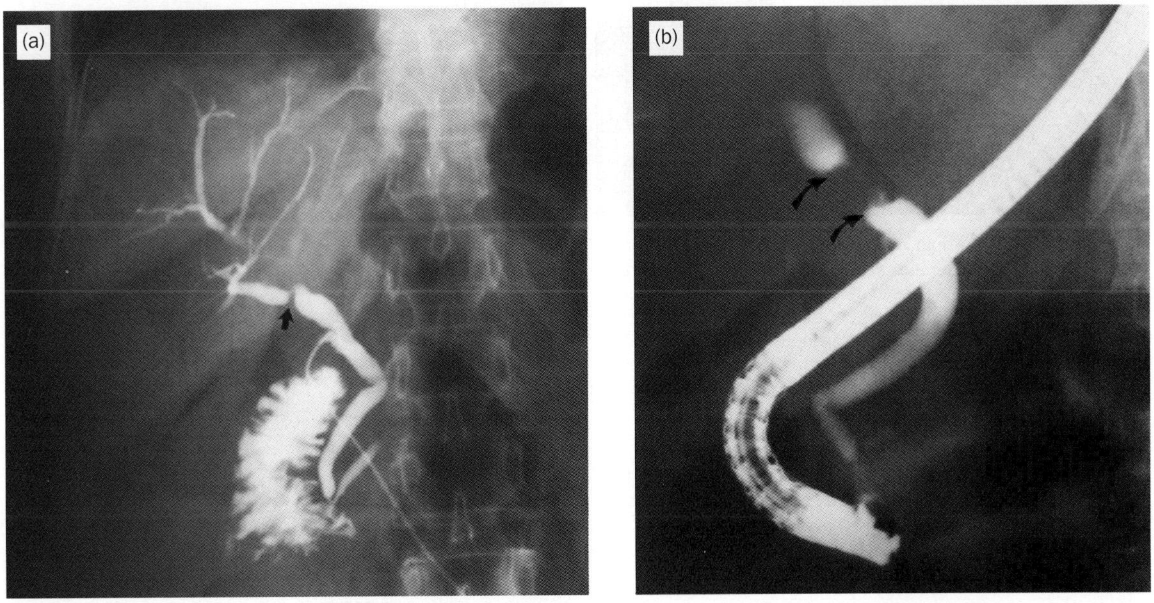

Figure 10.27 Narrowing (arrowed) in the common hepatic duct was thought to be the result of an impression caused by the right hepatic artery. Aside from the obvious stricture, the left intrahepatic ductal system is not visualized. Regrettably, this was overlooked. (b) The patient was referred to the author's unit 3 months later with deep jaundice. The ERCP showed an undoubted large carcinoma of the common hepatic duct (outlined between arrows) which proved inoperable.

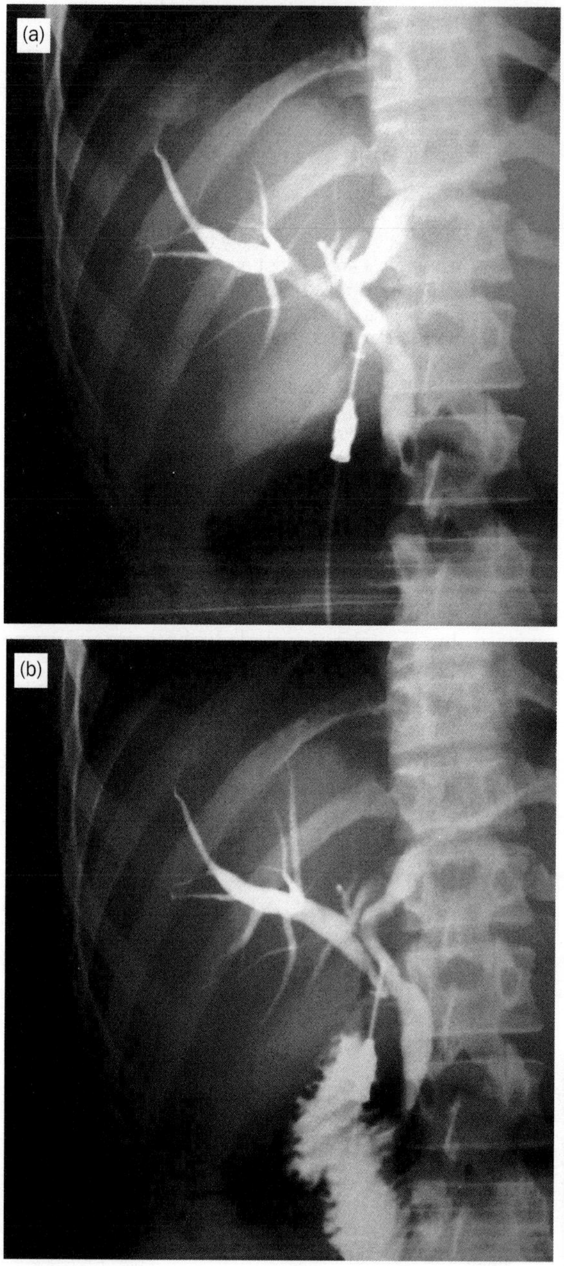

Figure 10.28 (a) Completion intra-operative cholangiogram – there is an apparent hold-up at the lower end which could be due to either spasm or a missed calculus. (b) Repeat cholangiogram in the same patient after administration of 1.0 μg ceruletide as an antispasmodic intravenously. There is now free flow of contrast medium into the duodenum. Alternatively glucagon may be used.

material or an excessive injection pressure. The latter can result in cholangiovenous reflux and bacteraemia especially in patients with cholangitis.

Other methods of intra-operative fluorocholangiograpy

Cholecystocholangiography

This is a simple technique that is primarily indicated when the surgeon is uncertain that the gallbladder needs removal but requires anatomical information of the extrahepatic biliary tract during the operation. Although it has been advocated as an easier alternative to transcystic fluorocholangiography during laparoscopic cholecystectomy, this practice is ill advised, since forceful injection of large amounts of contrast in the gallbladder may dislodge small stones down a wide cystic duct into the common bile duct. During laparoscopic cholecystectomy the technique is reserved for when dissection of the triangle of Calot proves difficult.

A cholecystocholangiogram is also indicated if a cholecystojeunostomy is being considered as a palliative procedure in patients with inoperable carcinoma of the pancreas/duodenum with severe obstructive jaundice and itch. The cholecystocholangiogram is performed to determine the patency of the cystic duct and the distance from its entry into the common bile duct and the upper limit of the tumour (Figure 10.29). Only if this distance is greater than 1.5 cm will cholecystojejunostomy suffice as an adequate palliation for jaundice and itching during the patient's lifetime (Figure 10.30). The method involves simple puncture of the gallbladder, using a sharp Veress needle attached by tubing to two 50 ml syringes (saline and diluted contrast). Usually some 40 ml have to be injected before contrast starts exiting the gallbladder into the biliary ducts. At the end of the procedure as much contrast is aspirated as is possible and the puncture site in the gallbladder is sutured with 3/0 absorbable material.

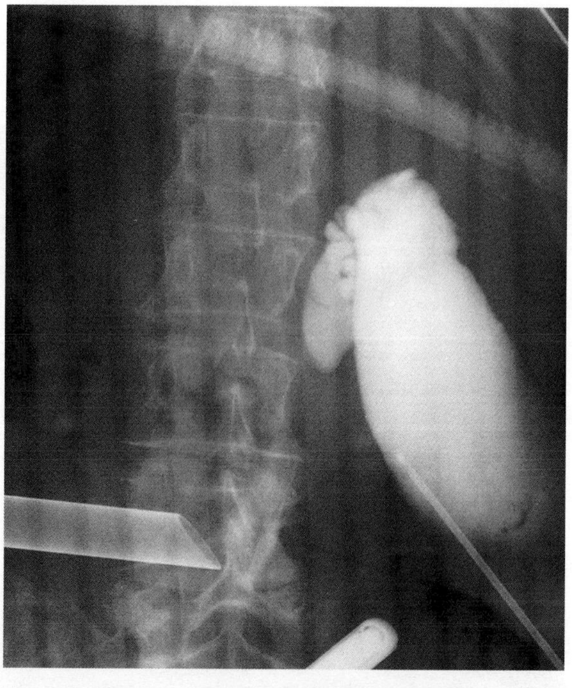

Figure 10.29 Laparoscopic cholecystocholangiogram in a patient with inoperable carcinoma of the pancreas. As the distance between the entry of the cystic duct into the bile duct is more than 1.5 cm from the upper limit of the tumour occlusion, a cholecystojejunostomy will provide adequate palliation of the jaundice and itching during the patient's lifetime.

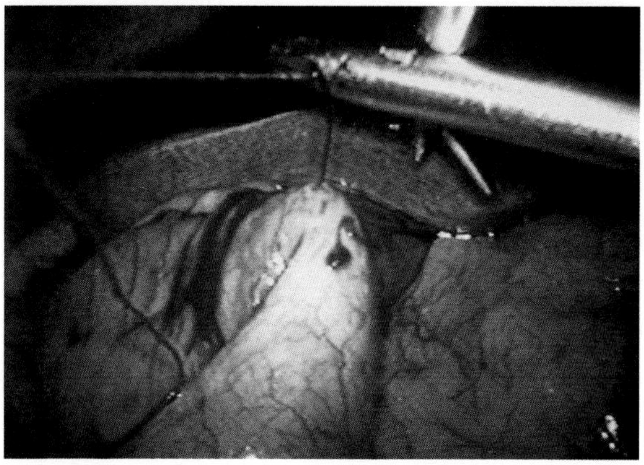

Figure 10.30 Laparoscopic palliative sutured cholecystojejunostomy.

Direct puncture

In post-cholecystectomy patients, IOFC may be carried out by direct puncture of the common bile duct using a fine intravenous cannula.

Transhepatic operative cholangiography

This is a valuable method that provides very useful information in patients with hilar tumours and during surgery for iatrogenic high bile duct injuries. A Chiba needle is used to puncture an intrahepatic bile duct under contact ultrasound control. When bile is aspirated, contrast is injected into the intrahepatic biliary tree. The technique can also be undertaken laparoscopically (Figure 10.31).

Choledochoscopy (cholangioscopy)

Operative choledochoscopy is well-established in biliary tract surgery and is considered an integral part of common bile duct exploration. Two types of choledochoscopes are available: the flexible fibre-optic instrument and the rigid Berci-Shore choledochoscope, which incorporates the Hopkin's rod lens system (Figure 10.32).

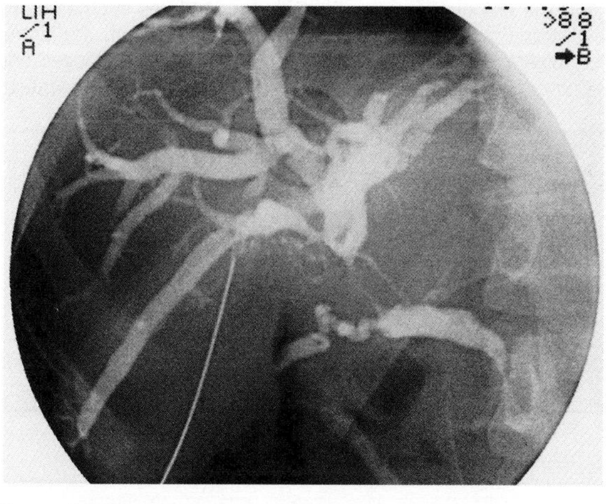

Figure 10.31 Laparoscopic transhepatic cholangiogram showing obstruction of the extrahepatic biliary tract by a large hilar tumour that appeared to originate from the gallbladder.

Berci-Shore rigid choledochoscope

This can only be used in open surgery. The rigid instrument is easy to deploy and permits therapeutic manoeuvres, such as the removal under visual guidance of calculi impacted at the lower end of the common bile duct. Saline irrigation to distend the biliary tract is needed. In most instances, gravity feed using a litre bag of saline suspended on a drip stand provides sufficient flow for adequate visualization. If not, a Fenwal pressure cuff is applied to the saline bag and insufflated to a pressure of 150–200 mmHg. However, care must be taken with this system since high pressures may be generated in the biliary tract causing cholangiovenous reflux and bacteraemia. An adequate mobilization of the first and second part of the duodenum is essential for choledochoscopic inspection of the distal common bile duct with the rigid instrument. As the mobilized duodenum is put on the stretch, it straightens the lower end of the common bile duct (which normally curves acutely to the right) and this facilitates choledochoscopic inspection.

The choledochoscope is introduced through a small choledochotomy in the supraduodenal part of the common bile duct. The initial inspection establishes the pathology, e.g. stones, tumour, etc. Removal of the stones can be performed under vision by the rigid instrument following attachment of the instrument channel. Either a biliary balloon catheter or a Dormia basket is introduced and the stone extracted under visual guidance. For impacted stones, the stone-grasping forceps are attached to the rigid instrument, which is then reintroduced and the stone dislodged and retrieved or crushed under vision. Once all the stones have been removed, a completion choledochoscopic examination of the entire biliary tract is performed before the insertion of a T-tube. Completion choledochoscopy is an alternative to completion T-tube cholangiography.

Flexible choledochoscopes

Flexible choledochoscopes do not require preliminary Kocherization of the duodenum for full inspection of the biliary tract and can be passed proximally to visualize the secondary and tertiary intrahepatic ducts. The standard choledochoscope has an external diameter of 4.0–4.5 mm and was designed for insertion into the common bile duct through a small choledochotomy (open or laparoscopic). The smaller ones (outer diameter of 2.8–3.0 mm) are referred to as mini-choledochoscopes and are used for transcystic duct extraction of ductal calculi during laparoscopic surgery. Often this entails prior dilatation of the cystic duct with a cylindrical balloon dilator. All mini-choledochoscopes used for laparoscopic extraction of ductal calculi through the cystic duct approach must have an instrument channel of 1.0 mm diameter or larger to enable insertion of small wire baskets (3 Fr) and balloon catheters and at the same time leave enough space for effective irrigation. During laparoscopic choledochoscopy, the endoscope is attached to a second charge-coupled device

(a)

(b)

(c)

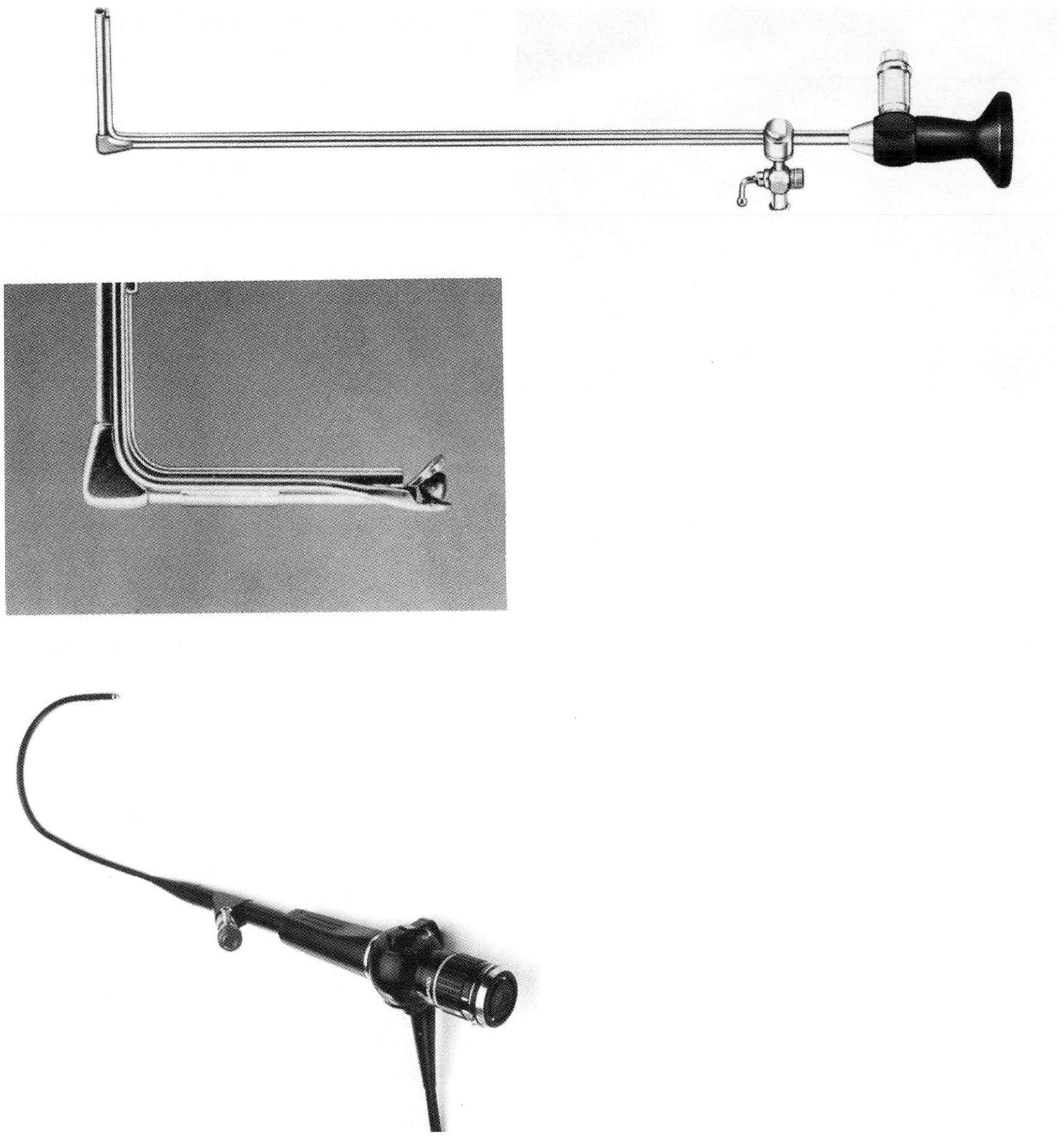

Figure 10.32 (a) The rigid choledochoscope (Berci-Shore) – it has an attachable instrument channel through which biopsy forceps, biliary balloon catheters and Dormia baskets can be passed into the bile duct for visually guided procedures such as stone extraction and biopsy of lesions. (b) In addition, it has an attachable strong stone forceps which moves together with the instrument and is extremely useful for dealing with impacted stones at the lower end of the bile duct. The stone can be dislodged and retrieved or crushed under vision. (From Cuschieri and Berci (1984) *Common Bile Duct Exploration*, Martinus Nijhoff, Dordrecht, by permission.) (c) The Olympus flexible choledochoscope.

(CCD) camera and with a picture-in-picture display (if available) both the laparoscopic and the endoscopic image are seen on the one monitor. This dual imaging greatly facilitates manipulations, especially extraction of ductal calculi

The advantages of choledochoscopy are:

- it provides the best evaluation of intracholedochal pathology
- it allows biopsy of suspicious lesions (Figure 10.33)
- it enables visually guided extraction of floating and impacted ductal calculi during both open and laparoscopic surgery
- the routine use of completion choledochoscopy results in an almost negligible incidence of retained ductal calculi
- it reduces the incidence of trauma, especially to the lower end of the bile duct caused by blind instrumentation with metal sounds and forceps
- the flexible endoscope provides an effective method of stone extraction of retained ductal calculi through the T-tube tract.

Biliary manometry

Biliary pressure studies can be undertaken intra-operatively or endoscopically during ERCP using a special perfusion catheter.

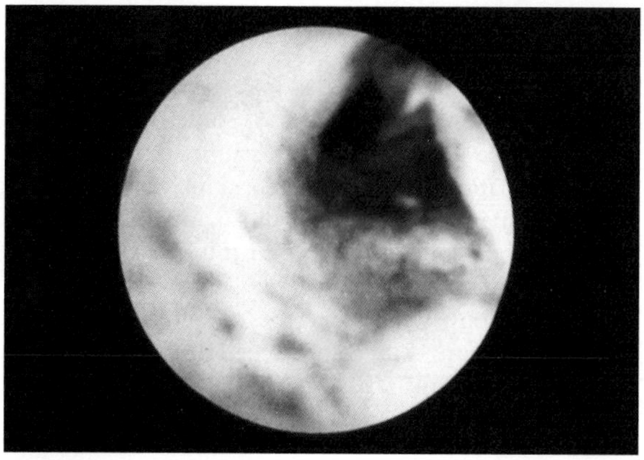

Figure 10.33 Choledochoscopic view of a stenosing lesion of the common hepatic duct. An endoscopic biopsy confirmed the presence of a cholangiocarcinoma.

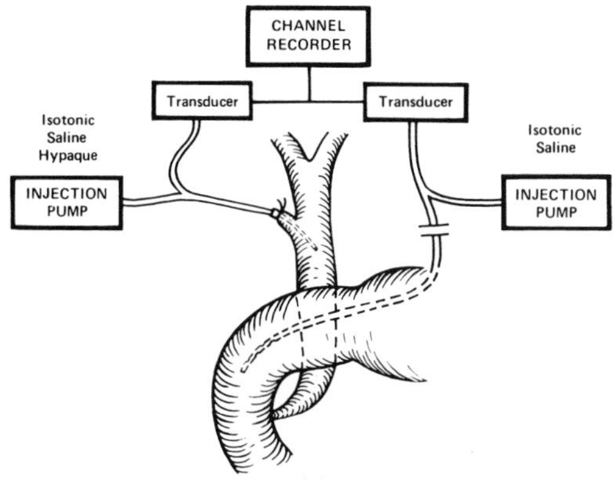

(a)

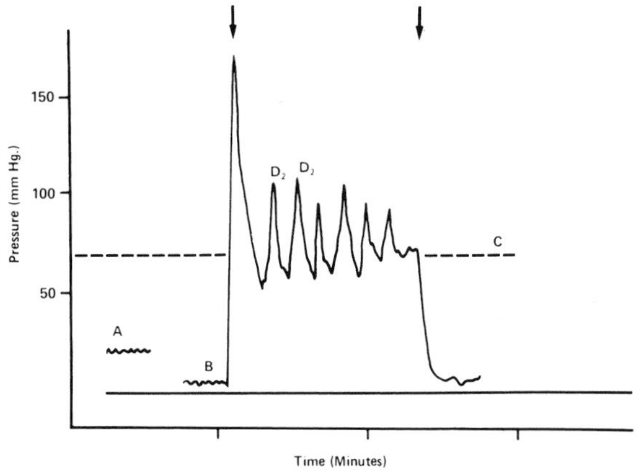

(b)

Figure 10.34 Peroperative radiomanometry: (a) apparatus; (b) normal pressure profile of the common bile duct during constant pump infusion of isotonic saline. A = pressure generated by the pump and intrinsic resistance of the system, B = basal bile duct pressure, C = filling pressure during injection, D = contractions of the sphincter of Oddi.

Intra-operative biliary manometry

This can be performed by the use of a pressure transducer connected to the cannula, which is inserted into the common bile duct via the cystic duct. The transducer is attached to a channel recorder which gives an instant display of the biliary pressure. This technique is known as radiomanometry and permits the measurement of the basal (resting) pressure and the filling pressure during the constant infusion of saline (5.0 ml/min). In addition, it demonstrates the sphincteric contractions and may be used to document the effect of spasmolytic drugs on the choledochal sphincter in patients with biliary dyskinesia (Figure 10.34). Operative biliary manometry is, however, seldom used nowadays except for research purposes.

The other technique used during biliary tract surgery is known as mano-debimetry. This measures the passage (yield) pressure at the choledochal sphincter and the flow rate through the common channel into the duodenum. The technique was first described by Caroli (Figure 10.35). The modern modification of the Caroli instrument is known as the Tondelli mano-debitometer. After measurement of the passage pressure, the upper limit of which is 25 cmH_2O, the calibrated reservoir (filled with saline or contrast medium) is raised to a standard height of 30 cm above the level of the common bile duct and the flow rate through the common channel measured from the rate of emptying of the reservoir per unit time. The normal flow rate measured in this way should exceed 12.0 ml/mm. A high passage pressure and a diminished flow rate are indicative of obstructive disease.

Endoscopic biliary manometry

Endoscopic biliary manometry is now an established diagnostic procedure in specialized units. It is performed by the use of a special perfusion catheter attached to an external transducer and has been used in the investigation of patients with persistent symptoms and pain after cholecystectomy in an attempt to characterize abnormalities of the sphincter (stenosis, dyskinesia). The procedure measures the basal sphincter pressure, the rate and propagation of sphincteric contractions and the response to pharmacological agents such as morphine and CCK. In patients with dyskinesia, increased basal pressure, altered frequency and amplitude of phasic contractions, and reversal of the normal peristaltic direction (retrograde propulsion) have been reported.

Laparoscopy

This procedure should be used routinely by surgeons in all patients with jaundice of malignant origin. It usually provides a direct visualization of the underlying pathology and the exact cause of the jaundice can be determined in all patients if ancillary techniques such as laparoscopic ultrasonography, cholangiography (transhepatic or transcholecystic) and targeted biopsy or cytology are employed. The liver, gallbladder, extrahepatic biliary tract and pancreas are directly visualized, as is the peritoneal lining and most of the intraperitoneal contents. Aside from detecting hepatic disease,

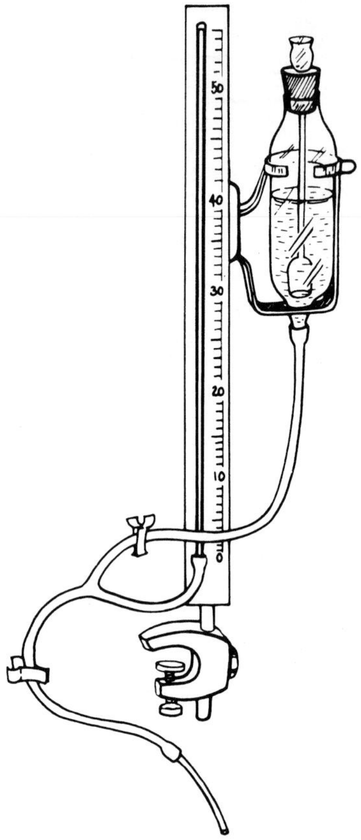

Figure 10.35 The Caroli instrument for mano-debimetry. The technique measures the passage (yield) pressure of the choledochal sphincter and the flow rate through the common channel into the duodenum.

primary neoplasms, secondary tumour deposits in the liver and peritoneal dissemination, all of which can be biopsied for histological confirmation, laparoscopy is invaluable in the staging of hepatobiliary and pancreatic tumours. Thus it avoids unnecessary laparotomy in patients with inoperable disease and can now be used to construct laparoscopic bilio-enteric and gastrojejunal bypass procedures for advanced inoperable pancreatic cancer. In patients with chronic liver disease and a bleeding tendency, laparoscopic liver biopsy is undertaken in preference to the blind percutaneous procedure as bleeding from the biopsy site can be controlled by electrocoagulation.

Section 10.4 • Jaundice

Bilirubin is produced in the reticuloendothelial system from the enzymic breakdown of haem, which is derived from effete red blood corpuscles. As it is water insoluble, bilirubin is carried bound to albumin in the plasma and is taken up by the hepatocytes by means of specific membrane carriers. Within the hepatocytes, the bilirubin is stored bound to specific binding proteins (ligandins Y, Z) and then conjugated by a specific enzyme (glucuronyl transferase) to the water-soluble bilirubin glucuronide (conjugated bilirubin) that is then secreted by means of specific carriers into the bile canaliculi, and finally excreted into the biliary tract and intestine. Bacterial degradation of some of the excreted conjugated bilirubin in the distal small bowel results in the formation of urobilinogen, which is reabsorbed and subsequently excreted in the urine and bile. The normal upper limit of serum bilirubin is 17 μmol/l.

Jaundice (hyperbilirubinaemia) is a syndrome of varied aetiology which may be recognized clinically when the serum bilirubin exceeds 40 μmol/l. The hyperbilirubinaemia may be either conjugated or unconjugated and may result from:

- Excess bilirubin production.
- Impaired uptake by the hepatocyte.
- Failure of conjugation.
- Impaired secretion of conjugated bilirubin into the bile canaliculi.
- Impairment of bile flow subsequent to the secretion by the hepatocytes – *cholestatic or obstructive jaundice* **[see Module II, Vol. I]**

The defect may be congenital (benign congenital hyperbilirubinaemias) but much more commonly, it is acquired as a result of haemolysis, liver disease, adverse drug reaction and biliary tract obstruction which may be intra- or extrahepatic. The early diagnosis and prompt treatment of patients with jaundice reduces both the morbidity and mortality of the underlying disease. In clinical practice, the largest groups by far are those with hepatocellular and cholestatic jaundice **[Module 11, Vol. I]**

Hepatocellular jaundice

This is due to parenchymatous liver disease which may be acute (viral hepatitis, liver cell necrosis, acute alcoholic hepatitis, etc.) or chronic (chronic active hepatitis, the various types of cirrhosis, primary biliary, etc.). The principal defect is the failure of secretion of the conjugated bilirubin into the bile canaliculi. The serum transaminases are grossly elevated especially in acute disease. In patients with alcohol-related liver disease, the gamma-glutamyl transpeptidase is elevated as a result of microsomal induction rather than cholestasis. Acute hepatitis due to viral infection or drugs may also cause a cholestatic picture, in which case the alkaline phosphatase and the 5-nucleotidase are elevated. The hyperbilirubinaemia is always (predominantly) of the conjugated variety with the presence of bilirubin in the urine even in the absence of a cholestatic component.

Cholestatic jaundice

This is the result of impaired bile flow to the duodenum subsequent to the secretion of conjugated bilirubin into the bile canaliculi. The block may be intrahepatic when it may be functional (e.g. drugs, hepatitis, etc.) or organic (obstruction of the intrahepatic biliary tree) or extrahepatic, also known as large bile duct obstruction which constitutes the most important surgical subgroup of cholestatic jaundice as it is always the result of organic disease, e.g. ductal calculi, pancreaticobiliary cancer, etc.

The biochemical features of cholestasis are:

- Conjugated hyperbilirubinaemia.
- Elevation of alkaline phosphatase, 5′-nucleotidase and gamma-glutamyl transpeptidase (gamma-GT). The enzyme 5′-nucleotidase is the most reliable since its level is not influenced by bone disease and the enzyme is not induced by alcohol.
- Minimal or no elevation of the serum transaminases.
- Presence of bilirubin in the urine as the conjugated bilirubin is water soluble and is therefore filtered in the glomerulus.
- Elevation in the serum cholesterol and bile acid levels although these are not routinely measured in patients with cholestatic jaundice.

It is important to stress that the above biochemical markers of cholestasis do not distinguish between intra- and extrahepatic obstruction.

Haemolytic jaundice

The unconjugated hyperbilirubinaemia results from excess haemolysis. Bilirubin is not present in the urine as the unconjugated pigment is water insoluble and is carried in the plasma bound to albumin. The excess bilirubin production is accompanied by an increased secretion of the conjugated pigment in the bile and therefore increased production of urobilinogen by bacterial decomposition in the distal small intestine. The urine, therefore, contains an excess amount of urobilinogen and urobilin. A cholestatic component may develop in patients with prolonged and recurrent haemolysis (e.g. congenital haemolytic anaemias).

In some patients excess bilirubin production is present in the absence of overt haemolysis. The excess unconjugated bilirubin is thought to result from breakdown of precursor/immature red cells in the bone marrow. This form of benign non-familial congenital hyperbilirubinaemia is referred to as *shunt hyperbilirubinaemia.*

Benign familial congenital hyperbilirubinaemias

This group includes Gilbert's disease, Dubin–Johnson syndrome and the Rotor syndrome. All three conditions are congenital and familial. Gilbert's disease is due to a defect in the uptake of bilirubin by the hepatocytes and results in mild unconjugated hyperbilirubinaemia. Both the Dubin–Johnson and Rotor syndromes are caused by a secretory defect of conjugated bilirubin by the hepatocytes into the bile canaliculi and therefore lead to a conjugated hyperbilirubinaemia. In addition, patients with the Dubin–Johnson syndrome are unable to excrete contrast media into the biliary tree and for this reason, the gallbladder is not visualized by oral cholecystography and intravenous cholangiography. Despite the accumulation of conjugated bilirubin in the blood and its appearance in the urine, there are no other biochemical markers of cholestasis in both conditions.

Section 10.5 • Management of patients with large bile duct obstruction

The investigation of the jaundiced patient is discussed in **Module 11, Vol. I**. It is important to reiterate that a properly taken history and physical examination will allow a correct diagnosis to be made in some 80% of patients. Surgical obstructive jaundice (or large bile duct obstruction) is always accompanied by dilatation of the biliary tract. In essence, the management entails establishing the cause, the general condition of the patient, and in the case of tumours, the stage of the disease. Malignant large bile duct obstruction may be inoperable either because the lesion is not resectable or because the patient's ASA grade or POSSUM risk assessment score precludes major surgical intervention. In this situation management is directed towards palliation by endoscopic/radiological stenting or laparoscopic bypass procedures.

Dilatation of the biliary tract

The common bile duct dilates more rapidly than the intrahepatic biliary tree. Thus, instant passive dilatation of the common bile duct demonstrated fluoroscopically can be produced by excessive filling of the biliary tract by contrast media. Dilatation of the intrahepatic biliary tree always signifies prolonged obstruction and, experimentally, it requires a minimum of 3 weeks of obstruction for the production of demonstrable intrahepatic duct dilatation. By convention, the diameter of the common bile duct is measured just above the junction of the cystic duct. A common bile duct whose diameter exceeds 10 mm after contrast injection (during cholangiography) is considered dilated. In the absence of contrast injection, e.g. ultrasound or MRCP, a diameter above 7 mm indicates dilatation.

Dilatation of the common bile duct signifies existing or recently relieved obstruction, the most common cause of which is calculous disease. There is an established positive correlation between the duct diameter and the incidence of ductal stones. On the other hand, stones may be present in a normal-sized common bile duct and in several reported series a 5–10% incidence of ductal stones has been reported in patients with common bile ducts of 5 mm. Other causes of duct dilatation include pancreaticobiliary cancer, chronic pancreatitis, congenital cystic disease and parasitic infestation. Controversy persists regarding dilatation of the bile duct after truncal vagotomy. Some studies have demonstrated abnormal gallbladder emptying after this procedure but not following highly selective vagotomy.

Although there are no intrahepatic communications between the right and the left intrahepatic ductal trees in the normal state, communications between the two systems develop following the onset of extrahepatic large bile duct obstruction.

Pre-operative management of the patient with obstructive jaundice

Adequate timing of the surgical intervention and preparation of the patient for surgery are essential in the management of patients with obstructive lesions of the biliary tract. Undue delays exceeding 3–4 weeks increase both the morbidity and mortality rates following surgical intervention. Adequate preparation entails the correction of metabolic abnormalities, improvement of the general condition and the institution of specific measures designed to minimize the incidence of complications associated with prolonged or severe cholestasis. These include:

- infections: cholangitis, septicaemia, wound infections
- disorders of the clotting mechanism
- renal failure
- liver failure
- fluid and electrolyte abnormalities.

Furthermore, the conjugation and metabolism of drugs and anaesthetic agents is impaired because of the hepatocyte malfunction. Contrary to popular belief, there is no evidence to support the view that wound healing is impaired in the presence of jaundice. Wound healing problems are largely confined to patients with malignant obstruction and are the result of the underlying disease and its association with a poor nutritional state. The nutritional deficits of these patients vary with the underlying pathology, age and social class of the patient. In general, parenteral nutrition should be used selectively, and only in those patients who are grossly malnourished, because of infective risks. A high intake of carbohydrates is essential and amino acid solutions containing aromatic amino acids (phenylalanine, tyrosine and tryptophan) should be used sparingly as these may precipitate encephalopathy in susceptible patients. An oral diet is the safest and should be used whenever possible. It may be supplemented by elemental diets in nutritionally compromised patients. Enteral nutrition is considered essential for the maintenance of the mucosal integrity of the gut against bacterial translocation. Some advocate the oral administration of bile salts or lactulose to reduce the intestinal absorption of endotoxin from the intestinal microflora and thus minimize the incidence of renal failure following surgical intervention.

Hypokalaemia is frequently present and should be corrected. In general, intravenous isotonic saline administration should be restricted in the jaundiced patients and those with liver disease as the total exchangeable body sodium is elevated. The low normal values of the concentration of the serum sodium frequently encountered in these patients are due to expansion of the intra- and extravascular fluid compartments consequent on the excessive retention of water (dilutional hyponatraemia). A viral screen should be is necessary in these patients and when the serology is positive, special precautions must be taken both in the ward and in the operating theatre to avoid spread of the infection to the attending medical staff.

Prevention of infective complications

Whereas the normal biliary tract and bile in the human is sterile, bacteria are frequently present in biliary tract disorders and may lead to septic complications, particularly cholangitis and septicaemia. Infection of the biliary tract is much more commonly present in ductal calculous disease than in patients with malignant obstructive jaundice. Anaerobes are less frequently found in the biliary tract and duodenum than aerobic bacteria even in the presence of pathological states. Thus, in the absence of stenting, the majority of infections associated with biliary tract disorders are aerobic in origin and most commonly due to Gram-negative bacilli. Endoscopic stenting of patients with malignant large bile duct obstruction results in infection of the biliary tract and is unwise if the patient is deemed operable.

A number of clinical trials have shown that the postoperative sepsis in patients having biliary tract surgery is generally due to bacteria in the bile and the use of short-term prophylactic antibiotics (three-dose regimen peri-operatively: immediately before surgery to 24 hours later) significantly lowers the incidence of sepsis only in patients who have bacteria in the bile at the time of surgery. Prophylactic antibiotics are therefore not advised in all patients undergoing surgery on the biliary tract but should be administered to those patients who are likely to have bacteria in the bile. The higher risk groups have been identified and include:

- all jaundiced patients
- patients with rigors and pyrexia
- patients undergoing emergency biliary procedures/operations
- elderly patients
- patients with common duct stones even if not jaundiced
- patients undergoing secondary biliary intervention.

Some advocate the use of Gram's staining of the bile at the time of surgery to determine both the presence and the Gram staining characteristics of the organisms in deciding on the appropriate antibiotic. The use of prophylactic antibiotic therapy with a cephalosporin, or aminoglycoside or pipericillin (three doses) in the high-risk groups outlined above has been shown to reduce the incidence of postoperative wound infection, cholangitis and septicaemia.

Bacterial proliferation in the bile following exploration of the common bile duct and insertion of a T-tube is extremely common and may become a source of infection or lead to the formation of calcium bilirubinate stones as a result of the deconjugation of the bilirubin-glucuronide by glucuronidase-producing bacteria, particularly *Escherichia coli*. Thus, a closed system of T-tube drainage should always be used and a bile culture performed a few days before the removal of the T-tube. A course of the appropriate antibiotic should be administered if the culture is positive.

Correction of disorders of coagulation

The most common disorder of coagulation encountered in patients with large bile duct obstruction is a prolonged prothrombin time resulting from a deficiency of vitamin K-dependent factors consequent on the malabsorption of this vitamin which occurs in cholestatic jaundice. The intramuscular injection of phytomenadione (10–20 mg) will reverse the multifactorial clotting deficiency within 1–3 days. Severe hepatic disease, usually with a poor prognosis, is present if the prothrombin time remains abnormally prolonged despite this treatment. If these patients require surgical intervention, administration of fresh frozen plasma is necessary to cover the peri-operative period.

A more serious bleeding disorder may arise usually in the severely jaundiced patient who may develop a consumptive coagulopathy from a disseminated intravascular coagulation due to the presence of circulating endotoxin. This serious haematological complication requires careful monitoring of fibrinogen levels, fibrinogen degradation products and platelet counts. It may improve with control of the infection but often requires specific treatment with fresh frozen plasma alone or in combination with heparin.

Prevention of renal failure

The association between post-operative renal failure and severe conjugated hyperbilirubinaemia is well known but the underlying mechanism of the renal impairment is inadequately understood, although a reduced glomerular filtration is usually present. Even in the absence of infection, endotoxinaemia is frequently present in jaundiced patients when it results from absorption of endotoxin produced by the intestinal microflora. There appears to be a relationship between impaired renal function and the presence of circulating endotoxin in jaundiced patients. Irrespective of the exact cause of the renal damage, there is now good evidence that adequate hydration and pre-operative induction of a natriuresis/diuresis reduces the incidence of renal failure after surgical intervention in jaundiced patients. It is current routine practice to administer intravenous fluids (5% dextrose saline) for 12–24 hours before surgery. This is followed by an osmotic diuretic (mannitol) or a loop diuretic (frusemide) administered intravenously at the time of induction of anaesthesia. All patients undergoing surgery should be catheterized and the urine output measured hourly. Further administration of diuretics (mannitol or frusemide) is indicated if the urine output falls consistently below 40 ml/h (despite adequate hydration and normovolaemia) during operation and subsequently thereafter.

Pre-operative administration of oral chenodeoxycholate commencing a few days before surgery is practised in some centres and one clinical trial has shown a reduction in the incidence of renal failure, although a second trial with the epimer, ursodeoxycholate, did not report any benefit. More recently, the administration of oral lactulose has been shown to reduce the incidence of renal failure in jaundiced patients undergoing surgical treatment but this requires confirmation.

Prevention of hepatic encephalopathy

Liver failure is usually encountered in patients with prolonged complete large bile duct obstruction or those patients with pre-existing chronic hepatocellular disease, such as cirrhosis, chronic active hepatitis, etc., who undergo surgery. If the jaundice is severe (above 150 μmol/l) or the patient shows signs of impending liver failure, a period of decompression is indicated. This is nowadays achieved by insertion of a plastic endoprosthesis for patients with malignant obstruction. Alternatively an endoscopic sphincterotomy is performed in patients with periampullary cancer. External percutaneous decompression via a transhepatic tube draining into an external collecting system is no longer advocated since it predisposes to infection and leads to a loss of bile acids unless the bile is returned to the gastrointestinal tube via a nasogastric tube. The correction of hypokalaemia, the restricted use of sedatives, hypnotics and potent analgesics, and the prompt treatment of infection cannot be overemphasized. If sedation is required, small doses of promethazine or chlorpromazine can be administered.

Section 10.6 • Post-operative jaundice

Jaundice occurring for the first time in the post-operative period may be due to a variety of causes (Table 10.1) and always requires detailed investigation to establish the cause and outline the necessary course of action. Mild self-limiting conjugated hyperbilirubinaemia, sometimes referred to as benign post-operative cholestasis, may follow prolonged operations and fever caused by chest infections. It is caused by a reactive hepatitis, which is probably multifactorial in origin, resulting from a combination of reduced liver blood flow, hypoxia, hypercarbia, breakdown of transfused cells and temporary hepatocellular dysfunction. Initially, it warrants observation with repeated assessment of the patient's condition and sequential biochemical profiles, as the majority of cases with this syndrome subside within 3–4 weeks.

Marked cholestatic jaundice develops after extensive hepatic resection, especially right hepatectomy and extended right hepatectomy. The serum bilirubin rises over a period of several days to reach a plateau at 7–10

Table 10.1 Causes of post-operative jaundice

- **Benign reactive hepatitis** – self-limiting
- **Sepsis** – leaking anastomosis, abscess formation, septicaemia, pneumonia, etc.
- **Pre-existing primary disease** – known or suspected liver disease
- **Major hepatic resections**
- **Drug-induced liver disease**
- **Biliary pathology** – residual stones, bile duct trauma and missed tumours pathology of the biliary tract
- **Massive blood transfusion** – each unit of blood provides a bilirubin load transfusion of 250 mg/100 ml when fresh.
- **Haemolysis** – unconjugated hyperbilirubinaemia, positive Coombs' test
- **Residual haematomas** – unconjugated hyperbilirubinaemia

days after which it should start to decline. In view of the extensive hepatic resection (low residual liver parenchyma), the rise in the serum alkaline phosphatase is small.

Severe or progressive jaundice in the post-operative period is always sinister and usually indicates a primary biliary tract problem, or significant liver disease or severe sepsis such as that resulting from an anastomotic dehiscence. Aside from the usual liver function tests, the following may be required:

- blood culture
- ultrasound/CT scanning for the detection of collections/bilomas/abscesses
- EHIDA scintiscanning
- ERCP
- contrast radiological examination of recently constructed gastrointestinal anastomoses
- liver biopsy if the above are negative or if hepatocellular disease or drug-induced jaundice is suspected.

Hepatitis B is rare nowadays because of better screening for the viral antigens and improved blood donor selection. Most instances of infection caused by blood and blood products are due to hepatitis C virus and other non-A non-B viruses. Drug-induced jaundice is common in hospital practice. Some of the important drugs which may give rise to this adverse reaction are listed in Table 10.2.

Severe hepatotoxicity can follow halothane anaesthesia. In the majority of patients (over 80%), this follows repeated exposure usually within 28 days (75%). The disease is usually severe and is accompanied by an overall mortality of 40%. The following recommendations have been issued by the Committee on the Safety of Medicines:

- A careful history to determine previous exposure and reactions to halothane should be obtained from every patient.
- Repeated exposure to halothane within a period of at least 3 months should be avoided if at all possible.
- A history of unexplained jaundice or pyrexia following exposure to halothane is an absolute contraindication to further use of halothane in that individual patient.

Clinical management of post-operative jaundice

In the first instance, a full examination of the patient and a careful reappraisal of the pre-operative liver function tests are carried out. If liver function was normal prior to operation, the following are performed in a sequential order.

Determination of the nature of the jaundice by the liver function tests and urine testing for bilirubin – post-operative unconjugated hyperbilirubinaemia is commonly due to large/massive transfusion. Each unit of blood provides a bilirubin load of 250 mg/100 ml of fresh blood. Unconjugated hyperbilirubinaemia may also result from resorption of residual haematoma/haemoperitoneum or haemolysis. Haemolytic reactions resulting from minor/major incompatibilities are accompanied by systemic signs. When suspected, screening tests for haemolysis should be performed.

If the jaundice is cholestatic, an assessment of all the drugs and anaesthetic agents used is followed by the

Table 10.2 Drug-induced liver damage

Category	*Example*	*Hepatic lesion*
Antibiotics	Tetracyclines, especially i.v. – dose related	Fatty infiltration
	Penicillins – hypersensitivity	Hepatitis
	Chloramphenicol	Hepatitis
	Sulphonamides – hypersensitivity	Granulomas, focal hepatocellular necrosis
Analgesics and anti-inflammatory drugs	Paracetamol – dose dependent	Centrilobular necrosis, massive liver necrosis
	Phenylbutazone – hypersensitivity	Hepatitis with granuloma may progress to cirrhosis
	Carbamazepine	Cholestasis
	Salicylates – dose related	Focal hepatic necrosis
Psychotropic drugs	Monoamine oxidase inhibitors	Hepatitis, may progress to massive hepatic necrosis
	Phenothiazines – hypersensitivity	Hepatitis and cholestasis
	Tricyclic antidepressants	Cholestatic hepatitis, more usually mild elevation of transaminases
Steroids	Testosterone and anabolic steroids	Cholestasis, peliosis hepatis, hepatic tumours
	Oestrogens	Cholestasis, gallstones, hepatic tumours
Anaesthetic agents	Halothane	Hepatitis which may progress to massive liver necrosis
Antituberculous drugs	PAS – hypersensitivity	Hepatitis
	INAH – related to acetylator status	Focal to severe hepatic necrosis
	Rifampicin – dose related	Defective bilirubin transport, mild hepatitis
Cytotoxic and immunosuppressive drugs	Azathioprine	Cholestasis and peliosis hepatis
	6-Mercaptopurine – dose related	Hepatitis
	Methotrexate – long-term therapy	Fatty change, fibrosis of the portal tracts and cirrhosis
Others	Benzothiazine diuretics	Cholestatic hepatitis
	Phenindione	Cholestatic hepatitis
	Chlorpropamide	Cholestatic hepatitis
	Phenytoin	Hepatocellular necrosis

withdrawal of any drug known to cause hepatotoxicity. A thorough search for sepsis by the appropriate tests (including blood cultures) is made and an ultrasound/CT examination carried out. External leakage of bile or evidence of anastomotic dehiscence in a jaundiced patient is always serious and establishes the cause. Cholestatic jaundice accompanied by sepsis and abdominal signs is always indicative of a major surgical complication, e.g. bile duct injury, cholangitis or anastomotic dehiscence, and requires urgent radiological investigation. In the absence of sepsis and if the ERCP confirms integrity of the biliary tract, the liver function tests are repeated daily to determine the course of the biochemical profile. If the cholestasis is seen to be resolving, an expectant policy is adopted, otherwise a liver biopsy is undertaken.

Section 10.7 • Jaundice in infancy and childhood

Apart from the physiological jaundice, the aetiology of hyperbilirubinaemia in infancy may be due to haematological disorders, enzymatic defects, inborn errors of metabolism, infections and obstructive disease. The causes of jaundice in infancy and childhood are shown in Table 10.3. Whereas unconjugated hyperbilirubinaemia may be physiological, all causes of conjugated hyperbilirubinaemia are abnormal. Inflammatory disease of the gallbladder and cholelithiasis are rare but do occur, including acalculous cholecystitis. A higher percentage of gallstones in the paediatric age group is associated with haemolytic disorders than in the adult population. An increased incidence of gallstones is also found in patients with cystic fibrosis. Children with gallstones present with an atypical history of vague abdominal pain and distress. Classical biliary colic is rare. An ultrasound examination of the gallbladder or oral cholecystogram should be performed in all children undergoing splenectomy for haemolytic anaemia.

Biliary atresia and neonatal hepatitis

The concept regarding the pathophysiology of these disorders proposed by Kasai has received widespread acceptance and they are now considered to be different manifestations of the same process, with atresia developing in infants who have a component of cholangitis which then progresses to fibrosis and obliteration of the extrahepatic ductal system. Experimentally, infection of mice and Rhesus monkeys with retrovirus III results in congenital biliary atresia that is indistinguishable from the human disease in its pathological features and clinical course. Both biliary atresia and neonatal hepatitis present with jaundice (conjugated) at birth. Untreated biliary atresia leads to irreversible cirrhosis, often within 2–3 months of onset.

The diagnostic protocol carried out in these infants is designed to differentiate neonatal hepatitis from biliary atresia and the standard work-up, apart from liver function tests, includes screening for infectious, genetic and enzymatic disorders. Studies required include the Rose Bengal or EHIDA scan (in which there is no bile passage into the duodenum over 3–4 days in biliary atresia as assessed by faecal radioactivity), liver biopsy and serial total bilirubin levels. A rising or flat bilirubin curve over several weeks is found in atresia, whereas in neonatal hepatitis there is a gradual fall in the serum bilirubin after an initial peak. Other congenital abnormalities, such as situs inversus and intestinal malrotation, may occur in association with biliary atresia.

The treatment of biliary atresia is surgical and must be carried out within 60 days of birth, otherwise the prognosis is poor from irreversible cirrhosis. At operation a cholecystocholangiogram (if the gallbladder is present) and a wedge liver biopsy are performed. If an extrahepatic stump of the common hepatic duct is present, a Roux-en-Y jejunal anastomosis is carried out. Hepatic portoenterostomy (the Kasai procedure) is performed if no extrahepatic ducts are discernible. The procedure consists of the progressive excision of fibrosed remnants of the ducts anterior to the portal vein at the porta hepatis together with a 1 cm ring of adjacent liver substance, advancing to some 2–3 cm in depth using the operating microscope until biliary structures are identified: bile ducts, collecting tubules of biliary glands or biliary glands. The excised scar tissue is subjected to histological examination to identify these structures. A modified Roux-en-Y anastomosis (Suruga II procedure) is then performed at the periphery of the saucerized area surrounding the bile ductules (Figure 10.36). This has an access jejunostomy placed subcutaneously which allows irrigation,

Table 10.3 Causes of jaundice in infancy and childhood

- Physiological jaundice
- Haematological disorders – inspissated bile plug
- Enzymatic defects
- Inborn errors of metabolism
- Hepatitis and other infections
- Biliary atresia
- Biliary hypoplasia
- Cystic disease of the bile ducts
- Congenital perforation of the common bile duct

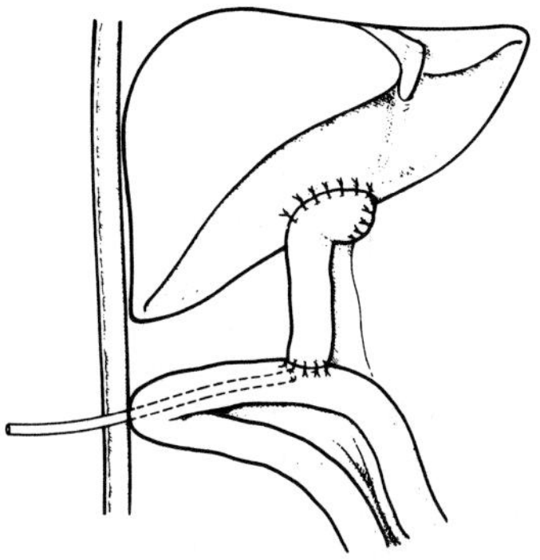

Figure 10.36 The Suruga II procedure of intubated access jejunostomy in patients with biliary atresia.

evaluation of post-operative bile flow and, if necessary, introduction of a paediatric flexible endoscope to inspect the porta hepatis. In an effort at reducing post-operative cholangitis due to reflux of intestinal contents, various valve constructions have been advocated between the portoenterostomy and the enteroenteric anastomosis. Some favour an isoperistaltic jejunal loop with a nipple valve interposed between the porta hepatis and the duodenum instead of the Roux-en-Y reconstruction.

An 80–90% successful outcome is obtained in infants in whom bile ducts communicating with the intrahepatic system have been identified at operation provided this is performed within 60 days of birth. These infants require vitamin E supplements to minimize the development of neurological sequelae. Overall, some 25% of these children develop cirrhosis and portal hypertension. Hepatic transplantation is now accepted as the treatment of choice in infants and children with biliary atresia in whom a portoenterostomy has failed and who develop cirrhosis. Recently the argument has been made for proceeding to primary liver transplantation instead of a portoenterostomy on the grounds that the majority of infants treated by the latter procedure develop biliary cirrhosis and portal hypertension with bleeding particularly when a cutaneous stoma leading from the portoenterostomy loop is employed. While primary hepatic transplantation may be appropriate in a small subset with adverse scoring system based on multiple liver function tests, for the majority of infants this policy is generally considered to be inappropriate. The Kasai operation works best at an age less than 6–8 weeks (when the results of hepatic transplantation are not optimal) and imparts long-term control in 30% of patients. Transplantation success improves considerably when the operation is performed after the age of 12 months. Thus a portoenterostomy buys time, allows patient growth, enhances the donor pool available to the patient and increases the chance of successful transplantation. In a recent large reported experience based on this policy, the 1-year transplant survival rate was 87%. Poor results were encountered only in patients in whom a portoenterostomy had been revised prior to transplantation. Thus a non-functioning portoenterostomy is an indication for hepatic transplantation and attempts at revision are unwarranted. The problem with transplantation in children relates to the scarcity of appropriate-size livers (which can be housed in the small subdiaphragmatic space), since the vast majority of donors are adults. The size disparity is being resolved by recourse to split liver or segmental hepatic transplantation either from brain-dead donors or living related donors.

Biliary hypoplasia

This is usually secondary to another primary disorder, such as extrahepatic biliary atresia, choledochal cyst, neonatal hepatitis and α_1-antitrypsin deficiency. Early surgical treatment, when indicated, is designed to correct the primary abnormality.

Inspissated bile plug syndrome

This condition is usually secondary to haemolytic disorders. The diagnosis is made by operative cholangiography and treatment, which is curative, consists of irrigation of the extrahepatic ducts.

Congenital perforation of the common duct

This condition presents with jaundice during the first to the third month of life. The perforation which occurs at the junction of the cystic with the common duct leads to the formation of a pseudocyst. Surgical treatment consists of transperitoneal drainage which is usually followed by spontaneous closure of the perforation.

Section 10.8 • Cystic disease of the biliary tract

Cystic disease of the biliary tract is rare and in the USA accounts for 1 in 13 000 hospital admissions. The aetiology remains unknown. Most instances are thought to represent congenital weakness of the common bile duct with distal obstruction caused by an anomalous acute or right-angle junction between the pancreatic duct and the common bile duct resulting in an abnormally long common channel (>0.6 cm). Another theory postulates an unequal proliferation of the duct epithelium. Several types are recognized (Figure 10.37):

- Type I diffuse choledochal cystic dilatation, commonest.
- Type II localized dilatation of the supraduodenal bile duct.
- Type III supraduodenal diverticulum.
- Type IV intraduodenal diverticulum or choledochocele.
- Type V solitary intrahepatic cyst.
- Type VI multiple intrahepatic cysts (Caroli's disease).
- Type VII multiple intra- and extrahepatic cysts.

Type VI (Figure 10.38), which is a hereditary disorder (autosomal recessive), is known as Caroli's disease and carries a poor prognosis from recurrent cholangitis and the development of intrahepatic stones, liver abscess formation and, eventually, cirrhosis. In some patients, multiple intrahepatic cystic disease is accompanied by congenital hepatic fibrosis. This condition is known as Grumbach's disease [see also Disorders of the Liver, Vol. II].

Clinical features

There appears to be a high incidence of cystic disease in the Japanese. There is a strong female predominance world-wide (70% of reported cases in the West) and 25% of the reported cases have been diagnosed during the first year of life. Another 35% become clinically manifest over the next 10 years. The symptoms include cholestatic jaundice, abdominal mass and pain. Complications of the disease include recurrent cholangitis and pancreatitis, hepatic abscess formation, calculous disease, biliary cirrhosis, rupture of the cyst with biliary peritonitis (rare) and portal vein thrombosis. There is also an increased risk of cholangiocarcinoma, which usually develops in the posteromedial wall of the cyst.

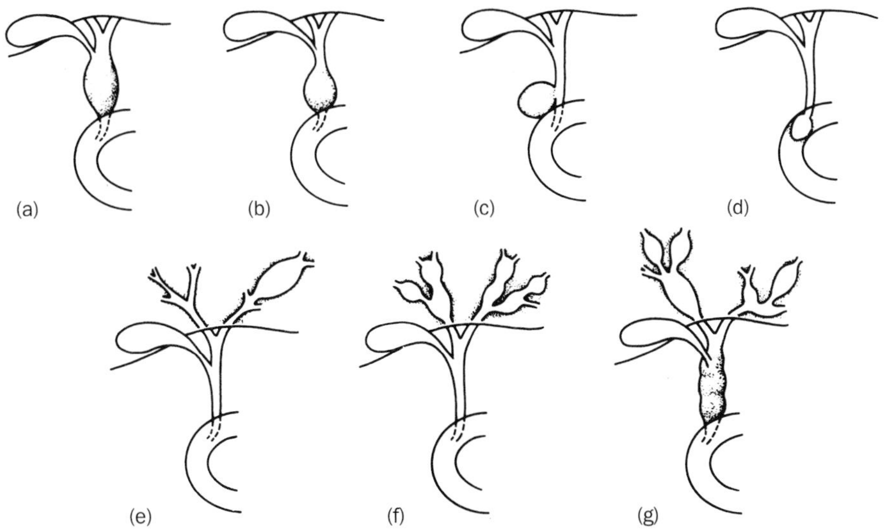

Figure 10.37 Diagrammatic representation of the types of cystic disease of the biliary tract: (a) type I – diffuse choledochal dilatation; (b) type II – localized choledochal dilatation; (c) type III – supraduodenal diverticulum; (d) type IV – intraduodenal diverticulum (choledochocele); (e) type V – solitary intrahepatic cyst; (f) type VI – multiple intrahepatic cysts (Caroli's disease); (g) type VII – multiple intra- and extrahepatic cysts.

The diagnosis can be established non-invasively with ultrasound and CT scanning. Better definition of the pathological anatomy is, however, obtained with MRCP or ERCP which also demonstrates the anomalous junction of the bile and pancreatic ducts and its angle (Figures 10.39 and 10.40). Type IV (intraduodenal diverticulum, choledochocele) can be recognized endoscopically as a smooth compressible elevation associated with an enlarged papilla which protrudes into the duodenum.

Treatment

The treatment of choice is surgical excision with a Roux-en-Y anastomosis. This gives much better results than drainage procedures and avoids or minimizes the risk of carcinoma. The excision is however, difficult as the cyst is often adherent to the other structures of the porta hepatis and is best performed in centres with biliary surgical expertise. The treatment of patients with intrahepatic cystic disease is difficult. When localized, partial liver resection is advisable. It is doubtful whether distal

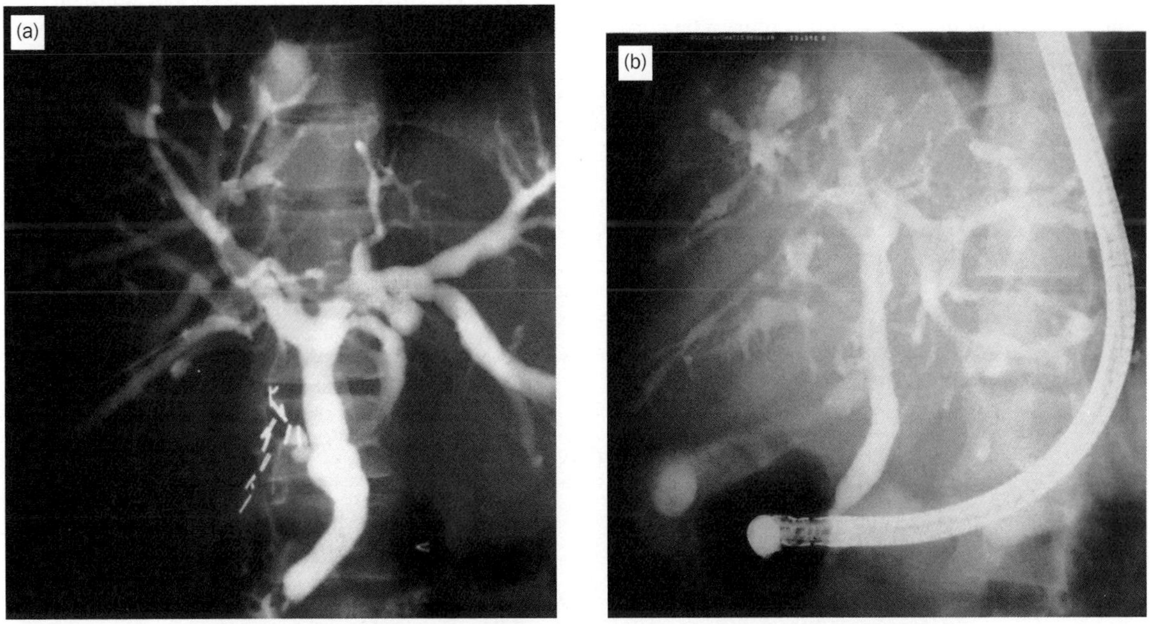

Figure 10.38 Caroli's disease: (a) PTC showing multiple intrahepatic cysts; (b) ERCP showing multiple intrahepatic cysts. The patient presented with bleeding from oesophageal varices. Liver biopsy showed hepatic fibrosis. The combination of diffuse intrahepatic cystic disease and hepatic fibrosis is known as Grumbach's disease.

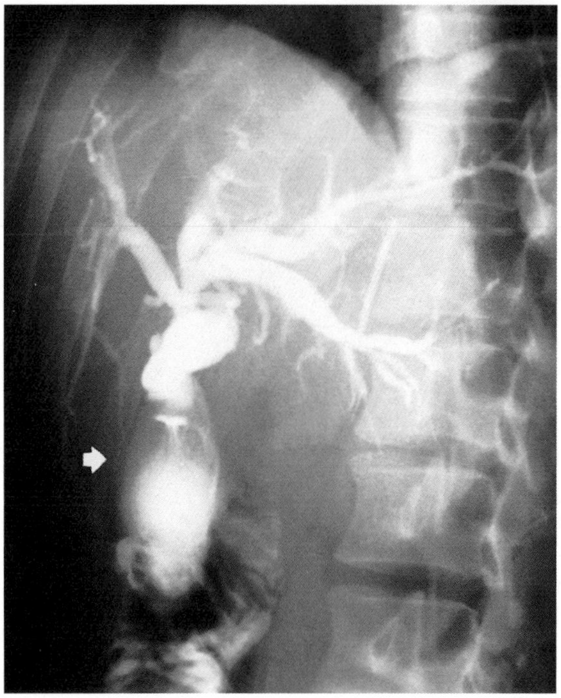

Figure 10.39 ERCP outlining diffuse choledochal dilatation (type I). This is the commonest variety and accounts for 80% of cases.

drainage, such as choledochoduodenostomy or transduodenal/endoscopic sphincterotomy, materially influences the course of the disease of the widespread intrahepatic variety and may indeed enhance the risk of cholangitis.

Section 10.9 • Gallstones

There has been a marked rise in the incidence of gallstones in the West during the past century. The current mean prevalence in Europe obtained from autopsy studies is 18.5% with the lowest prevalence being reported from Ireland (5%) and the highest from Sweden (38%). In the UK, USA and Australia, the prevalence rates vary from 15 to 25%. In every Western country, the prevalence of gallstones in females is approximately twice that of the male population. The highest prevalence is found in the Pima Indian tribe of Arizona with total and female prevalences of 49% and 73%, respectively. A high prevalence rate is also found in South American countries. Gallstones are rare in Africa and most recorded rates in this continent are below 1%. The prevalence of gallstones in Japan has also risen since the early twentieth century from 2 to 7%. In addition, the composition of stones in Japan has changed during the same period such that cholesterol stones now predominate over pigment stones.

Classification

The old classification of Aschoff into inflammatory, metabolic, static and mixed does not correlate with the present pathophysiological information relating to the formation of gallstones and is not currently used. Likewise, the classification into 'pure' and 'mixed' stones is inaccurate as the overwhelming majority of stones are composed of more than one component. The accepted current classification recognizes three main types of gallstones: cholesterol, black pigment and brown pigment stones.

Cholesterol stones

These form in the gallbladder and are preceded by the formation of biliary sludge (see below). They account for the vast majority (75%) of gallstones encountered in the West. They have a protein matrix and although they are composed predominantly of cholesterol, they con-

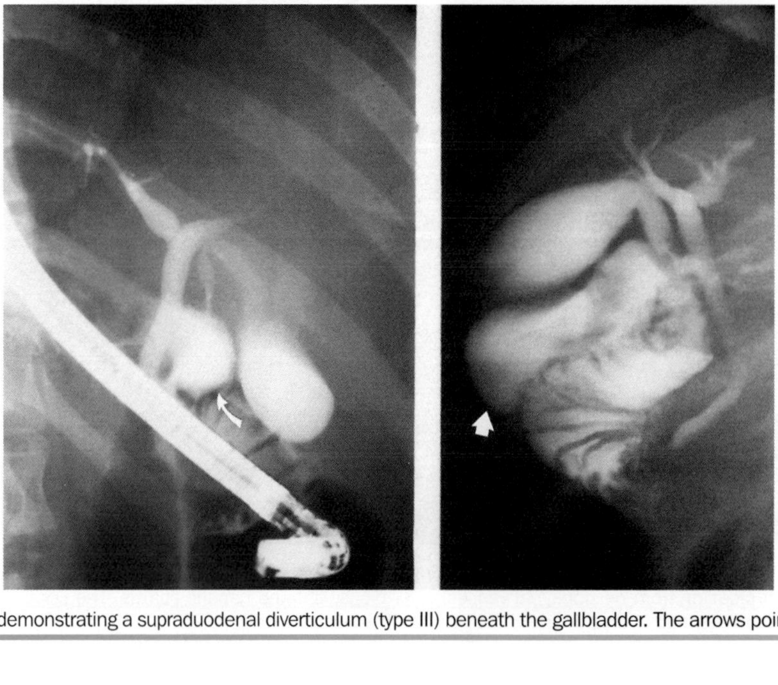

Figure 10.40 ERCP demonstrating a supraduodenal diverticulum (type III) beneath the gallbladder. The arrows point to the diverticulum.

tain bile pigments and varying amounts of calcium carbonate and palmitate. These calcium salts are deposited on the periphery of the stones and their amounts determine the radiodensity of these yellow gallstones. Cholesterol gallstones do not commonly harbour bacteria (10%) and are not usually associated with infected bile. They are often radiolucent and cast strong acoustic shadows on ultrasonography. Cholesterol stones are often multiple and medium-sized, but when solitary, they attain a large size and have a radiating crystalline cross-sectional appearance.

Black pigment stones

Black pigment stones form in the gallbladder and account for 25% of stones in the West although their prevalence is higher in Asian countries. They are composed of bilirubin polymers without calcium palmitate, varying amounts of cholesterol (3–25%) and a matrix of organic material. Associated infection is present in less than 20% of patients. Black pigment stones are usually multiple, small, irregular and dark green to black in colour. Although haemolytic states predispose to the formation of black pigment stones, the vast majority occur in patients without detectable chronic haemolysis. Their consistency is hard and they have a layered cut surface.

Brown pigment stones

In contradistinction to the above types, brown pigment stones form in the bile ducts (primary ductal calculi) and are associated with infection of the biliary tract. Scanning electron microscopy of fresh specimens demonstrates bacteria inside crevices and pits of these amorphous soft stones in 98%. Brown pigment stones contain calcium bilirubinate, calcium palmitate and only small amounts of cholesterol bound in a matrix of organic material.

Aetiology

There is an increased prevalence of gallstones in females and the frequency of gallstones increases with age in both sexes. Although familial incidence remains unproven, a positive family history of gallstones is more often obtained from patients with symptomatic gallstone disease than in controls. The importance of genetic and ethnic factors is exemplified by the unusually high prevalence of gallstones in the American Indians, particularly the Pima tribe. The genetic disorder in this ethnic group results in the production of a supersaturated bile and a deficient secretion of bile acids by the liver. Certain risk factors are known to increase the prevalence of gallstones; others induce symptomatic disease in patients with silent gallstones without necessarily enhancing the overall frequency (Table 10.4).

Although it is generally stated that the gallstones which form in patients with ileal disease or after ileal resection are of the cholesterol variety, recent studies have demonstrated that a substantial number of these stones are of the pigment variety. The enhanced lithogenicity and increased incidence of gallstones in the obese are the consequence of an increased hepatic synthesis and secretion of cholesterol. The supersaturation of bile with cholesterol is found in maturity-onset diabetes but not in the juvenile type. The exact mechanism responsible for bile lithogenicity in maturity-onset diabetes is not known. The enhanced incidence of gallstones in children with cystic fibrosis has been attributed to the abnormal mucus that impairs bile flow and favours nucleation.

Early reports demonstrated an increased incidence of symptomatic gallstones in females on the oral contraceptive pill, the relative risk being estimated at 2.5. However, more recent studies have been unable to confirm this finding. This discrepancy has been attributed to the lower oestrogen component of the modern 'mini' contraceptive pill. Studies on the prevalence of gallstones in asymptomatic populations with ultrasound scanning have shown no difference between women on the contraceptive pill and those who are not. Some reports have indicated that the modern 'mini' contraceptive pill may be associated with an increased risk of symptomatic disease in young women (aged 29 years or less).

Table 10.4 Risk factors for gallstone prevalence and symptomatic gallstone disease

Increased prevalence	*Precipitation of symptomatic disease*
Female sex[a]	Pregnancy
Obesity[a]	Clofibrate
Age[a]	Thiazide diuretics
Genetics and ethnic factors[a]	?Oral contraception
Highly refined, fibre depleted, high animal fat diet[a]	
Diabetes mellitus[a]	
Ileal disease and resection	
Haemolytic states[b]	
Infections of the biliary tract[b]	
Parasitic infestations[b]	
Cirrhosis[b]	
Cystic fibrosis	

[a]Increased prevalence of cholesterol stones.
[b]Increased prevalence of pigment stones.

Pathogenesis of gallstones

Our knowledge of the pathogenesis of gallstone formation remains incomplete although there has been considerable progress on the mechanisms involved during the past two decades. Undoubtedly the pathogenesis of cholesterol stones is different from that of black pigment stones, and brown pigment stone formation differs from both.

Cholesterol stones

The formation of cholesterol stones involves seven processes:

- supersaturation of bile with cholesterol
- incomplete transfer of cholesterol from the biliary vesicles to the bile salt-micelles
- formation of abnormal high cholesterol-containing biliary vesicles
- aggregation and fusion of unstable vesicles
- cholesterol crystallization: nucleating and anti-nucleating factors
- biliary sludge formation
- stone growth.

Supersaturation with cholesterol

The outstanding biochemical abnormality associated with the formation of cholesterol gallstones is the secretion of bile that is supersaturated with cholesterol. Under normal physiological conditions, cholesterol is secreted by the hepatocytes into the hepatic bile as cholesterol-phospholipid vesicles. Within the bile a phase change occurs due to the relative high concentrations of bile acids, and micelles form. These are essentially molecular aggregates in which the cholesterol and phospholipid molecules form a central core surrounded by bile salt molecules. This mechanism is invoked to maintain cholesterol (which is water insoluble) in solution. Within the narrow range of water content of bile (80–95%), the solubility relationships of the biliary lipids can be expressed by plotting their relative molar concentrations on triangular coordinates (Figure 10.41). In the micellar zone, which represents the normal, the cholesterol is in solution as micelles and the bile is unsaturated with respect to cholesterol. Thus cholesterol precipitation and stone formation do not occur. Other methods are used to express the solubility of cholesterol in bile. These include the percentage saturation, the lithogenic index and the ratio of the concentrations of bile salts and phospholipids over the concentration of cholesterol. The lithogenic index is the ratio of the actual amount of cholesterol that can be dissolved in the bile sample using the triangular coordinate plots. A lithogenic index of unity or greater indicates that the bile is supersaturated with respect to cholesterol. The normal ratio: conc. bile salts + conc. phospholipids/conc. cholesterol = 10:1.

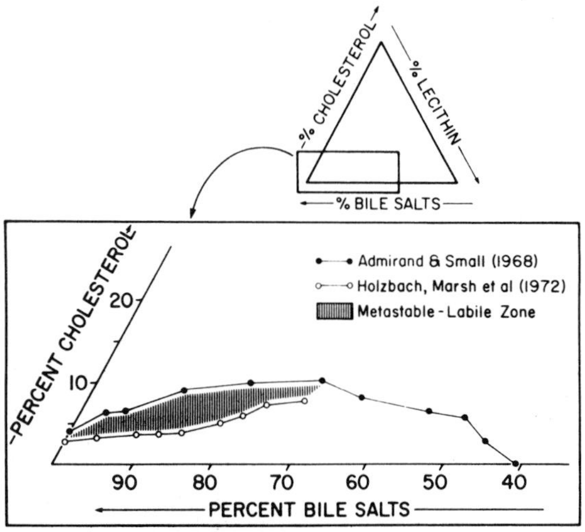

Figure 10.41 Solubility relationships of cholesterol, bile salts and lecithin (phospholipid) expressed by plotting their relative molar concentrations on triangular coordinates. Points below the metastable–labile zone indicate unsaturated bile. (From Popper, H. and Schaffner, F. (eds) (1976) *Progress in Liver Disease*, Vol. V. Grune and Stratton. New York.)

The source of the supersaturated bile is the liver, from either increased synthesis of cholesterol or a decreased synthesis/secretion of bile salts and phospholipids. Excess cholesterol secretion in the bile is well documented in obese patients and is thought to result from the increased activity of the enzyme hydroxymethylglutaryl coenzyme A (HMG CoA)-reductase resulting from the chronically elevated levels of insulin found in overweight individuals. Most non-obese patients with cholesterol gallstones have a reduced absorption as the cause of the diminished bile salt pool in these patients. The most likely explanation of the smaller pool (and supersaturated bile) is an exaggeration of the normal feedback mechanism between the bile salt return and the hepatic synthesis of bile acids together with an increased enterohepatic cycling possibly consequent on abnormal excessive gallbladder contractility. Although gallstones develop only in individuals with supersaturated bile, many patients with this abnormality never develop gallstones. Thus other factors are involved. These include the persistence of biliary vesicles and kinetic factors.

Biliary vesicles

Under normal conditions, the cholesterol-phospholipid vesicles are relatively stable and disappear as micelles form and take up their cholesterol and phospholipid constituents. In the pathological state, the phase change to micelles is incomplete and as more phospholipid than cholesterol is extracted into the micellar aggregates with bile salts, biliary vesicles with an abnormally high cholesterol–phospholipid ratio are produced. These abnormal vesicles are unstable and are the source of cholesterol monohydrate crystals in the bile. The crystallization is preceded by aggregation and fusion of the high cholesterol-containing vesicles.

Kinetic balance between nucleating and anti-nucleating factors

Bile contains substances which either inhibit (alipoprotein A1) or promote (mucin) the growth of cholesterol crystals. Thus the development of cholesterol gallstones is influenced by the balance between these two kinetic factors. An anionic polypeptide fragment (APF) of high-density lipoprotein occurs in bile and together with immunoglobulin A constitutes the lipoprotein complex of bile. It is thought that absolute or relative decrease in the amount of APF favours nucleation and growth of cholesterol monohydrate and pigment crystals.

The biliary proteins include enzymes, transport proteins, hormones, plasma proteins and mucin. The evidence for the important role of mucin in the nucleation and growth of cholesterol crystals is overwhelming. Hypersecretion of densely glycosylated mucin is observed in experimental models of gallstone formation, mucin is a major component of biliary sludge and stone formation appears to start in the mucous gel. Thus gallbladder mucus is thought to be involved both as a nucleation-promoting agent and in providing the right milieu which encourages stone growth. Recently a protein with marked nucleation promotion activity for cholesterol crystals that binds to concavalin A has been isolated from the bile of patients with and without gallstones. Its activity was found to be increased in patients harbouring gallstones.

Biliary sludge

Biliary sludge is composed of mucin, calcium, monoconjugated bilirubin and cholesterol and is now thought to be the direct precursor of gallstones. A number of reports have documented symptoms including biliary-type pain in patients who were found to have biliary sludge but no gallstones.

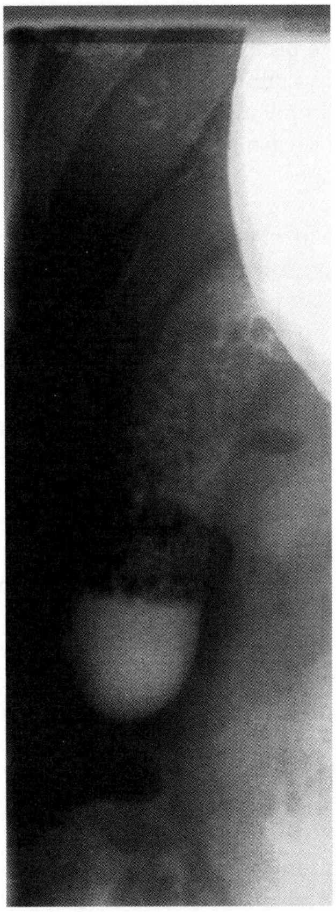

Figure 10.42 Stratification of bile with floating gallstone layer.

Other factors

There is no doubt that the above account presents an incomplete picture of the pathogenesis of cholesterol stones. The role of calcium is indicated by the presence of calcium salts in the majority of stones and the experimental demonstration in the prairie dog model that cholesterol vesicle aggregation and the induction of cholesterol gallstones is associated with an increase in the total and free ionized calcium concentrations in the gallbladder bile.

That the gallbladder plays an important role in gallstone formation (both cholesterol and black pigment) is evident by the fact that 85–90% of stones are encountered in this organ rather than in the bile ducts. It has been postulated that the gallbladder may alter the physicochemical composition of bile, favouring nucleation and crystal growth by abnormal absorption/secretion, defective surface pH, stasis resulting from impaired gallbladder emptying and stratification of bile (Figure 10.42) or by providing essential nucleating factors including mucin, desquamated cells, bacteria and refluxed intestinal contents. It is probable that gallstones are formed at different occasions depending on the balance between nucleation inhibition and promoting factors at different time periods (Figure 10.43).

Black pigment stones

Much less is known about the pathophysiology of black pigment stones. In cirrhotic patients who have a high prevalence of these stones, an elevated concentration of monoconjugated bilirubin and a lower bile salt concentration than normal has been documented. The hypothesis that patients with black pigment stones have a bile which is supersaturated with calcium bilirubinate has had some experimental backing in a dietary model of pigment stones by which a significant increase in the gallbladder concentrations of unconjugated bilirubin

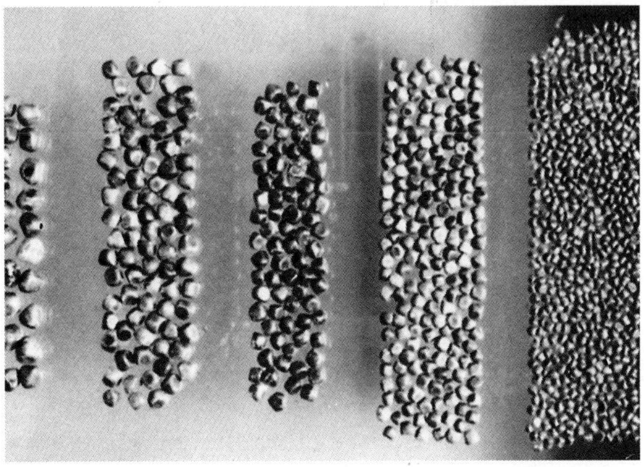

Figure 10.43 Several generations of cholesterol stones removed from a gallbladder after cholecystectomy. The factors within the gallbladder which favour precipitation of cholesterol crystals and the growth of cholesterol microliths into discernible stones are outlined in the text.

and calcium were documented. Calcium is a universal component of black pigment stones and both free and total ionized calcium is increased in canine models of pigment gallstone disease. As the hepatic bile concentration is unchanged, the altered chemical composition is thought to be secondary to altered gallbladder function.

Patients with bile acid malabsorption (after ileal resection) have low biliary cholesterol in addition to a reduced bile salt pool. They exhibit an increased risk of gallstone formation, predominantly of the black pigment kind. This observation has led to the hypothesis that biliary cholesterol may exert a protective action on the gallbladder mucosa and, accordingly, a low biliary cholesterol renders the mucosa susceptible to direct injury by bile acids as these are concentrated in the gallbladder. There is no proof for this hypothesis.

There is increasing evidence for the important role of some mucins (especially MUC3 and MUC5B) in the development of pigment stones, especially those forming in the intrahepatic ducts. The peribiliary glands are the source of the mucins. A recent study has demonstrated an increased mRNA expression of MUC3 and MUC5 in the cells of the peribiliary glands of stone-harbouring intrahepatic ducts compared to normal controls.

Brown pigment stones

These ductal calculi are caused by infection by Gram-negative bacteria such as *E. coli* and *Bacteroides fragilis*, which elaborate and release beta-glucuronidase in the bile. Recent studies have documented infection in 80–98% of cases. In many Eastern countries where infestation with *Ascaris lumbricoides* is endemic, the eggs of this parasite have been repeatedly identified in the nucleus of brown pigment stones, but the cause is the associated bacterial infection of the biliary tract. Likewise, the formation of both intrahepatic and extrahepatic ductal calculi in recurrent pyogenic cholangitis is due to infection of the biliary tract by Gram-negative bacteria. The bacterial beta-glucuronidase is implicated in the hydrolysis of conjugated bilirubin with consequent precipitation of insoluble calcium bilirubinate. Brown pigment stones are encountered in biliary tract conditions associated with stasis and infection such as chronic obstructive disease, indwelling biliary endoprostheses and around non-absorbable suture material or metal clips used in biliary tract surgery.

Clinical syndromes of gallstone disease

The symptomatology of gallstone disease is varied. Often non-specific, the symptoms may be acute, chronic or totally absent when gallstones are diagnosed as an incidental finding during the investigation of patients for unrelated disorders. The differentiation between silent and symptomatic gallstones is important since this affects management in the individual case.

In patients with chronic symptoms, it is important to stress that the demonstration of gallbladder disease by oral cholecystography/ultrasound scanning does not exclude other disorders being responsible for the symptoms, and a careful clinical evaluation, together with the appropriate investigative protocol, is essential in all patients with chronic symptoms and ultrasonically confirmed gallstone disease. This is especially important in the selection of patients for elective cholecystectomy. The common coexisting diseases include:

- colonic motility disorders and diverticular disease
- gastritis and peptic ulceration
- reflux oesophagitis and hiatal hernia
- pancreatitis
- colonic cancer
- renal disease
- ischaemic heart disease.

In addition to gallbladder imaging, an upper gastrointestinal endoscopy or barium series and, in certain situations, a barium enema, is advisable in all patients undergoing elective cholecystectomy for chronic symptoms.

Symptomless (silent) gallstones

Most surveys have shown that silent gallstones heavily outnumber the symptomatic ones. Silent gallstones are diagnosed as incidental findings most commonly by abdominal radiographs. The previous controversy regarding the management of asymptomatic gallstones has been resolved by prospective studies which have shown that the vast majority of silent gallstones will not cause symptoms or complications during life. Comparative evaluation of expectant versus surgical management of asymptomatic gallstones has shown that cholecystectomy reduces marginally the life expectancy in addition to being substantially more costly. Another argument for cholecystectomy in the past has been the prevention of gallbladder cancer, the development of which is known to be associated with the presence of gallstones. However, carcinoma of the gallbladder is rare and the overall operative mortality with the widespread adoption of prophylactic cholecystectomy in patients with silent gallstones would certainly exceed that due to cancer of the gallbladder by a significant margin. The evidence linking cholecystectomy with the development of colon cancer remains conflicting and cannot be used as a further argument against prophylactic cholecystectomy. The consensus of current surgical opinion is that there is no indication for cholecystectomy in the management of patients with asymptomatic gallstone disease.

There are four exceptions to this policy. The first relates to patients undergoing surgical intervention for other conditions in whom gallstones are found at laparotomy. In one report, 50% of these patients developed complications or symptomatic disease subsequently and 12% required cholecystectomy within 30 days after the operation. On the other hand, concomitant cholecystectomy increases the post-operative morbidity. Thus if incidental gallstones are found at operation, cholecystectomy is indicated if the patient's general condition is good (ASA I, II). The second group which merits cholecystectomy for asymptomatic gallstones is made up of acromegalic patients on long-term treatment with somatostatin analogue which often produces large gallstones. As somatostatin treatment has to be continued indefinitely, laparoscopic cholecystectomy is indicated in these patients, once stones are documented by ultrasound. Presently, prophylactic removal of the gallbladder (prior to stone formation) is not practised in these patients. Patients with a calcified gallbladder have a significant risk of developing cancer of the gallbladder and for this reason, cholecystectomy is indicated even if the condition is asymptomatic. Diabetic patients with gallstones are more prone to develop symptoms and complications and for this reason some advocate laparoscopic cholecystectomy in this group although this remains debatable.

Symptomatic gallstone disease

The clinical presentation varies and may be acute or chronic (Table 10.5).

Chronic cholecystitis

Chronic inflammation of the gallbladder is most commonly due to stones and the term 'chronic cholecystitis' should be restricted to gallbladders containing gallstones with varying degrees of inflammation, from mild mucosal/submucosal changes to gross transmural fibrosis leading to a contracted fibrous encasement of the biliary calculi.

Symptoms and signs

Most commonly, patients with chronic cholecystitis complain of recurrent attacks of epigastric or right hypochondrial pain, often radiating to the right side of the back and, less commonly, to the shoulder blade. The pain is more often persistent than intermittent. Episodes of biliary colic with severe intermittent peaks of pain lasting a few minutes to several hours may subside spontaneously or progress to cystic duct obstruction and acute cholecystitis. Nausea and vomiting may accompany both episodes of persistent pain and the severe attacks of biliary colic. Jaundice and dark urine may follow an attack and indicate common bile duct obstruction by a calculus. The jaundice often subsides after a few days but may persist as a major presenting symptom. It is now established that indigestion, dyspepsia, flatulence, intolerance to fatty foods, abdominal distension and belching occur with the same frequency in the general population as they do in patients with chronic gallstone disease.

Table 10.5 Spectrum of symptomatic gallstone disease

- Chronic cholecystitis
- Acute biliary colic/acute cholecystitis
- Jaundice due to large bile duct obstruction
- Cholangitis/septicaemia
- Acute gallstone pancreatitis
- Biliary fistulous disease
- Gallstone ileus

The only reliable sign, which is infrequently found on clinical examination, is tenderness in the right upper quadrant. More often than not, the clinical features of chronic cholecystitis are non-specific and confirmation by imaging tests (usually ultrasonography) is essential for diagnosis in the vast majority of cases.

Treatment

Cholecystectomy

The treatment of chronic cholecystitis is surgical – cholecystectomy. There is little doubt that these patients should have their gallbladder removed as approximately 30% of them will develop complications if surgical treatment is delayed. Furthermore, the morbidity and mortality following surgical intervention are enhanced in those patients who develop complications necessitating surgical intervention. In practice, the problem concerns the selection of patients, which should be based on establishing that the gallstones are the cause of the patient's symptoms since these are by no means specific and can be caused by other common gastrointestinal disorders. Poor case selection accounts for a large cohort of those patients who continue to experience symptoms after cholecystectomy (post-cholecystectomy syndrome). Some of these patients are subsequently found to have disease outside the biliary tract.

Per-operative cholangiography should be considered as an integral part of cholecystectomy. The cholangiographic findings, the presence of jaundice together with the operative appearances, dictate the need for exploration of the common bile duct. Exploration of the common bile duct is usually followed by the insertion of a T-tube even in those patients who are found to have a negative exploration, although some surgeons would opt not to insert a tube in patients with a negative exploration and simply close the choledochotomy. Others insert a small cannula through the cystic duct remnant to enable the performance of post-operative cholangiography before discharge from hospital. The T-tube should not be smaller than 14 Fr and its long limb should be brought out by the shortest route well laterally in the right subcostal region. These measures facilitate considerably the removal of retained ductal stones through the T-tube tract by means of the flexible choledochoscope (see below). The Whelan–Moss T-tube was specially designed to create a wide tract between the bile duct and the abdominal parieties and thus facilitate percutaneous stone extraction via the T-tube tract. Its long limb is wider than the intra-choledochal portion.

Opinion on the need for drainage of the gallbladder fossa remains divided. The argument against drainage has been strengthened by the results of several prospective clinical trials since these have either failed to show a difference between the drained and the undrained groups, or indicated that drainage increases the post-operative sepsis and morbidity. It seems likely that the routine uneventful cholecystectomy without exploration of the common bile duct does not require the insertion of a subhepatic drain, but most biliary surgeons would still recommend drainage for the following:

- Difficult cholecystectomy.
- Early cholecystectomy for acute cholecystitis.
- In patients who require exploration of the common bile duct.

The mortality of elective open cholecystectomy for chronic cholecystitis is low (0.3–1.0%) but is higher in the elderly (5–6%). Laparoscopic cholecystectomy (LC) is now firmly established as the gold standard therapy for symptomatic gallstone disease. With experience and training, it is applicable to over 95% of patients. The procedure reproduces all the steps of the traditional open cholecystectomy, which it has largely replaced because of its well-documented advantages. Conversion to open surgery is indicated if a safe dissection of the structures in the triangle of Calot cannot be performed because of dense fibrosis, severe adhesions from previous surgery, the presence of a Mirizzi syndrome and severe acute disease with gross inflammatory oedema. Conversion to open cholecystectomy may also be necessitated because of the onset of a complication (severe bleeding, bile duct injury, etc.) which cannot be safely dealt with by the laparoscopic approach.

The advantages of laparoscopic cholecystectomy over the conventional operation include less post-operative pain, virtual absence of ileus, short hospital stay (1–2 days) and accelerated return to full activity or work (within 10–14 days). In addition, there is an overall reduction of the incidence of post-operative wound and chest infections, wound dehiscence, incisional hernia and deep vein thrombosis. The post-operative mortality appears to be lower than that of open cholecystectomy. Other advantages include reduced adhesion formation and wound complications. The downside is an increased incidence of iatrogenic bowel, vascular and biliary injuries. The importance of routine IOFC during laparoscopic cholecystectomy must be stressed. The overriding reason for routine IOFC is the provision of a road map of the biliary anatomy and the determination of a safe site for medial ligature or clipping of the cystic duct without compromise of the extrahepatic bile conduit. The other reasons for routine IOFC are similar to those for open cholecystectomy: detection of biliary tract anomalies and unsuspected ductal calculi. If the surgeon is experienced, these calculi are best removed during the operation either by extraction through the cystic duct or by direct laparoscopic common bile duct exploration.

Mini-cholecystectomy

This implies performance of cholecystectomy through a small (5 cm wound) that should be placed in the midline and not in the right subcostal region. Proponents recommend this technique for both elective cholecystectomy and patients with acute cholecystitis. The procedure uses standard operating techniques with certain modifications such as the use of a headlight, a ring retractor, clip applicators and long instruments. The need to extend the incision is encountered in 15% of patients. A more recent modification has been described as 'cylindrical cholecystectomy'. The operation is based on the introduction of a 3.8–5.0 cm diameter cylinder that is 10 cm long which isolates the hepatocystic region from the surrounding structures, and thus facilitates the intervention.

In general, mini-cholecystectomy is associated with a shorter hospital stay (3.5 days versus 8.5–11 days) as compared to patients undergoing cholecystectomy through an unrestricted incision and some have reported an earlier return to work after the procedure.

The procedure can be technically difficult especially in patients with excessive fat in the triangle of Calot and most surgeons have abandoned it in favour of the endoscopic approach.

Partial cholecystectomy

This technique was first described by the group at Cape Town for cholecystectomy in patients with cirrhosis. Many variations of this technique have been described involving a subtotal (fundus first) resection of the gallbladder but leaving the posterior wall attached to the hepatic bed. More recently, the Cape Town group reported on this technique performed by the laparoscopic approach for patients with complicated acute cholecystitis or fibrosis and encountered one post-operative death (myocardial infarction) and three bile leaks in 29 patients. Thus suction drainage of the gallbladder bed is necessary after subtotal cholecystectomy (open or laparoscopic).

A modification using a 1 cm rim of Hartmann's pouch to buttress and occlude the internal opening of the cystic duct and leaving the structures of Calot's triangle undisturbed was described by Schein, who reported favourably on the technique in 16 elderly/high-risk patients. This author emphasizes its speed (mean operating time of 40 min), technical safety in obviating a difficult dissection of the liver bed and the practical advantage in comparison to other conservative surgical procedures that leave the gallbladder *in situ*, of preventing gallstone formation.

Cholecystolithotomy

Patients with previous vagotomy for ulcer disease frequently develop symptomatic gallstones. Cholecystectomy in vagotomized patients with a functioning gallbladder incurs the risk of severe explosive diarrhoea in a high percentage of cases. For this reason, cholecystectomy is not warranted in this subset of patients and removal of the gallstones (cholecystolithotomy) constitutes the appropriate treatment. This may be followed by maintenance therapy with oral bile salt in an attempt to prevent recurrence if the stones are of the cholesterol variety (see below). The best approach is laparoscopic cholecystolithotomy with closure of the gallbladder with absorbable suture after gallstone clearance has been achieved. Others favour radiological guided stone extraction, fragmentation or dissolution. A cholecystectomy is the right treatment in vagotomized patients if the gallbladder is non-functioning.

Dissolution by MTBE and percutaneous lithotripsy
Methyl tert-butyl ether (MTBE) is a powerful organic solvent which dissolves cholesterol gallstones within hours. It is administered locally via a pig-tail or other self-retaining catheter introduced percutaneously (usually through the hepatic substance) into the gallbladder under radiological control. MTBE is then instilled and left in the gallbladder for several hours. When dissolution is achieved, the gallbladder liquid contents are aspirated and the catheter is removed. MTBE is toxic following systemic absorption and can cause local damage if it escapes into the common duct and duodenum (erosions). For this reason, microprocessor controlled pump delivery systems (pressure and volume controlled) are used to obviate spillage of the solvent into the ductal system. MTBE dissolution is rarely used nowadays and is indicated as one of the alternatives when removal of the gallbladder is contraindicated (poor-risk patients, previous vagotomy) or the patient specifically requests removal of the stones but not the gallbladder.

Alternatively, a rotary mechanical lithotriptor (Kinsey–Nash) can be inserted percutaneously under radiological control into the gallbladder. This device operates by creating a vortex that draws stones to a high-speed rotating impeller that fragments the calculi. Although effective, this technique results in damage to the mucosa by the bombardment with stone fragments and the limited reported literature on its use indicates a high incidence of complications. This method has largely been abandoned.

Extracorporeal shockwave lithotripsy (ESWL)
With these devices, extracorporeal shockwaves produced by spark-gap (Dornier system), piezoceramic (Wolf system) or electromagnetic (Siemens system) generators are focused by a concave reflector and targeted under ultrasound guidance to the stones, thereby inducing fragmentation. The third-generation machines avoid the need for immersion in a water bath and general anaesthesia. Although ESWL can achieve successful stone fragmentation in 80% of patients with solitary small gallstones at 1 year, it often fails if the stones are large (>3 cm), multiple and calcified. It is thus applicable to only 19% of patients with symptomatic gallstones. Furthermore, repeated treatment is often necessary to achieve complete fragmentation and this has to be followed by maintenance therapy with oral bile salts, despite which, stone recurrence occurs in 50% at 5 years. Compared to surgical treatment, ESWL is costly, unreliable and has a limited applicability. Contrary to its established value in the treatment of renal calculi, ESWL is seldom used in the treatment of gallstones and its current role seems restricted to fragmentation of occluding ductal calculi in jaundiced patients. Even this indication is not established and remains to be defined in large patient studies. Currently, fragmentation of ductal calculi by ESWL can be achieved in 70–90% of patients with an average of two lithotripsy sessions. However, some 50% of patients require additional procedures (endoscopic extraction) to achieve stone removal, including operative intervention in 10%. Complications such as haematuria, biliary pain, sepsis and haemobilia are encountered in 15% of patients.

Oral bile salt therapy
Oral dissolution is applicable only to patients with cholesterol stones in a functioning gallbladder. The administration of the primary bile acid chenodeoxycholic acid (CDCA) and its 7-beta epimer, ursodeoxycholic acid (UDCA), reduces the cholesterol saturation of bile and prolongs nucleation time, thereby resulting in stone dissolution after several weeks/months of therapy. Following successful dissolution, maintenance therapy with low-dose UDCA is required. Despite this, the risk of gallstone recurrence is 12.5% after the first year and 61% by the eleventh year. Oral dissolution fails if the gallstone load is large (larger than 3 cm or multiple) and if the stones are calcified. The disadvantages of this treatment of gallstones include high cost, high recurrence rate and limited applicability. Currently, the place of bile salt therapy is restricted to patients in whom cholecystectomy is contraindicated, either as primary treatment or after gallstone extraction, fragmentation or dissolution by MTBE. Another important indication of oral bile salt therapy is in patients with endoscopic stents as a prophylactic measure to reduce the incidence and severity of stent encrustation with calcium bilirubinate.

Chemical sclerosis
Experimental sclerosis of the gallbladder (chemical cholecystectomy) after occlusion of the cystic duct has been achieved by instillation of various sclerosants in various animal models. However, none of the agents used to date is safe enough to use clinically. The other problems with this approach include regeneration of the gallbladder mucosa from the cystic duct remnant and the possible late risk of malignant change. Physical methods of destruction of the gallbladder mucosa are currently being studied in animal experiments. These include photodynamic laser treatment.

Acute biliary colic and acute cholecystitis

Acute biliary colic results in severe colicky abdominal pain usually accompanied by nausea and vomiting. The duration of the severe pain, which makes the patient restless, varies from 30 min to several hours. Biliary colic often merges into acute obstructive cholecystitis. However, resolution of the severe colicky painful episode either spontaneously or as a result of analgesic medication/anti-spasmodic without the development of acute cholecystitis is common and many patients give a history of recurrent episodes of biliary colic before the development of acute cholecystitis.

Between 10 and 30% of patients undergoing cholecystectomy present with acute cholecystitis. This is most commonly obstructive in nature (>95%) from impaction of a stone in Hartman's pouch/cystic duct.

Much less commonly, acute cholecystitis is acalculous although the incidence of this complication in critically ill patients is diagnosed more frequently nowadays. Acute cholecystitis in the elderly may result from cystic duct obstruction due to carcinoma of the gallbladder. Whereas patients harbouring residual infection of the gallbladder with *Salmonella typhi* as typhoid carriers may cause sporadic outbursts of typhoid, acute salmonella cholecystitis is very rarely encountered in the West.

Acute obstructive (calculous) cholecystitis

Pathology

The attack develops when the cystic duct becomes obstructed by a gallstone impacting in Hartmann's pouch. Following obstruction of the cystic duct/Hartmann's pouch, the gallbladder becomes hyperaemic, oedematous, tense and distended. The initial inflammation is chemically induced and is not of bacterial origin although sepsis is an important feature of the established disease and its complications. Cultures of gallbladder bile taken during open cholecystectomy are positive in only 15–30% of cases and in only 3% of patients undergoing LC for the same disease. The predominant microorganisms isolated from the gallbladder bile in these patients are *E. coli* (60%), *Klebsiella* spp. (22%) and *Streptococcus* spp. (18%). There appears to be no relation between positive gallbladder cultures and post-operative wound infections for both open and laparoscopic cholecystectomy but the overall incidence of wound infection is much higher after the open procedure (14% versus 5%) and serious wound infections after LC are very rare. Thus the small incisions used in laparoscopic gallbladder surgery may be less susceptible to infective complications.

These observations indicate that the initial inflammatory process following obstruction of the cystic duct is of a chemical nature with infection supervening in some patients during the later stages of the disease. It is believed that trauma, secondary to gallstone impaction, leads to mucosal damage through the release of phospholipases that convert lecithin (a mucosal protective factor against bile acids) to lysolecithin, a known mucosal toxin. Alternatively, the release of the prostaglandin precursor arachidonic acid by the action of phospholipase A on lecithin may mediate the inflammatory response by producing prostaglandins. In the first few days, the bile appears macroscopically normal and is sterile, but with the progress of the inflammation, absorption of pigments and bile salts takes place, and the contents then vary from a thin mucoid material to frank pus. The histological changes of the established condition involve the mucosa, fibromuscular wall and serosa and vary from mild acute inflammation with transmural oedema to severe disease with patches of necrosis usually in the fundal region of the gallbladder, which becomes wrapped by the greater omentum.

With conservative treatment, the inflammation resolves in some 80% of patients as the rising tension in the gallbladder lumen from the outpouring of the inflammatory exudate lifts the walls of Hartmann's pouch off the impacting stone. When this disengages and drops into the gallbladder lumen, cystic duct drainage leads to resolution. This fortuitous sequence is not encountered in 20% of patients, usually elderly, in whom patchy gangrene and/or perforation with a large inflammatory phlegmon or peritonitis supervene.

The subsequent sequence of events following the acute inflammatory process may vary from:

- Resolution (most common) with scarring, abnormal function or non-function of the gallbladder.
- Persistence of the infection: the gallbladder becomes distended with pus (empyema of the gallbladder).
- Resolution of the inflammatory process within the gallbladder with persistence of the cystic duct obstruction – mucocele (hydrops) of the gallbladder.
- Gangrene and acute perforation leading to localized (pericholecystic) abscess or frank biliary peritonitis.
- Chronic perforation with the development of bilio-enteric and bilio-bilial fistulas.

Whereas the majority of patients diagnosed as acute cholecystitis have the classic acute cystic duct obstruction and its associated inflammatory condition of the gallbladder, others are instances of chronic cholecystitis presenting with acute pain or biliary colic. Although acute cholecystitis is often suspected on clinical grounds, a definitive diagnosis can only be obtained by specific investigations (EHIDA scintiscanning, ultrasonography). The serum amylase should always be performed in addition to the liver function tests. Scout abdominal plain and film chest radiographs are used to exclude perforation and the presence of gas in the biliary tract.

Symptoms and signs

The clinical picture varies with the severity of the inflammatory process. Known pre-existing gallbladder disease may be present or chronic symptoms over several months to years may precede the acute presentation. Alternatively, acute obstructive cholecystitis may be the first intimation of gallstone disease.

In mild cases, the patient complains of right upper quadrant pain and tenderness. Pyrexia, severe pain and tenderness in the right hypochondrium with rebound reflect more severe degrees of gallbladder inflammation. In these instances, Murphy's sign (inspiratory arrest due to pain on inspiration during gentle palpation of the right subcostal region) is usually present. Nausea, vomiting, ileus, mild abdominal distension and toxicity are encountered in the severe forms of the disease. Jaundice is present in 20–25% of patients with acute obstructive cholecystitis but common duct stones are found in only 12% of these patients. In the absence of ductal calculi, jaundice has been ascribed to reactive hepatitis or oedema of the common bile duct. A tender palpable mass in the right subcostal region is found in 25% of cases and signifies one of the following:

- empyema of the gallbladder
- omental phlegmon
- abscess due to localized perforation
- carcinoma of the gallbladder, especially if the patient is elderly.

Laboratory tests are frequently non-specific, their greatest value being to rule out other important conditions in the differential diagnosis, particularly acute pancreatitis. Most patients will have a neutrophil leucocytosis ($>10 \times 10^9$/l) together with some abnormality of the liver function profile. The levels of serum bilirubin and alkaline phosphatases do not invariably correlate with the presence of ductal calculi but are suggestive and clinical jaundice warrants investigation with endoscopic retrograde cholangiography (ERC) or magnetic resonance cholangiopancreatography (MRCP). Other laboratory findings include raised transaminases and minor elevations of the serum amylase, below the diagnostic threshold for acute pancreatitis.

Differential diagnosis

Usually the diagnosis of acute cholecystitis is not difficult, but other common intra-abdominal conditions, e.g. perforated peptic ulcer, acute pancreatitis or a retrocaecal appendicitis associated with a high caecum and viral hepatitis, need to be considered in the individual case. Enterally transmitted non-A, non-B viral hepatitis can simulate acute cholecystitis quite closely as may right-sided pyelonephritis, lobar pneumonia and myocardial infarction. Aside from routine chest radiography and plain abdominal films, an electrocardiogram is advisable in the elderly and in those patients with a known history of ischaemic heart disease.

Imaging tests

The yield from a plain abdominal X-ray, though limited, may be important Calcified gallstones will be detected in 10–20% of patients. Gas in the gallbladder lumen and biliary tract caused by emphysematous cholecystitis (*vide infra*) is encountered infrequently but is obviously very important. Absence of free air under the diaphragm is useful for excluding perforated ulcer.

Real-time ultrasonography and biliary scintiscanning form the mainstays in the confirmatory diagnosis of acute cholecystitis. Grey-scale B-mode ultrasound is the most commonly used test since it is readily available, non-invasive, quick and easy to perform. Furthermore, it has the advantage of providing information about the liver, biliary tract and pancreas together with other sources of non-biliary right upper quadrant pain. The sonographic features include a positive Murphy's sign, calculi or sludge, thickened gallbladder wall and pericholecystic oedema. The examination is hampered by obesity and overlying bowel gas and is, of course, observer dependent. There is now good evidence from reported studies that the diagnostic accuracy of ultrasound for the diagnosis of acute cholecystitis is considerably improved with colour velocity imaging and especially with power Doppler when compared to grey-scale imaging (sensitivity = 95% vs 86%, accuracy = 99% vs 92%). However, the high susceptibility of power Doppler to motion artifacts requires expert adjustments of the technical parameters, and if anything, increases the observer dependency. The resistive index within the intramural vessels of the gallbladder which can now be measured by ultrasound techniques does not differentiate between inflamed and non-inflamed gallbladders.

Gallbladder scintiscanning using iminodiacetic acid derivatives (HIDA, PIPIDA scans) can be used to confirm non-functioning gallbladder and is regarded as the most accurate test of acute cholecystitis with a sensitivity of 97% and a specificity of 87%. A normal gallbladder scintiscan is virtually 100% accurate in excluding acute cholecystitis. The presence of pericholecystic uptake of the isotope is a valuable secondary sign in the diagnosis of acute cholecystitis and correlates with the presence of gangrenous cholecystitis or gallbladder perforation.

Intravenous cholangiography has been superseded by sonography in the diagnosis of acute cholecystitis. CT scanning is useful in complicated cases but ill advised in the majority in view of the radiation dosage. Good diagnostic accuracy for acute cholecystitis has been reported with MRI.

Acute acalculous cholecystitis

In a small percentage, usually in critically ill patients, the acute inflammation of the gallbladder arises in the absence of gallstones although biliary sludge is often present – acute acalculous cholecystitis. The incidence of this condition appears to be increasing and it now accounts for up to 8% of patients with acute cholecystitis. It is usually encountered in critically ill, elderly patients but acute acalculous cholecystitis has also been reported in children. The disorder usually occurs during the course of a prolonged serious illness, e.g. multiple trauma, following major surgical intervention, in patients with extensive burns, severe sepsis and drug overdosage. The risk factors that predispose to the development of acute acalculous cholecystitis are:

- blood volume depletion
- prolonged ileus
- morphine administration exceeding 6 days
- intravenous hyperalimentation
- multiple blood transfusions
- sepsis
- starvation.

However, acute acalculous cholecystitis does not always arise on a background of a critical illness, and in one report more than 70% of patients suffering from the condition presented *de novo*. Most of these patients were elderly men with atheromatous vascular disease and 15% were diabetic. The exact pathology is not known but the available evidence suggests that the inflammation develops as a consequence of prolonged distension of the gallbladder, bile stasis and inspissation (biliary sludge) which results in mucosal injury and thrombosis of vessels of the seromuscular layer of the gallbladder. The thrombosis is thought to be initiated by the activation of factor XII. Some have suggested that the development of acute acalculous cholecystitis may be related to a hypersensitivity reaction to concomitant antibiotic therapy because of the frequent presence of substantial eosinophilic infiltration of the mucosa of the gallbladder. Culture of the aspirated gallbladder bile from these patients is positive in only 38% of cases. Thus the inflammation is predominantly chemical in origin. In the fully developed condition, the gallbladder shows marked oedema of the seromuscular layer, mucosal ulceration, sloughing and focal necrotic areas. Substantial gangrene is encountered in 25%.

The diagnosis of acute acalculous cholecystitis is often difficult, especially in critically ill patients receiving narcotics and on artificial ventilation. The early manifestations include fever, leucocytosis and tenderness in the right hypochondrium. The diagnostic methods used are CT scanning, ultrasonography and isotope scintiscanning, although the latter two investigations are less accurate for this condition compared to their diagnostic yield for acute calculous cholecystitis. The ultrasonographic or CT findings indicative of acute acalculous cholecystitis include gallbladder wall thickness greater than 4 mm, pericholecystic fluid or subserosal oedema without ascites, intramural gas or sloughed mucosal membrane. Emergency surgical therapy is essential for survival. In the absence of significant gangrene, cholecystostomy (performed percutaneously, laparoscopically or by mini-cholecystostomy) is increasingly favoured, particularly in critically ill patients. Follow-up of patients treated with cholecystostomy has confirmed return to normal gallbladder function in the majority of these patients. Established gangrene requires total or subtotal cholecystectomy. Some advocate change of antibiotic regimen in view of the hypersensitivity theory.

Acute emphysematous cholecystitis

This fulminant form of acute cholecystitis is fortunately rare. It is caused by a mixed polymicrobial infection which includes gas-forming bacteria (*E. coli, Clostridium welchii*, aerobic and anaerobic streptococci). The gallbladder may or may not contain stones. Acute emphysematous cholecystitis occurs predominantly in males (70%) and has a special predilection for diabetic individuals. Thrombosis of the cystic artery has been implicated in the development of acute emphysematous cholecystitis.

The presence of air within the gallbladder lumen, its wall or the biliary tree on the plain radiograph of the abdomen is characteristic of the condition which often leads to gangrene (75%) and perforation (15%) by the time the diagnosis is made. The clinical picture is that of severe rapidly oncoming upper abdominal peritonitis with prostration and marked toxicity. Urgent surgical intervention is imperative. The antibiotic regimen of choice in these patients is a combination of penicillin and aminoglycoside.

Complications of acute cholecystitis

The important complications of all forms of acute cholecystitis are empyema, perforation and gangrene. All require urgent surgical intervention.

Empyema (suppurative cholecystitis)

Empyema of the gallbladder is an uncommon complication and has a reported incidence of 2–3% of all patients with gallstone disease. It presents as a tender mass in the right hypochondrium and usually affects elderly patients in whom systemic signs, including pyrexia and leucocytosis, may be minimal. Cultures of the gallbladder contents are positive in 80%. Empyema of the gallbladder doubles the mortality figures of cholecystectomy.

Gangrene

Patchy gangrene of the fundus of the gallbladder is encountered in 5–7% of patients with obstructive cholecystitis. It is more commonly encountered in elderly patients, diabetics, and in patients with empyema of the gallbladder, acute acalculous cholecystitis and, especially, emphysematous cholecystitis. It may lead to localized or free perforation of the gallbladder.

Perforation

Perforation may be localized with the development of a pericholecystic abscess or free, resulting in generalized infected biliary peritonitis which carries a high mortality, variously reported as 30–50%. A localized perforation may involve the duodenum with the development of a cholecystoduodenal fistula and resolution of the inflammatory episode. However, this bilio-enteric fistula persists and passage of a large stone through this fistula may eventually cause gallstone ileus.

Treatment of acute cholecystitis

Initial management

This consists of intravenous fluid and electrolyte replacement, nasogastric suction, systemic antibiotics and parenteral analgesia. The patient is kept fasted to reduce the cholecystokinin release from the upper small bowel in order to minimize gallbladder stimulation. Although the inflammation is initially chemical, most surgeons will choose to use systemic antibiotics because of the risk of progression to an empyema and septic complications. Also, if surgery is performed, antibiotic prophylaxis will reduce the wound infection rate although this has recently been questioned in patients undergoing LC. As the organisms cultured from gallbladder bile are predominantly Gram-positive aerobes (*E. coli*, *Klebsiella* spp., *Streptococcus* spp.), a third generation cephalosporin is the antibiotic of choice. Anaerobes such as *Bacteroides fragilis* and *Clostridium perfringens* are associated with more severe, mixed infections particularly in the elderly. These require combination chemotherapy using metronidazole with an aminoglycoside and/or penicillin. The diagnosis of acute cholecystitis should be confirmed during this initial 12–24 hour period of stabilization by ultrasonography or gallbladder scintiscanning.

Opinions still differ regarding the definitive treatment of acute cholecystitis. The management depends on whether the inflammatory condition is progressive and life-threatening or the cholecystitis is mild and resolving.

Table 10.6 Indications for emergency surgical intervention in patients with acute cholecystitis

- Progression of the disease despite conservative treatment
- Failure to improve within 24 hours especially in patients >60 years
- Presence of an inflammatory mass in the right hypochondrium
- Detection of gas in the gallbladder/biliary tract
- Established generalized peritonitis
- Development of intestinal obstruction

Severe progressive disease

The timing of surgery is dictated by the severity of the attack. Table 10.6 summarizes the indications for emergency or urgent surgical intervention. In these patients surgical intervention is carried out under antibiotic cover active against both Gram-negative aerobes and anaerobes (cephalosporin + metronidazole or piperacillin, etc.). Traditionally, such patients have been managed by laparotomy using a midline epigastric incision and the open approach is still favoured by many in critically ill elderly patients. Hitherto, less than 10% of cases fell into this severe category but more recent reports from North America and Europe have highlighted an increasing proportion of acute severe cases requiring urgent surgical intervention (from 6–10% up to 25%). This has been attributed to a decrease in the number of patients undergoing elective cholecystectomy though this has been reversed with the advent of LC, an increasingly aged population, and a rise in the actual incidence of acute complications of gallstone disease.

The exact procedure depends on the operative findings. In patients with a tense empyema, preliminary decompression of the gallbladder contents using a Mayo–Ochsner suction trocar-cannula inserted through a purse-string suture in the fundus should precede the cholecystectomy which, in the acute situation, is best performed by the retrograde technique (starting at the fundus). This allows easier identification of the cystic duct and, thereby, reduces the risk of bile duct damage. At times, the precarious condition of the patient precludes a lengthy operation or the anatomy may be so obscured by the inflammatory mass as to render the cholecystectomy hazardous. In these situations, a cholecystostomy should be performed. The gallbladder contents are evacuated, any gangrenous patches of its walls are excised and a 22–24 Fr Malecot catheter is inserted into the organ, which is closed round it by a purse-string suture. The catheter is then brought out through a separate stab wound. In these patients a cholecystectomy is advisable at a later stage unless the patient is elderly or has severe comorbid cardiorespiratory disease, because of the risk of recurrence of gallstones and symptoms. Moreover, the incidence of carcinoma of the gallbladder in patients who had previously undergone cholecystostomy is appreciable (7%).

Subtotal cholecystectomy is performed as an alternative approach to cholecystostomy in patients in whom formal cholecystectomy is considered hazardous. In this procedure, the posterior wall of the gallbladder is left *in situ*, attached to the liver bed, and the cystic duct is secured from within the gallbladder lumen by a purse-string suture (Figure 10.44).

In all instances specimens of bile and pus are obtained for bacteriological culture. Pus is thoroughly evacuated and peritoneal lavage, preferably with an antibiotic solution, carried out when gross peritoneal sepsis is found. Adequate drainage of the gallbladder bed is still considered advisable but is no substitute for thorough peritoneal toilet. All these patients are at risk from Gram-negative bacteraemia. They require a full

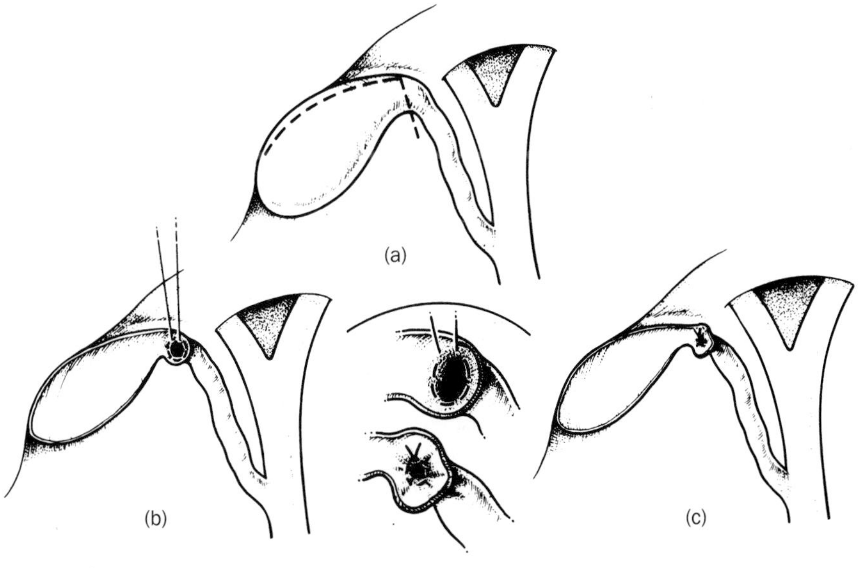

Figure 10.44 Technique of subtotal cholecystectomy described by Bormann and Terblanche: (a) the broken line shows the extent of the cholecystectomy – the posterior wall of the gallbladder is left attached to the liver; (b) a purse-string suture is inserted around the cystic duct orifice; (c) the purse-string suture has been tied with closure of the cystic duct orifice.

course of antibiotic therapy for a minimum of 7 days. The results of the culture of operative specimens of bile and pus may dictate changes in the antibiotic regimen.

Laparoscopic management of severe acute disease

Although the open surgical management outlined above is still considered by many to be the standard surgical management of these severely ill patients, there is a strong case, and indeed an increasing trend, for laparoscopic management. This is intended in the first instance as a diagnostic inspection to assess the severity of the disease. In the presence of established gangrene and perforation, open surgical management as outlined in the preceding section is indicated. Otherwise, a laparoscopic insertion of a self-retaining catheter will effectively drain the inflamed gallbladder and tide the patient over a critical illness. Once this has resolved and if the patient's condition permits, a cholecystectomy (laparoscopic or otherwise) is performed. If the patient's cardiorespiratory status precludes an elective surgical intervention, then gallstone extraction, fragmentation or MTBE dissolution through the established cholecystostomy tract is performed.

Mini-cholecystostomy of Burhenne and Stoller

This is an equally valid approach in poor-risk patients with severe acute disease. After the position of the fundus of the inflamed gallbladder is located by ultrasound, a small incision is made over it. Stay sutures are inserted. The gallbladder contents are aspirated and sent for culture and a Foley catheter is inserted into the gallbladder lumen and held in place by a purse-string suture. This approach, which can be performed under local anaesthesia and sedation, is quick and extremely safe.

Mortality of severe acute cholecystitis

The overall reported mortality of acute cholecystitis is 3%. The mortality in the elderly is higher (10%) and more than half of the deaths in patients over 65 years are secondary to cardiovascular and respiratory complications.

Established non-progressive disease

These form the majority and the acute obstructive cholecystitis usually resolves with conservative treatment. There are two management options:

- Delayed (interval, subsequent admission) cholecystectomy.
- Early (same admission) cholecystectomy.

The interval approach is the traditional one and entails conservative management of the acute episode with discharge of the patient after complete resolution of the attack. Subsequently, the patient is admitted some 2–3 months later for an elective cholecystectomy. The rationale for this treatment is that in most instances the raised pressure within the gallbladder lumen lifts the walls of the organ off the impacted stone which then dislodges and falls into the lumen with resolution of the inflammation, the view being held that it is safer to operate several weeks after the acute inflammatory episode has subsided.

Early cholecystectomy is increasingly favoured in the management of acute cholecystitis. It must be distinguished from emergency cholecystectomy. Following initial conservative management and confirmation of the diagnosis as outlined previously, the patient is operated electively (scheduled urgent) on the next available operating list or within a few days of admission. The results of several prospective clinical trials comparing early versus interval cholecystectomy have shown clear benefits from early cholecystectomy performed during the same hospital admission in fit patients (ASA I and II). These include less time spent in hospital and lower cost of treatment. Fears that an early cholecystectomy is a more hazardous procedure have proved groundless, in particular the incidence of complications including missed common duct stones and mortality rates reported in these prospective trials have been similar. On the other hand, the latter has several disadvantages which include:

- Failure of conservative treatment in 13%.
- Premature re-admission with a further attack while waiting for elective cholecystectomy (13%).
- Patient defaulting after discharge (10%).

More recently, a randomized trial of early versus interval laparoscopic cholecystectomy for acute cholecystitis has demonstrated similar results. In particular there was no significant difference in the conversion rates (early 21% vs interval 24%), similar morbidity but a significantly ($p < 0.001$) shorter hospital stay, 7.6 vs 11.6 days, although the operating time was longer for the early group, i.e. 122 vs 106 min. Similar benefits have been reported by another randomized trial comparing early versus interval LC for acute cholecystitis. Thus early LC carries both medical and socioeconomic benefits over interval LC for acute cholecystitis.

An aggressive policy of early cholecystectomy is indicated in the elderly and diabetic patients unless they have comorbid significant heart, disease as these patients often have gangrenous disease.

Laparoscopic versus open cholecystectomy

As with the elective situation, laparoscopic cholecystectomy offers significant advantages over open cholecystectomy for acute cholecystitis and early LC has rapidly become the treatment of choice for this condition. Aside from several retrospective reports indicative of reduced morbidity and hospital stay, the benefit of LC versus open cholecystectomy for acute cholecystitis has been confirmed by a prospective randomized clinical trial. This study showed a significant reduction in the post-operative morbidity in the LC arm (only 3% minor complications versus 23% major complications and 19% minor complications in the open cholecystectomy group). In adopting LC as the routine option, it must be stressed that the need for conversion is encountered in 20–25% of cases and an early decision should be made to convert electively in the presence of obscured anatomy. This is far better than persistence with a difficult operation with enforced conversion because of the onset of an intra-operative complication. These patients are at risk of severe post-operative complications.

Thus the valid approach is a flexible one. The procedure starts with an exploratory laparoscopy to assess technical difficulty of the operation with particular reference to the structures in the triangle of Calot. A large distended gallbladder should be aspirated and lifted by a retractor rather than grasped. Large stones impacted in Hartmann's pouch that cannot be dislodged may prove problematic. The practical axiom is a simple one, i.e. if adequate exposure for a safe dissection cannot be obtained, the case should be converted. In some cases, a fundus first dissection of the gallbladder may be required.

The case for routine fluorocholangiography is much stronger when cholecystectomy is performed for acute cholecystitis as these patients are much more commonly jaundiced (the inflammatory oedema or by concomitant ductal calculi). The cholangiogram should outline the entire biliary tract (intra- and extrahepatic). It ensures safe occlusion of the cystic duct stump without compromise of the common hepatic or common duct and differentiates stones from distortion caused by the inflammatory oedema.

Mucocele of the gallbladder

This is often confused with empyema. However, the grossly distended gallbladder associated with cystic duct obstruction, usually by a stone, is not inflamed and is filled with white mucoid material. Mucocele of the gallbladder is usually encountered in elderly patients and presents with a painless mass in the right hypochondrium. There may or may not be a history of acute pain indicative of biliary colic or mild acute cholecystitis. The treatment is cholecystectomy which can be performed safely by the laparoscopic approach.

Section 10.10 • Acalculous chronic gallbladder disease

Chronic inflammation of the gallbladder in the absence of gallstones is due to adenomyomatosis or cholesterolosis of the gallbladder and these may be conveniently grouped as acalculous chronic gallbladder disease. This can give rise to vague symptoms not dissimilar to those of chronic cholecystitis. Oral cholecystography shows no abnormality of the gallbladder in 50% of these patients, or is reported as demonstrating poor function or unusual appearances. Thickening and 'polypoid' lesions/diverticula may be documented by high-resolution ultrasound. In many instances, the diagnosis is made on pathological examination of the excised gallbladder. In general, the results of cholecystectomy for these conditions have been difficult to evaluate but in the presence of persisting symptoms, most surgeons would advise operation.

Adenomyomatosis of the gallbladder

This is variously named as adenomatous hyperplasia, diverticulosis of the gallbladder and cholecystitis glandularis proliferans. It is thought to represent a developmental defect that results in hyperplasia of the smooth muscle bundles with sacculation or diverticulum formation of the epithelial lining (Rokitansky–Aschoff sinuses). The cholecystogram may be normal or the late film taken after a fatty meal may demonstrate either the mural diverticula (Figure 10.45) or a concentric narrowing of the fundus.

Cholesterolosis of the gallbladder

In this condition, the epithelial cells and macrophages within the gallbladder mucosa become laden with cholesterol and lead to the formation of numerous lipid deposits. Chronic inflammation of the adjacent mucosa then leads to a striking appearance of the interior of the gallbladder, which has been aptly described as the 'strawberry gallbladder'.

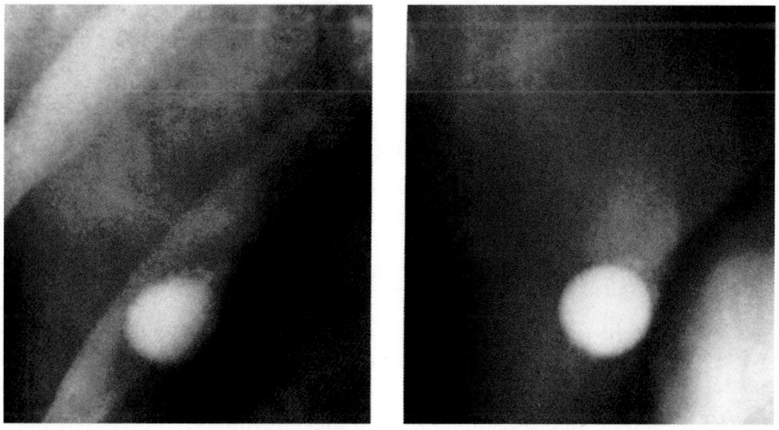

Figure 10.45 Oral cholecystogram: a concentric narrowing of the fundus is the striking feature but on closer inspection, intramural diverticula are discernible. When encountered, these are pathognomonic of adenomyomatosis of the gallbladder. Often, however, the oral cholecystogram is normal.

Section 10.11 • Ductal calculi and cholangitis

The majority of ductal calculi are found in the common bile duct and, in the West, only an estimated 5% of ductal calculi are located in the intrahepatic ducts (more commonly the left), although multiple intrahepatic calculi are common in Eastern countries, especially where parasitic infestations and recurrent pyogenic cholangitis are endemic. Ductal calculi may arise as follows:

- as secondary calculi from migration of gallstones
- as primary calculi arising *de novo* within the bile ducts.

Primary ductal calculi are brown pigment stones. Their composition and infective aetiology are discussed earlier in this module. In surgical practice, brown pigment stones are often encountered in the following conditions:

- stasis in the biliary tract caused by strictures, tumours and sclerosing cholangitis
- parasitic infestations
- recurrent pyogenic cholangitis (Asia)
- indwelling endoprostheses/internalized clips and non-absorbable sutures.

Less commonly, pigment stones form around metal clips and non-absorbable sutures when these become incorporated inside the bile duct. The important predisposing condition to infection and brown pigment stone formation is stasis and this requires correction in addition to removal of the calculi and eradication of any infection.

Clinical manifestations of ductal calculi

Although 15–20% of patients with stones in the common bile duct are asymptomatic, the majority present sooner or later with severe symptoms, and by and large incur a significant morbidity as the pathological potential of ductal calculi is high and may contribute to the death of the patient. Ductal calculi may present with:

- recurrent bouts of biliary colic accompanied by intermittent jaundice
- episodic upper abdominal pain and dyspepsia (Figure 10.46)
- stone impaction with progressive jaundice
- cholangitis
- gallstone pancreatitis
- secondary biliary cirrhosis and portal hypertension.

Management of ductal calculi

Role of endoscopic sphincterotomy and stone extraction

The current orthodox treatment for ductal calculi is by endoscopic sphincterotomy and stone extraction; in patients requiring cholecystectomy for symptomatic gallstone disease, endoscopic stone extraction is performed before the operation preferably during the same hospital admission. However, the increasing efficacy and usage of laparoscopic stone clearance for patients harbouring ductal calculi is challenging the role of pre-operative endoscopic stone extraction in centres with the necessary expertise. In addition, there is increasing concern regarding sphincterotomy in patients below the age of 50 years. The short-term morbidity of endoscopic stone extraction ranges from 5 to 10%. It has a median failure rate of 10% and a mortality of 0.5–1.0%. In addition, endoscopic sphincterotomy carries a long-term morbidity that includes recurrence of common duct stones (average of 11%), and stenosis (3% in the absence of papillitis and 30% if papillitis is present). Further, the sphincterotomy results in bacterial colonization of the extrahepatic biliary tract.

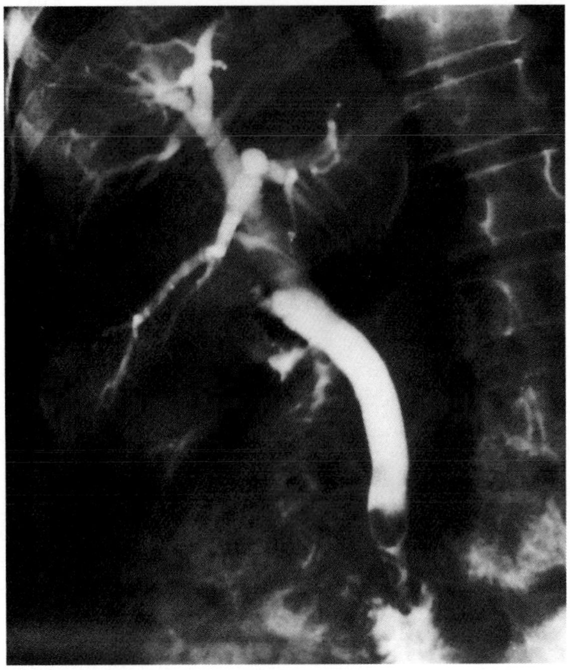

Figure 10.46 Primary ductal calculi situated at the lower end of the bile duct 13 years after a cholecystectomy. The patient complained of dyspepsia and episodic abdominal pain. Although the patient was not jaundiced, the liver function tests showed a mild elevation of the serum bilirubin and raised alkaline phosphatase.

There is agreement that the two-stage approach is indicated in poor-risk patients including those with established cholangitis or severe pancreatitis, but these constitute only 30% of patients with ductal calculi. In fit patients with ductal stones, single-stage laparoscopic surgical treatment (laparoscopic stone extraction and cholecystectomy) is gaining favour among laparoscopic surgeons especially as the evidence from four randomized clinical trials is that the two-stage sequential management of patients with ductal stones is inferior (increased overall morbidity) to single-stage surgical treatment. A recent large clinical trial involving 300 randomized patients showed the same efficacy, morbidity and mortality but a significant reduction in the hospital stay in the single-stage laparoscopic arm.

Undoubtedly, the single-stage laparoscopic approach requires a lesser resource and should replace the two-stage approach on the grounds of equal efficacy and safety but diminished costs. On average in 50% of patients undergoing ERCP for suspected ductal calculi, the ERCP is normal. The persistence of the two-stage approach is attributed to reluctance of gastroenterologists to relinquish this treatment and the limited number of centres undertaking laparoscopic ductal stone extraction routinely – regrettably the two are inter-linked. If evidence based treatment is to be followed, then endoscopic stone extraction should reserved for:

- poor-risk patients
- patients with cholangitis
- patients with severe pancreatitis
- some patients with failed laparoscopic stone extraction as an alternative to conversion
- retained or recurrent stones after cholecystectomy.

In elderly or poor-risk patients, endoscopic sphincterotomy alone leaving the gallbladder *in situ* has been recommended in the past. However, subsequent clinical trials comparing this approach with definitive single-stage treatment (open or laparoscopic) have shown similar morbidity and mortality rates and a high incidence (30%) in patients with *in situ* gallbladder of biliary symptoms/cholecystitis requiring subsequent cholecystectomy. Thus endoscopic sphincterotomy alone is no longer favoured unless the patient is totally unfit for surgery (Figure 10.47).

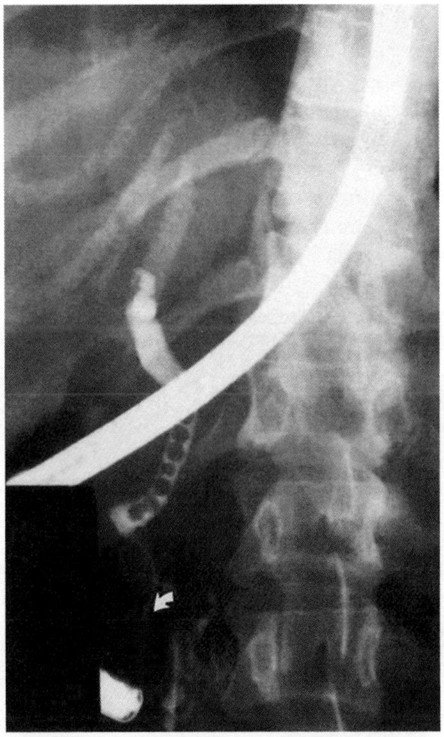

Figure 10.47 Endoscopic papillotomy for multiple ductal calculi in an elderly patient. The wire of the sphincterotome is visible above the tip of the endoscope.

Laparoscopic extraction of ductal calculi

The techniques of laparoscopic ductal stone clearance include:

- transcystic duct extraction
- direct supraduodenal common bile duct exploration
- rendez-vous laparo-endoscopic approach.

Transcystic duct extraction

This is the least invasive technique and has the undoubted merit of leaving the extrahepatic biliary tract including the choledochal sphincter intact. Thus its morbidity is low and the average post-operative hospital stay is short (3 days). It is indicated for small floating stones up to 7 mm diameter, where its reported efficacy in achieving ductal stone clearance ranges from 80 to 95%. There are two commonly used techniques:

- the choledochoscopic visually guided method
- the radiologically guided wire basket trawling technique.

The choledochoscopic technique requires dilatation of the cystic duct before insertion of the mini-choledochoscope through the cystic duct into the common bile duct. The stones are visualized and trapped using a wire basket introduced through the instrument channel of the endoscope and extracted through the cystic duct (Figure 10.48). Some advocate delivering the trapped stones through the sphincter of Oddi into the duodenum where they are released. This is, however, not generally recommended because of the risk of pancreatitis. A completion cystic duct cholangiogram is performed, and if this is normal, the cystic duct is ligated and the gallbladder removed. If there is any doubt about residual fragments, a cystic duct drainage cannula (Cook) is inserted into the common bile duct and tied to the cystic duct with two Roeder catgut extracorporeal slip knots. A post-operative cholangiogram is performed 24 hours later. If this is normal, the cystic duct drainage cannula is capped with a Luer lock and covered with an occlusive dressing before the patient is discharged usually on the third post-operative day. The cannula is removed as an outpatient 10–14 days later.

The radiologically guided trawling technique is quicker and simpler than the above. Furthermore, it has the added advantage of obviating the need for dilatation of the cystic duct. It consists of the insertion of a soft pleated four-wire basket in the closed position through the cystic duct into the lower end of the common bile duct. Once in position with the tip among the stones, the basket is fully opened and then withdrawn slowly. No attempt is made to close the basket as the wires of this are folded over the stones by the narrow cystic duct during the trawling process (Figure 10.49). With experience, the radiological exposure is minimal. The trawling process is repeated until complete stone clearance is achieved.

Laparo-endoscopic approach

This combined approach entails insertion of a guide wire by the laparoscopic surgeon through the cystic

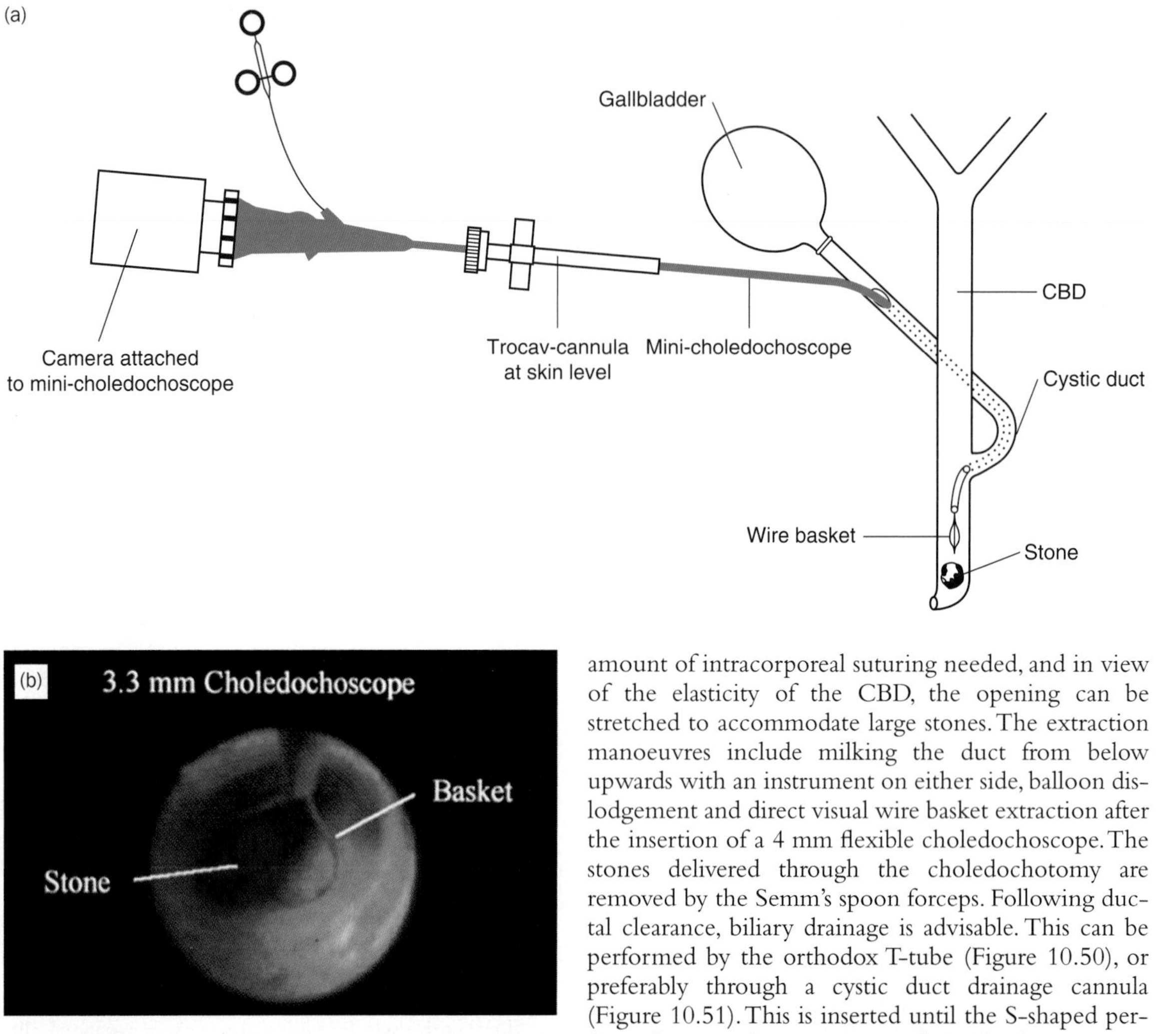

Figure 10.48 Visually guided transcystic laparoscopic duct extraction: (a) diagrammatic representation, (b) mini-choledochoscopic view of the trapped stone.

duct down the common bile duct (CBD) into the duodenum. The endoscopist then performs a sphincterotomy and stone extraction with the patient in the supine position. The reported experience with the laparoendoscopic technique is limited because of the additional resource needed. There is also a risk of acute post-operative pancreatitis with this technique.

Direct supraduodenal common bile duct exploration

This is indicated for large or occluding stones. The technique is similar to open exploration of the common bile duct. The dissection is minimal and consists of exposure of the anterior wall of the common bile duct after downward displacement of the duodenum. No stay sutures are inserted. A choledochotomy is made in the supraduodenal segment. The size of the choledochotomy should be approximately half to three-quarters the maximum diameter of the largest stone. Avoidance of a large choledochotomy reduces the amount of intracorporeal suturing needed, and in view of the elasticity of the CBD, the opening can be stretched to accommodate large stones. The extraction manoeuvres include milking the duct from below upwards with an instrument on either side, balloon dislodgement and direct visual wire basket extraction after the insertion of a 4 mm flexible choledochoscope. The stones delivered through the choledochotomy are removed by the Semm's spoon forceps. Following ductal clearance, biliary drainage is advisable. This can be performed by the orthodox T-tube (Figure 10.50), or preferably through a cystic duct drainage cannula (Figure 10.51). This is inserted until the S-shaped perforated terminal segment is well inside the common bile duct, after which it is secured to the cystic duct by two Roeder catgut sutures. Primary closure of the choledochotomy is carried out during which the CBD is constantly irrigated with saline via the cystic duct drainage cannula.

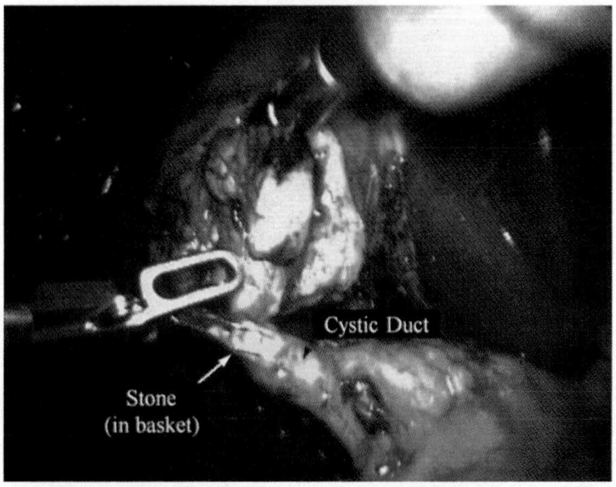

Figure 10.49 Trawling technique for transcystic laparoscopic ductal stone extraction.

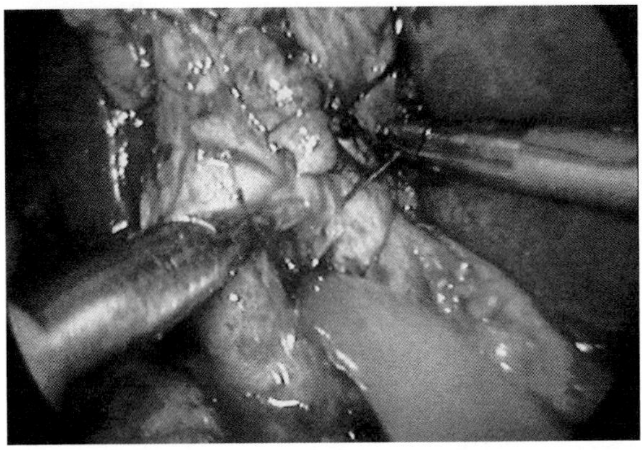

Figure 10.50 Laparoscopic common bile duct exploration with closure of the common bile duct around a T-tube.

In either case, a completion cholangiogram is essential to ensure ductal clearance and a subhepatic drain is necessary. The cystic duct drainage cannula or the T-tube is firmly anchored to the abdominal wall and connected to a biliary drainage bag. When a cystic duct drainage cannula is used, the post-operative cholangiogram is carried out on the second day and if this is normal, the cannula is sealed with a Luer lock and covered with an occlusive dressing. In the absence of any bile leakage from the subhepatic drain over the next 24 hours, the drain is removed and the patient discharged the next day with the cystic duct drainage cannula *in situ*. This is removed 7 days later as an outpatient. If a T-tube has been inserted, the post-operative cholangiogram is carried out on the seventh post-operative day, and if normal, the tube is clamped and provided there is no leakage from the subhepatic drain and the patient has no symptoms or fever over the next 24 hours, the T-tube is removed. The subhepatic drain is removed a day later. In the elderly, diabetics and patients on immunosuppressive drugs, the T-tube is kept in place for at least 2 weeks as the maturation of the T-tube tract is impaired in these patients. Thus early removal may lead to biliary peritonitis.

Patients with ductal calculi discovered during elective cholecystectomy (unsuspected ductal calculi)

These account for 4–10% of cases and are discovered by routine IOFC. They are usually small floating calculi

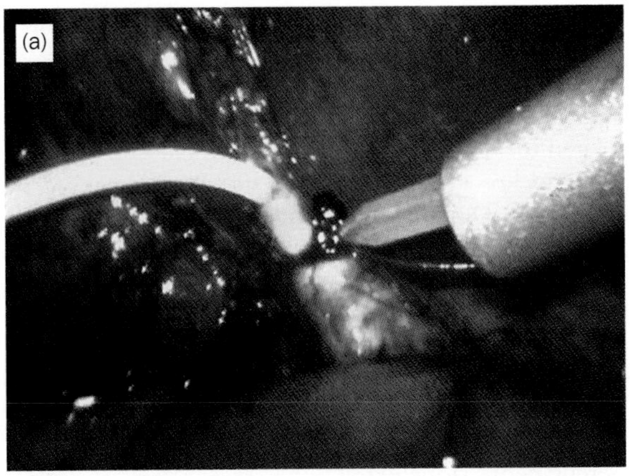

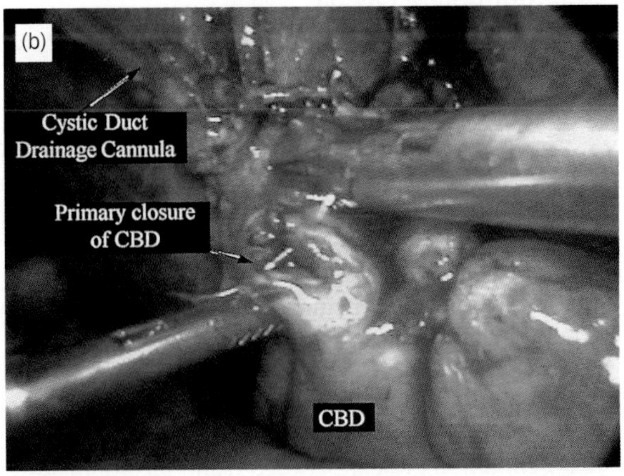

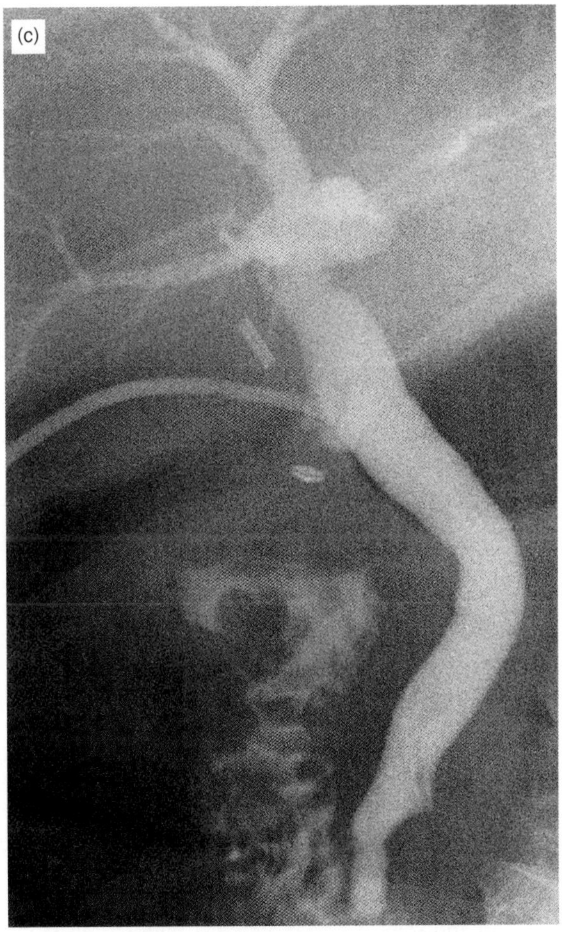

Figure 10.51 Decompression of the extrahepatic biliary tract by the Cuschieri cystic duct drainage cannula with primary closure of choledochotomy: (a) drainage cannula inserted and fixed to the cystic duct stump; (b) primary closure of the choledochotomy; (c) completion cholangiogram through the cystic duct drainage cannula.

without dilatation of the common bile duct. As these patients have no obstruction and normal liver function tests, some surgeons have advocated no intervention other than the cholecystectomy on the grounds that some of these calculi will pass spontaneously and if and when they become symptomatic or complications arise after surgery, endoscopic sphincterotomy can be performed. This policy is ill founded for several reasons. In the first instance, there are no hard data as to the frequency of spontaneous passage without complications. Furthermore, it is impossible to predict uncomplicated stone passage in the individual patient. This expectant policy will incur a definite morbidity from jaundice, cholangitis or pancreatitis and some (albeit few) patients will die as a result of one of these complications. The appropriate management of these patients, based on the known pathogenic potential of ductal calculi, is removal either at the time of laparoscopic cholecystectomy (transcystic duct extraction) or by post-operative endoscopic sphincterotomy.

Ductal calculi discovered soon after cholecystectomy and exploration of the common bile duct

These are referred to as missed, retained or residual stones. The incidence varies from 2 to 15% and averages 8%. Routine completion choledochoscopy/cholangiography virtually abolishes this complication. Retained ductal calculi following biliary tract surgery are either diagnosed in the immediate post-operative period by the post-operative T-tube cholangiogram or present with recurrent symptoms usually within 2 years of cholecystectomy without exploration of the common bile duct. Ductal stones presenting beyond this interval are generally considered to be of the primary variety.

Certain general considerations apply with regard to the management of patients with residual calculi following biliary tract surgery. Urgent intervention is not indicated if the liver biochemistry is normal, the patient is asymptomatic, and the T-tube cholangiogram shows no organic disease or significant dilatation. Spontaneous passage is likely if the calculi are small (less than 3 mm) and may be aided by simple measures such as T-tube clamping. If the patient tolerates clamping and providing no untoward symptoms or complications develop, such a conservative approach can be continued for a few weeks, at the end of which time the situation is reviewed radiologically.

The various methods available for the non-surgical management of retained stones are:

- flushing
- dissolution
- percutaneous stone extraction via the T-tube tract
- endoscopic sphincterotomy and stone extraction.

The first three options are applicable only to patients with an indwelling T-tube whereas endoscopic stone extraction can be used in all patients. All the above methods are performed under antibiotic cover because of the risk of cholangitis and septicaemia.

Flushing is usually carried out with saline, heparinized saline, or lignocaine–saline solution. The technique, which is simple and effective if the stones are small (<0.3 mm), is performed by infusing the solution through the T-tube under manometric control to ensure that the pressure does not exceed 30 cmH_2O, as this can lead to cholangio-venous reflux and septicaemia. The efficacy of this simple method of treatment, which does not require any special expertise, can be enhanced when it is accompanied by pharmacologically induced relaxation of the sphincter of Oddi.

Cholate infusion can dissolve cholesterol stones but its efficacy is low and it has been replaced by mono-octanoin which acts more rapidly and achieves complete stone clearance in 40%. The most effective agent for the dissolution of ductal calculi is MTBE, which is capable of achieving gallstone dissolution within hours of instillation.

Percutaneous stone extraction via the T-tube tract was initially performed by the Burhenne technique using a Dormia basket introduced via a specially designed steerable catheter to capture and extract the stone under fluoroscopic control. It has largely been replaced by the flexible choledochoscopic technique which is successful in 90–95% of cases. A 4–6 week period of maturation of the T-tube tract is required before the procedure can be performed safely. A guidewire is introduced into the common bile duct and the T-tube removed. Thereafter, the T-tube tract is dilated to allow the introduction of the narrow flexible choledochoscope. The retained stones are removed by means of a Dormia basket under visual control.

Endoscopic sphincterotomy with stone extraction is the most effective method of dealing with the problem of retained stones and can be performed in patients with and without T-tubes. Surgical management of missed stones is reserved for those patients in whom the above methods have failed or complications have developed during or after attempted endoscopic or percutaneous stone extraction.

Recurrent ductal calculi

Ductal calculi presenting 2 years or more after an operation are generally regarded to be primary. One study has identified suture material in 30% of cases. This finding stresses the importance of avoiding non-absorbable material during operations on the biliary tract. Internalization of metal clips used to secure the medial end of the cystic duct during laparoscopic cholecystectomy is now a well-recognized complication of this procedure. The exact pathology remains unclear, but it seems likely that the clip is placed too close to the common bile duct resulting in localized pressure necrosis. The internalized clip becomes covered with calcium bilirubinate to form a brown pigment stone. The patients who develop this condition present between 6 and 12 months after the procedure with jaundice and/or cholangitis. The condition is easily diagnosed on the ERCP films as the stone has a characteristic 'cat's eye' appearance.

The management of patients with recurrent ductal calculi depends on their age and general condition. Endoscopic sphincterotomy and stone extraction is the first-line treatment and surgery (open or laparoscopic) reserved if this approach fails. During surgery, the stones are removed atraumatically by means of biliary balloon catheters, stone-grasping forceps or Dormia baskets as described previously. A completion check by means of a choledochoscopic inspection or cholangiography abolishes the incidence of residual stones. Temporary biliary drainage by means of a T-tube is advisable.

In other situations, recurrent ductal calculi are often multiple and associated with gross dilatation of the bile duct and in some cases obvious distal ductal stenosis. This may be primary (papillary stenosis) or be secondary to trauma inflicted by metal bougies introduced through the sphincter region at the time of exploration of the common bile duct. In patients with multiple ductal calculi, grossly dilated bile duct (>2 cm) or papillary stenosis, a drainage operation is indicated: choledochoduodenostomy or transduodenal sphincteroplasty. Opinions are divided as to the relative merits of these two procedures. However, sphincteroplasty carries a significant risk of pancreatitis and involves a sizeable duodenotomy. A transection choledochoduodenostomy (Figure 10.52) is preferable to the side-to-side anastomosis as it provides dependent drainage and avoids the complication of the inspissated sump syndrome.

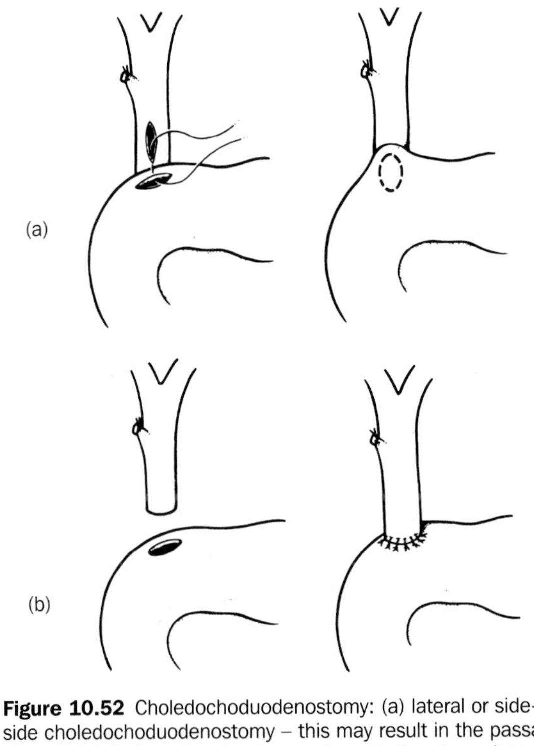

Figure 10.52 Choledochoduodenostomy: (a) lateral or side-to-side choledochoduodenostomy – this may result in the passage of food debris from the duodenum through the stoma into the lower end of the bile duct (distal to the anastomosis with the development of the inspissated sump syndrome which presents with cholangitis); (b) diagrammatic technique of the procedure of transection choledochoduodenostomy – the bile duct is mobilized from the portal vein and hepatic artery. It is then transected as it enters the pancreas. The distal end is closed with a running suture and the proximal end is anastomosed in an end-to-side fashion to the duodenum at the junction of the first with the second part.

Multiple intrahepatic calculi

Although rare in the West, these are common in Eastern countries and often pose serious management problems. The majority are associated with stricture formation of the hepatic ducts. If the stones are floating and located in the major intrahepatic bile ducts, removal may be possible through a standard choledochotomy with introduction of the flexible choledochoscope and visually guided extraction by balloon catheters or a wire (Dormia) basket.

Transhepatic lithotomy is necessary when stones are impacted above a strictured intrahepatic duct (usually left). The hepatic parenchyma of the involved liver segment is divided down to and including the involved duct. Thereafter, the stones are removed and, following irrigation, the stricture is dilated with a balloon dilator. A silicone T-tube is then inserted into the affected intrahepatic duct and the liver parenchyma is sutured around it. Resection of the involved lobe is reserved for cases with severe disease, i.e. multiple stones associated with extensive stricturing, fibrosis, gross destruction of the hepatic parenchyma and abscess formation.

Section 10.12 • Cholangitis

Acute bacterial cholangitis is a serious, life-threatening emergency caused by infection of an obstructed biliary tract. The systemic manifestations of the acute illness result from bacteraemia secondary to cholangiovenous reflux induced by the biliary hypertension (<20 cmH_2O). The most common obstructing agent is an occluding stone in the common bile duct, followed by bile duct strictures (including sclerosing cholangitis) and tumours of the bile ducts, pancreatic head and periampullary lesions. Less commonly, cholangitis is secondary to bilio-enteric anastomoses, spontaneous bilio-enteric fistulas, cystic disease of the biliary tract and duodenal diverticula. Cholangitis may also occur following instrumentation of the biliary tract. Thus, it is encountered in 7% of patients undergoing ERCP. The risk factors for cholangitis following this investigation are the presence of fever before the procedure and malignant biliary obstruction. Thus early decompression is indicated in these patients soon after the endoscopic retrograde cholangiography. Cholangitis caused by contamination of the endoscopes (*Pseudomonas* spp.) has also been reported. Cholangitis occurs frequently (38%) as a complication of percutaneous transhepatic biliary drainage and is the main reason for abandoning pre-operative decompression by this technique prior to surgical treatment in patients with severe obstructive jaundice. In Asia, recurrent pyogenic cholangitis is a frequent cause of recurrent bacterial cholangitis.

In severe cases of cholangitis there is neutrophilic infiltration of the sinusoids and microabscess formation in the hepatic lobules. Portal thrombi and areas of hepatic necrosis are present in patients with severe disease accompanied by hypotension (Figure 10.53). The infection is most commonly caused by Gram-negative organisms. The classical triad of symptoms consists of pain in the right hypochondrium, intermittent fever and jaundice (Charot's biliary fever) but the complete triad is present in only 70% of cases. Aside from toxicity, the high intermittent pyrexia is accompanied by severe rigors. The pain varies in intensity and may be severe. There is usually tenderness in the right hypochondrium, which if marked, suggests the presence of abscess formation (honeycomb liver). The liver is often enlarged although this may be difficult to ascertain because of the abdominal tenderness. Nausea and vomiting are frequent accompaniments. Hypotension is present in patients with severe cholangitis, when renal failure is usually present.

Prompt and energetic treatment is mandatory. Resuscitative measures include cystalloid and colloid solutions. A blood culture is taken and systemic antibiotics are commenced (cephalosporin with metronidazole or piperacillin, or imipenim). The majority respond to this treatment but some (up to 30%) do not and these patients require emergency biliary decompression. The patients who do not usually respond to conservative therapy include:

- females
- patients aged >50 years
- patients with acute renal failure
- patients with liver abscesses
- patients with bile duct stricture
- cirrhotic patients
- patients in whom the cholangitis is secondary to biliary instrumentation.

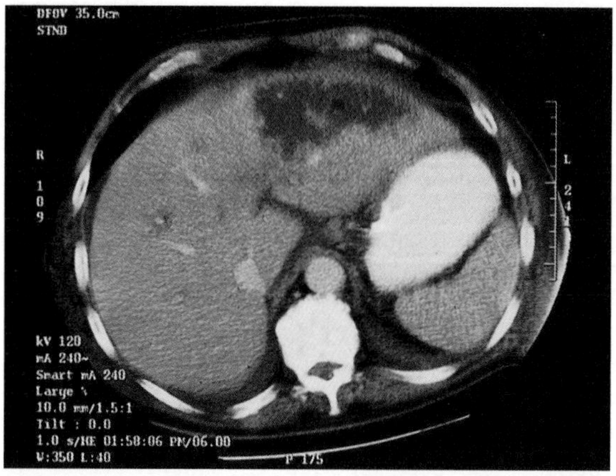

Figure 10.53 Intrahepatic segmental portal vein thrombosis with necrosis and abscess formation (central gas shadow) in a patient with severe cholangitis following pre-operative stenting of a cholangiocarcinoma. The infected segmental necrosis developed after resection of the tumour. At operation gross purulent cholangitis was observed as the biliary tract was transected above the tumour. The condition proved fatal despite resection of segments II and III.

Biliary decompression may be accomplished surgically, endoscopically or by percutaneous techniques. For most patients with cholangitis and ductal calculi, endoscopic decompression by sphincterotomy and extraction of calculi is generally favoured, especially if the patient is elderly. If the calculi cannot be extracted a temporary pigtail stent draining the proximal biliary tree into the duodenum is inserted endoscopically. The alternative is surgical exploration with ductal clearance and insertion of a T-tube. Surgical intervention is the treatment of choice if the stones are large. Cholangitis secondary to biliary instrumentation often requires operative treatment. Percutaneous transhepatic drainage is useful in patients with cholangitis complicating strictures and malignant obstruction. The overall reported mortality of patients requiring urgent decompression for severe cholangitis is 15–20%.

Sclerosing cholangitis

This is an obscure disorder of uncertain aetiology, which results in a progressive fibrous obliteration of the biliary tract. The prevalence of primary sclerosing cholangitis (PSC) approximates to 20–40 per million population. Although sclerosing cholangitis has well-recognized histological, radiological and clinical features, there are no pathognomonic findings that reliably differentiate this disease from other hepatobiliary disorders. The distinction between primary and secondary types is no longer held to be valid. The term primary was formerly used to indicate no previous biliary surgery or biliary tract disease. Often, however, sclerosing cholangitis occurs as a secondary complication of inflammatory bowel disease, usually ulcerative colitis and, much less commonly, Crohn's disease. The condition is currently regarded as an immune-complex disorder evoked by endotoxin–antibody complexes that have been identified in the peripheral blood of patients with inflammatory bowel disease.

The classification of the disorder is based on the extent of involvement of the biliary tree by the fibrous obliterative process (Table 10.7). The disease results in extensive fibrosis which extends beyond the confines of the biliary ductal walls. Histologically, the fibrosis is concentric (onion shell) with patchy, chronic inflammatory infiltrate consisting of mononuclear cells and polymorphs (Figure 10.54). In addition, changes of cholestasis are seen. The gross fibrous thickening results in localized or multiple stricture formation. Although

Table 10.7 Sclerosing cholangitis: classification based on extent of involvement of the biliary tree

Type	*Incidence (%)*
Total diffuse	50
Localized hilar	25
Diffuse intrahepatic	10
Diffuse extrahepatic	10
Localized extrahepatic (distal)	5

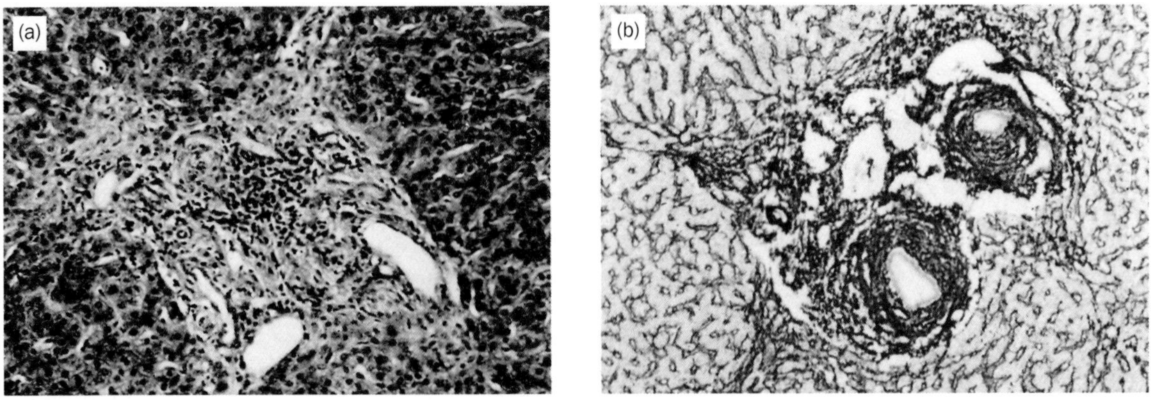

Figure 10.54 Sclerosing cholangitis: (a) histology of wedge liver biopsy (H&E) showing narrowing of the intrahepatic ducts, fibrosis and cellular infiltrate; (b) reticulin stain of the same biopsy illustrating concentric deposition of fibrous tissue around the bile ducts.

the ductal epithelium is frequently normal, it may become ulcerated and exhibit saccule formation. The disease progresses invariably to cirrhosis and the development of portal hypertension.

Sclerosing cholangitis occurs more commonly in males (3:2) and usually presents in the fifth decade. The symptoms include vague ill-health, asthenia, pain in the right hypochondrium, jaundice and itching, pyrexia and attacks of rigors. The liver is often palpable and tender. The liver function tests demonstrate a cholestatic picture and bilirubin is detected in the urine. The serum transaminases are mildly elevated. The majority of patients are hepatitis B surface antigen (HBsAg) negative. The anti-mitochondrial, anti-smooth muscle and anti-nuclear antibodies are absent. Contrast radiological visualization shows pruning of the biliary tree (scanty ducts) and stricture formation which may be localized or diffuse (Figure 10.55). Globular dilatations (sacculations) are often seen in patients with diffuse disease. Differentiation from hilar disease and cholangiocarcinoma is often difficult on radiological grounds and may not be possible even after histological examination of biopsy specimens. In these patients, only the subsequent clinical outcome can identify the true diagnosis.

The majority of patients are symptomatic at the time of presentation. However, the correlation between symptoms and liver histology and disease progression is weak. In general, the median survival between presentation and the development of end-stage liver disease is 12 years. However, rate of progression of the disease is very variable and is influenced by the frequency of episodes of bacterial cholangitis and the development of cholangiocarcinoma (central or peripheral), the diagnosis of which is often difficult in these patients. The most commonly used prognostic model is that of the Mayo clinic.

Mayo clinic prognostic model:

- 0.535 $\log_e$ serum bilirubin (mg/dl)
- + 0.486 histological stage
- + 0.041 age (years)
- + 0.705 if splenomegaly is present.

Unfortunately, there is no effective medical therapy for the condition. The pruritus may be controlled by cholestyramine. Episodes of cholangitis are managed by antibiotic therapy. Surgical intervention may be considered when adequate control of symptoms is not achieved by medical therapy, the specific indications being progressive jaundice and recurrent cholangitis. Surgical treatment gives best results for localized hilar disease. The hilar bifurcation is accessed through an anterior segmentectomy IV and a Roux-en-Y hepaticojejunostomy to the right and left hepatic ducts performed proximal to the stricture. Direct surgical intervention on the biliary tract for predominantly hilar disease is contraindicated in the presence of cirrhosis as the results are poor and the mortality is high.

For diffuse disease, intra-operative dilatation of the intrahepatic biliary tree via a choledochotomy using both metal and balloon dilators is followed by a large silicone stent introduced transhepatically down the bile

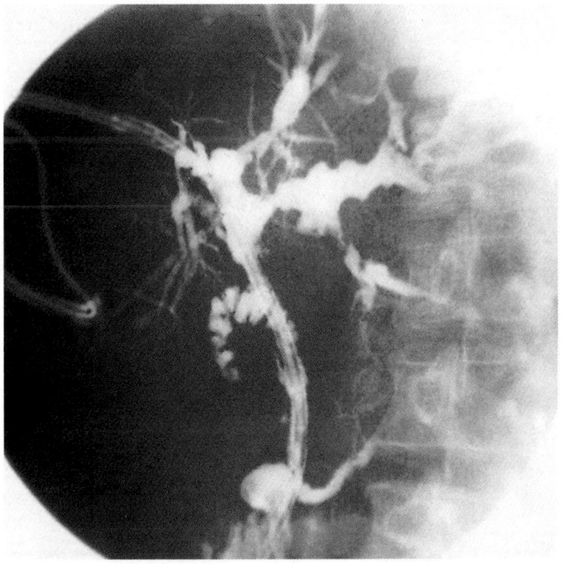

Figure 10.55 Sclerosing cholangitis: total involvement of the biliary tract.

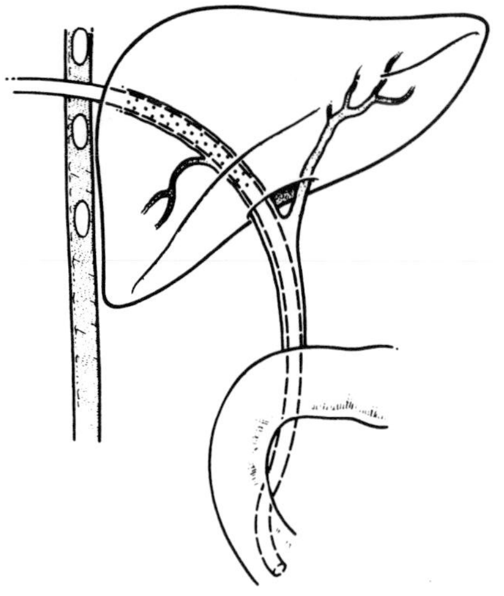

Figure 10.56 Technique of transhepatic stenting for total diffuse sclerosing cholangitis.

duct into the duodenum (Figure 10.56). The stent is exteriorized through the right lowest intercostal space in the anterior axillary line. Daily irrigation with heparinized saline and prolonged antibiotic therapy are essential components of the postoperative management. The stent is left in place for at least 12 months and progress is assessed by repeat cholangiograms carried out through the stent (Figure 10.57). Replacement of the stent may be necessary if it becomes blocked by encrustation with calcium bilirubinate. Both percutaneous transhepatic and endoscopic balloon dilatation and stent insertion have been employed to deal with strictures in patients with sclerosing cholangitis. Generally the results have been inferior to those achieved in patients with iatrogenic strictures following bile duct damage.

However, the results of surgical treatment for diffuse disease have been disappointing and these patients are better served by hepatic transplantation. The optimal timing of hepatic transplantation for PSC has not been defined and thus early referral to a transplantation centre is currently recommended. Certainly a Mayo score of ≥5 or Child C constitute definite indications for transplantation. The problem in these cases is the exclusion of a superadded cholangiocarcinoma, the presence of which is accompanied by a dismal prognosis and is a contraindication to transplantation.

Recurrent pyogenic cholangitis

This condition, which is prevalent in south-east Asia, is characterized by recurrent attacks of bacterial cholangitis which lead to the formation of pigment stones and strictures in the biliary tract. Although the exact aetiology is unknown, infection of the biliary tract with enteric organisms (*E. coli*, *B. fragilis*, *Klebsiella* spp. and *Clostridium* spp.) in debilitated (immunocompromised) patients is regarded to be the primary event. Although parasitic infestation with *Clonorchis sinensis* and *Ascaris lumbricoides* is found in some patients, there is little evidence that these parasites play an important role in the development of recurrent pyogenic cholangitis although they may predispose to it. The disease affects both the intrahepatic and the extrahepatic bile ducts. It has a well-established predilection for the left lobe of the liver. The early changes include ductal proliferation of the intraheptic tree on the affected side. The established disease is characterized by stricture formation with proximal dilatation. Multiple pigment stones form within the dilated ducts. There is a gradual destruction of the hepatic parenchyma which is replaced by fibrosis. The disease may be further complicated by hepatic abscess formation.

The condition presents with recurrent episodes of cholangitis and the diagnosis is confirmed by ERCP. Emergency treatment is by endoscopic stone extraction/stenting at the time of severe cholangitis. Definitive surgical treatment depends on the site, severity and extent of the disease. It entails bile duct exploration with removal of calculi and insertion of a T-tube,

Operative cholangiogram | Post-operative cholangiogram (4 weeks later) | Post-operative cholangiogram (19 weeks later)

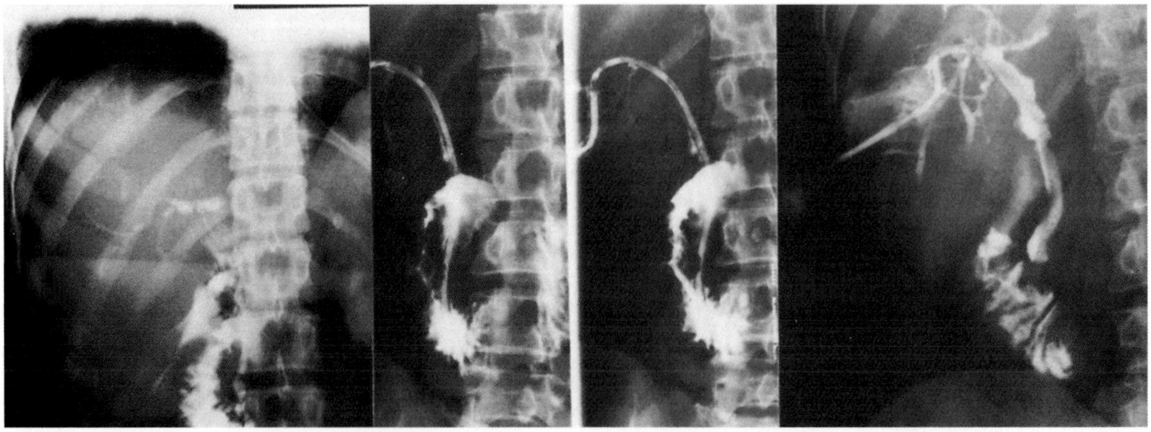

Figure 10.57 Marked radiological improvement in a patient with sclerosing cholangitis following prolonged stenting of the intra- and extrahepatic biliary tract. The patient showed a dramatic clinical and biochemical improvement.

sphincteroplasty or bilio-enteric anastomosis for strictures and hepatic resection for advanced disease of one lobe with atrophy of the liver parenchyma, multiple strictures and stones.

Biliary disorders in AIDS

Patients suffering from the acquired immunodeficiency syndrome (AIDS) are prone to develop acute acalculous cholecystitis, papillary stenosis and a cholangiopathy which simulates closely sclerosing cholangitis. Several hypotheses have been put forward for the high prevalence of acute acalculous cholecystitis in AIDS patients. These include anorexia, dehydration and cachexia due to multisystem disease, thrombosis of the cystic artery and infection with opportunistic pathogens such as cytomegalovirus (CMV) and cryptosporidium. The treatment is cholecystectomy although the mortality from sepsis is high and averages 40%.

Both papillary stenosis and cholangiopathy with intrahepatic and extrahepatic strictures are frequent and are thought to be caused by infection with CMV and cryptosporidium, although in some patients these pathogens are absent. In these cases, the biliary tract changes may be caused by direct invasion of the bile duct mucosa by the immunodeficiency virus (HIV). Both sclerosing cholangiopathy and papillary stenosis cause pain and are accompanied by raised alkaline phosphatase activity and mild hyperbilirubinaemia. The diagnosis is confirmed by ERCP. Biochemical improvement and relief of pain is obtained in patients with papillary stenosis by endoscopic sphincterotomy.

Section 10.13 • Duodenal diverticula

The prevalence of periampullary duodenal diverticula in patients undergoing ERCP is 12.5% and appears to increase with age. Their importance is two-fold. In the first instance, they predispose to bacterial infection. Thus patients with duodenal diverticula have a higher incidence of infected bile than normal subjects and the bacterial count of their duodenal contents is elevated (with proliferation of *Enterobacteriaceae* spp.) compared to patients without diverticula. Secondly, duodenal diverticula increase the difficulty of cannulation of the papilla during ERCP and thus the failure rate of this procedure, especially when the opening of the duodenal papilla lies inside a diverticulum.

Section 10.14 • Haemobilia

Major (profuse) haemobilia is rare and when it occurs spontaneously, it is caused by rupture of an intrahepatic aneurysm.

Nowadays, significant haemobilia is most commonly encountered as a complication of percutaneous radiological interventions on the liver and following hepatic trauma. The vascular injury within the hepatic parenchyma caused by transhepatic radiological interventions results in an arterio-venous fistula or pseudoaneurysm or direct vascular–biliary connection. If the bleeding is marked, blood clots with biliary colic complicate the clinical picture. Treatment is by percutaneous embolization of the bleeding site.

The second most common cause is blunt or penetrating hepatic trauma. Traumatic haemobilia may be treated by direct ligation of the vessels inside the liver haematoma or by percutaneous selective arterial embolization.

Minor haemobilia may also be caused by stones, primary hepatic tumours including angiomas, gallbladder and bile duct polyps, parasitic infestations, severe cholangitis and coagulation disorders. Haemobilia may complicate ESWL for ductal calculi.

Section 10.15 • Bilio-enteric fistulas

The various types and causation of biliary fistulas are shown in Table 10.8.

Spontaneous external biliary fistulas are exceeding rare and the few reported cases have been instances of neglected empyema of the gallbladder or extensive carcinoma of the gallbladder invading the abdominal wall. The vast majority of external biliary fistulas occur in the post-operative period and may result from the following:

Table 10.8 Biliary fistulas

Category	*Type*	*Causation*
External		Trauma and operative injuries therapeutic (T-tube, stents, cholecystostomy)
Internal	*Bilio-enteric*:	
	Cholecystoduodenal	Gallstones
	Cholecystocolic	Gallstones, Ca
	Cholecystogastric	Gallstones, Ca, peptic ulceration
	Choledochoduodenal	Ductal calculi, iatrogenic, duodenal ulcer, Ca
	Bilio-bilial:	
	Cholecystocholedochal	Gallstones (Mirizzi syndrome)
	Others:	
	Broncho/pleuro-bilial	Trauma, operative injuries, liver abscesses/hydatid, subphrenic abscesses
	Cholecystorenal	Gallstones

- leakage of bile from a slipped cystic duct ligature or cut accessory bile duct
- trauma to the extrahepatic biliary tree during cholecystectomy, gastric surgery or pancreatectomy
- dislodged T-tube after common bile duct exploration.
- leakage from bilio-enteric anastomosis
- hepatic resections.

Leakage of bile after removal of a T-tube is short-lived and requires investigation by ERCP if it persists beyond 2–3 days. Other external biliary fistulas may follow blunt or penetrating hepatic trauma. The external biliary fistula usually occurs after the surgical treatment of the hepatic injury and is then often accompanied by sepsis. External biliary fistulas do not result in skin excoriation but may cause significant fluid and electrolyte depletion if the output is high and prolonged. They are not usually accompanied by systemic manifestations unless sepsis is present. Abdominal tenderness and rebound indicates the concomitant presence of bile in the peritoneal cavity. Post-operative external biliary fistulas occurring in association with jaundice indicate bile duct trauma or a missed obstructive lesion of the biliary tract. These patients require urgent investigation with ultrasonography/CT and ERCP. Otherwise, a conservative management regimen is adopted as the biliary fistula usually closes spontaneously. Persistence of the fistula beyond a reasonable period (7–10 days), the development of jaundice, pyrexia or deterioration of the patient's condition are indications for urgent reassessment and investigation.

Internal fistulas are usually spontaneous and arise from chronic or acute perforation of the gallbladder into an adjacent organ. Others are due to malignant infiltration arising from or involving the gallbladder, e.g. carcinoma of the hepatic flexure, duodenum or gallbladder. The symptoms of the non-malignant internal fistulas involving the gallbladder are similar to those of chronic cholecystitis but jaundice and cholangitis are more common and radiology of the abdomen shows gas or barium in the biliary tree. The most frequent of the internal fistulas is the cholecystoduodenal fistula followed by cholecystocolic and cholecystogastric fistulas. The Mirizzi syndrome refers to a condition characterized by obstructive jaundice caused by a stone impacted in the neck of the gallbladder which compresses the common hepatic duct and which eventually ulcerates through into the common hepatic duct causing a cholecystocholedochal fistula (Figure 10.58).

A fistulous tract between the lower end of the bile duct and the duodenum (choledochoduodenal fistula) may arise spontaneously (secondary to ductal calculi or chronic duodenal ulcer) or be the result of iatrogenic injury from ill-advised probing of the Vaterian segment of the common bile duct during biliary surgery. Biliopleural and bronchobilial fistulas are usually the result of hepatic abscesses (Figure 10.59) and hydatid disease of the liver, though some follow hepatic injuries complicated by the development of subphrenic abscesses.

The treatment of bilio-enteric fistulas due to gallstone disease consists of a cholecystectomy and closure of the fistulous communication. Exploration of the common bile duct is frequently necessary and is dictated by the findings at peroperative cholangiography. Unless the Mirizzi syndrome is recognized at operation, damage to the common hepatic duct is inevitable. The surgical treatment of this condition entails leaving a small cuff of gallbladder wall, which is used to close the fistulous opening. The common bile duct is explored (if necessary) through a choledochotomy lower down. The management of bronchobiliary fistu-

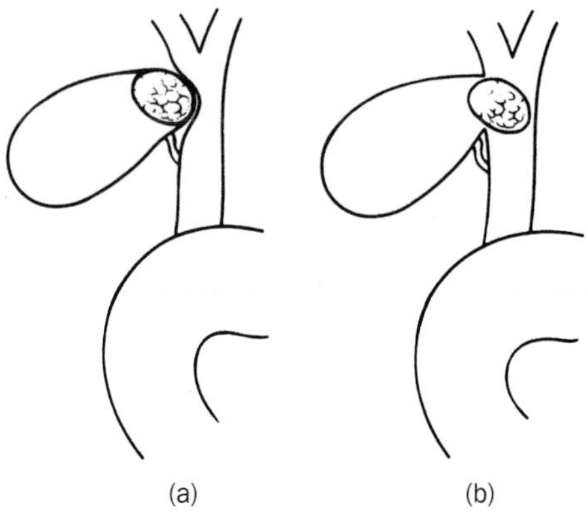

Figure 10.58 The Mirizzi syndrome: (a) a stone impacted in the neck/Hartmann's pouch causes extrinsic compression of the common hepatic duct followed by (b) fistula formation between the gallbladder and the common hepatic duct.

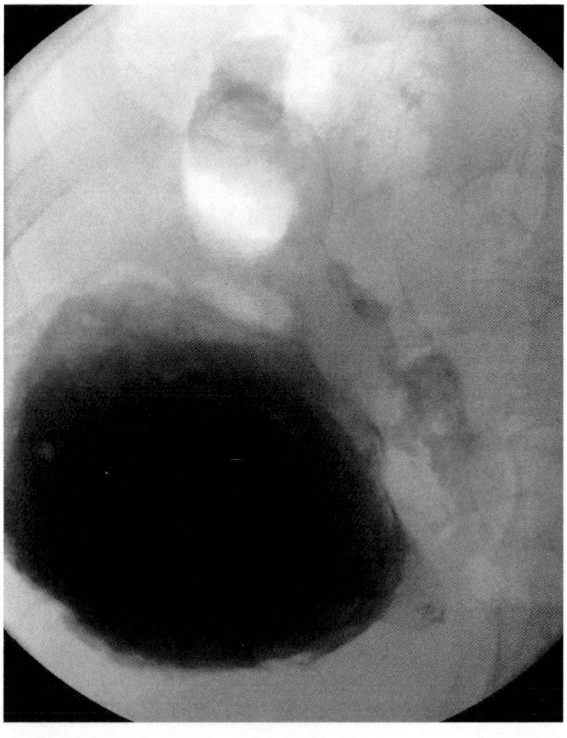

Figure 10.59 Contrast study of a large hepatic abscess with communication with the bronchial tree. At operation the abscess had burrowed through the diaphragm to involve the lower lobe of the lung which required resection.

las consists of adequate drainage of the underlying hepatic/subphrenic abscess and decompression of the biliary tract when necessary.

Gallstone ileus

This condition, which characteristically affects the elderly, is due to intraluminal intestinal obstruction by a large gallstone that enters the intestinal tract subsequent to the establishment of a fistula, usually between the gallbladder and the duodenum and, less commonly, the gallbladder and the colon. Rarely gallstone ileus may occur as a complication of endoscopic sphincterotomy with stone extraction. Naturally occurring gallstone ileus occurs in 2% of patients with gallstone disease and, in some reports, accounts for up to 20% of mechanical intestinal obstruction in the elderly.

The patient, who may give a history of gallbladder disease, presents acutely with acute intestinal obstruction, which in the vast majority of cases, affects the small bowel, colonic obstruction being distinctly uncommon. Characteristically, the level of the obstruction is changing until the stone becomes firmly impacted, usually in the terminal ileum (70%) as this is the narrowest part of the intestinal tract and much less commonly in the duodenum. Colonic obstruction due to impaction in the colon is the result of a cholecystocolic fistula.

The condition should be suspected in the elderly patient with mechanical intestinal obstruction in the absence of the more common causes of this condition. It can be diagnosed pre-operatively if gas can be demonstrated in the biliary tract or the gallstone is visualized, usually in the right iliac fossa (Figure 10.60).

The treatment requires emergency surgical intervention in all patients. The operative management depends on the findings and the general condition of the patient. In the elderly and frail patient with ileal obstruction, removal of the impacted calculus through a small enterotomy is performed and the cholecystoduodenal fistula is dealt with at a subsequent operation. A one-stage enterolithotomy with cholecystectomy and closure of the duodenal fistula can be performed in patients who, despite their age, are considered fit enough for this procedure. The treatment of patients with colonic obstruction and a cholecystocolic fistula consists of removal of the calculus through a colotomy, cholecystostomy (cholecystectomy if the patient is fit) and exteriorization of the colotomy as a temporary proximal (diverting) colostomy.

Section 10.16 • Post-cholecystectomy syndromes

These refer to the persistence of symptoms referable to the biliary tract after cholecystectomy. As currently defined, the syndromes exclude those patients whose symptoms are due to organic disease outside the biliary tract. These constitute a significant percentage of patients with persistent symptoms after cholecystectomy and they are usually a reflection of failure of proper

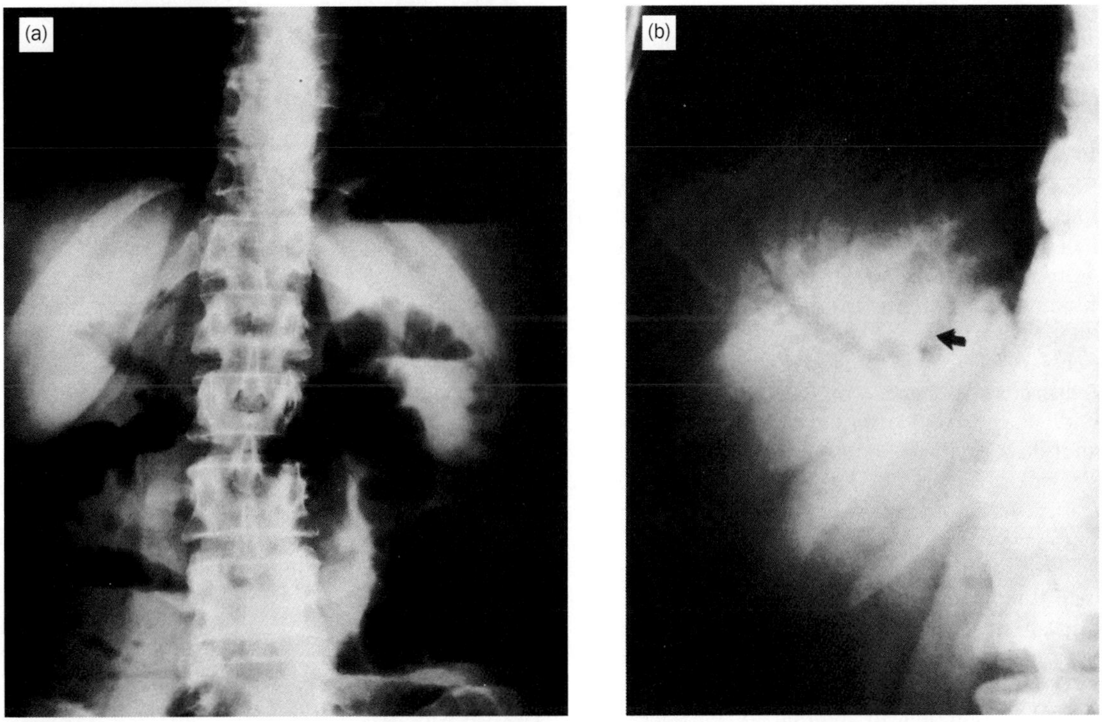

Figure 10.60 (a) Plain radiograph of the abdomen – gas outlines the common bile duct. The patient presented with cholangitis and gallstone ileus. A spontaneous cholecystoduodenal fistula was found at operation. (b) Gas outlining the right hepatic duct. The patient had an empyema of the gallbladder and a cholecystocolic fistula due to a carcinoma of the hepatic flexure.

evaluation and investigation of patients prior to the cholecystectomy.

The reported incidence of post-cholecystectomy syndromes varies widely and correlates with the duration of follow-up. There is a female preponderance, particularly in the 40–50 years age group. A careful evaluation and a full investigation of the biliary tract including an ERCP is advisable in all patients with persistence or recurrence of symptoms after cholecystectomy. The common causes of post-cholecystectomy syndromes are:

- retained or recurrent calculi
- gallbladder/cystic duct remnants
- bile duct strictures and other unrecognized iatrogenic injuries (choledochoduodenal fistula)
- papillary stenosis and biliary dyskinesia.

Persistent or recurrent symptoms after cholecystostomy are common and are one of the reasons for subsequent cholecystectomy in all patients who are considered fit for surgery. Controversy still exists regarding the role of a 'long cystic duct remnant' as a cause of persistent symptoms after cholecystectomy. There are undoubtedly patients in whom a dilated long cystic duct remnant containing stones is demonstrated on investigation and its removal together with the stones results in sustained symptomatic improvement. However, these cases are few and far between and at present there is no evidence to incriminate an otherwise normal long cystic duct remnant as one of the important causes of the post-cholecystectomy syndrome.

Papillary stenosis (also known as choledochoduodenal junctional stenosis) is nowadays regarded as a rare but definite entity, which results from fibrosis or fibro-muscular hyperplasia of the sphincter of Oddi. An associated duodenal diverticulum is common and cannulation of the papilla is difficult. In addition to pain in the upper abdomen, the patient may exhibit slight abnormalities in the liver function tests, including mild hyperbilirubinaemia and elevated alkaline phosphatase activity. The resting sphincter pressure is elevated as is the passage pressure and there is loss of the normal phasic sphincteric activity. At operation, papillary stenosis is best demonstrated radiologically by the technique of contact selective cholangiography. In addition to duct dilatation, there is a characteristic alteration in the configuration of the infundibulum (transduodenal segment) which loses its conical shape and becomes wider than the intrapancreatic segment (Figure 10.61). Biliary sludge and small ductal calculi are often present. Reflux into a dilated pancreatic duct is also observed in some cases.

The treatment of papillary stenosis is equally controversial. Endoscopic sphincterotomy or surgical transduodenal sphicteroplasty is recommended by the majority although there has not been an adequate long-term assessment of these procedures for this rare and elusive condition. In addition to the sphincteroplasty, Moody advocates the excision of the septum between the pancreatic duct and the bile duct in patients with chronic pain which he maintains is of

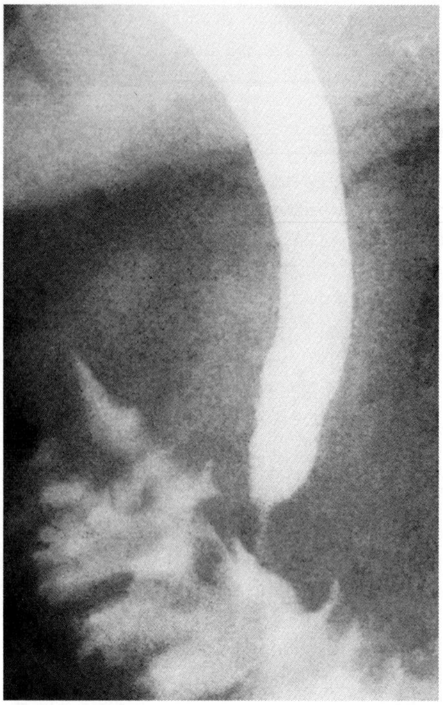

Figure 10.61 Operative contact selective cholangiogram demonstrating papillary stenosis. There is minimal dilatation of the bile duct and the infundibulum becomes globular. Biliary sludge/small ductal calculi are often present.

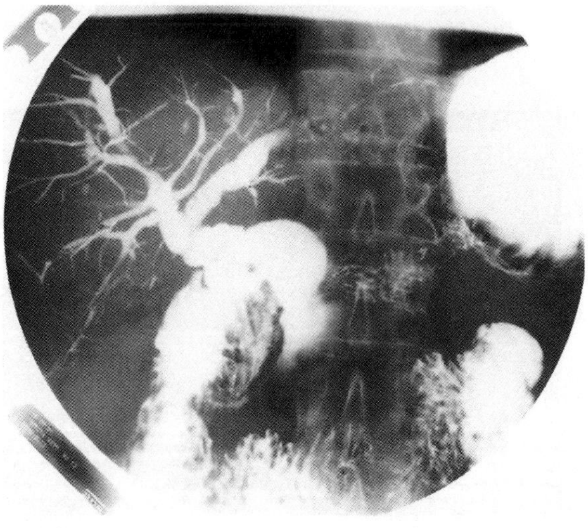

Figure 10.62 Barium meal contrast study after transection choledochoduodenostomy performed for papillary stenosis 3 years previously.

pancreatic origin. An alternative surgical treatment for papillary stenosis favoured by the author is transection choledochoduodenostomy with re-implantation of the mobilized duct into the junction of the first with the second part of the duodenum (Figure 10.62).

The term biliary dyskinesia is used to denote those patients who have persistent pain after cholecystectomy and no other abnormality on physical examination and routine testing but who exhibit the following abnormalities during ERCP manometry:

- elevated resting pressure
- tachyarrhythmia (increased phasic activity of the sphincter)
- retrograde contractions of the sphincter
- paradoxical response to cholecystokinin.

Treatment with endoscopic sphincterotomy has been advocated for these patients but the efficacy of this in the long-term relief of symptoms remains to be ascertained.

Section 10.17 • Benign bile duct strictures

The causes of benign bile duct strictures are shown in Table 10.9.

In the clinical context, benign strictures of the extrahepatic bile ducts do not exhibit a benign course since they are always attended by significant symptoms and serious complications that are life-threatening both in the short and the long term and carry a definite mortality. Thus they pose serious health and economic problems and may expose the surgeon to expensive medico-legal litigation. In addition, they increase substantially the economical burden to the patient, hospital and the community, and some have needed hepatic transplantation for survival. The costs of repair of cholecystectomy-related bile duct injuries is high, varying from 4.5 to 26 times the cost of the uncomplicated procedure. In one reported series, patients with LC-related bile duct injuries were billed a mean of $51 411 for the remedial surgery and incurred an average of 32 days of inpatient hospital stay. Both the costs of treatment and the outcome (mortality) of bile duct injury are related to early recognition. Thus in one large reported series, bile duct injuries recognized immediately at the time of the initial surgery incurred a significantly lower cost and reduced hospital stay than those in whom recognition was delayed. As the surgical management of these injuries requires special multidisciplinary expertise, referral to and treatment in specialized centres offers the best chance of reversal from a potentially fatal condition to long-term restoration of good health with freedom from symptoms and return to normal liver function.

A long stricture of the lower end of the common bile duct, which characteristically forms an angle with the proximal dilated duct, is encountered in 15–20% of patients with chronic pancreatitis (Figure 10.63a). However, the differentiation between this disease and pancreatic carcinoma is often difficult in these patients. Bile duct strictures are also a feature of recurrent pyogenic cholangitis and sclerosing cholangitis. A similar long but less angulated stricture of the distal common bile duct may be caused by trauma inflicted with metal bougies during open common bile duct exploration (Figure 10.63b).

Table 10.9 Causes of benign bile duct strictures

- Operative bile duct injury (iatrogenic)
- Penetrating and non-penetrating abdominal injuries
- Chronic duodenal ulcer
- Chronic pancreatitis
- Recurrent pyogenic cholangitis and parasitic infestations
- Sclerosing cholangitis

Incidence of bile duct injury

In the West, the vast majority of bile duct strictures are the result of preventable injuries to the extrahepatic biliary tract, usually during the operation of cholecystectomy and, less frequently, gastrectomy. Blunt and penetrating trauma accounts only for a small minority [see Trauma Module, Vol. II]. It is difficult to estimate the real incidence of bile duct injury after both open and laparoscopic cholecystectomy from published retrospective series. Accurate incidence can only be gathered from data of regional or national prospective audits that ensure complete data collection. Surveys from different countries reviewed by Strasberg *et al.* in 1995 showed an incidence of iatrogenic bile duct injury of 0.125% and 0.55% during open and laparoscopic cholecystectomy respectively. Based on this review, the incidence of bile duct injuries during sustained LC is 2–4.5 times higher than in the open technique. There is some evidence that the incidence decreases with increasing surgeons' experience. This is suggested by the data of a national prospective audit in Switzerland where the incidence of bile duct injury following LC fell from 0.6% to 0.3%. More recent reported series seem to confirm this positive trend and indicate that the incidence of biliary injury during open and laparoscopic cholecystectomy may be converging. The reason for this is probably two-fold: increased experience with the laparoscopic technique and allocation of the more difficult cases to the open technique. In a recent population-based study of iatrogenic injury associated with cholecystectomy in Western Australia the risk of iatrogenic injury during LC was found to be 1.79 times that of open cholecystectomy.

Classification of bile duct injuries

The most commonly used classification of bile duct injuries is that reported by Corlette and Bismuth in 1981 based on an analysis of 643 cases of post-operative biliary strictures. The basis of this classification is the length of the proximal biliary stump, since this is the most important factor in determining the nature of the biliary repair.

- *Type 1* – low common hepatic stricture, length of common hepatic duct stump >2.0 cm (Figure 10.64)
- *Type 2* – middle stricture, length of hepatic duct stump <2.0 cm.
- *Type 3* – high (hilar) stricture – no serviceable common hepatic duct but the confluence of the right and left hepatic ducts is preserved (Figure 10.65).
- *Type 4* – high stricture where the confluence is involved and there is no communication between right and left hepatic ducts. The thickness of the fibrosis separating the two branches depends on the extent of the injury, i.e. thin or thick septum (1–2 cm) (Figure 10.66).
- *Type 5* – combined common hepatic and aberrant right hepatic duct injury separating both from the distal biliary tract.

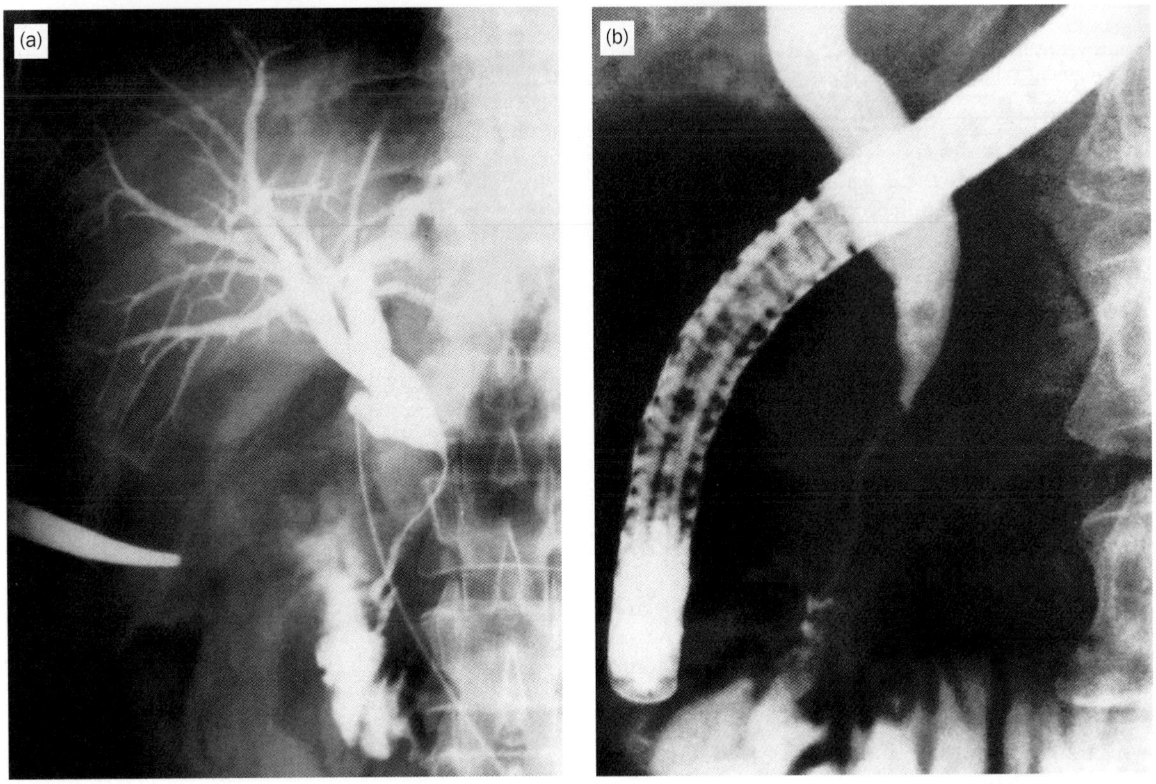

Figure 10.63 (a) Long stricture of the distal bile duct in a patient with chronic alcoholic pancreatitis of 12 years' duration. There is an angle between the stricture and the proximal dilated duct. The stenosis is due to the pancreatic fibrosis which constricts the transpancreatic segment of the common bile duct. (b) Stricture of the lower end of the common bile duct following blind stone fragmentation of an impacted stone and forcible passage of metal bougies.

The Corlette–Bismuth classification has proved useful because it provides essential information on the nature, risks and prognosis after the repair. There is an established correlation between the types of injury and the morbidity, mortality, success and recurrence after repair. However, the Corlette–Bismuth classification does not stipulate the length of the injury. This information is becoming increasingly important as nowadays, short strictures can be managed by non-operative treatment, such as percutaneous or endoscopic dilatation or stenting. A subclassification that indicates the extent of the lesion is desirable, i.e. discontinuity following excision of bile duct, short or long segment stenosis.

The more recent Strasberg classification considers bile injuries from a clinical perspective and includes biliary complications excluded in the Corlette–Bismuth types, e.g. bile leaks and bilomas, and isolated occlusion of the right hepatic duct. In essence it distinguishes two main categories:

- injuries that separate hepatic parenchyma from the biliary tract and
- those where the continuity is maintained.

The classification also groups together injuries that have similar presentation and management, as distinct from those that require different management despite having similar presentations.

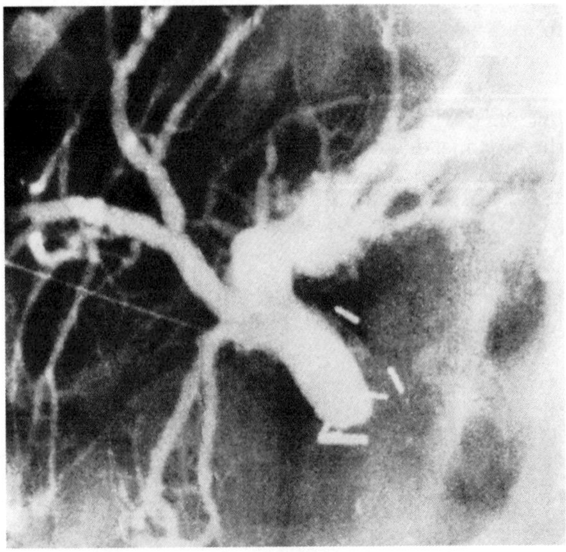

Figure 10.64 Type 1 Corlette–Bismuth injury.

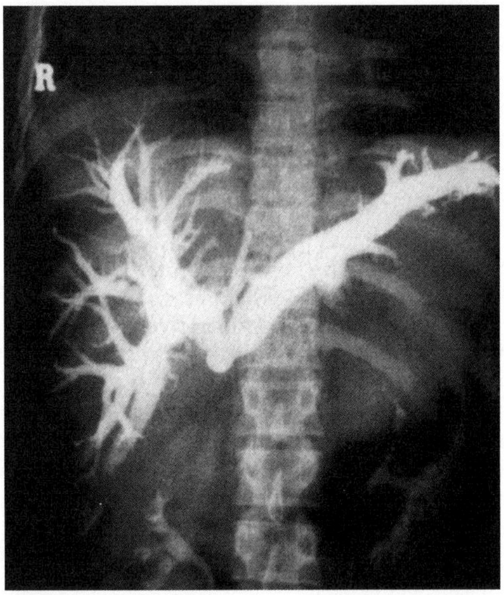

Figure 10.65 Obliteration of the hepatic duct with an intact confluence of the right and left hepatic ducts – type 3 stricture.

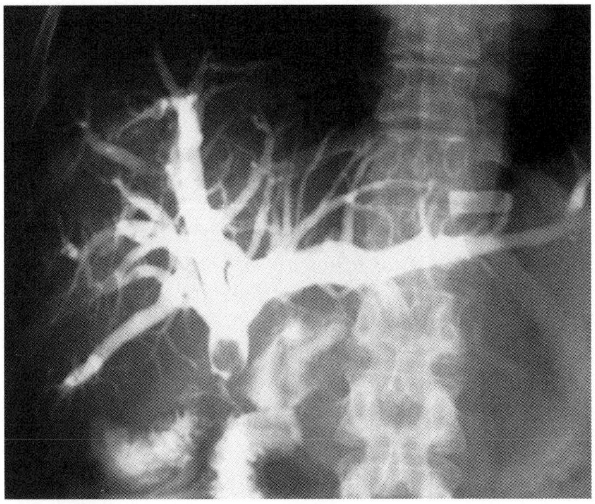

Figure 10.66 High stricture with destruction of hilar confluence. A primary ductal stone straddles the two ducts – type 4 stricture.

- *Type A* is a bile leak from a minor duct that is still in continuity with the common bile duct. These leaks occur either from the cystic duct stump or from the liver bed. These are not really bile duct injuries. Their importance lies in early recognition and appropriate management. They do not cause strictures or require tertiary referral.
- *Type B* is occlusion of part of the biliary tree – usually occlusion of an aberrant right hepatic duct mistaken for the cystic duct. In 2% of patients the cystic duct enters the right hepatic duct instead of the common hepatic duct. These injuries are often asymptomatic, or may present later with pain or cholangitis. The related hepatic segments drained by the occluded duct atrophy with variable hypertrophy of the rest of the hepatic parenchyma (disconnecting injury).
- *Type C* injury is bile leak from duct not in communication with the distal common bile duct. It is usually the result of transection of an aberrant right hepatic duct with drainage of bile into the peritoneal cavity. This lesion usually presents in the early post-operative period (disconnecting injury).
- *Type D* is lateral injury to extrahepatic bile ducts. The hepatic parenchyma remains in communication with the distal end of the biliary tree and duodenum. Unlike type A, however, the consequences of type D injuries are potentially more serious. They require laparotomy for repair, and may result in stenosis. Type D injuries may involve the common bile, common hepatic, right and left hepatic ducts.
- *Type E* is circumferential injury of major extrahepatic bile ducts with separation of liver parenchyma from the lower ducts and duodenum (major disconnection injury).

The Strasberg classification is more suited to a multidisciplinary approach to the management of bile duct injury and for this reason is gaining wider acceptance.

Pathology of bile duct injuries

There is little doubt that the majority of bile duct injuries sustained during operation result from failure of appreciation of the precise anatomy of the area. The situations which predispose to or result in damage to the bile ducts at operation are varied and usually but not always related to the degree of technical difficulty of the operation. Moossa *et al.* identified four mechanisms of bile duct injuries in open cholecystectomy, and later added a fifth one for LC:

- ligating or transecting the wrong duct
- occluding the lumen of the common bile duct during 'flush ligation' of the cystic duct
- compromise of the blood supply of the duct by excessive dissection
- trauma to the lumen of the common bile duct during exploration by manipulation or forceful 'dilatation'
- injury due to inappropriate application of energy source.

Although these are important, a more practical consideration of the mechanisms involved in bile duct injuries during LC identifies two basic error groups:

- misinterpretation of the anatomy and
- technical errors.

Misinterpretation of the anatomy

All the available evidence indicates this as the dominant factor in the aetiology and it accounts for 70% of biliary duct injuries sustained during LC. This primary error is related to the fact that during LC the surgeon is operating on images of the operative field rather than reality. Visual psychological studies have shown that humans scan pictures by slow pursuit eye movements and on the basis of the visual information relayed on the retina by this scanning process, the brain makes an interpretation. If the surgeon makes a snap interpretation, success or disaster depends on whether this is right or wrong. The vast majority of bile duct injuries during laparoscopic cholecystectomy would be avoided if the surgeon questioned the initial identification of key structures to the point of absolute certainty. In one report based on review of operative videotapes of patients who sustained a duct injury, various misinterpretations were identified.

Technical errors

The most important technical error is hilar bleeding. This may result from failure to secure the cystic artery or damage to the right hepatic artery that is particularly at risk when it is looped towards the gallbladder neck. As frantic attempts are made to control bleeding, adjacent structures may be injured by electrocautery or clips. These injuries can be prevented if the surgeon has a strategic plan for this eventuality. The first step is to apply pressure on the bleeding area using adjacent tissues that can be easily grasped and laid over the bleeding area. Two instruments are then used: an atraumatic grasper and suction irrigation. When these are in the operative field, the compression is relaxed and the bleeding point identified by suction and grasped. If control is not achieved within a few minutes, conversion with application of the Pringle's manoeuvre is mandatory.

Other technical errors include excessive tenting of the cystic duct–common bile duct junction by too much traction on the gallbladder such that a clip used to secure the cystic duct grips the lateral wall of the bile duct resulting in a lateral injury/partial occlusion. Bile leakage and bilomas in the absence of significant bile duct injuries are due to slippage of a clip on the cystic duct or too deep a plane of dissection on the liver bed during the detachment of the gallbladder.

Risk factors

These relate to surgeon, patient and local pathology.

Training and experience – the learning curve

Studies in the pre- and post-laparoscopic era found this to be a more important risk factor than local operative factors such as inflammation or bleeding. The fact that iatrogenic injuries can still be inflicted by experienced surgeons if they ignore basic surgical principles has been documented by reports in both open and laparoscopic cholecystectomy. In laparoscopic surgery experience is important not only in respect of technical competence but also in terms of correct visual perception and interpretation of the image displayed on the monitor. The *learning curve* appears to affect the risk of bile duct injury. For open cholecystectomy a large Swedish survey showed that most biliary injuries were made between the 25–100th operation per surgeon. The Southern Surgeons Club reported an initial high rate of bile duct injury (2.2%) during the first 13 laparoscopic cholecystectomies per surgeon. This rate fell to 0.1% for subsequent operations. Although experience is important in the reduction of bile duct injuries, it is clear that in the laparoscopic era there is no norm and the learning curve is surgeon related. Thus bile duct injuries sustained during LC occur over a larger spectrum of experience by individual surgeons.

Improper use of energized dissection systems

With the deployment of energized systems, the important fact is that any thermal source (whether high-frequency-electrocoagulation, laser or ultrasonic dissection) can cause damage to the portal structures if used incorrectly. The damage may not be apparent during the operation but can be severe and cause intractable strictures later. The perceived notion that ultrasonic dissection does not cause collateral proximity damage is not supported by experimental studies.

Patients' factors

The problem of morbid obesity in the laparoscopic era varies considerably from patient to patient. Some present fewer problems than with open surgery, whereas others are less easy because of their internal fat deposition that obscures the anatomy of Calot's triangle. Fatty livers may be difficult to elevate and are easily lacerated. Although increased age and male gender are associated with increased post-operative mortality after cholecystectomy, they are not significant risk factors for major bile duct injuries.

Anomalous and morbid anatomy

This includes 'dangerous anatomy' and 'dangerous pathological conditions' predisposing to biliary injury. These are present in 15–35% of injuries.

Dangerous anatomy embraces aberrant (anomalous) anatomy, pathological conditions that obscure the view of vital structures such as adhesions, inflammatory phlegmon and excessive fat in the porta hepatis. Anomalies of the biliary tree are present in 10–15% of patients and are not usually identified pre-operatively. The anomaly most likely to be involved in ductal injury is when an aberrant right hepatic duct inserts low into the common hepatic or bile duct, and is mistaken for the cystic duct. Another important anomaly is a short cystic duct. Variations in vascular supply also present dangerous situations, not only from the risk of compromise of the hepatic arterial supply (usually right hepatic) but also by increasing the likelihood of haemorrhage during the course of the operation. Adhesions from previous abdominal operations and pathological conditions such as inflammation can distort the anatomy and predispose to injury.

Dangerous biliary pathology includes chronic inflammation with dense scarring (the Mirizzi syndrome and the scleroatrophic gallbladder), fibrosis in the triangle of Calot and acute cholecystitis. A significant iatrogenic injury rate has been documented in patients undergoing LC for acute cholecystitis. Oozing of blood during the procedure with impaired visualization and anatomical distortion associated with the acute inflammation contribute to this increased risk. Nonetheless, the benefit of LC versus open cholecystectomy for acute cholecystitis has been confirmed by a prospective randomized clinical trial. This study showed a significant reduction in the post-operative morbidity in the LC arm (only 3% minor complications versus 23% major complications and 19% minor complications in the open cholecystectomy group). In adopting LC as the routine option, it must be stressed that the need for conversion is encountered in 20–25% of cases and early decision should be made to convert electively in the presence of obscured anatomy. Thus the valid approach to LC for acute cholecystitis is a flexible one. The procedure starts with an exploratory laparoscopy to assess the technical difficulty of the operation with particular reference to the structures in the triangle of Calot. A large distended gallbladder should be aspirated and lifted by a retractor rather than grasped. Large stones impacted in Hartmann's pouch that cannot be dislodged may prove problematic. The practical axiom is a simple one, i.e. if adequate exposure for a safe dissection cannot be obtained, or the gallbladder is gangrenous or perforated, the case should be converted. In some cases, a fundus first dissection of the gallbladder may be required. Dangerous biliary pathology also includes polycystic disease of the liver and portal hypertension caused by cirrhosis or schistosomiasis.

Prevention of bile duct injuries

Prevention of iatrogenic injuries to the bile ducts during laparoscopic cholecystectomy relies on (i) thorough understanding of the anatomy, risk factors and the mechanisms of injury described, (ii) image interpretative skills, (iii) meticulous technique and (iv) timely decision for elective conversion in the presence of difficult anatomy. There are no reliable pre-operative indicators of the risks of biliary and vascular injuries during LC. Prevention of these complications, therefore, depends on the adoption of correct surgical technique and a low threshold for conversion. Since the major direct causes of biliary injury are misidentification of anatomy and technical errors, safety is entirely dependent on complete visualization, display and identification of the structures in the triangle of Calot. In this respect, the 30° laparoscope provides a better view of the anatomy, especially the common bile duct.

The vast majority of surgeons use clips to secure the medial end of the cystic duct, and only a minority ligate this duct. Bile leakage without bile duct damage is usually due to slippage of the clip. There are well-documented reports of internalization of these cystic duct clips into the bile duct where the clip acts as a nidus for stone formation several months later. These patients usually present with jaundice and cholangitis suggestive of bile duct stricture. The diagnosis becomes apparent on ERCP. These problems can be prevented by use of absorbable clips or ligation of the medial end of the cystic duct.

During the detachment of the gallbladder from its liver bed the dissection should be kept close to the gallbladder and above the fascial covering of the gallbladder bed. This avoids both bleeding from the hepatic parenchyma and injury to segmental ducts in segments IV/V of the liver. This is a much commoner cause of post-operative bile leakage than damage to a duct of Lushka, which is a very rare anomaly.

Differences between open and laparoscopic bile duct injuries

There are some important differences between the pathology of bile duct injuries sustained during open versus laparoscopic cholecystectomy. The laparoscopic injuries tend to be more extensive involving excision of a segment of the common bile duct, and extend to higher levels often involving proximal hepatic ducts (Figure 10.67). The majority (60–75%) are not immediately recognized during surgery. The average age of patients with laparoscopic bile duct injury is 43 years, compared to 56 years in open cholecystectomy. Instances of combined bile duct and vascular injuries have been reported after LC and they carry a poor prognosis. In one reported series four patients had simultaneous occlusion or extirpation of the right hepatic or common hepatic artery. In the immediate post-operative period, three of four patients with combined injuries had hepatic necrosis and/or abscesses with two patients requiring percutaneous or operative drainage. None of the remedial biliary anastomoses failed in the patients with isolated bile duct injuries. By contrast two patients with combined injuries have had recurrent stenosis following reconstruction. Thus patients with major bile duct injuries should be evaluated for concomitant hepatic arterial injury as management and outcome are influenced by the absence of arterial blood flow to the injured bile ducts and to the liver.

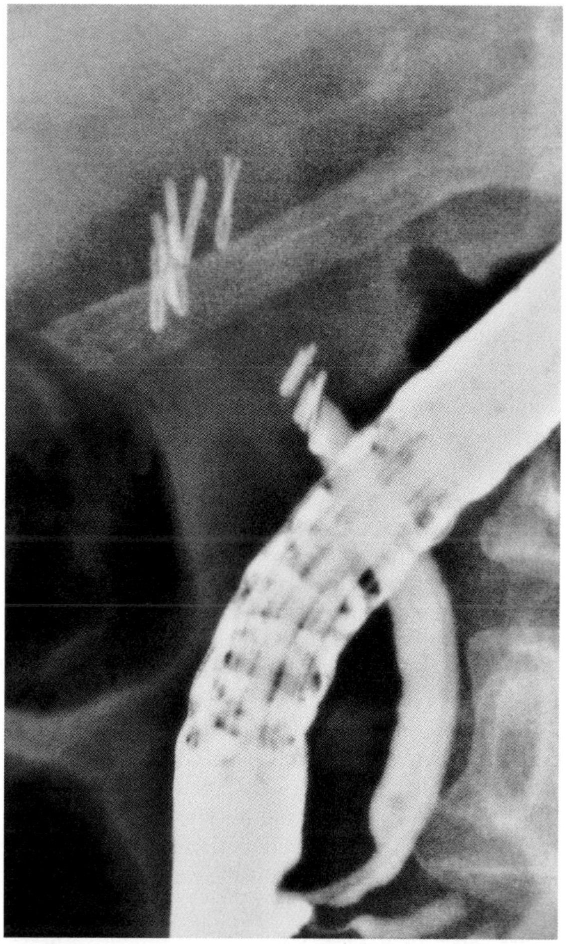

Figure 10.67 Bile duct injury after laparoscopic cholecystectomy: resection of the common hepatic duct. Note excessive shrapnel!

Clinical features

Only one-third of bile duct injuries sustained during LC are detected at the primary operation with the majority being discovered at an average of 10 days post-operatively. If the lesion is not recognized at operation, the bile duct injury usually declares itself post-operatively by the development of pain, fever and external biliary fistula if a drain had been placed at operation. Evidence of peritoneal irritation with guarding and rebound is present due to leakage of bile in the peritoneal cavity, and subphrenic/subhepatic collections are detected on ultrasound. Overt signs of sepsis including positive blood cultures rapidly supervene and the patient develops jaundice but this may not be severe or progressive in the presence of an external biliary fistula. Apart from liver function tests and culture of the discharge and blood, visualization of the biliary tract by an ERCP to ascertain the presence of bile duct damage and its severity is mandatory and should be performed without any delay. MRCP is inferior to ERCP in this situation as despite documenting the damage and collection of bile, it does not determine whether the leak is active. If the ERCP establishes the diagnosis, the patient should be referred to a tertiary hepatobiliary centre.

Some patients are actually discharged from hospital after LC and then admitted as an emergency with established sepsis and peritonitis. If a laparotomy is needed, the general surgeon should simply insert a self-retaining catheter into the proximal biliary tree through the defect in the bile duct, place a subhepatic drainage, evacuate any peritoneal bile collections and wash the peritoneal cavity. *Attempts at repair should be resisted at this stage.* As soon as the patient has recovered from the laparotomy, urgent referral to a tertiary unit is the appropriate course of action.

Treatment

Early recognition

Early recognition of the injury can be achieved by investigating the source of any biliary leak observed during the operation and routine IOFC. Only a few some surgeons use IOFC routinely during LC, some only selectively and the majority not at all. Proponents of the routine use argue that IOFC delineates the biliary anatomy and provides a 'road map' of the entire biliary tree. Failure to outline the entire extra and intrahepatic biliary tract with the patient in the Trendlenberg position is an indication for conversion. Although there are no firm data to confirm that IOFC reduces the bile duct injury rate, there is evidence that it reduces injury severity, and leads to detection at the time of surgery. Post-operative surveillance is crucial. Although bile duct injuries usually present post-operatively with a bile leak with or without jaundice and sepsis, some have only vague symptoms initially, e.g. persistent abdominal pain, anorexia, unwillingness to leave the bed. Abdominal pain persisting more than 12 hours after LC always requires investigation.

Definitive treatment

This depends on whether the injury is recognized at operation or subsequently because the patient either develops serious complications post-operatively or presents after discharge from hospital with recurrent episodes of pain, fever and jaundice.

Injuries recognized at operation

The treatment depends on the site and extent of the damage. For high complete transections, a Roux-en-Y hepaticojejunostomy is considered preferable to a difficult direct suture repair as this usually becomes strictured in time. For lower complete injuries with a serviceable proximal duct stump, primary suture repair with fine interrupted absorbable sutures over a T-tube is the treatment of choice (Figure 10.68). The long limb of the T-tube must not be exteriorized through the repair site as this enhances the risks of stricture formation. Partial (lateral) injuries are often treated by the insertion of a T-tube and a Roux-en-Y serosal patch. The long limb of the T-tube is exteriorized through the mobilized jejunum (Figure 10.69). Other techniques include repair with a vein patch over a T-tube (Figure 10.70).

There is an undoubted high incidence of stricture formation following primary repair of bile duct injuries (up to 60%). All these patients, therefore, require long-term follow-up with radiological assessment if they develop symptoms or abnormalities of the liver function tests.

Injuries recognized in the post-operative period

The initial management is supportive. Fluid and electrolyte disorders, if present, are corrected and the patient is put on systemic antibiotics. Surgical intervention is required for drainage of collections/abscesses and development of peritonitis. Otherwise, the patient is initially managed conservatively. An ostomy bag is used to collect the bile leakage from the fistula which may close. Persistence of the external biliary fistula does not constitute a serious problem since skin excoriation does not occur and the daily losses are sel-

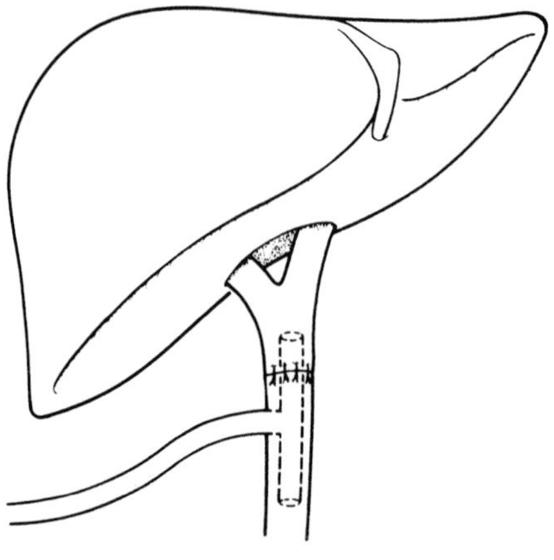

Figure 10.68 Primary repair of a complete injury recognized at operation. The long limb of the T-tube is exteriorized below the suture repair. The risk of stenosis is considerably enhanced if the long limb of the T-tube is brought out at the site of repair.

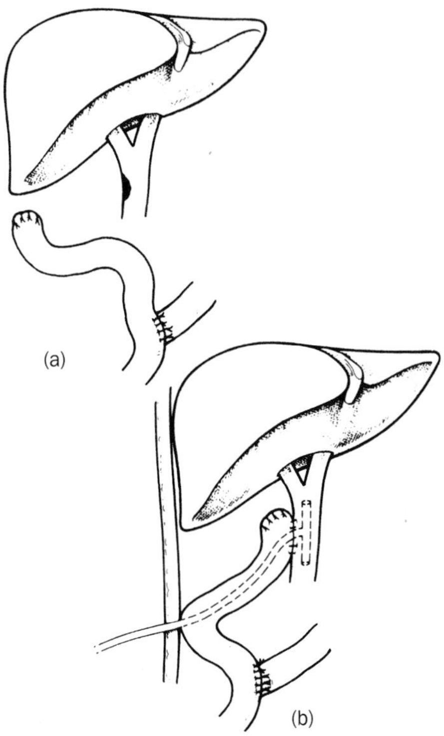

Figure 10.69 Serosal patch Roux-en-Y technique with T-tube intubation for lateral injuries discovered at operation. (a) Construction of a Roux-en-Y loop. (b) The Roux loop is sutured over the defect after the insertion of a T-tube, the long limb of which is brought out through the jejunal loop.

dom severe enough to cause significant fluid and electrolyte depletion. The bile collected in the bag is returned to the gastrointestinal tract via a naso-enteral tube which is also used for feeding. Surgical intervention to deal with the bile duct injury at this stage is ill-advised as the repair is difficult due to the inflammatory oedema and because the proximal ductal system is not yet dilated. Repair is, therefore, best postponed for several weeks, by which time the intra-abdominal sepsis has subsided, the stricture has matured and the proximal ducts have dilated, thus facilitating the procedure.

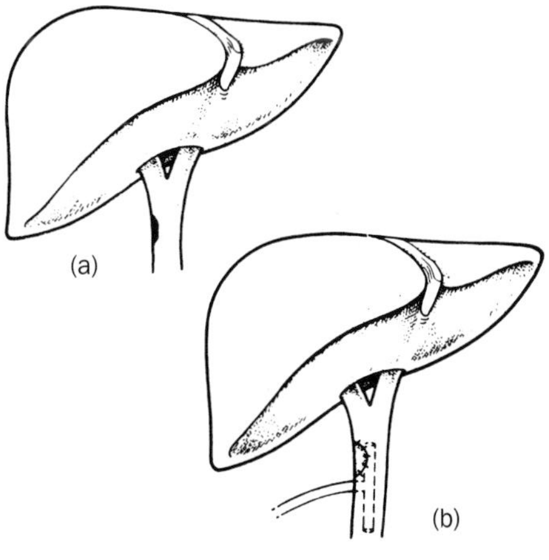

Figure 10.70 Repair of lateral injury recognized at operation by a vein patch. The T-tube is inserted via a small choledochotomy lower down.

The definitive treatment of bile duct strictures is best carried out in specialized centres where the overall results, in terms of long-term freedom from jaundice and cholangitis and maintenance of good to normal liver function, are excellent (85–90%) and the operative mortality is low (1–5%). The exact treatment depends on the pathological anatomy of the stricture.

For type 1 injuries, the choice is between Roux-en-Y jejunostomy and choledochoduodenostomy (of the transection type). For common hepatic duct strictures with a serviceable extrahepatic duct stump (type 2), a Roux-en-Y hepaticojejunostomy is indicated (Figure 10.71). The establishment of a mucosa-to-mucosa anastomosis using absorbable fine sutures between the bile duct remnant and the jejunal mucosa is the single most important factor in the prevention of recurrent stricture formation. If good mucosal coaptation is achieved, there is no indication for stenting of the anastomosis and indeed this is undesirable under these circumstances. Some prefer to use an isolated jejunal isoperistaltic segment interposed between the stump of the common hepatic duct and the duodenum (Figure 10.72) instead of the Roux-en-Y loop.

For high strictures with no residual stump but with an intact hilar confluence (type 4), dissection of the liver plate (Glissonian sheath) to enter the hilum of the liver enables downward displacement of the hilar biliary confluence for a good mucosa to mucosa anastomosis between the bifurcation and the Roux-en-Y jejunal loop (Figure 10.73). The inside spur of the bifurcation is divided transversely and the edges are

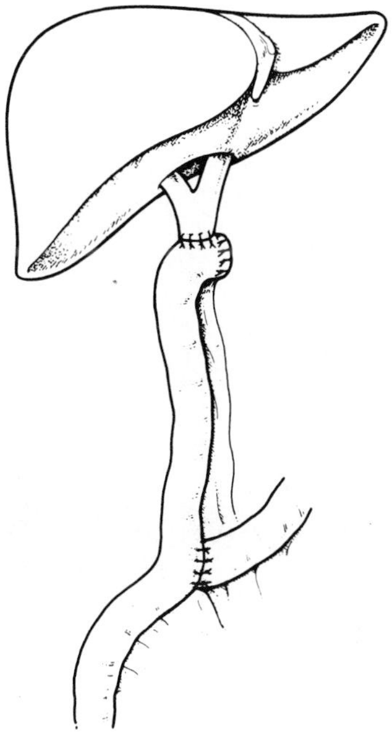

Figure 10.71 Roux-en-Y hepaticojejunostomy for a type 1 bile duct injury.

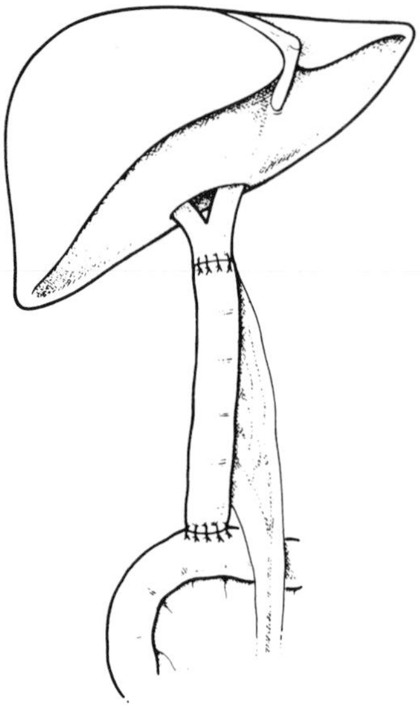

Figure 10.72 Isoperistaltic jejunal loop between the stump of the common hepatic duct and the duodenum.

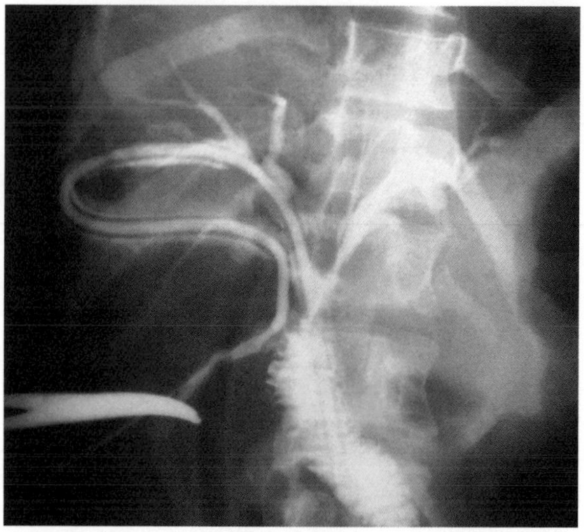

Figure 10.74 Post-operative cholangiogram through a transhepatic stent after Roux-en-Y hepaticojejunostomy for type 3 injury.

then sutured vertically to displace the junction of the two ducts proximal to the anastomosis. This technique does not require any splinting or resection of the liver parenchyma (Figure 10.74).

Destruction of the hilar confluence (type 5) constitutes the most difficult stricture to deal with and usually requires resection of the quadrate lobe to access the right and left hepatic ducts within the liver substance. Each duct is then anastomosed separately to the jejunal loop (Figure 10.75). In these high strictures, a silicone stent is placed across each anastomosis. These stents may be exteriorized transhepatically (Figure 10.76a) or preferably through the jejunal loop (Figure 10.76b) that is sutured to the abdominal wall at the exit site of the tube. The site of fixation of the jejunum is marked with metal clips. This allows easy identification of this access jejunostomy, thereby permitting the introduction of fine flexible endoscopes and balloon catheters for percutaneous dilatation in the event of re-stricturing after surgical repair. In the worst case scenario when this technique is not technically possible because of dense fibrosis, the round ligament approach with anastomosis to the segment III duct (Figure 10.2) is

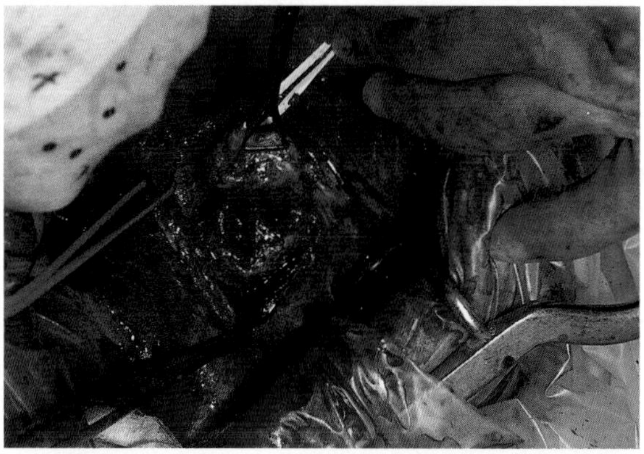

Figure 10.73 Operative photograph: repair of high stricture with no residual stump but with an intact hilar confluence (type 3). The liver plate (Glissonian sheath) has been divided anteriorly and posteriorly to enable entry into the hilum of the liver and downward displacement of the hilar biliary confluence for a good mucosa to mucosa anastomosis between the bifurcation and the Roux-en-Y jejunal loop.

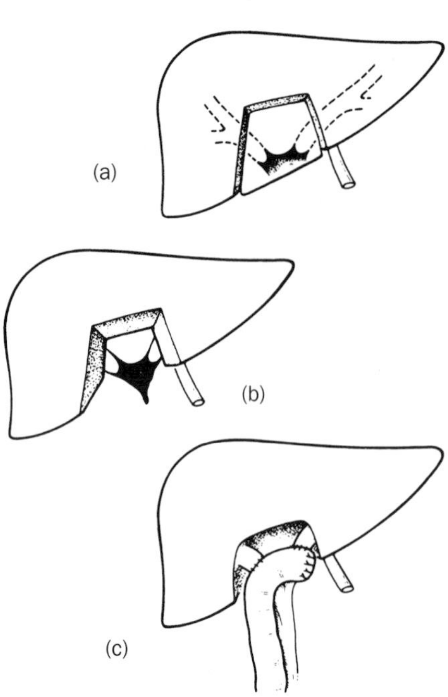

Figure 10.75 Hepaticojejunostomy for lesions with obliteration of the hilar confluence of the right and left hepatic ducts (type 4 injury): (a) the quadrate lobe (segment IV) anterior to the hilus is excised; (b) exposure of the obliterated confluence and identification of the right and left hepatic ducts; (c) the right and left hepatic ducts are anastomosed separately to the Roux-en-Y loop.

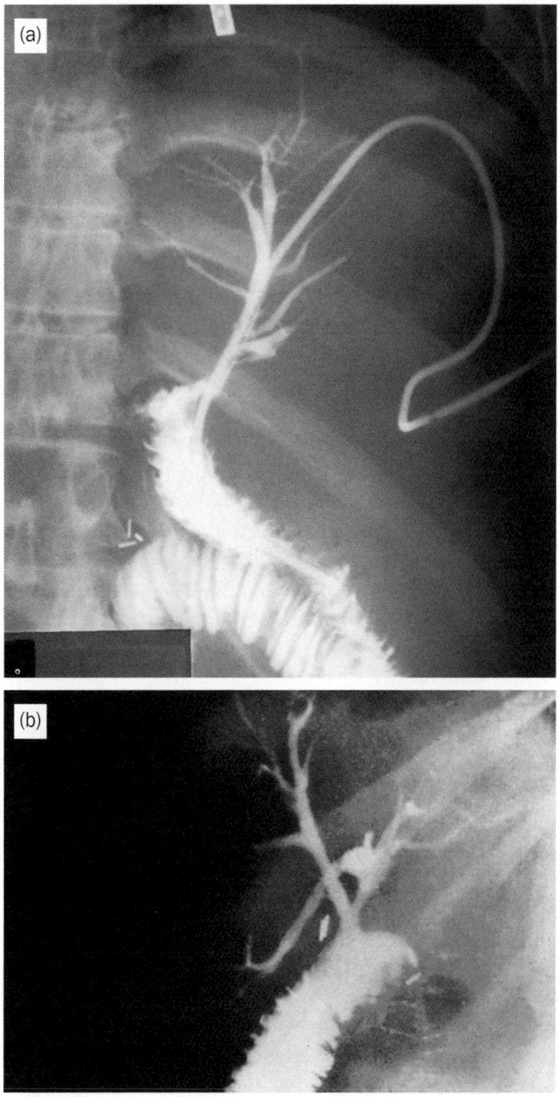

Figure 10.76 Post-operative cholangiograms after repair of type 4 injuries: (a) intrahepatic bilio-jejunal anastomosis has been stented transhepatically; (b) anastomosis has been stented through the jejunal loop.

used. This functions well provided there is a communication between the right and the left ductal systems.

Endoscopic treatment of bile leaks, clipped ducts and benign strictures

Bile leaks

Bile leakage from slippage of the cystic duct ligature or clips (after laparoscopic or open cholecystectomy) is best treated by endoscopic means. Three methods are available:

- insertion of a stent which traverses the papilla and the origin of the cystic duct
- sphincterotomy to reduce the outflow resistance
- nasobiliary drainage with low negative pressure suction.

All appear to be equally effective. Endoscopic cannulation of the common duct has been used to dislodge clips partially occluding the common bile duct after laparoscopic cholecystectomy. If successful, this is followed by stent insertion. It is not known at present how many of these patients will go on to develop bile duct strictures.

Bile duct strictures

Two techniques have been developed for the non-operative treatment of bile duct injuries:

- endoscopic balloon dilatation followed by stenting for 9–12 months
- percutaneous transhepatic biliary drainage (PTBD) using the Yamakawa prosthesis.

The ERCP-endoscopic technique is used whenever possible. A guidewire is passed through the stricture which is balloon dilated until the waist disappears, after which a plastic stent (10–11.5 Fr) is inserted. The stent is replaced every 3 months. Although metal stents have been used in the past, these have been abandoned because of two deaths associated with uncontrolled biliary sepsis. The reported long-term success of endoscopic stenting (stricture resolution) is 43% with a morbidity of 14% and mortality of 5%.

The PTBD is used when the ERCP-endoscopic technique is not possible. A special Yamakawa prosthesis is used. A peripheral bile duct is needled percutaneously under radiological control and a guidewire passed through the stricture into the duodenum (or jejunum following hepatojejunostomy). Initially a 10 Fr percutaneous drain is inserted over the guide wire. The drain is removed and the track dilated to 16 Fr some 7–10 days later when the Yamakawa prosthesis is inserted. The prosthesis is replaced every 3 months or sooner if it blocks and the treatment continued for 12 months. The original Yamakawa prosthesis was manufactured from polyvinyl chloride. This material becomes brittle and breaks in bile. The new version made from Tecothane does not have this problem. PTBD is more effective than the endoscopic technique is achieving stricture resolution but carries a higher morbidity (26%).

Obviously the results of non-operative treatment of bile duct strictures have steadily improved and there is now sufficient follow-up evidence to document stricture resolution by these methods. The treatment is however protracted and accompanied by a significant morbidity and a mortality of around 2–5%, i.e. similar to that of expert remedial surgery. The indications for non-operative treatment have not been clearly defined but recourse to endoscopic management seems sensible for:

- partial injuries
- poor-risk patients
- patients with portal hypertension
- failed surgical correction.

Late bile duct injury

Rarely, there is no record of any untoward mishap during the operation and the patient has a smooth

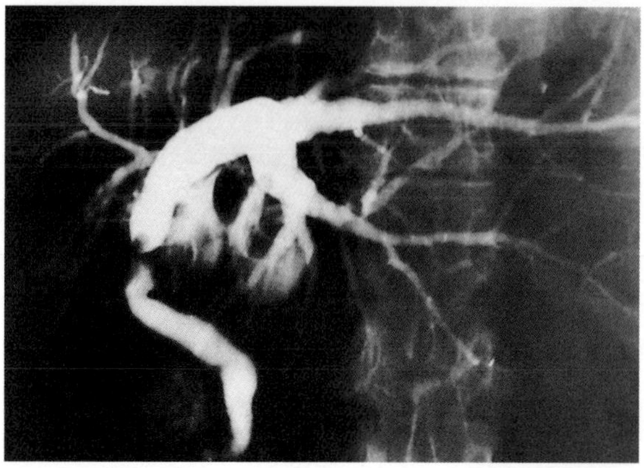

Figure 10.77 Localized stricture of the lower hepatic duct with ductal stones 10 years after cholecystectomy and exploration of the common bile duct. The patient had been completely symptom free until then and presented acutely with cholangitis. Some have ascribed these localized late strictures to impairment of the vascular supply.

postoperative period and is discharged from hospital without symptoms or complications. Attacks of pain in the right hypochondrium with episodes of jaundice and cholangitis develop several months to years later. The majority of these cases are the result of unrecognized partial injuries sustained during the cholecystectomy. A vascular element due to damage to the ascending arteries of the bile duct has been postulated by some in the pathogenesis of some of the strictures. This is more likely to be the case in patients in whom a supraduodenal common bile duct exploration has been performed with T-tube drainage in addition to the cholecystectomy (Figure 10.77). Another cause of jaundice and cholangitis several months after cholecystectomy is internalization of metal clips used to secure the medial end of the cystic duct into the common bile duct. The clip acts as a nidus for the deposition of calcium bilirubinate. The biliary tract is infected in these patients. Not all 'strictures' of the bile duct presenting several years after a laparoscopic cholecystectomy are the result of iatrogenic damage. The cholangiogram shown in Figure 10.78 of a patient who had undergone LC at Ninewells hospital 5 years previously was misdiagnosed as a late stricture but turned out to be a cholangiocarcinoma at operation.

Section 10.18 • Tumours of the biliary tract

Tumours of the gallbladder

These consist of benign lesions and carcinoma of the gallbladder.

Benign tumours

These include adenomas and papillomas. Most are discovered in clinical practice following pathological examination of the excised gallbladder although some are identified as a fixed isolated shadow seen on the oral cholecystogram or gallbladder ultrasound scan in patients with unexplained right hypochondral discomfort or pain. There is some evidence that adenomas may progress to carcinoma and if the polyp is 10 mm or more, cholecystectomy is considered advisable because of the uncertainty of the diagnosis and the possibility of malignant change.

Carcinoma of the gallbladder

Carcinoma of the gallbladder is the most common malignancy of the biliary tract and accounts for 3–4% of all gastrointestinal malignancies. The reported autopsy incidence is 0.6–1%. The disease is most commonly seen in elderly women (average age of 65 years) and affects females three times as commonly as males. Death from carcinoma of the gallbladder appears to be declining in many Western countries. This has been attributed to the increased cholecystectomy rate. The exact aetiology is unknown but gallstones are present in 75–90% of reported series of gallbladder cancer. Although the association with gallstones is well established, evidence that the stones are responsible directly for the cancer is not available. The role of infection and the consequent production of carcinogenic bile acid derivatives has been suggested but remains unconfirmed. There is undoubt-

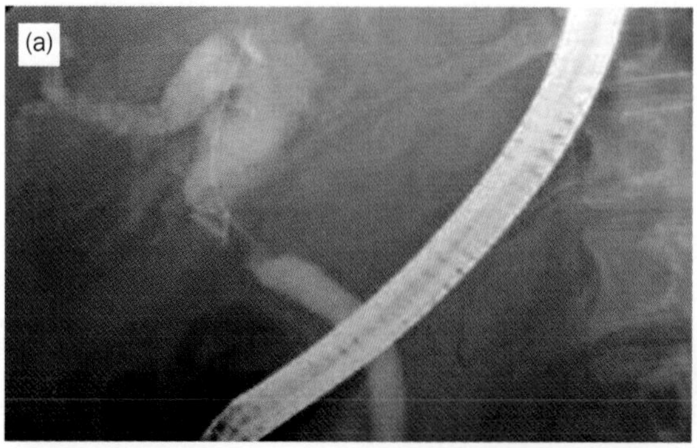

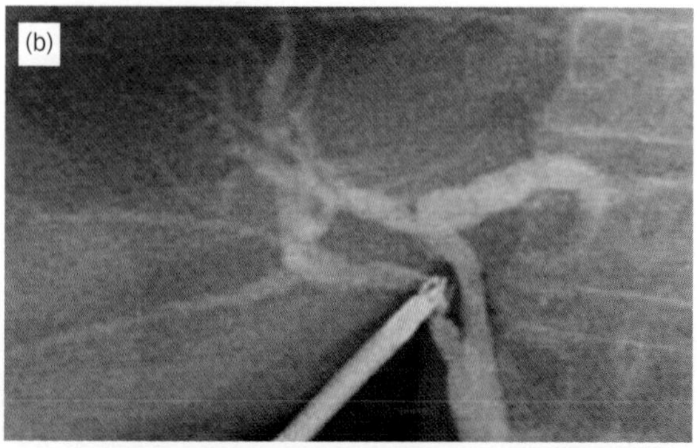

Figure 10.78 (a) Stricture of the common hepatic duct 5 years after laparoscopic cholecystectomy diagnosed pre-operatively as iatrogenic injury with delayed presentation. (b) The operative cholangiogram at the time of surgery was normal. A cholangiocarcinoma was found and resected at operation.

edly an increased risk in patients with calcified gallbladder irrespective of whether this is patchy or diffuse (porcelain gallbladder). The increased risk is sufficiently great to warrant a cholecystectomy, even if the patient is asymptomatic. An increased incidence of gallbladder cancer is found in chronic typhoid carriers, South American Indians and obese individuals.

The ras family of genes consists of three functional genes that encode highly similar, guanine nucleotide-binding proteins (p21) with GTPase activity. The p21 protein is present on the inner aspect of the plasma membrane of a variety of cells. Strong ras p21 immunoreactivity has been documented in most gallbladder carcinomas (62%) but not in gallbladder dysplasia or chronic cholecystitis. By contrast, ras p21 overexpression is encountered only in a minority of the cases of ampullary carcinoma and cholangiocarcinomas. In gallbladder cancer, there is no significant correlation between ras p21 expression and patient survival or between ras p21 expression and p53 immunoreactivity. Furthermore there is no relationship to tumour grade. This suggests that ras p21 may be important in the development of gallbladder carcinomas but not in its progression. The lower rate of ras p21 overexpression in cholangiocarcinomas and ampullary tumours indicates that these tumours probably have a different molecular origin.

The majority of gallbladder tumours are adenocarcinomas, with papillary, undifferentiated, squamous and adenoacanthoma constituting a minority. Rare tumours include carcinoid, melanoma and adrenocorticotropic hormone (ACTH)-secreting apudomas. The UICC staging of gallbladder cancer is based on the depth of invasion as follows:

- stage I – confined to the mucosa/submucosa
- stage II – involvement of the muscle layer
- stage III – serosal involvement
- stage IV – spread to the cystic node
- stage V – invasion of the liver and adjacent organs.

Stage V is referred to as advanced gallbladder carcinoma and is classified into four types in accordance with the extent of involvement of adjacent organs:

- type I – hepatic involvement with or without gastrointestinal invasion (Ia, Ib)
- type II – bile duct involvement with or without gastrointestinal invasion (IIa, IIb)
- type III – hepatic and bile duct involvement with or without gastrointestinal invasion (IIIa, IIIb)
- type IV – major gastrointestinal involvement without hepatic or bile duct invasion.

Clinical features

The disease is either discovered accidentally during cholecystectomy or presents with non-specific symptoms or acutely with an inflammatory mass in the right hypochondrium (acute cholecystitis). The non-specific symptoms include upper right abdominal pain, which is the commonest symptom (76%), anorexia, nausea and vomiting (32%) and weight loss (39%). Jaundice is present in 38% at the time of presentation and is due to involvement of the common hepatic duct. The liver may be enlarged or the gallbladder may be palpable. Ascitis is encountered in advanced disease. Anaemia is present in 50% of patients and is due to chronic haemobilia. Even in the presence of a normal serum bilirubin, the majority of patients have an elevated alkaline phosphatase activity. Few patients with stage I or II disease are diagnosed pre-operatively.

Although ultrasound examination of the gallbladder readily identifies advanced disease, it misses the early potentially curable lesions. Oral cholecystography may show a non-functioning gallbladder or a filling defect projecting into the lumen. Useful diagnostic information is obtained by angio-CT or MRI scan. The highest diagnostic yield is obtained by laparoscopy with contact ultrasonography and this is nowadays regarded as the gold-standard method for the diagnosis and staging of this tumour.

Treatment

The treatment of cancer of the gallbladder is surgical though opinions vary as to the exact operative procedure that should be done. For stages I–III, the best results are reported with extended cholecystectomy. Initially, the gallbladder is removed and the diagnosis is confirmed by frozen section. If this is positive and the tumour is stage I–III, a 3.0 cm resection of surrounding hepatic parenchyma is performed together with lymph node clearance. Resection of the extrahepatic bile duct in continuity is performed if the tumour encroaches the common hepatic duct.

If the tumour is advanced (stage V), some advocate an aggressive approach with right lobectomy or excision of segments IV and V together with extensive lymphadenectomy (cystic, hepatoduodenal, retroduodenal and coeliac nodes) and claim reasonable disease-free survival periods. Long-term survival has been reported after aggressive major resections of this nature only in patients with type I advanced gallbladder cancer. The other types of advanced disease, even if resectable (II–IV), are generally regarded as incurable and only palliative treatment is indicated in view of the uniformly poor prognosis.

A frequently encountered problem relates to patients in whom an unsuspected gallbladder cancer is found after laparoscopic cholecystectomy on pathological examination of the resected specimen. Most would agree that the port wound through which the gallbladder was extracted should be excised full thickness. Thereafter, there are no firm guidelines, but it would seem sensible that if the cancer is pT1 (confined to mucosa/submucosa) then no further action is needed except for careful follow-up of the patient. If the tumour involves the muscularis or serosa, then hepatic resection (segments IV, V) and lymph node clearance is wise provided the patient's general condition is good.

In inoperable patients with jaundice and itching, palliation can be achieved either by endoscopic/radiological stenting with metal expanding endoprostheses or surgically by the round ligament segment III bypass.

The palliation produced by this simple surgical bypass that is well tolerated is very good. The response of gallbladder cancer to radiotherapy and chemotherapy is poor.

Survival

The overall 5 year survival of patients with gallbladder cancer is 4%. The reported cumulative 5 year survival after extended cholecystectomy is 90–100% for stage I and 50–65% for stage II disease. Long-term survivors may also be encountered in patients with stage III, node negative tumours (T3N0).

Tumours of the bile ducts

Benign tumours

A variety of benign tumours of the bile duct including adenoma and papilloma have been reported but they are rare and far less common than cholangiocarcinomas. Benign bile duct tumours have a tendency to recur after excision and some have been reported to undergo malignant change. Benign bile duct tumours present with jaundice and occult chronic gastrointestinal haemorrhage (haemobilia).

Malignant tumours

The reported autopsy incidence of malignant bile duct tumours ranges from 0.01 to 0.5%. The prevalence of carcinomas of the biliary tract and gallbladder in England and Wales is 2.8/100 000 in females and 2.0/100 000 in males. These figures underestimate the true incidence of bile duct cholangiocarcinoma since the intrahepatic ones arising from the minor bile ducts are often classified with liver tumours in many census surveys. Contrary to gallbladder cancer, there is a slight preponderance of males (1.5:1). The age at presentation varies but the peak incidence is in the sixth decade. Bile duct carcinoma is very common in Asian countries where parasitic infestation with liver flukes is endemic (bistomiasis, *Clonorchis sinensis*, *Opisthorchis viverrini*). The median age at presentation of cholangiocarcinomas in areas of endemic infestation with *O. viverrini* is 52 years (range 32–69) and the majority of patients are male. Infestation with *O. viverrini* is a major public health problem in north-east Thailand, where approximately one-third of the population is infected. The infestation is acquired by eating raw fish, which harbour the infective stage of the fluke. Cholangiocarcinoma is one of the leading causes of death in this region. Population-based studies using ultrasonography to visualize early tumours have documented the close association between cholangiocarcinoma and heavy infestation with this parasite. Survival after surgical treatment of cholangiocarcinoma in patients with opisthorchiasis is broadly similar to that reported for cholangiocarcinoma without liver fluke infestation.

The aetiology of bile duct cancer is unknown. The association with gallstones is much less marked than it is with carcinoma of the gallbladder, but ductal calculi are found in 20–50% of patients who develop cholangiocarcinoma. Bacterial-induced endogenous carcinogens derived from bile salts (e.g. lithocholate) have been implicated and their role is supported by the findings of some epidemiological studies and the higher incidence in typhoid carriers. Cholangiocarcinoma is seen with increasing frequency in certain clinical groups (Table 10.10).

The majority of cholangiocarcinomas (85%) express p53 to a varying extent. By contrast the bile duct epithelium adjacent to the tumour and displastic areas do not. Thus overexpression of p53 is thought to play an important role as a late event in the pathogenesis of theses tumours. Marked diffuse p53 staining encountered in 30–40% of cholangiocarcinomas is associated with a significantly poorer survival than tumours with low/focal positivity. This adverse effect of high p53 expression on survival is reported to be independent of age, sex, tumour size, radicality of resection, histopathological grading, lymph-node status, perineural invasion and vasoinvasive growth.

Pathology

The tumours are best classified into the anatomical site of origin:

- Intrahepatic from the minor hepatic ducts (intrahepatic cholangiocarcinomas, ICCs).
- Proximal from the right and left hepatic ducts, hilar confluence and proximal common hepatic duct (Klatskin tumours) (Figure 10.79).
- Middle from the distal common hepatic duct, cystic duct and its confluence with the common bile duct (Figure 10.80).
- Distal from the distal common bile duct, ampullary and periampullary regions (Figure 10.81).

The classification of ICCs and their treatment remains controversial. Some are indeed diffuse (multicentric) and difficult to differentiate from primary hepatocellular carcinomas with which they are grouped because of similar clinical course and poor prognosis. However, the majority of ICCs fall into two macroscopic forms: *mass-forming type* (the majority) and the *periductal infiltrating type*. ICCs of the periductal infiltrating type have a marked tendency to spread along the nerves and lymphatics of the Glissonian sheath; whereas ICCs of the mass-forming type tend to invade the hepatic parenchyma via the portal vein, and exhibit perineural and lymphatic invasion of the Glissonian sheath only when large. Both types can produce satellite hepatic deposits. Therefore, major hepatectomy with combined resection of the extrahepatic bile duct is recommended for all ICCs of the periductal infiltrating type and for those of the mass-forming type with invasion of Glissonian sheath.

Table 10.10 High-risk groups for the development of cholangiocarcinoma

- Parasitic infestation of the biliary tract
- Cystic disease of the biliary tract
- Chronic typhoid carriers
- Ulcerative colitis
- Sclerosing cholangitis

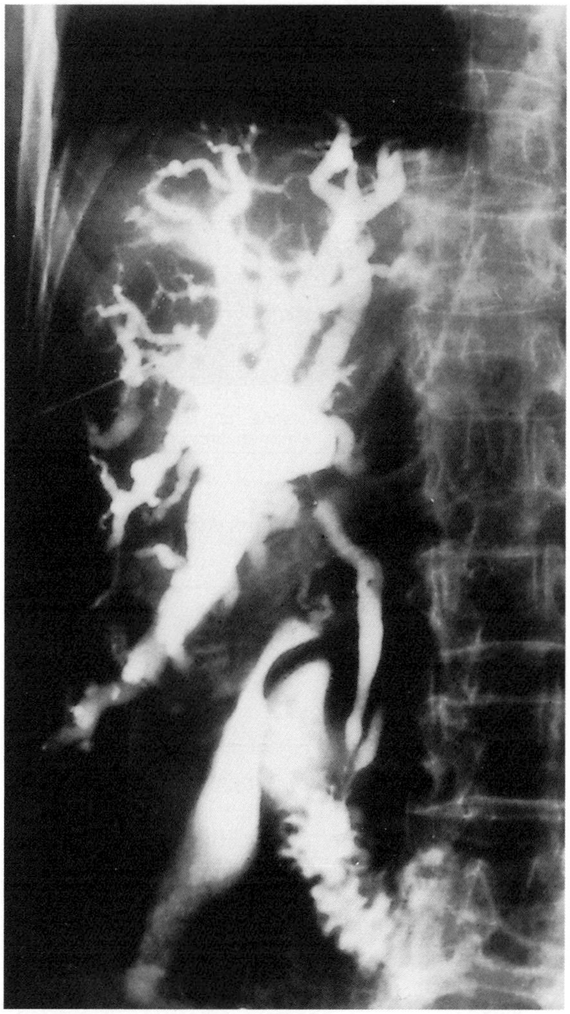

Figure 10.79 Percutaneous transhepatic cholangiogram in a 75-year-old female who presented with marked cholestatic jaundice showing a hilar (Klatskin) tumour.

The gross appearances of extrahepatic cholangiocarcinomas assume one of three forms: stricture (scirrhous variety); nodular; or papillary. The scirrhous variety can be very difficult to distinguish from sclerosing cholangitis even on histological grounds. These tumours are generally confined to the proximal ducts (hilar) and form grey annular thickenings with clearly defined edges. The nodular tumours form extraductal nodules in addition to intra-luminal projections. The papillary variety is most commonly found in the distal bile duct and periampullary region. These lesions are friable and may fill the duct lumen with vascular neoplastic tissue and tend to bleed in the ductal lumen causing haemobilia. The majority of tumours are adenocarcinomas of varying differentiation. The scirrhous variety is intensely fibrotic and relatively acellular, often with a few well-differentiated ductal carcinoma cells grouped as acini in a dense connective tissue stroma. Rare types include squamous cell carcinoma, adenosquamous carcinoma, adenoacanthoma, lymphoma, carcinoid tumours and melanoma. Malignant smooth muscle

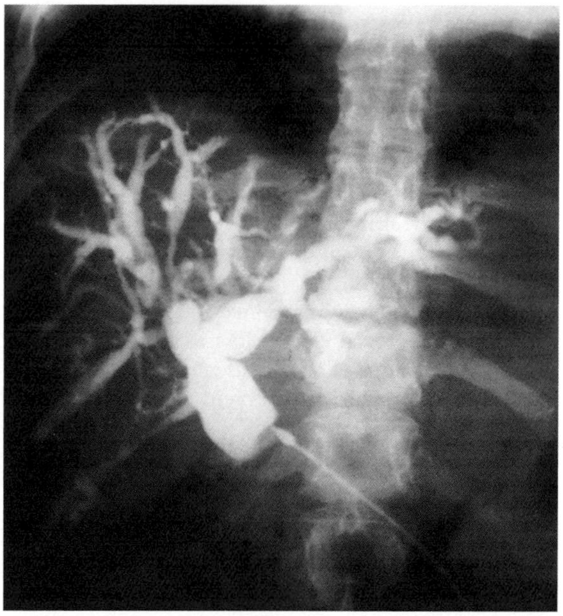

Figure 10.80 Operative cholangiogram showing a tumour at the junction of the cystic duct with the common bile duct. The patient presented with jaundice and acute cholecystitis.

tumours of the bile duct have also been reported as have instances of primary non-secreting apudoma of the hilar region. All cholangiocarcinomas are slow growing, locally infiltrative and metastasize late. Cholangiocarcinomas have a special predilection for perineural spread and do not metastasize beyond the liver. The best prognosis is encountered after resection especially of the distal ampullary and periampullary lesions.

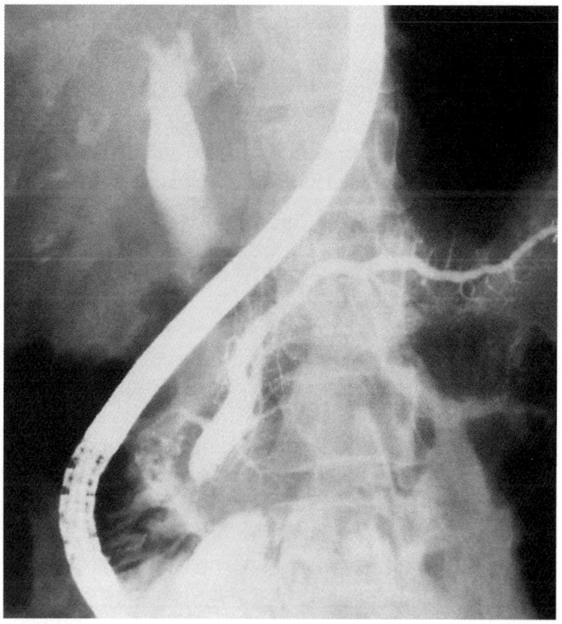

Figure 10.81 ERCP showing a papillary tumour of the distal bile duct extending to the periampullary region.

Clinical features

In patients with ICCs, mild abdominal pain is the most frequent presenting clinical sign and always warrants investigation. Presentation with jaundice in uncommon (13%). If a mass lesion is detected by imaging (CT, MRI, etc.), pre-operative biopsy is ill-advised since it may result in local implantation and in one reported series was correct in only 40%.

By contrast, the main presentation (90%) in patients with extrahepatic cholangiocarcinomas is with obstructive jaundice which is progressive and accompanied by itching and anorexia. Weight loss is not evident until the disease is advanced and is usually accompanied by evidence of hepatic involvement and ascites. Dull upper abdominal pain is a frequent symptom. Some patients present acutely with cholangitis or acute cholecystitis. The duration of symptoms is usually short and measured in months. In high prevalence areas such as Taiwan, the pre-operative diagnosis of ICCs is difficult because of the frequent association with hepatolithiasis (43%) and the high incidence of hepatocellular carcinoma (HCC). Thus in one large reported series of 125 patients from Taiwan, 25% of these patients underwent surgery for chronic cholangitis and 12.5% for HCC rather than cholangiocarcinoma.

In the West, distal bile duct stones and proximal extrahepatic malignant biliary obstructions may coexist. These stones probably pre-date the development of the malignant obstruction and are found in 12–18% of patients with proximal tumours, especially cholangiocarcinomas. In most instances the stones are distal to the malignant obstruction. They may interfere with stent function in inoperable cases (*vide infra*).

Physical examination reveals hepatomegaly. Anaemia is present in patients with papillary tumours especially at the lower end of the bile duct and periampullary region. It is caused by chronic blood loss. The faeces of these patients have a characteristic silvery appearance due to a combination of steatorrhoea and altered blood. A palpable gallbladder is present in patients with distal tumours. A significant percentage of patients with hilar tumours have previously undergone recent cholecystectomy (within 6–12 months of diagnosis). Regrettably, these tumours are missed at operation since the small nodule in the porta hepatis is not easily palpable, the common bile duct is not dilated and there is free flow of contrast into the duodenum. Often the surgeon concerned ignores the fact that there is poor filling of the intrahepatic biliary tree or interprets a localized narrowing as extrinsic vascular compression. An operative cholangiogram should never be passed as normal unless there is adequate and complete filling of the intrahepatic biliary tree.

Although ultrasound identifies dilatation of the biliary tree, it seldom localizes the tumour. CT scanning, likewise, does not permit sufficiently precise anatomical localization to predict the exact site and resectability of the tumours. It can, however, demonstrate atrophy of the left lobe consequent on vascular involvement by the tumour. The definitive investigation is MRCP

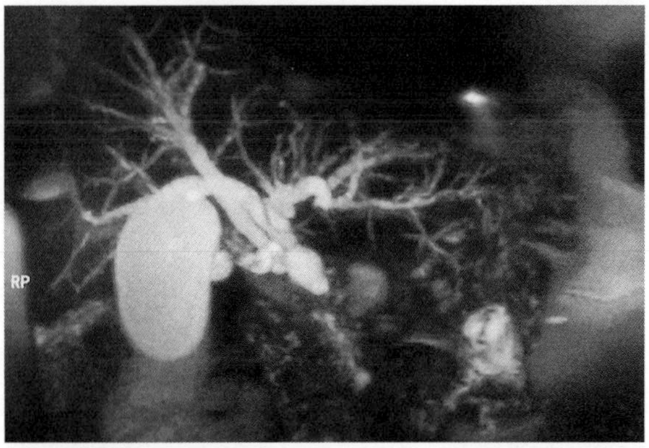

Figure 10.82 MRI/MRCP showing an advanced cholangiocarcinoma with involvement/thrombosis of portal vein. The patient was treated by stenting.

(Figure 10.82) which should precede an ERCP. ERCP is indicated:

- if the lesion shown on the MRCP is distal when the ampullary and periampullary region require to be visualized or biopsied
- if the patient is judged to be inoperable and requires endoscopic palliation
- if MRCP is not available.

The proximal (hepatic) longitudinal extension of extrahepatic cholangiocarcinomas is difficult to predict before surgery. In this respect, the cholangiographic findings may be misleading. In one reported study of 54 patients, histological examination of specimens indicated proximal longitudinal spread of the tumour in 41%. Cholangiography was unreliable in detecting this spread (63% accuracy). A significantly higher frequency of longitudinal spread was observed when the cholangiographic images showed a main tumour with collapsed edges as distinct from tumours with sharp edges on the cholangiographic films. These authors recommend a mapping biopsy performed by percutaneous transhepatic cholangioscopy to establish the limit of the proximal spread but this is not practised in other centres.

Treatment

The treatment of cholangiocarcinomas remains controversial and non-standardized, varying from therapeutic nihilism with the emphasis on palliation, to an aggressive surgical approach in patients judged to be fit for major surgery. Undoubtedly resection (for both intra- and extrahepatic lesions) is the best method of treatment and is indicated for all operable tumours in fit individuals. The reported resectability rate varies widely but averages 20%. The benefits of resection are:

- the possibility of cure and probability of long-term survival
- resection provides the best form of palliation in terms of duration and freedom from infective complications.

Furthermore, resection is now attended with a small mortality (around 5%) and an acceptable morbidity. If a patient with cholangiocarcinoma is judged to be potentially resectable, peroperative endoscopic stenting is contraindicated as this results in infection of the obstructed biliary tract. Cholangitis in these patients is often fatal. The surgical procedure depends on the location of the tumours.

Patients with operable ICCs require major hepatic resections. Excision of the extrahepatic bile duct in continuity is necessary for all periductal infiltrating tumours and for those of the mass-forming tumours with invasion of Glissonian sheath. Hepatic transplantation is contraindicated for diffuse inoperable disease, even if the patient is fit, as the results have been uniformly dismal. The median reported survival after resection of ICCs is 15 months, with actuarial 1, 2 and 5 year survival rates of 67, 40 and 32%, respectively. Thus the contention that these tumours carry a uniformly bad prognosis is not justified and a selective aggressive surgical approach constitutes the correct management.

For hilar lesions, an anterior segmentectomy IV provides good access to the confluence, allows good clearance proximal to the tumour and facilitates the hepaticojejunostomy. Often the caudate lobe is involved by hilar tumours (45%) and for this reason, it should be resected routinely in hilar tumours. When the tumour extends along the right or left duct with extension to the respective lobe, the resection includes a lobectomy in continuity with the main tumour mass. Thus curative resection often requires a major hepatectomy with caudate lobectomy. The reported 1 and 5 year survival rates after curative resection (as judged by specimen histology) average 60% and 45%, respectively. These survival data contrast with a median survival of 7 months in patients treated by surgical bypass or endoscopic/radiological stenting. Regrettably pathological examination of the specimen often shows tumour at the resection margins especially in patients in whom a hepatic resection is not performed.

Tumours arising from the middle third (close to the cystic duct) are excised from just below the confluence down to the duodenum (pancreaticoduodenectomy in continuity) together with the associated hepatoduodenal and retroduodenal lymph nodes. The standard surgical treatment of operable ampullary and periampullary cancers is with pancreaticoduodenectomy.

If at operation the tumour is found to be inoperable, a bilio-enteric bypass is performed. Anastomosis of a Roux loop to the segment III duct using the round ligament approach gives the best results for inoperable hilar lesions. A choledochojejunostomy is performed for inoperable distal tumours. A gastroenterostomy is added if duodenal obstruction is present or considered imminent in patients with inoperable periampullary tumours.

The percutaneous insertion of iridium-192 wire has been used to provide local irradiation (brachytherapy) with good results and reported median survival of 11–23 months. Iridium-192 brachytherapy administered via the transhepatic approach has been shown to provide worthwhile palliation in patients with unresectable disease and after recurrence following previous complete or partial resection. The most common acute complication after brachytherapy is cholangitis followed by duodenal ulceration.

A recent report from Holland on a large series of 71 patients has documented a survival benefit from post-operative radiotherapy after resection of hilar (Klatskin) tumours. Radiotherapy was administered externally (55 Gy) or in combination with internal radiotherapy (45 Gy external, 10 Gy internal with iridium-192 introduced along the bile duct anastomosis via the Roux-en-Y jejunal loop). The combined regimen caused more complications without any survival benefit over external radiotherapy alone, which is therefore the recommended regimen. Although adjuvant post-operative radiotherapy is not routinely administered after resection of bile duct tumours, this and other reports document that recurrences are reduced or delayed by post-operative external beam supervoltage radiotherapy and this should now be administered routinely after resection of these tumours.

Cholangiocarcinomas of the bile ducts are generally regarded to be unresponsive to chemotherapy although response rates have been documented with mitomycin C, doxorubicin and FUDR.

Non-surgical palliation

In patients who are considered inoperable on pre-operative assessment and those who are too old and frail or have serious cardiorespiratory disease, palliation of the jaundice is best achieved by percutaneous transhepatic or endoscopic stenting. The endoprosthesis has to be large (8–10 Fr) and may require replacement if it becomes blocked with calcium bilirubinate encrustation. Self-expanding stainless steel wire biliary endoprostheses are now used frequently for these malignant strictures. The big advantage of this type of endoprosthesis over plastic stents is that it can be introduced through a small-calibre sheath. When the latter is removed, the stent expands to achieve an internal diameter much greater than that of conventional plastic endoprostheses. In addition, the wire framework of the stent becomes buried in the wall of the duct and is thus less liable to cause infection and encrustation with calcium bilirubinate. This contributes to their high patency rate, which is reported to be 90%. These self-expanding metal stents are, however, contraindicated in patients with polypoid tumours as the fronds of the neoplasm project through the wire framework into the lumen. In addition, there is a risk of haemorrhage in these cases.

The controversy in the management of cholangiocarcinomas has until recently even extended to the endoscopic palliation in respect of the choice of stent (plastic versus metallic). This has now been resolved by a large prospective study of 101 patients who were followed until death or at least 1 year after inclusion into the study. By multivariate analysis, only tumour size predicted survival. Thus, a threshold of 30 mm at diagnosis distinguished two survival profiles: the median survival of patients with a tumour greater than 30 mm was 3.2 months as distinct from 6.6 months for patients with tumour size <30 mm. The recommended strategy involves the use of metal stents for patients with an inoperable tumour smaller than 30 mm, while larger tumours are efficiently palliated by a plastic stent.

Approximately 15% of patients develop stent occlusion at a mean interval of 4 months after insertion of metal stents. In 80% occlusion is due to tumour overgrowth and in 20% to debris. When the occlusion is caused by tumour ingrowth, the survival is limited to a maximum of 3 months and these patients are best treated by internal plastic stents. Occlusion of metal stents by debris is effectively cleared by sweeping the stent with a balloon catheter.

Distal tumours

These include:

- distal bile duct tumours
- ampullary tumours
- periampullary carcinoma
- primary duodenal carcinoma [see Disorders of the stomach and duodenum].

Ampullary tumours

These can either be adenomas or adenocarcinomas. Some ampullary tumours arise in association with familial polyposis coli. In general, ampullary carcinomas have a higher resectability rate and better prognosis than other periampullary carcinomas, although the prognosis is poor when the disease is advanced. Several studies have now shown that the pre-operative staging is best achieved by endoscopic ultrasound (EUS) which has an overall accuracy of tumour (T) staging of 75%, although it is less reliable in detecting lymph node involvement (60%). Its most important contribution, however, is in the detection of pancreatic invasion for which EUS has an accuracy of 86%, a sensitivity of 83% and a specificity of 87%.

The options for treatment of ampullary tumours include local excision, pancreaticoduodenectomy and endoscopic management (endoscopic papillectomy and debulking, endoscopic stenting). If the lesions can be confidently diagnosed as benign by endoscopic biopsy, treatment is by transduodenal excision of the ampulla of Vater. This can be performed surgically or by endoscopic papillectomy. Local excision is also used for malignant ampullary lesions if:

- the patient is unfit for major surgery
- the tumour is limited to the ampulla of Vater as diagnosed by pre-operative EUS (uT_1) and UICC-staging (pT_1); and the histological grading is G1 or G2 without lymphatic infiltration.

Close post-operative follow-up with duodenoscopy and ERCP are necessary in all patients treated by local excision. For all other operable tumours in fit patients the best treatment is obtained by pancreaticoduodenectomy.

Endoscopic management (laser debulking and stenting) is reserved for patients who are unfit for surgery and for advanced inoperable disease.

Periampullary tumours

These are generally more advanced than ampullary lesions and include ampullary carcinomas that have spread to involve the adjacent mucosa but they are considered to be distinct from primary duodenal carcinoma (*vide infra*). By definition these includes tumours that are located within 1.0 cm of the papilla. When operable and in fit patients, the treatment is excision by pancreaticoduodenectomy. Local excision (transduodenal papilloduodenectomy) is indicated in frail patients. The resection includes the papilla, the distal bile duct and pancreatic duct with surrounding pancreatic tissue. Following excision, the pancreatic and common bile duct are sutured together and then to the defect in the medial wall of the duodenum. The reported experience with this procedure is limited but the operation appears safe.

Section 10.19 • Parasitic infestations of the biliary tract

In addition to infestations with schistosomes and the larvae of *Taenia echinococcus*, the liver and biliary tract are involved with various other parasitic disorders. Some infestations, such as toxocariasis, remain subclinical in the majority of cases. Children usually acquire infection with *Toxocara canis* from their pets. In addition to hepatic granulomas, there may be CNS and eye involvement. The latter is serious and leads to endophthalmitis which can be mistaken for retinoblastoma in these children.

The parasitic disorders which are of significance in surgery of the biliary tract include infestation with *Ascaris lumbricoides*, *Clonorchis sinensis* and *Fasciola hepatica*.

Ascaris lumbricoides

Infestation with this nematode is endemic and prevalent in Asia, China and Africa. It is also found in the rural areas of Europe, the USA and Latin America. The adult worms live in the upper reaches of the small intestine but migrate to and from the bile duct through the ampulla of Vater, up the oesophagus and down to the appendix. The ova are excreted in the stools of infected individuals and contaminate soil and vegetables. Following ingestion of the encysted larvae and dissolution of the cyst wall by the gastric juice, the free larvae penetrate the intestinal mucosa to reach the portal venous system and thus the liver or the lung via the intestinal lymphatics and the thoracic duct. The pulmonary larvae are carried from the alveoli to the pharynx and then swallowed to reach the upper part of the small intestine where they mature into adult worms. The larval migration may involve other organs, e.g. CNS and kidneys.

The majority of adult worms migrating into the biliary tract die after a few weeks and may form a nidus for stone formation. Secondary infection of the bile with *E. coli* and other enteric organisms is common and is thought to play a role in the formation of calcium bilirubinate stones. Pyogenic liver abscess may complicate the disease. The usual hepatic lesions are granulomas surrounding the ova, which are deposited in the smaller bile ducts.

Clinical features

The stage of larval migration is accompanied by systemic symptoms: rigors, generalized aches, malaise, cough and asthmatic attacks. Eosinophilia is invariably present. Migration of the adult worms into the bile duct induces episodes of pain in the epigastric region. Jaundice is encountered in 20%. *Ascaris lumbricoides* infestation is one of the commonest causes of jaundice in children and young adults in Africa. At this stage, the clinical picture is usually dominated by recurrent attacks of cholangitis due to calculus formation and secondary infection.

Treatment

Surgical intervention is necessary to deal with the biliary complications. An initial laparotomy is required to look for and remove (by enterotomy) adult worms which can be easily palpated through the intact bowel wall. Exploration of the bile duct, and removal of stones and worms is performed next. A completion cholangiogram or, preferably, an inspection with the choledochoscope, is advisable at the end of the duct exploration T-tube drainage is essential in all cases and should be carried out with a large tube (16–18 Fr) to enable subsequent percutaneous stone and parasite extraction through the T-tube tract, if necessary. Surgical intervention should be followed by antihelminthic therapy.

Clonorchis sinensis

Man is the definitive host of this trematode which is widely distributed in China and East Asia. The adult worms live in the biliary tract and occasionally in the pancreatic duct. The eggs are excreted in the faeces and ingested by freshwater snails (e.g. *Parafossarulus manchouricus*) where they develop into cercariae. The free-swimming cercariae then penetrate freshwater fish and encyst themselves in the muscles of the host as metacercariac. Man becomes infected by eating contaminated fish, the encysted metacercariae being released in the duodenum. They then migrate into the biliary tract via the ampulla of Vater and mature into adult worms. These cause dilatation of the biliary tract with fibrosis of the ducts and adenomatous bile duct hyperplasia. Secondary infection of the biliary tract with enteric organisms is extremely common and results in death of the worm and stone formation. Recurrent episodes of cholangitis and septicaemia, and the development of bile duct carcinoma, account for the appreciable mortality of this parasitic infestation. The diagnosis is confirmed by the demonstration of the typical ova in the faeces.

Treatment

Mild cases can be managed conservatively with chloroquine (300 mg for 2–6 months). Surgical intervention is needed for jaundice and cholangitis. In addition to removal of worms and calculi from the bile duct, an internal biliary drainage (choledochoduodenostomy/jejunostomy or sphincteroplasty) is performed.

Fasciola hepatica

This is primarily an infestation of sheep and cattle. Man is an accidental host, acquiring the disease by eating wild watercress contaminated with metacercariae. The disease has a world-wide distribution and is common in Latin America and the USA. In the UK outbreaks of the disease occur in Hampshire and the Lake District (Silverside). The ova are excreted in the faeces of infected animals, develop into miracidia in freshwater and subsequently colonize the intermediate host, a freshwater snail (*Lymnae truncatula*). Within this host, they mature through various stages into metacercariae which become encysted on neighbouring water plants. Subsequent to ingestion, the free metacercariae are released in the upper part of the small intestine and penetrate the bowel to reach the peritoneal cavity. They then migrate across the peritoneal cavity and enter the liver parenchyma after penetration of the liver capsule. Maturation occurs in the bile ducts. Migration of the metacercariae may occur to other organs: kidneys, muscles, brain and subcutaneous tissue.

Clinical features

The disease is often asymptomatic if the infestion is mild. Systemic symptoms signify heavy infestations and include malaise, anorexia, nausea, vomiting, fever and weight loss. An urticarial rash, jaundice or hepatosplenomegaly may develop. Diagnosis is confirmed by the demonstration of ova in the stool.

Treatment

The disease is usually treated medically with bithionol (50 mg daily for 3 weeks). Surgical intervention is indicated only in cases of biliary obstruction and cholangitis.

Further reading

Imaging

Bret, P. M. and Reinhold, C. (1997). Magnetic resonance cholangiopancreatography. *Endoscopy* **29**: 472–86.

Clair, D. G. and Brooks, D. C. (1994). Laparoscopic cholecystectomy: the case for a selective approach. *Surg Clin North Am* **74**: 962–6.

Coakely, F. V. and Schwartz, L. H. (1999). Magnetic resonance cholangiopancreatography. *J Magn Reson Imaging* **9**: 157–62.

Cuschieri, A., Shimi, S., Banting, S. *et al.* (1994). Intraoperative cholangiography during laparoscopic cholecystectomy. Routine versus selective policy. *Surg Endosc* **8**: 302–5.

Flanebaum, L., Aldsen, S. M. and Trooskin, S. Z. (1989). Use of cholescintigraphy with morphine in critically ill patients with suspected cholecystitis. *Surgery* **106**: 668–74.

Flowers, J. L., Zucker, K. A., Graham, S. M. *et al.* (1992). Laparoscopic cholangiography: results and indications. *Ann Surg* **215**: 209–16.

Kullman, E., Borch, K., Lindstrom, E. *et al.* (1996). Value of routine intraoperative cholangiography in detecting aberrant bile ducts and bile duct injuries during laparoscopic cholecystectomy. *Br J Surg* **83**: 171–5.

Lai, E. C, S., Lo, C. M., Choi, T. K. *et al.* (1989). Urgent biliary decompression after endoscopic retrograde cholangiopancreatography. *Am J Surg* **157**: 121–5.

Lorimer, J. W. and Fairfull Smith, R. J. (1994). Intraoperative cholangiography is not essential to avoid duct injuries during laparoscopic cholecystectomy. *Am J Surg* **169**: 344–7

Phillips, E. H. (1993). Routine versus selective intraoperative cholangiography. *Am J Surg* **165**: 505–7.

Pu, Y., Yamamoto, F., Igimi, H. *et al.* (1994). A comparative study of usefulness of magnetic resonance imaging in the diagnosis of acute cholecystitis. *J Gastroenterol* **29**: 192–8.

Soyer, P., Brouland, J. P., Boudiaf, M. *et al.* (1998). Color velocuity imaging and power Doppler sonography of the gall bladder wall: a new look at sonographic diagnosis of acute cholecystitis. *Am J Roentgenol* **171**: 183–8.

Uggowitzer, M., Kugler, C., Schramyer, G. *et al.* (1997). Sonography of acute cholecystitis: comparison of color and power Doppler sonography in detecting a hypervascularized gallbladder wall. *Am J Roentgentol* **168**: 707–12.

Gallstone disease

Bragg, L. E. and Thompson, J. S. (1989) Concomitant cholecystectomy for asymptomatic cholelithiasis. *Archives of Surgery*, **124**: 460–2.

Carey, M. C. and Cahalane, M. J. (1988). Whither biliary sludge? *Gastroenterology* **95**: 508–23.

Cetta, F. (1991). The role of bacteria in pigment gallstone disease. *Ann Surg* **213**: 315–26.

Cetta, F. (1993). Do surgical and endoscopic sphincterotomy prevent or facilitate recurrent common duct stone formation? *Arch Surg* **128**: 329.

Cuschieri, A. and Berci, G. (1997). *Bile Ducts and Bile Duct Stones*, Philadelphia, PA: W. B. Saunders, pp. 33–42.

Cuschieri, A., Croce, E., Faggioni, A. *et al.* (1999). EAES multicentre prospective randomized trial comparing two-stage vs single-stage management of patients with gallstone disease and ductal calculi. *Surg Endosc* **13**: 952–7.

Dogra, R., Singh, J. and Sharma, M. P. (1995). Enterically transmitted non-A, non-B hepatitis mimicking acute cholecystitis. *Am J Gastroenterol* **90**: 764–6.

Groen, A. K., Noordam, C., Drapers, J. A. G. *et al.* (1990). Isolation of a potent cholesterol nucleation-promoting activity from human gallbladder bile: role in the pathogenesis of gallstone disease. *Hepatology* **11**: 525–33.

Hensman, C., Crosthwaite, G. and Cuschieri, A. (1997). Transcystic biliary decompression after direct laparoscopic exploration of the common bile duct. *Surg Endosc* **11**: 1106–10.

Holzbach, R. T. (1990). Current concepts of cholesterol transport and crystal formation in human bile. *Hepatology* **12**: 26-32S.

Kiviluoto, T., Siren, J., Luukkonen, P. and Kivilaakso, E. (1998). Randomised trial of laparoscopic versus open cholecystectomy for acute and gangrenous cholecystitis. *Lancet* **351**: 321–5.

Lai, P. B., Kwong, K. H., Leung, K. L. *et al.* (1988). Randomized trial of early versus delayed laparoscopic cholecystectomy for acute cholecystitis. *Br J Surg* **85**: 764–7.

Lo, C. M., Fan, S. T., Liu, C. L. *et al.* (1997). Early decision for conversion of laparoscopic to open cholecystectomy for treatment of acute cholecystitis. *Am J Surg* **173**: 513–17.

Lo, C. M., Liu, C. L., Fan, S. T., Lai, E. C. and Wong, J. (1998). Prospective randomized study of early versus delayed laparoscopic cholecystitis. *Ann Surg* **227**: 461–7.

Poole, G., Waldron, B., Shimi, S. M. and Cuschieri, A. (1997). Laparoscopic common bile duct exploration after failed endoscopic stone extraction. *Endoscopy* **29**: 609–13.

Smith, B. F. (1990). Gallbladder mucin as a pronucleating agent for cholesterol monohydrate crystals. *Hepatology* **12**: 183–8S.

Southern Surgeons Club (1991). A prospective analysis of 1518 laparoscopic cholecystectomies performed by Southern US surgeons. *N Engl J Med* **324**: 1073–8.

Tagle, F. M., Lavergne, J., Barkin, J. S. and Unger, S. W. (1997). Laparoscopic cholecystectomy in the elderly. *Surg Endosc* **11**: 636–8.

Taragona, E. M., Perez Ayuso, R. M., Bordas, J. M. *et al.* (1996). Randomised trial of endoscopic sphincterotomy with gallbladder left *in situ* versus open surgery for common bile duct calculi in high-risk patients. *Lancet* **347**: 926–9.

Tokunaga, Y., Nakayama, N., Ishikawa, Y. *et al.* (1997). Surgical risks of acute cholecystitis in the elderly. *Hepatogastroenterology* **44**: 671–6.

Trias, M., Taragona, E. M., Ros, E. and Bordas, J. M. (1997). Prospective evaluation of a minimally invasive approach for treatment of bile-duct calculi in the high-risk patient. *Surg Endosc* **11**: 632–5.

Villanova, N., Bazzoli, F., Taroni, F. *et al.* (1989). Gallstone recurrence after successful bile acid treatment. A 12-year follow-up study and evaluation of long-term postdissolution treatment. *Gastroenterology* **97**: 726–31.

Bile duct injuries

Adamsen, S., Hansen, O. H., Funch Jensen, P. *et al.* (1997). Bile duct injury during laparoscopic cholecystectomy: a prospective nationwide series. *J Am Coll Surg* **184**: 571–8.

Andren Sandberg, A., Alinder, G. and Bengmark, S. (1985). Accidental lesions of the common bile duct at cholecystectomy. *Ann Surg* **201**: 328–32.

Bismuth, H. (1982). Postoperative strictures of the bile ducts. In *The Biliary Tract V* (ed. Blumgart, L. H.), New York: Churchill-Livingstone, pp. 209–18.

Born, P., Rösch, T., Brühl, K. *et al.* (1999). Long-term results of endoscopic and percutaneous transhepatic treatment of benign biliary strictures. *Endoscopy* **31**: 725–31.

Carrol, B, J., Birth, M. and Phillips, E. H. (1998). Common bile duct injuries during laparoscopic cholecystectomy that result in litigation. *Surg Endosc* **12**: 310–14.

Chartrand-Lefebvre, C., Dufresne, M. P., Lafortune, M. *et al.* (1994). Iatrogenic injury to the bile duct: a working classification for radiologists. *Radiology* **193**: 523–6.

Collet, D. (1997). Laparoscopic cholecystectomy in 1994. Results of a prospective survey conducted by SFCERO on 4624 cases. Societe Francaise de Chirurgie Endoscopique et Radiologie Operatoire. *Surg Endosc* **11**: 56–63.

Collet, D., Edye, M. and Perissat, J. (1993). Conversion and complications of laparoscopic cholecystectomy: results of a survey conducted by the French Society of Endoscopic Surgery and Interventional Radiology (SFCERO). *Surg Endosc* **7**: 334–8.

Davidoff, A.M., Pappas, T. N., Murray, E. A. *et al.* (1992). Mechanisms of major biliary injury during laparoscopic cholecystectomy. *Ann Surg* **215**: 196–202.

Deziel, D. J. (1994). Complications of cholecystectomy: incidence, clinical significance and diagnosis. *Surg Clin North Am* **74**: 809–23.

Fletcher, D. R., Hobbs, M. S., Tan, P. *et al.* (1999). Complications of cholecystectomy: risks of the laparoscopic approach and protective effects of operative cholangiography: a population-based study. *Ann Surg* **229**: 449–57.

Gouma, D. J., Rauws, E. A., Keulemans, Y. C. *et al.* (1999). Bile duct injuries after a laparoscopic cholecystectomy. *Ned Tijdschr Geneeskd* **143**: 606–11.

Greenen, D. J., Greenen, J. E., Hoagen, W. J. *et al.* (1989). Endoscopic therapy for benign bile duct strictures. *Gastroint Endosc* **35**: 367–71.

Gupta, N., Solomon, H., Fairchild, R. and Kaminski, D. L. (1998). Management and outcome of patients with combined bile duct and hepatic artery injuries. *Arch Surg* **133**: 176–81.

Kadesky, K. M., Schopf, B., Magee, J. F. and Blair, G. K. (1997). Proximity injury by ultrasonically activated scalpel during dissection. *J Paediatr Surg* **32**: 878–9.

Kern, K. A. (1994). Medicolegal perspective of laparoscopic bile duct injuries. *Surg Clin North Am* **74**: 979–84.

MacFadyen, B. V., Vecchio, R., Ricardo, A. E. and Mathis, C. R. (1998). Bile duct injury after laparoscopic cholecystectomy: the United States experience. *Surg Endosc* **12**: 315–21.

Martin, R. F. and Rossi, R. L. (1994). Bile duct injuries: spectrum, mechanism of injury, and their prevention. *Surg Clin North Am* **74**: 781–803.

Meyers, W. C. and Southern Surgeons Club (1991). A prospective analysis of 1518 laparoscopic cholecystectomies. *N Engl J Med* **324**: 1073–8.

Moore, M. J. and Bennett, C. L. (1995). The learning curve for laparoscopic cholecystectomy. The Southern Surgeons Club. *Am J Surg* **170**: 55–9.

Moossa, A. R., Easter, D. W., Sonnerborg, A. *et al.* (1992). Laparoscopic injuries to the bile duct: a cause for concern. *Ann Surg* **215**: 203–8.

Moossa, A. R., Mayer, A. D. and Stabile, B. (1990). Iatrogenic injuries to the bile duct: who, how, where? *Arch Surg* **125**: 1028–31.

Regoly Merei, J., Ihasz, M., Szeberin, Z. *et al.* (1998). Biliary tract complications in laparoscopic cholecystectomy. A multicenter study of 148 biliary tract injuries in 26 440 operations. *Surg Endosc* **12**: 294–300.

Richardson, M. C., Bell, G., Fullarton, G. M. and the West of Scotland Laparoscopic Cholecystectomy Audit Group (1996). Incidence and nature of bile duct injuries following laparoscopic cholecystectomy: an audit of 5913 cases. *Br J Surg* **83**: 1356–60.

Robertson, A. J., Rela, M., Karani, J. *et al.* (1998). Laparoscopic cholecystectomy injury: an unusual indication for liver transplantation. *Transpl Int* **11**: 449–51.

Rossi, R. L., Schirmer, W. J., Braasch, J. W. *et al.* (1992). Laparoscopic bile duct injuries. Risk factors, recognition, and repair. *Arch Surg* **127**: 596–601.

Russel, J. C., Walsh, S. J., Mattie, A. S. and Lynch, J. T. (1996). Bile duct injuries, 1989–93: a statewide experience. *Arch Surg* **131**: 382–8.

Savader, S. J., Lillemoe, K. D., Prescott, C. A. *et al.* (1997). Laparoscopic cholecystectomy-related bile duct injuries: a health and financial disaster. *Ann Surg* **225**: 268–73.

Schol, F. P., Go, P. M. and Gouma, D. J. (1995). Outcome of 49 repairs of bile duct injuries after laparoscopic cholecystectomy. *World J Surg* **19**: 753–6.

Stewart, J. and Cuschieri, A. (1994). Adverse consequences of cystic duct closure by clips. *Minim Invasive Ther* **3**: 153–7.

Stewart, L. and Way, L. W. (1995). Bile duct injuries during laparoscopic cholecystectomy. Factors that influence the results of treatment. *Arch Surg* **130**: 1123–8.

Strasberg, S. M., Hertl, M. and Soper, N. J. (1995). An analysis of the problem of biliary injury during laparoscopic cholecystectomy. *J Am Coll Surg* **180**: 101–25.

Targarona, E. M., Marco, C., Balagne, C. *et al.* (1998). How, when, and why bile duct injuries occur: a comparison between open and laparoscopic cholecystectomy. *Surg Endosc* **12**: 322–6.

Trondsen, E., Ruud, T. E., Nilsen, B. H. *et al.* (1994). Complications during the introduction of laparoscopic cholecystectomy in Norway. A prospective multicentre study in seven hospitals. *Eur J Surg* **160**: 145–51.

Vincent Hamelin-E., Pallares, A. C., Felipe, J. A. *et al.* (1994). National survey on laparoscopic cholecystectomy in Spain. Results of a multi-institutional study conducted by the Committee for Endoscopic Surgery (Association Espanola de Cirujanos). *Surg Endosc* **18**: 770–6

Z'graggen, K., Wehrli, H., Metzger, A. for the Swiss Association of Laparoscopic and Thoracoscopic Surgery (1998). Complications of laparoscopic surgery in Switzerland: a prospective 3-year study of 10 174 patients. *Surg Endosc* **12**: 1303–110.

Tumours

Alstrup, N., Burcharth, F., Hauge, C. and Horn, T. (1996). Transduodenal excision of tumours of the ampulla of Vater. *Eur J Surg* **162**: 961–7.

Arora, D. S., Ramsdale, J., Lodge, J. P. and Wyatt, J. I. (1999). p53 but not bcl-2 is expressed by most cholangiocarcinomas: a study of 28 cases. *Histopathology* **34**: 497–501.

Berdah, S. V., Delpero, J. R., Garcia, S. *et al.* (1996). A western surgical experience of peripheral cholangiocarcinoma. *Br J Surg* **83**: 1517–21.

Chijiiwa, K. and Tanaka, M. (1996). Indications for and limitations of extended cholecystectomy in the treatment of carcinoma of the gall bladder. *Eur J Surg* **162**: 211–16.

Farrell, R. J., Noonan, N., Khan, I. *et al.* (1996). Carcinoma of the ampulla of Vater: a tumour with a poor prognosis? *Eur J Gastroenterol Hepatol* **8**: 139–44.

Klein, P., Reingruber, B., Kastl, S. *et al.* (1966). Is local excision of pT1-ampullary carcinomas justified? *Eur J Surg Oncol* **22**: 366–71.

Kubo, H., Chijiiwa, Y., Akahoshi, K. *et al.* (1999). Pre-operative staging of ampullary tumours by endoscopic ultrasound. *Br J Radiol* **72**: 443–7.

Lee, C. S. (1997). Ras p21 protein immunoreactivity and its relationship to p53 expression and prognosis in gallbladder and extrahepatic biliary carcinoma. *Eur J Surg Oncol* **23**: 233–7.

Lee, M. J., Dawson, S. L., Mueller, P. R. *et al.* (1994). Failed metallic biliary stents: causes and management of delayed complications. *Clin Radiol* **49**: 857–62.

Leung, J., Guiney, M. and Das, R. (1996). Intraluminal brachytherapy in bile duct carcinomas. *Aust N Z J Surg* **66**: 74–7.

Miyazaki, M., Itoh, H., Ambiru, S. *et al.* (1996). Radical surgery for advanced gallbladder carcinoma. *Br J Surg* **83**: 478–81.

Nichols, D. M. and Macleod, A. J. (1998). Choledocholithiasis associated with malignant biliary obstruction – significance and management. *Clin Radiol* **53**: 49–52.

Ogura, Y. and Kawarada, Y. (1998). Surgical strategies for carcinoma of the hepatic duct confluence. *Br J Surg* **85**: 20–4.

Parc, Y., Frileux, P., Balladur, P. *et al.* (1997). Surgical strategy for the management of hilar bile duct cancer. *Br J Surg* **84**: 1675–9.

Prat, F., Chapat, O., Ducot, B. *et al.* (1998). Predictive factors for survival of patients with inoperable malignant distal biliary strictures: a practical management guideline. *Gut* **42**: 76–80.

Rijken, A. M., Offerhaus, G. J., Polak, M. M. *et al.* (1999). p53 expression as a prognostic determinant in resected distal bile duct carcinoma. *Eur J Surg Oncol* **25**: 297–301.

Sasaki, A., Aramaki, M., Kawano, K. *et al.* (1998). Intrahepatic peripheral cholangiocarcinoma: mode of spread and choice of surgical treatment. *Br J Surg* **85**: 1206–9.

Scott-Coombes, D. M. and Williamson, R. C. (1994). Surgical treatment of primary duodenal carcinoma: a personal series. *Br J Surg* **81**: 1472–4.

Sithithaworn, P., Haswell-Elkins, M. R. *et al.* (1994). Parasite-associated morbidity: liver fluke infection and bile duct cancer in northeast Thailand. *Int J Parasitol* **24**: 833–43.

Tamada, K., Yasuda, Y., Nagai, H. *et al.* (1999). Limitation of cholangiography in assessing longitudinal spread of extrahepatic bile duct carcinoma to the hepatic side. *J Gastroenterol Hepatol* **14**: 691–8.

van Gulik, T. M., Rauws, E. A., Gonzalez Gonzalez, D. *et al.* (1997). Pre- and post-operative irradiation in the treatment of resectable Klatskin tumours. *Ned Tijdschr Geneeskd* **141**: 1331–7.

Wang, Y. J., Lee, S. D., Shyu, J. K. and Lo, K. J. (1994). Clinical experience in 126 patients with tissue-proved proximal cholangiocarcinoma. *J Gastroenterol Hepatol* **9**: 134–7.

Watanapa, P. (1996). Cholangiocarcinoma in patients with opisthorchiasis. *Br J Surg* **83**: 1062–64.

Miscellaneous

Cello, J. P. (1989). Acquired immunodeficiency syndrome cholangiopathy: spectrum of disease. *Am J Med* **86**: 539–46.

La Raja, L. A., Rothenberg, R. B., Odom, J. W. *et al.* (1989). The incidence of intra-abdominal surgery in acquired immunodeficiency syndrome: a statistical review of 904 patients. *Surgery* **105**: 175–9.

MODULE 11

Disorders of the spleen and lymph nodes

The spleen and lymph nodes combined constitute the bulk of the reticuloendothelial (monocyte–macrophage) system. During fetal development, the spleen serves a transient role of haematopoiesis. In adult life the spleen and lymph nodes share many functions with regard to immune processing, and are therefore, not surprisingly, commonly involved in similar disease processes.

Section 11.1 • Surgical anatomy of the spleen

The spleen is situated in the left upper quadrant tucked under and against the left dome of the diaphragm and overlain by the lower ninth to eleventh left ribs such that it is impalpable and has to enlarge two to three times before it becomes palpable on examination. It is overlapped anteriorly by the fundus of the stomach with its long axis lying along the line of the tenth rib. The normal dimensions of the spleen are 13 × 9 × 3 cm, although size even in healthy individual varies considerably. It has an anterior and posterior extremity (pole), superior and inferior borders and two surfaces: visceral facing antero-inferiorly and convex postero-superior (diaphragmatic). The visceral surface is in contact with the stomach, tail of the pancreas, left kidney (and adrenal) and splenic flexure of the colon, all of which cast impressions on this surface (Figure 11.1). The spleen is attached to the diaphragm and retroperitoneal organs by a fascia and peritoneal folds: splenocolic, diaphragmatic and lienorenal. The attachment to the fundus of the stomach is via the gastrosplenic section of the greater omentum that contains the short gastric vessels. Especially in obese subjects, the spleen is often covered with greater omentum, which indeed may be adherent to the surface of the organ.

The spleen varies in shape and three morphological types are described: crescentic (hilum extends from prominent superior to inferior poles), rhomboid (hilum forms a wide U) and triangular (with triangular hilum). It consists of red pulp (80%) made up of sinuses and sinusoids and cellular cords containing macrophages, and white pulp consisting lymphoid tissue (20%). The red pulp is concerned with maturation and the removal of damaged and senescent red cells, whereas the white pulp forms a major component of the cellular immune surveillance and protection of the body.

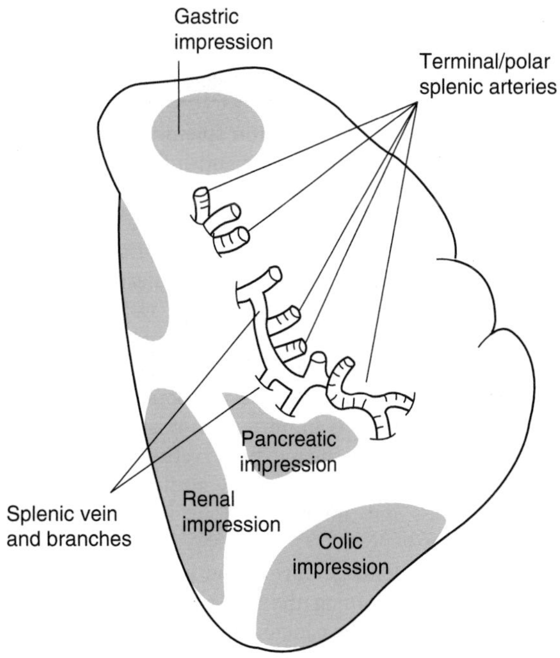

Figure 11.1 Visceral surface and hilum of the spleen.

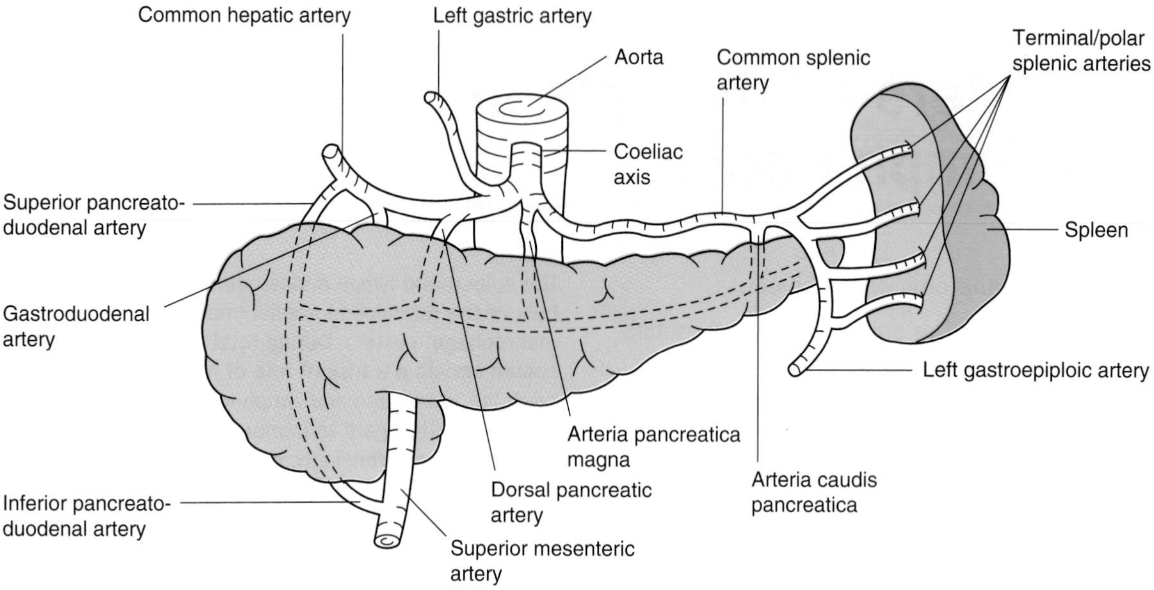

Figure 11.2 Arterial supply to the pancreas and spleen.

Blood supply of the spleen

The main arterial supply is from the common splenic artery (origin from the coeliac axis) which is tortuous and runs along the upper border of the pancreas. It gives rise to the following branches before dividing into its two terminal branches to the spleen (Figure 11.2):

- arteria colli pancreatis (pancreatica magna) – supplies neck of pancreas
- arteria corporis pancreatis – supplies the body of pancreas
- arteria caudis pancreatis – supplies tail of pancreas
- dorsal pancreatic artery – divides into right (to uncinate) and left (tail of pancreas) branches running transversely behind the pancreas
- short gastric vessels – to proximal stomach (two to four in number)
- left gastroepiploic – to greater curvature of stomach.

The division of the common splenic artery into its two terminal arteries (superior and inferior) occurs at a variable distance from the spleen. The two terminal arteries give off the segmental arteries to the spleen. The central segmental arteries always arise from the two terminal arteries, but the segmental arteries to the poles of the spleen (polar) have very variable origin (directly from common splenic artery, from terminal arteries and in the case of the lower polar artery, from the gastroepiploic artery). The segmental vasculature nature of the spleen is important in relation to partial splenectomy and to splenic preservation. The splenic segments, which are separated by avascular planes, are arteriovenous, and are usually four in number: two central and two polar.

The venous drainage mirrors the arterial supply with the splenic vein joining the superior mesenteric vein behind the neck of the pancreas to form the portal vein. The spleen also drains through the short gastric veins and these assume importance in two situations. In the first instance, they become varicose and lead to gastric varices when the splenic vein becomes thrombosed. Secondly, they provide the basis of transplenic decompression of oesophageal varices by the distal splenorenal shunt of Warren. The microcirculation of the spleen is unique and has two systems – closed and open circulation (Figure 11.3)

Accessory spleens

These are also known as splenunculi and are present in 10% of adults (Figure 11.4). They can be multiple but rarely exceed 10 and most are situated near the hilum (tail of the pancreas, gastrosplenic ligament, lienorenal ligament and greater omentum). However they can be located in other sites including the omentum along the

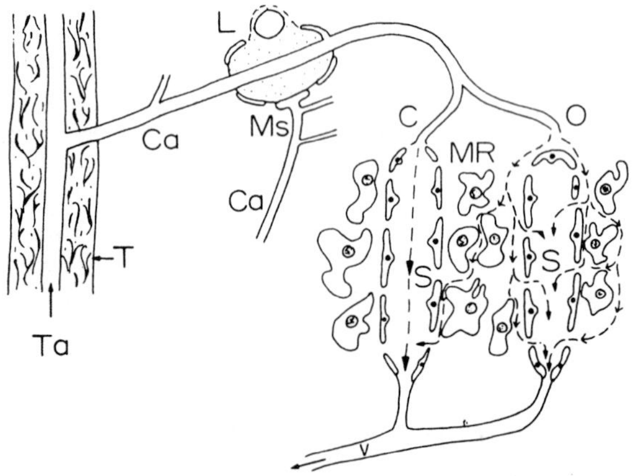

Figure 11.3 Splenic microcirculation: T = trabeculum, Ta = trabecular artery, CA = central artery, L = lymphoid tissue, Ms = marginal sinus, C = closed circulation, O = open circulation, MR = macrophages and reticulum of red pulp, S = sinus, V = collecting vein.

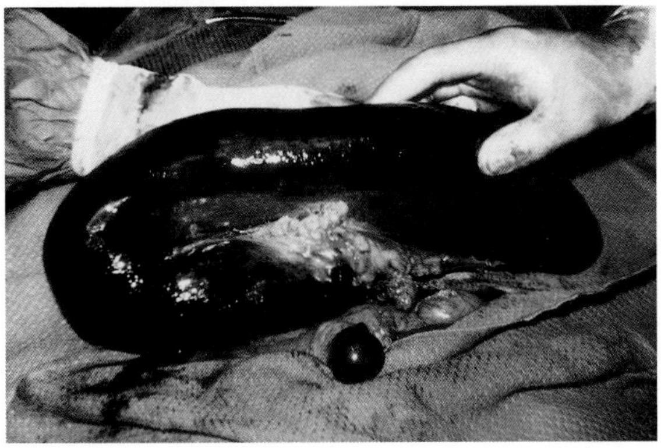

Figure 11.4 Accessory spleen during open splenectomy.

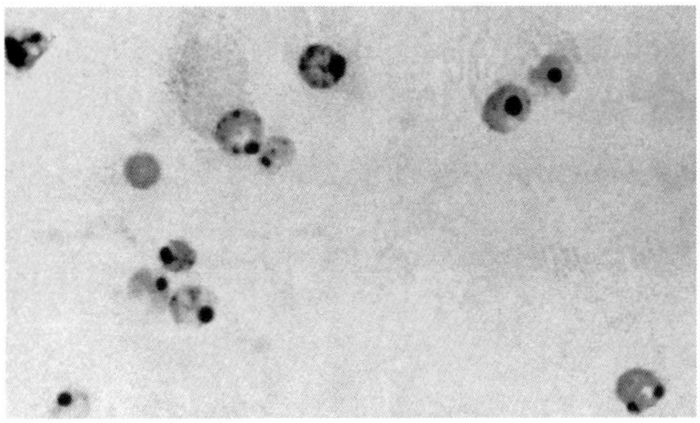

Figure 11.5 Blood film after removal of the spleen. The red cells contain ribonucleoprotein granules (Howell–Jolly bodies) which are normally pitted out by the spleen (Giemsa stain × 680).

greater curvature of the stomach, the mesenteries of the small and large intestine, the broad ligament of the uterus and the pouch of Douglas. They have even been reported in the left testis. Accessory spleens probably result from failure or incorporation of subsegments during embryological development. They have an organized splenic architecture and separate arterial supply usually from the inferior polar artery. Accessory spleens are important during splenectomy for haematological conditions such as immune thrombocytopenic purpura as if left behind, they may hypertrophy and cause recurrence of the disease. There is some evidence that accessory spleens are less easily identified during laparoscopic splenectomy.

Section 11.2 • Functions of the spleen and lymph nodes

Haematological functions of the spleen

Because of the peculiar anatomical arrangements of its blood vessels, the spleen is ideally suited as a site of 'quality control' of the erythrocyte population. It removes fragmented, damaged or senescent red cells from the circulation – a process known as culling. It also plays a role in the remodelling of the surface of maturing erythrocytes and in preserving the normal relationship between their membrane surface area and volume. Target cells, which have a relatively high ratio of membrane to intracellular haemoglobin, appear in the peripheral blood soon after splenectomy. A variety of intra-erythrocyte inclusions are removed by the spleen in a process known as pitting, after which the red cells are returned to the circulation. Among the inclusions removed are Howell–Jolly bodies which are probably nuclear remnants (Figure 11.5), siderotic granules (haemosiderin aggregates laid down during normal erythroid maturation) and Heinz bodies which are pathological aggregates of denatured haemoglobin. Thus after splenectomy, Howell–Jolly bodies and siderotic granules may be seen in the peripheral blood, and red cells show striking changes in shape and size, including the appearance of acanthocytes, irregularly crenated cells and target forms.

The spleen is very effective in the clearance of particulate matter from the circulation – an important function for the timely immune response to blood-borne antigens. The human spleen, contrary to that of other animals, holds relatively little blood in relation to the circulating blood volume, and as such has no significant role in blood storage. Within its volume, however, is a large number of sequestered platelets. Following splenectomy, there is a transient thrombocytosis that can lead to a clinically significant hypercoagulable state.

The spleen is involved with haemopoiesis only in fetal life with virtually no blood formation in the organ after birth. However, there may be a reversion to this fetal pattern of erythropoiesis in certain disease states and it is thought that the spleen may become an important organ of red cell production in at least some patients with progressive fibrosis of the bone marrow, i.e. myelosclerosis (Figure 11.6). A variable amount of splenic haematopoiesis also occurs in children with congenital haemolytic anaemia.

Immunological functions of the spleen and lymph nodes

The spleen and lymph nodes are shown diagrammatically and histologically in Figure 11.7. Each population of lymphocytes is in constant flux, with a continuous re-circulation of lymph into the blood stream at the thoracic duct. About one-half of the small lymphocytes of the spleen are migratory. Approximately one-quarter of the body's entire population of T-cells reside within the spleen at any point in time.

Lymphocytes enter the lymph nodes through the permeable walls of the post-capillary (epithelioid) venules of the paracortex; in the spleen, the site of transit is the marginal sinuses bordering the Malpighian corpuscles. T-cells tend to congregate in the paracortex of lymph nodes and form a periarteriolar lymphoid sheath in the spleen. B-cells congregate between the T-cells to form small clusters, or primary follicles, at the periphery of the outer cortex of nodes or in the spleen, adjacent to the marginal sinuses. A humoral response

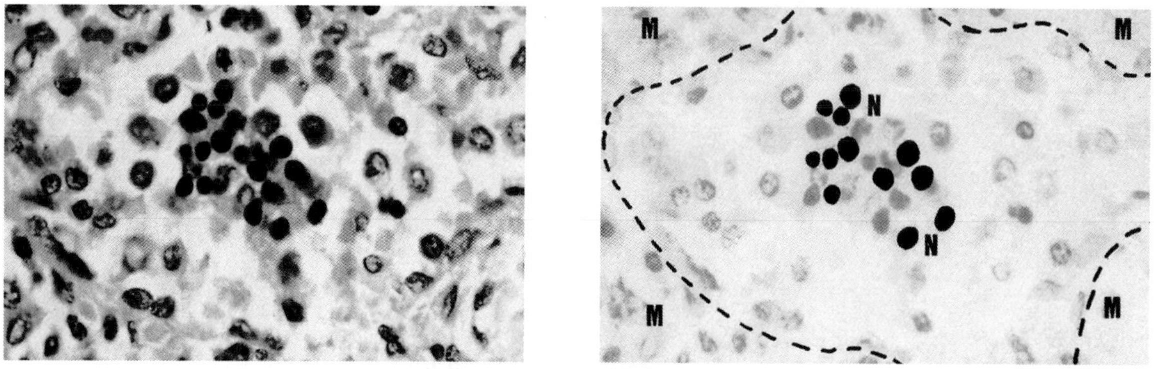

Figure 11.6 An erythropoietic island within a sinusoid in the red pulp of the spleen from a patient with myelosclerosis. N = normoblast, --- = wall of sinus, M = red pulp meshwork surrounding the sinus.

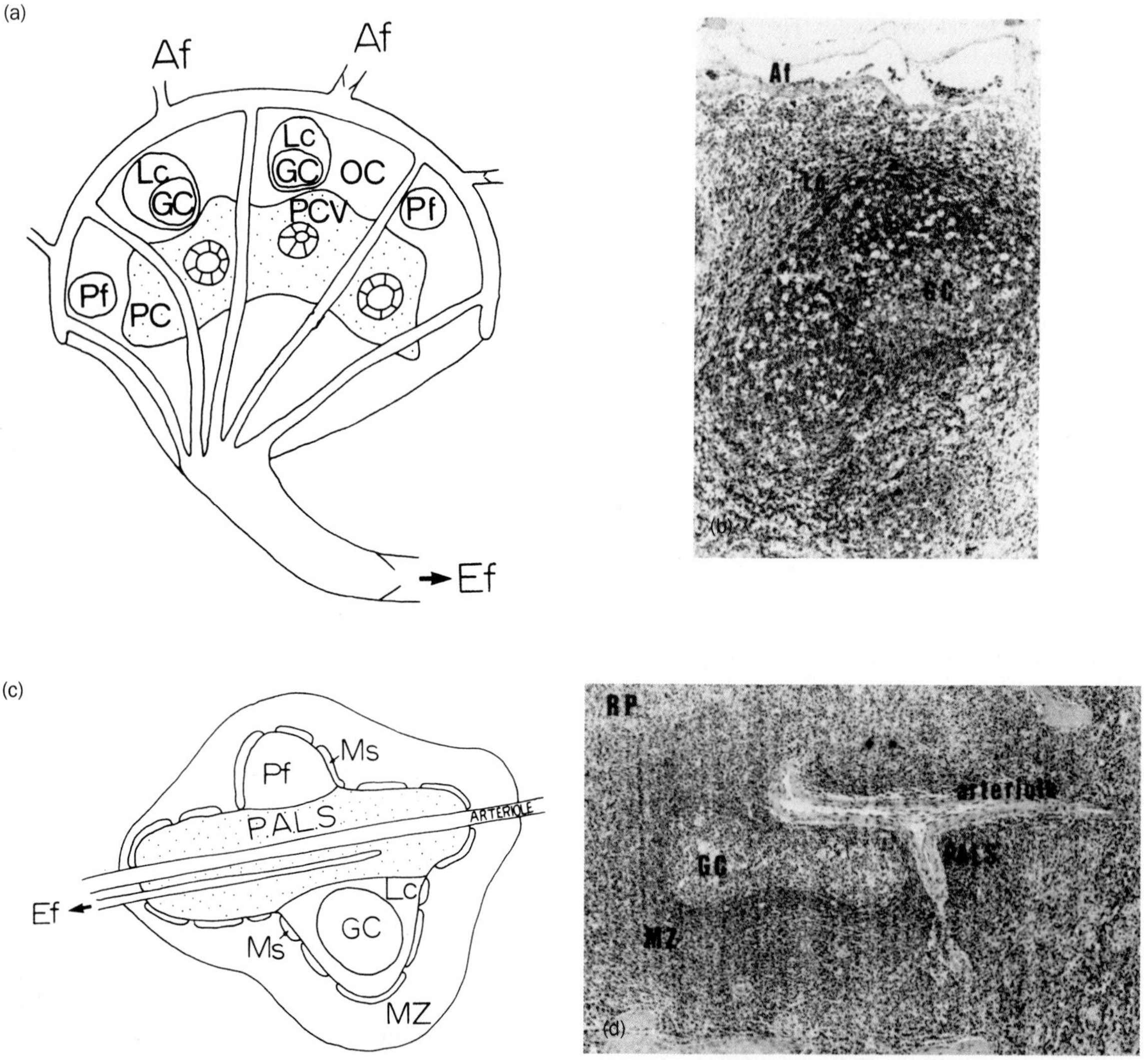

Figure 11.7 Basic arrangement of lymphoid tissue in lymph node and spleen. (a) Diagram of lymphatic arrangement in lymph node. (b) Photomicrograph of a section of the spleen showing some of the features illustrated in (a). (c) Lymphatic arrangement in the splenic Malpighian body. (d) Photomicrograph of a section of spleen illustrating some of the features shown in (c). Af = afferent lymphatic, OC = outer cortex, Pf = primary follicle, GC = germinal centre, Lc = small lymphocyte corona, PC = paracortex, PCV = post-capillary venule, Ef = efferent lymphatic, MZ = marginal zone of large lymphocytes, Ms = marginal sinus, PALS periarteriolar small lymphocyte sheath, RP = red pulp.

following antigenic stimulation involves co-operation between T- and B-cells possibly at the site of antigen localization on the surface of large dentritic cells. Immunoglobulin-synthesizing cells appear within days in the medullary cords of lymph nodes and in the red pulp of the spleen. Germinal centres, or secondary follicles, later appear within the primary follicles, and reach their maximum development about 8 weeks following antigenic stimulation. Mature lymphocyte populations exhibit numerous mitotic figures, and are enlarged and plump in comparison to senescent ones.

There is a described phenomenon of 'ineffective lymphopoiesis' within the spleen and lymph nodes. The nuclear remains of pyknotic cells are phagocytosed by macrophages, giving rise to so-called 'tingible bodies'. It may be that these represent 'forbidden clones' (capable of destroying self) and are recognized and destroyed at this stage within the spleen. The spleen may also be the major source for the production of suppressor T-cells. It is further thought that each secondary follicle produces polyclonal 'memory' B-cells. Such follicles may also be responding to more than one antigen.

A cellular immune response can be recognized by T-cell enlargement within the paracortex, cytoplasmic RNA synthesis, and cell division. Some cells leave the lymph nodes by way of the efferent lymphatics travelling up the thoracic duct to populate other lymphoid areas via the blood stream. Efferent lymphatics from the spleen run adjacent to the arterioles, but most lymphoid cells probably leave in vascular channels originating in the white pulp. These channels continue through the marginal zone and open into the red pulp sinuses.

These observations reinforce the fact that lymphoid tissues are not static collections of cells. There is a constant motion of cells through a reticulin scaffolding. Specific stimuli and reactions affect particular components of these populations. When clones of 'well differentiated' cells emerge, as for example, in chronic lymphatic leukaemia, they frequently retain the capacity to migrate, differentiate and form deposits in other distant body sites, e.g. the bone marrow. Structural tumours analogous to follicle centres can arise within a lymph node or group of nodes (follicle cell centre tumours of Luke), and as such may give rise to clones of circulating small cleaved cells that infiltrate and populate other lymphoid areas without causing architectural distortion. Such tumours of small, round, re-circulating lymphocytes and follicle centre cleaved cells account for 80% of the acute non-Hodgkin's lymphomas seen in the UK.

Monocytes are sequestered in the white pulp, the marginal sinuses and the red pulp of the spleen. It is in the red pulp where they are converted to fixed macrophages, endowing the spleen with its significant phagocytic capability. It is thought that the spleen, in disease states such as malaria, releases a humoral substance that acts on the bone marrow to cause release of additional monocytes. They eventually circulate to the spleen and can repopulate or further augment its phagocytic capabilities.

Table 11.1 Functions of the spleen and lymph nodes

- **Immunological (both spleen and lymph nodes)**
  - Antibody production and cell mediated responses
  - Phagocytosis
  - Maturation of lymphoid cells
  - Significant lymphopoiesis
  - Source of suppressor T-cells
- **Haematological (primarily spleen)**
  - Filtration of particles from blood: non-specific or antibody coated
  - Removal of red cell inclusions
  - Destruction of senescent or abnormal red cells
  - Compensatory haemopoiesis
  - Storage of platelets, iron and factor VIII

Following splenectomy, the primary antibody response is decreased compared to normal, and the secondary response is abnormal in that there is an impaired switching from IgM to IgG antibody subtypes. In addition to antibody synthesis, the spleen produces non-specific effectors of the immune response, such as the tetrapeptide tuftsin. Tuftsin (named after Tufts University where it was identified and characterized) opsonizes particulate matter, and as such facilitates phagocytic activity. It is virtually absent in the blood of asplenic patients. The spleen also influences the opsonization of pneumococci in non-immune individuals and is involved in the alternative pathway of complement activation. All these mechanisms probably account for the increased susceptibility to post-splenectomy sepsis especially in infants and children. The spleen and lymph nodes both contribute to the immunological surveillance of the host, whereas the spleen additionally performs an important haematological role (Table 11.1).

Section 11.3 • Disorders of the spleen

The most frequently recognized complication of the diseased spleen is the pathological destruction or pooling of blood elements. Splenic enlargement, as it occurs with venous thrombosis and congestion, causes entrapment and pooling that results in destruction of normal cells. This is an exaggeration of the normal function of the macrophage-laden vasculature of the spleen, i.e. the destruction of abnormal red cells, white cells or platelets as they are filtered through the spleen.

Hypersplenism

Hypersplenism is a syndrome of splenomegaly combined with decreased amounts of one or more circulating blood elements:

- anaemia – in patients with diseased bone marrow
- leucopenia < 4–$5000 \times mm^3$
- thrombocytopenia $< 100\,000 \times mm^3$.

Early on, hypersplenism was used to describe the essentially normal function of the spleen in destroying the abnormal cells of hereditary spherocytosis.

Damashek broadened this definition to include *all conditions of splenomegaly with decreased numbers of one or more of the blood elements.* Although he postulated that the spleen was active in the control of haemopoiesis via humoral mechanisms, this has no current scientific basis. Some distinguish between primary (due to haematological disease) and secondary (e.g. liver disease with portal hypertension) hypersplenism.

Work hypertrophy of the spleen occurs when the spleen enlarges due to the constant exposure of the spleen's phagocytic machinery to abnormal cells. This is distinctly different from splenomegaly, where destruction of normal blood elements occurs because of a *primary lymphoreticular* process. The term primary hypersplenism is usually reserved for this latter group of disorders as distinct from hyperactivity following splenic enlargement from other causes, e.g. liver disease – *secondary hypersplenism.* In hypersplenism states, the bone marrow is unable to maintain normal numbers of circulating cells or platelets, and splenic enlargement signals the site of destruction. Splenectomy is potentially curative of the cytopenias that occur in hypersplenic states but there are other alternatives (*vide infra*).

The exact cause of the cytopenia that occurs with splenic enlargement is a matter of some speculation. The pooling of blood cells is probably the most important mechanism. With increasing splenic size, up to 50% of the total red cell mass may reside in the spleen. This effectively sequesters red cells in a location 'outside' the circulation. The amount of this isolation of red cells can be estimated by measuring peripheral venous haematocrit and comparing that to the red cell volume obtained by isotope dilution techniques.

In a similar fashion, platelets are abnormally sequestered in states of splenomegaly. Approximately 10% of circulating platelets are contained within the spleen in the healthy state. With significant splenomegaly and pooling of blood elements, up to 90% of the circulating platelets are trapped within the spleen. The same can occur with circulating granulocytes and lymphocytes.

The overall effect of such congestive splenomegaly is a dynamic balance between the trapping of blood elements and the ability of the bone marrow to compensate. In disorders with a diminished bone marrow reserve, such as myelosclerosis or chronic myeloid leukaemia, severe anaemia, thrombocytopenia and/or neutropenia may result. If the marrow is healthy or minimally diseased, the peripheral smear may be quite normal.

Hypervolaemia is also a feature of splenomegaly. Where red cell production is limited, the expanded blood volume is mainly plasma volume, with a resultant dilutional anaemia that can compound the destructive anaemia. It is thought that a hyperkinetic portal circulation from an increased splenic blood flow somehow causes an expansion of the splanchnic blood volume. The exact mechanism is far from clear, however. Because of the expanded circulating volume, transfusion in an attempt to restore appropriate numbers of cellular elements can easily cause circulatory overload.

Destruction of blood cells by the spleen

In addition to pooling and trapping within the spleen, the survival of red cells is probably shortened because of 'metabolic stresses'. These include glucose deprivation, lactate accumulation and cellular acidosis due to abnormally close packing of the red cells. The haemolytic component of this specific type of hypersplenism is mild, however. There is less solid evidence for the thrombocytopenia and neutropenia due to these mechanisms.

The spleen routinely destroys abnormal red cells. The cytoskeletal defect manifest as hereditary spherocytosis causes these abnormal red cells to be particularly susceptible to destruction within the spleen. In addition to destroying senescent and diseased red cells, the spleen is active in policing for red cell inclusions such as Heinz bodies (haemoglobin precipitates), via selective membrane disruption and capture of these undesirable intracellular defects.

The spleen also maintains surveillance of surface abnormalities of cells and platelets. In this way, red cells coated with antibody are destroyed via macrophage recognition of the constant portion of the IgG, producing autoimmune haemolytic anaemia. A similar mechanism is probably responsible for the destruction of platelets in certain forms of idiopathic or drug-induced thrombocytopenic states. Additionally, the neutropenia seen in Felty's syndrome (rheumatoid arthritis and splenomegaly) has an immune basis, probably due to a circulating leucocyte-specific antinuclear factor. The conditions in which splenomegaly can occur with varying degrees of hypersplenism are listed in Table 11.2. *In practice however 45% of cases of hypersplenism are caused by haematological disease and 40% by liver disease with portal hypertension. Thus all the other causes together account for only 5%.*

Management of hypersplenism associated with chronic liver disease

Whereas splenectomy is the recognized treatment for hypersplenism due to haematological disease as it usually normalizes all the components of the cytopenia, the management of hypersplenism associated with chronic liver disease remains non-standardized and currently there are a number of options with no comparative data on efficacy and morbidity. To a large extent therefore, the treatment depends on local expertise and preferences. Factors that should influence management in the individual case include the severity (Child-Pugh stage) of the disease and the need for treatment of other complications, e.g. bleeding varices, the development of hepatoma in a cirrhotic patient, or an end-stage cirrhotic patient requiring liver transplantation.

The most important aspect of hypersplenism in patients with chronic liver disease is the thrombocytopenia and it is this that requires correction in these patients. Active management is considered only in patients in whom the splenic congestion and the thrombocytopenia are severe. In general, open splenec-

Table 11.2 Disorders producing splenomegaly

- **Infections**
  Acute: hepatitis, mononucleosis, salmonellosis, toxoplasmosis, cytomegalovirus, tularaemia, abscess
  Subacute: AIDS, bacterial endocarditis, tuberculosis, brucellosis, malaria, leishmaniasis, trypanosomiasis, histoplasmosis
  Chronic: fungal disease, syphilis, bacterial endocarditis
- **Congestive**
  Intrahepatic portal hypertension: cirrhosis, Wilson's disease, haemochromatosis, congenital hepatic fibrosis
  Pre-hepatic portal hypertension: portal vein thrombosis, obstruction, cavernoma, atresia
  Post-hepatic: Budd-Chiari, congestive cardiac failure
  Segmental (left sided portal hypertension): splenic vein occlusion by pancreatitis, pancreatic neoplasm, pancreatic pseudocyst, splenic artery aneurysm
- **Haematological**
  Haemolytic disorders: hereditary cell membrane defects, autoimmune haemolytic states (warm antibodies), thalassaemia, sickle cell disease, haemoglobin C disease
  Myeloproliferative disorders: myeloid metaplasia, polycythaemia vera, essential thrombocytaemia
  Miscellaneous: primary splenic hyperplasia, megaloblastic anaemia, iron deficiency
- **Malignant**
  Haematological malignancies: acute or chronic leukaemias, leukaemic reticuloendotheliosis, malignant lymphomas, malignant histiocytosis, myelomatosis
  Primary intrinsic malignancies: lymphosarcoma, plasmocytoma, fibrosarcoma, angiosarcoma
  Intrinsic secondary malignancies: carcinoma, melanoma
  Benign: hamartoma, fibroma, haemangioma, lymphangioma
- **Inflammatory or granulomatous**
  Felty's syndrome, systemic lupus, rheumatic fever, serum sickness, sarcoidosis, beryllosis
- **Storage disease**
  Gaucher's disease, Wilson's disease, Niemann–Pick syndrome, histiocytosis X, Hurler's syndrome, Tangier disease
- **Miscellaneous**
  Cysts: parasitic, pseudocysts, congenital, traumatic
  Others: hyperthyroidism, Osler-Weber-Rendu syndrome, splenic masocytosis, Albers-Schonberg disease

tomy is ill-advised in patients with liver disease and portal hypertension because it constitutes is a major high-risk operation and may be followed by thrombosis of the portal vein.

The options for the treatment of severe thrombocytopenia in patients with liver disease and portal hypertension are:

- distal splenorenal shunt (Warren procedure)
- transjugular intrahepatic portosystemic shunt (TIPSS)
- laparoscopic splenectomy
- partial splenic embolization.

Distal splenorenal shunt (DSRS) effectively reverses the profound thrombocytopenia resulting from presinusoidal portal hypertension or stable cirrhosis without sacrificing the spleen and in some centres is considered the treatment of choice for this condition in children. It is used as the only procedure (Child A/B patients) or before hepatic transplantation (Child C disease).

TIPSS appears to improve the hypersplenism in patients with portal hypertension. In one large reported series, the leucopenia was reversed in 50% and thrombocytopenia in 75% of patients. These early results indicate that TIPSS is a promising minimal access intervention that is effective in the treatment of complications of portal hypertension including secondary hypersplenism and may replace the use of DSRS in some adults. The problem with TIPSS is its poor long-term patency (beyond 6–12 months). The ideal indication seems to be patients with Child C disease awaiting liver transplantation.

In adult patients with end-stage liver disease and hypersplenism awaiting liver transplantation, and in patients with Child A/B disease requiring hepatic resection for small hepatoma, laparoscopic splenectomy prior to the liver resection/transplantation has been performed as an the alternative to TIPSS. Others advise concomitant splenectomy at the time of hepatic resection.

The fourth option in the management of patients with portal hypertension and hypersplenism is partial splenic embolization (PSE). This has to ablate 50% or more of the splenic parenchyma to be effective. It was initially reported to be successful in reversing the hypersplenism (thrombocytopenia and neutropenia) in 90% of patients undergoing embolization of hepatocellular carcinoma (HCC) and appears to be safe with a low reported incidence of severe complications including splenic abscess formation. PSE was subsequently extended to Child A or Child B (but not Child C) patients with liver disease, where it is reported to also normalize the levels of cholinesterase, total cholesterol and prothrombin time in addition to haematological improvement of the hypersplenism.

Hyposplenism

The more common causes of hyposplenism and the haematological features of such states are summarized in Tables 11.3 and 11.4. Hyposplenism is confirmed by the appearance of red cell defects (that normally would be culled from the circulation), and the degree of impairment may be qualitatively assessed by ^{99m}technetium-sulphocolloid scintiscanning. There is some evidence based on the percentage of pitted cells in the peripheral blood that splenic function is impaired in

Table 11.3 Causes of asplenism and hyposplenism

- Splenectomy
- Splenic agenesis
- Atrophy:
  Coeliac disease
  Inflammatory bowel disease and collagenous colitis
  Systemic amyloidosis
  Alcoholism (?)
  Old age
  Dermatitis herpetiformis
  Sickle-cell anaemia
  Systemic lupus erythematosus

Table 11.4 Haematological changes in hyposplenism

- **Abnormal red cells:**
  Burr cells
  Target cells
  Pitted cells
- **Red cell inclusions:**
  Howell–Jolly bodies
  Siderotic granules
- **Abnormal platelet morphology**
- **Thrombocytosis**
- **Leucocytosis:**
  Neutrophilia
  Lymphocytosis
  Monocytosis

the elderly and in alcoholics. Pitted erythrocytes are found in 40% of alcoholics and this functional hyposplenism as been attributed to a direct effect of alcohol on the spleen as the pitted erythrocyte count drops in patients who give up the alcohol habit. However, the possibility that the high pitted erythrocyte count is caused by a direct effect of the alcohol on the red cell membrane can equally account for these changes and the controversy remains unresolved.

The most frequent cause of hyposplenism is surgical splenectomy. Congenital asplenia (Ivemark syndrome) is a truly rare disorder, associated with complex cardiac, gastrointestinal, genitourinary and neuromuscular abnormalities. Survival in such cases is largely determined by the ability to recognize and correct the complex cardiac defects. Gastrointestinal anomalies such as malrotation and situs inversus are frequently seen in congenital asplenia. In surviving infants, a common cause of death is overwhelming sepsis due to encapsulated organisms, particularly pneumococcal.

Splenic hypoplasia can also occur from birth as part of the syndrome of Fanconi's anaemia, i.e. congenital hypoplastic anaemia. Acquired hyposplenism occurs in about 76% of patients with coeliac disease. The cause is unknown, but may be related to the increased absorption of dietary antigen and subsequent overload of the spleen with circulating immune complexes. The hyposplenic state improves with a gluten-free diet in these individuals. There has also been noted a relationship between the morphological state of the intestinal epithelium and splenic function. Hyposplenic states have also been described in other disorders involving the gastrointestinal mucosa including Crohn's disease, ulcerative colitis, collagenous colitis and intestinal lymphangiectasia.

Circulating autoantibodies and immune complexes in clinical autoimmune disorders, e.g. systemic lupus erythematosus, have been noted to cause a functional hypoplastic state secondary to Fc-receptor blockage. The hyposplenism of sickle-cell anaemia is related to the degree of splenic infarction. Hyposplenism is also a feature of systemic amyloidosis.

Hyposplenism can also occur in patients with full-blown human immunodeficiency virus (HIV) and these patients usually present with the *Mycobacterium avium* complex (infection) complicating HIV-related immune thrombocytopenic purpura. This combination is usually lethal, as the severe thrombocytopenia does not improve with corticosteroids, intravenous immunoglobulin and splenectomy. The peripheral blood smear shows Howell–Jolly bodies. Pathological examination of the spleen shows multiple granulomas with numerous acid-fast organisms.

Post-splenectomy sepsis

There is now uniform consensus that the risk of overwhelming sepsis is increased significantly after splenectomy. There is good evidence that the greatest risk is in infants and children (first 5 years of life), and to some extent, the risk in adults may have been overestimated in the past, although this is debatable. The problem of post-splenectomy sepsis has been compounded by the increasing incidence of penicillin-resistant pneumococci. The risk of post-splenectomy sepsis is also influenced by the nature of the disease for which the spleen is removed, with the lowest incidence of sepsis being reported after splenectomy for trauma as these individuals are otherwise healthy and have no other disease that impairs the immune defence against invading bacteria (Table 11.5).

Although the absolute lymphocyte count is increased after splenectomy for trauma, the peripheral blood lymphocyte subpopulations of these otherwise healthy subjects are distinctly abnormal. There is a significant reduction in the percentage of $CD4^+$ T-cells due to a selective and long-term decrease in the percentage of $CD4^+CD45RA^+$ lymphocytes. These decreased levels of $CD4^+CD45RA^+$ cells are accompanied by an impairment of the primary immune responsiveness both in terms of T-cell proliferation and antibody responses to newly encountered antigens. By contrast, levels of the reciprocal $CD45RO^+CD4^+$ T-cell subset, lymphoproliferative responses and IFN-gamma production to recall antigens remain normal. These findings suggest that the intact spleen is essential for the generation, maintenance and/or differentiation of unprimed T-cells or their precursors and may explain the impaired primary immune responses following splenectomy.

Table 11.5 Incidence of post-splenectomy sepsis in relation to indication

Indication for splenectomy	*Incidence of sepsis (%)*
Trauma	1.4
Immune (idiopathic) thrombocytopenia	2.0
Incidental (iatrogenic injury)	2.1
Congenital spherocytosis	3.5
Acquired haemolytic anaemia	7.5
Portal hypertension	8.2
Primary anaemia	8.5
Reticulosis/lymphomas	11.5
Thalassaemia	24.8

Modified from Singer, D. B. Postsplenectomy sepsis. *Perspectives in Pediatric Pathology* 1973; **1**: 285–311.

Splenectomy for trauma carries the lowest risk and thalassaemia the highest; but even for the lowest risk group, there is still a 40–50-fold increase in the incidence of overwhelming sepsis. Some of these estimates have been questioned largely because the majority of reported series have had small numbers, and indeed a substantial cohort of the data (on which estimates are based) are from single case reports of pneumococcal serious infections often with bacteraemia. It is an undeniable fact that community-acquired pneumococcal pneumonia with bacteraemia is common in patients with normal splenic function and is seldom reported because of its established occurrence in susceptible groups. Because of this, there are some who argue that the risk of post-splenectomy pneumococcal sepsis may have been exaggerated.

Although *Streptococcus pneumoniae* is implicated in over 55–60% of septic episodes in asplenic patients, infections by other encapsulated bacteria, e.g. *Haemophilus influenzae*, *Haemophilis pertussis* and *Neisseria meningitidis*, are also more commonly reported in these individuals, as indeed are infections by Gram-negative bacteria, e.g. *Escherichia coli*. The functional deficits in asplenic patients are numerous, but impaired filtration, diminished phagocytosis, decreased IgM levels and loss of the opsonic tetrapeptide tuftsin all contribute to the increased risk.

The syndrome of overwhelming post-splenectomy infection (OPSI) often begins insidiously. From a nonspecific viral-like illness or malaise, the course rapidly turns fulminant. High fever, nausea, vomiting, dehydration, hypotension and obtundation occur with alarming speed, death being the end result if the course of events is not quickly reversed by effective resuscitation and aggressive antibiotic therapy. Gram stain of the peripheral blood smears will occasionally reveal the causative organism and blood culture is invariably positive. The mortality rate of OPSI is 50–80% for all cases combined. Post-mortem examination often reveals bilateral adrenal haemorrhage (Waterhouse–Friedrichsen syndrome).

The treatment of suspected episodes of OPSI should be aggressive and without any delay. Broad-spectrum antibiotics effective against encapsulated cocci in the first instance are administered intravenously. Intravenous colloids are used to correct the hypovolaemia using CVP and urine output monitoring within an intensive care setting. Altered haemostasis and disseminated intravascular coagulation can occur, and replacement products (fresh frozen plasma, platelets) are often required.

The prevention of OPSI is imperfect at best and is based on vaccination, administration of oral penicillins and patient education. Prophylactic antibiotic therapy is recommended (together with vaccination) in children and some would extend it indefinitely to adults. Whilst this is sensible for the high-risk groups, there is less of an argument for long-term prophylactic antibiotics in adults undergoing splenectomy for trauma or iatrogenic injury sustained during abdominal surgery. The vaccination should be carried out at least 10–14 days prior to splenectomy for maximum effective immunization. The vaccination programme should always include the polyvalent pneumococcal vaccine and *Haemophilus* vaccines. Unfortunately the pneumococcal vaccine (against 23 most prevalent strains) does not provide immunity against all strains. Not all vaccinated patients develop immunity but the majority do, and the titres of anti-pneumococcal antibodies remain elevated for up to 42 months. The question of booster immunizations has not been resolved. Immunization after splenectomy (trauma cases) is much less effective but some advise it anyway.

Since no form of prophylaxis is completely effective, it is very important that all patients carry 'splenectomy' cards, and close surveillance and specific patient education are mandatory. At the first sign of infection, all patients with hyposplenic states should be strongly advised to seek medical attention and receive antibiotic therapy.

Splenic infarction

Infarction of the spleen is not uncommon and its clinical presentation is variable. Thus some patients have severe acute symptoms and signs, and may develop serious life-threatening complications (splenic rupture, splenic abscess), whereas others (up to 30%) have minor symptoms or are asymptomatic.

Aside from the predictable auto-infarction in patients with sickle-cell disease, splenic infarction occurs most commonly with splenomegaly due to congestive disorders such as chronic myeloid leukaemia and myelosclerosis. Thrombo-embolic disorders may cause splenic infarction, e.g. atrial fibrillation, arterial embolic (atheromatous) disease, diabetes-associated microvascular disease and acute torsion of an *ectopic (wandering) spleen*. A variety of other disorders may be complicated with the development of splenic infarction, e.g. falciparum malaria, Q fever, acquired immunodeficiency syndrome (AIDS), severe necrotizing pancreatitis, pancreatic pseudocysts. Splenic infarction has also been reported as a complication of injection of gastric varices with Histoacryl. The splenic infarction in patients with AIDS is associated with the development of high titres of anticardiolipin antibodies, thrombocytopenia and a coagulopathy. Episodes of cerebrovascular infarction may also occur in these patients. The cause of the splenic infarction in these AIDS patients is arterial thrombosis of the coeliac trunk.

The age range of splenic infarction varies widely (children to old age) and 70% are symptomatic. The most common symptoms are acute upper left quadrant abdominal pain, fever, chills and malaise. However a significant cohort are asymptomatic and these are usually patients with non-malignant haematological disorders. Fever and leucocytosis are especially marked in patients with thromboembolism as the cause for the splenic infarction. Physical examination reveals tenderness and guarding maximal in the left upper abdomen. Splenic infarction results in a capsular inflammatory reaction frequently causing irritation of the left diaphragm. This may result in left basal pleurisy/effusion and pain referred to the left shoulder (Kerr's sign). Confirmation of the diagnosis is usually achieved by abdominal angio-computed tomographic (CT) scan.

Initially, the management should be conservative with analgesia and antibiotics. Surgery is indicated if the diagnosis is in doubt or for complications (splenic abscess, bleeding from splenic rupture) when splenectomy is indicated. The morbidity (mainly pulmonary complications) is high and the mortality averages 5% overall.

Section 11.4 • Pathological changes in spleen and lymph nodes

The pathological processes affecting the spleen and/or lymph nodes can be categorized as:

- reactive
- non-Hodgkin's lymphomas
- Hodgkin's disease
- secondary tumour deposits.

Immunological reactivity

Reactive changes cause regional lymphadenopathy and, depending on the cause may be non-specific, granulomatous, epithelioid congeries and angioimmunoblastic with or without accompanying changes in the spleen (Table 11.6). The spleen and lymph nodes normally respond to antigen loads with an expansion of the mononuclear–macrophage and lymphocyte cell lines specific to the challenge. An antibody response results in the increased numbers of immunoglobulin-secreting B-cell proliferations in the medullary cords of the lymph nodes or red pulp of the spleen. Reactive follicle centres develop secondarily. Although bacteria that are coated with antibody are more rapidly cleared in the macrophage–monocyte/neutrophil systems than non-coated cells, it may be that such coating is counterproductive in the surveillance against tumour cells. Antibody-coated tumour cells may be less easily recognized as 'foreign' by cytotoxic T-cells.

T-cell proliferation follows vaccination or cellular challenges, and the result is expansion of the paracortex surrounding the epithelioid venules. This situation can simulate neoplasia even to the extent of producing binucleate, large cells resembling Reed-Sternberg cells. However, in this situation the architecture of the spleen or lymph node is maintained, and secondary follicle reactivation with plasma cells is usually seen.

Non-antigenic material within lymphatics, such as carbon pigment, is trapped in the medullary sinuses of lymph nodes. Blood-borne material, such as haemo-

Table 11.6 Reactive pathological changes caused by disease of lymph nodes and spleen

Reactive	*Lymph nodes*	*Spleen*
Non-specific – variable emphasis on:		
Sinus histiocytosis	Expansion of medullary cords by histiocytes. Removal of non-antigenic material, e.g. carbon, Hb or fat in dermatopathic lymphadenopathy, Gaucher's disease	Increased numbers of macrophages in red pulp
Follicle centre reactivity	Expanded reactive follicle centres. Numerous mitoses and tingible body macrophages	Development of reactive secondary follicles in Malpighian bodies
Paracortical	Expansion of paracortex by transforming T-cells, e.g. viral infections, post-viral infections	Expansion of periarterial lymphoid sheath by transforming T-cells
Plasma cell	Large numbers of polyclonal immunoglobulin-containing plasma cells in the medullary cords	Large numbers of plasma cells usually in the red pulp
Granulomatous:		
Non-caseating	Compact cortical epithelioid granulomas with Langerhans' giant cells, reticulin production and no necrosis in sarcoid, sarcoid reaction, e.g. draining tumours, beryllium poisoning	Similar granulomas, usually appearing first in the marginal zones
Caseating	Central caseous necrosis, often surrounding fibrosis, e.g. tuberculosis	May show amyloid deposition
Necrotising	Stellate micro-abscesses with polymorphs and peripheral pallisading of histiocytes, often with multinucleated giant cells, e.g. cat scratch fever, lymphogranuloma venereum	
Epithelioid congeries	Collections of small numbers of epithelioid histiocytes without caseation or giant cells in paracortex with active secondary centres, e.g. toxoplasmosis, visceral leishmaniasis (basophilic Leishman–Donovon bodies within histiocytes)	Red pulp greatly expanded by histiocytes containing L–D bodies in leishmaniasis
Angioimmunoblastic lymphadenopathy	Reactive hyperimmune state with proliferation of epithelioid venules, interstices filled with transforming lymphoid cells, polyclonal immunoblasts and mature plasma cells. May burn out leaving sclerotic nodes or progress to highly malignant immunoblastic sarcoma	

siderin, is trapped by splenic red pulp macrophages. Such non-antigenic entrapment can cause nodal enlargement, e.g. dermatopathic lymphadenopathy, Gaucher's disease (lipid storage disease) or thalassaemia/haemolysis. Expansion of the histiocytic elements of lymph nodes and spleen occurs with parasitaemia (leishmaniasis, malaria) and to a lesser extent with toxoplasmosis and systemic leprosy. Malarial infestation adds immunoproliferative responses to such histiocytic expansion.

Neoplasia

Lymphomas are the primary tumours and are classified as Hodgkin's and non-Hodgkin's. Secondary tumours (deposits) affect largely the lymph nodes, as although they may involve the spleen, splenic metastases are very rare. Secondary lymph node tumour deposits are considered later on in this module.

The spectrum of non-Hodgkin's lymphomas arises in cells that typically are migratory throughout the lymphatic system. As such, the more differentiated a tumour, the more difficult it may be to demonstrate malignancy before gross architectural distortion occurs. This spectrum is evident by describing two diseases: *chronic lymphatic leukaemia* where the overproduced small B-lymphocytes continue to circulate, and *lymphocytic lymphoma* where a small population remains confined to lymph nodes. This wide variety of pathological states certainly makes it difficult for the pathologist and clinician both diagnostically as well as in recommending therapeutic action.

It is possible to demonstrate a clone of abnormal cells within the circulating pool of lymphocytes. Thus peripheral blood can be diagnostic when architectural distortion of the lymph nodes or spleen is not diagnostic. This also serves to confirm that even in well-differentiated lymphomas, the disease is usually systemic, and not just confined to the enlarged lymph nodes/organs.

Intermediate and high-grade lymphomas more typically destroy locally and invade, rather than migrate widely. They are also often highly sensitive to radiotherapy and chemotherapy. As they can grow quickly, disseminate late and are often noticed early by the patient, local therapy alone may be effective. It is because of this wide spectrum of presentation and variable systemic involvement that accurate clinical staging is imperative in the choice of therapeutic regimens. This is especially true, paradoxically, for the cytologically more 'benign' lower grade tumours, which are often metastatic at the time of initial diagnosis. The histopathology/classification of Hodgkin's disease and non-Hodgkin's lymphomas is summarized in Tables 11.7 and 11.8. It is important to stress that in Hodgkin's disease, a portion only of the lymph node may be involved and typically the spleen shows scattered foci of the disease. This is in sharp contrast to non-Hodgkin's lymphomas where there is total involvement of the nodes or the spleen.

A special type of extranodal non-Hodgkin's lymphoma arises from the mucosa-associated lymphoid tissue found in the respiratory epithelium, salivary glands and the gut. This may give rise to MALT-lymphomas or MALTomas, most commonly of the stomach [see Disorders of the stomach].

Hodgkin's disease spreads less often along contiguous groups of lymph nodes as compared to non-

Table 11.7 Revised European–American classification of Hodgkin's disease

I	Lymphocyte predominance
II	Provisional entity: lymphocyteprich classical Hodgkin's disease
III	Mixed cellularity
IV	Nodular sclerosis
V	Lymphocyte depletion

Table 11.8 Revised European classification of non-Hodgkin's lymphoid (based on morphological, immunological and molecular data; likely to replace all other confusing classifications)

B-cell lymphomas

B-cell neoplasms: precursor B-lymphoblastic leukaemia/lymphoma

Peripheral B-cell lymphomas

1. B-cell chronic lymphocyic precursor leukaemia/small lymphocytic lymphoma
2. Lymphoplasmatoid lymphoma/immunocytoma
3. Mantle cell lymphoma
4. Follicle centre lymphoma
5. Marginal; zone B-cell lymphomas
   Extranodal (MALT type ± monocytoid B-cells)
   Provisional subtype: nodal (± monocytoid B-cells)
6. Provisional entity: splenic marginal zone lymphoma (± villous lymphocytes)
7. Hairy cell leukaemia
8. Plasmacytoma
9. B-cell large lymphoma
   Subtype: primary mediastinal (thymic) B-cell lymphoma
10. Burkitt's lymphoma
11. Provisional entity: high-grade B-cell lymphoma, Burkitt's-like

T-cell and putative NK-cell lymphomas

Precursor B-cell neoplasms: precuror T-lymphoblastic lymphoma/leukaemia

Peripheral T-cell and NK-cell neoplasms

1. T-cell chronic lymphocytic leukaemia'prolymphocytic leukaemia
2. Large granular cell lymphocytic leukaemia
3. T-cell
   NK-cell type
4. Mycosis fungoides/Sézary syndrome
5. Peripheral T-cell lymphoma, unspecified
   Provisional subtype: hepatosplenic T-cell lymphoma
   Provisional subtype: subcutaneous T-cell lymphoma
6. Angioimmunoblastic lymphoma (AILD)
7. Intestinal T-cell lymphoma (± enteropathy-associated)
8. Adult T-cell lymphoma/leukaemia
9. Anaplastic large-cell lymphoma, CD30, T- and null-cell types
10. Provisional entity: anaplastic large-cell lymphoma, Hodgkin's like

Hodgkin's lymphomas. The disease initially appears as a small focus within an otherwise reactive lymph node (Figure 11.8), and although it metastasizes widely like a carcinoma, actual invasion of the lymphatics rarely occurs. The more differentiated lymphocyte-predominant variety has a better prognosis than (in decreasing order) nodular sclerosing, mixed cellular or lymphocyte-depleted Hodgkin's. With the routine use of more aggressive radiotherapeutic and chemotherapeutic regimens, the exact cellular classification has become less important in the overall scheme of treatment. Secondary neoplasms, e.g. myeloid leukaemia, are a particular risk, however when radiotherapy and alkylating chemotherapeutic regimens are combined.

Familial erythrophagocytosis (of Claireaux and Farquhar) involves sinus histiocytes and splenic macrophages that abnormally engulf and destroy red cells. A severe anaemia occurs, but there is little, if any, architectural destruction of the involved organ. The end stage of this disease evolves into a monocytic leukaemia. A similar non-selective phagocytosis is seen in *histiocytic medullary reticulosis*. While centred in lymph nodes and or the spleen, the group of *histiocytosis X* diseases is probably not a primary disease of these organs.

Primary haematological disorders

Blood-borne 'haemic reticuloses' are less often found in biopsies of enlarged lymph nodes since such diagnoses are usually first made via other methods. Myeloid leukaemias may be associated with medullary lymph node proliferation or splenic red pulp enlargement and the diagnosis is readily made with stains specific to eosinophil granules (e.g. azo-eosin) or histochemical staining for chloracetate esterase (monocytes). In myelosclerosis, these same areas show a myeloid transformation with a high proportion of multinucleated giant cells, similar to those seen in bone marrow or to megakaryocytes. Erythroid cells, contrary to the lymphocyte lines, have a characteristically dense nucleus, so-called 'empty' cytoplasm, and a periodic acid–Schiff (PAS)-positive spherical cell membrane. Both familial and acquired haemolytic anaemias may produce myeloid metaplasia of the spleen and lymph nodes.

Section 11.5 • Splenomegaly

Although, as outlined in Table 11.2, there are numerous causes of splenomegaly, the relative incidence varies in different parts of the world, and in Western hospital practice, the distribution is as follows:

- patients with hepatic diseases, most commonly cirrhosis – 36%
- patients with haematological disease – 35%
- patients with infectious diseases – 16%, increasingly AIDS
- patients with inflammatory non-infectious disease – 5%
- patients with primary splenic disease – 4%
- others – 3%, e.g. congestive heart failure, endocarditis.

During the past 20 years, AIDS has come to account for 55–60% of patients with splenomegaly caused by infectious disease. The spleen may enlarge transiently in a variety of acute bacterial and viral infections, chronic infections and in subacute bacterial endocarditis. Parasitic infections, e.g. malaria, can result in massive congestive splenomegaly such that rupture is a very real and well-documented risk in those affected.

Portal hypertension causes mild to moderate splenomegaly unless it is post-hepatic (Budd–Chiari) or follows splenic vein thrombosis (sectorial, left-sided, sinistral portal hypertension) when massive splenomegaly may occur.

Splenomegaly accompanies both hereditary and acquired red cell defects. The increasing splenic size predisposes these patients to increased red cell surveillance and hence destruction on a volume basis alone. As such, a vicious cycle is established whereby increased destruction and splenomegaly produces even more rapid red cell destruction.

Splenomegaly occurs in about one-third of patients with megaloblastic anaemia, but less frequently in iron-deficiency anaemia. Splenomegaly is unusual in acquired aplastic anaemias, although for unexplained reasons it occurs in a significant number of children with congenital hypoplastic anaemia. It also occurs quite frequently in patients with dyserythropoietic anaemia or 'preleukaemic' states, e.g. sideroblastic anaemia.

Splenomegaly regularly accompanies myeloproliferative disorders. Although polycythaemia vera does not commonly exhibit extramedullary erythropoiesis, the process of myeloid metaplasia in myelosclerosis does and splenomegaly is often massive in this condition. Any form or leukaemia or lymphoma can also cause splenomegaly via the same mechanisms. As such, the splenomegaly that accompanies Hodgkin's disease or non-Hodgkin's lymphoma does not necessarily represent tumour involvement of the organ, raising the possibility of a false-positive clinical stage.

Clinical features

A left upper abdominal mass is often not splenomegaly. For this reason, a comprehensive history and good physical examination is necessary in the first instance to minimize the considerable expense and discomfort of a misdirected evaluation. The normal-sized spleen is not palpable but, when palpable, the spleen is at least two to three times the normal size. The important questions for history taking reflect the common causes of splenomegaly for the particular region. With the spectrum of diseases in mind, it is important to consider infectious (AIDS in particular) and neoplastic disease. A history of travel is often missed unless specifically questioned. Any suggestion of prior pancreatitis or abdominal pain with alcoholism should raise the suspicion of splenic vein thrombosis. The review of the systems enquiry should include questioning for pruritus, as this frequently accompanies myeloproliferative disorders.

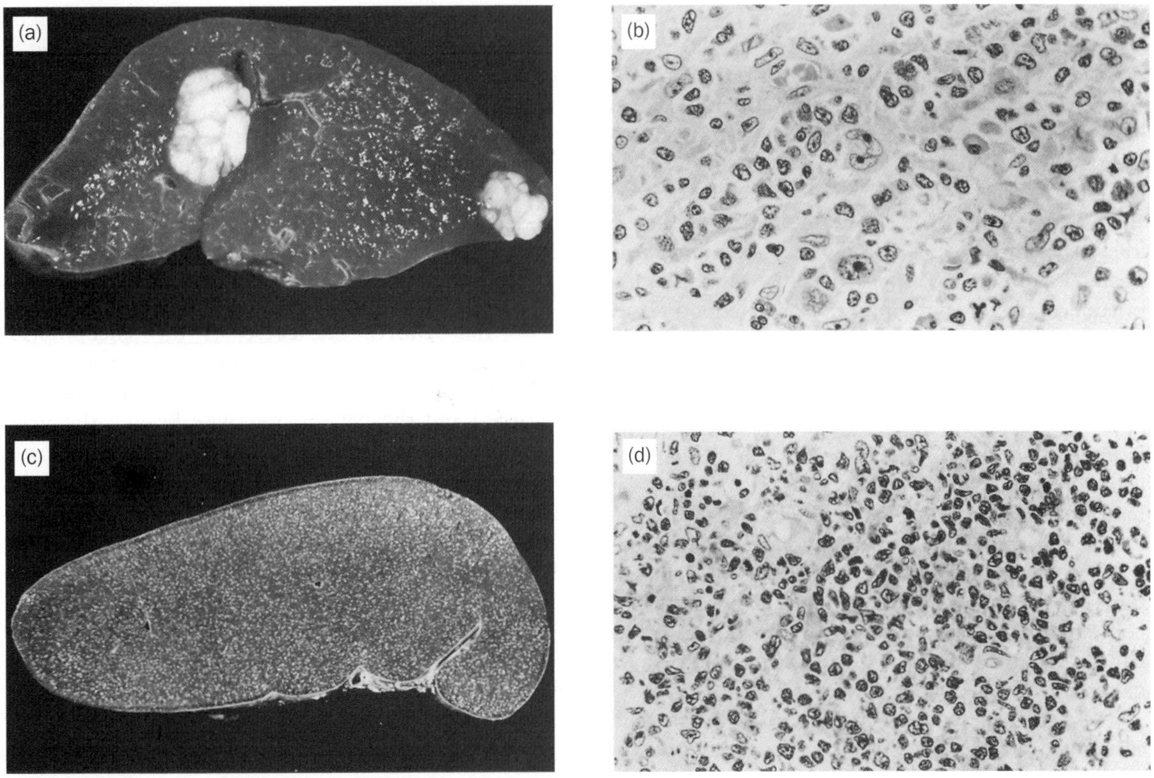

Figure 11.8 The spleen in Hodgkin's disease and non-Hodgkin's lymphoma: (a) transverse section of a 200 g spleen removed at laparotomy for staging Hodgkin's disease. Two discrete tumour foci are present and histology of the intervening tissue shows only non-specific reactive features. (b) Histology of one of the tumour nodules showing mixed cellular Hodgkin's disease, note the central diagnostic 'mirror image' binucleated Reed–Sternberg cell, eosinophils (with bilobed nuclei and granules in the cytoplasm, e.g. three cells from the R-S cell at one o'clock) and plasma cells (e.g. three cells away at three o'clock); the large cells with stippled nuclei are histiocytes. (c) Transverse section of a 400 g spleen from a patient with non-Hodgkin's lymphoma, note involvement of every Malpighian body, histologically there was minimal disturbance of architecture. (d) Tumour cells from the white pulp of the same spleen showing small cleaved follicle centre cells. This patient had a small number of similar cleaved cells circulating with his peripheral lymphocytes in the blood.

The symptoms of splenomegaly itself (irrespective of cause) do not correlate with size, but in practice they tend to be marked only when the spleen becomes massively enlarged since most are due largely to mechanical displacement of adjacent organs and weight of the congested spleen. The symptoms of splenomegaly, as distinct from the manifestations of the underlying disease, include chronic dragging abdominal pain, or pain when lying on the side, abdominal discomfort and early satiety. In addition patients may complain of attacks of acute (colicky) left upper quadrant pains. In general, the bigger the spleen the worse the cytopenia (from hypersplenism) although there are exceptions to this, e.g. marked thrombocytopenia/neutropenia in immune (idiopathic) thrombocytopenia purpura where the splenomegaly is invariably mild. Thus the significant correlation between splenic size and blood counts is not always clinically significant.

The physical examination of a left upper quadrant mass starts with the examiner's hand well inferior in the right iliac fossa probing gently through each exhaled breath of the patient. In addition, the examiner's left hand is cupped posteriorly on the patient's back and flank so as to produce a 'bimanual' feel to the mass in question. If the mass is an enlarged spleen, it will be impossible to appreciate its superior limit. In contrast to colon and stomach, the spleen lying against the abdominal wall is dull to percussion. Capsular inflammation of the spleen may produce a rub (with the stethoscope). Finally, the right lateral decubitus position may allow for easier examination of a left upper quadrant mass.

A renal mass can usually be distinguished from a splenic mass on physical examination since:

- the kidney moves inferiorly on respiration, whereas the spleen moves medially as well
- the organ shapes are quite different
- the colonic resonance in front of a renal mass is usually not present with splenic masses.

Colonic and gastric masses usually move less well with respiration as they are not as intimately attached to the diaphragm, are more irregular than splenic masses, and often have a superior limit that is palpable. The physical examination must also include a careful search for lymphadenopathy, including the tissues of the posterior pharynx. A search for the stigmata of chronic liver disease as well as evidence of purpura or bruising mandates a complete head-to-toe examination.

The investigation of splenomegaly

The cause of splenic enlargement can usually be identified by history, physical examination and a few appropriate tests. Those cases associated with haematological disorders are often fully characterized by a peripheral blood smear and a bone marrow biopsy. Lymphoreticular malignancies are defined by appropriate biopsy. Haematological or serological testing can identify most infectious causes of splenomegaly. Mononucleosis, a frequent cause, is diagnosed by the finding of atypical lymphocytes in the peripheral blood smear, a positive Paul–Bunnell test (or similar screen), and a rising anti-Epstein–Barr virus titre. Most patients with AIDS who develop splenomegaly are already known to have the disease, but when suspicion is aroused in previously undiagnosed patients, permission for the appropriate testing should be obtained. Patients with a history of travel or those living in endemic areas of disease should have blood smears looking for malaria or marrow for Leishman-Donovon bodies. Disseminated tuberculosis must be considered in all members of a community where there are also immigrants at risk. Laparoscopy may assist in this elusive diagnosis as the majority will have intestinal tuberculosis.

The size, shape and consistency of the spleen can be accurately visualized by either CT or ultrasonography. The determination of splenic size is of crucial importance in determining the surgical approach (open or laparoscopic) when splenectomy is indicated in the management of the patient (*vide infra*). The spleen's blood vessels can be imaged using either duplex ultrasound, high-dose contrast helical CT or (rarely nowadays) with selective visceral angiography. The latter is used almost exclusively for therapeutic embolization. It is no longer necessary to puncture the spleen directly for splenoportography, as other methods are usually sufficiently accurate. Fine ultrasound-guided needle splenic biopsy is carried out for specific lesions but only in specialized centres.

Ultrasound is the most widely used imaging modality in the investigation of patients with both acute and chronic disorders of the spleen. It is performed by scanning through the intercostal spaces with both grey scale and colour Doppler or power flow (splenic vasculature). Splenic ultrasound is useful for:

- detection of accessory spleens
- confirmation of splenomegaly but not the cause of the splenomegaly
- differentiation of solid from cystic intrasplenic focal masses
- detection of calcification, wall thickening, internal debris, and gas within cystic type lesions
- detection of splenic cavernous hemangiomas
- diagnosis of splenic infarction
- diagnosis of splenic trauma and monitoring patients with splenic injuries managed conservatively.

An accurate assessment of the spleen's function can be obtained through injection of labelled platelets, cells (red, white) or carrier molecules and radiotracer studies. The splenic uptake rate of Tc-sulphur colloid or Tc-tin colloid provides a sensitive and quantitative function of splenic function and is based on tracer uptake by the spleen (measured splenic uptake rate divided by measured injected activity). The normal splenic tracer uptake rate is 0.0002–0.0006/s. Values lower than 0.0002/s indicate hyposplenism and values >0.0006/s hypersplenism. There is good correlation between high splenic tracer uptake rates and the severity of the neutropenia and thrombocytopenia.

Undiagnosed splenomegaly

Patients are infrequently encountered where, despite all reasonable efforts, the cause of the splenomegaly remains cryptic. In an otherwise healthy person, this can be a vexing situation. If the organ is minimally enlarged and the patient otherwise healthy, the management consists of careful follow-up. If symptomatic, noticeably enlarging or already significantly enlarged at presentation (the more common situation), diagnostic splenectomy should be considered. In these patients, even if no specific pathological entity is found, one should continue careful surveillance as a lymphoma may develop years after such a splenectomy (possibly due to sampling error at pathological review). None the less, many of the patients who require splenectomy will be found to have an occult lymphoma.

Section 11.6 • Splenectomy and indications

Indications for splenectomy

There are definite, desirable and debatable indications for splenectomy (Table 11.9).

Definite indications

Neoplasms of the spleen should be removed for accurate diagnosis and staging. Septic emboli to the spleen

Table 11.9 Indications for splenectomy

- **Definite**
  - Non-salvageable spleen injury (see text)
  - *En-bloc* resection of adjacent neoplasms (usually proximal gastric cancer)
  - Neoplasms of the spleen – usually lymphomas
  - Splenic abscess
  - Echinococcal cysts
  - Bleeding gastric varices due to sinistral portal hypertension (splenic vein thrombosis)
  - Rupture of diseased spleen
- **Desirable – used selectively**
  - Hereditary spherocytosis
  - Immune (idiopathic) thrombocytopenic purpura
  - AIDS-related thrombocytopenic purpura
  - Autoimmune haemolytic anaemia
  - Sickling syndromes (sickle cell disease and sickle-beta thalassaemia)
- **Debatable**
  - Non-parasitic splenic cysts
  - Thalassaemia syndromes
  - Lymphoma with specific cytopenia or pancytopenia
  - Thrombotic thrombocytopenic purpura
  - Myeloproliferative disorders

do not require splenectomy, but when an abscess has formed, removal of the entire organ is the safest management course. Potential spillage of echinococcal cyst contents requires that the entire spleen be removed for this condition.

Bleeding gastric varices resulting from splenic vein thrombosis requires splenectomy as does rupture of a splenic artery aneurysm that can occur catastrophically during pregnancy. Splenectomy may be required (*de necessité*) during resection for proximal gastric cancer to obtain the necessary clearance and adequate regional lymphadenectomy. Although spontaneous rupture of the spleen does occur, it is most frequently seen at times of, or following an interval after minor abdominal trauma; or as the presenting symptom of previously silent splenomegaly in an already diseased spleen, e.g. malaria, mononucleosis, myelosclerosis, etc. Rarely, a rapidly enlarging spleen in the aggressive forms of non-Hodgkin's lymphoma may rupture spontaneously. Equally rare, a pseudocyst of the tail of the pancreas may cause splenic vein thrombosis, rapid enlargement and congestion of the organ and spontaneous rupture. In otherwise healthy patients, rupture of the spleen much more commonly follows blunt trauma of the chest and abdomen [see Trauma Module, Vol. II] or as an iatrogenic injury during abdominal surgery. Because of concerns regarding OPSIs, every reasonable effort should be made to salvage an injured spleen during surgery and emergency laparotomy (splenic suture, partial splenectomy, etc.). However, there are situations when splenic salvage is ill advised and splenectomy is the sensible option:

- hilar injuries or a shattered spleen (grade 4 or 5 injuries)
- blast injuries to the organs of the left upper quadrant
- multiple associated injuries where splenic salvage may prolong the procedure
- haemodynamically unstable and elderly patients
- marked intra-abdominal contamination
- rupture of a pathological spleen.

Non-operative conservative management of a known splenic injury, especially in the paediatric age group, is certainly an acceptable alternative to operative therapy in the first instance. Likewise, in an effort to avoid the many complications of splenectomy in patients with myelosclerosis, a small perisplenic haematoma may be closely observed in hospital, with frequent serial ultrasound examinations. But in either case, with any sign of haemodynamic instability or continued bleeding (persistent blood replacement need), laparotomy is clearly indicated. The disadvantage of conservative management is that in the event of failure, the potential for splenic salvage is reduced.

Desirable indications

In many of these patients, the need for splenectomy is made by the haematologist who refers the patient to the surgeon. It is usually desirable to perform splenectomy for hereditary spherocytosis, refractory immune (idiopathic) thrombocytopenic purpura and AIDS-related thrombocytopenia that have failed to respond to medical therapy (steroids and human IgG), and acquired haemolytic anaemia. Some cases of genetic red cell enzyme defects, such as pyruvate kinase deficiency, respond favourably to splenectomy. Splenectomy may reduce the blood transfusion requirements of haemoglobinopathies, such as the thalassaemia syndromes. It may also be useful in patients with neutropenia secondary to congestive splenomegaly, e.g. tropical or lymphomatous, for the same reason as in those with storage diseases.

In patients (usually children) with sickling disorders (sickle cell disease and sickle-beta-thalassaemia) splenectomy is beneficial in the management of patients who develop large spleens with hypersplenism, major splenic sequestration crisis, recurrent minor splenic sequestration crises, splenic abscess and massive splenic infarction. A high proportion (25%) of these patients have concomitant gallstones and cholecystectomy may be considered at the time of the splenectomy.

Debatable/controversial indications

Splenectomy in the treatment of myeloproliferative disorders is controversial. Its value in the management of chronic myeloid leukaemia remains unproven. It may be occasionally indicated in myelosclerosis with massive splenomegaly, but only if the sequestration of red cells exceeds the spleen's erythropoiesis as measured by isotope tests. The 'rebound thrombocytosis' often seen post-splenectomy is particularly severe in this situation. As myelosclerosis follows an unpredictable course of severity, splenectomy to avoid these complications is highly debated. Staging laparotomy for Hodgkin's and non-Hodgkin's lymphomas with splenectomy, lymph node harvest and liver biopsies is no longer performed, as accurate staging is possible with modern imaging tests (helical CT and magnetic resonance imaging (MRI)).

Splenectomy

The first splenectomy in the human is said to have been done by Zaccarelli of Naples in 1649, for splenomegaly in a 24-year old female. The truth of this report has been questioned, as have reports of splenectomy performed in the sixteenth and seventeenth centuries. The first successful splenectomy in the USA was reported by O'Brien in 1816 for splenic evisceration following a knife wound. In 1866, Spencer Wells performed the first elective splenectomy in England. Common knowledge at that time held that the spleen was expendable and splenectomy had no untoward side-effects. Laparoscopic splenectomy was first reported in several European and North American centres in 1989–1990.

Pre-operative management and preparation

As previously mentioned, all patients undergoing elective splenectomy should be immunized against *Streptoccoccus pneumoniae and Haemophilus* spp. and this should be carried out 2 weeks before surgery.

Otherwise, preoperative preparation for splenectomy should be routine as for any major abdominal operation and this includes prophylaxis against thromboembolic disease. Special consideration should be given to the patient's haematological findings, clotting parameters and liver enzymes. Patients with bone marrow dysfunction or with immune platelet destruction abnormalities may be markedly thrombocytopenic prior to operation. If the platelet count is low on the basis of bone marrow failure, then platelet transfusion to a level greater than 60 000 is indicated both prior to and following operation for the first few days, in an effort to prevent bleeding episodes. If the thrombocytopenia is on the basis of immune disease, e.g. immune thrombocytopenic purpura, then pre-operative platelet transfusions will be less useful, whereas human IgG will increase the platelet count. Coagulopathies due to liver disease require replacement therapy with fresh frozen plasma or cryoprecipitate as determined by factor assay.

In patients with massive splenomegaly, it may be useful to consider immediate pre-operative radiological embolization of the splenic artery. Otherwise, it is usually possible to ligate the splenic artery at the superior border of the pancreas via the lesser sac at the beginning of the operation. This allows for a period of 'autotransfusion' of the sequestered blood elements during the remaining dissection. As removal of a massive spleen may be accompanied by substantial blood loss, a cell-saver system for autotransfusion should be available. Particular attention should be made during the ligature and division of the splenic hilar vessels to avoid inadvertent damage to the tail of the pancreas.

Attention to exact haemostasis is critical for the reduction of post-operative complications. The bed of the spleen, especially the raw surface of the diaphragm, should be meticulously inspected for oozing and bleeders before closure. The use of the Argon spray coagulation is very effective in ensuring a dry splenic bed. Drains should not be inserted after splenectomy as they are ineffective and enhance the risk of subphrenic infection.

Laparoscopic splenectomy

Because of its advantages (fewer peri-operative complications, reduced morbidity and a shorter hospital stay), laparoscopic splenectomy is now preferable to open operation for some but not all disorders requiring splenectomy or splenic surgery. Laparoscopic splenectomy is recommended for benign disease when the spleen's largest diameter does not exceed 20–22 cm. This is usually the case in patients with immune thrombocytopenic purpura, AIDS-related thrombocytopenic purpura and acquired haemolytic anaemia. Although there are several techniques, the 'hanging spleen' method with the patient in the right lateral decubitus position is favoured by many. Initially, the laparoscopic approach took longer to perform than open splenectomy, but with increasing experience, operating times have become equivalent. There is some evidence, however, that accessory spleens are more difficult to identify laparoscopically. This may result in a recurrence of the thrombocytopenia although there are no comparative studies and the results of laparoscopic splenectomy in reversing the thrombocytopenia or acquired haemolytic anaemia have been equivalent to those obtained by open splenectomy. The laparoscopic approach is also safe and adequate for surgery on benign splenic cysts (*vide infra*).

Laparoscopic splenectomy is ill advised in patients with large spleens including those with hypersplenism and in patients with major traumatic splenic injury and haemodynamic instability. There are some concerns in relation to laparoscopic splenectomy for neoplastic disease as fragmentation/morcellation of the specimen may promote tumour spillage and implantation and also render pathological examination more difficult. However, with the advent of hand-assisted techniques larger spleens can be removed safely by the hand-assisted laparoscopic approach (HALS).

Complications of splenectomy

The complications of splenectomy include those commons to upper abdominal operations (wound and chest infections, etc.) in addition to specific early and late complications. Major complications are encountered in 10% of patients after open splenectomy reflecting the high-risk patients with serious haematological disease undergoing this procedure. The mortality varies with the nature of the underlying disease.

Early complications

Post-operative bleeding is most commonly due to oozing from the raw surface of the diaphragm and retroperitoneum especially after removal of large spleens and in the presence of low platelet counts or impaired platelet function. Additionally, patients with prior episodes of splenic infarction may have densely adherent yet vascular adhesions, which exacerbate the post-operative bleeding. A similar problem is encountered after splenectomy in patients with portal hypertension.

Minor post-operative bleeding results in a subphrenic collection and this complication is common in patients whose platelet count does not rise above 5×10^9/dl following the operation. Careful monitoring of the platelet counts and clotting parameters in those with hepatic dysfunction may prevent some of these collections which may become infected.

Thrombocytosis with a hypercoagulable state may occur after splenectomy. This 'rebound' phenomenon is more common following splenectomy for myeloproliferative disorders. If the platelet count is in excess of 100×10^9/dl, aspirin or anticoagulants should be administered. With adequate prophylaxis (heparin and graduated compression stockings) post-operative deep vein thrombosis and pulmonary embolism should be minimized.

Iatrogenic trauma to the surrounding viscera can occur during splenectomy. During the ligation of the short gastric vessels, if stomach wall is inadvertently included in the ligature, necrosis of the gastric wall with subphrenic abscess and gastric fistula formation will ensue. The tail of the pancreas is always intimately associated with the hilum of the spleen. For this reason, extreme caution must be exercised during dissection and ligature of the splenic hilar vessels. The current widespread practice, especially during laparoscopic splenectomy, of stapling the splenic arteries and veins together is particularly prone to this complication. Furthermore, this technique incurs the late risk of arteriovenous fistula. Surgical trauma to the tail of the pancreas during splenectomy may result in pancreatic ascites, subphrenic fluid collection/abscess and pancreatic fistula. Complications such as these can be life threatening in an already debilitated patient with serious underlying haematological disease. Prompt recognition with percutaneous CT/ultrasound guided drainage with appropriate antibiotic therapy and somatostatin (in the case of pancreatic ascites/fistula) is essential in these patients. A less common but equally disastrous complication is damage to the splenic flexure of the colon, which results in subphrenic abscess formation and faecal fistula.

Late complications

A small number of patients develop migratory thrombophlebitis or complications of deep vein thrombosis late after splenectomy. This is more likely to occur following splenectomy for haemolytic anaemia or myeloproliferative disorders. Especially in those patients in whom the anaemia does not respond (much like an inverse relationship), thrombocytosis and associated complications may ensue. These patients may require long-term anticoagulant therapy. Late recurrence of the disease may complicate splenectomy. The usual cause of recurrent anaemia or thrombocytopenia is hypertrophy of a missed accessory spleen. If suspected, the accessory spleen can be imaged with a radiolabelled nuclear scan, and curative surgical removal thereby planned. The most important late complication is, however, post-splenectomy overwhelming sepsis, which was discussed earlier in this module.

Section 11.7 • Miscellaneous disorders of the spleen

Splenic abscess

Splenic abscess may result from contiguous spread of infection from neighbouring viscera, e.g. diverticulitis or via infection of an infarcted spleen or post-traumatic splenic haematoma. Multiple abscesses may occur in the end stage of overwhelming sepsis or with bacterial endocarditis, in patients with leukaemia and in premature infants. Multiple splenic abscesses are often fatal, even with aggressive management.

The recognition of splenic abscess is commonly delayed. It should always be suspected in patients with established splenic infarction whose pain, fever and signs do not settle with conservative management. The clinical features of a splenic abscess are essentially non-specific, i.e. fever, pain and left upper quadrant tenderness. Splenomegaly is recognized in less than 50% of patients. The chest radiograph may show a left pleural effusion, and ultrasound scanning, an immobile hemidiaphragm and gas/debris in the abscess cavity. CT scanning is diagnostic. The management options include percutaneous drainage or splenectomy which is necessary if the abscess is large or multiple. Untreated, splenic abscesses can rupture with an invariably fatal outcome.

Ectopic (wandering) spleen

Ectopic (wandering) spleen is a rare condition, which seems to occur more commonly in women (7:1) between 20 and 40 years of age and is rarely encountered in children. It is due to lax attachments of the spleen to the retroperitoneum and long splenic vessels, such that the spleen 'wanders' and may become located in the lower abdomen. The diagnosis of the condition is difficult in view of its rarity. It may present acutely with abdominal pain due to torsion (which may progress to infarction, see Figure 11.9), with hypersplenism (due to congestion), or simply with an abdominal mass with or without associated pain. The diagnosis is confirmed by imaging studies, CT and duplex ultrasonography being the preferred modalities. Treatment of ectopic spleen is operative and consists of splenopexy (non-infarcted spleen). Splenectomy is only indicated (usually as an emergency) if splenic blood flow cannot be restored after de-torsion of the splenic pedicle.

Splenic cysts

Splenic cysts are primary or secondary. The latter constitute the common ones and these develop after splenic injuries, especially when treated conservatively, hence the name traumatic splenic pseudocysts (no lining epithelium).

Splenic traumatic pseudocysts may be totally asymptomatic but they have a tendency to enlarge although the natural history of these lesions is not fully under-

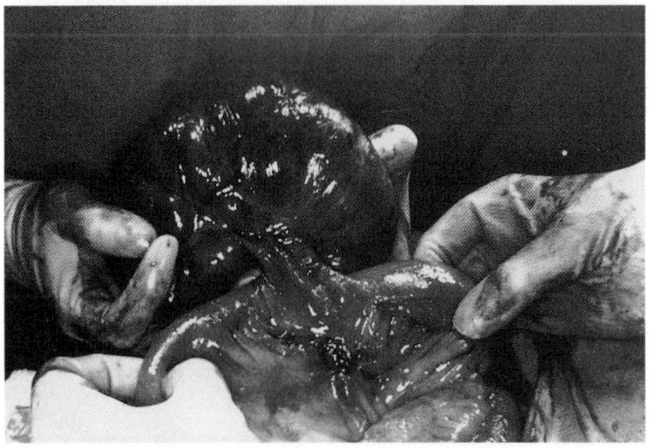

Figure 11.9 Infarcted wandering spleen. The patient presented as an emergency with acute upper abdominal pain.

stood. The time interval between the initial injury and presentation or diagnosis is extremely variable and cases are reported when this exceeded 30 years. Some traumatic pseudocysts of the spleen remain asymptomatic and are discovered accidentally during investigation by ultrasound. Others develop abdominal pain and a palpable mass or non-specific symptoms. Acute presentation with rupture is well documented. Surgical treatment is only necessary for large symptomatic cysts after confirmation of the diagnosis by ultrasound or CT. Spleen preserving excision is possible unless the cyst is very large or presents acutely with rupture and bleeding.

True splenic cysts have an epithelial lining. There are several types:

- epithelial
- epithelial in accessory intrapancreatic spleen
- dermoid
- lymphangiomatous
- mucinous cystic lesions
- parasitic – hydatid.

Epithelial cysts are the commonest (Figure 11.10). They are lined with epithelium and are filled with straw-coloured to brownish fluid. Immunohistochemical studies have shown that the epithelial cells of the cysts express keratin, epithelial membrane antigen, CEA, CA 19–9 but not BerEP4 (positive in cells of epithelial origin). These findings suggest that the origin is from epithelial metaplasia of the mesodermal undifferentiated cells from exposure to an unidentified irritant. Epithelial cysts can occur in both children and adults and can reach a large size. Some present with splenomegaly, others with left upper quadrant pain and/or non-specific symptoms (fever and non-bilious vomiting) and many are discovered accidentally during ultrasound scanning. Some have elevated serum levels of CEA and CA 19–9. Small asymptomatic cysts do not require treatment but should be followed up by serial ultrasound. Larger symptomatic cysts require treatment, and unless the cyst is very large, this should consist of partial splenic decapsulation with preservation of the spleen, especially in children. Similar epidermoid

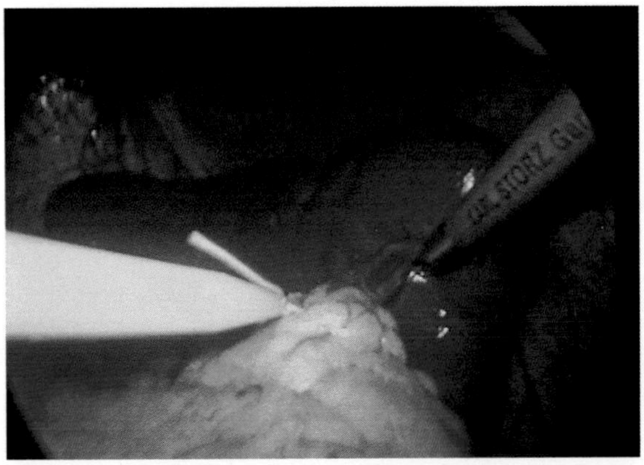

Figure 11.10 Laparoscopic splenectomy for epidermoid cyst of the upper pole of the spleen.

cysts have been reported in intrapancreatic accessory spleens. These are also lined by non-keratinizing stratified squamous epithelium and can be multilocular. They are thought to arise from embryonic inclusion cysts of the mesothelium.

Lymphangiomas of the spleen may occur as part of lymphangiomatosis or may be solitary lesions. Solitary splenic lymphangiomas tend to form subcapsular, multicystic proliferations that are often incidental findings. Some are not true lymphangiomas and immunohistochemical studies suggest a mesothelial derivation. Splenic lymphangiomas have a distinctive CT appearance with multiple, low-attenuation lesions that do not enhance with intravenous contrast material or a 'mottled spleen'. They rarely give rise to symptoms or splenomegaly and do not require treatment if the diagnosis is certain.

All mucinous cystic lesions of the spleen are associated with malignant pseudomyxoma peritonei (peritoneal mucinous cancinomatosis) with the immunophenotype (cytokeratin 7 negative; cytokeratin 20 and CEA positive) of the cystic splenic lesions indicative of a gastrointestinal primary, most commonly the appendix **[see Disorders of the abdomen and peritoneal cavity, Vol. II]**. The intrasplenic mucinous epithelial lesions cause splenomegaly and may thus be the presenting feature of malignant pseudomyxoma peritonei or develop as evidence of recurrent disease.

Splenic tumours

Apart from lymphomas, both primary and secondary tumours of the spleen are rare. The vascular tumours include primary angiosarcoma, haemangioma, haemangioendotheliomas and benign vascular neoplasms with myoid and angioendotheliomatous features. Splenic angiosarcomas constitute less than 1% of all sarcomas and less than 100 cases have been reported. They can present acutely with severe abdominal pain and intraperitoneal bleeding from spontaneous rupture (30%) and carry a uniformly poor prognosis.

Secondary tumour deposits are equally rare with a reported frequency of 2–5%. Although all malignant tumours can metastasize to the spleen, the most frequent site of the primary is the breast, lung, pancreas and ovary. Cutaneous melanoma has also been documented to metastasize to the spleen, and direct involvement from pancreatic and retroperitoneal sarcomas can occur.

Splenic vein thrombosis

This under-recognized condition occurs most often following either acute or chronic inflammation of the pancreas. It is also seen in infants who have had umbilical vein catheterization or from direct extension of a pancreatic neoplasm.

Isolated splenic vein thrombosis (i.e. without portal vein thrombosis) results in splenomegaly and sectorial or left-sided (sinistral) portal venous hypertension. This condition is characterized by the development of varices involving the short gastric and gastroepiploic veins. The most common presentation is with bleeding gastric varices in patients with normal or good liver function (Figure 11.11). As oesophageal varices may be absent, central portal pressures normal and gastric vessels easily overlooked at endoscopy, this condition can be easily missed. For this reason, gastrointestinal bleeding in the setting of prior pancreatitis should always raise the suspicion of splenic vein thrombosis. The diagnosis can be confirmed by high-dose helical CT or duplex ultrasonography, and these imaging tests have replaced direct visceral angiography and splenoportography.

Recognition of splenic vein thrombosis is critical, as otherwise the gastrointestinal haemorrhage may prove fatal. The treatment is splenectomy. Venous shunt procedures are contraindicated as central portal hypertension is not a feature of the disease, and the sectorial hypertension is not relieved by any type of central portosystemic shunt.

Splenosis

The peritoneum of patients who have sustained rupture or trauma to the spleen can be 'seeded' with splenic fragments that autotransplant. This pathological curiosity led to attempts at salvaging splenic function by intentional transplantation of fragments into the omentum. That such transplants survive is unchallenged, as demonstrated by animal studies, but the surveillance function of the spleen is lost. As such, the enthusiasm for surgical autotransplantation has declined in recent years.

Differentiating between splenosis and accessory spleens is not usually difficult. Accessory spleens are found in recognized locations, most often at the hilum of the spleen, tail of pancreas and omentum. They number less than 10 and have hilar vessels with normal splenic architecture. The splenic implants of splenosis often number more than 20, have antecedent traumatic events, are scattered over the surface of the peritoneum and do not have a co-ordinated circulation. Splenosis does not require treatment.

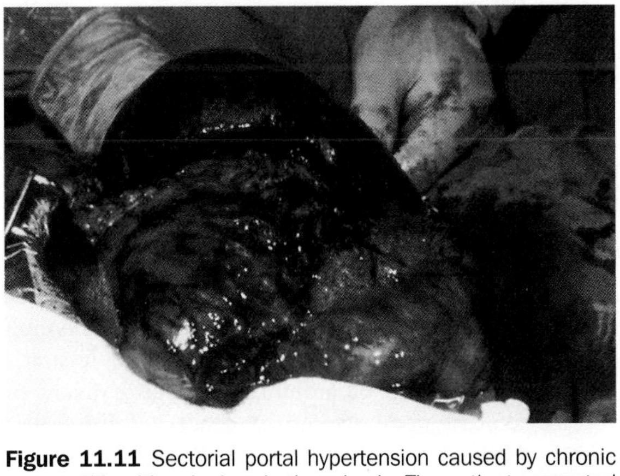

Figure 11.11 Sectorial portal hypertension caused by chronic pancreatitis with splenic vein thrombosis. The patient presented with severe haematemesis. The spleen was enlarged. Endoscopy showed bleeding gastric varices. Note the distended veins along the greater curvature and fundal region of the stomach (short gastric and left gastropepiploic).

Gaucher's disease

Hypersplenism and massive splenomegaly can occur due to this hereditary disorder of lipid metabolism. The three types of the disorder are due to a specific inherited enzyme defect (β-glucocerebrosidase). Type I is the most commonly encountered adult form, type II is the routinely fatal infantile form, and type III the intermediate form. Patients surviving into adulthood exhibit splenomegaly, thrombocytopenia, brownish discoloration of the limbs and pingueculae. The typical Gaucher's fat-laden cells can be found on marrow aspirate, and long bone abnormalities occur in approximately 50% of patients. Splenectomy is indicated for symptoms or complications of hypersplenism.

Section 11.8 • Disorders of lymph nodes

Palpable subcutaneous lymph nodes should be considered diseased until proved otherwise. The enlargement (lymphadenopathy) may be a transitory self-limiting process, or the harbinger of a life-threatening illness. Lymph node enlargement may be localized (regional) or generalized. It may be purely reactive (enlarged lymph nodes exhibiting sinus histiocytosis) or the nodes may be diseased (infection or involvement by tumour).

Localized lymphadenopathy

Many acute bacterial and viral infections produce localized tender lymphadenopathy. With streptococcal or staphylococcal infections the overlying skin and subcutaneous tissue is often inflamed and oedematous although antibiotic therapy usually prevents progression to suppurative lymphadenitis. By contrast, the periadenitis is minimal in lymphadenitis caused by viral disease, although the enlarged nodes are usually tender, e.g. infectious mononucleosis.

Chronic infections and parasitic infestations may produce considerable lymphadenopathy without or with minimal signs of acute inflammation. Primary bovine tuberculosis may produce a chronically enlarged group of matted deep cervical lymph nodes that suppurate and form a 'cold' collar stud abscess as it penetrates the investing layer of the deep cervical fascia, and eventually discharges through the skin forming a tuberculous sinus. Syphilis, leprosy, fungal infections and lymphogranuloma venereum can all produce chronic indolent lymphadenopathy.

The site of the enlarged lymph nodes may be of diagnostic help. Enlarged occipital nodes usually indicate a chronic scalp infection and posterior auricular node enlargement is common in rubella. Anterior auricular lymphadenopathy is most often bacterial in origin from infection of the eyelids and conjunctivae. Cervical painless lymphadenopathy is a frequent presentation of nasopharyngeal cancer and the commonest presentation of both Hodgkin's and non-Hodgkin's lymphomas. Axillary adenopathy is common in breast cancer and in upper limb infections, and less frequently Hodgkin's disease. Painless epitrochlear lymphadenopathy is commonly seen in childhood viral illness, secondary syphilis or generalized tuberculosis, but is rare in sarcoidosis. Palpable small 'shotty' lymph nodes in the groin do not necessarily signify disease, as they are often prominent in children and thin athletic adults. Larger fleshier nodes however should raise suspicion of disease and merit investigation.

In the chest, mediastinal or hilar lymph nodes do not become noticeably enlarged on the chest X-ray with bacterial and viral pneumonias, but pulmonary tuberculosis can produce unilateral hilar lymphadenopathy. Infectious mononucleosis may cause persistent mediastinal lymphadenopathy lasting for several months, but the most common causes of hilar lymphadenopathy are bronchial carcinoma and sarcoidosis.

Regional intra-abdominal lymphadenopathy is of paramount importance in all intra-abdominal cancers and may be due to sinus histiocytosis or secondary deposits (lymph node positive cancers). Secondary involvement of the lymph nodes (on pathological staging) is an important feature of the pathological staging of all cancers. It affects the prognosis and may indicate the need for adjuvant therapy.

Generalized lymphadenopathy

When there is noticeable lymph node enlargement in more than one drainage region, the most common cause is a viral infection. Common viral illnesses causing generalized lymphadenopathy include infectious mononucleosis, viral hepatitis, influenza, cytomegalovirus infection, rubella, infectious lymphocytosis and AIDS. Excision biopsy of the affected node or nodes is often useful in AIDS patients in directing supportive therapy. The findings in AIDS patients having lymph node biopsy in decreasing order of frequency, include tuberculosis, Kaposi's syndrome, reactive hyperplasia, cryptococcus, *Mycobacterium avium* complex, lymphoma and lymphoepithelial cysts.

Fever and generalized lymphadenopathy occurs in patients with secondary syphilis, acute leptospirosis, salmonellosis, typhoid, paratyphoid and generalized haematogenous tuberculosis. Protozoal infections, e.g. toxoplasmosis, can resemble illnesses such as infectious mononucleosis.

Non-infective and non-neoplastic illnesses producing generalized lymphadenopathy include the autoimmune haemolytic anaemia, collagen vascular disorders, hypersensitivity reactions, hyperthyroidism and a variety of skin disorders, e.g. exfoliative dermatitis.

Lymph node imaging studies

The early attempts at lymph node imaging to detect nodal involvement were performed in relation to staging of Hodgkin's disease and non-Hodgkin's lymphomas

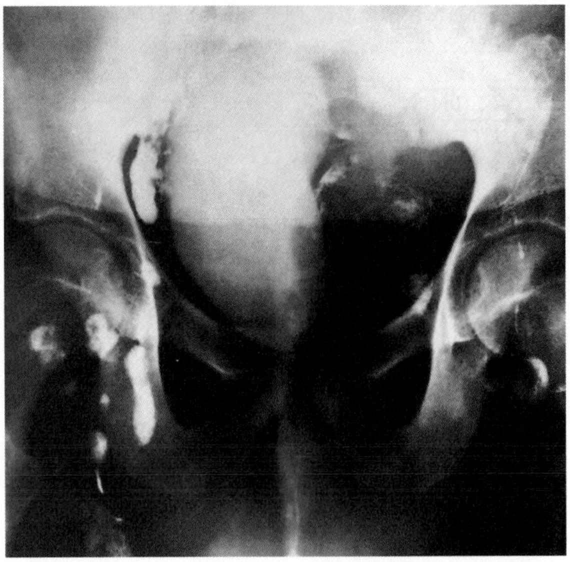

Figure 11.12 Lymphangiogram and intravenous pyelogram in a patient with non-Hodgkin's lymphoma. The very large lymph nodes on the left have filled poorly and are demonstrated as large masses indenting the urinary bladder.

using pedal lymphangiography. The lymphatics in the webs of the toes were identified after intradermal injection of a vital blue dye and then cannulated for contrast injection. In this fashion, proximal pelvic and abdominal lymph nodes could be imaged and involvement detected (Figure 11.12). This method of staging of lymphomas is rarely used nowadays, but the related technique of *sentinel lymph node mapping* is practised and has been shown to provide accurate nodal staging in patients with melanoma, and more recently, in patients with breast cancer. The original technique described by Morton *et al.* used a vital blue dye injected intradermally at the periphery of the primary tumour and this resulted in the sentinel node becoming stained blue and thus easily identified with minimal dissection. The technique has been modified by use of ^{99m}Tc-labelled human albumin colloid, 0.3 ml of which is injected intradermally at the edge of the tumour. Lymphoscintigraphy is then performed using an external dual-head gamma camera at 30 min and 2 hours and the site of the sentinel node marked on the skin. A special sterile radio probe connected to Geiger counter is also used to aid in precise location of the node during surgical harvest. The combined technique where the vital blue dye is mixed with the radiolabelled albumin colloid gives the best results. Sentinel node biopsy has been shown to yield an accurate assessment of the nodal status of the regional lymph nodes and to provide a strong prognostic factor. It carries a false-negative rate of around 10% and is likely to replace axillary node staging in cancer of the breast [Disorders of the breast, Vol. II]

Hodgkin's disease

Hodgkin's disease typically presents in middle-aged male adults. The neck is the most common site of primary presentation, as a group of painlessly enlarged anterior cervical nodes. Because of the dominant lymphatic drainage, the left side is the more common side of presentation. Axillary nodes are the site of presentation in less than 20% of patients, with the mediastinal or inguinal nodes being the first site in less than 15% of patients.

Hodgkin's disease is considered to be unicentric in origin and spreads via contiguous lymphatic channels to adjacent lymph nodes or lymphoreticular organs. The rate of growth of the involved lymph nodes varies between patients, and pain is uncommon in those patients with a slow-growing lymphoma. Enlarged nodes may fluctuate in size with inflammation or necrosis, but rarely shrink enough to escape careful palpation. Systemic symptoms may appear early or late, and variably include general malaise, listlessness, anorexia, weight loss, sweating, intermittent fever and pruritus. Clinically apparent hepatosplenomegaly appears late. Unchecked, the disease may involve any organ system. It is not uncommon to discover obscure involvement of the retroperitoneal, para-aortic, iliac and deep inguinal nodes, as well as diffuse infiltration of the bone marrow. In the late stages of the disease, lymphomas may spread to the meninges, pleura, thyroid, breasts, kidneys, urinary tract and gonads. Local node masses or organ involvement may produce mediastinal obstruction, neurological syndromes, e.g. Horner's, intestinal obstruction or renal failure.

The diagnosis of Hodgkin's, as with any lymphoma, begins with biopsy of a diseased lymph node. The biopsy should be excisional since the histological pattern of the disease is critical to the management of the individual patient. The corollary to exact pathological diagnosis is accurate staging of the disease, i.e. deciding on objective evidence based on staging tests, which nodal areas require treatment. For all patients this includes bone marrow biopsy, full blood count and biochemistry and high quality imaging with helical CT or MRI of the chest and abdomen. In the past laparotomy was an integral part of staging and included lymph node harvest, liver biopsies and splenectomy. Although it yielded valuable information that altered the stage of the disease, and hence influenced the nature of the treatment, it was attended by a significant morbidity. The very significant improvement in CT and MRI imaging has now virtually abolished the need for staging laparotomy and lymphangiography.

The clinical stages of Hodgkin's disease are given in Table 11.10. Stages I–IV are further subdivided into asymptomatic patients (A), and those with systemic symptoms (B). Clinically apparent hepatomegaly does not necessarily represent infra-diaphragmatic disease unless accompanied by elevated liver enzymes or abnormal scan, but a palpable spleen nearly always represents involvement. Questionable involvement of the spleen is confirmed by CT/MRI. In the past patients deemed to be in clinical stage I or IIa were subjected routinely to staging laparotomy which revealed stage III disease in up to 20% of patients. As mentioned previously, this is rarely undertaken nowadays because of the increased reliability of clinical staging. Splenectomy is, however carried out for splenic involvement as this removes a radiotherapy portal that is potentially very morbid, avoiding radiation injury to the lung, kidney and intestines in the left upper quadrant.

Table 11.10 Clinical staging of Hodgkin's disease

- **Stage I**
  Involvement of a single lymph node region, or a single extra-lymphoid organ or site (IE)
- **Stage II**
  Involvement of two or more lymph node groups on the same side of the diaphragm; or localized involvement of an extralymphoid organ or site and one or more lymph node groups on the same side of the diaphragm (IIE)
- **Stage III**
  Involvement of lymph node groups on both sides of the diaphragm, which may be accompanied by localized involvement of an extralymphoid organ (IIIE), spleen (IIIS) or both (IIISE)
- **Stage IV**
  Diffuse involvement of one or more extralymphoid organs with or without associated lymph node involvement: sites denoted: N (lymph nodes), H (liver), M (marrow), P (pleura), S (spleen), L (lung), O (bone), D (skin)
  A = asymptomatic
  B = weight loss > 10% body weight in 6 months, unexplained fever above 38°C, or night sweats

Non-Hodgkin's lymphomas

Non-Hodgkin's lymphomas (NHLs) are a heterogeneous group of tumours of the immune system with different origins, different natural histories and different prognoses. This diversity requires multiple treatment strategies. In contrast to Hodgkin's disease, NHLs tend to present more insidiously, with up to 25% of patients harbouring abdominal complaints because of retroperitoneal adenopathy. The majority of these patients present with painless enlargement of one or more superficial node groups. Less commonly, extranodal regions are the primary site of the disease, including the skin, orbit, pituitary, thyroid, tracheobronchial tree, gastrointestinal tract and central and peripheral nervous system. Approximately one-half of patients at presentation have no systemic complaints, but with disease progression, similar complications and symptoms may occur as in Hodgkin's disease.

In 1956, Rappaport proposed a classification scheme that proved both reproducible to pathologists and prognostically relevant. This system was used through the 1970s, when at least five new schemes were introduced with no scheme being clearly superior. Increasingly, the joint American–European classification is used for classification of the tumours based on morphological, immunological and molecular characteristics of the tumours. Two broad types are recognized: (i) B-cell lymphomas, and (ii) T-cell and putative natural killer (NK)-cell tumours. Within each category, some subtypes are still regarded as 'provisional entity'.

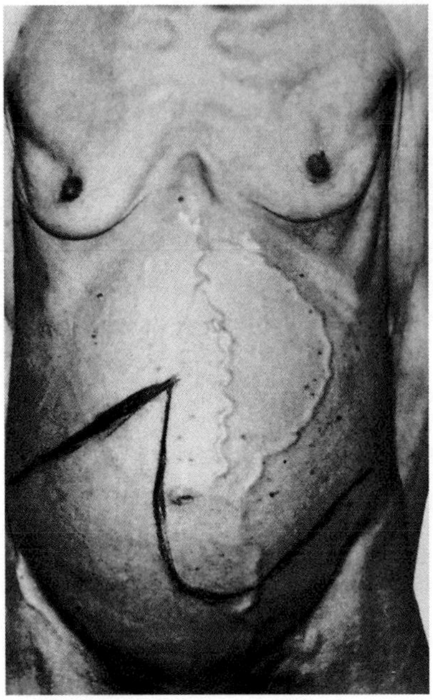

Figure 11.13 Patient with a low-grade malignant non-Hodgkin's lymphoma. Note enlargement of the left groin nodes and hepatosplenomegaly. Clinically there was obstruction of the left common iliac vein with dilatation of veins on the anterior abdominal wall.

Unlike Hodgkin's disease, the stage of the disease and spectrum of NHLs are accurately predicted on clinical grounds and staging laparotomy has never been proven to be of value, and for this reason, is not practised. Patients whose tumours show histiocytic morphology tend to develop systemic symptoms earlier than other varieties of lymphoma. Malaise, weight loss, superficial lymphadenopathy and hepatosplenomegaly occur early in this form of the disease. In 'fulminant' cases, fevers, rapid tissue wasting, massive lymphadenopathy and marked hepatosplenomegaly occur with alarming speed (Figure 11.13). There is a significant danger of spontaneous rupture of the spleen in some of the more clinically aggressive forms of NHLs, e.g. histiocytic medullary reticulosis. Mycosis fungoides and Sézary syndrome are two forms of NHLs that present with early cutaneous manifestations and later with generalized lymphadenopathy and/or systemic complaints.

Treatment strategies for NHLs and Hodgkin's disease

The treatment options for Hodgkin's disease and NHLs are multiple and varied. Indeed, treatment of these disorders is one of the relatively few areas where recent advances have had a major impact upon survival and cure rates (up to 90% 5 year survival for Hodgkin's disease). Critical to successful management is the accurate staging of the disease. This is especially true for patients with Hodgkin's disease.

Patients with stages I and II Hodgkin's disease are treated initially with wide-field megavoltage radiotherapy. This is in the form of 'mantle' and 'inverted Y' fields to cover the known areas of the disease. Patients with IIIA and more advanced disease are treated with combination chemotherapy. The early stages of NHL are treated in similar ways to Hodgkin's disease. Local radiotherapy is the first-line treatment of stage IA, or stage II with extranodal disease, bone lesions and/or some of the lymphomas of the gastrointestinal tract. In addition, NHLs of the mediastinum in children and adolescents are offered radiotherapy as a first-line therapy. Wide-field radiation is given, totalling 3000–4000 cGy over a 4 week period. Relapses occur most commonly within the first 2 years following such therapy. More advanced stages and patients with recurrent disease are given combination chemotherapy. There is no one 'standard' regimen for the treatment of NHLs, but combinations of cyclophosphamide, vincristine and predisone are usually employed in pulses over several months. The nodular and diffuse lymphocytic varieties carry a more favourable prognosis than the histiocytic malignancies. Patients with stage I histiocytic lymphomas, therefore, usually receive primary radiotherapy to the affected region but, because of the poorer response rates, patients with stage II or greater disease are also given chemotherapy in the first instance.

All regimens of chemotherapy produce varying degrees of neutropenia and/or thrombocytopenia. Severe, life-threatening infections are frequent. All neutropenic patients need regular oral inspection and maintenance hygiene with a prophylactic fungicide mouthwash. Rectal infections must be recognized early and treated with broad-spectrum antibiotics and surgical drainage as required. Bleeding during thrombocytopenic episodes must be treated with platelet transfusions. Often, anaemia complicates the clinical picture because of bleeding complications, underlying disease and or bone marrow suppressions. Replacement component therapy is therefore given as needed.

It should be remembered that some chemotherapeutic agents, notably vincristine, cause peripheral as well as autonomic neuropathies. As such, paralytic ileus with constipation is common, and should not be confused with mechanical obstruction; nor should it be ignored. Typhlitis is a condition of these patients where transmural necrosis of the caecum occurs, probably as a result of bacterial overgrowth within the setting of a paralytic ileus. Patients requiring surgery for this complication have a mortality exceeding 50%.

Mediastinal obstruction

Mediastinal lymph node involvement with lymphoma can occasionally cause mediastinal obstruction. This is particularly true of Hodgkin's disease, diffuse histiocytic tumours, or undifferentiated lymphomas of childhood. Highly differentiated mediastinal tumours in children (Sternberg's sarcoma) frequently develop into acute lymphoblastic leukaemia after initial treatment.

Patients with mediastinal obstruction present a therapeutic challenge. It is very important to obtain sufficient tissue for accurate histological diagnosis (anterior mediastinotomy, mediastinoscopy, thoracoscopy). If respiratory distress complicates the presentation, urgent treatment with corticosteroids, radiotherapy or vinca alkaloids may be necessary during the staging process. Hodgkin's disease presenting in this way is often associated with a good outcome. However, childhood lymphomas that are complicated by the development of acute lymphoblastic leukaemia carry a particularly poor prognosis.

Further reading

General

Andrews, M.W. (2000). Ultrasound of the spleen. *World J Surg* **24**: 183–7.

Gielchinsky, Y., Elstein, D., Hadas-Halpern, I. *et al.* (1999). Is there a correlation between degree of splenomegaly, symptoms and hypersplenism? A study of 218 patients with Gaucher disease. *Br J Haematol* **106**: 812–16.

Jansen, L., Nieweg, O. E., Peterse, J. L. *et al.* (2000). Reliability of sentinel lymph node biopsy for staging melanoma. *Br J Surg* **87**: 484–9.

Klingler, P. J., Tsiotos, G. G., Glaser, K. S. and Hinder, R. A. (1999). Laparoscopic splenectomy: evolution and current status. *Surg Laparosc Endosc* **9**: 1–8.

O'Reilly, R. A. (1996). Splenomegaly at a United States County Hospital: diagnostic evaluation of 170 patients. *Am J Med Sci* **312**: 160–5.

Rutland, M. D. (1992). Correlation of splenic function with the splenic uptake rate of Tc-colloids. *Nucl Med Commun* **13**: 843–7.

Secondary hypersplenism

Han, M. J., Zhao, H. G., Ren, K. *et al.* (1997). Partial splenic embolization for hypersplenism concomitant with or after arterial embolization of hepatocellular carcinoma in 30 patients. *Cardiovasc Intervent Radiol* **20**: 125–7.

Lin, M. C., Wu, C. C., Ho, W. L. *et al.* (1999). Concomitant splenectomy for hypersplenic thrombocytopenia in hepatic resection for hepatocellular carcinoma. *Hepatogastroenterology* **46**: 630–4.

Murata, K., Shiraki, K., Takase, K. *et al.* (1996). Long term follow-up for patients with liver cirrhosis after partial splenic embolization. *Hepatogastroenterology* **43**: 1212–17.

Pursnani, K. G., Sillin, L. F. and Kaplan, D. S. (1997). Effect of transjugular intrahepatic portosystemic shunt on secondary hypersplenism. *Am J Surg* **173**: 169–73

Shilyansky, J., Roberts, E. A. and Superina, R. A. (1999). Distal splenorenal shunts for the treatment of severe thrombocytopenia from portal hypertension in children. *J Gastrointest Surg* **3**: 167–72.

Hyposplenism

Brigden, M. L. and Pattullo, A. L. (1999). Prevention and management of overwhelming postsplenectomy infection – an update. *Crit Care Med* **27**: 836–42.

Cavenagh, J. D., Joseph, A. E., Dilly, S. and Bevan, D. H. (1994). Splenic sepsis in sickle cell disease. *Br J Haematol* **86**: 187–9.

Corazza, G. R., Addolorato, G., Biagi, F. *et al.* (1997). Splenic function and alcohol addiction. *Alcohol Clin Exp Res* **21**: 197–200.

Grotto, H. Z. and Costa, F. F. (1991). Hyposplenism in AIDS. *AIDS* **5**: 1538–40.

Khan, A. M., Harrington, R. D., Nadel, M. and Greenberg, B. R. (1998). Hyposplenism. In *Scintigraphic functional hyposplenism in amyloidosis* (eds Powsner, R.A., Simms, R.W., Chudnovsky, A. *et al.*). *J Nucl Med* 1998; **39**: 221–3.

Markus, H. S. and Toghill, P. J. (1991). Impaired splenic function in elderly people. *Age Ageing* **20**: 287–90.

Muller, A. F., Cornford, E. and Toghill, P. J. (1993). Splenic function in inflammatory bowel disease: assessment by differential interference microscopy and splenic ultrasound. *Q J Med* **86**: 333–40.

Wolf, H. M., Eibl, M. M., Georgi, E. *et al.* (1999). Long-term decrease of CD4+CD45RA+ T cells and impaired primary immune response after post-traumatic splenectomy. *Br J Haematol* **107**: 55–68.

Splenic infarction

Al-Salem, A. H., Naserullah, Z., Qaisaruddin, S. *et al.* (1999). Splenic complications of the sickling syndromes and the role of splenectomy. *J Pediatr Hematol Oncol* **21**: 401–6.

Cappell, M. S., Simon, T. and Tiku, M. (1993). Splenic infarction associated with anticardiolipin antibodies in a patient with acquired immunodeficiency syndrome. *Dig Dis Sci* **38**: 1152–5.

Cheng, P. N., Sheu, B. S., Chen, C. Y. *et al.* (1998). Splenic infarction after histoacryl injection for bleeding gastric varices. *Gastrointest Endosc* **48**: 426–7.

Nores, M., Phillips, E.H., Morgenstern, L. and Hiatt, J.R. (1998). The clinical spectrum of splenic infarction. *Am Surg* **64**: 182–8.

Ectopic (wandering) spleen

Allen, K. B., Gay, B. B. Jr and Skandalakis, J. E. (1992). Wandering spleen: anatomic and radiologic considerations. *South Med J* **85**: 976–84.

Dawson, J. H. and Roberts, N. G. (1994). Management of the wandering spleen. *Aust N Z J Surg* **64**: 441–4.

Desai, D. C., Hebra, A., Davidoff, A. M. and Schnaufer, L. (1997). Wandering spleen: a challenging diagnosis. *South Med J* **90**: 439–43.

Hon, T. Y., Chan, C. C., Loke, T. and Chan, C. S. (1998). Torsion of the wandering spleen. *Australas Radiol* **42**: 258–61.

Splenic cysts

Arber, D. A., Strickler, J. G. and Weiss, L. M. (1997). Splenic mesothelial cysts mimicking lymphagiomas. *Am J Surg Pathol* **21**: 334–8.

Du Plessis, D. G., Louw, J. A. and Wranz, B. P. A. (1999). Mucinous epithelial cysts of the spleen associated with pseudomyxoma peritonei. *Histopathology* **35**: 551–7.

Sasou, S., Nakamura, S. I. and Inomata, M. (1999). Epithelial splenic cysts in an intrapancreatic accessory spleen and spleen. *Pathol Int* **49**: 1078–83.

Sinha, P. S., Stoker, T. A. and Aston, N. O. (1999). Traumatic pseudocyst of the spleen. *J R Soc Med* **92**: 450–2.

Touloukian, R. J., Maharaj, A., Ghoussoub, R. and Reyes, M. (1997). Partial decapsulation of splenic epithelial cysts: studies on etiology and outcome. *J Pediatr Surg* **32**: 272–4.

Wadsworth, D. T., Newman, B., Abramson, S. J. *et al.* (1997). Splenic lymphangiomatosis in children. *Radiology* **202**: 173–6.

Yavorski, C. C., Greason, K. L. and Egan, M. C. (1998). Splenic cysts: a new approach to partial splenectomy – case report and review of the literature. *Am Surg* 1998; **64**: 795–8.

MODULE 12

Disorders of the pancreas

Section 12.1 • Surgical anatomy of the pancreas

Durmen has summarized the anatomical relationship of the pancreas as follows: 'The pancreas cuddles the left kidney, tickles the spleen, hugs the duodenum, cradles the aorta, opposes the inferior vena cava, dallies with the right renal pedicle, hides behind the posterior parietal peritoneum of the lesser sac and wraps itself around the superior mesenteric vessels.'

The pancreas is relatively inaccessible and, without some dissection, very little of it can be seen or palpated even at laparotomy. For this reason, it is much more difficult to manage surgically than all other abdominal viscera. Its retroperitoneal location in the upper abdomen means that it is almost completely hidden by the stomach, transverse colon and mesocolon (Figure 12.1). It derives its blood supply from numerous arteries arising from major branches of the coeliac and superior mesenteric arteries. A full understanding of the local vascular anatomy and its possible variations is essential for any surgeon operating on the pancreas.

In the thin patient, a part of the head of the gland may be seen directly behind the peritoneum of the supracolic and right infracolic compartments, and the inferior border of the body and tail may be visualized from the left infracolic compartment at the root of the transverse mesocolon. These views are very limited and are usually obscured by mesocolic and omental fat. The neck of the pancreas may be palpated by a finger passed through the epiploic foramen and directed inferiorly.

In order to inspect and palpate the pancreas properly, three surgical manoeuvres are necessary:

- The hepatic flexure of the colon is mobilized downwards and medially by dividing its attachments to the duodenum and anterior aspects of the pancreatic head. The peritoneum lateral to the second part of the duodenum is incised and the duodenum and pancreatic head are elevated by blunt dissection (Kocher manoeuvre) from the posterior parietal structures. In this way, the right kidney, right renal vein, inferior vena cava and the root of the left renal vein are exposed. The head of the pancreas, the duodenum and retroduodenal and pancreatic portions of the common bile duct can thus be palpated between thumb and finger.
- Limited visualization of the superior part of the body of the pancreas may be obtained by opening an avascular part of the lesser omentum and retracting the lesser curvature of the stomach inferiorly. This manoeuvre also brings the coeliac axis into view. The body of the pancreas can only be adequately visualized by widely opening the gastrocolic omentum, retracting the transverse colon and mesocolon inferiorly and the greater curvature of the stomach superiorly. By extending this opening to the right, into the pyloric region, the right gastroepiploic vessels can be divided near their origins and the anterior aspect of the neck of the pancreas can be visualized. Care must be taken to avoid damage to the middle colic vessels in this region. The opening can also be extended to the left and the gastrosplenic ligament with its contained short gastric vessels can be divided to permit complete visualization of the anterior surface of the tail of the pancreas at the splenic hilum.
- Downward and medial retraction of the dome of the spleen will tense the peritoneal leaf known as the lienorenal ligament and this can be divided to allow the spleen, splenic vessels and tail of the pancreas to be mobilized *en bloc*, allowing inspection of the posterior aspect of the body and tail of the pancreas and more careful palpation of the distal portion of the gland.

All three manoeuvres should be carried out safely, quickly and with little risk of damage to vital structures or troublesome bleeding. They will allow evaluation of all areas of the pancreas except the region of the neck

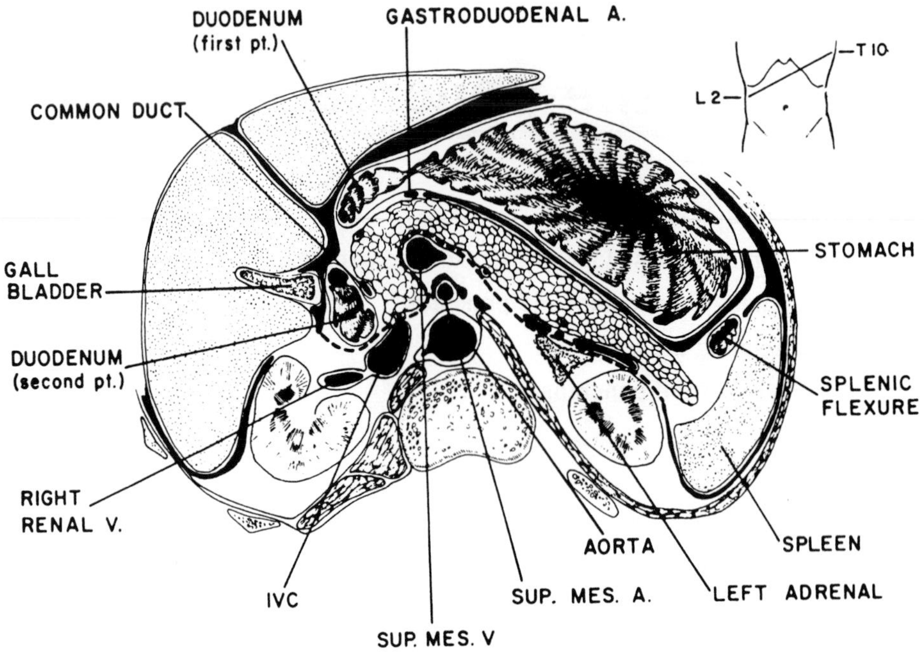

Figure 12.1 Oblique transverse cross-section of the upper abdomen viewed from below. Section passes through the long axis of the pancreas at approximately the levels indicated in the inset figure. The disposition and relations of structures shown approximate those seen in the oblique tranverse scanning.

and uncinate process. Further dissection and mobilization is usually necessary to assess the resectability of a pancreatic tumour. For this, a detailed knowledge of the pancreas and peripancreatic vasculature and its variations is essential.

The coeliac axis and the superior mesenteric artery and their branches vary a great deal in both their site of origin and their direction. The same applies to the venous drainage of the foregut, its appendages and the midgut into the portal venous trunk. The most demanding part of a pancreatic resection is dissection of the neck and head of the gland from the superior mesenteric and portal veins and the uncinate process from the superior mesenteric artery. Hence, it was formerly considered mandatory to have a coeliac and a superior mesenteric arteriogram (as well as a venous phase) prior to planning any major pancreatic resection. Recent refinement in computed tomography (CT scan) and magnetic resonance imaging (MRI) has rendered *diagnostic pancreatic angiography largely obsolete*.

As with the blood vessels, pancreaticobiliary ductal anatomy is very variable and the concept of a 'normal duct anatomy' should be abandoned. The terminology which is widely applied to describe the main pancreatic ductal system is explained in Figure 12.2. The variations in termination of the main and accessory pancreatic ducts and their relationship to the lower end of the common bile duct are depicted in Figure 12.3.

The pancreas occupies a central position at a complex anatomical crossroads and its lymphatic drainage is radially disposed along several major routes, namely, the coeliac, splenic, hepatic and superior mesenteric nodal

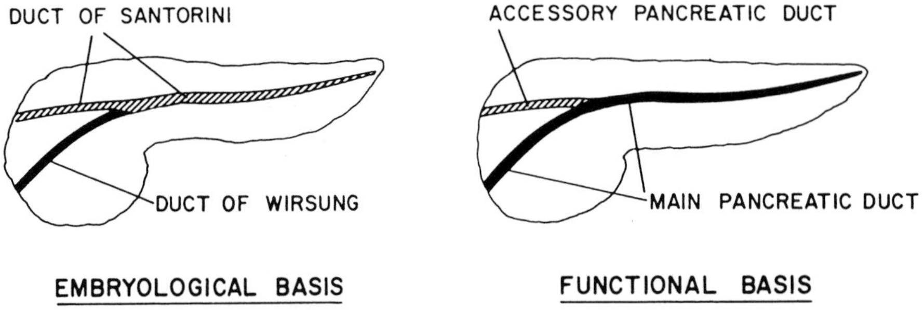

Figure 12.2 Terminology variously applied to describe the pancreatic ductal system. An understanding of ductal embryology, particularly with regard to the development of the more unusual variation, may be served by the terms given in the left diagram. For clarity and practicality the terms given in the right diagram are preferred.

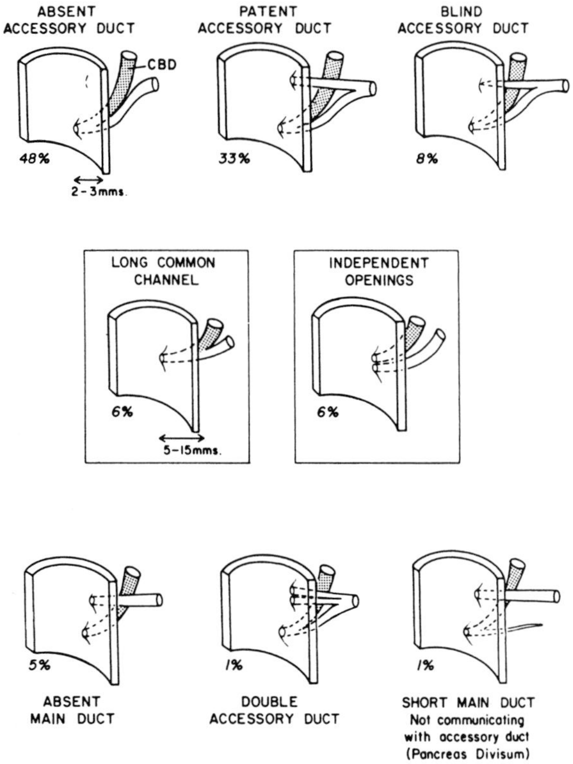

Figure 12.3 Variations of main and accessory pancreatic ducts and their relationship to the common bile duct (CBD).

basins. It is thus hard to design an adequate 'cancer-operation' which, in an orderly manner, removes the primary tumour *en bloc* with primary, secondary and tertiary lymphatic nodal territories. Moreover, the intimate anatomical association of the pancreas with major vessels at once limits the extent of the procedure and dictates what must be removed. Thus, when a tumour of the pancreas spreads a short distance, it involves the portal vein, superior mesenteric artery or coeliac axis, and usually becomes incurable. Similarly, if the gland is removed in radical fashion, the need to excise the vessels and lymph nodes associated with it makes removal of the spleen, duodenum, gallbladder, common bile duct, upper jejunum and part of the stomach necessary.

Where only part of the pancreas is excised or even if the gland is incised, safe management of any draining pancreatic juice becomes a matter of primary importance since enzymes, if allowed to accumulate in the peritoneal cavity, may cause local damage. A first principle of pancreatic surgery is the provision of adequate drainage. Similarly, the collection of serum, lymph and blood following a pancreatic resection needs to be drained. Secondly, the protein nature of catgut makes it vulnerable to digestion by trypsin. It should not, therefore, be used as ligature of major vessels, as a suture material for anastomosis, or for closure of the abdomen during pancreatic surgery. Non-absorbable material, such as silk, cotton, nylon or prolene, is essential for safety.

Section 12.2 • Cellular composition and physiology of the exocrine pancreas

The exocrine pancreas consists of acinar and ductal systems which drain its secretions into the duodenum. The exocrine tissue accounts for 98% of the pancreas by weight. Under the influence of neural and hormonal controls, the exocrine pancreas secretes water and bicarbonate from the ductal system and enzymes from the acinar cells. The parasympathetic vagal fibres have ganglia in the interlobular septa and post-ganglionic fibres are distributed to acinar cells and to smooth muscle cells in the ducts. The sympathetic fibres appear to be entirely distributed to the blood vessels and to be concerned solely with regulation of pancreatic blood flow rather than in the direct control of pancreatic secretion.

Fluid and electrolyte secretion from the pancreas is a ductal function and is an energy requiring process. The cationic composition of pancreatic fluid is similar to that of plasma. Sodium and potassium concentrations are identical to those in plasma and are independent of flow. During states of fluid and electrolyte secretion, calcium appears to enter the ducts passively. However, under the influence of cholecystokinin (CCK), it appears to be actively secreted in parallel with enzyme secretion. Anionic secretion consists almost entirely of bicarbonate and chloride. The sum of concentrations of these two anions remains constant – a high chloride concentration occurs at low flow rates and chloride is replaced by bicarbonate as the flow increases.

Pancreatic enzyme secretion originates in the acinar cell and accounts for virtually all the protein (2–8 g/day in man) in pancreatic juice. Many of the enzymes are secreted in their inactive or zymogen forms together with inhibitors. This mechanism protects the pancreas from autodigestion by its own proteolytic enzymes. Enzyme activation begins after the zymogen enters the duodenum, where mucosal enterokinase cleaves trypsinogen into trypsin, leaving trypsin to activate the other enzymes. The large list of enzymes secreted in pancreatic juice includes amylase, lipase, cholesterol ester hydrolase, phospholecithinase A, trypsin, chymotrypsin A and B, elastase, carboxypeptidase A and B, collagenase, leucine aminopeptidase, ribonuclease and, undoubtedly, other enzymes for which a function has yet to be described.

Control of pancreatic exocrine secretion

Basal pancreatic secretion results from either an intrinsic autonomy of the gland or a low level of activity of neurohormonal regulators. A complete neurohormonal control mechanism is at work and secretin, CCK and gastrin play the dominant roles. Secretin is released in response to duodenal acidification and there is also an increase in secretin release in man in response to alcohol and, to as lesser extent, after a meal. Secretin produces a secretion of fluid and electrolytes which is initiated within 30 s of an administered dose, the bicarbonate concentration of the fluid increasing as flow increases. It is now generally accepted that secretin is also a weak stimulant of enzyme secretion.

The stimulus for release of CCK appears to be entry of amino acids, fatty acids, hydrochloric acid and food into the duodenum. It causes an increase in the release of enzymes and a small increase in fluid and electrolyte output. In man, pancreatic secretion is initiated by CCK at a dose lower than that required for gallbladder contraction.

Gastrin has a varying effect on pancreatic secretion but, in man, it causes an increase in enzyme secretion. The action of glucagon and vasoactive intestinal peptide (VIP) on human pancreatic secretion has yet to be defined. Chymodenin appears to selectively induce chymotrypsin secretion. Somatostatin, pancreatic polypeptide and motilin have unidentified roles, but may act as a feedback control.

Hormonal and neural interaction

Combinations of two or more hormones have differing effects on the acinar and ductal cells. Secretin is a strong stimulant of fluid and electrolyte secretion and a weak stimulator of enzyme secretion; acting with CCK, however, marked augmentation occurs. These hormones have different receptor sites on the acinar cell and the site of interaction is probably intracellular. Such augmentation probably has an important physiological role since only small amounts of secretin are released into the circulation in response to a meal.

The interaction between the exocrine and endocrine cells of the pancreas is currently being elucidated. Insulin is trophic to the peri-insular cells and a loss of insulin secretion in diabetes mellitus results in progressive damage to the acinar cell. The blood supply to the human pancreas first passes the islets and then forms a capillary network around the acinar cells, allowing maximal effects of islet hormones on the acinus. Thus, insulin, glucagon, somatostatin and other islet cell secretions may affect exocrine pancreatic secretion.

In man, vagal reflexes in response to gastric distension result in a juice rich in enzymes, and this effect is abolished by truncal vagotomy. It is likely that the role of vagal stimulation is a permissive one, allowing secretin and CCK to exert their full effect. Thus, atropine, by blocking acetylcholine, depresses the responsiveness of the acinar and ductal cells to CCK in animals.

Section 12.3 • Anatomy and physiology of the exocrine pancreas

The islets of Langerhans form the endocrine portion of the mammalian pancreas and consist of cells arranged in spherical or ovoid clusters which are well circumscribed and irregularly distributed throughout the gland. Although variable, the total number of islets in the adult human pancreas is estimated to be one million. The average weight of the entire pancreas in the adult approximates 100 g. The islets weigh about 1–2 g and thus form, at best, only about 2–3% of the weight of the whole gland.

Our knowledge of the cellular composition of the islets is still incomplete but the existence of four cell types has been largely accepted in mammalian islets based on ultrastructural characteristics of their secretory granules (Figure 12.4). These are A, B, D and F cells. A cells form approximately 20% of the normal islet cell population, B cells 75%. In the various pathological conditions affecting the islets, including diabetes mellitus, the proportion of different cell types varies. A cells (alpha cells) synthesize, store and secrete glucagon. They are concentrated in the periphery of the islets. B cells (beta cells) synthesize, store and release insulin. Islet amyloid associated polypeptide (IAPP), or amylin, and pancreastatin are also formed in the pancreatic B cells. The physiological function of former is unclear. However, pancreastatin has a known inhibitory role on insulin secretion as well as glucagon and pancreatic acinar cell secretion in animal models. The role in humans is not well defined. B cells are concentrated in the centre of the islets. D cells supply the tetradecapeptide somatostatin and also probably gastrin. They tend to be located in the periphery of the islets. F cells are the rarest cell type encountered in normal islets and they are possibly responsible for the secretion of pancreatic polypeptide (PP). The F cells compromise approximately 15–20% of cells within the islets of the ventral pancreas but are uncommonly

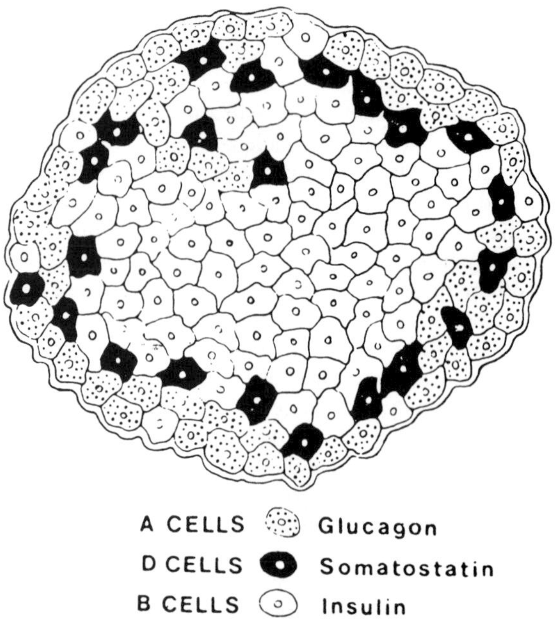

Figure 12.4 Schematic representation of an islet of Langerhans showing distribution of the three main cell types. (From Orci, L. and Unger, R. H. (1975). *Lancet* **ii**: 1243, by permission.)

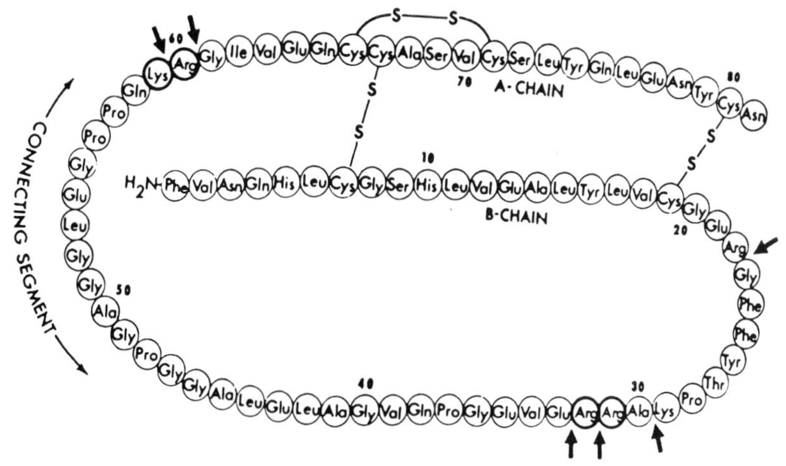

Figure 12.5 Covalent structure of bovine pro-insulin. Arrows indicate sites of tryptic cleavage.

found in the dorsal pancreatic islets. The number of F cells probably increases with age and in association with injury to pancreatic tissue. An increase in the number of F cells has been documented in such conditions as diabetes, pancreatitis, mucoviscidosis, haemochromatosis and various exocrine or endocrine pancreatic tumours.

Insulin has a molecular weight of 5800 and consists of two peptide chains A and B which are connected by two disulfide bridges (Figure 12.5). In man the A chain has 21 amino acids and the B chain is composed of 30 amino acids. There are structural variations from species to species. It is known that insulin is formed in a precursor form, pro-insulin, which compromises the insulin A and B chains linked by a polypeptide segment consisting of 30–35 amino acids. This connecting peptide (C-peptide) helps in the formation of the native structure of the insulin molecule by ensuring the correct pairing of the cysteine residues during formation of the disulfide linkages between the A and B chains. Proteolytic cleavage of pro-insulin by enzymes in the secretory granules results in the separation of insulin from the C-peptide. These two products are thus released in equimolar amounts from the B cells. Pro-insulin-like components (PLC) comprise 15% of the immunoreactive insulin concentration. The kidney is an important site of pro-insulin degradation; hence levels of PLC are markedly elevated in chronic renal failure. Raised serum pro-insulin concentrations have been found in both benign and malignant insulinomas. Neither insulin nor insulin antibodies interfere in the immunoassay for the estimation of C-peptide concentration. Since insulin and C-peptide are formed in equimolar amounts following cleavage of pro-insulin, the circulating levels of C-peptide provide a measure of B cell secretory activity, especially in the presence of circulating insulin antibodies produced in response to exogenous insulin. Thus it gives an indication of endogenous insulin production from the beta cell. C-peptide measurement therefore has a vital role in the diagnosis of surreptitious injection of insulin and in the follow-up evaluation of patients who have undergone total or near-total pancreatectomy for nesidioblastosis or a malignant insulinoma. Following resection of the latter, significant C-peptide levels indicate residual pancreatic tissue or the presence of functioning metastases. Recurrence may be heralded by a rise in C-peptide levels.

The main stimulus to insulin secretion is an increase in glucose levels. The insulin will thus cause a fall in glucose concentration and, by a negative feedback effect, this leads to a decrease in insulin release. Other stimuli for insulin release are the amino acids arginine and lysin, glucagon, growth hormone, cortisol, placental lactogen and the sex hormones (especially oestrogens). Glucagon releases insulin both by direct stimulatory effect on the B cells and also indirectly by mobilizing glucose from the liver. The remaining hormones mentioned above act by causing resistance to the actions of insulin and thus generate a compensatory increase in insulin secretion. A number of gastrointestinal hormones including gastrin, secretin, gut glucagon, CCK-PZ and gastric inhibitory polypeptide (GIP) may also be stimulants for insulin secretion. Insulin release is also enhanced by free fatty acids to prevent ketoacidosis which would otherwise occur during fasting in normal individuals.

Vagal stimulation is also a potent stimulus to insulin release although no impairment in the insulin release can be demonstrated following vagotomy. Adrenergic beta receptors also stimulate insulin release, but adrenaline and noradrenaline, acting via alpha receptors, have an inhibitory effect on insulin secretion. The ventromedial nucleus of the hypothalamus is believed to be important in the cephalic phase of insulin release. Finally, insulin secretion is influenced by various drugs. Tolbutamide and chlorpropamide have a stimulatory effect while alloxan and streptozotocin impair insulin secretion by directly damaging the B cells.

Glucagon

Glucagon is a secretory product of the A cell and is a linear peptide composed of 29 amino acids with a molecular weight of approximately 3500. Gel filtration of acid alcohol extracts of pancreatic tissue has revealed two peaks of immunoreactivity, one with a molecular weight in excess of 9000 (believed to represent proglucagon) and another which is a globulin-sized fraction that has been referred to as big plasma glucagon which may be a precursor of glucagon or simply glucagon bound to a larger protein.

Glucagon has catabolic actions. Hypoglycaemia (a fall below 90 mg/dl) produces a rise in plasma glucagon concentration and an increase in glucose concentration leads to a drop in glucagon levels. Glucagon activates adenyl cyclase which increases hepatic cyclic AMP to initiate breakdown of glycogen into glucose (glycogenolysis). It also inhibits the process of glycogenesis. It increases glucose formation from non-glucose precursors, e.g. glycerol, lactate and amino acids of the glycogenic type. Glucagon also enhances the breakdown of fat into free fatty acids and glycerol. It stimulates gluconeogenesis and, thus, its infusion lowers plasma amino acids. Finally, glucagon inhibits protein synthesis. There is evidence that glucagon, through its gluconeogenic, ketogenic and lipolytic effects, and not insulin lack alone, is partly responsible for the development of fulminant diabetic ketoacidosis in man.

The inter-relationship between insulin and glucagon is a complex one which is only partly understood. In general, an inverse relationship exists between insulin and glucagon levels. When glucose is needed, insulin levels fall and glucagon levels rise, producing an increased hepatic glucose production. The reverse is true in states of hyperglycaemia. Following a protein meal, a parallel change is observed in the levels of insulin and glucagon. The rise in glucagon level prevents the hypoglycaemia that would result from enhanced insulin secretion alone by amino acids. CCK-PZ, which stimulates insulin secretion, is also believed to facilitate glucagon secretion following the stimulus of a protein meal and is responsible for the buffer mechanism against hypoglycaemia arising from ingestion of protein.

Somatostatin

This tetradecapeptide is secreted by the D cell. It inhibits the release of growth hormone from the anterior pituitary and was first isolated from the hypothalamus. Its other actions include inhibition of insulin and glucagon secretion, gastrin secretion, acid and pepsin secretion from the stomach, as well as the release of pancreatic enzymes. It suppresses intestinal motility and contraction of the gallbladder. It also has a suppressive effect on glucose uptake from the gut and on appetite and may play a role in nutrient homeostasis. Infusion of somatostatin diminishes splanchnic blood flow. In view of its inhibitory effect on the exocrine pancreas, the long-acting somatostatin analogue (octreotide) has been tried in the treatment of patients with pancreatic fistula and acute pancreatitis. Somatostatin has been isolated from a variety of tissues and organs, including the gastrointestinal tract and pancreatic islets. Its exact and full spectrum of function is as yet unknown.

Human pancreatic polypeptide (HPP)

HPP consists of 36 amino acids in a straight chain. The ultrastructural identification of the HPP-producing cell is not definitely settled but the F cells are the prime candidates. The physiological role of HPP is unknown. It is almost totally confined to the pancreas and is thus undetectable in pancreatectomized patients. Its secretion is believed to be largely due to vagal cholinergic stimulation and, in part, by gastrointestinal humoral stimulation. It is released by ingestion of fat and protein but not by intravenous nutrients. In pharmacological doses, HPP inhibits pancreatic secretion caused by CCK-PZ and secretin, stimulates gastric emptying and intestinal transit, inhibits relaxation of the gallbladder and increases the tone of the choledochal sphincter. It has been suggested as a possible causative agent in the watery diarrhoea, hypokalaemia achlorhydria (WDHA) syndrome. Significant elevated levels of HPP are found in both maturity onset and juvenile diabetics. This observation has also been extended to patients with chronic pancreatitis. Many endocrine tumours of the pancreas and their metastases have also been found to contain numerous HPP cells and also to have a high tumour content of HPP. If this finding is substantiated, elevated circulating HPP levels in patients with these tumours may serve as an aid in diagnosis and in the monitoring of therapy in such patients.

Conclusions

The pancreatic islets consist of cell types in close topographical relationship which produce hormones with different but related actions. Gaps and tight junctions have been demonstrated between islet cells of the same as well as different types. This arrangement may play a role in co-ordinating the activity of the different cell types, e.g. somatostatin-containing cells are topographically closely related to B and A cells. As somatostatin inhibits insulin and glycogen release, it is possible that it serves a paracrine function by regulating the local (within the islet) release of these hormones from the appropriate cells. It is likely that the islets function as a well-integrated unit and further elucidation of such mechanisms will enhance the understanding of various pathological conditions arising in this endocrine organ.

Section 12.4 • Methods of investigating the pancreas

Introduction

Because of its deep-seated and inaccessible location, the pancreas is a difficult organ to investigate and to visualize. A precise diagnosis of pancreatic disease is often only possible through the use of a wide battery of tests. The results of such tests should be viewed in the light of the clinical information since all available procedures may not yield concordant data.

Procedures which are employed in the investigation of patients with suspected pancreatic disorders may be classified into five groups:

- Procedures which outline the gland to delineate enlargement, masses, irregularities in contour and calcification. These include:
  - (a) Indirect imaging of the pancreas:
    Standard radiological studies to visualize the effect of the pancreas on adjacent organs such as stomach, duodenum, small bowel, transverse colon and bile duct. These studies are largely outdated and have been replaced by other more modern imaging techniques.
  - (b) Direct imaging techniques to visualize:
    The pancreatic parenchyma, e.g. ultrasonography, computed tomography, magnetic resonance cholangiopancreatography (MRCP), endoscopic ultrasound (EUS).
    The pancreatic duct system – ERCP (endoscopic retrograde cholangiopancreatography).
    The pancreatic and peripancreatic vasculature – angiography, contrast CT scan, MRI.
- Procedures to define pancreatic exocrine function:
  - (c) Faecal fat excretion.
  - (d) Pancreatic function tests.
- Procedures to define pancreatic endocrine function:
  - (e) Measurement of fasting blood levels of glucose and/or hormones which are secreted by the pancreatic islets under normal and/or abnormal conditions. These include serum insulin, pro-insulin, C-peptide, glucagon, somatostatin and gastrin.
  - (f) Provocative tests to measure the serum level of the above substances if the fasting levels are not conclusive:
    Calcium infusion test (insulinoma and gastrinoma).
    Tolbutamide tolerance test (insulinoma).
    Glucagon test (insulinoma).
    Insulin suppression test (insulinoma).
    Secretin test (gastrinoma).
- Analysis of serum for markers of pancreatic disease:
  - (g) Enzymes, such as amylase, lipase, trypsin, ribonuclease.
  - (h) Tumour-associated antigens, such as carcinoembryonic antigen (CEA), pancreatic oncofetal antigen (POA) and CA 19-9.
- Pancreatic biopsy and cytology:
  - (i) Percutaneous fine-needle aspiration cytology using ultrasonography or computed tomography for guidance.
  - (j) Endoscopic transgastric or transduodenal needle aspiration cytology or brush cytology.
  - (k) Laparoscopic visualization and direct vision biopsy or aspiration cytology of the pancreas.
  - (l) Operative visualization, palpation and biopsy of the pancreas.

Standard radiological investigations

Standard or routine radiological investigations rely on the detection of anatomical abnormalities by the displacement or distortion of adjacent viscera, such as the pancreas. Maximum information may be obtained from each type of examination if the radiologist involved is alerted to the possibility of pancreatic disease prior to the actual procedure. The main value of the various investigations to be described is that they provide important information in a clinical setting suggestive of disease in the upper abdomen. They should be employed principally to identify and/or to exclude common disorders such as peptic ulcer, gallstones, hiatus hernia, gastric cancer and colon cancer. They may, however, show a wide range of abnormalities suggestive of pancreatic disease. Two common pitfalls need to be emphasized: (a) the presence of a common benign disorder, such as hiatus hernia or gallstones does not preclude the simultaneous presence of pancreatic disease; (b) normal routine radiological studies do *not* necessarily signify the absence of pancreatic disease.

A *plain radiograph of the abdomen* may show changes suggestive of *pancreatic disease*, the most important of which is pancreatic calcification. Radiating 'sun-burst' calcification is pathognomonic of cystadenomas or cystadenocarcinomas of the pancreas. Numerous other lesions of the pancreas may also show calcifications. These include chronic pancreatitis, with or without pancreaticolithiasis, lymphangiomas, haemangiomas and, occasionally, mucin-secreting adenocarcinoma or islet-cell carcinoma. In hereditary pancreatitis, the incidence of pancreatic calcification is higher than in other types of pancreatitis and the incidence of pancreatic malignancy is also increased. In general 2–4% of all patients with pancreatic calcification have a co-existing pancreatic carcinoma but, conversely, over 95% of all patients with pancreatic calcification will have benign disease.

Contrast studies of the gastrointestinal tract

Pancreatic disease may reflect changes in the oesophagus, stomach, small bowel and colon. A pancreatic pseudocyst may present in the posterior mediastinum and compress the oesophagus. Occasionally, a tumour arising in the tail of the pancreas will also deform and involve the distal oesophagus. Alternatively, metastatic lymphadenopathy in the posterior mediastinum may also occlude the oesophagus. Gastric and/or oesophageal varices occasionally accompany pancreatitis or any type of pancreatic cancer as a result of splenic vein occlusion.

Radiological examination of the stomach and duodenum

Changes produced in the stomach and duodenum can be considered under the headings of extrinsic compression and indentation, rugal and mucosal abnormalities, enlarged retrogastric space and gastric varices. If a double contrast examination is performed, some of the more subtle mucosal changes may be seen to better advantage. Motility changes of the stomach, particularly the antrum, may be seen when the posterior stomach wall is invaded by an inflammatory process or a malignant disease of the pancreas.

Pancreatic disease may reflect on the duodenum in a number of different ways and these may be seen on contrast radiography as pressure defects, abnormalities of duodenal fold pattern, widening of the duodenal

C-loop, displacement of the angle of Trietz, postbulbar ulceration of the duodenum (Zollinger–Ellison syndrome), disorders of duodenal motility under fluoroscopy, enlargement of the ampulla of Vater and duodenobiliary reflux.

It should be emphasized that by the time the presence of a pancreatic carcinoma is reflected by diagnosable changes on contrast radiology of the gastrointestinal tract, the lesion is advanced and incurable.

Radiological examination of the small bowel

Mass lesions of the pancreas may produce displacement of the duodenojejunal area and of the small bowel. These appearances are usually seen with pancreatic pseudocysts and large tumours. Chronic pancreatic disease associated with exocrine insufficiency and steatorrhoea may show a malabsorption pattern of the small bowel with thickened, clubbed or effaced folds. The classic appearance is seen in cystic fibrosis. Patients with the Zollinger–Ellison syndrome may show thickening of the folds in the duodenum and proximal jejunum and hypersecretion of fluid with dilution of the barium. Multiple peptic ulcerations may also be seen.

Radiological examination of the colon

In pancreatitis, characteristic changes have been described in the transverse colon and the region of the splenic flexure. These include ileus of the transverse colon (colon cut-off sign), displacement of the transverse colon and, sometimes, colonic strictures, fistulas and necrosis. Some of these appearances may simulate carcinoma of the colon. Rarely, a pancreatic pseudocyst may present in an unusual location and has even been described presenting as a pre-sacral mass indenting the rectum. Intraperitoneal seeding from metastatic pancreatic carcinoma may cause indentation of any part of the colon.

Cholangiography and isotope biliary excretion scan

Patients with pancreatic disease (cancer and/or pancreatitis) may present with biliary tract obstruction and jaundice. If the serum bilirubin exceeds 51 μmol/l (3 mg/100 ml), then the outdated oral or intravenous cholangiography and Tc-HIDA scan no longer play a role in the investigation. If ultrasonography or CT shows dilated biliary radicles, then percutaneous transhepatic cholangiography has a place in the investigation of biliary obstruction. However, when the biliary obstruction is suspected to be in the pancreatic region, endoscopic retrograde cholangiopancreatography (ERCP) is a preferred method of visualizing the biliary tree since it can provide valuable additional information.

Direct imaging of the pancreas

Ultrasonography

Ultrasonography is probably the most important advance in pancreatic investigation of the past two decades. The following features are indicators of pancreatic disease on ultrasonography:

- Diffuse or localized enlargement of the gland may be due to inflammation, tumour or pseudocysts. Atrophy of the entire pancreas usually indicates chronic pancreatitis.
- Alteration of the texture or 'pattern of internal echoes' within the pancreas may provide a *subjective* impression of pancreatic disease.
- Indirect signs outside the pancreas but readily traced to the pancreatic area are dilatation of the biliary system and displacement of the vessels adjacent to the pancreas.
- Abnormal dilatation of the pancreatic duct may be the result of cancer or chronic pancreatitis.
- Metastases and ascites are also indirect signs of pancreatic disease which by themselves do not necessarily imply the presence of an abnormal pancreas.

The distinction between pancreatic cancer, chronic pancreatitis and a variety of other pancreatic tumours can be difficult without knowledge of the clinical situation. Ultrasonography is relatively inexpensive, non-invasive and free of radiation hazards. It can be repeated as often as necessary but requires good equipment and enthusiastic, expert staff for its performance and its interpretation. In spite of this, technical failure which prevents proper visualization of the whole pancreas occurs in about 10–15% of patients and can be attributed to obesity, gastrointestinal gas and previous operations in the upper abdomen as well as massive ascites.

Computed tomography (Figures 12.6 and 12.7)

The CT scan is highly successful in demonstrating the pancreas and allows complete visualization of between 93–100% of all glands. The most valuable sign of disease shown by CT scan is the presence of localized or diffuse enlargement of the gland. As with ultrasonography, this finding is non-specific as to the type of disease. The pancreas may be abnormal without recognizable enlargement and, conversely, normal variants of size exist which may suggest abnormalities when none is present. An abnormally small pancreas may be a sign of chronic pancreatitis. The lower limit of normal is said

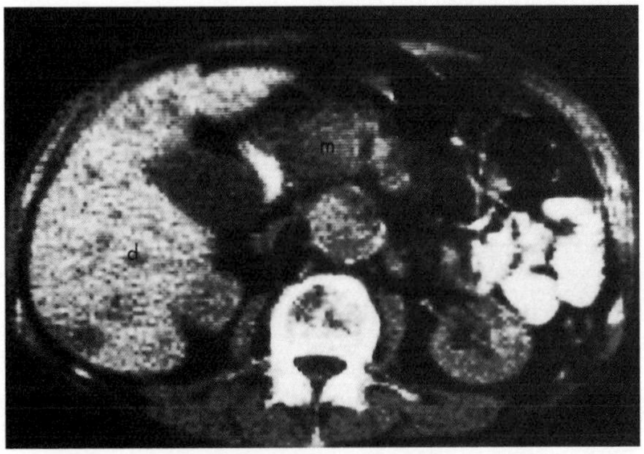

Figure 12.6 CT scan showing typical appearance of carcinoma of the pancreas, consisting of a mass (m) in the head of the pancreas, a distended gallbladder (g) and dilated intrahepatic ducts (d). Incidental note is made of an aortic aneurysm which was better seen in more caudal sections.

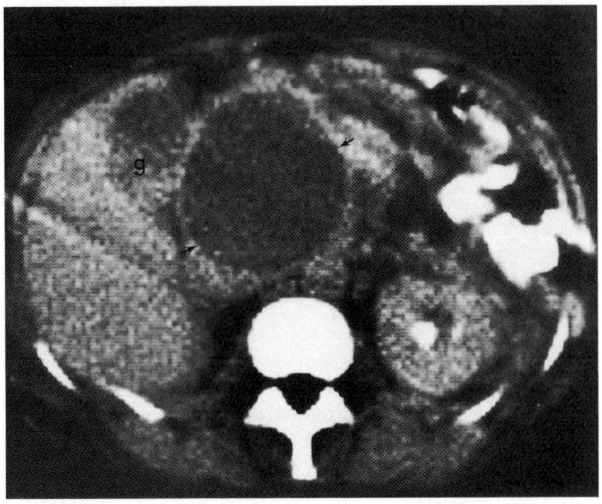

Figure 12.7 CT scan showing typical pseudocyst (arrows) near the head of pancreas. The gallbladder (g) is also visualized.

to be one-half of a vertebral body width for the head of the pancreas and one-third for the body of the gland. Nevertheless, when the size of the gland falls below these standards, the pancreas is often actually normal. Calcifications are readily identified by CT scanning. Other signs of pancreatic disease include dilatation of the hepatobiliary tree, dilatation of the pancreatic duct and liver metastases.

The accuracy of ultrasonography and CT scan in detecting abnormalities in the pancreas varies. The reported figures are dependent on the type and spectrum of diseases included in the population studied, on the nature of the equipment employed, and on the skill of the individuals involved in the study. Chronic pancreatitis produces more problems for ultrasonic detection – only about 50% of cases of chronic pancreatitis may show changes detectable by ultrasound. One major difference between ultrasonography and CT scan is the frequency with which the gland can be seen. Ultrasonography has a non-visualization rate that averages 15–20% when conventional techniques are used. What is more subtle, and not known, is the frequency with which significant portions of the pancreas are hidden even though the investigator thinks the entire gland is seen. Cases of non-visualization are often excluded when an investigator tabulates his figures – the test is thus made to appear more useful than it actually is. On the other hand, failure rates for CT are significantly lower and range from 0 to 10%. CT scan has a higher chance of visualizing the gland when ascites or extreme obesity is present. On the other hand, when the patient cannot remain motionless or suspend respiration during the scanning, CT study is usually inadequate but the ultrasound examination may produce diagnostic results. Recognition of pancreatic calcification and small intrapancreatic pseudocysts is clearer with CT scan and this facilitates diagnosis of pancreatitis. Finally, detection of gas and of the thicker walls of pancreatic abscesses is easier with a CT scan.

CT examinations are two to four times more expensive than pancreatic ultrasound. When serial or multiple studies are required, the small but potential risk of radiation exposure has to be taken into account with the CT scan.

Endoscopic retrograde cholangiopancreatography (ERCP)

Endoscopic diagnosis at ERCP

ERCP endoscopy provides direct visual observation of the oesophagus, stomach, duodenum and ampulla of Vater. Inflammatory or neoplastic lesions visualized in any part of the upper gastrointestinal tract may entirely explain the clinical picture.

Tissue diagnosis at ERCP

Conventional endoscopic biopsy with forceps, brush cytology, aspiration of pancreatic juice for cytology or direct transduodenal needle aspiration cytology may be possible and provides valuable information if positive for malignant disease. In addition, aspirated pancreatic juice may be assayed for research into tumour markers such as CEA and POA.

Radiological diagnosis at ERCP (Figures 12.8–12.10)

Retrograde pancreatogram and/or retrograde cholangiogram often provide information indicative of the presence of tumour, inflammatory disorders or stone disease.

The main disadvantage of ERCP is that it requires the combined team effort of an endoscopist, an assistant who is thoroughly familiar with the equipment and technique (including disinfection procedures and the handling of specimens), a radiology technician and, ideally, a radiologist. It is time-consuming and expensive. It is an invasive procedure which carries a small but definite risk of complications. ERCP is unsuitable for screening patients with unsuspected pancreatic disease.

Complications of ERCP

These are:

- Injection pancreatitis – this can be prevented by careful injection of the medium into the pancreatic duct without too much pressure and without attempting to obtain an acinar phase of the pancreatogram.
- Sepsis – pancreatic and biliary sepsis can be induced or precipitated by ERCP. Whether the sepsis is of endogenous or exogenous origin is a debatable and academic point. Suffice to say that ERCP sepsis is most frequently related to injection into an obstructed pancreatic duct, a pseudocyst or an obstructed common bile duct.

ERCP sepsis can be largely prevented or abolished if the following precautions are taken:

- Disinfection of the endoscope tip and the cannula with 2% glutaraldehyde.
- Prophylactic systemic antibiotics intravenously for 24–48 hours.
- Addition of antibiotics (chloramphenicol or gentamicin) to the contrast material.
- The patient should be operated on within 24 hours of ERCP if a pseudocyst or an obstructed duct is demonstrated.

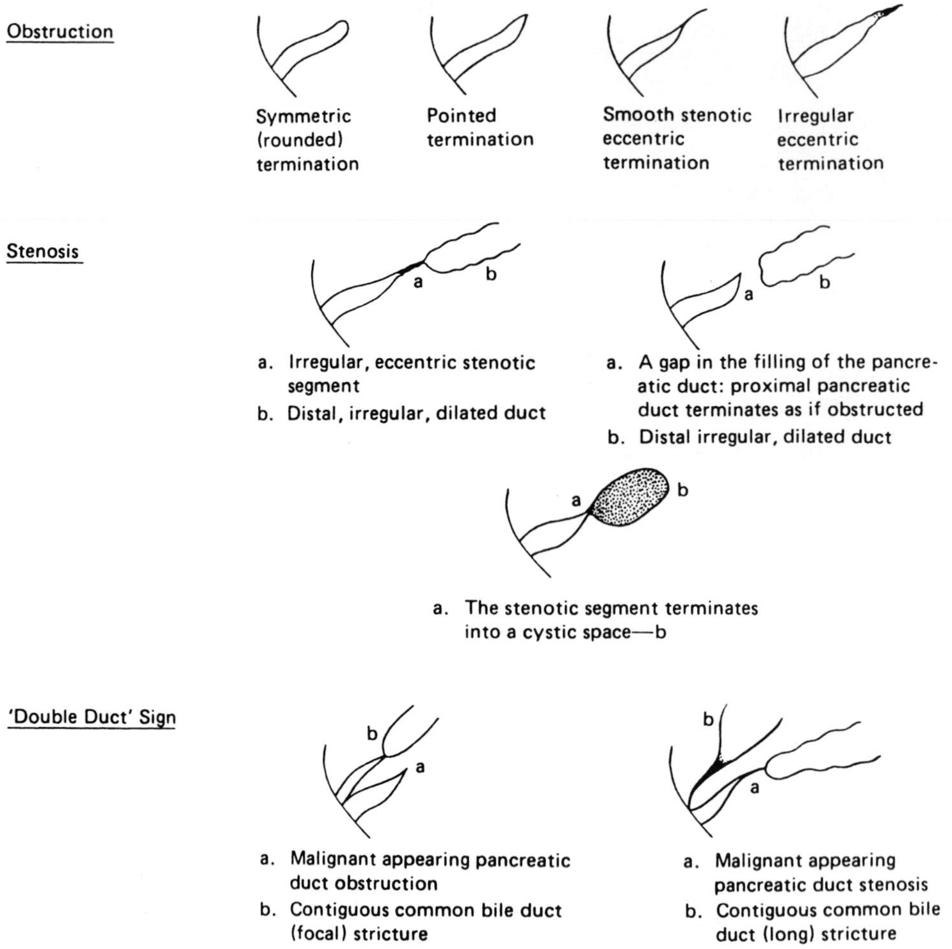

Figure 12.8 Diagram of typical radiographic appearances of the main pancreatic duct as demonstrated by ERCP in patients with cancer of the head of pancreas.

Other rare complications of ERCP are drug reactions, instrumental injury to the upper gastrointestinal tract and aspiration pneumonia which is associated with the amount of sedatives given to the patient.

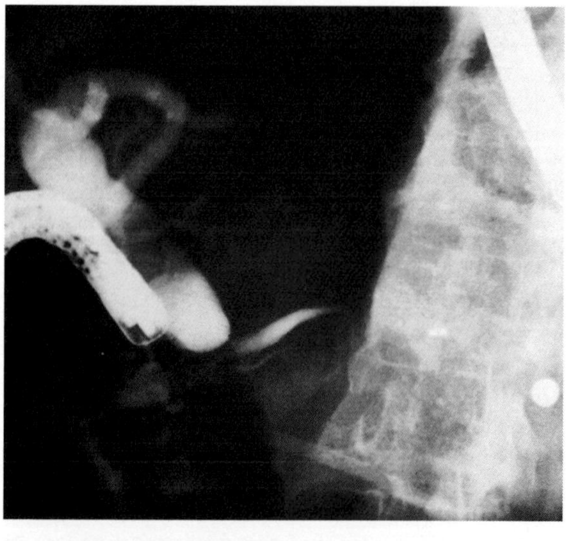

Figure 12.9 ERCP showing 'rat tail' appearance due to obstruction of the main pancreatic duct by a carcinoma. The common bile duct is dilated. The 'double duct' sign is highly suggestive of unresectablility of the cancer.

Angiography

Percutaneous transfemoral catheterization for coeliac and superior mesenteric angiography is, occasionally, a valuable method of studying the vasculature of the pancreas. With improvement in and refinement of catheter design, various techniques of super-selective catheterization may be enhanced by magnification radiography and, in some instances, by the intra-arterial injection of various drugs which improve the visualization (pharmacoangiography) of pancreatic vessels. Vasodilators (bradykinin, tolazolin) and/or vasoconstrictors (epinephrine, norepinephrine, angiotensin) and hormones (secretin and pancreozymin) have all been tried.

The single most useful and reliable angiographic sign of a malignant tumour of the pancreas is arterial encasement. Encasement is seen as a narrowing and/or

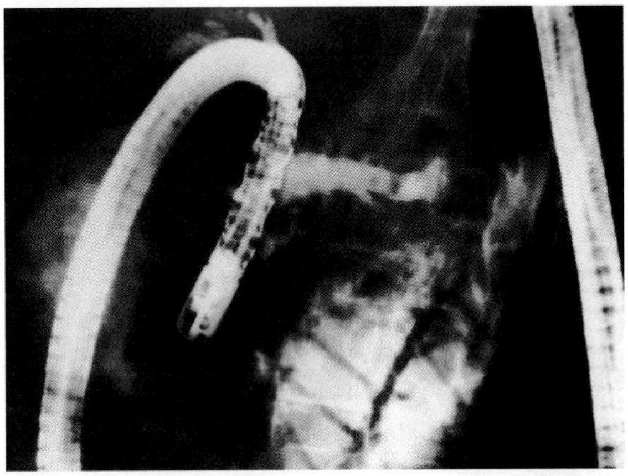

Figure 12.10 ERCP showing grossly dilated main pancreatic duct due to chronic pancreatitis.

irregularity of a vessel and is caused by invasion of the vessel by tumour or its compression by surrounding tissues. Arterial encasement may be irregular or smooth or may be serrated or serpiginous. The smooth encasement is much less specific for cancer and may be seen in pancreatitis. Large artery (splenic, hepatic, superior mesenteric, left gastric) encasement is highly suggestive of an unresectable tumour. Small artery encasement is a term applied when more distal branches supplying the pancreas are involved. In connection with the assessment of tumour resectability, the gastroduodenal artery is considered to be borderline between the two groups. A second angiographic sign of unquestionable value in the diagnosis of pancreatic cancer is the presence of major venous involvement. An adequate venous phase angiogram frequently reveals obstruction and narrowing or deformity of the veins. However, non-visualization of the splenic or portal vein alone, although suggestive, is not diagnostic of venous obstruction. Arterial occlusion or arterial displacement may also be caused by pancreatic tumours. Neovascularity is only *rarely* seen in pancreatic carcinoma because the cancer is avascular. However, hyperaemia or increased vascularity in the region of the pancreas may be seen in cases of pancreatic cancer and is usually due to secondary inflammatory changes around the tumour. Finally, an angiogram may occasionally disclose the presence of hepatic metastases, thereby suggesting the malignant nature of a pancreatic abnormality.

Islet cell tumours are typically vascular. A fine network of small vessels may be seen in the early arterial phase and, occasionally, feeding arteries and draining veins may be identified. With larger tumours, displacement of neighbouring arteries may be seen and larger, irregular 'tumour vessels' have been reported. It is difficult to correlate angiographic visualization of islet cell tumours with their malignant potential unless hepatic metastases are obviously seen or encasement (or occlusion) of arteries are striking features. When angiography does demonstrate a solitary islet cell tumour, the surgeon must be aware that there may be a second lesion not shown angiographically. When angiography shows multiple islet cell tumours, the likelihood of there being others not shown is very real. In this respect, angiography does not remove the surgeon's obligation to carry out a complete exploration of the whole pancreas.

A major value of angiography is to delineate variations in the foregut vasculature, especially the hepatic blood supply. The desirability of obtaining angiographic studies before embarking on a major pancreatic resection has previously been emphasized since ligation of a major hepatic arterial blood supply in a jaundiced patient may lead to fatal liver ischaemia.

Complications of angiography

Complications at the femoral puncture site include haemorrhage, haematoma, arterial occlusion, pseudoaneurysms and arteriovenous fistula. Embolization of thrombus formed at the puncture site, subintimal dissection of an atheromatous plaque with secondary thrombosis, distal embolization of catheter or guidewire fragments, have all been described. Post-angiographic renal failure is well documented, especially in patients with pre-existing renal disease. The injected contrast media are hypertonic and may be a real hazard, especially if the patient has been dehydrated for several hours. The jaundiced patient is particularly at risk from both bleeding problems and renal failure. They should be kept well hydrated and their coagulation abnormalities should be treated prior to angiography. The spectrum of adverse sequelae is indeed very broad and this invasive procedure should not be undertaken without good indication, by inexperienced personnel or where facilities are inadequate; but when planned and performed with care, abdominal angiography is an acceptably safe procedure. It is occasionally a useful part of diagnostic armamentarium in patients with pancreatic disorders, but its value has dwindled and its place has been usurped by the recent improvements of other less invasive imaging techniques such as the modern CT scan, MRI and endoscopic ultrasonography (EUS).

Pancreatic angiography remains of value in two preoperative situations, namely:

- Arterial embolization of feeding vessels to large vascular tumours.
- Splenic artery embolization for lesions around the tail of the pancreas obstructing the splenic vein and causing splenomegaly and left-sided portal hypertension.

In both instances, the angiographic manoeuvre facilitates the subsequent surgical excision by significantly reducing intra-operative blood loss.

Endoscopic ultrasonography (Figure 12.11)

EUS has emerged as a very useful tool for visualizing the pancreas and peripancreatic structures by combining the advantages of endoscopy with ultrasonography. It can detect small tumours that are not visible on a CT

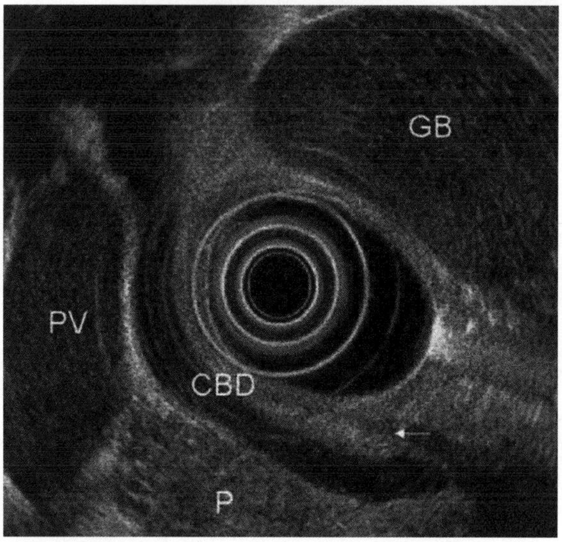

Figure 12.11

scan and helps in assessing resectability of larger tumours by delineating their relationship to adjacent major vessels. It has all the risks of upper gastrointestinal endoscopy and is very dependent on the technical expertise and interpretation of an experienced individual. EUS, when available, has clearly replaced diagnostic ERCP in the evaluation of the jaundiced patient. EUS-guided fine-needle aspiration of pancreatic masses and enlarged lymph nodes, and coeliac plexus nerve block are also being widely practised.

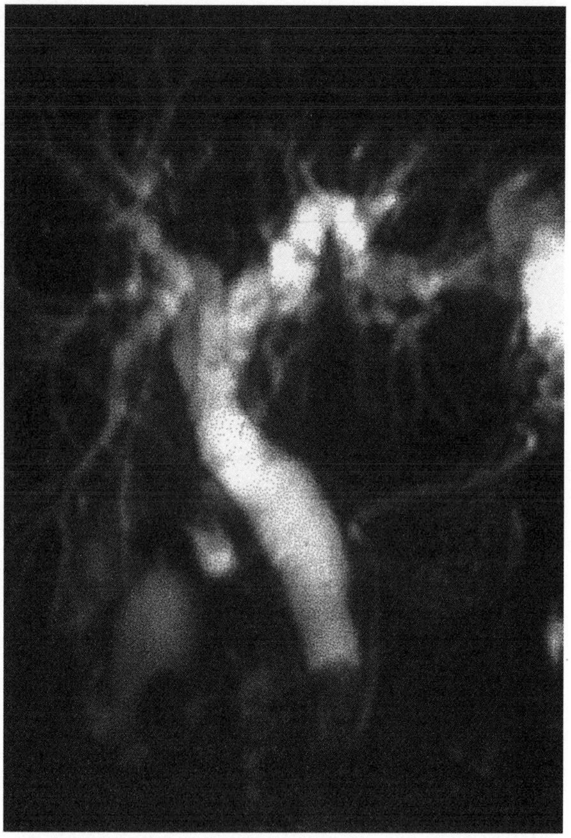

Figure 12.12 MRCP showing an impacted stone obstructing the distal common bile duct. Note a normal duct of Wirsung.

Magnetic resonance cholangiopancreatography

Magnetic resonance cholangiopancreatography (MRCP) is the latest imaging modality based on heavily weighted T2 imaging. It is non-invasive and provides excellent images with clear definition of structures (Figure 12.12). However, it is expensive and the equipment is not yet available at most medical centres.

Chemical analysis of the stool to demonstrate steatorrhoea

Stool examination for fat content is only useful as a screening test for malabsorption. Faecal fat excretion is not a valid measure of pancreatic dysfunction since about 80% of pancreatic secretory capacity may be lost without any detectable change in the test. In clinical practice, pancreatic secretory deficiency states and malabsorption syndromes co-exist in about 10–20% of patients. Even with more sophisticated tolerance tests, there is an overlap of the results obtained in malabsorption states and pancreatic insufficiency.

Direct measurement of pancreatic digestive and secretory capacity

Direct duodenal intubation and collection of pancreatic juice for analysis (duodenal drainage studies) following various stimuli is still widely practised largely as a research tool. The exact technique varies from institution to institution. In the Lundh test, a meal of fat is given and the output of pancreatic lipase in the aspirated duodenal content is determined. The pancreatic secretory response to an injection of secretin (measurement of volume of juice and bicarbonate output) is often studied, but data interpretation is sometimes difficult. However, they are the most reliable tests in detecting pancreatic exocrine insufficiency due to chronic pancreatitis or pancreatic carcinoma. Cytological examination of the duodenal aspirate during these maximal secretory tests sometimes documents the presence of malignancy in cases of pancreatic cancer.

Section 12.5 • Congenital anomalies of the pancreas

There are three congenital anomalies of the pancreas which are of potential surgical importance. They are ectopic pancreas, annular pancreas and pancreas divisum.

Ectopic (heterotopic, dystopic, aberrant) pancreas

Pancreatic tissue has been documented in ectopic sites in the gastrointestinal tract and even elsewhere. The most common site for nodules of aberrant pancreatic is on the wall of the stomach, duodenum or jejunum.

The nodules may be found in submucosa (75%) and in the muscular layer or subserous coat in the remainder. The overall incidence and relative frequency with which it causes symptoms varies. Autopsy studies have found heterotopic pancreatic tissue in the duodenum in as high as 14% of individuals. Scattered pancreatic tissue has been found in Meckel's diverticulum, gallbladder, colon, spleen, liver, bile ducts, mesentery or even omentum. Enterogenous cysts of the thorax have been reported to contain typical pancreatic tissue, including islets.

With the advent of widespread upper gastrointestinal endoscopy and improvements in contrast studies of the alimentary tract, ectopic pancreas of the stomach and duodenum is being more frequently recognized. The pathognomic radiological finding is a smooth, rounded or negative shadow with evidence of a tiny umbilication or even a small duct which may be outlined by a line of barium. Probably most individuals with ectopic pancreas have no symptoms whatsoever. However, abdominal pain suggestive of peptic ulcer disease sometimes occurs. Interference with gastric emptying by lesions situated in the pyloric region, direct production of a peptic ulcer, gastrointestinal haemorrhage, intussusception, and development of benign or malignant neoplasm arising in the pancreatic rest, have all been documented. Even an islet cell adenoma producing bouts of hyperinsulinism has been reported to be cured by resection of the ectopic pancreatic tissue from the duodenum.

Annular pancreas

The exact embryological explanation for this malformation is debatable. The classic description of annular pancreas is almost invariably a ring of pancreatic tissue, continuous with the head of the pancreas, surrounding the second part of the duodenum proximal to the ampulla of Vater. However, the infra-ampullary location has also been documented. Eighty-five per cent of cases occur around the second portion of the duodenum and the remaining 15% are scattered around the first or third part of the duodenum. The pancreatic tissue is generally firmly attached to and embedded into the duodenal musculature; only rarely is it loosely attached and readily separable from the duodenum. There is usually a variable amount of hypertrophy of the proximal duodenal wall resulting from obstruction. Half of the reported cases have manifested themselves in the first year of life. Some believe that there is invariably an associated intrinsic atresia or stenosis of the duodenum. Other developmental anomalies are also associated in about 60–70% of cases. They include Down's syndrome, non-rotation and incomplete rotation of the mesentery, pre-duodenal portal vein, imperforate anus, oesophageal atresia with tracheo-oesophageal fistula, and congenital heart disease. There is a high frequency of polyhydramnios in the mother of those children who have significant duodenal obstruction at birth.

Vomiting is the main symptom of annular pancreas. It may begin as soon as the infant starts feeding or may appear several days later. Bile may or may not be present in the vomitus. Jaundice may be present and has been explained by back pressure of the distended duodenum on the common bile duct or involvement of the ampulla of Vater by oedema at the level of the stenosis. A plain film of the abdomen may show a distended stomach and a 'double-bubble' sign at the level of the duodenum. Contrast studies may be necessary to diagnose the condition.

About one-half of the cases reported present for the first time with symptoms between the ages of 21 and 70 years. The reason for such late manifestations of symptoms is generally attributed to inflammatory changes in the pancreatic ring. Duodenal ulcer, frequently reported with annular pancreas in the adult, has not been observed in infancy. The differential diagnosis in infancy rests between annular pancreas and other causes of duodenal obstruction, all of which require urgent operative relief, namely, duodenal stenosis or atresia, compression of the duodenum by Ladd's bands, pyloric stenosis or volvulus in association with malrotation. An absolute differentiation between annular pancreas and duodenal atresia or stenosis is not possible without operation.

The operation of choice is either duodenoduodenostomy or duodenojejunostomy performed through the retrocolic route. Attempts at division of the pancreatic ring are attended with complications, including pancreatitis, pancreatic fistula, duodenal wall perforation and failures. Gastrojejunostomy is not a satisfactory operation since it inadequately decompresses the duodenum and has a high incidence of marginal ulceration. In patients with concomitant jaundice, an operative cholangiogram is mandatory before a decision about the need for and type of biliary diversion can be made.

Pancreas divisum and its implications are discussed in the section on pancreatitis.

Section 12.6 • Injuries to the pancreas

Pancreatic injuries occur infrequently in patients with abdominal trauma of all types and this may be accounted for by the relatively protected position of the gland in the retroperitoneum beneath the thoracic cage. Pancreatic trauma is often classified according to the source of the injury: (1) penetrating trauma; (2) blunt trauma; and (3) iatrogenic trauma.

Although the pancreatic injury rarely, if ever, accounts for the early death of a patient, it adds significantly to the morbidity and late mortality, especially if it is recognized late.

Injuries to the pancreas are being encountered more frequently today than 30 years ago. This may be attributed to the increasing incidence of motor vehicle accidents and civil violence. It is plausible that the increasing and often compulsory use of seat belts may further increase the incidence of blunt pancreatic trauma since the gland may be ruptured by sudden compression against the lumbar spine.

The overall mortality rate from pancreatic trauma is about 20%. Stab wounds have a mortality rate of about 8%, gunshot wounds 25% and shotgun wounds 60%. The mortality following blunt trauma from steering wheel injury is still approximately 50%. One-third of all pancreatic injuries are secondary to blunt trauma and two-thirds are due to penetrating trauma in the USA. Most of the early deaths result from massive haemorrhage and shock due to the associated injuries to major vascular structures.

Diagnosis

In less than 10% of patients with pancreatic trauma of all types is the pancreas found to be the only injured organ. This implies that over 90% of patients will have further internal injuries. In the clinical situation, patients with definite evidence of an injured intra-abdominal viscus and/or intra-abdominal haemorrhage following blunt or penetrating trauma to the abdomen are in need of an emergency laparotomy following adequate resuscitation. They should not be investigated further.

The initial emphasis is placed on adequate resuscitation rather than an elaborate, time-consuming and often unrewarding investigation. The diagnosis and the extent of the injury is made intra-operatively.

On the other hand, patients with doubtful evidence of intra-abdominal injury after blunt trauma should be observed and carefully investigated as dictated by clinical circumstances. There are a small group of patients in whom an isolated pancreatic injury may easily be missed.

Classification of pancreatic injuries

Pancreatic injuries can be classified as: (1) simple contusion, (2) parenchymatous laceration without major ductal injury, (3) major ductal disruption, and (4) combined pancreatoduodenal injury.

Penetrating pancreatic trauma

Isolated pancreatic injury is very rare. Associated injuries include liver, stomach, major vascular structures, spleen, duodenum, colon and kidney. Early death is invariably due to the associated injuries which can lead to catastrophic, often uncontrollable, haemorrhage. Late death accounts for some 41% of all mortality and is attributable to the pancreatic injury, leading to intra-abdominal abscess, sepsis and multi-organ system failure.

The emphasis in the management of penetrating injuries of the abdomen is on resuscitation with minimal essential investigations. The diagnosis is made at laparotomy. A long midline laparotomy is performed to provide access, exposure and assistance. Management of associated injuries takes precedence over any pancreatic injury. The underlying principles are: (1) arrest haemorrhage, (2) control contamination from the gastrointestinal tract, and (3) once the patient is stabilized, the lesser sac is widely opened and all peripancreatic haematomas are explored. If there is no major ductal disruption, selective pancreatic and peripancreatic debridement is performed only as necessary. Adequate external drainage is instituted and, if the patient develops a pancreatic fistula, it can be treated conservatively with a combination of total parenteral nutrition and Sandostatin.

Blunt pancreatic trauma

About 50% of patients with blunt pancreatic trauma will have an isolated pancreatic injury. If the patient is stable and the diagnosis of significant injury is doubtful, then the patient is observed and is investigated rationally. The only test that is of definite diagnostic value is computed tomography with intravenous and oral contrast. *Occasionally*, a flat X-ray plate of the abdomen, endoscopic ultrasound, ERCP and abdominal angiography may be useful. Serum amylase and lipase elevation or lack thereof, are not usually helpful in this clinical situation, although if these enzymes are highly elevated, they will strengthen a diagnostic suspicion of pancreatic injury.

If the patient is unstable and there is evidence of an injured abdominal viscus, the patient should be rapidly resuscitated and explored as for a penetrating pancreatic injury.

Treatment of major pancreatic ductal disruption

If the injury is well to the left of the mesenteric vessels, the simplest manoeuvre is to perform a distal pancreatectomy and splenectomy with oversewing of the cut end of the proximal pancreas. In children under 16 years of age, one may elect empirically, if conditions are favourable, to attempt preserving the spleen with its blood supply based on the short gastric vessels.

If the injury is close to or to the right of the superior mesenteric vessels, pancreatic preservation may be considered. The preservation of pancreatic tissue is often desirable, but should not become an irrational obsession. A partial pancreatic transection may be completed and the area debrided as necessary. The right side of the transection may be oversewn as before and the cut end of the left pancreas may be implanted into a Roux-en-Y loop of jejunum.

The decision to preserve pancreatic tissue and perform a pancreato-enteric anastomosis is based on: (1) the magnitude of the associated injuries, (2) the general condition of the patient, (3) the degree of contamination, and (4) the surgeon's expertise and experience in pancreatic surgery.

Pancreatoduodenal injuries

The duodenal injury has to be repaired on its own merits. Following duodenorraphy, the injury to the pancreatic head has to be evaluated. Minor lacerations with or without ductal injury can be appropriately debrided and drained. If the ductal injury and the trauma to the head parenchyma appear extensive, a

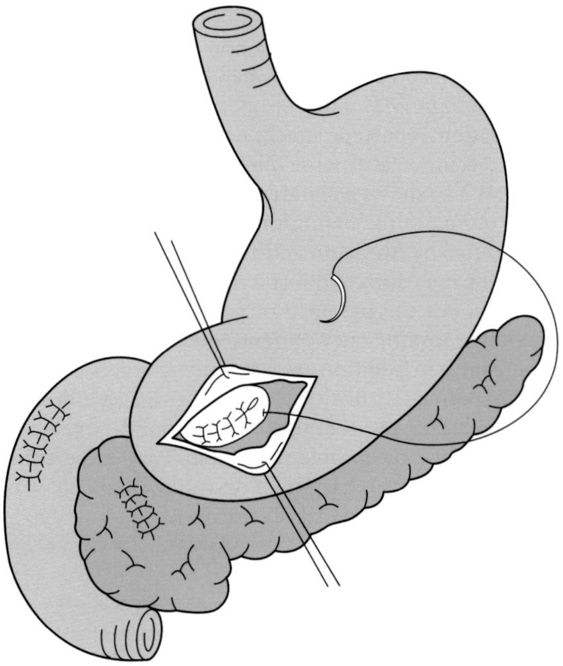

Figure 12.13 Pyloric exclusion procedure. The pylorus is oversewn through an antral incision.

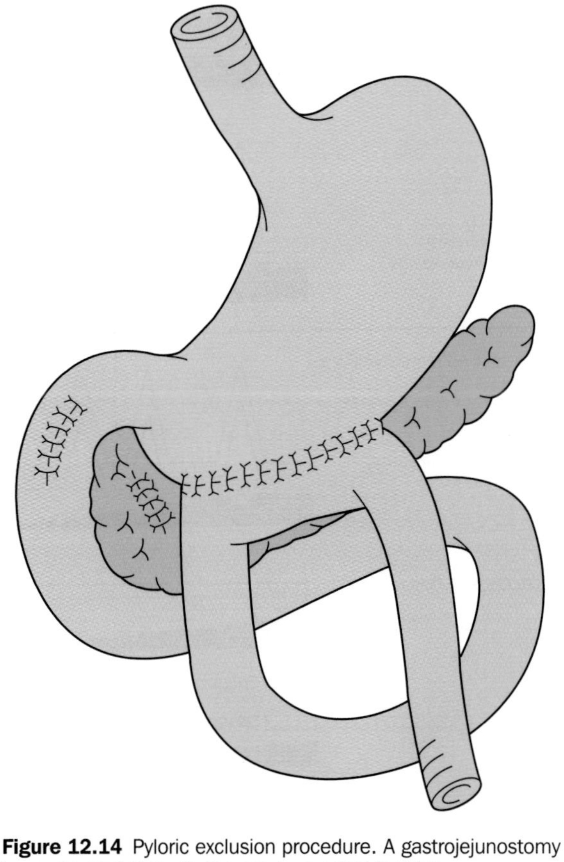

Figure 12.14 Pyloric exclusion procedure. A gastrojejunostomy is constructed through the previous antral incision.

duodenal diversion procedure can be performed. An incision is made in the distal antrum and the pylorus is closed with a running catgut suture. A distal gastrojejunostomy is performed using the antral incision to 'protect' the duodenal repair (Figures 12.13 and 12.14).

For more extensive trauma, the duodenal diverticulization procedure of Berne is sometimes advocated. This entails a distal gastrectomy, Billroth II gastrojejunostomy, T-tube insertion for drainage of the common bile duct, and duodenostomy tube drainage (Figure 12.15).

In all these extensive injuries, a duodenal and/or pancreatic fistula will eventually develop and this can be treated conservatively with TPN and Sandostatin (Octreotide). If the fistula does not spontaneously close after a few months, then a secondary attempt to drain it into an isolated bowel loop can be considered.

Occasionally, especially with gunshot wounds to the right upper abdomen, extensive devitalization of the duodenum and pancreatic head is seen with avulsion of the common bile duct and uncontrollable haemorrhage. In such a situation, the surgeon may have no choice but to 'complete' the pancreatoduodenectomy if only to control haemorrhage, usually from the superior mesenteric vessels, the renal vessels and the inferior vena cava. It is not unusual in such situations to be forced to perform a concomitant right nephrectomy. An experienced surgical team is needed for this type of injury since the mortality is in excess of 30%.

Iatrogenic pancreatic trauma

The commonest cause of iatrogenic pancreatic trauma is ERCP with or without associated sphincterotomy

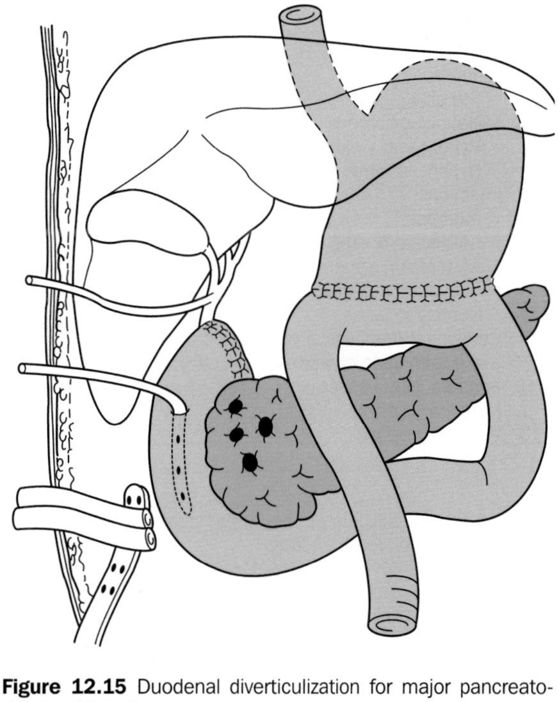

Figure 12.15 Duodenal diverticulization for major pancreatoduodenal injuries.

and stent placement. Multiple pancreatic biopsies are another cause, whether performed percutaneously or intra-operatively. Occasionally, surgical operations on a large penetrating duodenal ulcer may also lead to severe pancreatic injuries. Other surgical procedures which may lead to inadvertent pancreatic trauma are splenectomy, inexpert exploration of the common bile duct and transduodenal sphincteroplasty. All these invasive manoeuvres may lead to a fulminant pancreatitis with serious sequelae.

Section 12.7 • Pancreatitis

Definition and classification

The term 'pancreatitis' implies the presence of pancreatic inflammation and autodigestion. It can be classified according to its clinical presentation, according to the aetiological factors (Table 12.1) or according to the severity of the pathological process (Table 12.2). Clinically, pancreatitis is referred to as acute or chronic. Restitutio ad integrum is the hallmark of the acute form whereas persistence or progression of the disease or residual damage to the pancreas indicates the chronic variety. Nevertheless, if a patient recovers from acute necrotizing pancreatitis, normal recovery of pancreatic (endocrine and exocrine) function or morphology may never occur and the patient may be rightly labelled as having 'progressed' into chronic pancreatitis. Similarly, on occasion, recurrent attacks of acute pancreatitis due to any cause may merge into the chronic varieties. Figure 12.16 shows a clinical classification of pancreatitis according to the definition of Marseilles symposium as modified by Ammann and Trapnell. The emphasis on chronic pancreatitis is the absence of pain and enzyme elevation but the presence of pancreatic exocrine and endocrine insufficiency. Patients with chronic relapsing pancreatitis, in addition to the same disorders of function, experience pain which, in the overt case, is constant with relapses against the background of pain. All types of acute or chronic pancreatitis may cause complications such as biliary tract obstruction, splenic vein thrombosis and duodenal obstruction.

Acute pancreatitis

Although, experimentally, acute pancreatitis has been produced in various animal models by promoting duo-

Table 12.1 Classification of pancreatitis according to aetiological factors

1. Alcoholism
2. Biliary tract disease
3. Trauma
   - Surgical
   - Blunt
   - Penetrating
   - ERCP
   - Aortography
4. Drugs
   - Thiazides
   - Steroids
5. Metabolic disorders
   - Hyperparathyroidism
   - Hyperlipidaemia
6. Infections
   - Mumps
   - Coxsackie B virus
   - *Mycoplasma pneumoniae*
   - Infectious mononucleosis
   - Septicaemia
7. Congenital mechanical obstruction of pancreatic duct, e.g. pancreas divisum
8. Periampullary cancer
9. Hereditary pancreatitis
10. Vascular disease

Table 12.2 Classification of acute pancreatitis according to severity of pathological process

1. Acute oedematous pancreatitis – mild, self-limiting
2. Acute persistent – unresolving, subacute – pancreatitis – suspect development of complications
3. Acute haemorrhagic – necrotizing, fulminant – pancreatitis

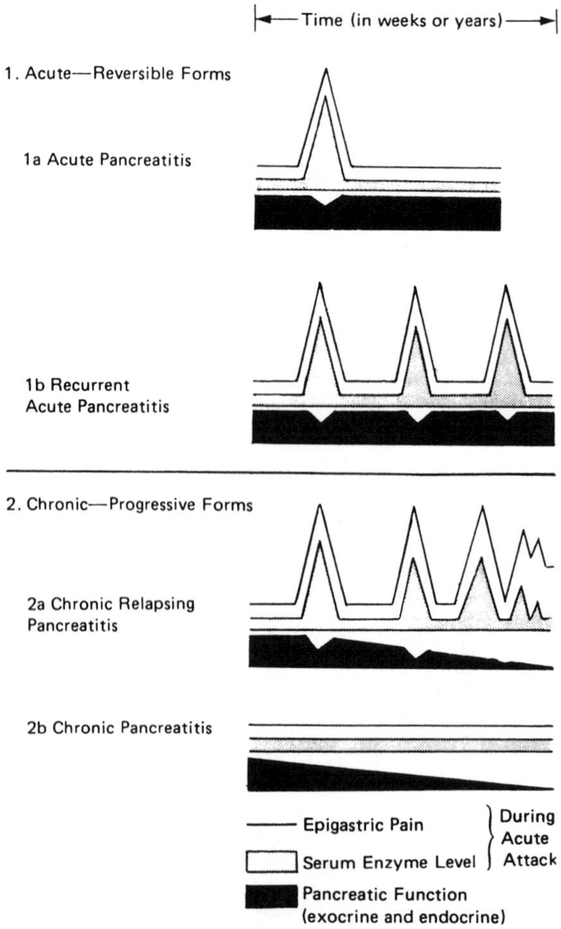

Figure 12.16 Clinical classification of pancreatitis, according to the definition of Marseilles, as modified by Ammann and Trapnell.

deno-pancreatic reflux, by the injection of bile salts, trypsin, etc., into the pancreatic duct, or by the occlusion of pancreatic arterial blood supply, the relevance of these models to the human clinical situation is still uncertain. Acute pancreatitis has been associated with a variety of clinical disorders, but the actual cause or mechanism which initiates the pancreatic autodigestion or which makes it either a self-limiting disease or a progressively fatal disease remains unclear. Acute pancreatitis developing in the course of viral infection, such as mumps and Coxsackie B viruses, is usually self-limiting. So is the acute pancreatitis in association with mycoplasma pneumonia. Metabolic disorders, such as hypercalcaemia (usually associated with contraceptive pills) have been well documented. So is acute pancreatitis resulting from drug therapy, such as diuretics and steroids. Autopsy examination of patients dying of such conditions as fulminant liver failure, hypovolaemic shock with renal tubular necrosis, transplantation and cardiac bypass surgery have revealed fulminant pancreatitis in a significant number of these patients. From the practical point of view, the two conditions most commonly associated with acute pancreatitis are alcoholism and biliary tract stone disease. The prognostic and therapeutic implications of acute pancreatitis due to these two associations are different. Gallstone pancreatitis usually occurs in patients older than 60 years, tends to be severe and is frequently accompanied by serious complications in the acute stage. However, recurrences may be prevented by early operative intervention or, if the patient recovers quickly, by appropriately timed elective surgical treatment of the biliary tract. By contrast, alcohol-associated pancreatitis tends to be recurring. Although the first attacks are usually quite severe, and can be fatal, subsequent attacks are commonly mild and carry low mortality. As time passes, the recurring attacks lead to progressive destruction of the gland and eventually the clinical picture merges into that of chronic pancreatitis or chronic relapsing pancreatitis.

Acute pancreatitis may be secondary to blunt or penetrating abdominal injury or may follow some invasive clinical test, such as endoscopic retrograde cannulation of the papilla (ERCP), and the now rarely performed translumbar aortography. Post-operative acute pancreatitis most commonly occurs after exploration of the common bile duct and is invariably due to injudicious, inexpert, forceful dilatation of the sphincter of Oddi or transduodenal sphincteroplasty. Distal pancreatitis may follow splenectomy.

Two morphological forms of acute pancreatitis are generally distinguished – the oedematous mild form and the severe, necrotizing, haemorrhagic, or suppurative type. The oedematous variety can progress to the necrotic type for reasons not well understood. Distinction between the two major forms of acute pancreatitis on the basis of the clinical features and conventional laboratory studies may be *impossible* at the *onset* of the disease. Indeed, the diagnosis itself may remain uncertain for several hours after presentation. It is not sufficiently emphasized that the diagnosis of acute pancreatitis is, at best, a shrewd guess based on clinical probabilities and backed by elevation of serum or urinary amylase levels, or serum lipase levels. The renal amylase:creatinine clearance ratio, iso-amylase measurements and determination of serum trypsin have not been generally helpful in doubtful cases and are not widely available.

Clinical features

The clinical manifestations of acute pancreatitis are protean since it can mimic any other abdominal emergency. In fact, it can co-exist with some such as acute cholecystitis. It can occur at any age, but is rare in children and in very young adults. In the latter group, it is usually associated with infections, trauma, parasites or drugs or is hereditary. Alcohol-related pancreatitis is usually found in the young adult less than 40 years of age, whereas the form associated with biliary tract disease manifests itself mainly in middle-aged and older persons.

The onset of symptoms may follow excess intake of food or alcohol but this is not invariable. Pain is the major initial symptom in over 90% of patients. It may vary in degree from mild to severe and is characteristically sudden in onset persisting for 12–48 hours or more. The wide spectrum of the intensity of the pain should be emphasized. Like many patients with pancreatic pain, there is a tendency for the patient to bend forward and assume various postures in order to obtain relief. Occasionally, even the severe fulminant fatal pancreatitis may be totally painless. The location of the pain is usually in the mid-epigastrium but can occur or radiate anywhere and may be diffuse or confined mainly to the back. Other common symptoms are nausea, vomiting, retching and hiccups. Less frequently, diarrhoea, dyspnoea, cyanosis, haematemesis and melaena may appear early. The bleeding may be due to erosive ulcers, bleeding diathesis, left-sided portal hypertension or erosion of the inflammatory process into the gut.

The physical findings may be minimal, in striking contrast to the severity of the symptoms. Obtundation, fever, tachycardia, epigastric tenderness and muscle guarding are frequent. Shock may be the initial symptom and, in severe cases, may be profound. Mild jaundice may be observed. Abdominal distension is often present in the early phase of the disease and is the result of a diffuse or localized paralytic ileus. Several days later, a palpable epigastric mass may be felt, indicating the development of a pseudocyst or marked peripancreatic fat necrosis. Other late signs include bluish discoloration of the skin around the periumbilical area (Cullen's sign) or in the loins (Grey Turner's sign); these indicate ecchymosis caused by seepage of blood arising from acute necrotizing pancreatitis along fascial planes. Another rare skin manifestation is nodular fat necrosis simulating erythema nodosum or Weber–Christian disease. Rarely, polyarthritis or bone pain may be observed and is also attributable to fat necrosis. Thrombophlebitis of the leg veins is only rarely seen. Abnormal physical findings on chest examination are found in less than one-third of cases, but a plain chest radiograph may reveal abnormalities in a greater proportion of patients. These include elevation of the diaphragm, basal atelectasis or pneumonitis, left-sided or bilateral pleural effusion.

Diagnostic procedures

The haematocrit is high in most patients at the onset of the disease, reflecting fluid loss related to the inflammatory process and vomiting. Leucocytosis with a white blood count of 10–20 $\times$ 10^9/dl is almost invariably present.

Serum enzyme elevations

The key to the diagnosis of acute pancreatitis remains an elevation of pancreatic enzymes in the circulating blood or urine. Although hyperamylasaemia is a nonspecific finding, the level of the serum amylase in various extrapancreatic conditions rarely attains a value five times above normal and this is commonly seen in primary acute pancreatitis. Normal serum amylase levels may be obtained if the determination is carried out 3 days or more after the onset, if previous attacks have completely destroyed the glandular tissue, or if the current attack is associated with massive destruction of the gland. Persistence of hyperamylasaemia for 10 days or longer may indicate a continuation of the acute inflammation or the development of local complications such as pseudocyst formation, pancreatic abscess or pancreatic ascites.

In view of the problems involved in the interpretation of hyperamylasaemia, measurement of isoenzymes of amylase and determinations of the renal amylase:creatinine clearance ratio have recently been advocated. The P-type isoamylase cannot be detected after extirpation of the pancreas and hence is only of pancreatic origin. Its measurement is unnecessary and time consuming for routine purposes but it is useful in establishing the cause of a persistent hyperamylasaemia.

In acute pancreatitis, the relative renal clearance of amylase increases compared to that of creatinine. It has been suggested that a clearance of amylase over the clearance of creatinine of greater than four is found in the first few days after an attack of acute pancreatitis and that this elevated ratio persists longer than abnormalities of blood or urinary enzyme levels. The view that the amylase:creatinine clearance is specific for acute pancreatitis has now been shown to be untrue since an elevated clearance ratio is found in numerous other conditions, such as diabetic ketoacidosis, burns and chronic renal failure, while many patients with acute pancreatitis may have normal clearance ratios.

Estimation of lipolytic activity in the blood, urine, pleural and peritoneal effusions has been advocated on the grounds that lipase is more specific for pancreatic disease than amylase and its level remains elevated for longer periods. The recent introduction of radoimmunoassay for trypsin has resulted in reports demonstrating high levels of immunoreactive trypsin in the circulation and in serous effusions in patients with acute pancreatitis. The diagnosis or prognostic value of immunoreactive trypsin assays compared with other enzymes has yet to be reported. Immunoreactive elastase levels have also been reported and are said to be elevated in patients with acute pancreatitis showing good correlation with levels of amylase.

Urinary amylase and lipase

Amylase clearance is increased about three-fold for 1–2 weeks in patients with acute pancreatitis whose renal function is unimpaired. Thus, increased urinary output of amylase may persist for several days after normalization of the serum amylase levels. Determination of the ratio of amylase:creatinine clearance permits the diagnosis of acute pancreatitis even in the presence of renal insufficiency. Timed urinary amylase output (usually expressed in terms of total activity per hour) and amylase clearance studies are particularly of diagnostic value after serum amylase has returned to normal. Urinary lipase determination has been abandoned since it is debatable whether lipolytic activity is detectable in the urine.

Hyperglycaemia and glycosuria

Transient hyperglycaemia has been observed in a varying proportion of patients with acute pancreatitis. One of the mechanisms may be the release of glucagon from the damaged pancreatic cells. Usually the hyperglycaemia disappears with remission of the acute pancreatits but, occasionally, following extensive parenchymal damage, diabetes mellitus may ensue.

Hypocalcaemia

The incidence, mechanism and prognostic implications of hypocalcaemia, serum calcium below 1.9 mmol/1 (7.5 mg/100 ml), are still controversial. Some believe that hypoalbuminaemia accounts for most of the measured hypocalcaemia. Deposition of calcium in areas of fat necrosis, release of glucagon with secondary hypercalcitonaemia and hypomagnesaemia have all been suggested as pathogenetic factors. Impairment of parathyroid gland function has also been reported.

Whatever its mechanism, hypocalcaemia complicating acute pancreatitis is occasionally manifested by tetany and usually denotes the presence of the severe form of the disease.

Methaemalbuminaemia

The presence of this haemoglobin derivative in the serum suggests severe haemorrhagic pancreatitis rather than the oedematous variety. Elevated methaemalbumin levels, however, are not specific for necrotizing pancreatitis, because they can occur with other necrotizing intra-abdominal processes.

Blood coagulation tests

A rise in circulating trypsin may result in an increased antithrombin activity, but this is not a reliable test for acute pancreatitis. The persistence of elevated serum fibrinogen levels, especially after the second week, is said to indicate either a severe form of acute pancreatitis or the onset of complications.

Hyperlipidaemia

Hyperlipidaemia, especially hypertriglyceridaemia, occurs in about 5–10% of patients with acute pancreatitis. The lipid rise may be primary and/or the cause of the acute pancreatitis may be secondary, resulting from the pancreatitis. Long-term studies of blood lipids after subsidence of acute pancreatitis may be necessary for the differentiation of primary and secondary hyperlipidaemia. It has been suggested that many of the patients with so-called 'secondary hyperlipidaemia' may have a primary disorder of lipid metabolism which is unmasked by the attack of pancreatitis.

Electrocardiogram (ECG)

ECG changes simulating myocardial infarction have been reported in patients with acute pancreatitis. The commonest ECG changes are S-T segment elevation or depression, inversion of T waves, and extended T wave negativity. These changes disappear rather quickly unless there is co-existent myocardial ischaemia or infarction or there are other cardiac complications of acute pancreatitis, such as pericarditis. The exact mechanisms underlying the ECG changes include several factors, such as myocardial damage due to shock, electrolyte disturbance, excessive parental fluid replacement, effect of severe pain on coronary artery disease, influence of circulating pancreatic trypsin, and vagally mediated reflexes from the pancreas to the heart.

Plain abdominal and chest radiography

A plain radiograph of the abdomen and chest may show evidence of pneumoperitoneum, thus excluding the diagnosis of acute pancreatitis and indicating the need for emergency operation for a perforated viscus. It may show abnormalities suggestive of acute pancreatitis in about 50% of cases. The radiological signs include intestinal distension in the region of the pancreas (sentinel jejunal loop, colon cut-off, duodenal ileus) or a generalized paralytic ileus. Haziness in the flat plate of the abdomen is caused by retroperitoneal fluid accumulation and may be associated with obliteration of the psoas outline. Other signs are elevation of the left diaphragm, caused by basal atelectasis or subdiaphragmatic fluid collection, and pleural effusions.

Differential diagnosis

The clinical picture of acute pancreatitis tends to change with evolution of the disease. Early (2–3 hours) after the onset, symptoms are often suggestive of acute cholecystitis – indeed, acute cholecystitis may co-exist with acute pancreatitis. After 6–8 hours a perforated duodenal ulcer or acute appendicitis may be simulated. After 2–3 days, the clinical features may mimic those of an intestinal obstruction because there is marked abdominal distension and ileus. If the patient presents with profound cardiovascular collapse, myocardial infarction, acute aortic distension, ruptured aortic aneurysm, mesenteric infarction or even massive pulmonary embolism may be initially suspected. Most of these conditions may be associated with elevation of serum amylase and often of lipase. Improved diagnostic ability will result if the clinical limitations in assessment are fully appreciated. Thus, the diagnosis of acute pancreatitis is based on 'thinking about it as a possibility' and excluding other sources of abdominal pain.

Clinical predictors of severity of acute pancreatitis

It is important to identify patients with severe acute pancreatitis early (day 1 or 2 of admission) because timely administration of broad-spectrum, pancreas-penetrating, antibiotics decreases the incidence of pancreatic and peri-pancreatic infection. Two well-controlled studies have shown a convincing benefit of Imipenim when administered within 48 hours of onset and maintained for 10 days to 2 weeks in patients with severe (necrotizing) pancreatitis. The incidence of pancreatic/peripancreatic infection is halved, from 40 to 20%.

The sensitivity of clinical judgement, even in experienced hands, is low (about 40%) for predicting the severity of an acute attack of pancreatitis. Because of the subjective nature of the clinical acumen, Ranson developed 11 objective criteria and postulated that the risk of death and/or developing major complications may be estimated objectively by five parameters on

Table 12.3 Clinical predictors of severity of acute pancreatitis

	Ranson criteria	
Admission	*Non-biliary*	*Biliary*
Age (years)	>55	>70
WBC	>16 000	>18 000
Glucose	>200	>220
LDH[a]	>350	>400
AST[a]	>250	>250
First 48 hours		
↓Hct	>10	>10
↑Urea	>5	>2
Ca^{2+}	<8	<8
PaO_2	<60	<60
Base deficit	>4	>5
Fluid requirement	>6	>4

[a]International units/ml.

Table 12.4 Clinical predictors of severity of acute pancreatitis

	Glasgow criteria
Age (years)	>55
WBC	>15 000
Glucose	>180
LDH[a]	>600
Urea	>96
Ca^{2+}	<8
PaO_2	<60
Albumin	<3.2

[a]International units/ml.

Table 12.5 APACHE II scoring system

Column A		*Column B*		*Column C*	
Parameter	*Points*	*Age*	*Points*	*Chronic health*	*Points*
Temperature	0–4	<44	0	Cirrhosis	2 or 5
Blood pressure	0–4	45–54	2	Immunosuppression	2 or 5
Heart rate	0–4	55–64	3	NY Heart Assoc. Class IV	2 or 5
Respiratory rate	0–4	65–74	5	COPD	2 or 5
PaO_2	0–4	≥ 75	6	Renal dialysis	2 or 5
Arterial pH	0–4				
Na^+	0–4				
K^+	0–4				
Cr	0–4				
Hct	0–4				
WBC	0–4				
HCO_3^-	0–4				
Glasgow coma score					

APACHE II score: A points + B points + C points > 9 points suggests severe pancreatitis.

admission to hospital and six parameters within the initial 48 hours of admission (Table 12.3). In patients with fewer than three of these 11 prognostic factors, the mortality rate was 0.9%; with three or four factors, 18%; with five or six factors, 50%; and with more than six factors, 90%.

Imrie proposed the Glasgow criteria (Table 12.4) based on eight of Ranson's factors. The presence of any three of the eight signs at anytime within the 48 hours of admission indicates a severe form of the disease.

While these combined criteria are better than clinical judgement at predicting the severity and prognosis of acute pancreatitis, they pose some difficulties: (1) they are somewhat difficult to memorize; (2) they require data from the initial presentation and 48 hours to mature; (3) evaluation of the patient after 48 hours is highly problematic; and (4) the criteria are not pancreas specific. They measure the systemic response to an inflammatory process in and around the pancreas and do not predict specific complications, e.g. severe necrosis, infection, pseudocyst and renal failure.

The APACHE II system is currently the best and easiest scoring system available to assess the severity of acute pancreatitis and can be used *at any time* in the course of the disease (Table 12.5). It is more sensitive and specific than the Ranson or Imrie criteria and is the scoring system of choice. The APACHE II system allocates three sets of points: A, B and C. The A points assess clinical parameters, e.g. vital signs, electrolytes and arterial blood gases. The B points are allocated according to chronological age. The C points take into consideration comorbidity or chronic health of patient. The APACHE II score is the sum of A, B and C points. If it exceeds 9, the patient has severe acute pancreatitis. If the score increases after admission, the mortality is extremely high.

Several other biochemical 'markers' of the severity of acute pancreatitis have been studied (Table 12.6). Ideally, any serum or urinary marker must be pancreas specific, originating from the organ producing the marker. Serum amylase or lipase are of *no* value. Thus far, four pancreas specific markers appear promising in discriminating between mild and severe (necrotizing) pancreatitis: (1) trypsin activated peptide (TAP) is a five amino-acid peptide released by activation of trypsinogen and can be measured in the urine. Early reports indicate a sensitivity of 80% and specificity of 90%; (2) phospholipase A_2 tends *not* to decrease in severe acute pancreatitis but the methodology of the assay has been questioned and its value is uncertain; (3) the pancreatitis associated protein (PAP) is a novel protein purified from the pancreatic juice of rats with experimental pancreatitis. The human counterpart correlates well with the severity of pancreatitis, but the changes in concentration take days to a week to become established; and (4) serum trypsinogen-2 is the newest marker which is reported to be 91% sensitive and 71% specific as an index of severe disease, but further confirmation is needed. At present, none of these pancreas-specific markers can be considered to be of value in routine clinical practice.

The most extensively studied non-specific marker of acute pancreatitis is the C-reactive protein (CRP). This

Table 12.6 Biochemical markers of severity of acute pancreatitis

Pancreas specific
- Trypsin activated peptide (TAP)
- Phospholipase A_2 (PLA_2)
- Pancreatitis associated protein (PAP)
- Trypsinogen-2
- Ribonuclease (RNase)
- Elastase 1
- Antichymotrypsin
- Carboxylic ester hydrolase (CEH)
- Procarboxypeptidase β

Non-pancreas specific
- C reactive peptide (CRP)
- PMN elastase
- α_1-Antitrypsin
- α_2-Macroglobulin
- Methaemalbumin

Table 12.7 Interleukins – a monitor of the local and systemic inflammatory response to acute pancreatitis

Tumour necrosis factor (TNF)
Interleukin-2
Interleukin-6[a]
Interleukin-8[a]
Serum complement factor C3
Serum complement factor C4

[a]Markers of macrophage activation.

acute phase protein can reliably differentiate mild from severe acute pancreatitis but it is only useful after the second or third day of the disease. Its sensitivity is high (about 95%) but its specificity is low (about 50%). CRP concentration in excess of 100 mg/dl usually indicates necrotizing pancreatitis. However, the assay is not routinely available in most medical centres and its clinical value is diminished because it requires a few days to help in the identification of severe disease.

Another approach to staging acute pancreatitis is to monitor interleukins (IL) or complement activation (Table 12.7) as a monitor of the local and systemic inflammatory response. Tumour necrosis factor (TNF), IL-2, IL-6 and IL-8 have been extensively studied in experimental pancreatitis. Clinically, IL-6 and IL-8 seem to be as useful as CRP levels and peak about 1 day earlier. However, their value in routine clinical practice is as yet highly uncertain. Clinical studies with complement activation factors C3 and C4 have thus far been disappointing.

Medical management

The mainstay of the medical treatment of acute pancreatitis entails correction of hypovolaemia by replacement of fluid, electrolytes, blood or plasma. The continuing activity of the pancreatitis and/or the development of complications may be assessed by serial clinical examination, monitoring of serum and/or urinary amylase, and by regular CT scan of the pancreas. Current evidence suggests that anticholinergics, glucagon, or trasylol, and octreotide have no place in the management of patients with acute pancreatitis.

Nasogastric suction is currently used for all patients except those with a very mild attack of pancreatitis. Oral feeding should not be instituted until 7 days (in the mild case) to 14 days (in the severe case) after the attack of pancreatitis, as measured by all parameters, has subsided. Premature feeding is probably the commonest cause of exacerbation of pancreatitis. A period of parenteral hyperalimentation may be needed.

Medical management also includes close monitoring of vital signs, hourly urine output and central venous pressure measurements. Arterial blood gases must be frequently measured during the first few days as clinically occult respiratory failure is common. Pulmonary arterial pressure monitoring is valuable in patients with large volume requirements and especially in those with associated cardiopulmonary disease or respiratory failure.

Such careful and repeated evaluation will also permit accurate differentiation between acute pancreatitis and other acute illnesses in the majority of cases. Selected patients may also need additional investigations, such as contrast studies of the alimentary tract, isotope biliary scanning, transhepatic cholangiography, or angiography to exclude with absolute certainty gastrointestinal perforation or obstruction, acute biliary tract disease, or mesenteric infarction. An even smaller group of patients will need a diagnostic laparotomy.

Early surgical intervention

There are three situations when early operative intervention is indicated in a patient with suspected acute pancreatitis:

- When the diagnosis is in doubt and a perforated or a gangrenous viscus cannot be excluded.
- Failure of the patients to improve on medical management indicates acute necrotizing pancreatitis and is often an indication for operative intervention.
- Patients with known biliary stone disease who develop an attack of acute pancreatitis which does not improve within 48–72 hours, especially if there is evidence of biliary obstruction and/or cholangitis. In this clinical setting, one must suspect an impacted stone at the ampulla and emergency ERCP with endoscopic papillotomy and stone extraction must be seriously considered. If this fails or if an experienced endoscopist is not available, then early operation to relieve ampullary obstruction is mandatory. The patient who recovers following non-operative management of acute gallstone pancreatitis has a high risk of recurrence. Operative correction of the cholelithiasis should be undertaken as soon as the pancreatitis has subsided, preferably during the same hospitalization.

When laparotomy is performed early in the course of acute pancreatitis, one or more of the following procedures may be advisable depending on the clinical situation and the surgeon's expertise:

- inspection only
- placement of catheters for peritoneal lavage
- biliary decompression via a cholecystostomy or a T-tube in the common bile duct
- operative cholangiogram
- cholecystectomy, common bile duct exploration, and choledocholithotomy with or without a sphincteroplasty
- pancreatic and retroperitoneal debridement (necrosectomy) and drainage
- decompressing gastrostomy and feeding jejunostomy.

Early abdominal exploration with pancreatic drainage or resection has an increased mortality in patients with severe pancreatitis, defined by the presence of three or more positive Ranson prognostic signs, from 18 to 67%. Peritoneal lavage by catheters placed percutaneously, coupled with adequate resuscitation, has been extremely effective in the management of early cardiovascular–respiratory renal complications of severe pancreatitis, virtually preventing all early deaths from those causes. It should be emphasized that peritoneal lavage and laparotomy are emergency resuscitative measures for the patient who is in refractory cardiovascular collapse and respiratory embarrassment. They should not be used indiscriminately for all cases of acute pancreatitis. If laparotomy is performed, the addition of a gastrostomy and jejunostomy confers several advantages. The former always allows gastric decompression and drainage which may be needed for several weeks without the discomfort of a nasogastric tube. The latter provides a route for enteral nutrition with minimal stimulation to the pancreas and obviates the use of intravenous alimentation which has the potential risk of catheter sepsis. Improvement in overall mortality following peritoneal lavage has been disappointing since lavage does not reduce the late deaths from pancreatic and peripancreatic necrosis and sepsis. It was rightly pointed out that the two surgical pitfalls in acute pancreatitis are:

- to operate too early and do too much
- to operate too late and do too little.

Any patient who has persistence or reappearance of inflammatory manifestations of acute pancreatitis must be suspected of developing a pancreatic pseudocyst or a pancreatic abscess. Clinically, fever, pain, tenderness, a palpable mass, leucocytosis and hyperamylasaemia are inconstant features. A positive blood culture is not usually obtained in the early development of a pancreatic abscess. If antibiotics are used, the fever may be partly masked. A plain radiograph of the abdomen may demonstrate the mottled 'soap bubble' appearance suggestive of a retroperitoneal abscess in less than 20% of cases. CT is an invaluable tool in these cases and obviates the need for contrast studies of the gastrointestinal tract.

Late surgical intervention

Apart from the eradication of biliary tract disease following an attack of acute pancreatitis which has subsided, the role of operative intervention late in the course of acute pancreatitis is for the treatment of complications. These are:

- pseduocyst formation
- abscess formation
- haemorrhage resulting from pseudoaneurysms or sectorial (left-sided) portal hypertension.

A pancreatic pseudocyst is a collection of fluid, serum and haematoma in the lesser sac and its walls have no recognizable epithelial lining. However, at some point, most pseudocysts connect with the pancreatic glandular tissue or ductal system and the discharge of fluid into the cyst is maintained via the connection. Microscopic examination of this area of a pseudocyst will reveal some epithelial lining. The majority of pancreatic epithelial cysts are neoplastic (Table 12.8). The differentiation between a true cyst and a pseudocyst is only histological. The epithelial lining of true cysts may atrophy due to overdistension or infection. Hence, the absence of histologically recognizable epithelium in the cyst wall on biopsy may be of no significance.

Management of pancreatic pseudocyst

Two types of pancreatic pseudocysts can be differentiated. Acute pseudocysts (acute peripancreatic effusions) follow an established acute attack of pancreatitis. They should be managed expectantly for 4-6 weeks. Spontaneous resolution often occurs and surgical therapy is more satisfactory if the cyst wall is allowed to mature. *Chronic pseudocysts* are usually asymptomatic and, often, no recent attacks of acute pancreatitis can be identified. Spontaneous resolution is rare and delay only invites the high risk of complications. The commonest cause of pancreatic pseudocysts in children is blunt abdominal trauma.

Other parameters which are helpful in the management of pancreatic pseudocysts are:

- *Size*. Pseudocysts less than 5 cm in diameter may be observed and expected to resolve in many instances. Those greater than 7.5 cm in diameter will probably need surgical drainage.
- The development of symptoms is indicative of an impending complication such as rupture, haemorrhage and infection.
- Maturity. As previously mentioned, an acute pseudocyst should be allowed to mature for 4–6 weeks to allow the cyst wall to mature since this facilitates internal drainage.
- Vascular complications. Recent advances in visceral angiography and its widespread practice have delineated a subgroup of patients with vascular complications associated with acute pancreatitis. These include pseudoaneurysms

Table 12.8 Cysts of the pancreas

True cysts	*Pseudocysts*
Benign cysts	
Enterogenous cyst	(1) Acute pseudocyst following acute pancreatitis
Retention (solitary) cyst	(2) Chronic pseudocyst following acute pancreatitis
Dermoid cyst	(3) Chronic pseudocyst associated with chronic pancreatitis
Lympho-epithelial cyst	(4) Miscellaneous peripancreatic cysts
Cystic fibrosis	– hydatid cyst
Von Hippel–Lindau disease	– choledochal cyst
Endometrial cyst	– post-pancreatitis necrotic collections
Neoplastic cysts	
Serous cystadenoma	
Mucinous cystadenoma	
Cystadenocarcinoma	
Papillary cystic neoplasm	
Solid malignancies with central necrosis and cavitation	

and left-sided portal hypertension from splenic vein thrombosis. If arterial complications are suspected, an arteriogram is helpful especially if pre-operative arterial embolization is contemplated. The presence of portal hypertension is an indication for splenectomy with or without gastric devascularization.
- The site of the pseudocyst is another important parameter which helps the surgeon decide on the method of internal drainage. Retrogastric cysts which are enlarging anteriorly are best treated by a posterior cystogastrostomy. Cysts around the head of the pancreas close to the duodenum can easily be drained by cystoduodenostomy. Large cysts which enlarge through and bulge inferiorly into the transverse mesocolon are best drained by cystojejunostomy with Roux-en-Y. Cysts located in the tail or body of the pancreas are technically more amenable to a resection (distal pancreatectomy and splenectomy) than cysts in the head and neck of the gland.

While internal drainage into the upper gastrointestinal tract is the preferred method of treating pseudocysts, there are some exceptions. Infected or ruptured cysts or the acute cysts with thin, friable walls are best drained externally with wide-bore sump suction drains. In many instances, the resulting pancreatic fistula will gradually close spontaneously. Occasionally a second procedure is needed to implant the fistulous tract into Roux-en-Y loop of jejunum. Two additional precautionary measures should be taken whenever a pancreatic cyst is drained:

- The cyst fluid must be routinely sent for cytological examination and a representative sample of the cyst wall must be excised for histological examination. The injudicious drainage of a cystadenoma or a cystadenocarcioma may thus be spotted and a planned reoperation for wide local excision entertained.
- The cavity of the cyst must be explored with the index finger and septa gently divided. The cyst must be thoroughly irrigated prior to anastomosis with adjoining bowel or external drainage.

Percutaneous drainage of a pseudocyst under CT scan or ultrasound guidance is often advocated indiscriminately. It definitely has a temporizing role in some specific situations such as:

- A patient who is unfit for or who refuses an operation.
- An acute pseudocyst which is rapidly enlarging and needs external drainage.
- An infected pseudocyst which needs external drainage in a very sick septic patient.
- A pseudocyst which is in an unusual location (e.g. mediastinum, pelvis) and is not readily amenable to internal drainage.

Endoscopic internal drainage of pseudocysts is too new a procedure to be evaluated. Early experience suggests that the hazards of bleeding and stenosis of the stoma are too prohibitive for the technique to be widely accepted.

Management of pancreatic abscess (infected pancreatic/peripancreatic necrosis)

The term 'pancreatic abscess' should not be used to connote a localized collection of pus in the lesser sac (infected pancreatic pseudocyst) which is easily drained externally with good results. A pancreatic abscess implies the presence of extensive pancreatic and peripancreatic necrosis with secondary infection. It has a very high mortality and morbidity and usually occurs after the second week of the onset of pancreatitis. The incidence of massive haemorrhage and injury to adjacent organs is also high. Drainage of the pancreatic bed alone is ineffective unless it is combined with wide retroperitoneal debridement to remove the pancreatic and peripancreatic slough. In most instances, additional necrosis and abscess formation occur and reoperation for further debridement, lavage and drainage must be instituted.

Since pancreatic abscess formation follows an attack of acute fulminating pancreatitis and is associated with a prohibitive mortality and morbidity, some have advocated early (within a few days of onset) total pancreatectomy to control fulminant pancreatitis. The mortality for this extensive procedure in seriously ill patients is also prohibitive and all patients with the severe disease do not invariably progress to abscess formation.

Recurrent pancreatitis

Any patient who has recovered from one or more attacks of pancreatitis must be investigated to identify and, if possible, to eliminate the aetiological factors. The need to identify surgically remediable problems, most commonly gallstones, is obvious. Ultrasonography of the biliary tract can be used even in the acute stage.

Stenosis of the sphincter of Oddi, often called papillitis, is without doubt a rare cause of recurrent pancreatitis. The stenosis is rarely of a primary nature and is probably due to a temporary impaction and later passage of a gallstone. Confidence in the diagnosis is strengthened by:

- Documented episodes of biliary obstruction or cholangitis.
- The endoscopic visualization of an inflamed papilla.
- Demonstrated tightness of the ampullary orifice when it is cannulated endoscopically.
- Documentation of delay in emptying of the common bile duct.
- Intermittent elevations of liver enzymes, especially serum alkaline phosphatase.
- Positive morphine-prostigmine (Nardi) test – reproduction of pain and enzyme elevation.
- Documentation of elevated pressures in the common bile duct by ERCP.

Treatment is sphincteroplasty which includes division of sphincter of Oddi and the septum between the common bile duct and the pancreatic duct to relieve both biliary and pancreatic outflow obstruction. The situation should be suspected in patients who have had more than one attack of pancreatitis and/or cholangitis without any other discernible cause. One word of caution – the condition of 'primary papillitis' has been overdiagnosed without adequate documentation of unexplained abdominal pain which is often not even of pancreatic or biliary origin. In such situations, the indiscriminate use of sphincteroplasty, often wrongly performed, has led the operation into disrepute. Endoscopic papillotomy has a definite place when the biliary sphincter alone needs to be divided.

Congenital malformations in the pancreas or duodenum around the ampullary region can cause recurrent pancreatitis in both children and adults. Endoscopic ultrasound and ERCP are invaluable in delineating these abnormalities, some of which may be amenable to surgical correction. Probably the commonest congenital abnormality leading to recurrent pancreatitis is the pancreas divisum which is an anatomical variant occuring when there is failure of the two embryonic pancreatic ductal systems to unite. In this situation, the duct of Wirsung is very small and may measure no more than 1–2 cm in length while the duct of Santorini becomes the major ductal drainage system of the pancreas and maintains its communication with the duodenum through the minor papilla. Following secretin administration, large volumes of juice can be visualized endoscopically from the minor papilla with little or none coming from the main papilla or aspirated from the duct of Wirsung during cannulation. The high incidence of recurrent pancreatic pain in patients with pancreas divisum may well be due to the very small papilla of the duct of Santorini which, in these patients, drains the majority of the pancreas, creating a marked relative stenosis of the ampulla.

The relief of pain by all treatment modalities is unsatisfactory leading one to question the proposed pathophysiological explanation. Endoscopic papillotomy, with or without stenting of the duct of Santorini, and surgical transduodenal sphincteroplasty of both the minor and major papilla, have not yielded favourable long-term results. Eventually, the recurrent pancreatitis coupled with the trauma induced by repeated endoscopic and/or surgical approaches, force the surgeon to consider a Whipple pancreatoduodenectomy or a duodenum-preserving proximal pancreatectomy for pain relief.

Left-sided (sectorial) portal hypertension due to pancreatitis

This occurs from occlusion by compression or by thrombosis of the splenic vein and is discussed in elsewhere [**Disorders of the liver and disorders of the spleen, Vol. II**].

Acute pancreatitis in children

In recent years, acute pancreatitis is being recognized with greater frequency in infancy and childhood. Although the treatment is not substantially different from that of adults, the aetiological factors are totally different. Biliary tract disease is not usually an aetiological factor; nor is alcoholism. A large number of mild acute pancreatitis causes results from viral infections such as mumps. Blunt abdominal trauma, resulting from relatively minimal injury, is probably the most common cause. Unlike the situation in adults, isolated pancreatic injury is commonly reported. A trifling fall upon a toy, such as a tricycle handlebar, may result in pancreatic trauma sufficient to induce a traumatic pancreatitis. Two clinical pictures emerge: (1) an acute abdominal emergency necessitating exploratory laparotomy when the pancreas is found to be inflamed. In such situations, care must be taken to exclude a complete pancreatic transection or major ductal injury; (2) the initial symptoms are mild and often the child is not even taken to the hospital for several days or weeks when a pancreatic pseudocyst or pancreatic ascites has developed.

Drug-induced pancreatitis, familial pancreatitis (usually associated with hyperlipidaemia or amino aciduria) and calculous disease of the biliary tree are all uncommon in children, although occasional cases with pigment stones due to congenital spherocytosis have been described. Obstruction of the ampulla of Vater due to a congenital anomaly of the pancreatic ductual ampulla has also been documented and has been corrected by an adequate sphincteroplasty. Roundworms entering into the pancreatic duct and causing pancreatitis have also been reported from time to time. Duodenal obstruction due to an annular pancreas may lead to current acute pancreatitis which responds to duodenal decompression.

The management of acute or recurrent acute pancreatitis in children is essentially the same as in adults. The prognosis is much better even in the presence of complications. If the aetiological factors are removed, recovery is complete. Acute or recurrent acute pancreatitis does not progress into the chronic or chronic relapsing form in the vast majority of children.

Surgical treatment of chronic pancreatitis and chronic relapsing pancreatitis

Chronic pancreatitis or chronic relapsing pancreatitis is not generally considered a surgical disease. Maintenance of adequate nutrition, enzyme replacement and/or insulin supplements may be necessary in the management of exocrine and/or endocrine insufficiencies. The input of social services and of an interested psychiatric team is essential to manage the drug addiction and alcoholic problems which are often present. Direct operative procedures on the parenchyma of the gland and/or its ductal system are indicated almost exclusively for the relief of pain. The limits and hazards of surgical treatment of these patients must be emphasized.

- No surgical procedure can restore either the endocrine or exocrine function of the pancreas. Nor is it likely to prevent further loss of glandular function.
- The conversion of a non-reformed alcoholic or drug addict into an insulin-dependent diabetic by major pancreatic resection is likely to be lethal and must be avoided.
- Rehabilitation of the patient must be planned well in advance, otherwise surgical intervention for pain is doomed to failure. The life expectancy of the non-reformed alcoholic drug addict is extremely limited and is often shortened by the complications and late sequelae of operations.
- Avoidance of alcohol is a more important determination of outcome after operation than the type of procedure performed.

There are two indications for surgical treatment:

- *Intractable pain* – it is crucial to delineate the frequency, persistence and degree of pain. The decision to advise operation is influenced by several factors including the degree of disruption of the patient's life, the narcotic need, the control of alcoholism, the age and general condition of the patient and, often, the surgeon's personal preferences.

- *The development of complications* – these include: (i) lower bile duct obstruction; (ii) duodenal obstruction; (iii) vascular involvement; (iv) pancreatic cysts, pseudocysts, pancreatic ascites, and pleural effusions; and (v) the presence of a dominant mass leading to the fear or suspicion of cancer.

It is important to emphasize that correction of a complication does not invariably relieve any associated pain.

Lower bile duct obstruction

The lower portion of the common bile duct passes through the head of the pancreas and is at risk of being narrowed by inflammation and fibrosis in this region. If frank obstructive jaundice is present, the onus is on the surgeon to exclude pre-operatively and operatively the presence of an underlying cancer. On occasions, this may only be possible after a total pancreatoduodenectomy. More commonly, the patient has low-grade cholangitis and pain indistinguishable from pancreatic pain. Frank suppurative cholangitis and secondary biliary cirrhosis have also been described. In the mild case, serum alkaline phosphatase elevation is the most consistent although non-specific effect of biliary obstruction. As a rule, investigation of the biliary tree (by endoscopic retrograde cholangiogram) is mandatory whenever surgical treatment of chronic pancreatitis is being considered. Relief of the partial common bile duct obstruction is, in some instances, all that is needed to relieve the pain.

Duodenal obstruction

This rarely occurs in patients with severe chronic pancreatitis and enlargement of the head of the pancreas. Here again a concomitant pancreatic cancer must be excluded by appropriate biopsies (in the young patient or by pancreatoduodenctomy (in the older patient). Vagotomy and gastrojejunostomy will adequately relieve the duodenal obstruction.

Development of vascular complications

These include multiple pseudoaneurysms and sectorial portal hypertension. These have been discussed in the section on acute pancreatitis.

Surgical treatment

Once a decision for surgical treatment has been made, the two most important pre-operative investigations are ERCP and angiography. ERCP will delineate the state of the main pancreatic duct and common bile duct and helps in the planning of surgical therapy. However, the findings on ERCP often do not correlate with the patient's symptoms. ERCP does not indicate the state of the parenchyma; nor does it indicate the need for operative intervention except if cytological examination of the pancreatic duct aspirate is positive for cancer. However, ERCP provides a good indication of the choice of operation. Similarly, angiography delineates the anatomy of the foregut vasculature as well as vascular complications which may necessitate an alteration in surgical strategy.

Although ERCP is often used as the gold standard for defining chronic pancreatitis, it is an invasive test that carries the risk of cholangitis and acute pancreatitis (approximately 4%). Angiography is also invasive and usually reserved for therapeutic embolization in cases of bleeding. Therefore, it is not surprising that newer imaging modalities such as magnetic resonance cholangiopancreatography (MRCP) and endoscopic ultrasonography are redefining the indications for ERCP and angiography in the evaluation of chronic pancreatitis.

MRI is capable of generating images non-invasively and without ionizing radiation. Heavily T2-weighted imaging allows reconstruction of ductal structures, including pancreatograms. MRCP rivals endoscopy in its visualization of the main pancreatic duct (98% in the head in one study) but detects secondary ductal branches only 10–25% of the time. Therefore, MRCP appears unable to approach the sensitivity of ERCP for early stage disease.

EUS allows viewing of the pancreas through the duodenal and gastric wall with high-frequency ultrasound probes, which are capable of much greater resolution of fine structural detail than conventional abdominal ultrasound. In addition, intestinal gas does not provide a barrier to the pancreas. Multiple criteria for the diagnosis of chronic pancreatitis have been proposed, including parenchymal changes described as hyperechogenic foci, hyperechogenic stranding, lobularity of the gland and cyst formation. Ductal changes include hyperechoic thickening, irregularity, dilatation, visible side branches and calcified duct stones. The EUS technology has the limitations of being operator dependent and therefore the exact role of its use in the diagnosis of chronic pancreatitis needs to be answered ultimately by long-term, careful follow-up of patients with suspected mild disease.

As a general rule, surgery should be conservative when:

- there is no endocrine or exocrine insufficiency
- a dilated duct of Wirsung is present.

Dilatation (diameter > 3 mm) of the main pancreatic duct, with or without partial stenosis of the duct at a number of points producing a 'chain of lakes' appearance, may be associated with pancreatic stones in the duct. In this situation, longitudinal filleting of the main pancreatic duct and side-to-side anastomosis to a Roux-en-Y loop of jejunum (modified Puestow operation) is highly appropriate after removing any stones if present. Relief of pain is accomplished in about 70% of patients who stop consuming alcohol although recurrence of pain is common after variable intervals.

Surgery should be radical when:

- Pancreatic cancer is suspected and/or cannot be excluded.
- There is established endocrine and exocrine insufficiency.
- There is extensive pancreatic destruction by ductal sclerosis, glandular fibrosis, calcification and multiple pseudocysts.

A single pseudocyst may be drained internally as a preliminary step to see if the patient's pain is relieved. The presence of multiple cysts or the re-formation of cysts is an indication for pancreatic resection. The 95% distal pancreatectomy (Child's procedure) is not uniformly successful and recurrent pain associated with pancreatitis in the region of the head and the uncinate process then necessitates a second-stage pancreatoduodenectomy which can be technically difficult and hazardous. When pancreatic cancer is not suspected, total pancreatectomy can be performed in one stage with preservation of the whole stomach, pylorus and first part of the duodenum by careful preservation of the blood supply to the pyloroduodenal area. This diminishes post-operative problems associated with reduced gastric reservoir capacity and dumping syndrome.

Because 40–60% of patients with painful chronic pancreatitis exhibit a ductal ectasia, decompression of the pancreatic ductal system has become one of the main therapeutic principles, based on the assumption that ductal ectasia indicates intraductal hypertension. Many different approaches to decompressing the pancreatic duct have been described. In 1956, Puestow and Gillesby described a technique in which drainage of the main pancreatic duct was accomplished by performing a longitudinal laterolateral pancreaticojejnunostomy after resection of the pancreatic tail and splenectomy. Although the procedure met with some success, 15–40% of patients did not experience permanent pain relief. In an effort to improve results with drainage alone, several surgeons including Beger and Frey have combined resection with drainage. The Beger procedure includes a subtotal resection of the pancreatic head following transection of the pancreas anterior to the portal vein. The gastroduodenal passage and common bile duct continuity are preserved. The body of the pancreas is drained by an end-to-end or end-to-side pancreatojejunostomy using a Roux-en-Y loop. The Frey procedure differs from the Beger in that there is no transection of the pancreas in front of the portal vein. For reconstruction, a longitudinal pancreaticojejunostomy is used draining the resection cavity of the head, body, and tail of the pancreas.

A less radical approach which has been reported to be occasionally successful is the performance of a truncal vagotomy, antrectomy and gastrojejunal (Billroth II or Polya) anastomosis. The rationale of this operation is the elimination of neural and hormonal stimuli to pancreatic secretion, especially those normally triggered by eating. No convincing data are available to support these contentions.

Two other indirect operations, namely cholecystectomy (for established gallbladder disease) and parathyroidectomy (for proved hyperparathyroidism), are sometimes advocated to reduce the severity of chronic pancreatitis. The incidence of gallstones in patients with chronic pancreatitis is the same as that in the general population. Cholecystectomy should be advised based on symptoms of gallbladder disease and on the risk of complications. It will not affect the natural history of chronic pancreatitis. Similarly, hyperparathyroidism should be treated to avoid the sequelae of severe hypercalcaemia without influencing the course of any incidental chronic pancreatitis.

Splanchnic neurectomies and coeliac ganglion block have generally been disappointing in the control of chronic pancreatic pain.

First reported in 1943, splanchnicectomy for the management of intractable pancreatic pain was practically forgotten because of the invasiveness required (laparotomy or thoracotomy in patients with limited survival) and the inconsistent results achieved. With the evolution of minimal access surgery, however, interest has been rekindled. The first thoracoscopic splanchnicectomy for pancreatic cancer pain was performed in 1993 and was soon followed by numerous other reports advocating its use for chronic pancreatitis pain. In this procedure, four trocars are optimal: camera, lung retraction and two working ports. After transecting the inferior pulmonary ligament, the lung is retracted anteromedially. The sympathetic trunk is identified as a guide to the greater splanchnic nerve, which lies medial to it close to the aorta on the left and the oesophagus on the right. The overlying pleura is incised, and the nerve is dissected free and transected sharply. Left-sided splanchnicectomy alone seems effective in most patients. Preliminary studies indicate that the procedure is effective, but long-term follow-up is lacking at the present time. Promising results have been obtained recently with thoracoscopic bilateral splanchnicectomy although the reported experience is limited and the follow-up short.

Section 12.8 • Neoplasms of the non-endocrine pancreas

Benign neoplasms of the non-endocrine pancreas are exceedingly rare and are of no clinical significance unless they become large enough to be palpable or to impinge on adjacent structures (common bile duct, duodenum, stomach or main pancreatic duct) and cause symptoms. Since both solid and cystic benign tumours are rarely found at laparotomy or at necropsy, there is no evidence to suggest that they represent an early phase in the development of the more common malignant neoplasms. The reported benign tumours of the non-endocrine pancreas include adenoma, cystadenoma, lipoma, fibroma, leiomyofibroma, myoma, haemangioma, lymphangioma, haemangioendothelioma and neuroma. These diagnoses should only be made after exclusion of the more frequent malignant tumours by some form of representative (preferably excisional) biopsy.

Pancreatic cancer

The term 'pancreatic cancer' is sometimes used to include all types of malignant neoplasms of the non-endocrine pancreas (which are classified in Table 12.9) as well as malignant islet cell tumours (Table 12.10). In clinical practice, pancreatic cancer is synonymous with

Table 12.9 Pathological classification of primary malignant neoplasms of the pancreas (non-endocrine)

1. *Duct (ductular) cell origin*	90%
Duct cell adenocarcinoma	10%
Giant cell carcinoma	
Giant cell carcinoma (epulis-osteoid)	
Adenosquamous carcinoma	
Microadenocarcinoma	
Mucinous (colloid) carcinoma	
Cystadenocarcinoma (mucinous)	
2. *Acinar cell origin*	<1%
Acinar cell carcinoma	
Cystadenocarcinoma (acinar cell)	
3. *Connective tissue origin*	<1%
'Osteogenic' sarcoma	
Leiomyosarcoma	
Haemangiopericytoma	
Malignant fibrous histocytoma	
4. *Uncertain histogenesis*	8%
Pancreaticoblastoma	
Papillary and cystic neoplasm	
Mixed type: duct and islet cells	
Unclassified	
5. *Miscellaneous others*	<1%
Malignant melanoma	
Oncocytoma	
Neuroblastoma	
Plasmacytoma	
Lymphoma	

pancreatic ductal adenocarcinoma (arising in the exocrine pancreas) which constitutes 90% of all primary malignant tumours arising from the gland. When the cancer originates in the head of the pancreas (in about 70% of cases) it must also be differentiated from cancer arising from the ampulla, duodenum or lower common bile duct which has a much better prognosis that true pancreatic adenocarcinoma. The incidence of pancreatic cancer has tripled over the past 40 years throughout the West. It is highly fatal and has one of the lowest 5 year survival rates (1–2%) of all cancers. About 29 000 new pancreatic cancers are diagnosed each year in the USA and the disease now accounts for 10% of all the cancers of the digestive tract (second behind colorectal cancer). It is the fourth most common cancer of all sites as a cause of death (behind lung, colorectal, and breast).

Cancer of the pancreas is distinctly more common in older people and is relatively uncommon, but not altogether rare, below the age of 55 years. It occurs more frequently in men than in women but the male-to-female ratio has decreased in recent years, suggesting that more women are now being diagnosed with this cancer.

The exact causative factors responsible for the increase in incidence of pancreatic cancer are unknown. A high-protein and high-fat diet, characteristic of the Western population, has been implicated epidemiologically as a possible factor. The strongest association is between pancreatic cancer and cigarette smoking. Exposure to industrial carcinogens, especially betanaphthylamine and benzidine, has been documented in pancreatic cancer patients. A higher than normal incidence rate of the neoplasm has also been reported in chemists, workers in metal industries, and coke and gas plant employees. In interpreting these retrospective epidemiological data, it must be remembered that the general class of 'labourer' has, both in the USA and in Britain, an

Table 12.10 Islet cell tumours and associated clinical syndromes

Cell type	*Peptide product*	*Tumour*	*Clinical picture*
A cell	Glucagon	Glucagonoma	Diabetes, necrolytic migratory erythema, stomatitis, glossitis Weight loss, weakness
B cell	Insulin	Insulinoma	Neuroglycopenia Clouded sensorium Behaviour disturbance Seizures Transient neurological deficit Adrenaline discharge Sweating Tremulousness Palpitation Hunger
D cell?	Gastrin	Gastrinoma	Fulminant peptic ulceration Diarrhoea Malabsorption
D cell?	Somatostatin	Somatostatinoma	Diabetes, pancreatic malabsorption with steatorrhoea, gallstones Weight loss
D_1 cell?	Vasoactive intestinal polypeptide (VIP)	VIPoma	Fulminant diarrhoea, hypokalaemia, hypercalcaemia, diabetes, flushing
D_1 cell?	Human pancreatic polypeptide	HPPoma	Uncertain
?	ACTH	?	Cushing's syndrome
?	Hydroxyindole	Carcinoid	Carcinoid syndrome?
?	Prostaglandin	?	Same as VIPoma?
?	ADH	?	?
?	None	Non-functioning islet cell tumour	Same as exocrine tumour but slow growing

excessively high incidence of pancreatic cancer so that occupational risk is mixed with social class risk.

Industrial causes of pancreatic cancer are probably less important than is believed or the causative exposures are far more widespread in most occupations that is generally accepted.

Molecular biology of pancreatic cancer

Sporadic cancers of the pancreas are frequently associated with the activation of an oncogene, K-ras, and the inactivation of multiple tumour suppressor genes, including p53, DPC4, p16 and Rb (Table 12.11).

Oncogenes of the ras family (e.g. H-ras, N-ras and K-ras) are among the most common activated oncogenes found in human cancer. The K-ras gene, on chromosome 12, encodes a 2.0 kb transcript that is highly conserved across species and is translated into the p21-ras protein. These proteins are located in the plasma membrane and transduce growth and differentiation signals from activated receptors to protein kinases within the cell. Up to 90% of human pancreatic cancers have ras gene mutations, most of which are K-ras mutations and these seem to be an early event in pancreatic carcinogenesis.

The p53 gene is the most frequently mutated gene identified in human cancers. The p53 tumour suppressor gene encodes a 393 amino acid phosphoprotein that acts as a potent transcription factor regulating a myriad of cellular functions. It inhibits oncogene-induced transformation, blocks progression through the G1 phase of the cell cycle, modulates the expression of growth control genes and maintains genome stability. Mutations in the p53 gene result in an abnormal protein unable to carry out its regulatory functions, leading to cell transformation and neoplasia. A number of studies have indicated that p53 mutations are relatively common in adenocarcinoma of the pancreas, occurring in 70% of patients. In addition, p53 mutation may be an independent prognostic factor in patients with pancreatic ductal adenocarcinoma.

The p16 gene, which is located on chromosome 9p, encodes a protein that binds cyclin D-cdk4 complexes. When p16 binds to these complexes, it inhibits the phosphorylation of a number of growth and regulatory proteins, including the retinoblastoma protein (Rb). Hypophosphorylated Rb binds to and sequesters transcription factors that would otherwise promote the G1/S transition in the cell cycle. Inactivation of p16 therefore inactivates another important cell cycle checkpoint. Mutations in the p16 gene are found in approximately 60% of pancreatic adenocarcinomas and may be associated with short patient survival.

A new tumour suppressor gene, DPC4 (deleted in pancreatic carcinoma, locus 4), which resides on chromosome 18q, has recently been identified. DPC4 has homology to a family of proteins called the Mad proteins which play a role in signal transduction for the transforming growth factor-β (TGF-β) family of cell surface receptors. TGF-β can downregulate the growth of epithelial cells and stimulate differentiation and apoptosis. Therefore, it is reasonable to expect that the loss of DPC4 would promote cell growth. DPC4 is inactivated in approximately half of all pancreatic cancers and, in contrast to p53 and p16, appears to be relatively specific to pancreatic cancer.

Pancreatic cancer and diabetes mellitus

There is no doubt that there is an association between pancreatic cancer and diabetes mellitus. Two hypotheses have been put forward. First, diabetes mellitus is an aetiological factor in the development of pancreatic cancer. The evidence for this theory is rather confusing. When recent diabetes was eliminated, some studies found as high as a six-fold risk for pancreatic cancer in diabetic women but not in diabetic men. Several uncertainties result from the fact that there has been no strict delineation of the type of diabetic who is prone to develop pancreatic cancer and no sorting out of the genetic aspects of the disease in the population studied. In addition there have been varying definitions of

Table 12.11 Genetic alterations in pancreatic cancer

Genes	*Chromosome*	*Mechanism of inactivation*	*Frequency (%)*
Oncogenes			
K-ras	–	Point mutations codons 12,13	80–100
Tumour suppressor			
p53	17p	LOH + IM	50–75
p16	9p	Homozygous deletion Hypermethylation	LOH + IM 40 40 15
DPC4	18q	Homozygous deletion LOH + IM	 30 20
RB1	13q	Mutation/small deletion	0–7

LOH + IM = loss of heterozygosity and intragenic mutation.
Modified from: Hruban, R. H., Peterson, G. M., Ha, P. K., Kern, S. E. (1998). Genetics of pancreatic cancer: from genes to families. *Surg Oncol Clin North Am* **7**: 1–23.

diabetes in all reported studies. We therefore do not know if all diabetics or a special subset are at risk from pancreatic cancer. It may well be that diabetics have so many other complications that few actually live long enough to develop pancreatic cancer.

The second hypothesis is that the presence of pancreatic cancer is some way induces glucose intolerance. This is supported by the fact that in many cases the diabetes is diagnosed within 2 years before the cancer is discovered. Thus, there may be two types of diabetes mellitus in pancreatic cancer; patients: (1) in a group of individuals in whom the hereditary type is present with its possible increased risk of pancreatic cancer, and (2) in another set of patients in whom the hyperglycaemia is of shorter duration and is a result of the pancreatic cancer. There is a definite suggestion of a bimodality of duration of clinical diabetes mellitus in several series of pancreatic cancer patients (40% of patients with a duration of greater than 2 years, and 50% with a duration of less than 1 year).

Alcoholism and chronic pancreatitis

Retrospective epidemiological data regarding an association between alcoholism and pancreatic cancer are inconclusive. As with diabetics, alcoholics have so many other problems that pancreatic cancer is one of their lesser worries. The main reason for considering an alcohol–pancreatic cancer association is that pancreatitis (which can be induced by alcohol) has been associated with pancreatic cancer. However, it must be emphasized that 'pancreatitis' may have three different meanings: (1) histological pancreatitis invariably coexists with pancreatic cancer, presumably due to ductal obstruction and/or direct destruction of parenchymatous tissues; (2) the acquired variety of chronic pancreatitis (clinical entity) does not seem to be related to pancreatic cancer; and (3) the hereditary type of chronic pancreatitis seems to have a higher predisposition to pancreatic cancer than the general population.

Clinical features of pancreatic cancer

The diagnosis of pancreatic cancer varies from the simple and clinically obvious to the most difficult and almost impossible. The initial symptoms and signs depend on the site and extent of the pancreatic cancer.

Cancer of the head of the pancreas

As previously mentioned, this has to be differentiated from cancer of the ampulla, lower common bile duct and/or duodenum since these latter tumours may present with similar features. The term 'periampullary carcinoma' is often used to denote tumours in this region irrespective of the exact site of origin. Progressive jaundice occurs in over 75% of patients with carcinoma of the head of the pancreas and the incidence of jaundice decreases as the location of the lesion progresses to the left towards the tail of the pancreas. Occasionally, a tumour may invade and compress the third or fourth parts of the duodenum without actually obstructing the common bile duct. Pain is extremely frequent and the classic description of painless jaundice is rarely encountered. Weight loss and anorexia are also common symptoms even in early stages. Nausea, epigastric bloating, change in bowel habits and vomiting are occasionally present. Haematemesis and melaena occasionally occur in late cases as a result of direct invasion the duodenal or gastric mucosa by tumour or superior mesenteric-splenic vein compression by the tumour. Chills and fever due to ascending cholangitis can occur in long-standing biliary obstruction. A palpable gallbladder (Courvoisier's sign) is noted in only about a quarter of patients with resectable tumours. The liver is usually enlarged on palpation.

Cancer of the body and tail of the pancreas

Pain and weight loss are the two main consistent symptoms. The pain may initially be dull and vague, localized to the epigastrium or to the back, or it may move to either upper quadrant. It may be episodic and related to meals or it may become constant and severe. In late cases, the patient learns to obtain partial relief by flexing the trunk forward. Severe pain invariably indicates extension of tumour into the perineural lymphatics and the posterior parietes. Weight loss is rapid and severe by the time the patient presents to the hospital. Again, haematemesis and melaena may be late features due to mucosal invasion or portal hypertension. Migratory thrombophlebitis (Trousseau's sign) can be present in any patient with advanced cancer, is not specifically indicative of pancreatic carcinoma and, by itself, does not merit diagnostic laparotomy or laparoscopy.

Physical examination in the early stages may reveal surprisingly few abnormal physical signs. In late cases, abdominal masses or liver metastases may be palpable. A rectal shelf may be evident on rectal examination in the rectovesical or rectovaginal pouch (Blumer's shelf), there may be evidence of ascites, and distant metastases may be present in the supraclavicular fossa (Troisier's sign).

Delay in diagnosis

Over 90% of patients with pancreatic cancer present in the late stage of their disease at a time when there is no chance of cure and, often, even meaningful palliation cannot be achieved. The factors responsible for late diagnosis are:

- The tumour is asymptomatic in the early stages. There is some evidence that the pre-clinical phase of pancreatic cancer may be present for months or even years before the tumour 'appears'.
- 'Patient delay' – the early symptoms are often vague and non-specific and the patient tolerates the discomfort.
- 'Physician delay' – the physician often does not have a high index of suspicion and fails to properly 'evaluate' the patient in the face of a vague history and normal physical examination.
- The patient may not have ready and easy access to competent diagnostic centres. Centralization or regionalization of the management of difficult pancreatic problems is long overdue because of the dependence on sophisticated diagnostic and therapeutic methods.

Positive physical signs in a patient with pancreatic cancer often reflect incurability. The diagnosis therefore needs to be made before the appearance of abnormal physical signs. The clinician should always consider the diagnosis of pancreatic cancer in any patient presenting with seemingly genuine recent symptoms, absent physical signs and negative routine radiological investigation. These are the very patients in whom maximum benefit may be gained by applying the more sophisticated investigative techniques.

The evaluation of diagnostic tests

It is no great triumph to diagnose incurable advanced pancreatic cancer. Any particular technique must be assessed on its ability to diagnose potentially curable lesions of the pancreas. A rational sequence of testing is as follows. CT is the best initial test in the evaluation of a patient with suspected pancreatic cancer. Thin section CT scanning through the pancreas with an i.v. bolus injection of contrast can delineate the pancreatic mass, the relationship of the tumour to the superior mesenteric artery and vein and to the coeliac axis, the patency of the portal vein, and the presence of distant metastastic disease.

Until recently, ERCP combined with cytology has been used to differentiate choledocholithiasis from malignant obstruction of the distal common bile duct when a mass is not seen on CT. With the advent of EUS, the rare but real complication of pancreatitis secondary to injection of contrast into the pancreatic duct during ERCP may be avoided. However, EUS takes a dedicated and skilled endoscopist with the appropriate equipment to be successful and may not be available at all medical centres.

It has become obvious that the diagnosis of *advanced* pancreatic cancer can be made after a careful history and routine physical examination. If obvious metastases are present such as seedings in the retrovesical pouch or the pouch of Douglas on rectal or pelvic examination or large left supraclavicular nodes (Troisier's sign) and/or obvious nodular hepatomegaly, careful consideration should be given in avoiding prolonged and unnecessary investigations and even a diagnostic laparotomy. This logic pertains especially to cancer of the body and tail of the pancreas which is rarely, if ever, curable in a symptomatic patient. Percutaneous needle biopsy of any accessible lesion, including the pancreatic mass, can achieve the diagnosis in many cases and the duration of hospitalization can be appreciably shortened. The frail elderly patient with clinically obvious cancer of the body or tail of the pancreas should be spared the mortality and morbidity of a diagnostic laparotomy. Direct percutaneous needle aspiration of the mass with ultrasound or CT scan for guidance should be attempted (Figures 12.17 and 12.18). Another way of obviating laparotomy in these seriously ill people is to perform laparoscopy and direct vision biopsy. ERCP with stent placement can be performed if the patient is jaundiced, or if the patient is fit and relatively young, exploration with a view to internal biliary drainage should be performed as described later. The technology of imaging methods is advancing rapidly. MRCP and three-dimensional CT scan appears to be the way of the future, but they are not readily available in most medical centres.

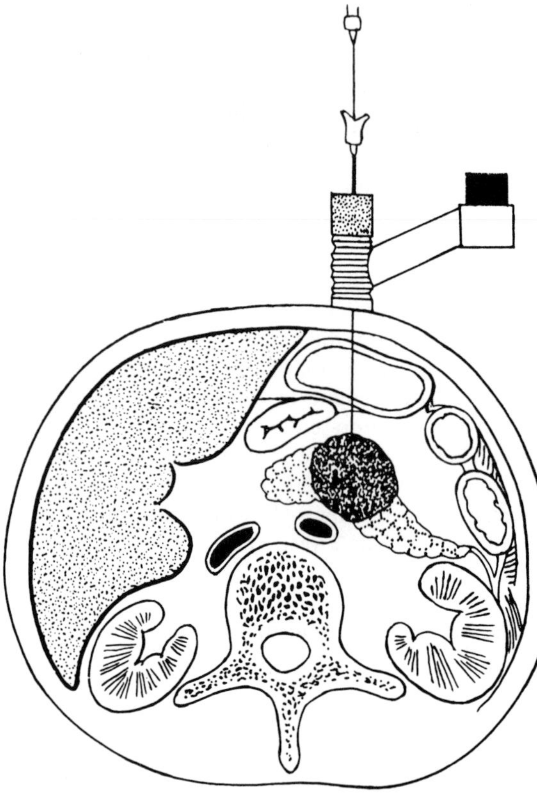

Figure 12.17 Schematic representation of percutaneous fine needle aspiration technique of a pancreatic mass under ultrasound or CT scan control. The aspirated material is smeared on glass slides and fixed and stained by the Papanicolaou or Giemsa method for microscopic examination.

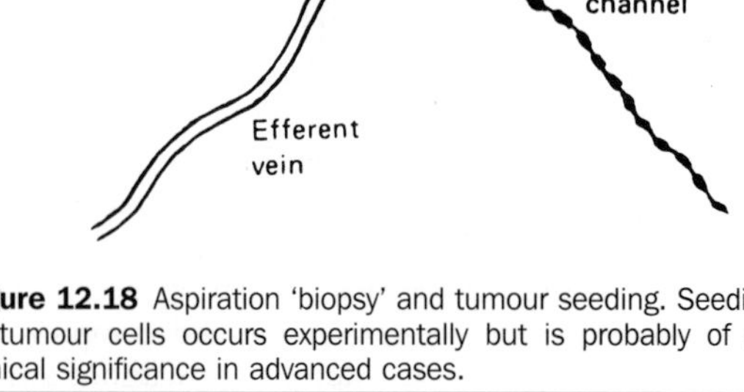

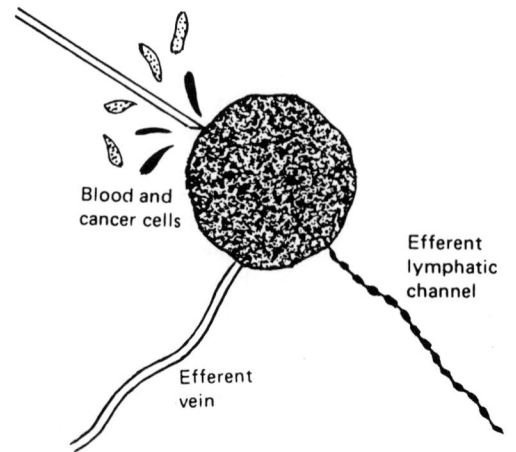

Figure 12.18 Aspiration 'biopsy' and tumour seeding. Seeding of tumour cells occurs experimentally but is probably of no clinical significance in advanced cases.

Surgical treatment of pancreatic cancer

Emphasis must be placed on pre-operative evaluation and adequate preparation of patient with pancreatic cancer. As mentioned earlier, CT scan, EUS and, in some instances, ERCP and fine-needle aspiration for cytology, provide the surgeon with valuable pre-operative information and obviate the need for time-consuming manoeuvres on the operating table. It cannot be overemphasized that pancreatic exploration with a view to resection should not be performed by the occasional surgeon or the resident-registrar in training or in institutions where there is not all the back-up expertise (endoscopy, radiology, cytology, endocrinology) necessary for the care and management of these difficult problems.

Pre-operative preparation

- All jaundiced patients must be kept in a good state of nutrition and hydration with supplemental intravenous fluids, elemental diet and multivitamins as deemed necessary. Injudicious use of i.v. contrast for CT scanning may precipitate renal failure which can also occur post-operatively due to hypovolaemia. A continuous diuresis must be maintained at all times. If the patient is grossly malnourished, a period of parenteral hyperalimentation both before and after operation may be beneficial.
- Blood clotting deficiencies must be corrected. Anaemia is corrected by blood transfusion. Daily injections of vitamin K are administered, preferably for 4–5 days prior to operation. Six units of fresh frozen plasma, six units of platelets and at least six units of blood should be made available. It must be emphasized that pancreaticoduodenectomy can now be safely performed without blood transfusion in many instances.
- Cardiopulmonary function should be carefully assessed by pulmonary function tests, chest X-ray and electrocardiogram as deemed necessary. Smoking is prohibited. Intensive pulmonary physiotherapy, active mobilization and leg exercises are strongly encouraged pre-operatively. The question of prophylactic digitalization and diruretic therapy is considered in individual patients to achieve maximum cardiovascular compensation.
- If a patient is critically ill with one or more of the following parameters: (a) a highly elevated serum bilirubin (greater than 200 μm/l (12 mg %); (b) sepsis; (c) hepatorenal failure; (d) severe cardiopulmonary disease which is expected to respond to medical management; or (e) severe malnutrition, a percutaneous transhepatic or endoscopic biliary decompression may be attempted to tide over the patient for 2 or 3 weeks until his/her general condition improves adequately for him/her to be considered for a major pancreatic resection. If the technique of percutaneous biliary drainage or endoscopic stenting is not available, a simple cholecystotomy using ultrasound for guidance may be undertaken under local anaesthesia. *Routine* biliary pre-operative decompression is *not* recommended. It increases the post-operative mortality and morbidity and should be undertaken only if the patient has septic cholangitis.

Selection of patients for pancreatic resection

Except under unusual circumstances, a major pancreatic resection should not be performed in the elderly (older than 80 years), in frail patients with multiple systemic disorders, or in those with an estimated life expectancy of less than 3 years. The operation should be reserved for the relatively fit patient under the most favourable circumstances. The surgeon must use clinical judgement in the determination of the relative indications and contraindications for each procedure. The operative mortality should not exceed 5%. A frank discussion must take place between the surgeon, the patient and his or her relatives prior to embarking on a potentially hazardous operation.

Surgical options

For curative surgical treatment of a cancer in the head of the pancreas, four options are available:

- The **Whipple operation** (pancreaticoduodenectomy) in which the head and neck of the pancreas together with the duodenum, the distal half of the stomach, lower common bile duct and gallbladder and upper jejunum are removed with as much of the regional lymph nodes as possible.
- **Pylorus-preserving pancreaticoduodenectomy** as introduced by Traverso and Longmire in 1978 in an attempt to eliminate the post-gastrectomy symptoms seen with antrectomy. This operation technically differs from the standard Whipple procedure only in the preservation of the blood supply to the proximal duodenum.
- **Total pancreatectomy** (total pancreaticoduodenectomy) includes, along with the contents of the Whipple operation, excision of the spleen, body and tail of the pancreas, and a more thorough regional lymphadenectomy.
- **Regional pancreatectomy** as proposed by Fortner entails extirpation of the transpancreatic portion of the portal vein, the coeliac axis, the superior mesenteric artery and the middle colic vessels, together with structures included in a total pancreatectomy.

Of these four alternatives, the Whipple operation is most commonly employed for tumours of the head of the pancreas. The operation is optimal for malignant tumours that are confined to the duodenum, ampulla of Vater or lower common bile duct. The neck of the gland is divided to the left of the superior mesenteric vein and the body and tail of the pancreas and spleen are left undisturbed. *En bloc* excision of the regional lymph nodes from the porta hepatis, aortocaval and superior mesenteric regions again forms part of the operation. With the Whipple operation, diabetic function can be preserved. Although there is the possibility of an anastomotic leak from the pancreaticojejunostomy, this complication occurs in less than 10% of patients at centres experienced with pancreatic surgery. Also, more effective management of pancreatic anastomotic leakage with hyperalimentation, percutaneous drainage and somatostatin analogue has reduced the magnitude of this problem. Total pancreatectomy should be reserved for situations when there is tumour at the pancreatic margin on serial frozen sections or if the pancreas is not suitable for an anastomosis, especially if the patient is already an insulin-requiring diabetic. Pylorus preserving Whipple operation is a reasonable alternative but may result in transient gastric stasis.

The concept of extended resection for pancreatic cancer with resections of one or more of the major vessels (regional pancreatectomy) is uniformly attended by an increased morbidity and mortality without a concomitant improvement in cure rate. When such extensive procedures are needed to resect the local tumour, occult metastatic disease is usually present and the disease is incurable. Several authors have advocated a selective approach to venous resection when the lesion has been deemed resectable, the pancreatic neck is divided, and while dissecting the uncinate process from the superior mesenteric vein the tumour is found to be adherent to the posterior-lateral portion of the vein. The venous segment can be replaced with an internal jugular vein interposition graft. It must be emphasized that resection of the portal-superior mesenteric venous axis is only recommended if it is relatively minor (less than 1 cm in length and less than half of the venous circumference) and it helps in achieving adequate clearance of soft tissue margins.

The operative diagnosis of pancreatic cancer and its differentiation from chronic pancreatitis

The jaundiced patient nowadays is well investigated pre-operatively and usually a diagnosis is made prior to laparotomy. A general rule is as follows: hard, non-cystic masses in the head of the pancreas which are associated with obstructive jaundice and dilatation of the common bile duct are usually carcinoma, especially if acute inflammation and/or gallstones are absent. Conversely, hard, non-cystic masses involving a major part of the retroampullary part of the gland and unassociated with jaundice or dilatation of the biliary tree are usually pancreatitis.

It is important to remember that pancreatitis of varying degree invariably co-exists with all carcinomas and that patients with gallstones may have a concomitant pancreatic cancer. In doubtful situations, the surgeon must decide whether to try to establish a tissue diagnosis by frozen section histology of biopsies prior to assessing resectability of any pancreatic mass. Every surgeon is influenced by his own philosophy, his experience and expertise, his pathologist's experience and by the clinical situation. Hence, any decision in such a clinical setting can easily lead to controversy when discussed retrospectively or hypothetically. The author's general policy about pancreatic biopsy can be summed up as follows:

- Since over 75% of all cancers in the head of the pancreas are identified pre-operatively by a positive cytology (at ERCP or percutaneous biopsy), it is preferable to assess the resectability of all such masses in the first instance. If conditions are favourable, they are resected without a preliminary biopsy.
- A suspected cancer of the body and tail of the pancreas is 'biopsied' by a distal pancreatectomy and splenectomy provided that the lesion is localized and resectable. If frozen section histological examination reveals a cancer, the 'excision biopsy' is converted to a total or near-total pancreatectomy with regional lymphadenectomy.
- On the other hand, all unresectable and/or metastatic tumours of the pancreas are diagnosed before the surgeon leaves the operating room even if the job is time-consuming. This takes the matter out of the realm of doubt, an especially important point when a palliative procedure restores the patient to relatively good health for a long period and doubt is raised as to the true diagnosis. A known positive biopsy for adenocarcinoma of the pancreas will then prevent a fruitless second laparotomy.
- Frozen sections and histological examination of lymph nodes peripheral or adjacent to delineated pancreatic masses are acceptable if unresectability and/or the presence of metastatic disease is documented. However, a positive regional node *per se* is not an absolute criterion of unresectability. Many patients have survived longer than 3 years following pancreatoduodenectomy in the presence of regional lymph node involvement.

These policies are supported by the following arguments:

- Truly representative needle biopsies of the pancreas are often hard to obtain because of sampling error and confusion between tumour and associated pancreatitis (Figure 12.19).
- The establishment of diagnosis by means of biopsies for frozen section histology is sometimes time-consuming and traumatic. Factors which influence the biopsy policy of surgeons include personal experience of complications, interpretative histological errors and traditional teaching. Many senior surgeons still regard pancreatic biopsy as inaccurate and dangerous. Pancreatitis, fistula formation, haemorrhage and infection have all been reported following all biopsy techniques. However, it is often difficult to decide whether such complications are directly attributable to the biopsy itself or to the concomitant surgical manoeuvres and manipulations. The consensus of opinion is that all surgeons involved in the practice of pancreatic surgery should be willing and able to perform pancreatic biopsy safely if it is indicated. When this is done, the surgeon should make great efforts to avoid major pancreatic ducts and vessels, the typical anatomy of which must be well fixed in his mind. A good Kocher manoeuvre between his fingers and thumb of the left hand will guide the biopsy needle through the duodenum into the appropriate suspicious area of the pancreas. The disposable Travenol 'Tru-Cut' needle is very suitable for this purpose. A less traumatic alternative is to employ a long no. 21 needle, pushing it in a similar fashion through the duodenum, and attaching a 10 ml syringe for aspiration in order to provide a smear for cytology. This is gaining in popularity with the

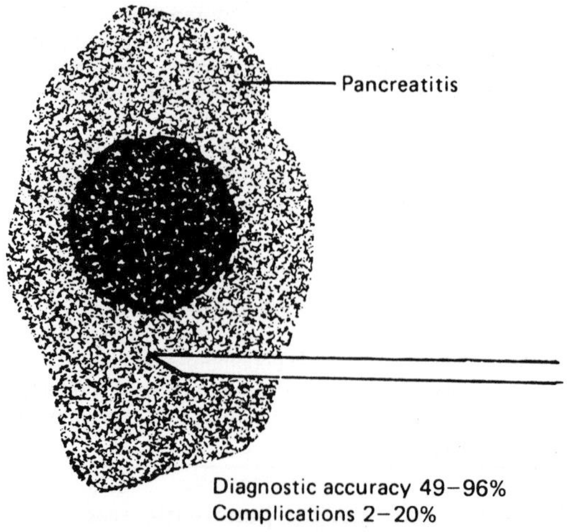

Figure 12.19 Per-operative pancreatic biopsy. A variable degree of pancreatitis surrounds any pancreatic cancer leading to a 'sampling error' with needle biopsies. The number of biopsies taken is limited because of potential morbidity and even mortality and the biopsies may miss the cancer altogether.

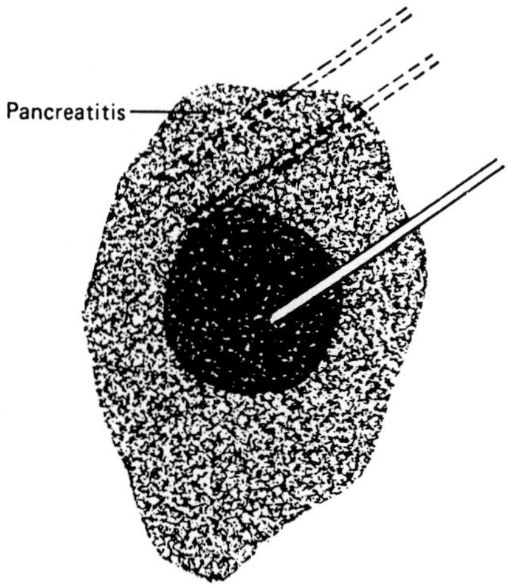

Figure 12.20 Fine needle aspiration 'biopsy' for cytological examination. Multiple punctures may be performed with minimal risks and increase the chance of obtaining material from the cancer.

more widespread availability of, and co-operation with, skilled cytopathologists (Figure 12.20). Haemorrhage, when encountered, can be controlled by finger pressure. Occasionally, silk mattress sutures are needed for haemostasis of the pancreatic capsule following direct pancreatic puncture.
- Errors in interpretation of frozen section biopsy specimens of the pancreas are sometimes made by the inexperienced histopathologist because some desmoplastic carcinomas closely resemble chronic pancreatitis.

Assessment of resectability

A cancer of the pancreas is considered unresectable if there are distant (liver or peritoneal) metastases, invasion of major vessels (portal vein, hepatic artery, superior mesenteric vessels, or coeliac axis) or any extension beyond the area of usual total pancreatectomy specimen. The possible exception is the case of isolated portal vein invasion provided the vein is patent. In these selected cases, portal vein resection with interposition venous graft placement has been described. Puckering of the transverse mesocolon *per se* does not always indicate unresectability since the transverse mesocolon and, if necessary, the transverse colon can be excised in a pancreatoduodenectomy specimen if there are no other contraindications to a resection.

Immediate post-operative care and complications

Following a major pancreatic resection, the patient should be transferred to an intensive care unit where experienced nursing care and sophisticated monitoring techniques are readily available. Patients may require respiratory assistance for the first 12–24 hours. For the first 3–4 post-operative days, the patient's blood sugar is checked every 3–4 hours and small doses of regular insulin (2–5 units) are given intravenously as boluses. Alternatively, a continuous intravenous infusion of insulin can be given. It is important to maintain the blood sugar between 75 and 150 mg% (4–8 mmol/l).

Haemorrhage is still the commonest intra-operative and post-operative complication encountered with pancreatoduodenectomy or total pancreatectomy. However, the incidence of this complication has decreased from about 10% to less than 1% in experienced hands. Meticulous pre-operative preparation, careful haemostasis, and adequate replacement of blood and clotting factors during the operation are essential. In spite of these precautions, the patient may occasionally continue to bleed at a fairly alarming rate from all raw areas in the abdominal cavity during the first 24 hours. The indications for reoperation are:

- If there is reason to suspect a major bleeding site.
- When clot accumulation in the abdomen causes distension and tamponade.
- When a consumption coagulopathy is recognized.

In most cases a discrete bleeding point is never found at reoperation. The clots are gently evacuated and the whole abdomen is irrigated prior to closure with drainage. Haemobilia following biliary decompression is not unusual. It invariably stops spontaneously.

Whenever haemorrhage is suspected, the patient must be kept normovolaemic by adequate blood and fluid replacement and by maintaining a continuous diuresis. Intermittent doses of diuretics may be given as necessary. Hepatorenal failure is the commonest sequence of events leading to post-operative death in this group of patients.

Other complications which may also be fatal include sepsis, mesenteric thrombosis, uraemia, liver insufficiency, myocardial infarction, cerebrovascular accident, congestive heart failure and pulmonary embolism. Leakage from the biliary enteric anastomosis or from the gastrojejunostomy are largely preventable by careful and proper construction of both anastomoses. Anastomotic leaks from the pancreaticojejunostomy occur in less than 10% of patients at centres experienced with pancreatic surgery. Management of pancreatic anastomotic leakage with hyperalimentation, percutaneous drainage and somatostatin analogue has reduced the magnitude of this problem. Complications that are usually non-fatal include pneumonitis, gastric retention, paralytic ileus, bowel obstruction, wound infection, wound dehiscence, atrial fibrillation, faecal fistula and gastrojejunal fistula.

Recurrence of jaundice after pancreatoduodenectomy for cancer of the pancreas

Recurrence of jaundice and/or cholangitis may be seen after pancreatoduodenectomy and may be due to small bowel obstruction. Nausea and vomiting are usually prominent features. The obstruction may be due to recurrent tumour or simply to adhesions. Laparotomy may be indicated to establish the diagnosis and to relieve the obstruction.

Post-operative chemoradiation for resectable cancer of the pancreas

Data from several randomized trials have shown a significant survival benefit in patients treated with infusional 5-fluorouracil (5-FU) and external beam radiation following pancreatectomy. Therefore, in patients who are well enough to tolerate it, adjuvant chemoradiation is recommended. Newer agents such as gemcitabine are currently being studied in combination with radiation as an alternative to 5-FU.

Monitoring of recurrence

A small number of patients with resectable pancreatic cancer have elevated levels of tumour markers such as CA 19-9, POA or CEA pre-operatively. When this is the case, serial monitoring of either marker may be useful in confirming the completeness of surgical excision and in the detection of recurrent pancreatic cancer.

Management of pancreatic endocrine insufficiency

This is discussed elsewhere [Module 20, Vol. I].

Replacement of pancreatic exocrine function

Adequate pancreatin tablets (Viokase, Pancrease, Creon) must be taken with each meal. The number of tablets must be increased if steatorrhoea develops. The patient is advised to take a low-fat, high-protein and carbohydrate diet in the form of frequent regular small meals. Patients must take acid-reducing agents (H_2 blockers) half an hour before taking the pancreatic enzymes to prevent acid inactivation.

Factors influencing prognosis after resection for ductal adenocarcinoma of the head of the pancreas

The mortality for major pancreatic resection is between 0 and 5% in specialized centres. Death as a result of operative complications usually occurs within the first 2 months of operation. After 2 months and up to 2 years, death is usually due to metastatic pancreatic cancer although a few individuals can present as late as the end of the third year with metastatic disease. If the patient has survived 3 years, the cause of death is usually unrelated to pancreatic cancer.

Three major factors appear to determine survival after pancreatoduodenectomy:

- The site of origin of the cancer. Ampullary and distal bile duct tumours have a better prognosis than pancreatic cancer (Figure 12.21).
- The operative mortality and morbidity of the surgical team. It is well established that the operative mortality, morbidity and eventual survival of patients following this and other major operations are dependent on the experience and expertise available in the institution where the operation is performed. Hospitals where a large volume of the operation is performed have much better overall results than those where the operation is performed occasionally.
- The stage of the tumour.
- The biological behaviour of the tumour.

Whether these last two factors are independent variables or are different manifestations of the same variable is debatable.

It is generally agreed that a uniform staging system for pancreatic cancer is clearly desirable. However, a major problem in staging the disease is that it can only

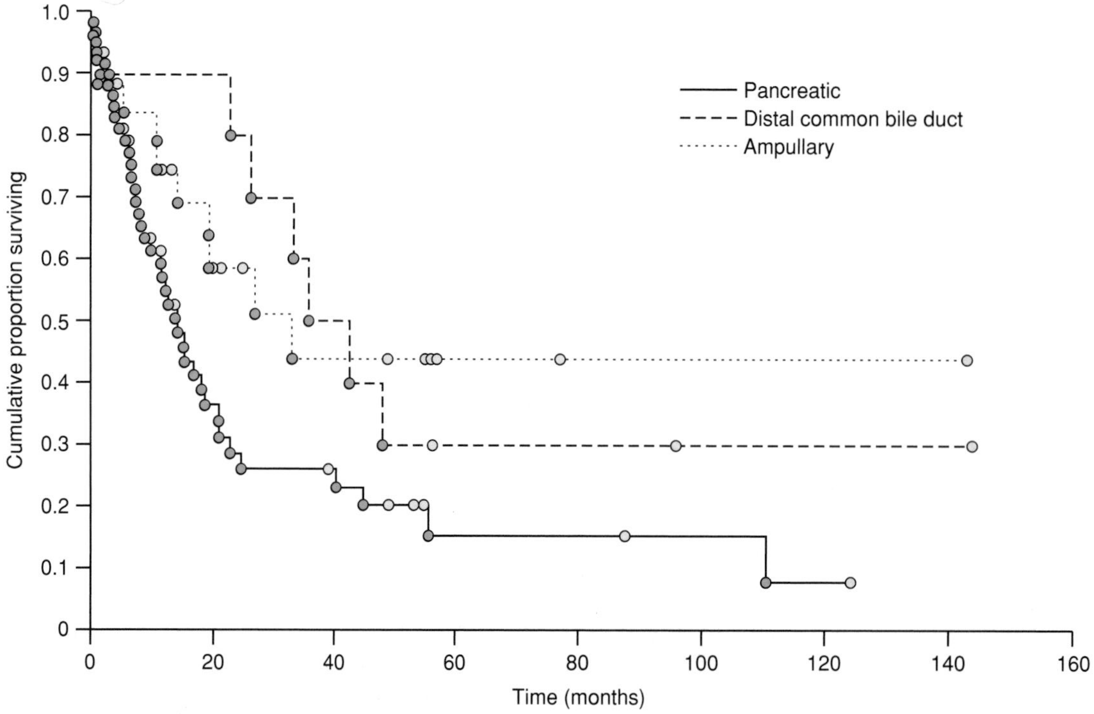

Figure 12.21 Different survival rates after resection of pancreatic cancers, cancers of the distal common bile duct and peri-ampullary cancers.

be performed retrospectively after an extensive pancreatoduodenal resection. The following parameters are considered important:

- The size of the tumour. In general, lesions less than 2 cm in diameter have a higher resectability rate and the best overall survival. Lesions greater than 4 cm have the lowest resectability rate and the lowest overall survival. Caution must be expressed here concerning intra-operative decision making based on size alone. It is not unusual for a small lesion to induce a substantial of surrounding pancreatitis and create a larger mass effect which impinges on neighbouring structures.
- Positive lymph nodes for tumour is an important negative prognostic factor. Hence, it is important to perform an adequate lymphadenectomy *en bloc* with the pancreatoduodenectomy specimen to ensure appropriate staging by the pathologists. How extensive should the lymph node dissection and excision of surrounding soft tissues be is debatable.
- Extrapancreatic invasion adversely affects survival. Since microscopic peripancreatic invasion appears to be important, the extent of the peripancreatic excision leading to skeletonization of the major vessels as advocated by several Japanese surgeons makes sense in order to provide a microscopically curative dissection. Whether a pylorus-preserving pancreatoduodenal resection can be achieved at the same time is debatable.
- Major vascular involvement. This is also an adverse prognostic factor. In most instances, this has the connotation of unresectability if the hepatic artery, coeliac axis or superior mesenteric artery is invaded. However, a short segment of portal vein–superior mesenteric vein (PV–SMV) axis is not necessarily incompatible with long survival, provided that *en bloc* excision of the adherent venous segment helps achieve a microscopically curative surgical resection.
- Histological grade of the tumour. In most series, poorly differentiated tumours are associated with lower survival than well-differentiated ones. Using absorption cytometry to measure DNA content of cells, patients with diploid cancers have a 50% 5 year survival compared to no 5 year survival among those patients with aneuploid cells.
- The amount of blood transfusion in the peri-operative period. Just like in the case of colon cancer, this factor has been proposed as an independent variable affecting survival. Patients who underwent pancreatoduodenectomy with 2 units or less of blood transfusion have a median survival of 24.7 months, whereas those who required 3 units or more in the peri-operative period survive only a median of 10.2 months.
- Perineural involvement. Extensive microscopic involvement of perineural lymphatics is usually associated with a poor prognosis, but such tumours are, by and large, extensive in terms of both peripancreatic involvement and nodal metastases.
- Sex of the patient. As with most other cancers, women appear to live longer than men after pancreatoduodenal resection for pancreatic cancer.

Palliation of pancreatic cancer

The surgeon can palliate incurable pancreatic cancer in several ways:

- Relief of jaundice, pruritus and impending cholangitis. The biliary tract decompression can be done either by cholecystojejunostomy or by hepaticojejunostomy (each with a diverting entero-enterostomy), depending on whether the cystic duct is widely patent and is in full communication with the biliary tree proximal to the obstructing cancer.
- Relief of duodenal obstruction. If the patient lives for more than a few months, duodenal obstruction invariably occurs. It is therefore advisable to perform a gastrojejunostomy at the primary operation.
- Relief of pain. The coeliac plexus can be infiltrated with 50 ml of 50% alcohol or with 20 ml of 6% phenol. This may be helpful in patients with cancer of the body of pancreas when the pain is a prominent feature. Cordotomy, extensive sympathectomy and sterotactic thalamotomy have all been tried with minimal or no objective response. More recently, thoracoscopic splanchnicectomy has been shown to achieve substantial pain relief in inoperable pancreatic cancer.

All locally unresectable or metastatic masses must be biopsied until a definite histological diagnosis is made on frozen section histology. The main tumour mass must be outlined with silver clips to provide a possible radiation port. Post-operative chemoradiation for locally advanced, unresectable tumours is indicated. If liver metastasis or carcinomatosis is found at laparotomy, single agent chemotherapy with gemcitabine may provide palliation and improve the patient's quality of life.

When a patient is unfit for, or refuses, operation, an alternative method of palliating the obstructive jaundice is by endoscopic sphincterotomy and placement of biliary stent. This approach does not relieve any duodenal obstruction which may be present. If the patient survives for more than a few months, recurrent cholangitis associated with stent blockage is a problem that necessitates regular endoscopic removal and replacement of the stent. Newer self-expandable metallic devices such as the Wall stent may prove to provide improved patency rates over plastic stents.

Percutaneous transhepatic placement of an internal expandable metal stent is being tried by the interventional radiologists and offers yet another option for palliation of the jaundiced patient with malignant biliary obstruction.

Section 12.9 • Lesions of the endocrine pancreas

Pancreatic islet cells are components of the gastroentero-pancreatic part of the diffuse neuroendocrine system. Cells belonging to this system are commonly referred to as APUD cells because they share the following cytochemical characteristics: a high amine content (A); the capacity for amine precursor uptake (PU); and the property of decarboxylation (D) of these precursors to form amines. Tumours arising from the APUD series of cells are called APUDomas. Although Pearse originally suggested that all APUD cells were probably derived from neural crest cells, it is now generally recognized that the gastroentero-pancreatic APUD cells (including pancreatic islet cells) probably arise from endoderm (dedifferentiation theory). Regardless of their origin, the APUD cells share similarities in structure, properties and potential. All have characteristic histological, histochemical, immunocytochemical and electron microscopic appearances and all contain the enzyme neurone-specific enolase that is the universal marker for such cells and their hyperplastic and neoplastic lesions.

APUD cells are capable of synthesizing and secreting a great variety of peptides which exert regulatory effects by four main modes of action:

- endocrine, i.e. involving secretion into the circulation to affect distant target sites
- paracrine, i.e. involving local secretion to act on adjacent cells
- neurocrine, i.e. involving secretion at neuronal synapses to act as a neurotransmitter; and
- neuroendocrine, i.e. involving release of a peptide product of the neurone into the circulation to act on other tissues.

Clinical syndromes may develop as a result of either inadequate or excessive production and release of the potent chemical messengers (e.g. inadequate insulin causes diabetes mellitus and excessive insulin leads to hypoglycaemia). The development of radioimmunoassays for a number of the gastroenteropancreatic peptide hormones has led to the understanding that hyperplastic as well as neoplastic pancreatic islet cells are capable of producing recognizable syndromes of hormone excess. Pancreatic tumours of the islet cell type may in fact secrete two or more identifiable peptide hormones although the threshold for the appearance of their respective clinical symptoms varies greatly and elevated levels of one hormone may be compensated by regulatory hypersecretion of other hormones. Endocrine tumours of the pancreas can be referred to as entopic if they produce hormones normally secreted by the pancreas (e.g. insulinoma, glucagonoma) and ectopic if they produce non-pancreatic hormones (e.g. gastrinoma, VIPoma). There is little correlation between tumour size and plasma hormone concentration or severity of clinical symptoms. Some 10–25% of patients harbouring pancreatic APUD tumours will have the multiple endocrine neoplasia type 1 (MEN 1) syndrome. The clinical syndromes associated with overproduction of identified pancreatic islet cell peptides are shown in Table 12.10.

The overwhelming majority and perhaps all islet cells additionally co-synthesize and co-secrete the protein chromogranin along with their peptide products. Elevated plasma levels of chromogranin or neurone-specific enolase are useful markers for pancreatic endocrine tumours and the MEN syndromes even in the absence of clinical symptoms or demonstrable hormonal excess. Immunohistochemical staining for these proteins confirms the endocrine nature of otherwise obscure pancreatic tumours.

With the exception of insulinoma, most endocrine pancreatic tumours are frankly malignant or at least have a high potential for metastatic spread. Compared to their non-endocrine pancreatic counterparts, the endocrine cancers are relatively slow-growing and many apparently metastasize only to regional lymph nodes. This characteristic allows curative surgical therapy in a sizeable proportion of patients.

Historically, the symptoms, morbidity and mortality of the pancreatic endocrine tumours have been due primarily to hormonal hypersecretion but earlier detection and more effective treatment now can often minimize symptoms and forestall death until the advanced stages of malignant spread. Some important characteristics of the more common tumours are presented in Table 12.10.

Hyperinsulinism

Hyperinsulinism in its primary form embraces several different varieties of pancreatic islet cell disease which include B cell hyperplasia/microadenomatosis and B cell neoplasia (insulinoma). These conditions manifest as symptomatic hypoglycaemia. Insulinomas are the most common of pancreatic APUDomas (75% of symptomatic cases) and the most frequent cause of organic primary hyperinsulinism. In the adult, approximately 80% of insulinomas are benign solitary tumours. There is an even distribution of tumours in the head, body and tail of the pancreas. Multiple tumours are usually present in patients with MEN 1 syndrome and are found in about 10% of cases. B cell carcinoma occurs in 5–10% and is characterized by local invasion and metastatic spread to regional lymph nodes and liver. Primary hyperinsulinism is rare in infants and children but, when encountered, a form of B cell hyperplasia (nesidioblastosis) is seem much more frequently than neoplasia. In contrast, microadenomatosis or islet cell hyperplasia is only very rarely found in adults.

Clinical features and diagnosis of hyperinsulinism

Hypoglycaemia induces a constellation of symptoms reflecting activation of the autonomic nervous system and release of epinephrine together with cerebral dysfunction related to insufficient glucose oxidation to meet energy needs. The symptoms of adrenergic hyperactivity are more apt to occur with rapid falls of plasma glucose and include weakness, sweating, hunger, palpitations and tremulousness. Neuroglycopenia manifests as headache, visual distrubance, dizziness and confusion and may progress to abnormal behaviour, seizures and coma. Hypoglycaemic episodes are often misinterpreted as suggesting brain tumour, epilepsy, alcoholism or drug abuse, psychosis or even hysteria. Delays in diagnosis and treatment of hypoglycaemia are common and contribute to the morbidity and mortality of the condition. The most important clue to early correct diagnosis is the relationship of the symptoms to periods of food deprivation or physical exercise and the relief of symptoms following food ingestion. In cases where diagnosis is long delayed, patients often develop obesity from increased carbohydrate intake as a behavioural adaptation to repeated episodes of symptomatic hypoglycaemia. Thus, it is not surprising that the diagnosis of hyperinsulism is often delayed for several years following the onset of symptoms. Patients are often 'shunted' from neurologist to cardiologist to psychiatrist.

Differential diagnosis of hypoglycaemia

Hypoglycaemia may occur in the fasting state or may be post-prandial (reactive) in nature. In the latter condition, low plasma glucose concentrations occur only in response to meals. In fasting hypoglycaemia a period of hours to a few days is required to precipitate hypoglycaemia. While patients with fasting hypoglycaemia (particularly insulinomas) may also exhibit a reactive component, patients with reactive hypoglycaemia never have symptoms when food is withdrawn. Fasting hypoglycaemia usually indicates a specific underlying disease process while symptoms suggestive of post-prandial hypoglycaemia are often found in the absence of an identifiable organic lesion.

Post-prandial hypoglycaemia

The more common causes of post-prandial hypoglycaemia are shown in Table 12.12. Alimentary hypoglycaemia is the most common type seen clinically and is usually found in patients who have undergone gastrectomy, pyloroplasty, gastrojejunostomy or, rarely, proximal gastric vagotomy. Symptoms occur within a few hours post-prandially and are particularly prominent after meals of high carbohydrate content in the form of mono- and disaccharides. Although the exact pathophysiological mechanisms remain to be defined, it is clear that rapid gastric emptying of simple sugars by the post-operative stomach with brisk absorption of glucose and excessive insulin release are of central importance. The attacks can be provoked in affected individuals by oral ingestion of 100 g of glucose in water. A rapid abnormal rise in plasma glucose together with a parallel, and often exaggerated, plasma insulin response occur following glucose challenge. Hypoglycaemic symptoms appear within 1–2 hours as the insulin response and/or effect exceeds the requirement of euglycaemia. True alimentary hypoglycaemia may occur in the absence of gastrointestinal surgery but is rare.

Reactive hypoglycaemia is often misused as a diagnostic label in patients suffering from anxiety states rather than true idiopathic reactive hypoglycaemia. Although some of these individuals manifest a very mild and asymptomatic depression in plasma glucose during the 5 hour glucose tolerance test, hypoglycaemia cannot be documented after normal meals not containing 100 g of rapidly absorbable carbohydrate. This is in contrast to the occasional case of true idiopathic reactive hypoglycaemia where spontaneous symptomatic episodes are reproducible and accompanied by demonstrably low plasma glucose levels. Most patients without true hypoglycaemia have post-prandial adrenergic discharge as a result of underlying anxiety and stress. The epinephrine-mediated symptoms suggest hypoglycaemia but occur in its absence and are presumably psychogenic in origin.

Table 12.12 Causes of post-prandial (reactive) hypoglycaemia

1. Alimentary hyperinsulinism
2. Hereditary fructose intolerance
3. Galactosaemia
4. Leucine sensitivity
5. Idiopathic
   - True hypoglycaemia
   - Non-hypoglycaemia

Fasting hypoglycaemia

The major causes of fasting hypoglycaemia are shown in Table 12.13. In this condition one or both of the following mechanisms may be operative: (1) hepatic glucose production is not adequate to meet ordinary tissue demands; (2) peripheral glucose utilization is increased to such a degree that maximal hepatic production is insufficient to match glucose egress from the plasma component. Since hepatic glucose output in normal fasting man is between 100 and 200 g per day, a requirement for greater than 200 g of intravenous glucose over a 24 hour period to prevent hypoglycaemia can be taken as evidence for overutilization of glucose.

From the practical standpoint, fasting hypoglycaemia in an otherwise healthy individual is always due to hyperinsulinism that is attributable to an insulinoma in the adult or islet cell hyperplasia in the neonate or

Table 12.13 Major causes of fasting hypoglycaemia

Conditions primarily due to underproduction of glucose
1. Hormone deficiencies
   - Hypopituitarism
   - Adrenal insufficiency
   - Catecholamine deficiency
   - Glucagon deficiency
2. Enzyme defects
   - Glucose-6-phosphatase
   - Liver phosphorylase
   - Pyruvate carboxlase
   - PEP-carboxykinase
   - Fructose-1,6-diphosphatase
   - Glycogen synthetase
3. Substrate deficiency
   - Ketotic hypoglycaemia of infancy
   - Severe malnutrition, muscle wasting
   - Late pregnancy
4. Acquired liver disease
   - Hepatic congestion
   - Severe hepatitis
   - Cirrhosis
5. Drugs
   - Alcohol
   - Propranolol
   - Salicylates

Conditions primarily due to overutilization of glucose
1. Hyperinsulinism
   - Insulinoma
   - Exogenous insulin
   - Sulfonylureas
   - Immune disease with insulin antibodies
2. Appropriate insulin levels
   - Extrapancreatic tumours
   - Cachexia with fat depletion
   - Carnitine deficiency
   - Carnitine acyltransferase deficiency

infant. Although patients with hyperinsulinism classically describe or manifest symptoms under fasting conditions in the early morning hours before breakfast or in the late afternoon following exertion, attacks may be highly unpredictable and distributed randomly throughout the day. While it is obvious that the development of fasting hypoglycaemia in insulinoma patients is due to excessive insulin secretion, the hypoglycaemia may result from insulin-mediated suppression of hepatic glucose production as well as augmentation of glucose utilization. Most patients learn quickly that symptoms can be relieved by intake of food or sweetened drink. Accordingly, a proportion of patients gain substantial amounts of weight.

In 1935, Whipple and Franz reviewed 35 cases of insulinoma and enunciated the primary diagnostic criteria which became known as Whipple's triad:

- Hypoglycaemic symptoms are produced by fasting.
- Hypoglycaemia is documented during symptomatic episodes (blood glucose level below 50mg/dl).
- Symptoms are relieved by glucose intake.

While the presence of Whipple's triad strongly suggests the presence of an insulinoma, differentiation from other causes of fasting hypoglycaemia is crucial. Factitious hypoglycaemia due to surreptitious self-administration of insulin must always be considered in cases posing diagnostic difficulty. Currently, the diagnosis of insulinoma is based upon three elements:

- Recognition of the probable nature of the patient's symptoms.
- Presence of Whipple's triad.
- Demonstration that the plasma insulin concentration is inappropriately high for the existing level of plasma glucose.

Thus, it is not the absolute level of insulin but its concentration relative to the plasma glucose that is diagnostic. Although absolute elevation of the insulin level is present in many insulinoma patients, rapid degradation of insulin by the liver is probably responsible for the normal absolute levels seen in others with functioning islet cell tumours. For this reason, the ratio of plasma immunoreactive insulin to plasma glucose is considered of greater diagnostic accuracy than absolute levels of insulin and glucose. An insulin (μg/ml) to glucose (mg/dl) ratio of greater than 0.3 indicates insulinoma. It is therefore essential in the investigation of suspected or documented hypoglycaemia to measure simultaneous insulin and glucose levels from the same plasma sample obtained at the time of hypoglycaemia.

Virtually all insulinoma patient will develop symptomatic hypoglycaemia during a diagnostic 72 hour fast. About 90% will manifest symptoms within 48 hours, 80% within 24 hours and 40% within 2 hours of fasting. The plasma glucose level at the time of symptoms is almost invariably less than 40 mg/dl (2.2 mmol/l). In normal individuals the level of immunoreactive insulin during fasting is very low to almost undetectable. At the time of fasting hypoglycaemia almost all insulinoma patients have basal insulin levels greater than

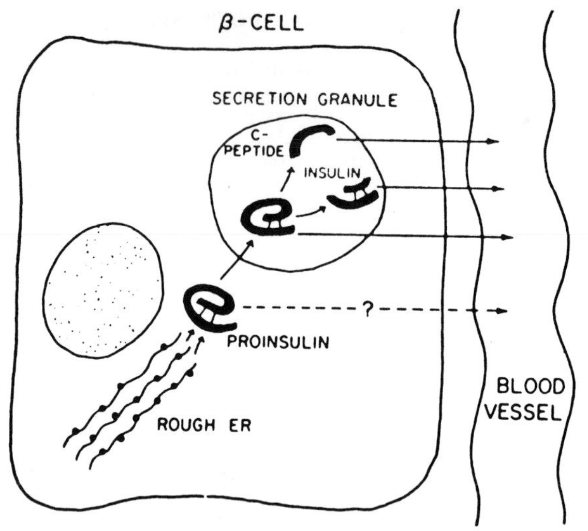

Figure 12.22 Conversion of pro-insulin to insulin and C-peptide within the pancreatic B-cell. Equimolar amounts of insulin and C-peptide are liberated during exocytosis. ER signifies endoplasmic reticulum. In normal circumstances only small amonts of the precursor, pro-insulin, are released into the bloodstream, while insulinomas release pro-insulin into the circulation in larger amounts.

5 μg/ml. Other causes of fasting hypoglycaemia such as fibrosarcoma and other non-pancreatic tumours, glucocorticoid deficiency or diffuse liver disease may exhibit a positive Whipple's triad but in none will the associated immunoreactive insulin level be increased.

Plasma pro-insulin levels are also helpful in the diagnosis of insulinoma. Pro-insulin is the single chain precursor of insulin and is normally present to an extent of 20% or less of the total immunoreactive insulin. Under ordinary circumstances, pro-insulin is split into C-peptide (connecting chain) and insulin prior to storage in B cell granules, with only a small percentage being secreted into the portal venous circulation (Figure 12.22). Because insulinoma tumour cells are usually less differentiated than normal B cells, they secrete more pro-insulin. Simple determination of pro-insulin in overnight fasted plasma provides good separation of patients with islet cell tumour from normal individuals in 90% of cases. Pro-insulin can be expressed as the absolute level or as a percentage relative to total insulin concentration in plasma. Occasionally, some well-differentiated insulinomas may have normal pro-insulin secretion. Greatly elevated values (greater than 50% of total immunoreactive insulin) are often associated with malignant tumours.

Provocative tests in the diagnosis of insulinoma

While no other test is as simple, safe and accurate as prolonged fasting with measurement of glucose and insulin, on rare occasions provocative testing may be needed. A variety of such tests have been advocated and all can be misleading and some potentially dangerous. The glucose tolerance test and the leucine infusion test are mentioned only to be condemned because of their inaccuracy. None of the others is diagnostic in more than 70% of cases. Their further disadvantage is the provocation of occasionally severe hypoglycaemic reactions resulting from release of substantial amounts of insulin from the tumour.

The calcium infusion test has been used as a provocative test for a number of APUDomas including gastrinoma, medullary thyroid carcinoma and carcinoid tumours as well as insulinomas. Patients with insulinomas release insulin and pro-insulin with resultant hypoglycaemia after calcium infusion. In order to avert the hypoglycaemic attack attending calcium infusion-stimulated insulin release, a combined glucose calcium infusion has been devised in which insulin release after glucose alone and after glucose plus calcium is compared. This, like all stimulation tests, suffers from a relatively low diagnostic accuracy and is indicated only when diagnostic difficulties arise.

The tolbutamide and glucagon tolerance tests are performed by intravenous administration of the respective drug followed by plasma collections for glucose and insulin determinations over a 1 hour period. In the tolbutamide test, a plasma insulin level of 195 μg/ml or greater is considered diagnostic. The critical insulin value in the glucagon test is 160 μg/ml.

A useful suppression test involves infusion of fish insulin to produce hypoglycaemia. While normal subjects respond with suppression of endogenous insulin secretion, patients with insulinoma fail to suppress because of the autonomous nature of hormone release by the tumour cells. Porcine insulin may be used instead of fish insulin but C-peptide must then be measured as a marker of endogenous insulin release. While the non-suppressibility of endocrine tumours is often interpreted as a sign of malignancy, caution in this regard should be exercised with respect to insulinomas where a different degree of suppressibility reflects a different degree of functional dedifferentiation but not necessarily malignancy.

Newer tests for insulinoma which may have good diagnostic accuracy without danger of hypoglycaemia are the sequential suppression tests using somatostatin followed by diazoxide with measurement of insulin levels and glucose consumption and the computer-controlled glucose infusion system which measures the glucose infusion rate required to maintain plasma glucose constant at 80 mg/dl (4.4 μmol/l).

Factitious hypoglycaemia must always be considered and this is especially true in individuals having access to insulin or oral hypoglycaemic agents. Concomitant measurement of plasma levels of C-peptide is critical in such circumstances as insulin and C-peptide are secreted in equimolar amounts by both the normal B cell and the insulinoma cell. C-peptide level thus serves as a direct marker of endogenous insulin release. Since all of the diagnostic tests presented can be positive following administration of exogenous insulin, the finding of an inappropriately depressed level of C-peptide can readily identify the surreptitious insulin user.

Pre-operative tumour localization

Most insulinomas are small benign adenomas with over 75% being less than 1.5 cm in diameter. They may be wholly embedded in the pancreas and not visible on its exposed surface. Moreover, they may be difficult to distinguish by palpation from a normal lobule of pancreas or a peripancreatic lymph node. Since intra-operative definition of the lesion is often problematic and occasionally impossible, pre-operative localization studies are mandatory once the definite diagnosis of hyperinsulinism has been made.

Angiography remains the most readily available and reliable method of delineating insulinomas. The use of superselective injection of contrast with subtraction technique and magnification allows confident identification of tumour 'blush' due to the hypervascularity. Care must be exercised to avoid false-positive localization related to presence of accessory spleens, large peripancreatic lymph nodes and hypervascular segments of normal pancreas.

The calcium arteriogram appears to be the most sensitive test. Feeding pancreatic arteries are selectively catheterized. Calcium stimulates insulin release. A catheter positioned in the hepatic vein is used to measure insulin levels 30–60 s following calcium injections. This permits a regional localization.

Pancreatic ultrasonography and CT are less efficient than angiography at localizing insulinomas but recently detection rates as high as 60% and greater have been realized. Rapid sequence CT scanning after a bolus of intravenous contrast has allowed improved definition of small slightly hypervascular tumours relative to normal pancreas. In general, however, lesions less than about 7–8 mm are poorly detected by currently available scans. The sensitivity of MRI appears to be equal to that of CT.

Octreoscan is a non-invasive, relatively new modality in which intravenously injected octreotide, labelled with radioactive tracer, binds to tumours with somatostatin receptors. The sensitivity is related to expression of somatostatin receptors; some 50–80% of insulinomas are imaged and specificity is virtually 100%.

EUS is a new method to detect pancreatic tumours. Tumours as small as 2–3 mm in diameter can be identified. The sensitivity for EUS ranges from 70 to 90% and is a highly observer-dependent technique that demands special expertise of the examiner.

In spite of their great utility in the localization of these small tumours, the results of imaging techniques cannot be interpreted as definitive information. When a solitary adenoma is defined, the surgeon must remember that a second tumour not seen may still be present. Likewise, when several tumours are defined, the probability of additional lesions not seen is very real. Hence, positive pre-operative localization studies in no way remove the surgeon's obligation to carry out a complete exploration of the entire pancreas. Intra-operative real time ultrasonography of the gland appears to hold considerable promise for facilitating the search.

When imaging techniques fail to identify any pancreatic or peripancreatic tumour mass, measurement of immunoreactive insulin in blood sampled from selective catheterization of small pancreatic veins via the percutaneous transhepatic route is indicated. In a few small series of insulinoma patients, this modality has correctly localized tumours with impressive regularity. At the time of portal sampling, samples are also drawn from the hepatic veins to detect metastatic or rare primary sources from within the liver. In addition, arterial samples are drawn periodically to detect any potentially confusing variations in systemic concentrations. These highly invasive procedures are not without risks and should be confined to centres with very experienced angiographers and to patients who are candidates for abdominal re-exploration following an unsuccessful prior operation.

Surgical management

Without positive pre-operative localization of a suspected insulinoma, the surgeon must be totally convinced that the diagnosis is correct before embarking on an operative search. However, with sufficiently strong biochemical evidence supporting the presence of an insulinoma, exploratory surgery is always indicated unless the patient cannot withstand the procedure. The entire pancreas and peripancreatic area must be examined visually and by palpation at operation. This requires access, exposure, assistance and gentle technique. Full mobilization of the gland should always be performed so that careful palpation between thumb and fingers is possible. Intra-operative ultrasonography has proved to be of some use in finding small, deeply situated tumours. To palpation, insulinomas characteristically are slightly firmer than normal pancreas. Enlarged lymph nodes in the peripancreatic region and any liver lesions found should be submitted for frozen section histological evaluation to exclude metastic disease. Histological examination of primary endocrine lesions in the pancreas is unreliable in the detection of malignancy unless obvious perineural or vascular invasion is present.

Solitary insulinomas should be enucleated whenever possible as a good cleavage plane is usually easily established between tumour and adjacent normal pancreas. Care must be taken to avoid injury to the pancreatic duct. Since the great majority of insulinomas are solitary and benign, distal pancreatectomy or, very occasionally, a Whipple type pancreaticoduodenectomy with pyloric preservation is justified for deeply situated tumours that cannot be safely enucleated. Very rarely is a Whipple operation justified for multiple tumours in the head of the pancreas since the likelihood of occult additional tumours being present in the body and tail of the gland is very substantial. Subtotal distal resection for multiple tumours throughout the gland, as seen in MEN 1 patients, is appropriate.

When malignant disease is encountered which can be extirpated by total pancreatectomy and regional lymphadenectomy, this should be done. Even if the tumour is inoperable, as much tumour mass is removed as is safely possible since debulking may provide good palliation with resolution of hypoglycaemic symptoms and increased efficiency of chemotherapy.

With a negative exploration, management options depend upon the clinical situation and the informed consent obtained pre-operatively. If not contraindicated by these consideration, it is appropriate to perform pancreatectomy distal to the superior mesenteric vessels. If immediate examination of the thinly sliced resected specimen reveals no tumour and the patient's blood glucose exhibits no rise within 1 hour, it may be elected to perform 90% or even total pancreatectomy. Arguments in favour of the lesser procedure include:

- a small tumour may be overlooked and subsequently found in the resected specimen
- symptoms of hypoglycaemia can be controlled by this procedure alone (in absence of tumour resection) in 20% of cases
- diazoxide therapy is often successful in controlling symptoms in those uncontrolled by the operation; and
- the procedure usually does not cause permanent diabetes mellitus.

The benefits of blind total pancreatectomy include:

- removal of an occult lesion that could be an early malignancy
- elimination of the possible need for re-exploration that is difficult and hazardous; and
- omission of drug therapy for prolonged periods with its undesirable side-effects.

It should be mentioned that patients not evaluated pre-operatively with percutaneous transhepatic portal venous sampling for insulin levels perhaps should be referred to a specialized centre for this test and then a second, more directed operation. Blind Whipple operations are likewise not recommended.

The results of surgical treatment of insulinoma suggest that about 75% of patients are cured with some 10% developing diabetes following extensive pancreatic resection. About 10–15% of patients have persistent or recurrent hypoglycaemia requiring reoperation at some time. The overall surgical mortality is between 0 and 10% and is related to the extent of resection and expertise of the surgeon. The major operative complications are pancreatitis, abscess, fistula and pseudocyst formation.

Neonatal and infantile hyperinsulinism

Excessive insulin secretion accounts for 20–30% of all cases of unremitting hypoglycaemia in neonates and infants. Such hypoglycaemia can lead to irreversible central nervous system (CNS) damage and thus requires early recognition, thorough investigation and expeditious treatment. A high intravenous and/or oral glucose intake is mandatory. Additional treatment with diazoxide, somatostatin or a variety of other agents (epinephrine, diphenylhydantoin, glucocorticoids, glucagon, growth hormone) is often required. When hypoglycaemia due to documented hyperinsulinaemia cannot be adequately controlled with medical therapy, urgent operation must be undertaken. Since the overwhelming majority of neonates and infants with hyperinsulinism have nesidioblastosis (B-cell adenomatosis or islet cell hyperplasia) as the cause, imaging techniques such as arteriography, ultrasonography and computed tomography have no place in the evaluation of these cases. Likewise, palpation of the pancreas at operation and biopsies for frozen section histological examination are non-contributory. The appropriate procedure is 80–90% extended distal pancreatectomy with splenic preservation. If careful post-operative monitoring of glucose levels indicates inadequacy of the resection, medical therapy should be reinstituted and consideration given to reoperation in cases of further unremitting hypoglycaemia. Reoperation consists of near total (95%) pancreatectomy with preservation of the distal bile duct and duodenum. Permanent exocrine or endocrine insufficiency is unusual in infants less than 3 months of age. This relates to the considerable regenerative capacity of the infantile pancreas.

Medical treatment

Antisecretory therapy with diazoxide is indicated for persistent hypoglycaemia in the pre-operative phase and when operation is unsuccessful or contraindicated because of the poor condition of the patient. Diazoxide is a non-diuretic benzothiadiazine which inhibits the release of secretory granules from normal islet B cells and from insulinoma cells. Dosage is individualized based on effectiveness. Because of side-effects such as oedema, bone marrow depression, hyperuricaemia, cardiomyopathy and hirsutism in females, patients on diazoxide require close medical supervision. Long-acting analogues of somatostatin (Octreotide) may hold considerable promise in the treatment of hyperinsulinism in inoperable patients with insulinoma. Octreotide both inhibits secretion of peptide by the hyperfunctioning islet cells or tumour and reduces target organ receptivity. In insulinoma patients, two-thirds have obtained good symptomatic relief despite much lower rates of control of insulin levels. Few or no antitumour effects have been demonstrated with the use of Octreotide in malignant insulinoma. Streptozotocin, an antibiotic which selectively destroys pancreatic islet cells by inhibiting DNA synthesis, is the chemotherapeutic agent of choice for metastatic insulinoma. Objective tumour regression occurs in about 60% of patients and longevity is doubled in those who respond to the drug. Streptozotocin is highly nephrotoxic and hepatotoxic and is thus not used as routine adjunctive therapy. Combinations of octreotide, streptozotocin and diazoxide are often useful in treating functioning malignant insulinoma.

Gastrinoma (Zollinger–Ellison syndrome)

In 1955, Zollinger and Ellison described two patients, each having a syndrome consisting of fulminant intractable peptic ulcer disease, massive gastric acid hypersecretion, and a non-beta islet cell tumour of the pancreas. Although the same clinical triad had been reported previously, Zollinger and Ellison postulated that the gastric acid excess was caused by a humoral factor released from the tumour. While their original supposition had been that glucagon was the responsible factor, the peptide hormone gastrin was subsequently extracted from such tumours which were found to be of the non-beta, non-alpha cell type. A radioimmunoassay was developed for gastrin and the hormone was found to be markedly elevated in the plasma of patients with Zollinger–Ellison (ZE) syndrome.

Clinical features and diagnosis of gastrinoma

The incidence of ZE syndrome by best estimate is approximately 1 in 100 000, although the exact incidence is impossible to determine since no large population has been screened for the disease. The disease is more common in men than women with the male-to-female ratio being 3:2. The ZE syndrome has been reported in patients ranging in age from 7 to 90 years but the majority of patients have been diagnosed between the third and fifth decades. Only approximately 1 in 750 patients with the peptic ulcer disease will have gastrinoma as the aetiology.

About one-quarter of ZE syndrome patients have their gastrinoma as part of the MEN 1 syndrome. MEN 1 is inherited as an autosomal dominant syndrome and the lesions most commonly associated with gastrinoma are parathyroid hyperplasia and pituitary prolactinoma. Gastrinomas in MEN 1 patients are less likely to be malignant but are almost always multifocal. This is in contrast to patients with sporadic gastrinoma in whom the disease is more often malignant but somewhat less frequently multifocal in origin. Overall, the gastrinoma is malignant in about one-half of patients and arises in the pancreas in about 75%. Even when benign, gastrinomas are more often multiple than solitary. The most common extrapancreatic primary tumour site is the duodenum. Tumours in this location are solitary in about one-half of cases. Much less commonly, primary gastrinomas are found in the omenta, lymph nodes, liver and gastric antrum. Malignant gastrinomas metastasize to regional lymph nodes and liver.

Peptic ulcer disease is present in over 90% of gastrinoma patients. Almost all patients with ulcers have typical dyspeptic pain which is more severe and less responsive to medical treatment than in routine peptic ulcer disease.

Co-existing diarrhoea is a significant complaint in about one-third of gastrinoma patients. About 5–7% of patients have diarrhoea as their sole presenting complaint. Large volumes of watery stools may result in dehydration, potassium loss, weakness and wasting. The diarrhoea is of the secretory variety and frequently accompanied by steatorrhoea. A multifactoral aetiology has been elucidated but the basic underlying abnormality is acid hypersecretion. With the accompanying rapid gastric emptying, the large acid load in the duodenum and upper jejunum lowers the pH to cause inactivation of pancreatic lipase and other enzymes. This, in addition to the mucosal injury imparted by the large acid load, leads to malabsorption and steatorrhoea. There is also increased intestinal motility and inhibition of salt and water absorption from the jejunum due to the hypergastrinaemia. When severe, the mucosal injury of the distal duodenum and proximal jejunum manifests as frank peptic ulceration at these atypical sites.

The majority of patients with ZE syndrome are diagnosed only after several years of symptoms although increasing awareness of the disease is lowering the time between symptom onset and diagnosis. In the past, the majority of patients were diagnosed only after one or more failed operations for presumed routine peptic ulcer disease. Currently, many patients are being dignosed prior to being subjected to ill-fated standard ulcer operations.

All of the complications of peptic ulcer disease are encountered in ZE syndrome patients and acute haemorrhage and perforation are each noted in approximately 20%. Vomiting and other symptoms of gastric outlet obstruction are distinctly less common as the fulminant nature of the ulcer diathesis more often precipitates acute complications. Wilfred Sircus of Edinburgh referred to patients with ZE syndrome as 'recurrent ulcerators, persistent perforators, and bleeders unto death.' Severe, refractory reflux oesophagitis has been an under-appreciated manifestation of the disease.

Patients with gastrinoma most often have no abnormal physical finding. However, signs of weight loss, epigastric tenderness and intestinal hypermotility are relatively common. Intra-abdominal tumour masses are rarely palpable but hepatic enlargement secondary to massive metastatic deposits is occasionally seen at initial presentation.

The diagnosis of ZE syndrome should be considered in any patient having:

- severe peptic ulcer disease refractory to histamine H_2-receptor antagonists
- multiple peptic ulcers or ulcers in unusual locations such as the distal duodenum or jejunum
- peptic ulcer disease associated with diarrhoea
- recurrent peptic ulcer disease following an acid-reducing operation;
- peptic ulcer disease in association with a strong family history of ulcer disease of MEN 1 syndrome or
- peptic ulcer disease without prior diagnosis or MEN 1 syndrome but in association with any other component of MEN 1 syndrome (e.g. hypercalcaemia).

In addition, findings of large gastric mucosal folds and diffuse inflammation or frank ulceration distal to the duodenal bulb on endoscopic or radiological examination of the upper gastrointestinal tract are suggestive of the ZE syndrome.

In the presence of peptic ulceration and/or a secretory diarrhoea, radioimmunoassay of fasting plasma gastrin level remains the key to diagnosis of ZE syndrome. A basal gastrin level greater than 100 pg/ml strongly supports the diagnosis of gastrinoma. The majority of patients have fasting levels greater than 200 pg/ml and not infrequently 1000 pg/ml or greater. It must be remembered that hypergastrinaemia can occur in association with gastric hypochlorhydria or achlorhydria from a variety of conditions not associated with gastrinoma. Patients with pernicous anaemia, chronic atrophic gastritis, gastric cancer, prior vagotomy or histamine H_2-receptor antagonist or omeprazole therapy may manifest hypergastrinaemia as a physiological response to an elevated antral pH. Thus, it is important to measure basal acid output in all patients suspected to have gastrinoma based on clinical presentation and an elevated plasma gastrin level.

The principal circulating form of gastrin in patients with gastrinoma is G-34 or 'big gastrin', a situation analogous to insulinomas and other peptide-producing endocrine tumours where elevated levels of precursor forms of the respective hormones are often found. The measured circulating gastrin level does not reflect the degree of gastric acid stimulation by the tumour, nor is there good correlation between gastrin level and tumour mass. Plasma gastrin levels normally rise following a meal and thus measurements must be made in the fasting state. Gastric outlet obstruction secondary to ordinary duodenal ulcer disease, antral G-cell hyperfunction or hyperplasia, and retained gastric antrum after Billroth II gastrectomy are other conditions associated with peptic ulcer in which elevated basal plasma gastrin levels may be found (Table 12.14). In order to differentiate these entities from gastrinoma and also to establish the diagnosis of gastrinoma in ulcer patients with borderline elevated basal gastrin levels, a number of provocative tests have been devised. The best of these is the secretin stimulation test. Following intravenous injection of secretin (2 u/kg), the plasma gastrin level rises within 5–10 min to a level 200 pg/ml greater than the basal level in patients with gastrinoma, but not in those with other conditions. The calcium stimulation test has also been used to differentiate gastrinoma from ordinary peptic ulcer disease. In this test calcium is infused at 5 mg/kg/hour for 3 hours and a positive test requires that the stimulated gastrin increases by 100% over basal level. Because of untoward side-effects of hypercalcaemia, long duration of the test and slightly lower accuracy, the calcium infusion test has been almost entirely supplanted by the secretin injection test. The meal provocation test may be used to differentiate gastrinoma from antral G-cell hyperfunction. In this

Table 12.14 Differential diagnosis of hypergastrinaemia

With acid hypersecretion
Zollinger–Ellison syndrome
Retained gastric antrum after Billroth II gastrectomy
Antral G-cell hyperplasia
Gastric outlet obstruction
With acid hyposecretion
Pernicious anaemia
Atrophic gastritis
Gastric cancer

test, a standard meal is ingested by the patient and causes a marked rise in plasma gastrin levels in those with G-cell hyperfunction but no rise or only a minimal one in gastrinoma patients.

In order to secure the diagnosis of gastrinoma in patients demonstrated to have hypergastrinaemia, gastric acid secretory testing is necessary. A basal level ouput greater than 15 mmol/hour strongly supports the diagnosis as does a value greater than 5 mmol/hour in the patient who has had previous acid reducing gastric surgery for peptic ulcer disease. A ratio of basal acid output to maximal acid output following stimulation with pentagastrin, histamine or betazole of greater than 0.6 has also been used as a discriminatory criterion for gastrinoma. However, this ratio is no more sensitive or specific than is the basal acid output alone. Upper gastrointestinal endoscopy and a standard barium upper gastrointestinal radiological series should be performed in all patients thought to harbour a gastrinoma. In addition to the mucosal abnormalities often found with these studies, on rare occasions a duodenal or antral polypoid lesion has proved to be a gastrinoma on biopsy.

All patients diagnosed as having ZE syndrome should be further investigated for the presence of MEN 1 syndrome. In addition to the plasma gastrin determinations, several serum calcium and phosphate measurements and a plasma prolactin level constitute the absolute minimal work-up for the most commonly associated endocrine lesions. A family history of refractory ulcer disease, hyperparathyroidism or other endocrine lesions warrants endocrinological screening of the immediate family as well as the patient. The diagnostic approach to the patient with suspected gastrinoma is summarized in Figure 12.23.

Tumour localization techniques

Pre-operative techniques to localize gastrinomas have not been particularly successful. Since gastrinomas may be small and deeply embedded in the pancreas, ultrasonography and CT have not been very sensitive. Recent information, however, would suggest that up to two-thirds of gastrinomas can be identified with the state-of-art CT scanners. However, tumours smaller than 7 mm are virtually never identified. MRI has not had wide application to gastrinoma patients but since islet cell tumours in general produce an unusually intense signal, this modality may prove particularly sensitive in their detection. Since most gastrinomas are hypovascular, visceral angiography has been much less useful in localizing gastrinomas as compared to insulinomas. There has been some anecdotal experience that simultaneous secretin injection enhances the angiographic tumour blush and may allow detection of otherwise non-hypervascular gastrinomas.

Both EUS and octreoscan have been useful in detection of gastrinomas and other neuroendocrine

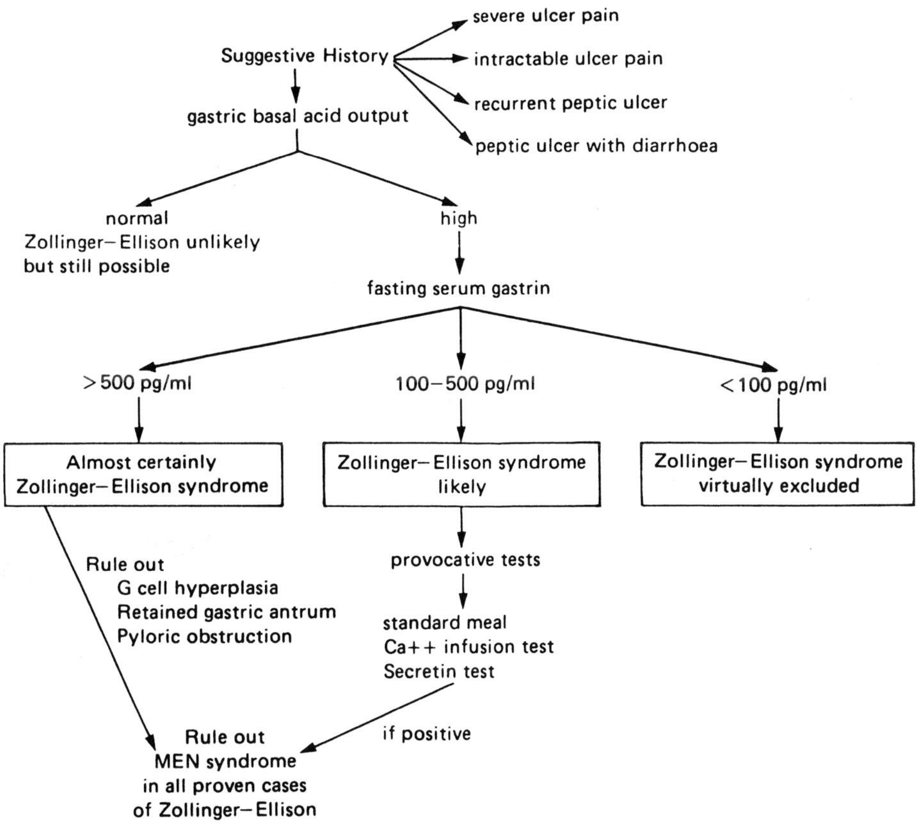

Figure 12.23 An approach to the investigation of patients with suspected ZE syndrome.

tumours. The combination of both can increase the sensitivity. The sensitivity of EUS is endoscopist dependent and can be in the range of 70–94%, which is much higher than that of CT scanning. Octrescan has its limitations; a high density of somatostatin receptors is a necessity. Other tumours or tissues may create a false-positive result. Active infection, inflammation or recent abdominal surgery limits the utility of octrescan. However, these diagnostic tests, if available, can be invaluable pre-operatively.

Percutaneous transhepatic selective sampling of the portal venous system for gastrin levels has been touted to be of value in gastrinoma patients. In theory, the technique is intended to localize the source or sources of hypergastrinaemia and, when combined with hepatic venous gastrin level sampling, predict the location of tumours and the presence or absence of hepatic metastases. Since up to 85% of gastrinomas have been found to reside within the anatomic gastrinoma triangle containing the duodenal C-loop, the head of the pancreas and their associated regional lymph nodes, transhepatic portal venous sampling can only be expected to determine if the tumour is within the triangle but not to localize it more precisely. Therefore, the test is of limited practical utility for gastrinoma. In general, presently available pre-operative tests do not appear capable of localizing the tumour any more reliably than careful intra-operative exploration by the experienced surgeon. Intra-operative ultrasonography may prove valuable in the localization of small tumours within the pancreatic gland. The experience with this technique remains limited at present but suggests that one-half of non-palpable tumours can be successfully imaged. Intra-operative upper endoscopy with transillumination of the duodenal wall has recently been reported to greatly facilitate the search for duodenal gastrinomas. It should be a routine part of the exploration and may obviate the need for duodenotomy in some cases.

Medical treatment

Until recently, medical therapy for control of the acid hypersecretion in patients with ZE syndrome consisted primarily of the histamine H_2-receptor antagonists cimetidine, ranitidine and famotidine. Unfortunately, these drugs were proved to be more effective in symptom control than in ulcer healing. Approximately one-third of patients were found to fail cimetidine treatment even when large doses were prescribed. Results with the newer histamine H_2-receptor antagonists have not been significantly better. To be effective the dose of H_2-receptor antagonist must be individually titrated to ensure that basal acid output immediately prior to the next dose does not exceed 10 mmol/hour. Many patients with gastrinoma require H_2-receptor antagonist drug doses two to four times that normally recommended for duodenal ulcer disease. The acid reducing effect of the drugs may be augmented and prolonged by concomitant administration of anticholinergics. The antimuscarinic drug pirenzipine has been shown to be effective in this role and does not have the untoward anticholinergic side-effects of earlier drugs of the same family. Antacids may be useful in treating dyspeptic symptoms but when given alone are entirely incapable of controlling the acid hypersecretion of gastrinoma patients.

A new class of antisecretory agents, the substituted benzimidazoles, act as potent inhibitors of the potassium-hydrogen ATPase of the parietal cell and as such are an important addition to the medical treatment regimen for gastrinoma. Experience with one of these new agents (omeprazole) suggests that this drug is by far the most powerful and specific gastric antisecretory agent yet developed. The acid hypersecretion in approximately 98% of gastrinoma patients can be successfully controlled with once or twice daily dosing. Experience with over 200 patients indicates that the dose required is highly variable with a range from 10 to 180 mg/day with about 40% needing a split dosage regimen. An increase in dose appears necessary over time in one-quarter of patients. Adverse effects have been extremely infrequent and mild (rash, constipation, headache) and there has been no evidence to implicate the drug as a risk factor for the development of gastric carcinoid tumours. Pharmacokinetic studies show that oral and intravenous omeprazole have the same duration of action and that intermittent bolus administration of parenteral drug obviates the need for continuous infusion of H_2-receptor antagonists in patients requiring parenteral antisecretory therapy. Because of its superior efficacy and extreme safety, omeprazole and the other new proton-pump inhibitors are now considered the antisecretory drugs of choice for all gastrinoma patients.

Surgical treatment

Prior to the advent of effective antisecretory therapy, total gastrectomy was required in virtually all gastrinoma patients in order to prevent mortality from the acute complications of peptic ulceration. With current medical therapy, satisfactory control of acid secretion and the ulcer diathesis is possible in a majority of patients. The focus of the surgeon has thus shifted somewhat from control of the ulcer diathesis to control of the tumour itself. Recent experience suggests that earlier pessimism regarding surgical curability of the tumour may have been unjustified. It appears, in fact, that at least one-third of patients are curable by tumour excision. For example, a recently reported 10 year prospective study of 73 gastrinoma patients surgically explored the cure resulted in an immediate disease-free rate of 58% and a 5 year disease-free rate of 30%. A similar but much smaller prospective series has documented an 82% surgical cure rate on short-term follow-up. The vast majority of these patients have undergone enucleation or local excision of tumours rather than radical pancreatic or pancreatoduodenal resections.

An approach to the management of newly diagnosed gastrinoma patients is summarized in Figure 12.24.

Patients with pre-operatively demonstrated liver metastases and/or MEN 1 syndrome are treated medically. This is particularly true if patients with metastatic disease are found to have multiple liver deposits or if patients with MEN 1 are found to have multiple primary tumours. If such patients fail medical therapy total gastrectomy should be performed. Whenever possible, confirmation of the multifocal nature of the disease is obtained by thorough biopsy of suspected tumours. Young and middle-aged patients without known liver metastases are subjected to the tumour localization techniques now available. These patients are offered elective laparotomy with the specific intent of accomplishing complete tumour excision. Experience suggests that even patients with regionally metastatic disease to lymph nodes can be cured and thus an aggressive approach to lymph node excision is always undertaken. Adequate exploration requires full mobilization of the pancreatic gland and the duodenum. All identified lymph nodes and palpable masses within and around the pancreas are removed and submitted for frozen section histological examination. Pancreatic tumour removal is accomplished by enucleation or distal pancreatectomy only and major resections are not performed. If pre-operative localization techniques have been unsuccessful, and extensive operative search for tumour is unrewarding, blind distal pancreatectomy is not performed as most tumours occur in and around the head of the pancreas and there is no evidence that islet cell hyperplasia has any aetological role in ZE syndrome. Proximal gastric vagotomy has been advocated as an adjunctive procedure to tumour removal but its efficacy remains unproved and the issue has become moot with the advent of omeprazole. Patients who are well controlled on medical therapy are thus not subjected to any gastric procedure even if no tumour is found. In contrast, patients responding poorly to antisecretory drugs, or who are non-compliant, and at exploration are found to have either no tumour or multifocal disease are treated by total gastrectomy in order to prevent life-threatening peptic ulcer complications. Contrary to the early experience with total gastrectomy for ZE syndrome, recent reports indicate that under elective circumstances the operative mortality is below 3% and the long-term sequelae are infrequently severe.

Successful removal of all gastrin-secreting tumour is confirmed by serially negative plasma gastrin responses to secretin stimulation. Long-term surveillance is required as tumour recurrences may be late and manifest as basal hypergastrinaemia (Figure 12.25).

Results with chemotherapy for advanced hepatic metastases from gastrinoma have not been very encouraging. Streptozotocin and 5-FU have been the only drugs to show therapeutic efficacy. There may be some advantage to delivering these drugs directly into the hepatic arterial circulation rather than intravenously but data remain sparse. Similarly, hepatic artery ligation or embolization has not been adequately evaluated.

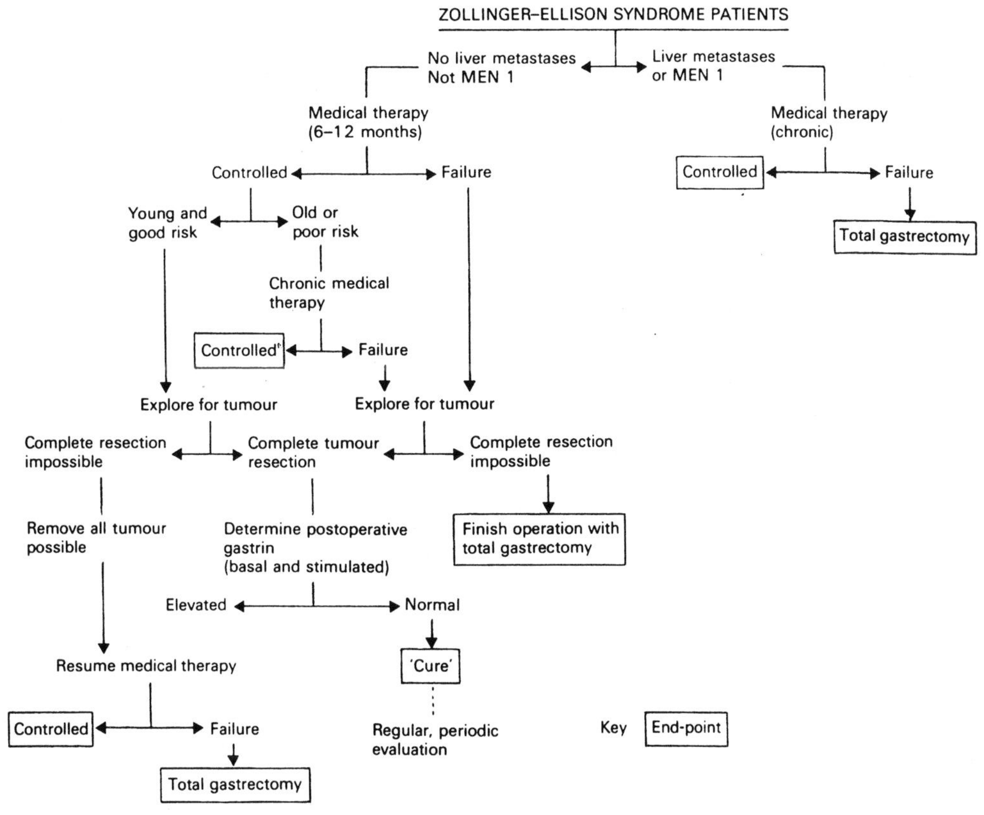

Figure 12.24 Management of newly diagnosed patients with ZE syndrome.

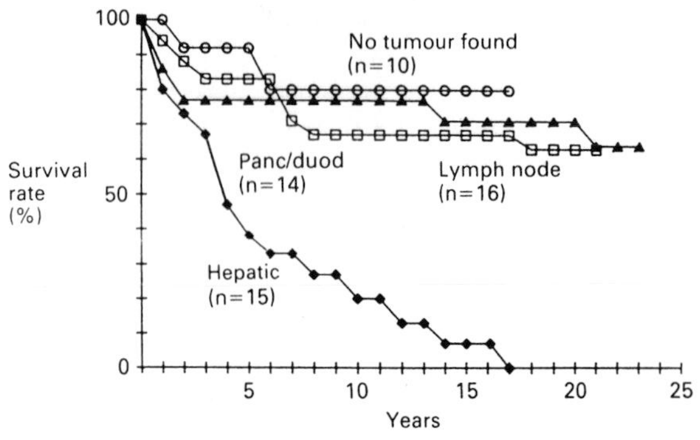

Figure 12.25 The dichotomous behaviour of gastrinoma. Patients with tumour in the lymph nodes have a prognosis very similar to those with tumour confined to the pancreas or duodenum. Patients with hepatic involvement have a predictably poor long-term survival.

Recently, octreotide has been used successfully to control the symptoms and hypergastrinaemia due to gastrinoma not amenable to surgical excision. Subjective and objective responses have been achieved in a small series of patients.

Gastrinoma patients with MEN 1 syndrome and documented hyperparathyroidism should have parathyroid surgery performed prior to any attempt at gastrinoma removal. In some such patients parathyroidectomy provides marked amelioration of ulcer symptoms and concomitant decreases in gastric acid secretion and plasma gastrin levels. These salutary effects are usually transient, however, and a definitive approach to the gastrinoma is still required and should not be unduly delayed.

Vipoma (Werner–Morrison syndrome; WDHA syndrome; pancreatic cholera)

The syndrome of watery diarrhoea, hypokalaemia and achlorhydria in association with an islet cell tumour of the pancreas was initially described by Werner and Morrison in 1958. A number of hormones have been identified in these tumours (including secretin, glucagon, gastric inhibitory polypeptide, pancreatic polypeptide and gastrin). However, VIP has been convincingly shown to be the causative agent in the majority of cases.

Patients afflicted with this condition have a secretory diarrhoea which is profuse and causes severe dehydration and loss of potassium. Acidosis almost invariably attends the hypokalaemia and patients suffer from lethargy and weakness as a result of the dehydration and electrolyte abnormalities. Virtually all patients incur significant weight loss, a majority have abdominal colic and a minority experience cutaneous flushing. Slightly less than half of the tumours are malignant and metastases to the liver are often found at the time of diagnosis. The primary tumour is located in the body and tail of the pancreas in approximately 75% of cases and is almost always solitary. Forty per cent are malignant and usually larger then 3 cm before causing symptoms. The extrapancreatic vipomas include ganglioneuromas and neuroblastomas and are capable of causing the identical clinical syndrome. Unlike the 75% of pancreatic tumours which also secrete pancreatic polypeptide, the extrapancreatic tumours do not.

VIP stimulates pancreatic, intestinal and gallbladder water and electrolyte secretions as well as pancreatic enzyme secretion and colonic potassium secretion. VIP inhibits absorption of water and electrolytes (sodium, chloride, bicarbonate and potassium) in the small intestine and colon and also inhibits acid and pepsin secretion in the stomach.

There are occasional patients, however, who have the identical clinical syndrome but with normal plasma VIP levels. In these cases, prostaglandin E is the most likely aetiological candidate.

In the setting of the proper clinical symptoms the diagnosis is made by demonstration of elevated plasma levels of VIP, exceeding 190 pg/ml. Fasting has no major effect on the diarrhoea. Localization of the primary tumour is not difficult in view of its large size and solitary nature. Ultrasonography, EUS, CT and angiography have all been effective. Tumours less than 1 cm are difficult to detect by CT scan. The technique visualizes only 30% of tumours in the 1–3 cm range.

Medical treatment consists of fluid and electrolyte resuscitation and support. Five or more litres of volume replacement may be required per day. Glucocorticoids or the somatostatin analogue Octreotide have been helpful in antagonizing the diarrhoeagenic effects of the tumour. Octreotide offers rapid symptomatic control in 90% of patients with marked amelioration of the diarrhoea, dehydration and their attendant metabolic sequelae. Typically, VIP levels decrease but do not fall to within the normal range, suggesting that the attenuation of symptoms is due in considerable degree to reduced target receptivity to the hormone.

The definitive treatment of vipoma is surgical excision of the tumour whenever possible. Debulking of metastatic disease often provides effective palliation. Since the majority of non-metastatic cases are caused by large solitary pancreatic tumours, enucleation or distal pancreatectomy is often curative. Blind distal or subtotal pancreatectomy in the absence of tumour localization is probably unwarranted since islet cell hyperplasia is an unproved cause of the syndrome.

Patients who cannot be significantly benefited by surgical resection, or who recur with multiple metastatic deposits, may have symptomatic responses to long-acting somatostatin analogues. Streptozotocin has been reasonably effective in palliation but immediately following administration, diarrhoea and electrolyte losses may be exacerbated for several days, necessitating aggressive replacement. The prognosis is poor with advanced disease, and thromboembolic complications due to excessive dehydration are often responsible for major morbidity and mortality. The occasional patient with pancreatic cholera secondary to prostaglandin E_2 hypersecretion may have dramatic relief with indomethacin therapy.

Glucogonoma

Glucagonomas are tumours of the A-cell of the pancreatic islet and are responsible for a characteristic syndrome consisting of severe skin rash, weight loss, diabetes mellitus, deep venous thrombosis, anaemia and hypoaminoacidaemia. The tumour is very rare and because its most salient feature, the skin rash, is frequently misdiagnosed, its true significance and the correct diagnosis are often made very late in the course. As expected, it is virtually always first seen in the dermatology clinic. Glucagonoma is considerably more common in females and is a disease of middle age. At the time of diagnosis approximately 60–70% of cases have already metastasized. The most common site of metastasis is the liver (50%). The typical clinical features are summarized in Table 12.15.

The typical skin rash is termed necrolytic migratory erythema. The lesions are characteristically symmetrical and erythematous with crusted erosions involving the perineum, groins, thighs, buttocks and distal extremities. The systemic manifestations of weight loss, weakness and lethargy are due to a combination of the catabolic effects of high plasma glucagon levels and the extensive malignant disease which is often present. Hyperglycaemia results from increased hepatic glycogenolysis and gluconeogenesis. Most patients are frankly diabetic but ketonaemia rarely develops because circulating insulin levels are increased. Panhypoaminoacidaemia is a uniform finding and may be responsible for the skin rash as well as the neurological deficits that are occasionally seen. The anaemia is characteristically normocytic and normochromic and although serum iron levels may be low, the anaemia does nor respond to iron and vitamin replacement.

The diagnosis is usually made upon recognition of the typical cutaneous manifestations in combination with diabetes mellitus in the setting of a chronic wasting disorder. The diagnosis is confirmed by finding an elevated plasma glucagon level. Normal values range between 50 and 150 pg/ml. Values of glucagon greater than 1000 pg/ml are often seen with glucagonoma but interpretation should be cautious in the absence of the typical skin rash or other suggestive signs. Numerous other conditions associated with hyperglucagonaemia are enumerated in Table 12.16. In most glucagonoma patients glucagon release from the tumour can be induced by the administration of arginine or tolbutamide. Pancreatic polypeptide levels are elevated in one-half of patients.

Since many cases are diagnosed in an advanced metastatic stage, tumour localization is not normally difficult. CT, angiography, EUS, MRI and Octreotide scintigraphy have all been used successfully in localizing tumours. While topical steroids and intravenous amino acid administration have been effective in ameliorating the skin eruption in some patients, definitive treatment is surgical. Operative exploration is indicated even for advanced metastatic disease as debulking procedures may significantly alleviate the debilitating catabolic effects of the excess glucagon. When surgical resection is not an option, selective arterial embolization and chemotherapy are indicated. Streptozotocin combined with 5-FU can produce reduction in both tumour size and glucagon levels. Dimethyltrizenoimidazole carboxamide has been effective in providing symptomatic relief and alleviation of skin rash.

Octreotide has proved highly efficacious both in the pre-operative management and as palliative therapy in glucagonoma. Octreotide reduces circulating glucagon levels, dramatically improves the skin rash, attenuates the systemic symptoms and augments the anabolic effects of intravenous hyperalimentation. Use of the somatostatin analogue is probably indicated in all cases regardless of the stage of disease or surgical plan. Unfortunately, no effects on tumour size or growth have been demonstrated. Similarly, interferon-alpha has been used with

Table 12.15 The glucagonoma syndrome: clinical features and incidence

Sex	*Female/male > 1*
Age range (mean)	20–71 (57)
Malignancy	70–80%
Clinical diabetes (abnormal glucose tolerance test)	70% (95%)
Skin lesions	80%
Glossitis/cheilitis	90–100%
Weight loss	90–100%
Diarrhoea	50–60%
Coarse intestinal mucosal folds	50–60%
Anaemia, normocytic, normochromic	70–80%
Hypoaminoacidaemia	80%
Neurological deficit	Unusual (incidence uncertain)
Marked hyperglucagonaemia	100%
Survival	80% more than 2 years 23% more than 5½ years

Table 12.16 Conditions associated with hyperglucagonaemia

1. Diabetes
   - Ketoacidosis
   - Hyperosmolar syndrome
2. Chronic renal failure
3. Shock states
   - Myocardial infarction
   - Septicaemia
   - Burns
   - Hypovolaemia/haemorrhage
4. Acute pancreatitis
5. Cirrhosis
   - Portosystemic shunting (natural, surgical)
6. Glucagonoma
7. Familial hyperglucagonaemia (asymptomatic)
8. Exercise
9. Antiglucagon antibodies in diabetics treated with insulin[a]

[a]These may be induced by slight glucagon impurities in commercially available insulins and manifest as hyperglucagonaemia when glucagon is measured by a double antibody immunoassay method.

some success. This induces an autoimmunity against the tumour. This treatment is not curative, but it can prolong survival and control the symptoms of the disease. Combination treatment with interferon-alpha and Octreotide or chemotherapy has shown synergistic or additive beneficial effects in some patients witih glucagonoma and other neuroendocrine malignancies.

Somatostatinoma

Somatostatinoma is a very rare tumour with less than 90 cases reported to date. The patients have been mostly middle-aged. The patients with pancreatic somatostatinoma are predominantly female. Over 80% of the tumours have been associated with liver metastases at the time of diagnosis. Along with somatostatin production most tumours have also elaborated other hormones such as VIP, pancreatic polypeptide, gastrin, calcitonin or cortisol.

Despite the potent inhibitory nature of somatostatin, the usual clinical syndrome is non-specific. Abdominal pain is the most common presenting symptom and this may relate to the high prevalence of cholelithiasis in these patients. Gallbladder stasis is thought to be of aetiological importance. Other symptoms and signs commonly associated with somatostatinoma are diarrhoea, diabetes mellitus (25%), weight loss, anorexia, hypochlorhydria, steatorrhoea and anaemia. Symptoms not related to excessive somatostatin levels such as tachycardia, flushing, hypertension, hypokalaemia and hypoglycaemia are also present in some patients. The diagnosis is made by chance in most cases although a radioimmunoassay for plasma somatostatin is available. Somatostatin released by the tumour may be stimulated by tolbutamide; however, the utility of this provocative test is unknown at present.

Ideally, treatment is by surgical excision of the pancreatic or duodenal lesion. Debulking of advanced tumours may be efficacious and some patients have benefited from adjunctive therapy with streptozotocin and 5-FU. The 5 year survival rate after diagnosis of somatostatinoma is only about 15%.

Human pancreatic polypeptide tumour (HPPoma)

HPPomas are rare and arise from PP-secreting cells (also referred to D2 cells or F cells). They have been associated with no apparent symptom complex and the clinical and metabolic characteristics of the tumour remain to be defined. In a few instance, HPPomas have been associated with diarrhoea and pruritic rash.

Elevated plasma levels of pancreatic polypeptide have been found in many patients with various islet cell tumours of the pancreas (gastrinoma, glucagonoma, etc.) and carcinoid tumours. It has been suggested that elevated pancreatic polypeptide levels be used as a marker for endocrine pancreatic tumours but only approximately one-half of all patients with such tumours have abnormal elevations of the hormone. Similarly, high levels are found in approximately 50% of patients with carcinoid tumours at all sites. While plasma pancreatic polypeptide levels may be used as a screening test for tumours in patients with MEN 1 syndrome and their relatives, high levels must be interpreted with caution as they may be found also in elderly patients, and those with renal failure, diabetes mellitus and certain inflammatory diseases. Atropine suppression of pancreatic polypeptide has been suggested as a method of determining whether the elevated hormone is the result of tumour secretion. At present it would appear that measurement of pancreatic polypeptide is of limited utility in screening for pancreatic endocrine tumours.

Whenever possible, treatment should be surgical and, since most HPPomas are large and located in the head of the pancreas, pancreaticoduodenectomy is typically required. Chemotherapy with streptozotocin may benefit patients with unresectable and/or metastatic disease.

Non-functioning endocrine pancreatic tumours

Approximately 10–15% of islet cell tumours have been diagnosed without any accompanying symptoms or signs other than those relating to a mass lesion. Such tumours are usually diagnosed late in their course, often after metastatic disease is present in the liver. A number of pancreatic tumours thought to be adenocarcinomas have, on histological examination, proved to be of the islet cell type. Some of these tumours have been found to contain pancreatic polypeptide and although this tumour is no longer regarded as biochemically silent, its clinical syndrome has yet to be defined.

Without measurable hormonal markers clinically non-functioning tumours will continue to be diagnosed by virtue of their large size. Thus, ultrasonography, CT, EUS, MRCP and, occasionally, angiography remain useful in their localization. As additional islet cell hormones are detected by new radioimmunoassays, other specific tumours will be described.

The best treatment currently available for non-functioning islet cell tumours is surgical resection of the primary tumour and of as much of the metastatic tumour as possible. Chemotherapy has been useful in a number of these cases but even without response the progression of tumour growth has, in general, been relatively slow.

Further therapeutic possibilities for the treatment of advanced islet cell malignancies

Many islet cell tumours have a high concentration of somatostatin receptors, pick up radiolabelled Octreotide, and can be localized by scintigraphy. The radiotherapeutic value of radiolabelled Octreotide is under investigation. There are reports of successful outcome of metastatic glucagonoma treated with peptide receptor radiotherapy demonstrating decrease in tumour burden and in circulating glucagon levels. If all extrahepatic tumours can be eradicated, there are successful instances of orthotopic liver transplantation for multiple liver metastases. Cryotherapy and radiofrequency thermal ablation of liver metastases and percutaneous injection of the lesions with ethanol under ultrasound guidance are being evaluated.

Multiple endocrine neoplasia type 1 syndrome (MEN 1; MEA 1; Wermer's syndrome)

The MEN 1 syndrome is inherited as an autosomal dominant disorder but considerable phenotypic variability exists even within an individual family. However, recent evidence suggests that the pancreas, parathyroid glands and pituitary are involved in all patients if examined pathologically. It is also now understood that the pancreas is inevitably involved with diffuse islet cell disease consisting of micronodular and macronodular hyperplasia, and often multiple tumours secreting multiple peptide hormones.

The parathyroid glands are most frequently involved in MEN 1 syndrome with hyperparathyroidism being present in 85% of cases. In the vast majority of these all four glands are affected. This is in contrast with the very low incidence of parathyroid hyperplasia in isolated primary hyperparathyroidism. Pancreatic abnormalities occur in over 80% in MEN 1 patients, with non-B cell tumours being most common. The most common pancreatic tumour found in MEN 1 syndrome patients is gastrinoma, and in virtually all such patients multiple pancreatic tumours are found.

Of the pituitary lesions, chromophobe adenomas and particularly prolactinomas are the most frequent lesions encountered. When small, these tumours may be without symptoms but, in male patients, they are associated with manifestations of the antiandrogenic effect of prolactin. Tumours producing growth hormone and leading to acromegaly are the next most frequently encountered variety.

While the MEN 1 syndrome is classically associated with lesions of the parathyroid glands, pancreatic islets and pituitary gland, an increasing number of adrenocortical lesions have been recognized in recent years. Many of these lesions are non-functioning adenomas; however, glucocorticoid excess has been noted in some. Other occasional associations of MEN 1 include thyroid nodules, bronchial and intestinal carcinoids and lipomas.

All patients with endocrine pancreatic tumours should be carefully investigated for additional manifestation of MEN 1 syndrome. Thus, estimations of serum levels of calcium and phosphate as well as plasma assays for parathormone, insulin, gastrin, glucagon, somatostatin, pancreatic polypeptide, prolactin, growth hormone, adrenocorticotropic hormone and cortisol constitute a relatively complete though by no means exhaustive endocrine evaluation for the MEN 1 syndrome. Whenever a patient is diagnosed as having MEN 1 syndrome, screening of all available family members is indicated.

Multiple endocrine neoplasia type 2 syndrome (MEN 2; MEA 2; Sipple's syndrome)

MEN 2 is another discrete endocrine syndrome which is inherited as an autosomal dominant with variable expressivity. It is not associated with pancreatic disease. It consists of hyperparathyroidism, medullary carcinoma of the thyroid gland and phaeochromocytoma. MEN 2b is a variant which is also inherited as an autosomal dominant but unlike in MEN 2, the incidence of parathyroid disease is extremely low. The syndrome consists of multiple mucosal neuromas, intestinal ganglioneuromatosis leading to megacolon and constipation, a Marfanoid habitus and characteristic facies with thickened lips and alae nasi, along with medullary carcinoma of the thyroid and phaeochromocytoma.

Further reading

Beger, H. G., Krautzberger, W., Bittner, R. *et al.* (1985). Duodenum preserving resection of the head of the pancreas in patients with severe chronic pancreatitis. *Surgery* **97**: 467–73.

Bouvet, M., Gamagami, R. A., Gilpin, E. A. *et al.* (2000). Factors influencing survival after resection for periampullary neoplasms. *Am J Surg* **180**: 13–7.

Bradley, E. L. III, Reynhout, J. A. and Peer, G. I. (1998). Thoracoscopic splanchnicectomy for 'small duct' chronic pancreatitis: case selection by differential epidural analgesia. *J Gastrointest Surg* **2**: 88–94.

Burns, G. P. and Bank, S., eds (1992). *Disorders of the Pancreas*, New York: McGraw-Hill.

Cuschieri, A., Shimi, S. M., Crosthwaite, G. *et al.* (1994). Bilateral endoscopic splanchnicectomy through a posterior thorascopic approach. *J R Coll Surg Edinb* **39**: 44–7.

Frey, C. F. and Smith, G. J. (1987). Description and rationale of a new operation for chronic pancreatitis. *Pancreas* **2**: 701–7.

Moossa, A. R., Robson, M. C. and Schmipff, S. C., eds (1992). *Comprehensive Textbook of Oncology*, 2nd edn. Baltimore, MD: Williams & Wilkins.

Mozell, E., Stenzel, P., Woltering, E. A. *et al.* (1990). Functional endocrine tumors of the pancreas: clinical presentation, diagnosis, and treatment. *Current Problems in Surgery*, Chicago, IL: Year Book.

Puestow, C. B. and Gillesby, W. J. (1958). Retrograde surgical drainage of the pancreas for chronic pancreatitis. *Ann Surg* **76**: 898–906.

Wiersema, M. J., Hawes, R. H., Lehman, G. A. *et al.* (1993). Prospective evaluation of endoscopic ultrasonography and endoscopic retrograde cholangiopancreatography in patients with chronic abdominal pain of suspected pancreatic origin. *Endoscopy* **25**: 555–64.

Yamaguchi, K., Dhijiwa, K., Shimizu, S. *et al.* (1998). Comparison of endoscopic retrograde and magnetic resonance cholangiopancreatography in the surgical diagnosis of pancreatic diseases. *Am J Surg* **175**: 203–8.

MODULE 13

Disorders of the small intestine and vermiform appendix

Section 13.1 • Anatomy

The small intestine is divided into two anatomical portions. The jejunum, which constitutes the proximal two-fifths, is normally situated in the upper left part of the infra-colic compartment, whereas the ileum tends to be situated in the right iliac fossa and pelvis. There is no clear demarcation line between the jejunum and the ileum but the proximal jejunum is thicker than the ileum with prominent plicae circulares and with an overall diameter which is twice that of the distal ileum. The mesentery of the jejunum contains less fat and the mesenteric vasculature consists of prominent arteries and veins which join to form one or two arcades in the mesentery before giving rise to the terminal intestinal branches. The mesenteric vasculature of the ileum is more complex with the vessels forming four or five levels of arcades before the origin of the terminal intestinal branches. The whole of the small bowel is supplied by the superior mesenteric artery (Figure 13.1). An understanding of the anatomy of the mesenteric vascular arcades of the small intestine is essential for the safe execution of reconstructive procedures on the gastrointestinal tract involving small bowel segments, e.g. ileal pouch construction.

The arteriolar supply to the small bowel is of particular surgical interest. Each arteriole and accompanying venule supply and drain one half of the circumference of the small intestine and the vessels are distributed to alternate sides of the bowel wall in regular sequence (Figure 13.2). This arrangement forms the basis of intestinal lengthening operations in infants and children with the short gut syndrome as the residual bowel can be split longitudinally with each half retaining an adequate blood supply (see the treatment of short-gut syndrome).

The length of the small bowel is highly variable and difficult to estimate. Post-mortem studies indicate that the length of the human small intestine stripped of its mesentery varies from 3.5 to 9 m with an average of 5 m. However, the tone of the smooth muscle reduces

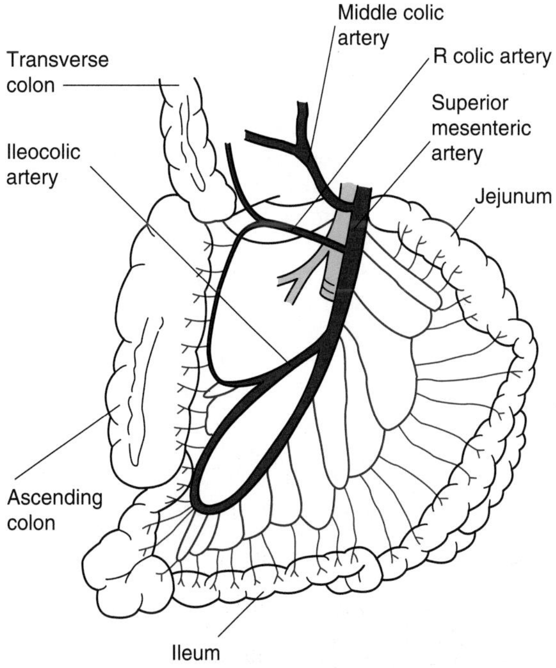

Figure 13.1 Blood supply of the small bowel.

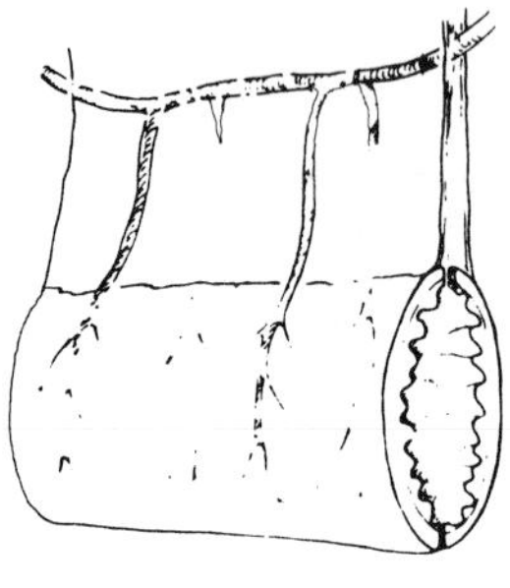

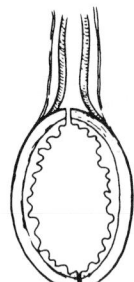

Figure 13.2 Diagrammatic representation of the distribution of the terminal branches of the mesenteric vessels to the small intestine. These are distributed to alternate sides of the gut.

the small bowel length considerably during life. Accurate assessment of intestinal length at operation is difficult owing to the changing state of the intestinal loops due to peristaltic activity, handling and exposure. In the adult the length of the small bowel measured along its anti-mesenteric border and in the unstretched state after a preliminary laparotomy averages 3.5 m. If a substantial portion of the small bowel is resected, it is important to record how much viable small intestine is left behind. Owing to the degree of variation it is not useful to record the amount resected.

Micro-anatomy

The small bowel mucosa is arranged in villi, which are finger like projections measuring 0.5–1.5 mm in length (Figure 13.3). These are covered by tall columnar absorptive cells (enterocytes) which have micro-villi at their luminal surfaces (brush border). These enterocytes rest on a thin basal membrane (lamina propria) and their micro-villi are kept lubricated by a surface mucus know as the glycocalyx which separates the brush border from the intestinal contents. Goblet cells, found interspersed among the enterocytes, synthesize the mucinous glycoprotein essential for maintaining the glycocalyx. At their bases the villi are surrounded by intestinal crypts that contain the stem cells from which the surface epithelium is constantly replaced by a process of cell division and migration.

The other cells found in the crypts are goblet cells in the upper half, Paneth cells at the base and endocrine cells. The Paneth cells are pyramidal in shape, and have abundant RNA rich cytoplasm and refractile granules containing lysosomes. The exact function of Paneth cells is unknown but they are thought to be capable of phagocytosing bacteria from the crypt lumen. The endocrine cells are also known as APUD cells. This term is derived from a basic characteristic of these entero-endocrine cells: the uptake and decarboxylation of amine precursors. These gut endocrine cells were once thought to be of ectodermal origin but are now thought to arise from the undifferentiated crypt stem cells. A separate group of gut endocrine cells stain with potassium chromate and silver dyes. These are known as enterochromaffin cells or argentaffin cells. These synthesize and secrete 5-hydroxytryptophan and 5-hydroxytryptamine (5-HT) in addition to a variety of peptide hormones such as motilin, substance P and others. The other important cellular components of the villus are lymphocytes which are subdivided into those in the basal lamina (lamina propria lymphocytes) and those found among the epithelial cells covering the villus (intra-epithelial lymphocytes).

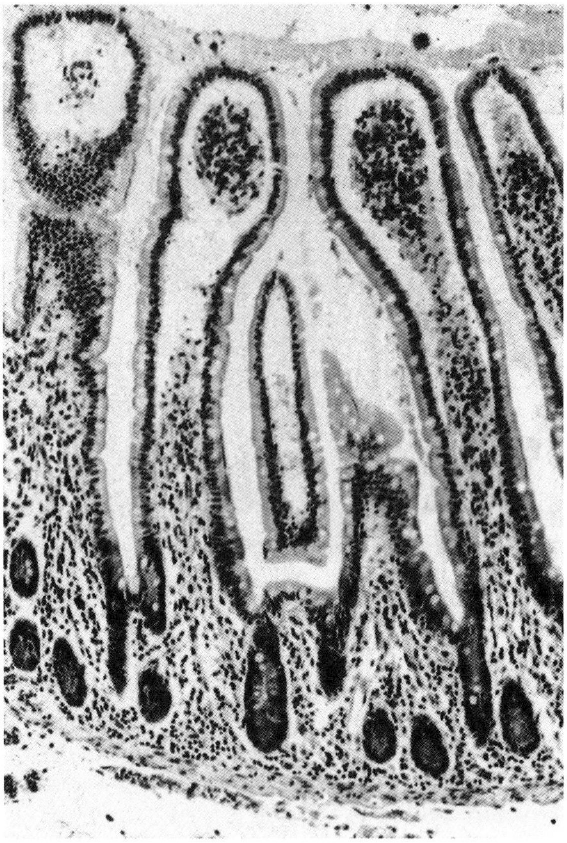

Figure 13.3 Normal appearance of jejunal mucosa.

Section 13.2 • Physiology

The primary function of the small intestine is the absorption of nutrients but it also has a role in digestion. Carbohydrate and protein digestion by the pancreatic enzymes is incomplete and brush border enzymes are essential for the final hydrolysis to tripeptides and dipeptides and monosaccharides. The dipeptides and tripeptides which have a high affinity for the brush border peptidases are hydrolysed to individual amino acids before absorption. Those with a low affinity for the surface enzymes are absorbed intact by the enterocytes. Triglyceride digestion and absorption requires the presence of co-lipase and lipase which convert the triglycerides to a mixture of free fatty acids and monoglycerides. These are then rendered water soluble by combining with bile acids to form micelles. At the surface of the enterocytes the monoglycerides and free fatty acids separate from the micelles leaving the bile acids within the intestinal lumen.

Following absorption the fatty acids are bound to fatty acid binding proteins (FABP) and are transported to the smooth endoplasmic reticulum where they are re-esterified. Within the Golgi apparatus of the endoplasmic reticulum, the triglycerides are converted to chylomicrons consisting of cholesterol and triglyceride surrounded by phospholipids, free cholesterol and apoproteins. These chylomicrons together with lipoproteins are transferred via the lacteals and lymph channels to the venous blood. Cholesterol behaves in a similar way except that it does not bind to FABP and is released slowly from the enterocyte. The absorption of medium-chain triglycerides (MCT) on the other hand is different. A significant percentage of MCT is absorbed intact into the portal blood. The rest is broken down by pancreatic lipase to medium-chain fatty acids which are readily absorbed by the intestinal cells after micellar aggregation with bile acids. These are then transferred as free fatty acids into the portal venous blood without chylomicron formation.

Under normal circumstances the digestion and absorption of fluid, electrolytes, iron, folates, carbohydrates, fat and proteins is completed in the jejunum. However, the effective absorption of bile salts and vitamin B_{12} can only occur in the terminal ileum as these substances require specific transport sites which are located in this region. In the absence of ileum the critical length of jejunum required for the absorption of water-soluble substances is somewhere between 30 and 120 cm. However, the absence of the ileum will produce malabsorption of fat from a diminished bile salt pool and of vitamin B_{12}. The ileum on the other hand is able to perform all the absorbative functions of the jejunum if the proximal small bowel is excised.

Another function of the small intestine is the synthesis of high-density, low-density and very low-density lipoproteins (HDL, LDL, VLDL). These are closely related to the chylomicrons and contain the same apoproteins. The intestinal lipoproteins reach the plasma via the thoracic duct. Although there are other tissues which synthesize these lipoproteins, e.g. the liver, the gastrointestinal tract is a major site of production and therefore plays an important part in the metabolism of plasma lipoproteins. The synthesis of these lipoproteins by the small intestine is impaired in kwashiorkor.

Yet another function of the small intestine is the synthesis of peptide and amine intestinal hormones. These are located within the entero-endocrine cells and in the neurones of the myenteric plexus. These modulate intestinal activity in three ways:

- as classic endocrine hormones
- as neurotransmitters
- as hormones with a paracrine action.

These hormones influence intestinal secretion and transport, growth and differentiation, the splanchic haemodynamic state and the release of insulin (Table 13.1). The complex hormonal interactions within the small intestine are closely linked with the activity of the enteric nervous system which is considered to act as an independent integrative system regulating reflex activity within the gut. Within the myenteric plexus neurones containing opioid peptides (enkephalins), substance P, VIP, serotonin and somatostatin have all been identified in addition to the better known adrenergic (noradrenaline) and cholinergic (acetylcholine) neurotransmitters.

Table 13.1 Hormones originating in the small bowel and their functions

Hormone	*Functions*
Acetylcholine	Neurotransmitter
Enkephalins	Neurotransmitter
Enteroglucagon	Growth and differentiation
GIP (gastric inhibitory peptide)	Glucose-dependent insulin release
Glucagon	Increased splanchnic blood flow
Motilin	Secretion and transport
Neurotensin	Increased splanchnic blood flow, secretion and transport
Noradrenaline (norepinephrine)	Neurotransmitter
Secretin	Secretion and transport
Serotonin	Neurotransmitter
Somatostatin	Neurotransmitter, secretion and transport
Substance P	Neurotransmitter
Vasopressin	Decreased splanchnic blood flow
VIP (vasoactive intestinal peptide)	Increased splanchnic blood flow

Small intestinal motility

Studies of gastrointestinal motility are difficult to undertake and to interpret. Most have been performed with multi-lumen fluid perfused catheters attached to external transducers linked to chart recorders. However, solid-state systems based on several miniature strain gauged transducers mounted at intervals on a fine catheter are now commonly used. The analogue signals (corresponding to the intestinal contractions) from these transducers are stored in a solid-state external portable logger. The data are then off-loaded onto a computer for analysis. Software systems are now available which are capable of sophisticated analysis of small bowel activity.

Using these new systems it has been possible to characterize small bowel motility both in normal and in pathological states. In the normal situation both fasting and fed patterns of intestinal activity are now recognized and the types of intestinal contractions fall into two categories, *mixing and propagating*. The mixing contractions include the *stationary ring contractions*, which occlude the lumen at one point and push the intestinal contents in both directions, and the *stationary cluster contractions*, which may occur at one or several sites simultaneously. The propagating contractions include *single propagated contractions, propagating power contractions, migrating cluster contractions and the phase III of the MMC.* The propagating power contractions (PPC) are also known as the giant migratory contraction (GMC). They correspond to the peristaltic rushes described by earlier workers and are effective at sweeping intestinal contents in a distal direction at a rapid rate. They are increased in patients undergoing radiotherapy and are now thought to be the cause of the nausea, vomiting, abdominal pain and diarrhoea which are often experienced by these patients.

Motility disorders may be functional (no definable organic cause) or secondary to myopathy (hollow visceral type), autonomic neuropathy, abnormalities of the enteric nervous system, endocrine disorders, tumours, drug induced and multiple endocrine neoplasia. The motility disorders of the small and large intestine that are of surgical importance include:

- adynamic ileus
- irritable bowel syndrome
- pseudo obstruction
- Hirshsprung's disease.

Microbiology

At birth the alimentary tract is sterile but becomes colonized by bacteria via the oral route so that within 3–4 weeks of birth the enteric microflora found in the adult is already established. The stomach, duodenum and proximal jejunum in the normal adult subject contains transient Gram-positive aerobes such as lactobacilli and enterococci in concentrations of less than 10^4 colony forming units (CFU) per ml of contents. In the terminal ileum however, the bacterial counts are higher (10^5–10^8 CFU) and the flora resemble that of the large bowel. The organisms encountered include coliforms and strict anaerobes (e.g. bacteroides). Substantially higher bacterial counts (10^5–10^{11} CFU) are found in the colon with bacteroides, anaerobic lactobacilli and clostridia predominating. It is thought that the small bowel microflora plays an important protective role against bacterial overgrowth and infection by preventing colonization of the surface epithelium by pathogenic bacteria. This is brought about by production of bacteriocins (antibiotics) and lowering of the oxidation–reduction potential by anaerobic metabolism which results in the production of substances which are toxic to bacteria.

Intraluminal bacteria produce endotoxin which is not absorbed into the blood stream in the presence of bile salts. However, absorption of endotoxin into the blood occurs whenever bile salts are prevented from reaching the small intestine as in obstructive jaundice. This endotoxinaemia may be responsible for the development of renal failure after surgical intervention in jaundiced patients.

The small bowel microflora plays an important role in intraluminal metabolism of various substances, particularly metabolized protein and other nitrogenous compounds the results of which are absorbed and used for synthesis of amino acids. For example, the excess ammonia produced by bacterial metabolism after an episode of gastrointestinal haemorrhage may precipitate encephalopathy in patients with chronic liver disease and portal hypertension.

Under normal conditions a symbiotic relationship exists between the gut and intestinal organisms and indeed the villous architecture and rate of regeneration of the intestinal mucosa depend on the presence of a normal resident microflora. However, in conditions of stasis and diminished or absent gastric secretary activity, bacterial overgrowth may occur leading to maldigestion and malabsorption.

Gut mucosal integrity and bacterial translocation

The normal intestinal mucosa in the presence of a competent immune system is able to resist invasion by pathogenic bacteria. This anti-microbial barrier can break down under certain pathological states with translocation of the pathogens to the blood and lymph with subsequent systemic invasion of tissues and organs. Such bacterial translocation underlies one of the hypotheses held responsible for systemic inflammatory response syndrome (SIRS), i.e. endotoxin induced activation of the cytokine cascade, which in turn leads to multi-organ failure (MOF) and death. This hypothesis has, however, been challenged recently because treatment with antibodies to the polysaccharide fraction of endotoxin has been shown to be ineffective in clinical trials, and other mechanisms, e.g. endothelial damage by activated neutrophils, may be responsible for MOF. The conditions that promote bacterial translocation are shown in Table 13.2.

In septic patients enteral feeding with complete diets may nonetheless protect the integrity of the gut barrier and improve the immune function and is thus superior to parenteral feeding. In patients where enteral nutrition is not possible specific amino-acid supplements (arginine and glutamine) in the parenteral feeding regimen may improve outcomes by restoring gut mucosal integrity and immune function.

The components of enteral feeds which have been shown to enhance the ability of the intestinal mucosa to resist bacterial translocation are arginine, glutamine and lipids (especially fish oil). Arginine, a dibasic amino-acid, can stimulate the secretion of insulin, prolactin and growth hormone and also has immunomodulatory effects. Thus in immunocompromised patients, arginine supplements have been shown to enhance

Table 13.2 Conditions promoting bacterial translocation

Bacterial overgrowth
Immunodeficiency
Physical disruption of the gut mucosa including ischaemia
Trauma
Burns
Sepsis
Endotoxinaemia and protein malnutrition

lymphocyte function in the post-operative period. There is also good evidence that dietary lipids may have a similar effect. This may act directly or indirectly via alterations in eicosanoid metabolism. The eicosanoids include prostaglandins and leukotrienes that modulate low inflammatory response and immune function.

Glutamine is the most abundant amino acid in the free amino acid pool and is essential for rapidly dividing cells including enterocytes. It thus plays an important role in maintaining the integrity of the intestinal mucosa. Although the glutamine pool is large it is labile and becomes rapidly depleted in injured and septic patients. Thus in the critically ill, glutamine may be regarded as an essential amino acid. There is good evidence that the translocation of bacteria encountered in sepsis, trauma and burns may be reversed by glutamine enriched intravenous or enteral nutrition. This positive effect is accompanied by a normalization of the secretary immunoglobulin A (IgA) levels and a decrease in the bacterial adherence to enterocytes.

Section 13.3 • Small bowel investigations

Specific investigation of the small intestine is indicated where small bowel obstruction, bleeding or malabsorption is suspected. The term malabsorption can be used to describe the failure to absorb specific substances, e.g. carbohydrates, fats, proteins and minerals, but when used unqualified it generally refers to fat malabsorption. This is frequently encountered in surgical practice as it may follow excisional and bypass procedures in the gastrointestinal tract which effectively shorten the small bowel. Clearly serum biochemistry, e.g. albumin, transferrin, electrolytes including calcium, iron, haemoglobin level and blood film are all necessary when malabsorption is suspected. There are, however, special investigations which may be of value. The investigations dealt with in this module are summarized in Table 13.3.

Radiology

The radiological investigations which are of value in the small bowel can be subdivided into plain radiography, barium studies, fistulography, ultrasound and computed tomography (CT) scanning, mesenteric angiography and isotope studies.

Plain radiography

A plain abdominal X-ray provides useful information in the diagnosis of the acute abdomen. As far as the small bowel is concerned, obstruction is diagnosed by visualizing dilated gas filled loops of small bowel. These can be distinguished from large bowel by the more central distribution and the ladder-like valvulae conniventes. Traditionally an erect abdominal film is obtained at the same time but this does not provide any extra information although it is only on the erect film that the typical fluid levels will be seen. Occasionally, however, obstructed small bowel may be so full of fluid that it will not be seen clearly on the supine film and it will only be the fluid levels on the erect film which will give the diagnosis. Thickening of the small bowel can be inferred when there is a significant gap between the gaseous outline lumen of adjacent loops of small bowel. Plain radiography is also very useful for identifying free air in the peritoneum but it must be remembered that an erect chest X-ray is more useful in this respect. With the erect abdominal film the diaphragm may not be included in the film.

Barium studies

The mainstay of the investigation of the small bowel is the barium small bowel follow through which is easy to perform as part of a barium meal study. However, a small bowel enema in which contrast medium is instilled via a Bilbao-Dotter tube directly into the upper jejunum carries a higher diagnostic yield, especially for small bowel tumours and in patients with suspected malabsorption. In particular, ulcers, sinuses and

Table 13.3 Investigations of the small intestine

Radiology	Plain abdominal films	Acute conditions
	Small bowel follow-through	
	Small bowel enema	
	Arteriography	Occult gastrointestinally bleeding
	CT scanning	Detection of fistulas and pre-operative staging of gastrointestinal malignancy
	Ultrasound	Diagnosis of cystic lesions
Isotope scintigraphy		Localization of gastrointestinal bleeding
		Estimation of intestinal transit
		Detection of inflammatory bowel disease
Faecal fat estimation		Diagnosis of steatorrhoea
Jejunal mucosal biopsy		In patients with malabsorption
Tests of terminal ileal function	Schilling	Absorption of vitamin B_{12}
	SeHCAT	Absorption of bile salts
Breath tests	^{14}C-Glycocholate/-D-xylose	Bacterial overgrowth
	^{14}C-Lactose	Lactose malabsorption
	Lactulose H_2	Small bowel transit and bacterial overgrowth
Enteroscopy		Obscure bleeding, small bowel tumours

fistulas are better visualized by a small bowel enema. The radiological criteria of malabsorption are flocculation and segmentation of the barium, thickening of the mucosal folds and dilatation of intestinal loops. It must be stressed however that these changes are non-specific and the diagnosis must be confirmed by other more specific tests.

There have been few comparative studies between barium meal and follow through and small bowel enema (enteroclysis) but available evidence indicates that the latter is superior except in Crohn's disease. The false negative rate for the detection of primary small bowel neoplasms is much higher (80%) for follow through examinations compared with small bowel enema (10%). Enterocylsis is better than follow through and even radionuclide studies for the detection of Meckel's diverticulum. Small bowel enema is useful in the diagnosis of partial/intermittent obstruction and is superior to both follow through and CT in these cases. By contrast, CT is accurate in showing site and cause in patients with established high-grade obstruction.

In the patient with obstruction due to adhesions where there are some doubts as to whether or not the obstruction will settle with conservative treatment, it is useful to give the patient a drink or nasogastric bolus of water-soluble contrast such as 40 ml of Urografin in 40 ml of distilled water. If the contrast has not reached the ascending colon within 24 hours, it is highly likely that the patient will require surgical intervention.

Injection of contrast into a fistula may also be of value (fistulography). This is particularly useful in Crohn's disease. Where enterocutaneous fistulas have formed, fistulography will permit the diagnosis of associated abscess cavities and strictures and will allow the planning of appropriate surgical intervention.

Ultrasound and CT scanning

Ultrasound scanning may be used in patients with intestinal obstruction and is capable of differentiating fluid-filled dilated intestinal loops from other cystic structures within the abdomen but its role in the investigation of small bowel disease is limited. CT scanning of the small intestine entails the use of a special barium sulphate suspension (E-Z-CAT) to opacify the lumen of the intestine. It is useful in detecting thickening of the bowel wall and in demonstrating the presence of enterocolic and enterovesical fistulas. However, indications for its use in small bowel disorders are limited since the information can often be obtained by standard contrast radiology.

Mesenteric angiography

Selective mesenteric angiography can be used to detect angiodysplastic lesions and vascular tumours in the small bowel which can lead to occult or frank bleeding from the gastrointestinal tract. It is also possible to detect an active bleeding site in the small intestine by this means if blood is being lost at more than 0.5 ml/min. If a bleeding point is identified during mesenteric angiography it is helpful if the radiologist

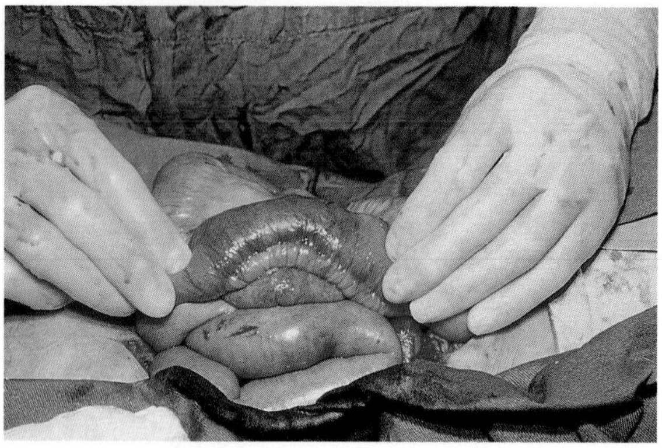

Figure 13.4 Segment of small bowel highlighted by intra-operative injection of methylene blue via a super-selective mesenteric angiogram catheter.

can place a super-selective catheter into the appropriate branch of the superior mesenteric artery to lie as close as possible to the lesion. The catheter is then left *in situ* when the patient goes to the operating theatre. The surgeon can then inject contrast (methylene blue) along the catheter and the segment of small bowel in which the bleeding lesion is present can easily be identified (Figure 13.4).

Isotope studies

External isotope scintigraphy following the intravenous administration of radio-labelled compounds or isotope-labelled autologous cells can be useful in the investigation of patients with occult gastrointestinal intestinal bleeding. It may also be useful in detecting inflamed intestine and in estimating the intestinal transit time.

Intestinal bleeding

Haemorrhage of small intestinal origin may be due to Meckel's diverticulum, polyps, tumours or vascular malformations. These may not be detectable using endoscopy, small barium studies or angiography. Under these circumstances, radionuclide methods may help to solve the problem. Basically three isotope methods are available. The first involves the injection of technetium pertechnetate. This is the method of choice for the detection of Meckel's diverticulum and carries an accuracy rate of 90%. The technetium is concentrated by ectopic gastric mucosa in the diverticulum which can be identified as a hot spot (Figure 13.5). For the detection of rapidly bleeding sites in the emergency situation 99m-sulfur colloid can be used following intravenous bolus injection. It is cleared from the circulation by the macrophage system within 15 min, at which point the blood radioactivity declines, but the extra vascular radioactivity at the bleeding site increases thereby allowing its detection as a hot spot by external scintigraphy. In practice this method is rarely used as mesenteric angiography gives a much more accurate anatomical localization. In the patient with intermittent gastrointestinal bleeding however, technetium

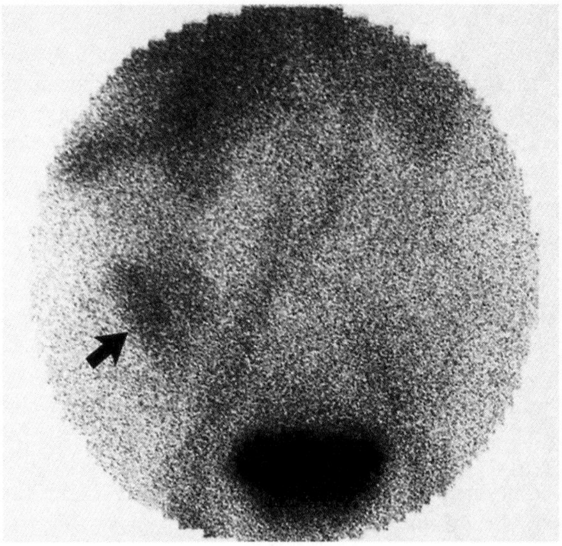

Figure 13.5 Ectopic gastric mucosa in a Meckel's diverticulum outlined by external scintiscanning after the intravenous administration of ^{99m}Tc.

labelled autologous red cells are useful. These are cleared much more slowly from the vascular compartment following their intravenous injection and it allows repeated examinations over a 24 hour period (Figure 13.6). Its main disadvantage is that it takes time to label the patient's red blood cells and it is therefore unsuitable for the actively bleeding patient.

Estimation of small bowel transit time

In the past, small bowel intestinal transit studies have been performed using radio-opaque solid, non-absorbable chemical markers. These however are generally regarded as being unphysiological and unsuitable for routine clinical practice. Estimation of the small bowel transit is best performed either by external scintigraphy after administration of isotope labelled meals or by breath tests (see below). Both liquid and solid meals labelled with TCSC or DTPA can be used to estimate simultaneously gastric emptying and small bowel transit time. The detection of caecal radioactivity is used as the end point for the estimation of the small bowel transit time.

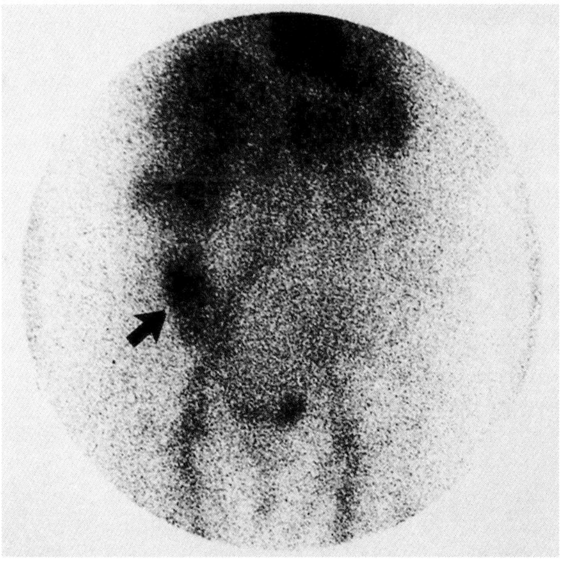

Figure 13.6 Occult bleeding site in the ascending colon located by the ^{99m}Tc-labelled autologous red cell technique. Selective arteriography was unhelpful in this elderly patient. The lesion proved to be an angiodysplasia.

Detection of small bowel inflammatory disease

Indium labelled autologous leucocytes when injected intravenously settle in areas of inflammation or abscess formation. This can be used to detect the extent of active inflammatory bowel disease and assess its severity. However, there can be great difficulty with interpretation because of the increased background radioactivity produced by the uptake of the radiolabelled leucocytes by the bone marrow, liver and spleen. Another approach is to use labelled sucralfate. Sucralfate is an aluminium salt of polysulfated sucrose which is used in the treatment of peptic ulceration. It binds selectively to areas of mucosal ulceration within the gastrointestinal tract and the use of labelled sucralfate has proved to be a useful technique in the detection of inflammatory bowel disease in both the large and small intestine. In view of its lower radiation dosage compared to barium studies it can be used as a screening test and in the serial assessment of disease activity. The labelled suspension of sucralfate is administered by mouth and serial isotope scans of the abdomen are carried out at 2, 6, 20 and 24 hours.

Investigations for malabsorption

Malabsorption implies the inability to absorb sufficient nutrient owing to disease of the gastrointestinal tract. It is most commonly due to dysfunction of the small bowel or the pancreas. The most common clinical feature is steatorrhoea owing to malabsorption of fat. Symptoms attributable to failure to absorb carbohydrate and protein are not so common and may consist of abdominal discomfort and bloating. Digested carbohydrate is fermented to lactic acid in the large bowel which can lead to diarrhoea. There are various methods of testing for the various causes of malabsorption (Table 13.4) which can be general or quite specific. These are dealt with below.

Estimation of faecal fat

The quantitative estimation of faecal fat remains the most sensitive and reliable test of disorders of digestion and absorption. The faecal fat output per day is estimated on a 3–5 day collection on a standard diet containing 80–100 g of fat. The normal is less than 6 g/day (80 mmol of triglyceride). Other tests such as the ^{14}C-triolein breath test and oxalate loading test are less reliable but are used in some centres as screening tests for steatorrhea.

Table 13.4 Investigation of a patient with suspected malabsorption

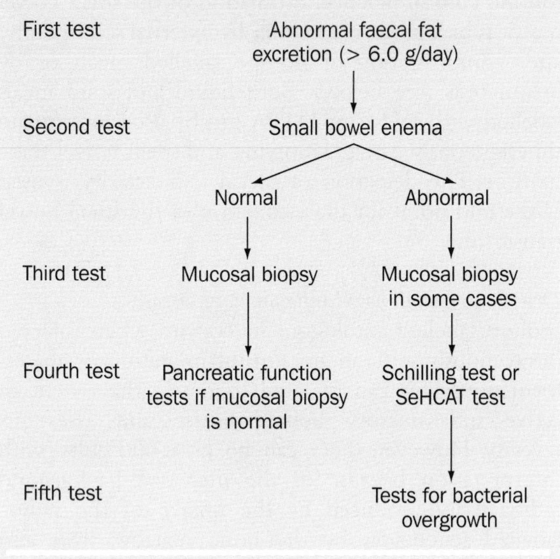

Duodenal mucosal biopsy

Biopsy taken at upper-gastrointestinal endoscopy of the distal duodenum can be used to look for abnormalities of villous architecture, e.g. subtotal villous atrophy in coeliac disease (Figure 13.7). In addition, abnormal mucosal pathogens may be detected as in Whipple's disease in addition to parasites, e.g. *Giardia lamblia* (Figure 13.8). Endoscopic duodenal biopsy has largely replaced the use of the suction Crosby capsule.

The Schilling test

The absorption of vitamin B_{12} by the terminal ileum requires the presence of intrinsic factor and to a lesser extent the R protein in the gastric juice. In the Schilling test radio-labelled vitamin B_{12} (1.0 μg) is administered orally immediately after a large parenteral injection of the unlabelled vitamin (1000 μg) to ensure saturation of the body stores. Under these conditions normal subjects will excrete 10% or more of the radio-labelled vitamin in their urine. If abnormally low excretion is found in a patient the test is repeated but the labelled vitamin B_{12} is given together with intrinsic factor. In the presence of ileal disease the abnormally low excretion of the labelled vitamin in the urine is not altered by the addition of the intrinsic factor. However, in patients with pernicious anaemia or after total gastrectomy the administration of intrinsic factor restores the urinary excretion of the labelled vitamin to normal. Both stages of the test are invalidated by dehydration and renal disease. Bacterial overgrowth may cause malabsorption of the vitamin and an abnormal Schilling test but this will revert to normal after a course of antibiotic therapy.

SeHCAT bile absorption test

This test estimates the ability of the terminal ileum to absorb bile acids. The synthetic selenium bile acid known as SeHCAT is used. A dose of this ^{75}Se-labelled compound is administered orally or intravenously and a gamma-counter is used to estimate the bile acid absorption. There is a very good correlation between the results of the SeHCAT test and faecal excretion of bile acids.

^{14}C-Glycocholate and the ^{14}C-D-xylose breath tests

The ^{14}C-glycocholate breath test is used to detect bacterial overgrowth in the small intestine. The glycine moiety of the conjugated bile salt is labelled with ^{14}C and ingested to mix with the endogenous bile salts in the intestine. Normally the bile salts are largely reabsorbed intact in the terminal ileum to enter the enterohepatic circulation and only a small amount reaches the colon where it is deconjugated by the colonic bacteria and the glycine metabolized to yield $^{14}CO_2$. This is absorbed and eliminated in the expired air. However, in the presence of bacterial overgrowth most of the ingested labelled salt is deconjugated by the small bowel bacteria and excess $^{14}CO_2$ is produced and eliminated in the expired air (Figure 13.9). False positive results are obtained with this test in the presence of ileal disease. The ^{14}C-D-xylose test is more reliable in this respect. D-xylose is a pentose, which is normally absorbed intact by the same transport mechanism as the hexoses.

Breath tests for carbohydrate malabsorption

The analysis of breath $^{14}CO_2$ following the ingestion of ^{14}C-lactose is a convenient test for lactose intolerance resulting from a deficiency of the brush border enzyme lactase. This test is easy to perform, is as accurate as the lactose tolerance test and agrees reasonably well with mucosal disaccharidase activity. Hydrogen is produced when carbohydrate is fermented by some bacteria. When there is lactose malabsorption the sugar reaches the colon where it is fermented with the production of hydrogen. A proportion of this gas is absorbed and excreted in the expired air. Using mass spectrometry it is possible to measure very low concentrations of hydrogen in a sample of end-expiratory air which has a similar composition to that of alveolar air. There is evidence that the breath hydrogen concentration is more accurate than $^{14}CO_2$ excretion in the diagnosis of lactase deficiency. Both tests give false positive results in patients with bacterial overgrowth.

Hydrogen breath tests for measurements of small bowel transit time and bacterial overgrowth

The hydrogen breath test is a useful and reliable method for determining small bowel transit time. Repeated measurements of the hydrogen in the end-expiratory air are taken every few minutes after the ingestion of a meal. The latter may be liquid in nature (drink of the non-absorbable sugar lactulose) or solid, usually mashed potatoes and baked beans which contain non-absorbable oligosaccharides. When the meal reaches the caecum the resulting bacterial fermentation

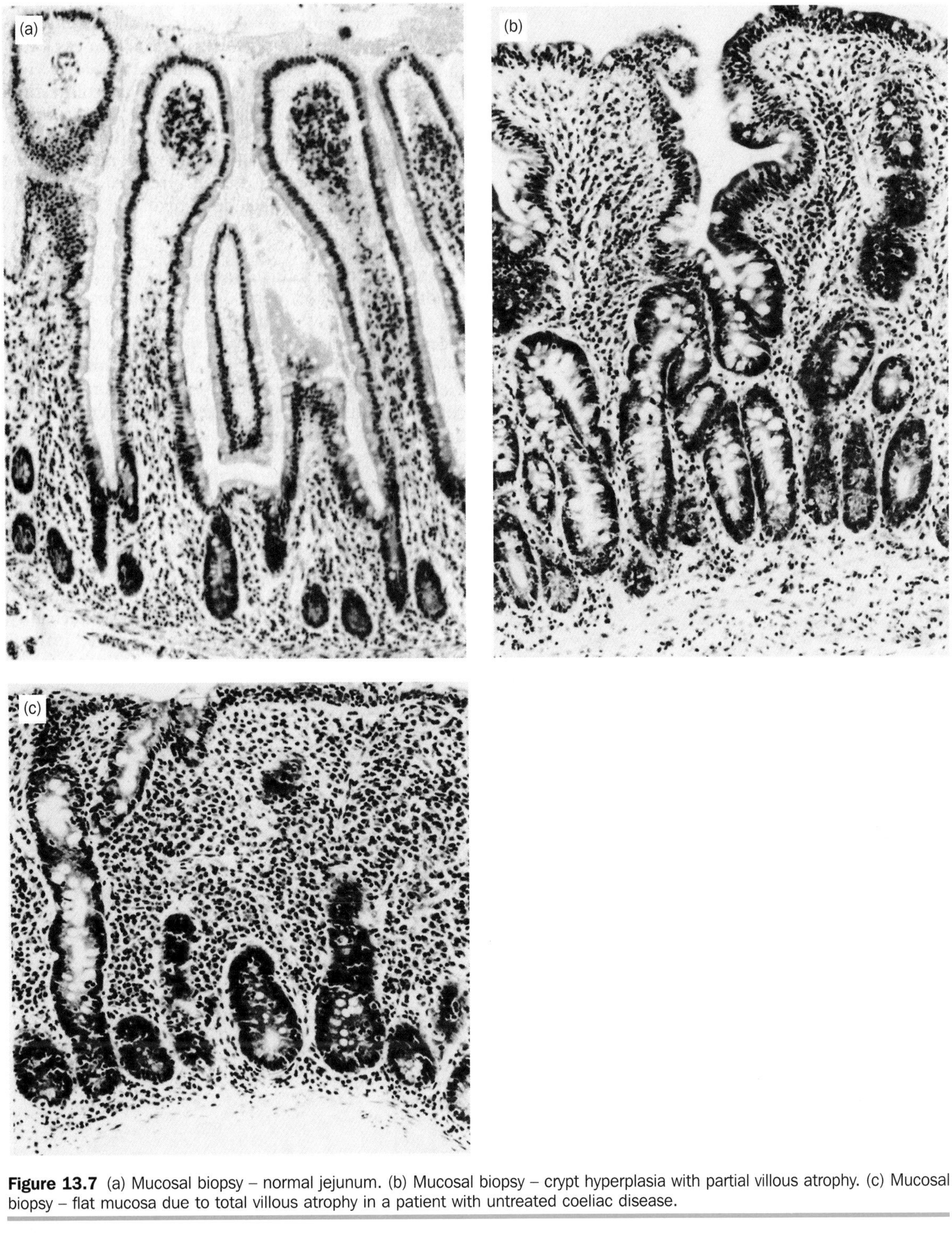

Figure 13.7 (a) Mucosal biopsy – normal jejunum. (b) Mucosal biopsy – crypt hyperplasia with partial villous atrophy. (c) Mucosal biopsy – flat mucosa due to total villous atrophy in a patient with untreated coeliac disease.

induces a sustained rise in the breath hydrogen concentration (Figure 13.10). Strictly speaking, the test measures the oral–caecal transit time which includes the gastric emptying time. However, if the meal is radio-labelled with technetium both gastric emptying and small bowel transit times can be calculated from a single investigation.

In patients with bacterial overgrowth the fasting hydrogen concentration in the expired breath is elevated. In addition there is an early rise in the hydrogen in the expired air following the administration of the lactulose solution (Figure 13.11). The investigation of a patient with suspected malabsorption should start with estimation of faecal fat. Once steatorrhea is confirmed

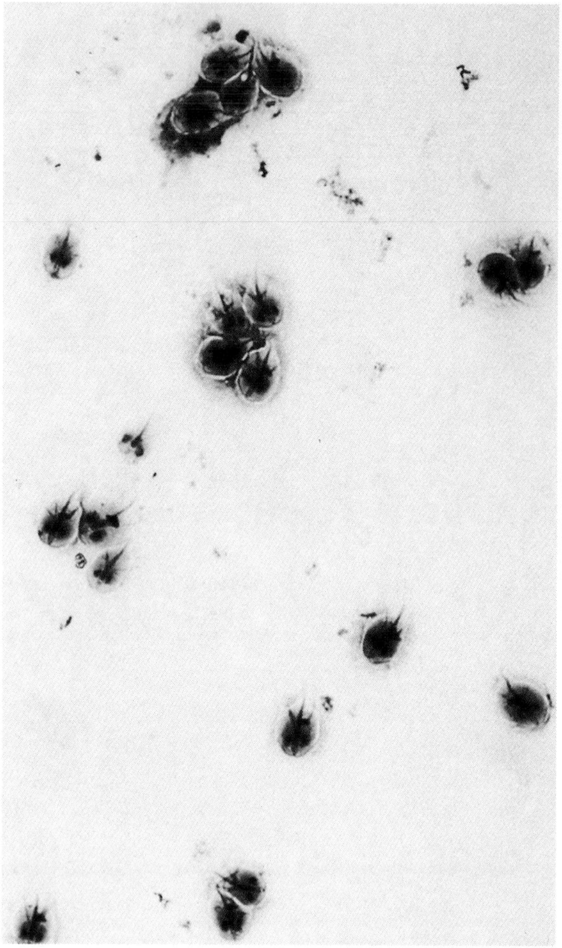

Figure 13.8 *Giardia lamblia* obtained from a jejunal mucosal biopsy.

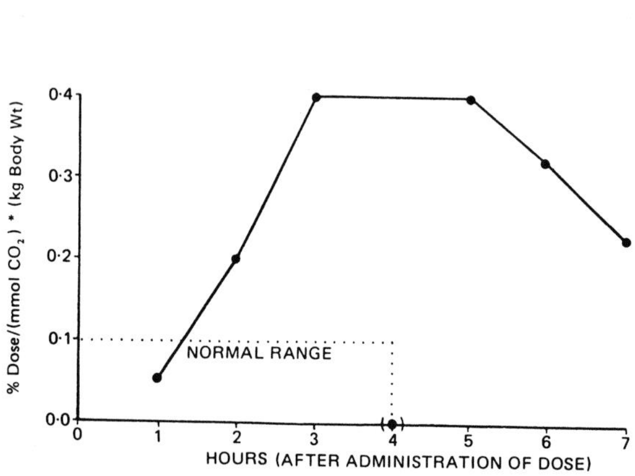

Figure 13.9 ^{14}C-Glycocholate breath test in a female patient with weight loss, hypoproteinaemia and moderate steatorrhoea. The investigation is clearly abnormal with an increased amount of labelled CO_2 being detected in the expired breath. Normally, less than 0.1% of the administered dose is recovered in the expired breath. The patient had had an ileotransverse anastomosis for Crohn's disease. The bacterial overgrowth subsided when the excluded diseased bowel was resected.

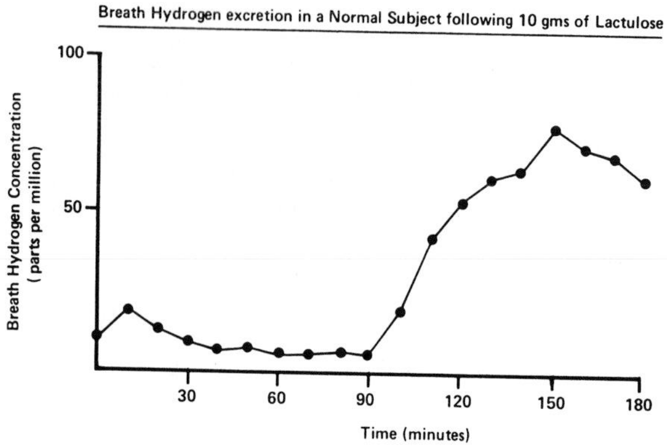

Figure 13.10 Determination of the oral–caecal transit time by the hydrogen breath test. Following the administration of lactulose solution, serial H_2 estimations are performed on samples of the end-expiratory air. A sustained rise in the H_2 in the expired air indicates that the head of the meal has reached the caecum where bacterial fermentation of the non-absorbable carbohydrate occurs.

further tests are required to establish the nature of the underlying pathology. An appropriate scheme is outlined in Table 13.4 and at the end of these tests the malabsorption will be found to be of small bowel (e.g. small intestinal disease or bacterial overgrowth) or the result of pancreatic exocrine insufficiency.

Tests of intestinal permeability

Various disorders including Crohn's disease and mucosal enteropathies are associated with abnormal permeability of the intestinal mucosa to macromolecules which are not absorbed by the intact normal mucosa. The methods used to test permeability are based on the absorption of substances that are normally excluded and if absorbed (because the gut permeability is pathologically enhanced) are not biodegraded and can thus be detected in the blood or urine. Clinically the pathological absorption of these substances is detected by analyses of urine samples for the specific agent used in the test. Examples of test substances include

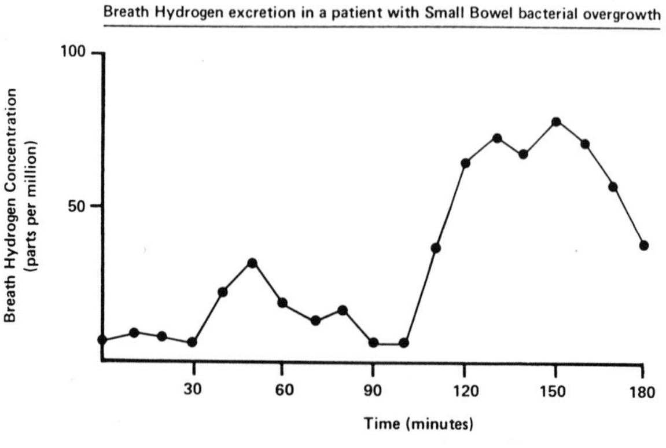

Figure 13.11 H_2 lactulose breath test in a patient with bacterial overgrowth. The fasting level of H_2 in the expired air is high and there is an early rise in the breath H_2 after the ingestion of the lactulose solution.

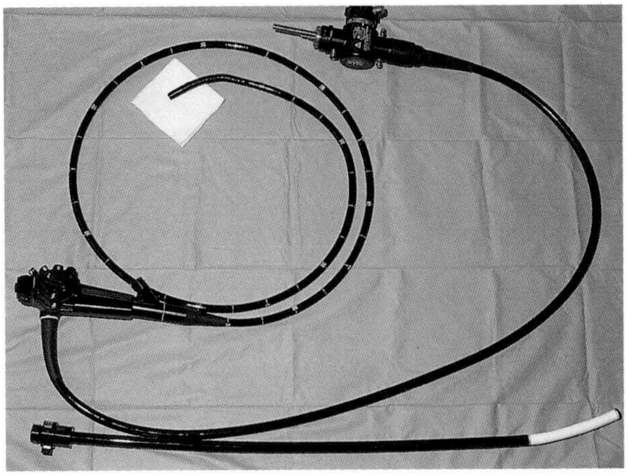

Figure 13.12 Small bowel enteroscope. Note the stiffening overtube at the bottom of the picture.

polyethylene glycol 400 and combinations of small and large compounds with differential absorption, e.g. mannitol and cellobiose. When differential studies using two substances are used the abnormal permeability is demonstrated by changes in the ratio of the urinary concentrations of high to low molecular weight test compounds. Recently, oral administration of ^{51}Cr-labelled EDTA has been used as a quick, non-invasive test of abnormal mucosal permeability.

Small bowel enteroscopy

Endoscopy of the small bowel can be performed either by means of a long balloon tipped small bowel enteroscope or by using a 'push' enteroscope. With the former the balloon is inflated after the endoscope has entered the duodenum and this enables gut peristalsis to carry the tip of the enteroscope to the caecum. This is established by radiological screening and inspection of the bowel is performed as the instrument is slowly withdrawn. This is useful in difficult diagnostic areas such recurrent obscure bleeding and has shown that many patients with bleeding from non-steroidal anti-inflammatory drugs have duodenal ulcers. The limitations of this type of equipment include the time required to carry out the procedure (in the region of 6 hours) and the inability to biopsy through the enteroscope (Figure 13.12). The push enteroscope on the other hand can be used to take biopsies, but only the first 60 cm or so of the small bowel beyond the duodeno-jejunal flexure can be visualized.

Section 13.4 • Small bowel neoplasia

Small bowel tumours are rare and collectively account for less than 10% of all gastrointestinal neoplasms. Although the aetiology is unknown, a number of gastrointestinal disorders are associated with an increased risk including Crohn's disease, coeliac disease, dermatitis herpetiformis, Peutz–Jeghers' syndrome and radiation enteritis.

Benign small bowel tumours

Pathology

Sixty-eight per cent of small bowel neoplasms are benign tumours and include epithelial tumours (tubular and villous adenomas), lipomas, haemangiomas and neurogenic tumours. The latter are subdivided into nerve sheath tumours (neurofibromas and neurilemmomas) and nerve cell tumours (ganglioneuromas, paraganglianomas and sympathicoblastomas). The neurofibromas may be solitary or multiple and associated with systemic neurofibromatosis and café-au-lait skin patches (von Recklinghausen's disease).

Aetiology

Although no definite aetiological factors have been identified, small bowel adenomas may occur in association with familial adenomatis polyposis (FAP).

Clinical features

Many benign small bowel tumours are asymptomatic but the commonest presentation is with intestinal obstruction due to intussusception. This should be distinguished from idiopathic intussusception, which commonly occurs in children under the age of 2 years. Tumour induced intussusception occurs later than the idiopathic variety and does not usually reduce by hydrostatic treatment. Chronic blood loss from a benign small bowel tumour may cause iron-deficiency anaemia and occasionally vascular tumours may give rise to overt gastrointestinal bleeding.

Diagnosis

The diagnosis may be made by small bowel follow through or small bowel enema or, in the case of vascular tumours, by mesenteric angiography. In the majority of cases however the diagnosis is made at laparotomy for small bowel obstruction.

Treatment

In the majority of cases, symptomatic benign small bowel tumours are treated by appropriate small bowel resection and primary anastomosis.

Malignant small bowel tumours

Malignant small bowel tumours are extremely rare, accounting for less than 5% of all malignant gastrointestinal neoplasms. Symptoms occur late and the tumour has usually spread beyond the confines of the bowel wall by the time of diagnosis. There are four important malignant small bowel tumours:

- adenocarcinoma (40%)
- carcinoid tumours (30%)
- lymphoma (25%)
- mesenchymal tumours (5%).

In most cases, diagnosis is usually made at laparotomy for small bowel obstruction, however, the diagnostic modalities which may be useful include small bowel follow through, small bowel enema, small bowel enteroscopy, mesenteric angiography and CT. In some cases laparoscopic examination of small intestinal loops may be useful and enables biopsy of serosal and mesenteric masses.

Adenocarcinoma

Pathology

Adenocarcinomas are usually well or moderately differentiated mucus secreting tumours and are commonest in the proximal part of the small intestine (duodenum 40%, jejunum 40%, ileum 20%). The majority of duodenal carcinomas are found in the periampullary region and in the third part of the duodenum. Intestinal adenocarcinomas spread primarily to the regional lymph nodes, liver and peritoneal cavity.

Aetiology

The aetiology is unknown but adenocarcinomas are seen in hereditary polypoid syndromes (FAP and Peutz–Jeghers syndrome). There is also an increased risk in Crohn's disease and coeliac disease.

Clinical features

The median age at diagnosis is 60 years with an equal sex distribution. The symptoms include abdominal discomfort which is usually post-prandial and colicky in nature, nausea and vomiting particularly in patients with duodenal carcinomas and weight loss. Gastrointestinal bleeding may be occult leading to iron-deficiency anaemia but may also be overt leading to melaena or frank rectal bleeding. Intestinal obstruction indicates advanced disease although a relatively small polypoid tumour may lead to intussusception. Patients with duodenal carcinomas usually present with obstructive jaundice. The carcinoma which develops in Crohn's disease differs in a number of ways from those arising *de novo*. It occurs in a younger age group (40–50 years) predominantly in males (3:1) and affects the ileum in 75% of cases.

Diagnosis

The diagnosis of duodenal carcinoma is usually established using duodenoscopy (endoscopic retrograde cholangiopancreatography, ERCP). Jejunal and ileal tumours are most commonly identified by a small bowel contrast enema.

Prognosis

The 5 year survival for adenocarcinoma of the small intestine is in the region of 15%, although it appears that carcinomas arising in patients with Crohn's disease have an even worse prognosis. Duodenal carcinomas appear to have a better prognosis **[see Module 8: Disorders of the stomach and duodenum]**.

Treatment

Surgical resection is the mainstay of treatment as chemotherapy or radiotherapy does not appear to have a significant role. Duodenal tumours are best treated by pancreatic or duodenectomy (Whipple's operation) although segmental resection may be possible (Figure 13.13). Jejunal and ileal tumours are resected with a minimum of 5 cm of healthy margin on either side of the lesion together with the associated mesentery and regional lymph nodes. Carcinomas of the terminal ileum usually require formal right hemicolectomy.

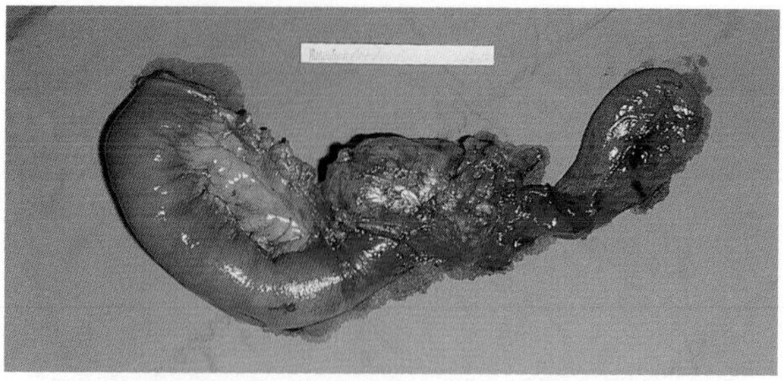

Figure 13.13 Segmental resection of carcinoma arising in the fourth part of the duodenum.

Carcinoid tumours

Pathology

Carcinoid tumours arise from the Kulchitsky cells of the crypts of Leiberkuhn. These are also referred to as the enterochromaffin cells as they stain with potassium chromate. Carcinoid tumours occur predominantly in the gastrointestinal tract and can be classified into three groups:

- *Foregut tumours* arise in the stomach, biliary tract and bronchus. These tumours consist of regularly shaped cells which assume a trabecular arrangement and contain round granules. They exhibit an argyrophilic reaction which indicates that the cells can only be stained with metallic silver in the presence of a reducing agent.
- *Mid gut tumours* are found in the jejunum, ileum and the right colon. The cells here are pleomorphic and are arranged in nests separated by connective tissue. These cells have both argentaffin (can be stained directly with metallic silver without reducing agent) and argyrophilic staining properties.
- *Hind gut tumours* occur in the left colon and rectum. The cells here are arranged in a trabecular pattern containing round granules but do not stain with silver.

Foregut tumours produce 5-hydroxytryptophan (5-HTP), 5-hydroxytryptamine (5-HT) (serotonin), histamine and substance P. Mid gut tumours produce 5-HT, kallikrein and possibly prostaglandins. Tumours of the hind gut do not usually secrete active peptides. In addition, mid gut and foregut tumours may contain and secrete a variety of hormones including insulin, somatastatin, adrenocorticotropic hormone (ACTH), gastrin, antidiuretic hormone (ADH), parathormone, glucagon, VIP, calcitonin, beta melanocyte-stimulating hormone (MSH), cholecystokinin and growth hormone. The cytology and histology cannot differentiate between benign and malignant carcinoid tumours. In general, tumours smaller than 1 cm are rarely malignant. Tumours between 1 and 1.9 cm may be malignant and tumours larger than 2 cm are usually invasive and exhibit metastatic spread. These more aggressive lesions invade the bowel wall mesentery, parietal peritoneum and adjacent organs. Metastatic spread involves the region lymph nodes and liver in particular but other sites such as the lung and the bones may be affected. The commonest sites of carcinoids of the gastrointestinal tract are the appendix, small intestine and the rectum in that order (see section on the appendix for further discussion of carcinoid tumour of the appendix).

Carcinoid tumours of the duodenum are rare. They tend to be similar in nature to other gastrointestinal carcinoids but there is an unusual type known as the carcinoid islet cell tumour which has the functional, morphological and histochemical features of both foregut carcinoids and pancreatic islet cell tumours (apudomas). In addition to serotonin, the tumour may also produce and secrete a variety of peptide hormones such as gastrin, insulin, parathyroid hormone and catecholamines causing bizarre clinical manifestations. Carcinoid tumours of the small intestine are most commonly encountered in the ileum. The majority are malignant, 40% are multiple and in 30% there is an associated malignant neoplasm, usually an adenocarcinoma.

Clinical features

The average age of reported cases of small intestinal carcinoid is between 45 and 55 years. Duodenal carcinoids may present with vomiting due to obstruction or as an endocrine syndrome. Carcinoids of the jejunum or ileum present with diarrhoea, intestinal obstruction, palpable abdominal mass and much less commonly, massive gastrointestinal haemorrhage or intestinal infarction. Occasionally the patient may present with symptoms of the carcinoid syndrome (see next section).

Treatment

Resection of the tumour with wide margins of healthy tissue, regional lymph nodes and associated mesentery is the standard treatment. Radiotherapy has been used for inoperable tumours but the results are disappointing.

Carcinoid syndrome

Pathology

The carcinoid syndrome is very rare, produced by less than 10% of all carcinoid tumours, and in the majority of cases the primary tumour originates in the small intestine. The syndrome is invariably associated with the presence of extensive hepatic involvement by tumour and the clinical manifestations are the result of inappropriate secretion of 5-HT, 5-HTP, kallikrein, histamine, prostaglandin and ACTH.

Clinical features

These include several types of flushing syndromes, intestinal colic and diarrhoea, bronchospasm, hypoproteinaemia oedema, cardiac lesions (tricuspid insufficiency or pulmonary stenosis), pellagra-like skin lesions (photosensitive dermatitis), neurological signs, peptic ulceration and neuralgia. The cutaneous flushing episodes affect the upper part of the body and are accompanied by sweating, itching, oedema, palpitations and hypotension.

Diagnosis

Biochemical confirmation of the diagnosis is achieved by the determination of the urinary metabolite of 5-HT and 5-HTP, 5-hydroxyindole acetic acid (5-HIAA). The intravenous administration of 2 μg of adrenaline results in a typical attack of flushing within 2 min of the injection but this test is no longer routine.

Treatment

Where possible hepatic deposits should be removed by segmental, lobar resection but this is not always feasible. Palliation can be obtained from reduction of the tumour volume by hepatic arterial embolization. Both resection and embolization should be covered with anti-serotonin therapy (cyproheptadine and parachlorophenylaline). Arterial embolization is performed percutaneously using a selective angiographic technique whereby the arteries feeding the metastases are blocked by gelatine sponge or human dura mater delivered in an antibiotic-containing solution and followed by steel coils. In addition to anti-serotonin therapy these patients must be covered by systemic antibiotics and steroids. More recently, *in situ* ablation of inoperable hepatic deposits by thermal ablation methods or cryotherapy has yielded excellent results [see Module 9: Disorders of the liver].

Lesser degrees of palliation can be obtained by chemotherapy. The drugs which have been shown to be useful are cyclophosphamide, adriamycin, 5-fluorourcil, 5-fluorodesoxyuridine and streptozotocin used singly or in combination. Good results are obtained by prolonged infusion chemotherapy through either the hepatic artery or a tributary of the portal vein. Prolonged access to the hepatic arterial tree is possible with the use of implantable subcutaneous chambers which have a silicone diaphragm allowing intermittent and prolonged infusions (Figure 13.14). Totally implantable infusion pumps are available but they are expensive and do not have any special advantage over implantable access systems connected to small portable battery power infusion pumps. Pre-treatment with anti-serotonin therapy is necessary to prevent a carcinoid crisis during chemotherapy. Anti-serotonin therapy can be undertaken with agents that either reduce the production of 5-HT or antagonize its effects. A combination of drugs tends to be more useful than single agent therapy (see Table 13.5 for anti-serotonin drugs).

Small bowel lymphoma

Pathology

An important distinction must be made between primary intestinal lymphoma and the much more common secondary involvement of the gastrointestinal tract by systemic nodal or extranodal disease. There are now agreed criteria for the diagnosis of primary intestinal lymphomas (Table 13.6) and it is likely that primary lymphoma accounts for less than 30% of all patients with intestinal involvement by lymphomatous disease.

Hodgkin's disease is extremely rare in the gut and accounts for only 1% of these tumours. Thus the vast majority of primary gut lymphomas are non-Hodgkin's and may be classified as B-cell lymphomas or T-cell lymphomas which can be further subdivided into low grade and high grade. The majority of these

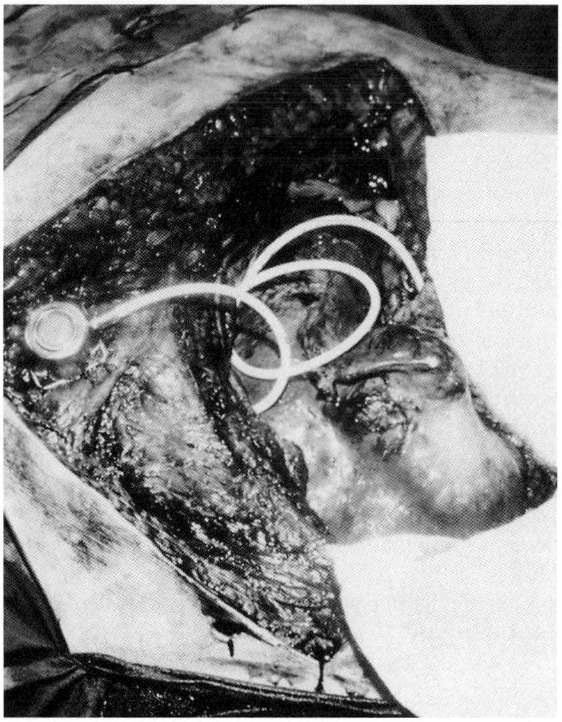

Figure 13.14 Port-A-Cath implantable venous/arterial access system. In this particular patient, the technique has been used for prolonged hepatic arterial infusion chemotherapy for hepatic secondary deposits. In between treatments, the system is left primed with heparinized saline.

are B-cell lymphomas arising from the centrocyte-like-cells of the mucosa associated lymphoid tissue (MALT) and referred to as MALT lymphomas. The classification of primary intestinal lymphomas is difficult and the Kiel classification is no longer considered appropriate. The suggested classification by Levison is shown in Table 13.7. The commonest types of intestinal lymphoma are the MALT lymphomas, the centrocytic lymphomas, Mediterranean lymphoma, Burkitt type lymphoma and the polymorphic T-cell lymphoma.

MALT lymphoma

Also known as polymorphic B-cell lymphomas, these are mostly low-grade tumours (predominantly small cell) with a tendency to remain localized for long periods and to metastasize late to other sites of mucosa-associated lymphoid tissue. Some tumours have a prominent large cell component. These are high-grade tumours and carry a less favourable prognosis. Microscopically the low-grade tumours form well-defined growths with deep invasion of the bowel wall and are usually single whereas the high-grade tumours involve extensive segments of the bowel and form large strictured lesions with a tendency to ulceration. Histologically the reactive B-cell follicles of the normal lymphoid tissue of the gut are surrounded by and infiltrated by neoplastic small to medium B-cells with an irregular nuclear contour which resemble centrocytes. For this reason they are known as centrocyte-like cells. The other characteristic feature of these tumours is the lympho-epithelial lesion which results when neoplastic centrocyte like cells invade and damage the crypt epithelium.

Centrocytic lymphomas

These account for 15% of primary intestinal lymphomas and form superficial diffuse lesions which do not invade deeply into the bowel wall. This results in a convoluted appearance of the mucosa suggesting multiple polyps and hence the alternative name of malignant lymphomatous polyposis. As opposed to other B-cell tumours surgical excision is not appropriate and the treatment is by chemotherapy. Another feature which distinguishes these primary gut tumours is the development of a centrocytic leukaemia and peripheral lymphadenopathy in most patients.

Mediterranean lymphoma

This is related to immunoproliferative small intestinal disease (IPSID) also known as alpha chain disease. IPSID occurs mainly in the Middle East, the Mediterranean basin and in South Africa. The diseased mucosa shows a heavy plasma cell and B-lymphocyte infiltration and the abnormal plasma cells secrete a fragment of IgA (alpha or heavy chain) which can be detected in the plasma and duodenal juice of affected patients. In some patients suffering from IPSID a malignant B-cell lymphoma develops but it is not clear whether IPSID is a benign disease which undergoes subsequent malignant change or whether lymphoma arises as a separate entity. Recent studies using molecular genetics show abnormal Ig gene rearrangement in both IPSID and

Table 13.5 Anti-serotonin drugs and their effects

Parachlorophenylalanie	Relieves diarrhoea
Phenoxybenzamine	Administered to achieve alpha blockade. It may relieve attack precipitated by emotion, diet, exercise and alcohol
Chlorpromazine	Has anti-kinin effects and may control flushing
Methysergide maleate	Most potent antagonist of 5-HT. May relieve flushing, diarrhoea and bronchospasm
Cyproheptadine	Less potent anti-serotonin agent. May relieve diarrhoea and less frequently reduce intensity of flushing
Prednisolone	May relieve facial oedema, diarrhoea and the flushing symptoms of bronchial carcinoids but not when the symptoms are caused by gastrointestinal tumours
Long-acting somatostatin analogue	Abolishes flushes due to gastrointestinal carcinoids and diarrhoea
Ketanserin	May reduce diarrhoea
Calcitonin	Same effects as somatostatin

Table 13.6 Criteria for the diagnosis of primary gut lymphoma

No palpable superficial lymphadenopathy
No mediastinal lymphadenopathy on chest radiograph/CT
Normal white cell count, normal bone marrow examination
Patient presents with gastrointestinal symptoms
Bowel lesion predominates at laparotomy and only regional lymph nodes are involved
Liver and spleen are not involved

Table 13.7 Proposed classification of primary gut lymphomas (Levison *et al.*)

B-cell lymphomas	
Low grade	*High grade*
Polymorphic B-cell[a]	Polymorphic B-cell[a]
Mediterranean lymphoma	Burkitt-type lymphoma
Centrocytic lymphoma[b]	Pure centroblastic
Plasmacytoma	Pure immunoblastic
Centroblastic–centrocytic	Unclassified
T-cell lymphomas	
Low grade	*High grade*
Small cell polymorphic[c]	Large cell polymorphic[c]
Epitheliotropic	Pure immunoblastic
	Large cell anaplastic
	Unclassified

[a]Also known as maltomas; low grade is predominantly small cell, high grade predominantly large cell. [b]Also known as malignant lymphomatous polyposis. [c]Can develop in patients with coeliac disease when it is referred to as enteropathy-associated T-cell lymphoma.

Mediterranean lymphoma indicting that IPSID is in fact a neoplastic condition.

The microscopic features of Mediterranean lymphoma are highly variable and range from diffuse thickening of the upper small intestine with enlargement of the associated mesenteric lymph nodes to localized, often multiple tumours. The histological features vary according to the stage of disease. Initially there is a diffuse infiltration of lamina propria by malignant plasma cells (stage A). Thereafter aggregations of centrocyte-like B-cells (stage B) and immunoblasts (stage C) appear and the picture becomes polymorphic. Although often extensive, Mediterranean lymphoma tends to remain confined until the late stages of the disease.

Burkitt type lymphoma

This primary high-grade B-cell lymphoma affects the ileocaecal region particularly in children, although other sites of origin may occur. It is an aggressive tumour which invades and permeates through the bowel wall at an early stage and is usually advanced at the time of presentation. There is a tendency to recur after surgical resection and for this reason resection should always be followed by adjuvant chemotherapy.

Polymorphic T-cell lymphoma

Formally known as malignant histiocytosis of the small intestine, this T-cell tumour is aetiologically related to coeliac disease. However, it can arise in the absence of this condition. The microscopic appearances are variable and although the tumour may occur in any part of the small bowel the jejunum is the commonest site. The lesion is often multi-focal and can form ulcers, strictures, plaques, nodules or diffuse thickening. In general the prognosis is poor and the disease tends to become disseminated at an early stage.

Staging of small bowel lymphoma

Small bowel lymphoma is commonly staged using the modified Ann Arbor clinical staging system (Table 13.8).

Aetiology

The aetiology of the majority of cases of small bowel lymphoma is unknown. However, certain predisposing disorders are well documented. These include coeliac disease, IPSID, ulcerative colitis and Crohn's disease, acquired immunodeficiency syndrome (AIDS) and other immunodeficiency states, e.g. transplant patients, chronic lymphatic leukaemia and long-term cyclophosphamide treatment for other forms of malignancy (e.g. carcinoma of the breast).

Clinical features

Small bowel lymphoma may occur at any age except in infancy but the peak incidence is in the sixth decade. A smaller peak is encountered in the first to third decades. In general, small bowel lymphomas are commoner in males with a reported sex ratio of 2:1. The presentation may be acute or insidious. In both the Middle East and the West these diseases often present as a surgical emergency with intestinal obstruction or a perforation leading to peritonitis. The intestinal obstruction may be due to intramural obstruction by a circumferential lesion or intussusception. The latter is particularly likely to occur with the ileocaecal tumours of childhood.

The chronic manifestations include malaise, abdominal pain, weight loss, diarrhoea and anaemia. The anaemia may be normochromic (chronic disease) or hypochromic microcytic (chronic occult bleeding). The erythrocyte sedimentation rate (ESR) is elevated and hypoproteinaemia is frequently present and results from a protein-losing enteropathy. In patients with coeliac disease the enteropathy associated lymphoma tends to occur in the fifth to the seventh decade. The symptoms of coeliac disease previously controlled by dietary management return and the patients complain of abdominal pain and diar-

Table 13.8 Modified Ann Arbor clinical staging of lymphoma

Stage I	Disease confined to a single extralymphatic organ
Stage II	Localized involvement of one organ or site + involvement of one or more lymph node groups on one side of the diaphragm:
II_1	Regional adjacent lymph node involvement
II_2	Regional but non-confluent lymph node involvement
Stage III	Localized involvement of organ or site + involvement of lymph node groups on both sides of the diaphragm
Stage IV	Diffuse disseminated disease with involvement of more than one organ + lymph node enlargement

rhoea with rapid weight loss. Perforation leading to peritonitis is a common presentation in these patients.

In the Middle East, IPSID is associated with growth retardation, malabsorption, bacterial overgrowth, hypoproteinaemia with oedema and ascites and parasitic infestations, particularly giardiasis. It can also present with intestinal obstruction, perforation and massive haemorrhage.

In all cases the commonest physical finding is a mobile abdominal mass.

Diagnosis

The diagnosis is often established by means of a small bowel contrast enema. More recently abdominal ultrasound CT scanning and laparoscopy have been useful diagnostic approaches. In IPSID the abnormal alpha chain is detected by immunocytochemistry of tumour sections and by immunoelectrophoresis with monospecific IgA antibody of serum and duodenal juice.

Treatment

Owing to its relative rarity, the treatment of gastrointestinal lymphoma is not standardized and there have been few clinical trials. All patients presenting with acute abdominal disease require surgical intervention and wherever possible the disease should be resected. Further treatment is then administered soon after recovery from the operation. This may consist of combination chemotherapy with drug regimens which are commonly used in Hodgkin's disease (CHOP, CMOPP, etc.) or radiotherapy. Radiotherapy is used less frequently as it is no more effective than chemotherapy and carries a high morbidity (bleeding and perforation in the early stage and radiation enteritis in the late stage).

In uncomplicated lymphoma, surgery followed by chemotherapy or radiotherapy is used for stage I and stage II of the disease. Chemotherapy alone is used for more advanced disease but the prognosis in these cases is extremely poor. Complete remissions have been reported in patients with IPSID whose biopsy shows plasmacytic infiltration after treatment with tetracycline or cytotoxic drugs but patients with established lymphoma are generally treated as outlined above. There is little role for surgical treatment in patients with malignant lymphomatous polyposis because of the widespread nature of the lesion, and reliance is placed on effective combination chemotherapy.

Mesenchymal tumours

Pathology

These include:

- smooth muscle tumours
- neurogenic tumours (Schwannomas)
- neoplasms of uncommitted mesenchymal cells, often considered as a less differentiated variant of leiomyomas.

More recently, the last group (tumours of uncommitted mesenchymal cells) has been classified as *gastrointestinal stromal tumours* (GISTs) separate from leiomyomas and leiomyosarcomas on the basis of their immunohistochemical staining characteristics. All are positive for c-kit (CD117) and CD34 and although some GISTs show positive staining for muscle actin, all are negative for desmin and S100-protein. The distinct genetic identity of GISTs has now been confirmed with DNA copy number losses in 14q not present in leiomyomas and leiomyosarcomas.

With all mesenchymal tumours the distinction between the benign and malignant forms is often impossible even on histological grounds. Mitotic activity is important in this respect although lesions with little or no mitotic activity have been known to recur or metastasize after excision. In general, however, malignant tumours are larger, more often ulcerated and exhibit marked cellularity and necrosis. The tumour can be confidently labelled as benign only if the patient is disease free for at least 3 years after surgical excision. Smooth muscle tumours may occur anywhere in the small intestine but are more commonly found in the jejunum and ileum.

The term *gastrointestinal sarcoma* covers smooth muscle, GIST and neurogenic tumours with malignant potential (as judged histologically). These sarcomas are rare. The commonest site is the stomach (50%), followed by small bowel and duodenum (30%).

Clinical features

The majority of tumours present in middle age (50–60 years) with a long history usually exceeding 12 months. The symptoms and signs including bleeding, abdominal pain, weakness and rarely weight loss. Acute presentation of intestinal obstruction or perforation can also occur. The most common clinical feature consists of repeated episodes of melena when the tumour is situated in the ileum or jejunum and frank haematemesis when it is in the duodenum. A palpable abdominal mass is present in about one-third of patients and this is usually mobile.

Some 20% are asymptomatic and may be found accidentally during operation, and 10–20% of gastrointestinal sarcomas present acutely with tumour perforation. Large tumours may cause massive intraperitoneal bleeding.

Diagnosis

Proximal lesions may be diagnosed by flexible endoscopy or push enteroscopy. Selective mesenteric angiography carries the highest diagnostic yield in patients with gastrointestinal bleeding as this may show either an abnormal tumour circulation or active haemorrhage into the small bowel lumen if the lesion is bleeding rapidly. A small bowel follow through or enema may also demonstrate the tumour.

Treatment

Smooth muscle tumours do not respond to radiotherapy or chemotherapy. The treatment is therefore surgical excision with a wide healthy margin together with the regional lymph nodes and associated mesentery.

Section 13.5 • Inflammatory conditions of the small bowel

Crohn's disease

Crohn's disease is an idiopathic chronic inflammatory condition which can affect any part of the gastrointestinal tract and may also be associated with systemic manifestations. The disease is localized in the ileocolic region in 60% of patients, to the small bowel alone in 20% and to the colon alone in a further 20%. Perianal disease is not uncommon and may accompany more proximal disease. Colorectal and perianal disease are dealt with in Module 14. Cases of Crohn's disease of the mouth, oesophagus and stomach are extremely rare.

The disease is most common in North America and Northern Europe and although the prevalence is increasing in Southern Europe it is relatively uncommon in other areas of the world. In the Far East it is almost never encountered.

Pathology

Irrespective of the site of involvement, Crohn's disease is a segmental condition with areas of involvement which are sharply demarcated from the contiguous normal bowel, at least on naked eye appearances. Particularly in small bowel disease, there may be several diseased segments with normal intervening bowel (skip lesions) but the number of such lesions is highly variable.

Macroscopic appearance

In early stages the disease appears as mucosal inflammation with small aphthoid ulcers. In more advanced disease the serosal surface of the affected bowel is granular and inflamed with a tendency for it to be encroached by mesenteric fat so that the intestine may at times by buried within a swollen oedematous and foreshortened mesentery. On palpation the involved areas feel heavy, thickened and firm as a result of the transmural inflammation which is usually associated with narrowing of the bowel lumen. Close inspection of the opened bowel reveals separation of the usual anatomical areas by fibrosis which is particularly marked in the submucosal and subserosal layers (Figure 13.15). The mucosal oedema accounts for the characteristic cobblestone appearance of the mucosa (Figure 13.16). This oedema is followed by sloughing and linear ulceration of the mucosa, particularly at the mesenteric attachements (Figure 13.17). Pseudopolyps and mucosal bridges may form and the ulcers which are typically deep and fissuring penetrate into the muscle layers and account for the tendency to localized perforation, adhesions and fistula formation. Regional lymphadenopathy is invariably present and usually the result of reactive hyperplasia.

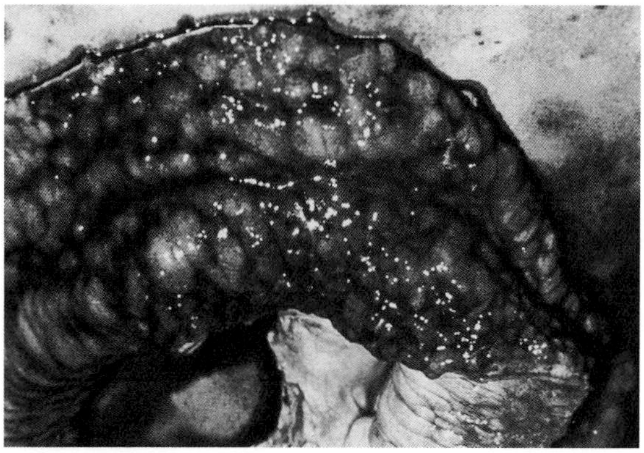

Figure 13.16 Diffuse mucosal/submucosal oedema resulting in the characteristic cobblestone appearance of the mucosa in Crohn's disease.

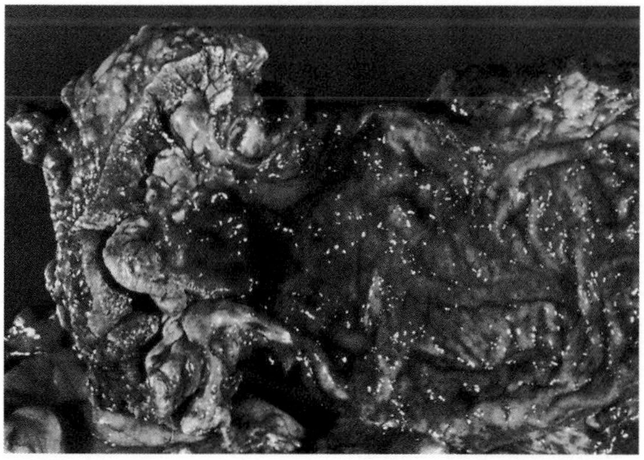

Figure 13.15 Crohn's disease of the ileocolic region. The affected bowel has been cut longitudinally to demonstrate the transmural fibrosis which is especially marked in the subserous and submucosal layers.

Fistula formation is an important feature of Crohn's disease and accounts for substantial morbidity, long periods of debility and a 5–10% mortality following surgical treatment. The fistulous tracts may be simple or complex and often incorporate intervening or associated abscesses. The important varieties of fistula encountered in Crohn's disease are:

- *Enterocutaneous fistulas*. Some 20–30% of these may heal with drainage of the associated abscess and parenteral nutrition.
- *Perianal fistulas*. These may be associated with severe anorectal disease but not in all cases.
- *Ileocolonic fistulas*. These can lead to diarrhoea and severe bacterial overgrowth of the small intestine leading to malabsorption and malnutrition.

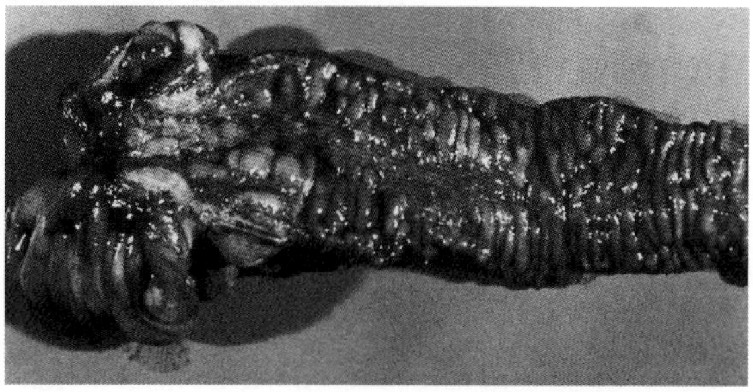

Figure 13.17 Extensive ulceration with stricture formation in Crohn's disease of the distal ileum. The longitudinal ulceration is more prominent along the mesenteric attachment.

- *Enterovesical fistulas*. These may involve the ileum or the colon or both and usually develop in patients with long-standing disease. Enterovesical fistulas are less common than the other varieties and have a reported incidence of about 5%. They usually follow a benign course and present with dysuria, pneumaturia and recurrent pyelonephritis. They do not respond to conservative measures and require surgical intervention.

Microscopic appearances

The histological features of Crohn's disease are characterized by a transmural inflammation consisting of chronic inflammatory cell infiltrates including eosinophils, crypt abscess formation, oedema, non-caseating epitheliod cell granulomas containing giant cells (Langerhans' cells), dilatation and sclerosis of the intestinal lymphatics and lymphoid aggregates with or without germinal centres. These are all found in the various layers of the bowel wall associated with epithelial regenerative changes and angiitis. These granulomas, which resemble those found in sarcoidosis, are found in the bowel wall in 50–60% of cases and to a lesser extent (25%) in the regional lymph nodes. The epithelial regenerative changes include the development of pseudopyloric gland metaplasia. The non-caseating granuloma is the most important criterion for the histological diagnosis of Crohn's disease and if this is not present it can be very difficult to make the distinction between Crohn's disease and ulcerative colitis when the disease affects the large intestine.

Aetiology

The aetiology of Crohn's disease remains obscure. However, the various hypotheses may be considered under the following headings: *genetic factors*, *environmental factors*, *infective agents*, *immunological factors* and *vasculitis*.

Genetic factors

There is a familial tendency to develop Crohn's disease and about 10% of patients have an affected first degree relative. There is no consistent human leucocyte antigen (HLA) association but patients with ankylosing spondylitis are at greater risk of Crohn's disease than the general population and this association appears to be linked with tissue type HLA B27. Recently, a susceptibility locus for Crohn's disease has been mapped on chromosome 16, and this has opened out exciting possibilities for both the diagnosis and treatment of this condition.

Environmental factors

The possible role of diet has been widely investigated and is thought to account for the large geographical differences in the prevalence of Crohn's disease. There do not appear to be reliable data linking fibre consumption with Crohn's disease but several studies show a high intake of refined carbohydrates by Crohn's patients compared with appropriate controls. Smoking is probably an important factor with smokers having a greater risk than those who have never smoked. This is in contrast with ulcerative colitis where smoking appears to be protective. There also appears to be an increased risk of Crohn's disease in women taking oral contraceptives.

Infective agents

There is little epidemiological support for the suggestion that Crohn's disease may be infective. Investigations for evidence of clustering in time or space have not been able to demonstrate any evidence of person to person transmission and studies on health care professionals dealing with Crohn's patients do not indicate an increased risk. However, some work suggests that low virulence bacterial yeast or chlamydia organisms may be responsible and two particular types of bacteria have been extensively investigated.

The variant or L-form bacteria have deficient cell walls and can develop from several bacterial species after exposure to antibiotics. The cell wall protein deficiency is accompanied by an alteration in virulence, antigenicity and pathogenicity. However, these variant bacteria which can pass through filters holding back normal bacteria can in time and under certain conditions revert back to their original form. *Pseudomonas maltophilia* is a variant bacterial species which has been isolated from intestinal Crohn's disease.

Mycobacterium paratuberculosis is an atypical mycobacterium which has been isolated from patients with Crohn's disease and on innoculation has been shown to produce granulomas in animals. In addition, patients with Crohn's disease have been shown to have IgG antibodies against this organism. However, the antibody levels do not bear any relation to disease activity and their level is not altered by resection of diseased bowel. Recent studies of DNA hybridization have revealed mycobacterial genomes in the tissues of patients with Crohn's disease providing further indirect evidence of the role of the organism in Crohn's disease.

Immunological factors

Although humoral immune responses appear to be normal in patients with Crohn's disease, cell mediated immune function may be defective. Some patients have impaired skin hypersensitivity, a reduction in circulating T-lymphocytes and a poor response to non-specific mitogens. It is quite possible however that these observed defects result from the disease itself or associated malnutrition rather than being aetiological factors. An abnormal permeability of the mucosal epithelium is well documented and it is possible that this could lead to exposure of the subepithelial immune cells to foreign protein, thus setting up an immune reaction in the wall of the intestine. This theory is supported by the favourable response of Crohn's disease to an elemental diet.

Vasculitis

A new hypothesis has emerged following the demonstration of intestinal vascular pathology (vasculitis) early in the evolution of Crohn's disease. These findings suggest that multi-focal gastrointestinal infarction may be the cause of Crohn's disease. This theory however remains unsubstantiated.

Clinical features

The peak incidence of Crohn's disease is in the third decade and it occurs with the same frequency in females as in males. It may however also affect children and the elderly. In the latter age group it is frequently colonic and accompanied by diverticular disease. The clinical manifestations of Crohn's disease are extremely varied and depend on the location and the extent of disease. There are also a number of complications which can determine the presenting features. The 'syndromes' by which Crohn's disease can present include the pseudo-appendicitis syndrome, small bowel obstruction, abscess formation, fistula formation, diarrhoea, growth retardation and portal venous gas.

Pseudo-appendicitis syndrome

Some patients with Crohn's disease of the terminal ileum develop acute abdominal pain, the severity and location of which simulate acute appendicitis. As many as 14% of children and young adults with Crohn's disease present in this manner. This clinical presentation is of particular importance as acute terminal ileitis often due to *Yersinia* infection is often encountered in many instances and has a very different natural history from that of Crohn's disease. Approximately one in eight cases of acute terminal ileitis are actually due to Crohn's disease. Accordingly, in the emergency situation the treatment should be conservative. The appendix should be removed if the caecum appears normal and swabs taken from the luminal contents for bacteriological culture. Appendicectomy will prevent further diagnostic dilemmas at a later stage. However, if the caecum and the base of the appendix appear to be affected by disease, appendicectomy should not be carried out as this may lead to fistula formation.

Small bowel obstruction

Crohn's disease of the small bowel gives rise to abdominal pain because of acute or subacute small bowel obstruction (Figure 13.18). Complete small bowel obstruction is relatively rare. Patients with intermittent self-limiting obstructive episodes invariably have gross bacterial overgrowth which may give rise to further malabsorption, hypoproteinemia and malnutrition.

Abscess formation

This is a common presentation. Abscesses may result either from bowel perforation which may occur at the site of a deep fissuring ulcer or proximal to a stricture. They can also arise in a mass of inflamed regional lymph nodes without perforation of the bowel. Apart from the local signs and symptoms, abscess formation leads to malaise, weight loss, fever and anorexia. The commonest site of abscess formation is in the right iliac fossa. This may track into the pelvis along the psoas muscle underneath the inguinal ligament and present as a tender groin mass (psoas abscess). Free perforation of Crohn's disease into the peritoneal cavity with widespread peritonitis is extremely unusual.

Fistula formation

The most common type is perianal which usually occurs in association with perianal abscesses and sinuses (Figure 13.19). These perianal complications are a significant feature of Crohn's disease and may be present months or years before intestinal symptoms are noticed. Enterocutaneous fistulas usually become evident following drainage of abdominal abscesses and can be classified as high or low-output in terms of the amount of intestinal contents which discharge everyday. Spontaneous closure with parenteral nutrition is more likely in the

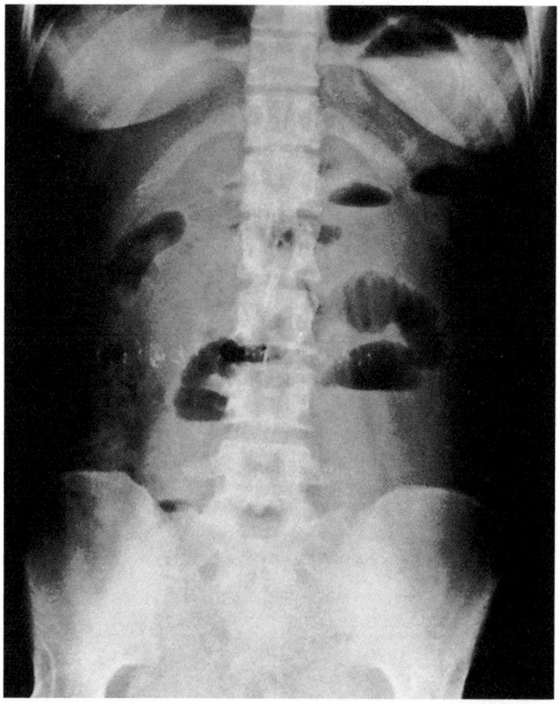

Figure 13.18 Plain erect abdominal film showing air/fluid levels in a stepladder pattern due to mechanical bowel obstruction. The patient had had a right hemicolectomy for Crohn's disease. Such an obstructive picture may be due to adhesions or recurrence which is most commonly situated at the level of the previous anastomosis.

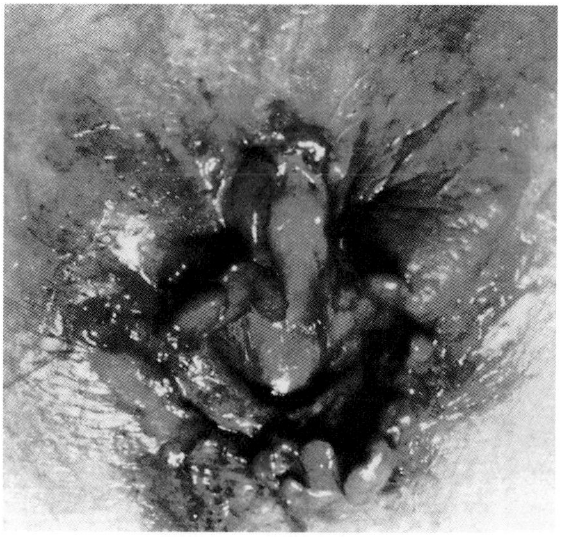

Figure 13.19 Extensive anal and perianal disease in a patient with Crohn's colitis. The patient had a high fistula-*in ano.*

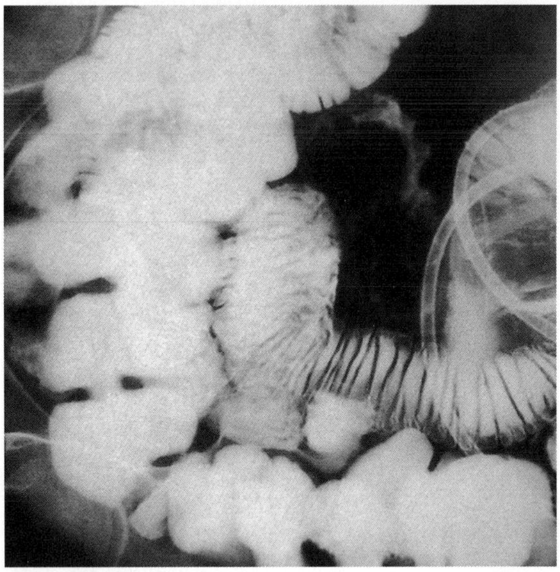

Figure 13.20 Barium study demonstrating a fistula between the small bowel and the colon in a patient with Crohn's disease.

low output variety. Enterocolic fistulas are associated with bacterial overgrowth, malabsorption and frequently diarrhoea (Figure 13.20). Enterovesical fistulas due to Crohn's disease do not usually cause severe systemic disturbance and present with urinary symptoms.

Diarrhoea

Diarrhoea occurs in about 70–80% of patients with Crohn's disease. It is particularly common in patients with terminal ileal involvement and this is thought to be related to the failure of the terminal ileum to reabsorb bile salts. Diarrhoea associated with colonic disease is accompanied by the passage of mucus and blood from the rectum and is very similar to the symptomatology of ulcerative colitis. Such diarrhoea is often accompanied by a protein-losing enteropathy and steatorrhoea due to bacterial overgrowth or bile salt malabsorption.

Growth retardation

This occurs in approximately 20% of all children with Crohn's disease. Failure to thrive in children with Crohn's disease has four basic components:

- Impairment of linear growth.
- Weight loss or failure to gain weight.
- Delayed sexual maturation and closure of the epiphyses
- Normal endocrinological parameters.

Thyroid function in these children is consistently normal and so is growth hormone secretion when several provocative tests are employed. The major factor in growth retardation is malnutrition which is due to failure to eat because of high-grade partial intermittent small bowel obstruction, protein and blood loss from the ulcerated inflamed areas of the small bowel and malabsorption due to bacterial overgrowth. When assessing the potential growth of these children it is crucial to evaluate their bone age and to note the stature of their parents. In this way it is possible to predict which children would be capable of responding to therapeutic intervention (including parenteral nutrition). Following an appropriate bowel resection growth resumes the normal pattern but compensatory growth does not occur. It is therefore essential to treat these children while their bones are still capable of growth. Fortunately in many of these teenagers closure of the epiphyses is delayed because of the associated malnutrition.

Portal venous gas

This potentially fatal complication has been described in patients with Crohn's disease. The patient develops severe toxicity with high fever and rigors and severe diarrhoea. The gas in the portal vein is best detected by abdominal CT scanning and indicates portal bacteraemia. All patients who develop this complication have active disease. Treatment of this complication is not standardized as it is a very rare complication but broad spectrum antibiotics active against both Gram-negative aerobes and anaerobes, steroids and intravenous fluids are generally recommended in the first instance with laparotomy and resection of the diseased segment of bowel if there is no improvement.

Diagnosis

The diagnosis of Crohn's disease rests on the evaluation of clinical signs and symptoms which are correlated with endoscopic, radiological and histological findings. In small bowel disease endoscopy and biopsy has a very small role to play, largely because enteroscopy is not widely available and biopsy via an enteroscope is not generally practical.

Certain laboratory tests are important to establish the nutritional state of the patients and as an index of disease activity. A full blood count, ESR, serum electrolytes, serum proteins and in particular serum albumin are important. Decreased serum albumin, hypochromic microcytic anaemia and low serum iron may be found in as many as 50% of untreated patients. Occasionally, a megaloblastic anaemia may be observed as a result of folic acid deficiency or impaired vitamin B_{12} absorption. Hypocalcaemia, hypomagnesaemia, low serum level of zinc and low serum vitamin A may also be present reflecting impaired absorption or decreased ingestion. Frank malabsorption with steatorrhoea may be present in patients with extensive small bowel disease or bacterial overgrowth. In these patients the Schilling test or the SeHCAT test may prove useful in defining the presence of malabsorption of vitamin B_{12} and bile salts respectively. Bacterial overgrowth is documented by the hydrogen breath tests and the oral ^{14}C-glycocholate test. Important indices of disease activity are:

- ESR
- serum alpha-1-glycoprotein level
- C reactive protein
- OKT9 lymphocyte positivity.

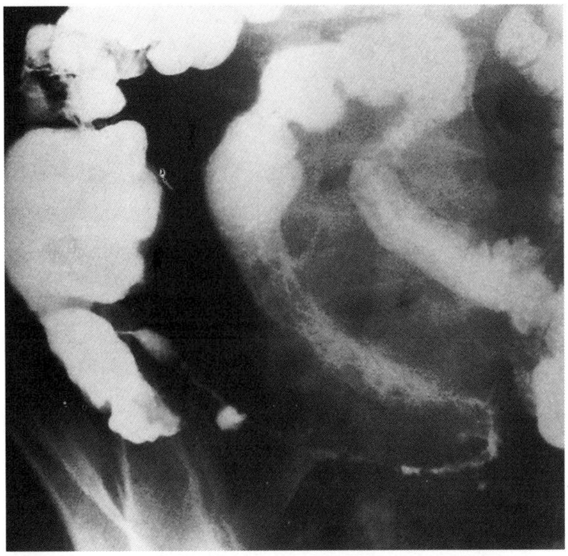

Figure 13.21 Small bowel enema showing several features of Crohn's disease of the distal ileum: stenosis (Kantor's string sign), cobblestoning of the mucosa, deep globular ulcer (pseudodiverticulum), deep penetrating fissure ulcers, wide separation of the intestinal loops due to thickening of the bowel walls and thickening of the ileocaecal valve due to lymphatic blockage and oedema. The patient presented with intermittent cramp-like abdominal pain after meals.

Radiological appearances
In small bowel disease affected segments are most commonly demonstrated by means of a small bowel enema or follow through. Narrowing of the lumen, nodularity of the mucosal pattern, thickening of the ileocaecal valve, mucosal irregularity and deep ulcerations perpendicular to the intestinal lumen (rose thorn ulceration) and fistula formation are all characteristic features of Crohn's disease. Long narrow strictures result in the well-known string sign of Kantor (Figure 13.21). Skip lesions are characteristic with normal bowel in between the strictured or diseased areas. Fistulas and sinuses may be evaluated by injection of contrast media following insertion of catheters of the appropriate size to ensure a close fit. More recently the use of magnetic resonance imaging (MRI) scanning has provided detailed appreciation of the pathological anatomy of the fistula and is especially useful in complex types with multiple and branched tracts.

Complications
Although intestinal obstruction abscess formation and fistula formation are technically complications of Crohn's disease, they are so common that they are usually regarded as integral clinical features of the disease. Crohn's disease may however be accompanied by systemic manifestations of inflammatory bowel disease. These include sclerosing cholangitis, skin problems such as pyoderma gangrenosum and erythema nodosum, arthritis and uveitis. A more detailed description of the systemic manifestation in Crohn's disease is given in the appropriate section of the colorectal module.

In addition to enterovesical fistulas the urological complications of Crohn's disease include an obstructive uropathy and an increased incidence of renal calculi. The obstructive uropathy is caused by retroperitonitis and fibrosis leading to obstruction of the ureter (usually on the right) and is more frequent than is clinically appreciated (Figure 13.22). Patients with obstructive uropathy are usually totally asymptomatic although occasionally pyuria, bacteriuria and pain in the renal angles are observed. If untreated obstructive uropathy can lead to severe hydronephrosis, recurrent pyonephrosis and loss of functional renal tissue. Imaging of the kidneys is therefore an important part of the work-up of patients with Crohn's disease using either intravenous urography or cross-sectional imaging (ultrasound or CT scanning). Renal calculi have been reported in 10% of patients with Crohn's disease and in most of these patients the duration of disease has been long standing. Calcium oxalate or phosphate stones account for 72% of cases and uric acid stones for 18%. Some 10% of the renal calculi cannot be classified. Only 36% of patients with renal stones have a predisposing urinary tract abnormality such as sponge kidney, obstructive uropathy or a metabolic disorder such as hypercalcaemia. Increased absorption of oxalate and increased cell turnover in the gut and a concentrated urine appear to be important factors in the formation of renal calculi in patients with Crohn's disease. A prevalence of renal stones in children with Crohn's disease is said to be as much as 25%.

There is also an increased incidence of gallstone formation in patients with severe ileal Crohn's disease or following ileal resections. This is attributable to malabsorption of bile salts with interruption of the enterohepatic circulation and a consequent reduction of the bile salt pool. In addition, there is now a well-established association between Crohn's disease and small bowel adenocarcinoma. These tumours occur at a younger age and are located predominantly in the distal ileum. Cases of small bowel lymphoma and carcinoid tumours have also been reported in patients with Crohn's disease.

Treatment
Owing to the fact that Crohn's disease is a chronic relapsing condition, its treatment is difficult and often unsatisfactory. In broad terms it can be divided into medical and surgical treatment.

Medical treatment
Medical treatment can be further subdivided into dietary modifications, parenteral nutrition and drug treatment.

Dietary modification
In patients with extensive disease the first priority is to correct deficiencies including vitamins (especially A), magnesium and zinc. Iron-deficiency anaemia is treated with oral supplements preferably in the glutamate form. There are various reports of benefit derived from

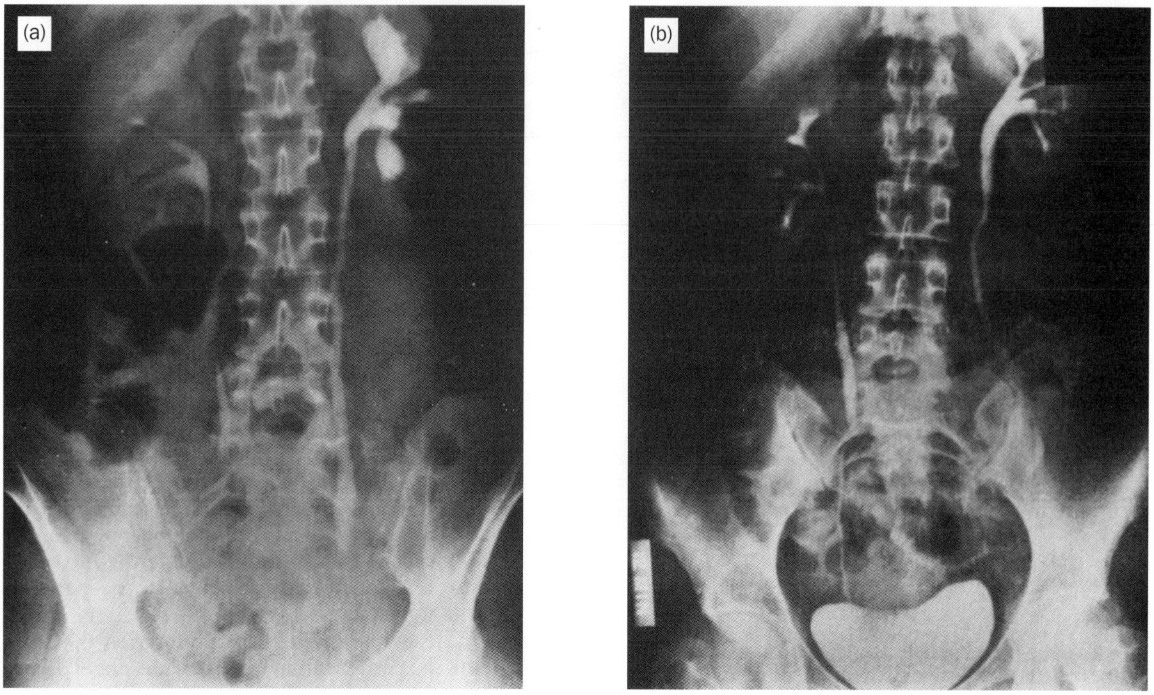

Figure 13.22 (a) Intravenous urogram demonstrating an obstructive uropathy on the left side. The patient had Crohn's disease of the ileum with fistula formation involving the sigmoid colon and resulting severe inflammation of the retroperitoneal tissue on the left side. (b) Same patients 1 month following bowel resection and ureterolysis. These is complete resolution of the left hydronephrosis and hydroureter.

high-fibre, low refined sugar diets and from the use of exclusion diets. In the latter, patients are started on distilled water and then items of food introduced and maintained or withdrawn according to whether or not they aggravate the condition. It appears that the most common dietary components which require exclusion are dairy products and wheat. There is some evidence for the benefit of an elemental diet (e.g. vivonex, flexical or ensure) in suppressing mucosal inflammation. The effect of elemental diets is thought to result from a reduction of the foreign protein load presented to the inflamed mucosa. The problems with long-term use of elemental diets include their expense and their unpalatability which reduces compliance in the long term.

Parenteral nutrition

This is of value in the following cases:

- Intestinal failure with gross nutritional deficiencies and severe hypoalbuminaemia.
- Malnourished patients prior to surgery.
- In obtaining remission in patients with severe active disease.
- In patients with enterocutaneous fistulas.

Long-term home parenteral nutrition is reserved for patients with extensive small bowel disease or resection and intestinal failure. The patients are taught to self-administer the parenteral feeds and to look after their central lines and it offers a reasonable quality of life. Some patients require only intermittent supplemental intravenous feeding and manage reasonably well with modified or elemental diets in the intervening periods. Home parenteral nutrition is supervised by the medical and nursing staff of specialized nutrition units.

Intravenous feeding is necessary on a short-term basis for patients with complications requiring elective surgical intervention but who are malnourished. Improvement to the nutritional status and elevation of the serum albumin above 3 g/l is essential for the safe healing of intestinal anastomoses. Some 30% of enterocutaneous fistulas due to Crohn's disease may heal spontaneously with the use of parenteral nutrition but persistence of a fistula beyond 6 weeks indicates failure of this approach and the need for surgical intervention.

Some advocate cessation of oral feeding and total parenteral nutrition for several weeks to achieve remission in active Crohn's disease. Although the immediate results of this approach are good, relapse is almost invariable within 3 months of resumption of oral intake.

Glutamine added to either parenteral or enteral diets improves intestinal healing and nitrogen utilization. In experimental colitis, glutamine also increases the survival rate. Folate requirements are increased by poor intake, malabsorption and faecal losses. Treatment with sulphasalazine (see next section) may aggravate folate deficiency. Supplemental folate therapy (0.2 mg/day) is indicated during acute exacerbations and particularly during parenteral nutrition. Reduced serum concentrations of trace elements (zinc, copper and selenium) are also found in patients with severe active inflammatory bowel disease and require correction as they are essential components of metalloenzymes and metalloproteins. Selenium is particularly important as it is an essential constituent of the detoxifying enzyme glutathione peroxidase and enhances the activity of the cytoprotective enzyme superoxide dismutase that has antioxidant activity against reactive radicals of oxygen.

Drug therapy

In the mild and moderately active Crohn's disease and for the maintenance of remission, the initial treatment of choice is 5-aminosalicylic acid (5-ASA). Salazopyrin, which is a combination of 5-ASA and sulphonamide, is inexpensive and effective for colonic disease but is not recommended for small bowel disease. In addition, it has quite prominent side-effects including headaches, nausea and oligospermia. Preparations containing 5-ASA alone are now widely used and are formulated to allow targeting of the drug at sites of active disease. Slow-release mesalazine (Pentasa) or pH-dependent release mesalazine (Asacol) are specifically designed for small bowel and right colonic disease. Although 5-ASA is now recognized as useful for the maintenance of remission in Crohn's disease its place after resection of all microscopically obvious disease in the small bowel is not clear.

Cortiscosteroids, both intravenous and oral, remain the most appropriate treatment for severe disease or cases not responding to 5-ASA therapy. They may also be necessary to maintain remission. Budesonide, a highly potent semi-synthetic steroid which exhibits considerable first pass metabolism in the liver, is highly effective and is now available in a controlled release preparation (Entocort) for the treatment of ileal and right colonic Crohn's disease. Trials have indicated that budesonide 5 mg/day as a single morning dose is as effective as 40 mg of prednisolone daily, and as budesonide has significantly reduced steroid associated side-effects it may become the drug of choice in the management of patients with active Crohn's disease.

It is important to appreciate, however, that both 5-ASA and corticosteroids are far from ideal and both are associated with significant failure and relapse rates, with only about 30% of patients achieving and maintaining remission for 2 years. Indeed with steroid treatment, although symptoms improve, there is little or no evidence to indicate that mucosal inflammatory disease itself resolves.

For particularly severe disease which relapses or is dependent on steroids there are a number of modulators of the cellular immune response which can be used. Azathioprine and 6-mercaptopurine are both useful in Crohn's disease and azathioprine can induce remission in approximately 70% of resistant cases. Other immune modulators which may be of value in unresponsive patients include cyclosporin and this appears to be particularly useful in fistulating Crohn's disease. Methotrexate has also been useful and may achieve remission in difficult cases.

All the widely used medications for Crohn's disease carry a significant risk of side-effects and for this reason there has been a lot of work in recent years to try to target therapy at more specific components of the immune response. Tumour necrosis factor alpha (TNFα) is a cytokine which appears to be central in the inflammatory response in Crohn's disease, and anti-TNFα monoclonal antibody therapy has been used in several studies. This antibody (infliximab) seems to be particularly efficacious in fistulating disease with a relatively low incidence of adverse effects.

Antibiotics have their place, particularly in the treatment of perianal Crohn's disease, but it has also been shown that broad spectrum antibiotics (ciprofloxacin and metronidazole) can induce symptomatic remission in active Crohn's disease with a similar efficacy to that of corticosteroids. Symptomatic treatment for diarrhoea includes the administration of loperamide or codeine phosphate and non-addictive analgesics for the abdominal pain. Cholestyramine may improve steatorrhoea in patients with extensive ileal disease or resection.

Surgical treatment

Owing to the chronic relapsing nature of Crohn's disease surgical treatment can never be regarded as curative but it has an extremely important role to play and it is important that all patients with Crohn's disease should have the benefit of a combined medical and surgical approach. Surgical intervention is indicated for the complications of the disease and for active disease which has not responded to medical therapy. It has to be borne in mind that there is considerable morbidity associated with the surgical treatment and about half of the deaths of patients with Crohn's disease are associated with operative intervention. It has to be appreciated, however, that patients coming to surgery for Crohn's disease often have serious complications of the disease.

In broad terms the indications for surgical intervention are as follows:

- Complications.
- Failure of medical management with persistence of severe symptoms.
- Complications of medical management and in particular steroid side-effects in patients requiring large doses to maintain remission.

Of the complications of small bowel Crohn's disease which require surgical intervention, the following are the commonest:

- Small bowel obstruction.
- Development of abscesses and fistulas.
- Growth retardation in children.
- Development of obstructive uropathy.
- Massive haemorrhage (rare).

Other factors which influence the decision to operate and the type of operative procedure include the anatomical site of the disease, the surgeon's preference and expertise and whether the operation is being performed as an emergency or as an elective procedure. The extragastrointestinal manifestations of Crohn's disease are rarely, if ever, an indication for operative intervention and certainly in small bowel disease resection does not appear to have a major effect in this respect.

When making an abdominal incision it should be planned with attention paid to previous incisions and the siting of a stoma. Laparoscopic assisted surgery is appropriate for a relatively small proportion of patients with isolated terminal ileal disease where a limited right hemicolectomy is required. The vast majority of patients, however, require open surgery. At laparotomy, an initial exploration is carried out to determine the extent and severity of the disease and to establish the state of the liver and the presence and otherwise of gallstones. Adhesions which are often present are taken down and the anatomy and the length of the small intestine is ascertained.

The emphasis of modern surgical treatment for small bowel disease is on the maximal preservation of intestine with resections being strictly limited to the diseased segment causing the symptom or complication. Bypass should only be carried out when there is no other alternative, as blind loops encourage bacterial overgrowth, increased incidence of abscess and fistula formation and risk of developing carcinoma. In deciding the extent of small bowel resection a balance must be struck between removing all grossly diseased bowel and retaining sufficient for adequate absorption and nutritional support. Macroscopic assessment of the disease is used to determine the extent of the resection and the important appearances include thickening of the bowel wall and mesentery, hyperaemia and oedema, fat encroachment of the bowel and the presence of ulcers at the resection line. It is now established that areas of minimal disease may be safely left as there is no evidence that microscopic disease at the resection margin reduces the recurrence rate. Skip lesions in the vicinity of the main disease process may be safely excised *en-bloc* but those at a distance should be resected separately if considered significant.

Conservative (non-resectional) surgery is particularly indicated in patients with multiple previous resections and in those with multiple strictures. In order to determine whether or not a small area of disease is causing a significant stricture, it is useful to manipulate the balloon of a Fogarty catheter along the lumen of the bowel introduced via an enterotomy. This will give some indication as to the size of the lumen at the strictured site. If the stricture admits the passage of an 18–20 mm inflated balloon, intervention is probably not necessary.

Stricturoplasty is now widely used for the treatment of strictures. The type of procedure used depends on the length of the stricture, a Heinecke–Mickulicz stricturoplasty being ideal for short stenotic areas (Figure 13.23) and the Finney equivalent for long strictures (Figure 13.24). The decision between a stricturoplasty and a resection for a long stenotic segment is dependent on surgical experience and expertise and it has to be remembered that stricturoplasty is associated with post-operative morbidity including a leak rate of around about 5%. Although there are no prospective randomized trials the immediate outcome of stricturoplasty appears to be similar to that encountered after resection for small bowel Crohn's disease and there is no evidence that there is a significant increased risk of recurrence after stricturoplasty.

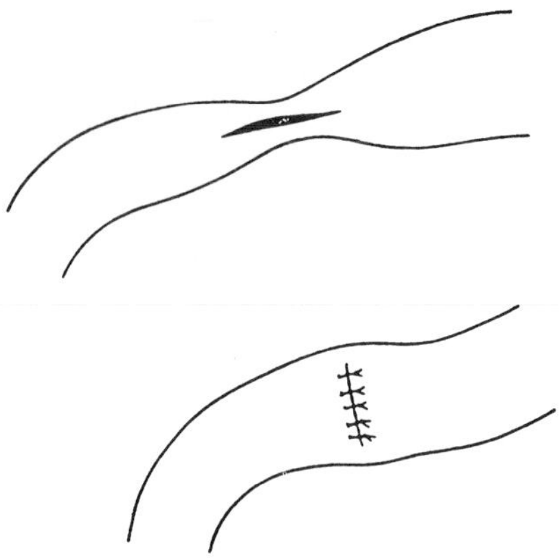

Figure 13.23 Diagrammatic representation of the technique of stricturoplasty. This operation is suitable for patients with short strictures in the absence of active inflammation. An operative biopsy of the stricture with frozen section histology is advisable to exclude carcinoma.

Compared to resection, stricturoplasty is not appropriate in the presence of sepsis (abscess) and fistula, both of which are best treated by resection. Adhesions and fistulas between diseased segments of bowel and adjacent hollow viscous are dealt with by careful separation of the diseased segment from the adjacent structure with debridement and primary closure of the latter. External fistulas are managed by similar excision with debridement and closure of the abdominal wall but not of the skin and the subcutaneous tissues. Secondary wound closure is performed several days later. If there is a mass involving several loops of bowel the surgeon must carefully identify and dissect healthy from diseased bowel. Provided that the length involved is not great a resection *en masse* may be performed. After the small bowel resections have been completed the length of the residual small intestine must be measured along the anti-mesenteric border and recorded.

Free perforation into the peritoneal cavity is rare in Crohn's disease and the commonest site is the ileum. Resection of the diseased segment with peritoneal

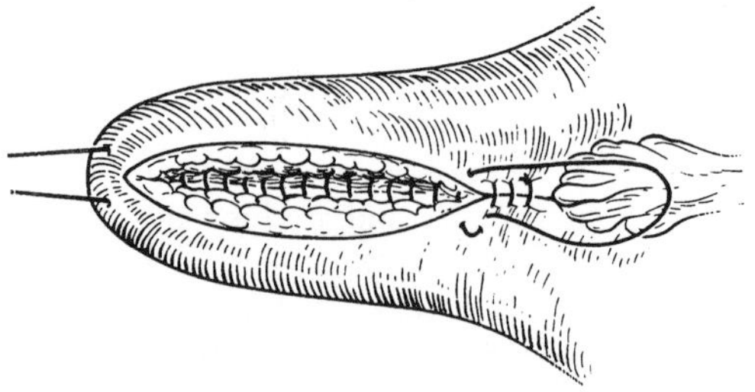

Figure 13.24 Diagrammatic representation of Finney-type stricturoplasty for long stenosed segments of Crohn's disease.

lavage and debridement is the treatment of choice. Primary anastomosis or exteriorization is performed depending on the duration and the severity of the peritoneal inflammation. Simple drainage of an abscess invariably results in a fistula. As described above, some 30% of enterocutaneous fistulas may heal with total parenteral nutrition but persistence of the fistula beyond 6 weeks is an indication for surgical intervention with excision of the diseased segment of bowel. Enterocolic and enterovesical fistulas never heal by conservative management and always require surgical intervention. Perforation of the diseased bowel into the retroperitoneal tissues causes intense fibrosis and retroperitoneal inflammation resulting in an obstructive uropathy. Although the obstructed ureter may be asymptomatic the renal impairment may be progressive and permanent. As a result, obstructive uropathy is an absolute indication for surgery and is best relieved by appropriate bowel resection and ureterolysis.

Operations for Crohn's disease are followed by a high incidence (10–15%) of post-operative complications such as anastomotic leakage, fistula formation, intra-abdominal abscess and haemorrhage. The overall reported mortality rate ranges from 2 to 8%. A high mortality is associated with emergency operations (up to 30%). Late post-operative complications include short bowel syndrome, urinary lithiasis, cholelithiasis, gastric hypersecretion and peptic ulcer disease.

One of the unresolved problems is the high incidence of recurrence following resection. The cumulative recurrence after resection of small intestinal Crohn's disease is 30% at 5 years, 50% at 10 years, and 60% at 15 years. Young patients and those with ileocolic disease have the highest and earliest recurrence and the worst ultimate prognosis. After resection, maintenance medical therapy does not appear to influence recurrence rate. The prognosis of patients with Crohn's colitis undergoing proctocolectomy is better in this respect as the development of ileal disease occurs in 10 and 20% of these patients at 5 and 10 years, respectively. After abdominal colectomy and ileorectal anastomosis the reported recurrence rate averages 50% at 5 years. The majority of recurrences occur at or near the anastomosis and in patients with ileorectal anastomosis the recurrent disease often involves the ileum and further resection does not necessarily require proctectomy and ileostomy. In assessing the divergent reported figures for recurrence rates after surgical intervention for Crohn's disease two points must be stressed.

- The recurrence rate rises gradually with the duration of follow-up.
- It is essential to differentiate patients with true recurrent Crohn's disease with those requiring re-operations for other complications including ileostomy revisions.

Many patients with Crohn's disease undergo multiple resections and a significant percentage of these develop the short gut syndrome. At present the majority of these patients are managed by home parenteral nutrition which may be complicated by catheter sepsis, venous thrombosis and parenchymal liver disease. Recently the development of more effective immunosuppressive drugs (cyclosporin especially) and the discovery of the protective effect of a concurrent liver transplant (especially on graft versus host disease) has led to the successful use of combined hepatic and small bowel transplantation. The early results have been encouraging but it has yet to become a routine procedure. One of the major concerns is the possibility of recurrence of Crohn's disease in the transplanted bowel but there are very few data to support this at present.

Polyarteritis

Pathology

This condition is characterized by a systemic necrotising vasculitis with fibrinoid necrosis and an inflammatory cell infiltrate affecting the blood vessels (arteries and veins) of several organs including the small intestine. The weakened vessels lead to aneurysm formation, which may rupture and bleed or thrombose causing multiple organ infarcts. There are several categories of polyarteritis but the two which effect the gut most frequently are polyarteritis nodosa (PAN) and the Churg–Strauss syndrome (CSS), also known as allergic granulomatous angiitis because of the eosinophilic infiltration and granuloma formation in the connective tissue in addition to the vasculitis.

Aetiology

Polyartertis is thought to be an immune complex mediated disorder.

Clinical features

In addition to systemic manifestations (fever, weight loss, malaise and hypertension) the symptoms emanating from involvement of the small intestine include nausea, vomiting, diarrhoea and steatorrhoea.

Complications

PAN and CSS can lead to life threatening complications such as intestinal infarction, perforation and massive gastrointestinal haemorrhage.

Treatment

Medical treatment with corticosteroids and either cyclophosphamide or azathioprine is the mainstay of therapy. Surgery is only undertaken for the major complications and entails resection of the affected segment of small bowel. Particularly in cases of infarction the ends should be exteriorized rather than attempting an anastomosis. Bowel continuity can be restored at a later stage.

Eosinophilic enteritis

Pathology

This is an extremely rare condition characterized by diffuse infiltration of the entire thickness of the small bowel wall with eosinophils. Microscopically the wall is thickened and there are small mucosal ulcers.

Aetiology

This is unknown but there are some reports which suggest that it may be related to infestation with certain nematodes or that it may reflect allergy to components of the diet, e.g. milk protein.

Clinical features

The clinical features depend on the distribution of the disease but when it affects the small bowel obstructive type symptoms are predominant.

Diagnosis

This is usually made at surgery for intestinal obstruction but a raised blood eosinophil count should alert the clinician to the possibility.

Treatment

When a short segment of small bowel is encountered at laparotomy this is usually resected. However, if the diagnosis is made pre-operatively or if the extent of the disease precludes surgery then corticosteroid therapy may be effective.

Radiation enteropathy

Pathology

The immediate effect of radiation on the gastrointestinal tract is arrest of cell division in the intestinal crypts. This effect is largely restricted to cells in the G1 phase. With greater radiation exposure, oedema and ulceration of the mucosa ensue. As a result of the diminished cell turnover the mucosa becomes thinner with stunted villi. If there is extensive small intestinal involvement, malabsorption of varying degrees will occur.

- The long-term effects are due to transmural fibrosis following the appearance of atypical fibroblasts in the submucosa and ischaemia from a proliferative endarteritis and vasculitis. Obliteration of the intestinal lymphatics with lymphatic ectasia complicates the pathological picture. The oedema is most marked in the submucosal layer. The fibrosis which affects all the coats is progressive and accompanied by hyalinization. The muscle layers exhibit areas of myofibrillar degeneration with atrophy of the muscle fibres, patchy hyalinization and disturbed motility. The serosa becomes thickened, opaque and greyish white and dense adhesions develop between adjacent intestinal loops.

Aetiology

Although the figure of 5% is often quoted for the incidence of intestinal radiation induced bowel disease in patients who receive radiotherapy to the abdominal and pelvic regions, the individual estimates vary from 3 to 25%. The most common situation is where the pelvis is irradiated, usually for rectal or gynaecological cancer. In the normal situation and particularly after rectal excision, loops of small bowel lie in the pelvis and are at great risk of irradiation.

Clinical features

Symptoms are encountered in the majority of patients during the first few weeks of radiotherapy. The anorexia, nausea and vomiting are central nervous system effects as these are often encountered in patients receiving radiotherapy in extra-abdominal regions. These early symptoms usually subside rapidly and do not necessarily indicate the development of late sequelae that characterize radiation induced bowel disease.

The commonest symptoms referable to chronic bowel damage are vague abdominal discomfort, diarrhoea, mild rectal bleeding and the passage of mucus. The interval between the time of radiation and onset of symptoms varies considerably from 2 months to 2 years. Intestinal obstruction may be acute or subacute and recurrent. Occasionally, acute presentation with infarction may occur and this carries a high risk of perforation and mortality. Most of the serious late complications tend to occur within 2 years of the initial treatment but may become progressively worse after this time.

Diagnosis

The investigative procedures used in the assessment of patients include contrast radiology of the small and large intestine and malabsorption studies. Sigmoidoscopy and colonoscopy may be appropriate in patients with large bowel disease.

Complications

As indicated above, the main complications are intestinal obstruction and perforation secondary to infarction (Figure 13.25). Fistula formation can also occur.

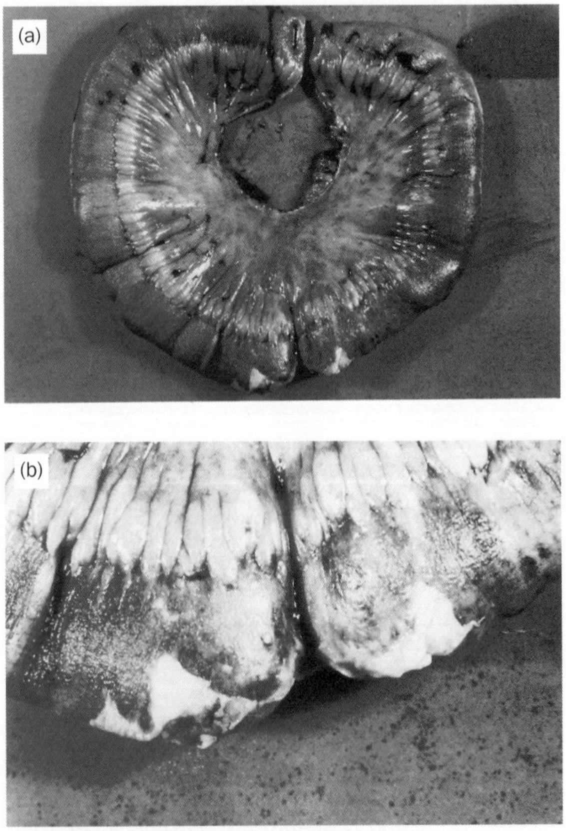

Figure 13.25 (a) Emergency resection of perforated small bowel Crohn's disease. (b) Close-up of perforation.

Treatment

Whenever possible, management should be conservative as surgical treatment has a high morbidity and an average reported mortality of 25%. Medical treatment involves the correction of nutritional deficiencies and the use of intestinal sedatives such as codeine phosphate, lomotil and diphenoxlate hydrochloride. There is no good evidence of 5-ASA or steroids having any beneficial effect, although it appears that prednisolone enemas may provide symptomatic benefit in patients with radiation proctitis. The presence of malabsorption necessitates further measures, such as antibiotics for bacterial overgrowth or bile salt binding agents (cholestyramine) for ileal disease together with careful dietary management, the use of elemental diets and oral supplements. Some patients with extensive small bowel disease and severe malabsorption require parenteral nutrition intermittently or indefinitely as in extensive Crohn's disease.

Emergency surgery is required for infarction with perforation or acute intestinal obstruction which does not resolve on conservative treatment. The radionecrotic bowel is ideally excised with primary anastomosis or exteriorization of the bowel ends in the presence of ischaemia and sepsis. Occasionally when the small bowel is firmly adherent into the pelvis, dissection of the affected segments may be hazardous and ileoileal or ileocolonic bypass may be more appropriate. Elective surgery may be undertaken for chronic severe symptoms due to stricture or internal fistula formation and the same considerations apply. In the performance of these operations only those adhesions which are in the operative field should be divided. Extensive adhesiolysis should be avoided as this is hazardous and can be complicated by perforation.

Infective conditions of the small bowel

Campylobacter infection

Infection with *Campylobacter fetus* is increasingly common in the UK.

Clinical features

It usually causes a self-limiting gastroenteritis leading to diarrhoea associated with abdominal pain.

Diagnosis

This can be made on stool culture but occasionally with severe abdominal pain and tenderness a laparotomy may be performed usually with negative results. However, there are rare instances of campylobacter appendicitis, cholecystitis and pancreatitis.

Treatment

This is supportive, ensuring that dehydration and electrolyte disturbances are corrected. Specific antibiotic treatment is not indicated.

Yersinia infections

These Gram-negative coccobacillary rods belong to the family Enterobacteriaceae which includes the organism responsible for the plague (*Yersinia pestis*). The two species which cause gastrointestinal infections particularly of the terminal ileum, appendix, ascending colon and mesenteric lymph nodes are *Y. enterocolitica* and *Y. pseudotuberculosis*. The infection sets up a granulomatous inflammatory picture with microscopic abscess formation which may simulate chronic inflammatory bowel disease. The ileum and ascending colon may become swollen, ulcerated and exhibit macroscopic appearances similar to Crohn's disease.

Clinical features

The most usual clinical syndrome is an acute febrile gastroenteritis which is self-limiting and does not require any treatment. However, chronic symptoms including diarrhoea and rectal bleeding may occur that are associated with persistent inflammation, particularly in children. The pseudo-appendicitis syndrome is also caused by Yersinia infection and is usually encountered in older children and adults.

Diagnosis

The diagnosis is established by recovery of the organism from the stool. However, in patients with chronic disease radiological investigation may show nodular filling defects in the terminal ileum which may look very like Crohn's disease. When operation is carried out the terminal ileum and mesenteric lymph nodes are found to be inflamed and swollen. Biopsy of the lymph nodes for Yersinia should always be performed in these patients.

Complications

Very occasionally *Y. enterocolitica* may give rise to severe ulceration with perforation and peritonitis. In addition, a septicaemic illness can result from Yersinia infection particularly in immunocompromised or elderly patients. Yersinia infections can also be associated with other intestinal manifestations including erythema nodosum and polyarthritis.

Treatment

Under most circumstances the disease is self-limiting and if a terminal ileitis is found, surgical resection should not be carried out unless complications have ensued. Normally, antibiotic treatment is not required but in severely ill patients or when symptoms persist appropriate antibiotics should be used and include chloramphenicol, co-trimoxazole and tetracycline.

Typhoid

Typhoid fever remains endemic in tropical and subtropical countries. It is caused by *Salmonella typhii* and is characterized by an early septicaemic phase with colonization of several organs such as liver, spleen, bones and small intestine. The terminal ileum in the region of the Peyer's patches is the commonest site for intestinal infection with the formation of a longitudinal ulcer on the anti-mesenteric border situated within 45 cm of the ileocaecal valve in the majority of patients.

Clinical features

The incubation period is usually between 10 and 15 days. The onset is insidious with a gradual rise in temperature over about 5 days. Presentation is usually as a pyrexia of undetermined origin. At the end of the first week a rash is seen over the trunk and splenomegaly may occur during the second week. Diarrhoea is usual as the disease progresses and there may be rectal bleeding. If untreated, septicaemia, coma and death may occur in the third week. When perforation of the terminal ileum occurs the patient will develop severe lower abdominal pain and will have signs of peritonitis on examination.

Diagnosis

Diagnosis is based on identifying the organism which can usually be found in faeces and urine in the second week. During the first week, blood culture and bone marrow culture may be positive. Liver function tests are often abnormal and if perforation has occurred a chest X-ray may show gas under the diaphragm. Serology (Widal's reaction) is of little value in the tropics as antibodies will be present from previous clinical or subclinical infection.

Complications

The main complication is perforation of the terminal ileum. This is solitary in 85% of cases and the incidence of perforation varies considerably from one endemic area to another. It is high in West Africa (15–33%) and low in Egypt and Iran (1–3%). The high incidence of perforation in West Africa has been attributed to late diagnosis and a particularly virulent strain of the organism.

Treatment

The treatment of typhoid perforation necessitates surgical intervention with antibiotic cover using chloramphanicol and gentamicin, thorough cleansing of the peritoneal cavity, and suture of the perforation with drainage. The edges of the perforation are trimmed before closure. Intestinal resection is contraindicated and carries a high mortality. Surgical intervention may also be indicated in typhoid fever for the following complications:

- Abscess formation which may occur in the septicaemic stage of the disease.
- Gangrenous typhoid cholecystitis.
- Chronic carrier state where cholecystectomy is indicated.

Intestinal tuberculosis

Intestinal tuberculosis can be classified into four macroscopic forms:

- hypertrophic
- ulcerative
- fibrotic
- ulcero-fibrotic.

The first two account for the majority of cases. The *hypertrophic type* affects predominantly the ileocaecal region and is characterized by the absence of gross caseation but with marked thickening of the submucous and subserosal layers. It can also involve the ascending and transverse colon and is generally regarded as a low-virulence infection in a patient with a high degree of immunological resistance from previous exposure to tubercles.

The *ulcerative type* affects predominantly the terminal ileum where multiple deep transverse ulcers develop and extend to the serosa and may give rise to perforation. The serosal surface is thickened and studded with tubercles. Healing may result in multiple strictures with intervening and dilated segments of ileum. Bacterial overgrowth may develop at this stage and cause diarrhoea and malabsorption. The *fibrotic variety* affects the terminal ileum, caecum and ascending colon. It leads to shortening and considerable narrowing of long segments of the bowel and may be accompanied by generalized peritoneal tuberculosis.

Clinical features

Patients with the hypertrophic type of intestinal tuberculosis are not usually very ill, although they exhibit the systemic manifestations of tuberculosis. The intestinal infection itself leads to recurrent episodes of subacute intestinal obstruction with colicky abdominal pain and vomiting or with a mass in the right iliac fossa. The ulcerative type leads to subacute intestinal obstruction with pain, vomiting and constipation. The fibrotic variety again presents with acute or subacute intestinal obstruction.

Diagnosis

The diagnosis of abdominal tuberculosis can pose difficulties even in endemic areas. The Mantoux test may be negative. Attempts should be made to culture the mycobacterium from gastric washings, faeces, peritoneal fluid and tissue biopsies including enlarged peripheral lymph nodes. It is important to realize however, that certain atypical mycobacteria (not responsible for tuberculosis) may be demonstrated in certain chronic inflammatory conditions including Crohn's disease. Plain radiographs of the abdomen may show extensive calcification. Barium studies show features of altered motility and stenotic radiological changes which may be indistinguishable from Crohn's disease. The best diagnostic procedure is laparoscopy with peritoneal biopsy and sampling of the ascitic fluid when present. In many instances however, the diagnosis is only made a laparotomy with subsequent culture and histology of resected intestine.

Treatment

In the absence of intestinal obstruction or perforation the treatment is conservative with rest, adequate nutritional intake and anti-tuberculous chemotherapy which is continued for 12 months. At the present time the favoured first line combination is rifampicin, isoniazid and ethambutol.

Surgical treatment is indicated for intestinal obstruction or perforation. Ileocaecal resection and right hemicolectomy are now the standard operations for ileocaecal disease and the results are excellent provided that chemotherapy is maintained for appropriately long periods of time after surgery. For disease in regions other than the terminal ileum and caecum, segmental resection of the bowel with end to end anastomosis is performed. More recently stricturoplasty has been introduced to deal with fibrotic strictures. Again this must be performed under anti-tuberculous drug therapy which has to be continued for some time after surgery.

Actinomycosis

Abdominal (ileocaecal) actinomycosis is rare and usually follows infection with *Actinomycosis israelii* following perforated appendicitis. Infection spreads mainly to the psoas muscle, abdominal wall and adjacent organs with the development of fistulas and multiple discharging sinuses. Spread of the infection by the portal venous system results in multiple intercommunicating loculated abscesses (honeycomb liver).

Clinical features

The patient usually presents some weeks following perforated appendicitis with a fixed indurated mass in the right iliac fossa with abscess and sinus formation.

Treatment

Treatment is conservation with prolonged penicillin and lincomycin therapy.

Human immunodeficiency virus (HIV) enteropathy

In patients with AIDS gastrointestinal problems are extremely common. In the majority of these patients the symptoms are caused by opportunistic infection with protozoal organisms, various bacterial species, viruses and fungi (Table 13.9). However, in a significant percentage of patients (about 30%) no identifiable pathogens can be isolated from the stool. This indicates that HIV1 may cause a specific enteropathy and recent studies using DNA probes have identified the presence of HIV1 in the base of the crypts and in the lamina propria. Most of the infected cells are enterochromaffin in nature.

Table 13.9 Opportunistic intestinal infections in patients with AIDS

Protozoal	
	Cryptosporidia
	Isopora belli
	Giardia lamblia
Bacterial	
	Salmonella
	Shigella
	Yersinia
	Mycobacterium avium intracellulare (MAI)
	Campylobacter
Viral	
	Cytomegalovirus
Fungal	
	Candida albicans
	Blastocystis hominis

Clinical features

The gastrointestinal symptoms which are common in AIDS are diarrhoea, weight loss and abdominal pain and they are often the presenting features. Other common symptoms are fever, sore throat, lymphadenopathy, arthralgia and an erythematous, maculopapular rash.

Diagnosis

The routine diagnosis of AIDS is based on the detection of antibodies to HIV. Following infection antibodies to the various antigens associated with the virus often do not appear for about 6 weeks so that there is a long window when an individual may exhibit negative antibody testing to HIV and yet still be infected. Other tests include detection of circulating viral p24 antigen and the use of polymerase chain reaction (PCR) by which very small amounts of viral are RNA in infected cells can be greatly amplified.

Treatment

There is little place for surgery in the treatment of the small bowel manifestations of AIDS, but infected patients with gastrointestinal symptoms may require endoscopy and stool culture. If a specific infection is established treatment is directed to eradicating the organism responsible. Symptomatic relief can be obtained using non-specific anti-diarrhoeal therapy.

Parasitic infestations of the small bowel

Ascaris (roundworm)

This infestation occurs directly from person to person without an intermediate host. The responsible parasite is ascaris lumbricoides which enters by the oral route. Ova do not require tropical conditions to survive and immediately after ingestion the larvae emerge and adult worms (up to 40 cm in length) develop in the jejunal lumen.

Clinical features

The majority of infested individuals are asymptomatic but obstruction of the gastrointestinal tract may occur leading to vomiting (sometimes of worms) and colicky abdominal pain. A palpable mass (worm bolus) may be felt and the patient may be pyrexial.

Diagnosis

The diagnosis is made by demonstrating ova in a faecal sample, and although adult worms are sometimes passed per rectum the worms may be seen on a small bowel follow through.

Complications

As well as intestinal obstruction, obstruction of the biliary tract, the pancreatic duct and the appendix may occur.

Treatment

Eradication treatment is with one of the benzimidazole compounds such as mebendazole or albendazole; piperazine is nowadays rarely used. Surgery is indicated for intestinal obstruction which does not resolve. At operation an attempt should be made to manipulate the mass of tangled worms into the caecum. If this fails, it may be necessary to extract the worm bolus via an enterotomy. Occasionally, a resection may be necessary if the viability of the bowel is in any doubt or if a perforation has occurred.

Ancylostomiasis (hookworm)

Ancylostomiasis is endemic in most tropical countries. It is caused by two filarial worms, *Ancylostoma duodenale* and *Necator americanus*. The larvae enter the body by penetrating into the skin and reach the lungs through the blood stream. They then ascend to the pharynx where they are swallowed. The adult worm lives attached by hooks to the mucosa of the jejunum and ova are excreted in the faeces.

Clinical features

Infestation is associated with severe dyspepsia and gastrointestinal bleeding causing a microcytic anaemia and frank gastrointestinal haemorrhage especially in children.

Diagnosis

The diagnosis is made by the identification of ova in the faeces or adult worms in duodenal or jejunal fluid. A peripheral blood eosinophilia may occur during the invasive stage.

Treatment

The first stage of treatment is the correction of anaemia using either oral or injectable iron. Benzimidazole compounds, mebendazole or albendazole are used as for ascaris.

Section 13.6 • Small bowel conditions causing malabsorption

Bacterial overgrowth

In this syndrome the small intestine becomes colonized by bacteria with an increase in the concentration of organisms which are usually confined to the lower small bowel and the colon. This is caused by surgery or disease which results in excess bacteria entering the small intestine or from delayed clearance of bacteria due to stasis (stagnant or blind loop syndrome). There are various reasons why this may occur and these are detailed in Table 13.10. In some cases bacterial overgrowth may develop in the absence of an obvious local cause particularly in patients with malnutrition or immune deficiency.

Table 13.10 Causes of bacterial overgrowth

Excessive entry of bacteria into the small intestine
Achlorhydria – absence of bacterial gastric acid
Gastrojejunostomy
Partial/total gastrectomy
Enterocolic fistulas
Cholangitis
Loss of the ileocaecal valve following right hemicolectomy
Intestinal stasis
Crohn's disease – stenosis
Tuberculosis – stenosis
Small bowel diverticulosis – stasis
Afferent loop stasis
Entero-enteric anastomosis and other intestinal bypass procedures
Subacute obstruction – adhesions, strictured anastomosis
Blind loops
Diabetes mellitus – autonomic neuropathy
Radiation enteritis – stenosis, impaired intestinal motility
Scleroderma – impaired intestinal motility
Amyloidosis

Pathophysiology

The bacterial overgrowth in the small intestine is usually in the order of 10^7–10^9 CFUs per ml of intestinal contents. Bacterial colonization results in intestinal mucosal injury characterized by patchy inflammatory changes in the lamina propria which is accompanied by alterations in the concentrations of the brush border enzymes. The increased bacterial population deconjugates the intraluminal bile salts by removing the glycine or taurine moiety. In addition the bacteria dehydroxylate the steroid nucleus at the C_7 position with the formation of deoxycholate and lithocholate which have a tendency to precipitate at the intraluminal pH levels of the small intestine. Thus these bile salts participate poorly in the emulsification of fat and they are passively absorbed to an extent by non-ionic diffusion through the small intestine. This leads to a net reduction of the concentration of effective bile salts in the lumen of the small bowel to levels below that required to form micelles. This in turn results in malabsorption of fats and fat-soluble vitamins.

The bacterial species which are responsible for bile salt deconjugation are eubacteria, bacteroides and corynebacteria. These bacteria also bind vitamin B_{12} and convert it to inactive derivatives (cobamides) which block the ileal receptors for the vitamin as well as for intrinsic factor. The resulting malabsorption of vitamin B_{12} may lead to megaloblastic anaemia. Often however, the anaemia has a dimorphic picture because of an iron deficiency component due to chronic blood loss from the primary lesion itself or from malabsorption of iron. Folate deficiency is rare as the bacteria synthesize folate in substantial amounts and some patients may in fact exhibit a high serum folate.

There is some malabsorption of carbohydrates and proteins although this is rarely significant. The main reason for malnutrition in patients with bacterial overgrowth is a diminished dietary intake, which accounts for growth retardation in children. The bacteria also metabolize triglycerides to free fatty acids which they hydoxylate to form hydroxy fatty acids. These impair the absorption of water and sodium by the intestinal mucosa of both the small and large intestine by acting as laxatives. This together with the action of the dehydroxylated bile salts, enterotoxin and osmotic load created by the fermentation of the major dietary components accounts for the diarrhoea which is seen in these patients.

Clinical features

The symptoms of bacterial overgrowth are varied. Initially the patients may exhibit symptoms referable to the underlying pathology, e.g. post-gastrectomy symptoms or recurrent intestinal colic due to subacute obstructing lesions. Patients with jejunal diverticulosis (Figure 13.26) are symptomless until the onset of malabsorption, although they may occasionally develop unrelated complications such as gastrointestinal bleeding or perforation of one the diverticula leading to generalized peritonitis. The symptoms and signs of bacterial overgrowth itself are often non-specific and include malaise, nausea and vomiting, excessive borborygmi and weight loss. Diarrhoea is extremely common and is usually watery, and frank steatorrhoea with bulky pale offensive stools which are difficult to flush is less common.

Diagnosis

A full blood count is essential to assess the extent and type of anaemia which is often present in these patients. Estimations of urea and electrolytes, albumin and total protein levels are also important. The most useful test for assessing the presence of bacterial overgrowth however, is the hydrogen breath test (see section on investigations).

Complications

The complications of bacterial overgrowth include glossitis, stomatitis, anaemia, hypoproteinaemia with peripheral oedema, tetany, osteomalacia and rickets and growth retardation in children. Occasionally neurological manifestations such as paraesthesiae and peripheral neuropathy may be found in association with vitamin B_{12} deficiency.

Treatment

Surgical treatment of the underlying conditions wherever possible is the definitive and curative treatment. However, situations are frequently encountered where surgical treatment is not possible or advisable because of the extensive or systemic nature of the underlying disease, e.g. extensive jejunal diverticulosis and scleroderma. In these cases intermittent therapy with oral antibiotics is often beneficial, the two most commonly used being tetracycline and metronidazole. As control of the anaerobic organisms seems to be the most helpful metronidazole is generally preferred, although tetracycline is also of value. A course of antibiotics is usually administered for about 2 weeks at a time and although repopulation of the intestine by bacteria occurs soon after discontinuation of the treatment, symptomatic improvement may last for several months. Intermittent therapy is therefore preferred to long-term treatment.

Short gut syndrome

This is the most serious form of intestinal decompensation and is encountered after extensive resection of the small bowel.

Pathophysiology

The outcome following intestinal resection depends on:

- The extent and site of resection.
- The age of the patient.
- The physical state and mental condition of the patient.

The intestinal decompensation that follows massive resection of the small intestine is due to a sudden reduction of the absorptive area and a greatly reduced transit time which further aggravates malabsorption and in extreme cases limits the extent of digestion.

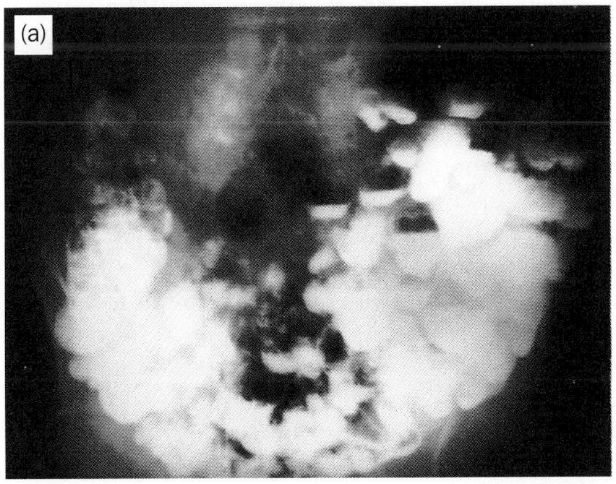

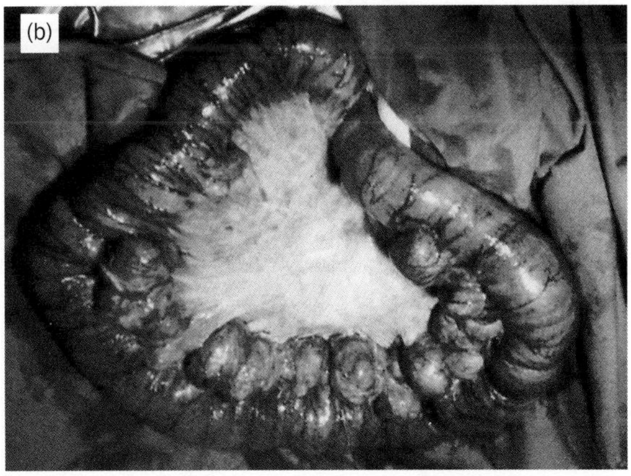

Figure 13.26 (a) Small bowel barium study showing extensive and multiple small intestinal diverticula in a 65-year-old female with severe malabsorption. The steatorrhoea improved considerably with oral tetracycline therapy. (b) Multiple jejunal diverticula localized to a segment of the upper small intestine. The patient's bacterial overgrowth syndrome resolved after excision of the affected bowel.

Malabsorption of fats and proteins is invariably present but its severity varies with the length and site of the residual bowel. Carbohydrate absorption is less severely affected and is the first to return to normal in 4–6 weeks. The improvement in the absorptive capacity for protein is more gradual and the absorption of fats remains impaired at a fixed percentage. This is the result of interruption of the enterohepatic circulation of bile salts after ileal resection and a diminished bile salt pool, as the increased hepatic synthesis is unable to compensate for the large daily faecal losses.

Spill over into the colon of primary bile salt conjugates, where bacterial action will convert them into deconjugated and dehydroxylated derivatives, contributes to the diarrhoea which is characteristic of the short gut syndrome. This is because some of these secondary bile salts block the absorption of water and electrolytes by the colonic mucosa. The hydroxylation of the unabsorbed fatty acids by colonic bacteria has also been implicated in diarrhoea. The malabsorption of fats and fat-soluble vitamins is accompanied by the malabsorption of calcium and magnesium which are precipitated as soaps with the unabsorbed fatty acids. The severe diarrhoea which can amount to several litres in the first few weeks after resection is further aggravated by the low pH of the stool and often causes severe perianal irritation.

Lactose intolerance may occur in some patients after extensive small bowel resection and this has been attributed to a rapid transit time allowing insufficient time for lactase to act and to a reduction of the total intestinal lactase activity.

Aetiology

The aetiology is essentially extensive resection of small bowel for any of the following reasons:

- Crohn's disease
- mesenteric infarction
- radiation enteritis
- mid gut volvulus
- multiple fistulas
- small bowel tumours.

Crohn's disease is by far the commonest cause as this often necessitates repeated resections over a number of years culminating in the short gut syndrome. Hence the reason for a conservative approach in these patients with limited resections and the judicious use of stricturoplasty for short fibrous strictures. While resection of more than half of the small bowel is frequently accompanied by serious malabsorption there is debate as to the extent of the small bowel resection which results in the short gut syndrome. An assessment of the length of the residual small bowel after resection is essential as there is a crucial length below which intestinal decompensation of varying degrees takes place. Patients with a residual small bowel length of less than 2 m have a diminished work capacity and those with less than 100 cm require home parenteral nutrition on an indefinite basis. Infants and neonates seem to tolerate extensive small bowel resections better than adults and a minimum of 30 cm of small intestine can support both nutrition and growth.

The critical length of residual small bowel necessary to prevent serious maldigestion and malabsorption depends on the site of resection and the retention or otherwise of the ileocaecal valve. Thus ileal resections are less well tolerated than jejunal resections, largely because the active transport sites for bile salts and vitamin B_{12} are localized in the ileum. The importance of retaining a terminal segment of ileum and ileocaecal valve whenever possible is well documented. An intact ileocaecal valve slows the transit time and limits the degree of colonization of the residual intestine by an overgrowth of colonic bacteria.

Clinical features

The main clinical features are weight loss and diarrhoea which is watery and frequently copious. Because of diarrhoea and the low pH of the stool, perianal irritation is common. In patients who develop lactose intolerance the consumption of fresh milk is followed by attacks of abdominal pain and an increase in the severity of the diarrhoea. Other clinical features depend on the development of complications (see below).

Diagnosis

Diagnosis is made on clinical grounds with a knowledge of the extent of small bowel resection. Other tests of malabsorption (see section on small bowel investigations) are helpful in the objective assessment of the severity of the malabsorption.

Course of condition

With time, structural and functional changes occur in the residual bowel as part of the process of adaptation to the reduced absorptive area. In the human, the structural changes consist of dilation of the remaining intestine and enlargement of the villi. An increase in the length of the bowel has also been reported in the neonate. These structural changes are accompanied by a gradual improvement in the absorption of water, electrolytes, carbohydrates and protein. The enhanced absorption of water-soluble substances per unit length of intestine is not the result of greater absorption by individual cells but rather from an increased cell population in the intestinal villi. Both luminal and humoral factors are involved in this adaptive hyperplasia. The luminal factors include alimentary secretions and ingested nutrients. Duodenal juice may be particularly important as a source of epidermal growth factor. The maintenance of an adequate intraluminal nutrition by the oral ingestion of appropriate food is essential for the adaptive response. Enteroglucagon is the most important humoral agent influencing the adaptive response. The stimulus for its release is thought to result from increased exposure of the residual bowel to luminal nutrition. The enteroglucagon then acts on the mucosal cells and stimulates an increased turnover of intracellular polyamines and cell growth. There is evidence however that the effect of intraluminal nutrition is also mediated through direct contact of the nutrients with the epithelial cells. Other factors which may contribute to compensation by the residual intestine include changes in the motility pattern leading to a gradual slowing of the transit time and increased absorption of water-soluble substances by the colon.

In cases of mesenteric infarction varying amounts of colon are frequently resected with the small intestine. It is not known whether the extent of the associated colonic resection influences the clinical outcome but colonic mucosa does absorb water and salt and to a lesser extent glucose and amino acids. Some reports indicate that residual colon minimizes the severity of diarrhoea and may assume some of the absorptive functions of the small intestine.

Complications

The complications which can be associated with short gut syndrome include:

- gastric hypersecretion
- cholesterol and pigment gallstones
- hepatic disease
- impaired renal function and stone formation
- metabolic bone disease.

Gastric hypersecretion

Gastric hypersecretion occurs transiently and bears no relation to the extent of the intestinal excision although it appears to be more common after proximal resections. It is caused by an increased rate of basal acid secretion consequent on delayed clearance of gastrin. Around 50% of patients with extensive small bowel resection are affected.

Gallstone formation

There is a well-recognized increase in the incidence of gallstones after extensive ileal resection and jejunoileal bypass for morbid obesity. Cholesterol stones are the result of a reduced bile salt pool which leads to the bile becoming lithogenic, i.e. supersaturated with cholesterol, which precipitates as cholesterol crystals. In addition however, pigment gallstones also occur after ileal resection.

Hepatic disease

Mild hyperbilirubinaemia, elevation of the serum transaminases and impaired excretion of bromsulfonphthalein (BSP) often occur after both massive intestinal resections and jejunoileal bypass. These are associated with fatty infiltration of the liver with or without hepatic atrophy. The increased deposition of fat in the liver after jejunoileal bypass occurs in patients while they are actively losing weight but not when the weight is stationary. Acute fulminate liver failure has been reported most commonly after jejunoileal bypass. The onset of the liver failure usually occurs within the first 6 months after operation and the clinical symptoms are those of a 'flu-like illness with anorexia, nausea, vomiting, rapid weight loss and a fall in the serum albumin. The onset of these manifestations is an indication for restoration of intestinal continuity. Cirrhosis may develop after jejunoileal bypass. Initially it causes no symptoms and its onset can only be detected by serial liver biopsies.

Impaired renal function and stone formation

The severe diarrhoea may lead to fluid and electrolyte losses and to a decrease in the glomerular filtration rate with a tendency to a low urine output and a concentrated urine. The consequent loss of electrolyte rich intestinal fluid causes hyponatraemia and hypokalaemia. A metabolic acidosis ensues from the fixed base losses into the gastrointestinal tract with the excretion of a persistently acid urine. The urinary calcium excretion is low but the oxalate concentration and excretion is high, especially in patients with an intact colon. Urinary calculi of all types (urate and oxalate) are very common in patients after small bowel resection and the vast majority of patients will develop this complication during their lifetimes.

The water and salt depletion results in increased secretion of aldosterone in an attempt at maximal renal salt conservation but at the expense of increased potassium loss. This chronic hypokalaemia apart from causing muscle weakness, anorexia and cardiac arrhythmias may limit protein synthesis and impair transport and utilization of carbohydrates. In addition it may lead to the development of a renal tubular nephropathy consisting of a characteristic patchy vacuolar change in the cells of the proximal convoluted tubules. This syndrome of hypokalaemic vacuolar nephropathy can complicate other disorders associated with diarrhoea including ulcerative colitis and coeliac disease.

Metabolic bone disease

Hypocalcaemia and hypomagnesaemia are common and often associated with neuromuscular symptoms, dehydration and other electrolyte abnormalities. Osteomalacia is common but difficult to confirm without a bone biopsy. These patients have bone pain and an elevated serum alkaline phophatase activity.

Treatment

The treatment of short gut syndrome is centred around supporting the patient during the initial stage of decompensation and through the critical stage of adaptation which may last up to 3 months. At the end of this time the stage of equilibrium is reached and the patient with residual small intestine enters the final stage of rehabilitation. In the patients with massive small bowel resection indefinite total parenteral nutrition via a permanent tunnelled silicon feeding line is the only option for survival. In these patients a programme of training with regard to the management of the intravenous feeds and the care of the feeding lines is essential so that they can eventually carry out the parental nutrition themselves in their own homes, usually at night.

In the immediate post-operative period total parenteral nutrition is essential and the regimen must provide 40 kcal/kg of body weight and 300 mg of nitrogen per kilogram of body weight, in addition to electrolytes, vitamins and trace metals, usually in a 3 litre single bag system administered over a period of 12 hours. Accurate fluid balance must be maintained by daily charting of the input versus the output which should include all measured losses. H_2 receptor blockade therapy (cimetadine or ranitidine) should be administered 6 hourly by the intravenous route to suppress gastric secretion. This avoids the necessity for nasogastric intubation and suction which should only be used if ileus is prolonged. Initially nothing other than weak hypotonic electrolyte solutions is tolerated orally and only small amounts (15–30 ml/hour) should be given to avoid a dry mouth.

When the patient's condition becomes stable (usually 3–6 weeks after the enterectomy) transition to an oral diet is started in those patients with an adequate length of small intestine. The feeding is started gradually, initially with isotonic carbohydrate and electrolyte solutions. Thereafter enteral diets are used. These are semi-synthetic fibre-free liquid diets containing all the basic components (protein, hydrolysates, simple carbohydrates, essential lipids, vitamins). The nitrogen component is available either as free amino acids (elemental) or as peptides (polymeric). There is some evidence that the peptide based polymeric diets lead to better nitrogen utilization than the elemental diets although this is controversial. The fats which contribute only a small amount of the caloric content of these artificial diets are necessary particularly as a supply of essential fatty acids.

The diet is administered via a nasogastric feeding tube, initially in a dilute form (1:4) and instilled by an infusion pump at a rate of 25 ml/hour. The rate and concentration are gradually increased until the patient is receiving 100–120 ml of full strength diet per hour. Care must be taken that gastric dilatation does not occur as pulmonary aspiration with a fatal outcome may occur during nasogastric enteral feeding.

One of the most common early problems is diarrhoea which is often accentuated at the start of enteral feeding. The most effective drugs to control this are loperamide hydrochloride, diphenoxylate hydrochloride and codeine phosphate. In patients with an intact colon, cholestyramine can be administered to limit the diarrhoea-inducing effects of the unabsorbed bile salts. In some patients the diarrhoea is so severe that it may be life threatening and requires control with a long acting analogue of somatostatin (octreotide).

Steatorrhoea is common in these patients and results from excess fat in the diet. Whenever possible dietary fats should be administered as medium-chain triglycerides which do not require the presence of salts for their absorption into the portal venous blood. Dietary supplements of calcium, magnesium, vitamins C, D and K and iron are all necessary. In patients in whom the ileum has been resected vitamin B_{12} is administered parenterally at 3 monthly intervals on an indefinite basis. The sequential medical management of patients after massive resection of the small intestine is summarized in Table 13.11.

Currently home total parenteral nutrition is the only option for the majority of patients with insufficient residual small bowel. This is costly and attended by significant complications. Although still in its infancy, combined hepatic and small bowel transplantation offers the best prospects for management of these patients in the long term.

Remedial surgical procedures

In adults, surgery is rarely indicated in patients with short gut syndrome unless intractable diarrhoea proves resistant to all forms of medical treatment including somatostatin. Under these cases reversed (antiperistaltic) segments can be employed. Although they do delay transit they can lead to intestinal obstruction and favour the development of bacterial overgrowth. In order to avoid risks of strangulation the antiperistaltic segment should be constructed without reversal of the mesenteric pedicle (Figure 13.27). In neonates and infants, the procedure of intestinal lengthening has given promising results (Figure 13.28). Truncal vagotomy and pyloroplasty although often used in the past is not indicated as patients who develop persistent gastric acid hypersecretion can be treated using H_2 receptor blockade or proton pump inhibitors on a long-term basis.

Coeliac disease

Pathology

Coeliac disease is the most common and most important cause of malabsorption in Western societies, but its prevalence varies considerably. In the UK, the overall prevalence in the population is about 1 in 1800. It is

Table 13.11 Sequential management of patients after massive resection of the small intestine

Stage of decompensation	Total parenteral nutrition, replacement of fluid and electrolyte losses, sips of oral hypotonic solutions
Transition to enteral feeding	(i) Parenteral nutrition + gradually increasing supplements of enteral feeds (ii) Full enteral feeding by chemically defined diets (elemental, polymeric)
Final stage	(i) Home parenteral nutrition (patients with no effective residual small bowel) (ii) Enteral feeding: intermittent parenteral feeding in patient with 100 cm or less of residual small intestine (iii) Normal low-fat (medium-chain triglyceride) diet + supplements in patients with > 1 m of residual small bowel

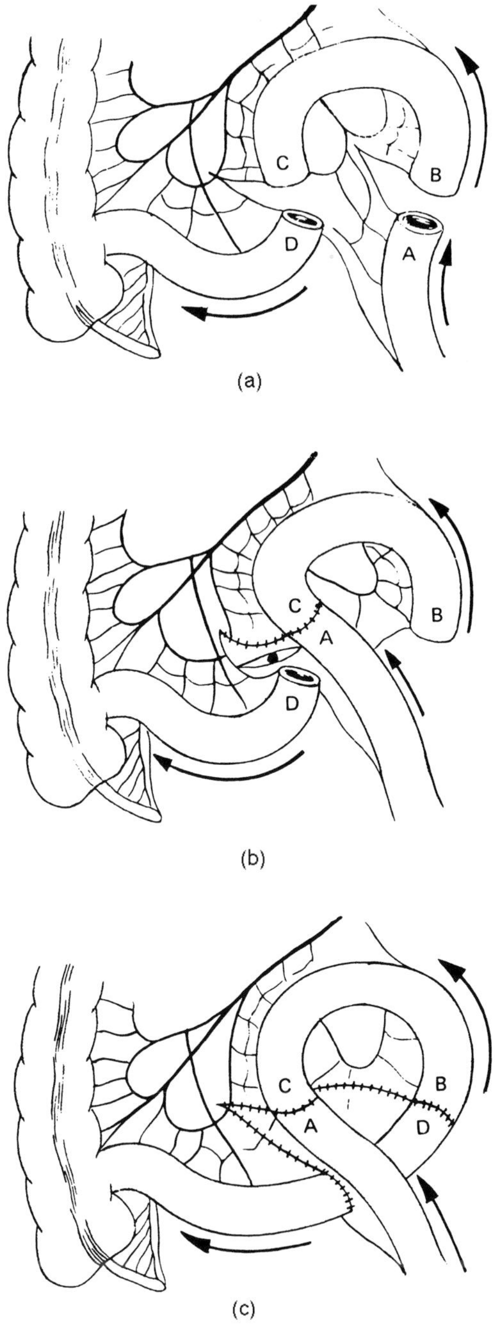

Figure 13.27 Technique of creating an antiperistaltic segment without reversal of the mesenteric pedicle.

characterized by a hypertrophic mucosa with shortened villi and lengthened crypts in the upper small intestine. As the severity of the disease increases the length of small intestine also increases but it is relatively unusual for the whole of the ileum to be involved. The malabsorption which occurs is complex and probably not entirely the result of mucosal damage. However, there is no doubt that loss of surface area and reduction in the brush border enzymes contributes significantly to the development of malabsorption.

Aetiology

Coeliac disease is caused by gluten, a water-insoluble protein contained in cereal, although how gluten actually damages the mucosa is not clear. It may be related to a defect of gluten digestion which leads to accumulation of a toxic factor. Other theories include an immunological reaction against gluten which damages the mucosa. There is clearly a genetic factor, as first degree relatives have a 2–5% risk of developing coeliac disease and a 10% risk of asymptomatic villous atrophy. In addition to this, there is a clear association between coeliac disease and HLA B8. It appears that the pattern of inheritance of coeliac disease is either modified dominant or polygenic.

Clinical features

The disease may present at any time of life from the first few months to extreme old age. In children the main features are growth retardation, abdominal distension, steatorrhoea and loss of appetite. In the adult, on the other hand, coeliac disease may present in a variety of ways. The peak age for presentation is between 20 and 40 years and the most characteristic features are diarrhoea, weight loss and anaemia. On examination the findings are non-specific but include weight loss, angular stomatitis, glossitis, oedema, pallor, skin pigmentation and abdominal distension with high-pitched bowel sounds.

Diagnosis

A small bowel follow-through shows an abnormal appearance in 90% of patients although the appearances are non-specific. The normal fine feathery appearance of the mucosa is no longer seen but is replaced by a course mucosal pattern with broad bars. As the disease becomes more severe the small bowel may appear as a featureless tube. Changes are mainly seen in the jejunum but distal spread is seen in more severe disease.

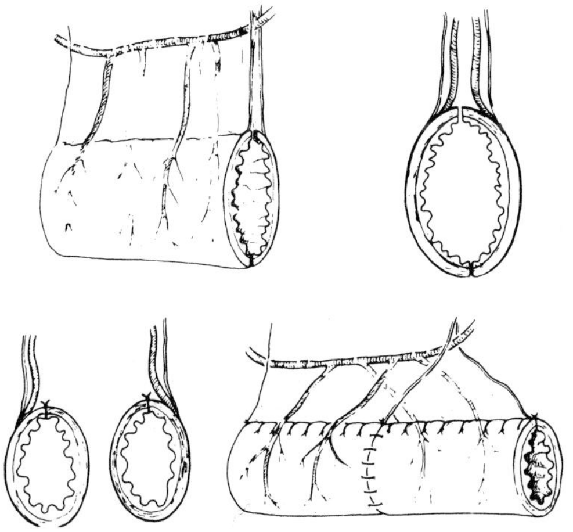

Figure 13.28 Diagrammatic representation of the intestinal lengthening operation developed by Bianchi. The bowel is split longitudinally into two halves, each retaining its blood supply. A tube is constructed from each half. The two tubes are then joined together.

The most important diagnostic test is jejunal biopsy which can be achieved either at endoscopy or using a suction (Crosby) capsule. At endoscopy it is common to see loss of the folds of Kerckring in the descending duodenum and this should alert the endoscopist to the possibility of coeliac disease.

Complications

To a certain extent, although the gut is the main target organ of gluten sensitivity, the condition can be systemic. The other most important manifestations are dermatitis herpetiformis and neurological dysfunction leading particularly to cerebellar ataxia often with a peripheral neuropathy. Many such patients will have histologically normal small bowel mucosa and little or nothing in the way of gastrointestinal symptoms.

The main complication of coeliac disease affecting the small intestine is small bowel malignancy. Lymphoma is more common but patients also have an increased risk of adenocarcinoma of the small intestine. Overall the incidence of malignancy in adult coeliac disease is in the region of 10%.

Treatment

The mainstay of treatment is withdrawal of gluten from the diet. This involves avoidance of wheat, rye, barley and all produce made from flour. Surgery only has a role in coeliac disease when intestinal malignancy intervenes.

Section 13.7 • Miscellaneous conditions of the small bowel

Vascular abnormalities

Aside from vascular tumours the small bowel can be affected by angiodysplasia, phlebectasia, telangiectasia and haemangiomas.

Pathology and aetiology

Angiodysplasias

Angiodysplasias are lesions which occupy the mucosa and submucosa of the gastrointestinal tract and consist of a cluster of arteriolar, venular and capillary vessels. Although this condition can occur in the small bowel it is most commonly seen in the right side of the colon. The aetiology is uncertain but theories include chronic mucosal ischaemia secondary to arterial venous shunting, decreased perfusion pressure and lowered oxygen tension in the terminal branches of the superior mesenteric arteries and chronic intermittent obstruction of the submucosal veins.

Phlebectasia

These lesions consist of a meshwork of dilated veins having a normal endothelial lining and situated in the submucosal layer of the intestine. They may be multiple and extensive.

Hereditary haemorrhagic telangiectasia (Osler–Weber–Rendu disease)

This rare inherited disorder leads to multiple telangiectasias of the lip, mouth, nasopharynx and gut. The lesion consists of arteriolar dilations due to a congenital weakness of the arterial muscle and absence of elastin in the medial coat.

Haemangiomas

These are rare congenital non-hereditary malformations of blood vessels (vascular harmartomas). They are classified into three types: capillary, cavernous and mixed. Most of the reported cases have been in the small and large intestine.

Clinical features

The basic clinical features of all of these lesions is gastrointestinal bleeding. Angiodysplasias and haemangiomas can lead to massive rectal bleeding and indeed the cavernous haemangioma carries a poor prognosis with an overall reported mortality of 30% usually from massive haemorrhage. In hereditary haemorrhagic telangiectasia gastrointestinal bleeding is rarely severe and the patients may present with anaemia or intermittent melaena. Likewise in phlebectasia the bleeding is usually mild although severe bleeding can occur.

Diagnosis

These vascular lesions are diagnosed by either endoscopy or mesenteric angiography. Angiodysplasias especially in the colon are cherry red in colour, each consisting of a central large vessel from which radiate multiple peripheral branches. In the small bowel however, mesenteric angiography is more likely to demonstrate the vascular malformation. In angiodysplasia the typical angiographic finding consists of a tortuous feeding artery and dilated veins with an intervening cluster of fine vessels. When there is active bleeding angiography may demonstrate extravasation of contrast into the small bowel lumen and scanning using labelled autologous red cells may be of value [**see Vol. I, module on gastrointestinal haemorrhage**].

Treatment

The treatment of lesions of the small bowel causing significant haemorrhage is resection of the affected segment of small bowel. Ideally, if mesenteric angiography has been carried out prior to surgery, the radiologist should leave a super-selective catheter in a mesenteric vessel as close to the lesion as possible. At surgery, the surgeon can then inject some dye (methylene blue) into the catheter and this will highlight the segment of small bowel to be resected (Figure 13.4). Alternatively, intra-operative endoscopy of the small bowel may be helpful as transillumination of the bowel can be very useful in identifying these vascular abnormalities.

Peutz–Jeghers syndrome

This is an inherited autosomal dominant disorder, characterized by jejunal or ileal polyps and mucocutaneous pigmentation. The polyps are hamartomatous in nature and consist of a fibromuscular stroma covered with well-differentiated epithelium. Rarely, the polyps may be localized in the stomach, duodenum or large bowel.

Clinical features

Attacks of intestinal colic may pre-date acute intestinal obstruction from intussusception or intraluminal obstruction by a large polyp. Bleeding from the polyps is common but is usually chronic, presenting with iron-deficiency anaemia rather than acute gastrointestinal haemorrhage. The patient will have pigmentation on the lips and buccal mucosa, but although this abnormal pigmentation usually appears in infancy, symptoms from polyps do not usually occur until the second decade.

Complications

Although malignant transformation may occur the risk is small and has been estimated at 2–3%. Cases of Peutz–Jeghers syndrome have been documented where the mucocutaneous pigmentation is associated with intestinal haemangiomas instead of hamartomatous polyps.

Diagnosis

This is made on clinical grounds, family history and the histology of resected polyps.

Treatment

In view of the small but definite risk of malignancy, all polyps greater than 2 cm should be removed. Surgical treatment is also indicated for intestinal obstruction and haemorrhage.

Section 13.8 • The vermiform appendix and Meckel's diverticulum

Vermiform appendix

Anatomy

The vermiform appendix is a narrow (around 5 mm) diverticulum of highly variable length (5–15 cm). The base of the appendix is attached to the postero-medial surface of the caecum approximately 3 cm inferolateral to the junction of the ileum and caecum. Its blood supply, which originates from the ileocolic artery, reaches it via a small extension of the mesentery of the small bowel, which passes posterior to the terminal ileum. The appendix is highly variable in position. Often it lies posterior to the caecum (retrocaecal) but it may also extend into the lesser pelvis and lie close to the ovary, fallopian tube and ureter. As with the small bowel the appendix is covered with peritoneum and has an external layer of longitudinal muscle and an internal layer of circular muscle. At the base of the appendix the longitudinal muscle is continuous with the three taeniae of the caecum and the colon. In the submucosal layer there are lymph follicles which are separated by crypts of the columnar epithelial lining that contains many goblet cells. When the submucosal layer becomes swollen it can readily block the lumen of the appendix.

Acute appendicitis

Pathology

Development of appendicitis appears to be related to swelling of the lymphoid tissue in the submucosa which is responding either to viral or bacterial infection. This may then proceed to gangrene of the appendiceal wall and perforation. The presence of gangrene or perforation seems to be associated with the presence of faecoliths, which are intraluminal laminated appendiceal calculi. These are usually radio-opaque. Approximately 50% of cases of gangrenous or perforated appendicitis are associated with a faecolith in contrast with uncomplicated appendicitis in which a faecolith is rarely present. It is thought that a faecolith increases the likelihood of obstruction of the appendix and thereby allows the accumulation of pus. Overall, about 20% of all patients with acute appendicitis have perforation at the time of operation. At the extremes of age (below 5 and above 60 years) the rate of perforation is in the region of 60%.

Aetiology

The aetiology of acute appendicitis is not at all clear. Its high incidence in the West and its relative rarity in Africa suggests a protective effect of a high-fibre diet. There is also evidence that appendicitis is commoner in urban society when compared with rural districts and this may be attributed to a high incidence of enteric infections related to crowded living conditions. Domestic and food hygiene has improved dramatically over the past 40 years and this has coincided with a significant fall in the incidence of appendicitis. There is also epidemiological evidence indicating that the consumption of green vegetables and tomatoes may be protective against appendicitis whereas potato consumption appears to be related to the disease. In elderly patients there is some evidence that chronic intake of non-steroidal anti-inflammatory drugs may increase the risk.

Clinical features

History

Owing to the embryological origin of the appendix as a mid-line structure the majority of patients with acute appendicitis first notice a pain which starts in the region of the umbilicus. This pain may be a dull ache or it may be colicky pain presumably owing to obstruction of the appendiceal lumen. After a variable period of time the pain shifts to the right lower quadrant of the abdomen owing to the inflamed appendix irritating the parietal peritoneum. It must be stressed, however, that approximately 30% of patients do not experience this shift of pain and their symptoms start with discomfort in the right lower quadrant.

Patients will usually report that movement, particularly coughing or laughing, leads to sharp exacerbations of the pain. Nausea and vomiting are common and anorexia is almost inevitable. It is important to appreciate that about 20% of patients will also have diarrhoea, particularly when the appendix lies in the pelvis, as this may lead to a mistaken diagnosis of gastroenteritis.

In taking the history it is important to ask questions which might alert one to possible alternative diagnoses. Particularly in children it is important to ask about a sore throat or 'flu-like symptoms as these often accompany mesenteric adenitis. The patient should be asked about dysuria, frequency and cloudy or strong smelling urine, as urinary tract infection can often lead to lower abdominal pain. In women, a menstrual history is essential. A missed period may point to an ectopic pregnancy. Pain at mid-cycle may indicate that the pain is due to ovulation (Mittleschmerz) and vaginal discharge may indicate pelvic inflammatory disease.

Examination

The first part of the examination should consist of general inspection of the patient's well being and measurement of their pulse and temperature. Patients with appendicitis may well have a normal pulse rate and temperature, but a sustained tachycardia is highly significant in the presence of abdominal pain and tenderness and should always be taken seriously. Likewise, the temperature may be normal but most patients with appendicitis have a low-grade pyrexia. A very high temperature (above 39°C) indicates probable abscess formation or some other diagnosis such as a viral illness.

The next stage is to observe the patient's abdomen and to look for movement with respiration. It is then useful to ask the patient to cough while watching their facial expression. If coughing produces obvious pain the patient should be asked to indicate the site of maximum pain. If this lies in the right iliac fossa this will indicate localized peritonitis in this area and is highly suggestive of appendicitis. The tongue, mouth and throat should be examined as a furred tongue and fetor oris will be present in about 50% of patients, particularly those with a long duration of illness. The tonsils should also be inspected particularly in children, as tonsillitis may be associated with mesenteric adenitis.

Attention should then be turned to palpation of the abdomen. The first point to establish is the site of maximal tenderness. In the majority of patients this is at or close to 'McBurney's point' which is situated at the junction between the upper two-thirds and lower one-third of a straight line joining the umbilicus and the anterior superior iliac spine. It must be stressed, however, that in patients with inflammation in a retrocaecal appendix the pain may be considerably higher and more lateral than this and in pelvic appendicitis the pain may be lower and almost mid-line. Indeed, with a low pelvic appendix tenderness may be only detectable by rectal examination. The abdomen should then be assessed for guarding or the involuntary contraction of the abdominal wall muscles over the area of inflamed peritoneum. Right lower quadrant guarding is found in about 90% of patients with acute appendicitis and if the appendix has perforated leading to generalized peritonitis the area of guarding may extend beyond the right lower quadrant. Rebound tenderness is another useful sign. This may be elicited by pressing gently but firmly into the right lower quadrant of the abdomen and then suddenly releasing the hand and watching the patient's face for signs of discomfort. Another approach is to use percussion which, in the presence of peritoneal irritation, will elicit the same response and is kinder.

When the amount of tenderness permits, careful palpation of the right iliac fossa for a mass should be carried out. This may indicate the presence of an appendiceal abscess or an appendix mass (phlegmon) created by omentum wrapped around the inflamed appendix. Of course, it may also indicate some other pathology such as a caecal carcinoma which is mimicking appendicitis in its presentation.

After careful examination of the abdomen, attention should be turned in the male to the testes as both acute torsion and orchitis may present initially with right lower quadrant pain. The hernial orifices should also be carefully examined for strangulated inguinal or femoral herniae and it should never be forgotten that acute appendicitis can occasionally occur in an appendix lying within a hernial sac.

Rectal examination can be extremely helpful in the clinical assessment of suspected appendicitis but in a patient with clear cut symptoms and signs it is unnecessary. However, particularly in a patient with diarrhoea and abdominal pain who does not have convincing abdominal signs, a rectal examination should always be carried out. The examining finger should be pressed on to the pelvic peritoneum first to the left and then to the right. When there is a pelvic appendicitis there will be more discomfort felt on the right. In the female the surgeon should then take opportunity of moving the cervix through the rectal wall as pain associated with this manoeuvre is highly indicative of pelvic inflammatory disease.

Diagnosis

The diagnosis of acute appendicitis is made largely on clinical grounds but there are some investigations which may be of value. These include:

- White cell count.
- A plain abdominal X-ray.
- Ultrasound and CT scanning.
- Aspiration cytology of the peritoneal cavity.
- Laparoscopy.
- Urinalysis.

White cell count

The majority of patients with acute appendicitis will have a polymorphonuclear leucocytosis and a white cell count of more than 14×10^9 per litre is suggestive of appendicitis. However, it must be remembered that various other causes of abdominal pain cause an increased white cell count and around 25% of patients with appendicitis have a normal pre-operative white cell count. For any patient in whom the diagnosis of acute appendicitis is doubtful and in whom a period of observation is felt to be appropriate it is worthwhile repeating the white cell count. A falling white cell count will strongly support the diagnosis of non-specific abdominal pain.

Plain abdominal X-ray

In a patient with clear cut symptoms and signs of acute appendicitis a plain abdominal X-ray is of little or no diagnostic value. However, it is clearly indicated if there is some clinical suspicion of intestinal obstruction or ureteric colic. An erect chest X-ray should always be requested when there is a suspicion of a perforated viscus.

Ultrasound and CT scanning

Ultrasound examination of the pelvis is particularly useful in female patients when a differential diagnosis of gynaecological pathology such as a twisted ovarian cyst is being entertained. It may also be useful in distinguishing between an appendix mass and an abscess. In addition to this there have been some reports indicating that ultrasound can be used to make the diagnosis of appendicitis with a high level of sensitivity and specificity. This has not become routine however owing to the fact that a high level of expertise is required. Such expertise is not routinely available for emergency situations in most institutions. CT scanning may occasionally be useful in establishing the diagnosis where a right lower quadrant mass is present. However, it does not have a place in the routine diagnosis of acute appendicitis.

Aspiration cytology of the peritoneal cavity

Using a 3.5 Ch umbilical artery catheter passed through a 14 Fr intravenous cannula introduced immediately below the umbilicus, it is possible to obtain samples of peritoneal fluid. If more than 50% of the cells found in the sample are neutrophils this indicates the presence of infection. This test is of particular value in distinguishing between acute appendicitis and non-specific abdominal pain but has not become routine.

Laparoscopy

Laparoscopy now has an established role in the diagnosis of acute appendicitis. It is particularly of value in women of child bearing age where there are a number of different causes of right lower quadrant pain and tenderness. Several studies now testify to the reduction in the negative appendicectomy rate in such patients. Use of laparoscopy in males and in children is less well established but whenever there is a diagnostic problem and the surgeon is unhappy about prolonged observation then laparoscopy is appropriate in any patient who has not had previous extensive abdominal surgery. During the procedure a probe should always be used in order to manipulate the caecum so that the appendix can be fully visualized.

Laparoscopy is greatly superior to a right lower quadrant gridiron incision for visualizing the abdominal and pelvic organs. For this reason it is particularly useful in planning incisions both for acute appendicitis and for other unsuspected intra-abdominal pathology. In expert hands, laparoscopy can also be used to carry out appendicectomy (see section on treatment).

Urinalysis

A urinalysis should always be carried out to exclude the possibility of urinary tract infection. It must be remembered however that about 20% of patients with appendicitis will have proteinuria and pyuria, although organisms will not be found.

Complications

Complications of acute appendicitis are secondary to gangrenous or perforated appendicitis and can therefore be avoided by prompt recognition of the condition and appropriate treatment. These are:

- Appendix abscess.
- Appendix mass.
- Generalized peritonitis, particularly in the very young or elderly.
- Intraperitoneal abscess formation, either subphrenic or multiple small intra-loop abscess.
- Faecal fistula usually following draining of an abscess.
- Recurrent intestinal obstruction due to the formation of adhesions.
- Portal pyaemia.
- Sterility in women of child bearing age. There is some debate as to whether perforation of the appendix increases the rate of infertility but recent studies indicate that it is probably not a major risk.
- Overwhelming sepsis and death.

Treatment

The mainstay of treatment in acute appendicitis is early appendicectomy. This is normally done through a small skin crease incision in the right iliac fossa, which involves splitting the underlying abdominal muscles rather than cutting them. After removal of appendix, the appendiceal stump is traditionally buried into the caecum but there have been trials to show that this manoeuvre is unnecessary. If the appendicitis is diagnosed at the time of a laparoscopy it is possible to carry out a laparoscopic appendicectomy if the surgeon has the necessary expertise. There have now been a number of randomized trials comparing conventional appendicectomy with laparoscopic appendicectomy which have produced conflicting results. The general consensus is that laparoscopic appendicectomy confers some advantage over the open operation in terms of time to mobilization and discharge from hospital. There is evidence that wound infection rate and post-operative pain are less with the laparoscopic procedure.

In all patients undergoing appendicectomy, prophylactic antibiotics should be used and a combination of metronidazole and cefuroxime is widely favoured. However, there is evidence that metronidazole alone, administered as a suppository, is appropriate. In the patient who has a perforated appendix, appendicectomy should be followed by peritoneal lavage with saline containing an antibiotic (cefuroxime or tetracycline). When perforation has occurred it is common practice to continue intravenous antibiotics for 5 days postoperatively. Clinical trials have shown that drains do not confer any benefit and may indeed increase the incidence of wound infection.

Appendicitis can be treated conservatively by means of bed rest and intravenous antibiotics (cefuroxime and metronidazole) but the risk of perforation and widespread peritonitis on this regimen is such that it cannot be recommended for routine use. However, in certain circumstances where surgery is impractical (e.g. on a ship without a surgeon on board), this may be the only feasible approach.

The treatment of patients presenting with an appendiceal mass is rather different. Although some surgeons favour an operative approach the majority will treat an appendix mass conservatively. If the patient has a fever and a high white cell count and the mass is tender these are indications that an abscess has formed. This can be confirmed by ultrasound or CT scanning and insertion of a percutaneous drain is the current treatment of choice. Occasionally this can be followed by the development of a faecal fistula but this is usually a low-output fistula which normally heals spontaneously. If percutaneous drainage is inadequate, it may be necessary to carry out operative drainage through an incision placed lateral to the mass.

If, on the other hand, a mass develops without the signs and symptoms of an abscess the best approach is conservative. However, it is important that the patient should be investigated and given a barium enema about 2 months after the development of the mass, to exclude other pathology, such as a caecal carcinoma. In patients who have had an appendix mass treated conservatively, about 15% will develop recurrent appendicitis. This should be explained to the patient and an interval appendicectomy can be carried out according to a decision made jointly by the patient and the surgeon.

When a patient has a laparoscopy or laparotomy which reveals an apparently normal appendix and no other pathology, there is some debate as to whether or not to carry out an appendicectomy. Given that the risk of developing appendicitis in adults is in the region of 0.04 and the risk from death from acute appendicitis is about 1 in 800, it seems reasonable to leave the appendix *in situ*. When a normal appendix is seen at laparoscopy this is the approach taken by most surgeons, although those skilled in laparoscopic appendicectomy may opt to remove the appendix. If on the other hand, a right iliac fossa incision has been made over the appendix it is reasonable to carry out an appendicectomy for the following reasons:

- If a scar is present in the right iliac fossa, a future assumption that appendicectomy has been carried out may be made.
- If the patient has recurring right iliac fossa pain, appendicectomy will rule out an important cause of the symptom.
- About 20% of normal appearing appendices show microscopic evidence of mucosal ulceration and pus in the lumen.
- The majority of cases of carcinoid of the appendix occur in organs which look macroscopically normal.

Neoplasms of the appendix

These are rare and include carcinoids, adenocarcinoma, mucinous neoplasms and lymphoma. The vast majority of tumours of the appendix present as acute appendicitis and the diagnosis is made on histology after appendicectomy.

Carcinoids

The appendix is the most common site for carcinoid tumour formation and carcinoid tumour of the appendix is the most common appendiceal neoplasm, accounting for 70% of tumours of this organ. The vast majority of appendiceal carcinoids are found incidentally at the time of appendicectomy, usually at the tip of the appendix. Rarely they arise at the base of the appendix and may then obstruct the lumen causing acute appendicitis. The vast majority of appendiceal carcinoids are less than 1 cm in diameter and there has never been a reported case of metastases occurring from a tumour of this size. However, when a carcinoid is greater than 1.5 cm in diameter there is a chance of metastatic disease occurring. Thus, for a carcinoid of less than 1 cm in diameter, appendicectomy is curative. If, on the other hand, the carcinoid is greater than 1.5 cm in diameter, then right hemicolectomy with radical removal of the ileocaecal lymph nodes is advisable. For tumours between 1 and 1.5 cm right hemicolectomy is probably unnecessary as long as the resection margins after appendicectomy are clear.

Adenocarcinoma

This is an extremely rare tumour and accounts for approximately 15% of all malignant tumours of the appendix. When it occurs at the base of the appendix, it may be difficult to be sure whether it has arisen in the appendix or the caecum. In all situations, the correct treatment is right hemicolectomy.

Mucinous neoplasms

A simple mucocele of the appendix is a rare condition, which is thought to arise as a sequel to obstruction of the appendix without the onset of infection. The appendix becomes distended by mucoid secretion and the normal mucosa becomes replaced by a single layer of mucus secreting cells. Eventually the lesion may calcify. Malignant mucocele on the other hand is a rare papilliferous cystadenoma or cystadenocarcinoma consisting of mucus secreting cells. It rarely metastasizes but may lead to pseudomyxoma peritonei following rupture and spillage of the mucus secreting cells **[see Module 6: Disorders of the abdominal wall and peritoneal cavity]**

Meckel's diverticulum

Anatomy

A Meckel's diverticulum is a remnant of the vitello-intestinal duct and is present in about 2% of the population. It arises from the anti-mesenteric side of the ileum. It has the same microscopic structure as the adjacent small bowel and it has a separate blood supply from the adjacent small bowel mesentery (the omphalomesenteric artery). Although it is frequently said that most Meckel's diverticula are situated 60 cm from the ileocaecal valve, as many as 25% may be situated more proximally in the ileum. The length and shape of the diverticulum is highly variable and although 85% are blind-ended, the rest have an attachment which is related to its embryological origin. Two per cent of these exist as a patent vitello-intestinal duct with a faecal fistula at the umbilicus. In 1% the diverticulum is attached to the umbilicus by a band and in about 10% of cases a band from the diverticulum is connected to the adjacent mesentery (a meso-diverticular band) (Figure 13.29).

Ectopic tissue is found within the Meckel's diverticulum in about 70% of cases. This is usually gastric mucosa, but it is also possible to find pancreatic, duodenal or colonic tissue. The presence of ectopic gastric mucosa has important implications for the clinical presentation of Meckel's diverticulum, as it is associated with peptic ulceration secondary to acid and pepsin secretion.

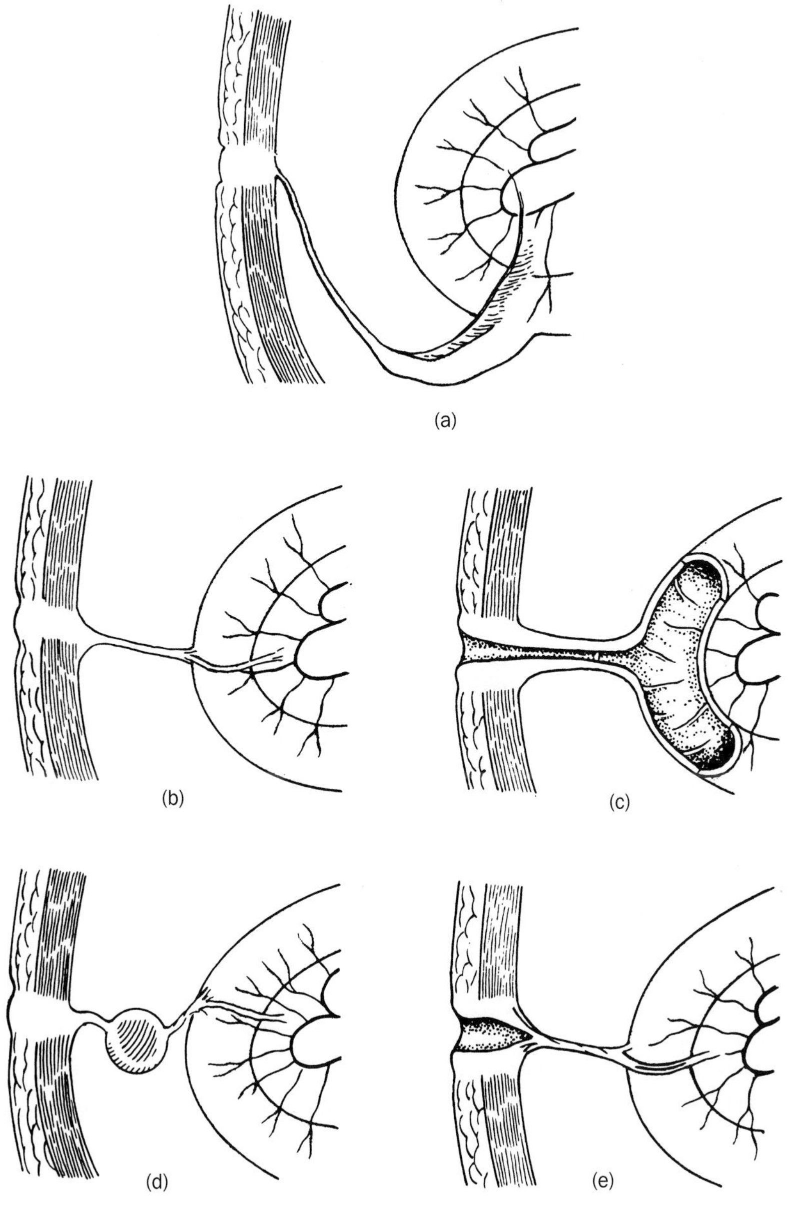

Figure 13.29 The vitello-intestinal duct may connect with the umbilicus as: (a) a fibrous cord extending from a Meckel's diverticulum; (b) a simple fibrous cord to a loop of ileum; (c) an umbilical intestinal fistula; (d) a fibrous cord with cyst; (e) an umbilical sinus.

Pathology

The majority of Meckel's diverticula do not cause problems and remain asymptomatic. However, the following three pathological processes may occur as a result of a Meckel's diverticulum:

- Inflammation of the diverticulum.
- Peptic ulceration of the small bowel.
- Intestinal obstruction.

Inflammation

Meckel's diverticulum can become inflamed in very much the same way as the vermiform appendix. Likewise, gangrene and perforation of the diverticulum may ensue.

Peptic ulceration

When there is heterotopic gastric mucosa within the lumen of the diverticulum (~40%) this secretes pepsin and hydrochloric acid. As a result peptic ulceration may occur, most commonly at the neck of the diverticulum or just distally in the ileum. The role of *Helicobacter pylori* in peptic ulceration related to a Meckel's diverticulum is not known.

Intestinal obstruction

Intestinal obstruction may result from intussusception occurring with the diverticulum acting as a lead point. It can also occur because of persistence of the band which was once the vitello-intestinal duct producing a small bowel volvulus. In addition, entrapment of small bowel can occur through a defect caused by a mesodiverticular band or the omphalomesenteric artery.

Clinical features

The clinical presentation of symptomatic Meckel's diverticulum depends on the underlying pathology.

Acute inflammation

Acute Meckel's diverticulitis produces a symptom complex which is very similar to appendicitis but normally the pain persists in the central abdominal area without a shift to the right lower quadrant. This usually occurs in children and frequently a diagnosis of acute appendicitis is made.

Peptic ulceration with bleeding

Peptic ulceration of the neck of the Meckel's diverticulum or the ileum can lead to bleeding which presents as either melena or fresh rectal bleeding. Again this nearly always occurs in children.

Intestinal obstruction

This may present with the typical clinical features of a small bowel obstruction. However, infarction of the bowel is likely with volvulus or entrapment of the small bowel by the band and in such cases the patient will become rapidly ill with a pyrexia and tachycardia, and be found to have peritonitis on examination.

Diagnosis

The diagnosis of Meckel's diverticulum is usually made at operation but in the child who is having repeated episodes of brisk rectal bleeding or melena, a technetium scan may be of value. In this test, intravenous administration of ^{99m}Tc is followed by external scintiscanning. The radionuclide is taken up by the ectopic gastric mucosa (see Figure 13.5). Mesenteric angiography may also be helpful in the presence of active bleeding.

Treatment

The standard treatment of a Meckel's diverticulum is excision of the diverticulum together with a wedge of the adjacent ileum. In some cases however, with extensive inflammation of the diverticulum a limited small bowel resection may be necessary. If a Meckel's diverticulum is found incidentally during the course of a laparotomy, removal is not necessary if the diverticulum has a wide base and feels soft on palpation. However, if the neck is narrow or nodules are palpable in the walls of the diverticulum, removal is advisable.

Further reading

Borley, N. R., Mortensen, N. J. and Jewell, D. P. (1997). Preventing postoperative recurrence of Crohn's disease. *Br J Surg* **84**: 1493–1502.

Bouchier, I. A. D., Allan, R. N., Hodgson, H. J. F. and Keighley, M. R. B. (1993). *Gastroenterology*, 2nd edn, London: WB Saunders.

Chen, S. C., Lin, F. Y., Lee, P. H. *et al.* (1998). Water-soluble constrast study predicts the need for early surgery in adhesive small bowel obstruction. *Br J Surg* **85**: 1692–4.

El-Rifai, W., Sarlomo-Rikala, M., Andersson, L. C. *et al.* (1998). DNA copy number changes in gastrointestinal stromal tumours – a distinct genetic entity. *Ann Chir Gynaec* **87**: 287–90.

Hugot, J. P., Laurent-Puig, P., Gomes-Rousseau, C. *et al.* (1996). Mapping of a susceptibility locus for Crohn's disease of chromosome 16. *Nature* **379**: 772–3.

Jones, P. F., Krukowski, Z. H. and Youngson, G. C. (1998). *Emergency Abdominal Surgery*, 3rd edn, London: Chapman and Hall.

Misewicz, J. J., Pounder, R. E. and Venables, C. W. (1994). *Diseases of the Gut and Pancreas*, 2nd edn, Oxford: Blackwell Science.

Morgan, B. K., Compton, C., Talbert, M. *et al.* (1990). Benign smooth tumours of the gastrointestinal tract. *Ann Surg* **211**: 63–6.

Nolan, D. J. (1997). The true yield of small-intestinal barium study. *Endoscopy* **29**: 447–53.

Present, D. H., Rutgeerts, P., Targan, S. *et al.* (1999). Infliximab for the treatment of fistulas in patients with Crohn's disease. *N Engl J Med* **340**: 1398–405.

Stebbing, J. F., Jewell, D. P., Kettlewell, M. G. W. *et al.* (1995). Long-term results of recurrence and reoperation after stricturoplasty for obstructive Crohn's disease. *Br J Surg* **82**: 1471–4.

MODULE 14

Disorders of the colon and rectum

Section 14.1 • Anatomy

The large intestine consists of the caecum, the vermiform appendix, the ascending colon, the hepatic flexure, the transverse colon, the splenic flexure, the descending colon, the sigmoid colon, the rectum and the anal canal (Figure 14.1). The anatomy of the appendix and anal canal is dealt with separately in the appropriate modules.

Originally a mid-line structure, the large intestine undergoes rotation during embryological development and as a result the ascending colon and the descending colon are essentially retro-peritoneal structures. However, the degree to which the large intestine has a mesentery is highly variable as is its total length that averages 1.5 m. The whole of the large intestine is capable of considerable distension although in the adult living in the Western world the left side of the colon tends to be less distensible than the right owing to muscular hypertrophy.

The caecum lies in the right iliac fossa and is approximately 7 cm in length and width. Proximally it becomes the ascending colon at its junction with the terminal ileum. The caecum lies on the iliac and psoas muscles and on the genitofemoral, femoral and lateral cutaneous nerves. It also lies anterior to the testicular or ovarian vessels and the ureter. The exact position of the caecum is variable and it may extend into the true pelvis. The caecum is almost completely surrounded by peritoneum but it is often attached to the iliac fossa medially and laterally. This can produce a retro-caecal peritoneal recess which may extend upwards posterior to the ascending colon.

The ileocaecal junction is extremely variable in appearance. In most circumstances the ileum enters obliquely into the large bowel through a horizontal slit and is partly invaginated into the caecum to form a fold (the ileocaecal valve). Reflux of caecal contents into the small bowel is prevented by contraction of the circular muscle of the ileum which leads to closure of the ileocaecal valve. However, the muscle in the valve

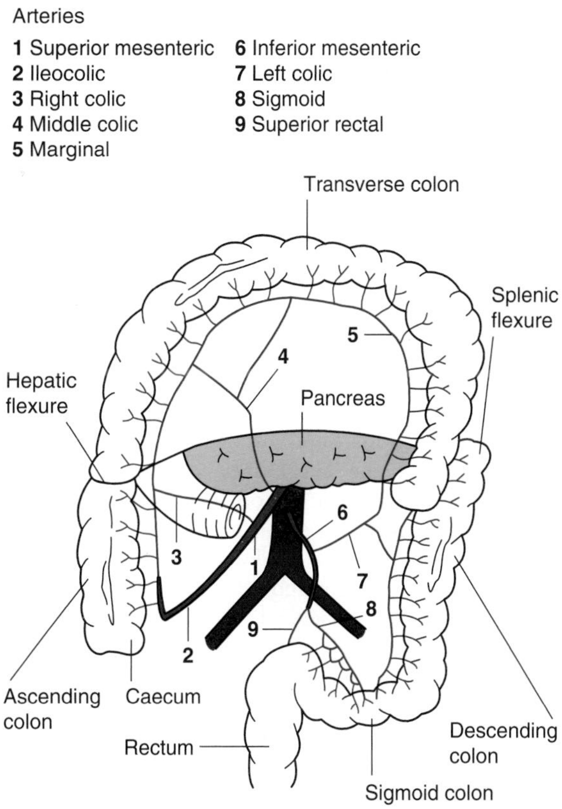

Figure 14.1 The large intestine and its blood supply.

is poorly developed and the ileocaecal valve is frequently incompetent.

The ascending colon varies from about 10 to 20 cm in length. It lies on the iliac muscle, the iliac crest and quadratus lumborum, crossing the lateral cutaneous nerve of the thigh, the ilioinguinal and iliohypogastric nerves. It ends at the hepatic flexure where the large bowel turns to the left on the lower portion of the right kidney posterior to the liver. Under most circumstances peritoneum covers the front and the sides of the ascending colon and fixes it firmly to the posterior abdominal wall, but occasionally there is a short mesentery.

The transverse colon is the longest section of the colon varying from 40 to 70 cm in length. It extends from the hepatic flexure to the splenic flexure and forms a dependent loop between both of these points. The lowest point of the transverse colon may reach below the umbilicus although it is usually just superior to it. The transverse colon is suspended by the transverse mesocolon which is fused to the posterior surface of the greater omentum. This transverse mesocolon is attached to the descending part of the duodenum, to the head and the lower aspect of the body of the pancreas and to the anterior surface of the left kidney. It contains both the middle colic vessels and branches of the right and left colic vessels with associated nerves and lymphatics. Thus the transverse colon starts immediately anterior to the descending part of the duodenum and the head of the pancreas, descends anterior to the small intestine and ascends to the splenic flexure. At this point it is anterior to the left part of the left kidney and immediately below the spleen. The splenic flexure is attached to the diaphragm by peritoneum (phrenicocolic ligament) and can be extremely close to the spleen. At this point the greater omentum frequently has attachments to the spleen and is closely associated with the colon. Traction on these splenic attachments may cause splenic bleeding in the course of mobilization of the splenic flexure.

The descending colon extends from the splenic flexure to the rim of the true pelvis close to the inguinal ligament. The descending colon is attached by peritoneum to the posterior abdominal wall in the left paravertebral gutter and iliac fossa. Superiorly it is anterior to the lateral surface of the left kidney and medial to the diaphragm, and then it lies on the same muscles and nerves as the ascending colon. At the anterior superior iliac spine, the descending colon turns medially superior to inguinal ligament and lies on the femoral nerve, psoas muscle and the genital vessels, and becomes the sigmoid colon immediately anterior to the external iliac vessels.

The sigmoid colon is the most variable part of the colon in terms of its length (50–80 cm) and its mobility. It extends from the end of the descending colon to the rim of the true pelvis where it becomes the rectum. It has a long mesentery (the sigmoid mesocolon) which has quite a short base starting at the end of the descending colon and ascending on the external iliac vessels to the mid point of the common iliac artery. At this point it turns downwards and to the right to the rim of the true pelvis. The mesocolon contains the sigmoid branches of the inferior mesenteric artery and associated nerves and lymphatics. Under normal circumstances the sigmoid colon lies free in the left iliac fossa and the true pelvis but it may also extend across to the right iliac fossa.

The rectum is that part of the large bowel which lies in the true pelvis at the point where the sigmoid mesocolon ends. Again, this is highly variable in length depending very much on the build of the individual but it is said to be 15 cm long as measured by a rigid sigmoidoscope. It follows the curve of the sacrum and the coccyx and then runs anteriorly and inferiorly to the central perineal tendon lying on the anococcygeal ligament and the levator ani muscles. It then ends by turning posteriorly and inferiorly as the anal canal, immediately posterior to the central perineal tendon and to the apex of the prostate in the male. The lowest part of the rectum is more capacious than the rest and is known as the ampulla. The rectum is not straight; in the sagittal plane it follows the curve of the sacrum and coccyx and in the coronal plane it is S shaped. This gives rise to prominent folds within the lumen of the rectum known as the valves of Houston. The front and the sides of the upper third of the rectum are covered with peritoneum but this gradually moves anteriorly and turns off the front of the rectum at the junction between its middle and lower thirds. This forms the rectouterine or rectovesical pouch by passing upwards on the back of the posterior fornix of the vagina or the back of the bladder respectively in the female and the male. In its lower third, the rectum lies behind the base of the bladder, the seminal vesicals and the prostate in the male and behind the vagina in the female.

In both sexes the rectum and its surrounding areolar tissue is separated from the anterior structures by a fascial layer known as Denonvilliers' fascia. Posteriorly the rectum is separated from the sacrum and the coccyx and anococcygeal ligament and the muscles attached to these (piriformis and levator ani) by a layer of pelvic fascia. This fascia is known as Waldeyer's fascia. In its upper two-thirds the actual muscular wall of the rectum is separated from the pelvic fascia by a posterior cushion of areolar tissue which becomes circumferential below the rectouterine or rectovesical pouch. This carries the blood supply to the rectum and its lymphatic drainage and is known as the mesorectum (Figure 14.2). Inferiorly and posteriorly the mesorectum has a bi-lobed structure.

Taeniae coli

The taeniae coli are three ribbon-like thickenings of the otherwise thin longitudinal muscle of the large bowel which arise from the longitudinal muscle at the root of the vermiform appendix and end by spreading out at the end of the sigmoid colon to become contin-

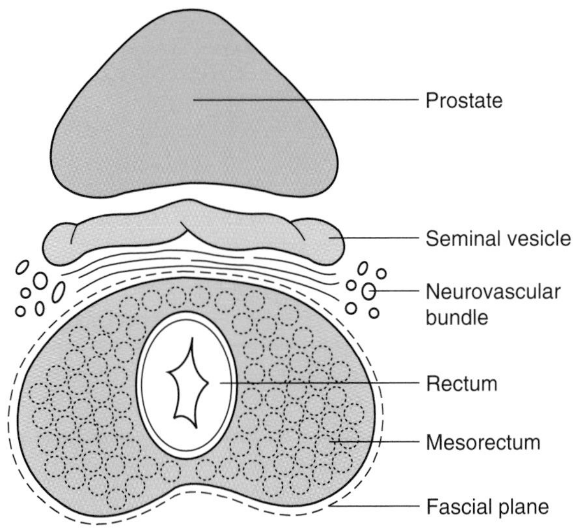

Figure 14.2 Cross-section of the rectum at the level of the seminal vesicles, showing the mesorectum.

uous with the thicker longitudinal muscle of the rectum. These three taeniae are spaced out uniformly around the circumference of the colon and between them the wall of the colon bulges outwards forming pouches or sacculations. In ascending colon and descending colon, the taeniae are anterior, posteromedial and posterolateral, whereas in the transverse colon the positions become posterior, superior and anterior.

Blood supply of the large intestine

The most important vessels involved in the blood supply of the colon are the superior mesenteric artery, the inferior mesenteric artery and the marginal artery which supplies an anastomosis between these two vessels (Figure 14.1). The superior mesenteric artery originates from the aorta just below the coeliac axis and passes posterior to the pancreas. Its terminal branch which supplies the caecum is known as the ileocolic artery. Its other named main branches which supply the colon are the right colic artery which supplies the ascending colon and the middle colic artery which runs in the transverse mesocolon to supply the transverse colon. The inferior mesenteric artery arises from the aorta just inferior to the third part of the duodenum and descends on the left side of the aorta posterior to the peritoneum. Its first branch is the left colic artery which passes to the left and divides into ascending and descending branches. The ascending branch supplies the left side of the transverse colon and the splenic flexure whereas the descending branch supplies the descending colon. The inferior mesenteric artery terminates at the base of the sigmoid mesocolon where it divides into sigmoid branches supplying the sigmoid colon and the superior rectal artery which descends in the mesorectum to supply the upper part of the rectum.

The marginal artery runs along the ascending transverse and descending colons, receiving branches from the other colic arteries so that under normal circumstances ligation of any one of the main colic arteries would not result in ischaemia of any part of the colon. It must be remembered, however, that the marginal artery can become quite tenuous at the splenic flexure and continuity of the blood supply may be maintained by the ascending and descending branches of the left colic artery. It is therefore imperative that these two vessels are preserved when dividing either the left colic artery or the inferior mesenteric trunk during mobilization of the colon.

As mentioned above, the upper part of the rectum derives its blood supply from the superior rectal artery which is a terminal branch of the inferior mesenteric artery, but the lower rectum receives blood from the two middle rectal (or haemorrhoidal) arteries coming from the internal iliac arteries and two inferior rectal arteries which originate from the internal pudendal artery in the ischiorectal fossa. The internal pudendal artery is itself a branch of the internal iliac artery.

The venous drainage of the large intestine follows its arterial blood supply but of course empties into the portal venous system. The inferior mesenteric vein diverges from the inferior mesenteric artery and passes up behind the pancreas to join the splenic vein. The superior mesenteric vein lies to the right of the superior mesenteric artery and joins the splenic vein at its junction with the portal vein behind the neck of the pancreas.

The lymphatic drainage of the large intestine also follows the blood supply. Small lymph nodes lie close to the marginal artery and also along the artery leading towards it. The lymph draining through the lymph nodes associated with the branches of the superior mesenteric artery passes into the intestinal trunk which lies in the root of the small bowel mesentery. The lymph nodes associated with the inferior mesenteric artery drain into the lumbar lymph nodes beside the aorta. Both of these empty into the cisterna chyli which enters the posterior thorax via the diaphragmatic hiatus.

Nerve supply of the large intestine

The nerve supply of the colon and the rectum, like the lymphatics, follows the course of the main vessels. The right colon receives sympathetic nerve fibres from the lower six dorsal ganglia via the superior mesenteric plexus and parasympathetic fibres from the coeliac branch of the posterior vagus nerve. The left colon and rectum are supplied through the upper three lumbar ganglia via the inferior mesenteric, superior hypogastric and inferior hypogastric plexuses (Figure 14.3). The latter plexus also receives branches from the sacral parasympathetic nerves (nervi erigentes). These nerves remain outside the pelvic fascia and are sometimes injured during mobilization of the rectum.

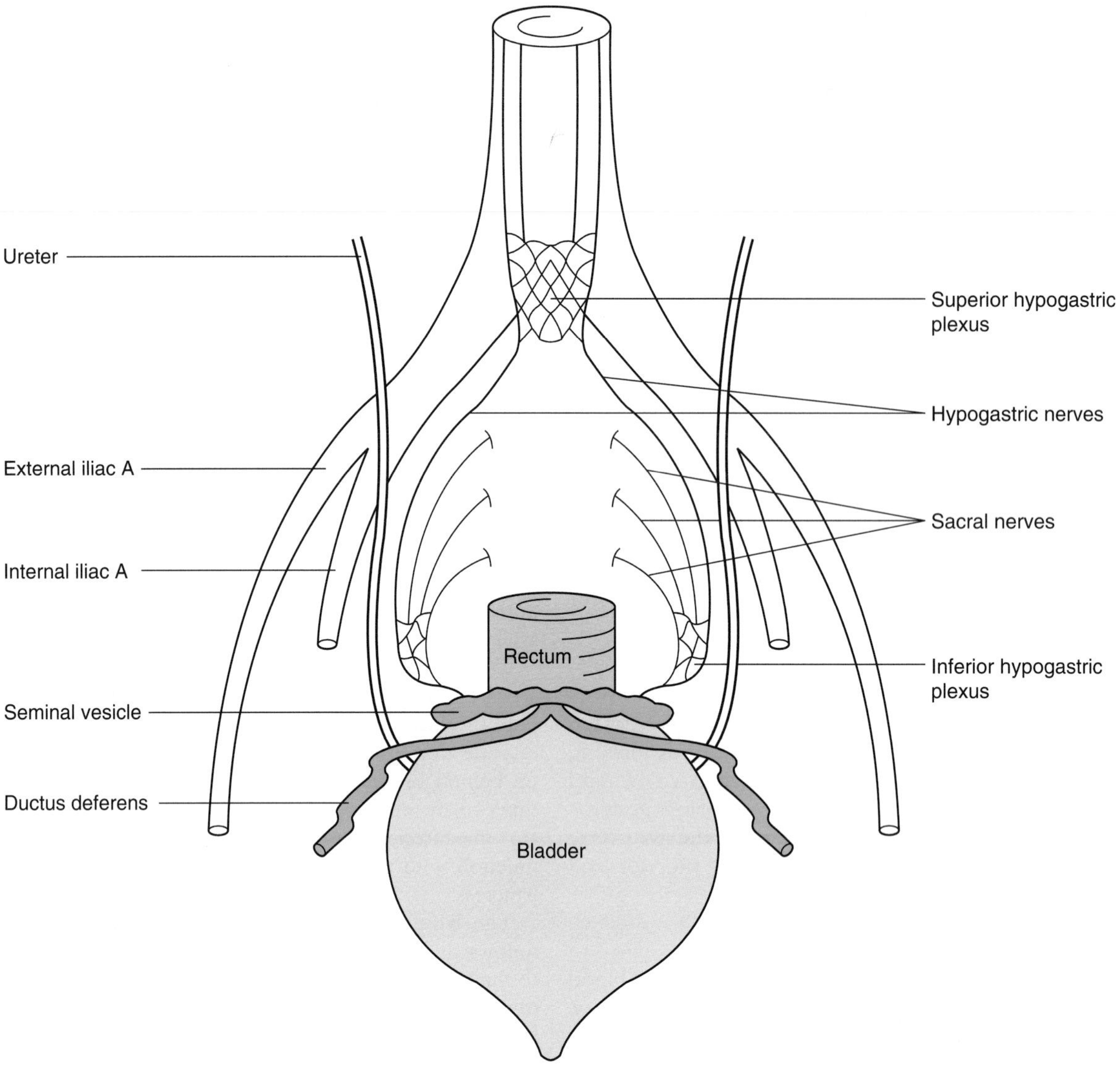

Figure 14.3 The autonomic nerves of the pelvis.

Section 14.2 • Physiology of the colon and rectum

Absorption and excretion

About 1000 ml of ileal contents containing 90% water are discharged into the caecum every day in the normal adult. Water absorption takes place during transit through the colon and only 100–200 ml of water are excreted in the faeces. The absorptive capacity of the colon depends on the rate at which ileal contents enter the caecum, and is greater in the right colon than in the left. Normal faeces are composed of 70% water and 30% solids; about 50% of the solids are bacteria and the remainder is composed of food waste and desquamated epithelium.

Nutrients such as glucose, amino acids, fatty acids and vitamins can be absorbed slowly through the colonic wall but only very small amounts of these substances actually reach the caecum under normal circumstances. Sodium absorption is very efficient and is maintained by an active transport mechanism enhanced by mineralocorticoids and glucocorticoids. A normal adult can remain in sodium balance with as little as 5 mmol of sodium per day in the diet but following total colectomy and ileostomy the minimum daily requirement increases to about 100 mmol to offset losses from the stoma. Chloride and water absorption is passive and follows electrical and osmotic gradients established by the sodium pump.

Potassium is actively excreted into the faeces against a concentration gradient and by secretion in mucus. Excessive mucus production (e.g. in colitis or in villous adenomas) may lead to enormous losses of potassium. Only a small amount of bicarbonate is secreted into the colonic lumen in exchange for chloride.

A normal bowel habit is hard to define since it is influenced by social and dietary customs. The frequency of bowel movement in Western countries ranges from every 8 hours to once every 2–3 days. Any persistent change in bowel habit is an indication for investigation to exclude organic disease. Diarrhoea may be defined as stools containing more than 300 ml of fluid daily, although again this is highly variable. When excessive, it may be debilitating and even fatal if associated with large losses of fluid and electrolytes which are not replaced. Inflammatory disease of the colon or small bowel mucosa may cause excessive exudation of fluid and also lead to diarrhoea as does anything that decreases the intestinal transit time and decreases absorptive surface area. The symptom of constipation has different meanings for different individuals. For some it implies infrequency of bowel movements, others hard consistence of the stool and others may use the term to indicate difficulty in evacuation. The pathologies leading to diarrhoea and constipation are dealt with later in the chapter.

Colonic motility

There are three patterns of motor activity in the colon:

- *Segmentation*. This is the most common type of motor activity seen in the transverse and descending colon and consists of annular contractions that divide the lumen into segments propelling faeces over short distances in both directions. Segmental contractions form, relax and re-form in different locations in a random fashion, three to eight times per minute.
- *Mass movements*. These consist of strong contractions moving distally over relatively short distances (30–45 cm) in the transverse and descending colon. These are infrequent and probably occur only a few times each day, often in response to a meal.
- *Retrograde peristalsis*. This consists of annular contractions moving proximally in the right colon and in the sigmoid and descending colon. This is more frequently seen in experimental animals than in man. The retrograde movement can be shown by observing the spontaneous movement of a radio-opaque marker from the left to right colon.

A complex neurohormonal mechanism is involved in the colonic response to eating which has been inaccurately described as the gastrocolic reflex. This response consists of increased ileal emptying, increased mass movements and an urge to defecate. Other factors influencing colonic motility are physical activity, emotional states and faecal bulk. Thus normal colonic emptying is slow, complex and exceedingly variable. It is difficult to define altered motility in diseased states. There is no orderly laminar flow; some of the material entering the caecum flows past faecal material which has remained from earlier time periods. In general, residue from a meal reaches the caecum after 4 hours and the rectosigmoid by 24 hours. Since there is a large amount of mixing of bowel contents in the colon, residue from a single meal may be passed in the stool for 3–4 days afterwards under normal circumstances.

Intraluminal pressure studies of the colon can be performed by the use of small balloons, fine open-ended catheters or telemetry capsules. Such studies indicate that although pressures of up to 100 mmHg can be generated, faecal transport can take place without a rise in intraluminal pressure. However, because specific patterns cannot be correlated with defined diseased states these investigations have little clinical significance. Rhythmic changes in the electrical potential in colonic muscle occur normally at two frequencies, 3 and 9/min, respectively. The frequency appears to be approximately 16/min in the sigmoid colon with diverticular disease.

Microbiology of the large intestine

The normal faecal flora exists in a symbiotic relationship with the human host and supports several physiological processes. Bile pigments are degraded by colonic bacteria to give the stool its brown colour. Characteristic faecal odour is due to the amines indole and skatole which are produced by bacterial action. Colonic bacteria also supply vitamin K to the host, alter both colonic motility and absorption and may be important in the defence against potentially more pathogenic organisms. Faecal bacteria deconjugate bile salts to produce free bile acids and also alter the steroid nucleus. These bacteria have been implicated in the pathophysiology of a variety of disease processes including the pathogenesis of carcinoma of the large bowel.

The colon of the fetus is sterile and bacterial colonization occurs soon after birth. The bacterial flora present in the colon varies with dietary and environmental factors, but over 99% of the normal flora is anaerobic. *Bacteroides fragilis* is the most prevalent. *Lactobacillus bifidus*, clostridia of various types and cocci of various types form the other common anaerobes. Aerobic bacteria can be divided into two groups, coliforms and enterococci. *Escherichia coli* is the predominant coliform and is present in counts of around 10^7 per gram of wet faeces. *Streptococcus faecalis* is the principal enterococcus and is present in similar numbers.

The bacterial flora of the colon is readily altered by antibiotic administration. Oral neomycin and tetracycline result in resistant R-factor enterococci and resistant staphylococci and bacteroides. Outbreaks of staphylococcal enterocolitis and more commonly pseudomembranous colitis from *Clostridium difficile* are frequently seen in surgical units.

Section 14.3 • Investigations

The main techniques used in the investigation of colorectal disease (excluding anorectal problems) can be subdivided into endoscopy and radiology. Under these headings the following procedures will be considered: rigid endoscopy, flexible endoscopy, barium enema, radio-opaque marker studies, colonic scintigraphy, ultrasound, computed tomography (CT) scanning and magnetic resonance imaging (MRI).

Rigid endoscopy

Rigid endoscopy is only of value in examining the anal canal and rectum and in the UK the nomenclature for describing the appropriate instruments is confusing. The term proctoscope refers to a short instrument which is only really of value in examining the anal canal and this will be described in the appropriate module. The term rigid sigmoidoscope is the term used to describe the 25 cm long instrument which is used in association with a fibre-optic light source and insufflating bellows (Figure 14.4). Although reusable metal instruments are available most outpatient departments now use disposable plastic instruments which can be self-lubricating. This allows multiple examinations to be performed without the risk of infection and without the need for cleansing and sterilizing the instrument. In addition, the attachment between the instrument and the bellows should be protected by a filtering device which will prevent infective agents being harboured in the bellows.

The term sigmoidoscope is misleading as only the very distal part of the sigmoid can be examined by the instrument and in most cases it is impractical to pass the instrument much beyond 15 cm. Under most circumstances the rigid instrument is used in unprepared bowel and although this may make the investigation difficult and sometimes impossible it is useful to be able to see whether there is any blood staining on the faecal material. The other major advantage of rigid sigmoidoscopy is that it allows the operator to determine the exact position of a rectal lesion, i.e. whether it is on the anterior, posterior, right or left lateral walls of the rectum. This is essential information when considering transanal excision of a rectal tumour as the positioning of the patient on the operating table will depend on the exact site of the tumour. Aside from this, rigid sigmoidoscopy has no advantages over flexible endoscopy and it has several disadvantages. First, it is more uncomfortable; secondly, examination is limited to the rectum; thirdly, it is difficult to see behind mucosal folds; and fourthly, it can be very difficult to see lesions just inside the anal canal.

Nevertheless, the instrument is widely used in outpatient departments as it offers the surgeon a rapid method of examining the rectum to look for tumours or mucosal inflammation. When carrying out an examination it is important to bear in mind the slightly anterior direction of the anal canal and then the sharp posterior angulation of the rectum, followed by the curve of the sacrum. Whenever pain is encountered the examination should be terminated immediately. When biopsies are taken using a rigid sigmoidoscope it must be remembered that the biopsy forceps are much larger than those used with flexible instruments and care must be taken not to cause full thickness damage to the rectal wall, particularly anteriorly where a perforation may occur.

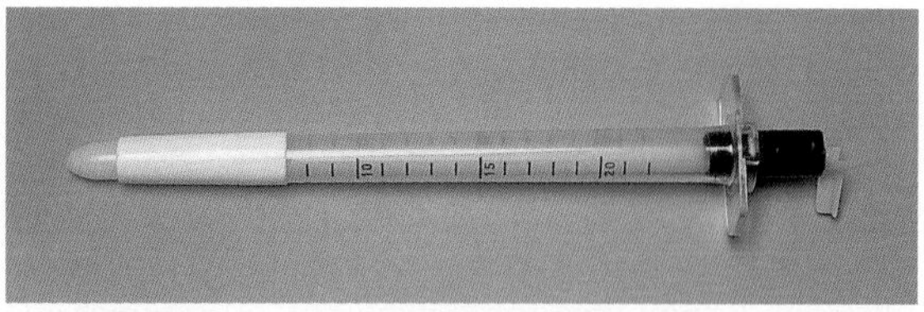

Figure 14.4 Rigid sigmoidoscope.

Flexible endoscopy

The two types of flexible endoscope available are the flexible sigmoidoscope and the colonoscope. The flexible sigmoidoscope is a 60 cm instrument which is designed to examine no further than the descending colon. The colonoscope (Figure 14.5), on the other hand, is a longer instrument, varying from 120 to 180 cm in length and this is designed to reach the caecum. The first generation of flexible endoscopes was based on fibre-optic technology, but more recently videoendoscopes which incorporate a chip camera in the distal end of the instrument have come to the fore. In the latter, a digital image is displayed on a video monitor without an eyepiece optical interface.

The technique of flexible sigmoidoscopy is essentially similar to that of the first part of colonoscopy and therefore separate descriptions of the two procedures are not necessary. However, it is conventional for flexi-

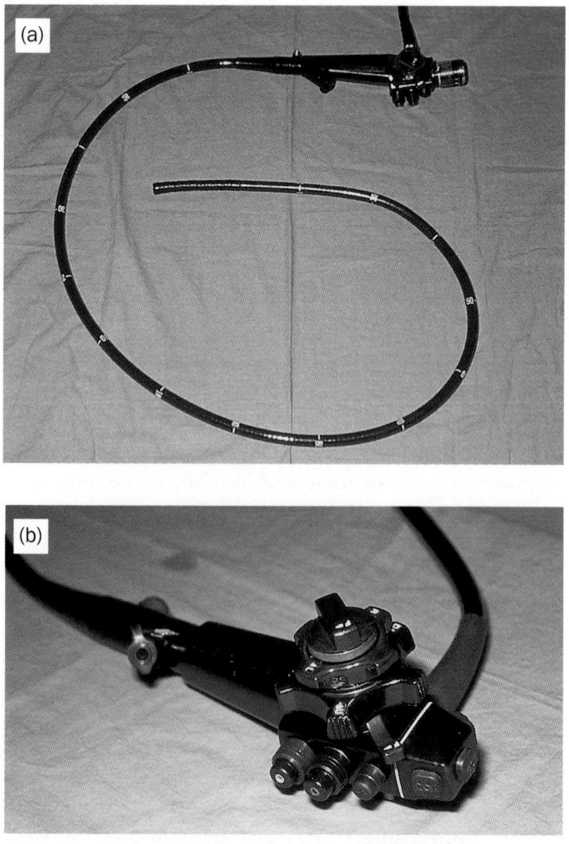

Figure 14.5 (a) A fibre-optic colonoscope. (b) The operating head of a video colonoscope. Note the absence of an eyepiece.

ble sigmoidoscopy to be done without sedation whereas most endoscopists will use some form of sedation for colonoscopy as both insufflation of the large bowel and stretching of the mesentery caused by looping of the colonoscope can cause considerable discomfort. It is however essential that the patient should be able to respond to pain as this is an important signal to the endoscopist that the procedure may be about to cause damage to the colon.

Although there are many different forms of sedation it is this author's preference to use a combination of an opiate (pethidine) and a benzodiazepine (diazemuls) given intravenously. Because the sedation produced is profound it is essential that secure venous access is obtained by means of an indwelling cannula and that the patient's oxygen saturation is continuously measured by pulse oximetry. It is also essential that antagonists to both opiates (nalaxone) and benzodiazepines (flumazenil) are readily available.

The examination begins conventionally with the patient lying in the left lateral position. The rectum is usually easy to negotiate but at the rectosigmoid junction it may be necessary to pass the tip of the colonoscope 'blindly' to gain access to the sigmoid colon. This is a hazardous manoeuvre, particularly in the patient who has had previous pelvic surgery leading to adhesions, as perforation of the colon can occur. It must therefore be carried out with the utmost gentleness. In the sigmoid colon the colonoscope may assume either an N loop or an alpha loop (Figure 14.6). Once a loop like this has formed it is necessary to straighten the endoscope by pulling back and applying clockwise torque (Figure 14.7). The colonoscope should then be advanced maintaining the torque. If clockwise torque does not work, it is worth trying anticlockwise torque.

It is then usually a straightforward procedure to reach the splenic flexure but advancing the endoscope along the transverse colon may be difficult because of the formation of a further loop (Figure 14.8). This again may be overcome by withdrawing the colonoscope and it often helps to turn the patient on to his or her back. Throughout this procedure it is important not to over-insufflate the colon and regular withdrawal of the colonoscope with suction will 'concertina' the colon over the colonoscope. When the hepatic flexure has been reached a useful manoeuvre is to angle the tip of the colonoscope into the ascending colon and apply suction. This will often bring the caecum up to the tip of the colonoscope. If this is unsuccessful then turning the patient on to their right side (facing the endoscopist) may be a useful manoeuvre.

It is very important to recognize when the caecum has been reached and the only two really definite land marks are the ileocaecal valve and the appendix orifice. Ideally the ileocaecal valve should be entered and a biopsy taken of the ileal mucosa to prove completion of colonoscopy but this is a tricky and time consuming manoeuvre and few endoscopists would recommend doing this routinely. It must be emphasized that the anal canal and the caecum are the only two parts of the large bowel which can be identified unequivocally during colonoscopy, and even the most experienced colonoscopist will have difficulty in identifying the exact anatomical location of a lesion lying within the colon if it is not in the lower rectum or the caecum.

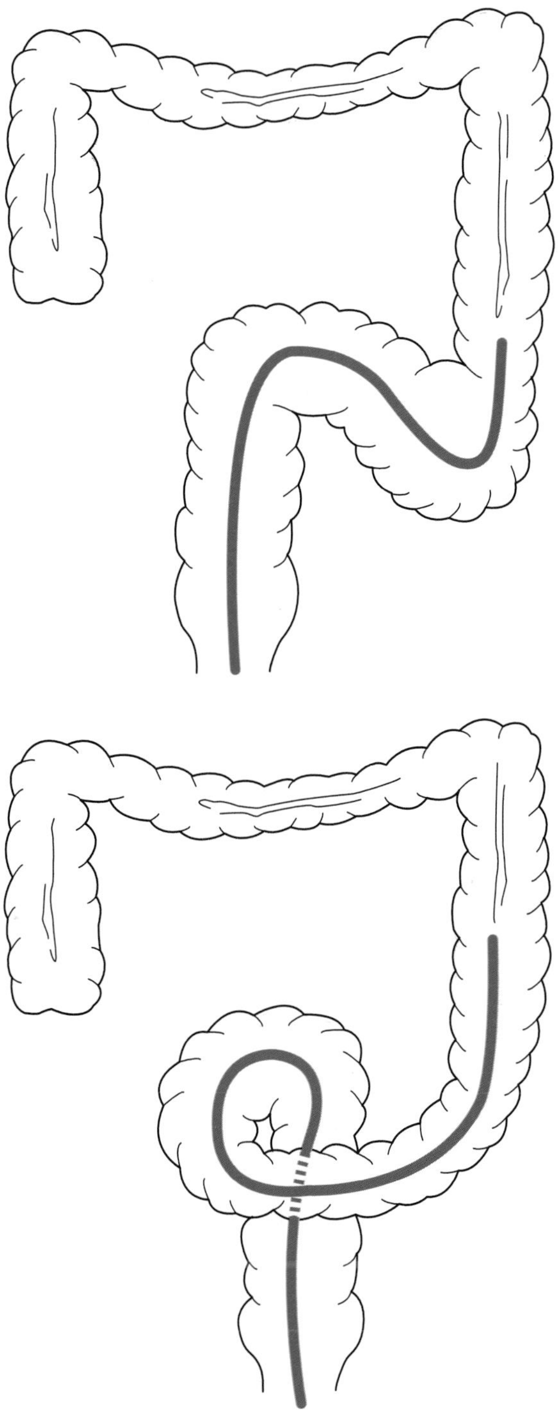

Figure 14.6 The N loop and the α loop.

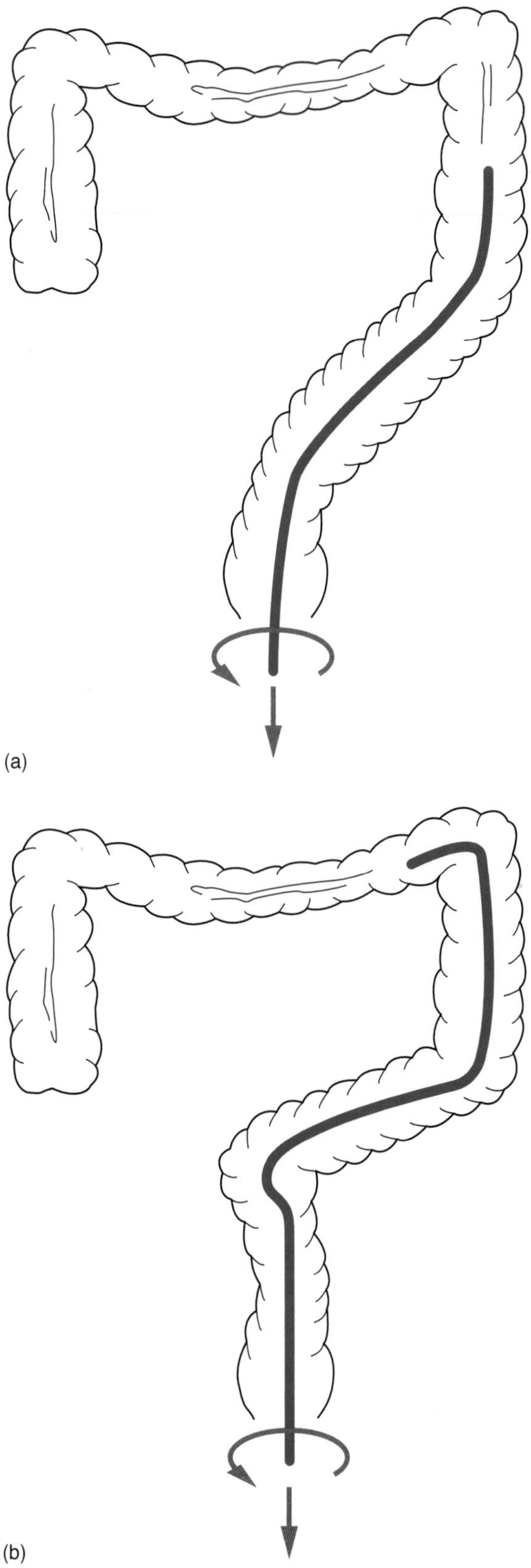

Figure 14.7 Straightening a sigmoid N loop (a) and α loop (b).

Complications of colonoscopy

The main complications of colonoscopy are perforation, haemorrhage, bacteraemia and cardiac arryhthmias. Perforation may result at the tip of the instrument or at the apex of a stretched loop (Figure 14.9). Perforation should always be suspected if there is bleeding or if fat can be seen through the wall of the colon. Obviously when small bowel loops can be seen the diagnosis is not in doubt. Perforation can also occur after polypectomy (see section on polyps) but this may be delayed. Likewise hot biopsy (see section on polyps) may lead to delayed perforation. The incidence of perforation is about 0.1% and all patients undergoing colonoscopy should have this risk explained.

Haemorrhage is nearly always a consequence of polypectomy. Significant haemorrhage after an ordinary colonocsopic biopsy is unlikely unless the patient has a coagulation disorder. Bacteraemia has been shown to occur after colonoscopy and it is therefore necessary to use intravenous antibiotics in patients with cardiac pacemakers, artificial cardiac valves or cardiac valve disease. Cardiac arryhthmias commonly occur during colonoscopy but they are usually insignificant and self limiting. It is however important that patients with cardiac disease should have continuous electrocardiogram (ECG) monitoring and it is essential that resuscitation equipment is present when colonoscopy is being performed.

Radiology

Plain radiology

Plain abdominal X-ray films are particularly useful in the emergency situation. In the patient with mechanical large bowel obstruction, a typical gas pattern will be seen with obvious haustration and a typical distributions of gas throughout the colon (Figure 14.10). Pseudo-obstruction may be difficult to distinguish from mechanical obstruction although, in the former, the colonic dilatation usually ends in the region of the proximal descending colon. Obstruction due to volvulus of the sigmoid colon or the caecum will show a typical pattern and in patients with ischaemic colitis typical 'thumb printing' is seen when plain abdominal X-rays are obtained. In the emergency situation an erect chest X-ray should also be carried out. This can be scrutinized for gas under the diaphragm. The plain abdominal X-ray is also essential in patients with an acute exacerbation of ulcerative colitis or Crohn's colitis as this will help in making the diagnosis of toxic megacolon.

Barium enema

The mainstay of radiological investigation of the large bowel is the barium enema. Nowadays, this is always carried out as a double contrast study, i.e. with barium and insufflated air. This coats the colonic mucosa with barium allowing radiologists to detect small lesions and mucosal ulceration. Barium enemas are excellent for diagnosing carcinoma of the colon (Figure 14.11) but

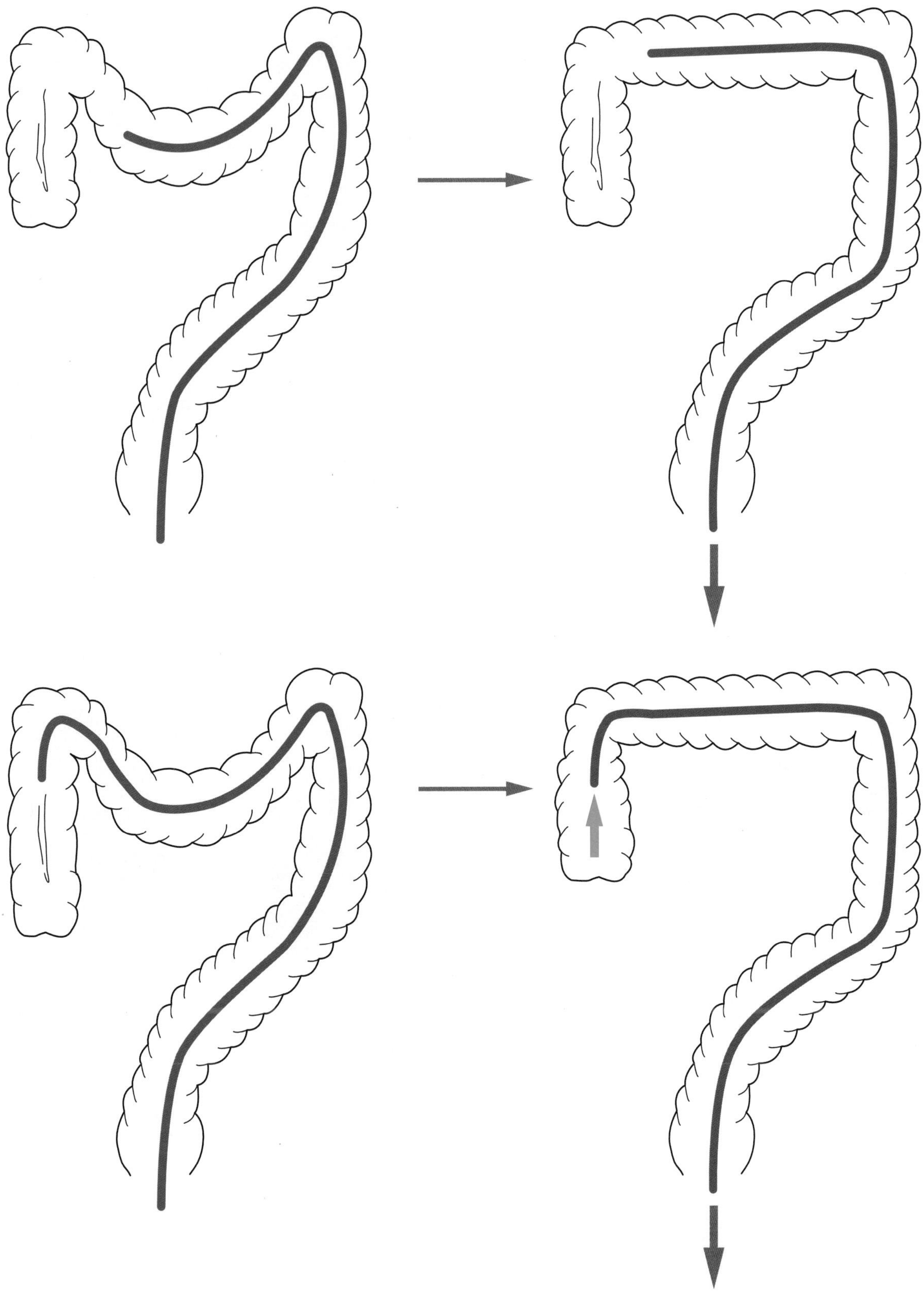

Figure 14.8 Progression of the colonoscope along the transverse colon.

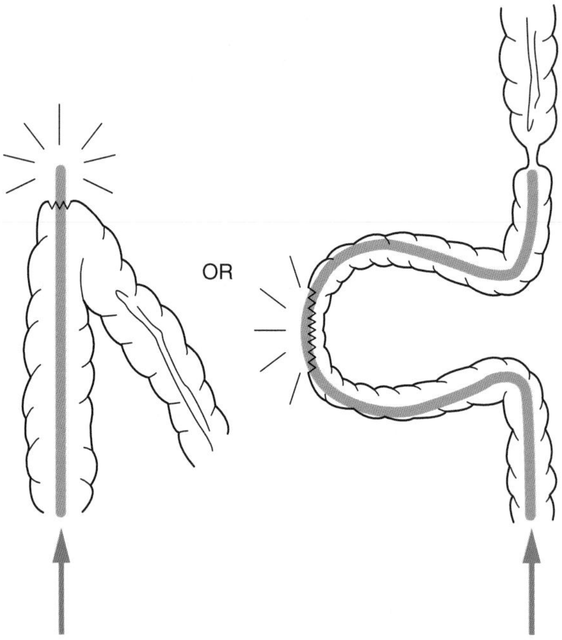

Figure 14.9 Colonoscopic perforation.

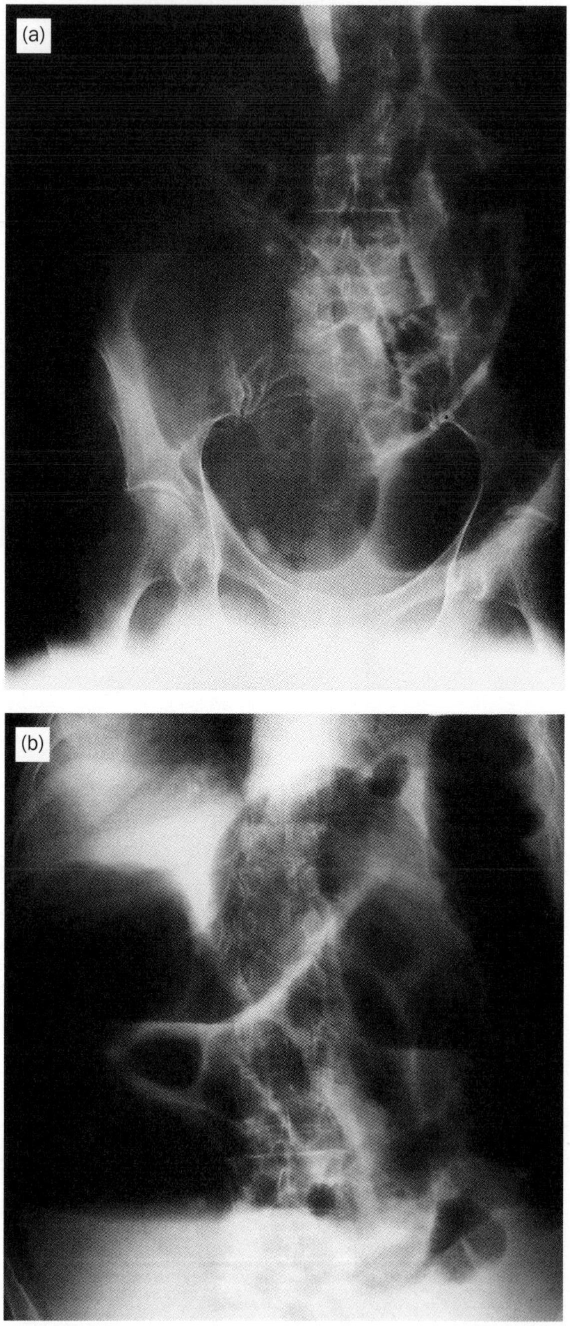

Figure 14.10 Plain abdominal X-rays showing large bowel obstruction: (a) supine film, (b) erect film, showing fluid level in the caecum.

caution must be exercised in interpreting appearances in the sigmoid colon and in the caecum. In a redundant sigmoid colon with multiple overlapping loops of bowel, particularly if affected by severe diverticular disease, lesions may be missed (Figure 14.12). Conversely, there tends to be a problem with over-reporting carcinomas in the caecum where prolonged spasm may mimic suspicious appearances (Figure 14.13). Thus in the patient with suspicious symptoms who has a normal looking sigmoid colon, a flexible sigmoidoscopy is mandatory. Likewise in the asymptomatic patient who is not anaemic, a diagnosis of carcinoma of the caecum should be confirmed by colonoscopy unless the appearances are absolutely unequivocal.

Strictures in the presence of diverticular disease are particularly difficult to interpret and may require direct endoscopic visualization and biopsy. Small polyps may be missed on barium enema and conversely diverticula or small particles of faecal matter may be misinterpreted as polyps. It should be stressed that both barium enema and colonoscopy are highly operator dependent and both can miss quite significant lesions. Thus in the patient who presents a diagnostic dilemma it may be quite justifiable to use both investigations.

Complications of barium enema

Serious complications are extremely rare. The incidence of perforation is approximately 1 in 25 000. When it occurs it is usually associated with passage of the rectal tube and it may occur proximal to a colostomy. Very occasionally perforation may result from preparation of obstructed bowel using a stimulant laxative such as Picolax.

Peroral enema

This technique is sometimes helpful where a standard barium enema has been unsuccessful in demonstrating the caecum. Barium is given by mouth and is monitored by fluoroscopy until it has reached the transverse colon. At this stage air is insufflated per rectum and the right colon is examined. Antispasmodics such as Buscopan may be useful in relaxing the colon for this examination.

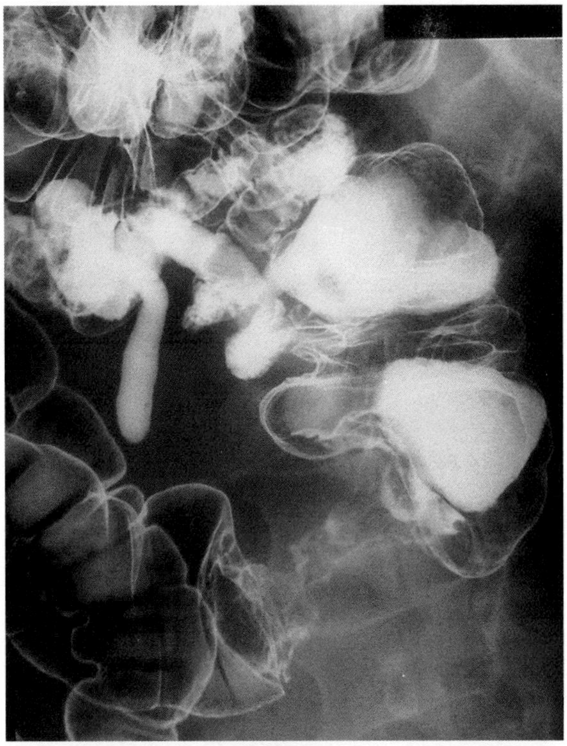

Figure 14.11 Barium enema appearances of a colonic cancer with typical 'apple core' shouldering.

Radio-opaque markers

In order to measure colonic transit radio-opaque markers can be used. Twenty markers are swallowed and in the normal individual the single abdominal X-ray taken on day 5 will show that at least 14 (80%) have been passed. For more detailed information daily X-rays can be taken or 20 markers of different shapes can be ingested daily on three consecutive days and a single X-ray taken on day 4. In normal individuals the mean total colonic transit time is 30 hours in males and 38 hours in females.

Colonic scintigraphy

Instead of radio-opaque markers it is possible to use material labelled with radioisotopes, e.g. ^{131}I bound to cellulose or indium^{111}DTPA. The isotope is ingested and the abdomen scanned using a gamma camera at 6, 24, 48, 72 and 96 hours.

Radiolabelled leucocyte scanning

Intravenous injection of autologous leucocytes labelled with ^{111}indium can be used to detect active colitis. The leucocytes accumulate in the inflamed mucosa and this relatively non-invasive procedure is useful in assessing the activity and extent of ulcerative colitis and Crohn's colitis. Technetium is an alternative to indium for labelling leucocytes.

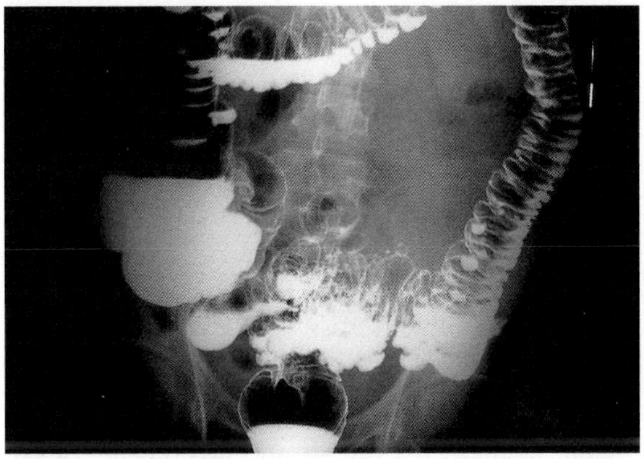

Figure 14.12 Severe sigmoid diverticular disease on barium enema. In this instance a carcinoma was missed.

Water-soluble enema

If there is a danger of barium entering the peritoneal cavity or if the bowel is obstructed then a water-soluble enema is a useful alternative to a barium. Gastrograffin or Niopam is frequently used. Indications for a water-soluble contrast enema include a suspected anastomotic leak, suspected perforation from diverticular disease or in the patient with a large bowel obstruction to exclude a pseudo-obstruction. Barium is avoided in the obstructed patient as the study may be followed by immediate surgery which may be compromised by the presence of barium in the colon.

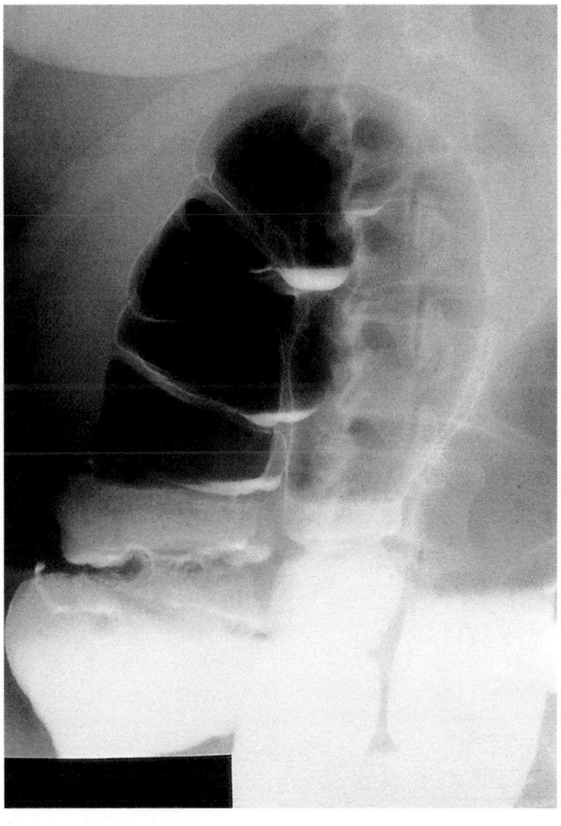

Figure 14.13 Spasm in the caecum interpreted as a stricture on barium enema.

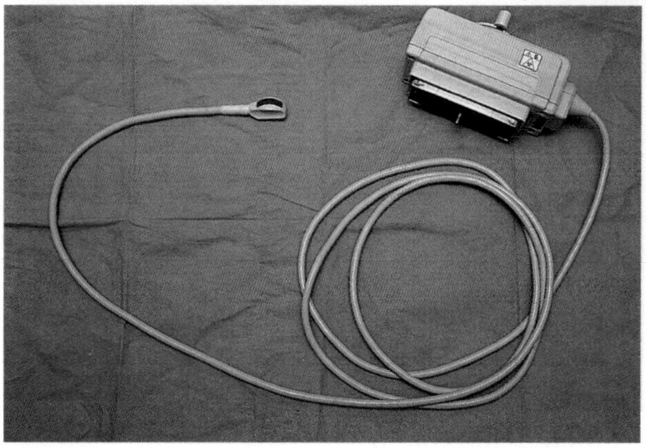

Figure 14.14 Intra-operative ultrasound probe.

Ultrasound

Abdominal ultrasound is widely used for the detection of hepatic metastases both pre-operatively and in follow-up for patients with colorectal cancer. It can also be used for the elucidation of abdominal masses and primary colorectal cancers have a characteristic ultrasound appearance. It is not, however, reliable enough to use as a standard investigative technique in a patient suspected to have the disease. Intra-operative contact ultrasound (Figure 14.14) can be used to screen the liver for metastatic disease and indeed this is the most sensitive available method for picking up hepatic deposits (Figure 14.15).

Transrectal ultrasound is an accurate method of pre-operative staging of rectal tumours. It may be used to distinguish between benign adenomas and invasive carcinomas and it may also be used to determine the extent of invasion through the bowel wall. It is particularly sensitive in distinguishing between T_2 and T_3 tumours but not quite so sensitive at distinguishing between T_1 and T_2 tumours (Figure 14.16). Unfortunately, its sensitivity for picking up lymph node metastases in the peri-rectal tissues is poor. The most useful rectal probe operates at 7 or 10 mHz and consists of a rotating probe inside a water-filled balloon which can be distended within the rectum to achieve

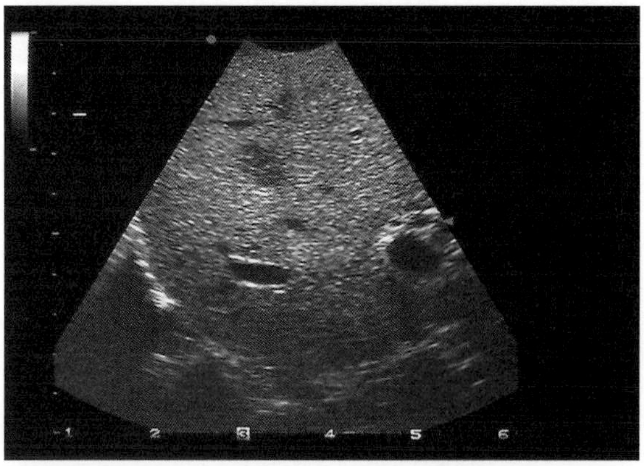

Figure 14.15 Ultrasound appearance of hepatic metastases – image obtained at intra-operative contact ultrasound.

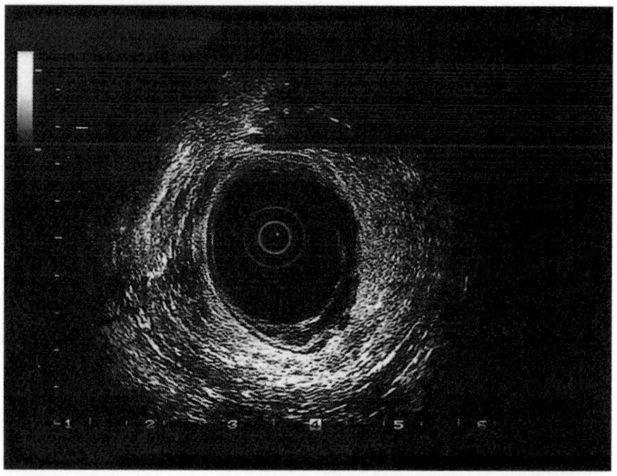

Figure 14.16 Transrectal ultrasound appearance of a rectal tumour. This is a T_2 tumour showing breaching of the muscularis propria.

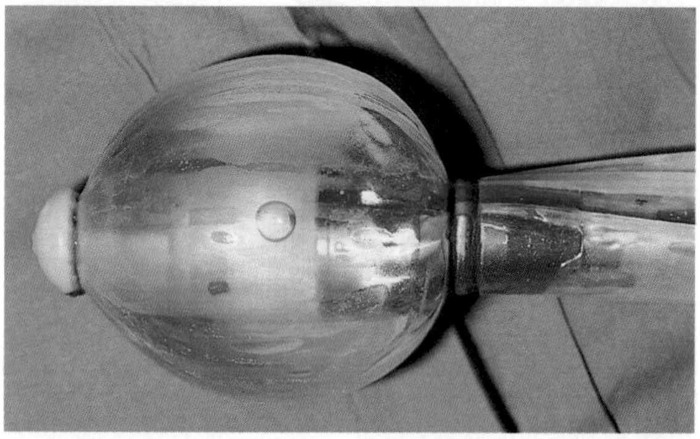

Figure 14.17 Head of a rectal ultrasound probe with balloon inflated to ensure contact with the rectal wall.

contact between the ultrasound probe and the rectal wall (Figure 14.17).

CT scanning

CT scanning is widely used for pre-operative staging especially of rectal cancer. It has advantages over ultrasound in that its sensitivity for liver metastases (Figure 14.18) is higher and an image of the primary tumour in the pelvis can be obtained (Figure 14.19). Again CT can also be used to diagnose abdominal masses and it is of particular value in elderly patients where barium enema and colonoscopy are impractical because of the patients' inability to retain either contrast or air.

A recent development has been virtual colonoscopy where the dataset acquired from a helical CT scan of the abdomen can be reconstructed in order to provide a 'fly through' view of the inside of the colon (Figure 14.20). This procedure shows great promise but like barium enema and colonoscopy it requires full bowel preparation and insufflation of air or CO_2. In addition, because of pooling of liquid in the colon, the CT has to be repeated once with the patient lying prone and again with the patient lying supine. Virtual colonoscopy has been quite widely studied but as

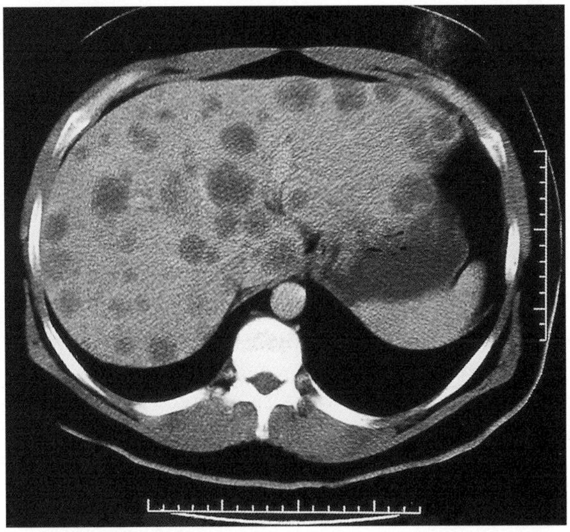

Figure 14.18 CT scan showing multiple hepatic metastases.

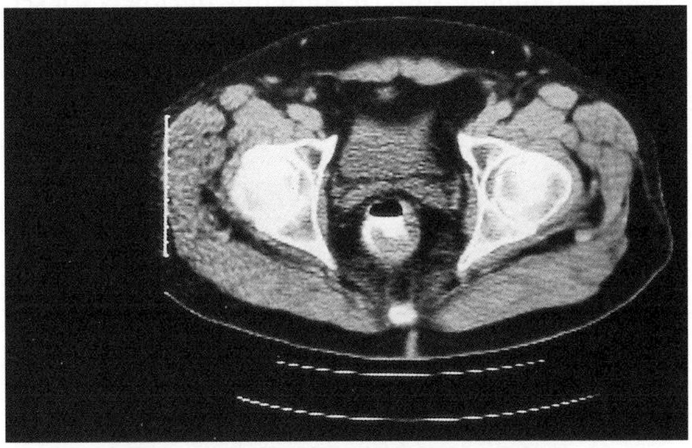

Figure 14.19 CT of rectal cancer showing posterior operable tumour.

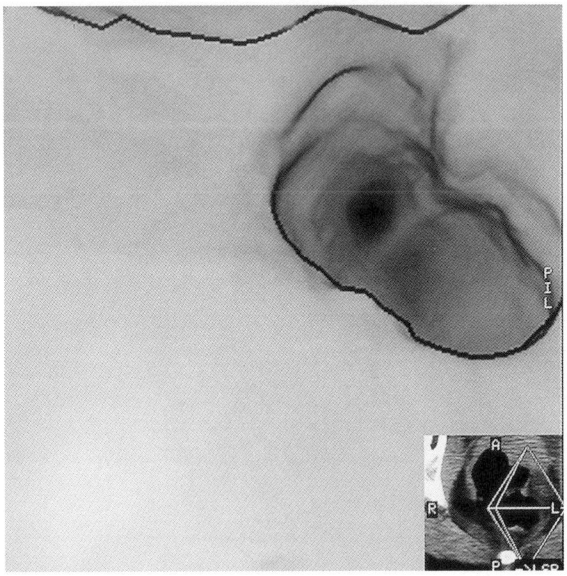

Figure 14.20 CT colography ('virtual colonoscopy').

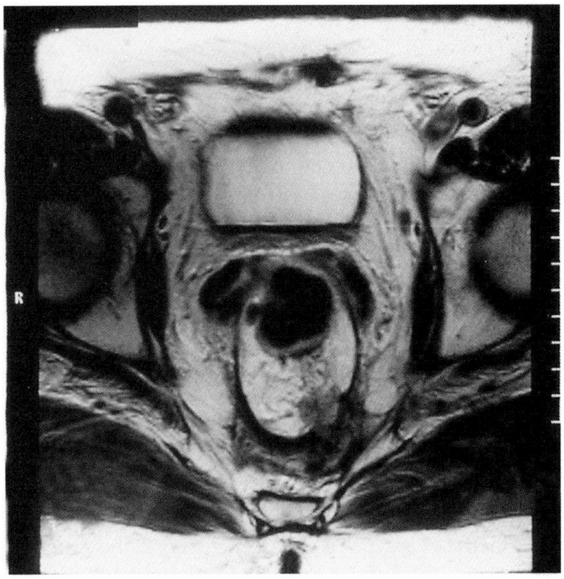

Figure 14.21 MRI image of the rectum obtained using phased array pelvic coils.

yet it has not been shown to be more sensitive or specific than either a high-quality barium enema or colonoscopy. However, future developments may lead to this technique being able to discriminate malignant lesions from non-malignant lesions with a high degree of accuracy.

MRI scanning

Because of the slow image acquisition time magnetic resonance imaging (MRI) scanning has not supplanted the much more rapid helical CT scanning. However, it does provide particularly good images of the rectum and the latest 1.5 tesla machines with pelvic coils provide very high-definition pictures of the rectum and the mesorectum which are likely to improve pre-operative staging considerably (Figure 14.21).

Section 14.4 • Large bowel neoplasia

Polyps

The term polyp is rather imprecise and in its broadest sense can be taken to mean a protuberant growth which can be either benign or malignant. As far as the colon and rectum are concerned however, the term is usually taken to mean a benign swelling arising from the colonic or rectal mucosa, although as it will be seen later on, certain types of polyp may contain a malignant or invasive focus and may indeed be an essential precursor in the development of colorectal cancer. Colorectal polyps may be inflammatory, hamartomatous, metaplastic or adenomatous. These will be dealt with in turn but particular attention will be paid to the adenomatous variety in view of their close association with colorectal cancer.

Inflammatory polyps

These occur in ulcerative colitis, Crohn's colitis, diverticulitis, chronic dysentery and in benign lymphomatous lesions of the colon. They are sometimes referred to as pseudopolyps as they are commonly formed from an island of hypertrophied mucosa in an area of inflammation and ulceration. These polyps tend to be small, rarely exceeding 0.5 mm in diameter and consist of inflamed congested mucosa with oedematous changes in the submucosa.

Hamartomatous polyps

Hamartomatous polyps may be found in two forms, as juvenile polyps and as the familial Peutz–Jeghers syndrome. Juvenile polyps are found in infants or children and are often multiple being round or oval with a smooth surface. At the time of diagnosis most lesions are pedunculated with a transition from normal colonic mucosa to a type of glandular tissue at the junction of the stalk and the polyp. The polypoidal substance consists of vascular tissue infiltrated by inflammatory cells and contains cystic spaces maintained by mucus-secreting columnar cells. There is a familial tendency in juvenile polyposis with the majority of patients presenting before the age of 10 years. Male children predominate over female. Fortunately they are single in 70% and 70% occur in the rectum and distal sigmoid colon.

The polyps occurring in the Peutz–Jegher syndrome are associated with pigmented lesions (a bluish brown discoloration) on the face and on the lingual and buccal mucosa. Here the familial tendency is very strong. The polyps are almost always multiple and are found more commonly in the small bowel than in the colon or rectum. On histological examination the basic malformation is found in the muscularis mucosae. Unlike juvenile polyposis there is a significant malignant potential and there are reports of carcinoma arising in young patients with this syndrome.

Metaplastic polyps

These are generally plaque-like growths which vary in size from 1 to 2 mm but rarely exceed 5 mm in maximum diameter. Although they are most commonly found in the rectum, the whole of the large bowel is susceptible. There is no specific age distribution or predisposing factor. On histological examination there is lengthening of the mucosal glands with dilatation of the goblet cells and evidence of inflammatory infiltration of the lamina propria. It is not understood why these lesions arise but they are very rarely symptomatic and do not appear to be pre-malignant. There is however some evidence that the presence of metaplastic polyps in the rectum or distal colon may be associated with an increased risk of adenomatous polyps or even carcinoma in the more proximal colon.

Adenomatous polyps

Pathology

Adenomatous polyps are benign neoplastic growths arising from the mucosa of the intestine and although they may occur anywhere between the stomach and the rectum, they are most common in the large intestine. In the Western world they are extremely common and post-mortem studies indicate that they are found in more than 30% of people over the age of 60 years. The distribution of polyps is similar to that of adenocarcinoma, i.e. commonest in the rectum and left side of the colon, rare in the transverse colon and with a slight increase in the incidence in the right side of the colon and caecum. Adenomas are highly variable in size and macroscopically may be pedunculated or sessile. Recently the concept of the flat adenoma, which can be defined as an area of adenomatous change barely discernible macroscopically, has emerged but the significance of these lesions has yet to be established. In the colon, adenomas are normally pedunculated whereas in the rectum they are commonly sessile. The villous papilloma is a sessile adenoma made up of frond-like strands which grows as a carpet on the rectal mucosa (Figure 14.22).

Histologically, the epithelium in an adenoma can be arranged in tubular pattern consisting of closely packed glands or a villous pattern where the epithelial cells are arranged on frond-like extensions from the surface of the tumour. In practice the majority of adenomatous

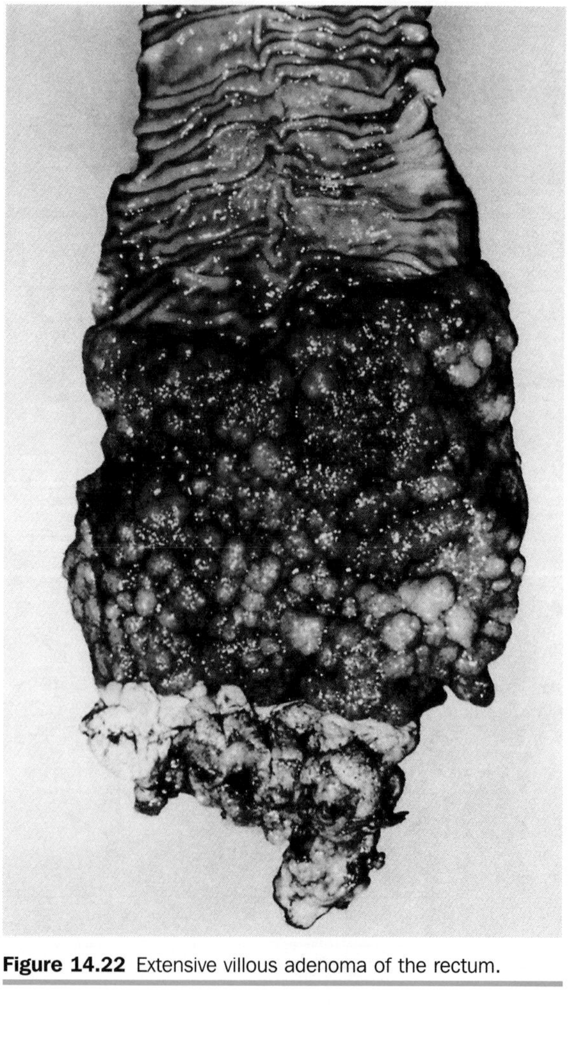

Figure 14.22 Extensive villous adenoma of the rectum.

polyps display a mixture of tubular and villous patterns and can be described as tubulovillous. When the pathologist examines an adenoma it is important to establish whether or not there are any areas of invasion where dysplastic cells have transgressed the basement membrane into the fibrous stalk of the polyp. This will be found in about 50% of all adenomas that are over 2 cm in maximum diameter. In general, villous adenomas are more likely to undergo malignant change than tubular adenomas but this is by no means an absolute rule.

Aetiology

The aetiology of adenomatous polyps is essentially the same as that of colorectal cancer, indeed it is believed that the majority of colorectal cancers arise from pre-existing adenomatous polyps (see next section). In summary, although environmental factors (probably mainly dietary) have important implications for the formation of polyps, the genetic background is crucial. Not only are there dominantly inherited mutations which predispose to the development of polyps and cancer (see sections on FAP and HNPCC) but there are also more subtle genetic variations which have an important impact on the predisposition to develop adenomatous polyps. This will be dealt with in detail in the section on colorectal cancer.

Clinical features

Most adenomatous polyps are asymptomatic and the diagnosis is made on routine examination. Nevertheless, both occult and frank bleeding can occur and patients may present with either rectal bleeding or anaemia. Occasionally, polyps may be extruded from the anal canal and may be misdiagnosed as prolapsing haemorrhoids. The retrograde propulsion of larger pedunculated polyps may produce abdominal pain and in extreme cases lead to the development of colocolic intussusception.

Rectal polyps may be accompanied by tenesmus and a change in bowel habit to diarrhoea. This may be the result of mucoid discharge from the surface of the polyps. This feature is particularly common with villous papillomas where spurious diarrhoea from the abundant mucus discharge leads to a failure in health, dehydration and electrolyte disturbance. In the mucus, sodium and chloride concentrations are similar to plasma but the potassium concentrations are between three and 20 times greater. Thus in the larger papillomas, hypokalaemia and metabolic acidosis may result in lethargy, muscle weakness, mental confusion and in some extreme cases renal failure. These metabolic disturbances require attention prior to any attempt at surgical treatment.

Diagnosis

The diagnosis of adenomatous polyps is made on either large bowel endoscopy or barium enema. Large bowel endoscopy (colonoscopy in particular) is more sensitive at identifying polyps but large polyps can easily be seen on a high-quality, double contrast barium enema (Figure 14.23). In some instances, it may be difficult to distinguish among a polyp, a diverticulum and faecal material and this gives rise to a significant false positive rate of polyp detection using barium enema. It must also be stressed, however, that colonoscopy is not 100% sensitive either and it has been demonstrated that repeat colonoscopy can often demonstrate lesions which were missed on the previous colonoscopy and miss lesions which had already been seen. One advantage of endoscopic diagnosis of polyps is that a biopsy can be taken of the larger polyps. This is important as it is often difficult to distinguish between a large benign adenomatous polyp and a polypoid carcinoma. Colonoscopy also offers the opportunity to remove the polyp using snare diathermy (Figure 14.24).

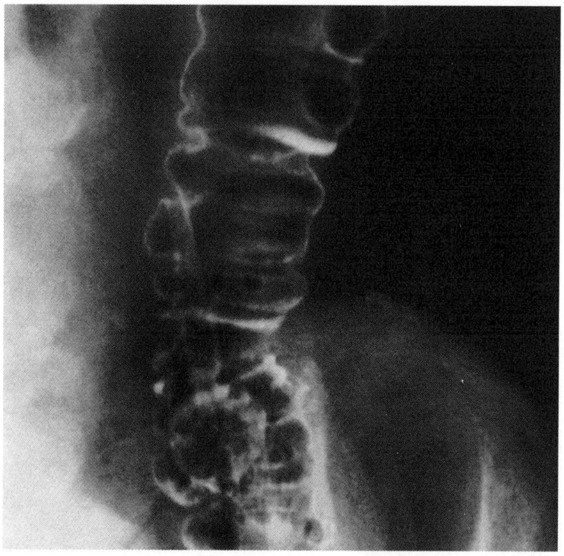

Figure 14.23 2 cm polyp on a stalk demonstrated by double contrast barium enema.

Prognosis

The prognosis of benign polyps in themselves is usually good with the proviso that large villous adenomas can be extremely debilitating (see above). However, as

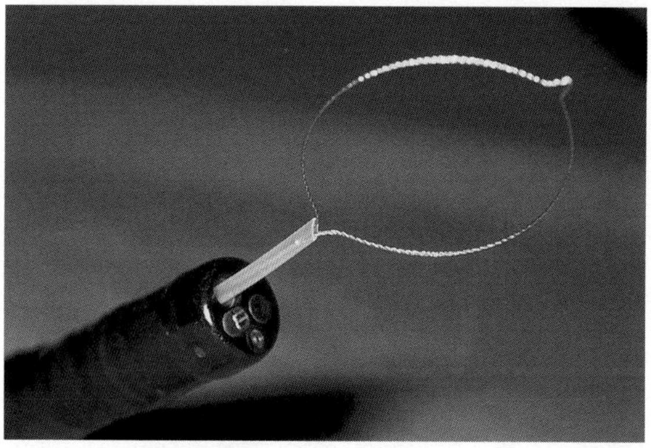

Figure 14.24 Colonoscopic snare.

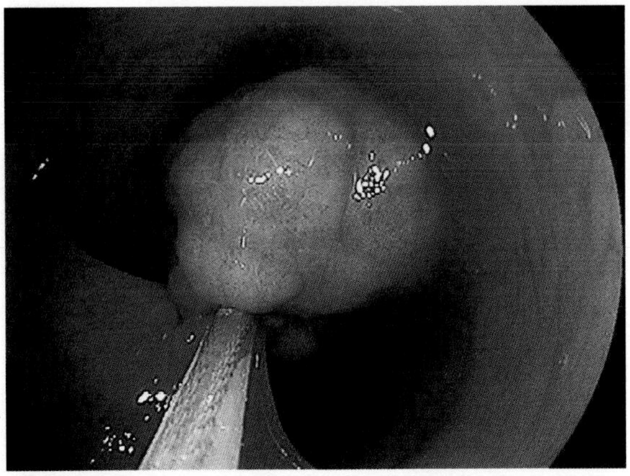

Figure 14.25 Snare excision of polyp.

most carcinomas are thought to arise from polyps, the potential for malignant change should never be ignored and wherever it is feasible benign adenomatous polyps should be removed.

Treatment

The mainstay of treatment of adenomatous polyps is endoscopic polypectomy. Using a colonoscope, a wire loop is placed around the stalk of a pedunculated polyp; a blended current is then passed along the snare which is gradually tightened until it cuts through the stalk (Figure 14.25). The polyp should then be retrieved for histological examination. Occasionally, polypectomy may be accompanied by brisk arterial bleeding. If this occurs, the endoscopist should grasp the bleeding stalk with the snare, tighten the snare and hold in place for about 5 min without using diathermy current. This will usually stop the bleeding.

Another important complication of polypectomy is perforation of the colon. All patients undergoing colonoscopy with polypectomy should be warned of the risks of bleeding and perforation, as both may require emergency surgery. When a colonic polyp is sessile or has a very broad stalk, then it may be hazardous to carry out a standard polypectomy owing to the risk of perforation. In this case it is possible to elevate the polyp by injecting saline into the submucosa (Figure 14.26). This will allow much safer polypectomy. In very large polyps, it may be possible to carry out piecemeal snare excision. This is a difficult and hazardous procedure and should only be carried out by experienced endoscopists.

When a polyp has been completely excised and sent for histology, a focus of invasion will occasionally be found within the polyp making it a polyp cancer. It is generally agreed that if the polyp has been removed in one piece and the invasion does not extend to the resection margin then further surgery is not required. However, if the resection margin is involved, the patient should then be offered a colectomy. For this reason, if an endoscopist is concerned that a polyp may in fact be a cancer, it is useful to mark the site of excision using an intramural injection of India ink via the colonoscope. Having said this, many surgeons will take the view that a large polyp in the colon is highly likely to be malignant, even in the absence of confirmatory biopsies and will advise the patient to go straight to colectomy.

Although these endoscopic approaches are suitable for the majority of colonic polyps, rectal polyps pose a different problem. Occasionally, a large pedunculated prolapsing rectal polyp can be pulled out through the anal canal and the stalk simply ligated and divided. However, the majority of rectal polyps are sessile and require a different approach. Traditionally a low sessile rectal polyp was treated by submucosal saline injection to lift it away from the muscle wall and then transanal excision using Park's anal retractors to gain access (Figure 14.27).

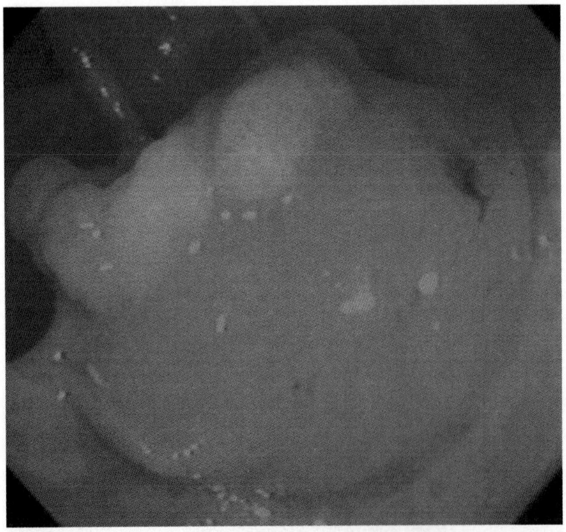

Figure 14.26 Elevation of polyp after submucosal saline injection.

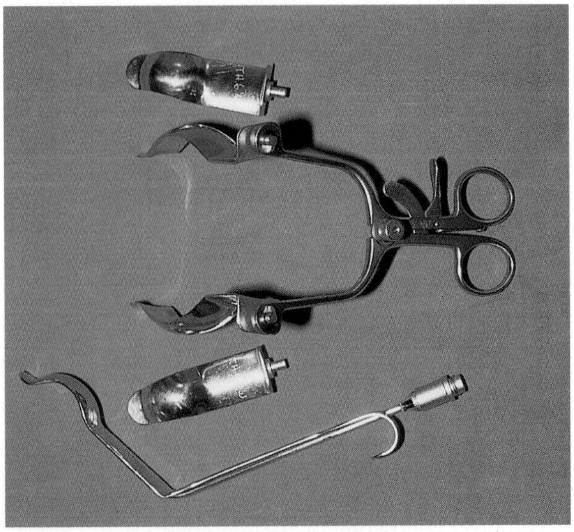

Figure 14.27 Park's anal retractor for local transanal excision of rectal tumours.

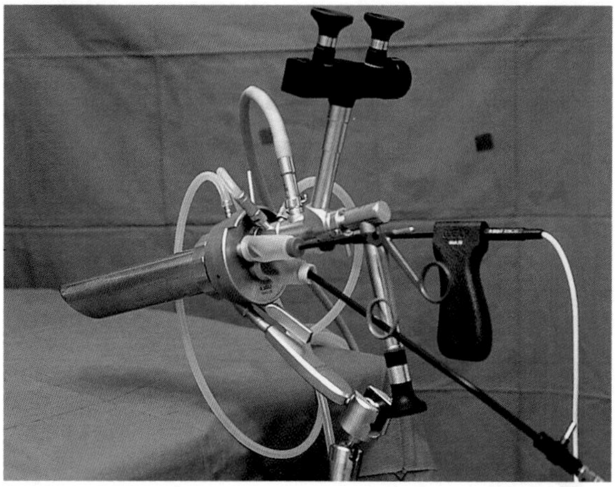

Figure 14.28 Operating protoscope for transanal endoscopic microsurgery.

For polyps which are higher in the rectum however, this is often not feasible and for this reason the technique of transanal endoscopic microsurgery (TEM) has been developed. This employs a sophisticated operating sigmoidoscope with a binocular optical system (Figure 14.28) which, by means of continuous insufflation and suction, offers an excellent operating environment to remove such polyps. When these polyps are situated posteriorly, it is safe to remove a full thickness disk of rectal wall and this is a sensible precaution as a proportion of such polyps will harbour invasive malignancy. However, anteriorly above about 10 cm this is hazardous as it may lead to perforation into the peritoneal cavity and a submucosal technique must be employed. An alternative procedure is the trans-sphincteric approach described by Yorke Mason which involves formal division of the anal sphincter mechanism in order to gain access to the rectum posteriorly. Owing to the currently available sophisticated techniques for transanal excision however, this approach is seldom used nowadays. Occasionally, a patient will have such an extensive carpet of adenoma throughout the rectum that a transanal approach is not feasible. In this case a total proctectomy (i.e. an anterior resection with a mucosectomy down to the dentate line) has to be carried out. Continuity can then be restored by means of a sutured coloanal anastomosis.

Adenocarcinoma of the colon and rectum

In the UK there are around 30 000 new cases of colorectal cancer each year and the disease accounts for about 20 000 deaths. This makes it the second commonest cause of cancer death in the UK exceeded only by lung cancer. In women breast cancer is more common but as colorectal cancer affects an almost equal proportion of men and women, its overall incidence is higher. The distribution of the disease world-wide seems to be related to industrialization and socioeconomic standards. There is a high incidence in industrialized countries including western Europe, Scandinavia and North America, whereas in the developing world (sub-Saharan, Africa, Asia and South America) the incidence appears to be lower. This has to be treated with some caution however, as registration of cancer in developing countries is considerably less reliable than in the developed world. Interestingly, within countries with a high incidence of colorectal cancer the disease is commoner amongst the lower socioeconomic groups which is in sharp contrast to breast cancer.

Colonic cancer deaths are more frequent in women than in men (11:7) but death from rectal cancer is slightly more frequent in men (6:5). Although colorectal cancer can occur at any age the incidence only starts to become appreciable over the age of 50 and the disease occurs maximally in the decade between 70 and 79 years (Figure 14.29).

Pathology

Macroscopic appearances

Traditionally, colorectal cancers are classified as polypoidal, ulcerating, annular and mucinous. The polypoidal variety takes the form of a fungating mass and is more common on the right side of the colon than on the left. The ulcerating type appears as a typical malignant ulcer with a raised everted edge and a necrotic base (Figure 14.30). These tumours predominate on the left side of the colon and in the rectum. The annular lesion, which encircles the colonic or rectal lumen, probably develops from a malignant ulcer that gradually extends around the bowel wall until the two edges meet. The mucinous or colloid carcinoma is a bulky tumour with a gelatinous appearance. It is said that the polypoidal lesion has the best prognosis, the ulcerating an intermediate prognosis and the mucinous the worst prognosis but, stage for stage, this does not hold up to rigorous scrutiny.

In Japan a system of macroscopic classification of early colorectal cancer has been developed which is similar to that used for early gastric cancer. This subdivides the tumours into pedunculated type, flat elevated type, flat type, depressed type and laterally spreading type. This system has not however found widespread acceptance in the Western World.

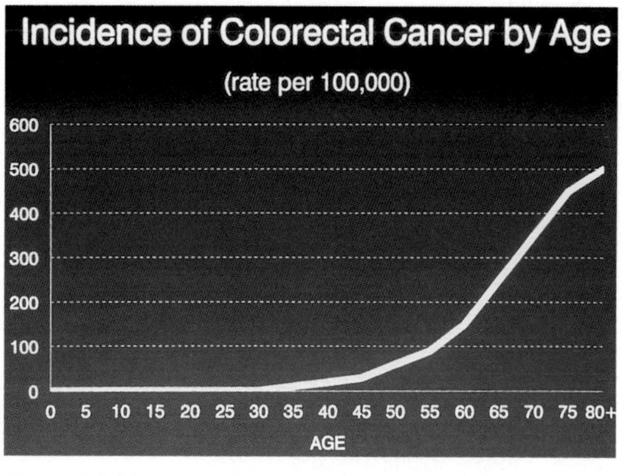

Figure 14.29 Age distribution of colorectal cancer.

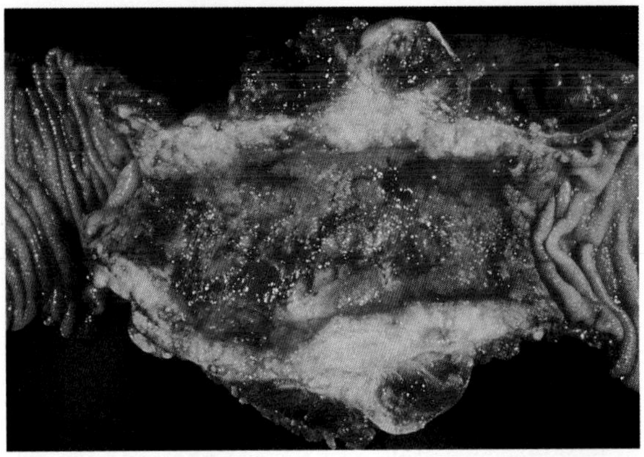

Figure 14.30 A typical ulcerating colonic cancer. (Courtesy of Dr F Carey, Department of Pathology, Ninewells Hospital, Dundee, UK.)

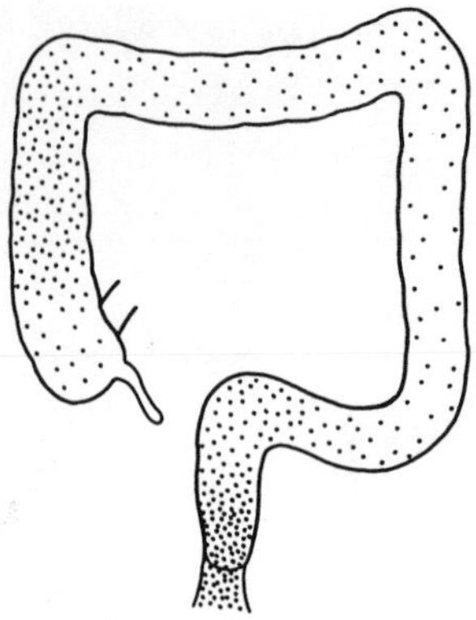

Figure 14.31 Anatomical distribution of colorectal cancer.

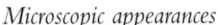

Microscopic appearances

In a vast majority of cases colorectal cancer is unequivocally an adenocarcinoma and it is commonly subdivided into well, moderately and poorly differentiated tumours on the bases of cellular atypia, mitotic rate and attempts at gland formation. In general, well-differentiated tumours have a better prognosis and the poorly differentiated tumours have a worse prognosis but as the majority of cancers are moderately differentiated relatively little store can be placed on the degree of differentiation. Various histological grading systems to describe the degree of differentiation (as opposed to the stage of the disease) have been described and the two best known are those of Dukes and of Broder (Table 14.1).

Distribution of colorectal cancer throughout the colon

The majority of colorectal cancers (75%) are in the rectum and sigmoid colon. The descending colon and transverse colon are relatively rare sites of tumour formation, whereas in the ascending colon and caecum the incidence is slightly higher (Figure 14.31). In recent years there appears to have been a slight change in this distribution with a slight increase in the proportion of tumours on the right side of the colon. The aetiology of the colorectal cancer also seems to be important as individuals with hereditary non-polyposis colorectal cancer (mutations in DNA mismatch repair genes) tend to have right-sided cancer (see below).

Histopathological staging

The purpose of histopathological staging which is carried out on resection specimens is to obtain an estimate of prognosis. This has three major advantages:

- It gives the clinician and the patient an estimate of likely long-term outcome.
- It provides a guide as to the potential usefulness of adjuvant therapy.
- It allows meaningful comparison between the results of different forms of treatment or treatment provided by different units. This is an essential component of case mix analysis.

In colorectal cancer the three most common types of staging system are the Dukes' system, the Jass system and the TNM system.

The Dukes' system

Initially described in 1929 by Cuthbert Dukes, this remains the most commonly used staging system for colorectal cancer. It is based on depth of penetration of the bowel wall and lymph node involvement and over the years Dukes modified his staging system from a simple ABC system to the following:

- Stage A, tumour confined to the bowel wall (including the muscularis propria).
- Stage B, tumour penetrating the muscularis propria.
- Stage C_1, regional lymph nodes involved by tumour but not affecting the node closest to the point of ligature.
- Stage C_2, lymph node at the point of ligature involved by tumour.

Table 14.1 The Dukes' and Broder systems of histological classification for colorectal cancer

Broder		*Dukes*
Grade I	Active epithelial proliferation with infiltration of muscularis mucosae – resembling an adenoma	Low-grade malignancy
Grade II	Crowded cells with regular arrangement, frequent mitosis	Average-grade malignancy
Grade III	Less differentiated with increased mitoses, crowded in irregular rings	High-grade malignancy
Grade IV	Anaplastic with no glandular arrangement; evidence of deep invasion with columns of cells	

It should be stressed that Dukes developed this staging for rectal cancer but it is now applied to all colorectal tumours. The prognosis associated with the various stages vary from series to series but cancer registry data indicate that the 5 year survival associated with stage A is 85%, for stage B 67% and for stage C 37%. It must be stressed however that these figures are susceptible to the 'Will Rogers' effect (stage migration owing to variable quality of pathology reporting). Thus if a pathologist is very assiduous in searching for lymph nodes, more patients will be shifted from the stage B category into the stage C category and the prognosis in both stages will improve.

Several pathologists have attempted to modify and improve on the Dukes system but none of these systems have gained widespread favour.

Jass classification

Some pathologists use the Jass classification which takes into account the degree of lymphocytic infiltration at the advancing margin of the tumour and the configuration of the advancing margin. It appears however that this classification is open to quite marked inter-observer variation and its prognostic usefulness appears to be restricted to rectal cancer.

TNM classification

The International Union Against Cancer has developed a TNM staging system for colorectal cancer. This system is gaining ground amongst pathologists as it provides a more comprehensive method of classifying the depth of invasion through the bowel wall. It also takes into account the presence or absence of distant metastases (Table 14.2).

Recently however, it has become clear that another histological parameter, lymphovascular invasion, is an extremely important prognostic factor which may be independent of lymph node involvement. This does not fit into any of the established staging systems, but pathologists are now encouraged to note this when it occurs. In the UK, the Royal College of Pathologists has agreed a minimum dataset which should be reported for all colorectal cancers (Figure 14.32).

Modes of spread

As with all cancers, colorectal cancer spreads by local extension, by lymphatic spread, by haematogenous spread and by spread through body cavities (in this case the peritoneum).

Intramural spread

Spread is three-dimensional, occurring in the longitudinal and transverse axes as well as radially through the bowel wall and into the tissues around the colon and rectum. The degree of longitudinal intramural spread is important as it determines what a safe margin of resection should be. Most surgeons will attempt to obtain at least 5 cm of longitudinal clearance and except for low rectal cancers this is easy to do. In point of fact however, microscopic intramural spread beyond the palpable tumour for more than 1 cm is unusual and when this occurs there are nearly always distant metastases. Thus for a low rectal cancer clearance of 2 cm is adequate.

Table 14.2 The TNM staging system for colorectal cancer

T – Tumour

- T_X – Primary tumour cannot be assessed
- T_0 – No evidence of primary tumour
- T_{is} – Carcinoma *in situ*
- T_1 – Tumour invades submuosa
- T_2 – Tumour invades but does not penetrate the muscularis propria
- T_3 – Tumour invades through muscularis propria into subserosa or into non-peritonealized pericolic or perirectal tissues
- T_4 – Tumour involves visceral peritoneum or directly invades other organs or structures

N – Regional lymph nodes

- N_X – Regional lymph nodes cannot be assessed
- N_0 – No regional lymph node metastases
- N_1 – Metastases in 1–3 pericolic or perirectal lymph nodes
- N_2 – Metastases in 4 or more pericolic or perirectal lymph nodes
- N_3 – Metastases in any lymph node along the course of a named vascular trunk

M – Distant metastases

RCS National Guidelines Minimum Data Set
Colorectal Cancer Histopathology Report

Patient Name: .... Date of Birth: ....
Hospital: .... Hospital No: ....
Histology No: .... Surgeon: ....

Gross Description
Site of Tumour ....
Maximum tumour diameter .... cm
Distance of tumour to nearest margin .... cm

For rectal tumours
Peritoneal reflection
above ☐ at ☐ below ☐

Distance from pectinate line .... cm

Histology
Type

	Yes	No
Adenocarcinoma	☐	☐

If No, Other ....

Differentiation by predominant area
poor ☐ other ☐

Local Invasion
Submucosa (pT1) ☐
Muscularis propria (pT2) ☐
Beyond Muscularis propria (pT3) ☐
Tumour cells have reached the serosal surface or invaded adjacent organs (pT4) ☐

Margins

Tumour involvement	Yes	No
doughnut	☐	☐
margin	☐	☐
circumferential margin	☐	☐

Histological measurement from tumour to circumferential margin .... mm

Metastatic Spread
No of lymph nodes examined ....
No of positive lymph nodes ....
(pN1 1-3 nodes pN2⊕4 nodes involved pN3 nodes along named vascular trunk)

	Yes	No
Apical node positive (C2)	☐	☐
Extramural vascular invasion	☐	☐

Background Abnormalities

	Yes	No
Adenoma(s)	☐	☐
Synchronous carinoma(s)	☐	☐
Complete a separate form for each cancer		
Ulcerative colitis	☐	☐
Crohn's	☐	☐
Familial adenomatous polyposis	☐	☐

Pathological Staging

	Yes	No
Complete resection at all margins	☐	☐

TNM
T ☐ N ☐ M ☐

Dukes
Dukes A ☐ (Growth limited to wall, nodes negative)
Dukes B ☐ (Growth beyond M. propria, nodes negative)
Dukes C1 ☐ (Nodes positive and apical node negative)
Dukes C2 ☐ (Apical node positive)

	Yes	No
Histologically confirmed liver metastases	☐	☐

Signature ....
Date ....

Figure 14.32 Royal College of Pathologists' minimum data set for reporting colorectal cancer.

More important, however, is circumferential clearance. With a tumour which has penetrated the muscular wall the pericolonic or perirectal tissues may be invaded and circumferential clearance is essential to avoid local recurrence. In the colon there is very little that the surgeon can do about this but in the rectum careful dissection of the entire mesorectum (see section on surgical treatment of rectal cancer) can make an immense difference to prognosis by ensuring adequate circumferential clearance of the tumour.

Involvement of adjacent structures

The entire length of the colon from the caecum to the distal sigmoid colon is located within the abdominal cavity. On the lateral sides the posterior halves of the circumference of the ascending and descending colon are usually embedded in the retroperitoneal space. The transverse colon and sigmoid colon are free in the peritoneal cavity on relatively long although variable mesenteries. Thus colonic cancer has a relatively small chance of invading into neighbouring structures. However, at the hepatic flexure the duodenum, biliary tree and liver may become involved and a tumour of the transverse colon may invade the stomach with the subsequent formation of a gastrocolic fistula. A large tumour of the splenic flexure may involve the spleen or the tail of the pancreas and tumours of the ascending or descending colons may involve the kidneys or ureters.

In contrast to the colon, the rectum is located in the true pelvis and thus has a close relationship to the neighbouring organs. Anteriorly the seminal vesicles and prostate in the male and the uterus and posterior vaginal wall in the female may become involved by an anteriorly situated tumour and in both sexes the bladder is similarly vulnerable. Posteriorly and latterly the rectum is surrounded by a layer of fatty tissue known as the mesorectum which is enveloped in a well-defined layer of fascia. It is relatively unusual for a tumour to penetrate this barrier but if it does then the sacrum and the iliac vessels may become involved. If this is the case then the tumour is usually technically inoperable unless it is possible to resect part of the sacrum. Inferiorly the levator ani muscles and the anal sphincter complex are at risk of involvement by a very low tumour.

Lymphatic spread

Lymphatic spread is the most common mode of spread of colorectal cancer at the time of diagnosis. The frequency of lymph node metastases varies from series to series and of course depends on the frequency of early diagnosis. Screen-detected cancers have a much lower incidence of lymph node metastases than those presenting with symptoms and there is evidence that lymph node metastases are commoner in individuals from lower socioeconomic groups which may reflect an effect of education on early recognition of symptoms. The lymphatic drainage of the colon follows its blood supply so that in caecal tumours the predominant site for lymph node metastases will be along the ileocolic vessel, for tumours of the ascending colon along the right colic vessel, for tumours of the transverse colon along the middle colic vessels and for tumours of the sigmoid and rectum along the inferior mesenteric vessels. In addition, rectal tumours will drain to lymph nodes embedded in the mesorectum. From an oncological point of view this anatomical distribution is important to the surgeon when planning the operation. Thus the above named vessels should be taken as close to their origins as possible when a tumour in that particular part of the colon or rectum is being resected. This will be dealt with in more detail in the sections on surgical treatment.

Haematogenous spread

As with most gastrointestinal tumours haematogenous spread occurs in the portal system and the organ most at risk is therefore the liver. Approximately 20% of cases of colorectal cancer will have liver metastases at the time of diagnosis. The other common site for haematogenous spread is the lung and this is commoner with rectal cancers than with colonic cancers. This may be related to the fact that the venous drainage of the lower rectum bypasses the portal system although this explanation may be somewhat simplistic.

Transperitoneal spread

Surprisingly transperitoneal dissemination of colorectal cancer is relatively unusual. When it occurs however, it is associated with a grave prognosis. Mucinous cancers are most prone to spread in this manner.

Aetiology

The aetiology of colorectal cancer can be seen as an interaction between genetic (inherited) and environmental factors but the basic underlying cause appears to be an accumulation of genetic mutations which leads to the development of benign adenomas with subsequent transformation to invasive malignancy (the adenoma–carcinoma sequence). The evidence that the majority of colorectal cancers arise from pre-existing adenomatous polyps is circumstantial but quite strong. The supporting evidence includes:

- The prevalence of adenomas is very similar to that of carcinomas and the average age of adenoma patients is about 5 years younger than patients with carcinomas.
- Cancers are often accompanied by adenomatous tissue and it is unusual to find small cancers without adjoining adenomatous tissue.
- Familial adenomatous polyposis (FAP) is unequivocally pre-malignant and the adenomas resulting from this condition are histologically identical to sporadic adenomas.
- Large adenomas are more likely to demonstrate cellular atypia and genetic mutations than small adenomas. When an adenoma is more than 2 cm in diameter there is a 50% chance that it contains foci of invasive cancer.
- The distribution of adenomas throughout the colon is almost identical to that of carcinomas.
- In about one-third of all surgical specimens resected for colorectal cancer, synchronous adenomas will be found.

In addition to these factors the adenoma–carcinoma sequence appears to be associated with an orderly progression of genetic mutations. Mutations of the adenomatous polyposis coli (APC) gene, the gene product of which is thought to be important in cell to cell adhesion, seem to occur early as they are found in 60% of all adenomas and carcinomas. Mutations of the K-ras gene are also commonly seen in both adenomas and carcinomas but they are much more common in large adenomas than in small adenomas and are therefore thought to represent a later event. The gene product of K-ras stimulates cell growth by activating growth factor signal transduction. The deleted in colorectal cancer (DCC) gene is a tumour suppressor gene which is thought to play a role in cell–cell or cell–matrix interactions and deletion of its function leads to further progression towards the malignant phenotype. Mutations in the p53 gene are commonly found in invasive colorectal cancers but they are relatively rare in adenomas. p53 mutation is therefore thought to be a late event as it accompanies the development of invasive cancer. The p53 gene product appears to be central in determining whether a cell undergoes repair or apoptosis in response to DNA damage.

This sequence of events is described in Figure 14.33 but it must be stressed that it represents only one possible scenario. Many other different genetic abnormalities have been observed in sporadic colorectal cancer and there is no single mutation that is common to all cancers. Thus there is a wide range of possible mutations, inactivations and deletions and there is no single pattern which is applicable to every tumour. Nevertheless with the rapid developments which are taking place in molecular biology, it is becoming easier to study a wide spectrum of genetic mutations and genetic 'finger printing' may have important implications for diagnosis, prognosis and gene therapy in the future.

These sporadic mutations may occur by chance or as a result of background radiation but there are certain inherited genetic abnormalities or polymorphisms which make the acquisition of these mutations more likely and there are a number of specific environmental carcinogens which have an important role to play.

Table 14.3 Family history and risk of colorectal cancer

Family history	*Lifetime risk*
None	1/30
One first degree relative	1/17
One first and one second degree relative	1/12
One first degree relative < 45 years	1/10
Two parents	1/8.5
Two first degree relatives	1/6
Three first degree relatives	1/2

Inherited genetic factors

Germline mutations of the APC gene lead to FAP and germline mutations of the DNA mismatch repair genes give rise to the hereditary non-polyposis colorectal cancer (HNPCC) syndrome. Both of these conditions display an autosomal dominant inheritance pattern and are dealt with separately. These syndromes aside however, colorectal cancer does display a familial tendency and the risk of developing the disease increases with increasing numbers of first degree relatives (Table 14.3). This statistical risk may in part be due to an admixture of very high-risk individuals with FAP or HNPCC. However, it is likely that there are genetic variations which put individuals at increased risk of developing colorectal cancer and, among a number of candidates, the genes coding for the drug metabolizing enzymes seem to be important in this respect. The drug metabolizing enzymes have evolved in order to protect living organisms from environmental toxins and there is good evidence that these enzymes can neutralize a variety of carcinogens.

Diet

Epidemiological evidence suggests that dietary fibre may be protective against colorectal cancer. This is supported by work on the effect of wheat fibre on mucosal cell turnover but recent prospective dietary studies

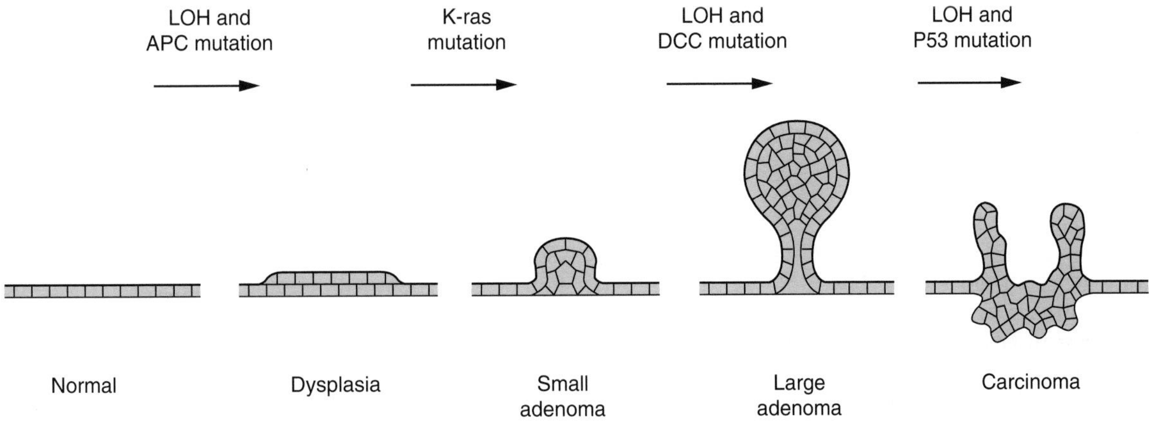

Figure 14.33 Possible series of genetic events leading to the development of invasive colorectal cancer via the adenoma-carcinoma sequence.

in women have been unable to demonstrate an effect of fibre in protecting against colorectal cancer. Animal fat may also be important as diets rich in animal fats increase the excretion of bile salts in the faeces and promote the growth of bacteria that are capable of degrading bile salts to carcinogens. Cooked meat may also have a carcinogenic influence on the colonic mucosa owing to high levels of heterocylic amines. There is now abundant evidence that a diet lacking in vegetables is a risk factor for colorectal cancer and there is increasing evidence that the cruciform vegetables (broccoli, brussels sprouts, cabbage, etc.) may induce drug metabolizing enzymes and stimulate apoptosis in tumour cells. The active ingredients in these vegetables are probably the isothiocyanates.

Bile acids

Bile acids may be carcinogenic and this is possibly related to calcium in the diet. Calcium binds bile acids and it has been shown that calcium supplements can reduce the rate of turnover of colonic mucosal cells. Secondary bile acid secretion is increased after cholecystectomy and having this operation may be a risk factor for developing colorectal cancer.

Bacteria

The faecal flora has been remarkably little studied with respect to the development of colorectal cancer. However, there is now some evidence that intraepithelial *E. coli* is strongly associated with the presence of polyps and colorectal cancer. There is also an association between *Helicobacter pylori* colonization of the stomach and colorectal cancer and this may be secondary to the helicobacter-induced hypergastrinaemia as gastrin can act as a growth factor for colonic mucosal cells.

Predisposing conditions

Long-standing inflammatory bowel disease (both ulcerative colitis and Crohn's disease) increases the risk of developing colorectal cancer although the underlying mechanism is not clear (see section on inflammatory bowel disease). Previous gastrectomy or vagotomy may also play a role and although the association is controversial, the risk may be as much as two-fold. Ureterosigmoidostomy is a well-established risk factor but this operation has now been superseded by the isolated ileal conduit for urinary divertion.

Clinical features

Symptoms

Colonic cancer can present either with chronic symptoms or as an emergency. The most well-recognized symptoms are rectal bleeding and change of bowel habit but in fact the most common presenting symptom is lower abdominal pain. Overt rectal bleeding is a relatively uncommon symptom of colonic cancer (as opposed to rectal cancer) and when it occurs it is usually dark red and mixed with the stool. It may also be seen on the surface of the stool.

Change of bowel habit usually presents itself as alternating constipation and diarrhoea. This tends to be a feature of left-sided colonic cancers. A right-sided colonic cancer usually presents late as the tumour can reach quite a large size without causing pain or change of bowel habit owing to both the distensible nature of the right colon and the fluid consistency of the stool. Commonly patients with right-sided cancers present with the symptoms of iron deficiency anaemia (fatigue, breathlessness, palpitations, etc.) and any individual over the age of 50 years with an unexplained iron deficiency anaemia must be assumed to have a caecal cancer unless proved otherwise.

The commonest mode of emergency presentation in colonic cancer is as intestinal obstruction. Here the patient notices colicky abdominal pain, constipation, abdominal distension and eventually vomiting. The patient may also present with colonic perforation either through the tumour itself or as a result of a closed loop obstruction when the ileocaecal valve is competent. Here the caecum becomes distended, ischaemic and eventually perforates. Under these circumstances the patient presents with right iliac fossa pain and tenderness when perforation has occurred and generalized peritonitis will ensue. This is usually a frank faecal peritonitis and the patient rapidly deteriorates with the onset of septic shock.

The symptoms of rectal cancer tend to be rather different. Rectal cancer very rarely presents as an emergency but rather with overt rectal bleeding, tenesmus or change of bowel habit. Rectal pain may occur but this is an ominous sign as it indicates a locally advanced cancer which is likely to be inoperable.

Physical signs

The vast majority of patients with colonic cancer have no physical signs at all but when examining the abdomen of a patient in whom this diagnosis is entertained the surgeon should search for a mass (indicative of the primary tumour) and hepatomegaly. It is also prudent to palpate the supraclavicular fossa for lymphadenopathy as this can be a sign of advanced intra-abdominal malignancy. General examination should take account of pallor, jaundice and cachexia.

Rectal cancer may be palpable by digital rectal examination. If the cancer is low a typical ulcerating lesion may be felt. If the cancer is high in the rectum it may be possible just to feel it with a tip of a finger. Occasionally a cancer of the sigmoid colon which has fallen down into the pelvis may be palpable through the rectal wall. It should be emphasized that a thorough digital examination is an essential part of the examination of any patient with rectal bleeding as up to 75% of all rectal tumours and 35% of all large bowel tumours can be palpated. It must also be stressed however that inability to palpate a rectal tumour should not preclude further investigation in a patient with suspicious symptoms. When a rectal tumour is palpated the surgeon must estimate its mobility in relation to the pelvis. This is usually classified as:

- *Mobile*: moves with mucosa.
- *Tethered*: does not move with mucosa but moves relative to the pelvis.
- *Fixed*: does not move relative to the pelvis.

These classifications have importance in determining the operability of tumours and indeed for adjuvant radiotherapy (see section on treatment).

Diagnosis

The correct use of diagnostic tests is of immense importance in the patient with suspected colorectal cancer. These can be subdivided into blood tests, endoscopy, radiology and staging investigations.

Blood tests

In a patient with suspected colorectal cancer a full blood count is mandatory as a proportion of such patients will be anaemic. Liver function tests may also indicate advanced metastatic disease but by the time the liver function tests are deranged for this reason, hepatomegaly is usually clinically detectable. Carcinoembryonic antigen (CEA) is an oncofetal protein which acts as a tumour marker. Serum levels are raised in about 60% of patients with colorectal cancer and they are also raised in a proportion of other cancers (e.g. gastric and pancreatic cancer). Owing to its lack of sensitivity and specificity CEA is not a particularly useful diagnostic test and a negative CEA should certainly not inhibit further investigations if there is a clinical suspicion. However, an elevated CEA may be of value when recurrence is suspected and a rising CEA level over a period of time is a very strong indicator of recurrent disease.

Endoscopy

There are basically three types of endoscopy which may be of value in the diagnosis of colorectal cancer: rigid sigmoidoscopy, flexible sigmoidoscopy and colonoscopy. These techniques have been described earlier in this chapter and all have their indications, advantages and limitations. The rigid sigmoidoscopy allows accurate localization of a rectal tumour in terms of both distance from the anal canal and quadrant (anterior, posterior, right lateral or left lateral). This cannot be achieved using a flexible instrument and is particularly important when planning transanal excision of a tumour. Rigid sigmoidoscopy is also useful for obtaining large biopsies.

Flexible sigmoidoscopy allows examination of the sigmoid colon and the descending colon in the majority of individuals although in a patient with a redundant sigmoid the 60 cm instrument may not be long enough. Three-quarters of colorectal tumours are within the reach of flexible sigmoidoscopy and it is therefore a very useful diagnostic test in patients with rectal bleeding. It is not however, a complete examination and it should be supplemented by a barium enema to visualize the whole of the colon.

Colonoscopy is regarded by some as the gold standard investigation of the colon as it is highly sensitive and specific for both cancers and adenomatous polyps. It has the advantage over barium enema of allowing biopsy and polypectomy but it has to be stressed that a caecal intubation rate of over 90% is exceptional and only achieved by the most expert colonoscopists. It must also be stressed that the location of a tumour in the colon is very difficult to estimate by colonoscopy.

Radiology

In the UK the double contrast barium enema remains the most widely used method of investigating the large intestine. It is not as accurate as colonoscopy but it is better tolerated, less dangerous and more widely available. Large cancers show up as typical apple-core deformities (Figure 14.11) but smaller lesions and polyps can be detected by high-quality examinations. Lesions can be missed, however, particularly in a tortuous sigmoid colon when there is diverticular disease present (Figure 14.12). Lesions are also apt to be missed in the caecum and occasionally a false diagnosis of cancer may be made because of spasm in the caecum (Figure 14.13). Although figures vary from series to series, it seems likely that false positive and false negative results may occur in up to 1% and 7% of cases respectively. Thus it is very important for the surgeon to look at the barium enema films personally to assess the quality of the pictures before relying too heavily on the radiologist's report. It is also essential that a patient who has had a normal barium enema but who continues to have suspicious symptoms should be investigated by flexible sigmoidoscopy, if this has not already been done, or by colonoscopy.

Staging investigations

Once a definitive diagnosis of colorectal cancer has been made it is generally agreed that investigations should be carried out to determine the extent of the tumour and particularly whether or not there are distant metastases. This involves organizing a minimum of a chest X-ray and an ultrasound of the liver. However, external liver ultrasound is not the examination of choice in detecting liver metastases as it is only about 85% accurate. For this reason, intra-operative contact ultrasound of the liver has been gaining favour recently as it seems to be the most sensitive modality for picking up liver metastases.

Many surgeons employ pre-operative CT scanning and in rectal cancer this is particularly useful as it will image not only the liver (Figure 14.18) but also the rectal tumour itself (Figure 14.19) and may give some information regarding potential operability. There is, however, very little evidence that CT scanning of the rectal tumour itself adds very much to clinical evaluation. Recently, MRI has become increasingly prominent. Contrast enhanced MRI particularly using superparamagnetic iron oxide which is selectively taken up by the reticuloendothelial cells in the liver provides an extremely sensitive means of detecting liver metastases. In addition, the use of phased array pelvic coils gives very high-definition images of the rectum and mesorectum (Figure 14.21) and may prove to be the most accurate method of pre-operative staging of rectal tumours.

Endorectal ultrasound carried out by means of a rotating probe in the centre of a balloon which is inflated with water to obtain circumferential contact can be used in staging rectal tumours. It is particularly useful in distinguishing between benign and malignant tumours and between T_2 and T_3 tumours. It is less accurate in distinguishing between T_1 and T_2 tumours (Figure 14.16) but it is nevertheless a useful means of assessing whether or not a rectal cancer may be suitable for transanal excision. Endorectal MRI coils are also available but at present these are rather bulky and of limited value.

Screening

It is well established that 'early' colorectal tumours (i.e. stage A) have a better prognosis than more advanced tumours, and it therefore makes sense to try to diagnose colorectal cancer at an early stage. Unfortunately the common symptoms of colorectal cancer (i.e. change of bowel habit, abdominal pain and rectal bleeding) only occur when the tumour is relatively locally advanced. The only way in which to reliably identify cancers at an early stage is to employ population screening and a great deal of research effort has gone into this approach over the past 20 years.

There are now three population-based randomized controlled trials which have demonstrated that screening asymptomatic populations with faecal occult blood testing can reduce disease specific mortality by 15–30%. Unfortunately, standard faecal occult blood testing, which is positive in about 2% of an unselected population between the ages of 50 and 75 years, is only about 50% sensitive. Thus a negative faecal occult blood test is not a guarantee that colorectal cancer is not present although a positive test is associated with a 50% chance of colorectal neoplasia and a 12% chance of having invasive malignancy. It is possible to increase the sensitivity of faecal occult blood testing but this reduces the specificity to such an extent that a large number of negative investigations would have to be carried out.

Another approach to screening is to use flexible endoscopy as the primary screening test. To use colonoscopy in this way would be impractical but flexible sigmoidoscopy is a more realistic proposition. As 75% of colorectal cancers are within the reach of this instrument and as the presence of an adenomatous polyp in the left colon is an indicator of possible neoplasia on the right of the colon then a 'once only' flexible sigmoidoscopy may be a useful screening test. This is the subject of a randomized trial carried out in the UK, but mortality data from this trial are not yet available. One of the problems with all forms of colorectal cancer screening is the low compliance rate which is presumably related to mixture of ignorance, fear and distaste.

Treatment

The mainstay of the treatment of colorectal cancer is surgical resection as this is the only therapeutic modality which can offer a cure. However, radiotherapy and chemotherapy both have important roles, both as adjuvant therapy and in the treatment of advanced disease. High-quality pathology reporting is essential for determining therapeutic strategy as is accurate pre-operative imaging. Colorectal cancer should therefore be managed by multi-disciplinary teams consisting of surgeons, oncologists, pathologists and radiologists. Stomatherapists and increasingly specialist nurses are important for ensuring good quality management and they should also be part of the team.

Surgical management of colonic cancer

The most appropriate method of obtaining local control of a colonic tumour is radical excision of the affected section of colon along with its vascular pedicle and accompanying lymphatic drainage (Figure 14.34). Thus a right hemicolectomy involves division of the right colic and ileocolic vessels close to their origins from the superior mesenteric artery and a formal left hemicolectomy involves division of the inferior mesenteric artery at its origin from the aorta. In tumours of the sigmoid colon, many surgeons will preserve the ascending branch of the left colic artery.

Transverse colectomy with division of the middle colic vessels has fallen out of favour owing to a perception of an unacceptably high leakage rate and for most surgeons the decision as to which operation to do for a colonic cancer lies between a right hemicolectomy and a left hemicolectomy with the extent of resection depending on the position of the tumour. There is some controversy surrounding the optimal surgery for tumours in the region of the splenic flexure. One option is to carry out a left hemicolectomy, dividing the inferior mesenteric artery at its origin and dividing the left branch of the middle colic artery. It is also possible to preserve the inferior mesenteric trunk but this is essentially a segmental resection which ignores the principles of radicality. The other main option is to carry out an extended right hemicolectomy, dividing the middle colic artery and the ascending branch of the left colic artery.

It should be pointed out that a formal left hemicolectomy will necessitate anastomosis between the splenic flexure and the rectum which may be technically difficult or even impossible. In addition, the blood supply of the colon is not constant. There is no left colic artery in 6% of cases and the blood supply to the splenic flexure therefore comes from the middle colic artery. In 22% of cases there is no middle colic artery and the splenic flexure derives its blood supply from both the left and right colic arteries. As the principles of cancer surgery in the colon involve removing the lymphatic drainage associated with a tumour and as the lymphatic drainage follows the arterial blood supply, it seems logical to ligate to the right colic, middle colic and left colic arteries and to carry out an extended right hemicolectomy.

When a colonic tumour is involving other structures it may still be possible to carry out a curative resection by *en-bloc* removal of the tumour along with the involved organ, e.g. ureter and kidney, duodenum, stomach, spleen or small bowel. Furthermore, about 5% of women have macroscopically evident ovarian metastases and a further 2% will have microscopic deposits. For this reason, a few surgeons will advise routine oophorectomy in all female patients with colorectal cancer. When a tumour of the colon is truly inoperable it may be appropriate to carry out an ileocolonic bypass for tumour on the right side and a defunctioning colostomy for tumours of the distal colon.

Surgical treatment for rectal cancer

The majority of rectal cancers are treated by either anterior resection (removal of the upper rectum with anastomosis of the colon to the rectal stump) or

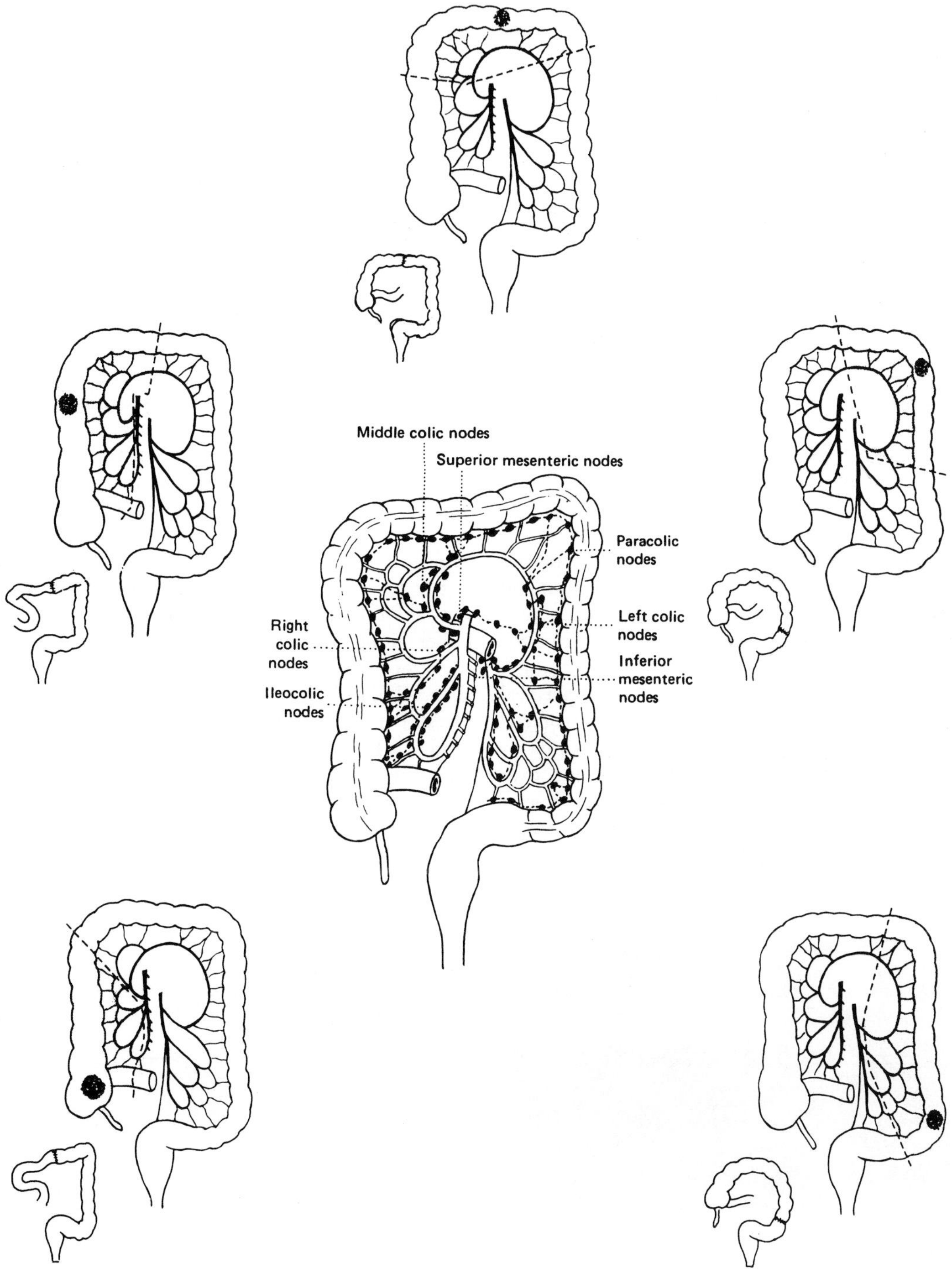

Figure 14.34 Colonic resections.

abdominoperineal excision of the rectum (complete excision of the rectum and anal canal with permanent end colostomy). For many years it was considered essential to have a least 5 cm of distal clearance of a rectal tumour before carrying out an anterior resection. However, the finding that distal intramural spread of rectal cancer for more than 1 cm is rare and nearly always associated with distant metastases has challenged this view and most colorectal surgeons will attempt anterior resection as long as the tumour is not involving the anal canal or the anal sphincter complex. Having said this, the patient's body habitus is important and a low anterior resection will be much easier in a thin female than in a well-built male.

Regardless of whether anterior resection or abdominal perineal excision is to be carried out, the most important principle of rectal cancer surgery is mesorectal excision. As mentioned above, rectal tumours have a tendency to spread into the surrounding mesorectum but it is relatively uncommon for them to transgress the fascial envelope which surrounds the mesorectum. Thus for tumours in the upper third of the rectum the mesorectum should be carefully dissected out of the pelvis and then the mesorectum and rectum transected at a point no less than 5 cm distal to the tumour. This will ensure that any distal spread within the mesorectum itself will be removed. If the tumour is situated in the lower two-thirds of the rectum, then a total mesorectal excision should be carried out (Figure 14.35). This means dissecting the rectum and the mesorectum right down to the pelvic floor. When this is done there is usually a muscular rectal tube of 1–2 cm in length between the end of the mesorectum and the pelvic floor. If it is possible to put a clamp or a stapler across this muscular tube below the tumour then an anterior resection may be carried out. If not, it is then necessary to perform an abdominoperineal resection. During the execution of a total mesorectal excision it is important to identify the inferior hypogastric sympathetic nerves as they descend over the lateral walls of the pelvis to form the inferior hypogastric plexuses. In this way it is possible to avoid damage to both the sympathetic and parasympathetic nerve supply to the bladder and sexual organs.

It will be noted that after total mesorectal excision, it is necessary to excise almost the whole of the rectum. This is usually done by placing a transverse row of staples across the rectal stump at the level of the pelvic floor and cutting above the staples. It is then possible to carry out an anastomosis between this ultra-short rectal stump and the proximal colon using a circular end to end stapler, fired through the transverse staple line on the rectal stump (Figure 14.36). Before doing this however, it is essential to make sure that the proximal colon is mobile enough to permit such an anastomosis without any tension. To do this it is usually necessary to mobilize the splenic flexure and divide both the inferior mesenteric artery and inferior mesenteric vein close to their origins. Thus the distal colon is dependent on the marginal artery, receiving its supply from the middle or right colic arteries and it is therefore important to assess the viability of the colon before performing the anastomosis. The functional result after such a low coloanal anastomosis is often far from perfect but it may be improved by forming a small (5 cm) colonic pouch with which to form the anastomosis (Figure 14.37).

In the female patient, an advanced rectal cancer may involve the uterus or the posterior wall of the vagina. When the uterus is involved, this is usually caused by a relatively high rectal cancer and the tumour can be removed *en-bloc* with the uterus and an anterior resection performed. In the case of vaginal involvement it is usually necessary to carry out an abdominoperineal excision of rectum along with the posterior wall of the vagina.

For small rectal cancers it may be possible to carry out a local excision transanally. This can be done either using special anal retractors (e.g. the Park's retractor) or using endoscopic equipment which allows TEM. Regardless of technique the aim is to excise the tumour with a full thickness disk of rectal muscle. Thus this technique is only suitable for posterior tumours up to about 20 cm or anterior tumours up to 10 cm. Attempts at local excision for tumours which are higher not only will be technically difficult but also may result in perforation into the peritoneal cavity.

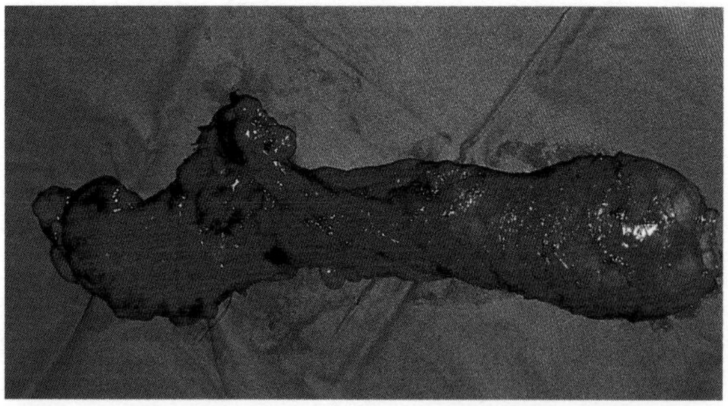

Figure 14.35 Posterior aspect of a surgical resection specimen after anterior resection with total mesorectal excision. Note the bulky mesorectum covered by smooth fascia and the distal staple line.

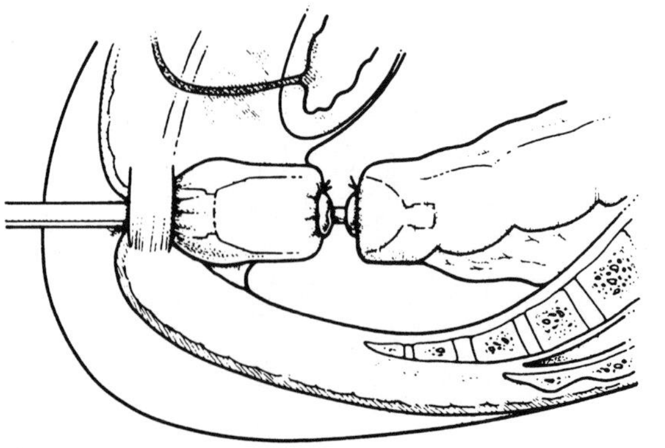

Figure 14.36 Low stapled anterior resection.

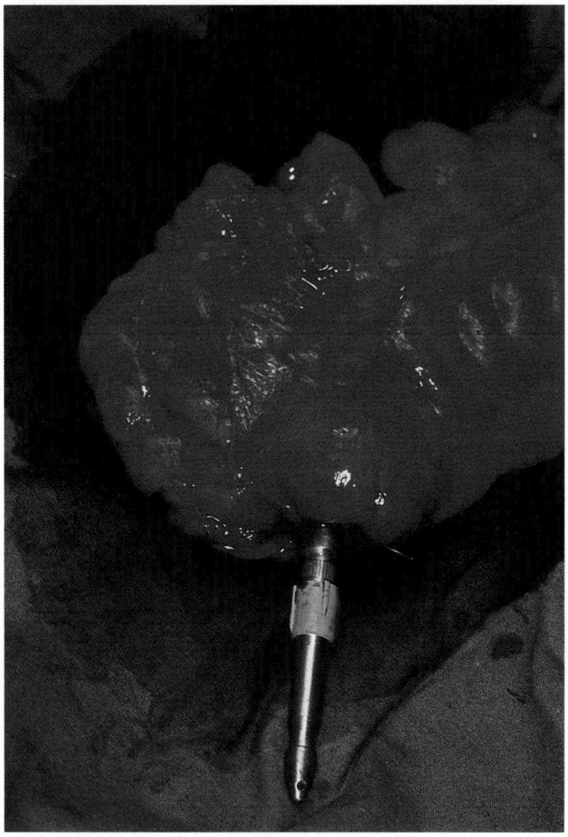

Figure 14.37 Colopouch with head of circular stapling gun in position.

Careful selection of tumours for local excision is essential. T_2 tumours (tumours invading the muscle wall) are associated with lymph node metastasis in approximately 20% of cases and will therefore be associated with a high risk of local recurrence. T_1 tumours (submucosal invasion only) are more suitable for this approach, but even so are associated with lymph node metastasis in about 4% of cases. Thus if local excision is used to treat T_1 or T_2 tumours, extremely careful follow-up must be employed using endorectal ultrasound and salvage surgery in the form of anterior resection or abdominoperineal excision carried out if recurrence occurs. Some centres using this technique also use adjuvant radiotherapy to reduce the risk of local recurrence.

It is generally regarded that T_3 tumours are unsuitable for local excision although it may be justifiable where patients are unfit for radical surgery. When a patient has a technically inoperable tumour (i.e. fixed to pelvic structures) the main role for surgery is the performance of a defunctioning colostomy which may improve the patient's quality of life, particularly if the tumour has rendered them incontinent by damaging the anal sphincters. However, this will not alleviate pain, bleeding or mucus discharge and endoanal ablation of the tumour using laser or a diathermy resectoscope may be of value.

Surgery for obstruction

About 20% of patients with colorectal cancer present as emergencies and the majority of these will have intestinal obstruction. This is usually caused by a left-sided cancer causing a large bowel obstruction but occasionally a caecal cancer will cause a low small bowel obstruction. In the case of the left-sided obstructing cancer there are various surgical options. The simplest procedure is to carry out a defunctioning transverse loop colostomy. This is a reasonable option in an unfit patient. When the patient has recovered and the bowel been prepared, the tumour can then be resected and an anastomosis performed. The loop colostomy can then be closed at a later stage. This is the classical three stage operation but is now rarely used.

Today, the most commonly used procedure is the Hartmann's operation where the tumour is resected, the rectum oversewn and the proximal colon brought out as a left iliac fossa colostomy. Re-anastomosis can be performed at a later stage. In recent years, however, there has been a tendency to carry out primary resection and anastomosis. This can be done either as a left hemicolectomy with on-table colonic irrigation as bowel preparation (Figure 14.38) or as a subtotal colectomy with anastomosis between the small bowel the remaining sigmoid colon. There is little to choose between these two approaches but a recent randomized trial has indicated that long-term bowel function is better after left hemicolectomy. It should be stressed that only relatively fit patients should be subjected to such an extensive procedure.

The most recent development in the treatment of obstructing left-sided cancers is the endoscopic or radiological insertion of an expanding metal 'wall' stent (Figure 14.39). This relieves the obstruction and, by allowing bowel preparation, allows the patient to undergo a semi-elective resection with primary anastomosis.

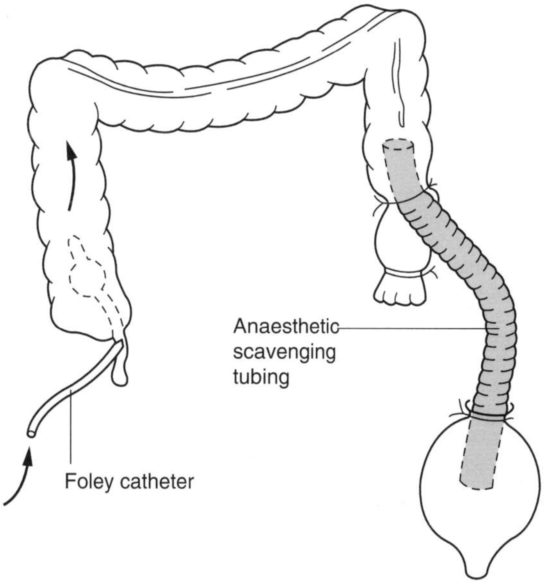

Figure 14.38 On-table colonic lavage.

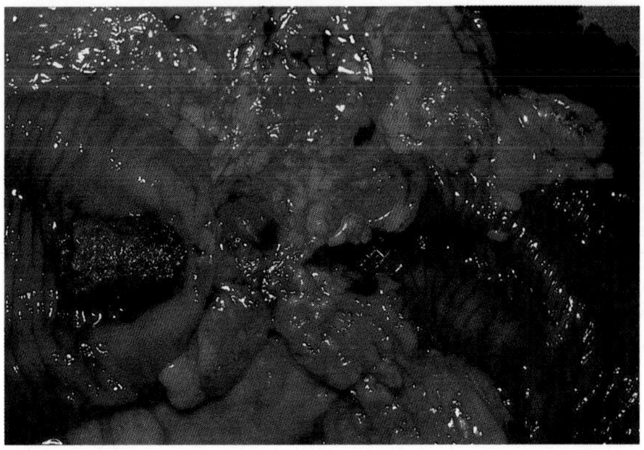

Figure 14.39 Wall stent across a malignant colonic stricture.

Surgery for metastatic disease

It is now recognized that a proportion of patients with hepatic metastases from colonic cancer are suitable for liver resection. Approximately 10% of all patients with colorectal cancer are found to have synchronous liver metastases and half of these (5% of the total) have resectable lesions. A further 10% of patients will develop metachronous liver metastases within about 2–3 years of resection of the primary colorectal cancer. The important criteria for resectability of hepatic metastases from large bowel cancer are as follows:

- The primary tumour must be controlled with no evidence of extrahepatic metastases.
- All of the hepatic metastases must be resectable with an adequate margin of at least 2 cm of normal liver tissue.
- The operation must be performed with an acceptable mortality and morbidity.

Although the best results are associated with solitary metastatic lesions it is possible to carry out extensive liver resections for multiple disease. Analysis of several large series indicates that multiple factors influence survival after hepatic resection. These are as follows:

- *Stage of the primary tumour*. The more advanced the stage of the primary lesion the worse the prognosis after liver resection.
- *Number of metastases and their location within the liver*. Patients with more than three metastatic lesions and those with bilobar disease tend to fare badly.
- *The interval of time between resection of the primary lesion and the appearance of the hepatic metastases*. The longer the period the better the prognosis.
- *Sex of the patient*. In general women live longer than men after resection of liver metastases.
- *The presence of extrahepatic metastases*. This adversely influences the results of liver resection.
- *The operative mortality*. Modern surgical standards dictate that this should be under 5% even for a major lobectomy or extended right hepatectomy.

Although there has been no randomized trial there is little doubt that resection of liver metastases confers a survival advantage. With careful patient selection, hepatectomy for colorectal metastases is associated with a 5 year survival around 30% which is the same prognosis as is associated with resection of a stage C cancer without evidence of distant metastases.

In patients with liver metastases which are not suitable for liver resection then *in situ* ablation using cryotherapy or radiofrequency probes may be of value. Currently this is performed under ultrasound control either at open surgery or laparoscopically. It seems to be associated with a modest prolongation of survival. Future developments include percutaneous *in situ* ablation using MRI guided probes in an open magnet and the use of extracorporeal high-energy focused ultrasound to destroy tumour deposits.

Minimal access surgery for colorectal cancer

Minimal access surgery in the form of endoscopic polypectomy or tumour excision has been available for many years. However, there has been increasing interest in laparoscopic or laparoscopy-assisted colonic resections for colorectal cancer. World-wide there is now a considerable experience of laparoscopic surgery for colonic cancer but there are still concerns regarding this type of surgery.

First, it is technically difficult to obtain the correct degree of traction required for a precise dissection and intracorporeal anastomosis is awkward leading most surgeons to use an extracorporeal method wherever possible. Another problem is specimen retrieval for which an abdominal incision has to be made. This negates a lot of the benefit of laparoscopic surgery and there is little evidence that in-hospital stay is any less after laparoscopic surgery when compared with conventional open surgery.

Port site tumour recurrence was a major concern in the early days of laparoscopic colonic cancer surgery, with the incidence varying from 1.5% to 21% depending on the series. However, it has been estimated that the local recurrence in the wound after open surgery is around 1% and recent experience would indicate that the port site recurrence rate may be as low as this if sensible precautions are taken (e.g. irrigating the port sites with cytocidal agents and making sure that the extraction site is properly protected before removing the tumour).

At present, the major concern regarding laparoscopic colonic surgery is the long-term recurrence rates as it is still not known whether these are comparable to open surgery. Currently, there are several randomized trials comparing open surgery and laparoscopic surgery and the results of these are awaited with interest. It will be important however, to make sure that the results of open surgery in these trials are comparable to the best results which can be achieved by specialist colorectal surgeons.

Chemotherapy

Adjuvant chemotherapy

There is now good evidence that patients with stage C colon cancer benefit from post-operative chemotherapy containing 5-fluorouracil (5-FU) as this leads to a 5–10% absolute improvement in survival. However, meta-analysis of the various trials has been unable to demonstrate an effect in stage A or stage B cancer or in rectal cancer. In addition, it cannot be shown conclusively that elderly patients benefit from adjuvant chemotherapy. Currently, the standard adjuvant chemotherapy consists of 5-FU and folinic acid (leucovorin). Folinic acid acts as a potentiator of the 5-FU and a recent randomized trial has demonstrated that low-dose folinic acid is as effective as high-dose folinic acid. For a number of years it has been considered that the immunomodulator levamisole conferred benefit when given with 5-FU, but this has now been disproven.

Palliative chemotherapy

Chemotherapy may also be used to treat disseminated colorectal cancer and there is now good evidence that with appropriate patient selection, significant prolongation of good quality life can be achieved. It has to be stressed however, that this is palliative only and prolongation of life for more than 6 months is unusual. Again the standard chemotherapy regimen consists of 5-FU and folinic acid but new drugs are on the horizon. The topoisomerase inhibitor irinotecan has been shown in a randomized trial to prolong survival in patients who have experienced a treatment failure with 5-FU. Another exciting development is the oral prodrug capecitabine which appears to have activity in colorectal cancer. Chemotherapy may be administered systemically or regionally and there has been considerable interest in delivering chemotherapy via a hepatic artery catheter for patients with liver metastases but as yet there is no convincing evidence that this is any better than systemic treatment.

Radiotherapy

Curative radiotherapy

Particularly in France there has been a vogue for treating small rectal cancers with contact radiotherapy and this approach has met with some success. There is no evidence however, that contact radiotherapy is any better than local excision for early cancers (see above).

Adjuvant radiotherapy

There is good evidence from several randomized trials that both pre-operative and post-operative radiotherapy can reduce the rate of local recurrence after resection of rectal cancer. In the USA, post-operative radiotherapy is favoured, usually combined with chemotherapy. The radiotherapy dose is usually in the region of 40 Gy given in about 20 fractions over 4 weeks. In Europe however, pre-operative radiotherapy given as 25 Gy in five daily fractions the week before surgery is favoured. This is based on the Stockholm trial which demonstrated not only a reduction in local recurrence but also an improvement in survival using this regimen.

It must be stressed however, that all the reported trials of adjuvant radiotherapy were conducted before the dramatic improvement in surgical technique which has occurred in recent years. The average local recurrence rate in the control arms of most trials was in the region of 20% which would now be considered unacceptable by specialist surgeons. It remains to be seen whether adjuvant radiotherapy confers any added benefit to high-quality specialist surgery for rectal cancer and trials are currently underway to look at this problem.

Adjuvant radiotherapy for rectal cancer is not without its problems as it is associated with significant degree of morbidity. This includes radiation damage to the residual rectum, radiation cystitis and radiation enteritis of irradiated small bowel which falls into the pelvis. Post-operative radiotherapy is sometimes used for colonic cancer where there is felt to be residual tumour, but this is associated with high morbidity because of radiation enteritis and not generally recommended.

Palliative radiotherapy

Palliative radiotherapy is used almost exclusively for inoperable rectal cancer but the response rates are not very high. Response is improved if chemotherapy is given at the same time but this is at the expense of markedly increased toxicity. In the case of fixed rectal cancer it is often worth giving a long course of radiotherapy (40 Gy in 20 fractions) with or without chemotherapy and reassessing the tumour about 6 weeks after the radiotherapy has been completed. Occasionally a fixed rectal tumour will be rendered operable by this approach.

Familial adenomatous polyposis

FAP is a dominantly inherited condition characterized by the appearance of multiple adenomatous polyps throughout the colon which inevitably leads to colorectal cancer by the fourth decade of life. It is caused by a germline mutation of the APC gene which is located on chromosome 5q and functions as a tumour suppressor gene with implications for cell-to-cell adhesion. The severity of the polyposis is variable and is related to the specific mutation, e.g. mutations at codon 1309 (exon 15) are associated with a very dense polyposis.

Although colonic polyps are the most important phenotypic manifestation of this condition, there are also extracolonic features which appear to a varying degree. These include adenomas and carcinomas of the small bowel and particularly the periampullary area of the duodenum, congenital hypertrophy of the retinal pigment epithelium (CHRPE) (Figure 14.40), and desmoid tumours. When FAP occurs in association with desmoid tumours, epidermoid cysts and bony exostoses it is termed Gardener's syndrome and this appears to occur in about 10% of cases.

Clinical features

Commonly this condition is picked up by surveillance as children of affected individuals have a 1:2 chance of developing colonic polyps. However, in an individual not suspected of having FAP, the most usual presenting

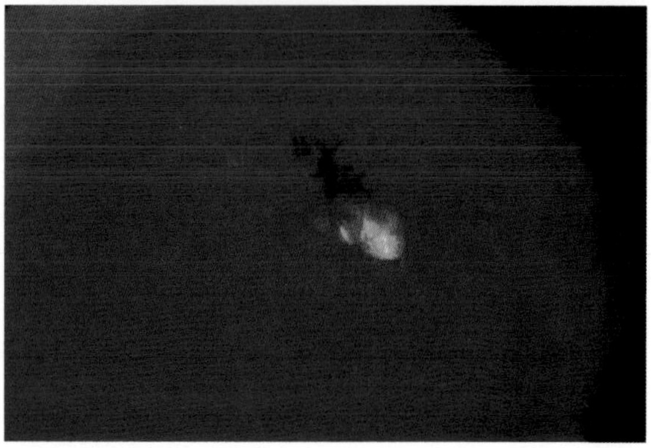

Figure 14.40 Congenital hypertrophy of the retinal pigment epithelium (CHRPE).

symptom is rectal bleeding. CHRPEs may be seen on retinoscopy and desmoid tumours usually present as abdominal wall or intra-abdominal masses.

Diagnosis

The age at which the polyps develop is variable but it is usually in the late teenage years and early 20s. For this reason, individuals at risk of FAP should undergo yearly sigmoidoscopy from puberty onwards. Genetic screening is now possible and once the specific mutation in the APC gene has been detected by genetic sequencing in an affected individual, his or her children can then be screened for that specific mutation. If they do not carry the mutation then endoscopic surveillance will not be necessary.

Treatment

The treatment for familial adenomatous polyposis is colectomy soon after the development of the adenomatous polyps (usually in the early 20s). There is some debate as to whether a total colectomy with ileostomy or ileo-anal pouch should be performed or whether it is safe to carry out a subtotal colectomy with ileorectal anastomosis followed by careful follow-up of the rectum with ablation of the polyps when they arise. Mutation analysis may help in this respect and it might be reasonable to plan the operation depending on the likely density of polyps (i.e. those with the mutation at codon 1309 at exon 5 might be best served by a total proctocolectomy, whereas in other mutations an ileorectal anastomosis may be appropriate). More work is required in this area.

Hereditary non-polyposis colorectal cancer (HNPCC)

While FAP probably accounts for 1–3% of all colorectal cancers, HNPCC, may account for 5–10%. Like FAP, HNPCC is a dominantly inherited condition but as it does not lead to multiple polyposis, it is more difficult to recognize. The germline mutations which lead to HNPCC are thought to occur in DNA mismatch repair genes and currently four are recognized – hMSH2, hMLH1, hPMS1 and hPMS2, but 90% of mutations in HNPCC are found in hMSH2 and hMLH1.

Clinically, the diagnosis of HNPCC depends on the 'Amsterdam criteria' which require three or more relatives with histologically verified colorectal cancer, one of whom is a first degree relative of the other two with at least one patient being less than 50 years of age. HNPCC is associated with an excess risk of extracolonic cancers and is classified into 'Lynch' syndromes 1 and 2 on the basis of extracolonic disease. In Lynch syndrome 2 there is a particularly strong association with endometrial and ovarian cancer but other malignancies which may occur include transitional cell carcinoma of the ureter and renal pelvis, gastric cancer, pancreatic cancer, biliary tract cancer and haematological cancers.

Clinical features

Clinical features are merely those of the cancer that develops, particularly colorectal cancer. It should be stressed that multiple polyps do not occur although small numbers of adenomatous polyps are a feature of this condition. The lifetime risk for colorectal cancer is about 85% of affected individuals which indicates incomplete penetrance of this inherited condition.

Diagnosis

In individuals at risk the current recommendations are that colonoscopy should be performed at the age of 25 years, then repeated every second year until the age of 35 and then repeated yearly. The reason for the increased frequency at 35 years is that the average age of developing colorectal cancer is around 40. Women with Lynch 2 syndrome may also be offered screening of the endometrium by endometrial aspiration and yearly measurement of the CA125 tumour marker. It is now possible to carry out mutation analysis for the known mismatch repair gene mutations. Once a specific mutation is known in an affected individual, their offspring may be offered genetic screening.

Treatment

When a cancer has been identified it is usual to offer a subtotal colectomy and ileorectal anastomosis in view of the high risk of metachronous tumours. Whether or not prophylactic colectomy should be carried in subjects known to be carrying a germline mutation in one of the appropriate genes is controversial but has its supporters. The main argument against this approach is the fact that the condition is not fully penetrant.

Unusual colorectal cancers

Squamous cell carcinoma

Squamous cell carcinoma of the colon or rectum is extremely rare and may be related to squamous metaplasia of existing adenomas or carcinomas. Chronic ulcerative colitis, schistosomiasis and radiotherapy are all other possible predisposing factors. This type of cancer presents as ordinary adenocarcinoma and the diagnosis is only made on histology. Squamous carcinoma of the colon and rectum must be differentiated from anal carcinoma which is a distinct clinical entity.

Carcinoid tumours

The most common site for carcinoid tumours is the appendix followed by the small intestine. The large bowel is the third most common site with the rectum or anus being the most frequent. The tumours are usually polypoid in nature and appear to be slow growing, remaining asymptomatic for long periods of time. Indeed about 50% of patients with colonic carcinoids have no symptoms attributable to the primary tumour at the time of diagnosis. Carcinoids are dealt with in more detail in the module on small bowel and appendix.

Lymphoma

Malignant lymphoma is the third most common malignant tumour of the large bowel after adenocarcinoma and carcinoid tumours but probably only represents about 1.5% of all colonic tumours. The commonest sites are the rectum and the caecum. The tumours are usually of the non-Hodgkin's variety. Because these tumours are rare, definitive guidelines on treatment are difficult to provide. However, it is generally recommended that colonic tumours should be treated by chemotherapy alone whereas rectal tumours should be treated by a combination of radiotherapy and chemotherapy. Surgical resection should follow unless there is a complete response to non-surgical therapy.

Sarcoma

Various types of sarcoma can arise in the colon and rectum and present in very much the same way as adenocarcinoma. Of particular note in recent years is Kaposi's sarcoma which is a feature of human immunodeficiency virus (HIV) infection. This tumour has been reported as being the presenting feature in the acquired immunodeficiency syndrome (AIDS) in about 25% of cases and is manifested by multiple lesions in the gastrointestinal tract and the skin. The rectum is a common site and this leads to symptoms suggestive of inflammatory bowel disease (diarrhoea and ulceration). Radiotherapy and chemotherapy may be used to treat Kaposi's sarcoma and occasionally surgery is required.

Section 14.5 • Inflammatory bowel disease

Ulcerative colitis

Ulcerative colitis is an idiopathic condition of the rectum and colon which has an incidence in the UK of about 10 new cases per 100 000 of the population per year. Prevalence is about 120 cases per 100 000 of the population.

Pathology

Ulcerative colitis tends to affect the distal large bowel and is confluent, in other words the rectum is nearly always involved (over 95% of cases) and extends in continuity to involve varying amounts of the colon (proctosigmoiditis, left colitis, subtotal colitis and total colitis). Segmental inflammation or skip lesions are not a feature of ulcerative colitis; these are typical of Crohn's disease.

Macroscopic appearances

The inflammatory process is largely confined to the mucosa and to lesser extent to the submucosa. Involvement of the muscularis and serosa is rare and lymph node enlargement is not a significant feature. Early disease consists of a haemorrhagic inflammation with loss of the normal vascular pattern, petechial haemorrhages and bleeding. Ulceration of the mucosa is seen in more advanced disease. Here, large areas may become denuded of mucosa and there is undermining of the mucosa which often results in the formation of mucosal bridges. This mucosal destruction is accompanied by the formation of excess granulation tissue and the development of pseudopolyps. As the mucosa heals these polyps become epithelialized and persist within either a normal looking or atrophic mucosa.

Microscopic changes

The disease starts with inflammation of the crypts of Lieberkühn and the development of crypt abscesses which result in necrosis of the crypt epithelium and the appearance of a more chronic inflammatory cell infiltrate, consisting of lymphocytes, plasma cells, eosinophils and mast cells in the adjacent submucosa. The inflammation and crypt abscess formation is accompanied by discharge of mucus from the goblet cells which become reduced in number as the disease progresses (Figure 14.41). Rupture of the crypt abscesses into the intestinal lumen gives rise to ulceration and the ulcerated areas rapidly become covered by vascular granulation tissue. Excessive fibrosis is not a feature of the disease. Very occasionally, the inflammatory process involves the whole thickness of the bowel wall including the muscle and serosa; this is a feature of toxic megacolon.

When remission occurs normal histological appearances may be restored but evidence of mucosal atrophy

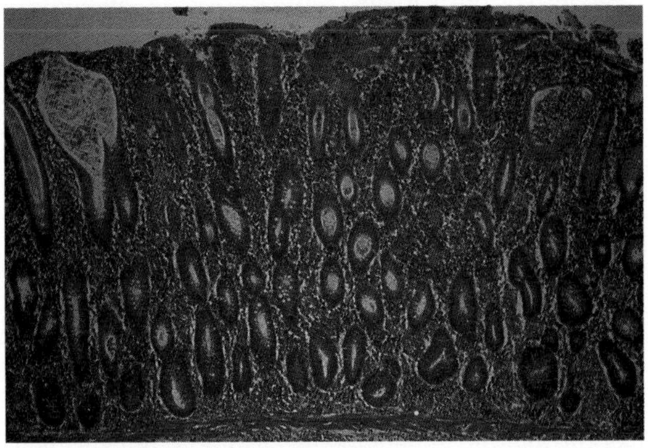

Figure 14.41 Histological appearances of ulcerative colitis. Note the crypt abcesses.

is often observed with a reduction in the number of colonic glands which are short (fail to reach the muscularis mucosae) and branched. Hypertrophy of the muscularis mucosae and Paneth cell hyperplasia may be encountered in long-standing ulcerative colitis. However, the most important long-term change is dysplasia which is thought to be a premalignant change. Hyperplastic areas are often widespread and may be accompanied by endoscopically and radiologically identifiable elevated plaques.

Aetiology

The aetiology of ulcerative colitis remains unclear. There is a marked geographical distribution with high prevalence in the USA and western Europe and very low incidences in the Far East. Males and females are affected to almost the same extent and although half of ulcerative colitis patients are aged between 20 and 40 years at diagnosis, it can occur in any decade of life.

As inflammation of the colonic wall seems to be the primary pathological feature, it is reasonable to look for an immunological cause but this has never been convincingly demonstrated despite the fact that about 50% of patients with ulcerative colitis have anti-colon antibodies detectable in the serum. It has also been suggested that there is a defect in the colonic mucus as there is evidence that there is a reduction in the production of type 4 mucin and this may represent loss of an important mucosal protective mechanism. Metabolic abnormalities include reduction in the ability of the colonic mucosa to utilize butyrate as an energy source and reduction in carboxypeptidase activity. This enzyme is needed to degrade bacterial chemotactic peptides that are important in the recruitment of inflammatory cells.

Specific aetiological factors can be divided into genetic and environmental.

Genetic factors

The first degree relatives of patients are 15 times at greater risk of developing ulcerative colitis than the general population but there is no clear cut Mendelian pattern of inheritance. Likewise, there is no consistent association with any human leucocyte antigen (HLA) type except in patients with associated ankylosing spondylitis where there is a high incidence of HLA B27.

Environmental factors

There have been suggestions that bacterial infection may play a role and there has been a report of an unexpectedly high frequency of ulcerative colitis or Crohn's disease after an epidemic of bacillary dysentery. However, there is no other epidemiological evidence to suggest an infectious agent. Smoking surprisingly appears to be protective against ulcerative colitis and there have been anecdotal reports of remissions after the use of nicotine but the underlying mechanism is unexplained. Dietary factors may be important but have yet to be identified. There is some evidence that patients with ulcerative colitis may benefit from avoiding cow's milk but there is no evidence from controlled trials to demonstrate that intravenous feeding has any effect on the course of the disease. Finally, it is often noted that patients with colitis are more likely to relapse when they experience periods of stress but detailed research work has been unable to show a significant association between life events and disease activity.

Clinical features

The clinical course of ulcerative colitis is variable and does not accurately reflect the extent of colonic involvement by the disease, although the severe intractable form which is attended by a reduced survival and a significant mortality is encountered in patients with total colitis. The severity of the disease can be roughly classified into mild, moderate and severe.

Mild ulcerative colitis

This is generally defined as disease which is associated with less than four bowel motions per day and the absence of systemic symptoms and signs. It is the most common form of the disease and in the majority of patients the mucosal inflammation is restricted to the rectum and distal sigmoid although a few patients may be found to have total colonic involvement. In addition to mild diarrhoea, mucus and some rectal bleeding, the patients often develop pruritus ani especially if they have haemorrhoids. They are also subject to the extracolonic manifestations especially uveitis, erythema nodosum and arthritis. Not infrequently these extracolonic manifestations constitute the main symptoms and may pre-date the onset of diarrhoea. In a small percentage of patients (10%) there is a slow progression of both the extent of the colonic involvement and the severity of the disease. Usually, however, the long-term prognosis of the mild disease is good, the patient rarely requiring hospitalization, and the overall life expectancy is not affected.

Moderate ulcerative colitis

In about a quarter of patients the disease is of an intermediate severity termed moderate colitis. Colonic involvement varies but is usually extensive or total. Diarrhoea is more marked (four to six times per day) and invariably contains blood. Abdominal pain, either mild colicky pain or lower abdominal discomfort, may be present and each attack is accompanied by a lowgrade fever. The patients often develop iron deficiency anaemia and may exhibit a loss of appetite and weight. The disease responds well to corticosteroid therapy. However, the long-term prognosis is not particularly good and rapid deterioration with the development of severe disease or acute local complications (toxic megacolon, massive bleeding or colonic perforation) may occur at some stage during the course of the disease.

Severe ulcerative colitis

Severe ulcerative colitis, which occurs in about 15% of cases, accounts for the vast majority of deaths from this disease. It may arise as a result of progression from mild or moderate disease but more usually it starts *de novo* with a severe attack with marked colonic symptoms and systemic manifestations. The diarrhoea is severe with tenesmus and profuse rectal bleeding. This is accompanied by severe water and electrolyte depletion. The patient become dehydrated, acidotic and anaemic. Hypovolaemic shock often develops. Pyrexia is present and is accompanied by a leucocytosis. Hypoproteinaemia and hypoalbuminaemia are invariable features of severe ulcerative colitis and are due to a combination of diminished protein intake, impaired synthesis and constant colonic loss. The patient complains of severe abdominal pain, there is general tenderness and there are varying degrees of abdominal distension. Often the response to medical treatment is poor and some of these patients require urgent or emergency colectomy for progressing disease or the onset of life-threatening complications. The mortality of a severe attack of ulcerative colitis is in the region of 5%.

Diagnosis

The diagnosis of ulcerative colitis is usually made on endoscopy and confirmed by mucosal biopsy. Although this can be done at rigid or flexible sigmoidoscopy a total colonoscopy is sometimes necessary to determine the extent of the disease. Colonoscopy is not advised in severe disease as this may lead to perforation. At endoscopy the earliest abnormality is loss of the vascular pattern in the mucosa which is caused by oedema obscuring the submucosal vessels. This progresses to a fine granularity, erythema, contact bleeding and frank ulceration. A biopsy is essential to demonstrate the histopathological features described above. Barium enema is also helpful but will not demonstrate mild disease as a degree of ulceration or granularity is necessary before the disease will show up on the barium enema films. In long-standing disease when there has been a degree of fibrosis, the colon appears featureless with loss of haustrations (Figure 14.42). A specimen of stool should always be sent for microbiological examination to exclude infective causes of colitis. If amoebiasis is suspected, the specimen should be examined in the laboratory by microscopy within a few hours. Other organisms which may cause an infective colitis include shigella, campylobacter and *Clostridium difficile*. These are dealt with later in this module.

When it is important to estimate the extent of colonic involvement, but colonoscopy or barium enema is inadvisable (i.e. in severe disease) a leucocyte scan can be helpful. This is carried out by re-injection of ^{111}indium-labelled autologous leucocytes, and external isotope scintiscanning. The leucocytes are concentrated in the areas of inflammation so that the involved colonic segment is demonstrated on the scan (Figure 14.43).

One of the biggest diagnostic challenges in ulcerative colitis is to distinguish it from Crohn's colitis. This

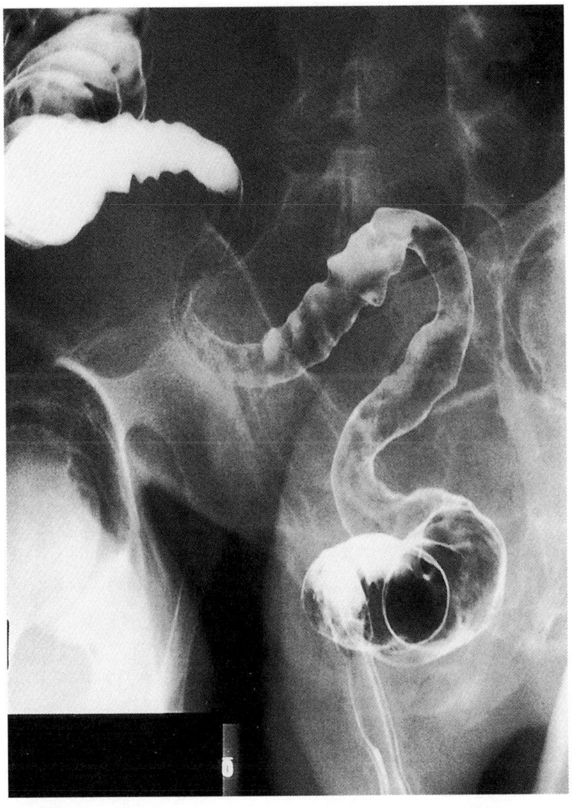

Figure 14.42 Barium enema appearances of long-standing ulcerative colitis.

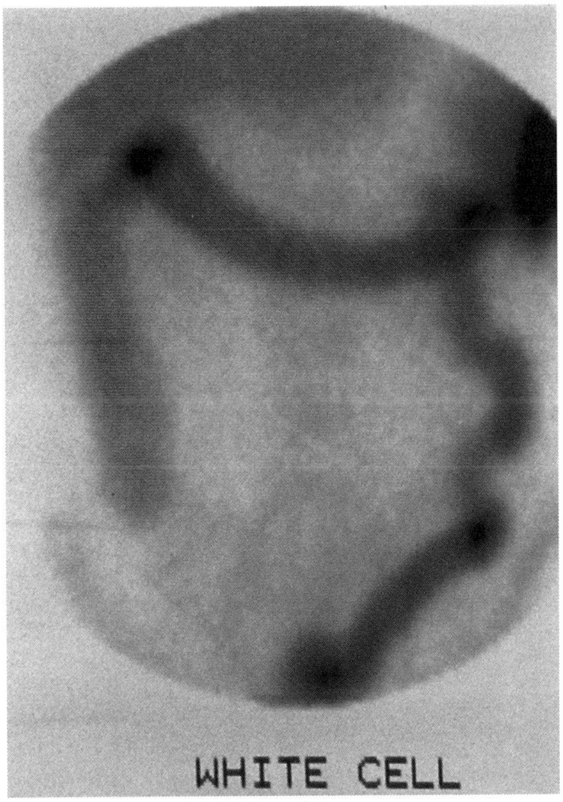

Figure 14.43 Labelled white cell scan showing active total colitis. (Courtesy Dr Norman Kennedy, Nuclear Medicine, Ninewells Hospital, Dundee, Scotland.)

may be possible on histological grounds but in some cases it is impossible to reach a firm diagnosis. When this is the case the patient may be labelled as having indeterminate colitis and it will be necessary to combine clinical histological and radiological features in order to come down more in favour of ulcerative colitis or Crohn's disease. The main factors which are used to distinguish between ulcerative colitis and Crohn's disease are shown in Table 14.4.

Complications

The complications of ulcerative colitis can be subdivided into local (large bowel) complications and systemic (extracolonic) complications. The systemic complications are similar to those seen in Crohn's disease and these are listed in the Table 14.5. Local complications include:

- toxic megacolon
- colonic perforation
- massive haemorrhage
- colonic stricture
- colonic carcinoma
- perianal suppuration
- giant inflammatory polyposis.

The relative incidence of these local complications is shown in Figure 14.44.

Toxic megacolon

This serious complication, which occurs in 2–10% of cases, carries a high mortality. It is not unique to ulcerative colitis and can occur in Crohn's disease, pseudomembranous colitis, bacterial colitis and amoebic colitis. It is more common in patients with extensive ulcerative colitis (total or subtotal) and tends to occur during the first attacks of the disease. Certain precipitating factors may be involved in some cases including metabolic alkalosis, hypokalaemia and the administration of drugs affecting intestinal motility, e.g. opiates and anticholinergic agents. The entire colon may be affected but more commonly it is the transverse colon which is predominantly involved. Histologically there is a transmural extension of the inflammatory process with deep ulcers reaching the serosa of the large bowel associated with vasculitis and inflammation of the myenteric and submucous nerve plexuses. This leads to thinning of the bowel wall. Clinically, toxic dilatation is characterized by abdominal distension, absent bowel sounds, severe systemic toxicity, fever, tachycardia, leucocytosis and marked fluid and electrolyte depletion. The diagnosis can usually be made on a plain abdominal radiograph (Figure 14.45) which shows a distended colon exhibiting loss of haustration mucosal irregularities in the colonic wall and in some instances intramural air (tramlining). Patients with this condition require very careful and frequent monitoring with daily abdominal X-rays. If the condition does not respond to intensive corticosteroid therapy within 72 hours, colectomy is mandatory because of the risk of colonic perforation.

Colonic perforation

Although colonic perforation is a feature of toxic dilation, it may occur in the absence of this complication. It carries a 50% mortality and accounts for about 30% of all deaths from ulcerative colitis. Although there is

Table 14.4 Essential differences between ulcerative colitis and Crohn's disease

	Ulcerative colitis	*Crohn's disease*
Clinical features		
Rectal bleeding	Very common	Unusal
Abdominal pain	Infrequent	Common
Abdominal mass	Rare	Sometimes
Spontaneous fistula	Very rare/never	Sometimes
Perianal infections	15%	30–40%
Rectal involvement	95%	50%
Carcinoma	Yes	Yes
Radiology		
Distribution	Continuous with rectum	Often discontinuous along and around colon
Rectum	Usually involved	Often normal
Strictures	Rare, usually Ca	Often present
Mucosa	Granular, shallow ulcers, pseudopolyps	Fissuring, deep undermining ulcers, cobblestone appearance
Small bowel	Backwash ileitis only	Discontinuous involvement by skip lesions
Histopathology		
Inflammation	Mucosal	Transmural
Vascularity	Often intense	Seldom prominent
Focal lymphoid hyperplasia	Restricted to mucosa/submucosa	Transmural
Mucus secretion	Grossly impaired	Less severe impairment
Paneth cell metaplasia	Common	Rare
Sarcoid granuloma	Absent	50–70%
Fissuring	Rare	Very common
Precancerous dysplasia	Yes	Yes
Lymph nodes	Reactive hyperplasia	Often sarcoid foci
Anal lesions	Non-specific	Often sarcoid foci

Table 14.5 Systemic complications of ulcerative colitis and Crohn's disease

Liver	Fatty change	Both Crohn's and UC
	Pericholangitis	Both Crohn's and UC
	Sclerosing cholangitis	Usually Crohn's
	Cirrhosis	Both Crohn's and UC
	Cholangiocarcinoma	UC
Skin	Pyoderma gangrenosum	More common in UC
	Erythema nodosum	Both Crohn's and UC
	Aphthous stomatitis	Usually Crohn's
	Finger clubbing	Both Crohn's and UC
Joints	Enteropathic arthritis	Both Crohn's and UC
	Sacro-ileitis/ankylosing spondylitis	Both Crohn's and UC
Eyes	Uveitis	Crohn's > UC
	Episcleritis	Crohn's > UC
	Corneal infiltrates	Both Crohn's and UC
Kidneys	Renal calculi	Both Crohn's and UC
	Pyelonephritis	Crohn's > UC
	Obstructive uropathy	Crohn's
Haemopoietic	Autoimmune haemolytic anaemia (rare)	UC
Cardiovascular	Systemic thrombosis	Both Crohn's and UC
	Vasculitis (rare)	Both Crohn's and UC
	Takayasu's disease	Crohn's
	Pericarditis	Both Crohn's and UC
Bronchopulmonary	Fibrosing alveolitis	Both Crohn's and UC
	Bronchiectasis	Both Crohn's and UC
	Pleural effusions	Both Crohn's and UC
Endocrine	Goitre and hyperthyroidism	UC
Other	Amyloid	Crohn's

UC: ulcerative colitis.

no evidence that corticosteroid therapy increases the risk of perforation, this type of treatment may mask the physical signs and delay the diagnosis. Perforation may be precipitated by the use of colonoscopy or barium enema during a severe attack of the disease. Clinically colonic perforation usually presents with sudden onset of abdominal pain and rapid deterioration as septic shock develops.

Massive haemorrhage
This is a rare complication and usually affects patients with severe and total colonic involvement by ulcerative colitis. It usually settles with conservative management and blood transfusion. Severe colonic bleeding may be associated with disseminated intravascular coagulation.

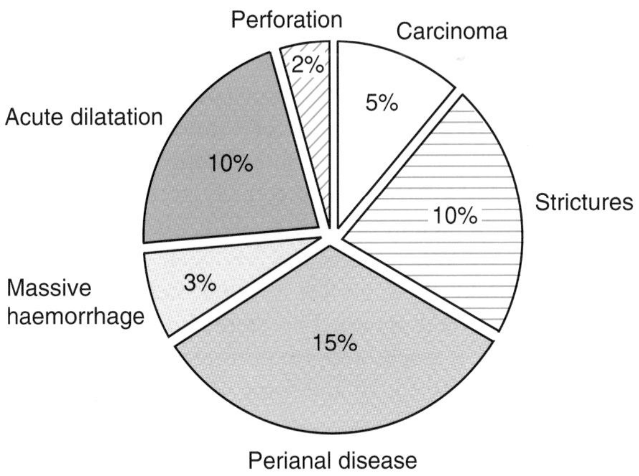

Figure 14.44 Incidence of local complications in ulcerative colitis.

Colonic stricture
Narrowing of the colon usually arises from submucosal fibrosis but may also be caused by hyperplastic mucosa and may therefore be reversible with medical treatment. Fibrous strictures, which occur most commonly in the rectum and transverse colon, are encountered in 5–10% of cases with ulcerative colitis with

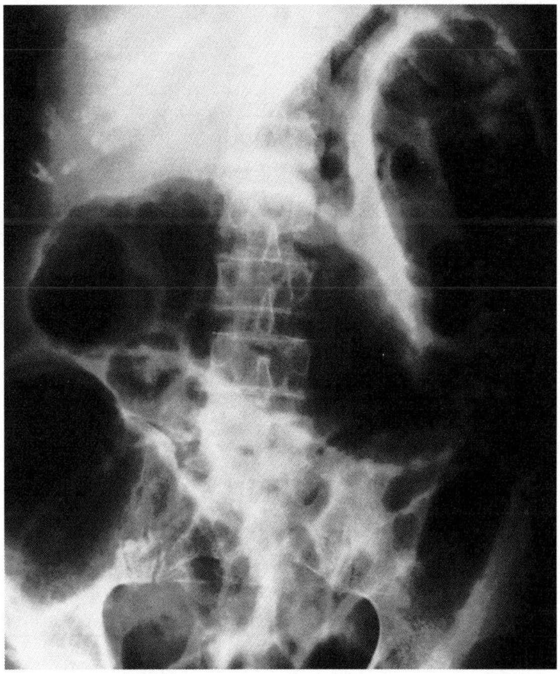

Figure 14.45 Plain X-ray appearances of toxic megacolon.

total colonic involvement. The radiological demonstration of a stricture is an indication for colonoscopy with multiple biopsies as it is impossible to exclude carcinoma on radiological grounds alone.

Colonic cancer

The increased risk of carcinoma of the large bowel in patients with ulcerative colitis is well established and the incidence is dependent on the duration of the disease. The exact risk varies from series to series but it seems to be about 1% at 10 years, 5% at 20 years and 10% at 25 years. The extent of the colitis also seems to be important with carcinoma usually occurring in patients with total or subtotal colonic involvement. Cancer in ulcerative colitis occurs at a younger age than in non-colitic patients. The tumours tend to be less well differentiated and are more often multiple than is normally the case.

It is now accepted that dysplasia of the colonic mucosa is a precursor of malignant transformation and for this reason colonoscopic surveillance is widely practised for patients with long-standing extensive colitis. There is, however, no firm evidence that this approach reduces mortality and there are no universally accepted guidelines which specify the indications for colonoscopy or the frequency with which the examination should be carried out. Presence of dysplasia in a patient with ulcerative colitis is an indication for colectomy. There is also an established association between ulcerative colitis and the development of cholangiocarcinoma. These tumours tend to be of the multiple peripheral (intrahepatic type) and occur in a younger age group than the usual type of bile duct tumour. Patients with ulcerative colitis have a 21-fold relative risk for bile duct carcinoma above the general population and because of its diffuse nature this tumour carries a very poor prognosis. Primary colonic lymphoma has been reported in patients with ulcerative colitis although a definite association has not been established.

Perianal disease

Apart from haemorrhoids which are frequently present, perianal disease (abscesses, fissures and sinuses) are encountered in patients with ulcerative colitis but very much less frequently than in Crohn's disease. The highest reported incidence of perianal sepsis in patients with ulcerative colitis is around 15% but this may represent underdiagnosis of Crohn's colitis.

Giant inflammatory polyposis

Although uncommon, this complication is important because it gives rise to a distinctive syndrome of abdominal pain and chronic iron deficiency anaemia. The transverse colon is most commonly affected. The polyps are multiple, often confluent and vary in size up to 2.5 cm in diameter. The polyps may have a complex structure with branching and bridging leading to trapping of inspissated mucus and faecal material. Resection is advisable in symptomatic patients.

Treatment

The treatment of ulcerative colitis can be divided into medical treatment and surgical treatment.

Medical treatment

The mainstay of medical treatment of ulcerative colitis remains 5-aminosalicylic acid derivatives and steroids. The regimen which is used depends on the severity of the attack.

Mild attack

Patients with mild ulcerative colitis can usually be managed as outpatients. The commonest form of treatment consists of steroid enemas either in an aqueous form or as a foam. This is particularly useful for proctitis and the foam formulations may be effective up to the mid sigmoid colon. Sulphasalazine and mesalazine enemas are also effective in active distal ulcerative colitis. However, if the patient has more extensive disease then topical treatment is not usually effective and oral prednisolone at 20–40 mg/day should be used in addition. The dosage of steroid should be kept constant until the symptoms and endoscopic appearance have improved and then they should be tailed off over a period of about 4 weeks. Oral sulphasalazine or mesalazine should be given at the same time.

Moderate attacks

Patients with moderate ulcerative colitis can be treated in much the same way as those with mild attacks except that an oral dose of prednisolone of 40 mg/day should be started immediately. If the patient is not too debilitated then outpatient management is appropriate but failure to respond promptly is an indication for admission to hospital.

Severe attacks

These patients require immediate admission to hospital with careful monitoring of their clinical condition. This includes pulse rate, blood pressure, temperature and urine output with clinical assessment on a regular basis. Plain abdominal radiography should be organized on admission and repeated daily. Intravenous hydrocortisone at 100–200 mg four times daily is the standard treatment and it is often necessary to give intravenous fluid and electrolytes and blood if the haemoglobin is less than 10 g/dl. If the patient's condition fails to settle within 5–7 days then emergency surgery should be seriously considered. In patients who show some improvement after 5 days but who have not actually gone into remission, it may be helpful to give azathioprine at a dose of 1.5–2 mg/day. When remission has been achieved the patients should then go on to oral steroids and 5-aminosalicylic acid agents. This steroid dose should be tailed off over 6 weeks and a typical regimen is 1 week each at 40, 30, 20, 15, 10 and 5 mg/day.

Maintenance of remission

One of the important aspects of treating patients with ulcerative colitis is to prevent relapse. There is good evidence that corticosteroids do not achieve this but sulphasalazine at 2 g/day has been shown in a placebo-controlled trial to be effective in maintaining remission. Chances of developing a recurrence are four times greater in individuals not taking sulphasalazine and the drug is effective for at least 5 years. In general it is recommended that sulphasalazine should be given for at least 1 year after the first attack and should given continuously in patients who have established recurrent disease. Sulphasalazine is made up of 5-aminosalicylic acid linked to sulphapyridine by an azo bond. This is split into the active salicylic acid and the inactive sulphapyridine by colonic bacteria and the sulphapyridine carrier molecule is responsible for most of the unwanted effects (gastrointestinal symptoms and headache). For this reason, different preparations of controlled release 5-aminosalicylic acid have been developed. These include mesalazine which is coated with a polyacrylic resin or ethylcellulose, olsalazine which consists of two aminosalicylic molecules linked by an azo bond and balsalazide, consisting of 5-aminosalicylic acid linked to an inert carrier. These new formulations are just as effective as salazopyrin but have fewer side-effects.

Other agents

There has been a lot of work in recent years looking at new agents. In particular, the steroid budesonide which is becoming established in Crohn's disease may be beneficial in patients with active ulcerative colitis. However, there is still no evidence that this is better than prednisolone. Owing to the reported protective effect of smoking, nicotine has been tried and there is evidence from a randomized trial that transdermal nicotine may be effective in mild and moderately active ulcerative colitis. Oral and rectal formulations have also been developed but there is little good evidence as to their efficacy as yet. Other medications which have been tried include anti-TNFα antibody, heparin and the cyclosporine-like drug FK_5O_6 but the role of these agents has yet to be established. Dietary folic acid supplementation may reduce the risk of development of cancer in patients with long-standing ulcerative colitis as initial studies indicate a reduction in the rate of proliferation of rectal cells using this approach.

Surgical management of ulcerative colitis

The surgical treatment of ulcerative colitis can be broadly divided into emergency treatment and elective treatment.

Emergency surgery

The indications for emergency surgery for ulcerative colitis are:

- Severe disease failing to respond to medical treatment.
- Perforation.
- Bleeding.

The first indication is by far the most common, and appropriate surgical intervention in these patients is dependent on close collaboration between gastroenterologist and surgeon. Essentially, if a patient does not respond to maximal medical treatment within 7 days then surgery should not be delayed. Toxic megacolon is an indication for urgent surgery, particularly if clinical signs of peritonism are present. Urgent surgery in this situation will usually avoid perforation but if this has occurred the mortality is in the region of 40%. It should be noted that in patients on large doses of steroids, perforation may not be clinically evident and only diagnosed when gas is seen under the diaphragm on plain chest or abdominal radiography. Bleeding as a reason for surgery is rare and usually rises from massive ulceration within the rectum.

When a patient is admitted to hospital with severe disease but without a toxic megacolon it can be difficult to predict whether surgery will be necessary. However, the risk factors include a frequency of defecation over 10 times per day with the passage of blood on each occasion, a low serum albumin, a low haemoglobin and a fall in lean body mass of greater than 10%. In deciding on whether or not to proceed to urgent surgery, it is also worthwhile taking into account the previous history. If a patient has had several relapses then the threshold for surgical intervention should be lower.

In the emergency situation the operation of choice is total colectomy with ileostomy and preservation of the rectum. The reasons for not removing the rectum in the acute situation are two-fold. First, it avoids a prolonged and potentially difficult dissection in an acutely ill patient. Secondly, it allows the option of construction of an ileoanal pouch at a later stage. Carrying out a primary ileoanal pouch in the acute situation is not recommended. The point of division of the rectum is important. A relatively long rectal stump (usually with a portion of the sigmoid colon still attached) is ideal. This will allow the stump to be brought up to the anterior abdominal wall where it can be either closed and stitched to the undersurface of the wound or left open and brought out as a mucous fistula. The latter is preferable if the bowel is very friable and a suture line unlikely to heal. The length of the stump will make it easy to find at subsequent proctectomy. The only situation where the rectum should be removed in the acute situation is where there is massive bleeding from rectal ulceration.

Indications for elective surgical treatment

The indications for elective colectomy in ulcerative colitis are less clear cut than in the emergency situation but the three main indications are:

- Failure of medical management.
- Growth retardation in young patients.
- Malignant transformation.

Failure of medical treatment is difficult to define and the decision to operate under these circumstances must result from a careful discussion among patient, the surgeon and the gastroenterologist. In general the main reasons for opting for surgical treatment are chronic colitis with long-standing persistent symptoms which are never fully resolved by medical treatment, frequent acute exacerbations requiring considerable time off work and perhaps hospitalization and steroid dependence where any attempt at withdrawing steroids results in relapse. In all three situations a balance must be made between the risks of surgery and the patient's quality of life. Extracolonic manifestations of the disease may be an indication for surgery when these are severe but it should be stressed that not all respond to removal of the large bowel, particularly sacroilitis and liver manifestations. However, pyoderma gangrenosum and arthropathy usually respond well to surgery although resolution of the symptoms may take many months. In children, severe ulcerative colitis may lead to retardation of growth and delay in the onset of puberty. Clearly it is a very difficult decision to subject a child to such a major procedure but it is sometimes necessary. Development of carcinoma in a patient with ulcerative colitis is a clear indication for colectomy. In addition a diagnosis of dysplasia made on colonoscopic biopsy is also regarded by most surgeons and gastroenterologists as a reason for proceeding to surgery.

Operative procedure

When a decision has been made to operate for ulcerative colitis there are essentially four options:

- Colectomy and ileostomy with preservation of the rectal stump.
- Colectomy with ileorectal anastomosis.
- Proctocolectomy with permanent ileostomy.
- Proctocolectomy with ileoanal pouch formation (restorative proctocolectomy).

It should be noted that there is no place in modern surgical practice for partial colectomy in ulcerative colitis even when the right side of the colon appears to be unaffected as such a policy will result in a very high rate of recurrence.

Colectomy with ileostomy and rectal preservation

Although this operation is usually reserved for the emergency situation, occasionally it may be indicated in a particularly frail patient who is considered unfit for proctectomy. It may also be used in the elective situation where a patient is undecided whether or not to have a permanent ileostomy or a pouch as it leaves the options open. Finally it may be valuable in a situation where there is doubt as to whether the patient is suffering from ulcerative colitis or Crohn's colitis. The pathologist will then have the whole colon to examine and if Crohn's colitis can be excluded then a second procedure to carry out an ileoanal pouch can be carried out with more confidence.

Colectomy with ileorectal anastomosis

This operation may be satisfactory in patients who have relative rectal sparing and an easily distensible rectum. If there is severe proctitis or if the rectum is relatively rigid owing to inflammatory change then the functional results will be very poor. Clearly if there is dysplasia in the rectum this option is contraindicated. If this operation is performed then the patient should undergo annual endoscopic inspection of the rectum with biopsies to exclude the development of malignancy and all patients should be warned of the possibility of failure owing to frequency of defecation or the symptoms of proctitis. If the operation fails however, the patient will still be a candidate for proctectomy with either an ileostomy or ileoanal pouch.

Proctocolectomy with permanent ileostomy

The advantage of a proctocolectomy is that the ulcerative colitis will be completely cured and in patients who have had severe symptoms the improvement in their quality of life more than compensates for the inconvenience of an ileostomy. In making the decision to carry out this operation it is important to consider the alternative procedure of an ileoanal pouch and in the vast majority of cases the decision as to which operation to opt for is determined by patient preference after a full discussion of the pros and cons of ileostomy and ileoanal pouch. In carrying out the proctectomy, care must be taken not to damage the presacral nerves and two approaches can be taken. As a radical clearance is not necessary it is possible to carry out a close rectal dissection which involves separating the muscular rectal tube from the mesorectum. This however, is a tedious and bloody operation and has largely given way to careful dissection in the plane just outside the mesorectum as for an anterior resection for cancer. When the anal canal is to be removed this should be dissected out in the plane between the internal and external sphincters so that the muscles of the pelvic floor are left intact. The ileostomy is normally performed in the right iliac fossa at a site which has been determined pre-operatively usually with the help of a stoma therapist.

The important factors in siting the ileostomy include avoidance of bony protuberances such as the iliac crest, avoidance of abdominal scars, accessibility for the patient and the patient's belt line. Normally the patient will wear an ileostomy appliance prior to surgery in order to determine the ideal site. The ileostomy is created by bringing the terminal small bowel through a trephine incision (preferably through the rectus muscle) and then creating an everted spout of 2–3 cm in length. This allows ileostomy effluent to drain into the appliance bag without causing skin excoriation. While a well-formed ileostomy will permit a good quality of life, patients have little control over when the ileostomy will function. For this reason Kock developed a continent ileostomy which incorporates a reservoir constructed from 30 cm of small bowel with the terminal 15 cm of ileum invaginated into the reservoir to form a nipple valve. This allows the ileum to be sutured flush to the skin and the reservoir is evacuated using a catheter at the patient's convenience. When the valve functions the patient does not need to wear an appliance. However, the results of this operation are variable with valve failure occurring in up to 40% of cases. Other complications include leakage from the reservoir, fistulation and pouchitis.

Proctocolectomy with ileoanal reservoir

Removal of the entire colon and rectum with preservation of the anal sphincter and 'straight' ileoanal anastomosis was first introduced by Ravitch and Sabiston. However, the functional results were poor and with the introduction of the Kock continent ileostomy it became clear that it was possible to form a reservoir with small bowel. Sir Alan Parks was the first to introduce the concept of the ileoanal pouch and this operation has become the gold standard surgical procedure for ulcerative colitis.

The pouch can be formed in various ways and the three commonest configurations are the J pouch, the S pouch and the W pouch (Figure 14.46). Owing to its simplicity of construction, the J pouch is by far the most commonly used. The limbs of the J pouch should be 20 cm in length and it can be constructed either by hand suturing or by stapling. The pouch can then be connected to the anal canal either by endoanal suturing after careful stripping of the rectal mucosa from the short rectal stump which is left after protectomy or by stapling on to the top of the anal canal. The former technique is more precise but technically more demanding and there is some concern that incontinence may be more likely after this procedure owing prolonged retraction of the anal sphincters. The stapling procedure however does involve the retention of a very short segment of inflamed rectal mucosa which can cause problems and has the potential of undergoing dysplastic change. Randomized trials have shown no major differences between the functional outcome following stapled and hand sutured anastomoses.

Complications of ileoanal pouch

The main short-term complication is suture or staple line leakage from the ileal pouch leading to pelvic sepsis. For this reason, many surgeons routinely defunction the pouch with a loop ileostomy which can be closed a few weeks later after a pouchogram has demonstrated integrity of the ileal pouch. Other complications of the ileal pouch include stricture of the anastomosis, intestinal obstruction and pouch–vaginal or pouch–perineal fistula.

The function of the pouch is highly variable but 20–30% of patients have a frequency of eight stools per 24 hours or more. Patients with poor sphincter function pre-operatively or a small reservoir may have more pronounced frequency. Surprisingly, frequency is often well tolerated by the patients as long as urgency (which only occurs in about 10% of cases) is absent. However, a combination of frequency and urgency may lead to pouch failure.

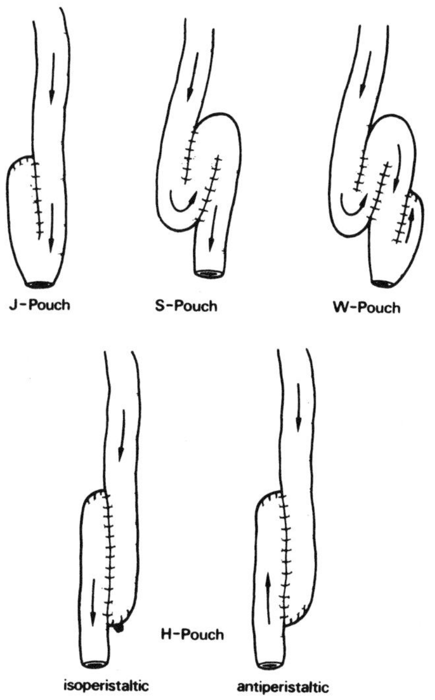

Figure 14.46 Diagrammatic representation of the various forms of pouches used after colectomy and mucosal proctectomy. The J Pouch is the most extensively used since it is the simplest to create, is attended with the lowest incidence of complications and functions best in the long term,

In the long term, deficiencies of iron and vitamin B_{12} may occur but in less than 10% of cases after 3 years of follow-up. This in turn may lead to anaemia. The most serious long-term complication, however, is pouchitis. This is idiopathic acute inflammation of the pouch leading to frequency, urgency, liquid stool and some extra-intestinal manifestations. No specific causative organism has been found but patients may respond to antibiotics, particularly metronidazole. Pouchitis causes significant problems in about 5% of all cases and leads to removal of the pouch in about 1–2% of cases. Interestingly, the endoscopic and histological appearances are very similar to ulcerative colitis and only seem to occur in patients who have had inflammatory bowel disease. Patients having a pouch after proctocolectomy for FAP almost never develop pouchitis.

Complications of ileostomy

The presence of an ileostomy entails a daily obligatory loss of 500–600 ml of ileostomy fluid containing 40–50 mmol of sodium. Thus there is a chronic salt-losing state. To a certain extent there is some compensation from increased renal tubular re-absorption of sodium and water which results in a lowering of the urinary sodium to potassium ratio. The altered chemical composition of the urine which becomes concentrated is thought to be responsible at least in part for the increased incidence of renal calculi in these patients. Adequate water and salt intake is essential in patients with an ileostomy, particularly in hot climates and during febrile illnesses. The local complications of a terminal ileostomy are:

- stenosis
- prolapse
- peristomal irritation
- fistulas
- para-ileostomy hernia
- ileostomy diarrhoea.

Stenosis of the ileostomy is now relatively uncommon owing to the modern technique of construction involving eversion and mucocutaneous anastomosis. If it occurs however, complete revision of the ileostomy may be necessary. Prolapse results from incomplete fixation of the small bowel to the abdominal wall and when marked may require surgical revision. Peristomal irritation is perhaps the commonest complication of an ileostomy (20–30%) and this can be minimized by regular cleaning of the surrounding skin and the use of skin barriers (stomadhesive, etc.). Occasionally irritation may be due to an inadequate spout and again ileostomy revision may be required.

Leakage from the ileostomy may lead to abscess formation in the abdominal wall and subsequent *fistula* formation. This almost always requires taking the ileostomy down, excising the affected bowel and recreating the ileostomy in a different site. Likewise, a *parastomal hernia* often requires resiting of the ileostomy, although a recent technique has been described which involves subcutaneous dissection around the ileostomy without disconnecting it from the skin and repair of the hernia with a mesh.

The occurrence of ileostomy diarrhoea is always an indication for thorough investigation as it usually signifies underlying pathology. The commonest causes of ileostomy diarrhoea are partial obstruction, internal abscess formation or the development of recurrence of ileal Crohn's disease. Essential investigations in all patients with persistent ileostomy diarrhoea include plain radiography of the abdomen, a small bowel enema through the stoma, and endoscopic examination of the small intestine through the ileostomy. Ileostomy cancer is a very rare complication which appears to develop in foci of dysplasia or colonic metaplasia in the ileal mucosa. Most of the reported cases have developed between 13 and 38 years after the formation of the ileostomy. Polypoid lesions developing in the mucosa of an ileostomy should always be biopsied.

Crohn's colitis

Crohn's colitis can be difficult to distinguish from ulcerative colitis, but it is usually possible to make a definitive diagnosis by employing a combination of histological and clinical features. Histologically, the inflammatory infiltrate tends to be transmural in Crohn's disease, whereas in ulcerative colitis it is normally confined to the mucosa and submucosa. The presence of non-caeseating granulomas is pathognomic of Crohn's disease, but their absence does not exclude the diagnosis.

Clinically, Crohn's colitis may be segmental, and if rectal sparing is observed, a diagnosis of ulcerative colitis can virtually be ruled out. In addition, if there are other features of Crohn's disease such as severe perianal fistulation and sepsis or small bowel disease, this will help the diagnostic process.

In many instances, Crohn's colitis behaves in a very similar fashion to ulcerative colitis, and the management is likewise similar. It can be subclassified as mild, moderate and severe, and the medical treatment parallels that of the same grades of ulcerative colitis. The indications for surgery are essentially identical with two important exceptions. If a patient has severe segmental Crohn's disease of the large bowel, then segmental resection is appropriate if the rest of the colon is unaffected. This is not the case with ulcerative colitis where total colectomy is always indicated owing to the high risk of recurrence if lesser degrees of surgical excision are employed. The other area of difference is in the use of the ileoanal pouch. As Crohn's disease always has the potential to affect the small bowel most surgeons regard this diagnosis as a contraindication to the formation of a pouch and will advise their patients to accept a permanent ileostomy when panproctocolectomy is necessary.

Radiation proctitis

The pathology of this condition is covered by the section on radiation enteropathy in the small bowel module. Clearly, radiation proctitis only occurs when the intact rectum is irradiated in the course of pelvic radiotherapy. This is usually delivered for the treatment of cervical, bladder or prostatic cancer. However, with increasing interest in the local treatment of rectal cancer, radiation proctitis can be a problem, especially when local excision is combined with external beam therapy. In addition, if pre- or post-operative radiotherapy is employed with anterior resection, the rectal remnant or (in the case of post-operative treatment) the colon used in the reconstruction can be affected. The main symptoms are rectal bleeding and diarrhoea, but in severe cases stricturing or fistulation into the vagina or bladder may occur. In extreme situations, a diversion colostomy or even rectal excision may be required.

Diversion colitis

When a section of the large bowel is isolated from the rest of the colon (usually the rectum and distal sigmoid after a Hartmann's procedure) the mucosa may become inflamed, causing mucus discharge, rectal bleeding and tenesmus. Histologically, this is indistinguishable from ulcerative colitis, but is thought to be due to a lack of intraluminal short-chain fatty acids. There is some evidence that the condition responds to butyrate-containing enemas.

Neutropenic colitis

This may occur as a complication of chemotherapy (especially for leukaemia or lymphoma), but it may also occur in other neutropenic patients and it has been reported in patients with large bowel and terminal ileal carcinoma. It is caused by superinfection by *C. septicum* or other clostridial species (*Clostridium sphenoides, C. perfringens, C. sordelli*, etc.), with the development of gas gangrene of the bowel and severe toxaemia. Fulminating neutropenic colitis carries a mortality of close to 100% as the only effective treatment is colectomy, and this is usually contraindicated by the underlying condition.

Collagenous colitis

Histologically, this disease is characterized by debasement of the epithelium, loss of goblet cells, neutrophil infiltration and subepithelial deposition of collagen which forms an irregular layer 7–25 mm in thickness. Its aetiology is unknown, and it presents with diarrhoea. The symptoms may respond to sulphasalazine, but in severe cases steroid therapy is required.

Section 14.6 • Infections and infestations of the large bowel

Amoebic dysentery

Amoebic dysentery is caused by *Entamoeba histolytica* which exists either as an active motile trophozoite or as a cyst. The former is characteristic of amoebic dysentery whereas the latter is more hardy and occurs in formed stool. The cysts are responsible for transmission of the infection. Amoebiasis is a common cause of diarrhoea in warm and humid parts of the world but sporadic cases may also occur in Europe and the USA. The amoebae cause colonic ulceration with the intervening mucosa being normal or hyperaemic.

Clinically the symptoms may be similar to ulcerative colitis and vary from mild diarrhoea to severe bloody diarrhoea. Metastatic amoebic infection may occur throughout the body with liver abscesses being the most common. These occur in 1–3% of cases and present with fever pain and tenderness in the right upper quadrant. Alternatively they may present with a pyrexia of unknown origin. Amoebic dysentery may also be complicated by colonic perforation, stricture formation or severe haemorrhage.

Definitive diagnosis is made by stool microscopy, rectal biopsy or serology. The stool is examined for trophozoites and cysts but the former are difficult to find unless fresh specimens are examined. Rectal biopsy is useful as amoebae may be seen in the surface exudate or within the lymphatics. Serology is most valuable in patients who have amoebiasis outside the intestine when the stool tests are often negative. Serology is also useful for patients with suspected inflammatory bowel disease in order to exclude amoebiasis. The drug of choice is metronidazole for acute amoebic dysentery whereas diloxanide furoate is effective in chronic intestinal infections associated with cysts in the stool.

Bacillary dysentery

This is due to infection with shigella organisms and four main serologically distinct groups are implicated in human disease: *Shigella dysenteriae, S. flexneri, S. boydii* and *S. sonnei*. The disease is spread by person to person contact, as faecal excretion of the bacterium continues for 1–4 weeks in untreated individuals. The organism invades the colonic wall leading to ulceration and the clinical features are characterized by fever, abdominal pain and watery diarrhoea leading to passage of blood and mucus. Complications include haemolytic uraemic syndrome, aseptic meningitis and Reiter's syndrome (arthritis, uveitis and conjunctivitis). This last complication is associated with HLA B27. The diagnosis is made by stool culture and serotyping for identification of the specific species. The disease is self-limiting and is usually quite mild but in severe cases ampicillin or co-trimoxazole should be used. It may also be necessary to apply specific re-hydration therapy, preferably orally although intravenous fluids are sometimes required.

Salmonellosis

Salmonella may cause simple gastroenteritis which is common in the developed world or typhoid which is common in areas with poor sanitation. Salmonella gastroenteritis is caused by *Salmonella typhimurium* and *S. enteritidis* and the major non-human reservoir of these organisms is in poultry and domestic livestock. Typhoid on the other hand is caused by *S. typhi* and *S. paratyphi* and humans are the only important reservoir for these organisms. Salmonella infections involve both the small intestine and the large intestine. The three major patterns of salmonella infection are:

- acute gastroenteritis
- typhoid (enteric) fever
- asymptomatic carrier state.

Salmonella gastroenteritis

This is relatively common with about 500 cases per 1 000 000 of the population occurring each year in the UK. The symptoms of gastroenteritis including headache, abdominal pain, fever and diarrhoea develop between 8 and 48 hours after eating contaminated food. The stool is watery and very rarely contains blood. The diagnosis can be made by culture of the stool. The disease is self-limiting and antibiotics are not valuable unless the patient is very ill with bacteraemia. In severe cases patients may require to be hospitalized and resuscitated with intravenous fluids.

Typhoid fever

Here the incubation period is in the region of 10–20 days and the clinical onset consists of progressive fever, vague abdominal pain, headache and cough. After about 5 days the patient develops abdominal distension, diarrhoea and splenomegaly. A cutaneous vasculitis occurs mainly on the abdomen giving rise to characteristic 'rose' spots. The disease may be complicated by intestinal haemorrhage and perforation and systemic problems including meningitis, encephalomyelitis, disseminated intravascular coagulation, hepatitis, pancreatitis and ectopic salmonella infections (e.g. in bone).

Diagnosis is made by culture of the organism from blood, stool, urine or bone marrow. Blood cultures are positive in 80% of patients in the first week of symptoms, whereas the stool cultures are usually positive during the second and third weeks. Serological tests can be useful when culture facilities are not available and a rising titre of O antibody indicates active infection. Typhoid fever should be treated with antibiotics and the most effective drug is chloramphenicol. However, drug-resistant organisms are becoming common and it may be necessary to use amoxycillin or co-trimoxazole. When perforation occurs laparotomy with peritoneal cleansing and simple closure of the perforation is necessary. This must be supplemented with antibiotic therapy.

Asymptomatic carriers

Carriers of *S. typhi* are important to identify as they represent a major source of the disease. The bacterium is commonly carried in the gallbladder and cholecystectomy may be necessary. Recently however, ciprofloxacin, with its good biliary penetration, has been shown to be reasonably effective in eliminating the carrier state.

Escherichia coli infections

Escherichia coli is a normal commensal of the gastrointestinal tract of human beings and most strains are harmless. Some strains however cause gastroenteritis. These are divided into four main groups:

- enteropathogenic
- enterotoxigenic
- enteroinvasive
- enterohaemorrhagic.

Pathogenic strains of *E. coli* can be spread by the ingestion of contaminated food (often cold meat) and by person to person transmission. Often both types of spread can be implicated in an epidemic with contaminated food being the initiating factor and a second wave of infection being caused by person to person transmission. The most common pathogenic serotype is 0157:H7 which produces cytotoxins and may lead to the haemolytic uraemic syndrome. This carries a high mortality particularly in elderly individuals. Diagnosis of *E. coli* infection is made by the isolation of the pathogenic strain from the stool but tests for verotoxin can be more sensitive than culture.

Campylobacter infection

In man, campylobacter infections are usually the result of ingestion of infected food, and poultry in particular. However, they may also be water borne, milk related and contracted from dogs. Campylobacter species affect both small and large intestine and most strains produce an enterotoxin and one or more cytotoxins. Clinically there is usually a self-limiting episode of diarrhoea which lasts for a few days and this may be preceded by fever, headache, myalgic malaise and abdominal pain. Rectal bleeding often follows the diarrhoea. Diagnosis is made by stool culture and the bacterium may be present in the stool for up to 5 weeks. Occasionally, infection may be complicated by massive lower gastrointestinal haemorrhage, Reiter's syndrome and Guillain–Barré syndrome. As the majority of infections are self-limiting, treatment is not usually necessary but in a prolonged illness, antibiotics such as erythromycin, tetracycline, chloramphenicol and gentamicin are appropriate.

Clostridium difficile infection

Clostridium difficile is a large Gram-positive anaerobic bacillus which produces two toxins, A and B. A is directly cytotoxic to colonic epithelial cells but the role of B is not completely clear. *Clostridium difficile* infection is important in both antibiotic-associated diarrhoea and the more serious pseudomembranous colitis.

Pseudomembranous colitis is a form of colitis in which a pseudomembrane is caused by surface inflammatory exudate. Both simple *C. difficile* infection and pseudomembranous colitis are associated with the use of almost all antibiotics, although lincomycin, clindamycin, ampicillin and amoxycillin account for about 80% of all cases. The pathogenesis of both forms of *C. difficile* infection is unclear. The organism is present under normal circumstances in the stools of about 2% of the population but it may be present in small numbers in a much larger proportion. The factors which favour proliferation of *C. difficile* in the colon are unclear but the administration of antibiotics is clearly of major importance.

Clinically, the disease varies from a mild illness with a moderate increase in bowel frequency to severe bloody diarrhoea associated with marked abdominal pain and tenesmus. Fever is present in the majority of cases and on examination there may be abdominal tenderness and peritonism. While the disease usually begins during a course of antibiotics, in about 30% of cases symptoms may start after the antibiotic has been discontinued.

The diagnosis is made by both culture of clostridium difficile from stool and from the demonstration of the toxin (usually B) in the stool. The diagnosis of pseudomembranous colitis depends on endoscopic appearances which consist of exudative punctate raised plaques with intervening areas of oedematous mucosa. Biopsy shows areas of focal necrosis with polymorphonuclear leucocytes forming characteristic 'summit' lesions. The most effective treatment is oral vancomycin at 2 g/day. Occasionally however, severe pseudomembranous colitis may not respond to antibiotic therapy and colectomy may be the only solution.

Chlamydial infection

The commonest type of chlamydial infection is a sexually transmitted urethritis but the rectum may also be affected particularly in homosexual men. This leads to an ulcerative proctitis characterized by rectal bleeding. The diagnosis depends on isolation of the organism from the rectum and treatment with tetracycline is usually effective.

Schistosomiasis

Schistosomiasis is dealt with in Volume 1. In the present context it should be remembered that the adult worms of *Schistosoma mansoni* reside mainly in the inferior mesenteric vein and *S. japonicum* in the supermesenteric vein. These worms produce large numbers of eggs which are retained in the wall of the intestine where they cause granulomatous reactions and some penetrate the intestinal wall and are passed with the faeces. The presence of the eggs in the intestinal wall may give rise to rectal bleeding and occasionally large polypoid lesions may occur and can be misdiagnosed as cancers, usually in the descending and sigmoid colon.

Cryptosporidiosis

The parasite *Cryptosporidium* causes diarrhoea and may be fatal in immunocompromised patients, particularly those with AIDS. The parasite infects the enterocytes of both small and large intestine and transmission appears to be either person to person or caused by ingestion of infected water. There is no known effective treatment although in normal individuals the gastroenteritis tends to be mild and self-limiting. In patients with AIDS however, *Cryptosporidium* causes protracted watery diarrhoea with severe weight loss.

Section 14.7 • Functional and structural colorectal disorders

Constipation

The term constipation is generally taken to mean the infrequent and/or difficult passage of small amounts of hard stool but a precise definition is clouded by the enormous variability of what is regarded as a normal bowel habit. In Western society 95% of the population defecate between three times per day and three times per week and so to a certain extent constipation is a subjective matter. Clearly constipation is a symptom rather than a disease and there are multiple causes. These can be divided into four main areas:

- structural pathology of the colon, rectum or anus
- aganglionosis and/or myenteric plexus lesions
- constipation due to extracolonic factors
- idiopathic constipation (no structural abnormality).

Structural pathology of the colon, rectum or anus

Constipation may be caused by any stricturing lesion and carcinoma of the colon is a particular concern. Other possible causes are strictures due to diverticular disease, ischaemia and ulcerative colitis or Crohn's disease. Painful anal lesions such as fissure, abscess or prolapsed haemorrhoids may also give rise to constipation by inhibiting the wish to defecate.

Aganglionosis and/or myenteric plexus lesions

Constipation may be caused by malfunction of the intrinsic nervous system of the large intestine and this in turn can be subdivided into Hirschsprung's disease and idiopathic megacolon and megarectum. These are dealt with as separate issues in following sections of this module.

Constipation due to extracolonic factors

Extracolonic factors that may give rise to constipation are listed in Table 14.6. Various drugs may give rise to constipation either through a local effect on the colon or through effects on the central nervous system. The main categories of relevant drugs are given in Table 14.7. The most common endocrine abnormality leading to constipation is hypothyroidism and individuals with myxoedema may develop megacolon. Hypercalcaemia may also present with constipation.

There are various neurological causes of constipation. Patients with diabetes mellitus may have severe constipation owing to an associated autonomic neuropathy. These patients demonstrate loss of colonic activity after a meal and this may be reversed by neostigmine indicating intact post-ganglionic neurones. It is therefore worth trying prokinetic drugs in these patients. Spinal cord injury can give rise to colonic problems which depend on the site and severity of the lesion. Spinal cord transection above L2 gives rise to decreased colonic compliance and the loss of conscious control of the external sphincter function. However,

Table 14.6 Extracolonic causes of constipation

Illness causing immobility (e.g. myocardial infarction)
Neurological disorders
– Multiple sclerosis
– Parkinson's disease
– Autonomic neuropathy (e.g. diabetes)
– Spinal cord injury
Endocrine disorders
– Hypothyroidism
Connective tissue disorders
– Systemic sclerosis

Table 14.7 Drugs causing constipation

Analgesics – particularly opioids such as morphine and codeine
Antacids – containing aluminium or bismuth
Anticholinergic agents – atropine and related substances
Anticonvulsants – carbemazapine
Antidepressants – most tricyclics, monoamine oxidase inhibitors
Antiemetics – ondansetrone, phenothiazines
Antipsychotics – e.g. chlorpromazine
Calcium channel blockers – verapamil
Cytotoxics – e.g. vinca alkaloids
Iron supplements
Lipid-lowering drugs – cholestyramine, simvastatin
Sedatives – benzodiazepines
Stimulants – barbituates

defecatory reflexes are intact. This leads to constipation, but reflex emptying of the rectum can be brought about using enemas or suppositories. Injuries of sacral nerves and the cauda equina give rise to lack of control and loss of tone of the external sphincter muscles and this may lead to both constipation and incontinence. Multiple sclerosis may lead to severe constipation via mechanisms similar to spinal cord transection. Finally, Parkinson's disease can be associated with constipation due to dystonia of the pelvic floor.

Psychological factors are clearly important in a proportion of patients with constipation. It may be a presenting feature of clinical depression and in patients with anorexia nervosa constipation may be a significant feature. However, there are a proportion of patients who complain bitterly of constipation but in fact when objective testing is carried out (see next section) normal colonic transit is demonstrated with normal passage of stool. If an individual perceives themselves to be constipated and yet objective evidence indicates that their defecatory habits are within the normal range, the best approach is a careful explanation of what can be regarded as normal.

Idiopathic constipation with no structural abnormality

A fairly high proportion of patients with constipation cannot be demonstrated to have any structural abnormality or any extracolonic cause for their constipation and yet have significant problems. Careful investigation is important in such patients and the simplest and most reliable way of assessing constipation is by the measurement of colonic transit using opaque markers (Figure 14.47). Alternatively, it is possible to use colonic scintigraphy. If colonic transit is delayed throughout the colon this indicates idiopathic slow transit whereas if there is slow transit in the distal left colon or rectosigmoid region this indicates obstructed defecation. On the basis of transit studies, idiopathic constipation may be divided into three main areas:

- slow colonic transit responsive to diet
- slow colonic transit unresponsive to diet
- obstructed defecation.

Slow colonic transit responsive to diet

The typical traditional Western diet is low in fibre leading to small hard stools which are difficult to pass. Patients with constipation should therefore be encouraged to change their diet so that they increase their intake of fruit, vegetables and unrefined carbohydrates. The aim should be to have a diet containing 20–30 g of fibre per day and dietary advice should include the use of wholemeal bread, a bran or oat-based breakfast cereal and a plentiful intake of fruit and vegetables. If a constipated individual finds this impossible it may be helpful to use a bulk laxative derived from ispaghula (a seed mucilage), sterculia (a plant gum) and methylcellulose.

Idiopathic slow colonic transit unresponsive to diet

In these patients increased dietary fibre does not help and often increases abdominal pain and distension. Transit studies show a uniform delay in colonic transit but the underlying aetiology is unclear. Some workers have demonstrated a decreased number of neurones in the myenteric plexus of the colon and abnormal concentrations of intestinal peptides. Very often these patients have a history of prolonged intake of stimulant laxative, especially Senna, and it is possible that some of these changes are related to the effects of these drugs. However, many of these patients show abnormalities of oesophageal, gastric, small bowel and bladder motility

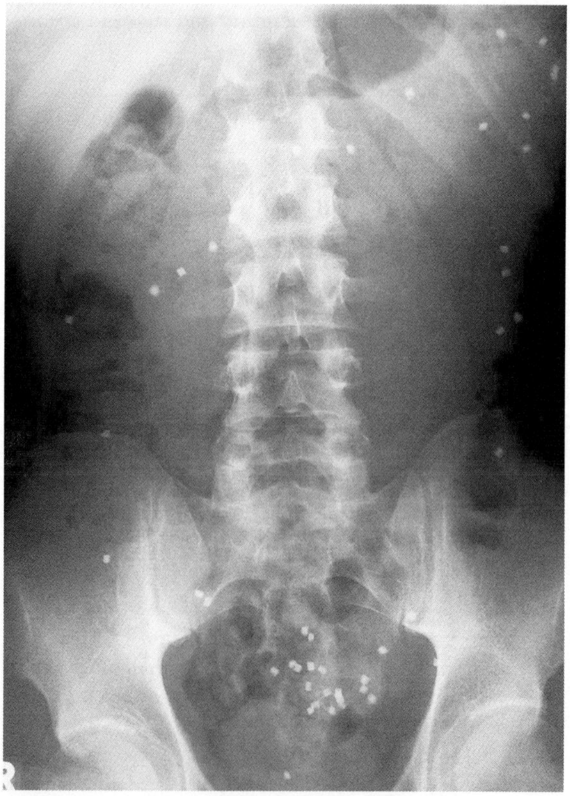

Figure 14.47 Plain abdominal radiograph showing radio-opaque markers distributed throughout the colon, but concentrated in the sigmoid. (Courtesy of Dr Tom Taylor, Radiology, Ninewells Hospital, Dundee, Scotland.)

so that prolonged laxative abuse cannot be the only causative factor. Treatment is extremely difficult as increased fibre or bulky agents merely exacerbate the symptoms and the majority of patients are resistant to stimulant laxatives. Osmotic purgatives may be helpful but again often cause abdominal bloating and occasionally prokinetics may be of value.

However, the majority of patients obtain little relief from medication and some will reach the surgeon. If marker studies indicate that there is no evidence of obstructed defecation and this is confirmed by normal anal manometry, normal electromyography and normal evacuation proctography (see next section) then total colectomy with ileorectal anastomosis may be valuable. Unfortunately, this will not always result in normal bowel function as 25% will be troubled with diarrhoea and a further 25% will continue to have constipation and abdominal pain. Occasionally it may be necessary to resort to an ileostomy although even here patients may continue to have abdominal pain and bloating as a result of small bowel motility problems. In a few patients restorative proctocolectomy using an ileal reservoir has provided good results but the outcome after this operation is highly unpredictable.

Obstructed defecation

When a patient with constipation has delayed transit in the left colon or rectosigmoid region, he or she is likely to be suffering from a defecatory disorder and careful assessment is indicated before advising treatment. Firstly, a careful history should be taken. Most of these patients are women and some will report using digital pressure within the vagina to assist defecation. This indicates the presence of a rectocele caused by weakness of the rectovaginal septum. As outlined above, investigations should include anal manometry, electromyography and evacuation proctography. Although the majority of patients will have normal resting and maximum squeeze pressures in the anal canal, some will have increased resting internal sphincter activity. In idiopathic constipation the rectoanal inhibitory reflex is always present in contrast to Hirschsprung's disease. Electromyography of the puborectalis and external sphincter muscles may demonstrate inappropriate activity during attempted defecation. Under normal circumstances these muscles become electrically silent during straining but failure of relaxation or increased activity is a feature of outlet obstruction or anismus. Evacuation proctography is carried out by fluoroscopic monitoring and videoing the evacuation of radio-opaque material. This will identify intussusception, rectocele and rectal prolapse. It will also demonstrate perineal descent.

The management of patients with obstructed defecation depends on the findings of the above investigations. When the main problem is a rectocele the patient should undergo a surgical repair. This is most commonly done using an endorectal approach in which a flap of mucosa is raised to expose the circular muscle of the anterior wall of the rectum to between 6 and 10 cm from the dentate line. This muscle is then plicated, the redundant mucosa excised and the mucosal defect closed. When the indications for this operation are correct, the results are usually very good.

Other forms of obstructed defecation are more difficult to treat. Anorectal myectomy in which a longitudinal segment of the internal anal sphincter is excised has been used for outlet obstruction particularly when there is a high resting internal sphincter pressure. This has been shown to be superior to anal dilatation but long-term results are disappointing. In patients with anismus partial division of the puborectalis muscle has been used, but again results are poor. Owing to the indifferent results of surgery, there has been a recent interest in biofeedback retraining in which patients with anismus are supplied with an anal probe that produces an audible and/or visual signal when the sphincter muscles are active. Patients are then taught to relax the sphincter muscles on attempted defecation and there is some evidence that this approach can achieve a successful outcome in 30–60% of cases.

Hirschsprung's disease

Hirschsprung's disease is caused by congenital aganglionosis of the intestine caused by a failure of intrauterine migration of ganglion cells from the neural crest. Embryologically the ganglion cells travel from proximal to distal along the vagus nerve pathways within the bowel wall, eventually reaching the anal canal around the time of birth. Arrest of migration at any point will result in aganglionosis of the bowel between that point and the anus. Frequently, the rectosigmoid segment of the large intestine is involved but any length of intestine may be affected, sometimes leading to total colonic aganglionosis or even very long segment Hirschsprung's disease affecting part of the small bowel.

Within the aganglionic segment of bowel there is associated proliferation of nerve fibrils some of which are hypertrophic with increased acetylcholinesterase activity. Failure of autonomic innervation to develop leads to absent peristalsis within the affected bowel and a consequent adynamic obstruction. Thus the bowel proximal to the aganglionic segment becomes markedly dilated and hypertrophic, eventually tapering distally into the affected region.

The underlying cause is unknown but it has an incidence of 1 in 4500 live births and appears to have a multi-factorial hereditary component. Eighty per cent of patients present in the neonatal period with abdominal distension, bile-stained vomiting and failure to pass meconium within the first 24 hours. However, in a few patients it may present in adult life where there is usually a history of infrequent bowel actions since birth and the need to use laxatives or enemas on a regular basis. In children the diagnosis should be suspected when no meconium is passed in the first 24 hours and in adults where there is evidence of chronically dilated intestine. A barium enema shows a typical narrowed distal segment with ballooning with megacolon above it. In adults anorectal manometry will demonstrate absence of the rectoanal inhibitory reflex and this is diagnostic of the condition unless the segment is extremely short.

Definitive diagnosis, however, depends on a full thickness rectal biopsy which shows an absence of ganglia associated with hypertrophy and proliferation of nerve fibrils and an increased acetylcholinesterase content in both Auerbach's and Meissner's neural plexuses. The treatment of Hirschsprung's disease is surgical and the same principles apply to neonates and adults with the exception that in neonates the first procedure is usually a temporary colostomy created in the normal ganglionic bowel. With the normal rectosigmoid distribution of affected bowel the appropriate treatment is resection of the aganglionic segment and anastomosis of ganglionic bowel to the anal margin. There are various ways of achieving this and the three most commonly used operations are the Swenson, the Soave and Duhamel procedures. In very short segment Hirschsprung's disease, an extended internal sphincterotomy may be adequate treatment. At the other extreme, patients with total colonic aganglionosis may require restorative proctocolectomy with ileal pouch formation and ileo-anal anastomosis.

Chagas' disease

This condition is caused by *Trypanosoma cruzi*, transmitted by the tiratomidae bug. This causes damage to the cells in the autonomic nervous system, most commonly affecting the heart and hollow abdominal organs, and can lead to both megaoesophagus and megacolon. The disease is endemic in South America, particularly Brazil. The acute phase of the disease consists of a febrile illness associated with lymphadenopathy, oedema and hepatosplenomegaly. The megacolon occurs as the chronic phase of the disease which presents with constipation. The diagnosis is made using the complement fixation test for *T. cruzi*. The megacolon may be complicated by stercoral ulceration, perforation and volvulus. Treatment depends on the extent of the disease but may require resection of the dilated segment of colon, usually the sigmoid.

Idiopathic megacolon and megarectum

Patients with this condition present with constipation and abdominal pain. They can be divided into two main groups. The first have symptoms going back to childhood and often have rectal impaction and soiling. This can be indistinguishable from Hirschsprung's disease. The second group develop their symptoms in later life usually without soiling. On examination faecal impaction is present and contrast studies reveal an enlarged rectum often associated with colonic distension. Anorectal manometry and full thickness rectal biopsy are necessary to exclude Hirschprung's disease.

The underlying cause is unknown and it may be associated with poor toilet training in infancy. In some cases it may be associated with a poorly defined abnormality of the myenteric plexus. Treatment is difficult and may involve regular enemas and washouts initially and then maintenance of a regular bowel habit with the use of laxatives. Magnesium sulfate and lactulose either alone or in combination are the most useful. It may also be necessary to use suppositories or enemas on a regular basis.

If a conservative approach fails surgical treatment may be necessary, but the precise operation will depend on the affected area of bowel. In the unusual situation where there is megacolon and no megarectum then colectomy and ileorectal anastomosis may be effective. If a megarectum is present then it will be necessary to carry out a proctectomy with coloanal anastomosis if the colon is normal. If the rectum and most of the colon are affected then restorative proctocolectomy with ileal pouch and ileoanal anastomosis may be effective.

Pneumatosis coli

This rare condition affects both the colon and the small intestine. It is usually discovered incidentally on abdominal X-ray. Gas-filled cysts are found in the subserosal and submucosal planes which are evident on plain films of the abdomen or as filling defects on barium enema or barium follow-through. The condition probably results from lymphatic stasis with subsequent filling of the lymph spaces with gas including nitrogen, carbon dioxide and hydrogen. The aetiology is unknown but there appears to be an association with chronic obstructive airways disease. Although it is often asymptomatic patients may suffer from frequent bowel action, large amounts of flatus, urgency, rectal bleeding, colicky abdominal pain and rectal mucus discharge. Surgical intervention is not indicated and the cysts can usually be induced to disappear with oxygen therapy over 3–4 days.

Volvulus

Colonic volvulus or twisting of the colon is a relatively uncommon cause of large bowel obstruction in Western society although it is much more usual in developing countries. The sigmoid colon is by far the most common site followed by the caecum. Very occasionally, volvulus of the transverse colon may occur.

Sigmoid volvulus

Sigmoid volvulus tends to affect elderly males and typically the patient will be institutionalized with a previous history of chronic constipation, laxative dependency and unrelated medical problems.

Pathophysiology

An anticlockwise torsion of 180° is considered to be physiological. It may cause no symptoms and usually reverts spontaneously. However, if the posterior loop gradually fills with gas and stool and becomes heavier, it then changes its position and falls anterior to the empty loop, leading to a 360° anticlockwise torsion. Sigmoid volvulus may affect an individual for many years in a subacute recurring form but acute sigmoid volvulus is a surgical emergency because of the tight compression of the mesocolic vessels and massive distension of the colonic lumen.

Aetiology

There are probably many aetiological factors but the most important is probably a long sigmoid loop with a narrow mesentery leading to a predisposition to torsion. In addition, chronic constipation, a high-fibre diet and systemic neurological disease are important. In South America there is an association with Chagas' disease.

Clinical features

In its chronic form the patient gives a history of intermittent lower colicky abdominal pain with abdominal distension which is relieved by the passage of flatus and loose stool. In the acute form, the patient will present as a large bowel obstruction with colicky abdominal pain, constipation and often massive distension. Vomiting is a late feature. On examination, the abdomen is distended and tympanic and may be tender over the dilated loop of colon. Tinkling bowel sounds can be heard initially but they vanish with either secondary ileus or perforation. Digital rectal examination reveals an empty distended rectum and there may be blood on the glove if gangrenous changes have set in.

Diagnosis

A plain abdominal X-ray (Figure 14.48) will confirm the diagnosis in 80% of cases. The diagnostic features include an enormously distended sigmoid colon arising from the left iliac fossa towards the right hypochondrium. It may lead to an elevated diaphragm. The loop has the appearance of a coffee bean and there is commonly a bird beak deformity at the site of the torsion. In late cases, peritoneal fluid is indicated by a ground glass appearance and there may be progressive distension of the small intestine with gas and fluid.

Complications

Acute sigmoid volvulus is complicated by gangrene and perforation of the twisted segment because of the tight compression of the mesocolic vessels and the massive distension. This may lead to faecal peritonitis. Occasionally, the massive distension may also lead to respiratory embarrassment.

Treatment

The first step should be to correct any fluid and electrolyte imbalance with intravenous replacement and then to attempt endoscopic reduction. This may be achieved by either a rigid sigmoidoscope or a flexible colonoscope and is successful in 80% of cases.

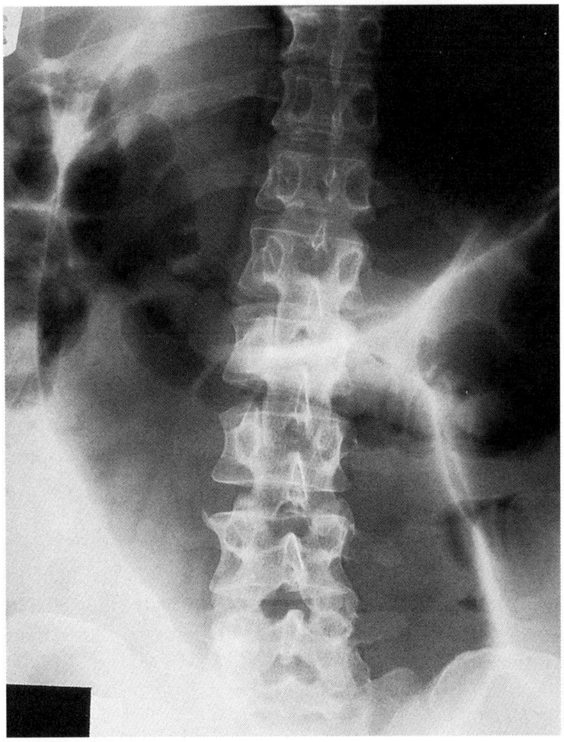

Figure 14.48 Plain abdominal X-ray of acute sigmoid volvulus.

A flexible instrument is preferable as the point of torsion may often be higher than the limit of the sigmoidoscope. Colonoscopy also allows for examination of the mucosal aspect for evidence of gangrene. If a flexible endoscope is not available and the rigid sigmoidoscope will not reach the point of torsion then it is possible to pass a blunt-ended flatus tube through the rigid sigmoidoscope to attempt a blind reduction.

It should be stressed that non-operative reduction does not constitute adequate treatment as the recurrence rate approaches 90%. Ideally, after successful endoscopic reduction, elective surgery should be carried out as quickly as possible as a one-stage sigmoid colectomy. However, if surgery is required urgently because of suspected strangulation or if non-operative decompression is unsuccessful, the standard treatment is resection of the sigmoid colon with a left iliac fossa colostomy and mucus fistula. Alternatively, the rectal stump may be oversewn as a Hartmann's procedure. In the relatively fit patient however, it may be possible to do a sigmoid resection with on-table colonic irrigation followed by primary anastomosis but this should only be attempted when there is no doubt about the viability of the involved colon.

Caecal volvulus

The term caecal volvulus is really a misnomer as 90% of the cases are more accurately described as ileocolic torsion with only 10% involving the caecum alone. The propensity for caecal volvulus depends on a congenital abnormality of intestinal rotation in which the right colon does not fuse with the posterior abdominal wall but rather remains on a mesentery and is therefore highly mobile. It should be stressed that caecal volvulus is uncommon accounting for less than 1% of all cases of large bowel obstruction and only about 10% of all cases of volvulus.

Clinical features
There are three well-recognized modes of presentation. First, the patient may present with acute intestinal obstruction and this accounts for about 50% of cases. Secondly, the patient may present with rapid onset of acute abdominal pain and peritonitis secondary to gangrene of the affected segment of intestine. Thirdly, a small number of patients present with chronic intermittent obstructive symptoms.

Diagnosis
Diagnosis in the acute stage is usually made on plain abdominal X-ray which reveals a large air-filled viscus with an air fluid level usually in the left upper quadrant (Figure 14.49).

Complications
The main complication as with sigmoid volvulus is gangrene leading to perforation and faecal peritonitis.

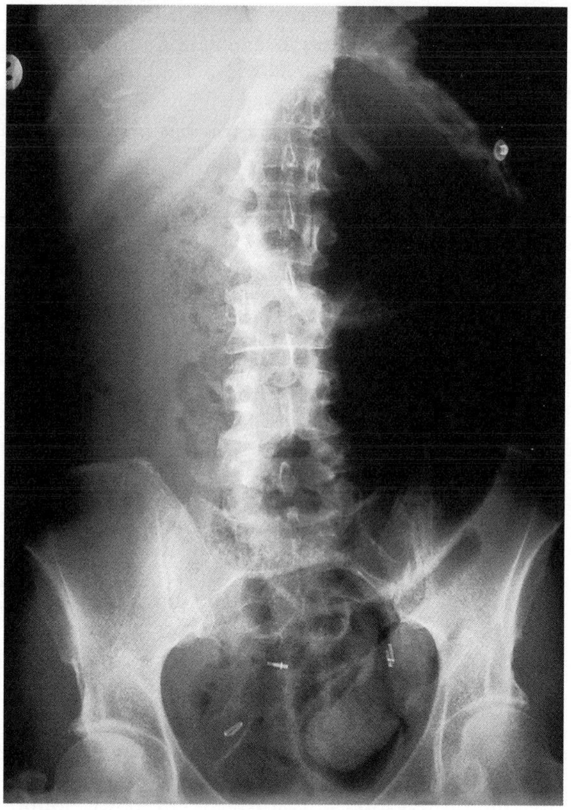

Figure 14.49 Plain abdominal X-ray of acute caecal volvulus.

Treatment
Colonoscopic decompression is not usually successful and the mainstay of treatment is laparotomy with right hemicolectomy. Primary anastomosis is appropriate if there is no peritoneal soiling but if there is any doubt about the safety of an anastomosis, an ileostomy and mucus fistula should be fashioned. Another surgical option when the affected segment of bowel is completely viable is to carry out a caecopexy. This involves mobilizing the peritoneum of the right paracolic gutter to form a pouch into which the caecum can be inserted and sutured into place.

Rectal prolapse

Rectal prolapse or protrusion of the rectum through the anal canal may be classified as partial or incomplete when the prolapse only involves the mucosa of the lower rectum or complete where the entire thickness of the rectal wall is involved. While prolapse can occur at any time, incomplete prolapse is more common in children and complete prolapse in the elderly. Prolapse in children is a feature of the first 2 years of life, being slightly more common in boys than girls. This contrasts strongly with complete prolapse in adults where females are four times more susceptible than males.

Aetiology
The aetiology of partial rectal prolapse is similar to that of haemorrhoids, i.e. laxity of the tissue in the rectal submucosa leading to abnormal mobility of the rectal mucosa on the underlying circular muscle. In complete prolapse, defecating proctography demonstrates that during straining the prolapse begins at about 6–8 cm above the anal verge as a circumferential intussusception. When the prolapse has passed through the anal canal and is fully descended the anterior segment is more prominent and contains a sac of peritoneum from the pelvic cavity which may contain loops of small bowel.

The most likely underlying cause is laxity of the pelvic floor musculature, as it has been shown that the resting activity of the sphincteric and levator ani muscles is profoundly reduced during defecation when compared with normal. There is also good evidence of somatic denervation of the sphincter and pelvic floor muscle but it is not clear whether this is a true aetiological factor of prolapse or a result of repeated episodes of prolapse through the anal canal.

Clinical features
In children the parents notice a reddened area of mucosa at the anal verge and may also notice excess mucus and occasional rectal bleeding. On examination it is possible that no abnormality will be detected but the prolapse may be precipitated by inserting a suppository. Once the prolapse has occurred careful palpation between the finger and thumb distinguishes between two layers of mucosa and a complete prolapse. After

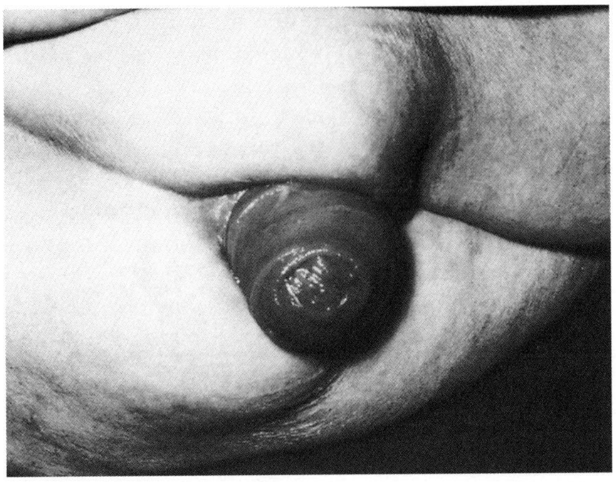

Figure 14.50 Rectal prolapse.

reduction of the prolapse, digital examination reveals no detectable abnormality of the anal sphincter.

In adults, the main symptoms are the prolapse itself and soiling of the underclothes from mucus, blood or faeces. The patient may also have frank faecal incontinence, but paradoxically some patients may have constipation as a prominent symptom. The prolapse tends to occur mainly at the time of defecation, but may also occur with coughing, laughing or even walking. On examination, the anus appears patulous and digital examination reveals that the sphincteric tone is deficient. On bearing down the prolapse will be produced and may reach as far as 12 cm from the anal verge (Figure 14.50). It is then possible to feel two complete layers of bowel wall between finger and thumb and even loops of small bowel may be palpable anteriorly. A prolapse greater than 5 cm is almost certainly complete although those less than 5 cm require careful examination to determine whether they are partial or complete.

Diagnosis

The diagnosis is essentially clinical although defecating proctography may be of value. However, in any patient with a rectal prolapse a complete colonic examination usually by means of barium enema is advisable before embarking on treatment. This is to exclude major colonic pathology which may have therapeutic implications.

Complications

The main complication of rectal prolapse is of course faecal incontinence although this may be seen as part and parcel of the whole pathological process. Rarely, the prolapse may become irreducible and progress to gangrene of the prolapsed segment.

Treatment

The mucosal prolapse seen in very young children is a self-limiting condition provided that a regular bowel habit can be established. Strapping the buttocks together after defecation may be required for a short period of time and occasionally in severe cases where constipation is a major factor daily enemas may be required. In slightly older children resolution of the prolapse may be hastened by the use of sclerosant injection into the lower rectal mucosa. In the adult patient with a partial prolapse the traditional approach was to carry out an extensive haemorrhoidectomy. However, the new procedure of stapled anopexy (see section on haemorrhoids) may be useful in these patients. For complete rectal prolapse, the available procedures can be usefully subdivided into perineal procedures and transabdominal procedures.

Perineal procedures

The simplest operation for rectal prolapse is the insertion of the so-called Tiersch wire. This involves the insertion of a subcutaneous circumferential suture around the anal canal to produce a form of anal stenosis. This is a simple procedure to perform and is a tempting solution in very elderly or unfit individuals. However, it is associated with a high rate of complications including sepsis, faecal impaction and a high rate of recurrence. It should now be regarded as obsolete. A much more satisfactory perineal procedure is Delorme's operation which involves excising a cuff of mucosa on the outer aspect of the prolapse and plicating the muscle layers with sutures to approximate the cut edges of mucosa. This often produces good results but does have a tendency to recurrence especially if insufficient mucosa has been excised. It is however, quite feasible to repeat a Delorme's procedure should a recurrence occur.

Another extremely effective procedure is a perineal procto-sigmoidectomy. Here the outer layer of the prolapse is completely transected close to the anal margin and as much rectum and sigmoid colon as possible is excised as it comes through the anus (Figure 14.51). The distal segment of the remaining sigmoid is then sutured to the anal canal.

Transabdominal procedures

The most widely performed transabdominal procedure is a rectopexy. Here the rectum is mobilized down to the pelvic floor and then fixed to the sacrum. The fixation may be achieved by simple suture or by the insertion of mesh or Ivalon sponge to create a fibrous reaction. This procedure is very effective at preventing prolapse but tends to cause constipation and should be avoided in the patient who has constipation as a prominent symptom. The reason for the constipation is not clear but it may be related to kinking of a redundant sigmoid loop just above the fixed rectum.

For this reason the operation of resection rectopexy has been developed. Here the rectum is mobilized down to the pelvic floor and then transected at the sacral promontory. The sigmoid colon is then resected and an anastomosis formed between the descending colon and the rectum. This operation has been associated with low rates of recurrence and relatively low rates of constipation. Both rectopexy and resection rectopexy can be achieved laparoscopically with a small

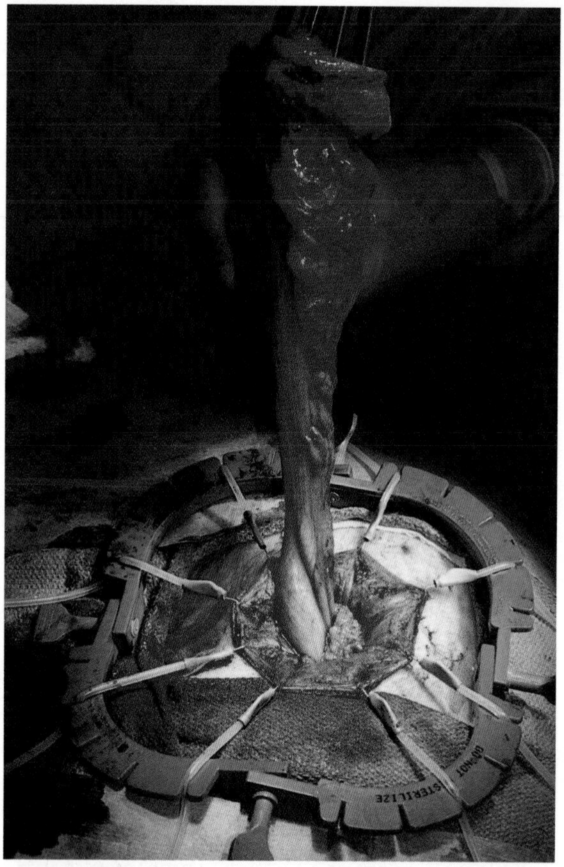

Figure 14.51 Perineal procto-sigmoidectomy. The rectum and a large portion of the sigmoid colon have been mobilized through the anal canal.

suprapubic incision required in the latter operation in order to removed the resected sigmoid colon. Other factors which may lead to constipation after rectopexy include damage to the nerve supply of the rectum and the intensity of the fibrous reaction induced by the introduction of foreign material into the pelvis.

In the patient with incontinence, repair of the prolapse by either a perineal or a transabdominal operation may improve matters considerably. However, a proportion of patients will continue to have faecal incontinence and under these circumstances a post-anal repair (see Module 15) may be of value.

Solitary rectal ulcer

The term solitary rectal ulcer is strictly a misnomer as the lesions may be multiple and ulceration may not necessarily be present. Although any age can be affected it is most common in young adults. The macroscopic appearance is of a red thickened area of rectal mucosa usually with a shallow ulcer in the centre. Classically it is positioned on the anterior wall of the rectum opposite the puborectalis sling 5–8 cm above the anal verge. Histologically the lamina propia is replaced by collagen and there is fibromuscular replacement of the mucosa. The aetiology is unclear but it is now believed that it is due to internal rectal prolapse or intussusception which causes trauma to the rectal wall.

Clinically, all patients have difficulty in defecation which involves going to the toilet several times a day but only actually defecating once or twice. Usually there is deep-seated perineal pain and blood and mucus are often passed. On digital examination there is usually an indurated area on the anterior aspect of the rectum. The diagnosis is made by endoscopy and biopsy. If a rigid sigmoidoscopy is being used, asking the patient to strain down during the procedure may reveal the intussusception. However, the only accurate way of demonstrating an intussusception is by using defecating proctography.

Treatment can be difficult and a conservative approach should be taken in the first instance. A high-fibre diet and the use of suppositories may prevent excessive straining and alleviate the symptoms. Biofeedback may also be useful if there is obstructed defecation. Topical steroids have been recommended but there is little evidence that these have any effect. In extreme cases surgery may be indicated. If there is complete rectal prolapse then abdominal rectopexy is indicated. However, for internal intussusception the results of this procedure are poor. Thus for patients with extreme symptoms who do not have a complete rectal prolapse, rectal excision with coloanal anastomosis or even abdominoperineal resection of rectum may be indicated.

Colonic pseudo-obstruction

Acute colonic pseudo-obstruction or Ogilvie's syndrome is characterized by marked dilation of the colon in the absence of mechanical obstruction. It nearly always occurs in hospitalized patients and the vast majority have an associated condition such as infection, widespread malignancy, recent surgery or trauma particularly to the spine. The underlying aetiology is not clear but it is a form of colonic dysmotility which is the final common pathway of a variety of physiological and biochemical disturbances. As it is often associated with pelvic pathology damage to the autonomic innervation of the distal colon has been implicated.

Clinical features

The clinical features of acute colonic pseudo-obstruction closely mimic acute large bowel obstruction. The patient often has colicky abdominal pain and progressive distension of the abdomen is the rule. Constipation is common although not absolute, as some patients will continue to pass a small amount of flatus or liquid stool. Nausea and vomiting are also common. On examination there is massive abdominal distension and if the caecum is distended to such an extent that its viability is compromised there will be right iliac fossa tenderness. Bowel sounds are variable and can be normal or obstructive in nature. Digital examination of the rectum usually reveals an empty rectum.

Diagnosis

The diagnosis is generally made on plain abdominal X-ray which shows the typical appearance of a distal colonic obstruction often with the cut-off in the descending colon. Measurement of the diameter of the caecum on the X-ray is important as perforation is common once this exceeds 12 cm. Unlike mechanical large bowel obstruction, the colonic haustral and mucosal pattern may be maintained and this also distinguishes it from the toxic megacolon of inflammatory bowel disease. However, the distinction between pseudo-obstruction and mechanical large bowel obstruction can be extremely difficult to make on plain abdominal X-ray and thus any patient with suspected mechanical large bowel obstruction should have this confirmed either by sigmoidoscopy or by water-soluble contrast enema before proceeding to surgery.

Complications

The main complication of pseudo-obstruction is faecal peritonitis secondary to perforation of the caecum.

Treatment

In the first instance, management consists of intravenous fluids, nasogastric aspiration and decompression with a flatus tube inserted at rigid sigmoidoscopy. Concomitantly, it is important to correct any metabolic disturbances, treat infections and stop any medications that may have an effect on colonic motility, e.g. narcotic analgesics, anticholinergic agents and calcium channel antagonists. If this does not bring about a rapid improvement, colonoscopy with decompression of the colon should be carried out. This reduces the diameter of the caecum in about 70% of cases but in about 40% repeated colonoscopy will be required. Recurrence of the pseudo-obstruction can be decreased by placing a drainage tube into the right side of the colon at the time of the first colonoscopy.

Recently, a randomized study has shown that 2.0 mg of neostigmine given intravenously over 3–5 min can resolve pseudo-obstruction in a substantial proportion of patients. When the neostigmine has been given the patient should lie supine for 60 min and continuous ECG monitoring should be used to detect a bradycardia. If this occurs 1.0 mg of intravenous atropine should be given.

Surgery for acute colonic pseudo-obstruction is indicated if all these conservative measures fail to bring about a reduction in the size of the caecum. In the absence of signs suggesting ischaemia or perforation of the bowel, the operation of choice is a tube caecostomy through a limited right iliac fossa incision to expose the caecum. A large Foley catheter can then be used to intubate the caecum and this should be retained for approximately 3 weeks. However, if there are signs of ischaemia or perforation, a midline laparotomy should be used. If the bowel appears to be viable then a tube caecostomy will be satisfactory. However, if there is extensive necrosis a right hemicolectomy should be performed. Under most circumstances an immediate anastomosis should be deferred and an ileostomy and mucus fistula fashioned. It should be remembered that the colonic pseudo-obstruction is associated with a significant mortality, largely owing to the underlying illnesses which are associated with this condition. In patients in whom conservative treatment is successful the mortality is about 15%, whereas in those undergoing surgical intervention it is in the region of 30%.

Irritable bowel syndrome

The irritable bowel syndrome (IBS) is not a precise diagnosis but rather a group of functional bowel disorders. It can be defined as abdominal discomfort or pain associated with defecation or a change in bowel habit and with an element of disordered defecation. In the West, IBS probably occurs in 15–20% of individuals with a higher prevalence in women. The course of IBS is highly variable, but essentially it is a chronic relapsing condition.

Clinical features

The clinical features of IBS vary in number and severity. They consist of an abnormal stool frequency (more than three times a day or less than three times a week), abnormal stool consistency (hard, loose or watery), abnormal passage of stool (urgency, straining or tenesmus), the passage of mucus and abdominal bloating or distension.

Diagnosis

Because of the imprecise nature of the symptom complex in IBS, many patients with this condition will require diagnostic tests to exclude organic disease. Normally this will take the form of barium enema and sigmoidoscopy or colonoscopy. Certainly, if a patient has irritable bowel-type symptoms associated with rectal bleeding, weight loss or other suspicious symptoms they should be thoroughly investigated. The diagnosis, however, rests on clinical features and the diagnostic criteria agreed at the multi-national consensus meeting on functional gastrointestinal disorders held in Rome in 1999 are as follows.

At least 12 weeks (not necessary consecutive) in the preceding 12 months of abdominal discomfort or pain that is associated with at least two of the following other features:

- relieved by defecation
- onset associated with change in stool frequency
- onset associated with change in stool consistency.

Treatment

The mainstay of treatment is a confident diagnosis coupled with reassurance. Other treatment strategies depend on symptom control. If constipation is a significant feature then dietary fibre should be increased by using wheat, bran or bulking agents. If diarrhoea is predominant then loperimide or diphenoxylate may be useful. For abdominal pain anticholinergic or antispasmodic agents such as mebeverine may be of value. There is also some evidence that low-dose antidepressants may help.

Proctalgia fugax

The term proctalgia fugax means 'fleeting rectal pain'. It is characterized by episodes of severe anal or lower rectal pain which last for a variable length of time ranging from a few seconds up to several minutes. Although it is a recurring condition, episodes may be separated by many days, weeks or months. The prevalence in a community is not clear but may be in the region of 20%. The pain can be extremely severe and cause considerable alarm and although there are no specific diagnostic features sigmoidoscopy should be carried out in order to exclude organic disease and to reassure the patient. The cause of the pain is probably smooth muscle spasm but the underlying cause is obscure. Treatment is usually unnecessary as the attacks are of short duration and infrequent but in patients with frequent proctalgia fugax inhalation of salbutamol may curtail episodes of pain. Clonidine or amylnitrate has also been recommended.

Diverticular disease

Diverticular disease is an extremely common condition in Western society and although the prevalence in those over 60 years of age approaches 30%, the disease remains asymptomatic in about 90% of cases. In some parts of the world, including areas of Africa, the condition is almost never seen. Acquired diverticular disease should be distinguished from congenital diverticula of the colon which are usually right sided. Unlike acquired diverticular disease, these are formed from the full thickness of the bowel wall and are wide necked. They are usually asymptomatic but may present with inflammation, mimicking acute appendicitis. The rest of this section will deal exclusively with acquired diverticular disease.

Pathology

Acquired diverticular disease may affect the whole colon but it always affects the sigmoid colon and this area is the only involved colonic segment in about two-thirds of cases. The diverticula consist of saccular prolapses of mucosa with its serosal covering at the point of entry of segmental blood vessels from the serosal to the submucosal layer (Figure 14.52). Diverticula never penetrate the taenia coli and usually prolapse between the antimesenteric and mesenteric taenia. In addition to these fully formed diverticula, it is common to find intramural and ridge diverticula which have an attenuated layer of circular muscle in the wall. The other main feature of diverticular disease is muscle thickening which affects both the circular and longitudinal muscle layers of the colon leading to a degree of shortening of the bowel. There appears to be genuine hypertrophy of the muscle fibres and the circular muscle and mucosa are projected as transverse folds into the lumen. When marked these folds may lead to partial obstruction of the colon.

Aetiology

Normal motility of the colon leads to segmentation of the large bowel with intervening sections subjected to intraluminal pressure which may reach as high as 90 mmHg. Persistent contraction rings may result, leading ultimately to thickening of the circular muscle, and the high pressures surrounded by these contraction rings cause herniation of the mucosa at weak points (i.e. where blood vessels penetrate the muscle wall).

The underlying factors responsible for this disordered colonic motility are not clear, however. There does not appear to be a racial predisposition, as all races living in the same cultural environment appear to have an identical prevalence of the condition. Conventionally it is considered that the widespread use of refined sugar and flour from which all cereal fibre has been removed is the main problem, as the colon is forced to propel contents of hard consistency leading to high segmentation pressures. It has been documented that the average daily stool weight of a rural African is 400 g with a transit time of 35 hours which compares with values in studies on Europeans of 150 g and 3–6 days, respectively. This difference is considered to be the result of differing intakes of dietary fibre and to account for the low incidence of diverticular disease in the African community.

Clinical features

As stated above the vast majority of individuals with diverticular disease remain asymptomatic and most of the important symptoms result from complications (see below). However, there is a small group of patients who

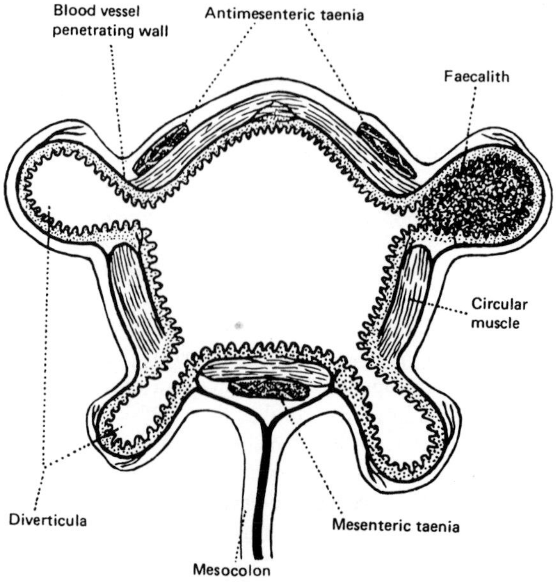

Figure 14.52 Structural abnormalities in diverticular disease.

have a condition known painful diverticular disease. This leads to chronic but intermittent lower abdominal pain mostly felt in the left iliac fossa. A feeling of distension is common, only relieved by passing flatus. Commonly, the patients are constipated and produce pellet-like stools although occasionally diarrhoea may be a feature. On examination, a thickened loop of bowel may be felt in the left iliac fossa in a thin individual but in the majority of cases with uncomplicated diverticular disease there are no physical finding. It should be noted that the symptoms of uncomplicated diverticular disease are similar to those of irritable bowel syndrome and clinically it can be impossible to distinguish between the two. This is further confounded by the fact that both conditions are extremely common and may easily co-exist.

Diagnosis

The diagnosis of diverticular disease is most commonly made on barium enema which shows the typical sacculations very clearly (Figure 14.12). The diagnosis may also be made on flexible sigmoidoscopy or colonoscopy where the typical diverticular mouths can be seen (Figure 14.53). Occasionally with severe diverticular disease it can be difficult to distinguish between the mouth of a diverticulum and the lumen of the colon and this can make endoscopy hazardous in these patients. Ultrasound examination and CT scanning of the abdomen may also be useful in patients with complications (see below).

Complications

The main complications of diverticular disease are acute diverticulitis, stricture formation, fistula formation and haemorrhage.

Acute diverticulitis

Acute diverticulitis occurs when one or more of the diverticula become inflamed, presumably as a result of obstruction by faeces. This may go on to perforation of the diverticulum leading either to paracolic abscess formation or more rarely faecal peritonitis. Peritonitis may also occur in the absence of faecal leakage if a paracolic abscess discharges pus into the peritoneal cavity. The patient with diverticulitis or a paracolic abscess typically presents with left iliac fossa pain and tenderness associated with malaise and fever, and examination will reveal localized peritonitis in the left iliac fossa. If there is generalized peritonitis, faecal or otherwise, there will be generalized peritonitis. Commonly, the diagnosis of acute diverticulitis is made on clinical grounds but if there is any doubt, a water-soluble contrast enema may be of value. This will also demonstrate whether or not there is leakage of colonic contents. Abdominal ultrasound or CT scanning is useful in demonstrating the presence of an abscess associated with diverticular disease.

Stricture formation

Stricture formation follows repeated attacks of acute diverticulitis with subsequent resolution by fibrosis. When severe, the patient will give a history of low abdominal pain and obstructive type symptoms often characteristic of the change of bowel habit seen with carcinoma of the sigmoid colon. These strictures show up on barium enema and can be distinguished from carcinomas by preservation of the mucosal pattern (Figure 14.54). Nonetheless it can sometimes be difficult to be absolutely certain of the

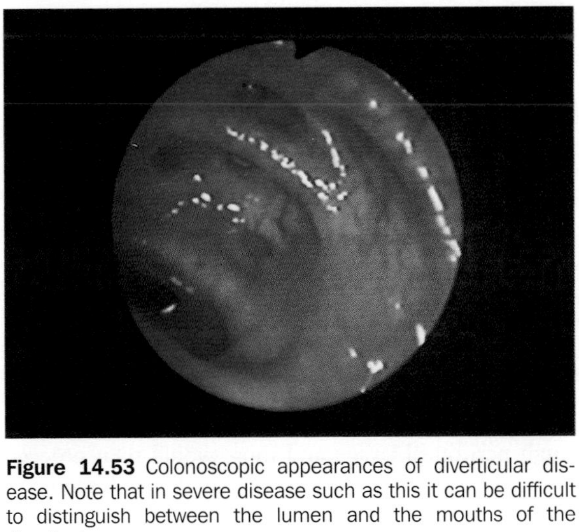

Figure 14.53 Colonoscopic appearances of diverticular disease. Note that in severe disease such as this it can be difficult to distinguish between the lumen and the mouths of the diverticula.

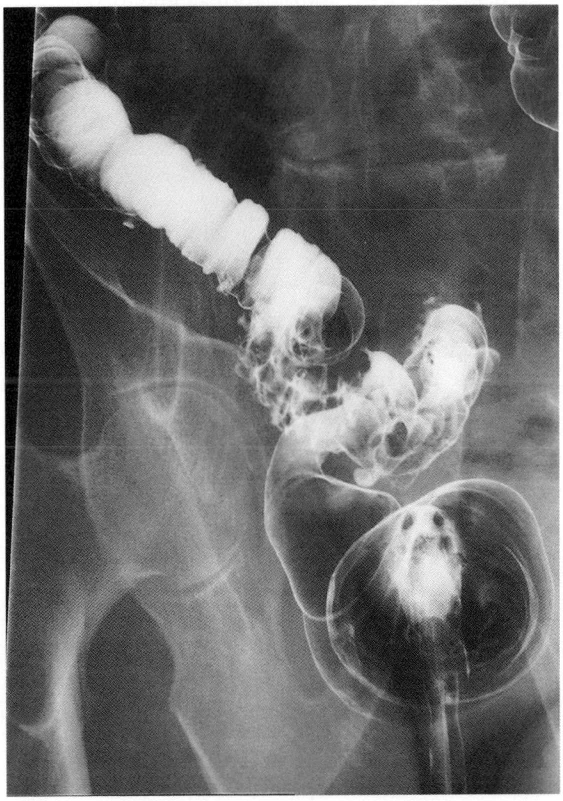

Figure 14.54 Barium enema showing a typical sigmoid diverticular stricture. Note that although the narrowing is marked, the mucosal pattern within the stricture is preserved,

diagnosis on radiological grounds alone, and follow-up endoscopy with biopsy of the stricture is often necessary to exclude carcinoma. Surprisingly, radiological strictures can sometimes resolve with time, presumably because a component of the stricture is due to spasm rather than structural changes in the bowel wall. In addition, paracolic abscess formation can cause stricture formation which may be reversible after treatment.

Fistula formation

Fistulas occur when a paracolic abscess forms next to an adjacent hollow organ and then discharges into that organ. The commonest sites for fistulation are between the sigmoid colon and the bladder (vesicocolic fistula), the vagina (colovaginal fistula) and the small bowel (enterocolic fistula). Colovaginal fistulas nearly always occur in women who have had previous hysterectomies. It is also possible to develop diverticular fistulas between the colon and the abdominal wall, the uterus and the perianal region leading to a complex fistula-in-ano. The patient with a vesicocolic fistula will present with recurring urinary tract infections, offensive urine and pneumaturia (passing bubbles of gas in the urine). Here the diagnosis can usually be confirmed by a contrast enema although sometimes cystoscopy may be necessary. Sigmoidoscopy rarely demonstrates a fistula. The patient with a colovaginal fistula will complain of passing faeces per vaginum and again a contrast enema may demonstrate the fistula. With an enterocolic fistula the patient will usually have diarrhoea as small bowel contents empty into the distal sigmoid colon. Either a small bowel follow-through or a barium enema may be of value in making the diagnosis here.

Haemorrhage

Haemorrhage from diverticular disease usually occurs in the absence of diverticulitis and is thought to be due to erosion of a vessel in the base of a diverticulum. Typically, patients present with massive sudden onset of rectal bleeding which usually stops spontaneously. Subsequent investigation then reveals diverticular disease. If the bleeding does not stop however, it may be necessary to carry out more sophisticated investigations and the procedure of choice is mesenteric angiography. If the bleeding is rapid enough (greater than 1 ml per min) active bleeding into the lumen of the colon will be seen. Occasionally it may be possible to carry out colonoscopy and to visualize bleeding from the mouth of a diverticulum but often the bleeding is too profuse for this to be feasible. Chronic blood loss is not a common feature of diverticular disease, and the presence of the condition should never be accepted as the cause of significant iron-deficiency anaemia.

Treatment

The treatment of diverticular disease is divided into the treatment of painful diverticular disease, diverticulitis, stricture formation, fistula formation and haemorrhage.

Painful diverticular disease

Traditionally, patients with diverticular disease are advised on a high-fibre diet and may be prescribed faecal bulk forming agents. If constipation is a major symptom then this is usually alleviated but there is no evidence that a high-fibre diet will actually cause regression of diverticular disease and there is little evidence that it reduces pain. Antispasmodic drugs such as mebeverine may be prescribed to good effect but the results are highly variable. The majority of patients with painful diverticular disease can be managed by a combination of reassurance and the above measures but occasionally surgical intervention will be necessary. For some years there was a vogue for carrying out a sigmoid myotomy in which the circular muscle of the sigmoid colon was incised down to the submucosa. This was shown to reduce intracolonic pressure but the symptomatic results were indifferent. Most surgeons would now recommend a sigmoid colectomy but even here patients may continue to have symptoms post-operatively. It has to be remembered that the symptoms may in fact be due to irritable bowel syndrome and patients should always be warned that there is no guarantee of relief of symptoms after surgical intervention for uncomplicated diverticular disease.

Diverticulitis

In the majority of patients with acute diverticulitis, when tenderness is confined to the left iliac fossa, conservative treatment with intravenous fluids and antibiotics will bring about resolution of acute diverticulitis. The patient should then be subsequently investigated with sigmoidoscopy and barium enema to exclude any other lesions. If the patient fails to settle and there is a swinging pyrexia then ultrasound or CT may reveal a paracolic abscess. It may then be worth attempting radiologically guided transcutaneous drainage of the abscess. If this fails however, or if a patient has acute diverticulitis without abscess formation which fails to resolve, then laparotomy may be indicated.

The usual operation would be a sigmoid colectomy in the form of a Hartmann's procedure (closure of the rectal stump and end colostomy), although if peritoneal contamination is minimal it may be possible to carry out a primary anastomosis after intra-operative colonic irrigation. In the patient who has widespread peritonitis, immediate laparotomy is mandatory. If there is faecal peritonitis then a Hartmann's procedure with thorough peritoneal lavage is indicated. These patients will almost all require post-operative intensive care and the mortality is extremely high. If, on the other hand, there is widespread purulent peritonitis without the presence of faeces, there is some controversy over ideal management. All surgeons would recommend thorough peritoneal lavage and most would then proceed to a Hartmann's resection of the diseased segment. Others, however, favour drainage and defunctioning using either a loop ileostomy or loop colostomy and yet others would recommend no specific intervention other than the peritoneal toilet. In the absence of randomized trials, treatment has to be tailored to the individual patient and will also be affected by the surgeon's experience and preference.

Stricture formation
In a patient with a diverticular stricture which has been proven to be benign histologically and which is causing little in the way of symptoms it is reasonable to treat as for painful diverticular disease. However, if there are significant obstructive symptoms then a sigmoid colectomy is the treatment of choice.

Fistula formation
A fistula requires the resection of the diseased segment of colon (nearly always the sigmoid colon) and repair of the fistula. It is usually possible to carry out a primary anastomosis following such a procedure.

Haemorrhage
As the majority of patients who bleed from diverticular disease stop bleeding spontaneously the majority can be managed with careful monitoring and blood transfusion. However, when the bleeding does not stop the ideal sequence is to carry out an upper gastrointestinal endoscopy to exclude upper gastrointestinal tract bleeding and then proceed to mesenteric angiography to try to identify the bleeding site. If this done, it is essential that the patient is accompanied to the radiology department by the responsible surgeon who will take charge of resuscitation as the radiologist carries out the procedure. As soon as the bleeding site has been identified the patient should be transferred to the operating theatre for resection of the appropriate segment of colon.

If, however, mesenteric angiography is unhelpful or unavailable, a laparotomy should be carried out with a view to on-table antegrade irrigation of the colon followed by intra-operative colonoscopy to try to identify the bleeding point. If this is unsuccessful or impossible or if the patient is bleeding too quickly to allow this to be done safely then a subtotal colectomy should be carried out. A blind left-sided colectomy is dangerous as the patient may be bleeding from an unrecognized angiodysplastic lesion on the right side of the colon. After subtotal colectomy, ileostomy or ileorectal anastomosis can be carried out according to the state of the patient.

Section 14.8 • Vascular disorders of the colon

Vascular disorders of the colon can be classified into three main categories:

- ischaemic colitis
- angiodysplasia
- visceral artery aneurysms.

Ischaemic colitis

The term ischaemic colitis can be used to cover ischaemic disorders of the large bowel caused by a number of different factors (Table 14.8). Generally speaking, ischaemia of the colon is caused by insufficient blood flow through the mesenteric vessels due to either thrombosis or embolus. Thrombosis of arteries to the colon is usually due to progressive narrowing of the vessels by atherosclerosis and may be accompanied by the development of a significant collateral blood supply. On the other hand, embolic occlusion of colonic vessels is usually sudden and therefore does not allow the development of collateral flow. In some cases ischaemia may occur in the absence of occlusive arterial disease, e.g. in patients with shock or congestive cardiac failure and following aortic reconstruction with ligation of the inferior mesenteric artery. This last cause is very unusual, however, as under most circumstances the entire colon can be adequately supplied by the superior mesenteric artery by way of the marginal artery. Various forms of vasculitis may also be responsible.

The degree of ischaemia in ischaemic colitis is highly variable and there are three clinical patterns:

- gangrenous ischaemic colitis
- transient ischaemic colitis
- stricturing ischaemic colitis.

Clinical features

Gangrenous ischaemic colitis
These patients are almost always elderly and usually have concurrent disease such as sepsis or cardiac failure.

Table 14.8 Causes of colonic ischaemia

Thrombosis – arterial or venous
Arteriosclerosis
Polycythaemia vera
Portal hypertension
Malignant disease of the colon
Hyperviscosity syndrome due to:
platelet abnormalities
high molecular weight dextran infusion
Emboli from:
Left atrium (atrial fibrillation)
Left ventricle (myocardial infarction)
Atheromatous plaque in aorta
Vasculitis
Polyarteritis nodosa
Lupus erythematosus
Giant cell arteritis (Takayasu's arteritis)
Buerger's disease
Henoch–Schönlein disease
Surgical trauma to vessels
Aortic reconstruction
Resection of adjacent intestine
Non-occlusive ischaemia
Shock – hypovolaemic or septic
Congestive heart failure
'Spontaneous' ischaemic colitis

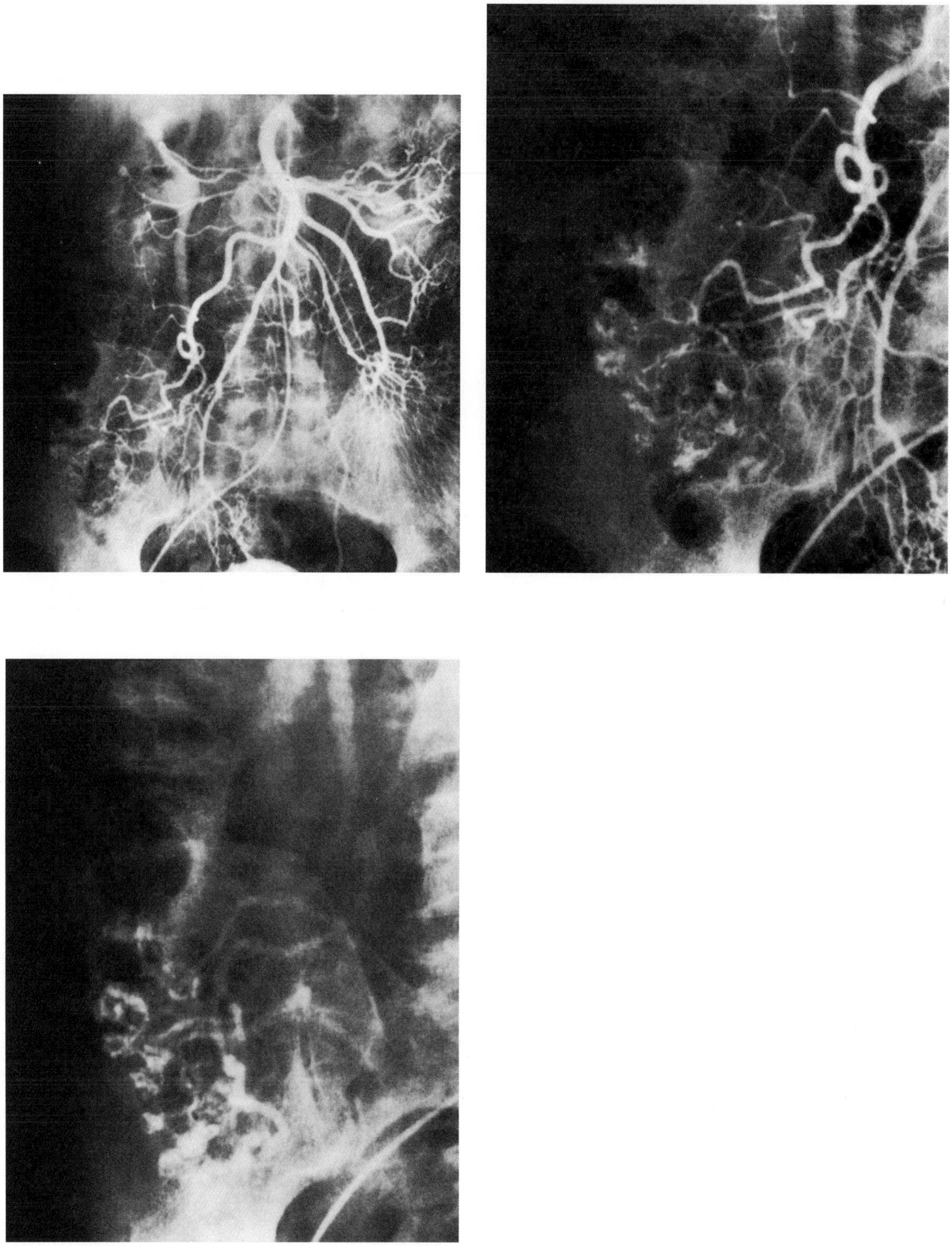

Figure 14.55 Angiographic appearances of angiodysplasia.

There is usually a history of acute onset of intense abdominal pain usually on the left side accompanied by bloody diarrhoea. On examination the patient is severely ill and the abdomen is usually extremely tender with peritonism.

Transient ischaemic colitis
In this less dramatic form of the disease, patients are usually middle aged and may have evidence of peripheral vascular disease. There is usually a history of abdominal pain of several days' duration and rectal bleeding is almost invariable. On examination there is mild to moderate abdominal tenderness.

Stricturing ischaemic colitis
In these patients the clinical presentation may be insidious although there may be a history of abdominal pain and rectal bleeding. Typically the patient will develop chronic abdominal discomfort and change of bowel habit and on examination there may be very little to find.

Diagnosis
Gangrenous ischaemic colitis
Plain abdominal X-rays in patients with colonic infarction show a blending of the mucosal folds, air in the wall of the colon and occasionally air in the portal venous system. If the colon has gone on to perforation, air under the diaphragm may be seen on an erect chest X-ray. Further investigation is usually not indicated as the patient will require urgent surgical intervention.

Transient ischaemic colitis
Here the abdominal X-ray will show 'thumb printing' which consists of multiple impressions of air due to submucosal oedema and haemorrhage. This is more clearly seen on a double contrast barium enema. If colonoscopy is carried out, haemorrhagic oedema of the colonic mucosa will be seen. However, owing to the possibility of perforation, colonoscopy is not to be recommended if the diagnosis of ischaemic colitis is suspected.

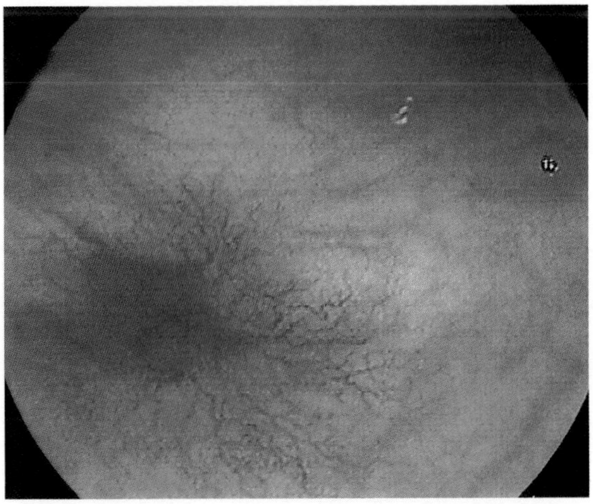

Figure 14.56 Colonoscopic appearances of angiodysplasia.

Stricturing ischaemic colitis
Here the barium enema may reveal a relatively smooth stricture of the colon and on endoscopy thickened mucosa will be seen. Biopsy will show damage to the underlying muscularis propia associated with fibrosis.

Treatment
Gangrenous ischaemic colitis
When gangrenous ischaemic colitis is diagnosed then urgent laparotomy after adequate resuscitation is mandatory. The infarcted segment should be resected and the healthy bowel ends brought out as a colostomy or ileostomy and mucus fistula. Because of the gross contamination which often accompanies this condition the mortality is high.

Transient ischaemic colitis
If laparotomy is not indicated, treatment consists of general supportive measures including intravenous fluids, parenteral nutrition where indicated and blood transfusion if the haemoglobin drops.

Stricturing ischaemic colitis
The treatment of this condition depends on symptoms and a colonic resection with primary anastomosis may be indicated.

Angiodysplasia

Angiomatous lesions of the bowel were first identified about 40 years ago with the introduction of angiography, and are now recognized to be relatively common. They characteristically occur in patients over the age of 60 years and are not usually associated with other angiomatous lesions of other viscera or of the skin. These lesions have been called angiodysplasias, angiomas, haemangiomas, arteriovenous malformations or vascular ectasias. Although they may occur anywhere in the gastrointestinal tract they are commonest on the right side of the colon and histologically they consist of thin walled vascular channels in the submucosa.

Aetiology
The cause of these lesions is unclear. They do not appear to be congenital and should be distinguished from hereditary haemorrhagic telangiectasia (Rendu–Osler-Weber syndrome). There are various theories as to the aetiology, including obstruction of submucosal veins as they pass through the muscle layers of the colonic wall and repeated episodes of bowel ischaemia with arteriovenous shunting. Both of these theories explain why the lesions should predominantly occur on the right side of the colon. This follows Laplace's law (tension is proportional to diameter and pressure) as the right colon has the widest diameter of the large bowel.

Clinical features

The clinical features of angiodysplasia depend on its tendency to bleed. Patients may present with anaemia or on some occasions with massive rectal bleeding.

Diagnosis

The main diagnostic modality is mesenteric angiography which characteristically shows an early draining vein parallel to a feeding artery (Figure 14.55). Colonoscopy may also detect the typical 'cherry red' spots which are characteristic of this condition (Figure 14.56).

Treatment

The most effective treatment for this condition is resection of the affected portion of bowel (usually a right hemicolectomy). In extreme conditions where the patient is actively haemorrhaging and the appropriate expertise is available, selective vasopressin infusion or transcatheter embolization with gelfoam at arteriography may stop major haemorrhage. If the lesion is detected at colonoscopy then grasping it with diathermy forceps, lifting it away from the muscular wall and applying diathermy current may coagulate the abnormal vessels and prevent recurrent bleeding.

Visceral artery aneurysms

Aneurysms of the visceral arteries are relatively common but aneurysms of the colonic arteries are uncommon. There are various aetiological factors including congenital abnormalities, atherosclerosis, trauma, medial degeneration and forms of arteritis. Rupture of these aneurysms gives rise to severe abdominal pain and signs of internal haemorrhage. Successful treatment depends on prompt operative intervention.

Further reading

General

Keighley, M. R. B. and Williams, N. S. (1999). *Surgery of the Anus, Rectum and Colon*, 2nd edn, Philadelphia, PA: W. B. Saunders.

Investigations

Cotton, P. and Williams, C. (1996). *Practical Gastrointestinal Endoscopy*, 4th edn, Oxford: Blackwell Science.

Fork, F.-Th. (1983). Reliability of routine double-contrast examination of the large bowel: a prospective study of 2590 patients. *Gut* **24**: 672–7.

Thomas, M. G. (1999). Obscure lower gastrointestinal tract bleeding. *Br J Surg* **86**: 579–81.

Neoplasia

Abulafi, A. M. and Williams, N. S. (1994). Local recurrence of colorectal cancer: the problem, mechanisms, management and adjuvant therapy. *Br J Surg* **81**: 7–19.

Bond, J. H. (1993). Polyp guideline: diagnosis, treatment and surveillence for patients with non-familial colorectal polyps. *Ann Intern Med* **119**: 836–43.

Fearon, E. R. and Vogelstein, B. (1996). A genetic model for colorectal cancer. *Cell* **87**: 159–70.

Hardcastle, J. D., Chamberlain, J. O., Robinson, M. H. E. *et al.* (1996). Randomised controlled trial of faecal occult blood screening for colorectal cancer. *Lancet* **348**: 1472–7.

Kronborg, O., Fenger, C., Olsen, J. *et al.* (1996). Randomised study of screening for colorectal cancer with faecal occult blood test. *Lancet* **348**: 1467–71.

Lynch, H. T., Smyrk, T. C., Watson, P. *et al.* (1993). Genetics, natural history, tumour spectrum and pathology of hereditary non-polyposis colorectal cancer: an updated review. *Gastroenterology* **104**: 1535–49.

McArdle, C. S. and Hole, D. (1991). Impact of variability among surgeons on postoperative morbidity and mortality and ultimate survival. *BMJ* **302**: 1501–5.

McFarlane, J. K., Ryall, R. D. H. and Heald, R. J. (1993). Mesorectal excision for rectal cancer. *Lancet* **341**: 457–60.

RCS (Royal College of Surgeons of England) and Association of Coloproctology. Guidelines on the Management of Colorectal Cancer. *RCS* 1996.

Scheele, J., Stang, R., Altendorf-Hofmann, A. and Paul, M. (1995). Resection of colorectal liver metastases. *World J Surg* **19**: 59–71.

Scott, N., Jackson, P., Al-Jaberi, T. *et al.* (1995). Total mesorectal excision and local recurrence: a study of tumour spread in the mesorectum distal to rectal cancer. *Br J Surg* **82**: 1031–3.

SIGN (1997). Colorectal Cancer – a National Guideline. Scottish Intercollegiate Guidelines Network, June 1997.

SRCT (Swedish Rectal Cancer Trial) (1997). Improved survival with pre-operative radiotherapy in resectable rectal cancer. *N Engl J Med* **336**: 980–7.

Inflammatory bowel disease

Elton, E. and Hannauer, S. B. (1996). The medical management of Crohn's disease. *Aliment Pharmacol Ther* **10**:1–22.

Present, D. H., Rutgeerts, P., Targan, S. *et al.* (1999). Infliximab for the treatment of fistulas in patients with Crohn's disease. *N Engl J Med* **340**: 1398–405.

Functional and structural disorders

Drossman, D. A., Corazziari, E., Talley, N. J. *et al.* (1999). Rome II: a multinational consensus document on functional gastrointestinal disorders. *Gut* **45** (Suppl II).

Krukowski, Z. H., Koruth, N. M. and Matheson, N. A. (1985). Evolving practice in acute diverticulitis. *Br J Surg* **72**: 684–6.

Laine, L. (1999). Management of acute colonic pseudo-obstruction. *N Engl J Med* **341**: 192–3.

MODULE 15

Disorders of the anal canal

Section 15.1 • Anatomy

The anal canal is about 3–4 cm long. It passes slightly posteriorly starting at the anal rectal angle and ending at the anal verge. In the male, anteriorly the anal canal is related to the bulb of the urethra and in the female to the perineal body and the vagina. Laterally it is related to the ischiorectal fossa containing the inferior haemorrhoidal vessels and pudendal nerve (Figure 15.1); posteriorly lie the coccyx and the puborectalis muscle. As described below, the anal canal is surrounded by the internal and external sphincter muscles.

The epithelium of the anal canal is columnar above the anal valves and squamous below them; the site of the anal valves is also known as the dentate or pectinate line and this indicates the mucocutaneus junction. The anal valves consist of pits which represent the openings of the anal glands, and the glands themselves lie in the plane between the internal and external sphincters, helping to lubricate the anal canal. The mucosa above the dentate line is arranged in longitudinal columns covering the internal haemorrhoidal plexus. This mucosa is loose but at the anal valves it becomes fixed to the internal sphincter by the mucosal suspensory ligament of Parks.

Strictly speaking the epithelium immediately above the anal valves is not columnar but cuboidal and this zone, which is between 0.5 and 2 cm in length, is known as the anal transition zone. Here there is a high density of sensory nerve endings. Although the epithelium is squamous below the dentate line there are no hair follicles, sebaceous glands or sweat glands in the anal canal. These only appear at the anal verge.

The internal anal sphincter is a downward, thickened extension of the circular muscle fibres of the rectum and extends about 1 cm below the anal canal. It consists entirely of smooth muscle and is innervated by the pelvic autonomic plexus. The external sphincter on the other hand is made up of skeletal muscle which is arranged around the anal canal outside the internal sphincter (Figure 15.1). Posteriorly the upper fibres of the external sphincter merge with those of puborectalis. Theoretically there are three components to the external anal sphincter complex but these are of little significance surgically. In the lower part of the anal canal there are longitudinal smooth muscle fibres and elastic tissue which extend through the lower fibres of the external sphincter to become attached to the perianal skin. These are extensions of the longitudinal muscle of the rectum.

As the pelvic floor is intimately related with the anal canal, it is also worth considering the anatomy of this structure. The pelvic diaphragm is formed by the levator ani which arises from the sides of the pelvis and allows the passage of the urethra, vagina and anal canal. The innermost fibres are called puborectalis. This arises from the symphysis pubis and surrounds the vagina or prostate and the anorectal junction just above the sphincters and is then inserted into the symphysis pubis on the opposite side. Thus it creates a sling which is deficient anteriorly. The rest of levator ani is made up of three parts: pubococcygeus, ileococcygeus and ischiococcygeus (Figure 15.2). Pubococcygeus arises from the pubis and is inserted into the coccyx. Ileococcygeus arises from the ileum and is inserted into the tissue between the anal canal and the coccyx (anococcygeal raphe) and into the coccyx itself. Ischiococcygeus arises from the ischial spine and is inserted into the coccyx and lower sacrum. Posteriorly, the pelvic floor is completed by piriforimis which arises on the pelvic surface of the sacrum and is inserted into the tip of the greater trochanter of the femur. On the perineal aspect of the pelvic floor is the central perineal tendon which is a mass of fibrous tissue lying between the anal canal and the bulb of the penis or vagina. Into this is attached the transverse perineal muscles which are divided into superficial and deep components. These muscles act as support for the pelvic floor. Deep to these structures lie muscle fibres joining the prostate or vagina to the anal canal known variously as levator prostatae, pubourethralis and pubovaginalis.

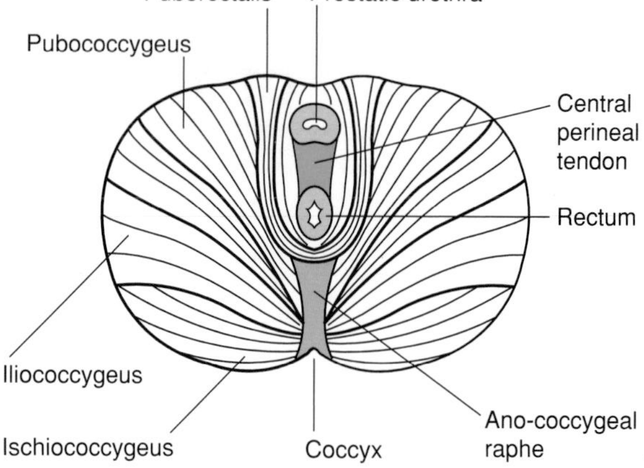

Figure 15.2 Anatomy of the pelvic floor.

Nerve supply

Levator ani derives its nerve supply from the third and forth sacral nerves as they pass from the pelvis through the pelvic floor. These nerves also supply the anal canal and perianal skin. The external anal sphincter complex is supplied by the pudendal nerve which is derived from S2 to S4. This nerve leaves the pelvis between piriforimis and ileococcygeus and re-enters it through the lesser sciatic foramen. It then runs forwards on the posterior surface of levator ani giving off the inferior haemorrhoidal nerve, the perineal nerve and the dorsal nerve of the penis. The inferior haemorrhoidal nerve supplies the external anal sphincter and perianal skin.

Blood supply

The blood supply to the anal canal comes from the inferior haemorrhoidal artery which is a branch of the anterior portion of the internal iliac artery. It passes out of the pelvis between piriformis and ileococcygeus and via the greater sciatic foramen and then re-enters by passing over the sacrospinous ligament. It then runs in the ischiorectal fossa to supply the levator ani and sphincter muscles as well as the lower rectum and anal canal. The branches of the vessel which supply the skin

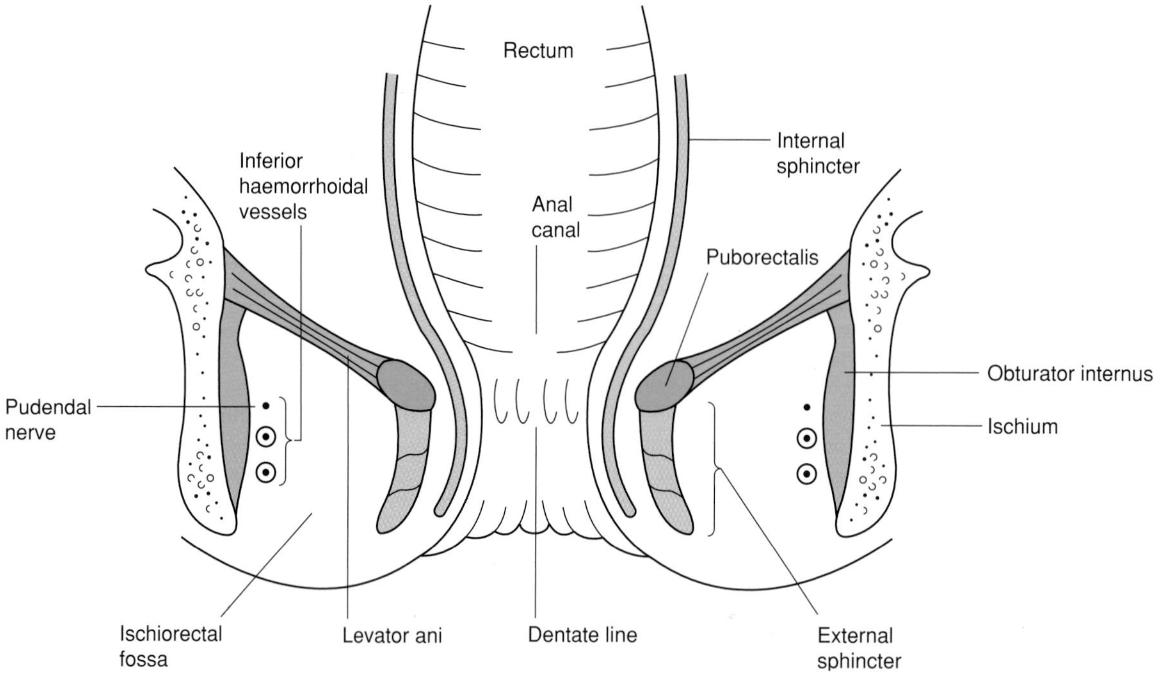

Figure 15.1 Anatomy of the anal canal.

of the anal canal have to pass through the internal sphincter muscle.

Venous drainage

The venous drainage very much follows the arterial supply but it is of interest to note that there is a very free communication between superior and inferior haemorrhoidal veins in the submucosal plexus of the anal canal and the rectum. Thus both the anal canal and the lower rectum can drain directly into the systemic circulation via the internal iliac vein rather than through the portal system.

Lymphatic drainage

The lymphatic drainage of the upper anal canal is via channels around the rectum and then along the inferior mesenteric artery to the pre-aortic nodes. However, the lower anal canal below the dentate line drains to the perianal plexus and then on to the inguinal lymph nodes.

Section 15.2 • Physiology

The anal canal is a highly complex mechanism which under normal situations allows the individual to control the retention and evacuation of gaseous, liquid and solid rectal matter. There is however, considerable individual variation and most people are sometimes incontinent to liquid faeces and slight leakage from the anal canal is common. When faecal material enters the rectum there are three phases:

- *Accommodation* where the rectum slowly expands but both the internal and external sphincters retain their tone.
- *Sampling* where the rectal contents come into contact with the sensory lining of the anal canal (transitional zone) after temporary relaxation of the internal sphincter.
- *Defecation*. Although this is under voluntary control to a certain extent, when the volume of rectal contents reaches a critical point the urge to defecate becomes overpowering and the tone in the external sphincter is inhibited.

The sensory component of incontinence is complex and most individuals are able to distinguish between gas, liquid and solid. Specialized nerve fibres are found within the anal canal and sensory endings in the levator ani complex of muscles have a role in controlling the urge to defecate. Motor control of continence is exerted by a high pressure zone in the anal canal (50–100 cmH_2O) produced by the combined tone of the internal and external sphincters. The angle of the anal canal and rectum is about 80° and is maintained by the action of puborectalis muscle. As indicated above the initial stimulus for defecation is distension of the rectum. This acts as a spinal reflex via a centre in the lumbosacral region but cerebral control is exerted over this centre if circumstances are not convenient. Conditioning leads to a degree of cerebral control so that defecation may take place only once a day even although the rectum contains faeces for much of the time.

During the act of defecation, particularly in the squatting position, the rectum and anal canal form a straight line owing to straightening out of the ano-rectal angle. Abdominal pressure is raised and the external sphincter muscle is inhibited allowing faeces to pass through the anal canal. This may be accompanied by a mass peristaltic action so that the whole distal colon is emptied. In some individuals however, repeated straining may be necessary to pass several smaller segments of stool.

Section 15.3 • Investigations

Owing to the complexity of the sphincter mechanism full investigation of the anal canal and its function requires considerable expertise and specialized equipment. The investigative procedures can be classified under the following headings.

- endoscopy
- ultrasound
- manometry
- electrophysiology
- radiology.

Endoscopy

The anal canal can be examined endoscopically by means of a short rigid endoscope called, in the UK, a proctoscope (Figure 15.3). This is something of a misnomer, however, and the North American term anoscope is more descriptive. This instrument allows visualization of the anal canal and lower rectal mucosa and is particularly useful for diagnosing internal haemorrhoids. It should not be used in the conscious patient when painful anal conditions such as fissure are present.

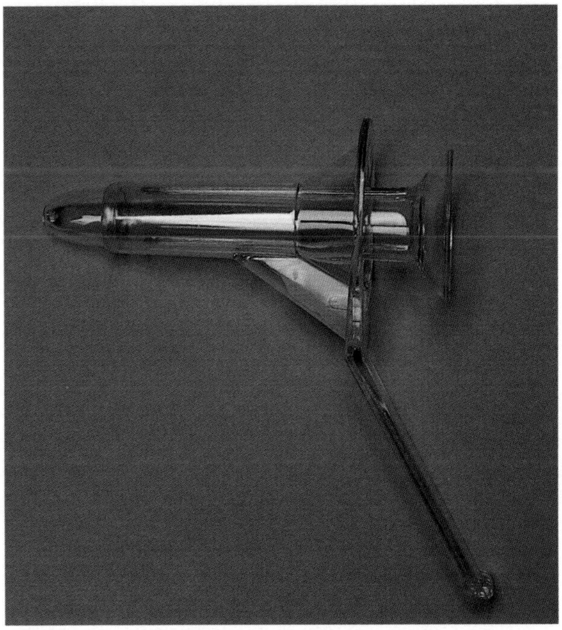

Figure 15.3 Proctoscope.

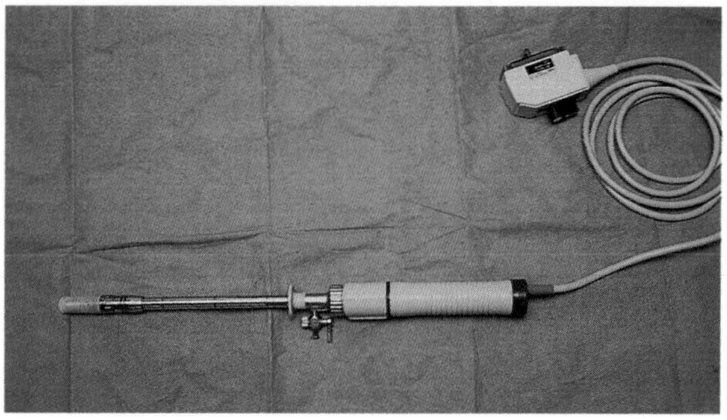

Figure 15.4 Anal ultrasound probe.

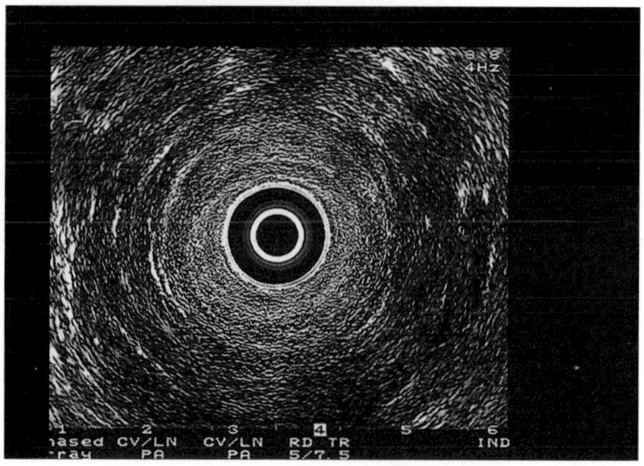

Figure 15.6 Normal ultrasound examination of the lower anal canal. At this level, the internal sphincter is absent.

Ultrasound

Ultrasound is useful for visualizing the anal sphincters. The most widely used probe is a rotating 7 or 10 MHz probe within a water-filled plastic cone (Figure 15.4). This produces a 360° cross-sectional image when inserted into the anal canal. The ultrasound image which is produced images the internal sphincter as a well-defined hypoechoic layer and the external sphincter as a thick echogenic layer (Figure 15.5). In the lower part of the anal canal the internal sphincter is absent (Figure 15.6) and in the upper part the puborectalis muscle is seen (Figure 15.7).

Anorectal manometry

Various devices are available for the measurement of pressures in the anal canal but the recording device should not be greater than 5 mm in diameter since larger catheters artificially raise anal pressure. The most modern devices are strain gauge catheters (Figure 15.8) which contain resistors on a metal diaphragm within a vacuum. Pressure on this diaphragm changes resistance which is then converted to a pressure measurement. This can be used to produce either a static or an ambulatory measurement. The resting anal pressure is largely due to the internal sphincter which is in a state of continuous contraction. This is highly variable but a pressure of 50–100 cmH_2O is generally regarded as normal. Resting pressure is lower in women than in men and tends to decrease with increasing age. A normal squeeze pressure is in the region of 250 cmH_2O for men and 100 cm H_2O for women. In general, patients with faecal incontinence have low resting and squeeze pressures but there is poor correlation between the pressures and the severity of symptoms, and the underlying cause for the incontinence cannot be diagnosed on pressure readings alone.

Another useful application of anorectal manometry is testing for the rectoanal inhibitory reflex in patients with intractable consiptation. This is tested by balloon distension of the rectum along with simultaneous recording of the anal pressure. A positive reflex leads to a fall in resting anal pressure of 20%. Although this reflex is absent for a variety of reasons, a positive result effectively excludes Hirschprung's disease.

Electrophysiology

Faecal or indeed urinary incontinence may be due to spinal or pelvic nerve damage and electrophysiological

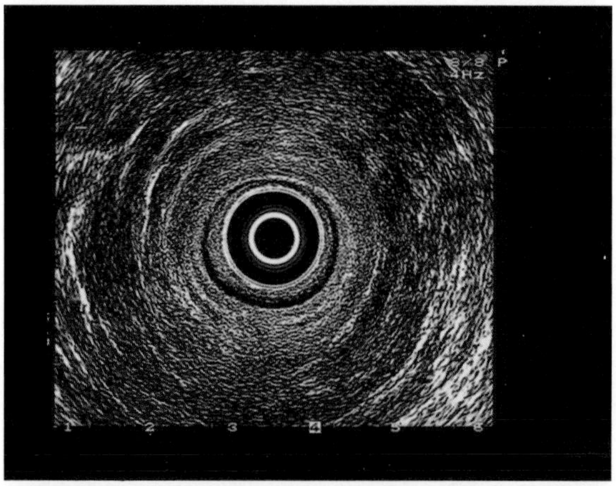

Figure 15.5 Normal ultrasound examination of the anal canal. The internal sphincter is seen as a hypoechoic (black) ring, and the external sphincer as an echogenic (white) ring.

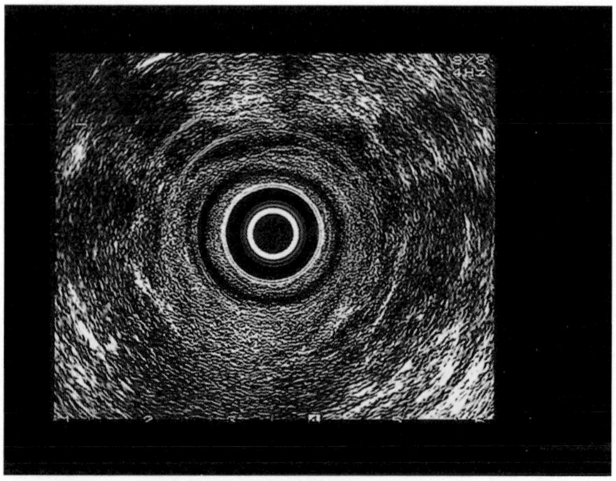

Figure 15.7 Normal ultrasound examination of the upper anal canal. Here the V-shaped fibres of the puborectalis muscle are seen posteriorly.

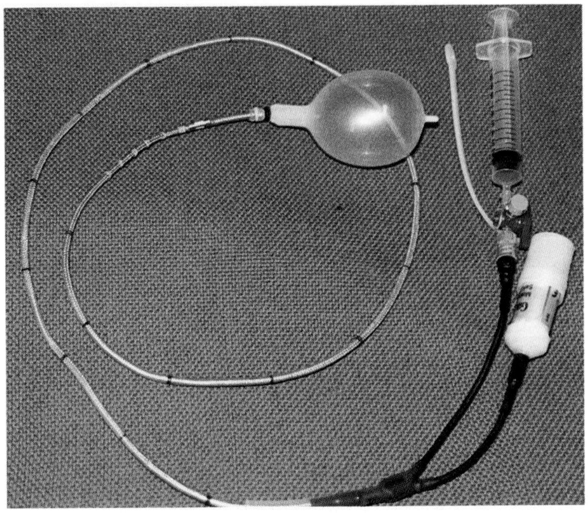

Figure 15.8 Anal manometry catheter.

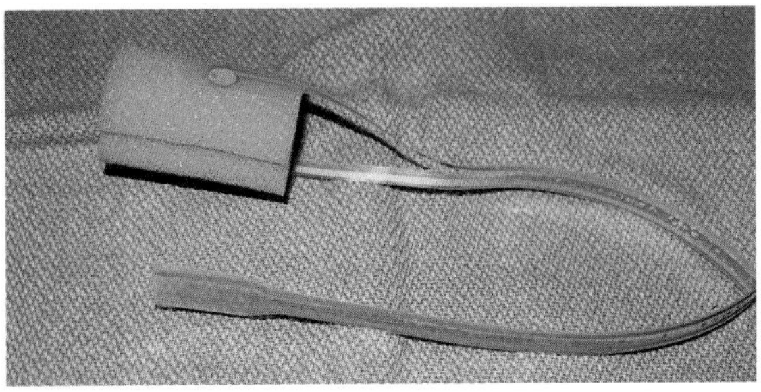

Figure 15.10 Sponge electrode for measuring puborectalis contraction.

studies may be useful under these circumstances. A common problem is incontinence related to child birth which may be caused by stretch-induced damage to the pudendal nerves. This may be detected by measuring pudendal nerve motor latency. Here a disposable electrode is attached to the gloved index finger (Figure 15.9) and the finger is inserted into the rectum. The pudendal nerves are then palpable as cord-like structures passing around the ischial spines. Latency is defined as the time between the stimulus being delivered to the nerve at the finger tip and the impulse reaching a recording electrode measuring external sphincter contraction at the base of the finger. Normal pudendal motor latency is around 2 (±0.2) ms. Prolongation beyond the normal range suggests neuropathy and this is associated with a poor outcome following sphincter repair. However, it must be stressed that prolonged latency does not absolutely preclude a good result from surgery. Perineal nerve motor latency can also be measured in a similar fashion. Spinal motor latency can be measured by transcutaneous stimulation at the L1 and L4 levels with recording of the impulse at the external sphincter. The latency from L1 is normally 5.5 ms and from L4 4.4 ms.

Electromyography involves measuring muscle activity and the most accurate method of testing for denervation is single fibre electromyography. This involves inserting a platinum wire into the muscle. The changes brought about by denervation or re-innervation are quantified by calculating the fibre density which is the average number of fibres recorded at 20 sites in the muscle. Needle electromyography is not used routinely in clinical practice owing to the discomfort of the test, and difficulty in interpretation. A simple sponge electrode (Figure 15.10) in the anal canal is useful in evaluating abnormal puborectalis contraction during straining (anismsus).

Radiology

The most useful form of radiology when considering anal function is defecating proctography (Figure 15.11). This involves using a thick paste impregnated with barium instilled into the rectum. The subject then

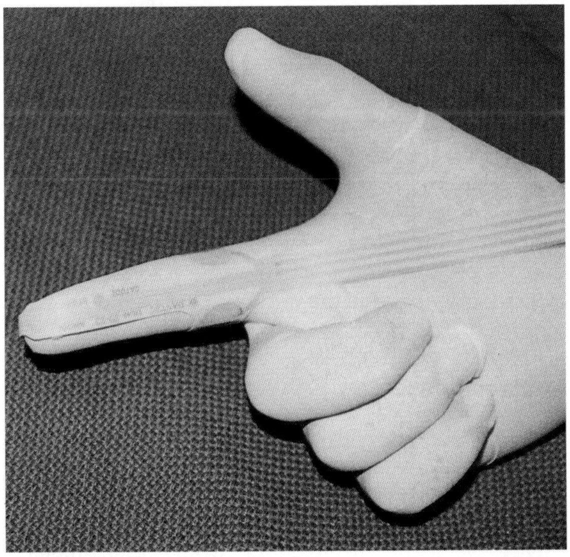

Figure 15.9 Finger mounted electrode for measuring pudendal nerve motor latency.

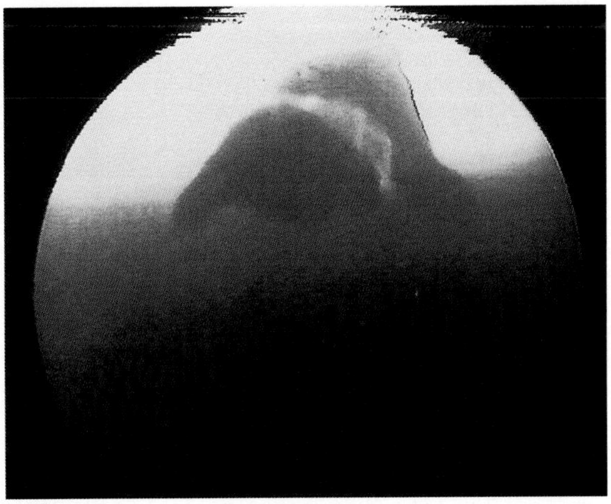

Figure 15.11 Defecating proctography showing a degree of recto-rectal intussusception.

sits on a commode and a video radiograph is taken during evacuation. Under normal circumstances as straining begins there is a slight concavity of the anterior rectal wall produced by abdominal pressure. The pelvic floor then descends and the anorectal angle widens, the anal canal begins to open, to shorten and to become funnel shaped. A slight degree of rectal wall intussusception can be accepted as normal. This investigation is useful for evaluating rectoceles and recto-rectal intussusception. Thus it is of value in investigating obstructed defecation but of limited use in the evaluation of incontinence.

Section 15.4 • Faecal incontinence

Faecal incontinence is potentially very disabling but is highly variable. It ranges from occasional soiling to regular incontinence to solid faeces.

Aetiology and pathology

Faecal incontinence can be due to various factors which are summarized in Table 15.1. It is worth noting that patients with haemorrhoids suffer a mild degree of incontinence, presumably due to a certain amount of sensory impairment in the anal canal due to loss or displacement of the anal cushions (see section on haemorrhoids). These patients do not usually require any intervention, however, and the vast majority of patients presenting with serious incontinence have either an obstetric injury or an iatrogenic injury after anal surgery.

Usually, the woman with incontinence after childbirth gives a history of prolonged labour or a traumatic vaginal delivery usually with forceps. When there has been a severe perineal injury with anal sphincter disruption (third degree tear) this is usually recognized at the time and immediate repair to the sphincter effected. If this is not recognized however, the patient will develop severe incontinence soon after delivery. More commonly the patient will gradually develop incontinence due to an occult sphincter injury being unmasked by a lax pelvic floor and neuropathic sphincter failure owing to stretching of the pudendal nerves. Thus, the majority of patients with incontinence following single or multiple vaginal deliveries are suffering from a combination of nerve damage and direct damage to the pelvic floor.

Incontinence following anal surgery is usually related to laying open of a fistula-*in ano* which has transgressed the external sphincter (see section on fistula-*in ano*). Lateral sphincterotomy for anal fissure, if done properly, is unlikely to give rise to frank incontinence but may lead to minor problems with control of flatus and mucus. Occasionally however, an overenthusiastic sphincterotomy may cause external sphincter damage. Vigorous stretching of the anal canal for fissure or haemorrhoids may also give rise to incontinence due to combined damage to the internal and external sphincters. Likewise, anal retraction of the sphincter to facilitate endorectal surgery is a risk factor.

Table 15.1 Factors leading to anal incontinence

Trauma
Obstetric injury
Surgical injury (after fistula surgery)
Accidental trauma (road traffic accident, war casualty)
Anorectal disease
Haemorrhoids
Rectal prolapse
Anal or low rectal cancer involving sphincter mechanism
Crohn's disease of anus
Factors causing diarrhoea
Inflammatory bowel disease
Infectious colitis
Malabsorption
Congenital disorders
Treated imperforate anus
Hirschsprung's disease
Spina bifida
Neurological disorders
Pudendal nerve damage
Peripheral neuropathy
Stroke
Multiple sclerosis
Spinal cord damage
Others
Behavioural
Faecal impaction
Encopresis

Clinical features

In the first instance it is important to establish the severity of the patient's symptoms. Intensive investigations and surgery for minor degrees of incontinence is not usually indicated as they are unlikely to be of value. A scoring system is useful for documenting the severity of incontinence and for estimating the response to treatment (Table 15.2). It is also important to establish whether or not there is co-existing urinary incontinence as this suggests a neuropathological cause, and to find out about previous surgery and obstetric history. On examination the patient should be ask to strain in order to assess the presence of a rectal prolapse and the degree of perineal descent. Digital rectal examination will give information regarding resting anal tone and squeeze pressure and it may also be possible to feel a defect particularly in the anterior part of the external sphincter.

Investigations

After a thorough clinical assessment it is important to carry out a sigmoidoscopy to exclude any rectal pathology and most surgeons would wish to investigate the entire colon with either a colonoscopy or a barium enema. Standard investigation would then include anorectal manometry, pudendal nerve latency and ultrasound of the anal canal (see section on investiga-

Table 15.2 Continence grading scale

Type of incontinence	*Never*	*Rarely*	*Sometimes*	*Usually*	*Always*
Solid	0	1	2	3	4
Liquid	0	1	2	3	4
Gas	0	1	2	3	4
Requires pad	0	1	2	3	4
Lifestyle alteration	0	1	2	3	4

Data from Oliveira, L., Pfeifer, J. and Wexner, S.D. (1996). Physiological and clinical outcome of anterior sphincteroplasty. *Br J Surg* **83**: 502–5.

tions). Ultrasound is perhaps the single most useful test as this will document defects in the external sphincter, measure their extent and reveal occult injuries (Figure 15.12).

Treatment

In many patients incontinence is related to loose stool and in such cases anti-diarrhoeal medication may be of value. In patients who are troubled by faecal leakage after defecation complete rectal emptying using suppositories (glycerine or bisacodal) may be helpful. Other conservative approaches include pelvic floor exercises and biofeedback retraining. A recent addition to the therapeutic armamentarium is the anal plug. This is a tampon-like device which is inserted into the rectum via the anal canal by the patient. At body temperature it expands to form a soft plug, and initial experience with this approach has been encouraging.

Surgery

In severe cases of faecal incontinence, surgery may be the only option. The main procedures are anterior sphincter repair, post-anal repair, total pelvic floor repair, gracilis neosphincter, gluteus maximus transposition and artificial sphincter insertion. Of course in some patients with intractable incontinence, particularly where multiple procedures have failed, the best option may be a permanent stoma – usually a colostomy. This option should always be discussed with patients before embarking on complex surgery which may not be successful.

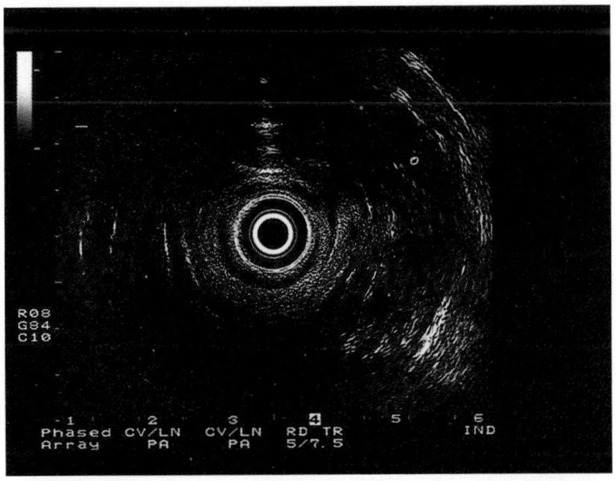

Figure 15.12 Anal ultrasound showing an anterior external sphincter defect. The crescentic echogenic band anteriorly is generated by the examiner's finger in the vagina.

Anterior repair

In the patient with an anterior sphincter defect, direct repair is usually effective. This involves making an incision anterior to the anal canal and carefully dissecting out the external sphincter. Usually there is a fibrous band at the site of the muscular defect (Figure 15.13). This is transected and the cut ends of the sphincter are overlapped and sutured together (Figure 15.14). Many surgeons will supplement this with an anterior levatorplasty which is carried out by suturing together the two sides of the levator ani muscle. Most surgeons leave the wound open to granulate.

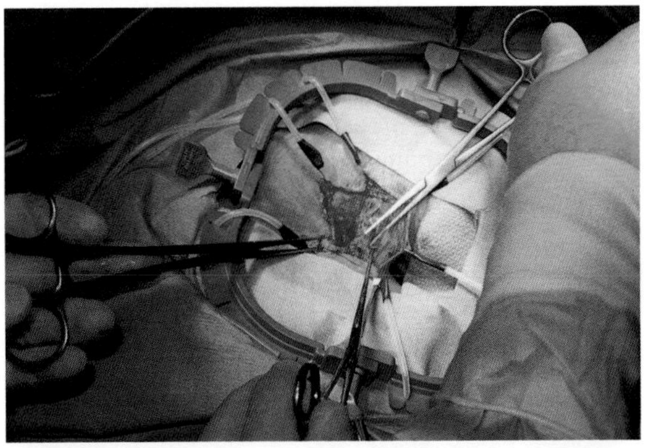

Figure 15.13 Fibrous band at site of anterior sphincter defect indicated by the Allis forceps.

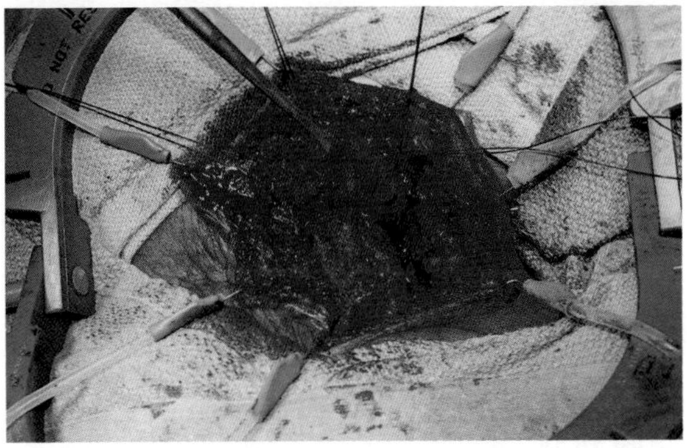

Figure 15.14 Overlapping anterior repair of the external anal sphincter.

Post-anal repair
This operation was originally devised in order to restore the normal angle between the anus and the rectum and involves making an incision posterior to the anal margin, dissecting in the intersphincteric plane and plicating the puborectalis muscle. This operation tends to be performed when the sphincter appears to be intact. The early results tend to be good although the mechanism whereby improvement occurs is controversial. However, long-term follow-up indicates that function deteriorates and the operation has lost favour in recent years.

Total pelvic floor repair
This operation combines a post-anal repair with anterior sphincter plication and levatorplasty. It may be more effective than post-anal repair, and can be performed in stages or as a single procedure.

Gracilis neosphincter
For many years the gracilis muscle has been used for anal sphincter supplementation (unstimulated graciloplasty), the operation having been originally devised for children with anorectal atresia. In adults, however, straightforward transposition is not associated with particularly good results because the external sphincter has resting tone which is not shared by the gracilis muscle. The operation of electrically stimulated gracilis neosphincter has therefore been developed (Figure 15.15). The stimulation is provided by an implanted electrode and a stimulator. This operation may be used for patients in whom sphincter repair has failed or is inappropriate, but it may also be used for those who do not have an anal sphincter, e.g. in anorectal agenesis or after abdominoperineal excision of the rectum. The results of this operation are difficult to assess objectively but about two-thirds of patients who have undergone the procedure appear to be satisfied with the results achieved.

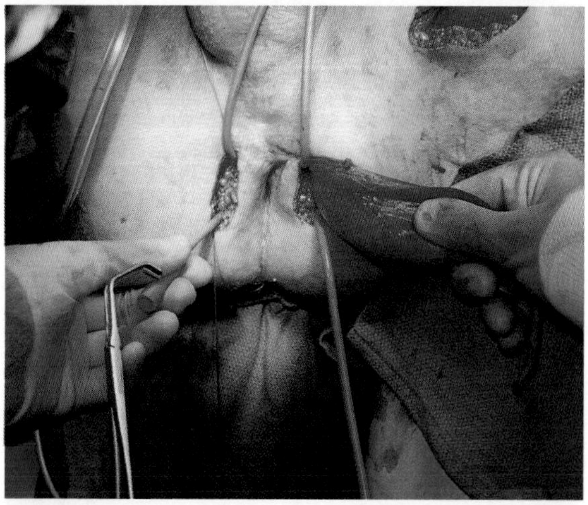

Figure 15.15 Electrically stimulated gracilis neosphincter. The photograph shows the gracilis muscle mobilized in preparation for plication around the anal canal.

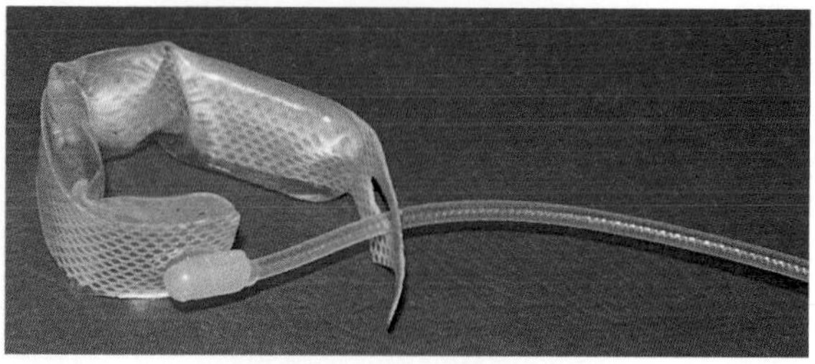

Figure 15.16 Artificial anal sphincter.

Gluteus maximus transposition
In this operation a strip of gluteus maximus is mobilized to allow transposition around the anal orifice. The results are variable and no one centre has extensive experience of this procedure.

Artificial sphincter insertion
An artificial plastic sphincter which can be inflated and deflated by the patient can be inserted around the anal canal (Figure 15.16). The most commonly used device is a modification of the artificial urinary sphincter which is inserted via the perineum. Early experience is encouraging, although infection requiring removal of the device occurs in around 20% of cases. Placement of the prosthesis via the abdomen with full mobilization of the rectum may be associated with a lower infection rate, but requires more major surgery.

Section 15.5 • Haemorrhoids

The term haemorrhoids or 'piles' means different things to different people and many patients will use these words to describe a wide variety of anorectal conditions. To the surgeon however, it refers to abnormalities of the vascular cushions of the anus.

Pathology and aetiology

The anal cushions consist of three spaces filled by arteriovenous communications supported by fibrous matrix and smooth muscle lying within the anal canal. This allows the anal lining to expand during defecation but yet to form a complete seal when the anal canal is closed. The arterial supply for these cushions comes from the superior, middle and inferior rectal arteries. Haemorrhoids are thought to result from degeneration of the smooth muscle and fibroelastic tissue which supports the cushions, allowing them to prolapse into the anal canal. However, the underlying reasons for this degeneration are not clear and although constipation and straining at stool have been implicated the evidence for this is patchy. There is a family history in about 50% of cases and it is therefore possible that a genetic predisposition exists.

Clinical features
The most common symptom is bleeding at defecation. Commonly this is bright red and follows immediately

after defecation. Typically this is painless but may be quite profuse and frightening for the patient. Other symptoms include perianal swelling, pruritus and minor soiling. Pain from haemorrhoids is associated with complications. Clinically, haemorrhoids can be classified into four groups:

- Internal haemorrhoids presenting with bleeding alone (first degree).
- Haemorrhoids which prolapse on defecation but reduce spontaneously (second degree).
- Haemorrhoids which prolapse and require manual reduction (third degree).
- Irreducibly prolapsed haemorrhoids (fourth degree).

Thus on examination the external appearances will depend on the degree of prolapse and the anal canal may in fact look normal. Skin tags around the anal orifice are common and mucosa may be seen to prolapse (Figure 15.17). Digital rectal examination is generally normal. The main diagnostic test is proctoscopy which gives a good view of the internal anal cushions. It is also essential to examine the rectum with a rigid sigmoidoscope at least to exclude other lesions.

Investigations

As far as making the diagnosis of haemorrhoids is concerned investigations other than those mentioned above are unnecessary. However, if there is any doubt about the source of bleeding then a full colonic examination in the form of a flexible sigmoidoscopy and barium enema or a total colonoscopy should be carried out. This would be indicated when there are other symptoms such as change of bowel habit or lower abdominal pain or if the patient is in the high-risk age range for colorectal cancer (i.e. over 50 years of age).

Complications

The complications of haemorrhoids include thrombosis, massive haemorrhage and faecal incontinence.

Thrombosis

When haemorrhoids become irreducible, intravascular thrombosis and oedema may ensue owing to strangulation of the blood supply. This gives rise to severe pain and on examination swollen bluish external haemorrhoids will be seen. Occasionally these may become gangrenous. Occasionally a small external haemorrhoid may become thrombosed without strangulation leading to the typical perianal haematoma.

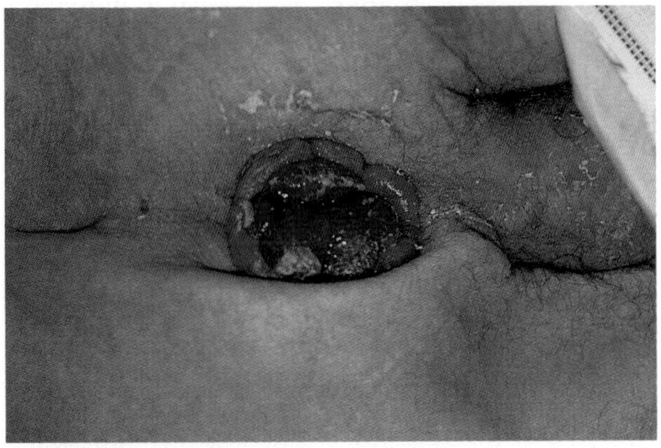

Figure 15.17 Prolapsing haemorrhoids.

Massive bleeding

Very occasionally patients may bleed so profusely from haemorrhoids that they become shocked and require resuscitation with blood transfusion. More commonly, although still relatively unusual, a patient may develop iron-deficiency anaemia because of regular bleeding episodes.

Incontinence

Pruritus and minor soiling are relatively common owing to leakage of mucus and liquid faeces from the rectum. This is thought to be due to a poor sealing mechanism owing to displacement of the anal cushions. This may be compounded by a certain amount of sensory impairment in the anal canal. Under most circumstances these symptoms are not particularly disabling but occasionally patients may find them extremely troublesome. If this is the case, then the patient should be fully investigated for incontinence as there may be some other underlying cause (see section on incontinence).

Treatment

The majority of patients with symptomatic haemorrhoids do not need active intervention. Often reassurance after exclusion of serious disease is sufficient. If the patient is finding that constipation or straining is an important feature then bulk laxatives may be of value. Topical ointments may help by providing lubrication but their value is unclear. Active intervention for haemorrhoids can be divided into two broad areas: (1) outpatient procedures and (2) surgery.

Outpatient procedures

Injection sclerotherapy

For many years injection of sclerosant (most commonly 5% phenol in almond or arachis oil) has been used for the treatment of haemorrhoids. This is injected using a long needle via a proctoscope and 3–5 ml of sclerosant should be injected into the submucosa well above the dentate line at each haemorrhoidal site. The underlying aim is to produce a fibrous reaction within the anal cushion to reduce the degree of prolapse. Care must be taken not to inject too superficially, as this will lead to ulceration, or too deeply as this will be ineffective. If the injection is too deep it is also possible to damage the prostate or the seminal vesicles and perirectal sepsis has been reported.

Rubber band ligation

An alternative to injection sclerotherapy is rubber band ligation and indeed in randomized trials it has been shown to be more effective. This involves placing tight rubber bands around the prolapsing cushion at least 1.5 cm above the dentate line. There are various devices for achieving this but most are used via a proctoscope. Perhaps the simplest device is a suction tube to which the band is mounted (Figure 15.18). The mucosa is then sucked into the tube and a special triggering device is used to push the band off the end of the tube. More than one band can be inserted at one time although it may be necessary to repeat the procedure. The surgeon should be very careful to apply the band above the dentate line as failure to do this will lead to immediate severe pain. If this happens it is necessary to remove the band by cutting on to it with the tip of a scalpel blade, and this may sometimes necessitate a general anaesthetic. After the procedure the patients should be warned to expect some bleeding at between 5 and 10 days when the necrotic cushion separates. They may also expect to have some aching which may be relieved by warm baths and non-steroidal anti-inflammatory drugs.

Other outpatient techniques

Bipolar coagulation, infrared photocoagulation, laser photocoagulation and cryotherapy have all been used but none has gained popularity.

The true efficacy of outpatient procedures is not clear. There have been a number of comparative randomized studies which tend to favour rubber band ligation but unfortunately stratification for severity of disease and the use of no-treatment controls has been lacking. There is little doubt that these procedures have a strong placebo effect and further research is required to establish their precise role in the management of haemorrhoids.

Surgery

In patients who have had failed to benefit from outpatient treatment, the surgical approach becomes necessary. In addition there is a feeling among many colorectal surgeons that patients with severely prolapsing haemorrhoids or in whom bleeding is a major concern should have primary surgical intervention. Currently there are two widely used surgical approaches: haemorrhoidectomy and stapled anopexy.

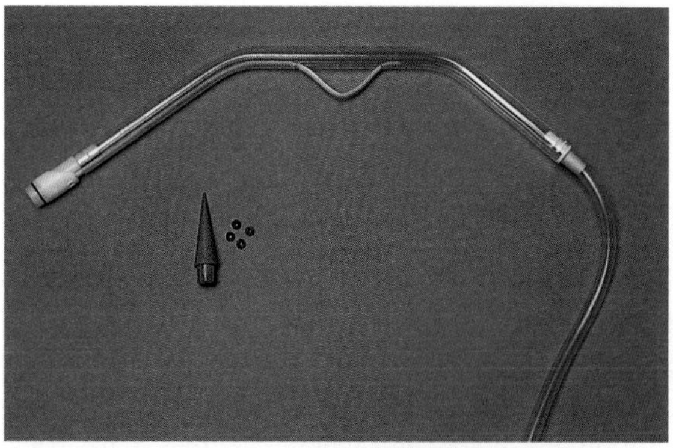

Figure 15.18 Rubber band ligation device for haemorrhoids.

Haemorrhoidectomy

There are many different varieties of haemorrhoidectomy but the basic principle is to excise the prolapsing anal cushions while maintaining mucocutaneous continuity between the areas of excision. The standard technique in many coloproctology centres is to operate on the patient in the prone jack-knife position. Each haemorrhoid is grasped close to the mucocutaneous junction in turn and excised in the plane immediately outside the internal sphincter using diathermy. If this is done carefully the pedicle will merely consist of a thin strip of mucosa and can be transected directly with diathermy although some surgeons still prefer to ligate the pedicle.

Traditionally, after haemorrhoidectomy patients were kept in hospital until their bowels had moved but with careful preparation and community support haemorrhoidectomy can be carried out as a day case. It is even possible to perform the procedure under regional anaesthesia although most British surgeons prefer general anaesthesia. There is good evidence that a regimen including lactulose prior to surgery and a course of metronidazole appears to reduce post-operative pain and facilitates day-case surgery.

Stapled anopexy

The procedure of stapled anopexy has attracted a great deal of interest in the last few years. The principle of this operation is to carry out excision of a circumferential strip of mucosa above the dentate line and to simultaneously close the defect. This pulls the mucosa and therefore the anal cushions back up into their normal position thus restoring the anatomy of the anal canal. This is done using a specially designed proctoscope and circular end-to-end anastomosing stapler.

A purse string is inserted in the rectal mucosa 4 cm above the dentate line, the stapler is inserted and the purse string tightened around the centre rod (Figure 15.19). The stapler is then fired, simultaneously excising the mucosa and stapling the two cut ends together. Immediately after the procedure the staple line must be inspected for bleeding points which can be oversewn. This procedure causes virtually no post-operative discomfort if the staples are placed in the correct position and it can be carried out as a day case with reasonable safety. Initial results seem to indicate at least equivalence with standard haemorrhoidectomy in the majority of cases and with considerably less discomfort. This procedure is still being evaluated however, and in the UK the current recommendation is only to carry out this procedure as part of a randomized trial.

Treatment of complications

The patient with thrombosed painful external haemorrhoids usually requires hospitalization for adequate analgesia and bed rest. Cold compresses applied directly to the haemorrhoids are also beneficial. Surgeons are divided as to whether or not early haemorrhoidectomy should be carried out in these patients and often an

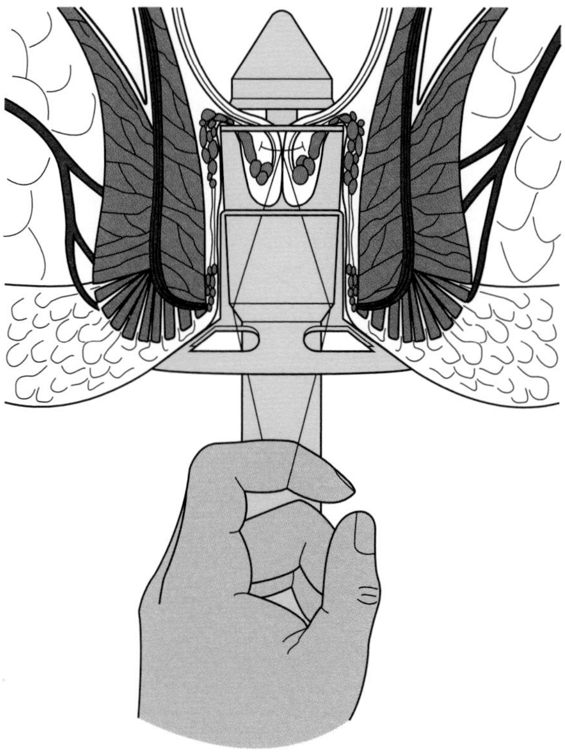

Figure 15.19 Stapled anopexy. Prolapsing rectal mucosa is drawn into a circular stapling gun. Simultaneous exision and stapling draws the anal canal back into an anatomical position.

individual decision has to be made on the basis of the severity of the haemorrhoids. Massive bleeding usually requires haemorrhoidectomy and minor degrees of incontinence usually respond well to haemorrhoidectomy or to stapled anopexy.

Section 15.6 • Perianal sepsis and fistula-*in ano*

Perianal sepsis and fistula formation may be associated with a number of disease processes including Crohn's disease, malignancy, tuberculosis, pilonidal sinus and trauma. In the majority of patients however, the condition is idiopathic.

Pathology and aetiology

Central to current thinking regarding perianal sepsis and fistula formation are the anal glands. These glands are situated in the intersphincteric space and open into the anal canal at the dentate line via a duct which transverses the internal sphincter. The function of these glands is not clear but as they secrete mucin they may have a lubricant function. It is thought these glands may become infected if the duct becomes blocked and when this occurs pus accumulates within the gland. The pus may then tract superiorly, inferiorly, latterly or circumferentially.

Most commonly, the pus will pass downwards in the intersphincteric plane to form a perianal abscess. It may also find its way through the external sphincter into the ischiorectal fossa and thus form an ischiorectal abscess. More rarely the pus may tract up in the intersphincteric plane and form an intersphincteric abcess or discharge down into the ischiorectal fossa through the levator ani muscles (Figure 15.20). When a perianal or ischiorectal abscess discharges through the skin, either spontaneously or as a result of surgical intervention, it may resolve completely. However, if the duct between the gland and the dentate line remains patent and becomes infected, the patient may then be left with a fistulous communication between the dentate line and the skin. According to the mode of spread the fistulous tracts can be classified in the following way (Figure 15.21):

- intersphincteric
- transsphincteric
- suprasphincteric
- extrasphincteric.

Intersphincteric fistulas make up about 50% of all fistulas and usually consist of a straightforward tract between the dentate line and the skin incorporating part of the internal sphincter. However, some of these can have a high intersphincteric extension and even a high opening into the rectum.

Transsphincteric fistulas account for about 30% and consist of a tract passing through the external sphincter. This may be low or high and occasionally may be associated with a blind high tract in the ischiorectal fossa which may even penetrate the levator ani muscles.

Suprasphincteric fistulas run above the puborectalis muscle and then descend down through the levator ani muscles into the ischiorectal fossa.

Extrasphincteric fistulas bypass the sphincter complex completely and extend from the lower rectum through the levator ani muscles and into the ischiorectal fossa.

This classification is important as it has implications for treatment.

Clinical features

The patient with a perianal sepsis usually presents with severe perianal pain, fever and malaise. The abscess may discharge spontaneously, but because of the severity of symptoms patients often present at hospital before this has occurred. On examination a perianal abscess is usually very obvious as a tender red swelling at the anal margin. The ischiorectal abscess however may be quite deep seated and more difficult to detect on clinical examination although pressure on the ischiorectal fossa will usually give rise to severe pain. In an advanced ischiorectal abscess a large area of tender induration will be seen. Occasionally a patient may present with an intersphincteric abscess which has not pointed at the anal canal and this can be very difficult to detect clinically. Thus in the patient with a severe acute anal or

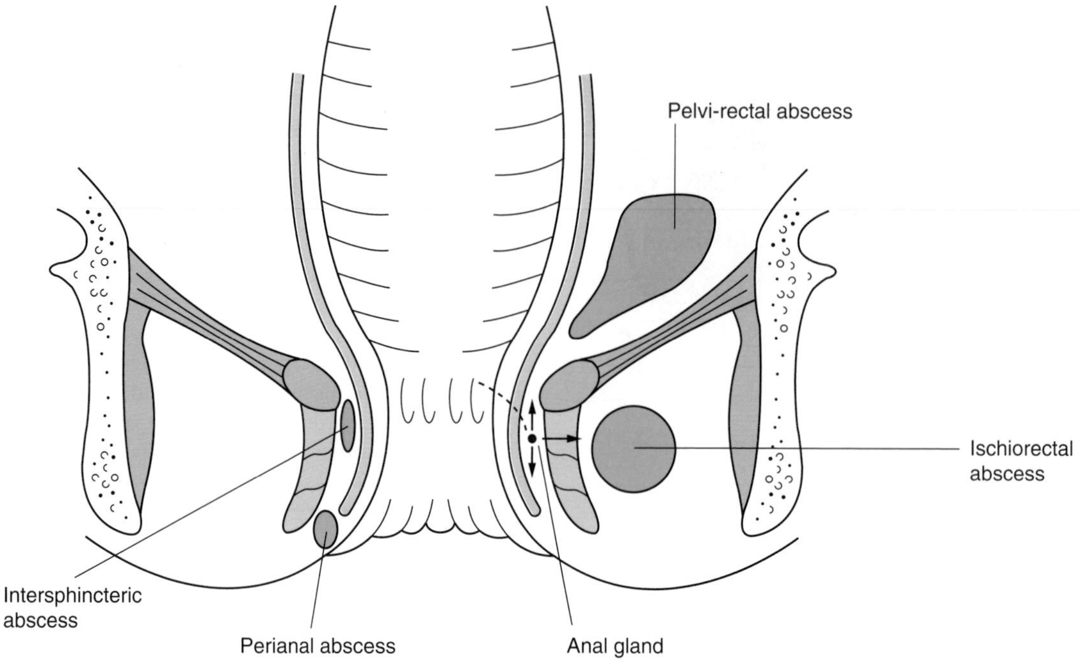

Figure 15.20 Anorectal abscesses.

perianal pain an examination under anaesthetic should be carried out. If there is an intersphincteric abscess this will be felt as induration through the rectal wall.

A fistula may present after discharge or incision of an abscess usually after all the inflammation and induration has settled down. Alternatively, there may be no history of abcess formation and the fistula may appear to arise *de novo*. The main symptoms are of discharge and pruritus, although occasionally a patient may notice the passage of flatus through a fistula track. There may also be a history of recurring episodes of pain relieved by discharge from the fistula.

On examination a punctate opening (or openings) can be seen, usually close to the anal verge although

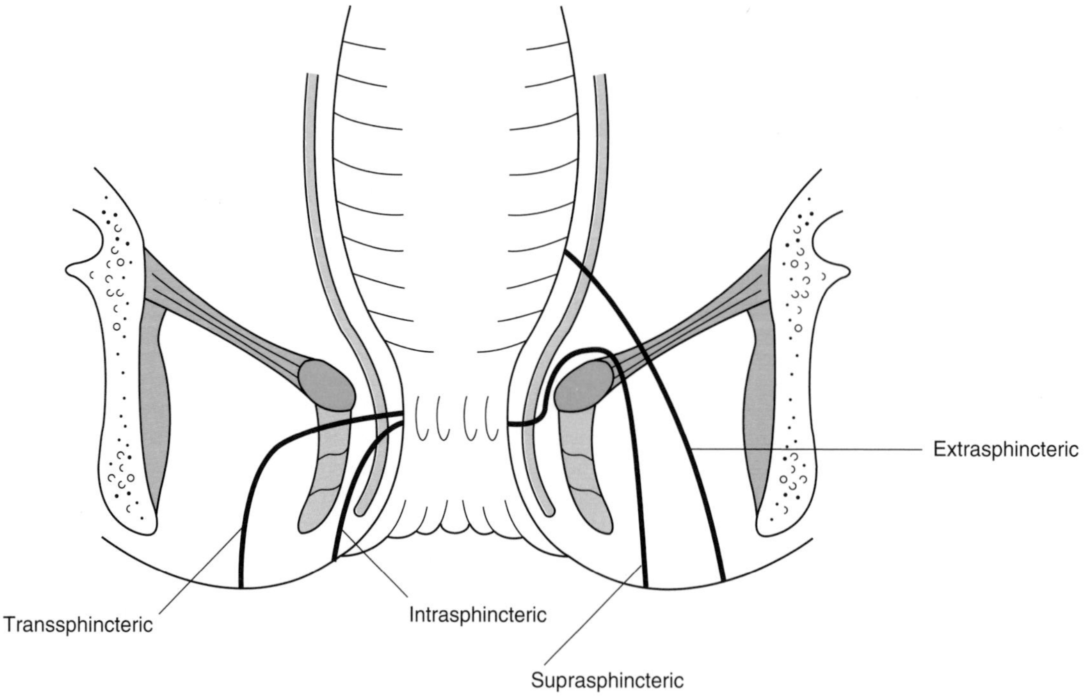

Figure 15.21 Anorectal fistulas.

sometimes a few centimetres away. Pus or serosanguinous discharge may been seen exuding from the opening particularly if digital pressure is applied over the fistula. Careful firm palpation between the opening and the anal canal will often reveal the fistulous track as a subcutaneous 'cord'. Goodsall's rule (Figure 15.22) is useful when estimating the course of a fistula; this states that if a fistulous opening is posterior to an imaginary line drawn transversely through the middle of the anus, the track will curve round so that it opens into the dentate line in the posterior midline, whereas if the opening is anterior, the track will be radial (i.e. follows a straight line from the opening to the dentate line). The main exception to this rule is the anterior opening which is 3 or more centimetres from the anal verge, as this may be 'horse-shoeing' round from the posterior midline.

Diagnosis

The diagnosis of an abscess is usually made clinically, and its exact position relative to the sphincter complex is made at operation. Likewise, the course of a fistula is usually established by examining the patient under general anaesthesia using specially designed fistula probes. The most widely used probes are those designed by Lockhart-Mummery; these are available in a variety of configurations, and the most useful are slightly curved (Figure 15.23). The flat handle allows for precise manoeuvring of the probe, and the groove is useful for laying the fistula open (see below).

Under normal circumstances it is relatively easy to pass the probe from the external opening along the tract to the internal opening at the dentate line (Figure 15.24). In doing this it is important not to use too much force, as it is possible to create a false tract in so doing. If it proves to be impossible to find the internal opening using this technique a valuable manoeuvre is to instil a very small amount of hydrogen peroxide into the external opening by means of a fine cannula. With an Eisenhammer retractor in place within the anal canal it is then usually possible to see bubbles appearing appearing at the site of the internal opening. This will guide further probing. In the process of probing a fistula it is important to look for extensions to the main tract. Indeed, if the probe cannot easily pass along the tract it is probably falling into a blind extension bypassing the main tract.

Although examination under anaesthetic with probing is the most useful diagnostic approach, some forms of imaging may also be of value. Fistulography has been used in the past, and is still important if an extrasphincteric fistula is suspected. However, under

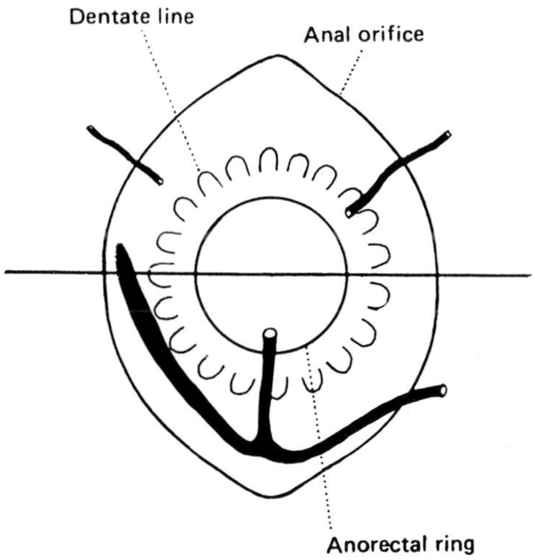

Figure 15.22 Goodsall's rule related to anal fistulas suggests that fistulas, with an external opening anterior to a line drawn horizontally through the anal canal, progress forwards in a radial fashion, whereas fistulas with external opening posterior to the horizontal line curve backwards and ultimately have an internal opening in the midline posteriorly. It is possible for fistulas to extend laterally on both sides, leading to the characteristic horse-shoe fistulas.

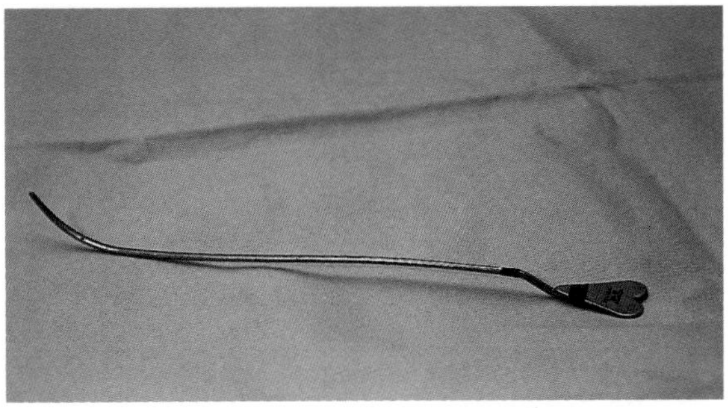

Figure 15.23 Lockhart-Mummery fistula probe.

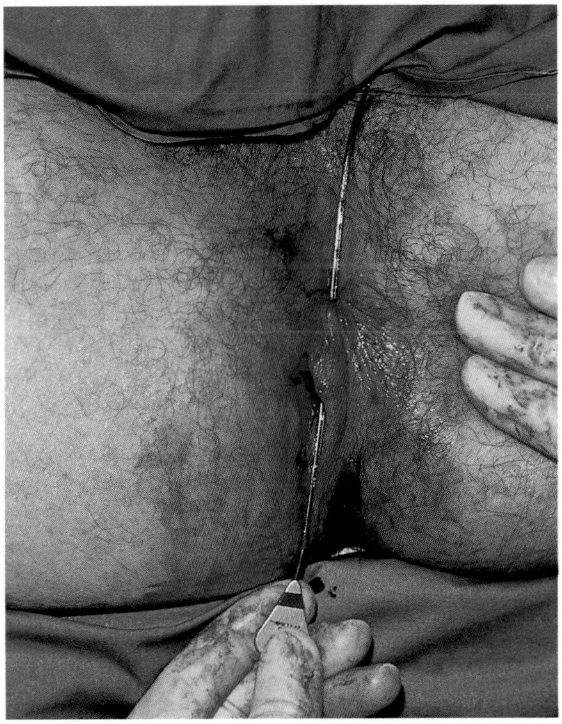

Figure 15.24 Probe in a fistula-*in ano*.

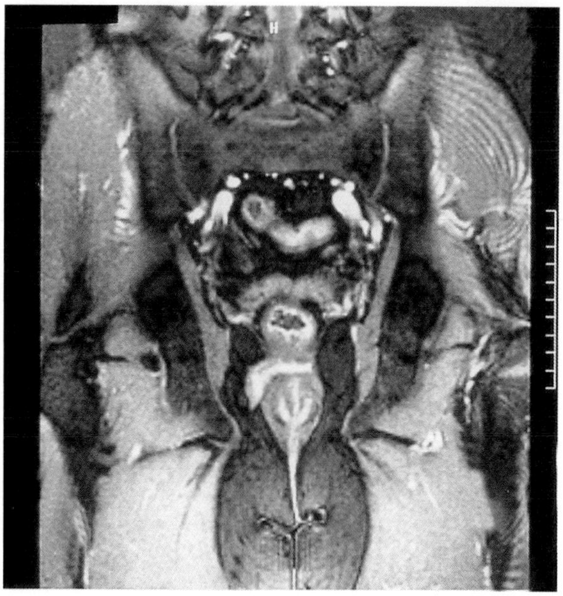

Figure 15.25 MRI scan of a fistula-*in ano*. The fistula is seen as a white track curving around the anal canal. (Courtesy of Dr Declan Shephard, Ninewells Hospital, Dundee, Scotland.)

most circumstances it does not yield particularly useful information. More recently the use of magnetic resonance imaging (MRI) has been finding a place in the evaluation of fistula-*in ano* (Figure 15.25). It appears to be particularly useful in complex fistulas with secondary extensions and abscesses and while it is perhaps no more accurate than an examination under anaesthetic by an experienced coloproctologist, a high-quality MRI of the sphincter complex may be useful as a 'road map' to guide the surgeon. Transanal ultrasound and anorectal physiology studies have been used in evaluation of fistula-*in ano* but have not found a routine place in the management of this condition.

Treatment

The initial treatment of a perianal or ischiorectal abscess which is pointing on to the skin is fairly straightforward. The abscess cavity should be incised and drained and an opening in the skin made which is large enough to allow continued drainage of the abscess. It is customary to place ribbon gauze soaked in antiseptic into the abscess cavity but it should not be packed tightly as this makes it uncomfortable for the patient and actually impedes drainage of the abscess cavity. Post-operatively the dressing should be changed daily in hospital until it can be managed by a district nurse. The patient should always be followed up at outpatients to look for the development of a fistula when the cavity itself has healed. One of the complications of incision and drainage of a perianal or ischiorectal abscess is the iatrogenic production of a high fistula by overenthusiastic curetting of the abscess cavity. This must be avoided at all costs.

The best treatment for fistula-*in ano* is undoubtedly laying open of the entire tract, curetting out of the granulation tissue and leaving the wound to granulate. This is done most easily by cutting down on to the groove on the concave aspect of the fistula probe, and then using a small Volkmann's spoon to curette. Some surgeons will marsupialize the tract by suturing the divided wound edge to the edges of the fibrous tract and this is said to result in faster healing. Laying open is perfectly safe with a simple intersphincteric fistula as the only muscle which will be divided will be the lower part of the internal sphincter. If, however, the fistula is transsphincteric then laying it open creates a risk of incontinence. Laying open of a suprasphincteric or extrasphincteric fistua will inevitably result in complete incontinence.

In the case of a low transsphincteric fistula which only involves a small part of the lower external sphincter, laying open is relatively safe. However, at the time of the initial examination it is important to assess exactly how much of the external sphincter is involved. It is therefore safer to establish drainage of the fistula by inserting a seton through the fistula tract. This can simply be a length of suture material or a vascular sling loosely tied. When the patient is awake after the procedure it is then easier to assess the anal sphincter and if the surgeon is confident that only a small part of the external sphincter is involved the patient can go back for laying open of the fistula.

If, however, a significant part of the external sphincter muscle is involved or if the fistula proves to be suprasphincteric then a more conservative approach must be taken. The most widely used approach is to ensure complete drainage of all the sepsis and to leave the seton in place for several weeks. When all the sepsis and inflammation has resolved the seton can then be removed and this will result in healing in about 50% of cases. If this fails then the seton must be reinserted and a careful discussion with the patient must take place. If laying open of the fistula will leave some external sphincter muscle intact then this is a feasible option as long as the patient is aware that a certain degree of incontinence may result.

Another approach is to use the so-called cutting seton where the seton is tied tightly and gradually cuts its way through the fistula tract leaving fibrosis behind it. This approach may be successful but does result in some degree of incontinence in about 60% of cases. Yet another approach for the transsphincteric fistula is fistulectomy and advancement flap repair. Here the fistula tract is excised by dissecting up through the external sphincter muscle. A flap of mucosa and internal sphincter is then raised above the internal opening and sutured down over it. This is successful in some cases but does not appear to carry any advantages over simple insertion of a seton and subsequent removal. The use of fibrin glue following fistulotomy appears to give good results in some hands.

With a high transsphincteric fistula or suprasphincteric fistula incontinence is inevitable with laying open, and one approach is to give the patient a temporary colostomy, lay open the fistula and then carry out a sphincter repair after healing has taken place. Alternatively the patient may be happy to live with a long-term seton in place, and this is also an option in patients with a high transsphincteric fistula.

The extrasphincteric fistula, which is usually secondary to Crohn's disease or trauma, is particularly difficult to deal with and particularly in Crohn's disease it may be better to avoid surgical interference. In such patients a long-term seton may be the answer and some patients may require a defunctioning colostomy. After resolution of the sepsis laying open of the fistula and subsequent sphincter repair may be possible but the ultimate results can be less than ideal.

Section 15.7 • Pilonidal sinus and abscess

Pilonidal sinus is a condition which occurs almost exclusively in the natal cleft of young males. It is characterized by multiple subcutaneous sinuses and abscess cavities containing hair.

Aetiology and pathology

There is very little evidence for a congenital origin in this condition and current consensus favours an acquired mechanism. It is thought that frictional forces generated in the depths of the natal cleft tend to drive hairs subcutaneously where they generate a foreign body reaction. Secondary infection may compound the problem leading to abscess formation.

Clinical features

Pilonidal sinus may be asymptomatic and only present on routine inspection. However, if the sinuses become infected the patient may have pain and discharge in the natal cleft. On examination there are a variable number of pits seen in the upper natal cleft (Figure 15.26) and in active inflammatory disease these may be seen to be exuding pus. When an abscess forms there will be a red tender swelling just to one side of the natal cleft. Although the appearances are typical occasionally a pilonidal sinus may be mistaken for a fistula-*in ano* and vice versa. The diagnosis is made on clinical grounds and specific investigations are not generally required.

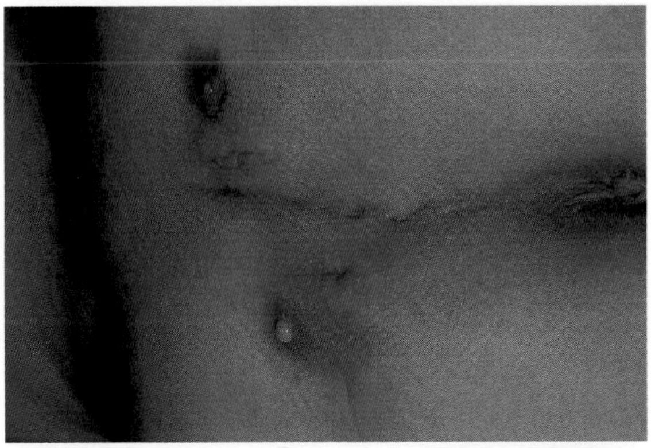

Figure 15.26 Pilonidal sinus. Midline pits in the natal cleft with distant fistulous openings. (Courtesy of Mr RAB Wood, Ninewells Hospital, Dundee, Scotland.)

Treatment

If asymptomatic pits are found then no treatment is required. If a patient presents with a pilonidal abscess then this should be incised and drained, and the patient kept under review until the wound has healed. The most difficult situation to treat is the patient with chronic discharging sinuses, and this requires a fairly radical surgical approach.

The most widely favoured procedure is excision of the sinus bearing area down to the deep fascia and removal of all sinuses and nests of hair. Surgical opinion is then divided as to whether this should be left open to granulate or whether primary closure should be attempted. If the latter approach is employed a proportion of the wounds will break down and healing by secondary intention will be necessary. In a patient who has pits which are some distance from the main disease in the natal cleft an elliptical excision of the main area may be carried out in association with 'coring out' of the long extensions. These need to be left open to heal by secondary intention. The long-term recurrence rate after excision of pilonidal sinus is in the region of 20%.

Section 15.8 • Hydradenitis suppurativa

Apocrine glands are found in certain zones including the axillae, the inguinoscrotal and perianal regions and the breasts. These glands develop from hair follicles and discharge a thick secretion into the follicle or on to the adjacent skin. As they are not active until puberty, inflammation of these glands (hydradenitis) does not usually appear until the third decade. Clinically the affected area becomes indurated then forms sinuses with the discharge of small amounts of pus. Although the axillae are the most predominantly affected areas the perianal region is involved in about 30%. When severe, treatment requires excision of the affected skin and subcutaneous tissue down to the deep fascia and when extensive, split skin grafting in necessary to provide cover. If the perianal region is extensively affected it may be necessary to carry out a temporary defunctioning colostomy to allow excision and skin grafting.

Section 15.9 • Perianal Crohn's disease

Anywhere between 30% and 70% of patients with Crohn's disease may have some involvement of the anal canal. This is more common in patients with colonic and particularly rectal Crohn's disease but it may occur in isolation or in association with Crohn's disease elsewhere in the gastrointestinal tract.

Table 15.3 Classification of Crohn's perianal lesions (after Hughes)

Primary lesions	
	Anal fissure
	Oedematous piles
	Ulceration
Secondary lesions	
	Skin tags
	Anal stricture
	Perianal abscess and fistula
	Anovaginal and rectovaginal fistula
	Carcinoma
Incidental lesions	
	Piles
	Skin tags
	Perianal sepsis
	Hidradenitis suppurativa

The perianal lesions are variable and have been classified by Hughes (Table 15.3) and according to this classification the primary lesions consist of anal fissure, ulcerated oedematous haemorrhoids and deep ulceration of the anal canal or lower rectum. These can lead to the secondary lesions of oedematous skin tags, anal or rectal stricturing, perianal abscess and fistula formation and rectovaginal or anovaginal fistula. It must also be remembered that Crohn's disease is potentially a pre-malignant condition and carcinoma of the rectum or anal canal may complicate this disease.

The severity of perianal Crohn's disease is highly variable and may cause only minor irritation. On the other hand in a patient with multiple fistulas ('watering can' anus) the severity of the symptoms may necessitate proctectomy. When assessing perianal Crohn's disease, examination under anaesthetic is the best approach although MRI may be of value.

The management of perianal Crohn's disease is conservative where at all possible. Metronidazole is widely used and ciprofloxacin has recently been associated with good results. Azathioprine, cyclosporin and anti-tumour necrosis factor antibodies have also been used. Surgical intervention is recommended for eradication of sepsis and this involves draining abscesses and inserting setons into fistulas. Frequently the fistulas are high and may be extrasphincteric so that laying open of a Crohn's fistula is usually contraindicated. Occasionally with severe disease, proctectomy is necessary but this should only be carried out after sepsis has been controlled; otherwise an infected perineal sinus is likely to result. Rectovaginal and rectoanal fistulas are particularly distressing and some surgeons will attempt repair with advancement flaps.

Section 15.10 • Anal fissure

An anal fissure is a linear ulcer which occurs in the anal canal just distal to the dentate line. This may be caused by Crohn's disease or trauma but most commonly it is a primary condition. It affects both men and women and the highest incidence is in the third and forth decades of life. It may occur soon after pregnancy and vaginal delivery.

Aetiology and pathology

The initiating factors in anal fissure are unclear although minor anal trauma caused by passage of a constipated stool has been suggested. The main underlying pathology, however, appears to be a high resting anal pressure caused by increased internal sphincter tone. The blood supply to the anal canal has to pass through the internal sphincter and therefore spasm of this muscle reduces the blood flow and the oxygen tension in the skin of the anal canal. Interestingly, the fissures tend to occur at the watershed of the blood supply, i.e. the anterior and posterior midline in women and the posterior midline in men.

Clinical features

The typical clinical features are of pain on defecation associated with bright red bleeding. This may be associated with pruritus ani and mucus discharge. On examination there is usually a skin tag overlying the fissure and the fissure itself can be seen by everting the anal canal using lateral traction (Figure 15.27). This will reveal a sharply defined ulcer and it may be possible to see the lower fibres of the internal sphincter at its base. Digital rectal examination or proctoscopy should not be attempted in the conscious patient as this will cause considerable discomfort.

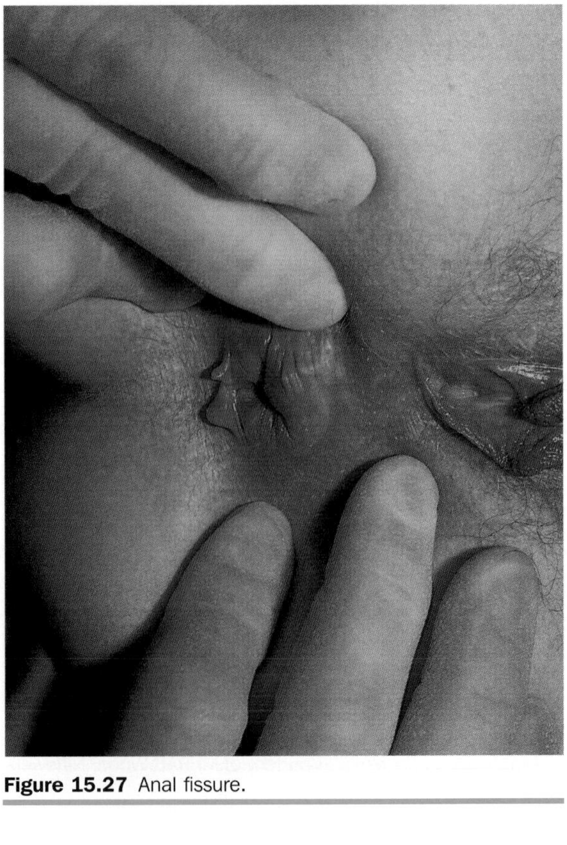

Figure 15.27 Anal fissure.

Diagnosis

In terms of making a diagnosis this is done clinically but it is important to exclude other conditions such as Crohn's disease or malignancy. This can be established by examination under anaesthesia and biopsy where appropriate.

Treatment

The underlying principle of treating anal fissures is to reduce the internal anal sphincter tone. In patients with minimal symptoms this may be achieved by topical application of a local anaesthetic and bulk laxatives. In patients with more severe symptoms however, the use of 0.2% glyceryl trinitrate (GTN) cream applied 2 or 3 times a day can produce healing of fissures in about 50% of cases.

If medical treatment fails then a surgical approach becomes necessary. Previously, forced anal dilatation was recommended and although effective this was associated with an unacceptable level of incontinence. The surgical treatment of choice is now a lateral sphincterotomy which involves dividing the internal sphincter at one point on the lateral wall of the anal canal up to the level of the dentate line. This is achieved by inserting a Park's anal retractor so that the internal sphincter is stretched and easily palpable. A small incision is then made on the lateral aspect of the anal canal just below the internal sphincter. Using scissors the intersphincteric plane is developed as is the plane between the anal skin and the internal sphincter. The scissors are then used to divide the sphincter and bleeding is controlled by firm finger pressure. Lateral sphincterotomy is said to be successful in about 95% of cases but patients should be warned that it can be associated with minor degrees of incontinence to flatus or mucus.

Section 15.11 • Pruritus ani

Pruritus ani or perianal itching is a common condition. There are a large number of anorectal and dermatological conditions which may give rise to this symptom but in the vast majority it is idiopathic. The primary cause is probably minor anal leakage as the result of internal sphincter dysfunction. This sets up an irritation which is exacerbated by brisk cleansing or scratching. This may then introduce fungal infection which intensifies the pruritus.

When taking a history it is particularly important to establish if the family includes small children as this would predispose to enterobius infestation (threadworm). On examination the perineal skin should be closely inspected to look for signs of dermatological disease. In idiopathic pruritus there is typically perianal excoriation and ichthyosis. Digital examination of the rectum should be carried out in order to assess the anal tone and proctoscopy to look for the presence of haemorrhoids. Perianal lesions or areas of abnormal skin should be biopsied and where appropriate skin scrapings should be examined for fungal infestation.

If enterobius infestation is suspected the Sellotape test should be carried out. This involves placing adhesive tape over the anus and then transferring it to a glass microscope slide. Histological examination will subsequently reveal the presence of ova which have been deposited on the perianal skin.

The treatment of pruritus ani depends on any underlying cause. Prolapsing haemorrhoids, anal polyps and skin tags should be treated surgically. Enterobius infestation can be treated using mebendazole. If there is a primary skin condition the patient should be referred to a dermatologist. In the case of idiopathic pruritus advice should be given in order to minimize anal leakage and damage to the perianal skin. This involves dietary modification to reduce excessive flatulence or loose stool. The patient should also be advised to keep as clean and dry as possible and to avoid scratching. When the pruritus is intense and particularly if a fungal infection is suspected then a cream containing steroid and an antifungal agent (e.g. Lotriderm) can be used in the short term to break the cycle of itching and scratching.

Section 15.12 • Perianal warts

Perianal warts or anal condylomata are caused by infection with human papilloma virus (HPV) and is a sexually transmitted disease. It is found in between 40% and 70% of homosexual men. Subtypes of the virus which are implicated in the development of these lesions are 6, 11, 16 and 18. The most common is subtype 6 but subtypes 16 and 18 are important in that they are associated with a high incidence of dysplasia and malignant transformation. In women about 80% will have associated warts on the external genitalia, vagina or cervix and about 20% of men will have warts on the penis.

Clinically, the patients tend to present with perianal itching and bleeding, and on examination warts are seen in the perianal region with varying degrees of confluence (Figure 15.28). In patients with the acquired immunodeficiency syndrome (AIDS), the warts tend to form a dense confluent sheet.

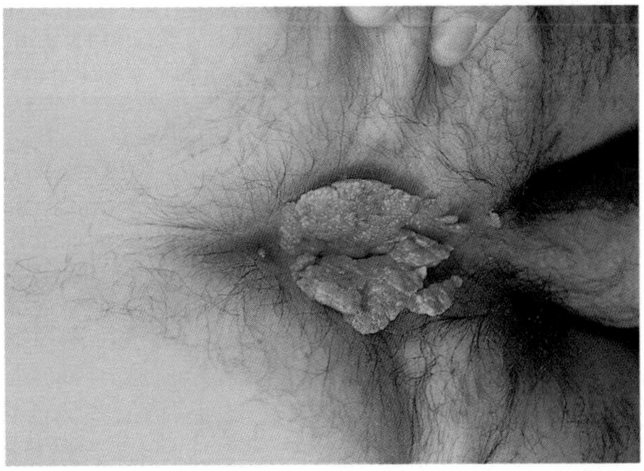

Figure 15.28 Perianal warts.

There are various methods of treatment, and for relatively mild disease with isolated warts, 25% podophyllin applied in either liquid paraffin or tincture of benzoin can be applied. Intervening normal skin should be avoided as podophyllin is very irritant and may give rise to skin necrosis. In general, although podophyllin treatment is effective the results are not as good as surgical excision which is the preferred method.

Excision involves operating on the patient in the prone jack-knife or lithotomy position and a 1:200 000 solution of adrenaline is injected subcutaneously. By causing swelling in the perianal skin, this separates the warts and they can be excised individually with scissors. The rate of recurrence after complete excision of all perianal warts is in the region of 10%. Unfortunately, this approach can be difficult when the warts are extremely confluent and it may be necessary to resort to electrocoagulation or cryotherapy. Both of these result in quite severe tissue damage and anal stenosis is a possible complication. Recently, an autologus vaccine prepared from the patient's own warts has been described and this appears to be highly effective not only in eradicating the warts but also in reducing the rate of recurrence. Interferon has also been used to good effect.

Anal intraepithelial neoplasia (AIN)

As is the case with perianal warts, AIN is caused by HPV and appears to be sexually transmitted. HPV types 6, 11, 16, 18, 31 and 33 can all be implicated. On histological examination epithelial dysplasia is seen and this is graded as 1–3 according to the epithelial depth of dysplasia. Thus, in grade 1 only the upper third is affected, in grade 2 the upper two-thirds and in grade three the whole thickness of the epithelium is dysplastic. Grade 3 AIN is also classified as carcinoma-*in situ*.

Clinically, the patients present with perianal discomfort, itching and bleeding and on examination the perianal epithelium is thickened and may have a whitish appearance. This may be exaggerated by the application of acetic acid which is useful in targeting areas for biopsy. In women it is important to appreciate that AIN may be associated with similar intraepithelial neoplasia of the cervix (CIN), vulva (VIN) and vagina (VAIN) and affected patients should be investigated appropriately.

The main risk associated with AIN is the development of invasive squamous carcinoma of the anus, and the treatment and follow-up of patients must be directed towards early detection of such a lesion. Unfortunately, surgical excision is not effective in eradicating the virus and for patients with AIN 1 or 2, a simple policy of regular observation is probably regarded as adequate. However, for AIN 3 the risk of developing carcinoma is thought to be much higher and if there is a small affected area then surgical excision would seem to be appropriate. However, where there is a large circumferential area of AIN 3, treatment is much more difficult. Some have recommended complete excision of the affected area with split skin grafting. However, this requires the formation of defunctioning colostomy and is associated with a high risk of anal stenosis. In addition it does not effectively eradicate the virus. Currently, therefore, it is recommended that such patients be followed up 6 monthly with careful inspection and biopsy with intervention only if invasive malignancy develops.

Section 15.13 • Anal cancer

Anal cancer only accounts for about 5% of all carcinomas of the large bowel and it is nearly always a squamous carcinoma. Rarely adenocarcinoma may be seen but this is usually a very low rectal cancer which is involving the anal canal. Another very rare condition is malignant melanoma of the anal canal. This section however will deal exclusively with squamous carcinoma. Histologically anal cancer is termed epidermoid and this may be subclassified as squamous cell, basaloid (or cloacogenic) or mucoepidermoid. This classification does not appear to have any prognostic significance. Local spread of an anal cancer tends to occur proximally and radially into the rectum and anal sphincters. In advanced cases it may also involve the vagina. Lymphatic spread is to the perirectal and inguinal lymph nodes. Distant metastases occur most frequently in liver, lung and bones but this is usually associated with advanced local disease.

Aetiology

It is now clear that the majority of anal cancers are associated with HPV infection although not all patients will have a clear cut history of perianal warts or AIN. The carcinogenic factors involved are not clear but immunosuppression or human immunodeficiency virus (HIV) infection appears to increase the incidence of anal cancer.

Clinical features

Patients tend to present with anal pain and bleeding and some will notice a mass in the anal canal. On examination the typical appearance is of a malignant ulcer at the anal margin or within the anal canal (Figure 15.29). It is also important to examine the inguinal region, although when inguinal lymph nodes are enlarged only about 50% will have metastatic spread on histological examination.

Investigation

Clearly the most important investigation is biopsy of the anal lesion but examination under anaesthetic is extremely important in evaluating the extent of disease. Ultrasound scanning may be useful in assessing involvement of the anal sphincters, and fine needle aspiration biopsy of enlarged inguinal lymph nodes is a useful staging investigation.

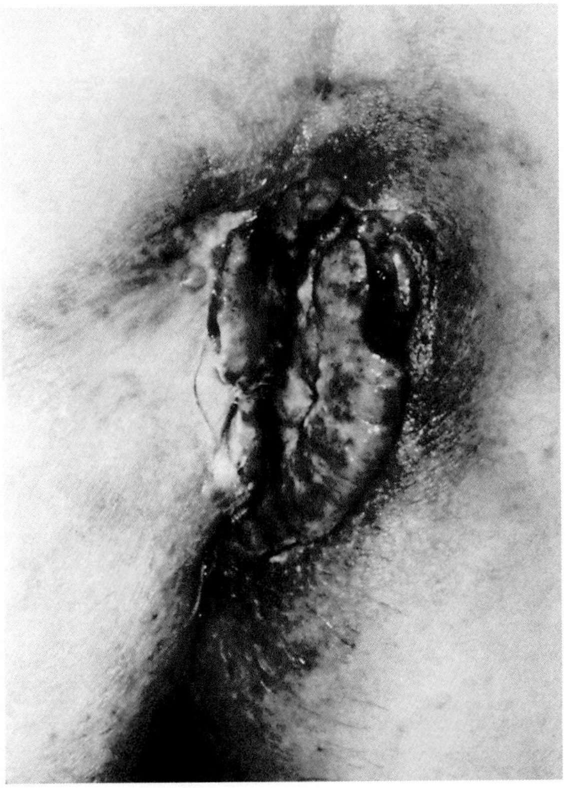

Figure 15.29 An advanced squamous cell carcinoma of the anal margin is demonstrated.

Treatment

For small mobile lesions at the anal margin the best treatment is still local excision but for larger lesions current recommendations for primary treatment consist of radiotherapy combined with chemotherapy (intravenous 5-fluorouracil plus mitomycin). This has been demonstrated to be preferable to radiotherapy alone in a recent randomized trial.

Surgery, however, retains an important role in the treatment of anal cancer. About 35% of patients undergoing combined radiochemotherapy will either experience recurrence or fail to fully respond to the treatment. In this case, radical surgery in the form of abdominoperineal excision of rectum is necessary. In addition, some patients may have such a debilitating tumour that defunctioning colostomy is necessary while they are having the radiochemotherapy. There is also a role for surgery in the treatment of inguinal lymph node metastases. If the nodes are found to be involved at the time of initial diagnosis there is some controversy regarding whether they should be treated by radiotherapy or radical groin dissection. If however lymph node metastases occur some time after primary therapy, it is generally agreed that radical groin dissection is clearly indicated and is associated with a 5 year survival in the region of 50%.

Further reading

Alexander-Williams, J. (1983). Pruritus ani. *BMJ* **287**: 159–60.

Henry, M. M. and Swash, M. (eds) (1985). *Coloproctology and the Pelvic Floor*. London: Butterworths.

Oliveira, L., Pfeifer, J. and Wexner, S. D. (1996). Physiological and clinical outcome of anterior sphincteroplasty. *Br J Surg* **83**: 502–5.

Parks, A. G., Gordon, P. N. and Hardcastle, J. D. (1976). A classification of fistula-in-ano. *Br J Surg* **63**: 1–12.

Phillips, R. K. S. and Lunniss, P. J. (1996). *Anal Fistula. Surgical Evaluation and Management*. London: Chapman & Hall.

Rowell, M., Bello, M. and Hemingway, D. M. (2000). Circumferential mucosectomy (stapled haemorrhoidectomy) versus conventional haemorrhoidectomy: randomised controlled trial. *Lancet* **355**: 779–81.

Wong, W. D., Jensen, L. L., Bartolo, D. C. and Rothenberger, D. A. (1996). Artificial anal sphincter. *Dis Colon Rectum* **39**: 1345–51.

MODULE 16

Vascular physiology

Transport between different areas of multi-cellular organisms is essential. This is generally accomplished by means of a vascular tree which, in all higher animals, has evolved into a highly efficient mechanism. An understanding of the structure and function of the vascular system is indispensable when treating patients with vascular disease and can help predict the success or otherwise of surgical manoeuvres. After briefly reviewing the anatomy and pathology of the peripheral vascular system (excluding the heart) this module will examine vascular physiology and how it relates to clinical practice.

Section 16.1 • Anatomy

The division of the vascular tree into arteries, veins and the microcirculation has been well known since William Harvey's time. On a microscopic level the structure of all these components follows a similar plan – the intima, the media and the adventitia – with variations reflecting function. All have a luminal lining comprising a single layer of endothelium.

Arteries

The major arteries are divided into those with primarily a transporting function (the elastic arteries) and those with primarily a distributive function (the muscular arteries). The elastic arteries such as the aorta and its major branches have a fairly complex intima comprising endothelium, several layers of elastin (the elastic laminae), smooth muscle cells and fibroblasts. In contrast, the intima of muscular arteries comprises simply the endothelium and a single elastic lamina. The media again reflects the functional difference between the two types of artery. It is predominantly comprised of elastic laminae with a few smooth muscle cells in elastic arteries and of smooth muscle cells with some elastin in muscular arteries. The adventitia is a layer of connective tissue and is thicker in muscular arteries than it is in elastic arteries. It provides up to 60% of the strength of the vessel, an important point to remember when suturing. The vasa vasorum penetrate into the media of both types of artery. The elastic arteries are well able to cope with rapid expansion during systole and their elastic recoil helps maintain blood pressure during diastole. The walls of muscular arteries contract and dilate as appropriate to help direct blood flow as required.

Microcirculation

As the muscular arteries branch successively they become smaller, and at the size of 0.1 mm they are called arterioles. These are characterized by an intima consisting of endothelium with a distinct elastic lamina and a media with one or two helical layers of smooth muscle. The adventitial connective tissue is thin. The thickness of an arteriolar wall is similar to that of its lumen. Some capillaries branch directly off arterioles and flow through them is controlled by a pre-capillary sphincter. More capillaries, however, originate off metarterioles (Figure 16.1). These are direct communications between arterioles and venules; they differ from arterioles in not having an intimal elastic lamina and in only having a discontinuous smooth muscle layer in the media. Capillaries branching off metarterioles are again regulated by pre-capillary sphincters. Flow through capillaries is well regulated and some capillary beds may be completely closed off at times; the metarterioles then act as arterio-venous shunts. As well as regulating blood flow through local capillary beds, the arterioles play an important role in overall vascular tone and so blood pressure control.

Capillaries have a diameter of 8–10 μm. Their endothelium is generally continuous (as in the rest of the vascular tree), although in specialized areas such as renal glomeruli there are fenestrations allowing more rapid transfer. They have no media and effectively no adventitia.

Veins

The venous side of the circulation is primarily characterized by its capacitance. This is reflected in the widely varying diameters of these vessels and in the absence of

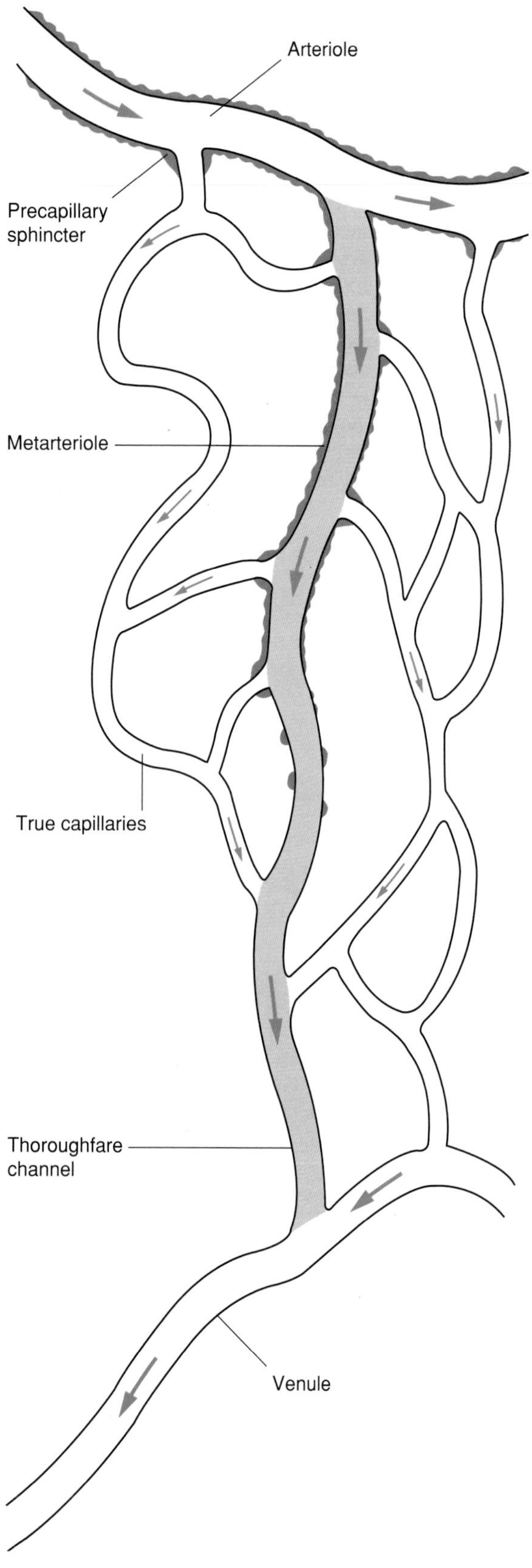

Figure 16.1 Schematic representation of the microcirculation. (From Cormack, D.H. *Clinically Integrated Histology*, 1998, page 135, Figure 5-18. Lippincott-Raven, Philadelphia, PA, USA.)

elastic tissue which would resist dilation. Venules collect blood from capillaries; their intima comprises endothelium only, their media a single layer of smooth muscle cells and their adventitia is very thin. They can vary in size from 8 to 100 μm. As venules combine, veins are eventually formed. In addition to endothelium, venous intima has a connective tissue component which becomes more important as the vein size increases. While large veins (such as the pelvic veins and inferior vena cava) have no valves, small and medium sized veins have semilunar valves to direct flow. The media of veins comprises smooth muscle cells while the adventitia is a relatively thick layer of connective tissue. As with arteries, vasa vasorum penetrate into the media.

Structure is therefore closely related to function across the whole vascular tree. In studying the applied physiology of the vascular system, however, it is not only normal structure that is involved. Atherosclerosis, the most common arterial disease, significantly affects arterial function. An understanding of this process is therefore important.

Section 16.2 • Atherosclerosis

The well-known derivation of 'atheroma' from the Greek for porridge relates to the advanced atheromatous plaque comprising, among other things, extracellular lipid. It is now recognized, however, that the early genesis of atheromatous plaques closely involves the endothelium and migration of cells into the intima. Much work is being carried out to elucidate the processes involved, with possible therapeutic potential in the future.

The primary event in plaque formation is endothelial dysfunction or damage. The well-known risk factors for atherosclerosis (diabetes, hypertension, smoking, low-density lipoprotein (LDL) cholesterol, homocysteine, loss of oestrogen) are directly involved at this level. Through changes in cell adhesion molecule expression monocytes, T-lymphocytes and LDL cholesterol bind to the endothelium and then transmigrate into the intima. A variety of cytokines and growth factors are then produced by the T-lymphocytes and monocytes. Endothelial dysfunction results in abnormalities of nitric oxide production with consequently diminished vasodilation. At this stage the lesion has the appearance of a fatty streak – a yellow minimally raised lesion, not uncommonly found at a young age.

As the process progresses smooth muscle cells migrate from the media into the intima. They accumulate lipid and develop the microscopic appearance of foam cells. Monocytes also continue to accumulate in the intima where they take on the phenotype of macrophages and accumulate lipid to become monocyte derived foam cells. The continuing production of cytokines and growth factors stimulates the cellular component of the plaque to produce an extracellular matrix of collagen, proteoglycans, elastin and glycoproteins. As lipid continues to accumulate in the plaque it becomes deposited in the extra-cellular matrix. At this

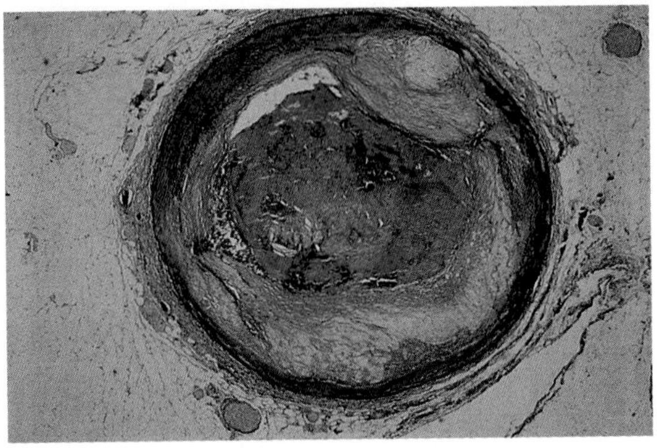

Figure 16.2 Atheromatous plaque with thrombosis nearly occluding the lumen.

stage the lesion is known as a fibrous plaque, with the fibrous component forming a 'cap' over a lipid core (Figure 16.2). The cellular component tends to lie between the fibrous cap and the lipid core. It is possible to see periarterial inflammation and even fibrosis.

Plaques are initially limited to the intima and can be of a very varied composition, with some being predominantly cellular while others have a significant fatty centre. With plaque enlargement there is extension into the media and the luminal cross-sectional area decreases. There is an initial compensatory enlargement of the whole vessel which results in a maintained blood flow. Eventually, however, this compensation is overwhelmed and luminal narrowing progresses.

As the plaque enlarges, the central portions become increasingly ischaemic and eventually a necrotic centre develops. The surface of the plaque ulcerates and the whole lesion becomes calcified. Haemorrhage may occur into the plaque and thrombosis on its surface. Such 'complicated' plaques result in regional symptoms, while the generalized process of intimal thickening has significant effects on the function of the normally compliant arterial tree.

Section 16.3 • Intimal hyperplasia

The white, firm, generally smooth raised lesion that develops following endothelial injury (most commonly surgery or balloon angioplasty) is known as intimal hyperplasia or occasionally as neointimal or myointimal hyperplasia. It consists almost entirely of smooth muscle cells and fibroblasts along with the extracellular matrix these cells manufacture – around 80% of the lesion is matrix. It starts developing within days of arterial injury but reaches a peak of clinical significance between 6 months and 2 years later. It can be responsible for late graft thrombosis secondary to luminal narrowing at anastomotic sites. After about 2 years its surface can become thrombogenic and the subsequent accumulated thrombus can result in the lesion appearing atherosclerotic.

Arterial injury results in platelet aggregation via the ADP pathway, with the presence of a prosthesis exacerbating this process. The aggregated platelets are activated and release growth factors (platelet-derived growth factor (PDGF) and transforming growth factor-β (TGFβ)) which attract smooth muscle cells into the intima from the media. The smooth muscle cells proliferate under the influence of growth factors and undergo a phenotypic change from their original contractile state to the synthetic and secretory state of fibroblasts. The lesion then grows and after several months can have clinical effects.

Balloon angioplasty can be an effective treatment for intimal hyperplasia, but it tends to be more durable when used for atherosclerotic lesions. In these latter lesions it is thought that an immunological process is involved in reducing the volume of the plaque following balloon angioplasty.

Section 16.4 • Arterial wall characteristics

Cardiac systole results in the ejection of about 80 ml of blood (the stroke volume) into the ascending aorta. This represents about 67% of the end diastolic volume of the left ventricle (left ventricular ejection fraction). The aorta is full of blood at the start of systole, so the extra volume pumped into it increases aortic pressure (blood, being a liquid, is non-compressible). The extra volume is partially accommodated by the propulsion of blood along the arterial tree through the capillary bed and into the venous side of the circulation, but is also partially accommodated by expansion of the elastic arteries. These vessels play no role in directing the distribution of blood flow – they simply accommodate the blood pumped into them and transport it. The muscular arteries, through their tone, have some control over the volume of blood they accept from the elastic arteries and so do not necessarily expand in the same way the elastic arteries do.

Compliance

Arterial expansion in systole is both in the longitudinal direction as well as in the more obvious circumferential direction – arteries get wider and longer in systole. The extent of the expansion obviously depends on the stiffness of the arterial wall, which is in turn determined by its composition and thickness. The thicker, stiffer walls of atherosclerotic arteries will expand less than healthy vessels. Stiffness is measured by the elastic modulus (*EM* – the ratio of the stress applied to a vessel wall to the strain that develops within it) and the greater the stiffness the higher the elastic modulus. Compliance is the reciprocal of the elastic modulus ($1/EM$), so a highly compliant vessel is not stiff and has a low elastic modulus. Age and atherosclerosis with its component fibrosis and calcification increase the stiffness of the artery wall – there is a higher *EM* and a lower compliance. A higher pressure within the vessel also tends to reduce compliance. Contraction of smooth muscle within the arterial wall also makes the vessel more stiff and less compliant – proximal elastic arteries tend to be more compliant than the more distal muscular varieties.

The reduced compliance of vessels in atherosclerosis prevents their expansion in systole. All the blood volume ejected in systole therefore has to be accommodated within the arteries by more rapid transit. The velocity of pulse wave transmission is, in fact, proportional to the elastic modulus. It is therefore faster in atherosclerotic vessels so enabling accommodation of the ejected blood of systole. The transmission of the pulse wave will be slowed down, however, by stenoses and more so by occlusions as it then has to pass via the more tortuous route taken by collaterals. This can place strain on the left ventricle.

Pulse wave transmission

During diastole the elastic arteries recoil and in so doing have the effect of maintaining diastolic pressure. As the more distal muscular arteries are less compliant they recoil less. There is therefore less support for diastolic pressure as distance from the heart increases. This effect is the opposite of what happens in systole: the compliant proximal arteries expand and so the pressure rise is less than in the more distal, less compliant arteries. Systolic pressure therefore increases with distance from the heart – explaining why the ankle:brachial index is a little greater than 1 in health – while diastolic pressure decreases. The overall effect is obviously an increase in pulse pressure. The pulse wave is also reflected off the peripheral vascular bed and has a further effect in modulating the shape of the pressure wave. The relatively flat pressure wave trace of the ascending aorta becomes more peaked by the radial artery with a slight fall in mean arterial pressure of a few millimetres of mercury (Figure 16.3). The pressure then falls more rapidly, reaching 40–60 mmHg by the arterioles and losing its pulsatility altogether by the capillaries.

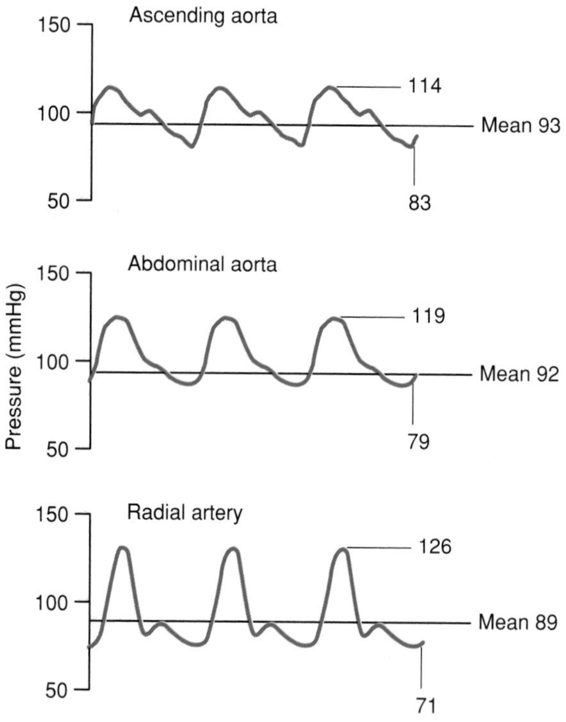

Figure 16.3 Arterial pressure waves. (From Smith, J.J. and Kampine, J.P., *Circulatory Physiology – The Essentials*, 3rd edn, 1990, page 93, Figure 6.3. Williams and Wilkins, Baltimore, MD, USA.)

Pressure is maintained in most peripheral vascular beds by a moderate peripheral vascular resistance with the result that blood flow reduces significantly and often stops by the end of diastole. The cerebral circulation, however, has a very low peripheral vascular resistance and the pressure within it is always lower than diastolic pressure. The result is constant forward flow of blood throughout the cardiac cycle – a feature which is obvious on duplex scanning. The same phenomenon can be seen in the radial artery in a hand demonstrating reactive hyperaemia.

Pulse palpation is an important part of clinical examination in vascular surgery. In experienced hands, the absence of a pulse suggests proximal arterial disease. The grading of the strength of a pulse is of little value, however. It is an entirely subjective phenomenon and is too much affected by vessel wall calcification which would reduce the strength of the palpated pulse, even though the pulse pressure is good. Furthermore, if there is a proximal stenosis within a compliant vessel whose pulse is being felt, then the palpated pulse will actually be good. If calculations are performed to predict how much the artery wall moves with each pulse wave the results are interesting – a normal circular femoral artery wall in a healthy young person will move less than 0.5 mm with each pulse – a degree of movement that would be very difficult to detect. When feeling a pulse, however, we compress the artery into an elliptical cross-section. It takes much less energy to move the wall of an ellipse so the pulse wave results in more movement of the wall making the pulse easier to feel. This explains why it can sometimes be difficult to feel a pulse in a mobile vessel or graft at operation – unless it is compressed against a rigid structure the movement of its wall with each pulse beat may not be detectable. Arterial lengthening with the pulse wave also makes the pulse easier to feel.

The palpation of a pulse should not necessarily be taken to imply patency of the vessel. Recent thrombus has a relatively low density compared to older, organized thrombus. The speed of transmission of a pulse wave is inversely proportional to the square root of the density. Lower density, fresh thrombus will therefore allow a pulse wave to pass slowly until it organizes into higher density thrombus through which the pulse wave is unable to pass at all. The clinical implication of this is that a pulse can sometimes be felt immediately distal to a recently thrombosed bypass graft. If there is any doubt about graft patency, flow should therefore be confirmed by Duplex scanning or angiography.

Section 16.5 • Flow dynamics

The flow dynamics of homogeneous liquids in rigid tubes is understood in rigorous mathematical fashion. Although blood is not a homogeneous liquid and it does not flow through rigid tubes, the principles of flow dynamics have been translated into haemodynamics. While the details of this topic are beyond the scope of this section, key concepts will be discussed.

Poiseuille's law and flow rates

Poiseuille described a fundamental law of fluid dynamics in the middle of the nineteenth century. It describes the relationship between the flow rate through a tube, the pressure gradient across the tube and the resistance to flow through the tube. In this manner it is analogous to Ohm's law governing the flow of electrical current:

$$\text{current} = \text{voltage/resistance}$$
$$\text{or } I = V/R$$

With respect to fluid flow:

$$\text{flow} = \text{pressure gradient/resistance}$$
$$\text{or } Q = \Delta P/R$$

Intuitively, the resistance to flow of a fluid is:

- directly related to the viscosity of the liquid – the stickier a liquid the harder it will be to get it to flow
- directly related to the length of the tube – it is harder to suck up a drink through a long straw of the same diameter as a short one
- inversely related to the radius of the tube – the narrower the tube the harder it is to force liquid through it.

Of these terms, the one with the greatest effect is the radius of the tube. Because it is the cross-sectional area of the tube and the rate of movement of a column of liquid that are being considered, it is the fourth power of the radius that is related to resistance.

Resistance to liquid flow is therefore:

$$\text{resistance} \propto \text{viscosity} \times \text{length/radius}^4$$
$$\text{or } R \propto \eta L/r^4$$

Placing this into the flow equation, $Q = \Delta P/R$:

$$Q \propto \Delta P r^4 \pi/\eta L$$

Poiseuille determined that the proportionality constant was $\pi/8$, making the flow equation:

$$Q = \Delta P r^4 \pi/8\eta L$$

The term 'resistance' refers to steady flow. In the circulation, however, flow is pulsatile and the correct term to use is impedance. This is difficult to measure, and in most circumstances approximations have been made to allow resistance to be used. It should be pointed out, however, that impedance to pulsatile flow is higher than resistance to steady flow, all else being equal. The reason for this is that some of the kinetic energy of the blood is used to expand the elastic arterial wall, making less available for forward blood flow. In patients suffering from generalized atherosclerosis with stiff, poorly compliant arteries and scattered stenotic or occlusive lesions the impedance of the aorta rises significantly – in order to help accommodate the volume of blood ejected during systole, much of the kinetic energy of the blood is used to expand the stiff aorta. This effect can even add to the strain on the left ventricle.

Resistance and flow rates

Poiseuille's equation explains how small changes in the diameter of arterioles can dramatically affect flow through a capillary bed. It is also of relevance in choosing the conduit for a bypass graft. If a vein is of small calibre then the flow through it may be insufficient to prevent thrombosis. In these circumstances it may be prudent to use a prosthesis if no other vein is available. When choosing a prosthesis, the largest practical size should be used – while 6 mm diameter tubes were generally used for infrainguinal bypasses in the past, many surgeons would now choose an 8 mm prosthesis to increase flow. Similarly, aortic bifurcation grafts should generally have a diameter of at least 14 × 7 mm for the same reason. The shorter the bypass, the less is its resistance – another factor in choosing anastomotic sites, and one reason why bypasses onto the above-knee popliteal artery tend to have longer patency times than those onto the below-knee popliteal.

As an atherosclerotic plaque starts narrowing the lumen of a vessel, the vessel itself enlarges so initially negating the effects on flow. Once the lumen is about 50% narrowed, however, vessel dilation is no longer able to compensate and the effects on flow and pressure become increasingly significant as the lumen narrows further. Balloon angioplasty would therefore not normally be considered for lesions causing less than a 50% stenosis.

When there are several stenoses in series along the length of a vessel the resistance of each is added together to give the total resistance. While each of the individual stenoses may not be critical, the effect of several in series can be. When there is an occlusion, the relevant resistance to include in this consideration is that of the collateral vessels – this will be high because of their small calibre and long length. It is therefore obvious that treating the lesion with the greatest resistance will have the greatest effect on improving distal blood supply. This should be remembered when planning treatment of multiple diseased arterial segments.

As blood viscosity increases, the flow rate decreases. This is of considerable importance when considering bypass surgery in conditions associated with a high blood viscosity, such as polycythaemia, myeloproliferative disorders or malignancy. Conversely, a slightly anaemic patient has a lower blood viscosity so enhancing the chances of graft patency.

Laminar and turbulent flow

Blood flow in most areas of the circulation is laminar – blood in contact with the vessel wall is stationary but as the centre of the vessel is progressively approached blood moves with greater velocity. This produces the well-known parabolic profile of blood flow. Under certain circumstances, however, blood flow will become turbulent with the associated random directions of movement superimposed on the overall pattern of forward blood flow. The blood flow profile in turbulence is blunt (Figure 16.4). The circumstances in which turbulence occurs are described by the Reynolds number:

$$\text{Reynolds number} = \frac{\text{diameter} \times \text{mean velocity} \times \text{blood density}}{\text{blood viscosity}}$$

or

$$Re = dv_{\text{mean}}\rho/\eta$$

As blood density and viscosity are stable, Reynolds number is directly related to the vessel diameter and mean velocity. In health, turbulence will only occur in the ascending aorta during the peak of systole. At a stenosis, however, blood velocity will often increase sufficiently to produce turbulence distal to the stenosis, even though the vessel may still be narrowed at this site. This will increase the shear force on the endothelium and so may result in further atherosclerosis arising from endothelial injury. Resistance to turbulent flow is also higher than it is to laminar flow, so compounding the effect of the stenosis itself. Turbulent flow can be detected clinically as either bruits or thrills because the vibrations created in the vessel wall result in noise production. It is possible that the normal laminar flow in arteries adopts a spiral pattern and there is some evidence that the spiral nature of the flow may reduce the risk of turbulence developing.

The increase in blood velocity at a stenosis can be used as a measure of the degree of the stenosis. Duplex scanning can determine this non-invasively and velocity measurements are used particularly in determining the severity of a vein graft stenosis – if the velocity at the stenosis is 2.5–3 times the proximal velocity then the stenosis should be considered significant.

Laplace's law

It is well recognized that the pressure required to blow up a balloon is greatest at the start of inflation and decreases as the balloon enlarges. Once an artery starts dilating, the force required to continue the dilation decreases. This is Laplace's law:

$$\text{pressure} = \text{wall thickness} \times \text{wall tension/radius}$$
$$\text{or } P = \mu T/R$$

When this equation is applied to aneurysm formation, it is clear that wall tension has to increase if blood pressure is to remain stable while the aneurysm radius increases and wall thickness decreases. This increase in tension is not of great clinical significance below a diameter of 5.5 cm, up to which size the annual rupture rate is only 1%. Over 6 cm, however, the rupture rate increases exponentially and the tension in the wall clearly becomes significant.

Section 16.6 • Prosthetic arterial graft characteristics

The two materials currently in popular use for the manufacture of arterial prostheses are Dacron (a polyester material) and PTFE (polytetrafluoroethylene).

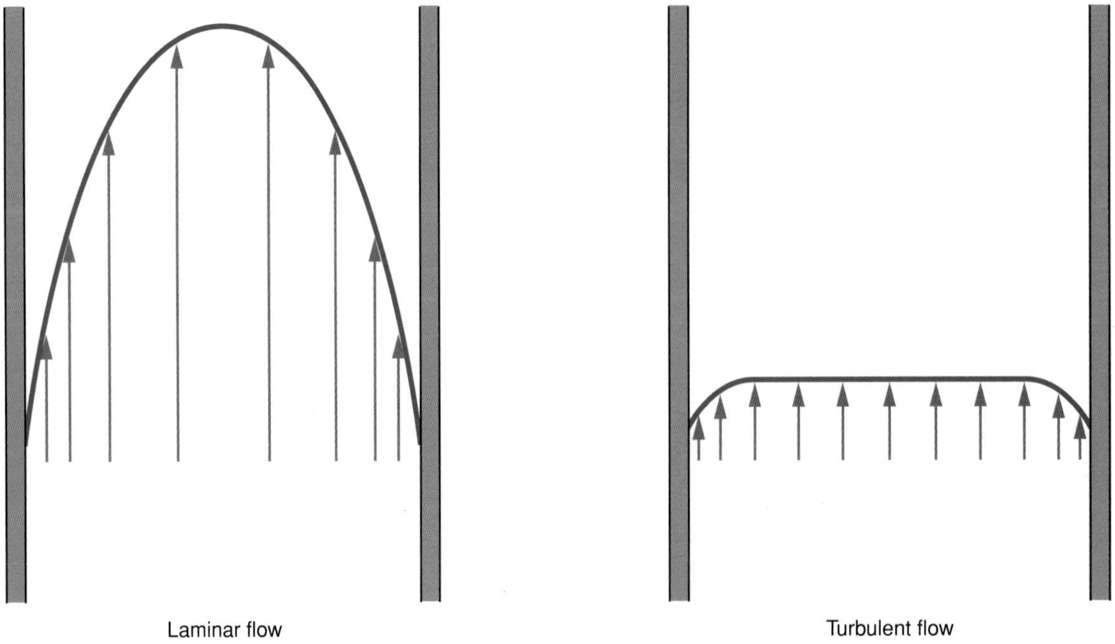

Figure 16.4 Flow profiles of laminar and turbulent flow. (From Callow, A.D. and Ernst, C.B. eds. *Vascular Surgery – Theory and Practice*, 1995, page 303, Figure 20.3. Appleton and Lange, Stamford, CT, USA.)

The interstices between the strands of PTFE are blood tight, but the material has little elastic recoil following the passage of a needle, explaining the needle hole bleeding that is common with this product. Dacron is either knitted or woven. While the woven material is blood tight, it frays at cut edges and generally requires heating to fuse the fibres. For this reason it is not in common use today. Knitted Dacron is much easier to work with as it does not fray when cut and holds its strength very close to the cut edge, allowing small needle bites to be taken. Knitted Dacron is not blood tight and in the past had to be 'pre-clotted' with some of the patient's own blood being forced under pressure into the fabric and being allowed to clot before suturing the graft into place. This drawback has now been overcome by coating the material with, for example, gelatine during manufacture. This results in a blood-tight graft that retains the handling characteristics of knitted Dacron. Recent work would suggest that there is little to choose between PTFE and Dacron in terms of infra-inguinal graft patency.

Both types of material are stiffer than native artery wall (higher elastic modulus, lower compliance) and this greater stiffness increases further with time after implantation as fibrous tissue forms a sheath around the graft and grows into the interstices of the material. Resistance to steady flow through a prosthetic graft is similar to that through native artery. However, the greater stiffness of a prosthesis increases its impedance (resistance to pulsatile flow) compared to native artery. The reason for this is intuitive – a stiff wall will resist deformation with each pulse wave and so energy is diverted away from the forward flow of blood into deforming the graft wall. Knitted Dacron, in fact, has the least compliance of the commonly used grafts. PTFE and woven Dacron are more compliant, but autologous vein is the most compliant bypass material of all. As a result, vein has the least impedance – an important factor (along with a viable endothelial lining) in explaining its superior patency rates compared to prostheses.

Anastomoses between prostheses and native arteries

There are potential problems at anastomoses between prostheses and arteries because of the different compliances of the two components of the anastomosis. The degree of expansion and movement of the prosthesis and artery wall with each pulse wave is determined by the compliance of each. Because arterial wall is more compliant than a prosthesis it will expand and move more than the prosthesis. This potentially places strain on the suture line as the artery moves a greater distance than the prosthesis with each pulse. It is not possible to make allowances for this by placing loose sutures – the anastomosis would obviously leak! Further potential problems at anastomotic lines arise from a partial reflection of energy due to the change in compliance and from vibrations and shear stresses which originate from the change in direction of blood flow. While an elastic suture might solve the risk of suture line disruption, it is fortunate that these potential difficulties translate only infrequently into the clinically significant events of anastomotic breakdown with early bleeding or late false aneurysm formation. Nevertheless, anastomotic false aneurysms are far more commonly associated with prosthesis/artery anastomoses than they are with vein/artery anastomoses – not only is there a much better compliance match between vein and artery, but the vein actually heals to the artery with scar tissue formation; a prosthesis never truly heals to an artery, so placing long-term reliance on the non-absorbable suture line.

Vein cuff interposition

There are a variety of techniques (Figure 16.5) which involve the placement of a vein cuff at the distal anastomosis between a prosthesis and a native artery (Miller cuff, Taylor patch, St Mary's boot) and there is evidence that these can improve patency of prosthetic below-knee femoro-popliteal bypasses. How they work, however, is not clear. It is apparent that the greatest effect on patency is in the first 30 days, suggesting that technical factors play the greatest role. Other possible reasons for improved patency have been suggested. While there is a much better compliance match at the vein cuff/artery suture line, there is still a mismatch at the prosthesis/vein cuff suture line. This latter anastomosis is wider, however, and the effects of the mismatch may be less. The width of the anastomosis at this site may mean that neointimal hyperplasia, should it develop, will have less of a haemodynamic effect. It is also possible that the altered pattern of blood flow reduces the overall formation of neointimal hyperplasia or alters the position at which it forms. The larger cuff can accommodate a similar volume of neointimal hyperplasia than a conventional anastomosis with less risk of occlusion.

There is work which shows that the impedance of an end to side anastomosis between a prosthesis and a native artery is lowered by the presence of a vein cuff. This is shown in Figure 16.6, where it can be seen that the presence of a cuff lowers the impedance of an anastomosis at a given flow rate. Figure 16.6 also confirms intuition by showing that impedance is lower for acute angle anastomoses than for those fashioned at 90 degrees or greater. This fact is of value in deciding whether to carry out a femoro-femoral cross-over (where the anastomotic angle of donor side is greater than 90°) or an ilio-femoral cross-over (where the donor side has a much more favourable acute anastomotic angle).

Graft endothelialization

Prosthetic grafts generally do not have as long a patency expectation as autogenous vein. Decreased compliance and increased impedance is likely to play some part in this but another important aspect is the absence of a full endothelial layer. The endothelium is now recognized as an essential component in the control of vascular tone, platelet aggregation and clotting. An

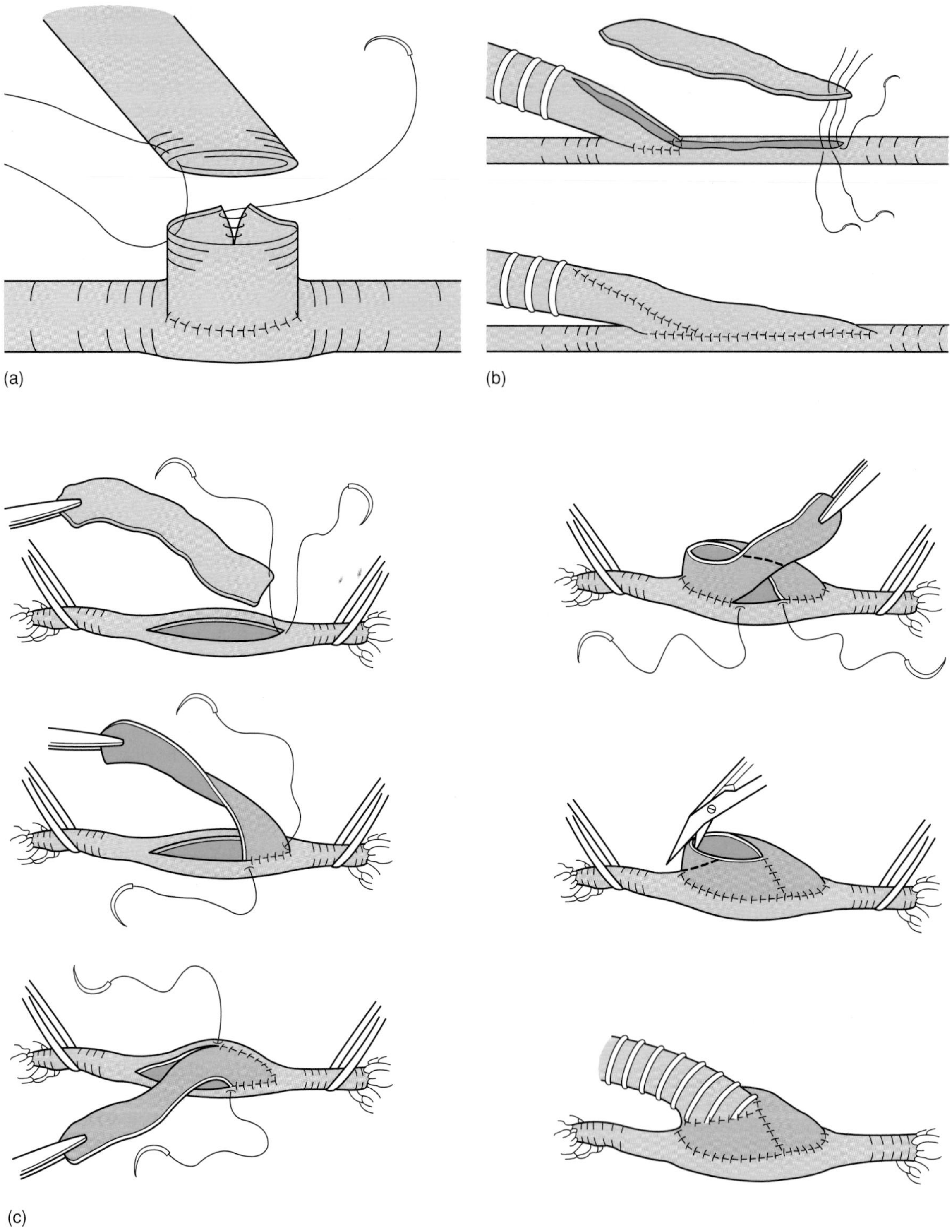

Figure 16.5 Vein augmentation of anastomoses between a prosthesis and an artery. (a) Miller cuff. (From Raptis, S., Miller, J.H. Influence of a vein cuff on polytetrafluoroethylene grafts for primary femoropopliteal bypass. Figure 2. *Br J Surg* 1995; **82**: 487–91. Blackwell Science, London.) (b) Taylor patch. (From Taylor, R.S., Loh, A., McFarland, R.J. *et al*. Improved technique for polytetrafluoroethylene bypass grafting: long term results using anastomotic vein patches. Figures 1 to 5. *Br J Surg* 1992; **79**: 348–54. Blackwell Science, London.) (c) 'St Mary's boot'. (From: Tyrrell, M.R. and Wolfe, J.H.N. New prosthetic venous collar anastomotic technique: combining the best of other procedures. Figures 1 to 6. *Br J Surg* 1991; **78**: 1016–17. Blackwell Science, London.)

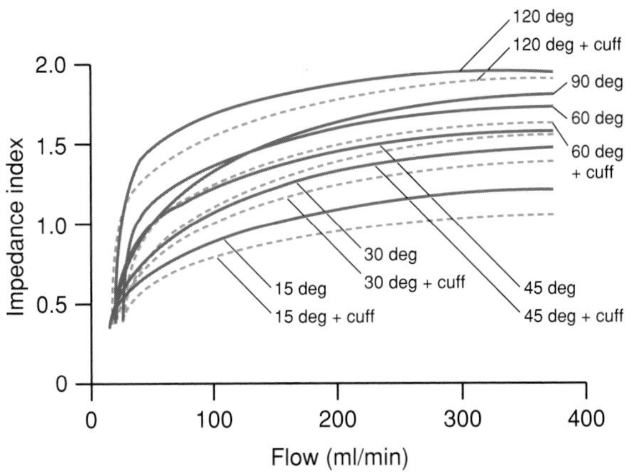

Figure 16.6 Effect of anastomotic angle and vein cuff on impedance and flow. (From Wijesinghe, L.D., Smye, S.W. and Scott, D.J.A. Impedance index measurements of *in vitro* PTFE end to side anastomoses: effect of angle and Miller cuff. *Eur J Vasc Endovasc Surg* 1998; **16**: 65–70. W.B. Saunders, London.)

experimentally denuded aorta re-endothelializes from the orifices of the intercostal and lumbar arteries at the rates of 0.07 mm per day circumferentially and nearly 0.5 mm per day longitudinally. Areas that are not endothelialized after a week tend to be invaded by smooth muscle cells which eventually create a multilayered fibrocellular lesion.

The extent to which a prosthesis endothelializes depends on the graft material, its porosity and on the species in which is implanted. The process starts at the border between the native artery and the graft and spreads by cell proliferation and migration as a single sheet of cells. In Dacron and expanded PTFE (the standard type of the material used in grafts) endothelialization ceases a few millimetres from the artery/graft interface. Why this happens is not clear, although the endothelial cells continue to proliferate. At the leading edge this can result in a raised ridge, while in the remainder of the sheet there is a generalized increase in endothelial cell turnover. This may be due to chronic cell injury induced by the graft or by growth factor production by adjacent white cells or smooth muscle cells. If porous PTFE is used then capillaries grow into the graft wall from the perigraft tissue. Much greater endothelialization of the graft surface occurs due to the presence of these capillaries. Clinically, however, this is of little value due to the porosity of the material at implantation. Endothelialization for a few millimetres from each edge of a prosthesis is a useful clinical fact, however, as it means that a prosthetic patch up to 7 or 8 mm wide will fully endothelialize. This supports the use of prosthetic patches in, for example, carotid endarterectomy.

Section 16.7 • Regulation of blood flow

Blood flow varies not only between different regions and organ systems but also within individual organs. Flow to a single organ can also change with time. These variations reflect the differing needs for blood by various tissues. The kidneys, for example, require a steady, high blood flow (around 420 ml/100 g/min) to carry out their excretory functions; skeletal muscle needs only a low blood flow at rest (around 4 ml/min/100 g) but this requirement increases significantly during exercise (around 50 ml/min/100 g). If the normal cardiac output of 5 litres per minute were evenly distributed, then muscle flow would be about 7 ml/min/100 g – clearly considerable control is exerted over blood flow distribution.

While muscular arteries play some part in control of blood flow to different regions, it is the arterioles which exert most influence through the degree of vasodilation or vasoconstriction they exert. Organs with a generally low arteriolar resistance such as the kidney, heart and brain are 'vascular' and have a high blood flow per unit weight. Resting muscle and skin are much less 'vascular', have a high arteriolar resistance and a consequently low blood flow per unit weight. In the face of a relatively constant blood pressure, it is the varying regional arteriolar resistances that determine flow – intense vasoconstriction can virtually shut off flow while vasodilation can allow up to a 20-fold increase in flow.

Control of arteriolar resistance is exerted either centrally or locally. Central control is either neural or humoral while local control is generally humoral. The most important aspect of central control is neural via the autonomic nervous system. Some areas (such as skin) have a high resting sympathetic tone, a tendency to vasoconstriction and a low flow. Other areas (kidney, brain and heart) have very little resting sympathetic tone and so have a high flow at rest. Central humoral control of blood flow is less tissue specific. It is exerted via angiotensin, 5-hydroxytryptamine or the metabolic gases (oxygen and carbon dioxide). Local tissue production of substances such as prostaglandins, histamine and lactate will affect blood flow over a limited area. It is now recognized that endothelial production of nitric oxide (endothelial derived relaxing factor) plays an important role in local regulation of flow – it is an active vasodilator and inhibits platelet aggregation. Reactive hyperaemia is an example of a locally controlled increase in blood flow following the production of lactate (a vasodilator) during a period of ischaemia. This is the basis of Buerger's test, in which a critically ischaemic foot is rendered more ischaemic by elevation and the reactive hyperaemia observed when the limb is then placed in a dependent position.

Autoregulation

Autoregulation is an aspect of blood flow control which deserves special mention. While central blood pressure generally remains fairly constant there are physiological and pathological circumstances in which it varies. Flow to many organ systems will vary directly with central blood pressure. If this were to happen in

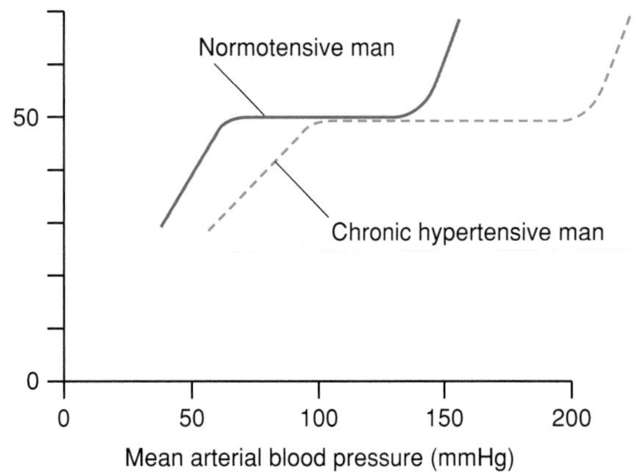

Figure 16.7 Autoregulation of blood flow. (From Smith, J.J. and Kampine, J.P. *Circulatory Physiology*, 3rd edn, 1990, page 189, Figure 11.5. Williams and Wilkins, Baltimore, USA.)

flow sensitive vital organs (brain, heart or kidneys) there could be catastrophic results. These areas demonstrate autoregulation – flow is kept relatively constant across a fairly wide range of blood pressure (Figure 16.7). In this way vital organ function is maintained across a range of blood pressures. In chronic hypertension, autoregulation is set at a higher level of blood pressure. It is interesting to note that organs which show the most autoregulation also have the least resting sympathetic tone – blood flow at low pressure will therefore be relatively high.

There are two possibilities as to how autoregulation occurs – both involve negative feedback. One suggestion is that stretching of the muscle of arterioles with a higher blood pressure results in vasoconstriction (stretching a muscle cell stimulates it to contract) so keeping flow constant. As pressure decreases, the stimulus to vasoconstriction is reduced, there is vasodilation and higher flow. The other possibility relates to carbon dioxide build up or hypoxia in low pressure states – this will result in vasodilation and higher flow. When the metabolites are washed away and tissue oxygenation returns to normal, there is a return to a more constricted state and flow falls. Either way, autoregulation is very efficient and plays an important part in cerebral protection during carotid endarterectomy.

Cerebral circulation

In addition to efficient autoregulation, there are other special aspects to the cerebral circulation. Cerebrospinal fluid (CSF) is formed in the choroidal plexuses of the ventricles at a rate of about 400–600 ml per day. It is resorbed via the arachnoid villi in the dural sinuses. It normally exerts a pressure of about 120–180 mm water. If this is elevated then there is a tendency for cerebral and spinal cord blood flow to fall due to the rise in pressure within the enclosed space of the cranium. In fact, blood flow will not fall significantly until CSF pressure reaches 50–60 mmHg due to the reflex rise in blood pressure secondary to a rise in intracranial pressure – the Cushing reflex. Along with this rise, there is a reflex bradycardia due to baroreceptor action.

When CSF pressure falls, however, the opposite occurs and there is a tendency for cerebral and spinal cord blood flow to increase. This fact is often used during surgical repair of thoracoabdominal aortic aneurysms – a procedure with a 10% risk of paraplegia due to spinal cord ischaemia. There is some evidence that a catheter draining CSF from the spinal canal and maintaining a low CSF pressure reduces the risk of cord ischaemia by increasing its blood flow.

Anaesthesia and atherosclerosis reduce cerebral blood flow, while cerebrovascular disease reduces the capacity for autoregulation. During carotid endarterectomy, the brain is therefore susceptible to changes in blood pressure – these will result in greater changes in cerebral blood flow than they would under normal circumstances. Blood pressure should therefore be maintained at a steady level at or slightly above the patient's normal pressure and wild swings should be avoided.

Circulation to other regions

The other circulatory regions which exhibit autoregulation include the heart and kidney – organs which cannot tolerate a fall in blood flow. The heart at rest receives about 70 ml/100 g/min (5% of cardiac output) and the kidney about 420 ml/100 g/min (20% of cardiac output). The high renal blood flow is essential in order to maintain its clearance functions. At rest, skeletal muscle blood flow is about 4 ml/100 g/min and skin 3 ml/100 g/min. With exercise or a rise in temperature, blood flow to these tissues can increase by 12-fold and 30-fold respectively. A lower limb bypass graft therefore carries a greater flow if it supplies more muscle and this flow is increased with exercise. This should be taken into consideration when deciding whether to perform a distal bypass graft – the small weight of tissue these bypasses perfuse can sometimes result in low bypass flows. This may predispose to early bypass thrombosis.

Section 16.8 • The endothelium

Over the past decade it has become apparent that the endothelium is fact more than an inert monolayer of cells lining all blood vessels. It has been described as one of the largest organs in the body – it is certainly the most extensive. It has been estimated that there are over a million million endothelial cells weighing about 1.8 kg (a greater weight than the liver). It is now known that healthy endothelium plays an important role in maintaining a vasodilated state, in preventing thrombosis and platelet aggregation and in regulating vascular permeability and leucocyte adhesion.

Permeability

Endothelial cell surface receptors are intimately associated with a complex of structural proteins lying inside the cell membrane (the cortical web – made of actin and other proteins). When healthy and intact this complex controls the adhesion of leucocytes, platelets and plasma proteins so regulating endothelial permeability. The cortical web controls the shape and stiffness of endothelial cells. If an increased shear stress is applied to the cells then the cortical web stiffens the cell membrane and with it the whole cell becomes rigid. In this state the cell is less able to control intercellular passage of materials. In health the gaps between endothelial cells are regulated by reactions within the cells involving actin, cAMP, cGMP, calcium and nitric oxide. Under the action of certain stimuli, these reactions can also change the overall shape of the cell, altering it from its flattened state to become more globular – blood flow may even be impaired in capillaries. The cytoskeleton is therefore active in controlling not only cell shape but also transcellular and intercellular permeability.

Vascular tone and blood flow

Endothelial cells are capable of secreting a wide variety of substances which can result in vasodilation or vasoconstriction, growth stimulation or inhibition, activation or inhibition of inflammation and thrombosis or its prevention. As has been mentioned, healthy endothelium maintains a vasodilated, antithrombotic and anti-inflammatory state. Nitric oxide (previously known as endothelium derived relaxing factor) is now known to be intimately involved in this. Normal endothelium constantly secretes small quantities of nitric oxide. The nitric oxide produces vasodilation by increasing smooth muscle cell cGMP, inhibiting smooth muscle cell growth, inhibiting leucocyte adhesion and inhibiting platelet aggregation.

Endothelial production of vasoconstrictor substances is normally kept in abeyance, but when it occurs it is secondary to arachidonic acid metabolism and the production of thromboxane A2, endothelin production and occasionally angiotensin or superoxide formation. The first three of these compounds cause direct vasoconstriction, but superoxide destroys nitric oxide so leading to indirect vasoconstriction.

The well-known risk factors associated with atherosclerosis (hypertension, diabetes, LDL cholesterol and smoking) all damage endothelial cells and there is inhibition of nitric oxide synthetase. The normal homeostatic balance is then shifted towards vasoconstriction, leucocyte adherence, platelet aggregation and thrombosis. The platelet and leucocyte adherence paves the way for the formation of atherosclerotic plaques.

It is now becoming understood how control of the atherosclerotic risk factors can prevent endothelial cell damage and so limit the development of atherosclerosis. Furthermore, the role of drug therapy in preventing or reversing these changes is being explored. Currently available drugs such as angiotensin-converting enzyme (ACE) inhibitors, calcium antagonists and statins all improve endothelial cell function by enhancing nitric oxide production via different mechanisms. Newer drugs such as nitric oxide donors, antioxidants (oxygen radical stress limits nitric oxide availability), endothelin antagonists and specific prostacyclin antagonists (COX-2) may also have a role to play in the future.

Section 16.9 • Oedema

Starling's law of capillary filtration (Figure 16.8) relates hydrostatic pressure within the capillary (which tends to force liquid out into the tissues) to plasma oncotic pressure (which tends to attract liquid back into the capillary). The principle states that at the arteriolar end of a capillary the hydrostatic pressure (32 mmHg) exceeds the oncotic pressure (25 mmHg) and liquid moves into the tissues. At the venular end of the capillary the hydrostatic pressure (15 mmHg) is lower than the oncotic pressure (25 mmHg) so liquid moves back into the capillary. The great majority of filtered fluid is resorbed into the capillaries by this mechanism, but that which is not (2–4 litres per day) is collected by the lymphatics.

Situations in which more fluid is filtered than reabsorbed result in oedema. The extra fluid in the tissues increases the diffusion distance from the capillaries to cells requiring nutrients. Effective tissue perfusion is therefore diminished in oedematous areas and wounds in these areas rapidly become sloughy and infected. Considerable improvement will result with elevation of the limb and reduction in the oedema.

Oedema of the lower leg is very common following infra-inguinal bypass, particularly when the bypass was carried out for critical ischaemia. The aetiology is probably multi-factorial and is not fully understood, particularly as the oedema can persist for many years post-operatively. Impaired deep venous return (with or without deep venous thrombosis) may contribute; the use of the long saphenous vein as the bypass conduit is less likely to contribute as this vein carries relatively little of the total venous return and post-bypass oedema also occurs after prosthetic bypass. Reperfusion of ischaemic tissues may also play a role.

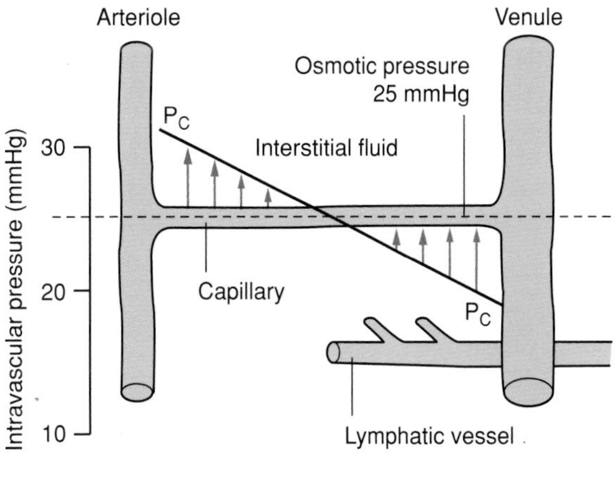

Figure 16.8 Starling's law of capillary filtration. (From Smith, J.J. and Kampine, K.P., *Circulatory Physiology – The Essentials*, 3rd edn, 1990, page 134, Figure 8.4. Williams and Wilkins, Baltimore, MD, USA.)

Ischaemia–reperfusion injury

Endothelium is damaged by ischaemia resulting in an increase in capillary permeability. Under these conditions, white cells marginate and become activated. The superoxides and other substances so released further increase capillary permeability and can cause direct tissue damage. When such tissue is reperfused there is an increase in oedema formation which may contribute to limb swelling, at least in the early stages.

A more sinister clinical feature of ischaemia-reperfusion injury is the release of myoglobin from ischaemia-damaged muscle cells in a severely ischaemic limb. The myoglobin enters the general circulation after reperfusion and precipitates in renal tubules resulting in renal failure. This effect can be minimized by ensuring good hydration at the time of and following reperfusion and possibly by using mannitol as a free radical scavenger and so reducing cellular damage. The clinical implication of this type of ischaemia-reperfusion injury is the need to be vigilant when considering and attempting salvage of severely ischaemic legs – preliminary fasciotomy should be considered to examine the viability of muscle, renal function needs close monitoring and primary amputation may be the appropriate course of action in the most ischaemic of limbs.

Further reading

Abbott, W. M., Green, R. M., Matsumoto, T. *et al.* (1997). Prosthetic above-knee femoropopliteal bypass grafting: results of a multicenter randomized prospective trial. Above-Knee Femoropopliteal Study Group. *J Vasc Surg* **25**: 19–28.

Callow, A. D. and Ernst, C. B. (1995) *Vascular Surgery – Theory and Practice,* Stamford, CT: Appleton and Lange.

Estes, J. E. (1950). Abdominal aortic aneurysms: a study of 102 cases. *Circulation* **2**: 258.

Johnson, W. C. and Lee, K. K. (1999). Comparative evaluation of externally supported Dacron and polytetrafluoroethylene prosthetic bypasses for femorofemoral and axillofemoral arterial reconstructions. Veterans Affairs Cooperative Study #141. *J Vasc Surg* **30**: 1077–83.

Noori, N., Scherer, R., Perktold, K. *et al.* (1999). Blood flow in distal end-to-side anastomoses with PTFE and a venous patch: results of an in vitro flow visualization study. *Eur J Vasc Endovasc Surg* **18**: 191–200.

Robinson, B. I., Fletcher, J. P., Tomlinson, P. *et al.* (1999). A prospective randomized multicentre comparison of expanded polytetrafluoroethylene and gelatin-sealed knitted Dacron grafts for femoropopliteal bypass. *Cardiovasc Surg* **7**: 214–18.

Smith, J. J. and Kampine, J. P. (1990). *Circulatory Physiology – The essentials*, 3rd edn. Baltimore, MD: Williams and Wilkins.

Stonebridge, P. A., Hoskins, P. R., Allan, P. L. and Belch, J. F. (1996). Spiral laminar flow *in vivo*. *Clin Sci* **91**: 17–21.

Stonebridge, P. A., Prescott, R. J. and Ruckley, C. V. (1997). Randomized trial comparing infrainguinal polytetrafluoroethylene bypass grafting with and without vein interposition cuff at the distal anastomosis. The Joint Vascular Research Group. *J Vasc Surg* **26**: 543–50.

UK Small Aneurysm Trial Participants (1998). Mortality results for randomised controlled trial of early elective surgery or ultrasonographic surveillance for small abdominal aortic aneurysms. *Lancet* **352**: 1649–55.

Wijesinghe, L. D., Smye, S. W. and Scott, D. J. (1998). Impedance index measurements of in vitro PTFE end-to-side anastomoses: effect of angle and Miller cuff. *Eur J Vasc Endovasc Surg* **16**: 65–70.

MODULE 17

Epidemiology of peripheral arterial occlusive disease

1 • Risk factors

2 • Prevalence and incidence

Peripheral arterial occlusive disease (PAOD) is a significant cause of morbidity in the Western world. PAOD may be asymptomatic or manifest as intermittent claudication or critical limb ischaemia. Patients with PAOD have an increased risk of cardiovascular and cerebrovascular death. Epidemiological studies have shown that certain diseases, lifestyles and habits increase the risk of developing atherosclerosis. Smoking, hypertension, hyperlipidaemia and high-fat diets appear to be high risk factors to the development of atherosclerosis. Conversely, low-fat diets, exercise and high levels of high-density lipoproteins reduce the risk of developing atherosclerosis.

The Framingham study was the first large-scale cardiovascular survey, which included peripheral arterial disease. More recently the Edinburgh Artery study, also examined a range of risk factors in over 1500 patients as a longitudinal study. Major population studies have also been performed in Europe and North America.

Section 17.1 • Risk factors

Smoking

Cigarette smoking is probably the single most important risk factor. Between 80% and 100% of people attending vascular outpatient clinics are current or recent smokers. The relative risk of smoking and developing peripheral arterial disease ranges from 1.4 to more than 10.0, and it is believed to be responsible for up to 53% of the disease in the community. The Framingham study indicated that nearly 80% of cases of intermittent claudication could be attributed to smoking. Autopsy studies suggest that cigarette smoking is a more important risk factor in peripheral arterial disease than it is in coronary arterial disease. PAOD associated with smoking may be related to deficiencies in antioxidants. The resulting increased free radical load then results in increased oxidation of fatty acids and atherogenicity of low-density lipoprotein (LDL) cholesterol. There is variance as to the time taken for an ex-smoker to normalize their risk.

Lipids

Abnormalities in cholesterol, lipoproteins and triglyceride metabolism occur in patients presenting with PAOD. The relationship between serum cholesterol and arterial disease is generally independent of other risk factors. In the Framingham study a cholesterol of >7 mmol/l was associated with a doubling of the risk of intermittent claudication.

Low levels of high-density lipoprotein (HDL)-cholesterol have been related to poor physical activity and smoking. HDL-cholesterol levels are generally lower in patients with PAOD. The Edinburgh Artery study reported an inverse relationship between PAOD and HDL-cholesterol that was independent of smoking, diabetes, obesity, exercise and alcohol consumption.

Apolipoprotein B, lipid-free protein components of plasma lipoproteins, may be involved in the development of peripheral arterial disease. Apolipoprotein A may play a role in coronary artery disease but no association has been reported with peripheral arterial disease.

Serum triglyceride levels have been observed to be associated with PAOD. However, serum triglyceride does not appear to be independently related to

PAOD. The Edinburgh Artery study demonstrated the disappearance of the univariate relationship between PAOD and serum triglyceride on multivariate analysis.

Essential fatty acids have been shown to reduce LDL cholesterol and platelet aggregation and may prevent atherosclerosis. The Edinburgh Artery study demonstrated reduced levels of the essential fatty acids docosapentaenoic and eicosapentaenoic acid in PAOD.

The Edinburgh Artery study demonstrated significantly reduced vitamin C intake in cases of PAOD. Other studies have also related reduced vitamin C and E intake to intermittent claudication. Antioxidants such as vitamins A, C and E protect polyunsaturated fatty acids from peroxidation. Lipid peroxides appear to correlate with severity of aortic atherosclerosis. Plasma lipid peroxide levels are elevated in both PAOD and ischaemic heart disease.

Diabetes

Peripheral vascular, cerebrovascular and cardiovascular diseases are all more common in diabetics than in the normal population. The risk of amputation for a diabetic is 15–70 times that for a non-diabetic. In the Framingham study the age adjusted incidence of intermittent claudication in males was 12.6 and 3.3 per 1000 person years for diabetics and non-diabetics, respectively. However, the role of glucose intolerance in the aetiology of PAOD is less clear. The Edinburgh Artery study observed a significant association between impaired glucose tolerance and intermittent claudication. The Aachen study and cross-sectional Moscow and Berlin studies reported impaired glucose tolerance to be impaired more commonly in claudicants. In contrast, cross-sectional surveys from Oxford, Finland and Jerusalem found no link between prevalence of intermittent claudication and impaired glucose tolerance.

Hypertension

Many studies have observed an association between PAOD and hypertension. Patients with intermittent claudication generally have higher mean arterial pressures than normal controls. The Framingham study has shown after 26 years of follow-up that hypertension increases the risk of claudication by a factor of three.

Haematological factors

Blood viscosity and plasma fibrinogen have consistently been found to be higher in patients with intermittent claudication than in control subjects. Increased haematocrit has also been shown to be related to peripheral arterial disease, although the Framingham study did not find any relationship with the development of intermittent claudication. It may be that these factors are co-incidental because they are all also related to smoking. Other factors such as fibrinolysis time, decreased fibrinolytic activity and raised factor VIII, factor XIII, plasminogen and platelet function have also been implicated. The incidence of hyperhomocysteinaemia is also substantially greater in a pool of patients with PAOD (up to 60%) than in a normal population (1%) with a higher incidence in patients with premature PAOD. The role of a hypercoagulable state has been questioned with an increased hypercoagulability in patients with claudication over controls.

Other factors

Personality type, alcohol consumption and exercise may be risk factors in the development of PAOD but some of the evidence is conflicting. The Edinburgh Artery study observed associations between hostile personality and both asymptomatic and symptomatic disease. Type A personality individuals are at increased risk of developing both cerebrovascular and PAOD. The role of alcohol consumption is controversial. The Edinburgh Artery study observed that patients with PAOD had higher alcohol consumption when compared to matched controls. By contrast, a study from Jerusalem found no such association. Furthermore, the consumption of small amounts of alcohol may reduce the risk of PAOD. Exercise may prevent peripheral vascular disease and the Edinburgh Artery study observed a higher risk in those who performed low levels of physical activity. However, the Framingham study did not observe any association with low levels of exercise and PAOD.

Section 17.2 • Prevalence and incidence

Asymptomatic disease

The prevalence and incidence of asymptomatic disease have been studied usually using an ankle brachial pressure index (ABPI) with a ratio of ≤0.9 as a marker for the presence of disease. A resting ABPI of 0.9 has been suggested to be 95% sensitive in detecting angiogram-positive arterial disease and up to 100% specific in identifying apparently healthy individuals. These studies suggest the prevalence of peripheral arterial disease ranges from 7–15% of the middle-aged and elderly population. The 5 year cumulative incidence of asymptomatic disease has been shown to be 18% in those aged 65 years or over in Switzerland and 14% in Denmark in a survey of 60-year-old patients. Patients with low ABPI (≤0.9) appear to have increased relative risks of death from ischaemic heart disease and other cardiovascular causes. Progression from asymptomatic disease to claudication is thought to occur in up to 15% of patients within 5 years.

Intermittent claudication

The diagnosis of intermittent claudication requires a careful history, clinical examination and verification by non-invasive tests. The most widely used questionnaire for identification of patients with intermittent claudication is the WHO/Rose questionnaire but it may still underestimate the true prevalence. History and examination alone are not completely reliable. Clinical examination of the peripheral pulses may also be misleading as the dorsalis pedis and posterior tibial pulse may be congenitally absent in up to 12% and 0.2%, respectively.

Between 2 and 7% of the populations of Western countries suffer from intermittent claudication. The Edinburgh Artery study showed the prevalence to be 4.6% in a population aged 55–74 years though it has been reported to be 10% in Scandinavia. In the Framingham study the biennial incidence rate was 7.1 per 1000 men and 3.6 per 1000 women, with women having the incidence of men 10 years younger and the difference reducing with advancing age. The Edinburgh Artery study, however found an identical prevalence in the sexes. This may have been a product of the older age group studied. The occupation of the patient has an impact on incidence possibly by influencing whether a patient will complain of claudication or not, farmers having a higher incidence than civil servants. Claudication increases with age.

Studies assessing the progression of intermittent claudication have shown 56–71% remained stable or improved and that 29–44% became worse. This symptomatic stabilization may be due to the development of collaterals, metabolic adaptation of ischaemic muscle by an increase in aerobic enzyme content and capillary density, or the patient altering gait to use non-ischaemic muscle groups. Deterioration of claudication is most frequent during the first year following diagnosis (7–9%) compared with 2–3% per annum thereafter. Bad prognostic indicators for limb survival include age over 65 years and distal vessel disease. Major amputation is a rare outcome of claudication, with only 1–3% of patients needing major amputation over a 5 year period. In the unselected populations in the Basle and Framingham studies only 2% proceeded to amputation. The amputation rate is related to the presenting symptom, 3% with claudication and 9% with rest pain. This is reflected by an ABPI of <0.5 being a strong predictor of local deterioration. The incidence of lower limb amputations increases from 0.3 per 100 000 per year for those younger than 40 years to 226 per 100 000 per year for those older than 80 years. The most important predictor is smoking. It has been reported that claudicants who stopped smoking did not require amputation, while 11.4% who did not stop smoking lost a limb. Smoking in excess of 40 pack-years (number of packs of cigarettes per day multiplied by the number of years smoked) triples the likelihood of surgery. Diabetes increases the risk of amputation five-fold with one study reporting that diabetic claudicants have a 21% risk of amputation. If patients progress to amputation between 15% and 50% will require a contralateral limb amputation within 2 years.

Comorbid vascular disease

As mentioned earlier there is an increased incidence of occlusive disease at other sites. The average prevalence of coronary disease derived from 10 studies was 44%, partly depending on the method of diagnosis, while the prevalence of cerebrovascular disease was between 4% and 52%, again depending on whether it was diagnosed by clinical history or objective investigation. Clinical history and electrocardiogram reveal that ischaemic heart disease is present in 40–60% of patients with leg ischaemia. Coronary angiography shows that 90% of patients have disease there, it being severe in 28%. Both the prevalence of cardiac disease and the frequency of cardiac events are related to the severity of the peripheral disease. Furthermore, the severity of coronary artery disease has been shown to be related to the resting ABPI. Life expectancy of patients with intermittent claudication is decreased by 10 years. The average mortality rate of patients with claudication appears to be 2.5 that of non-claudicants. This equates to a 30, 50 and 70% mortality rate at 5, 10 and 15 years after diagnosis and a 5–10% rate of non-fatal cardiovascular events in 5 years. An ischaemic electrocardiogram (ECG) in a claudicant confers a life expectancy similar to that of one who has survived a myocardial infarction, but if the ECG is normal life expectancy is similar to controls. Coronary heart disease accounts for 30–60% of deaths, cerebrovascular disease for 10–20% and other vascular events (i.e. ruptured abdominal aortic aneurysms) approximately 10% of deaths. The outlook for patients with critical limb ischaemia is as grim as for Dukes 'C' carcinoma of the colon, with 20% dying in 1 year.

Critical limb ischaemia

Critical limb ischaemia is a difficult definition; the implication is a clinical state that will lead to amputation if not improved. Critical limb ischaemia has been defined by a European consensus conference as: persistently recurring rest pain requiring regular analgesia for more than 2 weeks, or ulceration, or gangrene of the foot; plus an ankle systolic pressure less than 50 mmHg, or absent peripheral pulses in diabetics. The incidence of critical limb ischaemia is approximately 500–1000 patients per million per year. The annual prevalence of critical limb ischaemia in the UK and Ireland is around one in 2500.

Progression of critical limb ischaemia to amputation is not inevitable with 30–75% of patients with rest pain improving spontaneously. Assessment of the true natural history of this condition is no longer possible because 50–60% undergo some sort of limb salvage procedure, although 20% still require an amputation. Randomized placebo-controlled drug trials have provided data on patients with unreconstructable critical limb ischaemia: 35% will lose the leg within 6 months and 15% will die. Not unexpectedly ulceration and gangrene carry a greater risk of amputation. The 5 year mortality rate of patients with rest pain is 50%, and 95% of patients with gangrene are dead within 10 years.

Of particular concern is the mortality rate of major amputees (Table 17.1).

Table 17.1 Mortality after first amputation

Hospital/1 month	*1 year*	*3 years*
14%	32%	61%

The most important risk factor is again smoking which may increase the mortality rate three-fold. Diabetes is also a risk factor for death as are hypertension and concomitant coronary or cerebrovascular disease. The site of the peripheral lesion also has an impact on mortality, with popliteal trifurcation disease being associated with a doubling of the 5 year mortality rate, although this may more reflect the pattern of diabetic vascular disease. In addition, the mean survival of patients with aorto-iliac disease has been shown to be longer (10.7 years) than those with femoro-popliteal disease (7.2 years).

The risk factors for peripheral arterial disease are also those for coronary artery disease and vascular disease at other sites. Carotid artery disease, as measured by duplex scanning, is present in 25–50% of claudicants. Renal artery disease is also associated with PAOD, with 15% of patients having a stenosis greater than 50%. Patients with both PAOD and hypertension are three times more likely to have renal artery stenosis. There is a significant overlap with multiple areas of vascular disease. In patients with PAOD between 4 and 8% will have cerebrovascular and coronary artery disease.

Lower limb PAOD is a disease of the middle aged and elderly with prevalence increasing with advancing age. Men are more commonly affected than women. Mortality is increased in both symptomatic and asymptomatic patients with PAOD from cardiac and cerebrovascular causes. Most patients with intermittent claudication plateau and some may improve. However, smoking and diabetes accelerate disease progression. The risk of amputation is low and has decreased in recent years. The risk factors of PAOD are similar to coronary artery disease. However, smoking is particularly important for lower limb disease and is potentially the most preventable cause. Hypertension, hypercholesterolaemia and diabetes are independently associated with this disease. Correcting these abnormalities may also reduce the incidence of PAOD. The role of antiplatelet agents and antioxidants in primary prevention requires further investigation.

Further reading

Fowkes, F. G. R., Housley, E., Cawood, E. H. H. *et al.* (1991). Edinburgh Artery Study: Prevalence of Asymptomatic and Symptomatic Peripheral Arterial Disease in the General Population. *Int J Epidemiol* **20**: 384–92.

Kannell, W. B. and Shurtleff, D. (1973). The Framingham study, cigarettes and the development of intermittent claudication. *Geriatrics* **28**: 61–8.

Leng, G. C. and Fowkes, F. G. R. (1998). Epidemiology and risk factors for peripheral arterial disease. In: Beard, J. D. and Gaines, P. A. eds. *Vascular and Endovascular Surgery*. London: W. B. Saunders, pp. 1–23.

Management of Peripheral Arterial Disease (PAD). (2000). Trans-Atlantic Inter-Society Consensus (TASC): A2 Epidemiology, Natural History, Risk Factors. *J Vasc Surg* (suppl) **31**: 5–34.

MODULE 18

Vascular risk reduction

1 • 'Population' versus 'individual' strategies
2 • Risk factors for vascular disease and vascular risk assessment
3 • Lifestyle measures
4 • Drugs for lipid lowering
5 • Antihypertensive drugs
6 • Aspirin
7 • Special cases

The UK has one of the highest rates of coronary heart disease (CHD) in the world and this is mirrored by high rates of other atherosclerotic vascular disease including peripheral vascular disease (PVD). Over a period of decades the major risk factors, both modifiable and unmodifiable, for CHD have been well delineated, although in recent years additional risk factors such as elevated plasma homocysteine levels have been added to the list. Although the evidence is most convincing for CHD similar risk factors apply, although possibly in different proportions, to peripheral vascular disease. In recent years a remarkable body of evidence has accumulated on the benefits of treatment of some of these risk factors in reducing CHD risk. There is scope for further elucidation of the details of this, but there is widespread consensus about the main issues involved. The evidence for risk factor modification for reduction of PVD is less striking, with the exception of promotion of exercise and smoking cessation.

Section 18.1 • 'Population' versus 'individual' strategies

Overall reduction in vascular risk involves strategies directed both at the whole population and at individuals. The nature of risk distributions means that there are very many more individuals with only modestly elevated risks for cardiovascular events than there are with markedly elevated risks. The consequence of this is that a large proportion of individuals suffering a cardiovascular event have only modestly elevated risks and may therefore not be picked up as meriting treatment of their risk factors in advance of the event. Influencing vascular risk in this group involves population interventions including health education and promotion, fiscal measures to discourage smoking and encourage healthy eating, and the promotion of increased levels of activity. In time this will decrease the overall population risk and reduce the need for treatment in the future. In contrast, the strategy targeted at the individual involves finding and treating the relatively small proportion of individuals who are at highest risk of future cardiovascular events. This is considered in more detail in this chapter. These two strategies are clearly complementary.

Section 18.2 • Risk factors for vascular disease and vascular risk assessment

Vascular risk factors

Vascular risk factors can be divided into those which are unmodifiable, such as being male or having a strong family history of ischaemic heart disease, and those that can be modified, such as cigarette smoking, hypertension, diabetes mellitus, elevated plasma total or low-density lipoprotein (LDL) cholesterol, and a low high-density lipoprotein (HDL) cholesterol (Table 18.1). The importance of these risk factors for vascular disease has been delineated over many years, firstly by epidemiological studies, which quantified their importance in comparisons of populations between and within countries. Their importance has been confirmed in many observational studies. More recently further knowledge has accumulated from intervention studies, which, for at least some of these risk factors, have demonstrated that intervening to lower that risk factor improves the outcome, in terms of morbidity and mortality, both from vascular disease and from all causes.

There is overwhelming evidence implicating cholesterol as a cardiovascular risk factor. In recent years a particularly potent piece of accumulating evidence has

Table 18.1 Risk factors for cardiovascular disease

- Age
- Male sex
- Family history of premature CHD (<55 years in men, <65 years in women)
- Personal history of cardiovascular disease

- Obesity*
- Cigarette smoking*
- Diet high in saturated fats, calories and cholesterol*
- Diet low in fruit and vegetables*
- Physical inactivity*

- Hypertension*
- Raised total or LDL cholesterol*
- Low HDL cholesterol*
- Raised triglycerides
- Hyperglycaemia, diabetes*
- Homocysteine
- Lipoprotein(a)
- Raised fibrinogen

*There is a well-established role for intervening to improve these risk factors.

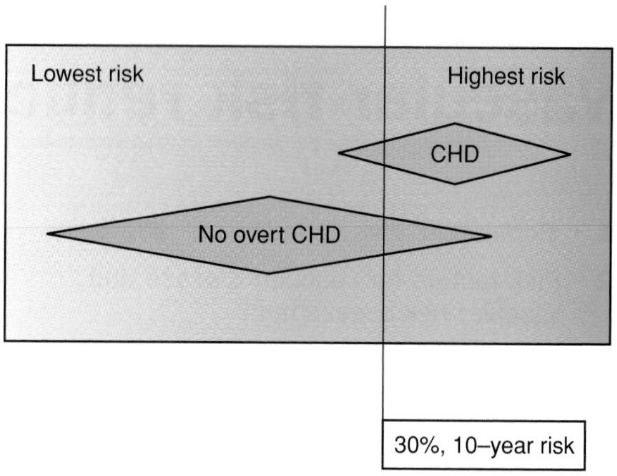

Figure 18.1 Risk of coronary disease. (Adapted, with permission, from Isles, C., ed. Consensus Conference on Lipid Lowering to Prevent Vascular Events. *Proceedings of the Royal College of Physicians of Edinburgh* 1999; **29** Suppl 5, p. 2.)

been the reversibility of vascular risk by the use of cholesterol lowering drugs (see below). Furthermore, a number of other vascular risk factors, including cigarette smoking, hypertension and diabetes mellitus, have a stronger association with CHD in populations with a high prevailing cholesterol than in those with lower levels.

When assessing cholesterol levels it is important to remember that following a myocardial infarction total cholesterol, LDL cholesterol and HDL cholesterol decrease within about 24 hours, and can take up to 6 weeks to return to pre-infarction levels. Other types of physical stress have a similar effect. A lipid profile taken up to about 24 hours after the onset of chest pain will provide a reasonable indication of the usual cholesterol level, but a further sample should be taken at 6 weeks either to confirm the need or lack of need for treatment, or to adjust the dose of treatment if this has already been started.

Hypertension is an important risk factor for stroke and for CHD, and its reduction by lifestyle measures and drugs has been shown to reduce the risk of stroke at all ages, and of CHD in the elderly. Although the reduction in stroke risk is greater than for CHD risk, the higher incidence of CHD than strokes means that treatment of hypertension may prevent as many CHD deaths as strokes.

Consideration of vascular risk reduction has frequently been considered under the headings of primary and secondary prevention, that is the prevention respectively of an initial or a recurrent vascular event. However, there is in fact a continuum of risk for patients from the lowest risk, in patients with very few risk factors, all the way through to the highest risk in patients who already have overt CHD. In the middle of this risk distribution there is considerable overlap between the highest risk primary prevention subjects who have multiple cardiovascular risks but no overt CHD and those with established CHD but who are at relatively low risk for further events (Figure 18.1).

Division into primary and secondary prevention is therefore fairly arbitrary, and may not best describe the future risk of a cardiovascular event, but remains a convenient way of identifying at least a proportion of individuals likely to be at the highest end of the risk spectrum, because of a pre-existing vascular event, and who therefore stand to gain the greatest benefit from intervention. It also reflects the reality of clinical practice, since these are individuals who will have already presented themselves to medical services, and who are already receiving care. These patients are also a priority for treatment because the quality of evidence for the benefits of treatment in reducing their morbidity and mortality is among the best available for any aspect of medical practice.

For primary prevention, subjects have no symptomatic disease, and high-risk individuals have to be sought out by screening, whether this is opportunistic or systematic. There is now widespread agreement that risk reduction treatment in these individuals should be aimed at their overall cardiovascular risk rather than at any single risk factors taken in isolation, such as a high cholesterol level. This will ensure that treatment will be given to those who will benefit most from intervention. The elevated risk in that person may be the result of a marked elevation of a single risk factor, such as in familial hypercholesterolaemia or accelerated hypertension. However, frequently it is the consequence of the combination of more modest increases in a number of different risk factors, each of which individually may not be sufficiently elevated to be an obvious candidate for treatment.

This targeting of treatment at those at highest risk derives from the results of intervention trials, which show that those at highest overall vascular risk have most to gain from treatment. A given reduction in cholesterol or in blood pressure produces a constant proportional reduction in risk whatever the absolute risk. This means that an individual at high baseline risk has more to gain from a particular intervention than one at low baseline risk. For example, statins reduce relative risk by about one-third. A 45-year-old man with a cholesterol of 6.0 mmol/l but no other vascular risk factors will have a risk of CHD in the next 10 years of <10%. A similarly aged man with the same cholesterol level but who smokes, has diabetes, hypertension and left ventricular hypertrophy will have a risk of CHD in the next 10 years of >30%. Treatment of these two men with a statin would provide the same relative benefit in each, but a <3% absolute benefit in the first and a >10% absolute benefit in the second.

Vascular risk assessment

Clinical judgement has repeatedly been shown to be a poor way of assessing overall vascular risk. Some means of estimating overall risk is therefore required. A number of methods are available, but most are based on the wealth of epidemiological data that has been gained from the Framingham study. In this study a large proportion of the population of the US town of Framingham has been assessed in detail for a wide variety of potential cardiovascular risk factors, and then followed up for many years, recording subsequent cardiovascular morbidity and mortality. These data have been embodied in a series of equations that allow calculation of the risk of a variety of cardiovascular events on the basis of information about risk factors such as age, sex, blood pressure, cholesterol, HDL cholesterol, the presence of electrocardiogram evidence of left ventricular hypertrophy, cigarette smoking and diabetes. The data derived from this study, initiated many years ago, of the population of a single US town have been demonstrated to be applicable in the present to a number of European populations, including that of the WOSCOPS study, which originated from Glasgow in Scotland. The risk factor information can be presented in the form of a table (for example the 'Sheffield' table) or a chart (for example the 'New Zealand' charts or the joint British recommendations charts), or is available on a number of calculators that can be integrated into computer based patient databases. All of these aim to take the known information about an individual's risk factors, and provide an indication of the future risk of CHD or cardiovascular disease.

The Framingham equations underestimate risk in some patients, for example those with type I diabetes mellitus (in whom elevated HDL cholesterol levels confer less benefit than in the non-diabetic population), patients with proteinuria, those with familial hypercholesterolaemia or those with a family history of premature CHD.

The question of who should be considered for risk assessment is an important one. There is little evidence on the consequences of routine population screening in terms of the balance of benefit and harm, or of cost-benefit at an individual or at a population level. A pragmatic approach is to pre-select for screening those individuals who are most likely to have an elevated risk, and who are most likely to benefit from drug treatment. In practical terms this sets a lower age limit for screening of perhaps 40 years, since below this age the proportion of the population with an elevated risk is small, and an upper limit of perhaps 70, since above this age the proportion will be very high but the evidence for the benefit of treatment is less clear. However, these limits can only be a guide, and individuals outside these limits may merit assessment of risk factors, and hence overall risk, for example because of a family history of premature vascular disease, or because of chance detection of an elevated vascular risk factor. Furthermore, decisions about whether to screen or to start drug treatment should be reviewed regularly. The absolute risk associated with a risk factor (or combination of risk factors) increases with advancing age, and may over a period of years become great enough to justify treatment when this was not considered justified previously.

Vascular risk thresholds for treatment with lipid lowering or antihypertensive drugs

Lifestyle changes can influence cholesterol, blood pressure and overall cardiovascular risk, and should be initiated in all patients (see below). However, many will require the use of drugs in order to reach treatment targets.

The level of risk that merits drug treatment is determined by a balance between the level at which treatment has been shown to be beneficial, potential side-effects of the drugs used, the cost of treatment (both of the drugs used and of the screening and monitoring of patients), and of the number of individuals in the population who are above the risk threshold. The trials of thiazide diuretics and β-blockers in the treatment of hypertension, and of statins in the treatment of elevated cholesterol, have shown that they cause few major adverse effects, so there is little to clinically offset against the potential benefits.

The recently published joint recommendations of the British Cardiac Society, British Hyperlipidaemia Association and the British Hypertension Society on prevention of CHD suggest that, initially, patients without known CHD or other major atherosclerotic disease should receive statin therapy if their CHD risk is 3% per year or greater. This was proposed as the minimum acceptable standard of care that should be initiated at the time of publication, but the eventual stated aim was to treat patients above a threshold of 1.5% annual CHD risk. This is because the available evidence shows an unequivocal benefit in individuals with this lower level of absolute risk, but the magnitude of the task of identifying and treating all such individuals is such that it should be approached in stages, and treatment initially targeted at those with most to gain. The joint recommendations of these organizations are to begin lipid-lowering treatment with a statin in patients above the threshold risk and with a cholesterol concentration >5 mmol/l. As described above, the risk of future CHD in some patients considered for primary prevention overlaps with the risk in some patients with established CHD, so it is reasonable to apply the same cholesterol threshold in each group.

An elevated cholesterol and low HDL remain risk factors for recurrent CHD events after a myocardial infarction. In patients with established vascular disease (i.e. in secondary prevention), the trials of statin drugs provide strong evidence for the benefit of lowering cholesterol when this is over 5 mmol/l (see below). The event rate in the groups receiving placebo in the lower risk secondary prevention trials was around 3% per year, in turn confirming the logic of the initial threshold for treatment in primary prevention.

An overview of trials of antihypertensive agents has shown that an average fall in diastolic blood pressure of 5–6 mmHg over 4.9 years was associated with a highly significant 38% reduction in stroke, 16% reduction in myocardial infarction and 12% reduction in all cause mortality. Cardiovascular risk increases across the whole range of observed blood pressures, but the thresholds recommended for intervention are based on the levels above which treatment has been shown to be beneficial. In addition, although the entry criteria for many of the earlier trials of antihypertensive treatment were based on diastolic pressures, systolic pressures are at least as closely related with cardiovascular disease as diastolic pressures.

A number of national and international sets of guidelines for hypertension management are available. They differ in detail, but are broadly comparable. The recommendations here derive from the British guidelines.

Blood pressure measurements should be standardised, and use a properly validated, maintained and calibrated device. The subject should be seated, with the arm at the level of the heart. The cuff size should be appropriate to the arm circumference, since a size that is too small will give artefactually high blood pressure readings. Blood pressure should be recorded to the nearest 2 mmHg, and diastolic pressure recorded as the disappearance of the sounds (Korotkoff phase V). At least two measurements should be made at each of several visits over a period of time (see below) to determine blood pressure thresholds for treatment.

Under some circumstances ambulatory blood pressure monitoring can be useful. These include unusual variability in clinic pressures, suspected 'white coat hypertension' (when clinic pressures are markedly higher than those recorded under more normal circumstances), when hypertension is resistant to drug treatment and when symptoms suggest the possibility of periods of hypotension.

All adults should have their blood pressure measured at least every 5 years until the age of 80 years. Those who have had previous high readings and those with pressures in the higher part of the acceptable range (135–139/85–89 mmHg) should have yearly checks.

At the high end of the blood pressure range, those with initial pressures ≥220/120 mmHg should be treated immediately. Those with pressures ≥199/109 mmHg should have these confirmed over 1–2 weeks, unless in the malignant phase of a hypertensive emergency, and should then be treated. In the initial blood pressure range 160–199/100–109 mmHg, if there are cardiovascular complications or target organ damage (Table 18.2), or diabetes, blood pressure should be checked over 3–4 weeks, and if sustained at these levels should be treated. In the absence of these factors it is acceptable to measure blood pressure weekly and treat if these levels persist over 4–12 weeks.

In the intermediate initial blood pressure range 140–159/90–99 mmHg, if cardiovascular complications, target organ damage or diabetes are present, blood pressure should be confirmed over 12 weeks, and if sustained should be treated. If these features are absent and these blood pressures are maintained over a period of months, the CHD risk over 10 years should be assessed, and treatment initiated if this is ≥15%. If the CHD risk is <15% over 10 years, the patient should be observed and the CHD risk reassessed annually.

The best available evidence on optimal blood pressure targets in treated hypertension comes from the hypertension optimal treatment (HOT) trial. Major cardiovascular events were lowest at a blood pressure of 139/83 mmHg, and blood pressures reduced below this level caused no harm. Patients with blood pressure below 150/90 mmHg were not significantly disadvantaged. Patients with diabetes benefited from diastolic blood pressure below 80 mmHg rather than below 90 mmHg. From these data suggested optimal targets for blood pressure lowering with antihypertensive drugs are <140/85 mmHg, and <140/80 mmHg in patients with diabetes. The minimum recommended levels of blood pressure control are <150/90 mmHg, and <140/85 mmHg in diabetes. However, even with best practice these targets will not be achieved in all hypertensive patients.

There is virtually no clinical trial evidence on risk factor management in patients with cerebral vascular and peripheral vascular disease. However, the limited

Table 18.2 Complications of hypertension and target organ damage

- Stroke, transient ischaemic attack, dementia
- Left ventricular hypertrophy, heart failure
- Myocardial infarction, angina, coronary artery bypass graft or angioplasty
- Peripheral vascular disease
- Fundal haemorrhages or exudates
- Proteinuria
- Renal failure

trial data that are available support the treatment of hypertension, serum cholesterol and blood glucose as risk factors for the development of atherosclerotic disease in these as in other vascular territories. The statin trials of cholesterol lowering for secondary prevention of CHD also showed a reduction in the risk of strokes, so patients with cerebrovascular disease could also potentially benefit. In addition, patients with cerebrovascular and peripheral arterial disease are potentially at as high risk of developing or dying from CHD as many patients who have already suffered a myocardial infarction. So, treatment can be justified as reducing coronary as well as other vascular risks.

Section 18.3 • Lifestyle measures

There is no doubt that lifestyle interventions can have a beneficial impact on individual vascular risk factors and on overall vascular risk. However, a number of randomized trials performed in the community and aiming at multiple risk factors have concluded that the benefits are relatively modest, with small reductions in smoking, blood pressure and cholesterol, and non-significant falls in CHD mortality. This may be as a result of lack of motivation causing poor compliance, possibly in turn linked to poor socio-economic status. However, this small average reduction in risk factors conceals much greater reductions in some of those at the highest risk, which reinforces the need to attempt appropriate lifestyle measures before resorting to the use of drug therapy. An additional benefit is that these measures may benefit the whole family and not just the individual at risk.

Smoking

Smoking is a major risk factor for an initial cardiovascular or peripheral vascular event and is also a major risk factor for fatal and non-fatal recurrences. Observational data demonstrate that those individuals with established CHD who stop smoking have approximately one half the risk of future fatal events of those who continue to smoke. Stopping smoking probably has a greater effect on the risk of future vascular disease than cholesterol reduction, antihypertensive treatment or aspirin. Many strategies to help people to stop smoking have been tested. The highest success rates come from a combination of both individual and group smoking cessation advice, reinforced on multiple occasions and backed up by nicotine replacement therapy. Weight gain is common after stopping smoking so dietary advice is also needed to limit the subsequent weight gain.

Diet and obesity

Body mass index (BMI) is a significant predictor of coronary events and central obesity (reflected in the waist/hip ratio) may be even more important. A BMI greater than 24 is associated with increases in blood pressure, cholesterol and glucose and a reduction in HDL cholesterol, and increases in risk of coronary events, strokes and diabetes. Between BMIs of 24 and 30 cardiovascular mortality increases by 40%, and above a BMI of 30 it increases by 100%. Waist circumferences of 102 cm or more in men and 88 cm or more in women indicate a substantially increased risk.

Obesity is associated with a number of risk factors for CHD, including hypertension, high cholesterol, low HDL cholesterol and diabetes, and these all improve with weight reduction. If the ultimate goal is to reduce CHD levels, weight reduction may therefore be a more logical aim than intervening with single risk factors such as lipids or blood pressure by other means. However, it may be difficult to achieve. Advice to patients should include realistic targets for final weight and rate of weight loss. These may be in the region of 5–10 kg weight loss, at a rate of 0.5–1.0 kg per week.

The relationship between diet and vascular disease is complex, and compounded by the association of obesity with dyslipidaemia, hypertension and type II diabetes mellitus. Dietary advice has been demonstrated to be a relatively ineffective way of lowering cholesterol levels, with a reduction of about 5% being the best that can be achieved. Blood pressure falls by about 2.5/1.5 mmHg for every 1 kg of weight loss. Moderate salt reduction to less than 6 g per day lowers blood pressure by 7/3 mmHg, and the response may be greater in older patients and those with higher blood pressures. In view of these beneficial, albeit modest effects, dietary advice to lose weight and to modify the diet should not be abandoned.

The main dietary determinant of serum cholesterol is not its cholesterol content but saturated fat. There are many other components of a healthy diet not directly related to changes in serum lipid levels, including fruit and vegetables, dietary fibre, oily fish and monounsaturated fatty acids. A healthy diet may also contribute to reducing the risks of a variety of cancers.

A reduced saturated fat and supplemented polyunsaturated fat intake is the prime dietary intervention in patients with hyperlipidaemia. Obese individuals should not replace this reduced dietary energy intake with energy from other sources, in order to encourage weight loss which can in turn improve insulin sensitivity. There are no controlled clinical trials of the effect of reducing obesity following the development of vascular disease, but it would seem reasonable for dietary advice to include weight reduction, in view of the associations of obesity with vascular risk factors such as dyslipidaemias, hypertension and type II diabetes mellitus. For those who are not overweight, or who have succeeded in reducing weight, the reduction in dietary energy intake can be replaced with other energy sources such as unrefined carbohydrate and mono- and polyunsaturated fats, derived from oily fish and olive or rape seed oils.

Dietary goals for the healthy population include a dietary fat intake of 35% or less of total energy intake, with saturated fat amounting to no more than one-third of the total fat intake. Cholesterol consumption should be less than 300 mg daily. Increased use of monounsaturated and polyunsaturated fats and an increase in fresh fruit and vegetable intake to five portions per day is recommended. These recommendations were developed by the Committee on Medical Aspects of Food (COMA) panel on diet and cardiovascular diseases and were intended for the healthy population. A more rigorous approach is required for many patients with established CHD, or who are at high risk of CHD. Dietary intervention in patients with hypertension includes weight loss, reduction in salt intake, increased fruit and vegetable intake, and an alcohol consumption of less than 21 units per week in males and less than 14 units per week in females. There is also evidence that vegetarian diets and diets high in potassium may reduce blood pressure.

Early randomized controlled trials of diet in secondary prevention used a reduced fat intake and, in particular, a reduction in saturated fat, and failed to convincingly show an overall benefit in the reduction of cardiac events or mortality. More recent trials have investigated diets both low in saturated fats and supplemented with polyunsaturated fatty acids. These have in particular been the omega-3 fatty acids derived from an increased fish intake or the use of fish oil capsules and from α-linolenic acid margarine. These trials have demonstrated a significant reduction in coronary mortality and improved survival. The patients in these studies were not selected because of hyperlipidaemia and the interventions used had a minimal effect on the lipid profile, so it is unlikely that the observed benefits were achieved through quantitative changes in the cholesterol level. More subtle changes in lipoprotein composition or reduction in thrombotic tendency remain possible mechanisms.

Oxidized LDL is highly atherogenic and there is experimental evidence that antioxidants can have a beneficial effect on this process. Fruit and vegetables contain naturally occurring antioxidants and are important components of a healthy diet. Trials of the use of antioxidant supplements in primary and secondary prevention have given conflicting results and at present there is no clear evidence for benefit.

Plant sterols and stanols in the diet reduce the absorption of cholesterol from the gut and lower cholesterol concentrations. A number of food products, such as margarines and yoghurts, which incorporate these compounds in a lipid-soluble form are now available. These can lower the cholesterol by a modest but useful amount, for example by 0.54 mmol/l in those aged 50–59 years. They are relatively expensive. They may be useful in those who are willing to buy them and who are close to a threshold for treatment, or as an adjunct to statins, with which they have an additive effect. They should not, however, be considered as a substitute for statins, because of the much greater cholesterol-lowering effect of the statins.

Epidemiological studies have shown a linear independent relationship between serum levels of the amino acid homocysteine and cardiovascular risk. Homocysteine levels can be effectively reduced by supplementation of the diet with folic acid. A number of trials of the effect of folate supplementation on reducing CHD are in progress.

Dietary and other lifestyle advice should be given to all individuals considered for primary or secondary prevention of vascular disease. However, relatively few will achieve target cholesterol concentrations of <5 mmol/l on diet alone, and many will require statin treatment. Likewise, those with mild hypertension may achieve target blood pressures, but many patients with hypertension are likely to require treatment with antihypertensive drugs.

Exercise

Epidemiological studies show that a sedentary lifestyle is associated with an increased risk of CHD, but there is no outcome trial evidence that increasing the amount of exercise taken results in a reduction in CHD. However, taking up moderate physical activity in middle age appears to have a beneficial effect on risk, with a reduction in total and LDL cholesterol, an increase in HDL cholesterol, and reduction of blood pressure. In patients with pre-existing CHD, exercise programmes result in a reduction in coronary and total mortality when incorporated into lifestyle interventions including smoking reduction and diet improvement. Pragmatic advice is for those who are inactive to aim to accumulate 30 min of moderate intensity physical activity on most days. Those who are already active should in addition aim for 20–30 min of vigorous aerobic exercise three times per week.

Alcohol

Heavy drinking (greater than 21 units per week) raises blood pressure and triglycerides, contributes to obesity, and increases cardiac and total mortality. Smaller amounts of alcohol appear to protect against CHD, with light to moderate drinkers (1–2 units per day) having a lower CHD incidence and mortality than non-drinkers. A number of mechanisms for this protective effect of a moderate intake of alcohol have been suggested, including an increase in HDL. Although moderate alcohol intake appears to be beneficial, the effect is not so large that non-drinkers should be encouraged to drink.

How long to persist with lifestyle measures

There is no available evidence on how long lifestyle measures should be continued before considering drug therapy. Patients at very high risk are unlikely to achieve a sufficient risk reduction from lifestyle measures alone such that their risk is lowered to below the threshold for intervention, and may justify drug treatment at an early stage. Individuals who are closer to decision thresholds should pursue lifestyle measures for 3–6 months. Lifestyle measures should continue long term, irrespective of the need for drug treatment.

Section 18.4 • Drugs for lipid lowering

A number of classes of drug with lipid-lowering effects are available, but the majority of the evidence for benefit comes from studies using 3-hydroxy-3-methylglutaryl coenzyme A (HMG-CoA) reductase inhibitors (statins).

Statins

These drugs inhibit HMG-CoA reductase, a rate-limiting enzyme in the pathway of cholesterol synthesis. They lower total and LDL cholesterol concentrations, with a more modest reduction in triglyceride and increase in HDL concentrations. Their main role is therefore in patients whose primary lipid abnormality is an elevated total or LDL cholesterol, although there is also evidence of benefit in patients with an 'average' cholesterol but a low LDL cholesterol (Table 18.3). They are well tolerated, with a low incidence of side-effects. A rare side-effect is myositis or rhabdomyolysis, and patients should be warned to stop the drug if they experience muscle pains.

The publication of the 4S trial in 1994 represents a landmark in the accumulation of evidence for the benefits of treatment. This trial demonstrated that in a group of patients, aged 35–70, with a high risk of future CHD, on the basis of their pre-existing CHD and cholesterol levels between 5.5 and 8.0 mmol/l, cholesterol lowering with simvastatin 20–40 mg per day resulted in a 34% reduction in coronary events and a 30% reduction in overall mortality. This trial has been extended by further trials in secondary prevention (CARE, LIPID) to demonstrate benefits at lower levels of cholesterol (Table 18.3).

In summary, these trials of lipid lowering with statins in secondary prevention show that reduction of total and LDL cholesterol by 20–25% reduced CHD mortality by about 25–30%, regardless of age, sex or the presence of diabetes mellitus. Patients with unstable angina benefited as much as post-infarction patients. A pragmatic approach is to offer all patients with a vascular event dietary advice. In addition, all patients with cholesterol clearly above 5 mmol/l should receive a statin before discharge. Those with more borderline elevations of cholesterol should have this checked at 6 weeks, and a statin should be started if it remains above 5 mmol/l.

The WOSCOPS trial was a trial of primary prevention conducted in the west of Scotland, and demonstrated that individuals, mainly without pre-existing CHD but at a high risk of events because of their high cholesterol levels could, if treated with pravastatin, have the risk of a future myocardial infarction reduced by 31% (Table 18.3). Again this trial has been extended by a further trial to demonstrate a benefit in lower risk individuals (AFCAPS/TexCAPS, Table 18.3).

These large well-conducted trials have convincingly demonstrated that lipid lowering treatment with statins reduces cardiovascular morbidity and mortality in both primary and secondary prevention. Issues in treatment have therefore moved on from consideration of efficacy and safety to those of treatment targets, cost-effectiveness and patient selection.

The goal of statin treatment

The statin trials have all produced similar relative reductions in CHD, despite using either a fixed dose of drug or titrated doses to achieve predefined treatment targets based on either total or LDL cholesterol. A pragmatic approach to statin treatment is therefore to

Table 18.3 Selected outcome rates from the major trials of lipid lowering drugs[a]

Study	*Drug*	*Baseline cholesterol (mmol/l)*	*Mean % reduction in total cholesterol*	*Reduction in CHD events*	*Reduction in overall mortality*
Primary prevention					
4S	Simvastatin 20–40 mg	6.7	29%	34% ↓ in major coronary events	30%
CARE	Pravastatin 40 mg	5.4	20%	24% ↓ in fatal or non-fatal MI	Not designed to detect difference in overall mortality
LIPID	Pravastatin 40 mg	5.6	18%	29% ↓ in fatal or non-fatal MI	22%
Secondary prevention					
WOSCOPS	Pravastatin 40 mg	7.0	20%	31% ↓ in non-fatal MI	22%
AFCAPS/TexCAPS	Lovastatin 40 mg	5.7[b]	18%	37% ↓ in first acute coronary event[c]	Not designed to detect difference in overall mortality
VAHIT	Gemfibrozil 1200 mg	4.5[d]	4%[e]	22% ↓ in non-fatal MI or death from coronary causes	Not designed to detect difference in overall mortality

[a]For references to these trials see text. Follow-up ranged from 4.9 to 6.1 years.
[b]Patients selected to have 'average' total cholesterol and 'below average' HDL cholesterol (mean HDL cholesterol 0.94 mmol/l).
[c]First acute coronary event in this trial defined as sudden cardiac death, fatal and non-fatal MI, new unstable angina.
[d]Patients selected to have a low level of HDL as primary lipid abnormality (mean HDL cholesterol 0.8 mmol/l).
[e]HDL increased by 6%, triglycerides decreased by 31%.

base the target of treatment on a total cholesterol of 5 mmol/l, and to titrate the dose to achieve this. If the cholesterol was relatively low before statin treatment (5–6 mmol/l) a 30% decrease in cholesterol may be a more logical treatment target. Treatment should normally be considered to be lifelong.

Fibrates

The fibric acid derivatives include gemfibrozil, bezafibrate and fenofibrate. Their effect on reduction in total and LDL cholesterol is typically more modest than that of the statins, but they have more marked effects on reducing triglycerides and increasing HDL. Evidence from early trials of fibrates in primary prevention suggested that there was a beneficial effect on CHD, but there were doubts raised by non-significant increases in non-coronary mortality, such that all-cause mortality was not reduced.

A more recent trial of gemfibrozil in secondary prevention (VAHIT, Table 18.3), in patients whose primary lipid abnormality was a relatively low HDL, has demonstrated a substantial reduction in CHD events. There was no increase in non-CHD adverse events. The trial was not designed to be large enough to establish a benefit on overall mortality, but there was a non-significant trend in favour of gembibrozil, which was reassuring in view of the outcomes in earlier trials.

Fibrates may be expected to have a particular role in reducing vascular risk in patients with type II diabetes, where the typical adverse lipid profile includes a reduction in HDL and an increase in triglycerides. As yet there is no evidence to support this suggestion but a number of trials are in progress.

Other lipid-lowering drugs

These include the bile acid sequestering resins such as cholestyramine. They promote increased cholesterol conversion to bile acids by breaking the enterohepatic circulation of bile acids, achieving reductions in total and LDL cholesterol. Studies of the effects of the resins in primary prevention have shown reductions in CHD events, but small non-significant increases in non-coronary mortality. They are inconvenient to take, and not well tolerated due to a high incidence of gastrointestinal side-effects. They are, however, safe to use in pregnancy and in children, because they are not systemically absorbed. They may be considered when statins or fibrates are not tolerated or are contraindicated.

Other drugs with lipid lowering effects include the nicotinic acid group, fish oils and soluble fibre. Although there is evidence to show variable (often modest) effects on lipid levels, there is little or no evidence of a benefit on cardiovascular outcome to support their use.

Section 18.5 • Antihypertensive drugs

The majority of the evidence of the outcome benefit of antihypertensive drug treatment comes from trials using thiazides or β-blockers. However, studies comparing the major classes of antihypertensive drugs (thiazides, β-blockers, calcium antagonists, angiotensin converting enzyme inhibitors and α-blockers) have shown no major differences in antihypertensive efficacy, side-effects or quality of life. Despite this, there are often large individual variations in response to the different classes of drug, and significant variations among different ethnic and age groups. There may also be particular indications or contraindications for the use of one or other of these classes of drugs in an individual patient (see below). If none of these applies it is appropriate to use the drugs which have the most supportive trial evidence and are the least expensive, which are low dose thiazides or β-blockers, with thiazides being the least expensive option. Long-acting dihydropyridine calcium antagonists are a good alternative for isolated systolic hypertension in the elderly when a low dose thiazide is not tolerated or is contraindicated.

Unless it is necessary to lower blood pressure urgently, a period of at least 4 weeks should be allowed to assess the full response to a drug. If required and appropriate the dose should then be increased. If the first drug chosen results in an insufficient response, an alternative drug should be substituted if the hypertension is mild and uncomplicated. If the hypertension is more severe, or there are cardiovascular complications, it may be safer to add further drugs to the initial treatment rather than substitute.

Over half of patients with hypertension will require more than one drug, with up to one-third requiring three or more drugs. Submaximal doses of two drugs are likely to give a larger blood pressure lowering effect and fewer side-effects than a maximal dose of one drug. Drugs from different classes usually have additive effects when prescribed together, but it is rational to combine classes with different modes of action. Examples include diuretics with β-blockers, diuretics with angiotensin converting enzyme inhibitors, β-blockers with calcium antagonists, and calcium antagonists with angiotensin converting enzyme inhibitors. Some combinations should be avoided, including β-blockers with verapamil or diltiazem, angiotensin converting enzyme inhibitors with angiotensin II antagonists, and angiotensin converting enzyme inhibitors with potassium sparing diuretics.

With regard to drug choice, there is particularly good evidence for the use of thiazides in the elderly. During and after myocardial infarction β-blockers reduce mortality in survivors, and are the drug of choice here and in angina. Rate limiting calcium antagonists also improve outcome, although this benefit is restricted to patients without left ventricular impairment. Dihydropyridine calcium antagonists have good evidence of benefit in the elderly with isolated systolic hypertension and a role in the treatment of angina. Angiotensin converting enzyme inhibitors have a clearly established benefit for patients with heart failure, including those who have had a myocardial infarction, and in diabetic nephropathy. Angiotensin II receptor antagonists may be an alternative if an angiotensin converting enzyme is indicated but its use limited by causing a cough. They also have a particularly good side-effect profile and may be tolerated when other antihypertensive drugs are not. The presence of prostatism may make α-blockers an appropriate choice of antihypertensive drug.

Thiazides and β-blockers may have an adverse effect on the lipid profile (although this effect is usually small at currently recommended doses), so may not be the best choice of antihypertensive drug in the presence of dyslipidaemias. Thiazides are clearly contraindicated in patients with gout, and β-blockers in patients with asthma, chronic obstructive pulmonary disease and heart block. β-Blockers may worsen heart failure, but in specialist hands in low doses may be used in its treatment. In peripheral vascular disease, β-blockers may exacerbate symptoms and angiotensin converting enzyme inhibitors and angiotensin II antagonists should be used with caution because of its association with renovascular disease, in which they can cause severe deterioration in renal function.

Section 18.6 • Aspirin

Aspirin treatment at a dose of 75–300 mg is indicated for secondary prevention in patients with no contraindications, since the benefits are sufficiently high as to clearly outweigh the risks. Its place in primary prevention is less clear, with a number of trials showing varying reductions in CHD events, but no benefit on CHD or all-cause mortality, and all showing an excess of gastrointestinal bleeding. The interpretation of these trials remains controversial. However, it may be reasonable to consider the use of low dose aspirin in patients whose risk of a CHD event is high enough as to justify the use of lipid lowering drugs, and in patients with well controlled hypertension, and either target organ damage or diabetes, or a 10 year CHD risk >15%.

Section 18.7 • Special cases

Women

Vascular disease is commoner in men than in women, at all ages. However, it remains a major cause of death and morbidity in women and the same risk factors apply as in men. The onset of CHD in women lags about 10 years behind that in men with the result that up to the age of 65 years women have one-third the CHD mortality of men. There is no evidence that they do not derive benefit from intervention to lower vascular risk, through treatment of risk factors in the same way as for men.

Fewer women have been entered into trials than men, so there is less evidence for the benefit of lipid lowering drugs, but what there is suggests that women are at least as likely to benefit as men.

There is observational evidence of a benefit from oestrogen replacement therapy in reducing cardiovascular disease. However, this evidence is of lower quality than that coming from placebo-controlled trials of lipid-lowering and anti-hypertensive drugs. Placebo-controlled trials of oestrogen replacement have yet to demonstrate any clear-cut evidence of benefit, so it cannot be considered as an adequate means of reducing CHD risk in women.

Elderly

Cholesterol, hypertension, smoking, diabetes and physical inactivity remain risk factors in older people, although the relative risk declines with age. However, CHD is much more common in the elderly, so the attributable risk (the amount by which CHD would be reduced in the absence of that risk factor) is increased, so a larger proportion of the population are at least as likely to benefit as younger people. The statin trials only recruited patients up to the age of 75 years, but there was no suggestion from the results that the benefit of treatment diminishes with age. The secondary prevention studies (4S, CARE and LIPID) showed that patients in the 60–75 years age group achieved similar benefits to younger patients. In the primary prevention studies, WOSCOPS only enrolled patients up to the age of 65 but the risks and benefits appeared greater in the older than the younger age groups; AFCAPS/TexCAPS enrolled patients up to the age of 73 years, but there were few CHD events in this age group in this low risk trial and there was no conclusive evidence of benefit. The results of further trials are awaited.

In contrast there is good evidence that the treatment of hypertension in the elderly reduces CHD as well as cerebrovascular disease and is probably the most important modifiable CHD risk factor in this age group.

Diabetes and impaired glucose tolerance

Patients with diabetes have a two to four times higher risk of CHD than those without. The total cholesterol level in diabetics is similar to that in the general population, but their LDL tends to be smaller and more atherogenic. The more typical and readily measurable lipid abnormalities, especially in type II diabetes, are elevated triglycerides and a low HDL level, and this dyslipidaemia is linked to CHD in both male and female type I and type II subjects.

Relatively small numbers of patients with diabetes were entered into the statin trials, but subgroup analysis suggests that diabetic patients benefit from treatment at least as much as non-diabetic patients. Prospective studies of lipid lowering in patients with diabetes are in progress. Risk should be assessed and treatment initiated as for non-diabetic patients, with the caution that all of the risk assessment tools available tend to underestimate CHD risk in patients with type I diabetes and in those with nephropathy. Also, before initiating lipid lowering drug treatment it should be remembered that improved glycaemic control by whatever means (diet, oral agents or insulin) reduces cholesterol and triglyceride levels.

A lower target blood pressure than in non-diabetics, of <130 mmHg systolic and <80 mmHg diastolic, may be justified from the trial evidence for reduction of macrovascular and microvascular complications.

Familial hypercholesterolaemia

Patients presenting with a myocardial infarction at an early age (men aged less than 55 years and women aged less than 60 years) with cholesterol >5 mmol/l or any patient with cholesterol greater than 8 mmol/l may have familial hypercholesterolaemia or another inherited dyslipidaemia. Consideration should be given to further investigation and the need for aggressive lipid lowering therapy, and first degree relatives should be invited for screening.

Heterozygous familial hypercholesterolaemia has a prevalence of 1 in 500, making it one of the most common inherited metabolic disorders. It is caused by a deficiency in the number of LDL receptors or defects in their function. Tendon xanthomas in the patient or a relative are virtually pathognomonic of the condition if present, but up to 20% of patients do not have them. They are found particularly over the knuckles and in the Achilles tendons.

Familial hypercholesterolaemia can be more formally classified as 'definite' or 'possible'. Definite familial hypercholesterolaemia is defined as total cholesterol >7.5 mmol/l in adults or >6.7 mmol/l in children (or LDL cholesterol >4.9 mmol/l in adults or >4.0 mmol/l in children) plus tendon xanthomas in the patient or a first or second degree relative. Possible familial hypercholesterolaemia requires the same cholesterol levels plus a family history of either a myocardial infarction before age 60 in a first degree relative or age 50 in a second degree relative, or a total cholesterol >7.5 mmol/l in a first or second degree relative.

The cumulative risk of a fatal or non-fatal coronary event in heterozygous familial hypercholesterolaemia by the age of 60 is at least 50% in men and about 30% in women. Clinical events can occur as early as the mid-twenties, and there is an approximately four-fold increase in the risk of CHD in both sexes.

Patients with familial hypercholesterolaemia have been excluded from the statin trials because their risk of CHD precluded the possibility that they may be randomized to receive treatment with placebo. There is therefore no evidence from randomized trials for the benefit of treatment. However, evidence from the long-term follow-up of cohorts of patients with familial hypercholesterolaemia suggests that their prognosis has improved in recent years, and this is almost certainly because of more effective treatment with statins. All patients with heterozygous familial hypercholesterolaemia should be strongly discouraged from smoking and given intensive dietary advice, but are likely to require drug treatment to achieve an adequate reduction in cholesterol.

Further reading

Anderson, K. M., Odell, P. M., Wilson, P.W. and Kannel, W. B. (1991). Cardiovascular disease risk profiles. *Am Heart J* **121**: 293–8.

Bloomfield Rubins, H., Robins, S. J., Collins, D. *et al.* for the Veterans Affairs High-Density Lipoprotein Cholesterol Intervention Trial Study Group (1999). Gemfibrozil for the secondary prevention of coronary heart disease in men with low levels of high-density lipoprotein cholesterol. *N Engl J Med* **341**: 410–18.

Collins, R. and Macmahon, S. (1994). Blood pressure, antihypertensive drug treatment and the risks of stroke and of coronary heart disease. *Br Med Bull* **50**: 272–98.

Downs, J. R., Clearfield, M., Weis, S. *et al.* (1998). Primary prevention of acute coronary events with lovastatin in men and women with average cholesterol levels: results of AFCAPS/TexCAPS. *JAMA* **79**: 1615–22.

Hansson, L., Zanchetti, A., Carruthers, S. G. *et al.* for the HOT Study Group (1998). Effects of intensive blood pressure lowering and low dose aspirin in patients with hypertension: principal results of the hypertension optimal treatment (HOT) randomised trial. *Lancet* **351**: 1755–62.

Jackson, R. (2000). Updated New Zealand cardiovascular disease risk-benefit prediction guide. *BMJ* **320**: 709–10.

Law, M. (2000). Plant sterol and stanol margarines and health. *BMJ* **320**: 861–4.

Long-term Intervention with Pravastatin in Ischaemic Disease (LIPID) Study Group (1998). Prevention of cardiovascular events and death with pravastatin in patients with coronary heart disease and a broad range of initial cholesterol levels *N Engl J Med* **339**: 1349–57.

Ramsay, L. E., Williams, B., Johnston, G. D. *et al.* (1999). Guidelines for management of hypertension: report of the third working party of the British Hypertension Society. *J Hum Hypertens* **13**: 569–92.

Ramsay, L. E., Williams, B., Johnston, G. D. *et al.* (1999). British Hypertension Society guidelines for hypertension management 1999: summary. *BMJ* **319**: 630–5.

Sacks, F. M., Pfeffer, M. A., Moye, L. A. *et al.* (1996). The effect of pravastatin on coronary events after myocardial infarction in patients with average cholesterol levels. *N Engl J Med* **335**: 1001–9.

Scandinavian Simvastatin Survival Study Group (1994). Randomised controlled trial of cholesterol lowering in 4444 patients with coronary heart disease: the Scandinavian Simvastatin Survival Study (4S). *Lancet* **344**: 1383–9.

Shepherd, J., Cobbe, S. M., Ford, I. *et al.* (1995). Prevention of coronary heart disease with pravastatin in men with hypercholesterolaemia. *N Engl J Med* **333**: 1301–7.

Silagy, C., Mant, D., Fowler, G. and Lodge, M. (1994). Meta-analysis on efficacy of nicotine replacement therapies in smoking cessation. *Lancet* **343**: 139–42.

Tang, J. L., Armitage, J. M., Lancaster, T. *et al.* (1998). Systematic review of dietary intervention trials to lower total cholesterol in free-living subjects *BMJ* **316**: 1213–20.

Wallis, E. J., Ramsay, L. E., Haq, I. U. *et al.* (2000). Coronary and cardiovascular risk estimation for primary prevention: validation of a new Sheffield table in the 1995 Scottish health survey population. *BMJ* **320**: 671–6.

Wood, D., Durrington, P., Poulter, N. *et al.* (1998). Joint British recommendations on prevention of coronary heart disease in clinical practice. *Heart* **80** (Suppl 2): S1–29.

MODULE 19

Thrombophilia

Over the past 10–15 years the term thrombophilia has become increasingly familiar to clinicians working in all specialities. There is no internationally accepted definition of thrombophilia, but broadly the term is used to describe a 'tendency to thrombosis' and in practice the term is usually restricted to a tendency to develop venous thrombotic events. In North America the term thrombophilic is frequently used by clinicians to describe patients who appear to have developed venous thrombosis either spontaneously or of a severity out of proportion to any recognized stimulus. The term thrombophilic is also sometimes used for patients who have recurrent venous thrombotic events and patients who develop venous thrombosis at an early age.

In 1990 the British Committee for Standards in Haematology suggested that the term thrombophilia should be used to describe 'the familial or acquired disorders of the haemostatic mechanism which are likely to predispose to (venous) thrombosis'. This definition is widely used but it has several serious disadvantages. First, it has become evident as new thrombophilias have been described that many individuals who carry these defects remain asymptomatic. Secondly, even though the number of haemostatic abnormalities recognized as thrombophilic has increased since 1990, detailed laboratory investigation fails to detect any abnormality in at least half of the patients who present with a history of thrombosis – including many who appear clinically thrombophilic.

Thrombophilias, or thrombophilic defects, may be inherited, acquired or mixed – the result of environmental factors such as diet or other lifestyle factors interacting with genetic background. The abnormalities at present accepted as thrombophilic are listed in Table 19.1.

Table 19.1 Thrombophilic defects

Heritable
Antithrombin deficiency
Protein C deficiency
Protein S deficiency
Factor V Leiden
Prothrombin 20210A
Dysfibrinogenaemia
Acquired
Antiphospholipid syndromes
Mixed
Factor VIII elevation
Hyperhomocysteinaemia (?)

Section 19.1 • Heritable thrombophilic defects

To date a limited number of genetic abnormalities are accepted as independent risk factors for venous thromboembolism (VTE). These defects include mutations in the genes encoding the natural anticoagulants antithrombin, protein C and protein S and the clotting factors fibrinogen, prothrombin and factor V.

Antithrombin deficiency

Antithrombin (previously called antithrombin III) is a single chain plasma glycoprotein. Antithrombin is synthesized in the liver. In adult humans, it is the primary inhibitor of thrombin and other activated clotting factors of the intrinsic coagulation cascade (e.g. factors Xa, XIa, XIIa, IXa). It is therefore one of the most important physiological regulators of fibrin formation (Figure 19.1).

Antithrombin inactivates thrombin and other activated clotting factors by forming irreversible complexes – the reactive site of the antithrombin molecule forming a stabilized bond with the active site of the activated clotting factor. The rate of inhibition of activated clotting factors by antithrombin is accelerated at least 1000-fold by the binding of heparin (unfractionated heparin, low molecular weight heparin or heparin-like compounds such as endothelial heparin sulfate) to antithrombin.

Two major types of heritable antithrombin deficiency are recognized. Type I defects are characterized by a quantitative reduction of qualitatively (functionally)

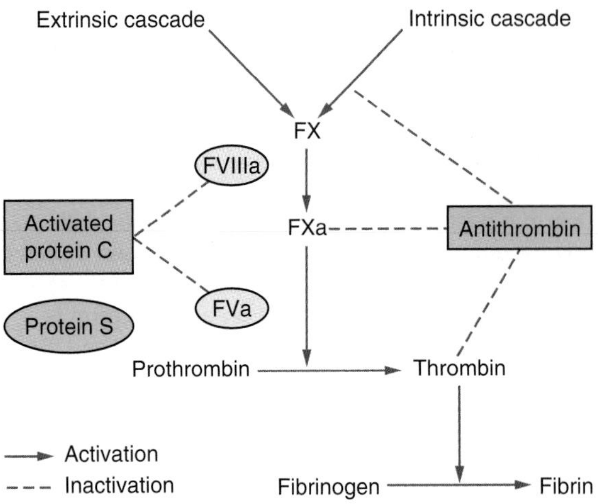

Figure 19.1 Regulation of the clotting cascade.

normal antithrombin protein. Type II antithrombin deficiency is due to the production of a qualitatively (functionally) abnormal protein. In both types antithrombin activity is reduced to a greater or lesser extent. In type I defects the quantity of antithrombin measurable on functional and immunological assay is concordantly reduced, whereas in type II defects the immunological assay result is discordantly high compared to the functional assay result and may be normal or near normal. Type II defects are further subclassified according to the site of the molecular defect, e.g. at the reactive (activated clotting factor inhibiting) site or at the heparin binding site. The incidence of thrombosis is higher in association with type I defects and type II defects where the mutation affects the reactive site than in type II defects where the mutation affects the heparin binding site.

For routine clinical purposes it is generally recommended that a functional antithrombin assay which measures the ability of heparin to bind to antithrombin and catalyse the neutralization of thrombin or factor Xa (an antithrombin heparin cofactor assay) is used since only functional assays will detect all type I and type II antithrombin deficiencies. If it is considered that a reduced antithrombin activity is possibly the result of a heritable defect, further investigation is merited including immunological assays (to allow initial classification into type I or type II defect) and progressive functional assays which measure antithrombin activity in the absence of heparin acceleration. Although many mutations associated with antithrombin deficiency have been identified, identification of the mutation is not necessary for clinical purposes. In patients where there is doubt about whether reduced antithrombin activity is inherited it may be useful to test other family members.

Antithrombin levels are slightly lower in premenopausal females than in males of similar age and are slightly lower in women using combined oral contraceptive pills than in non-pill using women. More significant decreases in antithrombin activity are observed in patients on heparin and in patients with a current thrombosis. Significant, and sometimes profound, decreases in plasma antithrombin levels are seen in disseminated intravascular coagulation (DIC), liver disease and the nephrotic syndrome. In interpreting the results of an antithrombin assay it is essential to take into account the patient's general clinical condition.

The prevalence of type I antithrombin deficiency in the general population is of the order of 1 in 5000 (0.02%). Type II defects are more common. In a review of studies of young patients with VTE, 4.5% were found to be antithrombin deficient but in general about 1% of unselected patients presenting with a first VTE have antithrombin deficiency. In selected patients with a family history of VTE in addition to their personal history of thrombosis, 4–5% will be found to be antithrombin deficient (Table 19.2).

From a clinical point of view, inherited antithrombin deficiency is heterogeneous. Deep vein thrombosis of the leg is the most common presentation although thrombosis may occur at a variety of other sites including renal veins, mesenteric veins and cerebral veins. Antithrombin deficiency seems to be a more severe defect than deficiencies of protein C or protein S.

Thrombosis may occur at a very young age. About half of the individuals with type I or type II reactive site defects will have already had a thrombotic event by the age of 25 years.

Protein C deficiency

Protein C is a vitamin K-dependent glycoprotein synthesized in the liver. It circulates in plasma as an inactive precursor. During coagulation it is activated by thrombin to activated protein C (APC). APC with its cofactor, protein S, inactivates the activated clotting cascade cofactors, activated factor VIII (FVIIIa) and activated factor V (FVa) by selective proteolytic cleavages inhibiting the activation of (respectively) factor X and prothrombin (Figure 19.1).

Like antithrombin deficiency, protein C defects have been classified into type I (quantitative) defects and type II (qualitative) abnormalities. The genetic defect has been characterized in a large number of patients with protein C deficiency. In contrast to antithrombin deficiency where the prevalence of type II defects vastly outweighs that of type I defects, type I protein C defi-

Table 19.2 Prevalences[a] of heritable thrombophilic defects

	General population	*Patients with VTE*	
		Unselected	*Selected*[b]
Factor V Leiden	3–7%	20%	50%
Prothrombin 20210A	1–2%	6%	18%
Antithrombin deficiency	0.02%	1%	4–5%
Protein C deficiency	0.30%	4%	6–8%
Protein S deficiency	?	1%	3–6%

[a]Approximate prevalences in UK.
[b]Positive family history of VTE in addition to personal history of VTE.

ciency is much more common than type II. From population based studies the relative risk of VTE for heterozygous protein C deficient carriers is around 6.5 times that of non-carriers. Unlike antithrombin deficiency where the level of antithrombin activity and the site of the mutation on the antithrombin gene appear to be useful in predicting the risk of thrombosis, there is no clear correlation between the level of protein C activity or the mutation site and the risk of VTE. Deep vein thrombosis of the leg is the most common presentation but thrombosis may occur at a variety of other sites including portal, mesenteric or cerebral veins.

Functional protein C assays using amidolytic or clotting endpoints are widely available. Amidolytic assays are simple to perform and will detect all type I defects and the vast majority of type II defects. Increased plasma clotting factor VIII may produce a falsely low protein C activity result in clotting endpoint assays. Clotting assays may also give artefactually low results in patients who carry the factor V Leiden mutation.

It is suggested that the initial screen for protein C deficiency is performed using an amidolytic functional assay. Where the possibility of an inherited protein C defect is being considered it may be helpful to test other family members. An immunological assay of protein C antigen will help distinguish between type I and type II defects but since there appears to be no clear relationship between the type of the protein C defect and the risk of clinical symptoms there is no clinical justification for this extra investigation or for molecular studies to identify the specific mutation.

There is a wide overlap in observed protein C activity levels in families with protein C gene variants between heterozygous carriers and their unaffected relatives. Protein C activity levels appear to be related to age and gender. However, a positive correlation between protein C activity levels and plasma lipid levels has been reported and when the relationships between protein C activity and age and gender are adjusted for lipid levels they are no longer significant. Protein C activity may increase slightly in women using combined oral contraceptives. Protein C activity is markedly reduced in patients using oral anticoagulants. Significantly reduced levels of protein C activity are observed in patients with DIC and in patients with liver disease. The prevalence of heritable protein C deficiency in the general population is approximately 0.3% and protein C deficiency is reported in around 4% of unselected patients with a history of VTE (Table 19.2).

Protein S deficiency

The vitamin K-dependent protein S is synthesized in the liver, endothelial cells and megakaryocytes. In the circulation 60% of protein S is bound to C4b binding protein, a regulatory protein of the complement pathway, and the remaining 40% is free. Free protein S acts as a cofactor for APC in the proteolytic cleavage of the activated coagulation cascade cofactors – FVa and FVIIIa. The exact mechanism of action of protein S remains incompletely understood but its importance as an anticoagulant is clearly demonstrated by the association of protein S deficiency with an increased risk of VTE. The prevalence of protein S deficiency in the general population remains unknown so the 'size' of the risk of thrombosis associated with protein S deficiency cannot be calculated. In addition to deep vein thrombosis and pulmonary embolism, patients with protein S deficiency may suffer recurrent episodes of superficial thrombophlebitis.

The diagnosis of protein S deficiency is difficult and fraught with pitfalls. Functional protein S assays are based on the cofactor activity of protein S to APC. These functional assays detect all types of protein S deficiency but some functional assays of protein S are non-specific and have been shown to be sensitive to the inherited APC resistance associated with the factor V Leiden mutation and the acquired APC resistance observed in some patients with antiphospholipid syndrome. It is not therefore possible at present to recommend the use of a functional protein S assay as a screening test for protein S deficiency. Instead it is suggested that immunological assays of protein S are included in the initial thrombophilia screen. Enzyme-linked immunosorbent assays (ELISAs) using polyclonal antibodies are widely used to measure total protein S antigen and, after polyethylene glycol (PEG) precipitation of the protein S complexed to C4b binding protein, free protein S antigen. Identification of precise molecular defects in individual patients is difficult and time consuming because the protein S gene is very large and complex.

Previously three types of protein S deficiency were recognized. In accord with the classification of antithrombin and protein C deficiencies, type I protein S deficiency is a quantitative defect caused by genetic defects which result in the reduced production of structurally normal protein. In type I protein S deficiency both total and free antigen levels are reduced. Type II protein S deficiency was characterized as a qualitative (functional) defect but as previously mentioned, it has been shown that some individuals with inherited or acquired APC resistance have been incorrectly diagnosed as having a type II protein S deficiency. In type III defects, although free protein S is reduced, the total protein S level is normal. It has been suggested that type I and type III protein S deficiencies may be phenotypic variations of the same underlying genetic disorder.

Protein S levels are slightly higher in males than in females. Protein S levels fall progressively during pregnancy and fall, but to a lesser extent, in women using oestrogen containing oral contraceptives or hormone replacement therapy (HRT). Acquired protein S deficiency is seen in patients on oral anticoagulants and in patients with DIC, renal disease or liver disease. Low levels of protein S have also been reported in patients with lupus inhibitors or other antiphospholipid antibodies. About 1% of patients presenting with a first VTE are found to be protein S deficient (Table 19.2).

APC resistance and factor V Leiden

APC resistance is assessed by measuring the anticoagulant effect which results from adding (*in vitro*) to patient plasma a standardized amount of APC. The anticoagulant effect is quantified by measuring the activated partial thromboplastin time (APTT) in the patient's sample tested before and after the addition of APC. The resultant APTT clotting times are expressed as a ratio (APTT with APC/APTT without APC): the so-called APC sensitivity ratio (APC:SR). Care must be exercised in interpreting APC:SR results since, confusingly, it is as the APC:SR decreases that the patient is becoming increasingly APC resistant.

The phenomenon of APC resistance first attracted widespread attention when it was reported that APC resistance cosegregated with thrombosis in three unrelated families with familial VTE in whom no other thrombophilic defect had been identified. Shortly thereafter it was demonstrated that the majority of patients with familial APC resistance have the same single point mutation in their gene for clotting factor V. This mutation, which is widely known as the 'factor V Leiden' mutation, destroys one of the APC cleavage sites in FVa, causing it to be relatively resistant to inactivation by APC.

Although the factor V Leiden mutation is the most common cause of inherited APC resistance, a number of other changes in haemostasis can result in acquired APC resistance, e.g. increased plasma levels of genetically normal factor VIII or factor V, severely decreased levels of protein S or the presence of antiphospholipid antibodies. APC resistance increases with increasing age and in women who use oestrogen containing contraceptive pills or HRT. APC resistance also increases during normal pregnancy and at term 45% of women will have an APC:SR which falls beneath the 95th percentile of the normal reference range for non-pregnant women of similar age.

The originally described APC:SR test is abnormal in patients with acquired APC resistance and it is not a reliable screen for the factor V Leiden mutation in these patients or in patients who for any reason have a prolonged baseline APTT – in other words patients who have clotting factor deficiencies, patients with lupus inhibitors or elevated anticardiolipin levels, or patients currently using anticoagulants. A modified APC resistance test which includes sample dilution in factor V deficient (but otherwise normal) plasma prior to testing increases the sensitivity and specificity of the APTT based APC:SR as a screen for factor V Leiden and must be used in patients who are anticoagulated or who for any reason have a prolonged baseline APTT.

Detection of the factor V Leiden mutation includes amplification of the nucleotide region close to the exon–intron boundary in exon 10 of the factor V gene either from genomic DNA or from mRNA followed by a mutation detection step.

In Caucasian populations heterozygosity for the factor V Leiden mutation is the most common heritable thrombophilic defect, being found in between 3 and 7% of healthy populations – and being more prevalent in individuals of northern European extraction than in those from southern Europe. Depending on patient selection it is found in 20–50% of patients presenting with a first episode of VTE. Heterozygous carriers have a seven-fold increased risk of venous thrombosis and homozygotes have an 80-fold increased risk.

There is evidence that the APC:SR as determined with the basic (unmodified) test correlates with VTE risk irrespective of whether or not the patient carries factor V Leiden. The specificity of the modified APC:SR (pre-dilution in factor V deficient plasma) test and the polymerase chain reaction (PCR) studies means that individuals who have increased APC resistance for reasons other than the possession of the factor V Leiden mutation will be overlooked if the basic (unmodified) APC:SR test is omitted from the screening procedure. It is therefore recommended that for initial thrombophilia screening in non-anticoagulated patients the original unmodified APC:SR test is employed. Samples which give low or borderline results can be retested after pre-dilution in factor V deficient plasma. If molecular techniques are available the presence of the factor V Leiden mutation should be confirmed with genetic testing.

Prothrombin 20210A

The most recent heritable thrombophilic defect to be described is a polymorphism in the gene for clotting factor II (prothrombin) – prothrombin 20210A – a G to A transition at nucleotide 20210 in the 3′ untranslated region of the prothrombin gene. This polymorphism is associated with increased plasma levels of prothrombin and an increased risk of VTE. The association between the defect and plasma prothrombin levels is however not strong enough to allow prothrombin levels to be used as a screening test for this mutation and genetic testing is essential.

The prevalence of this defect in northern Europe is 2% in the healthy population and about 6% in patients with a first episode of VTE but higher prevalences have been reported in southern Europe where the prothrombin 20210A polymorphism is the most prevalent heritable thrombophilia. The risk of VTE in heterozygous carriers of the 20210A allele is estimated to be around 2.8 times that in non-carriers, i.e. less than the risk associated with deficiency of antithrombin, protein C or protein S or factor V Leiden.

Combinations of defects

Heritable thrombophilic defects are much more prevalent than was originally anticipated and it is not at all unusual to find individuals and families with more than one identifiable thrombophilic defect. Combinations of deficiencies of the natural anticoagulants – antithrombin, protein C and protein S – are rare due to the low allelic frequency of each of these defects but factor V Leiden and prothrombin 20210A are common and combinations of these defects with deficiencies of a natural anticoagulant are not infrequently found, e.g. factor V Leiden plus prothrombin 20210A, antithrombin deficiency plus factor V Leiden. Combinations of inherited thrombophilic defects with acquired thrombophilia due to the presence of antiphospholipids or complex defects such as elevated factor VIII levels are also frequently observed.

Heritable thrombophilia is a multigene defect

It is now recognized that the vast majority of individuals who have laboratory evidence of a thrombophilic defect remain asymptomatic. In symptomatic kindred (families with familial thrombosis and identified heritable thrombophilic defects), the incidence of thrombosis is higher than expected in the genetically unaffected family members (those without the thrombophilic defect on laboratory testing). It has to be assumed that in these families other (as yet unidentified) genetic factors which increase thrombotic risk are involved. Presumably this is also the case in families in whom there is clear clinical evidence of familial thrombosis but in whom no laboratory defect can at present be found. This polygenetic background in addition to a variable exposure to environmental risk factors may explain the variability in the clinical expression of the major thrombophilic gene defects.

Section 19.2 • Clinical presentation of heritable thrombophilia

The heritable thrombophilias are associated with an increased risk of venous thrombosis. Events occur at a relatively early age and may be recurrent. Around half of the initial events appear to have arisen spontaneously without any identifiable trigger. In some, an acquired prothrombotic stimulus such as surgery or trauma or some physiological challenge such as pregnancy or combined oral contraceptive pill use can be identified but in many patients the provocation may be extremely minor and the only possible identifiable trigger no more than a long journey, mild dehydration or an apparently trivial injury or infection. Often there is a family history of VTE.

Cross-sectional studies of symptomatic families have shown that heterozygous antithrombin, protein C or protein S deficient individuals in general remain asymptomatic until about the age of 15 years – although occasionally patients with type I or type II reactive site antithrombin deficiency present with a first thrombotic event at an earlier age. After the age of 15 years venous thrombotic events occur at the rate of 2–4% per year until, by the age of about 50 years, 50–70% of the heterozygotes in symptomatic families will have had an event.

Factor V Leiden and prothrombin 20210A heterozygotes appear to have a rather lower thrombotic risk than antithrombin, protein C or protein S deficient patients. Individuals with combined defects are at higher risk than those with single defects.

Section 19.3 • Management of heritable thrombophilia

Management of acute venous thrombosis

First event

The initial management of a first deep vein thrombosis or pulmonary embolus event in patients with heritable thrombophilic events does not differ from the management of a first VTE in any other patient. For a few patients thrombolytic therapy may be appropriate but for most initial anticoagulation with unfractionated or low molecular weight heparin is followed by oral anticoagulation for 3–6 months at a target international normalized ratio (INR) of 2.5 (range 2.0–3.0).

In all patients with a history of VTE the intensity and duration of anticoagulant treatment must be determined on an individual patient basis taking into account other remediable or short-term thrombotic risk factors, the severity of the VTE event and the risk of bleeding on anticoagulants.

Fewer than 1% of VTE events are fatal. The rate of life threatening haemorrhage in patients on warfarin is at least 0.25% per year but rises with increasing age or if the INR exceeds 4.0. There is at present no evidence to support long-term or more intensive anticoagulation after the first thrombotic event for the majority of patients with heritable thrombophilia, but where the first event has been life threatening or limb threatening a longer period of anticoagulation or indefinite anticoagulant prophylaxis may be reasonable providing there are no contraindications.

Patients with severe antithrombin deficiency type I or type II reactive site may occasionally merit, in addition to their anticoagulant treatment, replacement therapy with antithrombin concentrate if there is difficulty obtaining adequate heparinization or if a recurrent event has occurred despite apparently adequate anticoagulation. Usually a dose of 0.65–0.75 units per kilogram body weight will raise the plasma antithrombin level by 1 unit per ml. It is usually necessary to continue replacement for a few days only and for most patients once daily dosing is adequate. However, some patients require longer periods of treatment and severely ill patients who are consuming antithrombin at an increased rate require more frequent dosing. In any case it is important that the response to dosing is monitored by checking plasma antithrombin activity.

Recurrent events

In general, patients who have had two or more apparently spontaneous thrombotic events require indefinite thromboprophylaxis. Occasionally where a patient has had recurrent events at times when it was possible to identify a temporary and no longer present acquired risk factor (such as pregnancy, combined oral contraceptive use or surgery) it may be possible to avoid long-term anticoagulation. Vigorous thromboprophylaxis is required for these patients at times of increased thrombotic risk (e.g. surgery, trauma, pregnancy, puerperium, immobilization, long journeys).

Prevention of thrombosis

General advice

Patients who have heritable thrombophilic defects and who are either personally symptomatic or belong to symptomatic kindred should be fully informed of the nature of their defect and they should be instructed to warn medical attendants that they may be at increased risk of thrombosis. Patients should have direct and rapid access to informed advice about the potential thrombotic risk associated with surgery, trauma, immobilization, pregnancy, contraceptives, hormone replacement therapy, travel, etc. If possible they should be referred to a specialist thrombophilia clinic. It may be helpful to issue them with a card stating their defect and giving contact telephone numbers for their thrombophilia clinic or other responsible clinician.

Short-term thromboprophylaxis

Consideration should be given to their possible requirement for short-term anticoagulation at times of increased thrombotic risk such as immobilization due to severe medical illness, surgery or trauma, pregnancy, etc. Patients with thrombophilic defects may merit a longer period of post-operative anticoagulation than other patients and in some, for example those with type I or type II reactive site antithrombin deficiency, a more intensive regimen may be appropriate. In patients with antithrombin deficiency requiring moderate or high-risk surgery prophylactic use of antithrombin concentrate peri-operatively may be a useful adjunct to anticoagulant prophylaxis.

Contraception and pregnancy

Women who have thrombophilic defects identified as a result of screening either because they have a personal or family history of proven VTE should if possible avoid combined oral contraceptives. Depending on their clinical history and their thrombophilic defect they may warrant post-natal and in addition, in some, antenatal anticoagulant treatment. Women with antithrombin deficiency may be given antithrombin concentrate around the time of their delivery to allow a reduction in the dose of their prophylactic anticoagulation at this time of high bleeding risk.

Section 19.4 • Acquired thrombophilic defects

The most common and important acquired thrombophilic abnormalities are those broadly grouped together as 'antiphospholipids' – lupus inhibitors and elevations of anticardiolipin levels. Antiphospholipid antibodies comprise a family of antibodies reactive with epitopes on proteins (e.g. beta-2-glycoprotein-1, prothrombin) which are complexed with negatively charged phospholipids.

Antiphospholipid syndrome may be diagnosed when persistent evidence of a lupus inhibitor and/or elevated IgG or IgM anticardiolipin levels are found in an individual with arterial or venous thrombosis or recurrent fetal loss. The presence of antiphospholipid must be confirmed in two separate blood samples collected at least 6 weeks apart.

Lupus inhibitors

A large number of diagnostic tests for lupus inhibitors have been described and a number of commercial kits and reagents have been introduced. Despite this the criteria for the diagnosis of lupus inhibitor remain:

- prolongation of a phospholipid dependent coagulation test, for example an activated partial thromboplastin time (APTT) or a dilute Russell's viper venom time (DRVVT)
- evidence of inhibitor activity in mixing studies
- confirmation of the phospholipid dependent nature of the inhibitor.

Accurate detection of a lupus inhibitor is not possible in patients using oral anticoagulants.

Anticardiolipins

ELISAs for anticardiolipins are widely available and the results are not affected by clotting factor deficiency or the use of anticoagulants. The detection of elevated IgG or IgM anticardiolipin allows the diagnosis of antiphospholipid syndrome in a patient with the appropriate clinical history even when there is no evidence of a lupus inhibitor. However, anticardiolipin assays are not a substitute for lupus inhibitor testing, nor does the presence of anticardiolipins confirm the presence of a lupus inhibitor – since different antibodies appear to be responsible.

Section 19.5 • Clinical presentation of antiphospholipids

The most frequent clinical presentations of the antiphospholipid syndrome (APS) are VTE and arterial occlusive events, including stroke and recurrent miscarriage. Antiphospholipid antibodies are not infrequently identified incidentally in healthy subjects – as a result for example of finding a prolonged APTT on preoperative coagulation screening.

Antiphospholipid antibodies are found in patients with systemic lupus erythematosus (SLE), in patients with lupus-like disorders who do not meet the full criteria for SLE and in patients with other autoimmune disorders where they are associated with thrombosis or fetal loss (see Table 19.3). Patients with the clinical symptoms of APS and evidence of antiphospholipid antibodies on laboratory testing but no evident underlying disease are said to have primary antiphospholipid syndrome. Antiphospholipid antibodies also occur in relation to the use of certain drugs, particularly chlorpromazine and transiently in association with many infections. Persistent antiphospholipid antibodies may be seen in patients with chronic infections such as hepatitis C or human immunodeficiency virus (HIV) infection.

Thrombocytopenia is frequently present in APS. The low platelet count is usually due to an immune mechanism, analogous to that in idiopathic immune

Table 19.3 Antiphospholipid antibodies – clinical associations

1. *Primary antiphospholipid syndrome*		
	Venous of arterial thrombosis or recurrent fetal loss with persisting evidence of antiphospholipids but no evident underlying pathology	
2. *Secondary antiphospholipid syndrome*		
	Venous or arterial thrombosis or recurrent fetal loss with persisting evidence of antiphospholipids in association with underlying connective tissue disorder	
		Systemic lupus erythematosus
		Rheumatoid arthritis
		Systemic sclerosis
		Behçet's syndrome
		Psoriatic arthropathy
		Sjögren's syndrome
3. *Other associations*		
	Evidence of antiphospholipids in	
	Infections	Viral – HIV, hepatitis C, chicken pox
		Bacterial – syphilis
		Malaria
	Drug exposure	Procainamide, phenothiazines, phenytoin, hydralazine, quinidine
4. *Incidental finding of antiphospholipids*		

thrombocytopenia (ITP). In spite of the prolonged APTT and frequently associated thrombocytopenia it is unusual for patients with APS to haemorrhage.

Section 19.6 • Management of patients with antiphospholipids

Patients with an incidental finding of antiphospholipids

Where antiphospholipids are found by chance, clinical assessment including screening to exclude connective tissue disorder is indicated. The thrombotic risk associated with an incidental finding of antiphospholipids in apparently healthy individuals is relatively low although some reports have suggested an increased risk over the general population risk. Antithrombotic prophylaxis is not therefore generally indicated providing there is no history of thrombosis. However, since this group will include some subjects who will in time have a first thrombotic event, a low threshold for the use of thromboprophylaxis at times of increased thrombotic risk (e.g. peri- and post-operatively) is indicated.

Management of acute venous thrombosis

First thrombosis

The initial management of acute VTE, with intravenous unfractionated or low molecular weight heparin, is no different in patients with APS than in the generality of patients. Warfarin should then be introduced in the usual manner. There continues to be some controversy about the optimal INR range for patients with APS who have had a venous thrombosis. There is evidence that the rate of recurrent VTE is relatively high in patients with APS. Three retrospective studies suggested ongoing risk of VTE in APS patients if the INR was less than 3.0 and a target INR of 3.5 has been recommended. The British Committee for Standards in Haematology (BCSH) Guidelines (1999) on the other hand suggest that for many patients with a deep vein thrombosis and APS, treatment for 6 months with an INR target of 2.5 (range 2.0–3.0) and management of additional reversible risk factors is reasonable.

Recurrent venous thrombosis

Recurrent thrombosis in patients with APS is usually an indication for long-term thromboprophylaxis with oral anticoagulants. Recurrence whilst the patient is on anticoagulants with an INR between 2.0 and 3.0 is uncommon and would suggest the dose of anticoagulant should be increased to raise the target INR to 3.5 (range 3.0–4.0).

Management of arterial thrombosis

Because of the high risk of recurrence and the likelihood of consequent permanent disability or death, stroke due to cerebral infarction in APS should be treated with long-term oral anticoagulant treatment, target INR 2.5 (range 2.0–3.0). Higher intensity anticoagulation for some patients has been recommended by some authors. Recurrence whilst on anticoagulants with an INR between 2.0 and 3.0 would dictate the use of a more intensive anticoagulant regimen (INR target 3.5).

Extracerebral arterial thromboembolic events in patients with APS also merit consideration of long-term anticoagulant treatment with warfarin in many patients. As in patients with VTE attention should be paid to avoiding or correcting added acquired thrombotic risk factors.

Section 19.7 • Mixed thrombophilic defects

In some patients it is evident that the thrombophilic changes observable in their blood are the result of complex interactions between genetic and environmental factors and not simply the product of either alone.

Factor VIII activity

There is clear and increasing evidence that plasma clotting factor VIII levels are directly related to thrombotic risk. Factor VIII levels above 150 IU/dl are associated with a six-fold increased risk of VTE compared with patients with factor VIII levels of less than 100 IU/dl. Factor VIII levels are in part under genetic control and partly a response to environmental factors – stress, oestrogens, etc.

High factor VIII levels are very frequent – 11% of the healthy population and 25% of patients with a first VTE – and the relative risk of VTE associated with elevated factor VIII is high, thus high factor VIII levels are an important cause of VTE.

Hyperhomocysteinaemia

Two case control studies demonstrated a 2.5-fold increased risk of VTE in individuals with homocysteine levels exceeding 18.5 μmol/l and a 3–4-fold risk associated with levels exceeding 20 μmol/l.

Hyperhomocysteinaemia may be the result of a number of abnormalities, genetic or environmental. Classic hyperhomocysteinaemia due to heterozygosity for cystathionine beta-synthase is uncommon but the more recently described variant in the gene for methylene tetrahydrofolate reductase (MTHER), which leads to the production of a thermolabile variant of the enzyme and mildly elevated homocysteine levels, is common.

Environmental causes of hyperhomocysteinaemia include reduced vitamin B_6, vitamin B_{12} or folic acid levels. The mechanism of the relationship between hyperhomocysteinaemia and venous thrombosis is not clear. It has been suggested that the homocysteine levels associated with the thermolabile MTHFR variant are not in themselves sufficiently increased to cause thrombosis or that the elevated homocysteine levels observed in some thrombotic patients with this variant are a result rather than a cause of the thrombosis.

In the meantime hyperhomocysteinaemia cannot be disregarded as a potential risk factor for VTE since between 5 and 10% of Europeans have homocysteine levels over 18.5 μmol/l. There is no simple screening test. Testing for the presence of the MTHFR variant is unhelpful and at present there is no widely available method for measuring homocysteine levels.

The treatment and prevention of VTE in patients with mixed thrombophilic defects is similar to that in patients with heritable thrombophilias. Patients with hyperhomocysteinaemia should be prescribed vitamin supplements.

Section 19.8 • Thrombophilia screening

Clinical assessment

The investigation of any patient presenting with a clinical picture suggestive of thrombophilia must commence with a carefully taken history and family history followed by a full clinical examination with appropriate laboratory, imaging and other investigation. The initial investigations should include a full blood count and clinical chemistry including urea and electrolytes, liver function tests and a random glucose assay.

The thrombophilia screen

Formal thrombophilia screening should include a routine coagulation screen – an APTT, prothrombin time and thrombin clotting time. The thrombin clotting time will allow identification of patients with rare fibrinogen defects (dysfibrinogenaemias), some of which are associated with an increased risk of venous thrombosis, and the APTT may identify some patients with antiphospholipids (depending on the sensitivity of the APTT reagent used).

The thrombophilia screen must include tests for the common heritable defects – deficiency of antithrombin, protein C or protein S and for the factor V Leiden and prothrombin 20210A mutations. Currently most thrombophilia clinics would also include an assay of clotting factor VIII but only research groups could justify including an assay of homocysteine. A thrombophilia screen must also include a search for acquired thrombophilic defects, screening for lupus inhibitor activity and assays of IgG and IgM anticardiolipins (Table 19.4).

When to collect samples for thrombophilia screening

Some thrombophilia screening tests are affected by the acute post-thrombotic state and some are influenced by heparin or oral anticoagulant use. Finding a thrombophilic abnormality rarely influences the management of an acute thrombotic event. Therefore there is little point in striving to obtain samples for thrombophilia screening when the patient presents with an acute thrombotic event and screening is usually best delayed until at least a month after completion of the course of anticoagulation. If possible thrombophilia screening should also be avoided when the patient is for any reason 'unwell', or is pregnant, or is using a combined oral contraceptive pill or hormone replacement therapy. If this is impossible, then it is essential that the individual interpreting the screen is aware of the presence and potential influence of these various acquired factors on the components of the thrombophilia screen. PCR based tests for factor V Leiden and prothrombin 20210A and ELISAs of anticardiolipins are unaffected by anti-coagulant use and PCR based tests can be done on samples taken even when the patient is unwell.

Who should be screened for thrombophilic defects?

Inevitably with the developing interest in the role of thrombophilic defects in thrombosis risk, haematologists and other clinicians have come under pressure to screen an increasing number of patients for defects. Identifying a defect seldom alters the management of an acute thrombotic event. However, knowledge that a patient has a thrombophilic defect may lower the threshold for suggesting an extended period of anticoagulation after a thrombotic event or for offering thromboprophylaxis to cover minor surgery or lengthy journeys.

Table 19.4 Basic thrombophilia screen

Coagulation screen	– APTT, PT, TT
Antithrombin activity	– amidolytic
Protein C activity	– amidolytic
Protein S antigen	– total – ELISA
	– free – ELISA
Unmodified APC sensitivity ratio	
Factor V predilution APC sensitivity ratio	
Factor V Leiden	
Prothrombin 20210A	
Lupus inhibitor screen	
IgG and IgM anticardiolipin antibodies – ELISA	

APTT = activated partial thromboplastin time; PT = prothrombin time; TT = thrombin time.

There is a case for thrombophilia screening selected patients, including any patient who has a VTE at a relatively young age (arbitrarily 50 years or under); any patient who has had recurrent idiopathic events; any patient who has a thrombosis at an unusual site; any patient who gives a clear family history of proven VTE – at a young age, or spontaneously or recurrently, etc., as above. It is now widely accepted that women with a history of three or more consecutive pregnancy losses should be screened for antiphospholipids but consideration should be given to extending screening to include women who have had two consecutive miscarriages or three non-consecutive pregnancy losses. Increasingly also women who have a history of recurrent fetal loss are being screened not only for acquired thrombophilic defects but also for heritable thrombophilias (Table 19.5).

Although in many cases finding a heritable thrombophilic defect may have few implications for the patient him or herself it may be information which is potentially important to other family members. There is evidence that the risk of VTE is increased in women with thrombophilic defects when they use combined oral contraceptives and there is compelling evidence that at least in the case of the factor V Leiden mutation this genetic defect interacts with combined oral contraceptives to preduce a relative risk of VTE that is considerably greater than would be predicted from the additive effect of the relative risks of VTE associated with contraceptive use and factor V Leiden. Heritable thrombophilia seems to play a role not only in the pathogenesis of pregnancy associated VTE but also in pre-eclampsia and in increasing the risk of fetal loss. Women from symptomatic families may merit screening to identify whether or not they are affected. Knowing that they have a defect may influence their choice of contraceptive or may alert their antenatal care team to a potentially complicated pregnancy and influence decisions about where and how the pregnancy is managed.

Patients with SLE should be screened for antiphospholipids as part of their autoantibody profiling as the risk of thrombosis is higher in those found to be positive.

Subjects who have a stroke or a peripheral arterial occlusive event at a young age (less than 50 years) merit screening for antiphospholipids – especially when risk factors for atheromatous arterial disease are not prominent – and a case can be made for screening older subjects who are non-smokers and who do not have other significant risk factors such as hypertension, diabetes mellitus or dyslipidaemia. Where recurrent arterial occlusive events recur despite antithrombotic prophylaxis, APS should be excluded.

It must however be re-emphasized that the majority of individuals with single heritable thrombophilias who belong to asymptomatic kindred will themselves remain asymptomatic. Thus in spite of the growing information about the role of heritable thrombophilia in the aetiology of a range of clinical problems, widespread population screening for heritable thrombophiilic defects is not currently recommended.

Table 19.5 Patients who may be considered for thrombophilia screening

VTE under 50 years
Spontaneous VTE
Recurrent VTE
Family history of VTE at young age, or recurrent or spontaneous VTE
Thrombosis in unusual site
Stroke or peripheral arterial thrombosis under 50 years
Recurrent arterial thrombosis despite anticoagulation
Recurrent fetal loss
Systemic lupus erythematosus

Further reading

Allaart, C. E., Poort, S. R., Rosendaal, F. R. *et al.* (1993). Increased risk of venous thrombosis in carriers of hereditary protein C deficiency. *Lancet* **341**: 134–8.

Bertina, B. M., Koeleman, B. P. C., Koster, T. *et al.* (1994). Mutation in blood coagulation factor V, association with resistance to activated protein C. *Nature* **369**: 64–7.

British Committee for Standards in Haematology (BCSH) (1990). Guidelines on the investigation and management of thrombophilia. *J Clin Pathol* **43**: 703–10.

British Committee for Standards in Haematology (BCSH) (1998). Guidelines on oral anticoagulation: 3rd edition. *Br J Haematol* **101**: 374–87.

British Committee for Standards in Haematology (BCSH) (1999). Guidelines on the investigation and management of the antiphospholipid syndrome. In Press.

Clark, P., Brennand, J., Conkie, J. A. *et al.* (1998). Activated protein C sensitivity, protein C, protein S and coagulation in normal pregnancy. *Thromb Haemost* **79**: 1166–70.

Conard, J., Horellou, M. H., van Dredan, P and Samama, M. M. (1987). Pregnancy and congenital deficiency in antithrombin III or protein C. *Thromb Haemost* **58**: 39 (Abstract).

Conard, J., Horellou, M. H., van Dredan, P. *et al.* (1990). Thrombosis and pregnancy in congenital deficiencies of antithrombin III, protein S or protein S: study of 78 women. *Thromb Haemost* **63**: 319–20.

Dahlback, B., Carlsson, M. and Svensson, P. J. (1993). Familial thrombophilia due to a previously unrecognized mechanism characterized by poor anticoagulant response to activated protein C. Prediction of a cofactor to activated protein C. *Proc Natl Acad Sci USA* **90**: 1004–8.

D'Angelo, A. and Selhub, J. (1997). Homocysteine and thrombotic disease. *Blood* **90**: 1–11.

De Moerloose, P., Reber, G. and Bouvier, C. A. (1998). Spuriously low levels of protein C with Protac activation clotting assay (Letter). *Thromb Haemost* **70**: 281–5.

Den Heijer, M., Koster, T., Blom, H. J. *et al.* (1996). Hyperhomocysteinaemia as a risk factor for deep vein thrombosis. *N Engl J Med* **334**: 759–62.

De Ronde, H. and Bertina, R. M. (1994). Laboratory diagnosis of APC resistance. A critical evaluation of the test and the development of diagnostic criteria. *Thromb Haemost* **72**: 880–6.

De Stefano, V., Leone, G., Masterangelo, S. *et al.* (1994). Thrombosis during pregnancy and surgery in patients with congenital deficiency of antithrombin III, protein C-protein S. *Thromb Haemost* **71**: 799–800.

Faioni, E. M., Franchi, F., Asti, D. *et al.* (1993). Resistance to activated protein C in 9 thrombophilic families. Interference in a protein S functional assay. *Thromb Haemost* **70**: 1067–71.

Faioni, E. M., Franchi, F., Asti, D. and Mannucci, P. M. (1996). Resistance to activated protein C mimicking dysfunctional protein C: a diagnostic approach. *Blood Coag Fibrinol* **7**: 349–52.

Faioni, E. M., Valsecchi, C., Palla, A. *et al.* (1997). Free protein S deficiency is a risk factor for venous thrombosis. *Thromb Haemost* **78**: 1343–6.

Finazzi, G., Caccia, R. and Barbui, T. (1987). Different prevalence of thromboembolism in the subtypes of congenital antithrombin III deficiency: review of 404 cases (Letter). *Thromb Haemost* **58**: 1094.

Finazzi, G., Branaccio, V., Moia, M. *et al.* (1996). Natural history and risk factors for thrombosis in 360 patients with antiphospholipid antibodies: a four year prospective study from the Italian Registry. *Am J Med* **100**: 530–6.

Frosst, P., Blom, H. J., Milos, R. *et al.* (1995). A candidate genetic risk for vascular disease: a common mutation in methylene tetrahydrofolate reductase. *Nat Genet* **10**: 111–13.

Ginsburg, K. S., Liang, M. H., Newcomer, L. *et al.* (1992). Anticardiolipin antibodies and the risk for ischemic stroke and venous thrombosis. *Ann Intern Med* **117**: 997–1002.

Ginsberg, K. S., Wells, P. S., Brill-Edwards, P. *et al.* (1995). Antiphospholipid antibodies and venous thromboembolism. *Blood* **86**: 3685–91.

Griffin, J. H., Evatt, B., Wideman, C. and Fernandez, J. A. (1993). Anticoagulant protein C pathway defective in a majority of thrombophilic patients. *Blood* **82**: 1989–93.

Hellgren, M., Tengborn, L. and Abildgaard, U. (1992). Pregnancy in women with congenital antithrombin III deficiency: experience of treatment with heparin and antithrombin. *Gynaecol Obstet Invest* **14**: 127–41.

Hirsh, J., Piovella, F. and Pini, M. (1989). Congenital antithrombin III deficiency. Incidence and clinical features. *Am J Med* **87** (Suppl 3B): 34–8S.

Kang, S. S., Zhou, J., Wong, P. W. K. *et al.* (1988). Intermediate homocysteinaemia: A thermolabile variant of methylene tetrahydrofolate reductase. *Am J Hum Genet* **48**: 536–45.

Khamashta, M. A., Cuadrado, M. J., Mujic, F. *et al.* (1995). The management of thrombosis in the antiphospholipid–antibody syndrome. *N Engl J Med* **332**: 993–7.

Koster, T., Rosendaal, F. R., de Ronde, H. *et al.* (1993). Venous thrombosis due to a poor anticoagulant response to activated protein C: Leiden thrombophilia study. *Lancet* **342**: 1503–6.

Koster, T., Rosendaal, F. R., Briet, E. *et al.* (1995). Protein C deficiency in a controlled series of unselected outpatients: an infrequent but clear risk factor for venous thrombosis (Leiden thrombophilia study). *Blood* **85**: 2756–66.

Koster, T., Blann, A. D., Briet, E. *et al.* (1995). Role of clotting factor VIII in effect of von Willebrand factor on occurrence of deep vein thrombosis. *Lancet* **345**: 152–5.

Lane, D. A., Mannucci, P. M., Bauer, K. A. *et al.* (1996). Inherited thrombophilia: Part 1. *Thromb Haemost* **76**: 651–62.

Lowe, G. D. O., Rumely, A., Woodward, M. *et al.* (1999). Activated protein C resistance and the FV:R506Q mutation in a random population sample. *Thromb Haemost* **81**: 918–24.

Mateo, J., Oliver, A., Borrell, M. *et al.* The EMET Group (1997). Laboratory evaluation and clinical characteristics of 2132 consecutive unselected patients with venous thromboembolism – results of the Spanish Multicentre Study on Thrombophilia (EMET-Study). *Thromb Haemost* **77**: 444–51.

Mathonnet, F., de Mazancourt, P., Bastenaire, B. *et al.*, (1996). Activated protein C sensitivity ratio in pregnant women at delivery. *Br J Haematol* **92**: 244–6.

Nordstrom, M., Lindblad, B., Bergqvist, D. and Kjellstrom, T. (1992). A perspective study of the incidence of deep vein thrombosis within a defined urban population. *J Intern Med* **323**: 155–60.

Pabinger, I. and Study Group on Natural Inhibitors (1996). Thrombotic risk in hereditary antithrombin III, protein C or protein S deficiency. *Arterio Scler Thromb Vasc Biol* **16**: 742–8.

Palareti, G., Leadi, N., Coccheri, S. *et al.* (1996). Bleeding complications of oral anticoagulant treatment: an inception cohort prospective collaboration study (ISCOAT). *Lancet* **348**: 423–8.

Poort, S. R., Rosendaal, F. R., Reitsma, P. H. and Bertina, R. M. (1996). A common genetic variation in the 3′ untranslated region of the prothrombin gene is associated with elevated plasma prothrombin levels and an increase in venous thrombosis. *Blood* **88**: 3698–703.

Rees, D. C., Cox, M. and Clegg, J. B. (1995). World distribution of factor V Leiden. *Lancet* **346**: 1133–4.

Ridker, P. M., Hennekens, C. H., Lindpainter, K. *et al.* (1995). Mutation in the gene coding for coagulation factor V and the risk of myocardial infarction, stroke and venous thrombosis in apparently healthy men. *N Engl J Med* **332**: 912–17.

Ridker, P. M., Miletich, J. P., Hennekens, C. H. and Buring, J. E. (1997). Ethnic distribution of factor V Leiden in 4047 men and women. *JAMA* **277**: 1305–7.

Rosendaal, F. R. (1997). Risk factors for venous thrombosis; prevalence, risk and interaction. *Semin Haematol* **34**: 171–87.

Rosendaal, F. R. (1999). Risk factors for venous thrombotic disease. *Thromb Haemost* **82**: 610–19.

Rosendaal, F. R., Koster, T., Vandenbroucke, J. P. and Reitsma, P. H. (1995). High risk of thrombosis in patients homozygous for factor V Leiden (activated protein C resistance). *Blood* **85**: 1504–8.

Schulman, S., Svenungsson, E. and Granqvist, S. (1998). Anticardiolipin antibodies predict early recurrence of thromboembolism and death among patients with venous thromboembolism following anticoagulant therapy. *Am J Med* **104**: 332–3.

Simioni, P., Prandoni, P., Burlina, A. *et al.* (1996). Hyperhomocysteinaemia and deep vein thrombosis: a case control study. *Thromb Haemost* **76**: 883–6.

Simioni, P., Prandoni, P., Zanon, E. *et al.* (1996). Deep venous thrombosis and lupus anticoagulant. *Thromb Haemost* **76**: 187–9.

Souto, J. C., Coll, I., Llobe, D. *et al.* (1998). The prothrombin 20210A allele is the most prevalent genetic risk factor for venous thromboembolism in the Spanish population. *Thromb Haemost* **80**: 306–9.

Tait, R. C., Walker, I. D., Islam, S. I. A. M. *et al.* (1993). Influence of demographic factors on antithrombin activity in a healthy population. *Br J Haematol* **84**: 476–8.

Tait, R. C., Walker, I. D., Islam, S. I. A. M. *et al.* (1993). Protein C activity in healthy volunteers – influence of age, sex, smoking and oral contraceptives. *Thromb Haemost* **70**: 281–5.

Tait, R. C., Walker, I. D., Perry, D. J. *et al.* (1994). Prevalence of antithrombin deficiency in the healthy population. *Br J Haematol* **87**: 106–12.

Tait, R. C., Walker, I. D., Reitsma, P. H. *et al.* (1995). Prevalence of protein C deficiency in the healthy population. *Thromb Haemost* **73**: 87–93.

Ubbink, J. B., Vermaak, W. J., van der Merwe, A. and Becker, P. J. (1993). Vitamin B12, vitamin B6 and folate nutritional status in men with hyperhomocysteinaemia *Am J Clin Nutr* **57**: 47–53.

Vandenbroucke, J. P., Koster, T., Briet, E. *et al.* (1994). Increased risk of venous thrombosis in oral contraceptive users who are carriers of the factor V Leiden mutation. *Lancet* **344**: 1453–7.

MODULE 20

Microvascular disease

1 • Obstructive microvascular disease

2 • Vasospastic microvascular disease: Raynaud's phenomenon

Patients with disease in the microvasculature provide only a minor proportion of the surgeon's workload. However, when they are encountered, they can present the most strenuous challenge to the surgeon's diagnostic and therapeutic skills. The microvasculature, commonly defined as vessels <8 μm in diameter, can be affected by many disease processes. The end result is common to all, however, i.e. vascular damage and ischaemia. The challenge for the clinician is not in making the diagnosis of ischaemia but in determining which processes are ongoing, thus allowing speedy and effective management of the underlying pathological condition.

For classification purposes, microcirculatory disorders can be divided into two broad categories: obstructive and vasospastic. Some overlap does occur between these two groups, for example in the connective tissue disorders (CTDs) where severe vasospasm can be complicated by vascular obstruction, but this division has practical implications and can usefully be employed here. Figure 20.1 shows the full spectrum of microvascular diseases, some of which will be covered in this module and others elsewhere within the book. This module aims to classify microvascular disease into diagnostic groups, allowing appropriate investigation and management to be determined for patients presenting to the surgeon with microvascular ischaemia.

Section 20.1 • Obstructive microvascular disease

Embolus

Embolus is a major cause of acute limb ischaemia contributing to its aetiology in approximately 40% of cases. Its diagnosis and management, where it affects the macrovasculature, are dealt with elsewhere. Occasionally, however, microemboli shower into the microcirculation and they can be an important cause of microvascular obstruction. Small areas of palpable purpura are seen (Figure 20.2). Often the tissue round the lesions is healthy and vascularized with no decrease in capillary return. In clinical situations where peripheral pulses distal to a stenosis are felt then embolus should be considered. Sources of microemboli include the heart, aorta and proximal peripheral vessels (Table 20.1). Emboli from plaque consist predominantly of cholesterol, and those from thrombus contain fibrin, platelets and other blood cells in varying proportions. Infected embolus occurs in septicaemia, e.g. meningococcal. Embolism secondary to septicaemia is usually associated with fever, malaise and widespread rash though it may present early with only a few spots. Particularly troublesome microembolization is caused

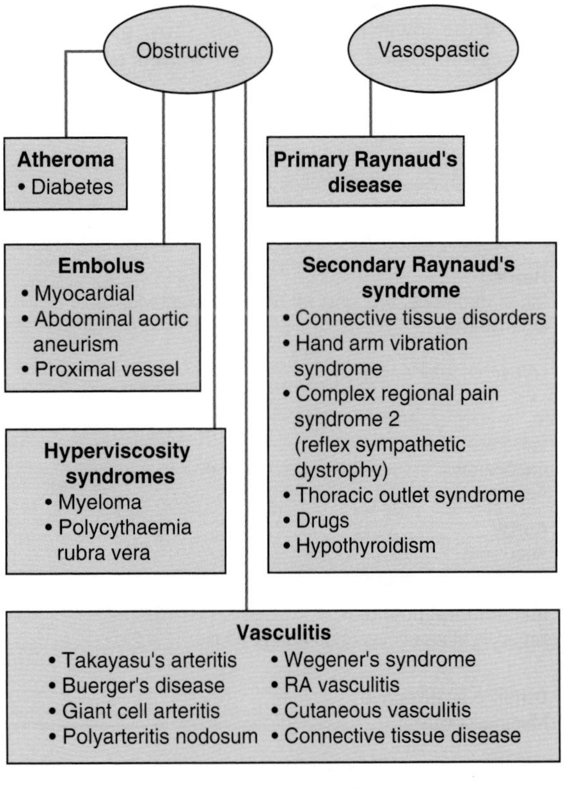

Figure 20.1 Causes of microvascular disease.

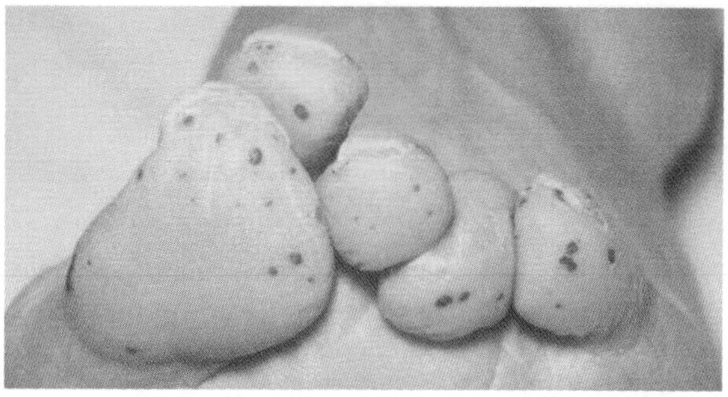

Figure 20.2 Microembolism.

by intra-arterial drug abuse. This is due in part to the chemical irritation produced by the injected drug itself, to the solid matter injected, e.g. chalk, in addition to the microvascular occlusion. In the majority of cases microembolization resolves with the therapy described below. However, complications include tissue loss if the ischaemia is severe, compartment syndrome (common with intra-arterial drug abuse) and subsequent sepsis within the ischaemic lesions.

Investigations include a standard 12-lead electrocardiogram (ECG) and 24 hour ECG recording to detect myocardial infarction and dysrhythmia. Echocardiography, particularly using the transoesophageal approach can detect intracardiac clot related to an infarct site, left ventricular aneurysm, defective or infected valves, endocarditis and, rarely, atrial myxoma. Abdominal ultrasound, computed tomographic (CT) scanning or magnetic resonance imaging (MRI) of the abdomen will detect aortic aneurysm and duplex scanning of the lower limb vessels will show pathology in this region. Blood cultures are required to diagnose septicaemia.

In the majority of cases the lesions will heal over time, especially emboli composed of thrombus. These can rapidly resolve due to the fibrinolytic potential of the intact local endothelium. In general, however, if no contraindication exists, short-term anticoagulation with heparin is appropriate to enhance microcirculatory flow and help prevent recurrence. Warfarin can be introduced if this is appropriate management of the underlying cause. Care should be taken to ensure patients with aortic aneurysm are diagnosed prior to this decision as this finding may be a contraindication to such therapy. Anecdotally, iloprost infusion has been given with some success in these patients, particularly in those cases associated with intra-arterial drug abuse. Longer term management depends on the underlying cause. Disease of the peripheral vessels or the aorta should be managed in the standard way with anticoagulants being continued until the surgical or endovascular procedure can be undertaken. Embolization from the myocardium is best managed in conjunction with the physician as anti-arrhythmic treatment may be required in addition to anticoagulants. Antiplatelet treatment may be more appropriate long term for some elderly patients, and silent myocardial infarction needs to be considered. The management of septic patients is with parenteral antibiotics initially. Long-term anticoagulation for intra-arterial drug abuse is not appropriate.

Atheroma

Damage to the microcirculation occurs in atheromatous disease. Whilst this is accepted for diabetes, it is less well recognized in the non-diabetic patient. Atherosclerotic microvascular disease usually manifests as vasospasm and is therefore covered later.

Table 20.1 Sources of emboli and their investigation

Source	*Investigation*
Heart	
Mural thrombus, e.g. post MI (especially anterior)	ECG, transoesophageal echocardiogram
Dysrhythmia	ECG
	24 hour ECG
Left ventricular aneurysm	ECG
	CXR
	Echocardiogram
Valve vegetations	Echocardiogram
Endocarditis	
Atrial myxoma	Echocardiogram
Aorta	
Aneurysm	Abdominal ultrasound/MRI
Atheromatous plaque	
Iliac/femoral/popliteal	
Stenosis/plaque/intra-arterial drug abuse	ABPI
	Duplex scanning + angiography if required
Other, e.g. infective	
Meningococcal	Blood cultures

MI = myocardial infarction, ECG = electrocardiogram, CXR = chest X-ray, ABPI = ankle brachial pressure index, MRI = magnetic resonance imaging.

Hyperviscosity syndromes

Hyperviscosity syndromes contribute to microvascular disease by impeding flow within the microcirculation. Blood viscosity is dependent both on plasma and blood cell determinants, and also on shear stresses. Diseases associated with hyperviscosity, such as multiple myeloma and dysfibrinogenaemias can be detected by the simple measure of plasma viscosity. Cryoglobulinaemia and cryofibrinogenaemia are more difficult to detect, requiring a temperature-regulated sample of blood. These diseases should be suspected if cold-induced cyanotic areas or lesions occur in the extremities. Raynaud's phenomenon (RP) can be a component of these disorders. Their investigation and management should be discussed with the appropriate specialist.

Blood cell abnormalities contributing to microvascular disease include polycythaemia. Secondary polycythaemia is common in patients with peripheral arterial disease, resulting from a cigarette smoking habit. Although this type of polycythaemia may contribute to decreased flow in the microcirculation, occlusion rarely occurs unless the haematocrit becomes very high. In contrast, polycythaemia rubra vera, and various other myelodysplastic disorders such as the leukaemias and thrombocythaemias, can cause microvascular occlusion. A full blood count for haemoglobin, packed cell volume, white cell count and platelet count provide a core screen for these disorders. Rare causes of microvascular occlusion include sickle cell disease and other haemoglobinopathies but these usually present early with other manifestations and the diagnosis is already known.

Vasculitis

Vasculitis is characterized by inflammation within the blood vessel wall, with impairment of blood flow and possibly damage to vessel integrity. This inflammatory process may involve only one or many blood vessels and therefore organ systems. The clinical features result from ischaemia to the tissues supplied by the damaged vessel and are often accompanied by the constitutional systemic features of weight loss, fever, malaise and anorexia which result from widespread inflammation. These conditions produce a range of symptoms from a mild obliterative disorder to necrotizing vasculitis. Vessels of predominantly one or many types may be affected (Table 20.2). While cutaneous vasculitis, rheumatoid arthritis (RA) vasculitis and vasculitis associated with the CTDs affect mainly the microvasculature, vasculitis affecting the larger vessels must be considered in cases of unexplained vascular pathology. These include Takayasu's arteritis, Buerger's disease, giant cell arteritis, polyarteritis nodosa and Wegener's granulomatosis. The vasculitides, once thought to be rare, are now recognized with increasing frequency and represent a clinical challenge for many disciplines. Some are unlikely to present with vascular insufficiency, e.g. Churg–Strauss (lungs), Beçhet's syndrome (oral and genital ulceration), but others can do and if not treated effectively or rapidly may carry a poor prognosis. Reassuringly, relatively few patients do present with acute life-threatening vasculitis. However, those with peripheral ischaemia as a major manifestation of their disease can do, so it is appropriate to have a knowledge base in this area.

Cutaneous vasculitis

The vessels primarily involved in cutaneous vasculitis are the post-capillary venules, though capillaries and arterioles may also be inflamed. Often occurring as a result of hypersensitivity, a leucocytoclastic (necrotizing) appearance is seen on microscopy. The most common causes/agents implicated in the pathogenesis of these diseases are listed in Table 20.3.

Henoch–Schönlein purpura (HSP)

This is a distinctive syndrome of acute systemic vasculitis characterized by non-thrombocytopenic purpura, skin lesions, joint involvement, colicky abdominal pain with gastointestinal haemorrhage, and renal disease. While more common in the paediatric population, it is also observed in adults. The clinical presentation of HSP is fairly standard and this allows the diagnosis to be made on clinical criteria. Purpura affects the skin, usually in a symmetrical fashion. The extremities (Figure 20.3), particularly distally and on the extensor surfaces often have a covering of rash. Joint pains occur in over two-thirds of patients, usually

Table 20.2 The vasculitides and vessel size

Vasculitides	*Microcirculation, i.e. arterioles, capillaries and venules*	*Small muscular arteries*	*Medium sized arteries*	*Large and medium sized arteries*	*Aorta and branches*
Cutaneous vasculitis (leucocytoclastic)	×				
Rheumatoid vasculitis	×	×			
Connective tissue disease	×	×			
Wegener's granulomatosis		×	×		
Kawasaki arteritis		×	×		
Polyarteritis nodosa			×	×	
Giant cell arteritis				×	×
Buerger's disease				×	×
Takayasu's arteritis					×

Table 20.3 Cutaneous vasculitis

Immunological disorders
- Connective tissue disorders
- Churg–Strauss syndrome
- Cryoglobulinaemia
- Henoch–Schönlien purpura

Infections
- Upper respiratory tract viruses, e.g. mycoplasma
- Streptococcus
- Hepatitis B/C virus
- Epstein–Barr virus

Drugs
- Antibiotics (e.g. penicillins/sulphonamides)
- Diuretics
- Non-steroidal anti-inflammatory agents
- Anticonvulsants

affecting the large joints. It is often more extensive in the adult. The gastrointestinal tract is involved in >50% of the patients, most commonly presenting as abdominal pain. Similarly the kidneys are affected in half the cases of HSP presenting with haematuria.

In this vascular purpura the platelet count is normal. The erythrocyte sedimentation rate (ESR) or plasma viscosity is usually increased but not in all cases. Biopsy confirms a leucocytoclastic vasculitis affecting the small vessels. Standard immunopathological tests are negative.

The outlook for children with HSP is excellent, but amongst adults nephritis can contribute to a poorer prognosis. Therapy consists of supportive care and symptomatic relief. Some workers advocate steroid therapy if there is a progressive deterioration of renal function. Because of the characteristic nature of the purpura, the patient is unlikely to be referred to a surgeon unless gastrointestinal problems are a presenting feature. Symptoms of colicky abdominal pain, with the rare occurrence of pancreatitis and intersusseption, can come the surgeon's way.

Idiopathic mixed cryoglobulinaemia

In this condition the symptoms include cutaneous vasculitis, arthralgias, weakness of the muscles and renal disease. Cutaneous involvement, though most often manifest by purpura, can also include presentation with RP. Purpura is usually non-pruritic and involves

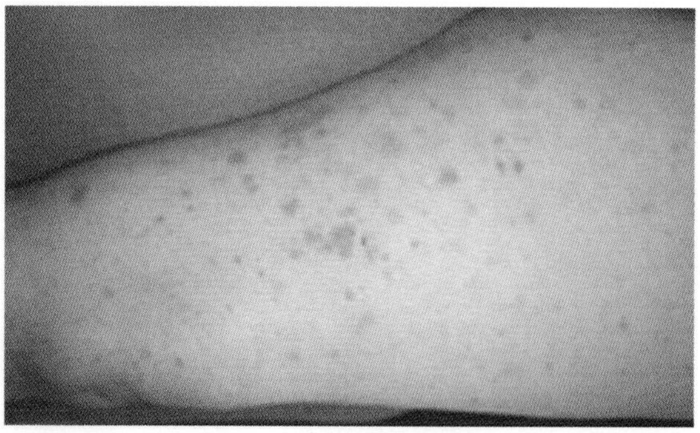

Figure 20.3 Henoch–Schönlein purpura.

the lower extremities. It occurs in crops lasting for 3–10 days and leg ulcers develop in over 20% of patients, thus this patient may present to the surgeon. The next most common presentation is with arthralgia. Nephritis is seen in 50% of patients and may present as nephrotic syndrome. Hepatomegaly and splenomegaly are often found, as are abnormal liver function tests. Over two-thirds of patients are anaemic. There tends to be a mild leucocytosis with an elevated ESR or plasma viscosity. Occasionally there is an eosinophilia. Plasma complement levels may be low. A diffuse hypergammaglobulinaemia without any homogeneous band is found on serum electrophoresis. Cryoprecipitation is found when the patient's blood is incubated at 4°C. Up to 60% of patients have an associated infection such as hepatitis B or C virus or Epstein–Barr virus. Histology of skin lesions shows a small vessel vasculitis affecting mainly small arterioles and capillaries characteristic of the hypersensitivity vasculitides.

The long-term prognosis is influenced by the degree of renal involvement. Treatment is usually supportive but immunosuppressive agents and plasmapheresis can be used for patients in whom there is severe organ involvement.

Other cutaneous vasculitides

Table 20.3 gives a list of common causes of cutaneous vasculitis. Vasculitis often affects the extremities, particularly in the dependent areas. Questioning as to drug therapy and recent infections should always be carried out. Diagnosis is usually by biopsy. Treatment is by withdrawal of the pharmaceutical agent if this is the cause and supportive therapy. The diagnostic algorithm of Figure 20.4 may be useful in cases of suspected vasculitis.

Rheumatoid vasculitis

Systemic vasculitis is a serious complication of RA with a mortality as high as 40%. The incidence in the total rheumatoid population is approximately 2–5%. The most common clinical manifestations of RA vasculitis are cutaneous skin lesions with leg and foot ulceration (Figure 20.5) being found in approximately 75% patients. Gangrene of the extremeties, palpable purpura and occasionally pyoderma gangrenosum can also be found. Neuropathy is a common feature of vasculitis with mononeuritis multiplex being a common presentation. Other life-threatening complications can occur following organ involvement in the vasculitic process. These include gastrointestinal bleeding, bowel infarction and perforation, myocardial infarction and pleurisy.

The diagnosis can be easy if the patient has clinical RA where the index of suspicion for vasculitis will be high. Occasionally, however, the vasculitis presents in someone with minimal joint disease or indeed no obvious joint disease at that moment in time. Laboratory investigations show high titres of rheumatoid factor with low levels of complement. C-reactive protein (CRP) and plasma viscosity are elevated.

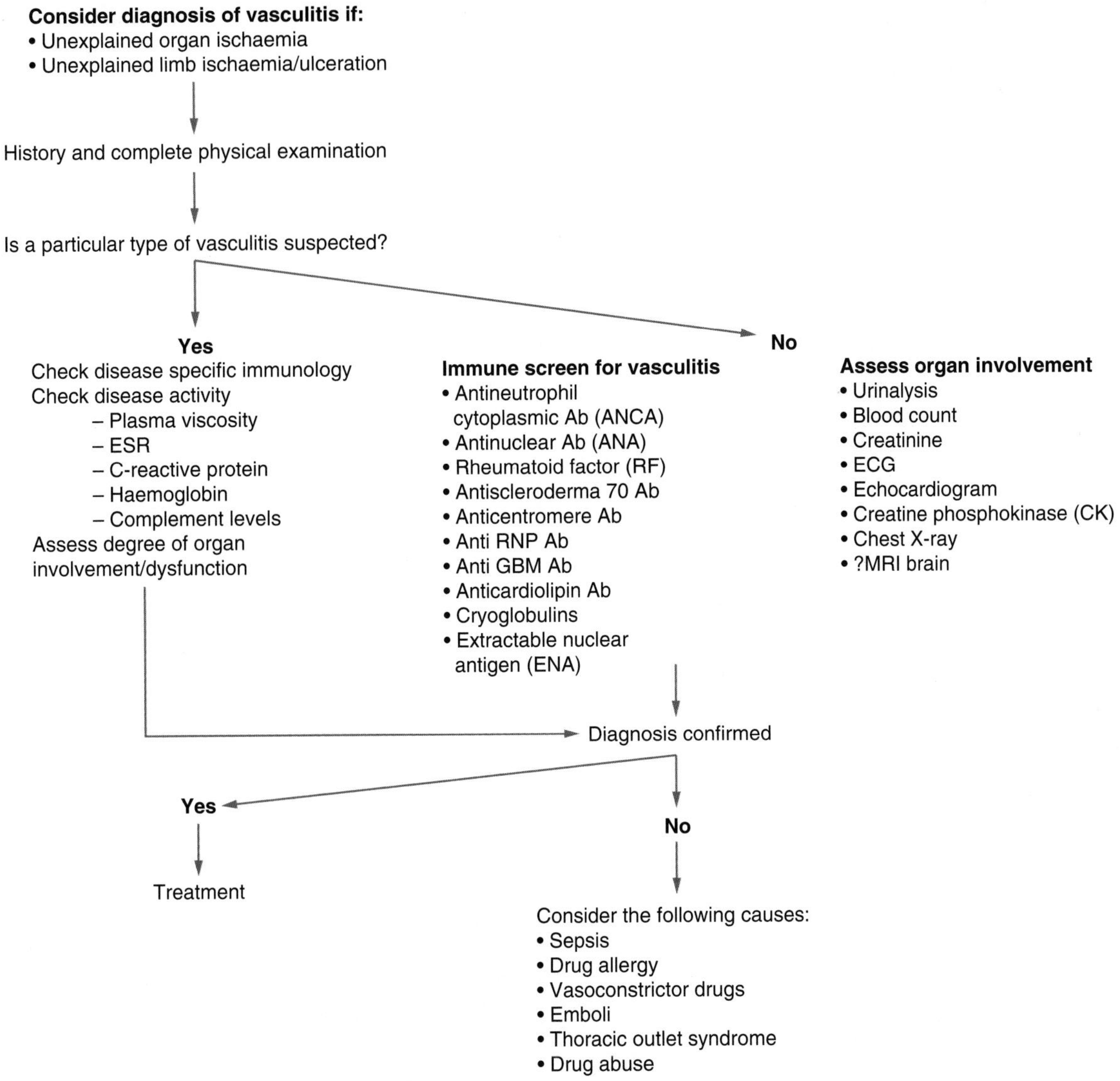

Figure 20.4 Diagnostic algorithm for vasculitis.

Therapy is dependent on the clinical manifestations of the RA. Severe disease manifest by unresponsive vasculitic ulcers may require treatment with corticosteroids and immunosuppressive therapy. This should be planned in conjunction with the rheumatology team.

Connective tissue disorders

This term covers a wide variety of disorders including systemic lupus erythematosus (SLE), antiphospholipid syndrome (APS), Sjögren's syndrome (SS), systemic sclerosis (SSc), polymyalgia rheumatica (PMR), giant cell arteritis (GCA), and polyarteritis nodosum. These latter three affect the larger vessels and are not covered here. Most of the CTDs are associated with Raynaud's syndrome (RS) and come through this symptom to the vascular surgeon.

Systemic lupus erythematosus

Systemic lupus erythematosus is a chronic autoimmune disorder with a wide spectrum of clinical manifestations. It characteristically affects younger women but all age groups can be affected. The prevalence is thought to be between 4 and 280 cases/100 000, with a sex ratio of 13:1 in favour of females. The disease can produce pathology in any organ (Table 20.4). The clinical features which lead to presentation to the surgeon are noted below.

Raynaud's syndrome is associated with SLE in approximately 25–45% of cases. It can be severe, with associated digital ulceration and gangrene. Diagnosis and management of RS associated with the CTDs is covered under vasospasm.

Apart from RS, the likeliest reason for presentation to the surgeon is through vasculitis of the small blood vessels producing skin microinfarcts, particularly affecting the hands and feet (Figure 20.6). Bowel infarcts from gastrointestinal vasculitis may present as an acute abdomen. When these appearances are seen, then SLE should be suspected and the appropriate testing carried

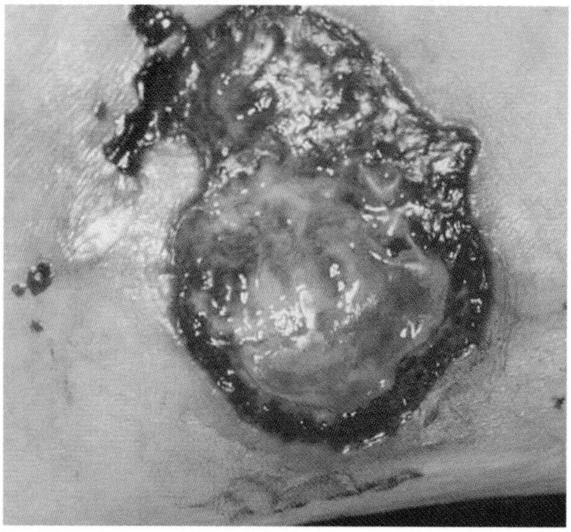

Figure 20.5 Rheumatoid vasculitis.

out (Figure 20.4). On initial screening, blood should be taken for plasma viscosity/ESR measurement and also for CRP titres as these are usually increased in active disease. The full blood count (FBC) may show a leucopenia despite the inflammation present and/or a secondary anaemia. The antinuclear antibody screen is the best screening test but is non-specific so, if positive, most laboratories will automatically measure antibodies against double-stranded DNA. Between 5% and 10% of SLE patients do not have high titres of anti-double-stranded DNA Ab so a negative test does not exclude SLE if clinical suspicion is high. In the presence of SLE, antibody markers for other associated autoimmune diseases should be sought. These include extractable nuclear antigens (ENAs) for anti Ro and La to diagnose Sjögren's syndrome and anticardiolipin antibodies to diagnose APS. APS was previously called by the misnomer lupus anticoagulant. It is a true misnomer as the disease confers prothrombotic tendencies and often occurs as an isolated syndrome in the absence of lupus (see later).

Table 20.4 Frequency of symptoms in SLE

Symptoms	*Percentage (approximate)*	*Comment*
Fatigue	80–100	
Fever	80	
Weight loss	60	
Arthralgia or arthritis	95	Non-deforming
Skin involvement		
Butterfly rash	50	
Photosensitivity	60	
Mouth ulcers	40	
Alopecia	70	
Raynaud's	30	
Purpura	15	
Urticaria	8	
Renal impairment	68	
Gastrointestinal problems	38	Mild
Pulmonary involvement		
Pleurisy	45	
Effusion	24	
Cardiac		
Pericarditis	30	
Murmurs	23	
Lymphadenopathy	50	
Splenomegaly	10	
Hepatomegaly	25	
Central nervous system		
Mood disturbance	50	
Convulsions	15	
Stroke	?1–2	

With permission from Professor P. Emery and the Arthritis Research Campaign.

The management of active SLE is complex and involves immunosuppressant agents such as corticosteroids and cyclophosphamide. Organ screening is essential and patient care should be undertaken in conjunction with the rheumatologist. Vascular occlusive lesions/thrombosis require treatment with anticoagulants in the acute phase which may need to be lifelong in duration in some SLE cases with APS.

Antiphospholipid syndrome

Antiphospholipid syndrome requires identification by the surgeon for two main reasons. First, *de novo* thrombosis may occur in APS and present to the vascular surgeon acutely. Additionally, APS is associated with unexplained blockage of vascular grafts and post-operative deep vein thrombosis (DVT). Table 20.5 shows

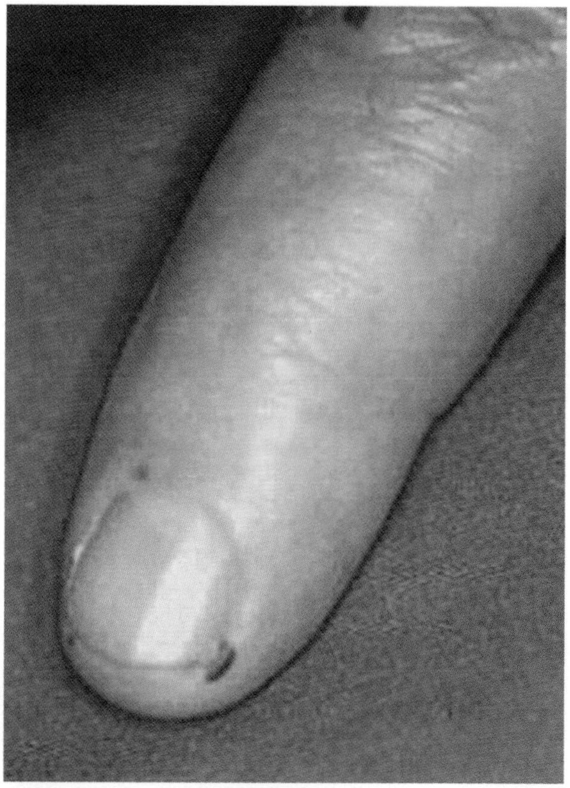

Figure 20.6 SLE digital micro-infarct.

Table 20.5 Thrombotic presentation associated with the antiphospholipid syndrome

Arterial	*Venous*
Acute limb ischaemia (unusual) Unexplained graft failure Unexplained stroke or TIA (particularly if <60 years of age) Recurrent fetal loss Intracardiac thrombus (leading to distal emboli)	Deep vein thrombosis (upper and lower limb) Mesenteric, hepatic, splenic, caval thrombosis

TIA = transient ischaemic attack.

the potential thrombotic syndromes associated with APS. Diagnosis is made both by measurement of anticardiolipin antibodies and through coagulation tests specifically designed to detect the lupus anticoagulant. 30% of patients may only have one or other of the tests positive so both screens should be carried out.

In the presence of arterial thrombosis anticoagulants are used as treatment if there are no contraindications to this therapy. Long-term anticoagulants are frequently indicated in some but not all cases, where aspirin may be the treatment of choice, e.g. the elderly or when a high risk of haemorrhage is present. Specific antithrombotic/anticoagulant regimens are available for treatment of APS in pregnancy associated with fetal loss which include aspirin and low molecular weight heparin therapy.

Sjögren's syndrome

Sjögren's syndrome represents a group of disorders characterized by inflammation and subsequent destruction of, particularly, the salivary and lacrimal glands. The symptoms of dry eyes and mouth (sicca syndrome) are well recognized. Less well recognized are the extraglandular manifestations of SS and the fact that SS can occur as an overlap with other CTDs such as SLE, SSc and RA.

Its importance to the surgeon lies in the fact that, like SLE, it can be associated with unexplained vascular events, particularly in the younger than expected patient. Thus SS should also be sought in cases of purpura, digital infarcts and cutaneous ulcers. Testing for the disease includes measurement of specific autoantibodies, the extractable nuclear antigens Ro and La, and the usual non-specific screen for inflammation, such as plasma viscosity/ESR and CRP measurements. Treatment, when required for active disease, is with immunosuppressant regimens such as corticosteroids. Thromboses should be managed by anticoagulation if no contraindications to such treatment exist.

Systemic sclerosis

Systemic sclerosis is the CTD most commonly associated with chronic persistent digital ischaemia. Its early diagnosis in cases of RP presents the biggest challenge to the clinician involved with the care of this disease. SSc can be classified as either limited SSc (lSSc) or diffuse SSc (dSSc). lSSc was previously called CREST syndrome. This latter term was discarded as not all patients have calcinosis or telangiectasia, and the other symptoms of oesophageal dysfunction and sclerodactyly can appear at different timepoints in the disease process, and can be features of dSSc. dSSc is the new term for progressive systemic sclerosis, which again lost favour as a poor descriptor of the pathology. The disease is not always progressive and this term was frightening for patients. SSc was thought to occur with an incidence of 10 cases per million but is now recognized as being much more common. This is due in part to better epidemiological studies, but also to more sensitive laboratory tests for the disease. In any case of severe RP, and particularly if associated with digital ulceration, SSc must be suspected. There is a female prevalence of 7:1 and patients tend to present in middle age. Table 20.6 lists the symptoms particularly associated with either lSSc or dSSc. In lSSc the RP may precede other symptoms of the disease such as sclerodactyly by many years, whereas in dSSc the skin changes (Figure 20.7) usually become apparent within 1 year of onset of RP. It is therefore the limited form that is the more difficult to diagnose. Certain clinical features are linked to the RS associated with SSc and can be helpful in differentiating primary Raynaud's disease (RD) from RS; these include presenting with isolated features of CTD such as sclerodactyly or pitting digital scars. It is reasonable to suspect that such patients will evolve into fully established SSc and indeed this impression is supported by prospective clinical studies. Another warning sign is digital ulceration which does not occur in RD and heralds the later development of CTD. Thus isolated features of CTD occurring in association with RP should alert clinical suspicion to an underlying disorder.

The age of onset of RP may also be important. RP is a frequent finding in young women and most have RD. When RP develops at an older age the likelihood of later CTD development is increased. Women in their thirties are more likely to have an underlying connective tissue disease associated with their Raynaud's rather than primary RD. About 80% of patients over 60 years of age presenting with RP for the first time will have an associated condition but, as the incidence of SSc remains the same as the general population, the higher number of secondary cases is likely to merely reflect the large number of atherosclerotic Raynaud's and to a certain extent some of the hyperviscosity syndromes which may be associated with malignancy.

Severe RP symptoms occurring all year round are also suspicious, as is the recurrence of chilblains in adults. Patients with asymmetrical colour change

Table 20.6 Clinical features of limited and diffuse systemic sclerosis

Limited SSc	*Diffuse SSc*
Vascular	
Raynaud's (preceding skin changes by many years, often decades)	Raynaud's (with subsequent skin changes within 1–2 years)
Skin	
Sclerodactyly (severe)	Sclerodactyly (Fig. 20.8)
Scleroderma limited to hands, feet, face or forearms, or absent	Scleroderma truncal and sacral in distribution
Nailfold capillary abnormalities	Nailfold capillary abnormalities with capillary destruction/dropout (Fig. 20.9)
Lungs	
Pulmonary hypertension + fibrosis	Early and significant pulmonary fibrosis
Gut	
Oesophageal symptoms from hiatus hernia/dysmotility	Widespread gastrointestinal involvement with significant dysmotility, diverticulae ± malabsorption
Renal	
Mild disease	Potential for significant and severe renal failure
Blood tests	
CRP/PV/ESR often normal	CRP/PV/ESR often normal
FBC often normal	FBC often normal
Anticentromere Abs positive in 70–80%	Anticentromere Abs negative
Scleroderma 70 Abs (Anti-topoisomerase Ab) negative	Scleroderma 70 Abs positive in 30–50%

CRP = C-reactive protein, PV = plasma viscosity, ESR = erythrocyte sedimentation rate, FBC = full blood count.

suggest RS as opposed to RD. Thus a high index of clinical suspicion for SSc can be raised during the first clinical assessment of a patient. This can be further augmented by capillary microscopy. Recent software development for this technique has led to the availability of very sophisticated machines and these can be used very effectively in research projects. However, less sophisticated apparatus such as simple microscopes or a hand-held ophthalmoscope can be used satisfactorily as a screening tool for the nailfold vessels. If one uses a hand-held ophthalmoscope, the magnifying power should be adjusted to the maximum and the scope held about 0.25 cm from the nailfolds. Abnormal vessels can usually be seen clearly (Figure 20.8a). It should be noted that no vessels are detectable in the normal person. Whilst this technique will miss early abnormalities, detection of such vessels in a patient with RP is a marker for later development of CTD. Nailfold capillary abnormalities are found in a number of diseases but most characteristically in the scleroderma spectrum of disorders (Figure 20.8b).

The diagnosis of SSc rests heavily on clinical findings but auto-antibody tests can be helpful. Anticentromere antibody is found in patients with lSSc, and scleroderma 70 (isotopoisomerase) in those with dSSc. Anticentromere antibody has a predictive value for pSSc (sensitivity 60%, specificity 98%) and scleroderma 70 for dSSc (sensitivity 38%, specificity 100%). It has been suggested that abnormal nailfold capillaries plus the finding of a positive antibody in the serum will detect over 90% of patients destined to have SSc.

Treatment of SSc is based on organ screening to ensure that the lung, kidneys and pulmonary blood pressure do not deteriorate. This is combined with symptomatic treatment. Thus a proton pump inhibitor is given for dyspepsia. Constipation, diverticulitis and possible malabsorption secondary to the bowel motility problems are treated appropriately as is the Raynaud's phenomenon. Immunosuppression is required for progressive disease. This can include corticosteroids if an inflammatory element such as myositis is present but more usually comprises azathioprine or cyclophosphamide. Treatment should be undertaken in conjunction with the rheumatologist.

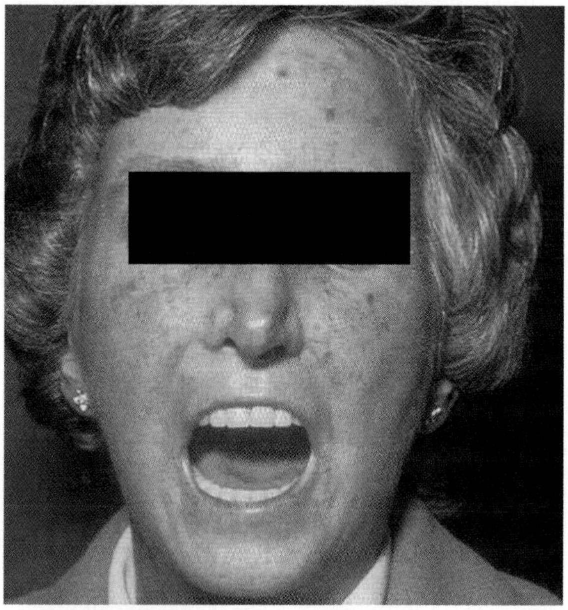

Figure 20.7 Scleroderma in systemic sclerosis.

(a)

(b)

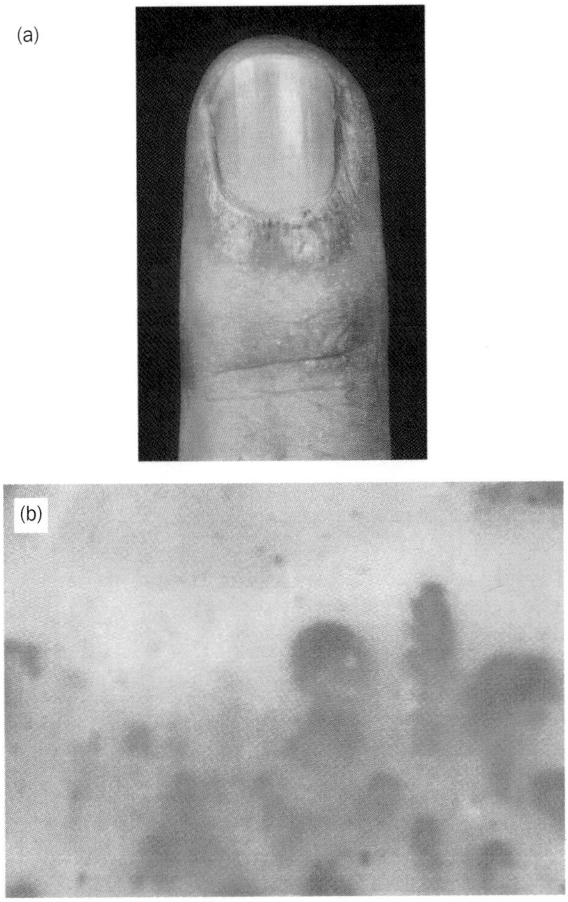

Figure 20.8 **(a)** Abnormal nailfold capillaries in systemic sclerosis. (b) Capillary microscopy showing abnormal nailfold capillaries in systemic sclerosis.

Section 20.2 • Vasospastic microvascular disease: Raynaud's phenomenon

The best recognized of the cold-related disorders is Raynaud's phenomenon which affects 10–20% of young women. It is nine times more prevalent in women than in men. Raynaud's phenomenon is subdivided into Raynaud's syndrome where there is an associated disorder and primary Raynaud's disease where there is not. In 1862 Maurice Raynaud first described this clinical syndrome associated with his name. He defined it as episodic digital ischaemia provoked by cold and emotion. It is classically manifest by pallor of the digits (Figure 20.9), followed by cyanosis and rubor. The pallor reflects vasospasm in the digital vessels, the cyanosis results from deoxygenation of static venous blood, and the rubor is caused by reactive hyperaemia following the return of blood flow.

Raynaud's original definition is now known to require modification; for example the full triphasic colour change is not essential for diagnosis. A number of patients have blanching alone. Furthermore, the tip of the nose, tongue and earlobes may also be involved. We now know that more widespread vasospasm occurs in this disorder with decreased oesophageal and myocardial perfusion after cold challenge. Some workers have speculated that the lesions of the kidney and lung that are seen in severe cases of RS associated with SSc may be accounted for in part by vasospasm. Moreover, stimuli other than cold and emotion can provoke an attack, for example trauma, hormones and various chemicals including those in tobacco smoke. A wide spectrum of disease may be associated with Raynaud's phenomenon (Table 20.7).

Nomenclature

Raynaud's phenomenon is the blanket term used to describe cold-related digital vasospasm. Raynaud's phenomenon is divided into Raynaud's syndrome and primary disease (described above). However this European classification is not globally accepted and workers in the USA tend to use the term syndrome and phenomenon interchangeably. Consequently assessment of the literature may be difficult. The situation is further complicated by the fact that long-term studies have shown that Raynaud's phenomenon may be the precursor of systemic illness by over 20 years, and recently developed sensitive laboratory procedures such as autoantibody testing have shown that more than one-half of patients referred to hospital for management of

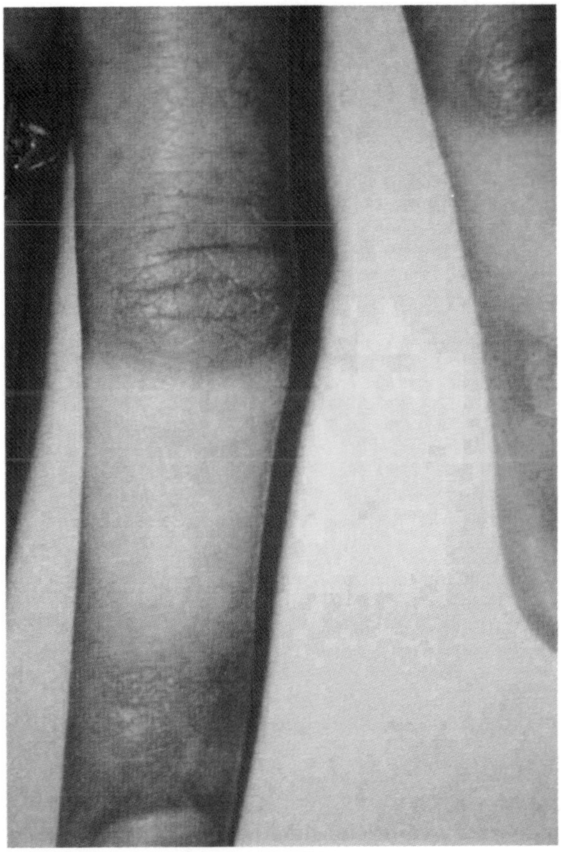

Figure 20.9 Raynaud's phenomenon.

their RP may have an associated systemic disease. Clearly this latter figure depends on local referral patterns but the clinician seeing a patient with severe RP must have a high index of suspicion for an associated disorder.

Pathophysiology of Raynaud's phenomenon

Maurice Raynaud postulated hyperreactivity of the sympathetic nervous system in RP causing an increase in the vasoconstrictor response to cold. This theory is supported by the fact that emotional stimuli can provoke attacks and lumbar sympathectomy can ameliorate symptoms in the lower limb. Others however, prefer a local fault theory suggesting that cold hypersensitivity of the pre-capillary resistance vessels cause the symptoms. Subsequent work has shown that many of these findings may be related to abnormalities of the peripheral sympathetic nervous system. There are three areas which should be considered as having aetiological importance in Raynaud's: (i) neurogenic mechanisms, (ii) blood and blood vessel wall interactions, and (iii) abnormalities of the immunological and inflammatory responses.

Neurogenic mechanisms

Published work in this area tends to focus on the peripheral sympathetic nervous system. Abnormalities described include increased alpha-adgenergic receptor sensitivity and/or density and also an increase in the responsiveness of β-presynaptic receptors in the peripheral vessels of the RS patient.

Table 20.7 Disorders associated with Raynaud's syndrome

Connective tissue diseases and other immunological disorders
- Systemic sclerosis
- Systemic lupus erythematosus
- Sjögren's syndrome
- Dermatomyositis and polymyositis
- Mixed connective tissue disease
- Rheumatoid arthritis

Occupational conditions
- Hand–arm vibration syndrome (proscribed industrial disease A11)
- Work with polyvinyl chloride
- Cold injury (e.g. frozen food packers)

'Obstructive' vasospastic disease
- Atherosclerosis (elderly)
- Thoracic outlet syndrome
- Emboli

Drug induced Raynaud's phenomenon
- Non-selective β-blockers
- Ergot and other anti-migraine drugs
- Cytotoxic agents
- Sulphasalazine
- Bromocriptine
- Ephedrine

Miscellaneous
- Cold agglutinins/cryoglobulins
- Hypothyroidism
- Neoplasm (usually with hyperviscosity syndrome)
- Idiopathic Raynaud's disease

The role of the central sympathetic system is unknown. There is some support for its involvement coming from work showing that local vibration of one hand induces vasoconstriction of the other, which is abolished by proximal nerve blockade. It is further supported by body cooling which induces central nervous system mediated vasoconstriction and may produce vasospasm in one hand when only the other is being exposed to local digital cooling. The literature is not agreed on this point, however, and though abnormalities of the nervous system probably exist in RP they are at present not clearly defined. This should be an area for focused research. One new finding relates to a potential dysfunction of the calcitonin gene-related peptide (CGRP)-dependent neurovascular access. CGRP is a potent vasodilator and early work suggests that digital skin CGRP-containing neurones may be decreased in RP when compared to normal subjects.

Blood and blood vessel wall interactions

The nervous system mediated changes in vascular tone described above do not, however, explain all the features of RP. In particular they cannot explain the systemic nature of RP with its widespread effects on blood flow affecting many organs when control of blood flow to all organs is not regulated by the same mechanisms. It is therefore likely that blood-borne factors or endothelial dysfunction are also involved. Flow in the microcirculation depends not only on the size of the blood vessel lumen but also on the integrity of the endothelium and the various cellular elements and plasma factors in the blood.

It has been known for some time that the cellular components of blood are abnormal in certain forms of RP, in particular in RS associated with CTD. The platelet is more aggregatable and releases increased amounts of vasoconstrictor and platelet aggregating substances such as thromboxane A_2. The red blood cell (RBC) is less deformable in RS, and the cold temperature in association with the acidosis present in cold ulcerated fingers will further increase RBC stiffness. More recently the important role that the white blood cell (WBC) has in maintaining flow in small vessels has been recognized. WBC activation, with increased release of prothrombotic free radicals, and increased WBC aggregation forming microemboli has been reported in RS and these may contribute to the decreased flow seen in this disorder.

The importance of the endothelium as a functional organ has also been increasingly recognized. The endothelium releases many vasoactive chemicals such as prostacyclin (PGI_2), a potent antiplatelet agent and vasodilator. PGI_2 may be elevated in the early stage of vascular disease although in the later stages PGI_2 stimulating factor may be decreased, facilitating platelet aggregation and vasoconstriction. Similarly nitric oxide (NO) is also an important endothelial vasodilator. Abnormalities of its production and in vascular sensitivity to NO have been described in RS. The damaged endothelium releases factor VIII von Willibrand factor antigen (vWF) which can have pro-thrombotic effects via its participation in the coagulation cascade and in mediating platelet aggregation. Endothelin, another endothelial product, causes vasoconstriction and has been found to be increased in RP, increasing further following a cold challenge. Impaired fibrinolysis has also been reported as a further manifestation of endothelial cell dysfunction.

It should be noted that RD patients do not show these blood and endothelial abnormalities whilst the majority of RS patients do. Interestingly this is true for both CTD-associated RS and that associated with hand–arm vibration syndrome/vibration white finger disease. Thus, while these changes are likely to be a consequence of the underlying disorder, they may augment the symptoms of vasospasm and their attenuation is an important feature in the pharmacological management of RP.

Immunological inflammatory responses

Activation of the WBC also has profound effects on inflammation and immunity. The endothelium is also involved in these processes by the production of chemo-attractant agents, growth factors and growth inhibitors. Disordered immune/inflammatory responses occur in the majority of severe cases of RS via their association with the CTDs, but also in hand–arm vibration syndrome which has no clear immune/inflammatory basis. Tumour necrosis factor, lymphotoxin, phagocytes, macrophages and T-cell derived proteins, along with immune complex deposition in the vessel wall, are all likely to be involved in the vascular damage seen in RS.

Treatment of Raynaud's phenomenon

There is no cure for Raynaud's phenomenon, but much can be done to alleviate symptoms. With the diverse pathophysiology associated with RP one of the key arms of treatment must be detection of underlying disease. This must, however, be combined with symptomatic treatment. In this case treatment is aimed at one or several of the mechanisms which have been implicated in contributing to symptomatology. As our knowledge of the pathophysiology improves so will our management of the condition. A diagram giving a suggested algorithm for the management of RP is shown in Figure 20.11.

Supportive measures

Much can be done for patients with mild disease without recourse to drug treatment. As many patients are apprehensive about their fingers turning white or blue, reassurance is often required and information regarding both their disease and self-help groups such as the Raynaud's and Scleroderma Association, Alsager, is often gratefully received. This group provides information booklets about various disorders associated with RP which can be requested by both doctor and patient. It is also important to advise patients on protecting themselves from cold. Even patients with primary RD are at risk of cold injury if exposed to severe conditions. Practical solutions to these problems include ensuring maintenance of body heat, hand warmers, battery-heated gloves, etc.

Smoking is known to provoke attacks in susceptible people and therefore advice about stopping smoking should always be given. This also applies to passive smoking and patients and their relatives should be aware of this and advised accordingly. In the occupational forms, a change in occupation can be required. The withdrawal of drugs known to be associated with RP can also be useful, e.g. β-blockers. It has been suggested that the oral contraceptive pill is implicated in provoking attacks but, in our experience, we have not usually found this to be the case. Our current accepted practice is to discontinue the contraceptive pill only if there is a clear association with the development of vasospasm. Hormone replacement therapy is not contraindicated by the presence of RP. Some well-motivated people may benefit from bio-feedback techniques with the suggestion that bio-feedback induced vasodilatation is mediated through a non-neural decrease in β-adrenergic stimulation.

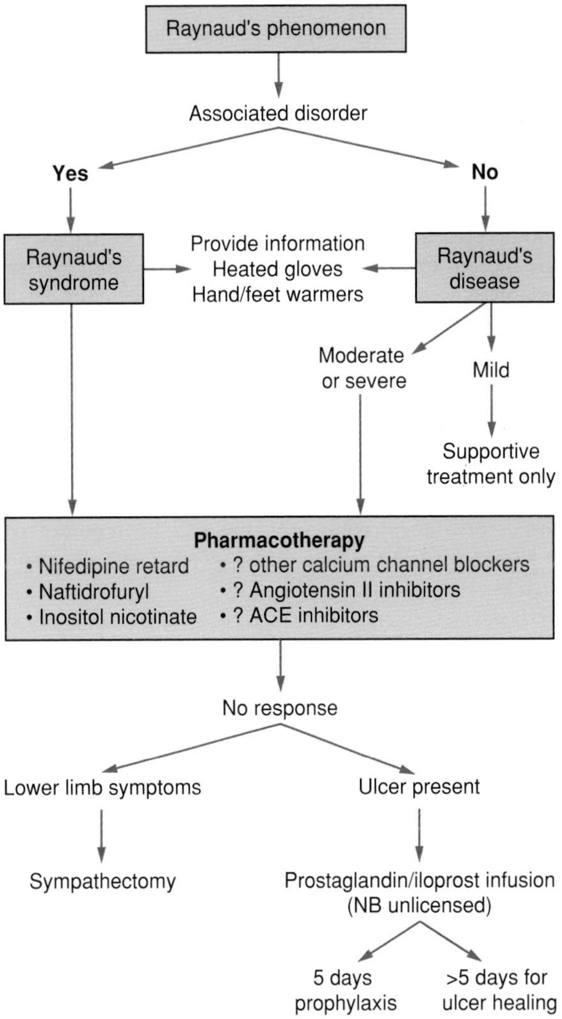

Figure 20.10 Therapeutic algorithm for Raynaud's phenomenon.

Battery-heated gloves and socks are the perfect solution for some patients with mild disease. There are a number of types available, including one with a rechargeable battery fixed on a belt providing up to 3 hours of warmth, with the wires from the belt concealed beneath the clothing. They can, however, be a little bulky and heavy for the elderly. Skiing-type battery powered gloves are available where the battery is attached at the wrist and patients find these more user-friendly. It should be noted that the irritation of ulcers by the added heat has been found to be an infrequent problem. Chemical hand warmers obtained from local chemists and sports shops provide a satisfactory alternative source of heat. These come in both disposable and reusable forms. Surgical shoes such as comfort shoes, or ABEL shoes can be obtained from surgical appliance departments and these can also be useful. The padded soles keep the feet warm and relieve the pressure on the toes which can result in vasospasm. Pressure is well recognized as causing vasospasm and the patient generally learns to avoid such things as carrying hand-held plastic shopping bags. It is, however, less well recognized that properly designed padded footwear can relieve the pressure over the digital vessels and spread the pressure more evenly throughout the foot thus attenuating the vasospastic symptoms.

When ulcers are present, good footcare should also be undertaken. Any ulcer that is moist should be swabbed and cultured. A major pitfall in the management of digital ulceration in severe RP is the failure of the clinician to detect infection. Significant infection can be present even in the absence of warmth, erythema and pus formation since blood flow to initiate these responses is impaired. One should perhaps consider a trial of antibiotics in patients where healing is a significant problem. The organisms detected are usually staphylococcus, but infection by less common organisms can also occur.

Drug therapy

If symptoms are recurrent and severe, it is likely that some form of pharmocotherapy will be required to reduce both the frequency and severity of vasospastic attacks.

Calcium channel blockade

Calcium channel blockers are the most frequently prescribed drugs for RP. Nifedipine is now the treatment of choice for symptoms of RP. Its mechanism of action is thought to be predominantly vasodilatory but it also has antiplatelet and anti-white cell activities. Its use, however, can be limited by the vasodilatory side-effects to which the RP patient appears very susceptible. They commonly include flushing and headache but also palpitations, dizziness and ankle swelling. Nifedipine, in the preferred Retard preparation can be introduced slowly to attenuate these vasodilatory responses. It is our current practice to start 10 mg of the Retard preparation at night then shifting the dosing regimen to the morning and then, if tolerated, increasing to 10 mg twice a day, then three times a day increasing to a total of 60 mg/day. This latter dose, however, can provoke ankle swelling. It is important to reassure the patient that the vasodilatory side-effects usually disappear with continued treatment, so unless they are intolerable the patient should persevere for 10–14 days before discontinuing the therapy. The drug has not, however, been passed for use in pregnancy and the patient must be advised to avoid pregnancy when this drug is prescribed. If side-effects require discontinuation, one can consider the other calcium channel antagonists although none have a licence for use in RP and the patient should be informed about this. Amlodipine, diltiazem and asradipine have all been studied in placebo-controlled trials in RP. Verapamil has been found to be ineffective.

If a calcium channel blocker is not tolerated because of side-effects, Nifedipine capsules can be used as rescue medication during a severe spasm attack, with the capsule being pierced with a pin, crushed by the teeth and placed below the tongue, in an effort to alleviate acute symptoms.

Other vasodilators

Use of other vasodilators in RP has been evaluated in predominantly Raynaud's disease populations. Four compounds do merit consideration. Inositol nicotinate (Hexopal) has produced encouraging results in mild to moderate RD. The drug may take a number of weeks to produce its effect. Similarly, naftidrofuryl may produce benefit over a number of weeks. Although these drugs are known vasodilators, their action in RP may be through other mechanisms which include modification of some of the rheological abnormalities mentioned earlier. Thymoxamine is a selective α_1-blocker which may also be tried initially for a period of 2 weeks. A trial of these treatments given in sufficient dosages for a sufficient period of time may be worthwhile. It is unusual, however, for the more severely affected patient to benefit from these treatments, most of which will have been prescribed by the general practitioner before hospital referral. Thus in such a severely affected population, simple vasodilators are often ineffective with the limiting factor being the development of side-effects at high dosage.

Prostaglandin therapy

The vasodilator antiplatelet prostaglandins PGE_1 and PGI_2 have been evaluated in the management of Raynaud's phenomenon. These drugs are given by intravenous infusion (PGE_1 by central line) and therefore require at least hospital attendance if not admission. Recent studies with the prostacyclin derivative Iloprost have proven successful in the management of RP. This drug, however, is not a licensed preparation and appropriate information must be provided to the patient. Five-day treatment periods appear optimum, with the infusion being given for approximately 5 hours each day. The dose is slowly increased to ensure tolerability. Side-effects include headache, flushing and nausea and are related to the vasodilatation. Blood pressure should be monitored throughout the infusion.

The vasodilator and antiplatelet effects appear short-lived following prostaglandin therapy. However the duration of response can be for many months. The prostaglandin infusions should be reserved, however, for patients who are severely affected and for those with digital ulceration.

Alternative approaches are being investigated (such as the use of orally and transdermally absorbed stable analogues) which may allow more prolonged treatment.

Future trends

Local application of glyceryltrinitrate cream was tried with some success but limitation of its use occurred because of side-effects. More recently studies of NO and NO donors have proven interesting and may well be therapies for the future. Similarly, angiotensin-2 inhibitors have been evaluated in one placebo-controlled double-blind trial and if this work is confirmed it will open up a further avenue for treatment. Relaxin, a potent vasodilator, did show some exciting responses in this group of patients but the potential for intra-uterine side-effects has prevented this compound's effective development.

Sympathectomy

Upper limb sympathectomy gives a high relapse rate and an especially poor response in RS. It is therefore no longer indicated for RP of the upper limb. It should be noted, however, that the more selective laparoscopic thoracic sympathectomy operation has not yet been critically assessed in RP although it is possible that it will fail in the same way. Similarly the more localized digital sympathectomy has shown encouraging early work but current reports suggest a similar failure rate to conventional upper limb sympathectomy. Long-term follow-up assessments are essential in assessing these latter two procedures. In contrast, sympathectomy still has an important role in the treatment of RP affecting the feet when results may be rewarding. Lumbar sympathectomy is usually carried out using needle injection of phenol into the ganglia rather than open operation.

Amputation

Very occasionally, in order to alleviate pain or intractable gangrene, it becomes necessary to amputate the digit. Fortunately, today, this is rare. Usually it becomes necessary after long-term medical treatment has failed to salvage the digit. Thus it is always important to instruct the patient to present early to the clinic. In systemic sclerosis where skin tightening over the finger pulp causes ischaemia, operations to remove part of the terminal phalanx to relieve pressure may be useful. Tissue viability and potential for wound healing must be carefully assessed.

Other surgical procedures

Any local pressure on the arterial supply to the limb should be removed if possible. This includes consideration of the removal of cervical ribs and fibrous bands (discussed elsewhere).

Conclusion

Microvascular disorders are common and until recently management has been difficult. Part of this relates to the poor clarity of diagnosis. However, as research into the field continues and our knowledge of the pathogenesis of these disorders improves, so have our management and diagnostic techniques. With the help of a careful clinical history and examination and a selection of specific blood tests, it is now possible to correctly diagnose the different vasculitides, connective tissue disorders and types of Raynaud's phenomenon. Although a cure is not available in the majority of these conditions, many patients with these disorders can achieve a satisfactory amelioration of their symptoms. Finally it should be remembered that the prognosis of Raynaud's syndrome is determined by that of the underlying disorder which must first be detected, then monitored and treated.

Acknowledgement

Professor Jill J. F. Belch receives support from the Raynaud's and Scleroderma Association, Alsager, UK.

Further reading

Belch, J. J. F. and Zurier, R. B., eds (1995). *Connective Tissue Diseases*. London: Chapman and Hall.

Butler, R. C. and Jayson, M. I. V. (1995). *Collected Reports on the Rheumatic Diseases*. Arthritis and Rheumatism Council.

Tooke, J. E. and Lowe, G. D. O., eds (1996). *A Textbook of Vascular Medicine*. London: Arnold.

Yao, J. S. T and Pearce, W. H., eds (1995). *The Ischemic Extremity: Advances in Treatment*. Stamford, CT: Appleton and Lange.

MODULE 21

Non-invasive vascular assessment

1 • Ultrasound
2 • Pressure measurements
3 • Doppler velocity waveforms
4 • Duplex scanning applications
5 • Plethysmography
6 • Other techniques
7 • Future directions in vascular technology

Quantitative non-invasive vascular assessments can aid clinicians in their assessment of the functional severity of arterial and venous disease and facilitate monitoring of disease progression in the longer term. A plethora of techniques have been developed over the past 30 years, many of which are both complex and time-consuming and have been made obsolete by the availability of rapid and accurate duplex ultrasound scans. However, several simple and well-validated techniques still have a valuable role in vascular assessment. This chapter covers ultrasound and its use in pressure measurements, Doppler waveform analysis and duplex scanning; other techniques, including plethysmography, will also be discussed.

Section 21.1 • Ultrasound

Continuous wave Doppler

Ultrasound beams are generated by piezoelectric crystals resonating at a particular frequency. Ultrasound beams reflected from a stationary object will return with the same frequency. However, ultrasound beams reflected from moving objects, or from moving fluids containing scatterers such as red blood cells, will be shifted in frequency. The frequency shift, or Doppler shift, is determined by the velocity with which the object is moving and the frequency of the emitted signal. If the angle between the direction of movement and the ultrasound beam is known, the frequency shift can be converted into velocity using the Doppler equation

$$F_d = \frac{2vF_t \cos \Phi}{c}$$

where F_d is the Doppler shift, v is the velocity of blood flow, F_t is the frequency of the transmitted ultrasound, c is the velocity of ultrasound propagation in tissue (1540 m/s) and Φ is the angle between the ultrasound beam and the direction of blood flow.

The simple hand-held Doppler velocimeters used in the majority of vascular and diabetic clinics are continuous wave (CW) systems, with separate transmitting and receiving piezoelectric elements. The frequency shifts recorded represent movements along the whole length of the ultrasound beam, and the depth examined cannot be adjusted.

Pulsed wave Doppler

Pulsed Doppler systems transmit short bursts of ultrasound, and the receiving crystal can be set to only recognize signals returning after a selected delay. Since the speed with which ultrasound travels in human tissue is known, the timing of this delay allows the user to specify the depth, or range, from which the returning signal is received. This means that the Doppler shift at a particular site can be evaluated simultaneously with the image obtained from a B-mode scanner, a feature of the duplex scanner. It also allows signals from different sites within the lumen of an artery to be analysed. Pulsed wave Doppler is generally used for transcranial Doppler evaluations and duplex scans.

Duplex scanners

B-mode scanners convert ultrasound echoes from tissue interfaces into dots on a two-dimensional (2-D) display; the brightness of each dot is proportional to the intensity of the reflected signal. The reflected ultrasound beam also contains information about movement within the sampled tissues, for example the blood flow within arteries insonated by the beam, but these data are not used when a B-mode image is formed. Duplex scanners (see Figure 21.1) process this additional information and add pulsed Doppler and colour flow data to the B-mode image. The instantaneous mean velocity at each sampled volume within a specified area is determined and displayed as colour superimposed on the simultaneous 2-D image. Doppler shifted signals from scatterers moving towards the transducer will have a higher frequency and

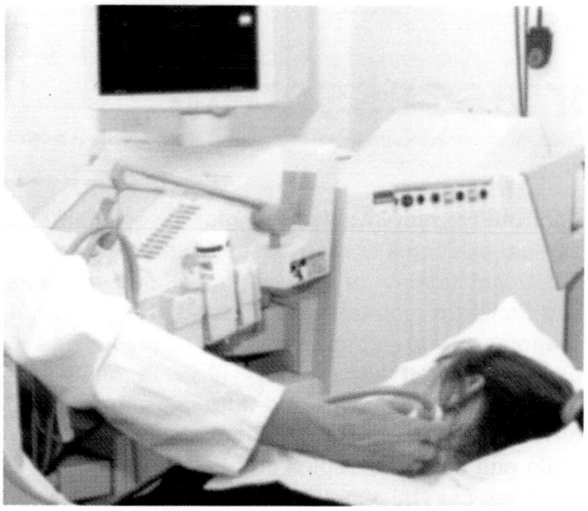

Figure 21.1 A duplex scan of the carotid arteries.

are traditionally displayed as 'red' on the image; similarly if the reflector is moving away from the beam the frequency shift is displayed as 'blue'.

Power Doppler

The power or intensity of the back-scattered Doppler signal can also be displayed on the grey scale image. The intensity of the signal is a function of the number of scatterers rather than the speed and direction in which they are travelling, and is independent of the Doppler angle. This modality is more sensitive than colour for demonstrating filling in tortuous vessels or low flow situations, and can improve visualization of flow at the artery wall, particularly around plaques.

Section 21.2 • Pressure measurements

Ankle/brachial pressure indices (ABPIs)

Patients rest supine for at least 10 min before pressure measurements are made; if the patient has been walking for any significant distance, this resting time may need to be increased. A suitably sized sphygmomanometer cuff is placed around the ankle just proximal to the malleolus (see Figure 21.2). The width of the cuff bladder should be approximately 20% greater than the diameter of the limb at the site of the cuff. If the cuff used is too small, erroneously high readings may be obtained. For most patients an adult cuff with a standard bladder measuring approximately 12 cm wide and 22 cm long can be used for both upper arm and ankle measurements. A CW Doppler pencil probe is used to detect blood flow in the posterior tibial artery (PT), using aquasonic gel to ensure a good contact with the skin. This probe should be held at about 60° to the presumed direction of blood flow, and gently moved until the strongest Doppler signal is obtained. The occluding cuff is then inflated above systolic pressure, and allowed to deflate slowly. The pressure is noted at the first reappearance of the Doppler signal. This method should also be used to obtain the systolic blood pressure in the dorsalis pedis arteries (DP) and brachial arteries bilaterally. It is also possible to measure the blood pressure at the ankle using Doppler signals from the pedal arch should this be necessary.

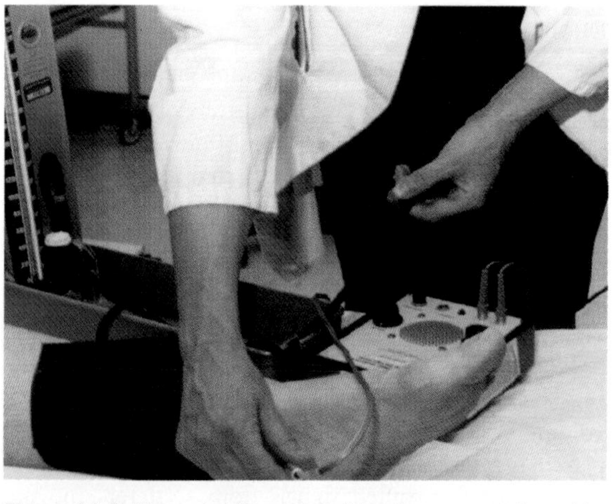

Figure 21.2 Measuring the systolic blood pressure at the ankle.

The ankle/brachial pressure index (ABPI) is defined as:

$$\text{Right ABPI} = \frac{\text{Highest right ankle pressure (PT or DP)}}{\text{Highest brachial pressure (right or left)}}$$

Arterial compliance reduces with distance from the heart, so the pedal artery systolic pressure should be higher than that in the arms.

In normal subjects:

- the ankle systolic pressure should be equal to or greater than the arm pressure, i.e. ABPI ≥ 1.0 (normal range 0.9–1.2)
- there should be pressure symmetry between both limbs at the same level.

Exercise tests

A reduced ABPI ratio is usually seen in patients with intermittent claudication, although occasionally the pressures at rest can approach normal levels. If the ABPI is less than 0.8 at rest there will undoubtedly be a fall in the ankle pressure after exercise, therefore this test is often reserved for claudicants with ABPIs in or just below the normal range. The standard patient exercise regimen is to walk for 1 min at 4 km/hour on a 10% gradient, but some centres prefer to exercise the patient to claudication. A treadmill is normally used for these studies, but it is possible to obtain adequate data by walking the patient for a measured distance in a corridor. The ABPIs are recorded at rest, and the patient is exercised for a standard time or to claudication. After exercise, ABPI measurements are repeated until the

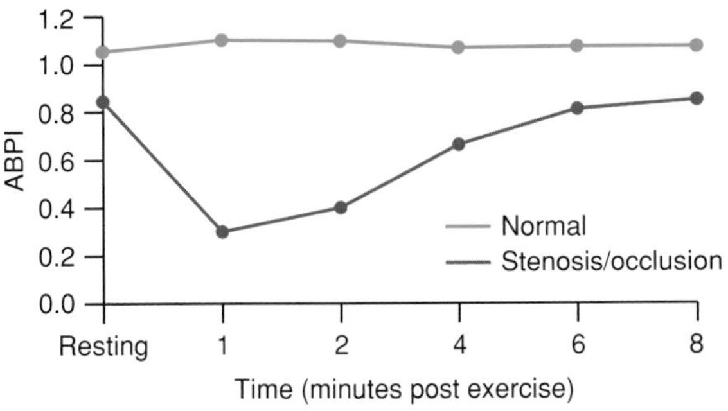

Figure 21.3 Post-exercise ABPIs in a patient with PVD and a normal subject.

ratios have returned to pre-exercise levels (Figure 21.3). The pedal artery with the strongest signal and/or highest pressure, and the arm with the highest brachial pressure reading are generally used to facilitate rapid post-exercise pressure recordings.

In normal subjects:

- the ankle systolic pressure after exercise should be equal to or greater than the arm pressure i.e. ABPI ≥ 1.0 (normal range 1.0–1.2)
- the extent of the pressure drop post-exercise and the time taken to return to resting values are dependent on the number, severity and level of atheromatous lesions in the limb studied.

If the ABPI studies suggest distal artery calcification, a limited duplex scan of the popliteal and crural arteries, noting the Doppler waveforms in each vessel, is usually helpful. If any abnormality is detected, a more comprehensive scan may be required.

Critical limb ischaemia

Vascular assessment can provide a functional assessment of disease severity. Patients with critical limb ischaemia will normally have ABPIs <0.5, and occasionally it will be impossible to detect any blood flow in the pedal arteries. However, patients with 'trash foot' may have normal ABPIs, and a duplex scan including an assessment of the abdominal aorta should be performed to identify any source of emboli.

Problems

- ABPI measurements may be unreliable if calcification of the arterial wall makes the underlying vessel difficult to compress, leading to an overestimation of pressure. Ankle systolic pressure measurements of >300 mmHg are not uncommon in diabetics and patients with renal disease. The strength and quality of the Doppler signal should help to alert the investigator to potential problems, and the pressure should be checked against measurements made in the thigh, calf or toe.
- The width of the occluding cuff can be very important. A narrow arm cuff placed around a large or swollen ankle will give an erroneously high reading.
- Venous and arterial Doppler signals can be confused, especially in the presence of congestive cardiac failure. If the signal obtained is venous, it should augment with distal manual limb compression.

Ulcers

A thorough clinical examination is usually sufficient to establish the aetiology of a leg ulcer. In areas where the aetiology is unclear, or where healing is delayed, ABPIs may be helpful. It is also important to assess the state of the arterial system before compression bandaging is applied, in order to minimize the likelihood of exacerbating any pre-existing ischaemia. Generally an ABPI ratio of <0.8 would preclude this method of treatment.

The pole test

The pressure within an artery should remain relatively constant with positional changes. However, in the presence of critical ischaemia the pressure within the vessel will drop when it is elevated above the heart. Doppler signals are obtained from a pedal artery, and the effect of elevation of the limb is monitored. Historically a pole was used to measure the height at which the Doppler signal disappeared – hence the name of this test.

Problems

- Signal loss may be due to Doppler probe movement rather than atheromatous disease.
- Data obtained are qualitative rather than quantitative, although calibration of the measuring pole can be helpful.

Segmental pressures – lower limb

The systolic blood pressure can also be measured in the thigh and upper calf using appropriately sized cuffs (see above). A pressure drop of more than 20 mmHg across any segment is usually regarded as clinically significant.

Pre-operative assessment of amputation level

If amputation becomes necessary, a below-knee procedure (BKA) is the preferred option for most patients. However, unless primary healing is likely to be achieved, an above-knee procedure (AKA) is likely to give a better eventual outcome. An absolute thigh pressure reading of >60 mmHg is usually consistent with primary BKA healing (see also 'thermography' and 'spectrophotometry').

Digital pressures

Toe pressure measurements may be helpful in patients with calcified lower limb arteries or in the assessment of small vessel disease. The normal toe blood pressure is less than that in the brachial artery, but the toe/brachial pressure ratio should be greater than 0.7 in a normal study. The systolic blood pressure in the digital arteries of the toes and fingers (see Figure 21.4) is measured in a similar way to the ABPI. The patient lies supine and small pneumatic cuffs of the appropriate size (usually with a bladder size approximately 40 mm × 12 mm) are placed around the base of the digit. In the lower limb the great toe is generally used, but other toes may also be assessed.

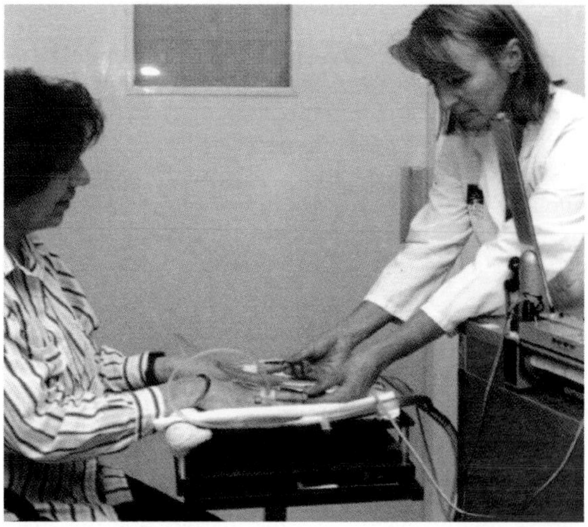

Figure 21.4 Digital pressure measurements using a strain gauge plethysmograph.

The flow to the pulp of the toe is usually detected with a mercury-in-silastic strain gauge plethysmograph (SGP) or with a photoplethysmographic (PPG) sensor (see below, 'plethysmography'). CW Doppler may be used, but it is difficult to maintain a clear signal due to the small size and low flow in the arteries insonated. In each case the baseline signal is recorded, and the pneumatic cuff inflated to a pressure just above systolic so that flow ceases. The cuff is then gradually deflated until flow returns when the systolic pressure is reached, denoted by arterial pulsations on the recorder. If SGP is used, it is helpful to gently squeeze the toe distal to the pneumatic cuff to facilitate venous emptying. This gentle pressure is maintained while the suprasystolic cuff is inflated, preventing arterial inflow to the toe. This technique maximizes the increase in blood volume, and hence toe diameter, seen when the occlusive cuff pressure is reduced to that in the digital arteries and the arterial inflow is re-established.

In normal subjects:

- the toe systolic pressure is usually lower than the arm pressure, i.e. toe/brachial pressure index normal range is 1.0–0.7.

Problems

- The toe studied must be long enough to accommodate both an occlusive pressure cuff and a flow detector.
- Cold sensitivity in the toes is very common, and may produce abnormal toe pressure ratios. If this problem is suspected, the studies should be repeated after the feet have been warmed.

Segmental pressures – upper limb

Systolic blood pressure can be measured at several sites in the upper limbs. A sphygmomanometer cuff is placed around the upper arm, and a CW Doppler is used to obtain the systolic blood pressure in the brachial artery (see ABPIs above). The cuff may then be moved to the forearm, and the pressure in the radial and ulnar arteries noted. If the patient has symptoms affecting the hand or digit, the systolic blood pressure in the digits can be recorded using strain-gauge or photoplethysmography (see 'digital pressures' and 'plethysmography'). It may also be useful to perform digital mapping studies, documenting the patency of the digital arteries in each finger using a CW Doppler.

In normal subjects:

- there should be pressure symmetry between both limbs at the same level
- the digital pressures should be similar to the radial and ulnar systolic pressure (normal digital/radial pressure ratio is 0.9–1.1).

Digital cooling

In the investigation of Raynaud's, hand–arm vibration syndrome (HAVS) and erythromelalgia it is important to establish both the severity of any vasospasm and the degree of permanent damage to the digital arteries. A technique that is commonly used is to measure the digital pressure pre- and post-cooling of the hands.

The systolic blood pressure in the digital arteries is recorded in both arms and the digits of both hands as described above. The hands are then placed in cold water for 5 min, after which the digital pressure readings are repeated. The pressure in the digital arteries should be unaltered by cooling, and a drop of >20% is considered diagnostic of severe vasospasm. Reduced digital artery pressure at rest suggests that permanent damage to the digital arteries may have occurred. This can be confirmed by digital mapping studies, using a CW Doppler to document the presence or absence of flow in all the digital arteries, at both the base and tip of the finger.

In normal subjects:

- the digital pressures should be similar to the radial and ulnar systolic pressure (normal digital/radial pressure ratio is 0.9–1.1)
- the digital pressure should not drop post-cooling (a pressure drop of >20% is usually considered to be diagnostic).

Problems

- If the patient has had a vasospastic attack on the day of their investigation, a positive response to the test is unlikely to be obtained.
- No vasodilating medication should be taken during the 24 hours preceding the test.
- No drinks containing caffeine (coffee, tea, etc.) should be taken on the day of the test, and smoking should be discouraged.
- In patients with Raynaud's disease, testing is less likely to be positive in the summer months, even if a temperature-controlled room is used for the investigation.

Section 21.3 • Doppler velocity waveforms

A CW or pulsed Doppler with directional information and spectral analysis capabilities (usually Fourier analy-

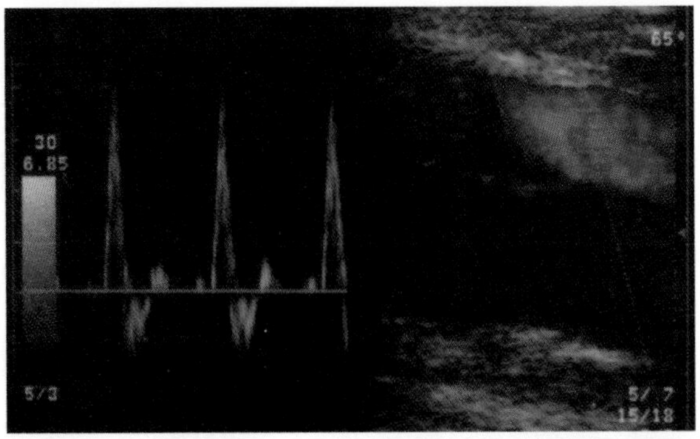

Figure 21.5 A normal triphasic waveform in a superficial femoral artery.

sis) may be used to study the Doppler waveforms at different sites in the body. In vessels that supply vascular beds with high peripheral resistance a waveform with three distinct phases, or triphasic waveform, is normally seen. High velocity forward flow in systole is followed by flow reversal in early diastole, and a low velocity forward component late in diastole (Figure 21.5). This triphasic waveform becomes monophasic (lower amplitude antegrade flow with no reverse component) distal to a tight stenosis or occlusion (Figures 21.6 and 21.7). Organs such as the brain and kidneys generally offer less resistance to arterial blood flow, and have similar waveforms to those found with peripheral vasodilation (Figure 21.9). At the site of a stenosis, the velocity will generally increase. This can be used to classify the severity of the lesion. If the peak systolic velocity demonstrates an increase of more than 100% at the site of maximum stenosis, a narrowing of at least 50% of the lumen diameter is likely to be present.

Problems

- In the presence of vasodilation the resistance of the distal bed is reduced; this may reduce or abolish flow reversal in diastole.
- Cardiac arrhythmias may make the waveform difficult to interpret.

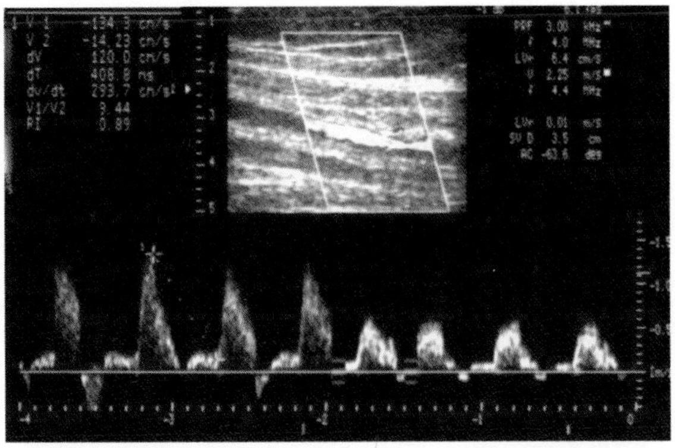

Figure 21.6 The triphasic waveform in a superficial femoral artery becomes damped and monophasic distal to a significant lesion.

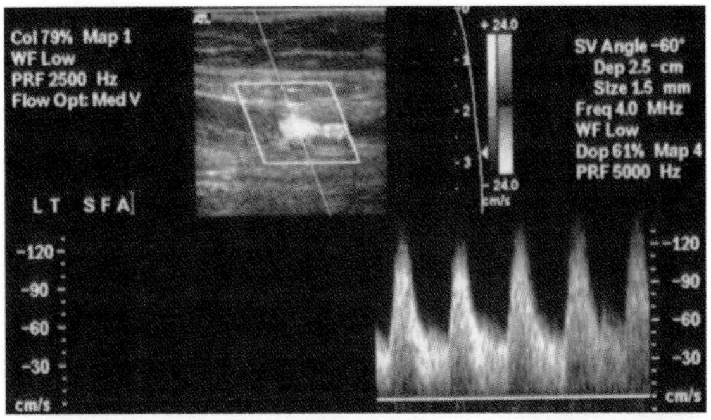

Figure 21.7 Waveform in a superficial femoral artery stenosis. The waveform is monophasic, indicating significant proximal disease. Peak systolic velocity is only slightly elevated (1.3 m/s), but spectral broadening associated with turbulence is seen.

Transcranial Doppler (TCD)

TCDs use low frequency (usually 2 MHz) pulsed Doppler to examine the intracranial arteries. The four commonly used approaches are the transtemporal, transorbital, suboccipital and submandibular techniques. TCD is useful for detecting severe disease in the major basal intracranial arteries, assessing collateral circulation in patients with severe cerebral vessel disease, and detecting arteriovenous malformations. However, it also has an established role in per-operative monitoring during carotid endarterectomy. The middle cerebral artery (MCA) is usually insonated at 50–55 mm depth. Baseline recordings are made, and the effect of clamping the internal carotid artery is observed. MCA flow is usually only slightly affected. A reduction in MCA mean velocity of greater than 65% has been suggested as a useful indication for shunt insertion, but no clear correlation between MCA flow during surgery and peri-operative stroke has been demonstrated, suggesting that most peri-operative strokes may be embolic.

Problems

- The accuracy of this technique relies heavily on the skill of the technologist, and a good knowledge of the anatomy of the cerebral arteries is vital. Interpretation of results is frequently influenced by the clinical picture.

Section 21.4 • Duplex scanning applications

Cerebrovascular assessments

Duplex scans of the extracranial carotid and vertebral arteries have become the primary investigation of choice for patients with cerebrovascular symptoms in most vascular centres (see Figure 21.8). The accuracy of these studies is such that angiography is rarely performed, most patients proceeding directly to surgery, where appropriate, on the basis of their ultrasound assessment.

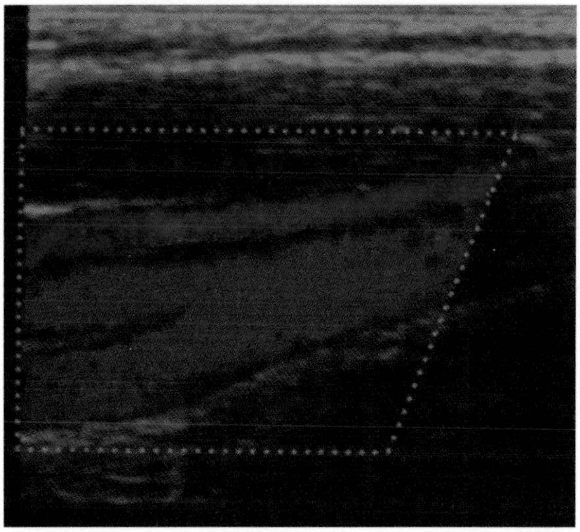

Figure 21.8 A normal carotid artery bifurcation. The internal jugular vein can be seen lying superficial to the carotid artery.

The most common site for a carotid artery stenosis is at the origin of the internal carotid artery (see Figures 21.9–2.11). When the stenosis approaches 50% of the vessel diameter, laminar flow will gradually be disrupted, and the resulting turbulence will be seen as a broadening of the Doppler velocity spectrum, with subsequent obliteration of the clear systolic window (Figure 21.10). When the lumen is reduced by more than 50%, the velocity of blood through the stenosis will increase (Figure 21.11). These increases are used to quantify the extent of the disease (Table 21.1). It is particularly important to differentiate between stenoses of >70% and those below this level, as this is the criterion on which surgical intervention is currently based. Most vascular centres record the maximum peak systolic and end diastolic velocities, which are generally located at, or just distal to, the site of maximum stenosis. It is also usual to record the peak systolic and end diastolic velocities in the common carotid artery, as these data can be helpful in the accurate determination of stenoses of 50–70% of the vessel diameter. Spectral Doppler information should always be used in conjunction with the B-mode image to minimize errors due to increased velocities in young subjects, ectopics, reduced cardiac output and common carotid artery disease.

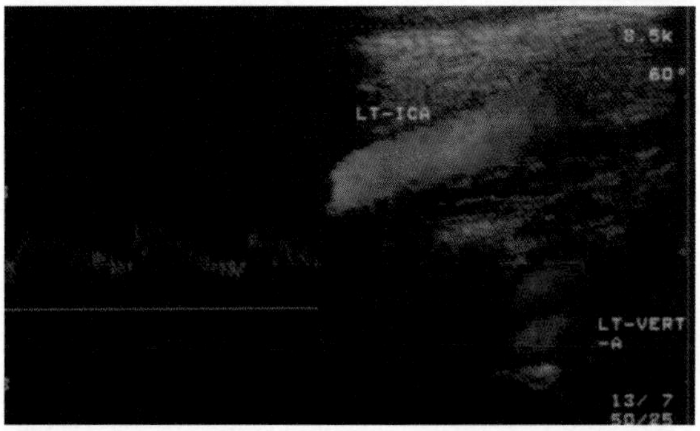

Figure 21.9 A normal low resistance internal carotid artery waveform. The vertebral artery and vein can be seen lying deep to the carotid.

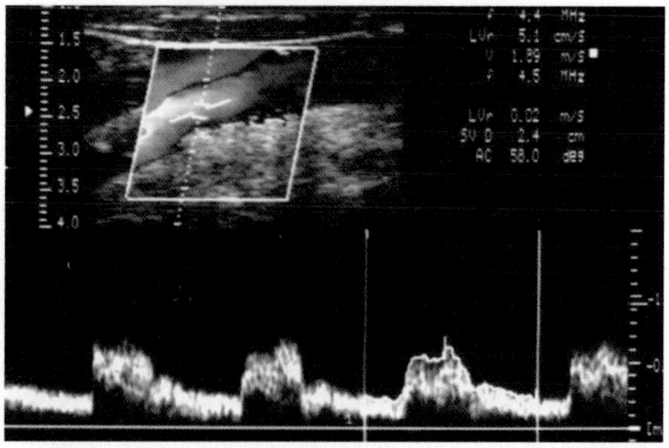

Figure 21.10 A small plaque near the origin of the internal carotid artery has produced some spectral broadening, but the clear spectral window during systole is still present.

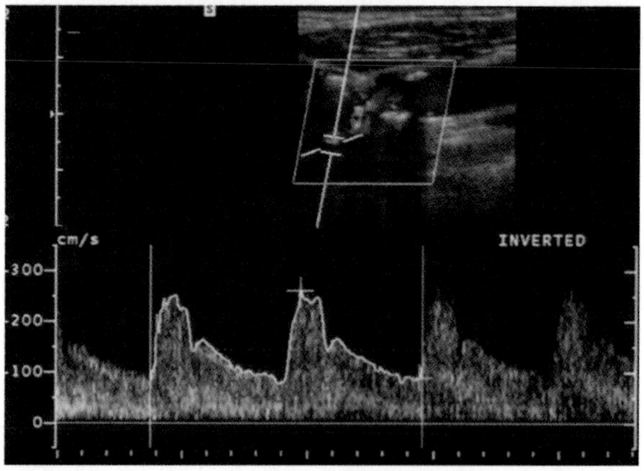

Figure 21.11 Severe stenosis at the origin of the ICA. PSV is 2.6 m/s, and the waveform demonstrates spectral broadening and abolition of the systolic spectral window.

The vertebral arteries are always examined, paying particular attention to the direction of flow, which should be cephalad. The Doppler spectrum is normally similar to that seen in the internal carotid artery, i.e. low resistance with forward (cephalad) flow in diastole.

Problems

- It is difficult to confirm accuracy and perform quality control studies since angiography is not usually performed.
- Calcification of the carotid arteries can reduce accuracy.
- Intracranial lesions cannot be demonstrated, although significant vascular problems such as occlusion of the ipsilateral middle cerebral artery may affect the Doppler waveform seen in the extracranial internal carotid artery, reducing the amplitude or introducing high resistance characteristics.
- Significant disease of the proximal CCA can reduce the PSV and EDV in both the CCA and ICA. Asymmetry of the CCA waveforms should alert the investigator, and the use of velocity ratios will help in the identification of any tandem ICA stenosis.

Table 21.1 Criteria currently used in the Vascular Laboratory in Ninewells Hospital for the determination of severity of carotid artery stenoses. Lesions are graded using the peak systolic velocity (PSV) and end diastolic velocity (EDV) measured in the internal carotid artery (ICA) and ipsilateral common carotid artery (CCA)

Percentage ICA stenosis	*Peak systolic velocity ICA (m/s)*	*Peak end diastolic velocity ICA (m/s)*	*Systolic velocity ratio PSV ICA/PSV CCA*	*Diastolic velocity ratio EDV ICA/EDV CCA*
0–29%	<1.25	<0.4	<1.8	<2.4
30–49%	<1.25	<0.4	<1.8	<2.4
50–59%	>1.25	<0.4	<1.8	<2.4
60–69%	>1.25	>0.4	>1.8	>2.4
70–79%	>2.30	>0.4	>3.0	>2.4
80–99%	>2.30	>1.0	>3.7	>4.0
ICA occlusion	n/a	n/a	n/a	n/a

- Young patients often have elevated Doppler velocities in their carotid arteries, invalidating velocity criteria.
- The diagnostic criteria used in many vascular laboratories are based on Strandness's work, with subsequent local validation. In the United Kingdom the indications for surgical intervention have altered, and ultrasonographers have had to adjust their reporting appropriately, often without angiographic validation.

Carotid body tumours

The examination is performed with a duplex ultrasound scanner in the usual way. The tumour is usually seen as a vascular mass distorting the carotid bulb into a classic wineglass shape. Small, tortuous vessels are often demonstrated within the tumour.

Carotid and subclavian artery aneurysms

The majority of patients referred with a suspected carotid or subclavian artery aneurysm have a pulsatile mass in the base of the neck. Ultrasound examination of elderly patients commonly demonstrates a tortuous artery of normal diameter. However, if the artery is enlarged the diameter should be noted. Tortuous displacement of the brachial artery can also occur, becoming more common with increasing age.

Lower limb arterial assessments

Duplex scanning is frequently used in the assessment of the arteries of the lower limbs. It is sometimes difficult to obtain adequate views of the common iliac arteries, but most centres would expect to visualize the external iliac, common femoral, superficial femoral and crural arteries accurately. The value of duplex scanning for ultrasonic angiography is widely recognized, but its main value is in the identification of stenoses which might be amenable to angioplasty, to document occluded arteries and grafts, to confirm calf vessel patency, and to identify and evaluate aneurysms or pseudoaneurysms. The severity of a stenosis can be evaluated by identifying the maximum increase in velocity associated with it (see 'Vein graft surveillance' below). It is also usual to assess the iliac and femoral arteries and veins using duplex ultrasound in patients being considered for renal transplantation.

Vein graft surveillance

If vein has been used for a bypass graft, most centres advise regular duplex scans (usually at 6 weeks, 3 months, 6 months and one year post-operatively, and then annually as required) to identify any stenoses that are developing within the graft. These narrowings can occur at any point, and are often amenable to angioplasty or surgical patching. The maximum velocity within the stenotic section is usually indicative of the extent of narrowing. The technologist should note the peak systolic velocity (PSV_1) proximal to the stenosis, the peak systolic velocity (PSV_2) seen within the stenotic area, and the peak systolic velocity (PSV_3) distal to the stenosis. If $PSV_2 > 2 \times PSV_1$ the stenosis is likely to be at least 50% of the graft diameter, and intervention should be considered to maintain graft patency. The maximum PSV seen within the graft distal to a stenosis should always be recorded, since if this falls below the critical level of 0.45 m/s the graft is at risk of occluding due to low flow.

Upper limb arterial assessments

The distal subclavian, axillary, brachial, radial and ulnar arteries are readily assessed using duplex scanning. However, the innominate and proximal subclavian arteries may be difficult to visualize. If subclavian steal is suspected, the brachial systolic blood pressure should be noted in both arms using a CW Doppler. If these readings demonstrate reduced pressure in the affected limb, the direction of flow in the ipsilateral vertebral artery should be documented by duplex scanning. If flow in the vertebral artery is caudad, either continuously or during diastole, the effect of occluding the brachial artery with a suprasystolic blood pressure cuff should be noted. Retrograde flow in the vertebral artery should diminish or cease during this manoeuvre.

Thoracic outlet syndrome

The brachial systolic blood pressure should be recorded in both arms, and a pressure drop of >20 mmHg is usually seen on the affected side. The subclavian arteries should be examined with a duplex scanner for any evidence of stenosis or post-stenotic dilatation.

Problem

- It is difficult to assess flow in the subclavian arteries using ultrasound during patient manoeuvres (see below).

Surgical formation of arteriovenous fistulas for haemodialysis

The veins in the forearm (usually the cephalic vein), the radial and ulnar arteries, the brachial artery and vein, and the proximal cephalic and basilic veins are readily evaluated using a duplex scanner. It is particularly important to assess the subclavian veins if the patient has had an ipsilateral central line in the past. Once the fistula has been created, duplex scanning can be used to estimate the suitability of flow in a vein for haemodialysis, to record the position and diameter of vessels suitable for cannulation, and to document stenoses in the arterial or venous component of the fistula.

Abdominal aortic aneurysms (AAAs)

Ultrasound scans can visualize the aorta in most people, allowing measurement of the size and location of any aneurysm present. Involvement of the renal and iliac arteries can also be assessed. Duplex examination of the femoral and profunda arteries should also be considered, and conversely if a popliteal aneurysm is identified, the contralateral popliteal, the aorta and the femoral vessels should also be examined.

Asymptomatic AAAs should be assessed at regular intervals. The authors' practice is to perform a second scan 6/12 after initial assessment, and decide the appropriate frequency of follow-up (usually from 6-monthly to biennially) according to the size and rate of growth. Colour and Doppler are not essential for these studies, but they can be helpful in demonstrating leaks, particularly following endovascular repair.

The measurement recorded is usually the trans AP diameter, but it is also helpful to record the length of the aneurysmal segment and the proximity to the renal arteries. Visualizing the renal arteries accurately and consistently with ultrasound can be difficult, but the superior mesenteric artery (SMA) is usually seen. Studies suggest that if the neck of the AAA is more than 2.5 cm below the SMA origin, it is very unlikely that the renal arteries will be involved. Involvement of the iliac arteries can also be established. Ultrasound is of limited value in identifying rupture of an AAA but may have a role in identifying endoleaks as part of the follow-up of patients treated by endovascular repair (EVAR).

Pseudoaneurysms

Duplex scanning is the ideal modality to assess both the size of pseudoaneurysms and whether there is still an active leak. If the scan identifies a discrete neck between the collection and the leaking artery, it may be possible to apply external compression with the ultrasound transducer to eliminate the leak. This technique can be both time-consuming and uncomfortable for the patient, and should not be attempted if the patient has been anticoagulated. It is also possible to thrombose the aneurysm using coils or thrombin under ultrasound guidance. Again, a discrete neck to the pseudoaneurysm is vital if the risk of thrombosing the artery itself is to be minimized.

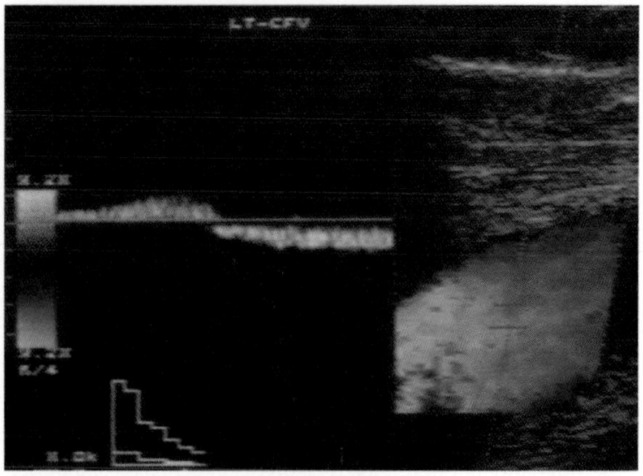

Figure 21.12 The Doppler waveform demonstrates significant reflux in the common femoral vein.

Lower limb venous assessments

Assessment of the deep veins in the lower limbs usually involves compression manoeuvres to exclude the presence of thrombus, documenting the effects of respiration, noting spontaneous flow and evaluating the response to distal compression. The presence of thrombus in a vein is indicated by failure to compress and absence of colour in the vein both spontaneously and with augmentation manoeuvres. Any significant reflux in the deep veins should also be documented (Figure 21.12), particularly if the investigation is being performed in a patient with ulcers or a post-phlebitic limb.

Duplex ultrasound examination of the superficial veins is usually reserved for patients with recurrent varicose veins. It is not uncommon to visualize an incompetent long saphenous vein in patients who have had a previous high tie of this vessel, although it may be difficult to establish whether this is the result of an unrecognized pairing of the long saphenous, or of the surgical technique used. Incompetent perforating veins should always be documented.

Duplex scanning is also used to establish the presence, diameter, length and condition of the long saphenous vein prior to femoropopliteal bypass surgery. If the ipsilateral vessel is unsuitable, the contralateral LSV, the short saphenous veins or the cephalic veins in the arms may be evaluated for possible use.

Section 21.5 • Plethysmography

The term 'plethysmograph' is derived from the Greek word for increase, *plethysmos*, and the word to write, *graphein*, and simply means the measurement of changes in volume of a portion of the body.

Mercury strain-gauge plethysmography

Mercury-in-silastic strain gauges are fine-bore silicone rubber tubes completely filled with mercury that makes contact with copper electrodes at either end. The tube is wrapped around the part of the body (usu-

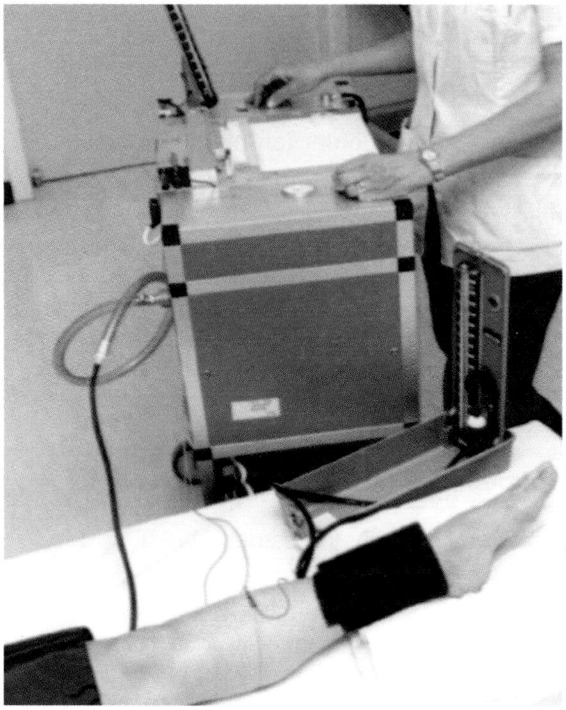

Figure 21.13 Venous occlusion plethysmography. A thin silastic tube filled with mercury is placed around the calf, and the thigh cuff is rapidly inflated to abolish venous outflow.

ally forearm, calf or digit) being investigated, with just enough stretch to ensure good contact (Figure 21.13). As the part expands or contracts, the length of the gauge is changed by a corresponding amount. This produces a measurable change in the resistance of the mercury within the gauge, which in a limb or digit is proportional to the change in circumference. The gauges can be used as simple pulse detectors when digital pressure measurements are being made, but they are also used in the measurement of limb blood flow, as described below.

Venous outflow is occluded using cuffs inflated rapidly to just above the normal level of venous pressure, but below arterial diastolic pressure. This will cause an increase in limb circumference proportional to the change in limb volume as venous outflow ceases. Measurements are made a few seconds after the venous cuff is inflated, as the pressure in the veins distal to the cuff will gradually increase until the pressure within the cuff is exceeded, and some outflow will occur. Thus the technique gives us a measure of volume blood flow in the limb, and is useful as a research tool. Its clinical use is limited by the complicated and time-consuming nature of both the study and the analysis of the results.

Photoplethysmography

Photoelectric plethysmographs (PPGs) do not measure volume changes, but detect changes in the blood content of the skin using photoelectric cells, so they are not true plethysmographs. Changes in the blood content of the dermis are detected by measuring the infrared light reflected from the dermal microcirculation of the skin. Digital photoplethysmography (D-PPG) uses a microprocessor to facilitate calibration, enabling corrections to be made for skin pigmentation and skin thickness.

The pulse contours obtained are quite similar to those recorded by other methods. The ease with which they can be used makes PPGs valuable for clinical investigation, especially when the presence or absence of pulsatile flow is the only critical issue. They are commonly used as pulse detectors in the measurement of digital pressures.

Venous refilling times

It is not uncommon for patients with venous ulcers of the lower limb to have reflux in both the deep and superficial veins, and it is helpful to perform a functional test to determine whether surgical treatment of the superficial veins is likely to benefit the patient. This can be evaluated using a PPG to measure the venous refilling time (Figure 21.14).

The PPG sensor is usually positioned about 10 cm superior to the medial malleolus. The patient performs foot dorsiflexions (usually between eight and 12 times), which should reduce the blood volume in the dermis of the calf. The amount of light absorbed will be reduced, resulting in an increase in the reflected light detected by the sensor. As venous refilling occurs, the reflected light will reduce until the baseline level is reached, usually after 18–40 s (Figure 21.15a). In the presence of venous reflux this refilling time is reduced (Figure 21.15b). An occlusive cuff is then positioned above the knee, and inflated to occlude the superficial veins without compromising the deep veins or the arterial inflow. If the refilling time

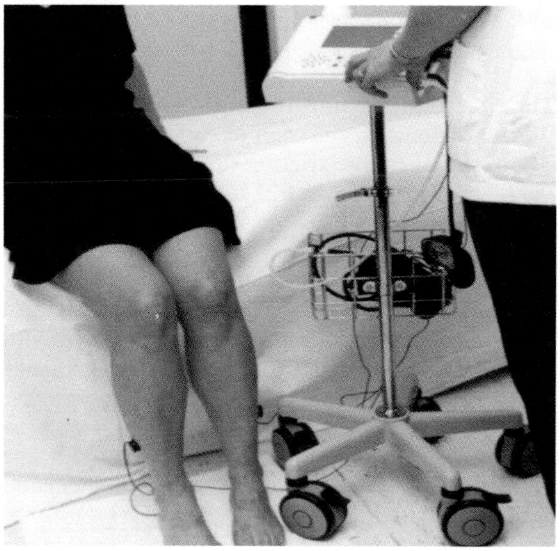

Figure 21.14 Venous refilling times using a photoplethysmograph.

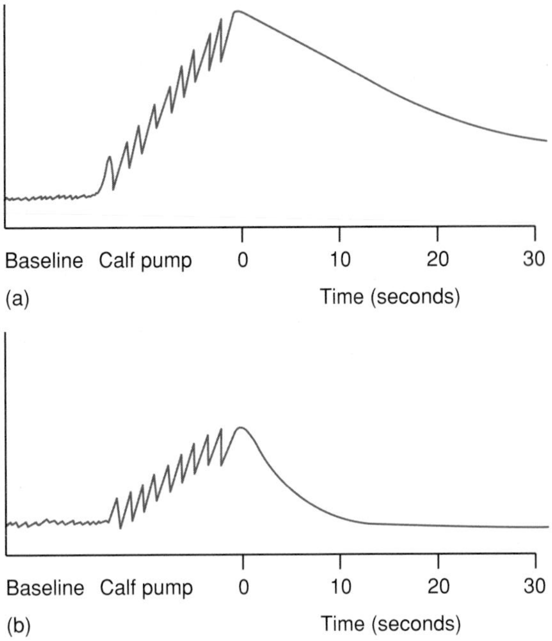

Figure 21.15 (a) Normal venous refilling study. The recording has not returned to the baseline level after 20 s. (b) Abnormal venous refilling study. The recording has returned to the baseline level after 12 s.

improves significantly when the cuff is inflated, surgical treatment of the incompetent superficial veins is likely to be of some benefit to the patient.

Deep vein thrombosis (DVT)

Plethysmography was a popular method of screening for DVT until accurate duplex scanning made other non-invasive investigations largely redundant. However, in recent years there has been renewed interest in using plethysmography for rapid screening when an ultrasound scan is not readily available. Data suggest that venous refilling times using a D-PPG have good sensitivity and negative predictive value for DVT, although the specificity is poor.

Thoracic outlet syndrome and cervical ribs

When positional compression or entrapment of a subclavian or innominate artery is suspected, PPG sensors can be used to obtain arterial readings from the digits of both hands. Since these devices are relatively insensitive to movement, and may be secured on the digits using clips, Velcro bands or adhesive pads, the patient can perform various manoeuvres whilst the arterial waveforms are recorded. Readings are obtained with the arm in the neutral position; the arm is then gradually raised, in the same plane as the trunk, until it is over the head, and any changes in the PPG signal are documented. The studies should be repeated with the patient adopting Adson's position (i.e. hyperabduction of the arm with external rotation, followed by rotation of the head towards and away from the arm). If the arterial signal detected by the PPG disappears in any of these positions, the test is positive.

Problem

- Approximately 30% of the population will have a positive test with no associated symptoms.

Pulse volume recorder (air plethysmograph)

A pneumatic cuff is placed around the site of investigation, usually the calf or thigh. This cuff is inflated to a pre-determined pressure (65–70 mmHg), and a sensitive pressure transducer records the change of pressure within the cuff during the cardiac cycle or in response to the inflation or deflation of pneumatic cuffs at other sites on the limb. These devices can also be used to assess venous emptying.

Section 21.6 • Other techniques

Ambulatory venous pressures (AVPs)

This technique is similar to the venous refilling times described above (see 'Photoplethysmography') in that it provides a functional assessment of the competency of the veins in the lower limb. A vein on the dorsum of the foot of the affected leg is cannulated, and the resting pressure is recorded using a pressure transducer. The patient performs various manoeuvres to exercise the calf muscles. These exercises are limited by the cannulating needle and also the requirement for proximity to the measuring system. The effect of exercise and the time to return to baseline levels are noted.

Problems

- It may be difficult to cannulate a suitable vein in patients with longstanding venous disorders.
- The cannula may become displaced during the exercise manoeuvres.

Transcutaneous oxygen tension ($TcpO_2$) and spectrophotometry (SaO_2)

Both these techniques assess the oxygen content in the skin, and can be used to evaluate tissue viability at the proposed level of a lower limb amputation. $TcpO_2$ and $TcpCO_2$ electrodes to monitor oxygen and carbon dioxide transcutaneously were originally developed for neonatal monitoring, but have been adapted for vascular applications. $TcpO_2$ monitors give an indirect electrochemical measurement of arterial partial pressure of oxygen (PaO_2) by heating the skin to induce hyperperfusion. This heating can cause tissue damage in the ischaemic limb, and readings can be unreliable in severe ischaemia.

Spectrophotometers (Figure 21.16) monitor arterial oxygen saturation (SaO_2), which is related to PaO_2 through the oxyhaemoglobin dissociation curve. This S-shaped curve becomes flatter at higher pO_2, with a corresponding reduction in accuracy of SaO_2. However, for PO_2 between 20 and 60 mmHg (the steep portion of the curve) saturation is more sensitive in assessing tissue oxygenation. Light is transmitted to the skin

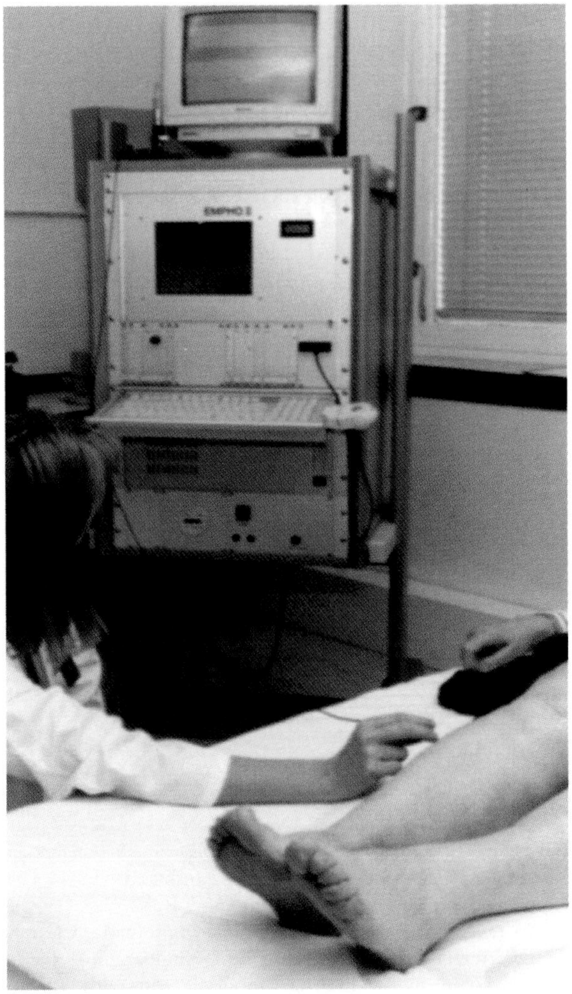

Figure 21.16 Spectrophotometry can be used to measure the oxygen saturation at different sites on the lower limbs.

through a light-guide, the scattered light returning along the same route. The absorption wavelength bands for oxyhaemoglobin are examined and compared to internal references to give a value for the oxygen saturation within the tissue. The saturation is the ratio of the amount of oxygen bound to haemoglobin and the capacity to bind oxygen, expressed as a percentage. SaO_2 studies are non-invasive and do not involve any heating of the tissues. However, dark skin pigmentation can invalidate results. The standard pulse oximeter measures oxygen saturation using a sensor on the earlobe or the finger, but equipment that does not require direct skin contact can be more useful in the vascular laboratory.

Thermography

Thermographic cameras focus the infrared thermal energy radiated from the surface of the body onto a cooled point detector to form an image of the heat distribution across the area of interest. It is important that the temperature of the room in which the examination takes place is controlled, and the patient must be

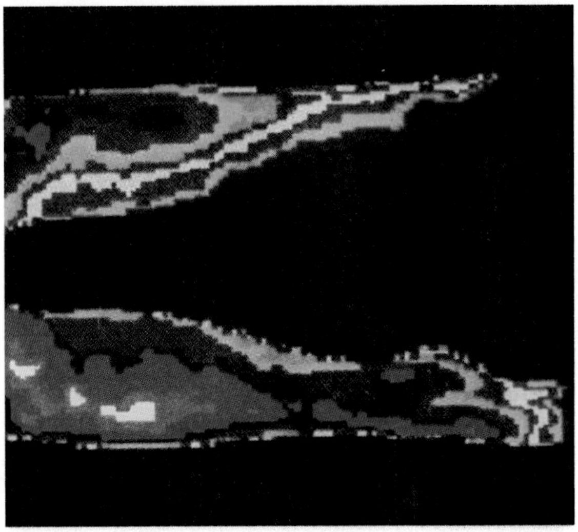

Figure 21.17 Thermography can demonstrate temperature differences between normal and ischaemic tissue.

allowed to acclimatize to this. If the patient is uncomfortably warm, sweating may cause local cooling which can invalidate the data recorded. There is a good correlation between skin blood flow and thermography, but the technique is prone to interpretation difficulties, and is generally only used in conjunction with other measurements. It can be a valuable guide to changes in perfusion across the limb at a particular level, facilitating optimal selection of skin flaps in below-knee amputations (Figure 21.17).

Capillary microscopy

A detailed examination of the microvasculature of the nailbed using a microscope can be helpful in patients with Raynaud's or connective tissue disorders. A small drop of special oil is placed on the area to be examined, to ensure that the incident light is reflected off a smooth surface (Figure 21.18). A simple ophthalmoscope can also be used to give a less detailed picture of the nailfold capillaries. In secondary Raynaud's an increase in the size of the capillary loops is often accompanied by a reduction in the number of loops seen. The picture is less clear in primary Raynaud's, with the different findings reported between groups of researchers suggesting that any changes are likely to be minor.

Tactile thresholds for thermal and vibration stimuli

These tests may be used to detect any sensory changes associated with neurological dysfunction. The patient places their finger on a vibrating plate and presses a button when vibrations of different frequencies or amplitudes are detected. Similarly, a temperature-controlled plate may be used to detect responses to thermal stimuli. These tests are being used increasingly for medicolegal evaluations of HAVS.

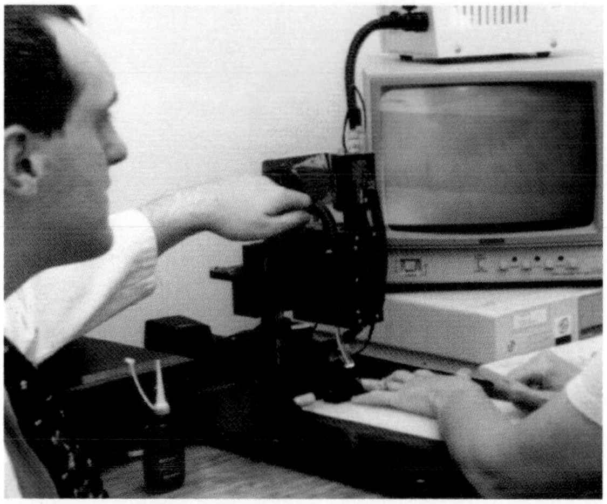

Figure 21.18 Capillary microscopy being used to examine the nailbed.

Scanning laser Doppler

Laser Doppler monitors use optical fibre light guides to transmit laser light to the tissue, where the light is both scattered and partly absorbed. The laser light which interacts with moving red cells will undergo a Doppler shift in wavelength related to the number and velocity of the red cells, but independent of the direction of their movement. Tissue perfusion can be continuously monitored in a small tissue volume, but tissue contact and an associated heating element are usually required. Scanning laser Dopplers process the scattered laser light from a larger area, without the necessity for tissue contact. An image representing both the flux (proportional to the blood flow in the tissue) and the concentration of the moving red blood cells is formed.

Section 21.7 • Future directions in vascular technology

In all fields of medicine the emphasis is shifting from treatment to early diagnosis with a view to prevention. This is particularly true of cardiovascular medicine, but in general a symptomatic patient presenting with peripheral vascular disease will already have associated damage to the arteries of the heart and brain. An increased thickness of the intima-media layer of the carotid artery wall and an ABPI of less than 0.9 may prove to be markers for increased risk of stroke and heart disease, and are being evaluated in populations known to be at increased risk of cardiovascular disease. The stiffness or distensibility of arteries also promises to be a useful prognostic indicator of cardiovascular risk, and several techniques for investigating this parameter have been developed. Specialized ultrasound scanners incorporating a sensitive echo-tracking system, which will accurately follow the movement of the arterial wall during each cardiac cycle, give a direct measure of arterial compliance at specific sites and have also been used to investigate flow-mediated arterial dilatation. Indirect systems include pulse wave analysis of arterial signals obtained using radial artery tonometry, analysis of PPG waveforms, and measurement of pulse wave velocity, which should increase as the artery wall becomes less compliant. If patients at high risk of developing peripheral arterial disease can be identified before the onset of symptoms, it may be possible to reduce the impact of this debilitating disease.

Further reading

Bernstein, E. F. (1978). *Noninvasive Diagnostic Techniques in Vascular Disease*. St Louis, MO: CV Mosby.

Moneta, G. L., Edwards, J. M., Chitwood, R. W. *et al.* (1993). Correlation of North American Symptomatic Carotid Endarterectomy Trial (NACSET) Angiographic Definition of 70 to 99% Internal Carotid Stenosis with Duplex Scanning. *J Vasc Surg* **17**: 152–9.

Pemberton, M., Nydahl, S., Hartshorne, T. *et al.* (1996). Can lower limb vascular reconstruction be based on colour duplex imaging alone? *Eur J Vasc Endovasc Surg* **12**: 452–4.

Thrush, A. and Hartshorne, T. (1999). *Ultrasound – How, Why and When*. London: Churchill Livingstone.

Zwiebel, W. J. (1992). *Introduction to Vascular Ultrasonography*. Philadelphia, PA: W. B. Saunders.

MODULE 22

Anaesthesia for vascular surgery

Anaesthesia for vascular surgery demands meticulous attention is given to pre-operative assessment, peri-operative management and post-operative care.

Discussion with medical and surgical colleagues is important to ensure intercurrent disease is optimized and that the nature and timing of surgery are appropriate to the general health of the patient. This module aims to outline anaesthetic management of the patient undergoing major vascular surgery.

Section 22.1 • Pre-operative assessment

Patients with vascular disease are regarded as being at higher risk of peri-operative complications than those in the general surgical population. They have a high incidence of coronary artery disease, which may be asymptomatic, as well as hypertension, chronic obstructive pulmonary disease and diabetes mellitus. In addition many patients are heavy smokers. Pre-operative evaluation and preparation comprises identification and quantification of co-existing medical problems. If necessary, interventions can then be made in order to improve the patient's pre-operative condition in order to minimize the risks associated with anaesthesia and surgery.

Ischaemic heart disease

A number of studies show that 50–70% of patients requiring surgery for peripheral vascular disease (PVD) have evidence of ischaemic heart disease (IHD). The leading cause of peri-operative mortality after vascular surgery is myocardial infarction, which accounts for 40–60% of peri-operative deaths. Therefore determining the presence and severity of coronary artery disease pre-operatively enables decisions on the nature of the surgery, the safest anaesthetic technique and level of monitoring required intra- and post-operatively to be made.

Hypertension

Hypertension may be present in up to 60% of patients with PVD. Those with untreated or poorly treated hypertension exhibit marked vascular hyper-reactivity. They are subject to exaggerated responses to induction of anaesthesia, regional blockade and intermittent positive pressure ventilation (hypotension) and to laryngoscopy and surgical stimulation (hypertension). As a result of this lability, rapid changes in coronary perfusion can occur resulting in peri-operative ischaemia.

Congestive cardiac failure

This may be present in up to 15% of patients with PVD and if decompensated, mortality can be as high as 15–20%. A left ventricular ejection fraction of less than 35% is associated with a high risk of peri-operative myocardial infarction.

Diabetes mellitus

The prevalence of diabetes is higher in the vascular surgical population than in the general surgical population. A number of the complications associated with diabetes, if present, may increase the risks of surgery and anaesthesia, e.g. autonomic neuropathy, silent myocardial ischaemia and vascular hyper-reactivity.

Respiratory disease

As many as 90% of patients with PVD are smokers and chronic pulmonary disease may be present in up to 60%. Simple spirometric tests can be performed pre-operatively to quantify the extent of lung disease and a chest X-ray should be carried out. The chest X-ray is mainly of use post-operatively as it serves as a baseline to which changes after surgery can be compared. Arterial blood gas analysis can also be performed in those undergoing major surgery with a history of pulmonary disease. This gives a useful baseline measurement of PaO_2 and $PaCO_2$. Measures should then be taken to aggressively treat any reversible component of lung disease with bronchodilators and infection with physiotherapy and antibiotics in order to optimize the patient pre-operatively.

Section 22.2 • Investigation

The routine history and examination should be used to guide the need for further investigations. Not all patients will require special investigations and the decision to further investigate someone should be based on an indication in the history and the likelihood that a given test will quantify the extent of a problem and allow the anaesthetist to act on the information provided. The nature of the proposed surgery will also have a bearing on the need for further investigation.

A wide range of tests exists to assess myocardial function and there is considerable variation in their invasiveness and cost.

Electrocardiogram

Abnormalities on the standard 12-lead electrocardiogram (ECG) have been used to try to predict the likelihood of an adverse cardiac outcome post-operatively. Although the changes of previous myocardial infarction and ST segment depression are suggestive of ischaemic heart disease other abnormalities, e.g. arrhythmias or conduction defects may have another cause.

Ambulatory ECG monitoring has established a high incidence of silent myocardial ischaemia in the vascular surgical population. This in turn has been associated with an increased risk of post-operative adverse cardiac events.

The exercise ECG has the patient exercising at a gradually increasing work rate in order to achieve a maximum heart rate or ischaemia. The development of ischaemia on exercise has been shown to have a correlation with the occurrence of myocardial ischaemia peri-operatively. However, many patients awaiting vascular surgery are unable to complete the exercise protocol due to claudication and its use may therefore be limited.

Echocardiography

Visual imaging of the heart by echocardiography is probably the most frequently undertaken additional investigation in vascular surgical patients, being non-invasive and relatively cheap. An assessment of ventricular filling and contractility can be made, an estimate of ejection fraction given and areas of ischaemia are shown as abnormalities in ventricular wall function. It is also possible to perform stress echocardiography by infusing either dobutamine to increase heart rate or dipyridamole, a vasodilator, while looking for abnormalities in wall motion. This method has good correlation with other methods used to detect coronary artery disease pre-operatively.

Nuclear imaging

Dipyridamole-thallium-scintigraphy involves scanning for the radioisotope thallium in the myocardium in the presence of the coronary artery vasodilator, dipyridamole.

Ischaemic areas are poorly perfused and show up as a defect in the normal pattern. A repeat scan is performed after 4 hours and defects can then be classed as reversible (ischaemia) or irreversible (infarction). Thallium scanning is non-invasive and highly sensitive for the detection of myocardial perfusion abnormalities but it is very expensive and is associated with some complications (bronchospasm, myocardial infarction).

Equilibrium radionuclide ventriculography (MUGA scan) uses red blood cells labelled with ^{99m}technetium to estimate left ventricular end diastolic and end systolic volumes, ejection fraction and cardiac output. This method is currently the standard for assessing ejection fraction which if less than 35% is associated with a high incidence of peri-operative myocardial infarction.

Coronary angiography

In certain US centres it has been routine practice to recommend that patients requiring vascular surgery have coronary angiography first with recourse to cardiac surgery prior to vascular surgery if there was a correctable lesion. One group performed coronary angiography on 1000 consecutive patients requiring vascular surgery. They showed that even in those with no clinical or ECG features suggestive of coronary artery disease, 30% had severe stenosis of one or more coronary arteries. However, angiography is invasive, expensive and not without risk and may not be justified on a routine basis.

In summary, good communication between surgeon, physician and anaesthetist is essential in the pre-operative decision making process. There are no hard and fast rules regarding the investigations a patient will require before undergoing major vascular surgery. However, given the high incidence of IHD and pulmonary disease in the vascular surgical patient population a few generalizations can be made.

All patients are likely to require a full blood count, urea and electrolytes, ECG and chest X-ray as a minimum. Patients with symptoms of IHD may then need further cardiac investigation if they are having carotid surgery. Patients undergoing aortic surgery are exposed to a major cardiac stress at the time of aortic clamping and unclamping. In this case it is useful to have some measure of left ventricular contractility and so echocardiography or some form of nuclear imaging should be obtained. For those undergoing lesser interventions such as infra-inguinal bypass surgery, further investigation of cardiac function is necessary only if symptoms are severe. In all cases if symptoms have increased in recent times review by a physician should be obtained to ensure medical optimization prior to surgery.

Section 22.3 • Anaesthetic technique

The findings from pre-operative assessment and investigation may influence not only surgical decision making, e.g. when to operate and what operation to perform, but also choice of anaesthetic technique, peri-operative monitoring and the level of post-operative care required. The choice between general anaesthesia, regional anaesthesia or a combination of the two still causes controversy.

As patients presenting for major vascular surgery frequently have a high incidence of intercurrent disease it is often maintained that regional anaesthesia may be safer and associated with fewer complications than general anaesthesia alone. However, there are risks associated with regional anaesthesia and it may be important to weigh up the risks and benefits in each individual case.

Central neural blockade

Central neural blockade (CNB) in the form of epidural or spinal anaesthesia can be used as the sole anaesthetic for infrainguinal vascular surgery and in combination with general anaesthesia it is suitable for aortic surgery.

The sympathetic block that occurs in conjunction with sensory and motor block is largely responsible for the cardiovascular changes associated with epidural anaesthesia. The result is vasodilatation and increased venous pooling in the lower limbs leading to a reduction in venous return and a fall in cardiac output. Above the level of the block there will be compensatory increase in vasoconstrictor activity. If the block level is sufficiently high to block the cardiac sympathetic outflow (T1–T4) there will be a further drop in cardiac output and a reduction in heart rate.

The haemodynamic changes discussed above normally develop during the first 20 min after the onset of the block. In patients with IHD the reduction in afterload and pre-load associated with CNB may improve ventricular function while coronary vasodilatation may improve myocardial oxygen supply. However, when combined with the myocardial depression seen with general anaesthesia, vasodilatation due to CNB can lead to marked hypotension. Therefore meticulous attention to fluid administration and careful use of vasopressor agents is required when using a combined technique.

Controversy still persists as to whether cardiac outcome is improved by the use of CNB. In 1987, one group showed improvement in survival and less morbidity in patients undergoing major surgery with a combined epidural and general anaesthetic technique. Another group in 1993 showed that there was no difference in cardiac morbidity after lower extremity vascular surgery when epidural or general anaesthesia was carefully executed. However, in this study and in another epidural anaesthesia and analgesia conferred a benefit in terms of fewer peri-operative thrombotic events. There appears to be no consistent evidence for improved cardiac outcome in those receiving CNB but a recent meta-analysis showed significant reductions in peri-operative mortality, pulmonary morbidity and thrombotic complications in patients receiving epidural or spinal anaesthesia.

The use of epidural anaesthesia may improve respiratory function post-operatively by attenuating diaphragmatic dysfunction after upper abdominal surgery. Reduced post-operative pain also enables patients to cough effectively thereby maintaining PaO_2 in the early post-operative period. In contrast general anaesthesia can lead to atelectasis, mucociliary dysfunction and ventilation/perfusion mismatching in the lung with resultant hypoxaemia.

After lower abdominal or lower limb surgery the use of CNB can reduce the stress response to surgery and may attenuate the hypertension, tachycardia and increased myocardial oxygen demand with which it is associated. This reduction in stress response may be in part responsible for the beneficial effects on coagulation seen with CNB.

As mentioned above epidural and spinal anaesthesia are also associated with a number of complications. **Hypotension** is related to the extent of the sympathetic block and is likely to be more severe in the presence of cardiac disease and hypovolaemia. Careful monitoring, judicious use of intravenous fluids, gradual extension of the block and appropriate use of vasopressors should limit the extent of this potential complication.

Instrumentation of the vertebral canal may cause some bleeding and there are concerns that during vascular surgery, when anticoagulation is often used, the likelihood of developing a **vertebral canal haematoma** (VCH) is high enough to advocate avoidance of CNB. However, many VCH occur spontaneously with no apparent risk factors. Every unit should have a protocol for the management of patients who are to receive CNB and who will require anticoagulation.

It has been advocated that in those receiving unfractionated low-dose heparin, institution of CNB should be avoided for 4–6 hours after a dose and that removal of a catheter should take place at least 1 hour before the next dose is given.

For those being given low molecular weight heparin (LMWH), 10–12 hours should elapse between a dose of drug and insertion or removal of an epidural (or spinal). In addition at least 1 hour should pass after insertion or removal before the next dose of LMWH is given.

For patients who are to receive intra-operative systemic heparinization it has been suggested that skilled personnel should perform the CNB and that 1 hour should elapse before heparin is administered.

Regional anaesthesia in the form of cervical epidural or cervical plexus block has also been advocated as the technique of choice for carotid endarterectomy. It has been argued that it allows continuous neurological assessment of the patient but evidence from a number of trials fails to show a reduction in peri-operative stroke rate. However, it may be that there is a reduction in peri-operative myocardial complication rate if a regional as opposed to general anaesthetic technique is used.

Anaesthesia for infra-renal aortic surgery

Given the complex and often prolonged nature of aortic surgery, the choice of anaesthetic technique is between general anaesthesia with or without a regional technique.

General anaesthesia

The aim here is to provide a balanced combination of sleep, muscle relaxation and analgesia. Sleep can be maintained either using volatile anaesthetics such as isoflurane with or without nitrous oxide, or using total intravenous anaesthetic techniques with propofol. Analgesia is provided by relatively high doses of opioid agents which must be continued post-operatively. Intra-operative muscle relaxation is provided using either boluses or an infusion of non-depolarizing muscle relaxants, e.g. atracurium, vecuronium.

In order to maintain adequate pulmonary gas exchange during surgery, the trachea is intubated and intermittent positive pressure ventilation (IPPV) is established. Most anaesthetists advocate maintenance of normocapnia during surgery.

General anaesthesia with regional blockade

The use of a combined technique allows a lighter plane of anaesthesia to be maintained while the regional block provides analgesia and attenuation of the sympathetic response to surgical stimulation. This should enable rapid recovery of consciousness at the end of surgery but with maintenance of profound analgesia into the post-operative period.

Insertion of a thoracic epidural catheter at the level of T8/9 or T9/10 and use of 5 ml of local anaesthetic will provide a somatic segmental blockade of the anterior abdominal wall sufficient to allow surgery to proceed. The associated sympathetic block is responsible for the haemodynamic changes mentioned above and as such meticulous attention to fluid balance is required when using a combined technique.

Monitoring

Due to the potential for rapid alterations in cardiovascular function and fluid balance during aortic surgery, a number of haemodynamic variables need to be monitored constantly.

It is normal practice to have a continuous display of at least one ECG lead in order to detect myocardial ischaemia or arrhythmias. Many monitors now have the capability to perform on-line ST segment analysis alerting to impending ischaemia.

Intra-arterial pressure monitoring, usually from the radial artery, gives rapid warning of haemodynamic changes associated with anaesthesia and surgery. This should be instituted prior to induction of anaesthesia.

Continuous measurement of central venous pressure (CVP) aids in the assessment of fluid balance during surgery.

In a relatively few patients presenting for aortic surgery who are known to have poor ventricular function pre-operatively, a pulmonary artery catheter can be placed to guide ventricular filling.

In addition to the above pulse oximetry should be monitored. As well as information on oxygenation and heart rate it provides a rough estimate of pulse volume and adequacy of tissue oxygenation.

Continuous capnography ensures adequacy of ventilation and allows the surgeon to see appropriate rises in carbon dioxide load after the period of arterial clamping.

Special considerations

Temperature

Inadvertent hypothermia after prolonged surgery is a potential problem especially in the elderly. The increased energy expenditure required to return temperature to normal post-operatively can lead to myocardial ischaemia and hypoxaemia. Core temperature should be monitored during surgery and active steps taken to prevent heat loss. Intravenous fluids should be warmed, anaesthetic gases should be delivered through a heat and moisture exchanger and warming blankets should be used to cover those parts of the body away from the operative site.

Aortic cross-clamping

Application of the aortic clamp increases the resistance to blood flow in the lower half of the body. Both systolic and diastolic pressures increase but stroke volume and cardiac output fall due to a reduction in myocardial contractility. In the upper body arteriolar resistance will fall due to the baroreceptor reflex. Over a period of about 10 min the normal heart will accommodate these changes by implementing the Frank–Starling response.

However, patients with coronary artery disease may develop signs of ischaemia due to the increased left ventricular load. In those with reduced ventricular contractility aortic clamping can lead to a rapid rise in pulmonary artery occlusion pressure with incipient left ventricular failure.

These changes in blood pressure associated with cross-clamping may be attenuated somewhat in the presence of thoracic epidural blockade. If a reduction in aortic pressure is required an intravenous infusion of glyceryl trinitrate can be commenced producing arteriolar and venous dilatation and coronary artery dilatation.

Release of the aortic clamp

Below the level of the aortic clamp the vascular bed becomes maximally vasodilated due to the build up of vasoactive metabolites during the period of aortic occlusion. These changes are less marked in those undergoing surgery for aortic occlusive disease due to the presence of a collateral arterial supply. Before the aortic clamp is released replacement of clear fluids and blood volume should have taken place in an attempt to ensure CVP is slightly higher than the pre-clamping value. As the clamp is released the left ventricle ejects into a maximally dilated vascular tree and there is washout of vasoactive metabolites, which can lead to myocardial depression. The result can be marked arterial hypotension and further myocardial ischaemia. In order to minimize these changes many surgeons apply clamps to the common iliac arteries which they release in turn after a period of stabilization. If the surgeon communicates to the anaesthetist that he is about to release the clamps, steps to ensure the patient is well filled prior to removal can be taken. The judicious use of methoxamine (a vaso- and venoconstrictor) before the clamp is released also helps to prevent huge swings in blood pressure.

Post-operative management

Invasive monitoring of the patient should continue into the post-operative period while there is still likely to be some cardiovascular instability. Attention should be paid to adequacy of oxygenation and prevention of hypotension and hypertension. The use of epidural infusion techniques allows excellent analgesia to be provided during the first post-operative days and may reduce respiratory complications. The effectiveness of the epidural infusion may be enhanced if the surgeon uses a transverse approach at surgery rather than a midline incision.

Anaesthesia for carotid surgery

A variety of techniques have been used to provide anaesthesia for patients undergoing surgery of the carotid artery. Most studies have been unable to show a difference in peri-operative stroke rate between regional and general anaesthetic techniques. However, there may be a lower incidence of myocardial complications when regional anaesthesia is employed.

Regional anaesthesia

Carotid endarterectomy can be performed using either superficial and deep cervical plexus blocks or cervical epidural anaesthesia. Proponents of these techniques claim that the ability to carry out neurological testing during the period of carotid artery occlusion makes them the anaesthetic method of choice. The tachycardia and hypertension, which may develop during surgery performed under regional block, may be problematic given the high incidence of associated coronary artery disease. They can, however, be attenuated somewhat by pre-treatment with a beta-blocker.

General anaesthesia

Use of a general anaesthetic technique allows the anaesthetist to control certain physiological variables in order to improve cerebral blood flow. The choice of specific anaesthetic agents is probably less important than ensuring peri-operative haemodynamic stability and an adequate supply of oxygen to the brain during the period of carotid cross-clamping.

Anaesthesia is usually induced with an intravenous induction agent while a non-depolarizing muscle relaxant is used to facilitate endotracheal intubation. Volatile anaesthetic agents can be used to maintain anaesthesia or a total intravenous technique using propofol can be employed. Ventilation is controlled during surgery and the use of capnography allows the anaesthetist to maintain normocapnia. Hypercapnia, which was advocated in the past as increasing cerebral blood flow (CBF), is now out of favour. It is believed to lead to intracerebral steal with blood being diverted away from already poorly perfused areas. In addition, an elevated $PaCO_2$ can lead to increased myocardial work and arrhythmias.

At the end of surgery, anaesthesia should be discontinued and muscle relaxation reversed in order to facilitate a rapid, smooth and clear-headed recovery.

Special considerations

Circulatory instability frequently arises during carotid surgery. Carotid sinus baroreceptors lie in the bifurcation of the common carotid artery and respond to stretching of the vessel wall by reducing blood pressure and heart rate. If exposed to lower than normal pressures there is an increase in sympathetic tone resulting in increased blood pressure. Thus at application of the carotid arterial clamps marked arterial hypertension can arise, while hypotension as the clamps are removed is often seen. Injection of local anaesthetic into the region of the carotid sinus in order to block the sinus nerves may attenuate these effects but blood pressure often remains labile due to loss of normal autoregulation. In the author's practice injection of the sinus nerves is rarely required.

Monitoring

Routine monitoring for carotid surgery includes ECG, pulse oximetry, capnography and intra-arterial blood pressure measurement. In addition, a number of techniques have been advocated for use to assess the adequacy of cerebral perfusion during the period of carotid artery occlusion. However, the only completely reliable way of ensuring continued adequacy of cerebral perfusion is with a conscious patient.

With the patient awake a test period of carotid clamping usually lasting 2 min takes place. The patient is continually assessed for changes in contralateral motor power, mental status and speech. If symptoms arise a temporary indwelling arterial shunt may be inserted. Testing should continue throughout the period of arterial clamping as late symptoms can occur.

The electroencephalograph (EEG), which monitors cortical activity, has been used to predict the likelihood of cerebral ischaemia during carotid surgery resulting in a post-operative neurological deficit. However, both false positives and false negatives arise in many studies. In addition the EEG only detects activity in the superficial layers of the cortex and may be normal in the presence of significant ischaemia in the deeper cortex and internal capsule. Patients with a pre-existing stroke may have an abnormal EEG and further changes may be difficult to interpret.

Somatosensory-evoked potentials (SSEP) monitor deeper cerebral pathways in brain or spinal cord and have also been used to detect ischaemia. Like the EEG they only reflect integrity in a small part of the nervous system.

The pressure in the internal carotid artery distal to the arterial clamps (stump pressure) has been used to reflect the adequacy of the collateral circulation through the circle of Willis. They noted that brisk backbleeding from the internal carotid artery was associated with tolerance of carotid clamping and went on to measure stump pressure. A number of 'safe' levels of stump pressure above which the patient would tolerate arterial clamping have been postulated ranging from 25 to 70 mmHg. Awake patient studies have shown great variability in the level of pressure associated with ischaemia. There is also poor correlation between stump pressure and other monitors used to assess the adequacy of cerebral perfusion. Although easy to perform, both stump pressure measurement and assessment of backbleeding are single measurements and will not reflect changes during the whole period of carotid clamping.

Transcranial Doppler monitoring (TCD) is used to measure changes in blood flow velocity in the middle cerebral artery at the time of carotid clamping. However, velocity of flow does not necessarily equate with actual blood flow. The TCD may, however, alert to potentially dangerous embolic events occurring during shunt insertion and removal and other manipulations of the carotid artery.

The cerebral oximeter, which uses similar principles to pulse oximetry, appears to be a reliable indicator of cerebral oxygen saturation. However, there is a wide variation between patients in the measured value of cerebral oxygen saturation. As such a level of cerebral oxygen saturation below which there is a high chance of a neurological deficit arising cannot be predicted.

Post-operative management

Anaesthesia should be discontinued and muscle relaxation reversed and the patient allowed to wake up smoothly. An assessment of neurological function should be made in the operating theatre.

Lability of blood pressure is common in the early post-operative period. Hypertension is often self-limiting but treatment may reduce the likelihood of myocardial and neurological complications. Hypotension is thought to be the result of exposure of carotid baroreceptors to increased pressure though the endarterectomized vessel. Increased baroreceptor activity leads to a reduction in sympathetic tone and an increase in vagal activity. Judicious use of vasopressors may be required in the first 24 hours after surgery.

Section 22.4 • Summary

Patients requiring vascular surgery present a challenge to surgeon, anaesthetist and physician. Inter-speciality co-operation is essential for the optimum management of these patients.

There are a number of approaches to investigating the patient presenting for vascular surgery. Some centres take a minimalist approach where special cardiac investigations are performed only on those with severe symptoms. In some areas all patients have either echocardiography or ventriculography as a routine.

In any given area it is probably best that the clinicians involved discuss the approach that best suits their patient population, facilities and financial situation.

Likewise, little evidence exists for the superiority of one anaesthetic technique over another for all the major vascular surgical procedures. More important is an understanding of the potential problems and meticulous attention to detail.

One cannot emphasize enough the need for informed discussion with surgical colleagues, physicians from the relevant specialities as well as with the patient in order to ensure appropriate management.

Further reading

Blomberg, S., Emanuelsson, H., Kvist, H. *et al.* (1990). Effects of thoracic epidural anesthesia on coronary arteries and arterioles in patients with coronary artery disease. *Anesthesiology* **73**: 840–7.

Bunt, T. J. (1992). The role of a defined protocol fo cardiac risk assessment in decreasing peri-operative myocardial infarction in vascular surgery. *J Vasc Surg* **15**: 626–34.

Christopherson, R., Beattie, C., Fank, S. *et al.* (1993). Perioperative morbidity in patients randomised to epidural or general anaesthesia for lower extremity vascular surgery. *Anesthesiology* **79**: 422–34.

Cunningham, A. J. (1989). Anaesthesia for abdominal aortic surgery – a review. *Can J Anaesth* **36**, 568–77.

Davies, M. J., Dysart, R. H., Silbert, B. S. *et al.* (1992). Prevention of tachycardia with atenolol pre-treatment for carotid endarterectomy under cervical plexus block. *Anaesthesia and Intensive Care* **20**, 161–4.

Hertzer, N., Beven, E. G., Young, J. R. *et al.* (1983). Coronary artery disease in peripheral vascular patients. A classification of 1000 coronary angiograms and results of surgical management. *Ann Surg* **199**: 223–33.

Lalka, S. G., Sawada, S. G., Dalsing, M. C. *et al.* (1992). Dobutamine stress echocardiography as a predictor of cardiac events associated with aortic surgery. *J Vasc Surg* **15**, 831–42.

Moore, W. S. and Hall, A. D. (1969). Carotid artery back pressure. A test of cerebral tolerance to temporary carotid occlusion. *Arch Surg* **99**: 702–10.

Muir, A. D., Reeder, M. K., Foex, P. *et al.* (1991). Preoperative silent myocardial ischaemia: incidence and predictors in a general surgical population. *Br J Anaesthesia* **67**: 373–7.

Rodgers, A., Walker, N., Schug, S. *et al.* (2000). Reduction of postoperative mortality and morbidity with epidural or spinal anaesthesia: results from overview of randomised trials. *BMJ* **321**: 1493–7.

Tangkanakul, C., Counsell, C. and Warlow, C. (1996). Carotid endarterectomy performed under local anaesthetic compared to general anaesthetic: a systematic review of the evidence. In: Warlow, C., Van Gijn, J. and Sandercock, P,. eds. *Stroke module of the Cochrane Database of Systematic Reviews.*

Tuman, K. J., McCarthy, R. J., March, J. *et al.* (1991). Effects of epidural anesthesia and analgesia on coagulation and outcome after major vascular surgery. *Anesth Analg* **73**: 696–704.

Yeager, M. P., Glass, D., Neff, R. K. and Brink-Johnsen, T. (1987). Epidural anesthesia and analgesia in high-risk surgical patients. *Anesthesiology* **66**: 729–36.

MODULE 23

Carotid artery disease

1 • Radiation injury to the carotid artery
2 • Fibromuscular dysplasia
3 • Carotid artery dissection
4 • Arteritis
5 • Carotid artery aneurysm
6 • Occlusive carotid artery disease
7 • Carotid body tumour

Section 23.1 • Radiation injury to the carotid artery

Incidence

There are no reliable data regarding the incidence of arteritis following therapeutic neck irradiation. Uncontrolled studies suggest that the incidence of moderate to severe stenosis is probably increased, particularly in those with hypercholesterolaemia. However, there is little evidence that the incidence of ipsilateral symptoms is any different to that of patients with asymptomatic atherosclerotic disease

Pathology

The immediate effect of radiation to the carotid artery is fibrin deposition and endothelial swelling together with intimal necrosis. Over the subsequent few weeks or months, there is endothelial regeneration and proliferation with destruction of the internal elastic lamina, while the media/adventitia develop focal areas of necrosis and oedema with an associated inflammatory cell infiltrate which might be potentiated by a parallel injury to the vasa vasorum. In the chronic phase of the injury, the intima becomes thickened with evidence of accelerated atherosclerosis while the media and adventitia become increasingly fibrotic. Accordingly, histological examination of the carotid plaque following onset of symptoms can show varied combinations of active inflammation, atherosclerosis and fibrosis.

Clinical features

Radiation arteritis can produce symptoms due to: (i) vessel rupture, usually in association with skin necrosis and infection, (ii) stroke due to carotid thrombosis in the subacute phase of the disease process, i.e. not usually associated with atherosclerosis, and (iii) thrombo-embolic stroke/transient ischaemic attack (TIA) in patients with radiation arteritis and accelerated atherosclerosis. The latter may occur several decades following exposure to the radiation making accurate aetiological differentiation impossible.

Investigation

Although some believe that all patients undergoing neck radiotherapy should be serially imaged with duplex ultrasound, this is neither practical nor cost-effective. In the UK, duplex imaging is the first line investigation in any patient with ipsilateral cerebral ischaemic symptoms who should otherwise undergo routine blood, chest X-ray and electrocardiogram (ECG) investigations. Contrast angiography (MRA) or magnetic resonance angiography may also be necessary as the disease process may be more extensive than was initially thought.

Management

Asymptomatic stenoses should be left alone, especially if they are unilateral, while symptomatic severe stenoses warrant intervention. The decision to operate should take into account the potential risks associated with secondary skin necrosis, infection, tracheostomy, cranial nerve injury following radical neck dissection and tissue plane obliteration. In the past, endarterectomy and patch or saphenous vein bypass were the options of choice but these have been superseded by balloon angioplasty.

Prognosis

Radiation arteritis in the presence of overlying skin necrosis and adjacent infection carries a poor prognosis. There is no evidence that the risk of recurrent stenosis or symptoms is any higher following surgery for arteritis as opposed to pure atherosclerotic disease.

Section 23.2 • Fibromuscular dysplasia

Incidence

The incidence of fibromuscular dysplasia (FMD) is unknown but is noted in about 0.5% of patients undergoing angiography for symptomatic cerebral vascular disease. However, 10% of patients with carotid artery dissection will have evidence of FMD in the contralateral internal carotid artery (ICA).

Pathology

FMD is a rare non-inflammatory, non-atheromatous segmental arteriopathy of unknown aetiology which primarily affects the renal, carotid and mesenteric vessels. Although a number of reports have recently highlighted a causal association with alpha-1-anti-trypsin deficiency this remains unproven.

There are four subtypes of FMD: intimal fibroplasia, medial hyperplasia, medial fibroplasia and peri-medial dysplasia. Two forms predominate in the extracranial carotid arteries; intimal fibroplasia is usually associated with elongation or kinking/coiling of the carotid arteries. The more common medial fibroplasia predominantly affects women and is characterized by alternating segments of hyperplasia (stenosis) and medial destruction (dilatation). Medial fibroplasia does not affect the origin of the ICA, but localizes to the mid-upper section of the ICA opposite to the bodies of C-2 and C-3. The disease process is bilateral in up to 60%. One quarter of patients with FMD of the carotid arteries will have renal artery involvement, 25% will have FMD of the vertebral arteries while up to 20% will also have intra-cranial aneurysms.

Clinical features

Intimal fibroplasia is rarely symptomatic and the kinks/coils can co-exist with atherosclerotic disease. The majority of patients with medial fibroplasia remain asymptomatic although true natural history data are unavailable. Symptoms can arise through: (i) embolism or rupture of focal aneurysms, (ii) cerebral ischaemia and/or local rupture following spontaneous dissection, (iii) arteriovenous fistula formation, (iv) embolism from a chronic dissecting aneurysm, and (v) haemodynamic cerebral infarction.

Investigation

The commonest reasons for suspecting FMD include a duplex scan of the carotid arteries (i.e. a beaded appearance) and the fact that FMD of the renal arteries has already been diagnosed thereby raising the possibility of ICA involvement. Whenever FMD is suspected and being considered for treatment, the next line of management is contrast angiography in order to define the upper limits and extent of the disease process. To date, MR angiography has not been able to replace contrast angiography because of problems with flow definition that cause the luminal undulations to be less apparent.

Management

There is no evidence that intervention is appropriate in asymptomatic individuals, especially those with localized coiling or kinking. However, patients in whom a diagnosis of carotid FMD has been made should be serially followed up. Once symptoms develop it is important to expedite investigation and management as up to 20% may suffer a stroke if left untreated. As a general rule, therefore, management decisions should be based on the same clinical and investigative criteria as if the patient had presented with atherosclerotic disease. As a general rule, if the disease process is readily accessible to surgery then it is probably best treated by resection and interposition vein graft. If the disease process extends towards the more distal reaches of the ICA, the standard treatment to date has been exposure of the ICA to the level of the styloid process followed by open, graduated balloon dilatation of the segmental web-stenoses. The reason for mobilizing the carotid artery is to enable it to be straightened out, thereby minimizing the risks of perforation and dissection. To date, percutaneous carotid angioplasty (± stent) has rarely been utilized in this situation but could be of considerable benefit in the future, especially in those with distal aneurysm formation and dissection.

Prognosis

The long-term prognosis for asymptomatic individuals remains unknown. Surgical intervention caries a 5% risk of procedural stroke and a higher risk of cranial nerve injury than conventional CEA because of the more distal location of the disease. Following a successful surgical intervention, the 10 year stroke free survival rate is about 90%, but about 5% will require re-operation over a 5 year period. No long-term data are available regarding the prognosis following percutaneous angioplasty. Irrespective of the method of treating the carotid lesion, one should always bear in mind that long-term survival may be more dependent on appropriate treatment of hypertension secondary to renal artery involvement and prevention of subarachnoid haemorrhage secondary to intracranial aneurysm rupture.

Section 23.3 • Carotid artery dissection

Incidence

Carotid artery dissection (CAD) accounts for 2% of all strokes, with the highest incidence amongst younger stroke sufferers. Traumatic CAD complicates about 1% of all head injuries but about one quarter of trauma patients with an unexplained focal neurological deficit will be found to have a dissection following angiography.

Pathology

Carotid dissection can occur spontaneously (although minor preceding trauma can never be excluded) and tends to affect patients with Marfans or fibromuscular dysplasia. A second form of CAD follows iatrogenic dissection, e.g. following cannulation, wire manipulation, angioplasty, etc., whilst the third type follows trauma. The latter is usually associated with forced lateral rotation and hyper-extension which causes the ICA to be crushed between the skull base and the transverse process of C2. Alternatively, a seemingly trivial hyper-extension injury may be the only cause of the transverse intimal tear. The dissection usually starts 2–3 cm beyond the origin of the ICA but then extends over a variable distance towards the petrous bone. The dissection can cause: (i) complete vessel occlusion through compression by mural haematoma, (ii) a source of embolism from the mural haematoma, (iii) formation of an aneurysmal dilatation of the distal ICA, and (iv) distal re-entry with an intervening double lumen.

Clinical features

An indeterminate number will be asymptomatic. The presentation of traumatic cases will be largely directed by the extent and severity of other injuries which may mask subtle or more overt signs of cerebral or ocular ischaemia. Ipsilateral headache and/or neck pain occurs in 80% of patients with spontaneous dissection. Ocular signs and symptoms are present in 60% and may be one of the initial features in up to 50%. Overall, 50–75% of patients will present with a TIA or stroke (usually embolic), syncope, pulsatile tinnitus, isolated or multiple cranial nerve injuries or ocular signs. The latter include miosis, painful Horner's syndrome, hemianopia, ischaemic optic neuropathy and III, IV or VI nerve palsies. The association between spontaneous CAD and presenting ocular features is important as up to 25% of these patients are destined to suffer a stroke within the following 2 weeks.

Investigation

A diagnosis of CAD should be considered in any patient with neurotrauma and unexplained cerebral infarction on computed tomography (CT). Thereafter, angiography or duplex can exclude or confirm this diagnosis. In spontaneous CAD, the diagnosis may be suspected clinically and a high resistance signal demonstrated on duplex ultrasound, but the gold standard remains contrast angiography. Angiography is able to confirm the extent of the dissection and will provide information on the presence or absence of intimal flaps, stenoses, aneurysmal dilatations, the string sign and any double lumen. Similarly, orbital Doppler studies may show reversed flow in the ophthalmic artery.

Management

There is controversy regarding the management of CAD. To date, the majority of patients with an asymptomatic or symptomatic dissection have been managed conservatively with bed-rest and anti-coagulation (initially heparin followed by warfarin). Evidence suggests that a significant proportion will recanalize and clinically improve. Surgery (ICA ligation, venous bypass, EC-IC bypass) tends to be reserved for patients with recurrent symptoms despite anticoagulation. Traumatic CAD poses a more difficult problem and complex carotid reconstructions involving exposure of the petrous section of the ICA have been advocated in patients with a stenosis >70% or a 50% dilatation of the ICA. However, in the future most of the surgical strategies may become replaced by endovascular techniques which avoid the need for a difficult high carotid dissection and lessen the risk of cranial nerve injury.

Prognosis

Strokes following CAD have a high morbidity and mortality. Once a diagnosis of CAD has been made, it is essential to commence anticoagulation to reduce the risk of secondary embolic stroke.

Section 23.4 • Arteritis

Incidence

The commonest forms of arteritis affecting the extracranial carotid arteries include Takayasu disease (TD) and temporal arteritis (TA). Both predominantly affect women but TD primarily affects females <40 years while TA is principally found in women >50 years.

Pathology

Both TA and TD are associated with a transmural inflammatory cell infiltration which frequently contains giant cells during the acute phase. TD comprises four principal subtypes (Table 23.1). Types 1 and 2 account for 35% of cases, 55% are type 3 and only 10% type 4. TA principally affects the extracranial vessels but not the intracranial arteries. As a rule, TA is associated with bilateral symmetrical lesions. During the quiescent phase of TD, arteries undergo circumferential sclerosis which precedes occlusion.

Clinical features

In both TD and TA, there is a prodromal phase comprising a systemic illness with fever, malaise, myalgia and, in the case of TA, headache. Thereafter, 50% of TA patients will complain of jaw claudication and 50% of pain over the temporal artery. The feared ocular symptoms (including blindness) tend to occur 1–4 months after onset of the prodromal period. In TD, the symptoms depend on the location and severity of vessel occlusion/stenosis/aneurysm formation. Accordingly, TD can present with any combination of asymptomatic pulselessness, renovascular hypertension, stroke/ TIA and mesenteric ischaemia.

Table 23.1 Patterns of involvement in Takayasu disease

Type 1 =	aortic arch plus principal branches
Type 2 =	descending aorta and abdominal aorta
Type 3 =	combination of types 1 and 2
Type 4 =	patients with types 1 to 3 and pulmonary artery disease

Investigation

The current gold standard technique for TD is contrast angiography which can delineate the areas of involvement, etc. There may, however, be an increasing role for duplex ultrasound in the future because of its ability to non-invasively monitor disease activity, stenosis and aneurysm development at anastomoses and the intima-media thickness. TA is diagnosed with a combination of a raised erythrocyte sedimentation rate (ESR) and temporal artery biopsy.

Management

In TD, active disease is managed with high dose prednisolone plus long-term maintenance therapy until the active phase has resolved. The response to steroids can be monitored using duplex measurement of the intima-media thickness. Those resistant or unable to take steroids can try cyclophosphamide or methotrexate. As a rule, surgery should be avoided in the active phase unless absolutely necessary and any bypass should arise from uninvolved vessels, e.g. the ascending aorta. There is no role for endarterectomy in TD. Percutaneous angioplasty may be of benefit in treating renal artery stenoses but because the common carotid artery tends to be affected over a long length, it is unlikely to be of value in this location. The mainstay of treating TA is prednisolone, using the ESR as a guide to disease activity. Surgery is almost never indicated in TA.

Prognosis

Patients with TD require long-term clinical and duplex surveillance (some centres even advocate 6 monthly angiography). The aim is to anticipate and prevent disease activation.

Section 23.5 • Carotid artery aneurysm

Incidence

Aneurysms of the extracranial carotid artery comprise <1% of all arterial aneurysms and <2% of all carotid operations. The true incidence is unknown but is determined by the choice of definition. At present, the threshold is 150% of the common carotid artery diameter and 200% of the ICA diameter.

Pathology

Carotid aneurysms are predominantly atherosclerotic with other less common causes including fibromuscular dysplasia, dissection, trauma, mycotic and post-endarterectomy.

Clinical features

Up to two-thirds of carotid aneurysms are asymptomatic at the time of diagnosis. Common presentations include a pulsatile mass in the neck, thrombo-embolic stroke, tenderness over the carotid artery, cranial nerve dysfunction, dysphagia and, very rarely, rupture.

Investigation

The majority presenting with a pulsatile neck mass will be found to have prominence, ectasia or coiling of the common carotid or innominate arteries. Thus the first line investigation is a duplex scan. Thereafter, investigations are directed towards ascertaining the probable underlying cause (dysplasia, trauma, etc.) as management strategies will vary. Contrast angiography is usually performed to evaluate the upper limits of the aneurysm and to aid in the planning of surgical strategies. A CT scan may also be necessary to aid in the differential diagnosis of other neck lumps (e.g. carotid body tumour).

Management

Management will depend on the underlying aetiology, urgency of symptoms and the level and distal extent of the aneurysm. The principal reason for actively treating carotid aneurysm is to prevent thrombo-embolic stroke. The main surgical options include exclusion/resection with either primary end-to-end anastomosis, interposition saphenous vein bypass or transposition of the distal ICA to the origin of the ECA (Figure 23.1). Ligation is now rarely employed but may still be indicated in patients with bleeding or whose aneurysm extends to the skull base. If ligation is to be considered, some means of testing the adequacy of the collateral circulation is necessary (e.g. regional anaesthesia, transcranial Doppler) so as to minimize the risk of haemodynamic stroke. Newer alternatives such as endovascular coiling/balloon occlusion (which will also enable test occlusions to be performed) or the insertion of covered stents have the potential to replace surgery in the management of many patients.

Prognosis

Most patients with carotid aneurysm will become symptomatic with time. Surgery, however, carries the risk of procedural stroke and cranial nerve injury in 5–7% of patients. Management decisions must therefore balance the risks and benefits associated with intervention which may mean adopting a more conservative strategy in selected elderly asymptomatic patients with distal internal carotid aneurysms.

Section 23.6 • Occlusive carotid artery disease

Incidence

Stroke is defined as a focal (or occasionally global) loss of cerebral function lasting for >24 hours which, after investigation, is found to have a vascular cause. A TIA carries the same definition but a time scale of <24 hours. The overall annual incidence of first-ever stroke is 2.4/1000, with the rate increasing with age. The annual incidence of TIA is 0.5/1000. Stroke is the third commonest cause of death in the UK (accounting for

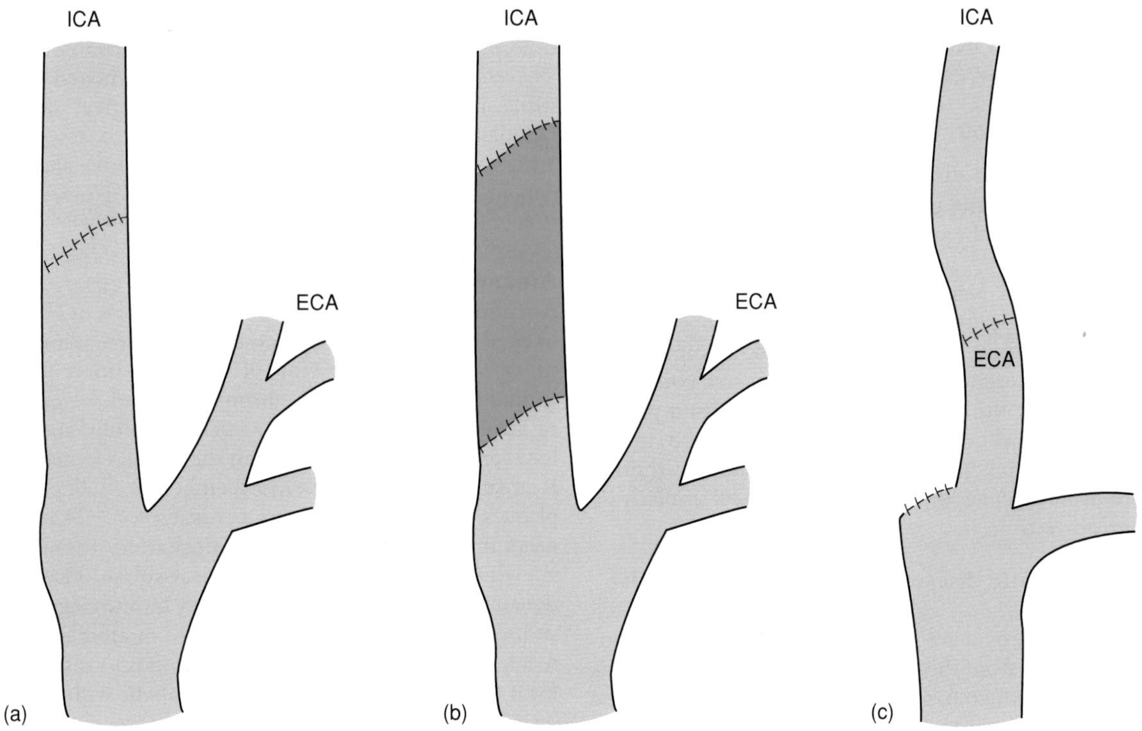

Figure 23.1 Surgical options for reconstruction following resection/exclusion of a carotid aneurysm: (a) spatulated end-to-end anastomosis, (b) reversed interposition vein graft, (c) oversewing of ICA origin with transposition of the distal ICA to the ECA mainstem.

12% of all deaths), is the principal cause of permanent neurological disability and consumes 5% of health resources annually.

Pathology

Eighty per cent of strokes are ischaemic and 20% are haemorrhagic (intracranial or subarachnoid). The principal causes of carotid territory ischaemic stroke include infarction due to thrombo-embolism of the ICA and/or middle cerebral artery (MCA) (50%), lacunar infarction due to small vessel occlusion of the deep penetrating end-arteries (e.g. the lenticulostriate arteries) in patients with hypertension and diabetes (25%), cardiac embolism (15%), haematological disorders (myeloma, polycythaemia, thrombocytosis) in 5%, whilst 5% comprise an assortment of less common conditions including tumour, arteritis, oral contraceptive related, etc. The main risk factors for stroke include hypertension, ischaemic heart disease, smoking, hyperlipidaemia, TIA, diabetes and hyperfibrinogenaemia.

Thus, the commonest single cause of ischaemic stroke is thrombo-embolism from an atherosclerotic stenosis at the origin of the ICA (Figure 23.2). The carotid bifurcation is particularly prone to atherosclerosis formation particularly on the outer aspect of the carotid sinus (opposite to and just distal to the origin of the external carotid artery). In this region there is an area of flow separation and low shear stress which predisposes to the formation of atheroma. These haemodynamic phenomena together with hyperlipidaemia and other risk factors contribute towards the activation of endothelial cells which become increasingly permeable to low-density lipoproteins whilst also promoting the adhesion of platelets and neutrophils. Smooth muscle cells lose their contractile function and assume a more secretory role which facilitates further smooth muscle cell proliferation and cholesterol accumulation. Thus the initial intimal fatty streak becomes a mural plaque which thereafter progresses onto an eccentric lesion which variably protrudes into the vessel lumen. Histologically, the plaque is composed of variable amounts of cholesterol, calcium, fibroblasts and other inflammatory cells.

Quite why some plaques should remain asymptomatic while others cause a TIA or stroke remains unknown. However, evidence suggests that acute changes in plaque morphology predispose to fissuring, ulceration or intraplaque haemorrhage. The net result is either thrombosis of the extracranial ICA or adherent thrombus which may embolize thereafter. The plaque is very high risk for embolization for about a month (which accounts for the phenomenon of TIA clustering) and then starts to heal. Recent evidence suggests that the onset of symptoms may be associated with increased expression and production of matrix metalloproteinase (MMP9) from macrophages within the plaque. MMPs are a family of enzymes which regulate the extracellular matrix and inhibition of this enzyme offers the prospect of plaque stabilization in the future.

Although infection of the plaque by *Helicobacter pylori* and *Chlamydia pneumoniae* has also been implicated, there is no proof of causation.

Clinical features

Asymptomatic disease

About 0.5% of the population under 50 years have an asymptomatic atherosclerotic stenosis in excess of 50% luminal diameter at the carotid bifurcation. Asymptomatic stenoses become apparent through auscultation of a cervical bruit or by the patient becoming aware of pulsatile tinnitus. However, the term 'asymptomatic' may be misleading as the patient may not consider a recent funny turn or transient episode of hand paraesthesia or weakness to be of importance and it will therefore go unreported. Similarly, because one-third of our lives is spent asleep, nocturnal TIAs will similarly go unreported.

Symptomatic disease – predicting the vascular territory

Table 23.2 provides a guide to the more typical symptoms arising from the carotid and vertebrobasilar territories. Homonymous hemianopia is never a carotid symptom in its own right but does occur in large volume infarctions (usually in association with conjugate gaze deviation) when there is invariably a severe motor and sensory deficit and evidence of higher cortical dysfunction. Similarly, 10% of vertebrobasilar strokes will present with hemisensory/motor signs. In the past, there has been a tendency to ascribe a diagnosis of cerebrovascular insufficiency to patients with blackouts, isolated diplopia, isolated vertigo, isolated dizziness, presyncope and syncope. In reality, these should never be considered to be carotid or vertebrobasilar in origin unless they co-exist with more typical symptoms. As a rule, there is usually another cause.

Transient ischaemic attacks

According to the definition, TIAs can last for up 24 hours but, as a rule, they have usually resolved within an hour or two and most within minutes. Carotid TIAs tend to be embolic whilst vertebrobasilar TIAs tend to be haemodynamic. TIAs often exhibit the phenomenon of clustering whereby recurrent TIAs occur within the first month after onset. This is attributed to the presence of overlying thrombus on the plaque during this period. Crescendo TIAs occur when repeated focal neurological events occur within a very short period of time, e.g. several per day or one per day for some days. The entity is poorly defined but is differentiated from stroke-in-evolution because the neurological deficit completely resolves between each attack. Crescendo TIAs are highly predictive of impending stroke and the patient should be admitted immediately for investigation and management.

Amaurosis fugax

Amaurosis fugax is a transient monocular loss of vision, likened to a shutter or curtain coming down although, on occasions, only greying of the vision may occur. Embolic amaurosis has an abrupt onset and the extent of involvement reflects the size of the embolus and the location of the occlusion within the retinal circulation. Retinal examination may reveal emboli or Hollenhorst plaques. Complete visual loss persisting for >24 hours raises the likelihood of central retinal artery thrombosis which is analagous to a cortical stroke. Haemodynamic amaurosis can be triggered by moving from sitting to standing, following hot baths or after a heavy meal. In this situation, the visual loss tends to disappear from the periphery first. Rarely, the patient with a very severe carotid stenosis will also display signs of rubeosis iridis (network of tiny blood vessels over the outer surface of the iris).

Stroke

A completed stroke is the term relating to the final neurological deficit following a cerebral infarction. In contrast, a stroke-in-evolution represents an evolving phenomenon wherein a pre-existing neurological deficit does not completely resolve before the next one intervenes. On occasions this can be a surgical emergency and urgent investigation is required.

The Oxfordshire Community Stroke Project developed a classification of acute ischaemic stroke that enables a bedside prediction of outcome. Patients with total anterior circulation infarction (TACI) present with the triad of hemiplegia/sensory loss, homonymous hemianopia and evidence of higher cortical dysfunction. TACI usually follows major vessel occlusion (ICA and/or MCA) and has the worst outcome with a 30 day mortality of 39% and a 30 day independence rate of 4%. Patients with partial anterior circulation infarction (PACI) present with one or more components of the TACI triad but never all three. PACI

Table 23.2 Cerebral vascular symptoms by territory

Carotid	*Vertebral*	*Non-hemispheric*
Hemisensory/motor signs	Hemisensory/motor signs (10%)	Isolated vertigo
Unilateral visual loss	Bilateral motor/sensory signs	Isolated diplopia
Higher cortical dysfunction	Bilateral visual loss	Isolated dizziness
	Dysarthria	Presyncope
	Gait and stance problems	Syncope
		Nystagmus
		Homonymous hemianopia

patients usually have branch occlusion(s) of the MCA and have the best prognosis with a 4% mortality at 30 days while 56% are independent by this time.

Investigation

The investigation of patients with carotid artery disease primarily revolves around identifying correctable risk factors and determining the degree of stenosis.

Risk factor analysis

All patients should undergo a series of baseline investigations comprising urea and electrolytes, lipids, glucose, full blood count, plasma viscosity, chest X-ray and ECG. These can be undertaken in the outpatient clinic. More specialized investigations including thrombophilia screening, autoantibodies, homocysteine levels, echocardiography and 24 hour tapes should be reserved for selected cases.

Diagnosis of carotid stenosis

With the rapid advances in duplex ultrasound and MRA, fewer centres now advocate routine carotid angiography. This does, however, remain a point of controversy and the benefits/disadvantages of each modality are reviewed. One factor that should be borne in mind when interpreting the results of comparative studies is that because angiography is invariably deemed the gold standard against which duplex and MRA must be compared, it is impossible for the latter to be better than the gold-standard!

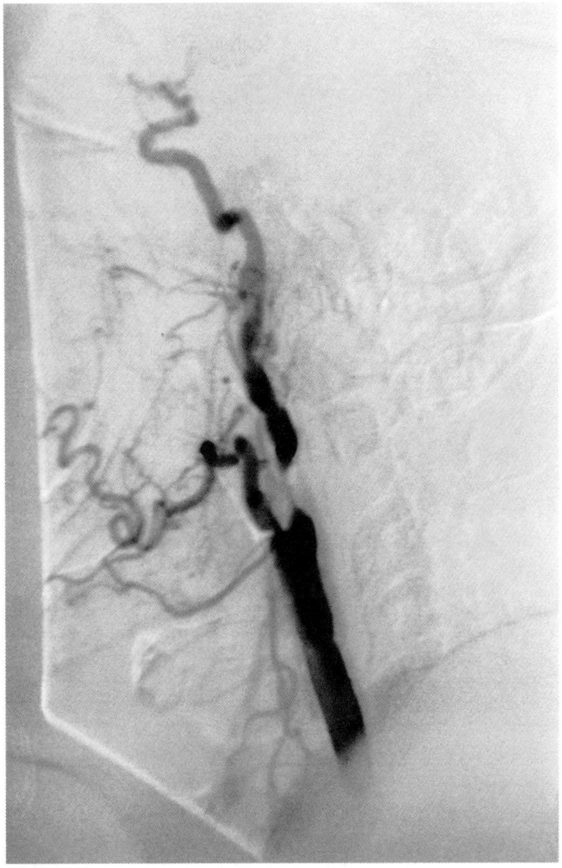

Figure 23.2 Selective IADSA demonstrating a severe stenosis at the origin of the ICA with evidence of mural plaques extending into the distal ICA.

Carotid angiography

The aortic arch, carotid and vertebral arteries can be imaged by digital subtraction angiography (DSA). Intravenous DSA, with contrast injected into the cephalic vein, is rarely used nowadays because of poor overall image quality. Intra-arterial DSA (IADSA) requires Seldinger catheterization of the femoral artery with passage of a guidewire and catheter to the arch. Selective images thereafter require passage of the catheter into each artery in turn (Figure 23.2). The principal advantage of IADSA is the ability to produce a hard-copy of the arterial system which many surgeons prefer.

However, angiography carries a 1–2% risk of procedural stroke. Accordingly, an increasing number of surgeons are now looking towards non-invasive methods of pre-operative imaging (see below). However, supporters of angiography note the fact that angiography formed the basis upon which measurements of stenosis were quantified in the international trials and that it should therefore remain the gold standard. Angiography has also been recommended as being the only method capable of evaluating: (i) inflow disease at the aortic arch, (ii) the upper limit of the carotid plaque, (iii) outflow disease in the carotid syphon, (iv) differentiation between subocclusion and complete thrombosis, and (v) intracranial images. As will be seen, however, most of these criteria no longer apply and most centres currently employ a policy of selective angiography following duplex ultrasound or MRA. Moreover, angiography does not provide reliable data on plaque morphology, particularly the presence of luminal thrombus. Those who continue to advocate routine angiography prior to carotid endarterectomy (CEA) must add the 2% angiographic stroke risk to the operative risk when discussing management with the patient. The measurement of stenosis using IADSA was different in the European and American studies (Figure 23.3), which accounts for the apparent discrepancies in the calculated values and prognoses. For example, a 70% European stenosis is equivalent to a 50% American stenosis.

Magnetic resonance angiography

MRA is a non-invasive means of imaging the extracranial circulation. Its principal advantage is that it can be combined with MR functional imaging of the brain (as well as providing intracranial vascular images) thereby obviating the need for any additional CT scan. MRA traditionally provides two- (2-D) or three-dimensional (3-D) images. In 2-D MRA, a large number of thin tomographic slices are generated in sequence which are then combined to provide a 12 cm field of view. The

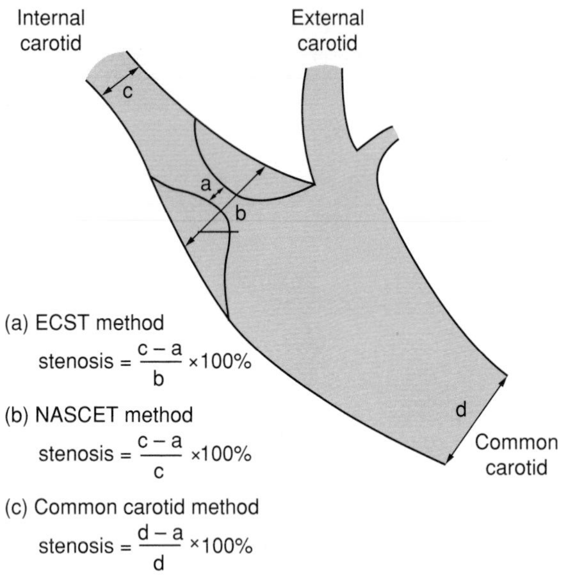

Figure 23.3 Schematic representation of the different methods for measuring the degree of stenosis in (a) the European Carotid Surgery Trial and (b) the North American Symptomatic Carotid Endarterectomy Trial. The third method, based on the diameter of the common carotid artery, is demonstrated in equation (c).

main advantage of 2-D MRA is the ability to differentiate subocclusion from total occlusion because of its ability to detect trickle flow. However, 2-D MRA is limited by the creation of flow voids in areas of turbulence and non-laminar flow which can give rise to overestimation of the degree of stenosis. Similarly, 2-D MRA will have trouble interpreting loops and kinks in the distal carotid artery. Three-dimensional MRA images the block of tissue at one time and thereafter generates tomographic slices. Three-dimensional MRA provides better spatial resolution but has a smaller field of view. However, the principal advantage of 3-D MRA is that flow voids are almost always diagnostic of a severe carotid stenosis.

To date, MRA has assumed an increasing role in the investigation of patients with carotid artery disease. However, there is no evidence that imaging the intracranial circulation alters decision making in a clinical and cost-effective manner. The main potential advantage of MRA over duplex is the ability to image the inflow vessels of the aortic arch. As with IADSA, MRA todate has not provided clinically useful information regarding plaque morphology.

Duplex ultrasound

The rapid evolution of colour flow duplex ultrasound technology over the last decade has contributed towards its ascendancy over contrast angiography in the investigation of patients with carotid artery disease. Fewer than 2% of all extracranial lesions responsible for ischaemic stroke now lie outside the scanning range of the state-of-the-art machines which use a combination of B-mode imaging, colour flow and Doppler waveform analysis to diagnose occlusive plaques (Figure 23.4). Damped signals in the common carotid artery warn of the probability of inflow disease while high resistance or reverberent signals in the ICA suggest outflow or syphon disease. Both are indications for either MRA or contrast angiography. Similarly, it may not be possible to image above or below the carotid plaque using ultrasound and these patients should undergo some form of angiographic examination prior to surgery. In the authors' practice, <5% of patients now undergo IADSA prior to carotid surgery. Before instituting a policy of operating upon the basis of duplex ultrasound alone it is important that each centre validates its duplex findings against angiographic and operative features. Only when reliability and quality is assured is it appropriate to delete routine IADSA from the pre-operative protocol.

CT scanning

Despite the attractive logic, there is little cost-based or clinical evidence to support a routine policy of CT scanning patients prior to carotid surgery. Common arguments supporting routine CT scanning include exclusion of tumours, AVMs and other rare causes of stroke whilst enabling a better prediction of operative risk. However, the likelihood of encountering a concurrent tumour in a TIA patient with classical carotid territory symptoms and a severe ipsilateral ICA stenosis is remote and does not justify a policy of routine CT scanning. Similarly, the time to perform a CT scan following a stroke is in the first 14 days so as to differentiate haemorrhage from infarction. There seems little point in performing this investigation some weeks or months later as it is unlikely to alter surgical decision making.

Management

Optimal medical therapy

Irrespective of presentation, all patients should receive optimal medical therapy which does not just mean tak-

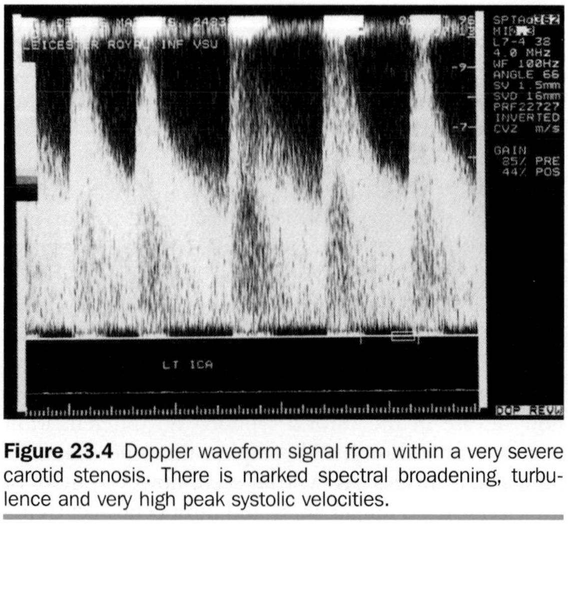

Figure 23.4 Doppler waveform signal from within a very severe carotid stenosis. There is marked spectral broadening, turbulence and very high peak systolic velocities.

ing aspirin. Optimal medical therapy requires treatment of ischaemic heart disease and control of hypertension. Although the optimal levels for blood pressure remain the subject of debate, it seems reasonable to aim for <150/85 mmHg for those aged <60, <160/90 mmHg for patients aged under 70 years, while allowing up to 170/95 mmHg in older age groups. To date, primary care doctors have been very reluctant to adhere to the British Heart Foundation guidelines for blood pressure control, but evidence suggests that the lower the diastolic pressure the lower the stroke risk. Similarly, there is considerable debate regarding the role of lipid lowering therapy. To date, no published series have specifically compared targeted lipid lowering in stroke prevention but evidence from parallel trials in ischaemic heart disease suggests that the risk of stroke will reduce.

Other important aspects of optimal medical therapy include ensuring normoglycaemia, stopping smoking, recommending exercise and moderating alcohol intake. Finally, all patients should be on anti-platelet therapy. In the past, almost all patients received aspirin (75–150 mg/day) with no systematic evidence that higher aspirin doses reduced stroke risk. However, there remains controversy over the role of the newer antiplatelet agents including dipyridamole, ticlopidine (disadvantaged by 1% incidence of neutropenia) and clopidogrel (disadvantaged by price). These newer agents act to a greater (or lesser) extent via the ADP receptor on the platelet, whilst aspirin acts via the cyclo-oxygenase pathway. Despite evidence of a marginal benefit in favour of ADP antagonists in clinical trials, the current advice is to continue with aspirin and reserve clopidogrel for patients who are genuinely intolerant or unable to take aspirin.

Symptomatic carotid artery disease

The European Carotid Surgery Trial (ECST) has shown that CEA is not indicated in symptomatic patients with an ipsilateral 0–69% stenosis. The only exception might be the highly symptomatic patient with a 60%+ stenosis with recurrent symptoms despite best medical therapy. CEA is however indicated in patients with a severe (70–99%) stenosis. The overall benefit is greatest in patients with an 80–99% stenosis where the benefit of CEA extends for up to 12 months following the most recent event, as opposed to 6 months for those with a 70–79% stenosis. The risk of operative death/stroke in symptomatic patients with a 70–99% stenosis in the ECST was 7.5%. The latest data from the ECST suggest that predictive factors such as hemispheric versus ocular, male versus female gender, stenosis severity and plaque irregularity may help to identify the 20% subgroup who really need to undergo CEA. This hypothesis is currently being tested on the NASCET database for validation.

The North American Symptomatic Carotid Endarterectomy Trial (NASCET) reported that CEA was not indicated in patients with a symptomatic 40–50% stenosis, but that CEA conferred a small but significant benefit in patients with a 50–69% stenosis. The most significant benefit was observed in patients with a 70–99% stenosis despite a 5.8% operative risk. The apparent differences between the ECST and NASCET are explained by the methods of quantifying stenosis (Figure 23.3). NASCET also confirmed the long-term durability of CEA and that surgery was beneficial for up to 12 months after a TIA or minor stroke in patients with severe disease.

Emergency carotid surgery

There is no randomized trial evidence supporting the use of emergency CEA in clinical practice. However, current opinion supports the role of urgent CEA in selected patients with crescendo TIAs or stroke in evolution. There is no evidence of any role for emergency surgery in acute completed stroke but this may change in the future as trials examine the combined role of surgery and thrombolysis in this situation. Finally, the traditional view that CEA should be deferred for 6 weeks following a stroke because of the risk of transforming an ischaemic stroke into a haemorrhagic stroke is no longer so rigidly adhered to. Evidence suggests that patients making a good neurological recovery are candidates for surgery after 2–3 weeks have elapsed. Patients with large volume infarcts and severe persisting deficits are never candidates for urgent or emergency surgery.

Asymptomatic carotid disease

If the role of CEA in symptomatic disease has been clarified, it would be fair to say that the same does not easily apply to asymptomatic disease. A number of randomized trials have addressed this issue but only the Asymptomatic Carotid Atherosclerosis Study (ACAS) has come close to providing an answer. ACAS demonstrated that CEA was associated with a 5.9% absolute risk reduction in stroke risk (from 11% to 5.1%) in favour of CEA in patients with an asymptomatic stenosis >60%. The ACAS study was associated with a 2.3% operative risk (1.2% angiographic risk, 1.1% surgical risk) which also reinforces the fact that the participating surgeons were highly selected from the outset. However, ACAS has been criticized for having stopped too early (the median follow-up was only 2.7 years), for having generated a projected 5 year stroke risk on relatively limited data, for not having shown any evidence of benefit in women or for preventing disabling stroke and for showing no evidence of any association between stroke risk and stenosis severity.

A recent overview of all published data confirms a small but significant benefit in favour of surgery, but for methodological reasons that was confined to those with a stenosis >50%. Thus although the ACAS findings have become readily adopted by colleagues in the USA, the same is not true in the UK. Here the policy is either to randomize patients into the ongoing Asymptomatic Carotid Surgery Trial or to adopt a more selective policy of operating such as only those with severe bilateral disease.

Carotid endarterectomy

General or local anaesthesia?

In the past, the majority of CEAs were done under general anaesthesia. This was partly because of surgeon convenience (i.e. the patients lie still and do not swallow or speak) but also because there was a belief that general anaesthesic agents reduced cerebral metabolic requirements and thus might be cerebrally protective. Over the past 5 years, however, there has been a vogue towards performing CEA under local anaesthesia on the bases that: (i) awake testing is the only infallible method of knowing whether a stroke has occurred or whether a shunt is necessary, (ii) it may reduce intensive therapy unit and overall hospital stay, and (iii) the incidence of myocardial infarction and pulmonary complications might be reduced. To date, no randomized trials have demonstrated that either is preferable.

CEA under local anaesthesia requires an anaesthetist or surgeon who is experienced in the performance of superficial and deep cervical plexus blockade and an anaesthetist should always be available to intubate a restless or deteriorating patient. Finally, awake testing will only inform the surgeon that a neurological deficit has occurred. It will not prevent an embolic stroke due to surgeon error.

Shunt or no shunt?

Along with carotid patching, this has become another of the 'single issue' topics that has dominated the practice of CEA. The simple rationale underlying shunting is that it prevents haemodynamic stroke during clamping. Surgeons, therefore, tend to fall into three camps. The two largest comprise the routine shunters (i.e. you have to shunt everyone because it is not possible to reliably predict those at risk unless you use awake testing) and the selective shunters (i.e. shunts interfere with the performance of CEA, cause intimal injury and embolization and should only be used in the 10–15% of patients who really need them). The third group, the never shunt surgeons, comprise the minority who believe that shunts cause as many strokes as they prevent and if you do the operation quickly enough they are not necessary. The few available randomized trials suggest that a policy of routine shunting is safer than never shunting. No trial has ever compared a policy of routine with selective shunting. The Javid shunt permits higher flow rates than the Pruitt–Inahara, but the latter does not require external clamps to hold it in place. This is of particular benefit should the stenosis extend high into the neck.

Patch or no patch?

The rationale underlying patching is that it widens the carotid bulb, improves haemodynamic flow, prevents distal stenosis formation at the time of surgery and reduces the risk of peri-operative thrombosis. Long term it should also reduce the risk of restenosis and stroke. As with the shunt, surgeons tend to be routine patchers, selective patchers or routine primary closers. Overviews of the randomized trials indicate that routine patching confers a three-fold reduction in peri-operative stroke and/or thrombosis as well as late stroke and/or restenosis as compared with routine primary closure. No randomized trials have compared selective patching (usually patients with an ICA diameter <5 mm) against routine patching. Similarly, there is no evidence from the overviews that prosthetic patching is preferable to saphenous vein patching provided the latter is harvested from the groin.

Monitoring or no monitoring?

There are a plethora of monitoring modalities and each have there own advantages and disadvantages. Most importantly, no single monitoring method is superior or infallible and methods capable of monitoring should not be confused with quality control (QC). At present, only transcranial Doppler (TCD) is capable of diagnosing embolization. Reduced cerebral perfusion can be monitored using stump pressure, ICA backflow, near infrared spectroscopy (NIRS), jugular venous oxygen saturation and TCD. Loss of cerebral electrical activity can be monitored using electroencephalography or evoked potentials, but only awake testing will tell you that a neurological deficit has occurred (but not necessarily why). From the QC point of view, TCD warns of embolization and is the easiest method for diagnosing shunt malfunction. Angioscopy, angiography or colour flow duplex will identify luminal thrombus, intimal flaps and residual stenoses. To date, no randomized trial has demonstrated that monitoring and QC assessment reduces the operative risk. In Leicester the authors have adopted a policy of intra-operative TCD and completion angioscopy plus 3 hours of post-operative TCD to guide selective Dextran therapy in patients with high rates of embolization. This policy has resulted in a 60% reduction in the operative risk over the past several years.

How to manage a peri-operative neurological deficit

This will depend on the timing of the event and the availability of duplex and TCD ultrasound. In the absence of these, the patient recovering from anaesthesia with a new neurological deficit has to be assumed to have suffered an on-table thrombosis until proven otherwise. Failure to clear the thrombus within 1 hour significantly increases the rate of disability. Similarly, within the first 24 hours of surgery one should otherwise assume that any neurological deficit is thromboembolic and the patient re-explored to exclude either an occluding thrombus or underlying technical error. Thereafter there is an increasing likelihood of intracranial haemorrhage and the patient should undergo a CT scan.

In Leicester, the policy is to monitor all patients intra-operatively with TCD and completion angioscopy. The latter identifies the 3–4% of patients with retained luminal thrombus prior to restoration of flow. Similarly, TCD allows a speedy diagnosis of on-table thrombosis to be made (i.e. flow levels similar to that observed during clamping) and the artery can be re-opened immediately. Since introducing this policy, the rate of intra-operative stroke (i.e. apparent upon recovery from surgery) has dropped from 4 to 0.25% and the authors have not had to re-explore any patient following recovery from anaesthesia in the last 600 CEAs. Early post-operative thrombosis can be prevented by the selective use of dextran and, to date, they have not had to re-explore any patient with a symptomatic thrombosis. It is the authors' opinion that prevention is easier than treatment.

Carotid angioplasty

Angioplasty has emerged as a potential alternative to endarterectomy in the management of patients with carotid artery disease. The procedure traditionally uses the Seldinger approach via the femoral artery although direct carotid puncture is an alternative. The pioneers of this technique practised balloon angioplasty alone but there is currently an increasing vogue towards primary stenting (Figure 23.5). Excellent results have been published around the world but neither of the available randomized trials has demonstrated that angioplasty confers any overall benefit. The potential advantages of angioplasty include no wound complications or cranial nerve injuries, possibly fewer cardiovascular problems and the potential for day case treatment. However, its principal problem remains procedural embolization. In the future, this may be circumvented by the use of distal 'umbrella' protection systems but none of these techniques has been subjected to large scale review. At present, angioplasty should only be used routinely within the setting of a randomized trial. However, there are several situations where angioplasty may be of considerable benefit including the post-endarterectomy or carotid bypass restenosis (Figure 23.6), radiation injury and open angioplasty of inflow lesions at the aortic arch via controlled exposure of the carotid artery.

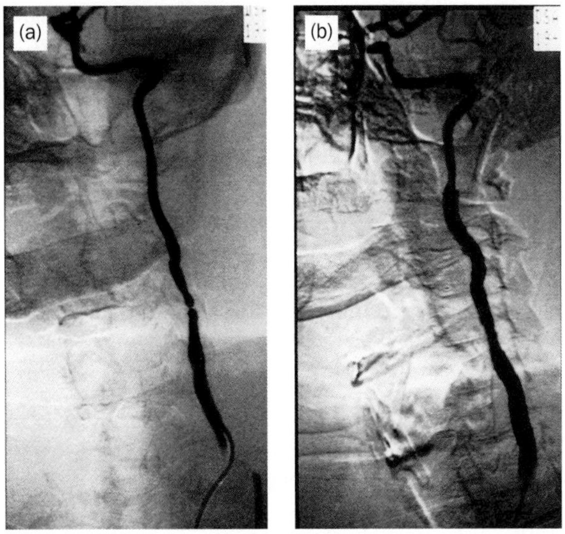

Figure 23.6 This patient underwent a carotid vein bypass because of marked coiling of the ICA immediately distal to the stenosis. Twelve months post-operatively, duplex surveillance revealed a focal web-like restenosis (a) which was successfully treated by balloon angioplasty (b). As with lower limb vein grafts, all carotid vein bypasses should be regularly surveyed as up to 30% will develop restenoses.

Section 23.7 • Carotid body tumour

Carotid body tumours are uncommon. They are paraganglionomas, derived from neural crest tissue, which migrate in close association with autonomic ganglion cells. Other examples of paraganglionomas include tumours of the vagal body and phaeochromocytomas.

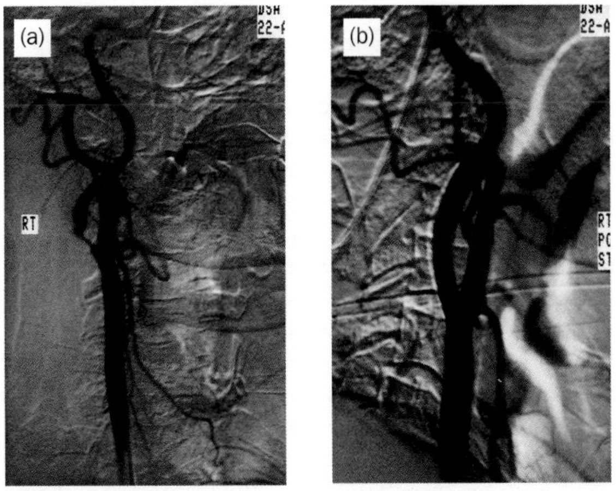

Figure 23.5 Diagnostic IADSA of severe ICA stenosis (a), subsequently treated by carotid angioplasty and primary stenting (b).

The carotid body is a small chemoreceptor organ located in the adventitia of the posterior aspect of the common carotid bifurcation. It is primarily responsive to hypoxia and to a lesser degree hypercapnia and acidosis. The blood supply of the carotid body is derived from the external carotid artery in most individuals. Carotid body tumours consist of epitheliod 'chief' cells and well-vascularized fibrous tissue components. Although chemoreceptors are able to secrete catecholamines, carotid body tumours are mainly non-secretory. The majority of carotid body tumours are benign. However, 20% will exhibit local invasion, lymph node and haematogenous metastases. Histological markers of malignancy appear to be unreliable in predicting tumour behaviour. The aetiology of this condition is unknown. However, hypertrophy of the carotid body is documented in chronic hypoxia and an increased incidence of these tumours is reported in patients living at high altitude. Carotid body tumours may be sporadic or familial. In the more common sporadic form, 5% of cases may be bilateral. The familial form accounts for 10% of cases and is bilateral in approximately 30%. These are inherited as an autosomal dominant trait and screening of family members is recommended.

Carotid body tumours are slow growing and usually present as an asymptomatic neck lump located below the angle of mandible. Patients can present at any age, however the fifth and sixth decades are more common. On examination, although carotid body tumours appear pulsatile they are non-expansile. They can be moved from side to side but not up and down because of their attachment to the carotid bifurcation.

Most carotid body tumours increase in size and cause symptoms secondary to pressure on adjacent structures – pain in the neck or ear is common while hoarseness, dysphagia and cough are seen in 10% of cases. Non-specific symptoms such as headache, dizziness and syncope may be mediated by tumour secretion of hormones. Cranial nerves (the vagus, glossopharyngeal and hypoglossal) and sympathetic nerves are involved in 20% of patients. Carotid body tumours are usually confined to the adventititial layer and derive their blood supply from this. However, 5–10% are considered to be malignant because of local infiltration and distant metastases.

Diagnostic studies

The possibility of carotid body tumour should be considered in any patient with a lump in the anterior triangle of the neck. Errors in referral diagnosis occur in about 30% of cases and an unexpected finding of this lesion at surgery should be avoided. duplex ultrasound scanning will demonstrate both the relationship between the mass and the carotid bifurcation and the highly vascular nature of this lesion. CT and MR imaging scanning are useful in providing information about size and extent of local infiltration. Angiography should be performed when the former investigations suggest the diagnosis of a carotid body tumour and is required for operative management. Selective carotid angiography should demonstrate the tumour arising at the carotid bifurcation producing the characteristic saddle or splaying deformity. A late phase angiogram will demonstrate blushing indicative of the highly vascular nature of this lesion. Large tumours may demonstrate principal feeding vessels that may be amenable to embolization. Furthermore, bilateral angiography is important for the evaluation of concurrent atherosclerosis and identification of multicentric disease.

Surgical management

The majority of asymptomatic patients will eventually develop symptoms from local compression and local invasion if the tumour is managed conservatively. Furthermore, 30% will die from the effects of local invasion or metastatic disease. Therefore, all but the asymptomatic elderly patient should be considered for resection before the tumour becomes large or locally invasive. The aims of surgery are removal of tumour, preservation of cerebral function and protection of vital adjacent nerves.

Pre-operative management

Cranial nerve function should be evaluated. Furthermore, examination of the pharynx for invasion is important before surgery. The risks of hemiplegia and cranial nerve damage should be explained to the patient. Catecholamine screening should be reserved for patients with a history suggesting endocrine activity and those with bilateral tumours. Because these tumours are highly vascular, resection may result in excessive blood loss and 6 units of blood should be cross-matched. Although the role for pre-operative embolization is controversial, it may be considered for lesions larger than 3 cm. The external carotid artery usually provides the main feeding vessels for the tumour but there is also a contribution from the vertebral arteries. Brain embolization with consequent stroke or death is therefore a risk of therapeutic embolization. Successful embolization should be followed by surgery within 2–3 days because of potential tumour revascularization. Pre-operative radiotherapy makes the operation more difficult and therefore has no role.

Operative management

This operation is performed under a general anaesthetic; the use of nasal intubation may improve access in tumours extending high into the neck. The operator should be a vascular surgeon. The assistance of a head and neck surgeon may be helpful in lesions extending high in the neck. In addition to the operative field, the groin should be prepared as long saphenous vein may be needed. The positioning of the patient and incision are identical to those used during carotid endarterectomy. The common, internal and external carotid arteries are dissected and controlled with slings. The tumour is then mobilized circumferentially to assess the extent of the disease. The vagus and hypoglossal nerves are identified as they may be adherent or invaded by tumour. Bleeding may be reduced by clamping or dividing the external carotid artery. The Shamblin classification of carotid body tumours relates to resectability and is based on degree of arterial wall invasion. Group 1 lesions are small tumours with minimal involvement of the internal carotid artery and are relatively easy to remove. Group 2 tumours are larger. They demonstrate partial incorporation of the internal carotid artery requiring subadventitial dissection and the use of a temporary intraluminal shunt. Group 3 lesions encircle and invade the carotid bifurcation requiring *en bloc* removal of both tumour and internal carotid artery with autogenous vein interposition graft. Around 50% of carotid body tumours belong to Shamblin group 2, 25% to group 1 and 25% to group 3. For Shamblin groups 1 and 2 tumours, dissection begins at the bifurcation and displacement of the lesion upwards allows visualization of cranial nerves that lie beneath. The tumour is dissected along a white line that separates it from the adventitial layer of the artery. The media should not be resected as this leads to a weakened vessel wall with increased risk of intra-operative haemorrhage or post-operative carotid blowout. Dissection should be careful and haemostasis meticulous in order to see and preserve cranial nerves. Bipolar diathermy is recommended to reduce the risk of nerve damage. Exposure of lesions extending high in the neck may be improved by mobilization of the parotid gland and division of the digastric and stylohyoid muscles. In addition the styloid process may be fractured. Finally forward dislocation of the temporomandibular joint may be necessary. With very large tumours, the distal internal carotid artery may not be accessible and requires ligation following resection. This is associated with a stroke rate of up to 50% and mortality of up to 64%.

The patient should be managed post-operatively in a high dependency unit and monitored for neurological deficits and blood pressure control. Oral fluids are introduced cautiously in case cranial nerve injury causes aspiration. The incidence of nerve defects (mainly the mandibular branch of the facial nerve, the glossopharyngeal, the vagus, the hypoglossal and cervical sympathetics) ranges between 20 and 40% of cases and occurs more frequently in large tumours. However, the majority of these will resolve in several weeks. Patients with bilateral carotid body tumours should have each tumour excised at separate operations because of the risk of bilateral recurrent laryngeal and hypoglossal nerve damage. Patients with previous nerve damage following carotid body tumour resection are at high risk during surgery on contralateral lesions and radiotherapy or embolization may be an alternative. In most series stroke occurs in less than 3% of cases and mortality should approach zero.

Radiotherapy

Radiotherapy appears to slow the progression of carotid body tumours when used as primary treatment. However, there are few data available comparing the efficacy of this modality with surgery. Post-operative radiotherapy may be used in incomplete resections, histologically malignant lesions and in disease recurrence.

Prognosis

Surgery offers the only permanent cure for carotid body tumours. Survival of patients after 'curative' resection is similar to sex and age-matched controls. Metastatic disease develops in up to 2% of patients and disease recurrence in only 6% of patients following 'curative' resection. Patients with malignant tumours survive many years because of the characteristic slow growth of these lesions even in the presence of metastatic disease.

Further reading

European Carotid Surgery Trial

European Carotid Surgery Trialists' Collaborative Group (1991). MRC European Carotid Surgery Trial: interim results for symptomatic patients with severe (70–99%) or with mild (0–29%) stenosis. *Lancet* **337**: 1235–41.

European Carotid Surgery Trialists' Collaborative Group (1996). Endarterectomy for moderate symptomatic carotid stenosis: interim results from the MRC European Carotid Surgery Trial. *Lancet* **347**: 1591–3.

European Carotid Surgery Trialists' Collaborative Group (1998). Randomised trial of endarterectomy for recently symptomatic carotid stenosis: final results of the MRC European Carotid Surgery Trial (ECST). *Lancet* **351**: 1379–87.

Rothwell, P. and Warlow, C. P. (1999). Prediction of benefit from carotid endarterectomy in individual patients: a risk modelling study. *Lancet* **353**: 2105–10.

North American Symptomatic Carotid Endarterectomy Trial

Barnett, H. J. M., Taylor, D. W., Eliasziw, M. *et al.* (1998). Benefit of carotid endarterectomy in patients with symptomatic moderate or severe stenosis. *N Engl J Med* **339**: 1415–25.

North American Symptomatic Carotid Endarterectomy Trial Collaborators (1991). Beneficial effect of carotid endarterectomy in symptomatic patients with high grade carotid stenosis. *N Engl J Med* **325**: 445–53.

Asymptomatic Carotid Atherosclerosis Study

Barnett, H. J. M., Eliasziw, M., Meldrum, H. E. and Taylor, D. W. (1996). Do the facts and figures warrant a tenfold increase in the performance of carotid endarterectomy in asymptomatic patients? *Neurology* **466**: 603–8.

Executive Committee for the Asymptomatic Carotid Atherosclerosis Study (1995). Endarterectomy for asymptomatic carotid artery stenosis. *JAMA* **273**: 1421–8.

Carotid endarterectomy in general

Counsell, C., Salinas, R., Naylor, A. R. and Warlow, C. P. (1997). A systematic review of the randomised trials of carotid patch angioplasty in carotid endarterectomy. *Eur J Vasc Endovasc Surg* **13**: 345–54.

Eckstein H. H., Schumacher, H., Ringleb, P. and Allenberg, J. R. (1998). Indications for surgery in neurologically unstable patients. In: Branchereau A. and Jacobs M., eds. *European Vascular Course: New Trends and Developments in Carotid Artery Disease.* Armont: Futura, 77–92.

Hsai, D. C., Krushat, W. M., Moscoe, L. M. (1998). Epidemiology of carotid endarterectomy among Medicare beneficiaries: 1985–96 update. *Stroke* **29**: 346–350.

Naylor, A. R., Hayes, P. D., Allroggen, H. *et al.*. (2002). Reducing the risk of carotid surgery: a seven year audit of the role of monitoring and quality control assessment. *J Vasc Surg* (in press).

Angiography and angioplasty

Brown, M. M. (1992). Balloon angioplasty for cerebrovascular disease. *Neurol Res* **14**(Suppl): 159–63.

Davies, K. N. and Humphrey, P. R. (1993). Complications of cerebral angiography in patients with symptomatic carotid territory ischaemia screened by carotid ultrasound. *J Neurol Neurosurg Psych* **56**: 967–72.

Carotid body tumours

Whitehill, T. A. and Krupski, W. C. (2000). Uncommon disorders affecting the carotid arteries: carotid body tumors. In: Rutherford, R. B., ed. *Vascular Surgery*. Pennsylvania: W. B. Saunders, 1856–62.

MODULE 24

Renovascular disease and mesenteric ischaemia

1 • Epidemiology and pathology of renovascular disease

2 • Mesenteric ischaemia

Percutaneous transluminal angioplasty (PTA) for ostial atherosclerotic renal-artery stenosis has poor results. Angioplasty with stent placement (PTAS) is a better technique than PTA to achieve vessel patency in ostial atherosclerotic renal-artery stenosis. Primary PTAS and primary PTA plus PTAS as rescue therapy have similar outcomes. However, the burden of reintervention after PTA outweighs the potential saving in stents, so primary PTAS is a better approach to use.

Section 24.1 • Epidemiology and pathology of renovascular disease

There are two main causes of renal artery stenosis, fibromuscular dysplasia (FMD), which is relatively uncommon and seen mainly in young to middle-aged women, and atheromatous renovascular disease (ARVD), an increasingly common disease seen in the older patient (>50 years). Although stenosis of the renal artery is common to both pathological types, they differ dramatically in their epidemiology, clinical presentation and prognosis. Since ARVD is now such a commonly encountered finding this section will concentrate mainly on this cause of renal artery stenosis and on its presentation and clinical management.

Fibromuscular dysplasia

FMD is the most common cause of renovascular hypertension in young people and has been classified according to four different pathological types (see page 716). However, the most common type in adults (accounting for over 70% of cases) is medial fibroplasia which produces the classical beading pattern on angiography due to areas of medial thickening interspersed with aneurysmal dilatation. By contrast with atherosclerosis, patients with FMD very rarely progress to complete occlusion. FMD is usually managed very successfully by angiographic transluminal dilatation leading to a reduction in blood pressure and need for antihypertensive drugs. Recurrent disease is not common but renal artery duplex scanning can be done at regular intervals to determine if further intervention is required.

Atheromatous renovascular disease

The prevalence of ARVD in the population is unknown but there are various sources of data suggesting it is common, particularly in patients over the age of 50 years with other risk factors for generalized atherosclerosis. Post-mortem studies report an overall prevalence of 4–20%, but this rises to 25–30% for those over 60 years and 40–60% for those over 75 years. Patients undergoing investigation for vascular disease elsewhere have a high prevalence of ARVD; in an American review of three studies involving 1600 patients undergoing cardiac catheterization, 11–23% of patients were found to have renal artery stenosis (defined as >50% in at least one kidney) at aortography.

In contrast with FMD, the renal ostium is involved in ARVD in 85% of patients and in less than 5% the second or distal third of the main renal artery is involved. It is also important to be aware that bilateral ARVD is common (30–80% of patients) and a shrunken, atrophic kidney on ultrasound has an approximately 70% chance of being associated with a significant renal artery stenosis.

Clinical presentation of atheromatous renal artery stenosis

ARVD can present in several different ways which in turn demand different clinical management strategies.

Incidental non-significant renal artery stenosis

Non-haemodynamically significant stenosis (<60–65%) can present as a 'silent finding' whilst investigating other types of vascular disease. ARVD is a progressive disease and these patients need follow-up and monitoring of blood pressure and renal function. Repeat imaging is indicated if there is deterioration in these parameters.

Significant stenosis with normal range serum creatinine

Haemodynamically significant stenosis can present with isolated hypertension and apparently normal renal function (i.e. serum creatinine within the normal range). However, more sensitive measures of renal function based on radioisotope glomerular filtration rate (GFR) measurements often show diminished function. The management of this group of patients is controversial in that improvement in blood pressure control following renal artery angioplasty is usually modest and its value in preservation of renal function, especially in unilateral disease is uncertain.

Ischaemic renal disease

Ischaemic renal disease (IRD) is a term sometimes used to describe the group of patients presenting with renal impairment, usually also with hypertension due to atheromatous stenotic narrowing of the renal artery. The reduced perfusion to the renal parenchyma results in shrinking of renal size, patchy cortical scarring, and at a histological level, glomerular involution and sclerosis with renal tubular drop-out or atrophy. There are three main anatomical variations of IRD:

- stenosis or occlusion in a single kidney
- bilateral critical stenosis or occlusion
- unilateral critical stenosis with a contralateral non-functioning kidney.

It is important to realize that the pathological end result in IRD may also be as a result of other comorbid conditions. These would include cholesterol athero-emboli, worsening hypertensive damage and the co-existence of other renal parenchymal disease, for example due to diabetes mellitus. IRD results in progressive renal impairment and is currently an important cause of end-stage renal failure. It has been estimated that 14–20% of all patients entering dialysis programmes have ARVD as the primary cause of renal failure.

Diagnosis of atheromatous renal artery stenosis

When deciding on which screening and diagnostic tests are most appropriate to diagnose or exclude ARVD it is important to realize the specificity and sensitivity of the test depends the mode of presentation of the disease as noted previously.

Suspected renovascular hypertension with normal range creatinine

A patient presenting in this way is more likely to have unilateral ARVD disease and although GFR may be reduced, the serum creatinine is likely to be within the normal laboratory range. In this situation isotope renography is very useful as a screening test, it may be used alone or combined with an angiotensin converting enzyme (ACE) inhibitor (commonly captopril) which enhances any difference in functional activity between the two kidneys in the presence of renal artery stenosis. The most common isotopes used are technetium-99m labelled diethylenetriamine pentaacetic acid (DTPA), a marker of glomerular filtration, and technetium-99m labelled mercaptoacetyl-triglycine (MAG3), a marker of renal blood flow. These tracers are injected twice, with and without prior administration of oral captopril (25–50 mg) and sequential scintigrams are recorded. Patients must stop taking diuretics and ACE inhibitors 3–5 days prior to the investigation. This test is very useful in that it has a high negative predictive value if the scan is completely normal in this situation. Another common screening method used in some centres is renal artery duplex scanning. This method is highly dependent upon local radiological expertise and as such does not have universal appeal. However, in experienced hands has been reported to have a sensitivity of 84% and a positive predictive value of 76% in detecting a greater than 50% stenosis of a single renal artery.

Renal arteriography remains the gold standard diagnostic test but because of its invasive nature particularly in this situation, magnetic resonance angiography (MRA) and spiral computer tomography (spiral CT) are commonly employed with very good results.

Diagnosis of ischaemic renal disease

In this situation, where there is by definition impaired renal function, non-invasive screening tests are generally less useful. Isotopic scans are particularly difficult to interpret because they rely on the comparison of an involved with an uninvolved kidney. In ischaemic renal disease there is almost always bilateral disease even if this is not entirely due to renal artery stenosis. These tests are particularly insensitive and difficult to interpret where there is significant uraemia and a raised serum creatinine. Therefore in clinical practice, a high degree of clinical suspicion, in for example a patient with widespread evidence of vascular disease and renal impairment, would provoke the clinician to proceed with the investigations outlined below.

MRA and spiral CT, which are non-invasive, have been shown to be useful for screening and diagnosis of ARVD. However, accessory renal arteries and other small lesions can be missed with MRA, and the very nature of the computerized image production utilized in this method can also lead to over-interpretation of some lesions which may not in fact be significant. Spiral CT requires the peripheral intravenous injection of a large volume of contrast which is potentially nephrotoxic, however studies have shown results that are comparable with intra-arterial digital subtraction angiography.

Intra-arterial digital subtraction angiography provides the best images to support or refute the diagnosis of IRD and it also provides additional useful information such as the presence or absence of accessory arteries and collateral blood supply. There is a risk associated with the catheterization of a major artery. The risk associated with angiography via femoral artery puncture is about 0.5–2%, but depends on the degree of generalized atherosclerotic disease in the vessels, obesity and blood pressure. Most of the risk is associated with the formation of haematoma at the puncture site, but more serious events such as cholesterol emboli, false aneurysms and arterial dissection and thrombosis may occur.

Treatment of atheromatous renovascular disease

The benefit of any intervention for unilateral disease with a normal, functioning contralateral kidney is unproven. Revascularization has been only modestly effective in treating hypertension associated with the hyper-reninaemic state in this situation. In most studies only approximately one-third of patients treated by percutaneous angioplasty show an improvement in blood pressure. This improvement in blood pressure is often only manifest in a reduction in the number of antihypertensive agents required and a 'cure' (diastolic <90 mmHg on no treatment) is seen in less than 10% of patients.

However, more generally agreed aims of treatment in ischaemic renal disease are stabilization or reversal of renal impairment. The rationale for surgical or radiological intervention in patients with ARVD has developed from studies of the natural history of the condition, which have shown that 5% of patients with >60% arterial narrowing will progress to renal artery occlusion each year. The main treatment options for ischaemic renal disease are as follows: percutaneous transluminal angioplasty with or without endovascular stenting, surgical revascularization, or 'medical' therapy. The best approach for the patient with IRD should be determined by: the site and the nature of the lesion, any comorbid disease/anaesthetic risk and most importantly local experience and expertise in any one method.

Percutaneous transluminal renal angioplasty

Percutaneous transluminal renal angioplasty (PTRA) became a commonly used treatment strategy for renal artery stenosis in the 1980s and is the treatment of choice for fibromuscular dysplasia where the technical success rate is very near to 100% in most series. The advantages of PTRA over surgery include: (1) avoidance of risk associated with a general anaesthetic, (2) shorter inpatient stay times, (3) lower cost, and (4) low mortality and relatively low morbidity rates. The complications relate to the site of arterial puncture and damage to the renal artery. Those complications most commonly encountered are haematoma and false aneurysm, arterial dissection and thrombosis, cholesterol embolization, and rarely arterial rupture. The overall complication rate of PTRA is 5% in most series, it varies depending on case mix and the experience of the centre but in general this means it can be carried out as an outpatient.

Results of percutaneous transluminal renal angioplasty in atheromatous renal artery stenosis. Comparison of results between series is again difficult because of variations in the severity of ARVD, the site of the stenosis as well as inclusion of cases of fibromuscular dysplasia. However, it is accepted that there is a high (approximately 85%) initial technical success rate in most series. PTRA has a lower initial success rate when the atherosclerotic lesion is longer or ostial or when the vessel is occluded. The main draw back to this treatment is the high restenosis rate which occurs in up to 35% of cases. There are few long-term follow-up studies of patency but at 12 months following PTRA, restenosis is more common in ostial lesions (65%) compared with proximal or truncal lesions (25–35%). Despite this high restenosis rate, repeat PTRA is usually possible with reasonable results. Therefore cases at high risk of restenosis should be followed clinically and, with the imaging techniques detailed above, long-term reasonable results are therefore expected.

The impact of PTRA on renal function in ischaemic renal disease is more controversial. While observational data exist, there has not been a randomized controlled trial comparing PTRA (with or without stenting) with medical management alone. Sos studied 55 patients with 70% bilateral stenosis and a mean pre-treatment creatinine of 3.1 mg/dl (280 mmol/l). PTRA was successful in 45 patients, renal function improved in 47% and worsened in 9%, and acute renal failure requiring dialysis resulted in five patients. Follow-up to 2 years showed only 47% of patients remained dialysis independent, 27% were dead and 25% were on dialysis. Many authors report that the most encouraging results are seen where there has been a relatively rapid decline in renal function without evidence of co-existent disease and preserved renal parenchymal thickness. The question of functional improvement in renal function after intervention versus 'best medical management' for ischaemic renal disease is being addressed by the forthcoming ASTRAL trial (Angioplasty and Stent for Renal Artery Lesions).

Endovascular stents

The disappointing long-term results with PTRA, particularly for ostial lesions provoked the use of endovascular stents in an attempt to improve patency. Proof that primary and long-term patency is improved has recently been shown by van de Ven and colleagues. Forty-two patients with atherosclerotic ostial stenosis underwent PTRA and PTRA with stenting; primary patency rates (<50% residual stenosis) were achieved in 57% and 88% of patients respectively. Furthermore at 6 months patency was only 29% with PTRA but was 75% with endovascular stenting. A more recent study compared stent placement in ostial and non-ostial stenosis and found that stent placement considerably improved patency in ostial lesions but compared with successful PTRA had no benefit on proximal and isolated truncal lesions.

Surgical treatment of atheromatous renal artery stenosis

Surgical techniques are now really only indicated for the preservation or restoration of renal function. Where hypertension appears to be the only factor complicating renal artery stenosis, percutaneous transluminal renal artery angioplasty is used when intervention is warranted. The main indications for surgical treatment are as follows: ostial stenosis of the renal artery; failure of PTRA; severe contrast hypersensitivity; renal artery occlusion; aneurysmal renal artery; simultaneous aorto-iliac reconstruction and impossible percutaneous access due to aorto-iliac disease.

Reconstructive techniques currently used include: (1) aortorenal bypass using saphenous vein, hypogastric artery or in selected cases, synthetic material, (2) re-insertion of the renal artery onto the aorta, (3) thrombo-endarterectomy via arteriotomy or by a transaortic approach, and (4) extra-anatomical bypass procedures, e.g. splenorenal bypass on the left side and hepatorenal bypass on the right. Comparison of different surgical techniques is difficult as case mix is often not well matched between groups and also definitions of 'improvement' are not consistent and often refer to hypertension as well as renal function. The question of deciding the best timing for surgical intervention or indeed PTRA is a difficult one. ARVD is undoubtedly a progressive disease, and intervention where there is renal impairment, hypertension and preserved renal size is common. Intervention before this time is controversial mainly due to a significant complication and mortality rate.

Results of surgical treatment. A cure of hypertension in ARVD has been reported in 25–60% of patients, and 'improvement' reported in a further 30–35% of patients. In patients with IRD, functional improvement occurs in 50–70% of cases depending on the centre and presumably case mix. Examples of recent studies are shown below (Table 24.1). In the study by Cambria, operative management consisted of aortorenal bypass in 47%, extra-anatomic bypass in 45% and endarterectomy in 8% of patients. Improvement in function was defined as a 20% reduction in serum creatinine; it is also worth noting that the actuarial survival in this high-risk group of patients was 52 ± 5% at 5 years post-procedure.

Medical treatment

Hypertension is often present in cases of renal artery stenosis. Control of blood pressure is an important factor in reducing the decline in renal function with time. Angiotensin II is involved in the maintenance of GFR through its constrictive effects on the efferent arteriole. Therefore angiotensin converting enzyme inhibitors (ACEI) whilst being effective in controlling blood pressure are usually best avoided as they can precipitate acute renal failure which may be irreversible. Although there are no randomized controlled trials to support the use of cholesterol lowering and the use of aspirin, many clinicians would recommend lowering cholesterol with a statin. Similarly no specific targets have been recommended but many would aim to lower cholesterol to secondary cardiovascular prevention levels and prescribe aspirin at 150 mg/day.

Summary

Atheromatous renovascular disease is an increasingly important cause of chronic renal failure and end stage renal disease. Revascularization is indicated in ischaemic renal disease where there is good preservation of renal parenchymal thickness. Intervention for HT alone is improven. Surgical results are currently superior to PTRA but recent evidence suggests PTRA with endovascular stenting may be able to achieve similar results. Currently the method of revascularization will be determined by local expertise and facilities as well as patient factors.

Section 24.2 • Mesenteric ischaemia

The overall volume of blood supplied to the splanchnic bed is approximately 1.5 l/min. The blood supply to the gut is via three anterior branches of the intra-abdominal aorta: the coeliac, superior mesenteric and inferior mesenteric arteries. There is a rich collateral system linking the above arteries and other vessels (especially the middle rectal arteries, branches of the internal iliacs) which allows the gut to survive even when one and occasionally two of these major aortic branches are occluded. For this to be possible there must be a slow progressive stenosis leading to occlusion rather than an acute event such as an embolus. The venous return is via the portal system. Mesenteric ischaemia may arise from acute or chronic arterial or venous disease.

Arterial anatomy

The **coeliac artery** arises as the first anterior branch of the abdominal aorta immediately below the median arcuate ligament. The coeliac artery is short and divides into three branches: the hepatic, the left gastric and the splenic artery. The coeliac artery supplies the foregut:

Table 24.1 Effect of surgical revascularization procedures on renal function in ischaemic renal disease

Author	*No. of patients*	*Improved (%)*	*Stable (%)*	*Worse (%)*	*Mortality (%)*
Novick (1987)	161	58	31	11	2.1
Messina *et al.* (1992)	17	77	12	11	0
Cambria (1996)	139	54	19	27	8
Darling *et al.* (1999)	176[a]	26	68	6	5.5

[a]Subgroup of 'symptomatic patients' with raised serum creatinine ± hypertension.

the lower oesphagus, the stomach and duodenum proximal to the ampulla of Vater. It collateralizes with the superior mesenteric artery via the hepatic artery through the gastroduodenal artery.

The **superior mesenteric artery** arises usually within 1 cm below the coeliac artery. It anastomoses with the coeliac artery via the pancreaticoduodenal artery. It passes over the uncinate process of the head of the pancreas, anterior to the left renal vein. It supplies the midgut: the duodenum distal to the ampulla of Vater, the jejunum, the ileum and the large bowel as far as the mid-transverse colon. The superior mesenteric supplies the proximal and distal parts of its territory via proximal branches and the middle of its territory via its more distal branches. The result of this is that emboli, which usually pass beyond the first few centimetres of its length, spare the proximal small bowel and the transverse colon, but do affect the ileum and caecum. There are collaterals with the inferior mesenteric artery via the middle colic artery.

The **inferior mesenteric artery** arises anteriorly below the renal arteries a few centimetres above the aortic bifurcation. It gives rise to the left colic artery early, which itself divides into ascending and descending branches.

Venous anatomy

Veins draining the gut initially follow the arterial supply but eventually they all drain into the portal vein which carries the blood into the liver. From the liver blood drains via the hepatic veins into the inferior vena cava.

The **superior mesenteric vein** is formed by tributaries which follow the arterial supply of the midgut. After passing over the third part of the duodenum and uncinate process of the pancreas, it runs behind the body of the pancreas and is joined by the **splenic vein** to form the **portal vein**. This runs up the free edge of the lesser omentum to the liver. The other foregut veins follow their respective arteries and take the shortest route to drain directly into the portal vein. The **inferior mesenteric vein** starts at the pelvic brim as the continuation of the **superior rectal vein**. This receives tributaries corresponding to the branches of the inferior mesenteric artery and runs up the retroperitoneum to the left of the midline. After passing to the left of the duodenojejunal flexure it runs behind the pancreas and drains into the splenic vein.

Acute mesenteric ischaemia

There has been little improvement in the management of this condition over the last few decades with the mortality rate for acute mesenteric infarction varying between 60 and 85%. The reasons for this are two-fold: the condition is not common, accounting for only 1–2% of patients with acute abdominal pain, and it is usually diagnosed late. This results in as many as 40% of patients receiving either no operation or an 'open and close' laparotomy.

Pathology

Acute arterial ischaemia may arise from an embolus or from the formation of *in situ* thrombus on an underlying stenosis. It may also occur as a result of a low cardiac output state (non-occlusive infarction). Other rare causes include aortic disection, fibromuscular dysplasia, intimal hyperplasia associated with the oral contraceptive, arteritis associated with rheumatoid arthritis, systemic lupus erythematosus and polyarteritis nodosa. Mesenteric ischaemia may also occur in Takayasu's and Behçet's diseases. Thrombosis of aortic and visceral aneurysms may also be responsible.

Clinical features

The distinction between an embolic and a thrombotic cause of acute mesenteric ischaemia is often difficult. However, classically a mesenteric embolus would present as acute colicky central abdominal pain of abrupt onset in a patient with atrial fibrillation or recent myocardial infarction with no antecedent history of gastrointestinal upset or weight loss. A more insidious onset suggests mesenteric artery thrombosis. As this is superimposed on chronic occlusive disease there may be a prior history of post-prandial abdominal pain ('intestinal angina'), weight loss and diarrhoea indicating pre-existing mesenteric ischaemia.

A history of minor gastrointestinal bleeding is a late symptom occurring in approximately a quarter of patients. Abdominal pain may be mild or more classically out of proportion to the physical findings. Onset of signs of peritoneal irritation or frank peritonitis is usually a late sign and indicative of irreversible bowel ischaemia.

Investigations

The plain abdominal radiograph may be normal. A markedly elevated white cell count is suggestive of severe mesenteric ischaemia. In a review of 103 patients with acute mesenteric ischaemia 44% had a white cell count above 20 000. An unexpected acidosis can also be a clue. A raised serum phosphate has been reported to be diagnostic, though this has not been confirmed by other studies. A raised serum amylase is common in mesenteric infarction, but is again not diagnostic. The use of intraluminal pH tonometry has been explored but not fully evaluated. Angiography is a diagnostic investigation of both arterial and in the venous phase, venous infarction. Superior mesenteric artery thrombosis is seen as a tapering of the origin of the vessel, whilst embolic occlusion shows an abrupt blockage, often at a branching point.

Management

The key to successful management is a high index of suspicion. By the time the diagnosis is clear it is usually too late for the patient. There is massive fluid loss as a consequence of mesenteric ischaemia/infarction. The adequate replacement of this dramatic and often underestimated fluid loss (2–3 litres) is of prime importance. As the patients are often elderly with cardiovascular disease the replacement should be closely monitored.

Early operation in the hope of removing an embolus or bypassing an atheromatous occlusion is the key. The first successful mesenteric embolectomy was carried out in 1951. Embolectomy is performed by incision over the superior mesenteric artery in the root of the small bowel mesentery. The superior mesenteric artery is controlled, an arteriotomy is made and thrombus removed by suction and a balloon embolectomy catheter. Any non-viable bowel is excised. If the embolus is lodged beyond the major early branches of the superior mesenteric artery simple bowel resection may be enough. Patients who undergo bowel resection without revascularization not infrequently die of ischaemia of the remaining intestine. Despite revascularization the mortality rate is reported between 20 and 70%.

Acute mesenteric ischaemia secondary to arterial thrombosis rather than embolus may be diagnosed radiographically or intra-operatively. The site of occlusion is usually at the origin of the artery rather than at its first major bifurcation. At operation this is manifest by no pulse being palpable in the proximal portion of the artery in contrast to embolic disease where a pulse may be present proximally. The treatment of choice is a short aorto-superior mesenteric artery bypass, preferably with saphenous vein because of the risk of prosthetic graft infection in the presence of ischaemic bowel. The superior mesenteric artery is exposed in the root of the small bowel mesentery and the graft routed round its free edge to the aorta.

Non-occlusive mesenteric ischaemia is a very uncommon condition. It is normally a product of end stage cardiovascular collapse secondary to a low cardiac output. The condition carries a high mortality.

An important aspect of the surgical management of patients with acute mesenteric ischaemia is the 'second look' laparotomy within 24 hours of the first procedure, as a high proportion (40%) of patients require a further bowel resection at the second operation. In the intervening time the patient's overall condition can be also improved.

The role of free radicals in the sequelae of intestinal ischaemia has been the subject of much animal experimentation. There is little evidence for their role in humans. However, as allopurinol, a xanthine oxidase inhibitor, is an effective protector of reperfused animal bowel, and as it is relatively free of side-effects it has been suggested that it should be used in humans following revascularization. The local catheter infusion of papaverine has been shown to be effective in overcoming precapillary vasospasm associated with mesenteric occulsion; however, it has not gained much acceptance.

Acute mesenteric venous thrombosis

Primary acute mesenteric vein thrombosis is usually diagnosed late, but as it causes less widespread ischaemia it is associated with a lower mortality rate (around 40%) than arterial occlusion. However, when it occurs secondary to another event (visceral infection, systemic hyper-coagulability or portal hypertension) its outlook is similar to mesenteric arterial occlusion. The 'acute' history may be prolonged with a reported average of 14 days – up to three-quarters of patients have a history longer than a week and a quarter longer than a month. A previous episode of deep venous thrombosis or pulmonary embolus may be present in up to 50% of such patients, with up to 75% of cases being associated with hypercoagulability, portal hypertension or visceral infection. Some patients may complain of a preceding flu-like illness. A plain abdominal radiograph may show a dilated or thick-walled small bowel with an irregular mucosal pattern. CT scan features have been used to diagnose the condition (Table 24.2). Acute mesenteric venous thrombosis may result in infarction or it may run a more benign course.

Table 24.2 CT scan features of acute mesenteric vein thrombosis

- Enlargement of mesenteric or portal vein
- Sharp definition of venous wall
- Hyperlucency of venous wall
- Central venous low density (thrombus)

The diagnosis is more usually made at laparotomy, but if it is made by other means the patient should be heparinized to prevent further thrombus propagation and bowel necrosis. Nevertheless all patients should be explored with a view to resecting non-viable bowel as without this precaution mortality rates of 100% have been reported. Post-operatively the patient should be heparinized and life-long anticoagulation has been advocated. During the post-operative period the patient should be investigated for coagulopathic conditions.

Chronic mesenteric ischaemia

There is no doubt that chronic mesenteric ischaemia exists as a clinical entity. However, it is an uncommon diagnosis and, as with acute mesenteric ischaemia, is often diagnosed late. It is unusual for a single vessel occlusion to be responsible, unless previous surgery has interrupted the collateral pathways.

Clinical features

The patient is usually female and complains of abdominal pain, classically related to eating, which may cause fear of eating and consequent weight loss. Numerous investigations have usually been carried out including, occasionally, a negative laparotomy. As the patient is generally elderly, other disease processes such as diverticulosis may mislead the clinician. There may be nausea, vomiting and alteration in bowel habit. On examination, the patient will have lost weight and may exhibit an epigastric bruit. In this age group, however, a bruit is not unusual.

Investigation

This is usually a diagnosis of exclusion, the common causes of abdominal pain having been investigated.

Any patient being considered for an investigative laparotomy for chronic abdominal pain and weight loss should have arterial investigations prior to operation. The initial investigation of choice is non-invasive duplex ultrasound scanning which may show abnormal velocity waveforms and flow, especially in the superior mesenteric artery. The definitive investigation, however, is a transfemoral angiogram. Lateral and oblique views are required to demonstrate the origins of the anteriorly arising arteries followed by selective catheterization and imaging of each artery in turn. The presence of large collateral vessels may indicate a missed occlusion/stenosis.

Management

The lesions are usually ostial and are often extensions of aortic atheroma. The management options are balloon angioplasty with or without stenting, transaortic endarterectomy or bypass grafting.

Balloon angioplasty

Balloon angioplasty is a less invasive procedure than open surgery and consequently morbidity and mortality is likely to be lower. Primary technical and clinical success rates have been reported to be good, with success also being possible for repeat angioplasty. It is difficult to recommend angioplasty as first-line treatment, however, until more evidence is available – the consequences of failure can be catastrophic with acute mesenteric arterial occlusion requiring emergency surgical revascularization. Angioplasty should be considered in malnourished, poor-risk patients, particularly if the lesion is a stenosis rather than an occlusion.

Transaortic endarterectomy can be used for combined occlusions of the superior mesenteric, coeliac and occasionally renal arteries and requires supra-coeliac aortic clamping. This is a large undertaking and carries a peri-operative mortality of around 10%. In the hands of enthusiasts the results can be good but, in general, the procedure is less commonly used than bypass grafting.

There are many technical variations of visceral artery bypass with respect to the graft used (saphenous vein, Dacron or externally reinforced polytetrafluoroethylene), graft configuration (antegrade 'wide-sweep', retrograde, multiple vessels) or direct reimplantation. Which approach is best has not been proven, although in a limited comparison of Dacron and vein grafts, the former produced long-term patency in five out of six compared with a patency of one out of six vein grafts. Antegrade bypass (taking the origin of the bypass proximal to the coeliac artery) is a greater untaking than retrograde bypass (where the origin of the bypass is from the infra-renal aorta) but it does result in a better configuration for the graft with less risk of kinking. Antegrade bypass also allows revascularization of the coeliac and superior mesenteric arteries at the same time. This is generally recommended although there is no hard evidence to support it. If a single vessel is to be revascularized then it should usually be the superior mesenteric. This can be very successful, particularly in emergency cases, and can be performed in retrograde fashion so avoiding the risks of supra-coeliac cross-clamping.

From time to time mesenteric vessel occlusion is discovered in a patient undergoing angiogram prior to aortic reconstructive surgery There is little guidance in the literature as to the appropriate action in these circumstances. One author does advocate the addition of a mesenteric bypass, and in a limited retrospective analysis there appeared to be a benefit.

Colon ischaemia

Ischaemia of the large bowel is essentially an acute phenomenon, although it may have late sequelae. Boley introduced a useful classification of this condition based on the depth of the ischaemia:

- Type 1. Transient mild mucosal ischaemia with complete return to normal appearance and function.
- Type 2. Muscle and mucosal ischaemia, which may lead to chronic stricture formation.
- Type 3. Full thickness ischaemia, gangrene and perforation.

The classically affected site is the splenic flexure, which is a 'watershed' between the superior and inferior mesenteric arterial supply. Depending on the severity of the Boley type the patient may mimic acute diverticulitis with mild abdominal pain or bloody diarrhoea or may present with collapse and peritonitis. What determines the severity is uncertain but poor cardiac function and large bowel distension may have a role. The diagnosis is made by colonoscopy or barium enema, both of which may be hazardous in the acute phase. Treatment is by circulatory support in types 1 and 2 with the possibility of elective colonic resection for a symptomatic stricture. Type 3 requires urgent colonic resection with formation of a colostomy.

Colonic ischaemia following aortic reconstruction

Ischaemic colitis is a not uncommon and much feared complication following aortic reconstruction. Ernst and co-workers prospectively recorded the incidence of ischaemic colitis by routine colonoscopy following aortic reconstruction and found it to be 6%, although ischaemic changes are present in 30% when biopsies are examined histologically. Ischaemic changes were noted in 4.3% of patients undergoing aortic surgery for occlusive disease and 7.4% for aneurysmal disease. Patients with ruptured aortic aneurysm have been reported to have an incidence as high as 60%. The overall mortality rate when colon ischaemia follows aortic reconstruction is approximately 50% and approaches 90% when there is transmural involvement.

Peri-operative ligation of a patent inferior mesenteric artery with poor back flow is believed to be the main factor in the development of the condition, although other risk factors have been identified, including previous symptoms of visceral ischaemia and flow from the inferior mesenteric to the superior mesenteric in the marginal artery. An awareness of the collateral circulation to the left colon is vitally important, especially the role of the mid-colic branch of the superior mesenteric artery and the internal iliac arteries.

Prevention

The use of intra-operative techniques to assess the adequacy of the left colonic blood supply has been advocated. Sterile intra-operative hand-held Doppler probe signal, an inferior mesenteric artery stump pressure less than 40 mmHg, an intramural pH measurement using balloon catheter tonimetry of less than 7, a reduced pulse oximetry and a loss of photoplethysmographic pulsatility have all been advocated as predictive of ischaemia.

Clinical features

A high index of suspicion is the most important factor in the diagnosis of this complication. The most common symptom is diarrhoea, with or without frank blood. Diarrhoea usually begins 24–48 hours after operation. There is debate as to whether bloody diarrhoea is a worse prognostic sign. Nevertheless, the presence of diarrhoea mandates a careful colonoscopy. Other symptoms include abnormal post-operative pain, particularly left sided, and progressive abdominal distension with increasing peritonism. Unexplained sepsis (i.e. a white cell count over 20×10^6 cells/l), acidosis, progressive oliguria and severe thrombocytopenia (less than 90×10^9 platelets/l) may suggest bowel infarction. Reversible lesions should improve within 7–10 days.

Prevention of ischaemic colitis is by far the best management, as diagnosis can be difficult and subsequent treatment carries a high mortality.

Coeliac axis compression syndrome

This is a contentious condition, in that reduction of flow through a single gut artery is not expected to produce symptoms. It is suggested that the coeliac axis is compressed and narrowed as it passes under the median arcuate ligament. The largest series with the longest follow-up is reported from San Francisco. Fifty-one patients underwent 16 simple decompressions with long-term symptomatic success in 53%. Thirty-five had additional flow enhancing procedures such as dilatation or reconstruction of whom 76% had a long-term relief of symptoms. The best correlation with success was women who had lost more than 9 kg in weight.

Summary

The early consideration of the diagnosis and its objective investigation appears to be the key to success in the treatment of this difficult group of patients.

Further reading

Abdu, R., Zakhour, B. J. and Dallis, D. J. (1987). Review: Mesenteric venous thrombosis. *Surgery* **101**: 383–8.

Baumgartner, I., von Aesch, K., Do, D. -D. *et al.* (2000). Stent placement in ostial and nonostial atherosclerotic renal arterial stenoses: a prospective follow-up study. *Radiology* **216**: 498–505.

Bergan, J. J., Dean, R. H., Conn, J. Jr and Yao, J. S. T. (1975). Revascularisation in the treatment of mesenteric infarction. *Ann Surg* **182**: 274–81.

Bergan, J. J., Flinn, W. R., McCarthy, W. J., Yao, J. S. T. (1987). Acute mesenteric ischaemia. In: Bergan, J. J. and Yao, J. S. T., eds. *Vascular Surgical Emergencies*. Orlando: Grune and Stratton, 401–13.

Bergan, J. J., McCarthy, W., Flinn, W. R. and Yao, J. S. T. (1987). Non-traumatic mesenteric vascular emergencies. *J Vasc Surg* **5**: 903–9.

Black, H. R., Bourgoignie, J. J., Pickering, T. *et al.* (1991). Report of the working party group for patient selection and preparation: captopril renography. *Am J Hypertens* **4**: 745s–6s.

Boley, S. J., Brandt, L. J. and Veith, F. J. (1978). Ischaemic disorders of the intestines. *Curr Prob Surg* **15**: 1–85.

Boley, S. J., Feinstein, S. R., Sammartano, R. *et al.* (1981). New concepts in the management of emboli of the superior mesenteric artery. *Surg Gynecol Obstet* **153**: 561–9.

Breslin, D. J., Swinton, N. W., Libertino, J. A. and Zinman, L. (1982). *Renovascular Hypertension*. Baltimore, MD: Williams and Wilkins.

Brooks, J. and Carey, L. C. (1973). Base deficit in superior mesenteric artery occlusion: an aid to early diagnosis. *Ann Surg* **177**: 352–6.

Clark, A. Z. and Gallant, T. E. (1984). Acute mesenteric ischaemia: angiographic spectrum. *Am J Radiol* **142**: 555–62.

Clavien, P. A. (1990). Diagnosis and management of mesenteric infarction. *Br J Surg* **77**: 601–3.

Clavien, P. A., Durig, M. and Harder, F. (1982). Venous mesenteric infarction: a particular entity. **154**: 205–8.

Clavien, P. A., Muller, C. and Harder, F. (1987). Treatment of mesenteric infarction. *Br J Surg* **74**: 500–3.

Darling, R. C., Kreienberg, P. B., Chang, B. B. *et al.* (1999). Outcome of renal artery reconstruction: analysis of 687 procedures. *Ann Surg* **230**: 524–30.

Ernst, C. B., Hagihara, P. F., Daugherty, M. E. *et al.* (1976). Ischemic colitis incidence following abdominal aortic reconstruction: a prospective study. *Surgery* **80**: 417–21.

Grim, C. E., Yune, H. Y., Donahue, J. P. *et al.* (1982). Unilateral renal vascular hypertension: surgery vs. dilatation. *Hypertension* **4**: 367–8.

Hagihara, P. F., Ernst, C. B. and Grifen, W. O. Jr (1979). Incidence of ischemic colitis following abdominal aortic reconstruction. *Surg Gynecol Obstet* **149**: 571–3.

Harding, M. B., Smith, L. R., Himmelstein, S. I. *et al.* (1992). Renal artery stenosis: prevalence and associated risk factors in patients undergoing cardiac catheterization. *J Am Soc Nephrol* **2**: 1608–14.

Isles, C. G., Robertson, S. and Hill, D. (1999). Management of renovascular disease: a review of renal artery stenting in ten studies. *Q J Med* **92**: 159–67.

Jamieson, W. C., Marchuk, S., Ronsom, J. *et al.* (1982). The early diagnosis of massive acute intestinal ischaemia. *Br J Surg* **69**(Suppl): 552–3.

Johansson, M., Jensen, G., Aurell, M. *et al.* (2000). Evaluation of duplex ultrasound and captopril renography for detection of renovascular hypertension. *Kidney Int* **58**: 774–82.

Johnson, W. C. and Nabseth, D. C. (1974). Visceral infarction following aortic surgery. *Ann Surg* **180**: 312–18.

Kaatee, R., Beek, F. J. A., de Lange, E. E. *et al.* (1997). Renal artery stenosis: detection and quantification with spiral CT angiography versus optimised digital subtraction angiography. *Radiology* **205**: 121–7.

Kwaan, J. H. M., Connolly, J. E. and Coutsaftides, T. (1980). Concomitant revascularisation of intestines during aorto-iliac reconstruction: deterrent to catastrophic bowel infarction. *Can J Surg* **23**: 534–6.

Levy, P. J., Krausz, M. M. and Manny, J. (1990). Acute mesenteric ischaemia: improved results – a retrospective analysis of ninety-two patients. *Surgery* **107**: 372–80.

Mailloux, L. U., Belluci, R. O., Napolitano, B. *et al.* (1994). Survival estimates for 683 patients starting dialysis from 1970 through 1989: identification of risk factors for survival. *Clin Nephrol* **42**: 127–35.

Matsumoto, A. H., Tegtmeyer, C. J., Fitzcharles, E. K. *et al.* (1995). Percutaneous transluminal angioplasty of visceral artery stenosis: results and long term clinical follow up. *J Vasc Intervent Radiol* **6**: 165–74.

Matthews, J. E. and White, R. R. (1971). Primary mesenteric venous occlusive disease. *Am J Surg* **122**: 579–83.

Naitove, A. and Weisman, R. E. (1965). Primary mesenteric venous thrombosis. *Ann Surg* **161**: 516-23.

Novick, A. C., Ziegelbaum, M., Vidt, D. G. *et al.* (1987). Trends in surgical revascularisation for renal artery disease: ten years' experience. *JAMA* **257**: 498–501.

Ottinger, L. W. (1978). The surgical management of of acute occlusion of the superior mesenteric artery. *Ann Surg* **188**: 721–31.

Pederson, E. B. (1994). Angiotensin-converting enzyme inhibitor renography. Pathophysiological, diagnostic and therapeutic aspects in renal artery stenosis. *Nephrol, Dial Transplant* **9**: 482–92.

Peterson, R. A., Baldauf, C. G., Millward, S. F. *et al.* (2000). Outpatient percutaneous transluminal renal artery angioplasty: a Canadian experience. *J Vasc Interv Radiol* **11**: 327–32.

Preston, R. A. and Epstein, M. (1997). Ischaemic renal disease: an emerging cause of chronic renal failure and end stage renal disease (Editorial) *J Hypertens* **15**: 1365–77.

Rapp, J. H., Reilly, L. M., Qvarfordt, P. G. *et al.* (1986). Durability of of endarterectomy and antegrade grafts in the treatment of chronic visceral ischaemia. *J Vasc Surg* **3**: 799–806.

Reilly, L. M., Ammar, A. D., Stoney, R. J. and Ehrenfeld, W. K. (1985). Late results following operative repair for coeliac artery compression syndrome. *J Vasc Surg* **1**: 79–81.

Rogers, D. M., Thompson, J. E., Garrett, W. V. *et al.* (1982). Mesenteric vascular problems. A 26-year experience. *Ann Surg* **195**: 554–65.

Rosen, A., Kobin, M., Silverman, P. M. *et al.* (1984). Mesenteric vein thrombosis: CT identification. *Am J Roentgenol* **143**: 83–6.

Sachs, S. M., Morton, J. H. and Schwartz, S. I. (1982). Acute mesenteric ischaemia. *Surgery* **92**: 646–53.

Schroeder, T., Christoffersen, J. K., Andersen, J. *et al.* (1985). Ischemic colitis complicating reconstruction of the abdominal aorta. *Surg Gynecol Obstet* **160**: 299–303.

Sos, T. A. (1991). Angioplasty for the treatment of azotemia and renovascular hypertension in atherosclerotic renal artery disease. *Circulation* **83**: 162–6.

Tegtmeyer, C. J., Selby, J. B., Hartwell, G. D. *et al.* (1991). Results and complications of angioplasty in fibromuscular disease. *Circulation* **83**: 155–61.

Umpleby, H. C. (1987). Thrombosis of the superior mesenteric vein. *Br J Surg* **74**: 694–6.

van de Ven, P. J., Kaatee, R., Beutler, J. J. *et al.* (1999). Arterial stenting and balloon angioplasty in ostial atherosclerotic renovascular disease: a randomised trial. *Lancet* **353**: 282–6.

Welch, M., Baguneid, M. S., McMahon, R. F. *et al.* (1998). Histological study of colonic ischaemia after aortic surgery. *Br J Surg* **85**: 1095–8.

Zierler, R. E., Bergelin, R. O., Isaacson, J. A. and Strandness, D. E. Jr. (1994). Natural history of atherosclerotic renal artery stenosis: a prospective study with duplex ultrasonography. *J Vasc Surg* **19**: 250–8.

MODULE 25

Aneurysm

1 • Definitions
2 • Epidemiology
3 • Aetiology
4 • Diagnosis

Section 25.1 • Definitions

An aneurysm can be defined as an abnormal dilatation of a blood vessel. Aneurysms can be separated into true, false, dissecting and mycotic. The wall of a true aneurysm comprises all layers of the normal arterial wall. True aneurysms can be divided morphologically into two types; fusiform, a symmetrical swelling, and saccular, an asymmetric localized bulge. False aneurysms arise from a defect in the arterial wall, due to trauma at the site of an anastomosis, and the wall of such a false aneurysm is comprised of adventitia or fibrous tissue. Dissecting aneurysms arise from a defect in the intima with formation of a false channel tracking in the media which may re-enter the true lumen more distally. Mycotic aneurysms are caused by embolism of infective material which lodges in an artery. Bacterial proliferation and inflammation cause weakness and subsequent dilatation of the wall. Mycotic aneurysm is also widely used to describe any infection associated with the presence of an aneurysm.

The stage at which the increase in diameter of a blood vessel becomes abnormal is debatable. Arterial diameter within a population is a continuum and the measurement at which an artery becomes aneurysmal is arbitrary. Some authors have defined aortic aneurysm according to the ratio of the infra-renal aorta to the supra-renal aorta but this carries its own problems as the supra-renal aorta may also be abnormal. In practice most surgeons would consider an aorta greater than 30 mm in diameter or double the diameter of the adjacent aorta to be aneurysmal. Similar arguments can be applied to aneurysms at other sites.

Section 25.2 • Epidemiology

True aortic aneurysms are predominantly a condition of the elderly with a marked male sex bias. The Oxford screening programme of men aged 65–74 years reported a 2.3% prevalence of aortic diameter > 4.0 cm. The Birmingham Community Aneurysm Screening Project examined a similar population and reported 8.4% and 3.0% prevalence of aortic diameters >2.9 and >4.0 cm respectively. The mortality from aortic aneurysm in men aged >80 years is ten times that of men aged 55–64 years and 100 times than of men aged <55 years. The reported incidence is increasing. In Scotland the incidence in the general population has risen from 25.8 per 100 000 in 1971 to 63.6 per 100 000 in 1984. In England and Wales the mortality rate per 100 000 population has risen from 15.7 to 17.5 and 18.0 in 1988, 1992 and 1997, respectively. Similar increases have been reported in many other countries. The reported increasing incidence is partly due to an ageing population and better detection rates, due to greater awareness of the disease and increased use of ultrasound and computed tomographic (CT) scanning for other medical conditions. However, there is also a true underlying increase in the incidence of the condition.

Screening

There is ongoing debate as to whether screening programmes for the detection of asymptomatic abdominal aortic aneurysm (AAA) are worthwhile. There are a number of pilot studies and the evidence in support of screening is strengthening. The arguments for screening are that AAA rupture has an approximately 90% mortality rate while elective repair carries a mortality rate of only about 5% and if successful is essentially curative returning patients to a normal life expectancy. Screening by means of ultrasound scanning is non-invasive, is acceptable to patients and has excellent sensitivity and specificity. Economic studies have estimated that cost per life year saved is between £450 and 1500 which is considerably less than that calculated for breast cancer screening (approximately £4000). Aortic aneurysm screening meets the WHO criteria for a screening programme.

The counter-arguments are that most detected AAA will be small and are unlikely ever to require repair. Patients with such aneurysms would require frequent follow-up and may suffer anxiety about the diagnosis. Such anxiety may lead to inappropriate surgery on a small aneurysm which carries a significant mortality rate and may not be of benefit to the patient. Surveillance programmes for these small screen detected aneurysms would require significant resources. Some patients with larger aneurysms will be unfit for surgical repair and these patients will also be exposed to the anxiety of being diagnosed with a life-threatening condition which could kill them at any moment and for which nothing can be done. In one study of community screening only 7% of screen detected aneurysms were greater than 6 cm and only a further 19% reached 6 cm during a median follow-up of 85 months. Of these patients 28% did not undergo operation. Thus only 19% of those diagnosed with aortic aneurysm actually underwent operative repair.

Despite these concerns the results from two studies show a benefit from screening. The first, conducted in Chichester, showed a reduction in the incidence of rupture and aneurysm mortality in a screened population compared with an unscreened population. The second, a larger study conducted in Gloucester but with no control group, reported a steady decrease in rupture rate and aneurysm mortality following the introduction of the screening programme. A multicentre UK study of aneurysm screening is currently in progress and should report shortly.

Section 25.3 • Aetiology

True aneurysm is a disease of the arterial tunica media. The normal media is comprised of concentric bands of collagen, smooth muscle cells and elastin fibres. The important abnormality in the wall of the aneurysmal aorta is reduced elastin content. The normal arterial wall is compliant due to the elastin content and this allows the wall to absorb the energy of the systolic pulse pressure wave. Loss of elastin makes the wall less compliant (i.e. stiffer) and thus less capable of withstanding pulsatile increases in intraluminal pressure which in turn leads to stretching of the wall. Elastin degradation in the aortic wall appears to be due to excess metalloproteinase activity but the reason for this remains obscure. The abnormalities in the arterial wall are present throughout the arterial system but only certain sites become aneurysmal. The inference from this is that there are additional local haemodynamic factors present at these sites which in combination with the abnormal wall lead to aneurysm formation. For example the pulse pressure is maximal in the infrarenal aorta due to the gradual distal tapering of the aorta and reflected waves from the aortic bifurcation add further haemodynamic stress in this area, which is the commonest site of aneurysm formation. Hypertension is another important haemodynamic factor. Hypertension is associated with both aneurysm formation and increased rate of expansion of established aneurysms. The only pharmacological intervention which has been shown to slow the rate of expansion is beta-blockers, presumably due to their effect on blood pressure.

Microscopic examination of the aneurysm wall reveals a marked chronic inflammatory cell infiltrate which may play a role in the pathogenesis. Some patients may have very marked inflammation which leads to macroscopic changes (see below – Inflammatory aneurysm). The role of atherosclerosis in aneurysm formation remains debatable but current opinion supports the view that the two conditions are merely commonly associated and are not causally linked.

A small percentage of patients with aneurysm have a recognized collagen defect due to an inherited condition such as Ehlers–Danlos type IV or Marfan's syndrome. Ehlers–Danlos is a heterogeneous group of conditions with varied patterns of inheritance and patients with Ehlers–Danlos type IV, inherited in an autosomal dominant manner, have abnormal type III collagen. Patients commonly develop aneurysms often at an early age and may also rupture non-aneurysmal vessels. Marfan's syndrome is inherited in an autosomal dominant manner but about 25% of cases are spontaneous mutations. Patients have abnormal fibrillin, a component of the arterial wall, and Marfan's is particularly associated with aortic dissection and thoracic and abdominal aortic aneurysm. Behçet's disease is a rare cause of aneurysm. Patients with Behçet's disease may develop aneurysms at almost any site but most commonly in the thoracic and abdominal aorta. False aneurysm and recurrence after operation is a particular problem.

Some patients have widespread arteriomegaly, multiple aneurysms and young age at the onset of disease and it seems probable that these patients have some, as yet unrecognized, connective tissue disorder. There is undoubtedly a genetic basis to aneurysmal disease: about 25% of first degree male relatives will develop an aneurysm. Several candidate genes have been investigated, e.g. the type III collagen gene and alpha-1-antitrypsin gene, but these studies have not as yet identified the responsible genes.

The risk factors for aneurysm development are family history, smoking and hypertension. There is an association with emphysema and inguinal hernia. It has been suggested that this association is due to some weakness of connective tissue but it may simply be that smoking is a common risk factor for emphysema and aneurysm and that coughing due to smoking and emphysema is responsible for the higher than expected incidence of inguinal hernia.

Section 25.4 • Diagnosis

The mainstays in the diagnosis and assessment of aneurysmal disease are ultrasound and CT scanning. These modalities can determine the size and anatomical position of the aneurysm. Ultrasound scanning is cheap, portable, non-invasive and does not expose the patient to ionizing radiation or contrast agents. It is highly operator dependent but in experienced hands it has good reproducibility with margins of error as little as 3 mm. In the case of false aneurysms duplex ultrasound can demonstrate the presence of turbulent flow within the sac which distinguishes it from a simple haematoma with transmitted pulsation. Ultrasound scanning is not useful for imaging the thoracic aorta and it can be difficult to determine the relationship of aortic aneurysms to the renal and visceral arteries. For these indications CT scanning is more useful (Figure 25.1). Computerized three-dimensional reconstruction of spiral CT scans can provide more detailed information on the anatomy of the neck of the aneurysm (Figure 25.2). Magnetic resonance imaging is also useful but is not widely available. Angiography cannot reliably determine the size of aneurysms as the sac usually contains thrombus and the apparent lumen on angiography is therefore much smaller than the true internal diameter of the sac. However, angiography can provide information regarding the presence of concomitant occlusive disease in other vessels such as the renal and iliac arteries and can help determine the relationship of the aneurysm to the renal and visceral arteries. If endovascular repair is to be undertaken then calibrated angiography may be required to provide accurate sizing of the length of the aneurysm in order to select the appropriate sized device.

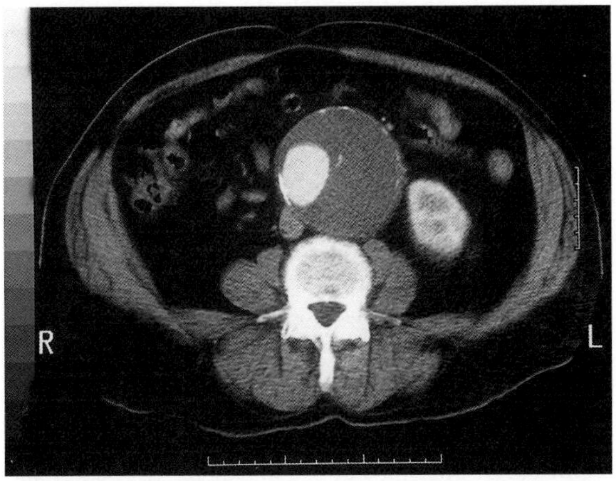

Figure 25.1 Contrast enhanced CT scan demonstrating 7 cm infrarenal abdominal aortic aneurysm.

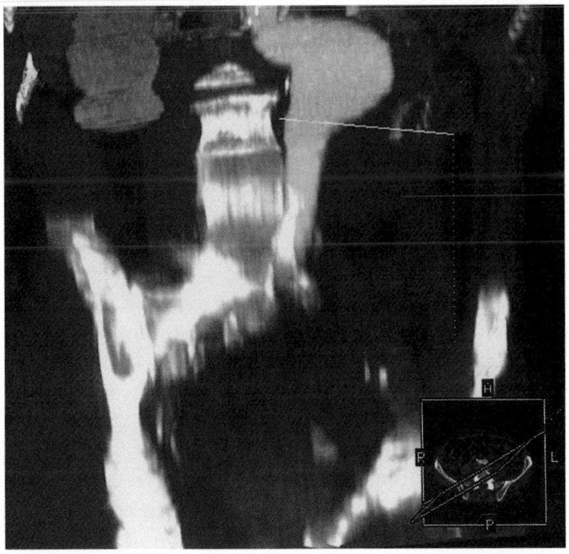

Figure 25.2 Computerized reconstruction of spiral CT scan of infrarenal aortic aneurysm. This demonstrates severe angulation at the neck of the aneuysm which makes it unsuitable for endovascular stenting.

Infrarenal abdominal aortic aneurysm

The commonest form of aneurysm arises in the abdominal aorta below the level of the renal arteries extending equally commonly to the aortic bifurcation or bifurcation of the common iliac arteries. These aneurysms are mostly fusiform though occasionally saccular aneurysms are found. The natural history of infrarenal AAA is that they gradually expand and eventually rupture unless the patient dies from some other cause. The mean growth rate is 3 mm per year and larger aneurysms grow more quickly. The growth rate is highly variable both between different patients and within the same patient over different time periods. Hypertension and smoking are associated with an increased rate of growth. Most aneurysms remain asymptomatic until they rupture and are usually only detected during abdominal examination, ultrasound or CT scanning for some unrelated condition.

Asymptomatic abdominal aortic aneurysm

Elective repair of AAA is a prophylactic operation undertaken with the aim of prolonging life by preventing death from ruptured AAA. Therefore to determine whether operation is indicated the risk of death or major morbidity from operation must be balanced against the risk of death by rupture. The mortality rate from elective operation is in the region of 3–8%. The factors associated with increased risk of death are age, ischaemic heart disease, chronic obstructive pulmonary disease and renal impairment.

Estimation of the risk of rupture for an individual patient within a given time period is difficult. The major determinant for rupture is the maximum diameter of the aneurysm but precise rupture rates for different sizes of aneurysms are not clearly defined. Rupture of small aneurysms, <4 cm diameter, has been reported but this is a very rare occurrence. Aneurysms of 4–5.5 cm have an annual rupture rate of 1% per year. Large aneurysms, >6 cm diameter, carry a significant risk of rupture in the order of 10–20% per year. The risk of rupture has been shown to be related to the rate of expansion. Aneurysms that are rapidly expanding, 5 mm or greater over 6 months, are generally regarded as being at high risk for rupture and most surgeons would undertake early surgery.

Life expectancy must be taken into consideration; for example a patient with disseminated malignancy and a life expectancy of 1 year would not be considered for elective surgery even if the aneurysm was large and the patient otherwise fit for surgery because the patient would be unlikely to gain enough benefit of extended years of life to justify the risks of surgery.

The UK Small Aneurysm Trial randomized 1090 patients aged 60–76 years fit for surgery with asymptomatic aneurysms 4–5.5 cm maximum diameter on ultrasound scan to early surgery or ultrasound surveillance until the aneurysm either grew to 5.5 cm or became symptomatic when operation was undertaken. The outcome was similar in both groups and the conclusion is that asymptomatic aneurysms less than 5.5 cm maximum diameter should be treated expectantly by 6 monthly ultrasound surveillance and should be operated on if growth exceeds 5 mm in 6 months or if they become symptomatic and the patient is fit. Asymptomatic aneurysms >5.5 cm maximum diameter should undergo operation unless there are contraindications.

When weighing up the evidence for and against surgery the clinician must not forget that the final decision lies with the patient and his or her personality has a part to play. Some patients find it intolerable to live with a 'time-bomb' in their abdomen that may go off at any moment. Such patients may prefer to get the surgery over with, even when it involves considerable risk, so that they can get on and enjoy their lives. In the UK Small Aneurysm Trial patients undergoing early surgery had an improvement in health perception compared with those undergoing surveillance.

Operation

Careful pre-operative assessment is required to determine fitness for surgery and to optimize concurrent medical conditions. History and clinical examination can identify most problems and can evaluate general fitness for operation. Most patients unfit for operation can be identified by these means alone. Patients not ruled out at this stage require further investigations which are to a large extent tailored to the individual patient depending on findings on history and examination. All patients require screening tests of cardiac, respiratory and renal function such as electrocardiogram (ECG), chest X-ray, full blood count, urea and creatinine and pulmonary function tests. Patients with a history of cardiac disease require careful assessment as myocardial infarction accounts for approximately 50% of peri-operative mortality. Echocardiography is the minimum required and exercise stress ECG, dypiridamole thallium stress testing and coronary angiography should be considered. Review by a cardiologist is recommended to determine whether cardiac function can be optimized pre-operatively by altering drug therapy, performing coronary angioplasty or even coronary artery bypass grafting. Some authors advocate extensive cardiac screening even in asymptomatic patients because of the significant contribution of myocardial infarction to peri-operative mortality. Respiratory complications are common post-operatively and patients with chronic bronchitis may benefit from early admission for pre-operative chest physiotherapy. All patients should be encouraged to stop smoking prior to surgery. Renal impairment should be investigated to determine whether there is a renovascular component.

Operation is performed under general anaesthetic often with thoracic epidural anaesthesia. Invasive monitoring of arterial blood pressure is required as there may be rapid fluctuations at the time of aortic clamping and unclamping. Prophylactic antibiotics are administered.

Operation is performed through a midline or transverse supra-umbilical incision. The fourth part of the duodenum and duodeno-jejunal flexure are mobilized and the inferior mesenteric vein may need to be divided. The neck of the aneurysm is dissected out taking care not to injure the left renal vein which normally crosses the aorta at this level. The iliac arteries are dissected out taking great care not to injure the iliac veins. The patient is normally heparinized. Some surgeons do not use heparin but a randomized trial has shown a reduced rate of post-operative myocardial infarction in those patients given intra-operative heparin. There is debate about whether the proximal or distal clamps should be applied first. The argument for distal clamping first is that it reduces distal embolism. The arguments for proximal clamping first are that this reduces visceral and renal embolization, that the aneurysm may rupture due to the sudden increase in pressure when the distal clamps are applied and that blood loss from the aneurysm sac is greater when the distal clamps are applied first. There is no good evidence that either approach is superior. The aneurysm sac is opened and the lumbar back-bleeders are oversewn. The inferior mesenteric artery is commonly occluded but if it back-bleeds then it can usually be safely oversewn. Should the left hemicolon or sigmoid appear ischaemic later in the procedure it may be re-implanted onto the graft with a patch of aortic wall. The graft is sewn in using an inlay technique with non-absorbable sutures. It is important to cover the graft, usually with the sac, to isolate it from the gut and thus prevent potential graft infection and aorto-enteric fistula. If the aneurysm extends into the iliac arteries then a bifurcated graft is used. It is preferable to perform the distal anastomoses within the abdomen to avoid groin incisions. Aneurysms rarely extend into the external iliac artery and the distal anastomosis can usually be performed at this level. It is important to perfuse at least one internal iliac artery to avoid pelvic ischaemia and buttock claudication.

The quoted 30 day mortality rate is about 5–8% although many centres have reported a mortality rate of 1–2%. The commonest cause of death is myocardial infarction. Other common early complications include chest infection, stroke and renal failure. Lower limb ischaemia can occur; this may be due to embolism of clot formed while the aorta and iliac arteries are clamped and is treated by femoral embolectomy. Patchy ischaemia of the feet, especially the toes, may occur due to multiple embolism of small fragments of the aneurysm contents and is known as 'trash foot' or 'blue toe syndrome'. Colonic ischaemia occurs uncommonly and spinal cord ischaemia has been reported but it is rare.

Long-term outcome after successful aneurysm repair is good. Patients have similar actuarial survival to age-matched controls. Late complications are uncommon. Graft infection is a serious complication which necessitates removal of the graft, oversewing of the aortic stump and insertion of extra-anatomic axillo-bifemoral bypass. Some surgeons have advocated removal of the infected graft and replacement with a rifampicin bonded graft. Another option is to fashion an aorto-bifemoral graft from autogenous vein. Aorto-enteric fistula may occur between the proximal aortic anastomosis and the third or fourth part of the duodenum. Patients present with massive haematemesis and melaena. The fistula may seal spontaneously after an initial bleed. The diagnosis can be made on endoscopy if the endoscope can be passed as far as the third part of the duodenum. Angiography may not confirm the diagnosis if the patient is not actively bleeding. It is assumed that there is an associated graft infection and the graft should be excised and revascularization performed with bilateral axillo-femoral grafts.

Endovascular repair

In 1991 Parodi first described the repair of an aortic aneurysm by means of transfemoral intraluminal placement of a stent-graft device. Since then there has been considerable technological development and there are now many commercially available devices. The rationale of endovascular repair is that the operative mortality and morbidity of open operation is due to the cardiac stress of aortic cross-clamping, the large abdominal incision, extensive dissection and large blood loss. Endovascular repair avoids these factors and thus the early outcome of aneurysm repair should be improved.

Endovascular repair consists of intraluminal delivery via the femoral artery of a graft which is secured to the artery wall above and below the aneurysm with metal stents which are attached to, or part of, the graft. A certain length of normal aorta is required to anchor the graft proximal and distal to the aneurysm. Proximally this means that the neck of the aneurysm must be a few centimetres below the renal arteries which excludes a large number of aneurysms. Recently techniques have been described for fixing the proximal stent across the ostia of the renal arteries but the long-term effect on renal function is yet to be determined. The need for a few centimetres of normal artery distal to the aneurysm means that tube grafting is rarely possible. The options are therefore to use a bifurcated device or to use a uni-iliac device, which occludes the contralateral iliac artery, and perform a femoro-femoral cross-over graft. If both common iliacs are aneurysmal then the point for distal fixation, the 'landing site', must be in the external iliac arteries. This means that the graft will cover the origins of both internal iliac arteries which can cause buttock claudication. Other anatomical features that can preclude endovascular repair include stenosed or tortuous iliac arteries and severe angulation at the neck. Careful assessments by means of CT scanning and calibrated angiography are therefore required to assess suitability for stent grafting.

Low mortality rates have been reported but have not yet been proved to be better than open repair in case-controlled or randomized trials. There are concerns about long-term outcome. Pressurization of the aneurysm sac by leak at the proximal or distal end of the graft, by leakage through the graft or by perfusion via lumbar vessels may occur and is known as endoleak. Expansion of the aorta above the aneurysm, where the graft is secured, may cause proximal endoleak. The graft material used is thinner than that used in conventional repair to allow greater ease of delivery and this may predispose to tearing and leakage through the graft. The metal components of the stent-graft are subject to repeated stresses which can cause metal fatigue with subsequent loss of fixation. Endoleak may lead to continued expansion of the aneurysm sac and even rupture. Late ruptures of previously stent-graft repaired aneurysms have been reported even when no endoleak is present. Endovascular repair is now being performed in a large number of centres but until good quality long-term outcome data are published it must still be considered to be an experimental procedure.

Symptomatic abdominal aortic aneurysm

Abdominal aortic aneurysm may cause symptoms of pain or distal embolization. Pain is usually felt in the abdominal or lower lumbar region and is constant in nature. Painful or tender aneurysms should be repaired in patients fit for surgery both for humanitarian reasons of pain relief and also because of the perceived threat of impending rupture. The major difficulty in a patient with pain and an aneurysm is to determine whether the aneurysm is indeed the cause for the pain rather than some other intra-abdominal pathology or musculoskeletal disorder. Alternative diagnoses such as renal colic, pancreatitis, duodenal ulcer and myocardial infarction should be rigorously investigated. If no indisputable cause for the pain is found then the aneurysm should be repaired urgently. CT scanning has been shown to be unreliable in discerning the presence of a leak in symptomatic patients and surgery should not be delayed.

Distal embolism usually presents with multiple small infarcted patches on the feet, commonly described as 'trash foot'. Operation is indicated to prevent tissue loss. Rarely AAA can thrombose and present with critical ischaemia of the lower limbs. Urgent aorto-bifemoral grafting is necessary, usually with distal embolectomies, to restore the distal circulation. Very rarely intact aneurysms can cause disseminated intravascular coagulation which can present as a bleeding disorder. Such patients can be stabilized on low dose heparin prior to operation.

Inflammatory aneurysms

Approximately 3–10% of aortic aneurysms are inflammatory. The inflammation occurs through all layers of the aneurysm wall, which is thickened, and extends into the peri-aortic tissues, obscuring tissue planes and occasionally involving and obstructing the ureters, inferior vena cava and neighbouring structures. Inflammatory aneurysm is not a distinct clinical entity but rather it appears that patients develop non-inflammatory aneurysms which subsequently for unknown reasons become inflammatory. About 50% of patients have an elevated erythrocyte sedimentation rate and the appearances of thickened aortic wall can usually be seen on CT scanning. Such aneurysms are often symptomatic but are considered to be at slightly lower risk of rupture than other aneurysms. The clinical significance of inflammation is that operation is technically more difficult due to the obscured tissue planes. Ureteric obstruction may necessitate pre-operative ureteric stenting. In over 70% of cases aortic replacement is followed by complete resolution of the peri-aortitis.

Ruptured abdominal aortic aneurysm

Ruptured abdominal aortic aneurysm is a common cause of death, accounting for 1.5% of deaths in men over the age of 55 years. Community mortality for rupture is 90–95%. About 50% of patients die in the community and about 50% of those that reach hospital are unfit for surgery and the mortality rate for those who do undergo operation is about 50%. The reason that some patients survive long enough to undergo surgical repair is due to the fact that many aneurysms rupture postero-laterally into the retroperitoneum where tamponade combined with hypotension slows blood loss and may even temporarily seal the rupture. Anterior rupture into the peritoneal cavity usually causes devastating blood loss and successful repair is uncommon.

Aortic aneurysm rupture is a clinical diagnosis based on a triad of conditions: pain, collapse and the presence of an aneurysm. Pain is usually constant, located in the centre of the abdomen or lower back. Often the pain is situated in the flank radiating to the groin mimicking renal colic. Patients usually present in varying degrees of shock and even those who are normotensive usually give a history of collapse or light-headedness with subsequent recovery. The presence of an aneurysm can be difficult to detect clinically, especially in the obese, and where there is clinical suspicion of rupture an ultrasound or CT scan should be undertaken urgently to detect the presence of an aneurysm. Neither ultrasound nor CT scanning can reliably confirm or exclude the diagnosis of rupture and should only be used to confirm the presence, size and anatomy of the aneurysm.

When the diagnosis is made the management is either palliative or immediate operation. The decision not to operate can be difficult but generally operation should not be offered to those with very little chance of surviving. Factors associated with poor outcome are age, profound hypotension, conscious level, coagulopathy, and pre-existing cardiac, pulmonary or renal disease.

Operation should not be delayed unnecessarily even if the patient appears to be stable; sudden collapse can occur at any moment. In collapsed patients resuscitation should be carried out synchronously with operation. Successful outcome requires both speed and an experienced surgical and anaesthetic team. If an experienced team is not available locally then the patient should be transferred to a suitable hospital. Some patients will die during transfer but it is argued that these patients are unstable and would also be unlikely to survive operation at the referring hospital, especially if operated on by a surgical team which does routinely perform aortic surgery. Those who are likely to survive operation should be stable enough to survive transfer. During the transfer period the patient's blood pressure should not be raised excessively by over-enthusiastic transfusion as this may precipitate further rupture and collapse; a blood pressure adequate to maintain consciousness is sufficient for transfer. The use of an anti-shock suit does not appear to confer any benefit and can hamper preparation for surgery.

The induction of anaesthesia can cause sudden hypotension and even cardiac arrest. It is therefore customary to induce anaesthesia in the operating theatre with the patient prepared and draped and the surgical team ready to start. Operation proceeds much as described above for elective repair. The neck is dissected out and clamped before the iliac arteries are dissected and systemic heparin is not administered. To reduce the risk of lower limb arterial thrombosis some surgeons inject heparinized saline down the iliac arteries. Release of the distal clamps and reperfusion of the lower limbs is often associated with profound hypotension. This is due to suddenly reduced peripheral vascular resistance and washing out metabolites from ischaemic tissues which have a myocardial depressant effect. The clamps are therefore removed from one limb at a time and the graft may need to be compressed to maintain a satisfactory blood pressure. Emergency aortic surgery is often complicated by the presence of a coagulopathy and clotting factors and platelets should be ordered routinely. When post-operative haemorrhage occurs it is usually due to diffuse bleeding, associated with coagulopathy, and is only rarely due to a simple technical error. Other post-operative complications are similar to, but more common than, those described for elective repair. The long-term outcome for those that survive aneurysm repair is good with similar actuarial survival rates and quality of life to age-matched controls. Of course those that survive the rigors of emergency operation are a select group of robust patients who might be expected to have a good long-term survival rate.

Aorto-caval fistula

Aneurysms which rupture on the right lateral side may do so into the inferior vena cava. This is usually associated with rupture into the retroperitoneal tissues. Venous engorgement in a patient with a rupture may raise suspicion pre-operatively but the diagnosis is often only made on encountering profuse venous bleeding after opening the aneurysm sac. If the fistula is present for some time then high pressure in the inferior vena cava may cause acute renal failure with associated haematuria. At operation the fistula should be compressed and the defect sutured from inside the aneurysm sac. Very rarely the aneurysm may rupture into the cava alone and present with high output cardiac failure and venous engorgement.

Thoracic and thoraco-abdominal aneurysm

Thoracic aortic aneurysms are seldom isolated but are usually associated with aneurysms at multiple sites or the presence of an underlying connective tissue disorder. Patients are usually asymptomatic and the aneurysm is detected by chance on chest X-ray or CT scanning undertaken for some other reason. Very large aneurysms may cause symptoms, such as dysphagia, recurrent laryngeal nerve palsy or Horner's syndrome by compressing adjacent structures. Rupture is often immediately fatal but patients may present with chest pain and collapse.

Thoraco-abdominal aneurysms are classified according to the Crawford classification of type I–IV (Figure 25.3). Type I is aneurysmal from the descending thoracic aorta to above the level of the coeliac artery, type II is aneurysmal from the descending thoracic aorta to the aortic bifurcation, type III is aneurysmal from mid descending thoracic aorta to the aortic bifurcation and type IV is aneurysmal from the level of the diaphragm to the aortic bifurcation. As with infrarenal aneurysm repair the risks of operation must be balanced against the risks of rupture. Studies of patients unfit for or refusing elective repair with aneurysms greater than twice the normal aortic diameter indicate a 39% mortality from rupture at 2 years with a further 29% dying from other causes. Unfortunately, detailed natural history studies have not been undertaken to provide guidance on the expected rate of rupture with any given size of aneurysm. As the risks of operation are considerable, especially in types I–III, operation should only be considered in fit patients with large aneurysms, probably in excess of 6 cm maximum diameter. Type IV aneurysms should be considered separately as the operation required is far less hazardous than that for types I–III and in expert hands the morbidity and mortality approaches that of infrarenal AAA repair.

The major difficulties with operation for types I–III thoraco-abdominal aneurysms are the significant increase in peripheral vascular resistance after proximal

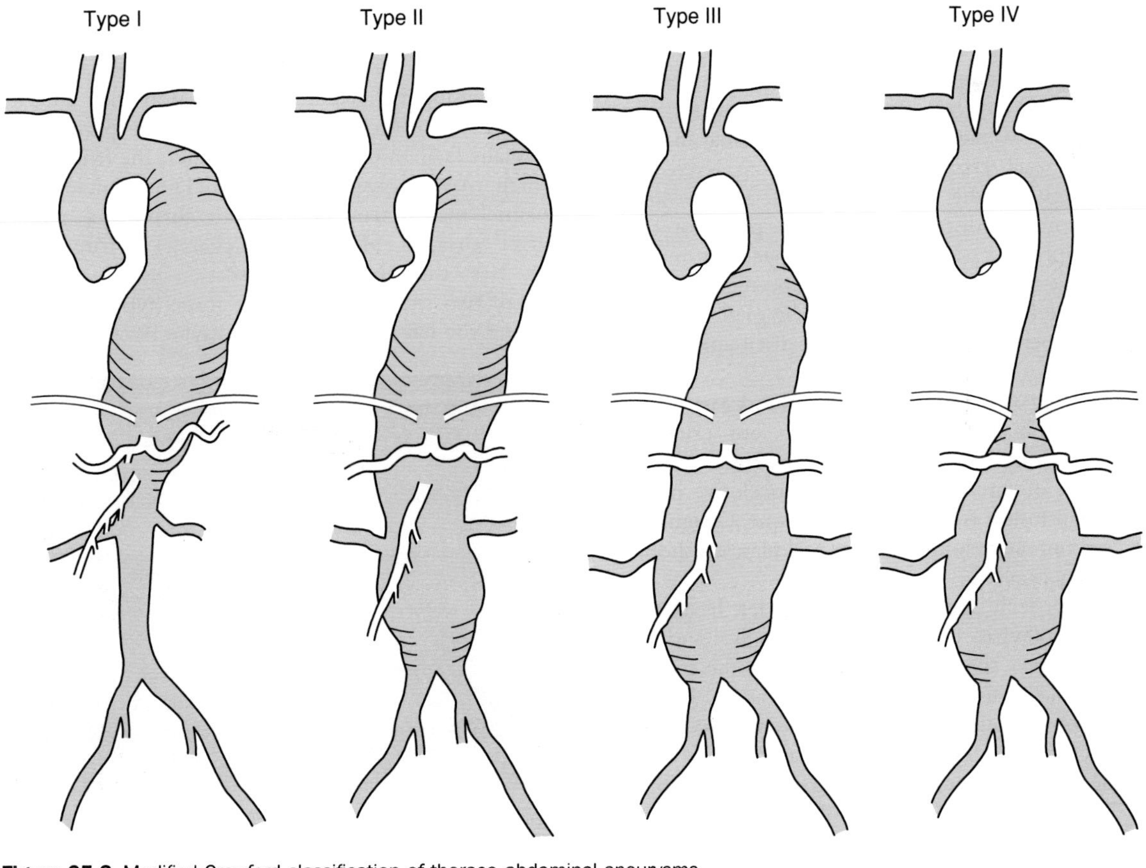

Figure 25.3 Modified Crawford classification of thoraco-abdominal aneurysms.

cross-clamping, prolonged visceral and renal ischaemia, possible interruption of arterial supply to the spinal cord, large blood loss and coagulopathy and the overall trauma of a long procedure requiring a thoraco-laparotomy and extensive dissection. Various strategies can be employed to overcome these problems. There is no standard approach and different surgeons use different techniques according to local experience, resources and expertise.

The effects of cross-clamping on peripheral vascular resistance can be offset by pharmacological means such as vasodilators. Left heart bypass with inflow from the left atrium and outflow pumped into the femoral or iliac artery or temporary bypass from the proximal aorta or subclavian to femoral can be employed. These latter methods also have the advantage of providing distal and retrograde visceral perfusion.

Spinal cord ischaemia is a not uncommon and serious complication. The problem may be partly due to interruption of the arterial supply from intercostal arteries. Large intercostal arteries should be re-implanted into the graft on a patch of surrounding aorta. Spinal cord ischaemia may also be caused by inadequate perfusion pressure during operation. Perfusion pressure is the arterial pressure minus the cerebro-spinal fluid (CSF) pressure. To increase perfusion pressure a CSF drain can be inserted, the CSF pressure monitored and if the pressure is high CSF can be drained off to lower CSF pressure and thus increase perfusion pressure. Despite these techniques even in the best hands the rate of post-operative paraplegia remains up to 20%.

Visceral and renal ischaemia may be reduced by employing a temporary shunt. If left heart bypass is being employed then a policy of sequential clamping can be used. While performing the proximal anastomosis the distal clamp is placed at the level of the diaphragm and the renal and visceral arteries are perfused from the distal inflow via the pump or bypass. Some surgeons simply rely on speed to minimize ischaemic time. Once the visceral and renal arteries are implanted the clamp is placed on the graft below them to allow perfusion while the final distal anastomosis is being performed.

Bleeding is a major problem. Blood loss from the visceral and renal arteries, which are usually not clamped, may be reduced by sequential clamping, insertion of shunts or insertion of occlusive balloons. Autotransfusion is a valuable technique. Coagulopathy is common and clotting factors and platelets should be routinely available.

A 'high tech' approach employing left heart bypass, temporary bypass or shunts appears logical and attractive. However, these techniques increase the complexity of what is already a major undertaking. It may be preferable to adopt a simpler approach and rely on speedy operating: the so-called 'clamp and sew' technique. For an operating team frequently performing these operations the problem of increased complexity may be overcome by familiarity with the techniques.

Type IV aneurysm repair is a less complex and hazardous procedure. The risk of spinal cord ischaemia is much less and cross-clamping at the level of the diaphragm produces less increase in peripheral vascular resistance. The overall mortality rate is approximately 10% and paraplegia rate 5%. The operation can be carried out without the need for thoracotomy via a subcostal incision although the benefits of this approach are not proven. A retroperitoneal approach is made to the aorta on the left side by rotating the viscera medially. The aorta is clamped proximally at the diaphragm and distally at the iliac arteries. The aneurysm is opened longitudinally posterior to the left renal artery. Back-bleeding from the renal and visceral arteries can be recycled by autotransfusion or the vessels can be occluded with balloon catheters. The proximal anastomosis is fashioned obliquely with the suture line starting from the neck on the left postero-lateral corner and running obliquely posterior to the orifices of the renal and visceral arteries. A clamp is then placed on the graft and the renal and visceral arteries are reperfused. The distal anastomosis is performed as for standard infrarenal repair.

Aortic dissection

The underlying defect in many patients with dissection is weakness of the tunica media, most commonly cystic medionecrosis. Most patients with dissection have significant hypertension and this is an important pathogenic factor. A tear in the intima allows entry of blood under high pressure to the media and the haemorrhage tracks along and dissects the weakened layer (Figure 25.4). There are several possible sequelae of dissection. The dissection may proceed along side branches of the aorta causing ischaemia. The dissection may rupture externally into the pericardium or pleural space which is usually fatal. In other cases it re-enters the true lumen which may resolve the problem. The resultant false channel may remain permanently, forming a 'double barrel' aorta, or either the false channel or true lumen may later thrombose. The dissection usually starts at one of two sites; the ascending aorta: (type A) or just beyond the left subclavian artery (type B).

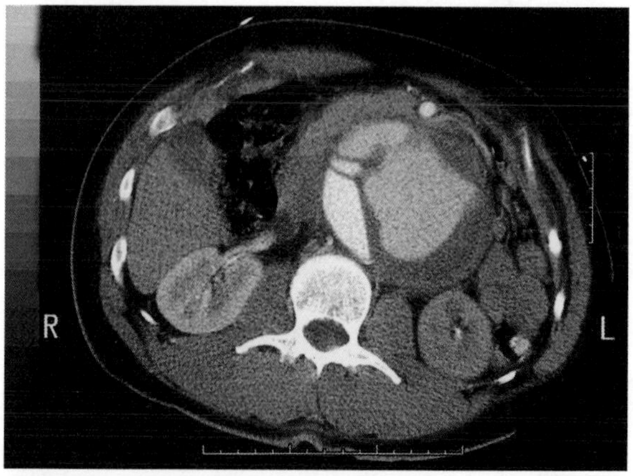

Figure 25.4 CT scan demonstrating chronic dissection and aneurysm formation in the proximal abdominal aorta of a patient with Marfan's syndrome.

Patients commonly present acutely with severe 'tearing' chest pain radiating to the back associated with shock. However, patients usually have underlying hypertension unless rupture has occurred. Dissection is often initially misdiagnosed as myocardial infarction. Less commonly it may present with ischaemic phenomena such as stroke, paraplegia, renal, mesenteric or lower limb ischaemia. Clinical suspicion of rupture may be raised by the presence of unequal or asynchronous pulses, but usually the first clue is a widened mediastinum on plain chest X-ray which is present in about 85% of patients. The diagnosis can be confirmed by contrast enhanced CT scanning or aortography. Aortography is invasive but can give useful information such as whether the aortic valve is competent and can more accurately localize the entry and exit sites of the dissection.

Type A dissections are a surgical emergency with a very high early mortality rate unless operated on successfully. Operation requires cardiopulmonary bypass using femoral cannulation and may also require a period of total circulatory arrest with hypothermia. Replacement or resuspension of the aortic valve may also be required. The major technical problem is the friable nature of the dissected tissues which makes anastomosis extremely challenging.

Type B dissections have a better prognosis unless there is some ischaemic complication. Initial management is usually medical with the aim of rendering the patient relatively hypotensive by pharmacological means such as glyceryl trinitrate or sodium nitroprusside infusions. It is hoped that good blood pressure control will limit the extent of the dissection and its attendant complications. The situation may stabilize and many patients will not require operation. The development of ischaemic complications, either of the lower limbs or abdominal viscera, is an indication for operation. Operation requires clamping of the aorta proximal to the entry point of the dissection and this may need to be between the innominate and left common carotid artery. Left heart bypass may be useful to reduce heart strain and allow perfusion of the kidneys, gut and lower limbs. The distal thoracic aorta is clamped, the aorta opened and a graft is inlaid into the true lumen. Large intercostals should be re-implanted or incorporated into a bevelled distal anastomosis. Even when dissection has extended into the abdominal aorta replacement of the abdominal aorta is not undertaken unless there is visceral compromise. Obliteration of the false lumen at the level of the distal anastomosis in the thoracic aorta should restore flow to the true lumen and the false channel within the abdominal aorta should thrombose and obliterate.

Conservative management may be followed by the formation of a thoraco-abdominal aneurysm. Successful operative repair may also be complicated by late aneurysm formation or further dissection above or below the graft.

Popliteal artery aneurysm

The popliteal artery is the commonest site for true aneurysms apart from the aorta. As with AAA the diameter at which the popliteal artery is considered aneurysmal is debatable but a popliteal artery >2 cm is widely accepted to be an aneurysm. There is an association with AAA; 10% of patients with AAA have a popliteal aneurysm and 40% of patients with popliteal aneurysm have an AAA. Popliteal aneurysms are bilateral in 50% of cases. The risk associated with popliteal aneurysm is thrombosis with distal embolism usually causing severe acute ischaemia. Rupture is a rare complication. Compression of neighbouring structures, especially the popliteal vein, can occur. Patients may present subacutely with progressive intermittent claudication secondary to calf vessel embolization.

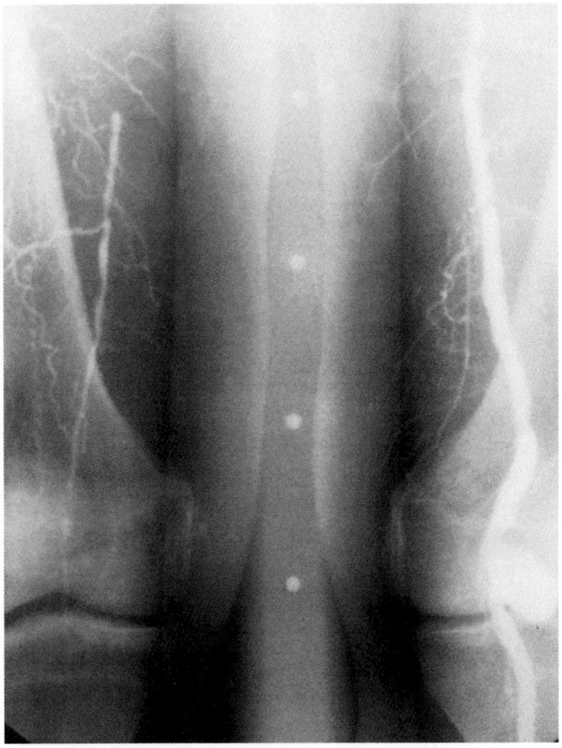

Figure 25.5 Transfemoral angiogram of a patient who presented with an acutely ischaemic right leg secondary to a thrombosed popliteal artery aneurysm. An asymptomatic popliteal artery aneurysm is present in the left leg.

In the acute situation the diagnosis can be difficult as the aneurysm may have thrombosed and thus be impalpable (Figure 25.5). Distal embolism of the contents of the sac into the tibial vessels usually causes devastating ischaemia. Limb loss is common and even in the case of successful revascularization the degree of ischaemia is such that fasciotomy is commonly required. Emergency treatment requires exposure of the above and below knee popliteal arteries, embolectomy of the tibial vessels, construction of a bypass graft (preferably reversed vein) and ligation of the popliteal artery above and below the aneurysm. On-table thrombolysis, by instilling either streptokinase or tissue plasminogen activator down the tibial vessels, is commonly used to clear thrombus from branch arteries and the distal circulation (Figure 25.6).

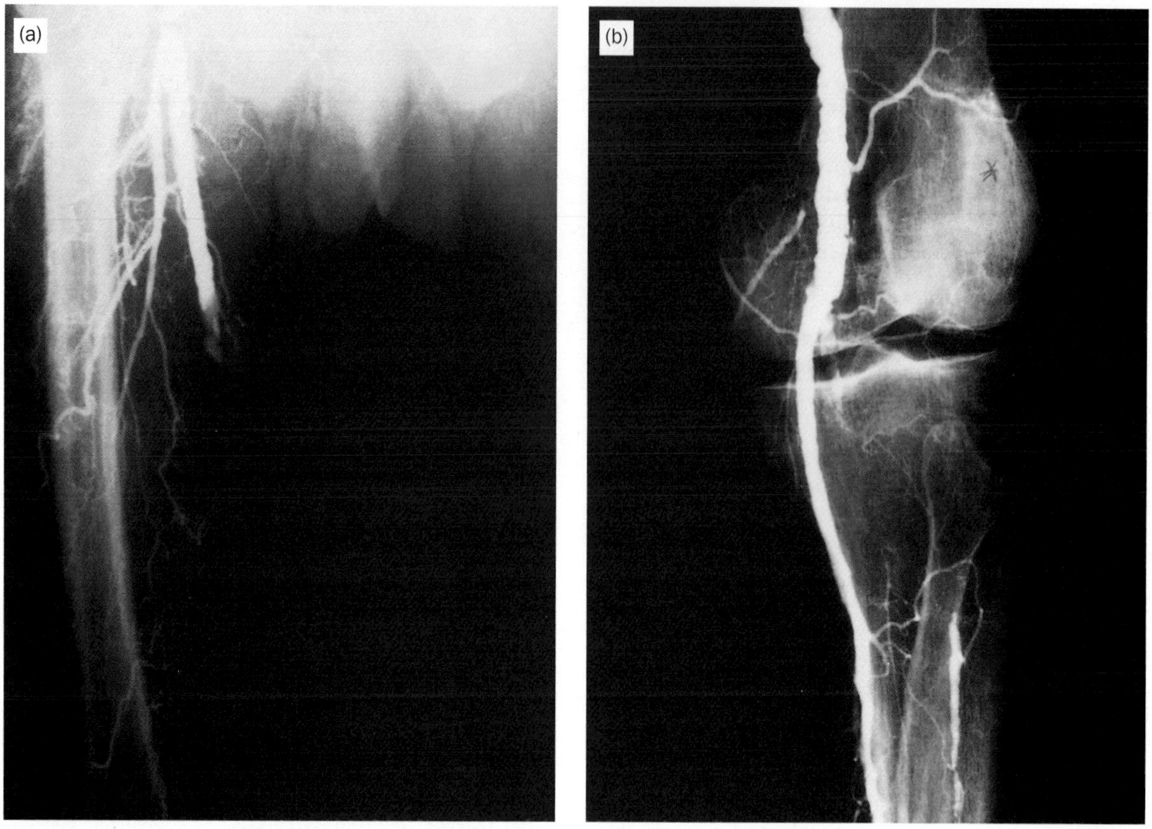

Figures 25.6 (a) Transfemoral angiogram of a patient who presented with acutely ischaemic left leg secondary to thrombosed popliteal artery aneurysm. (b) Completion angiogram of same patient as (a) after treatment with thrombolysis and aneurysm ligation and bypass grafting from above knee popliteal to tibio-peroneal trunk using reversed saphenous vein.

The natural history and risk of thrombosis of asymptomatic popliteal aneurysms is not clearly understood but the serious consequences of thrombosis and the low risk of elective operation means that most surgeons advise elective repair. Elective operation consists of bypass graft and ligation of the popliteal artery above and below the aneurysm.

Femoral artery aneurysm

The femoral artery is the commonest site for false aneurysm (see below) but true aneurysms are much less common. These usually occur in conjunction with aneurysms at multiple sites. Femoral aneurysm can compress local structures, such as femoral vein and nerve, are at risk for rupture and can be a source of emboli. Operation is often undertaken in conjunction with other procedures such as aorto-bifemoral grafting for aortic and iliac aneurysms. When operated on in isolation a bypass graft can usually be taken from the external iliac, which is rarely affected by aneurysm, to the profunda femoris and superficial femoral arteries.

Visceral artery aneurysm

Aneurysms in the visceral vessels are rare. The most common site is in the splenic artery but aneurysms in the hepatic, superior mesenteric and coeliac arteries are occasionally seen. These aneurysms are usually impalpable and asymptomatic unless they rupture and the diagnosis is usually an incidental finding at the time of angiography, CT scanning or ultrasound. When these aneurysms rupture the diagnosis is usually only made at laparotomy. Hepatic arteries seem to be particularly prone to rupture and operation should be considered in all patients.

Splenic artery aneurysms are usually saccular and commonly calcify in later years. They are more common in females and are associated with multiple pregnancies. Most are asymptomatic and are usually an incidental finding on plain X-ray. Rupture is uncommon but aneurysms presenting at a young age, in pregnancy and symptomatic or large (>2.5 cm) aneurysms should be considered for operation. The surgical options are either splenectomy or proximal and distal ligation without reconstruction. Collateral supply via the short gastric arteries is sufficient for splenic survival.

False aneurysm

False aneurysm is caused by a defect in the vessel wall. Bleeding is tamponaded by the adventitia and surrounding tissues but continuing turbulent flow in the centre of the haematoma prevents clotting and sealing of the defect. The aneurysm can then slowly expand.

The initial defect may be caused by trauma to the native vessel or may arise at vascular anastomosis. Those caused by trauma are most commonly iatrogenic. Small iatrogenic false aneurysms, less than 2 cm diameter, thrombose spontaneously and can be encouraged to thrombose by prolonged application of pressure sufficient to stop flow in the sac as demonstrated on ultrasound scanning. Larger false aneurysms are unlikely to thrombose and require surgical repair to prevent blood loss, breakdown of the overlying skin, compression of neighbouring structure and distal embolization. Non-iatrogenic false aneurysm caused by penetrating trauma can be dealt with in a similar way. Unfortunately many non-iatrogenic false aneurysms are caused by inadvertent arterial puncture in intravenous drug abusers. Local infection in these patients may make arterial repair impossible and the relevant artery may need to be ligated with a high risk of limb loss.

Anastomotic false aneurysm can arise many years after arterial surgery. Such aneurysms, especially when occurring at an early stage, raise the suspicion of graft infection. Infection is the commonest aetiology but other causes include the use of absorbable suture material, such as silk, simultaneous endarterectomy and anastomosis under excessive tension. Surgical repair in the absence of infection usually entails taking down the anastomosis and inserting a short interposition graft. If infection is present the graft must be excised, infected tissue debrided and revascularization undertaken using autogenous vein or by routing a new prosthetic graft through sterile tissue planes.

Further reading

Crawford, E. S. and DeNatale, R. W. (1986). Thoraco-abdominal aortic aneurysm: observations regarding the natural course of disease. *J Vasc Surg* **3**: 578–82.

Dawson, I., Sie, R. B. and van Bockel, J. H. (1997). Atherosclerotic popliteal aneurysm. *Br J Surg* **84**: 293–9.

Law, M. (1998). Screening for abdominal aortic aneurysms. *Br Med Bull* **54**: 903–13.

Panayiotopoulos, Y. P., Assadourian, R. and Taylor, P. R. (1996). Aneurysms of the visceral and renal arteries. *Ann R Coll Surg Edinb* **78**: 412–19.

Rasmussen, T. E. and Hallet, J. W. (1997). Inflammatory aortic aneurysms. A clinical review with new perspectives in pathogenesis. *Ann Surg* **225**: 155–64.

Scott, R. A., Wilson, N. M., Ashton, H. A. and Kay, D. N. (1995). Influence of screening on the incidence of ruptured abdominal aortic aneurysm: 5 year results of a randomized controlled study. *Br J Surg* **82**: 1066–70.

UK Small Aneurysm Trial Participants (1999). Mortality results for the randomised controlled trial of early elective surgery or ultrasonographic surveillance for small abdominal aortic aneurysms. *Lancet* **352**: 1649–55.

Wills, A., Thompson, M. M., Crowther, M. *et al.* (1996). Pathogenesis of abdominal aortic aneurysm – cellular and biochemical mechanisms. *Eur J Vasc Endovasc Surg* **12**: 391–400.

Wilmink, A. B. and Quick, C. R. (1998). Epidemiology and potential for prevention of abdominal aortic aneurysm. *Br J Surg* **85**: 155–62.

Woodburn, K. R., May, J. and White, G. H. (1998). Endoluminal abdominal aortic aneurysm repair. *Br J Surg* **85**: 435–43.

MODULE 26

Acute limb ischaemia and thrombolysis

Patients presenting with acute limb ischaemia can present a challenge to the most seasoned vascular surgeon. The therapeutic window to allow successful restoration of arterial blood supply without tissue loss can be quite small, and is highly dependent on any pre-existing peripheral arterial disease. It is ironic that the patient with a preceding history of intermittent claudication or even early rest pain will be seemingly able to tolerate a longer period of ischaemia due to the existence of collaterals compared to the patient with previously normal vessels who having occluded their major inflow has no effective pre-established collaterals. It is generally accepted that skeletal muscle can withstand up to 6 hours of total ischaemia before irreversible muscle damage will occur. The time commences from the time of injury, embolic occlusion or *in situ* thrombosis – not from the time of admission.

In the days of rheumatic heart disease, the classic 'white leg' was invariably caused by a major proximal embolus which was readily amenable to a balloon catheter thromboembolectomy. Once successful extraction of the thrombus was achieved, one could expect relatively normal underlying vessels and satisfactory limb salvage. However, today most patients presenting with acute or acute on chronic ischaemia will have underlying peripheral vascular disease. Their acute episode is more likely to represent an *in situ* thrombosis superimposed on a pre-existing stenosis, or indeed embolism in the presence of pre-existing peripheral stenotic disease. Injudicious use of the balloon embolectomy catheter can cause intimal disruption and put the limb at further risk rather than saving the limb.

It is therefore essential that a full history and examination are carefully performed. Pre-existing history of intermittent claudication, whether it was progressive, degree of severity, presence of rest pain and tissue necrosis should all be noted. Other risk factors such as hypertension, smoking, diabetes, cholesterol/triglyceride, angina, myocardial infarction and cerebrovascular disease including transient ischaemic attacks will need to be modified wherever possible and may point to the underlying aetiology of the current presentation. Even if the pulse is regular, the patient may have still suffered a transient arrhythmia (e.g. paroxysmal atrial fibrillation) leading to embolism. Similarly transient arrhythmias may also cause transient hypotension sufficient to occlude critical peripheral arterial stenoses whether these are in native vessels or within peripheral arterial bypass grafts. The presence of mitral stenosis may also be an aetiological factor in embolism. Multiple small embolic episodes may present as the 'blue toe syndrome'. In the upper limb, proximal constriction or aneurysmal changes as a result of thoracic outlet compression can give rise to peripheral embolism. The presence of cervical ribs or bands must be considered (Figure 26.1).

With the increasing application of percutaneous techniques, the risk of intimal dissection flaps, pericatheter thrombosis and embolism may also require urgent or emergency intervention by the vascular surgeon.

Section 26.1 • Examination

Traditional teaching refers to the six Ps – pain, pale, pulseless, perishing cold, paralysis and paraesthesia as clinical characteristics of the acutely ischaemic leg (Table 26.1). Not all of these will necessarily be present in all patients due to the presence of collaterals, due to pre-existing disease and due to incomplete occlusion. They are still invaluable to help determine the viability and urgency of intervention. In addition to the above findings, the presence of venous guttering, tenderness and suppleness of the calf muscles and anterior compartment may all contribute to determine the urgency of the situation. The presence or absence of Doppler signals and their pressure at the ankle level in dorsalis pedis, posterior tibial and peroneal vessels need to be recorded. The absence of Doppler detectable venous flow at the ankle level is a particularly poor prognostic sign.

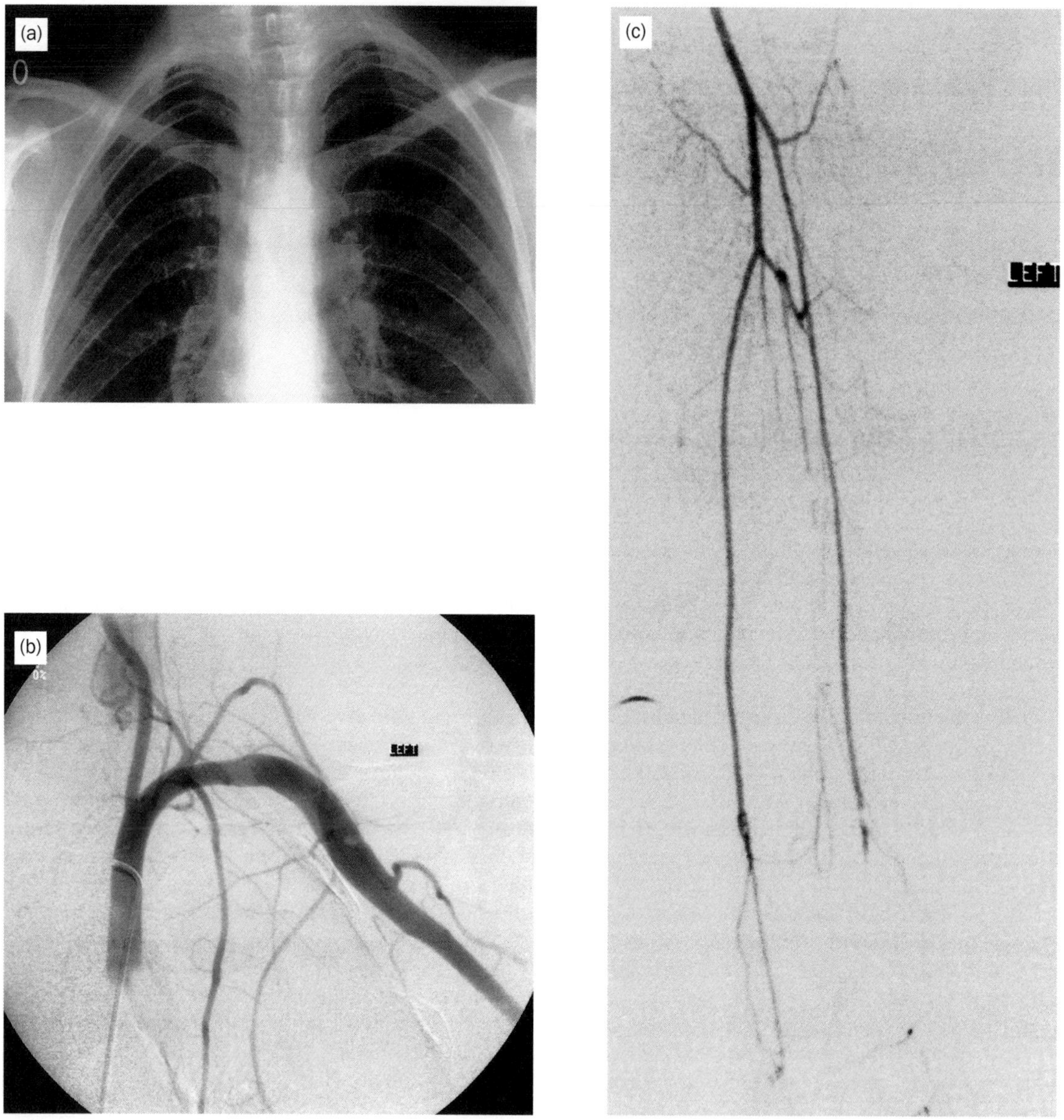

Figure 26.1 (a) Bilateral cervical ribs (complete on left). (b, c) Intra-arterial digital subtraction angiogram (IA DSA) showing thrombus within a post-stenotic dilatation aneurysm (b) of the third part of the subclavian and proximal axillary arteries, with distal embolization (c).

A long duration of total ischaemia, i.e. >6 hours from time of onset to time of flow restitution, should demand a call for a four compartment fasciotomy. In other less acute situations, it may be preferable to test and if necessary continually monitor the compartment pressures. Any value above 30 mmHg should progress to fasciotomy, as should any progressive increase in pressure above 20 mmHg. If in doubt it is probably safer to perform a fasciotomy rather than risk losing a leg or a permanent foot drop due to compartment syndrome.

Table 26.1 Presenting symptoms of acute ischaemia

Symptoms/signs:
Pain
Pallor
Pulselessness
Paraesthesia
Paralysis
Perishing cold

The attempted revascularization of an irreversibly ischaemic leg may cause the death of the patient. This situation should be avoided by careful examination of the patient and their affected limb and a realistic assessment of outcome. The categories of acute limb ischaemia have been described and recently modified (Table 26.2).

Table 26.2 Clinical categories of acute limb ischaemia

Category	*Description*	*Muscle weakness*	*Sensory loss*	*Doppler signals* *Arterial*	*Venous*
(i) Viable	Not immediately threatened	None	None	Audible (>30 mmHg)	Audible
(ii) Threatened					
(a) marginally	Salvageable if promptly treated	None	Minimal (toes) or none	Inaudible	Audible
(b) immediately	Salvageable with immediate revascularization	Mild, moderate	More than toes, associated with rest pain	Inaudible	Audible
(iii) Irreversible	Major tissue loss or permanent nerve damage inevitable	Profound, paralysis (rigor)	Profound, anaesthetic	Inaudible	Inaudible

Reproduced with permission from Rutherford *et al*. Recommended standards for reports dealing with lower extremity ischemia: Revised version. *J Vasc Surg* 1997; **26**: 517–38.

Section 26.2 • Investigations

Baseline investigations should include a full blood count to check haemoglobin, white cell and platelet counts, all of which can adversely effect the outcome if deranged. Renal function and electrolytes, especially the potassium level, must also be optimized as many patients will be on diuretics, inhibitors, digoxin; angiotensin converting enzyme (ACE), etc. A 12-lead electrocardiogram should be routinely performed. Baseline clotting studies would also be prudent.

The urgency of the situation and the availability of local resources will determine which investigations are appropriate and indeed likely to be helpful. Waiting for several hours for an arteriogram may lose the opportunity to save the limb. The patient with no preceding history of claudication, a full complement of contralateral lower limb pulses and a pulseless, white leg with paraesthesia and paralysis should be taken to theatre otherwise delays in performing an arteriogram could well render the limb irrecoverable before the patient has even reached theatre. Other patients may also benefit from an immediate approach such as those patients with a saddle embolus. The desirability for high quality intra-arterial digital subtraction imaging (Figure 26.2) along with the interventional expertise of the vascular radiologist need to be balanced against the 'therapeutic window' available. In other words, image and consider all possibilities including thrombolysis providing the limb is thought able to withstand the time expected to return at least partial arterial inflow to that limb. It is inappropriate to consider lysis in a limb with sensory and motor deficit as the time taken to achieve lysis, even using high dose bolus or 'pulse-spray' techniques, will be considerably longer than the limb can be expected to endure. Modern units now have the facilities to perform on-table angiography including digital subtraction and road-mapping techniques.

Duplex imaging in the acute situation can still provide very useful and potentially rapid information including the presence or absence of aortic and popliteal aneurysms. Injudicious use of a thromboembolectomy catheter in an acutely ischaemic limb secondary to a thrombosed popliteal aneurysm is unlikely to be successful and may render attempts at surgical reconstruction futile. The presence of a thrombosed or embolizing popliteal aneurysm should be raised by the presence of an easily palpable mass or a prominent pulse in either popliteal fossa, and also in the presence of a known femoral or aortic aneurysm.

Rapid duplex scanning will confirm or refute the diagnosis quickly. If the limb is still viable, percutaneous thrombolysis can be used to lyse the run-off vessel(s) with the catheter passed through and beyond the aneurysm itself. Lysis within the aneurysm is likely to cause further embolization which may not be

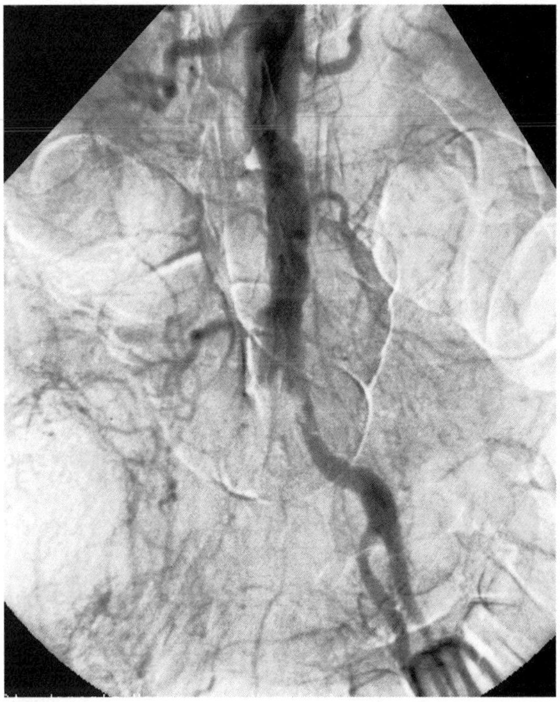

Figure 26.2 IA DSA showing right common and external iliac artery occlusion and partially occlusive thrombus within left common iliac artery.

amenable to lysis or surgical extraction. Once the run-off vessel(s) have been identified, then surgical proximal and distal ligation of the aneurysm together with a reversed saphenous vein bypass graft should be performed.

In the more severely affected cases, intra-operative lysis through the distal popliteal artery or tibio-peroneal trunk can be utilized whilst vein harvesting is being performed. Proximal and distal ligation of the aneurysm, and the proximal anastomosis can all be performed whilst lysis is continuing. Once a suitable run-off vessel is confirmed with on-table digital subtraction angiography, the distal anastomosis can then be performed. In severe cases, a four compartment fasciotomy should also be considered.

Section 26.3 • Management (Table 26.3)

On presentation, the patient should ideally be reviewed by the vascular surgical registrar or equivalent. The administration of 5000 units of intravenous heparin will help to reduce further propagation of thrombus while awaiting definitive treatment with either thrombolysis or surgery. Following resuscitation and appropriate imaging as mentioned previously, the patient can be considered for thrombolysis, balloon catheter thromboembolectomy or surgical reconstruction. In reality, the patient should be continually assessed throughout which ever treatment modality is chosen, to ensure that it remains the preferred option, and that circumstances have not changed to make an alternative approach more likely to be beneficial to the patient.

The patients should be kept well hydrated and careful control of blood glucose, potassium, haemoglobin and oxygen saturation will all contribute to protect and salvage the acutely ischaemic limb and indeed the patient. Reperfusion syndrome can be severe and cause arrhythmias due to the release of potassium, hydrogen ions and lactate. Alkalization of the urine may be helpful to attempt to reduce the incidence and severity of myoglobin induced renal failure.

Heparin therapy

Heparin therapy as an alternative to surgical intervention has been advocated for patients with acute ischaemia especially in the presence of comorbidity. While a controversial, limb salvage rate of approximately 60% with a cumulative mortality of 27% could be achieved. In the severely compromised patient it may be a safer option than inappropriate attempts at reconstruction.

Surgical thromboembolectomy (Figures 26.3 and 26.4)

Balloon catheter thromboembolectomy was pioneered by Thomas Fogarty in 1963. He showed that with careful use, thromboembolic material could be removed

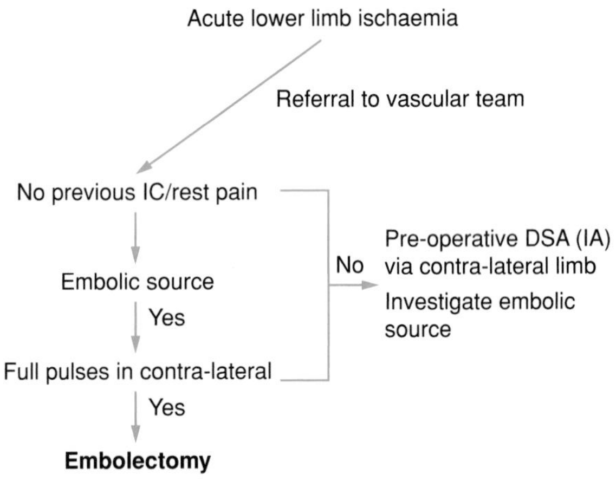

Figure 26.3 Initial flow diagram for the management of acute lower limb ischaemia.

Table 26.3 Management options in acute limb ischaemia

Heparin

Thrombolysis:
- Agents
  Streptokinase
  r-Tissue plasminogen activator
  Urokinase
- Techniques
  High-dose bolus
  'Pulse-spray'
  Low-dose infusions

Surgery:
- Fogarty embolectomy
- Intra-operative thrombolysis
- Intra-operative angioplasty
- Atherectomy
- Reconstruction/fasciotomy

Amputation

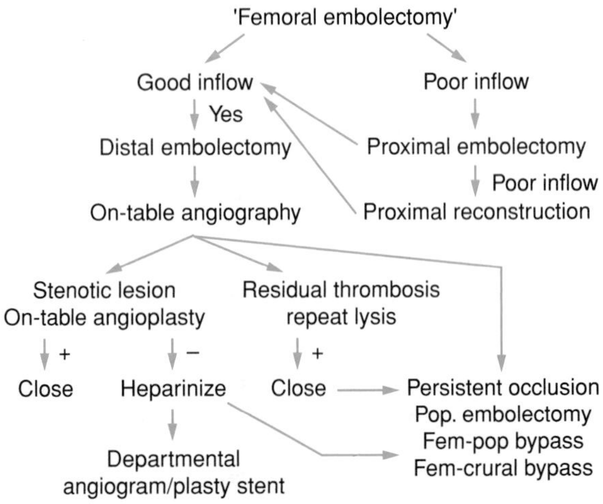

Figure 26.4 'Femoral embolectomy' flow diagram – suggested intra-operative strategy.

from remote sites with a significant increase in limb salvage. This procedure may only be the preliminary to a more radical surgical reconstruction if necessary. Patients may have recently suffered a myocardial infarction and this needs to be remembered in the management plan to avoid death of the patient – a local anaesthetic balloon extraction may be insufficient. Whenever possible general or regional anaesthesia will allow an uninhibited approach to attempting limb salvage for the patient. The surgeon should be prepared to perform on-table imaging (preferably digital subtraction angiography) to assess the efficacy of each intervention.

Using a 30° coude tip on the embolectomy catheter, anatomical studies have shown that the posterior tibial artery can be entered in approximately 75% of cases. It is the peroneal artery that is usually entered (85%) with a direct in-line catheter.

For crural emboli, the surgeon may need to consider the relative merits of popliteal/tibial embolectomy against per-femoral catheter directed thrombolysis. The latter technique is less invasive, can be beneficial and is readily checked using repeat on-table angiography.

It is known that up to 30% of patients will have residual thrombus following balloon catheter thromboembolectomy. These patients can then receive on-table thrombolysis with either streptokinase 100 000 units in 100 ml (in normal saline) over 20 min or recombinant tissue plasminogen activator 5 mg boluses (in 20 ml normal saline) up to three times over 30 min. Repeat angiography can then be performed to ensure clearance. Further gentle thromboembolectomy can then be performed which will probably be able to extract the less adherent thrombus. Other devices which can be utilized include the 'adherent clot removal catheter' and 'graft thrombectomy catheters' (Baxter Healthcare Corporation, Irvine, California, USA) which consist of a helical design to allow extraction of adherent clot from the side walls of native vessels and of prosthetic grafts respectively. Angioscopy can directly visualize the effects of these catheters to ensure complete clearance. Distal use of balloon thromboembolectomy catheters can be performed with some contrast in the balloon and the use of on-table image intensification to help reduce multiple passages likely to damage the intima. This will allow directed extraction and monitoring of the efficacy and deformation of the balloon itself. Careful manipulation of the balloon and the catheter itself under vision should help to keep intimal damage to a minimum and avoid limb threatening intimal or pseudointimal flaps which will either dissect and cause occlusion or be the focus of further embolization.

Saddle embolus at the aortic bifurcation requires a simultaneous bilateral femoral approach. Good quality image intensification is essential to confirm adequate visualization of clearance. Some vascular units have sterile facilities within the vascular radiological suite to allow departmental quality imaging. However, with modern carbon fibre operating tables and mobile image intensifiers with digital subtraction facilities, very good imaging is possible within the theatre suite. Following this procedure the patient should remain on heparin until all sources of embolization have been adequately investigated with the use of echocardiography, spiral computed tomography examination and arteriography as necessary. The type of echocardiography should also be considered as only transoesophageal will adequately visualize the left atrium and auricle to fully exclude left atrial thrombus or myxoma. Patients should then be warfarinized unless the underlying aetiological problem (e.g. critical stenosis) has been corrected, when anti-platelet therapy alone may be deemed sufficient.

Upper limb thromboembolectomy

Due to the excellent collateral circulation, embolism in the upper limb does not usually present as a white limb. Embolic material will usually lodge within the brachial artery or its division. A lazy 's' incision centred on the antecubital fossa will allow good visualization of brachial, radial and ulnar arteries. Pre-operative digital subtraction angiography should be performed to allow confirmation of diagnosis, to allow recognition of the extent of the embolus or thrombus and potential intervention for any significant proximal lesions including non-occlusive thrombus material proximally.

The results following brachial embolectomy, which can easily be performed under local anaesthesia, are usually excellent even in the most frail patients. Closure of the arteriotomy should be performed with loop magnification using 6/0 or 7/0 sutures, augmented in small vessels with an autogenous vein patch.

Due to the underlying concurrent cardiac pathology, the death rate following major arterial embolism is still approximately 20–30%.

Thrombolysis

Percutaneous thrombolysis can offer an alternative therapy for the management of acute and acute-on-chronic limb ischaemia (Figure 26.5). Particular indications include thrombosed grafts, native vessel thromboses, distal emboli, thrombosed popliteal aneurysms and post-procedural thromboses. The duration of history is still debatable, although data from the STILE study suggest that the more recent lesions fare better with thrombolysis (less than 14 days and 7 days, respectively). Most centres within the UK have limited the technique to those lesions less than 30 days old. Due to increased cross-linking of fibrin, thrombus becomes more resistant to lysis with lesions older than 6 months associated with a 24% recanalization rate, compared to 72% in lesions less than 1 week old. Patients need to be selected to exclude patients with a history of cerebrovascular accident within the previous 2 months, neurosurgery including spinal surgery within the previous 3 months, a bleeding diathesis, recent trauma including cardiopulmonary resuscitation within the previous 10 days, pregnancy or those unable to

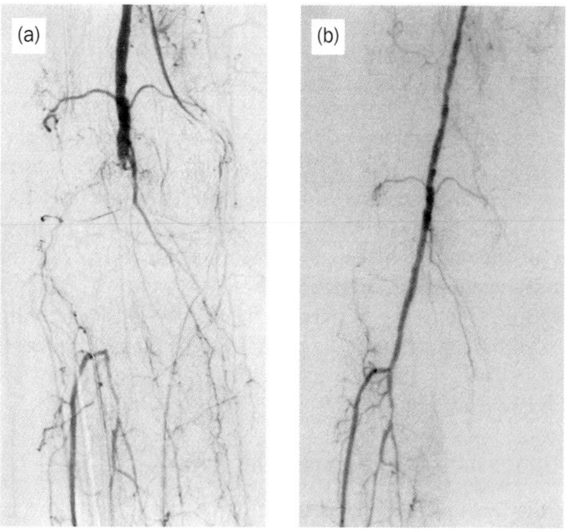

Figure 26.5 (a) IA DSA showing occlusion of the popliteal artery and proximal crural run-off vessels. (b) IA DSA following rt-PA and angioplasty of a residual popliteal proximal stenosis. (Mosby Year Book, St Louis, USA.)

give informed consent or likely to be potentially uncooperative. Age itself is not a bar, but in the very elderly (over 75 years of age) is associated with a higher haemorrhagic complication rate.

While thrombolysis can produce impressive clearance of thrombus, it can be associated with an overall stroke rate of 1–3%, a major haemorrhage rate of 10% and a minor haemorrhage rate of up to 25%. Distal embolization can occur in approximately 2% of patients during peripheral arterial thrombolysis, but is more likely in cases of thrombosed popliteal aneurysms (12%), especially when the catheter is not placed within the distal popliteal artery beyond the aneurysm itself. Other, though less frequent complications include peri-catheter thrombosis, anaphylaxis and reperfusion injury. Informed consent must include a discussion of these specific risks with the patient.

Which drug?

Streptokinase was initially used systemically but was associated with unacceptable haemorrhagic complication rates. Local low-dose regimens were more successful (streptokinase 5000 units/hour), and within strict protocols very encouraging results were obtained and continued to be shown long term. Later experience with urokinase and recombinant tissue plasminogen activator (rt-PA) suggested that increased efficacy and reduced complications might be achievable with these two agents compared to streptokinase. Graor *et al.* in an open comparison suggested a significant advantage of urokinase and rt-PA over streptokinase. Streptokinase excites an antibody response and therefore may be ineffective in patients who have previously received streptokinase for coronary thrombolysis or peripheral arterial thrombolysis, and even in those patients with a recent past history of streptococcal infection. Subsequent reuse may therefore be completely ineffective and may cause allergenic reactions including, rarely, anaphylaxis. Few randomized trials are available to allow a definitive conclusion. Berridge *et al.*, in a small randomized comparison of intra-arterial streptokinase and intra-arterial recombinant tissue plasminogen activator, showed a reduced haemorrhagic complication rate and an increased patency sustained at 3 months. Streptokinase was used at 5000 units/hour, intra-arterial rt-PA was used at 0.5 mg/hour. In another small randomized comparison of rt-PA and urokinase, faster lysis and more frequent lysis was seen with rt-PA compared to urokinase but this did not achieve statistical significance possibly due to a type II statistical effect. There is insufficient evidence to differentiate efficacy and safety between rt-PA and urokinase.

Which technique?

Local low-dose thrombolysis was the initial method of choice. It allowed accurate delivery of the thrombolytic agent directly into the thrombus. The end of the catheter was buried distally into the thrombus and then sequentially retracted in stages as thrombolysis progressed. Other centres would advocate lysing proximally and then repositioning under image intensification more distally as necessary. It is essential that the catheter tip remains embedded in the thrombus to allow local high concentrations of lytic agent and to minimize systemic loss and therefore creating a systemic lytic state. It was originally thought that this method of local delivery would allow a purely local lytic process, however it was subsequently shown that even with low doses such as 0.5 mg/hour rt-PA or 5000 units/hour streptokinase, a systemic effect could be detected. This was more rapid and more severe in the streptokinase group compared to the rt-PA group. The mean time to lysis was approximately 22 hours which meant that for the severely acute limb, there would be insufficient time to allow lysis and still be able to realistically expect limb salvage. To attempt to widen the scope of thrombolysis, multi-side hole catheters were used to allow a greater surface area of thrombus to be exposed to the lytic agent simultaneously. This progressed to the concept of the 'pulse-spray' technique which involved multi-side hole catheters and high velocity spraying of the thrombus with the lytic agent. Initially the technique was a manual process, but later an automated device became available. Initial work suggested that lysis could be achieved at a much faster rate, with no apparent increase in the complication rate including the concern of distal embolization. However, in the only randomized comparison of pulse-spray and local low dose infusions, Kandarpa *et al.* did not show any benefit over the standard method following an initial bolus. Similar claims were suggested with high dose bolus techniques. Braithwaite *et al.* performed a randomized trial comparing local low dose infusions with high dose bolus infusions. There was no overall difference in efficacy between the two groups although approximately half of the high dose bolus group achieved lysis within 4 hours. Complications were higher in the high dose bolus group although these did not reach statistical significance possibly due to a type II statistical error (i.e. insufficient numbers). The choice of technique therefore lies with the experience of the institution performing thrombolysis.

Initial thrombolysis or initial surgery in the treatment of the acutely ischaemic limb?

To justify the use of thrombolysis the limb must be potentially recoverable and be able to withstand a further period of ischaemia which may be up to 24 hours before significant antegrade pulsatile flow is restored. Even with pulse-spray and high-dose bolus techniques, half of the patients will still need continuing of lysis beyond 4–6 hours. The classical 'white leg' should therefore not be treated with this technique.

There are few randomized studies comparing surgery with thrombolysis. In a small study of 20 patients of less than 14 days' duration randomized to surgery or lysis, Nilsson *et al.* demonstrated a higher patency (65% vs 40%) in the thrombectomy group – although one must exercise caution in the interpretation due to the low numbers. The STILE trial recruited 393 patients, the majority of whom were actually acute-on-chronic or chronic as their duration of history was up to 6 months. Lysis was performed either using rt-PA at 0.05 mg/kg/hour for up to 12 hours or urokinase in an initial bolus of 250 000 units followed by 4000 units/min for 4 hours then 2000 units/min for up to 36 hours. There was no difference between rt-Pa and urokinase in terms of safety or efficacy. Of those patients with a duration of history of less than 14 days, initial lysis was associated with significantly lower amputation rates at 6 months and approximately half (56%) had a reduction in the magnitude of their anticipated initial surgical procedure. It should be noted that 30% of patients did not receive thrombolysis as intended due to the inability to be able to place the catheter within the thrombus. Two further publications from the same trial have allowed a greater analysis of the groups of patients most likely to benefit. Weaver *et al.* specifically looked at those patients with native (non-embolic) occlusions. At 1 year follow-up, patients randomized to initial lysis had a higher incidence of major amputation or continuing ischaemia (59.8% vs 33.8%) compared to the surgical group, but there was no significant difference in mortality. Twenty-two per cent of patients randomized to lysis were unable to have the catheter positioned correctly to allow thrombolysis. Comerota *et al.* analysed thrombosed lower limb bypass grafts. Those patients with a duration of ischaemia of less than 14 days had a lower amputation rate at 1 year compared to the surgical group ($p = 0.03$). Conversely, those patients with a duration of ischaemia in excess of 14 days fared worse with lysis, with similar amputation rates but significantly more ongoing or recurrent ischaemia ($p < 0.001$). However, 39% of those randomized to receive thrombolysis received surgical revascularization as a direct result of failure of catheter placement. Patients with occluded prosthetic grafts were associated with significantly greater morbidity than those with occluded autogenous grafts.

Ouriel *et al.* studied 114 patients with short duration of history of less than 7 days, using a regimen of urokinase 4000 units/min for 2 hours, followed by 2000 units/min for a further 2 hours, and then 1000 units/min up to a maximum lytic duration of 48 hours. All patients were also given 325 mg aspirin on entry into the study. Follow-up at 1 year showed a significant survival advantage in the lysis group (84% vs 58%, $p < 0.01$). This was probably due to the marked difference in in-house cardiopulmonary complications seen at the time of the initial admission (49% vs 16%, $p = 0.001$).

The TOPAS trial phase I consisted of 213 patients of less than 14 days' duration of ischaemia, who were randomized to either surgery or one of three thrombolytic regimens using urokinase at 2000, 4000 or 6000 units/min for 4 hours followed as necessary with 2000 units/min for up to 48 hours. The most optimal dose regimen occurred using 4000 unit/min urokinase, with a 1 year mortality of 14% and amputation-free survival of 75%. These results did not differ significantly from those obtained in the surgical group. There was a significant reduction in the frequency and severity of open surgery at 1 year. In the subsequent phase II study 544 patients with limb ischaemia of less than 14 days' duration were entered from 113 centres within North America and Europe. The urokinase dose was fixed at 4000 units/min. Again there was no significant difference in the amputation-free survival at 1 year (65% thrombolysis; 70% surgical). However, there were substantially fewer open procedures performed at 6 months in the group initially treated with lysis (315 vs 551). There were four strokes (1.6%), one of which was fatal, all occurring in the lysis group.

In carefully selected and monitored patients, thrombolysis can reduce the need for or severity of open vascular surgery required with acceptable limb salvage and haemorrhagic complication rates. It is a useful further treatment and diagnostic modality in modern vascular and endovascular units.

Post-thrombolysis

After successful thrombolysis, it is essential to correct the underlying aetiological factor that precipitated the acute event: achieved with balloon angioplasty, stents, corrective bypass surgery or treatment of medical factors such as atrial fibrillation or an inherent thrombophilia. Gardiner *et al.* have shown widely disparate patencies depending upon whether an underlying stenosis is corrected. Providing this factor(s) is corrected it would be reasonable to treat the patient initially with heparin (to counter the post-lysis prothrombotic state) and then follow with aspirin. For those patients still at substantial risk, including those in atrial fibrillation, poor run-off, slow-flow states and thrombophilia, warfarinization should be used.

Long-term results

Providing that the catheter can be adequately sited and especially if the underlying aetiological factor has been corrected then good long-term results can be expected. Giddings *et al.* reported a 4 year limb salvage rate of 68% with the majority of those requiring amputation occurring within the first 30 days. A 2 year cumulative patency of 81% was found in the Nottingham series.

Further reading

Berridge, D. C., Makin, G. S. and Hopkinson, B. R. (1989). Local low-dose intra-arterial thrombolytic therapy: the risk of stroke or major haemorrhage. *Br J Surg* **76**: 1230–3.

Berridge, D. C., Gregson, R. H. S., Hopkinson, B. R. and Makin, G. S. (1991). Randomised trial of intra-arterial recombinant tissue plasminogen activator, intra-venous recombinant tissue plasminogen activator and intra-arterial streptokinase in peripheral arterial thrombolysis. *Br J Surg* **78**: 988–95.

Blaisdell, F. W., Steele, M. and Allen, R. E. (1978). Management of acute lower extremity arterial ischaemia due to embolism and thrombosis. *Surgery* **84**: 822.

Braithwaite, B. D., Buckenham, T. M., Galland, R. B. *et al.* (1997). Prospective randomised trial of high-dose bolus versus low-dose tissue plasminogen activator infusion in the management of acute limb ischaemia. *Br J Surg* **84**: 646–50.

Braithwaite, B. D., Davies, B., Birch, P. A. *et al.* (1998). Management of acute leg ischaemia in the elderly. *Br J Surg* **85**: 217–20.

Campbell, W. B., Ridler, B. M. F. and Szymanska, T. H. (1998). Current management of acute leg ischaemia: results of an audit by the Vascular Surgical Society of Great Britain and Ireland. *Br J Surg* **85**: 1498–503.

Comerota, A. J., Weaver, F. A., Hosking, J. D. *et al.* (1996). Results of a prospective randomised trial of surgery versus thrombolysis for occluded lower extremity bypass grafts. *Am J Surg* **172**: 105–12.

Dawson, K., Armon, A., Braithwaite, B. D. *et al.* (1996). Stroke during intra-arterial thrombolysis: a survey of experience in the UK. *Br J Surg* **83**: 568 (Abstract).

Decrinis, M., Pilger, E., Stark, G. *et al.* (1993). Simplified procedure for intra-arterial thrombolysis with tissue-type plasminogen activator in peripheral occlusive disease. Primary and long-term results. *Eur Heart J* **14**: 297–305.

Fogarty, T. J., Cranley, J. J., Krause, R. J. *et al.* (1963). A method for extracting arterial emboli and thrombi. *Surg Gynaecol Obstet* **2**: 241–4.

Fogarty, T. J. and Hermann, G. D. (1991). New techniques for clot extraction and managing acute thromboembolic limb ischaemia. In: Veith, F. J., ed. *Current Critical Problems in Vascular Surgery*. St Louis: Quality Medical Publishing, **3**: 197–203.

Galland, R. B., Earnshaw, J. J., Baird, R. N. *et al.* (1993). Acute limb deterioration during intra-arterial thrombolysis. *Br J Surg* **80**: 1118–20.

Gardiner, G. A., Koltun, W., Kandarpa, K. *et al.* (1986). Thrombolysis of occluded femoro-popliteal grafts. *Am J Roentgenol* **147**: 621–6.

Giddings, A. E. B., Quraishy, M. S. and Walker, W. J. (1993). Long term results of a single protocol for thrombolysis in acute lower-limb ischaemia. *Br J Surg* **80**: 1262–5.

Graor, R. A., Olin, J., Bartholomew, J. R., Ruschhaupt, W. F. and Young, J. R. (1990). Efficacy and safety of intra-arterial local infusion of streptokinase, urokinase or tissue plasminogen activator for peripheral arterial occlusion: a retrospective study. *J Vasc Med Rev* **2**: 310–15.

Gwynn, B. R., Shearman, C. P. and Simms, M. H. (1987). The anatomical basis for the route taken by Fogarty catheters in the lower leg. *Eur J Surg* **1**: 129–32.

Kakkar, V. V., Flanc, C., O'Shea, M. J. *et al.* (1969). Treatment of deep-vein thrombosis with streptokinase. *Br J Surg* **56**: 178–83.

Kandarpa, K., Chopra, P. S., Aruny, J. E. *et al.* (1993). Intra-arterial thrombolysis of lower extremity occlusions: prospective, randomised comparison of forced periodic infusion and conventional slow continuous infusion. *Radiology* **188**: 861–67.

Lonsdale, R. J., Whitaker, S. C., Berridge, D. C. *et al.* (1993). Peripheral arterial thrombolysis: intermediate-term results. *Br J Surg* **80**: 592–5.

Meyerovitz, M. F., Goldhaber, S. Z., Reagan, K. *et al.* (1990). Recombinant tissue-type plasminogen activator versus urokinase in peripheral arterial and graft occlusions: a randomised trial. *Radiology* **175**: 75–8.

Nilsson, L., Albrechtsson, U., Jonung, T. *et al.* (1992). Surgical treatment versus thrombolysis in acute arterial occlusion: a randomised controlled study. *Eur J Vasc Surg* **6**: 189–93.

Ouriel, K., Shortell, C. K., DeWeese, J. A. *et al.* (1994). A comparison of thrombolytic therapy with operative revascularisation in the initial treatment of acute peripheral arterial ischaemia. *J Vasc Surg* **19**: 1021–30.

Ouriel, K., Veith, F. J., Sasahara, A. A. for the TOPAS Investigators (1996). Thrombolysis or peripheral arterial surgery: phase I results. *J Vasc Surg* **23**: 64–75.

Ouriel, K., Veith, F. J., Sasahara, A. A. for the TOPAS Investigators (1998). A comparison of recombinant urokinase with vascular surgery as initial treatment for acute arterial occlusion of the legs. *N Engl J Med* **338**: 1105–11.

Pemberton, M., Varty, K., Nydahl, S. and Bell, P. R. F. (1999). The surgical management of acute limb ischaemia due to native vessel occlusion. *Eur J Vasc Surg* **17**: 72–6.

Rutherford, R. B., Baker, J. D., Ernst, C. *et al.* (1997). Recommended standards for reports dealing with lower extremity ischaemia: Revised version. *J Vasc Surg* **26**: 517–38.

STILE Investigators (1994). Results of a prospective randomised trial evaluating surgery versus thrombolysis for ischaemia of the lower extremity – the STILE trial. *Ann Surg* **220**: 251–68.

Tawes, R. L., Harris, E. J., Brown, W. H. *et al.* (1985). Arterial thromboembolism. A 20 year perspective. *Arch Surg* **120**: 595–9.

Walker, W. J. and Giddings, A. E. B. (1985). Low-dose intra-arterial streptokinase: benefit versus risk. *Clin Radiol* **36**: 345–3.

Walker, W. J. and Giddings, A. E. B. (1988). A protocol for the safe treatment of acute lower limb ischaemia with intra-arterial streptokinase and surgery. *Br J Surg* **75**: 1189–92.

Weaver, F. A., Comerota, A. J., Youngblood, M. *et al.* and the STILE Investigators (1996). Surgical revascularisation versus thrombolysis for nonembolic lower extremity native artery occlusions: results of a prospective trial. *J Vasc Surg* **24**: 51–3.

Working Party on Thrombolysis in the Management of Limb Ischaemia (1998). Thrombolysis in the management of lower limb peripheral arterial occlusion – a consensus document. *Am J Cardiol* **81**: 207–18.

MODULE 27

Chronic lower limb occlusive disease

1 • Aetiology
2 • Risk factors
3 • Pathophysiology of chronic lower limb ischaemia
4 • Risk factor management
5 • Pharmacotherapy
6 • Endovascular interventions in the management of intermittent claudication
7 • Surgery for intermittent claudication
8 • Non-vascular management

The term chronic lower limb ischaemia should be used in clearly defined terms to differentiate between the two major spectra of the disease (i.e. intermittent claudication and critical limb ischaemia). Since the management and the outcome of these two conditions are different, the impact on the individual and the resources required for management differ.

Intermittent claudication is used to describe patients in whom the degree of ischaemia does not constitute an immediate threat to the limb. In critical limb ischaemia, the limb is threatened by the degree of ischaemia as determined by rest pain and/or tissue loss.

Section 27.1 • Aetiology

The most important cause of peripheral vascular disease is atherosclerosis giving rise to stenosis or occlusion of the arterial supply to a limb resulting in chronic ischaemia. Atherosclerosis is considered to be a dynamic condition with periods of quiescence and increased activity. It is a generalized disease affecting the macrocirculation and microcirculation. Its effect on the macrocirculation involves mainly the coronary, carotid bifurcation, aorto-iliac and femorodistal segments. The main effect on the microcirculation is reduction in the perfusion pressure and increased interaction of cellular elements with the endothelium due to increased transit time. There is local release of adenosine diphosphate (ADP) and activation of platelets. In addition there is activation of neutrophils and release of endothelial-damaging substances (interleukins, tumour necrosis factor, etc.) with a net result of damage to vascular endothelium and worsening ischaemia.

Section 27.2 • Risk factors

The major risk factors for the development of atherosclerosis appear to be smoking, elevated blood lipids, hypertension and diabetes mellitus (Table 27.1). Nevertheless, many others exist, although they probably have less influence on the development of atherosclerosis in most individuals.

Smoking

Cigarette smoking appears to be the single most important risk factor in chronic limb ischaemia, with smokers having a four-fold increased risk of developing peripheral arterial occlusive disease over non-smokers. Current smokers account for an estimated 14–53% of disease; if ex-smokers are included this figure increases. The Framingham study has suggested that three-quarters of cases of intermittent claudication can be attributed to smoking.

The exact mechanisms by which smoking causes atherosclerosis are unknown, but may be associated with lower intakes of antioxidants (β-carotene and vitamin C). A low antioxidant intake may lead to increased oxidation of fatty acids and atherogenecity of low-density lipoproteins (LDL). Other mechanisms including platelet and neutrophil activation also seem to be involved, but further studies are needed to elucidate the precise mechanism(s) by which smoking causes its deleterious effects on the arteries.

Smoking is a controversial issue in patients with chronic limb ischaemia who are believed to be less than open regarding their smoking status. Using objective evidence of cessation of smoking (carboxyhaemoglobin concentrations and cotinine levels), no short-term (1–3 years)

Table 27.1 Major risk factors for peripheral arterial occlusive disease

Positive	Men over 45 years
	Women over 55 years or premature menopause (no HRT)
	Family history of premature atherosclerosis
	Smoking
	HDL < 35 mg/dl
	Diabetes mellitus
	Hypertension

benefit in the progression of the disease or symptoms was found. However, clear trends show that smoking is associated with a higher graft failure rate. A smoking cessation period of more than 7 years was found to be associated with diminished progression to critical limb ischaemia.

Hyperlipidaemia: cholesterol and lipoproteins (low- and high-density lipoproteins)

The importance of elevated cholesterol levels in the development of atherosclerosis has been examined and a strong association implicated. The LDLs carry cholesterol from the liver to the peripheral tissues and the high-density lipoproteins (HDLs) return cholesterol to the liver. Low levels of HDLs have been shown in patients with chronic lower limb ischaemia compared to controls.

Apolipoproteins

Apolipoprotein B is a large protein contained within the LDL particles and a high level of apolipoprotien B has been associated with the development of atherosclerosis. The apolipoprotein levels in the peripheral circulation may discriminate between patients with atherosclerosis and controls better than cholesterol or lipoproteins.

Elevated levels of triglycerides appear to correlate more with the development of peripheral vascular disease than cholesterol. In the Edinburgh Artery Study, this strong univariate association disappeared on multivariate analysis.

Hypertension

Elevated mean blood pressure is more common in patients with intermittent claudication compared to normal controls. Hypertension seems to have a synergistic effect with smoking by increasing the movement of nicotine across the endothelial cell membrane.

Diabetes mellitus

Most studies support the view that progression of atherosclerosis is more rapid in diabetics. The age-adjusted prevalence of intermittent claudication was three to four times and 5.7 times higher in diabetic men and women respectively in a study from Finland. The most distinguishing feature in diabetics with peripheral vascular disease is the distribution of the pattern of lower limb arterial disease. The occlusive disease tends to involve the infrageniculate arteries sparing the proximal and often pedal arteries. Glucose intolerance may play a role in the aetiology of atherosclerosis although reports are conflicting. Further studies will be needed to evaluate the role of glucose intolerance.

Antioxidant vitamins

Polyunsaturated fatty acid peroxidation seems to play a significant role in the genesis and progression of peripheral vascular disease. Antioxidants prevent the oxidative damage to polyunsaturated fatty acids and the naturally occurring antioxidants are vitamins A, C, E and β-carotene, a provitamin. Patients with intermittent claudication have been shown to have lower levels of antioxidants and raised levels of plasma lipid peroxide. A large randomized controlled trial is required to support the above findings.

Fibrinogen and rheological factors

Reports have shown that elevated levels of fibrinogen are a significant risk factor for myocardial infarction. In patients with intermittent claudication elevated plasma levels of fibrinogen have also been found, suggesting that fibrinogen may play an important role in atherosclerosis.

In the Edinburgh Artery Study, the odds ratio for peripheral artery disease in relation to the plasma fibrinogen was highly significant. However, fibrinogen levels may be affected by smoking and population studies have shown that cessation of smoking leads to a fall in the fibrinogen level. There is also an elevated level of other factors including factors VIII and XIII, plasminogen and antiplasmin in these patients. This study also found that mean levels of von Willebrand factor, β-thromboglobulin (a marker of platelet release), plasminogen activator inhibitor and cross-linked fibrin degradation products were each significantly raised. When adjusted for smoking an even greater impact on the odds of the disease was found. Blood viscosity has been found to be raised in patients with intermittent claudication.

It would appear from these results that patients with peripheral vascular disease have an increased tendency towards thrombogenesis, but how these various haemostatic factors contribute to chronic vessel wall damage is unclear.

Other risk factors

A sedentary lifestyle has been shown to be a risk factor for ischaemic heart disease. The relation between exercise and peripheral vascular disease is less certain. People who walk for half an hour a day have half the cardiovascular mortality rate of those who lead a sedentary life. In the Edinburgh Artery Study, male smokers with less physical activity had a higher risk of peripheral vascular disease. The relationship of obesity and peripheral vascular disease is controversial.

Personality type IA has been associated with an increased risk of developing cardiovascular disease. These people are competitive and have less ability to control anger.

Homocysteine

Elevation in the levels of homocysteine has been recently shown to be associated with all forms of peripheral vascular disease. Homocysteine is an amino acid that reacts with LDL cholesterol to form oxidized LDL – a component of foam cells which are found in early atheromatous plaques. A high level of this amino acid is also a risk factor for thrombophlebitis and is

Table 27.2 Risk factors grouped according to whether they are modifiable

Fixed	*Modifiable*
Age	Smoking
Sex	Lipids
Diabetes	Hypertension
	Exercise
	Obesity

associated with accelerated progression of atherosclerosis. The genetic deficiency of the enzyme cystathionine β-synthetase is thought to lead to the elevated levels of homocysteine. Dietary deficiency of folic acid or vitamins B_2 and B_6 may also cause raised homocysteine levels.

A combination of risk factors rather than a single dominant risk factor seem to be important in the development of peripheral vascular disease (Table 27.2).

Section 27.3 • Pathophysiology of chronic lower limb ischaemia

For a long time the attention of the vascular surgeon was focused on the large vessel changes giving rise to occlusion or stenosis seen in atherosclerosis. Although this is important as the primary cause of chronic limb ischaemia, recent studies have increasingly recognized the role of microvascular millieu changes in the pathophysiology of chronic limb ischaemia. The pathophysiology of chronic limb ischaemia in humans is not fully understood but it appears that atherosclerosis is a dynamic process involving haemodynamic, biochemical and haematological disturbances. The atheromatous plaque may undergo periods of increased activity associated with deterioration of limb ischaemia or it may heal and regress. There may be development of collateral blood flow. The ability of the microcirculation to respond to the reduction in blood flow may ultimately determine the outcome of the limb.

Macrocirculation

The fundamental process in the pathogenesis of chronic limb ischaemia is atherosclerosis. In general, the development of an atherosclerotic plaque can be divided into three stages: early lesions, fibrous plaques and complicated lesion.

Early lesions

Fatty streaks appear early in life as minimally raised yellow lesions and represent lipid laden foam cells in the intima. On microscopy, these show lipids deposited in macrophages and smooth muscle cells. These have been shown experimentally to progress to fibrous plaques.

Fibrous plaques

These are more advanced atheromatous lesions composed of large numbers of smooth muscle cells and connective tissue forming a fibrous cap over an inner yellow core of mainly cholesterol esters (Figure 27.1). Alterations may occur in the composition of the fibrous plaque with advancing disease. The fibrous cap may become thin and ulcerate or there may be associated intraplaque haemorrhage. Generally, the fibrous plaque with time causes partial or complete obstruction of the lumen of the artery resulting in diminished blood flow.

The complicated lesion

Fibrous plaques complicated by ulceration, haemorrhage, calcification or extensive necrosis comprise end-stage atherosclerosis. Thinning of the fibrous cap and a

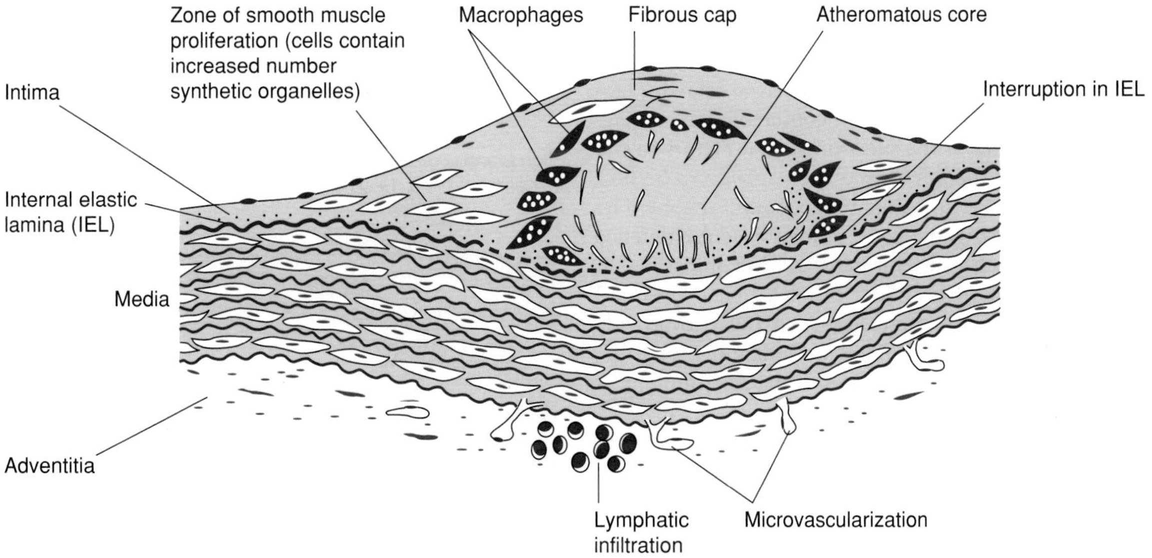

Figure 27.1 Diagram showing the composition of a fibrous atheromatous plaque. (Reproduced with permission from DePalma, R. G. The pathology of atheromas. In: Bell, Jamieson and Ruckley (eds). *Surgical Management of Vascular Disease*. London: WB Saunders, 1992.)

larger lipid core are characteristics of an unstable lesion. This unstable plaque may rupture or ulcerate exposing a highly thrombogenic surface which may lead to activation of platelets and formation of a thrombotic plug. Plaque rupture may also give rise to thrombotic occlusion or distal small vessel embolization. This corresponds to clinical events of stroke, myocardial infarction and gangrene. There is evidence to indicate that the risk of clinical cardiovascular events is associated with the number of unstable plaques.

The macrocirculation has compensatory mechanisms which can help with limiting the effects of atherosclerosis. Probably the most important mechanism in chronic ischaemia is the presence of a collateral circulation. These are pre-existing blood vessels which form alternate channels for blood reaching the extremity. The anastomosis between the profunda femoris artery and the geniculate arteries is an example of a well recognized collateral pathway. Collaterals probably develop as a result of a pressure gradient across the collateral bed in the presence of occlusion of the main artery to the limb. There has been recent experimental evidence suggesting that some factors may promote the growth of new blood vessels (angiogenesis), but more work is needed before any definite conclusions can be drawn.

Microcirculation

In health

The microcirculation is composed of the arterioles, capillaries, venules and the interstitial spaces as well as the lymphatic channels. In health, vascular endothelial cells form a non-thrombogenic barrier between the blood and the tissue and are the final arbiter of tissue nutrition. The normal function of the microcirculation is under a complex control by extrinsic neural mechanisms and intrinsic local factors as well as modulation by circulating humoral and blood-borne factors. In healthy tissue, the endothelium is involved with the regulation of flow across it to the tissues by the release of vasodilatory (e.g. endothelium-derived relaxing factor, nitric oxide (NO)) and vasocontractile factors (e.g. endothelin). One of the most important factors in the maintenance of the microcirculation appears to be NO which plays a role in maintaining vasomotor tone. The endothelium also participates in microvascular defence mechanisms such as haemostasis and inflammation. In the normal microcirculation, platelets, leucocytes and vascular endothelium interact in such a way to provide appropriate reactions to injury and inflammation without compromising the nutrition of the micromilieu.

Chronic ischaemia

The main stimulus to changes in the microcirculation in chronic ischaemia seems to be a reduction in perfusion pressure. A reduction in perfusion pressure leads to compensatory vasodilation and abnormal vasomotion and there is maldistribution of nutritive blood flow. This makes the skin prone to minor injuries. The transit time of cells passing through the microcirculation is increased allowing greater interaction with the endothelium. There is also an increase in plasma viscosity in the microcirculation. Red cells are more rigid and, with increased plasma viscosity, they tend to clump together and release ADP which promotes platelet aggregation. Neutrophils are important in the damage that occurs to the microcirculation and neutrophil counts have been found to be elevated in patients with atherosclerosis. The neutrophils '*roll*' along the vessel wall and are arrested. The neutrophils are activated and may release injurious substances like collagenase, gelatinase and elastase which damage the endothelium and cause increased endothelial permeability. The activation of platelets and neutrophils and the damaged endothelium may result in a vicious cycle of damage by way of a complex and incompletely understood mechanism. The damaged endothelium becomes swollen and permeable (Figure 27.2). The increased permeability further reduces tissue nutrition and the damaged endothelium is less capable of producing endothelium-derived relaxing factor (NO) and endothelium-derived vasorelaxant prostacyclin. Prostacyclin inhibits mediator-induced vasospasm and increases cyclic adenosine monophosphate in endothelial cells thereby possibly counteracting increases in endothelial permeability. It also inhibits platelet activation. Following reperfusion of ischaemic limbs, an ischaemia–reperfusion injury may occur and this injury may also occur in remote organs such as the lung and kidney.

Diabetes

The pathophysiology of chronic limb ischaemia in diabetic patients appears to be different. In diabetic patients, the above described changes are more exaggerated with greater platelet adhesion and aggregation, decreased fibrinolytic activity, increased leucocyte free radical production, decreased red cell deformability and increased plasma viscosity. Peripheral neuropathy has a high prevalence in diabetic patients. As a consequence

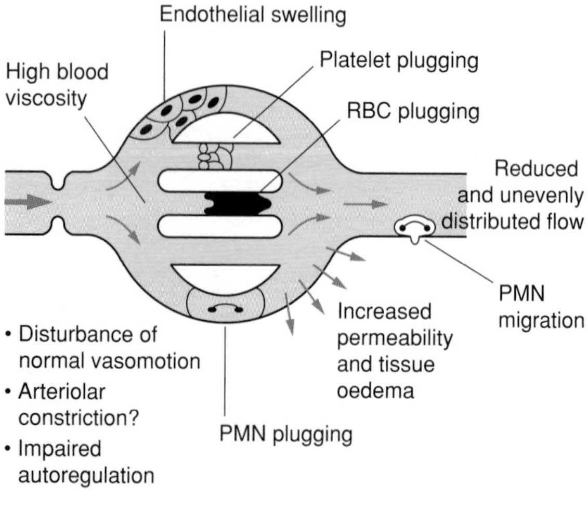

Figure 27.2 Possible causes for microvascular flow obstruction in critical leg ischaemia. RBC, red blood cell; PMN, polymorphonucleocyte.

of reduced pain and thermal sensation, diabetic patients may not notice noxious stimuli and may develop ulcers, gangrene and infection. There is controversy about the vascular changes in diabetic patients with atherosclerotic disease. However, the site of atherosclerotic disease is more distal and more diffuse in diabetics than in non-diabetics. It is also agreed that diabetic angiopathy manifests at an earlier age than in non-diabetics. Poorly controlled diabetics are more prone to infections than those well controlled. Advanced glycosylation end products of proteins in diabetic patients result in the loss of plasticity of these structures. This may lead to alteration of metabolic processes. Also, the glycosylated structures may become antigenic and trap immunoglobulins. This may result in production of immune complexes that enhance platelet aggregation and endothelial damage. Acting together, neuropathy, infection and angiopathy contribute to the sequence of tissue necrosis, ulceration and gangrene seen in the diabetic foot.

The progression of the disease in an ischaemic leg may be stepwise. Therefore, reports dealing with management of chronic leg ischaemia should avoid mixing the different categories. A classification for grading the severity of chronic leg ischaemia has been proposed by the Society for Vascular Surgery and the International Society for Cardiovascular Surgery/North American Chapter (SVS/ISCVS) in 1986 and revised in 1997 (Table 27.3).

Conclusion

The primary cause of chronic limb ischaemia is arterial occlusion. The response of the circulation to arterial occlusion involves both macrocirculation and microcirculation. The direct role of many of the complex rheological factors involved in the pathophysiology of chronic limb ischaemia remains to be fully established and more work is required to elucidate these areas.

Intermittent claudication

Intermittent claudication affects at least 5% of men over 50 years of age, and is twice as common in men as in women. Patients with intermittent claudication are at two to four times greater risk of dying from the complications of generalized atherosclerosis than similar people without claudication. A history of extremity pain, discomfort or weakness that is consistently produced by the same amount of exercise or walking and that is promptly relieved by rest is strongly supportive of the diagnosis.

Claudication implies ischaemic muscle pain induced by exercise, and can be described as hip, buttock, thigh or calf claudication. Calf claudication is due to disease of the superficial femoral artery in the presence of absent popliteal and foot pulses. Thigh and buttock claudication is generally associated with aorto-iliac disease in the presence of a weak or absent femoral pulse and a possible femoral bruit.

In normal individuals, one pedal pulse may be absent and many patients with aorto-iliac disease will present with calf claudication. For these reasons, clinical examination is not infallible. The decision to consider a patient with intermittent claudication for treatment is made by balancing the existing disability against the procedural risk and likelihood of long-term success of an intervention. The patient's disability should be assessed in terms of both the claudication distance and the patients occupation and preferred everyday activities.

Disability is relative, being governed by age, occupation and leisure interests. Therefore, a short claudication distance may be acceptable in a retired elderly patient with very few recreational needs while a 500 m distance may be disabling in a young employed engineer.

Qualifying patients with claudication for intervention as 'disabled' patients or with 'less than one

Table 27.3 Clinical categories of chronic limb ischaemia

Grade	*Category*	*Clinical description*	*Objective criteria*
0	0	Asymptomatic – no haemodynamically significant occlusive disease	Normal treadmill or reactive hyperaemia test
	1	Mild claudication	Completes treadmill exercise[b] and AP after exercise > 50 mmHg but at least 20 mmHg lower than resting value
I	2	Moderate claudication	Between categories 1 and 3
	3	Severe claudication	Cannot complete standard treadmill exercise[b] and AP after exercise <50 mmHg
II[a]	4	Ischaemic rest pain	Resting AP < 40 mmHg, flat or barely pulsatile ankle or metatarsal PVR and TP < 30 mmHg
III[a]	5	Minor tissue loss – non-healing ulcer, focal gangrene with diffuse pedal ischaemia	Resting AP <60mmHg, ankle or metatarsal PVR flat or barely pulsatile and TP < 40 mmHg
	6	Major tissue loss – extending above TM level, functional foot no longer salvageable	Same as category 5

AP, ankle pressure; TP, toe pressure; TM, transmetatarsal; PVR, pulse volume recording.
[a]Grades II and III, categories 4–6, are embraced by the term chronic critical ischaemia.
[b]Five minutes at least at 2 mph on a 12% incline.

block' claudication is convenient and adequate for clinical practise but not precise enough for categorizing patients in clinical research studies. Disability is better assessed by a more detailed analysis of activities and capabilities, such as community-related activity, walking impairment questionnaires, Nottingham Health Profile or other similar quality of life instruments. Quality of life (QOL) measurements assess the functional impairment of claudication on various indices of perceived health. Therefore, 'disabling' claudication, although an acceptable indication for intervention in carefully selected patients, is not an acceptable categorizing criterion in clinical trials. These scores may be helpful in identifying the patients who need intervention, in stratifying patients for therapeutic clinical trials and in monitoring the efficacy of therapy.

Differential diagnosis

There are many possible causes of claudication-like symptoms of the leg which can co-exist with asymptomatic peripheral vascular disease. The absence of pulses in the leg does not necessarily prove the diagnosis of claudication. On the other hand, the presence of pulses in the leg especially in a young patient does not prove the absence of peripheral vascular disease. Therefore, a careful history and detailed examination of the peripheral pulses is important.

Popliteal artery entrapment syndrome

First described by a medical student who dissected an amputated leg in Edinburgh in 1879, the syndrome was thought to be a rare phenomenon by early authors. A greater awareness of the popliteal artery entrapment syndrome as a possible diagnosis in young adults seen by sports medicine specialists and better investigation and screening techniques have led to a more frequent diagnosis and treatment of this condition. The entrapment arises as a result of the popliteal artery coursing around the medial head of the gastrocnemius muscle rather than between the two heads. The natural history of the popliteal artery with unrelieved compression is thought to be an aggressive one. There is progressive fibrosis of the entrapped vessel wall leading to aneurysmal formation and thrombosis. One-third of cases are bilateral and the popliteal vein is involved in 10%. In young athletes with claudication-like symptoms, popliteal artery entrapment syndrome may be the underlying cause in about 60% of cases.

The popliteal entrapment syndrome has been classified into types I–IV on the basis of the developmental anomaly (Figure 27.3).

The syndrome has been reported to occur in more than one individual in a family. The diagnosis of this syndrome should be suspected in a young and often athletic individual presenting with claudication-like symptoms, in whom ankle pulses are normal at rest (if the distal arteries are not yet occluded). On examination, the popliteal artery blood flow is occluded or reduced by forced active plantar flexion or dorsiflexion of the foot against resistance. The diagnosis can be confirmed by duplex scanning or arteriography using the above manoeuvre to demonstrate the abnormality of the popliteal artery (Figure 27.4).

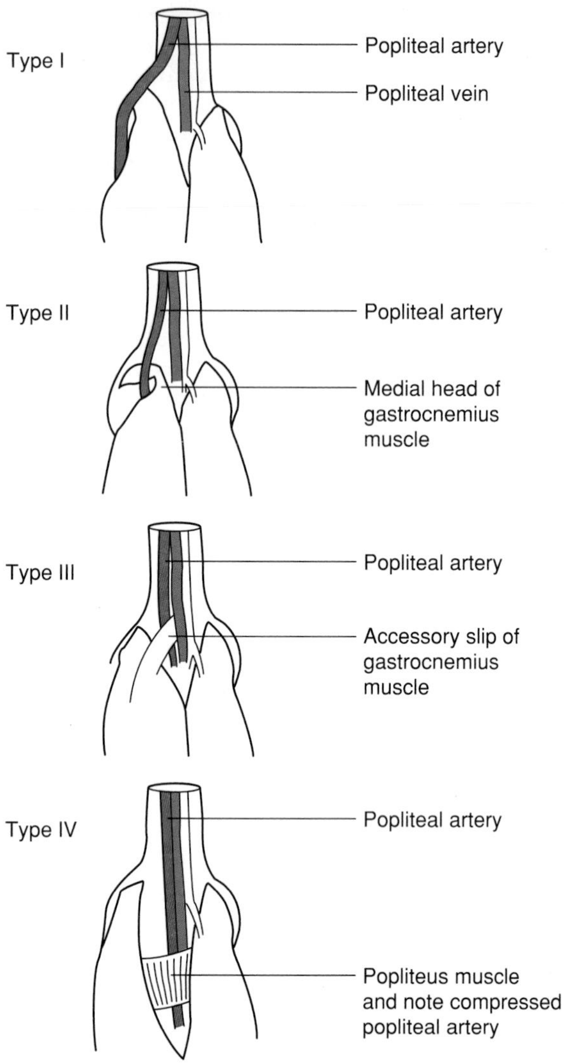

Figure 27.3 Classification of popliteal entrapment syndrome.

Magnetic resonance angiography and computerized axial scanning can be used for diagnosis. Contrast arteriography is important in planning surgery. The treatment of this condition before occlusion of the popliteal artery should be by release of the compressing mechanism. In the presence of occlusion of the popliteal artery, replacement of the popliteal artery is the preferred choice. Other interventions in the form of angioplasty, thrombolysis or thrombectomy give a poor medium-term result. The medial head of the gastrocnemius muscle is divided by the posterior approach and an interposition vein bypass graft performed when the popliteal artery is occluded.

Persistent sciatic artery

This is a congenital abnormality involving the embryonic axial artery of the lower limb, the sciatic artery.

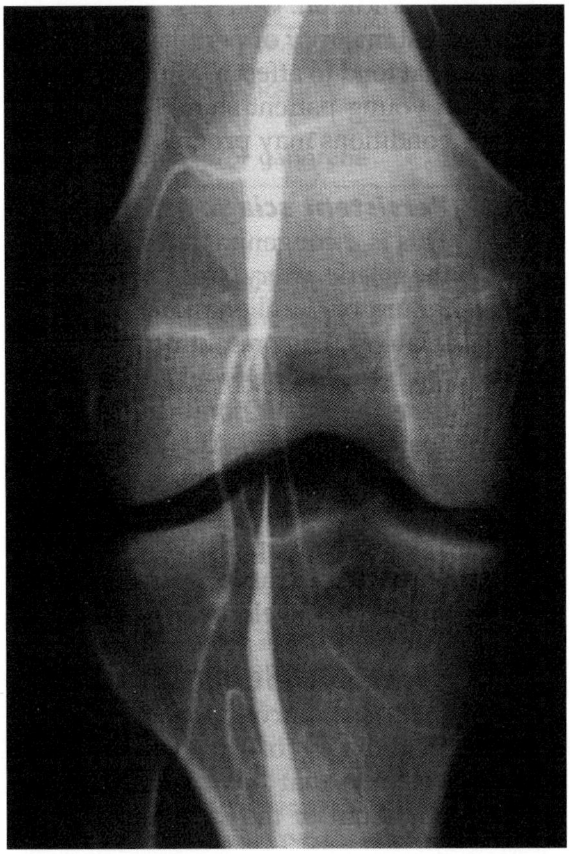

Figure 27.4 Arteriogram of popliteal entrapment syndrome showing occlusion of popliteal artery with passive foot dorsiflexion.

This artery becomes persistent, replacing the ilio-femoral system. The condition is often bilateral and the patients present with intermittent claudication affecting the buttocks and thigh. The persistent sciatic artery may become aneurysmal and cause peripheral embolization. The treatment is excision of the aneurysm and a bypass procedure.

Fibromuscular dysplasia

This is a rare cause of intermittent claudication in young patients. Fibromuscular dysplasia commonly affects the renal or carotid arteries but can affect the limb arteries, with the external iliac artery being the commonest site. The treatment of the symptomatic patient is angioplasty.

Cystic adventitial disease

This is also a rare cause of claudication and is due to cystic abnormality of the adventitia of the popliteal artery. The symptoms of claudication may come on suddenly and on examination there may be a palpable pedal pulse which disappears on knee flexion. The diagnosis can be confirmed on duplex scan, computed tomogram (CT) or magnetic resonance which shows a cystic abnormality of the popliteal adventitia that may be connected to the knee joint synovium. An arteriogram may show a smooth hourglass abnormality of the popliteal artery. The treatment of choice is surgical excision of the cystic abnormality and vein replacement of the arterial segment.

Other differential diagnosis

Spinal canal stenosis causing a cauda equina compression could be mistaken for claudication due to peripheral vascular disease. A careful history of pain associated with change in posture as well as associated neurological deficit will help to differentiate the two. A magnetic resonance scan may reveal stenosis of the spinal canal. The compartment syndrome (shin splints) is a condition occurring in athletes after prolonged exercise such as jogging. The anterior compartment becomes painful and on examination it may be tense or tender with an elevated compartment pressure. Fasciotomy may give rise to symptomatic relief. Venous claudication may occur after extensive ilio-femoral deep vein thrombosis.

Investigation of chronic leg ischaemia

The ankle brachial pressure index

The hand-held continuous-wave (CW) Doppler ultrasound allows measurement of the ankle brachial pressure index (ABPI). The principle of the CW Doppler is that the frequency of the emitted sound from a moving source increases when the source of sound moves towards the receiver and decreases when the source moves away. In the Doppler ultrasound, a beam of high frequency ultrasound is transmitted into the tissues and in return, part of the energy is reflected back at an acoustic boundary detected by the Doppler probe. The Doppler probe contains two piezoelectric crystals which continuously transmit and receive. The ABPI is measured by placing the pneumatic cuff around the ankle and inflating this to above the systolic pressure. The cuff is deflated and the probe used to detect the pressure at which there is return of the Doppler signal. The Doppler probe is similarly used for the brachial pressure which is compared to the ankle pressure. A ratio greater than 1 is normal and less than 0.9 is suggestive of peripheral vascular disease. Differences of 0.15 in the ABPI fall into the limits of the standard error of measurement. The clinician should interpret the above ratio with caution in patients with calcified arteries (diabetics and chronic renal failure) in whom the artery may be incompressible. Toe pressures are more reliable in diabetics because the digital arteries are usually unaffected by arterial medial calcification. The toe pressures are measured by a smaller pneumatic cuff and the toe brachial index is greater than 0.7 in normal subjects.

Exercise tests

Stressing the peripheral arterial system by exercising could allow evaluation of lesions which are asymptomatic at rest. This allows the clinician to decide whether a lesion is functionally related to the claudication symptoms. It may also be useful in determining the

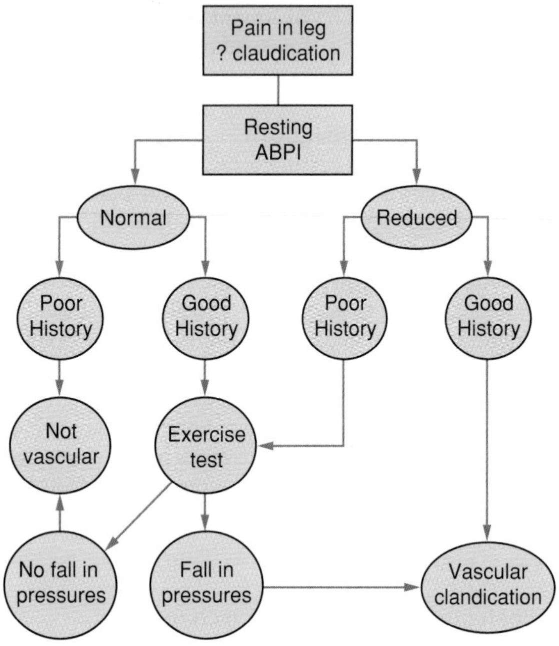

Figure 27.5 Algorithm for the investigation of pain on walking. ABPI, ankle brachial pressure index. (Reproduced with permission from Clifford, C. P. and Beard, J. D. Chronic leg ischaemia. In: Davies, A. H., Beard, J. D. and Wyatt, M. G. eds., *Essential Vascular Surgery*. Philadelphia, PA: WB Saunders, 1999.)

extent to which claudication and breathlessness (in a patient with chronic obstructive airways disease) contributes to the patient's disability. During the exercise, the increased blood flow to the muscle leads to a fall in the ankle pressure in the presence of arterial disease. The most widely used exercise protocol consists of resting the patient for at least 20 min before the commencement. The patient walks on a treadmill at 2 mph (3.5 km/hour) up to a 10% grade for 5 min or until the patient's walking is limited by their symptoms. The ABPI is measured again and the magnitude of the drop in ABPI is indicative of the degree of ischaemia. An algorithm for the investigation of pain on walking is given in Figure 27.5.

Blood investigations

A full blood count (haemoglobin, haematocrit, platelet count and white cell count) should be done. A low haemoglobin, high haematocrit or high platelet count may all worsen the degree of ischaemia. The serum cholesterol and triglycerides as well as glucose, electrolytes and urea estimation are important in overall and risk factor management of the patient. Homocysteine levels should be measured in younger patients with peripheral arterial disease (PAD).

Plethysmography

Several types of plethysmography are available but they all measure the volume change in a limb. For the routine assessment of chronic leg ischaemia plethysmography is not widely used. It is used mainly as a research tool.

Transcutaneous oxygen tension

The transcutaneous oxygen tension ($tcpO_2$) is a measure of the metabolic state of the tissues. Measurements may be obtained from the dorsum of the foot, the calf or the thigh a hand's breadth below or above the patella respectively. In the elderly $tcpO_2$ tends to decrease due to a fall in arterial partial pressure. Changes in the $tcpO_2$ are not detected normally in patients with a mild degree of ischaemia because the oxygen supplied to the tissues exceeds the metabolic demand. In exercise, the oxygen requirement of the tissues increases exponentially and a large proportion of the available oxygen is used up, resulting in a fall of the measured $tcpO_2$. In patients with severe ischaemia, the amount of oxygen reaching the sensor is reduced and the $tcpO_2$ falls. The probe used for the measurement consists of a Clark-type oxygen electrode with a heating element and a temperature sensor. The probe is clipped to a ring which is attached to the skin and filled with an electrolyte solution. The $tcpO_2$ may fall to zero in tissues that are still perfused by oxygen detectable by other methods. This does not imply that there is no oxygen reaching the tissues but that all the available oxygen is being utilized with none diffusing to the sensor.

The resting $tcpO_2$ is approximately 60 mmHg and younger subjects tend to have a level about 10 mmHg higher than in elderly subjects. Patients with claudication tend to have normal $tcpO_2$ values but patients with critical limb ischaemia have reduced levels. Measuring the $tcpO_2$ is particularly useful in determining the site of an amputation.

Isotope blood flow

^{99m}Technetium-labelled radioisotope clearance studies have been used to measure blood flow but are used more as research tools.

Duplex ultrasonography

Duplex ultrasonography has become an essential part of the investigation of peripheral vascular disease. The duplex scanner generates three types of image information based on grey-scale B-mode ultrasound, colour flow and pulsed Doppler spectral analysis. The B-mode ultrasound provides information on the grey scale of the tissues interrogated. The pulsed Doppler flow detector provides the opportunity to interrogate a small sample of tissue, guided by the B-mode and colour flow images. The colour duplex encodes the Doppler information with regard to the velocity and presents the image visually as a colour display within the grey-scale vessel image. The blood moving towards or away from the probe is coloured red or blue. Turbulence in blood flow due to disease in the vessels is shown in golden yellow or orange colours.

The duplex scanning of the aorta and iliac arteries employs a 2–3 MHz transducer and a 5–7 MHz transducer is used for interrogating the infrainguinal arteries.

The most widely accepted criterion for making a diagnosis of peripheral arterial stenosis is a 100% peak systolic volume rise (velocity ratio ≥ 2.0) compared with a normal area of artery proximal to the narrowed segment. This has been shown to correlate with a 50% or greater degree of stenosis in the blood vessel. Spectral broadening and loss of end-systolic reverse-flow known to be previously present are also considered in making a diagnosis of 50% stenosis. The duplex scan report should aim to establish whether the artery is patent without significant stenosis, patent with stenosis greater than 50% or occluded. Duplex scanning is used to screen for haemodynamically significant stenoses in the aorto-iliac segment but it may underestimate the degree of stenosis in up to 25% of cases. The duplex scan can be used to select patients suitable for antegrade superficial femoral angioplasty.

The duplex scan is also used in pre-operative marking of the long saphenous vein for femoropopliteal bypass and for post-operative surveillance of vein grafts.

Duplex scanning is operator dependent, and hence the skill of the vascular technologist is essential to the results obtained.

Arteriography

Arteriography remains the gold standard by which the lower limb arteries are assessed (Figure 27.6). It gives accurate information about anatomy which is invalu-

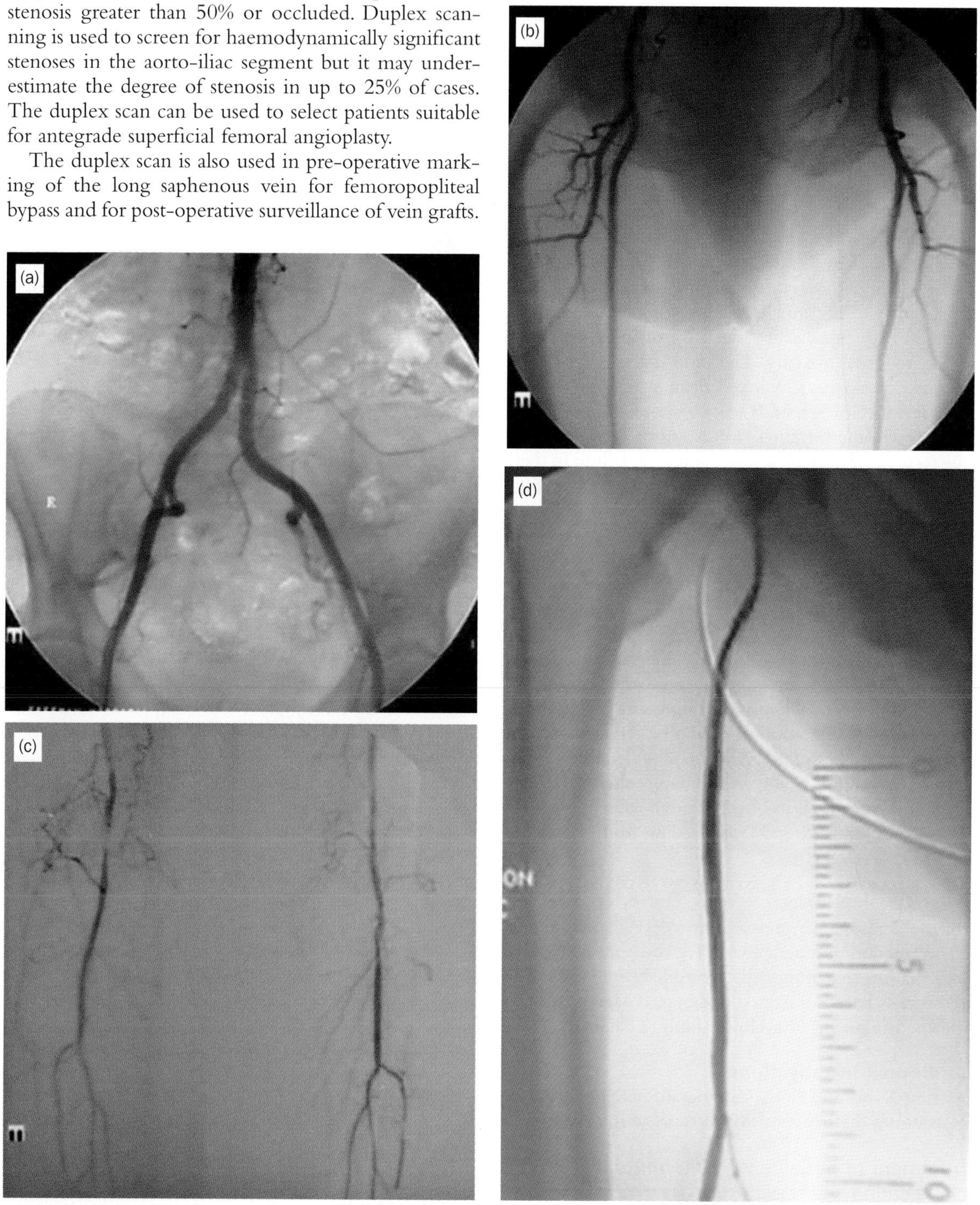

Figure 27.6 Digital subtraction arteriogram (DSA) showing: (a) normal proximal aortoiliac segment, (b) normal proximal superficial femoral arteries (SFA), (c) short segment of occlusion of right distal SFA and (d) successful technical outcome following angioplasty.

able in planning vascular reconstructions. The basic conventional angiogram is done through the femoral artery using the Seldinger approach. A digital subtraction angiogram (DSA) is a more advanced method of arteriography in which a computer subtracts the pixels of a first image of the series (the mask image) from the subsequent images. The result is an image of the contrast within the lumen of the artery without the surrounding tissues. Movement of the patient including breathing and peristalsis can interfere with the images obtained.

Other possible routes used for arteriography are the brachial artery and the common femoral vein. Intravenous DSA uses a comparatively larger volume of contrast. Modern contrast agents are non-ionic (i.e. the benzene ring of the contrast does not dissociate) and have reduced osmolality. These are more benign than the previous iodine-based contrasts. Patients may develop major reactions to contrast but the most common reactions are nausea and vomiting. The renal function of patients may deteriorate following arteriography since all contrast agents are cleared by glomerular filtration. Patients with pre-existing renal impairment are more prone to renal toxicity after arteriograms and such patients should be rehydrated prior to the procedure. The Royal College of Radiologists recommend that patients stop metformin 48 hours prior to arteriography due to the risk of lactic acidosis and renal failure in these patients. It is recommended that such patients should have electrolytes and urea checked before restarting metformin. Hypertension should be controlled as much as possible prior to routine arteriograms. The risk of bleeding from the puncture site may be minimized by stopping oral anticoagulation 1–2 days prior to routine arteriography to bring the international normalized ratio (INR) to normal while the patient is heparinized.

Basic techniques for radiation protection should be strictly adhered to when performing any arteriogram. The output of the radiation should be reduced and the operator and all assisting personnel shielded from exposure. Patients undergoing arteriography should be kept on bed rest for a period of 2–6 hours after the procedure to minimize the risk of bleeding from the puncture site.

Other imaging modalities

Magnetic resonance angiography (MRA) and computed tomogram angiography (CTA) can provide useful information regarding the aortoiliac segment. The above tests have not gained widespread acceptance as a routine use for investing lower limb ischaemia.

Additional investigations

A chest X-ray and electrocardiogram may be indicated in assessing the patient prior to surgical intervention.

Treatment of patients with intermittent claudication

Intermittent claudication is thought to be benign in nature but these patients are at a high risk of developing life-threatening cardiovascular and cerebrovascular complications. Patients with claudication have a two to four times greater risk of death from these complications compared with age-matched control subjects. Therefore, in the overall management plan of these patients, priority should be given to modifying the risk factors which lead to progression of generalized atherosclerosis.

The next step in the management should be directed at exercise programmes to increase the walking distance. Interventional treatment for claudicants should be carefully balanced and tailored to individual patients. The disability against the risks of the procedure should be considered.

Section 27.4 • Risk factor management

Cigarette smoking

Smoking is associated with progression of atherosclerosis and risk of myocardial infarction, stroke and death as well as a higher likelihood of limb loss. The cessation of smoking is very important in the risk management of the patient. Cessation of smoking is associated with increased treadmill walking distance. Following intervention, the patients who have stopped smoking are more likely to have a successful outcome (Table 27.4).

The TransAtlantic Inter-Society Consensus (TASC) in 2000 recommended that all patients with peripheral vascular disease should have repeated and strong advice to stop smoking. The advice should be detailed, continuous and supportive. Setting up of smoking cessation clinics where specialist nurse practitioners counsel the patients may be helpful. The relatives of the patients may be involved in such clinics, in particular where both spouses smoke. Finally, nicotine replacement therapy should be used in addition to modification of life-style.

Diabetes mellitus

Diabetes mellitus is clearly a significant contributing factor to limb loss due to a combination of ischaemia, infection and neuropathy. According to the United Kingdom Prospective Diabetes Study (UKPDS), aggressive glycaemic control is associated with a significant fall in diabetes end points and myocardial infarction. However, intensive glycaemic treatment did not appear to reduce the risk of PAD, underpinning the importance of cessation of smoking and other risk factor management. The TASC has recommended that patients with diabetes and PAD should have intensive glycaemic control and normal blood glucose achieved.

Hyperlipidaemia

Elevations in total cholesterol and LDL, and reduction in HDL cholesterols are associated with cardiovascular mortality. There is a 10% increase in the risk of PAD for every 10 mg/dl elevation in total cholesterol. An elevated level of lipoprotein(a) is an independent risk factor for peripheral arterial and coronary artery disease. A

Table 27.4 Effects of tobacco on outcomes of peripheral occlusive arterial disease (POAD)

Clinical event	*Tobacco use (%)*	*Abstinence (%)*
Revascularization procedure success rates		
Vein graft patency at 1 year	70	90
'Reconstruction success'	19	81
Vein graft patency at 3 years	50	90
Patency rate at 3 years	78	94
Prosthetic graft patency rate at 1 year	65	85
Cumulative patency rate		
1–12 months	66.7	75.4
1–2 years	55.2	65.5
2–3 years	52.6	63.6
3–4 years	48.6	60.8
4–5 years	48.6	55.7
Secondary graft patency		
1 month	70	91
12 months	40	75
Vein graft patency (femoro-popliteal) at 2 years	60	90
Vein/Dacron graft patency (aortofemoral) at 4 years	75	90
Vein graft patency at 1 year	63	84
Amputation rates		
Amputation rate	23	10
Cumulative limb loss rate		
1–12 months	2.7	2
1–2 years	14.9	3.3
2–3 years	22.8	6.5
3–4 years	28.1	6.5
4–5 years	28.1	10.9

Adapted from Hirsch, A. T., Treat-Jacobson, D., Lando, H. A. *et al.* The role of tobacco cessation, antiplatelet and lipid-lowering therapies in the treatment of peripheral arterial disease. *Vasc Med* **2**: 243–51, 1997.

lipoprotein(a) level greater than 30 mg/dl is considered to be abnormal. Unfortunately, treatment options for this lipoprotein are non-specific and involve control of other lipid fractions. There is evidence to suggest that lipid modification is associated with stabilization of both coronary and PADs. In the Scandinavian Simvastatin Survival Study (4S), there was a 38% risk reduction in the development or progression of claudication in patients treated with simvastatin.

Currently, all patients with PAD who have elevated serum lipids should be placed on dietary restrictions as a first line of management. Restriction of cholesterol and saturated fats as well as weight reduction could achieve better reduction in lipid levels. The National Cholesterol Education Programme (NCEP) has recommended that a lipid profile be done in all patients with PAD and lipid-lowering treatment started if the LDL cholesterol is higher than 130 mg/dl. The goal of treatment should be to reduce the level of LDL cholesterol to below 100 mg/dl. Treatment with statins leads to a reduction in levels of LDL cholesterol and it could avoid one death/year in 640 treated patients. The treatment of a low HDL cholesterol level by niacin is limited by the side-effects of liver function abnormality, development of glucose intolerance and increased uric acid concentration. Subjects with low HDL and high triglyceride in whom dietary control has failed, could be treated with fibrates.

In summary, patients with PAD who have elevated levels of lipids should be placed on a dietary restriction and a lipid-lowering agent to achieve an LDL cholesterol level below 100 mg/dl.

Hypertension

In patients with PAD, treatment of hypertension is directed at reducing the associated risks of cardiovascular morbidity and mortality. The Joint National Committee (JNC) provides guidelines for the treatment of hypertension. Although there was initial concern that the use of β-adrenergic blockers was associated with worsening of intermittent claudication, evidence now supports the safe use of these drugs in the claudicant.

Obesity

Obesity, in general, is a risk factor for most fatal conditions, but specifically aggressive weight reduction may result in improved claudication distance.

Homocysteine therapy

Homocysteine may be important as a risk factor in patients younger than 50 years who present with PAD. Elevated levels above 5 mmol/l should be considered for treatment particularly when associated with folic acid or vitamin B_{12} deficiency. Lowering of homocysteine levels could be achieved by treatment with B vitamins and folic acid. Elderly patients should not be treated with folic acid alone, but in combination with vitamin B_{12} to avoid development of peripheral neuropathy. More studies are needed to evaluate the place of vitamin treatment in the prevention of PAD.

Exercise programmes

Most patients with chronic lower limb ischaemia are likely to reduce their daily walking distance due to discomfort. Therefore, simply telling these patients to stop smoking and start walking is not likely to achieve the desired beneficial effects of exercise. There is strong evidence to suggest that structured exercise programmes are needed to achieve optimal results. The improvement in walking distance from exercise programmes could range from an increase of 80% to over 200%. A high level of claudication pain during training programmes and training programmes lasting 6 months are associated with good response. Exercise programmes may also lead to improvements in the risk factors for cardiovascular disease. Patients with impaired left ventricular function, chronic obstructive airways disease and severe chronic arthritis are unable to tolerate exercise programmes. Some patients may willingly opt out of exercise programmes. A study from Germany has shown that in a group of 201 patients recommended for exercise, 34% had contraindications and 36% declined participation. The mechanism responsible for the improvement in the walking distance noticed during exercise programmes is not fully established. The development of collateral vessels has been suggested but not supported by studies. Exercise programmes should be adapted to the patients' needs. In general, the programme should last for an hour a day, one to three times weekly, running for a period of 6 months.

In summary, a supervised exercise programme should be considered for all patients with intermittent claudication.

Section 27.5 • Pharmacotherapy

There is no pharmacotherapeutic agent that has been shown to significantly increase walking distance in patients with intermittent claudication. Therefore, modification of risk factors remains an essential part of treatment that should not be replaced by pharmacotherapy in the medical management of the claudicant.

Established drugs with proven but small benefit in improving claudication

Pentoxifylline

Pentoxifylline improves red cell deformability, lowers serum fibrinogen levels and reduces platelet aggregation. A large American placebo-controlled trial in 128 patients treated over 6 months using a dose of 1200 mg/day has shown a 56% improvement over a 38% placebo improvement in absolute claudication distance. A more recent study has shown that the benefit from treatment is better in a subgroup of patients with duration of symptoms longer than 12 months and ABPI less than 0.8. The actual clinical benefit of pentoxifylline remains undefined. Further trials looking at the quality of life are needed to determine the clinical benefit of pentoxifylline in patients with intermittent claudication.

Naftidrofuryl

Naftidrofuryl, a 5-hydroxytryptamine (5-HT) antagonist, has been in use for over 20 years for treatment of intermittent claudication. Its mechanism of action may involve reduction of platelet aggregation. Four placebo-controlled trials have shown that naftidrofuryl is more effective than placebo in improving walking distance but one study has not shown a significant difference.

Cilostazol

Cilostazol is a phosphodiesterase III inhibitor with antiplatelet and vasodilator activity. Randomized multicentre studies have shown a consistent improvement in absolute claudication disease in patients treated with cilostazol compared to placebo.

Established drugs with minimal or no benefit in improving claudication

Antiplatelet therapy

Antiplatelet drugs are important in the long-term reduction of morbidity and mortality from cardiovascular disease (Figure 27.7).

Aspirin, the most commonly used antiplatelet drug, has not been shown to be of direct benefit in the treatment of claudication. Aspirin inhibits the synthesis of the platelet activator thromboxane A_2 by irreversible acetylation of the cyclo-oxygenase enzyme. This indirectly inhibits the release of ADP and reduces platelet aggregation. The inhibition of the cyclo-oxygenase also leads to reduction of synthesis of prostaglandin E_2 which has a cytoprotective effect on the gastric mucosa. This produces the side-effects of gastric erosion or ulceration. There is emerging evidence that aspirin in combination with other newer antiplatelet drugs may be more effective than aspirin alone. Dipyrimadole, another antiplatelet therapy, has been found to lead to a reduced stroke rate when used in combination with aspirin. Ticlopidine is a potent inhibitor of platelet aggregation which has been shown in a randomized placebo-controlled trial to lead to a reduction in claudication pain and to an increase in exercise performance. Clopidogrel, a non-competitive, selective ADP inhibitor, inhibits the GpIIbIIIa expression, hence preventing platelet activation and aggregation. Clopidogrel and ticlopidine are similar in chemical nature, belonging to the thienopyridine group of substances. Both drugs exert their action after metabolism by the P450 enzyme system in the liver.

The CAPRIE trial has shown the beneficial effects of clopidogrel in PAD and the lower rate of associated gastric mucosa ulceration. The benefit is demonstrated with prolonged treatment.

Prostaglandins

The prostaglandins have been used in the intravenous form (iloprost) in several studies for the treatment of critical limb ischaemia. More recently, oral preparations have now been developed and results of trials using these preparations are awaited. The adverse reactions of prostaglandin include headaches, flushing and nausea which may limit their use in patients with claudication.

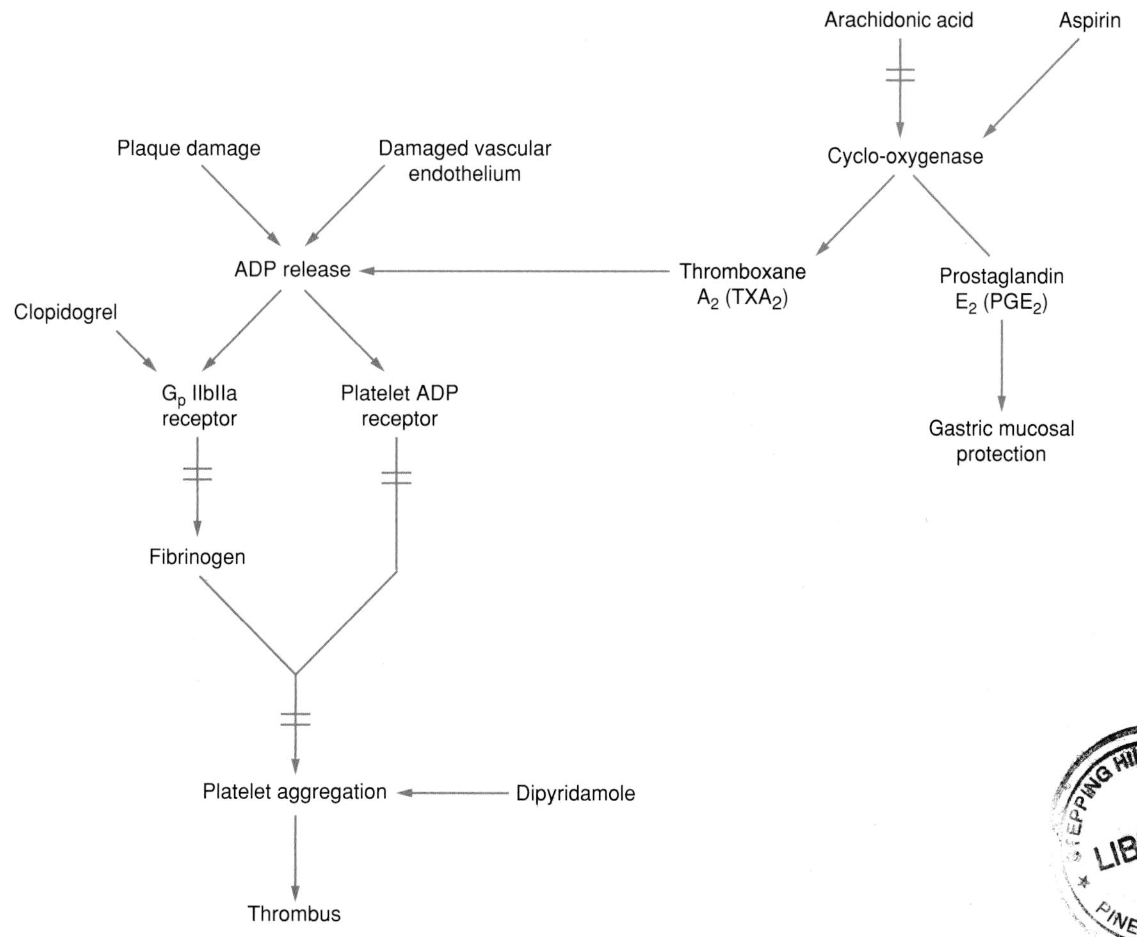

Figure 27.7 Antiplatelet mechanisms of action of aspirin, clopidogrel and dipyridamole.

A study has shown that treatment with the calcium channel blocker verapamil led to a significant improvement in the absolute claudication distance in treated patients compared with the placebo group. The criticism of this study was the period, lasting only 2 weeks. Several other drugs have been investigated but their efficacy remains unestablished.

In summary, the critical issue in patients with intermittent claudication is the identification and modification of cardiovascular risk factors to reduce death due to coronary and cerebrovascular disease. Further studies are needed to establish the role of pharmacotherapy in patients with PAD.

Section 27.6 • Endovascular interventions in the management of intermittent claudication

Since the original report of percutaneous transluminal balloon angioplasty (PTA) over 30 years ago, the technique and instruments have been modified, more practitioners have been trained and stenting has been introduced. The technique has now become more widely applicable.

The management of a patient by catheter techniques is influenced by the site of the lesion, the type of lesion, available interventional equipment and the expertise of the personnel. The interventional treatment of claudicants varies from centre to centre and within centres for the above reasons.

In general, aorto-iliac lesions give better results compared to femoro-popliteal lesions. The outcome of treatment for single focal lesions with good calf vessel run-off is better. Improvements in endovascular practice have allowed a more widespread use of the technique. The availability of better (low profile) catheters has resulted in improved technical success rates and lower complication rates.

The introduction of stents has allowed the treatment of more complex infrarenal occlusive disease. These stents could be balloon-expandable and rigid (Palmaz) or flexible and self-expanding (Wall).

Factors affecting outcome

Characteristics of the lesion

The long-term results of PTA for larger arteries are better. At 5 years, the mean patency rate for aortic lesions following angioplasty was 80% and iliac 69%. The results of PTA for stenosis have been shown to be better than for occlusion due to a higher technical failure rate associated with the latter. However, once the occlusion has been successfully traversed the outcome following intervention is the same as in stenosis. Longer lesions are more difficult to traverse and multiple areas of stenosis present more potential sites for complications. Calcified arteries are more prone to dissection and eccentric plaques may require stenting in the iliacs to eliminate a residual pressure gradient.

Patient factors

Good run-off into the calf is associated with improved results following PTA. Female gender appears to be associated with lower patency rates from iliac PTA and diabetic patients show poorer results. The degree of disability remains the most important factor in the consideration for intervention in claudicants. However, the short- and long-term benefits are the key factors guiding the decision to embark on endovascular treatment.

The TASC has defined and broadly categorized arterial lesions into four groups for the purpose of intervention (Tables 27.5 and 27.6). Lesions in the same group are usually treated by a similar method. Type A lesions are treated radiologically and type D surgically. The tendency is for type B lesions to receive radiological and type C surgical treatment.

Endovascular treatment of aorto-iliac disease

Aorto-iliac angioplasty

PTA is best applied to a focal stenosis of the aorta and iliacs (type A – Table 27.5).

Isolated aortic stenosis is relatively uncommon but treatable by angioplasty, particularly in females.

The technical success rate for PTA of iliac stenosis is greater than 90% and 1 and 5 year patency rates of 90% and 80% are achieved. The technical success rate for PTA of iliac occlusion and the 1 year patency rate is up to 80%. The patency rate following recanalization of an iliac occlusion is similar to that of PTA of iliac stenosis. The results of common iliac angioplasty are better than external iliac angioplasty. Angioplasty in patients with IC should be restricted to suitable lesions although selective stenting may extend the indication.

Aorto-iliac stenting

The use of stents in aorto-iliac occlusive disease may improve technical success rates by allowing effective treatment of problems of recoil and dissection flaps. In iliac occlusion, stenting is ideal for recanalizing the artery since angioplasty alone may give rise to problems with elastic recoil, dissection or a residual pressure gradient. The 1 and 3 year patency rates for iliac stents are 90% and 80%, respectively. The recommended indications for aorto-iliac stents are as follows:

- pressure gradient following PTA
- massive, lumen-obstructing dissection
- treatment of chronic occlusions
- restenosis following previous PTA
- symptomatic ulcerated plaques in the iliac artery
- complex lesions that may give a more satisfactory result with stenting.

In addition, PTA or stenting may be used to treat the proximal disease to allow a femoro-femoral or femoro-popliteal bypass graft. The place of primary stents in the iliac artery requires evaluation by clinical trials (Figure 27.8).

Femoro-politeal angioplasty (PTA)

The ideal intermittent claudication patient for angioplasty is one with type A lesion (Table 27.5). The longer lesions are less suitable for conventional transluminal angioplasty. The technical success rate for stenosis is 90% and for occlusion 80%. Studies using Cox stepwise multiple regression analysis have shown that claudication, good run-off, proximal short stenosis and non-diabetic patients fare better following PTA. The patency rate at 1 year for infra-inguinal angioplasty is about 47% to 71%.

Table 27.5 Morphological stratification of iliac lesions

TASC type A iliac lesions:
Single stenosis < 3 cm of the CIA or EIA (unilateral/bilateral)
TASC type B iliac lesions:
Single stenosis 3–10 cm in length, not extending into the CFA
Total or two stenosis < 5 cm long in the CIA and/or EIA and not extending into the CFA
Unilateral CIA occlusion
TASC type C iliac lesions:
Bilateral 5–10 cm long stenosis of the CIA and/or EIA, not extending into the CFA
Unilateral EIA occlusion not extending into the CFA
Unilateral EIA stenosis extending into the CFA
Bilateral common iliac occlusion
TASC type D iliac lesions
Diffuse, multiple unilateral stenosis involving the CIA, EIA and CFA usually >10 cm
Unilateral occlusion involving both the CIA and EIA
Bilateral EIA occlusions
Diffuse disease involving the aorta and both iliac arteries
Iliac stenosis in a patient with an abdominal aortic aneurysm or other lesion requiring aortic or iliac surgery

CIA, common iliac artery; EIA, external iliac artery; CFA, common femoral artery.

Table 27.6 Morphological stratification of femoro-popliteal lesions

TASC type A femoro-popliteal lesions: Single stenosis up to 3 cm in length, not at the origin of the superficial femoral artery or the distal popliteal artery
TASC type B femoro-popliteal lesions: Single stenosis or occlusions 3–5 cm in length, not involving the distal popliteal artery Heavily calcified stenosis up to 3 cm in length Multiple lesions, each less than 3 cm (stenosis or occlusion) Single or multiple lesions in the absence of continuous tibial run-off to improve inflow for distal surgical bypass
TASC type C femoro-popliteal lesions: Single stenosis or occlusion longer than 5 cm Multiple stenosis or occlusion, each 3–5 cm, with or without heavy calcification
TASC type D femoro-popliteal lesions Complete CFA or SFA occlusions or complete popliteal and proximal trifurcation occlusions

CFA, common femoral artery; SFA, superficial femoral artery.
Changes suggested by CIRSE (Cardiovascular and Interventional Radiology Society of Europe).
Type B(2) lesions classified as 3–10 cm stenosis or occlusion and type C (6) as stenosis or occlusions longer than 10 cm. The suggested changes were based on the fact that newer catheters and techniques of intervention have led to better technical success rates.

The outcome of the use of stents in femoro-popliteal occlusive disease has so far been disappointing.

Long lesions of the superficial femoral artery normally treated surgically could be treatable by subintimal angioplasty. The results of clinical trials are awaited. PTA of infrapopliteal arteries is usually undertaken only for critical ischaemia.

Complications of endovascular procedures

These include the complications of the procedure and the interventional modalities utilized. Major complications resulting in surgical intervention, delayed hospitalization and possible death occur in about 5.6%. The risk of major amputation is 0.2%. The complications could occur at the time during the procedure due to distal embolization or soon after at the site of the arterial puncture causing bleeding or false aneurysm.

Section 27.7 • Surgery for Intermittent claudication

General considerations

Surgery should be reserved for critical limb ischaemia and avoided initially in patients with intermittent claudication, where the emphasis should be on risk factor modification and pharmacotherapy. This group of patients has a high prevalence of ischaemic heart disease and they are more at risk from cardiovascular complications of atherosclerosis than from claudication. Surgery should be considered in patients in whom other non-surgical options have failed in the presence of severe disabling claudication.

The decision to operate should be individualized, based on the risks (morbidity/mortality/graft failure) and benefits (symptomatic relief/employment needs/quality of life) to the patient. Overall the benefit should outweigh the risks for surgery to be justified in claudicants. Patients undergoing bypass procedures for intermittent claudication should have shown commitment to rehabilitation programmes and given time to carefully consider the pros and cons of reconstructive surgery. Young patients with isolated aorto-iliac disease are the ideal patients for consideration for surgery but they are at risk of cardiac morbidity and mortality from aortic clamping.

Most surgeons would consider femoro-politeal bypass to the above knee segment of the popliteal artery for claudication while distal reconstructions to the calf vessels would be reserved for limb threatening ischaemia.

Suprainguinal reconstructions

Aorto-bifemoral bypass is regarded as the gold standard for proximal disease (Figure 27.9). The pre-operative assessment of these patients should aim to detect cardio-pulmonary disease and renal impairment, which should be treated optimally before surgery. Pre-operative chest physiotherapy, bronchodilator and oxygen therapy, and chest physician review may be necessary. 40% of patients with PAD have associated coronary artery disease (CAD). Therefore, patients with CAD should be referred for a cardiology opinion and considered for appropriate intervention before peripheral bypass operation. Prophylactic antibiotics should be given to patients having a bypass graft. A cephalosporin antibiotic is generally used along with metronidazole when groin exposures are involved.

Direct anatomical surgical reconstruction

The results of aortic reconstruction are good with 5 and 10 year patency rates of 90% and 80%, respectively. The associated mortality from the procedure is 1–2%. The main complication of this procedure in men is sexual dysfunction from injury to the hypogastric plexus. These nerves should be identified and preserved during the procedure and sexually active men should be counselled pre-operatively about this. The proximal aortic anastomosis can be made end-to-end or end-to-side. The end-to-end anastomosis should be performed

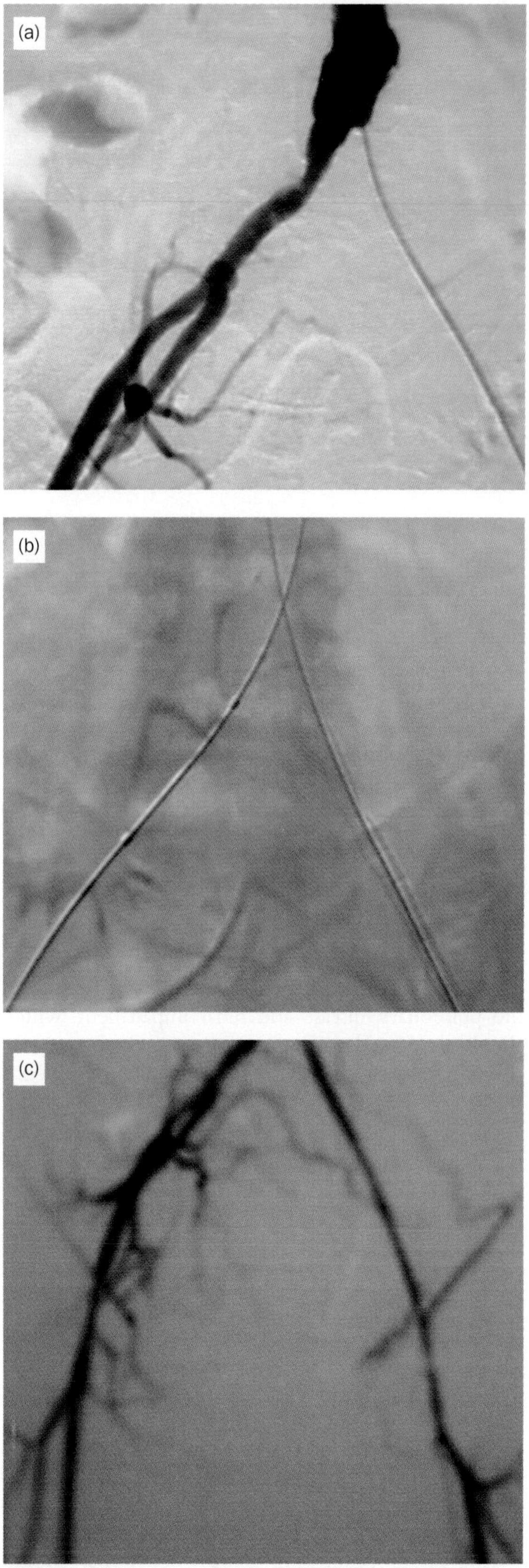

Figure 27.8 Arteriogram showing iliac stent: (a) occluded left common iliac artery, (b) stent deployed, (c) recanalized left common iliac artery.

in the presence of aneurysmal dilatation of the aorta. This anastomosis is a haemodynamically sound reconstruction with a potential benefit of less turbulent blood flow. Side-clamping of the partially occluded aorta could result in distal embolization. Finally, transsecting the aorta and resection of a short segment gives access for an anatomical anastomosis. The end-to-side anastomosis is preferred when the common to internal iliac axis is patent and the EIAs are occluded, to allow pelvic visceral perfusion. This may also minimize the complication of post-operative erectile dysfunction. The distal anastomoses are usually constructed to the common femoral artery to keep the profunda in circulation. Distal anastomosis to the external iliac artery is technically feasible when this option is available. In cases where the anastomosis is to the groin, wound problems remain a source of concern.

Aorto-iliac endarterectomy

In the type A TASC aortic lesions, aortic endarterectomy could be performed avoiding the potential problems of prosthetic graft complications in the aorta, the most disastrous of which is infection. Iliac artery lesions suitable for endarterectomy are now being treated successfully by endovascular intervention.

Extra-anatomical reconstruction

The extra-anatomical graft avoids the risks of aortic dissection and clamping but it offers inferior results of patency rates in comparison to aorto-bifemoral grafts.

Axillo-bifemoral graft has a 5 year patency rate of 33–85%. It should be reserved for critical limb ischaemia (CLI). It is indicated in patients with severe cardiac or pulmonary disease for CLI. The femorofemoral bypass is technically the easiest to perform of the extra-anatomical bypass grafts. It has a 5 year patency rate of 80%. The ideal indication for this procedure would be a unilateral iliac artery occlusion in an elderly patient. Ilio-femoral bypass could also be performed in cases of unilateral iliac occlusion. The obturator bypass is a procedure of choice in cases of graft infection in the groin and crushing injuries to the groin.

In summary, proximal reconstructions have good patency rates of 80% or more in intermittent claudicants and an acceptably low morbidity rate.

Infra-inguinal reconstructions

Infra-inguinal bypass to the popliteal artery is infrequently employed in the treatment of intermittent claudication. The ideal subject would be a short distance claudicant with patent above knee segment of the popliteal artery and good run-off vessels to the calf. The 2 year patency rate of above knee femoropopliteal graft is 80%. There is controversy as to the choice of the grafts (prosthetic versus vein grafts) in the above knee segment (Table 27.7).

The comparison of the results of studies on different grafts is difficult due to variability of procedures and lack

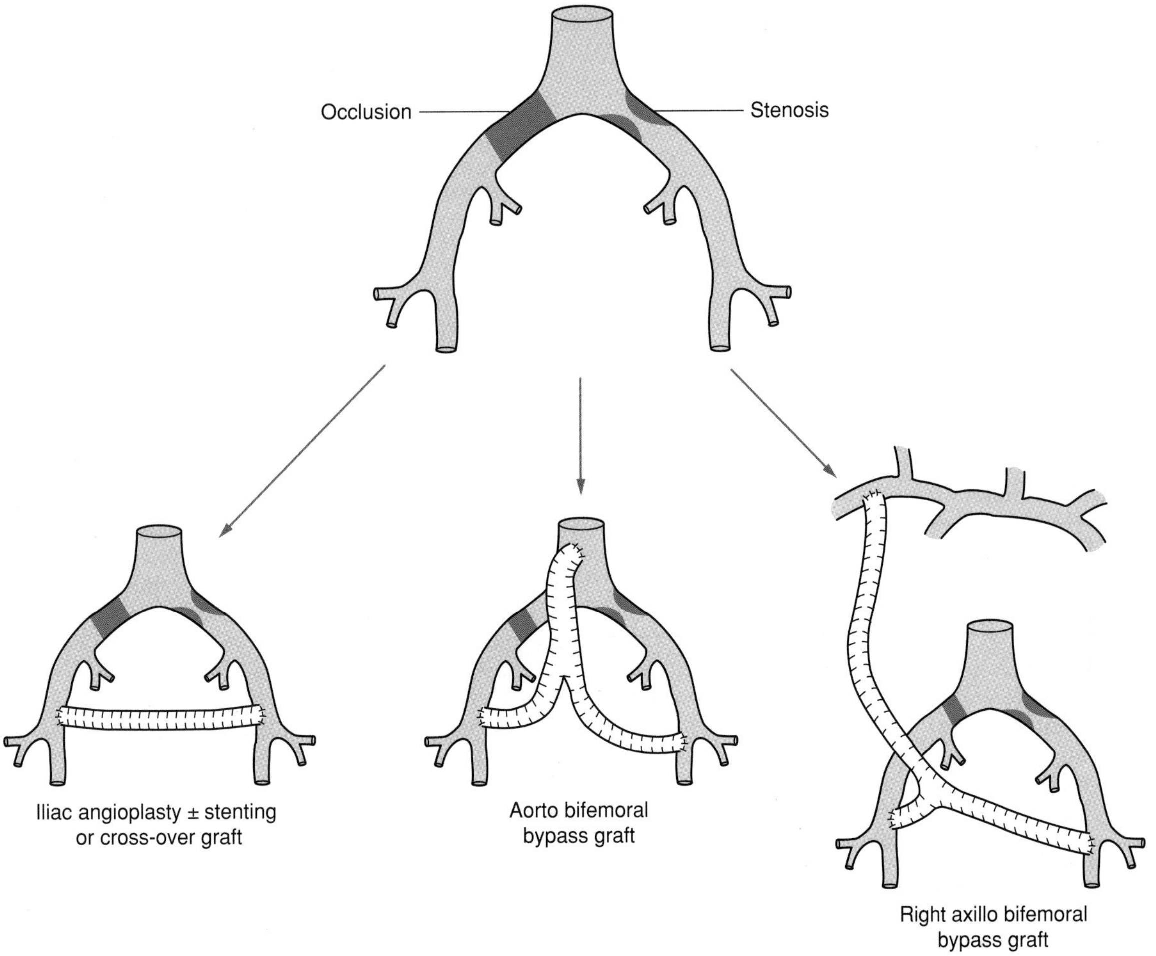

Figure 27.9 Treatment options for aorto-iliac disease.

of consensus in reporting indications for the procedures. A large randomized trial comparing vein to expanded polytetrafluoroethylene (PTFE) graft has shown identical patency rates at 2 years but different rates at 4 years. The 4 year patency rate was significantly different for below knee bypass with vein (76%) compared with PTFE (54%). Infra-inguinal bypass in intermittent claudication patients is therefore difficult to justify. The technique of infra-inguinal bypass will be discussed under the section on critical limb ischaemia.

In summary, surgical reconstruction for intermittent claudication can only be justified by a high patency rate and low operative mortality and morbidity. At present surgery plays a very selective role in the treatment of claudicants.

Critical limb ischaemia

General considerations

CLI (Figure 27.10) is commoner in males (the ratio is 1.48:1), has a peak age incidence between 70 and 79 years, and an equal sex distribution in the octogenarian. The annual incidence is 50–100 per 100 000 in the UK and the total national workload is very high. About 50% of patients with CLI have severe multilevel occlusive disease. The patients have a high risk of major amputation and death (>10% per year). Patients who undergo revascularization have a shorter hospital stay and lower mortality rate compared to those having major amputation. Also, revascularization is more cost-effective than amputation. One-third of patients have diabetes mellitus and they are less likely to have revascularization procedures. The majority have associated cardiovascular disease and this is a common ultimate cause of death. A multidisciplinary approach, in a specialist centre should be adopted for the management. With more resources and increasing expertise in treating CLI, more patients will receive treatment especially in the elderly population. This has significant implications for health care resources.

Diagnosis

The audit committee of the Vascular Surgical Society of Great Britain and Ireland has shown that 50% of patients develop symptoms for 3 or more weeks before presentation. The commonest complaint is rest pain (74%), followed by gangrene (34%) and ulcers (32%).

Table 27.7 Benefits of vein versus prosthetic grafts for the above-knee femoro-popliteal bypass

In favour of vein	*In favour of prosthesis*
Better long-term patency rates	Close to equivalent long-term patency rates
Lower risk of graft infection	Better combined patency rates with prosthesis first, vein second if the need for secondary reconstruction is considered
Avoidance of 'staged' approach to femoropopliteal reconstruction (i.e. best operation first time)	Fewer wound complications but risk of graft infection
Other graft material (i.e. internal mammary arteries) is available for those patients requiring coronary artery bypass	Vein available for secondary or coronary bypass
Need for other use overestimated	Shorter operative time

The Fontaine classification, which has been in use for a long time, has defined the severity of chronic ischaemia as follows:

- Stage 1: Asymptomatic.
- Stage 2: Intermittent claudication limiting lifestyle.
- Stage 3: Rest pain due to ischaemia.
- Stage 4: Ulcer/gangrene due to ischaemia.

A suggested classification for grading the clinical severity of chronic limb ischaemia for the purpose of standardizing reports is outlined in Table 27.3. In addition, the consensus document of the European working group has defined CLI in either diabetics or non-diabetics by either of the following two criteria:

- persistent rest pain that requires regular adequate analgesics for at least 2 weeks, with resting ankle pressure of <50 mmHg or a toe pressure of <30 mmHg; or
- presence of gangrene/ulcer of the foot/toes with the same resting pressures.

Ischaemic rest pain is characterized by severe pain in the foot/toes not readily controlled by analgesics, brought on or made worse by elevation, relieved by dependency and typically occurring at night. The term 'non-healing ischaemic ulcer' is used for cases in which, irrespective of the original cause of the ulcer, there is insufficient tissue perfusion to heal the ulcer. The European consensus document has encouraged a standardized way of reporting CLI. However, there are drawbacks in this definition of CLI. For an instance, diabetic patients may not experience any pain in the foot due to neuropathy. On the other hand, a sensory diabetic neuropathy alone could cause pain at rest not due to ischaemia. Diabetic patients could also have false elevation of their ankle pressure due to calcified ankle arteries. For this reason, toe pressures should be taken in the base of the great toe using an appropriate toe cuff.

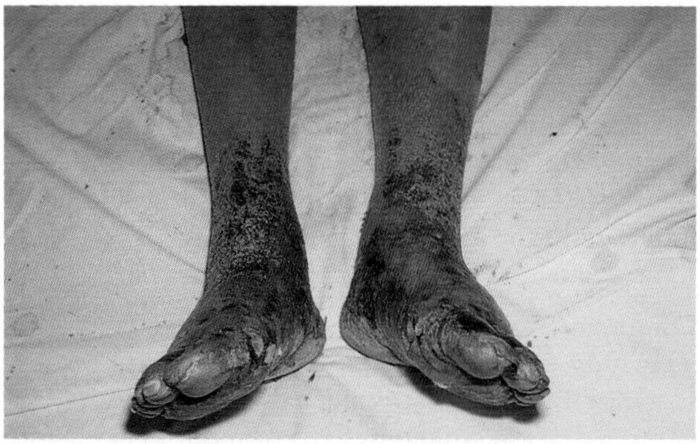

Figure 27.10 Photograph showing a patient with chronic limb ischaemia.

The ABI is useful to follow up the response to intervention in a patient but the absolute pressure is a more reliable measure of the actual perfusion pressure in an ischaemic limb.

Investigation for CLI

In addition to the investigations outlined above in the section on intermittent claudication, patients with ulcer or gangrene should have a wound swab for bacteriology and radiograph of the leg and/or foot to look for osteomyelitis or dystrophic changes.

Patients with CLI should be admitted urgently for full lower limb vascular assessment and intervention where appropriate.

Management

All patients should be considered for vascular reconstruction if at all possible because of the risk of major amputation. However, the success of any revascularization procedure carried out for CLI will depend on careful patient selection and good surgical/radiological technique. Primary amputation should be considered in elderly infirm patients with a short life expectancy in whom a good outcome of reconstruction is doubtful.

Patient considerations

In general, proximal lesions are treated before more distal ones in peripheral vascular disease. There should be at least a run-off vessel in the calf to serve as outflow for the graft. Sometimes, a combination of a bypass and angioplasty is employed in the treatment of CLI.

Treatment options

Endovascular treatment

The principles of endovascular treatment are the same for both intermittent claudication and CLI (see the TASC guidelines above). The initial success and patency rates for femoro-popliteal PTA are not as good as for aorto-iliac PTA. This is due to the fact that disease in the femoro-popliteal segment in patients with CLI is often multiple and crural vessels are often involved. Previously, a major limiting factor in the use of endovascular techniques for the treatment of infra-popliteal disease was the fact that the vessels are of small calibre and conventional catheters were of a large calibre. More recently, catheters with smaller diameter shafts and low profile balloons have become available. These allow intervention for a wider range of lesions in the distal vessels. The technique of subintimal angioplasty, where a plane of dissection is deliberately created as a point of entry above an occlusion and re-entry into the lumen distally in a patent segment, is currently undergoing evaluation. This method may allow treatment of longer lesions by angioplasty. The reports of endovascular stenting for infra-inguinal lesions have so far been disappointing.

Infra-inguinal percutaneous angioplasty

A successful outcome from infra-inguinal PTA for suitable lesions depends largely on paying attention to important technical details during the procedure. Selecting the approach to the lesion that gives the shortest and most direct route, in the case of infra-inguinal lesions an antegrade ipsilateral approach, is important. Intra-arterial heparin should be given prior to angioplasty. The lesion should be crossed by a floppy-tip or steerable guidewire under fluoroscopy before angioplasty is attempted. The position of the guidewire should be checked before angioplasty and use of a 'road map' facilitates the procedure. The diameter of the balloon chosen should not greatly exceed the diameter of the 'normal' segment of the artery measured on the 'road map' to avoid arterial rupture. When dilating the lesion, the balloon is inflated with contrast under fluoroscopy. The 'waist' of atherosclerosis should be dilated for 30–60 s about two or three times. A completion angiogram should be done to check the site of angioplasty as well as patency of the distal run-off. In the common femoral artery, PTA is usually performed from the contralateral side over the aortic bifurcation but patients fare better with surgery (endarterectomy) because the lesions consist of a heavy eccentric plaque. Overall, the results of PTA of the femoro-popliteal segment show a 1 year patency rate of 47–71%. PTA of long extensive femoro-popliteal occlusions has a poorer outcome. Recently, due to advances in the catheters, angioplasty of more distal infra-popliteal lesions is being performed. These are often reserved for patients with CLI in whom severe co-morbid factors make reconstruction hazardous. There are few reports in which distal PTA has been performed in patients with intermittent claudication but there is concern that this may jeopardize any prospect of subsequent revascularization. The complications of PTA are classified in Table 27.8.

Complications following PTA can often be treated with the following adjunctive techniques. Thrombolysis using catheter-directed streptokinase or tissue plasminogen activator can be utilized in patients with distal embolization or early graft thrombosis. Catheter suction embolectomy and rotablator (atherectomy) are newer techniques which avoid the bleeding complications of thrombolysis. Clinical trials are required to evaluate the role of these newer techniques in the treatment of lower limb ischaemia.

Surgical treatment

Endarterectomy

Operatively removing plaques in the artery was a popular procedure about two decades ago, but it has become largely replaced by bypass and endovascular procedures. Endarterectomy is a relatively safe procedure with mortality of 0.8%, complication rate of 10% and a 3 year primary patency rate of 87%. Anatomically, the arterial wall consists of three layers which are the intima, media and externa (adventitia). Also, there are three natural cleavage planes in the arterial wall named subintimal, transmedial and subadventitial. Endarterectomy should be performed in the transmedial plane to avoid the potential problem of arterial perforation associated with subadvential plane or early thrombosis of the vessel wall in subintimal plane. Endarterectomy can be performed open or semiclosed using the Vollmar ring stripper.

In patients with infrainguinal lesions, endarterectomy may be performed as a primary or secondary procedure in addition to a bypass. Following endarterectomy, the arteriotomy could be closed primarily or using a patch (venous or prosthetic). Localized lesions in the common femoral artery are ideal for endarterectomy with a cumulative patency rate of 94% reported over 10 years.

In summary, endarterectomy is a safe local procedure with a comparatively good result that should be used selectively in the armamentarium of the surgeon treating lower limb ischaemia.

Infra-inguinal reconstructions

Infra-inguinal reconstruction techniques have resulted in increased limb-salvage rates and reduced amputation rates. However, secondary procedures are often necessary to maintain graft patency and many of these patients often require life-long treatment. Therefore, the initial emphasis on limb salvage and amputation rates for patients with CLI is changing towards maintaining and improving the quality of life.

Table 27.8 Complications of angioplasty

Puncture site	*Catheter-related*	*Systemic*
Haematoma False aneurysm Arteriovenous fistula	Dissections, Distal embolization	Vasovagal syncope Nausea and vomiting Contrast reaction Renal impairment Cardiac arrest Death

Primary amputation may be the appropriate choice of treatment in patients with a short life expectancy in whom revascularization may not be successful.

Operative management

A wide range of procedures is available for infra-inguinal reconstruction and the reported patency rates vary greatly (Table 27.9). In some groups of patients treated by bypass, graft patency rate is not equivalent to limb loss because the ulcer may heal before the graft occludes. However, early graft occlusion may lead to premature amputation.

Autogenous vein bypass

Autogenous vein has been shown to be superior to other conduits for use in vascular reconstruction because it acts as a living structure that participates to a degree in homoeostasis. The greater saphenous vein has been found to be the most suitable for crural reconstructions.

The ipsilateral vein may be unavailable for use in 10–30% of cases due to congenital absence or abnormality, previous harvest for other bypass, removal in varicose surgery or thrombophlebitis. The contralateral greater saphenous vein is the preferred next choice unless there is evidence of chronic ischaemia of this limb that may imminently require revascularization.

Other alternative sources of autogenous vein include the lesser saphenous vein, cephalic and basilic vein. The cephalic vein is used by most surgeons as an alternative to the grater saphenous vein. The common femoral vein has been used anecdotally to replace infected aorto-bifemoral grafts.

When harvesting veins for use as a conduit a pre-operative duplex scan is useful. This not only enables pre-operative determination of vein suitability (size and quality), but also allows precise vein localization, enabling accurate cutdown and avoidance of skin edge undermining (a possible cause of wound dehiscence).

Autogenous vein can be harvested by open or endoscopic techniques. The open technique utilizes a long incision for harvesting which is prone to healing problems and which may subsequently influence the outcome of wound healing if amputation becomes necessary.

More recently, endoscopic vein harvesting by minimally invasive approaches has been used but clinical trials are necessary to evaluate its place. The controversy continues as to whether the *in situ* or reversed venous bypass is better. Up to now there is no clinical evidence to suggest that one is superior to the other. In general, veins smaller than 3 mm in diameter are considered unsuitable for use as a conduit except in patients having *in situ* venous bypass where a better size match exists. Irrespective of the method of harvest, the size or the surgical orientation of the vein, meticulous techniques of vein handling and preparation should be maintained. The use of magnification for anastomosis, smaller sutures, intra-operative quality control and postoperative graft surveillance have resulted in improved long-term patency rates.

Table 27.9 Typical patency rates of surgical reconstructions for CLI

Procedure	*1 year patency rate*
Aorto-iliofemoral	90%
Femoro-popliteal above knee (vein)	75%
Femoro-popliteal above knee (prosthetic)	65%
Femoro-popliteal below knee (vein)	70%
Femoro-popliteal below knee (prosthetic)	60%
Femoro-tibial (vein)	70%
Femoro-tibial (prosthetic)	40%

After European consensus document (*Eur J Vasc Surg* **6**, Suppl. A, May 1992).

Reversed autogenous greater saphenous vein

A suitable greater saphenous vein will be available in more than 55% of cases. An adequate length of the vein is harvested and all its tributaries are ligated. It is gently flushed through using heparinized Ringer's lactate and any leaks are ligated usually with a 5/0 or 6/0 prolene suture. The vein is reversed, tunnelled carefully to avoid a kink and the proximal and distal anastomoses are constructed end-to-side onto the common femoral artery and the popliteal or distal arteries respectively. Intravenous heparin is usually given after the vein is tunnelled and before clamping of the arteries.

In situ autogenous greater saphenous vein

Since the technique of *in situ* bypass was introduced by Hall in 1962, it has undergone technical improvements. The basic principle of the technique involves the ligation of tributaries and disruption of the valves to allow antegrade flow of blood. A major advantage of this method is the better size match. The distal artery for anastomosis is determined from the pre-operative arteriogram but it is good practice to explore this vessel first as disease may have progressed since the angiogram or it may have been underestimated. Also, the length of the vein harvested could be adjusted to reach the site of distal anastomosis.

The vein is usually exposed through a full incision along its length but multiple incisions with skin bridges may be used. Regular moistening of the vein is necessary to avoid desiccation. The tributaries are ligated to prevent arteriovenous fistulas which could precipitate cardiac failure. The cusps of the first valve should be disrupted before the proximal anastomosis is constructed to the common femoral artery by end-to-side technique. Valvulotomy is performed blind using a valvulotome (Figure 27.11) or under direct vision using an angioscope (Figure 27.12). When using the valvulotome, it should not be introduced up to the proximal anastomosis to prevent anastomotic disruption. All the valves are destroyed to allow pulsatile flow to the distal end of the vein before the distal anastomosis is constructed.

Angioscopy

The angioscope was introduced by Vollmar *et al.* in 1969 and it offers the opportunity to see the valves and ensure their complete removal as well as demonstrate unsuspected endoluminal abnormalities. The angioscope utilizes a closed irrigation system, a sheath and a video camera. While the angioscope is introduced from the proximal end of the venous graft, the valve cutter is introduced from the lower end towards the scope and the valves are disrupted under vision. Traditionally, the side branches are ligated as the vein is dissected out through a full length incision along its course. However, using the angioscope, the side branches can be identified, transilluminated against the skin and marked out for ligation through a small skin incision. This could potentially minimize the problem of wound dehiscence associated with long incisions in the lower limb.

Prosthetic bypass

When the saphenous or other autogenous veins in the body are unavailable for use, a prosthetic graft may be used. When these grafts have been used to replace large arteries (aorto-iliac segment), they produce good results but the results with smaller calibre vessels (femoro-crural arteries) have not been so good (Table 27.9). Broadly, prosthetic grafts are classified as synthetic, biological or composite grafts.

Biological grafts (human umbilical vein) are no longer used for bypass as they are tedious to prepare and give rise to problems with post-operative aneurysmal change.

The most commonly used prosthetic grafts are the synthetic ones which could be further classified as textile (Dacron) and non-textile (expanded polytetrafluoroethylene (ePTFE)) grafts. There is controversy regarding the best prosthetic graft available, but Dacron and PTFE are the most widely used. The patency rates for PTFE and Dacron grafts in the above knee femoro-popliteal segment are similar (3 year patency rates 55% for PTFE and 62% for Dacron) according to a prospective, randomized multicentre trial from the Netherlands in 1999.

Areas of continuing controversy

Vein versus prosthetic in the above knee bypass

Although there is little doubt that the autogenous vein is superior to the prosthetic graft in below knee reconstructions, there is debate as to the most appropriate material for above knee bypass. The long-term graft patency rates are similar for above knee femoro-popliteal bypass using either prosthetic or vein. Surgeons who advocate using prostheses for above knee bypass claim that reports have demonstrated similar patency rates between the two. Using a prosthesis will preserve vein for use in the event of graft failure or coronary bypass. On the other hand, the need for a coronary bypass and infra-popliteal bypass is low (5–10%) and this does not justify preserving a suitable vein.

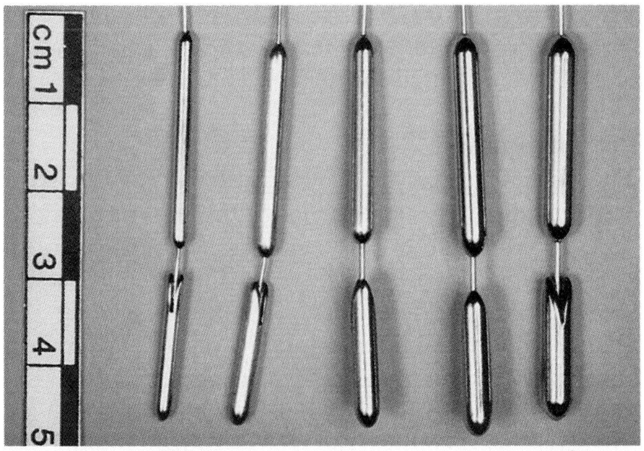

Figure 27.11 Photograph showing a set of Hall valvulotomes. (Note the varying sizes for the use with different sized veins.)

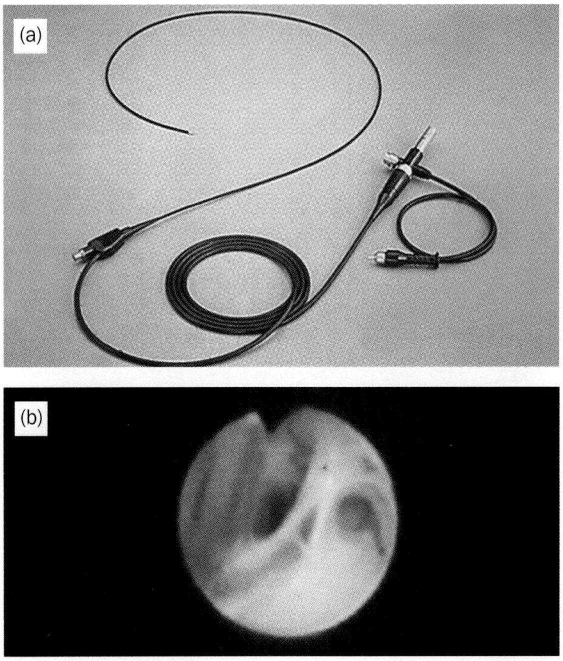

Figure 27.12 Photographs showing: (a) a typical angioscope and (b) the view obtained. Note the presence of a single side branch and a valve.

Reversed versus in situ

The patency rates for reversed and *in situ* venous grafts are similar and the surgeon's preference usually determines the procedure of choice.

PTFE versus Dacron

There is no significant difference in patency rates between PTFE (55%) and Dacron (62%) grafts at 3 years.

Adjunctive techniques

To minimize the occurrence of graft failure due to intimal hyperplasia, vein cuffs may be interposed between the artery and the prosthesis. The Miller cuff technique consists of incorporating a circumferential collar of vein to the arteriotomy before the prosthesis is anastomosed end-to-end to the vein. In the Taylor patch, a vein patch is incorporated in the distal end (Figure 27.13).

Composite or sequential prosthetic–vein grafts give similar results to vein cuffs. This involves a segment of

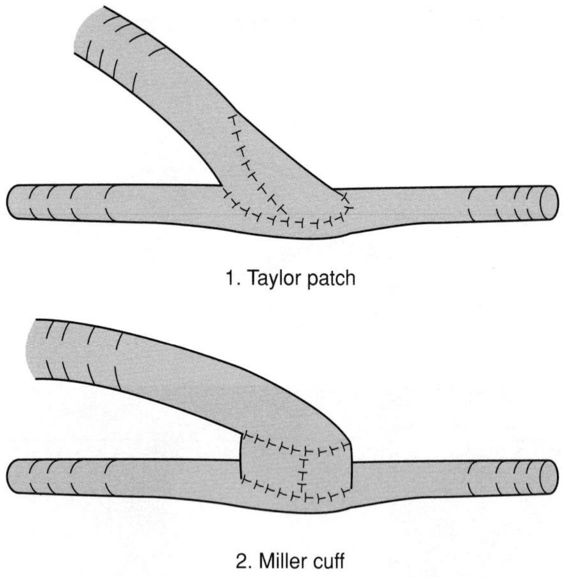

Figure 27.13 Diagrams showing a Taylor patch and Miller cuff.

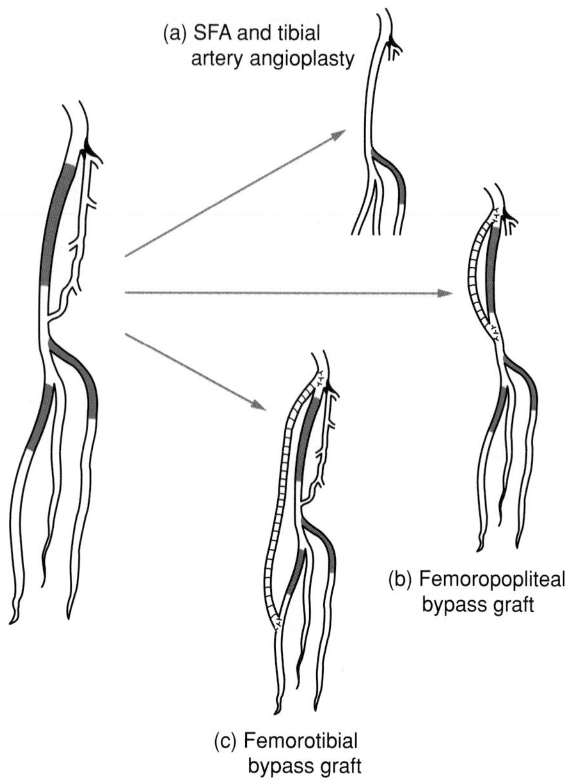

Figure 27.14 Techniques available for infra-inguinal reconstruction in a patient with CLI.

vein for the below knee part of the graft while the proximal portion is prosthetic. An arteriovenous fistula can be created to lower the peripheral resistance in the graft, increase its flow and reduce the risk of occlusion, but there is little evidence for the use of this adjunctive technique.

Quality control

Following a femoro-distal bypass, an objective evaluation of the graft and prompt correction of technical defects could improve the graft patency rate and reduce the incidence of early graft failure. An on-table completion arteriogram is performed to visualize the distal anastomosis and run-off vessels. Angioscopy is better in detecting endoluminal abnormalities but gives no information regarding the run-off state. Intra-operative duplex scanning could be performed to detect areas of flow disturbance or an OPDOP flowmeter could be used to measure the flow and resistance in the graft.

Papaverine, a vasodilator, is given intra-arterially in cases of high peripheral resistance.

Infra-inguinal bypass options

There is a wide variety of procedures that can be performed for critical lower limb ischaemia (Figure 27.14).

Femoro-popliteal (above knee or below knee)

The proximal anastomosis is to the common femoral artery but the superficial femoral artery could be used as a take-off of the graft when it is patent and of good calibre. The common femoral artery is usually approached through a vertical incision in the groin centred over the inguinal ligament. The above knee popliteal artery is approached by a vertical medial incision above the knee and the below knee through a similar incision below the knee.

Tunnelling of the graft is done subsartorially and the anastomoses are done end-to-side. Before commencing the distal anastomosis below the knee, the knee should be straightened and a good length of the graft obtained to avoid shortening. Autogenous vein bypasses fare better than prosthetic ones for below knee femoro-popliteal bypass and should be used if possible.

Femoro-tibial/peroneal

When there is occlusion of the distal popliteal artery, a femoro-distal bypass should be performed using vein if possible. The posterior tibial artery is approached through a vertical incision above the medial malleolus while the anterior tibial is approached by an incision 4 cm lateral to the anterior tibial border. A magnification of at least 2.5 is used for the distal anastomosis.

Profundaplasty

The profunda artery has been described as the 'back door' to the leg in patients with femoro-popliteal occlusion. Since the introduction of femoro-popliteal bypass, profundaplasty has become limited in its use for lower limb ischaemia. Also, the introduction of the oblique view in addition to antero-posterior views on lower limb arteriograms has led to increasing recognition of profunda origin stenosis or occlusion which are amenable to percutaneous transluminal angioplasty. Profundaplasty is combined with the procedure of aorto-bifemoral bypass when the superficial femoral artery is occluded. It is performed, infrequently, as an isolated procedure for lower limb ischaemia instead of femoro-popliteal bypass in frail patients not fit for major revascularization.

In summary, infra-inguinal reconstruction should be undertaken in patients with CLI who have favourable technical factors (i.e. suitable vein and distal run-off vessels) in the absence of confounding comorbidities. Autogenous vein should be used as much as possible for femoro-crural bypass.

Complications of bypass grafts

By the nature of vascular surgery, it is very prone to complications which may lead to re-operation, prolonged hospital stay, permanent disability and death.

Graft failures

Graft failure could be classified as early (<30 days) or late (Table 27.10). Operative technical errors are the commonest causes of early graft failures while progression of atherosclerosis and development of intimal hyperplasia are often the cause of late graft occlusions. Progressive atherosclerosis leading to graft failure has been significantly correlated with continued smoking and high plasma level of fibrinogen. The majority of graft failures occur within 1 year with approximately 10% developing in 1 month. Because many infra-inguinal vein grafts are performed for critical limb ischaemia, when they fail the limbs may become threatened by ischaemia. The results of attempts to salvage grafts are poor, hence efforts should be directed at identification and treatment of failing grafts.

Graft surveillance

Many patients with failing grafts are asymptomatic and clinical examination may be normal. Ancillary tests are therefore needed for the early detection of this group. Symptomatic patients should be referred promptly by family doctors for evaluation.

The post-exercise ankle-brachial pressure index may be useful in detecting failing grafts. Duplex scanning, particularly colour duplex, is being used widely for surveillance of grafts with good sensitivity. For the diagnosis of stenosis in vein grafts, the peak systolic velocity in the area of stenosis compared to an adjacent normal area of vein has been shown to have the best correlation to angiographic results. A peak systolic velocity ratio greater than 2.5 suggests stenosis. Patients should be entered into a duplex scan surveillance programme and those with failing grafts should undergo an arteriogram with a view to treatment.

Table 27.10 Aetiology of graft failures

Early (<30 days)	Incorrect operation Poor operative technique Inadequate run-off Small calibre or diseased vein Prosthetic graft thrombogenecity
Intermediate (<1 year)	Neointimal hyperplasia Vein graft stenosis
Late (>1 year)	Progressive atherosclerosis Deterioration of graft

Treatment of graft failure

The treatment of graft failure due to stenosis is usually accomplished by percutaneous angioplasty. Failing this, a patch open angioplasty or jump graft could be performed. Anastomotic strictures are difficult to treat by angioplasty and an open procedure should be considered. When the graft is occluded, thrombolysis with subsequent treatment of the underlying factor or re-do bypass where at all feasible should be performed.

Graft infection

Graft infection may lead to catastrophe. The overall incidence of graft infections varies from 0.5 to 5% depending on the site of the bypass, host defence mechanisms and indication for intervention. The true incidence is difficult to determine because of the late occurrence of many graft infections. There has been a reduction in the incidence since the introduction of prophylactic antibiotics and improvement in surgical techniques. The dreaded consequence of aortic graft infection is death while for infra-inguinal graft infection it is limb loss.

Microbiology of graft infection

The commonest cause of graft infection is contamination of the prosthesis at the time of implantation. The commonest organism causing graft infection is *Staphylococcus aureus*. *Staphylococcus epidermidis* and Gram-negative infections have increased in frequency. Infections with *Candida* organisms are commoner in immunocompromised patients. Szilagyi types I and II wound infections are associated with a higher risk of late graft infection.

Diagnosis

The diagnosis of graft infection can be difficult, particularly in the abdominal cavity, and a high index of suspicion is important in all patients with previous aortic grafts. The clinical presentation is usually late, occurring after 3–4 months, and it may be subtle. The patients may present with fever, malaise, weight loss, loss of appetite and abdominal pain in aortic graft infection. The heralding symptom may occasionally be prolonged paralytic ileus or gastrointestinal bleeding in aortic graft sepsis. Patients with infra-inguinal graft infection may present with local redness, pain, swelling due to false aneurysm or haemorrhage.

Laboratory tests may show an elevated white cell count and erythrocyte sedimentation rate and both may be contributory to making a diagnosis. A blood culture should always be done and if positive patients should be given the appropriate antibiotics based on sensitivity. A contrast-enhanced CT scan may show perigraft fluid or gas collection suggestive of graft infection in the delayed post-operative period (Figure 27.15).

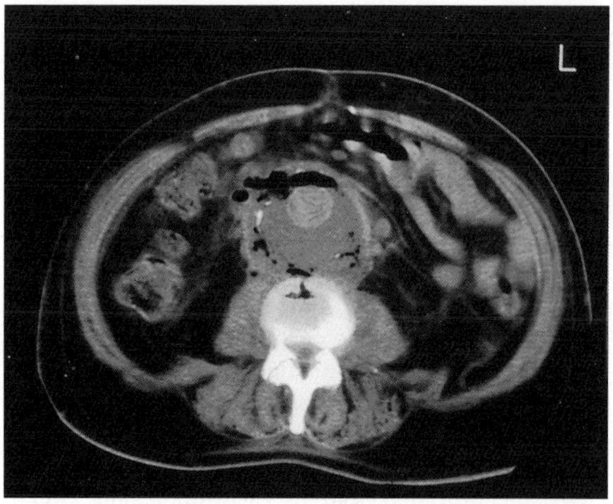

Figure 27.15 Computed tomogram showing an infected aortic graft. Note the bubbles of gas anterior to the graft.

Magnetic resonance imaging can also be used to detect perigraft collections. Functional white cell scans are useful for showing sites of white cell accumulation which may indicate infection. The labelled white cell scans (indium-111-labelled leucocyte) are more reliable in the late post-operative period.

Duplex scan and angiography are important in determining the patency of the graft and in planning the surgical treatment. Endoscopy is important in patients who present with gastrointestinal bleeding as a result of aorto-enteric fistula. However, a negative endoscopy does not exclude the possibility of aorto-enteric fistula.

Management

When a patient presents with shock they should be resuscitated as much as possible prior to surgical intervention. Patients who present more insidiously should have pre-operative optimization of pulmonary, cardiac and renal functions before surgery. Antibiotic therapy should be commenced pre-operatively parenterally and patients should be counselled with regard to the morbidity and mortality of the condition.

Aorto-bifemoral graft infections

The graft infection could be treated by complete excision of the graft and extra-anatomical bypass. In carefully selected cases when the graft infection is localized and limited to the femoral region only with no involvement of the anastomosis, local treatment of the graft could be performed by drainage of the abscess and irrigation with povidone-iodine. The patients should be on long-term antibiotic treatment.

Infra-inguinal graft infection

Infected grafts in the groin should be excised and all perigraft infected tissue should be debrided. When available an autogenous vein graft should be used to replace the graft but this is not usually a feasible option. A prosthetic graft could be used for reconstruction via a remote anatomical pathway (obturator bypass). The patients should also be on long-term antibiotic treatment.

Aorto-bifemoral bypass complications

The results following occlusive aortic reconstruction have improved due to improved surgical technique, invasive intra-operative monitoring and post-operative intensive care. The major cause of post-operative death following aortic surgery remains myocardial ischaemia, which is responsible for up to 40–60% of deaths.

Local vascular complications

Anastomotic false (pseudo)aneurysms

These commonly occur at the femoral anastomosis but could also occur at any anastomosis. The predisposing factors are infection, technical failure due to excessive tension from a short graft length or poor suturing technique and weakened arterial wall from over-enthusiastic endarterectomy. Suture line disruption was common with silk sutures leading to false aneurysms. The aneurysm is usually palpable in the groin and can be investigated by duplex ultrasound and angiography. Treatment is advised to prevent rupture and distal embolization. Occult infection should always be suspected and cultures taken for microbiology at the time of repair.

Renal impairment

Some patients having aorto-bifemoral bypass grafts have underlying renal impairment which may deteriorate post-operatively. The leading cause of post-operative acute renal failure is hypovolaemia leading to poor renal perfusion. The incidence of post-operative acute renal failure in patients undergoing aortic reconstructive surgery is 2–6%.

Atheroembolization is another important cause of peri-operative renal failure which could occur during clamping, clamp release or removal of thrombus from the juxtarenal diseased aorta. Myoglobinuria from ischaemic reperfusion injury may also precipitate acute renal failure in the early post-operative period. Important peri-operative measures to minimize renal insult include catheterization to monitor urine output, adequate volume replacement, invasive monitoring of arterial and pulmonary wedge pressures and close co-ordination with the anaesthetist at the time of clamping or slow release of clamps. The administration of diuretics, dopamine or mannitol to induce diuresis may be beneficial but their role in preventing renal failure is doubtful. Treatment with temporary renal replacement therapy may be necessary but permanent dialysis is rarely required.

Colon ischaemia

This is an unusual complication of aortic surgery and is commoner following aneurysm repairs. It is more common in those patients with concomitant inferior mesenteric artery and bilateral internal iliac artery occlusions with the sigmoid colon most commonly affected. Lesser degrees of intestinal ischaemia leading to ischaemic colitis are identified more commonly at colonoscopy. The prediposing factors to colonic ischaemia peri-operatively are hypotension, ligation of collaterals of the inferior mesenteric artery and atheroembolization. A widely patent inferior mesenteric artery (IMA) should be incorporated into the repair or re-implanted and an occluded artery should be ligated from within the aorta or the sac in aneurysm repair. The left colon must be inspected for viability before closing the abdomen. When colonic ischaemia is suspected at the time of surgery, the IMA should be re-implanted if not previously done. Post-operatively, a high index of suspicion is the key to diagnosis and prompt laparotomy with exteriorization of the left colon could be life-saving.

Spinal cord ischaemia

This is fortunately a very uncommon complication following aortic reconstruction for occlusive disease. The precise aetiology is not known and its occurrence is unpredictable post-operatively following infrarenal aortic surgery. The aggressive treatment of intra-operative hypovolaemia may reduce the risk of developing post-operative spinal cord ischaemia.

Local non-vascular complications

The ureters are prone to injury during aortic surgery because they cross the anterior aspect of the bifurcation of the common iliac arteries. Hence, at the time of difficult dissection of the iliacs and retroperitoneal tunnelling of the bifurcating graft, they should be identified and kept under vision to avoid injury. Tunnelling should be done immediately anterior to the iliac vessels. When injury is recognized at the time of operation, repair should be undertaken. Post-operative ureteral obstruction may develop due to fibrosis and often does not require treatment. When indicated, treatment with placement of ureteric stents usually suffices.

All male patients having aortic reconstructive surgery should be warned about the risk of post-operative impotence. Damage to the autonomic plexus of nerves should be avoided by careful dissection at the aortic bifurcation and preservation of the nerves. The treatment of this condition involves a careful assessment to determine the cause of the impotence. If it is due to reduced pelvic blood flow, revascularization of the dorsal penis artery can be undertaken, but the outcome is poor particularly in elderly men with widespread atherosclerosis. More frequently, this condition is treated with drugs (Viagra) or prosthetic placement.

Section 27.8 • Non-vascular management

Pharmacological therapy

The indications for medical therapy of CLI are limited due to improvement in both surgical and radiological interventions for lower limb vessels. Medical treatment is indicated in patients in whom prospects of distal revascularization are deemed to be poor due to severe distal disease. The main drugs in use are the prostanoids. Prostacycline (PGI_2) is the most widely used prostanoid and iloprost, its stable analogue, has been in use for over a decade. It is usually administered intravenously but an oral preparation is currently undergoing trial. Iloprost is given over a period of 2–3 weeks as a daily 6 hour continuous infusion in hospital. The patients could develop complications of facial flushing, headaches, nausea and arterial hypotension. The initial dose of 2 ng/kg/min is gradually increased to a maximal tolerated dose by the patient. The results of randomized studies suggest that iloprost may be beneficial in patients with CLI who have irremediable distal disease.

Lumbar sympathectomy

Sympathectomy increases the flow of blood to the extremity by peripheral vasodilatation of arterioles in the skin bed. This may be sufficient to heal small superficial ulcers or relieve ischaemic rest pain in patients not fit for vascular reconstruction or those with severe distal disease. Diabetic patients with autonomic denervation are unlikely to benefit from sympathectomy. Chemical lumbar sympathectomy could be performed by the open surgical technique or radiologically using a translumbar approach with the image intensifier. The injection of alcohol or phenol has been used for the ablation of the sympathetic nerves. The morbidity associated with the surgical approach makes the radiological translumbar approach, which is as effective, more widely acceptable.

Diabetic foot

The treatment of the diabetic foot should be multidisciplinary involving the vascular surgeon, diabetologists and chiropodist. The main pathophysiology of the diabetic foot involves a combination of neuropathy, infection and ischaemia. The goal of medical management should be control of blood glucose and health education directed at preventing foot trauma. Infection in the diabetic foot is often caused by multiple organisms and osteomyelitis frequently occurs. Prolonged combination antibiotic therapy should be used in the event of osteomyelitis. Prompt surgical drainage of abscesses should be undertaken. Full vascular assessment should be carried out and revascularization performed where feasible.

In summary, the treatment of the diabetic foot should involve adequate control of blood glucose, prompt control of sepsis, vascular assessment and appropriate revascularization, and further debridement including minor amputations where indicated. Major amputation should be undertaken for severe spreading uncontrollable limb infection threatening life or where revascularization is not possible and the limb is severely ischaemic.

Amputations

In some patients amputation should be considered to relieve pain and remove a life-threatening ischaemic-limb. In the patients with severe medical problems in whom the risk of anaesthesia is very high or in those with severe dementia, analgesia might be more appropriate.

Major amputations performed below the level of the knee joint have a great advantage for rehabilitation but they have more problems with wound healing. However, above knee amputation has better prospects of wound healing but only a 40% chance of successful rehabilitation compared to 80% following below knee amputation.

Below knee amputation

This should not be performed when the calf muscles are infarcted or in a bed-ridden patient with fixed-flexion deformity of the knee. The techniques of skew flap and long-posterior flap (Burgess) have been used with good results. The skew flap is based on the arteries that accompany the short and long saphenous veins and the posterior flap is based on the artery to the gastrocnemius/soleus mass.

Through knee Gritti–Stokes amputation

This is a good option in patients who are unlikely to be rehabilitated and are not suitable for below knee amputations. It provides a longer lever for transfer compared to above knee amputation.

Above knee amputation

The main advantage of this method is better wound healing. The results of rehabilitation are poor compared to below knee.

Further reading

Audit Committee of the Vascular Surgical Society of Great Britain and Ireland (1996). Recommendations for the management of chronic critical lower limb ischaemia. *Eur J Vasc Endovasc Surg*, **12**: 131–5.

Beard, J. D. and Gaines, P. A. (1998). *Vascular and Endovascular Surgery*. Philadelphia, PA: W. B. Saunders.

Bell, P. R. F., Jamieson, C. W. and Ruckley, C. V. (1992). *Surgical Management of Vascular Disease*. Philadelphia, PA: W.B. Saunders.

Branchereau, A. and Jacobs, M. (1999). *Critical Limb Ischaemia*. Armonk, NY: Futura.

Consensus Document: Chronic Critical Leg Ischaemia. (1992). *Eur J Vasc Surg* **6** (Suppl): 1–32.

Davies, A. H., Beard, J. D. and Wyatt, M. G. (1999). *Essential Vascular Surgery*. Philadelphia, PA: W.B. Saunders.

Rutherford, R. B. (2000). *Vascular Surgery*, 5th edn. Philadelphia, PA: W. B. Saunders.

TransAtlantic Inter-Society Consensus. (2000). Treatment of intermittent claudication. *J Vasc Surg* Part 2, **31**, 1–40.

MODULE 28

Diabetic foot disease

Diabetic patients have always suffered from foot ulceration. This complication has become more prevalent since advances in the general medical care of diabetes, particularly the discovery of insulin, have prolonged the life expectancy of patients with this disease. Despite progress in the treatment of ulcers, prevention and achieving healing of established ulcers remains a considerable challenge. This challenge is compounded by a number of misconceptions that have entered medical lore which can result in an attitude of therapeutic nihilism. With enthusiasm and the application of basic principles, however, much can be achieved in treating patients with this common complication of diabetes.

Section 28.1 • Epidemiology

The epidemiology of diabetic foot disease has been reviewed in detail by others, and a summary is presented here. It is correctly pointed out that great difficulties exist in comparing different studies because of variations in the definitions used and differences in the case loads of individual clinics. What is clear, however, is that the morbidity of foot disease in diabetes extracts a considerable toll, not only on health care provision, but especially on patients.

Diabetes is a common disease affecting over one million patients in the UK – around 2% of the whole population – and accounting for an estimated £1 billion of health care spending in 1986/87. It has been estimated that approximately 10–25% of all diabetics develop some foot problems during the course of their illness, ranging from simple calluses to major abscesses and osteomyelitis. Complications of diabetes affecting the lower limb are among the most common these patients suffer and often lead to inpatient hospital treatment – between 1 in 10 and 1 in 5 of all diabetes related admissions are a direct result of foot ulceration, infection or gangrene. More in-hospital days are spent treating foot-related problems than any other complication of diabetes. The costs of treating these complications account for about 25% – around £12.9 million in the UK in 1986/87 – of the hospital costs of diabetes. The indirect costs in loss of earnings and productivity can only be guessed at – it is thought these amount to about 50% of the total direct costs of treating diabetes.

As may be inferred from these figures, a large number of diabetic patients are at risk of foot problems. The Oxford Community Diabetes Study found that the prevalence of neuropathy (reduced vibration perception threshold) in diabetic patients was 23% and the incidence of peripheral vascular disease was 146 per 1000 person years. The same study found a 7% prevalence of active ulceration and a 3% prevalence of amputation of all or part of a foot. Extrapolating these figures to the whole country would suggest about 70 000 patients have diabetic foot ulcers and 30 000 have had a minor or major lower limb amputation. It is likely that greater numbers than these are in fact at risk as some newly diagnosed diabetic patients have detectable neuropathy and some of these will have actual foot problems.

It has been estimated that about 1 in 100 diabetic patients per year will require an amputation of some sort – figures which agree well with the Oxford Diabetes Study where the amputation rate was 8 per 1000 person years. The US National Commission on Diabetes estimates that 5–15% of all diabetics will require a lower extremity amputation at some time in their lives. A comprehensive study of hospital discharges has shown that 45% of all lower limb amputations are performed on diabetics. The annual major amputation rate (below or above knee) was 41.5 per 10 000 in diabetics, and 2.0 per 10 000 in non-diabetics. Among diabetics, it is those over 65 years and males who face the highest risk of amputation. Once one limb has been amputated, not only is there an increased risk that the other limb will also require amputation, but the patient's 5 year survival rate is only about 30%.

While progress has been made in the treatment of diabetic foot ulceration, particularly by the establishment of dedicated diabetic foot clinics which have reduced bed usage by up to 38% over the decade from 1980 to 1990, there remains much morbidity and no measure of economics can reflect the misery suffered by these patients.

Section 28.2 • Aetiology

It is firstly important to appreciate that the aetiology of diabetic foot disease is truly multifactorial. Within any individual patient one factor may predominate over all or some of the others, but generally foot disease arises from more than one cause. Factors to consider include neuropathy, macrovascular disease, microvascular disease, infection, connective tissue abnormalities and haematological disturbances. Identification of the dominant causative factors in each case is essential in planning treatment and the concept of the neuropathic foot, the neuroischaemic foot and the ischaemic foot is very useful (Figure 28.1). The use of blanket terms such as diabetic gangrene, however, is no longer acceptable.

Neuropathy

The glove and stocking distribution of diabetic somatic sensory neuropathy is well known. What is not so commonly appreciated is that the neuropathy also affects somatic motor nerves, visceral sensory nerves and the autonomic nervous system. Each has a contribution to make in the formation of a neuropathic ulcer.

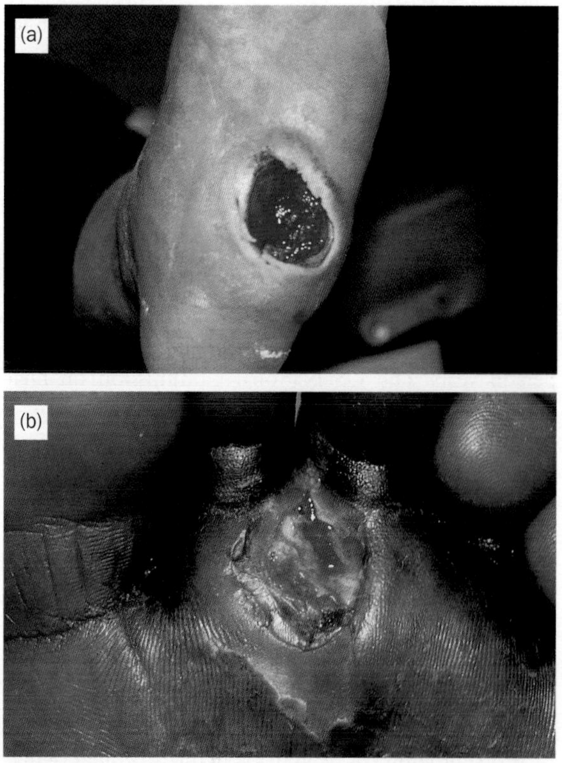

Figure 28.1 (a) A neuropathic ulcer. (b) A neuroischaemic ulcer.

Causes of neuropathy

There are essentially two theories as to the causation of diabetic peripheral neuropathy – one related to metabolic factors and the other associated with microvascular disease. The metabolic theory suggests that peripheral nerve damage arises from abnormalities of sugar-alcohol metabolism (Figure 28.2). Hyperglycaemia results in increased levels of intraneural sorbitol, which may be directly toxic to neural tissue. Hyperglycaemia also reduces the sodium-dependent uptake of myoinositol by competitive inhibition. The reduction in myoinositol levels impairs the action of the membrane bound sodium–potassium-dependent ATPase. This is responsible for maintaining the electrochemical gradient across the cell membrane and also assists in the transport of myoinositol into the cell by moving sodium out of it. A vicious cycle is therefore established, the result of which is a decrease in the activity of the sodium–potassium pump and a reduction of nerve conduction velocity. Microcirculatory changes which are described below may have an adverse effect on nerve metabolism. As discussed, however, the exact nature of these changes and how they may affect tissue function remains to be elucidated.

Effects of neuropathy

Extrinsic neuropathic foot ulceration

Loss of somatic sensation over the plantar aspect of the foot can lead to extrinsic neuropathic foot ulceration following trauma. The trauma can be varied – ill-fitting footwear, thermal, foreign bodies in shoes and toenail cutting are merely examples. The initial trauma is often minor and a person with intact sensation would naturally tend to protect the injury until it healed. In the absence of somatic sensation, however, areas which would normally be painful are not perceived as such, so allowing tissue damage to continue, once started. An established ulcer is the end point of this process.

Intrinsic neuropathic foot ulceration

The aetiology of intrinsic neuropathic ulcers is more complex. Somatic motor neuropathy results in weakness

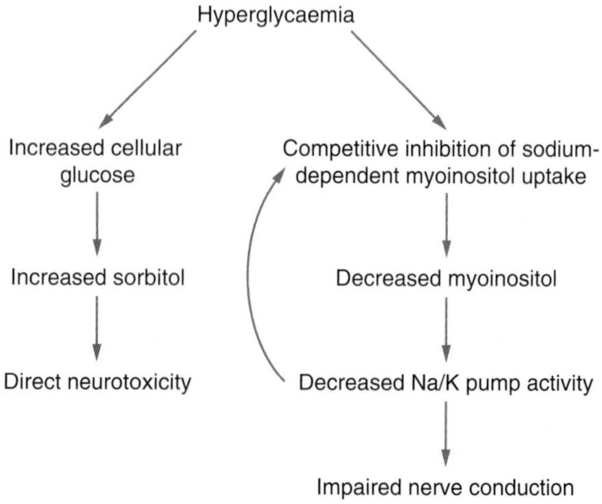

Figure 28.2 The altered sugar-alcohol pathway in diabetes.

of the intrinsic muscles of the foot, which in turn allows abnormal movement of the small bones of the foot and joint subluxation occurs. Weakness of foot ligaments due to abnormalities of collagen metabolism (see below) contributes to this effect. The early bone movements are small but would normally cause an aching foot which a person with intact proprioception would rest. Visceral sensory neuropathy reduces or abolishes proprioception, however, and the patient continues to walk on the foot. Ligaments and joint capsules are stretched further and the bony structure of the foot is altered permanently. As time goes on, these changes lead to foot deformities such as a claw foot with prominent metatarsal heads, or a rocker-bottom foot with collapse of the longitudinal arch and prominence of the tarsal bones (Figure 28.3). Should these subluxed joints become inflamed, Charcot's arthropathy is the result.

The bony changes produce localized areas of high pressure on the sole of the foot, particularly under the metatarsal heads, on the tips of toes, on the heel and under the midfoot. These high pressure areas are associated with ulceration – around three quarters of neuropathic ulcers occur in the forefoot, while the remainder occur under the midfoot and on the heel. The initial response to this high pressure is the formation of protective callus. In addition to the vertical load force resulting from the patient's weight acting on the callus, transverse and longitudinal shear forces are also established. These shear forces, particularly those in the longitudinal plane, traumatize the subcutaneous tissues between the underlying bone and overlying callus, producing cavities containing serum or blood. The cavities under the callus coalesce, and eventually the callus breaks down resulting in an ulcer. The breakdown tends to occur centrally and the defect in the callus is

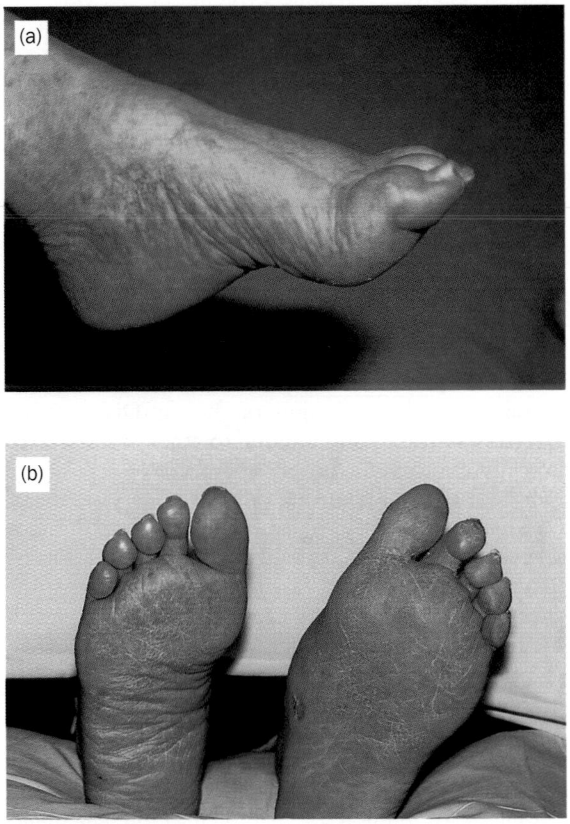

Figure 28.3 Neuropathic foot deformity: (a) claw foot, (b) rocker bottom foot.

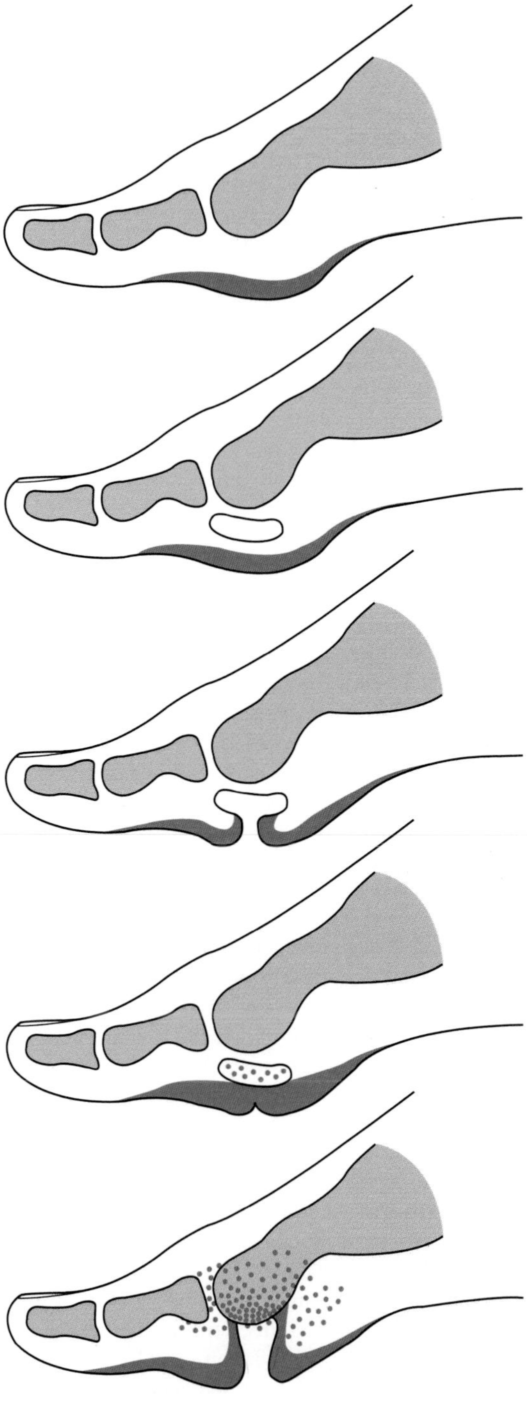

Figure 28.4 The process of callus and neuropathic ulcer development. (Reproduced with permission from Delbridge, L., Ctercteko, G., Fowler, C. *et al*. The aetiology of diabetic neuropathic ulceration of the foot. *Br J Surg*, 1985; **72**: 1–6.)

much smaller than the cavity underneath (Figure 28.4). This pattern of deep tissue destruction preceding epithelial breakdown is typical of neuropathic ulceration and differs from most other forms of ulcer.

Autonomic neuropathy also contributes to the formation of calluses through a reduction in sweating. Sweat contains keratinolytic enzymes which help break down hyperkeratotic areas. In their absence, the callus shows unimpeded growth. The absence or reduction of sweating also results in skin that is dry, inelastic and more prone to trauma.

Vascular disease

A belief in 'diabetic small vessel disease' – a supposed occlusive arteriolar phenomenon – is the greatest misconception when discussing vascular disease in diabetes and the commonest cause of therapeutic nihilism. There is no occlusive arteriolar disease in diabetes; diabetic patients do, however, suffer from atherosclerosis, from poor neural control of the microcirculation secondary to neuropathy and from abnormal transcapillary diffusion. It is better to abandon the term 'diabetic small vessel disease' and to restrict discussion to macrovascular disease and microvascular disease. A historical explanation is worthwhile.

Forty years ago, peripheral vascular disease rose to prominence as a principal aetiological factor in diabetic foot ulceration following the publication of a paper retrospectively examining amputated limbs from diabetic patients. A material that stained positive with the periodic acid–Schiff reaction was found to occlude the arterioles in the specimens studied and this was interpreted as a specific arteriolosclerosis associated with diabetes. This led to the widely held belief that diabetics suffer from an occlusive arteriolar disease that produces small areas of gangrene. This concept was propagated and became accepted knowledge. The work could not be repeated, however. Indeed, two prospective studies, one using standard histology to study serial sections of progressively smaller arteries and arterioles and the other using delicate casting techniques down to 10 μm, failed to demonstrate any arteriolar luminal occlusion. A subsequent study in which diabetics and non-diabetics undergoing femoro-popliteal bypass grafting showed similar degrees of vasodilatation in response to papaverine provided further evidence contradicting the presence of an occlusive arteriolar disease.

Diabetic microvascular disease

There are structural abnormalities of the capillary basement membrane in diabetes. The basement membrane is thickened as part of the general abnormality of extracellular matrix components, and its composition is altered by excessive glycosylation of collagen and proteoglycans. This glycosylation may take place by either enzymatic or non-enzymatic means and reduces the charge on the membrane. These changes may explain the increase in capillary permeability to highly charged molecules such as albumin. They do not appear to affect the diffusion of oxygen, however, as determined by transcutaneous measurement of oxygen tension in diabetic and non-diabetic patients. The basement membrane abnormality may still affect transcapillary movement of leucocytes and macromolecules.

Diabetics have been shown to have abnormal function of, and increased flow through the distal arteriovenous shunts proximal to the dermal capillary bed. There is an increased capillary luminal diameter secondary to basement membrane thickening and there is also an increase in capillary flow. The effect of this absolute hyperperfusion, however, is to raise tissue temperature and there is a consequent increased metabolic rate. Because of this it appears that there remains a relative hypoperfusion of tissues.

Although there is an absolute overperfusion at rest, there is less ability to vasodilate and increase blood flow in response to various stimuli. Vasodilatation is an important response to infection and trauma. Diabetics have been shown to lack such a response and are therefore at a disadvantage compared to non-diabetics when it comes to reacting to such stimuli. Furthermore, the vasoconstrictor response to the vertical posture is reduced with the result that capillary pressure rises. This increases oedema formation with the effect of impairing tissue perfusion.

Endothelial function is disturbed in diabetes. There is normally a fine balance in favour of vasodilatation over vasoconstriction and an anti-thrombotic tendency brought about by reactions involving nitric oxide (the endothelium-derived relaxing factor). Diabetes impairs this function of the endothelium with the result that blood flow through the microcirculation can be impaired. How these findings relate to those describing overperfusion remains to be elucidated. What is clear, however, is that the functional abnormalities of the microcirculation in diabetes have a real effect on tissue perfusion and potentially play an important role in ulceration.

Diabetic macrovascular disease

Atherosclerosis in diabetes is the same condition as it is in the absence of diabetes. Where it differs is in the prevalence and distribution of disease. Diabetics are four to seven times more prone to atherosclerosis than non-diabetics and the process appears to be accelerated – diabetic patients requiring vascular surgery are therefore likely to be younger than non-diabetics. Atherosclerosis tends to affect the tibial and peroneal arteries in diabetes, in contrast to non-diabetics, where the affected vessels tend to be above the knee. The vessels of the foot tend to be affected to a greater extent in non-diabetics than in diabetics. This difference in disease distribution demands more distal bypasses, but otherwise lower limb ischaemia in diabetes can be treated in the same way as it is in the absence of diabetes.

One caveat to this is vascular calcification. The media of arteries in diabetes tends to become calcified, often in excess of the degree of atherosclerosis that is present.

The calcification is often visible on plain radiography or on angiography. While this calcification *per se* does not result in vascular obstruction, it increases the impedance of the vessel, can make surgery difficult and makes measurement of ankle brachial indices unreliable. The pressure required to obliterate the ankle Doppler signal in such cases is often falsely high and in some patients it is not possible to obliterate the signal. A more realistic measure of perfusion pressure may be obtained by using toe digital artery pressures – the vessels within the toes can be spared the effects of calcification.

It may be thought that measurement of tissue oxygen partial pressure would overcome these difficulties of non-invasive arterial pressure assessment. However, this is not always reliable either, particularly in the presence of neuropathic ulceration where tissue oxygen partial pressure is often elevated above normal levels. If there is any doubt regarding the peripheral circulation in a diabetic patient, angiography should be performed.

Infection

Infection is not generally a primary cause of foot lesions in diabetes, with the exception of fungal infections between the toes which can lead to skin breakdown and secondary bacterial infection. Once a lesion has developed infection plays an important role in determining its outcome, whether the primary aetiology is neuropathic, ischaemic or a combination of the two (the neuroischaemic lesion).

When infection is secondary to a primary neuropathic or ischaemic lesion, it may remain superficial and localized. A spreading cellulitis can develop, however, or the infection can spread into the deeper tissues. Deep spread is less likely as long as the lesion can drain. Drainage is most problematic in neuropathic ulcers with a small defect in the overlying callus. If this defect is blocked, either by hyperkeratinization or by inspissated contents, then the infection is likely to spread into the deeper tissues and bone. This may result in osteomyelitis or abscess formation with possible spread along the planes between the anatomical layers of the foot and along the long tendon sheaths. In this way, infection is responsible for most of the tissue destruction seen in complicated diabetic foot lesions. Once infection is established a vicious cycle is set up in which areas immediately surrounding the infection become oedematous. The small vessels within this area are prone to thrombosis and occlusion as a result of sluggish flow due to platelet and leucocyte adhesion to vessel walls. These two factors may combine to produce localized tissue ischaemia and even gangrene, particularly in presence of macrovascular disease.

There are several reasons for an increased propensity to infection in diabetes. These include intrinsic abnormalities of the immune system with deficiencies in cell mediated immunity, impaired leucocyte chemotaxis, phagocytosis, intracellular bactericidal activity and serum opsonization. The infection is virtually always polymicrobial with Gram positive and negative aerobes and anaerobes, including *Staphylococcus aureus*, *Bacteroides*, *Proteus*, *Enterococcus*, *Clostridia* and *Escherichia coli* being present. Antibiotic treatment can be valuable when the infection is local or superficial. The choice of drug should take account of the polymicrobial nature of these lesions. There is some evidence that prolonged antibiotic treatment for small ulcers results in a more favourable outcome, although there is some debate on this issue. Once there is tissue destruction secondary to infection surgical debridement is required, although broad spectrum antibiotics still have an important role to play.

Connective tissue abnormalities

The hyperglycaemia of diabetes can significantly affect the structure and function of proteins. This is most commonly brought about by non-enzymatic glycosylation, a process in which glucose first binds reversibly with amino groups on proteins. These then irreversibly bind more glucose to form advanced glycosylation end products. These can then form covalent cross-links with amino groups on other matrix proteins or on extravasated plasma proteins. These reactions are seen with haemoglobin, where the glycosylated product is haemoglobin A1c – a well-known marker of the plasma glucose level over the previous 6 weeks.

The structural proteins, collagen and keratin, are also subject to these changes, and, as a result, the inter-molecular cross-linking produces tissues that are rigid, inflexible and resistant to digestion by proteases. The rigidity of the subcutaneous tissue between a callus and underlying bone renders it more likely to be torn by the shear forces referred to above. The resistance of the keratin to keratinases helps explain the production of callus, both at sites of high pressure and at the edges of open ulcers. The protein cross-linking makes this callus hard, and at the edge of an ulcer this can delay healing by preventing wound contraction. The collagen of the ligaments and joint capsules of the foot is affected in the same way. These structures then become weak and inelastic and the process contributes to the deformation of the bony structure of the foot. It is this collagen cross-linking which also contributes to the thickening and subsequent dysfunction of the basement membrane discussed above.

Haematological disturbances

Rheological abnormalities in diabetes contribute to ischaemia, ulcer formation and to the spread of infection. While details are beyond the scope of this section, it is appropriate to include a summary of the relevant points. Red cells are less deformable possibly due to glycosylation of their cell membrane. This, along with a tendency towards hypercoagulability and increased plasma viscosity, may play a part in reducing capillary circulation, so contributing to any ischaemia that is present. White cell function is impaired (as discussed above) with the resultant decreased resistance to infection.

Patient evaluation

All diabetics should undergo daily examination of their feet, either by themselves or by a relative. Who should carry out this inspection will be determined by the patient's general state of health, their visual acuity and their mobility. In addition, all diabetic patients should have regular inspections of their feet by a trained health care professional. How frequently there should be a medical examination is determined by the patient's degree of risk of developing foot ulceration. This introduces the concept of the 'at risk' foot – assessing this degree of risk is central to the examination of a diabetic patient. During this assessment, attention must be paid to determining the presence and degree of neuropathy, peripheral vascular disease, a history of previous ulceration and the foot's appearance. With this information a patient's foot can be described as normal, ischaemic, neuropathic or neuroischaemic. This information is essential in determining the appropriate treatment plan.

Neuropathy

Neuropathy may be tested by the traditional clinical methods examining the various sensory modalities, muscle power and the knee and ankle reflexes. More reproducible and meaningful information can be collected by assessing pain sensation with nylon monofilaments and vibration with a biosthesiometer. Nylon monofilaments are 5–10 cm lengths of nylon (similar to, but thicker than, a suture) of two differing thicknesses – one which will buckle when a load of 80 g is applied and the other at 10 g. The 10 g monofilament is pressed onto the skin of the foot until it buckles. If the patient is unable to feel this then it is assumed that protective sensation is lost. If the patient is unable to feel the 80 g monofilament then a severe neuropathy is present. The biosthesiometer allows the vibration perception threshold to be measured. The device is placed on the great toe tip or onto a malleolus and the voltage increased until the patient can feel the machine vibrating. A threshold greater than 25 V indicates significant neuropathy.

Peripheral vascular disease

Peripheral vascular status is assessed clinically by eliciting any history of claudication (which may present as weakness rather than pain due to the neuropathy) or rest pain and by examination of foot pulses and any foot colour changes with elevation and dependency. The presence of gangrene and the appearance of any ulcers are noted. This is supplemented by ankle-brachial pressure index (ABPI) measurement. However, up to 10% of diabetic patients will have falsely high ABPIs due to vascular calcification in the arterial media and so caution is required in their interpretation. Significant peripheral vascular disease (PVD) is unlikely if a foot pulse is palpable; if the ABPI is low, however, PVD is still possible in the presence of palpable pulses. Similarly, an elevated ABPI suggesting vascular calcification also makes PVD possible, even in the presence of a palpable pulse. Absent foot pulses make PVD likely and, in this context, the foot should be labelled 'ischaemic' – a term which implies any degree of vascular insufficiency rather than the more significant manifestations with which the term is normally associated. Because of the increased vascularity of the microcirculation at rest (see above) the foot may appear inappropriately warm in the presence of PVD. There should therefore be a high index of suspicion for the presence of PVD and if this possibility is raised in the presence of an ulcer then further assessment in the form of Doppler waveform analysis, duplex scanning and angiography should be considered. Digital subtraction angiography gives excellent images of distal vessels, but may not always demonstrate a patent vessel if flow is very low. In these circumstances, duplex scanning or magnetic resonance angiography may demonstrate a patent vessel not seen on catheter angiography (Table 28.1).

Previous ulceration

Previous ulceration is one of the most significant risk factors for the development of subsequent ulcers. A careful history regarding the development, location, treatment and eventual healing of the ulcer will give strong pointers as to its aetiology and to the pattern of possible future ulceration.

Foot appearance

The feet should be examined for any change in shape which may lead to the development of areas of high pressure – prominent metatarsal heads, hammer toes or a collapsed midfoot (Figure 28.3). Such areas may be identified by the presence of callus or by excessive wear on the sole of the shoe at that site. These areas are particularly prone to ulceration and should be watched carefully. If the skin of the foot is very dry then sweating has been reduced by the autonomic neuropathy. Such skin cracks easily lead to a site of entry for infection. The toes and interdigital spaces are examined for

Table 28.1 ABPI and diabetic foot disease

	ABPI < 0.9	*ABPI 0.9–1.1*	*ABPI > 1.1*
Palpable foot pulse	PVD possible assess further	PVD unlikely	Calcification present – PVD possible, assess further
No palpable foot pulse	PVD probable, assess further	PVD likely, assess further	Calcification present – PVD probable, assess further

Table 28.2 Risk of ulcer development for individual patients

	Low risk	*Moderate risk*	*High risk*
Sensation	Normal	Neuropathy or/	Neuropathy or/
Vascularity	Palpable pulses	absent pulses	absent pulses
History	No previous ulcer	No previous ulcer	Previous ulcer
Appearance	No deformity	No deformity	Deformity
Vision/mobility	Normal	Normal	Impaired, with any of the above

fungal infection and for small ulcers which may not be immediately apparent. The shoes should be looked at to determine their fit and any sites which may rub.

Risk assessment

It is useful to stratify the information obtained and grade the degree of risk of ulcer development for individual patients. This helps determine how intensive foot observation has to be and can impress on high-risk patients the need for vigilance. The following is a pragmatic stratification (Table 28.2).

Treatment methods

General issues

Patient education is central to the management of the diabetic foot with the emphasis on prevention. The importance of daily self-examination and careful hygiene is stressed along with the need for good, well-fitting shoes with sufficient depth. The patient should always look and feel (with their hand) in the shoe before putting it on in case any object has fallen in which may cause foot trauma. Patients with foot deformities should have shoes which accommodate the foot without creating abnormally high pressure areas – this may mean simply obtaining extra depth shoes or formally fitted orthoses may be required. Hand cream without perfume or colouring should be used daily or twice daily to prevent dry skin from cracking. Toenail cutting should only be carried out by patients if they are low risk (as defined above) – for all others regular chiropody is advised. Patients should be told never to attempt trimming of calluses themselves. Above all, the patient should be told to seek advice as soon as any problem with the foot develops.

The neuropathic ulcer

The principal aim in treating neuropathic ulcers is relief of pressure – assuming infection and ischaemia are not playing any significant role. The ultimate method of achieving this aim is bed rest, but this is not practical for the majority of patients who want to retain some degree of mobility. The realistic options available range from chiropody through special footwear to surgery. Conservative methods are used initially, with surgery being reserved for cases which do not respond.

Chiropody

In addition to cutting toenails and foot inspection for medium- and high-risk patients, removal of callus is an important part of diabetic foot treatment. This is done with a scalpel and has been shown to reduce the pressure exerted at these sites. By doing this the risk of ulceration is reduced. Padding for prominent areas or overlapping toes is provided. If a neuropathic ulcer develops then removal of callus from its edge is important to allow free drainage and also to enable wound contraction – the callus can be so hard as to prevent this.

Orthotics

In addition to providing appropriate footwear for the non-ulcerated foot, orthotists play a very important role in achieving the healing of neuropathic ulcers by providing footwear which reduces the pressure at the site of ulceration. This will involve tailor-made temporary shoes or total contact plaster casts which very effectively reduce pressure and allow ulcers to heal. The latter can only be used on stable ulcers where there is no infection or ischaemia as they stay on for a week or more at a time. They are excellent at relieving pressure and allowing ulcer healing but have the drawback of making ulcer inspection difficult. To get around this various custom-built devices such as Scotch cast boots and healing sandals have been developed which also relieve pressure but which allow easy access to dressings. These are widely used and enable the healing of the majority of neuropathic ulcers.

Surgery

In a small number of cases conservative measures fail to heal the ulcer. A decision must then be made regarding surgery. The options available depend on the ulcer. Assuming there is a good vascular supply and no infection requiring debridement (see below) surgery can relieve pressure on an ulcer by excision of the prominent bone through an incision away from the ulcer site. In this way metatarsal heads and even prominent tarsal bones can be removed with the effect of reducing pressure at the ulcer site (Figure 28.5). Although chronic ulcers will heal surprisingly quickly after such procedures, caution must be exercised before performing these operations. Pressure can be transferred to other areas of the foot with subsequent secondary ulcer development, the vascularity of the foot has to be adequate and the patient has to understand the need for close follow-up. These operations should only be performed by those with a particular interest in the diabetic foot.

Eradication of infection

Outpatient debridement by the chiropodist and oral antibiotics may be all that is required for superficially

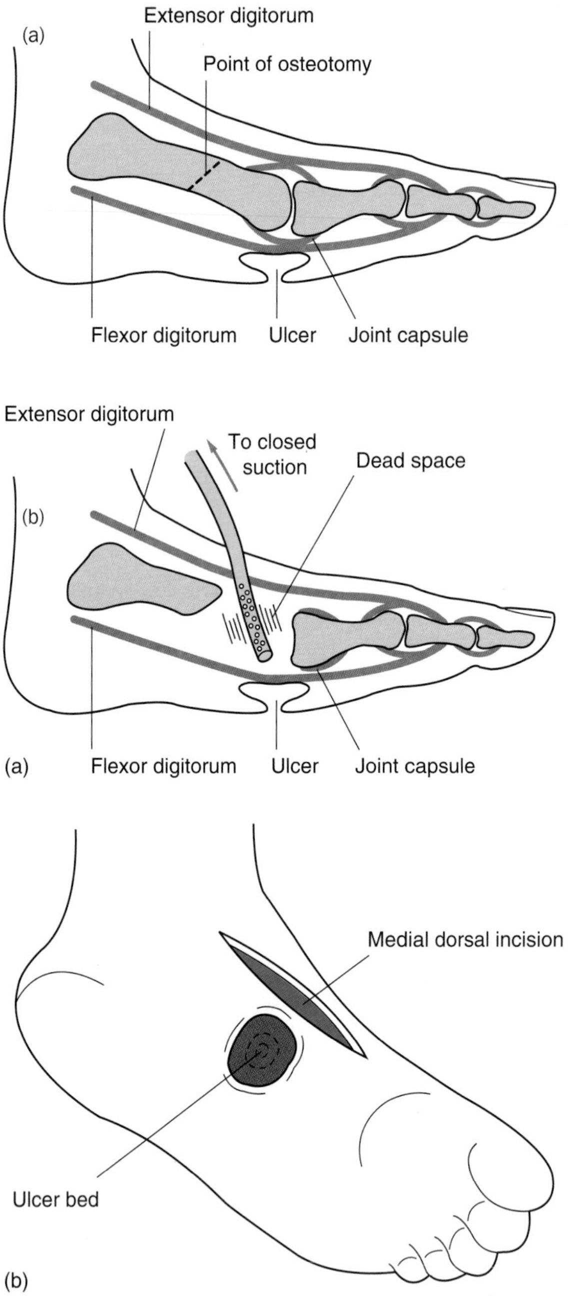

Figure 28.5 (a) Metatarsal head resection – this is performed through a dorsal incision. (Reproduced with permission from Griffiths, G. D. and Wieman, T. J. Metatarsal head resection for diabetic neuropathic foot ulcers. *Arch Surg* 1990; **125**: 32–5.) (b) Incision through which prominent tarsal bones and metatarsal bases can be excised for midfoot ulcers. (Reproduced with permission from Wieman, T. J., Griffiths, G. D. and Polk, H. C. Jr. Management of diabetic midfoot ulcers. *Ann Surg* 1992; **215**: 627–32.)

infected ulcers. The debridement has to be regular and antibiotic choice is dictated by sensitivities.

Superficial neuropathic ulcers will generally heal with a combination of chiropody, orthotics and eradication of infection. Larger or deeper ulcers, however, are more often associated with tissue necrosis and abscess formation. In these cases there is an urgent need for surgical debridement which should open all deep abscesses and excise all necrotic tissue. Deep specimens are sent for bacteriology as the organisms can be very different from superficial swabs. Broad spectrum intravenous antibiotics are required.

Dressings

Although a wide variety of dressings is available, none is particularly superior to any others with the possible exception of enzymatic preparations (streptokinase) which can be effective at superficial debridement or anti-pseudomonal chemicals (acetic acid). The important principle is that the dressing should absorb any exudate which may be produced and it should be non-adherent.

The neuroischaemic or ischaemic ulcer

General measures in the management of PVD are employed, particularly the treatment of risk factors. If the ulcer is small and superficial then a trial of conservative treatment under close supervision is appropriate. Measures similar to those used for neuropathic ulcers are employed. If there is no rapid improvement then further investigation of the vascularity of the foot should be undertaken with angiography. Vascular reconstruction is carried out to enable ulcer healing when appropriate. This may involve angioplasty, stenting, bypass surgery or a combination. Distal bypasses onto tibial or pedal vessels are often required and autogenous vein should be used whenever possible. The results of bypassing in patients with diabetes are as good as those in non-diabetics. The inflow for such bypasses can often be taken more distally than the common femoral – it is not uncommon for there to be a palpable popliteal pulse in the presence of occluded proximal calf vessels. Taking the bypass origin more distally allows a shorter bypass with the advantages of requiring less vein, a shorter anaesthetic and reduced bypass resistance. The results of such bypasses are as good as those taking origin from the common femoral artery, with 3–5 year patency rates of 80–90% when autogenous vein is used.

Surgical debridement

There is often discussion as to the relative timing of vascular reconstruction and surgical debridement. Generally speaking, reconstruction should take place first. Debridement or minor amputation can be carried out at the same time if the line of demarcation is clear. If tissue viability is not clearly determined at the time of reconstruction then debridement should be deferred as it may be possible to salvage more of the foot than is first apparent. Small patches of dry gangrene may be left to autoamputate – the larger the gangrenous area the less likely this is to be successful. Wet gangrene and infected tissue should generally be debrided at the time of vascular reconstruction. There is evidence that carrying out the two procedures simultaneously does not impair graft patency. If a

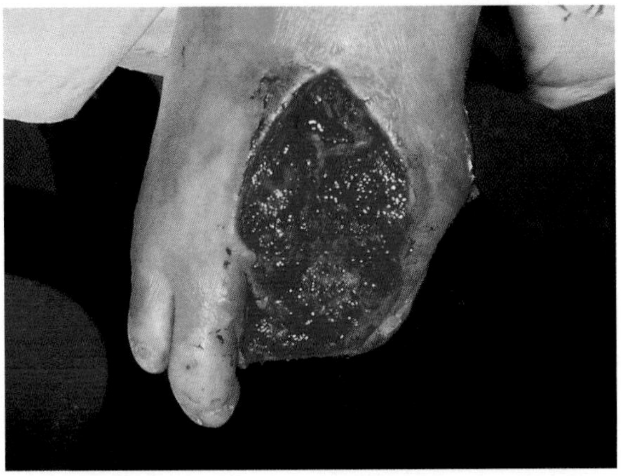

Figure 28.6 Foot after debridement of necrotic tissue.

patient presents with rampant and rapidly spreading foot infection then surgical debridement should be carried out as an emergency for two reasons – firstly to minimize the degree of foot destruction and secondly to treat the systemic effects of the infection which are generally present in such cases. These patients often have a neuroischaemic foot but may only have neuropathy. If there is a degree of ischaemia than it can be formally assessed once the infection is under control.

When debriding diabetic feet it is important to remove all infected and necrotic tissue (Figure 28.6). This often requires more extensive surgery than may be predicted pre-operatively and the patient should be warned of this and appropriate consent obtained. The necessary debridement may result in a foot of bizarre shape, but as much tissue should be preserved as is practicable: loss of the great toe is not a catastrophe; two central toes may be amputated as a single ray and the wound often heals very well; there is generally no advantage in preserving a little toe if the three central toes are amputated.

The future

It is apparent that successful management of diabetic foot disease is a multidisciplinary process with input from a variety of health care workers. While much of this is carried out at the primary care level, co-ordination is best achieved with the establishment of a diabetic foot clinic. Through this, each specialty can provide their input in the most effective manner. Such clinics improve the outcome of patients and ensure the most efficient use of resources. Patients with an ischaemic component should have aggressive vascular investigation and treatment with the recognition that distal bypass procedures can improve limb salvage rates. In the future it is to be hoped that the preventive measures discussed can be taken one step further with the successful prevention of neuropathy – such a breakthrough would greatly reduce the burden of diabetic foot disease.

Further reading

Barner, H. B., Kaiser, G. C. and Willman, V. L. (1971). Blood flow in the diabetic leg. *Circulation* **43**: 391–4.

Boulton, A. J. M., Connor, H. and Cavanagh, P. R. eds, (2000). *The Foot in Diabetes*, 2nd edn. Chichester: Wiley.

Brownlee, M., Cerami, A. and Vlassara, H. (1988). Advanced glycosylation end products in tissue and the biochemical basis of diabetic complications. *N Engl J Med* **318**: 1315–21.

Brownlee, M., Vlassara, H. and Cerami, A. (1984). Nonenzymatic glycosylation and the pathogenesis of diabetic complications. *Ann Intern Med* **101**: 527–37.

Conrad, M. C. (1967). Large and small artery occlusion in diabetics and non-diabetics with severe vascular disease. *Circulation* **36**: 83–91.

Ctercteko, G. C., Dhanendran, Hutton, W. C. and Le Quesne, L. P. (1981). Vertical forces acting on the feet of diabetic patients with neuropathic ulceration. *Br J Surg* **68**: 608–14.

Delbridge, L., Ellis, C. S. and Le Quesne, L. P. (1983). Nonenzymatic glycosylation of keratin in the diabetic foot. *Br J Surg* **70**: 305.

Flynn, M. D., Edmonds, M. E., Tooke, J. E. and Watkins, P. J. (1988). Direct measurement of capillary blood flow in the diabetic neuropathic foot. *Diabetologia* **31**: 652–66.

Foot Subgroup of Tayside Diabetes Advisory Group (2000). Guidelines for diabetic foot care in Tayside.

Glynn, J. R., Carr, E. K. and Jeffcoate, W. J. (1990). Foot ulcers in previously undiagnosed diabetes mellitus. *BMJ* **300**: 1046–7.

Goldenberg, S. G., Alex, M., Joshi, R. A. and Blumenthal, H. T. (1959). Non-atheromatous peripheral vascular disease of the lower extremity in diabetes mellitus. *Diabetes* **8**: 261–73.

Griffiths, G. D. and Wieman, T. J. (1990). Metatarsal head resection for diabetic neuropathic foot ulcers. *Arch Surg* **125**: 832–5.

Griffiths, G. D. and Wieman, T. J. (1992). Meticulous attention to foot care improves the prognosis in diabetic ulceration of the foot. *Surg Gynaecol Obstetr* **174**: 49–51.

Hamlin, C. R., Kohn, R. R. and Luschin, J. H. (1975). Apparent accelerated ageing of human collagen in diabetes mellitus. *Diabetes* **24**: 902–4.

LoGerfo, F. W., Gibbons, G. W., Pomposelli, F. B. *et al.* (1992). Evolving trends in the management of the diabetic foot. *Arch Surg* **127**: 617–21.

Menzoian, J. O., LaMorte, W. W., Paniszyn, C. C. *et al.* (1989). Symptomatology and anatomic patterns of peripheral vascular disease: differing impact of smoking and diabetes. *Ann Vasc Surg* **3**: 224–8.

Most, R. S. and Sinnock, P. (1983). The epidemiology of lower extremity amputations in diabetic individuals. *Diabetes Care* **6**: 87–91.

Neil, H. A. W., Thompson, A. V., Thorogood, M. *et al.* (1989). Diabetes in the elderly: the Oxford Community Diabetes Study. *Diabetic Med* **6**: 608–13.

Patel, V. G. and Wieman, T. J. (1994). Effect of metatarsal head resection for diabetic foot ulcers on the dynamic pressure distribution. *Am J Surg* **167**: 297–301.

Pollard, J.P. and Le Quesne, L.P. (1983). Method of healing diabetic forefoot ulcers. *BMJ* **286**: 436–7.

Pomposelli, F. B., Jepsen, S. J., Gibbons, G. W. *et al.* (1990). Efficacy of the dorsal pedal bypass for limb salvage in diabetic patients: short term observations. *J Vasc Surg* **11**: 745–52.

Rayman, G., Hassan, A. and Tooke, J. E. (1986). Blood flow in the skin of the foot related to posture in diabetes mellitus. *BMJ* **292**: 87–90.

Ruderman, N. B. and Haudenschild, C. C. (1984). Diabetes as an atherogenic factor: progress in cardiovascular disease. *Diabetes* **26**: 373–412.

Songer, T. J. (1992). The economics of diabetes care. In: Alberti, K. G. M. M., DeFronzo, R. A., Keen, H. and Zimmet, P. eds. *International Textbook of Diabetes Mellitus*. Chichester: Wiley, 1643–54.

Stokes, I. A. F., Faris, I. B. and Hulton, W. C. (1975). The neuropathic ulcer and loads on the foot in diabetic patients. *Acta Orth Scand* **46**: 839–47.

Strandness, D. E., Priest, R. E. and Gibbons, G. E. (1964). Combined clinical and pathologic study of diabetic and non-diabetic peripheral vascular disease. *Diabetes* **13**: 366–72.

Tooke, J. E. (1979). A capillary pressure disturbance in young diabetics. *Diabetes* **29**: 815–19.

Schnider, S. L. and Kohn, R. R. (1980). Glycosylation of human collagen in ageing and diabetes mellitus. *J Clin Invest* **66**: 1179–81.

Shah, D. M., Chang, B. B., Fitzgerald, K. M. *et al.* (1988). Durability of tibial artery bypass in diabetic patients. *Am J Surg* **156**: 133–5.

Stonebridge, P. A., Tsoukas, A. I., Pomposelli, F. B. *et al.* (1991). Popliteal-to-distal bypass grafts for limb salvage in diabetics. *Eur J Vasc Surg* **5**: 265–9.

Tannenbaum, G. A., Pomposelli, F. B. Jr, Marcaccio, E. J. *et al.* (1992). Safety of vein bypass grafting to the dorsalis pedis artery in diabetics with foot infections. *J Vasc Surg* **15**: 982–90.

Waugh, N. R. (1988). Amputations in diabetic patients: a review of rates, relative risks and resource use. *Community Med* **10**: 279–88.

Wieman, T. J., Griffiths, G. D. and Polk, H. C. Jr (1992). Management of diabetic midfoot ulcers. *Ann Surg* **215**: 627–32.

Williams, D. R. R. (1984). Hospital admissions of diabetic patients: information from Hospital Activity Analysis. *Diabetic Med* **2**: 27–32.

Williams, D. R. R. (2000). The size of the problem: epidemiological and economic aspects of foot problems in diabetes. In: Boulton, A. J. M., Connor, H. and Cavanagh, P. R. eds, *The Foot in Diabetes*, 2nd edn. Chichester: Wiley, 15–24.

Williams, D. R. R., Anthony, P., Young, R.J. and Tomlinson, S. (1994). Interpreting hospital admissions across the Korner divide: the example of diabetes in the North Western Region. *Diabetic Med* **11**: 166–9.

Young, M. and Matthews, C. (1998). Neuropathy screening, can we achieve our ideals? *Diabetic Foot* **1**: 22–5.

Young, M. J., Cavanagh, P. R., Thomas, G. *et al.* (1992). Effect of callus removal on dynamic foot pressures in diabetic patients. *Diabetic Med* **9**: 75–7.

Zlatkin, M. B., Pathria, M. and Sartoris, D. J. (1987). The diabetic foot. *Rad Clin North Am* **25**: 1095–105.

MODULE 29

Amputation

Amputation is undoubtedly one of the oldest surviving surgical procedures, although the indications for amputation have changed with time. Traditionally surgeons have tended to adopt a negative approach to amputation surgery, which thus has suffered in terms of attention, financial support and application of technology. The most difficult and demanding aspects of amputee care frequently relate to decision-making, rehabilitation and psychological factors rather than surgical technique. The amputating surgeon must be attentive and meticulous during surgery, whilst optimistic and dogmatic with the patient following surgery. It is essential for the amputating surgeon to realize that their responsibility for the amputee does not diminish with wound healing but must continue during post-operative psychological and physical rehabilitation as part of the multidisciplinary team. This chapter will review the history and epidemiology of amputation surgery, discuss the clinical aspects of amputee management, detail the technical aspects of amputation surgery and finally examine the rehabilitation process.

Section 29.1 • Historical overview

Amputations, of one kind or another, have been performed since time immemorial. Evidence of amputations, perhaps performed for ritual reasons, can be found in the drawings of Neolithic man. The writings of Hippocrates (460–377 BC) refer to surgical amputation as a medical therapy, emphasizing the need to ablate gangrenous tissue. A bronze lower limb protheses, dated 300 BC, was found at Pompeii and for many years was housed at the Royal College of Surgeons of England until it was destroyed in an air-raid in 1940. The techniques involved in amputation surgery were brutal and crude, until the time of Ambrose Paré (1510–1590). Paré is considered to be the originator of the modern principles of amputation surgery and is credited with the popularization of vascular ligatures, vessel transfixion, haemostats and tourniquets, replacement of cautery with bland dressings and the aggressive rehabilitation of amputees. John Hunter (1729–1793) held a conservative approach to amputation surgery, recommending elective late amputation through the necrotic rather than the living tissue. The wars and military campaigns of the late eighteenth and early nineteenth century focused attention on amputation surgery. In 1797, during an attempted boat landing at Santa Cruz, Tenerife, Admiral Lord Nelson received a severe musketshot injury to his right arm, which ultimately necessitated a right above elbow amputation. His nephew, Lt Josiah Nesbit, probably saved the admiral's life by applying a tourniquet at the time of the injury, thus enabling the admiral to survive the time taken to refloat his grounded boat and row back to the fleet anchored offshore. The Earl of Anglesey was another famous amputee. He underwent an above knee amputation after being struck on the leg by a cannon ball when stood next to Lord Wellington at the Battle of Waterloo in 1815. He made a complete recovery and was fitted with an elegant wooden prosthesis. During the Napoleonic wars, Dominique Jean Larrey (1776–1842) continued and expanded the principles of amputation championed by Paré. He recognized the importance of early treatment with his concept of 'flying horse' ambulances to snatch the sickest casualties from the battlefield. Larrey advocated the early mobilization of amputees, the use of ice for analgesia and the coverage of the transected bone with muscle in addition to skin. Improvements in anaesthesia, reorganization of hospitals and the introduction of aseptic Listerian techniques are responsible for progress in amputation surgery during the first half of the nineteenth century.

Around this time Lisfranc, Chopart and Syme described the operations that have subsequently come to bear their names, Pean introduced his locking scissor haemostat, Esmarch introduced his atraumatic tourniquet and Rocco Gritti described his supracondylar femoral amputation, which was later applied by William Stokes. During the First World War, huge numbers of compound fractures were treated by primary amputation. Gas gangrene and sepsis were common, often fatal, complications of amputation surgery and this fuelled a return, during the Spanish Civil and Second World Wars, to the concept of debridement rather than amputation. This approach to trauma management, together with the availability of antibiotics, greatly reduced the number of military amputees in these and future military campaigns. In the past 50 years, the main advances in the field of amputation surgery have included the rapid rehabilitation and limb fitting of amputees, the refinement of amputation level selection, and the incorporation of new designs and materials into the construction of prosthetic limbs.

Section 29.2 • Epidemiology

The reported incidence of lower limb amputation varies considerably (Table 29.1). The incidence of amputation increases exponentially with age, with 75% of patients undergoing amputation being over 60 years old. Men have an amputation rate two to three times higher than women, but with increasing age there is closer parity. The aetiology of amputations varies with age and geography. Congenital deformity is the commonest cause of amputation in children who, fortunately, account for <1% of all amputees. In Western society, trauma is the most common cause of amputation in patients below the age of 40 years, with 40% of cases involving a motorcycle road traffic accident. In patients over 40 years of age, critical lower limb ischaemia secondary to peripheral vascular disease accounts for over 90% of amputations. Approximately 10–20% of patients with critical lower limb ischaemia will require major amputation.

Malignancy and industrial accidents are rare causes of amputation, which would appear to be decreasing. In developing countries, trauma secondary to war injuries, in particular anti-personnel mines, remains an important cause of amputation. The geographic and ethnic variations observed in the incidence of amputation reflect differences in the prevalence of peripheral vascular disease and its predisposing factors (e.g. diabetes), variation in culture and access to medical care, including vascular services. The impact of lower limb revascularization on amputation rates is disputed. There can be no doubt of the exponential increase in the number of revascularization procedures performed for

Table 29.1 The epidemiology of lower limb amputation

Study	*Date*	*Country*	*Incidence of amputation (per 100 000 population/year)*	
Tunis *et al.*, 1991	1979 1989	USA	28 32	
Gutteridge *et al.*, 1994	1983–87 1988–91	UK	7.8	
Lindholt *et al.*, 1994	1986–87 1989–90	Denmark	30.9	
Ebskov *et al.*, 1994	1983 1990	Denmark	25	
Humphrey *et al.*, 1994	1945–79	Rochester, USA	375 (diabetics)	
Huber *et al.*, 1999	1992–95	USA	50 (African–Americans) 25 (White Americans)	
Pohjolainen *et al.*, 1999	1995	Finland	28	
Feinglass *et al.*, 1999	1996	USA	25	
Global LEA study, 2000	1995–97		*Men*	*Women*
		Leeds, UK	19.9	10.2
		Leicester,UK	7.2	4.3
		Middlesborough, UK	27.8	8.4
		Newcastle, UK	20.2	8.8
		Madrid, Spain	3.7	0.5
		Vicenza, Italy	9.6	7.0
		Montgomery, USA	34.9	17.0
		Navajo, USA	58.7	32.0
		Ilan, Taiwan	11.3	8.3

critical ischaemia over recent decades. In published case series from specialized tertiary centres, this increase in 'limb salvage' procedures is associated with a decline in the need for major amputation. These series are undoubtedly affected by case mix and referral patterns and therefore suffer from selection bias. However, population studies after the late 1980s do begin to support the hypothesis that increased rates of attempted lower limb revascularization are associated with a reduction in amputation rates. The delay between the increased rates of revascularization and fall in amputation rates may reflect the time lag phenomenon associated with arterial reconstruction in patients with earlier stages of lower limb ischaemia. Progression of disease may be prevented or postponed by intervention at an earlier stage thus inevitably reducing the requirement for amputation. Distal surgical reconstructions in patients with diffuse disease, previously considered only for primary amputation, specifically seem significantly associated with lower amputation rates.

Pre-operative assessment and management (Table 29.2)

Initial assessment of a patient with critical lower limb ischaemia involves a detailed history and thorough examination, together with a few basic investigations. The pathological decision to amputate is often an easy one, however, difficulties are commonly encountered on an ethical or humane basis. Honest, open discussion with patients and relatives generally reveals the most appropriate course of action in the majority of cases and later dissatisfaction is usually a result of poor communication.

Primary amputation may be defined as amputation of an ischaemic limb without attempted antecedent revascularization. It is indicated in advanced distal ischaemia with uncontrollable pain or infection in the specific settings of non-reconstructable occlusive arterial disease; necrosis of significant areas of the weight bearing portion of the foot; fixed, irremediable flexion contracture of the leg; or a very limited life expectancy due to comorbid illness.

Secondary amputation, or amputation following revascularization, is indicated when revascularization has failed and no further revascularization is possible. Less commonly, secondary amputation may be indicated when there is continued deterioration of a limb (e.g. progressive sepsis) despite a patent reconstruction. The effect of previous reconstructive surgery on amputation level remains a topic of debate. Some authors claim that secondary amputations are performed at a higher level than primary amputations, while others have found no significant difference between the eventual level of primary and secondary amputations.

Generally, the indications for amputation are relatively obvious, however, on occasion the appropriateness of amputation is unclear. Two areas of difficult decision making are commonly encountered. The first is the choice between amputation and reconstruction. If the patient is sufficiently fit to survive revascularization and a previously useful limb is salvageable, then every effort should be made to revascularize the limb. Purists would argue that no limb should be amputated without the patient being offered angiography and the chance of reconstruction, and amputation should then only be performed if two vascular specialists agree reconstruction is not possible. Frequently, however, the vascular surgeon is faced with an elderly, medically unfit patient with a borderline arterial tree. In such cases, personal audit is essential. The surgeon's own experience and record of success with distal arterial revascularization are pivotal in this decision-making process. If a surgeon thinks reconstruction is advisable and possible but beyond his or her own technical ability, referral to a specialist unit is recommended.

The second area of difficulty arises when a very elderly or debilitated patient, in whom arterial reconstruction is impossible or inappropriate, presents with a critically ischaemic leg. Management options in such cases are amputation or conservative, symptomatic treatment. Pain control can usually be achieved by appropriate analgesics and the involvement of the specialist pain team, thus amputation should very seldom be necessary. After receiving appropriate medical advice, the ultimate decision to consent for amputation lies with the patient. This medical advice may be flavoured by the patient's current quality of life, medical, psychiatric and social history, the details of which may require discussion with the patient's friends, relatives and primary care team.

The majority of lower limb amputations are best performed on elective operating lists. This allows ample time for pre-operative optimization of the patient's medical and psychological condition. Pre-operative assessment and support from physicians, anaesthetists, physiotherapists, occupational therapists, pain specialists

Table 29.2 Essential aspects of amputee management

Pre-operative management	*Post-operative management*
Vascular assessment	Post-operative pain control
Assess urgency of amputation	Wound management
Adequate pain relief	Nutrition
Infection control	Treatment of concurrent medical disease
Nutrition assessment	Management of contralateral limb
Cardio-respiratory assessment	Early mobilization
Anaesthetic consultation	Attention to psychological problems
Amputation level assessment	Rehabilitation assessment

and other amputees are often helpful. Emergency amputation should be reserved for gangrene resulting in septicaemia or irreversible acute ischaemia involving large muscle masses. The surgeon should approach an amputation as a reconstructive procedure, and the procedure is therefore best performed by an interested and experienced surgeon, who is prepared to take the time and trouble to get it right and who has some accountability for the patient's post-operative rehabilitation. To view amputation surgery as uninteresting and unrewarding and to delegate the procedure to a junior or inexperienced surgeon is to the patient's detriment.

The selection of amputation level should involve consideration of maximum mobility and wound healing. Improved post-operative rehabilitation and mobility following amputation is associated with preservation of the knee joint. These advantages, however, are lost in the presence of poor stump healing and revisional surgery. Trans-tibial to trans-femoral amputation ratios average at <1.0 in England and Wales; however, surgeons with an interest in amputations achieve a higher ratio. Simple clinical assessment of the patient and the limb is essential, as in 50% of trans-femoral amputations, co-existent medical problems (e.g. stroke and flexion contractures) are more influential than concerns regarding wound healing. In all cases of amputation, the implicit goal is to obtain primary healing, and in those with a potentially useful limb this should be at the most distal level possible. Numerous methods have been used to try and accurately identify this site. Clinical examination of the leg, with assessment of warmth, skin integrity and capillary refill time has been proven to be of little value. The presence of a palpable pulse in the major artery immediately above the proposed level of amputation is a strong predictor of primary healing, however the absence of a pulse in this artery does not exclude primary healing. The ideal test for selecting amputation levels would be sensitive, specific, quick, non-invasive, inexpensive and acceptable to both patients and staff. Needless to say, such a test does not exist, but in a review of investigations aimed at predicting primary healing, arterial pressures and indices measured using a handheld Doppler probe proved to be the most useful. No healing was found in diabetics following foot amputations with an ankle pressure less than 50 mmHg and no healing of toe amputations with toe pressures less than 15 mmHg. Systolic toe pressures were found to correlate with healing rates more closely than ankle pressures or skin perfusion pressures following digital and trans-metatarsal amputations. In these patients, healing rates of 17%, 59% and 78% were observed with toe pressures of less than 20, 20–29 and greater than 30 mmHg, respectively. In a study of 236 trans-tibial amputees, healing was observed in 93% of patients in whom pre-operative popliteal occlusion pressure exceeded 50 mmHg. Healing was by primary intention in 64% and by secondary intention or following local wedge resection in 29% of cases. Other investigations including skin blood flow measurement using iodo-antipyrine and xenon; skin perfusion pressure using radioactive tracers and photoplesthsmography; laser Doppler flowmetry; fluorescein uptake; transcutaneous oxygen pressure; thermography; and capillary microscopy have all been used to predict primary healing with variable results. They have not, however, been widely used, mainly because of technical complexities, cost and result variability. The value of these more specialized tests, therefore, remains to be established and they should probably be confined to specialized centres.

General pre-operative preparation of a patient for amputation has both physical and psychological considerations and in many areas these may overlap. Patients requiring amputation frequently suffer with multiple medical conditions including ischaemic heart disease cerebrovascular disease, diabetes, hypertension, hypercholesterolaemia, chronic obstructive pulmonary disease and malnutrition. It is essential that any such conditions are appropriately treated and stabilized prior to amputation and the involvement of an interested physician is often beneficial. Dietary assessment and, if required, supplementation by a dietician is also often advantageous. Pre-operative pain control is essential for the patient's physical and psychological well being and may reduce post-operative flexion contractures and phantom pain. The anaesthetist responsible for the amputation anaesthetic or the specialist hospital pain team should assess and treat pre-operative pain. Probably the most effective means of pre-operative pain control is by epidural infusion, which can then be supplemented as necessary by oral medication. Pre-operative involvement of the physiotherapist and occupational therapist responsible for post-operative rehabilitation is also advantageous to prepare the patient physically and psychologically for amputation. A pre-operative visit from a well-rehabilitated amputee or a member of an amputee support group often helps allay the patient's fear and reduce anxiety.

Section 29.3 • Amputation surgery

General principles

The exact choice of anaesthetic for amputation surgery will vary according to the condition of the patient, available local skills and the preferences of the anaesthetist. In general terms, however, it is probably preferable to do major amputations under epidural anaesthesia, which ideally should be sited 24–48 hours pre-operatively. Prophylactic antibiotics should be given immediately prior to surgery and continued post-operatively according to unit protocol. Once the patient is ready for surgery, the planned skin incisions should be marked with an appropriate pen. In patients undergoing amputation for peripheral vascular disease, a tourniquet should virtually never be used but may be useful in amputations performed for trauma or tumour.

Gentle tissue handling is by far the most important technical principle of successful amputation surgery.

Minimal manipulation of the tissues with instruments is recommended and where possible the use of only fingers to manoeuvre skin flaps is promoted. It is essential to understand that the blood supply to the skin of the lower leg is dependent upon the integrity of the vascular plexus immediately superficial to the deep fascia. This fascia, therefore, must be protected and treated as one with the skin, especially in trans-tibial amputations. Mass ligation of neurovascular bundles should be avoided and the artery and veins should be ligated separately to avoid the possibility of arteriovenous shunts. Nerves should be dissected from the vessels, drawn down and transected under tension. Terminal neuromas form at the end of every cut nerve, thus it is important to try to keep the ends of transected nerves away from weight bearing areas, sites of compression and areas of scar formation. Transected bone also requires specific attention. The periosteum should only be elevated the minimal distance above the level of transection to avoid damage to the nutrient vessels, and a cuff of periosteum can be dissected off below the intended level of amputation and used to seal the medullary cavity. Bone wax should be avoided. Sharp spicules and bone edges should always be smoothed with a bone rasp or file.

Digital amputation

The most common amputation performed in vascular units is probably the digital amputation.

These amputations will only heal in the presence of reasonable blood supply and thus frequently are performed in conjunction with limb revascularization, either bypass or angioplasty.

Diabetics may on occasion present with isolated small vessel disease and a black toe that may be suitable for amputation without the need for improvement in regional blood supply. The requirement for digital amputations can be drastically reduced by the introduction of a dedicated foot clinic involving dedicated podiatrists, prosthetist/shoe fitter, nurse and physician.

The level of digital amputation is dependent on the degree of infarction/infection but often amputation through the proximal phalanx using equal anterior and posterior flaps is possible thus preserving foot architecture, which is important for proper function. In cases of more extensive disease disarticulation at the metatarso-phalangeal (MTP) joint using a 'racquet' incision may be possible. The 'handle of the racquet' is placed on the dorsum of the foot for the second, third and fourth toes but on the medial and lateral aspect of the foot for the first and fifth toes. If disarticulation through the MTP joint is possible the articular cartilage should be shaved off to allow granulation tissue to evolve from the bone. Some authors would advocate resection of the metatarsal head to remove this articular cartilage. Resection of the metatarsal heads of the second, third or fourth digits results in a lack of support of adjacent digits leading to inward displacement, reduced stability and often more discomfort. If gangrene has spread

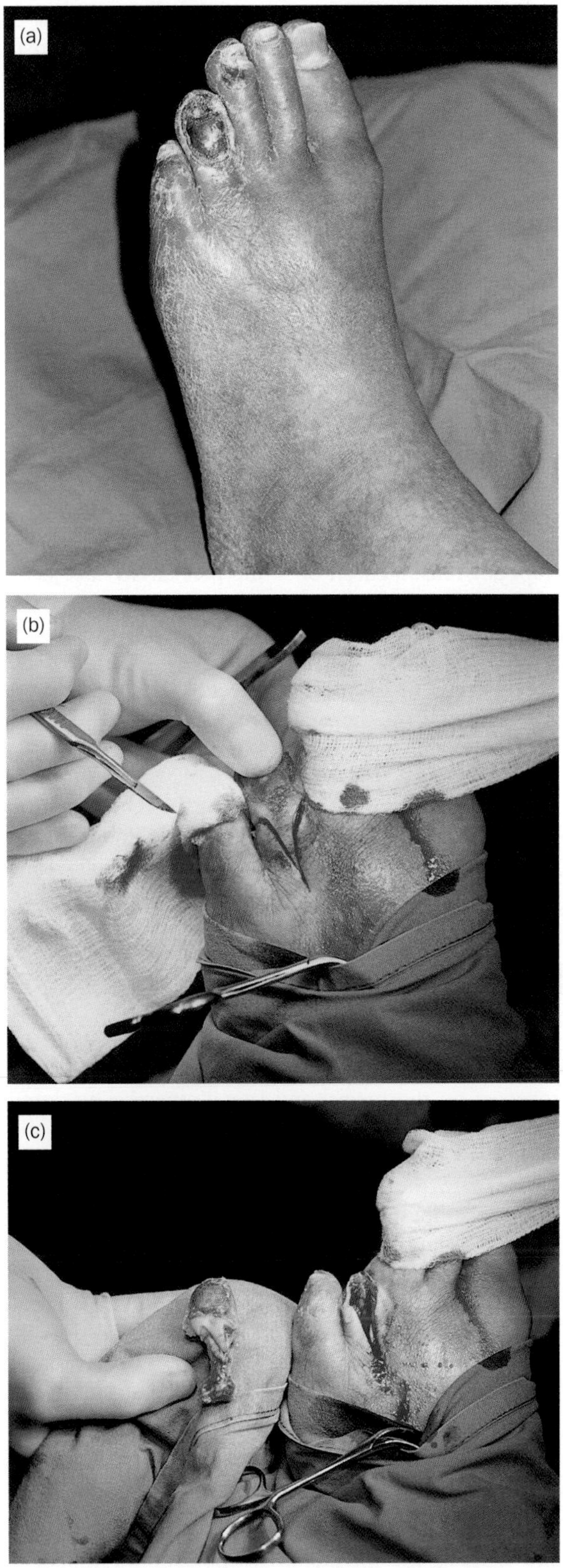

Figure 29.1 (a) Dry digital gangrene of the fourth toe in a diabetic who has previously undergone percutaneous transluminal angioplasty of the superficial femoral artery. (b) Racquet incision used for digital amputation. (c) Amputation of the fourth toe by disarticulation through the metatarsophalangeal joint. The articular cartilage of the metatarsal head was subsequently removed and the wound left open.

proximal to the MTP joint then a ray amputation of the digit and accompanying metatarsal bone is optimal. The proximal resection should then be performed through the cancellous bone at the base of the metatarsal. Most surgeons advocate avoidance of skin sutures in digital amputations for vascular disease, preferring to leave the wound open, especially in cases of marginal viability. While this inevitably means a longer healing time, the chances of complete healing and the avoidance of infective complications usually more than justify this approach (Figure 29.1).

Foot amputations

Apart from the trans-metatarsal amputation, partial foot amputations result in a surprisingly high degree of disability and the provision of appropriate footwear is often difficult. Some vascular surgeons would therefore argue that a trans-tibial amputation provides the best hope for rehabilitation once the metatarsals have been lost.

Trans-metatarsal amputation

When gangrene or infection affects several toes and/or the great toe on the same foot, but the plantar skin beneath the metatarsal heads is viable, consideration should be given to a trans-metatarsal amputation. It is essential in order to obtain healing in these amputations to ensure an adequate proximal blood supply. They can be of particular value in the patient with a previously revascularized leg or in the diabetic patient. Contraindications include gangrene or infection proximal to the MTP crease. The dorsal skin incision is made side to side, approximately 1 cm distal to the intended site of bony transection, at the level of the metatarsal shafts. The plantar incision is made in the MTP skin crease and the two incisions are joined together on the medial and lateral aspects. The dorsal incision is continued down to the metatarsal bones and each metatarsal shaft is transected approximately 1 cm proximal to the skin incision. This is generally most easily accomplished using an air-driven oscillating saw. Using a scalpel, the tissues in the plantar aspect of the forefoot are dissected from the metatarsal shafts and the plantar flap is thinned. After obtaining absolute haemostasis with ligatures, the plantar flap is rotated dorsally and sutured in position using a deep layer of absorbable interrupted sutures and monofilament interrupted vertical mattress sutures for skin closure. In the presence of infection or when the viability of the plantar flap is in doubt, a simple trans-metatarsal 'guillotine' forefoot amputation may be performed at the level of the dorsal incision. In such cases, no plantar flap is fashioned and there is no attempt at wound closure, which is achieved by secondary intention. Once healed, a trans-metatarsal amputation provides excellent prospects for rehabilitation with minimal prosthetic requirements. Problems include non-healing, haematoma, infection and oedema, which may necessitate revision to a higher amputation level.

Lisfranc's amputation

Using equal transverse dorsal and plantar skin incisions, the tarso-metatarsal joints are disarticulated, and the cartilage is shaved away, or excised with a saw cut through the distal tarsal bones (Hey's modification). Another option is the disarticulation of the medial tarso-metatarsal joints combined with transection through the bases of the lateral metatarsals, disregarding the anatomy of the articulations but preserving uniform foot length. Care must be taken to preserve the plantar arteries that lie very close to the second and third cuneiform bones. Lisfranc's amputation produces a relatively unstable foot, as it is difficult to ensure the line of bone section obtains uniform contact with the ground. There is a tendency to develop an equinus deformity due to the unopposed actions of peroneus longus, brevis and tertius.

Chopart's amputation

Similar to Lisfranc's amputation but at a slightly more proximal level, this amputation is performed using equal transverse dorsal and plantar flaps. The tarso-tarsal joints are disarticulated and the articular surfaces of the talus and calcaneous bones are rounded off to obtain a well-rounded stump. Stump contractures in equinus and supination may be prevented by external ankle fixation, or treated by lengthening of the Achilles tendon, transfer of the tibialis anterior tendon to the lateral border of the stump, or wedge osteotomy and fusion of the subtalar joint. That which pertains to Lisfranc's amputation applies to a greater degree to Chopart's trans-tarsal amputation. It is probably best avoided, as the majority of tendinous attachments around the ankle have been lost and thus it is an unstable amputation.

Syme's amputation

James Syme, a professor of surgery in Edinburgh, first described this amputation in 1843. Harris later highlighted the commonly encountered problems and advised on their avoidance and management. Syme's amputation is essentially an ankle disarticulation, modified to remove the protruding malleoli and the cartilage of the tibio-talar articulation. The skin incisions are plantar and dorsal. The plantar skin incision begins at the tip of the lateral malleolus, runs inferiorly curving slightly forwards, across the sole, to a point just below the medial malleolus. The dorsal skin incision joins the ends of the plantar incision at an angle of 45° from the line of the tibia. On the dorsum the extensor retinaculum is divided and the extensor tendons divided as high as possible. The anterior capsule of the ankle joint is opened, the foot plantar is flexed and the medial and lateral collateral ligaments are divided from within. Great care must be taken to avoid damage to the calcaneal branches of the posterior tibial and peroneal arteries or the vessels themselves. The posterior capsule of the ankle joint is now opened, and the medial, lateral and eventually the inferior surface of the os calcis are dissected, keeping close to the calcaneal periosteum to enucleate the bone from the fatty tissue. During this dissection it is necessary to detach, firstly, the long plantar ligament from its tuberosity on the os calcis and then secondly, the insertion of the tendo Achilles, taking care to avoid button holing the skin. The foot is now removed. With the heel flap turned backwards and upwards the malleoli and a thin slice of distal tibia are removed with a saw, ensuring the cut is at right angles to the tibia and the subarticular bone is preserved. The bone edges are smoothed with a file. The amputation is then closed in two layers over a drain.

The Pirogoff–Boyd amputation is similar to the Syme's amputation but a variable amount of calcaneum is retained in the plantar flap, which is then used to form an arthrodesis with the lower end of the tibia.

The Syme and Pirogoff–Boyd amputations have a relatively small place in the management of patients with peripheral vascular disease, because the bulky heel flap has a tenuous blood supply from the medial and lateral calcaneal arteries, which are frequently affected by atherosclerosis. The heal flap also tends also to be thick and therefore folding it is difficult and may further impair the blood supply. The rigidity of the plantar flap also results in a large volume of dead space related to the cut bone and thus the incidence of haematoma and infection is significant. It is a useful amputation in highly specific circumstances. In cases of forefoot trauma or critical ischaemia due to small vessel occlusive disease when the circulation around the ankle is not compromised it can provide a good weight-bearing stump. With modern-day prosthetic fitting, a fully functional and cosmetically acceptable limb can be provided following Syme's amputations.

Trans-tibial amputation

In the patient with non-reconstructable critical ischaemia, when the blood supply is inadequate to ensure healing at more distal levels, the trans-tibial (or below knee) amputation is undoubtedly the gold standard of management. Healing rates of over 80% can be expected for all patients undergoing amputation at the trans-tibial level. This may be increased to 93% using objective amputation level selection with arterial pressures. Contraindications to trans-tibial amputations include proximal extension of the disease process to the tissues of the posterior flap or within close proximity of the tibial tuberosity anteriorly; a fixed flexion contracture of the knee joint; spasticity (e.g. due to previous stroke), as unopposed muscle action following amputation will pull the knee into flexion; and finally occlusion of the profunda femoris artery without objective amputation level selection data supporting healing.

The two methods of trans-tibial below knee amputation are distinguished only by their different choice of placement of fasciocutaneous flaps.

The 'long posterior flap' trans-tibial amputation was first described by Heister in 1739, but failed to gain popularity until its refinement by Burgess and Romano. The rationale behind the 'long posterior flap' technique is that the best blood supply to the posterior skin of the calf is from the sural artery which may be supplemented by perforating arteries from the gastrocnemius/soleus muscle mass. The anterior skin incision is made 8–12 cm distal to the tibial tuberosity and encompasses two-thirds of the circumference of the calf at this level. The length of the posterior flap should be is approximately one-third the circumference of the calf at the level of the anterior skin incision (Figure 29.2a). The skin incision is deepened to include the subcutaneous fat and deep fascia.

The 'equal skew flap' trans-tibial amputation was described later and popularized by Robinson. In this case, two equal fasciocutaneous flaps are fashioned, with the antero-medial flap based on the saphenous artery and the postero-lateral flap based on the sural artery. The potential benefits claimed for the 'equal skew flap' trans-tibial amputation include an improved blood supply to the wound and therefore a higher primary healing rate; a wound sited away from the prominent crest of the subcutaneous tibia which is therefore less prone to wound dehiscence; a less bulky amputation stump more suited to early use of a patellar tendon bearing prosthesis; and finally, a less technically demanding procedure to perform than a 'long posterior flap' trans-tibial amputation. The skin flaps are based at a level 8–12 cm below the tibial tuberosity. At this level, 2.5 cm lateral to the subcutaneous crest of the tibia, the anterior intersection of the two flaps is marked. The posterior intersection of the two flaps is then marked at distance of half the circumference of the calf at this level. The midpoint of the base of the two flaps is marked a quarter of a circumference from each intersection. The same quarter circumference is then used to mark the length of each flap. The skin, subcutaneous fat and deep fascia are incised along these marked lines.

Whichever method of fasiocutaneous flap fashioning is used, the procedure from this point is essentially the same. The long and short saphenous veins are identified and ligated. The saphenous and sural nerves are separated, pulled down and divided under tension. The sural nerve artery and saphenous nerve artery may require ligation. The muscles in the anterior tibial compartment are divided, and the anterior tibial artery and vein ligated. The tibia is isolated 10 cm distal to the tuberosity and, after stripping the periosteum, it is divided with either a hand or pneumatic saw. The fibula is likewise exposed and divided slightly proximal to the level of the tibial transection. Following this, the myocutaneous flap consisting of skin, subcutaneous fat, deep fascia and gastrocnemius is developed, with excision of the other muscles. The peroneal and posterior tibial arteries and veins are ligated and divided. The posterior tibial nerve is distracted downwards, transected and allowed to retract again. The myocutaneous flap is then sculpted to fit over the stump end without tension (Figure 29.2b). The distal end of the tibia is bevelled by using a saw to cut obliquely across the anterior tip and the edges are smoothed with a file. Following

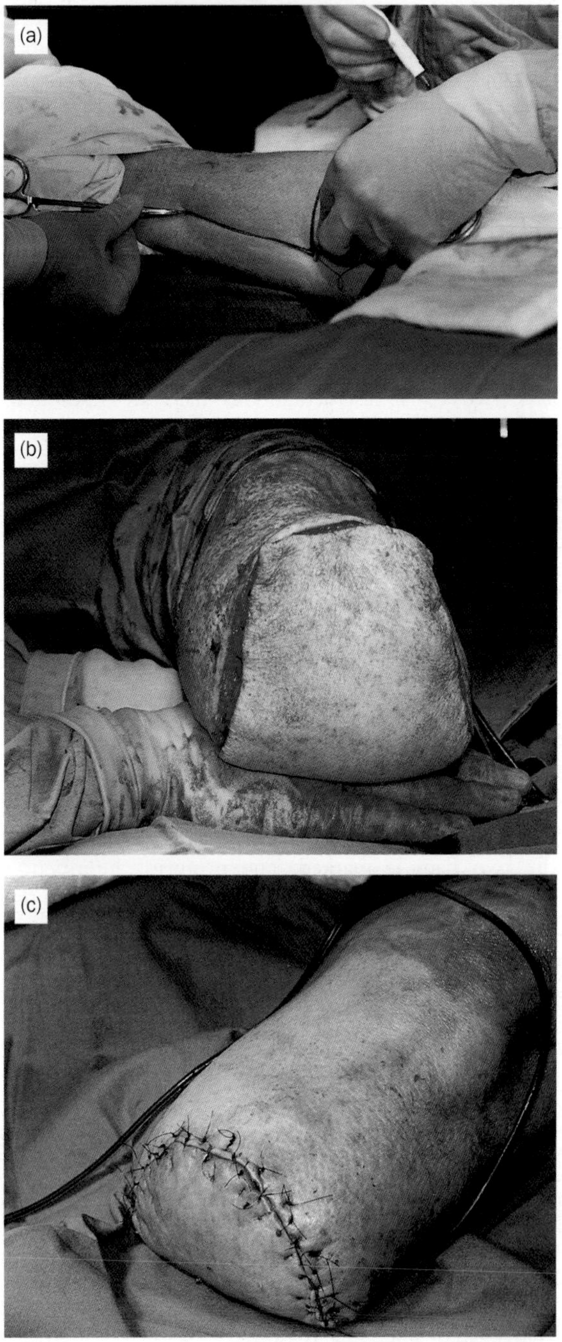

Figure 29.2 (a) Marking of skin flaps for a trans-tibial amputation. (b) The posterior and anterior flaps are brought together. (c) A completed trans-tibial amputation closed with interrupted vertical mattress monofilament sutures, over a suction drain.

this the deep fascia of the posterior flap is approximated over a suction drain to either the bone or the anterior deep fascia and periosteum. The skin edges are then approximated with simple interrupted sutures (Figure 29.2c). The stump is then ideally encased in a layered dressing and plaster of Paris cast incorporating the knee joint. This rigid dressing protects the stump, prevents flexion contracture and promotes healing and early mobilization. It may be split and temporarily removed for physiotherapy. Severe stump pain or evidence of infection should prompt the removal of the plaster cast to inspect the stump.

The trans-tibial amputation, when correctly performed, provides a pain free and infection free stump which maximizes the chances of patient mobility whilst preserving limb length and most importantly knee proprioception. In addition, trans-tibial amputees have considerably less energy expenditure than trans-femoral amputees. Oxygen consumption increases by about 9% in unilateral trans-tibial amputees compared to about 50% in trans-femoral amputees. These facts combine to mean that patients with a trans-tibial amputation are very much more likely to rehabilitate well compared with trans-femoral amputees. They also tend to live longer and have an improved quality of life, although some of these differences may well be due to natural case selection with trans-femoral amputees having more severe arterial disease. The trans-tibial to trans-femoral ratio attainable with appropriate patient selection should approach 3:1 and trans-tibial amputation failure rates should be less then 10%, although some patients may require local revision to obtain healing. Randomized controlled trials comparing the 'long posterior flap' and the 'skew flap' techniques have demonstrated small improvements in healing and rehabilitation rates with the latter technique.

Through knee amputations

Indications for through knee amputations include sufficient proximal progression of the disease process (e.g. gangrene) to preclude below knee amputation, or involvement of the knee joint in the disease process rendering it non-salvageable. A through knee amputation provides a durable stump capable of end weight bearing. Through knee amputations are associated with better rehabilitation rates than trans-femoral amputation, which reflects better stump stability and prosthetic suspension. In those patients unable to mobilize following amputation, a through knee amputation results in a long, powerful muscle stabilized lever and therefore a mechanical advantage compared to a trans-femoral amputation. Hence, through knee amputations should be performed, if possible, in preference to trans-femoral amputations in most circumstances.

Knee disarticulation

One of four commonly used skin incisions may be used for knee disarticulation, depending on the availability of suitable skin: the classical long anterior flap (Figure 29.3a); equal anterior and posterior flaps; equal sagittal flaps; or the 'no flap' technique utilizing a circumferential incision made 1 cm below the tibial tuberosity. These various skin flaps have been employed in an attempt to minimize delayed wound healing, the major complication encountered with knee disarticulation. The dissection commences anteriorly with the detachment of the patellar tendon from its insertion. The hamstrings medially and the biceps femoris and ileotibial band laterally are dissected, divided and allowed to retract. The knee joint is entered anteriorly and, with the knee in flexion, the tibial insertions of the cruciate ligaments are detached. The posterior capsule of the joint is then carefully opened from the front, and the popliteal artery and vein are individually dissected, clamped and suture ligated. The tibial and peroneal nerves are pulled down under tension, divided and allowed to retract into the proximal muscle mass. The patellar tendon, semitendinosus and biceps tendons are sutured to the cruciate ligaments improving muscle stability. The superficial fascia is approximated over a suction drain and the skin closed with monofilament vertical mattress sutures. Alternatively skin staples may be used.

Supracondylar amputation

This was introduced in vascular patients in 1969 by Weale. It is performed in a similar fashion to the above using the long anterior skin flap technique. The patella, however, is enucleated from its periosteum, and the residual defect in the patellar tendon sutured. The femoral condyles are then transected transversely 1.5 cm above the knee joint using a saw, and the sharp bony edges filed smooth. The myoplasty, fascia and skin closure are then performed as for a disarticulation.

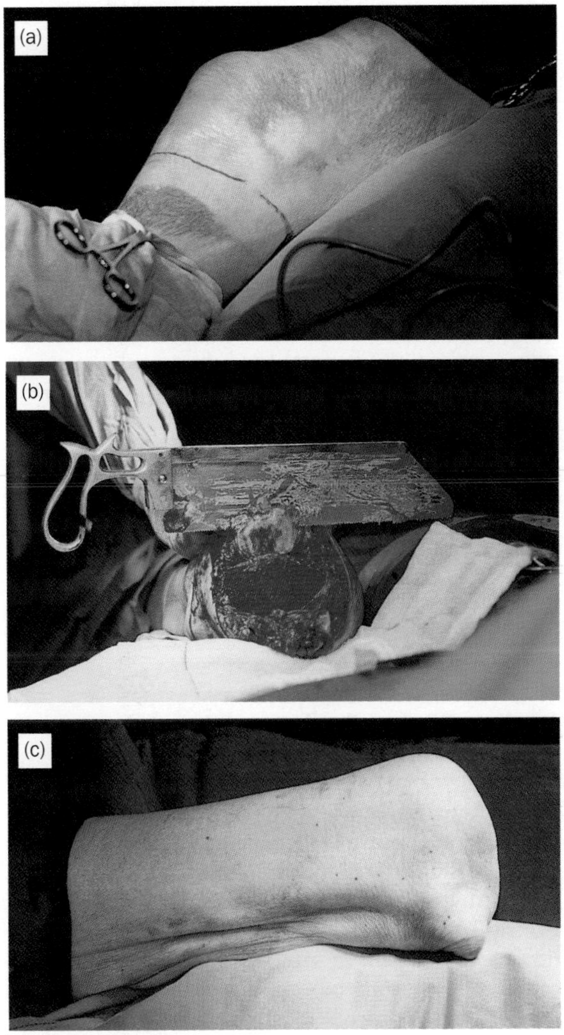

Figure 29.3 (a) Marked skin incision for a Gritti–Stokes amputation using the 'long anterior flap' technique. (b) A Gritti–Stokes amputation. The femoral condyles and articular surface of the patella are excised. (c) A completed Gritti–Stokes amputation.

Gritti–Stokes amputation

This amputation, described by Gritti in 1857 and subsequently modified by William Stokes, has become an increasingly popular amputation in the management of lower limb ischaemia. The femoral condyles are removed as for a supracondylar amputation but the patella is not excised. Its articular femoral surface is removed with a saw and the patella is fixed to the cut end of the femur (Figure 29.3b). Several methods of anchoring the patella to the femur have been described including periosteal sutures, sutures or wires passing through drill holes in the cortex of the distal femur and patella and transfixion screws. Whichever method is used it is essential that the patella is firmly fixed and does not become dislodged. The myoplasty, fascia and skin closure are then performed as for a disarticulation (Figure 29.3c).

Trans-femoral amputation

Historically, trans-femoral amputation was the most commonly performed major amputation for end-stage vascular disease because primary healing can be virtually assured regardless of the patient's general status. There is now clear evidence that most major amputations will heal at the trans-tibial level with all the associated advantages in mobility and rehabilitation. We would suggest that trans-femoral amputations should only be performed if disease extends above the knee joint precluding a more distal amputation, or when objective evaluation of perfusion supports clinical suspicion that a more distal amputation is unlikely to heal (i.e. thigh pressure less than 50 mmHg). In general, a trans-femoral amputation stump should be made as long as possible with the usual level of bony transection being the junction of the proximal two-thirds with the distal third of the femur. Occasionally, in patients with very severe ischaemia, a shorter stump is necessary. In such cases the level of bony transection is the junction of the proximal third with the distal two-thirds of the femur. Following skin marking, myocutaneous flaps are fashioned. Transverse flaps are commonly used with the anterior flap made a little shorter than posterior, but sagittal flaps or circular incisions may be used. In general, flaps should be 4–5 cm in length and based at the level of proposed bone transection. It is wise to leave flaps longer than appears necessary leaving final trimming until the end of the procedure. Skin incisions are carried through subcutaneous fat and fascia. The anterior, medial and lateral muscle groups are divided in the same line as the skin but the plane of incision is angled towards the level of bone section. This slanted cut facilitates adequate bony coverage and effective

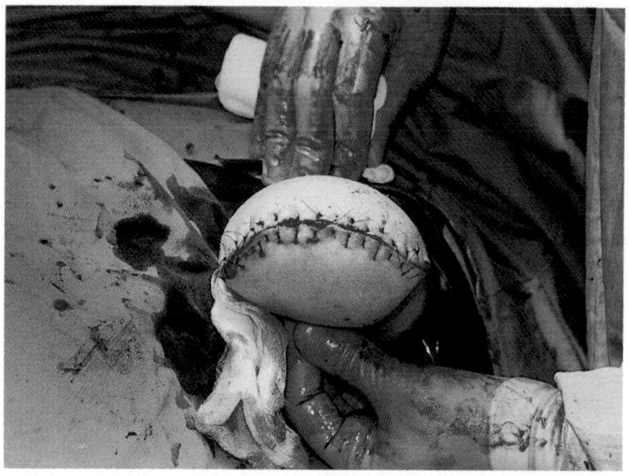

Figure 29.4 A completed trans-femoral amputation using transverse flaps.

myodesis. The femoral artery and vein are then dissected in the subsartorial canal and individually clamped, divided and suture ligated. The sciatic nerve is identified posteriorly, transected under tension and allowed to retract. The femur is exposed, the periosteum elevated and the bone transected. The bone edges are carefully smoothed with a rasp or file. Holes are then drilled through the anterior, lateral and posterior aspects of the distal femoral cortex for myodesis. The adductor magnus is then passed posteriorly around the femur and sutured to its lateral aspect to maintain adduction. Ensuring the hip is in extension, the quadriceps is then sutured to the posterior femoral cortex. The remaining posterior muscles are then sutured to the posterior aspect of the femur. Myodesis is preferable to myoplasty of opposing muscle groups, as the latter may dislocate leading to subcutaneous protrusion of the bone within the stump. The superficial fascia is approximated over a suction drain and the skin closed with monofilament vertical mattress sutures (Figure 29.4). The stump is then bandaged with a hip spica in extension. Some units will apply special customized elastic bandages called shrinkers to control the post-operative swelling though these are not strictly essential. Unfortunately, trans-femoral amputations are frequently poorly performed, leaving the patient with a substandard stump and thus the prosthetist with a difficult limb fitting. The required energy expenditure for mobilization, already far greater for trans-femoral than trans-tibial amputees, is made considerably worse by a technically inadequate operation. The most common mistake is inadequate myodesis, which results in a stump that lacks control and which lies with the hip flexed and abducted. Many patients undergoing trans-femoral amputation are, however, frequently afflicted with concomitant severe systemic disease, which limits function and quality of life. In many cases, therefore, the solitary goal of rehabilitation is adjustment to a wheelchair existence and no attempt at limb fitting is made. It is important that these aims and goals are assessed and recorded prior to amputation.

Hip disarticulation

Fortunately, amputation at this level is seldom required, as it generally reflects massive ischaemia associated with an aortic or iliac thrombosis, falling cardiac output and approaching demise. A hasty operation at this stage may simply accelerate this outcome and thus careful judgement is required. The indications for this procedure are therefore severe ischaemia extending above the level of an above knee amputation in a patient who is expected to survive surgery. With the patient supine on the operating table, a sandbag is placed under the ipsilateral sacroiliac joint, the hip is flexed and the skin incisions are marked. The wide posterior flap begins 3 cm below the pubic tubercle and passes around the buttock to the anterior superior iliac spine. The anterior incision is made 2 cm below and parallel to the inguinal ligament. Once the skin and fascia have been incised, the femoral vessels are dissected, clamped, divided and suture ligated. The femoral nerve is transected under tension and allowed to retract. Sartorius is detached from the anterior superior iliac spine and the anterior hip joint capsule exposed. With the hip in abduction, the adductors are divided, the obturator vessels are suture ligated and the obturator nerve is transected under tension. Hip flexion, adduction and internal rotation facilitate development of the posterior flap. The gluteus maximus is divided, the hamstrings are cut close to the ischial tuberosity, and the sciatic nerve is transected under tension and allowed to retract into the sciatic notch. The gluteus medius and minimus muscles are divided and the superior and inferior gluteal vessels transfixion ligated. With the limb laid flat the anterior hip joint capsule is incised, the femoral head dislocated, the round ligament divided and the posterior capsule incised. Division of the obturator tendons and piriformis allows removal of the limb. Following careful ligature haemostasis and with a suction drain in the acetabulum, the posterior flap is sutured to the inguinal ligament and anterior aspect of the pelvis. The skin is then opposed with interrupted non-absorbable monofilament sutures and a crepe bandage applied as a hip spica to eliminate potential dead space.

Section 29.4 • Post-operative management

Several key areas in the post-operative care of patients following major amputation demand attention (Table 29.2). These key areas represent a continuation of the care pathway initiated at the original consultation. Primary management goals following major amputation include patient survival, the avoidance of complications and the provision of a well-healed, pain free, useful stump in order to maximize subsequent function and mobility. Patients are ideally managed in a single rehabilitation unit with support staff on site. Systemic complications are common in the early post-operative period following major amputation, exemplified by an early mortality rate which approaches 10%. The majority of these early deaths are due to cardiovascular complications (e.g. myocardial infarction, congestive cardiac failure, stroke, mesenteric ischaemia). Centres with a special interest in amputation often report very low mortality rates which have been attributed to aggressive, multidisciplinary, high dependency peri-operative care. Concomitant medical conditions therefore demand vigilant attention in the early post-operative period. Diabetes necessitates close monitoring and may require insulin sliding scale regimens. Any reports of chest pain, palpitations or shortness of breath must be thoroughly investigated. Pneumonia and atelectasis frequently affect patients undergoing major amputation and are second only to ischaemic heart disease as a cause of morbidity and mortality. Adequate pain relief, frequent aggressive physiotherapy and appropriate targeted use of antibiotics are the mainstay of treatment. The factors that predispose to pulmonary sepsis (immobility and dehydration) also predispose to thromboembolic phenomena. Pulmonary embolus and deep venous thrombosis following major amputation are serious problems and thus early mobilization, active and passive physiotherapy, low molecular weight heparin and an anti-thromboembolic stocking for the non-amputated lower limb are recommended. Renal insufficiency is also a common complication following amputation, usually precipitated by dehydration and nephrotoxic medication (e.g. diuretics, non-steroidal anti-inflammatory agents, antibiotics), and is therefore generally preventable. Malnutrition is frequently encountered in patients with critical ischaemia. Dietary assessment and supplementation if necessary is essential and some cases may warrant naso-gastric feeding.

The psychological response of the patient to major amputation is variable but often follows the pattern of a normal grief reaction. There are three main stages to this reaction, which may overlap and last a variable length of time. The first stage is one of numbness and disbelief. This generally lasts 1–2 days. The second phase of despair is a very painful stage, involving peaks of distress, anguish and anxiety. Somatic symptoms such as constipation, chest tightness, throat dryness and insomnia are also common during this phase. The third and final stage is recovery where the patient begins to adapt and rebuild in order to accommodate the required changes associated with their loss. It is thus favourable to warn patients as early as possible when amputation is a probability, to allow the first two phases of the grief reaction to pass before surgery is performed. The positive aspects of the amputation should be stressed to the patient. The benefits of an amputation service skilled in the management of physical and psychological problems are inestimable. Psychologists, psychiatrists and amputation support groups may be of particular value in such circumstances.

There are also early complications specifically related to the amputation stump, the most important of which is the inevitable pain that accompanies major amputation. Patients frequently require opiate analgesics in the pre-operative and early post-operative periods. They can, however, be quickly reduced and stopped following this. Ideally, patients will have had a spinal or epidural anaesthetic, which provides excellent immediate post-operative pain relief. Some surgeons advocate the use of an epidural catheter placed alongside the sciatic nerve for post-operative rehabilitation and this does seem to work well in most cases. Patient controlled analgesia (PCA) is possible in many patients, especially after the first 24 hours, and allows better titration of analgesia according to needs. The concurrent administration of a non-steroidal anti-inflammatory drug (NSAID) often dramatically improves initial pain relief. Most patients will have some degree of 'phantom limb' which will vary from a feeling of the leg still being present to severe pain. Fortunately with aggressive post-operative analgesia, often supplemented with carbamazepine, these sensations usually gradually disappear. True chronic severe phantom limb pain is thankfully relatively uncommon, but when it does occur is often difficult to manage and frequently requires the input of a pain specialist.

Reported healing rates, as may be expected, vary widely. Common causes of delayed or non-healing include ischaemia, trauma, haematoma and infection. Non-healing secondary to ischaemia may be minimized by objective amputation level selection. Minimal tissue handling during surgery, the use of plaster of Paris dressings and controlled environmental treatment regimens reduce wound trauma. Skin sutures are generally left in for an extended period (about 3 weeks) in most patients, as wound healing is inevitably slow. Peri-operative prophylactic antibiotics are recommended, as is the use of micro-organism specific antibiotics for stump infections in the early post-operative period. The authors would also recommend, if possible, the removal of all prosthetic material in secondary amputations. It is also important to note that a wound which initially does not appear to be healing does not necessarily equate to amputation revision to a higher level. With appropriate support, sometimes necessitating re-casting or local resection, many of these wounds will undergo delayed healing by secondary intention. Healing rates of over 90% are attainable for trans-tibial amputations whilst still maintaining high trans-tibial to trans-femoral ratios. Hip or knee contractures occur quickly in the early post-operative period and can become irreversible, precluding successful rehabilitation and possibly necessitating amputation at a higher level. Rigid dressings, immediate use of mobility aids and both active and passive physiotherapy reduce the incidence of contractures.

Section 29.5 • Rehabilitation

Amputation rehabilitation may be defined as retraining in physical, functional and social activities and thus effective rehabilitation demands a team approach and includes many of the areas previously discussed (Figure

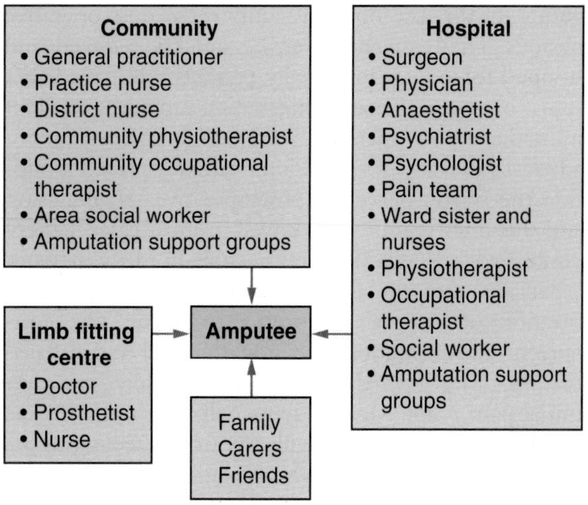

Figure 29.5 The multidisciplinary team involved in the management of the amputee.

29.5). Within this team the physiotherapist and occupational therapists play pivotal roles. The physiotherapist predominantly directs physical rehabilitation whilst the occupational therapist oversees functional and social training but inevitably overlap exists. The therapists' role in amputee rehabilitation may be viewed in three phases: the pre-operative phase; the post-operative phase, early and late; and the prosthetic phase.

The pre-operative phase

This should cover three areas including an introductory visit, assessment and operative preparation. The therapists' introductory visit to the patient and their carers should include a brief explanation of the roles of the members of the rehabilitation team and reassurance that amputation is a positive step towards discharge back into the community. Pre-operative assessments of physical, psychological and social status are essential in order to set realistic goals. The physical assessment should include all aspects of the patient's health and physical condition which may affect mobility, e.g. angina, chronic obstructive airways disease (COAD) or arthritis. Muscle strength and range of joint movement are assessed. The presence of contractures and the skin condition, especially pressure areas, are assessed and recorded. The patient's balance, co-ordination and mobility are also recorded. It is important to note maximum walking distances if the patient is mobile, or wheelchair abilities if not. Dressing, toileting and bathing abilities should also be noted. Social assessment includes recording accommodation type and access, stairs, toilet facilities and any help the patient requires with cooking, laundry or shopping. Psychological assessment includes analysis of the patient's moods, attitudes and hopes and fears. This may be more accurately performed with the help of patients' carers as frequently toxaemia, confusion and pain may colour this picture. Preparation for the operation involves, if time allows, visits to the environments in which the patient will spend much of their post-operative time, i.e. gymnasium and occupational therapy department. If the patient is to be fitted with a prosthesis post-operatively, it is useful to show the patient a prosthesis similar to the one they may receive. Patients and their families often find it helpful to speak to other amputees, especially if the amputee is of similar age and has the same level of amputation as projected for the patient. If this is not possible on the ward, amputation support groups are often invaluable in this regard. Minutes of physical therapy in this pre-operative period, to maintain both upper and lower limb strength and to reduce or prevent contractures, are worth hours of therapy after the operation.

The post-operative phase

In the early post-operative phase physiotherapy should be directed at reducing retention of chest secretions and preventing the development of pulmonary sepsis, the prevention of flexion contractures and maintenance of muscle strength. The important exercises are the movements opposite to those producing contractures; these are knee extension for trans-tibial and hip extension for the trans-femoral amputations. When the patient begins to sit out, stump boards are recommended for use with trans-tibial amputees in the absence of rigid dressings, to ensure the stump is kept horizontal, therefore avoiding flexion contractures and local oedema.

Once the patient's drips and drains have been removed and the patient is medically sufficiently fit and well, treatment may be continued in the gymnasium. These treatment sessions ideally should be performed twice per day, and their length gradually increased as the patient becomes fitter and stronger. The occupational therapist aims to improve upper and lower limb muscle strength, balance and co-ordination and thus maximize the level of daily living activities attainable. It is important in this early post-operative period to ensure bed equipment aids are available (e.g. monkey poles, rope ladders, cot sides). The therapist also works with the nursing staff to ensure the patient returns to self care of personal needs (e.g. washing, shaving and dressing) as soon as possible. This may require assistance, aids, advice and practice.

It is essential patients are taught essential wheelchair technique including brake application and release, foot rest rotation and release, arm rest removal, safe chair to bed/toilet transfer, chair propulsion and turning. Patients and carers must be taught how to fold and lift the chair for transportation and storage. Bilateral amputees have their centre of gravity shifted backwards and thus require a wheelchair with the rear wheels set further back to prevent them tipping backwards. Appropriate wheelchair cushions and wheelchair seat belts should be supplied if required.

Psychological support may be required in order to enable patients to overcome the bereavement process associated with amputation, which may otherwise impair progress. Therapeutic activities such as cooking, woodwork or even providing the patient with the opportunity to do their own washing may also be helpful.

An early home visit without the patient is arranged during the first post-operative week. With the patient's knowledge and consent, the physiotherapist, occupational therapist and social worker visit the patient's home to assess the accommodation, noting the equipment, aids and adaptations that will be required prior to discharge. It is often helpful if a member of the patient's family is also present. A report of this visit is then distributed to all members of the multidisciplinary team and a copy filed in the notes. Weekly team meetings are essential if the multidisciplinary approach is to be successful. At such meetings, each patient is appraised and individual long- and short-term goals are identified and reviewed.

Aggressive early mobilization on two limbs using a bipedal gait is essential for successful maximal rehabilitation. Early walking aids are therefore vital in the rehabilitation of patients deemed suitable for prosthetic fitting by enabling this early mobilization, while allowing assessment of the ability, physical capability and motivation for prosthesis use. They also reduce stump oedema and pain. Once the stump is healing and without complications, generally 5–10 days post-operation, early walking aid use can begin. Daily inspection of the wound following this is essential to ensure healing continues.

Various early walking aids exist including pneumatic devices, vacuum devices and pre-formed sockets. Pneumatic aids are commonly used, with the Vessa pneumatic post-amputation (Ppam) mobility aid being one of the most popular (Vessa Ltd, Alton, Hampshire, UK). It consists of a small inner air-filled cushion and larger above and below knee bags. An outer metal frame encases the bags. These frames have a crucible sling support and a shoulder support strap. At the first sitting, the appropriate length bag with the small cushion is applied. The pressure is slowly increased to the maximum the patient can tolerate, which at this initial sitting is generally 15–25 mmHg, for 5–10 min. When the patient can tolerate 40 mmHg, standing balance exercise and walking between parallel bars can begin (Figure 29.6). The amount of time the patient uses the device thereafter is increased in conjunction with, and not instead of, routine mobilizing and strengthening exercises. During gait training it is important to lead with the unaffected leg, to maintain an even step length and to maintain an upright posture.

Vacuum devices are also used as early mobilization aids. The LIC Tulip limb (LIC Orthopaedic, Solna, Sweden) is one such vacuum device. It consists of an inner cushion containing small plastic pellets and an outer, adjustable, rigid, polypropylene frame. Attached to the polypropylene frame is an adjustable tube with a single axis foot. The inner cushion is wrapped around the dressed stump, evacuated of air, and then wrapped with a bandage. The polypropylene frame is then applied using Velcro bands and the tube adjusted to the correct length. This vacuum device serves as a semi-rigid support, used for 30–60 min at a time, until the patient takes possession of a definitive prosthesis.

Pre-formed socket prostheses are generally used with trans-femoral amputees. The LIC femorett (LIC Orthopaedic) has three different sizes of adjustable sockets for left and right fittings with a shoulder strap. This is fitted within an adjustable thigh section, above a single axis knee joint and a tubular lower leg section with a neutral uniaxial ankle and foot. It is light and easy to fit, and provides rigidity during mobilization.

At this stage, the social worker should aim to relieve and prevent social distress, by helping with social and personal problems linked with the amputation. They can counsel on residential and nursing homes if required, and advise on welfare and benefit entitlement. The social worker is also generally heavily involved in the patient's discharge planning. The aims include physical and psychological preparation of patient and family for discharge; promotion of the highest level of independence attainable; and provision of continuity of care to make the transfer from hospital to community as smooth as possible.

During the late post-operative period, once the stump has healed and the sutures have been removed, full weight bearing can commence. It is important to continue specific hip and knee exercises. Exercise diaries, group therapy, sport and recreational activities (e.g. swimming), and periods of home leave help

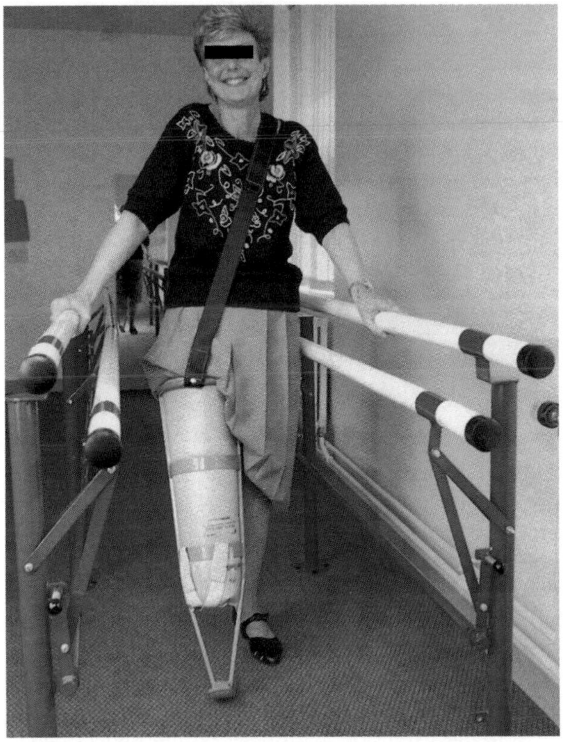

Figure 29.6 The Vessa pneumatic post-amputation mobility aid.

motivation and relieve monotony. A prosthetic referral is performed only when the multidisciplinary team agree that this is appropriate for a specific patient. It is essential that only patients who are able to use a prosthesis are prescribed one. These patients are ready for their first prosthetic measurement only when the wound is satisfactory and the stump volume is stable.

The occupational therapist at this stage should reassess the patient's activities of daily living (washing, dressing, etc.), perform a kitchen appraisal and arrange a final home visit. The purpose of this visit, when the patient is almost fully independent is to ensure the patient is safe, independent and fully supported in their home environment. It is essential to assess and request necessary aids and accommodation adaptations. A home visit report is compiled and circulated to the multidisciplinary team members. Once the patient is fully independent and all requests have been delivered, a discharge date is planned and the patient's general practitioner informed. One week's notice of discharge date is recommended and discharge on Fridays is best avoided in patients requiring high levels of social service support.

The prosthetic training phase

Over 50% of amputees are referred to a prosthetic centre, and over 90% of those referred are fitted with a prosthesis. Daily gait training begins once the patient receives his prosthesis and includes periods of rest and walking. Gait training should begin between parallel bars and then progress to one bar and a stick or two sticks. Training should include sitting to standing, balancing, weight transference, hip hitching, stance and swing phase control, stepping forward with the good leg, ensuring upright posture, and even stride length and timing. Once good balance and gait are achieved, the programme continues with functional exercises and practice, e.g. stairs, inclines, getting up from the floor and picking up objects. Regular stump inspection for signs of irritation is essential. The various types and uses of different stump socks should also be explained. The majority of prostheses are constructed for trans-femoral (49%) or for trans-tibial (42%) amputees and thus we will concentrate on the prosthetics associated with these two groups of patients.

Trans-femoral prosthesis

The trans-femoral prosthesis has six main components: suspension, socket, knee joint and knee control mechanism, shank and the ankle and foot device.

Six methods of suspension are commonly used. The pelvic band is a metal (generally aluminium) belt usually covered with leather, which has a lateral extension that attaches to the inferolateral aspect of the socket. The rigid pelvic band (RPB) incorporates a uniaxial hip joint within the extension, which permits only flexion and extension, whilst the double swivel pelvic band (DSPB) allows multiaxial movement. The pelvic band provides prosthetic support, controls rotation and thus gives a more rigid gait but is heavy weighing up to 1.5 kg, and can be uncomfortable when sitting. It is useful when suction is difficult, i.e. with a short stump. The Silesian belt is a non-elasticated belt worn around the hips between the iliac crest and the greater trochanter. It is attached to the prosthesis posteriorly with a strap passing from the middle of the belt to the lateral aspect of the socket, and anteriorly with a strap passing from the belt at the level of the contralateral iliac crest to the socket anteriorly at the height of the ischial tuberosity. The Silesian belt is lighter and more comfortable than the pelvic band and does not resist hip mobility. It is often used in conjunction with a suction socket, especially in the early stages of suction use. The total elastic suspension (TES) belt, made of neoprene, is pulled over the socket; then pulled up onto the pelvis when donning is complete. It closes anteriorly with Velcro, comes in various sizes and is washable. Suction (or self suspension) sockets have one way valves incorporated into the socket, through which the patient passes the stump sock and pushes the stump into the socket; on weight bearing the remaining air within the socket is expelled through the one way valve creating a negative pressure or suction effect. Suction sockets are relatively contraindicated in patients with peripheral vascular disease, or a stump that fluctuates in size. They cause stump oedema and increase sweating, thus they can precipitate skin problems. They require an intimate fit and thus it may not be possible with a short stump to achieve sufficient suction. In the right patient, however, they are very comfortable and cosmetically excellent. Shoulder harnesses and straps are almost obsolete in modern prosthetics and only used as a last resort.

Sockets commonly used with trans-femoral prostheses include quadrilateral, conventional, 'H', flexible and ischial containment sockets. The socket must supply comfortable, stable support for the weight-bearing area, which in trans-femoral amputees is mostly supplied by the pelvis. Quadrilateral and ischial containment sockets are the most commonly encountered trans-femoral prostheses sockets. Controversy exists over the advisability of flexible versus rigid socket walls. The flexible sockets provide greater comfort and proprioception, are more pliable when sitting and dissipate heat faster than traditional sockets. They are, however, less durable.

Knee joints and their control mechanisms can be complex as the requirements of the prosthetic knee joint vary according to phase of gait. During the stance phase stability is important, whilst during the swing phase flexibility is the key. In single or uniaxial knees, the joint rotation centre is fixed in all knee positions. In polycentric knees, however, the joint rotation centre varies with different knee positions. Different systems use different designs. For example, the four-bar linkage knee joint has a centre of rotation which projects proximally and posteriorly in the stance phase for stability, but moves anteriorly or distally in the swing phase to provide shank shortening.

Knee joint controls may be divided into stance and swing phase mechanisms. There is a vast array of stance phase stability controls including a variety of locking mechanisms. Swing phase control mechanisms aim to control the forward motion of the shank during this phase of gait. They function, therefore, as shock absorbers or damping units, and various designs are available including pneumatic and hydraulic dampers, and internal and external extension bias systems.

Modern shanks tend to be endoskeletal, modular shanks as they reduce costs, are more cosmetic and are easily exchanged or adjusted.

Several ankle and foot devices are commonly used today including the solid ankle cushion heel (SACH) foot, articulated ankle and foot devices (uniaxial or multi axial) and energy storing ankle/foot devices. The SACH device combines the ankle and foot into one unit, thus no ankle articulation is required. The soft rubber heel compresses under loading and provides the required movement. It is light, robust and low maintenance, whilst providing a smooth heel strike and toe off. The uniaxial foot is a hinge joint whose movements are restricted to 15° of plantar flexion and 5–7° of dorsal flexion by rubber bumpers. This device thus permits a large range of adjustable movement, is easy to maintain and improves stability. It is, however, heavy, cosmetically poor and the rubber bumpers quickly wear and become noisy. The multiaxial device allows some movement in all three planes of ankle movement. Energy storing ankle/foot devices incorporate mechanisms providing a natural lift and thrust to the foot during the 'toe off' phase, e.g. the Delrin heel in the Seattle foot. These mechanisms facilitate more effective and less tiring walking and running.

Trans-tibial prosthesis

The trans-tibial prosthesis has four main parts: the suspension, socket, shank, and ankle and foot mechanism. The shank and the ankle and foot mechanisms have been described with the trans-femoral prostheses, thus only suspension mechanisms and sockets will be described here.

Two suspension mechanisms are commonly used with trans-tibial prostheses: thigh corsets used with older plug fit sockets and the supracondylar cuffs or straps used with patella tendon bearing sockets. The leather thigh corset has metal sidebars with knee joints, which attach to the prosthesis socket and shank. This partially weight-bearing corset adds stability and therefore is useful when there is muscle weakness. The thigh corset can be uncomfortable, bulky and cosmetically poor, and may cause atrophy.

Supracondylar or suprapatella cuffs pass around the thigh above the femoral condyles and patella, and are closed with a buckle or Velcro laterally. The cuff is attached to the socket medially and laterally with studs. The cuff supports the prosthesis in the swing phase and stops hyperextension in the stance phase.

Trans-tibial prostheses have inner and outer sockets, commonly referred to as the liner and shell respectively. Traditional below knee plug shaped sockets were often used with a thigh corset. More modern patella tendon bearing sockets are total contact sockets which fit intimately. This increases weight-bearing capacity, controls oedema and improves proprioception. The socket is triangular, has high medial and lateral walls, and has a posterior flare to accommodate knee flexion. The socket ensures weight bearing takes place on the pressure tolerant areas (the patella tendon, the medial tibia, the pretibial muscles and the posterior aspect of the stump) and relieves the pressure intolerant areas. Suction sockets are available.

During the prosthetic phase of rehabilitation it is essential to ensure that patients understand their prostheses. It is critical to make certain that the socket is smooth, and that shoes are appropriate and not worn out. It is important to check application or donning and to perform a static and dynamic check out. The static check out ensures that weight is taken only on the weight tolerant areas, the prosthesis is the correct length and the suspension is adequate. The dynamic check out involves observation of the patient during mobilization from the front, back and side to assess any gait deviations.

A follow-up visit by the occupational therapist, 1 or 2 weeks following discharge, may be necessary to assess new practical problems or anxieties. Outpatient physiotherapy should only be necessary if patients are discharged from hospital before becoming fully independent, or in other specific circumstances, e.g. the fitting of a new prosthesis. Surgical outpatient follow-up is essential.

Section 29.6 • Prognosis

The long-term prospects of the amputee are poor, reflecting the systemic nature of the underlying atheromatous disease, which remains a constant threat, not only to life but also to contralateral and ipsilateral limbs. In hospital, mortality following trans-tibial amputation is 5–10%, while that following trans-femoral amputation is closer to 20%. This higher mortality rate probably relates to the selection of older, 'higher risk' patients in to the latter group, rather than the higher amputation level. Myocardial infarction is the commonest cause of death in the early post-operative period. The difference in mortality rates between trans-tibial and trans-femoral amputees does, however, appear to be maintained, as 2 year motality rates are reported at 30% and 45% for the two groups, respectively. Post-amputation mortality is higher in diabetics than in non-diabetics. Myocardial infarction, stroke and other cardiovascular events are common causes of significant morbidity, in addition to mortality, following major amputation. Progression of peripheral vascular disease in unilateral amputees results in an annual risk of contralateral limb loss of approximately 10%. The risk of patients requiring a higher ipsilateral amputation in a limb following stump healing is much lower, in the order of 1–2% per year. Following digital amputation, revisions or further digital amputations are common, especially in diabetics, and up to 40% of patients will require a more proximal amputation.

The ultimate aim for the majority of patients undergoing a major lower extremity amputation is to achieve independent mobility. Rates of independent ambulation with a prosthesis fall with increasing proximity of amputation level. Independent ambulation rates with a prosthesis of up to 80% are reported for trans-tibial amputees, which is two to three times better than the rates achieved with trans-femoral amputees. Better rehabilitation results are obtained following knee disarticulation procedures than following trans-femoral amputations. Poorer rehabilitation results are also observed with increasing age and in bilateral amputees. Amputation for critical ischaemia results in an improvement in overall quality of life, but in order to obtain independent existence over 30% require alterations to their homes, whilst over 10% require re-housing.

Section 29.7 • Conclusions

It is essential to realize that patients with end-stage peripheral vascular disease necessitating amputation have a very limited life expectancy. The primary aims of management, therefore, are to rehabilitate as quickly as possible thus minimizing hospital stay whilst maintaining maximal independence and a reasonable quality of life. Systemic arteriosclerosis is the major threat to life and remaining limb in both the early and late post-operative periods. There is some evidence that aggressive management of risk factors such as hypertension and cholesterol with cessation of smoking and treatment with low-dose aspirin will improve prognosis, but many of these patients are unwilling to comply with such management even if recommended and equally unwilling to give up smoking which is often their one significant remaining pleasure! Aggressive pre-operative management of comorbid conditions, careful and attentive surgery by an interested surgeon, aggressive management of post-operative complications and early diligent rehabilitation are all essential to achieving the best possible results. These patients are best managed if possible in a single surgical/rehabilitation unit by an enthusiastic committed multidisciplinary team. The reality of life, however, dictates that the standards of care provided to the vascular patient with end-stage disease vary considerably. Different surgeons and different units have varying rates of revascularization, primary amputation and trans-tibial amputation to trans-femoral amputation ratios. Furthermore, regions vary enormously in the final fitting and utilization rates for prosthetic devices. Some of these differences will reflect local variations in disease patterns but they are so great that sadly it appears that the main elements in the variation are a lack of adequate resources and expertise. In the future, it is essential to develop the expertise in order to ensure appropriate resources are requested and utilized.

Further reading

Bloom, R. J., Stevick, C. A. (1988). Amputation level and distal bypass salvage of the limb. *Surg Gynecol Obstet* **166**: 1–5.

Burgess, E. M. (1977). Disarticulation of the knee. A modified technique. *Arch Surg* **117**: 1250–5.

Burgess, E. M., Romano, R. L., Zettl, J. H. and Schrock, R. D. Jr (1971). Amputations of the leg for peripheral vascular insufficiency. *J Bone Joint Surg* **53A**: 874–89.

Chetter, I. C., Spark, J. I., Scott, D. J. A. *et al.* (1998). Prospective analysis of quality of life following infrainguinal reconstruction for chronic critical ischaemia. *Br J Surg* **85**: 951–5.

Cumming, J. G. R., Spence, V. A., Jain, A. S. *et al.* (1988). Further experience in the healing rate of lower limb amputations. *Eur J Vasc Surg* **2**: 383–5.

de Cossart, L., Randall, P., Turner, P. and Marcuson, R. W. (1983). The fate of the below knee amputee. *Ann R Coll Surg Engl* **65**: 230–2.

Dormandy, J. A. and Thomas, P. R. S. (1988). What is the natural history of a critically ischaemic patient with and without his leg. In: Greenhalgh, R. M., Jamieson, C. W. and Nicolaides, A. N. eds., *Limb Salvage and Amputation for Vascular Disease*. Philadelphia, PA: W. B. Saunders, Chapter 2: 11–26.

Dwars, B. J., van den Broek, T. A., Rauwerda, J. A., Bakker, F. C. (1992). Criteria for reliable selection of the lowest level of amputation in peripheral vascular disease. *J Vasc Surg* **15**: 536–42.

Ebskov, L. B., Hindso, K. and Holstein, P. (1999). Level of amputation following a failed arterial reconstruction compared to primary amputation – a meta-analysis. *Eur J Vasc Endovasc Surg* **17**: 35–40.

Ebskov, L. B., Schroeder, T. V. and Holstein, P. E. (1994). Epidemiology of leg amputation: the influence of vascular surgery. *Br J Surg* **81**: 1600–3.

Edmonds, M. E., Blundell, M. P., Morris, H. E. *et al.* (1986). Improved survival of the diabetic foot: the role of a specialised foot clinic. *Q J Med* **232**: 736.

Evans, W. E., Hayes, J. P. and Vermilion, B. D. (1990). Effect of failed distal reconstruction on the level of amputation. *Am J Surg* **160**: 217–220.

Fagrell, B. and Lundberg, G. (1984). A simplified evaluation of vital capillary microscopy for predicting skin viability in patients with severe arterial insufficiency. *Clin Physiol* **4**: 403–11.

Feinglass, J., Brown, J. L., LoSasso, A. *et al.* (1999). Rates of lower extremity amputation and arterial reconstruction in the United States, 1979 to 1996. *Am J Public Health* **89**: 1222–7.

Global Lower Extremity Amputation Study Group (2000). Epidemiology of lower extremity amputation in centres in Europe, North America and East Asia. *Br J Surg* **87**: 328–37.

Gottschalk, F. (1992). Transfemoral amputation – surgical procedures. In: Bowker, J. H., Michael, J. W., eds. *Atlas of Limb Prosthetics. Surgical, Prosthetic and Rehabilitation Principles.* St Louis: Mosby Year Book, 501–8.

Gregory-Dean, A. (1991). Amputations: statistics and trends. *Ann R Coll Surg Engl* **73**: 137–42.

Gutteridge, B., Torrie, P. and Galland, B. (1994). Trends in arterial reconstruction, angioplasty and amputation. *Health Trends* **26**: 88–91.

Ham, R. and Cotton, L. (1991). *Limb Amputation. From Aetiology to Rehabilitation*. London: Chapman and Hall.

Harris, R. I. (1956). Syme's amputation: technical details essential for success. *J Bone Joint Surg* **31A**: 639–49.

Heister, L. (1778). *General System of Surgery*. London: W Innes.

Holstein, P. (1984). The distal blood pressure predicts healing of amputations on the feet. *Acta Orthop Scand* **55**: 227–33.

Holstein, P., Sager, P. and Lassen, N. A. (1979). Wound healing in below knee amputations in relation to skin perfusion pressure. *Actra Orthop Scand* **50**: 49–58.

Houghton, A., Allen, A., Luff, R. and McColl, I. (1989). Rehabilitation after lower extremity amputation: a comparative study of above knee, through knee and Gritti–Stokes amputations. *Br J Surg* **76**: 622–4.

Huber, T. S., Wang, J. G., Wheeler, K. G. *et al.* (1999). Impact of race on the treatment for peripheral arterial occlusive disease. *J Vasc Surg* **30**: 417–25.

Humphrey, L. L., Palumbo, P. J., Butters, M. A. *et al.* (1994). The contribution of non-insulin dependant diabetes to lower extremity amputation in the community. *Arch Intern Med* **154**: 885–92.

Kram, H. B., Appel, P. L. and Shoemaker, W. C. (1989). Prediction of below knee amputation wound healing using non invasive laser Doppler velocimetry. *Am J Surg* **158**: 29–32.

Larsson, J., Apelqvist, J., Castenfors, J. *et al.* (1993). Distal blood pressure as a predictor for the level of amputation in diabetic patients with foot ulcers. *Foot Ankle* **14**: 247–53.

Lindholt, J. S., Bovling, S., Fasting, H. and Henneberg, E.W. (1994). Vascular surgery reduces the frequency of lower limb amputations. *Eur J Vasc Surg* **8**: 31-5.

McCollum, P. T., Spence, V. A., Swanson, W.F. *et al.* (1984). Experience in the healing rate of lower limb amputations. *J R Coll Surg Edinb* **29**: 358–62.

McCollum, P. T., Spence, V. A. and Walker, W. F. (1985). Circumferential skin blood flow measurements in the ischaemic limb. *Br J Surg* **72**: 310–12.

McCollum, P. T., Spence, V. A. and Walker, W. F. (1986). Oxygen inhalation induced changes in the skin as measured by transcutaneous oxymetry. *Br J Surg* **73**: 882–5.

McCollum, P. T., Spence, V. A. and Walker, W. F. (1988). Amputation for peripheral vascular disease: the case for level selection. *Br J Surg* **75**: 1193–5.

Miller, N., Dardik, H., Wolodiger, F. *et al.* (1991). Transmetatarsal amputation: the role of adjunctive revascularization. *J Vasc Surg* **13**: 705–11.

Moore, W. S., Hall, A. D. and Lim, R. C. (1972). Comparative results of conventional operation and immediate operative fitting technique. *Am J Surg* **124**: 127–134.

Moore, W. S., Henry, R. E., Malone, J. M. *et al.* (1981). Prospective use of xenon clearance for amputation level selection. *Arch Surg* **116**: 86–8.

Pedersen, A.E., Bornefeldt, Olsen, B. *et al.* (1994). Halving the number of leg amputations: the influence of infrapopliteal bypass. *Eur J Vasc Surg* **8**: 26–30.

Pohjolainen, T. and Alaranta, H. (1999). Epidemiology of lower limb amputees in Southern Finland in 1995 and trends since 1984. *Prosthet Orthot Int* **23**: 88–92.

Robinson, K. P. (1988). Skew-flap below knee amputation. In: Greenhalgh, R. M., Jameison, C. W. and Nicolaides, A. N., eds., *Limb Salvage and Amputation for Vascular Disease.* Philadelphia, PA: W. B. Saunders, 373–82.

Robinson, K. P. (1991). Historical aspects of amputation. *Ann R Coll Surg Engl* **73**: 134–6.

Robinson, K. P. (1992). Amputations in vascular patients. In: Bell, P. R. F., Jameison, C.W. and Ruckley, C.V. eds., *Surgical Management of Vascular Disease.* London: W. B. Saunders, 609–35.

Sarin, S., Shami, S., Shields, D. A. *et al.* (1991). Selection of amputation level: a review. *Eur J Vasc Surg* **5**: 611–20.

Silverman, D. and Wagner, F. W. (1983). Prediction of leg viability and amputation level by fluorescein uptake. *Prosthet Orthot Int* **7**: 69–71.

Syme, J. (1843). Amputation at the ankle joint. *London and Edinburgh Monthly Journal of Medical Science* **2**: 93.

TASC Working Group (2000). Management of peripheral arterial disease (PAD). TransAtlantic Inter-Society Consensus (TASC). *Eur J Vasc Endovasc Surg* **19** (Suppl. A): S24.

Tunis, S. R., Bass, E. B. and Steinberg, E. P. (1991). The use of angioplasty, bypass surgery and amputation in the management of peripheral vascular disease. *N Engl J Med* **325**: 556–62.

Van den Broek, T. A. A., Dwars, B. J., Rauwerda, J. A. and Bakker, F.C. (1988). Photoplethysmographic selection of amputation level in peripheral vascular disease. *J Vasc Surg* **8**: 10–13.

Vascular Surgical Society of Great Britain and Ireland (1995). Critical limb ischaemia: management and outcome. report of a national survey. *Eur J Vasc Endovasc Surg* **10**: 108–13.

Wagner, W. H., Keagy, B. A., Kotb, M. M. *et al.* ((1988). Noninvasive determination of healing of major lower extremity amputation: the continued role of clinical judgement. *J Vasc Surg* **8**: 703–10.

Weale, F. E. (1969). The supra-condylar amputation and patellectomy. *Br J Surg* **56**: 589.

White, S. A., Thompson, M. M., Zickerman, A. M. *et al.* (1997). Lower limb amputation and grade of surgeon. *Br J Surg* **84**: 509–11.

MODULE 30

Upper limb ischaemia

1 • Relevant anatomy
2 • Pathophysiology of upper limb vascular insufficiency
3 • Assessment
4 • Investigations
5 • Clinical presentations and management

Ischaemia of the upper limb occurs considerably less frequently than in the lower extremity, accounting for less than 5% of all peripheral ischaemic episodes. Furthermore, acute arm ischaemia accounts for approximately 15% of all acute peripheral ischaemic events. However, labelling ischaemic episodes of the upper limb as acute or chronic is of academic interest only as it is often difficult to differentiate between the two as the extensive nature of collateral vessels can leave an arm asymptomatic despite quite severe disease. Moreover, the effect of normal or abnormal vasospasm exacerbating any existing arterial insufficiency deepens this diagnostic dilemma. Patterns typical of lower limb ischaemia are rarely seen in the upper limbs where coldness and discoloration of the digits are the most common presenting symptoms and ulceration and gangrene less frequent. If left untreated, ischaemia of the upper limb often results in severe functional impairment even in the absence of overt tissue loss, threatening both the livelihood and independence of the person. While identifying the level of the arterial disease is usually straightforward, establishing the underlying aetiology is often more complex, particularly in chronic disease when it may be a manifestation of a systemic disorder. In contrast, acute ischaemia is generally a result of trauma or embolic disease. In the case of the latter, emboli commonly originate from the heart or large proximal vessels and are associated with atrial fibrillation, mural thrombus and myocardial infarction. Acute thrombosis is less common in the upper limb occurring in proximal vessels and usually secondary to an atherosclerotic stenosis, subclavian aneurysm or extrinsic compression within the thoracic outlet. Furthermore, while digital vessel occlusion may be a result of micro-emboli from diseased valves or atherosclerotic plaques, collagen vascular disorders present in a similar fashion.

Section 30.1 • Relevant anatomy

The upper limb is supplied by a single subclavian artery arising from the aortic arch on the left immediately behind the left common carotid artery and from the innominate on the right at the level of the sterno-clavicular joint (Figure 30.1). Both subclavian arteries leave the chest via the thoracic outlet, where they lie on the first rib behind the clavicle and in between scalenous anterior and medius. Scalenus anterior divides this vessel into three parts. Three branches arise from the first part. The second part gives two branches and lies close to the trunks of the brachial plexus behind the subclavian vein. The third part of the artery extends to the lateral border of the first rib, where it may be palpated and continues as the axillary artery and usually has no branches. The axillary artery lies mainly under

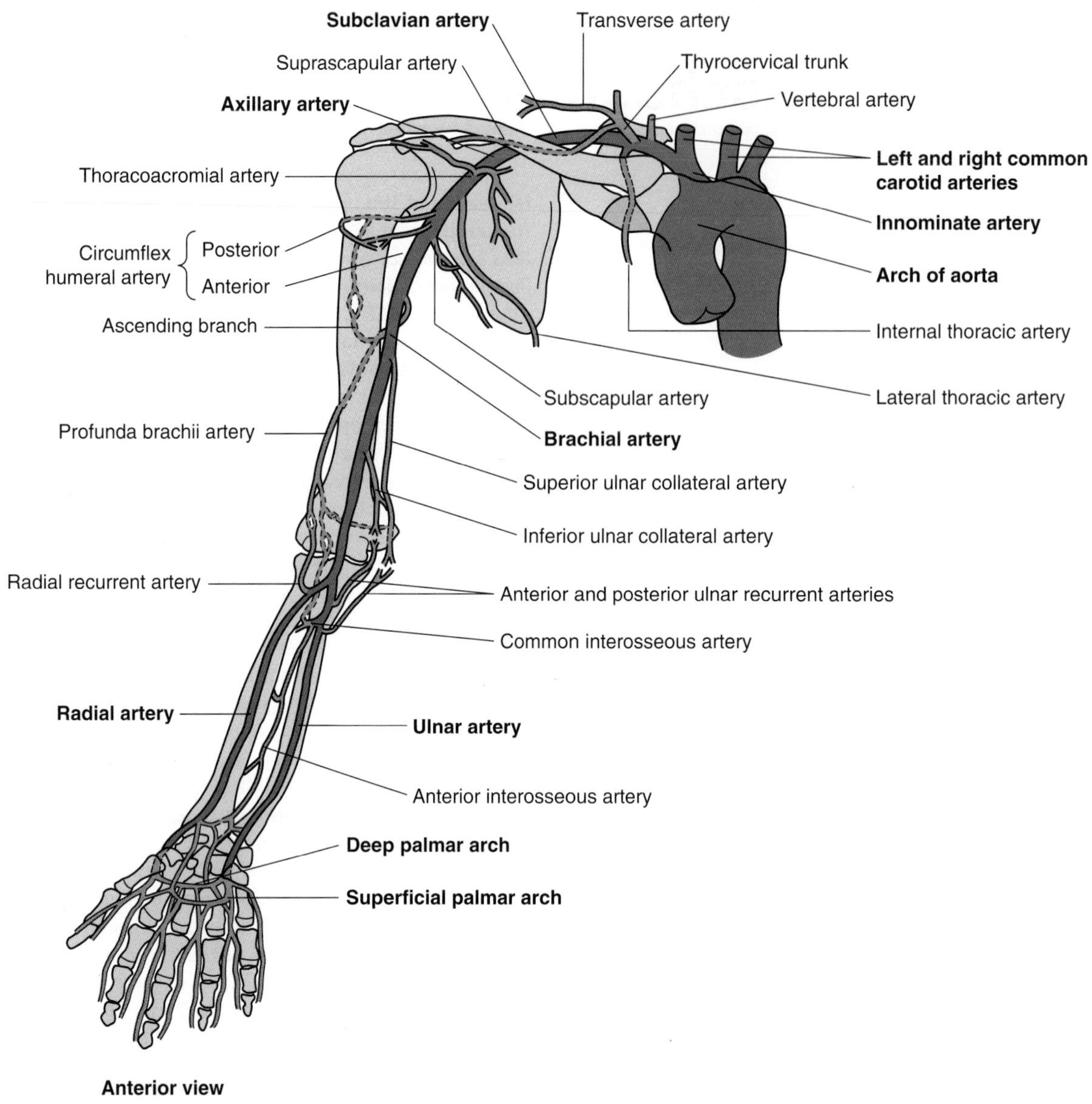

Figure 30.1 Right upper limb arterial tree. (From Moore, K., ed. *Clinically Orientated Anatomy,* 3rd edn. Lippincott Williams & Williams, Baltimore, 1992, p. 526.)

the cover of pectoralis major and ends at the lower border of teres major. It is divided into three parts by pectoralis minor giving rise to one artery from the first, two from the second and three from the third. Throughout its course the artery is closely associated with the cords of the brachial plexus. It continues as the brachial artery at the lateral border of teres major muscle. It then runs superficially throughout its course and is crossed by the median nerve at the mid-arm level. It finally splits into its two terminal branches at the neck of the radius. The radial artery is the smaller of two and is covered by brachioradialis in its proximal part. It lies on muscle throughout its length except at the wrist where it is in contact with the radius and easily palpated. Having given off the superficial palmar branch which joins the superficial palmar arch, it then winds around the radius laterally, crosses the floor of the anatomical snuff box and ends by forming the deep palmar arch. The ulnar artery gives off the common interosseous artery in the cubital fossa and then passes deep to the muscles emanating from the common flexor origin and is crossed by the median nerve. It becomes superficial in the distal half of the forearm and crosses the flexor retinaculum to form the superficial palmar arch which gives rise to three common palmar digital arteries which anastomose with three palmar metacarpal arteries arising from the deep palmar arch. Each common palmar digital artery finally divides into a pair of proper palmar digital arteries.

It is important to note that major collateral arteries exist around all major joints in the upper limb and vessels are paired below the elbow. This accounts for the low incidence of symptomatic upper limb arterial insufficiency despite the presence of occlusive lesions.

Section 30.2 • Pathophysiology of upper limb vascular insufficiency

To understand why the terms acute and chronic ischaemia are of academic interest in upper limb vascular insufficiency, it is important to recognize the compensatory mechanisms that come into play. Firstly, numerous collateral channels exist around the shoulder, elbow and wrists avoiding the situation of single vessel dependence. Furthermore, paired forearm vessels, palmar arches and digital arteries provide parallel circuits that are able to compensate in the event of an occlusion of one or other channel.

Fixed arterial obstructions such as atherosclerosis, emboli and those associated with connective tissue disorders create a drop in flow and pressure across a lesion. However, while isolated lesions in the lower limbs are unlikely to result in significant haemodynamic consequences unless there is a diameter compromise of greater than 50%, a similar stenosis in the upper limb is unlikely to result in symptoms. However, the consequence of sequential stenoses in the upper limb and particularly those at a more distal level results in a greater degree of flow limitation often producing symptoms on minimal exertion or possibly at rest as is the case in lower limb peripheral vascular disease.

Finally, to appreciate vasospastic disorders it is crucial to understand what is normal or abnormal vasospasm. Hands, like the head and face, have an important thermoregulatory role and as such have several arteriovenous shunts. These shunts regulate blood flow to the digits and are exquisitely sensitive to sympathetic control. Cold conditions and strong emotional stimuli affect these shunts resulting in a decrease in digital blood flow. The degree of flow resistance varies between individuals; however, complete cessation of blood flow is abnormal vasospasm.

Therefore, the clinical manifestation of upper limb vascular insufficiency results from a combination of all the above mechanisms and this must be born in mind when considering its underlying aetiology.

Section 30.3 • Assessment

Clinical assessment

History

Assessing the level of arterial occlusion, limb viability and underlying aetiology demands careful history taking and thorough physical examination. The presence of swelling, wrist pulses and a generalized blue discoloration aids in the differentiation between arterial and venous ischaemia. On establishing an arterial aetiology, it is important to identify whether symptoms are unilateral or bilateral. Symmetrical symptoms are frequently part of a more generalized disease process and have a significant vasospastic element, while unilateral ischaemia is often a result of fixed arterial lesions occurring *in situ* or originating from a proximal source. Indeed, in the case of unilateral digital ischaemia, a proximal source of embolization such as an ulcerated atherosclerotic plaque or subclavian aneurysm must be sought. Occupational factors are important to record, particularly if they involve the use of vibrating tools or exposure to ergot or vinyl chloride. Furthermore, risk factors commonly associated with lower limb peripheral vascular disease such as smoking, diabetes, generalized atherosclerotic disease and a history of other connective tissue disorders or haematological disorders are also noted. It is also important to remember that intermittent obstructions such as those caused by extrinsic compression within the thoracic outlet or vasospasm of digital arteries may occur as isolated events or in conjunction with fixed arterial lesions.

Presenting symptoms may indicate an underlying vasospastic disorder with patients reporting repetitive symptoms with exacerbations in cold conditions or by emotional stimuli. They may demonstrate typical triphasic colour changes in the fingers. The initial pallor on vasoconstriction is soon followed by cyanosis, as restored blood is rapidly desaturated and finally rubor as a result of a reactive hyperaemia. However, it is wise to remember that these symptoms may also be encountered as an early manifestation of true occlusive disorders of the upper limb. True vasospasm is invariably intermittent with a lack of symptoms and signs between attacks. An exception to this is chemical induced vasospasm such as in the case of ergotism, toxins or various substances used by intravenous drug abusers. In these situations, prolonged vasospasm may result in irreversible damage. On the other hand, while true occlusive disease may present with a vasospastic element, there is no return to normality between exacerbations.

Physical examination

Inspection of both hands may demonstrate colour changes such as blanching, erythema, or cyanosis (Figure 30.2) as well as areas of digital ulceration

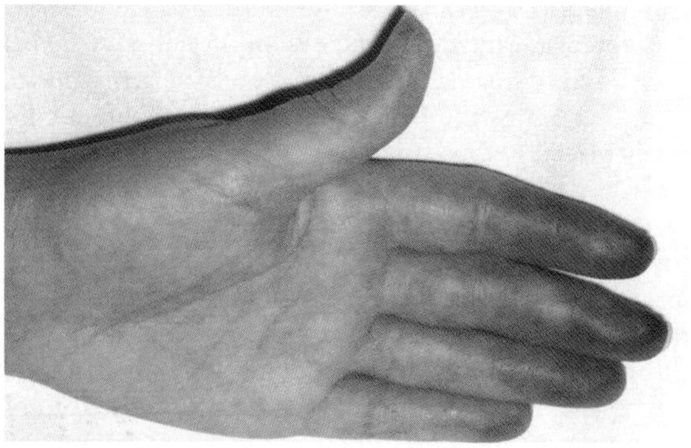

Figure 30.2 Unilateral digital ischaemia associated with a brachial embolus.

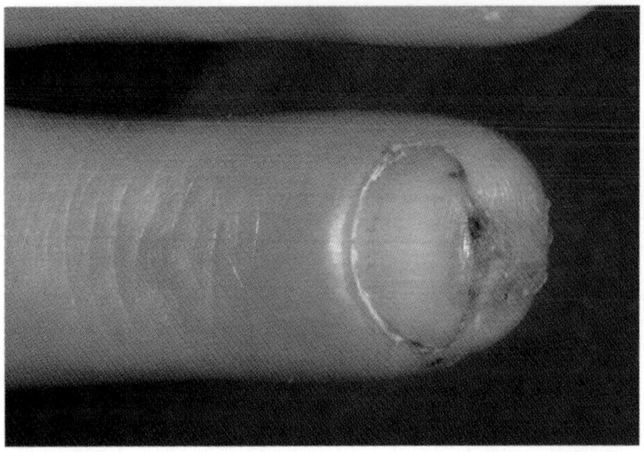

Figure 30.3 Digital infarct associated with a collagen vascular disorder.

(Figure 30.3). Signs of venous congestion may be evident in an oedematous discoloured arm by the presence of large upper arm collateral veins.

Following palpation of both radial and ulnar pulses, the brachial artery can be examined both in the antecubital fossa and also at the level of the mid upper arm where it can be compressed against the medial aspect of the humerus. The axillary artery can be easily felt within the axilla and a prominent subclavian pulse may occasionally be palpated in the supra-clavicular region. It is prudent to compare pulses and blood pressure between both arms at each level.

The competence of the palmar arch can be assessed by Allen's test. Performed one hand at a time, the subject is asked to clench their hand to make a fist. This allows most of the blood to be expelled. The examiner then occludes both radial and ulnar pulses and asks the patient to open their fist. The hand will remain white and mottled until one or other pulse is released at which point blood rushes in and a reactive hyperaemia ensues. If the released artery is occluded, the hand will remain mottled and in the presence of an incomplete palmar arch, only the side of the hand with the released artery will regain colour.

While palpating the neck, one should always look for a cervical rib within the supraclavicular fossa. There may be tenderness noted on palpation over the rib. Auscultation over both carotids and subclavian arteries may reveal a bruit and in the case of the subclavian, this may be accentuated at different levels of arm adduction. This forms the basis of Adson's test where a correctly placed stethoscope, below the middle third of the clavicle, may identify a bruit that is loudest at a particular degree of arm abduction and external rotation. At the same time the radial pulse may be noted to weaken. There may be a specific range of abduction where the bruit disappears signifying either a total occlusion or in fact a total lack of any compression. Further clinical evaluation such as Tinel's test, reproduction of symptoms by direct pressure over the brachial plexus or by 90° abduction and external rotation may aid the diagnosis of thoracic outlet syndrome.

Section 30.4 • Investigations

While a reasonable evaluation of the level of disease and sometimes the underlying cause can be made by a careful clinical assessment, simple non-invasive measurements can provide valuable information for diagnostic purposes as well as monitoring the progress of specific therapies. These include those directed at ascertaining the level and significance of stenosing or occlusive lesions as well as those aimed at identifying and quantifying vasospastic elements. For precise location of stenoses and collaterals in the face of significant arterial insufficiency, angiography is essential in order to plan surgery or radiological intervention.

Non-invasive

As with the lower limbs, non-invasive methods of evaluating the arterial supply to upper limbs are first line investigations. However, there are two further areas of interest in the upper limbs, namely the thoracic outlet and the evaluation of vasospastic disorders.

Segmental pressures

Segmental pressures are measured in a similar fashion as for the lower limbs by placing arm cuffs at the above elbow, below elbow and above wrist positions and insonating over the radial and ulnar arteries using a Doppler flow detector. Arterial waveforms are also assessed. A significant drop in pressure noted at any level indicates proximal stenotic/occlusive disease such as the subclavian or axillary artery at the above elbow position, brachial at the below elbow and radial or ulnar at the above wrist. In general, a pressure drop of greater than 20 mmHg between the two arms at a specific level or between two levels on the same arm is considered significant. Furthermore, abnormal arterial waveform profiles indicate proximal stenotic or occlusive disease and occasionally, in cases of increased peripheral resistance, distal occlusive disease.

Digital plethysmography

Measurement of digital pressures and pulse waveforms is useful in investigating vasospastic disorders as well as in identifying fixed stenotic/occlusive lesions of the small vessels. These data can be acquired by means of a Doppler probe, photoplethysmography (PPG) or mercury strain gauge plethysmography. A small 1 inch cuff is applied around the base of the proximal phalanx to allow pressure measurements to be taken. A Doppler probe is then applied to the volar aspect of a digit at the distal interphalangeal joint to record flow restoration. Alternatively, a photocell is applied to the fingertip pulp and secured by means of adhesive tape or a mercury strain gauge is placed around the fingertip (Figure 30.4). It is crucial to record a finger temperature of greater than 25°C before confirming a diagnosis, as there is a high false positive rate if cold induced vasospasm is encountered. Warming the hands in warm water and recording the digital temperature may be

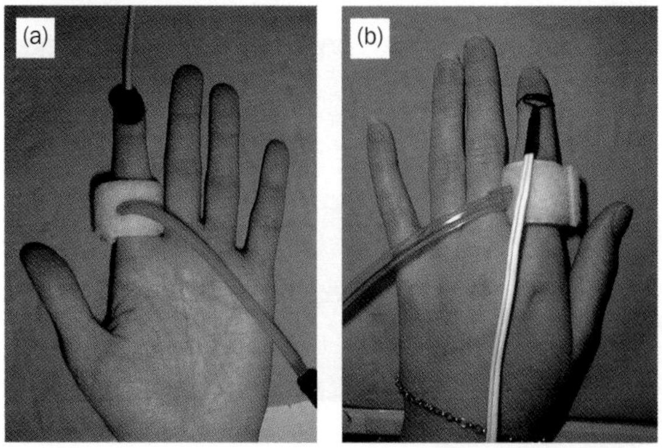

Figure 30.4 (a) Photoplethysmography, (b) mercury strain gauge.

required prior to performing the analysis. The absolute pressure is noted as well as the ratio between digital and brachial pressures, which are usually within 20–30 mmHg of each other. Digital waveforms can then be analysed. The length of time to complete the upstroke provides an indication of the peripheral resistance. A normal waveform is recorded if the upstroke time is less than 0.2 s and obstruction diagnosed if it is slower. In primary vasospastic disorders, the digital arteries have greater elasticity resulting in a very short upstroke time termed a 'peaked pulse'. Waveform analysis is not highly sensitive in determining the presence of fixed arterial disease, as it is unable to determine if only one of the two paired digital or forearm vessels is occluded. However, by assessing all digits on both hands and finding normal waveforms and pulse volumes, it is highly unlikely that the underlying aetiology is secondary Raynaud's. The pulse amplitude response to a short period of ischaemia is a useful test when determining the likely benefit of vasodilatory treatment whether by drugs or sympathectomy. This involves applying a pressure cuff around the arm and inflating to a suprasystolic pressure for 5 min prior to rapid deflation. The pulse volume and contour are then measured and compared

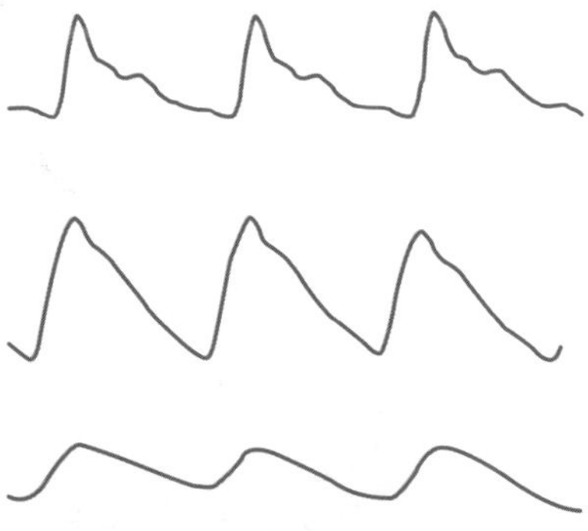

Figure 30.5 Comparison of velocity waveforms between primary and secondary Raynaud's phenomenon. Note damped signal in the case of secondary and the sharp upslope and high dichrotic notch in cases of primary Raynaud's.

to pre-ischaemia levels. In those with a normal response or primary Raynaud's, the pulse amplitude can be seen to increase following reactive arteriolar dilatation. In the case of the latter, the amplitude may double and demonstrate a 'peaked' pulse contour. Those with fixed distal arterial lesions achieve a poor response (Figure 30.5).

Cold challenge test

For further analysis of vasospastic disorders, a 'cold challenge test' can be performed. For this test, finger temperature is measured first and warmed as necessary to ensure a temperature of greater than 30°C and the resting pressure and waveform are recorded using digital plethysmography. The hands are then immersed in ice-cold water for up to 1 min and the measurements are repeated at regular intervals. A test is reported normal if the post cold challenge pressures return to normal within 10 min. This is a reliable and reproducible test but has limited diagnostic abilities in that half the normal population will have an abnormal test despite being asymptomatic.

Other forms of 'cold challenge testing' include measuring finger temperatures using a thermistor at regular intervals for up to 1 hour following immersion into ice-cold water. Digital hypothermic challenge can also be performed using a finger cuff that allows perfusion of cold fluid.

Scanning laser Doppler

Quantifying blood flow within the digital microcirculation has challenged physicians for some time. Accurate and reliable data would allow objective measures of treatment progress to be evaluated. Furthermore, it may assist in differentiating between primary and secondary Raynaud's. Technology has advanced considerably overcoming many of the limitations of the single channel laser Doppler probe. Using a scanning laser Doppler, it is now possible to build up a map of perfusion detailing regions of interest. Furthermore, as there is no contact with the patient, there is no artefact in the scans (Figure 30.6). While other modalities for measuring digital blood flow have failed to provide reliable quantifiable data, scanning laser Doppler has proved a promising technique. Nevertheless, more validation work is required with direct comparisons with nailfold microscopy, thermography and the effect of vasodilatory therapy.

Thermography

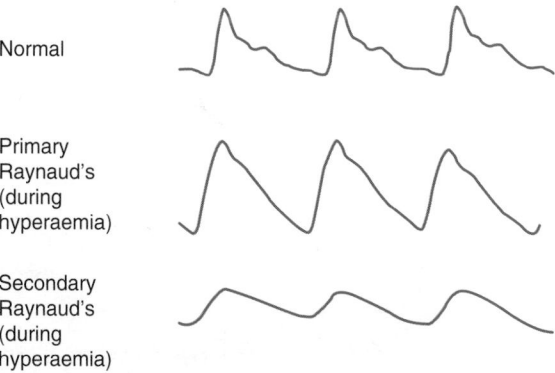

The pattern of hand rewarming after a cold challenge has been used to differentiate between primary and secondary Raynaud's phenomenon. However, its use is limited to specialist centres with a specially adapted room with temperature and humidity control. The patient must first acclimatize at a room temperature of 23 ± 0.5°C and humidity 45 ± 5% for 20 min before a thermal image can be recorded (Figure 30.7). Following immersion in water at 15°C for 1 min the patient's hand (wearing protective gloves) is allowed to rewarm while

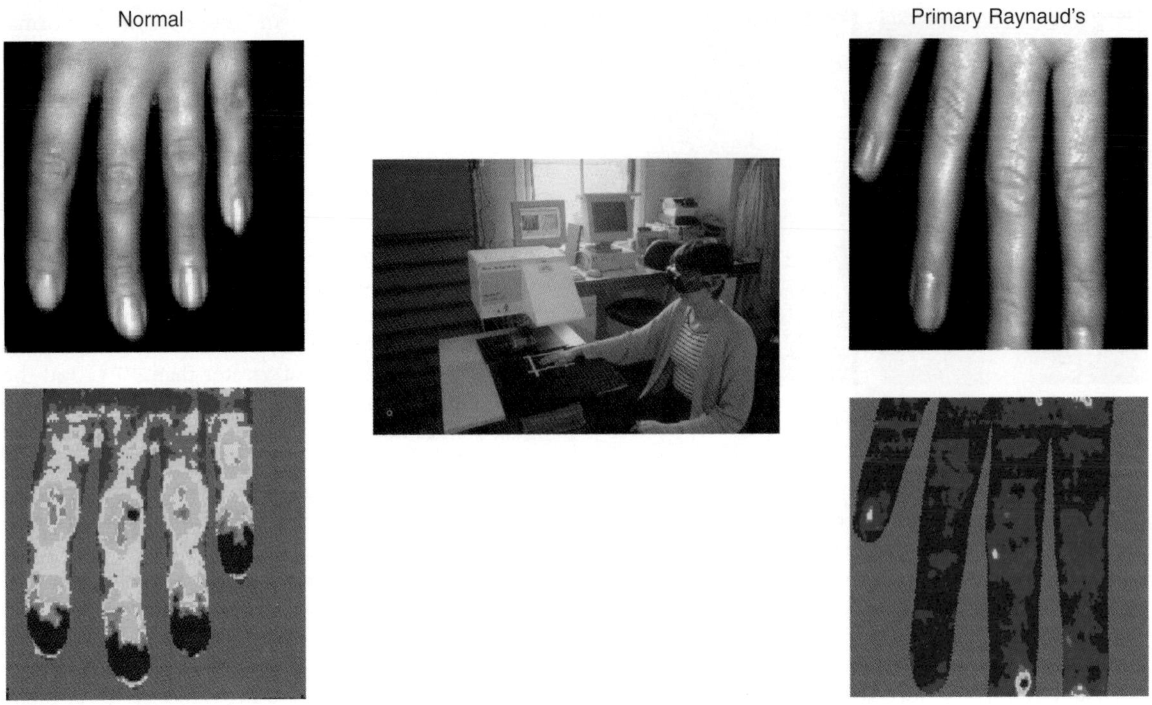

Figure 30.6 Scanning laser Doppler. Note poor digital perfusion in hands with Raynaud's phenomenon.

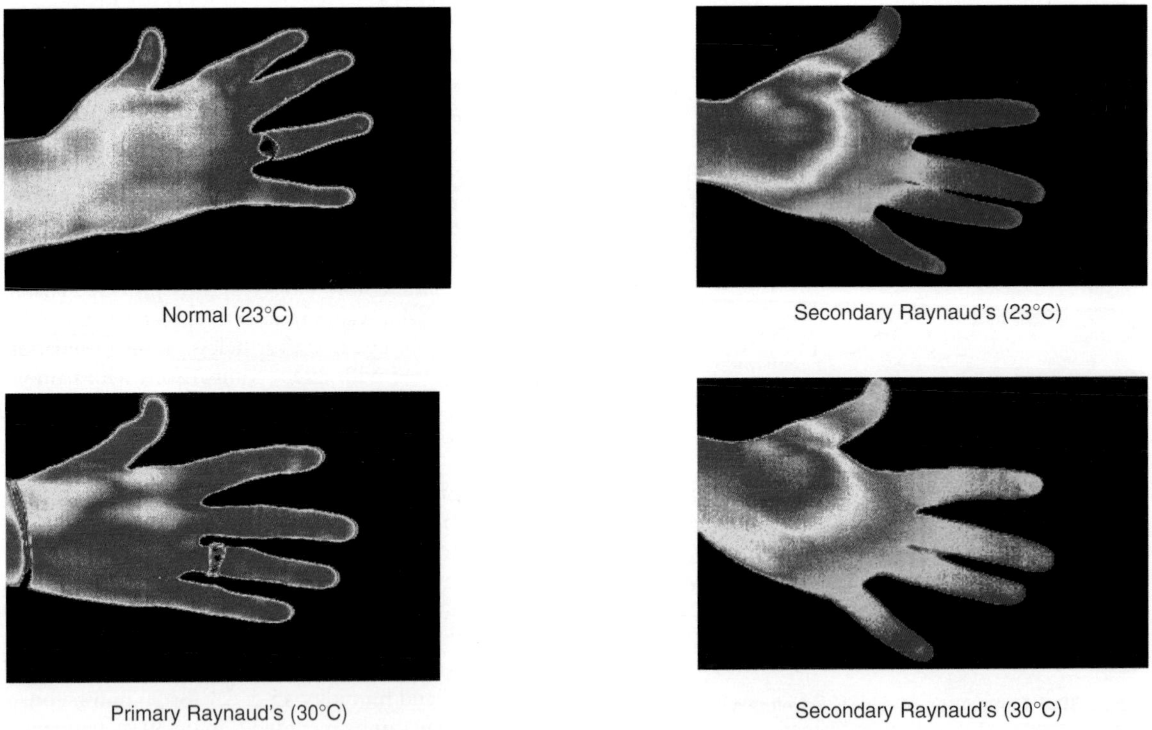

Figure 30.7 Thermography demonstrating the difference between primary and secondary Raynaud's disease. (Courtesy of Dr A.L. Herrick and Mrs T.L. Moore, Rheumatic Diseases Centre, University of Manchester, Hope Hospital.)

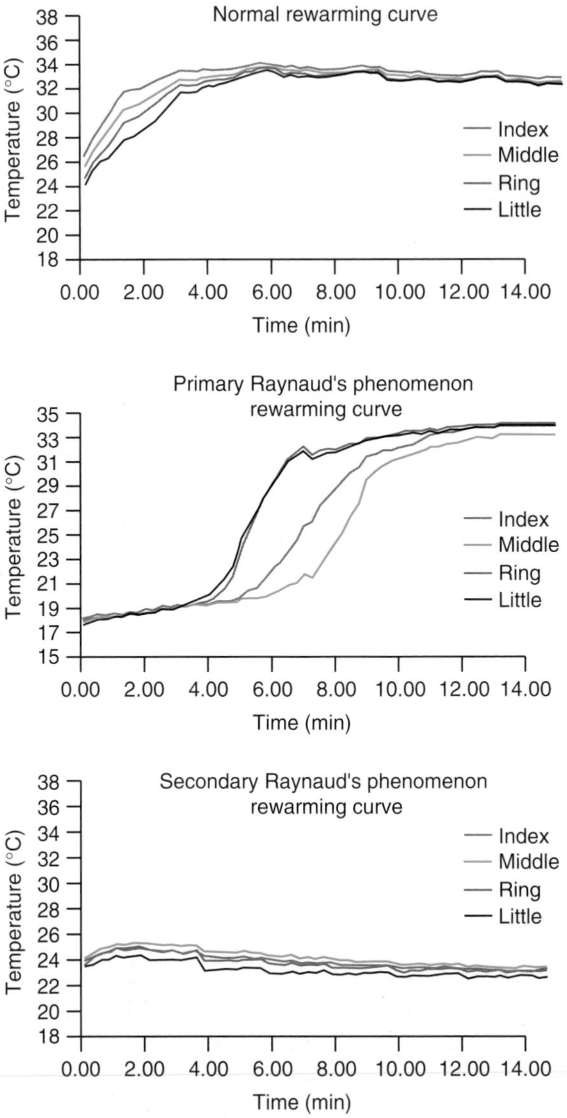

Figure 30.8 Rewarming curves demonstrate the failure of patients with secondary Raynaud's phenomenon to return to normal temperature within 14 min. Primary Raynaud's results in delayed digital rewarming. (Courtesy of Dr A.L. Herrick and Mrs T.L. Moore, Rheumatic Diseases Centre, University of Manchester, Hope Hospital.)

images are captured over 15 min to measure the speed at which the skin temperature returns to baseline. A normal response is recorded if the temperature returns to baseline within 10 min. Fingertip temperature over the test period may be extracted from the thermal images and plotted on a graph to allow comparison between patients, or of the same patient before and after therapy. Patients with primary Raynaud's demonstrate delayed rewarming curves while those with secondary Raynaud's phenomenon do not return to baseline temperature for over an hour (Figure 30.8).

The disadvantage of thermography is the need for a high level of operator and interpreter competency and an adherence to established protocols. The results of infrared imaging must be interpreted in context. This involves correlating the findings with a thorough history, relevant clinical examination and other diagnostic studies as may be clinically indicated. In this way, infrared imaging may be an aid in differentiating between diagnoses and determining prognosis.

Nailfold microscopy

The dimensions and morphology of nailfold capillaries are a reliable way to differentiate between primary and secondary Raynaud's. In normal people, the capillaries are numerous and evenly distributed parallel to the skin. On viewing with a microscope at 200–600× magnification, normal nailfold capillaries can be seen to be of similar sizes and morphology. However, they may be enlarged and distorted in patients with connective tissue disorders and there may be a non-uniformity in their distribution with areas of avascularity (Figure 30.9).

Duplex ultrasound

Arteries in the upper limb apart from the subclavian are generally superficial and thus amenable to duplex ultrasound. Even in the case of the subclavian arteries, it is still possible in some patients to identify their origin from the aortic arch on the left (Figure 30.10) and innominate on the right. While stenotic regions cannot easily be visualized behind the clavicle, Doppler wave patterns above and below the lesion can indicate a nearby stenotic region. Subclavian vessels are best viewed using a 4 or 5 MHz probe, unlike the more distal superficial vessels which require a 7.5 or 10 MHz probe. The same factors apply to upper limb ultrasonography as to the lower limb: a doubling in peak systolic velocity across a lesion indicates a 50% diameter reduction. In conjunction with provocative positioning of the affected arm at various levels of abduction and external rotation, duplex ultrasound plays an important role in evaluating symptoms attributable to thoracic outlet syndrome. It is important that when viewing a subclavian stenosis or occlusion, carotid and vertebral vessels are also viewed. The recognition of subclavian steal syndrome is crucial and is demonstrated by retrograde flow in a vertebral artery that 'steals' blood from the circle of Willis.

Invasive angiography

In many cases, sufficient information can be obtained through clinical examination and non-invasive tests to enable a diagnosis to be made and allow appropriate treatment to be instigated. However, when surgery or some form of radiological intervention is proposed, angiography is essential to accurately locate stenotic or occlusive segments and associated collateral vessels. A femoral approach is usually necessary for imaging the aortic arch, innominate and subclavian vessels. However, if views are to be limited to forearm and distal vessels, then a direct axillary or brachial puncture provides a simple approach.

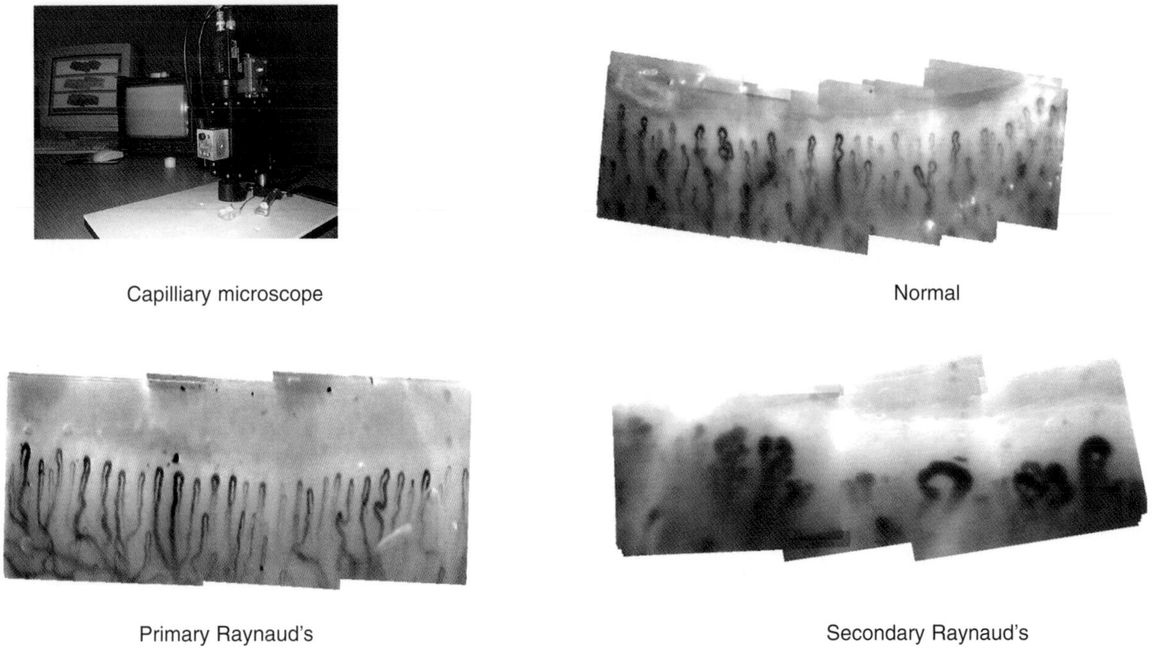

Figure 30.9 Capillary microscopy demonstrating the difference in appearances between primary and secondary Raynaud's. Note non-uniformity of capillaries and area of avascularity in the case of secondary Raynaud's. (Courtesy of Dr A.L. Herrick and Mrs T.L. Moore, Rheumatic Diseases Centre, University of Manchester, Hope Hospital.)

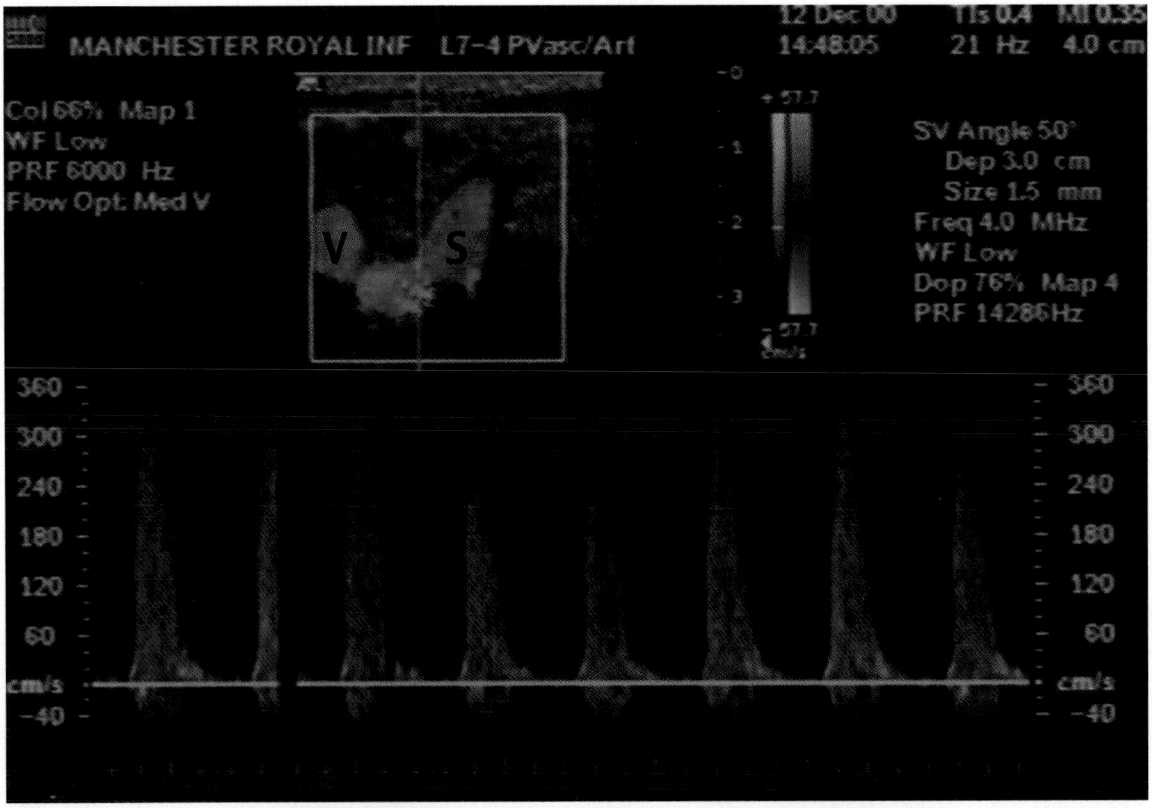

Figure 30.10 (V) Vertebral artery, (S) right subclavian artery. (Courtesy of Dr A.L. Herrick and Mrs T.L. Moore, Rheumatic Diseases Centre, University of Manchester, Hope Hospital.)

Section 30.5 • Clinical presentations and management

Proximal vessel disease

With respect to the upper limb, proximal vessels include those originating from the aortic arch and continuing to the wrist. Distal vessels within the hand will be considered separately.

Vasospasm rarely affects the proximal vessels with the exception of ergot poisoning, a chemical found in some medications or less commonly as a fungal contamination of some strains of grain. When symptoms of ischaemia are confined to the upper arm and forearm, the level of arterial occlusion will be at the radial/ulnar, axillary or subclavian arteries. The innominate artery may also be the site of occlusive disease on the right side. In most cases, reduced resting segmental pressures and damped Doppler waveforms will locate the problem without the need of any digital plethysmographical studies. Occasionally it may not be possible to demonstrate a significant difference in pressures between the two arms in those patients in whom symptoms are only brought on by vigorous exercise. In these cases, it is still possible to measure post-exercise pressures or compare resting pressures with those following a 5 min brachial artery occlusion during the hyperaemic phase. A significant pressure drop of greater than 20 mmHg between the two arms following exercise or hyperaemia is considered significant if the symptomatic arm is the lower of the two readings. Doppler flow studies and duplex ultrasonography can further isolate the diseased segments and clarify the quality of run-off vessels. Atherosclerosis is often the cause of innominate or subclavian arterial obstruction but rarely extends more distally. Thoracic outlet syndrome (TOS) is a separate entity that can present with a positional type of upper limb ischaemia through intermittent subclavian or axillary arterial compression. However, it is important to note that pure arterial compromise in the thoracic outlet is rare as neurological and venous elements are also frequently involved. Emboli and trauma are the more common features of forearm vessel obstruction. Certainly with the increasing use of brachial access for coronary angiography, iatrogenic trauma resulting in arterial dissection and acute thrombosis is unfortunately becoming a more frequent presentation. Less common causes of proximal vessel occlusive disease include the arteritides such as giant cell arteritis or Takayasu's disease, which often affects the large aortic arch branches, and subclavian disease. Thromboangiitis obliterans (Buerger's disease), another uncommon aetiology, tends to affect the middle-sized arteries in the forearm of heavy smokers.

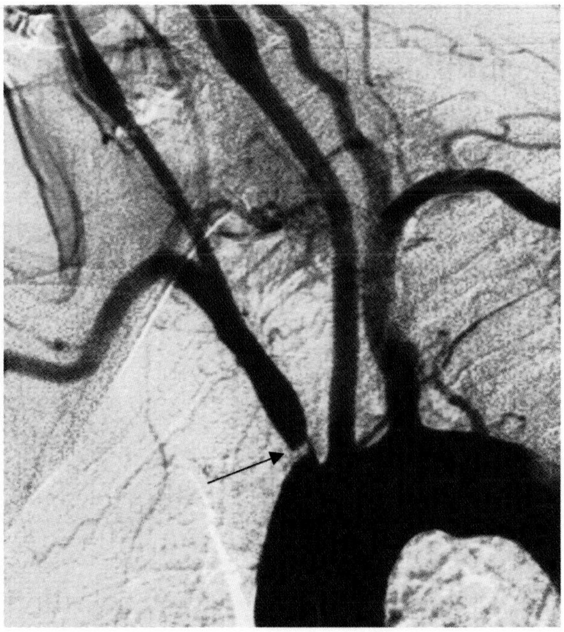

Figure 30.11 Black arrow indicates a tight innominate artery stenosis.

Innominate and subclavian arterial occlusive disease

Many patients with stenotic or occlusive disease in the innominate or subclavian arteries will remain asymptomatic. They are predominantly within their sixth decade and are thus a slightly younger group than those with vascular disease elsewhere. While it is only marginally more common in men, a greater proportion of women with peripheral vascular disease have this pattern of atherosclerosis. A report by the Joint Study of Extracranial Arterial Occlusion showed that occlusive disease of these vessels could be found in up to 17% of all angiograms performed for cerebrovascular disease. Symptoms reported included unilateral digital ischaemia as a result of atheroembolic episodes to distal vessels; arm claudication following thrombosis of an ulcerated plaque and subclavian steal syndrome where retrograde filling of the ipsilateral vertebral artery occurs. In the case of innominate and proximal subclavian disease, focal hemispheric and non-hemispheric symptoms may occur. While atherosclerotic disease can present with both atheroembolic and occlusive symptoms, Takayasu's disease, giant cell arteritis and radiation-induced arteritis seldom present with embolic episodes. These less common aetiologies are more predominant in younger females and often affect multiple vessels.

Innominate artery reconstruction

Surgical reconstruction still remains the mainstay for treatment of debilitating symptomatic innominate artery occlusive disease and particularly for atheroembolic complications. Arch aortography accurately delineates the extent of the disease (Figure 30.11) and also confirms the anatomy, which may be abnormal in a quarter of all patients. Atheroma most commonly occurs at the bifurcation or the origin of the innominate artery. Before the advent of prosthetic grafts, sympathectomy and thrombectomy were attempted but results were poor. Extra-anatomical bypass such as axillo-axillary and femoro-axillary bypass procedures became more popular especially since the high perioperative mortality associated with direct reconstruction, at that time, deemed direct reconstruction not feasible. However, with the major advances in perioperative management, thromboendarterectomy, aorto-innominate, aorto-subclavian and aorto-carotid bypass have been increasingly performed with excellent results. Innominate artery endarterectomy is still offered at some centres with good results, but difficulty with selective innominate artery clamping and satisfactory termination of the endarterectomy has led to this technique being superseded by prosthetic bypass. Recent advances in interventional radiological techniques and imaging have also allowed more complex and challenging lesions to be tackled without the need for surgery. This is certainly the case with percutaneous transluminal angioplasty (PTA) with or without stenting of the large aortic arch branches. Early results have been promising in selected groups of patients but as yet there is a paucity of data. It is likely that short isolated lesions will be amenable to this technique but complex and multiple lesions will continue to require formal surgical reconstruction.

Innominate artery bypass

The patient is placed supine and a midline sternotomy approach is used. Cervical or lateral extensions may be required for better access to the right common carotid or subclavian respectively. The thymus can be separated through its midline or reflected to one side and should be preserved to interpose between graft and sternum for closure. The pericardium is then opened over the ascending aorta below the left innominate vein. The dissection is then continued along the innominate artery to its bifurcation and the right common carotid and subclavian arteries are then controlled using slings (Figure 30.12). Care is taken to avoid damage to the recurrent laryngeal nerve during dissection. A side-biting clamp is then applied to the aorta and a longitudinal arteriotomy fashioned. A prosthetic graft is then bevelled at one end and an end-to-side anastomosis performed using a continuous 3-0 Prolene suture. The innominate artery is then clamped in its mid-portion and non-traumatic clamps are applied to the common carotid and subclavian arteries. The innominate artery is divided distal to the proximal clamp and the stump closed securely in two layers. The bypass graft is led anterior or posterior to the left innominate vein and cut to length. The graft is then anastomosed to the distal innominate artery as an end-to-end anastomosis with a continuous 5-0 Prolene suture (Figure 30.13). Prior to completion of the anastomosis, the proximal end of the graft is flushed through and then washed out with heparinized saline. Flow is then restored to the subclavian and common carotid artery in turn. An arterial trace of the blood flow in the right arm indicates the return of normal waveforms (Figure 30.14). Where the left common carotid artery also requires revascularization, a bifurcated graft can be used with additional side branches as required (Figure 30.15). The perioperative mortality is in the region of 5% as is the perioperative stroke or transient ischaemic attack (TIA)

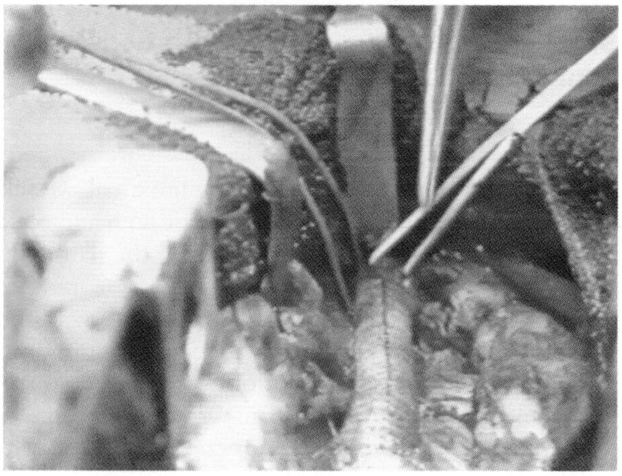

Figure 30.13 Distal anastomosis of aorto-innominate bypass.

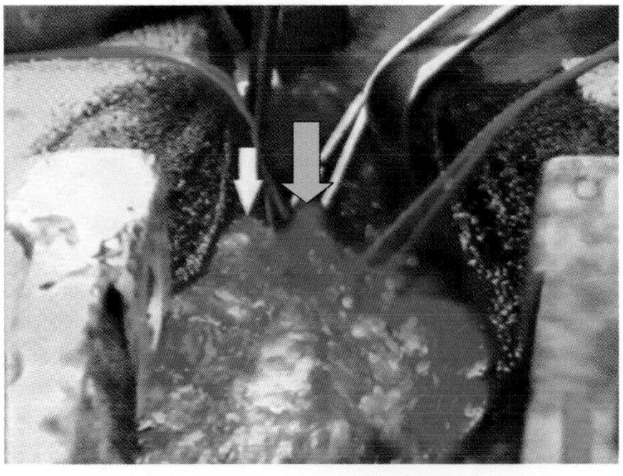

Figure 30.12 Right common carotid (green arrow) and subclavian artery (white arrow) are controlled with slings. (Courtesy of Mr T.O. Oshodi, Oldham Royal Infirmary.)

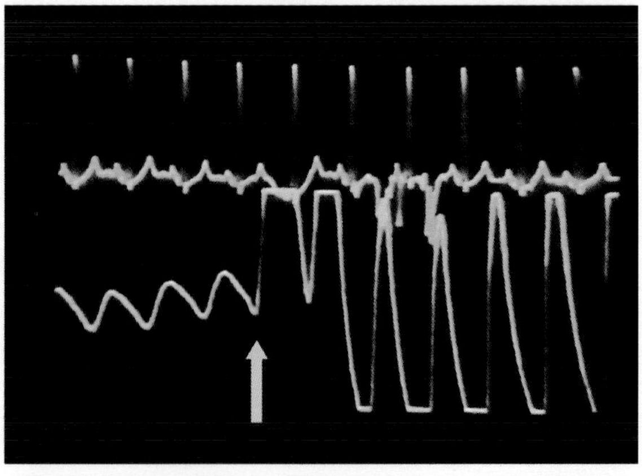

Figure 30.14 Yellow arrow represents the time at which blood flow is restored to the right arm.

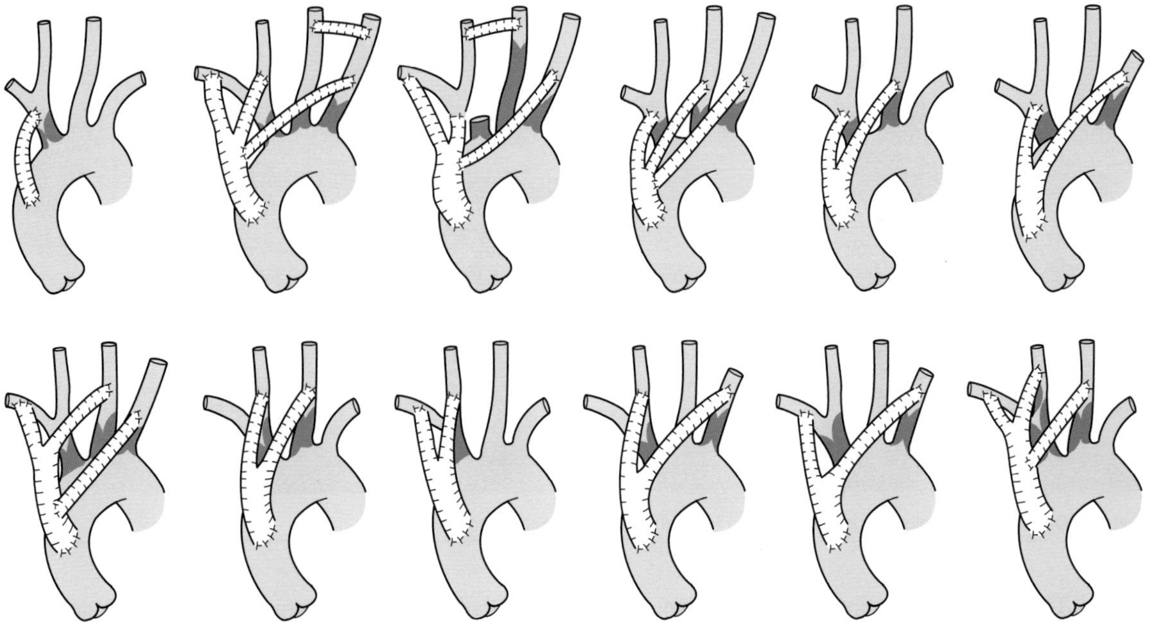

Figure 30.15 Variations of innominate artery and great vessel reconstructions. (From Reul, G.J., Jacobs, M.J., Gregoric, I.D. *et al.* Innominate artery occlusive disease. Surgical approach and long-term results. *J Vasc Surg* **14**: 405–12, 1991.)

rate. However, results of this type of surgery are excellent with long-term graft patency and freedom of symptoms in 90% of patients. Results vary considerably between centres and reflect both experience and extent of disease treated.

Subclavian steal syndrome

Atherosclerotic lesions in the subclavian artery are more common than those of the innominate artery and much more frequently encountered on the left side. However, fewer isolated subclavian stenoses or occlusions are symptomatic because of the rich collateral supply, particularly around the neck and shoulder.

Fisher first coined the term subclavian steal syndrome in 1961 to describe the reversal of blood flow within a vertebral artery when associated with a proximal subclavian artery occlusion (Figure 30.16). The theory behind its name comes from the fact that when the ipsilateral arm is exercised, it 'steals' blood from the circle of Willis via the ipsilateral vertebral artery. This simplistic view is not entirely factual. Indeed this classical presentation is seen in very few patients. Furthermore, the radiological finding of reversed vertebral artery flow is seen in many asymptomatic individuals. Therefore it is believed that symptoms occur in those patients with additional extracranial vascular

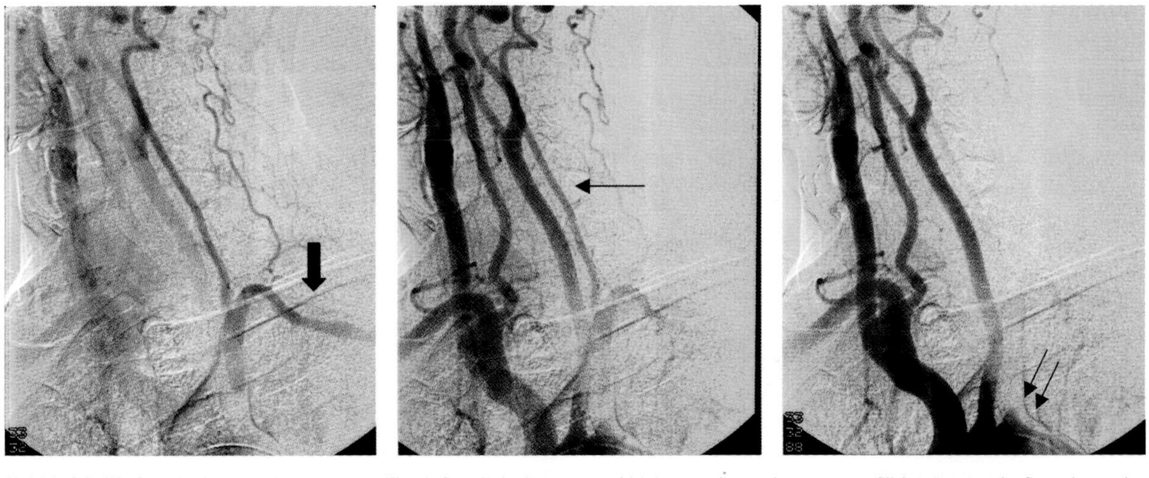

Figure 30.16 Subclavian steal syndrome. The left subclavian artery (thick arrow) can be seen to fill by retrograde flow down the ipsilateral vertebral artery (thin arrow), thereby bypassing the occlusion at the subclavian origin (double arrow). (From Reul, G.J., Jacobs, M.J., Gregoric, I.D. *et al.* Innominate artery occlusive disease. Surgical approach and long-term results. *J Vasc Surg* **14**: 405–12, 1991.)

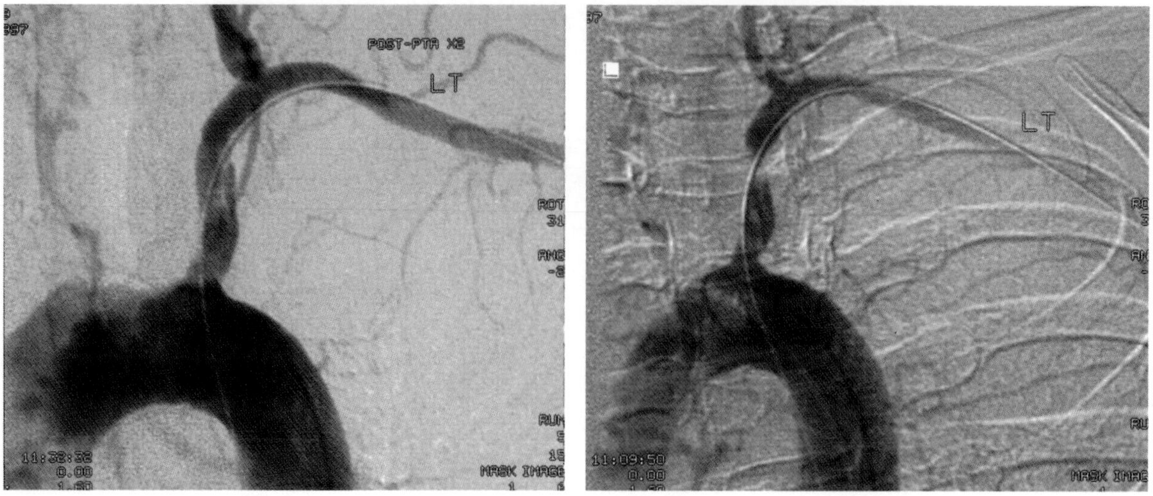

Figure 30.17 Good radiological result following left subclavian artery balloon angioplasty.

disease. This is the case in up to 85% of patients with symptomatic subclavian artery lesions. Therefore an incidental finding of reversed vertebral artery flow is not an indication for intervention.

Symptoms attributable to subclavian artery occlusive disease include non-hemispheric neurological conditions such as vertebro-basilar insufficiency resulting in vertigo, dizziness, bilateral visual disturbances and ataxia and arm ischaemia akin to claudication of the lower limb. Recurrence of angina in patients who have undergone coronary artery bypass using an internal mammary artery (IMA) and who subsequently develop proximal subclavian artery disease is an indication for intervention. Focal hemispheric symptoms are less common but nonetheless are an absolute indication for intervention. However, there are few data regarding the true incidence of stroke in these patients. It is likely to be very low unless other significant extracranial disease is also present.

Management of subclavian artery occlusive disease

When symptomatology demands revascularization of a stenotic or occluded subclavian vessel, the preferred surgical options include carotid–subclavian bypass or subclavian artery transposition onto the common carotid artery. Both these treatment options produce excellent results with patency rates in excess of 90% at 10 years. In the case of the former, the performance of prosthetic grafts is superior to vein, possibly due to size mismatch of vein grafts and subsequent tension on neck movements. While an advantage for subclavian artery transposition is that it avoids the need for a prosthetic graft, the downside is that it involves more dissection behind the sternum to reach the proximal end of the subclavian artery. However, while the reported stroke rate for carotid–subclavian bypass is 1-5%, the incidence is much lower for transposition in which it is has been reported to be less than 1%. A reason for this difference may be the fact that early thrombotic occlusion of a bypass graft may propagate into the common carotid artery and embolize. The mortality rate for either procedure is very low at less than 1%.

Endarterectomy of the subclavian artery is not ideal but may be useful in managing the symptoms of myocardial ischaemia in patients with IMA coronary artery grafts where subclavian artery transposition is not an option.

PTA is also increasingly being employed to treat short subclavian artery stenoses (Figure 30.17). Short-term results are promising but once again paucity of long-term data prevents appropriate comparison with surgical reconstruction. Results for occlusion are somewhat disappointing even in the short term. The morbidity and mortality associated with PTA is low in most series. Embolization to the brain is avoided despite the proximity to the vertebral artery as orthograde flow is delayed for up to a minute following PTA. The long-term data available so far indicate a less than 50% patency rate following angioplasty. Indeed there is a recurrence rate of up to 20% within 2 years. As techniques and devices improve it will undoubtedly be the treatment of choice in selected patients. However, as the results and durability following surgical reconstruction are excellent, it is likely that interventional radiological procedures will remain a useful adjunct particularly for complex lesions.

Middle-sized upper limb arteries

Seventy per cent of cases of acute non-traumatic upper limb ischaemia are secondary to emboli originating from the heart and in other instances from large proximal vessel atherosclerotic plaques or aneurysms. In 10–20% of cases, the source of emboli is not found. Recent investigations have also implicated paradoxical embolism via a patent foramen ovale. Clinical features include a cold, painful, pulseless arm with paraesthesia and decreased motor function. Rarely does a patient present with a non-viable arm. Findings of atrial fibrillation or recent myocardial infarction support the diagnosis of an embolism. Clinical assessment will usually identify the level of occlusion and allow a decision for where to access the artery for radiological or surgical intervention. If there is any doubt, Doppler flow studies and duplex ultrasonography will often confirm the diagnosis. Pre-operative angiography is advisable if an embolic source is not likely to be cardiac in origin so as to identify the proximal source. However, on-table angiography following surgical embolectomy is prudent to confirm vessel patency. Emboli tend to lodge at one of three sites: in the proximal brachial artery at the level of the profunda branch; mid-arm level at the origin of the superior ulnar collateral; and at the brachial bifurcation. It is unusual for the subclavian or axillary artery to be involved. Furthermore, embolization into the radial or ulnar artery is more common when originating from a proximal arterial source.

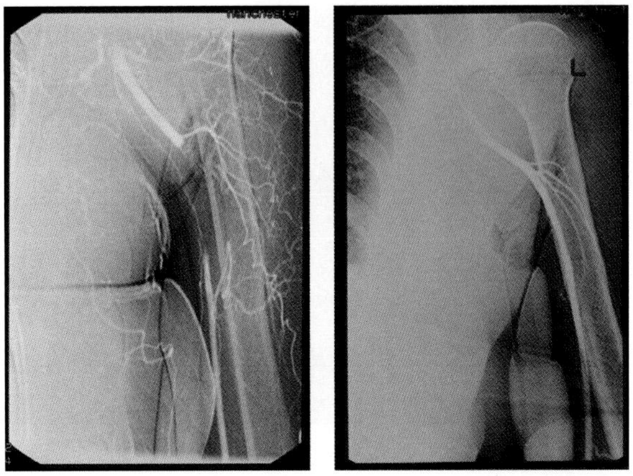

Figure 30.18 Brachial artery embolus is successfully thrombolysed.

Management of acute embolic occlusion

Revascularization of a severely acutely ischaemic arm or hand is indicated in all patients unless the individual is moribund. Patients should be systemically heparinized as soon as possible to prevent thrombus propagation as well as reduce the risk of further embolic episodes. In most cases, surgical embolectomy can be performed under local anaesthetic. An axillary approach can be performed by making an incision in the upper third of the arm and is the preferred technique for proximal brachial artery embolic occlusion. An antecubital fossa approach is indicated to extract emboli at the mid-arm level or at the bifurcation. Control of the radial and ulnar branches is necessary in the case of the latter. Transverse arteriotomies are preferred to reduce the chance of narrowing the vessel on closure. Embolectomy is performed using a 3 or 5 Fr catheter proximally and a 2 or 3 Fr catheter distally. Arteriotomies should be closed using an interrupted 7-0 monofilament suture. If there are any concerns regarding arterial narrowing on closure, then a vein patch technique should be employed.

Conservative management using systemic heparinization is an acceptable option in selected cases where the viability of the limb is not in doubt. In such cases, Doppler signals are present at the wrist and forearm pressures usually exceed 60 mmHg. In these cases a careful observation period is crucial as the clinical state may deteriorate rapidly. Less invasive techniques such as intra-arterial clot aspiration, various hydrolyser catheters and thrombolysis catheters are also available in many institutions. Over recent years, selective intra-arterial thrombolysis has gained widespread acceptance as first-line therapy for acute lower limb ischaemia. However, there have been few reports on its use in acute upper limb arterial occlusion. A potential benefit is that it may reveal underlying stenoses that may be amenable to angioplasty or surgical reconstruction as secondary adjunctive procedures. While in the authors' experience, it is an effective initial treatment for acute upper limb ischaemia, caution must be exercised in selecting patients (Figure 30.18). Those who present late with markedly threatened limb viability are unsuitable for thrombolysis and require surgical intervention for limb salvage. It is important to note that the overall mortality following an embolic episode remains in the region of 20% regardless of initial management. This is in part related to underlying comorbid features in this group of patients, particularly cardiac morbidity. However, limb salvage is usually possible with 80–100% success rates reported.

Trauma

Both iatrogenic and non-iatrogenic trauma can result in acute arm ischaemia. With the increasing use of brachial catheterization for coronary angiography, as well as cannulation of the radial artery for blood pressure monitoring, iatrogenic trauma is becoming more common. The incidence of trauma to the brachial artery resulting in acute thrombosis is 1–4%, which is in contrast to that of the femoral approach, which remains at 0.4%. This relates to the technique of arteriotomy closure, such as purse-string or longitudinal closure, and degree of technical expertise. In short segment thrombosis, the patient may remain asymptomatic through adequate collateral channels. Symptoms akin to claudication may be experienced following the patient's discharge, particularly as the right brachial is commonly catheterized and thus results in dominant arm claudication. In contrast, extensive segmental occlusion compromising major collaterals will result in acute and profound ischaemia necessitating urgent repair. Often there is arterial damage to the posterior wall of the artery at the site of arteriotomy. The dissection flap should be noted and following open thrombectomy, closure should be made by means of a generous vein patch. Occasionally the arterial injury is remote to the arteriotomy in which case a dissection flap may have been created through difficult catheterization. In this situation, a formal reconstruction using a vein graft to bypass the occlusion will be necessary. If the level of dissection is very proximal, an axillary-brachial or even a carotid-axillary bypass may be required.

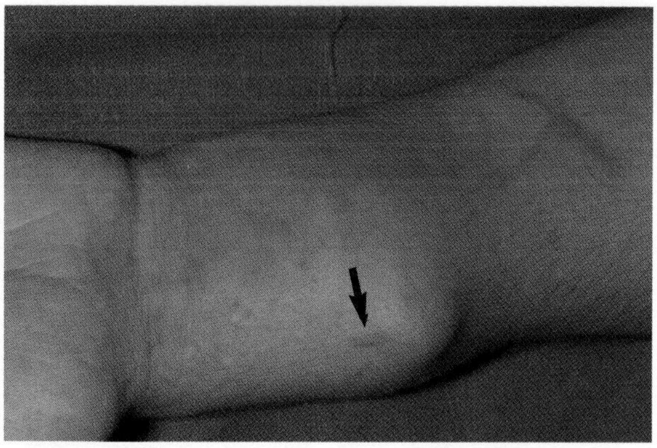

Figure 30.19 False aneurysm of left radial artery 8 weeks following a penetrating injury (arrow).

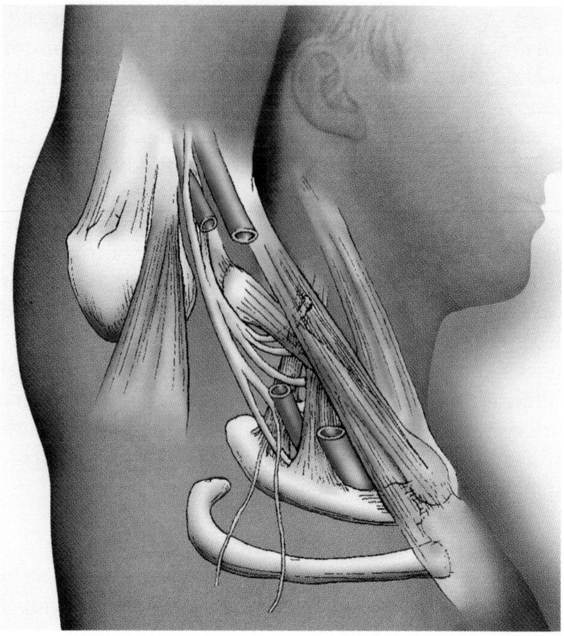

Figure 30.20 Anatomy of the thoracic outlet.

Non-iatrogenic trauma commonly affects the brachial, radial or ulnar arteries. Limb viability will not be threatened when injury occurs to one of the two distal vessels. In this situation the vessel may simply be ligated. However, brachial artery injury will require repair. If a localized procedure is not possible because of extensive damage and tissue loss then a bypass using a vein graft will be necessary. The subclavian and axillary arteries are less commonly involved as they are protected to some degree by the shoulder girdle. Situations in which these vessels may be injured include gunshot, stabbing, deceleration trauma and laceration by bony fragments from a fractured clavicle. Injury at this level can be easily missed on initial presentation, especially if the patient is in shock. Unless there is heavy bleeding and the site of injury is obvious, then pre-operative angiography is crucial especially as the presence of wrist pulses does not exclude significant proximal arterial injury. Injury to the axillary or subclavian vessels invariably involves concomitant brachial plexus damage due to its close proximity. Nevertheless, penetrating injuries of any artery should be explored to avoid later complications such as false aneurysm formation (Figure 30.19), delayed haemorrhage and haematoma compression of neighbouring nerves.

Thoracic outlet syndrome

Although the role of the scalene triangle in the causation of neurovascular symptoms was first recognized by Murphy in 1910, when he described first rib resection, it was not until 1956 that the term 'thoracic outlet syndrome' (TOS) was first used by Peet. Thoracic outlet syndrome is defined as symptoms in the arm and hand due to compression of nerves or blood vessels within the thoracic outlet (Figure 30.20). These symptoms include paraesthesia and pain in the distribution of specific nerves arising from the brachial plexus, particularly the ulnar nerve arising from the lower plexus. Referred pain in the form of occipital headaches is commonly reported. Arm weakness (particularly of the hands) is associated with nerve compression. Obstruction of the subclavian artery or vein is less frequent and often present in conjunction with nerve compression. Intermittent cold discoloration of the hands, in the presence of normal distal pulses, is frequently a result of increased sympathetic activity as these fibres travel with the lower plexus. Symptoms are often of a positional nature and frequently worse at night. Compression is usually due to the scalene muscles or tendons, fibrous bands or bony abnormalities such as a cervical rib (Figure 30.21). Cervical ribs are present in less than 1% of the population but these patients are 10 times more likely to develop TOS. Infrequently a post-stenotic arterial dilatation is noted just distal to the point of arterial compression. This can be a source of distal embolization.

There is frequently a history of a hyperextension neck injury such as whiplash or occupational repetitive strain injury. This is thought to be the likely initiator of TOS, a theory that has gained support following the identification of histological changes consistent with increased muscle fibrosis in patients with this condition.

While much has been written about the subject, accurate diagnosis and thus correct patient selection for treatment remains a core problem due to the wide range of symptoms with which TOS may present. This is compounded by the fact that there is no one diagnostic test specific to the syndrome. Some clinicians even doubt its existence. It is believed by some investigators that scalene muscle block is a highly sensitive method for diagnosing patients who will benefit from surgery. This involves local anaesthetic infiltration into the tender area of the anterior scalene muscle and observing for symptomatic improvement. Electromyography (EMG) and nerve conduction tests have

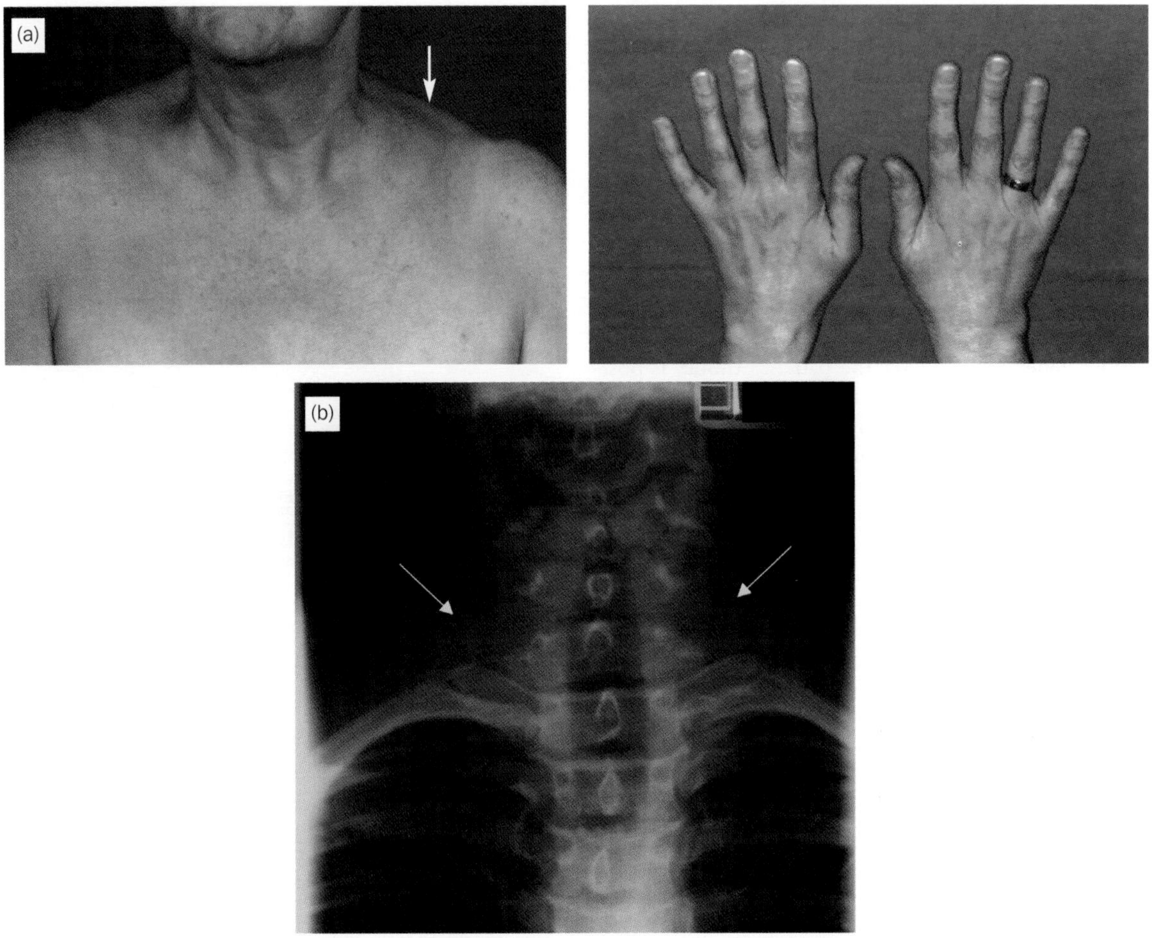

Figure 30.21 (a) This 64-year-old woman presented with bilateral TOS associated with cervical ribs. An area of fullness associated with a prominent cervical rib was identified in the left supraclavicular fossa (white arrow). This resulted in significant wasting of the small muscles of the hands, particularly on the left. (b) Bilateral cervical ribs (yellow arrows) are clearly seen in the radiograph. (Courtesy of P. and R. Fulford.)

both proved non-specific and are seldom used in this practice. Angiography or venography is only indicated when a vascular origin is suspected. In these patients, non-invasive tests such as Doppler flow studies and duplex ultrasound may provide the necessary information. In the authors' practice, patients suspected of having TOS are examined independently by a vascular surgeon and neurologist. The diagnosis is thus mainly based on clinical grounds.

Patients are selected for surgery if, in the absence of other neurological disease, three of the following four criteria are present: (1) a history of aggravation of symptoms with the arm in the elevated position, (2) a history of paraesthesiae in the distribution of C8–T1, (3) tenderness over the brachial plexus superiorly, and (4) a positive 'hands-up' test. (The Roos test – reproduction of symptoms on repeated hand clenching with both shoulders abducted to 90° and elbows flexed to 90°.)

Management of thoracic outlet syndrome

A period of conservative management should always be employed first. This involves gentle neck stretching exercise routines, relaxation therapy as well as adequate analgesia and occasionally muscle relaxants. Modification of their work place may also help posture. Over 50% of patients will benefit with this type of conservative therapy and avoid surgery. Those patients who fail to improve and in whom symptoms are severe enough to affect their ability to work or carry out social activities should be referred for surgery. There is much controversy regarding the optimal surgical procedure for relieving the symptoms. While current debate is largely focused on whether a transaxillary or supraclavicular approach for resection of the first and/or cervical rib gives better results, other procedures are well described such as total scalenectomy. A supraclavicular approach is best suited to repair a concurrent aneurysm and occasionally resection of the middle third of the clavicle is necessary to gain better access to the subclavian artery. Simple post-stenotic dilation does not necessarily warrant reconstruction and should be managed on an individual basis. In many cases, the dilatation reverts to normal once decompression has been achieved.

There is much variation in the reported post-operative outcome, whichever procedure is used. This can be attributed to varying patient selection for surgery, combined with the lack of scientific methods for quantifying symptoms and outcome. The success rate for TOS surgery regardless of technique is in the range 43–78%. In the authors' experience of 61 patients undergoing 83 transaxillary rib resections, 74% reported an improvement in symptoms at a median of 4 years following surgery of which 58% had complete resolution.

Transaxillary first rib resection

Under general anaesthesia, the patient's thorax is positioned at 60° and an assistant supports the arm, applying traction to open up the axilla and allow clear visualization of the structures. An incision is made along Langer's lines at the lower border of the axillary hairline. During axillary dissection the intercostobrachial nerve is identified and preserved. Division of the superior thoracic artery and vein allows full exposure of the first rib and its related structures. Scalenus anterior is divided at its insertion, avoiding damage to the phrenic nerve and pleura. Scalenus medius is then carefully dissected from the rib, avoiding damage to the nerve to serratus anterior. The isolated rib is then divided close to the transverse process and sternum, taking care to avoid damage to the T1 root (Figure 30.22). The space so created allows resection of a cervical rib when appropriate.

Aneurysmal disease

Aneurysms are uncommon in the upper limb and are most frequently a result of trauma, both iatrogenic (Figure 30.23) and non-iatrogenic. Other causes such as atherosclerosis, Takayasu's disease and fibromuscular dysplasia are less common. In the vast majority of cases, patients are symptomatic on presentation, especially in the case of aneursym of the larger vessels. Embolization to the brain or arm is a common mode of presentation. Larger aneurysms may also present with upper limb and chest pain or neurological compromise through compression of neighbouring structures. Rarely, upper limb aneurysms, particularly atherosclerotic or traumatic cases, present as a rupture. The most common site for

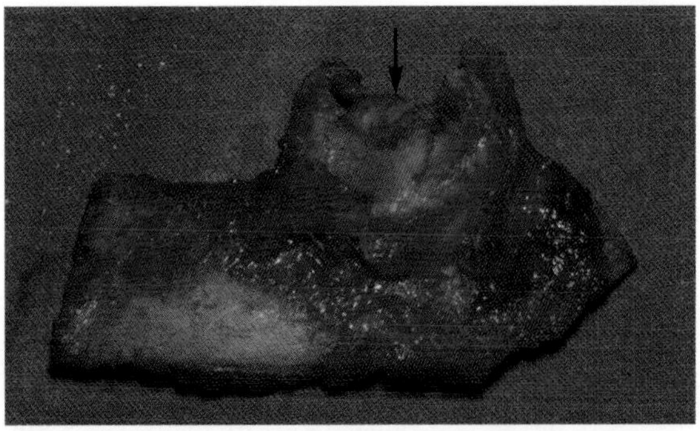

Figure 30.22 First rib resection. The attachment of scalenus anterior tendon to the scalene tubercle is clearly seen (arrow).

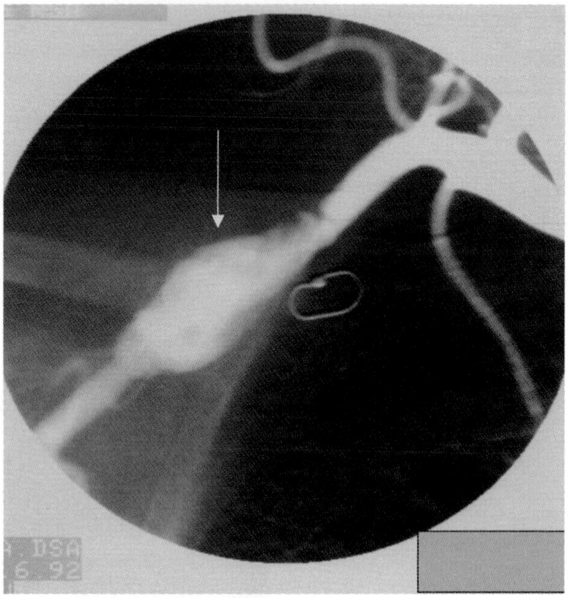

Figure 30.23 Aneurysm of subclavian vein graft for subclavian artery aneurysm 28 years post-surgery (yellow arrow).

non-traumatic upper limb aneurysms is the subclavian artery followed by the innominate artery. Amongst the causes are thoracic outlet obstruction (for distal subclavian artery aneurysms) and atherosclerosis, which is the underlying aetiology in up to 50% of proximal and mid subclavian artery aneurysms. While the incidence of an aberrant subclavian artery is less than 1%, it remains an important site of a subclavian artery aneurysm. Often patients will present with signs of obstruction to either the oesophagus, trachea or neck veins. Furthermore, these aneurysms have a greater propensity to rupture.

Distal vessel disease (vasospastic and small vessel occlusive disorders)

Small artery vasospastic disease is by far more common than occlusive disease. Maurice Raynaud first reported Raynaud's syndrome in 1888 as 'episodic digital asphyxia due to arterial insufficiency'. However, since then it has become readily apparent that symptoms and signs of this syndrome covered a wide variety of aetiologies from the benign vasospasm that is never associated with tissue loss to the connective tissue disorders with small vessel occlusive lesions. While some have divided this syndrome into two subcategories, Raynaud's phenomenon and Raynaud's disease or primary and secondary Raynaud's, the division is somewhat arbitrary. Indeed, late manifestation of an associated systemic disease in patients originally diagnosed as primary Raynaud's has been reported up to two decades following initial presentation. A classification of conditions associated with Raynaud's syndrome is listed in Table 30.1. These groups of patients have diffuse obstructive small vessel disease within the palmar and/or digital vessels and by far the most common underlying aetiology is the connective tissue disorders.

Table 30.1 Conditions associated with Raynaud's syndrome

Connective tissue disorders	Scleroderma
	Systemic lupus erythematosus (SLE)
	Mixed connective tissue disease
	Rheumatoid arthritis
	Dermatomyositis
	Polymyositis
	Sjögren's syndrome
Vasculitis	Polyarteritis
	Hypersensitivity vasculitis
	Giant cell arteritis
	Takayasu's arteritis
	Drug induced vasculitis
Obstructive disease conditions	Thoracic outlet syndrome (TOS)
	Atherosclerosis
	Buerger's disease
Drugs	Beta-blockers
	Ergot containing drugs
	Cytotoxic drugs
Occupational	Vibration injury
	Exposure to vinyl chloride
	Arterial trauma
Miscellaneous	Cryoglobulinaemia
	Cold agglutinins
	Polycythaemia
	Neoplasia
	Heavy metals
	Nicotine
	Hypothyroidism
	Hemiplegia

The theoretical mechanisms that are thought to be active in patients with Raynaud's syndrome include increased sympathetic nerve activity, increased density of alpha-adrenoreceptors in digital vessels as well as increased basal levels of endothelin-1. More recently interest has focused on the deficiency of calcitonin gene-related peptide (CGRP), which is an endogenous vasodilator. In addition, prostaglandins as vasoconstrictors and nitric oxide as a potent vasodilator have also been implicated.

The true incidence of this syndrome is difficult to ascertain, however, it has been reported that it can be found in up to 25% of young adults living in countries with a cool climate. Young females under the age of 45 years are predominantly affected. Furthermore, various occupational factors predispose individuals to Raynaud's syndrome, particularly those involved with vibratory tools.

Symptoms experienced as a result of exposure to cold or emotional stimuli include an initial pallor in one or more fingers of both hands up to the metacarpal phalangeal joints and seldom more proximal. This is soon followed by cyanosis and finally a hyperaemic rubor. Patients do not always demonstrate this classical triphasic colour changes and may indeed only experience an initial pallor or a biphasic response. Associated with these colour changes are symptoms of coldness, pain and paraesthesia. Symptoms usually settle within 15–20 min. Approximately 50% of patients will experience these symptoms in their hands alone while a further 50% get symptoms in both their fingers and toes. Very seldom are symptoms solely in the toes.

Diagnosis

Diagnosis of Raynaud's syndrome is based on clinical history and examination. On close questioning, it is usually possible to ascertain a history of episodic vasospastic attacks precipitated by cold or emotional stimuli. Other symptoms of systemic illness may also be revealed such as arthritis, skin rash, myalgia and dysphagia. Examination should specifically search for signs of arthritic changes, sclerodactyly, telangectasia and skin rashes as well as for evidence of past or present digital ulceration and gangrene.

Non-invasive investigations have been discussed earlier and are invaluable in the diagnosis of this syndrome and in the differentiation between primary or secondary Raynaud's. In brief, no one test is 100% specific and sensitive but a combination of investigations, including capillary microscopy, thermography and cold challenge testing using PPG, may assist the clinician in the diagnosis and direct future therapy. Also these non-invasive modalities aid in monitoring the progress of the disease.

The role of angiography in the management of Raynaud's syndrome is not for assessing the digital vessels but mainly to exclude pathologies in the proximal vessels that may be contributing to the symptoms and may be amenable to reconstruction. These include subclavian aneurysms, proximal vessel stenoses and TOS. In the case of the latter, a thoracic outlet radiograph is useful.

In addition to the usual haematological blood tests, specific serological tests are useful in identifying an underlying cause of Raynaud's syndrome. These include markers for systemic illness such as erythrocyte sedimentation rate, which is usually elevated in patients with connective tissue disorders and vasculitis, antinuclear antibodies (ANA), anti-centromere antibodies (ANCA), rheumatoid factor, cold agglutinins and cryoglobulins.

Treatment

In most cases, the best course of treatment is avoidance of any initiating factors such as cold weather by wearing thermal gloves and socks. An understanding that further vasoconstriction by specific drugs and nicotine should be avoided is important. Also behavioural therapy in the form of biofeedback has proved promising in selected groups of patients.

However, in patients where conservative therapy is not adequate, then first line medical treatment includes calcium channel blockade with drugs like nifedipine. While this is reported to be useful in select groups of patients by reducing smooth muscle tone, the side-effects of headaches and postural hypotension prevent up to a quarter of patients from continuing on this treatment.

Prostaglandin analogues have been used for the treatment of those cases resistant to the above treatments. Results have been variable with a benefit in acute and prolonged attacks by intravenous infusions. Newer oral formulations have yet to be tested in formal trials.

Other pharmaceutical drugs that have been used at some time or other for the management of symptoms have included angiotensin-converting enzyme inhibitors, alpha-blockers and vasodilators such as nitroglycerine. While there are theoretical benefits with all these agents, as yet results are not consistent and side-effects of some of these drugs are prohibitive in a substantial number of people.

Surgical treatment options for resistant and severe symptoms of Raynaud's syndrome are limited to thoracic sympathectomy, as distal vessel reconstruction and local denudation of small vessel adventitia have produced generally unsatisfactory results.

While thoracic sympathectomy was commonly used for symptomatic relief of angina, its use is more common for the treatment of upper limb disorders such as ischaemia and hyperhidrosis as well as for facial blushing. It can be performed as an open procedure using a transaxillary, supraclavicular or extrapleural approach. However, more frequently an endoscopic approach is used. Results are variable with some patients having relief of symptoms for several years. In others the effect lasts for a few months with symptoms slowly returning thereafter.

Acknowledgements

We are grateful to Dr A. L. Herrick and Mrs T. L. Moore at the Rheumatic Diseases Centre, University of Manchester, Hope Hospital and Helena Boddil and Charis Richards, from the Vascular Laboratory at Manchester Royal Infirmary, for their valuable contribution to the section on non-invasive investigations.

Further reading

Baguneid, M. *et al.* (1999). Management of acute non-traumatic upper limb ischemia. *Angiology* **50**: 715–20.

Fulford, P. E., Baguneid, M. S., Ibrahim, R. *et al.* (2001). Outcome of transaxillary rib resection for thoracic outlet syndrome – a 10 year experience. *Cardiovasc Surg* **9**: 620–4.

Machleder, H. I. (1998). *Vascular Disorders of the Upper Extremity*, 3rd edn. Armonk, NY: Futura.

Rutherford R. B. (1977). *Vascular Surgery*, 5th edn. Vol. 2, Section XI, Chapters 78–87. Philadelphia, PA: W.B. Saunders.

MODULE 31

Vascular access surgery

Chronic haemodialysis as a practical treatment for endstage renal failure only became a reality in the 1960s despite the commercial availability of dialysis machines since 1956. These could only be used for intermittent dialysis in patients with acute renal failure whose renal function was expected to recover. Access to the blood stream was by a 'cut-down' on an accessible artery and vein and insertion of glass cannulae which were heparinized and sealed after each session. The expected life span of this form of access was at most 10 days. The limiting factor therefore, was reliable long-term access to the circulatory system.

The introduction of a Teflon–silicon rubber (Silastic) external arteriovenous shunt in 1960 by Scribner and his colleagues provided a solution. Tapered Teflon cannulae with Silastic extensions were inserted into the radial artery at the wrist and the adjacent cephalic vein. Dialysis sessions lasted from between 24 and 60 hours at a time and were performed every 4 to 21 days. Despite the common complications of infection thrombosis and haemorrhage, long-term survival was possible. Of the original four cases reported, one died of cardiac disease 11 years later and another survived 8 years on dialysis until successfully transplanted.

The external shunt was superseded in 1966 when Brescia, Cimino and co-workers in New York described the creation of an internal arteriovenous fistula by a side-to-side anastomosis of the radial artery at the wrist and the cephalic vein. Arterialization of the proximal arm veins allowed repeated insertion of dialysis needles and dialysis blood flows in excess of 400 ml/min. This remains the primary procedure of choice and the 'gold standard' by which alternatives are compared.

The external shunt continued to be used for acute access until suitable long-term catheters were developed in the late 1970s and early 1980s. The introduction of a single lumen Silastic catheter by Broviac in 1973 for parenteral nutrition led to development of larger catheters with multiple lumens (Hickman 1979, Francis 1983, PermCath 1985) which were capable of providing sufficient blood flows to be a practical alternative in haemodialysis. The technological advances in catheter design have been matched by the expanding number of clinical applications which now include adjuvant chemotherapy, stem cell harvesting for bone marrow transplantation, chemoprophylaxis for infection, administration of blood products and total parenteral nutrition as well as blood monitoring.

Section 31.1 • End-stage renal disease statistics

Over the past 20 years there has been a major expansion in the provision of health care for renal failure patients. This is most clearly seen in wealthy developed countries such as the USA and Japan, with much smaller incidence rates in western Europe and Australia. The incident rate in the USA in 1997 was 296 patients per million population (pmp) per year while in the UK, and in particular England, the take on rate was estimated at 89 pmp. The increase in new end-stage renal disease (ESRD) patients in the UK has been slower than in the USA, increasing from 55 pmp in 1988 to 89 pmp in 1997. This is mainly due to the increased uptake of patients over 65 years of age, now comprising 43% of new cases. It was realized during the 1980s that patients over the age of 65 years tolerate dialysis as well as younger patients and provided they receive adequate dialysis their survival rates did not differ significantly from age-matched individuals without renal failure. The resistance to treating this group, particularly in the UK, reflected limited health care resources but

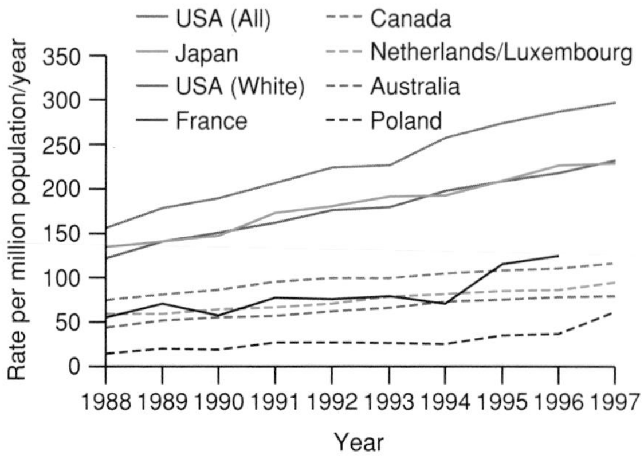

Figure 31.1 International comparison of the incidence of new end-stage renal failure patients, 1988–97. (Source: United States Renal Data System Annual Report 1998.)

with improved funding for renal replacement therapy growth has been rapid and is predicted to continue at between 8 and 10% per annum, which will double the numbers on dialysis within 7 years. Similar trends are being observed throughout western Europe and are most pronounced in the wealthier northern European countries with Germany, France and the Benelux countries reporting incidence rates of between 100 and 140 pmp/year (Figure 31.1).

As expected, the aetiological causes in the over 65s are related to the ageing process, notably hypertension, atherosclerotic reno-vascular disease and more importantly type II diabetes. Diabetic patients (types I and II) account for approximately 17% of patients presenting with ESRD in the UK but the proportion is increasing. In some units diabetes accounts for 30% of new cases and almost all are type II. The situation is more extreme in Europe with regions such as Alsace and Lower Necker reporting incidences of over 50 pmp/year, i.e. comparable to figures for whites in the USA. The reason appears to be that type II diabetes is becoming more common because of an ageing population and that the survival of these patients has greatly improved over the past 15 years with many now living

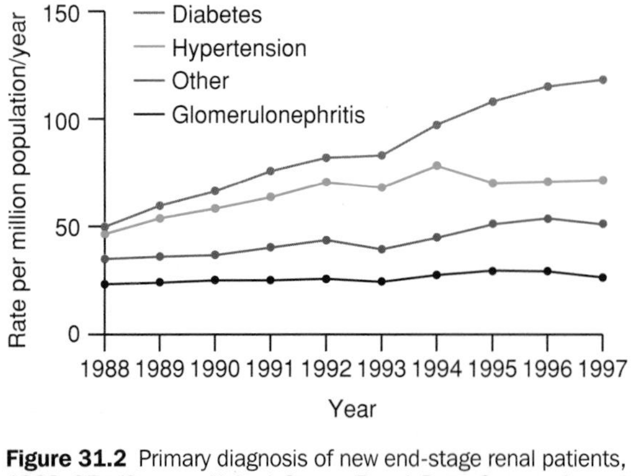

Figure 31.2 Primary diagnosis of new end-stage renal patients, 1988–97. (Source: United States Renal Data System Annual Report 1998.)

long enough to develop ESRD. However, because of comorbid conditions such as cardiac disease, peripheral vascular disease and obesity relatively few type II diabetics are suitable for renal transplantation and are destined to remain on dialysis for the remainder of their lives (Figure 31.2). The implications are that the need for vascular access surgery will more than double in the next 10 years with proportionately more elderly and diabetics with pre-existing vascular disease adding to the complexity of procedures required and presenting a challenge in maintaining vascular access.

Importance of the quality of vascular access to haemodialysis adequacy

The effectiveness of dialysis is dependent on adequate removal of fluid and solutes such as urea, creatinine and other undetermined small molecular weight molecules as well as correction of acid base balance and mineral concentrations. How this is achieved is known as the dialysis prescription and is individual to each patient. Factors affecting delivery of the prescribed dose relate to the amount of time on dialysis, i.e. number of sessions per week and length of session, size of dialyser and permeability of the membrane, dialysate fluid characteristics and flow rate, and blood flow rate. The efficiency of dialysis is primarily determined by the removal of urea and with it other low molecular weight toxins, and the concept of urea kinetics has developed to enable accurate calculation of the desired 'dialysis dose'.

Two aspects have particular importance to the vascular surgeon:

- calculation of urea clearance
- estimation of re-circulation.

Haemodialysis removes urea principally by diffusion from blood into the dialysate fluid. Many kinetic models have been developed but the most commonly used is the variable volume, single pool model which in its simplest form derives to

$$\ln C_t/C_0 = K_d \times t_d/V$$

where C_t is the post-dialysis urea concentration, C_0 is the pre-dialysis urea concentration, K_d is the dialyser clearance (ml/min obtained from manufacturer), t_d is the treatment time (min) and V is total body water in ml (0.6 × body weight).

In practice, the prescribed urea clearance ratio K_t/V is rarely achieved. Clinical guidelines suggest that there should be a minimum K_t/V of 1.2. If urea clearance falls below this level an adjustment in the dialysis prescription is required. Because the volume of distribution of urea (V) is essentially fixed for a given patient, K_t/V can be increased only by increasing the urea clearance (K_d) by increasing the blood flow or by prolonging the treatment time (t_d) (Table 31.1). Increasing the treatment time has major logistical implications for dialysis units as well as not being popular with patients. It is important to verify that the prescribed dialyser urea clearance is being achieved. Actual blood flow rates are frequently

Table 31.1 Example of the calculation of dialysis requirement

Example: 70 kg man dialysed with a dialyser clearance of 245 ml/min at a blood flow of 300 ml/min

$$-\ln C_t/C_0 = K_d \times t_d/V$$

Total body fluid volume (V)	=	$(70\,\text{kg} \times 1000) \times 0.6 = 42\,000\,\text{ml}$
Dialyser clearance (K_d)	=	245 ml/min
Pre-dialysis [urea] (C_0)	=	40 mmol/l
Post-dialysis [urea] (C_t)	=	10 mmol/l

$$-\text{logn}\ (10/40) = (245 \times t_d)/42\,000 = 1.38$$

Required dialysis time (t_d) = 237 min

less than that displayed by the dialysis machine, particularly at higher flow rates, leading to lower than expected urea clearances (Figure 31.3).

Re-circulation is the return of dialysed blood from the venous line directly back, via the arterial line, to the dialyser, bypassing the systemic circulation, thereby diluting waste-rich undialysed blood and compromising the efficiency of dialysis. Falsely high re-circulation rates may result from placing the arterial and venous needles too close together or by inadvertent reversal of the blood lines but given that there are no technical errors the significance of re-circulation in the clinical situation is that it may be a warning of pending access failure. Re-circulation as a result of access dysfunction may be caused by either inadequate arterial flow (arterial disease, anastomotic stenosis or poor cardiac output) or venous obstruction (stenosis or thrombosis). The blood pump on the dialysis machine will attempt to draw blood at the set rate. If inflow is inadequate,

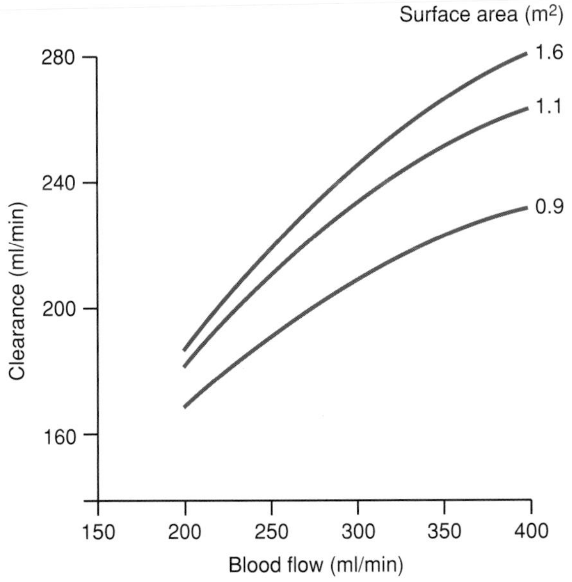

Figure 31.3 Illustration of the dependence of urea clearance on access blood flow for three different surface areas of dialyser. Standard dialysate flow of 500 ml/min.

returned dialysed blood will be drawn back into the dialysis circuit and similarly with a venous stenosis dialysed blood is prevented from rapid return to the systemic circulation and is drawn back into the arterial limb of the circuit.

A false negative result may be obtained if the venous return needle is placed proximal to a stenosis effectively using the dialysis circuit to bypass the lesion. In this circumstance reversal of the blood lines will clarify the situation. Blood now drawn from the vein proximal to the stenosis will have a low inflow and the venous return will be to the vein distal to the lesion, i.e. closer to the arteriovenous anastomosis and will have a high resistance to flow as measured by the pressure monitor.

Classically, re-circulation is determined by the equation:

$$\text{Access re-circularization} = \frac{(P-a)}{(P-v)} \times 100$$

where P is the systemic concentration of urea usually taken as a venous sample from the contralateral limb, a is the arterial blood line concentration of urea and v is the venous blood line concentration of urea.

This 'three needle technique' has been criticized because during dialysis venous blood has a higher urea concentration than systemic arterial blood. This inaccuracy is thought to arise by removal of excess body fluid during dialysis (ultrafiltration) leading to progressive peripheral vasoconstriction and slowing of venous blood flow allowing more time for urea to diffuse into the venous blood; in addition there is a lower concentration in arterial blood because of cardiopulmonary re-circulation. In this latter situation dialysed blood is returned to the heart, transits the lungs and returns to the arteriovenous access without passing through major tissue beds.

A newer validated method for measurement of access blood flow uses an indicator dilution technique, with the indicator being the change in ultrasound velocity induced by the dilution of blood with normal saline. Saline injected into the venous blood line if re-circulated will appear in the arterial line where the dilution results in a change in the velocity of ultrasound transmission. With clinical equipment the proportion of blood re-circulated is automatically calculated. Any reading in excess of 10% is considered clinically significant and warrants investigation.

The utility of these techniques is in the ability to detect access dysfunction before it progresses inevitably to total occlusion and thrombosis. Poorly functioning or failure of access has a major impact on the morbidity and mortality associated with ESRD. Numerous peer-reviewed studies have confirmed the association between the adequacy of the delivered dose of haemodialysis and patient survival. It has been estimated that for every 0.1 higher K_t/V up to a value of 1.2, mortality is reduced by 7%. This is now regarded as the recommended minimum though in practice is achieved in less than 70% of patients.

Vascular access dysfunction is now the leading cause of admission to hospital with approximately 25% of dialysis patients annually requiring treatment for catheter associated sepsis, revisionary surgical procedures or thrombolysis. As such, it has a substantial impact in terms of cost and labour as well as disrupting elective surgery and dialysis schedules.

Section 31.2 • Clinical strategy and assessment

In an ideal situation all chronic renal failure patients should have some form of permanent access established and matured prior to reaching a requirement for dialysis. In most patients who are referred from a chronic renal failure programme the rate of progression of renal disease has been monitored and a prediction of end stage can be made reasonably accurately. In patients with good quality arteries and veins and an expected high initial success rate, the fistula should be created about 2 months before it is needed. Those with evidence of arterial disease or damaged veins should be assessed at least 6 months prior to needing dialysis to allow time for investigation, surgery and possible slow development. The importance of allowing sufficient maturation cannot be overemphasized. A fistula in an active young adult male with prominent vessels will mature within 6 weeks but the majority of patients will take 2–3 months. Early needling causes haemorrhage, venous rupture, perivascular scarring and progression to stenosis or occlusion.

Unfortunately, 30–40% of patients reaching end stage do not come through a chronic renal failure programme and present acutely with signs and symptoms of severe uraemia or with cardiac embarrassment. These patients require immediate inpatient assessment and establishment on haemodialysis usually through temporary central venous catheters. Despite prompt treatment these patients are generally more debilitated, have multiple comorbid conditions and are more likely to be elderly. Reports from European registries suggest that these 'late referrals' have a 2 month mortality approaching 25%. There is no reliable method of differentiating potential survivors from those who will succumb. Therefore creation of permanent vascular access should be delayed until they are stable and established on outpatient haemodialysis. Priority may then be given to them by virtue of having a temporary central venous catheter because of the high frequency of complications associated with this mode of access.

In general, survival on dialysis is improving but the patients are increasingly elderly or diabetic and vascular disease whether pre-existing or arising *de novo* will lead to some failures in the medium to long term. Planning suitable access must therefore take into account the individual condition of each patient to optimize primary success rates but also to preserve options for likely subsequent access procedures.

Table 31.2 Strategy for vascular access placement

1. Access should be created in the upper limbs
2. The non-dominant arm should be the first option
3. Access should be constructed as distally as possible
4. The cephalic vein in the forearm is preferred
5. Avoid venepuncture or cannulation in **both** arms in renal failure patients
6. For central venous access use the internal jugular or femoral veins

Several principles apply in vascular access surgery and are applicable to all patients irrespective of age, aetiology or mode of presentation (Table 31.2). Access should preferentially be created in the upper limbs to reduce the incidence of infection and as distally as possible to preserve more proximal sites for subsequent procedures. Accessibility of the fistula or graft is important to facilitate needling but also for patient comfort. The cephalic venous system, which runs subcutaneously on the radial side of the forearm and arm, is preferred as this allows the arm to rest in a semi-prone position. Additionally, the non-dominant arm should be the first option as immobilization during dialysis will be less inconvenient to the patient. It should be made aware to the patient at the earliest opportunity of the need to avoid venepuncture or cannulation in *both* arms. Medical and nursing staff at all levels of seniority and not only within the field of nephrology need to be made aware of the need to preserve veins of any patient with chronic renal failure. Much damage however antedates the development of renal failure. If central venous access is required, the internal jugular or femoral veins are preferred. The subclavian vein should be not be used if possible because of the high incidence of thrombosis (up to 50%). Stenosis or occlusion will preclude the use of the ipsilateral limb for subsequent access.

It should be possible to create an autologous arteriovenous fistula in the majority of patients presenting for primary vascular access. The decision to be made is where to place a fistula in order to maximize the chance of successful development. Clinical examination is sufficient in the vast majority of cases in determining the patency of the cephalic venous system. With a tourniquet applied to the upper arm it should be possible to see or palpate the vein from the radial side of the wrist to the elbow where it gives off a large median cubital branch before continuing up the lateral aspect of the arm. Difficulties arise when the vein is not palpable throughout its length. This is common in obese patients and in those who have an history of venous cannulation. Occasionally, the cephalic vein dilates well just above the wrist and then disappears to re-form from side branches a few centimetres proximally. Spasm of the vein to this extent is uncommon and a stenosis or occlusion should be presumed. If the anatomy cannot be accurately defined it is essential to have upper limb venography performed with imaging of the whole length of the cephalic venous system to its confluence with the axillary vein. If there is any history of central venous catheterization the central veins should also be included to exclude a central stenosis. The basilic vein which originates at the ulnar aspect of the wrist and passes up the medial side of the forearm is more commonly spared from venepuncture or cannulation. Although not as convenient for needling, the ulnar-basilic fistula can provide satisfactory flows and is underutilized.

Arterial quality is as important as venous integrity. The artery chosen for formation of an arteriovenous fistula must be capable of dilatation and high blood flow. The blood flow in the normal radial artery is 20–30 ml/min rising to 200–300 ml/min following formation of an arteriovenous fistula and up to 1200 ml/min in a mature fistula. Small vessels or those affected by atherosclerosis or diabetes will never enlarge sufficiently to sustain flow. Clinical evidence of marginal flow is easily determined by hardness with lack of compressibility on palpation of the artery, a weak pulse, pallor of the hand and poor capillary return. If there is any doubt Doppler flow measurements should be performed. Collateral circulation from the ulnar artery may be clinically assessed by Allen's test but absence of ulnar arterial flow does not preclude the formation of a radio-cephalic fistula. However, if present the risk of digital ischaemia is reduced.

Section 31.3 • Central venous access

The principal sites are the jugular and femoral veins. Subclavian veins should not be used unless other sites are contraindicated. Access via subclavian veins has a higher insertion complication rate and results in thrombosis of the vein in up to 50% of cases. This precludes the use of the ipsilateral limb for any further access procedure (Figure 31.4).

The external jugular vein is formed by the confluence of the posterior facial and posterior auricular vein. It lies superficial to the sterno-mastoid muscle and passes inferiorly across the posterior triangle before entering the deep fascia approximately 2 cm above the clavicle. It is usually of small calibre and is only useful for insertion of thin-walled Silastic catheters such as Hickmann or Port-a-Cath. These types of catheters because of their flexibility should ideally be placed with X-ray screening as malposition is not uncommon.

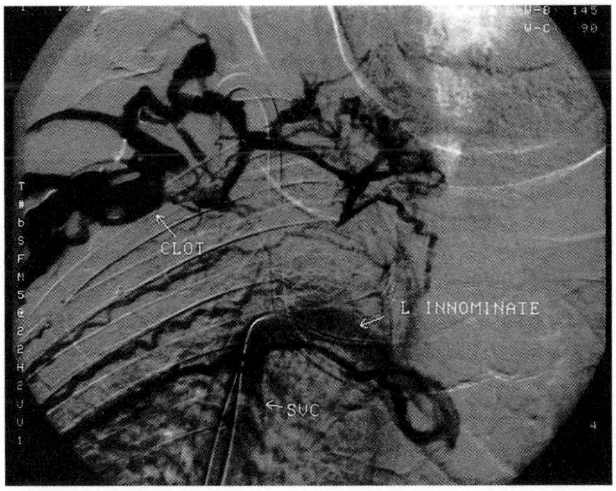

Figure 31.4 Venogram of right arm: view of central veins showing occlusion of subclavian vein secondary to previous subclavian insertion of central venous catheter. Note extensive intercostal collaterals.

The internal jugular vein is the preferred insertion site for the larger catheters required for haemodialysis and is used for both temporary and permanent venous access. The right side is generally preferred because of its short straight course to the superior vena cava and right atrium reducing the incidence of misplacement. Most catheters are inserted by a percutaneous technique. The patient is placed in a Trendelenburg position and the introducer needle is inserted at a 45° angle to the skin surface just lateral to the carotid pulsation between the sternal and clavicular heads of the sterno-mastoid muscle and directed towards the ipsilateral nipple. Following venepuncture a guidewire is fed down the lumen of the needle over which track dilators and a peel away introducer sheath are advanced. Location of the internal jugular veins has been simplified by the introduction of hand-held real-time ultra-sound devices with a guide channel along which the introducer needle may be advanced. This is particularly recommended in patients who have had a number of catheter insertions because scarring may distort the normal anatomical arrangement. Repeated passes in an attempt to locate the vein increase the likelihood of traumatic injury to structures in the thoracic outlet. Temporary access catheters which are semi-rigid are inserted directly over the guidewire through the neck incision and are held in place by either a skin suture or an adherent dressing. Permanent Silastic cuffed catheters are tunnelled from the lateral chest wall to the neck incision and fed into the peel-away sheath. Occasionally, in patients who have exhausted all peripheral access and had repeated central venous cannulae, it is advisable to perform an open insertion of a dialysis catheter. Vein stenoses or angular distortion may prevent accurate placement of a guidewire and passage of a rigid track dilator or peel-away sheath may be misdirected. Forceful attempts at insertion may rupture the jugular vein or more seriously cause open penetration into the mediastinum or pleura. The approach through the sterno-mastoid heads has usually been used previously and therefore a more cephalic skin incision should be made to enter virgin tissue.

Complications of central venous access

It has been estimated that the major complication rate for central venous access approaches 10% and is directly related to the experience of the operator. Most occur at the time of insertion and are the consequence of technical failure or iatrogenic injury. Renal failure patients more than any other group of patients are subjected to multiple catheter insertion and removal, usually because of infection or thrombosis. Trauma caused by these procedures or inflammation associated with the infection and physical intra-luminal damage may result in distortion or stenosis of the jugular or central veins. Careful assessment of past patient history and operative records should alert the operator to potential problems.

The use of percutaneous techniques has gained universal popularity because they substantially reduce operating time and are available to physicians, and radiologists as well as surgeons. However, it must be realized that virtually all the complications reported have been with this technique. The potential for major vascular injury is substantial with catheters that are used for dialysis; some, for example PermCath, are over 5 mm in diameter. The blind insertion of a guidewire and rigid dilators is acceptable in a patient presenting for the first time with virgin tissues but if it is a repeat catheterization it is prudent to use ultrasound location of the jugular vein and X-ray screening for placement of the guidewire and catheter. If difficulties are encountered, the operation should be abandoned in favour of an open exploration and placement under general anaesthetic. On no account should an attempt be made on the contralateral side until a pneumothorax has been excluded.

The list of reported complications is extensive (Table 31.3); these have resulted in considerable morbidity and occasional mortality. Monitoring of the patient during the intra- and post-operative period is recommended and a post-operative chest X-ray is mandatory. The elderly and those with cardiac or respiratory disease are at greatest risk and prompt recognition of complications may be life saving.

Table 31.3 Complications of central venous access

1. Catheter malposition
2. Venous:
   (a) Venous laceration
   (b) Air embolism
   (c) Subcutaneous haematoma
3. Arterial:
   (a) Arterial laceration
   (b) Traumatic arteriovenous fistula
   (c) Carotid/subclavian pseudo-aneurysm
4. Thoracic:
   (a) Pneumothorax/tension pneumothorax
   (b) Haemo-thorax
   (c) Haemo-mediastinum
   (d) Hydro-thorax
   (e) Thoracic duct laceration
5. Cardiac:
   (a) Right ventricular infarction
   (b) Cardiac tamponade
   (c) Dysrhythmia
6. Neurological:
   (a) Brachial plexus injury
   (b) Phrenic nerve injury
   (c) Vagus nerve injury

Pneumothorax

Puncture of the pleura and lung with the introducer needle is the commonest complication. It usually occurs when multiple passes have been made in an attempt to locate the jugular (or subclavian) vein. The diagnosis is generally made with the post-operative chest X-ray in those without respiratory compromise. Those with less than 15% lung collapse and no symptoms may be managed conservatively. Large pneumothoraces can occur if an apical bulla has been ruptured and may progress to a tension pneumothorax with respiratory distress and cardiovascular collapse. If the pneumothorax is large, with or without symptoms, the safest course is to insert a chest drain.

Haemorrhage

A minor haematoma is to be expected as the inserted catheter is slightly smaller than the peel-away sheath through which it is introduced. Local pressure and sitting the patient up is sufficient treatment. More serious bleeding may be caused by forceful dilatation resulting in splitting of the jugular vein. Deaths from cerebral infarction have been reported following posterior rupture of the jugular vein causing retropharyngeal haematomata with compression of the common carotid artery. Dilators and the peel-away sheath or semi-rigid temporary catheters should be advanced gently over the guidewire with a rotating action and preferably a number of graded dilators should be used.

The soft J-tipped guidewires are probably not responsible for many perforating injuries, these being more likely with straight guidewires. The wire should pass easily without resistance and confirmation of the correct placement of the guidewire in the right atrium by X-ray screening is preferred. If screening is not available advancement into the right side of the heart may elicit electrocardiogram (ECG) abnormalities which will confirm its position, but the wire should be immediately withdrawn a few centimetres until the dysrhythmia settles.

Most injuries result from forceful insertion over a misplaced or coiled guidewire. Venous bleeding into the mediastinum is usually self-limiting but if the rupture is into the pleural cavity free bleeding may occur. A chest X-ray will confirm the presence of fluid and, if significant or progressive, a chest drain must be inserted to allow lung re-expansion and prevent clot formation. If drainage persists endovascular stenting of the superior vena cava (SVC) or a thoracotomy and repair will be required. It must be emphasized that the dilator and peel-away sheath used for Silastic catheter insertion need only be introduced into the jugular vein and should not be advanced into the central veins. The tips of temporary dialysis catheters, however, have to be placed at the junction of the SVC and the right atrium and care must be taken not to advance the catheter too far. Tears in the right atrium with haemo-pericardium and cardiac tamponade have occurred. Cardiovascular collapse may rapidly ensue and tamponade must be treated immediately by pericardiocentesis or a pericardial window. If this does not resolve the situation a formal repair via a median sternotomy will be required.

Commonly the carotid artery is punctured while locating the jugular vein. Provided a small gauge needle is used for initial localization digital pressure for 5 min will suffice. Puncture with the large-bore introducer needle or worse with a dilator will cause substantial damage requiring open repair or endovascular stenting. Pseudo-aneurysm formation and carotid-jugular fistulas have been reported even after unsuspected arterial injury.

Air embolism

The Trendelenburg position and high central venous pressure in fluid loaded renal patients makes air embolism a relatively uncommon complication during insertion of central lines. Forced inspiration during a coughing fit when the catheter is about to be fed down the peel-away sheath will cause a massive influx if it is not rapidly occluded with a finger. No indwelling cannula should be left open to the air for more than a fraction of a second. It is more common for massive air influx to occur from a split in the catheter tubing caused by either degeneration or sharp damage during removal of adherent dressings. Mortality from air embolism is directly related to the size of the embolus and the rate of entry. Volumes of air greater than 50 ml cause hypotension and dysrhythmias whereas 300 ml of air can be rapidly fatal. A large volume of air in the right atrium can cause an air lock which leads to obstruction of the right ventricular outflow tract, decreased venous return and decreased cardiac output. Clinically significant venous air embolism presents with respiratory distress followed by cardiovascular collapse. Bronchoconstriction is often an early feature and may result from release of vaso-active substances causing an increase in airway pressure, and wheezing. Air in the pulmonary circulation causes microvascular occlusion resulting in effectively increased dead space causing hypoxia and hypercapnia. If the patient is anaesthetized and being monitored a fall in end tidal CO_2 will be recorded. Hypotension, cardiac dysrhythmias and cardiovascular collapse follow. The classic finding of a 'millwheel murmur' indicates a massive air embolism and cardiovascular collapse is imminent.

Treatment of air embolism is largely supportive. FiO_2 should be increased to 100%. The blood pressure should be supported with fluid and vasopressor agents. Positioning the patient in the left lateral decubitus position will help to keep air in the right atrium from entering the ventricle. If the right atrial catheter is *in situ* it should be aspirated until no more air can be obtained. If closed methods of resuscitation are to no avail with progression to a cardiorespiratory arrest, a left anterolateral thoracotomy with right ventricular needle aspiration and cardiac massage will be necessary. Despite intervention the mortality is still approximately 50%.

Nerve injuries

Nerve injuries, and in particular brachial plexus injuries, have become less common since the use of the subclavian approach for central venous access has been discouraged. Temporary sensory dysfunction can occur as a consequence of local oedema or haematoma but permanent injury is rare. Trauma to the vagus, recurrent laryngeal or phrenic nerves is unusual because of their small size and posterior position relative to the internal jugular vein.

Infection

Silastic cuffed central vein catheters are increasingly being used as permanent vascular access in elderly patients or those who have exhausted all surgical options. They are popular with patients and nursing staff because connection for dialysis is via a simple Luer-lock. There is no maturation period, no needling and very little skill required in their management. Unfortunately in common with all intra-vascular devices they are prone to clotting and are a pathway for introduction of bacteria with a very high risk of becoming infected, complications which often require their premature removal.

The incidence of serious infective complications has been reported as 3.9 per 1000 patient catheter days. Effectively, 40% of patients have a significant bacteraemia within 9 months and of those affected 20–25% will develop major complications or die.

Catheter-related infection is commonly categorized as exit site, tunnel or bacteraemia. Exit-site infection is defined as a localized reaction with no systemic symptoms and negative blood cultures. There may or may not be a purulent exudate. The treatment is to take a swab for culture, empirically treat with anti-staphylococcal antibiotics and await sensitivities. There is no need to change the catheter unless there is a worsening of the local signs or a failure to respond to treatment. Tunnel infection is infection above the Dacron cuff but with negative blood cultures. Because there is no barrier between the infection site and the vein, inevitably the infection will progress to bacteraemia. It is best to arrange early replacement at a different site. Presentation of catheter-related bacteraemia ranges from low-grade spiking fever to rigors and septic shock. The exclusion of other causes of sepsis is imperative but can often be inconclusive. However, attributing all systemic infection to the catheter will result in unnecessary loss of vascular access. Two methods have been developed to distinguish between catheter related and other sources. Endoluminal brushings may help in detecting bacteria adherent to the lumen walls or in the biofilm around the tip of the catheter. This method has a reported sensitivity of 95%. Secondly, simultaneous blood cultures may be taken from the catheter and also from a peripheral site. The time taken to obtain a positive culture is recorded and if the catheter-derived specimen produces a positive result more than 2 hours in advance of the peripheral specimen this may be designated as the infection source. Specificity and sensitivity have been reported to be 100 and 96%, respectively.

Attempts have been made to reduce the number of infective episodes associated with catheters. Results are on the whole inconclusive. The route of infection differs depending on the duration of insertion. Infection originating from the track generally occurs early before incorporation of the cuff into surrounding tissue providing a physical block, while hub and lumen contamination, which account for the majority of infections, reflect poor aseptic technique. Topical application of antiseptics such as povidone-iodine or Mupirocin around the exit site, impregnation of the cuff with silver sulphadiazine and avoidance of impermeable adhesive dressings have all been shown to be beneficial. Bonded coatings to catheters using bacteriostatic agents such as rifampicin, minocycline or silver sulphadiazine have been reported to reduce the incidence of bacteraemia.

Thrombosis

Occlusion, whether partial or complete, is the commonest long-term complication of central vein catheters. The mean patency is between 68 and 84 days. Early dysfunction presenting as poor or intermittent flow is due to incorrect placement and is entirely preventable with X-ray screening. Late flow problems are related to thrombosis and may be considered as either extrinsic or intrinsic.

Extrinsic thrombosis occurs as a result of damage to the venous endothelium. Predisposing factors include the size of the catheter relative to the vessel, length of time it has been *in situ*, composition of the catheter, presence of infection or any condition causing hypercoagulability. Most are asymptomatic because of the extensive venous collateral network in the neck and shoulder, and only discovered when repeat catheterisation fails or when formation of an arteriovenous fistula results in major swelling of an ipsilateral limb. The diagnosis is confirmed by duplex ultrasound or venography.

Thrombosis of the catheter itself, either intra-luminal or around the catheter tip, is not particularly common and is due to inadequate filling with heparin. The intra-luminal clot is easily displaced by aspiration while the clot localized at the tip may be part of a much larger clot that cannot be aspirated. Instillation of 5000 IU of urokinase into the catheter lumen will dissolve part of the clot as it diffuses out. The success rate is 40–50% and the benefit is only temporary as the clot will rapidly re-form.

The most frequent cause of catheter occlusion is the formation of a fibrin sheath that encases the catheter from its entry at the venotomy site to the tip where it acts as a flap valve. It often presents with decreasing flows followed by an inability to withdraw blood while retaining the ability to infuse fluids. Because of the extent of the sheath and its location on the outer surface of the catheter heparin or urokinase intra-luminal locks cannot be expected to have a prolonged effect. Systemic urokinase infusions were introduced in the early 1990s and the use of high dose infusions (125 000 IU per lumen over a 2 hour period) has raised the success rate to around 80% with one infusion and 99% with two. Patients who require repeated infusions should be commenced on warfarin to maintain the International Normalized Ratio (INR) between 1.5 and 2.5. In patients in whom thrombolysis or warfarinization is contraindicated mechanical stripping may be attempted. An endovascular loop inserted via the femoral vein is used to ensnare the catheter. The stripped fibrin sheath is embolized to the lung. Initial results have been acceptable but recurrence has been common.

Section 31.4 • Arteriovenous fistulas

Autologous arteriovenous fistulas are recognized as closest to the ideal form of vascular access that is likely to be achieved. They have a low infection rate, are capable of supplying blood well in excess of the 400 ml/min required for dialysis and, once established, are not prone to thrombosis even at low flow rates caused by hypotension or rapid ultrafiltration.

Demographic changes in many countries have seen a rise in the proportion of patients aged over 65 years and in those presenting for renal replacement therapy the proportion is even greater. Many present with histories of repeated hospital admissions for whatever cause and inevitably in this interventionist age peripheral veins have been irreparably damaged. An absolute requirement for successful fistula formation is uninterrupted venous outflow. Multiple stenoses or occluded segments in the forearm cephalic vein from previous intravenous access preclude the formation of distal fistulas. The principle is that access should be created as distally as possible initially preserving proximal sites for future procedures (Table 31.4).

Distal arteriovenous fistulas

Forearm fistulas may be fashioned by direct anastomosis of either the radial or ulnar arteries to a suitable

Table 31.4 Preferential order of vascular access procedures

Primary procedure	
Non-dominant arm	Radio-cephalic fistula (wrist) Snuff box fistula Radio-cephalic fistula (forearm) Ulnar-basilic fistula (wrist) Brachio-cephalic fistula Brachio-basilic fistula with transposition of vein
Dominant arm	Repeat above list
Secondary procedure	
	Straight forearm PTFE graft (radial artery to patent ante-cubital vein) Looped forearm PTFE graft (brachial artery to patent ante-cubital vein) Upper arm PTFE graft (brachial artery to proximal basilic, cephalic or axillary vein) Looped PTFE graft femoral artery to saphenous or femoral vein)

adjacent vein. Distal fistulas have a higher primary failure rate (7–27%) than more proximal fistulas or polytetrafluoroethylene (PTFE) grafts, primarily because of thrombosis or failure to develop. Studies with duplex ultrasound on the influence of the vessel size on subsequent patency have shown that success is significantly more likely (8.3% primary failure) if the artery diameter is >2 mm and the vein diameter is >2.5 mm.

The radiocephalic arteriovenous fistula is the preferred procedure. It may be performed under local anaesthesia as a day case. A longitudinal incision of about 5 cm is made roughly midway between the cephalic vein and the radial artery at the wrist. The distal cephalic may be left intact if a side-to-side anastomosis is planned, which is the classic Brescia-Cimino, but most divide the vein to perform an end vein to side artery anastomosis. The advantage of this method is that the extent of mobilization is reduced and there is no risk of venous hypertension in the hand. A small feeding tube is passed up the vein to test its patency with instillation of heparinized saline. If an unsuspected venous stenosis is found it may be repaired with a vein patch angioplasty through an overlying incision. Not all surgeons give heparin but the authors have found that 2000 IU intravenous is sufficient to prevent thrombus formation in the artery prior to resolution of vessel spasm.

The artery is located under the deep fascia which is easily recognizable by its transverse fibres. Care must be taken to avoid damage to the lateral branch of the superficial radial nerve as it emerges from under the brachioradialis tendon. Damage will affect sensation of the dorsum of the thumb. The artery is mobilized by gently separating it from the venae commitantes which surround it like a plexus. Only 1.5–2 cm of artery need be mobilized and flow is controlled by Silastic slings. An 8–10 mm longitudinal arteriotomy is made and the anastomosis commenced at the proximal corner and heel of the vein using a double-ended 6/0 polypropylene suture. If a thrill is not felt following restoration of flow there is a likely technical problem. This may be due to rotation of the vein, or angulation of artery or vein and a check should be made that both lie in an easy curve with no compression. Alternatively, it may be due to thrombus formation in the proximal artery. In this event the anterior wall anastomosis should be taken down, patency of all limbs confirmed and proximal and distal arterial lumina irrigated with heparinized saline. Frequently one finds that a bruit may be heard once the patient is mobile and may reflect resolution of vessel spasm or an increase in blood pressure.

In patients who have had a previously functioning radiocephalic fistula that has failed, a more proximal anastomosis may be performed. The vein is kept patent by collaterals usually within 5–8 cm of the old anastomosis. The radial artery in the distal forearm lies under the brachioradialis tendon and in some patients this may need to be partially divided but in most, adequate mobilization of both the artery and vein will allow anastomosis. In this situation the outflow vein is already arterialized and may be accessed within 2 weeks.

The snuff box fistula is constructed by anastomosis of the radial artery where it lies between the tendons of extensor pollicis longus and brevis and the overlying cephalic vein. It is less commonly created as a first choice because in many the radial artery is of insufficient size, but can be successful particularly in adult males. Of the reported series, patency rates of 65% at 1 year and 45% at 5 years have been achieved. Of those that failed, 45% could still have a radiocephalic fistula constructed.

The ulnar-basilic fistula is much underused because it is perceived as being more technically difficult and the developed fistula is not as convenient to needle. The artery lies on flexor digitorum profundus with the ulnar nerve on the medial side and therefore the basilic vein requires more mobilization to reach it. The vein is more thin walled than the cephalic with multiple branches and is easily damaged. If the ulnar artery is poorly developed or a pulse is absent and the basilic vein is of good calibre it may be mobilized throughout its length in the forearm and tunnelled subcutaneously across to the radial artery.

Proximal arteriovenous fistulas

Proximal autogenous arteriovenous fistulas are formed at the ante-cubital crease by anastomosis of either the cephalic, median cubital (cephalic) or basilic veins to the brachial artery. Indications for a primary fistula at this site include diseased distal arteries, occluded forearm veins or as a secondary procedure following failure of a distal fistula. The disadvantage of using the brachial artery is that excessive fistula flow will result in steal from both the radial and ulnar arteries rendering the hand ischaemic. The arteriotomy should be limited to 5–6 mm in length.

The brachiocephalic fistula is preferred because the cephalic vein is subcutaneous throughout its length on the antero-lateral aspect of the arm which facilitates needling for dialysis. The median cubital when present joins the laterally placed cephalic venous system to the basilic system and overlies the brachial artery. It may be divided proximally and anastomosed end to side to the artery perfusing the cephalic system alone. Valves are not usually found within this segment except where the median vein of the forearm vein enters the cubital fossa. At this confluence there is usually a large calibre perforating vein connecting to the deep system. If left intact it will enlarge substantially and delay development of the fistula.

The forearm cephalic should be left in continuity if possible because as the venous complex dilates under arterial pressure the valves will become incompetent allowing retrograde perfusion of the proximal forearm cephalic, increasing the area of vein available for needling. Alternatively, if there is a long patent segment of forearm cephalic, the valves may be disrupted with a valvulotome passed to the distal forearm and retrieved via a cut down. The lower venotomy is then closed. This retrograde fistula has not found much favour because of the high incidence of venous hypertension and oedema.

In the absence of a median cubital vein it may be possible to mobilize the proximal forearm and distal arm cephalic in continuity, performing a side-to-side anastomosis to the brachial artery or end to side using the divided perforating vein. If it is not possible to perform a tension free side-to-side anastomosis the cephalic vein may have to be divided, with loss of potentially useful forearm vein, and swung across end to side on the artery. A recently reported alternative is to interpose a short length of 6 mm PTFE between the artery and the vein. One and 3 year primary patency rates of 85 and 67%, respectively have been reported.

Frequently the cephalic vein is not well developed, presenting initially high outflow resistance with a high probability of failure. A side-to-side anastomosis of the median cubital and brachial artery will allow flow into both the cephalic and basilic systems maintaining patency while the cephalic enlarges. The preferential drainage and therefore development will be via the larger basilic system. This may be retarded by placing a restriction band of loosely tied suture material around the median cubital vein proximal to the anastomosis. The risk is that if it is applied too tightly it can cause the vein to thrombose.

Brachio-basilic arteriovenous fistula with vein transposition

Brachio-basilic fistulas are increasing in popularity as an alternative to prosthetic grafts. The basilic vein by virtue of its short subcutaneous path before it enters the deep fascia rarely has suffered iatrogenic damage and its large capacitance is capable of sustaining high flow rates. The procedure is similar to formation of a brachiocephalic fistulas except the proximal median cubital is anastomosed to the brachial artery. The short subcutaneous segment is only suitable for single needle dialysis. The remainder lies under the deep fascia alongside the neurovascular bundle, too deep for safe needling. The classical single-stage management is for the vein to be mobilized throughout its length, detached at the elbow and tunnelled in a loop anteriorly and superficially being anastomosed to the brachial artery at a convenient level (Figure 31.5).

The two-stage procedure is initially to form the arterivenous fistula in the usual manner and leave the vein to arterialize for about 6 weeks. The second stage involves mobilization of 12–15 cm of the vein up towards the axilla and transposing it in continuity into a more anterior and superficial plane. The deep fascia is closed underneath it to prevent retraction. The advantages of this latter method are the vein is more durable and less easily damaged and spiral rotation cannot occur. Reported patency rates at 1 year and 2 years of 86 and 73% are typical.

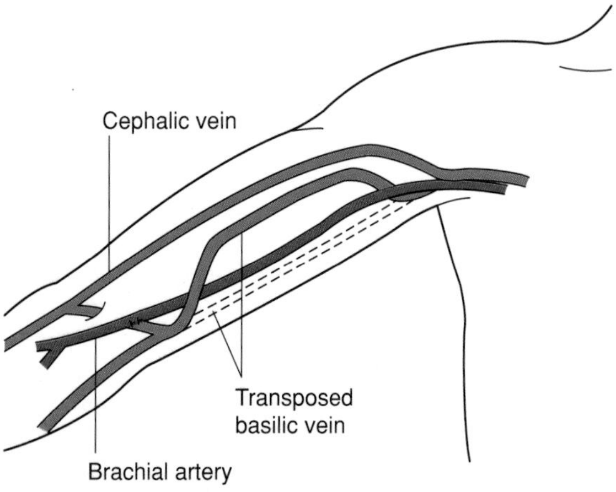

Figure 31.5 Diagram of brachio-basilic vein transposition arteriovenous fistula.

Section 31.5 • Interposition grafts

Interposition grafts are used to form an arteriovenous conduit between anatomically discrete regions. As the sites of inflow and outflow are determined by the surgeon the permutations are enormous and only limited by the ingenuity of the surgeon. They may be derived from autogenous vein, usually saphenous, or more commonly one of a variety of prosthetic materials. There are fundamental differences in the application of these grafts in Europe and North America. European surgical practice in the main reserves interposition grafts for patients in whom all autogenous arteriovenous fistula sites have expired while in North America there is a strong tendency to use them as a primary access procedure. Comparison of outcomes therefore must be approached with caution.

Graft materials

Interposition grafts for haemodialysis were first described in 1969 when autogenous saphenous vein was used as a forearm loop graft from the brachial artery to an ante-cubital vein. It is still used for this purpose but the indications for its use have become less clear with the advances made in synthetic and biological grafts. The advantage of autogenous vein was its better primary patency, i.e time to first revision, and a much reduced incidence of infection compared to biological or synthetic grafts. It has the disadvantage of requiring a second operation site for retrieval, it is prone to stenosis at needle puncture sites and of course it is variable in size and quality. Most surgeons would now limit its use to thigh loop grafts, the distal end being looped around to the superficial femoral artery with the sapheno-femoral junction left intact. Another consideration should be whether it is likely to be needed for coronary bypass grafting.

Similar 12 month cumulative patency (~70%) has been reported for saphenous vein, PTFE, bovine carotid artery and human umbilical vein. The latter two were prone to aneurysm formation and to dissolution if infected and are no longer used. Newer heterografts using bovine mesenteric vein and the most recent polyurethane prosthetic graft are both claimed to perform better than PTFE. The flexibility afforded to the surgeon by a graft that can be produced in different lengths, lumen diameter, wall thickness and tapered conformations has seen PTFE being adopted as the interposition graft of choice.

Choice of site

The site chosen for insertion of an interposition graft follows the same principles as placement of arteriovenous fistulas, namely upper limb and start as distally as possible. These considerations are more apposite with prosthetic grafts because of their propensity to infection, which is difficult or even impossible to eliminate, and intimal hyperplasia at the venous anastomosis which occurs in all cases eventually requiring proximal revision. Prosthetic grafts require a greater blood flow to maintain patency than arteriovenous fistulas. Flows less than 750 ml/min after construction are associated with a 50% thrombosis rate within 6 months. Placement of a graft onto a small or diseased artery which is incapable of sufficient dilatation will fail. Flow according to Poiseuille's law is dependent on the diameter and length of the graft. The longer the graft the greater the diameter required to achieve the same flow. The diameter however has to be tailored to the size of the vessel to make anastomosis practical and must be large enough to be easily located and needled with 15 G dialysis needles. If too large a diameter graft is used the resistance in the graft will be substantially less than the distal artery and blood will preferentially flow into the graft resulting in distal ischaemia. The standard size used in the upper limb is 6 mm but tapered versions 4 mm arterial to 7 mm venous are available.

Straight forearm graft

The use of straight grafts in the forearm is best reserved for failed radiocephalic or ulnar-basilic fistulas that have a well developed distal radial or ulnar artery. An occasional patient with obliterated forearm veins may have a sufficiently large radial artery to warrant an attempt as a primary procedure. The venous anastomosis should be to a large ante-cubital vein just distal to the elbow crease so as not to interfere with future arteriovenous fistula placement at this site. The graft preferably should be tunnelled subcutaneously as a gentle curve along the radial border of the forearm towards the ante-cubital fossa. This allows the patient to maintain the forearm in a neutral position during dialysis.

Looped forearm graft

The decision to use a forearm loop graft is not as clear cut. If the vessels are capable of sustaining a prosthetic graft in most cases it is possible to form a brachio-cephalic or brachio-basilic fistula which has superior long-term patency. Any surgical intervention in this area must be considered with the prospect of further explorations and revisions being required. It should be considered in: (1) grossly obese patients in whom no vessels are palpable and (2) those with an occluded cephalic vein but well developed forearm basilic vein just distal to the elbow. It may be possible to create an arteriovenous fistula in an obese patient but the primary requirement is that the arterialized outflow vein should be easily palpable for needling. Vein transposition or superficialization works well in the upper arm and may be considered as a subsequent procedure to a subcutaneous forearm loop.

Veins in the ante-cubital fossa should be left intact so as not to jeopardize future fistula formation and the venous anastomosis should be performed distal to the elbow crease. Drainage can often be obtained via the proximal forearm cephalic running off via a large perforating vein or median cubital or alternatively via the basilic vein in the upper forearm.

Brachio-axillary graft

If the upper arm veins have been previously used for access a more proximal venous anastomosis to the axillary vein is often possible. The patency and size of the vein should be determined in advance, especially if there is a history of central venous cannulation or signs of collateral venous circulation. Grafts originating from the brachial artery should be anastomosed as distally as possible on the vein, preferably just proximal to the confluence of the basilic, brachial and cephalic. If any of these is of a substantial size they should be used preserving axillary vein for future use. Results with this graft have been excellent due to the high flow and low resistance run-off. In some patients it may be necessary to restrict inflow with a tapered graft because of potential distal ischaemia. An upper arm loop graft from the origin of the brachial artery to the axillary vein is another option if the distal brachial has been used for previous access attempts.

Groin access grafts

If upper limb access sites have been exhausted use of the lower limb vessels should be considered. The larger vessels in the groin are capable of sustaining higher flows and an 8 mm diameter graft is most commonly used. While this may provide excellent flow for dialysis purposes it may render the distal limb ischaemic if there is pre-existing distal vascular disease. Pulse pressures should measured and if the ankle–arm index is less than 0.8 an arteriogram should be obtained and remedial procedures, such as angioplasty, performed to improve inflow. Larger grafts based on the femoral vessels have a particular benefit in patients who are prone to hypotensive episodes which lead to thrombosis of the smaller lower flow grafts in the upper limb.

The common configurations are:

- superficial femoral artery to sapheno-femoral junction (SFJ) loop graft
- superficial femoral artery to femoral vein loop graft
- distal superficial femoral artery to SFJ straight graft.

If possible the graft should be tunnelled towards the lateral side of the thigh and of sufficient length to facilitate needling as far away from the groin crease as possible. Infection remains the main drawback of grafts in this region with between 10 and 35% subsequently becoming infected from needling.

Alternative configurations

Numerous other permutations are possible and are only limited by the ingenuity of the surgeon. Among those described are axillary artery to contralateral axillary vein, axillary artery to femoral vein, femoral artery to contralateral saphenous or femoral vein and iliac artery to axillary vein. None of these is widely used and enthusiasm for esoteric arrangements has to be tempered by consideration of how to manage subsequent complications as, and indeed when, they arise.

Section 31.6 • Complications of arteriovenous access

Complications arising from vascular access procedures are common and are associated with considerable morbidity and occasional mortality. It has been estimated that over 20% of the prevalent renal failure population require inpatient hospital treatment each year for access-related problems. The majority of these relate to infection and thrombosis. Units in which a there is a greater dependence on central venous catheters or prosthetic shunts for arteriovenous access have a significantly greater revision workload than those who primarily use autogenous arteriovenous fistulas.

Thrombosis

Thrombosis of fistulas or prosthetic shunts is the most frequent complication of arteriovenous access though the incidence, timing and aetiology differ between the two groups. Complications are generally subdivided into early (within 30 days) and late (beyond 30 days). Early thrombosis occurs more frequently with autogenous arteriovenous fistula and the majority of these occur within the first 5 days. In established units with dedicated surgeons few of these can be ascribed to operator error but represent a multitude of factors many of which are difficult to predict. Quoted early failure rates range between 7 and 27% with 10–15% being the norm.

Most surgeons rely on clinical assessment of the patient to decide where to place the fistula or graft. Pre-operative radiological evaluation by venous mapping or venography has not been shown to be cost effective except in cases with specific clinical indications such as those with a history of multiple venous cannulation or those requiring access revision. Frequently at operation the vessels are found to be patent but of inadequate size (artery <2 mm or vein <2.5 mm), limiting flow or, as in the elderly and diabetic population, atherosclerosis of the artery may result in insufficient pressure to maintain patency. Passage of a 6 Fr umbilical catheter up the vein often reveals an unsuspected stenosis and despite being able to infuse heparinized saline, outflow is restricted. These justify exploration and repair if limited in extent. Re-exploration of a fistula created with suboptimal vessels that fails within hours of surgery is not indicated. Grafts are subject to the same limitations as fistulas but the outflow vein needs to be >4 mm in diameter and in patients prone to hypotension long-term anti-coagulation should be considered.

An increasing number of patients presenting for access surgery are already established on dialysis via temporary catheters and have anaemia corrected by erythropoietin replacement. They have usually had dialysis within the previous 24 hours with substantial amounts of fluid ultra-filtrated to achieve their 'dry weight' in an attempt to control hypertension. These patients are in a hyper-coagulable state and uraemic coagulopathy cannot be relied upon to maintain fistula or graft patency. Intra-operatively every patient receives heparin i.v. (2000 IU for fistula, 3500 IU for grafts) and post-operatively patients should be maintained at least 1 kg above their normal 'dry weight' and not be ultra-filtrated greater than 2 litres at any dialysis session for the first 2–3 weeks. If they are non-compliant with oral fluid restrictions with large inter-dialytic weight gain they may require daily dialysis/ultrafiltration in the short term to control fluid overload.

Late thrombosis

Native fistulas, once established, have a superior long-term patency compared to prosthetic grafts (Figure 31.6). The commonest cause of dysfunction in either fistulas or grafts is venous stenoses, though the site of occurrence differs. Fistulas are prone to two types of venous stenosis: (1) within 10 cm of the arteriovenous

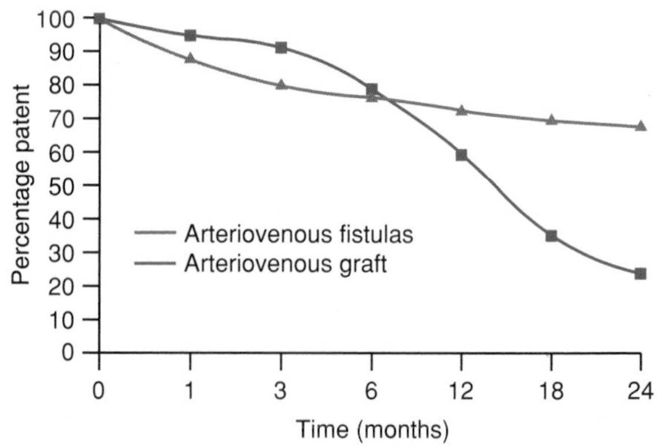

Figure 31.6 Patency of arteriovenous fistulas versus prosthetic arteriovenous grafts over a 24 month period.

anastomosis and (2) more commonly at needle puncture sites, while prosthetic grafts almost invariably develop venous anastomotic stenoses and less commonly intra-graft stenoses. In both cases previous central venous cannulation may give rise to stenoses in the subclavian vein. Normal dialysis pressures may be maintained if there is adequate run-off via collateral veins but with high flow fistulas or arteriovenous grafts based on the brachial artery distal venous hypertension is common. Arterial stenosis in both types of access is relatively uncommon.

Stenosis occurring in proximity to an arteriovenous fistula anastomosis tends to occur within a few months of formation and often before it has been used for dialysis. It tends to be progressive eventually leading to thrombosis. The cause is unknown but turbulent flow causing intimal hyperplasia or damage to the vein by stripping of adventitia during mobilization has been suggested. This type of stenosis may account for some of the 10% of cases that have poor development (Figure 31.7).

The vast majority of native fistula stenoses relate to injury of the arterialized vein. Needling the vein before it has had adequate time to hypertrophy causes perivascular bleeding and fibrosis; recurrent needling at 'easy' sites has the same effect. Probably the commonest cause of thrombosis is unskilled personnel transfixing the vein during access causing a 'blow-out' characterized by extensive bruising which leads to compression of the vein, markedly reduced fistula flow and thrombosis (Figure 31.8).

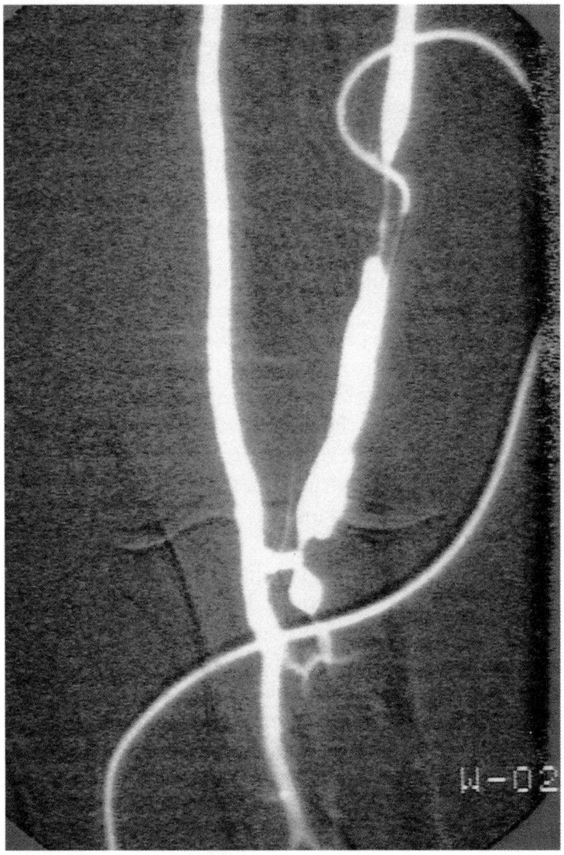

Figure 31.8 Fistulogram of brachio-cephalic arteriovenous fistula showing peri-anastomotic stenosis and critical proximal stenosis caused by needling injury.

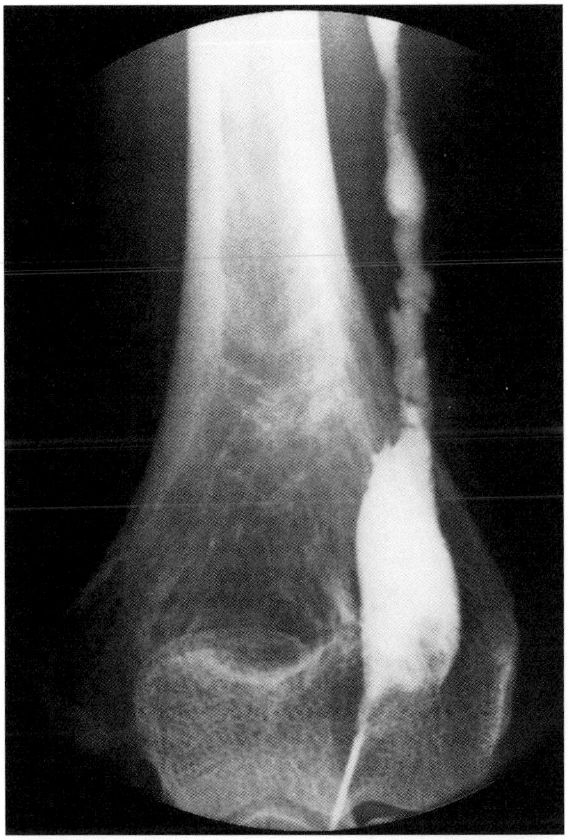

Figure 31.7 Fistulogram of left arm brachio-cephalic arteriovenous fistula. Note peri-anastomotic venous dilatation with more proximal multiple stenoses secondary to intimal hyperplasia.

There are fewer problems related to needling of prosthetic grafts as their path is predictable and easily palpable. However, repeated needle puncture of the same area can give rise to intra-luminal organized laminated clot which disturbs flow and is thrombogenic. Fibrosis eventually leads to luminal narrowing and thrombosis.

Venous stenoses, whether anastomotic or in the outflow tract, are the primary cause of prosthetic graft failure (0.5–1.3 events per patient year) and are the main reason why grafts have a poor primary patency rate compared to arteriovenous fistulas. Neointimal hyperplasia leads to progressive occlusion with associated increase in resistance and fall in flow leading eventually to thrombosis. Clinical features that suggest the development of a stenosis are prolonged bleeding from needle sites, difficulties in needling, a change in character of the associated thrill or bruit and, with more proximal stenoses, oedema of the limb may be a feature. These are all late features and the emphasis recently has been on the assessment of surveillance methods for early detection of stenoses. The weight of evidence favours monitoring the functional status of the graft whether by venous pressure changes, access blood flow, efficiency of dialysis (K_t/V) or percentage re-circulation. Selection of patients at risk on the basis of intragraft venous pressure alone has been shown to reduce the thrombosis rate to 0.2 episodes per patient year. Studies which have controlled for venous pressures have shown that a more sensitive predictor of graft stenoses is a progressive reduction in flow rates measured by ultrasound dilution methodology. Clinical guidelines from North America now recommend monitoring arteriovenous fistulas every 2 months and arteriovenous grafts monthly. The indications for angiography in arteriovenous fistulas are an access flow within 100 ml/min of the dialysis circuit blood flow and for grafts an access flow less than 650 ml/min. A drop in flow greater than 20% from baseline in either case carries a greater than four-fold relative risk of subsequent access failure.

Prevention of stenosis by pharmacological intervention has not been investigated to any great extent in dialysis patients. The limited evidence available is that drugs that inhibit vascular smooth muscle proliferation, e.g. dipyridamole, are beneficial while anti-platelet drugs such as aspirin are beneficial in the post-operative period only and subsequently (beyond 3 months) have a detrimental effect. It has been proposed that by its effect on the cyclo-oxygenase pathway aspirin promotes the production of 12-HETE which is a potent inducer of vascular smooth muscle cell proliferation. A number of trials are under way which will hopefully clarify this issue.

Treatment of stenosis and thrombosis

The aim of early detection and repair of venous stenoses is to maintain good quality dialysis, preservation of access vessels and prevention of thrombosis. Treatment of stenoses and thrombosis of fistulas or grafts may be by surgical or radiological intervention. The indications for radiological intervention have not been clearly defined but results in selected cases can approach those of surgical management.

Surgical management of thrombosis or stenosis

Ideally, stenoses should be detected and corrected before thrombosis occurs. The majority of stenoses in autologous arteriovenous fistulas occur in proximity to the arteriovenous anastomosis while with prosthetic grafts the predominant site is at the graft-venous anastomosis. Unfortunately most patients still present following acute thrombosis. The emphasis should be on a rapid correction of the underlying problem and restoration of arteriovenous blood flow with minimal disruption of dialysis schedules and avoidance of central venous catheters if possible.

Stenosis occurring at or within a few centimetres of a radiocephalic or ulnar-basilic anastomosis are best dealt with by forming a new fistula just proximal to the obstruction. This preserves the matured draining vein and allows early re-use. Longer stenotic segments arising within the first 10 cm should also be managed by a new proximal anastomosis or in some cases if there is normal vein immediately adjacent to the arteriovenous anastomosis a 6 mm PTFE 'jump graft' may be inserted from normal peri-anastomotic vein to normal proximal vein beyond the diseased segment. More often florid intimal hyperplasia is found extending from the anastomotic site and it is better abandoned in favour of a more proximal site. If thrombosis has occurred in an autologous arteriovenous fistula surgical thrombectomy with a Fogarty balloon catheter via a transverse venotomy may restore flow. Thrombus present for more than 6 hours is usually very adherent and difficult to clear by mechanical means alone. Instillation of urokinase or tissue plasminogen activator (t-PA) into the efferent vein with a dwell time of 5–10 min followed by repeated balloon thrombectomy has a higher rate of clearance. Once outflow is restored, on-table angiography should be performed to determine the underlying cause. Occasionally no clinically significant stenosis is found and thrombosis may be attributed to hypotension, excessive ultrafiltration or prolonged compression of needle sites following dialysis.

Stenoses related to needling sites are not as common as one would expect given the repeated trauma the vein is subjected to. Short fibrous stenoses, associated with peri-venous scarring caused by haematoma, do not respond well to angioplasty. There is a high early failure rate with this technique due to elastic recoil and stenosis recurrence. They can be repaired by a vein patch angioplasty (Figure 31.9) or if longer (>2 cm), bypassed with a PTFE 'jump graft' (Figures 31.10 and 31.11). Significant pre-stenotic dilatation may allow the use of a larger 8 mm graft which will maximize flow to the draining vein. Occasionally, if it is a mature fistula the draining vein may be tortuous and it may be possible to mobilize the vein sufficiently to excise the stenotic segment and perform an end-to-end anastomosis abrogating the need for prosthetic material. Multiple stenoses in forearm veins are best managed by a PTFE graft from the radial artery to a suitable large

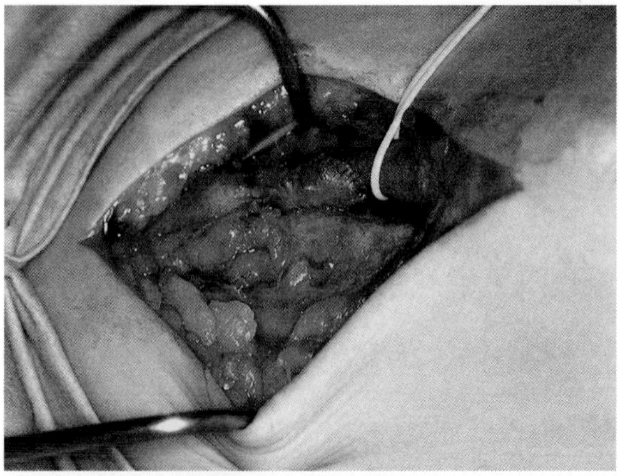

Figure 31.9 Vein patch angioplasty repair of proximal stenosis shown in Figure 31.8.

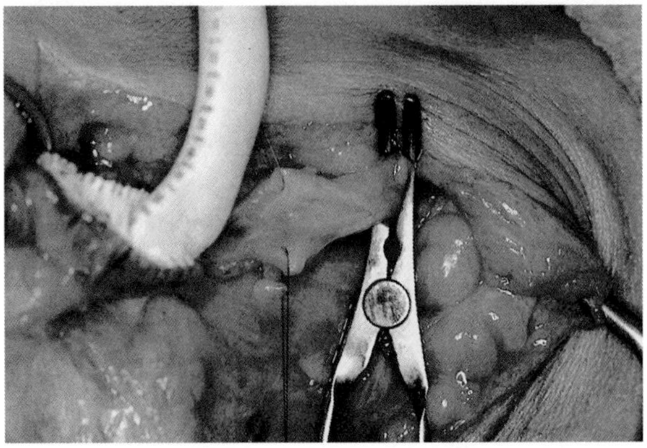

Figure 31.10 Repair of venous stenosis by 6 mm PTFE 'jump graft'. Proximal anastomosis completed and graft retracted to show pale fibrous stenosis.

vein in the ante-cubital fossa provided that arterial inflow is sufficient. If not, a new fistula based on the brachial artery will be necessary.

In a small number of cases intimal hyperplasia may result in total occlusion of the proximal radial artery, the matured vein being kept patent by retrograde flow from the palmar arch. This flow is usually inadequate for dialysis but may be augmented by a 6 mm PTFE bypass graft from the brachial artery to the distal cephalic vein. Needling should be restricted to the venous component. An alternative is to perfuse the vein retrogradely by anastomosis of the median cubital vein and the brachial artery or interposition of a short segment of 6 mm PTFE between the brachial artery at the elbow to adjacent matured cephalic vein. Flow will be directed both distally, because of incompetent valves, which may be used as arterial supply, and proximally which may be used for venous return. Provided the graft is not used for needling, 1 and 5 year primary patencies of 85 and 48% have been reported.

Stenoses occurring close to arteriovenous anastomoses in the ante-cubital fossa are more difficult to refashion because the length of superficial vein is limited or patent segments lie too far from the brachial artery for direct anastomosis. When the artery and vein do not lie in close proximity a 'jump graft' of 6 mm PTFE may be interposed between brachial artery and more proximal cephalic vein or alternatively one may opt for formation of a brachio-basilic fistula with transposition of the vein to a more superficial and anterior position.

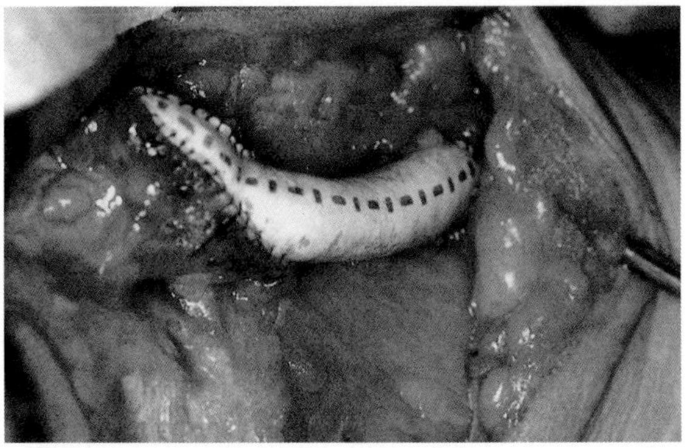

Figure 31.11 Completed repair of stenosis shown in Figure 31.10.

Approximately 50% of prosthetic grafts will fail within 18 months and in 70% of cases the cause is a venous anastomotic stenosis with arterial stenosis, infection and pseudo-aneurysm accounting for the remainder. Unless a surveillance programme has detected a rise in intra-graft pressure or increasing recirculation, the majority present with graft thrombosis. The primary treatment is a surgical thrombectomy with angiography to delineate inflow, outflow and intra-graft stenoses which may be multiple in up to 36% of cases. Acceptance of return of arterial inflow or venous backflow as an indication of adequate treatment is unreliable with between 40 and 50% of haemodynamically significant stenoses being missed. Simple thrombectomy has a patency rate of only 10% at 120 days while intra-operative angiography will detect 90–95% of underlying stenoses and will define any residual thrombus. Invariably as some form of revision is necessary, both the arterial and venous anastomoses should be exposed with thrombectomy performed through a transverse incision close to the venous anastomosis. The arterial limb can be opened in a similar manner if there is difficulty in dislodging the arterial anastomotic plug.

Intimal hyperplasia at the arterial anastomosis forms as a ring, progressively occluding the proximal and distal artery as well as the graft mouth. Repair requires a patch angioplasty extending from normal artery on both sides of the anastomosis as well as widening the graft lumen. Failure to include the distal artery will create a low resistance outflow through the graft and poor distal flow, rendering the distal limb ischaemic. The patch should be of PTFE or bovine pericardium to preserve vein (particularly saphenous) for future access.

Radiological treatment of stenosis and thrombosis

Interventional radiology has become an accepted alternative to surgical management of dysfunctional vascular access. Perceived benefits include less invasive procedures, preservation of the patient's veins and the convenience of day case procedures. The published reports are predominantly from North America and therefore reflect the current emphasis on prosthetic grafts for dialysis access. Relatively few European centres have reported their experience with percutaneous management of autologous arteriovenous fistulas stenosis or thrombosis.

Angiographic detection of stenoses in peripheral veins can be more difficult than in arteries because of widely variable calibre, multiple vessels, superimposition or tortuosity. The most reliable method is to perform pull back pressure measurements from the SVC to the arterial anastomosis. Differences of more than

50% in systolic pressure across a segment indicate the presence of a functionally significant stenosis. The presence of collateral circulation on the arterial side of the stenosis may reduce the pressure difference but the presence of collaterals, particularly in the subclavian region, should alert the radiologist to a likely underlying stenosis. Agreement has yet to be reached concerning the need for dilatation of asymptomatic stenoses. American guidelines suggest that angioplasty should be performed in stenoses greater than 50% when there is a history of access thrombosis or if there is evidence of re-circulation, raised venous pressure or an unexplained decrease in dialysis dose.

Standard techniques of percutaneous angioplasty are employed with the exception that access stenoses because of their rigidity almost invariably require high pressure or even cutting balloons. Balloon diameters approximately 1 mm greater than the adjacent normal vessel are used initially, though larger ones can be used if there is residual stenosis after repeated inflation. Upper arm and central veins are prone to elastic recoil and placement of an intravascular stent may be required. Venous stenoses are generally approached antegradely but those near to the arterial anastomosis or involving the anastomosis may be approached retrogradely. Complications of dilatation are fairly common and rupture of veins most commonly occurs where there is angulation of the vein such as the proximal upper arm cephalic arch or peri-anastomotic vein at the wrist. Treatment by prolonged balloon inflation is adequate in most cases though on occasion a stent may be required. A rupture that reopens or leakage from the cannulation site can lead to pseudoaneurysm formation which again may be treated by placement of a stent. All invasive procedures in renal failure patients should be covered by anti-staphylococcal antibiotics as at least 60% of patients are colonized. Infection of post-procedural haematomata has been reported in all series and infection in or surrounding a prosthetic graft may necessitate its removal. Local infection or anti-coagulation is an absolute contraindication for angioplasty.

The long-term success rate of angioplasty is generally poor and experience has shown that long stenoses (>5 cm) or those in proximity to wrist fistulas fare particularly badly and surgical management is recommended. The best results are obtained with forearm autologous arteriovenous fistulas with patency rates of around 40% at 1 year. Stenoses related to prosthetic grafts or upper arm fistulas have 1 year patency rates of around 20–25%. Simple dilatation of central veins has been shown to have similar 1 year patencies to dilatation and stenting (10%). Repeated intervention has been successful in maintaining access patency in approximately 85–90% at 1 year in the few reported series.

Percutaneous management of thrombosed access involves two stages: (1) removal of thrombus and (2) treatment of the underlying disorder which is most commonly an outflow stenosis. Simple thrombolytic therapy has been abandoned because the process is too slow and incomplete, and haemorraghic complications are common. They have been replaced by pharmacomechanical techniques using a combination of thrombolytic therapy and clot removal by either thromboaspiration or Fogarty balloon.

The pulse-spray technique requires placement of an introducer sheath in both the arterial and venous limbs of the thrombosed graft through which two multiholed catheters are passed, one antegradely from the arterial side to the venous anastomosis and the other retrogradely. Forceful injection of small volumes of a urokinase/heparin mixture are made every 30 s for about 15 min then followed by contrast to evaluate clot lysis. If the graft is cleared the outflow stenosis is dilated and then any residual clot including the arterial plug dislodged into the circulation with a Fogarty balloon catheter. Some North American centres have used balloon clearance alone with intentional embolization of graft thrombus to the lungs. Deaths from cardiorespiratory arrest, hemiplegia from paradoxical emboli and septic emboli have been reported.

Concerns about the effect of deliberate pulmonary embolization lead to the development of the thromboaspiration technique where following a 2 hour infusion of urokinase the remaining clot is aspirated through a large bore catheter. Results are comparable to the pulse spray technique. Experience with more recently developed thrombectomy devices is limited. They are designed to macerate intra-graft clot using either a high speed rotating cage or devices based on a vortex or Venturi effect. The resultant slurry is aspirated through the introducer sheath.

Treatment of thrombosed autologous fistulas is more difficult because of the varied anatomy. Often stenoses in the arterialized vein are very tight and multiple with aneurysmal dilatation in the intervening segments. Clots developing in this situation may be massive and well organized and therefore resistant to thrombolysis and if dislodged into the circulation may prove to be fatal. Partial thromboaspiration followed by placement of a wide mesh puncturable stent across the stenosis has had some success.

Even in centres that use these techniques regularly the reported procedure times are between 90 min and 2 hours. Reported assisted primary patency rates at 1 year range from 4 to 39% for PTFE grafts. Very few reports on the use of percutaneous techniques in autologous fistulas are available but the impression is that currently results are not as good as in grafts and surgical revision remains the treatment of choice.

Infection

Infection is second only to cardiovascular disease as the major cause of death in renal failure patients, accounting for 15% of deaths. The increasing reliance on temporary or 'permanent' central venous catheters in patients with multi-system disease with compromised immunity has meant that far from improving, the incidence of bacteraemia is increasing and is now the primary cause of hospital admission. Timely provision of permanent vascular access prior to establishment on dialysis would prevent much of the associated morbidity and mortality.

The presence of uraemia is associated with an increased incidence of infection at all sites (chest, urinary, gastrointestinal, wound) as well as peritonitis and septicaemia and is thought to be a reflection of overall impaired immunity. There appears to be an altered immune response with a direct effect of uraemia on the cellular function of neutrophils, natural killer cells, monocytes and T-lymphocytes. Specific biochemical abnormalities contribute to immune dysfunction. Excess intracellular calcium ion concentration secondary to parathyroid hormone inhibition of the Ca^{2+}/Mg^{2+}-ATPase pump inhibits phagocytosis, chemotaxis and intra-cellular killing of organisms, while zinc deficiency and iron overload both impair cellular motility and the development of cell-mediated immunity.

The greatest risk of infection of either graft or fistula is from failure of aseptic technique when performing needle puncture. Relatively few infections arise at operative sites but if a bacteraemia occurs in the early post-operative period prior to development of a neo-intima, infection of the graft tunnel or anastomotic site may ensue. Over 70% of graft and 90% of autologous fistula infections are caused by staphylococcus species. Up to 50% of dialysis patients are colonized by *S. aureus* and a growing proportion of these are methicillin resistant. The risk of graft infection is also influenced by placement site. Grafts based on the femoral vessels have been reported to have a higher infection rate than forearm grafts and have a significant incidence of limb loss or mortality.

Infections of fistulas or of grafts may be diagnosed by the classical signs of inflammation. Fistula infections are generally related to infection of a peri-venous haematoma and may be treated by local drainage and antibiotics. Rarely infection may arise from the operative procedure and if treatment is inadequate anastomotic infection and pseudoaneurysm formation may occur. Likewise, infections in incorporated prosthetic grafts are usually localized but treatment with antibiotics is usually unsuccessful and chronic discharge with skin breakdown commonly occurs. It must be appreciated that patients with prosthetic grafts usually have few options left in terms of vascular access and therefore an aggressive approach to graft salvage should be undertaken.

Under cover of systemic anti-staphylococcal antibiotics (vancomycin, teicoplanin) the graft should be transected through clean skin incisions and an interpostion graft tunnelled through a clean track circumventing the infected site. When graft continuity has been re-established the wounds are closed and isolated. The infected segment can then be removed and the wound treated as any chronically infected wound and left to heal by secondary intention. Salvage rates up to 90% have been reported using this technique in isolated infections but success in more extensive tunnel infections is poor and the best approach is total graft excision. Management of the arteriotomy in this situation is controversial. Attempts at repair either by primary suturing or by vein patch repair will result in arterial rupture in up to 50% of cases. The safest approach is to ligate the artery and if debilitating limb ischaemia results (which is uncommon) a revascularization procedure may be performed when the infection has been eradicated.

Ischaemia

Construction of an arteriovenous fistula causes a substantial increase in arterial flow which is dependent on the pressure gradient between artery and vein. This in turn is related to the size of the arteriotomy, i.e. anastomotic length. The in-flow from the proximal artery increases as the anastomosis is enlarged until the arteriotomy exceeds 75% of the proximal artery diameter whereupon no further significant increase is obtained. In small fistulas, the flow in the artery distal to the anastomosis is sustained in an antegrade manner throughout systole and diastole. As the size of the anastomosis increases, the diastolic antegrade flow in the distal artery decreases until it eventually reverses, directing blood from the distal vascular tree towards the fistula. This may cause symptoms of steal particularly with brachial fistulas where blood flow is reversed in both the radial and ulnar arteries. If excessive it may lead to ischaemic necrosis of the digits. The distal vasculature can compensate to a certain extent by vasodilatation, development of collateral circulation and a decrease in the diameter of the distal artery due to lower flow and pressure.

Ischaemic symptoms in limbs with fistulas or grafts are regarded as an uncommon side-effect but can range from debilitating digital paraesthesia to devastating critical ischaemia. The incidence with wrist fistulas is reported as being 1–2% while with more proximal access the incidence rises to over 30%. There are two main groups of patients: (1) with a steal syndrome because of a high outflow fistula and (2) with normal or low flow fistulas and peripheral arterial disease of the forearm.

Fistulas formed on the brachial artery are particularly prone to distal ischaemia as collateral circulation around the elbow is often not well developed and a mature fistula commonly has a flow in excess of 1 l/min. Conditions which result in narrowing of distal vessels such as diabetes, atherosclerosis or vasculitis predispose to the development of hand ischaemia.

Symptoms may be mild, only precipitated or exacerbated by dialysis, with coolness of the fingers and mild paraesthesia. The radial pulse is usually present and these cases may be expected to resolve with the opening up of collateral circulation. In more severe cases the radial pulse is absent and the symptoms are present at rest. Sensation may be completely lost and pain is a major feature. Late manifestations are trophic changes progressing to gangrene.

The type of fistula created may contribute to steal. A side-to-side fistula at the wrist may cause digital ischaemia by providing such a low resistance outflow that blood from the ulnar artery preferentially supplies it via the palmar arch. Combined with this, elevation of venous pressure in the hand will aggravate the already compromised digital perfusion. This can be avoided by forming end-to-side fistulas. However, even with end-to-side fistulas if the arteriotomy is too large (>1 cm) steal may occur.

The diagnosis of steal syndrome is easily made by digital occlusion of the venous outflow. The radial pulse will become palpable, there may be immediate relief of symptoms and there is a characteristic palmar flush. If the diagnosis is not clear cut, measurement of digital blood flow by plethysmography, distal arterial flow and direction by Doppler ultrasound or tissue perfusion by pulse oximetry have all been shown to be satisfactory methods of determining augmentation of the pulse pressure with fistula occlusion. Failure to show an improvement with occlusion suggests distal arterial disease or embolism and angiography should be obtained. If diffuse distal arterial disease is found the only safe treatment is ligation of the fistula.

Treatment of steal syndrome may be approached in a number of ways:

- prevention of retrograde flow to the fistula
- avoidance of distal venous hypertension
- reduction of fistula outflow
- improvement of distal arterial blood flow
- ligation of access.

Retrograde flow can be prevented by ligation of the artery distal to the arteriovenous fistula. It is essential to ensure that the correct diagnosis has been made and there is sufficient collateral circulation from (usually) the ulnar artery. It therefore can only be applied to wrist or distal forearm fistulas. The brachial artery, being an effective end artery, does not have a corresponding collateral vessel.

As outlined above, avoidance of side-to-side anastomoses will ensure that all fistula outflow is directed centrally. With fistulas formed at the elbow, the penetrating branch to the deep venous system should be ligated at the initial operation. Often the median vein of the forearm is left intact to provide additional needling area when the vein dilates and the valves become incompetent. It may, however, develop substantially in the presence of a stenosis in the upper arm outflow vein. It may be necessary to sacrifice the vein if the condition does not resolve following correction of the proximal stenosis.

Methods used to restrict fistula flow are notoriously problematic. If the flow-limiting procedure is inadequate, ischaemic symptoms will persist, while if overdone the access will thrombose. The commonest method is to band the outflow vessel with a piece of PTFE approximately 3 cm from the arterial anastomosis. Digital pressures are measured intra-operatively and graft flow should be reduced to around 800 ml/min as measured by a Doppler probe. Patients with more severe early ischaemia benefit from revision of the anastomosis to no more than 4 mm in length.

Patients with normal flow fistula but with ischaemic symptoms are usually diabetic with peripheral arterial disease. Two procedures have been described which permit access flow while preserving distal arterial perfusion. A prosthetic graft may be inserted as either a straight or loop graft onto one of the axillary artery branches which by virtue of their smaller size will limit inflow. The alternative approach is the distal revascularization interval ligation (DRIL) procedure. The fistula is left intact but an arterio-arterial bypass is taken from proximal artery to distal artery beyond the access anastomosis. Reversed saphenous, cephalic or basilic vein or prosthetic graft may be used. The native artery is then ligated between the fistula and the distal arterial anastomosis to prevent retrograde flow (Figure 31.12). Of the small numbers reported, 100% of bypasses were patent at 1 year and 82–94% of fistulas.

Ischaemic neuropathy

The carpal tunnel syndrome is the commonest presentation of neuropathy following creation of vascular access. Compression of the median nerve may be related to congestion within the carpal tunnel secondary to oedema or venous hypertension, but the majority of patients have histological evidence of α_2-microglobulin amyloid, which is a well-known cause of carpal tunnel syndrome in long-term dialysis patients. It is likely that in only a few cases is ischaemia a precipitating cause. The diagnosis may be confirmed by nerve conduction studies which will show slowing of nerve conduction velocity limited to the wrist. Treatment is by surgical release of the transverse carpal ligament.

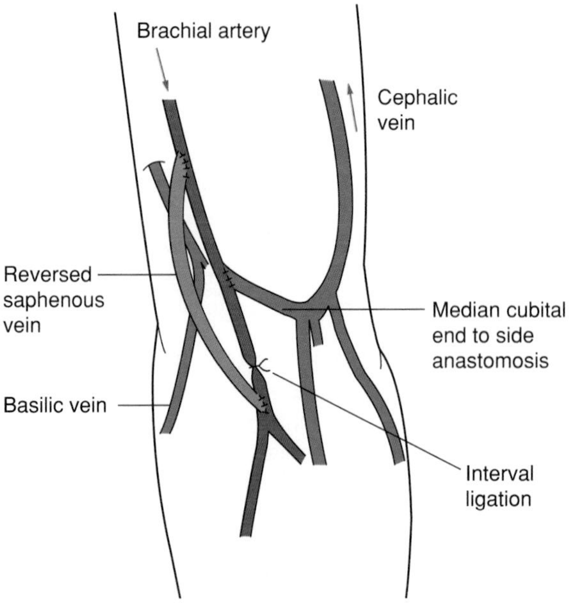

Figure 31.12 Schematic representation of the distal revascularization interval ligation (DRIL) procedure.

A more serious condition related to ischaemic damage is ischaemic monomelic neuropathy (IMN) and should be regarded as a surgical emergency. It is seen exclusively in diabetics who have fistulas created on the brachial artery. There is usually a pre-existing neuropathy or evidence of peripheral vascular disease. Symptoms present acutely, within hours of formation of a fistula, and are characterized by severe pain, paralysis and sensory loss in the forearm affecting all nerve distributions. There is usually little evidence of hand ischaemia and the radial pulse may be present. It is thought that ischaemia preferentially affects nerve tissue because of its higher metabolic activity and its limited blood supply. Rapid axonal loss occurs which is maximal distally. Despite early reversal of the fistula, pain and paralysis may be permanent.

Venous hypertension

Excessively elevated venous pressure may occur in two circumstances:

- retrograde (distal) flow when valves are rendered incompetent by venous dilatation and
- major central venous thrombosis.

The condition is characterized by swelling and blue discoloration and in more protracted cases pain, pigmentation and skin ulceration. Oedema resulting from central venous occlusion may be so severe as to render the limb non-functional. The effects of distal side-to-side fistulas are confined to the hand and may be alleviated by ligation of the vein distal to the anastomosis effectively converting it into an end-to-side fistula. Central venous stenoses are less amenable to surgical treatment. Percutaneous balloon dilatation with or without stenting is generally successful in the short term, but there is a high incidence of recurrent stenosis. In a few selected cases it may be possible to bypass short stenoses of the subclavian vein by direct anastomosis of the internal jugular vein to the distal subclavian/axillary vein or by inserting a PTFE graft from the axillary vein either to the internal jugular or in rare cases to the contralateral subclavian vein.

Aneurysm and pseudo-aneurysm

Aneurysmal dilatation is relatively common in autologous fistulas which have been needled over a prolonged period. They are almost invariably found associated with partial stenosis of the draining vein and repeated needling of easy sites causing weakening of the vessel wall in the presence of high intra-luminal pressures. Focal swellings of prosthetic grafts are technically pseudo-aneurysms caused by disruption of the graft wall from repeated puncture at one site. Anastomotic pseudo-aneurysms do occur in autologous fistulas and are most commonly associated with infection or technical failure.

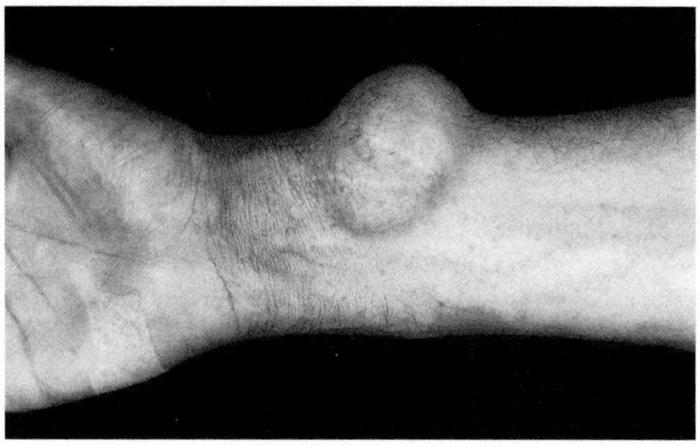

Figure 31.13 Aneurysmal dilatation of cephalic vein caused by proximal stenosis.

Surgical repair is recommended because of the high incidence of thrombosis, infection, pressure necrosis of the overlying skin and rupture. Chronic fistulas frequently have blood flows in excess of 2 l/min and exsanguination can occur rapidly. Prosthetic grafts are easily repaired by insertion a new segment of PTFE bypassing the affected area. Long-term fistulas are more difficult as the vein may have deteriorated over a considerable length with multiple stenoses. The most prudent approach is to ligate the fistula and form new access at a more proximal site. If the problem is restricted to a short segment (Figure 31.13) the aneurysm may be resected and continuity restored with a PTFE jump graft.

Further reading

Freischlag, J. (1997). Angioaccess: an update. *Semin Vasc Surg* **10**(3).

Henry, M. L. ed. (1999). *Vascular Access for Haemodialysis VI.* Chicago, IL: Bonus Books.

NKF-DOQI (1997). Clinical practice guidelines for vascular access. *Am J Kidney Dis* **30**: S150–91.

Wilson, S. E. ed. (1996). *Vascular Access: Principles and Practice*, 3rd edn. St Louis, MO: Mosby.

MODULE 32

Diagnostic radiology and endovascular techniques

Section 32.1 • Diagnostic radiological techniques in vascular surgery

Plain films

The limitation in contrast differences between soft tissues and vessels restricts the value of plain films in the investigation of arterial disease. The presence of calcification in the arterial wall may indicate atheroma and is a common finding in elderly patients while a tubular pattern of calcification is seen in patients with diabetes mellitus, particularly in the tibial and pedal vessels. Curvilinear calcification may be seen in the wall of aneurysms such as in the abdominal aorta or splenic aneurysms. This may be associated with a soft tissue mass. Calcification may also be seen in phleboliths often seen within the pelvis while an unusual site may suggest an underlying arterial-venous malformation.

Catheter angiography

The gold standard of diagnostic radiology in vascular surgery has relied on catheter angiography to provide assessment of the luminal integrity of the vascular territory under investigation. The indications are summarized in Table 32.1. In summary, placement of an angiographic catheter proximal to the vascular territory under investigation is achieved under fluoroscopic guidance, usually by the transfemoral access route. A bolus injection of radiographic contrast media, through injection holes distally placed on the catheter, at a prescribed rate and volume suitable for the territory under examination provides the radiographic contrast depiction of the luminal pathological anatomy. Advances in technique have resulted in reduction of complications as given in Table 32.2. The procedure is normally performed as a day-case.

The aim of the angiographic assessment is to determine the state of the vascular anatomy and identify the possible treatment options in terms of surgical vascular reconstruction, or interventional radiological (endovascular) treatment possibilities (Figure 32.1). The use of dynamic angiographic assessment in different anatomical positions may assist in the diagnosis of underlying vascular entrapment (Figure 32.2). There is an increasing tendency to perform both the diagnostic and an endovascular therapeutic procedure at the same examination where possible.

Arteriography is best performed by the transfemoral route because of the low complication rate of 1.7% and a mortality rate of 0.03%. Alternative routes have higher complication rates (transaxillary 3.3%, translumbar 2.9%). Direct puncture of the carotid or subclavian arteries is generally no longer performed.

Arteriotomies, previously commonly performed for coronary angiography, are now increasing as combined surgical/radiological procedures for deployment of stent grafts or combined angioplasty with bypass procedures.

The femoral vein may be catheterized in the groin, in a similar technique to arterial puncture giving access to the iliac, vena cava, renal, adrenal, heart and pulmonary vessels. The internal jugular vein or other upper extremity vein may be catheterized for diagnostic assessment or intervention in the superior vena cava or hepatic veins, or as a means of establishing vascular access.

All modern angiographic units are digital, allowing subtraction of the background data prior to contrast

Table 32.1 Indications for catheter arteriography

Peripheral vascular disease	90%
Ischaemic heart disease	
Cerebral vascular disease	
Upper limb ischaemia	
Reno-vascular hypertension and chronic renal failure	
Mesenteric ischaemia	
Abdominal aortic and other aneurysm	
Localization of the site of bleeding – such as trauma	
Investigation of pulmonary emboli	
Assessment of arteriovenous malformations	

Table 32.2 Complications of catheter angiography

Arterial puncture site: (0.2% require surgical treatment)	5%	Immediate	Haemorrhage/haematoma Arterial spasm Subintimal dissection Thrombosis Nerve trauma
		Delayed	Local sepsis Arteriovenous fistula False aneurysm formation
Within region examined: (0.1% require surgical treatment)	0.5%		Embolization Subintimal dissection Arterial spasm Thrombosis Perforation Vasovagal reaction Septicaemia
Contrast media reactions			

injection from that with contrast (Figure 32.3). This gives greater contrast and image definition but relies on a co-operative patient and absence of involuntary movements such as bowel gas. In addition the volume of contrast, length of the procedure, diameter of catheters (allowing day-case angiography) and film used are reduced. The digital images may be used as a reference or 'roadmap' for further manipulations or interventions. The post-processing of digital data allows estimation of the degree and length of stenoses or geometry of an aneurysm to be assessed to guide intervention and the appropriate size of stent or stent graft.

The alternative intravenous injection with imaging delay to allow transit to the arterial segment under investigation is an alternative method of arterial angiography which may be of value in patients with limited arterial access or increased risk of bleeding. However, the images obtained are generally not of the same quality as those provided by an intra-arterial injection at the site of the arterial territory under investigation. They may however provide sufficient information as a screening examination for renal arterial or carotid disease, follow-up after intervention, examination in patients with difficult femoral access or venous assessments.

Doppler ultrasound

Real-time ultrasound, complemented by pulsed Doppler and continuous wave Doppler have become established methods of assessing specific vascular territories by colour flow mapping and spectral analysis (Figure 32.4). Doppler ultrasound may also be applied for venous assessments, particularly of the lower limb and inferior vena cava. Transthoracic access limits the technique in the thorax.

The non-invasive nature of the technique makes Doppler ultrasound most suitable for initial assessment where possible and follow-up of surgical and endovascular procedures such as graft patency or infra-inguinal angioplasty.

The percutaneous placement of small-bore catheters with distal ultrasound transducers has allowed intravascular ultrasound to be performed. While a useful adjunct particularly in the research capacity, its widespread use as a diagnostic tool has not fulfilled its potential.

Real-time ultrasound is commonly used to assess the size, extent and rate of growth of abdominal aortic aneurysm or any other peripheral aneurysm. It may be used in the follow-up of aortic grafts, in the investigation of pulsating masses in the neck groin axillae or peripheries may be used as an aid to performing an arterial venous puncture under image guidance.

Duplex ultrasound combining pulse Doppler and real time ultrasound may be used to detect and assess the severity of stenoses in peripheral arteries and femoro-popliteal grafts, stenoses in the extracranial carotid arteries and renal and mesenteric arteries in the abdomen. It may be used in the assessment of peripheral graft patency (Table 32.3).

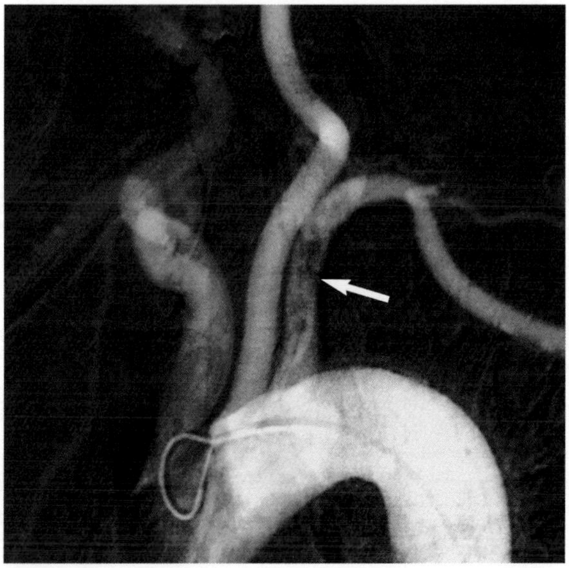

Figure 32.1 Digital subtraction arch aortogram demonstrating an embolus in the left subclavian artery (arrow).

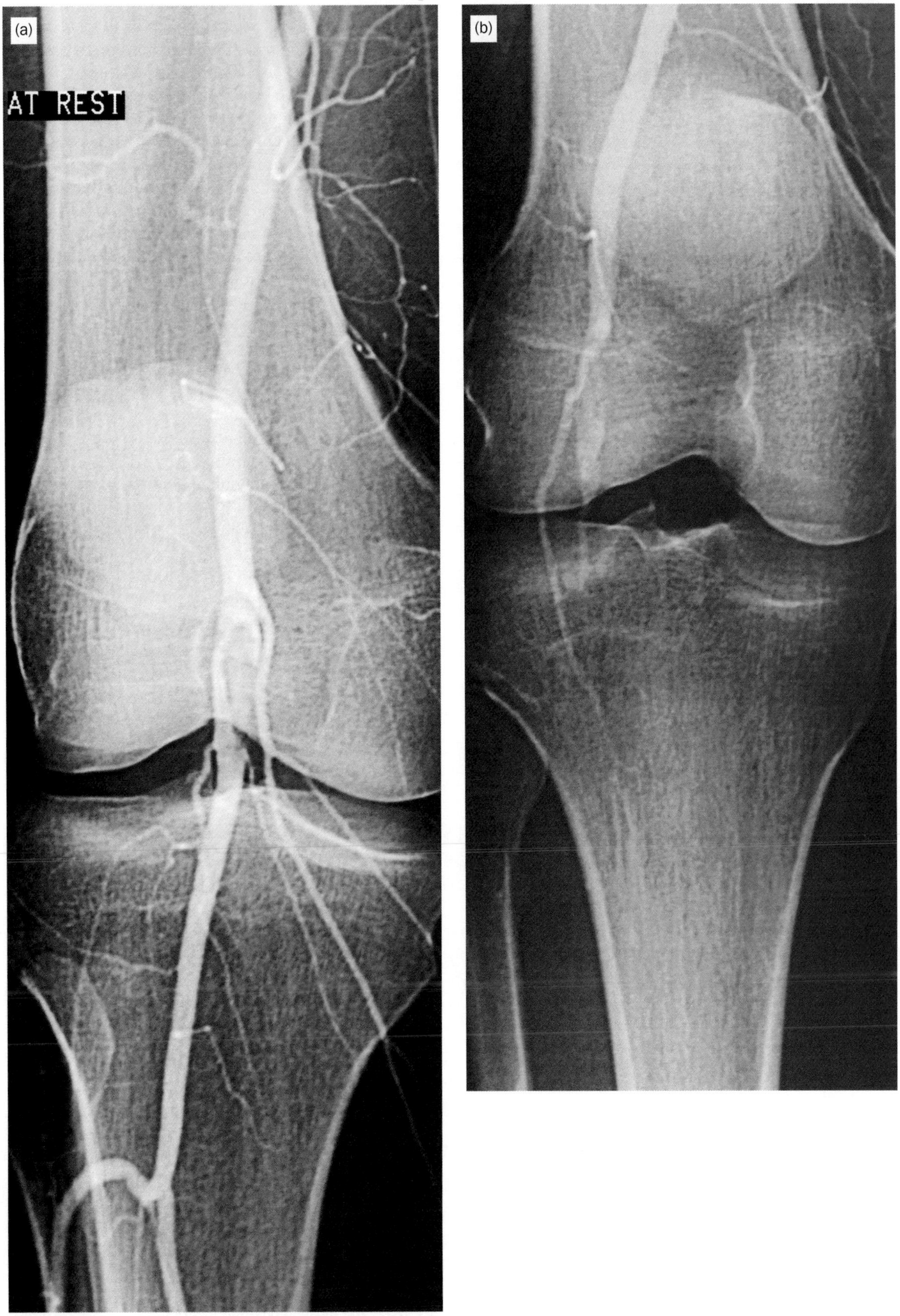

Figure 32.2 Angiography of the popliteal artery in (a) neutral and (b) active plantar flexion demonstrating popliteal artery entrapment syndrome.

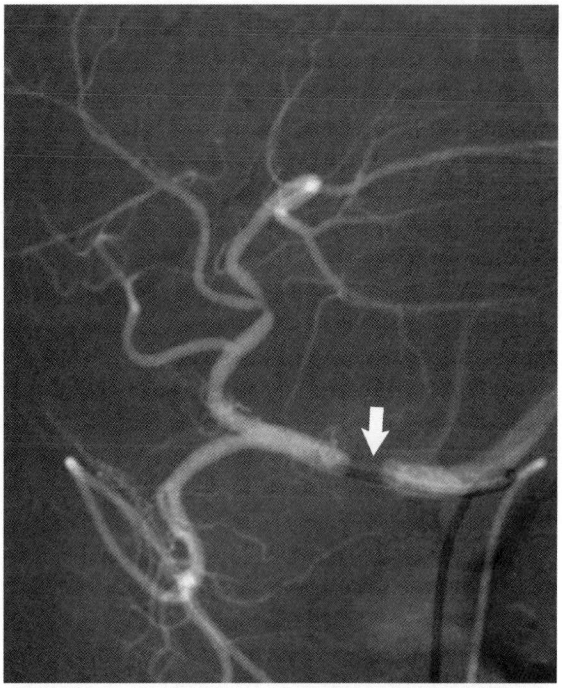

Figure 32.3 Digital subtraction angiogram of the hepatic artery demonstrating stenosis (arrow) suitable for angioplasty.

Computed tomographic angiography

With the advancing technology in computed tomography (CT) allowing subsecond rotations, spiral acquisitions augmented by bolus intravenous contrast media has allowed CT angiography (CTA) to give diagnostic information in a less invasive way than catheter angiography. The area examined demonstrates both luminal three-dimensional (3D) anatomy and also luminal and extraluminal pathologies not seen on standard catheter angiography. Its use therefore is an expansion of vascular assessment beyond the field of catheter angiography and may provide additional information of diagnostic value. The area of examination is limited by the number of rotations and therefore elongated vascular anatomy such as limbs is less acceptable on the basis of significantly increased radiation dosage. A further complication is the depiction of vascular calcification of a similar density to the lumen contrast which requires careful attention to distinguish these entities.

As the images are acquired in a 3D data set these may be manipulated by multi-plane reformat or maximum intensity projection to provide further diagnostic information not easily achieved by catheter angiography (Figure 32.5).

The typical examinations performed by CTA are given in Table 32.4.

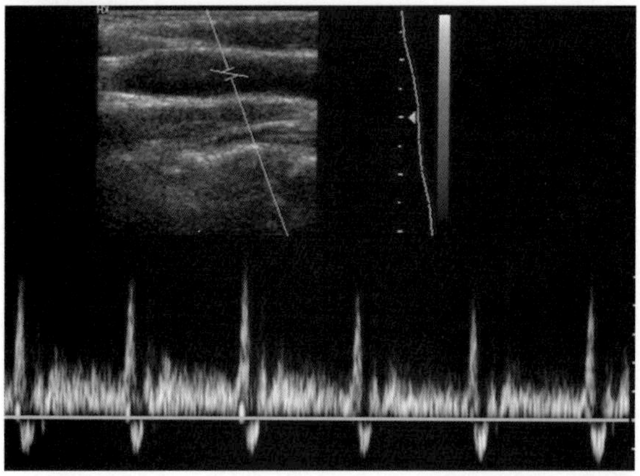

Figure 32.4 Doppler ultrasound of the common carotid artery demonstrating velocity waveform.

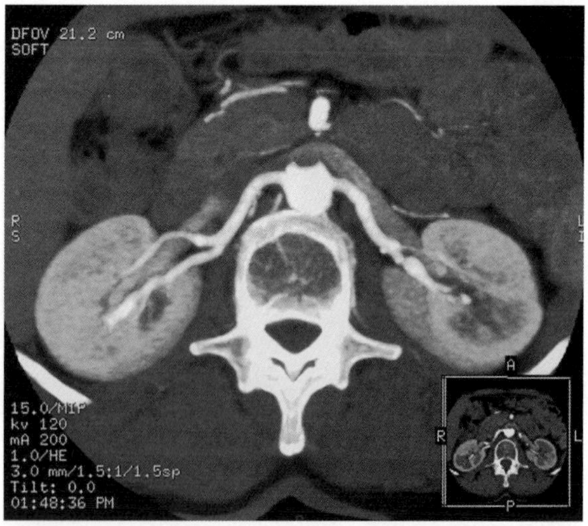

Figure 32.5 CT angiogram of the renal arteries showing single normal renal arteries bilaterally.

Table 32.3 Commonest indications for vascular ultrasound

Aorta	Aneurysm size, extent and rate of growth Aortic graft follow-up
Carotid	Bifurcation stenosis/occlusion
Upper extremity	Vascular access/fistula assessment
Renal	Arterial stenoses, renal size
Mesenteric	Arterial stenoses/occlusion
Femoro-popliteal	Mapping and degree of stenoses
Tibial	Patency prior to distal grafting

Table 32.4 Commonest indications for CTA

The size and extent of a thoracic aneurysm
Confirming the diagnosis of a ruptured thoracic aorta
Follow-up of aortic graft complications
Investigation of a pulsating mass
Quantitatively assessing dimensions of aortic aneurysm for appropriate stent graft placement and suitability of an access route
CT, renal and mesenteric arteriograms
Pulmonary angiograms

Magnetic resonance angiography

Advances in magnetic resonance imaging (MRI) such as reduced acquisition time, improved sequences, gradient subsystems, phased array coil technology and intravenous pump injectors with integrated table movement have recently greatly expanded the role of MR angiography (MRA) in the diagnostic assessment of vascular disease. Like CT the information gained is a 3D dataset of luminal, wall and extraluminal anatomy which may be of diagnostic superiority over catheter angiography in certain clinical situations. The luminal signal is achieved using time of flight (2D or 3D techniques), contrast enhanced 3D MRA or phased-contrast imaging. Three-dimensional contrast enhanced MRA is becoming established as the optimum MRA sequence for vascular luminal assessment while phase contrast angiography can provide flow quantitation.

MRI is a less invasive technique than catheter angiography although there are particular contraindications which may exclude some patients. These are given in Table 32.5.

Like CT, the dataset is 3D and therefore may be manipulated in multi-plane reformat or maximum intensity projection. In addition, as the orientation of acquisition may be in any direction (while CT may only be acquired in the axial orientation), there are particular advantages of MRA in vascular territories that are tortuous or are more appropriately examined with non-axial acquisition (Figures 32.6 and 32.7). The area examined in one sequence may be limited by the receiver coil geometry available. Multiple acquisitions may be achieved with sequential boluses of contrast for extensive peripheral vascular assessment. The recent addition of integrated bolus tracking and table movement may achieve a peripheral angiogram in a single acquisition. The types of examination regularly examined under MR angiography are given in Table 32.6.

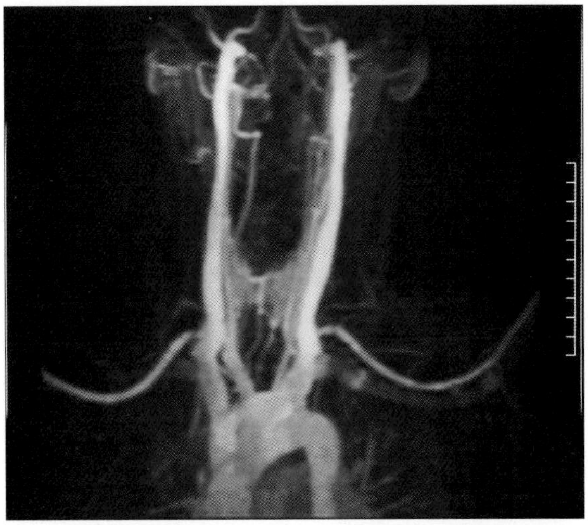

Figure 32.6 MRA of the aortic arch and great vessels.

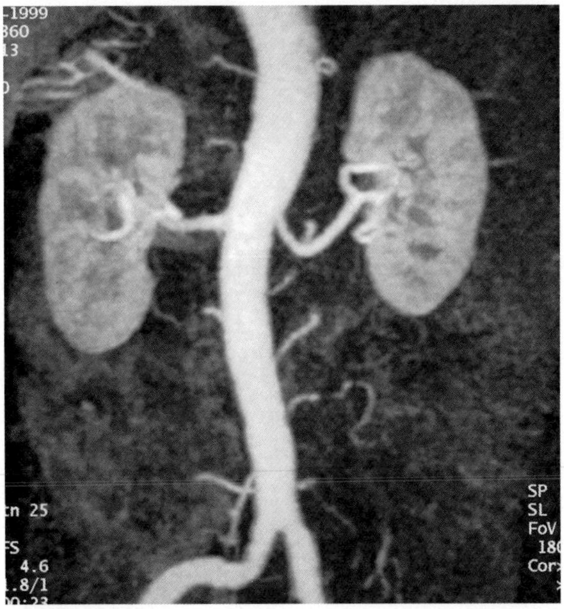

Figure 32.7 MRA of the renal arteries.

Radionuclide imaging

Although the spatial resolution of radionuclide studies does not compare with that of angiography or CT, the targeted use of radiolabelled white cells may be used to confirm the diagnosis of an infected arterial graft, technetium labelled red cells or labelled colloid may be used to determine the site of active bleeding from the gastrointestinal tract and may be a useful adjunct to guiding arteriography.

Table 32.5 Contraindications to MRI

Electrical implanted device	Cardiac pacemaker
	Electrical nerve stimulator
	Cochlear implant
	Other electrical device implanted
Metallic devices at risk in field	Aneurysm clips
	Certain heart valves
Metallic fragments	Fragments in eyes
General state	Cardiac failure, thermoregulatory disorder
	First trimester pregnancy
	Claustrophobia

Table 32.6 Commonest indications for MRA

Intracranial	Arteriovenous malformations
	Venous sinus thrombosis
Carotid	Stenosis/occlusion
	Carotid body tumour
	Pulsatile swelling in the neck
Upper extremity	Thoracic outlet syndromes
	Arteriovenous malformations
Aorta	Chronic thoracic dissection
	Coarctation
	Mycotic/inflammatory aneurysm
	Aortic aneurysm assessment
Renal/mesenteric	Stenoses/occlusion
Iliac	Stenoses/occlusion
Peripheral	Absent femoral arteries
	Popliteal artery entrapment
	Arteriovenous malformations

Other techniques

Intravascular ultrasound (IVUS) uses a minute transducer at the tip of an arterial device to produce ultrasound images of the arterial wall and perivascular anatomy.

Angioscopy using optical fibres in a catheter delivered through a vascular sheath may be used to directly visualize the intima. The field of view is continually obscured by blood which has to be flushed away. Its value in routine practice is unclear.

Section 32.2 • Applications of diagnostic and endovascular techniques

Haemorrhage

Arteriography can be used in localizing the site of bleeding in the gastrointestinal tract, the urinary tract and the respiratory tract and in patients following severe trauma.

Gastrointestinal haemorrhage

The initial investigation of acute gastrointestinal haemorrhage using endoscopy has a diagnostic accuracy of 90% and flexible sigmoidoscopy and colonoscopy has a diagnostic accuracy of 50–90%. Arteriography is indicated in patients who continue to bleed severely, particularly when the initial investigations have failed to demonstrate the site of bleeding. Arteriography has a diagnostic accuracy of 50–75% but this is increased if the patient is actively bleeding at the time of the examination. It has been calculated that arteriography demonstrates active bleeding when the rate of blood loss exceeds 0.5–1.0 ml/min while radionuclide studies using technetium-labelled colloid or red cell can detect active bleeding when the rate of blood loss is as low as 0.1–0.5 ml/min.

Arteriography in acute upper gastrointestinal haemorrhage may show extravasation of contrast medium from a gastric or duodenal ulcer, gastro-oesophageal varices, a false aneurysm and pancreatitis or unusually aortoenteric fistula. In acute lower gastrointestinal haemorrhage arteriography may show a small intestinal arteriovenous malformation, angiodysplasia, or more commonly extravasation into a colonic diverticulum or ulcer. Small bowel leiomyomata or Meckel's diverticulum may be seen as a site of bleeding from small bowel sources. Sites of bleeding may be treated by intra-arterial infusion of vasoconstrictors such as vasopressin. Dependent on vascular anatomy, embolization with coils or temporary embolization may be employed. Arteriovenous malformations may also be embolized permanently.

Urological haemorrhage

Renal arteriography may be indicated in patients with severe haematuria following renal biopsy, in patients with recurrent haematuria after a normal intravenous urogram and cystoscopy (Figure 32.8). In particular, findings of an angiomyolipoma on ultrasound or CT may allow embolization as an alternative to surgery (Figure 32.9). In uncontrolled haematuria in patients with inoperable renal or bladder carcinoma embolization may be used as palliative treatment.

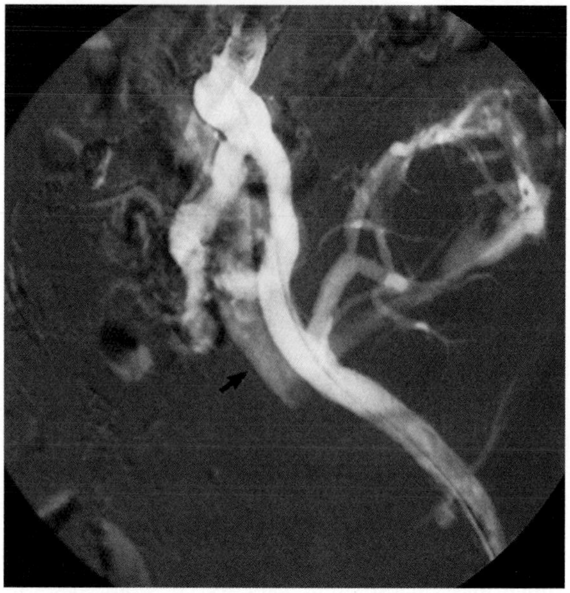

Figure 32.8 Subtraction angiogram of the transplant renal artery demonstrating early venous filling (arrow) in keeping with an iatrogenic post-biopsy arteriovenous fistula.

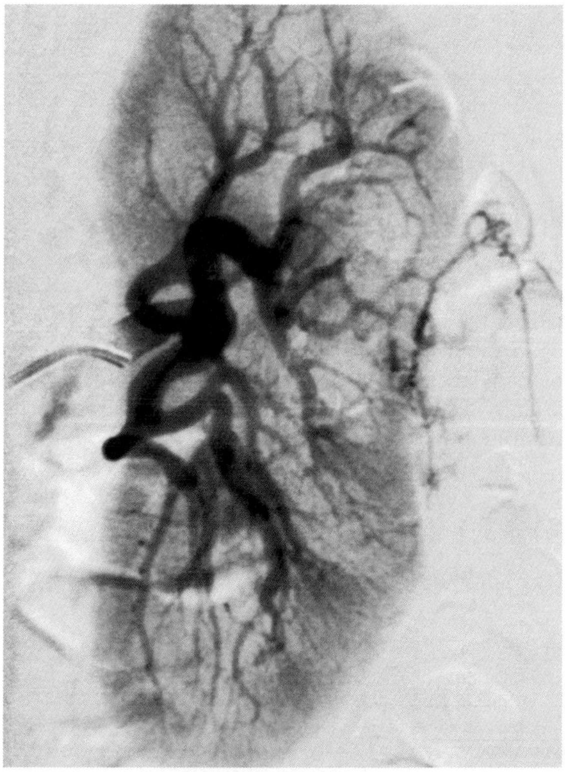

Figure 32.9 Subtraction angiogram of the left kidney allows embolization of an angiomyolipoma with polyvinyl alcohol.

Respiratory tract haemorrhage

While upper respiratory tract haemorrhage from the nasal cavity usually is controlled by conservative measures of packing or cautery, if severe haemorrhage persists then selective catheterization and embolization of the maxillary artery may be undertaken as an alternative to external carotid branch ligation.

Lower respiratory tract haemorrhage in patients with chronic fibrotic lung disease, bronchiectasis, cystic fibrosis and aspergilloma (Figure 32.10) may be treated by selective bronchial artery catheterization and embolization.

Traumatic haemorrhage

Arteriography may be required to characterize the nature of the vascular injury in patients with uncontrolled haemorrhage due to blunt or penetrating trauma. Occasionally it may be used to assess the blood supply to a limb in a patient who requires orthopaedic surgery and in whom the peripheral vessels are suspected to have been compromised.

Arterial injuries that can occur in acute trauma include arterial spasm, extrinsic compression from a haematoma, intramural bleeding partial or complete trans-section of the artery, and the formation of a false aneurysm or arteriovenous fistula (Figure 32.11).

Blunt trauma to the chest may produce a partial tear in the artery with the formation of a false aneurysm. CT and angiography may confirm the diagnosis of a false aneurysm (Figure 32.12). Chest injury may also result in venous haemorrhage which may also show as superior mediastinal widening.

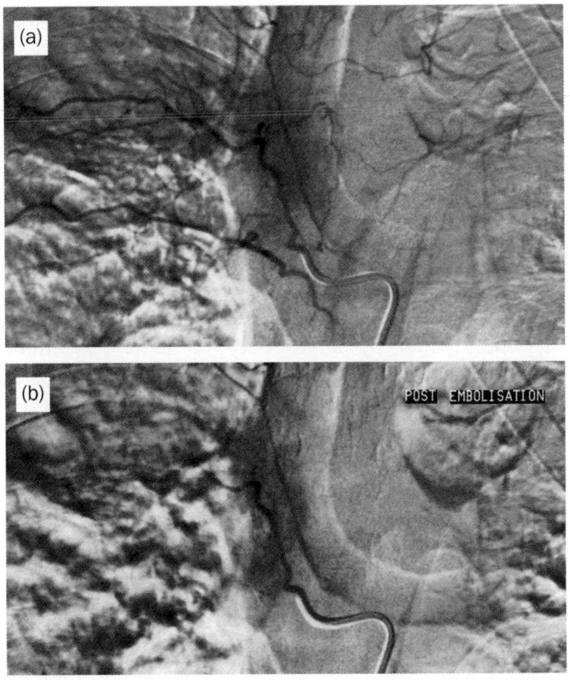

Figure 32.10 Right bronchial artery angiogram (a) before and (b) after embolization in a patient with recurrent haemoptysis due to aspergilloma.

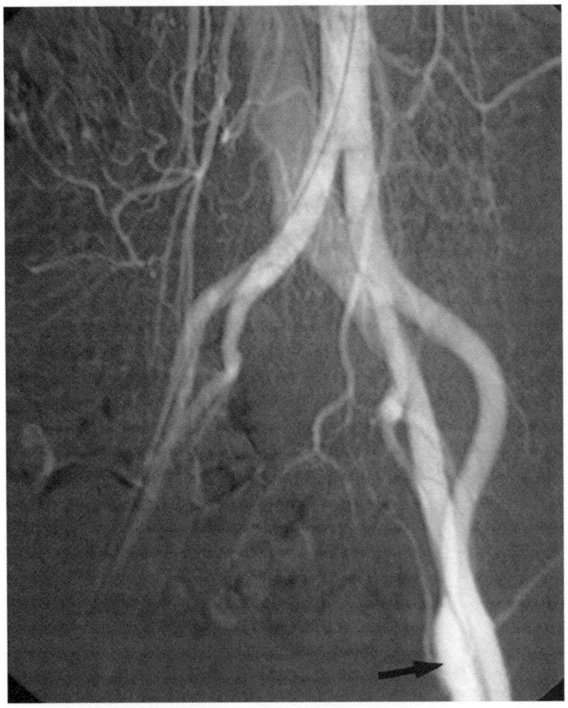

Figure 32.11 Iatrogenic common femoral arteriovenous fistula (arrow) after cardiac catheterization.

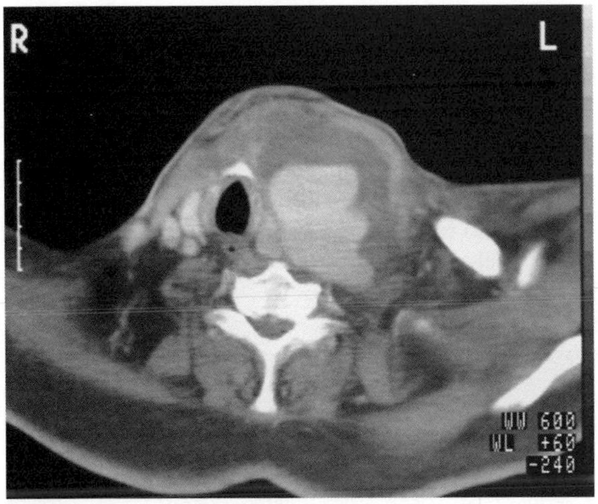

Figure 32.12 Dynamic contrast-enhanced CT showing a false aneurysm of the left subclavian artery.

Blunt trauma to the abdomen may cause solid organ trauma particularly to the spleen, liver or kidneys while tears in the mesentery may also produce mesenteric haematoma (Figure 32.13).

Pelvic fractures commonly cause extensive blood loss and where there are partial tears of the iliac arteries embolization may be life saving.

Vascular malformations

Congenital vascular malformations are classified according to the angiographic characteristics into high flow arteriovenous malformations and low flow capillary

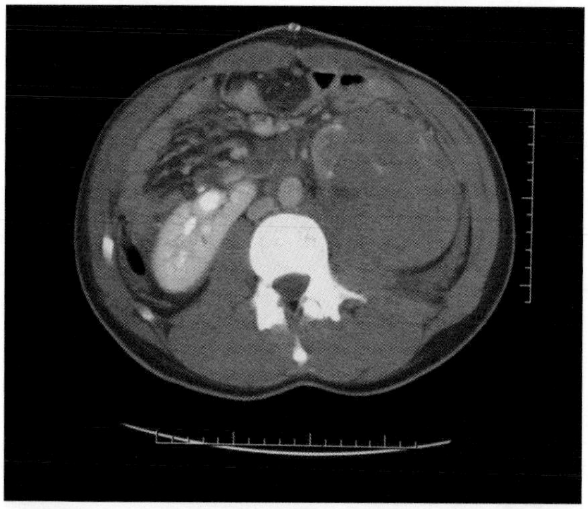

Figure 32.13 Dynamic contrast enhanced spiral CT showing left renal transection and haematoma after a sledging accident.

venous malformation or venous haemangioma. Arteriovenous malformations may present as soft tissue pulsatile masses while they may occur in any internal organ.

Arteriography of arteriovenous malformation may show hypertrophic tortuous feeding arteries, a network of abnormal smaller vessels (the so-called nidus) and early prominent venous filling due to shunting with associated aneurysm formation. Arteriovenous malformations may be treated by catheter embolization with permanent embolization as an alternative to surgery (Figure 32.14).

Capillary venous malformations may show angiographically as normal arteries with abnormal venous pooling or enlarged veins in the venous phase with no early shunting. While difficult to treat surgically they tend to recur and do not respond to embolization. The vessels and soft tissue components may be best demonstrated with MRI.

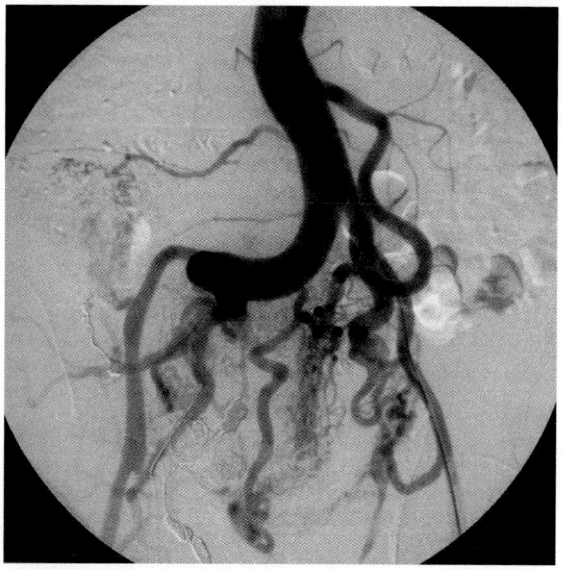

Figure 32.14 Pelvic arteriogram demonstrating a large arteriovenous malformation.

Atheromatous occlusive disease

The combined approach of arterial surgery with associated interventional radiology or endovascular techniques is widely used for atheromatous occlusive disease affecting large vessels.

Cerebrovascular disease

Carotid arterial stenosis due to atheromatous disease may present as either transient ischaemic attacks or strokes. Initial investigation usually consists of duplex ultrasound. The alternative non-invasive technique of MRI particularly using 3D contrast enhanced techniques is an alternative. Angiography is reserved for those patients where the duplex findings are difficult to interpret particularly in differentiating high-grade stenoses from occlusions. MRI also tends to over estimate stenoses.

Angiography carries a risk of permanent neurological damage of approximately 1%; while the risks are lower with arch aortography which is primarily aimed at assessment of the common carotid arteries, in cases of possible internal carotid occlusion, selective injection may be required with the attendant high risk. Stenoses in other great vessels such as subclavians may produce steal syndromes with reversal of flow in the vertebral arteries.

While patients with low-grade stenosis (less than 30%) and middle-grade stenosis (30–70%) are treated conservatively with anteplatelet therapy, high-grade stenosis (>70%) should be considered for surgery or possible angioplasty and stenting. While carotid angioplasty is currently under active evaluation the lack of a general anaesthetic may be balanced by an apparent increase in peri-procedural stroke (Figure 32.15).

Upper limb vascular disease

Patients presenting with acute or chronic upper limb ischaemia may be investigated initially by Doppler, but the lack of access to the origins of the great vessels limits its value. Non-invasive assessment with MRA (Figure 32.16) is increasingly being used to avoid the cerebrovascular complications. Following diagnostic assessment, focal stenoses or short occlusions may be treated by angioplasty or stent placement with due consideration of the risks of cerebrovascular complications, e.g. in lesions of the inominate or subclavian vessels proximal to the vertebral artery origins, care must be taken not to compromise these vessels.

Mesenteric vascular disease

The presence of occlusive disease of the mesenteric vessel origins may be determined by Doppler ultrasound, CTA, MRA or catheter angiography. In those patients with symptoms suggestive of chronic mesenteric ischaemia, and occlusion of two of three mesenteric vessels, with stenotic disease of the remaining vessel, angioplasty and stenting may be of value.

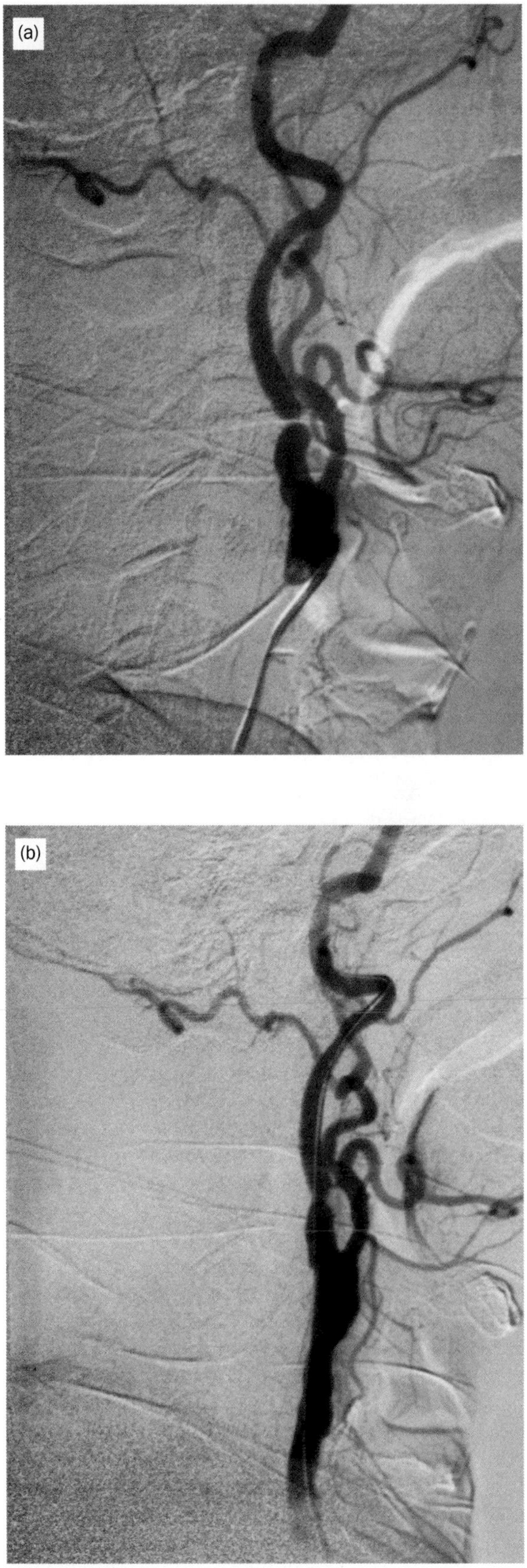

Figure 32.15 Subtraction right carotid arteriogram (a) before and (b) after carotid angioplasty.

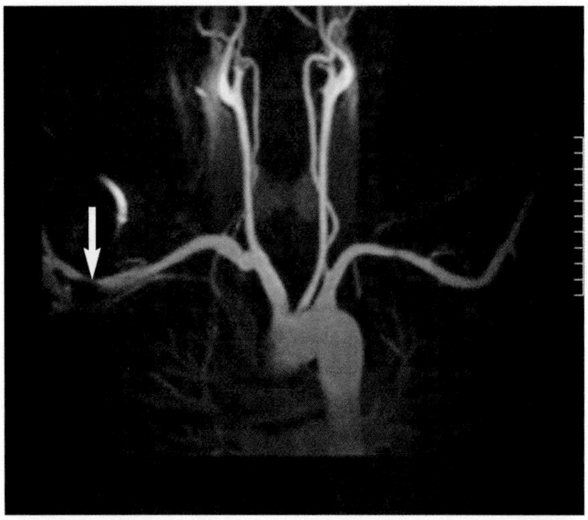

Figure 32.16 MRA demonstrating a right axillary stenosis (arrow).

Renovascular disease

Renal ischaemia is the cause of hypertension in approximately 5% of hypertensive patients. Investigation of patients with hypertension with angiography, CTA or MRA is limited to those patients in whom the blood pressure is difficult to control with conventional treatment.

There is increasing recognition that ischaemia is a component of chronic renal failure in 25% of cases and patients showing deterioration in renal function may benefit from intervention. Other indicators of underlying renal arterial stenosis may be deterioration of renal function on an angiotensin-converting enzyme inhibitor, poor hypertensive control in patients with previously well controlled hypertension and flash pulmonary oedema.

Investigation of renal artery stenosis using angiography has been partly replaced by CTA and MRA. Although duplex ultrasound is a non-invasive method of imaging the renal arteries, due to patient habitus it may be difficult to demonstrate this in all patients.

Definitive investigation by intra-arterial renal arteriography may show an atheromatous stenosis at the origin of the vessel (ostial) which may be associated with aortic atheroma or aneurysm formation. Angioplasty in these types of lesions is more likely to result in recoil and restenosis and therefore stent placement is often required (Figure 32.17). Post-ostial stenosis and fibromuscular disease is more amenable to angioplasty alone. In addition, other causes of renovascular hypertension such as renal artery aneurysm, arteriovenous fistula, embolus or renal vasculitis such as polyarteritis nodosa will be demonstrated at arteriography. Arteriography in transplant renal arteries may also show stenoses at the time of transplantation in cadaveric kidneys (Figure 32.18) while arterial stenosis may recur in long-term transplants.

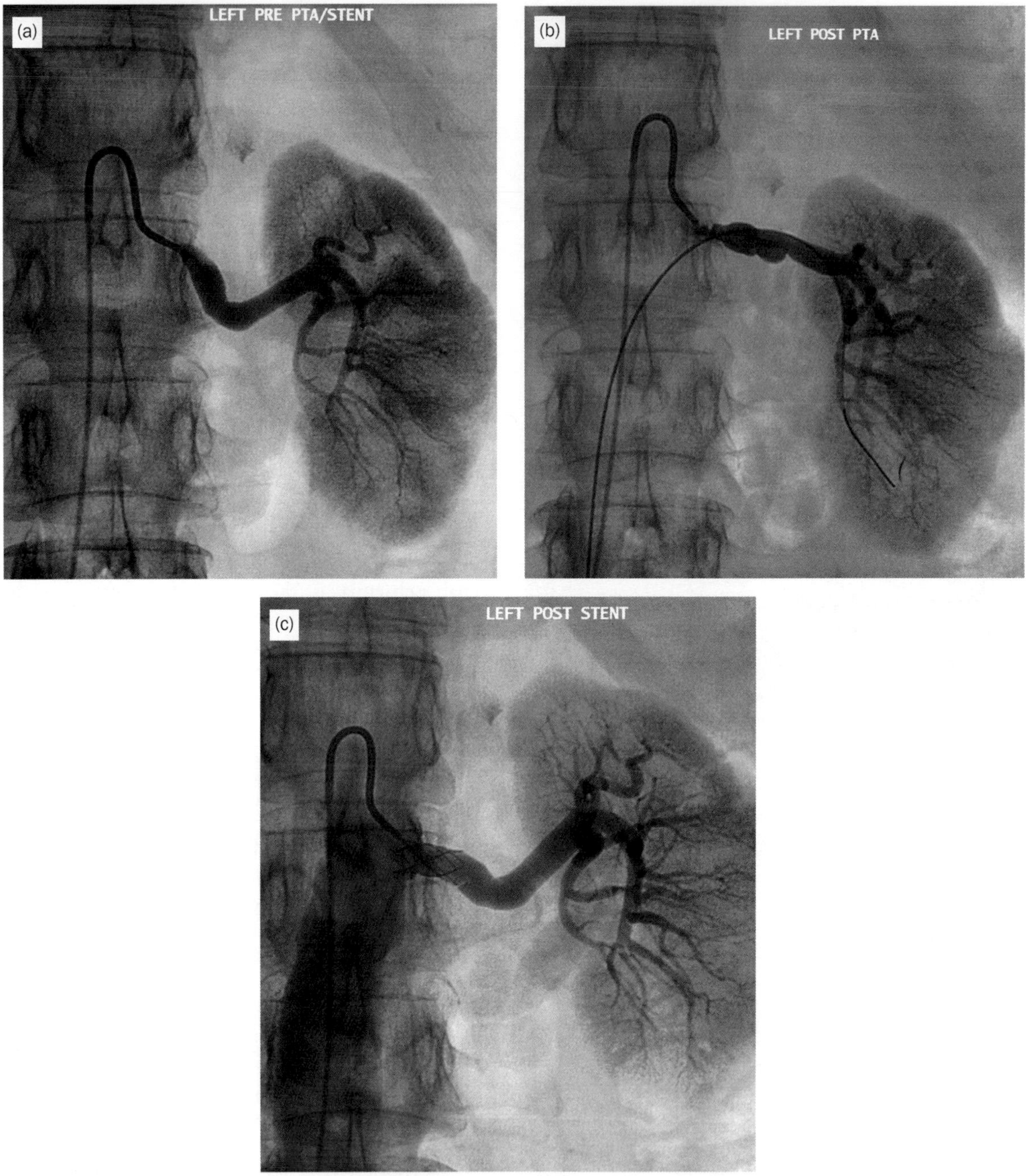

Figure 32.17 Renal arteriogram: (a) before, (b) after angioplasty and (c) after stent placement.

Peripheral vascular disease

Diagnosis and management planning

The assessment of patients presenting with chronic lower limb ischaemia includes clinical examination, simple investigations such as blood tests, urine analysis, electrocardiography, Doppler arterial pressure measurements, treadmill testing and imaging with either duplex ultrasound, catheter or MRA. There is an increase in use of duplex examination of the lower limb to map the stenoses, or occlusions and the assessment of aneurysms. While this may be time consuming, the ability to non-invasively assess the lower limbs in the presence of good femoral pulses and reduced ankle brachial pressure indices has reduced the need for catheter angiography in some centres. Duplex ultrasound is however most useful in the follow-up of patients who have had surgical bypass grafts or angioplasty and in the assessment of possible aneurysms and soft tissue masses. Vein mapping prior to surgical bypass is useful. The weakness of duplex is the relatively poor access to iliac vessels and therefore the inability to exclude stenotic disease in the segment.

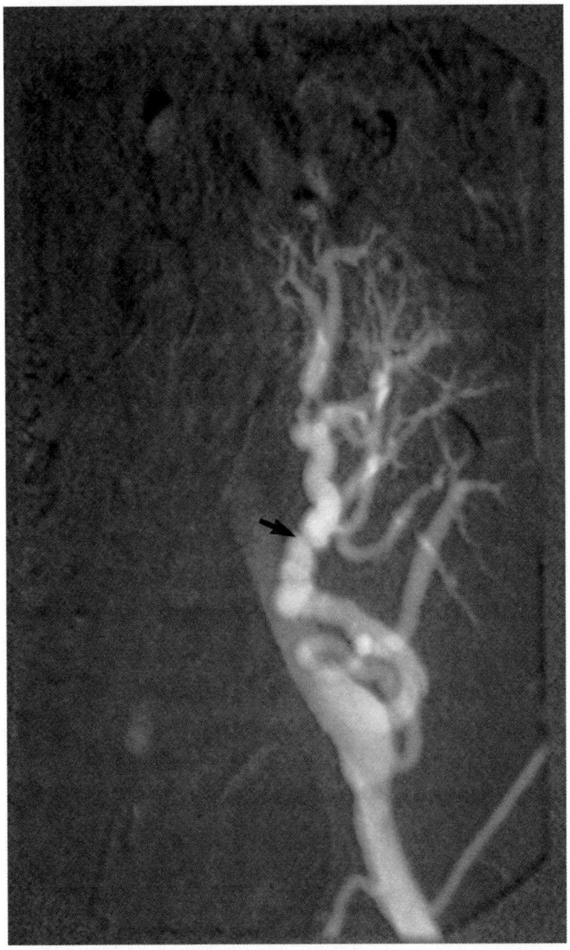

Figure 32.18 Cadaveric transplant arteriogram demonstrating fibromuscular dysplasia (arrow).

MRA can produce excellent images of the peripheral vasculature from the aortic bifurcation to the pedal arch. There is no doubt the techniques of bolus tracking, moving table and advanced contrast injection will reduce the examination time and improve image quality.

Catheter angiography remains the optimal method for imaging the lower limb vessels and was described previously. Femoral angiography reveals various patterns of atheromatous disease or thrombotic occlusion in the aorto-iliac segment, superficial femoral artery, the popliteal artery and distal vessels. In severe chronic ischaemia, combinations of these patterns in one or both legs may be present. While the images provide an overview, additional information in relation to the rapidity of flow particularly in ectatic vessels, or suspected aneurysms and in patients with poor cardiac function, is displayed which is not readily achieved from duplex ultrasound. Its particular strength is the assessment of the aorto-iliac segment and the ability, where conditions allow, to proceed directly to a therapeutic procedure at the time of angiography, i.e. the ability to perform diagnostic examinations with therapeutic procedures at the same appointment on a day-case basis.

Endovascular therapy: angioplasty and stenting in chronic ischaemia

Following a diagnostic assessment to determine the sites of occlusive disease, intervention will depend on the symptomatology and the degree and morphology of the lesion. The degree of stenosis that is taken to be significant is greater than 70%. At this level there is an associated haemodynamic effect with an associated pressure gradient and impaired flow. The lesions most suitable for angioplasty are focal concentric stenoses or short segment occlusions of up 5 cm in length in the iliac arteries and femoro-popliteal segments. These limitations have been extended by more enthusiastic use of long segment angioplasty, particularly involving the subintimal technique in which the intentional subintimal passage of guidewire through the occlusion is followed by angioplasty. Such techniques may be augmented by the use of vascular stents, particularly in relation to stabilizing the upper or lower extent of the subintimal angioplasty site.

Angioplasty requires an experienced vascular radiologist not only to recanalize the occlusion and to inflate/deflate the balloon safely but also to be able to deal quickly with the complications of intervention such as occlusion and distal embolization. High quality angiographic equipment is required, preferably with digital subtraction facilities (Figures 32.19 and 32.20). The contraindications to angioplasty are the presence of fresh thrombus which should be treated by thrombolysis, increased risk of haemorrhage due to a bleeding diathesis and local sepsis.

The approaches are usually from the common femoral artery. While either common femoral artery may be used for aortic, renal, upper limb, mesenteric or carotid angioplasty, an ipsilateral approach is usually performed for iliac and femoro-popliteal segments with an antegrade approach being used for the femoro-popliteal and distal angioplasties. During the angioplasty patients should receive intra-arterial heparin. The choice of balloon size is based on the size of the native vessel and if stent placement is required this is usually chosen to be 1 mm greater than the previously used balloon size. The choice of stent, i.e. balloon expandible, self-expandable, design and length will depend on the segment of vessel, tortuosity, lesion morphology, proximity of branches and access limitations.

Assessment of a segment that shows equivocal angiographic features is improved by using pressure gradient measurement with a pull-back or dual pressure recording technique. A pressure gradient of >15 mmHg at rest in an iliac artery or stenosis is taken to be significant. If >10 mmHg, a vasodilator such as papaverine, tolazoline or glyceryl trinitrate should be injected. This reduces the peripheral resistance and increases the gradient. An increase to >15 mmHg indicates that the stenosis is likely to be haemodynamically significant on exercise and therefore might be expected to benefit from angioplasty. In the femoro-popliteal segment pressure gradients are not frequently assessed. (Pressure measurements in the renal artery have been used widely while those in the mesenteric, carotid and upper limb are less often employed.)

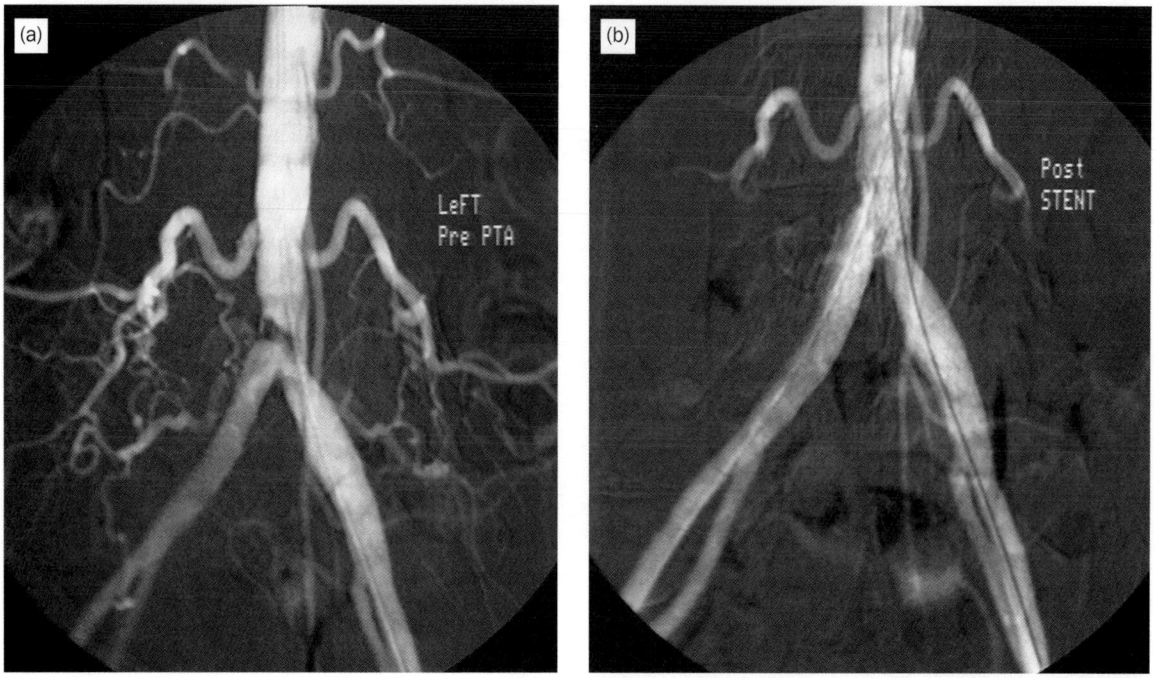

Figure 32.19 Iliac arteriogram (a) before and (b) after bilateral common iliac stent placement.

In the assessment of the result of angioplasty, suboptimal results are usually categorized as those in which there is greater than 30% recoil, a residual pressure gradient of 5 mmHg, extensive dissection or reocclusion. In these situations the deployment of an intravascular stent may result in maintenence of the lumen and stabilization.

The expected results of angioplasty are given in Table 32.7.

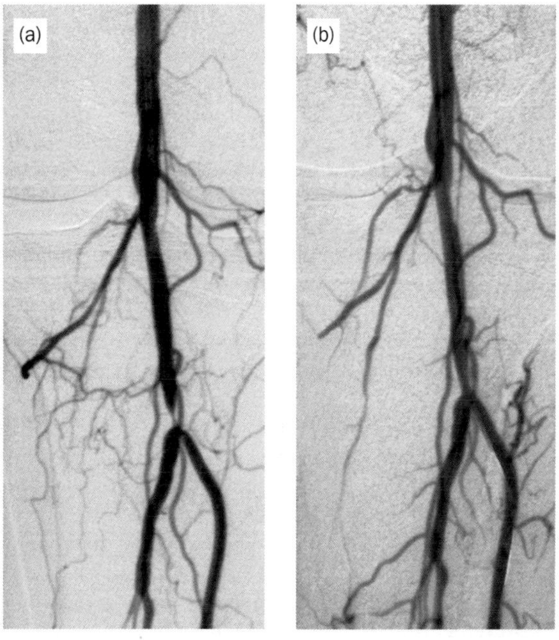

Figure 32.20 Tibial arteriogram (a) before and (b) after balloon angioplasty.

Endovascular therapy: atherectomy

The mechanical removal of atheroma or neointimal hyperplasia has been employed in cases in which conventional angioplasty or stent placement has failed or is unlikely to succeed. Various devices have been designed using rotational cutting edges to remove or macerate the stenosis (Figure 32.21). They have not gained widespread use due to the sizes of the delivery systems but do offer alternative approaches in selected cases.

Endovascular therapy: thrombolysis and angioplasty in acute ischaemia

In patients with acute limb ischaemia catheter directed thrombolysis may be of value as a means of lysing thrombus prior to treatment of the underlying stenosis in native vessels or graft by angioplasty stent placement or surgical revision. Following a diagnostic catheter angiogram, the placement of an infusion catheter into the thrombosed segment allows infusion of thrombolytic agent under a controlled and regularly monitored coagulation regimen, with frequent check

Table 32.7 Typical results of angioplasty and stent placement

	Technical success	*Complication*	*12–24 month patency*
Carotid	>80%	<5%	70–80%
Great vessel	>85%	<3%	70–80%
Renal	>90%	<3%	65–80%
Mesenteric	>80%	<5%	55–70%
Iliac	>95%	<3%	85–95%
Femoro-popliteal	>95%	<3%	50–65%

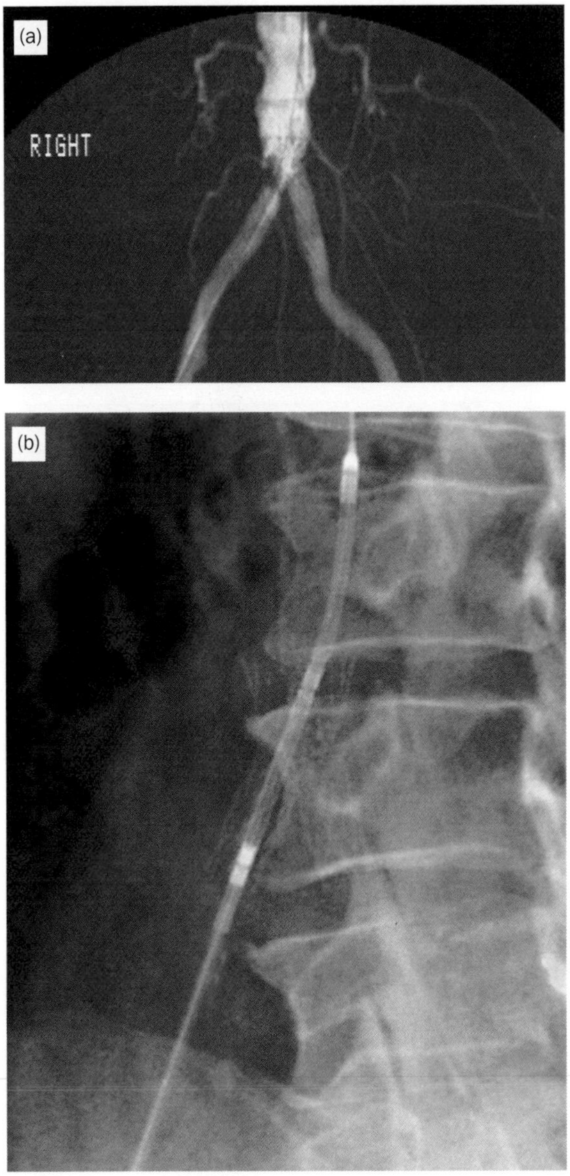

Figure 32.21 Iliac arteriogram showing: (a) restenosis in a right common iliac stent and (b) during atherectomy.

angiograms to achieve optimal lysis while minimizing complications (Figure 32.22). The thrombolysis should always be followed immediately by attempts to correct the underlying abnormality.

Aneurysmal disease

Intracranial aneurysms

Saccular aneurysms of the circle of Willis are the commonest cause of subarachnoid haemorrhage. The standard diagnostic technique is selective catheter angiography of the cerebral vessels. They may be displayed on MRA or CTA, and with improvements in technique this may provide an alternative. There is increasing evidence that endovascular coiling of aneurysms may be of value in selected patients.

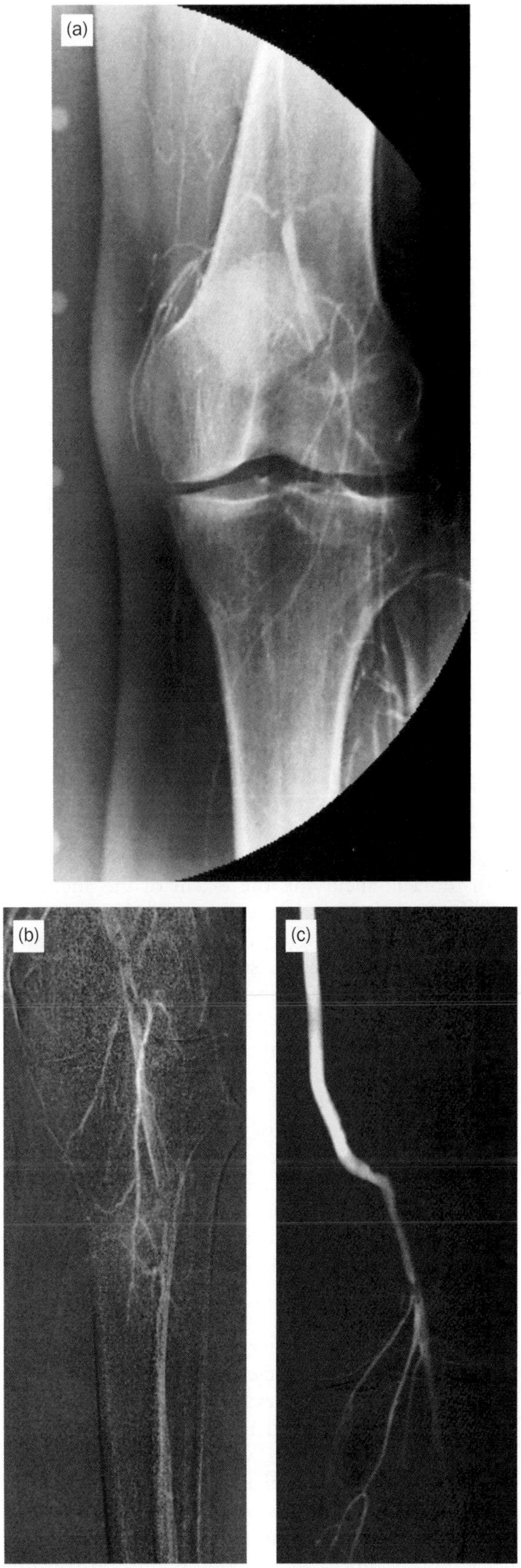

Figure 32.22 Femoral arteriogram: (a) before, (b) during and (c) after thrombolysis of a right femoro-popliteal graft.

Aortic aneurysms

One-quarter of aortic aneurysms occur in the thoracic aorta, 70% being atherosclerotic, 15% traumatic and the remainder predominantly associated with Marfan's syndrome or inflammatory causes (either mycotic, Takayasu's arteritis or syphilitic). Abdominal aortic aneurysms are predominantly atherosclerotic but 5–15% may be inflammatory.

Traumatic thoracic false aneurysm

A false aneurysm may follow blunt decelerating injury such as a road traffic accident. The chest radiographic signs are superior mediastinal widening, left apical pleural shadowing, downward displacement of the left main bronchus or tracheal displacement. CT is particularly relevant in the context of trauma due to its ability to determine other thoracic injuries such as pneumothorax, pericardial effusion or lung contusion. The diagnosis is made on arch aortogram and this examination should be performed without delay. Disruption of one or more layers of the aortic wall, usually at the site of the ligamentum arteriosum just distal to the left subclavian artery or occasionally at the aortic root is found (Figure 32.23).

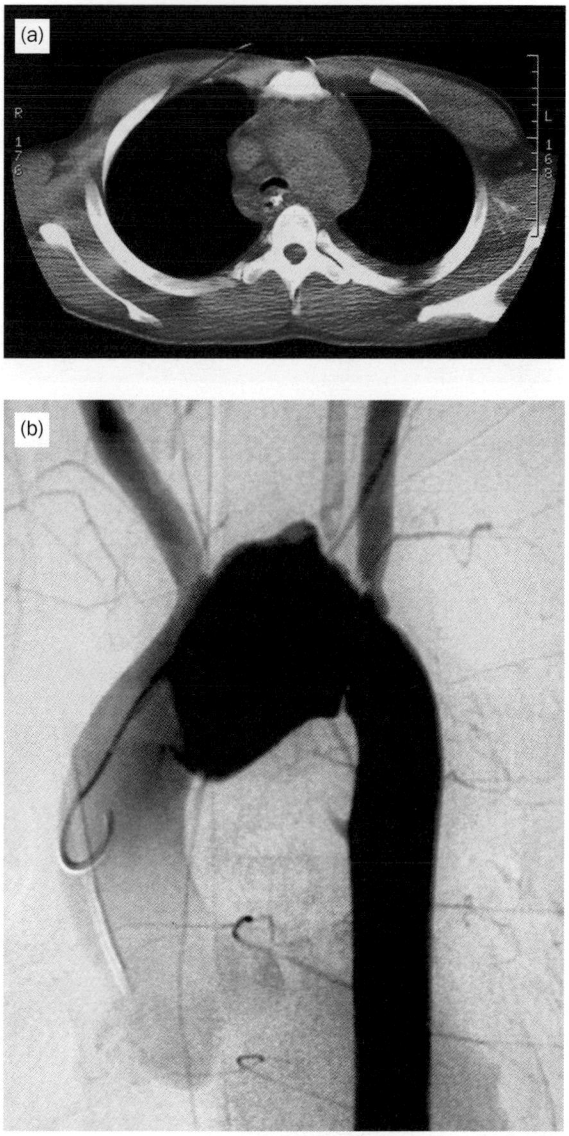

Figure 32.23 (a) Thoracic CT demonstrating a mediastinal haematoma and (b) arch aortogram demonstrating a traumatic false aneurysm following a road traffic accident.

Atherosclerotic aneurysms

The diagnosis of thoracic aortic aneurysm may be indicated on the chest radiograph, but cross-sectional imaging using CT or MRI is required to assess the site and extent of the aneurysm in order to plan management. The CT assessment of thoracic aneurysms allows surgical planning. In particular in patients presenting with thoracic aneurysms the extent of the aneurysm and subdiaphragmatic involvement will determine the approach. Catheter angiography may be used to assess the lumen for possible stent graft placement or assess the coronary arteries for necessary myocardial revascularization.

While aortic aneurysmal wall calcification may be seen on abdominal radiograph, the standard assessment of abdominal aneurysms includes ultrasound to determine the size and extent of the aneurysm, to measure renal sizes and exclude renal pathology or horseshoe kidney that may complicate surgery. CTA or MRA may determine the level in relation to the renal arteries and measure the geometry for possible aortic stent graft placement (Figure 32.24). Catheter angiography may clarify any renal artery stenosis or multiple renal arteries.

Endovascular aortic aneurysm repair may be undertaken in either the thoracic or abdominal aorta. The technique remains under evaluation but is being more extensively employed particularly in the elective repair of aneurysms in patients with poor operative risk (Figure 32.25). There remain technical problems of delivery in certain patients with extreme angulation or tortuosity and in follow-up there is a significant number requiring further intervention due to proximal or distal leaks around the graft ('endoleaks'). Improvements in devices may increase the number of suitable patients, and reduce the requirements for surgical arteriotomy and the failures of the device to exclude long-term endoleaks. The potential exists for extension of the technique into emergency aortic rupture.

Other aneurysms

Atherosclerotic, post-traumatic and inflammatory aneurysms in other arterial sites (commonly iliac (Figure 32.26), splenic, hepatic and gastroduodenal arteries) may be treated by endovascular stent graft or coil embolization.

Venous disease

Commonly the venous system will be assessed by venography or ultrasound, while CT or MRI may be

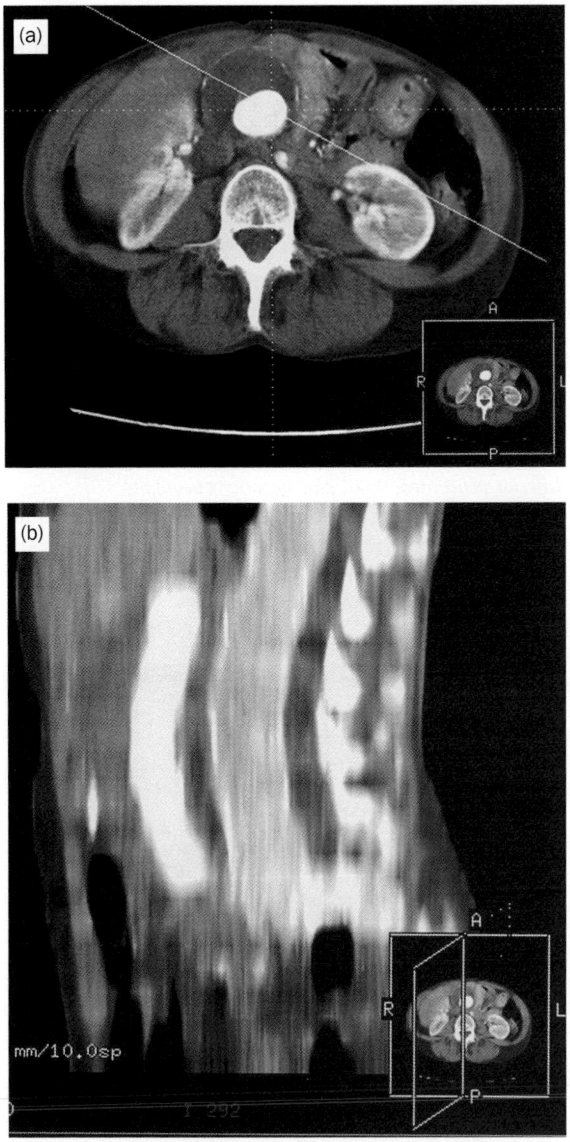

Figure 32.24 CTA allows: (a) axial measurements and (b) reconstructions of an abdominal aortic aneurysm prior to aortic stent graft placement.

of value when the vein is less accessible or the structures adjacent to the vein require evaluation. The presence of thrombus may be assessed with nuclear medicine.

Venography

Similar to angiography, venography depends on visualization of intraluminal contrast medium on X-rays using the normal flow of venous blood from a puncture site or catheter.

Lower limb venography

Using a tilting table and after applying a tourniquet around the ankle, a cannula in a vein on the dorsum of the foot allows injection of contrast and diversion of blood flow to the deep veins under examination.

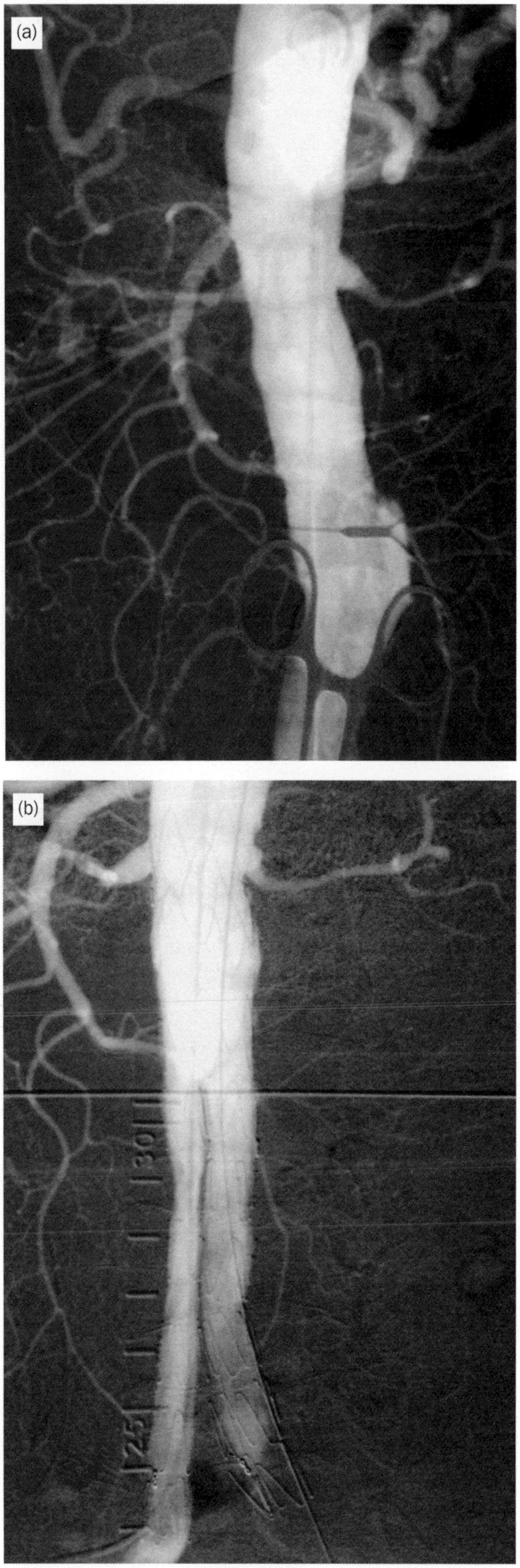

Figure 32.25 Aortic angiogram: (a) before and (b) after stent graft for a 9 cm aortic aneurysm.

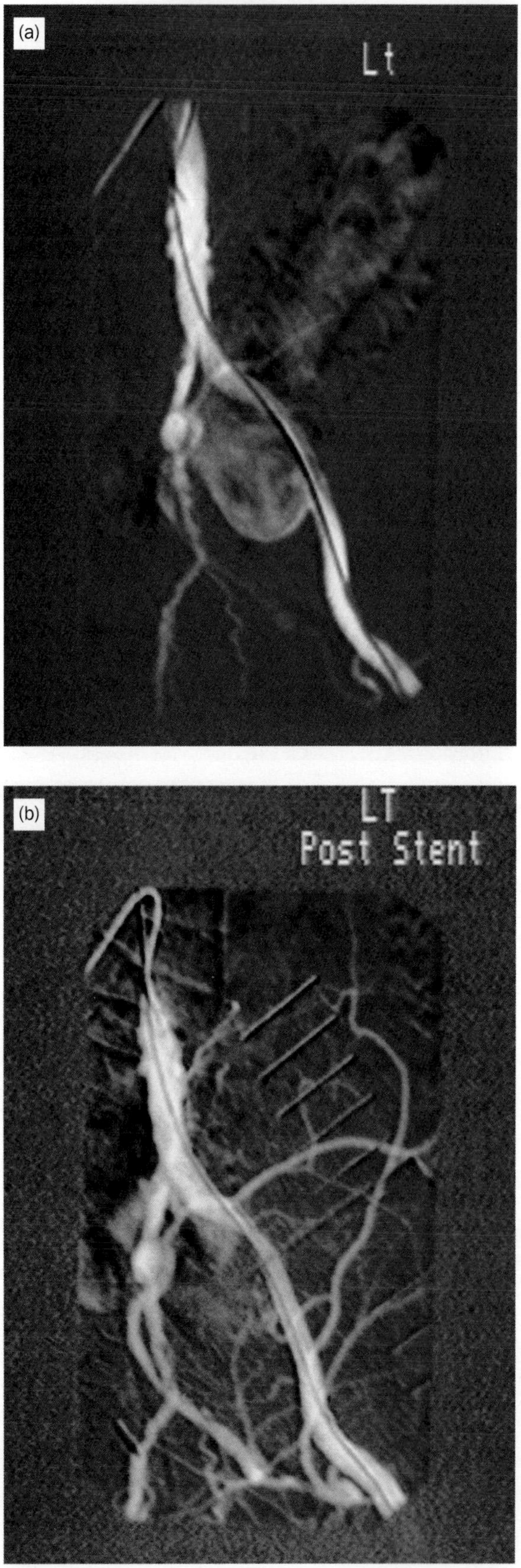

Figure 32.26 Left Iliac arteriogram: (a) before and (b) after stent graft placement for a 5 cm external iliac aneurysm.

This is commonly performed for suspected deep venous thrombosis. Using the tilting table to slow the transit of contrast, images of the lower limb, including the iliac veins and inferior vena cava are obtained (Figure 32.27). Alteration of the technique may be used to assess incompetent perforators by the use of various tourniquets or direct superficial varix injection.

Upper limb venography and superior vena cavography
A similar technique is applied to the upper limb, except the tilting table is not required and there is a need for subtraction images during suspended respiration to achieve adequate views of the innominate veins and superior vena cava.

Inferior vena cava, renal and hepatic venography
Similar to catheter angiography, assessment of the inferior vena cava, renal and hepatic veins requires a Seldinger technique and catheter placement to inject contrast into the required vessel.

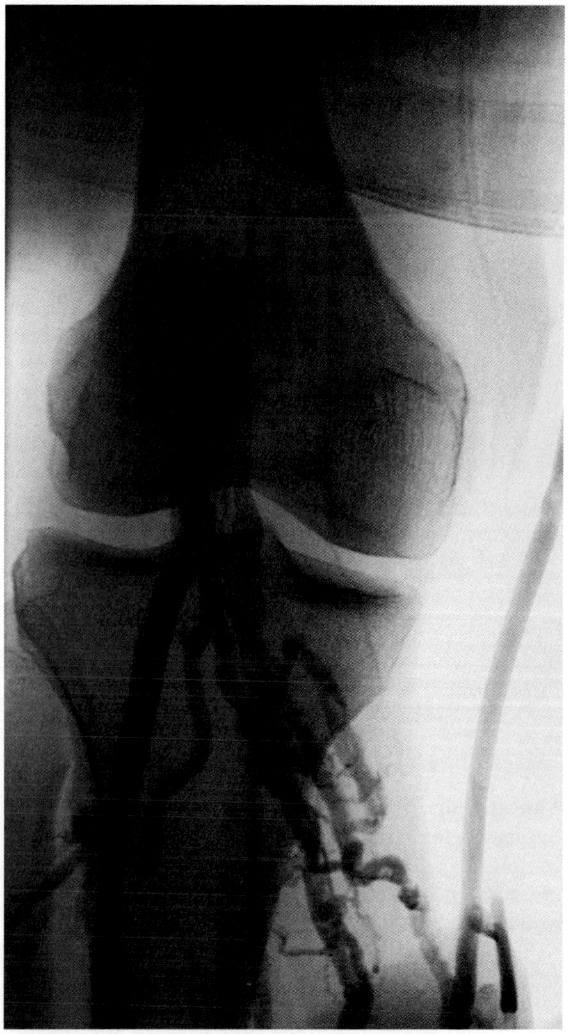

Figure 32.27 Contrast venogram demonstrating an occluded popliteal vein due to thrombosis.

Ultrasound

The addition of colour Doppler and continuous wave Doppler to conventional grey-scale Doppler, and the accessibility of veins, except in the thorax, .has established ultrasound as the primary imaging modality for venous disease (Figure 32.28). In certain obese patients abdominal assessment of the iliac veins and inferior vena cava is difficult. The superior vena cava is not accessible to transthoracic ultrasound.

CT and MRI

Contrast-enhanced CT may be used to show veins and neighbouring structures, particularly the inominate veins, superior vena cava (Figure 32.29), inferior vena cava and portal vein. Thrombus is identified as a filling defect in an enlarged vein and underlying compressive aetiology may be identified. MRI may offer similar information and is of particular value in intracranial thromboses and characterization of pelvic compressive causes of iliac vein thromboses.

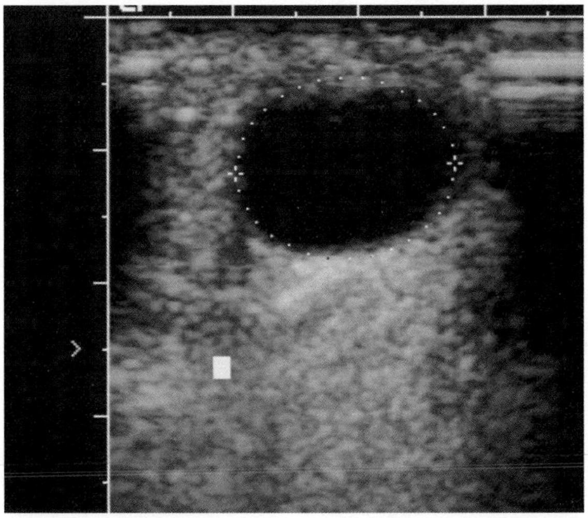

Figure 32.28 Doppler ultrasound of the common femoral vein to assess thrombosis.

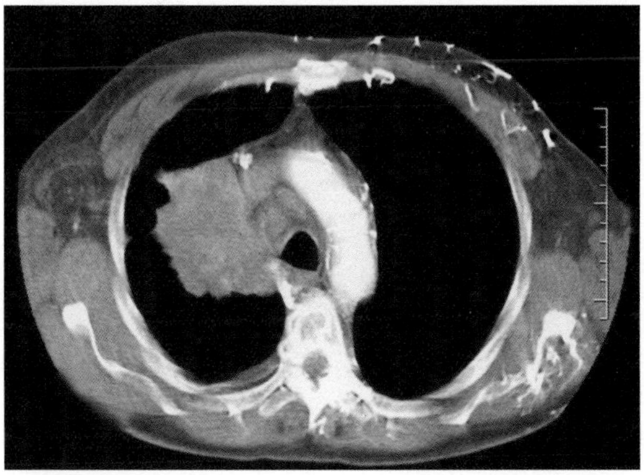

Figure 32.29 CT venogram of the thorax demonstrating superior vena cava obstruction due to a bronchial carcinoma.

Radionuclide scanning

Isotope techniques have been used to demonstrate the venous system and, in particular, ^{99m}Tc-labelled macrophages may be used to demonstrate lung perfusion, as part of the ventilation perfusion study for suspected pulmonary thromboembolism.

Endovascular therapy in venous disease

Venous occlusive disease

Superior vena cava obstruction

In patients with symptomatic superior vena caval obstruction commonly due to a compressive malignant aetiology, such as bronchial carcinoma or mesothelioma, the use of catheter recanalization with or without thrombolysis, from either a basilic or common femoral vein approach may bring symptomatic relief. The use of balloon angioplasty with stent placement is commonly undertaken (Figure 32.30).

Iliofemoral venous thrombosis

Deep venous thrombosis extending into the iliac segments rarely may result in phlegmasia and limb threatening ischaemia. Catheter-directed thrombolysis, from an arterial or a venous route, may be used to restore venous drainage. More commonly the iliofemoral thrombosis may result in chronic venous insufficiency. The use of thrombolysis and venous angioplasty of underlying stenotic disease is at present controversial.

Upper limb venous thrombosis

The swelling resulting from axillary vein thrombosis with extension may limit the function of the limb acutely such that thrombolysis may be used in a similar technique to arterial thrombolysis.

Venous embolic disease

In cases of pulmonary thromboembolism from lower limb deep venous thrombosis, despite anticoagulants or in patients in whom anticoagulation is contraindicated, an inferior vena cava filter, either temporary or permanent, should be considered.

Vascular access

There is an increasing role of interventional radiology in the placement and maintenance of venous vascular access for renal dialysis or chemotherapy ports. The image guidance employed reduces complication rates. The malposition of central lines, placed without imaging assistance, may be corrected using repositioning techniques (Figure 32.31).

The maintenance of venous access, in particular for renal dialysis patients, is important in prolonging the durability of access routes. Shunt or fistula stenosis may be treated by balloon angioplasty with or without stent placement, while acute occlusion of shunts may be treated with thrombolysis, mechanical thrombectomy and subsequent angioplasty.

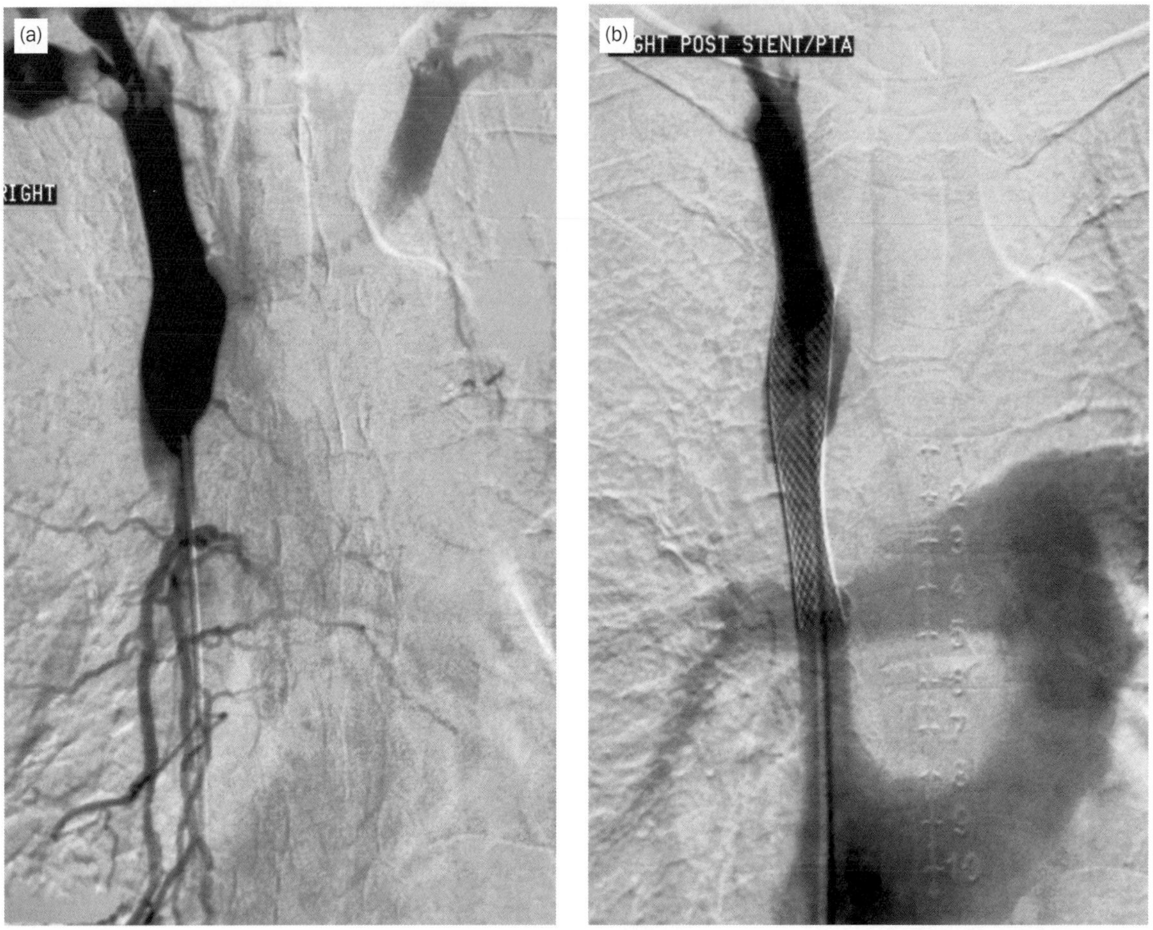

Figure 32.30 Venogram: (a) before and (b) after superior vena cava angioplasty and stenting.

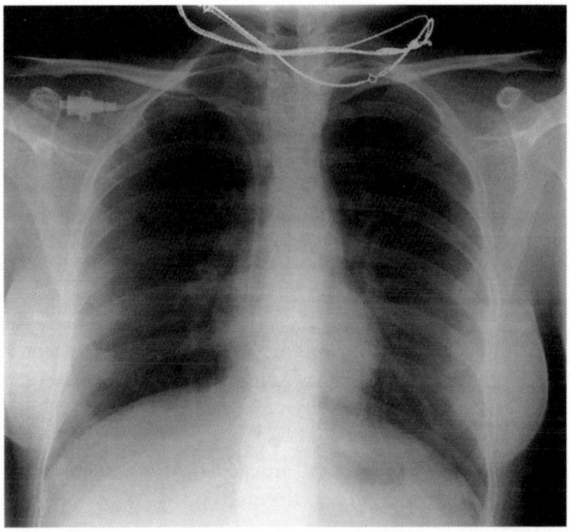

Figure 32.31 Chest radiograph demonstrates a temporary dialysis catheter malpositioned in the pulmonary artery.

Further reading

Baum, S. (1997). *Abram's Angiography: Vascular and Interventional Radiology*, 4th edn. Boston, MA: Little, Brown.

Body, M. R. (1998). *Angiography. MRI Clinics of North America*. Philadelphia, PA: W.B. Saunders.

Darcy, La Berge (1994). *Peripheral Vascular Interventions*. SCVIR Syllabus.

Edelman, R. R., Hesselink, J. R. and Zlatkin, M. B. (1996). *Clinical Magnetic Resonance Imaging*, 2nd edn. Philadelphia, PA: W.B. Saunders.

MODULE 33

Venous thrombo-embolism

1 • Aetiology

2 • Clinical features

3 • Investigation

4 • Treatment

5 • Thrombo-embolic prophylaxis

Throughout this module the term venous thrombo-embolism (VTE) will be used to describe the disease which may present as deep venous thrombosis (DVT) alone or in combination with pulmonary embolism (PE) or occasionally as PE with no detectable DVT. The more carefully PE is looked for in patients with DVT the more often it will be found. In clinical practice it is still not unusual to see PE managed without regard to the source (most patients who die from PE have had 'herald' emboli) or the late risk of post-thrombotic syndrome. Equally, DVT is often managed without consideration of the presence of or potential for embolism. They are one and the same disease, and should be managed as such.

VTE is responsible for considerable morbidity and mortality, both in hospital and in the community. The impact of VTE on morbidity and mortality is largely unrecognized in daily practice because of low autopsy rates. In the USA, it estimated that DVT and PE occur in over two million people each year. The incidence of inpatient PE is estimated as 23 per 100 000, with an associated mortality rate of approximately 12%. In the UK, it is estimated that PE is responsible for 30 000–40 000 deaths each year. Despite thrombo-embolic prophylaxis, symptomatic and asymptomatic PE occurs in approximately 25% of surgical patients, and is responsible for 3% of surgical inpatient deaths. Approximately 25% of patients who have a fatal PE have had recent surgery. The principal late complication of DVT is the post-thrombotic syndrome. Destruction of the valves or residual obstruction of the deep veins of the leg causes deep venous insufficiency which is manifest as swelling, venous claudication, lipodermatosclerosis and leg ulceration. The post-thrombotic syndrome will not be discussed in this module.

Section 33.1 • Aetiology

Virchow was the first to demonstrate that venous thrombo-embolism was principally due to the interaction of three factors: reduced or static venous blood flow, injury to the vein wall and a hypercoagulable state (Virchow's triad). This remains a useful starting point in understanding the pathogenesis. Almost invariably, when a patient presents with VTE several predisposing factors will be present. While reduced blood flow may be an important initiator of DVT in an immobile post-operative patient, autopsy and experimental data have been unable to demonstrate that the combination of reduced blood flow and vein wall injury alone can lead to thrombosis. Experimental data, however, suggest that reduced blood flow combined with a local and/or systemic hypercoagulable state can initiate thrombosis. It has been postulated that a number of factors such as activation of the coagulation cascade and/or endothelial cell injury secondary to hypoxia, and thromboxane and thrombin release may lead to the formation of a nidus of thrombus in the stagnant region of the vein deep within the venous valve pocket. As the thrombus forms it either attaches to the vein wall beyond the valve and occludes the vein, or propagates proximally to become free-floating and non-occlusive. Venous thrombosis can occur in any part of the venous system but most commonly originates in the soleal veins of the calf.

Primary deep venous thrombosis

A primary hypercoagulable state or thrombophilia is a specific abnormality of the coagulation system which results in increased risk of thrombosis. In a patient with such an abnormality, DVT may occur without any obvious precipitating cause. The number of factors recognized as responsible for thrombophilia has increased steadily in recent years. Over half of these abnormalities are due to genetic mutations.

Antithrombin (AT) III deficiency

AT III inactivates thrombin to form thrombin–antithrombin (TAT) complex, and also inhibits coagulation factors IXa, Xa, XIa and XIIa. The natural and exogenous heparins bind to AT III to increase the antithrombin effect. Patients are at increased risk of DVT, mesenteric vein thrombosis and arterial thrombosis rarely before the second decade of life and usually in association with other risk factors such as surgery or trauma. The risk of thrombosis increases as the functional AT III activity falls to less than 80% of normal. Secondary AT III deficiency occurs in liver dysfunction, disseminated intravascular coagulopathy, DVT and sepsis syndrome.

Protein C and S deficiencies

Proteins C and S are vitamin K-dependent proteins. Thrombin binds to thrombomodulin (TM) on the surface of endothelial cells and this activates protein C which is released and binds to the co-factor protein S to form a complex which inactivates coagulation factors Va and VIIIa. Protein C also enhances fibrinolytic activity by decreasing plasminogen activator inhibitor (PAI) activity. Plasma levels are reduced in liver dysfunction, chronic renal failure, disseminated intravascular coagulation (DIC), major surgery and in association with thrombotic events. In families with a history of DVT, about 50% of patients with heterozygous protein C deficiency will have had a DVT before 40 years of age. Venous thrombosis also occurs in the mesenteric, renal and cerebral circulation. Arterial thrombotic events are uncommon. Activated protein C resistance (APCR) is the commonest risk factor for VTE, characterized by the inability of activated protein C to degrade an altered form of coagulation factor Va (factor V Leiden). APCR accounts for up to 64% of inherited causes of thrombosis. Heterozygous and homozygous APCR are associated with a seven-fold and an 80-fold increased risk of VTE, respectively.

Antiphospholipid syndrome

This syndrome occurs in 1–5% of the population and increases with age such that 50% of patients aged 80 years and over have antiphospholipid antibodies. The syndrome occurs in patients with lupus anticoagulants and anticardiolipin antibodies. The antibodies are directed against protein–phospholipid complexes and inhibit the antithrombotic effects of endothelial cells and increase platelet activation. Patients have a high incidence of venous and arterial thrombotic events including recurrent DVT, PE, inferior vena cava (IVC) thrombosis, myocardial infarction, stroke and failure of vascular reconstruction.

Hyperhomocysteinaemia

Homocysteine is an amino acid formed during methionine metabolism. Abnormal methionine metabolism may be inherited or secondary to deficiencies of vitamins B_{12}, B_6 and folate. Hyperhomocysteinaemia is associated with increased risk of recurrent arterial and venous thrombo-embolic events.

Hypofibrinolytic state

Several abnormalities of the fibrinolytic system exist, but elevated PAI activity is the most important. PAI is the naturally occurring inhibitor of tissue plasminogen activator (t-PA) which converts plasminogen to active plasmin which causes lysis of fibrinogen, fibrin and fibrin clot. The hypofibrinolytic state, characterized by elevated PAI and reduced t-PA activities, occurs in 30–40% of patients with DVT, and is probably a major factor in primary DVT and in secondary DVT where it constitutes part of the acute phase response to trauma and surgery.

Secondary deep venous thrombosis

DVT is usually of this variety: a multifactorial condition which is the result of a combination of venous stasis and/or vessel wall damage and a secondary hypercoagulable state with activation of the coagulation cascade, platelet activation and impaired fibrinolysis. Thus, there will almost invariably be an obvious precipitating cause or event consistent with Virchow's triad. Patient risk factors include previous VTE, age greater than 40 years, prolonged surgery; trauma; sepsis; malignancy and chemotherapy; inflammatory bowel disease and other chronic inflammatory conditions; immobility due to for example recent surgery, obesity, stroke and paralysis, cardiac failure, diabetes and pregnancy. After surgery, there is increased activation of the coagulation system and a hypofibrinolytic state for at least 10 days. Risk factors for post-operative VTE include those listed above and in addition, thrombophilia, cardiovascular complications, major joint replacement, peripheral vascular reconstruction, and surgery for cancer and inflammatory bowel disease.

Section 33.2 • Clinical features

Patients with suspected DVT or PE may have a family history or past history of VTE. There may also be a history of recent trauma, surgery, immobility, pregnancy, malignant disease or air travel. DVT in its early and most dangerous stage is asymptomatic. The great majority of patients who die of pulmonary embolism will have had no prior signs or symptoms in their legs. Why is this? Newly formed thrombus is soft, friable and, for most of its length, free floating. It is the inflammatory change associated with early organization of thrombus which not only gives rise to clinical symptoms but also anchors the thrombus to the vein wall.

Deep venous thrombosis: lower limb

The main symptoms, once they develop, are calf pain and swelling, usually unilateral. When DVT originates in the ilio-femoral segment, as is commonly the case in association with pelvic or femoral trauma, hip surgery or pregnancy, the swelling starts in the thigh and the pain in the groin or iliac fossa. Sometimes it will have a marked inflammatory component. Signs include pitting oedema, tenderness, erythema, increased temperature and dilated collateral superficial veins. Severe and extensive ilio-femoral DVT may be complicated by the development of phlegmasia alba dolens (PAD), phlegmasia caerulea dolens (PCD) and venous gangrene.

PAD is characterized by a swollen, painful, pale or erythematous limb and this may progress to PCD within 24–48 hours. PCD is usually found in patients with advanced malignant disease. It is characterized by a severe 'bursting' pain, cyanosis and extreme swelling of the entire limb, and in 50% of patients venous gangrene develops affecting the toes and foot initially within 24–48 hours of onset. PCD is an aggressive form of the thrombotic process in which thrombosis extends from the major veins into the venules and capillaries resulting in secondary arterial insufficiency. The resultant increased capillary hydrostatic pressure leads to interstitial oedema which may be so massive that the patient develops hypovolaemic shock. The increase in the interstitial pressure compresses the capillaries and further compromises capillary flow. PCD is associated with considerable morbidity and mortality – 50% of patients require an amputation, 12–40% develop PE and the mortality rate is 20%. Although the appearances of the limb may be alarming, it is a mistake to embark on early amputation (unless there is compartment syndrome with impending muscle necrosis) since tissue loss can often be minimized by aggressive medical treatment.

Deep venous thrombosis: upper limb

Venous compromise of the upper limb may present as the end result of chronic thoracic outlet compression as a consequence of ligamentous or bony abnormality; or it may arise out of the blue, often precipitated by physical activity in a young person, the so-called 'effort syndrome'.

Indwelling catheters in any of the great veins of the upper limb or neck may give rise to thrombosis as may malignancy in the area. Sudden swelling and cyanosis of the arm occurs and is accompanied by engorgement of the collateral veins of the upper arm, shoulder and chest wall.

Pulmonary embolism

Lower limb DVT is responsible for more than 90% of PE, but is clinically apparent at the time of the PE in only 10% of patients. If the patient survives leg symptoms commonly emerge later. Symptomatic PE is associated with acute onset dyspnoea, pleuritic chest pain and haemoptysis. Clinical signs include a low-grade pyrexia, cyanosis, tachycardia, hypotension, tachypnoea and a raised jugular venous pulse. The symptoms and signs may be subtle, insidious and non-specific and are commonly mistaken for chest infection. Thus, VTE should always be suspected in a patient who is in a high-risk situation and whose condition is deteriorating for no obvious reason. Massive PE may present as sudden cardiovascular collapse and cardiac arrest. The initial diagnosis is based on the context in which it occurs. Autopsy series and lung scanning studies have shown that in patients with a proven PE, half will have a proximal DVT and half will have thrombosis originating in calf veins.

Section 33.3 • Investigation

The purpose of investigations is not simply to confirm or exclude the presence of DVT or PE.

It is to identify the location of the thrombus, to ascertain the degree of risk to life, to determine the probability of later post-thrombotic syndrome and to provide a basis for selective treatment. Diagnostic imaging should be performed within 24 hours in patients with suspected VTE to minimize exposure of the patient to the potential adverse effects of anticoagulant therapy if no VTE is diagnosed. Pending definitive diagnosis, if consistent clinical signs of DVT or PE are present, then full anticoagulation with heparin should commence on the basis of clinical diagnosis. One possible algorithm for the investigation and treatment of DVT is shown in Figure 33.1.

Before commencing heparin, however, a thrombophilia screen is recommended in the following situations: VTE before 45 years or arterial thrombotic events before 40 years of age; VTE occurring without any apparent precipitating factor or high-risk circumstances, recurrent VTE or thrombophlebitis; venous thrombosis in an unusual site; warfarin or heparin-induced skin necrosis and a family history of VTE or thrombophilia.

As sophisticated diagnostic methods such as radiolabelled fibrinogen and ultrasound become available, it has been fashionable to state that clinical diagnosis is extremely inaccurate. In broad terms this is quite true given that DVT is silent in its early stages and given the number of conditions which give rise to leg pain and swelling. In fact it has been shown that if patients are classified into categories of high, medium and low

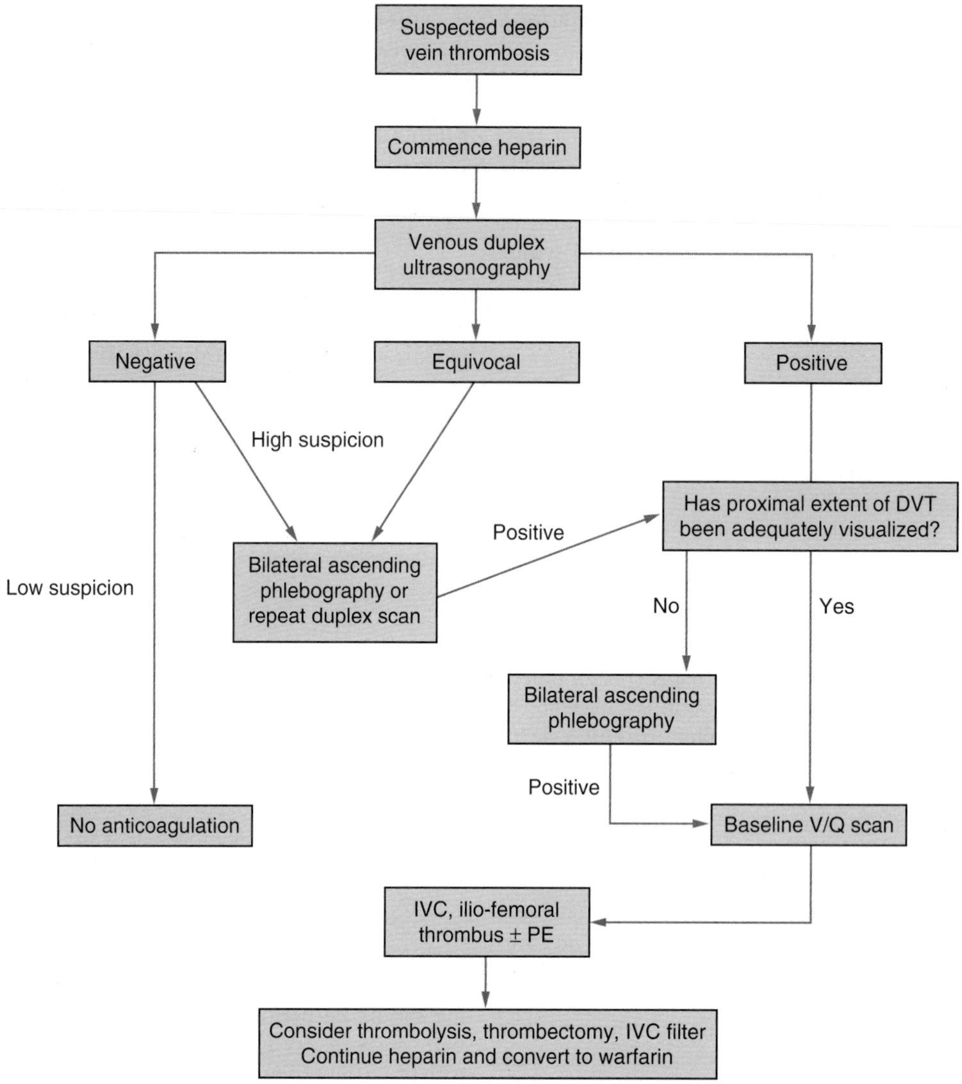

Figure 33.1 Algorithm for the investigation and treatment of clinically suspected DVT.

probability of DVT on clinical grounds this corresponds to diagnostic accuracies of 85%, 33% and 5%, respectively. A diagnostic policy can therefore be rationalized and made cost effective on the basis of clinical acumen.

Deep venous thrombosis: lower limb

Ascending contrast phlebography

This is the reference standard for the diagnosis of DVT, but being invasive it is now regarded as a second line investigation in cases where duplex ultrasonography is inadequate or equivocal. Its major advantage is that the tibial, popliteal, femoral and iliac veins and IVC can all be imaged. DVT is manifest as a filling defect within the deep veins. In approximately 10% of patients, imaging is inadequate. It should not be assumed that failure to get contrast into a vein means that it is thrombosed.

An important point, often ignored, is that when iliac vein thrombosis is suspected clinically ascending phlebography should be performed by the bilateral route, and if gross thigh swelling is present it should only be performed by the contralateral route (see below). In ilio-femoral DVT injection of contrast medium into the veins of the opposite leg is the only way (other than upper limb catheterization) to provide adequate visualization of the IVC. In addition clinically important DVT may be discovered in the asymptomatic leg. Morbidity associated with phlebography includes tourniquet discomfort if the limb is very swollen and, in rare instances, contrast reactions, DVT and PE. Ascending phlebography should not be attempted in a leg which is grossly swollen with proximal DVT, particularly in a patient with suspected thrombophilia. Such an intervention, even with modern non-ionic contrast media, carries the serious risk of extravasation of contrast medium into the tissues, aggravation of the DVT and conversion of PAD into PCD. Duplex scan will reveal whether the ilio-femoral segment contains thrombus. The important question in such a case is whether the thrombus is extending up the IVC. Contrast should therefore be injected via the contralateral foot or groin.

Venous duplex ultrasonography

This is now regarded as the first-line diagnostic method in symptomatic patients with DVT and as such has placed difficult demands on imaging services in many hospitals. A carefully constructed diagnostic protocol is therefore essential. The method relies on the ability to visualize luminal thrombus, interference with flow or non-compressibility of the vein by pressure from the ultrasound probe. In patients with no leg symptoms, as for example when the patient presents with PE or when attempts are made to use duplex for screening at-risk populations, duplex has lower success rates in detecting DVT because early thrombus may not impede blood flow and soft, fresh thrombus in the vein may be readily compressible.

Although non-invasive, duplex scanning is more technically demanding to perform and interpret than phlebography. The superficial femoral, profunda femoris and popliteal veins are readily imaged, but the iliac and tibial veins are difficult to assess. Consequently, if duplex is negative then venography may be performed in order to detect tibial or iliac vein thrombosis, or duplex can be repeated after 7 days to detect proximal extension of tibial DVT. DVT is manifest as an inability to compress the vein and flow within the vein suggests that the thrombus is non-occlusive. Duplex is associated with a sensitivity and specificity of 95 and 98%, respectively, for femoral and popliteal DVT. The sensitivity for asymptomatic patients at risk of DVT, i.e. as a screening method, is considerably lower at 38–83%.

D-dimer

This fibrin degradation product is elevated in VTE. It may also be elevated in a number of other conditions. A negative test is very valuable as it excludes VTE. A positive value must be considered in the light of other clinical evidence.

Deep venous thrombosis: upper limb

The condition appears to present earlier than is the case with lower limb DVT and the diagnosis is usually clinically obvious. Duplex ultrasonagraphy is not going to provide the additional information needed. Phlebography is required, followed by catheter-delivered thrombolysis. As soon as lysis has been achieved films should be obtained without delay, with a range of arm positions, to demonstrate any underlying anatomical abnormality giving rise to venous compression, i.e. one of the family of thoracic outlet compression syndromes. Venous compression most commonly occurs as a result of bony compression in the apex of the pincers formed by the clavicle and the first rib. Abnormal ligamentous bands may also cause compression. Many different anatomical varieties have been described, the commonest of which is a costocostal band running between the neck of the first rib and the posterior aspect of the scalene tubercle. A cervical rib can also cause thoracic outlet compression but is more likely to present with neurological or arterial symptoms. If the thrombosis has been precipitated by an indwelling catheter it should temporarily be left in place and utilized for phlebography and delivery of a lytic agent.

Pulmonary embolism

Plain chest radiography

Although seldom diagnostic of PE a plain chest X-ray is valuable as it may help to exclude alternative pathology as a cause of the patient's symptoms and signs. Features suggestive of PE include atelectasis, prominent hilar markings, pleural effusion, oligaemic lung fields, elevated hemidiaphragm and cardiomegaly.

Electrocardiography (ECG)

Features suggestive of PE include signs of right heart strain and/or ischaemia. T-wave inversion in one or more precordial leads closely matches the severity of PE, and reversibility of this ECG sign after thrombolysis for PE has been reported to be a predictor of good outcome.

Arterial blood gas analysis

The degree of hypoxia and hypocarbia roughly correlates with the size of PE. However, a large minority of patients with PE have normal arterial blood gases.

Echocardiography

Intracardiac clot is associated with a mortality rate of approximately 50% and consequently routine pulmonary embolectomy or thrombolysis has been advocated. Signs indicating right ventricular dysfunction (such as right ventricular and pulmonary artery dilatation, right ventricular wall dyskinesia, tricuspid regurgitation) are associated with a mortality rate of approximately 13%.

Pulmonary arteriography

This is the reference standard for the diagnosis of PE. It is invasive and is best performed through a pulmonary artery catheter. It is the first-line investigation if there is cardiovascular collapse or hypotension and PE is suspected. PE is manifest as intraluminal filling defects and abrupt cut-offs of the pulmonary arterial tree. The investigation is associated with a mortality rate of less than 1%, and major morbidity of 1%. It is not recommended in patients with renal failure, cardiac failure or pulmonary hypertension.

Pulmonary radio-isotope ventilation perfusion scan (V/Q scan)

Lung scans are valuable as long as they are interpreted in the clinical context and in the light of other key investigations, particularly duplex leg scans or phlebography. Very low, low and high probability scans in patients who have consistent clinical findings are of most value. In 25% of cases, V/Q scans are diagnostic of PE, and in 25% the scans exclude PE. The results are unreliable if the patient has had recent major surgery, lower limb trauma or a prolonged period of immobility. In these circumstances, and where an indeterminate probability scan has been reported (50% of patients), further investigation for co-existing DVT or pulmonary arteriography are recommended.

Spiral computed tomography CT angiography

This is a recent development which is not in general use. The sensitivity and specificity of spiral CT for PE is 94 and 96% respectively, compared with pulmonary arteriography. It is more sensitive than V/Q scan, but less accurate in detecting peripheral emboli.

Section 33.4 • Treatment

The treatment of DVT has three principal aims – prevent clot propagation, reduce the risk of PE and enhance the resolution of the clot to minimize the post-thrombotic syndrome. Recent trials suggest that active treatment of DVT by means of thrombolysis or thrombectomy offers better long-term outcome than anticoagulation alone. However, this only applies to carefully selected patients presenting with severe and extensive proximal thrombus. Hospital protocols should identify the phlegmasia group and these patients should be admitted to the vascular service for selective active intervention.

The majority of patients with DVT will be treated with anticoagulation, limb elevation when resting, calf exercises and compression stockings. Compression stockings should be worn on the affected limb for at least 2 years after ilio-femoral DVT to reduce the incidence of severe post-thrombotic syndrome from 23 to 11%. Knee length class II hosiery is usually the most appropriate. The treatment of calf vein DVT is controversial. In 20% of patients, the thrombus extends to the popliteal vein and 40–50% will have clinically detected PE. Calf vein DVT alone is associated with PE in 10% of patients and 25% of patients will develop chronic venous insufficiency after 1 year follow-up. Currently, therefore, full anticoagulation is recommended. Patients with PCD will require treatment with anticoagulation, high limb elevation and fluid resuscitation for hypovolaemic shock which will improve limb perfusion. The early removal of the thrombus is considered the most effective means of preventing the early and late complications of DVT. Thrombolysis and venous thrombectomy are discussed below.

In patients with symptomatic PE, the mortality rate is 30% without treatment and 2% with treatment. In a patient with suspected PE, analgesia should be prescribed for chest pain and supplemental oxygen administered for hypoxia. If there is a moderate or high suspicion of PE, then the patient should be anticoagulated before investigation using intravenous heparin (following the same regimen as described below for DVT) to achieve an activated partial thromboplastin time (APTT) of 1.5–2.5 as soon as possible to reduce the risk of recurrent PE. If the patient is haemodynamically compromised, then fluid resuscitation, central venous pressure monitoring and inotropic support may be required. If PE is confirmed and the patient is stable, intravenous or low molecular weight heparin (LMWH) should be continued and warfarin should be commenced within 3 days, overlapping with heparin for at least 4 days (because warfarin takes several days to achieve its full therapeutic effect) and continued for 4 weeks if the PE has occurred postoperatively. Thrombolysis, pulmonary embolectomy and IVC filtration for PE are discussed below.

Sixty per cent of patients with a first episode of proximal DVT develop post-thrombotic syndrome within 2 years and virtually all will do so within 5 years. These figures can be halved by compression therapy. Late follow-up of patients with proximal DVT is therefore essential to ensure attention to high quality compression hosiery if deterioration of post-thrombotic symptoms is to be avoided.

Out-patient management of deep venous thrombosis

This important recent development is based on clinical trials which have shown that selected patients with DVT can be maintained as ambulant outpatients without detriment to outcome in terms of post-thrombotic problems or PE. The outpatient with suspected DVT has blood taken for routine blood tests plus D-dimer and coagulation screen. He or she is clerked and scored for DVT probability. A negative D-dimer plus a low probability score excludes DVT. Positive D-dimer or negative D-dimer plus medium or high probability score is the indication for duplex ultrasonography. If this is a suboptimal study the patient goes on to phlebography. A good quality duplex study rules out DVT. A clearly positive study leads to evaluation for outpatient management. Exclusion criteria leading to inpatient management include phlegmasia, thrombus in or extending above the common femoral vein, significant co-morbid disease active risk factors (listed in Table 33.1), suspected or confirmed PE, bleeding tendency or recent gastrointestinal bleed and medical or social reasons for non-compliance.

Patients selected for ambulatory treatment are entered into a formal outpatient programme. They are commenced on LMWH and warfarin and fitted with elastic compression hosiery. LMWH is continued for a minimum of 6 days and until the international normalized ratio (INR) has been >2.0 for 2 consecutive days. Patients are also carefully counselled and provided with an information booklet and an anticoagulation log. Active and regular walking while wearing compression hosiery is encouraged as the most effective means of reducing swelling. Close liaison is essential with the general practitioner who undertakes the INR

Table 33.1 Risk factors for venous thrombo-embolism

Primary hypercoagulable state
Antithrombin (AT) III deficiency
Protein C deficiency
Activated protein C resistance (APCR) (factor V Leiden)
Protein S deficiency
Antiphospholipid syndrome
Lupus anticoagulant
Anticardiolipin antibodies
Hyperhomocysteinaemia
Hypofibrinolytic state
Elevated plasminogen activator inhibitor (PAI) activity
Secondary hypercoagulable state
Previous venous thromboembolic event
Age > 40 years
Obesity
Surgery
Trauma
Sepsis
Malignancy and chemotherapy
Inflammatory bowel disease
Immobility
Stroke and paralysis
Cardiac failure and recent myocardial infarction
Pregnancy
Oestrogen therapy
Central venous catheters

monitoring. Warfarin is continued for a minimum of 3 months. Hospital follow-up at 6 weeks is arranged and arrangements are made for a thrombophilia screen if appropriate when the course of warfarin has been completed.

Anticoagulation

Anticoagulant therapy discourages further clot formation while facilitating endogenous clot lysis. Before commencing anticoagulation, blood should be sampled for baseline urea, electrolytes, liver function tests, coagulation screen and thrombophilia screen if indicated. In clinically suspected DVT or PE, heparin should be commenced, unless contraindicated, until the diagnosis is excluded. There is considerable evidence to support the fact that, for a first episode of DVT or PE, especially if of the secondary variety, adequate anticoagulation is: 4–6 days of heparin (either intravenous unfractionated, LMWH or subcutaneous miniheparin) and early institution of warfarin and discontinuation of heparin when the INR is >2.0 on 2 consecutive days. As noted earlier the full therapeutic effect of warfarin takes several days to achieve, and it should therefore be overlapped with heparin for at least 4 days. Thereafter warfarin should be continued for a minimum of 3 months to maintain an INR of 2.0–4.5. Patients with suspected primary DVT or in particularly high-risk situations should be maintained on heparin until propagation of thrombus and continuing PE have been excluded. For patients with continuing risk factors at 3 months, warfarin therapy may be continued. This regimen is associated with an 80% reduction in the risk of recurrent VTE to between 5 and 7%. During adequate anticoagulation, the risk of fatal PE is 0.3–0.4% for patients who are being treated for DVT, and 0–1.5% for patients treated for PE. After 3 months of adequate anticoagulation, the incidence of symptomatic recurrent VTE is 25% at 5 years and 30% at 8 years. Anticoagulation may be withheld in patients with an indeterminate probability V/Q scan and negative ascending contrast phlebography as the risk of subsequent VTE is considered to be similar to that in patients with a normal V/Q scan.

Unfractionated heparin

The principal mode of action is by increasing the binding of coagulation factors IXa, Xa, XIa, XII and thrombin to antithrombin III. Intravenous administration has an immediate effect with a half life of 90 min, and subcutaneous administration results in a peak at 4–6 hours and lasts for up to 12 hours. The intravenous regimen comprises a bolus dose of 5000 IU or 75 IU/kg body weight followed by 1000–2000 IU/hour to maintain an APTT of 1.5–2.5. It is recommended that an APTT > 1.5 should be achieved within 24 hours of commencing treatment as this reduces the risk of recurrent VTE from 23% if this is not achieved to 4–6%. Subcutaneous unfractionated miniheparin 5000 IU given 12 hourly is as effective and safe as intravenous unfractionated heparin in preventing recurrent VTE in patients with acute DVT. The risk of bleeding with intravenous unfractionated heparin is approximately 10% after 5–10 days of treatment. A major advantage of intravenous heparin is that its anticoagulant effect is easily reversed by stopping the infusion and administering intravenous protamine. Heparin should be given for at least 5 days, oral anticoagulation should be commenced after 24 hours and heparin should then be stopped when the INR is at a therapeutic level.

Heparin-induced thrombocytopenia (HIT)

During heparin therapy the platelet count should be monitored every 3 days. HIT occurs due to heparin-associated antiplatelet antibodies. Clinical manifestations include abdominal and/or back pain, heparin-induced skin necrosis, heparin resistance (inability to achieve a therapeutic APTT despite increased dose), falling platelet count (PC), and thrombo-embolic complications in 10–20% of patients (mainly arterial but also VTE and PCD) and to a lesser extent haemorrhagic complications, both of which occur due to intravascular platelet clumping and occasionally activation of the coagulation cascade.

Type I HIT is characterized by a transient fall in PC to 100–150 ($\times 10^9$) between 1 and 5 days after starting heparin, and this returns to normal without stopping treatment and is rarely associated with complications. Type II HIT is characterized by heparin resistance and a falling PC to less than 50 usually more than 6 days after starting heparin or within hours of re-exposure to heparin. PC returns to normal within 1 week of stopping heparin. The risk of HIT is lower with subcutaneous miniheparin, LMWH and low doses of intravenous unfractionated heparin.

The treatment is as follows:

- If the PC is less than 50 and the INR is subtherapeutic then stop all heparin and start a different anticoagulant. Warfarin is not appropriate because it reduces protein C and promotes thrombin generation in the presence of platelet depletion. Hirudin or danaparoid is an appropriate alternative.
- If the PC is approximately 100 and INR is subtherapeutic, then continue heparin and warfarin and monitor PC until INR reaches a therapeutic level.
- If the haemorrhage risk is high and the PC is less than 50, then give platelet transfusion once the heparin has been cleared from the circulation.

Low molecular weight heparin

The mode of action of LMWH is that it binds with factor Xa. The treatment regimen consists of a single weight-dependent daily subcutaneous dose which does not require monitoring of the APTT except in special circumstances such as renal failure, as LMWH is renally excreted. LMWH and warfarin are started simultaneously and LMWH is stopped when the INR is therapeutic. As LMWH cannot bind to antithrombin III and thrombin, the anticoagulant activity and bleeding complications are reduced compared to unfractionated heparin. LMWH is less easily reversed than unfractionated intravenous heparin. PC should be monitored as the incidence of HIT is approximately 1%. LMWH has similar efficacy to unfractionated heparin with regard to reducing extension of DVT and recurrent VTE, risk of major bleeding and mortality. In patients with DVT, LMWH treatment is associated with reduced hospitalization and increased outpatient treatment (achieved in up to 80% of patients) with cost savings. Outpatient treatment is not recommended for young adults with extensive iliofemoral DVT, extensive PE, PCD and patients at increased risk of active or major bleeding.

Warfarin

Warfarin acts by reducing the activity of the vitamin K-dependent coagulation factors VII, IX, X and thrombin, and reducing the levels of proteins C and S. Warfarin has a half life of 36–40 hours, and a reduced dose should be considered in patients with liver failure and those on parenteral nutrition or antibiotic therapy. Heparin should always be administered before commencing warfarin and the two should be overlapped by 4–6 days as thrombin has a half-life of 36 hours and so warfarin is ineffective for approximately 48 hours. In addition, warfarin initially leads to a reduction in the levels of proteins C and S which produces a temporary hypercoagulable state for approximately 24–72 hours. The target INR should be >2.0.

Lifetime warfarin should be considered for patients with a second VTE, those with thrombophilia, and patients with a first VTE and malignancy until this has been resolved. Six months of warfarin therapy is associated with a 21% incidence of recurrent VTE at 4 years compared with 2.6% for lifetime therapy. The risk of major bleeding with therapeutic warfarin therapy is approximately 0.5–1% per month. Warfarin-induced skin necrosis occurs due to thrombosis and haemorrhage of the venules and capillaries within the subcutaneous fat and skin, mainly affecting the breasts, thighs, buttocks and legs.

Catheter-directed intra-thrombus thrombolysis

Lower limb

If phlebography demonstrates fresh, free-floating iliofemoral or caval thrombus then a V/Q scan should be performed and an IVC filter inserted. Thrombolysis can performed via the internal jugular vein, contralateral common femoral vein or ipsilateral popliteal, deep tibial or calf perforating veins. Some authorities prefer to administer it intra-arterially. It has been suggested that infra-popliteal venous access may lead to improved patency and competence of the superficial femoral and popliteal veins although the long-term results of thrombolysis are largely unknown. Placement of the thrombolysis catheter within the clot allows an increased drug concentration to be delivered directly into the clot which results in rapid clearance of the DVT with improved valve function, reduced bleeding and reduced costs. In PCD, combined intra-arterial and venous thrombolysis may reduce micro- and macrovascular thrombosis and reduce the pain, swelling and hypotension within 12 hours of starting treatment. Contraindications to thrombolysis include recent surgery, biopsy or trauma; recent or active bleeding and a bleeding diathesis; pregnancy; and cerebral abnormalities such as stroke, tumour or arteriovenous malformation. A US national registry of venous thrombolysis has reported complete lysis in 31% of patients with a greater probability of complete lysis occurring in patients with an acute DVT and no history of previous DVT. Major bleeding requiring blood products has occurred in 11% and minor bleeding in 16% of patients with a mortality rate of 0.4%. The 1 year patency was 79% for complete lysis and 32% for less than 50% lysis. Vein competence at 1 year was 42% for the total cohort and 72% in those with complete lysis.

Upper limb

There is a higher success rate with thrombolytic therapy in the upper limb than the lower. The lytic agent t-PA should be delivered into the thrombus by catheter as otherwise it will bypass the thrombus via the collaterals. In most cases, once the thrombus has been cleared, an underlying anatomical cause of thoracic outlet compression will become apparent. The patient should be maintained on heparin therapy pending further investigation such as CT or magnetic resonance imaging (MRI) and surgical correction by first rib resection. This is not an area where endoluminal angioplasty or stenting is recommended unless the external cause of compression has been surgically corrected first. Alternatively, conservative therapy, with 6 months of anticoagulations as detailed above, is also associated with a good clinical response and few long-term complications.

Pulmonary embolism

In PE, intravenous thrombolysis is advocated in the haemodynamically unstable patient where the benefits of PE resolution outweigh the risks of bleeding. In the patient presenting with cardiorespiratory collapse thrombolytic therapy should be administered without delay on the basis of clinical diagnosis without waiting for definitive investigations. Thrombolysis can be commenced up to 14 days after the onset of PE. It is associated with improved PE resolution and outcome compared with heparinization alone, and achieves maximum benefit in patients with massive PE. In the post-operative patient, a lower dose of the thrombolytic agent can be delivered using catheter-directed intra-thrombus thrombolysis (CDITT) within 14 days of surgery.

Venous thrombectomy

Venous thrombectomy is performed more frequently in many European countries than it is in the UK. It requires considerable expertise. The aim is to prevent the crippling consequences of severe post-thrombotic syndrome. Indications for venous thrombectomy include PAD, PCD with impending venous gangrene threatening to the patient's life and limb, and failed or contraindicated anticoagulation and thrombolysis. Firstly, however, it should be borne in mind that PCD means that the entire venous system down to capillary level is thrombosed and therefore effective clearance is unlikely. However, if partial clearance can be maintained by physical measures and effective anticoagulation, it may permit limb survival. Secondly, PCD is usually a manifestation of widespread malignancy. A failed thrombectomy is likely to leave the patient with a complicated leaking wound in a grossly swollen leg. The indication for thrombectomy in PCD therefore would be early intervention in the rare case of the relatively young patient who has a cause other than malignant disease for the DVT.

In the case of PAD or PCD if pre-operative phlebography demonstrates IVC or ilio-femoral vein involvement, then a V/Q scan should be performed and an IVC filter may be inserted.

Intravenous heparin is administered throughout the operation. The femoral vein is exposed and under image intensification, the common iliac vein (CIV) is thrombectomized and while the CIV is occluded by a balloon catheter, the internal iliac vein is cleared by suction thrombectomy. Manual massage from the foot proximally removes distal thrombus. If an IVC filter has not been inserted, the risk of intra-operative PE can be reduced by performing all venous manipulations while the anaesthetist applies positive end-expiratory pressure (PEEP) and by using a separate IVC occlusion catheter. As backbleeding is an unreliable sign, vein patency is confirmed by ascending iliac phlebography. If ilio-femoral vein thrombosis appears to be secondary to ascending thrombosis from the calf, and thrombus in the femoral vein is considered too chronic to remove, then iliac and profunda vein thrombectomy combined with superficial femoral vein (SFV) ligation has been advocated as theoretically recanalization of the SFV will be associated with venous reflux. Completion phlebography may demonstrate a venous web, a radiation stricture or extrinsic compression of the iliac veins which should be corrected by open surgery or angioplasty and stent placement to prevent re-thrombosis. If the iliac vein occlusion cannot be cleared and the IVC and contralateral iliac veins are patent, then cross-pubic venous bypass (the Palma operation) is indicated. This is performed with the contralateral long saphenous vein or 8 mm externally reinforced polytetrafluoroethylene (PTFE) graft from the ipsilateral common femoral vein (CFV) to the contralateral iliac vein. A temporary arteriovenous fistula (AVF) between the ipsilateral CFV and superficial femoral artery has been advocated. This increases blood flow in the thrombectomized vein segment and reduces early re-thrombosis from 18–34% to 12–13%, it allows the venous endothelium time to heal and it promotes venous collateral formation if incomplete iliac vein clearance has been achieved or immediate re-thrombosis occurs. The AVF can be occluded by endovascular therapy after 6 weeks. If venous thrombectomy has been performed for PCD and impending venous gangrene then calf fasciotomies may be performed. Post-operative management includes high limb elevation, calf exercises, compression stockings, antibiotic therapy, heparin for at least 5 days and warfarin for 6 months or lifetime if cross-pubic bypass has been performed. With careful patient selection and in the most experienced hands, the mortality rate from modern series is less than 1%. Intra-operative PE occurs in approximately 20% but these events are usually subclinical and asymptomatic. The clinical success rates are reported to be 42–93% with re-thrombosis occurring in approximately 20% of patients. Successful venous thrombectomy and AVF has good long-term results especially if performed within 7–10 days of the event. At 10 year follow-up, iliac vein patency of 77% and popliteal vein reflux of 32% have been reported which compares with 47% and 67% respectively for conservative management alone. Although improved iliac vein patency, reduced reflux and reduced venous hypertension are achieved, the post-thrombotic syndrome is not convincingly prevented. In patients with severe PCD and venous gangrene, the outcome is poor as it is not possible to clear the microvascular thromboses.

Pulmonary embolectomy

Indications for pulmonary embolectomy include failed or contraindicated thrombolysis, and massive PE with hypotension and rapid deterioration requiring inotropic support. Catheter suction embolectomy can be performed via the internal jugular or common femoral vein under local anaesthesia and image intensification. The best results are achieved in patients with major and massive PE with poor results in patients with chronic PE. The 30 day survival rate is reported as approximately 70%.

Open pulmonary embolectomy is performed via median sternotomy with or without cardiopulmonary bypass, and is indicated if catheter embolectomy has failed or cardiac massage is required for hypotension. The 30 day survival rate is reported as 60–84% with pre- and peri-operative cardiac arrest a major predictor of mortality.

Inferior vena caval filtration

The commonest type of IVC filter is the conical Greenfield filter. This traps emboli as small as 3 mm diameter and almost 85% of the device length can contain clot while maintaining peripheral bloodflow which allows endogenous clot lysis. The devices are made of titanium or nickel titanium alloy and are placed percutaneously under local anaesthesia via the common femoral, internal jugular or antecubital veins. The filter is normally positioned in the infra-renal cava but it can, with safety, be sited above the renal veins if necessary.

Some authors recommend the use of temporary filters which are removed endoluminally once the acute episode is relieved. This presupposes that the period of risk can be defined. Patients who have had an episode of VTE are at increased risk of a subsequent episode. The long-term patency for the Greenfield filter at follow-up of up to 20 years is 96% independent of anticoagulation, and the recurrent PE rate is 3–4%. There seems little case therefore for the use of temporary filters.

Absolute indications for insertion of an IVC filter are recurrent PE despite effective anticoagulation, complications of VTE or anticoagulation which prevent further anticoagulation, where anticoagulation is contraindicated due to an increased risk of bleeding, and the prevention of early recurrent PE associated with pulmonary embolectomy. Relative indications include recurrent chronic PE with pulmonary hypertension and cor pulmonale; extensive pulmonary emboli; ilio-femoral thrombus propagation despite effective anticoagulation; free-floating IVC thrombus, extensive free-floating ilio-femoral DVT and bilateral free-floating femoral DVT, which despite effective anticoagulation are associated with PE in 30–60%, 43% and 27% of patients, respectively. A caval filter has also been recommended as a prophylactic measure in patients undergoing venous thrombolysis where 20% of patients develop PE, and controversially as prophylaxis in major hip and knee replacement surgery and multiple trauma where the risk of PE is considerable.

Section 33.5 • Thrombo-embolic prophylaxis

Without thrombo-embolic prophylaxis, the risk of DVT is 25% for major general and cardiovascular surgery, and 40–80% for major hip and knee surgery, and the risk of fatal PE is 0.7% and 1–10%, respectively. There is no association between increased risk of VTE and uncomplicated varicose veins in the absence of other risk factors and where no surgery is performed. Superficial thrombophlebitis, however, may be associated with a slightly increased risk of DVT. The incidence of VTE in routine varicose vein surgery is approximately 0.2%. The risk of post-operative VTE in patients taking the low-dose oral contraceptive pill (OCP), combined OCP or hormone replacement therapy (HRT) is increased 2–4-fold but remains so small that the OCP or HRT should be stopped 4–6 weeks before elective surgery only if there are additional risk factors for VTE. The Thrift risk assessment protocol allows thrombo-embolic prophylaxis to be adjusted relative to the individual patient's risk. Prophylaxis in low-risk groups (minor surgery or trauma, major surgery in patients <40 years old, and minor medical illness) consists of leg elevation and early mobilization. Prophylaxis in moderate risk groups (major trauma, burns or medical illness, major surgery in patients >40 years, minor surgery in patients with additional risk factors, and patients with inflammatory bowel disease) consists of leg elevation, early mobilization, and either graduated compression stockings (TEDs) or subcutaneous unfractionated miniheparin 5000 IU twice daily (reduces risk of VTE by two-thirds) or LMWH once daily. Prophylaxis in high-risk groups (major cancer, pelvic and lower limb joint surgery, those undergoing surgery or suffering illness associated with previous VTE or thrombophilia) consists of leg elevation, early mobilization, TEDs, subcutaneous miniheparin 5000 IU twice or three times daily or LMWH, and mechanical calf compression. In some areas of surgery, particularly where the surgeon wishes to avoid intra-operative anticoagulation, mechanical compression is a useful option for the medium- and high-risk groups.

Further reading

Hamilton, G. and Platts, A. (1998). Deep venous thrombosis. In: Beard, J. D. and Gaines, P. A., eds. *Vascular and Endovascular Surgery. A Companion to Specialist Surgical Practice*. Philadelphia, PA: W.B. Saunders.

Scottish Intercollegiate Guidelines Network (1999). Venous thromboembolism. In: *Antithrombotic Therapy*. Scottish Intercollegiate Guidelines Network (SIGN) publication No. 36 (March 1999). Edinburgh: Royal College of Physicians.

Silver, D. and Vouyouka, A. (2000). The caput medusae of hypercoagulability (Review article). *J Vasc Surg* **31**: 396–405.

Tai, N. R. M., Atwal, A. S. and Hamilton, G. (1999). Modern management of pulmonary embolism (Review article). *Br J Surg* **86**: 853–68.

Wakefield, T. W. (2000). Treatment options for venous thrombosis (Review article). *J Vasc Surg* **31**: 613–20.

MODULE 34

Varicose veins

The spectrum of venous disease in the leg ranges from venous telangiectasia through to chronic venous insufficiency and the post-thrombotic syndrome. This chapter focuses on varicose veins, with the more advanced venous pathology being covered in greater detail elsewhere, although there is inevitably some overlap.

Section 34.1 • Definition and classification

There is no universally accepted definition of a varicose vein. However, the following definition incorporates the important elements: 'a superficial vein of the lower limb, which has permanently lost its valvular efficiency, and as a product of the resultant venous hypertension in the standing position becomes dilated, tortuous and thickened'. This definition excludes the 'muscular veins' seen in thin patients who have simply got prominent but normally functioning veins without venous reflux.

There is also no universally accepted classification of venous disease of the lower limb. An ideal classification should be easy to apply, should not require information which is only obtained on some patients and should not depend on inconsistent assessment techniques. Widmer described a simple clinical classification based on the appearance of the limb, which he used in his seminal work on the epidemiology of varicose veins (Table 34.1). Although this has been widely used in the past and is easy to apply, it has been increasingly criticized for the fact that it did not take account of any haemodynamic and imaging data. Classifications proposed by Sytchev in 1985 and Porter in 1988 amongst others did include some imaging or haemodynamic data, but did not find general acceptance. The more recent and comprehensive CEAP classification, devised at the American Venous Forum Meeting in 1994, is based on four elements: the **C**linical presentation, a**E**tiology, **A**natomical areas affected and the **P**athophysiology found (Table 34.2). The CEAP classification is not only difficult to use in routine clinical practice, owing to the extent of investigation required in every patient, but also ends up with so many different subgroups that analysis is of limited value, even when the classification has been fully applied. At present most venous specialists have concluded that CEAP in its present form is too complex for routine use and have suggested simplification. A simplified version of the CEAP classification has been proposed by Bergan and is currently under assessment.

Table 34.1 Widmer classification of venous disease

Category	*Description*
Hyphen webs	Venous telangiectasia, spider veins
Reticular veins	Dilated tortuous subcutaneous veins, not major trunks or branches
Truncal veins	Dilated tortuous LSV or SSV or main branches
CVI grade 1	Venous flare at the ankle, 'corona phlebectatica'
CVI grade 2	Hyper- or depigmented area in gaiter area
CVI grade 3	Open or healed venous ulcer

Section 34.2 • Epidemiology

Varicose veins are common. The prevalence has been variously reported from as little as 2% to over 60% in population studies. This enormous variation results from the different populations studied, different definitions applied and the different assessment or examination techniques used. The Edinburgh Venous Study (EVS) published in 1998 examined over 1500 adults and gives the best current data on the prevalence of varicose veins in the UK. In that study 39.7% of men and 32.2% of women had a dilated tortuous trunk of the long and/or short saphenous vein and their first or second order branches. The prevalence of hyphen webs

Table 34.2 CEAP classification

Clinical	*(a)Etiology*	*Anatomical*	*Pathophysiology*
None	Congenital	Superficial	Reflux
Telangiectasia or reticular	Obstruction	Primary	Perforating
Varicose veins	Secondary	Deep	Reflux + obstruction
Oedema	– Post-thrombotic	Leg veins are classified into segments 1–18 if more detail required	
Venous eczema	– Post-traumatic		
Pigmentation	– Other		
Lipodermatosclerosis			
Healed ulcer			
Open ulcer			

or small reticular varicosities was even higher at over 80% for both males and females. Although it was previously widely believed that varicose veins are more common in women, the few other general population studies confirm that varicose veins are at least as common in men.

The prevalence of varicose veins rises with age in virtually all published studies; the prevalence of trunk varicosities in the EVS rose from 11.5% in the 18–24 year old group to 55.7% in those aged 55–64. Although there is considerable anecdotal evidence to suggest that varicose veins are less common in developing countries, the absence of adequate epidemiological data leaves the question open.

Section 34.3 • Pathophysiology

The deep, superficial and perforating veins of the leg contain valves, which allow flow from distal to proximal and from superficial to deep as appropriate, but prevent retrograde flow (reflux). The presence of these valves as well as patent veins and a working calf muscle pump are required for normal venous function. Anatomical studies have shown that there is considerable variation in the number and position of the vein valves in the leg between individuals and that most people do not have venous valves above groin level. Although these valves may appear to be very flimsy, tests have suggested that they can resist pressures of up to 300 mmHg.

It is generally accepted that primary varicose veins are caused by failure of these vein valves which leads to reflux into the superficial leg veins. There is an unresolved controversy as to whether the valve failure is due to degenerative changes/failure in the valves themselves, or whether there is a degenerative change in the vein wall leading to dilatation of the vein and secondary valve failure. The following mechanisms have been suggested.

Hydrostatic pressure

The hydrostatic effects of gravity in the upright position are thought to be of great importance in valvular failure. The pressure in the superficial leg veins depends on the relative positions of the right atrium and the leg. Pressure in the superficial veins will be near zero when the patient is lying down and the foot is at the same level as the heart, but in the standing position, the hydrostatic pressure rises and puts stress on the proximal vein valves. Factors such as standing for long periods, obesity and pregnancy or indeed any condition which increases intra-abdominal pressure will lead to an increased hydrostatic pressure. However, if the hydrostatic pressure is the main causative factor, one would expect to always see a progressive cascade of valve failure from proximal to distal down the superficial vein from the point of 'leakage' from the deep venous system. In some cases valvular failure appears to begin distally and spread proximally and this has led some authors to question the importance of the hydrostatic pressure as an aetiological factor. They suggest that local changes in the vein wall are the cause of the valve failure as dilatation of the vein wall below the valve has been observed in some instances to precede the vein valve incompetence and proximal dilatation of the vein.

Family history

There is some evidence that hereditary influences are involved. Studies have suggested that children of parents who both had varicose veins are at least twice as likely to have varicose veins, compared with children whose parents had no varicosities. Studies of identical and non-identical twins also support this view. The hereditary effect may be on the vein wall or the valves themselves or even on the number and placement of the valves in the venous system. The early onset of severe and intractable varicose veins in the very young person often indicates that they have relatively few valves in the venous system of the leg.

Hormonal factors

Hormonal influences may also play a part in pathogenesis of varicose veins. Varicose veins often occur during the first few weeks of pregnancy. The effect of increased blood volume and blood flow and the pressure effects of the enlarged uterus in the pelvis, which may account for the development of veins later in pregnancy, are absent at this early stage. It is thought that the changes in hormone levels, particularly progesterone, have an effect on the vein wall. Changes in the hormone levels during the menstrual cycle will also affect the veins and could account for the increased symptoms which trouble many female patients in the pre-menstrual period.

Ageing

As the prevalence of varicose veins increases with age, it has been postulated that structural changes occur within the vein or valve, perhaps to elastin or collagen, as part of the ageing process. Evidence that these changes actually occur is scanty and may be a consequence of other factors apart from age.

Secondary veins

Secondary varicose veins have a different pathogenesis and occur as a consequence of other venous abnormalities; the commonest of which is deep vein thrombosis (DVT). In the early stages, the occlusion of deep veins may lead to the rapid distension of superficial veins resulting in the appearance of varicosities. These veins may well demonstrate valvular incompetence as the dilatation stretches the valves. At a later stage the occluded veins usually recanalize, but with damaged valves, resulting in reflux and incompetence in the deep veins, which can also give rise to secondary varicosities. Although secondary varicose veins can also occur as the result of congenital malformations such as the Klippel–Trenaunay syndrome or acquired arteriovenous fistulae, the evidence to support the theory that abnormal arteriovenous communications are the cause of primary varicose veins is scanty.

It is likely that the pathogenesis of varicose veins in an individual is the combination of a number of factors. Factors such as hormones and aging acting on the vein wall, hereditary factors such as the number and position of the veins and the original strength of the vein wall and the effect of lifestyle factors such as pregnancy, occupation and obesity will all interact to produce the pattern of varicosities found in that individual.

Section 34.4 • Venous anatomy

A detailed understanding of the venous anatomy of the lower limb and its variations is essential for the diagnosis and management of varicose veins. The veins of the lower limb can be divided into three groups: the deep veins, which lie within the deep fascia, the superficial veins lying outside the deep fascia and the 90 or so communicating/perforating veins, which pass through the deep fascia and connect the deep and superficial systems. Although a detailed knowledge of the deep veins and perforating veins is required, it is beyond the scope of this module, which will concentrate on those points of anatomy of the superficial veins and their anatomical variants which are of clinical importance.

Long saphenous vein

The long saphenous vein (LSV) originates on the medial border of the foot and passes superiorly, just anterior to the medial malleolus. It passes upwards over the distal third of the tibia and then proximally along the medial margin of the tibia to knee level. The LSV is accompanied by the saphenous nerve below the knee. This nerve is therefore at considerable risk of damage during ligations or stripping of the main saphenous trunk below the knee and can even be damaged by sclerotherapy. Anterior and posterior branches join the main trunk of the LSV just below the level of the knee. This trifurcation is an important point to control in patients with LSV incompetence as it is usually these branches or their tributaries which are visibly varicose.

At the level of the knee, the LSV lies superficially in a posterior position, approximately 10 cm from the front of the patella. Trainee surgeons may have difficulty in identifying the LSV at this level by exploring too anteriorly. In the thigh, the LSV passes antero-superiorly up the medial side of the thigh, often lying deep to the superficial fat, to reach the saphenous opening in the deep fascia through which it passes to join the femoral vein. A communicating vein (Giacomini vein) comes off the LSV in the thigh, passes postero-inferiorly around to the popliteal fossa and joins the short saphenous vein a little below its insertion into the popliteal vein. The vein of Giacomini can transmit LSV incompetence and thus give the spurious appearance of short saphenous incompetence even when the sapheno-popliteal valve is entirely competent.

The surface marking of the LSV at its termination in the femoral vein is 3 cm below and lateral to the pubic tubercle. This point may well lie above the inguinal skin crease, particularly in an obese person. It is a common surgical error to make the skin incision for sapheno-femoral ligation at or below the skin crease in such patients. The proximal centimetre of the LSV is covered with an extension of the fascia of the femoral sheath. Dissection inside this sheath makes the exposure of the sapheno-femoral junction much easier and safer. The superficial external pudendal artery usually runs across superficial to the femoral vein and deep to the LSV just below the angle created at the junction of the two veins and can be a very helpful landmark.

Surgeons should be alert to the possibility of a double LSV, as they are not uncommon in the thigh, and failure to identify the duplication is a cause of early recurrence after surgery.

The LSV is usually joined in the upper thigh a few centimetres below its termination by antero-lateral and postero-medial thigh branches. The postero-medial branch, in particular, is often found just below the level of dissection in the groin. It is therefore advisable to clear the saphenous trunk for a few centimetres and identify and divide this branch separately before stripping. This branch is a common cause of haematoma in the groin wound if not ligated, as it is usually above the level of compression applied after surgery and is therefore poorly controlled.

The anatomy of the branches of the LSV at the groin is very variable. The superficial external pudendal vein, the superficial inferior epigastric vein and the superficial circumflex iliac vein all join the LSV as it passes through the saphenous opening. The deep external pudendal vein usually joins the femoral vein, close to the sapheno-femoral junction. There is considerable variability in the way that these four vessels and the previously mentioned antero-lateral and postero-medial thigh veins join the saphenous vein or each other. Failure to be aware of the eight or more possible variations may lead to an inadequate sapheno-femoral ligation. Common variants include the postero-medial thigh tributary joining the femoral vein separately or through a short common stem or alternatively the antero-lateral branch joins the superficial circumflex iliac vein directly to form a common trunk. Ligation of this common stem close to the saphenous vein will leave the two branches in continuity and lead to a high risk of recurrence.

Short saphenous vein

The short saphenous vein (SSV) arises on the lateral border of the foot and passes upwards behind the lateral malleolus and then across to the midline, initially lateral to the tendo calcaneus and then up the midline posteriorly. It then pierces the deep fascia in the upper part of the calf and enters the popliteal fossa, where in most cases it terminates in the popliteal vein. Although its course in the popliteal fossa can be variable, it can be identified very easily at operation lying deep to the fascia in the midline approximately 4 cm below the popliteal skin crease. The SSV is accompanied for most of its length by the sural nerve, which is at risk during surgery.

The level of entry of the SSV into the popliteal vein is very variable. The most common level is 2–3 cm proximal to the transverse skin crease at the back of the knee. In one-third of cases the entry level is more proximal and the SSV may rarely join the femoral vein near the groin. Conversely in 15% of cases the entry level is distal to the popliteal skin crease. Very occasionally there is no communication with the deep vein at all and the SSV then drains via the vein of Giacomini into the LSV or terminates amongst the vasa vasorum of the sciatic nerve or one of its branches. The entry point into the popliteal vein is most often not, as one might expect, on the posterior surface of the popliteal vein, but usually on the medial or lateral side of the vein. Rarely the SSV enters the deep anterior surface of the popliteal vein.

Section 34.5 • Presentation

Patients with varicose veins present in one of three categories: cosmetic, symptomatic or with one of the complications of venous disease (Table 34.3). The assessment of patients in the cosmetic group 1 is relatively simple as the problem can be clearly seen. Although investigation may need to be more comprehensive in the complicated group 3 patients, there are clinical signs present indicating that there is a problem in the venous system. It is the large number of patients presenting in the symptomatic group 2 who present the greatest challenge in identifying those patients whose symptoms are of venous origin and correctable.

Section 34.6 • Assessment

Although it would be ideal to assess patients with varicose veins fully at a single visit to the clinic, this is not always possible at present. However, a one-stop clinic with the facility to carry out non-invasive investigations such as duplex scanning is more efficient for both the hospital and the patient.

Clinical assessment

Many specialized venous clinics now use a standardized recording form to record both the clinical history and examination. The use of such a form ensures that all the necessary venous symptoms and signs and appropriate past medical history are obtained *and recorded* in a consistent manner. A well-designed form should also include other factors which might affect subsequent management, such as medication with aspirin or oestrogens.

Patients should be examined standing, preferably on a plinth, in a warm and well-illuminated room. The

Table 34.3 Varicose vein presentation

Group 1 *Cosmetic only*	*Group 2* *Symptomatic*	*Group 3* *Complications*
Venous telangiectasia	Aching on dependency or before periods	Bleeding from trauma
Visible varicose veins	'Heaviness' in the legs	Superficial phlebitis
	Itching	Ankle venous flare
	Cramps	Atrophie blanche
	Swelling	Venous eczema
	Restless legs	Lipodermatosclerosis ± inflammatory component
	Tenderness	Venous ulcers
	Paraesthesia	

patient should rest most of his/her weight on the leg which is not being examined. The presence of any of the signs of venous insufficiency listed in group 3 as well as the site and distribution of any visible varicosities should be noted. Patients presenting with primary varicose veins are most likely to have long saphenous incompetence (70%) with visible varicosities on the medial side of the leg and in many cases extending above the knee. Short saphenous incompetence is much less common (15%) and usually is associated with varicosities lying on the posterior aspect of the calf. However, the pattern of varicosity in an individual limb is only a guide to the sites of incompetence. Studies have shown that simple inspection has an unacceptably high error rate and it has to be supplemented by further tests. Traditionally this has been done using either local compression or a tourniquet to control proximal reflux to assess the level and site of incompetence. However, such techniques still have a significant error rate.

Continuous wave Doppler

Most vascular surgeons now routinely use continuous wave (CW) hand-held Doppler to assess patients with varicose veins. Careful insonnation at the groin and down the inside of the thigh can demonstrate the presence and duration of reflux in the LSV and may also pick up reflux in the femoral vein. The technique is less accurate in the obese patient. Insonnation of the popliteal fossa can confirm patency of the veins and detect the presence of reflux. If reflux is detected it may be difficult to identify which vein(s) (popliteal, gastrocnemius, SSV) are at fault. However, the absence of reflux is a reliable guide to the absence of a SSV problem, particularly if insonnation is carried out over the SSV 2–4 cm below the popliteal skin crease as well as in the popliteal fossa. Several studies have shown that CW Doppler is an effective assessment tool for patients with varicose veins and will improve diagnostic accuracy when compared with simple clinical examination. However, the more complex patients will require more specialized assessment.

Colour duplex

The advent of colour-flow duplex scanning has revolutionized the assessment of venous disease. There is still considerable debate as to which patients with varicose veins should be scanned. A case can be made for scanning all patients before surgical intervention because even the most experienced clinician will have an error rate of about 5% using clinical tests and CW Doppler only. A duplex scan provides the following information, which will have an effect on the decision to operate and the nature of the procedure.

Patency and competence of the deep veins

If the deep veins are occluded, removal or interruption of the superficial veins is likely to cause deterioration and is usually contraindicated. Major incompetence in the deep venous system also calls into question the benefits of surgery. If a patient has both deep and superficial incompetence, surgery may well be less effective and the patient will still have to wear elastic compression to prevent symptoms and deterioration post-operatively.

Site and level of major incompetence identified
Scanning proximally from the visible or symptomatic veins confirms that they communicate with the point of incompetence.

Additional points of incompetence identified
In the authors, series of over 2000 duplex scans for varicose veins an unsuspected additional point(s) of incompetence was detected in approximately 10% of cases.

Anatomy of the popliteal fossa identified accurately
The exact level and point of insertion of the SSV into the popliteal vein is very variable and accurate identification enables a proper flush ligation of the SSV with minimal dissection and risk to adjacent structures.

Anatomical abnormalities identified
Abnormal venous channels or vein duplication if identified pre-operatively are likely to be more effectively controlled. The demonstration of an incompetent vein of Giacomini (see venous anatomy section) will avoid unnecessary surgery in the popliteal fossa.

Duration and velocity of venous reflux
A knowledge of the duration and velocity of reflux at a given site can be useful in determining whether intervention is likely to be helpful in the relief of symptoms and to an extent the degree to which a patient's symptoms may be attributable to their venous disease.

However, in many centres the availability of duplex is limited and not all patients will be scanned. If a patient with primary varicose veins has visible varicosities within the long saphenous territory on the medial side of the leg, has demonstrable reflux with CW Doppler in the LSV at the groin and in the thigh, has no incompetence at all in the popliteal fossa and has no history of DVT it is reasonable to proceed to intervention without a duplex scan. This will comprise 40–50% of patients presenting with primary varicose veins.

However, if a patient has recurrent varicose veins, an unusual pattern of varicosities which cannot be elucidated by hand-held Doppler, a history of DVT *or any incompetence in the popliteal fossa on hand-held Doppler* then a duplex is advisable as the probability of an incorrect assessment increases.

Varicography

In the rare case (approximately 1 in 100) where clinical/Doppler/duplex examination cannot identify the point of reflux from the deep to superficial circulation, the use of local varicography can be helpful. This applies particularly to patients with vulval varicosities or those who have abnormal refluxing veins, often on the posterior surface of the thigh, which arise from the profunda vein or more proximally.

Venography

The use of duplex has largely replaced venography in the investigation of patients with varicose veins. There is an occasional indication in a patient in whom it has been impossible to image the deep vein system with duplex and there is residual doubt about the patency of the deep system.

Venous function tests

Venous function tests such as plethysmography or volumetry have little place in the routine clinical assessment of patients with simple varicose veins. Their use is confined to research studies to assess the results of treatment and in the assessment of patients with more complex venous problems.

Section 34.7 • Treatment

As a substantial percentage of the population have varicose veins, the selection of cases for treatment becomes very important. Within the context of the British National Health Service (NHS) resources are limited, and even in countries where insurance funded health care systems are the norm, the funding agencies are increasingly expecting the clinician to justify treatment in terms of health gain. Unfortunately there are few robust data with long-term follow-up to provide such a justification. A reasonable approach in an individual patient is to consider the likely benefits of a particular intervention in three areas: cosmetic benefit, symptomatic benefit and the prevention of progression of venous insufficiency and venous ulceration.

It is the symptomatic category which presents the greatest difficulty. In experienced hands it is relatively easy to predict the likely cosmetic benefit, allowing for the risks of complications which may affect the cosmetic appearance. Similarly one can make a reasonable estimate of the benefit of an intervention to control reflux and prevent further deterioration in the venous system. However, the correlation between symptoms and varicose veins is so poor, it is not surprising that it is difficult to predict the likely outcome after intervention as far as symptoms are concerned. As a general observation, patients who obtain benefit from properly fitted graduated elastic hosiery are likely to benefit from intervention in appropriate cases, whereas those who do not benefit symptomatically are unlikely to do so.

If the funding is not an issue and the purpose of the intervention is cosmetic, and there is a high expectation of a satisfactory result, then it is reasonable to go ahead after careful discussion with the patient about the risks and benefits, as with any other cosmetic procedure. Similarly if the purpose of the procedure is to control gross superficial venous reflux in a patient who has already developed some of the signs of chronic venous insufficiency, and the patient is judged fit for treatment then once again the decision is straightforward. For the symptomatic patient, particularly if they have benefited from compression and have a normal deep venous system, and are reluctant to wear long-term support, intervention is reasonable, provided that they have correctable disease.

A proportion of patients present primarily with concerns about the risk of DVT, bleeding or eventual ulceration. It is reasonable to reassure these patients if they have asymptomatic minor varicose veins only. Clearly patients whose symptoms are not related to their varicose veins will need alternative treatment.

Careful consideration should be given to the necessity to operate on patients with recurrent veins as the risk of complication is increased and the chance of an excellent result reduced.

Section 34.8 • Treatment options

Drug therapy for varicose vein symptoms

An extensive international review of the data on the use of drugs in venous disease concluded that a few drugs could have a modest effect on some of the symptoms such as heaviness of the legs, discomfort, cramps and swelling associated with varicose veins when compared with placebo. The international task force stated that most of the studies had been carried out many years ago and rarely complied with current scientific standards for clinical trials and the lack of standardized outcomes limited any comparability between results. These factors, compounded by small sample size, poorly defined study populations, high dropout rates and absence of control groups, meant that no clear recommendation on the use of any drug for varicose vein symptoms could be made.

Compression hosiery

Graduated compression hosiery is often the first line of treatment in the management of varicose veins. Graduated compression has several effects on the venous system in the leg, including decrease in oedema, increase in venous velocity, decrease in venous volume and decrease in venous reflux. There are studies demonstrating that the use of compression will ameliorate the symptoms associated with varicose veins, and delay the progression of the changes of chronic venous insufficiency. One study has even shown that the use of compression hosiery after varicose vein surgery will reduce the risk of varicose vein recurrence. Many patients may well have tried commercially available 'support tights' even before consulting their medical practitioner. However, many of these garments provide only very mild compression which in some cases has little graduation. In consequence properly fitted elastic compression hosiery may still be an option for patients whose symptoms have not responded to 'support tights'. For graduated compression to be effective in the treatment of varicose veins, a pressure of 30–40 mmHg is required at the ankle becoming less at more proximal levels. In most cases a below knee stocking is adequate, and it should be replaced regularly (a minimum of two stockings every 6 months).

Compliance is a major problem. At least 10% of patients will not tolerate the use of stockings at all and a further 25% will abandon the use of compression within a few months. This lack of compliance may be due to vanity, discomfort or allergy, inability to apply the stockings due to poor grip, or even the cost of replacement. Unfortunately, stockings are worn least in the hot weather, when thanks to vasodilatation, the need is greatest. Where compliance is a problem, it is worth looking for the underlying reasons, which may be surmountable.

Graduated compression is a reasonable first line of treatment for symptomatic varicose veins, but if the patient's primary concern is cosmetic, then the provision of a thick stocking is unlikely to be acceptable. A trial of graduated compression is a useful diagnostic tool in a case with varicose veins and leg symptoms, which may or may not be due to the varicosities; if controlled by the compression, the symptoms are likely to be due to the varicose veins. The use of compression routinely after 'curative' surgery may be of benefit, and for patients who have residual deep vein incompetence is advisable to prevent further deterioration.

Graduated elastic compression is effective but can cause damage. The compression exerted by the stocking is not uniform, but over areas of prominence will be much higher and may cause damage in a patient with arterial insufficiency. The presence of normal foot pulses or adequate ankle/brachial pressure ratio should be confirmed before compression is prescribed.

Sclerotherapy

Sclerotherapy has been used in the treatment of varicose veins for at least two millennia. It is therefore chastening to have to state that the evidence in terms of its efficacy remains scanty. The use of sclerotherapy in recent times was popularized in the UK by Fegan (Ireland) and in continental Europe by Sigg (Switzerland) and Touunay (France). Although there are differences between the three techniques, the basic principles remain the same. The objective of sclerotherapy is to ablate the superficial veins. The injection of a small amount of sclerosant solution, such as sodium tetrodecyl sulfate (STD) or polydocanol, into an empty vein will produce an endothelial reaction and a chemical phlebitis very rapidly, provided that the sclerosant does not get diluted or displaced by venous flow and the endothelial walls are kept approximated. It was originally believed that siting the injection close to the point where a perforating vein joined the superficial varicosity was extremely important. However, as belief in the importance of perforators has waned, siting the injection close to the perforator is now considered to be much less important.

Most experts recommend compression after injection to keep the sclerosant at the site of injection and to maintain the endothelial wall approximation. Opinion is divided as to the duration of post-sclerotherapy compression. However, as the vein becomes occluded very rapidly, compression is likely to be necessary for a few days only.

The exact choice of sclerosant and technique varies widely between practitioners and reflects where a practitioner was trained rather than any scientific trials comparing different methods. The key points are the careful placement of the needle within the vein, ensuring the vein is empty, the correct choice of concentration and volume of sclerosant for the size of vein and adequate compression of the vein for sufficient time for vein occlusion to occur. Some authors have recommended the use of duplex guided sclerotherapy to ensure more accurate placement of the sclerosant, but evidence that the long-term results are improved or the complications less is awaited. A very recent development of sclerosant 'foam', which sets on contact with blood and is claimed to prevent the sclerosant from migrating away from the site of injection even in larger veins, has still to be extensively tested in clinical trials.

Complications of sclerotherapy

Excessive concentrations of sclerosant, especially if injected outside the vein will lead to the formation of a deep and painful ulcer, which will be slow to heal and leave a cosmetically unsightly mark on the leg. A little extravasation from the vein puncture is unlikely to cause ulceration. If a large haematoma occurs from the site of injection, this can be aspirated under local anaesthetic to relieve pain.

If the vein being injected is not empty or refills after injection, then a thrombophlebitis ensues leaving pain and a line of discoloration along the vein, which is usually permanent. The bigger the vein being injected, the more likely this complication is to occur. The incidence of DVT after sclerotherapy is not known but is believed to be rare in the UK, where more extensive varicose veins tend to be treated surgically. Ambulation after sclerotherapy is encouraged to reduce the risk further, and is probably wise, although direct evidence to support the practice is lacking. It is not current practice to stop the contraceptive pill or hormone replacement therapy (HRT) prior to sclerotherapy.

Rare complications of sclerotherapy include anaphylactic reactions to the sclerosant, accidental intra-arterial injection (usually involving the posterior tibial artery close to the medial malleolus) or neurological damage either due to injection close to the head of the fibula or from over enthusiastic compression. Sensible precautions are to ensure that the necessary requirements for treating anaphylaxis are available, avoidance of injection close to the medial malleolus or near the head of the fibula, and advising patients to report pain in the leg or foot after sclerotherapy immediately. In cases where pain is reported the compression should be removed and the leg examined. If an arterial injection is suspected, urgent referral to a vascular surgeon and admission to hospital are recommended.

In the absence of robust trial data, the choice of patients suitable for sclerotherapy depends on the individual view of the practitioner consulted. Some phlebologists, particularly in continental Europe, take the view that almost all varicose veins, including long saphenous truncal varicose veins, are suitable for sclerotherapy. Although the available evidence would suggest that the long-term results from surgery for truncal varicosities are superior, sclerotherapy enthusiasts hold that repeated courses of injections can achieve similar results without surgery. Such an extreme view is rarely held in the UK, where most patients with varicose veins consult a surgeon who has the option of both surgery and sclerotherapy. Most UK practitioners use sclerotherapy in a much more limited role to treat isolated below knee reticular varicosities, in the absence of truncal disease or to 'tidy up' any distal varicosities left after surgery. The treatment of thigh varicosities is much less successful because of the difficulty in applying adequate compression, particularly in the obese patient.

The treatment of thread veins (venous telangiectasia/dermal flares) with microsclerotherapy is more controversial. Thirty per cent of these cosmetic blemishes are associated with underlying varicosities, which can be treated with good results by standard sclerotherapy. The remaining 70% have no underlying venous problem. Some authors have suggested that these blemishes can be treated with specially modified 32 gauge needles and a very dilute concentration of sclerosant such as polydocanol. A very slow injection and a meticulous technique is required and as a result it is a very time consuming procedure. Complications of skin pigmentation and even ulceration can occur and the thread veins are likely to recur even after successful treatment. As this procedure is being done almost entirely for cosmetic benefit, it is vital that the patient is made fully aware of the possible complications and the chances of success. An advice sheet and the use of a consent form, which indicates that the patient has read and understood the advice sheet, is a sensible precaution in this area where dissatisfaction with the cosmetic results is not uncommon. Similar precautions are advisable even with 'standard' sclerotherapy. More recently the use of laser in the treatment of thread veins has been suggested. However, as the equipment is costly, the treatment often results in depigmentation/hyperpigmentation of the skin, and the results are no better than microsclerotherapy the practice has not been widely adopted.

Surgery

The general indications for surgical intervention for varicose veins have already been discussed. However, there are a number of specific issues to consider if surgery is being contemplated.

Pregnancy

Many surgeons in the past have advised female patients to wait until they have completed their pregnancies before having surgery for their veins, on the grounds that the veins will recur after subsequent pregnancies. Varicose veins which appear during pregnancy may improve after the child is born, but if they do not, then the possibility of a further pregnancy should not debar the patient from surgical treatment. Intervention prior to the first pregnancy is often necessary as many women are now delaying their pregnancies until over the age of 30.

Obesity

Many patients with varicose veins are obese. Although it is suggested that obesity will make the severity of the symptoms and the appearance worse in a patient who has a predisposition to varicose veins, the evidence that obesity is a direct aetiological factor remains scanty. There does not appear to be any compelling evidence to suggest that obese patients are more likely to get recurrence either. Some surgeons refuse to operate on the obese patient with varicose veins because of concern about the increased risks. Although one should encourage the obese patient to lose weight prior to surgery, and every effort should be made to aid them in achieving weight loss, most will never reduce their weight to a point where these risks will be substantially reduced. In those patients who have started to develop skin changes, it is reasonable to weigh up the anaesthetic and surgical risks against the risk of intractable ulceration and consider surgery even for the obese patient.

Operative risk

Studies have shown that well over 95% of patients with routine varicose veins fall into ASA grades 1 and 2. Surgery is a therefore a reasonable option for the vast majority of such patients. Clearly the requirement for surgery should be reconsidered for any higher ASA grade and these cases can be managed with compression hosiery or even sclerotherapy. A further option for the elderly and unfit patient with actual or incipient leg ulceration, where the main problem is primary long saphenous incompetence, would be a simple flush ligation of the LSV under local anaesthetic combined with compression hosiery.

Day case surgery and anaesthesia

Many patients with varicose veins (up to 75%) are suitable for day case surgery, but it must be stressed that if carried out appropriately there is little cost saving. Some costs are merely transferred from the secondary to the primary sector. Dedicated day care units with consultant-led operations and suitable pre-admission and post-operative follow-up services are essential, if the use of day case surgery is to be maximized in safety. The majority of patients treated as day cases have unilateral long or short saphenous surgery. If the LSV is being stripped then the procedure should be carried out early in the day to allow maximum time to recover before discharge. Although some surgeons are prepared to do bilateral primary varicose vein surgery as a day case, most still admit them overnight or do one limb at a time. However, as most patients prefer to have a single procedure, the authors' practice is to admit such patients overnight. At present most surgeons will admit patients for recurrent vein surgery. The availability of 24 hour stay units or patient hotels would allow almost all patients for varicose vein surgery to be treated as 'day cases'.

There has been a modest increase in the use of local anaesthesia for varicose vein surgery but the vast majority are still done under a general or occasionally a regional anaesthetic. Even if a general anaesthetic is given, infiltration of the wounds with 0.5% bupivicaine at the end of the procedure will improve pain control especially for day cases.

Patient information sheets

All patients selected for surgery should be given, at the clinic, an information sheet describing the risks and benefits of the intended procedure. Many patients have unrealistic expectations as far as outcome is concerned and some may well decide not to have surgery after all. In the event of a significant delay between the clinic and surgery, which is often the case, the information sheet should be reissued to the patient at the time of pre-admission or admission. The information sheet can be an integral part of the operative consent form and when consent for the procedure is given, can help ensure that the patient *has read and understood* the advice sheet.

Pre-operative marking

It is advisable that pre-operative marking of the patient's leg is carried out by the surgeon who is going to undertake the procedure, using an indelible marker with the patient standing. Each surgeon tends to mark in a different manner and this can give rise to confusion.

Tourniquets

The use of an exsanguinating bandage and a tourniquet or more recently a pneumatic ring tourniquet, which acts as both tourniquet and exsanguinator, has been advocated. A tourniquet does limit blood loss but prolongs the procedure and can cause difficulty when passing the stripper, if applied before the stripper is passed. The leg will swell after removal of the tourniquet and this can cause problems with the post-operative compression. The use of a pneumatic tourniquet can be recommended for patients who require very extensive varicose vein surgery, even if not for routine use.

Operative procedures

Although a full description of all the operative procedures available is beyond the scope of this chapter, the following sections contain points of technique for the common operations. Attention to technical details will decrease the regrettably high rate of recurrence after sapheno-femoral ligation and render safer the exploration of the popliteal fossa for sapheno-popliteal ligation.

Sapheno-femoral ligation

Accurate siting of the incision

The anatomical landmarks for the sapheno-femoral junction have been covered in the section on superficial venous anatomy. It is worth delineating the line of the LSV at the groin during the pre-operative marking as this ensures that the incision is centred on the sapheno-femoral junction. Although this will limit the length of the incision, it should be stressed that the incision must be of an adequate length to allow safe visualization of the anatomy.

Identification of the sapheno-femoral junction

The sapheno-femoral junction must be identified before any significant vein is divided. The femoral vein needs to be identified on both medial and lateral sides to confirm that there is a deeper vein before the LSV is divided. Although the superficial external pudendal artery is a useful landmark, lying normally between the LSV and femoral vein just inferior to the sapheno-femoral junction, it can occasionally lie anterior to the LSV and mislead the unwary surgeon.

Surgery for recurrence

Re-exploration of the sapheno-femoral junction for recurrent disease requires particular care. It is advisable to approach the sapheno-femoral junction as far as possible through tissue which has not previously been dissected. Exposure of the femoral artery lateral to the femoral vein allows the sapheno-femoral junction to be displayed and controlled at a level posterior to the previous dissection. Once it has been controlled then the scarred recurrent veins can be dealt with safely.

The anatomical variation of the venous anatomy at the groin, the possibility of venous duplication, the necessity to ligate the postero-medial thigh branch separately and the importance of following out and dividing the branches of the LSV have all been addressed in the anatomy section.

Stripping of the long saphenous vein

There is still some debate as to whether it is necessary to strip the LSV. The available data suggest that stripping does indeed reduce the risk of recurrence, but the opponents of stripping argue that it increases the risk of nerve damage and haematoma as well as increasing the amount of pain. However, as most vascular surgeons now strip only from the groin to just below the knee the risk of nerve damage is already greatly reduced. It is the authors' practice to pass the stripper from the groin down to knee level. Although it is slightly more difficult to manoeuvre the stripper past the valve cusps retrogradely, it ensures that the stripper is in the main LSV trunk and is less likely to pass into the deep system. The stripper can be easily palpated at the knee level and brought out through a small stab incision just at the level of the trifurcation. If the vein is stripped in a retrograde manner, the groin wound can be closed before stripping, thus ensuring that compression can be applied as soon as possible after the stripping has been done. If the stripped vein is brought out in a controlled manner, any substantial residual branches attached to the lower part of the vein will come into the wound and can be ligated and divided, reducing the risk of haematoma. The alternative to stripping the thigh LSV is to remove it in segments through small incisions but although this may reduce the risk of haematoma it tends to give a poorer cosmetic result.

Sapheno-popliteal ligation

Identification of the sapheno-popliteal junction

The question of identification of the sapheno-popliteal junction has already been partially covered in the anatomy section. It is essential that the surgeon is aware of the level and point at which the SSV enters the deep system. One option is to mark the site with the aid of duplex just before surgery but this requires the ready availability of duplex at the time of surgery. An alternative approach, which has been found to be satisfactory, is to identify the level of the sapheno-popliteal junction in relation to the skin crease at the back of the knee at the time of the diagnostic duplex. This ensures that the incision is made at the correct level. The sapheno-popliteal junction is not as obvious as the sapheno-femoral at operation and the anatomy can be confusing. In most cases there is a continuation of the SSV in a superior direction joining the LSV system, profunda vein or even accompanying the sciatic nerve up the leg.

Communication(s) between the SSV and one of the gastrocnemius veins can also complicate the findings. In difficult cases a pre-operative review of the duplex scan video can be very helpful. If difficulty is experienced in identifying the SSV in the popliteal fossa, a small incision in the midline approximately 4 cm below the skin crease will allow easy and safe identification. A gentle pull on the vein through this incision allows the SSV to be identified in the popliteal incision easily. Care must be taken during the dissection as both the SSV and the popliteal vein are far more fragile than the veins in the groin.

Nerve damage

The popliteal vein lies deep to the popliteal artery and the nerves. The common peroneal nerve is the branch most likely to be damaged. Careful dissection, identification of structures before division and the avoidance of excessive retraction will all help to prevent damage. It is unwise to strip the SSV as it is likely to lead to sural nerve damage.

Perforator surgery

The significance of incompetent calf perforators found in patients with varicose veins remains unclear. The use of duplex scanning has demonstrated that many patients who previously would have been diagnosed as having perforator disease only are now found to have clinically occult proximal saphenous incompetence. Duplex has also shown that incompetent calf perforators, found in patients with calf perforator incompetence and long saphenous incompetence, frequently become competent after sapheno-femoral ligation without any surgery to the perforators. It is reasonable to ligate separately any large perforators which are found to be grossly incompetent despite proximal control of the saphenous system, but widespread ligation of perforators does not seem to be justified for patients with simple varicose veins. Extensive open surgical interruption of the perforating veins in the calf was advocated for some patients with chronic venous insufficiency but had a formidable complication rate. The advent of minimally invasive subfascial endoscopic perforator surgery (SEPS) has raised the issue again as it allows the procedure to be carried out with much greater safety. However, the evidence that the widespread interruption of perforators will give benefit even in patients with advanced venous disease remains scanty.

Avulsions/ligations

Most patients expect that the unsightly veins will be removed by surgery. After control of the main stem proximal incompetence, there is still a need to ablate the smaller subcutaneous veins. Some surgeons prefer to treat these by sclerotherapy at a subsequent visit but this does prolong the treatment period for the patient and has cost implications. If the leg has been carefully marked pre-operatively, the use of a limited number of avulsions/ligations at strategic sites can achieve the same result. In the authors' practice using this technique, only 1 in 20 patients require follow-up sclerotherapy. An alternative method of achieving a good cosmetic result is to use multiple stab incisions and pin strippers to remove all the varicose superficial veins, although this can be very time consuming.

Post-operative compression

It is advisable to apply compression after varicose vein surgery, particularly when stripping or avulsions are carried out. Although some surgeons apply anti-embolism stockings at the end of the procedure, they tend to get blood stained and may not give adequate compression. The application of cohesive bandages from the base of the toes proximally can be recommended as they maintain compression much longer than the traditional crepe bandage. After 24 hours they can be removed and replaced with an anti-embolism stocking. As already mentioned care should be taken about applying compression to any limb where there is evidence of ischaemia and the bandage should be removed immediately if the patient gets disproportionate pain after surgery.

Alternative approaches to vein ablation

There has been much research into different methods of ablating the main superficial veins either as an alternative to surgery altogether or as an adjunct to sapheno-femoral ligation. The use of cryotherapy, radiofrequency ablation, diathermy or extensive intra-operative sclerotherapy amongst others has been proposed but has not as yet gained widespread support. Evidence for the long-term results of these newer techniques is very limited.

Complications of varicose vein surgery

The potential for litigation after varicose vein surgery is considerable as demonstrated by the recent review by Tennant and his colleagues. The crucial importance of full documented discussion with the patient of the aims, likely symptomatic and cosmetic outcome and possible complications of any procedure cannot be overemphasized. Although it will not necessarily prevent legal action if there is an operative mishap, it will certainly decrease the number of lesser complaints about outcome. Trainee surgeons should have adequate supervised experience and the availability of consultant assistance before being allowed to operate independently as the review demonstrates that varicose vein surgery is not for the inexperienced surgeon.

Damage to major venous, arterial and nerve structures

Venous damage to the femoral and popliteal veins usually occurs either from a failure to recognize the anatomy or due to attempts to control bleeding blindly. Adequate identification of the venous anatomy before any major structure is divided will reduce the risk of accidental damage to the deep veins. In the event of uncontrolled bleeding, application of local digital pressure and tilting the operating table head down will allow enough time to dissect out the anatomy and get good control. The blind application of haemostats or blind suturing is dangerous and may increase the risk of damage. Repair of any deep vein damage should be carried out with a fine Prolene monofilament stitch. Simple pressure and the assistance of a more experienced vascular surgeon should be sought if bleeding cannot be controlled. If it is felt that the deep veins have been compromised then the venous system should be assessed early as the chances of a successful outcome are reduced if delay occurs.

The risk of arterial damage is small, but there are cases where the femoral artery has been divided and on at least one occasion stripped during a varicose vein operation! Damage to the popliteal artery is very rare, as is damage to the posterior tibial artery above the ankle during ligation of perforators.

Injury to the common peroneal nerve and the sural nerve during short saphenous surgery has already been discussed, as has the risk to the saphenous nerve from stripping or avulsions below the knee. Damage to branches of the femoral nerve can occur during a lateral approach to a recurrent sapheno-femoral junction.

Wound complications

The incidence of wound haematoma and bruising, particularly in the thigh segment, depends on the surgical technique and the compression applied post-operatively. The use of a small stripper head (or none at all with inversion stripping), stripping just before the application of compression, as well as elevation of the limb post-operatively are all thought to decrease the risk. It is important to ensure that any major branches close to the groin and knee wounds are identified and ligated separately as bleeding from these branches may be profuse.

Wound infection in the groin is a relatively rare but troublesome complication. It is often associated with a wound haematoma. A lymphocele may occur after revisional surgery in the groin but is fortunately very rare. Aspiration may be necessary but carries the risk of introducing infection.

Thrombo-embolism

The risk of DVT after primary varicose vein surgery in a patient with no specific risk factors is low. It is not the authors' routine practice to stop HRT or the oral contraceptive pill (OCP) in such patients, although they would give them subcutaneous low molecular weight heparin. For patients with other additional risk factors such as advanced age, obesity or a history of previous thrombosis or embolism the authors would advocate stopping the OCP or HRT and use a higher dose heparin. Patients with known or suspected thrombophilia or recurrent DVT are at high risk of thrombo-embolism and therefore the need for surgery should be reviewed and only undertaken if strictly essential.

Recurrent varicose veins

The chance of developing further varicose veins after surgery is considerable. Follow-up studies have reported clinical recurrence rates from 20 to 60% after 5 years or more. These high figures are supported by the fact that 15–20% of varicose vein operations are undertaken for recurrence. Although some of these cases are due to the development of new varicosities due to progress of disease, the majority are preventable (Table 34.4).

The risk of a complication is greater after surgery for recurrence so that careful assessment and attention to the technical points alluded to throughout this chapter are particularly important for recurrent surgery.

Table 34.4 Causes of varicose vein recurrence

Cause		*Preventable*
Inadequate assessment	Deep venous incompetence	Yes
	Deep venous occlusion	Yes
	Missed point(s) of incompetence	Yes
	Anatomical abnormality	Yes
Inadequate surgery	Inadequate LSV ligation	Yes
	Residual branch at groin	Yes
	Thigh LSV not stripped	Yes
	Duplicate LSV not removed	Yes
	Inadequate SSV ligation	Yes
Progress of disease	New valvular incompetence	No

Labial varicosities

Patients occasionally present with vulval varicosities; these may give rise to pain or heaviness and occasionally to bleeding during or after intercourse. In almost all cases these arise from within the pelvis from branches of the internal iliac vein and may communicate through the obturator foramen or directly via the vulval veins. It often requires varicography to demonstrate the point(s) of communication with the pelvic veins. They are rarely improved by high saphenous ligation. Surgical treatment and/or sclerotherapy are advocated for the most severe cases, but the results are often poor due to the extensive venous intercommunications within the pelvis. Interventional radiology with embolization or even direct intra-pelvic surgery have also been proposed in very severe cases but there is little evidence available on the long term results.

Klippel–Trenaunay syndrome

Patients with this congenital syndrome often present to a vascular surgeon at an early age. They have varicose veins, haemangiomata, frequently excess growth of bone and soft tissues and may be associated with other congenital abnormalities. Referral may simply be a result of the cosmetic appearance but can be due to pain, bleeding, ulceration, phlebitis or even thromboembolism. Treatment is usually conservative using compression stockings. If surgery is being considered then a full imaging of the venous tree is essential, as there may be abnormalities of the deep as well as the superficial veins

Summary

Varicose veins affect at least one quarter of the adult population and present a substantial socio-economic burden to the health services. Although many are asymptomatic, large numbers present with symptoms or clinical signs caused by their venous pathology. Many could benefit from appropriate intervention but resource limitations have restricted the availability of treatment. Efficient assessment clinics to evaluate the patients and select those who would benefit from intervention are essential to make best use of limited resources. A thorough understanding of the underlying anatomy and pathophysiology is necessary not only for case selection but also to ensure that the operative procedures are carried out safely and with good outcomes. The development of vascular subspecialization should help to ensure that surgeons in training will have the opportunity to obtain the necessary knowledge and supervised experience.

Further reading

Ruckley, C. V., Fowkes, F. G. R. and Bradbury, A. W., eds. (1999). *Venous Disease. Epidemiology, Management and Delivery of Care.* London: Springer.

The management of chronic venous disorders of the leg: an evidence based report of an international task force. *Phlebology,* Volume 14, 1999.

Callam, M. J. (1998). The peripheral vascular system. In: Glasby, M. A., Owen, W. J. and Krismundsdottir, F., eds. *Applied Surgical Anatomy – A Guide for the Surgical Trainee.* Oxford: Butterworth-Heinemann.

Tennant, W. G. and Ruckley, C. V. (1996). Medicolegal action following treatment for varicose veins. *Br J Surg* **83**: 291–2.

MODULE 35

Chronic venous insufficiency

Chronic venous insufficiency (CVI), culminating in chronic venous ulceration (CVU), is the most common vascular disease affecting the lower limb and represents a major health and socio-economic problem for many patients in many countries. In the UK, the treatment of CVI is estimated to consume 2% of all National Health Service funding (c. £600 million per annum) and up to one-third of all community nurse resources. Despite this, CVI appears to receive a low priority in terms of research funding when compared, for example, to arterial disease.

Section 35.1 • Definitions and classification

Definitions

There is no universally accepted definition of 'chronic venous insufficiency'. Some authorities use the term CVI to describe any chronic disorder of the veins of the limbs. However, more usually, the term is restricted to those patients who have developed irreversible skin damage as the result of sustained ambulatory venous hypertension. Chronic venous ulceration (CVU) may be defined as a break in the skin, present for more than 6 weeks, between the malleoli and tibial tuberosity, that is presumed to be wholly or partly due to venous disease.

Classification

CVI has proved difficult to classify for the purposes of scientific reporting. A lack of consensus in this area has hampered research because it has obfuscated attempts to directly compare the findings of different epidemiological, pathophysiological and clinical studies. To date, three classifications have predominated in the literature.

The Basle classification (Widmer)

Widmer concentrated on the outward clinical appearance of the lower limb:

- CVI I – corona phlebectatica (venous, or malleolar, flare)
- CVI II – hyper- or depigmented areas (lipodermatosclerosis, atrophe blanche)
- CVI III – open or healed ulceration.

The SVS/ISCVS classification

The Society for Vascular Surgery/International Society for Cardiovascular Surgery classification was first developed in 1988 (Table 35.1) and includes information regarding anatomical region, clinical severity, physical examination and assessment of function.

Table 35.1 SVS/ISCVS classification

Class	*Current clinical symptoms*	*Prior*	*Anatomical location*	
0	Asymptomatic	Same	0	Unknown
1	Mild	Same	1	Superficial
2	Moderate	Same	2	Perforators
3	Severe (ulceration)	Same	3	Deep-calf
			4	Deep-thigh
Origin			5	Deep-iliofemoral
			6	Deep-caval
0	Unknown		7	Combination of 2–5 (any)
1	Congenital			
2	Post-thrombotic			

Table 35.2 CEAP classification

Clinical[a]	
Class 0	No visible or palpable signs of venous disease
Class 1	Telangiectasia[b] or reticular veins[c]
Class 2	Varicose veins[d]
Class 3	Oedema
Class 4	Skin changes (lipodermatosclerosis, atrophe blanche, eczema)
Class 5	Healed ulceration
Class 6	Active ulceration
(a)Etiological	
E_C	Congenital (may be present at birth or recognized later)
E_P	Primary (with undetermined cause)
E_S	Secondary (with known cause): post-thrombotic, post-traumatic, other
Anatomical	
A_S	Superficial veins (numbered 1 to 5)[e]
A_D	Deep veins (numbered 6 to 16)[f]
A_P	Perforating veins (numbered 17 and 18)[g]
Pathophysiological	
P_R	Reflux
P_O	Obstruction
$P_{R,O}$	Both

[a]Supplemented with (A) for asymptomatic or (S) for symptomatic, e.g. $C_{6,A}$.
[b]Intra-dermal venules up to 1 mm in diameter, [c]subdermal, non-palpable venules up to 4 mm, [d]palpable subdermal veins usually larger than 4 mm.
[e]Telangectasia/reticular veins (1); greater (long) saphenous vein above (2) or below (3) knee; lesser (short) saphenous vein (4); non-saphenous (5).
[f]Inferior vena cava (6); common (7), internal (8), external (9) iliac; pelvic (10); common (11), deep (12), superficial (13) femoral; popliteal (14); crural (15); muscular (16).
[g]Thigh (17), calf (18).

The CEAP classification

Both these classifications have now been largely superseded by CEAP (Clinical, (e)Atiological, Anatomical and Pathophysiological) (Table 35.2) which was drawn up under the auspices of the American Venous Forum in Hawaii in 1994. Weaknesses of this classification include:

- its exhaustive anatomical classification, especially given the fact that the majority of patients have no venous investigation performed above the level of the common femoral vein
- patients with oedema are given a separate clinical class (class 3) despite the fact that oedema is variable in these patients and, of course, may be due to non-venous disease
- the sheer complexity of the system makes it impractical for day-to-day clinical use and even for research purposes if the number of subjects being studied is large.

The utility of CEAP has already been the subject of debate and controversy. It is expected that an improved, and simplified, version will be forthcoming.

The CEAP scoring system

The CEAP classification has been used as the basis for a scoring system based upon the number of venous segments affected (anatomical score), grading of symptoms and signs (clinical score) and disability (disability score) (Table 35.3). The utility of the this system requires to be determined.

Section 35.2 • Epidemiology

When discussing any medical condition, it is important to know the number of patients affected, which groups are particularly are at risk, and why. Furthermore, by understanding the natural history of CVI, it may be possible to recognize and treat the condition at an earlier stage. A number of epidemiological studies have been carried out in the field of CVI over the past 30 years. Unfortunately, a lack of uniformity of methodology, study population, definitions and reporting means that the conclusions reached by these studies have not always been in accord. It is also possible that the epidemiology of the condition may have changed over the last three decades. However, it can be concluded with some confidence that:

- with regard to a randomly selected sample of a typical adult Western population
- using the Widmer classification
- on the basis of clinical examination

Table 35.3 CEAP severity scoring

Anatomical score	Sum of the anatomical segments, each scored as 1 point
Clinical score	
Pain	None (0), moderate not requiring analgesia (1), severe requiring analgesia (2)
Oedema	None (0), mild/moderate (1), severe (2)
Venous claudication	None (0), mild/moderate (1), severe (2)
Pigmentation	None (0), localized (1), extensive (2)
Lipodermatosclerosis	None (0), localized (1), extensive (2)
Ulcer	
size (largest)	None (0), < 2cm (1), $\geq$ 2cm (2)
duration	None (0), < 3 months (1), $\geq$ 3 months (2)
recurrence	None (0), once (1), more than once (2)
number	None (0), single (1), multiple (2)
Disability score	
0	Asymptomatic
1	Symptomatic but can function without support device
2	Can work 8 hour day but only with support device
3	Unable to work even with support device

at any one point in time:

- a third to a half will have trunk varicose veins
- 7% will have CVI I
- 1–3% will have CVI II
- 1% will have CVI III. Of these, approximately 10% of ulcers will be open at any one time, giving a point prevalence for open CVU of 0.1%.

Typically, recurrent episodes of CVU affect patients for decades. Thus, the point prevalence for open/healed CVU quoted above will be quite different from the period prevalence (the number of ulcer episodes occurring over any given time period) and the incidence (the number of patients developing their first episode of ulceration over a given period of time). Only longitudinal epidemiological studies, where the same population is repeatedly sampled, are able to relate these different variables in a coherent way and thus map out the natural history of this chronic condition.

Age

The point prevalence of CVU increases exponentially with age, rising to 3.6% in those over 65 years. However, it is important to note that up to 25% of patients develop their ulcer before the age of 45 years.

Gender

CVU is frequently stated to be commoner in women, although epidemiological studies suggest that, once prevalence is corrected for age, men and women are affected almost equally. The excess of women observed in clinical practice is largely due to their longevity, together with an apparent reluctance on the part of working men to seek medical attention.

Social class

Varicose veins do appear to be commoner in people from the lower social classes. There is no clear evidence that low socio-economic class predisposes to CVI, although healing rates of CVU may be poorer. In one study, failure of ulcer healing in the community was significantly related on multivariate analysis to the absence of central heating in the patients' homes. The environmental and socio-economic factors contributing to the development and persistence of CVI require further study, and are often overlooked by those caring for such patients.

Occupation

Certain occupations, specifically those that involve prolonged standing, are more frequently associated with varicose veins. Although it has not been possible to prove that these occupations are associated with disease progression to CVI, clinical experience suggests that they do have a bearing on ulcer healing. Data on the relationships between physical activity and CVI are conflicting.

Weight and height

There does not appear to be a relationship between weight, height and the development of CVI in men, but the severity of venous disease in women was related to body mass index (BMI) in the Edinburgh vein study. Increased BMI may also be associated with delayed CVU healing.

Diet

It has been hypothesized that a fibre-deficient diet and constipation aggravate the onset of varicose veins. However, a definite link with CVI has not been established.

Smoking

There is no known association between smoking and the development of CVI, although it is, of course, related to the presence of arterial disease which may have a bearing on the prognosis and treatment of CVU (see below).

Parity

VV are frequently said to be associated with pregnancy and multiparity, although the epidemiological evidence for this is inconsistent and the association often disappears following an adjustment for age. It is not unusual to obtain a history of post-partum venous thrombosis (DVT) in the patient with CVU. Having said that, many female patients afflicted by CVU are elderly spinsters.

Heredity and race

It is frequently said that varicose veins 'run in families', especially where the condition develops in the teenage years. CVI and CVU may also have a familial tendency in some cases through an association with the inherited thrombophilias that predispose to DVT. There is an increased prevalence of varicose veins in Caucasians compared with native black populations. However, no difference has been shown between black and white Americans.

Trends over time

The number of completed consultant episodes of care for CVI has increased markedly in the UK in recent years, although this may reflect an increased awareness of the condition rather than a true increase in prevalence. Historical data suggest CVU used to be very much more common that it is today. It is hoped better prophylaxis and treatment for DVT, as well as the more widespread use of compression hosiery, will lead to a reduction in future prevalence. However, these beneficial affects may be overshadowed by the effects of an ageing population.

Section 35.3 • Pathophysiology

Introduction

CVI, culminating in CVU, is the end-result of sustained ambulatory venous hypertension acting upon a dermal microcirculation designed to operate in the presence of low venous pressure. A clear grasp of the macrovascular and microvascular pathophysiological mechanisms leading to CVI is essential to an understanding of the symptoms, signs and medical and surgical treatment of the condition. First, however, it is necessary to describe, briefly, the normal macro- and microvascular systems as they pertain to lower limb venous function.

Macrovascular system – normal

Venous blood from the lower limbs returns to the right heart against gravity through the deep and superficial venous systems. The deep veins follow the named arteries and are often paired from the popliteal down (Figure 35.1). The superficial system comprises the long (LSV) and short (SSV) saphenous veins and their tributaries (Figure 35.2). There are numerous communications between the long and short saphenous systems, as well as between the superficial and deep veins through junctional and non-junctional (eponymous) perforators (Figure 35.3). As such, these three elements are highly interdependent, both anatomically and functionally, in health and in disease.

The LSV has a number of reasonably constant tributaries in the thigh and calf. It is worth noting that it is these tributaries, not the main trunk (which is invested

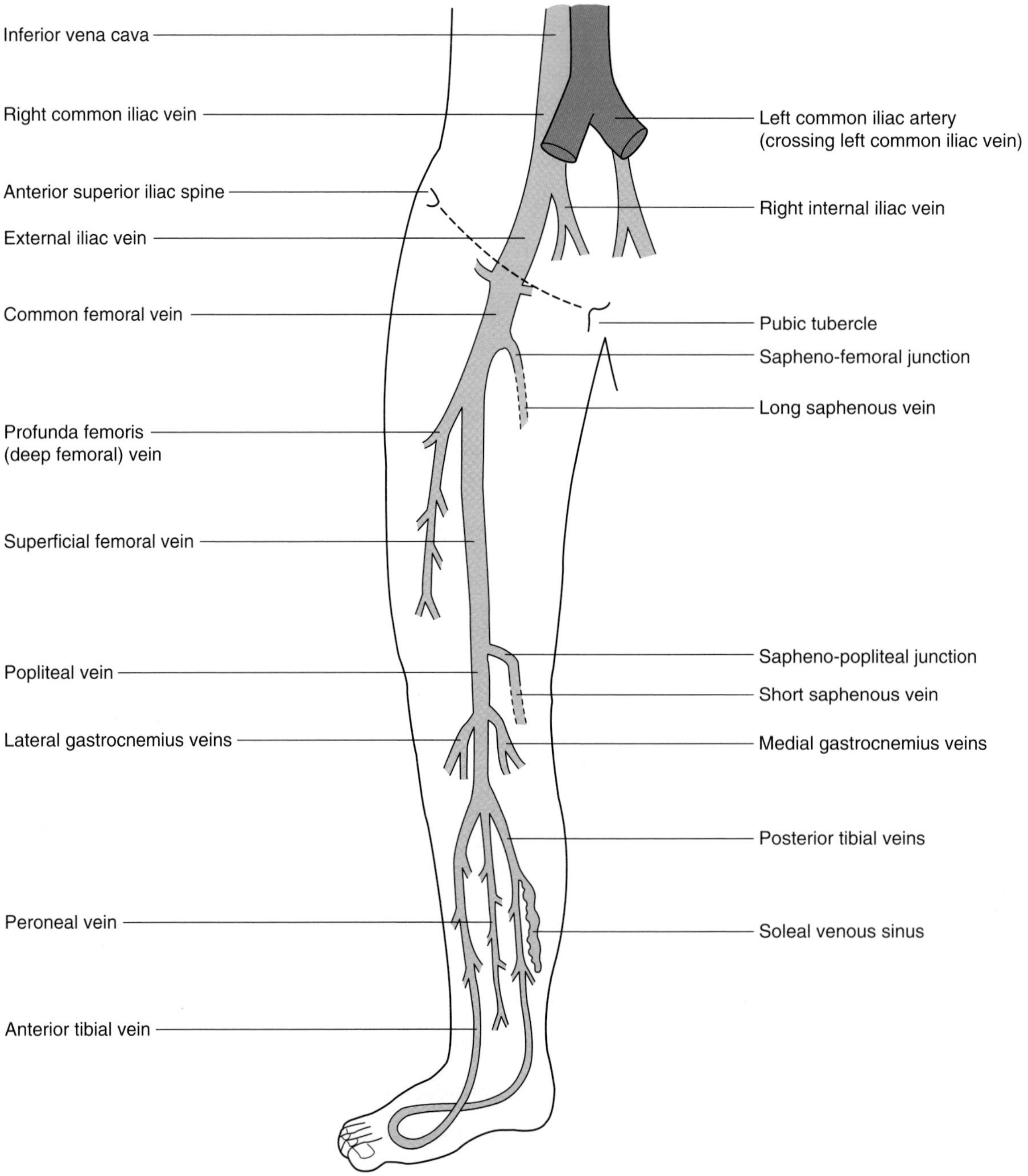

Figure 35.1 Deep veins of the lower limb.

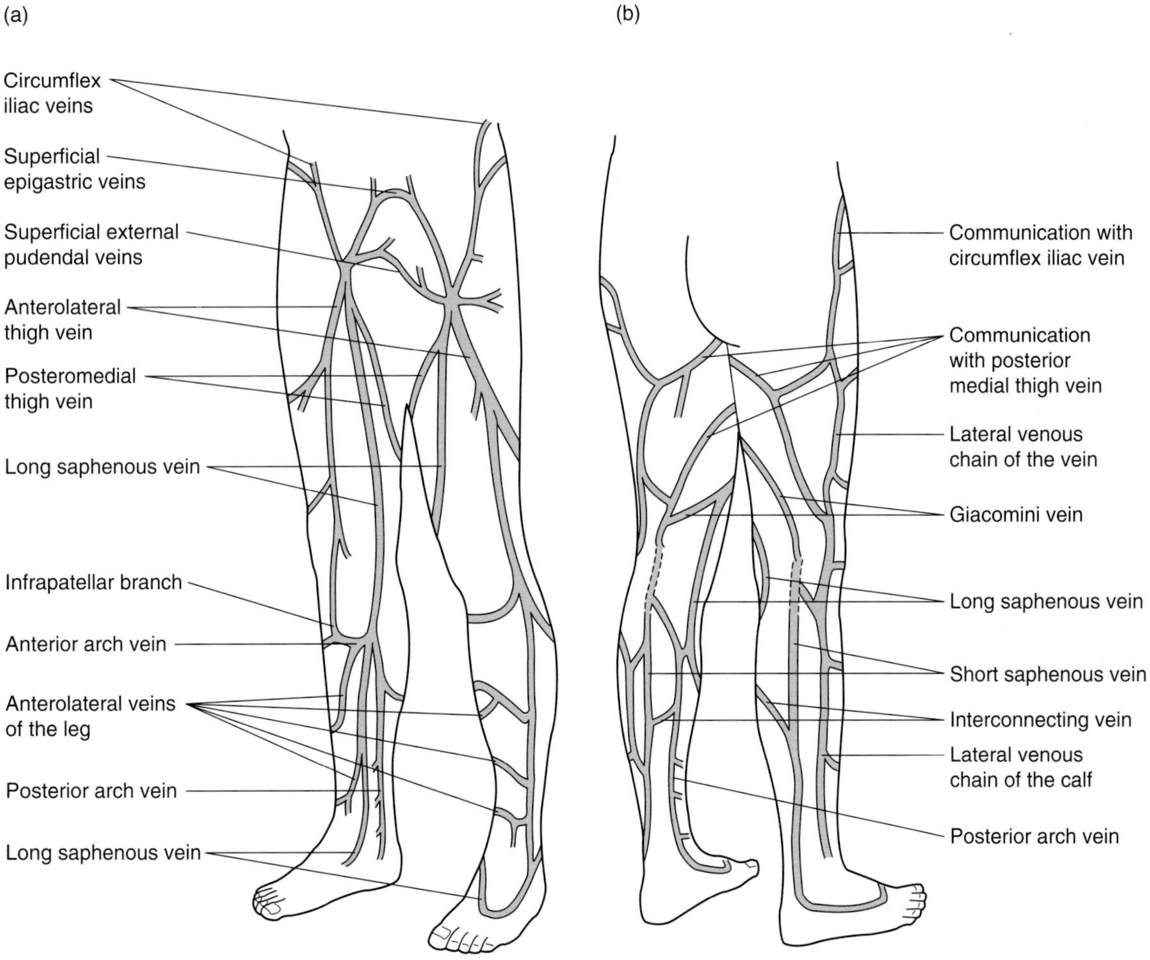

Figure 35.2 Superficial veins of the lower limb. (a) Anterior aspect. (b) Posterior aspect.

in supporting fascia), which become varicose. It is also important to note that it is the posterior arch vein, and not the main LSV, that is in direct continuity with the posterior tibial veins via the medial calf perforating veins.

Superficial veins drain blood from the tissues superficial to the deep fascia. Most of this blood immediately enters the deep venous system via perforators in the foot, calf and thigh. In health, less than 10% of the total venous return from the lower limb passes through the LSV and SSV to the sapheno-femoral (SFJ) and sapheno-popliteal (SPJ) junctions respectively. The apparent overdevelopment of the superficial venous system is explained teleologically by its thermoregulatory role in furred animals. Failure of the superficial system to involute, together with our bipedal posture, may explain the uniquely human predisposition to CVI.

Blood is forced back up the leg during leg muscle 'systole', and prevented from flowing back down the leg under the influence of gravity during 'diastole', through the actions of the muscle pumps and closure of venous valves respectively (Figure 35.4). The act of walking sequentially compresses venous sinuses in the sole of the foot, the calf (soleus, gastrocnemius) and to a lesser extent the thigh and buttock. During relaxation these sinuses fill from the deep and superficial venous systems and valves close in the superficial and axial veins to prevent reverse flow (reflux). In both the superficial and deep systems, the density of valves is greatest in the calf and gradually diminishes in the thigh. The iliac veins and inferior vena cava are frequently valveless (Figure 35.5).

When standing completely motionless, with all the leg muscles relaxed, the venous valve leaflets come to lie in a neutral mid-position. As a result, the venous pressure in the dorsal foot veins comes to represent the hydrostatic pressure exerted by the unbroken column of venous blood stretching up from the foot to the right atrium (approximately 90–100 mmHg in a person of average height). Contraction of the leg muscles immediately leads to the compression of deep veins and sinuses and to the movement of venous blood both cranially and caudally. The latter is terminated by valve closure, usually within 0.5–1.0 s Nor does blood leave the deep compartment via perforators to enter the superficial system. Conventionally, this has also been ascribed to the closure of valves within the perforators.

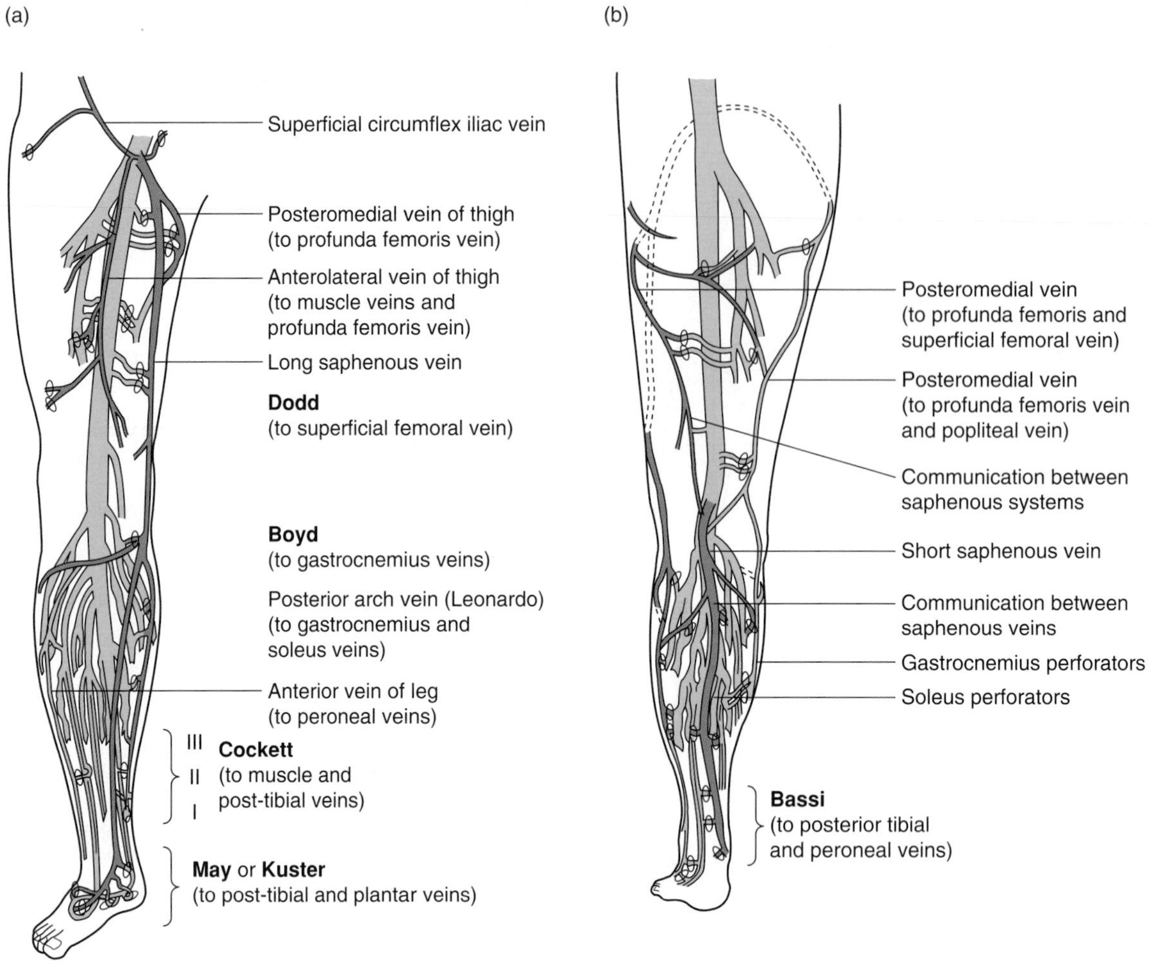

Figure 35.3 Connections between the superficial and deep venous systems of the lower limb. (a) Anterior aspect. (b) Posterior aspect.

However, several studies have shown that many perforators are devoid of valves. Instead, outward flow through perforators may be limited by external compression from contracting muscle and a 'pinch-cock' mechanism involving the deep fascia (Figure 35.6). The importance of these mechanisms is that the very high pressures (up to 200 mmHg) generated within the calf muscle pump are used exclusively to propel blood back up the leg against gravity, and are not transmitted to the superficial or distal deep systems. When the muscle pump relaxes, the previously expelled venous blood will tend to flow caudally under gravity but is prevented from doing so by valve closure. This has the effect of dividing a single long (and heavy) column of blood into a series of shorter columns lying between closed valves. The pressure within each of these segments is low and the ambulatory venous pressure (AVP) in the dorsal foot veins will fall typically to <25 mmHg (Figure 35.7). An AVP above 30 mmHg is associated with an increasing incidence of CVU: 31–40 mmHg 15%; > 90 mmHg 100%. During muscle pump diastole, blood in the superficial system flows in to the deep system along a pressure gradient.

Microcirculation – normal

The microcirculation is the site of fluid and molecular exchange between the vasculature and the interstitium. Filtration of fluid at the arteriolar end of the capillary, in response to hydrostatic pressure, is followed by re-entry of fluid at the venular end due to the osmotic effects of the plasma proteins (oncotic pressure). Normally, around 10% of the filtered fluid is reabsorbed by the lymphatic system (Figure 35.8). Any change in arteriolar and/or venular hydrostatic pressure will clearly have a marked effect on the balance of these, so-called, Starling's forces.

When one moves from the supine to the standing position there is an immediate rise in arterial and venous hydrostatic pressure in the lower limb. However, in health, the veno-arteriolar reflex (VAR) leads to arteriolar constriction in the skin of the lower leg in response to venous distension such that skin blood flow actually falls. This reflex has an important role in preventing oedema as well as protecting the dermal microcirculation against excessively high pressures. The VAR may be impaired in patients with

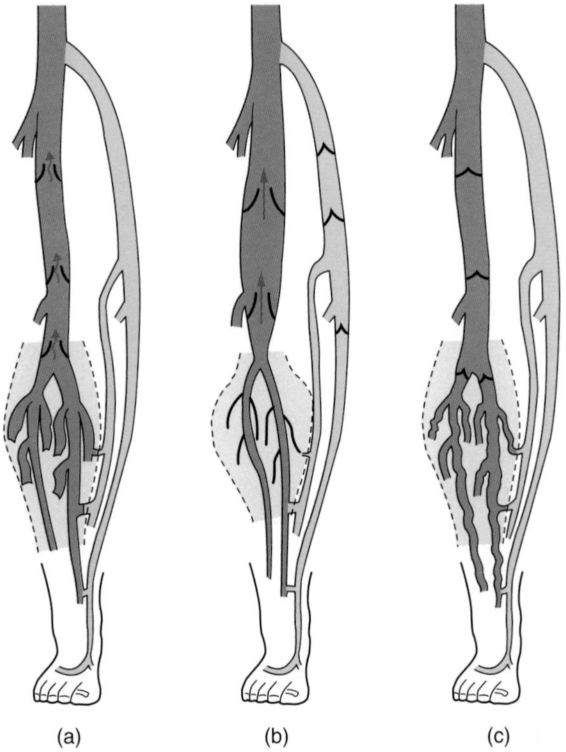

Figure 35.4 The calf muscle pump of the lower limb. (a) During calf muscle pump diastole the deep veins and sinuses fill from arterial inflow and from the superficial venous system via perforating veins. (b) During systole blood is ejected cranially and prevented from moving distally, or back into the superficial system through the closure of valves. (c) During diastole, ejected blood is prevented from re-entering the calf muscle pump though the closure of valves.

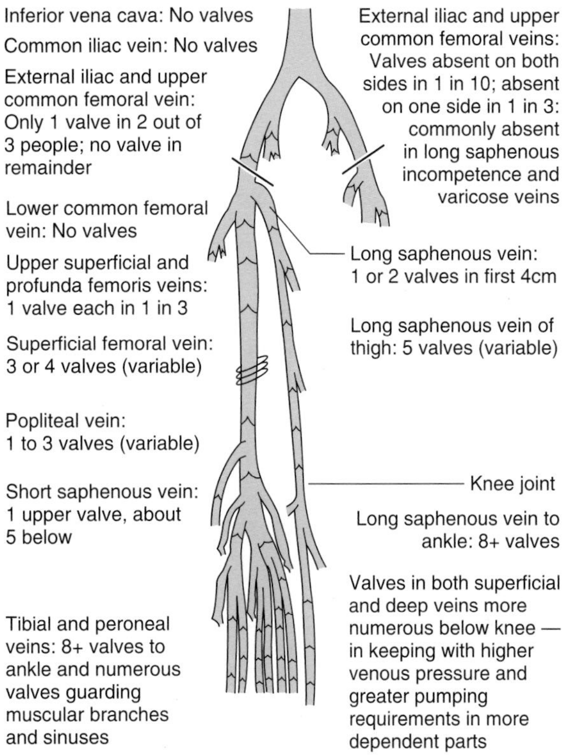

Figure 35.5 Venous valves of the lower limb.

CVI although the reasons for this are unclear. Similarly, any condition that impairs the calf muscle pump and/or valvular function described above will lead to abnormally high back-pressure on the microcirculation. It is generally believed that it is this sustained venous hypertension which leads to the skin changes of CVI.

Macrovascular system – abnormal

There are three basic mechanisms that lead to the sustained venous hypertension and thus the skin changes characteristic of CVI; namely, muscle pump dysfunction, valvular reflux and venous obstruction.

Muscle pump dysfunction

Ageing, general debility and a range of musculo-skeletal and/or neurological lower limb pathologies can impair the ability of the calf muscle pump to expel venous blood. Perhaps the most obvious and clinically apparent example is the patient with a fixed ankle; perhaps due to arthritis or following trauma. Loss of the longitudinal and transverse arches of the foot also impairs the venous foot pump, which can be likened to the atrium priming the ventricle (the calf pump).

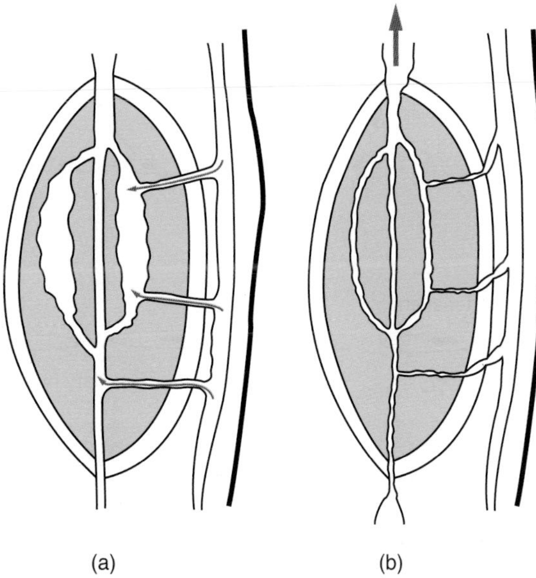

Figure 35.6 Mechanisms of perforator competence. (a) During calf muscle diastole blood enters the deep compartment from the superficial system via perforating veins. (b) Larger perforating veins have valves that prevent outward flow during calf muscle pump systole. Other factors ensuring competence include compression by contracting muscle and a pinch-cock mechanism as the veins pass through the fascia.

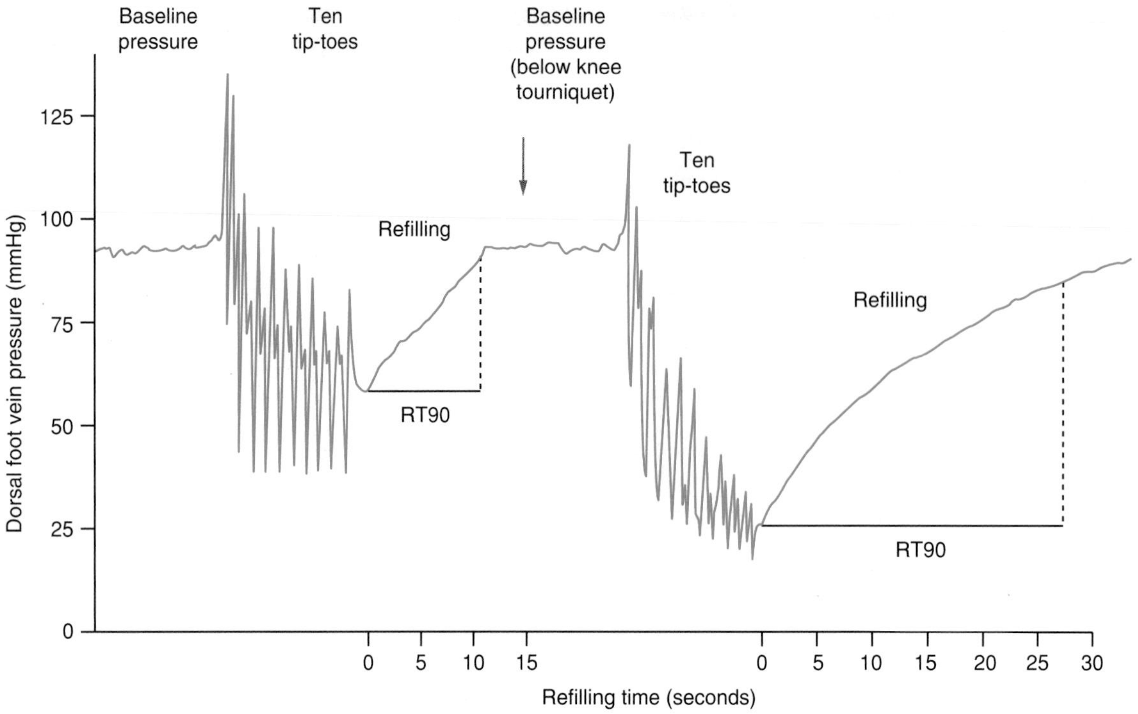

Figure 35.7 Ambulatory venous pressure. Standing motionless, baseline pressure rises to 90 mmHg. Ten tip-toe movements will reduce the pressure to normal in the absence of venous disease. In this patient, normal post-exercise pressures and refilling times are only attained once superficial reflux down the long saphenous vein has been abolished by means of a below knee tourniquet.

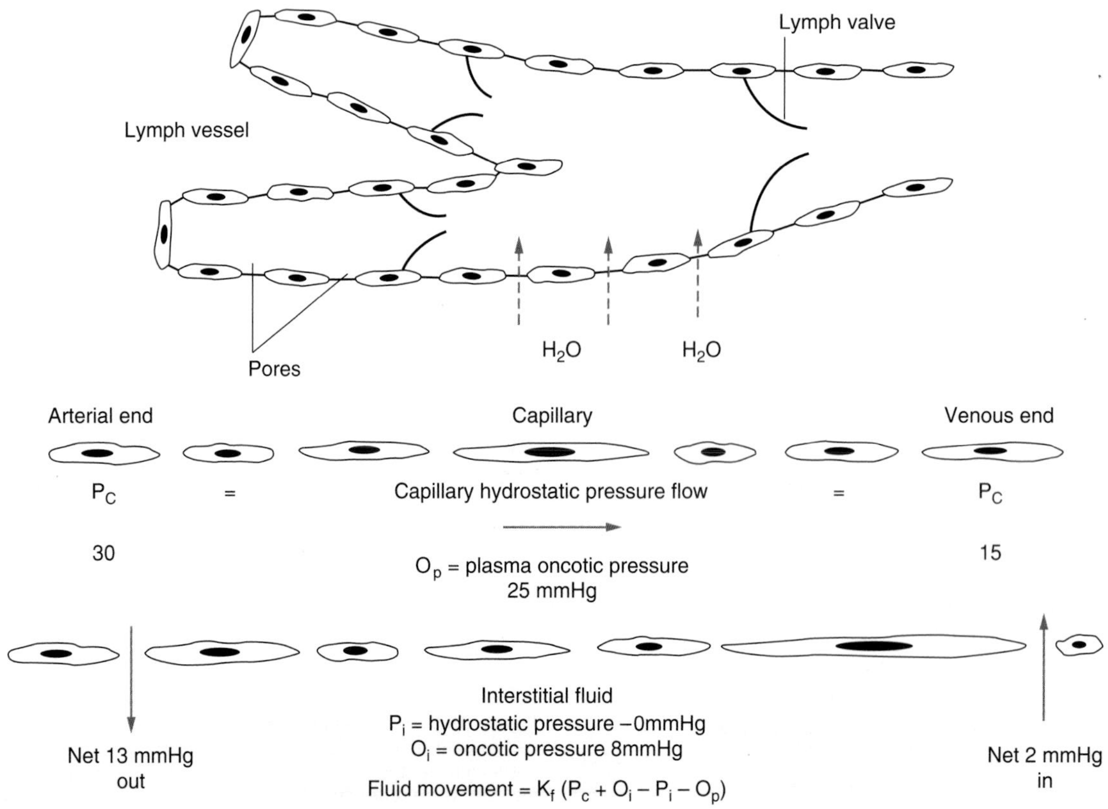

Figure 35.8 Starling's forces. The formation and clearance of interstitial fluid is dependent on hydrostatic and osmotic forces across the capillary endothelium, as well as lymphatic function.

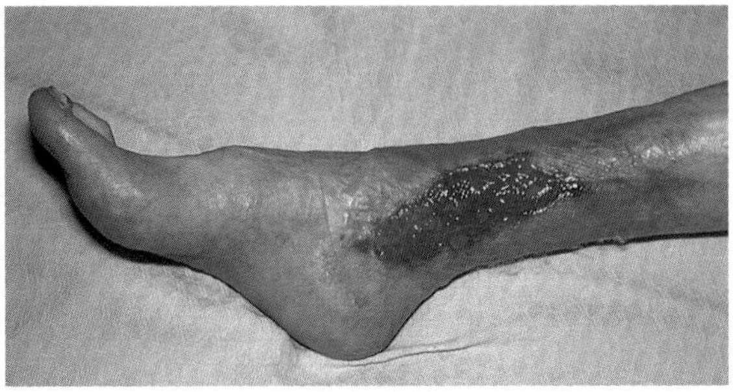

Figure 35.9 Fixed ankle. This patient had a fixed ankle following trauma and developed a venous ulcer despite the absence of significant reflux on duplex ultrasonography.

Muscle bulk and tone are also important in the maintenance of perforator competence (see above). Failure of perforator competence leads to calf pump inefficiency (akin to mitral regurgitation), as well as the transmission of the high deep pressure directly to the skin of the gaiter area.

Although most discussions of CVI focus on valve function, it is possible to develop the skin changes of CVI in the absence of reflux simply as a result of poor muscle pump function (Figure 35.9). Such a situation may be encountered in elderly patients after stroke (in whom DVT is also common) as well as in younger patients with, for example, multiple sclerosis or muscular dystrophy.

Valve reflux

Valvular reflux in the deep and/or superficial veins is present in more than 90% of patients with CVI. In approximately a third to a half of cases this is confined to the superficial system. In the remainder, both systems are affected. If patients have previously undergone superficial venous surgery then only the deep system may be involved. In general, the prognosis of patients with isolated superficial reflux is better than that of those with deep reflux, particularly if the latter is secondary to DVT. Furthermore, distal (crural, popliteal) reflux appears to have a greater adverse haemodynamic and clinical effect than proximal (thigh) reflux. Valvular reflux can arise in three ways.

Primary valvular incompetence

In this condition, loss of elastin and weakening of collagen in the vein wall, particularly around the valve commissures, leads to dilatation, separation of the valve leaflets and reflux. Because of the dilatation, and as the vein is no longer divided by competent valves into a series of low pressure segments, tension on the vein wall increases according to Laplace's law. The end result is an incompetent, varicose, elongated and thus tortuous venous segment. While this process is most commonly seen in relation to the superficial system to produce varicose veins, it is also believed to affect the deep venous system.

In some circumstances, a (relatively) normal venous segment may be rendered incompetent because of excessive distending pressures elsewhere in the patient's venous system. The importance of this mechanism is that the incompetence may be reversible; that is, if the distending pressure is removed then the vein segment, which may be structurally (near)-normal, may regain competence. For example, in a proportion of patients with varicose veins and accompanying deep vein reflux, surgical correction of the superficial venous incompetence may restore competence to the femoro-popliteal segment. Furthermore, in the absence of popliteal and/or crural vein reflux, eradication of superficial venous incompetence may lead to restoration of competence in previously incompetent medial calf perforating veins. These observations impact directly upon the selection of patients for surgery, as well as the nature of the surgery undertaken (see below).

Post-phlebitic (secondary) valvular incompetence

Lower limb DVT is a common clinical entity and a clear history of DVT is found in about 20% of patients with CVU. In addition, an unknown, and probably unquantifiable number, of people develop asymptomatic DVT without ever knowing it.

The presence of thrombus within a vein, especially where it is occlusive, leads to an inflammatory, possibly ischaemic, phlebitis. This is thought to be due to obstruction of the vena venorum and direct humoral and/or cellular damage to the endothelium. It is important to note that the classical symptoms and signs of the 'medical' DVT (pain, redness, tenderness, swelling and distension of superficial veins) are all manifestations of occlusive thrombophlebitis. At this point the thrombus is adherent to the vein wall and no longer juxtaposed to a flowing venous stream; as such, the risk of pulmonary embolus (PE) is low. Conversely, most surgical patients suffering a major or fatal PE have normal legs on clinical examination because their DVT is non-occlusive, non-adherent (non-inflammatory) and lies within a flowing blood stream. Both types of DVT can lead to the post-thrombotic syndrome through valvular damage although it is more likely with more extensive disease.

In the short term, partial or complete occlusion of the deep venous system with thrombus leads to flow through collaterals that are:

- valveless, thus permitting reflux
- of narrow diameter, so increasing the resistance to venous outflow.

Later, the thrombus undergoes 'organization' that is accompanied by an inflammatory infiltrate, neovascularization, fibrinolysis and partial or complete recanalization of the affected segment. However, even the though the segment may no longer be physically obstructed it:

- will have no functional valves, so permitting reflux
- may pose a functional obstruction to venous outflow because of its reduced diameter and compliance; that is, its thickened fibrotic wall may lead to stricturing at rest and prevent the vein distending in response to the ejection of blood from the calf muscle pump, or increases in blood flow with exercise.

Physical and functional deep venous obstruction leads to the formation of collaterals and the establishment of venous return through pathological channels. Thus blood may return from the leg by being forced out from the calf deep compartment via perforators to the skin of the gaiter area and through distended so-called secondary varicose veins. Failure of haemodynamic compensation may quickly lead to the development of the post-thrombotic syndrome (PTS). This comprises the skin changes of CVI leading to ulceration, swelling and a bursting discomfort in the leg following exercise relieved only by resting and elevating it (venous claudication).

The incidence of PTS quoted in the literature varies considerably. However, following standard treatment of DVT with heparin and 3 months of warfarin the risk of recurrence and PTS at 2, 5 and 8 years is probably in the region of 20, 25 and 30%, respectively. There is, therefore, a very clear association between recurrent thrombosis and PTS. However, the risks for an individual patient are difficult to define because the development of PTS is affected by a number of different factors, not all of which are easy to recognize, quantify or control.

Extent and resolution of thrombus. Many patients with CVI have no remembered episode of DVT. Resolution is a dynamic process that can occur over months, even years, and thus is difficult to define unless repeated imaging or physiological testing is undertaken.

Age. The risk of DVT increases exponentially with age.

Malignancy. Some of the most extensive DVTs are associated with (advanced) malignancy (Figure 35.10). However, because of their limited life expectancy, relatively few patients go on to develop PTS.

Inherited thrombophilia. Genetically determined, congenital, abnormalities of haemostasis that predispose to DVT – the so-called inherited or 'classical' thrombophilias (Table 35.4) – are increasingly recognized as an importance cause of (recurrent) thrombosis, and thus PTS, in often young, otherwise healthy, individuals. The 'classical' thrombophilias should be suspected if:

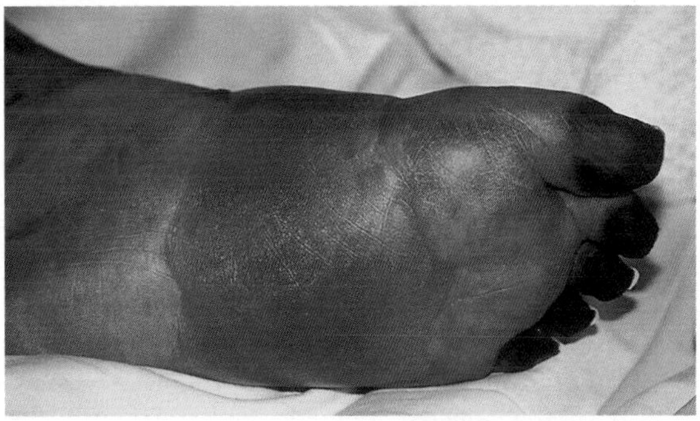

Figure 35.10 Venous gangrene. This patient has advanced pancreatic malignancy.

Table 35.4 Risk factors for venous thrombosis

Congenital patient factors	Protein C, protein S and antithrombin III deficiency Activated protein C resistance (factor V Leiden) Antiphospholipid antibodies Hyperhomocyteinaemia
Acquired patient factors	Antiphospholipid antibodies Increased factor VIII and fibrinogen Age Obesity Immobility Pregnancy Puerperium Varicose veins Oestrogen therapy Previous venous thrombo-embolism
Disease/surgical factors	Pelvic, hip and lower limb trauma and/or surgery Malignancy Paralysis Sepsis Dehydration Nephrotic syndrome Inflammatory bowel disease Cardiac failure

- the patient suffers their first DVT under the age of 45 years
- there are recurrent episodes (especially in the absence of clear 'triggering' events)
- there is a family history of thrombotic disease, especially if it was recurrent, of early onset, or in unusual places
- there is a history of recurrent fetal loss.

In the Leiden study of almost 500 patients with a first DVT under the age of 70 years and without malignancy, 8% had anti-thrombin III, protein C or protein S deficiency compared with 3% of the normal population. Factor V Leiden genetic mutation leading to activated protein C resistance (APCR), was present in 19% of the patients and 3% of the controls. Thus, up to one-fifth of DVT are associated with an identifiable inherited predisposition. The link between thrombophilia, DVT and venous ulceration is demonstrated by one study that has shown an increased prevalence of factor V Leiden in CVU patients. CVI patients also tend to have high fibrinogen levels and impaired fibrinolysis but it is difficult to know whether these changes represent the 'chicken' or the 'egg'.

Acquired thrombophilia. Many and varied conditions predispose to DVT (Table 35.4). Some are clinically obvious, others occult. The total thrombotic risk for an individual patient can be estimated by summating all the identifiable inherited and acquired thrombophilic factors, e.g. hormone replacement therapy plus a long bone fracture requiring immobilization plus a, hitherto unknown, classical thrombophilia is likely to lead to a very high risk of DVT.

Treatment. The quality of the immediate treatment received by a patient for DVT has a marked affect on the propagation and resolution of thrombus, the risk of rethrombosis and presumably the incidence of PTS. Furthermore, in the medium to long term, compliance with compression hosiery undoubtedly limits the progression of the symptoms and signs of PTS. This aspect of prevention is often overlooked.

Of all the patients with CVI and CVU, those with the PTS have the worst prognosis and are the most refractory to treatment. The importance of ensuring that all patients at risk are provided with adequate DVT prophylaxis and, if necessary, treatment, in order to prevent this very condition developing in the future cannot be overemphasized.

Valvular hypoplasia/agenesis

This is an extremely rare condition, individuals developing gross varicosities and CVU.

Microvascular system – abnormal

It is generally accepted that CVI and CVU are due to sustained ambulatory venous hypertension. However, there is still uncertainly as to how a raised AVP actually leads to the pathological changes observed in the affected skin. Furthermore, for reasons that are as yet unclear, individual susceptibility to venous hypertension appears quite variable.

Venous stasis and hypoxia

At one time it was believed that varicose veins contained slow flowing, 'stagnant' blood that was low in oxygen and that ulceration of the overlying skin was due to hypoxia. Unfortunately, the term 'stasis ulcer' is still used in some texts to describe CVU. However, modern studies have shown that this is not the case.

pO_2 measurements in varicose veins. In the supine position, the pO_2 of blood in varicose veins is higher than that observed in non-varicose superficial veins. Although varicose veins pO_2 does fall on standing, it is still similar to that seen in normal individuals.

Transcutaneous oximetry (tc-pO_2). The Clark electrode was originally used in neonates to measure arterial pO_2 because, when the skin is heated to 43°C to produce maximal vasodilatation, there is little or no gradient between skin and arterial pO_2. At 43°C, the tc-pO_2 of CVI skin is lower than controls; but, paradoxically, at 37°C, it is higher. Recovery of tc-pO_2 after 5 min of arterial occlusion with a tourniquet is also similar in CVI and normal skin.

Direct needle measurements. These have shown moderate decreases in oxygen tension within skin affected by CVI. It was concluded that these levels were not low enough to cause tissue breakdown but might impair healing once ulceration is already present.

Positron emission tomography (PET). This technique has revealed a marked increase in the blood flow through skin affected by CVI but a reduced oxygen extraction, leading to no overall change in oxygen delivery.

Xenon clearance studies. These have shown no difference between normal controls and CVI patients.

Arteriovenous fistula

The increased oxygen tension observed in the superficial veins of legs affected by venous disease led to the suggestion that CVI, and specifically ulceration, might be associated with the development of arteriovenous fistula which were 'stealing' blood from the skin. This hypothesis has not been supported by recent studies using microspheres and macroaggregates.

Peri-capillary fibrin cuff

Browse and Burnand suggested that the fibrin cuffs they had observed on histological sections surrounding the dermal capillaries of skin affected by CVI were acting as a barrier to oxygen diffusion and leading to local tissue ischaemia. These cuffs develop because of disturbed Starling's forces that lead to the deposition of peri-capillary protein and because of the reduced fibrinolytic activity observed in both the endothelium and vein wall of CVI patients. It is important to note that 'fibrin' cuff is a much more complex structure than was originally imagined. For example, it also contains abnormal depositions of laminin, fibronectin, tenascin and type IV collagen. Theoretical data suggest that the cuff is not a significant barrier to gaseous exchange. However, the cuff, basement membrane and surrounding extracellular matrix (ECM) may yet turn out to have a pathophysiological role in terms of its interaction with leucocytes, cytokines, polypeptide growth factors and proteases (such as the metalloproteinases, urokinase and tissue plasminogen activators).

Leucocyte activation

Margination of leucocytes in post-capillary venules is a normal physiological response to microvascular 'stress', e.g. inflammation, infection, ischaemia. It had been observed that, following a period of enforced motionless dependency, about 25% of the leucocytes entering the legs of normal volunteers were trapped. On moving the leg and regaining the supine the position, these leucocytes were 'washed out' of the leg and re-entered the systemic circulation. This 'white cell trapping' was greatly exaggerated in patients with CVI and the trapped leucocytes took much longer to leave the leg. This led Coleridge-Smith to propose that leucocytes were blocking the capillaries of the skin and causing skin damage by interrupting nutritive flow, as well as by becoming activated and releasing harmful moieties. Subsequent studies with laser Doppler fluxmetry suggested that leucocytes were not blocking capillaries in sufficient numbers to reduce overall blood skin flow.

Histological sections indicate that most of the chronically trapped leucocytes are mononuclear cells – macrophages and lymphocytes. Immunohistochemistry also shows increased expression of factor VIII antigen and adhesion molecules as well as certain cytokines.

In patients with CVI, the creation of acute venous hypertension in the leg by motionless dependency leads to:

- neutrophil activation as shown by the release of neutrophil elastase and lactoferrin, as well as changes in the expression of the neutrophil activation marker CD11b
- endothelial cell activation and injury, as shown by the release of soluble adhesion molecules involved in leucocyte binding and von Willebrand factor.

While it is clear that CVI is associated with trapping of activated leucocytes within the leg, it is not certain whether this is a cause or an effect of the skin pathology.

Capillary proliferation

Histological sections of skin affected by CVI show an increase in capillary cross-sections suggesting capillary proliferation. Capillary microscopy shows a reduction in visible capillary loops due to capillary 'thrombosis'. However, the remaining capillaries are elongated, tortuous and dilated. This is possibly secondary to the upregulation of various growth factors such as vascular endothelial growth factor (VEGF). Loss of capillaries, especially marked in areas of atrophe blanche, may lead to localized areas of tissue hypoperfusion, contributing to tissue loss and poor healing, even though the overall skin blood flow is normal, even increased.

CVU as a 'failing' wound

It remains unclear why the above factors should lead to CVU or why venous ulcers fail to heal. The venous ulcer can be seen as a model of the 'failing wound'. A number of studies have shown ulcer exudate to inhibit keratinocyte migration and fibroblast activity, even in rapidly healing ulcers, in comparison with controls. Proteolysis is increased, and the activity of matrix metalloproteinases is upregulated, along with numerous cytokines. Considerably more research is required before it can be determined with certainty how the macrovascular venous abnormalities so easily observed in the leg affected by CVI lead to the less easily observed microvascular abnormalities. However, such research does hold out the promise of novel therapeutic avenues.

Clinical assessment

History

Taking a careful history will often reveal factors that are thought to lead to or exacerbate venous disease. Enquiry should be made as to duration of the present ulcer as well as the length of ulcer disease, the number of episodes and any precipitating factors. Previous treatment history and contact allergies to dressings and bandaging materials are often found. Peripheral artery disease (20%), diabetes mellitus (5%) and rheumatoid arthritis (8%) often co-exist in patients with CVU. It is important to appreciate that many ulcers, particularly those that are resistant to treatment, are multi-factorial in origin, and that sustained healing will only be achieved once all the aetiological factors have been addressed. One also needs to be aware that certain socio-economic factors such as social class, housing, nutrition and occupation have a bearing upon both aetiology and prognosis. A full past medical history should be taken, particularly with regard to diabetes mellitus, rheumatoid arthritis, vasculitis and malnutrition.

Physical examination

Patient mobility and gait

It is important to assess the patient's mobility and to watch how the patient walks. Is there evidence of neurological and/or locomotor disease? Flat feet, a fixed ankle and reduced mobility at the knees or hips will markedly impair the ability of the foot and calf pump to expel blood from the leg, exacerbating venous hypertension.

Patient positioning

The patient should be examined in a warm room, standing (preferably on an elevated platform for the benefit of the examiner) with the hip and knee flexed to allow venous filling. It is not unusual for patients to feel dizzy or faint during the examination and adequate care and support must be provided. The examiner must be able to see the whole leg and lower abdominal wall.

Inspection

Note the following:

- *Varicose veins*: Are these primary or recurrent? If the patient has had previous venous surgery, where are the scars? Has the patient had their long saphenous vein stripped? (Ask the patient, they may know.) Are the veins primarily long or short saphenous, or both? Are these true varicose veins or secondary veins acting as collaterals bypassing an obstructed deep venous system? Dilated veins running across the lower abdomen between the groin(s) and the umbilicus are likely to be collaterals bypassing an occluded iliac system.
- *Scars*: Note the presence and position of scars; not just those related to venous surgery. Has the patient had a hip and/or knee replacement, or an arterial bypass procedure?
- *Oedema*: There are several causes of generalized oedema that may co-exist in a patient with CVI, e.g. right heart failure, renal disease and hypoproteinaemia. Is the oedema unilateral or bilateral? Does it pit? A degree of lymphoedema is quite common in CVI and, except in its earliest stages, will not pit.
- *Skin changes of CVI*: Record the presence of telangectasia, ankle flare (also called a malleolar flare or corona phlebectatica), lipodermatosclerosis (LDS), venous dermatitis and ulceration, healed or active.
- *Additional features*: Are there signs of rheumatoid arthritis (Figure 35.11), vasculitis (Figure 35.12) or neuro-ischaemia associated with diabetes (Figure 35.13)?

Description of ulcer

In Western countries approximately 80% of all leg ulcers are primarily venous in aetiology. However, it is important to realize that, in most cases, especially where ulcers are refractory to standard therapy, there

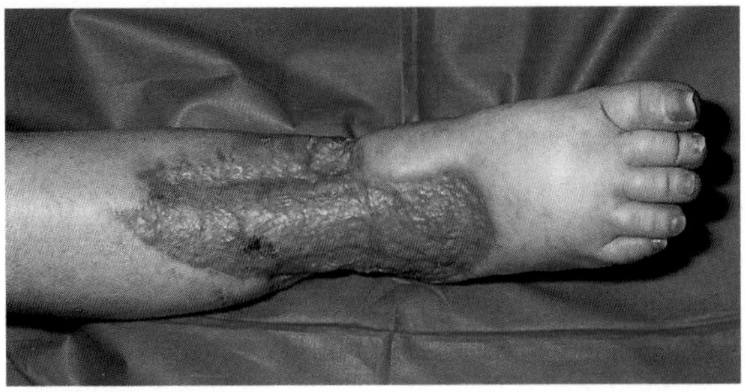

Figure 35.11 'Rheumatoid' ulcer. This patient with rheumatoid arthritis presented with a large necrotic ulcer thought initially to be venous in aetiology. However, a venous duplex was normal. The patient was treated successfully with surgical debridement and skin grafting.

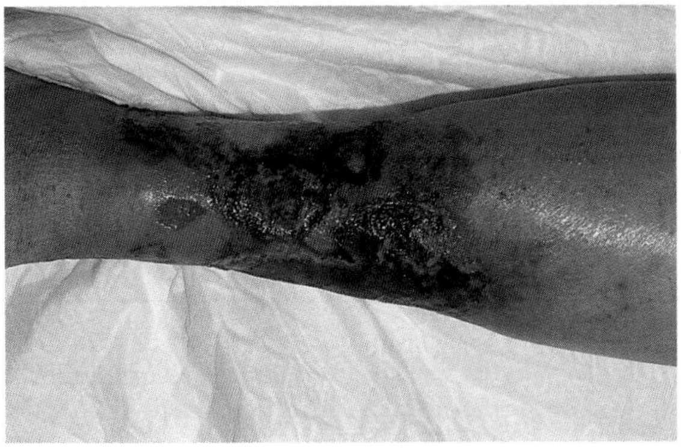

Figure 35.12 Pyoderma gangrenosa.

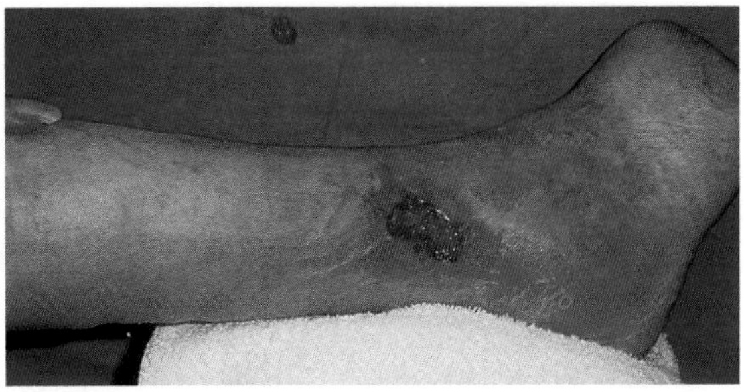

Figure 35.13 Venous ulcer in a diabetic patient with neuro-ischaemia.

are one or more comorbid pathologies contributing to the ulcer and/or limiting its ability to heal. An accurate description of the ulcer is important for both diagnosis (Table 35.5) and assessment of healing. The taking of a clinical photograph with a simple Polaroid camera can be invaluable.

Position

Most venous ulcers are on the medial side of the leg just above the malleolus (the gaiter area). However, 20% are laterally placed and may be associated with reflux in the SSV (Figure 35.14). Less than 5% are circumferential. Ulcers on the feet are almost never venous and are due to atherosclerotic arterial disease, with or without (diabetic) neuropathy, in the great majority of cases. Ulcers above the gaiter area are unusual; consider trauma, vasculitis or malignancy (if in doubt biopsy).

Table 35.5 Distinguishing features of arterial and venous ulcers

Clinical features	*Arterial ulcer*	*Venous ulcer*
Gender	Men > women	Women > men
Age	Usually presents > 60 years	Typically develops 40–60 years but patient may not present for medical attention until much older, multiple recurrences are the norm
Risk factors	Smoking, diabetes, hyperlipidaemia and hypertension	Previous DVT, thrombophilia, varicose veins
Past medical history	Most have a clear history peripheral, coronary and cerebrovascular disease	More than 20% have clear history of DVT, many more have a history suggestive of occult DVT, i.e. leg swelling after childbirth, hip/knee replacement or long bone fracture
Symptoms	Severe pain is present unless there is (diabetic) neuropathy, pain may be relieved by dependency	About a third have pain but it is not usually severe and may be relieved on elevation
Site	Normal and abnormal (diabetics) pressure areas (malleoli, heel, metatarsal heads, 5th metatarsal base)	Medial (70%), lateral (20%) or both malleoli and gaiter area
Edge	Regular, 'punched-out', indolent	Irregular, with neo-epithelium (whiter than mature skin)
Base	Deep, green (sloughy) or black (necrotic) with no granulation tissue, may comprise major tendon, bone and joint	Pink and granulating but may be covered in yellow-green slough
Surrounding skin	Features of severe limb ischaemia	LDS, varicose eczema, atrophe blanche
Veins	Empty, 'guttering' on elevation	Full, usually varicose
Swelling	Usually absent	Often present

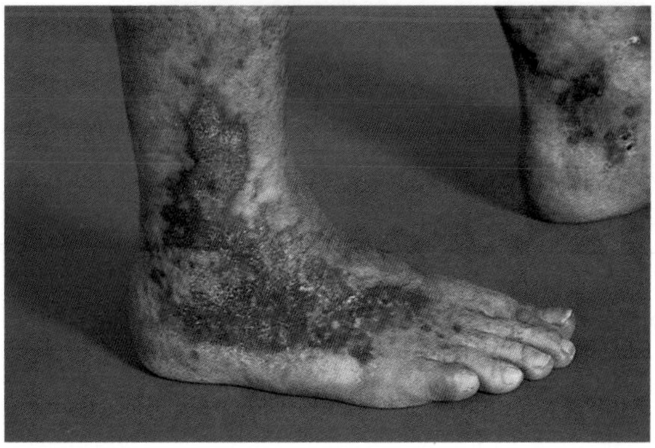

Figure 35.14 Laterally placed lipodermatosclerosis and healed ulceration associated with short saphenous vein reflux.

The base
Venous ulceration is a failure of epithelialization. Thus, although many venous ulcers are sloughy, underneath there is usually a base of pink granulation tissue. A necrotic base suggests an alternative diagnosis or co-existing pathology, e.g. arterial disease.

Depth
Venous ulcers are shallow. Deep and punched out ulcers suggest arterial disease; exposure of tendon and/or bone is a grave prognostic sign.

Margin
Venous ulcers are have an irregular margin. The edge is often associated with a strip of neo-epithelialization that appears white or pale lilac.

Surrounding tissue
The skin around a venous ulcer is invariably affected by the other skin changes of CVI. Acute LDS can be difficult to distinguish from acute cellulitis although the later is unusual in venous ulcers unless there is associated arterial disease. Unlike LDS, cellulitis is associated with marked pain and tenderness, constitutional symptoms, pyrexia, leucocytosis and sometimes lymphadenitis or lymphadenopathy.

Size
The total area of ulceration should be measured rather than simply the greatest dimension of the largest or 'index' ulcer. This is best accomplished by tracing the ulcer outline onto a transparent sheet and 'counting squares' using graph paper.

Adhering to this pattern of description will aid not only in establishing the ulcer aetiology, but also in assessment of healing progress, especially when a number of carers are involved over a long period.

Assessment of the arterial circulation
All patients must have their pulse status recorded and, if pedal pulses are not easily palpable, the ankle-brachial pressure index (ABPI) must be measured. An ABPI of <0.8 at rest indicates haemodynamically significant lower limb arterial disease and mandates referral to a vascular surgeon. Diabetic patients may have incompressible, calcified vessels leading to abnormally high pressure readings.

Investigations

Overview
Virtually every patient referred to a vascular surgeon with CVI undergoes some form of further investigation. The most obvious conclusion to be drawn from this practice is that most surgeons believe history and examination alone to be inadequate, even misleading in the assessment of CVI. By arranging one or more tests the surgeon hopes to be able to answer the following questions:

- Are the symptoms of which the patient complains, and the signs that have elicited on clinical examination, due to venous disease?
- Are there other pathological processes contributing to the clinical presentation?
- What are the anatomical and functional venous abnormalities responsible for this patient's symptoms and signs?
- Will this patient benefit from surgical intervention and, if so, what form should the surgery take?

Although these are important questions, and in most cases can only be answered by further investigation(s), it is important not to order investigations as a thoughtless 'knee-jerk' response. The investigation(s) must be chosen with care to maximize the chances of getting a reliable answer, with minimum discomfort and inconvenience to the patient, and with minimum expenditure; while, at the same time, being sensitive to the availability of equipment and/or expertise in the unit. It perhaps goes without saying that the yield of useful information is likely to be much greater if one takes the trouble to explain the clinical situation and questions posed to the doctor or technologist who is going to perform the test.

Handheld Doppler studies

Handheld Doppler (HHD), also known as continuous wave (CWD), is increasingly replacing the use of tourniquet (Trendelenberg, Perthes) tests in the clinic. It is quick, easy to learn, non-invasive and inexpensive. One technique for using the HHD is now described.

Superficial veins
Long saphenous system
The examination begins with the patient standing holding on to a frame to prevent inadvertent calf muscle contraction. The probe is placed at an angle of 45° over the SFJ which is found by insonating the femoral artery and moving medially. Squeezing the calf will result in a prograde signal. In the presence of SFJ incompetence, release of calf compression, or a Valsalva manoeuvre, will result in a retrograde signal (greater than 0.5 s) that is abolished by LSV compression (using

either a finger or a tourniquet). Persistence of reflux, despite compression of the LSV below the probe, suggests deep venous reflux in the femoro-popliteal segment. By moving the probe down along the course of the LSV, while compressing the LSV above the probe, one can locate incompetent thigh perforator(s). Tapping the varix elicits a signal over the SFJ and indicates an anatomical connection.

Short saphenous system

Venous reflux in the popliteal fossa may be detected by finding the arterial signal, moving laterally, and using the calf-squeeze-release manoeuvre. It is not possible to reliably differentiate SPJ from popliteal and/or gastrocnemius vein incompetence because it is difficult to reliably occlude the SSV with a finger or a tourniquet, and because the anatomy of the popliteal fossa is complex and variable. Nor is HHD a reliable means of determining the level of the SPJ. Nevertheless, HHD examination does provide a useful screening test. If no reflux is found in the popliteal fossa, this is fairly strong evidence that the SSV, popliteal and gastrocnemius veins are competent; by contrast, detection of reflux should prompt consideration of duplex scanning and/or varicography.

Deep veins

Opinions vary as to whether HHD can provide reliable information about the deep veins. With the patient supine, and in the presence of a normal unobstructed deep system, the Doppler will usually detect spontaneous cranial flow in the popliteal and femoral veins. This flow is phasic (varies with respiration), and can be halted by a cough or Valsalva manoeuvre, and augmented by a calf squeeze or forced inspiration against a closed glottis. However, these are all qualitative observations and, while they may exclude gross deep venous obstruction, patients thought to have deep venous pathology should undergo further investigation.

Duplex ultrasonography

Duplex ultrasound allows Doppler information regarding the velocity of arterial and venous blood to be superimposed upon a grey-scale (B-mode) image in real time. Colour duplex, also known as triplex, ultrasound entails the representation of different velocities, moving towards or away from the transducer, by means of different colours (blue and red scales).

It is probably no exaggeration to say that the advent of duplex ultrasound has revolutionized our understanding of the pathophysiology of venous disease. Because of its widespread availability, ability to provide anatomical as well as physiological information, and obvious advantages over invasive imaging methods requiring ionizing radiation, duplex has virtually replaced all other tests of venous function for the purposes of day-to-day clinical practice in most units. While the images and information provided by duplex are indeed impressive, we must not let its convenience and utility obscure its short-comings. Thus duplex:

- measures blood velocity, not flow or volume
- measures valve closure time, which is not closely related to volume of blood refluxing through that valve.

This may explain the inconsistent relationships observed between patterns and severity of reflux as demonstrated by duplex, the results of plethysmographic and pressure tests (see below) and the symptoms and signs of venous disease. The latter are related to changes in venous volumes and pressures, not velocities. There is an increasingly held view, shared by the authors, that for most patients with CVI, duplex should be supplemented by a functional test

- cannot reliably distinguish deep venous incompetence due to primary valvular incompetence from that which arises secondary to post-phlebitic damage. these two entities may have very different natural histories, prognoses and responses to treatment and, as such, this 'blind spot' may be a serious deficiency of duplex
- cannot reliably determine the presence or functional severity of venous outflow obstruction
- may be unreliable in the assessment of the supra-inguinal venous system
- is time-consuming and highly operator dependent
- does not provide a 'road-map' for the surgeon
- may be over-sensitive to clinically insignificant degrees of reflux.

Thus, there has been considerable debate over what constitutes a normal duplex scan based upon different thresholds for valve closure. Bearing in mind the comments made above, it is important to note that more than 20% of normal individuals, with no symptoms of signs of venous disease whatsoever, will have an 'abnormal' duplex scan; that is, reflux >0.5 s will be detected somewhere within their deep and/or superficial systems. Whether such individuals will ultimately develop clinically apparent venous disease is unknown; that question can only be answered by longitudinal epidemiological studies.

Notwithstanding, duplex should remain the first-line investigation for virtually all patients with CVI and will provide the following information with a high degree of reliability:

- whether there is significant reflux (usually taken as >0.5 s) at the SFJ, SPJ and in the main stem and tributaries of the LSV and SSV.
- the position of the SPJ. The SPJ most commonly lies 2 cm above the popliteal skin crease but does so in less than half of all patients. It is, therefore, mandatory to mark the junction pre-operatively
- whether the deep vein are patent and competent. A number of studies have suggested that the presence of popliteal vein reflux is an adverse prognostic feature in patients with CVU in terms of their response to both surgical and medical (compression bandaging) therapy (Figure 35.15)
- the site of incompetent medial calf perforators permitting outward or bidirectional flow.

The advent of subfascial endoscopic perforator surgery (SEPS) has re-opened the controversy surrounding

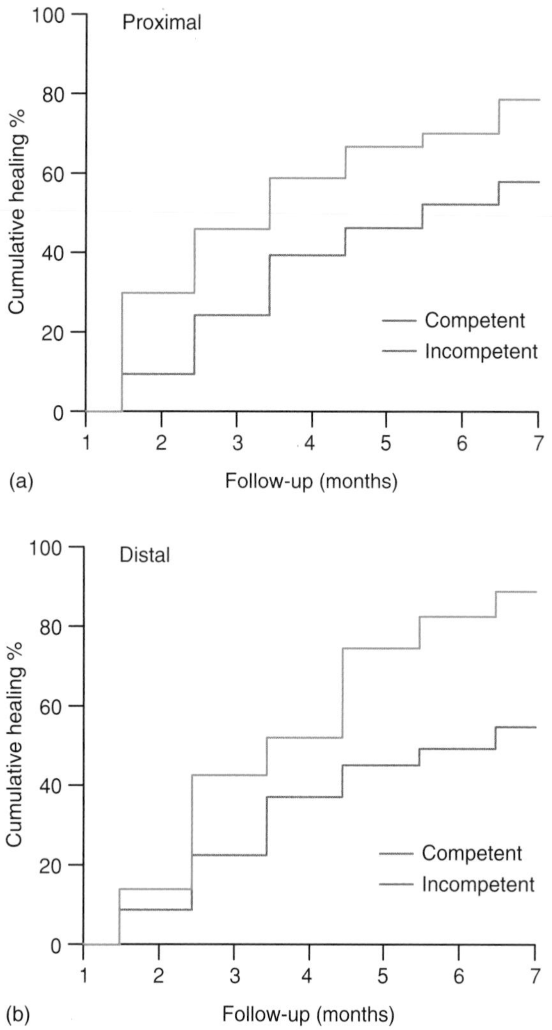

Figure 35.15 Effect of popliteal vein reflux on the healing of venous ulceration treated with multi-layer graduated compression bandaging: (a) proximal and (b) distal show the relationship between venous incompetence and ulcer healing of the popliteal vein.

the benefits of interrupting incompetent medial calf perforating veins (see below). However, if SEPS is to be performed, then duplex is a reliable way of marking the position of the perforators to be divided so as to allow optimal placement of the operating scope and minimize the extent of subfascial dissection required.

Numerous studies have used duplex to define the pattern of reflux in patients with different severities of venous disease. In general, skin changes are associated with mixed superficial and deep disease, although in most series a proportion (on average about 30%) of patients appear to have reflux limited to the superficial system. The more distal the reflux the greater the haemodynamic effect appears to be. Thus popliteal, crural (particularly posterior tibial), below-knee LSV and SSV reflux are more closely associated with CVI than above-knee LSV or ilio-femoral reflux. However, it is worth noting that less than 50% of patients with apparently maximal superficial and deep reflux have skin changes. This may be because of:

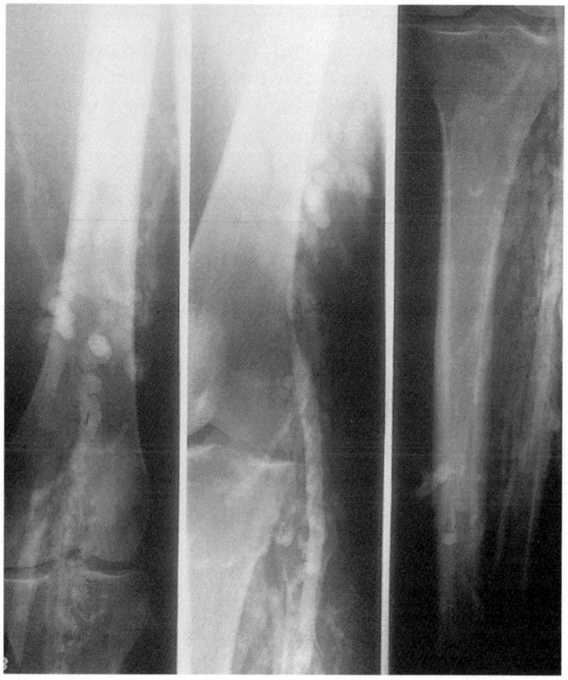

Figure 35.16 Ascending venogram showing post-phlebitic changes.

- the short-comings of duplex discussed above
- chronicity i.e. given time all the patients would eventually develop skin changes
- the differential susceptibility of individuals to venous hypertension
- other, as yet unidentified, factors important in the pathogenesis of skin disease.

Phlebography

Ascending phlebography

Ascending phlebography is primarily performed to obtain information about the anatomy of the deep venous system (Figure 35.16); specifically, to determine the:

- presence of residual thrombus
- extent of recanalization
- distribution of collaterals.

Contrast medium is injected into a vein on the dorsum of the foot and is directed into the deep veins by the placement of a 2.5 cm tourniquet (80 mmHg) just above the ankle. To prevent the contrast from dissipating too quickly the examination can be performed with the patient 60° head-up and/or by using another tourniquet around the thigh. The iliac system and the vena cava may not be visualized, even if the patient is positioned head down, in which case a separate injection can be made in the common femoral vein (CFV) (cavography).

Although the presence of venous outflow obstruction can be inferred from the images, as the examination does not provide any physiological information, the functional severity of the obstruction cannot be quantified. For this reason, the technique has been largely replaced by a combination of duplex and plethysmography in this regard.

The technique can also be modified, so-called 'functional' ascending phlebography, to enable the presence and site of incompetent calf perforating veins to be established. While contrast is being injected, and with the patient in a 60° head-up tilt, the subject is asked to plantar flex the ankle. In certain circumstances, contrast is seen to leave the deep venous compartment of the calf and enter superficial varices through 'incompetent' medial calf perforators whose positions can be noted in relation to bony landmarks and/or radio-opaque markers. It is now known that this manoeuvre does not reproduce the physiological closing mechanisms of the perforating veins. There are, therefore, a significant number of false positives and negatives when the result of functional phlebography are compared with duplex. Duplex provides better functional information and also allows the position of the perforators to be marked on the skin immediately prior to surgery, if required.

Descending phlebography

Descending phlebography involves injecting contrast medium into the CFV with the subject positioned 60° head-up. The competence of the long saphenous and the deep system is determined by the distal extent of the contrast both spontaneously in response to gravity and following a Valsalva manoeuvre. Five grades of reflux have been defined: grade 0 being no reflux and grade 4 being reflux to the ankle. However, if there is a competent segment above a refluxing segment, the latter will not be visualized. The correlation between the images obtained from descending phlebography, symptoms and signs and the results of functional tests is poor. Once again, for the great majority of patients, duplex a more useful alternative. Descending phlebography should be reserved for those patients who are being considered for deep venous reconstruction.

Varicography

This technique involves injecting contrast medium directly into varices. It is particularly useful in patients with recurrent varicose veins for delineating the anatomy of previously operated SFJ and SPJ.

Computed tomography and magnetic resonance venography

Both techniques are commonly used in the imaging of the large central veins. However, they are not yet widely employed in peripheral venous disease because the spatial and temporal resolution are sufficient to compete with duplex and phlebography and because, at present, patients cannot be tilted into the vertical position required for optimal assessment.

Ambulatory venous pressure (AVP) measurement

The superficial venous pressure at the ankle can be directly measured by cannulating a vein on the dorsum of the foot and connecting it to a pressure transducer and recorder (Figure 35.7). The patient:

- stands motionless, holding on to a frame to prevent inadvertent calf muscle contraction, until the venous pressure reaches a steady state. This is usually about 90 mmHg depending upon the height of the subject
- performs 10 tip-toe movements, one per second to a metronome, to simulate walking. In health this is associated with a fall in pressure to around 15–30 mmHg – the AVP
- once again stands still. The venous pressure gradually returns to baseline. The time taken to regain 90% of the baseline level is called the 90% refilling time (RT 90); this is usually 18–40 s.

By repeating the procedure with tourniquets, the superficial and deep systems may be distinguished, although some workers have found this unreliable. There is a close relationship between AVP and the prevalence of ulceration: < 30 mmHg – none; 41–50 mmHg – 22%; 61–70 mmHg – 57%; and > 80 mmHg – 73%. Having said that there is considerable overlap in the AVP of patients with simple varicose veins, skin changes and ulceration. As suggested above, this may simply be a manifestation of chronicity; that is, those patients with simple varicose veins and a high AVP will eventually develop CVI and possibly ulceration. Alternatively, it may be that for unknown reasons, the dermal circulation of different individuals varies considerably in its susceptibility to venous hypertension. AVP measurement is invasive and not therefore suitable for routine clinical use. However, it appears to remain the reference standard for research purposes.

Arm and foot vein pressures

In patients with venous outflow obstruction the AVP may actually be higher following tip-toe exercises than at baseline. The ratio between the arm and foot vein pressures can also be used to assess the severity of this obstruction. The method involves simultaneous recording of the venous pressure in a dorsal foot vein and the hand while the patient lies supine at rest and following reactive hyperaemia in the leg. Normally, the arm/foot differential at rest is < 5 mmHg, and a rise of < 6 mmHg is observed following hyperaemia. In general, the more proximal the obstruction, the greater the adverse haemodynamic effect. Such patients may have an arm/foot differential of 15–20 mmHg even at rest. This information is important if venous bypass is being considered. Unless a pressure gradient can be demonstrated across the obstructed segment, it is doubtful whether the bypass will relieve the patient's symptoms, or remain patent.

Photoplethysmography (PPG)

The amount of blood present in the dermal circulation affects how much light falling upon the skin is absorbed and how much is reflected (backscatter). The PPG comprises a light source and a light sensitive receptor that is attached with double-sided adhesive tape about a hand's breadth above the medial malleolus, either anterior or posterior to the LSV. The patient is asked to sit with the legs hanging over the edge of the couch, feet just touching the floor, taking care not to obstruct the popliteal artery or vein.

After calibrating the baseline to read near the top of the recording screen or paper, the patient briskly plantar flexes the foot five to ten times to empty the calf, and thus the dermal circulation of the gaiter area, of blood. Following this manoeuvre, the recording trace falls to a stable low level and the patient relaxes the calf musculature. The time taken for the trace to return to the upper baseline is measured, a normal refilling time (RT) being greater than 20 s. The simplicity of PPG has made it popular as a screening test for venous disease but has not found much use beyond that because:

- the refilling time has not been shown to correlate with AVP
- the technique cannot reliably distinguish reflux in the superficial and deep systems.

Thus, if the RT is normal (>20 s) then it effectively excludes venous disease, but if it is not then further venous investigations should be performed.

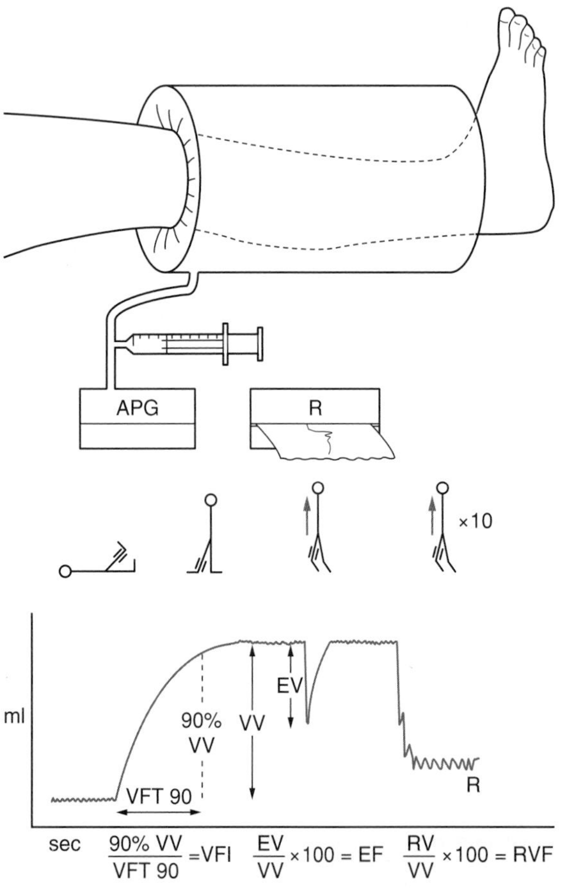

Figure 35.17 Air plethysmography. See text for explanation.

Air plethysmography (APG)

The APG can be used to determine changes in whole leg volume (ml) in response to exercise and posture and can be used to quantify venous reflux, calf pump function and venous outflow obstruction. The APG comprises a 40 cm tubular polyvinyl air chamber that is fitted around the leg. The technique proceeds as follows (Figure 35.17), although not every variable will be measured in every patient:

- The patient lies supine with the leg elevated, motionless, at 45° on a heel rest. With the veins of the leg empty, a stable baseline recording is obtained.
- The chamber is inflated to a pressure of 6 mmHg. This ensures good contact with the leg is ensured while minimizing any effect the chamber itself might have on leg volume.
- The device is calibrated by withdrawing 100 ml of air and noting the pressure drop.
- The patient stands with their weight on the opposite leg, holding on to a frame, and keeping the leg under examination as still as possible. Venous filling under the influence of gravity leads to an increase in venous volume (normal 100–150 ml, CVI up to 350 ml) and so the chamber pressurizes. This is the venous volume (VV) and the time taken to reach 90% of the VV (VV 90) is termed the venous filling time 90 (VFT 90). The venous filling index (VFI) is defined as VV 90/VFT 90. A VFI of <2 ml/s is normal. By using one or more tourniquets, reflux in the deep and superficial system can be distinguished. However, a VFI > 7 ml/s appears to be associated with a high incidence of CVI and CVU, regardless of which systems are involved.
- The patient takes one tip-toe and the ejected volume (EV) is noted. The ejection fraction (EF) is defined as EV/VV × 100.
- The patient is asked to perform 10 tip-toes and the residual venous volume (RV) is noted. The residual volume fraction (RVF) is RV/VV × 100. The RVF is perhaps the single most useful non-invasive index of calf pump function and can be abnormal (>40%) due to: (i) reflux (VFI > 2 ml/s), (ii) weak calf muscle (EF < 60%) or both. There appears to be a close relationship between AVP, RVF and the clinical status of the leg; if the RVF is >80% then the prevalence of CVU is almost 90%.
- The patient is returned to the supine position with the leg elevated to 10° so that a baseline level is regained.
- A thigh tourniquet (10–12 cm width) is placed as proximally as possible and inflated to 80 mmHg. Leg volume increases to a new plateau. The cuff is suddenly released and the venous outflow curve is recorded. The outflow fraction at 1 s (OF1) is defined as the percentage of the total venous volume expelled in 1 s. In the normal limb OF1 is >38%; 30–38% denotes mild and <30% denotes severe outflow obstruction. The use of occluding tourniquets can be used to determine the proportion of the venous outflow that is conducted by the superficial veins. The slope of the initial part of the outflow curve is termed the maximum venous outflow (MVO) and should be >45 ml/100 ml/s.
- If dorsal foot vein pressure is measured directly at the same time, the venous outflow resistance (VOR) can be measured where VOR = pressure/flow (mmHg/ml/min). VOR changes as the leg empties, being low at first when pressure is high and the veins are distended, and then falling.

Haematological and biochemical testing

Ideally, all patients with CVI should undergo baseline biochemical and haematological assessment to exclude anaemia and hepatic and renal impairment. A fasting blood glucose should be performed to exclude diabetes. Patients with an arterial component should also have a fasting lipid screen. Other blood tests, such as rheumatoid factor, auto-antibody and thrombophilia screening are performed as clinically indicated.

Bacteriological examination

Most venous ulcers are colonized with bacteria rather than infected. However, it is worth taking a swab for culture if the ulcer has an arterial component, the patient is diabetic, or the ulcer site appears 'infected' (cellulitis or systemic upset) or is slow to heal. Furthermore, a swab should always be taken prior to skin grafting, arterial bypass or venous surgery (especially if a prosthetic bypass graft is being considered).

Biopsy

Ulcers which fail to heal with conventional therapy, which have a tendency to bleed, or which have unusual features should undergo biopsy. This can easily be performed under local anaesthetic. The tissue removed should include both the margin and the base of the ulcer.

Which test, and when?

There is no single test that can provide all of the information required for a full investigation of every patient with CVI. Ideally tests performed should be rapid, inexpensive and of minimal inconvenience to the patient.

The basic questions that need to be answered are:

- Are the symptoms due to venous disease?
- What is the anatomical extent and severity of reflux and/or obstruction?
- Are there any other contributory factors?
- What treatments are being considered and how much anatomical detail is required?
- How should the results be interpreted?

Medical management

Overview

The optimal management of CVI rests upon the ability of a highly motivated, multi-disciplinary team of doctors, nurses and other healthcare professionals to deliver a complex, multi-modality package of care that is specifically tailored to the individual patient and treats that patient in a holistic manner. Failure on the part of individual doctors, including vascular surgeons, to understand this paradigm, and to deliver it to the patient, inevitably leads to a poor outcome, a disaffected patient and a demoralized clinical team. The patient must be viewed on a number of different levels.

Social circumstances. Are the patient's living circumstances and/or lifestyle leading to progression of disease and/or failure of treatment? Would the provision of central heating, social support and/or mobility aids, for example, improve the prognosis?

Medical comorbidity. Most patients with CVI are elderly and have comorbidity which is likely to impact negatively on their disease and its response to treatment; for example, cardiac failure, oedema, nutritional status (malnutrition or obesity). As many of these factors as possible need to be corrected, or at least improved, in order to achieve optimal healing rates.

Other pathologies. Many patients with CVU, particularly those with ulcers that are refractory to standard treatments, have other pathology in the leg; for example, arterial, locomotor and/or neurological disease. This needs to be recognized and if possible treated.

The venous disorder. Only once the above factors have been considered should the clinician begin to focus on the anatomical and physiological venous abnormalities and their treatment.

Patient satisfaction, compliance and outcome. Unless a patient:

- understands why a particular treatment is being recommended
- accepts that the benefits of the treatment outweigh the associated risks and discomforts
- sees some improvement in their symptoms and signs having embarked upon the treatment

they will cease to be compliant and the treatment plan will fail. The poor compliance observed with compression bandaging and/or hosiery, despite its proven efficacy, is an obvious example. A knowledgeable, satisfied patient is a compliant patient and is likely to do well. Although sometimes difficult, it is vital to keep the patient 'on board'.

Dressings and topical agents

Aims of a dressing

The age-old ritual of dressing wounds continues today in order to:

- control (absorb) odour, exudate and/or bleeding
- exclude pathogenic bacteria and minimize colonization
- relieve pain
- enhance the wound environment to speed up healing (see below)
- protect the wound from further environmental (or iatrogenic) injury
- maintain the wound at body temperature
- reduce excessive scarring and/or recurrence
- hide the wound from sight.

However, in the context of venous ulceration, no particular dressing or topical agent has been shown unequivocally to significantly hasten healing. But, dressings do have different physical properties, and an understanding of these properties in relation to ulcer healing enables the carer to determine their usefulness in different patients and at different times in the healing process. Although nurses apply most dressings and bandages, they will often look to medical staff to direct their efforts, particularly when things are not going well. It is important therefore that the surgeon has a basic grasp of the underlying science (and art) of wound care.

Wound healing

Dermal wound healing, including that of a CVU, comprises four stages:

- *Inflammatory phase*: following the arrest of any bleeding by vasoconstriction and the haemostasis, an inflammatory phase, characterized by vasodilatation, increased capillary permeability and the ingress of polymorphonuclear leucocytes, develops over the first 24 hours. Within days, mononuclear cells, specifically macrophages, come to dominate the infiltrate, having been attracted into the wound by cytokines released from polymorphs and endothelial cells. These phagocytes digest bacteria and devitalized tissue, and release growth factors that attract and stimulate fibroblasts, smooth muscle and endothelial cells.
- *Synthetic or proliferative phase*: These cells support angiogenesis and the development of granulation tissue.
- *Epithelialization*: In response to poorly understood signals, presumably from the bed of granulation tissue, epithelial cells migrate across the wound to restore dermal continuity.
- *Maturation*: 'Remodelling' of collagen and other structural proteins leads to wound maturation and strengthening over many months.

The first two stages appear intact in CVU in that most ulcers have beds of well developed granulation tissue; indeed over-granulation is not an uncommon problem. The failure of venous ulcers to heal, and their propensity to recur, is primarily a failure of stages three and four respectively. Much current research is devoted to defining the characteristics of the failing wound. It is hypothesized that important growth factors necessary for epithelialization may be broken down by wound proteases or bound, inactive, to a disordered ECM. Alternatively epithelial cells in patients with CVI may be refractory to the normal signalling processes.

Factors influencing wound healing

Wound healing depends on:

- *Moisture*: Keeping a wound moist rather than allowing a dry eschar to form enhances the first three phases of wound healing.
- *Oxygenation*: Perhaps surprisingly, the development of a low oxygen tension in a wound appears to be an important stimulus for the early stages of wound healing
- *Microflora*: With the exception of certain pathogenic micro-organisms such as pseudomonas and β-haemolytic streptococci, most studies suggest that the colonization of chronic wounds with a mixed growth of commensal bacteria does not impair healing. However, by excluding pathogenic bacteria and maintaining a moist acidic wound environment dressings can inhibit the growth of bacteria.
- *Devitalized tissue*: The presence of 'slough' comprising bacteria and particularly devitalized tissue does appear to inhibit wound healing.
- *Temperature*: Little is known about the effects of temperature on wound healing but extremes are likely to be detrimental by altering blood supply and cellular metabolism.
- *Systemic factors*: Ischaemia, poor nutritional status, anaemia, any form of immunodeficiency, uncontrolled venous hypertension and/or oedema will obviously impair wound healing.

Antiseptics

Even in very low concentrations these agents (e.g. hypochlorite, povidone iodine and hydrogen peroxide) are toxic to tissues as well as bacteria, which are believed anyway to be largely harmless. Experimental data have shown them to inhibit all the phases of wound healing. As there is no evidence of clinical benefit, they should be avoided. CVU should be washed in warmed tap water instead.

Enzymatic debridement

These agents (e.g. streptokinase-streptodornase) undoubtedly digest the constituents of 'slough'. However, they are relatively ineffective against deep necrosis or hard eschar, and there is little or no evidence that they speed up healing. They may, in fact, have an adverse effect on the wound environment. For these reasons, and because of their expense, they are best avoided until further evidence is forthcoming.

Hydrocolloid dressings

These dressings are extremely popular for the treatment of CVU. There are many different types, brands and formulations available but they share the following properties:

- they are generally impermeable to gases, water vapour and bacteria
- they produce a moist, acidic, low oxygen tension wound environment (see above) that has been shown experimentally to enhance the inflammatory and proliferative phases of wound healing
- they absorb exudate and do not require frequent changing. This will reduce costs and possibly the risks of cross-infection
- the patient can bathe with the dressing *in situ*
- several trials have suggested that hydrocolloid dressings may provide superior pain relief
- they are very easy to use and are popular with patients which aids compliance.

However, in randomized controlled trials where both treatment arms a have received equal and adequate compression, hydrocolloid dressings have not be shown to improve overall healing compared with non-adherent dressings, tulle, paste bandage, Unna boot or alginates. Nor is there any evidence that one hydrocolloid dressing is superior to another.

Bead dressings

The two preparations available in the UK (cadexomer iodine and dextranomer) are both hydrophilic, polysaccharide materials that absorb large amounts of fluid and slough. The former also releases iodine into the wound. While these agents may speed up desloughing they have not been shown to enhance healing.

Paste bandages

These comprise a plain weave cotton fabric impregnated with zinc oxide paste either alone or with calamine, calamine and clioquinol, coal tar or icthamol. These additives are designed to soothe venous eczema. How-

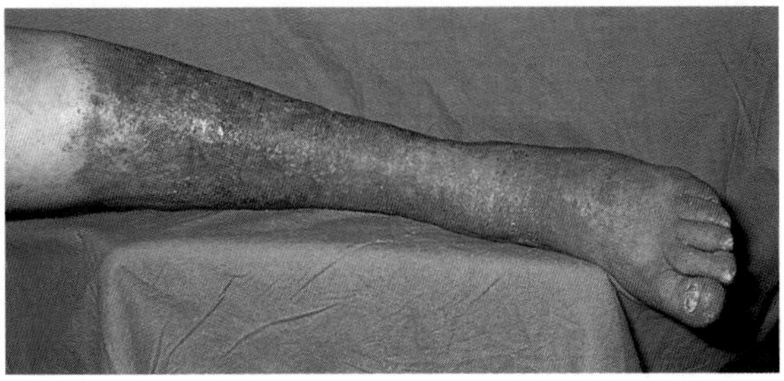

Figure 35.18 Contact dermatitis following treatment with a paste bandage.

ever, these substances and preservatives contained within paste bandages are a common cause of contact allergy (Figure 35.18). Patch testing with a small square of material is strongly recommended. Paste bandages do not retain moisture and for this reason, as well as to apply compression, additional layers of bandaging are required. The Unna boot is a paste bandage that contains glycerin and thus hardens into semi-rigid dressing. In trials where equal amounts of compression are applied, no form of paste bandage has been shown to improve healing when compared to other forms of dressing. No particular form of paste dressing has been shown to be superior to any other. The principal benefit of paste bandages is probably that (because they are cohesive) they provide a form of inelastic compression.

Alginate dressings

These dressings are produced from seaweed and contain calcium and/or sodium alginates. On contact with the wound the dressing becomes a hydrophilic gel which absorbs exudate and creates a moist healing environment. However, once again, there are no data to suggest that alginate dressings are superior to any other type of dressing in terms of ulcer healing.

Biological dressings

Several types of biological dressing comprising cultured human epithelium and/or fibroblasts are under development and/or being trialled at the present time. It is suggested that such 'living' dressings act as a source of growth factors that are deficient within the wound, as well as a scaffold for the ingrowth of the patient's own cells. It has yet to be demonstrated that these dressing significantly increase ulcer healing when compared to other forms of treatment. Even if they do show a healing advantage, their use may not be cost-effective because of their expense. However, this is the subject of ongoing investigations.

Summary

There is ample evidence to show that there is no advantage in using expensive drug- or antibiotic-impregnated dressings over a simple, occlusive, non-adherent pad. However, in the case of the painful ulcer, hydrocolloid dressings may be beneficial. The simplest dressings are the best, e.g. paraffin emollients and gauze, alginates and zinc, which do not appear to be frequent sensitizers, thereby reducing venous dermatitis.

Dermatitis

Dermatitis (this term is preferable to eczema), characterized by weeping, scaling and intensely pruritic skin, is common in patients with CVI and is considered here because it is germane to the choice of topical treatment and dressings. Dermatitis may be:

- endogenous – due to patient factors (varicose or venous stasis dermatitis)
- exogenous – due to the application of external substances (contact dermatitis).

Varicose dermatitis

The mechanisms underlying the development of varicose dermatitis are not understood. However, it may represent an inflammatory and/or immunological response to substances not usually found in the skin, and which are present due to venous hypertension.

Contact dermatitis

Contact dermatitis is a common problem in patients being treated for chronic venous ulceration. Not only is it intensely uncomfortable for the patients, it is also frustrating for the carer who may have difficulty in identifying the specific allergen(s) and continuing treatment. Dermatitis is, not surprisingly, associated with non-healing and may be irritant (exudate, antiseptics and bandages) or allergic due to cell mediated, delayed hypersensitivity to a specific antigen. Sensitization can occur following a short exposure (10–14 days) to the allergen or may develop after many years of exposure. Patch testing should be considered if there is surrounding dermatitis, the ulcer is failing to heal or there is a past history of dermatitis. The specific allergens and protocol for patch testing are clearly defined and well within the capability of all dermatology units. The commonest allergens in leg ulcer patients are:

- *Lanolin (wool alcohols)*: This is still widely used as an emollient and moisturizer. Products containing lanolin should be avoided.
- *Topical antibiotics (e.g. neomycin, soframycin, framycetin)*: These are sometimes found impregnated into dressings. They are not effective and not only cause sensitization but also encourage the emergence of resistant bacteria and should not be used.
- *Perfumes (Balsalm of Peru, fragrance mix)*: These are commonly found in commercial moisturisers, even baby products, and should be avoided. White soft paraffin is preferable.
- *Preservatives and antiseptics*: These are found in some paste bandages, dressings and creams and include parabens, phenosept, quinoline mix, chlorxylenol (Dettol) and chlorhexidine.
- *Vehicle (cetylstearyl alcohol)*: This is present in many topical preparations and some paste bandages.
- *Rubber*: This is present in many elastic bandages and stockings and the mercapto/thiuram xix/carba mix used as an accelerator in its manufacture can sensitize the skin.
- *Adhesives (colophony/gum resin)*: These materials may be found in the adhesive backing of tapes and bandages.

Management

Virtually every material brought in contact with the skin of a patient with CVI has been reported to result in contact sensitivity. However, the use of bland paraffin cream, gauze or non-adherent dressings will greatly reduce the risks. In patients with marked exudate zinc oxide paste can be used to protect the surrounding skin. Acute dermatitis must be treated with removal of the offending allergen and topical steroid therapy (see below). Allergens identified by patch testing must be recorded conspicuously in the notes and the patient informed. Products containing these substances, whether they be prescribed or bought over the counter, must be avoided. This is not as easy as it sounds because the quality of labelling is generally poor. It is possible for a patient to become sensitive to a substance that was negative on previous testing so that repeat patch testing may be indicated. To summarize, the risks of dermatitis can be minimized by using:

- tap water or saline only to irrigate the wound
- zinc oxide paste to protect the skin from exudate
- 50/50 mixture of soft and liquid paraffin
- a layer of gauze or tubular cotton bandage beneath elastic and/or adhesive bandages
- rubber free compression hosiery after healing (if the patient has a rubber allergy)
- patch testing (liberally).

Section 35.4 • Pharmacotherapy

Veno-active drugs

Veno-active drugs are a heterogeneous group of naturally occurring and synthetic compounds that are believed to improve the symptoms and haemodynamic abnormalities, specifically oedema, associated with venous disease. The principal members of the group are:

- *Horse chestnut extract*: The active ingredient is believed to be aescin, a mixture of triterpenoid saponins.
- *Flavonoids*: This group comprises rutin and its derivatives, principally O-(β-hydroxylethyl)-rutosides. Diosmin is a synthetic flavonoid.
- *Calcium dobesilate*: Synthetic.
- *Tribenoside*: Synthetic.
- *Dihydroergotamine*: Ergot derivatives are rarely used because of their narrow therapeutic index and severe side-effects.

Several studies have shown these compounds to be localized in and around endothelial cells. Their precise mode(s) of action are unclear but may include:

- closure of inter-endothelial capillary pores, so reducing capillary filtration
- improving venous tone (particularly ergot derivatives)
- free radical scavenging and inhibition of lipid peroxidation
- inhibition of leucocyte activation and the release of inflammatory mediators such as interleukins and tumour necrosis factor
- inhibition of thromboxane production
- improvement in skin Tc-pO_2 and laser Doppler flux.

None of these compounds is currently licensed in the UK, although they are widely prescribed in continental Europe. Unfortunately, the literature in this field is dominated by small, poorly conceived, conducted and reported, commercially driven studies. More recently, however, a number of double-blind, randomized, controlled trials have shown a benefit both subjectively in terms of symptoms relief, and objectively in terms of plethysmographic assessment and oedema reduction. Some studies also suggest an adjuvant effect on ulcer healing when used with compression, and that flavonoids may retard the development of the post-phlebitic syndrome when commenced immediately following a first episode of DVT. At present, it is difficult to draw any definite conclusions about their efficacy in patients with CVI. However, this is an area of active research and the use of these compounds may become more accepted in the future.

Antibiotic therapy

Most venous ulcers are colonized with bacteria rather than infected. When there is no evidence of clinical infection, i.e. cellulitis, systemic antibiotic therapy is not indicated. Topical antibiotics should not be prescribed as they are frequent sensitizers. A swab should, however, be taken prior to skin grafting, arterial bypass or venous surgery (especially if a prosthetic bypass graft is being considered). Systemic antibiotic treatment is required for a heavy growth of *Pseudomonas* species or *Staphylococcus aureus* or β-haemolytic streptococcus prior to surgery or grafting.

Topical applications

No large, randomized, controlled, clinical trials have shown improvement in CVU healing using topical applications, including zinc, selenium, antibiotics and various growth factors, although growth factor therapy has been shown to be effective in both arterial and diabetic ulceration. Many trials are at present underway in this area.

Section 35.5 • Physical therapies

Elevation and bed rest

Elevation and bed rest will eventually heal virtually all CVU. However:

- in a modern health service, it is impractical to admit patients to hospital for long periods of bed rest
- confining elderly patients to bed in hospital is associated with a wide range of iatrogenic complications: colonization of the ulcer with resistant bacteria, thrombo-embolism, loss of mobility, disorders of bowel and bladder function, confusion and depression
- as soon as the patient leaves hospital, if no other measures are taken, the favourable haemodynamic environment is lost and early recurrence is inevitable.

Having said that it is essential that whenever the patient is not walking, he or she should rest with the ankles above the hips to lower venous pressure. Short periods of hospital admission for the optimization of the wound environment with intensive nursing care may be clinically beneficial and cost-effective in certain circumstances, especially prior to surgery.

Exercise therapy

Poor calf muscle pump function is often overlooked as an important factor in the pathogenesis of CVU. Improvement in muscle function through (supervised), regular exercise will improve the AVP even if venous reflux and/or obstruction remain unchanged. This is an area where further research and trials are urgently required.

Compression therapy

Overview

Compression therapy has been the mainstay of treatment for CVI for at least 2000 years. Today, there remains general agreement that compression retards the development and progression of CVI, and heals CVU. However, bandaging is still more of an art than a science. For example, in a systematic review conducted to Cochrane Collaboration standards, of the 132 studies relating to compression therapy for CVU, only eight (total 750 patients) fulfilled the inclusion criteria. Concerns relating to the excluded trials were small sample size, no power calculation, short duration, method of randomization not stated, no blinding, inappropriate end-points (i.e. reduction in ulcer size and not ulcer healing), no quality of life or health economic analysis, and the inclusion of ulcers of mixed aetiology. Furthermore, most of the trials were (single) hospital, as opposed to community based, raising questions about their wider validity and applicability. The most popular bandaging system in the UK, the Charing Cross four-layer system, which is described in detail below, was first adopted on the basis of a small number of uncontrolled observational studies. Its efficacy, and superiority over other forms of compression, has since been demonstrated in several larger studies.

While support stockings can be used to heal ulcers, the need for accurate fitting, the difficulty of applying stockings over dressings and the tendency for the stocking to become soiled with exudate, mean that most centres favour the use of bandaging until ulcer healing is achieved. Thereafter compression hosiery is used, hopefully, to maintain healing.

The skill that is required to correctly bandage a leg affected by CVI should not be underestimated. In the past, the standard of bandaging has frequently been poor and, predictably, so has the healing. More recently, great efforts have been made to educate nurses in the theory and practice of compression therapy. It is hoped that these initiatives will enhance the application and results of this proven method of treatment.

Mechanisms of action of compression therapy

Numerous mechanisms have been proposed to explain the benefits of compression therapy.

Macrovascular: the superficial and deep veins are compressed which may:

- decrease wall tension and thus further damage to the elastin and collagen structure of the wall
- increase the velocity of flow
- force blood from the superficial to the deep system and prevents the reflux of high pressure blood through medial calf perforating veins
- abolish the recirculation of refluxing blood down the superficial vein and into the deep system which may overload the calf muscle pump
- reduce reflux by apposing the vein wall and restoring valvular competency, and limiting the distensibility of the calf veins and sinuses
- reduce oedema and thus skin tension
- improve refilling times
- reduce AVP.

Microvascular: returns Starling's forces, haemostasis and leucocyte margination at the capillary towards normal by:

- preventing excessive fluid and protein filtration
- decreasing pressure in the post-capillary venules
- augmenting lymphatic clearance of excess filtrate
- augmenting the release of prostacyclin and plasminogen activator from the endothelium
- increasing the velocity of flow through the nutritional capillaries.

Terminology: types of bandage

Several terms are used to describe the properties of bandages:

- *Conformability*: The ability to follow the contours of the limb; this depends upon its density of weave/knit and its extensibility. Knitted bandages are generally more conformable.
- *Extensibility*: The change in length produced by a given extending force. This is described in terms of the percentage increase in length achieved at the point of 'lock out', i.e. when the bandage can extend no more.
- *Power or modulus*: The amount of extending force required to bring about a given percentage increase in length.
- *Elasticity*: The ability of an extended bandage to return to its original length when the extending force is removed.
- *Cohesion/adhesion*: Adhesive bandages stick to each other and to the skin. Cohesive bandages stick to each other but not the skin. They are less prone to slippage while at the same time do not damage the skin upon their removal.

On the basis of these and other material properties, bandages can be divided into the following types (Thomas):

- *Type 1, lightweight conforming stretch bandages*: These comprise lightweight elastomers with high elasticity but little power; they are mainly used to retain dressings.
- *Type 2, light support bandages*: These are sometimes called short or minimal stretch and include the familiar crepe/cotton/viscose bandages. They exhibit limited elasticity and tend to lock out on minimal extension (short-stop). In the ambulant patient with CVI they form an essentially inelastic covering to the leg which will tend to exert pressure during calf systole but not during diastole; or when the patient is supine. They do not, therefore, exert sustained pressure and, as they will not 'follow in' are unsuitable for control of oedema.
- *Type 3, compression bandages*: These are extensible (long-stop), elastic and powerful to a varying degree. They provide and maintain pressure of different strengths depending upon their class (see below).

Tubular bandages are quick and easy to apply but may produce a reverse pressure gradient. Shaped tubular support bandages are therefore to be preferred. However, as they exert only a low pressure (< 20 mmHg), they can only usually be used as part of a multi-layer system, often forming the outer layer holding the rest of the bandages in place.

Elastic or inelastic compression?

Much has been written about the theoretical and actual advantages and disadvantages of elastic versus non-elastic compression. All types of compression exert their maximal effect when the patient is ambulant. Elastic compression also exerts compression in the supine position and tends to exert more sustained pressure. Once applied elastic (long-stretch) bandages maintain a better pressure profile over the next 24 hours than short-stretch bandages, which, in turn, are better than inelastic materials.

For these reasons, it is often said that non-elastic is safer and is to be preferred in patients with arterial and/or sensory impairment, e.g. diabetics (see below). However, it is certainly possible to generate local areas of inappropriately high pressure over bony prominences with inelastic bandages, which tend to give a less even pressure than elastic bandages. In fact, during walking the pressure exerted by inelastic compression may be higher. Randomized controlled trials have shown greater healing rates with elastic bandaging. Elastic compression is popular in the UK and France, while the Germans prefer inelastic compression.

How much compression?

Measuring pressures under bandages is more difficult that one would imagine. Because the shape of leg is obviously not a simple cylinder or cone, and varies enormously between individuals, large differences in pressure can be exerted by the same stocking or bandage. Due to Laplace's law, the pressure will be highest over parts with a small radius of curvature; for example, the shin, malleoli and Achilles tendon. Pressure will be lowest over the flatter areas and may be non-existent in hollows such as that found behind the medial malleolus. This is an area frequently affected by CVI and a retromalleolar foam pad may be required to ensure adequate compression at that site.

Early work in otherwise healthy supine subjects with normal venous anatomy and function showed that modest compression (< 20 mmHg) could markedly enhance deep venous blood flow. These data proved the basis for the low-pressure thrombo-embolic deterrent (TED) stockings used in everyday surgical practice. However, for the ambulant patient with a disordered venous system much higher pressures are required to achieve the same effects. The British Standard for compression hosiery (BS 6612:1985) describes four classes:

- Class I: < 25 mmHg (at the ankle): Thrombo-embolic prophylaxis or early varicose veins
- Class II: 25–35 mmHg: Advanced varicose veins, oedema, early CVI
- Class III: 35–45 mmHg: Moderate to severe CVI, lymphoedema
- Class IV: > 45 mmHg: Severe CVI and lymphoedema.

These recommended pressures are based more on theoretical considerations than on the results of scientific observation. Furthermore, for the reasons outlined above, the pressures specified by the manufacturers for their products are seldom the actual pressures exerted on the patient. Lastly, many patients with these conditions can neither apply nor tolerate pressures above 30 mmHg and non-compliance is a major issue. Any compression is better than no compression and there is no point adopting an unrealistic approach. For most CVI patients class II compression represents a reasonable compromise between efficacy, compliance and patient comfort. Tall, heavily built or obese patients are often best treated with two stockings, i.e. a class I is worn over a class II. While ambulant during the day both stockings are worn simultaneously; in the evening, when the patient is sitting, the outer one can be removed. Patients should not wear their stockings in bed at night but should don them as soon as they rise.

Above or below knee compression?

Compression should commence at the metatarsal heads and in most cases terminate at the tibial tuberosity. There is no need to exert large pressures on the foot as it is already supported by footwear and bony prominences are at risk. Excessive pressure around the foot may even compromise rather than enhance venous return by inhibiting the foot pump mechanism (which is often preserved in CVI as long as the foot is structurally normal) and preventing ankle movement. There is no evidence that extending compression above the knee confers benefit in patients with CVI. Compliance also tends to be lower with above knee compression. It is important to note that excess bandage should be cut off, not wound around the leg as extra layers as this may cause a tourniquet effect. One of the most common bandaging errors, and one that causes non-compliance, is the production of a reversed gradient (tourniquet effect). This will cause discomfort, particularly upon walking, and may result in oedema of the foot and ankle.

Single or multiple layers?

The advantages of a multi-layer over a single layer bandaging system include:

- The shape of the leg ensures that, provided the bandages are applied with equivalent tension throughout their length, graduated compression (40 mmHg ankle, 15–20 mmHg upper calf) will be obtained.
- The use of several layers, each of which on its own would exert a relatively low pressure, means that the pressure on the leg tends to be distributed more evenly.
- If put on with uniform stretch, the pressure under a bandage is proportional to the number of layers. A figure of eight is said to provide approximately 1.5–2 times more pressure than a simple spiral with 50% overlap; so care must be exercised when using the former technique.

- Multi-layer bandaging, presumably because of the cohesion between its different layers, means that little pressure is lost following application, even over a few days. A figure of eight, as opposed to a simple spiral appears to offer more sustained pressure.
- This together with the absorbency of the orthopaedic wool means the bandaging only needs to be changed once or twice weekly.

Perhaps the single most important layer is the inner wool as it evens out the pressure, protects prominences from damage and absorbs moisture. Drawbacks of multi-layer, elastic bandaging include increased cost and the danger of exerting excessive pressures. Specially trained nurses are required to ensure that the multi-layer bandage is applied correctly.

In the future it may be possible to design single-layer bandages that incorporate most of the advantages seen with multi-layer systems.

Control of oedema

Many patients with CVI and CVU have severe oedema. Until it is controlled, ulcer healing will not be achieved. Although compression is effective at relieving oedema of venous and/or lymphatic aetiology, it is important to realize that compression alone will not abolish severe oedema; indeed attempts to do so while the patient remains ambulant may be dangerous. High elevation, often with bed rest and expert physiotherapy is usually required in the initial stages. Many older patients with venous oedema have a degree of heart failure that contributes to the condition. The rapid redistribution of fluid that occurs when a patient is confined to bed, and has the legs elevated and compressed may precipitate pulmonary oedema. In such patients, a limited course of diuretic therapy may be indicated or as prophylaxis. Some patients may also require temporary catheterization to avoid discomfort and/or incontinence, particularly at night. Apart from measuring calf circumference and keeping a careful eye on the overall fluid balance, weighing the patient is a good way of establishing the success of therapy. As oedema is controlled so the patient will have to be refitted for their stockings at fairly frequent intervals.

The 'four-layer' bandage

In the UK, it is generally believed that optimal compression and healing is obtained with a multi-layer graduated, elastic compression bandaging system (Figure 35.19). The original four-layer bandage described below emanated from Charing Cross. Since then, several groups have modified the original components although the underlying principles and properties of the system remain the same. The term is now used, almost generically, to describe multi-layer elastic compression bandaging comprising:

- a wound dressing
- orthopaedic wool: to protect the bony prominences and to absorb any exudate
- a crepe bandage: to compress and shape the wool, and to provide a firm base for the compression bandages
- a long stretch elasticated bandage (e.g. Elset™, Seton): applied at 50% stretch
- a self adhesive elasticated bandage (e.g. Coban™, 3M): to add to compression and fix the bandaging in place.

The Charing Cross four-layer bandage described above was found to exert 42 mmHg at the ankle and 17 mmHg just below the knee. The final layer can be replaced with a shaped tubular bandage (e.g. SSB™, Seton). This can be removed by the patient in the evening and replaced in the morning if he or she finds high compression throughout the 24 hours intolerable.

How often should compression be changed?

Correct application of a bandage which retains graduated pressure is a skill which requires training, supervision and practice. The frequency of bandage change depends on:

- the amount of exudate, 'strike-through', from the ulcer
- the type of bandaging being used: elastic multi-layer exerts its pressure for longer than single-layer, non-elastic bandaging
- the adequacy of the arterial circulation (see below).

When compression therapy is first initiated, it is important for the nurse to review the patient regularly to check for any discomfort, and confirm that the bandage is staying in place and that the bandage is neither too tight nor too loose.

With regard to compression hosiery, patients should be provided with two pairs to allow frequent washing, and these should both be replaced at least every 6 months. Washing has a variable effect on the properties of compression bandages and the manufacturer's instructions should be followed.

Paste bandages

Paste bandages are always used in conjunction with compression bandages so they should be viewed primarily as a dressing. However, they:

- do provide some inelastic compression. As they are completely inelastic, care must be taken not to apply them too tightly; they should be applied with frequent folds or by cutting the fabric into strips
- can improve the maintenance of compression
- convert overlying elastic bandages to inelastic bandages.

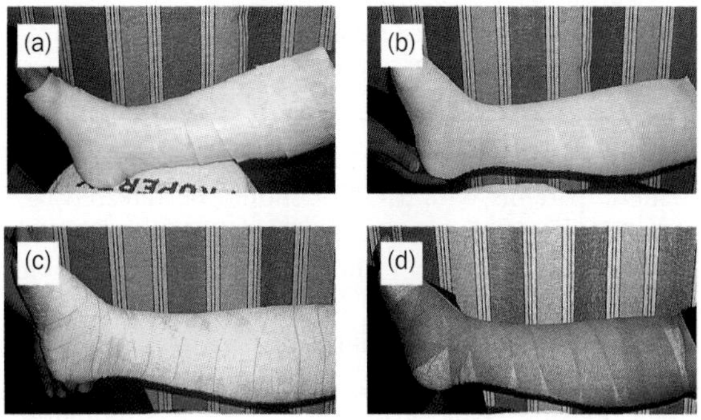

Figure 35.19 The 'four-layer' bandage. (a) Orthopaedic wool. (b) Crepe. (c) Elasticated bandage. (d) Cohesive bandage.

The main problem with paste bandages is the relatively high incidence of contact dermatitis (Figure 35.18). For this reason it is wise to test the patient with a patch of material prior to applying the whole bandage.

The Unna boot is a rigid paste bandage popular in the USA and mainland Europe. It gives inelastic compression and favourable healing rates, but pressures beneath it fall rapidly as oedema decreases, and it therefore requires more frequent bandaging changes, often every 24 hours. It is infrequently used in the UK.

Healing and recurrence rates

In the absence of compression, healing rates of less than 30% at 10–12 weeks are typically reported from community studies. By contrast, several groups using the four-layer bandage have reported healing rates of up to 74% healing over the same time period. Other authors reported healing rates of 30–60% at 3–6 months with various other forms of elastic compression. In Edinburgh, most of the trials were associated with a healing rate of around 50% at 3–6 months in the most favourable arm. So, while compression is better than no compression, even in the idealized circumstances found within clinical trials (highly selected, generally favourable and well motivated patients cared for by interested and experienced nurses) the healing rates are often disappointing. Non-compliance with compression hosiery following ulcer healing was about 30%.

Compression in patients with arterial disease

Approximately 25% of patients with CVI will have coexistent arterial disease as defined by an ABPI of <0.8. Although this prevalence is not significantly different from an age and sex matched population without CVI, it has an impact upon treatment and prognosis because:

- ischaemia may impair CVU healing
- it limits the use of compression therapy
- it is a marker for widespread atherosclerotic disease.

Arterial impairment is particularly significant in the diabetic patient because:

- the ABPI may be falsely raised due to medial calcification
- despite the presence of extensive crural artery disease, the popliteal pulse may be easily palpable and thus give a false impression of the adequacy of arterial inflow
- there may be associated neuropathy which predisposes to painless, neuroischaemic tissue damage under compression bandaging.

All patients with CVU and an ABPI < 0.8, and all diabetic patients with a CVU, should be referred to a vascular surgeon for assessment.

Patients with an ABPI of 0.6–0.8 can be treated with compression, provided that an expert fits it and they are closely supervised. Vulnerable areas must receive extra padding; beware excessive pressure at the edge of a thick dressing. Avoid a figure-of-eight technique and excessive overlap as this will increase the pressure exerted. In patients with mixed ulcers, a three-layer bandage system may be preferred. There are many variations but one option would be orthopaedic wool, a conformable elastic bandage and an SSB.

Compression is contraindicated if the ABPI is <0.6. Such patients should be assessed for angioplasty and/or arterial reconstruction. Failure to observe these principles may lead to major limb amputation from pressure necrosis (Figure 35.20).

Problem legs

'Champagne-bottle' leg

- Pad the narrow part of the leg with plenty of wool to make the leg more cone-shaped; be extra vigilant for areas of pressure necrosis
- use a figure of eight as it is less prone to slippage
- use a narrower bandage (i.e. 7.5 rather than 10 cm) as it may conform better to the 'steep' part of the leg
- use a cohesive bandage.

The large leg

Due to the law of Laplace, normal bandaging techniques may not be able to exert adequate pressure; so:

- use a more powerful bandage
- use a figure of eight technique
- consider adding an extra layer.

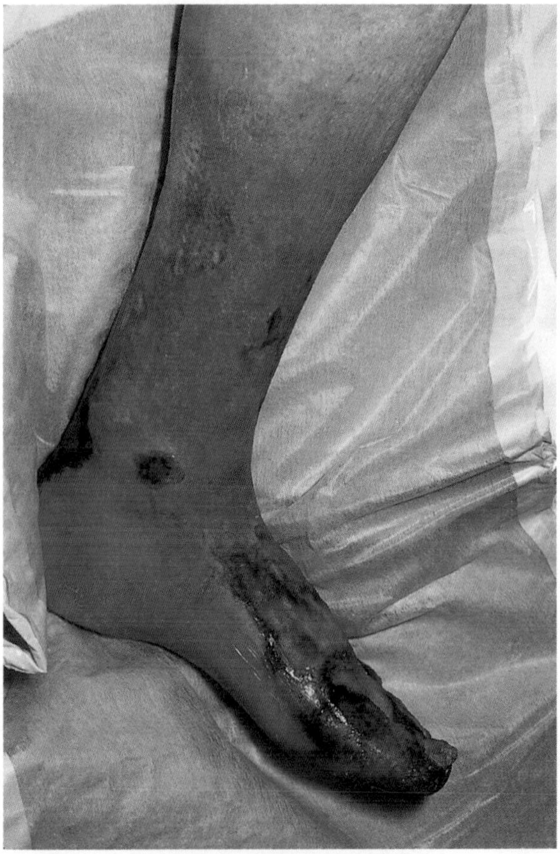

Figure 35.20 Ischaemia necrosis in a patient treated with compression bandaging for venous ulceration. The patient required an above knee amputation.

The thin leg
The thin elderly female patient with little subcutaneous tissue over bony prominences and tendons is at particular risk of pressure necrosis. Extra padding is required.

The oedematous leg
Compression therapy alone will not control severe oedema and other measures must be taken (see above).

Compression hosiery
As discussed above, most UK centres prefer to use bandaging rather than compression stockings until the ulcer is healed. However, there are compression systems, such as Jobst UlcerCare, which are stocking based. This system comprises an inner liner that exerts about 15 mmHg at the ankle and an outer stocking, zipped posteriorly for easier donning and doffing, which increases ankle pressure to about 40 mmHg. Healing rates appear to be as high as with compression bandaging and compliance may be better, although it is only really suitable for ulcers that are relatively dry.

Two studies have shown that compression should be continued in the form of elastic stockings for at least 5 years after healing, if not for life. There is no evidence that class III stockings are superior to class II.

A number of patients simply cannot tolerate multilayer bandaging, due to itching or the inherent bulkiness of the bandages. They may complain that it is 'too hot' or that they cannot find a shoe to fit, and may remove the bandages themselves. In these cases a certain degree of compromise is required and a compression stocking over a dressing may be more acceptable to the patient.

Other physical therapies

Massage
Although frequently advocated in lymphoedema, massage is seldom used in CVI. This is surprising given what we know about the macro- and microvascular changes that occur in CVI and the fact that a degree of lymphoedema, or at least lymphatic dysfunction, often co-exists. However, the authors are not aware of any studies in this area.

Pneumatic compression devices
Two small studies have suggested that intermittent pneumatic compression might improve ulcer healing, although this needs to be confirmed in larger trials. Devices that provide sequential compression appear to be superior. Mechanistically, one would expect such compression to be of benefit but, of course, there are issues of expense and patient compliance. However, if patients suggest self-purchasing a device, it is generally worth encouraging. At the very least it means the patient will be sitting with the leg elevated for a couple of hours each day and it also shows a high level of patient motivation. As with any compression therapy, arterial disease must be excluded.

Other physical methods

Several other physical therapies have been advocated; for example, hydrotherapy, radio-frequency and electrical therapy, and hyperbaric oxygen. There is a considerable body of work on the effects of ultrasound on wound healing where it is thought to increase blood flow and stimulate fibroblasts, macrophages and angiogenesis. Three small and imperfect studies have suggested ultrasound might speed the healing of CVU. However, further evidence is required before ultrasound, or any of these therapies can be recommended for routine use.

Sclerotherapy
Injection sclerotherapy is not effective in the treatment of varices in the presence of main-stem long or short saphenous vein reflux. It is, however, useful for the treatment of isolated calf varices without main-stem incompetence and can be performed in infirm patients who are unfit for surgery. The authors are not aware of any trials examining the effect of sclerotherapy on ulcer healing.

Section 35.6 • Surgical management

Overview

The role of surgery in the management of CVI, and specifically CVU, has not been defined because, to date, no randomized, controlled trial has compared best medical therapy and best medical therapy plus surgery. However, a substantial amount of uncontrolled data suggests that surgery is of benefit in selected patient groups.

The surgical treatment of CVI is significantly different from that of uncomplicated varicose veins in a number of important ways:

- The patients are older and often have multi-system, medical comorbidity. The risks of anaesthesia and surgery are, therefore, higher.
- They run a higher risk of thrombo-embolic complications, especially those with post-thrombotic syndrome. This mandates meticulous prophylaxis.
- CVU and skin affected by CVI are frequently colonized by bacteria, some of which are pathogenic. Peri-operative antibiotic prophylaxis against wound infection is important.
- Patients often require a period of inpatient treatment before they are suitable for surgery; for example, to optimize cardiorespiratory function, to treat 'weeping' eczema, to reduce oedema or to deslough an ulcer. Although it is not necessary for an ulcer to be healed prior to surgery, the ulcer bed and surrounding skin should be optimized.
- Patients may also undergo adjuvant procedures such as skin grafting or SEPS.

The result is that few patients are suitable for day-case treatment and the hospital stay, and thus the costs, associated with surgery for CVI are considerably greater than for straightforward varicose veins patients:

- Patients frequently have deep venous disease and, not infrequently, have had their veins operated previously. A full anatomical and functional pre-operative venous assessment is mandatory. It is also important to determine the arterial status of the limb.
- Surgery that might be considered incomplete in terms of eradicating simple varicose veins may still achieve a worthwhile haemodynamic result in patients with CVI. Thus, several groups have advocated SFJ and SPJ ligation, without stripping or avulsions, under local anaesthesia.

Patient selection

Once the anaesthetic and surgical risks have been found acceptable, the decision to offer surgery is usually based upon the nature and extent of the underlying venous abnormality. From a surgical perspective, patients with CVI and/or ulceration can be divided, usually on the basis of duplex ultrasonography, into four groups:

- Isolated superficial venous reflux (40%).
- Combined deep and superficial reflux (50%).
- Isolated deep venous reflux (10%).
- Deep venous obstruction (co-existing with any of the above) (10%).

The proportion of patients falling into each of the above categories varies considerably between different series. The figures given are based on an average taken from the literature as well as the authors' personal experience.

Isolated superficial reflux (40%)

Several uncontrolled series suggest that the surgical eradication of such reflux though standard saphenous surgery: (1) retards the development of skin changes and (2) augments the healing, and reduces the recurrence, of CVU.

Is post-operative compression necessary?

Opinions vary as to whether such patients should receive post-operative compression therapy as well. Those who believe it is unnecessary argue:

- The only abnormality was the superficial reflux and that has been corrected.
- Why subject the patient to the worst of both worlds; that is, the morbidity of surgery and the discomfort and inconvenience of compression hosiery?
- It is not cost-effective.
- Excellent long-term healing in this group without the use of compression has been demonstrated.

By contrast, others, including the authors, would argue that:

- Superficial venous surgery is rarely complete. Residual reflux is inevitable, particularly in the below knee tributaries of the LSV and SSV, and especially in this patient group where there is understandable reluctance to perform numerous avulsions through the damaged skin of the lower leg.
- The development of further superficial reflux is likely. There are data to suggest that, following simple varicose vein surgery, compression hosiery prevents the emergence of further varices.
- Compression will augment the function of the calf muscle pump. Although these patients only had reflux demonstrable in their superficial system, in order to develop CVI it is generally believed that a degree of calf muscle pump dysfunction must co-exist and should be treated.
- Compared with the cost of recurrent ulceration, the cost of stockings is minimal.
- Stockings protect the leg from injury. This is perhaps the weakest argument, although at least 30% of CVU follow an episode of trauma.

Combined superficial and deep reflux (50%)

Several groups have suggested that, in the presence of deep venous reflux, particularly that affecting the popliteal vein, the results of superficial venous surgery are much less encouraging. This has led some authorities to conclude that surgery should never be contemplated in this group. However, others argue that:

- Although the results of surgery in this mixed group are disappointing there is some evidence to suggest that they are better than those achieved by best medical therapy alone. Clearly, this needs to be tested by means of a randomized, controlled trial.
- The outcome of surgery in this group may depend upon the aetiology of the deep venous reflux. If deep reflux is due to calf muscle pump overload secondary to superficial reflux then eradication of the latter may reverse the former. The same may hold true, or at least superficial surgery may improve the overall haemodynamics of the leg, if the deep reflux is due to primary valvular insufficiency. By contrast, if the deep reflux is due to extensive post-thrombotic damage, then it is unlikely that superficial surgery will be of benefit.

Isolated deep venous reflux (10%)

This unusual situation usually arises because the superficial veins have previously been removed. Such patients might be considered for perforator ligation or deep venous reconstruction (see below).

Deep venous obstruction (10%)

In about 10% of patients with CVI, deep venous obstruction co-exists with deep venous reflux, and often superficial reflux as well. These are a difficult group to manage because they are often highly symptomatic, have a poor prognosis, and if superficial veins are acting as collaterals they may be made symptomatically and haemodynamically worse by compression hosiery and/or superficial venous surgery. The standard teaching has been to avoid surgery because the severity of outflow obstruction was difficult to quantify, as was the contribution being made to the venous outflow of the leg by the superficial veins. However, a number of authorities believe that it is, in fact, rare for superficial varices to be contributing positively to the overall venous haemodynamics of the leg and have suggested a more aggressive approach to the eradicating of superficial reflux in this group. Before considering surgery on this group:

- Perform a full functional assessment of the leg; for example, with APG.
- Consider measuring arm/foot pressure differential.
- Consider ascending venography to define the anatomy of any deep venous obstruction and the nature of any collaterals.
- Duplex the LSV and SSV. If this shows continuous upward flow and/or minimal reflux, they are likely to be acting as collaterals.

Section 35.7 • Perforating vein surgery

Overview

Open ligation of medial calf perforating veins (Homan's, Cockett's procedure) (Figure 35.21) has been largely abandoned because of the high associated complication rate (mainly wound breakdown and infection and thrombo-embolism), and because of a lack of proof that the operation was beneficial.

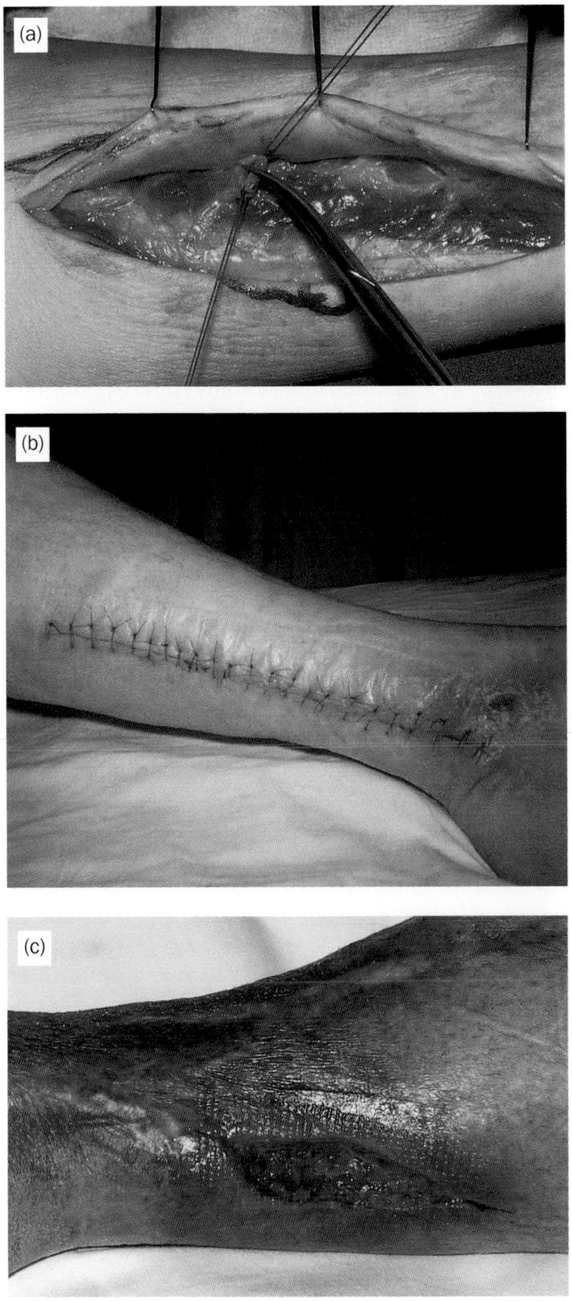

Figure 35.21 Open perforator ligation (Linton's procedure). (a) Direct ligation of medial calf perforators through a longitudinal incision. (b) Immediate post-operative appearance of the wound. (c) Recurrence of venous ulceration in the surgical wound.

The advent of SEPS (Figure 35.22), together with the ability to mark precisely the site of incompetent perforating veins (IPV) with duplex immediately prior to surgery, has re-awoken the debate regarding the role of perforator surgery. SEPS can be performed with little additional morbidity over and above that which might be expected following standard saphenous surgery in this patient group. It can also be used to divide perforators underlying open ulcers. When duplex clearly shows jets of high velocity, and presumably high pressure, blood leaving the deep compartment through an IPV underlying such an ulcer it is difficult to believe, intuitively, that dividing that perforator would not be beneficial. However, it has proved surprisingly difficult to prove that performing SEPS, in addition to saphenous surgery, has any adjuvant effect upon ulcer healing or recurrence and a randomized controlled trial is required.

Pathophysiology

The key to understanding the benefits and shortcomings of SEPS lies, as always in venous disease, with an understanding of the anatomy and pathophysiology. In health, perforators direct blood from the superficial to the deep compartments of the calf during calf muscle diastole. Valves and other mechanisms discussed above normally prevent that blood from escaping the deep compartment through perforators during calf muscle systole. Outward or bidirectional (inward and then outward) flow in medial calf perforators is gener-

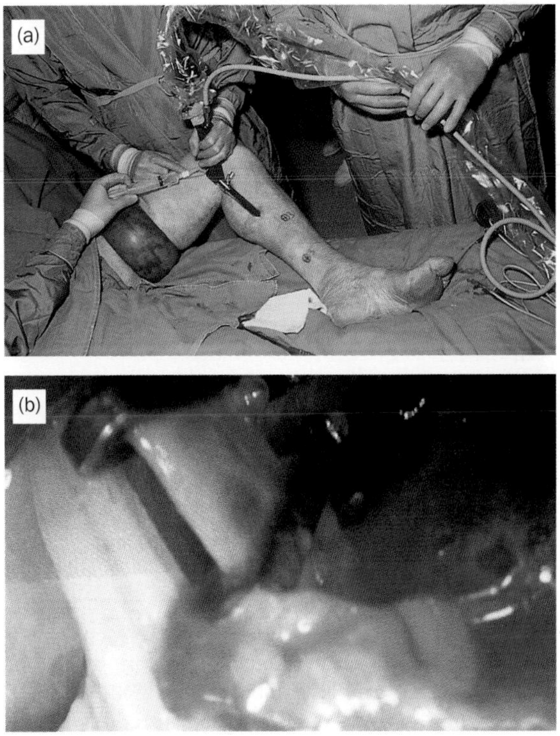

Figure 35.22 Subfascial endoscopic perforator surgery (SEPS). (a) Endoscopic division of previously marked (duplex) medial calf perforators using a single port technique and an exsanguinating tourniquet. (b) Application of two clips to a perforator.

ally believed to be pathological. Such IPV are rare in healthy individuals but their prevalence and size increases as the clinical status of the leg deteriorates. They are virtually ubiquitous in the leg affected by CVU. The question remains, however, whether these IPV cause ulceration or whether they are simply a manifestation of disease elsewhere in the system. Isolated IPV are rare (< 5% of patients with CVU) and are almost always found in association with superficial but more especially deep reflux. Perforators can therefore become incompetent through one or both of two mechanisms: (1) deep venous reflux and/or calf muscle pump dysfunction causes a 'blow-out' of high pressure blood through IPV during calf systole; (2) superficial reflux leads to excessive inflow of blood from the superficial to the deep compartment during calf diastole which stretches the perforator and overloads the calf muscle pump such that blood refluxes back out during calf systole.

The importance of appreciating the latter mechanism is that it is reversible. Thus, if the deep veins are normal, eradication of superficial reflux leads to 80% of IPV regaining competence.

Classification of perforators

On the basis of these and other pathophysiological and clinical studies, the author's group have attempted to classify IPV on the basis of their underlying aetiology and suitability for SEPS:

- Type I IPV: occur with isolated superficial reflux; 80% will return to normal following standard saphenous surgery; SEPS is not normally indicated.
- Type II IPV: occur with isolated deep reflux; SEPS may be indicated.
- Type III IPV: occur with mixed deep and superficial reflux; saphenous surgery will not correct IPV; SEPS may be indicated.
- Type IV IPV: occur with deep venous obstruction; care must be exercised in case IPV are acting as part of a collateral pathway (see above), SEPS may be harmful.
- Type V: no detectable deep or superficial reflux; this is a rare group and it may be that small segments of deep and/or superficial reflux are simply being missed SEPS may be indicated.

Experience with SEPS

SEPS is undoubtedly safe and feasible. Several groups have published encouraging results with early ulcer healing following the procedure. However:

- SEPS has nearly always been performed at the same time as saphenous surgery making it impossible to distinguish the effects of the two procedures.
- Follow-up has been short.
- There has been no control group.

The North American SEPS register has recently published its medium-term results and unfortunately the ulcer recurrence rate is disappointingly high, especially in the group with deep vein (popliteal) reflux. Clearly, the only way to resolve this issue is to perform a randomized, controlled trial. In such a trial, it would be important to ensure that the two arms are balanced with regard to the different types of IPV classified above.

Section 35.8 • Deep venous reconstruction

Overview

Several procedures have been advocated to reverse deep venous incompetence. These procedures have not gained widespread acceptance and are not, to the authors' knowledge, being performed in the UK in any significant number. However, the various options are briefly described here for the sake of completeness.

Vein diameter reduction

Reducing the vein diameter around an incompetent valve by the use of vein wall plication or placement of a synthetic cuff around the valve can restore competence with little or no endothelial damage.

Vein valve repair

The edges of floppy valve cusps can be sutured to the vein wall by either an open or closed technique, thus rendering the valve competent. The open technique was first described by Kistner in 1968 and involved a longitudinal venotomy directly through a commissure. A transverse incision above the level of the valve can also be used, or commissural reefing can be performed without opening the vein. A number of small series have shown good long-term results.

Vein valve transplantation

Autologous valve transplantation interposes a segment of axillary or brachial vein, containing a competent valve, into an incompetent deep, usually the popliteal, vein. Results are variable, the world-wide experience is small and the transplanted vein segment has a tendency to dilate. Procedures using synthetic, mixed and animal valves are still experimental.

Vein transposition

An incompetent superficial femoral vein can be transected and anastomosed end-to-end or end-to-side to a profunda femoris or long saphenous vein that has a competent valve. With end-to-side anastomosis, there requires to be a competent valve below the anastomosis as well as above. In most series, a high proportion of patients have recurrent incompetence at 1 year postoperatively.

Veno-venous bypass

Palma procedure

This operation is designed to bypass unilateral iliac vein occlusion. The patent LSV on the contralateral side is tunnelled suprapubically to the affected side and anastomosed to the patent common or superficial femoral vein below the obstruction. In carefully selected patients, this procedure produces satisfactory long-term clinical and haemodynamic results.

Saphenopopliteal bypass

An obstructed femoral segment may be bypassed by anastomosing a transected, competent LSV to the side of the popliteal vein. Again, satisfactory long-term patency rates have been reported in small series.

Other surgical interventions

Ulcer debridement

One intuitively feels that debriding an ulcer back to a healthy (bleeding) tissue will encourage the formation of granulation tissue. There are also theoretical grounds for believing that 'freshening' the edges of the ulcer will promote epithelialization. However, these practices have not been subjected to trials and are, therefore, based upon clinical experience.

Skin grafting

Split-skin and pinch grafting (Figure 35.23) can be used to speed up epithelialization and may reduce pain. However, it is important that before a graft is placed:

- a healthy, well vascularized, granulating base is available
- pathogenic bacteria (*Pseudomonas aeruginosa*, *Staphylococcus aureus*, β-haemolytic streptococcus) have been eradicated
- wound exudate, which tends to lift off the graft, has been minimized
- the haemodynamic venous abnormality has been normalized as far as is possible.

If these criteria are not met then there is a high probability of the graft not 'taking' and of the ulcer recurring. Split-skin grafting requires admission to hospital and a period of post-operative bed rest but with 'meshing' can be used to cover a large area. Pinch grafting can be performed as an outpatient under local anaesthetic but is only suitable for small ulcers.

Pinch grafting has been shown to improve early healing rates, but it is unclear whether this remains so later. This can be performed as an outpatient procedure. Pinch grafting produces an aesthetically ugly cobbled surface, each 'pinch' being full thickness in the centre, but this is better than an open wound requiring frequent dressings in the long term. Even if not all 'take', the gaps can be filled in at a later date, and the process of re-epithelialization is hastened.

Split-skin grafting can be used, meshed or perforated, the fenestrations allowing passage of exudate into the dressing. Recent studies have shown good short-term healing rates after grafting with meshed or fenestrated bioengineered skin. An area of multiple ulcers is best excised and the whole area covered with a split skin graft. Pedicle and free flaps are sometimes useful in highly selected patients.

Arterial reconstruction

Patients with an ABPI of < 0.8 should be considered for angiography with a view to reconstruction or angioplasty. Compression therapy can then be applied under a careful surveillance programme.

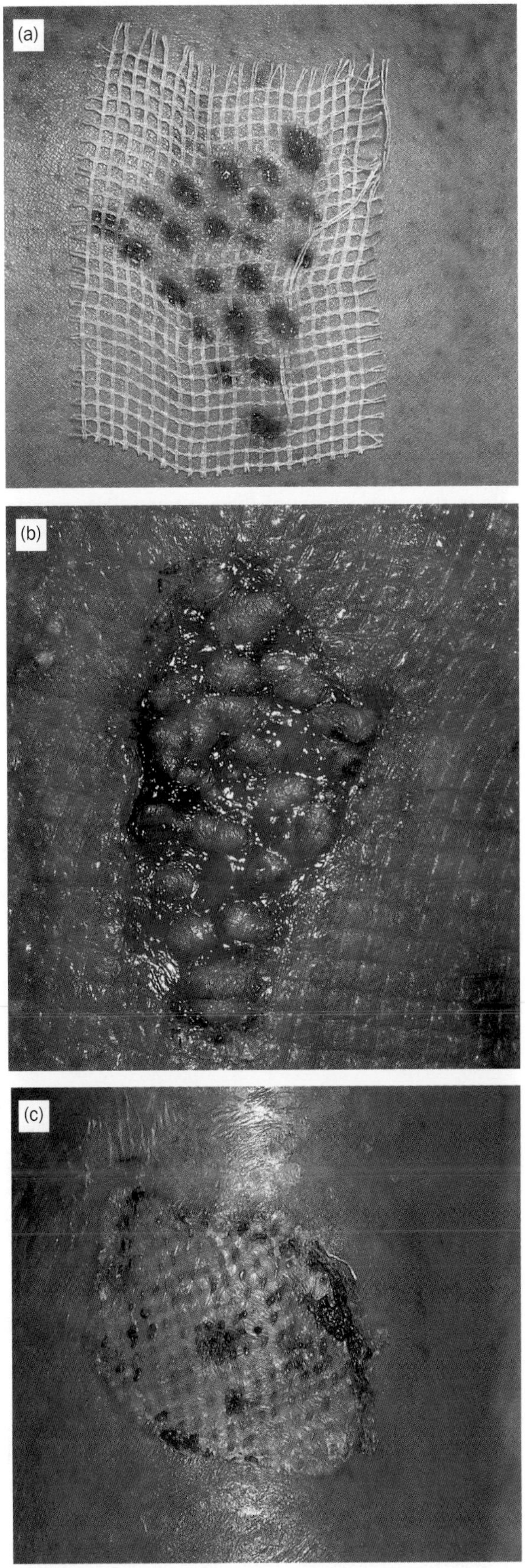

Figure 35.23 Skin grafting. (a) Pinch graft donor site. (b) Pinch grafts 6 weeks after application. (c) Meshed split-skin graft.

Amputation

In patients with severe intractable ulceration whose quality of life has become intolerable, amputation may have to be considered as a last resort. These patients usually have ulcers of mixed aetiology, particularly arterial disease and vasculitis.

Section 35.9 • Models of care provision

Overview

Nurses and general practitioners manage approximately 80% of patients with CVU solely within the community. A range of hospital specialists such as dermatologists, physicians and vascular surgeons treats the remaining 20%. Increasingly, community and hospital-based specialist leg ulcer nurses are taking a lead role in the management of these patients. Provision of care will obviously depend on local resource availability and expertise. However, it is important to ensure that:

- The overall treatment package is delivered by an interdisciplinary team of interested doctors and nurses who communicate readily with each other and have ready access to the skills of other disciplines such as physiotherapist and occupational therapists.
- Carers understand the multi-factorial aetiology of most leg ulcers and are capable of identifying, early in the course of the disease, those patients who might benefit from surgical correction of underlying venous and arterial disease and/or other specialist input.
- Patients are treated according to evidence-based guidelines derived from a systematic review of the available literature. The Scottish Leg Ulcer Project, still underway, is evaluating the impact on leg ulcer healing rates of national guidelines.
- The patient's treatment is viewed as a joint effort between primary and secondary care.

The 'one-stop' clinic

The optimal management of leg ulceration rest crucially upon gaining a precise understanding the aetiology early in the course of the disease. One way of achieving this aim is to refer patients to a 'one-stop' clinic where they undergo physical examination, measurement of ABPI and duplex ultrasonography. On the basis of this information:

- recommendations for treatment in primary care can be made
- patients who might benefit form surgery can be identified at an early stage
- complex ulcers can be distinguished at an early stage and, if resources allow, their treatment can be shared between primary and secondary care.

It has yet to proved that such an arrangement increases healing and reduces recurrence rates. However, one feels intuitively that an organized, protocol driven 'one-stop clinic' approach where patients in need of special expertise can be identified sooner rather than later will be both clinically effective and cost-effective (Tables 35.6 and 35.7).

Community versus hospital-based care

There has, understandably, been a move away from specialist-run hospital-based leg ulcer clinics towards nurse-led community-based treatment. Nevertheless, it is important to realize that the excellent healing rates achieved with compression in clinical trials of highly selected patients in centres of excellence are never going to be matched in the typical patient population found in the average community setting.

Conclusions

Although the most 'difficult' cases of leg ulceration are multi-factorial in origin, CVI is the single most

Table 35.6 Summary of recommendations for the management of chronic venous ulceration (adapted from the SIGN guidelines)

- Measurement of ABPI is an essential part of the assessment; patients with an index < 0.8 should be assumed to have significant arterial disease and referred to a vascular surgeon
- The total surface area of all the ulcers on the limb, not just the largest (index) ulcer should be measured
- All patients should be considered for duplex ultrasonography of the deep and superficial veins
- Bacteriological swabs should be obtained only when there is clinical evidence of infection (excessive pain, cellulitis, pyrexia, lymphangitis/adenitis) or when surgery (skin graft, bypass surgery) is being contemplated
- Topical antibiotics should never be used; systemic antibiotics should only be prescribed when there is evidence of infection
- No specific systemic therapy is of proven benefit
- Ulcers which fail to show signs of healing after 3 months should be biopsied to exclude malignancy
- Leg ulcer patients with associated (contact) dermatitis should be referred to a dermatologist for patch testing with an extended leg ulcer series
- Venous ulcers should be washed in tap water and then carefully dried prior to dressing; no other cleaning agent has been shown to be superior
- Simple non-adherent dressings are recommended; no other form of dressing has been shown to be superior, except hydrocolloid or foam dressings may be of benefit in ulcers that are particularly painful
- Multi-layer graduated elastic compression is the most effective method of healing uncomplicated venous ulcers
- Superficial venous surgery should be considered in patients with superficial reflux, especially when the deep veins are normal
- Large ulcers should be considered for skin grafting
- Graduated compression hosiery should be fitted to all patients with uncomplicated venous ulceration after healing and should be worn for life to reduce the risk of recurrence

Table 35.7 Suggested criteria for early specialist referral (adapted from the SIGN guidelines)

- Uncertain aetiology
- Atypical ulcer distribution
- Suspicion of malignancy
- Arterial disease (ABPI < 0.8)
- Surgically correctable superficial venous reflux
- Diabetes mellitus
- Rheumatoid arthritis or other condition associated with vasculitis
- Dermatitis refractory to topical steroids
- Failure to shows signs of improvement after 3 months

common underlying pathology. As such, there is some hope that the prevalence of ulceration may decline in future as a result of improved thrombo-embolic prophylaxis and treatment. For the moment, however, venous ulceration is a common and disabling condition that is often resistant to conservative therapy, prone to recurrence and very expensive to manage.

There needs to be a low threshold for referral to a vascular surgeon, preferably through a 'one-stop' assessment clinic where a thorough venous and arterial duplex-based assessment can be performed. This will allow patients who might benefit from surgical intervention to be identified and treated early on. It will also allow ongoing community based treatment to be based upon an in depth understanding of the pathophysiological mechanisms responsible in each individual patient.

Great progress in the management of CVU has been made over the past decade because of:

- an increased understanding of the pathophysiology
- an improvement in the provision of community care for the condition, specifically through the training of nurses with a special interest in this field
- the availability of data from clinical trials that have provided a scientifically robust platform on which to base treatment algorithms.

Despite all this, there is yet much to be learnt, and there is no room for complacency. Further research is required into the epidemiology and natural history of CVU, models of care, primary prevention and pathogenesis. We need to examine the effect of evidence-based treatment regimens and published guidelines on prevalence and incidence in the future. Large-scale, multi-centre trials are required, aimed at smaller groups of patients, particularly those undergoing deep venous surgery, those with mixed ulcer disease and those with intractable ulceration.

However, we are now able to offer these patients more effective treatment than ever before and there has never been a time when the management of these challenging patients has been more interesting and fulfilling.

Key points

- Although most leg ulcers are multi-factorial in aetiology, CVI is the single commonest underlying pathology.
- Multi-layer, elastic, graduated compression therapy is the single most effective means of healing venous leg ulcers.
- Compression hosiery reduces recurrence and stockings should be worn for life once the ulcer is healed.
- Compression therapy should never be prescribed without first establishing the arterial status of the patient. If pedal pulses are not readily palpable, measure the ABPI. If it is less than 0.8, do not apply compression and refer to a vascular surgeon
- Remember 1–2% of leg ulcers are malignant and even 'experts' miss the diagnosis.
- No effective pharmacotherapy has been found for venous ulceration.
- Do not prescribe antibiotics unless there is a specific reason, i.e. for frank infection, preferably after the results of swabbing, or before skin grafting.
- The management of leg ulcers is best conducted jointly between primary and secondary care with specialist community and/or hospital based nurses playing a major role in the day to day provision of care.

Further reading

Bergan, J. J. and Yao, J. S. T. eds, (1991). *Venous Disorders*. Philadelphia, PA: W.B. Saunders.

Negus, D. (1991). *Leg Ulcers. A Practical Approach to Management*. Oxford: Butterworth-Heinemann.

Ruckley, C. V., Fowkes, F. G. R. and Bradbury, A. W. eds, (1999). *Venous Disease – Epidemiology, Management and Delivery of Care*. London: Springer.

Scottish Intercollegiate Guidelines Network Publications. Edinburgh: Royal College of Physicians.

MODULE 36

Arteriovenous fistulas

The term arteriovenous fistula (AVF) can be simply defined as an abnormal communication between the arterial and venous systems other than the normal pulmonary and systemic capillary bed. It encompasses a bewildering variety of lesions most of which are abnormal and can be broadly classified as congenital or acquired. The former includes haemangiomas and arteriovenous malformations (AVM) (Figure 36.1) whereas the acquired lesions are traumatic fistulas, erosions between an artery and a vein secondary to infection, tumour or pressure and surgically created shunts. These lesions can appear in any part of the body. Signs and symptoms depend on the location of the fistula, the amount of blood shunted from the arterial to the venous system and the duration of this communication.

Section 36.1 • Introduction

Whenever the subject of AVF is addressed an inadequacy of vocabulary, an inconsistency of nomenclature and an absence of a satisfactory classification suitable for all purposes become evident. The congenital AVF comprises a spectrum of developmental abnormalities that may involve all components of the peripheral circulation i.e. arteries, veins, capillaries and lymphatics. A number of classifications have been proposed based on clinical lesions, developmental abnormalities *in utero*, correlation of clinical and angiographic findings and the type of anatomical/pathological features. The most widely accepted classification is by Mulliken which is based on cell kinetics and is now the official nomenclature used by the International Workshop of Vascular Anomalies. According to this classification congenital AVF are divided into two major types: haemangiomas and malformations. Haemangiomas demonstrate endothelial hyperplasia with abundant mast cells. They are not visible at birth, grow in the early life, tend to regress and in 90% of cases involute naturally by the age of 5–10 years. Malformations have normal endothelial turnover. These lesions are invariably present at birth, usually grow with age and in women may enlarge dramatically during puberty or pregnancy. Mast cells are rarely seen in these lesions. A simple classification is given in Figure 36.2.

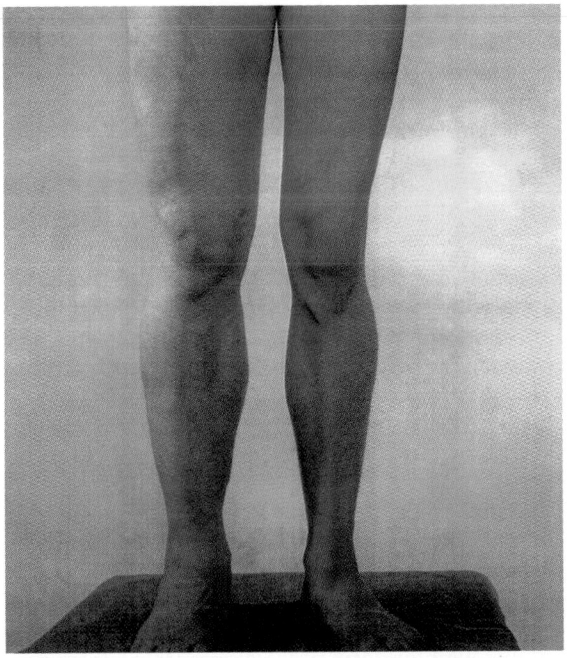

Figure 36.1 Arteriovenous malformation of right leg.

The aims of this module are: (1) to describe the aetiology, pathophysiology and clinical presentation of AVF, (2) to propose the diagnostic approach; and (3) to discuss various therapeutic options.

Section 36.2 • Aetiology

Acquired fistulas most often result from trauma. Penetrating injuries from knives, bullets, needles and catheters injure adjacent arteries and veins. Blunt trauma that causes fracture or joint dislocation may lead to the

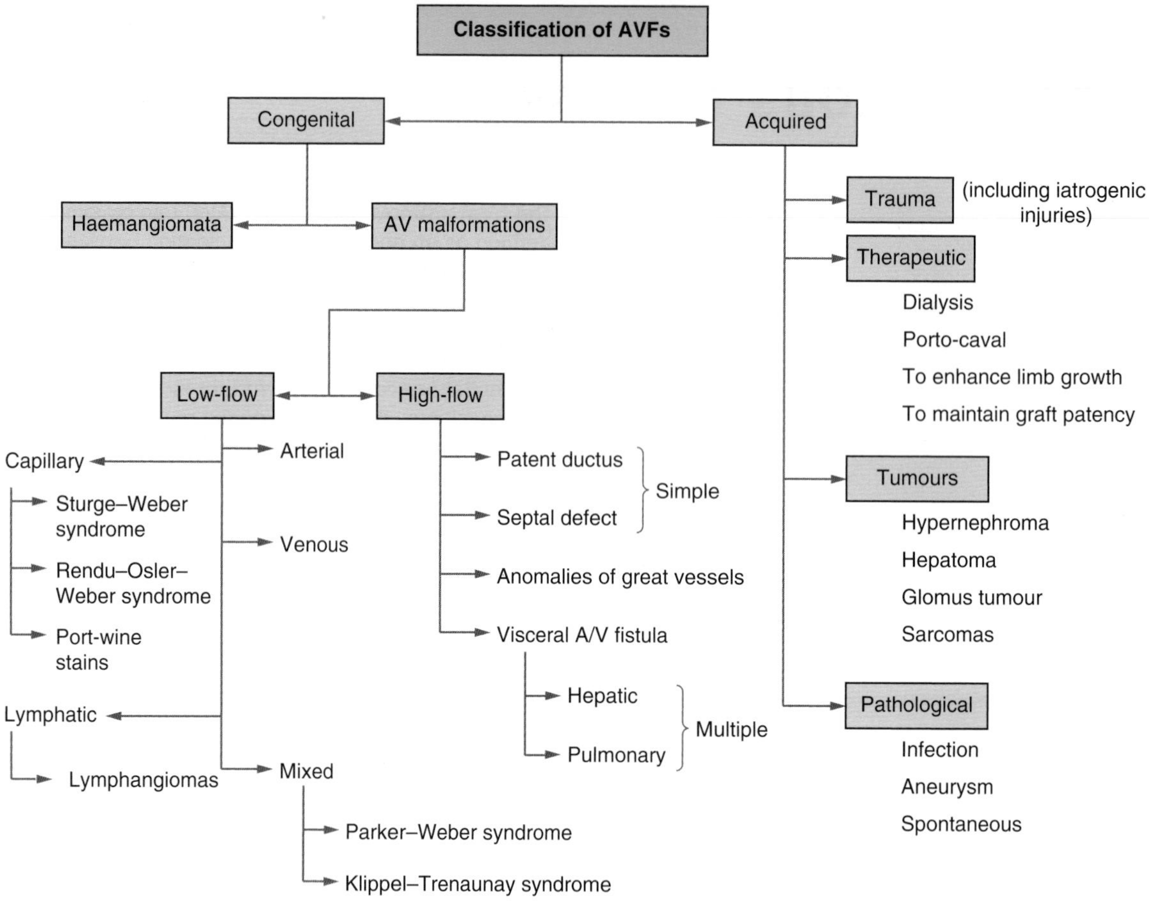

Figure 36.2 Classification of AVFs.

development of an AVF, e.g. hypogastric artery fistulas from pelvic fracture and carotid cavernous fistula from facial injuries. About 60% of traumatic fistulas will have an associated false aneurysm. Occasionally the injury is iatrogenic. The most common responsible procedures are femoral arterial access and lumbar discectomy. In the latter, the close relationship of the aorta and the inferior vena cava (IVC) to the level of the L4–L5 disc space and iliac vessels at L5–S1 disc space can lead to injury and formation of an AVF. Mass ligation of the major arteries and veins during splenectomy or nephrectomy can result in fistulas. Needle biopsy of the kidney can lead to an intra-renal fistula.

Spontaneous weakness of the wall of the aorta or one of its major branches or the erosion of a false aneurysm secondary to sepsis and aortitis can cause an AVF. A rare cause is the erosion of intra-vascular appliances such as IVC filters. Rupture of an atherosclerotic aortic aneurysm into the IVC is another common cause of acquired fistulas.

Fistulas are also created for therapeutic purposes such as dialysis, portal hypertension, maintenance of arterial bypass and venous repairs and to enhance limb growth.

The cause of congenital AVF is unknown, but a widely held view is that it is the arrest or misdirection of the normal development of the vascular tree that takes place during one of the three stages of vasculogenesis which is at fault. These three stages were described by Wollard as: (1) the stage of undifferentiated capillary networks; (2) the retiform stage consisting of large plexiform structures formed by coalescence of the original equipotential capillaries; and (3) the stage of appearance of mature vascular stems after the disappearance of the primitive element. Thus congenital AVF occur purely by chance during the extremely complex development of the vascular system. Occasionally these congenital lesions are familial and recent work by Boon *et al.* and Gallione *et al.* has identified a locus on chromosome 9p for these malformations. AVF involving the pulmonary circulation may occur in association with hereditary haemorrhagic telangiectasia (HHT) which is an autosomal dominant trait. Genetic linkage for this condition has been established on the long arm of chromosome 9 and the gene at this site codes for endoglin, an endothelial protein involved in the growth and function of blood vessels. Patients with this disease (HHT1) have approximately a 30% chance of developing pulmonary AVF. Genetic linkage of HHT has also been established on chromosome 12 and families with this form of the disease (HHT2) are considerably less likely to develop pulmonary AVF (3%)

but are at greater risk of fistulas on the systemic side of the circulation, notably within the liver. In most circumstances however the cause of congenital AVF is unknown.

Whenever an AVF appears later in life (an inexplicable, but frequent clinical scenario) a malignant lesion should be excluded, usually by biopsy. Highly vascular tumors such as sarcomas or secondaries from hypernephroma must always be considered in the differential diagnosis.

Section 36.3 • Pathophysiology

AVF, by connecting the high-pressure arterial system to the low-pressure venous system, short circuits the circulation and prevents blood from reaching the capillary bed. This short circuiting has effects at three levels, locally (at the fistula site), peripherally (distal to the fistula) and centrally. The severity of the pathophysiological changes depends upon the magnitude and location of the leak and longevity of the fistula.

Locally the blood vessels leading to and draining the fistula can undergo hypertrophy or degeneration, giving rise to varicose veins and arterial aneurysms. Such patients may develop peripheral effects like distal ischaemia. To prevent ischaemia the peripheral vascular bed vasodilates which in turn produces excessive demands on the heart and if longstanding results in central effects, i.e. cardiac failure.

The location of the fistulas is also important. Those closer to the heart are more likely to produce central effects, whereas those located in the extremities are more likely to cause ischaemia. Because of their complexity and low flow, congenital AVF produce more local effects than the high flow acquired fistulas which produce more central and peripheral effects.

AVF can be typically side-to-side or H-shaped (bridge fistula). The side-to-side fistula has no intervening bridge, e.g. Brescia–Cimino fistula for haemodialysis and aortocaval fistula, whereas the H-type fistula has a finite length of a graft interposed between the artery and the vein. Polytetrafluoroethylene is widely accepted as the conduit of choice for this bridge. The haemodynamics of these fistulas are different. A typical AVF has the following components: a proximal artery and vein, a distal artery and vein, collateral vessels – arteries connecting the proximal and distal arteries bypassing the fistula and veins connecting the distal and proximal vein, a peripheral vascular bed supplied by the involved arteries and finally heart and great vessels that feed and drain the fistula. As in any blood conduit the resistance in a fistula is directly proportional to its length and inversely proportional to its diameter. Although according to Poiseuille's law:

$$R_{\min} = 8hL/\pi r^4$$

there should be no resistance in a side-to-side fistula (zero length offer no resistance) some resistance is always present owing to the inertial factors. On the other hand both length and diameter of the conduit affect the resistance of H-type fistulas. Hence H-type fistulas always have a greater resistance than side-to-side fistulas of equal diameter.

Local effects

Blood flow in the proximal artery is always increased and depends on the size of fistula, venous outflow resistance, collaterals and the peripheral vascular bed. Because of the fall in resistance caused by the AVF, diastolic blood flow in the proximal artery increases reducing the pulse pressure. Blood flow in the proximal vein is also markedly increased and becomes pulsatile. Because of the great compliance of the venous system these pulsations rapidly dampen out and within 1 cm proximal to the fistula mean pressure ranges between 0 and 15 mmHg and pulse pressure is seldom over 5 mmHg. The continuation of the pulsation beyond that point would mean stenosis or occlusion of the proximal vein and in the case of obstruction the venous pressure will approach that on the arterial side of the fistula. The key to understanding the haemodynamic effects of an AVF is the direction of blood flow in the various components of this circuit.

The flow in the proximal artery is always towards and in the proximal vein always away from the fistula. The arterial collateral flow will always be towards the peripheral vascular bed bypassing the fistula and venous collateral flow will also bypass the fistula but in the opposite direction. However, the direction of blood flow in the distal artery and vein varies. To understand the flow patterns in these segments of the fistula two reference points should be remembered – the arterial and venous ends of the fistula and the site of collateral in-flow and out-flow distal to the fistula.

Three possibilities exist for the flow in the distal artery:

- Flow in the normal peripheral direction – when the pressure at the arterial end of the fistula is greater than the pressure at the site of collateral inflow. This occurs in small high resistance fistulas with not well-developed collaterals. In this situation the blood pressure will gradually decrease from the proximal artery past the fistula to the distal artery.
- Flow in retrograde direction – when the pressure at the site of collateral inflow is greater than the pressure at the arterial end of the fistula. This occurs in large chronic low resistance fistulas with well-developed collaterals. This situation will cause distal ischaemia in addition to overburdening the heart. The blood pressure will decrease from the proximal artery to the fistula but will rise again from the fistula to the distal artery. In chronic fistula as collateral arteries dilate, pressure in the distal artery rises causing a dual effect of encouraging retrograde flow in the distal artery and of facilitating flow to the peripheral tissues.
- Stagnant flow – this rare situation occurs when both pressures are equal. This is seen in large acute fistulas before collaterals are well developed. In this situation blood will flow in the normal direction during systole and reverse direction during diastole.

If the fistula is small, blood in the distal vein will flow in the normal direction past the fistula because the pressure at the venous end of the fistula is less than that at the site of collateral outflow. The pressure gradient will be normal, i.e. there will be a slight but progressive fall in pressure from the periphery towards the fistula. On the other hand if the fistula is large the pressure at the venous end of the fistula will be higher than the site of collateral out-flow, hence there is a retrograde flow in the distal vein. This flow will be prevented if a competent valve is present between these two points. In such a case the distal venous pressure may equal or even exceed that of the distal artery. With time and continued pressure the valve will become incompetent and then the blood will flow down the distal vein until it is diverted into the collateral vein. In chronic fistulas the excess pressure in the distal vein segment will neutralize and retrograde flow will cease.

The thrill and bruit so characteristic of an AVF are the results of turbulent flow that cause vibrations in the wall of the associated blood vessels. The factors responsible for these flow disturbances are: (1) increased velocity of blood flow, (2) abrupt change in the luminal diameter at the entrance to and exit from the fistula, and (3) arterial and venous flow streams either bifurcating at the entrance to and exit from the fistula or meeting the head on stream flow from the distal artery and distal vein respectively. Thus it is not surprising that the flow patterns are markedly disturbed and set up vibrations in the wall of the contributing vessels.

In addition to haemodynamic and flow changes, morphological changes also occur in the vessels. The proximal artery becomes elongated and tortuous. The arterial wall may initially become thickened but it eventually degenerates with atrophy of the smooth muscle, decrease in the quantity of the elastic tissue and formation of atheromatous plaques. These changes are irreversible if the fistula is allowed to persist for more than 2 years. The proximal vein similarly dilates and becomes tortuous. The internal elastic lamina tends to fragment and disappear, hence the term arterialization of the vein is inappropriate. Like the proximal vein the distal vein dilates and elongates and its valves become incompetent. The distal artery in contrast tends to remain the same size.

AVF constitute the most powerful stimulus to collateral development. Two major theories have been proposed: (1) collateral development is a function of an increased velocity of blood flow; or (2) it is a function of an increased pressure differential across the collateral bed. The weight of evidence appears to favour the former theory.

In summary, the local effects of AVF could be due to blood flow, pressure changes, turbulence, morphological changes or development of a collateral circulation around the fistula.

Peripheral effects

The peripheral effects of AVF are due to the lack of blood supply to the peripheral tissues. Low volume pulse, pallor, cyanosis and oedema are common. The temperature of the skin muscles and bone is elevated near the fistula and below normal distal to it. The venous blood draining these tissues shows an increased concentration of lactic acid owing to decreased oxygen tension. Such patients describe pain and paraesthesia and many develop ulceration and gangrene of the digits distal to the fistula. If the fistula is located proximally in the limb, patients may complain of intermittent claudication.

Systemic effects

The single most important change responsible for all the systemic effects of AVF is a drop in the total peripheral resistance. This in turn causes a fall in central arterial pressure, a rise in the central venous pressure, a reduction of systemic blood flow and shunting of blood from the arterial to the venous side of the circulation. Compensatory mechanisms come into action to avert these changes. The first change is an increase in the stroke volume, which is initiated by a rise in the central venous pressure. At the same time heart rate is increased by baroreceptor reflexes in response to the fall in arterial pressure. An increase in heart rate and stroke volume augments cardiac output (CO). In addition catecholamines and sympathetic discharges strengthen the myocardial contractility. This sympathoadrenal effect causes systemic arteriolar constriction which, although further reducing peripheral blood flow, increases peripheral resistance and helps to maintain central arterial pressure. The constriction of veins on the other hand facilitates venous return. Collectively these compensatory mechanisms increase and maintain the cardiac output hence increasing central arterial pressure. The CO is further augmented by an increase in blood volume mediated by the renin-angiotensin-aldosterone system which results in sodium and water retention.

When cardiac function is good the CO will increase sufficiently to bring the central arterial pressure to normal pre-fistula levels. This in turn switches off the sympathoadrenal effect, allowing the pulse rate to return to near normal and alleviating the peripheral vascular constriction. Systemic blood flow also returns to an adequate although somewhat reduced level. On the other hand, if the myocardium is damaged or the fistula is massive (e.g. aorto-caval) the compensation will be incomplete. Cardiac failure ensues and the increased CO will not be sufficient to maintain central arterial pressure and peripheral blood flow in the face of massive shunting from the arterial to the venous side of the circulation.

In compensated patients with the passage of time the fistula circuit continues to expand and arterial and venous collaterals continue to develop. The end result is a further drop in total peripheral resistance and increased cardiac output. Depending upon the state of the heart, patients may decompensate due to depletion of cardiac reserves; hence cardiac failure occurs.

Section 36.4 • Clinical presentation

As is evident from Figure 36.2, AVF can be classified into two basic types, acquired and congenital. Despite the same fundamental pathophysiological abnormality, the clinical presentation of AVF is extremely variable and depends upon the tissues involved, anatomical location, contiguous structures and the amount of blood shunted from the arterial to the venous circulation.

Acquired AVF

The diagnosis of acquired AVF is not usually difficult. A careful history and clinical examination are the key to the diagnosis. In the case of a major AVF between the aorta and its major branches there may or may not be a history of trauma. The symptoms of congestive cardiac failure may be evident. The patient may have abdominal pain secondary to visceral ischaemia, hypertension due to renal ischaemia and cerebrovascular insufficiency. In the case of an aorto-caval or ilio-caval fistula patients may experience intermittent claudication or critical leg ischaemia.

The classic signs are a bruit over the fistula, peripheral oedema, diminished distal pulses, increased venous pressure, pulsatile veins and increased pulse pressure. A clinical triad of sudden high output cardiac failure, lower limb ischaemia or venous engorgement and a thrill or bruit over the abdominal mass is diagnostic of an aorto-caval fistula. In the case of a fistula associated with an abdominal aortic aneurysm the symptoms may be intermittent as the thrombus in the aneurysm may cover the fistulous opening from time to time.

In peripheral AVF a history of penetrating injury is usually obtained which may be forgotten in long-standing chronic fistulas. Patients usually present with a pulsatile mass, which may be apparent by a vibrating sensation or buzzing sound over it. It is rare that the diagnosis has not been made before the symptoms of ischaemia and heart failure develop. Examination reveals the site of injury or old scar, a machinery murmur best heard over the fistula, elevated skin temperature over and reduced temperature distal to it. Veins are distended and may be varicose, and in long-standing fistulas chronic venous hypertension may cause skin changes characteristic of the post-phlebitic state. Tachycardia observed in these patients may be decreased by applying pressure to the proximal artery of the AVF (Branham's sign). According to Branham the heart rate slows down by more than four beats per minute and blood pressure temporarily increases. Atropine abolishes this reflex which is mediated by the vagus nerve.

Congenital AVF

Though present from birth, congenital AVF often may not become symptomatic until later in life. Those lesions with major AV shunting have a predilection to more rapid progression during adolescence and pregnancy. Those with a dermal component are easily visible although it is important to remember that the clinically obvious cutaneous mark may represent only a small part of the total lesion. The lesions may occur virtually anywhere. Fistulas within the chest, abdomen or brain are only detected when complications arise. The pelvis is one of the more common sites of vascular malformation whereas involvement of the extremities is rare. The history of onset of the lesion is the single most important question and will differentiate the AVM from haemangiomata that present a few weeks after birth and which have a far greater likelihood of spontaneous regression. The age at the time of first clinical presentation is inversely related to the severity of the lesion.

Young children present with obvious swelling, disfigurement, discoloration (birthmark) or limb enlargement. Adults more often complain of varicose veins, swelling, limb length discrepancies, aching and a heavy sensation in the affected extremity and in the pelvis in the case of pelvic lesions. They usually have a previously recognized birthmark. Women might have noticed exacerbation of their symptoms at menarche or during pregnancy. The most common presenting symptoms of AVM are a birthmark (70%) closely followed by varicose veins (60%). Pain, which can be severe, is often the reason for the request for treatment. Occasionally the pain is due to pressure on the local structures such as the brachial plexus. Ulceration and bleeding are late presentations. Ulceration occurs due to venous hypertension. The venous hypertension of AVM is never totally relieved by elevation and healing may be further impaired by a degree of superimposed ischaemia. Bleeding, fortunately rare, can be severe if there is a major arterial component to AVM. Bleeding can also occur from the low flow venous lesions but this is virtually never life threatening and is easily controlled by elevation or by direct pressure.

Asymmetric limb length can result from significant regional arteriovenous shunting by an incompletely understood mechanism or it may indicate significant osseous involvement. The changes in the soft tissues of the affected limb go hand in hand with osseous changes, but it must be remembered that giant hypertrophy of one limb can occur without an underlying AVM.

Physical examination of such lesions may reveal skin discoloration or an abdominal mass, which is usually firm, spongy and non-compressible except in predominantly venous lesions. Prominent pulsation and a thrill are characteristic findings and on auscultation a continuous or oscillating bruit can be found. Enlarged draining veins are characteristic and may or may not be pulsatile. Varicose veins are present in long-standing lesions and are not infrequently complicated by superficial phlebitis or even thrombosis. Many lesions are silent on auscultation but in some cases a fistula can be detected using handheld Doppler. Extremity lesions presenting with overgrown bone and soft tissues are disfiguring. Often the limb is not only longer but larger overall, hence recording serial measurements may be helpful in determining the rate of growth and the need for intervention as timing may be critical. Ischaemic ulceration with bleeding is sometimes seen in association with extremity lesions. The predominantly venous lesions empty completely on gentle compression and refill slowly. Venous lesions are most obvious when the affected area is dependent and on elevation it may appear completely normal. When close to the skin surface they have a distinct bluish discoloration and the overlying skin may be thinned even to the extent that ulceration and spontaneous bleeding occur. Venous lesions are usually asymptomatic. Mixed lesions such as the Klippel–Trenawnay syndrome, which in 95% of the cases affects the lower limb, present with bone and soft tissue hypertrophy. These lesions also consist of venous anomalies (varicosities), cutaneous capillary haemangiomas (port-wine stains) and lymphatic abnormalities. Some authors have postulated that congenital microscopic AVF (which are not visible on angiograms) are the cause of this syndrome. When these fistulous communications are demonstrable angiographically the condition is termed Parker–Weber syndrome.

Another lesion which warrants recognition is the Rendu–Osler–Weber syndrome which has an autosomal dominant pattern of inherentence. The characteristic lesions are discrete bright red maculopapules, which are typically located on the face, tongue, lips, nasal and oral mucous membranes. They are also seen on conjunctiva, palmar aspect of the fingers and in the nailbeds. These lesions involve the mucosal surface of the gastrointestinal tract, respiratory and genitourinary tract. Internally they may be found in the liver, spleen, pancreas, kidney and brain. In 50% of cases pulmonary AVF are present and may be complicated by cyanosis, finger clubbing and polycythaemia due to marked arteriovenous shunting.

Haemangiomas on the other hand appear 4 weeks after birth and 10–20% of Caucasian children have these lesions on their first birthday. They are more common in girls (3:1), in 8% of the cases are single and in 20% multiple. The commonest site of appearance is the head and neck (60%), followed by the trunk (25%) and the extremities (15%). They grow in the dermis (strawberry naevus) or deep in the lower dermis. The latter are best referred to deep haemangiomas and not by the old term cavernous haemangiomas. The history of onset is important. The lesions are bright scarlet in colour, and the colour deepens in the first year of life. On examination they are firm and rubbery in consistency and cannot be emptied of blood on compression. After an initial phase of rapid growth, involution of the lesions starts between 6 and 10 months. These regressing lesions present with deepening of the crimson colour to purple with greyish or white flecks and patches appearing in the lesion which become softer with slight wrinkling of the overlying skin. By the age of 5 years, 50% of the lesions are completely resolved, 70% at 7 years of age and 90% are gone by the age of 10 years. About 10% of haemangiomas do not resolve completely. Patients may present with ulceration or bleeding, primarily during the proliferative phase. Some lesions may present with visual interference or with subglottic haemangiomas. In the case of multiple cutaneous, hepatic, pulmonary or gastrointestinal tract haemangiomas, infants of 2–8 weeks may present with congestive heart failure and anaemia.

Section 36.5 • Diagnosis

In majority of individuals the diagnosis of an AVF is simple and requires nothing more than a good clinical history and physical examination and any further investigations are then part of the treatment process (as shown in Figure 36.3). Angiography is said to be the 'gold standard' for evaluating AVF, but with the advent of new non-invasive diagnostic techniques (particularly magnetic resonance imaging (MRI) angiography can now be limited to those patients who are likely to undergo interventional therapy.

Non-invasive tests

Doppler velocity waveforms (VWFs)

Use of handheld Doppler should be the part of examination. Using Doppler waveform analysis, the velocity of the blood flow can be recorded. Because of its greater peripheral resistance the velocity pattern in a resting extremity artery is normally tri-phasic with major forward flow in early systole, some flow reversal in late systole, minor forward flow in early diastole and negligible forward flow in late diastole. As a result of the latter the normal VWF rests on (or lies close to) the zero line. Significant AVF flow eliminates any end-systolic flow reversal and produces significant flow through diastole so the VWF tracing proximal to the fistula never drops near the zero line (Figure 36.4). In fact the degree of elevation of the velocity tracing above the baseline is directly proportional to the fistula flow. The VWF is the most sensitive and least specific non-invasive vascular test for AVF.

Duplex scanning

Duplex allows the nature and extent of more localized lesions to be well characterized. Examination of the venous system can largely be made by duplex-scanning, in particular the patency or otherwise of the deep venous system. In cases of traumatic AVF, particularly the iatrogenic variety produced by the percutaneous introduction of catheters via a femoral vessel, it readily detects the communication between the artery and the vein.

Measurement of mean arterial blood pressure

As pointed out earlier, the mean arterial blood pressure distal to an AVF is always reduced to some degree. The magnitude of the pressure drop across a fistula can provide the surgeon with an objective assessment of its

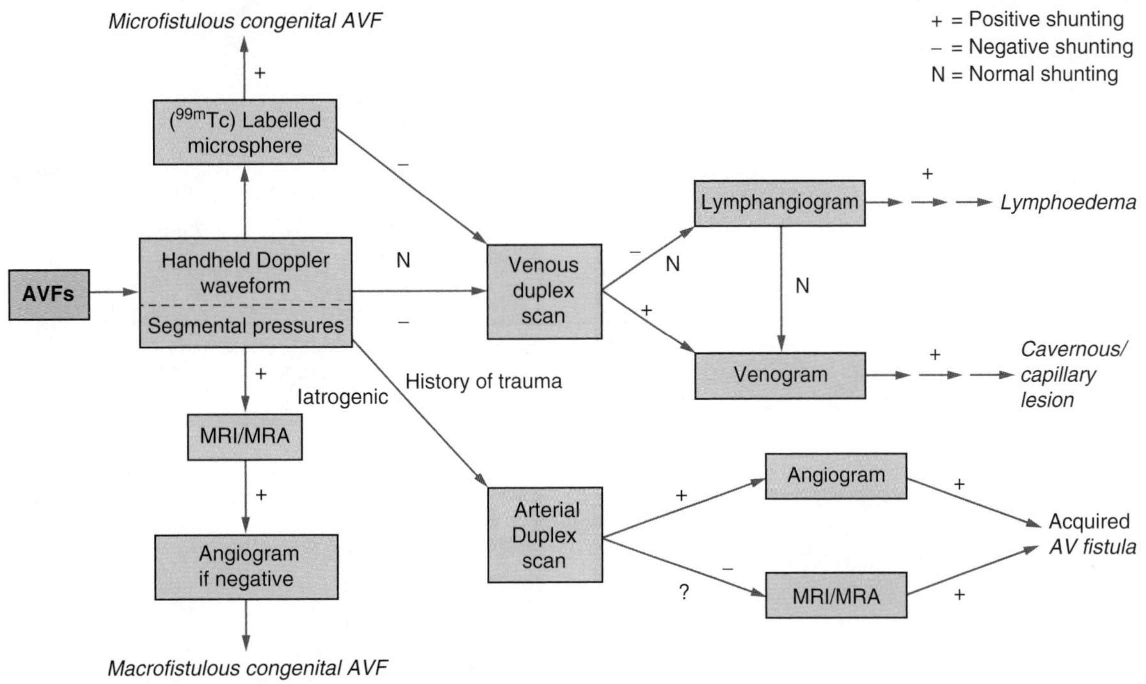

Figure 36.3 Investigation of microfistulous and macrofistulous congenital AVF.

haemodynamic consequences. A low peripheral pressure is not diagnostic of an AVF. If however the pulsatile mass is compressed and peripheral pressure rises, the diagnosis of AVF is established.

Segmental limb pressure

Proximal to the fistula the systolic pressure is often increased and distal to it the pressure may be normal or decreased. Segmental limb pressure may help locate an AVF by demonstrating a reduction in systolic pressure from above the fistula to below it when compared with the normal contralateral extremity.

Plain X-ray

This is of limited value but may reveal the extent of soft tissue swelling and calcification due usually to phleboliths within the lesion. Phleboliths are normally only seen in venous lesions. A chest X-ray is important in arterial lesions in order to monitor heart size.

Computed tomography and magnetic resonance imaging

The anatomical location, extent and involvement of important surrounding structures determine the resectability of a congenital AVF. Computed tomography (CT) and MRI both help define the anatomical involvement of such lesions. CT will usually demonstrate the location and extent of the lesion and even the involvement of specific muscle groups and bone. With contrast it provides a clear picture of the vascularity of the lesion.

MRI possesses a number of distinct advantages over CT in evaluating congenital AVF. There is no need for contrast; it differentiates muscle, bone, fat and blood vessels and thus demonstrates the anatomical extent more clearly. Longitudinal as well as transverse sections may be obtained and the flow patterns in the fistulas can be characterized. As a result, MRI has become the pivotal diagnostic study in the evaluation of most congenital AVF. Its current major drawback is a lack of universal availability.

Magnetic resonance angiography (MRA) is also employed in congenital AVF. With this technique vascular contrast is produced non-invasively by the phase response of moving protons and holds the promise of three-dimensional reconstruction. A recent study from South Manchester University Hospital did not find any additional practical information to the diagnostic process on MRA and recommended catheter angiography for congenital AVF.

Invasive tests

Labelled microspheres

Technetium (^{99m}Tc)-labelled human albumin microspheres can be used to diagnose and quantify arteriovenous shunting. The rationale is quite simple: microspheres too large to pass through capillaries are introduced into an artery. Those passing through an AVF are trapped in the lungs and the fraction reaching the lungs is determined by gamma camera. Naturally occurring arteriovenous shunts divert less than 3% of the blood flow. When the fraction of microspheres reaching the lung exceeds this value, abnormal shunting is present. This technique is useful as an initial diagnostic test and to evaluate therapy.

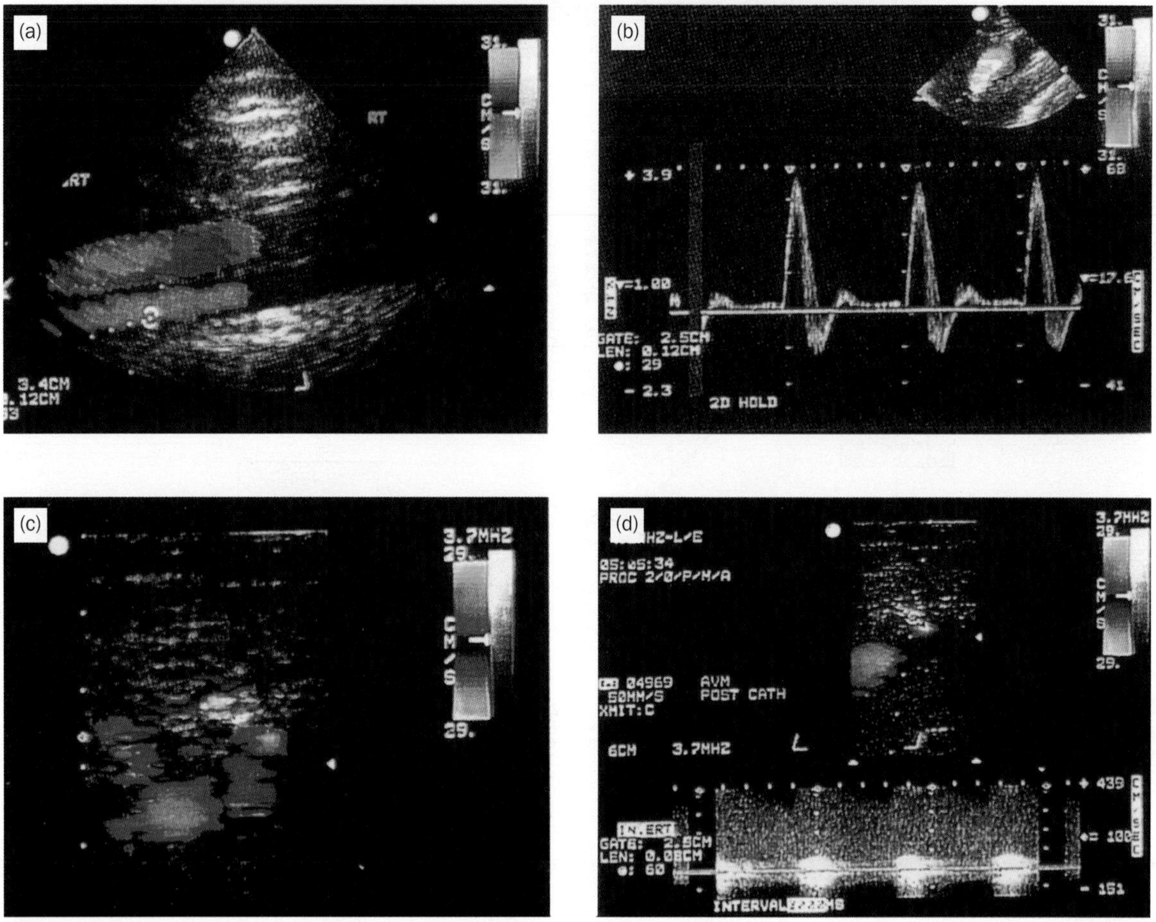

Figure 36.4 (a) Superficial femoral artery. At rest, flow is characterized by rapid changes of flow magnitude and direction. At this point in the cardiac cycle, the image shows flow reversal at the artery walls while there is still forward flow in the centre of the vessel as a result of the different momentum of blood at these two sites. (b) Flow waveform: common femoral artery. The waveform is described as triphasic with reversed flow following the systolic peak and a period of forward flow in late diastole. This waveform is typical of a healthy peripheral artery under at-rest conditions. (c) Arteriovenous malformation (fistula): the femoral artery and vein are imaged in a transverse view. There is a flow channel not normally seen at this site. (d) Pulsed wave Doppler showing a very high velocity dampened pulsatility waveform in the abnormal flow channel. The waveform is typical of flow in a small conduit with very low distal resistance – in this case forming part of an arteriovenous shunt.

Venography

This is still useful in order to visualize the venous system when surgical intervention is planned. It is particularly useful in Klippel–Trenaunay syndrome and demonstrates absence of deep veins.

Angiography

Angiography is necessary in most acquired AVF (Figure 36.5). In cases of congenital AVF it is employed in arterialized lesions with an intent to treat. It is often possible to proceed to treatment at the same time.

In acquired AVF the actual communication may be apparent, otherwise the point of initial venous filling indicates the site of the fistula. Not uncommonly, aneurysms are found in the vicinity of the fistula.

In cases of congenital AVF which require treatment, angiography is performed in lesions with a dominant arterial contribution. It should not be employed for diagnosis and should be delayed as long as possible to avoid angiography in children. The route of injection should be arterial, as intravenous studies are confusing. The angiographic appearance of such lesions is complex owing to multiple feeding and draining vessels and because the communications may be quite small and often are of microscopic size.

An angiogram is carried out usually from the groin and selective arterial injections are required. More than one source of supply should be investigated and any treatment must be directed at all of these sources otherwise the lesion will rapidly be revascularized from alternative vessels.

Lymphangiography

This is rarely indicated and is used for lesions with low flow where Doppler examination has ruled out a significant venous contribution. The lymphatic component of some mixed congenital AVF can be assessed. In one study, 84% of the patients with mixed lesions demonstrated abnormal lymphangiograms.

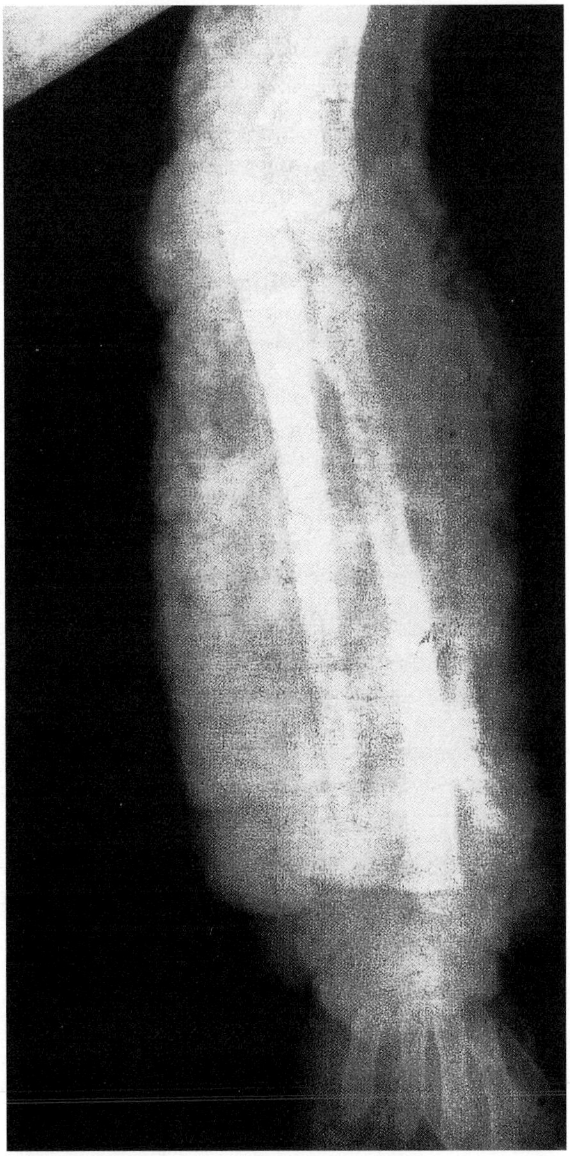

Figure 36.5 Angiography: arteriovenous malformation of left arm.

There are three basic diagnostic goals in evaluating patients with congenital AVF: (1) to establish diagnosis and categorize the dominant lesion, (2) to define anatomical the extent of the lesions and (3) to determine the local and systemic haemodynamic effects.

The first two goals are directed to define the lesion and the third goal is to help establish the need for intervention. The recommended diagnostic approach is shown in the algorithm in Figure 36.3. It is worth mentioning that angiography, venography and lymphangiography should be undertaken only when intervention is required for significant functional or cosmetic disability.

Other tests which can be useful in the diagnosis of AVF are: plethysmography, volume flow measurement, direct measurement of skin temperature, cardiac output and venous oxygen tension.

Section 36.6 • Management

As is evident from the previous discussion, acquired and congenital AVFs are two different entities, so their management is also different. In acquired AVF the goal of treatment should be early, complete closure either surgically or by percutaneous techniques, whereas the most frequently chosen treatment option in congenital AVF is conservative management.

Acquired AVF

The history of the treatment of such lesions is a fascinating tale of clinical frustration, scientific observation and surgical ingenuity. William Hunter in 1762 described the AVF for the first time. The management options of conservative treatment, ligation of the proximal and distal arteries or opening of the sac and tying off the feeding vessels were debated until the 1900s. After the experience of World War II and the Vietnam war, it became clear that early surgical treatment of traumatic fistulas with establishment of arterial and venous continuity is the best therapeutic option for such fistulas.

AVF of the aorta and its major branches present an unparalleled challenge because of their central location, amount of blood shunted, associated complications which are dramatic and extensive haemorrhage during operation. It is imperative to establish a pre-operative diagnosis in such fistulas. The surgeon should also be aware that patients with chronic AVF are usually hypervolaemic and do not need volume blood replacement. On the other hand patients with acute fistulas may be hypovolaemic due to blood loss despite the presence of pulsating veins. As the central venous pressure is elevated, this cannot be used as a guide for fluid replacement – a Swan–Ganz catheter (pulmonary artery flotation catheter) should be used for this purpose. When surgery is performed enough blood must be available and auto-transfusion is highly recommended in such cases. The goal of surgical therapy is to close the fistula, to restore normal haemodynamics and to re-establish vascular continuity. In case of aorto-caval fistula the closure of the fistula is achieved from within the aorta. The IVC is compressed both proximal and distal to the fistula and non-absorbable sutures are used to close the communication. After the IVC is repaired the aortic continuity is restored with a Dacron graft. Special care should be taken when manipulating the aortic aneurysm (if present) which is filled with thrombus. If the thrombus is dislodged, it will embolize to the pulmonary artery through the fistula and IVC. Occasionally, abdominal aortic aneurysm can rupture into the left renal vein, most commonly when it is retro-aortic. Such communication is managed as an aorto-caval fistula.

In cases of AVF in the base of the neck between suclavian artery and vein or carotid artery and internal jugular vein, there is little place for non-operative therapy. Their natural history is that the false aneurysm continues to grow and will rupture or the patient will develop symptoms of cardiovascular insufficiency. The fistulas at the base of the neck are approached by a trap door incision but the left subclavian artery is best controlled through left anterior thoracotomy.

In cases of peripheral AVF (particularly congenital), ligation of the proximal artery should be avoided at all costs not only because of its failure to cure the fistula but also because it closes the avenue for interventional radiology techniques. The choice of surgery or interventional radiology depends on the site and size, accessibility and aetiology of the fistula. Using interventional radiology, the arteries can be obliterated by percutaneously placed detachable balloons or embolic agents (i.e. stainless steel coils), liquid embolic agents like cyanoacrylate tissue adhesive, polyvinyl alcohol particles (Ivalon) and liquid silicone. When embolic agents are used to obliterate the fistula, care is taken to avoid loss of embolic agent into the venous circulation by the use of an occlusive balloon catheter. Whether the fistula is closed surgically or by percutaneous techniques, it is important to be sure of the distal circulation. When major vessels are involved, sacrifice of the major feeding artery is not an option. In such cases the treatment of choice is direct surgical repair and arterial and venous reconstruction using saphenous vein when possible.

Finally, if the fistula occurs in an area that is surgically inaccessible, e.g. carotid-cavernous fistula, interventional radiology is the treatment of choice.

Congenital AVF

Management of congenital AVF presents an extremely difficult therapeutic challenge. The management options vary widely ranging from counselling to complex excisional surgery. The most frequently chosen course is conservative. Absolute indications for treatment include haemorrhage, distal ischaemia due to arterial steal, congestive cardiac failure and refractory ulceration due to venous hypertension. Relative indications for treatment are pain, limiting claudication, functional impairment of the extremity and significant cosmetic deformity.

The basic approach is to use the minimal intervention compatible with control of symptoms and prevention of complications. The patient's family usually requires considerable time and support as many parents have a sense of guilt believing that AVF appear as the result of some event during pregnancy. Most parents and patients hope for a cure and it is difficult to explain that the basis of treatment is to control rather than cure. For peripheral lesions, deformity and pain can sometimes be simply managed with a class III compression stocking.

A multidisciplinary approach to the management is mandatory. A surgeon should see such patients in the outpatient clinic with an interventional radiologist who has an interest in congenital AVF. A cardiologist may be needed to assess the heart, an orthopaedic surgeon may be required for the management of limb length, a plastic surgeon may have to deal with disfigurement and a facio-maxillary surgeon can deal with common oral and facial lesions.

The conservative management includes support stockings and elevation of the extremity to control the complications of venous hypertension. Follow-up is important as intervention may become necessary at a later date because conservative treatment only delays the progression of symptoms.

The appearance of vascular tumours and secondary deposits may be similar to a congenital AVF, so the possibility must be kept firmly in mind and when in doubt biopsy must be undertaken. The goal of surgery should be complete resection of the lesion. If it is possible and safe this is an attractive proposition in the hope of preventing the need for further treatment. Such an opportunity is, however, rare (10% or less). More often partial excision is achieved by removing the area that is most disfiguring. Ligation of feeding arteries is only temporarily effective due to rapid development of the collaterals and should be avoided as it makes further treatment, especially embolization, impossible. Surgical skeletonization involves the ligation of all supplying vessels coming off the adjacent main artery. It has now been superseded by therapeutic embolization and is not recommended. Surgical intervention is made easier by prior embolization, which is performed as near to the time of surgery as feasible in order to prevent recurrence or enlargement of collateral vessels. Amputation is occasionally necessary but is only required on rare occasions when other methods of control have failed to control the pain, bleeding or ulceration. On occasions, especially in previously treated fistulas where the feeding vessel has been ligated, it becomes impossible to obtain a route of access for embolization. In such cases access may be provided by vein bypass or direct repair of the vessel. On occasions where embolization fails and excision is not possible intra-tumoral ligation (sutural compartmentalization) is performed. In this technique a large handheld needle is used to under-run the lesion in a criss-cross fashion, either externally or subcutaneously. This results in a cobblestone appearance, which induces thrombosis in all of the compartmentalized segments of the lesion because of the obliteration of blood flow. It may appear rather ugly but the procedure can be life saving. In very extensive lesions where the only hope is control, total circulatory arrest and cardiopulmonary bypass may be considered.

Therapeutic embolization is the mainstay of treatment in most high flow lesions but although excellent palliation may be achieved using this technique, a cure is unlikely. Thus embolization therapy necessitates a commitment to long-term follow-up and repeated intervention as required. Great care has to be taken when planning embolization to anticipate the resulting flow changes which might jeopardize an adjacent organ. Hands and feet are particularly difficult to treat because of the risk of blocking digital arteries with embolic material. Embolization is performed under general anaesthesia to obviate pain and intolerance for an often lengthy procedure and is always necessary in children. The treatment usually has to be repeated at least once and sometimes multiple sessions are required. The principle of treatment is to fill the lesion from within by selective catheterization of the feeding artery. The embolic materials most appropriate for embolization include microparticles or liquids that can reach the small calibre vascular bed. Ivalon (polyvinyl alcohol) particles ranging in size from 100 to 500 μm are useful for precapillary occlusion. Absolute ethanol and cyanoacrylate adhesive can also be used.

Low flow lesions are impossible to treat with embolization. It may be possible to treat them by direct pressure sclerotherapy, which is performed under imaging control. Direct puncture of one of the varicosities is made, note is made of the venous drainage and the volume of contrast used is measured. Direct pressure or temporary occlusion is applied to occlude important outflow veins. The lesion is then compressed to collapse and the sclerosant injected to a volume approximating the volume of contrast required for obtaining the diagnostic image. Of the variety of agents used for venous sclerotherapy the most commonly used are absolute alcohol, 3% sodium tetradecyl sulfate (STD) and Ethibloc. Lymphatic lesions can be treated by percutaneous sclerotherapy and this may be usefully combined with surgery in certain individuals.

Embolization is not without complications. Minor complications include leucocytosis, pyrexia, mild to moderate pain, tissue necrosis and sensory or motor deficits that do not require specific treatment. Major complications include extensive tissue and skin necrosis requiring skin grafting, inadvertent embolization of normal vessels especially of hands and feet, necessitating amputation, pulmonary embolization and permanent neurological deficit resulting from embolization of critical vasa nervosum. In general, procedures in the hands and feet are reserved for patients in whom the only alternative is amputation.

Haemangiomas resolve spontaneously in 90% of the children by the age of 10 years. The remaining 10% may develop problems and treatment is reserved for lesions producing functional impairment or life-threatening complications. Even in these, therapeutic options are limited. Corticosteroids and radiotherapy are inconsistently effective whereas embolization has been used successfully in some patients to speed the process of involution. Surgery in such cases is difficult and potentially disfiguring and is reserved for lesions producing life-threatening complications.

Conclusion

In conclusion, acquired AVF usually result from trauma and in most cases consist of a single fistula associated with high flow. They respond well to surgical closure, which is necessitated by the local and systemic complications. On the other hand congenital AVF represent a diverse group of lesions, which in the majority of cases are treated conservatively. Whenever treatment is required it is extremely difficult and should be directed at eradication of the lesion. This can be achieved by embolization, surgical excision or a combination of the two. Low-flow lesions can be treated successfully by direct puncture and sclerotherapy. The complexity of the congenital lesions demands a multidisciplinary approach to achieve best results.

Further reading

Barker, W. H., Sharzer, L. A. and Ehrenhaft, J. L. (1972). Aortocaval fistula as a complication of abdominal aortic aneurysm. *Surgery* **72**: 933.

Belov, S. (1993). Anatomopathological classification of congenital vascular defects. *Semin Vasc Surg* **6**: 219.

Berenstein, A. and Kricheff, I. I. (1997). Catheter and material selection for transarterial embolization. Technical consideration. II. Material. *Radiology* **132**(3): 631.

Berenstein, A., Scott, J., Choi, I. S. and Persky, M. (1986). Percutaneous embolization of arteriovenous fistulas of the external carotid artery. *Am J Neuroradiol* **7**: 937.

Bernardino, M. E., Jing, B. S., Thomas, J. L. *et al.* (1981). The extremity soft tissue lesions: a comparative study of ultrasound, computed tomography and xeroradiography. *Radiology* **139**: 53.

Boon, L. M., Mulliken, J. B., Vikkula, M. *et al.* (1994). Assignment of a locus for dominantly inherited venous malformations to chromosome 9p. *Hum Mol Genet* **3**: 1583.

Branham, H. H. (1890). Aneurysmal varix of the femoral artery and vein following a gun shot wound. *Int J Surg* **3**: 250.

Cohen, J. M., Weinreb, J. C. and Redman, H. C. (1986). Arteriovenous malformations of the extremities: MR imaging. *Radiology* **158**: 475.

Connall, T. P. and Wilson, S. E. (1995). Vascular access for haemodialysis. In: Ratherford, R. B. ed. *Vascular Surgery*, 4th edn. Philadelphia: W. B. Saunders, 1233.

Cotton, L. T. and Sykes, B. J. (1969). The treatment of diffuse congenital arterivenous fistulae of the leg. *Proc R Soc Med* **62**: 245.

de Takats, G. (1931). Vascular anomalies of the extremities. *Surg Gynecol Obstet* **55**, 227.

Derbun, G., Lacour, P., Caron, J. P. *et al.* (1975). Inflatable and released balloon techniques. Experimental in dog, application in man. *Neuroradiology* **9**: 267.

Dobson, M. J., Hartley, R. W. J., Ashleigh, R. *et al.* (1997). MR angiography and MR imaging of symptomatic vascular malformations. *Clin Radiol* **52**: 595.

Erdmann, M. W. H., Davies, D. M., Jackson, J. E. and Allison, D. J. (1995). Multidisciplinary approach to the management of head and neck arteriovenous malformations. *Ann R Coll Surg Engl* **77**: 53.

Fishman, S. J. and Mulliken, J. B. (1993). Hemangiomas and vascular malformations of infancy and childhood. *Pediatr Clin North Am* **40**: 1177.

Gallione, C. J., Pasyk, K., Boon, L. M. *et al.* (1995). A gene for familial venous malformations maps to chromosome 9p in a second large kindred. *J Med Genet* **32**: 197.

Graham, J. M., McCollum, C. H., Crawford, E. S. *et al.* (1980). Extensive arterial aneurysm formation proximal to ligated arteriovenous fistula. *Ann Surg* **191**: 200.

Halliday, A. W. and Mansfield, A. O. (1993). Congenital vascular malformations. *Br J Surg* **80**: 2.

Hunter, W. (1762). Further observations upon a particular species of aneurysm. *Med Observ Inquiries* **2**: 390.

Ingebrigtsen, R. and When, P. S. (1995). Local blood pressure in congenital arteriovenous fistulae. *Acta Med Scand* **163**: 169.

Ingebrigtsen, R., Krog, J. and Leraand, S. (1963). Circulation distal to experimental arteriovenous fistulas of the extremities: a polaragraphic study. *Acta Chir Scand* **125**: 308.

Jackson, J. E. (1998). Vascular malformations. In: Beard, J. D. and Gaines, P. A. eds. *Vascular and Endovascular Surgery*. London: W. B. Saunders, 461.

Jackson, C., Greene, H., O'Neill, J. *et al.* (1977). Hepatic haemangioendothelioma: angiographic approaches and apparent prednisone responsiveness. *Am J Dis Child* **131**: 74.

Jamison, J. P. and Wallace, W. F. M. (1976). The pattern of venous drainage of surgically created side to side arteriovenous fistulae in the human forearm. *Clin Sci Mol Med* **50**: 37.

John, H. T. and Warren, R. (1961). The stimulus to collateral circulation. *Surgery* **49**: 14.

Lauigne, J. E., Mesinna, L. M., Golding, M. R. *et al.* (1977). Fistula size and haemodynamic events within and about canine femoral arteriovenous fistulas. *J Thorac Cardiovasc Surg* **74**: 551.

Lie, M., Sejerated, O. M. and Kiil, F. (1970). Local regulation of vascular cross-section during changes in femoral artery blood flow in dogs. *Circ Res* **27**: 727.

Lough, F. C., Giordano, J. M. and Hobson, R. W. II (1976). Regional haemodynamics of large and small femoral arteriovenous fistulas in dogs. *Surgery* **73**: 346.

Malen, E., ed. (1974). Vascular malformations. *Milan Carol Erba Foundation* 41.

Mansfield, A. O. (1994). Arteriovenous malformations. In: Galland R. B. and Clyne C. A. C., eds. *Clinical Problems in Vascular Surgery*. London: Edward Arnold, 242.

McAuley, C. E., Peitzman, A. B., deVries, E. J. *et al.* (1986). The syndrome of spontaneous iliac arteriovenous fistula: a distinct clinical and pathophysiologic entity. *Surgery* **99**: 373.

McCue, C. M., Hartenberg, M. and Nance, W. E. (1984). Pulmonary arteriovenous malformations related to Rendu-Osler-Weber Syndrome. *Am J Med Genet* **19**: 19.

McDonald, M. T., Papenberg, K. A., Ghosh, S. *et al.* (1994). Genetic linkage of hereditary haemorrhagic telangiectasia to mark on 9q. *Nat Genet* **6**: 197.

Meuli, R. A., Wedeen, V. J., Geller, S. C. *et al.* (1986). MR gated subtraction angiography: evaluation of lower extremities. *Radiology* **159**: 411.

Mulliken, J. B. (1988). Classification of vascular birthmark. In: Mulliken, J. B. and Young, A. E. eds, *Vascular Birthmarks Haemangiomas and Malformations*. Philadelphia: W.B. Saunders, 24.

Mulliken, J. B., Zetter, B. R. and Felkman, J. (1982). *In vitro* characterization of endothelium for haemangiomas and vascular malformations. *Surgery* **92**: 348.

O'Donnel, T. F. Jr, Edwards, J. M. and Kinmonth, J. B. (1976). Lymphangiography in congenital mixed vascular deformities of the lower extremities. *J Cardiovasc Surg* **17**: 535.

Popesco, V. (1985). Intratumoral ligation in the management of orofascial cavernous haemangiomas. *J Maxillofasc Surg* **13**: 99.

Reilly, D. T., Wood, R. F. M. and Bell, P. R. F. (1982). Arteriovenous fistulas for dialysis: blood flow, viscosity and long term patency. *World J Surg* **6**: 628.

Riles, T. S., Rosen, R. J. and Berenstein, A. (1995). Peripheral arteriovenous fistulae. In: Rutherford, R. B. ed, *Vascular Surgery*, 4th edn. Philadelphia: W.B. Saunders, 1211.

Rosen, R. J., Riles, T. S. and Berenstein, A. (1995). Congenital vascular malformation. In: Rutherford, R. B. ed, *Vascular Surgery*, 4th edn. Philadelphia: W. B. Saunders, 1218.

Rotan, M., John, M., Stowe, S. *et al.* (1980). Radiation treatment of pediatric hepatic hemangiomatosis and coexisting cardiac failure. *N Engl J Med* **302**: 852.

Rozin, L. and Perper, J. A. (1989). Spontaneous fatal perforation of aorta and vena cava by Mobin-Uddin umbrella. *Am J Forensic Med Pathol* **10**: 149.

Rutherford, R. B. and Sumner, D. S. (1995). Diagnostic evaluation of arteriovenous fistulas. In: Rutherford, R. B., ed. *Vascular Surgery*, 4th edn. Philadelphia: W.B. Saunders, 1192.

Rutherford, R. B., Anderson, B. O. and Durham, J. D. (1998). Congenital vascular malformations of the extremities. In: Moore, W. S., ed. *Vascular Surgery A Comprehensive Review*, 5th edn. Philadelphia: W. B. Saunders, 191.

Schwartz, R. S., Osmundson, P. J. and Hollier, L. H. (1986). Treatment and prognosis in congenital arteriovenous malformation of the extremity. *Phlebology* **1**: 177.

Shovlin, C.L., Hughes, J. M. B., Tuddenham, E. C. D. *et al.* (1994). A gene for hereditary haemorrhagic telangiectasia maps to chromosome 9q3. *Nat Genet* **6**: 205.

Silverman, R. A. (1991). Haemangiomas and vascular malformations. *Pediatr Clin North Am* **38**: 811.

Simkins, T. E. and Stehbens, W. E. (1974). Vibrations recorded from the advential surface of experimental aneurysms and arteriovenous fistula. *Vasc Surg* **8**: 153.

Stanley, P., Grinnell, V.S., Stanton, R. E. *et al.* (1983). Therapeutic embolization of infantile hepatic hemangioma with polyvinyl alcohol. *Am J Roentgenol* **141**: 1047.

Stehbens, W. E. (1974). The ultrastructure of the anastomosed vein of experimental arteriovenous fistulae in sheep. *Am J Pathol* **76**: 377.

Szilagyi, D. E., Elliot, J., DeRusso, F. *et al.* (1965). Peripheral congenital arteriovenous fistulas. *Surgery* **57**: 61.

Szilagyi, D. E., Smith, R. F., Elliott, J. P. and Hageman, J. H. (1976). Congenital arteriovenous anamolies of the limbs. *Arch Surg* **111**: 423.

Woollard, H. H. (1922). The development of the principal arterial stems in the fore limb of the pig. *Cont Embryol* **14**: 139.

Woolley, M. M., Stanley, P. and Wesley, J. R. (1977). Peripherally located congenital arteriovenous fistulae in infancy and childhood. *J Pediatr Surg* **12**: 165.

Young, A. E. (1988). Pathogenesis of vascular malformations. In: Mulliken, J. B. and Young, A. E., eds. *Vascular Birthmarks, Haemangiomas and Malformation*. Philadelphia: W.B. Saunders, 107.

Young, A. E. (1992). Congenital vascular anomalies. In: Bell, P. R. F., Jamieson, C.W. and Ruckley, C.V., eds. *Surgical Management of Vascular Diseases*. London: W.B. Saunders, 1069.

MODULE 37

Lymphoedema

1 • The lymphatic system
2 • Structure and function
3 • Lymph drainage of specific tissues and regions
4 • Lymphoedema

Section 37.1 • The lymphatic system

Overview of structure and function

Functions

The lymphatic system is absolutely vital for the normal functioning of the macrovasculature and microvasculature. Total lymphatic failure, for even a few hours, would lead to death. Despite this, the lymphatics are often given little consideration compared to the arterial and venous systems. The lymphatic system performs three key functions:

- it permits the circulation of immunologically competent cells, particularly lymphocytes
- intestinal lymph (chyle) transports cholesterol, triglycerides, medium chain fatty acids, and the fat soluble vitamins (A, D, E and K) directly to the circulation, bypassing the liver
- it removes water, electrolytes, low molecular weight substances (polypeptides, cytokines, growth factors) and macromolecules (fibrinogen, albumin, globulins, coagulation and fibrinolytic factors) from the interstitial space and returns them to the circulation.

Anatomy

Lymphatics accompany veins everywhere in the body except in the cortical bony skeleton and central nervous system, although the brain and retina possess analogous systems (cerebrospinal fluid and aqueous humour respectively). The lymphatic system comprises lymphatics, lymphoid organs (lymph nodes, spleen, Peyer's patches, thymus, tonsils) and the circulating elements (lymphocytes and other mononuclear immune cells) contained within it.

About 10% of lymph arising from a limb is transported in deep lymphatic ducts that accompany the main neurovascular bundles (Figure 37.1). The majority of lymph, however, is conducted in epifascial lymph ducts, against venous flow from the core of the limb to the surface. Superficial ducts form lymph bundles of various sizes that are located within strips of adipose tissue, and tend to follow the course of the major superficial veins (Figure 37.2).

Lymph from the lower limbs and abdomen drains to the cisterna chyli, which lies between the aorta and azygos vein, and then to the thoracic duct (see below). Lymph from the head and right arm drains, via the right lymphatic duct, into the right internal jugular vein. Lymph nodes develop as condensations along the course of these lymphatic highways.

Section 37.2 • Structure and function

Lymphatic capillaries

Lymphatic capillaries originate within the interstitial space either from specialized endothelialized blind-ended (initial) lymphatics, or from non-endothelialized pre-capillary channels such as the spaces of Disse in the liver. Initial lymphatic capillaries are unlike arterio-venous capillaries in that:

- they are blind-ended
- they are much larger (50 μm)
- they allow the entry of macromolecules up to 1000 kDa. This is because the basement membrane is fenestrated, even absent, and because the endothelium itself possesses intra- and intercellular pores
- endothelial cells overlap each other to form rudimentary inlet valves
- the abluminal surface of the endothelium is attached to the interstitial matrix through collagenous and elastic anchoring filaments. At rest, lymphatic capillaries are collapsed. However, when interstitial fluid volume and pressure increases, the interstitial space expands, and lymphatic capillaries and their pores are pulled open by these filaments to facilitate increased lymphatic drainage.

Collecting lymphatics

Lymphatic capillaries drain into pre-collectors, which in turn drain into collecting lymphatics that possess bicuspid valves and endothelial cells rich in the contractile protein actin. Larger collecting lymphatics are innervated and surrounded by smooth muscle. Valves partition these lymphatics into segments termed lymphangions, which are believed to contract sequentially to propel lymph into the lymph trunks. The area of skin drained by a single terminal lymphatic is termed an areola.

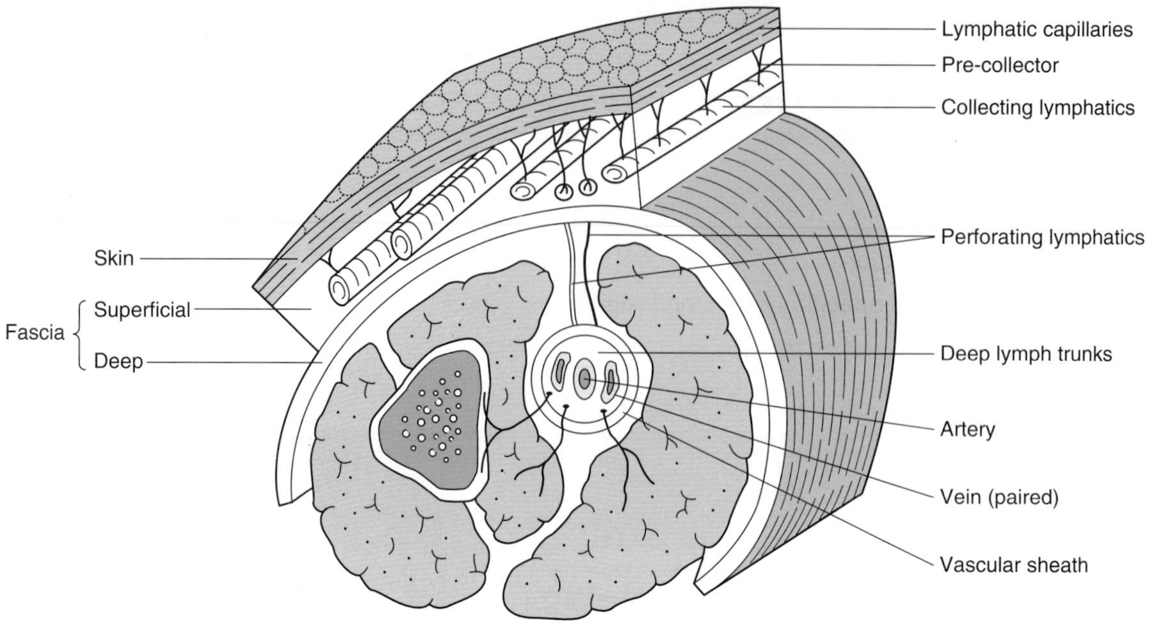

Figure 37.1 In the extremities two lymphatic pathways can be distinguished. The superficial system drains the skin, subcutaneous and epifascial layers. Superficial trunks tend to follow the course of the superficial veins. The deep system drains structures deep to the deep fascia. Bones may not have lymphatic vessels. Deep lymph trunks follow the neurovascular bundle of the limb. It is believed that arterial pulsation may promote lymphatic drainage. Lymph flows from the deep to superficial system through perforators that are found at the site of lymph nodes and may also run with perforating veins.

Lymphatic anastomoses

Although there is some overlap between adjacent areolata, there are lymphatic watersheds and there is limited capacity for bypass flow when a main collecting duct or lymph trunk is blocked.

Lymph trunks

Collecting lymphatics lead to lymph trunks which comprise a single layer of endothelial cells, a basement membrane and a media containing smooth muscle cells that are innervated by sympathetic and parasympathetic, motor and sensory nerve endings. These vessels possess inner longitudinal and outer circular muscle layers and an adventitia. This musculature allows the propulsion of lymph. There are generally few connections between the deep and superficial system except at the site of regional nodes. The larger trunks are supplied with their own vasa vasorum and are accompanied by a plexus of fine blood vessels. In lymphangitis, this plexus becomes congested and leads to the characteristic painful, red lines seen in the skin.

Lymph nodes

As well as the lymphatic vessels, the lymphoreticular system comprises condensations of the lymphoid tissue; namely:

- Primary: thymus and bone marrow.
- Secondary: lymph nodes, spleen, Waldeyer's rings (tonsils and adenoids) and lymphatic tissues of the mucous membranes (respiratory and alimentary tracts).

The function of the central or primary lymphatic tissues, the thymus and bone marrow, is the production of immunologically diverse and competent T- and B-lymphocytes. The secondary or peripheral lymphoid tissues are involved with the presentation of antigen.

Lymph nodes are present in groups or nodal chains situated alongside blood vessels. In total there are about 700 lymph nodes in the human body, of which approximately 150 are located in the mesentery. The number, size and distribution of lymph nodes varies considerably between different body regions. However, they can be classified into three main types:

- intermediate nodes: these lie alongside, or in the path of major lymph trunks from the extremity, e.g. nodes around the popliteal and antecubital fossae
- regional or primary lymph nodes: these drain large body territories, e.g. inguinal and axillary nodes
- central nodes: these lie between the regional nodes and the venous system.

Lymph nodes serve three main functions:

- filtration of potentially damaging material such as effete cells, bacteria and antigens
- presentation of antigen to lymphocytes which then undergo clonal expansion and leave the lymph node to mount a systemic immune response
- regulation of the protein content of efferent lymph. Excess protein leaves the lymphatic circulation through the nodal lymph–blood barrier.

The protein content of lymph arriving at lymph nodes from the periphery (afferent lymph) varies from about 2 g/dl for the extremities to 6 g/dl for the liver depending on the 'leakiness' of the capillary bed. As lymph passes through lymph nodes, it is exposed to a rich vascular capillary network. At this point fluid, elec-

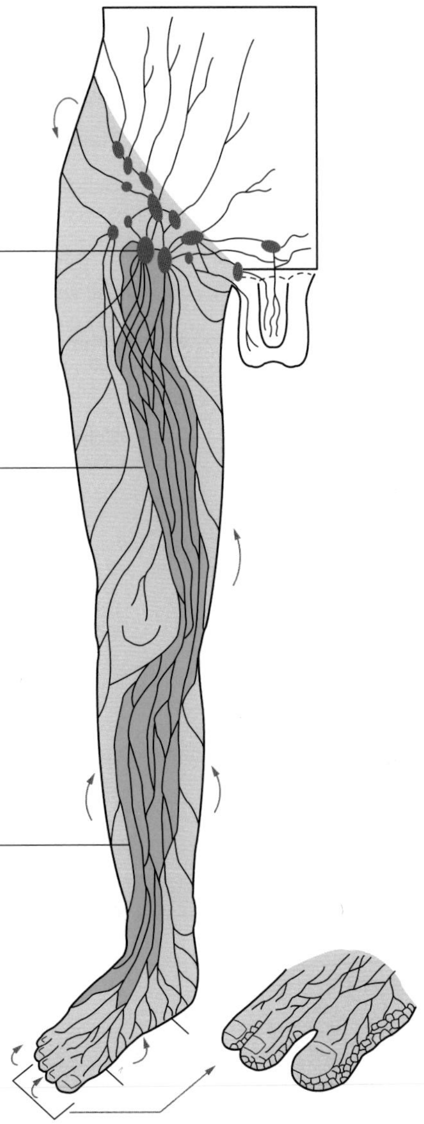

Figure 37.2 Most of the lymphatic outflow from the lower limb runs in the ventromedial bundle to the inguinal lymph nodes. This is wide in the calf and thigh and thus more resistant to injury. However, it is narrow at the level of the knee and at risk from surgical intervention; for example, stripping of the long saphenous vein.

trolytes and low molecular weight substances (but not protein) are exchanged to achieve hydrostatic and osmotic equilibrium. Thus, lymph leaving lymph nodes (efferent lymph) may have a quite different composition from afferent lymph. The protein content of lymph entering the thoracic duct is about 3–4 g/dl as, generally, lymph is concentrated via its passage through lymph nodes.

Lymph ducts

The thoracic duct returns about 80% of lymph to the circulation and the right lymph duct returns most of the remainder. The thoracic duct begins as the cisterna chyli, which lies on the bodies of the first and second lumbar vertebrae and receives the intestinal and lumbar lymph trunks (Figure 37.3). The duct proper begins at the lower border of the twelfth thoracic vertebra and enters the thorax alongside the aorta. It ascends the posterior mediastinum with the aorta on its left and azygos vein on its right. At the level of the fifth thoracic vertebra the duct inclines to the left and runs along the left side of the oesophagus through the superior mediastinum. It passes behind the aortic arch and left subclavian artery. The duct rises as high as the seventh cervical vertebra some 3–4 cm above the clavicle where it arches laterally across the vertebral vessels, the sympathetic trunk, the phrenic nerve at the medial border of scalenus anterior and the thyrocervical trunk and its branches. At this point it lies behind the common carotid artery, vagus nerve and internal jugular vein. It then descends anterior to the left subclavian artery and usually terminates at the junction of the left internal jugular and subclavian veins. The duct receives tributaries from the left chest, arm and head and neck. The duct varies from 2 to 5 mm in diameter and can be damaged in the course of operations in the abdomen, chest and neck. Injury can lead to chyloperitoneum or thorax. As such lymph contains protein and fat it is a source of nutrients for bacteria and secondary infection may occur. The right lymph duct is about 1 cm long and opens in a mirror image fashion into the great veins of the right neck having received tributaries from the right arm, head and neck and chest.

Function

Starling's forces

Starling described the balance of hydrostatic and oncotic pressures that, together with the relative impermeability of the blood capillary membrane to molecules over 70 kDa, determine the distribution of fluid and protein between the vascular and interstitial spaces. Briefly, water, low molecular weight substances and a small amount of protein enter the interstitial space at the arterial end of the capillary because of hydrostatic pressure. This leads to an increase in plasma oncotic pressure such that most (>90%) of the water re-enters the venous end of the capillary due to osmosis. The only way the remaining water, and importantly the accompanying micro- and macro-molecules can exit the interstitial space is via the lymphatics. This is termed the obligatory lymph load and is about 2–4 litres per 24 hours in health. Failure of the lymphatics to clear the interstitial space would lead to a build-up of protein rich fluid (lymphoedema) which, if complete and uncorrected would result in most of the intravascular fluid volume of the body transferring to the interstitial space within a few hours.

Transport of particles

The lymphatic system is also the only means of clearing the tissues of particulate matter. Particles enter the initial lymphatics through inter-endothelial openings

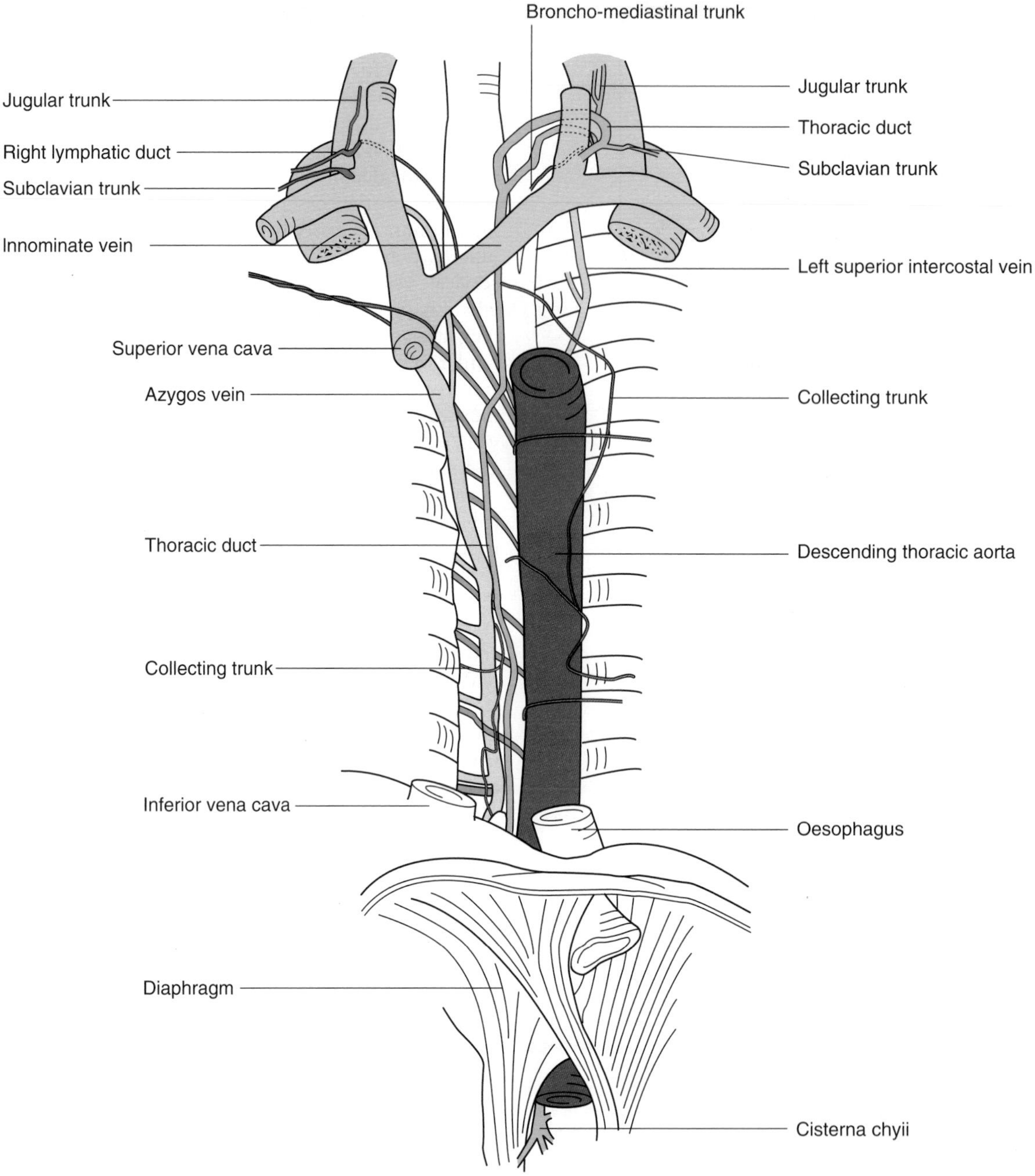

Figure 37.3 Anatomy of the cisterna chyli, thoracic duct and right lymph duct.

and via vesicular transport through intra-endothelial pores. Large particles are actively phagocytosed by macrophages and transported through the lymphatic system intracellularly.

Immune circulation

Mononuclear and polymorphonuclear leucocytes and lymphocytes also leave the circulation, particularly at sites of inflammation, and enter the interstitial space. These cells drain via lymphatics to lymph nodes, present antigen, and carry out other functions vital for the maintenance of immunocompetence, in terms of both infection and tumour surveillance. Some of these cells then return to the circulation and begin the cycle again.

Lymphovenous communications

These have been observed on lymphangiography and are thought to allow decompression of a hypertensive lymphatic system. These communications may be absent in some cases of lymphoedema, e.g. post-mastectomy lymphoedema. However, the pathophysiological consequence of this observation is unclear.

Mechanisms of lymph transport

Resting interstitial fluid pressure is negative (–2 to –6 mmH_2O), whereas lymphatic pressures are positive. This indicates that lymph flows actively against a pressure gradient because of

- transient increases in interstitial pressure secondary to muscular contraction and external compression
- the sequential contraction and relaxation of lymphangions
- the presence of valves that prevent retrograde flow.

Valves separate collectors and trunks into segments called lymphangions. These form a 'string-of-beads' appearance, which can be visualized easily on lymphangiography. Lymphatic valves are semilunar, paired, and comprise an endothelial covered flap of fine collagen and reticular fibres. Valves are situated 2–3 mm apart in the collectors and 6–8 mm apart in peripheral trunks. In the central lymph trunks such as the thoracic duct valves may be separated by up to 20 cm. Valves are found in both the deep and superficial systems but are more frequent in the latter. On average, lymph will pass through 80–100 lymphangions between the periphery and entering the venous system. Each lymphangion is reinforced with longitudinal, circular and spiral muscle layers, especially in its mid-portion. This muscle contracts spontaneously in response to dilatation. Through successive peristaltic contractions, occurring at rest some 10–12 times per minute, the lymph is moved from one lymphangion to the next. Valves open and close passively in response to hydrostatic forces to permit onward, but prevent backward, flow (reflux). For these reasons lymphangions used to be termed 'microlymph hearts'.

The continuous replenishment of lymph from the periphery, sometimes referred to as the vis-a-tergo (force from behind) leads to dilatation and contraction of lymphangions. In much the same way as venous return provides preload and, through Starling's law, determines the contractility of the heart so the lymphatic system can respond to increased lymph production in the tissues. In health, lymphangion contraction leads to pressures of 25–50 mmHg; much higher pressures (up to 200 mmHg) are observed in the presence of lymphatic obstruction.

Although, in health, the propulsion of lymph is primarily due to this intrinsic motility, other factors become increasingly important in disease states. Thus limb movement, either active or passive, and massage can propel lymph through stretching of the lymphatics and through compression of lymph trunks within fascial sheaths. Arterial pulsation may also augment lymph flow in the neurovascular bundles of the extremities and the thoracic duct. Respiration and gastrointestinal peristalsis may also play a part. Lymph flow increases markedly (10–30-fold) during exercise because of:

- increased capillary fluid filtration
- muscle contraction
- increased arterial pulsation
- augmented negative intra-thoracic pressures
- increased sympathetic tone, which may increase the contractility of lymphangions.

Conversely, lymph flow in the immobile limb is extremely sluggish and explains the oedema observed in patients with a range of conditions such as stroke, paraplegia, multiple sclerosis and trauma. Patients with lymphangitis and lymph leaks from proximal wounds should therefore be advised to rest the affected part.

Lymphangions respond to increased lymph flow in much the same way as the heart responds to increased venous return; that is, they increase their contractility and stroke volume. Noradrenaline, serotonin, prostaglandins, thromboxanes and endothelin-1 also enhance contractility. Lymphatics may also modulate their own contractility through the production of nitric oxide. Contractility appears to be inhibited by haemoglobin, haem-containing proteins and oxygen derived free radicals.

Transport in the thoracic and right lymph ducts is also dependent upon changes in:

- intra-thoracic pressure that occur with respiration
- central venous pressures through the cardiac cycle.

Cardiorespiratory disease may, therefore, have an adverse effect on lymphatic function.

In the normal limb, lymph flow is almost entirely dependent on intrinsic lymphatic contractility. However, in lymphoedema, where the lymphatics are constantly distended, exercise, limb movement and external compression do increase lymphatic return; this explains the success of physical therapy.

Section 37.3 • Lymph drainage of specific tissues and regions

The skin

Lymph from a 'lymph area' is collected in the dermis by a subpapillary capillary network (Figure 37.1). Although there is some overlap between lymph areas, each essentially drains into a single pre-collector. Several pre-collectors then coalesce to form a collector that serves a 'lymph zone'. Each collector drains into a lymph trunk running on the deep fascia, which serves a 'lymph territory'. There are very limited anastomoses between lymph trunks so that in the presence of disease there is limited capacity for lymph from one territory to be transported by the lymphatic system of an adjoining territory. Thus, with the exception of the dermal capillary plexus, where there is some overlap of drainage between lymph areas, a lymphatic end circulation essentially serves each lymph territory. This explains the phenomenon of 'dermal backflow' observed in patients with lymphatic obstruction. Perforators from deep lymph trunks, which run with minor and major neurovascular bundles, join superficial lymph trunks. Minor superficial lymph trunks from individual territories coalesce to form the major lymph trunks from the limb. One again, anastomoses between these lymph trunks, and so the possibilities for collateral flow in the presence of disease, are limited.

The lower limbs

Superficial lymph trunks

Major lymph trunks are situated so that the movement of joints does not put them under undue strain. For example, in the lower limb, the ventromedial bundle of trunks is concentrated on the antero-medial aspect of the ankle, the medial aspect of the knee behind the medial condyle, and the anterior aspect of the thigh and hip (Figure 37.2). These lymph trunks drain four lymph territories.

- Ventromedial territory: toes, most of the sole and the dorsum of the foot, the medial heel and ankle, and most of the calf. This is the largest territory and is drained by the so-called ventromedial bundle of lymph trunks that run up the medial aspect of the leg. The bundle is broad in the thigh and calf but narrow at the knee where it lies behind the medial condyle near the long saphenous vein and can be easily damaged by a transverse incision. The number and pattern of lymph trunks in this area is highly variable such that some individuals may be at greater risk of lymphoedema than others.
- Dorsolateral territory: lateral heel and ankle, middle of the posterior calf. Lymph trunks for this territory drain alongside the short saphenous vein and share its relationship to the deep fascia. These trunks drain to intermediate nodes in the popliteal fossa from which efferent lymphatics travel up the leg with the femoral vessels.
- Dorsomedial thigh territory: inner thigh, medial buttock and perineum.
- Dorsolateral thigh territory: lateral thigh and buttock.

The ventromedial bundle drains directly to the inguinal lymph nodes and failure of the bundle is equivalent to inguinal lymphadenectomy. Lymph can only leave the limb by refluxing back down the extremity through the dermal capillary plexus (dermal backflow) and hence into adjoining superficial territories or through deep lymph channels.

Deep lymph trunks

These are fewer in number and run with named arteries. Intermediate nodes are found along the course of these trunks. Superficial trunks from the dorsolateral territory join them in the popliteal fossa. Other anastomoses between the deep and superficial systems may follow the course of perforating veins.

Regional lymph nodes

These are situated in the inguinal region in the lower layer of the subcutaneous fatty tissue overlying the fascia lata. They surround the termination of the long saphenous vein and other venous tributaries of the sapheno-femoral junction. These lymph nodes have been subclassified in a number of different ways. They drain all four lymph territories of the leg together with the anterior abdominal wall and the perineum: penis, scrotum, vagina below the hymen, anus below the dendate line, but *not* the testes. They do however receive uterine lymph via lymphatics running with the round ligament. Efferent lymphatics from the inguinal nodes drain to the iliac nodes lying alongside the iliac arteries and veins and thence to para-aortic lymph nodes and trunks. These join with gastrointestinal trunks that run alongside the mesenteric arteries to form the cisterna chyli.

The upper limbs

Superficial lymph trunks

The hand is served by a fine meshwork of lymphatics, particularly on its dorsal aspect. In the forearm and arm the trunks run with the major veins. Trunks draining the posterior aspect of the arm tend to run spirally around to the anterior aspect where, above the elbow, they tend to coalesce into a medial bundle, which runs with the basilic vein, and a lateral bundle which follows the cephalic vein.

Deep lymph trunks

These are smaller and flow alongside the radial, interosseous, ulnar and brachial vessels. There are few communications with the superficial system.

Regional lymph nodes

Although there are a few nodes related to the:

- deep trunks
- basilic vein just above the elbow (supratrochlear nodes)
- cephalic vein at its termination (infraclavicular nodes)

most of the major lymph trunks drain directly into the axillary lymph nodes. These nodes also drain the breast and the postero-lateral chest wall as far down as the iliac crest. Efferents from the axillary nodes coalesce to form the subclavian lymph ducts on each side.

Section 37.4 • Lymphoedema

Pathophysiology

Oedema formation

Any pathological state that tends to increase interstitial fluid pressure will have a dramatic effect on lymph flow in the absence of lymphatic disease. For example:

- elevated capillary pressure (heart failure)
- decreased plasma colloid pressure (renal, hepatic and gastrointestinal disease)
- increased interstitial protein concentration, usually due to increased capillary 'leakiness' (inflammation, ischaemia)
- increased interstitial protein concentration due to lymphatic insufficiency.

However, once mean interstitial pressure rises above 0 mmHg, lymph flow begins to plateau and soon reaches its maximum limit because:

- lymphatics are maximally dilated so that their valves are held open and can no longer prevent reflux
- despite the presence of anchoring filaments, constant positive pressure causes lymphatics to collapse.

When the production of interstitial fluid exceeds the capacity of the lymphatic system to remove it oedema appears. Thus, to a certain extent all oedema is 'lymphoedema'. Nevertheless, if the primary problem is excess interstitial fluid production then the oedema fluid usually, but not always, has a low protein content. By contrast, if the primary problem is lymphatic insufficiency, then the oedema fluid has a high protein content and in this circumstance patients will develop the characteristic signs of lymphoedema (see below). However, it is worth noting two points:

- by the time oedema appears, the normal compensatory mechanisms designed to deal with excessive lymph production or insufficient lymph clearance are already exhausted
- in a significant proportion of patients with oedema both mechanisms are at work.

So long as the interstitial pressure remains negative there is little change in interstitial volume despite increases in pressure because the lymphatics remove the excess fluid and protein to keep the space 'dry'. However, once interstitial pressure rises above zero, a small increase in pressure leads to a marked increase in volume. In other words there is a marked (25-fold) increase in compliance. Oedema is not usually clinically detectable until there has been a 30% increase in interstitial fluid volume. As oedema becomes chronic so the interstitial space 'relaxes' and, in severe cases, there may be a 300% increase in interstitial fluid volume.

Normal safety mechanisms

Normally, interstitial fluid is trapped in a complex gel matrix comprising proteoglycan (complex polysaccharides of molecular weight >1 000 000) and structural proteins. As the space between these molecules is of the order of 20–40 nm, bulk flow of water through the interstitium cannot occur. As oedema begins to form so the gel takes up the excess fluid until the interstitium has swollen by 30–50%. Thereafter the capacity of the gel is exceeded and free fluid spaces begin to form. This leads to the accumulation of water that is highly mobile and moves to the most dependent region of the affected part; it also explains the phenomenon of 'pitting' observed in low protein oedema. By contrast, in lymphoedema, the high protein content leads to coagulation so that except in its very early stages it does not exhibit pitting and gives the skin a thickened, indurated, brawny appearance. It is assumed that the sequestration of polypeptide growth factors in the interstitium leads to the excessive skin thickening and papilla formation so characteristic of the disease. In time these processes only involve not the skin but also the subcutaneous tissues and deep fascia which can lead, in some cases, to a chronic compartment syndrome and secondary venous and even arterial insufficiency.

Underlying lymphatic abnormalities

Lymphoedema is due to defective lymphatic drainage in the presence of (near) normal net capillary filtration and is the result of lymphatic:

- aplasia or hypoplasia
- hypocontractility (with or without valvular insufficiency)
- obliteration (due to inflammation)
- dilatation and valvular failure (megalymphatics).

Whatever the underlying cause, lymphatic hypertension leads to distension with secondary impairment of contractility and valvular competence. Lymphostasis results in the accumulation of fluid, proteins, growth factors and other active peptide moieties, glycosaminoglycans and particulate matter, including bacteria, in the interstitial space. As a consequence, there is increased collagen production by fibroblasts, activation of coagulation, fibrin formation, an accumulation of inflammatory cells (predominantly macrophages and lymphocytes) and activation of keratinocytes. The end result is protein rich oedema fluid, increased deposition of ground substance, subdermal fibrosis and dermal thickening and proliferation.

Cross-sectional imaging of the affected limb by means of computed tomography (CT) or magnetic resonance imaging (MRI) clearly indicates that lymphoedema, unlike all other causes of oedema, is confined to the epifascial space comprising the skin and subcutaneous tissues. Although muscle compartments may be hypertrophied due to the increased work involved in limb movement, they are characteristically free of oedema.

Classification

There are several ways in which lymphoedema can be classified.

Primary vs secondary

Lymphoedema is most commonly classified (Table 37.1) into:

- primary lymphoedema, in which the cause is unknown (or at least uncertain)
- secondary lymphoedema, in which the aetiology is apparent.

Table 37.1 Aetiological classification of lymphoedema

Primary lymphoedema	Congenita (onset < 1 year old) – sporadic Congenita (onset < 1 year old) – familial – Milroy's disease[a]) Praecox (onset 1–35 years) – sporadic Praecox (onset 1–35 years) – familial (Meige's disease[a]) Tarda (onset after 35 years of age)
Secondary lymphoedema	Bacterial infection Parasitic infection (filariasis) Fungal infection (tinea pedis) Exposure to foreign body material (silica particles) Primary lymphatic malignancy Metastatic spread to lymph nodes Radiotherapy to lymph nodes Surgical excision of lymph nodes Trauma (particularly degloving injuries) Superficial thrombophlebitis Deep venous thrombosis

[a]These terms are used variably.

However, as will be discussed below, the distinction between primary and secondary disease is not always that clear-cut.

Age of onset

Primary lymphoedema is usually further subdivided on the basis of age of onset:

- lymphoedema congenita is present at birth or develops within the first year of life
- lymphoedema praecox develops between 1 and 35 years of age, most commonly during adolescence
- lymphoedema tarda develops after the age of 35 years.

Although these age limits are somewhat arbitrary, the three groups do manifest different aetiologies and clinical features, which makes the classification of some value.

Congenital vs acquired

In a proportion of patients, lymphoedema is present at birth or develops shortly thereafter. Even in adult patients, there is often a family history. This suggests that lymphoedema may be due to an underlying genetically determined abnormality of lymphatic development and/or function. However, such an abnormality may be multi-factorial, have variable penetrance and is clearly affected by environmental factors.

Underlying abnormality

Lymphoedema may also be classified on the basis of lymphangiographic and lymphiscintigraphic findings (see below).

Clinical severity

Lymphoedema may be classified according to its severity and extent regardless of the underlying cause (Table 37.2).

Clinical features

History

The patient usually complains of gradual painless swelling of one or both legs. It is normally possible to distinguish lymphoedema from other causes of leg swelling (Table 37.3), and to differentiate primary from secondary lymphoedema on the basis of:

- age of onset
- family history
- co-existent pathology.

Table 37.2 Clinical classification of lymphoedema

Grade (Brunner)	*Clinical features*
Subclinical (latent)	There is excess interstitial fluid and histological abnormalities in lymphatics and lymph nodes but no clinically apparent lymphoedema
Stage I	Oedema pits on pressure and swelling largely or completely disappears on elevation and bed rest
Stage II	Oedema does not pit and does not significantly reduce upon elevation
Stage III	Oedema is associated with irreversible skin changes: fibrosis, papillae

It is important to remember that, in developed countries, lymphoedema is a relatively uncommon cause of limb swelling. At first, lymphoedema is like other forms of oedema in that it is present only upon dependency; that is, worse at the end of the day, absent in the morning. However, as the condition develops and the oedema fluid becomes more protein rich and the tissues indurated, it is less and less affected by position and is there all the time. Lymphoedema nearly always commences distally on the foot and extends proximally, usually only to the knee. If it commences proximally then pelvic pathology, particularly malignant disease, must be excluded. This can be done with ultrasound or preferably CT. Similarly, lymphoedema beginning from middle age onwards may well signify underlying malignant disease and should be fully investigated.

Although, as discussed above, many cases of primary lymphoedema are thought to be due to an inherited underlying lymphatic defect, it is clear that in a proportion of patients so affected this congenital predisposition only leads to clinically apparent disease following exposure to an environmental trigger. Recognized precipitating event for the onset of lymphoedema include:

- infection, e.g. episode of cellulitis (to which such individuals may be especially prone (see below))
- trauma, e.g. soft tissue injury, long bone or pelvic fracture
- surgery, e.g. joint replacement, arterial and venous surgery, pelvis surgery
- venous disease, e.g. deep venous thrombosis, chronic venous insufficiency and the post-phlebitic limb

Thus, many patients with apparently primary lymphoedema also have a significant secondary component and, perhaps, vice versa (see below).

Some patients first present to medical attention because of acute cellulitis. Such patients are prone to recurrent episodes, each one of which damages still further the lymphatic system, leading to a vicious spiral (see below).

Signs

Foot changes

Unlike other types of oedema, lymphoedema characteristically involves the foot, as opposed to the lower calf and ankle (Figure 37.4). This is characterized by

- infilling of the submalleolar depressions
- the presence of a 'buffalo hump' on the dorsum of the foot
- a 'square' due to confinement of foot wear
- the skin on the dorsum of the toes cannot be pinched due to subcutaneous fibrosis (Stemmer's sign).

Lymphoedema usually spreads proximally to knee level and less commonly affects the whole leg.

Pitting

Lymphoedema will pit easily at first but with time fibrosis and dermal thickening prevent pitting except following prolonged pressure.

Table 37.3 Differential diagnosis of the swollen limb

Non-vascular lymphatic	General disease states	Cardiac failure from any cause. Liver failure. Hypoproteinaemia due to nephrotic syndrome, malabsorption, protein losing enteropathy. Hyperthyroidism (myxoedema). Allergic disorders including angioedema and idiopathic cyclic oedema Prolonged immobility and lower limb dependency
	Local disease processes	Ruptured Baker's cyst. Myositis ossificans. Bony or soft tissue tumours. Arthritis. Haemarthrosis. Calf muscle haematoma. Achilles tendon rupture
	Retroperitoneal fibrosis	May lead to arterial, venous and lymphatic abnormalities
	Gigantism	Rare. All tissues are uniformly enlarged
	Drugs	Corticosteroids, oestrogens, progestogens; monoamine oxidase inhibitors; phenylbutazone; methyldopa; hydrallazine; nifedipine
	Trauma	Painful swelling due to reflex sympathetic dystrophy
	Obesity	Lipodystrophy, lipoidosis
Venous	Deep venous thrombosis	There may be an obvious predisposing factor such as recent surgery. The classical signs of pain and redness may be absent.
	Post-thrombotic syndrome	Swelling, usually of the whole leg, due to ilio-femoral venous obstruction. Venous skin changes, secondary varicose veins on the leg and collateral veins on the lower abdominal wall. Venous claudication may be present
	Varicose veins	Simple primary varicose veins are not usually associated with significant leg swelling
	Klippel–Trenaunay syndrome and other malformations	Rare. Present at birth or develops in early childhood. Comprises an abnormal lateral venous complex, capillary naevus, bony abnormalities, hypo(a)plasia of deep veins, and limb lengthening. Lymphatic abnormalities often co-exist.
	External venous compression	Pelvic or abdominal tumour including the gravid uterus. Retroperitoneal fibrosis
Arterial	Ischaemia–reperfusion	Following lower limb revascularization for chronic and particularly chronic ischaemia
	Arteriovenous malformation	May be associated with local or generalized swelling
	Aneurysm	Popliteal. Femoral. False aneurysm following (iatrogenic) trauma

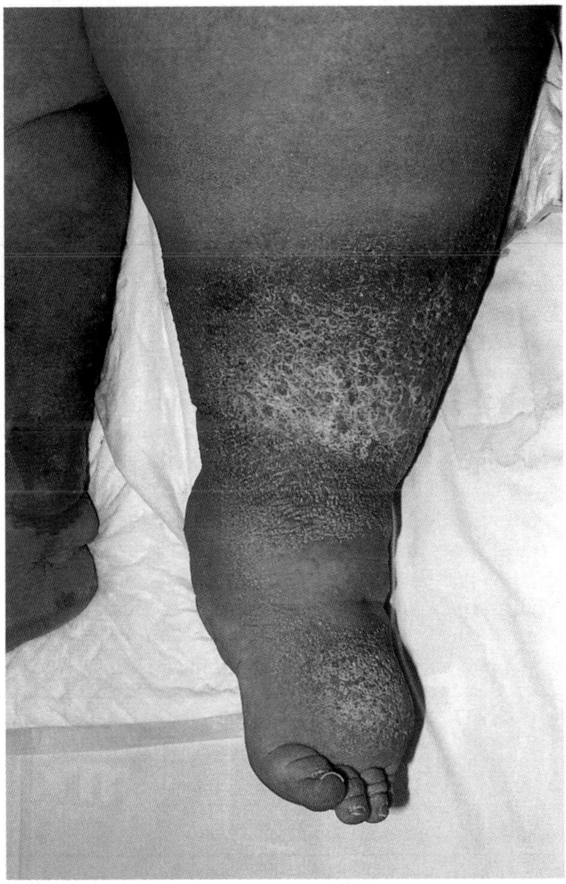

Figure 37.4 The lower leg of a patient with typical lymphoedema.

Skin changes

Chronic eczema, fungal infection of the skin (dermatophytosis) and nails (onychomycosis), fissuring, verrucae and papillae are frequently seen in advanced conditions. Frank ulceration is rare except in the presence of chronic venous insufficiency. However, the two conditions not infrequently co-exist and chronic venous insufficiency may actually lead to lymphatic insufficiency. Ulceration can also develop after minor trauma and be slow to heal, despite the lymphoedematous limb having an abnormally high blood flow.

Lymphangectasia

Protein-losing diarrhoea, chylous ascites, chylothorax, chyluria and discharge of lymph from skin vesicles (lymphorrhoeas, chylorrhoea) secondary to lymphangectasia (megalymphatics) and chylous reflux are rare.

Malignant change

Ulceration, non-healing bruises and raised purple–red nodules should lead to suspicion of malignancy. Lymphangiosarcoma was originally described arising in post-mastectomy oedema (Stewart–Treves syndrome) but can develop in any in long-standing lymphoedema. It is rare, aggressive, usually diagnosed late and frequently leads to loss of limb or life.

Primary lymphoedema

Epidemiology

Primary lymphoedema is estimated to affect 1–2 people per 100 000 under 20 years of age. Approximately

10% have a positive family history; that is, a first degree relative affected by the condition.

Non-familial primary lymphoedema

It has been proposed that all cases of primary lymphoedema are due to an inherited abnormality of the lymphatic system, sometimes termed dyplasia *in utero*. However, it is more likely that many sporadic cases occur in the presence of a (near) normal lymphatic system and are examples of secondary lymphoedema for which the triggering event has gone unrecognized. In animal experiments, simple excision of lymph nodes and/or trunks leads to acute lymphoedema that resolves within a few weeks, presumably due to collateralization. The human condition can only be reproduced when extensive lymphatic obliteration and fibrosis are produced; for example, by injecting silica particles. Even then there may be considerable delay between the injury and the onset of oedema. It is possible that a significant proportion of non-familial primary lymphoedema is due to chronic injury over many years due to seemingly trivial (but repeated) triggering events (see above) such as bacterial and/or fungal infections, barefoot walking (silica) and episodes of thrombophlebitis. Primary lymphoedema is far commoner in the legs than the arms. This may be due to gravity, a bipedal posture, the fact that the lymphatic system of the leg is less well developed than that of the arm, or because of the increased susceptibility to trauma and/or infection.

Familial primary lymphoedema

In familial cases it is assumed that there must be some, as yet undefined, genetic susceptibility of the lymphatic system to such injury. This may be:

- a structural problem such as aplasia or hypoplasia or dilatation
- a functional problem such as defective lymphatic contractility.

However, at the present time, the exact mechanisms causing familial primary lymphoedema remain largely speculative.

Lymphoedema congenita

Congenital lymphoedema (onset at or within a year of birth), also sometimes termed Milroy's disease (although this term is used variably), accounts for less than 5% of primary lymphoedema and:

- is commoner in males
- is more likely to be bilateral
- is more likely to involve the whole leg
- may be associated with other congenital abnormalities, e.g. Pierre–Robin syndrome.

Lymphoedema praecox

Lymphoedema praecox (onset from 1 to 35 years) accounts for about 65% of primary lymphoedema and:

- is three times commoner in females
- has a peak incidence shortly after menarche
- is three times more likely to be unilateral than bilateral
- usually only extends to the knee.

The familial form is referred to as Meige's disease and represents about a third of all cases.

Lymphoedema tarda

Lymphoedema tarda develops, by definition, after the age of 35 years, but in practice is a disease of middle age. It account for about 30% of cases. It is often associated with obesity and, histologically, lymph nodes are replaced with fatty and fibrous tissue. The cause is unknown. Lymphoedema developing for the first time in later life should prompt a thorough search for underlying malignancy, particularly of the pelvic organs, prostate and external genitalia; such malignancy may be found in up to 10% of patients. It is worth noting that in such patients lymphoedema often commences proximally in the thigh rather than distally.

Secondary lymphoedema

This is the most common form of lymphoedema. There are several well-recognized causes.

Filariasis

This is the commonest cause of lymphoedema worldwide, affecting up to 100 million individuals. It is particularly prevalent in Africa, India and South America where 5–10% of the population may be affected. The viviparous nematode *Wucheria bancrofti*, whose only host is man, is responsible for 90% of cases and is spread by the mosquito. The disease is associated with poor sanitation. The parasite enters lymphatics from the blood and lodges in lymph nodes where it causes fibrosis and obstruction, due partly to direct physical damage and partly to the immune response of the host. Proximal lymphatics become grossly dilated with adult parasites. The degree of oedema is often massive and is sometimes termed elephantiasis. Immature parasites (microfilariae) enter the blood at night and can be identified on a blood smear, a centrifuged specimen of urine or in lymph itself. A complement fixation test is also available and is positive in present or past infection. Eosinophilia is usually present. Diethylcarbamazine destroys the parasites but does not reverse the lymphatic changes, although there may be some regression over time. Once the infection has been cleared treatment is as for primary lymphoedema. Public health measures to reduce mosquito breeding and the provision of shoes are helpful.

Malignancy and its treatment

This is the commonest cause of lymphoedema in developed countries and may complicate:

- Hodgkin's and non-Hodgkin's lymphoma
- malignant melanoma that has metastasized to regional lymph nodes
- malignancy of the pelvic organs (ovary, uterus, bladder), anus, prostate, testes, penis
- breast cancer (peau d'orange).

More often lymphoedema is a result of treatment, either surgical excision of draining lymph nodes

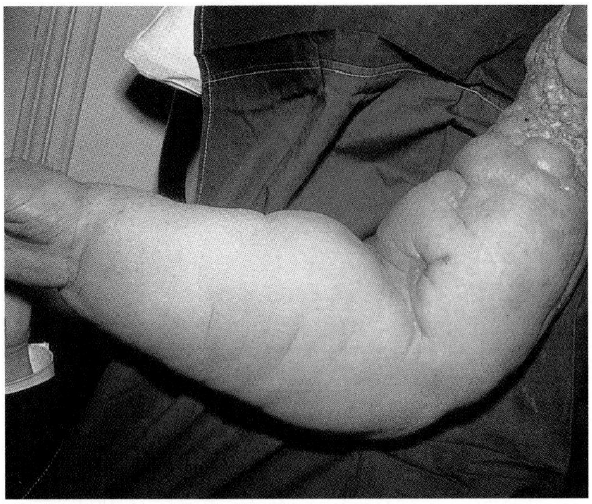

Figure 37.5 Lymphoedema of the arm following radical surgical treatment for advanced breast carcinoma.

and/or radiotherapy. Lymphoedema following treatment for breast carcinoma (Figure 37.5) is the commonest example but fortunately this is decreasing in incidence as surgery for the condition has become more conservative.

Trauma

This is an unusual cause of lymphoedema but is especially seen after degloving injuries of the extremities.

Acute cellulitis

As described above, acute bacterial lymphangitis is a frequently observed triggering event for secondary lymphoedema.

Venous disease

It is apparent that many patients with chronic venous insufficiency have a degree of lymphatic impairment that contributes to leg swelling. The nature of the link between these two processes is not clear but may include:

- shared risk factors such as age, obesity, immobility, pelvic pathology and previous surgery
- episodes of thrombophlebitis leading to secondary lymphatic injury
- lymphatic damage at the time of venous surgery
- shared underlying impairment of vascular wall structure and function.

Patients who present with leg swelling, thought to be due to lymphoedema, but who also have clinical and/or duplex evidence of venous disease are likely to be made worse rather than better by venous surgery. This is because surgery involves dissection around popliteal and inguinal lymph nodes and often stripping, which with regard to the long saphenous vein, for example, may damage the medial thigh lymphatic bundle. Such patients should be treated non-operatively if at all possible.

Factitious lymphoedema

This may be caused by application of a tourniquet (a rut and sharp cut-off are usually seen on examination) or 'hysterical' disuse.

Investigations

When are investigations necessary?

Lymphoedema can usually be diagnosed on the basis of history and examination alone, expecially when the swelling is mild and there are no apparent complicating features. Indications for investigation include:

- uncertainty about the diagnosis
- a suggestion that several pathologies are contributing to limb swelling
- concerns about underlying malignancy
- when consideration is being given to surgical bypass.

'Routine' tests

Depending on the circumstances any or all of the following may be indicated: full blood count, urea and electrolytes, creatinine, liver function tests, chest radiograph, auto-immune serology and midnight blood smear for microfilariae.

Venous investigations

Limb swelling of any description often leads to a 'reflex' request for venous duplex. While this will provide information about reflux in the superficial and deep venous systems, it is unlikely to alter management and, in the absence of skin changes of chronic venous insufficiency, is probably unnecessary. Venography should be avoided.

Arterial investigations

Blood flow through a leg affected by lymphoedema is increased. Nevertheless, as high grade compression is the mainstay of treatment, the adequacy of the arterial inflow must be established and documented, especially in older patients who are at greater risk for peripheral vascular disease. Pulses can be difficult to feel and measurement of ankle/brachial pressure index can also be problematic due to swelling and induration. An arterial duplex scan can usually exclude major arterial disease.

Direct contrast lymphangiography

Few centres now perform lymphangiography. However, it remains the standard by which all other lymphatic imaging is judged and provides precise anatomical information on the lymphatics. It is generally reserved for pre-operative evaluation of patients with megalymphatics who are being considered for bypass or fistula ligation.

Briefly, the patient is admitted for limb elevation to reduce swelling and facilitate lymphatic cannulation. Isosulphan blue is injected subcutaneously to identify the lymphatics. Under local or general anaesthesia, lymphatics are dissected out under loupe magnification and a 30 gauge needle is used to infuse lipid soluble contrast. Serial radiographs are taken during injection and at intervals up to 24 hours. In a normal limb the injection with usually fill 5-15 superficial valved medial thigh lymphatic vessels, as well inguinal lymph nodes, in about 20 min; iliac nodes fill at between 20 and 45 min. Deep lymphatics which are frequently paired and follow the deep vessels, as well as the lateral superficial lymphatics are not usually seen except in disease. Three main anatomical patterns of primary lymphoedema are identified by lymphangiography (Table 37.4, Figure 37.6):

- distal obliteration (hypo/aplasia)
- proximal obliteration
- hyperplasia (lymphangectasia).

Isotope lymphoscintigraphy

Technique

This has largely replaced contrast lymphangiography and is used in most centres as the primary diagnostic technique. Radioactive technetium-labelled antimony sulfide colloid particles (10 nm diameter) are injected into the web space between the second and third toes (or fingers) with a 27 gauge needle bilaterally. The particles are specifically taken up by lymphatics and about 30% of the tracer is absorbed in 3 hours. Immediately after injection a gamma camera is positioned to include the inguinal region in its upper field. During the first hour 12, 5 min dynamic anterior exposures are taken. The patient is requested to exercise with a foot ergometer (to permit reproducible exercise and tracer clearance) for 5 min initially, and then for 1 min out of every subsequent 5 min. At 1 and 3 hours, and in selected patients at 6 and 24 hours, 20 min whole body exposures are taken. Between exposures the patient is ambulant.

Normal examination

In a normal leg activity ascends the anteromedial aspect of the limb. Several lymph channels are seen in the calf but in the thigh they cannot usually be distinguished. Normally, radioactivity first appears in the inguinal (axillary) nodes at between 15 and 60 min and is symmetrical; individual nodes cannot usually be distinguished. At 60 min there is only faint uptake in the liver and bladder. At 3 hours there is intense activity over the liver and good symmetrical uptake in inguinal, pelvic and abdominal lymph nodes; the thoracic duct may also be seen. Most groups interpret lymphoscintigraphy qualitatively as attempts to perform quantitative assessment have produced inconsistent results. It is not possible to distinguish primary from secondary lymphoedema with certainty. However, lymphoscintigraphic patterns can be correlated to some extent with lymphangiographic findings.

Distal obliteration

This is associated with little or no removal of tracer from the injection site, little or no activity in the regional nodes at 1 or 3 hours and a cutaneous pattern of tracer distribution (dermal backflow). Although the time taken for radioactivity to reach the groin is prolonged, onward passage from there is usually normal.

Proximal obliteration

This is associated with normal uptake from the injection site and appearance of tracer in inguinal nodes. However, there is a failure of tracer to progress from the inguinal lymph nodes; collaterals crossing over to the other side are present.

Table 37.4 Lymphangiographic classification of primary lymphoedema

	Congenital hyperplasia (10%)	*Distal obliteration (80%)*	*Proximal obliteration (10%)*
Age of onset	Congenital	Puberty (praecox)	Any age
Sex distribution	Male > female	Female > male	Male = female
Extent	Whole leg	Ankle, calf	Whole leg, thigh only
Laterality	Uni = bilateral	Often bilateral	Usually unilateral
Family history	Often positive	Often positive	No
Progression	Progressive	Slow	Rapid
Response to compression therapy	Variable	Good	Poor
Comments	Lymphatics are increased in number although functionally defective; there is usually an increased number of lymph nodes. May have chylous ascites, chylothorax and protein losing enteropathy	Absent or reduced distal superficial lymphatics. Also termed aplasia or hypoplasia	There is obstruction at the level of the aorto-iliac or inguinal nodes. If associated with distal dilatation the patient may benefit from lymphatic bypass operation. Other patients have distal obliteration as well

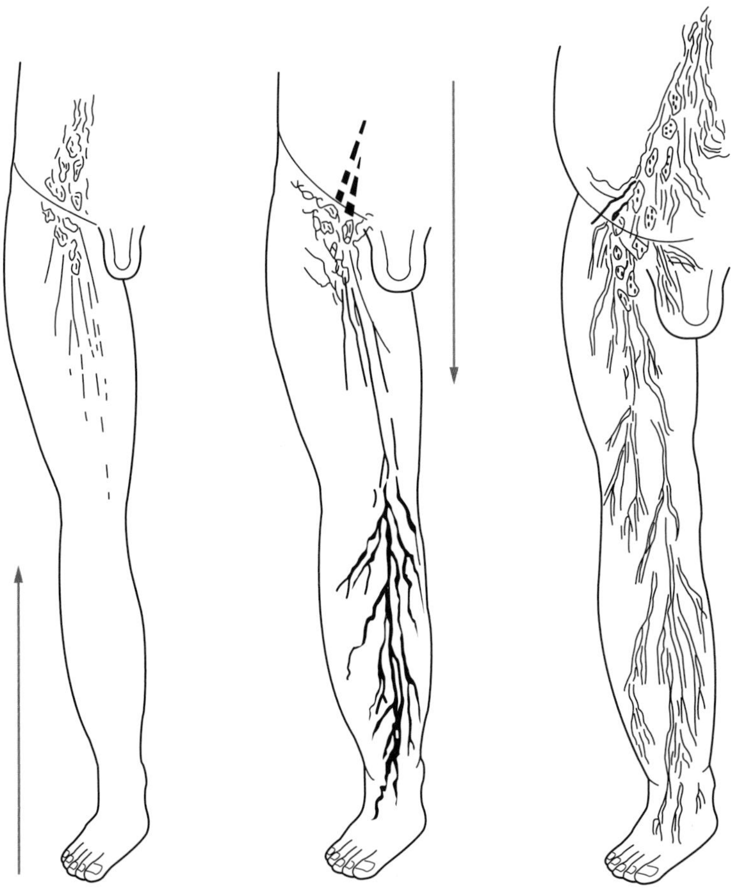

Figure 37.6 Lymphangiographic patterns of primary lymphoedema. (a) Distal obliteration which progresses proximally; this is the commonest pattern. (b) Proximal obliteration. This usually starts at the level of the inguinal lymph nodes and may progress distally. Lymphatics distal to the obstruction may become secondarily dilated. (c) Megalymphatics due to congenital lymphangectasia.

Lymphangectasia

This is associated with abnormal collections of tracer activity indicating extravasation into the peritoneal or pleural cavities or into viscera. Lymphoceles and dilated lymph channels (megalymphatics) are also seen.

Computed tomography

The main role of CT is to exclude pelvic or abdominal mass lesions. Although lymphoedema itself can be visualized on CT, it is of little diagnostic value in this respect

Magnetic resonance imaging

MRI can provide clear images of lymphatic channels and lymph nodes, and can also distinguish venous and lymphatic disease as the cause of a swollen limb. However, it cannot at present provide the information available from lymphoscintigraphy and as a cross-sectional imaging technique it appears to have little advantage over CT.

Pathological examination

In cases where malignancy is suspected, samples of lymph nodes may be obtained by fine needle aspiration, needle core biopsy or surgical excision.

Management

Physical methods

The patient should elevate the foot above the level of the hip when sitting, elevate the foot of the bed when sleeping and avoid prolonged standing. Various forms of massage are effective at reducing oedema. Single and multiple chamber intermittent pneumatic compression devices are also useful. In most clinics the mainstay of therapy is correctly fitted graduated compression hosiery. Pressures exceeding 50 mmHg at the ankle may be required to control oedema. The adequacy of arterial inflow must be established and documented. Below knee stockings are usually sufficient. The patient should don the stocking on first thing in the morning when the leg is at its least swollen and doff the stocking when retiring to bed. General advice regarding exercise and weight reduction, if necessary, is sensible.

Drugs

Diuretics are of no value in pure lymphoedema. Their use is associated with side-effects including electrolyte disturbance. The hydroxyrutosides are reported to be beneficial, as are the coumadins, but there are no scientifically robust data to support their use. Antibiotics should be prescribed promptly for cellulitis; penicillin V 500 mg four times daily for streptococcal infection and flucloxacillin 250 mg four times daily are suitable. In severe cases there should be no hesitation in admitting the patient to hospital, elevating the limb and administering antibiotics intravenously. Antibiotics should be continued for at least 7 days or until all signs and symptoms have abated. Erythromycin is a reasonable alternative for those who are allergic to penicillin. In patients who suffer recurrent spontaneous episodes of cellulitis, long-term prophylactic antibiotic therapy may be indicated. Fungal infection (tinea pedis) must be treated aggressively. Topical clotrimazole (1%) or miconazole (2%) used regularly are sufficient in most cases but in refractory situations systemic griseofulvin (250–1000 mg) daily may be required. The feet must be dried after washing and the skin kept clean and supple with water-based emollients to prevent entry of bacteria. The importance of good foot care cannot be overemphasized to the patient.

Surgery

Only a small minority of patients with lymphoedema benefit from surgery. Surgery for lymphoedema is increasingly rare in the UK, and only a small number of specialists now have any significant experience with the techniques. Operations fall into two categories: reduction procedures and bypass procedures.

Reduction procedures

Reduction surgery for lymphoedema can be a major undertaking and can expose the patient to significant risk which should not be entered upon lightly. Blood loss is considerable and the post-operative recovery may be long and fraught with complications relating to the wounds and the effects of prolonged bed rest. The long-term success of these operations can be excellent but depends crucially upon a high level of post-operative patient compliance with compression hosiery. If patients have not shown commitment and perseverance with compression therapy prior to surgery they are even less likely to do so after their operation. Such patients are not good candidates for operative intervention and the surgeon should not be 'bullied' into operating as an act of desperation. The best indication for reduction surgery is inability to mobilize because of the sheer bulk of disease.

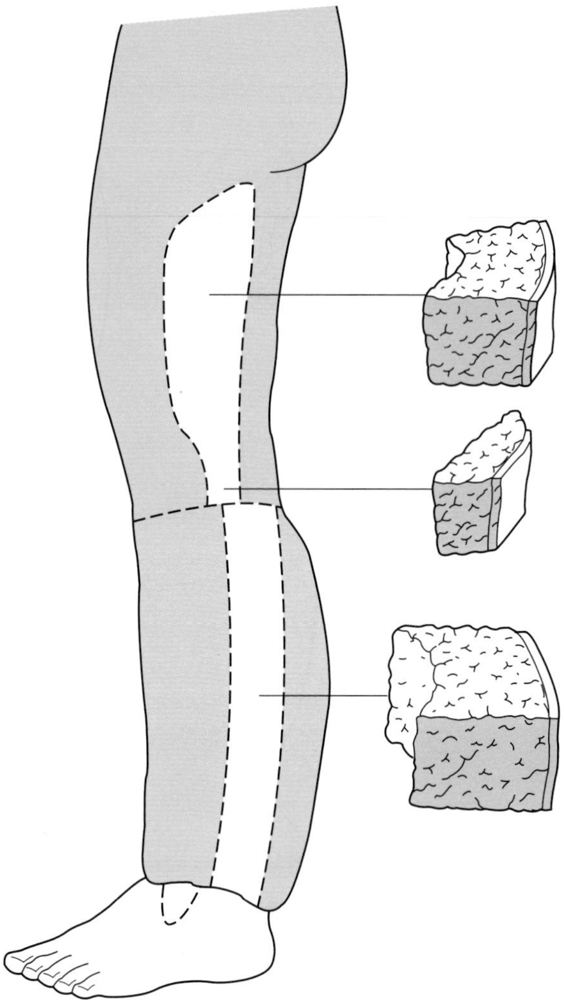

Figure 37.7 Homan's procedure involves raising skin flaps to allow the excision of a wedge of skin and a larger volume of subcutaneous tissue down to the deep fascia. Surgery to the medial and lateral aspects of the leg must be separated by at least 6 months to avoid skin flap necrosis.

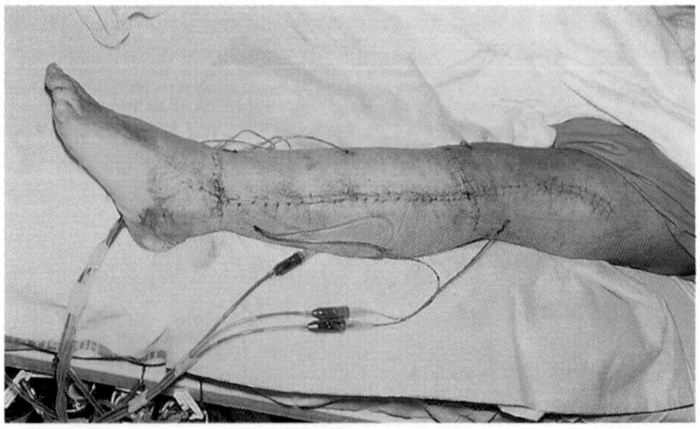

Figure 37.8 This patient underwent a Homan's reduction procedure on the medial aspect of his left calf 5 days previously. Note the presence of suction drains removing lymphatic fluid. Post-operatively, the patient also was placed in a multi-chamber sequential compression device to prevent re-accumulation of lymphoedema. Once the wounds are satisfactorily healed the patient is fitted with compression hosiery which should be worn indefinitely.

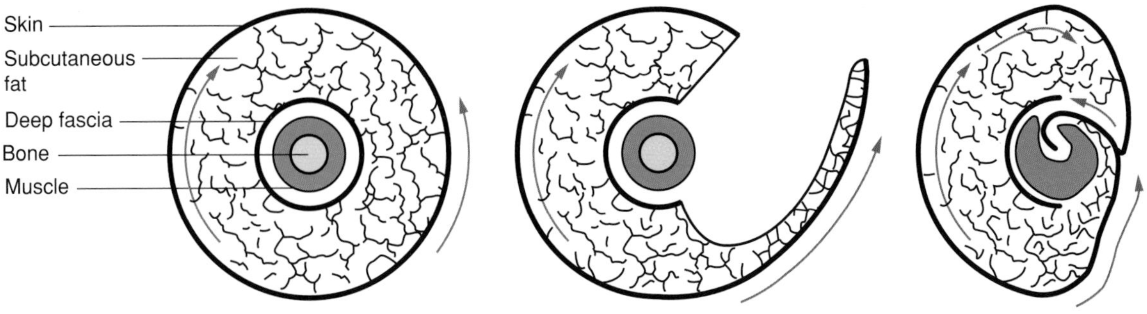

Figure 37.9 A cross-sectional representation of Thompson's reduction operation; the buried dermal flap.

Four operations have been described:

- *Sistrunk* – a wedge of skin and subcutaneous tissue is excised and the wound closed primarily. This is most commonly employed to reduce the girth of the thigh.
- *Homan* – skin flaps are elevated; subcutaneous tissue is excised from beneath the flaps which are then trimmed to size to accommodate the reduced girth of the limb and closed primarily. This is the most satisfactory operation for the calf (Figures 37.7 and 37.8). The main complication is skin flap necrosis. There must be at least 6 months between operations on the medial and lateral sides of the limb and the flaps must not pass the midline. This procedure has also been used on the upper limb but is contraindicated in the presence of venous obstruction or active malignancy.
- *Thompson* – one denuded skin flap is sutured to the deep fascia and buried beneath the second skin flap (the so-called buried dermal flap) (Figure 37.9). This procedure has become less popular as pilonidal sinus formation is common, the cosmetic result is no better than that obtained with the Homan's procedure and there is no evidence that the buried flap establishes any new lymphatic connection with the deep tissues.
- *Charles* – this operation was initially designed for filariasis and involved excision of all the skin and subcutaneous tissues down to deep fascia with coverage using split-skin grafts (Figure 37.10). This leaves a very unsatisfactory cosmetic result and graft failure is not uncommon. However, it does enable the surgeon to reduce greatly the girth of a massively swollen limb.

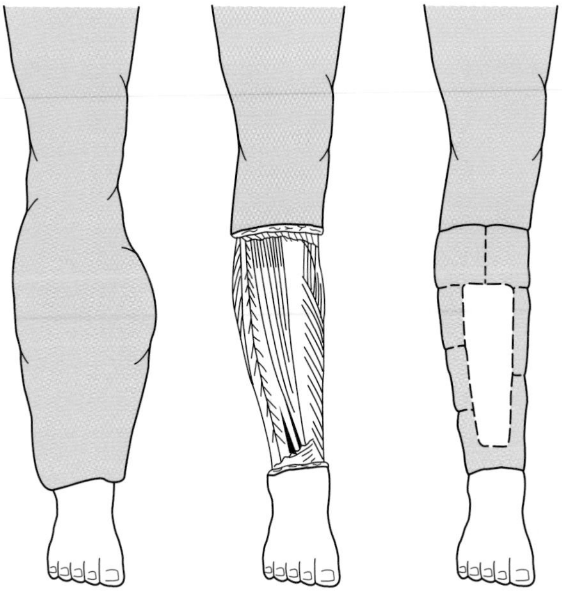

Figure 37.10 Charles' procedure involves circumferential excision of lymphoedematous tissue down to and including the deep fascia followed by split-skin grafting. This procedure gives a very poor cosmetic result but does allow the surgeon to remove very large amounts of tissue and is particularly useful in patients with severe skin changes.

Bypass procedures

In less than 2% of patients with primary lymphoedema, lymphangiography will demonstrate proximal lymphatic obstruction in the ilio-inguinal region with essentially normal distal lymphatic channels. In theory at least, such patients might benefit from lymphatic bypass. A number of methods have been described including the omental pedicle, the skin bridge (Gillies), anastomosing lymph nodes to veins (Neibulowitz), the ileal mucosal patch (Kinmonth) and, more recently, direct lymphovenous anastomosis with the aid of the operating microscope. Although the last two techniques do appear to lead to significant improvement in about 50% of patients it is not possible to predict which patients will benefit. The procedures are technically demanding, not without morbidity, and there is no controlled evidence to suggest that these procedures produce a superior outcome to best medical management alone.

Further reading

Browse, N. (1986). *Reducing Operations for Lymphoedema of the Lower Limb*. London: Wolfe.

Gloviczki, P. (1994). Direct operations on the lymphatics. In: Jamieson, C. W. and Yao, J. S. T., eds. *Rob and Smith's Operative Surgery: Vascular Surgery*. London: Chapman & Hall, 624–35.

O'Donnell, T. F. and Howrigan, P. (1992). Diagnosis and management of lymphoedema. In: Bell, P. R. F., Jamieson, C.W. and Ruckley, C.V. W.B., eds. *Surgical Management of Vascular Disease*. London: Saunders, 1305–28.

Szuba, A. and Rockson, S. G. (1997). Lymphoedema: anatomy, physiology and pathogenesis. *Vasc Med* **2**: 321–6.

Tibbs, D. J., Sabiston, D. C., Davies, M. G. *et al.* (1997). *Varicose Veins, Venous Disorders and Lymphatic Problems in the Lower Limbs*. Oxford: Oxford University Press.

Wolfe, J. H. N. (1994). Lymphography. In: Jamieson, C. W. and Yao, J. S. T., eds. *Rob and Smith's Operative Surgery: Vascular Surgery*. London: Chapman & Hall, 615–624.

MODULE 38

Mild and moderate head injury

Module 4 of *Essential Surgical Practice* (Volume I) described the principles of modern head injury care. An apparently minor blow on the head is a common event in everyday life, and the main reasons for assessment at hospital are a scalp wound that requires surgical repair, or the existence or threat of brain damage.

Section 38.1 • Introduction

General surgeons in many countries are involved in the initial assessment and treatment of patients with severe head injury, including those with multi-system trauma. This topic is dealt with in **Module 4, Volume I**. Equally important in current clinical practice in the UK are the many patients with less obviously serious head injuries who are admitted to surgical wards for 'observation' (a better term would be 'clinical monitoring'). This deceptively simple task is not always done well, and the consequences for some patients can be catastrophic. This module aims to help general surgeons to fulfil a role for which many have had little formal training.

Section 38.2 • Epidemiology of mild and moderate head injury

Around a million people in the UK attend hospital every year after a head injury, and an unknown number seek medical or paramedical advice without going to hospital. Around 1% have an obviously severe head injury and are rapidly triaged to neurosurgery or the intensive care unit. Up to 90% of the others need only reassurance and first aid for minor injuries before discharge from the accident and emergency (A&E) department or the minor injuries unit. Most do well, but some develop physical or neuropsychological symptoms similar to those seen after more serious head injury. General surgeons rarely become involved in the care of these mildly head injured patients.

In 10–15% of cases, the head injury is neither trivial enough to allow immediate discharge nor serious enough to involve a neurosurgeon or intensivist at once. These patients are admitted for observation to general surgical or orthopaedic wards, or to short-stay wards under the care of doctors working in A&E. Most can be discharged within a few days, but while being monitored a small minority develop delayed complications which worsen outcome if not detected promptly and dealt with properly.

Section 38.3 • Pathological processes in the injured brain

However mild or severe, traumatic brain injury is the sum of immediate (primary) damage and delayed (secondary) damage. From the moment of injury the emphasis must be on preventing or at least limiting secondary brain damage. Often what is needed is quite simple, but it may need to be done quickly to be effective.

Primary brain damage is the result of energy transferred to the brain at the time of injury. This damages

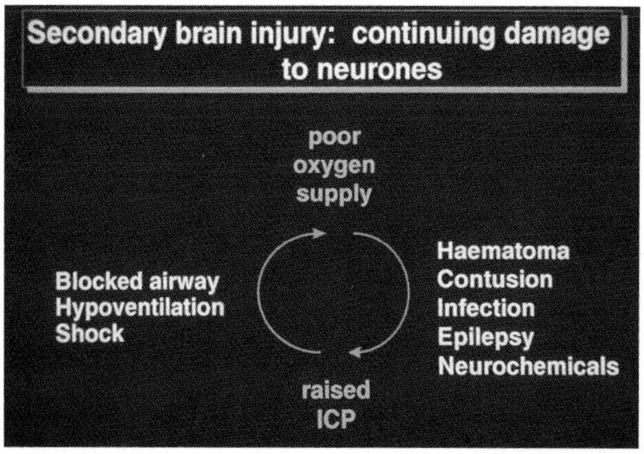

Figure 38.1 Diagram showing the inter-relationship between extracranial and intracranial causes of secondary brain damage and the crucial importance of oxygen and intracranial pressure.

neurones, other brain cells and the cerebral microvasculature. The amount of energy transferred determines the severity of brain damage, depth of altered consciousness and duration of post-traumatic amnesia, making it possible to define broad categories of patients with mild, moderate and severe head injuries – the rough and ready basis of early triage. *Secondary brain damage* is due to a reduced oxygen supply to injured neurones, which are highly susceptible to this further insult and can be damaged beyond hope of recovery. Lack of oxygen deprives them of a key metabolic fuel and leads to a hostile micro-environment rich in substances which cause further brain damage. Adequate cerebral perfusion and oxygenation must be maintained at all times, in the face of a variety of threats which can reinforce each other (Figure 38.1).

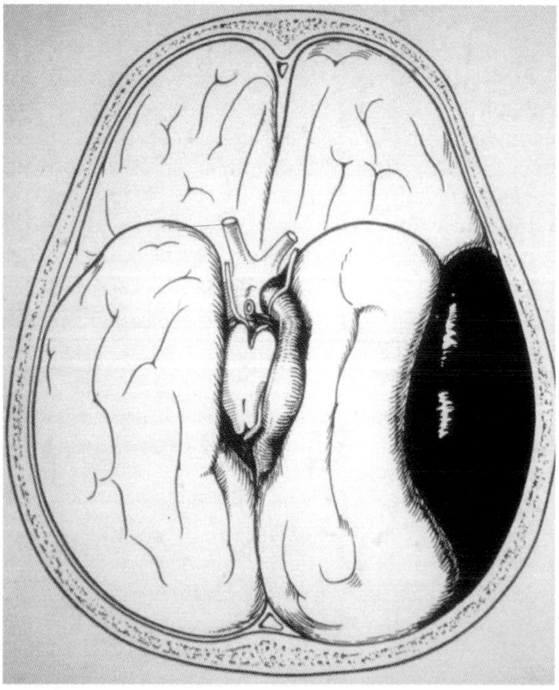

Figure 38.2 Diagram showing large acute extradural haematoma causing distortion and displacement of the brain structures and early tentorial herniation.

Cerebral perfusion pressure (CPP) is the difference between mean arterial pressure (MAP) and intracranial pressure (ICP), so that CPP falls when ICP rises or MAP falls. Normal CPP is about 70–80 mmHg (ICP 5–15 mmHg, MAP 80–90 mmHg). Brain injury damages or abolishes the normal autoregulatory mechanisms, and blood flow to the brain then varies in a linear way with CPP. Thus high ICP or low MAP can reduce the blood supply to the brain below critical levels. The skull is a rigid box of bone with little room to spare, and ICP can rise rapidly when a haematoma expands (Figure 38.2), or when contused brain swells as water and ions enter it through damaged vessels and cell membranes, or when all the cerebral vessels are engorged by hypercapnia. Uncontrolled haemorrhage from injuries of the trunk, pelvis or limbs can lower the MAP. Systemic hypoxaemia renders the brain's oxygen supply vulnerable just as its metabolic need for oxygen is raised by various consequences of brain injury: epileptic seizures, excitotoxic neurotransmitter activity and free radical damage to the integrity of the cell membranes.

Vigilance is needed to detect airway compromise, inadequate respiration and shock. These complications can develop insidiously in patients whose head injury does not seem serious at first, causing secondary damage and converting a drama into a crisis.

Section 38.4 • Clinical and radiological assessment of the patient

The assessment and treatment of any patient with a serious injury begins with a primary survey according to the principles of advanced trauma life support [Module 4, Volume I], with immediate action to resuscitate the patient from any life-threatening complications. Neurological assessment during the primary

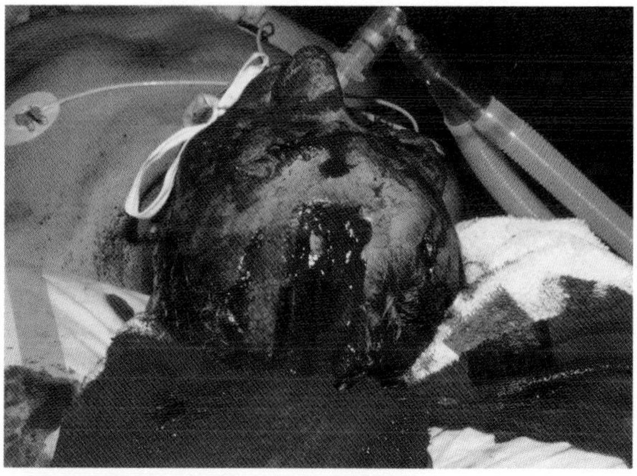

Figure 38.3 Major penetrating injury showing extensive scalp haemorrhage, bone fragments and almost certain brain penetration.

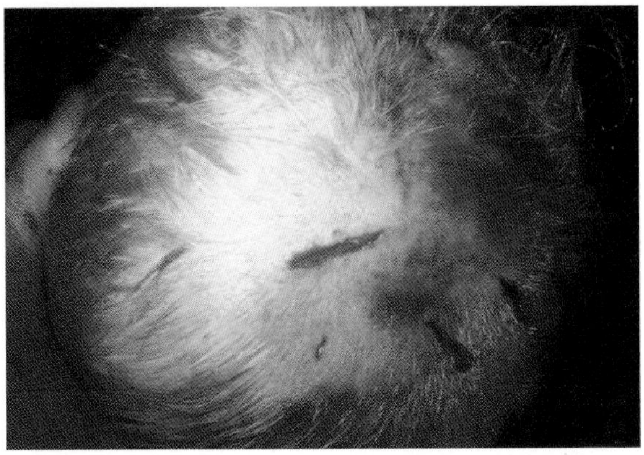

Figure 38.4 Penetrating brain injury. At initial presentation the fact that these apparently minor scalp lacerations were entry wounds for multiple stabs into the brain was not recognized, and the patient was discharged home, only to be re-admitted 4 days later with a cerebral abscess from which he later died.

survey should be confined to assessing conscious level by means of the Glasgow Coma Scale (GCS) (Figure 14.1 in Module 14) and the pupil size and responsiveness to light. These observations should be repeated at frequent intervals to establish a trend in the patient's neurological state (see below).

The secondary survey then follows: a head-to-toe assessment of the patient aimed at identifying and initiating treatment for all injuries. A detailed clinical examination of the head should be made, looking for external evidence of injury. A boggy haematoma or full thickness laceration of the scalp suggests an underlying skull fracture. Extensive scalp wounds (e.g. degloving injuries) can cause serious blood loss and may need to be dealt with in the primary survey under 'C for circulation' (Figure 38.3). External pressure controls nearly all scalp bleeding, allowing surgical repair to be deferred to a convenient time. Beware the unimpressive scalp injury which might have been caused by a sharp object; the brain may have been penetrated too (Figure 38.4).

Some skull fractures can be diagnosed clinically. The force needed to fracture the skull base also tears adjacent mucous membranes, and the result is a periorbital haematoma, haemotympanum (seen on auroscopy), mastoid haematoma (Battle's sign) (Figure 38.5a), or leak of cerebrospinal fluid (CSF) from the nose or ear (Figure 38.5b). Palpating the head may reveal a piece of skull broken off and displaced inwards by a hard object such as a hammer (Figure 38.6). The scalp wound overlying this depressed fracture may contain visible bone fragments or even brain tissue. A linear fracture (Figure 38.7) is unlikely to be diagnosed clinically unless it is exposed by extensive degloving of the scalp.

Which investigation for which patient?

Head injured patients at risk of intracranial complications must be urgently identified and treated. Pre-emptive investigation is far better than awaiting clinical deterioration. The risk of haematoma can be stratified by the conscious level and/or skull film appearances (Table 38.1). There is a shift away from using skull films for circumstantial evidence of intracranial damage to using a computed tomography (CT) scan to answer the question definitively.

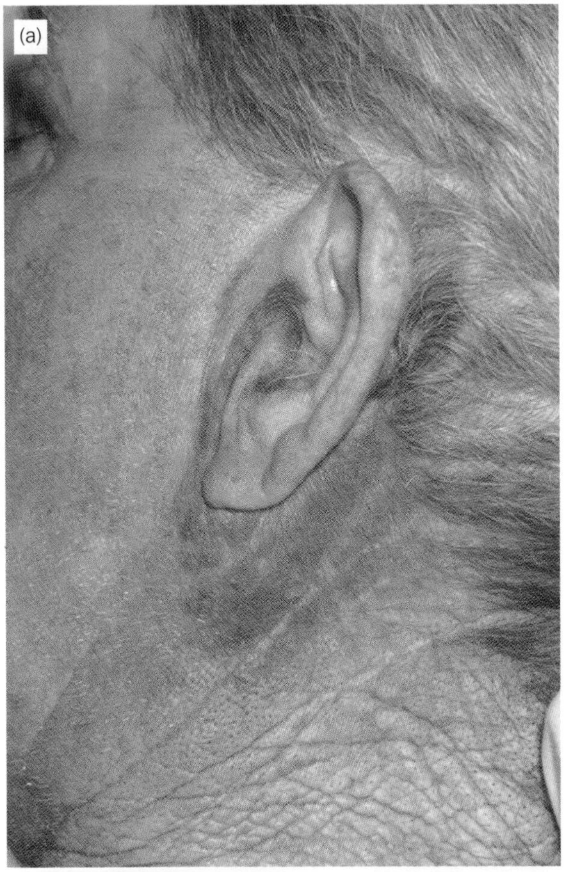

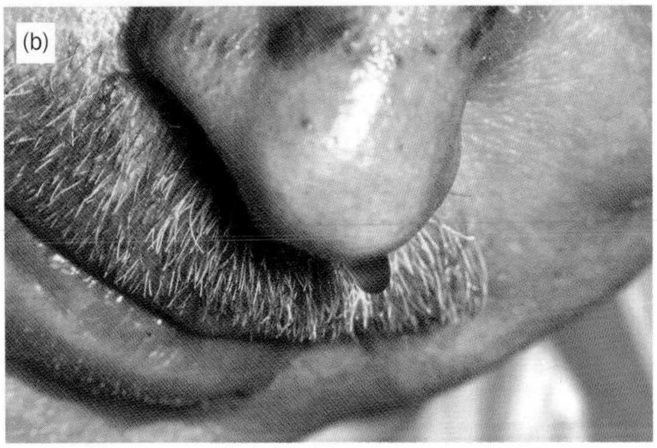

Figure 38.5 (a) Mastoid haematoma, indicating middle cranial fossa fracture. (b) CSF rhinorrhoea, demonstrated with the head forward in flexion.

Skull films – showing a fracture

If there is a skull fracture the patient – whatever the conscious level – is at much increased risk of intracranial complications, and should not be sent home

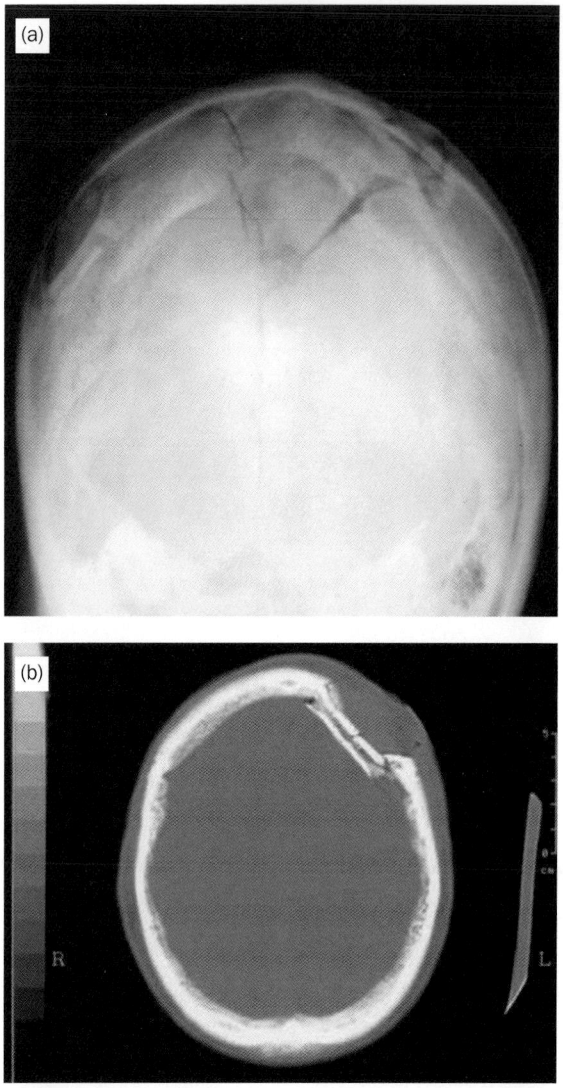

Figure 38.6 (a) Plain skull films: tangential view showing depressed fracture and also widely separated linear fractures. (b) CT scan (set to bone windows): depressed skull fracture of the left frontal bone.

Table 38.1 Risk of an operable intracranial haematoma in head injured patients (adapted from Teasdale *et al.*, 1990)

GCS	*Risk*	*Other features*	*Risk*
15	1 in 3615	None	1 in 31 300
		Post-traumatic amnesia (PTA)	1 in 6700
		Skull fracture	1 in 81
		Skull fracture and PTA	1 in 29
9–14	1 in 51	No fracture	1 in 180
		Skull fracture	1 in 5
3–8	1 in 7	No fracture	1 in 27
		Skull fracture	1 in 4

GCS = Glasgow Coma Scale.

Table 38.2 Indication for skull films

- The mechanism of injury has not been trivial
- Consciousness has been lost
- The patient is amnesic or has vomited
- The scalp has a full thickness laceration or a boggy haematoma

without a CT scan or a period of observation. The need for skull films to confirm or exclude a fracture depends on the mechanism of injury, extent of scalp trauma, neurological findings, and imaging resources available (Table 38.2). They have no added value when a decision has been made on clinical grounds that the patient should be scanned. If no scan is planned but the head injury has clearly not been trivial then a series of skull views – lateral, antero-posterior and Towne's views – is a useful triage tool.

A skull fracture can be missed because the clinician who reads it is inexperienced, the film is blurred due to patient movement during the exposure or too few views have been taken. A linear fracture forms a sharp-edged straight line across the skull vault where no markings should be seen (Figure 38.7). A depressed fracture causes a 'double density' as the bone fragment is seen through the skull vault, best seen on a tangential view (Figure 38.6). Occasionally a stab wound is seen as a 'slot' fracture on plain films, but this is easy to miss if the history is misleading or the entry wound apparently trivial.

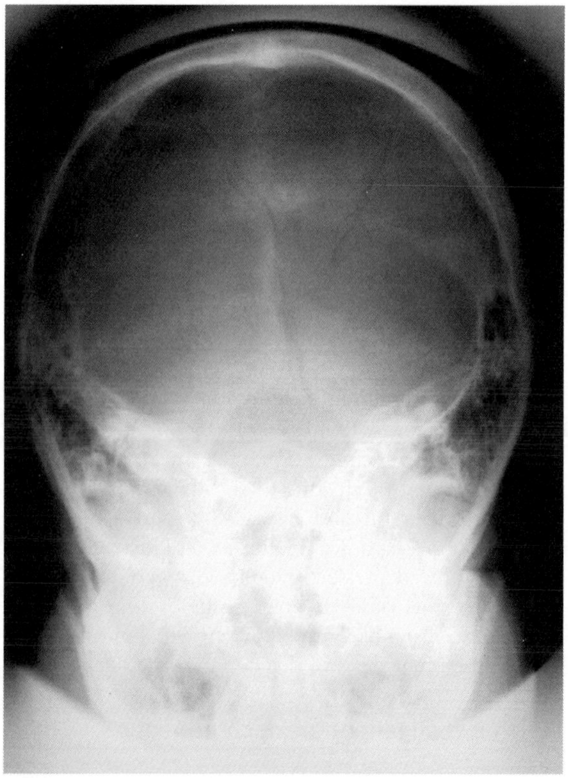

Figure 38.7 Skull films: Towne's view showing linear occipital fracture.

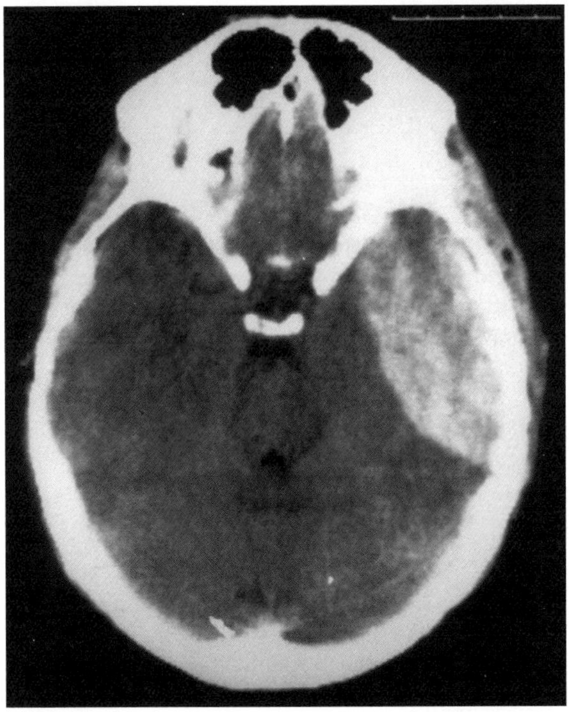

Figure 38.8 CT scan showing acute left temporal extradural haematoma.

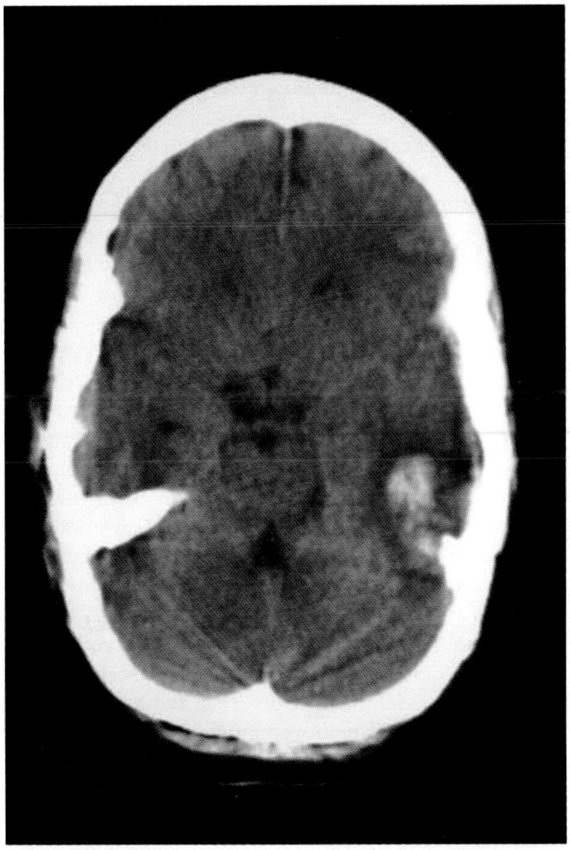

Figure 38.9 Cerebral contusion.

Table 38.3 Criteria for admitting a head injured patient to hospital

- The Glasgow Coma Scale (GCS) score is less than 15
- The GCS score is 15 but additional risk factors are present:
  - nausea and vomiting
  - persisting post-traumatic amnesia
  - a seizure at any time after injury
  - focal neurological signs in the limbs or pupils
  - irritability or abnormal behaviour
  - a recent skull fracture
  - an abnormal CT scan
- The patient has significant medical comorbidity or social problems

CT scanning – imaging the brain

CT scans show haematomas (Figure 38.8) and areas of contused and swollen brain (Figure 38.9), whose radiodensity differs from normal intracranial structures. The chief value of CT scanning is as a means of distinguishing patients at high and low risk of delayed deterioration, so that they can be sent to the most appropriate facility.

Section 38.5 • Deciding whether or not to admit the patient

Every hospital receiving trauma cases should use evidence-based criteria for admission after head injury (Table 38.3), taking into account its resources (staff numbers and skills, CT scanners) and its distance from neurosurgical services. Patients whose head injury is not trivial but who do not need immediate neurosurgical attention should be admitted for observation in order to detect the complications which a minority will develop and which can cause secondary brain damage. Admission may also be necessary if there is no reliable history or if there are other medical or social problems, e.g. extracranial injuries, alcohol abuse, anticoagulant therapy or concern about supervision at home. A senior doctor should be aware of the admission and approve the plan of management.

Section 38.6 • Neurological assessment on a surgical ward

A patient admitted to a surgical or short stay ward should be assessed *repeatedly and regularly* by staff familiar with the care of head injured patients, who understand the need to seek help early if deterioration occurs. Verbal and written communication must be of a high standard.

Neurological assessment tools for use after head injury need to be quick and simple, yet able to detect clinical change. Of greatest value are conscious level (measured by means of the GCS), pupil size and symmetry and light response, and the symmetry and

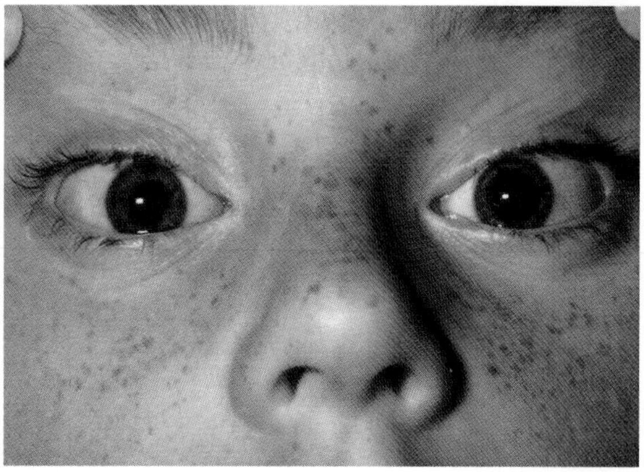

Figure 38.10 Dilated left pupil due to left extradural haematoma with tentorial herniation.

pattern of limb movements. Nurses should monitor and chart these, as well as respiratory rate, pulse rate, blood pressure and temperature.

The GCS is a simple yet powerful way to measure conscious level in any condition, and is as useful on general wards as in neurosurgical units. Module 14 of Vol. I describes the GCS and its use in more detail. The patients being considered in this module have a GCS of between 9/15 and 15/15, and the lower the initial GCS the greater should be the concern for the patient's safety and the readiness to obtain a CT scan and advice from a neurosurgeon. Patients thought to be under the influence of alcohol or other drugs need very careful observation, and the assumption that the drug is the cause of any deterioration or failure to improve must be resisted. If the alcohol level is below 200 mg% (43.5 mmol/l) persistent confusion and inability to obey commands warrants an urgent CT scan.

After a head injury there are several reasons why the pupils may be unequal in size or responsiveness to light (Figure 38.10), but a focal intracranial expanding lesion such as a haematoma must be assumed until proven otherwise. Limb responses are elicited by equal stimuli (verbal in a conscious patient, painful in an unconscious one) to the right and left sides. Again, any asymmetry should be ascribed to the head injury and appropriate action taken.

How often assessments are done depends on time since injury, GCS score, neurological progress, evidence of a skull fracture or CT changes, and specific risk factors like anticoagulant therapy. There is no magic 'recipe' for the frequency and duration of observation; what is needed is an intelligent awareness that even 'mildly' head injured patients can and do deteriorate as the result of intracranial events, and that vigilance is needed to detect this. It seems reasonable to recommend that a patient with an initial GCS score less than 13/15, or a skull fracture, or an abnormal CT scan with minimal neurological disturbance should be assessed every 15 min in A&E and in the ward until conscious level is normal, then hourly for at least 12–24 hours. If conscious level is not becoming normal within 4-6 hours the patient should have a scan or be discussed with a neurosurgeon. Even if he or she remains well, a doctor should carry out an assessment at least once in the first 24 hours after admission, looking at conscious level, limb power, signs of skull base fracture, cranial nerves, speech and cognitive function.

Section 38.7 • Recognizing and acting on deterioration

Urgent reappraisal by an experienced doctor is needed if there is a fall in the GCS (other than the normal variation in eye opening), increasing headache, persistent vomiting or a new neurological sign (e.g. limb or facial asymmetry or pupil inequality). Deterioration during clinical observation demands the same level of urgent attention as if the patient had just arrived in the resuscitation room in an unstable condition.

The priority is always to reassess the ABCs – airway, breathing and circulation – and to treat any problem found there. All trauma patients are 'dying for oxygen', and high flow oxygen should be given through a trauma (re-breathing) mask. Only when it is clear that deterioration is not explained by an ABC problem should attention turn to the head injury itself and the need for further action.

An important intracranial cause of deterioration is critically rising ICP from an occult haematoma. It is well known that outcome is closely related to how quickly the haematoma can be removed, and a patient in whom this complication is suspected must be referred immediately to a neurosurgeon with a view to arranging rapid transfer. In some areas limited neurosurgical resources may lead to a request to arrange a CT scan first, but if the decision to transfer is based on the clinical grounds that the patient has deteriorated neurologically then there is nothing to gain and potentially much to lose by exposing the patient to the delay and risk of an additional journey to the CT scan suite.

Head injury can cause generalized or focal epileptic fits. The risk is greatest when a depressed skull fracture or other wound has penetrated the dura and damaged the brain, post-traumatic amnesia (PTA) is prolonged, or there is a large haematoma. Generalized convulsive seizures are rare events on general surgical and orthopaedic wards, and alarm many doctors and nurses. As ever, the priority is to keep the airway open (either positionally or using an oral airway if this can be inserted) and to give high flow oxygen via a trauma mask. Intravenous or rectal diazepam is reserved for the few cases where the fit does not subside spontaneously after 1–2 min, and the dose given should be the least to abort the convulsive movements; 10 mg is a typical dose for an adult. Frequent neurological reassessment is done to monitor progress, and failure of the patient to recover within a few minutes demands immediate consultation with a neurosurgeon. As diazepam depresses respiration, it is wise to monitor the arterial blood gases after the fit and to seek anaesthetic help. Persistent or serial fits (status epilepticus) present an enormous threat to the brain; neurosurgical advice and anaesthetic help are needed to guide seizure control, definitive protection of the airway and decisions about the timing of transfer to neurosurgery.

Section 38.8 • Planning discharge

There are no rigid rules about how long observation needs to last, as the aim is to ensure that the patient has recovered enough to go home with no further fear of complications. CT scanners are increasingly used to confirm or exclude intracranial structural damage in patients still causing concern after observation for a day or two.

Before discharge from hospital every patient with mild head injury must be assessed by an experienced doctor, to establish that all discharge criteria have been met (Table 38.4). The patient should be given a head injury instruction card appropriate to their age (Tables 38.5 and 38.6), and a friend or relative must take responsibility for monitoring progress and reporting persistent or worsening symptoms. Enquiries about general health, medication, and home circumstances are important in the elderly, and referral to a geriatrician should be considered. The possibility of child abuse should be considered if the physical findings in a young child are not consistent with the explanation given, and a medical social worker should be consulted to allow investigation while observation continues on a paediatric ward.

Table 38.4 Pre-discharge examination of a head injured patient

Before discharge from the ward a patient with mild or moderate head injury must be critically assessed by an experienced doctor, who must confirm that:

- The GCS score has been 15 for at least 12 hours
- The patient is eating normally and not vomiting
- All neurological symptoms/signs have resolved or are minor, e.g.
  - mild headache relieved by simple analgesia
  - anosmia from olfactory nerve damage
  - positional vertigo from vestibular disturbance
- The patient is mobile/self caring or going to a safe environment with support
- There is no acute skull fracture or a CT scan has been done and is normal
- Extracranial injury has been excluded or treated

Table 38.5 Head injury instruction card (adults)

- Ensure a responsible person monitors you for the next 24 hours – show them this card
- Rest for the next 24 hours
- DO take painkillers such as paracetamol to relieve pain and headache
- DO NOT drink alcohol for the next 24 hours
- Take your normal medication, but DO NOT take sleeping tablets or tranquillizers without consulting your doctor first

If any of the following symptoms occur then you should return or be brought back to the hospital, or the hospital telephoned immediately (Telephone number: 1234 (24 hours)):

- Headache not relieved by painkillers such as paracetamol
- Vomiting
- Disturbance of vision
- Problems with balance
- Fits
- Unrousability

Table 38.6 Head injury instruction card (children)

- Your child has sustained a head injury, and following a thorough examination we are satisfied that the injury is not serious.
- Your child may be more tired than normal.
- Allow them to sleep if they want to
- Give Calpol or Disprol (paediatric paracetamol) for any pain or headache
- Try to keep your child resting for 24 hours.

If your child should develop any of the following, bring them back to the hospital or telephone for advice immediately:

- Headache not relieved by Calpol or Disprol
- Vomiting
- Altered vision
- Irritability
- Fits
- Becomes unrousable

Section 38.9 • Selecting patients for follow-up and rehabilitation

Even mild head injury can be followed by a wide variety of physical, cognitive and psycho-social symptoms (post-traumatic or post-concussional syndrome). Patients with PTA of over 1 hour, a skull fracture, or neuropyschological or neurological symptoms at discharge are more likely to have such problems.

Information on the common sequelae of head injury (e.g. memory problems, dizziness, attention deficits, anosmia), and advice on return to driving, work or sport should be available in hospital and be offered to patients at discharge. It may be helpful then or later to refer to a multidisciplinary team and/or a support agency (e.g. Headway). Advice on substance abuse and contact numbers of patient support groups can be offered if appropriate, either to the family or to the patient. The family in particular often needs much support and information during the difficult early months after a head injury.

It is good practice for a discharge letter to be sent to the general practitioner (GP), and this is a good time to offer to review the patient in an appropriate clinic if progress is not as expected or if new problems develop. In any event it should be made straightforward for the GP to seek a specialist opinion later, although expert resources are often scarce. In particular, some neuropsychological deficits may not be obvious at discharge, but only emerge later as the patient fails to readapt in the way that he and his family expected.

Advice may be available from various specialists, often working as a team: rehabilitation physician, clinical neuropsychologist, specialist liaison nurse, occupational therapist, physiotherapist, speech and language therapist, and medical social worker or care manager. Even mildly head injured patients can benefit from an interdisciplinary and goal-orientated approach to solving their problems. Continuity of care and information about the ability of patient and family to cope in the community can be obtained from home visits by social workers or occupational therapists, who often go on providing information and help long after other professionals have ceased to have any contact.

Conclusion

A recent report from the Royal College of Surgeons may have sounded the death knell for general surgical and orthopaedic involvement in the care of patients with recent minor and moderate head injury. However, this policy will only be complete after 10 years and is dependent on more resources being available to the two specialties whose workload will inevitably increase: neurosurgery and A&E. Meantime, there is a clear case for general and orthopaedic surgeons to put themselves in a position to look after patients with mild or moderate head injury according to the highest standards. As with anything in medicine, success is most likely when there is a clear understanding of roles and guidelines to help the non-expert clinician to make the best decision.

Further reading

American College of Surgeons Committee on Trauma (1993). *ATLS Course Manual*. Chicago, IL: American College of Surgeons.

Gentleman, D. (1999). Head and neck injuries. In: Greaves, I. and Porter, K. eds. *Pre-hospital Medicine – The Principles and Practice of Immediate Care*. London: Arnold.

Scottish Intercollegiate Guidelines Network (SIGN). *Guideline 46: Early Management of Head Injury*. SIGN, Royal College of Physicians of Edinburgh.

MODULE 39

Severe head injury

Head injuries are very common and their incidence is increasing throughout the world. Module 38 describes a pragmatic classification of head injury and discusses the clinical management of mild and moderate head injuries from the point of view of the general surgeon. This module looks at the early management of those head injuries which are clearly more serious from the outset.

Section 39.1 • Introduction

Severe head injuries occur either on their own or with other severe trauma. A thoracic injury is found in 40% of cases, long bone fractures in 60%, abdominal injuries in 20% and a spinal fracture in 15%. The presence of a head injury trebles mortality in multiply injured patients. Head injury is the main contributor to trauma-related mortality and long-term disability, and produces enormous social and economic costs to society as well as enormous suffering to the individual and their family.

Severe head injury is commonest in young adult men between the ages of 15 and 24 years. It is much less common in females (ratio 4:1). Motor vehicle accidents account for over 50% of cases, many of these related to alcohol. Other common causes are falls, assault and sport. Despite some variations this pattern is remarkably similar throughout the world, although the USA and some other countries have a particularly high incidence of gunshot wounds to the head. With the growing number of motor vehicles on the road world-wide, the incidence of vehicle-related trauma is expected to increase, and with it the overall number of severe head injuries. This is reflected in the importance that planners and clinicians give to the need for guidelines on the management of the severely head injured patient, from pre-hospital care through to rehabilitation (Table 39.1).

Table 39.1 The elements of good head injury care

- Injury prevention
- Pre-hospital care
- Organization of accident and emergency care
- Guidelines for imaging, especially computed tomography scanning
- Guidelines for referral and transfer to neurosurgery
- Standards for inter-hospital transfer
- Neurosurgical treatment
- Intensive care protocols
- Rehabilitation and follow-up

Section 39.2 • Classification of head injury

Brain damage from head injury can be classified by severity, mechanism or morphology (Table 39.2). *Initial severity of injury* is defined using the Glasgow Coma Scale (GCS) (Table 39.3), which is also the standard

Table 39.2 A classification of head injury

Severity of injury	Mild		GCS 13–15
	Moderate		GCS 9–12
	Severe		GCS 3–8
Mechanism of injury	Blunt trauma – high velocity		
	Blunt trauma – low velocity		
	Penetrating trauma		
Morphology	Skull fracture	Vault	Linear
			Depressed
		Base	
	Intracranial lesion	Focal	Haematoma
			Contusion
		Diffuse	

Table 39.3 The Glasgow Coma Scale

Eye opening	
	spontaneously
	to speech
	to pain
	none
Motor response (in upper limbs)	
	obeys commands
	localizes to pain
	withdraws to pain
	flexes to pain
	extends to pain
	no response
Verbal response	
	orientated
	confused
	inappropriate words
	incomprehensible sounds
	none

tool for monitoring the patient's neurological progress. Patients with severe head injury have a GCS score between 3 and 8 out of 15. A GCS score of less than 8/15 is the commonly used definition of coma.

The mechanism of injury produces a characteristic pattern of clinical imaging and pathological findings, so knowing it is of great clinical value. Blunt trauma at high velocity (e.g. a car crash) causes the brain to decelerate abruptly and imparts significant energy to it, resulting in a diffuse brain injury in which many neurones are irreparably damaged – 'diffuse axonal injury' (Figure 39.1a, b). The patient is in coma from the time of injury, and at the severe end of the spectrum may die immediately. Blunt trauma at low velocity (e.g. a fall in the street) is more likely to cause contusion of the brain surface as it strikes the inner surface of the skull (Figure 39.2). Penetrating injury (e.g. a gunshot wound) usually produces a track through the brain, with a varying extent of surrounding damage (Figure 39.3). High velocity bullets produce a shockwave, which causes 'cavitation' injury distant from the missile track and leads to a poor outcome.

Morphology is another way to classify head injuries. Fractures of the skull vault are either linear (Figure 39.4a) or depressed (Figure 39.4b). Fractures of the skull base are often easier to diagnose clinically than radiologically (Figure 39.5a, b). Intracranial lesions can be described as either focal or diffuse. Focal injuries are typified by intracranial haematoma (Figure 39.6) and cerebral contusions (Figure 39.2), while diffuse injury ranges from cerebral concussion in mild cases to widespread diffuse axonal injury in more severe ones (Figure 39.1).

Section 39.3 • Pathology of severe head injury

In the 1970s, Jennett and others introduced the concept of primary and secondary brain damage and focused attention on the avoidability of much death and disability after head injury. Intracranial and

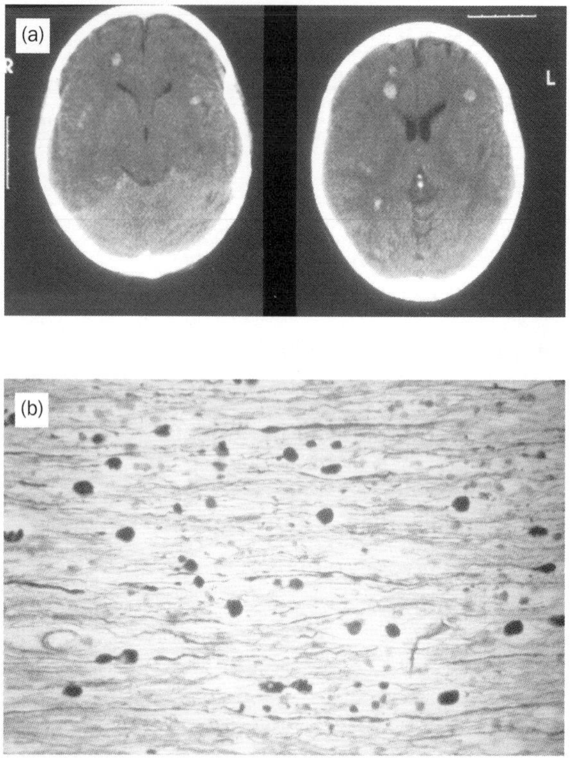

Figure 39.1 (a) CT brain scan showing severe diffuse brain injury with petechial haemorrhages throughout the grey and white matter of both cerebral hemispheres. (b) Photomicrograph of brain showing severe diffuse axonal injury with disruption of axonal structure and the formation of axon buds.

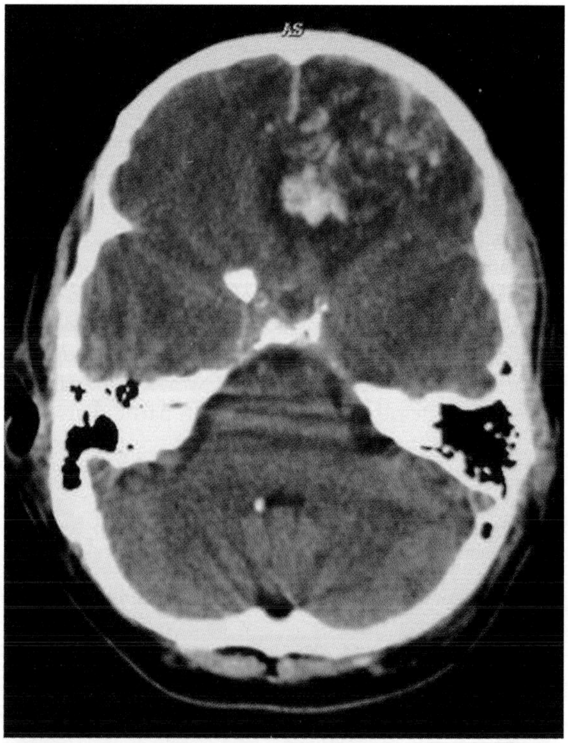

Figure 39.2 CT scan of brain showing left frontal contusions.

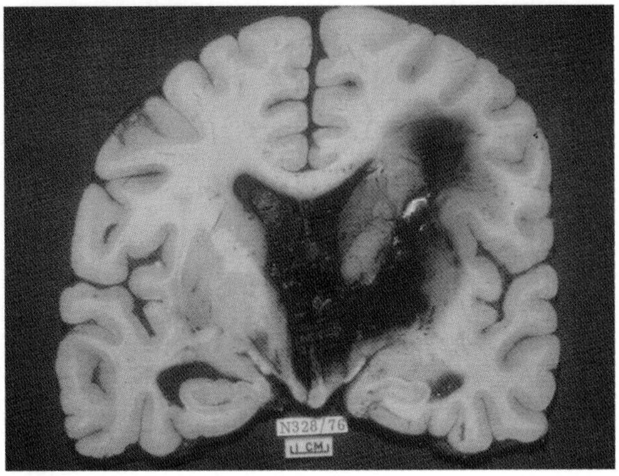

Figure 39.3 Coronal brain section showing missile track through right cerebral hemisphere into lateral ventricles, with haemorrhage into the track and ventricles.

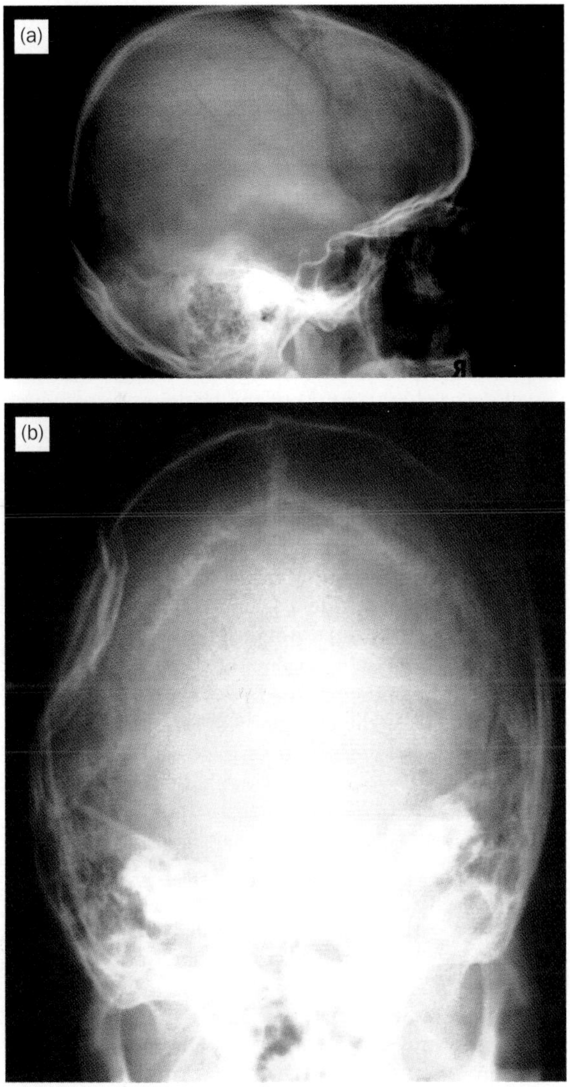

Figure 39.4 Plain skull films: (a) Lateral film showing linear fractures. (b) Towne's view showing tangential view of depressed skull fracture.

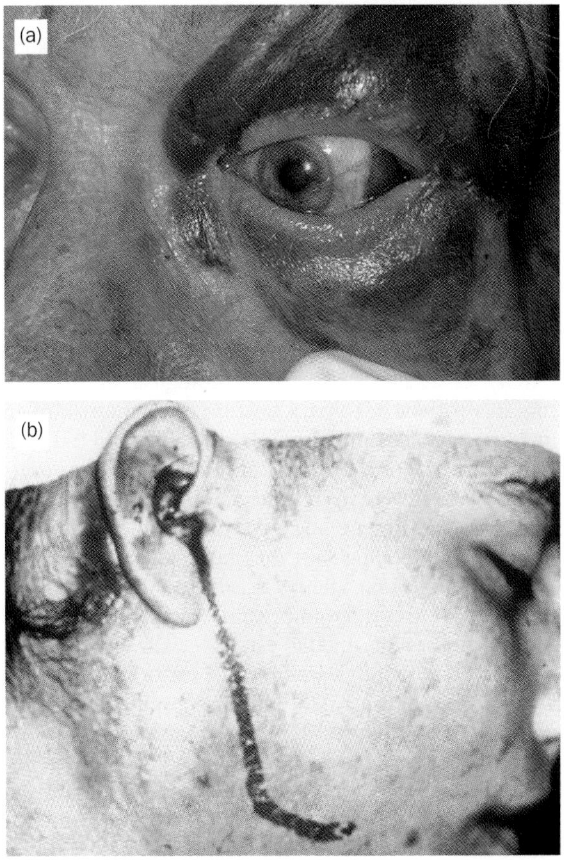

Figure 39.5 (a) Bilateral periorbital haematomas: fracture of anterior cranial fossa. (b) Cerebrospinal leak from the ear: fracture of middle cranial fossa.

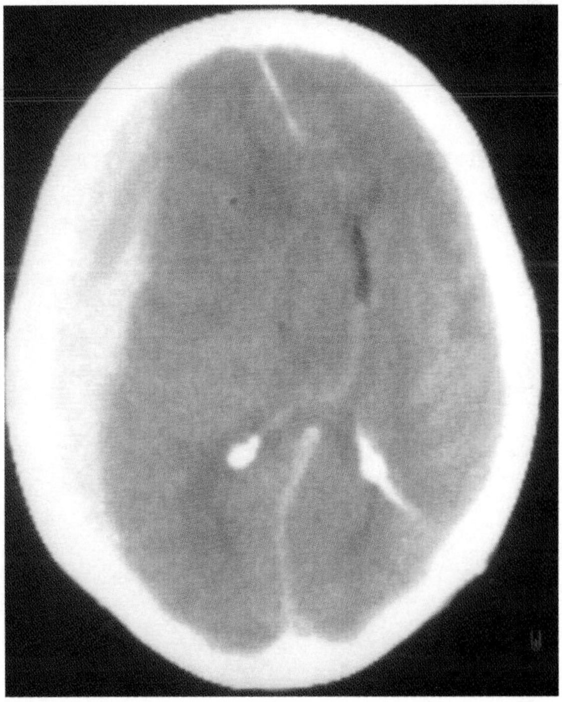

Figure 39.6 CT scan showing large acute right subdural haematoma, with severe midline shift to the left.

extracranial complications can threaten survival or the quality of that survival: haematoma, raised intracranial pressure (ICP), blood gas disturbances, and systemic shock. The attending doctor must be able to recognize these early on and follow established protocols of care to limit the risk of secondary injury and death.

Skull fractures

The importance of skull fracture is as a predictor of intracranial complications of head injury. An intracranial haematoma is more likely when there is a fracture (Table 38.1 in Module 38) on mild and moderate head injury), especially if there is neurological impairment too. In a patient in coma, a fracture raises the risk of an intracranial haematoma from 4% to 25%. Skull fractures occur in up to 65% of those admitted to a neurosurgical unit with severe head injury, and in as many as 80% of fatal cases. Most are linear fractures of the skull vault, sometimes extending into the skull base, and 4% have basal fractures alone. The latter carry the risk of delayed intracranial infection from organisms which spread from the air sinuses or middle ear, especially when cerebrospinal fluid (CSF) leaks from the ear or nose or there is intracranial air on a skull film or computed tomography (CT) scan (Figure 39.7). Depressed fractures of the vault usually have an overlying wound, and the penetrating bone fragment may tear the underlying dura and lacerate the brain. They too are an important route for intracranial infection, and also carry a significant risk of post-traumatic epilepsy. The risk of intracranial infection after head injury is low (3–5%) in the UK, but the resulting morbidity and mortality is high.

Intracranial haematomas and contusions

Extradural haematoma is found in 5–15% of patients with severe head injury, and usually results from bleeding

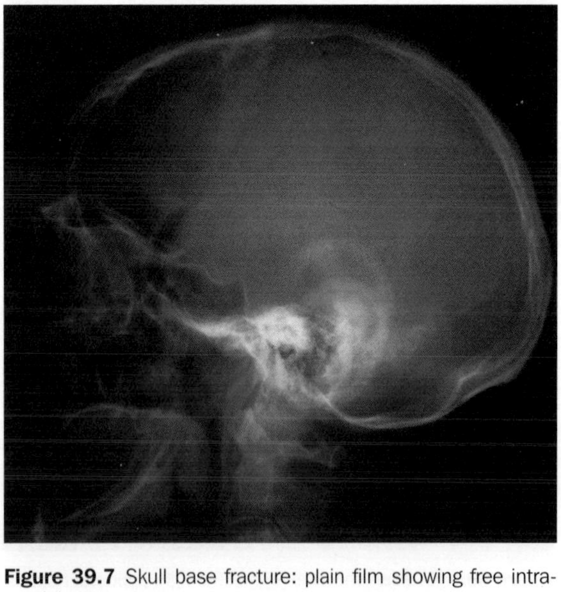

Figure 39.7 Skull base fracture: plain film showing free intracranial gas.

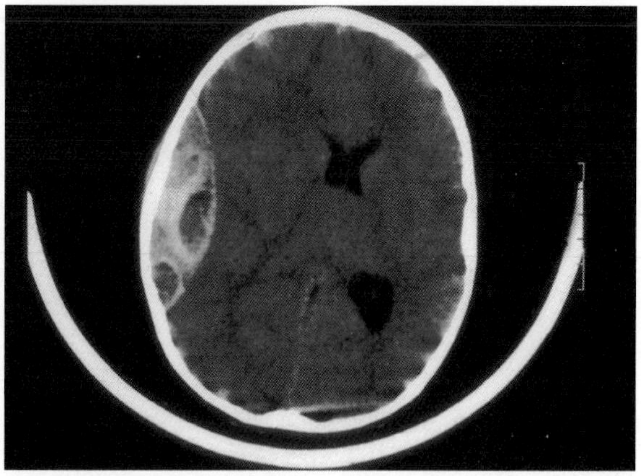

Figure 39.8 CT scan of acute right extradural haematoma, with displacement of the falx to the left.

from a tear of the middle meningeal artery, rarely a tear of a venous sinus. Small ones can arise from the fracture alone. As the haematoma enlarges, it gradually strips the dura from the inner table of the skull to form a large biconvex mass that progressively distorts the adjacent brain (Figure 39.8). Conscious level may remain more or less normal for some time (the 'lucid interval') before a rapid loss of consciousness, but more often the patient has been in coma from the time of injury due to significant primary brain injury. Extradural haematomas are most often found in the temporal region, but 30% occur elsewhere, including the posterior fossa.

Subdural haematoma has been reported in 26–63% of patients who sustain blunt trauma to the head. It is usually caused by rupture of the bridging veins which cross from the cerebral cortex to the inner surface of the dura mater, but can also result from a small tear in a cortical vessel on the brain surface. Low velocity blunt injury (such as occurs in assaults) may result in a lucid interval before conscious level deteriorates due to the expanding haematoma, but high velocity blunt injuries (e.g. road accidents) tend to cause coma from the outset due to primary brain injury.

An acute subdural haematoma is composed of clotted blood and appears hyperdense on CT scan (Figure 39.9a). As the clot gradually lyses over the next few days the scan starts to show hypo- and hyper-dense areas (Figure 39.9b), and once it has completely lysed its high osmotic pressure draws in water and produces a low density *'chronic' subdural haematoma* (Figure 39.9c). This gradually becomes encapsulated in a membrane and slowly grows in size as a result of repeated small haemorrhages into it, eventually distorting and compressing the brain. A chronic subdural haematoma often presents 1–4 months after an apparently trivial head injury, especially in the elderly. Subdural haematoma is the most common type of intracranial injury found in infants with non-accidental injury.

Intracerebral haematoma is found in 15% of patients who sustain a fatal head injury. It may be single or multiple and occurs mainly in a frontal or temporal lobe,

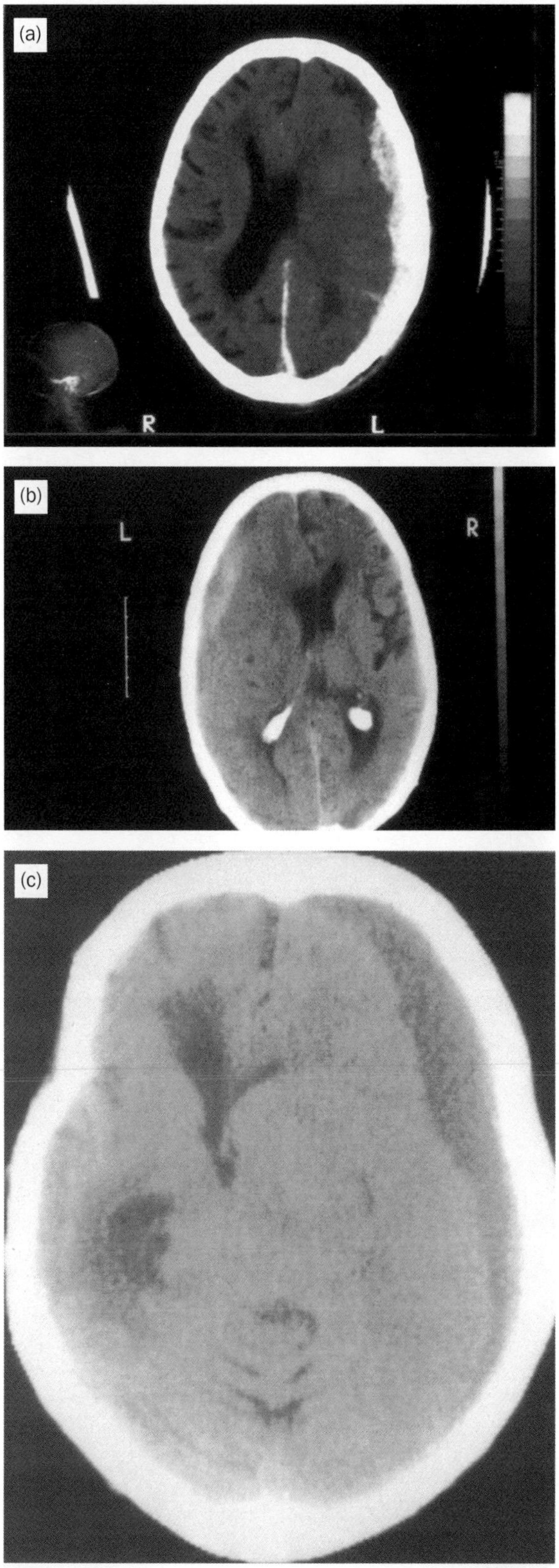

Figure 39.9 CT scan of acute left subdural haematoma with obliteration of sulcal pattern, midline shift to the left, and dilatation of the opposite lateral ventricle. (a) CT scan of subacute right subdural haematoma with mixed hyperdense and hypodense areas. (b) CT scan of left chronic subdural haematoma with midline shift.

less often in a cerebellar hemisphere (Figure 39.10a, b). They are caused by the direct rupture of blood vessels within the brain as it strikes the inner table of the skull at the moment of impact.

Cerebral contusions result from a similar mechanism. For example, in deceleration injuries the head is thrown backwards, the brain moves backwards, and the occipital lobes strike the inner table of the skull (a 'coup' injury). The brain then deforms and rebounds and the frontal lobes strike the inner table of the frontal bones (a 'contre-coup' injury). Contusions are most often seen in the frontal lobes, the temporal lobes (which impact against the sharp sphenoid wing) and the occipital lobes (Figure 39.11). Early on there is a variable degree of bleeding and swelling in the brain

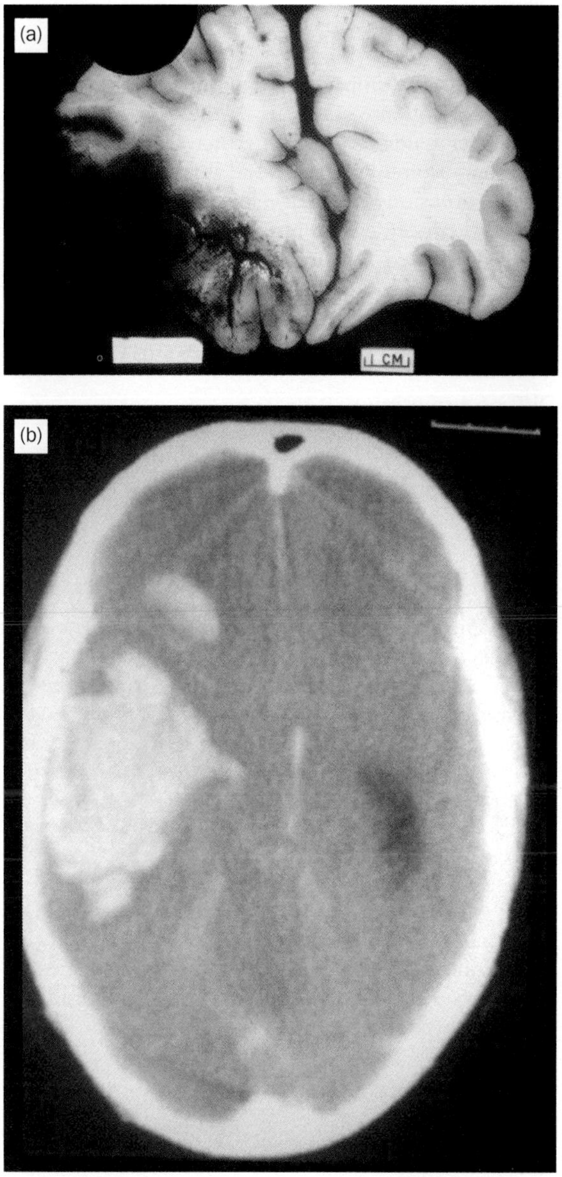

Figure 39.10 (a) Coronal brain slice showing large left temporal intracerebral haematoma. (b) CT scan showing large right fronto-parietal intracerebral haematoma with severe brain compression and midline shift to the left.

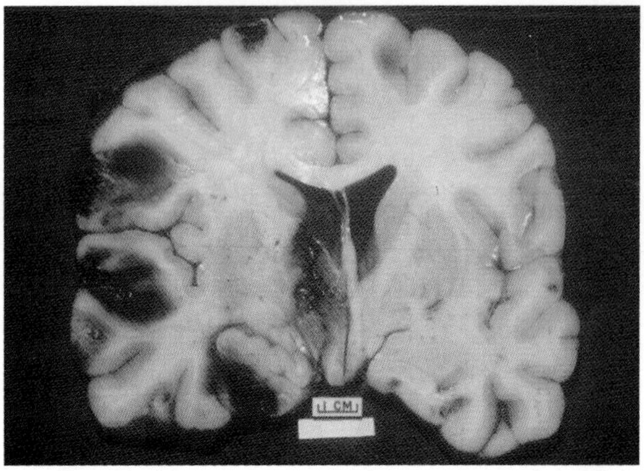

Figure 39.11 Coronal brain slice showing multiple cerebral contusions.

adjacent to the impact, and in the long term these lesions develop into glial scars. As the damage caused by contusions tends to be focal rather than diffuse, consciousness is often well preserved at first. However, even small contusions can develop significant swelling around them or develop into haematomas, and there is a risk of delayed deterioration on the third or fourth day after injury in a patient who has hitherto been well (Figure 39.12a, b). Despite this risk, even patients with severe contusions can make a good recovery.

Diffuse brain injury

Diffuse injury represents a wide spectrum of severity, which is not necessarily paralleled by the appearance of the brain on CT scan. In mild and moderate cases the clinical syndrome of cerebral concussion is associated with little structural damage and a normal CT scan. In severe cases diffuse axonal injury causes widespread brain damage (Figure 39.1b) and coma from the time of injury, but even so the initial CT scan may show little abnormality bar a few petechial haemorrhages in the corpus callosum or the midbrain (Figure 39.1a). Evidence of diffuse axonal injury is found in about 50% of severely head injured patients, and it causes one third of deaths from severe head injury.

Hypoxic/ischaemic brain injury

Autopsy studies show histological evidence of brain ischaemia in up to 97% of fatal severe head injuries, underlining the importance of rapid and effective resuscitation. Inadequate oxygenation or perfusion of the brain is associated with a very poor outcome.

Penetrating head injury

This can be caused by a low velocity object (such as a metal spike) or an object with higher velocity and imparting more energy (such as a bullet). Low velocity injuries can simply result in a compound depressed fracture, with or without tearing of the dura, but the missile may also penetrate the brain and produce a focal injury (Figure 39.13). This type of injury carries a high risk of brain swelling, seizures and delayed infection. Outcome from such injuries can be good if the rest of the brain is undamaged, but in high velocity missile injuries due to bullets or shrapnel a significant shock wave travels through the brain tissue (cavitation) and causes significant damage at a distance from the missile track (Figure 39.14). A high index of suspicion is needed to avoid missing penetrating head injuries, especially where the weapon has caused a small entry wound.

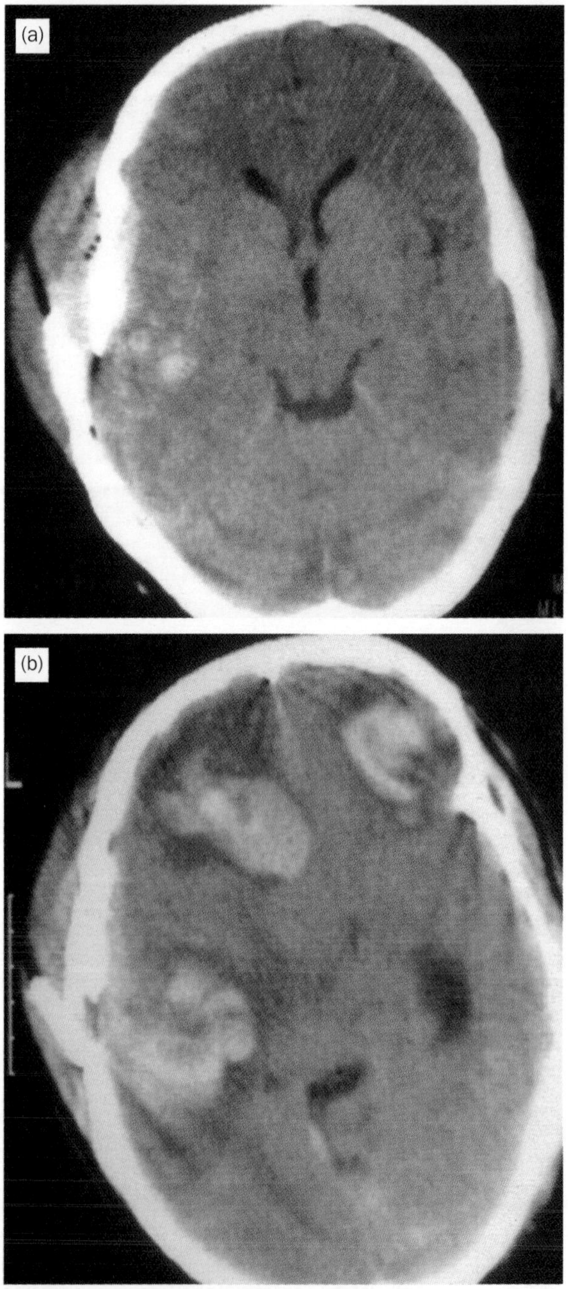

Figure 39.12 (a) CT scan showing right depressed skull fracture and minor cerebral contusions. (b) Increase in size of bilateral contusions after 3 days, with increased ICP (same patient as (a)).

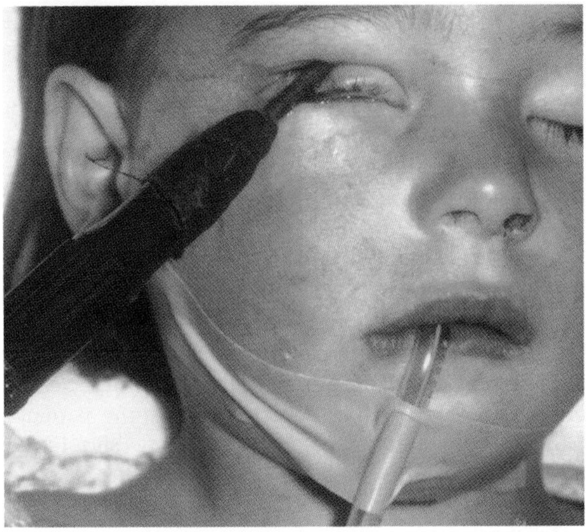

Figure 39.13 Accidental stab injury of right frontal lobe. If still embedded the weapon should not be withdrawn before theatre.

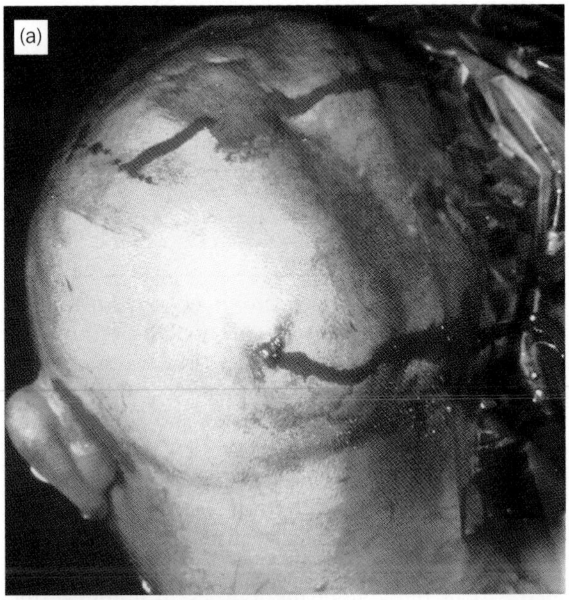

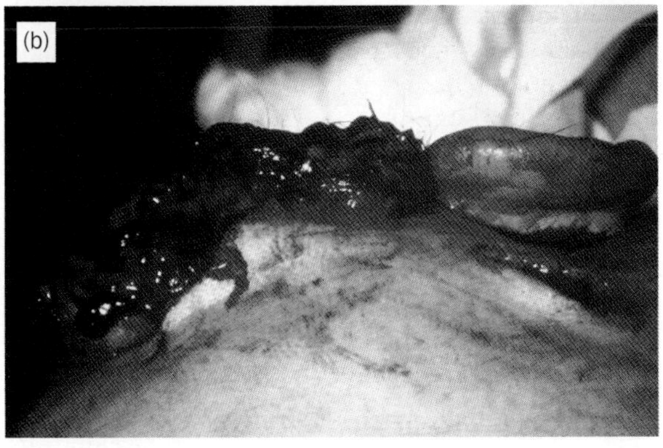

Figure 39.14 Gunshot wound of the head caused by a bullet from Kalashnikov rifle (AK47). (a) Entry wound, (b) exit wound.

Section 39.4 • Early clinical management

A head injured patient who cannot speak, obey commands or open the eyes to stimuli is by definition in coma, has sustained a severe head injury, and is at high risk of serious or even life-threatening complications.

Immediate priorities: oxygenation and perfusion

The immediate need is for clinical assessment and resuscitation, using a standard protocol such as the advanced trauma life support system described in **Module 39, Volume I**. Table 39.4 outlines the initial assessment and resuscitation of the head injured patient (the primary survey). Attention is directed to clearing and maintaining a patent airway, stabilizing the cervical spine, ensuring adequate chest movements, administering high flow oxygen by face mask or endotracheal tube, and maintaining adequate perfusion of the brain and other organs.

As brain injury is adversely affected by secondary insults such as hypoxaemia or shock, these require immediate attention if found. A significant proportion of patients are hypoxaemic, shocked or anaemic when they arrive in the accident and emergency (A&E) department – sometimes a combination of these. The presence of hypovolaemic shock doubles mortality when compared with normotensive patients (60% versus 27% mortality), and if there is also hypoxaemia mortality rises to 75% or even more. Restoring adequate oxygenation and circulation is therefore vital to a good outcome.

All head injured patients with a GCS score of 8 or less should undergo endotracheal intubation and ventilation. High flow 100% oxygen should be administered until the blood gases are known. Signs of shock should always be assumed to be due to systemic bleeding and not attributed to a brain injury, except in the occasional young child who has sustained significant blood loss from scalp injuries. Brain injury causes hypotension only in the late stages of brain stem failure, and it must not be assumed that low blood pressure or other signs of shock are due to a brain injury until thorough and conscientious searches for extracranial injuries have consistently revealed nothing.

Another important cause of hypotension is spinal cord injury (when the pulse rate is often paradoxically low). In these cases administering large volumes of fluid can cause increased mortality from pulmonary oedema, and a spinal cord injury should be ruled out as soon as

Table 39.4 Immediate priorities in the management of the severely head injured patient

A	clear and protect AIRWAY, control cervical spine
B	assess and maintain adequate BREATHING
C	assess and maintain adequate CIRCULATION
D	briefly assess neurological function – DISABILITY
E	EXPOSE the whole body, check the ENVIRONMENT

Table 39.5 Indications for consulting a neurosurgeon after severe head injury

- When a CT scan in a general hospital shows a recent intracranial lesion
- When a patient fulfils the criteria for CT scanning but this cannot be done within a reasonable period
- Irrespective of the result of any CT scan, when the patient has clinical features that give rise to concern that neurosurgical assessment, monitoring or management is required, e.g.:
  - GCS score deteriorating after admission (sustained drop of one point on the motor or verbal subscales, or two points on the eye opening subscale)
  - persisting coma (GCS score 8 or less) after initial resuscitation
  - progressive focal neurological signs
  - a seizure
  - confusion which persists for more than 6–8 hours
  - compound depressed skull fracture
  - definite or suspected penetrating injury
  - a CSF leak

possible before administering large volumes of fluid.

When blood pressure is low or is only restored temporarily by infusing intravenous fluids, or there are other signs of hypovolaemic shock, a search for the source of bleeding is the priority. Investigations and procedures such as the insertion of chest drains, diagnostic peritoneal lavage and CT of the chest or abdomen take priority over a CT scan of the head. However, as soon as the patient's blood pressure and oxygenation are stable, the exclusion of an intracranial haematoma by CT scan is necessary.

A CT scan of the head should not be performed until the patient's medical condition has been stabilized. Since the negative impact of hypoxaemia or shock on head injury outcome is so large, there is no benefit – and considerable risk – to the patient being taken to the CT scanner in an unstable condition.

Most A&E departments in the UK are in hospitals without a neurosurgical unit, so inter-hospital transfer becomes necessary for patients who require neurosurgery or neurointensive care. It is essential that the patients have been properly assessed and stabilized *first*, so that there is minimal risk of deterioration in transit. An abnormal CT scan of the head should be discussed with the local neurosurgical unit before transfer. Indications for consultation with a neurosurgeon are detailed in Table 39.5.

The secondary survey

After the primary survey (initial assessment and resuscitation) and the patient has been scanned, a secondary survey should be carried out. Up to half of patients with severe head injury have systemic injuries too, and some of these are easily overlooked at first. A complete examination of the patient should be carried out, including log rolling to examine the back and spine. The secondary survey should include tests for full blood count, urea and electrolytes, coagulation profile, blood group typing and cross matching of blood, arterial blood gases, hepatic enzymes, amylase, and in females a pregnancy test. Urinalysis should be done. X-rays of cervical spine, chest and pelvis should be done as a routine, but as the patient has had a CT scan, skull films are rarely useful.

Confusion can arise as to the relative priorities of a laparotomy or thoracotomy for truncal bleeding versus a craniotomy for intracranial haematoma. As a general rule, the thoracotomy or laparotomy should be done first in order to stabilize the patient and so protect cerebral perfusion. Where there is a neurosurgeon on site, a craniotomy can be performed simultaneously, but more usually transfer is necessary, and the patient must be stabilized *first*. During the secondary survey, the patient's GCS score and pupillary light response should be assessed. It is very important to carry out a reliable neurological examination to assess the patient's GCS score *before* intubation and ventilation, as this is extremely useful in guiding decision making later on. In patients who have been intubated but not yet sedated or paralysed it is usual to record verbal response as a 'T' on the chart. Where there has been a direct injury to the eye or a major facial injury with swelling a dilated non-reacting pupil *may* reflect local trauma, but the only safe practice is to assume that it is due to an intracranial complication until proved otherwise.

Often the need for urgent transfer prevents completion of the secondary survey at the referring hospital. It is then important that the neurosurgical team know this, so that they can complete the secondary survey as soon as possible.

Inter-hospital transfer

Patients who need urgent neurosurgery or admission to a neurosurgical intensive care unit (ICU) often require inter-hospital transfer. This carries risks for the patient and sometimes for the accompanying clinical staff too, and should not be undertaken unless and until the neurosurgical unit agrees that it is necessary. When it is, the clinical support for inter-hospital transfer should be of a high standard. The patient must be accompanied by an experienced doctor (usually an anaesthetist) and a nurse or paramedic. They must be able to monitor the ventilated patient throughout the journey, to minimize the risk of unrecognized systemic injuries, to prevent hypoxaemia and shock, to ensure that the cervical spine is safely immobilized, and to communicate effectively with the neurosurgical unit. The CT scan and cross-matched blood must be brought with the patient. Adherence to a recognized protocol reduces the risk of oversight and improves outcome for patients.

Therapeutic manoeuvres

Prior to transfer of the head injured patient, various interventions may be indicated. Mannitol has a high molecular weight, and its osmotic effect produces a rapid but short-lived reduction in brain swelling. Its main disadvantage is that it promotes a diuresis, and in patients who are shocked it may precipitate recurrent hypotension. Routine use of mannitol is not recommended, and it should be reserved for patients with clear signs of raised ICP, such as a dilated and unreactive pupil, bradycardia or an extensor motor response in the limbs. When these are absent and the CT scan shows no intracranial haematoma or other significant mass lesion, then mannitol should not be given. Hyperventilation has been used as a temporizing measure for patients with neurological deterioration due to raised ICP. However, aggressive hyperventilation has been shown to have an adverse effect on outcome after severe head injury, because it produces a metabolic alkalosis which causes cerebrovascular constriction and in turn cerebral ischaemia. There is no evidence that it reduces overall mortality, so pCO_2 levels should be kept within or just below the normal range in most cases. Steroids are still given to severely head injured patients in many countries, but there is no good evidence of either benefit or harm. The possibility of a small benefit has not been excluded, and the results of a large ongoing clinical trial (the CRASH trial) are awaited.

Section 39.5 • Imaging

Skull films

The place of skull films in the modern management of head injury remains controversial. As most cases of moderate and severe head injury fulfil the guidelines for a CT scan, skull films are usually unnecessary. However, they can be useful for quickly determining the site of skull fractures (especially depressed fractures) and whether or not there are significant injuries of the facial skeleton. If done they should be examined for evidence of linear or depressed fractures of the skull vault (Figure 39.4a, b) or skull base fractures (fluid levels in the sphenoid and maxillary sinuses, intracranial air) (Figures 39.5 and 39.7).

Computed tomography scan

CT scanning is well established as the investigation of choice in severe head injury. It is increasingly used too in moderate head injury and selected cases of mild head injury [see Module 40, Volume I]. Radiodensity is measured in Hounsfield units (HU), and the normal intracranial tissues have characteristic radiodensities: grey matter (36–60 HU), white matter (24–36 HU) and blood (40–80 HU). CT scans can be reconstructed in soft tissue, blood and bone window algorithms, allowing subtle details to be differentiated. For example, the 'slot' fracture caused by a stab injury is best seen on bone windows, while petechial haemorrhages within the brain substance are revealed by soft tissue settings.

When examining the CT scan of a patient with a severe head injury, it is important to look carefully for blood, contusions, and evidence of focal or generalized brain swelling. Acute haematomas (Figures 39.6, 39.8, 39.9a and 39.10b) are white (high radiodensity), but if managed without operation the blood gradually becomes isodense with brain (Figure 39.9b), then hypodense (Figure 39.9c), over a period of days as its chemical composition alters. An acute extradural haematoma forms a biconvex mass, often running from one suture line to another (Figure 39.8). An acute subdural haematoma tends to form an irregular crescentic shape conforming to the surface of most of one cerebral hemisphere (Figure 39.9a). An intracerebral haematoma appears as a rounded hyperdense area of variable size within the brain substance (Figure 39.10b). It is often associated with contusion of the brain, which if large can constitute a 'burst' frontal or temporal lobe (Figure 39.15).

Cerebral contusions are a trap for the unwary clinician. At first they can appear as small areas of high density on the surface of the brain, which seem harmless. However, even small contusions can enlarge significantly over the next few days, and this can go unrecognized unless the patient is carefully monitored and re-scanned (Figure 39.12a, b). The next scan may reveal patchy blood (hyperdense) within swollen brain tissue (hypodense). If the volume of blood and swollen brain involves most of a lobe (Figure 39.15) there is a risk of delayed clinical deterioration and even death.

Signs of diffusely raised ICP include obliteration of the third ventricle, narrowing or obliteration of the basal cisterns, and disappearance (effacement) of the normal pattern of cortical sulci (Figure 39.16a). An expanding haematoma or a large area of contused brain can also distort the underlying cerebral hemisphere and makes it swell, displacing midline structures such as the third ventricle (Figure 39.6). The swollen brain obliterates the third ventricle and the basal cisterns around the mid-

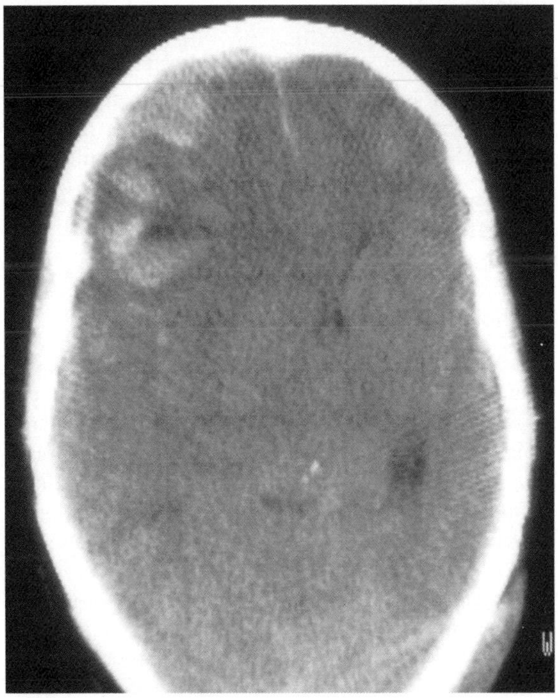

Figure 39.15 Axial CT scan showing burst right frontal lobe with brain distortion and raised ICP.

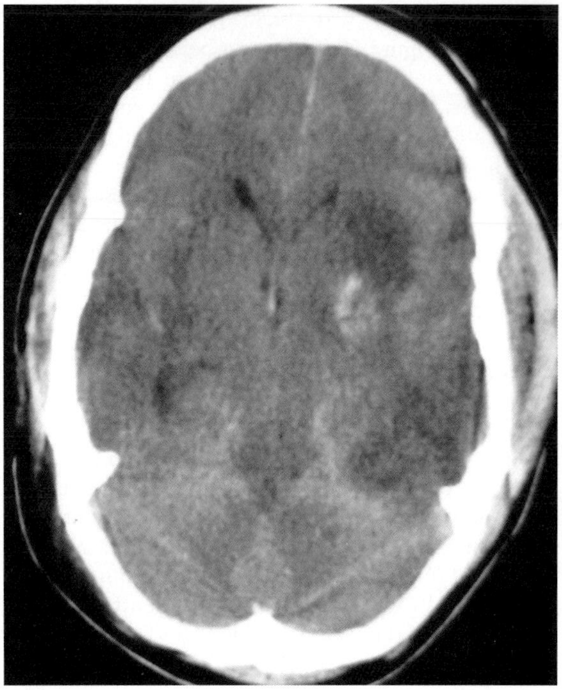

Figure 39.16 Diffusely swollen brain with raised ICP.

brain, eventually compressing the foramen of Munro and blocking normal CSF outflow from the contralateral ventricle, which dilates (Figure 39.9a) and further raises ICP. This is a late sign, and a worrying one.

CT scan data can help to predict outcome. The risk of death is considerably increased by an intracranial haematoma which is large enough to require surgery, especially if diagnosis and treatment are delayed for any reason. Smaller rises in mortality are seen with brain swelling and with traumatic subarachnoid haemorrhage. However, patients with abnormal CT scan appearances which do not include these features have a mortality rate which is no higher than those with a normal scan.

Section 39.6 • Operative surgical treatment

Burrhole drainage: crisis intervention

The one neurosurgical procedure which a general surgeon may occasionally be called on to perform is a burrhole to decompress an acute extradural haematoma. Any acute haematoma consists largely of *clotted* blood, so the definitive treatment is always to lift a craniotomy flap, evacuate the clot and control the point of bleeding – which clearly should be done by a trained neurosurgeon. Rarely, extremely rapid deterioration from a large expanding extradural haematoma justifies emergency burrhole decompression by a non-neurosurgeon, to buy time before embarking on transfer to a neurosurgical unit which may be some distance away or difficult to reach because of bad weather. This scenario is much less rare in countries where travel is longer or more difficult than in the UK, or where there are fewer neurosurgeons.

Skilful judgement about the best option may be needed in a head injured patient with a rapidly deteriorating conscious level who is developing signs of critical brain compression (e.g. a dilated and unreactive pupil). Neurosurgical advice should be sought whenever possible before the general surgeon embarks on a burrhole operation. Such intervention can be life-saving (especially if the clot is extradural) and achieve a temporary reduction in ICP, but continued bleeding can make it a potentially hazardous procedure for the inexperienced surgeon. In any event, a neurosurgeon should be involved in the decision-making process as early as possible, and will almost certainly wish to convert the burrhole into a craniotomy in due course.

The traditional temporizing measure in a patient with a suspected extradural haematoma is a burrhole over the likely site of the haematoma. Most often this is near the pterion or just above the origin of the zygoma (Figure 39.17). If more than one burrhole is made they should be placed along the line that will ultimately be used to fashion a craniotomy flap (Figure 39.18). A 3–5 cm skin incision is made, and the incision is carried through to the periosteum. Bleeding from galeal vessels is most conveniently and rapidly controlled by a self-retaining retractor. The periosteum is incised or diathermied and scraped off the bone, and a standard 14–16 mm perforator (Figure 39.19) is used to drill a conical hole in the bone. The burrhole is irrigated to remove bone dust and allow its depth to be judged by frequent direct inspection until the dura can be seen at its apex. It is crucial not to apply too much force in the latter stages of drilling with the perforator, to avoid the risk of plunging into the brain. Once the dura is seen, a burr (Figure 39.19) is used to enlarge the hole to about 16 mm diameter. Children have thinner skulls, and a rounded enlarged 'rose' burr can then be used on its own to fashion the hole.

An extradural haematoma appears at this stage as a dark and solidified blood clot at the base of the burrhole (Figure 39.20). It may issue under pressure or with *gentle* suction. Bone nibblers can be used to enlarge the opening into a small craniectomy to get better access to the clot, but the general surgeon should be satisfied at this stage with achieving a reduction in ICP, and not hunt around for the source of the haemorrhage. Bleeding from dura or bone can be stopped with judicious use of diathermy or bone wax, respectively.

Often the haematoma proves to be subdural, appearing as a blue discoloration beneath a tense dura. Unless experienced it is wise to stop there. The surgeon *may* consider making a small incision in the dura to release some of the subdural clot and relieve the raised ICP. Diathermy is useful for reducing haemorrhage from the exposed dura before it is nicked with a small scalpel and opened with scissors to reveal dark clotted blood, some of which may emerge under pressure, often mixed with disrupted brain tissue. Irrigation may release enough clot to reduce ICP temporaily, but without a craniotomy the haematoma is sure to reaccumulate

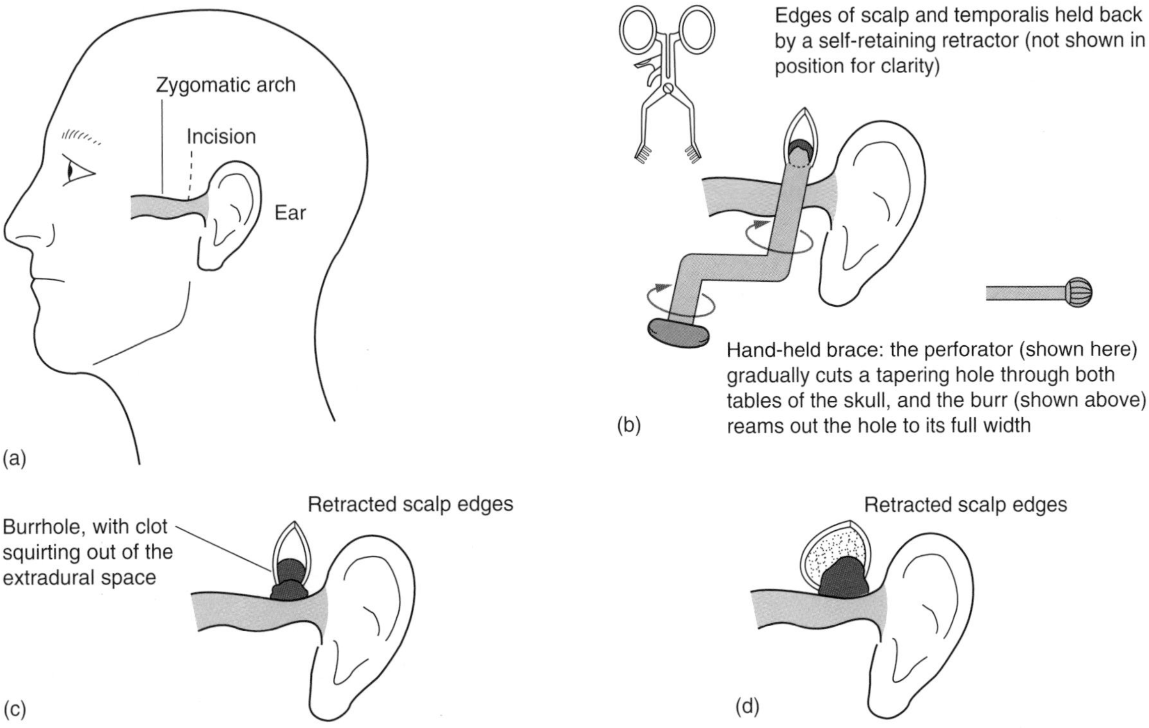

Figure 39.17 Burrhole drainage of an extradural haematoma: diagrams showing the technique for fashioning a burrhole.

quickly. It is vital *not* to put a sucker blindly into the dural opening, in case this further damages the brain. Sometimes the underlying brain lobe starts to bulge out through the dural opening, but it is then a bad mistake to open the dura further unless one has the ability to carry out a craniotomy.

Craniotomy: the definitive intervention

Few UK general surgeons ever undertake a craniotomy themselves in their professional lifetimes, but most will from time to time look after patients who have undergone craniotomy for haematoma by a neurosurgeon. In some countries such operations have to form part of the general surgical repertoire. For these reasons general surgeons should understand the principles of craniotomy for traumatic intracranial haematoma.

Definitive surgery for an extradural haematoma must allow access to the source of the bleeding as well as the clot itself. Often the culprit is the middle meningeal artery as it emerges from the foramen spinosum and runs beneath the squamous temporal bone. An extradural haematoma near a venous sinus needs expert attention, as torrential venous bleeding is possible during surgery. Craniotomy for an acute subdural haematoma must allow access to nearly the whole of the hemisphere, as the clot usually covers a wide area and its source is unknown before surgery. A large question-mark shaped scalp flap is progressively reflected, using arterial clips or skin edge haemostatic clips to

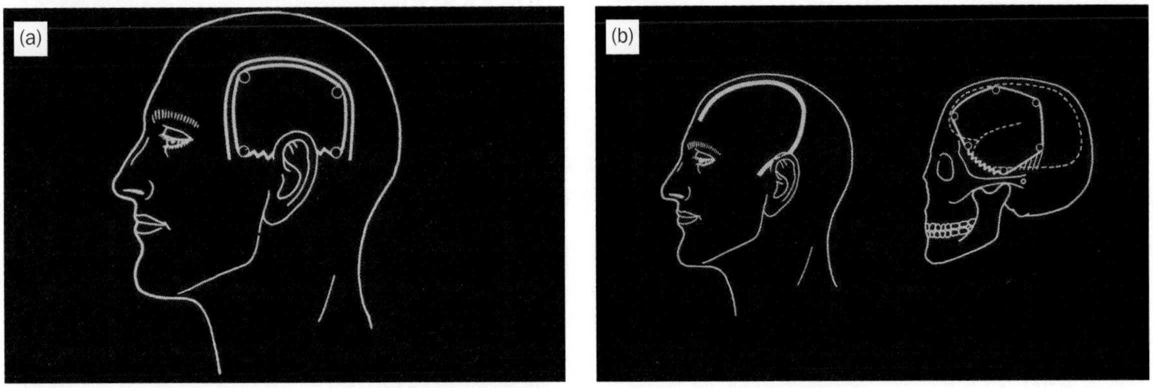

Figure 39.18 (a) Position of burrholes and craniotomy flap for temporal extradural haematoma. (b) Position of burrholes for craniotomy flap for fronto-temporal subdural haematoma.

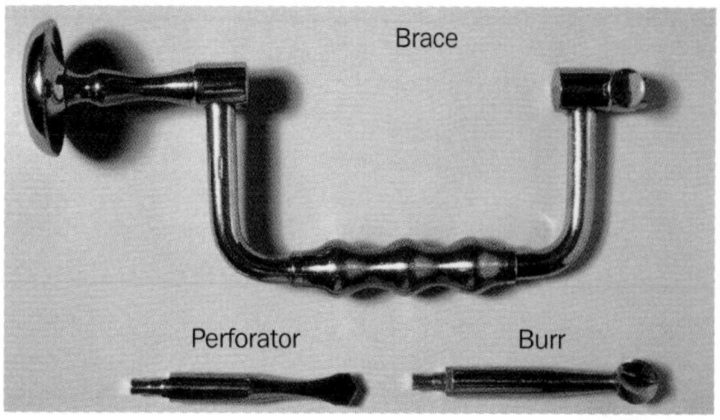

Figure 39.19 Hudson brace, with perforator and burr.

reduce blood loss (Figure 39.21a). Several burrholes are placed at the margins of the incision and joined with a flexible Gigli saw or a craniotome, allowing a large area of bone to be gently raised from the dura. Bleeding from the bone edges is controlled by bone wax, and from the dura by sutures placed around its exposed margins to tack it up to the periosteum. The dura is nicked with a scalpel and then widely opened to reveal the underlying haematoma (Figure 39.21b), which is gently removed by suction and irrigation so as not to damage the underlying cortex. A systematic search is made under direct vision or microscope illumination to find the source of bleeding (Figure 39.21c, d). Care must be taken to keep the anaesthetist well informed about blood loss and potential difficulties, so that clotting problems and hypotension can be prevented. Swollen brain may make it difficult or impossible to suture the dura or even replace the bone flap.

Many subdural haematomas are associated with brain contusion, intracerebral haematoma and brain swelling. As a general rule the surgeon must deal with all components that may contribute to a potentially lethal elevation in ICP, e.g. frontal lobectomy for a

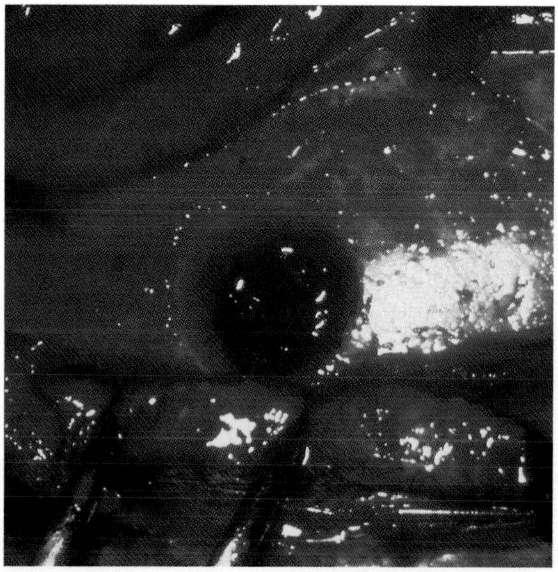

Figure 39.20 Burrhole with extradural haematoma visible at its base.

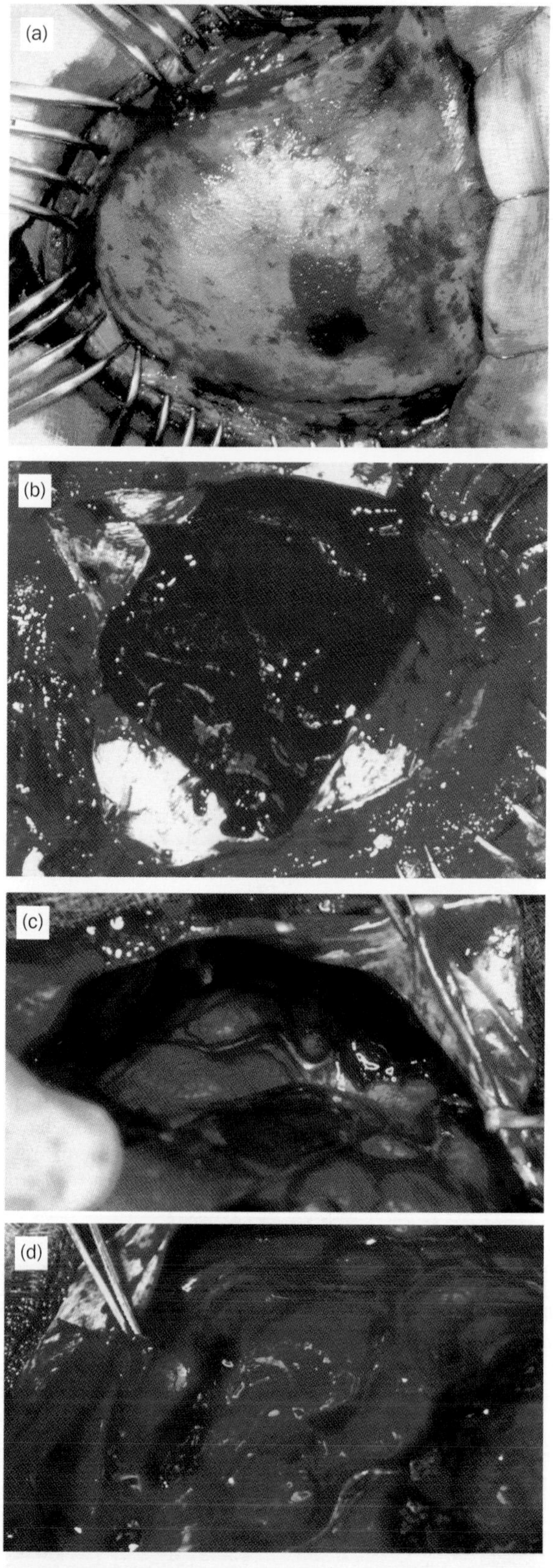

Figure 39.21 Evacuation of acute subdural haematoma. (a) Question-mark-shaped scalp flap being reflected. (b) Subdural haematoma exposed as the dura is opened. (c) Looking for the bleeding point. (d) Diathermy of vein causing the haematoma.

burst lobe. Wide craniectomy with dural incisions may be effective and should be considered as a prophylactic measure if further swelling is likely, but this decision should be made by a trained neurosurgeon.

During wound closure a subgaleal drain should be used to close the potential space beneath the scalp, and a gravity drain left in the extradural space may reduce reaccumulation. Patients who do not improve at the expected rate after decompressive surgery should be rescanned to exclude reaccumulation of the original clot, formation of a new clot or enlargement of a contusion. Reaccumulation has been shown to be more likely in patients with platelet counts below 100×10^9 and reduced fibrinogen levels, and in most cases it occurs within the first 6 hours after surgery.

Section 39.7 • Critical care

Patients who have sustained a severe head injury and have evidence of brain swelling and CT signs of raised ICP should be admitted to a neurosurgical ICU and intensively monitored. Monitoring various physiological parameters allows the early detection and treatment of rising ICP, falling cerebral perfusion pressure and secondary brain events due to changes in systemic blood pressure or oxygenation. Table 39.6 shows the types of monitoring that can be performed on patients in the ICU.

Clinical monitoring

In a sedated or anaesthetized patient neurological monitoring depends on examining the pupils. Intermittent reversal of anaesthesia can allow some assessment of conscious level or focal signs. This type of monitoring is important but limited, and not sufficient to monitor the severely injured brain.

Systemic monitoring

This usually includes blood pressure measurements via an arterial line. Systemic blood pressure must be maintained to ensure adequate cerebral perfusion, and CPP cannot be calculated without an accurate reading of systemic blood pressure. *Pulse oximetry* allows the early detection of hypoxia, which is associated with a poor prognosis in head injury. *Central venous access* allows monitoring of the adequacy of fluid administration, and provides a route for fluid and drugs, e.g. adrenergic drugs to raise blood pressure and improve cerebral perfusion. *Core temperature* should be monitored, as hyperthermia is associated with a poor prognosis in brain injury and should be treated aggressively. Clinical trials are under way to assess the usefulness of hypothermia in the treatment of severe brain injury. Cooling to 32°C within 10 hours of injury has been shown to improve neurological recovery in head injured patients with a GCS of 5–7, but not in those with a lower GCS. *Blood gas analysis* allows monitoring of pCO_2 levels. Routine hyperventilation is not advocated, as it produces a metabolic alkalosis which can trigger cerebral vasoconstriction and decrease cerebral blood flow. The advantages of a lower ICP are then offset by cerebral ischaemia, and outcome is poorer.

Table 39.6 Methods of monitoring in neurological critical care units

Clinical	Glasgow Coma Scale, pupil reactivity to light
Systemic monitoring	Blood pressure, pulse oximetry, central venous pressure, core temperature, blood gas analysis
Imaging	CT scanning
Cerebral perfusion	ICP monitoring to calculate cerebral perfusion pressure (CPP), transcranial Doppler scanning to measure flow velocity in cerebral arteries, xenon-enhanced CT scanning to measure global or regional cerebral blood flow
Cerebral oxygenation	Jugular bulb oximetry, brain tissue oxygenation, microprobes, near infrared spectroscopy
Electrophysiology	EEG recordings

Imaging

CT scanning allows assessment of change in focal lesions such as enlarging cerebral contusions, and can also reveal evidence of rising ICP. When ICP is monitored directly and shows a rise, CT scanning can be used to determine whether this has a reversible cause. Magnetic resonance imaging (MRI) is rarely used in critically ill brain injured patients, because of the logistics of scanning an unstable patient, but studies have shown that some head injured patients who fail to recover as expected have a brain stem injury which is seen on MRI but not on CT scan (Figure 39.22).

Monitoring intracranial pressure

The armamentarium available in neurosurgical ICUs to monitor severely head injured patients has grown in recent years, but ICP monitoring is still the most widely – often the only – technique used. It allows the early and rapid detection of high or rising ICP, so that action can be taken to restore normal intracranial conditions before irreversible damage is done. ICP can be monitored via a fluid-filled tube introduced through a burrhole into the subdural or extradural space, or via a fibre-optic transducer introduced into the brain substance via a twist drill. On-line ICP data are displayed on a liquid crystal display (LCD) or a paper roll, and can be linked to other data. For example, continuous monitoring of mean systemic arterial pressure (MAP) and ICP allows calculation of the cerebral perfusion pressure (CPP) by a simple formula:

$$CPP = MAP - ICP.$$

Maintaining an adequate CPP is essential for brain function, and high ICP and low MAP therefore both threaten the brain.

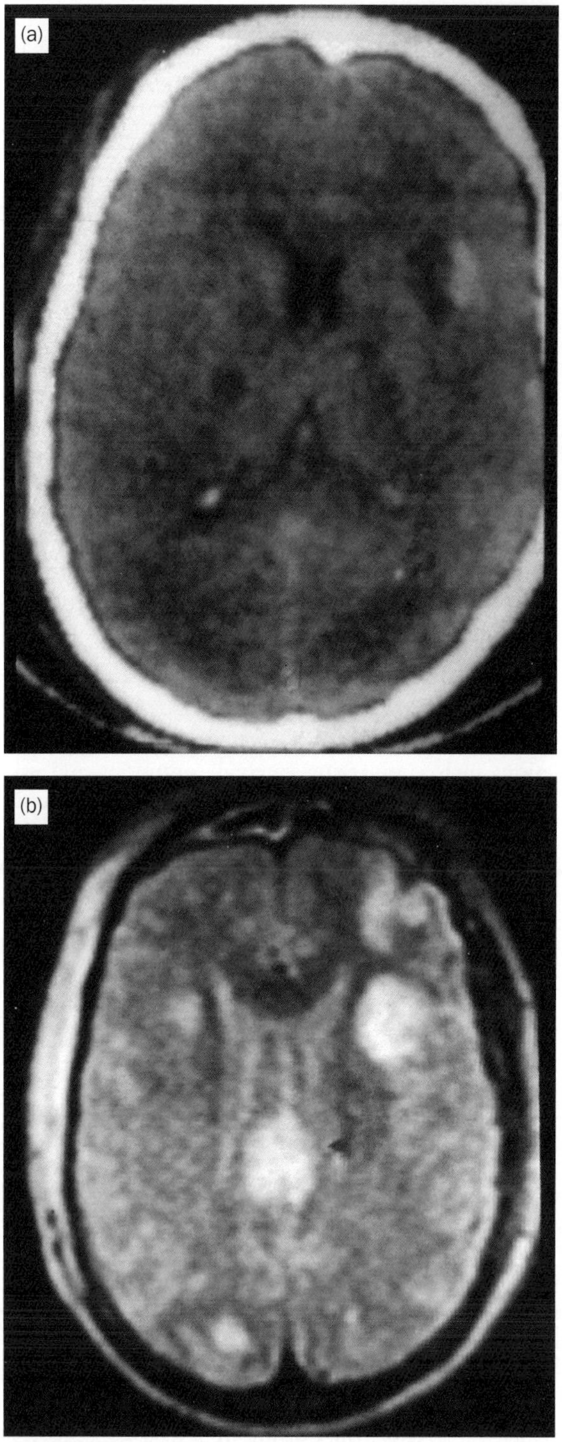

Figure 39.22 (a) CT scan of a patient in a deep coma after a road traffic accident. (b) Magnetic resonance scan of the same patient an hour later showing extensive high signal lesions in the cerebral hemispheres and brain stem.

The normal ICP is 10–12 mmHg and the usual threshold of clinical concern is 20 mmHg. Malfunction of the ICP monitoring system is common, and should always be checked before acting to lower an apparently high ICP. Causes of a genuine rise in ICP

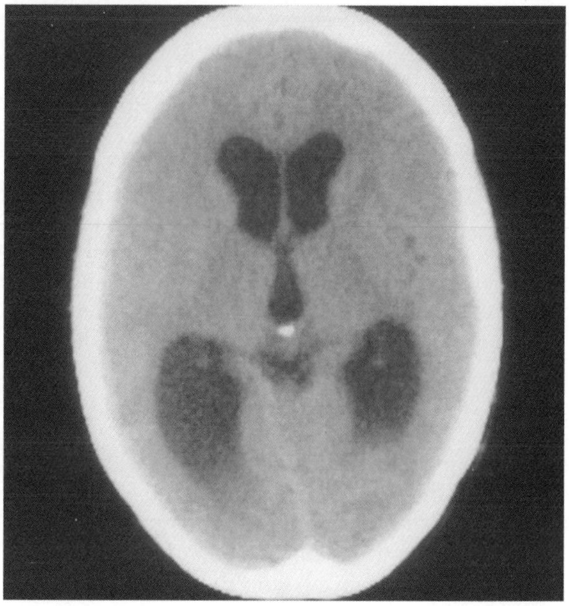

Figure 39.23 CT brain scan showing general dilatation of the ventricles secondary to severe traumatic subarachnoid haemorrhage 2 weeks previously.

include an expanding haematoma or contusion, hydrocephalus (Figure 39.23), and brain swelling due to poor cerebral perfusion or systemic blood gas disturbance. If the raised ICP does not fall by changing the ventilatory or circulatory parameters, a CT scan may be needed to identify the cause and allow it to be corrected.

There is still debate about the total impact of ICP monitoring on outcome after head injury. Definitive proof of its usefulness would require a very large prospective trial that would be difficult to do. However, clinical experience suggests that it is particularly useful when the CT leaves doubt about the need to evacuate a haematoma. If the ICP is persistently above 20–25 mmHg then the haematoma should be evacuated. The usefulness of ICP monitoring in a diffusely brain injured patient is rather less certain.

Other intracranial monitoring

Transcranial Doppler monitoring (TCD) is used in some neurosurgical ICUs to give information on middle cerebral artery blood flow velocity. Normal velocity is 55–65 cm/s, which is reduced immediately after head injury. Later rises in velocity may be due to hyperaemia or to vasospasm from traumatic subarachnoid haemorrhage. Cerebral autoregulation – the ability to keep cerebral blood flow within narrow limits across a wide range of systemic blood pressure – is often impaired after severe head injury, and this is associated with a poorer outcome. TCD can assess autoregulation by measuring changes in blood flow velocity induced by changes in end-tidal CO_2 or blood pressure.

Cerebral blood flow can be assessed by stable xenon-enhanced CT scanning. This involves the inhalation of radioactive xenon, which reaches a steady state within the brain within 5 min. Areas of decreased or increased perfusion can then be detected and the actual blood flow (ml/100 g/min) can be calculated.

Cerebral oxygenation

The ability to measure intracerebral oxygen levels is a further refinement of cerebral monitoring, and indicates whether cerebral perfusion and oxygenation are adequate. *Jugular bulb oximetry* is the most commonly used technique, and uses a fibre-optic probe placed in the jugular bulb via the internal jugular vein to measure the oxygen saturation (SJO_2) of the venous blood leaving the cerebral hemispheres. This reflects the balance between oxygen delivery, cerebral blood flow and oxygen demand. A *high* SJO_2 indicates cerebral blood flow in *excess* of the metabolic demand for oxygen. This may be due to hyperaemia ('luxury perfusion') from impaired autoregulation, or to reduced oxygen extraction from metabolic depression or cerebral infarction. A *low* SJO_2 occurs when oxygen delivery falls below the metabolic demands of the brain because of systemic hypoxaemia, impaired cerebral perfusion or hypermetabolism within the injured brain. The brain then extracts more and more oxygen from the blood. Eventually anaerobic metabolism begins and the production of lactate increases.

Microprobes which incorporate a Clark oxygen electrode can be inserted via a burrhole to make direct measurements of local cerebral oxygenation. However, this measures oxygenation within an area only a few micrometres in diameter and does not rule out significant ischaemia in other areas of the brain. *Near infrared spectroscopy* has aroused interest because of its potential as a non-invasive and portable monitor of cerebral oxygenation. It is based on the fact that infrared light penetrates tissues more readily than visible light. Oxyhaemoglobin, deoxyhaemoglobin and oxidized cytochrome 003 all have their characteristic absorption spectra, and measuring the tissue absorption of near infrared can be used to calculate their relative concentrations. However, this technique remains experimental and is not used routinely in head injury cases.

Nutrition in the head injured patient

Failure to provide nutritional support to a head injured patient by the end of the first week after injury is associated with an increased mortality rate. Metabolic expenditure in the comatose head injured patient increases to a mean of 140% of the expected value at rest (125% if the patient is pharmacologically paralysed), e.g. the resting metabolic expenditure for a 70 kg, 25-year-old male (1700 kcal/24 hour) rises to 2400 kcal/24 hour after a severe head injury. Ideally, nutrition should be started within 24 hours of injury. The preparation should contain at least 15% of calories in the form of protein, to replace the accelerated nitrogen loss after injury that results predominantly from muscle wasting.

Section 39.8 • Rehabilitation after severe head injury

After intracranial surgery or intensive care for a severe head injury, a mixture of physical, cognitive and psycho-social problems often stand in the way of a return to normal life. These can be far from obvious to the patient or even the non-specialist clinician, and are responsible for the reputation of brain injury as the 'hidden disability'. Most natural recovery of brain function is complete by the end of the first year, but there is now strong evidence that structured rehabilitation programmes are effective at reducing disability and handicap and helping the patient to recover function and independence. Rehabilitation is also cost-effective in reducing the overall health care burden.

Everyone who treats the head injured should understand the principles of rehabilitation. It should begin as soon as possible after injury, identify and pursue clear goals which the patient wants to achieve, and continue by whatever means until the goal is achieved or the patient reaches a plateau of function. The process of rehabilitation often continues in several settings over a long period: the acute ward, the rehabilitation unit, the outpatient therapy department and the patient's own home. Successful rehabilitation depends on a holistic and patient-centred approach, a set of consistent and achievable goals, an expert multi-professional team which works across administrative boundaries, and careful discharge planning and handover when the patient moves from one phase to the next.

In the acute stage, rehabilitation is targeted towards achieving adequate nutrition, skin care, bladder and bowel function, passive stretching of muscles, good posture and effective communication. An obvious goal in a conscious patient is to get co-operation and engagement. The family needs information and help – sensitively given – to understand the nature of brain injury and the rehabilitation process. The patient's immediate environment should minimize irritability and fatigue, avoiding unnecessary noise and over-stimulation. Often this requires tact in handling the family.

Many patients with serious brain injury have extensive neuropsychological deficits and benefit from skilled early assessment. They are usually disorientated from the start or when they emerge from coma, and re-orientation becomes an important goal. Memory is linked to orientation, and is also commonly affected. Post-traumatic amnesia (PTA) is the period after injury when the patient is conscious but cannot lay down new memories in a normal continuous way, although isolated events may be recalled and memory for distant events is often unimpaired. The duration of PTA reflects the severity of diffuse brain injury, but can only be measured retrospectively and is easy to under-estimate early on. Other common cognitive deficits involve the ability to focus or divide attention, and the ability to plan, initiate, sequence and monitor tasks ('executive' function).

Many patients lack insight into the extent of their deficits, fail to engage in rehabilitation, and are then labelled as 'awkward' and discharged home too soon on the basis of satisfactory physical progress, only to re-emerge later with established problems of mood and cognition. Irritability is common after brain injury, and can be hard for non-specialist staff to deal with effectively. Major behavioural disturbance is actually quite uncommon, but always difficult to deal with in an acute general ward, and requires early input from clinical psychology or liaison psychiatry, with transfer in some cases to an environment which can contain and manage such challenging behaviour.

As patients become more stable, their rehabilitation is best undertaken in specialized units with appropriate skills for managing physical, cognitive and behavioural problems and for actively involving family and carers. In the UK at least provision of these facilities across the country is patchy, and the needs of many patients are not met. Some do not need prolonged inpatient rehabilitation, and can be referred to community-based rehabilitation services which have outpatient and domiciliary therapy teams, or to the general practitioner and the primary care team. Involving the local authority social work department bridges the patient's clinical and social needs and broadens the scope of the rehabilitation process.

Few brain-injured patients need long-term institutional care. Most return home with support from social services, hospital or community health professionals, and voluntary sector organizations such as Headway (a national brain injury charity with branches around the UK). Outpatient rehabilitation programmes focus on improving mobility and stamina, independent living skills, family and social relationships, mood and cognition. They can also help with vocational rehabilitation, a return to leisure activities, or harm reduction from alcohol and drugs.

Section 39.9 • Mortality and outcome in survivors

Mortality is (and always will be) an important outcome measure after severe head injury. Most published series quote 30–40%, but several factors have significantly improved this over the past 30 years. Standards of prehospital care, resuscitation and transfer have all risen, and the need to be vigilant and vigorous in dealing with hypoxia and shock throughout acute care is well understood. The wider availability of CT scanning has led to the earlier identification of more patients with treatable lesions, and a fall in the number of avoidable deaths from late evacuation of haematomas or failure to control raised ICP. Neuro-intensive care continues to develop rapidly.

This fall in deaths has been accompanied by less morbidity in survivors, but many patients still have significant long-term disability, even when crude global outcome measures are used. A good outcome in terms of the Glasgow outcome score occurs only in about 40% of cases, and about 20% remain moderately disabled. Fortunately, only about 10% have severe disability and are dependent on others on a daily basis, and well under 1% become persistently vegetative. Nevertheless, the overall burden of long-term disability in severe head injury survivors is considerable, and is often largely hidden from view. Rehabilitation is now recognized as a clinically effective and cost-effective way to help these people to recover function, independence and quality of life.

Outcome after severe head injury can often be predicted early on. The presence of a fixed dilated pupil, a low motor score on the GCS, and age greater than 60 years – especially in combination – are associated with a high risk of death or severe disability. However, there is wide individual variation. One study has shown that predictions made in the first 24 hours after injury are correct in less than half of cases. Clearly, great caution is needed before basing clinical decisions on such predictions.

Section 39.10 • The future

There has been significant progress in our understanding of severe brain injury over the last two decades. Further improvement can be expected as we learn more about the role of ischaemia and of biochemical and cellular mediators of secondary brain injury. Future clinical trials will concentrate on evaluating experimental treatments. Assessment of outcome will become more sophisticated and focus increasingly on neuropsychological endpoints as recognition grows that even patients with an apparently good outcome have subtle cognitive deficits which seriously impact on function and quality of life.

Further reading

American College of Surgeons Committee on Trauma (1997). *ATLS Course Manual*. Chicago: American College of Surgeons.

Andrews, P. J. D., Piper, I. R., Dearden, N. M. and Miller, J. D. (1990). Secondary insults during inter-hospital transport of head injured patients. *Lancet* **335**: 327.

Gentleman, D., Dearden, N. M., Midgley, S. and Maclean, D. (1993). Guidelines for resuscitation and transfer of patients with severe head injury. *BMJ* **307**: 547.

Joint Working Party on Head Injury Transfer (1996). Recommendations for the transfer of emergency head injured patients to neurosurgical centres. London: Association of Anaesthetists of Great Britain and Ireland.

Marshall, L. F., Gauntilley, T., Klauber, M. R. *et al.* (1991). The outcome of severe closed head injury. *J Neurosurg* **75** (Suppl): 528.

Narayan, R. K., Wilberger, J. E. Jr and Poulishock, J. T., eds. (1996). *Neurotrauma*. New York: McGraw-Hill.

Scottish Intercollegiate Guidelines Network (SIGN). *Guideline 46: Early Management of Head Injury*. SIGN, Royal College of Physicians of Edinburgh.

MODULE 40

Spontaneous intracranial haemorrhage

Section 40.1 • Introduction: what causes bleeding inside the head?

The distributions of spontaneous and traumatic haemorrhage inside the head are quite different. The dura is so tightly attached to the skull that some force is needed to strip it away and produce an extradural haematoma, which hardly ever occurs without clear-cut trauma. By contrast, the brain and arachnoid membrane are easily displaced away from the dura and offer minimal resistance to the spread of blood in the subdural space, so that although a subdural haematoma often follows major trauma there are other cases where the injury is quite minor or even remains unidentified despite careful questioning. In some circumstances intermittent leakage of blood into the subdural space can progressively enlarge a subdural collection until symptoms appear. The diagnosis and management of traumatic intracranial haematoma is described in Module 39.

Chronic hypertension produces micro-aneurysms on the small vessels of the brain, most often on perforating arteries in the deep cerebral nuclei. This is why hypertensive haemorrhages are found mainly in the basal ganglia, internal capsule and thalamus – unusual sites for traumatic intracerebral haematoma, which mainly occur in the parts of the brain most vulnerable to mechanical injury – the frontal and temporal lobes.

Vascular anomalies – arterial aneurysms and a variety of malformations – are important causes of spontaneous intracranial haemorrhage and often produce a characteristic anatomical pattern of bleeding.

Less common causes of intracranial haemorrhage include brain tumours, and some (e.g. metastatic melanoma) have a particular propensity to bleed. Haemorrhage can follow even minor trauma if there is a disorder of clotting due to disease (e.g. liver failure) or to poor control of therapeutic anticoagulation. The fact that intracranial haemorrhage is more common in the elderly probably reflects the higher prevalence of hypertension, minor forgotten injuries and anticoagulant use in this age group.

A pragmatic approach is to classify spontaneous intracranial haemorrhage according to whether there is an underlying structural abnormality, or whether the haemorrhage is merely one incident in another disorder. In the first group surgical treatment may be needed to deal with the underlying structural cause, whereas in the second group it is limited to cases where the haematoma is large enough to threaten life.

Section 40.2 • 'Surgical' causes of haemorrhage

Arterial aneurysms

The main type is the saccular or 'berry' aneurysm (a name derived from its appearance). Probably multifactorial in aetiology, this arises where arteries branch, is more common in smokers and in females, and is multiple in 20% of cases. Up to 10% are familial, often associated with polycystic kidneys or aortic coarctation. Aneurysmal subarachnoid haemorrhage has an annual incidence of 10–12 per 100 000 in Western populations, and typically occurs in the 40–70-year age range. Although the aneurysm nearly always bleeds into the subarachnoid space, blood often also breaks through into the brain substance or even the subdural space. About 90% of aneurysms are found in the anterior (carotid) circulation, mainly on the internal carotid, middle cerebral and anterior communicating arteries. Most internal carotid aneurysms arise at the origin of the posterior communicating artery, others at the ophthalmic artery origin or the internal carotid bifurcation. Most middle cerebral artery aneurysms occur at its trifurcation. Posterior circulation (vertebro-basilar) aneurysms account for 10% of the total, and mostly arise at the basilar bifurcation, the superior cerebellar artery origin from the basilar trunk or the posterior inferior cerebellar artery origin from the vertebral artery.

At least 20% of aneurysmal haemorrhages are rapidly fatal, and the propensity for a ruptured aneurysm to re-bleed (20% within the first 14 days, with 50% mortality) is the reason for urgency in reaching a diagnosis and offering definitive treatment. Although the diagnosis is usually straightforward, it is occasionally delayed because the warning bleed has been minor and undramatic. Clinical acumen is needed to assess the symptom of sudden headache. Failing to make the diagnosis until a catastrophic bleed occurs is a clinical disaster and can be a medico-legal one too.

Other types of intracranial aneurysm are less common. **Intimal dissection** in the internal carotid or vertebral artery in the neck after direct trauma or in a hypertensive patient can present as a thrombo-embolic event. The mainstay of treatment is anticoagulation to prevent clot propagation, and most heal spontaneously. Occasionally a dissection in a neck artery extends intracranially to involve the posterior inferior cerebellar or middle cerebral artery, usually causing a haemorrhage because arteries are relatively thin walled once inside the dura. The treatment is vessel occlusion, usually by endovascular means. **Traumatic (false) aneurysms** are rare complications of penetrating trauma such as stab wounds of the head (occasionally skull base or depressed vault fractures), and are treated by excision or (for large vessels) proximal occlusion. Small peripherally located **bacterial (mycotic) aneurysms** usually occur in the context of infective endocarditis, with fever and cardiac murmurs punctuated by intracranial haemorrhage, and are usually excised. **Aneurysms associated with vasculitis** occasionally occur on peripheral cerebral arteries, and treatment is aimed at the underlying condition.

Vascular malformations

The prevalence of **arteriovenous malformations (AVMs)** in the general population has been estimated at 1%. In these high flow lesions arteriovenous shunting occurs within a tangle of abnormal 'nidal' vessels. Despite the classical view that AVMs are congenital, only one rare type (vein of Galen aneurysm) has ever been shown on the vast numbers of antenatal ultrasound examinations carried out over the years.

Large AVMs tend to be pyramidal in shape, with the apex reaching the ventricular system, so they tend to bleed into the brain substance or into the ventricle (Figure 40.1). Less often subarachnoid haemorrhage is the presenting feature. AVMs can also present with intractable 'migrainous' headaches or epilepsy, rather than haemorrhage.

The risk of haemorrhage from an AVM is estimated at 2% per annum, with a 10% risk of death at each bleed. After one bleed the risk of another is only modestly increased in the first year (6–10%), so there is much less urgency to treat an AVM than a ruptured arterial aneurysm. However, in at least 10% of cases arterial aneurysms occur along with the AVM (Figure 40.2), presumably because of haemodynamic stresses on the vessel walls. Either can bleed and it is important to establish which has done so. If it is the aneurysm, treatment is more urgent in view of the higher risk of re-bleed and the higher mortality from recurrent aneurysmal rupture.

Cavernous malformations (cavernomas) are low flow lesions consisting of endothelial-lined caverns with no intervening brain tissue. They are detectable by magnetic resonance (MR) scanning techniques but not cerebral angiography (Figure 40.3), and large MR studies from North America suggest that their prevalence is about 0.4%. It is still not known whether they

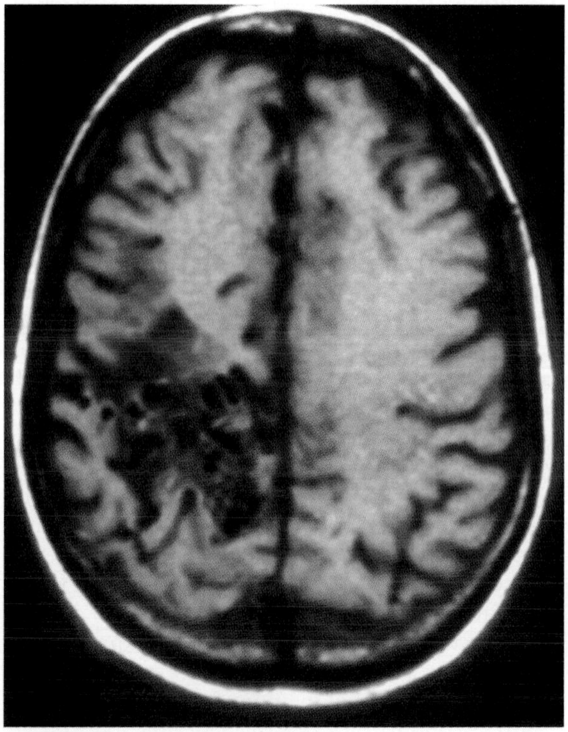

Figure 40.1 AVM. Axial MR scan.

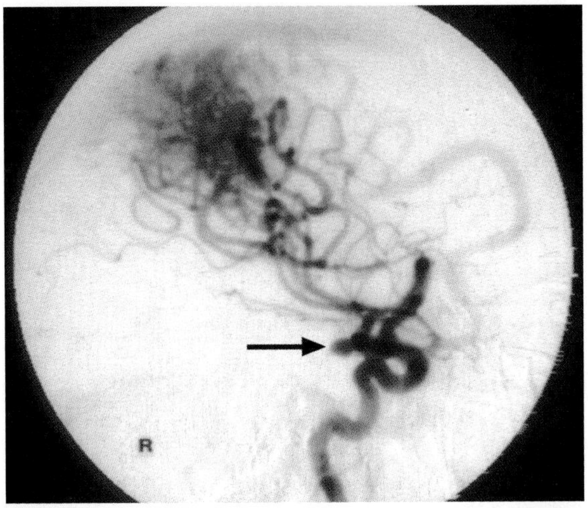

Figure 40.2 AVM. Lateral subtraction angiogram showing pathological circulation superiorly, and an internal carotid artery aneurysm (arrow).

are congenital or acquired, but rarely a dominant gene causes multiple lesions in families. Haemorrhage from a cavernoma can be minor and repeated, with a clinical presentation like that of a tumour, or acute and even devastating (especially if located in the brain stem). The haematoma can be within the lesion or in the surrounding brain. A previously unruptured cavernoma carries a risk of under 1% per annum of bleeding, but one which has already bled carries a 2% per annum risk. Whatever makes it bleed once clearly makes it more likely to bleed again.

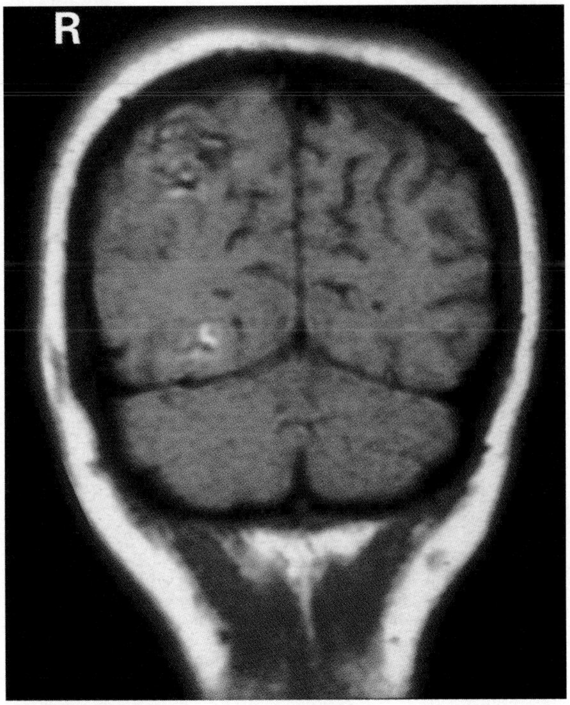

Figure 40.3 Cavernous malformations: two separate lesions are seen in the right cerebral hemisphere.

Capillary malformations are occasionally identified in the wall of a haematoma when an abnormal-looking area is biopsied at operation, but are otherwise only found at autopsy. They occur most often in the pons, are often multiple, and may be associated with hereditary haemorrhagic telangiectasia. Little is known about them, but they are thought to occur in 1 in 150 of the population. They have been speculatively linked with cavernomas as part of a spectrum of vascular change. **Venous angiomas and medullary venous malformations** are anomalous patterns of venous drainage from the brain found in 2% of people. They are sometimes visible on MR scan (even computed tomography (CT) scan), but angiography is the definitive way to diagnose them. They tend to be associated with cavernomas, which are almost always responsible for any haemorrhage which occurs and should be carefully sought. There is no alternative venous drainage pathway for the affected brain, so the anomalous veins must be spared when removing the cavernoma. **Arteriovenous fistulas** result from venous thrombosis in dural sinuses or intradural veins. Blood is shunted into subarachnoid or intracerebral veins, causing venous hypertension and bleeding into the brain or the subarachnoid or subdural space. Treatment is endovascular occlusion of the fistula – often requiring sacrifice of the vein – or open surgery to occlude the arterialized vein.

Brain tumours (also see Module 41)

Almost any intracranial tumour can bleed, but some have a particular propensity to do so. Malignant melanoma deposits are notorious for causing brain haemorrhage, and often reveal the presence of the primary tumour. However, it is commoner to encounter haemorrhage from primary brain tumours (especially malignant glioma), and it is wise to arrange a follow-up scan (allowing time for the blood to clear) whenever intracranial haemorrhage occurs at an atypical site and there are no vascular risk factors such as hypertension. Occasionally a meningioma bleeds into the subdural space, appearing on the CT scan as a 'filling defect' within a collection of fresh subdural blood (Figure 40.4). Spontaneous haemorrhage and haemorrhagic necrosis can occur in benign pituitary adenomas and mimic subarachnoid haemorrhage, with headache, loss of consciousness and loss of vision. Chiasmal compression from the enlarged gland can cause dilated unreactive pupils, but the rest of the patient's neurological profile will be out of keeping with this apparently ominous feature. Increased stress and the failure of the pituitary gland to produce adrenocorticotropic hormone (ACTH) lead to an Addisonian crisis, which responds dramatically to intravenous hydrocortisone. Emergency trans-sphenoidal surgery can salvage vision.

Spontaneous haemorrhage of no known cause

Up to 20% of non-traumatic subarachnoid haemorrhages have no identifiable cause despite investigation.

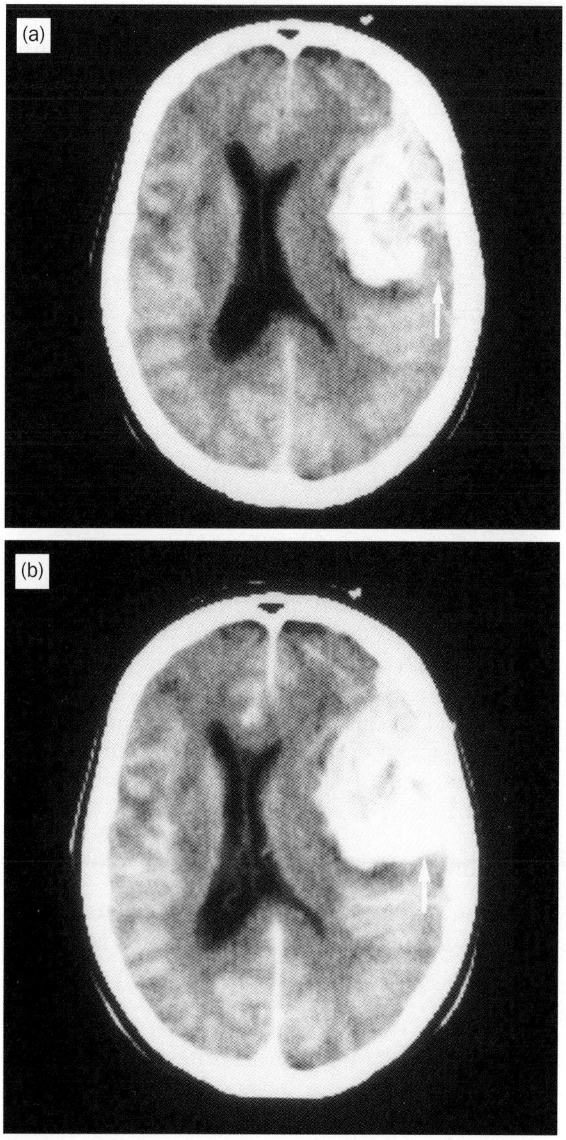

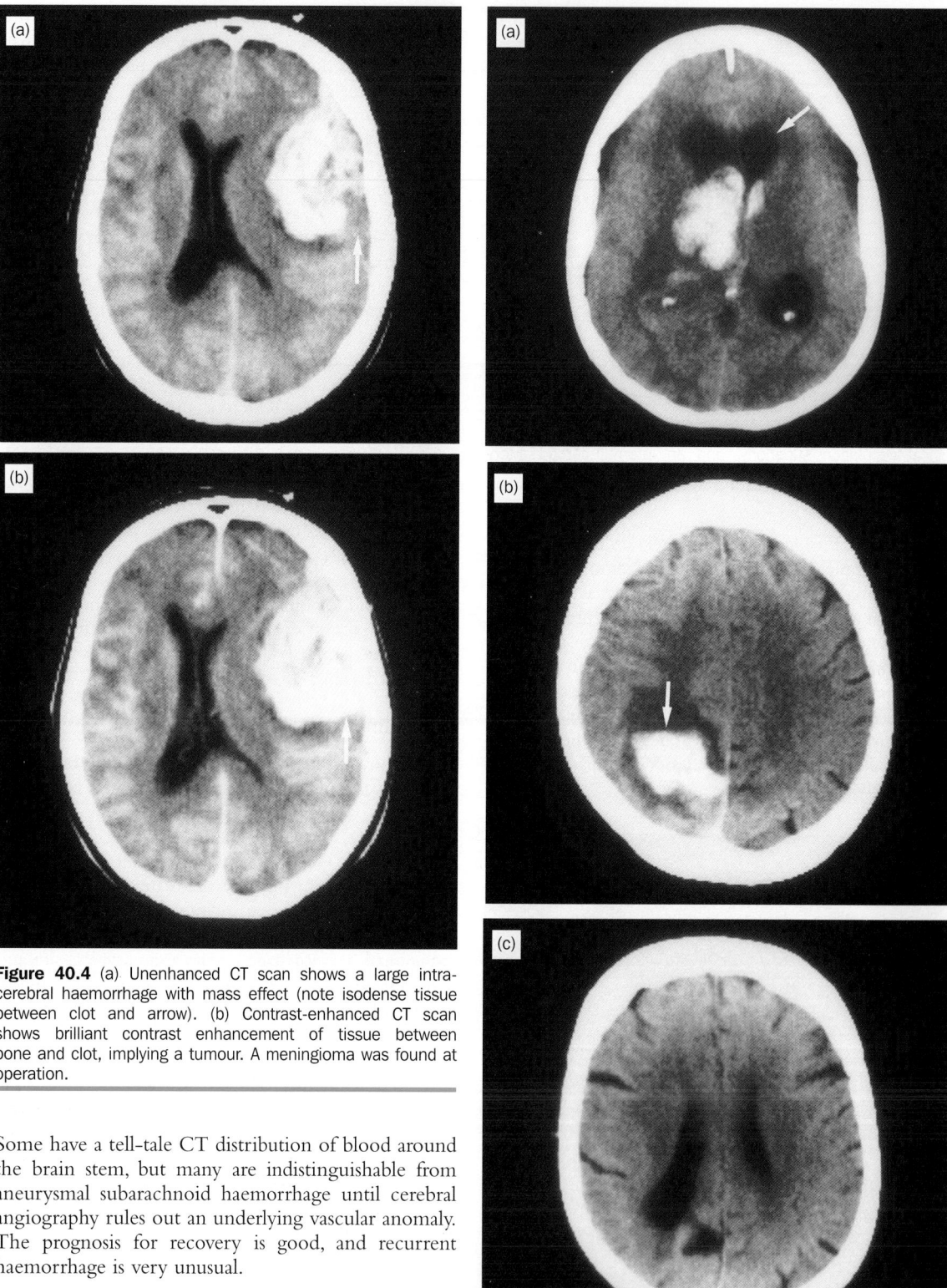

Figure 40.4 (a) Unenhanced CT scan shows a large intracerebral haemorrhage with mass effect (note isodense tissue between clot and arrow). (b) Contrast-enhanced CT scan shows brilliant contrast enhancement of tissue between bone and clot, implying a tumour. A meningioma was found at operation.

Some have a tell-tale CT distribution of blood around the brain stem, but many are indistinguishable from aneurysmal subarachnoid haemorrhage until cerebral angiography rules out an underlying vascular anomaly. The prognosis for recovery is good, and recurrent haemorrhage is very unusual.

Section 40.3 • 'Medical' causes of haemorrhage

In these disorders, surgical treatment can be needed to relieve the space-occupying effect of the haematoma, but is ineffective for its underlying cause.

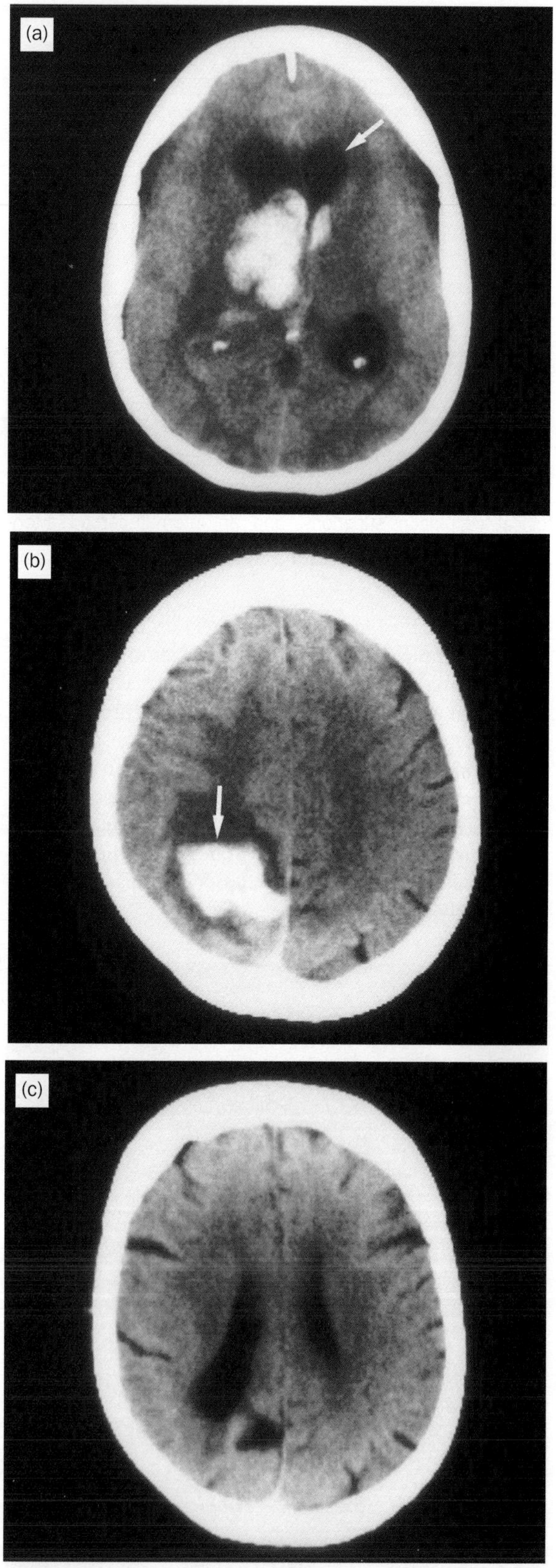

Figure 40.5 (a) CT scan of a haematoma centred on the thalamus, causing obstructive hydrocephalus (note dilated frontal horn – arrow). (b) Clot has broken into the ventricle, as shown by fluid level with CSF (arrow). (c) Late CT scan showing resorption of clot and residual CSF cavity communicating with the ventricle.

Hypertension

Hypertension is a major cause of intracranial haemorrhage. About 80% occur in the basal ganglia, internal capsule or thalamus, and little benefit has been shown from surgery in these deep locations, except where extension of blood into the ventricular system causes obstructive hydrocephalus (Figure 40.5). If the clot is large enough to threaten life from raised intracranial pressure (ICP), the extent of brain tissue destruction usually makes the expected outcome very poor, and most neurosurgeons are reluctant to operate. Another 10% of patients have a 'lobar' haemorrhage which approaches the surface of the brain, and the easier surgical access and better long-term outcome make the removal of these clots a more worthwhile surgical proposition if they cause mass effect (Figure 40.6). The remaining 10% of hypertensive haemorrhages occur in the posterior fossa, where a cerebellar haematoma only 20 ml in size can cause obstructive hydrocephalus and compress the brain stem (Figure 40.7). Evacuation of the haematoma is often life-saving if the patient still has brain stem function. Pure brain stem haemorrhages are almost never amenable to surgery and are often rapidly fatal, especially in the elderly.

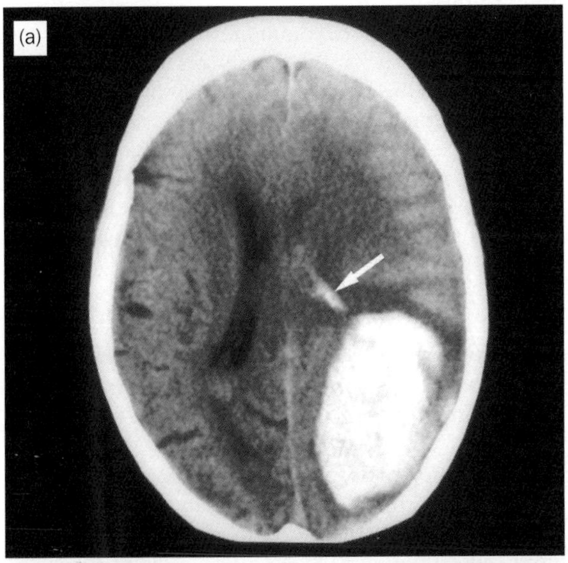

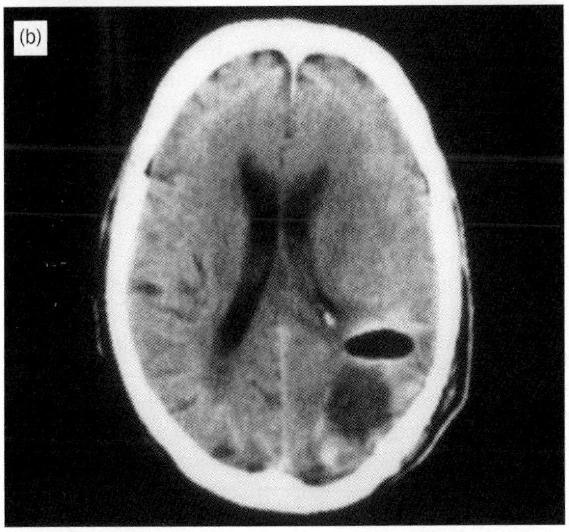

Figure 40.6 (a) Large clot almost reaching the brain surface, compressing the lateral ventricle, and displacing the choroid plexus (arrow) anteriorly. (b) Post-operative CT scan showing re-expansion of the lateral ventricle and residual air in the haematoma cavity.

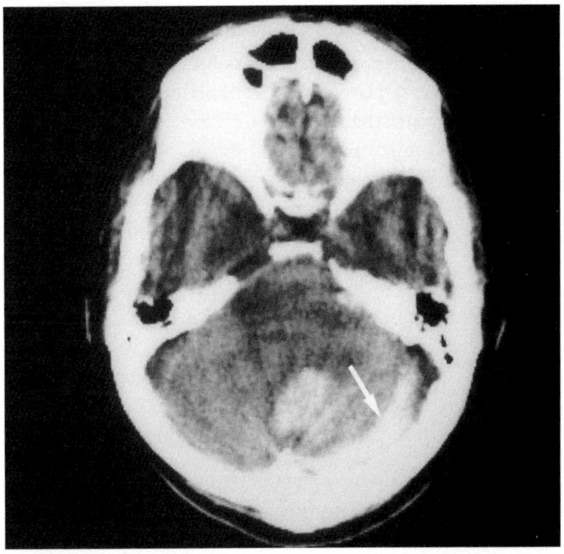

Figure 40.7 CT scan of a hypertensive cerebellar haemorrhage. Although the clot is not large it has a subdural component (arrow) and needs surgical evacuation.

Anticoagulation

Most intracranial bleeds after therapeutic anticoagulation are into the subdural space and need surgery. Clotting must be normalized first, to prevent intra-operative haemorrhage, although the risk of this is low with aspirin or non-steroidal drugs. Timing the re-start of anticoagulation needs careful judgement in each case, balancing the risks of the underlying disorder and of provoking another bleed.

Fibrinolytic therapy

A few spontaneous intracranial haemorrhages result from the growing use of streptokinase and other fibrinolytic agents to treat myocardial infarction. This number will grow further if fibrinolysis also becomes a common treatment for ischaemic stroke. General principles apply: restore normal coagulation, and if need be remove the clot.

Haemorrhagic infarction

About 10% of cerebral infarcts involve some bleeding into the infarcted tissue, presumably because perfusion is restored through vessels with necrotic walls. Treatment is as for a hypertensive bleed. When fibrinolytic agents have been used, the provisos above to restore normal clotting apply prior to any operation.

Amyloid angiopathy

This rare condition predisposes to haemorrhages at the margin between cortex and subcortical white matter. Previous haemorrhage in a different location is the usual clue, but sometimes a biopsy of the wall of a haematoma yields the diagnosis after the first haemorrhage. Occasionally repeated bleeds need evacuation.

Venous sinus thrombosis

Occasionally venous sinus thrombosis causes significant haemorrhage. The risk from using heparin (the usual treatment for venous infarction) or thrombolysis (increasingly used for extensive sinus thrombosis) is then high. These cases require careful judgment.

Section 40.4 • The site of haemorrhage in relation to its cause

Haemorrhage outside the brain

Extradural haemorrhage is so rarely spontaneous that blood in the extradural space should always be regarded as traumatic in origin, even with no history of trauma. In a child in particular, an extradural haematoma can present some time after quite trivial trauma with no skull fracture. *Subdural haemorrhage* too is usually of traumatic origin, but can follow aneurysm rupture if the arachnoid is torn where it adheres to the aneurysm sac, allowing blood to enter the subdural space at the base of the brain and spread over the brain convexity. Haemorrhage from a superficial AVM or a tumour attached to the dura can also do this, but usually there are pointers to their presence on the scan. Minor or repeated head injury can lead to the gradual accumulation of a chronic subdural haematoma days or weeks after the injury. In a patient on anticoagulant medication (including aspirin or non-steroidal drugs) minor head injury can lead to a substantial acute subdural haematoma within hours. The preceding injury may be so trivial as to be overlooked when the history is taken, but careful questioning may reveal a minor bump on the head. *Subarachnoid haemorrhage* is usually from an aneurysm, less often from an AVM, and 20% are idiopathic.

Ventricular dilatation (hydrocephalus) is often seen after intracranial haemorrhage. *Communicating hydrocephalus* can be marked when blood enters the ventricular system, which is more likely with aneurysms of the anterior communicating, terminal basilar and vertebral arteries. Less often a large intraventricular clot causes *obstructive hydrocephalus* at the level of the aqueduct.

Haemorrhage into the brain substance

Aneurysms may bleed into the brain but usually cause subarachnoid haemorrhage too. Any haematoma close to a major intracranial artery may have an aneurysmal origin, and it is then advisable to perform vascular imaging by conventional angiography or the less invasive techniques of CT angiography or MR angiography. A large *AVM* is usually evident on CT or MR scan, but a small one may only be visible by angiography. Early angiography may be falsely negative, because vessels are in spasm from the presence of blood and the AVM nidus is compressed in the wall of the haematoma, so that interval angiography is more reliable. Low flow lesions such as *cavernomas* tend to produce modest haematomas, often with an insidious presentation. They are difficult to identify on CT scan, and are best identified on delayed MR scan a few months after the acute event, by which time the high signal from methaemoglobin in the haematoma has faded. Blood may mask a *tumour*, but extensive oedema around the haematoma on the initial scan can hint at primary or secondary tumour, and the history may also point to this.

Hypertension is so common that finding it is no guarantee that it is the cause of an intracerebral haematoma. However, a haematoma in the capsular region, the putamen or thalamus is very suggestive of a hypertensive bleed, and many cerebellar bleeds are also caused by hypertension. If no major artery abuts the haematoma there is little likelihood of an aneurysmal origin, but finding fever and a cardiac murmur always raises the question of a mycotic (bacterial) aneurysm due to infective endocarditis.

Section 40.5 • Investigating the cause of intracranial haemorrhage

The vast majority of spontaneous intracranial haemorrhages can be confirmed by CT scan and the position and appearance of the blood may suggest the underlying cause (Figure 40.8). In a few cases of subarachnoid haemorrhage the scan is negative, especially after the first few days, and if the history strongly suggests a bleed, a negative CT scan must be followed by a lumbar puncture (at least 10 hours from the onset of symptoms). The cerebrospinal fluid (CSF) is diffusely bloodstained after a subarachnoid haemorrhage, while the supernatant is xanthochromic. A very high protein level can make the CSF seem xanthochromic to the naked eye but chemical analysis is helpful. Spectrophotometry is available in most neuroscience centres and can make the CSF analysis more precise.

The extent and timing of further investigation are closely linked to the suspected diagnosis and the patient's condition. It is important to confirm an aneurysmal haemorrhage promptly to allow appropriate treatment, but other types of haemorrhage can be investigated with less haste unless the patient is in a coma or has a major neurological deficit. MR scanning is nearly always needed to diagnose a cavernoma with confidence and can also help in the late diagnosis of a case of subarachnoid haemorrhage. However, a CT scan after an interval may be more useful for showing features of a tumour that has bled, as MR is too sensi-

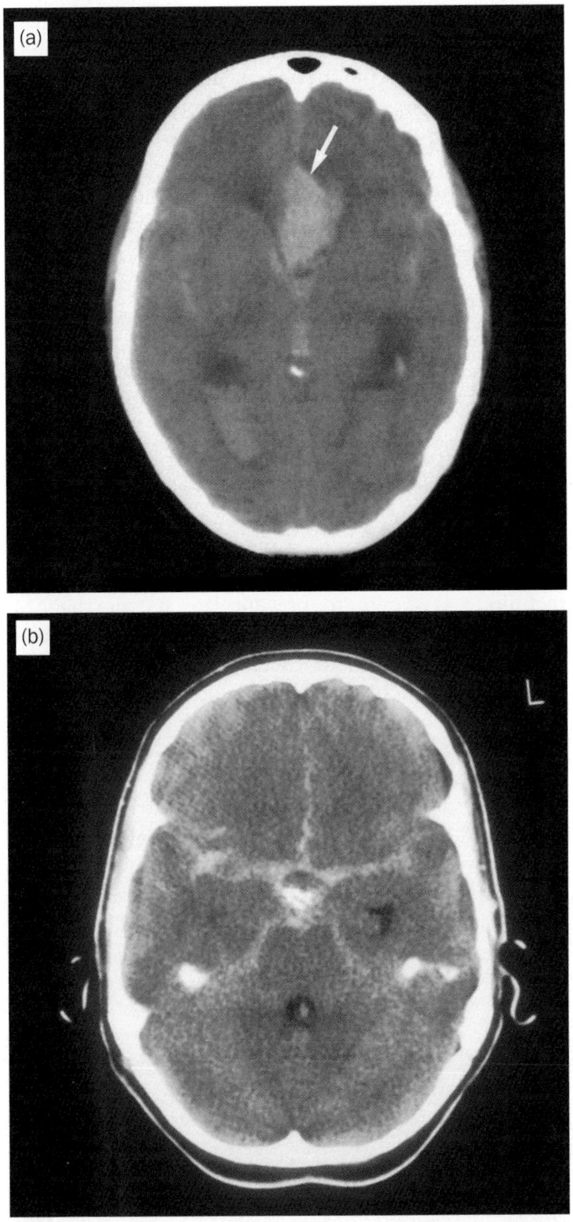

Figure 40.8 (a) Subarachnoid haemorrhage from a ruptured anterior communicating artery aneurysm. Intraventricular blood is seen, as well as a haematoma in the septum pellucidum (just above the anterior communicating artery). (b) CT scan soon after subarachnoid haemorrhage, showing diffuse blood throughout the basal cisterns.

tive to the methaemoglobin which persists for months after a major bleed and obscures underlying structural detail. After an intracranial haemorrhage it is important to carry out tests of clotting status and to correct abnormalities, especially if surgery is planned. Routine laboratory tests do not detect platelet malfunction due to aspirin or non-steroidal drugs.

After a subarachnoid haemorrhage cerebral arteriography (angiography) is needed to confirm or refute a structural abnormality – most often an aneurysm. This is done by intra-arterial injection in the groin, using a Seldinger technique to steer a catheter into the internal carotid and vertebral arteries, often using digital subtraction techniques to improve the definition on the films. Direct carotid artery puncture in the neck is much less often used nowadays, and carries greater risks. MR angiography or CT angiography is increasingly used in selected cases, but neither can yet exclude a small aneurysm and both can be difficult to interpret when there is much blood clot. The risk of a persistent ischaemic neurological deficit after cerebral angiography is 0.1% in young people, but higher with diseased arteries and hence in older people. For unknown reasons the risk of fatal anaphylaxis from iodinated contrast medium is higher for intravenous than for intra-arterial injection. A history of atopy or asthma raises this risk even further and justifies premedication with antihistamines and/or steroids when time allows.

When cerebral angiography is negative after a diffuse subarachnoid haemorrhage, it is wise to repeat the angiogram after a few days, particularly in a younger patient. This is because a previously ruptured aneurysm is likely to bleed again (4% per annum after the first 6 weeks), and it is necessary to be certain that there is no aneurysm. Repeat angiography is probably unnecessary when there is a perimesencephalic distribution of blood on the CT scan and the patient has remained conscious at the initial haemorrhage. Angiography must be comprehensive before being accepted as normal; an aneurysm arising at the origin of the posterior inferior cerebellar artery (PICA) from the vertebral artery can be missed unless both vertebral arteries are demonstrated. Delayed MR scan is occasionally done after two negative cerebral angiograms in young patients with diffuse subarachnoid haemorrhage, mainly to exclude a cavernoma on the brain surface.

Section 40.6 • Clinical management

General assessment and treatment

Resuscitation is the first priority for any unconscious or poorly responsive patient, irrespective of cause. A Glasgow Coma Scale score of 8/15 or less should make one consider sedation, intubation and ventilation. This protects the airway, and (if a normal or slightly raised blood pressure is maintained) tends to reduce ICP and maximize cerebral perfusion. Aggressive hyperventilation should be avoided, and the aim is to maintain a $PaCO_2$ of 4.5–5.0 kPa. Above this range the risk is CO_2-induced cerebral vasodilatation, and below it the risk is cerebral vasoconstriction and ischaemia.

Neurological evaluation prior to sedation is essential, and includes assessment of conscious level, pupillary size and reaction to light, and any major hemisphere deficits such as dysphasia or hemiparesis. Coma from haemorrhage in the posterior cranial fossa is a poor prognostic sign, as it may indicate brain stem involvement, but beware missing reversible damage due to obstructive hydrocephalus. Aneurysmal subarachnoid haemorrhage carries a risk of cerebral vasospasm and delayed ischaemic neurological deficits, but the calcium channel blocker nimodipine (orally or by nasogastric tube) can minimize this. Patients should be kept well hydrated and a coagulation screen done.

Once a CT scan and/or lumbar puncture have confirmed the diagnosis of intracranial haemorrhage, a neurosurgical opinion should be obtained about treatment. This consultation should take place without delay in any patient who is unconscious, or who has a cerebellar haemorrhage or a subarachnoid haemorrhage.

Definitive treatment

Haematomas

Operative treatment should be considered for any haematoma causing significantly raised ICP and located at an accessible site in a patient who has a reasonable prognosis. This includes the relatively small hypertensive haematomas of the cerebellar hemispheres, where surgical evacuation can pre-empt catastrophic deterioration and improve outcome (Figure 40.7). Very occasionally a tumour is found when the clot is removed, and can be definitively treated at the same operation.

Aneurysmal subarachnoid haemorrhage

The aim of treatment is to obliterate the aneurysm and forestall further haemorrhage. The options are surgery and interventional radiology by the endovascular route, and the anatomical details of the aneurysm as seen on angiography determine its suitability for either treatment as well as the risks. In the anterior cerebral circulation the two techniques carry similar risks, but with basilar aneurysms the risks of surgery are higher and for these lesions the endovascular route may offer attractions.

Most aneurysms are technically suitable for a direct surgical approach via a craniotomy, and most neurosurgeons now prefer to operate as early as possible if the patient's general condition allows. Surgery in the first few days has not been convincingly shown to be superior to delayed surgery in terms of outcome, but may be more efficient by allowing earlier definitive treatment and a shorter length of stay in hospital.

Endovascular techniques have been adopted with varying enthusiasm around the world, and in some units most aneurysms are now treated by this route. A common method is to pack the aneurysm sac with fine coils of pre-formed platinum wire (Figure 40.9). If this technique is shown to prevent late haemorrhage as effectively as surgery its use is likely to increase, but it requires great skill and there are recorded cases of aneurysms which re-emerge and require surgical treatment (Figure 40.10).

Malformations

Treatment depends on the location and structure of the lesion, and on the views of the surgeon and the patient about what risks are reasonable. Many AVMs and cavernous malformations can be excised surgically (Figure 40.11), sometimes combined with endovascular techniques to reduce blood loss. Stereotactic radiosurgery is being assessed as an option to treat small AVMs in sur-

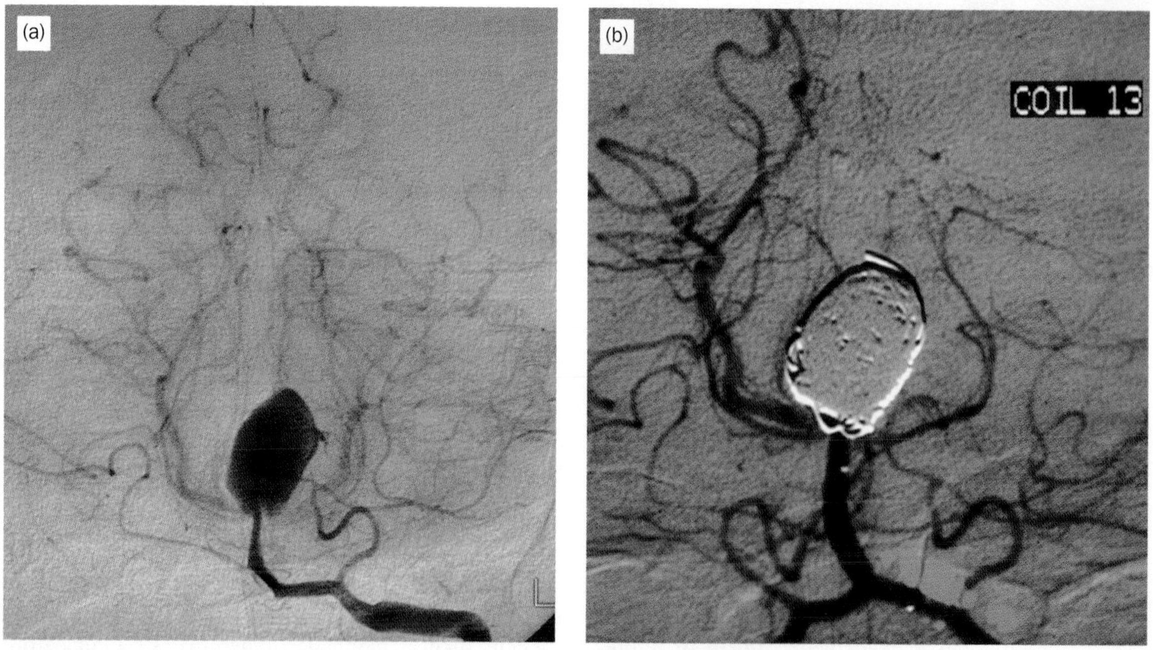

Figure 40.9 (a) Giant aneurysm of the basilar bifurcation (frontal projection): before endovascular treatment. (b) After packing with coils.

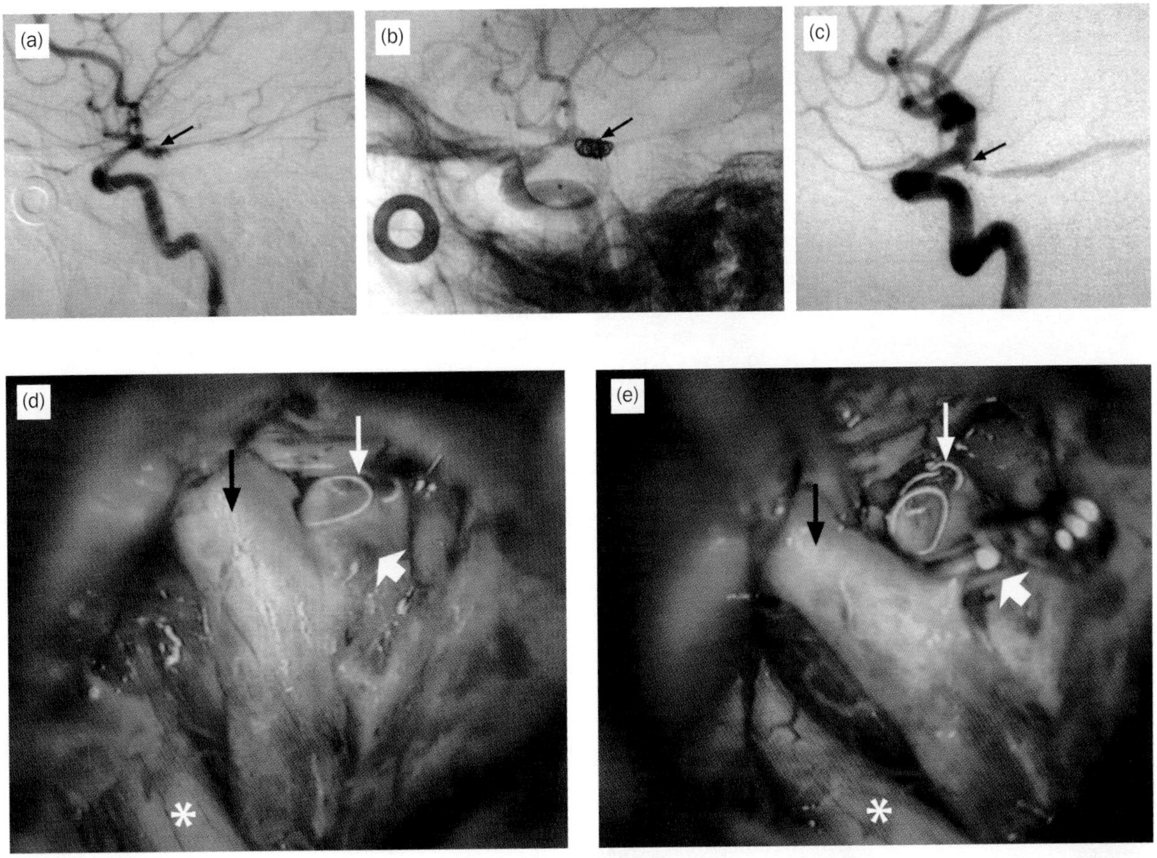

Figure 40.10 (a) Aneurysm of the internal carotid artery at the posterior communicating artery origin: left lateral carotid angiograms – subtraction view showing aneurysm (arrow). (b) Conventional view showing coils packed into the aneurysm sac (arrow). (c) Subtraction view 3 months later showing refilling of the neck of the aneurysm (arrow). (d) Intra-operative view before clipping the re-opened neck of the aneurysm. (e) After clipping the aneurysm neck. Asterisk = left optic nerve, black arrow = internal carotid artery, thin white arrow = coils in aneurysm fundus (visible through wall), broad white arrow = neck of aneurysm in (d) and clip across neck in (e).

gically inaccessible sites. Conservative management is sometimes imposed by the nature of the lesion or the condition of the patient, but can also be considered when the lesion has not bled.

Section 40.7 • Complications of intracranial haemorrhage

The risks of recurrent haemorrhage and delayed ischaemic deficits from a ruptured aneurysm or other vascular anomaly were considered earlier in this module.

A patient with an intracranial haemorrhage is often bed bound, and therefore at risk from the general complications of bed rest, including venous thromboembolism, chest infection and urinary tract infections from bladder catheters.

A strategically situated haematoma can cause acute obstructive hydrocephalus, usually in the third or fourth ventricle. This may need emergency surgery to relieve the rapidly rising ICP by draining the obstructed ventricle and (usually) removing the haematoma. Much more often, communicating hydrocephalus develops insidiously over days or weeks as the debris of the haemorrhage blocks the absorption of CSF. Up to 15% of patients with a subarachnoid haemorrhage develop this problem, which often requires the insertion of a CSF shunt.

Spontaneous intracranial haemorrhage is often followed by hyponatraemia (serum sodium below 130 mmol/l), due either to the cerebral salt wasting syndrome (CSWS) or the syndrome of inappropriate antidiuretic hormone secretion (SIADH). CSWS is the more common after aneurysmal subarachnoid haemorrhage, and probably occurs because a catecholamine surge after the bleed triggers excess secretion of the atrial natriuretic peptide in the brain. Its hallmarks are *reduced* intravascular and total body water, hyponatraemia and natriuresis, and the treatment is to replace the volume and sodium deficit. By contrast, SIADH *increases* intravascular water and total body water, causing dilutional hyponatraemia with natriuresis, so fluid restriction is the rational treatment. However, this is undesirable after aneurysmal subarachnoid haemorrhage because of the risks of vasospasm and delayed ischaemic deficits. Despite the biochemical abnormality it is then safer to maintain hydration and

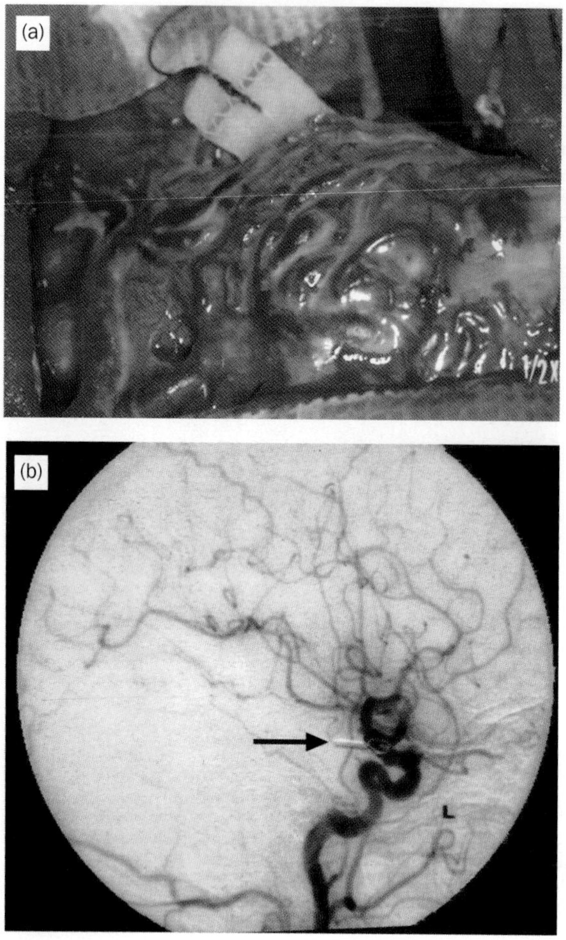

Figure 40.11 (*a*) AVM exposed at operation (white surgical pattie (12 mm wide) indicates size. (*b*) Post-operative angiogram without AVM, and clip on associated aneurysm (arrow).

give additional salt. The tetracycline derivative demeclocycline can also be used in SIADH to block the renal tubular action of ADH, but its effectiveness is limited by its delayed action. The central venous pressure is elevated in SIADH, which helps to distinguish it from CSWS.

Section 40.8 • The aftermath: rehabilitation and secondary prevention

Intracranial haemorrhage and its treatment often produce significant neurological deficits, and the patient's rehabilitation needs should be assessed and met. Even after mild subarachnoid haemorrhage without loss of consciousness it is common to find subtle problems such as poor concentration and persisting headache, which tend to improve with time. With larger bleeds the neurological and neuropsychological deficits caused by the initial haemorrhage and its ischaemic and metabolic complications tend to be more obvious to the patient and family as well as to the clinician, more disabling and less likely to improve without a rehabilitation programme. Evidence is growing to support the clinical effectiveness of rehabilitation after all forms of acquired brain injury, although what matters is not the style and location as much as simply having a well-organized, goal-orientated and individualized programme.

Rehabilitation is a team game. The physiotherapist and occupational therapist treat major physical deficits such as hemiparesis or incoordination, and restore mobility and personal independence. Improvement in these deficits can continue for many months, with functional gains continuing for up to 2 years. Visual field defects often improve spontaneously in the first few months after the bleed, and the patient can be also taught to scan by head movements to minimize the effect of the field defect. The speech and language therapist addresses communication (comprehension and expression) and swallowing. A dysphasic patient can go on making gains for a year or more after the bleed, and if necessary alternative and augmentative communication aids can be tried. A clinical neuropsychologist can diagnose cognitive deficits accurately and help plan and carry out a treatment programme which takes proper account of the emotional, psychosocial and behavioural factors which are common after acquired brain injury.

The underlying cause of the haemorrhage can be as important to the long-term outcome as the bleed itself. Definitive treatment of aneurysms, malformations and tumours is clearly important. Anticoagulant-related haemorrhage should be followed by a review of the need for the drug and close monitoring of its dose. Hypertension and other risk factors such as diabetes and hypercholesterolaemia must be optimally managed. Lifestyle changes may be crucial, such as persuading the patient not to smoke cigarettes.

There is a risk of late epilepsy following subarachnoid haemorrhage, and in the UK the Driving and Vehicle Licensing Agency should be notified of all intracranial bleeds. It will not normally suspend an ordinary (group 1) driving licence after aneurysmal haemorrhage unless a middle cerebral artery aneurysm has been treated surgically or there have been seizures, neurological deficits or an intracerebral haematoma. After non-aneurysmal intracerebral haemorrhage a driving licence suspension is to be expected, except after cerebellar haemorrhage with good recovery. The regulations are far more stringent for vocational (group 2) licence entitlement.

Section 40.9 • Conclusion

Spontaneous intracranial haemorrhage is common, usually dramatic in onset, and often disabling in its consequences. Prompt and appropriate early assessment and management can contribute greatly to an optimal outcome.

MODULE 41

Tumours of the brain and spine

1 • Epidemiology and incidence
2 • How does the patient with a brain tumour present?
3 • Brain tumour syndromes
4 • Investigations
5 • Types of brain tumour
6 • Treatment
7 • Outcome
8 • Tumours of the spine

Managing tumours of the central nervous system (CNS) presents unique challenges to the neurosurgeon and neuro-oncologist. As the CNS is enclosed in a rigid bony box, tumour growth is at the expense of invasion or compression of adjacent neural tissue.

The site and invasiveness of an intracranial or intraspinal tumour determines the scope for its resection, and the usual prognostic distinction between benign and malignant tumours becomes less important in such circumstances. For example, a tumour growing in the brain stem may be irresectable and ultimately fatal, even though it is histologically benign. The commonest primary brain tumour – the malignant astrocytoma – almost never metastasizes outside the CNS, yet is currently incurable and indeed is one of the most malignant of human tumours. However, systemic cancers (especially of the lung and breast) frequently metastasize to the brain, skull, meninges and vertebral column and are the commonest type of CNS tumour in the elderly.

Section 41.1 • Epidemiology and incidence

About 8% of primary cancers arise in the CNS. In adults they form the sixth largest groups of cancers, with a UK incidence rate of 4–10 per 100 000 (maximal in the sixth decade), while in children the CNS is the commonest site for solid tumours. Most adult brain tumours arise in the supratentorial compartment, but about 60% of those in children arise in the posterior fossa. Meningiomas and schwannomas are commoner in females but malignant primary CNS tumours are slightly more common in males.

Section 41.2 • How does the patient with a brain tumour present?

Table 41.1 summarizes the relative frequency of some common clinical features caused by brain tumours. The brain itself has no pain receptors, but raised intracranial pressure (ICP) can generate *headache* by distortion or compression of the dura, periosteum and cranial blood vessels. Over 50% of brain tumour patients have headache, although only 10% have the 'classic' presentation of headache (usually worse in the morning), associated with nausea and temporarily relieved by vomiting. In three-quarters the pain is similar to a benign 'tension-type' headache. Some patients have lateralized headache, and occasionally a tumour is found at the site of the pain.

Table 41.1 Clinical features of intracranial tumour at presentation

Progressive neurological deficit	68%
Headache	54%
Seizures	26%

Vomiting is not associated with abdominal pain. It is often worse in the morning and can be intractable in patients with posterior fossa tumours which directly infiltrate the brain stem or structures around the fourth ventricle.

Two-thirds of brain tumour patients have a *progressive neurological deficit* – usually focal motor weakness – making this the commonest presentation. This deficit arises from direct neuronal damage or the effects of tumour compression on brain or cranial nerves. Sudden change may be due to haemorrhage into a pre-existing tumour.

Generalized or focal epileptic *seizures* occur in about a quarter of patients. Focal seizures may help to localize the site of the tumour, particularly for those in the motor cortex. A high index of suspicion is required for patients past the second decade with recent onset of epilepsy. These patients should have brain imaging.

A pituitary tumour or other tumour near the midline can cause *papilloedema* and *visual disturbances* from compression of the optic nerves, chiasm or tracts. A tumour in the temporal, parietal or occipital lobes can produce a visual field deficit (homonymous hemianopia or quadrantanopia), which may only be noticed after the patient injures themselves while walking or driving. Visual failure from chronic papilloedema can occur whenever a tumour mass or obstructive hydrocephalus causes raised ICP.

Tumours of the frontal lobes can cause *mental changes* such as confusion, depression and apathy, and this can be a diagnostic trap for the unwary. The corpus callosum is the main connecting tract between the hemispheres, and a glioma there – the so-called 'butterfly glioblastoma' – commonly presents with dementia and incontinence.

Section 41.3 • Brain tumour syndromes

Frontal lobe

Frontal lobe tumours present with memory impairment, personality change and incontinence. The tumour may reach a large size due to the relatively 'silent' function of the anterior frontal lobe. Some patients show the primitive reflexes normally present only in babies, such as a grasp reflex and snout reflex. A tumour in the motor cortex at the posterior margin of the frontal lobe causes motor weakness of a spastic type, while one in Broca's motor speech area produces expressive dysphasia.

Parietal lobe

A parietal lobe tumour in the dominant hemisphere causes receptive dysphasia and weakness in the contralateral limbs. In the non-dominant hemisphere it can lead to hemisensory neglect and loss of visuo-spatial and body image. The patient may experience difficulty getting dressed (dressing apraxia), e.g. trying to put both legs in one trouser leg, or being unable to put on a shirt which has one sleeve outside in.

Temporal lobe

Temporal lobe tumours cause contralateral limb weakness, a homonymous (and contralateral) visual field loss and epilepsy. The epilepsy can feature olfactory phenomena or feelings of fear, pleasure, uncertainty or '*deja vu*'. Complex partial seizures with psychomotor movements can also occur.

Occipital lobe

An occipital lobe tumour causes a visual field defect, usually a homonymous hemianopia. This may not be noticed by the patient until it is relatively large.

Third ventricle

Tumours involving the hypothalamus, pineal region and optic chiasm are more common in children, in whom they cause endocrine disturbance, growth failure, visual loss and hydrocephalus.

Posterior fossa

Tumours here present with focal cerebellar signs (incoordination and ataxia) and with headache and vomiting from raised ICP caused by the hydrocephalus which follows blockage of the cerebral aqueduct or fourth ventricle. Compression of the cranial nerves and brain stem may also produce diplopia, disconjugate gaze, or difficulties with speech or swallowing.

Section 41.4 • Investigations

The best initial investigation is computed tomography (CT) scan of the head. This shows where the tumour alters the attenuation of the X-ray beam as it passes through the brain, and also distortion of the ventricular system or obliteration of the pattern of sulci. Iodinated contrast agent given intravenously leaks through the damaged blood–brain barrier (BBB) to show areas of increased attenuation of the X-ray beam (increased whiteness) on the scan (Figure 41.1). The area of enhancement does not correspond to the margin of the tumour, but where the brain capillaries have become 'leaky'. Particularly in glioma, tumour cells often extend far beyond the area of enhancement, and this fact has a major influence on treatment and prognosis.

Magnetic resonance imaging (MRI) often gives extra information and may eventually supersede CT completely. It is a tomographic imaging technique based on the response of body tissue protons when they are placed in a magnetic field and exposed to pulses of

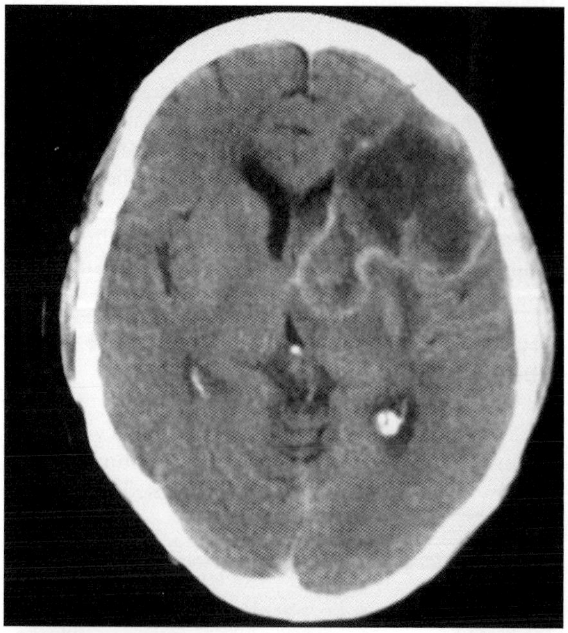

Figure 41.1 CT scan showing a large left frontal glioblastoma, extending medially and posteriorly and showing marginal enhancement with intravenous contrast.

radio-frequency energy. When the pulses cease, the protons 'relax' and release energy, which can be detected. The relaxation time is determined by the chemical and physical properties of the tissue containing the protons, and the MRI scanner can be adjusted to give the best signal contrast in various locations. Intravenous administration of chelated gadolinium (a paramagnetic substance) shortens the relaxation time in tissues which take it up and increases the signal. Gadolinium is not carried across the intact BBB, so enhancement tends to occur in tumours and in peritumoral brain tissue where there is BBB breakdown. MR has the advantage over CT of a volume acquisition, so that any plane of section can be used. It can 'see through' bone and so is the investigation of choice for imaging the posterior fossa and the spine. Its disadvantages are cost, availability and the time taken to acquire a sequence.

There is no indication for plain skull films nowadays and they are of historical interest only. Occasionally a skull film done for a different purpose (e.g. after a head injury) shows a calcified tumour or erosion of parts of the skull. Radioisotope scanning is generally only used for screening for metastatic lesions in the spine or skull.

Section 41.5 • Types of brain tumour

Table 41.2 shows the relative frequency of the types of tumour which occur in the brain.

Astrocytoma

This is the commonest primary brain tumour, arising from the supporting glial cells and diffusely infiltrating brain tissue early on. Two grading systems (WHO and St Anne/Mayo) are useful for treatment planning and prognostication. A grade I or grade II ('low grade') tumour is slow-growing and compatible with prolonged good quality survival, and a grade III or IV tumour is rapidly growing and frankly malignant. Grade IV tumours (glioblastoma multiforme) are highly radio-

Table 41.2 Incidence of commoner types of brain tumour

Tumour	*Overall percentage incidence* Adults	Children
Astrocytoma (all types)	40	50
Oligodendroglioma	6	1
Ependymoma	5	6
Medulloblastoma and PNET	2	25
Meningioma	18	3
Schwannoma (neurilemmoma)	8	
Craniopharyngioma	2	9
Haemangioblastoma	2	
Pituitary	10	
Pineal	<1	4
Lymphoma	1	–
Metastatic	5 (25% at post-mortem)	<1
Others	<1	3

resistant and chemoresistant, with median survival only 12 months even with optimum treatment.

Even low grade tumours often show genetic abnormalities such as mutation of the p53 and PGDF genes, and evolve over time into 'secondary' glioblastomas. Molecular genetic studies are revealing a cascade of genetic aberration during this process, shedding light on the natural history of malignant transformation of tumours in general. 'Primary' glioblastomas tend to occur in older patients than secondary ones (median 55 vs 40 years), and apparently arise *de novo* within a few months. Although histologically identical to secondary glioblastomas, their genetic aberrations are distinct and they have an even poorer prognosis. Molecular genetics may soon be able to define a 'family' of glioblastomas rather than a single entity.

The pilocytic astrocytoma is a distinct tumour within the WHO grading (WHO grade I). It does not progress into a more malignant grade and is curable by excision. It occurs anywhere in the CNS but especially the hypothalamus, optic nerves and cerebellum. It is commoner in children.

Oligodendroglioma

This type of glioma also forms a histological spectrum, ranging from well-differentiated to frankly malignant. The grading system for astrocytomas is not directly applicable to oligodendrogliomas, and only the extremes of the histological spectrum have prognostic significance. Oligodendrogliomas are usually slow-growing tumours and over half arise in the frontal lobes. There may be a history of epilepsy or even focal neurological signs of many years' duration. They grow diffusely within white matter tracts and may show calcification both microscopically and macroscopically.

Ependymoma

These glial tumours arise from the cells which line the ventricles of the brain and the central canal of the spinal cord (WHO grade II). They are most common in the fourth ventricle in children and young adults, where they block the flow of cerebrospinal fluid (CSF) and often present with hydrocephalus. Prognosis is more favourable in adults.

Choroid plexus tumours

These arise in the ventricles of the brain from the epithelium of the choroid plexus. Choroid plexus papilloma is a benign condition (WHO grade I), curable by surgical resection. It can present with raised ICP from obstructive hydrocephalus. Malignant transformation leads to choroid plexus carcinoma, a solid and locally invasive tumour which seeds throughout the CNS (WHO grade III).

Embryonal tumours

Primitive neuroectodermal tumours (PNET) are a group of highly malignant tumours of which the cerebellar

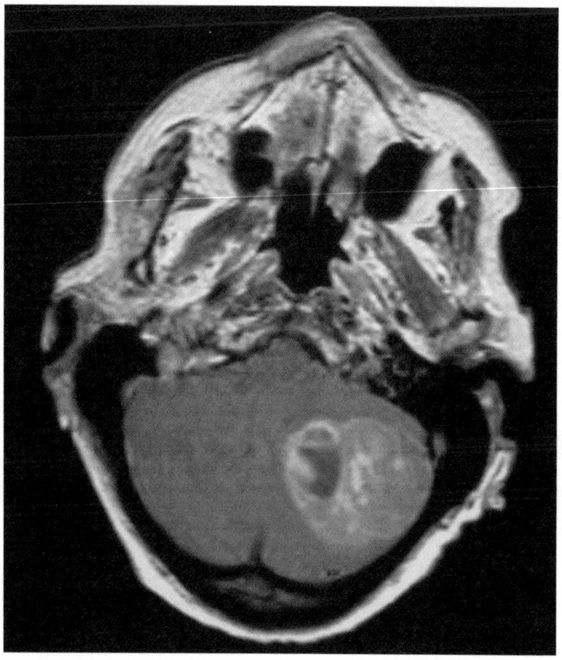

Figure 41.2 MR scan of the posterior fossa (axial view) showing a medulloblastoma extending into the left cerebellar hemisphere.

PNET or 'medulloblastoma' (Figure 41.2) is the archetype. A recent reclassification of CNS tumours has recognized that these histologically similar tumours, like the glioblastomas, have distinct genotypes. They are commonest in children and young adults, and may originate from primitive cell rests which have undergone malignant transformation. Medulloblastoma is the most common malignant brain tumour in children. The patient presents with truncal ataxia, headache, vomiting and sometimes diplopia. All PNETs are prone to spread within the CNS, producing 'sugar-coating' metastases which are best seen on an MRI of the spine.

Pineal region tumours

The pineal gland is a favoured site for supratentorial PNET ('pinealblastoma'). It also gives rise to a diverse group of germ cell tumours (germinoma, teratoma, choriocarcinoma, and embryonal carcinoma). Hydrocephalus is a common presentation, from blockage of the back of the third ventricle.

Pituitary adenomas

These benign tumours are often 'micro-adenomas', limited to the adenohypophysis and presenting with endocrine symptoms. Larger tumours have a suprasellar extension (Figures 41.3–41.5) and invade the adjacent cavernous sinus. Secretory tumours can produce hormones derived from their precursor cell type, often in large amounts leading to characteristic endocrine syndromes: adrencorticotropic hormone (ACTH) (Cushing's syndrome), prolactin (infertility/galactorrhoea), or

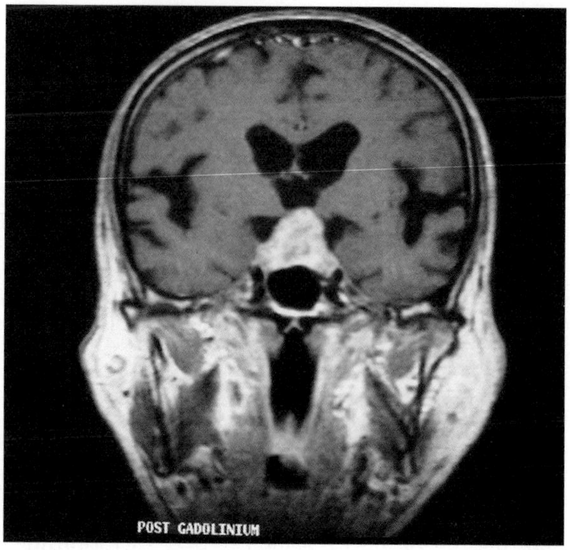

Figure 41.3 MR scan showing a pituitary adenoma with a suprasellar extension (coronal view).

growth hormone (acromegaly or gigantism). The non-secretory tumours cause pituitary insufficiency from compression or destruction of the normal gland tissue, and visual field defect from compression of the optic chiasm.

Craniopharyngioma

These tumours arise from the anterior border of the pituitary and cause visual failure and pituitary insufficiency. They are lined with stratified squamous epithelium and contain solid and cystic components. They do not undergo malignant transformation but they are difficult to resect because they grow widely under the frontal and temporal lobes and the capsule adheres tightly to the hypothalamus, optic nerves and carotid arteries. About half are calcified and visible on plain skull films.

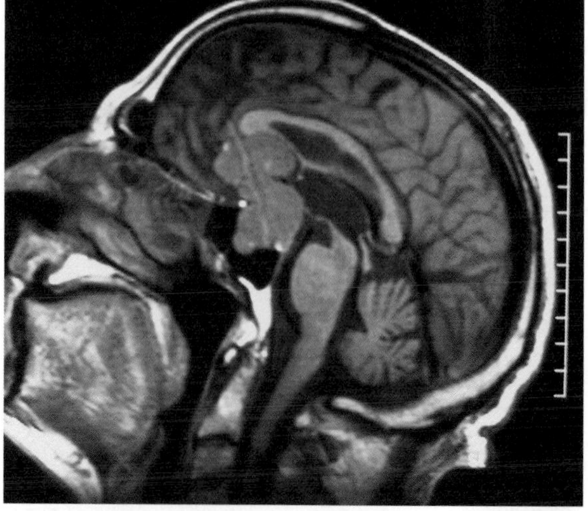

Figure 41.4 Same patient as Figure 41.3 – sagittal view showing the extent of suprasellar extension.

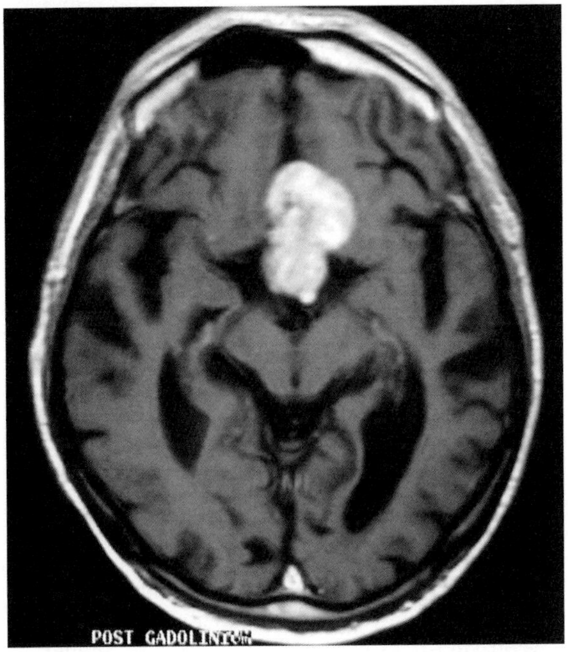

Figure 41.5 Same patient as Figure 41.3 – axial view at the level of suprasellar extension.

Schwannoma (neurilemmoma)

Peripheral neurones get their myelin sheaths from Schwann cells. Occasionally these form slow-growing benign tumours on cranial or spinal nerves. The cranial nerve most often affected is the vestibular division of the eighth nerve, and the tumour is usually then called an acoustic neuroma, even though it does not arise from the acoustic nerve and is not a neuroma! As this tumour enlarges it causes progressive deafness, but as it grows exceedingly slowly it can become very large and markedly distort the brainstem and cerebellum, causing hydrocephalus and ataxia. Less often schwannomas arise on the trigeminal or vagus nerves. Bilateral vestibular schwannomas are associated with the central form of neurofibromatosis (NF2). A tumour suppressor gene on chromosome 22q codes for a protein called merlin, and loss of merlin expression is a universal finding in schwannomas.

Meningioma

These tumours arise from the arachnoid layer of the meninges and the arachnoid villi. They are commonest over the falx and convexity of the skull, but may also arise from the skull base (especially the sphenoid wing and the olfactory groove) or inside a lateral ventricle. They are commonest in middle-aged women and may occur at the site of a previous radiation field. Most meningiomas are benign and grow very slowly. They can be clinically silent for many years and can reach a huge size before producing symptoms from raised ICP (Figures 41.6–41.8). Tumours over the convexity present with epilepsy or focal deficit. Anterior cranial fossa meningiomas stretch the olfactory nerves (causing anosmia) and the optic nerves (causing blindness). Meningiomas tend to provoke endosteal hypertrophy or exostosis in the overlying skull and are still occasionally detected on an incidental skull film or even by palpation of the skull. Although they tend to be histologically benign they may be inoperable due to their position, particularly if they invade the cavernous or sagittal sinuses or encase the carotid artery. Patients with neurofibromatosis type 2 (NF2) often have

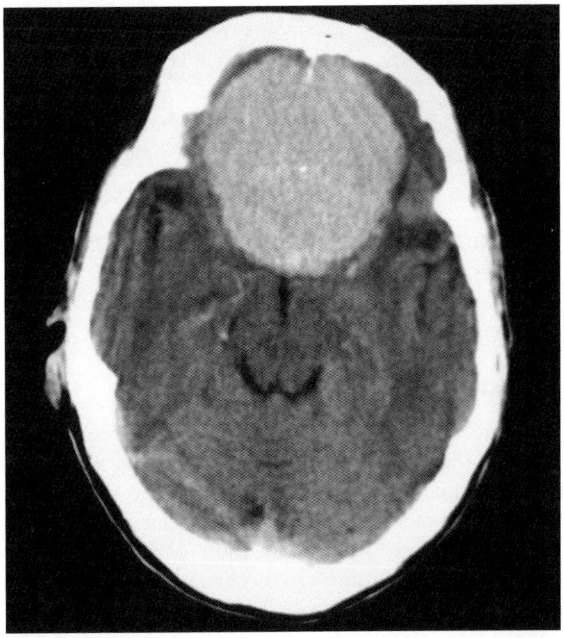

Figure 41.6 CT scan showing enormous homogeneously enhancing meningioma arising from the base of the anterior cranial fossa.

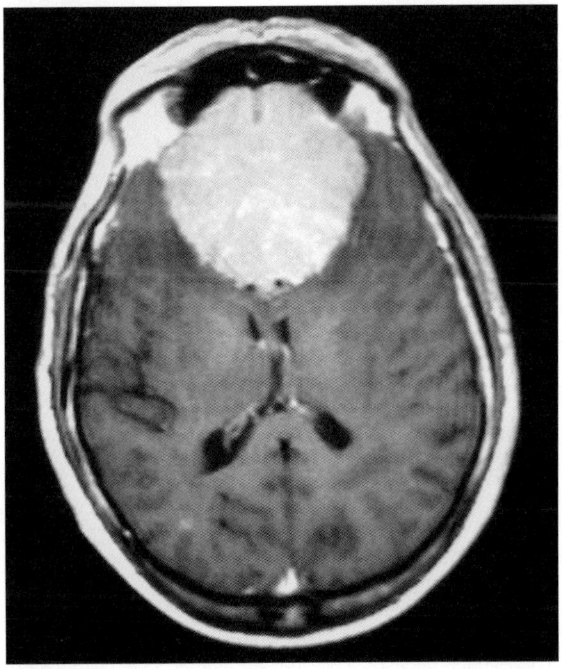

Figure 41.7 Same patient as Figure 41.6 – MR scan (axial view).

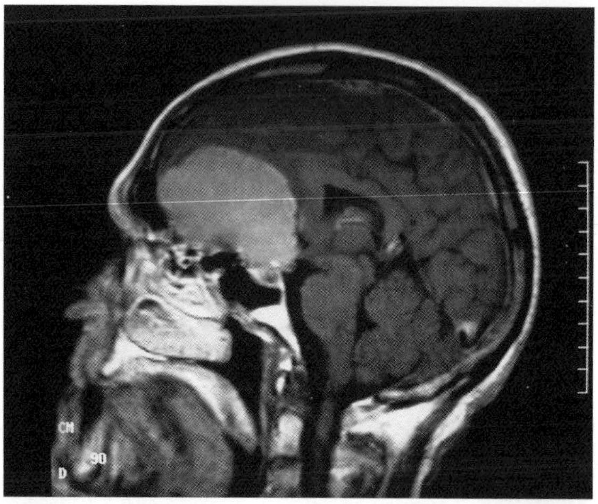

Figure 41.8 Same patient as Figure 41.6 – MR scan (sagittal view).

multiple meningiomas. Rarely they are malignant and require post-operative radiotherapy.

Metastases

A quarter of all cancer patients have intracerebral metastases at the time of death. The main primary sites are the bronchial tree (50%), breast (15%) and melanomas (10%), with clear cell carcinoma of kidney and gastrointestinal cancers making up most of the rest. Lymphoma and melanoma can occur either as a primary CNS tumour or as metastatic deposits (Figure 41.9). Only a small proportion of metastases are detected during life and even fewer are considered for neurosurgical treatment, so in operative series of intracranial tumours only 5% are metastases. Metastases may occur anywhere in the skull, meninges or brain. In the cerebral hemisphere they are found at the grey/white matter boundary and often provoke a disproportionate amount of brain oedema. Metastatic carcinoma can also cause a diffuse infiltration of the subarachnoid space ('meningeal carcinomatosis'), which presents with headache and a variety of cranial nerve palsies. Some cancers such as prostate tend to metastasize to the skull and meninges in preference to the brain.

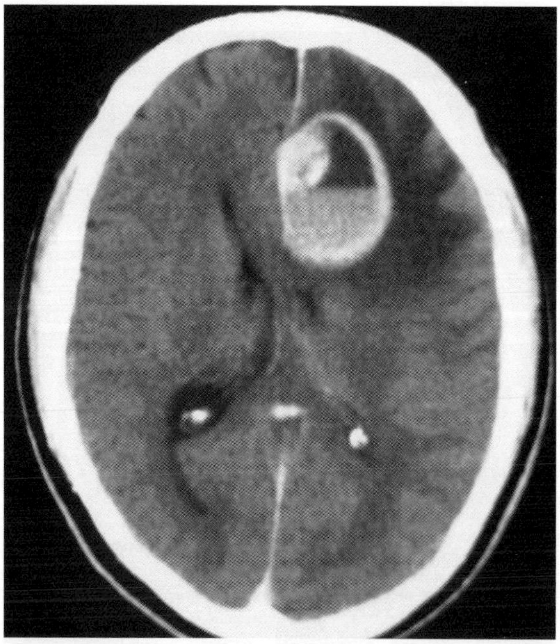

Figure 41.9 CT scan showing a large single metastasis from a malignant melanoma in the left frontal lobe, with recent haemorrhage within it.

Section 41.6 • Treatment

Immediate management depends on the severity and type of symptoms. Acutely raised ICP (intractable headache and decreasing conscious level) can be reduced quickly by giving intravenous (i.v.) mannitol 1 g/kg body weight, or by relieving hydrocephalus using a CSF diversion system (closed external ventricular drainage or a ventriculo-peritoneal shunt). A seizure should be aborted by i.v. or rectal lorazepam 0.1 mg/kg, given concurrently with a loading dose of i.v. phenytoin 18 mg/kg given as an infusion over 30 min. The patient should then be maintained on phenytoin 300 mg daily.

Corticosteroids are often given once cranial imaging has shown a tumour. Oral dexamethasone 4 mg q.i.d. reduces symptoms of raised ICP, which may make surgery easier. Mild opiates such as codeine or dihydrocodeine reduce headache without depressing conscious level.

Surgery

This remains the mainstay of treatment, as few CNS tumours are sufficiently sensitive to radiotherapy or chemotherapy to be treated effectively by non-surgical means. The aim of surgery is to obtain as complete a tumour excision as possible without producing a neurological deficit. This is not always possible due to the site of the tumour, in which case compromises must be made. For example, when a tumour arises from the brain stem the balance may favour leaving a small piece of it behind rather than risking a disastrous neurological deficit by attempting a complete removal. Even for benign tumours there is a trade-off between preventing recurrence and preserving function. For tumours where it is obvious that complete excision is impossible then a policy of biopsy and adjuvant treatment should be considered.

Localization of an intracranial tumour is critical if additional neurological deficit is to be avoided. Biopsy through a burrhole can be performed to an accuracy of 1 mm using a stereotactic frame attached to the patient. This method produces very small samples, but more recently frameless stereotaxy or image-guided surgery has been developed. This uses a computer to register the image data from a pre-operative CT or MR brain scan to create a virtual image of the head. The entry point and direction of approach can be viewed on the computer screen and the surgeon is 'guided' on the depth and direction of approach. The main problem is brain shift from loss of CSF and tumour resection, which limits the usefulness of image guidance during surgery. Real-time updates can be made using ultrasound, and open-coil intra-operative MR scanning is being developed. If the logistic and image quality problems can be solved then real-time image guidance with MRI should make open surgery safer and more efficient.

Astrocytomas and other malignant gliomas in the cerebral hemispheres are de-bulked if possible by open craniotomy. Even if the tumour is apparently well circumscribed and in a single lobe of the brain, a lobectomy will not remove it all. Astrocytoma cells produce a protein which allows them to grow and move with ease along the white matter tracts which interconnect the lobes of the brain. Malignant astrocytoma is really a whole-brain disease, and the aims of surgery are confined to diagnosis and palliation of the symptoms caused by the mass effect of the tumour. Brain stem astrocytomas in particular have a poor prognosis and biopsy is considered too dangerous in this region. However, these tumours usually have characteristic appearances on a CT or MRI scan.

For meningiomas and other benign supratentorial tumours, complete excision is the aim. At some sites, e.g. parts of the skull base, an attempt at this can lead to severe technical problems and unacceptable deficits, and in these cases a small remnant of tumour is deliberately left and either observed or treated by radiotherapy to delay recurrence. In vestibular schwannoma too the aim is to achieve complete excision, but the tumour's intimate relationship with the facial nerve influences whether only a subtotal resection is attempted. A complete facial nerve palsy is a serious complication, and some patients prefer to risk tumour recurrence than a facial nerve palsy from over-zealous surgery.

Pituitary tumours which are still contained within the pituitary fossa are approached from below via the trans-sphenoidal route. This avoids the risk of epilepsy and can often preserve some of the compressed pituitary tissue by removing only encapsulated tumour. Adenomas which have spread upwards towards the hypothalamus can also be approached this way, but if there is marked lateral extension a transcranial approach which splits the Sylvian fissure is preferable. Post-operative radiotherapy can be used to treat residual or recurrent tumour, but must be given very accurately with tightly collimated beams to avoid radiation damage to the optic tracts or hypothalamus. After surgically de-bulking the central part of a craniopharyngioma radiotherapy can slow down cell turnover in the capsule, which is often so densely adherent to surrounding vital structures that it cannot be separated from them safely and has to be left behind.

Pineal region tumours are difficult to approach due to their deep location and intimate relationship with

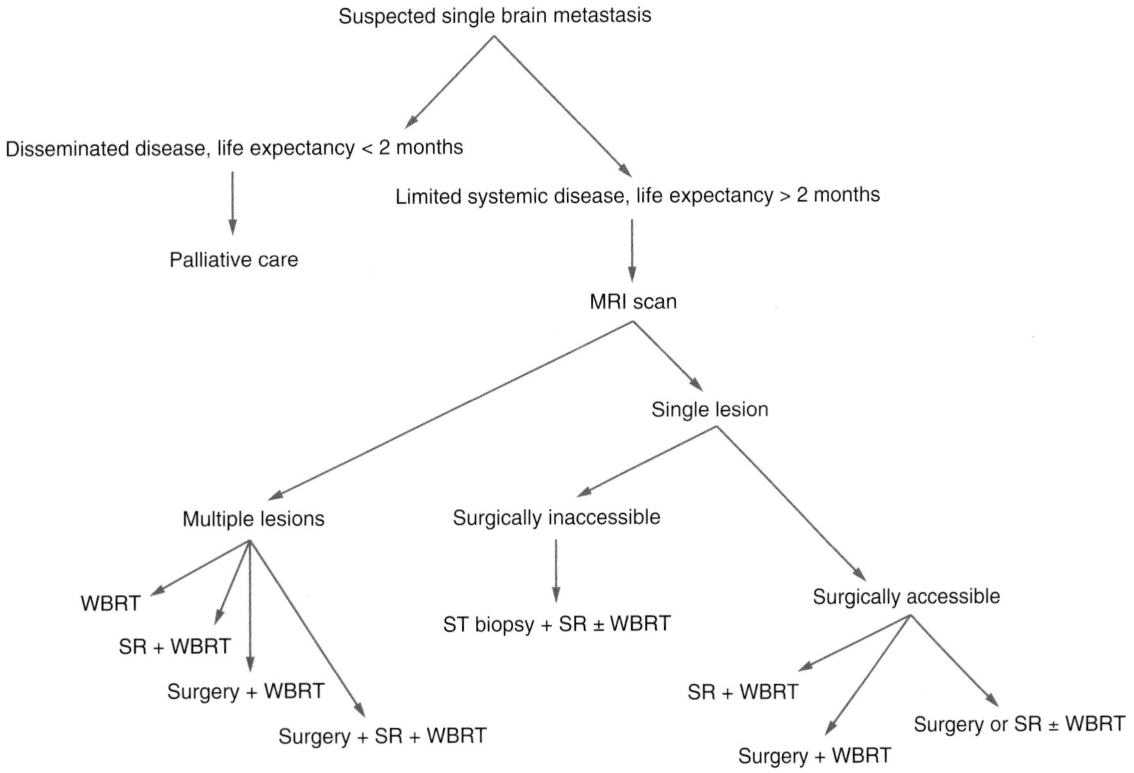

Figure 41.10 Flow chart for the management of cerebral metastases. (WBRT – whole brain radiotherapy; SR – stereotactic radiosurgery; ST biopsy – stereotactic biopsy.)

the deep cerebral veins. They can be biopsied by frame-based stereotactic biopsy or endoscopy. Fortunately, pineal germinoma is very radiosensitive and can be treated without the need for de-bulking surgery.

Medulloblastomas (and other malignant posterior fossa tumours) are best treated by de-bulking. Although a moderately radiosensitive tumour, the volume of residual tumour after surgery is the most significant prognostic variable for patients without metastases. Unfortunately this is often a midline tumour in children with invasion into the brain stem and cerebellar peduncles, thus precluding complete excision.

Radiotherapy

Intracranial tumours are relatively radio-resistant, and radiotherapy is primarily a palliative treatment. Malignant astrocytoma always recurs after surgery, but external beam whole brain radiotherapy can delay recurrence. The effect is related to the dose of radiation, with 5000–5500 cGy the minimum which will improve survival. Without radiotherapy median survival with glioblastoma is about 17 weeks, which can be increased to nearly 40 weeks with 5500 cGy radiotherapy. However, increasing the dose further to 7000 or 8000 cGy does not stop the tumour growing or improve survival.

Adjuvant treatment with radiotherapy in low grade astrocytoma has yet to be proven. Some series have shown a survival advantage at 5 and 10 years, but no randomized studies have shown a clear benefit for patients with grade I or II tumours. In selected cases where further surgery is not possible, such as the basal ganglia and brain stem, radiotherapy may be justified to try and improve function even if not survival.

Medulloblastoma and other PNETs have a tendency to seed within the CSF, and so need craniospinal irradiation to prevent a distant relapse. The posterior fossa also receives a boost dose. Inadequate dose of radiotherapy is correlated to local recurrence in some series of children with medulloblastoma.

Stereotactic radiosurgery

This technique uses a highly focused beam of radiation to produce an extremely high radiation dose to a target, with a rapid fall-off in the surrounding tissues. It is a single-dose technique, unlike fractionated conventional radiotherapy. So far it has shown promise for the treatment of metastatic tumours where there are up to three tumours each <3 cm in diameter. Early trials with vestibular schwannoma and meningioma are under way.

Chemotherapy

As yet there has been no well-designed randomized controlled trial to show that chemotherapy is of benefit in glial tumours. The most promising new agent, temozolomide, is currently undergoing clinical trials to assess its usefulness in glioblastoma and recurrent oligodendroglioma.

Table 41.3 Outcome for malignant CNS tumours

Tumour	*Median survival (adults)*
Astrocytoma WHO grade I	>10 years
Astrocytoma WHO grade II	7–8 years
Astrocytoma WHO grade III	2–3 years
Astrocytoma WHO grade IV	<1 year
Oligodendroglioma	3 years
Ependymoma	3 years
Medulloblastoma and PNET	2–3 years
Lymphoma	<1 year
Metastases (all types)	~9 months

Section 41.7 • Outcome

Surgery offers good prospects for the treatment of benign brain tumours such as meningioma or pituitary adenoma. Unfortunately the prognosis for most malignant CNS tumours remains dismal despite maximum therapy (Table 41.3).

Section 41.8 • Tumours of the spine

Most (55%) occur in the spinal extradural space, some (40%) are intradural but extramedullary, and a few (5%) are intramedullary tumours within the spinal cord itself. *Extradural tumours* may involve the vertebral bone or lie purely in the extradural space. Most are metastases from lymphoma (although some lymphomas are primary tumours) or from carcinomas of lung, breast or prostate. Benign *intradural extramedullary tumours* include meningioma, neurofibroma and dermoid/epidermoid tumours. Neurofibromas can grow out through the exit foramen into the paravertebral tissues and expand into large masses. A third each of *intramedullary tumours* are astrocytomas and ependymomas, less malignant than their intracranial counterparts but liable to cause significant cord compression because of the confined space within the vertebral canal. Astrocytomas occur anywhere in the spinal cord, while ependymomas arise from the lining of the central canal. The continuation of the spinal cord as the filum terminale can give rise to the myxopapillary variant of ependymoma, which has a good prognosis if completely excised.

The commonest presenting symptom of a spinal tumour is pain. When due to an intramedullary tumour it is unremitting, burning, often bilateral and poorly described by the patient. Local spinal pain in the neck or back that is worse on lying down and at night should raise the suspicion of spinal tumour. Radicular pain in a dermatomal distribution which is worse with coughing or movement may be due to a neurofibroma or meningioma irritating a nerve root. Spinal pain on movement, immediately relieved by rest, is indicative of spinal instability, often from metastatic disease.

Myelopathy (dysfunction from spinal cord compression) causes loss of sensation to pain, touch and motor power at and below the level of the lesion. The loss of

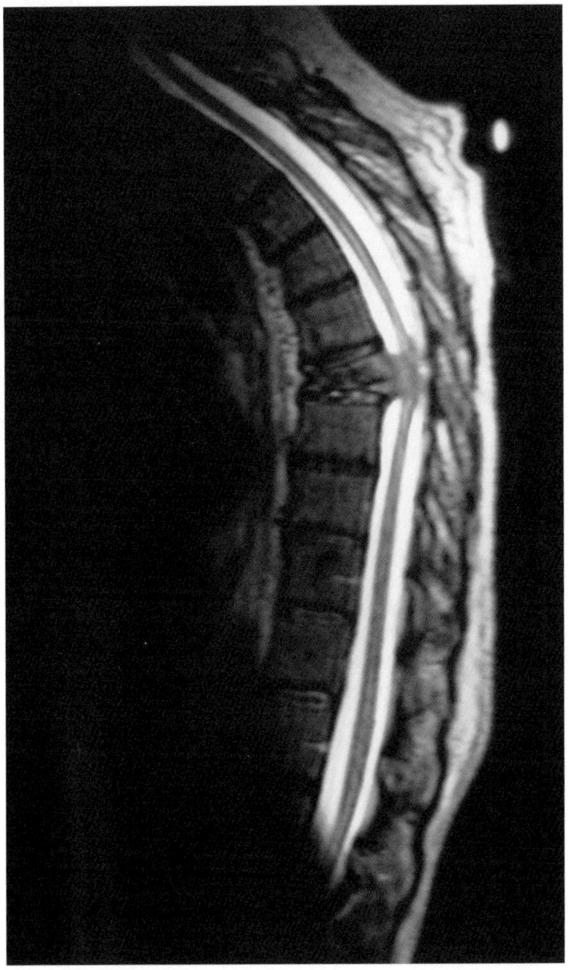

Figure 41.11 MR scan of the thoracic spine (sagittal view) showing destructive collapse of one vertebral body and posterior tumour extension into the spinal canal.

descending inhibitory inputs causes spasticity, hyperreflexia, sensory loss and bladder dysfunction below that level. The spinal cord ends at the level of the first lumbar vertebra, and compression below this level causes a *cauda equina syndrome*, with flaccid weakness and reduced lower limb reflexes.

Meningiomas of the spinal canal present with a slowly progressive paraplegia and are often diagnosed late due to their insidious onset. They occur most frequently in the thoracic area in postmenopausal women and produce a spastic lower limb weakness (paraparesis). Following excision of the tumour a gratifying improvement in symptoms may result even when the patient has a moderately severe myelopathy.

Spinal metastases are present in about 10% of cancer patients. Extradural tumour can directly compress the cord, and tumour invasion of the vertebral body and pedicles can cause the bone to compress or collapse against the cord (Figure 41.11). This can be a sudden event and occlude the blood supply to the cord, causing incontinence, limb weakness and a sensory level. There is usually marked tenderness to palpation over the back.

The investigation of choice for suspected spinal tumour is *MRI scan*. This is exquisitely sensitive to changes in signal from the marrow space in the vertebral bodies, and is a good screening investigation when there is no sensory level. Sometimes the spine is affected by direct extension of tumour rather than by blood-borne metastases, and tumour may then be traced from the spine into the retroperitoneum, mediastinum or pleura to give a clue as to the site of the primary. Intramedullary tumours appear as an expansion of the cord, sometimes with an associated syrinx, and may enhance with contrast. Meningiomas and neurofibromas also enhance strongly, but they are more discrete lesions and tend to displace rather than expand the cord. *Plain films* of the spine can show bony collapse or erosion of the pedicles. In a slow-growing benign tumour such as a dermoid the vertebral canal may be seen to be expanded, and there may be an associated spinal dysraphism such as spina bifida occulta.

The surgical treatment of intramedullary tumours ranges from simple diagnostic biopsy to internal de-bulking. Complete excision is possible in only 50%, as usually there is no plane of cleavage between the tumour and the spinal cord. Dermoid and epidermoid tumours have a capsule which is densely adherent to the spinal cord or cauda equina, and often it is safer to perform an internal de-bulking than to risk neurological deficit. All patients are given dexamethasone 4 mg q.i.d. as a neuroprotective agent before surgery, continued if adjuvant or palliative radiotherapy is to be given.

Surgery for spinal metastases is indicated where the primary is unknown and needle biopsy is not feasible, where decompression is likely to improve neurological function in a radio- and chemo-resistant tumour, where the compression is due to a retropulsed fragment of bone or disc, and where there is instability pain and the disease is limited to one or two vertebrae. If the primary tumour is known and there is no instability

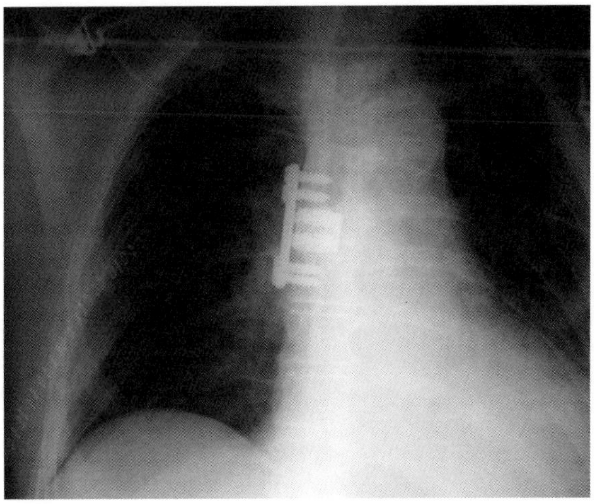

Figure 41.12 Plain chest film showing a plate and screws used to stabilize the spine after malignant collapse.

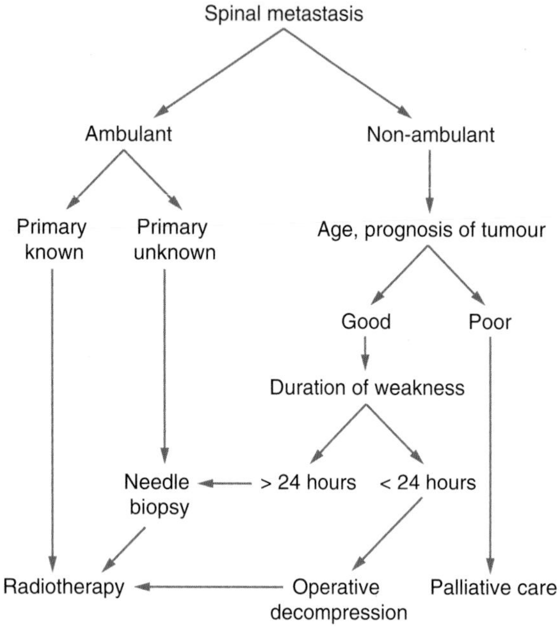

Figure 41.13 Flow chart for the management of spinal metastases.

pain, radiotherapy or chemotherapy is preferable to avoid a surgical wound; the results in terms of neurological outcome are not significantly different. Instability is treated by internal stabilization using several types of metallic construct, which can be attached posteriorly by wires or pedicle screws, or anteriorly by bone cages, plates and screws (Figure 41.12). Figure 41.13 shows a flow chart illustrating the management of spinal metastases.

Patients with spinal metastases have a median survival of less than 4 months, and any treatment is palliative. Avoiding surgery where possible lets them spend less of their remaining life in hospital. One factor is whether they can walk; about 60% of patients who are still ambulant at the time of surgery remain so afterwards, but those presenting with paraplegia (especially of more than 24 hours' duration) have only a 10% chance of walking again and virtually none of regaining full bladder control. Intradural tumours have a much better prognosis and the outcome for meningioma and neurofibroma is generally good. Astrocytomas and ependymomas are generally of lower grade than those affecting the brain, and the recurrence rate for astrocytoma is 30% at 5 years.

MODULE 42

Neurosurgical conditions of the skull base and spine

In much of medicine diagnosis is achieved by pattern recognition. We respond to a constellation of symptoms and/or signs that past experience has made familiar. In a busy medical practice with ever narrowing fields of expertise it is perhaps inevitable that we find it increasingly difficult to make a diagnosis in a specialist field different from one's own. Sadder still, we may increasingly fail even to consider such an alternative diagnosis.

It is intended that this module will expand the range of potential diagnoses that you might consider, and will help you from time to time to reach a diagnosis that has proved elusive to others. Who knows, it might also keep you out of court!

Section 42.1 • The oropharynx

Facial pain: trigeminal neuralgia

Surgical patients often present with facial pain. For example, pain in the region of the cheek may be due to infection (maxillary sinusitis, dental abscess) or neoplasia, and pain in the region of the jaw may be due to parotid or submandibular salivary gland stone.

There is an alternative diagnosis to consider. Trigeminal neuralgia is a form of facial pain confined to the distribution of the trigeminal nerve. This nerve has three divisions – ophthalmic (V1), maxillary (V2) and mandibular (V3) – and two-thirds of patients with trigeminal neuralgia have pain in V2 and/or V3; V1 involvement is distinctly less common. For unknown reasons women are more commonly affected than men and the right side of the face is more often affected than the left. Trigeminal neuralgia becomes distinctly more common with age, more than 70% of patients being 50 years or older at time of presentation.

The diagnosis lies in the history. Bouts of pain are usually severe, sudden, brief (typically a few seconds up to a minute), but can be repeated. The pain is often described as 'shooting' because of its abrupt quality, but prolonged and repeated attacks can leave a background aching discomfort in that part of the face. It can begin spontaneously or be associated with 'triggering', where pain is stimulated by actions as simple as touching the face, brushing the teeth, drinking hot or cold liquids, speaking or chewing. Patients frequently ascribe the pain to a dental cause and some undergo a dental clearance. It is frequently very severe, and if frequent and recurrent can be so intolerable that suicide is a real risk.

There are a number of causes of trigeminal neuralgia. Multiple sclerosis is present in 2–3%, a variety of benign tumours are found to be compressing the trigeminal nerve in 5–8%, but the commonest cause is an arterial or venous loop in contact with the trigeminal sensory root where it enters the pons at the root entry zone (REZ). It has been suggested that vascular contact with the trigeminal REZ is more likely to occur as vessels elongate and become ectatic with ageing, or as systemic hypertension develops.

Initial treatment makes use of the neuronal membrane-stabilizing effect of anticonvulsant drugs, especially carbamazepine (200 mg per day, rising every third or fourth day by 200 mg increments to 1000–1600 mg per day). Nausea and cognitive blunting are quite common at higher dosage, and it is also wise to monitor liver function tests and serum sodium.

If anticonvulsants fail to control pain, surgery is usually indicated. For most neurosurgeons nowadays the operation of first choice is microvascular decompression. Via a small suboccipital craniectomy the cerebellopontine angle is explored, and any vascular loop is mobilized from the trigeminal nerve and held away from the REZ by a piece of Teflon sponge. About 90% of patients do well when an arterial loop is identified, fewer if venous compression alone is found. In 10–15% of cases no vascular loop is found, and perhaps not surprisingly the results of surgery are poor in these cases.

An operation can also be done to divide part of the trigeminal sensory root (rhizotomy). An alternative approach, particularly useful in a patient unfit for open surgery, is to make a percutaneous lesion in the trigeminal ganglion by injecting glycerol, by making a radiofrequency lesion or by balloon compression of the ganglion. All forms of rhizotomy can improve trigeminal neuralgia either temporarily or permanently.

Pharyngeal pain: glosso-pharyngeal neuralgia

Rarely, patients presenting with pain in the pharynx have glosso-pharyngeal neuralgia. The general visceral afferent fibres of the glosso-pharyngeal nerve carry sensory information from the pharynx and tongue, and neuralgia causes bursts of pain in this distribution. Almost all cases are idiopathic, with no specific cause identified.

Apart from the location of pain the attacks are identical to those of trigeminal neuralgia. The pain is severe, shooting, like an electric shock in the posterior third of the tongue or in the tonsil, and virtually always unilateral. Typically, swallowing precipitates pain. Some glosso-pharyngeal fibres supply sensation to the back of the ear, and there may be ear pain.

Some patients respond to anticonvulsants like carbamazepine or phenytoin, but if that fails surgical treatment is indicated. The cerebello-pontine angle is explored, and the ninth cranial nerve and the upper one-sixth of the tenth cranial nerve are divided. This operation causes diminished sensation over the pharynx and abolishes the gag reflex on the ipsilateral side, often leading to transient problems with swallowing but usually no long-term effects.

Section 42.2 • Neurosurgical causes of dysphagia

Dysphagia is an important symptom in general surgery and can reflect pathology anywhere from the oropharynx to the stomach. By far the most common and important causes are intraluminal problems (e.g. a foreign body) and diseases of the oropharynx or oesophagus itself (e.g. a carcinoma or stricture). It is much rarer for dysphagia to be due to extrinsic compression from a condition of the skull base or cervical spine, and all other possible causes must be excluded before accepting extrinsic compression as the cause of dysphagia.

Tumours of the skull base

Any skull-base tumour can extend anteriorly, displace the pharynx and cause dysphagia, but the classical tumour to do so in this location is the cranial chordoma, an uncommon tumour which arises predominantly from the clivus, just posterior to the pharynx (Figure 42.1). Extension of a clivus chordoma anteriorly and inferiorly can cause dysphagia, while extension posteriorly or laterally causes cranial nerve and/or long tract symptoms and signs. The patient may therefore have lower cranial nerve palsies, dysarthria, vertigo, hyperreflexia, or ataxia as well as dysphagia, so take a history and listen to the patient! A clivus chordoma causes extensive bone destruction, which by the time a patient presents with dysphagia will be obvious on a lateral skull film.

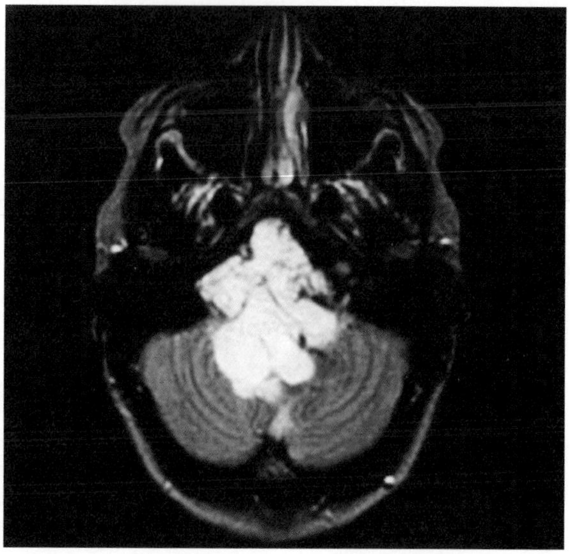

Figure 42.1 Chordoma arising from the clivus. Axial MR scan of posterior cranial fossa showing a large irregular tumour mass extending anteriorly from the clivus and causing dysphagia.

Surgical treatment is by attempted complete surgical excision, and a variety of approaches have been described. More often than not only an incomplete resection is achieved, and even where complete surgical resection is thought to have been achieved there are often residual remnants of chordoma. Long-term follow-up is therefore essential.

Cervical degenerative disease

Cervical degenerative disease (spondylosis) is very common. Osteophytic spurs of bone form, and if these project posteriorly they can compress either the laterally placed nerve roots or the spinal cord. Osteophytes can also project anteriorly (Forrestier's disease), often forming extensive bony spurs, compressing the oesophagus as it runs over the osteophytes. A lateral cervical spine plain film will demonstrate the extent of anterior osteophytes. However, it is wise to remember that cervical spondylosis is very common – 95% of people over the age of 60 years have some radiological evidence of it – whereas Forrestier's disease is an very uncommon cause of dysphagia. Unless the anterior osteophytes are gross they are unlikely to be responsible, and it is necessary to exclude all other potential causes of dysphagia before ascribing this symptom to Forrestier's disease. The diagnosis can be supported if a video fluoroscopy or radio-opaque swallow shows obstruction to the flow of contrast at the precise level of a large anterior osteophyte. The anterior cervical spine can be approached via an incision in the line of sterno-mastoid, retracting the carotid sheath laterally to expose the oesophagus as it lies on the osteophyte(s). The oesophagus is mobilized to the opposite side and the osteophytes are drilled off.

Section 42.3 • Hand–arm syndromes

A common cause of referral to a surgeon is pain in the upper limb, for example to consider whether a thoracic outlet syndrome may be responsible. However, this is only one of four important causes of shoulder/arm /hand symptoms:

- referred pain from cervical spondylosis
- radicular pain from cervical spondylosis
- peripheral nerve disorders
- thoracic outlet syndrome.

Referred pain

Cervical degenerative disease is extremely common and few people escape some degree of neck pain at some time in their lives. Pain may be felt not only in the neck itself, but *referred* to the cervical paraspinal muscles, to the shoulder, and into the upper arm – typically as far as but not below the elbow. Referred pain has similar qualities to degenerative neck pain, that is to say it is 'aching' and it tends to be 'mechanical', brought on for example by turning the neck, by carrying objects in the arms and the hands, or by holding the neck in a fixed position for some time. Referred pain can be unilateral or bilateral, or it can move from one side to the other.

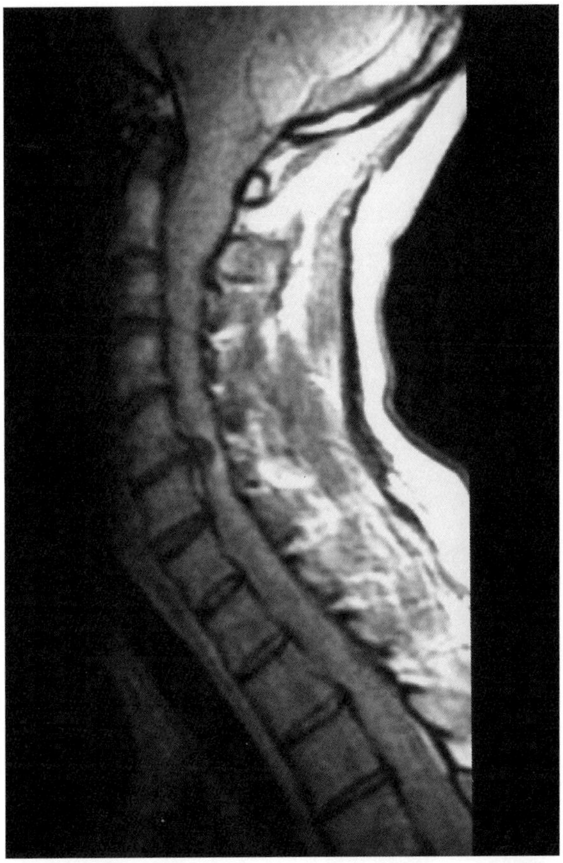

Figure 42.2 Sagittal MR scan of cervical spine: soft disc prolapse posteriorly at C5/6 causing spinal cord and nerve root compression.

Cervical radiculopathy

Cervical radiculopathy is caused by compression of a nerve root, typically where it emerges from the cervical spinal cord and passes through the nerve root canal to enter the brachial plexus. The vast majority of cervical radiculopathies are caused by cervical degenerative disease, either a soft disc prolapse (Figure 42.2) or more often a degenerative osteophyte ('hard disc').

Cervical radiculopathy is associated with *pain, sensory disturbance, reflex loss* and *motor weakness*. Radiating arm pain is almost always present, typically going below the elbow as far as the wrist or hand (whereas referred pain normally only radiates to the shoulder or upper arm). *Sensory disturbance* is almost as common; paraesthesia or numbness is felt in the thumb and index finger if the C6 nerve root is compressed, in the middle finger for the C7 nerve root, and in the ring and little finger for the C8 nerve root. The C6 nerve root contributes to the biceps reflex, and the C7 nerve root to the triceps reflex, which may then be reduced or absent. Motor weakness tends to be a late feature of cervical radiculopathy.

The diagnosis can almost always be made by magnetic resonance imaging (MRI). In a few cases computed tomography (CT) myelography is required, but this is invasive and can be unpleasant. The most important thing to bear in mind is that cervical degenerative disease is extremely common, lateral osteophytes being found in the vast majority of patients in their fifth and sixth decades. Before ascribing a hand–arm syndrome to a radiculopathy the neurological findings must be 'pure', i.e. there must be pain, the distribution of that pain must be appropriate to the root compressed, and any other neurological symptoms and signs must also be not only appropriate to the root compressed but exclusive to it. Patients who present with diffuse hand/arm pain and sensory disturbance that is not confined to a single dermatome (the area of skin supplied by a specific nerve root) should not have those symptoms described to a cervical radiculopathy unless there are compelling reasons to suspect a multi-level compressive radiculopathy. Objective neurological signs are not needed to make the diagnosis, but the pattern and distribution of pain and sensory disturbance must be as close to that expected anatomically if diagnostic and therapeutic success is to be achieved.

There are two approaches to decompressing a cervical nerve root: anterior or posterior. The former is usually via a small transverse anterior cervical skin crease incision, going medial to the carotid sheath to reach the anterior cervical spine. The appropriate cervical disc is confirmed by intra-operative films. A discectomy

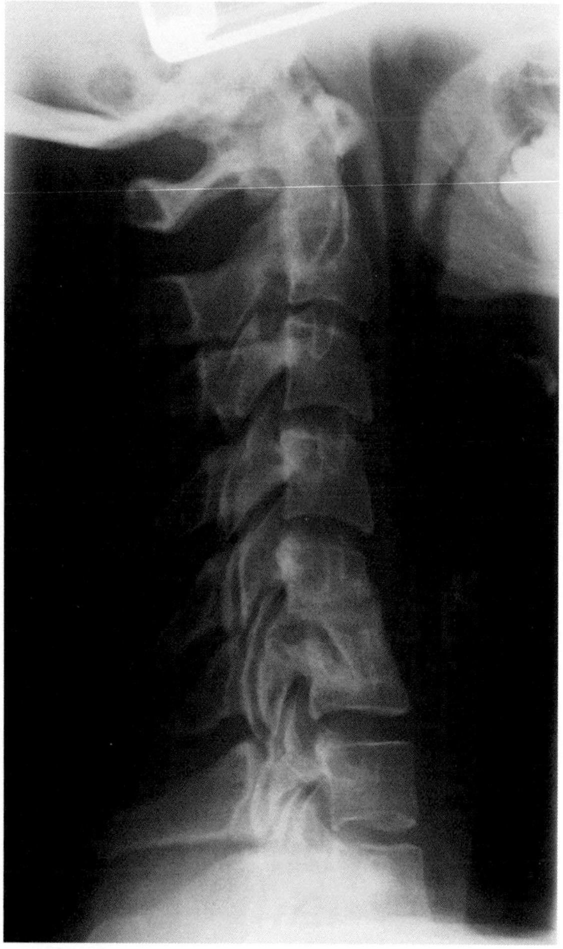

Figure 42.3 Lateral film of cervical spine: post-surgical fusion of the bodies of C5 and C6 vertebrae following anterior cervical decompression and fusion for spondylotic radiculopathy.

and/or osteophytectomy is done to decompress the appropriate cervical nerve root, which lies just behind the disc prolapse or osteophyte. The disc space can be fused with a graft of autologous bone or other material (Figure 42.3). The alternative approach (posterior foraminotomy) is usually as successful. Via a mid-line posterior cervical incision the paraspinal muscles are mobilized and retracted laterally to expose the laminae and facet joint at the appropriate level, again confirmed radiologically at operation. A very modest amount of lamina is excised, together with about 50% of the medial side of the facet joint, which 'unroofs' the cervical nerve root lying beneath.

Peripheral nerve syndromes

The three classical upper limb peripheral nerve syndromes are the carpal tunnel syndrome (median nerve compression), ulnar neuropathy and radial neuropathy (uncommon except after humeral fractures). A good description from the patient of the distribution of the sensory disturbance in the hand is usually diagnostic. Peripheral nerve syndromes can 'split' sensation in fingers, but cervical nerve root syndromes never do. The sensory disturbance from median nerve compression affects the thumb, index, middle, and half of the ring finger. In ulnar neuropathy it involves the little finger and half of the ring finger.

The diagnosis must always be a clinical one, but should be confirmed neurophysiologically with electromyography (EMG). The treatment is to decompress the appropriate nerve root, for a carpal tunnel syndrome dividing the flexor retinaculum at the wrist, and for an ulnar neuropathy mobilizing the ulnar nerve at the elbow.

Thoracic outlet syndromes

The brachial plexus and subclavian artery and vein leave the root of the neck and enter the arm through a triangle bounded posteriorly by the scalenus medius muscle, anteriorly by the scalenus anterior muscle, and based on the first rib. 'Positional' compression of the neurovascular bundle can occur, either by an actual cervical rib or much more commonly by a compressive band continuous with the medial edge of scalenus medius.

Clinical diagnosis is difficult. Symptoms can include arm pain (often rather non-specific in nature), and motor and/or sensory loss due to compression of the lower cord of the brachial plexus. There can be muscle wasting in the hands. Compression of the subclavian artery may cause a variety of vascular symptoms, including subjective coldness and easy fatiguability. Plain films may demonstrate a cervical rib (not an uncommon finding in asymptomatic individuals) but cannot show the much more common compressive fibrous band. EMG and nerve conduction studies may reveal abnormalities in the cords of the brachial plexus. The author has found dynamic subclavian angiography to be helpful, but not all would agree. Subclavian angiography is performed with the arm in the neutral and then the extended position, looking for subclavian artery compression in the extended position.

A variety of surgical approaches has been advocated. One of the commonest undertaken today is an endoscopic approach through a very small anterior cervical incision, releasing the fibrous band that lies medial to scalenus medius. The results are mixed.

Section 42.4 • Thoraco-lumbar mimics of abdominal conditions

General surgeons often consider retro-peritoneal diagnoses, but seldom remember that the spinal column lies just behind all the retro-peritoneal structures. Many pathological processes in the spine can cause spinal pain (which can mimic a number of abdominal conditions), radiculopathy (nerve root pain or loss of function) or myelopathy (loss of spinal cord function). Spinal pathology should be considered whenever entertaining a diagnosis such as pancreatitis, psoas abscess or hydronephrosis; the true diagnosis may be an osteoporotic fracture (Figure 42.4) or a metastatic tumour (Figure 42.5) involving the vertebral body, for example.

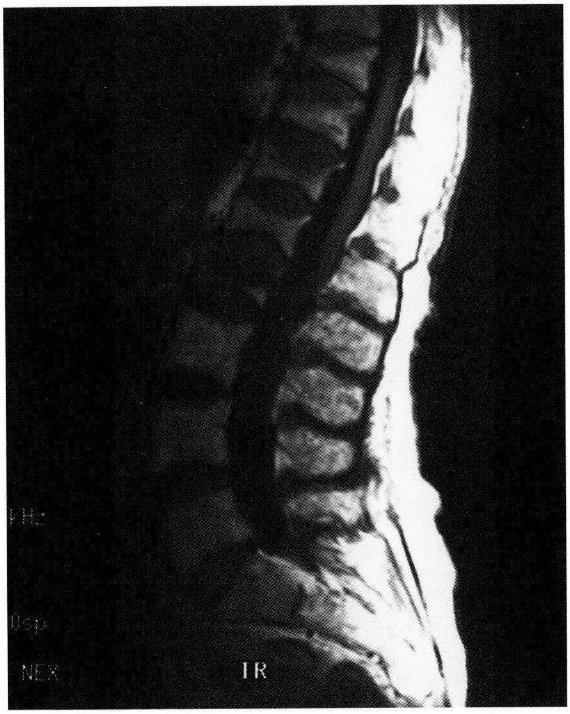

Figure 42.4 Sagittal MR scan of thoraco-lumbar spine: severe osteoporosis, with multiple compression fractures. The patient presented with severe back pain, which was initially thought to have a retro-peritoneal cause.

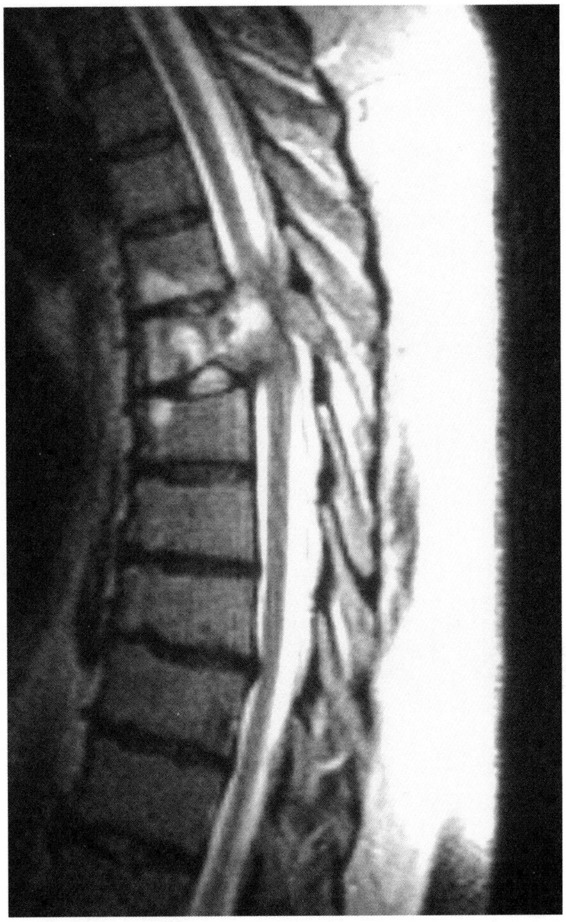

Figure 42.5 Sagittal MR scan of the thoracic spine showing destruction of a vertebral body by metastatic carcinoma. The tumour is extending posteriorly into the spinal canal and is distorting and compressing the spinal cord at the level of the bony destruction.

Spinal pain

Spinal pain is either bone pain or instability pain. **Bone pain** occurs when a vertebra has been invaded by a pathological process (usually tumour (Figures 42.6 and 42.7), occasionally infection). The patient has severe, relentless and gnawing back pain which seems to bore through from the back. **Instability pain** arises because replacement of bone (usually by tumour) compromises the structural integrity of the vertebral column and allows abnormal degrees of movement. This pain has a similar character to bone pain but typically is worse on movement, and when severe can make the patient terrified to move or even cough.

The quality of spinal pain is quite different to degenerative spinal pain, and after taking a careful history it is unlikely that one would label such a patient as simply having a 'bad back'. If the quality of the pain is such that you are considering a diagnosis, e.g. of pancreatic carcinoma, then think of the structures that lie just behind the pancreas and consider metastatic tumours of the spine as well.

One way to reach the right diagnosis is to look for other features of a spinal disorder in the clinical history and examination. Is there any evidence of spinal cord compression? Has the patient had problems with balance or walking? Do they walk as if drunk? Is there intercostal pain (see below)? There may be objective neurological signs in the lower limbs. MRI is usually diagnostic, but plain films of the spine may reveal radiolucent or radio-opaque metastases, or a pathological fracture. Myeloma can be associated with relatively normal plain films until a pathological fracture occurs, and diagnosis may require isotope bone scanning or MRI. Always ask for biplanar films (AP and lateral), and always *read the films* properly. The author has been involved in a number of medico-legal cases where a general surgeon got as far as thinking about a spinal cause for pain which was apparently retro-peritoneal, arranged for appropriate plain films, but failed either to read them or to think about the radiologist's report. As one might imagine, when the patient presents a few months later with acute spinal cord compression and ends up with a major long-term deficit the earlier failure to make a diagnosis is difficult to defend.

Intercostal nerve root pain

A thoracic dermatome (the area of skin supplied by a single intercostal nerve root) forms a band about 3 cm wide. Remember a few key dermatomes and the rest will follow logically: the nipple (T5), subcostal area (T8), umbilicus (T10) and inguinal ligament (L1).

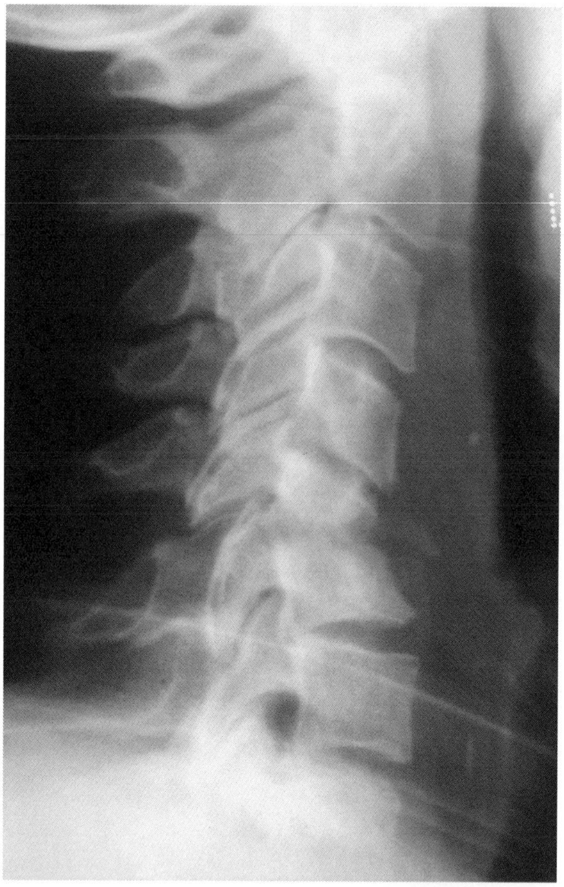

Figure 42.6 Lateral film of cervical spine showing anterior wedge fracture of the body of C5 vertebra with kyphotic angulation at the spine. Single metastasis of carcinoma of the thyroid presenting with acute neck pain.

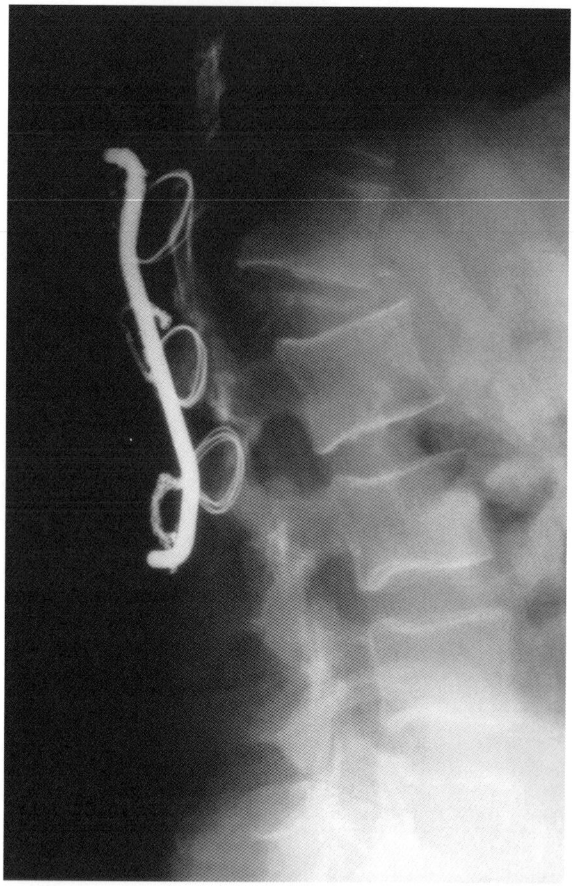

Figure 42.7 Lateral plain film of thoracic spine showing virtually complete destruction by a tumour of the body of one thoracic vertebra. A surgical procedure has been carried out to fuse the spine posteriorly at that level.

Intercostal pain normally arises posteriorly at the spine and radiates round the flank to the anterior abdominal wall. Subcostal (T8) pain on the right side can mimic gallstones, and on the left side a peptic ulcer. Para-umbilical pain can be mistakenly be ascribed to a wide variety of intra-abdominal disorders. Right iliac fossa pain (T11) can mimic appendicitis.

The best clue to the diagnosis is the distribution of pain. In most (but not all) cases it clearly radiates from the spine round to the anterior abdominal wall and follows a single dermatome. Careful neurological examination may demonstrate a band of hyperaesthesia or hypoaesthesia in the appropriate dermatomal distribution, but often there are no specific physical signs. If the intercostal nerve root irritation is due to shingles there may be a typical rash. Think about other features of spinal disorders: is there spinal pain, is there evidence of a myelopathy (unsteady gait, brisk lower limb reflexes)? Plain films should be performed in the out-patient clinic if there is any suggestion of a spinal source for pain. AP and lateral films are necessary in all cases, and *read the films or get a report*. MRI of the appropriate spinal region reveals the great majority of spinal pathologies (Figure 42.8).

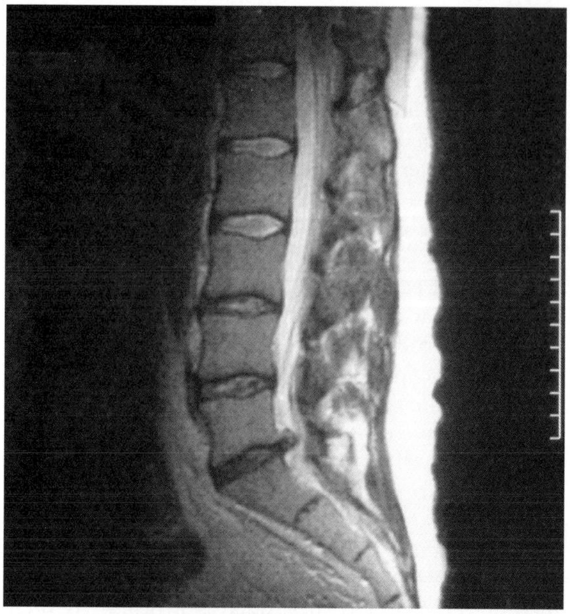

Figure 42.8 Sagittal MR scan of the lumbar spine showing a disc prolapse at the L5/S1 level with degenerative disc changes seen at the L3/4 and L4/5 levels.

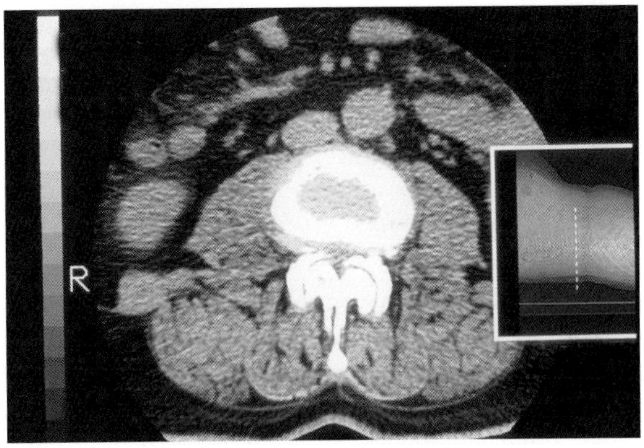

Figure 42.9 Axial CT scan of the lumbar spine showing severe facet joint hypertrophy and lumbar stenosis. This patient presented with low back pain and a gait pattern suggestive of neurogenic claudication.

Section 42.5 • Degenerative spinal pain mimicking disorders of the hip and thigh

Degenerative disease of the low back is extremely common (Figure 42.9). Very few individuals have not experienced low back pain at some times in their lives, and degenerative changes on a plain film of the lumbar spine are found in 90% of women and 95% of men over the age of 60 years. Low back pain is typically mechanical in nature, brought on by 'using' the lower back. Although it is perhaps obvious that activities such as bending and lifting heavy objects can generate mechanical low back pain, static activities such as standing or sitting can also bring it on. The lower back is made more for movement than for static activities, and most people with low back pain are better when 'pottering about'.

Mechanical low back pain is often referred to the paraspinal muscles, hip, groin, buttock or lower limb (typically as far as but not below the knee). The referred pain can be more severe than the low back pain itself, so that an alternative diagnosis such as osteoarthritis of the hip is thought more likely, and it may be necessary to investigate both possibilities. Referred pain can extend from the groin into the scrotum and testis, mimicking inguinal and scrotal disorders. In the author's experience referred pain in the thigh is almost always on its anterior, lateral or posterior aspect and virtually never on its medial aspect. In the patient who presents with pain on the medial aspect of the thigh beware instead of pelvic pathology (particularly malignancy) irritating the obturator nerve.

Lumbo-sacral radiculopathy

Irritation of a lumbo-sacral nerve root typically causes some combination of pain and sensory disturbance in one lower limb, sometimes with reflex loss and motor weakness. The pain typically radiates all the way down the limb as far as the foot. In an L4 radiculopathy it radiates only as far as the knee. In the much more common L5 or S1 radiculopathy it radiates to the lower leg and/or foot, with sensory disturbance over the dorsum of the foot (L5) or on the sole of the foot and the heel (S1). The dorsiflexors and plantarflexors of the foot are innervated by L5 and S1 respectively, so look for the appropriate loss of muscle power.

MRI of the lumbar spine is the preferred way to exclude or to confirm the diagnosis (Fig. 42.8). Plain X-ray films are an optional extra, to demonstrate excess mobility. Before diagnosing lumbo-sacral radiculopathy make sure that the clinical evidence of nerve root compression fits precisely with the MRI data. In older patients in particular, be wary of ascribing pain to degenerative disorders if it is new and/or severe. Degenerative disorders of the lumbar spine are usually chronic and one would expect a history of similar symptoms in the past. The author has seen two patients with an apparently clear-cut L5 radiculopathy, but much more severe pain than one would expect from the modest degree of nerve root compression seen on MRI. Both were later found to have a pelvic tumour irritating the lumbar plexus.

Proven lumbar radiculopathy which does not resolve quickly or which causes neurological deficits is almost always treated by decompressive surgery, using a posterior approach.

Neurogenic bladder dysfunction

Cauda equina compression, e.g. from a central disc prolapse, is a much-feared cause of bladder dysfunction – not least because the diagnosis is often made too late. The nerve roots of the cauda equina are exquisitely sensitive to compression, and if this is allowed to go on for more than 24 hours after sphincter control has been lost then even prompt decompressive surgery is unlikely to restore lost bladder – and bowel and sexual – function.

In the context of known degenerative low back pain the commonest cause of inability to pass urine is an acute exacerbation of the pain. Bladder sensation is preserved, but patients find it difficult to pass urine because straining increases their pain – whether in the low back, referred or radicular. The hallmark of neurogenic bladder dysfunction is painless retention of urine, associated in almost all cases with perineal sensory disturbance (usually bilateral). Low back pain is very common, as are disorders of pelvic musculature in women and prostatic symptoms in men, so the potential for overlap for these potential causes of bladder dysfunction is great.

Much can be learned from the history and physical examination. Does the bladder dysfunction occur in the context of acute and very severe low back pain? Is there radicular lower limb pain (sciatica), or sensory or motor disturbance in the legs or feet? Are there objective neurological signs? Is there perineal sensory loss? If in doubt sagittal MRI of the lumbar spine – an investigation taking perhaps 10 min – will exclude significant cauda equina compression.

Claudication: neurogenic or vascular?

Peripheral vascular disease is very common, and stenosis or occlusion of lower limb arteries at various levels can cause exercise-induced leg pain and/or weakness. By contrast, neurogenic claudication is found only with severe lumbar degenerative disease, especially spinal stenosis (Figure 42.9). Women are more often affected than men. The commonest level involved is L4/5, where the stenosis compresses the L5 nerve root and causes pain which radiates down the lateral aspect of the leg to the dorsum of the foot, sensory disturbance in the dorsum of the foot, and weakness of the dorsiflexors of the foot. Neurogenic claudication usually affects both legs, but if there is lateral nerve root canal stenosis then it may affect one leg only. It has features in common with vascular claudication; it is brought on by exercise, with the exercise limit less in cold weather or when walking uphill or over uneven ground. A period of rest eases the pain and lets the patient walk on for a shorter distance.

The dimensions of the central spinal canal and the lateral nerve root canal are dynamic, that is to say they vary in different positions of the spine. Classically a patient with major spinal stenosis walks or stands with the spine held flexed by 30° – the position which maximizes the space available for the central and lateral nerve roots. This is a good pointer to a spinal cause for claudication. If vascular examination points to a vascular cause and neurological examination to a neurological one, then clinical examination, Doppler studies of the lower limb vessels and MRI of the lumbar spine may all be needed for a diagnosis.

When the patient's lower limb pain is neurogenic, a relatively straightforward posterior decompression usually leads to good results.

Conclusion

It is hoped that reading this module will have brought to your attention (and even to your long-term memory) some neurosurgical conditions that can mimic disorders often seen by a general surgeon. Obviously the general surgical conditions are vastly more common, for example gallstones are a far more common cause of right subcostal pain than a metastatic spinal tumour. However, as ever the key to reaching the right diagnosis is to think about an alternative to the obvious one, perhaps especially where the patient's symptoms are not absolutely typical, where primary investigations (e.g. abdominal ultrasound or endoscopy) have not identified the expected condition, or where the patient has been back to the clinic several times with apparently progressive symptoms but a diagnosis that remains elusive. No surgeon can get it right all the time, but it is hoped that this module will help to trigger your memory when the diagnosis appears to be more difficult then usual.

MODULE 43

Surgery of the face

The face is the most aesthetically sensitive part of the body, being constantly exposed, and the first part of the body normally visualized in any encounter. Even small deformities, scars, etc. attract immediate attention. This can have a profound effect on the individual's perception of themselves, and whereas many aspects of facial anatomy are beyond the control of the surgeon, an appreciation of anatomy and function of the face can significantly influence the aesthetic outcome of surgery, whether this be elective (in the case of congenital anomalies, reconstruction following cancer excision) or as a result of trauma (following injury, burn, etc.). All the structures which go to make up the face have a bearing on the outcome of repair or reconstruction, e.g. skin, facial muscles, facial nerve, facial bones, mucosa of lips, etc. The blood supply to the face is especially good, and healing is usually rapid, with even very narrow pedicled flaps following injury surviving which in other parts of the body would necrose. This is particularly important in managing a patient with facial lacerations in which adequate debridement prior to suturing must not be compromised whilst at the same time preserving as much viable tissue as possible.

Section 43.1 • Pre-operative

Placing of incisions

Incisions should be made in or parallel to natural crease lines (or lines of'relaxed skin tension'). In older patients these are usually easy to identify, in younger patients, especially children, this is much more difficult. Gently pinching the skin in different directions can be helpful to define these lines. Failing this, where a lesion is to be removed from the face, excision should be carried out with a uniform margin all round; the orientation of the resulting defect will be dictated by the lines of tension, which enable the defect to be sutured, the 'dog ears' at either end being excised at the end of the procedure (see Figure 43.1). There are exceptions to this rule, however, particularly for elective excisions below the lower eyelid – unless the lesion to be excised is very small, excision should be carried out in a vertical orientation to avoid scar contracture and resulting ectropian (see Figure 43.2).

Some examples of correct placing of incisions for elective facial surgery are show below.

For more extensive exposure, e.g. craniofacial surgery for the forehead, and orbital region, a bicoronal incision is made. For maxillectomy, the standard approach is through the Weber–Fergusson incision, and for intraoral resections of tumours in posterior floor of mouth, tonsil area or posterior tongue, a lower lip splitting incision extending around the chin is made (this enables division of the mandible which facilitates access to the posterior oral cavity).

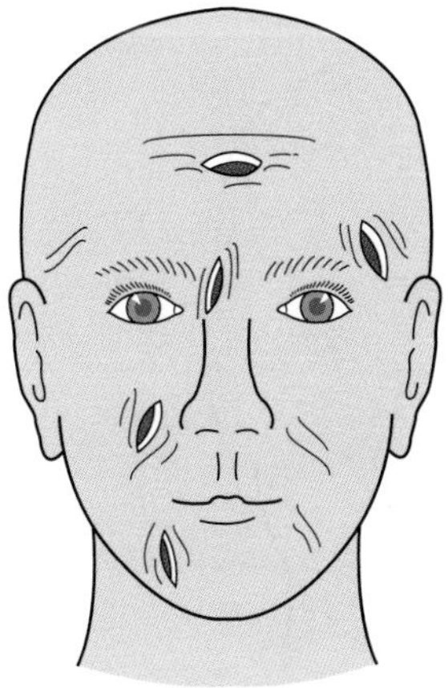

Figures 43.1 The importance of placing incisions in or parallel to natural crease lines.

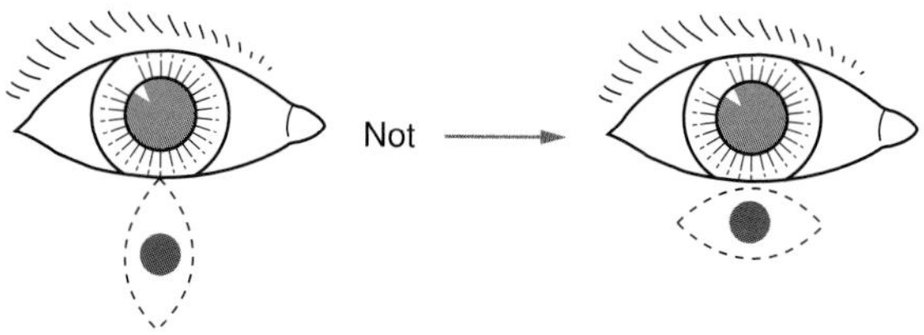

Figure 43.2 The importance of placing incisions in or parallel to natural crease lines.

Mark out incision with pen

This is usually helpful, but particularly important when excising lesions with indistinct margins to help avoid incomplete excision.

Repair 'like-with-like'

This principle of reconstructive surgery is particularly important when repairing defects of the face. Complex microvascular flap reconstructions, interesting and challenging to carry out, may not fulfil the optimum aesthetic outcome. Local tissue is usually best, e.g. a local rotation flap for defects in the cheek, rather than a distant flap from, for example, the chest wall. Use the simplest method which can achieve the optimum functional and aesthetic result. The experience of the surgeon and facilities available must be taken into account when planning reconstruction of the face (see Figure 43.3). Any potential donor site morbidity must be taken into consideration.

Section 43.2 • Operative

Tissue handling

Fine instruments, such as skin hooks and fine toothed forceps, should be used, and tissues handled gently. Incisions should be at right angles to the skin surface. In hair bearing areas such as the scalp, the incision should be bevelled, parallel to the direction of the hair follicles to minimize the area of alopecia in the vicinity of the scar.

Meticulous debridement of wounds with careful haemostasis is important in management of facial lacerations. Debridement should be thorough but not radical, as even small narrow flaps can survive in the face due to the excellent blood supply within the region.

Careful suturing of facial wounds can influence the quality of scar. Of particular importance are the following:

- Suture individual layers separately, e.g. in a full thickness defect of the lip, the mucosa, muscle and skin layers should be sutured individually.
- Deep sutures should take up the tension in the wound. Carefully placed absorbable sutures, e.g. 4/0 or 5/0 Vicryl, should be inserted with the knot buried deeply. When suturing the skin itself a well placed fine absorbable suture placed in the dermis will approximate and help to evert the epidermis. Fine 5/0 or 6/0 Nylon, or Prolene sutures cause less 'reaction' in the skin, than, for example, silk, and result in a better scar, and should be used for the final outer layer.
- Other tension relieving measures are helpful, for example, use of steristrips placed across the wound.

Section 43.3 • Post-operative

Early suture removal

In the face the outer sutures should be removed at 3–5 days. This is only possible, however, where deeper tension relieving sutures are in place, as otherwise the wound is likely to dehisce. After suture removal, steristrips should be placed across the wound for a further 3–5 days.

Regular massaging of the scar with a simple moisturizing cream can help in the ensuing months.

Patients should be advised that scars take up to 18 months to 'mature', i.e. fade and soften. Unless causing tethering to an important structure, e.g. ectropion on the eyelid, any revision of the scar should be left until the period of maturation is complete.

Scar revision can be beneficial, e.g. scars orientated across natural crease lines often stretch and become

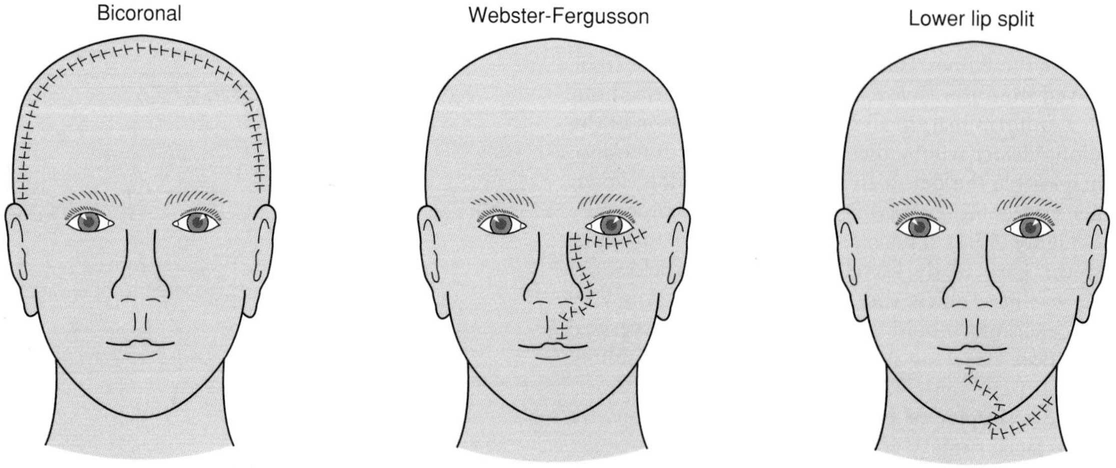

Figure 43.3 Examples of incisions for more extensive exposure for surgery of the face.

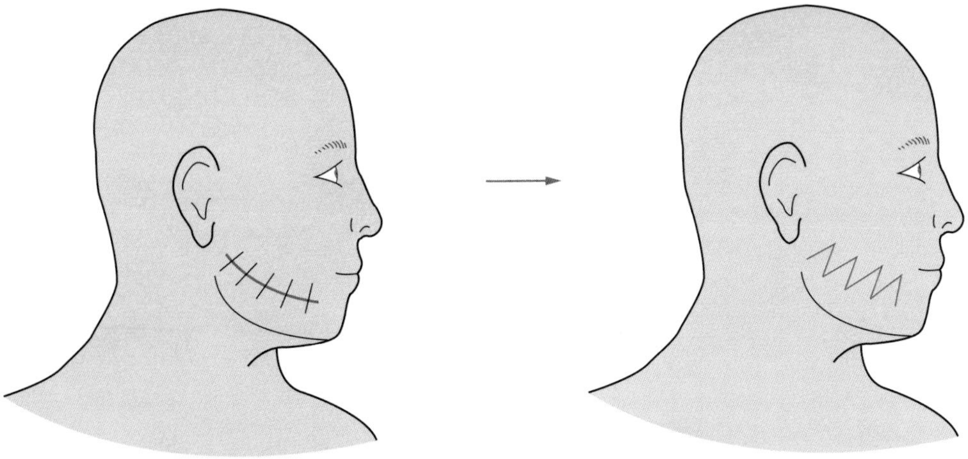

Figure 43.4 Scar revision using Z-plasties.

very noticeable. Realignment using either Z-plasty or W-plasty can result in a significant difference, though the full benefit will not be realized until the scar has once again matured (Figure 43.4).

Scar revision is contraindicated where the disfigurement is due to the colour of the scar. Laser treatment can be very useful in this difficult situation (see also Table 43.1).

Direct suture

Small wounds or defects following elective excision can be sutured. Excellent aesthetic results can be achieved. Attention to detail has already been alluded to.

Skin-graft

Split-skin graft

Split-skin grafts can be useful for extensive areas of skin loss on the face, e.g. following burns, but have significant drawbacks which include contraction, and poor colour and texture, resulting in an inferior aesthetic outcome in the face. Split-skin grafts are also used for secondary defect coverage as for the forehead following forehead flap use for intraoral or facial skin defect coverage. The deformity here can be reduced considerably by harvesting the forehead flap superficial to the frontalis muscle, where the graft adopts the normal pattern of forehead crease lines with time (Figures 43.5–43.9).

Split-skin grafts can be useful for intraoral defects particularly following excision of cheek mucosa, or repair of larger superficial defects on the dorsum of tongue. Small defects in the floor of mouth can also be

Table 43.1 Methods of repair

1. Direct suture
2. Skin graft
   - Split-skin graft
   - Full thickness skin graft
   - Composite graft
3. Skin flap – these can be local or distant, and subdivided as:
   - Random
   - Axial (pedicled or free microvascular)
   - Cutaneous
   - Muscle
   - Bone
   - Compound (e.g. myocutaneous, osteomyocutaneous)
4. Tissue expansion
5. Prosthesis
6. [Tissue culture]

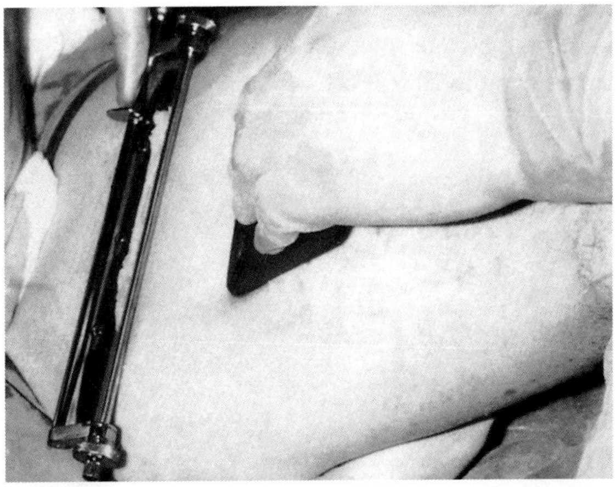

Figure 43.5 Split-skin graft being cut from thigh with hand-held knife.

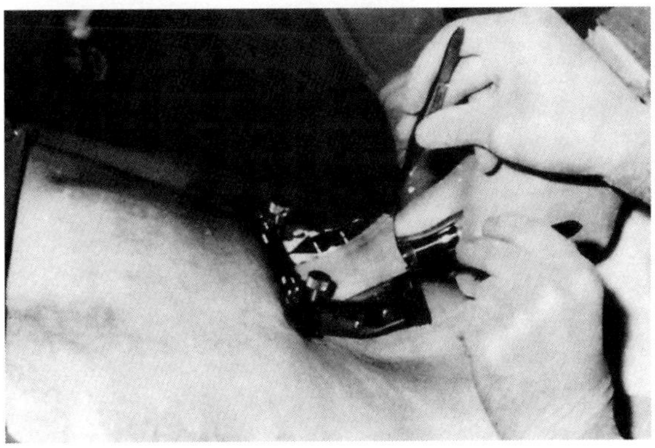

Figure 43.6 Split-skin graft being cut using an electrical dermatome.

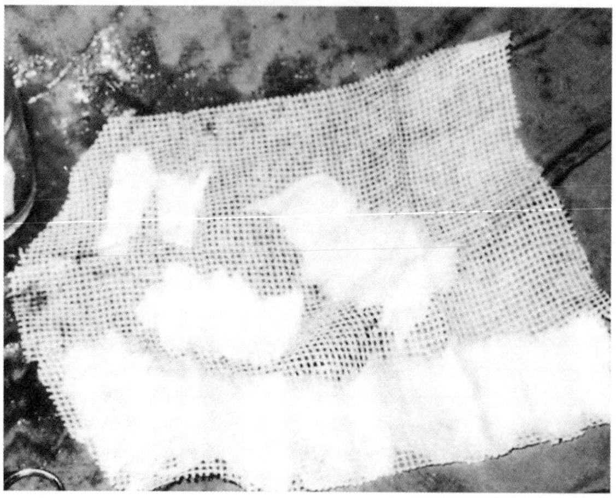

Figure 43.7 Skin graft laid out on tulle. It may be stored in a sterile container at 4°C for 2–3 weeks.

grafted (Figure 43.10), although regeneration of oral mucosa is surprisingly rapid and many defects will close in without any tissue transfer being required. Split-skin grafts should be avoided on the ventral surface of the tongue as contraction and subsequent tethering of the tongue will result.

Full thickness graft

Small full thickness skin grafts (epidermis and dermis) are useful in facial repair. They do not contract and can therefore be used in repair close to the eyelids. Further,

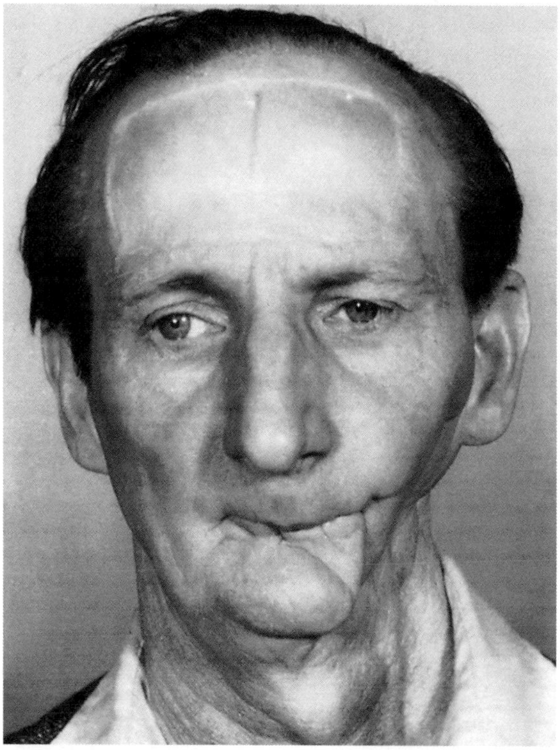

Figure 43.8 Skin-grafted forehead following use of a flap for intraoral reconstruction and partial mandibulectomy.

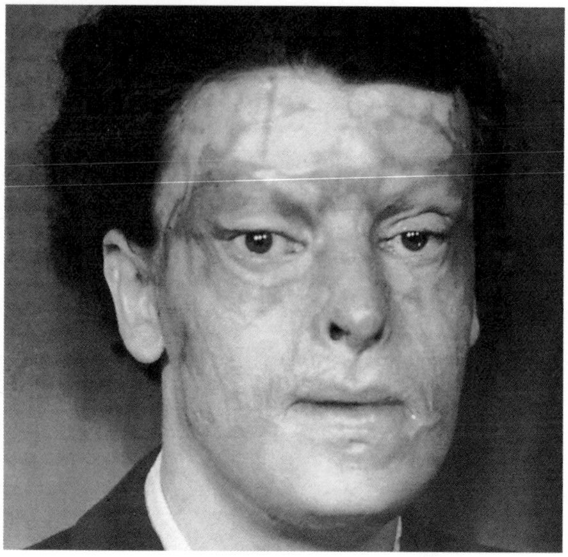

Figure 43.9 A severe burn of the face showing repair by skin grafting.

they result in minimal distortion of surrounding tissues; when harvested from the periauricular area, they provide a good colour and texture match. For small grafts, direct closure of the secondary defect behind or in front of the ear is possible. Careful preparation of the graft and defect bed is important for graft 'take'. Figure 43.11 shows a full thickness graft that has been used to repair a defect on the nose following excision of an enlarging pigmented naevus.

Composite grafts

These are grafts consisting of more than one tissue. Typically in facial reconstruction, grafts of skin and cartilage are used to reconstruct defects of the alar rim of nose, or mucosal cartilage grafts (from the septum of nose) to reconstruct eyelids. The success of these is conditional upon careful preparation of graft and recipient site and the contact area between graft and recipient area should be bevelled to maximize the contact interface between the two. Excellent results can be achieved.

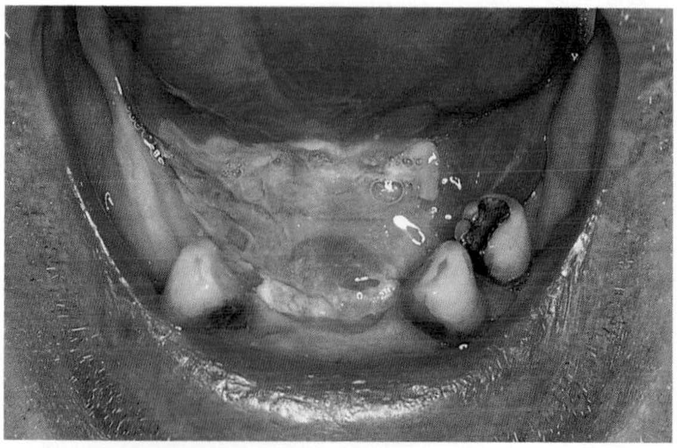

Figure 43.10 Intraoral split skin-graft.

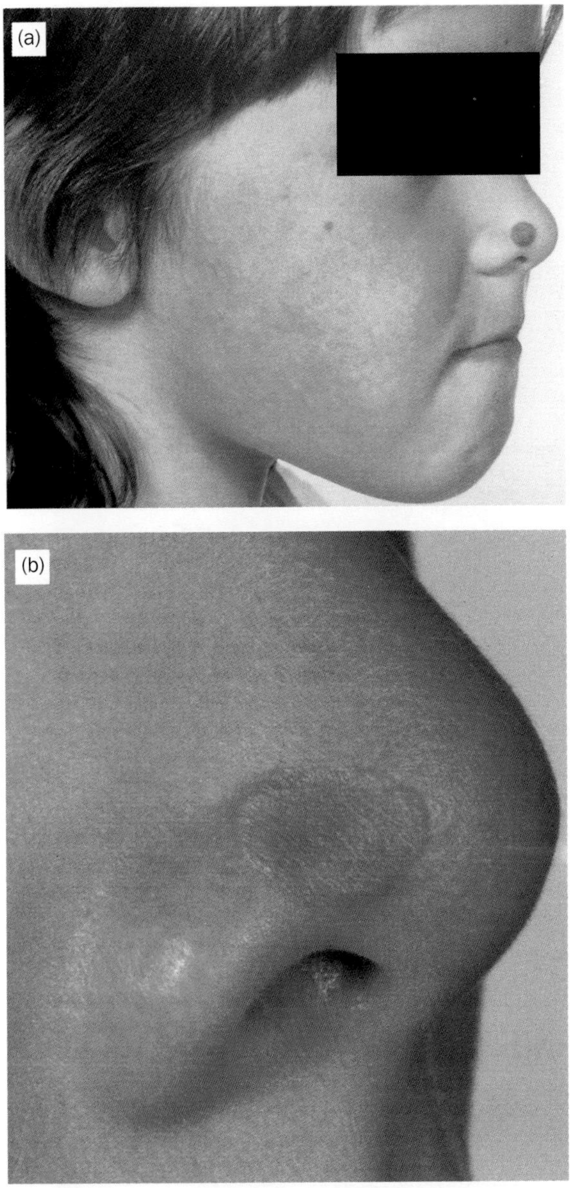

Figure 43.11 Full thickness graft following excision of naevus.

Flaps

The fundamental principle of a flap is that it retains its own blood supply, i.e. unlike a graft, it is not dependent on the bed of the defect for its survival. Local flaps have wide application in the face due to the excellent blood supply. Great versatility can be exercised in the design of these flaps, ensuring placement of resulting scars in natural crease lines, and observing the 'facial aesthetic units' (e.g. nose, cheek, forehead). Where possible, reconstruction using flaps should be confined to an aesthetic unit, as transgressing the boundaries can result in inferior outcome.

Random (i.e. with no named blood supply)

These flaps may be random, as shown in the cheek rotation flap used to reconstruct the defect following excision of a lesion on the cheek (Figure 43.12).

Axial (i.e. based on a particular vessel)

Cutaneous. The nasolabial island flap, based on the facial artery, is a good example of a cutaneous island flap. Figure 43.13 is an example of this used to reconstruct a defect resulting from excision of a basal cell carcinoma.

Another example in Figure 43.14, shows a full thickness defect of the right upper lateral lip following excision of a pleomorphic adenoma. The flap is based on the labial artery of the lower lip. In this reconstruction, it is important to achieve balance in the length of upper and lower lips, and in calculating the dimension of the flap, half the width of the defect is used as the flap width, thus resulting in upper and lower lips of similar width. Further, the natural crease lines are observed as far as possible, as illustrated by the donor scar around the chin.

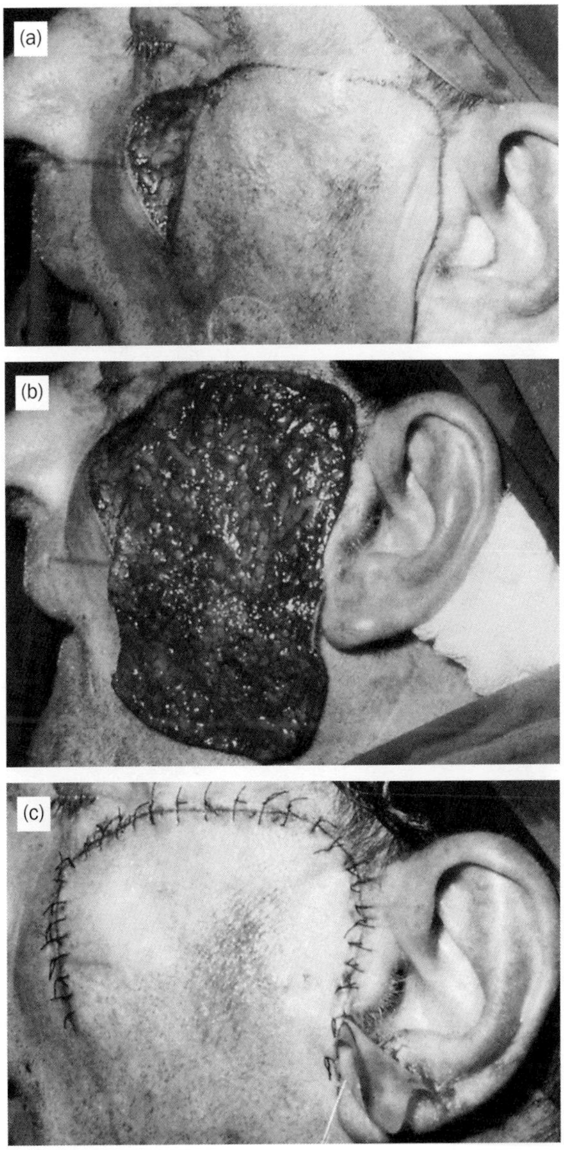

Figure 43.12 Resurface of a defect of the cheek by means of a transposition cheek flap.

Reconstruction may need to be carried out as a staged procedure. Figure 43.15 shows a defect on the nasal tip – following excision of a basal cell carcinoma reconstructed with a glabellar flap, based on the supratrochlear artery. After 3 weeks, the intervening bridge of the flap is divided and inset at which time the distal end of the

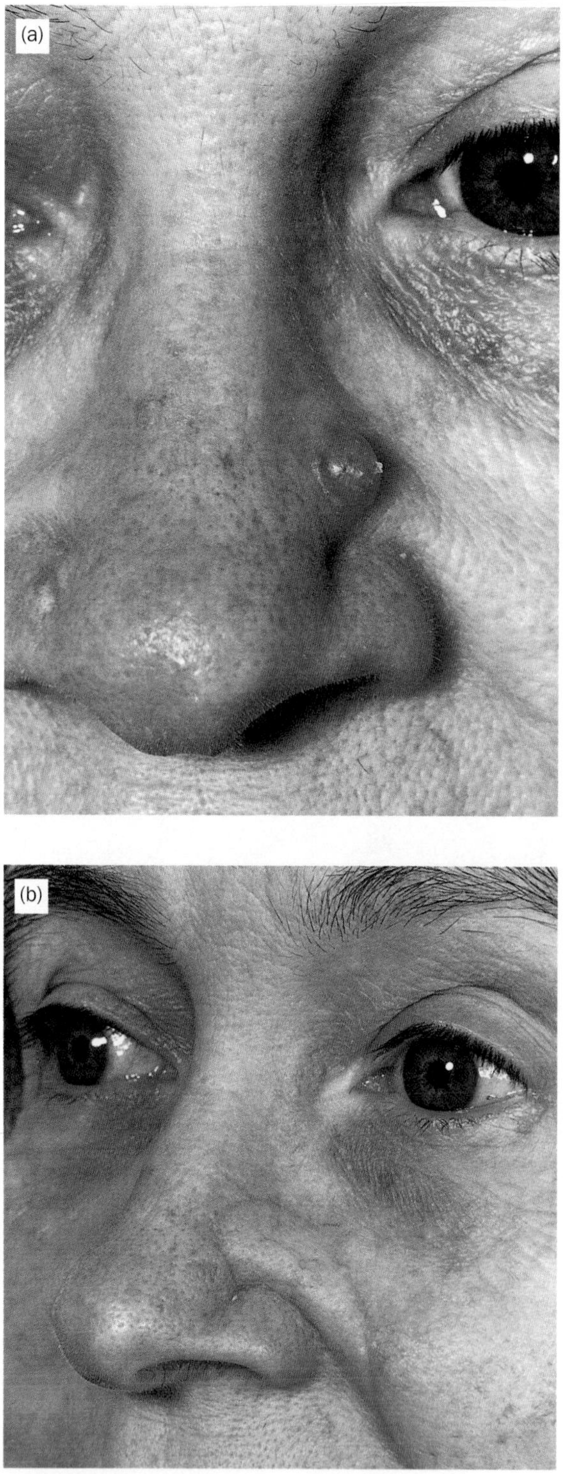

Figure 43.13 Nasolabial island advancement flap used to reconstruct defect following excision of BCC.

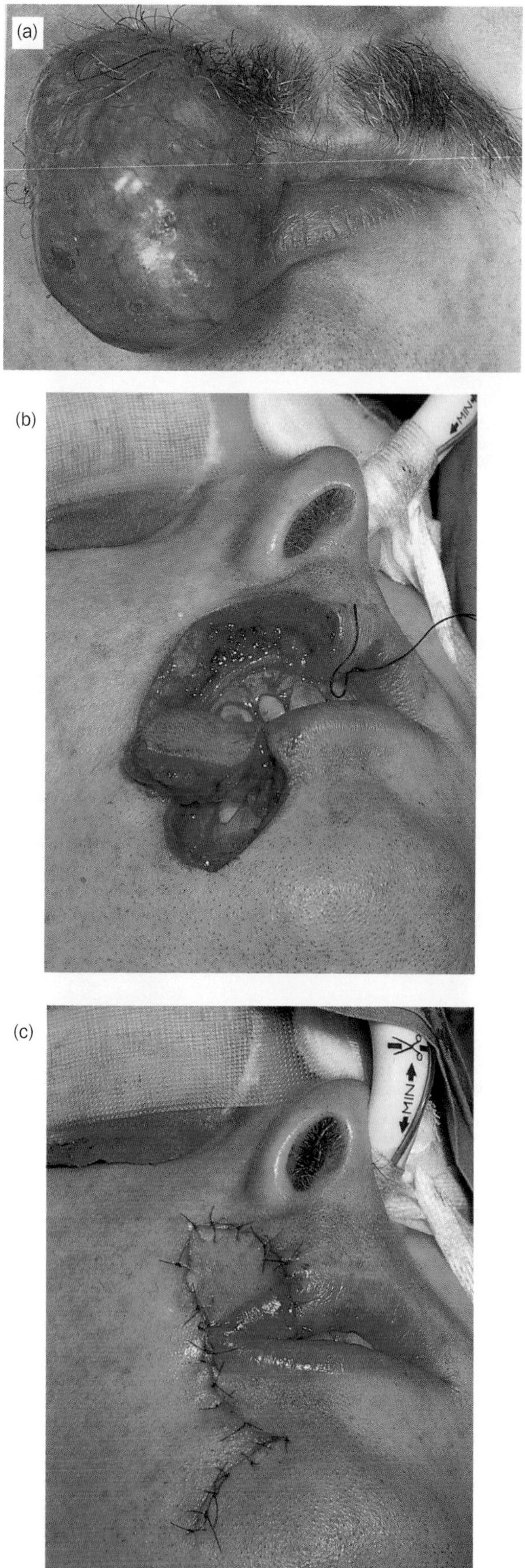

Figure 43.14 Axial flap for reconstruction defect of lip.

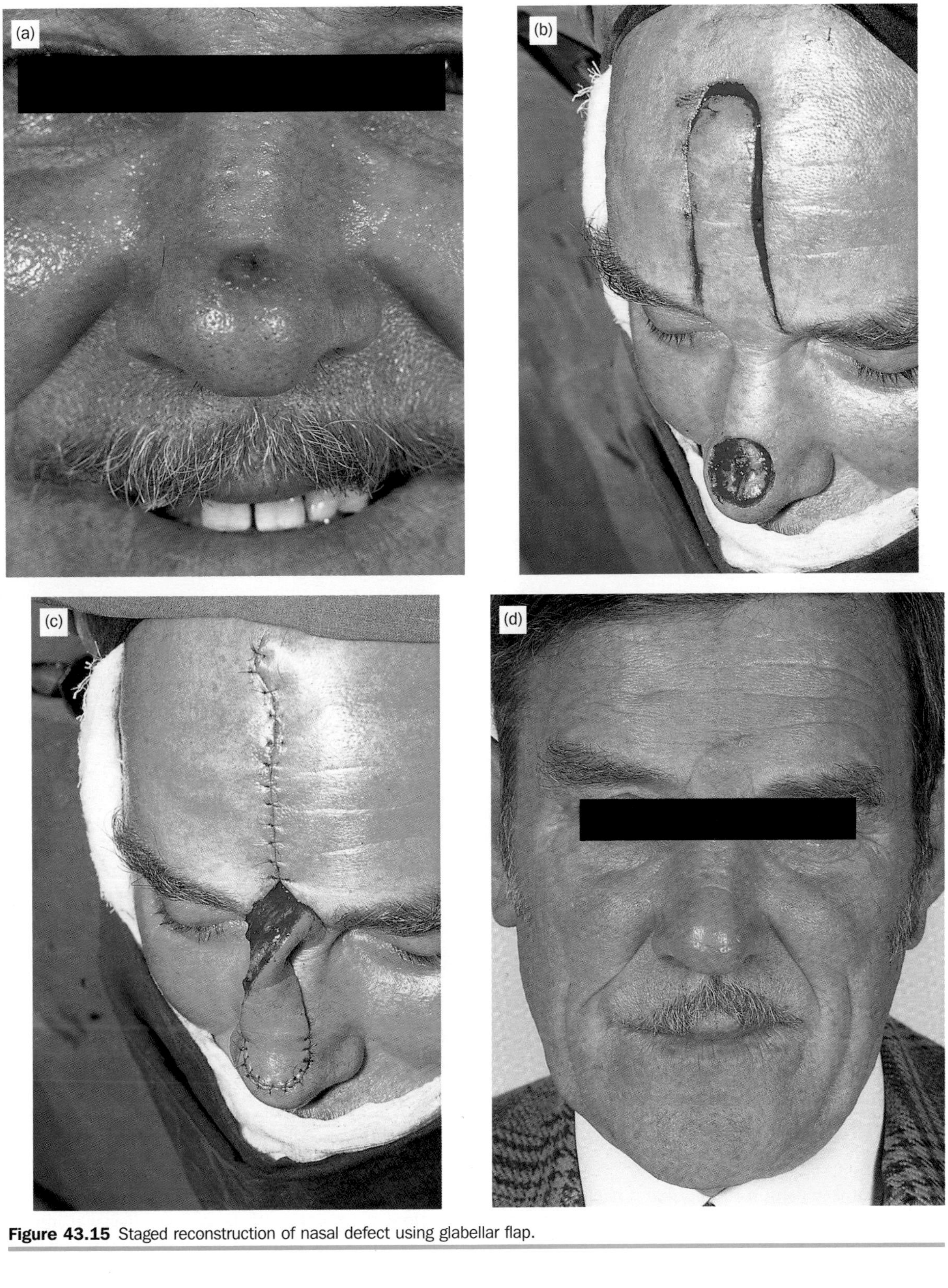

Figure 43.15 Staged reconstruction of nasal defect using glabellar flap.

flap has sufficient vascular input from the surrounding tissue to maintain viability. Larger defects can also be reconstructed on the face using local axial flaps, such as this full thickness defect of the whole lower lip (Figure 43.16) resulting from an aggressive tumour originally arising in the mucosa of the right commissure of the mouth treated with previous surgery and radiotherapy. This large island flap (i.e. no cutaneous bridge) is based on the left facial artery. It contains muscle which is still innervated by the facial nerve and these illustrations show function of the reconstructed lower lip (Figure 43.16).

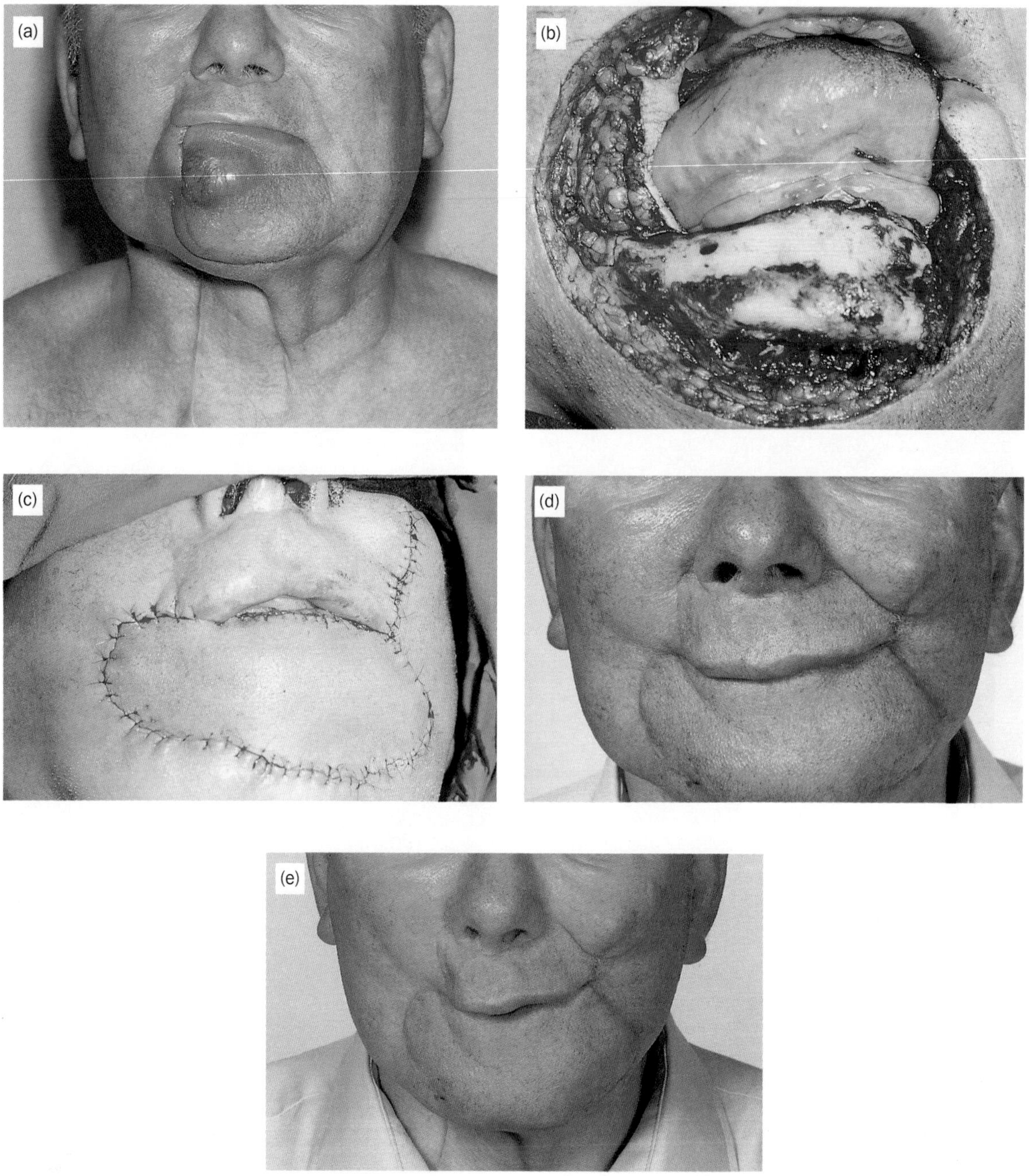

Figure 43.16 Total lower lip reconstruction.

Free flaps

The use of free flaps in the head and neck (including face) greatly increases the range of reconstructive options; a piece of tissue, based on a defined vascular axis, can be detached, transferred, and using microvascular anastomosis be incorporated into a defect. This is well illustrated in Romberg's disease, where several options of 'free flap' are available, e.g. omentum, latissimus dorsi muscle, or, as in the case illustrated, de-epithelialized groin flap (Figure 43.17). Reconstruction in a patient with bilateral disease using free groin flaps is shown in Figure 43.42.

Muscle

Functioning muscle flaps have a unique place in reconstruction of patients with facial palsy (facial reanimation). These can be pedicled (e.g. temporalis transfer) or free (e.g. pectoralis minor or gracilis). For free muscle flaps, an initial operation inserting a cross-facial nerve graft from the normal to the paralysed side is required, and an interval of approximately 6 months left for the nerve to regenerate to the paralysed side. The distal end of the nerve graft is then anastomosed to the muscle branch of the revascularized free muscle graft (Figure 43.18).

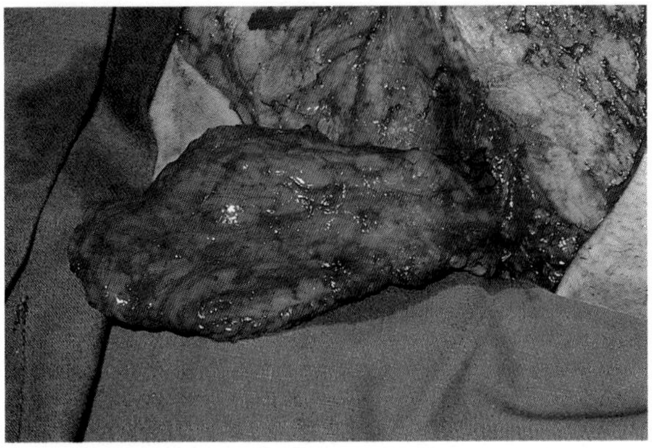

Figure 43.17 De-epithelialized free groin flap (used to augment cheek profile in Romberg's disease).

Early muscle function is usually seen within 6 months of transfer.

Bone
Bone grafts can be non-vascularized or vascularized. Free non-vascularized bone grafts are used in maxillofacial surgery (including alveolar bone grafting in cleft patients) and more extensively in advancement osteomies involving upper and lower jaws and around the orbit. Vascularized bone grafts are particularly useful in reconstruction following tumour ablation, particularly of the mandible. Where the field has been irradiated, non-vascularized bone grafts seldom heal due to the reduced vascularity of the bed consequent upon the radiotherapy. Vascularized bone grafts may be pedicled (as part of a pectoralis major myocutaneous flap) or free (e.g. free fibula, part of radius or iliac crest).

Compound
Any combination of skin, muscle or bone can be incorporated in a flap. With the advent of microsurgery, the ability to match flap tissue to the defect to be reconstructed has been greatly enhanced, e.g. for penetrating tumours of the floor of mouth, requiring resection of mucosa, bone and outer skin, flaps can be raised to reconstruct each of these layers; these can also incorporate cutaneous nerves which can be anastomosed to local nerves to reinnervate the flap (examples of these are shown below).

Tissue expansion
First introduced as a tool in reconstructive surgery in the 1970s, the main application of this technique is in delayed rather than immediate reconstruction. A deflated silicone balloon is inserted subcutaneously adjacent to the area to be reconstructed (previously grafted area, scar, etc.). Over a period of weeks, inflation of the expander with saline though a separate or integral injection port is carried out. The 'surplus' skin produced, following removal of the balloon, is then advanced to cover the defect. In the head and neck, resurfacing areas of alopecia on the scalp with normal hair bearing scalp tissue is currently the only way of restoring hair in significant defects and is particularly applicable in post-burn reconstruction.

Prosthesis
Replacement of facial bone structure with acrylic prostheses has a long tradition. The most common application is following maxillectomy, where the obturator, after impressions of the defect have been taken, can be incorporated into an upper denture, which lies in apposition to the grafted cheek flap restoring profile to the mid face region. (Figure 43.19a, b). More recently, osseointegrated prostheses (e.g. Bränemark), attached to the bony skeleton using titanium studs, have further increased the scope of this method of reconstruction. They are particularly applicable for patients with congenital auricular deformities and following total or subtotal removal of the nose for cancer where autogenous reconstruction is contraindicated (Figure 43.19c, d).

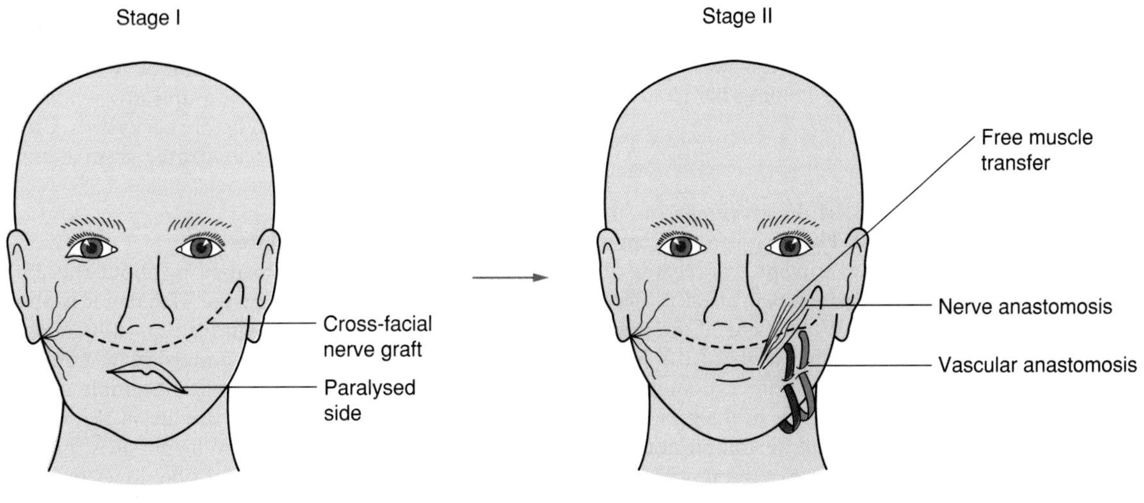

Figure 43.18 Facial reanimation using cross-facial nerve graft and free muscle transfer.

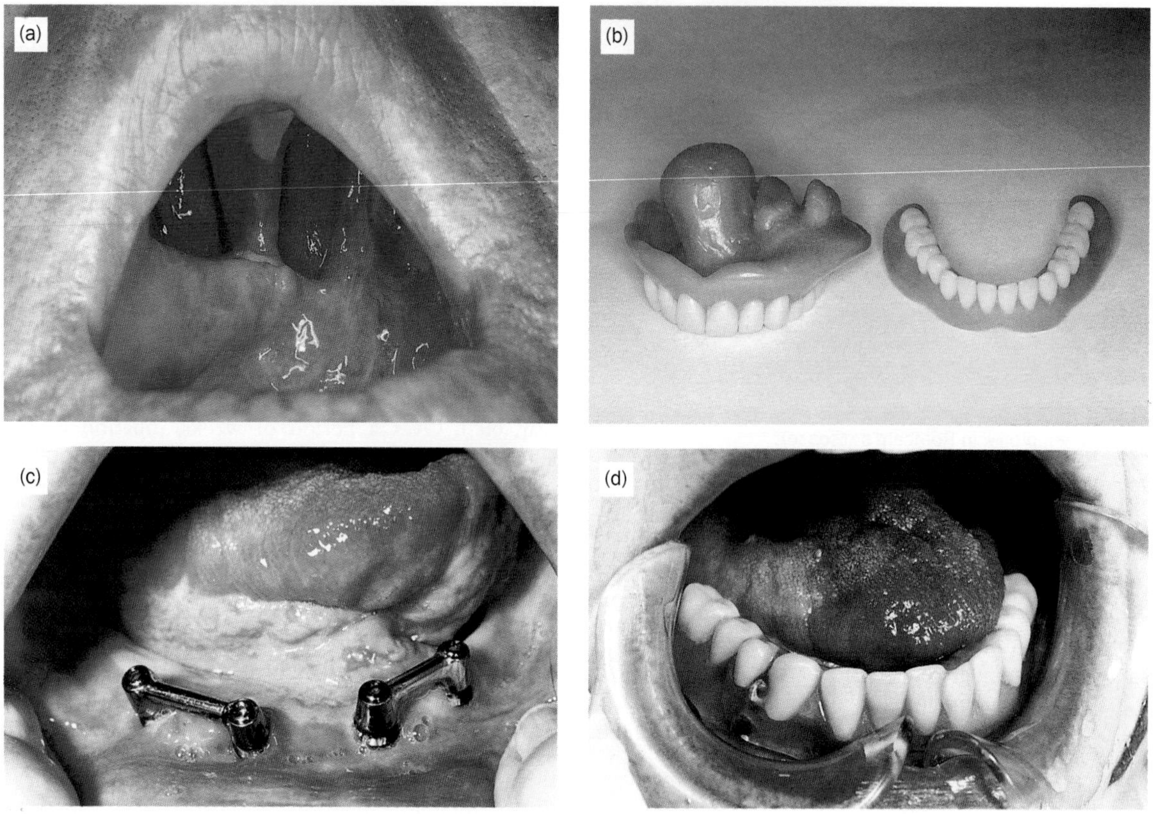

Figure 43.19 Prosthesis following maxillectomy.

Section 43.4 • Clinical applications

Congenital

Cleft lip and palate

Bearing in mind the complex functions which are concentrated in the face it is hardly surprising that the development of this region is subject to a bewildering assortment of anomalies. It is beyond the scope of this section to describe the detailed development of the face and related structures, though a few general points should serve as a basis for understanding the treatment of some of the major deformities.

Pathology

While there is a good deal of disagreement on the detailed formation of the face, His's original concept of the fusion of several processes is helpful as regards the position of the various clefts which may affect it. These are indicated in Figure 43.20. While clefts of the upper lip are relatively common, midline clefts of the lower lip and jaw and oblique facial clefts are extremely rare and are not considered further. Clefts of the lip may be uni- or bilateral and from a simple vermilion notch to a complete cleft involving the floor of the nostril. They also vary in the extent to which they involve the underlying hard tissues.

The palate may be divided into primary and secondary palates on embryological grounds. The primary palate consists of two parts: (a) the central lip; and (b) the premaxillae as far as the incisive foramen, so that a complete cleft of the primary palate involves the soft tissues of the lip and nostril floor as well as the alveolus and anterior portion of the hard palate, i.e. the structures formed from fusion of the medial and lateral nasal processes and the maxillary processes. The secondary palate is the rest of the hard palate and all of the soft palate and develops quite differently, 10–12 days later, by the fusion of two processes from the maxillae which swing upwards when the tongue descends and fuse from before backwards. Clefts of the secondary palate vary in degree from behind forwards.

Clefts of the primary palate

Since the primary palate is formed by about the 35th day and the secondary palate by the 47th day, it is obvious that clefts in this region will have an influence on subsequent development. This results in a complex deformity which comprises more than a simple cleft in the surrounding structures. Thus the lip on the medial side of the cleft is short in vertical height as is the columella. The alveolus on the medial side slopes upwards and tends to be rotated anteriorly and towards the normal side, while the alveolus on the lateral side is short

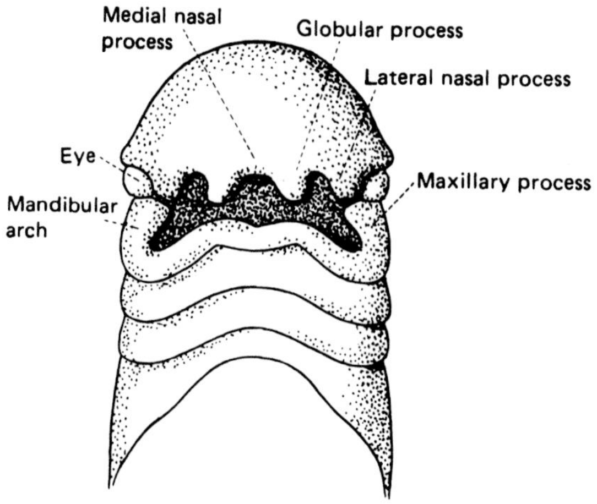

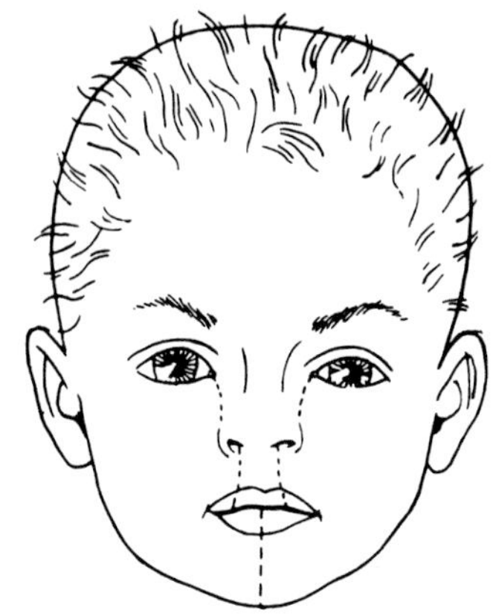

Figure 43.20 (a) His's concept of facial development. (b) Lines of cleft formation resulting from faulty fusion.

and retroposed. This causes a flaring or lateral displacement of the alar base while the nasal tip and septum are displaced towards the normal side (Figure 43.21). In bilateral clefts the philtrum or central lip is short in vertical height, as is the whole columella which pulls down the tip of the nose. Unrestrained growth of the central stem leads to the protrusion of the whole premaxillary complex (Figure 43.22). A further complicating factor in the treatment is the fact that these are not simple clefts in otherwise normal tissues. There is also a tissue deficiency, and a lack of growth potential persists throughout the growth period causing further deformity, such as maxillary retrognathism. In recent years attention has been focused on the absence of muscle in the central lip in complete bilateral clefts, and abnormal disposition and attachment of the fibres of the orbicularis oris in both unilateral and bilateral clefts (Figure 43.23).

Orthodontic treatment

The value of presurgical orthodontic treatment to reduce the size of the alveolar deformity has recently been questioned, and studies now suggest that this treatment may be less beneficial than previously thought. However, in bilateral cleft lip with a prominent central premaxilla segment orthodontic treatment prior to surgery is almost always worthwhile.

Cleft lip repair is usually carried out at 3 months and operation is usually combined with repair of the anterior palate, i.e. as much of the hard palate as is reasonably possible. Neonatal lip repair has been advocated by some, but long-term results have failed to show any benefits, and the anaesthetic risks at this age are significantly greater. Clefts of the secondary palate should be repaired at 6 months. This provides the child with an intact mechanism by the time he or she starts to speak and produces better speech.

Repair of cleft lip

There are many surgical techniques for cleft lip repair. For the unilateral cleft Millard's rotation/advancement operation is widely used and gives excellent results (Figure 43.24). This technique preserves the natural landmarks which are always present and places them in their normal position. It lengthens the medial side of the cleft as well as the columella on the cleft side, corrects the alar flare and provides a balanced lip and a greatly improved nose. The bilateral cleft is a different problem: attempts to increase the vertical height of the central lip cause horizontal tightness, for, while there is sufficient tissue available for this type of rearrangement

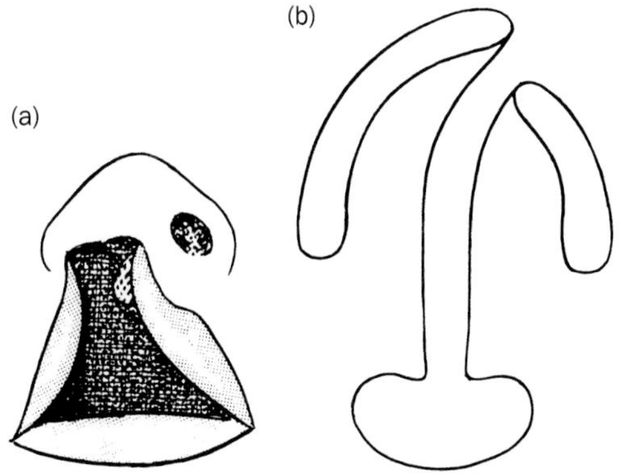

Figure 43.21 (a) External deformity in unilateral cleft. (b) Distortion of alveolar arches.

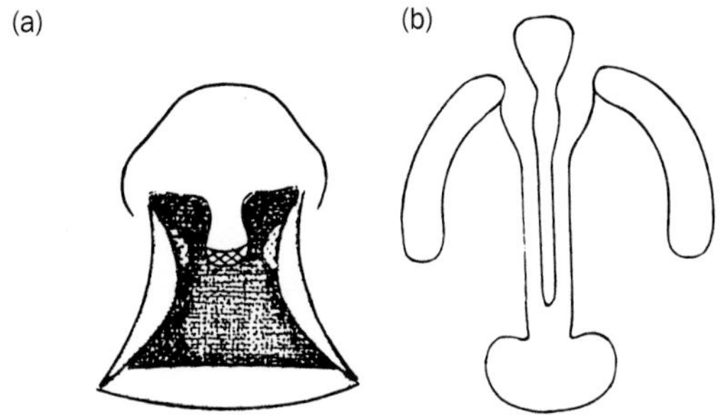

Figure 43.22 (a) External deformity in unilateral cleft. (b) Distortion of alveolar processes and protruding premaxilla.

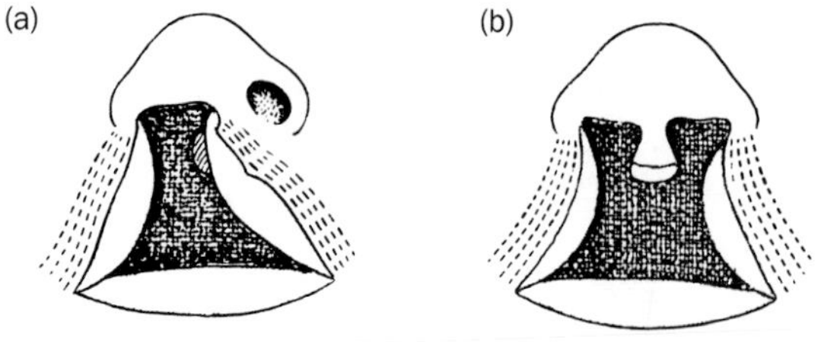

Figure 43.23 Disposition of fibres of orbicularis in (a) unilateral and (b) bilateral cleft lips.

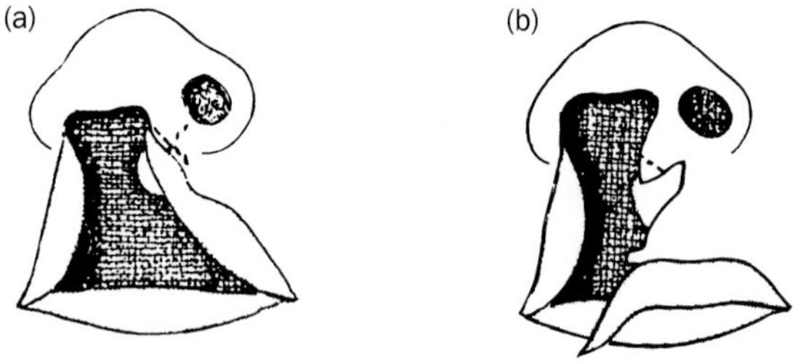

Figure 43.24 Millard's rotation/advancement repair.

in a unilateral cleft, there is not enough to do it on both sides. A lip which is symmetrical if slightly short, but slack enough horizontally must be accepted. Figure 43.25 indicates how this can be achieved while not discarding any tissue at all. This procedure does not lengthen the columella, and leaves an unnaturally square and wide philtrum with flaring alar bases. All of this is corrected at a second operation when the orbicularis muscle fibres can also be freed from the alar bases and sutured together to reconstruct the oral sphincter (Figure 43.26).

Repair of the secondary palate

Clefts of the secondary palate are repaired in two layers. The nasal layer consists of mucuous membrane which is mobilized from the upper surface of the hard palate by special dissectors and posteriorly from the soft palate. Additional mucosa, when required, is available on the vomer. The oral layer consists of mucoperiosteum anteriorly and of palatal mucosa on the soft palate. By raising flaps, as indicated in Figure 43.27, it is possible to achieve a V to Y lengthening of the palate to facilitate velopharyngeal closure which is vital if the typical speech deformity characterized by nasal escape is to be avoided. It is also vital to release the levators palati from their abnormal attachments to the posterior nasal spines and to unite them to each other, thereby reconstructing the normal levator sling mechanism.

The exposed bone on the hard palate lateral to the flaps granulates and epithelizes very rapidly. The area which presents most difficulty in closure is usually the junction between the hard and soft palates, and there are a number of more or less complicated flaps described to deal with this problem. Considerable controversy exists as to how much stripping mucosal flaps off the underlying bone interferes with bony (and therefore facial) growth. Minimal dissection is now performed by an increasing number of surgeons in this field.

Secondary corrective surgery

While it is usually possible to obtain an acceptable result on the lip at the primary operation for unilateral clefts, a secondary procedure is almost routine for bilateral clefts. Many minor 'trims' can be required for the perfect result, including correction of excess vermilion, marginal notches and irregularities of the mucocutaneous junction. Secondary procedures of the nose are also often required, including adjustment of the alar base, correction of tip asymmetry and straightening of the nasal septum and bony framework. To an increasing degree, secondary work is also being advocated for correction of the underlying maxillary deformities.

In some cases of cleft palate there are residual speech defects following the primary repair. The most usual and typical stigma is nasal escape due to inadequate closure of the velopharyngeal opening. This can be shown in some cases by lateral radiographs which show

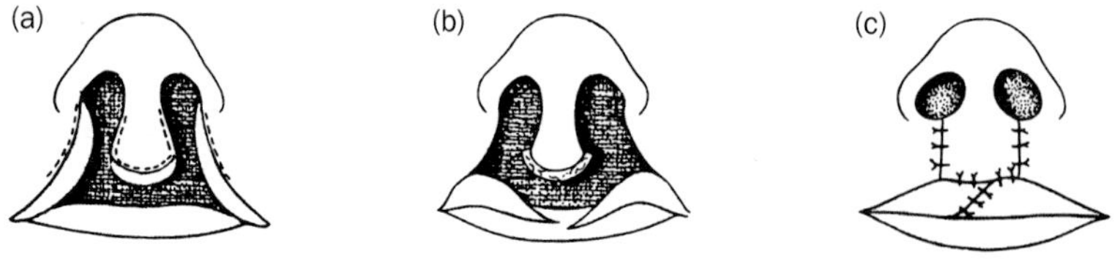

Figure 43.25 Simultaneous bilateral cleft lip repair.

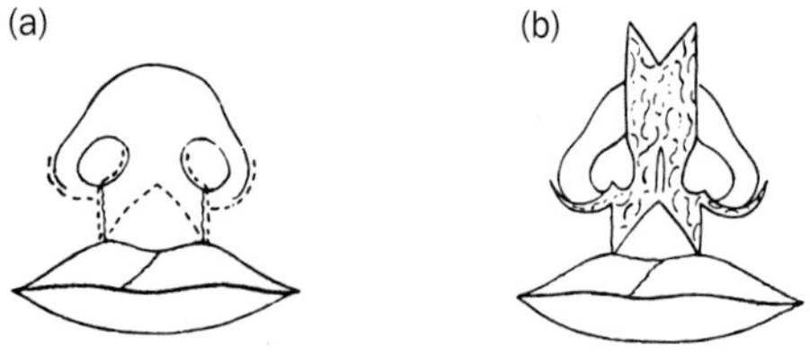

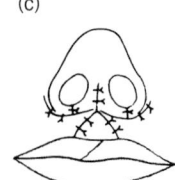

Figure 43.26 The fork flap procedure to lengthen the columella, correct the alar flare, reconstruct the muscle sphincter and improve the shape of the philtrum.

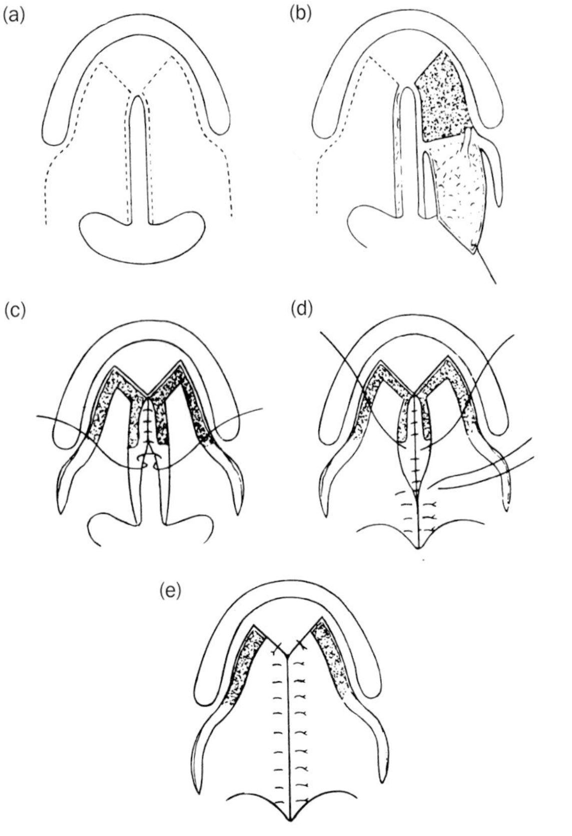

Figure 43.27 V to Y repair of cleft palate.

a failure of contact between the soft palate and the posterior pharyngeal wall, but obviously this will not be demonstrated where the gap is to each side of the midline. Direct observation and assessment of the function of this region is readily made during speech using nasendoscopy. Where there is nasal escape several operations are available for lengthening the soft palate and for building the posterior pharyngeal wall forward by implants or flaps. Other varieties of pharyngoplasties using flaps seek to narrow the gap or to improve the function in this area. Assessment of the merits of different operations is not easy.

Congenital deformity of the ears

Preauricular sinuses and accessory auricles

As a result of the complex development of the auricle from the first and second branchial arches, maldevelopment may give rise to sinuses and accessory parts of the cartilage. The latter are usually excised early (unless they are required to reconstruct a malformed ear). Recurrent abscesses may point to the presence of sinuses. Careful surgical excision is usually effective.

Prominent or bat ear

This is the commonest congenital anomaly and one which can cause considerable distress. The deformity occurs in varying degrees and may be associated with a failure of cartilage folding to create an antihelical fold or due to a relative excess of conchal cartilage. The former abnormality is treated readily by a variety of operations designed to create a new fold. The surgical approach is usually through the posterior skin. Folding the cartilage can be achieved by insertion of nonabsorbable horizontal mattress sutures and/or by scoring the anterior surface of the cartilage. This releases tension and enables the cartilage to bend in the opposite direction. Where the deformity is due to conchal excess, excision of an appropriate amount of conchal cartilage can give satisfactory correction (Figure 43.28).

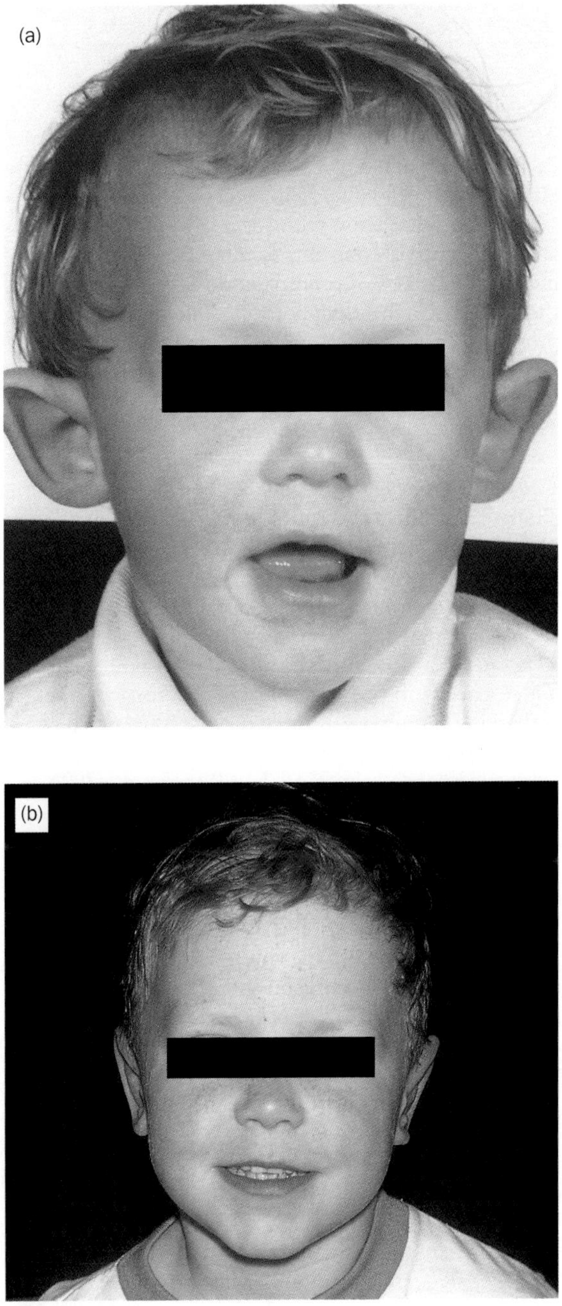

Figure 43.28 (a) Prominent (bat) ears. (b) Correction.

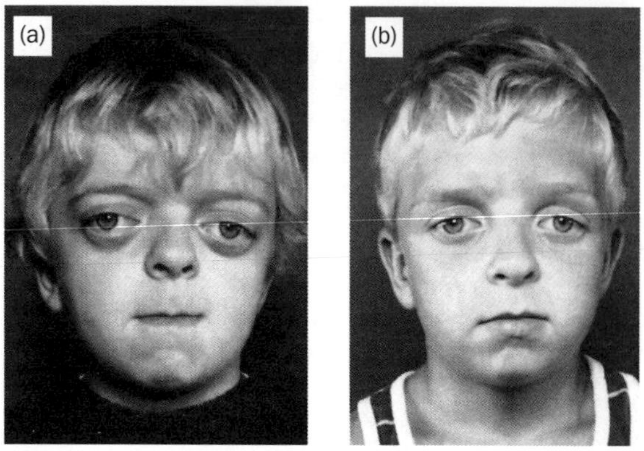

Figure 43.29 (a) Crouzon's pre-operative. (b) Crouzon's after Le Fort III advancement. (Courtesy of Dr I.T. Jackson.)

Cryptotia and microtia

These deformities occur less commonly. In the former the cartilage framework, though present, is partly buried under the scalp skin. Reconstruction involves release and resurfacing with local skin flaps. Microtia is where the ear is congenitally absent apart from rudimentary soft tissue. Reconstruction is very difficult and the results can be disappointing. The provision of a prosthetic ear may be a better solution, using the Bränemark technique. This may be performed in conjunction with a bone anchored hearing aid as appropriate.

Congenital anomalies of the nose

These defects may constitute part of a complex of congenital abnormalities of the adjacent face, as in cleft lip, or a more extensive craniofacial syndrome (e.g. Crouzon syndrome, where the bridge of the nose is recessed) (Figure 43.29).

Isolated nasal deformities include midline swellings. These need to be investigated thoroughly before embarking on surgery, as there may be intracranial communication, e.g. midline dermoid, encephalocele. A magnetic resonance imaging (MRI) scan is the definitive investigation. A small dermoid with no intracranial extension can be excised through an incision carefully placed on the nose; dissection needs to be meticulous in the event that a very small fistulous tract is encountered. For larger lesions, and all encephaloceles a bicoronal incision giving access to the anterior cranial fossa in conjunction with a neurosurgeon should be performed, e.g. Figure 43.30. In this example, the surgery was carried out at 2 weeks through a bicoronal approach. The medial orbital walls were cut and moved medially. A craniectomy bone graft was placed over the frontal bone defect.

Pigmented vascular naevi

Three types commonly occur.

Port wine stain

This well-recognized lesion is a capillary haemangioma lying in or just beneath the dermis (Figure 43.31). It is usually flat and skin texture is normal, but irregularities

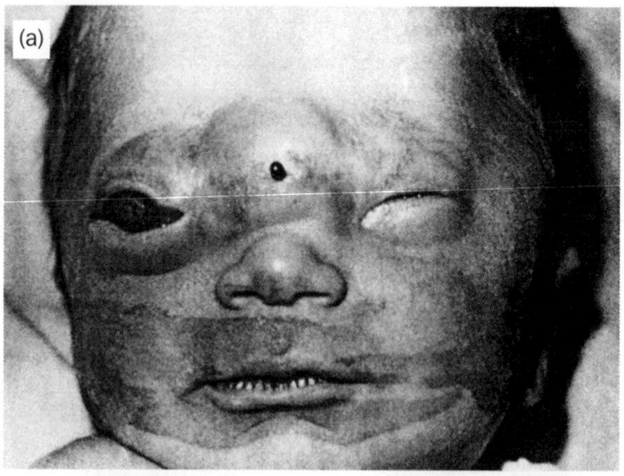

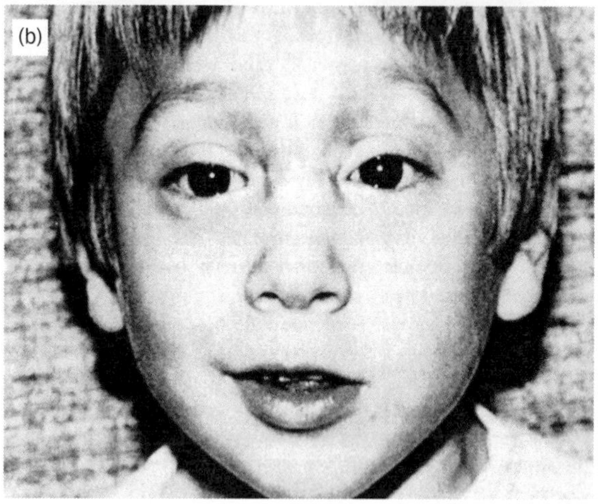

Figure 43.30 (a) This patient has a moderately severe nasofrontal encephalocele, protrusion of the conjunctiva of the right eye, and moderate orbital hypertelorism. (b) The same patient is shown 4 years following reconstruction and recent nasal scar revision. The reconstruction was done at age 2 weeks when the encephalocele was operated on. An intracranial approach using a binfrontal craniotomy provided exposure of the anterior cranial base. The medial canthal ligament on the right side could not be identified. Fibrous tissue on the right side was wired across the midline to the canthal ligament of the opposite side. The medial orbital walls were cut and moved medially. Craniectomy bone was placed inside the orbit laterally to help shift the eyes medially. A craniectomy bone graft was placed over the frontal bone defect.

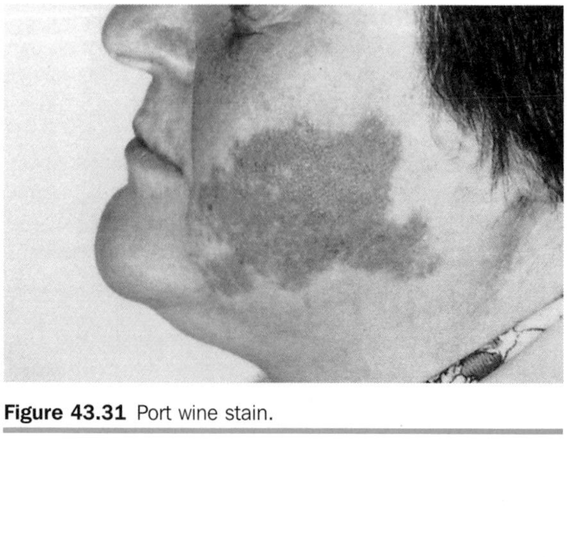

Figure 43.31 Port wine stain.

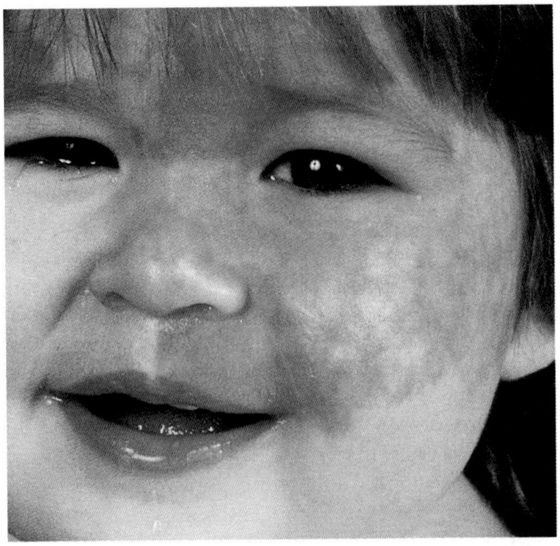

Figure 43.32 Port wine haemangioma of the face.

can occur, particularly later in life when the colour often darkens, taking on a purplish hue. Treatment with a tunable dye laser is now the preferred management with often excellent results. Figure 43.32 shows an early response to laser treatment.

Strawberry naevus

This usually appears shortly after birth and can enlarge at an alarming rate over a period of weeks. Histologically it presents a varied picture of large vascular spaces deep into the dermis with capillary elements. Spontaneous resolution normally occurs, generally over a period of years. Figure 43.33 shows an example of an extensive lesion which regressed over a period of 10 years, with some minor trimming of excess skin only being required at the end of this period of time. Reassurance rather than early surgery is advised unless the lesion is in the eyelids and threatens to occlude the vision. (Some reduction in size can occasionally be achieved with steroid use, either systemically or intra-

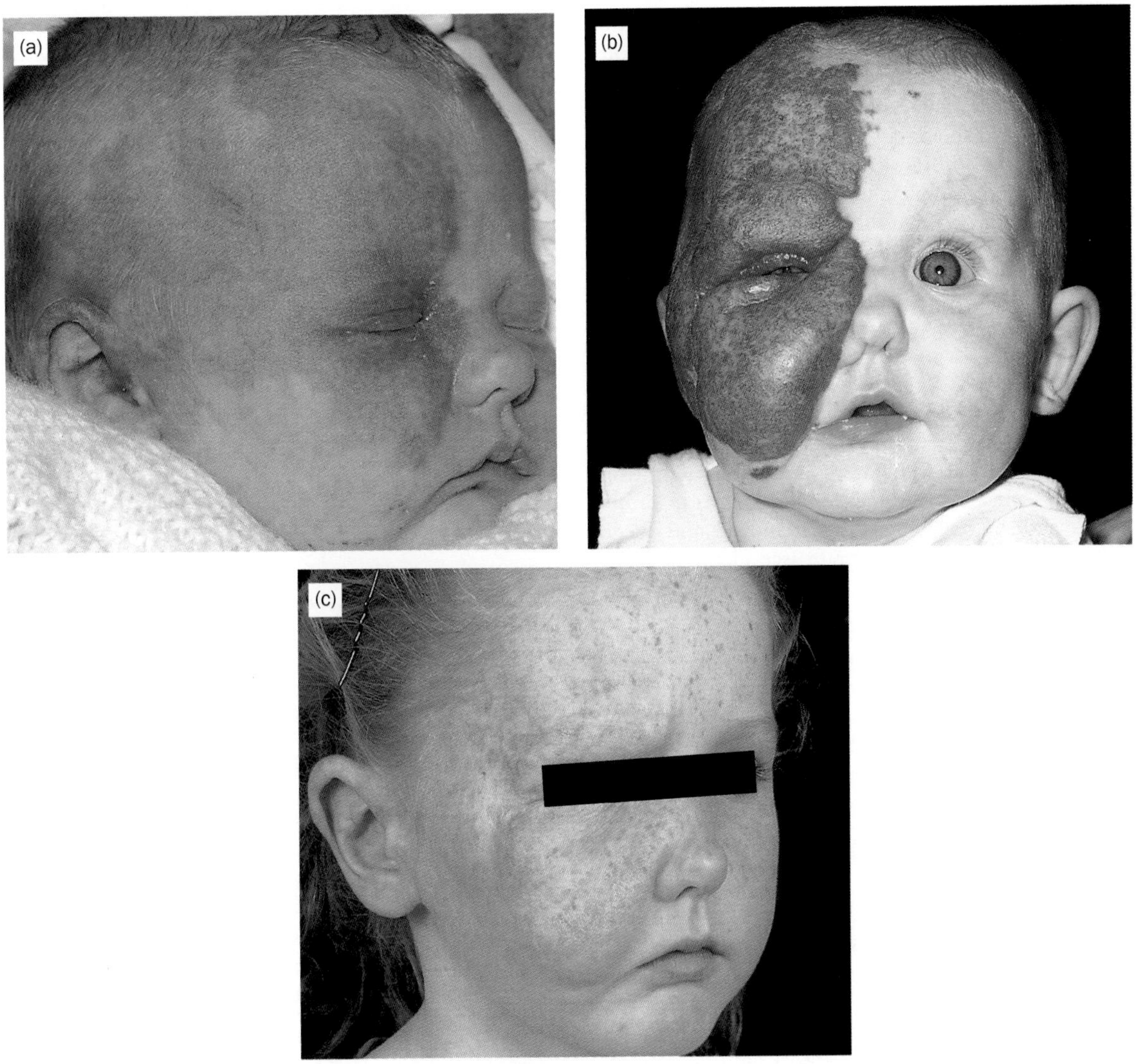

Figure 43.33 Strawberry haemangioma.

lesionally, but this should only be attempted in conjunction with an ophthalmologist and paediatrician.) Laser treatment can occasionally be helpful in reducing the size of these haemangiomas.

Cavernous haemangioma and arteriovenous malformation
These consist of large vascular spaces at the subdermis level usually of a venous nature. Sometimes there is an element of lymphangioma and overlying strawberry components and it is worthwhile allowing time for any spontaneous resolution. When the lesions persist there is a limited place for cryosurgery but the results can be disappointing. Surgery can be difficult and it is advisable to consider carefully the risks as opposed to the cosmetic deficit which may ensue. Angiography is itself not without risk but may be necessary to delineate the vascular channels and components, be they arterial or venous.

An arteriovenous malformation is a potentially dangerous lesion characterized by progressive enlargement which becomes pulsatile, usually with a bruit heard on auscultation and increased temperature on palpation. It may arise *de novo*, or from a pre-existing cavernous haemangioma. Arteriography and selective embolization (which often needs to be repeated on several occasions) is the initial treatment of choice. This needs to be done by a specialist radiologist, and in the head and neck region, can be associated with significant morbidity and even mortality (if intracranial vessels are involved). Proximal ligation of main arteries may be dangerous as well as inadequate since the result may be an opening up of alternative anastomotic pathways. Bone changes may occur in association with haemangiomas either through direct involvement or as a result of increased local vascularity.

Pigmented non-vascular naevi
Large congenital naevi result in significant cosmetic blemishes. Excision and repair by direct closure, grafts or flaps (which may be in conjunction with tissue expansion) may be required. Similar lesions in prominent places in children can be removed and reconstructed with full thickness grafts (see Figure 43.11).

Trauma

The compulsory wearing of seat belts for front-seat passengers in the UK and many other countries has reduced the incidence of facial injuries resulting from road traffic accidents. A careful, even if brief, history is essential to the correct assessment and management of face, head and neck trauma. Soft tissue injuries of the face can be classified as follows.

Laceration
Caused by a sharp object such as glass or a knife, these types of injuries tend to cause division of all soft tissue structures until bone is reached. A glass injury to the cheek, therefore, must be assumed to have divided skin, muscle, facial nerve, parotid gland or duct (depending on the site) until proved otherwise. Careful pre-operative assessment is mandatory. Repair of nerves and ducts should be carried out under magnification. As a general rule, for facial nerve injuries medial to an imaginary vertical line down from the outer canthus of the eye spontaneous recovery of function usually occurs. Lateral to this line, the nerve should be explored and repaired. A divided parotid duct should be repaired; if ignored, stenosis may occur which will result in recurrent parotititis. Lacerations of the neck (e.g. stab wounds) are particularly dangerous due to the important anatomical structures present. Particular attention must be directed to possible injuries of the airway and great vessels.

Crush
Caused by a blunt force; where severe, crush may be associated with soft tissue devitalization and necrosis and fractures of the underlying bony skeleton. Assessment of skin viability, X-rays and computed tomography (CT) scans are indicated in these injuries.

Degloving
This is caused by a shearing force. In the head and neck, this is most commonly seen in the scalp (e.g. hair caught in machinery). Careful assessment in conjunction with a good history is essential. Clinical examination may show a laceration, but closer inspection usually reveals extensive bruising in the surrounding area, and under anaesthetic, the tissues are found to have been undermined for often considerable distances. All devitalized tissue must be debrided, the wound irrigated and repair with grafts/flaps carried out.

Avulsion
This occurs where a piece of tissue has been forcibly removed. Most commonly seen resulting from a human or animal bite, and commonly occurs to prominent anatomical structures such as the nose or ear. Bite wounds are contaminated and thorough cleansing must be carried out before reconstruction, which may involve replacement of the avulsed segment as a free composite graft or use of a local flap. In favourable situations, these grafts can 'take' well. Antibiotic cover is advised which should cover the Gram-negative organisms commonly found in the mouth.

Burns
Deep burns to the face are fortunately rare in developed countries, but can result in considerable disfigurement. At presentation, it is very important to establish whether or not there is an associated inhalation injury (i.e. injury to the upper and/or lower respiratory tract caused by inhaled hot gases). This is a potentially life threatening condition and must be recognized early. Clinical findings which are suggestive of inhalation injury may include the following:

- burns to mouth, nose and pharynx
- sputum containing soot
- changes of voice, hoarseness
- stridor
- singed nasal hairs.

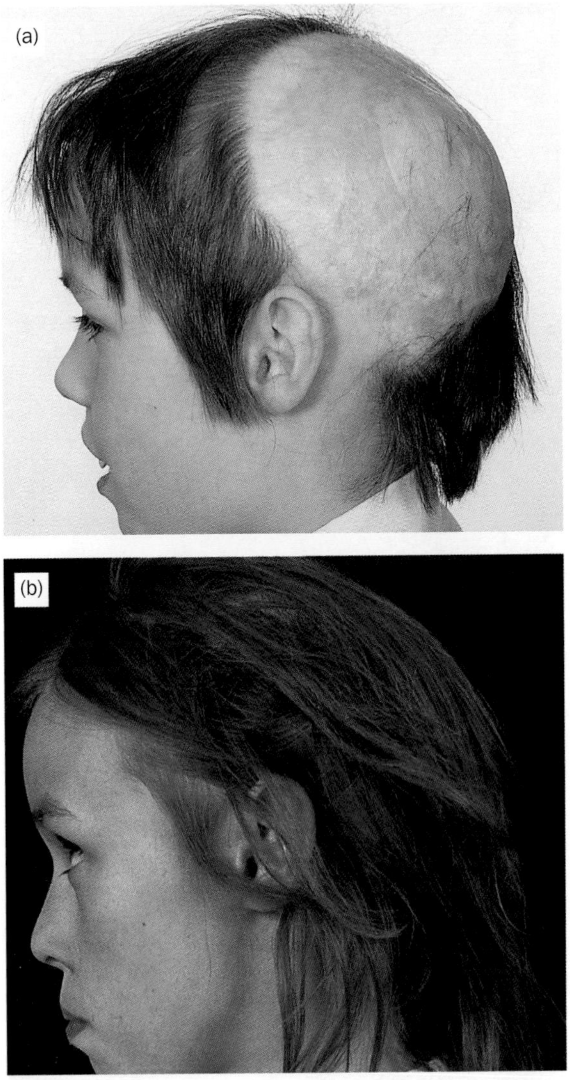

Figure 43.34 Tissue expansion to reconstruct extensive post-burn scald alopecia.

The usual presentation is of increasing respiratory distress over several hours. Investigations include chest X-ray and blood gases (including carboxyhaemoglobin levels). These patients may need to be intubated, and if left until the mucosa becomes oedematous this can be very difficult, tracheostomy occasionally being required. Facial burn wounds should be treated conservatively unless clearly full thickness, when grafting will be required (Figure 43.9).

Late reconstruction of burn wounds includes scar revision and release of contractures; reconstruction of large areas of scalp alopecia can be very successfully performed using tissue expansion (expanding healthy, hair bearing scalp adjacent to the 'bald' area) and then advancing flaps, as shown in Figure 43.34.

Neoplasia

Skin tumours of the face can be benign or malignant.

Benign

These lesions are similar to those found in the skin elsewhere in the body – papillomas, moles, etc. Greater care must be exercised in removal of these lesions on the face to achieve an optimal cosmetic result. Due respect should be paid to the natural crease lines, and sutures should be carefully placed, with removal by 5 days if possible. Solar keratoses can be treated with liquid nitrogen, and more recently PDT (photodynamic therapy) is proving useful in patients with multiple lesions.

Malignant

The common malignant skin tumours are basal cell carcinoma, squamous cell carcinoma and malig-nant melanoma. The incidence of all of these is rising and is likely to continue to do so with an increase in the percentage of older patients in the population.

Basal cell carcinoma (BCC)

Slowly growing, these tumours rarely metastasize but are capable of progressive local tissue erosion. There are several clinical types, the classical 'rodent ulcer' being a well-circumscribed lesion. They are usually painless and may present with bleeding or ulceration. Excision with a margin of 3–4 mm of healthy tissue around is advisable. The method of repair or reconstruction will depend on the site and size of the lesion, and will be governed by the criteria already mentioned earlier in the module. Some defects will require direct closure, others a more complex flap reconstruction, e.g. Figure 43.15 shows the use of a glabellar flap to reconstruct a large defect at the tip of the nose. Figure 43.13 shows the result following reconstruction of a defect on the upper nasolabial area with an island nasolabial advancement flap. A combination of techniques may be necessary following resection of a full thickness BCC of the lower eyelid. Conjunctiva, tarsal plate and outer skin need to be reconstructed: conjunctiva and tarsal plate can be replaced with a chondromucosal graft taken from the septum of the nose, and a cheek advancement flap then used to give skin cover. BCC are radiosensitive, but surgical excision has the advantage of being able to confirm removal of the lesion by histopathology; radiotherapy is extremely useful however, if the BCC is fixed to the bone.

Squamous cell carcinoma (SCC)

These lesions can metastasize, usually to the regional lymph nodes – these should always be palpated as part of the examination of a suspected SCC. Excision with a 1 cm margin all round (including the deep surface) should be carried out. Again, the options for reconstruction depend on the site and size of defect, taking the reconstructive principles already mentioned into consideration. The lower lip is a common site for SCC. Full thickness defects of up to one-third of the width of the lip can generally be closed directly, but for larger defects than this more complex flaps are required and several different techniques have been described.

One of the most widely used is the Karapandzic flap, which preserves as much functioning muscle as possible. Total lower lip reconstruction can also be managed using a modification of the McGregor flap, as in the example shown in Figure 43.16. This patient presented with a rapidly enlarging recurrent SCC arising in the mucosa of the lower lip. Tumours of the upper lip are much less common; Figure 43.14 shows a reverse Estlander flap based on the labial artery which is rotated through 180°. The width of this flap is calculated as half of the width of the defect, thus balancing the total widths of upper and lower lips.

Malignant melanoma

These potentially aggressive tumours also metastasize to the regional lymph nodes and/or via the blood

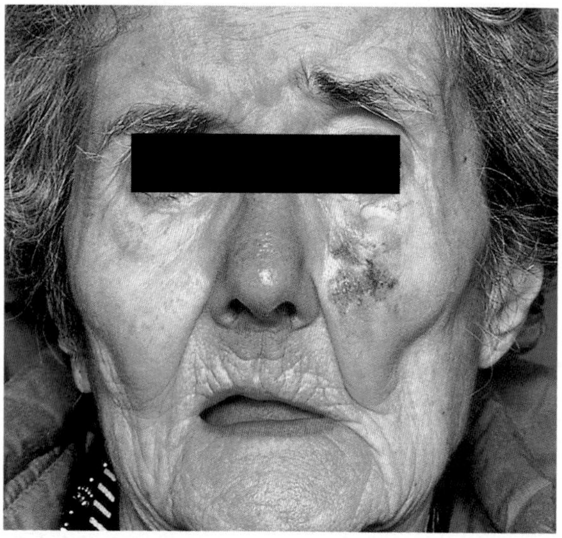

Figure 43.35 Lentigo maligna melanoma of cheek.

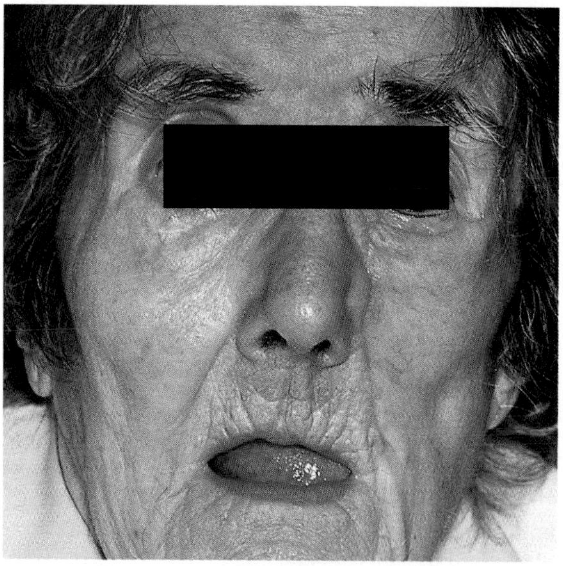

Figure 43.36 Cheek rotation flap repair following excision of the cheek.

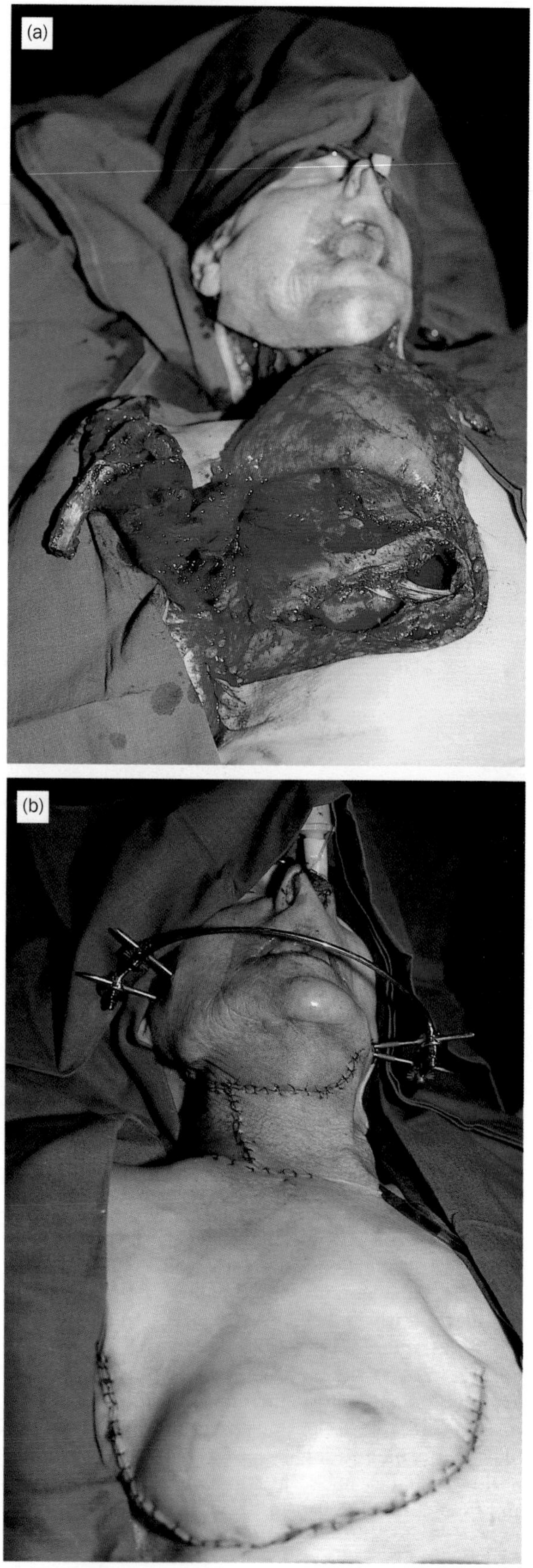

Figure 43.37 Pectoralis major osteomyocutaneous flap. (Courtesy of Mr A.J. Leonard.)

stream, especially to the lung, liver, brain and bone. Although the prognosis is most closely linked to the depth of invasion (Clark's level and Breslow thickness), there is some evidence that in the face the prognosis may be more favourable. Excision with a 1 cm margin and reconstruction is indicated. Lentigo maligna and lentigo maligna melanoma are most often seen in elderly patients. These lesions tend to grow slowly. Figure 43.35 shows a typical example; early changes of malignancy include an increase in size, alteration in shape, persisting itching and later bleeding. A large cheek rotation flap was carried out in this woman to repair the defect following resection (Figure 43.36).

Tumours of the oral cavity/sinuses

These tumours can cause facial distortion either before treatment, or as a consequence of it. Tumours arising in the maxilla are normally approached through the Weber Fergusson incision. The resulting contour defect on the face can be reconstructed with a prosthesis conveniently added as an obturator to an upper denture, or by a free vascularized bone graft (e.g. iliac crest or fibula). Figure 43.37 shows reconstruction of the body of the mandible following resection for SCC arising in the anterior floor of the mouth, with a pectoralis major osteomyocutaneous flap – an excellent chin can be achieved with this method, though the vascularity of the rib is suboptimal. Free vascularized grafts

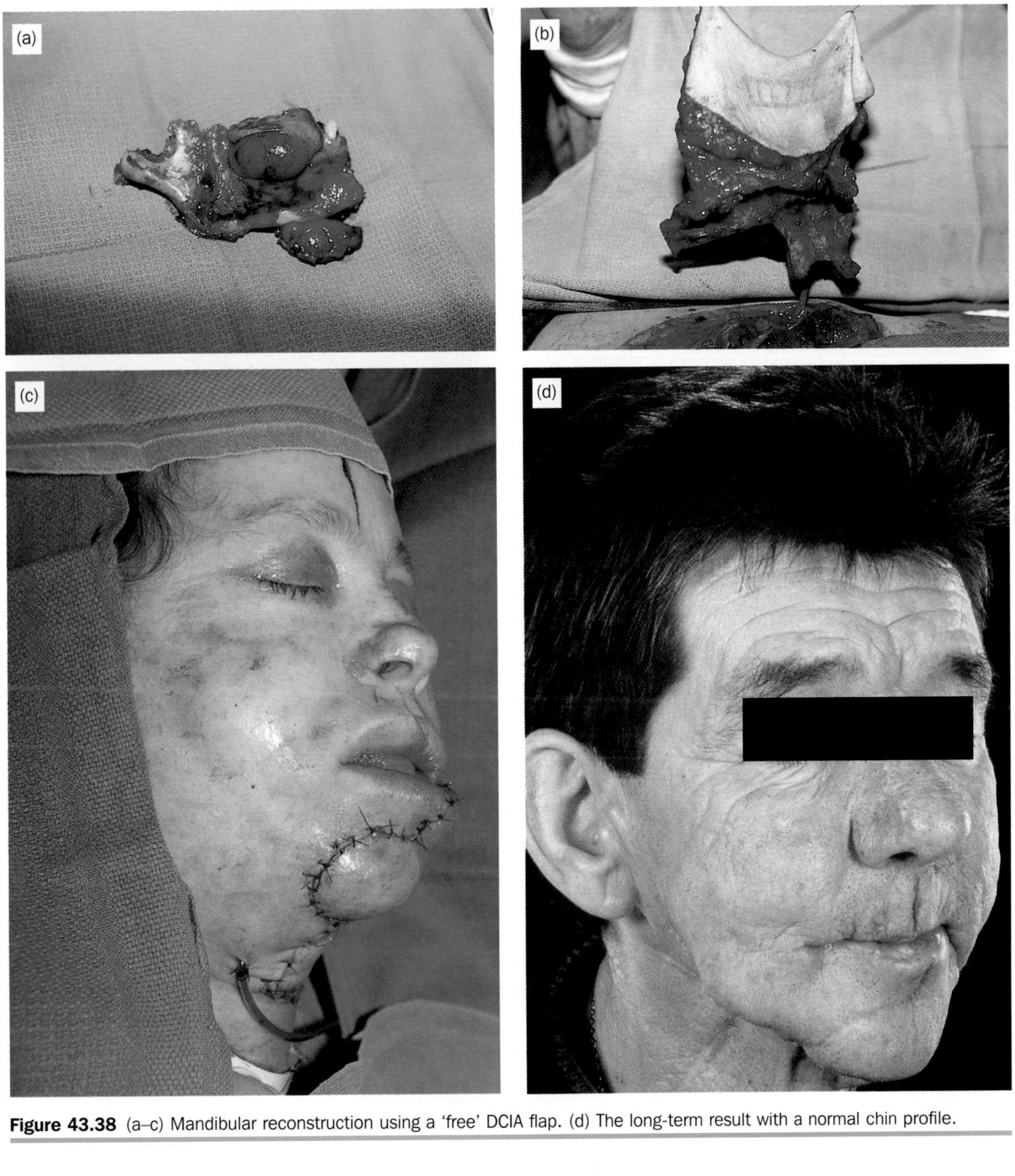

Figure 43.38 (a–c) Mandibular reconstruction using a 'free' DCIA flap. (d) The long-term result with a normal chin profile.

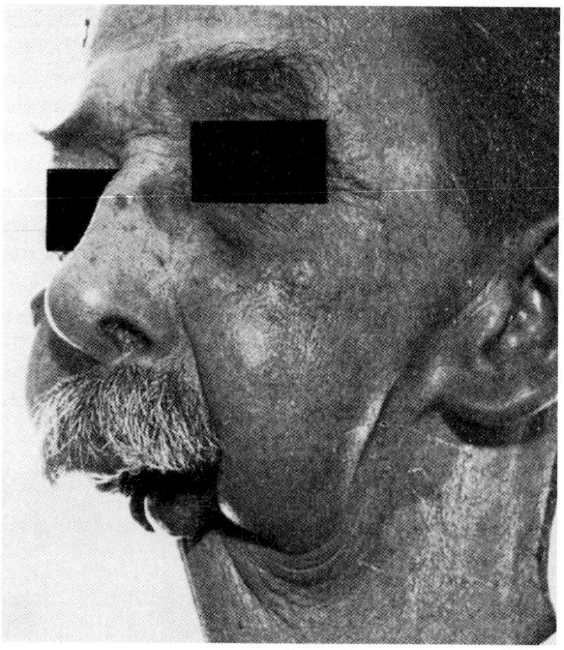

Figure 43.39 Absence of mandibular arch results in significant morbidity.

incorporating iliac crest (deep circumflex iliac artery flap – DCIA or fibula) offer much better vascularity, and this is important if the patient is to undergo post-operative radiotherapy (see Figure 43.38). This shows resection of a recurrent sarcoma involving mandible and reconstruction using a free DCIA flap. Figure 43.38(d) shows a similar case illustrating the chin profile achieved (long-term follow-up following radiotherapy). These options mark a significant advance on the earlier practice of simply suturing skin to mucosa, resulting in the so-called 'Andy Gump' (an American cartoon character) deformity, associated with significant morbidity (Figure 43.39). The free radial forearm flap, now the mainstay of intraoral reconstruction following excision of cancer, is a versatile flap which can be used to reconstruct not only mucosa but skin for outer cheek cover by simply de-epithelializing a short segment and folding the flap on itself. A portion of radius can also be incorporated in

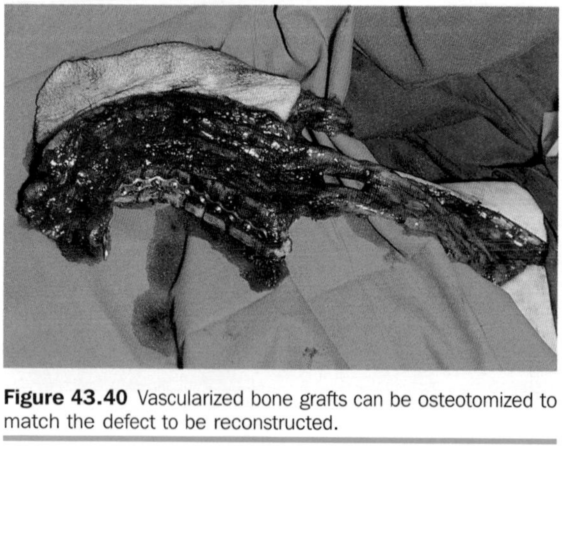

Figure 43.40 Vascularized bone grafts can be osteotomized to match the defect to be reconstructed.

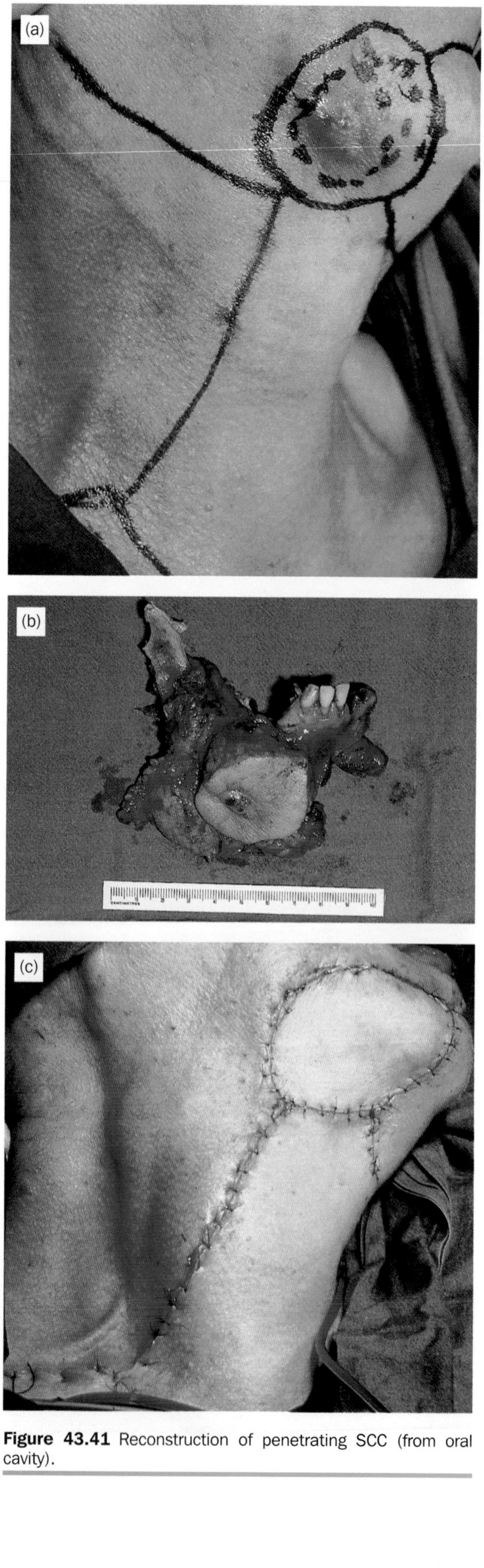

Figure 43.41 Reconstruction of penetrating SCC (from oral cavity).

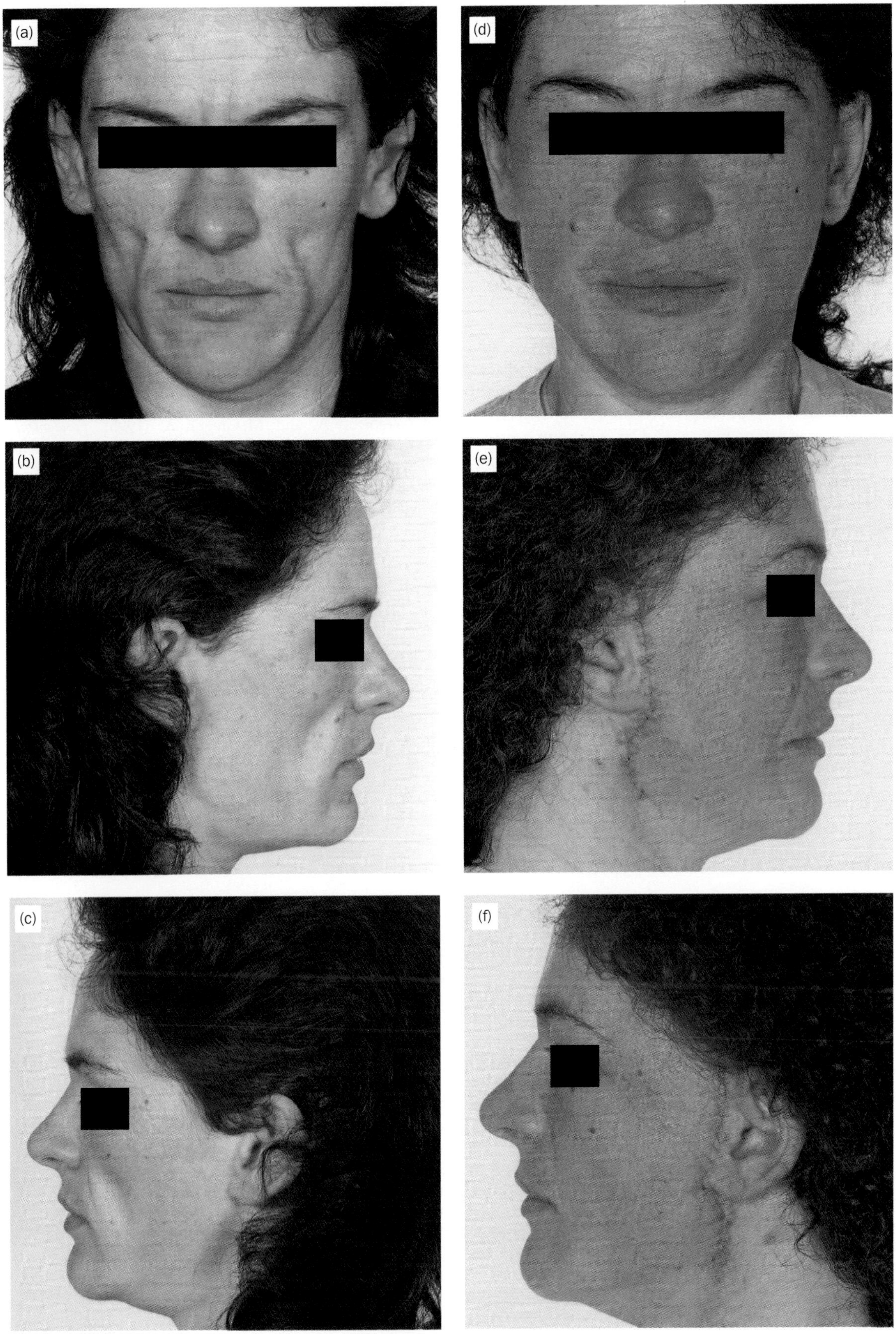

Figure 43.42 Facial contour restored with two de-epithelialized groin flaps, using microvascular surgery.

this flap for small mandibular defects, which can be osteotomized to reconstruct mandibular contour (Figure 43.40), but harvesting too much bone from the radius will result in fractures of the remaining bone in the forearm. The volume of bone available for this flap is usually insufficient to enable osseointegrated denture reconstruction to be carried out – a fibular or DCIA flap is necessary. Figure 43.41 shows a patient with a penetrating SCC arising in the cheek mucosa but involving overlying cheek skin, which has been resected and reconstructed with a radial forearm flap folded on itself.

Degenerative

Romberg's disease, in which there is a progressive atrophy of the subcutaneous fat (and on occasions, adjacent structures) can be reconstructed using free microvascular flaps, e.g. the groin flap based on the superficial circumflex iliac artery. Figure 43.42(a, b) shows a case in which bilateral flaps have been de-epithelialized, inverted and sutured beneath the cheek skin, the vessels being anastomosed to the superficial temporal vessels to maintain viability.

The future

Advances in tissue culture hold out the promise of being able to replace structures more accurately than at present, though this remains largely experimental. Composite tissue transplantation is another technique which may hold promise to enhance facial reconstruction in the future.

Further reading

Emmett, A. J. J. and O'Rourke, M. G. E., eds (1991). *Malignant Skin Tumours*, 2nd edn. Edinburgh: Churchill Livingstone.

Georgiade, G. S., Riefkohl, R. and Levin, L. S. (1997). *Plastic, Maxillofacial and Reconstructive Surgery*, 3rd edn. Baltimore, MD: Williams and Wilkins.

Mathes, S. J. and Nahai, F., eds (1982). *Clinical Applications for Muscle and Musculocutaneous Flaps*. St. Louis, MO: Mosby.

McGregor, I. A. and McGregor, A. (1995). *Fundamental Techniques in Plastic Surgery*, 9th edn. Edinburgh: Churchill Livingstone.

Strauch, B., Vasconez, L. and Hall-Findlay, E., eds (1990). *Grabb's Encyclopedia of Flaps*. Boston, MD: Little, Brown.

MODULE 44

Injuries of the maxillofacial skeleton

The face is the key part of the anatomy in a social animal such as *Homo sapiens*, and injuries to it are significant for a variety of reasons, both physical and emotional. The visage is extensively utilized for expressive purposes. It also harbours the entry to the respiratory and gastrointestinal tracts, together with the portals of vision, hearing and smell. Injuries may materially interfere with the functions of communication, breathing, eating, speaking, sight and hearing. Interference with the airway may be life-threatening in occasional instances.

Section 44.1 • Introduction

Deformity of the face, whether it is temporary or permanent, can be most distressing because it threatens to disrupt social contact so that the psychological management of the patient must be remembered, with reassurance playing a significant part. Maxillofacial injuries tend to incite more fear in the subject than trauma elsewhere as it is harder to divorce oneself from a condition which is so close to the centre of consciousness.

As the face is commonly unprotected by clothing, it is especially exposed to trauma. In addition, facial bones are vulnerable as they are quite thin because lightness is important in an animal which holds its head erect, such as man.

Fortunately, the area has an excellent blood supply, so that injuries heal well with a lack of secondary infection, and fractures unite far more quickly than in the long bones. However, at the time of the acute injury the abundant blood supply may create problems, particularly in the scalp, tongue and lips where haemorrhage can be profuse. Control is usually prompt, however, with conventional measures of pressure combined with clamping of any major arterial bleeding points. The speed of healing of facial bone fractures provides a minimum of inconvenience for the patient but does mean that definitive reduction should be carried out within 10 days, otherwise malunion may well occur.

All of the above features stress the importance of maxillofacial injury. It behoves any doctor to be beware of the signs and symptoms of such injuries and their initial treatment. This is especially true of the casualty officer.

Section 44.2 • History

As always, a good history can be most helpful in piecing together a picture of the accident, and with it an appreciation of the sort of injuries to be expected. It may not be possible to obtain this from the subject due to impairment of speech or defect of consciousness. A relative's testimony or that of an ambulance man may be very useful in filling in some of the missing data.

It is particularly important to establish the following.

Mechanism of injury

Information on this aspect can aid in determining the possible sites of injury and their severity and nature. It is meaningful to divide the various mechanisms into three main groups related to the causative kinetic (Lindahl's classification).

Kinetic energy of the individual exerted on to the facial structures

This is seen most typically in falls, and is commonest in the young and elderly. A typical example in the adult is shown in Figure 44.1(a), which illustrates the so-called 'parade ground fracture'. This occurs when someone faints, as for example a soldier on parade, and falls directly on to the point of chin. Here there may typically be a laceration below the chin, fractures of the thin condylar necks of the lower jaw, and often a midline fracture. In the elderly, one should be mindful of possible medical causes for such falls. Myocardial infarction or cerebrovascular accident particularly should be excluded as these may be of major importance, especially if an anaesthetic is planned. In the child the elasticity of the facial bones is remarkable but fractures can occur. The maxilla is relatively protected by the cranium as the face has as yet failed to grow downwards and forwards to its full degree. Fracture of the upper jaw in the young child, if it does occur, is often accompanied by a skull fracture for this reason (usually a group 3 causative mechanism).

Kinetic energy expended on to the individual

The causative incident here is a blow which most typically may be caused by a fist, kick or sporting equipment such as a tennis racket. Such incidents are commonest in young adolescents and adults. It is helpful to know whether a single blow was administered or whether multiple traumas occurred. Two typical examples are shown in Figure 44.1(b).

The first one comprises a localized blow, as by a racket in this case, over the zygomatic arch causing a fracture of its most prominent part.

The second example shows a more powerful and diffuse force in the form of a kick administered over the horizontal ramus of the jaw producing a direct injury at the site of impact and a contre-coup injury on the opposite side in the thin condylar region.

Combination of kinetic energy of the individual and kinetic energy exerted on to the individual

In this instance the body may be thrown against an object which has its own individual momentum. Such a combination produces a major degree of disruptive energy and can be responsible for severe and multiple injuries. The most common example is the road traffic accident which may of course occur in all age groups. Fortunately road traffic trauma is tending to decrease due to lowering of speed limits and the compulsory use of front seatbelts. It is in this group that the most severe injuries are likely to occur, and also that combination with injury in other regions is most likely. Figure 44.1(c) shows how a maxillofacial injury may be combined with other conditions in the context of a front-seat passenger without a seatbelt. The face is commonly impacted against the upper part of the dashboard resulting in skeletal injuries to any of the facial bones. Soft tissue laceration occurs due to the shattering of the windscreen. Impact of the thoracic region against the main dashboard can result in a variety of injuries, particularly rib fractures and sternal fractures. Air bags reduce the incidence and severity of these injuries.

The abdomen may also share in such trauma with the possibility of rupture of intra-abdominal organs, particularly the spleen.

Lastly, the lower limb may be thrust forcibly against the lower part of the dashboard structures, again with the possibility of a variety of lesions but perhaps most typically fractures of the patella or long bones.

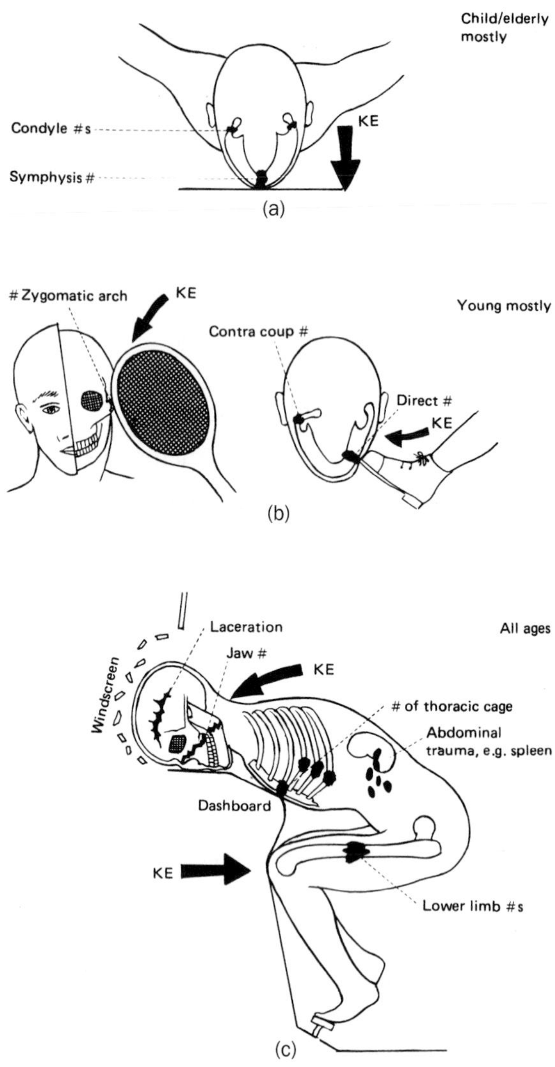

Figure 44.1 Mechanism of facial injuries: kinetic energy on to facial structures (Lindahl's classification), (a) of individual, e.g. fall, (b) on to individual, e.g. sports and assault, (c) combination, e.g. road traffic accident.

Functional deficit noted

One should record whether the patient has noted any particular problems since the incident or whether these have been observed by onlookers. One should know whether the patient was rendered unconscious at any time. Retrograde or post-traumatic amnesia should be enquired into as an indication of possible cerebral damage. Enquiries should be made as to whether any pain is noted in the facial region and for nasal discharge, failure of teeth to occlude, visual problems, particularly double vision and numbness of the facial dermatomes. One should also enquire for pain in other regions, and particularly for any difficulty in moving the neck. It is vitally important to pick up a cervical fracture early, as neurological damage can occur in an unstable case during further examination or, more particularly, as a result of administration of a general anaesthetic with relaxant during treatment of a facial fracture.

Previous treatment

If the patient has been seen at a previous hospital then normally a casualty card will accompany him. One should note whether any tetanus prophylaxis and fluid replacements have been given. The administration of antibiotics is also of significance.

General medical history

It has previously been mentioned that medical conditions may be significant as a cause of a fall so that enquiries should be made of any previous cardiac, neurological or endocrinological problems.

Other conditions which are particularly important in trauma patients include steroid medication or adrenal pathology as there is a danger of Addisonian crisis after trauma unless steroid supplements are adequate, and also diabetes because jaw injuries may preclude the taking of a full diet.

Section 44.3 • Examination

A number of schemes for examining a possible maxillofacial injury have been advocated. The simplest and the one most unlikely to miss signs, is to start at the top of the scalp and work down steadily level by level until the chin is reached. *Prior to detailed examination of the facial region, the neck should be checked as moving the head could produce neurological damage in undetected cervical fracture.* The hand should be gently run down the back of the neck palpating each neural spine and also searching for any areas of tenderness in the associated longitudinal muscles.

The following features should be specially looked for (Figure 44.2).

Tenderness and swelling

The tissues are likely to be tender to palpation and often swollen in an area of injury although this sign does not, of course, indicate definite skeletal damage. It does, however, alert one to the need for further checking at the particular site.

Deep bleeding

Facial lacerations will, of course, leave superficial traces of blood but there are certain sites where deep bleeding may be detected and these are particularly significant.

Haematoma of the scalp

This may indicate an underlying skull fracture, e.g. of the frontal bone.

Aural (Figure 44.3)

Bleeding from the ear may occur in a fracture of the middle cranial fossa or more locally a rupture of the tympanic membrane or disruption of the walls of the bony meatus. The latter can occur when the condylar head is driven forcibly back after a blow on the lower jaw.

Circumorbital (Figure 44.4)

Bleeding can arise within the orbit as a result of fracture of any of the bones contributing to this structure, particularly the frontal bone, ethmoids, nose, maxilla and zygoma. Deep bleeding tends to be confined to the limits of the orbit by the orbital septum which is a

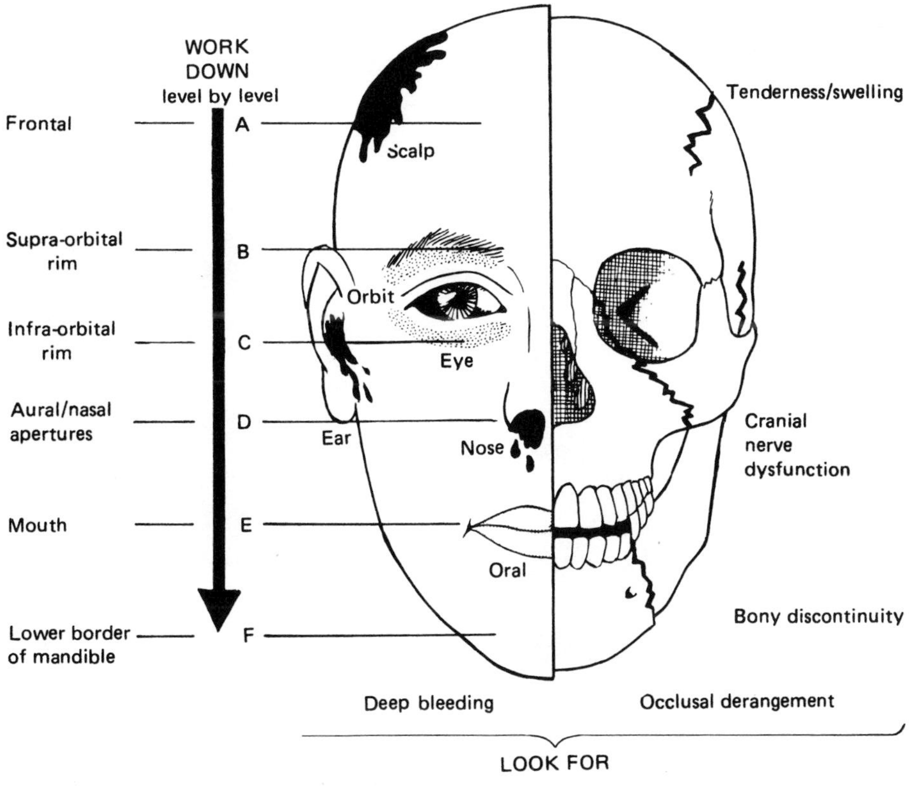

Figure 44.2 Examination of facial injury.

condensation of connective tissue in continuity with the tarsal plates. This characteristic distribution is known sometimes as 'panda eyes' or in the USA as 'racoon eyes'.

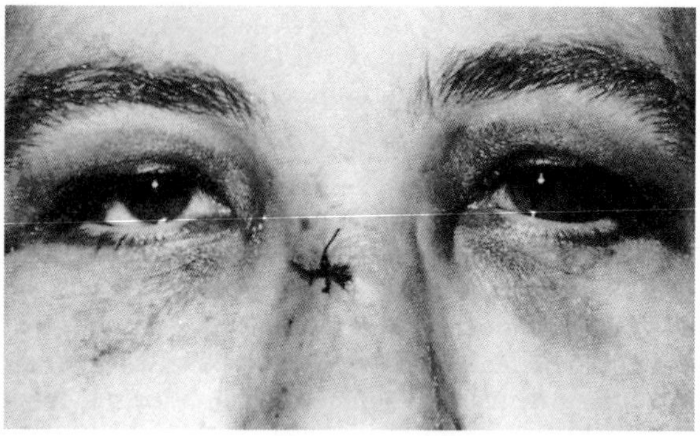

Figure 44.4 Circumorbital ecchymosis ('panda eyes') is due to bleeding within the orbit confined by the orbital septum and is seen in fractures of the maxilla, zygoma, ethmoids or frontal bone.

Subconjunctival haemorrhage (Figure 44.5)

Local trauma to the sclera can produce a small localized haemorrhage, but a haemorrhage where it is impossible to discern the posterior limit even when the eye is moved to the contralateral side indicates bleeding coming from within the orbit and spreading underneath the conjunctiva. This again indicates a fracture somewhere within the orbit, i.e. frontal bone, nasal bones, maxilla or zygoma. It may be either lateral or, less commonly, medial and this gives some indication of which bone is involved. Bilateral subconjunctival haematomas may also occur in strangulation.

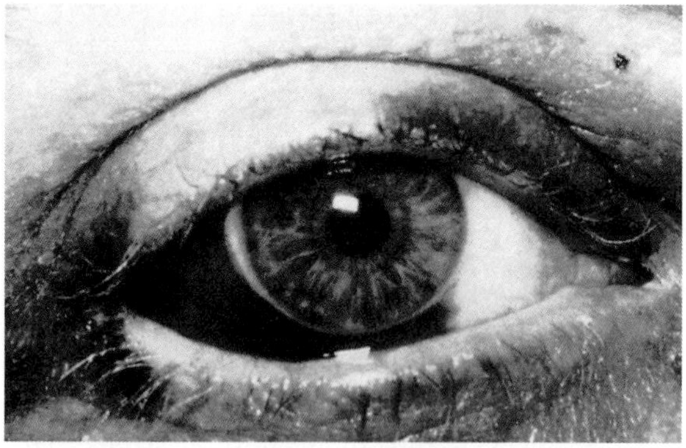

Figure 44.5 Subconjunctival haemorrhage without posterior limit is due to blood tracking forward under the conjunctiva from injury to the orbit, almost always a fracture.

Nasal bleeding (epistaxis) (Figure 44.6)

The nose may bleed after relatively minor trauma in some individuals. However, it should alert one to the possibility of skeletal fracture of the nose or of one of the bones which contribute to the maxillary sinus which is in continuity with the nose, particularly the maxilla and zygoma. Unilateral nose bleeding or epistaxis is particularly significant.

It is very important to differentiate epistaxis from leakage of cerebrospinal fluid (CSF) which may occur in high level maxillary and nasal fractures involving the region of the cribriform plate. Such leakage indicates the risk of meningitis. In the early

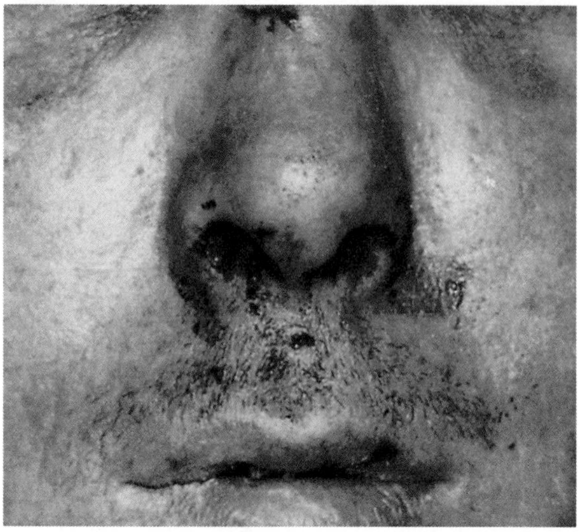

Figure 44.6 Epistaxis may be a result of trauma to the nose or bleeding from the nasal cavities in fractures of the maxilla or zygoma.

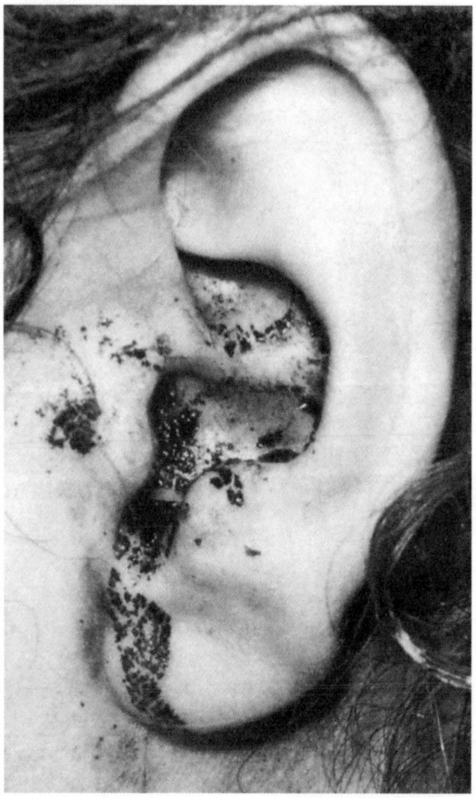

Figure 44.3 Aural bleeding indicates a fracture of the bony meatus or rupture of the drum. Middle cranial fossa fracture should be excluded.

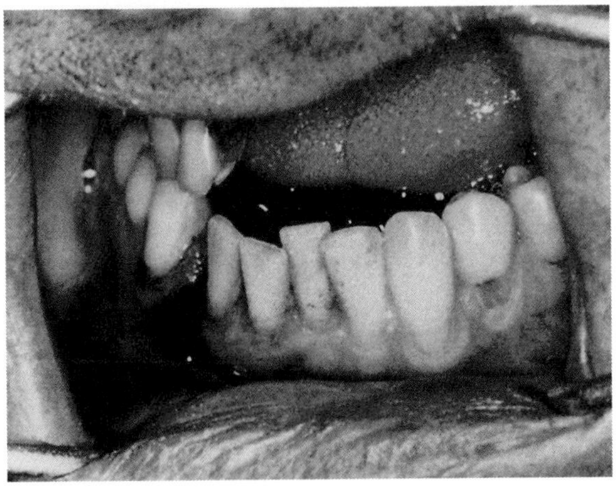

Figure 44.7 Lingual haematoma in mandibular fracture, between the lower right lateral incisor and canines.

stages CSF may be mixed with blood and nasal catarrh. Later it is present alone and has a characteristic pale amber appearance leaving a faint stain on the skin. Biochemical estimation of glucose and protein levels can be undertaken as confirmation. The detection of beta-2 transferrin in the nasal discharge confirms the presence of CSF.

Intraoral (Figure 44.7)

A haematoma in the lingual sulcus related to the mandible is said to be pathognomonic of fracture of the mandible as this area is protected from direct trauma and is only likely to be affected if the bone is fractured. Haemorrhage in the region of the greater palatine foramen is Guérin's sign and indicates a fracture through the region of the greater palatine canal, i.e. a maxillary fracture.

Bony discontinuity (Figure 44.8)

It may be possible to detect a step of a displaced fracture of the facial bones. However, oedema occurs very rapidly in the facial region so that after an hour or so post-injury, it may not be possible to detect lesser degrees of bony discontinuity. The following sites are particularly important.

Frontal bone

It may be possible to detect depressed fractures of this bone.

Supraorbital rim

Fracture of the frontal bone may give rise to a step at this site. Steps in the region of the frontozygomatic suture occur often in zygomatic fracture but can be very difficult to palpate.

Infraorbital rim

Steps at this site may occur in pyramidal fractures of the maxilla or zygomatic fracture.

Mandibular lower border

It is important to palpate the whole of the lower border of the mandible for any discontinuity. A useful adjunctive test is to place a finger in the external auditory meatus and ask the patient to open and close the jaw. Normally the condyle should be felt to move in and out of the fossa but in the case of a fracture-dislocation this will not be palpated.

Cranial nerve dysfunction

A simple rapid testing of cranial nerves should always be carried out in facial injury although the finer points of such an examination may not be practicable in an injured patient. The following findings are of particular importance.

Disturbance of extraocular movements

These can occur in orbital fractures where the most inferior muscles may be entrapped, notably the inferior oblique (Figures 44.9 and 44.14). More widespread disturbance can occur where the nerves of supply (cranial nerves III, IV and VI) together with the frontal branch of V are disturbed in fractures through the superior orbital fissure (superior orbital fissure syndrome).

Fortunately the optic nerve is usually well protected by a dense ring of bone but occasionally this may be disrupted in this so-called orbital apex syndrome. The significance of pupillary changes in cranial injury is

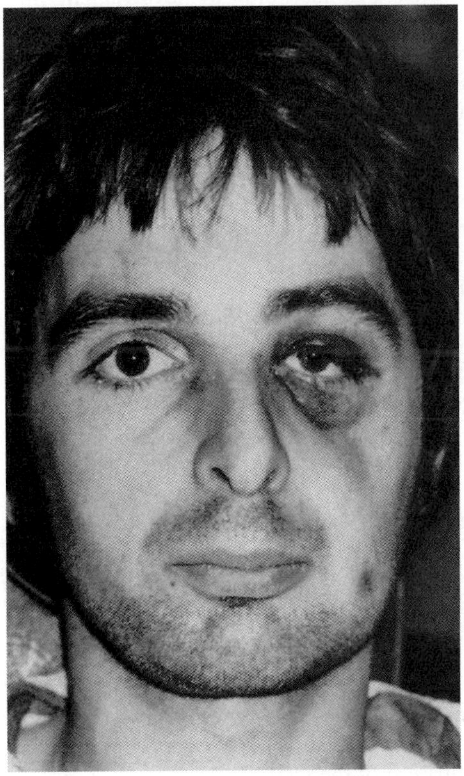

Figure 44.8 Obvious step over a depressed fracture of the left zygoma.

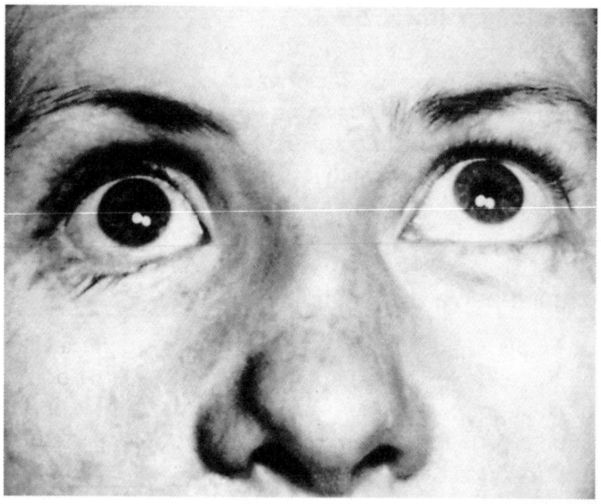

Figure 44.9 Failure of elevation of right eye on looking upwards due to entrapment of inferior oblique muscle in a fracture of the orbital floor.

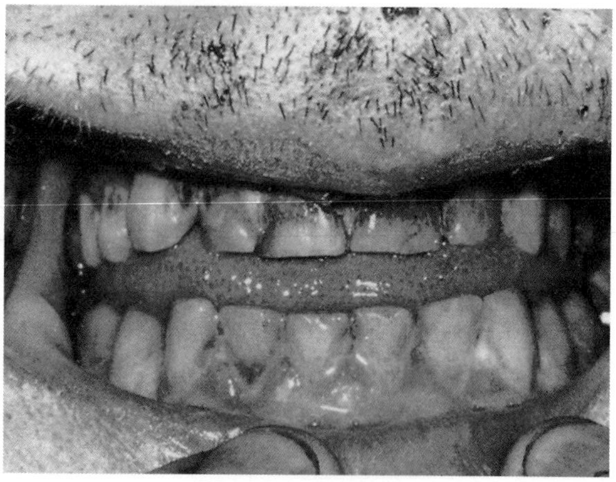

Figure 44.10 Disturbance of dental occlusion. Anterior open bite, as here, can occur in fractures of the maxilla or in bilateral fracture of the mandibular condyles.

well recognized. Local injury to the eye in the form of a traumatic iritis can also produce a sluggish or even dilated pupil. Testing both direct and consensual reflexes may help to determine in pupillary changes whether the basic defect is in the afferent limb, i.e. optic nerve, or in the efferent limb, i.e. oculomotor nerve.

Disturbance of Vth nerve function

Sensory loss should be sought over the main distribution of the trigeminal nerve. Disturbance in the infraorbital area may indicate involvement in either the nasal, labial or palpebral branches and may occur where any fracture extends through the region of the infraorbital foramen or canal, as in fractures of the maxilla or zygoma. Disturbance of mental sensation may well occur in fractures of the mandible as the inferior alveolar nerve traverses a large length of the lower jaw between the mandibular and the mental foramina.

Loss of facial nerve or auditory function

Disturbance in function of these may occur in fractures of the middle cranial fossa. It is important in cases of facial lacerations to check that there has been no loss of VIIth nerve function or related branches. If this has occurred then peripheral nerve repair is likely to be required.

Disturbance of dental occlusion

A displaced fracture of the jaws involving the dental alveolar segment is likely to cause a derangement of the occlusion of the teeth (Figure 44.10). There may well be a step in the occlusal plane. Some slight experience may be necessary in certain cases as one may not know in a particular case whether the patient has a pre-existing malocclusion, such as an open bite. In these cases examination of the teeth for wear facets is very helpful in determining where pre-existing contacts occurred. Where front teeth have never met, the small tubercles which are present at eruption may persist on the incisal edges. Particular occlusal disturbances seen in individual fractures are described in relevant sections.

Section 44.4 • Radiographic examination of maxillofacial injury

It is probably true to say that if a facial fracture is not detectable by clinical examination then there will be little indication for treatment. Radiographic examination is, however, an important investigation for any patient with a suspected facial fracture. It can be particularly helpful when facial swelling is at its height, obscuring bony deformity; it may take as long as 4 or 5 days for such swelling to regress after a major injury. Radiographs enable one to assess the full extent of injury and this is most valuable in treatment planning. It is important to detect stable undisplaced fractures which do not require treatment for medicolegal reasons. The fact that a blow occasioned in an assault was sufficiently powerful to cause bony injury has legal significance.

A word of caution is necessary in ordering detailed radiographic examination early in the management of patients with multiple injuries. A number of facial views, particularly those utilized in examination of the upper jaw (occipitomental views) require the patient to be turned on his face. This may be unsafe and impracticable in a severely injured patient, particularly one who is unconscious or who may have spinal injuries. Alternative views not requiring the prone position may have to be obtained in these cases, even though they prove somewhat inferior. Also in such instances, the emphasis is thrown on careful clinical examination to establish the fracture pattern. Tomography may be useful in complex cases as this can be carried out without the need for turning the patient.

A general principle of fracture radiography is that for certain diagnosis two views at right angles to each other are required. This should be observed in the maxillofacial region as far as possible, particularly in the mandible where an undisplaced fracture may be very hard to detect save in an angulation near to the plane of the discontinuity itself.

Mandible

Classically, lateral views of the lower jaw are provided by **right** and **left** lateral obliques (Figure 44.11) which are taken with the relevant side of the face against the film but rotated so as to throw the image of the opposite side of the mandible clear. A tomographic view requiring a special apparatus, the **orthopantomogram** (OPG) has tended to supplant lateral oblique views, where it is available, as it shows the whole of the lower jaw from condyle to condyle in one continuum (Figure 44.12).

In either case a further radiograph at right angles is needed to observe the principle previously stated. A **posteroanterior** view of the mandible is best as the vertical ramus areas show clearly being nearest to the film (Figure 44.13). This requires the subject to be face downwards, and if this is inadvisable an **anteroposterior** view may be substituted.

The midline region of the mandible is poorly seen on lateral obliques, while in the OPG or posteroanterior projections the image of the cervical vertebrae is superimposed. To overcome this, certain intraoral views, which involve placing a film in the mouth, are available, such as the **true occlusal** film showing the outline well and the **oblique occlusal** taken at an angle revealing bony detail well. Dental **periapical** films are useful in examining the relationship of a fracture to individual teeth and detecting root damage, but may be difficult to obtain in a severely injured patient due to the precision of placement necessary.

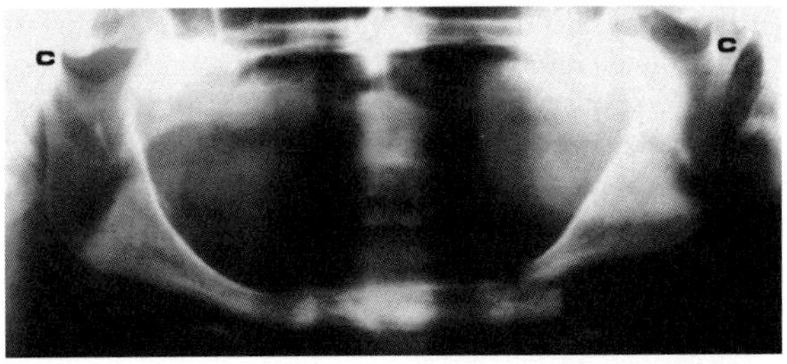

Figure 44.12 Orthopantomogram (OPG) showing fracture of the left body in an elderly subject with an atrophic mandible. The OPG, if available, is preferable to the lateral oblique views as it shows the whole mandible from condyle to condyle (c).

The condylar areas tend to be superimposed on the image of the base of a skull and a specialized anteroposterior view is helpful, namely the **Towne's view** or even better the **reverse Towne's**. In cases of difficulty **transcranial condylar** radiographs may be needed.

Maxilla

Standard anteroposterior views of the skull, such as the occipitofrontal view, cause superimposition of the dense petrous part of the temporal bones over the lower parts of the orbit and maxilla, so that their usefulness is limited, although the supraorbital margin and

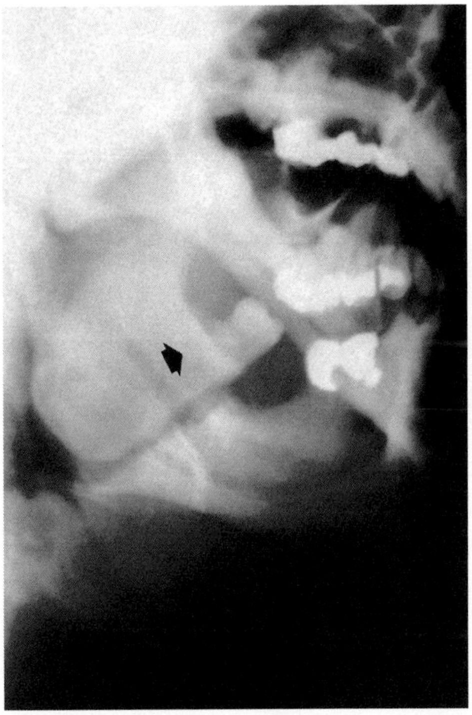

Figure 44.11 Lateral oblique radiograph of mandible showing fracture. This is 'horizontally unfavourable' in its obliquity allowing upward displacement of the proximal fragment under the influence of the elevator muscles (pterygomasseteric sling) as shown by the arrow.

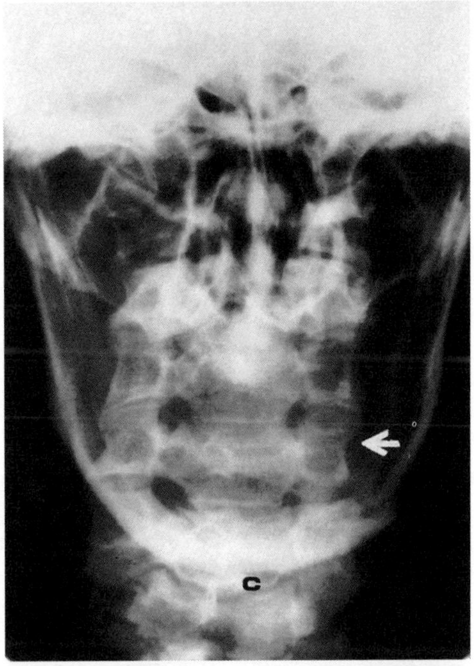

Figure 44.13 Posteroanterior view of the mandible of the same fracture as in Figure 44.12. This shows that the obliquity of the fracture is 'vertically unfavourable' allowing inward displacement of the proximal fragment under the influence of the pterygomasseteric sling (arrow). Cervical spine outlines (c) tend to be superimposed over the anterior mandible and here a dental occlusal film can be very helpful.

the area of the frontomalar sutures can be seen well. For proper delineation of the maxilla and zygoma it is necessary to displace the image of the petrous temporal bone away from the area of interest. The following radiographs are helpful.

Occipitomental (Figures 44.14 and 44.15)
This shows vertical displacement at the orbital margin.

Thirty degree occipitomental (Figure 44.16)
This view has greater 'tip' and one is viewing the inferior orbital margin almost from below so that horizontal displacement can be judged.

If the patient cannot be turned on his face for the occipitomental view, which involves placing the chin (mentum) and nose on the film while shooting the rays through the occiput (hence the term occipitomental) then a view may be taken with the patient lying face upward, but in the reverse direction, i.e. **mento-occipital**. Definition on this view is very much inferior to the true occipitomental as the facial structures are furthest away from the film and hence show magnification and lack of clarity. It is, however, well worthwhile undertaking in the circumstances indicated.

Lateral facial bones
This shows fracture lines running through the region of the frontomaxillary suture lines or nasal septum, and also any steps in the line of the pterygoid plates.

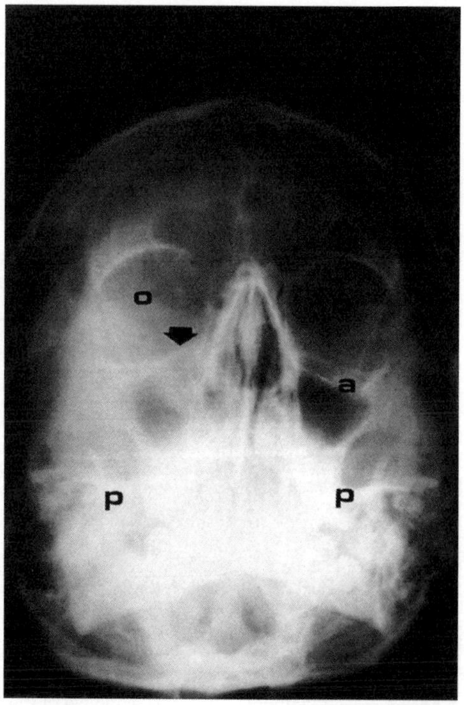

Figure 44.14 Occipitomental radiography showing right-sided orbital blow-out fracture (arrow). Note the clear antrum on the contralateral side (a). The orbits are indicated (o). In this view the dense petrous part of the temporal bone (P) is projected away from the mid-face whereas in a conventional posteroanterior view of the skull (occipitofrontal) there is superimposition.

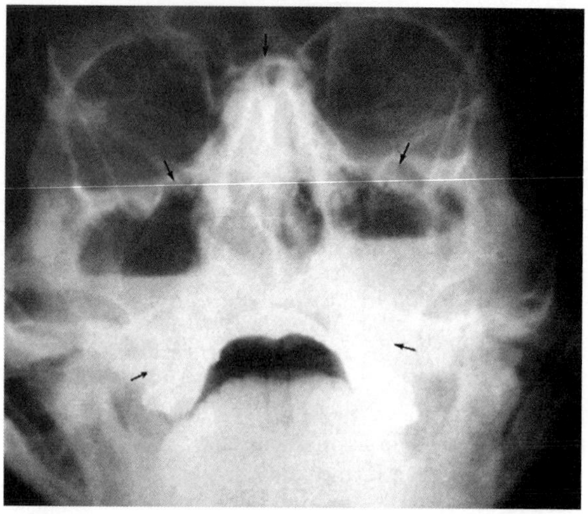

Figure 44.15 Occipitomental radiography showing blood in both antra as a result of a Le Fort II fracture of the maxilla. Arrows indicate the fracture sites.

Zygoma

The same views as for the maxilla are indicated, namely the **occipitomental** and 30° occipitomental with the addition of the **submentovertical** which is taken from below showing the zygomatic arch outlines. Occcasionally in a case where fracture is uncertain a **rotated occipitomental** taken from one side of the midline may help. In suspected 'orbital blow-out' tomography is usually needed.

Nose

Occipitofrontal
This shows mediolateral displacement of the nasal bones and the position of the nasal septum. An AP view of the skull is an alternative if the patient cannot be turned on his face.

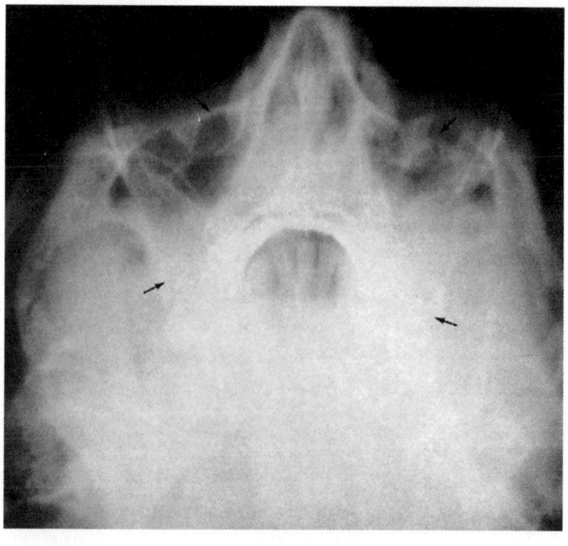

Figure 44.16 The same case of Le Fort II fracture as Figure 44.15 but occipitomental shows more angulation (30° occipitomental). Radio-opacity of the antra now appears more diffuse.

Table 44.1 Facial fractures

Site	*Signs (not always present)*	*X-rays*	*Treatment*	*Immobilization or union*
Mandible	Deranged dental occlusion Disturbed mental sensation Sublingual haematoma	1. Right and left lateral obliques of mandible or OPG 2. PA mandible (P) 3. Occlusal (true and oblique) 4. Towne's view for condyles (ideally Reverse (P))	Intermaxillary fixation (IMF) Skeletal fixation in unstable cases	Unilateral 4 weeks Bilateral 6 weeks Unilateral condyle 10 days
Maxilla Le Fort I	Anterior open bite I, II, III Circumorbital ecchymosis II, III Subconjunctival haemorrhage II, III	1. Occipitomental (P) 2. 30° Occipitomental (P)	Craniomaxillary Fixation, plus IMF	4 weeks
Maxilla Le Fort II Maxilla Le Fort III	Epistaxis I, II, III Disturbed infraorbital sensation II Guérin's sign I	3. Lateral of facial bones		
Zygoma	Circumorbital ecchymosis Subconjunctival haemorrhage Unilateral epistaxis Lack of cheek prominence Disturbed infraorbital sensation Trapped coronoid Diplopia	1. Occipitomental (P) 2. 30° Occipitomental (P) 3. Submentovertical	Elevation by temporal approach Skeletal wiring in unstable cases	4 weeks
Orbital blow-out	Disturbed infraorbital sensation Diplopia Muscle entrapment Enophthalmos	1. Occipitomental (P) 2. 30° Occipitomental (P) 3. CT scan orbits	Pack antrum and/or orbital floor implant or graft	3 weeks
Nasal bones	Epistaxis Asymmetry of nose Circumorbital ecchymosis Subconjunctival haemorrhage	Lateral nasal bones Occipitofrontal (P)	Reduction by: Walsham's forceps, Ashe's forceps POP splint or lead plates	3 weeks

NB: (P) indicates that this view requires the patients to be turned face downwards which may be contraindicated in a major trauma case. Alternative, if inferior, views in these cases are: PA mandible–AP mandible, Reverse Towne's view–Towne's view, Occipitomental–Mento-occipital, Occipitofrontal–AP skull.

Lateral nasal bones

This is useful in establishing the presence of a fracture, although care should be taken not to interpret the normal suture between the frontal and nasal bones as a discontinuity. Clinical examination is of more importance than radiographs in nasal fractures and the signs are detailed in the following section.

The various radiographs detailed above are summarized in Table 44.1. Those views requiring the patients to be in the prone position are marked with a P and alternatives are suggested if this is not advisable.

Section 44.5 • Computed tomography scanning (Figure 44.17)

CT scanning may provide useful information in relationship to injuries of the facial bones. It may be used in the following circumstances.

At time of brain scanning

Many cases of head injury will be examined by CT scanning for suspected intracranial injury or to exclude acute intracerebral pathology such as extradural haematoma. If clinical signs suggest fracture of the facial bones, particularly the nasoethmoidal complex and maxilla, it is advisable to ask the radiologist to extend the scan to include the facial region. This allows a more rapid and accurate diagnosis of maxillofacial injuries to be made in the severely injured patient who may be unfit for conventional radiography for some time.

As an extra investigation

Certain cases may prove difficult to diagnose with certainty on conventional radiographic views. This particularly applies to orbital injuries (such as the orbital floor blow-out and the much rarer medial blow-out) and nasoethmoidal injuries (such as those involving displacement of the bony attachments of the medial canthal ligaments). Tomography is often helpful in such cases but CT scanning may be even more definitive. For examination of the orbits and nasoethmoidal skeleton a coronal view is the ideal. The newer imaging modality of nuclear magnetic resonance (NMR) does not image bone and is therefore not utilized in the diagnosis of facial bone fractures.

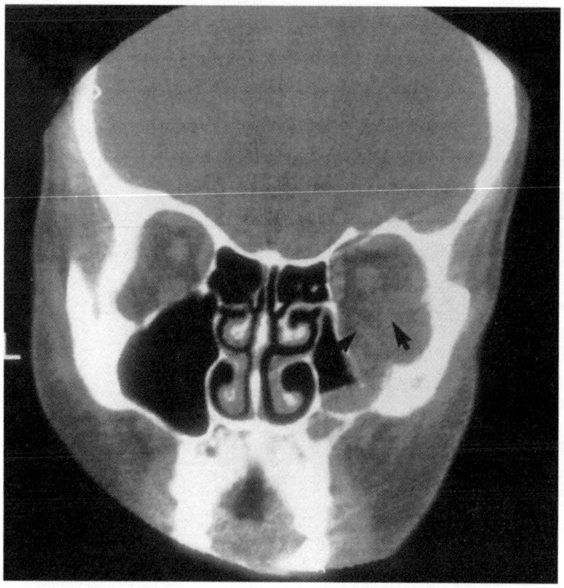

Figure 44.17 CT scan in the coronal plane of a patient who was complaining of double vision and numbness of the cheek after a fist blow to the left orbit 6 days previously. The scan showns a very large orbital blow-out fracture prolapsed into the left antrum (in which there is a fluid level due to blood). It is possible to discern the optic nerves near the mid-points of the orbits and the inferior oblique and inferior rectus muscles, which are involved in the blow-out on the left and indicated by arrows.

Section 44.6 • Signs of individual facial fractures

Mandible

The signs that may be seen in fracture of the mandible are summarized in Figure 44.18. Especially significant are the following.

Deranged occlusion

If the patient has teeth or wears dentures then in a displaced fracture it is likely that the dental occlusion will be altered. In the normal state the mandible is in a state of balance between the elevator muscles (pterygomasseteric sling) and the depressor muscles (digastrics and mylohyoids). When fracture occurs the mandible may be separated into different segments, each of which may be displaced by the actions of one group of muscles alone so that the normal balance is disrupted. A typical example of this is shown in Figure 44.18.

Fractures of the condyles, vertical ramus and angle region are prone to exhibit telescoping of the affected region by the pull of the pterygomasseteric sling. This causes premature contact of the posterior molar teeth which may be on both sides in bilateral fractures or unilateral in one-sided fracture. Fractures in the posterior body region of the mandible tend to have the minor fragment pulled upwards and inwards by the sling. Bilateral fractures of the anterior part of the mandible may allow the symphyseal region to be pulled downwards and backwards by the digastric muscles with a risk of airway obstruction. Midline fractures of the mandible may allow both sides to collapse in somewhat under the influence of the mylohyoid muscles. The degree of displacement that occurs depends on the mobility within the fracture site and also the obliquity of the fracture. A fracture may be described as horizontally favourable or unfavourable depending on whether displacement is discouraged or encouraged in the particular plane.

Deranged mental sensation

The inferior dental nerve runs through a large part of the lower jaw from the mandibular foramen to the mental foramen. It may be traumatized in this course by fractures and sensory impairment may occur. This may be total (anaesthesia) or partial where the patient has a sense of touch but cannot perceive pinprick (paraesthesia) or where light touch and pinprick can be felt but the sensation feels different from the other side (dysaesthesia). Occasionally sensation may be accentuated by comparison with the other side (hyperaesthesia) but this is more usually seen during a phase of nerve recovery.

Haematoma formation

It is usual to see some degree of haematoma formation in the region of a fracture. Lingual haematoma is almost certainly pathognomonic of fractured mandible, as this area is protected from external trauma.

Fractures of the condyle of the mandible usually exhibit tenderness over the pre-auricular region, and there may be unilateral premature contact of molar teeth on the affected side if telescoping of fragments has occurred. In fracture dislocation a finger in the

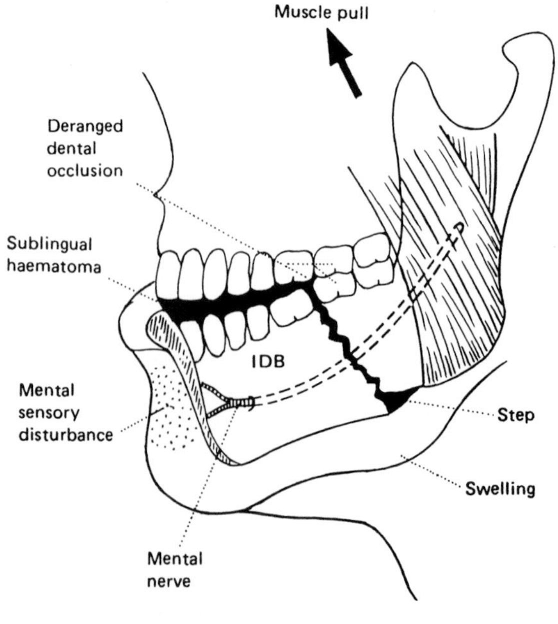

Figure 44.18 Signs of fracture of mandible. IDB, Inferior dental bundle comprising inferior dental nerve and vessels.

external auditory meatus while the patient opens and closes the mandible will detect that no movement is felt in the glenoid fossa on the affected side.

Maxilla

There are three classic fracture sites of the maxilla as described by Le Fort. They are shown in Figure 44.19 together with their associated signs. The classic Le Fort fracture lines are:

Le Fort (low level or Guérin) fracture

This fracture line starts at the lateral aspect of the pyriform fossa and extends above the roots of the teeth under the zygomatic buttress and across the pterygoid plates low down. It also traverses the lower part of the nasal septum. It separates the dentoalveolar part of the maxilla from the rest of the cranial skeleton. The fragment may be surprisingly mobile (floating maxilla). There is usually evidence of haematoma formation in the buccal sulcus throughout its extent. Epistaxis is common as the fracture lines run through the antral cavities which communicate with the nose. Dental occlusion may be deranged and the classic malocclusion is that of an anterior open bite, as with all maxillary fractures.

Le Fort II fracture (pyramidal)

A higher level fracture such as the Le Fort II is often characterized by major facial oedema. This fracture courses across the nasal bones into the medial part of the orbit and then across the anterior aspect of the maxilla in the region of the infraorbital foramen to cut across the pterygoid plates near their mid point. There is an associated fracture across the nasal septum. As the fracture runs through the orbit there is commonly circumorbital ecchymosis ('panda eyes') and subconjunctival haemorrhage. Epistaxis is likely to occur and CSF leak may be present. An anterior open bite is the classic occlusal deformity.

Le Fort III fracture (high level or craniofacial dysjunction)

This is a very major injury where the whole of the maxilla and the zygoma is sheared off the rest of the cranium. There is commonly major facial oedema. Circumorbital ecchymosis and subconjuctival haemorrhage are likely to occur. A hooded appearance of the upper eyelids may occur as the maxilla can be driven downwards and backwards along the plane of the sphenoids taking with it the suspensory ligaments of Lockwood which support the

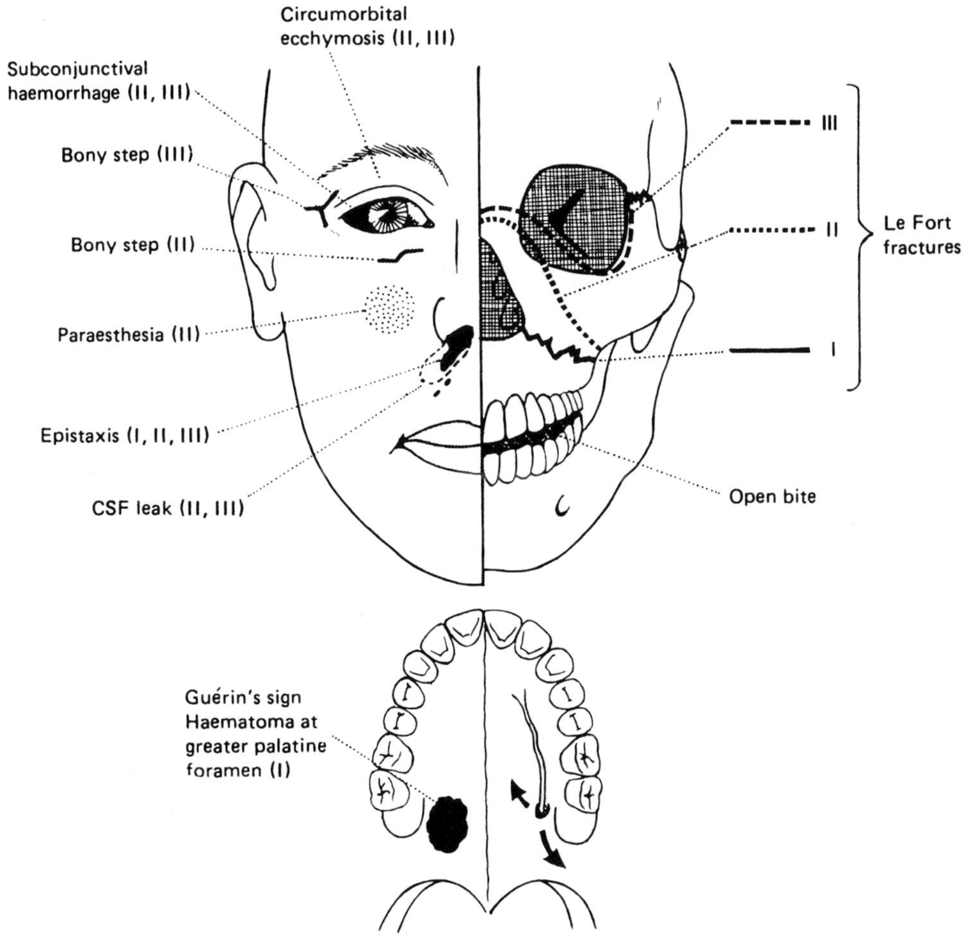

Figure 44.19 Signs of fracture of maxilla.

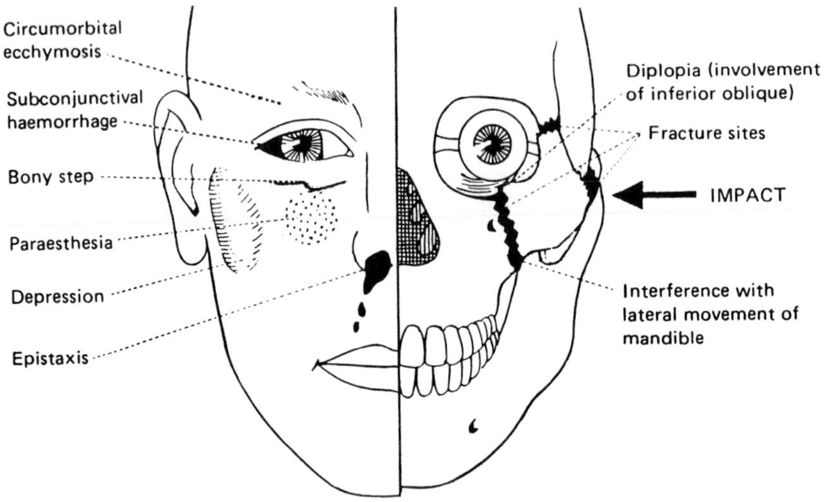

Figure 44.20 Signs of fracture of zygoma.

eyes. There is a great risk of CSF rhinorrhoea due to the high level fracture running through the region of the cribriform plate and posterior walls of the frontal sinuses.

It should be emphasized that the classic Le Fort fracture sites are not always found and it is not uncommon to see fractures at different levels on two sides or for fractures to be present at two or more sites.

Zygoma

In the USA this frature is often known as a 'trimalar' fracture as there are usually three main fracture sites, i.e. at the frontomalar suture, at the zygomatic arch and in the region of the zygomaticomaxillary suture close to the infraorbital foramen. The important signs are summarized in Figure 44.20. They are:

- circumorbital ecchymosis and subconjunctival haemorrhage
- sensory changes in the regions of the infraorbital nerve. These are also commonly seen in Le Fort's II fractures of the maxilla
- unilateral epistaxis
- lack of normal cheek prominence due to depression
- interference with lateral movement of the mandible due to impingement on the coronoid process (may occur in arch fractures particularly)
- ocular disturbance.

As part of the fracture site involves the orbital floor it is common for bruising to occur in the most inferior extraocular muscles, i.e. the inferior oblique and inferior rectus. This may produce some defect of function of these muscles with resulting double vision or diplopia. In simple bruising this will settle with time but if the muscles are actually entrapped in the fracture site such improvement does not occur and defective elevation of the eye is usually obvious.

One must be aware of the orbital 'blow-out' fracture where the floor of the orbit caves into the antral cavity (Figure 44.21). This may occur alone (pure 'blow-out') or in combination with other neighbouring fractures (impure orbital 'blow-out'). Entrapment of the inferior oblique may occur. In major 'blow-out' fractures where a major degree of orbital fat prolapses into the antrum, fat atrophy and scarring may produce a progressive diplopia and loss of prominence and lowering of the eye (enophthalmos). This may occur some weeks or even months after the actual fracture.

Nose

Lateral blows tend to displace the nose to the contralateral side. Anterior trauma tends to result in a depression of the nasal bridge and widening of the intercanthal distance. Circumorbital ecchymosis and medial subconjunctival haemorrhage is likely. Epistaxis is obviously very common and will be bilateral (Figure 44.22). Septal deflection may occur so that the interior of the nose should always be inspected to detect this fracture and also a septal haematoma which requires urgent drainage to prevent cartilage necrosis.

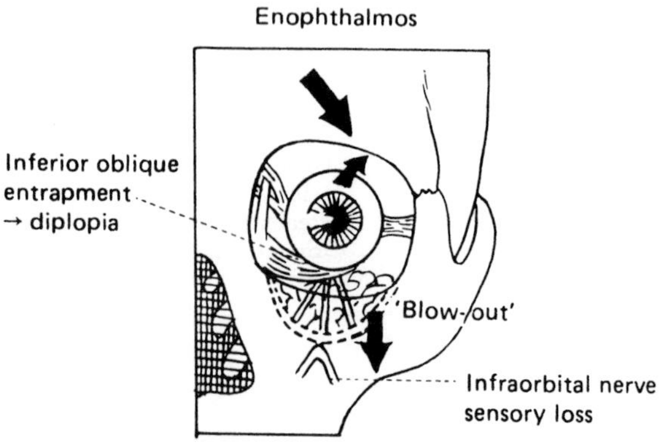

Figure 44.21 Orbital 'blow-out' fracture.

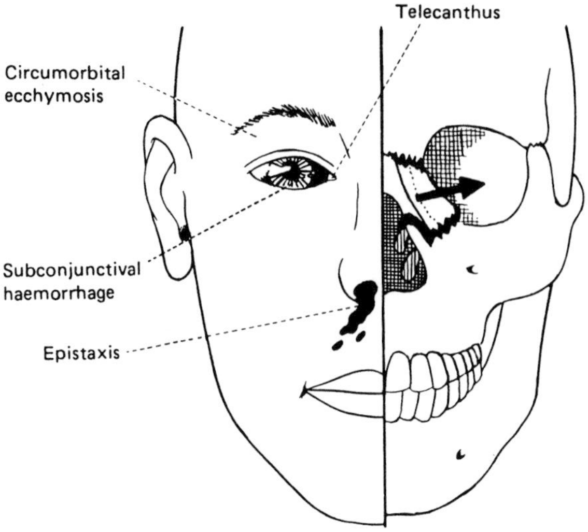

Figure 44.22 Nasal bone fracture.

Section 44.7 • Treatment of maxillofacial injuries

Primary treatment

It should be emphasized that a maxillofacial injury must be seen in the context of the patient's general status and other injuries. In multiple trauma cases it is often good policy to delay definitive treatment of the maxillofacial injury until the full extent of the patient's other injuries is established and stabilization is obtained of the major systems. There is a real danger in subjecting a patient to general anaesthesia shortly after major trauma unless this is necessary for life-threatening injury such as a ruptured spleen or a middle meningeal haemorrhage. One normally has about 10 days before a provisional union occurs in which definitive redution and fixation may be carried out. Simple maxillofacial injuries on their own can, of course, be treated without delay. There are, however, certain emergencies which may present initially in a maxillofacial injury and which require primary treatment.

Obstruction of the airway (Figure 44.23)

An unstable bilateral fracture of the anterior part of the mandible may allow the attachment of the tongue to be posteriorly displaced under the influence of the digastric muscles as shown in Figure 44.23(a). A fracture of the maxilla with gross posterior displacement may occlude the nasal airway and force the soft palate down on to the dorsum of the tongue, again with obstruction (Figure 44.23b). Such events require emergency measures. The mouth should be cleared of blood and debris manually and suction applied. If the tongue has fallen back it may be brought forward by pushing a finger behind it and inserting a large tongue suture through the dorsum of the tongue or grasping it with a towel clip. A posteriorly displaced maxilla may be brought forwards and upwards by two fingers passed behind the soft palate to quickly bring the jaw forward. After these initial measures attention must be given to obtaining a more permanent airway. In the case of maxillary injury nasopharyngeal airways may be passed through both nostrils and may suffice. An alternative measure, which is likely to be necessary with an unstable mandible or combination injuries is to intubate the patient. After this, consideration can be given to the need for tracheostomy although it should seldom be necessary to perform an emergency tracheostomy without the presence of an endotracheal tube.

Bleeding (Figure 44.24)

Major life-threatening haemorrhage is seldom a feature of maxillofacial injury. Indeed in a patient who shows signs of hypovolaemia, such as a lowered blood pressure, one should exclude other injuries more likely to give this picture, such as a ruptured spleen.

Arterial bleeders or a venous ooze may be encountered. Pressure packs held firmly in place for approximately 10 min will usually deal with the problem, but a persistent arterial bleeder requires clamping.

Occasionally in maxillary or nasal fractures, nose bleeding may be very profuse. Anterior nasal packing may be tried but often it is necessary to pass bilateral post-nasal packs. The technique for this is illustrated in Figure 44.24(c). It involves passing a soft rubber catheter down the nasal cavity so that it can be grasped behind the soft palate and pulled forward through the mouth. This enables a tape to be attached to it which connects with a post-nasal pack. Traction on the rubber catheter brings the pack round the back of the soft palate to lodge in the posterior nares. The traction tape is tied to the face as is also a small tape acting as a tail which is left tied to the corner of the mouth to enable eventual removal of the pack. A Foley type catheter can be used as an alternative or there are now purpose-designed inflatable nasal catheters on the market. Post-nasal packs should not normally be left for longer than 48 hour because of the risk of infection, although this is minimized by prescription of antibiotics. Following the insertion of the post-nasal pack, conventional anterior nasal packs should be inserted to reinforce their effect.

In a very occasional case even the above measures may fail to arrest bleeding, and consideration may need to be given to ligation of the external carotid artery on the affected side. This is often not as effective as might be hoped because of the cross-over circulation from the opposite side but may help in the overall control of a difficult situation.

Pain relief

Surprisingly many maxillofacial injuries are not very painful in the early stages. Presumably this is due to trauma of the peripheral nerve branches at the fracture site. Narcotics may be indicated, but great care should be given in administrating opiates in cases of head

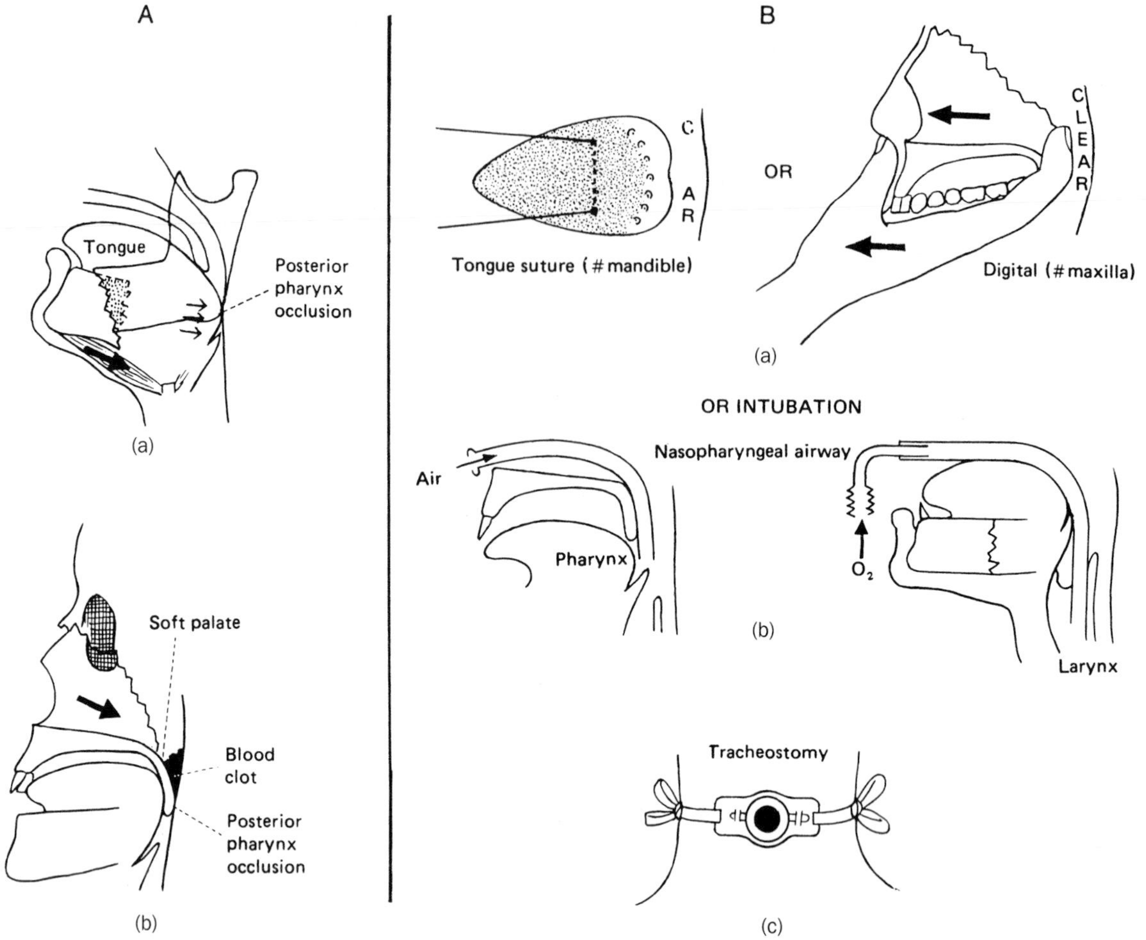

Figure 44.23 Airways obstruction. A, Problem. (a) Displaced bilateral fracture of mandible. (b) Fractured maxilla displaced backwards and downwards. B, Remedy. (a) Immediate. (b) Intermediate. (c) Definitive.

injury, lest changes of consciousness are obscured and pupillary changes masked. Conservative doses of pentazocine can be administered with caution.

The use of supportive bandages to help discomfort is a traditional first aid method. The Barton bandage has a time-established place in the history of primary treatment. Such supports, however, can provoke more pain and disturbance unless they are very carefully applied. A crêpe bandage gently taken from under the chin to over the crown of the head and then around tansversely, with turns going under the external occipital protuberance, can provide a gentle support in some cases. It can be reinforced with stretch Elastoplast. The majority of cases, however, do not need these measures.

Prevention of infection

In high level fractures of the maxilla and naso-ethmoidal fractures there is a risk of meningitis associated with CSF leak. Current neurosurgical practice is to withhold prophylactic antibiotics.

In compound fractures either externally or into the mouth antibiotic medication is indicated, usually with penicillin.

Where facial laceration may have been contaminated with dirt there is a need to provide protection against tetanus **[Module 5, Vol. I]**

Fracture of mandible

If the patient has teeth then intermaxillary fixation (IMF) is employed to fix the teeth of the mandible to those in the maxilla. Dental occlusion provides a good guide to accurate reduction. Eyelet wiring or the use of arch bars or the employment of cap splints (Figure 44.25) may be indicated. Eyelet wires are used where there is a good dentition, but arch bars will help where gaps are present. Cap splints are particularly helpful in more complex fractures. Where the patient has no teeth, Gunning splints can be constructed which are secured to the jaws themselves usually by peralveolar wires in the upper and circumferential wires in the lower. It is of great help in the construction of Gunning splints to have the patient's dentures, and the casualty officer should obtain these for the oral surgeon when he first sees the patient. Even if the dentures have been broken they can still prove of considerable use.

In unstable fractures, IMF alone may be insufficient for control, so that open reduction is indicated with

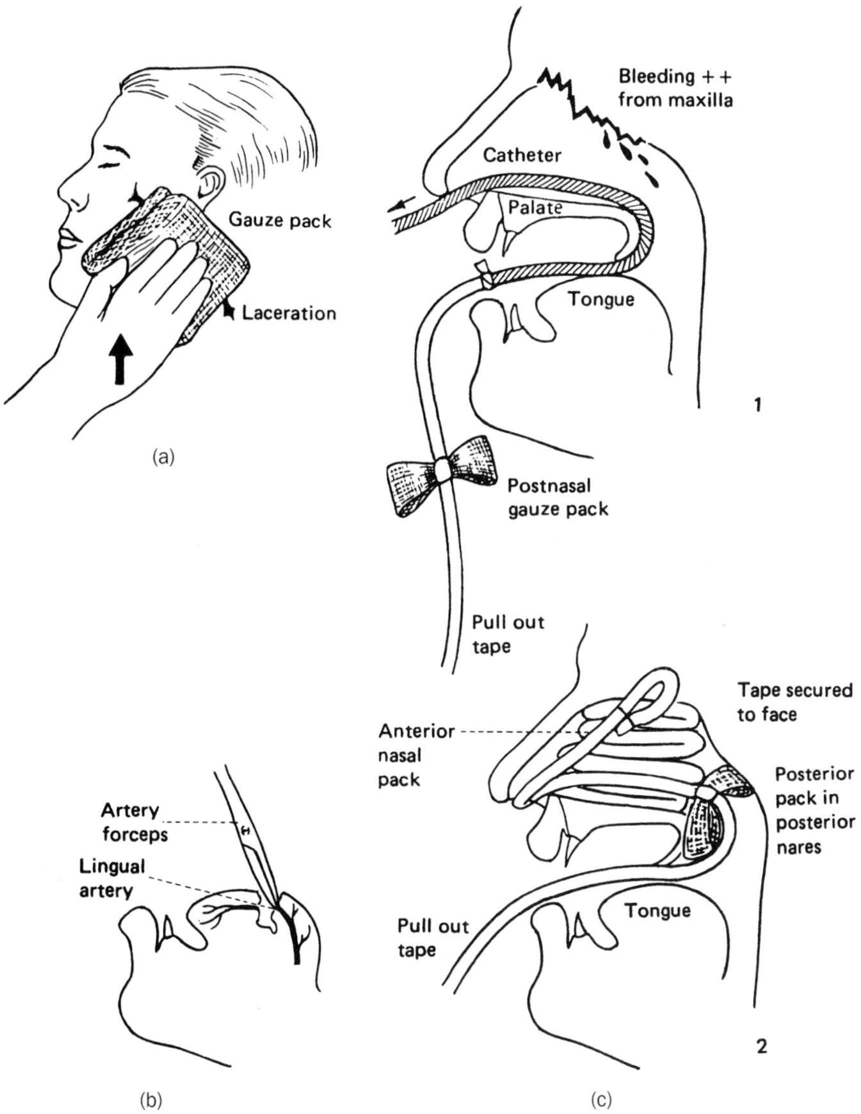

Figure 44.24 Control of bleeding. (a) Pressure. (b) Clamping arterial bleeders. (c) Nasal packing for persistent epistaxis, e.g. fracture of maxilla. 1. Introduction. 2. Secured (leave = 48 hours + antibiotic).

skeletal fixation by lower border or upper border wiring, bone plating or alternatively pinning. Fixation after mandible fracture is for approximately 4 weeks in unilateral cases but may require 6 weeks in bilateral cases or even longer in grossly comminuted fractures, atrophic mandibles or very elderly patients. Unilateral fractures of the condyle may only require 10 days' fixation. Fractures of the condyle normally only require treatment if the patient is unable to attain centric occlusion.

Fracture of maxilla

It is not sufficient in fractures of the maxilla to carry out intermaxillary fixation as mandibular movements will be transmitted to the maxilla and there is a real danger of pumping organisms through the region of the cribriform plate with a risk of meningitis. After reduction with Rowe forceps, cranial fixation should be undertaken and ideally this is to the maxilla

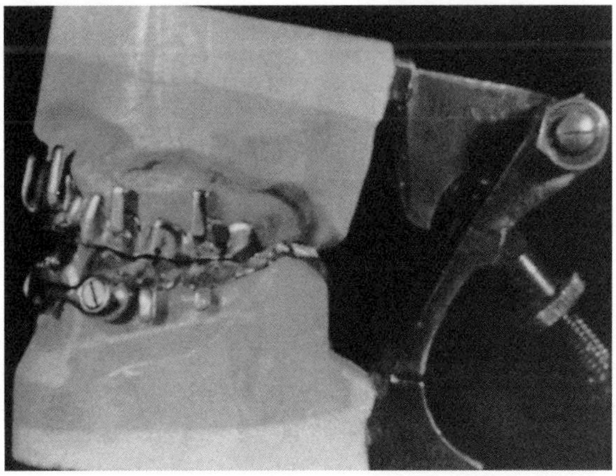

Figure 44.25 Cap splints. The jaws are immobilized together (intermaxillary fixation) by passing wires around the hooks on the upper and lower splints.

(craniomaxillary fixation). A 'halo' or Levant type frame (Figure 44.26) or plastic headcap is used and this is linked to the splint in the upper jaw via projection bars and universal joints. Alternatively, in minimally displaced fractures, internal suspension wires may be used and either attached to the pyriform aperture or over the zygomatic arches or from the frontal bone above the frontomalar suture. The site of the origin of the suspension wire must obviously be above the known fracture site. Four weeks is normally sufficient for union of a fractured maxilla.

Fracture of zygoma

The majority of simple zygomatic fractures can be reduced via an incision in the temporal region which passes through the temporalis fascia allowing an instrument to be slipped down beneath the zygomatic arch. The instrument (an elevator) can then lift up the displaced part (Figure 44.27). Union is normally complete in about 4 weeks. More complex fractures may require exposure of the fracture sites at the frontomalar suture and/or infraorbital margins with direct skeletal wiring.

An orbital blow-out fracture in isolation can often be remedied by direct surgical exposure of the orbital floor through an infra-orbital or eyelid incision with the insertion of an orbital floor implant.

Nasal fracture

Reduction is carried out with Walsham's forceps for the nasal bones and frontal processes of the maxilla (Figure 44.28). Ashe's septal forceps are used to attempt to reposition the displaced septum in the vomerine groove although this can be difficult. Immobilization of the fracture is obtained with a plaster-of-Paris nasal splint which is left on for 5–7 days. In unstable cases, lead plates and a vertical mattress suture of wire can be used.

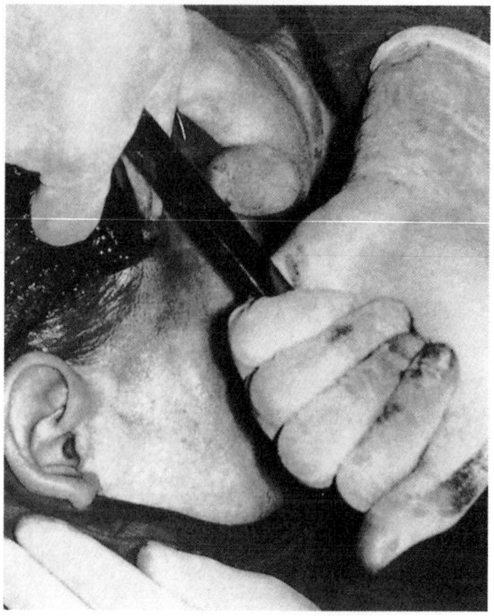

Figure 44.27 Elevating a fracture of the zygoma by the Gillies temporal approach.

It can be difficult to obtain adequate control of a displaced nasal septum, and if the healed position is inadequate then a subsequent operative procedure several weeks later can be carried out in the form of a nasal septoplasty or occasionally a submucosal resection of part of the nasal septum.

Occasionally the insertion of the medial canthal ligaments may be disrupted together with a small related fragment of bone. In these cases surgical exposure may be necessary together with wiring which needs to be carried out with a special technique in view of the thin nature of the bone.

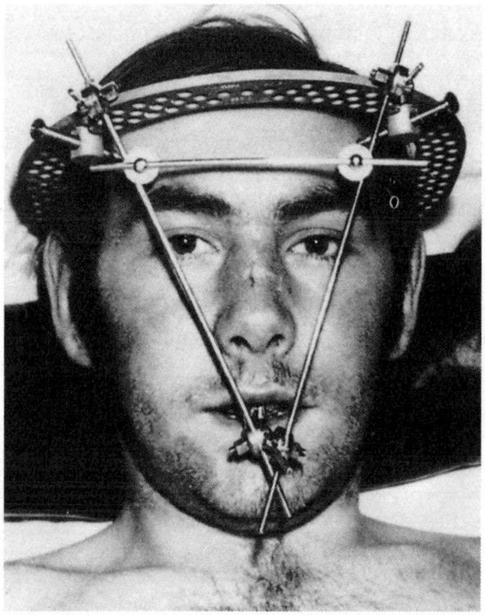

Figure 44.26 A 'halo' frame providing craniomaxillary fixation for a fracture of the maxilla.

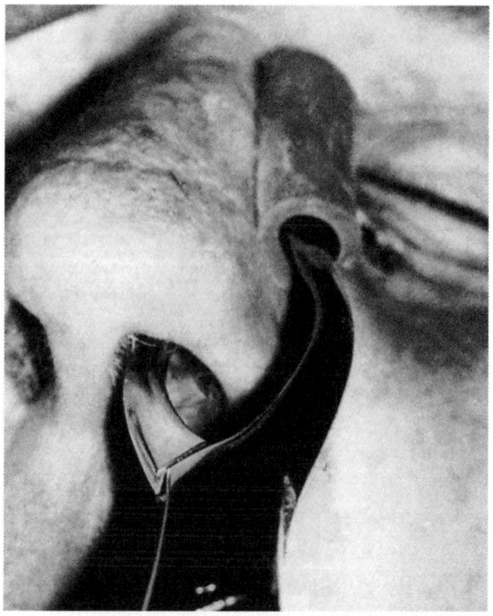

Figure 44.28 Reduction of a nasal bone fracture with a Walsham's forceps.

Section 44.8 • Conclusion

In general, fractures of the facial skeleton heal well due to the excellent blood supply of the area. Indeed, prompt recognition is necessary as definitive reduction needs to be undertaken within 10 days of injury because a degree of early union will be encountered after this time. This behoves a knowledge of the signs and symptoms of such injuries in those responsible for the management of trauma victims. It is, however, vital to take into account other co-existing conditions, particularly in the central nervous system, thorax and abdomen, which should take precedence because of their life-threatening nature. Facial injuries do not constitute an emergency unless they threaten the airway or are a source of haemorrhage. Should malunion occur due to inevitable delay, as for example in a severe head injury, a range of procedures is now available for eventual osteotomy and definitive reduction.

Prevention is obviously the ideal form of management. Legislation to ensure the wearing of front seatbelts has brought about a significant reduction in maxillofacial trauma and this may be enhanced further by the general use of rear seatbelts.

Management will be helped by extension of knowledge of the mechanisms of traumatic damage. For example, a better understanding of compartmentalization within the orbital fat is leading to improved insight into orbital blow-out fractures.

Accurate radiographic diagnosis is obviously a preliminary to good reduction. Tomography helps greatly in more difficult cases. CT scanning is finding an increasing role, as in orbital injuries where it may localize unusual sites of blow-out and of course, very importantly, in the evaluation of concomitant head injuries.

Bone plating techniques are becoming more widely used in maxillofacial practice. Compressive plates are now available (Figure 44.29) although their use requires very careful technique to avoid the creation of occlusal discrepancies. It may be possible to dispense with intermaxillary fixation in many cases. This may be very valuable in mentally compromised patients or where there is a risk of ankylosis due to prolonged immobilization as in intracapsular condylar fractures, or in the presence of other injuries as in the thorax requiring a free airway. Additionally, many subjects wish to return to activity as soon as possible in a time of economic recession where prolonged convalescence can lead to a deterioration in clientele in self-employed occupations or even job loss.

There is a growing awareness that a combined craniofacial approach may be necessary in certain instances. This particularly applies to severe nasoethmoidal injuries associated with damage to the anterior cranial fossa in the region of the posterior walls of the frontal sinuses and the cribriform plate. Co-operation between neurosurgeons and maxillofacial surgeons has led to improved management in this field. Indeed, growing mutual understanding between all those specialties dealing with the victims of trauma is a continuing aim to provide optimal therapy for patients.

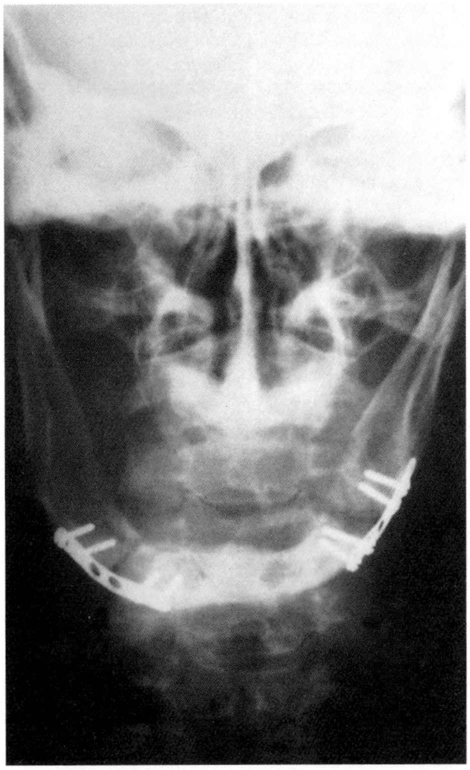

Figure 44.29 Fracture of an atrophic mandible on postero-anterior radiography showing treatment by compressive bone plating. Bone plates are particularly useful where one wishes to avoid intermaxillary fixation either because it would not give a precise reduction or because of poor patient compliance as in a mentally disturbed subject.

Modern trends

Several trends in modern regimens of management of maxillofacial injuries can be summarized:

- There is a tendency towards treatment of the majority of displaced bony injuries by osteosynthesis with titanium non-compressive mini-plates. In the case of mandibular fractures and low level maxillary fractures, these are inserted via an intraoral approach. In the case of high level maxillary injuries combined with severe involvement of the nasoethmoidal complex, the use of the bi-coronal flap gives greatly improved access; this may be shared with the neurosurgeons where there are associated fractures of the anterior cranial fossa requiring attention. The increased use of osteosynthesis has resulted in a much lesser need for long term intermaxillary fixation which reduces the need for special nursing care necessary where the airway is at hazard; it also reduces morbidity for the patient. However, the use of rigid bone plates allows much less adjustment post-operatively of any minor occlusal irregularities necessitating very accurate primary reduction to avoid dental malocclusion. The titanium bone plates do not require removal unless there are signs of infection in the long-term post-operative management.

- Pilot schemes involving helicopter evacuation of major trauma victims (e.g. Royal London Hospital HEMS) show the prospect for survival of subjects with very complex multi-system injuries including head and neck involvement. A number of these cases tend to show concomitant fractures of all the facial bones providing a challenge to reconstruction of the face. Often it is advisable to reconstitute the mandible by open reduction and bone plating as a first measure to provide a template to which the other bones may be reduced. A common order of procedure is frequently reconstitution of the mandible, elevation of zygomas, reduction of the maxilla with plating, final adjustment and plating of zygomatic complex, nasal reduction and lastly, repair of facial lacerations. Tracheotomy is frequently needed in the early management of these cases, which tend to hazard the airway.
- There is interest in the use of ultrasound as a screening method for detecting facial fractures. With the increasing use of small parts ultrasound apparatus, this trend may in the future offer possibilities in the accident & emergency department. Its role would be in confirming whether or not a fracture was present. Conventional radiography would still be necessary for those cases requiring operative intervention, as ultrasound would only detect the superficial aspect of a fracture line. The latter method is most applicable to relatively flat superficial bony surfaces and requires probes of a rating around 10 MHz.

Overall, the trend is for more accurate surgical reduction with less morbidity to the patient combined with a lesser demand on nursing services.

Further reading

Killey, H. C. (revised by P. Banks) (1983). *Fractures of the Mandible*. Bristol: Wright.

Killey, H. C. (revised by P. Banks) (1987). *Fractures of the Middle Third of the Facial Skeleton*. Bristol: Wright.

Rowe, N. L. and Williams, J. L. (1994). *Maxillofacial Injuries*, Vols 1 and 2. Edinburgh: Churchill Livingstone.

MODULE 45

Neck lumps

Section 45.1 • General considerations

Surgeons caring for patients with diseases of the head and neck need to be fully familiar with the complex anatomy and physiology of this region. Conventionally different aspects of care have been devolved to separate medical and dental disciplines, not always to the patient's benefit. No individual clinician possesses the multiplicity of skills necessary to undertake all aspects of diagnosis and treatment of head and neck disease. It is increasingly recognized that only interdisciplinary teams which include nurses and therapists are able to offer optimal care particularly for those patients afflicted by cancer of the head and neck.

Because the head and neck is such a visible part of the body and because the patient's sense of identity is so closely associated with his facial features it is important when operating in this area to take into account not only functional, but also cosmetic considerations. Functional disturbances in the head and neck include disordered breathing, speaking and swallowing. In the last 20 years or so reconstructive techniques have improved immeasurably although disappointingly overall survival rates for many head and neck cancers have not improved greatly during this period. The day of the mutilated patient who could neither speak nor swallow and was incontinent of saliva should now be long gone. This is not to say that all patients with head and neck cancer can be cured or even effectively palliated. Many such patients have multisystem disease. They often present late with advanced tumours and those charged with their care must ensure that if the patient is genuinely incurable their last few months of life are not rendered more miserable by inappropriate and futile therapy.

Major advances have been made in the outpatient endoscopic examination of the various cavities in the head and neck. The traditional armamentarium of the otolaryngologist/head and neck surgeon of head mirror, bullseye lamp and laryngeal and nasopharyngeal mirrors is used less and less as improved light sources

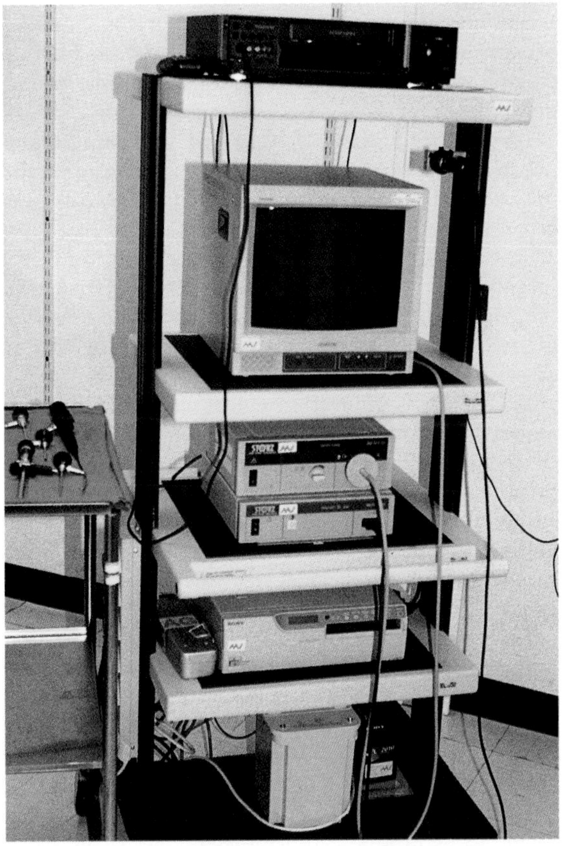

Figure 45.1 A typical 'tower' of equipment for outpatient use in examination and documentation of the head and neck.

and rigid and flexible endoscopes become more widely available (Figure 45.1).

These, combined with miniature cameras which can be attached to the endoscopes, together with high-resolution monitors, have revolutionized the outpatient examination of patients with head and neck disease. Not only are higher quality images available to the surgeon, but these can be captured in various ways and stored in the patient's records. They can be shown to and discussed with the patient and relatives as appropriate. They also provide an unsurpassed teaching resource for students and staff. An important economic benefit is that patients who previously would have required examination under anaesthesia can now be adequately assessed in the outpatient clinic.

Current imaging techniques of the head and neck have also resulted in greatly improved appreciation of the nature and the extent of head and neck disease. Computed tomography (CT) and magnetic resonance imaging (MRI) scans have resulted in improved appreciation of structural changes and are particularly valuable in the determination of the extent of head and neck cancers. Delineation of tissue masses has allowed the extent of the necessary surgery and if appropriate, reconstruction to be planned in detail prior to surgery. Conventional radiological techniques still have a place in the imaging of head and neck disease and examination by techniques such as videofluoroscopy and contrast swallow are invaluable in assessing disturbances of function. Ultrasound examination is useful in distinguishing between solid and cystic masses and may be used as one type of image guided technique for fine needle aspiration biopsy.

In the investigation of head and neck lumps fine needle aspiration cytology (FNAC) is now an established diagnostic technique. Dedicated cytopathologists or pathologists with a special interest in this area generate very high levels of diagnostic accuracy in FNAC specimens. Interpretation must always be undertaken in the context of the clinical findings and close communication between the clinician and the cytopathologist allows for high levels of accuracy in reporting.

Endoscopic examination under anaesthesia is still required in many patients to establish the extent and the nature of the disease process and to obtain adequate biopsy material for histological examination. However, as indicated above, because of the improved endoscopic visualization available on an outpatient basis fewer endoscopies under general anaesthesia are nowadays required.

Conventional blood tests rarely add greatly to the management of patients with head and neck disease. Standard biochemical parameters are rarely disturbed in such patients, unless there has been a period of dysphagia for solids and liquids when the patient may become dehydrated, hypoproteinaemic and hypokalaemic. More specific blood tests such as detection of autoantibody to neutrophil cytoplasmic antigens (ANCA) in Wegener's granulomatosis or angiotensin-converting enzyme (ACE) levels in sarcoidosis are helpful in the diagnosis in certain specific conditions.

The role of tumour markers in the investigation of head and neck cancer is still largely experimental. The main exception to this is the measurement of anti-Epstein–Barr virus antibodies in patients at high risk of developing nasopharyngeal carcinoma, such as the population of Hong Kong. A wide range of antigens in head and neck cancers have been studied using immunohistochemistry. These include p53, cyclin D1, epidermal growth factor receptor (EGFR) and proliferation markers. Tumours from different sites in the head and neck exhibit different biological behaviours and to make an accurate assessment of a factor's value requires a large scale study of a well-defined tumour population. These new techniques offer the potential of giving information about the likelihood of such clinically important issues as the chance of nodal metastases in a clinically negative neck, the chance of locoregion recurrence following therapy and the chance of developing a metachronous primary. It seems likely that the measurement of a number of such factors will provide more valuable prognostic information than any single marker alone.

Section 45.2 • Congenital neck lumps

Thyroglossal cyst

Embryology

The anlage of the thyroid gland arises as an outpouching from the floor of the primitive pharynx. It enlarges caudally as a diverticulum and as the heart and great vessels descend it develops as a bilobed structure leaving a tract behind. The distal bilobed end develops into the lobes of the thyroid gland and the stalk, when it persists, becomes the pyramidal lobe of the thyroid gland and the thyroglossal tract. The tract usually disappears leaving the foramen caecum at the tongue base as the only evidence in the adult of its site of origin. If the thyroid tissue fails to descend into the neck it persists as a lingual thyroid at the tongue base. The most common condition resulting from persistence of remnants of the thyroglossal tract is the thyroglossal cyst. There are no natural internal or external openings of the tract. A thyroglossal sinus may result from infection and subsequent rupture of a cyst, drainage of a cyst or incomplete removal of a cyst.

The thyroglossal duct tract is intimately related to the hyoid bone. Some embryological studies suggest that the developing hyoid bone is pulled downwards by the attached strap muscles resulting in indentation of the thyroglossal tract remnant. In the adult the persisting thyroglossal tract is described as passing down in front of the hyoid bone and then hooking up around its inferior border to lie posterior to the bone before finally descending to the thyroid isthmus. Others studies suggest that as the hyoid bone develops from lateral to medial the tract may lie in front, behind or even run through the hyoid bone. The important practical surgical consideration is that the tract cannot be successfully dissected from the hyoid bone at operation and the central part of the hyoid bone must be removed.

Clinical features

Thyroglossal cysts occur equally commonly in males and in females. They may present at any age, but usually do so in childhood or young adulthood. The cyst may occur at any point between the foramen caecum above and the manubrium below and the anterior borders of the sternomastoid muscles laterally. Most cysts lie in the midline with 10% being to one side of which the vast majority occur on the left. The most common site is just in front or slightly below the hyoid bone, but a few will present in the suprahyoid area or at the level of the thyroid or cricoid cartilage. Very occasionally a cyst will present at the tongue base.

The commonest presentation is as a symptomless lump in the midline of the neck (Figure 45.2). Thyroglossal cysts rarely produce pressure symptoms unless they are large and tense. The lump is freely mobile from side to side. It moves on swallowing and will also rise on protrusion of the tongue when the mouth is open. This latter sign is pathognomonic. Some patients present with a thyroglossal cyst abscess which may rupture resulting in spontaneous sinus formation. The cyst and duct are lined with squamous epithelium or sometimes pseudo-stratified ciliated columnar epithelium. Occasionally no epithelial lining can be identified. Thyroid tissue may be present in the cyst wall. Some cysts may form on both sides of the hyoid bone resulting in a dumb-bell shaped lesion. Most cysts contain thick, viscous mucus. The differential diagnosis includes dermoid cyst, sebaceous cyst, lipoma, enlarged lymph node, hypertrophic pyramidal lobe of the thyroid gland and choristoma.

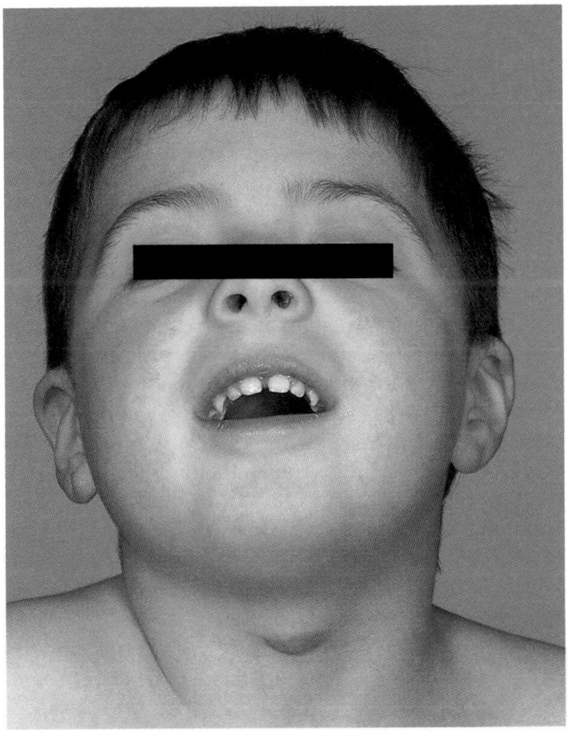

Figure 45.2 Thyroglossal duct cyst.

Investigation

The cystic nature of the lesion can usually be confirmed by ultrasound examination. This investigation will also allow the detection of a normally positioned thyroid gland. Thyroid function tests are usually normal. If there is any doubt about the presence of a normal thyroid gland an isotope scan will identify all functioning thyroid tissue.

Treatment

Thyroglossal cysts should be removed surgically if they are the site of recurrent infection, if they are cosmetically unacceptable or if they produce pressure symptoms. Very occasionally carcinoma may develop within the cyst or tract but this is usually only detected histologically. Although Sistrunk was not the first surgeon to remove the body of the hyoid in conjunction with excision of a thyroglossal cyst his name is given to the standard operation. A core of tissue between the hyoid bone and the foramen caecum should also be removed in continuity. A horizontal incision is made at the lower border of the cyst and the skin carefully dissected. Occasionally the skin is tightly adherent to the cyst wall and the cyst may rupture. The body of the hyoid bone should be divided between the lesser horns. More lateral dissection should be avoided to prevent damage to the hypoglossal nerves. Sometimes the tract is multiple. Once the core of muscle is followed up to the tongue base the tract can be divided. There is no need to enter the oral cavity. Loss of the central portion of the hyoid bone produces no disability. Haemostasis must be meticulous to avoid the risk of post-operative haematoma and the associated risk of respiratory obstruction. A suction drain should be placed. Recurrence following a Sistrunk operation is uncommon. If the central portion of the hyoid bone is not removed there will be recurrence in three out of four patients.

It is generally felt that the diagnosis of a thyroglossal duct cyst is easy to make given the classic clinical features. However, it may be difficult to differentiate thyroglossal duct abnormalities from other midline cervical masses pre- and intra-operatively. It is sometimes not possible, for example, to clearly distinguish even at operation between a thyroglossal duct abnormality and a dermoid cyst. If there is any doubt it is best that all midline cervical masses are treated using a Sistrunk procedure. The additional time required to undertake this procedure with its minimal morbidity is a small price to pay to prevent recurrence of a thyroglossal duct cyst.

An infected cyst should not be incised or excised. If it is very tense and painful and antibiotics have not proven effective, the cyst should be aspirated with a wide bore needle with removal of the cyst and tract some weeks or months later.

A thyroglossal sinus results from spontaneous or surgical drainage of a thyroglossal cyst. It is dealt with by excision of an ellipse of skin around the sinus followed by a Sistrunk operation.

Papillary carcinoma of thyroid tissue associated with the thyroglossal duct has been reported. Such lesions present usually in association with benign cysts and the diagnosis is only made by histological examination. Treatment is by a Sistrunk operation with suppressant doses of thyroxine post-operatively.

Branchial apparatus abnormalities

Embryology

During the third week of embryonic life a series of mesodermal condensations known as the branchial arches appear in the walls of the primitive pharynx. These condensations fuse ventrally producing U-shaped structures. Between the six branchial arches lie five pharyngeal pouches internally and five branchial clefts (grooves) externally. The fifth arch is vestigial and rapidly disappears. The branchial pouches are lined by endoderm and the branchial grooves by ectoderm and there is a thin layer of mesoderm between each pouch and groove. In fish this tissue breaks down to form a gill-slit.

The mesoderm of each arch differentiates into a central core of cartilage and muscle. Each arch is supplied by a cranial nerve and an aortic arch artery. The first branchial arch gives rise to the maxilla, malleus and its anterior ligament, incus, sphenomandibular ligament and the mandible. The nerve of this arch is the trigeminal nerve, the artery is the maxillary artery and the muscles are the muscles of mastication. The second arch gives rise to the stapes, styloid processs, stylohyoid ligament and the lesser cornu and upper body of the hyoid bone. The nerve is the facial nerve, the artery occasionally persists as the stapedial artery and the muscles differentiate into the muscles of facial expression.

The third arch gives rise to the remainder of the hyoid bone. The nerve is the glossopharyngeal nerve and the artery contributes to part of the internal carotid artery. The fourth and sixth arches differentiate into the laryngeal cartilages and the muscles of the pharynx and larynx supplied by the superior laryngeal nerve (fourth arch) and recurrent laryngeal nerve (sixth arch). The fourth arch artery forms the definitive aorta on the left and subclavian artery on the right while the sixth arch artery becomes the pulmonary trunk.

The second arch grows downwards on its lateral side to meet the fifth arch thus enclosing the second, third and fourth branchial clefts forming the sinus of His. By week 6 the branchial apparatus has disappeared.

Many theories of origin of so-called branchial arch abnormalities have been adduced. Many of the original papers regarding these theories do not withstand critical scrutiny and it is likely that the lesions termed branchial cysts, sinuses and fistulas do not all have a common origin from developmental abnormalities of the branchial apparatus.

A sinus is a blind ended tract leading from an epithelial surface into deeper tissues. A fistula is an abnormal communication between two epithelial surfaces. Branchial sinuses and fistulas are present at birth and most likely represent developmental defects of the branchial apparatus. However, the peak age incidence for branchial cysts is in the third decade suggesting a different pathogenesis. Some cysts may represent remnants of the pharyngeal pouches or branchial clefts which do not disappear in embryological life. Branchial cysts rarely have an internal opening and it seems likely that most cysts arise within lymph nodes. This theory of origin is supported by the fact that most branchial cysts have lymphoid tissue in their walls.

Clinical entities

Abnormalities of the first and second branchial arches may give rise to accessory tragi and peri-auricular cysts and sinuses. Most peri-auricular sinuses and cysts produce little in the way of symptoms, but if they become infected may require to be excised surgically. Apparently simple cysts and sinuses may have extensive and deep branching ramifications which pass in close proximity to the seventh cranial nerve. Most pre-auricular sinus tracts are only 1 cm or so in length, but occasionally a tract will pass deeply into the parotid gland and it may be necessary to perform a superficial parotidectomy with preservation of the facial nerve and its branches to completely eradicate the lesion.

Branchial fistula

A branchial fistula is presumed to occur when the cervical sinus of His persists and the layer of endoderm, mesoderm and ectoderm between the second pouch and groove breaks down. The fistula opens externally onto the lower third of the neck just anterior to the sternocleidomastoid muscle. The opening is present at birth. Occasionally branchial fistulas are bilateral. The fistula may be asymptomatic or there may be intermittent clear mucoid discharge often noticed particularly in children after a hot bath. If the fistula becomes infected an abscess may develop with discharge of pus. If the fistula is asymptomatic no treatment is required, but if there is repeated discharge this will soon become cosmetically unacceptable as the child grows. It is important pre-operatively to distinguish between a sinus and a fistula because all of the tract must be removed to prevent recurrence. A fistulagram will produce this information (Figure 45.3). The fistula consists of a epithelial lined tube, the epithelium being of either respiratory or squamous type. In the wall of the tube are muscle fibres and lymphoid tissue. The lumen of the tube is rarely uniform with frequent cystic dilatations. If the fistula has been repeatedly infected it may be tightly adherent to other cervical structures.

At operation an elliptical incision is made around the opening of the fistula and the tract is dissected through the deep cervical fascia and along the carotid sheath. It is often necessary to make further horizontal incisions higher in the neck as the dissection proceeds to allow

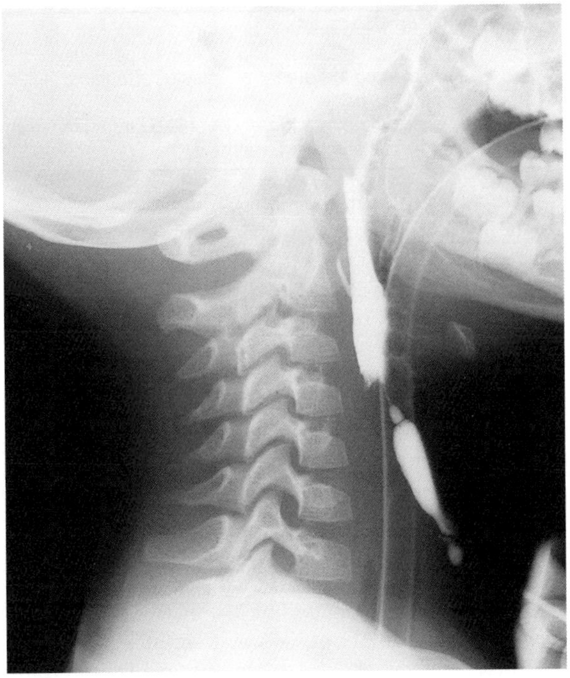

Figure 45.3 Fistulagram demonstrating connection between skin and tonsillar fossa.

the tract to be followed superiorly as it passes towards the pharyngeal wall (Figure 45.4). Many tracts do not reach as high as this, but the pre-operative fistulagram will demonstrate the relevant anatomy. The tract passes between the internal and external carotid arteries and anterior to the third and fourth arch nerves, i.e. the glossopharyngeal and vagus. If the tract extends to the pharynx any mucosal breach of the pharynx should be closed primarily. Other less invasive techniques have been described for dealing with branchial fistulas, but the operation outlined above is the safest and most reliable method of dealing with these abnormalities.

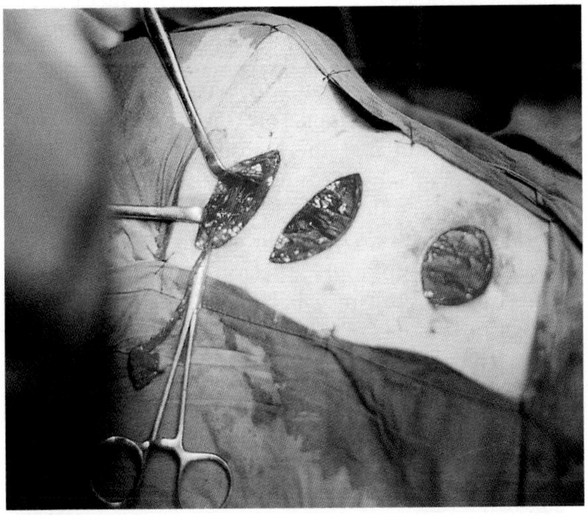

Figure 45.4 Step ladder incision used to excise a branchial fistula.

Branchial cysts

As indicated above most cervical cysts labelled branchial cysts probably result from epithelial inclusions within lymph nodes. Sixty per cent of such cysts occur in males and the peak age incidence is in the third decade. The age at presentation varies between 1 and 70 years. Sixty per cent occur on the left side with 2% being bilateral. Most occur in the classic position at the anterior border of the sternomastoid muscle at the junction of its upper one-third and lower two-thirds. Most cysts present as continually present swellings, but in about 20% of patients the swelling will be intermittent. Some cysts present very abruptly often with infection. Some are sufficiently large to produce pressure symptoms (Figure 45.5).

Two types of epithelial lining are seen in branchial cysts:

- stratified squamous epithelium
- non-ciliated columnar epithelium.

Differential diagnosis is to some extent dependent on the age of the patient. In the young child dermoid cyst or lymphangioma should be considered. In the older child the most common swelling is reactive lymphadenitis. Lymph node enlargement from various causes is the most likely alternative diagnosis in the teenager and young adult, but in the older adult the possibility of metastatic lymph node carcinoma has to be considered. Lymphoma, lipoma, neurogenic tumour, chemodectoma and tuberculosis should all be considered. Fine needle aspiration biopsy is often helpful, but if a paraganglioma is considered a possibility, a CT or MR scan should be requested.

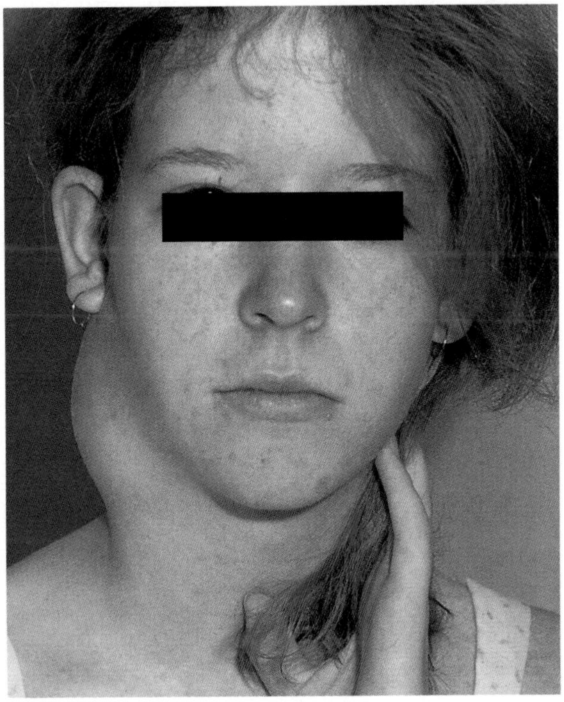

Figure 45.5 A large right-sided branchial cyst.

Branchial cysts should be removed for both diagnostic and cosmetic reasons. If left there is a risk that they will become infected. Tracts are rarely found and the cyst is usually readily mobilized from the underlying structures. If the cyst is large it may be decompressed with a large bore needle to facilitate dissection. If the cyst presents as an acutely infected mass, it should be aspirated and treated with antibiotics. It should be excised 2 or 3 months later.

Occasionally a cyst which was clearly present when the patient was listed for surgery may have disappeared by the time of operation. There is no place for exploring the neck in such circumstances. It is likely that the cyst will not be found or worse that it will be partially excised leading to a draining sinus. This also applies in the case of other lesions in the neck such as thyroglossal duct cysts.

Branchiogenic carcinoma

Ectotopic squamous epithelium may exist within lymph nodes and undergo malignant change. It is essential when faced with a potentially malignant cystic mass in the neck to exclude an undiagnosed primary tumour by panendoscopy and random biopsy. Most such malignant cystic lesions in the neck result from breakdown of necrotic tissue within a lymph node which contains metastatic carcinoma from a squamous cell primary in the head and neck.

Section 45.3 • Neurogenous tumours

These tumours arise from neural crest cells which differentiate into the Schwann cell and the sympathicoblast (Figure 45.6).

Neurofibromas may present as solitary tumours, but when associated with Von Recklinghausen's disease they are often multiple. They have a 1 in 10 chance of becoming malignant. Schwannomas, sometimes called neurilemmomas, present as solitary tumours; they are not associated with Von Recklinghausen's syndrome and seldom become malignant. Two histological types are described:

- Antoni A, where there are well-developed cylindrical structures which on cross-section produce a palisading pattern of nuclei around a central mass of cytoplasm (Verocay body).
- Antoni B, where there is a loosely arranged stroma in which the cells form no distinctive pattern.

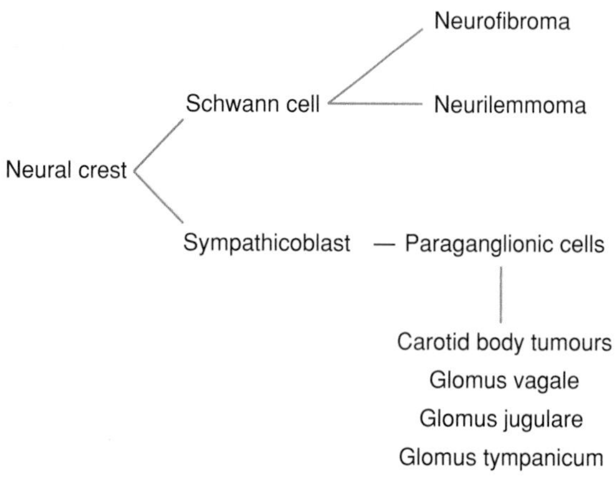

Figure 45.6 The tumour derivatives from the neural crest.

The two types may be mixed and the histological differentiation has no surgical or prognostic significance. Indeed the distinction between neurofibromas and Schwannomas is not absolutely clear cut histologically and features of each tumour can be seen in one specimen. From a prognostic point of view an important feature is the degree of cellularity of the tumour.

Neurofibromas may exhibit a plexiform pattern of growth where the abnormal nerve tissue grows into the adjacent tissue planes. This may present as a cutaneous or subcutaneous mass or arise in deep seated tissue. Such plexiform neuromas are difficult to remove and are liable to recur. Gangliomas or ganglio-neuromas are rare tumours which usually arise from the cervical sympathetic ganglia. They are firm, smooth and well encapsulated. About a quarter are malignant.

Post-operative or post-traumatic neuromas result from division of a nerve and resultant attempts by the damaged nerve to repair itself. Axons from the proximal stump become embedded in fibrous tissue. If the process is sufficiently active swelling develops at the end of the nerve and the patient experiences localized pain and tenderness.

Paraganglionic cells are derived from the sympathicoblast from the neural crest. They migrate in close association with autonomic ganglion cells. Their greatest concentration is in the adrenal medulla where they produce catecholamines and may give rise to phaeochromocytomas. Paragangliomas occur at various sites in the head and neck as well as in other parts of the body. Because carotid body tumours arise from paraganglionic cells rather than chemoreceptor cells, the term 'chemodectoma' should not be used to describe carotid body tumours. Some carotid body tumours contain secretory granules like those in the adrenal medulla and produce catecholamines. Carotid body tumours are sometimes associated with paragangliomas elsewhere in the head and neck and also with phaeochromocytomas.

Carotid body tumours are histologically poorly encapsulated and extremely vascular. They encroach upon and gradually surround the carotid bulb. They may extend along the carotid arteries for long distances and may ensheath the adjacent cranial nerves and base of skull. Glomus tumours in relation to the vagus nerve at the base of skull may behave in a similar fashion. There may be a family history of such tumours and 25% are bilateral in those with a positive family history. Sex incidence is equal and the average age of presentation is in the fifth decade.

Pathogenesis

Nerve sheath tumours grow in either a fusiform or plexiform pattern. The function of the nerve is rarely disturbed although at surgery the nerve may be found to be grossly distorted with fibres stretched over the tumour. Apart from the eighth nerve the vagus is more commonly affected than any other nerve in the head and neck. Involvement of the lower cranial nerves, the sympathetic chain and branches of the cervical plexus have all been described. Little is known about the aetiology of nerve tumours other than those that occur in association with Von Recklinghausen's disease. There is some evidence that radiation which used to be given for tonsil and adenoid enlargement leads to the development of larger numbers of such tumours in the head and neck than in the non-radiated population. Malignant change is suggested by pain, rapid growth and loss of function. Malignant neurogenic tumours of the head and neck tend to metastasize to the lungs rather than to the regional lymph nodes.

Clinical features

Nerve sheath tumours enlarge slowly over a period of years with little in the way of symptoms. A painless neck mass is usually the only sign. There is no interference with nerve function apart from when the sympathetic chain is involved when pressure may result in Horner's syndrome. Differential diagnosis is from other neck masses. If the tumour presents as a parapharyngeal mass the tonsil and soft palate may be displaced. In the parapharyngeal space nerve sheath tumours are usually fusiform producing an ill-defined firmness deep to the sterno-mastoid muscle. As the vagus lies posteriorly in the parapharyngeal space tumours arising from it tend to push the posterior tonsillar pillar and posterolateral oropharygneal wall medially and forwards. Tumours of the hypoglossal, accessory and cervical nerves generally present as neck lumps. Tumours of the facial nerve are most likely to be confused with parotid tumours.

Treatment

Solitary nerve tumours are dealt with by removal. The nerve with which the tumour is associated is commonly stretched over the capsule of the tumour or less commonly the tumour lies in the centre of the nerve with fibres spread around it. Every effort should be made to preserve the nerve although this is often not possible.

Malignant nerve tumours should be removed with a wide margin of adjacent tissue. Post-operative neuromas if symptomatic should be excised and the nerve sharply divided. The tissue should be examined to exclude recurrent tumour.

Paragangliomas

These tumours arise from aggregations of non-chromaffin paraganglionic cells adjacent to the carotid bulb, the jugular bulb, in the cavity of the middle ear, in the ganglion nodosum of the vagus and elsewhere in the body.

In the head and neck such tumours most commonly present as carotid body tumours at the bifurcation of the common carotid artery. This is a rare tumour, but has a relative high incidence in populations living at high altitudes. It is generally slow growing and transmitted pulsation may be present. The tumour most commonly arises from the inner aspect of the bifurcation of the carotid artery and may present as a pharyngeal mass with displacement of the tonsil. The differential diagnosis includes lymphadenopathy and branchial cyst. The mass is usually firm and a bruit may be present on ausculation. If the tumour is large pressure symptoms may be troublesome. The lower cranial nerves are occasionally involved.

Neither fine needle aspiration nor open biopsy is appropriate in view of the extremely vascular nature of the lesion. Imaging modalities include CT, MRI and angiography. It is necessary to check for the presence of other paragangliomas in the head and neck as there is a recognized incidence of associated ipsilateral and contralateral tumours. Angiography allows assessment of the tumour circulation and allows an assessment of cross-circulation through the circle of Willis should there be a need to resect and graft the artery.

If technically possible the tumour should be removed otherwise the patient is left with a progressively enlarging neck mass of uncertain behaviour. It is usually possible to dissect the tumour from the carotid arterial system. However, some tumours extend to the skull base and it is not possible to resect the tumour and attach a graft at this level. Resection should be undertaken only by or in conjunction with an experienced vascular surgeon and facilities should be available for immediate vascular grafting if required.

Radiotherapy is not appropriate as a primary treatment of paragangliomas. However, it may be appropriately used for patients with inoperable disease, malignant disease, those for whom surgery poses a very high risk and for those who refuse surgery.

Glomus vagale tumour

This rare tumour presents as a mass at the angle of the jaw. Occasionally it will present as a pharyngeal mass. Imaging will reveal the extent of the tumour. Because it is higher in the neck than the more common carotid body tumour resection is technically more difficult and dangerous. Removal of the tumour almost inevitably results in a vocal cord paralysis which may require a subsequent cord medialization procedure to provide glottic closure.

Section 45.4 • Lymphangiomas

Lymphangiomas arise from sequestration of lymphatic tissue derived from the primitive lymph sacs which have lost connection with the main lymphatic system. An alternative theory of origin suggests that they develop from endothelialial membranes which arise from the walls of the cyst, penetrate surrounding tissues, canalize and then produce more cysts. Pathologically they are classified into three groups:

- Lymphangioma simplex – composed of thin walled capillary sized lymphatic channels.
- Cavernous lymphangioma – composed of dilated lymphatic spaces often with a fibrous adventitia.
- Cystic hygroma – composed of cysts varying in size from a few millimetres to several centimetres.

Simple lymphangiomas and cavernous lymphangiomas occur most commonly in the oral cavity and the head and neck. They present usually as soft fluctuant lesions. At the base of tongue they need to be distinguished from lingual thyroid and internal laryngocele. In the floor of the mouth they may look like a ranula.

Cystic hygromas occur in the cervico-facial region and may involve the tissues of the neck, mouth and cheek (Figure 45.7). Histologically they are lined by a single layer of flattened endothelium. Most present at birth and 90% will declare themselves by the end of the second year.

Cystic hygromas form 30% of head and neck lymphangiomas. There is no sex or side predominance. Typically they appear as soft fluctuant masses which transilluminate readily. Regression may occur spontaneously, but this is rare. They may not enlarge in which case as the child grows they become relatively smaller, but others continue to grow producing increasing disfigurement and compromise of function. Large hygromas may press on vital structures including oesophagus, trachea and great neck vessels. They may interfere with swallowing and speech. Sudden enlargement of a hygroma may result from spontaneous or traumatic haemorrhage into the hygroma or acute infection. Such episodes may be life threatening. There may be extension of cervico-facial cystic hygroma into the thorax and axilla. Such extensions can readily be imaged by MRI or CT.

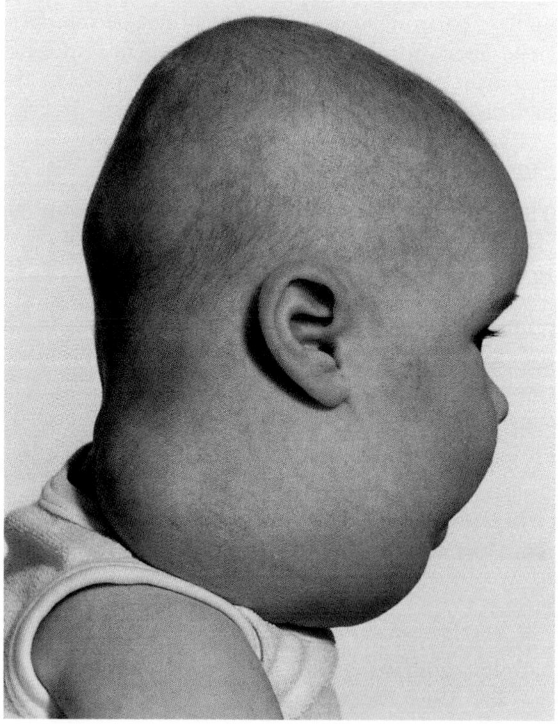

Figure 45.7 A large cervical facial cystic hygroma in an infant.

Treatment

Small cystic hygromas may be left until the child is 3 or 4 years old. A child of this age is more able to withstand a prolonged anaesthetic and the structures which need to be dissected from the hygroma are larger. However, if the hygroma is very large and disfiguring and vital structures are compromised surgery should not be delayed. It is impossible to remove all of the hygroma because of the way in which the hygroma infiltrates tissue planes. If 90% or so of the hygroma can be removed the remainder will, in most cases, involute spontaneously. It is essential not to damage the child. Structures such as the accessory nerve and marginal mandibular branch of the facial nerve are particularly at risk.

Incision and drainage is not appropriate treatment unless the cyst is infected as there will inevitably be re-accumulation of the cyst fluid. In the past injection of sclerosants was advocated, but this has now been abandoned. More recently a streptococcal product OK432 has been used mainly in Japan as an alternative non-surgical therapy for cystic hygroma. It appears to work best in children who have not undergone any other form of therapy and in whom the fluid content of large cysts can be aspirated and replaced by the agent. Following a brisk inflammatory response the hygroma undergoes fibrosis and shrinkage.

Section 45.5 • Dermoid cysts

The term dermoid cyst is used clinically to describe three distinct lesions:

- epidermoid cysts
- dermoid cysts
- teratoid cysts.

Epidermoid cysts

The epidermoid cyst comprises a lining of simple squamous epithelium surrounded by a fibrous wall with no adnexal structures. It usually contains desquamated keratinous material which clinically has the appearance of soft cheese or toothpaste. These are the most common type of cyst encountered in the head and neck.

Dermoid cysts

These cysts are lined by squamous epithelium. In the wall of these cysts are epidermal appendages such as hair follicles, sebaceous glands and sweat glands. These cysts also contain cheesy keratinous material in their cavities.

The congenital type of dermoid cyst arises in the midline and paramedian region of the neck and may be confused with a cyst of thyroglossal duct origin. The acquired type of dermoid cyst results from implantation of epidermis usually at the time of a puncture type of injury.

Teratoid cysts

A teratoma is a tumour composed of multiple tissues foreign to the part of the body in which it arises. These tumours present at birth. In the head and neck they commonly present in or adjacent to the midline and if large may result in aerodigestive tract compromise. They may be diagnosed pre-natally by ultrasound or MRI.

The term teratoid has been used to indicate teratomatous-like neoplasms that lack a trigerminal or complex histological appearance.

There is no sex predominance in these cysts. They usually present as painless swellings in the neck in or adjacent to the midline between the suprasternal notch and the submental region. Occasionally these lesions will present in the mouth either deep or superficial to the mylohyoid muscle.

Treatment

These lesions are usually easily excised and surgical excision should be undertaken for diagnosis and cosmesis.

Section 45.6 • Laryngocele

The laryngeal saccule is a blind pouch which arises from the laryngeal ventricle and passes between the false vocal cord and the inner surface of the thyroid cartilage. It is probably an atavistic remnant of the lateral laryngeal sac which is well developed in anthropoid apes. The saccule is lined by columnar ciliated epithelium with many mucous glands which provide lubrication for the true vocal cord. When the saccule becomes distended with air and expands a laryngocele is formed. Contrary to popular belief laryngoceles do not appear to be more common in patients who play musical instruments such as trumpets or bagpipes or who are involved in occupations such as glass blowing. They occur five times more commonly in men than in women and most commonly present in the sixth decade of life.

About one-third of laryngoceles present externally as a neck swelling. In this situation the laryngocele expands into the neck through the thyro-hyoid membrane. About one-fifth of laryngoceles are confined to the larynx and are known as internal laryngoceles. They may present as a swelling in the region of the vallecula. About half of all laryngoceles have both external and internal components.

In patients with laryngoceles it is essential to exclude a co-existing carcinoma or papilloma of the larynx. Such lesions can act as a one-way valve allowing air into, but not out of the ventricle. All patients with laryngoceles should have a direct laryngoscopy performed to exclude this possibility.

Clinical features

Most laryngoceles are associated with hoarseness and in external laryngoceles there is neck swelling. Sometimes a laryngocele will enlarge very rapidly and produce stridor. If they are sufficiently big they may produce dysphagia, throat discomfort and noisy respiration. Secondary infection of a laryngocele results in a laryngopyocele. The patient will present with pain in the throat and an enlarging swelling in the neck, if the laryngocele is external. Whereas laryngoceles are typically soft and compressible, laryngopyoceles are firmer and are tender on palpation. If sufficiently large a laryngopyocele can produce airway obstruction and stridor.

A plain X-ray of the neck with and without the patient performing a valsalva manoeuvre is diagnostic. A laryngocele shows up as a air filled sac. If the mouth of the sac is blocked it may be filled with inspissated mucus and is not radiolucent. MR scan is useful in this situation.

Treatment

It is essential to exclude an underlying lesion of the laryngeal ventricle. If the laryngocele is small and asymptomatic it requires no treatment. A laryngopyocele should be aspirated and the patient given antibiotics. When the infection has settled formal excision should be undertaken. Internal laryngoceles may be marsupialized, but if this does not improve the symptoms or if the lesion recurs the laryngocele should be excised by the approach used for an external laryngocele.

The operation for an external laryngocele involves excision of the laryngocele at its neck, i.e. at the saccule. This is best identified by removing or reflecting the upper half of the ala of the ipsilateral thyroid cartilage and following the neck of the laryngocele into the interior of the larynx as far as possible. The neck of the laryngocele is transected, the defect repaired and closed in layers. The thyroid ala may be replaced or if removed the thyroid perichondrium is sewn into the area. Care should be taken to avoid damage to the superior laryngeal nerve, although this is sometimes difficult in large, previously infected lesions. Occa-sionally a tracheostomy may be required to protect the airway either before or at the time of definitive treatment.

Section 45.7 • Infectious conditions

Deep neck infections

In the head and neck there are three major fascial layers, superficial fascia, deep fascia and visceral layer (Figure 45.8). The deep fascial layer subdivides further and there are several potential deep neck spaces between the various layers. Various classifications are used to describe the anatomy of the neck spaces depending on how many layers of fascia are defined. In practice knowledge of the anatomy of the parapharyngeal space, the retropharyngeal space and the submandibular space will allow appropriate surgical management of most deep neck space infections. The carotid sheath forms a potential space allowing infection to spread superiorly to the skull base and inferiorly to the mediastinum.

Microbiology

Aerobic streptococcal and non-streptococcal anaerobic infections account for the vast majority of deep neck space infections. Bacteria present in the normal oral flora may produce infection when normal mucosal barriers are breached. Deep neck space infections produced by Gram-negative organisms are relatively rare, but may be found in immunocompromised, debilitated, elderly and diabetic patients.

Clinical features

Patients with deep neck space infections are generally unwell with fever, chills, malaise and loss of appetite. There is often difficulty and pain swallowing, limitation of neck movement and sometimes torticollis and trismus. Depending on the site of the abscess there may be external neck swelling, swelling in the floor of the mouth or bulging of the pharyngeal wall. The airway may be compromised and immediate steps should be taken to evaluate and if indicated secure the airway. Physical examination of the pharynx and larynx may be difficult because of trismus and flexible fibre-optic nasopharyngoscopy is useful in this situation.

The great vessels may be involved particularly in deep neck space infections of more than a few days' duration. Thrombosis of the internal jugular vein may occur as may mycotic infection of the carotid artery with the risk of spontaneous haemorrhage.

Imaging

Plain X-rays are of limited value, but a lateral neck X-ray taken in inspiration may reveal retropharyngeal or prevertebral space involvement. In children, and in particular if the film is taken in expiration, the prevertebral soft tissue will appear thickened leading to incorrect interpretation. CT provides excellent imaging to confirm the extent of the deep neck space infection and relationship to the surrounding structures. MRI will also provide high quality imaging, but is often less readily available than CT scan. If there is any concern regarding the airway this must be controlled prior to any imaging being undertaken. A chest X-ray should be undertaken to exclude mediastinal widening, lung abscess and aspiration.

Initial antibiotic treatment is usually empirical, high dose intravenous penicillin or a third generation cephalosporin being commonly used. Clindamycin is an appropriate alternative and these antibiotics are often given in conjunction with metronidazole. The advice of the local microbiologist or infectious diseases specialist should be sought on an urgent basis and the microbiologist should be consulted as appropriate thereafter.

Specific neck space infections

Parapharyngeal space

The parapharyngeal space extends from the base of the skull at the petrous temporal bone to the hyoid bone. It is conical in shape with the apex at the hyoid bone. It is contiguous with the retropharyngeal space. Medially it is bounded by the lateral pharyngeal wall and laterally its boundaries are the mandible, parotid gland and medial pterygoid muscle. It is divided into an anterior and posterior compartment by the styloid process and associated muscles. The anterior compartment contains fat and connective tissue, but the posterior compartment contains the ninth, tenth and twelfth cranial nerves, the internal jugular vein, the internal

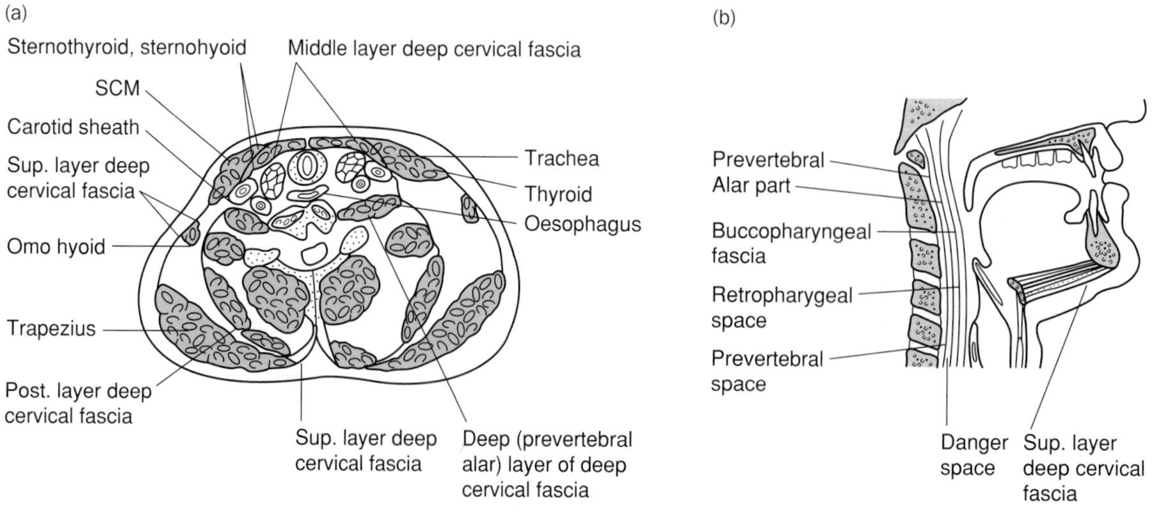

Figure 45.8 (a) Axial section of neck to show major fascial layers. (b) Coronal axial section of neck to show major fascial layers.

carotid artery and the cervical sympathetic chain. Antero-superiorly the space is bounded by the pterygomandibular raphe. The parapharyngeal space is prone to infection spreading from the tonsils, teeth, floor of mouth and the parotid and submandibular salivary glands. Abscesses of this space are more common in adults than in children. Most infections result from complications of tonsillitis or tonsillectomy with infection or extraction of the lower third molar making up most of the remainder. Infection of the temporal bone either at the petrous apex or at the mastoid tip can result in parapharyngeal space infection, but this is rare nowadays.

A patient with a parapharyngeal abscess is considerably iller than the patient with a quinsy. There will be trismus because of involvement of the medial pterygoid muscle, the tonsil or pharyngeal wall may be displaced medially and there may be an ill-defined swelling in the neck deep to the mid portion of the sternomastoid muscle. Typically a patient with a parapharyngeal abscess will experience pain on moving the head from side to side, unlike a patient with quinsy. If the abscess involves the posterior compartment of the parapharyngeal space there may be involvement of the cranial nerves and Horner's syndrome. The great vessels are at risk with thrombosis of the internal jugular vein and bleeding from the arterial system. Complications of internal jugular vein thrombosis include:

- bacteraemia
- septic pulmonary emboli
- metastatic abscess formation
- thrombosis of the lateral and cavernous sinuses.

Involvement of the carotid artery still carries a significant mortality rate because of bleeding and asphyxiation.

Definitive management of a parapharyngeal abscess involves control of the airway, intravenous antibiotics and surgical drainage. If the scan indicates that pus has not formed and the condition is a cellulitis of the parapharyngeal space surgical drainage need not be undertaken. When pus is present drainage by an external approach is indicated. This involves an incision along the anterior border of the sternocleidomastoid muscle to the mid portion of the submandibular gland. The fascia deep to the gland is divided and blunt dissection under the angle of the mandible releases pus from the lateral pharyngeal space. If there is concern regarding the integrity of the great vessels the incision along the anterior border of the sternomastoid muscle can be extended, the vessels identified and controlled with a vessel loop. The space should be drained with a corrugated drain and the incision loosely reapproximated.

Retropharyngeal space

This space extends from the base of the skull to the bifurcation of the trachea and is posterior to the pharynx and the oesophagus. It is sometimes therefore referred to as the retrovisceral space and lies anterior to the deep fascia which bounds the prevertebral space. It connects anteriorly with the pretracheal space and infections can pass by this route into the anterior mediastinum. Two chains of lymph nodes lie on each side of the midline raphe and usually involute by the age of 5 years. Infections in this space result from lymphadenitis secondary to an upper respiratory tract infection and are rare after the age of 5. This space can also be infected by penetrating trauma, blunt trauma and instrumentation such as oesophagoscopy, endotracheal intubation or passage of a nasogastric tube. It may also be infected by extension from adjacent spaces. It may be difficult to detect a retropharyngeal space infection in a young child. There may be no complaint of a sore throat, but the child is ill and refuses to eat. The temperature will be elevated. If the swelling occurs below the palate a mass may be seen on the posterior pharyngeal wall to one side of the midline. A superior swelling may result in obstruction of posterior nares and the soft palate may be displaced inferiorly. An inferior swelling may be associated with swelling in the supraglottis resulting in a 'hot potato' voice. There may be cervical lymphadenopathy and nuchal rigidity. Respiratory obstruction is unusual unless there is mediastinal extension.

Diagnosis may be aided by a lateral soft tissue X-ray of the neck but in infants a true lateral radiograph may be difficult to obtain and swelling of soft tissue anterior to the vertebral column difficult to interpret. Treatment of an uncomplicated retropharyngeal abscess is by trans-oral drainage and intravenous antibiotics. The patient is positioned as for adenoidectomy. Initial localization of the abscess may be performed using needle aspiration and the cavity can be incised vertically and then open widely. If there is lateral extension of the abscess an external approach via incision along the anterior border of the sternomastoid muscle is necessary. If mediastinitis supervenes the mortality rate is high with sepsis being the usual cause of death. Thoracotomy may be indicated if the infection is advanced.

Prevertebral space

The prevertebral space lies posterior to the retropharyngeal space and contains the longus colli muscle. Classically infection of this space results from tuberculosis involving a vertebral body and is known as a Pott's abscess. Other causes of infection in this space include trauma, surgery and extension from the retropharyngeal space. Presenting complaints are often vague and include neck and shoulder pain perhaps with some dysphagia. On examination a midline bulge of the posterior pharynx may be seen. If pus is present it may be drained trans-orally followed by appropriate chemotherapy.

Submandibular space

This space is bounded by the deep fascia which extends from the hyoid bone to the mandible inferiorly and superiorly by the mucosa which covers the floor of the mouth and tongue. The space is divided into a superior compartment lying above the mylohyoid muscle with an inferior compartment lying below this muscle. The superior space contains the sublingual salivary glands and the space inferior to the muscle contains the submandibular salivary gland. The anterior part of the submandibular salivary gland wraps around the anterior border of the mylohyoid muscle and extends into the superior compartment. Anteriorly the submental space lies between the two anterior bellies of the digastric muscles.

Infections frequently involve both parts of this space and there is communication at the posterior part of the mylohyoid muscle. Infections of this space are known as Ludwig's angina, Ludwig being a nineteenth-century German surgeon and angina referring to the spasmodic, choking or suffocating pain experienced in this condition. Over 80% of these infections arise from the teeth or mandible and most typically occur in 20–40-year-old adults. Tooth root abscesses are a common source of infection with alpha-haemolytic streptococcus being the most commonly isolated organism from this space. External swelling is limited because of the strength of the deep fascia which forms the inferior boundary of the space. The floor of mouth is usually very swollen, indurated and erythematous and fluctuance is rarely present. The tongue is pushed upwards and backwards and may obstruct the airway. As with other deep neck abscesses the patient is ill with associated fever and pain. Trismus is not common and if present suggests extension to the parapharyngeal space.

Treatment includes control of the airway, antibiotic therapy and surgical intervention. Inexperienced physicians and nurses may underestimate the danger to the airway in this condition. Respiratory obstruction is the commonest cause of death in Ludwig's angina. The airway may be secured by oral or nasal intubation or by tracheostomy. Such patients are best managed in a facility such as a high dependency or intensive care unit where control of the airway can be quickly achieved if the infection progresses rapidly. High dose intravenous penicillin with anaerobic coverage with clindamycin or metronidazole is appropriate until culture results can be obtained. If there is a poor response to antibiotic therapy or rapid progression of the infection threatening the airway, surgical drainage is required. Intra-oral drainage is indicated when a submandibular space infection is limited to the superior compartment and is uncomplicated. In all other cases an external approach is needed. A submental incision following a line parallel to the body of the mandible with preservation of the marginal mandibular nerves is used. The deep fascia is divided and the abscess drained using blunt dissection. The mylohyoid is usually very inflamed and oedematous and a drain should be placed through the mylohyoid muscle and the incision loosely closed.

Infective neck masses

Cat scratch disease

Cat (kitten) scratch disease results from infection by *Bartonella henselae*, an organism found in the mouth of kittens. It is suspected to be transmitted by flea faeces from under the claws of cats. Typically a 3–5 mm macule at the site of inoculation appears 3-10 days after animal contact. This evolves in a papule, pustule or vesicle. Inoculation papules can be found in over two-thirds of all patients. Regional lymphadenopathy proximal to the site of inoculation is observed 1–8 weeks later. This usually involves the head, neck or upper extremities. The lymph nodes are initially tender. Suppuration and association cellulitis are rare. Resolution occurs spontaneously in 2–4 months. The development of lymphadenopathy may be associated with constitutional symptoms, including headache, malaise and myalgia. Systemic involvement including encephalitis, osteomylitis, pneumonia, hepatosplenomegaly and thrombocytopenic purpura may occur.

Serological testing involving indirect fluorescent antibody tests for *Bartonella* species has recently been developed. Culture of the organism from lymph nodes in patients with clinical disease may be undertaken, but the organism can be difficult to isolate. Histopathologically the lymph nodes show granulomas, non-specific inflammatory infiltrate and stellate abscesses.

Macrolides, tetracyclines, refampicin, third generation cephalosporins, gentamicin and trimethophram-sulphamethoxazole have all been reported to benefit patients with this condition, although supportive therapy is often all that is required. There is no evidence that this disease is transmitted from human to human.

Toxoplasmosis

Toxoplasmosis is caused by the protozoon *Toxoplasma gondii* which is transmitted by ingestion of cysts from cat faeces or by ingestion of undercooked meat from pigs, sheep, poultry and goats. Toxoplasma in meat is killed by cooking at 66°C or higher or freezing for a day in a household freezer. The oocyst in cat faeces is very hardy and can survive freezing and several months of extreme heat and dehydration. Pregnant women and immunodeficient individuals are at risk. In the USA it is estimated that approximately 3000 children are born infected with toxoplasmosis every year. The majority show no symptoms of toxoplasmosis at birth, but may develop signs of infection later in life. This may involve loss of vision, mental retardation, loss of hearing and death in severe cases. Patients with acquired immune deficiency syndrome (AIDS) are susceptible to toxoplasmosis and may develop neurological symptoms. The acute infection may occur in a normal host and is manifested by cervical lymphadenopathy and associated malaise, low grade fever and possibly sore throat. Skin rash and hepatosplenomegaly may also exist. Diagnosis is made by specific serological tests. An atypical lymphocytosis may be seen in the peripheral blood. Biopsied lymph nodes show reactive follicular hyperplasia with epithelioid histiocytes and focal distension of sinuses. There may be granuloma formation, but this is not typical.

The clinical course is benign and self-limiting. Specific antimicrobial therapy is usually not necessary.

Actinomycosis

Actinomyces is an anaerobic organism present in the oral cavity. Infection in the cervico-facial region is usually associated with poor oral hygiene and generally follows dental manipulation or trauma.

Cervico-facial actinomycosis typically presents as a painless slowly enlarging bluish induration below the mandible. Occasionally it may present in a similar fashion to an acute pyogenic infection and it may occur elsewhere in the head and neck, including the salivary glands, facial skin and paranasal sinuses. Cervical lymph node involvement is unusual. Multiple draining sinuses develop which discharge pus containing sulphur granules. Diagnosis is made by examining the discharge microscopically and by anaerobic culture. The treatment of choice is high dose penicillin given intravenously. If the patient is allergic to penicillin, tetracycline may be given. Treatment is required for several weeks.

Brucellosis

Brucellosis is primarily a disease of animals particularly cattle, pigs, sheep, goats and dogs. In humans it occurs principally in farmers, veterinarians and slaughterhouse workers. The organisms (*Brucella abortus*, *B. suis* or *B. melletensis*) gain entry through the skin, conjunctiva or mucosa of the oropharynx. They then localize in tissues provoking a granulomatous reaction. The average incubation period is 1–3 weeks and the symptoms are highly variable including an acute pyrexial illness. The disease may present as lymphadenopathy in the neck and inguinal regions and there may be enlargement of the spleen and liver.

Diagnosis is made by detection of an elevated antibody titre and the organism may be isolated from blood cultures, cerebrospinal fluid or urine. Tissue specimens may also be cultured.

Many patients recover without treatment; if antibiotics are used tetracycline or tetracycline plus streptomycin is currently recommended. Brucellosis is now a rare infection with less than 200 cases per year being reported in the USA.

Infectious mononucleosis

An estimated 90% of mononucleosis cases result from Epstein–Barr virus infection. This virus is a member of the herpes virus group. Most of the remaining cases are caused by other herpes viruses particularly cytomegalovirus. Many Epstein–Barr virus infections occur without symptoms and the Epstein–Barr virus remains in the body for life after infection, usually controlled by a healthy immune system. About 80% of cases of mononucleosis involve young adults between the ages of 15 and 30 years. Among college students the rate is higher than in the general population. The virus infects and reproduces in the salivary glands and also infects B-cells. Direct contact with virus-infected saliva, such as through kissing, transmits the virus and may result in infectious mononucleosis. A patient is infectious for several days prior to symptoms appearing and the virus may continue to be excreted in the saliva for years after infection.

The illness is characterized by general malaise, headache, fatigue and loss of appetite. The conventional triad of fever, sore throat and swollen lymph glands may last for several weeks. High fever late in the illness suggests bacterial superinfection. Most lymphadenopathy in this condition involves the cervical lymph nodes, but the axillary and inguinal lymph nodes may also be enlarged. There is sphenomegaly in 50% of patients and hepatomegaly in 20%. The tonsils are often very swollen and there is pain and difficulty in swallowing. Rarely tonsillar enlargement is such that the airway is compromised. Complications include encephalitis, splenic rupture, cranial nerve palsies, pericarditis, auto-immune haemolytic anaemia and thrombocytopenia.

Diagnosis is made by detection of antibodies to the Epstein–Barr virus and detection of heterophile antibodies and atypical lymphocytes in the peripheral blood.

Infectious mononucleosis is usually an acute self-limited infection requiring only supportive therapy. Hospitalization may be required if the patient has severe difficulty and pain swallowing or there is a risk of airway obstruction. Bed rest may be required for a few days and thereafter the patient should avoid strenuous exercise for some weeks. Analgesics may be used for headache, myalgia and sore throat, and oral steroids may be used to reduce pharyngeal swelling when the airway is at risk and in the treatment of haemotological complications. Ampicillin should not be used as over 80% of patients with infectious mononucleosis will develop a rash.

Tuberculosis

Although now rare in western Europe and North America tuberculosis remains an important communicable disease in many countries. Entry of the tubercle bacillus into the body via the alimentary or respiratory tract is not necessarily followed by clinical illness. This depends on factors such as age and sex, host resistance, socio-economic circumstances and conditions resulting in immunocompromise such as diabetes, alcoholism, AIDS and treatment with immunosuppressive drugs. A primary tuberculous infection usually occurs in the lung but may occur in the tonsil. Such infection is often associated with caseous cervical lymph nodes.

Usually the primary infection and associated lymph node lesions heal and calcify. However, particularly in lymph nodes, healing may be incomplete and viable tubercle baccilli spread by the blood stream. When the primary infection does not heal in the neck it may be complicated by the development of a 'cold abscess' and a discharging sinus. When the primary infection involves the tonsil there is very low incidence of co-existing pulmonary tuberculosis. Cervical adenitis may be precipitated by an attack of acute tonsillitis. Usually only one cervical lymph node group is involved, most commonly the deep jugular chain. Other lymph groups in the anterior and posterior triangles are less commonly affected.

Diagnosis is made by a positive skin test and demonstration of acid and alkali fast bacteria in the biopsy or discharge. The bacterium may be cultured to determine sensitivity.

Atypical mycobacterial infection resulting in cervical lymphadenopathy is more common in children. Typically such organisms are not sensitive to the more commonly used anti-tuberculous agents.

Excisional biopsy should be followed by several months of appropriate chemotherapy. A specialist in infectious diseases should be involved in the patient's management. In the neck tuberculous lymph nodes are occasionally large and matted and adherent to adjacent structures. This makes excisional biopsy difficult and potentially dangerous as the nodes may be tightly adherent to the internal jugular vein. In this circumstance a modified neck dissection may be necessary. If chemotherapy is not given thereafter a sinus may form with a continual discharge with eventual healing by hypertrophic scar formation.

Section 45.8 • Malignant neck masses (Figure 45.9)

The main malignant problem to be considered is secondary carcinoma metastatic to the lymph nodes in the neck.

Squamous cell carcinomas of the head and neck are assigned a stage, which depends not only on the extent of the primary tumour (and the presence of distant metastases) but also on enlargement of the cervical lymph nodes. The current classification suggested by the UICC (International Union Against Cancer) and the AJC (American Joint Committee) is shown in Tables 45.1 and 45.2. CT or MRI scanning of the neck can be used in the staging system of neck nodal metastases and plays a useful part in the assessment of involved nodes including the relationship to the carotid artery, prevertebral space, skull base and mediastinum. As part of the TNM staging of cancer a chest CT scan is more accurate in

Table 45.1 UICC staging of nodes in cancer of head and neck

NX	– Regional lymph nodes cannot be assessed
N0	– No regional lymph node metastases
N1	– Metastases in a single ipsilateral lymph node 3 cm or less in greatest dimension
N2	– Metastases in a single ipsilateral lymph node more than 3 cm but not more than 6 cm in greatest dimension, or in multiple ipsilateral lymph nodes, none more than 6 cm in greatest dimension, or in bilateral or contralateral lymph nodes, none more than 6 cm in greatest dimension
N2a	– Metastases in a single ipsilateral lymph node, more than 3 cm but not more than 6 cm in greatest dimension
N2b	– Metastases in multiple ipsilateral lymph nodes, none more than 6 cm in greatest dimension
N2c	– Metastases in bilateral or contralateral lymph nodes, none more than 6 cm in greatest dimension
N3	– Metastases in a lymph node more than 6 cm in greatest dimension

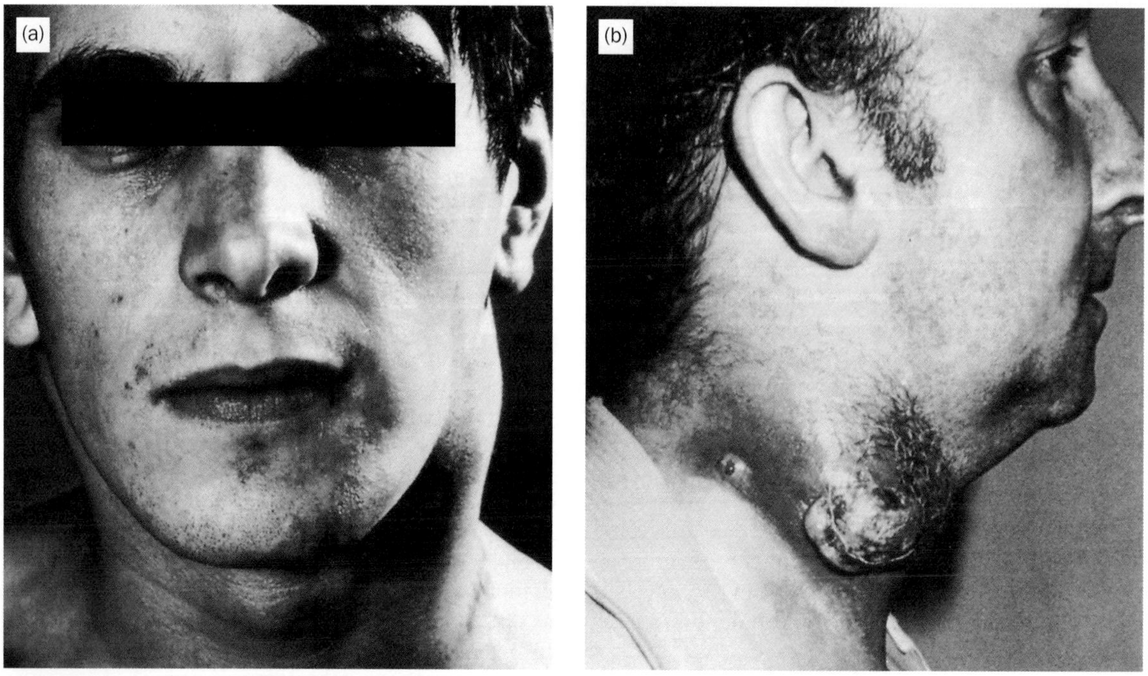

Figure 45.9 (a) Malignant neck nodes N2. (b) Malignant neck nodes N3.

Table 45.2 AJC staging of nodes in head and neck cancer

NX	– Minimum requirements to assess the regional nodes cannot be met
N0	– No clinically positive node
N1	– Single clinically positive homolateral node 3 cm or less in diameter
N2	– Single clinically positive homolateral node more than 3 cm but not more than 6 cm in diameter, or multiple clinically positive homolateral nodes, none more than 6 cm in diameter
N2a	– Single clinically positive homolateral node more than 3 cm but not more than 6 cm in diameter
N2b	– Multiple clinically positive homolateral nodes, none more than 6 cm in diameter
N3	– Massive homolateral node(s), bilateral nodes, or contralateral node(s)
N3a	– Clinically positive homolateral node(s), none more than 6 cm in diameter
N3b	– Bilateral clinically positive nodes (in this situation, each side of the neck should be staged separately; i.e. N3b; right, N2a; left, N1)
N3c	– Contralateral clinically positive node(s) only

Table 45.3 Approximate incidence of lymph node metastases

N0	70%
N1	20%
N2	5%
N3	5%

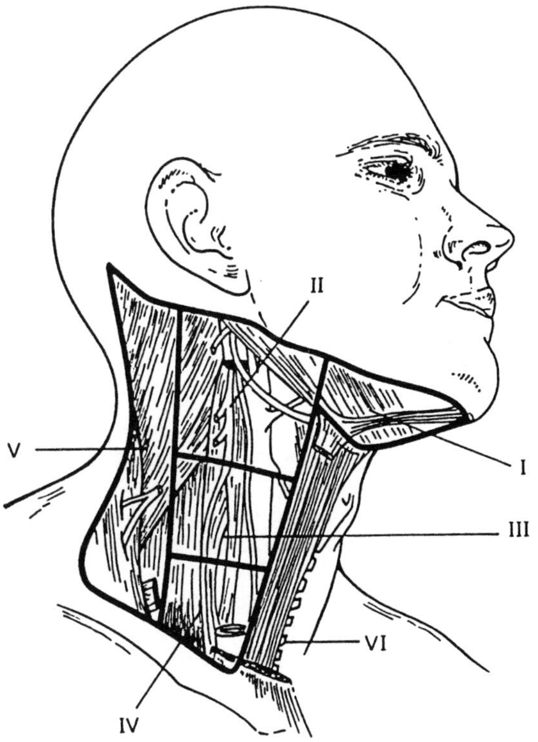

Figure 45.10 The level system for describing the location of lymph nodes in the neck. I = submental and submandibular group; II = upper jugular group; III = middle jugular group; IV = lower jugular group; V = posterior triangle group; VI = anterior compartment group.

diagnosing metastatic disease than routine chest X-rays or bronchoscopy and should be recommended in the staging process of all head and neck cancer patients. There is a great deal of observer variability in clinical examination such that different observers agree on the presence of palpable nodes in only about 70% of patients.

The approximate distribution of patients between four categories N0–N3 is shown in Table 45.3. The four categories of the classification will be used as convenient headings to discuss various aspects of the management of metastatic nodes in the neck.

Levels of neck nodes

It is now usual to describe nodes by levels (Figure 45.10).

Level I

This consists of the submental group of lymph nodes within the triangle bounded by the anterior bellies of digastric and the hyoid bone and the submandibular group of nodes bounded by the posterior belly of digastric and the body of the mandible.

Level II – upper jugular group

This consists of the lymph nodes located around the upper third of the internal jugular vein and adjacent spinal accessory nerve extending from the level of the carotid bifurcation to the skull base.

Level III – middle jugular group

This consists of lymph nodes located around the middle third of the internal jugular vein extending from the carotid bifurcation superiorly to the cricothyroid membrane inferiorly.

Level IV – lower jugular group

This consists of the lymph nodes location around the lower third of the internal jugular vein extending from the cricothyroid membrane to the clavicle inferiorly.

Level V – posterior triangle group

These nodes are located along the lower half of the spinal accessory nerve and the transverse cervical artery. The supraclavicular nodes are also included in this group. The posterior border is the anterior border of the trapezius and the anterior boundary is the posterior border of the sternomastoid muscle.

Level VI – anterior compartment group

This consists of lymph nodes surrounding the midline visceral structures of the neck extending from the hyoid bone superiorly to the suprasternal notch inferiorly. The lateral boundary in each side is the medial border of the sternomastoid. It contains the pretracheal, the paratracheal, and the perilaryngeal and precricoid lymph nodes.

Table 45.4 Incidence of occult nodes

Supraglottic larynx	15%
Pyriform sinus	40%
Base of tongue	20%
Transglottic	10%
Glottic with a fixed cord	5%

Patients with no palpable metastases (N0)

Over 40 years ago it was suggested that when an operation was carried out for a carcinoma of the oral cavity, the nodes in the neck should be cleared at the time without waiting for nodal involvement to become evident, i.e. a so-called elective neck dissection. The pathological argument supporting this concept is that lymph nodes may be involved by tumour (occult nodes) and still be impalpable. The incidence of such occult nodes at various sites is given in Table 45.4.

It may be that elective neck dissection has some place in the patient who is unlikely to return for follow-up or has a tumour with a known high incidence of occult nodes such as a pyriform fossa carcinoma, whereas there can be little or no reason to operate on a patient who can readily attend for follow-up and who has a tumour such as a laryngeal carcinoma where the incidence of occult nodes is low. In laryngeal carcinoma the incidence of occult nodes is in the region of 10–15% so that if all these patients are submitted to radical neck dissection 85–90% will suffer the increased morbidity and mortality associated with this operation to no purpose. Furthermore, there is some evidence that a patient with a laryngeal carcinoma with no palpable nodes in the neck is better treated by radiotherapy so that the issue of prophylactic neck dissection for laryngeal carcinoma scarcely arises.

All these arguments may now be becoming superfluous as it appears that elective irradiation of the entire neck can sterilize the vast majority of occult nodes. Elective neck irradiation drastically reduces recurrence in the same side of the neck in patients with carcinoma of the mouth, oropharynx, pyriform fossa and supraglottic larynx.

Patients with unilateral neck nodes under 3 cm (N1)

It is generally accepted, at least by surgeons, that surgery is required to control lymph node metastases in the neck. The standard operation for dealing with metastatic nodes in the neck is a radical neck dissection as described by Crile in 1906; a further classic paper decribing the indications, the technique and the complications was that of Hayes Martin.

Although the technique of radical neck dissection has been standard for many years several changes in management of metastatic cervical lymph nodes have taken place within the past 10 or 15 years, notably in the use of combined radiotherapy and surgery and various technical modifications of the classical operation to reduce the incidence of complications, and in the development of the so-called functional neck dissection.

Prevention of complications

The incidence of major complications after radical neck dissection is low. The major potentially lethal complications of radical neck dissection are wound breakdown and infection, necrosis of the skin flaps and rupture of the carotid artery. It is well recognized that these complications are increased by previous radiotherapy. Two major modifications of technique have been introduced over the past 20 years to combat lethal complications – modifications of the incision and protection of the carotid sheath.

In the patient who has been irradiated, particularly one in whom a fistula is likely to form because a carcinoma of the larynx, pharynx or mouth has been resected, the carotid sheath should be protected. Two methods have been described, muscle flaps and free dermal grafts. The former method is safer than the latter. The most commonly used muscle is the levator scapulae which derives its blood supply from superiorly and anteriorly. At the end of the radical neck dissection it can therefore be divided at its inferior and posterior limits and be turned forward to be stitched over the carotid sheath, protection being completed by stitching the muscle graft to the posterior belly of the digastric superiorly and the remnant of the sternomastoid muscle inferiorly. This technique, however, is rapidly becoming superfluous because of the excellence of the incisions and the excellence of modern radiotherapy. In order to minimize skin breakdown, skin incisions to maximize blood flow to the subdermal plexus include using curved, horizontal incisions and limiting the use of three point junctions. Wound breakdown rates after radiotherapy are now less than 5% and indeed if the wound breaks down the dehiscence is very seldom over the carotid artery. The carotid artery is most at risk from internal fistualization.

Functional neck dissection

Attempts have been made to reduce morbidity after a radical neck dissection by so-called functional, conservative techniques. The greatest long-term morbidity after radical neck dissection is caused by the removal of the accessory nerve. Removal of both internal jugular veins can cause a very unsightly swelling of the face which may be permanent, in addition to a dangerous increase in intracranial pressure on rare occasions. In a functional neck dissection the entire aponeurotic system of the neck, with its lymph nodes included, is removed preserving the sternomastoid muscle, the accessory nerve and the internal jugular vein. In the N0 neck it carries the same recurrence rate as the full radical neck dissection and does not leave the patient with a stiff, painful shoulder. On the other hand, surgery in the N0 neck has virtually been abandoned in favour of elective radiation. In the N1 neck, the recurrence rate after classical radical neck dissection is 25%. It has now been established that the true recurrence rate is very much higher after functional neck dissection in a node-positive neck and this procedure has largely been abandoned for node-positive necks. It is well recognized, however, that a restricted neck dissection is appropriate in metastatic papillary carcinoma of the thyroid gland.

Neck dissection classification

The following classification is now recommended for neck dissection.

Radical neck dissection

This is the classical operation which includes removal of the cervical lymph node groups extending from the inferior border of the mandible superiorly to the clavicle inferiorly and from the midline anteriorly to the anterior border of the trapezius muscle posteriorly. All the lymph node groups from levels I through to VI are included, as are the spinal accessory nerve, internal jugular vein and the sternomastoid muscle.

Modified radical neck dissection

This refers to the excision of all lymph node groups removed by the radical neck dissection with preservation of one or more of the following structures – spinal accessory nerve, internal jugular vein and sternomastoid muscle.

Selective neck dissection

This refers to any type of lymph node removal where there is preservation of one or more lymph node groups removed by radical neck dissection. The classification is as follows:

- Supra-omohyoid neck dissection refers to the removal of lymph nodes from levels I, II and III. The posterior limits of the dissection are the cutaneous branches of the cervical plexus and the posterior border of the sternomastoid muscle. The inferior limit is the superior belly of the omohyoid muscle where it crosses the internal jugular vein.
- Posterolateral neck dissection refers to removal of lymph nodes in levels II, III, IV and V. The procedure is mostly used to removal nodal disease from cutaneous melanoma of the posterior scalp and neck.
- Lateral neck dissection refers to removal of nodes in levels II, III and IV.
- Anterior compartment neck dissection refers to removal of lymph nodes from the anterior triangle of the neck, i.e. level VI.
- Extended radical neck dissection refers to the removal of one or more additional lymph node groups and/or non-lymphatic structures not encompassed by the radical neck dissection. This may include the parapharyngeal and superior mediastinal lymph nodes. Non-lymphatic structures may include the carotid artery, the hypoglossal nerve, the vagus nerve and the para-spinal muscles.

The occult primary

One further problem to be discussed is the pathology, diagnosis and treatment when a lymph node in the neck is found to contain carcinoma but the primary site is unknown.

Cancer presenting with a node in the neck is mainly a disease of men (male to female ratio of 4:1) with a maximum age incidence of 65 years on average in men and 55 years in women. Between one-third and one-half of all such nodes are replaced by squamous carcinoma, one-quarter by undifferentiated or anaplastic carcinoma and a similar number by adenocarcinoma if the supraclavicular nodes are involved, followed by a small number of miscellaneous tumours, such as melanomas and thyroid gland tumours. In about one-third of patients a primary tumour can be found by investigation at the time of presentation. The primary sites in order of frequency are: nasopharynx, tonsil, base of tongue, thyroid gland, supraglottic larynx, floor of mouth, palate and pyriform fossa (head and neck sites); bronchus, oesophagus, breast and stomach (non-head and neck sites).

Careful follow-up will later reveal a primary site in up to one-third of patients. These primary sites are rather more commonly found in the head and neck than anywhere else and the sites are again those in the above list. The relative frequency of the various sites is as shown in Table 45.5.

Investigations

The steps to be followed are those used in the investigations of any patient with an undiagnosed lump in the neck (Figure 45.11). In patients with suspected secondary malignancy in the cervical lymph nodes, the areas to be covered include:

- Primary sites; head and neck
  - inspection, palpation, radiology, endoscopy, biopsy
- Cervical lymph nodes
  - inspection, palpation, pattern, level, fine needle aspiration cytology (FNAC), excision, morphology, histology
- Other primary sites
  - general physical examination, imaging, laboratory tests, endoscopy, biopsy, cytology.

Fine needle aspiration is the initial investigation of choice as the aspirate often gives an indication of the underlying pathology.

The lists of radiological investigations were formidable at one time, but experience has shown that apart

Table 45.5 Relative frequency of primary sites

Oropharynx	15%
Nasopharynx	15%
Thyroid	20%
Hypopharynx	10%
Lung	20%
Gastrointestinal tract	10%
Miscellaneous distant sites	10%

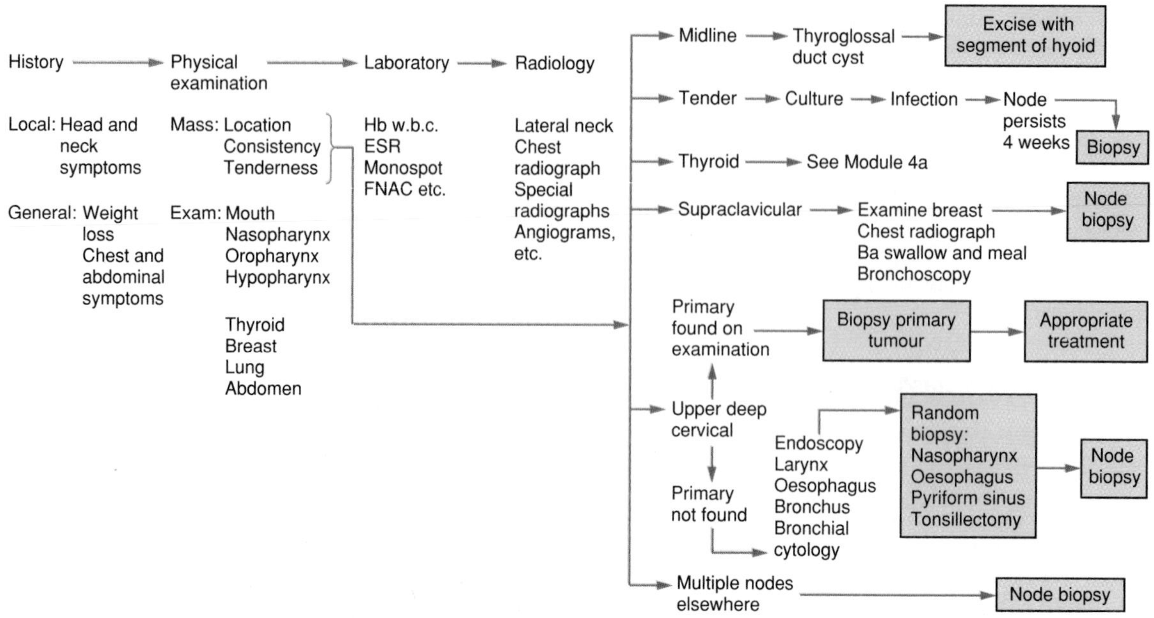

Figure 45.11 Flow chart for the investigation of a patient with a lump in the neck.

from the chest, imaging any area from which there are no symptoms or signs shows a very low yield and often results in unnecessary delay and expense.

Endoscopy must be meticulous, particularly when examining the nasopharynx, the bronchial tree and the oesophagus. If no primary tumour is found a random biopsy should be taken from the posterior wall of the fossa of Rosenmuller in the nasopharynx and from the pyriform fossa on the same side. It is also good practice to remove the tonsil on the same side and have it examined by multiple sections.

If aspiration biopsy does not give a satisfactory answer, excisional biopsy must be contemplated. Even then there may be serious consequences of excision including:

- local and possibly general spread of the disease
- compromise of a subsequent neck dissection or irradiation
- additional scar tissue causing difficulty in accurate palpation
- a false sense of security for the patient who feels that the lump has been removed.

It cannot be too strongly emphasized that excisional biopsy of a node in the neck should seldom be necessary and Hayes Martin's statement still holds true – 'an enlarged lymph node should never be excised as the first or even an early step in diagnosis'. A cervical node biopsy must be performed by a surgeon who is able and willing to treat the primary cancer if it is later found somewhere in the head and neck.

Management

In nearly all series, the treatment of the node with a truly occult primary has almost always been accompanied by post-operative radiotherapy. If the node is large and the biopsy shows a squamous carcinoma with extracapsular spread, radiotherapy should be given. If one discrete node in the upper part of the neck is involved a radical neck dissection should be carried out, whereas if more than one node is involved, or nodes in the lower part of the neck are involved, radiotherapy is given. Supraclavicular nodes are not treated further because it is presumed that they are secondary to a visceral carcinoma. This policy yields a survival rate of about 35%.

In those patients where the primary tumour is not found it is essential to repeat the search for a primary tumour at frequent intervals after the neck nodes have been treated. Large series have shown that the primary lesion was later found in about 30% of cases, whereas a further 40% die with metastatic disease and no evidence of a primary lesion. Of the survivors, 20% show no further evidence of any malignant disease at any time after treatment of the neck nodes. This again, however, raises the possibility of the existence of branchogenic carcinoma. It would be unlikely that a primary head and neck tumour would disappear on removal of the metastasis. Total removal of a cancer arising in heterotopic squamous epithelium in a lymph node could well result in a long-term cure. The follow-up needs to be continued for a very long time, since the primary tumour, particularly if it is in the tonsil, may not appear for many years and also patients with one head and neck squamous cancer have a higher chance of developing another one.

Metastases in multiple nodes (N2b) or nodes larger than 3 cm (N2a)

If there is more than one node in a neck and if there is extracapsular spread then the prognosis worsens by 100%. The treatment for an N2b or an N2a neck is a radical neck dissection followed by post-operative radiotherapy. It must be emphasized, however, that the prognosis for an N2a or an N2b neck is very different from an N1 neck.

Bilateral neck nodes (N2c)

Bilateral neck nodes are not common, occurring in about 5% of head and neck cancers at presentation overall, more commonly from tumours of the base of the tongue, the supraglottic larynx and hypopharynx. It is generally agreed that the presence of bilateral neck nodes at presentation is a very bad prognostic sign and the 5 year survival rate falls to about 5%. Despite this low survival rate many surgeons have advised staged or simultaneous bilateral neck dissection.

For the past 10 years or more it has been appreciated that it may not be necessary to stage the neck dissections. It is possible to carry out simultaneous bilateral neck dissections with reasonable safety, although the complication rate may be high. Formation of fistulas, sepsis, skin slough and facial oedema are the most important complications. The post-operative death rate is about 10% and half the patients die of uncontrolled local disease. Patients with supraglottic carcinoma and bilateral neck nodes have a reasonable prognosis, whereas nearly all other tumours, particularly of the mouth, the oropharynx and the hypopharynx, when associated with bilateral neck nodes, have an extremely bad prognosis, and surgery probably does not influence the natural history of the disease.

The most feared complication after bilateral neck dissection is increased intracranial pressure. It has been shown that tying one internal jugular vein produces a three-fold increase in the intracranial pressure, whereas tying the second side produces a five-fold increase; the intracranial pressure then tends to fall over about 8 days but not to normal. Furthermore, the pressure falls quite rapidly within the first 12 hours, so that it the patient can be managed safely over this period he or she is probably out of immediate danger. The methods to be used to avoid this complication include:

- removal of cerebrospinal fluid (lumbar drain)
- nursing the patient in the sitting position
- avoiding dressings which compress the neck
- infusion of mannitol.

It should be noted that the treatment and prognosis for a patient in whom a node appears on the second side of the neck some time later is quite different from the patient who suffers from bilateral neck nodes at the time of presentation, and a 5 year survival rate of 30% can be achieved in such cases.

Nodes greater then 6 cm (N3)

The presence of fixed nodes greater than 6 cm is an uncommon event occurring in about 5% of all patients with head and neck cancer. If a node is greater than 6 cm it will almost certainly be fixed to adjacent structures and will have exited from the node capsule. It has generally been thought that the presence of fixed nodes contraindicated surgery, but this is probably not absolutely true. If the tumour is fixed to, or invades the jugular vein, the patient is almost certainly incurable, since nearly all the patients will die of distant metastases and it must therefore appear that such invasion is indeed a contraindication to useful treatment.

Fixation to the base of the skull in the region of the mastoid process and to the branchial plexus is also almost certainly a contraindication to surgery. Fixation to the skin is not necessarily a contraindication and it is possible to resect the tumour with the overlying skin, which is replaced with a myocutaneous or free flap. On occasion, this has produced long-term survival and certainly may give very useful palliation.

When a tumour invades the carotid system, resection has been advocated. If the common carotid artery is replaced by a vein graft the operative mortality is high. Despite the occasional survivor reported by the highly skilled, this techniques does not appear to have been generally accepted.

As with the N2 neck, since the tumour has exited from the lymph node capsule, it is mandatory to follow any excisional operation with post-operative radiotherapy.

The way ahead

Benign neck masses

While it may produce little clinical dividend there is still a place for investigation into the anatomy and embryology of some of the benign diseases of the neck, notably branchial cyst. The most frequent opinion that this lesion is congenital in origin is almost certainly wrong.

Malignant neck nodes

No significant advance in the management of malignancy in the neck nodes can be expected from conventional surgery or radiotherapy or a combination of the two. The improvements in prognosis which were originally hoped for from prophylactic neck dissection have not occurred, although the real answer could only be provided by a controlled prospective trial, which remains to be done. Similarly prophylactic neck irradiation for the patient without palpable metastases offers promise, but again a controlled trial is lacking.

In the treatment of the patient with established lymph node metastases in one side of the neck the supremacy of surgery has recently been challenged by radiotherapists. It may be that radiotherapy can sterilize small nodes, but carefully controlled investigations are needed to determine the place of radiotherapy.

Another question to be answered by a trial is the place of pre- and post-operative radiotherapy. Despite initial enthusiasm for pre-operative radiotherapy for the majority of head and neck tumours, recent careful trials have shown that in fact the survival rate for tumours or all head and neck sites is not increased by pre-operative radiotherapy.

Trials are currently being undertaken to assess the benefit of combined chemotherapy and radiotherapy in head and neck cancer.

In summary, there are several forms of treatment which have been advocated very strongly, but which have not been subjected to a clinical trial before they were introduced. Because the number of patients with head and neck cancer is small, it is very difficult for one person to run a trial in one centre, so that multicentre trials are needed, with all the associated problems. Despite these difficulties such trials can be organized and it is a great pity that repeated attempts are made to introduce new forms of treatment without proper trials.

Perhaps the greatest advance which could be achieved in the next few years would be general acceptance of the fact that if a man over the age of 50 years presents with a single node in the upper part of the neck, the head and neck, the naso-, oro- and hypopharynx must be examined particularly carefully *before* a biopsy is always taken of the node. To do otherwise almost always leads to the death of a patient who otherwise had a reasonable chance of cure.

Further reading

Canadian Paediatric Society Statement (1997). Infectious Diseases and Immunisation Committee; Cat scratch disease: diagnosis and management. *Paediatr. Child Health* **2**: 275–8.

Jones, A. S., Phillips, D. I. and Hilgers, F .J. M. (1998). Diseases of the head and neck. *Nose and Throat*. London: Arnold.

Katz, A. D., Passy, V. and Kaplan, N. (1971). Neurogenous neoplasms of major nerves of the head and neck. *Arch Surg* **103**: 51–6.

Ogita, S., Tsuto, T., Nakamura, K. *et al.* (1996). *J Paediatr Surg* **31**: 477–80.

Spiro, R. H., Derose, G. and Strong, E. W. (1983) Cervical node metastases of occult origin. *Am J Surg* **146**: 441.

Wilson, J. A., Watkinson, J. and Gaze, M. N. (2000). In *Stell and Maran's Head and Neck Surgery*, 4th edn. Oxford: Butterworth-Heinemann.

MODULE 46

The salivary glands

1 • Surgical anatomy and physiology
2 • Benign salivary gland disease
3 • Tumours of the salivary glands
4 • Investigations
5 • Treatment policy

Section 46.1 • Surgical anatomy and physiology

Embryologically, salivary glands derive from ectodermal and endodermal invaginations and are classified as tubulo-acinar glands. The salivary glands are divided into two groups: the major salivary glands (parotid, submandibular, sublingual) and the minor salivary glands, consisting of 600 to 1000 small glands distributed mainly in the oral cavity but found throughout the upper aerodigestive tract.

Histologically, both major and minor salivary glands consist of two basic secretory cell types, mucinous cells and serous cells. Active salivation is stimulated by taste, touch, smell and hunger via neurological stimulation from the parasympathetic nerve supply. The parotid and submandibular glands account for 90% of total salivary secretion with the remainder contributed by sublingual and minor salivary glands. Adults secrete a total volume of approximately 1000 ml of saliva in every 24 hours.

The parotid gland (Figure 46.1)

The body of the parotid gland overlies the masseter muscle and the tail of the gland extends into the retromandibular fossa. The facial nerve passes through the parotid gland tissue dividing the gland into a superficial lobe and a deep lobe, which are not distinct structures. The superficial lobe, superficial to the facial nerve, comprises 80% of the gland and the deep lobe (deep to the facial nerve) makes up 20% of the parotid tissue. A fibrous capsule surrounds the parotid gland in continuity with the deep cervical fascia. Within the fascia lie 15–20 lymph nodes, which when swollen may mimic a parotid tumour. A further group of lymph nodes is embedded in the parotid glandular tissue. The parotid duct (Stensen's duct) runs horizontally, 1–2 cm below the zygomatic process and then turns medially to pierce the buccal mucosa opposite the second upper molar tooth.

Examination of the parotid gland should include the assessment of obvious masses, facial nerve function and an intraoral examination to exclude deep lobe parotid gland pathology affecting the parapharyngeal space. Two important nerves are related to the parotid gland, the facial nerve and greater auricular nerve. The latter comprises branches (C2 and C3) of the cervical plexus which supply sensation to the lower two-thirds of the pinna. The facial nerve exits from the stylomastoid foramen passing anteriorly above the upper border of the posterior belly of the digastric muscle. The nerve trunk is approximately 3 mm in diameter and measures 0.5–1.5 cm before entering the parotid gland and dividing into upper zygomatico-temporal and lower cervico-facial divisions.

There are several ways to identify the facial nerve trunk during parotidectomy; the two best are:

- The tragal cartilage pointer of the external ear canal. The facial nerve trunk lies approximately 1 cm inferior and 1 cm medial to this landmark.
- The upper border of the posterior belly of the digastric muscle at its junction with the bony tympanic plate is approximately 1–2 mm inferior to the nerve trunk.

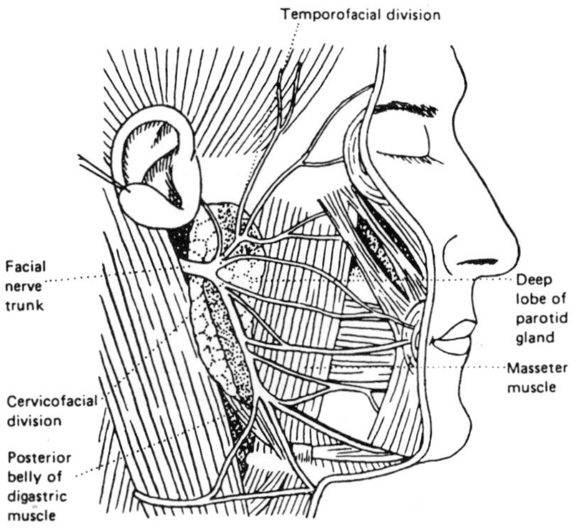

Figure 46.1 Surgical anatomy of the parotid salivary gland.

The terminal branches of the facial nerve may be located using the following landmarks:

- The zygomatico-temporal division crosses the zygoma midway between the tragus and the lateral canthus of the eye.
- The buccal branch runs parallel to the parotid duct and 1 cm superior to it.
- The mandibular branch of the facial nerve crosses the facial artery (which is 2.5 cm anterior to the angle of the mandible), 1 cm below the lower border of the mandible.

If the main trunk of the facial nerve cannot be readily identified during parotidectomy because of the location of a parotid tumour, retrograde dissection of a branch of the facial nerve can be used. The buccal branch is best for this approach, as loss of function in the distribution of this branch is less significant than damage to either the zygomatico-temporal or mandibular branches.

The retromandibular portion of the gland lies in the lateral wall of the parapharyngeal space in close association with the carotid sheath, vagus nerve, sympathetic chain and parapharyngeal space fat.

The submandibular gland (Figure 46.2)

The submandibular gland lies under the mandible on the mylohyoid muscle, with the bulk of the gland lying superficial to the mylohyoid muscle. The anterior part of the gland bends around the anterior border of the mylohyoid muscle. The submandibular duct (5 cm) runs in the floor of the mouth to open adjacent to the lingual frenulum in the anterior floor of mouth. The facial artery is intimately associated with the submandibular gland, which is covered with a layer of fascia in continuity with the deep cervical fascia. The marginal mandibular branches of the facial nerve, which supply the muscles at the corner of the mouth, lie just superficial to the fascia and may be easily damaged during surgical dissection of the submandibular gland. The lingual nerve and its associated submaxillary ganglion may be damaged during deep dissection of the submandibular gland and more rarely, the hypoglossal nerve may be injured in association with deep disease of the gland. There are numerous lymphatic channels in the submandibular gland region and lymph nodes are encountered overlying the submandibular gland fascia.

The sublingual glands

The sublingual glands are located just beneath the anterior mucous membrane of the floor of the mouth and are poorly encapsulated rather diffuse glands. The small ducts enter the floor of mouth directly or enter the submandibular duct.

Minor salivary glands

These occur in numerous locations in the upper aerodigestive tract and are poorly encapsulated small glands with small ducts draining directly into the oral cavity, pharynx and larynx.

Section 46.2 • Benign salivary gland disease

Sjögren's syndrome

Sjögren's syndrome may be divided into two types:

- Primary Sjögren's syndrome or the Sicca syndrome, consists of xerostomia and/or xerophthalmia without association with a connective tissue disorder.
- Secondary Sjögren's syndrome is an auto-immune disorder associated with connective tissue diseases (rheumatoid arthritis, system lupus erythematosis or polyarteritis nodosa).

Sjögren's syndrome is a multi-system disease mainly affecting the mouth, eyes and parotid gland and is usually associated with intermittent, unilateral or bilateral salivary gland enlargement. The diagnosis is made by screening laboratory tests for anti-nuclear factor, rheumatoid factor and protein electrophoresis. The pathological findings are of a lymphocytic infiltrate with acinar atro-

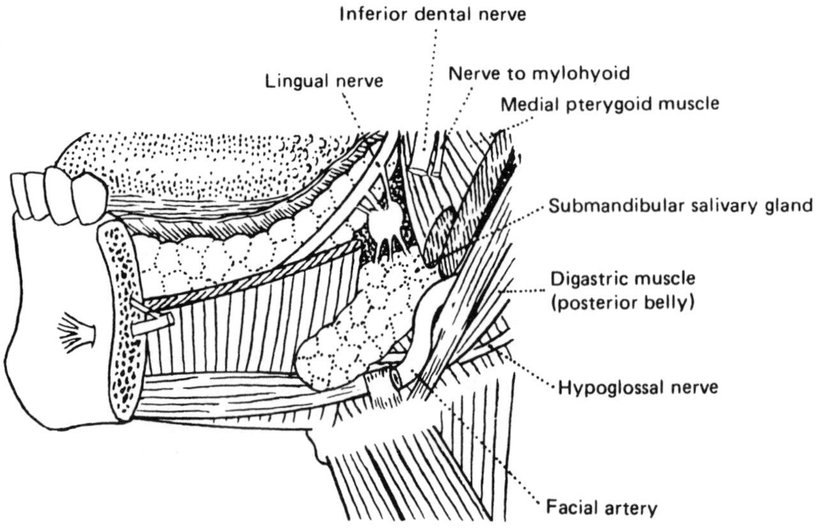

Figure 46.2 Surgical anatomy of the submandibular salivary gland.

phy with duct epithelial hyperplasia and metaplasia. A definitive diagnosis can be made by performing a biopsy where minor salivary glands are sampled from the inner surface of the lower lip. Current evidence indicates that Sjögren's syndrome results from a lymphocytic mediated destruction of exocrine glands which produces a reduction or absence of glandular secretion. Patients with primary Sjögren's syndrome are at risk of developing lymphomas (usually non-Hodgkin's). The benign lymphoepithelial lesion described by Godwin in 1952 is now considered to be a localized form of Sjögren's disease.

Infections

The commonest infection is due to the mumps virus. Other viruses implicated in salivary gland inflammation include the echo and coxsackie viruses. Bacterial parotitis, often associated with dehydration, causes intense pain and inflammation as the swollen gland is confined within the parotid capsule. Bilateral cystic enlargement of the parotid glands may be a presenting feature of patients with human immunodeficiency virus (HIV) infection.

Sialectasis

This is the salivary gland analogue of bronchiectasis, with areas of stenosis and dilatation of the ductal system. The condition may be congenital or follow infective or inflammatory changes in the duct system. The typical presentation is of painful enlargement of one salivary gland shortly after eating. It takes a few hours to regress and is made worse by eating again. Attacks come in runs lasting for days or weeks with long periods of remission. These attacks are thought to be due to blockage of the main ducts by either epithelial debris or calculi. The diagnosis is confirmed radiologically by sialography, which shows either a fusiform or globular (sacular) pattern to the duct system. An example of globular sialectasis is seen in Figure 46.3.

Salivary gland calculi

The submandibular gland is a mixed seromucinous gland with secretions high in calcium content.

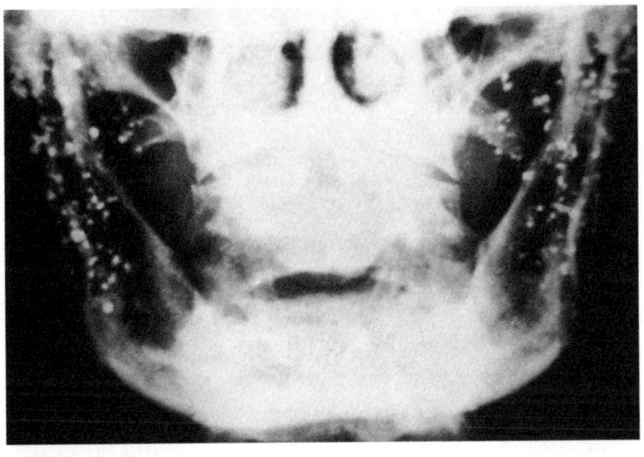

Figure 46.3 Bilateral parotid sialogram showing diffuse saccular sialectasis.

Epithelial debris here can calcify and form stones, which are often of high density and are radio-opaque. The parotid gland is a serous gland and has secretions which are low in calcium content. Stones form uncommonly in the parotid gland duct system but are low in density and usually radiolucent.

Section 46.3 • Tumours of the salivary glands

There are two features of salivary gland tumours, which make them unique. First, some tumours occur only in the salivary glands and nowhere else in the body and secondly, as well as benign and malignant tumours there are some which have very variable biological behaviour. These two facts and also the difficulty of histopathological interpretation have led to a profusion of classifications, none of which has been universally accepted.

The common benign tumours are the pleomorphic (mixed cell) and monomorphic adenomas and the common malignant ones, the adenoid cystic carcinoma and carcinoma arising in a pleomorphic adenoma. Adenocarcinomas are rare and there is considerable doubt as to whether squamous cell carcinomas exist at all in the salivary glands. Areas that look like squamous cell carcinoma occur in both malignant mixed cell tumours and mucoepidermoid tumours. Tumours of variable malignancy are the mucoepidermoid tumour and the acinic cell tumour. Rarer salivary gland tumours are haemangioma, lymphangioma, sarcoma, lipoma, lymphoma and metastatic tumours.

The commonest non-tumorous condition is sialectasis, which is the background in which calculi form. Some medical disorders and certain allergies can cause sialomegaly and a number of conditions can mimic sialomegaly with no actual abnormality of the glands.

Benign tumours

Pleomorphic adenoma

This is also known as a mixed cell tumour and comprises 60% of all salivary gland tumours. In the parotid it forms 90% of all benign tumours and in the submandibular and minor salivary glands it constitutes less than 50% of all tumours but is the commonest benign tumour. The sex distribution is equal and the peak age incidence is in the fifth decade. It is usually unilateral but bilateral tumours can occur. In the minor salivary glands the only site in which it presents with any frequency is the palate.

The tumour grows with long quiescent periods and short periods of rapid growth. Some patients may have ill-defined local discomfort but it is usually symptomless, apart from the presence of a lump. Rapid growth, pain, facial weakness or skin tethering should arouse the suspicion of malignancy.

The capsule of compressed normal parotid tissue varies in thickness and the tumour extends into the capsule in a lobulated fashion (Figure 46.4) This is why shelling out (enucleating) the tumour leads to the risk of local recurrence which may be in several sites since some of the lobules in the capsule can be left behind. The cut surface of the tumour is greyish white or blue with possible cyst formation and haemorrhage. Ten per cent of tumours are highly cellular and although showing no malignant propensity such tumours are more liable to recur.

The tumours contain epithelial and mesodermal elements (Figure 46.5). The mesodermal parts arise from the myoepithelial cell which is a contractile cell surrounding the tubules draining individual acini.

Pleomorphic adenoma is a tumour which is readily implanted. If the capsule is ruptured during removal then tumour will implant in the residual parotid or adjacent tissues. This will cause recurrences, which are apparently multi-focal, but this is geographical rather than a pathological notion. In the management of the recurrent tumour, the facial nerve is at greater risk of being damaged in tumour removal. Although these tumours are not very radiosensitive, surgery for recurrence may be followed by radiotherapy to limit further tumour recurrence.

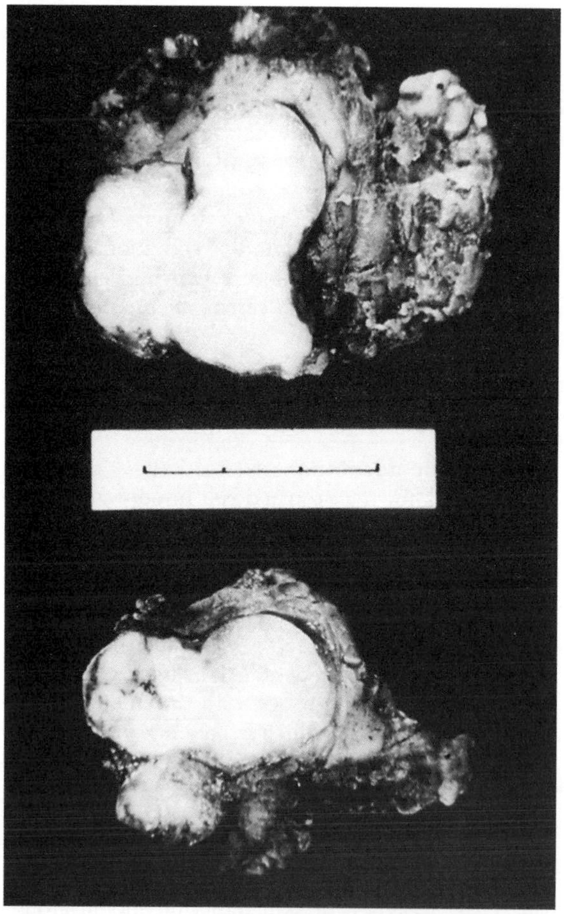

Figure 46.4 Pleomorphic adenoma. The tumour is seen to extend into the capsule which consists of compressed normal parotid tissue varying in thickness.

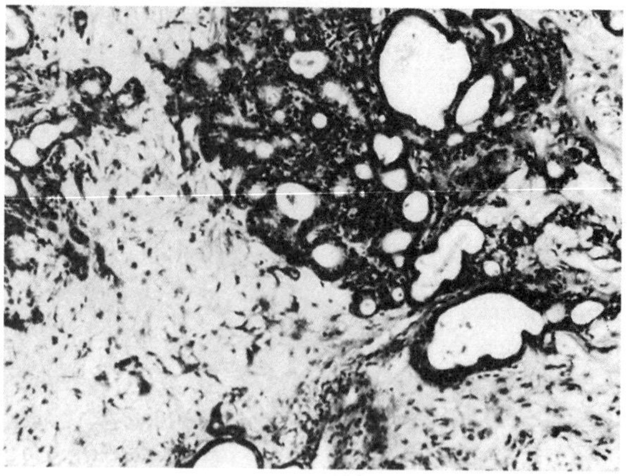

Figure 46.5 Photomicrograph of a pleomorphic adenoma showing epithelial and myoepithelial (mesodermal) components.

Monomorphic adenoma

Papillary cystadenoma lymphomatosum (Warthin's tumour) is invariably benign and is only seen in the parotid gland. It is much commoner in males, the male to female ratio being 7:1. The peak age incidence is in the seventh decade and 10% are bilateral but rarely synchronous. They are soft and cystic and are often fluctuant. The tumour probably arises from parotid tissue included in the lymph nodes, which are usually present within the parotid sheath.

Oncocytoma arises from oncocytes which are derived from intralobular ducts or acini. They may undergo a diffuse multinodular hyperplasia known as oncocytosis. This is seen most frequently in the sites of minor salivary glands and the diagnosis must be borne in mind in the differential diagnosis of lumps in the nasopharynx and larynx, especially in elderly males. The tumour is also known as an oxyphil-cell adenoma. It rarely undergoes malignant change.

Malignant tumours

Mucoepidermoid carcinoma

Since this was first described in 1945 debate has continued about its correct biological classification. This can be summarized as follows:

- One view is that it is always a carcinoma whose behaviour is related to its histology. Low-grade or well differentiated tumours act like benign mixed cell tumours – intermediate ones are more aggressive and high-grade or undifferentiated tumours metastasize early and carry a poor prognosis.
- A more recent view is that behaviour is not related to histological appearance and apparently benign ones may eventually metastasize while initially aggressive appearing ones can disappear with appropriate treatment. For this reason the word 'tumour' is applied rather than 'carcinoma'.

Mucoepidermoid tumours may arise in any salivary tissue and constitute 4–9% of salivary gland tumours. Nine out of ten involve the parotid gland. In minor salivary glands, the palate is the commonest site, followed by the buccal mucosa, the tongue, the floor of mouth, the lip and the tonsil. The age range at presentation is very wide and it is the commonest salivary gland tumour in childhood. The sex incidence is equal and the peak age incidence is in the fourth decade. If low-grade tumours are excluded there is almost a 50% incidence of lymph node metastases. Five-year survival rates of around 40% for intermediate and high-grade tumours are reported.

Adenoid cystic carcinoma

This comprises 30% of minor salivary gland tumours, 2% of parotid gland tumours and 15% of submandibular gland tumours. Five per cent of parotid tumours are malignant with 14% of these proving to be adenoid cystic carcinomas. Slightly less than half of all submandibular gland tumours are malignant and 30% of these are adenoid cystic carcinomas. Sixty-five per cent of minor salivary gland tumours are malignant and 40% of these are adenoid cystic carcinomas.

The maximum incidence is in the sixth decade and they occur equally in males and females. The commonest presenting feature is pain and the tumour may be present for some years before diagnosis. It is often some time before a mass becomes palpable or evident and the patient may spend some years visiting different specialists with the complaint of facial pain.

Adenoid cystic carcinoma tends to spread along nerve sheaths and this accounts for the large number of pre-operative facial paralyses (20%) when it involves the parotid gland. Distant metastases, especially to the lungs, are another feature of this tumour indicating that vascular dissemination is more important than lymphatic spread. Forty-three per cent of patients with adenoid cystic carcinoma develop distant metastases and two-thirds of these are in the lungs.

The 5 year survival rate varies from 60 to 80%, but few series record more than a 30% 10 year survival.

Adenocarcinoma

Adenocarcinomas account for 3% of parotid tumours and 10% of submandibular and minor salivary gland tumours. The sex incidence is equal and it is one of the more common salivary gland tumours in children. There are three basic histological patterns – tubular, papillary and undifferentiated. The last type is usually very biologically aggressive and metastasizes distantly. There is also a 25% incidence of pre-operative facial paralysis when the parotid gland is involved.

Squamous cell carcinoma

This is a rare tumour in the salivary glands and almost never occurs in the minor glands. Two-thirds of patients are men and the maximum age incidence is in the seventh decade. It is an aggressive tumour and shows no tendency to encapsulation. It grows rapidly causing pain, skin fixation, ulceration and facial paralysis when the parotid gland is involved. About one-half of patients have metastatic lymph glands when first seen. It appears to arise from the duct system and some pathologists deny its existence considering such tumours to be high-grade mucoepidermoid carcinomas. A possible source of diagnostic error in this situation is the tumour arising in a parotid lymph node as metastatic from another head and neck site.

Carcinoma in a pleomorphic adenoma (malignant mixed tumour)

This has been used synonymously with carcinoma ex-pleomorphic adenoma (carcinoma arising from a mixed tumour). The true malignant pleomorphic adenoma is very rare and presents in two forms: the first is the benign pleomorphic adenoma which inexplicably metastasizes and the second is the carcinoma which develops after a number of years in a previously benign tumour. The carcinoma arising in a mixed cell tumour is commoner and represents 1–6% of mixed cell lesions. It is commonest in the parotid gland, then the submandibular gland followed by the minor salivary glands of the palate, lip, paranasal sinuses, nasopharynx and tonsil. The original mass will usually have been present for 5–15 years and even when malignancy supervenes the tumour may remain grossly encapsulated. It has the worst prognosis of any salivary gland malignancy. There is an accelerated recurrence rate and a high incidence of metastases (30–70%). Most series report a 5 year survival rate of less than 40%.

Acinic cell carcinoma

This accounts for between 2% and 4% of all parotid gland tumours and like Warthin's tumour it may be bilateral (3%). It is rarely found outside the parotid gland. The peak age incidence is the fifth decade.

These tumours are derived from two cell sources: the reserve cells of the terminal tubules, or the intercalated ducts. They may also occur in intraparotid lymph nodes, a feature shared with Warthin's tumour. They exhibit variable biological behaviour but survival rates of around 90% at 5 years make acinic cell carcinoma a much more benign tumour than mucoepidermoid carcinoma. Attempts to predict biological behaviour from histomorphological findings have not been fruitful. About 10% metastasize.

Rare tumours

Haemangioma

Fewer than 20 cases of primary haemangiona of the parotid gland have been reported. The parotid may, however, be involved in haemangionas occurring primarily elsewhere, e.g. the skin overlying the gland and the infratemporal fossa. Spontaneous regression occurs in some tumours and therefore no treatment should be offered until the age of 7 or 8 years and then only if the tumour is enlarging.

Lymphangioma

There are three types of lymphangioma – simple lymphangioma, cavernous lymphangioma and cystic hygroma. These conditions are discussed in the module on benign neck disease.

Sarcoma

Sarcomas may be part of the rare malignant mixed cell tumour spectrum but salivary glands can also be involved in osteogenic sarcomas and chrondrosarcomas of the mandible.

Lipoma

This neoplasm must be differentiated from fatty infiltration, which is usually bilateral, while lipomas are usually unilateral. Lipomas usually lie lateral to the parotid but the rare tumour of brown fat, the hibernoma, can occur in the parapharyngeal space. Removal of a superficially placed lipoma is generally uncomplicated unless it extends into the anterior compartment of the face in which case the terminal branches of the facial nerve can be at risk.

Metastatic tumours

Metastases to the parotid gland may reach parotid lymphatics via drainage from the scalp usually from primary cutaneous malignancies such as squamous cell carcinoma or melanoma. Tumours in the external auditory canal often metastasize to paraglandular nodes whereas those originating in the mucosal lining of the oral cavity, sinuses or pharynx spread to the intraglandular nodes. Adenocarcinomas from the digestive tract or urogenital system may present as parotid gland metastases.

Salivary gland heterotopia

Heterotopic islands of salivary gland tissue may occur in a number of sites in the head and neck: pituitary gland, middle and external ear, temporal bones, thyroglossal duct remnants, capsules of the thyroid and parathyroid glands, mandible, lymph nodes and the sternoclavicular joints. If these develop to any size they become manifest as lumps or as interference with function.

Basal cell adenoma

Basal cell adenomas are composed of basaloid cells with a prominent basal cell layer and basement membrane. This tumour may be misdiagnosed as an adenoid cystic carcinoma. It can occur in any salivary tissue but usually occurs in the parotid. This possibly represents a dominance of myoepithelial cells in a mixed tumour. Malignant variants have never been described and such tumours tend to occur in young adults.

Lymphoma

Lymphomas of the salivary glands are rare and the prognosis is usually better for salivary gland lymphoma than for nodal lymphoma of similar histology.

Minor salivary gland tumours

Tumours in minor salivary glands account for 15% of all salivary gland tumours, with 55% being benign tumours usually in the form of pleomorphic adenoma. The commonest malignant minor salivary gland tumour is an adenoid cystic carcinoma followed by adenocarcinoma, mucoepidermoid carcinoma, malignant mixed tumour and acinic cell carcinoma.

Section 46.4 • Investigations

History

The age of the patient is obviously important because mumps is much commoner in children than in adults. Although mumps can be predominantly unilateral, such a presentation should make one suspect a diagnosis of congenital sialectasis rather than mumps – especially if glandular enlargement occurs more than once. It is important to establish if the condition affects only one gland or more than one. Tumours are unilateral (Figure 46.6) apart from Warthin's tumours on very rare occasions. Sialectasis also usually affects only one parotid gland although bilateral submandibular involvement is sometimes seen. Diffuse enlargement (sialomegaly) is caused not only by sialectasis but also by benign lymphoepithelial lesion, drug allergies and a number of systemic conditions (see below), while tumours are typically localized masses.

If salivary gland swelling is related to eating then it is likely to result from calculus disease secondary to sialectasis (Figure 46.7). No other sialomegalies are related to eating. The duration of swelling resulting from calculus disease is variable and may last from under an hour to several days. Benign tumours grow slowly, although if bleeding occurs inside a cystic tumour the patient may become alarmed at a growth spurt. Malignant tumours increase in size fairly rapidly and are often associated with facial weakness, skin infiltration and pain.

Acute pain is a characteristic feature of duct obstruction by calculus or infection (e.g. mumps). Benign lymphoepithelial lesion is often uncomfortable rather than painful, as are allergic reactions. Adenoid cystic carcinoma typically presents with pain, which may result in the patient seeing specialists in various disciplines such as neurologists and dentists.

Systemic conditions such as myxoedema, diabetes mellitus, Cushing's disease, hepatic cirrhosis, gout and alcoholism may rarely be associated with painless sialomegaly. More recently parotomegaly has been recognized as a feature of bulimia and also of HIV disease. Drugs such as thiouracil, phenylbutazone, isoprenaline, distalgesic (dextropropoxyphene) and high oestrogen contraceptive pills can also cause sialomegaly.

Finally, enquiry should be made into other symptoms the patient may have, because sarcoidosis, tuberculosis, actinomycosis and hydatid disease may result in glandular enlargement.

Examination

Inspection should reveal which area is involved and whether one or more glands are involved. Skin involvement should make one suspect a malignant tumour as should evidence of facial weakness.

Palpation should reveal whether the mass is solid or cystic, localized or diffuse. Cystic masses may be Warthin's tumours, cystic pleomorphic adenomas,

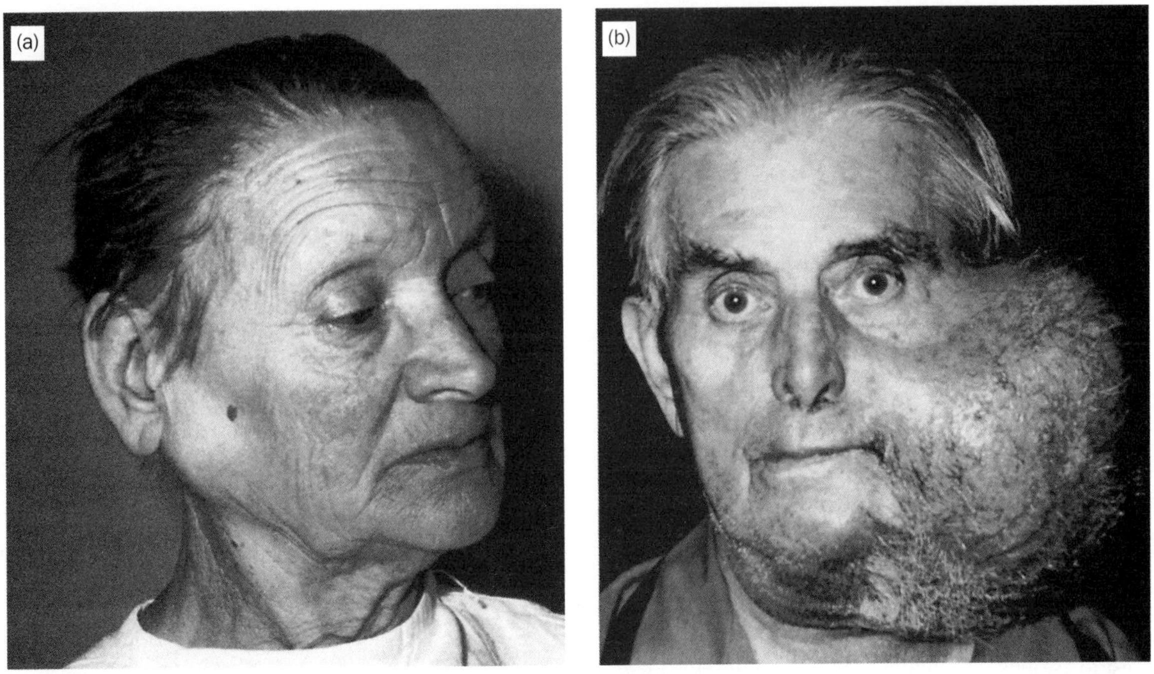

Figure 46.6 (a) Pleomorphic adenoma of the right parotid gland. (b) Large pleomorphic adenoma of the left parotid gland. Despite the size, there is no paralysis of the facial nerve.

branchial cysts or parasitic cysts. Solid tumours can be smooth or irregular, but this gives little help as to diagnosis because pleomorphic adenomas are often irregular and knobbly. Benign tumours are always mobile and any fixation should raise a strong suspicion of malignancy. In assessing a parotid mass one should ask the patient to clench the teeth so that the masseter muscle contracts; this allows one to assess if the swelling is in fact a hypertrophied masseter muscle and it also allows one to see whether the mass is within the muscle (haemangioma or myxoma) or outside it. Complete examination of all the salivary glands is essential to decide whether the mass is single or multiple and whether or not other glands are affected as in Sjögren's disease.

No examination of this area is complete without examination of the pharynx. Parotid tumours involving the parapharyngeal space are either dumb-bell shaped, in which case they present in the pharynx and also in the superficial lobe of the parotid, or deep lobe only, in which case they present primarily in the pharynx pushing the tonsil and/or soft palate medially. All salivary glands should be palpated bimanually. In the submandibular area stones may be felt or moved and in the parotid area pressure on a sialectatic gland may allow pus to be expressed from the duct.

The clinical diagnosis of a salivary gland mass is usually not difficult but the following rarities should be kept in mind as they may mimic sialomegaly:

- hypertrophy of the masseter muscle
- winged mandible (in the first arch syndrome)
- dental cysts
- branchial cysts
- myxoma of the masseter

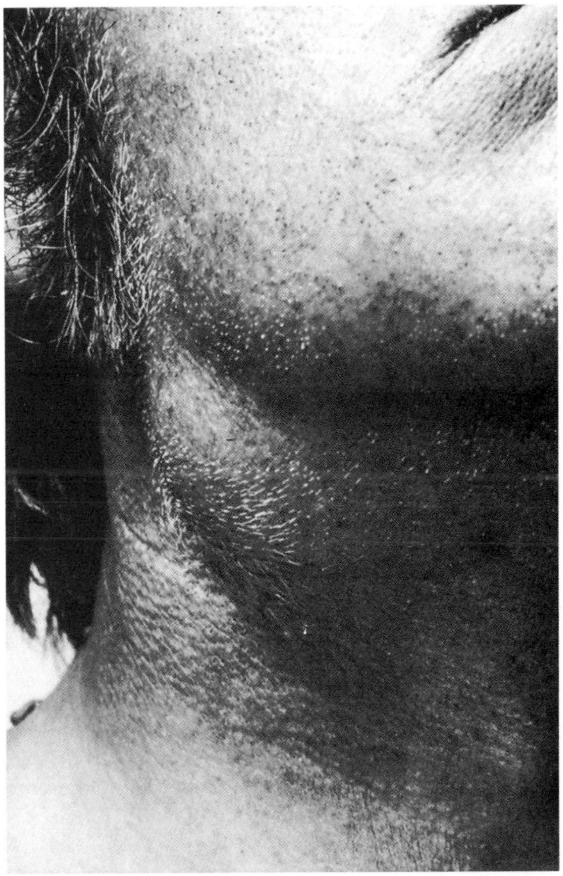

Figure 46.7 Enlargement of the right submandibular salivary gland due to calculous disease. Attacks of pain and swelling were precipitated by meals.

- lipoma
- neuroma of the facial nerve
- lymphangioma
- facial vein thrombosis
- mastoiditis
- temporal artery aneurysm
- mandibular tumours
- lymphadenitis of a pre-auricular node
- sebaceous cysts.

Laboratory tests

The appropriate tests should be done to exclude diabetes mellitus, myxoedema and Cushing's disease. Positive rheumatoid factor, antinuclear factor (ANF) and hypergammaglobulinaemia are often found in Sjögren's disease. If sarcoidosis is suspected, a chest X-ray and SACE (serum angiotensin-converting enzyme) should be requested. Less frequently used tests measure salivary flow and tearing.

Radiology

Plain films

Parotid stones are almost always radiotransluscent, while submandibular stones are nearly always radio-opaque. Intraoral films (occlusal) should be performed in both cases. Plain films are also sometimes useful in differentiating many of the extra-salivary causes of sialomegaly.

Sialography

Sialography is the most useful radiological investigation of salivary gland disease, but it must be performed by an experienced radiologist since artefacts can readily be created both by traumatic cannulation and by overfilling the gland with contrast material. Its main use is in the assessment of suspected sialectasis. In congenital saccular sialectasis the characteristic snow storm appearance is seen. There is extravasation of radio-opaque material at the intralobular duct level and strictures and clubbing of the duct system may be demonstrated. In advanced cystic sialectasis large collections of dye are seen in the cyst and this is most marked in the post-emptying films. Overfilling can mimic both of these types of sialectasis.

Isolated duct stenosis is nearly always an iatrogenic artefact caused by traumatic cannulation. Some patients may cause stenosis of their parotid duct by biting the buccal mucosa, but submandibular duct stenosis is usually caused by operative interference in the floor of the mouth or by traumatic cannulation.

Sialography in tumour assessment is generally of little value. It can, however, give some idea of deep lobe involvement and also whether or not a mass is indeed within the parotid, when combined with computed tomographic (CT) scanning.

Scanning techniques

The early promise of dynamic salivary gland scanning with technetium-99m pertechnetate has not been fulfilled. The finding that all tumours were 'cold' apart from Warthin's has not been substantiated in the longer term and the technique is accompanied by an unacceptably high number of false positive and false negative results. CT scanning with sialography shows up deep lobe displacement and also reveals filling defects in the superficial lobe. Magnetic resonance imaging (MRI) scanning is useful in determining the extent of deep lobe parotid tumours and any other associated soft tissue abnormalities such as extent of invasion by malignant tumours.

Angiography

This is sometimes required in the investigation of tumours of the parapharyngeal space in order to differentiate salivary gland tumours from paragangliomas of the carotid bodies or nerve sheath tumours, both of which have a characteristic tumour circulation. It also allows identification of feeding vessels. CT and MRI scanning have largely superseded angiography in this situation.

Biopsy

On no account should a discrete salivary gland mass be subjected to incisional biopsy. Since there is a nine out of ten chance that a solitary parotid mass is a pleomorphic adenoma, incising it is not only unnecessary but will almost certainly lead to later recurrence. The only acceptable biopsy in such cases is parotidectomy. If, however, there is skin involvement and probable malignancy then incisional biopsy is warranted. Many cytologists are expert in evaluating fine needle aspiration biopsy samples and this technique should be performed in every case of suspected tumour. However, cytology should only be interpreted in relation to the clinical history and findings as occasionally this technique can be inaccurate or misleading.

A parapharyngeal mass presenting in the oral cavity or oropharynx should not be biopsied through the pharynx. If the mass is a paraganglioma the bleeding will be uncontrollable and if it is a salivary gland tumour it is likely to recur.

On the other hand diffuse enlargement of a salivary gland is probably not due to a tumour and if a diagnosis has not been made after clinical, radiological and laboratory studies an incisional biopsy may be performed. If Sjögren's disease is suspected a sublabial minor salivary gland biopsy is necessary.

Minor salivary gland tumours presenting in the oral cavity and upper respiratory tract have a high chance of being malignant. They are surface tumours and therefore incisional biopsy is to be preferred to excisional biopsy. This policy carries no risk of implantation but it does mean that patients with benign tumours will be subjected to a later local excision. On the other hand this practice ensures that a correct treatment plan can be formulated and discussed with the patient if the tumour is malignant with no danger of a false sense of security being engendered that the tumour has been 'removed'.

Section 46.5 • Treatment policy

Benign conditions

Inflammatory or infective salivary gland disease should be treated with appropriate supportive management of pain and fluid intake and with appropriate antibiotic administration if required.

Sialectasis is usually managed conservatively but on occasions the parotid duct orifice or duct may be dilated in order to improve flow through the ductal system. Long-term antibiotic use has a part to play in the management of chronic sialectasis and is a useful form of management in young patients with this condition. The parotid duct orifice can be tied off surgically resulting in initial pain and swelling of the parotid gland which is managed symptomatically until the duct system and salivary gland tissue atrophies resulting in symptomatic improvement. Aggressive surgical intervention in the form of total parotidectomy should be resisted in sialectasis as the operation is often difficult to perform, runs a significant risk of damage to the facial nerve and often results in post-operative fistulas and ongoing pain and discomfort in the region. Other forms of treatment which have been used to treat this problematic clinical condition include radiotherapy and sectioning of the parasympathetic nerve supply to the gland.

Salivary gland calculi are managed by either removing the calculi from the ductal system or removing the gland if the calculi are well embedded within salivary glandular tissue. As the vast majority of calculi occur in the submandibular system management usually involves transoral removal of calculi which can be palpated within the floor of mouth, and surgical excision of the submandibular gland if calculi are found to be within the gland itself. Recurrence is likely and many advocate elective removal of the gland in these circumstances.

Sjögren's disease is managed symptomatically by providing adequate lubrication for the oral cavity mucosa and artifical eye drops to maintain adequate conjunctival lubrication. Many artificial saliva products are available but none is satisfactory. Recently pilocarpine has been used to stimulate the residual functioning salivary tissue.

Benign tumours

Parotid

Treatment of benign tumours of the parotid has passed through several phases during the past 30 years. Enucleation carried a high risk of recurrence and a policy of enucleation and post-operative radiation was adopted by some. This policy was often unacceptable in the young who were given a long-term risk not only of potential recurrence but also of radiation induced cancer. Recurrence rates were much lower in those series in which enucleation involved not merely the extracapsular removal of the tumour but removal of the mass together with a cuff of surrounding normal parotid tissue.

Since facial weakness was a risk of these techniques, especially extracapsular enucleation (as well as the other risks), superficial parotidectomy with identification of the facial nerve was next advocated. This was very successful in terms of prevention of recurrence and the nerve was safe in the hands of skilled operators as the first step in the operation is identification of the facial nerve and its two main branches. It became evident, however, that the procedure was often too extensive, e.g. removal of the upper portion of the parotid gland for a small tumour at the tail of the gland being unnecessary. Now, therefore, a hemisuperficial parotidectomy is often done (i.e. removal of all the parotid tissue lateral to one main branch, either upper or lower, of the nerve), to encompass the tumour with a cuff of surrounding parotid tissue.

Submandibular

Benign tumours in this gland are relatively uncommon and are often misdiagnosed – the cause of the mass being often an enlargement of one of the overlying lymph nodes. This does not alter the fact that the operation of choice is simple removal of the submandibular gland taking care to preserve the mandibular branch of the facial nerve, the lingual nerve and the hypoglossal nerve.

Parapharyngeal salivary tumours

The approach which is vetoed on grounds of risk of recurrence and also damage to surrounding structures is the intraoral one. If the tumour is of the dumb-bell variety then a standard superficial parotidectomy is commenced. The superficial lobe is left pedicled to the deep lobe at one of two places, depending on the site of the deep lobe tumour – either between the upper and lower division of the nerve or below the lower division. Thereafter the nerve and its branches, to the extreme periphery, are dissected from the medial surface of the superficial lobe so that either the upper and lower branches can be separated, giving access to the parapharyngeal space, or the lower branch is lifted up and access gained by this route. The deep lobe is removed by finger dissection quite easily because there is an area of very loose areolar tissue lateral to the pharyngeal mucosa. It is occasionally difficult to remove a bulky tumour behind the vertical ramus of the mandible. In this case, simple forward dislocation of the mandible doubles the retromandibular space; if, however, even more room is required then a mandibilar osteotomy can be performed with wiring or plating. This is rarely necessary.

Minor salivary gland tumours

Once the diagnosis has been established by incisional biopsy, the technique of removal depends on the site. In all sites, apart from the hard palate, local removal with or without primary closure is usually straightforward. In the hard palate there is always the possibility of extension into bone from the deep surface of the tumour. It is, however, unnecessary to make a hole in the palatal bone with the consequent necessity of wearing an obturator in every patient. This operation is used for highly cellular pleomorphic adenomas in which the recurrence rate is more than 50%. Other tumours are removed locally, the bare area of palatal bone being left to re-epithelialize.

Malignant tumours

Parotid

Primary radiation has little place to play in the treatment of malignant salivary gland tumours. It does, however, have an increasingly important part to play as an adjuvant to surgery, especially in adenoid cystic carcinoma which was traditionally considered to be radioresistant.

Whatever else is done in the management of malignant parotid tumours there is little doubt that the whole parotid must be removed. What else is removed with it depends on the size and position of the tumour. It will be clear whether or not to remove the temporomandibular joint, the vertical ramus of the mandible, the mastoid, the external auditory meatus or skin. What is not so well established is what to do about the facial nerve. If the nerve is free of tumour then is should be dissected out and left intact. This is rarely possible, however, because the nerve is often totally enmeshed in tumour often with no apparent facial weakness. When the nerve is removed an immediate attempt should be made to bridge the gap with a nerve graft using either the sural nerve or the medial antebrachial nerve of the forearm, both of which have a similar diameter to the main trunk of the facial nerve. If this fails then later attempts to rehabilitate the facial paralysis can be undertaken, provided there is no evidence of residual or recurrent tumour, using a cross-face anastomosis technique. It is very rarely possible in parotid surgery for malignancy to carry out a facio-hypoglossal anastomosis because the necessary main trunk of facial nerve is almost always removed proximal to its bifurcation.

In adenoid cystic carcinoma, the nerve excision should be wide because the tumour infiltrates nerve sheaths and travels intracranially. The facial nerve should be removed well into the mastoid by drilling it out of its bony canal. The greater auricular and the auriculotemporal nerves should be removed.

In the rare case of nodes being palpable in the neck a radical neck dissection is performed but if no nodes are palpable elective neck dissection is contraindicated.

The role of post-operative radiotherapy is not defined but consideration should be given to its use if clearance margins are in doubt. A facial nerve graft however will not be affected by post-operative radiotherapy but in animal experiments pre-operative radiotherapy has been shown to adversely affect the success of nerve grafts.

Submandibular

The operation indicated here is wide removal of the submandibular gland, including the submental fat, the digastric muscle and the tail of the parotid. Depending on the extent of the tumour the mandible or skin may have to be removed also. A supra-omohyoid neck dissection should be performed in continuity with the gland excision if no nodes are clinically palpable. If palpable lymph nodes are present a radical neck dissection should be performed. If the tumour is an adenoid cystic carcinoma the lingual and hypoglossal nerves should be excised as far proximally as possible. Post-operative radiotherapy should be given.

Parapharyngeal tumours

These tumours will almost certainly affect the superficial lobe of the parotid and therefore the same considerations apply as laid down in the section on benign tumours (see above).

Minor salivary gland tumours

The treatment of malignant tumours of minor salivary glands, which are almost invariably adenoid cystic carcinoma, depends on the site. If the tumour arises in the oral cavity a very extensive excision and reconstruction will be required. Adenoid cystic carcinoma is traditionally thought to have a good 5 year survival but poor 10 year survival. It is now considered that this is because most of the large series in the literature originate from specialist centres where there are large numbers of tertiary referrals. This means that the tumour has been inadequately treated for some years prior to onward referral. It has now been shown that if these tumours are treated by wide excision when first seen, the prognosis is good not least because this group of patients do not have the risk of developing further tumours in the head and neck, in contrast to patients with squamous carcinoma.

Tumours of variable malignancy

Low-grade mucoepidermoid carcinomas and acinic cell carcinomas can usually be managed by simple excision and close follow-up of the primary site and neck. However, intermediate and high-grade mucoepidermoid carcinomas should be treated with post-operative radiotherapy.

Rare tumours

Haemangioma

Fewer than 20 of these have been described in the parotid and excision by means of a parotidectomy is usually possible. Careful pre-operative assessment and imaging is essential prior to considering surgery for this condition as intra-operative bleeding can complicate the surgery and risk damage to surrounding structures.

Lymphangioma

This usually forms part of a previously treated cystic hygroma. The lymphangioma is usually superficial to the parotid and is easily removed without the usual exposure of the facial nerve.

In the submandibular region a lymphangioma is usually a cavernous lymphangioma of the submaxillary space and is best approached intraorally if it lies above the myelohyoid muscle.

Lipoma

These tumours generally lie superficial to the salivary gland and are easily removed without nerve damage although in the face they may extend anterior to the parotid putting the terminal branches of the facial nerve at risk.

Sarcoma

This tumour usually arises from the mandibular bone and displaces one of the salivary glands laterally. Osteogenic sarcomas should be excised, irradiated and treated with long-term cytotoxic chemotherapy.

Lymphoma

If a lymph node removed from a salivary gland region proves to be lymphomatous then the usual steps of staging the disease by clinical examination, bone marrow aspiration and chest and abdomen CT scanning are performed.

Complications of parotidectomy

Frey's syndrome

Frey's syndrome consists of discomfort, sweating and redness of the skin overlying the parotid area occurring during and after eating. It is caused by the severed ends of parasympathetic secretomotor fibres which innervated the salivary gland growing into the sweat glands of the skin. When the patient eats these fibres are stimulated resulting in vasodilatation and sweating.

If asked about the symptoms 60% of patients post-parotidectomy will admit to some degree of gustatory sweating but only 20% actually complain of it. Spontaneous resolution within 6 months is usual but a small number of patients require active treatment. This may take the form of a tympanic neurectomy, which divides the parasympathetic pathways, although this usually results in only temporary relief of symptoms. The simple use of a mild antiperspirant deodorant applied to the affected skin is usually all that is required to treat this condition.

Nerve damage

This is best avoided by using the landmarks previously mentioned to identify and preserve the facial nerve. In addition to these anatomical landmarks, a facial nerve stimulator aids identification of the nerve and some surgeons now routinely use facial nerve monitoring equipment during parotid surgery. If the nerve is deliberately sacrificed at the time of excision the gap should be bridged with a graft. If the main trunk is divided and only one, or at the most two, distal branches require joining proximally then a facial-hypoglossal anastomosis is advised. Other rehabilitative procedures are tarsorrhaphy, facial sling procedures and unilateral face-lift.

Salivary fistula

The development of a salivary fistula is a theoretical possibility in all superficial parotidectomies where a normal deep lobe with a cut surface is left *in situ*. In practice, however, is extremely rare and it only seems to occur if a sialectatic deep lobe is left behind. It also occasionally occurs after open biopsy.

Most cases settle in a few weeks and anticholinergic drugs to reduce secretion are of little value. Radiotherapy to destroy residual parotid tissue may be considered if the problem persists.

Cosmetic deformity

After a total parotidectomy a considerable retromandibular depression occurs. This usually does not trouble the patient, but can be filled by rotating a sternomastoid muscle flap to fill the defect.

Further reading

Da-Quan, M. and Guang-Yan, Y. (1987). Tumours of the minor salivary glands. *Acta Otolaryngol (Stockh)* **103**: 325–31.

Eveson, J. W. and Cawson, R. A. (1985). Salivary gland tumours. A review of 2410 cases with particular reference to histological types, site, age and sex distribution. *J Pathol* **146**: 51–8.

Jones, A. S., Phillips, D. I. and Hilgers, F. J. M. (1998). Diseases of the head and neck. *Nose and Throat*. London: Arnold.

Wilson, J. A., Watkinson, J. and Gaze, M. N. (2000) In *Stell and Maran's Head and Neck Surgery*, 4th edn. Oxford: Butterworth-Heinemann.

MODULE 47

Pharynx

Section 47.1 • Anatomy

The pharynx is made up of three parts (Figure 47.1):

- the nasopharynx
- the oropharynx
- the hypopharynx.

The **nasopharynx** is often referred to colloquially as the post-nasal space. It lies posterior to the nasal cavities and superior to the soft palate. It is a hollow air containing passageway with an expanded upper portion which tapers downwards like a funnel to the level of the soft palate where it becomes continuous with the oropharynx. It occupies the angle between the base of the skull above and the vertebral column behind. The roof and the posterior wall merge smoothly with one another and from above downwards are supported by the posterior part of the basi-sphenoid, the basi-occiput, the atlanto-occipital membrane and the anterior arch of the atlas. Anteriorly the nasopharynx communicates with the nasal cavities through the choanae. The medial end of the cartilaginous eustachian tube forms a prominent projection high up on the lateral wall of the nasopharynx. Above and behind the tubal elevation lies the pharyngeal recess or fossa of Rosenmüller. The fossa of Rosenmüller is of clinical importance as it is the commonest site of origin of nasopharyngeal carcinoma.

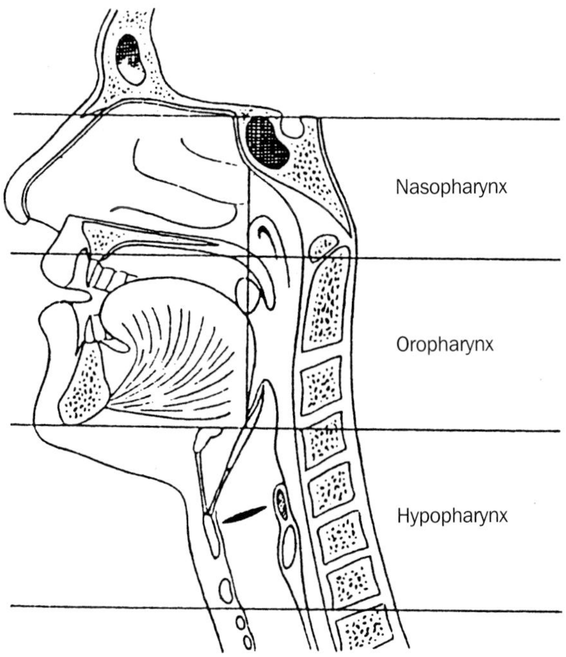

Figure 47.1 Divisions of the pharynx.

The **oropharynx** extends from the level of the junction of the hard and soft palates to the level of the floor of the valleculae. This corresponds to the level of the hyoid bone. The anterior wall of the oropharynx superiorly is in free communication with the oral cavity. Below this the anterior wall is made up of the tongue base, the valleculae and the epiglottis. The lateral wall is made up of the palatine tonsils and the anterior and posterior tonsillar pillars. The posterior wall of the oropharynx consists of the mucosa covering the superior constrictor muscles and the pre-vertebral fascia. The superior wall is formed by the inferior surface of the soft palate and the uvula.

The **hypopharynx** extends from the level of the hyoid bone to the lower border of the cricoid cartilage. It consists of that part of the pharynx lying behind and to each side of the larynx where it forms the pyriform fossae, also called the pyriform sinuses. It is continuous above with the oropharynx and below with the oesophagus. The anterior wall of the hypopharynx communicates directly with the oblique inlet of the larynx (Figure 47.2). Below the inlet the anterior wall is made up of the mucosa covering the posterior surfaces of the arytenoid cartilages and the posterior plate of the cricoid cartilage. On each side of the larynx are the pyriform fossae which are bounded laterally by the mucosa covering the medial surface of the thyroid cartilage and medially by the lateral surface of the fold of mucosa linking the arytenoid cartilage to the epiglottis. The posterior wall of the hypopharynx,

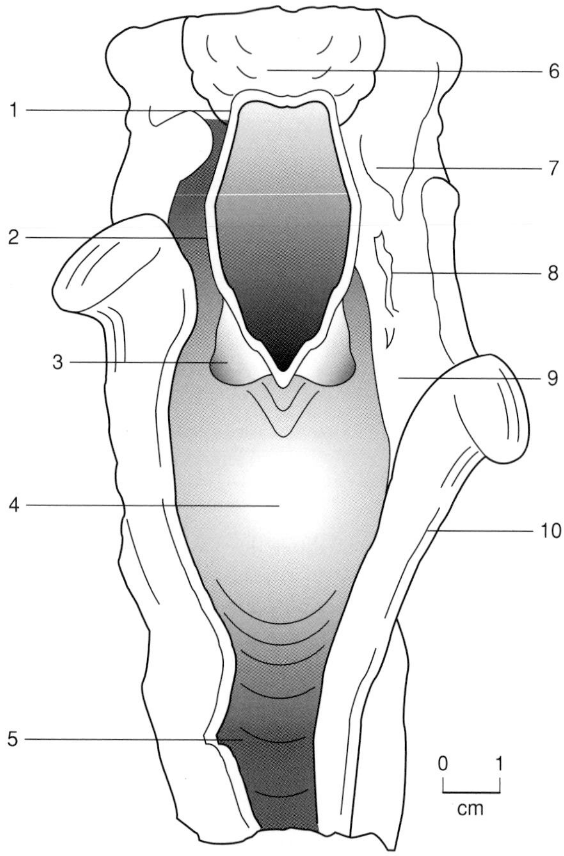

Figure 47.2 The lower pharynx, opened from behind, to show the valleculae, pyriform fossae and post-cricoid regions. Note the shallow upper and deeper lower parts of the pyriform fossae. (1 – Epiglottis; 2 – Aryepiglottic fold; 3 – Arytenoid cartilage; 4 – Post-cricoid region; 5 – Cervical oesophagus; 6 – Base of tongue; 7 – Vallecula; 8 – Upper pyriform fossa; 9 – Lower pyriform fossa; 10 – Posterolateral pharyngeal wall.)

from the level of the floor of the valleculae to the level of the cricoarytenoid joints, is formed by mucous membrane covering the pharyngeal constrictor muscles. The region below this, down to the level of the inferior border of the cricoid cartilage is the pharyngo-oesophageal junction (post-cricoid area) and is bounded anteriorly by the posterior plate of the cricoid cartilage and encircled by the cricopharyngeus muscle which constitutes the upper sphincter of the oesophagus.

Section 47.2 • Diseases of the nasopharynx

Adenoid hypertrophy

The lymphoid tissue in the nasopharynx (adenoid) appears deep to the mucous membrane during the fourth month of embryonic development. This tissue hypertrophies rapidly in early childhood followed by gradual regression after the age of 9–10 years. Enlargement of this lymphoid tissue may result in nasal obstruction which may be associated with recurrent infections of the nose and paranasal sinuses. It is generally assumed that enlarged adenoids may result in blockage of the eustachian tubes resulting in otitis media and deafness.

Children with obstructive adenoid hypertrophy may develop respiratory disturbances during sleep with snoring, restlessness and periods of apnoea. They may also be unable to eat and breathe simultaneously. Because the child is forced to breathe through the mouth the child may experience a sore throat resulting from pharyngeal dryness and inflammation. The voice is often hyponasal, as little or no air passes through the nose on phonation. Adenoidectomy is performed for relief of such obstructive symptoms and also in children with recurrent acute otitis media and otitis media with effusion.

Nasopharyngeal carcinoma

Aetiological factors

In most parts of the world nasopharyngeal carcinoma is a rare tumour with an incidence of less than one per 100 000 people per year. The highest incidence is in southern China where in males, 30–50 new cases are identified per 100 000 people per year. High frequencies of nasopharyngeal carcinoma are also seen in immigrant southern Chinese populations in south-east Asia, the west coast of North America and elsewhere. Aetiological factors include dietary and environmental factors, particularly the consumption of salted fish in childhood. Genetic factors are implicated with specific haplotypes in the human lymphocyte antigen (HLA) region being associated with an increased risk of nasopharyngeal carcinoma. The Epstein–Barr virus is a herpes virus closely implicated in the developed nasopharyngeal carcinoma. Natural primary infection with this virus usually takes place in childhood without any clinical manifestations and in developing countries virtually all children are infected by the age of 3 years. In developed countries the primary infection is less common in early childhood. If primary infection is delayed until adolescence or early adult life there is a 50% chance it will be accompanied by the clinical manifestations of infectious mononucleosis. The association of the Epstein–Barr virus with nasopharyngeal carcinoma is strong and consistent. Higher Epstein–Barr virus antibody titres occur in patients with nasopharyngeal carcinoma than in controls. These antibody levels rise with the tumour burden regardless of different geographical locations and ethnic groups. The Epstein–Barr virus genome and Epstein–Barr virus associated antigens have been consistently found in undifferentiated and in well differentiated nasopharyngeal tumours.

The incidence of nasopharyngeal cancer in both sexes begins to rise at the early age of 20 years, reaches a plateau between 35 and 65 years and declines thereafter. The male to female ratio is approximately 2:1.

There is continuing controversy regarding the exact pathological nature of the tumour commonly referred to as nasopharyngeal carcinoma. Many pathologists have reverted to the old term 'lymphoepithelioma' believing that this best describes the Epstein–Barr virus-related undifferentiated tumour arising deep to the surface epithelium of the nasopharynx. Other authorities feel that the term squamous cell carcinoma best describes the lesion.

Clinical picture

Presenting symptoms

These depend on the position of the tumour in the nasopharynx and the degree of direct and regional spread. In endemic areas the commonest presenting complaint is the presence of a mass in the neck and in this clinical situation it is essential that the possibility of metastatic disease is entertained. Nasal complaints including obstruction, discharge and epistaxis are the presenting features in about one-third of patients. Less than 20% of patients complain of ear symptoms and even fewer present with neurological deficits which tend to occur late in disease and result from extensive local spread.

Examination

Conventionally the post-nasal space is examined with a post-nasal mirror. The fossa of the Rosenmüller is difficult to examine using this technique and it is preferable to perform a direct nasopharyngoscopy using either a rigid or flexible endoscope. The latter technique allows a biopsy to be taken using topical local anaesthesia. Nasopharyngeal carcinomas are often friable and bleed when lightly touched by an endoscope. It is essential to conduct a full head and neck examination in all patients suspected of having nasopharyngeal carcinoma. In particular the tympanic membranes must be inspected for evidence of indrawing or middle ear fluid. The cranial nerves and the cervical sympathetic chain must also be assessed. The neck must be carefully palpated for metastatic cervical lymphadenopathy.

The detection of IgA antibodies to the Epstein-Barr virus specific antigens is helpful in the diagnosis of nasopharyngeal carcinoma.

Imaging

The main role of imaging in nasopharyngeal carcinoma is to delineate the exact extent of the tumour. Plain X-rays of the nasopharynx and base of skull are of limited value. Computed tomography (CT) scanning of the nasopharynx is particularly useful in demonstrating the exact extent of bone destruction and is particularly helpful in submucosal disease. Magnetic resonance imaging (MRI) is more accurate than CT in detecting and staging nasopharyngeal carcinoma, but its value is limited by the relative lack of bone detail. MRI is particularly helpful in its ability to differentiate tissue densities following radiotherapy, being useful in distinguishing tumour from inflammation or scarring. Both CT and MRI are useful in assessing cervical lymphadenopathy. Fine needle aspiration cytology is helpful in this regard. In nasopharyngeal carcinoma cervical nodal disease is typically undifferentiated.

Treatment

In patients without metastatic disease radiotherapy is the mainstay of curative treatment. External beam radiotherapy is most commonly used. In recurrent tumour a repeat course of external beam radiotherapy may be given. However, radiation associated damage to adjacent organs such as the temporal lobe of the brain carries a high morbidity and mortality.

Nasopharyngeal carcinoma is a chemo-sensitive tumour and chemotherapy has a defined role in the palliative treatment of metastatic disease and an increasing role in the primary treatment of locoregionally advanced disease. Drugs which are active and most commonly used in nasopharyngeal carcinoma patients include cisplatin, carboplatin, 5-fluorouracil and paclitaxel.

Lymph node metastases

Lymph node metastases in nasopharyngeal carcinoma are common. Despite the sensitivity of the tumour to radiotherapy there is a recurrence rate of around 10% in the neck after therapeutic or prophylactic neck irradiation. Radical neck dissection is used in patients where lymph node metastatic disease has not been controlled by radiotherapy or when lymph nodes appear after the primary lesion has been controlled.

Direct surgical approaches to the nasopharynx have limited use except to provide for local excision and implantation radiotherapy. Oncological resection with adequate margins is difficult because of the intimate proximity of the brain, skull base, eye and internal carotid artery to the nasopharynx.

Angiofibroma

Angiofibroma is a vascular benign tumour of the nasopharynx which occurs in pre-pubertal and adolescent males. It arises from the spheno-palatine foramen in the posterior part of the lateral wall of the nasal cavity. From there it extends into the nasopharynx and into the nasal cavities. It may extend laterally into the pterygopalatine fossa and to the infratemporal fossa.

In the nose and nasopharynx the tumour appears pink. If it extends into recesses at the skull base it appears grey. Histologically the tumour consists of thin walled sinusoidal vessels lined by flattened epithelium with no muscular coat. The tumour exhibits varying amounts of fibrous stroma. Although nasopharyngeal angiofibroma is benign it grows by local invasion and may invade intracranially. Angiofibromas do not metastasize.

Clinical presentation

Typically the pubescent or adolescent boy complains of recurrent nose bleeds and nasal obstruction. There may be associated facial pain related to infection in the paranasal sinuses. The voice is hyponasal. The eustachian tubes may be obstructed resulting in otitis media with effusion and associated hearing loss. If the orbit is

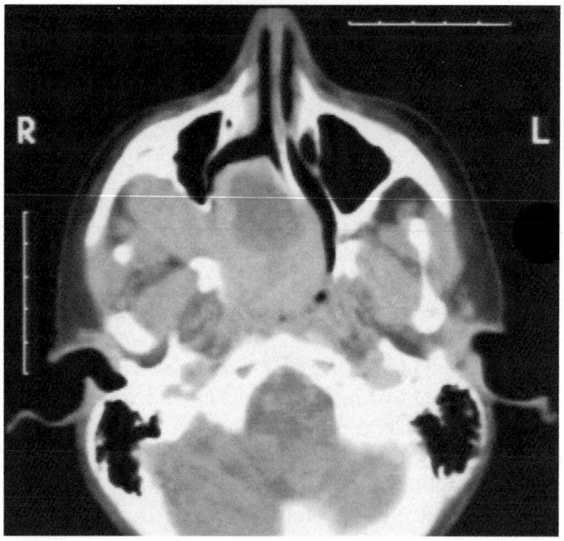

Figure 47.3 A large juvenile angiofibroma of the nasopharynx with lateral extension.

involved there may be proptosis. If the infratemporal fossa is involved there may be swelling in the cheek.

Investigations

Biopsy is generally contraindicated in view of the highly vascular nature of these lesions. High quality CT scans will show the extent of these and associated bony erosion (Figure 47.3). MR scans and angiography are useful adjuncts. In some centres it is common practice to embolize these tumours 2–3 days prior to surgery. Embolization as the only the treatment is seldom worthwhile.

Treatment

Surgical removal is the treatment of choice. A midfacial degloving incision extending from one maxillary tuberosity to the other allows excellent access to the tumour and its extensions and avoids a facial scar. Care should be taken to avoid rupture of the tumour as this can result in brisk bleeding. Radiotherapy has been used as primary treatment, but is usually reserved for treatment of intracranial extension. If radiation is used the pituitary may be damaged and hormonal supplementation or replacement required. There is also a risk of radiation induced tumour formation in later life.

Section 47.3 • Diseases of the oropharynx

The diseases of surgical interest which affect the oropharynx are recurrent infection of the tonsils and neoplasms.

Tonsils

The palatine tonsils lie between mucosal folds known as the anterior and posterior tonsillar pillars. They form part of a ring (Figure 47.4) of lymphoid tissue (Waldeyer's ring) which is made up also of the adenoid tissue and the tonsillar tissue at the base of the tongue (lingual tonsils). Recurrent tonsillitis is a common problem in children and teenagers. It rarely causes problems after the age of 25 years. The infection is short lived, lasting at the most 7–10 days and is characterized by fever, difficulty and pain on swallowing, and sore throat, and is frequently associated with malaise and enlargement of the upper cervical lymph nodes. It may be complicated by the development of peritonsillar abscess (quinsy), or more rarely the development of a parapharyngeal abscess.

Tonsillectomy remains the most common surgical operation undertaken in children in most Western countries and yet there are major differences in rates of surgery in apparently similar populations even within limited geographical areas. The currently accepted criteria for surgery have been arrived at arbitrarily. It is generally accepted that if episodes of tonsillitis have been occurring for at least a year and more than five such episodes have occurred per year with significant disruption of schooling or work, tonsillectomy is warranted. No randomized control studies of tonsillectomy against non-surgical management have been reported in adults. In children four such studies have been reported. They were all designed in the early 1970s and none would satisfy current criteria for design and

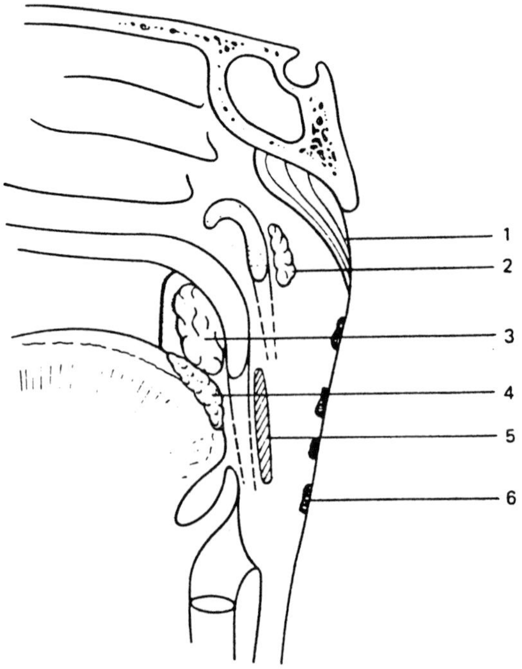

Figure 47.4 Diagram of the right lateral wall of the pharynx to show the aggregations of gut-associated lymphoid tissue that form Waldeyer's ring. (1 – Nasopharyngeal tonsil (adenoid); 2 – Tubal tonsil in fossa of Rosenmüller; 3 – Palatine tonsil; 4 – Lingual tonsil on base of tongue; 5 – Lateral pharyngeal band of lymphoid tissue behind palatopharyngeal fold; 6 – Lymphoid nodules on posterior pharyngeal wall.)

analysis. Nevertheless, despite this lack of high quality evidence many non-controlled studies indicate the benefit of tonsillectomy in children, not only in the reduction of number of sore throats, but also in improvement in general health. The Scottish Tonsillectomy Audit which reviewed tonsillectomy practice in Scotland over a 1 year period in the 1990s revealed a high satisfaction rate among patients and parents.

An increasingly common indication for tonsillectomy is sleep apnoea which occurs in children who develop episodes of respiratory obstruction during sleep. The main complication of surgery is haemorrhage, either primary or secondary which occurs in 1–2% of all patients undergoing the procedure.

Tumours

Tumours may arise in the oropharynx from the lining squamous epithelium, the lymphoid tissue and the minor salivary glands which occur at this site. Epithelial tumours, mainly squamous cell carcinomas, are by far the most common (80%), with non-Hodgkin's lymphomas (15%) and minor salivary gland tumours (5%) being much less frequent. In the upper aerodigestive tract as a whole squamous cell carcinomas account for approximately 90% of all epithelial tumours. The proportion is lower in the oropharynx because of the presence of the relatively large amounts of lymphoid tissue which give rise to lymphomas.

Pathology

Squamous cell carcinoma

The incidence of squamous cell carcinoma of the oropharynx varies greatly in different parts of the world. It is relatively uncommon in the UK, but much more so in the USA and parts of Europe. As elsewhere in the head and neck, these tumours arise more commonly in those who use tobacco and alcohol. In some parts of Asia there is a high incidence of squamous cell carcinoma of the soft palate in women because of their habit of reverse smoking. The male/female ratio of carcinoma of the oropharynx is around 3:1 with the maximum age incidence in the sixties. The site incidence is shown in Tables 47.1 and 47.2.

Cervical lymph node metastases from the oropharynx are common and may be the presenting clinical feature. Metastatic lymph nodes in the neck may be associated with an apparently occult primary tumour usually in the tonsil or the tongue base which is only identified following endoscopy and random biopsy. The degree of tumour differentiation does not appear to be associated with the development of lymph node metastases. Most lymph node metastases from oropharyngeal tumours develop in the jugulo-digastric lymph node at the angle of the mandible (level two). These lymph node metastases may grow to considerable size and outgrow their blood supply. This results in cystic degeneration of the central part of the lymph node and the patient may present with a cystic mass which in the past has been diagnosed as a branchial cyst carcinoma. True branchial cyst carcinomas, if they exist, are extremely rare. Histologically some oropharyngeal tumours are widely permeated by lymphocytes and are termed lymphoepitheliomata. The squamous component of such tumours is often undifferentiated and histologically these tumours may be confused with lymphoma. Immunocytochemistry and surface marker assessment of the lymphocytic population are helpful in establishing the true nature of the tumour.

Table 47.1 Site incidence of oropharyngeal tumours

Tonsil	70%
Base of tongue	20%
Posterior oropharyngeal wall	5%
Remainder	5%

Table 47.2 Incidence of nodes in the neck of oropharyngeal tumours

N0	*N1*	*N2*	*N3*
35%	30%	5%	30%

Lymphomas

These tumours in the head and neck may arise both in nodal and extranodal sites. Hodgkin's disease is extremely uncommon in the oropharynx, but non-Hodgkin's lymphoma accounts for up to 20% of tumours at this site. Most are B-cell lymphomas and like other mucosa associated lymphoid tissue (MALT) tumours remain localized longer than lymphomas arising intranodally. In the oropharynx the non-Hodgkin's lymphomas are usually solitary at the time of diagnosis, i.e. there is no involvement elsewhere in the body.

Salivary gland tumours

In the oropharynx these account for around 5% of all tumours. The commonest site is in the soft palate adjacent to the upper pole of the tonsil. Most of these tumours are malignant with adenoid cystic carcinoma being the most common variety. The 5 year survival rate of such tumours is around 80%, but most patients will eventually die of metastatic disease.

Clinical presentation

Most oropharyngeal tumours present with symptoms of pain and discomfort in the throat which is made worse by swallowing. There may be referred pain to the ear and more than half of all patients with oropharyngeal carcinoma will have lymph node metastases present at the time of diagnosis. Large tumours, particularly those involving the base of the tongue, alter the quality of the voice.

A detailed clinical examination of the upper aerodigestive tract including the neck is necessary. The laryngeal mirror gives a good view of the tongue base and the flexible nasopharyngoscope allows assessment of the lower extent of these tumours. The tumours are either exophytic or ulcerative, but a small number spread mainly submucosally and are often only identified by palpation using local or general anaesthesia. Metastases from squamous cell carcinomas are generally hard to firm in consistency and may be attached to adjacent structures. Cystic degeneration may occur in larger nodes.

Investigation

A chest X-ray should be performed in patients presenting with oropharyngeal carcinoma. A CT scan of the chest may detect metastatic disease not seen on standard chest X-ray. The extent of local and metastatic disease should be demonstrated by contrast CT scan or MRI. If lymphoma is diagnosed staging with CT scan of the thorax, abdomen and pelvis is necessary.

Fine needle aspiration cytology may be used in the clinic to obtain material from a neck swelling. Full examination of the upper aerodigestive tract should be undertaken under general anaesthesia to determine by inspection and palpation the extent of the primary lesion and to obtain an adequate biopsy specimen. It also allows for assessment of synchronous primary tumours in the upper aerodigestive tract or lung which in some series are reported to occur in as many as one in five patients.

Treatment of squamous cell carcinoma

Many patients presenting with oropharyngeal carcinoma are elderly, in poor general health and have advanced disease often with bilateral neck gland involvement and distant metastases. Such patients are incurable and only palliative treatment is appropriate. When treating for cure radiotherapy and surgery are used. Most patients presenting with oropharyngeal carcinoma without palpable lymphadenopathy are treated with radiotherapy. When metastatic lymph nodes are present, particularly if they are larger than 3 cm, the response to radiotherapy is poor and surgery offers better long-term survival. A composite resection involving the lateral wall of the oropharynx with part of the adjacent soft palate and tongue base in conjunction with the ramus of the mandible and a radical neck dissection is the classic operation described in the 1950s by Hayes Martin. Colloquially this operation is known as a Commando procedure, being an acronym for combined neck dissection, mandibulectomy and resection of the oropharynx. Initially such procedures were undertaken without any attempt at reconstruction with resultant variable cosmetic and functional compromise. Some patients suffered severe difficulties with function and appearance and the defect created by the Commando procedure is nowadays best repaired using a free radial forearm flap which may incorporate bone from the radius. This produces optimum results in terms of speech and swallowing. The pectoralis major myocutaneous flap may be used, but this flap tends to be more bulky and results in less mobility of the tissues.

Tumours which involve the base of tongue and vallecula are usually treated by radiotherapy. The base of the tongue cannot be removed in isolation and the only oncological procedure which is appropriate involves not only removal of the tongue but also removal of the larynx. A total glossolaryngectomy is an extremely mutilating procedure and not acceptable to many patients.

Treatment of non-Hodgkin's lymphoma

Localized lymphoma is potentially curable by radiotherapy. In some centres combined radiotherapy and chemotherapy are used. Systemic chemotherapy is the treatment of choice for disseminated non-Hodgkin's lymphoma.

Treatment of salivary gland tumours

Benign tumours which are mainly pleomorphic adenomas are readily treated by wide local excision. Malignant tumours which are generally adenoid cystic carcinomas have a tendency to spread by peri-neural invasion and require radical surgery which must be at least as extensive as for squamous cell carcinoma at the same site. Radiotherapy may be used if the surgical margins are in doubt and can be used for palliation.

Section 47.4 • Diseases of the hypopharynx

Globus pharyngis

This consists of a sensation of a lump in the throat, characteristically felt in the supra-sternal area and usually in females. There is a sensation of having to swallow over the lump but there is no true dysphagia. The symptom is not associated with weight loss, dietary restriction or hoarseness. There is often associated anxiety and depression. Patients with this condition are often predisposed to introversion and have an increased sensitivity to body sensations. The experienced clinician is often readily able to differentiate between the patient with globus and the patient with more sinister disease. There are, however, other causes of a sensation of a lump in the throat. Reflux oesophagitis is commonly implicated in the production of globus pharyngis, but the evidence that such patients suffer from reflux is weak. Other causes include goitre, cervical vertebral oestophytes, the Plummer-Vinson syndrome, oesophageal stricture and carcinoma. The difficulty is to know what, if any, further investigations should be undertaken in the patient presenting with symptoms of globus pharyngis when indirect laryngoscopy is normal. Hypopharyngeal carcinoma can present in this way and there is nothing in the history or physical examination which can eliminate this diagnosis with absolute certainty. Judgement is therefore required as to whether to proceed to barium swallow and/or endoscopy. Generally speaking if the history is suggestive of acid reflux a trial of a potent antacid such as Omeprazole is warranted. If this is ineffective, a barium swallow should be performed. If symptoms persist rigid oesophagoscopy with assessment of the hypopharynx is indicated. Most patients with globus pharyngis require strong reassurance that there is no serious disease present. In particular they require reassurance that they do not have cancer as for many patients this is the primary concern. It is important to emphasize to the patient that the more they try to clear the throat and dry swallow the worse and more persistent the sensation will become. It is helpful to draw the analogy with scratching of an itchy patch of skin. Most patients will accept that they have developed an increased awareness of their throat and that increasing worry can exacerbate the symptoms. It is helpful to explain that this is a common symptom which usually settles spontaneously with time.

Plummer-Vinson syndrome and pharyngeal pouch

These are dealt with in Module 7.

Tumours of the hypopharynx

Surgical anatomy

The hypopharynx is divided into three parts (Figure 47.2):

- pyriform sinuses
- posterior wall
- post-cricoid area.

Surgical pathology

Benign tumours of the hypopharynx are very rare. The most common are lieomyoma and fibrolipoma. These usually present as polypoid masses. Benign tumours of minor salivary gland origin also occur and usually present as diffuse submucosal masses.

Malignant tumours are virtually always squamous cell carcinomas and are usually poorly differentiated. Often they are well advanced at the time of presentation and the 5 year survival rate is generally less than 30%. Malignant tumours of salivary gland origin are rare.

Squamous cell carcinomas are usually classified according to the site of origin. When the tumour is large it is often difficult to be sure from which site in the hypopharynx the tumour has arisen. In very large tumours which involve the larynx it can be difficult to be certain whether the tumour is of laryngeal or hypopharyngeal origin. These tumours have a tendency to spread submucosally and this must be taken into account when planning treatment. Such tumours may spread directly into the neck particularly through the thyrohyoid membrane and this may be mistaken for nodal metastasis. Generally such a mass will move on swallowing whereas a metastatic lymph node will not. Medially the tumour may extend via the aryepiglottic fold to invade the larynx. The crico-arytenoid joint may be directly involved resulting in fixation of the vocal cord. Vocal cord paralysis may also result from direct invasion of the recurrent laryngeal nerve. The thyroid gland may be invaded directly and extension posteriorly may result in invasion of the prevertebral fascia.

Because of the very rich lymphatic drainage of the hypopharynx cervical lymph node metastases occur early and may be the presenting feature of the disease.

Table 47.3 Incidence of lymph node metastases at presentation

	No. (%)	*N1/2/3 (%)*
Pyriform fossa	35	65
Post-cricoid area	70	30
Posterior pharyngeal wall	60	40
Overall	55	45

This is particularly true of tumours arising in the pyriform fossa. The incidence of lymph node metastases in hypopharyngeal carcinoma is shown in Table 47.3.

Epidemiology

Post-cricoid carcinoma occurs more commonly in women than in men. This is in marked contrast to carcinomas arising in the oral cavity, larynx and remainder of the pharynx. Post-cricoid carcinomas account for up to half of all hypopharyngeal cancers in the UK and Canada, but occur rarely in the continent of Europe and the remainder of North America. Post-cricoid carcinomas appear to be associated with dietary risk factors, particularly iron deficiency anaemia, especially in patients with the Plummer-Vinson syndrome. Alcohol and tobacco are the principal carcinogens related to the development of carcinoma in the pyriform sinuses. Previous irradiation, particularly radiation of the thyroid gland, is also a recognized risk factor.

Clinical presentation

These tumours commonly present late as the tumour can grow asymptomatically, particularly in the pyriform sinuses. Patients usually complain of dysphagia, sore throat, weight loss, hoarseness and referred otalgia. A neck mass resulting from either direct extension of the tumour or metastatic lymph node involvement is a common presenting feature. In exophitic tumours clearing of blood from the throat may be the presenting symptom. Such symptoms can usually be differentiated from those in the patient with globus pharyngis. In patients with hypopharyngeal carcinoma there is true progressive dysphagia and often weight loss, pain is common and the symptoms are usually lateralized.

Examination

The hypopharynx and larynx are examined with either a laryngeal mirror, a rigid endoscope via the mouth or a flexible endoscope placed via the nose. Vocal cord mobility must be assessed as should any actual or potential airway obstruction. Pooling of saliva either unilaterally in the case of pyriform fossa tumours or bilaterally in post-cricoid lesions is an important physical sign. Examination of the neck should include not only assessment of cervical lymphadenopathy, but movement of the larynx over the vertebral column. Laryngeal crepitus is lost in patients with post-cricoid carcinoma and there may also be fixation to the prevertebral tissues. The neck must be carefully examined.

Imaging

A barium swallow should be performed in patients with symptoms suggestive of hypopharyngeal carcinoma. CT scan and MRI can identify extension into the larynx, tongue base and prevertebral areas. They are also helpful in assessing the size and relationships of involved cervical lymph nodes.

Endoscopy

Prior to endoscopy the patient's general and in particular nutritional status should be assessed. Endoscopy is necessary to assess the extent of the disease and to obtain a tissue biopsy. Assessment of the extension of tumour to the larynx, base of tongue and oesophagus should be made. The mobility of the pharyngeal mucosa over the pre-vertebral fascia should be evaluated. It is important to determine whether the tumour is operable and if so to determine the extent of the operation required and the type of reconstruction which will be necessary.

Treatment

Benign tumours can usually be removed via a lateral pharyngotomy with primary closure.

In patients with malignant hypopharyngeal tumours the decision to treat is often much more difficult. In some cases the condition may be incurable because of local extension of the tumour particularly posteriorly to involve the pre-vertebral area. Bilateral involved neck nodes and distant metastases indicate that the disease cannot be cured. The patient, and if relevant the family, should be made aware of the nature and extent of any proposed treatment. It is important for the surgeon to be clear in his own mind whether treatment is intended to be palliative or curative and it is important to avoid making the patient's last few months more miserable than they need be. If laryngectomy is contemplated as part of the treatment plan it is helpful for the patient to meet a laryngectomee prior to surgery.

Radiotherapy

Radiotherapy should be reserved for patients without involved lymph nodes and who present with small tumours. Surgery is the primary form of treatment for large tumours, for involved cervical lymph nodes and for recurrence following radiotherapy. Pre- and post-operative radiotherapy as part of planned combined treatment have been used in the management of these tumours. There is conflicting evidence regarding the benefit of such measures.

Surgery

In patients with cervical lymphadenopathy the primary tumour should be excised in continuity with a radical neck dissection. The operation necessary for resection of the primary tumour depends on its size and site. Tumours of the pyriform fossa may require a partial pharyngectomy and laryngectomy with preservation of residual pharyngeal mucosa. If the tumour is extensive a total pharyngolaryngectomy may be required. Occasionally if the tumour is small and confined to the posterior pharyngeal wall or the lateral wall of the pyriform fossa it is possible to resect the primary by a pharyngotomy approach with primary closure.

The prognosis in hypopharygneal carcinoma is generally poor and many patients will be dead within a year or 18 months of uncontrolled disease, second primary tumours or associated cardiovascular and respiratory problems. It is important to use a reconstructive technique which results in few complications and allows the patient to be rehabilitated rapidly and to return home. It is sometimes possible to preserve sufficient pharyngeal mucosa to obtain primary closure or to allow pharyngeal reconstruction with a pectoralis major myocutaneous flap or radial forearm flap.

If a total laryngopharyngectomy is needed the gap between the tongue base and the cervical oesophagus may be bridged with a free jejunal flap. A jejunal segment roughly 10 or 12 cm long can readily be inserted. It is important that the graft is orientated such that peristaltic movement occurs in the direction of swallowing. A feeding gastrostomy is required temporarily.

If a total pharyngolaryngectomy is required with resection of all or part of the oesophagus, which is often the case in post-cricoid carcinoma, the most satisfactory repair is by gastric transposition which allows a single high anastomosis rather than a visceral anastomosis in the mediastinum. By resecting the entire oesophagus the potential for skip lesions and a second oesophageal primary is eliminated. Gastric transposition is contraindicated in patients who have undergone previous gastric surgery. The stomach is transferred to the neck through the posterior mediastinum with two surgical teams working synchronously. The first two parts of the duodenum are mobilized and a pyloromyotomy is performed. An incision is made in the fundus of the stomach which is anastomosed to the base of the tongue.

Fistula and stricture formation are uncommon after these procedures. Normal swallowing is restored within a week or two following surgery and the patient is able to continue to swallow even if disease recurs locally in the neck. When local skin flaps were used to reconstruct the hypopharynx fistula and stricture formation were common and patients often spent many miserable months in hospital.

Further reading

Blair, R. L., McKerrow, W. S., Carter, N. W. and Fenton, A. (1996). The Scottish Tonsillectomy Audit. *J. Laryngol Otol* Suppl 20.

Van Hasselt, A. and Gibb, A. (1999). *Nasopharyngeal Carcinoma*, 2nd edn. London: Greenwich Medical Media.

MODULE 48
The oral cavity

Knowledge of the oral cavity and the diseases affecting it is important to the general surgeon. Many patients who present with oral disease will not have previously seen an oral specialist. Furthermore, many systemic conditions can manifest initially within the mouth. Indeed, features of oral disease may lead to the diagnosis of previously unrecognized systemic conditions.

Section 48.1 • Introduction

In considering the diagnosis of a lesion arising within the oral cavity, it is helpful to consider that this may derive not only from the soft tissues, e.g. mucosa, but also the hard tissues, e.g. tooth, bone. As a general rule any lesion that has failed to resolve or improve within 2–3 weeks should be biopsied to exclude malignancy. Early diagnosis and treatment is currently the best way to improve the relatively poor prognosis of oral cancer.

The following sections contain a general overview of either the more common or, if rare, more serious disorders that may affect the oral cavity. It is not an exhaustive list of all the conditions that can possibly arise within the mouth. The patient's presenting complaint, its manifestation and investigation, together with treatment are briefly reviewed. The effects of trauma and conditions occurring outside the oral cavity, e.g. salivary gland disease, are covered in other modules.

Section 48.2 • Tooth

Extraoral sinus, e.g. under chin

A history of trauma leading to a non-vital 'dead' tooth is often found. There is a history of local pain which remits when the infection is 'discharged', to create a sinus (Figure 48.1). The loss of pain explains why patients, who are often fearful, fail to seek dental treatment at the time. A frequent surgical error is to excise the sinus without treating the cause, i.e. the non-vital tooth. The vitality of the suspect teeth should be checked, e.g. the lower anterior teeth, using ethylchloride and if there is any doubt regarding vitality a dental periapical radiograph should be taken. Signs and symptoms of a chronic dental infection may include a darkened crown, tooth mobility and pus. Radiographically, there is often bone loss around the apex of the tooth. The patient should be referred to a dental specialist for root canal therapy or extraction, after which the sinus may resolve without the need for excision of the sinus tract

Dental abscess giving rise to facial swelling (Figure 48.2)

Often these patients are not registered with a dentist, attending only when in pain, have a neglected dentition, e.g. poor oral hygiene, halitosis and bleeding gums, and eat a poor diet with a high sugar content. On examination, there may be obvious cavitation

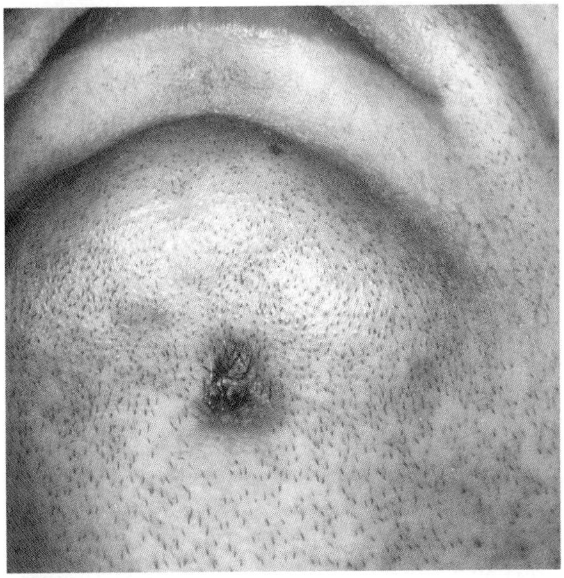

Figure 48.1 Illustration of an extraoral sinus resulting from a non-vital anterior tooth.

within a tooth often coloured brown, or around an existing restoration (filling). Pain on chewing is suggestive of an infection spreading beyond the apex of the tooth root into bone and leading to an abscess. This infection is painful, when enclosed in bone, with relief initially when spreading through the soft tissue spaces. Depending upon the tooth involved, this may present clinically as swelling around the eye, e.g. maxillary canine, facial swelling, e.g. mandibular molar, or palatal swelling, e.g. maxillary lateral incisor.

Fluctuant swellings require incision and drainage. However, it is rare for a swelling to be fluctuant if it has been present for less than 48 hours. A sample of the exudate should be sent for culture and antibiotic sensitivity. If the offending tooth is not extracted it requires root canal therapy. A drain should be sutured in place, intravenous antibiotics prescribed (if there is systemic involvement), pus sent for culture and sensitivity and the mouth examined to exclude a dental cause. It is often preferable to do this under general anaesthesia, although trismus may hinder the extraction of an abscessed tooth at this stage. The exception to a general anaesthetic is in Ludwig's angina, since respiratory paralysis (from a muscle relaxant) and a failure to intubate (due to the gross oedema) may prove fatal. Ludwig's angina is discussed in the section on deep neck abscesses.

Other dental anomalies

Malformations affecting the tooth may involve the cementum around the root apex, e.g. cementoma, dentine, e.g. dens invaginatus, or other tooth elements, e.g. odontome. In addition, there are numerous possible odontogenic tumours or cysts that can arise from these tooth elements, all of which are rare.

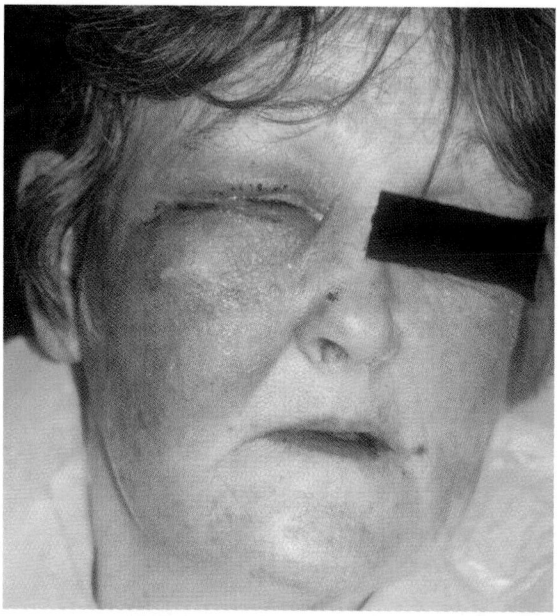

Figure 48.2 Typical facial appearance for a patient presenting with a severe dental abscess of a maxillary tooth resulting in closure of the eye.

Section 48.3 • Bone

Lesions affecting the bones of the facial skeleton may or may not be associated with expansion or facial swelling. An incidental finding on radiographic examination of a radiolucent lesion, particularly if well defined with a smooth, white sclerosed outline, is usually a cyst, e.g. odontogenic keratocyst – although other conditions exist (see below). A radiolucent lesion at the apex of a tooth root usually indicates a 'dead' tooth, for which referral to a dental surgeon is indicated. Developmental cysts usually arise in association with the crown of an unerupted tooth, or developmental absence of a tooth (Figure 48.3). Symptoms rarely arise and in general enucleation with primary closure is recommended to prevent cyst expansion and possible pathological fracture. Cysts arising within bone rarely cause obvious facial swelling.

Other lesions arising from bone can result in:

- **Facial swelling**
  A hard facial swelling in the absence of symptoms is usually due to a benign condition (although it is important to exclude early signs of malignant disease – see below).
- **Osteoma**
  This presents as a discrete bony hard expansion, fixed to the jaws. If multiple lesions are seen, then gastrointestinal investigation is required to exclude Gardner's syndrome (intestinal polyps with malignant potential).
- **Fibro-osseous lesion**
  Fibrous dysplasia usually affects the maxilla bilaterally. Radiographs reveal a 'ground glass' or 'orange peel' appearance. The teeth may be displaced. Surgical resection may be required for cosmetic reasons after childhood.
- **Paget's disease**
  Patients may complain of progressive facial anaesthesia, deafness and blindness secondary to nerve compression. It is rare under the age of 40 years, and may present with widespread enlargement and deformity of the bones. Jaw lesions are more common in the maxilla, with a 'cotton wool' appearance observed on radiographs. Serum alkaline phosphatase is often greatly raised with normal blood calcium and phosphate levels. Treatment is not indicated for asymptomatic cases. Surgery of the jaws and tooth extraction should be avoided if possible as profuse bleeding or infection may occur.

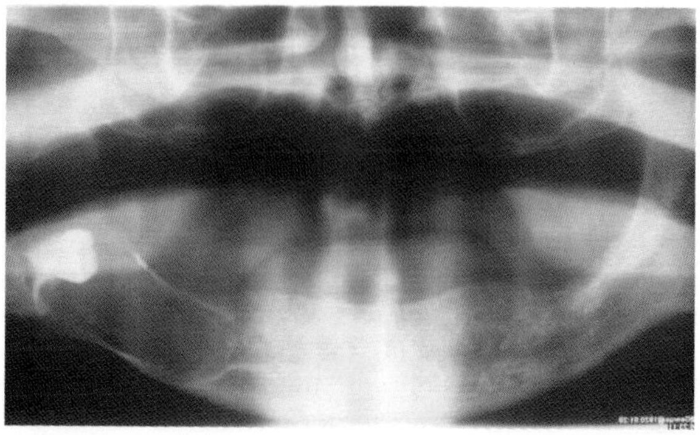

Figure 48.3 Panoramic radiograph depicting a radiolucent lesion (odontogenic keratocyst) affecting the posterior aspect of the body and ramus of mandible.

Ameloblastoma (Figure 48.4)

The molar region of the mandible is the most common site. If left untreated it can cause obvious facial disfigurement and derangement of the occlusion. Radiographically it may appear as a unilocular or multilocular radiolucency and thus may give the appearance of a cyst. It may cause resorption of adjacent tooth roots in which it mimics malignancy. It is often described as a locally invasive benign tumour as it can spread into surrounding soft tissues.

Curettage may be associated with recurrence. Excision of the lesion together with adjacent normal bone is preferable, with preservation of the lower border of mandible where possible. Bone grafts run the risk of tumour infiltration. Thus regular radiographic examination is required.

Haemangioma

Although very rare, haemangioma should be considered in the differential diagnosis of a radiolucent lesion of the jaw. Clinically, it may give rise to a progressive painless swelling, which if the overlying bone thins, may be pulsatile. Death from exsanguination following tooth extraction may occur.

Facial swelling due to malignant lesions

Invariably these lesions are characterized radiographically by tooth root resorption, with poorly defined 'moth eaten' boundaries.

Osteosarcoma

This is rare, but the jaws (usually mandible) are affected in about 7% of all cases. It may arise as a complication of Paget's disease. Characteristically it is a slow growing, painful lesion, giving rise to mobility of the teeth. If the mandible is affected it may cause paraesthesia of the lip. Radiographs may reveal loss of the lamina dura around the tooth root, irregular bone destruction (sometimes said to be like 'rays of sunlight') and tooth root resorption. Computed tomography (CT) films can be helpful in diagnosing the extent of the disease, as can a chest X-ray to exclude metastasis. Although they rarely metastasize to the regional lymph nodes, approximately 50% recur within 1 year. Aggressive therapy, e.g. mandibulectomy plus radiotherapy, is required as these tumours frequently extend further than their radiographic appearance suggests.

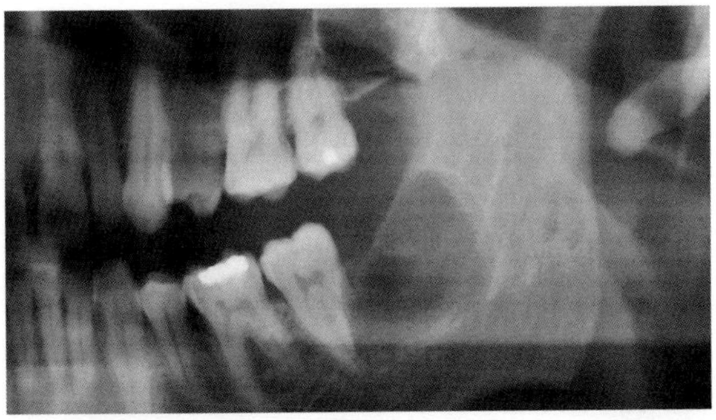

Figure 48.4 Radiograph showing a radiolucent lesion and absence of the wisdom tooth in the posterior aspect of the mandible (an ameloblastoma).

Langerhans' cell histiocytosis (histiocytosis X or eosinophilic granuloma)

This rare, osteolytic group of conditions is now thought to arise from the Langerhans' cell. These diseases range in severity from a solitary lytic lesion in bone to a fatal leukaemia-like disorder. The jaws, usually the mandible, are affected in over 10% of cases. The unifocal lesions are mostly seen in males under 20 years of age. Treatment consists of curettage, excision and/or radiotherapy with long-term follow-up. Multifocal disease may give rise to loss or loosening of teeth (radiographically teeth appear to be 'floating in air'), and spleen and liver enlargement. Hand–Schuller–Christian syndrome comprises skull defects, exopthalmos and diabetes insipidus.

Intraoral hard swellings

It is important to exclude malignant disease and infection. Developmental anomalies, such as a torus, occur commonly on either the midline of the hard palate or lingual aspect of the mandible. They are said to be more common in certain ethnic groups, e.g. Eskimos, Japanese. These harmless lesions do not increase in size and only require removal when interfering with a denture.

Section 48.4 • Orofacial pain

Pain in this region usually results from either infection (see Section 48.2), neurological causes or psychogenic reasons.

The key features of psychogenic pain are:

- patients often appear otherwise quite well
- the symptoms are often ill defined
- the patient is not awakened by the pain
- other psychogenic related complaints often co-exist
- objective signs are absent and investigations are negative.

It is important to exclude an organic cause for the pain.

Common complaints are considered below.

Atypical facial pain

This term is reserved for any facial pain for which no organic cause can be found. It is more common in females over age 30 years. They typically complain of a dull continuous ache, usually in the maxillary region, which rarely disturbs their sleep or appetite. It is important to exclude dental causes. Antidepressants sometimes help.

Burning mouth syndrome

Classically the tongue is most frequently affected, usually bilaterally, in the absence of any other clinical signs or symptoms of disease. Other oral mucosal sites can be similarly affected. Aetiologies includes xerostomia, mucosal disorders, e.g. geographic tongue, systemic diseases, e.g. haematological disorders, diabetes, psychogenic factors, e.g. cancer phobia, infection, e.g. candida, drugs and food allergy.

In half the cases a local cause such as ill-fitting dentures or tongue thrusting can be found. It is important to exclude nutritional deficiency states, diabetes and candidiasis. New dentures and vitamin B complex may help.

Trigeminal neuralgia

This condition is usually seen in middle aged and elderly people. It consists of a unilateral severe electric shock type of facial pain, usually confined to one division of the trigeminal nerve. It is often triggered by fine touch or even a blast of cold air. Neurological assessment is required to exclude other causes. Long-term prophylactic use of a membrane stabilizing drug such as carbamazepine is often helpful. Referral to a neurosurgeon for surgical decompression of the trigeminal nerve or another less invasive procedure (such as cryotherapy) should be considered if medical management fails.

Temporomandibular joint syndrome syndrome

The characteristics of this common condition may include: clicking or locking of the jaw joint, trismus and unilateral facial discomfort in people where no obvious organic cause can be found. It is frequently seen in young females, being attributed to stress, bruxism (grinding of teeth) or trauma. Treatment includes jaw exercises, the use of a bite raising appliance, non-steroidal anti-inflammatory agents and physiotherapy. The click is caused by the meniscus snapping back into position. Locking is more serious, indicating tearing and entrapment of the meniscus. Jaw surgery is very rarely indicated nor in the long run helpful, although initially it may bring relief of pain.

Other causes

Other disorders causing facial pain include diseases of the teeth, e.g. pulpitis, abscess, jaw fracture, maxillary infection, vascular disorders, e.g. giant cell arteritis, and referred pain, e.g. angina pectoris.

Section 48.5 • Soft tissues

Ulceration

Important questions to ask include: Is the ulcer painful? How many ulcers do you have? When did they first start? How long do they last? Which oral (and other body) sites are affected? Is it associated with anything such as food ingestion, trauma or menstrual period?

Possible causes

Trauma

This usually results from the dentition, e.g. sharp tooth or in edentulous patients from a poorly fitting denture. These painful areas should heal within 2–3 weeks, once the cause is removed. If not, a biopsy should be taken to exclude malignancy. A single ulcer is more likely to be malignant than multiple ulcers, particularly if asymptomatic.

Infection

Oral ulcers resulting from infection are usually of viral aetiology and arise as multiple lesions affecting a particular region, such as the soft palate in herpangina. Infection and ulceration due to herpes simplex virus may also occur. In primary infection there is widespread oral ulceration with systemic involvement. Secondary infection is characterized by small recurrent lesions on the lip (cold sores). Such lesions may also occasionally occur intraorally.

Recurrent apthous stomatitis

These may be classified into three types: minor, major and herpetiform. Minor apthae usually occur in young people, are less than 1 cm in diameter and consist of small yellowish ulcers surrounded by a red border (halo) affecting the non-keratinizing sites, e.g. ventral tongue, buccal mucosa. These ulcers disappear without scarring within 2 weeks. Local anaesthetic mouthwashes can help alleviate the discomfort, especially when used prior to eating. Possible aetiological factors include iron deficiency, stress, menstruation, allergy to certain foods and a genetic predisposition.

Major apthae (Figure 48.5) are larger, last longer and unlike minor apthae, may appear on the keratinized mucosa, e.g. dorsal tongue and hard palate, sometimes leaving a scar.

Herpetiform ulcers (Figure 48.6) present as multiple, pin-prick-sized ulcers which may coalesce to form larger ulcers. This may appear like a herpetic infection but the systemic upset is lacking. The ulcers are very painful and commonly appear on the tip of the tongue or inner lips. Tetracycline mouth rinses are helpful. Ulcers in association with other syndromes, e.g. Behçet's or gastrointestinal disease, may occur. Management involves

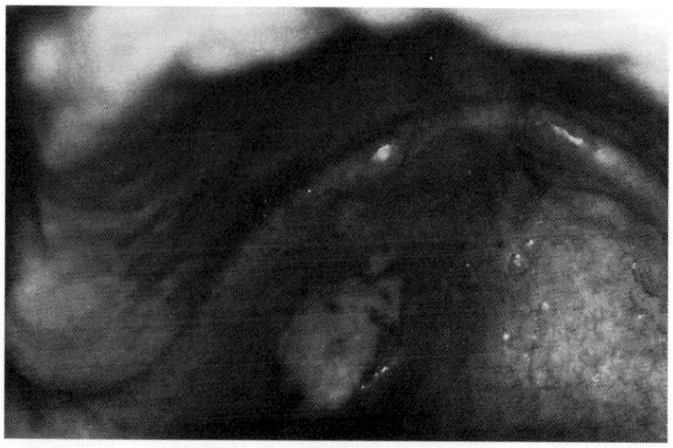

Figure 48.5 Recurrent aphthous ulceration (major type) affecting the soft palate.

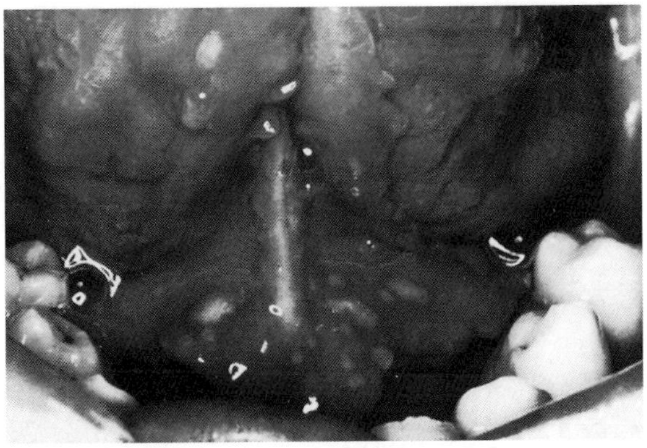

Figure 48.6 Recurrent aphthous ulceration (herpetiform type) affecting the anterior floor of the mouth and ventral surface of the tongue. (Courtesy of Professor D.M. Chisholm, Department of Dental Surgery, Dental School, University of Dundee.)

investigation for an underlying cause. Dietary advice (e.g. avoidance of chocolate or foods containing benzoates), correction of any deficiency state and the use of chlorhexidine mouthwash can be helpful.

Other systemic diseases

A number of conditions may present initially with oral ulceration. These include skin disorders, e.g. pemphigus, erythema multiforme, blood disorders, gastrointestinal disorders, e.g. Crohn's disease, coeliac disease and drugs.

Intraoral swelling

Torus

See Section 48.3.

Fibroma/papilloma (Figure 48.7)

Fibromas are normally sessile, smooth surfaced, rounded and firm. The overlying mucosa is usually pink. They tend to arise at sites of chronic irritation, e.g. buccal mucosa. Papillomas are predunculated, often with a rough surface, pink and usually affect non-keratinized sites.

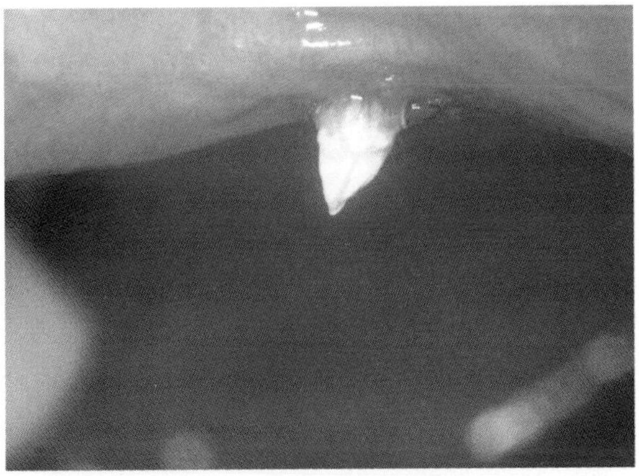

Figure 48.7 Squamous papilloma affecting the commissure of the mouth. (Courtesy of Professor D.M. Chisholm, Department of Dental Surgery, Dental School, University of Dundee.)

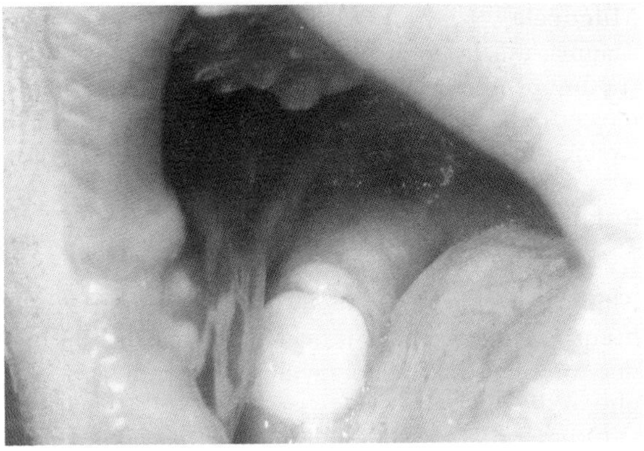

Figure 48.8 Illustration to show swelling and cobblestone appearance to the buccal mucosa in a patient with orofacial granulomatosis. (Courtesy of Professor D.M. Chisholm, Department of Dental Surgery, Dental School, University of Dundee.)

Orofacial granulomatosis (OFG) (Figure 48.8)

The clinical signs of OFG include facial or lip swelling, angular cheilitis, oral ulceration, mucosal tags and a 'cobblestoned' oral mucosa. Previously this condition was described as oral Crohn's disease or when associated with facial nerve palsy and fissured tongue, as the Melkersson-Rosenthal syndrome. Possible aetiological factors include allergy, foreign bodies, Crohn's disease and sarcoidosis. The term OFG is used to describe the various manifestations and should prompt further investigations such as biopsy and allergy testing for an underlying cause. Biopsy of the swollen lip should be avoided if possible so as to lessen post-operative discomfort. Gastrointestinal investigation is probably unnecessary in the absence of other gastrointestinal symptoms.

Gingival epuli (Figure 48.9)

Pyogenic granuloma, pregnancy, or drugs such as phenytoin and calcium channel blockers, may all cause gingival swelling. This is usually a reaction to chronic local irritation from dental plaque. Swollen, bleeding gums, although usually the result of poor oral hygiene, may occasionally be an early sign of leukaemia.

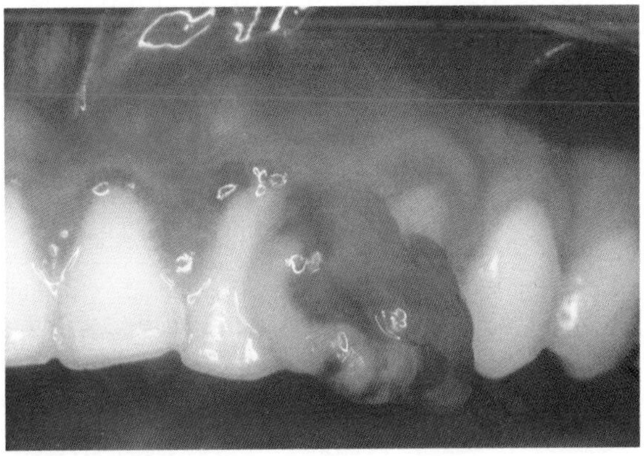

Figure 48.9 A gingival epulus resulting from poor oral hygiene in a pregnant patient. (Courtesy of Professor D.M. Chisholm, Department of Dental Surgery, Dental School, University of Dundee.)

Mucocele

Trauma, usually from biting the lower lip,can lead to rupture of minor salivary glands and the creation of a tense, rounded swelling of the lower lip. A similar swelling in the upper lip is likely to be a neoplasm.

Colour changes

Red lesions

Although a number of vascular lesions can arise, e.g. haemangioma, purpura, most red patches that are not due to candidal infection are due to thinning and atrophy of the oral mucosa.

Other causes of red lesions include the following.

Geographic tongue (erythema migrans), Figure 48.10

Irregular, partially depapillated red areas on the dorsal surface of the tongue with white, meandering boundaries that frequently change are observed. Patients should avoid hot, spicy foods if symptoms occur.

Candida infection – median rhomboid glossitis

Occurring in the posterior midline region of the tongue, median rhomboid glossitis is a smooth, red lesion.It is now thought to be due to candidal infection rather than a developmental disorder resulting from a remnant of the tuberculum impar. It has been reported in human immunodeficiency virus (HIV)-positive and immunocompromised patients.

Denture induced candidiasis (Figure 48.11)

This occurs as a red patch confined to the area of hard palate covered by the denture. Patients should be advised to leave the denture out at night, and to use appropriate denture cleaners. Rarely antifungal agents and a new denture may be required.

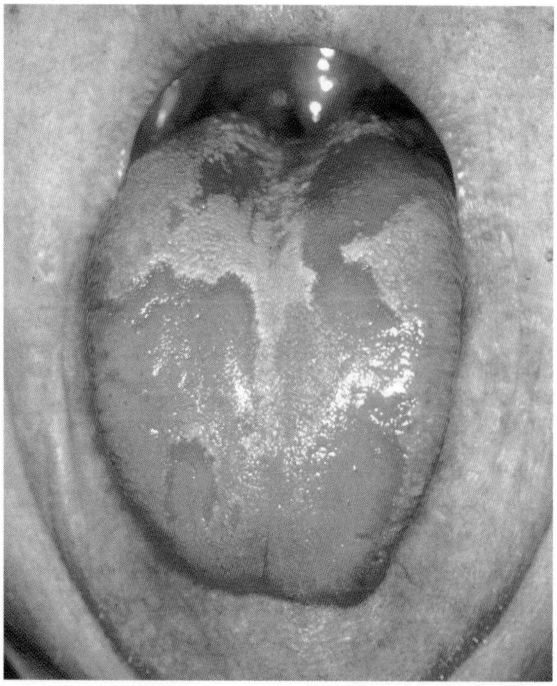

Figure 48.10 Erythema migrans (geographic tongue) affecting the dorsal surface of the tongue. (Courtesy of Professor D.M. Chisholm, Department of Dental Surgery, Dental School, University of Dundee.)

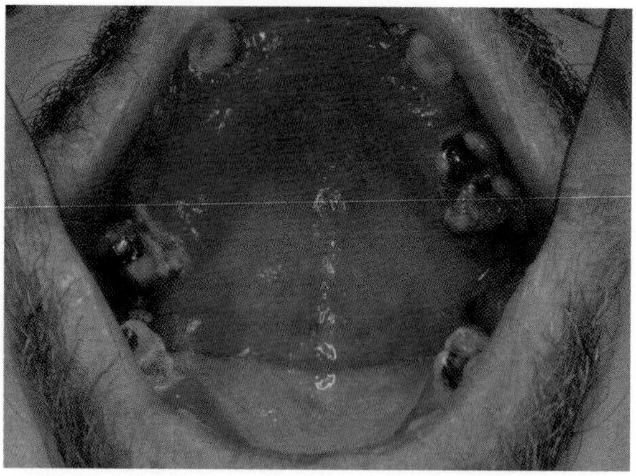

Figure 48.11 *Candida albicans* infection affecting the hard palate. Note that the area of erythema corresponds exactly to the fitting surface of the denture. (Courtesy of Professor D.M. Chisholm, Department of Dental Surgery, Dental School, University of Dundee.)

Erythroplasia

This has been defined by the World Health Organization as 'any lesion of the oral mucosa that presents as a bright red velvety plaque, which cannot be characterized clinically or pathologically as any other lesion'. High-risk sites include the soft palate and retromolar trigone. These lesions have a malignant transformation rate in excess of 80%. Excisional biopsy is usually indicated and patients who smoke should be told to stop (Section 48.7).

White lesions

Developmental anomalies

Fordyce spots are yellow/white lesions usually appearing on the buccal mucosa, and are intra-oral sebaceous glands. White sponge naevus (Figure 48.12) is another developmental lesion that usually presents as a rough, solitary white plaque, present from birth.

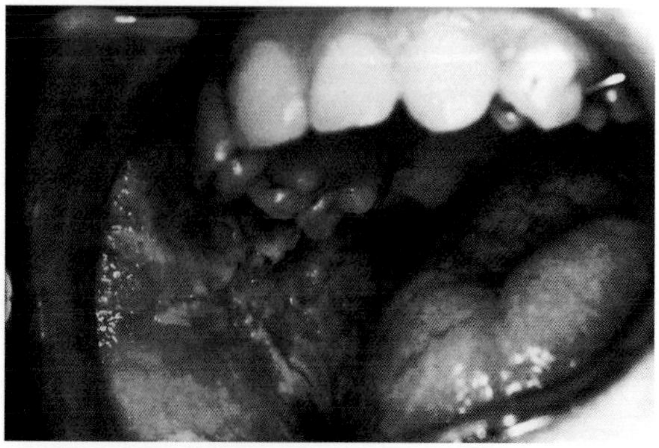

Figure 48.12 White sponge naevi (familial white-folded dysplasia). This is a developmental lesion affecting the buccal mucosa and is entirely benign.

Candida

Acute pseudomembranous candidiasis (thrush) presents as white plaques that can be rubbed off revealing an underlying erythematous base. It is rare in healthy patients but may arise following the use of broad spectrum antibiotics or steroid inhalation. It is associated with immunosuppressed states, e.g. HIV infection, leukaemia. Management includes investigation for the underlying cause and treatment with antifungal agents.

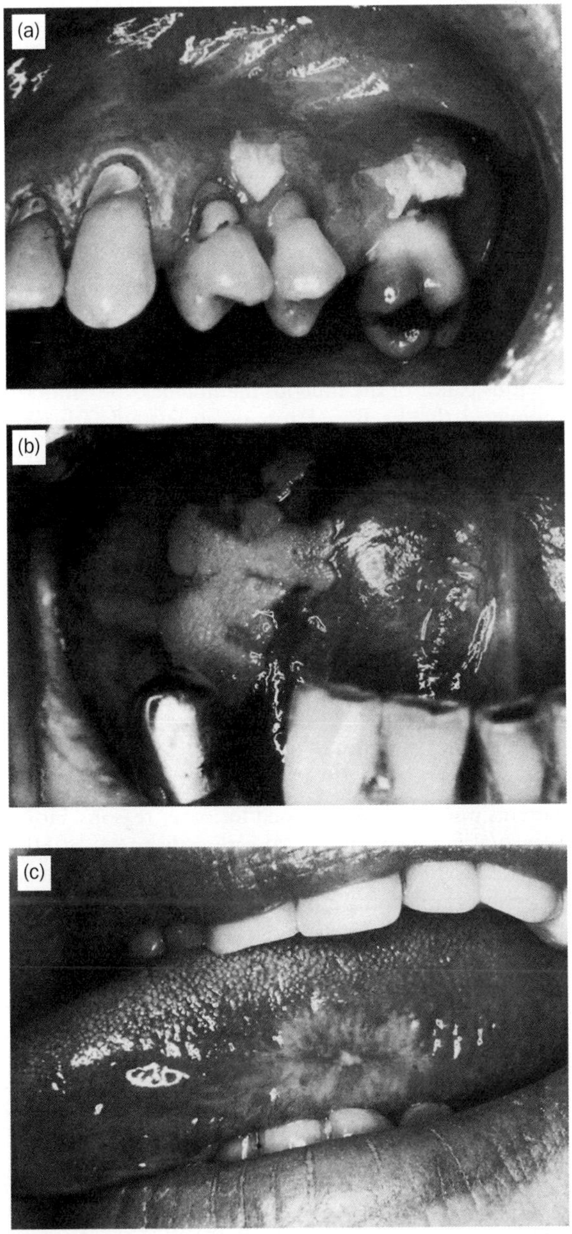

Figure 48.13 Simple keratosis (benign white patches) due to mild irritation. (a) Frictional keratosis of gingiva due to excessive toothbrushing. Note erosion at cervical margins of the teeth. (b) Frictional keratosis of the lateral border of the tongue due to ill-fitting gold crown. (c) Frictional keratosis of the lateral border of the tongue.

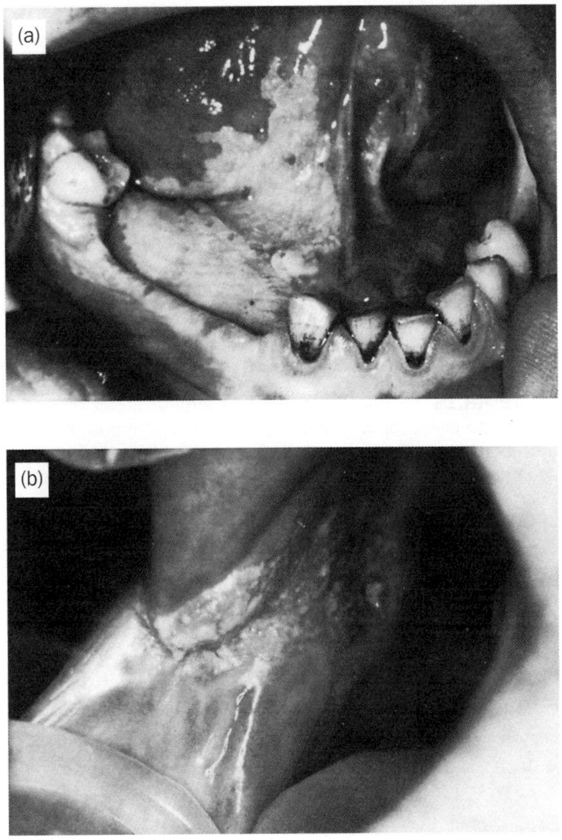

Figure 48.14 Pre-malignant white patches. (a) Sublingual keratosis affecting right surface and floor of the mouth. Aetiology was unknown. (b) Chronic hyperplastic candidosis (speckled leucoplakia) affecting right angle of the mouth.

Oral keratosis (Figure 48.13)

This may occur in response to tobacco, chronic trauma, drugs, lichen planus or of unknown cause, in which case it is termed leucoplakia. Leucoplakias have a low rate of malignant change (less than 5%) except when found in the floor of mouth or when infected with candida (Figure 48.14). Biopsy (to exclude malignancy) with long-term review is necessary.

Oral cancer

See Section 48.7.

Red/white lesions

Speckled leucoplakia (Figure 48.15)

This is a non-tender, red patch with white foci commonly affecting the non-keratinizing regions. It carries a high risk of malignant change, especially in smokers and when affecting the floor of the mouth. Biopsy and close follow-up are required.

Lichen planus

There are many variants of lichen planus, the erosive and atrophic ones being sometimes associated with cancer. It may also be associated with certain drugs (such as antihypertensive and hypoglycaemic agents)

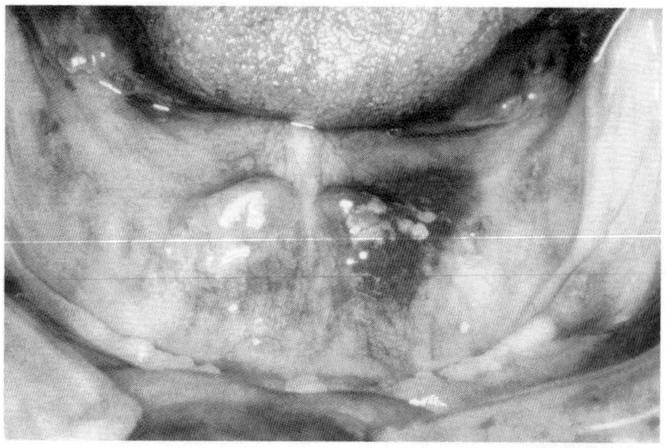

Figure 48.15 Speckled lesion (i.e. alternate areas of leucoplakia and erythroplakia) affecting right floor of mouth close to the submandibular duct orifice. Biopsy revealed early invasive squamous cell carcinoma. (Courtesy of Professor D.M. Chisholm, Department of Dental Surgery, Dental School, University of Dundee.)

when it is termed a lichenoid drug reaction. Skin lesions may be present, affecting the flexor surface of the arms. In the mouth, it classically affects non-keratinizing mucosa bilaterally, although it can occur on the lateral border of the tongue. Biopsy and steroids are indicated, particularly if the lesion is symptomatic.

Stomatitis nicotina

Pipe, cigar or reverse smoking may give rise to a characteristic white appearance of the hard palate, with numerous red dots secondary to blocked minor salivary glands. It is not considered to be potentially malignant, but since these patients smoke it does indicate that there is an increased risk of oral cancer.

Oral cancer

See Section 48.7.

Pigmentation

Amalgam tattoo

Previous dental treatment with amalgam filling material is the most common cause of isolated pigmentation which if large enough may show up on a plain radiograph. The lesions are asymptomatic, do not blanch on pressure or change shape. They usually persist for life.

Other causes of pigmentation include drugs (such as the contraceptive pill and antimalarials), endocrine disorders, e.g. Addison's disease, naevi, heavy metal poisoning and certain syndromes, e.g. Peutz–Jeghers as well as natural racial pigmentation.

Melanoma

This malignant lesion rarely occurs intraorally but when it does it usually affects the palate. The colour may vary from brown to black, grey or even white. It often has ill defined margins and satellite lesions. Recent change in size, shape or colour is very ominous. Excisional biopsy and investigation to exclude metastasis are required.

Section 48.6 • Oral manifestation of systemic disease

Gastrointestinal disease

Orofacial granulomatosis (OFG) (see Section 48.5)

The clinical signs of OFG include lip swelling, angular cheilitis, oral ulceration, mucosal tags and a cobblestoned appearance of the buccal mucosa. Oral ulceration in OFG can arise in association with coeliac disease, ulcerative colitis and Crohn's disease. In the absence of a history of weight loss or bowel symptoms patients need not be subjected to a full gastrointestinal screening.

Peutz–Jeghers syndrome

This is characterized by circumoral pigmentation in association with benign intestinal polyps and possible anaemia.

Haemopoietic

Anaemia

Profound deficiency is required to produce either obvious pallor of the mucous membranes, the 'smooth' tongue or the 'beefy red' tongue associated with vitamin B_{12} deficiency. Oral ulceration and glossitis are more frequently observed.

Leukaemia

Gingival enlargement and bleeding gums are frequently seen in acute leukaemia, as is oral ulceration, petechiae and infection (viral/candidal). Professional oral care is required.

HIV infection

No oral manifestation is pathognomonic of HIV infection. All of the following conditions may arise in patients immunocompromised for other reasons. However, oral lesions may lead to earlier diagnosis of HIV infection, which with the development of triple therapy, may significantly improve the patient's prognosis. For all conditions listed below, it is important to exclude other possible causes prior to considering testing for HIV infection.

Candida

Other causes (e.g. use of steroid inhalers or diabetes) should be excluded. It usually presents as white plaques (thrush) although red lesions can arise, particularly affecting the tongue.

- Oral ulceration – often appears like major apthae.
- Kaposi's sarcoma. This is characterized by purple, violet lesions which may be raised, usually affecting the hard palate.
- 'Hairy' leucoplakia. This results from Epstein–Barr virus infection it usually affects the lateral border of the tongue appearing characteristically as white striae and is strongly associated with HIV infection.

- Periodontal disease. Dental radiographs may show rapid bone loss around the teeth, especially the posterior teeth, sometimes in the absence of obvious poor oral hygiene.
- Gingivitis. This common condition can result in an exaggerated gingival response to dental plaque bacteria, in HIV patients.

Section 48.7 • Oral cancer

In the UK the incidence of oral cancer in males is similar to that of cervical cancer in women. Indeed, the death to registration ratio for oral cancer (0.43) is the same as that for breast and cervical cancer. In other parts of the world such as south-east Asia, oral cancer is the most common cancer and cause of death. In the UK it is responsible for approximately 1% of all UK deaths from cancer and has a 5 year survival rate of less than 50%. General medical and dental practitioners can help to improve the prognosis by detecting oral cancer at an earlier stage, for example by increasing their index of suspicion for early oral cancers, which are frequently asymptomatic. Noting any colour change is probably the single most important early finding, with referral if the lesion fails to resolve within 2–3 weeks. The site of occurrence is also important, as the prognosis deteriorates the more posterior the lesion is in the oral cavity.

Tumour biology

Tumour growth is a balance between rate of proliferation and cell death. Proliferation can be measured through the uptake of radioactive substances incorporated during DNA synthesis or the expression of markers present during certain aspects of the cell cycle, e.g. Ki67. Cell death may be through either necrosis or apoptosis. Apoptosis, defined as genetically programmed cell death in the absence of an inflammatory reaction, is thought to be a protective reaction when the cell is unable to effect DNA repair.

Proto-oncogenes are normal cellular genes, for example, involved in cell growth. When the protein products of these genes are overexpressed or excessive after mutation they are termed oncogenes. However, where genetic material is lost in tumour development, these regions are often found to harbour tumour suppressor genes (genes that protect the cell from cancer).

Mutations that result in malignant transformation may affect genes important for cell cycle control, DNA repair and differentiation. It has been estimated that between six and 16 mutations are required for this to occur. Like colorectal cancer, oral cancer is thought to progress through a series of clinical and histopathological stages. A sequence of mutations or deletions has been proposed that include chromosome 9p (containing the tumour suppressor gene p16), chromosome 3p and chromosome 17p (mutation or loss of p53), to transform normal mucosa into dysplastic mucosa. From there, further mutations on chromosomes 11, 14, 13, 6 and 8 (in order of frequency) have been found.

The presence of specific tumour markers in tissues can be assessed at the protein level(using monoclonal antibodies), the mRNA level (using *in situ* hybridization) and at the DNA level (through quantification of DNA using polymerase chain reaction (PCR) technology).

Other techniques include fluorescence *in situ* hybridization (FISH) in which a DNA probe can be coupled to a fluorescent chromophere that will bind specifically to a unique chromosomal region and identify specific alteration.

Samples can be screened for loss of heterozygosity (LOH) using microsatellite analysis. This technique amplifies the DNA, using PCR. These markers, termed microsatellite markers, are DNA repeats. The ratio of maternal and paternal alleles in normal tissue can be compared to the ratio of these alleles in the cancer cells, to observe either gain or loss of genetic material within the chromosome.

The most common deletion in head and neck cancers is on chromosome 9 and is an early event. It often affects the tumour suppressor gene p16, which normally inhibits cyclin dependent kinase (CDK) complexes. Its loss allows the cell to continue dividing, unchecked. Chromosome 3p loss is seen in approximately 60% of head and neck cancers.

Cyclin D1 protein (found on chromosome 11 and also known as CCNDI) is one of the cyclins involved in cell cycle regulation. Overexpression of cyclin D1 protein or mRNA is found in 30% of head and neck cancers, in association with tobacco exposure.

p53 is the most frequently mutated gene in cancers. It controls the cell cycle and activates DNA repair or apoptosis if the damage is too great to repair by arresting the cell cycle. Mutation of the p53 gene can lead to the production of dysfunctional protein (or its loss) or there may be post-translational modification of the protein, e.g. human papilloma virus (HPV) degrades p53 protein. At least 50% of all oral cancers harbour a p53 mutation, particularly in subjects who smoke and drink heavily. However, despite thorough investigation, there is little correlation between p53 and the natural history, prognosis and response to therapy of these tumours. Methods to transfect wild type p53 to restore normal function have involved liposomal transfection and the use of an oncolytic adenovirus that destroys mutant p53 containing cells, i.e. malignant cells, whilst leaving normal wild type p53 containing cells intact.

For the tumour to invade into the surrounding tissues, the collagenase type enzymes, now termed matrix metalloproteinases (MMPs) are important, particularly in breaking down the basement membrane. These MMPs can be induced within cancer cells as well as released by surrounding stromal cells.

In the future, molecular biology techniques will be used to: (1) create a genetic profile of a clinically suspicious lesion or cancer, (2) screen asymptomatic high-risk patients, (3) indicate whether the surgical margins really are clear of tumour, (4) indicate which novel form of therapy to use, and (5) guide gene therapy.

Aetiology of oral cancer

The vast majority of oral cancers arise in people who smoke tobacco and drink alcohol. Any form of tobacco use such as chewing, reverse smoking, betal quid and pipe smoking increases the risk for oral cancer thought to be largely due to the polycyclic aromatic hydrocarbons acting on the DNA. Smoking more than 20 cigarettes per day and drinking more than 6 units of alcohol per day increases the risk by a factor of 24. However, someone who has stopped smoking for over 10 years has the same risk as a non-smoker. Other possible causes for oral cancer include viruses, e.g. herpes, HPV 16 and 18. Although the evidence is not strong poor nutrition, particularly lack of vitamins A and C, is also thought to have a role.

In the Western world there has been a trend towards an increasing incidence in younger people often not in association with alcohol or tobacco use. Either aetiological agents exist that we are not aware of or there may be an unrecognized interaction between known risk factors and other states, such as nutritional deficiency. There is weak evidence for a familial link and no convincing evidence that poor dentition predisposes to oral cancer. However, a previous cancer in the region does increase the risk for a second malignant tumour in the upper aerodigestive tract.

An increasing number of women are affected; the male to female ratio is now 2:1, probably because proportionately more women are smoking now. The usual age of occurrence is over 60 years in non-smokers and non-drinkers and over 45 years in drinkers and smokers. However, it can arise at any age, hence the clinical signs and symptoms of malignant disease should be appreciated.

Clinical warning signs of malignant disease

Colour

- White patches have a malignant transformation rate of approximately 4%. Where no obvious cause is identified the lesion is termed 'leucoplakia'.
- Red patches (erythroplasia) due to thinning or erosion of the epithelial layers are very likely to become malignant (>80%), especially if also found in association with white patches (often termed 'speckled leucoplakia').
- Intraoral pigmentation is rarely due to malignant melanoma.

Ulceration

A single ulcer, in the absence of any obvious trauma, that has been present for at least 2 weeks without any sign of regression, should be suspected of being malignant and biopsied. Pain is a late symptom of oral cancer.

Surface texture

Early cancers are often smooth or possibly granular and rarely raised. Bleeding is considered to be a late sign of oral cancer, carrying a poorer prognosis, as does induration and fixation to the underlying structures.

Other signs and symptoms

As the lesion grows, it may involve blood vessels (giving rise to bleeding), sensory nerves (e.g. the lingual nerve, resulting in a numb tongue) and motor nerves (e.g. hypoglossal nerve, giving rise to deviation of the tongue on protrusion). Local growth of a tumour in the maxillary antrum can give rise to a blocked or bleeding nose, numb cheek or loosening of the teeth and lymph node spread.

Clinical assessment

History

The duration of symptoms and signs such as pain, numbness and any bleeding is important. Risk factors such as alcohol, tobacco and previous head and neck cancer should be noted. Possible causes of continued irritation, e.g. overextended denture, should be sought. In general, symptoms arise late in oral cancer.

Clinical examination

The site, size, colour and details of any regional lymphadenopathy should be recorded. A clinical photograph should be taken to allow assessment of rate of growth. The lesion should be palpated as oral cancers, other than early tumours, are usually locally invasive ('the tip of an iceberg') and are rarely exophytic. The extent of induration should be included in estimating size for staging purposes. The extent of spread of the disease can be recorded by using the TNM classification (Table 48.1) to stage the disease (which gives an indication of prognosis and potential form of therapy) (Table 48.2). However, tumours classified as being of the same TNM stage may have different genetic aberrations, and thus exhibit different forms of clinical behaviour and responses to therapy.

Staging is based on size of the lesion, with increasing nodal involvement (stage 3) and metastasis (stage 4) associated with a worsening prognosis.

Table 48.1 Tumour classification pretreatment

T1:	Tumour <2 cm diameter
T2:	Tumour between 2 and 4 cm
T3:	Tumour >4 cm
T4:	Tumour invading into adjacent structures, e.g. muscle, bone
N0:	No regional lymph node metastasis
N1:	Lymph nodes <3 cm diameter
N2:	Lymph nodes 3–6 cm diameter
N3:	Lymph nodes >6 cm diameter
M0:	No distant metastases
M1:	Distant metastases

Table 48.2 The UICC TNM staging system for oral cancer

Stage 1:	T1	N0	M0
Stage 2:	T2	N0	M0
Stage 3:	T3	N0	M0
Stage 4:	Any T classification with nodes >3 cm Any T metastasis	T4	

The tumour can spread to the regional lymph nodes, the submental, submandibular and deep cervical being involved. Posterior lesions can drain to the retropharyngeal nodes, which may put pressure on the sympathetic chain, giving rise to Horner's syndrome.

The use of 2% toludine-blue mouth rinse to detect dysplastic/malignant disease, which stains blue after rinsing the mouth out, may be helpful in deciding on the limits of excision or biopsy site. Photodynamic detection of malignant disease, based upon the uptake of a dye that is activated by a laser, is not yet in routine clinical practice. Oral lesions associated with HIV infection are not considered to be potentially malignant conditions.

Special investigations

Imaging techniques

Assessment of the depth of spread and whether the underlying structures are involved should include plain radiographs, with views at right angles to each other (e.g. for mandible, panoramic plus occlusal view of mandible, and for maxilla, panoramic plus maxillary occlusal or tomograms). In addition, the state of the dentition, e.g. caries, retained roots and teeth with poor prognosis needs to be assessed and treated, particularly if radiotherapy is to be used.

The radiological signs of malignant disease may include:

- a radiolucent lesion with an irregular margin
- bone loss around the roots of the teeth, i.e. 'floating' teeth
- resorption of tooth roots
- pathological fracture, e.g. of mandible.

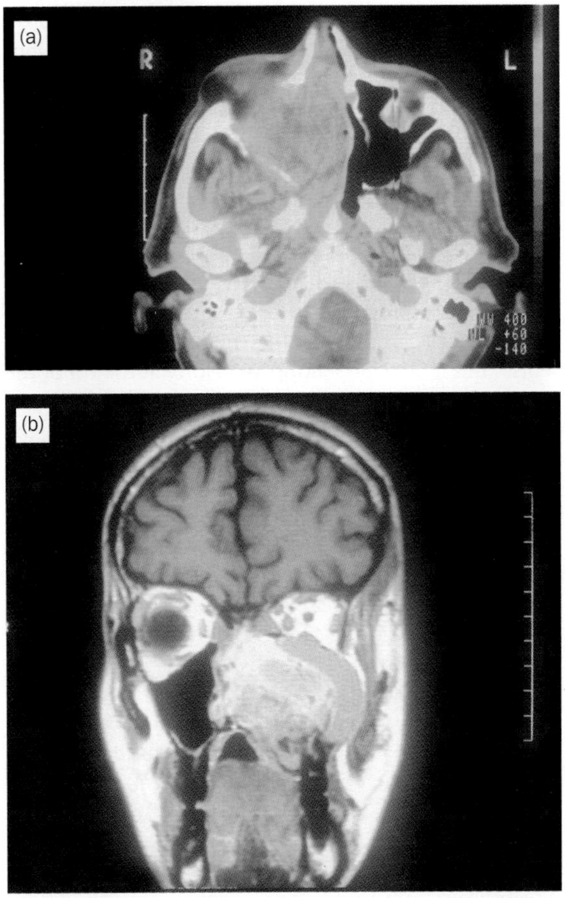

Figure 48.16 (a) CT scan illustrating a tumour involving the entire maxillary antrum on the right side. Note the radio-opaque lesion in contrast to the normal radiolucent antrum on the other side. (b) MR scan showing a tumour involving the left maxillary antrum.

CT scans are also helpful for constructing three-dimensional (3-D) views of bone invasion, whilst a magnetic resonance imaging (MRI) scan is better for showing soft tissue invasion (Figure 48.16). The extent of spread of the disease, together with the TNM classification, will help indicate the most appropriate form of treatment.

Biopsy

Biopsy is mandatory for all lesions that have failed to show signs of resolution after 2–3 weeks. A histopathologist familiar with oral pathology is necessary given that some oral lesions can mimic malignant disease, e.g. necrotizing sialometaplasia.

Prior to definitive therapy, histopathological confirmation of malignant disease is essential. Biopsy under general anaesthesia allows for better assessment of the extent of disease particularly where there is trismus or pain on movement of the jaw or tongue. Biopsies can then be taken from several sites, if the oral mucosa is deemed 'unstable'. Incisional biopsy is appropriate in lesions too large to excise prior to a definitive diagnosis of malignancy. An ellipse of normal mucosa should be included in the incision. Excisional biopsies should always include at least a 1 cm margin of normal mucosa. Areas of obvious necrosis should be avoided and steps taken to ensure that the biopsy is large enough and deep enough to provide information regarding involvement of underlying submucosa and the relationship to adjacent 'normal' mucosa. The biopsy specimen should be placed immediately in fixative and a record made of the exact site and size of the lesion.

Certain oral sites, e.g. soft palate and posterior tongue, are best biopsied under general anaesthetic to avoid the patient gagging and to ensure adequate control of tissues and haemorrhage. Other structures to note include: the greater palatine artery (at the junction of the hard and soft palate), the lingual nerve (on the posterior lateral surface of the tongue), the opening of the submandibular duct (in the anterior floor of mouth), the opening of the parotid duct (opposite the second upper molar tooth) and the mental nerve (buccal to the premolars).

Biopsies for diagnostic purposes rarely require elaborate suturing, with haemostasis best achieved using bipolar coagulation. Squamous cell carcinomas are frequently friable, such that sutures may pull out when attempting primary closure. Exfoliative cytology is still a research tool and cannot replace the need for biopsy. Where appropriate laboratory facilities exist, the application of molecular biology techniques may in the future help dictate the best form of treatment, based upon identification of various tumour markers, e.g. p53 or keratin expression or molecular profile.

Treatment

The treatment of oral cancer

Generally the prognosis of oral cancer becomes worse the further back in the oral cavity that the tumour presents. Thus lesions presenting anteriorly at the tip of the tongue have a better prognosis. They tend to present early while the tumour is still small. Those towards the base of the tongue are generally not noticed until they are much larger. Thus they tend to present late. The prognosis is worse, as would be expected, with more advanced disease. One of the key prognostic factors is whether palpable lymph nodes exist at presentation. Their size and number are also important. As with cancers elsewhere in the head and neck, extracapsular spread of lymph node disease results in a poorer prognosis.

Surgery, radiotherapy or a combination of both are the accepted treatment modalities for head and neck cancer. As elsewhere in the head and neck, it is essential to determine the extent of the disease prior to planning definitive therapy and to recognize that in some patients, particularly those with multisystem disease, very advanced local disease and/or distant metastases, no attempt at curative treatment may be appropriate. Chemotherapy, cryotherapy and electrocoagulation therapy have all been used in the treatment of mouth cancers, but have little if any place nowadays. On the other hand the carbon dioxide laser is a valuable tool for resection of localized disease, resulting in minimal bleeding, reduced pain and rapid healing. The carbon dioxide laser is particularly useful in the management of superficial dysplastic lesions of the oral mucosa.

Early disease

Early lesions, that is T1 (2 cm or less) or T2 (between 2 and 4 cm), may be treated by surgery or radiotherapy. In the absence of metastatic lymph nodes at presentation, 5 year survival rates of 80% are commonly obtained. Surgery for such lesions, particularly if the carbon dioxide laser is used, is straightforward involving a short hospital stay and none of the long-term sequelae of radiation treatment. Radiation may be given by external means or interstitial implant.

The defect resulting from surgery if the carbon dioxide laser is used may be left open, but otherwise is usually dealt with by primary closure. If a large area of oral mucosa is denuded of epithelium a split skin graft may be sutured and quilted in place. However, some surgeons prefer to allow the area to granulate and re-epithelialize naturally, as this leads to a return to a normal, pink appearance. For the latter approach a Whiteheads varnish pack is loosely sutured in place for a week or so.

About one-third of patients presenting with early oral cancers without lymph nodes will go on to develop metastatic cervical lymphadenopathy following successful treatment of the primary tumour. Several management options are available in this situation. In patients in whom there can be regular follow-up and hence early detection of metastatic disease, a policy of no treatment of the neck and watchful waiting is reasonable. Alternatively, particularly if regular follow-up is unlikely, treatment of the entire neck by prophylactic neck dissection or by radiotherapy is appropriate.

Advanced disease

Patients presenting with stage III and IV tumours of the oral cavity and those with metastatic neck disease have a significantly poorer prognosis than those with early disease without cervical lymph nodes. Such patients do best with surgical treatment. The evidence that combined surgery and radiotherapy is more effective than surgery alone is not good. In any event all such patients should be assessed pre-treatment by a surgeon and radiotherapist/oncologist to allow rational planning of treatment and to allow optimal management of any long-term complications and of recurrence. It is common practice in many centres to follow resection by planned radiotherapy.

Conventional radical neck dissection is the standard operation to deal with cervical metastatic disease. Preservation of the accessory nerve is often possible as disease is rarely found in the posterior cervical triangle. Suprahyoid neck dissection is not appropriate in oral cavity cancer as much of the lymphatic drainage of the tongue is directly to the lower neck, particularly to the jugulo-omohyoid group of nodes.

Surgical treatment of advanced cancers

The key to adequate surgical excision of advanced cancers of the oral cavity is adequate exposure. Contrary to the illustrations depicted in many surgical atlases such patients rarely have long swan-like necks and large oral commissures. Many patients with oral cancer are middle aged or elderly men with short thick necks and small oral commissures. In these patients adequate access and exposure may be difficult. Although most patients with oral cancers will have few if any remaining teeth, in those patients with a dentate mandible access, even anteriorly in the oral cavity, may be difficult and surgery must not be compromised by inadequate exposure. Splitting of the mandible, anterior to the mental nerve,can markedly improve the access for surgical excision (Figure 48.17). Residual cancer after surgical treatment is almost always fatal and therefore excision of the primary tumour with an adequate margin is mandatory.

The per-oral route is satisfactory for small anteriorly placed lesions. If access is at all limited, particularly in the anterior floor of mouth, splitting the lower lip in the midline inflicts minimal injury to the lower lip and

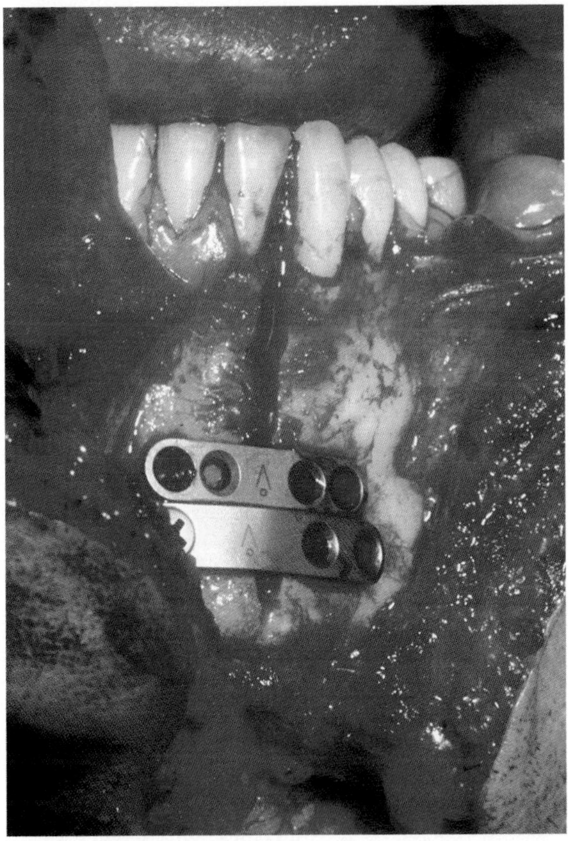

Figure 48.17 An example of the mandible being divided and subsequently repaired by the use of titanium miniplates. Note that this approach does not require the extraction of a healthy tooth and greatly aids access to the posterior tumour.

reconstruction with careful matching of the various anatomical points results in excellent functional and cosmetic results. The lip splitting incision may be extended to encircle the chin prominence and continued posteriorly to the submandibular component of a radical neck dissection. Once the lip has been divided further exposure depends on whether the mandible is being retained or resected and if it is being retained whether the disease is lateral or medial to it.

Pull-through procedures involve excision of the oral cancer by a combination of a per-oral and an external approach in which a cheek and upper neck flap are elevated, but the mandible and lip are not divided. This allows for the primary lesion to be excised in continuity with a neck dissection. This technique, while providing excellent cosmesis, generally gives poorer access than a lip splitting procedure, particularly when the mandible is left intact. In inexperienced hands there is a risk of inadequate excision and given the excellent cosmetic results from a properly reconstructed lip splitting procedure, the authors prefer the lateral approach.

A surgical margin of microscopically normal tissue must be included around the tumour. It is generally accepted that a 2 cm margin is the minimal requirement and this should be clearly marked out prior to resection. On the resected specimens the mucosa shrinks and the resection margin may appear to be much less than the original 2 cm, hence the importance of marking out the proposed incision lines prior to resection. It is important that the surgeon thinks in three dimensions and allows for a 2 cm margin all round. In infiltrating tumours, it can be particularly difficult to determine an adequate deep margin and frozen section control is a useful adjunct.

Squamous cell carcinomas of the oral cavity arising close to the mandible may invade bone. Pre-operative imaging will indicate the extent of such involvement, but the surgeon must be prepared to modify the operation depending on the findings at the time of surgery. Ideally a rim of mandible should be preserved as this has major functional and cosmetic advantages. However, if the inferior dental canal or the cancellous bone of the mandible is involved, full thickness resection is needed. The edentulous mandible is often very thin and it is sometimes not possible to remove the tumour without moving the entire thickness of the mandible.

Reconstruction

Split-skin grafts

These have limited use, but following removal of superficial lesions such grafts may be sutured to cover the defect using a quilting technique.

Primary closure

This is acceptable following resection of small lesions. However, if primary closure is used following resection of larger lesions, function will be compromised. Tongue mobility will be reduced resulting in tethering of the tongue with poor speech and difficulty swallowing.

A surprising amount of tongue can be excised without having a major effect on speech. Up to about half of the tongue can be removed provided the remaining tongue retains sufficient mobility. Reconstruction should be undertaken in such a way as to allow, if possible, the sulcus between the lip and tongue to be retained to prevent pooling and drooling of saliva.

Flap repair

Local flaps including buccal flaps, lingual flaps and nasolabial flaps have a limited role in the reconstruction of small defects. The forehead flap and the deltopectoral flap are now only of historical interest.

The pectoralis major myocutaneous flap is a useful work horse in oral cavity reconstruction. It provides a one stage repair and its bulk can be useful to fill a defect, particularly following neck dissection and mandibular excision. However, the bulk of the flap may result in decreased tongue mobility. Other myocutaneous flaps including the trapezius, latisssimus dorsi and the sternomastoid flaps are now rarely used in oral cavity reconstruction.

Free flaps with microvascular anastomosis provide optimum repair of oral cavity defects. The radial forearm flap which may incorporate bone from the radius provides mobile flexible skin which is readily incorporated into the oral cavity. Such reconstruction should be undertaken by a separate team of surgeons who can raise the flap during resection of the primary tumour. This shortens the operative time to the patient's and operating team's advantage.

Reconstruction of the mandible
Where possible a marginal mandibular resection should be undertaken providing continuity of the mandibular arch. When a full thickness section of mandible is removed, reconstruction is best undertaken using a free flap technique. If the mandible is not reconstructed the remaining segment of the mandible swings to the side of the excision when the patient opens his mouth. This results in cosmetic and functional problems. The fitting of a denture is rarely successful although implant retained protheses offer an improvement. Other techniques of replacing mandibular bone with an iliac crest graft, cancellous bone chips in a tray and incorporation of bone into a myocutaneous flap are generally less successful than microvascular techniques.

Radiotherapy is best avoided if the tumour invades bone as osteoradionecrosis of the mandible is likely to ensue and there is little chance of cure. Radiation of the oral cavity results in destruction of the minor salivary gland in the mucosa producing a distressing xerostomia.

Radiotherapy treatment including associated complications

Megavoltage radiotherapy, e.g. 5000–7000 rads over 5–7 weeks, is used in preference to interstitial radiotherapy (which is rarely used outside very specialist centres).

Oral complications of radiotherapy
Prior to radiotherapy, an oral examination is mandatory. Teeth of poor quality should either be extracted or restored. Side-effects of radiotherapy include the following.

Mucositis
This appears around day 12 of radiation treatment and if severe, may necessitate a break in treatment. Erythema, fibrous exudate and if severe, ulceration may occur. Treatment includes avoidance of smoking and of spicy food, together with the use of mouth rinses such as warm salt water, aspirin and antibacterial antiseptics. Mucositis is thought to result from superficial infection of the oral mucosa.

Xerostomia
This is a common and very unpleasant side-effect of irradiation to the oral cavity. If the major salivary glands are in the path of the radiation, a reduction of saliva which may thicken will result and there is an increased risk of dental caries. Once irradiated, the acini never fully recover. Oral pilocarpine may stimulate saliva production and saliva substitutes can be helpful. However, most patients find simply taking frequent sips of water to be just as effective.

Loss of taste
This is thought to be due to the reduction in saliva, although it may also result from structural damage to the taste buds.

Infection
Candidal infection as either a white or red lesion may occur, and may require antifungal agents.

Dental caries due to reduced saliva flow is a risk and requires fluoride therapy and excellent oral hygiene.

Osteoradionecrosis is a risk, particularly if teeth are later extracted from a previously irradiated site. In such cases antibiotics should be prescribed prior to tooth extraction.

Other treatment modalities

Chemotherapy
This is generally reserved for treatment of advanced disease, where no other options are available. Traditionally results have been poor, in part due to problems with toxicity, the patient's debilitated and malnourished state, and possibly reduced blood supply to the tumour after radiotherapy. A number of drugs have been employed, including methotrexate, cis-platinum, bleomycin and 5-fluorouracil. Combination therapy can be chosen to 'attack' the malignant cells at different stages of the cell cycle. Adjuvant chemotherapy (i.e. in combination with either surgery or radiotherapy) may also be helpful but may harm the host's immune defence response. Some examples include cyclophosphamide, vincristine and adriamycin. In theory, chemotherapy can eradicate cells that have metastasized, reduce tumour size to make inoperable tumours operable, and does not necessarily preclude other forms of therapy.

Chemotherapy (for malignant disease in any body site) may give rise to oral manifestations in approximately 40% of cases. These include ulceration, mucositis, xerostomia and opportunistic infection.

Photodynamic therapy
This technique relies upon the preferential uptake by malignant cells of a photosensitizer, e.g. porphyrin, which when activated by light of a certain wavelength in the presence of oxygen leads to the creation of singlet oxygen that is toxic to the cancer cells. Limitations of the technique include: limited depth of penetration by the laser to activate the drug and thus destroy malignant cells, time delay in optimal uptake of the photosensitizer by the cancer cells, rate of metabolism of the photosensitizer once taken up and avoidance of sunlight, until the drug is cleared and the skin is no longer sensitive. The short duration of treatment, relatively inexpensive equipment and lack of need for sophisticated hospital back-up suggest that this technique could be of particular value in developing countries or for those patients not suitable for conventional therapy.

Special problems

Field cancerization

Patients with head and neck cancers, including oral cancer, have a much greater risk of developing a second malignant tumour, particularly within the first 2 years of treatment. This is thought to be due to the widespread influence of the aetiological agents (alcohol and tobacco) on the upper aerodigestive tract, priming the mucosa and in susceptible patients creating satellites of potentially malignant disease, the field cancerization effect.

Two alternative theories for field cancerization have been proposed. First, that these areas of abnormality involve separate, independent clones, each with a unique genetic alteration. The second theory suggests that all tumours in that region are derived from expansion of a single malignant clone. Both states can however co-exist.

It is also possible that an existing tumour in that region can induce field change or field cancerization effects.

Analysis of surgical margins by constructing unique oligonucleotide (single-stranded DNA) probes, specific to the mutation found in the cancer, can determine whether there are cells at the boundary of the excision harbouring the mutation, that are not readily recognized morphologically, at light microscope level. Their detection and treatment might help prevent further tumours developing.

Second malignant tumours arise at a rate of approximately 4% per year for stage 1 and 2 disease and exert an adverse influence upon patient survival. Thus long-term follow-up is required, although the benefit of routine pan-endoscopy of this region remains controversial. The majority of patients with advanced disease do not survive long enough to develop further primaries.

Notwithstanding the above, the vast majority of people who smoke tobacco and drink alcohol do not develop oral cancer. So why do some people develop cancer and field change, following less exposure to risk factors than others? Are they prone to genetic damage?

In vivo analysis of chromatid breaks in chromosomes from lymphocytes exposed to bleomycin is said to give an indication of the host sensitivity to environmental carcinogens, genotoxicity and cancer risk. Another indication of cancer susceptibility is the rate at which the DNA is repaired. The ability to identify, for example, those smokers who have a genetic profile suggestive of greater risk for oral cancer, will in the future allow targeting of specific prevention programmes. Greater understanding of tumour biology should help determine not only how the tumour will grow, invade and metastasize but also its response to therapy.

Further reading

Cawson, R. A. and Odell, E. W. (1998). *Essentials of Oral Pathology and Oral Medicine*, 6th edn. London: Churchill Livingstone.

Harrison, L. B., Sessions, R. B. and Hong, W. K. (1999). *Head and Neck Cancer. A Multidisciplinary Approach*. New York: Lippincott-Raven.

Hermanek, P. and Sobin, L. H., eds (1992). *UICC TNM Classification of Malignant Tumors*, 4th edn. Berlin: Springer.

Langdon, J. D. and Henk, J. M. (1995). *Malignant Tumours of the Mouth, Jaws and Salivary Glands*, 2nd edn. London: Edward Arnold.

Langlais, R. P. and Miller, C. S. (1998). *A Color Atlas of Common Oral Diseases*, 2nd edn. Philadelphia, PA: Williams & Wilkins.

Ogden, G. R. and Macluskey, M. (2000). An overview of the prevention of oral cancer and diagnostic markers of malignant change: 1 Prevention. 2 Markers of Value in Tumour Diagnosis. *Dental Update* **27**: 95–9, 148–52.

Platz, H., Fries, R. and Hudec, M. (1986). *Prognosis of Oral Cavity Carcinomas: Results of a Multicentre Observational Study*. Munich: Carl Hanser.

Prabhu, S. R., Wilson, D. F., Daftary, D. K. and Johnson, N. W. (1992). *Oral Diseases in the Tropics*. New York: Oxford University Press.

Scully, C., Flint, S. and Porter, S. R. *Oral Diseases*, 2nd edn. London: Martin Dunitz.

Shah, J. P. (1996). *Head and Neck Surgery*, 2nd edn. New York: Mosby Wolfe.

MODULE 49

Applied anatomy and physiology of the respiratory system

Section 49.1 • Developmental abnormalities

The lung

During the fourth week of intrauterine development a midline groove appears on the ventral surface of the foregut immediately caudal to the hypobronchial eminence (future epiglottis) from which the respiratory tract will develop. Starting caudally a diverticulum becomes progressively separated from the foregut leaving only a small patent connection (the laryngeal aditus) just below the hypobronchial eminence. Maldevelopments during this phase may result in oesophageal atresia, tracheal stenosis or a tracheo-oesophageal fistula. The distal end of the diverticulum soon divides equally into the right and left lung buds. The respiratory epithelium and mucous glands arise from the diverticulum while the cartilage, muscle, elastic tissue, blood vessels and lymphatics develop from the splanchnic mesoderm on the ventral surface of the foregut into which the diverticulum grows. The developing trachea and bronchi derive their blood supply from the dorsal aorta and upper posterior intercostal arteries and autonomic innervation from the vagus nerves and sympathetic chains, an arrangement which persists into adult life.

Initially the two lung buds are symmetrical but by the 5 mm stage the adult asymmetry is evident with the left bud lying more transversely. Soon both tubes give off an anterior diverticulum (the right middle and the left upper/lingular divisions) and by the 15 mm stage the right bud has divided further giving a cranio-dorsal branch (right upper division) and the adult pattern of three right and two left lobes is laid down. Additional primary branching of the stem bronchi may give rise to an accessory lobe, e.g. a cardiac lobe, or a segmental bronchus may be derived directly from the trachea or stem bronchi, i.e. the apical division of the right upper lobe arising from the trachea. By birth, 18 bronchial generations have been formed by successive divisions, often unequal, of the daughter bronchi.

Among the types of accessory lobes described are:

- the tracheal lobe arising from and communicating with the trachea
- dissociated lung masses situated in the abdomen or neck
- interlobar sequestration (lower accessory lobe).

The third has the greatest clinical significance.

The sequestrated lobe may consist of a single large cyst or a mass of ill-defined tissue firmly adherent to the posterior segment of a normal lower lobe (90% left) and having its own blood supply from the aorta passing through the pulmonary ligament. The abnormality may present as a tension cyst soon after birth or as various radiological shadows. Opinions vary as to whether these are true accessory lobes with an independent origin or whether they represent a portion of lung which has become detached from a normal lobe. Rarely an extralobar sequestration of lung occurs which shares the pulmonary artery supply of its associated lung.

Early in fetal life deepening furrows (fissures) divide the lung mesenchyme into lobules around each primary bronchial division (future lobes). If separation is incomplete vascular bridges between adjacent lobes may persist into the adult and present problems at lobectomy. Failure of segregation results in a single-lobed lung.

Normally the azygos vein lies medial to the lung bud curling anteriorly above the right hilum. Occasionally the developing bud pushes the vein laterally where the vein becomes embedded within the right upper lobe and a deep fissure separates a segment of lung; the 'azygos lobe' may be visible radiologically.

Agenesis of one lung is compatible with normal life until the third or fourth decade when emphysema usually develops in the remaining lung. In true agenesis the ipsilateral pulmonary artery is absent but there is often a small bronchial stump surrounded by hypoplastic or cystic lung tissue. The remaining lung may lack lobulation and grows to twice its normal size displacing the heart and mediastinum to the contralateral side. Occasionally one lung may be hypoplastic.

The early lung buds contain a loose vascular network, which drains into the sinus venosus and cardinal veins, i.e. the future systemic venous system. Later, after the septum primum has divided the primitive atrium, a single vessel develops and connects the primitive pulmonary circulation with the left atrium. Maldevelopment at this stage may lead to persistence of some drainage into the systemic veins or right atrium. Scimitar vein syndrome is a common vein draining the right lung into the right atrium.

The common terminal veins and the origins of the primitive left and right pulmonary veins are progressively absorbed in the developing atrium until two veins from each side open separately into the fully developed left atrium. Anomalous venous drainage arises from a failure of the common pulmonary vein to fuse with the posterior wall of the left atrium.

The pulmonary arteries arise from the sixth branchial arch arteries and by the sixth week receive their blood supply wholly from the right ventricle. Soon the right artery only supplies the right lung but on the left the connection with the aorta persists until birth as the ductus arteriosus.

The primitive pleural spaces (the pericardioperitoneal canals) into which the lung buds grow are in continuity with the primitive pericardium and the peritoneal cavity. With the rapid growth of the lungs the pericardium becomes separated from the pleural cavity, a process that may be incomplete (usually on the left) or which may produce developmental abnormalities, i.e. pleuropericardial cysts. The development of the diaphragm gradually closes the pleuroperitoneal openings.

The diaphragm

The closure of the pleuroperitoneal canals completes the formation of the diaphragm which is a composite structure derived from several elements, some of them pairs, as shown in Table 49.1. The septum transversum forms the bulk of the adult diaphragm. The motor supply is entirely through the phrenic nerve (C3, 4 and 5, the segmental origin of the septum transversum) but the intercostal nerves carry some sensory fibres from the lateral aspects of the diaphragm. Any infection, injury or compression which involves the phrenic nerve during its extended course may cause diaphragmatic paralysis. Within the diaphragm, the phrenic nerves form a series of arcades (Figure 49.1) and these should be avoided during operations involving the diaphragm. The muscle fibres are situated peripherally around an unyielding central tendon forming a cupola, which flattens when the muscle contracts.

The developing diaphragm contains five major openings: three permanent – the oesophageal, the aortic and the inferior vena caval – and two transient – the pleuroperitoneal canals. The foramen of Bochdalek arises from inadequate development of the diaphragmatic muscle in the region of the lumbocostal trigone; the abdominal and thoracic contents may or may not be separated by the peritoneal and pleural membranes in this defect. Similar defects may occur in the region of the sternocostal triangles, i.e. herniation through the foramen of Morgagni, while muscular maldevelopment may be responsible for some para-oesophageal hernias. In eventration of the diaphragm, part or all of a hemidiaphragm, usually the left, is devoid of muscle fibres and moves paradoxically with respiration. Partial or complete eventration shows on chest X-ray as a lobulated or elevated hemidiaphragm. Ruptured diaphragm commonly involves the central tendon with herniation of the abdominal contents through a tear along the line from the anterior aspect of the oesophageal hiatus to where the phrenic nerve penetrates the diaphragm (Figure 49.1).

Lymphatics

Within the lungs there is a steady flow of filtrate from the pulmonary capillaries to the interstitium. This fluid drains via the parenchymal lymphatics at a rate of 10–20 ml/hour, i.e. a maximal flow of approximately 200 ml/day. The lymph drains to the peribronchial lymphatics then to the mediastinum. The lungs are

Table 49.1 Origin of components of the diaphragm

Source	*Structures derived*
Septum transversum	The central tendon and parts of the sternal, costal and lumbar muscle components
Pleuroperitoneal membranes	Small dorsolateral muscle segments
Costal and sternal chest wall	Varying amounts of sternal and costal muscular attachments
Dorsal mesentery	Muscle between the oesophageal and aortic orifices
Dorsal body wall	Part of the lumbar muscular segment
Mesoderm around the aorta	Parts of the posterior muscle bundles

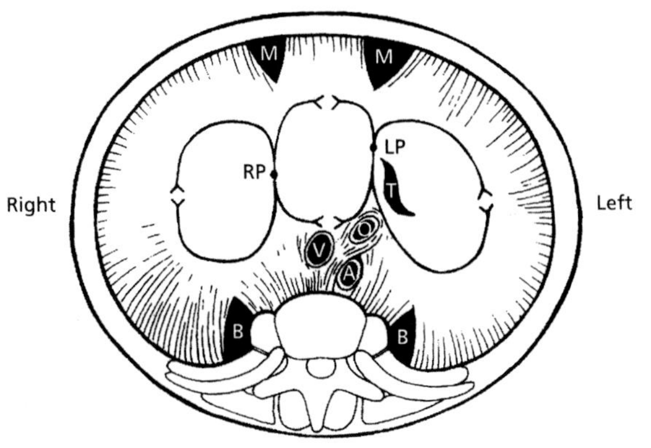

Figure 49.1 Schematic representation of the undersurface of the diaphragm to illustrate the phrenic nerve arcades and the various normal orifices and pathological defects. A, aortic orifice; LP, left phrenic nerve; RP, right phrenic nerve. The potential defects are B, lumbosacral trigone (Bochdalek's hernia); M, sternocostal trigone (Morgagni's hernia); and T, traumatic tears leading to diaphragmatic hernia.

richly supplied with lymphatic channels which surround; the bronchi and blood vessels, form a plexus beneath the visceral pleura and permeate the bronchial walls. The constant expansion and relaxation of the lungs help to pump the lymph towards the hilum, flow being directed by simple valves. The vessels communicate freely and some lymph flows outwards to the subpleural plexus before returning through the lung to the hilar region, this is important in the spread of bronchial carcinoma and explains the local spread within a lobe and possibly to pleural space. Lymphoidal tissue is found at each bronchial bifurcation from the respiratory bronchioles inward, although true lymph nodes only appear at the level of the segmental bronchi.

The lymph drains to the hilar nodes, then some drains to the carinal nodes from each side. The bulk of the lymph from right lung drains to the right paratracheal nodes. The aorta crosses over the left main bronchus and the lymph drainage from the left lung flows under and over the arch. There are subaortic nodes lying in the aortopulmonary window which drain lymph from both lobes of the left lung. Much of the lymph from the left upper lobe drains into the left paratracheal chain but still most of the lymph from the left lung drains across the midline to the right paratracheal nodes both under and over the aortic arch. The trachea, the oesophagus and the upper mediastinal structures send efferent vessels to the deep lower cervical nodes. The left recurrent laryngeal nerve and left vagus nerve at the aortic arch are closely related to the lymphatic drainage.

The lymph finally enters the venous system at the junctions of the subclavian and internal jugular veins either independently or having joined the right lymphatic or thoracic ducts. In addition to the principal drainage some lymph from the lower lobes passes via the pulmonary ligaments to nodes in the posterior mediastinum or through the diaphragm into the retroperitoneal chain. Some fluid and all the protein from the pleural space are drained principally through lymphatics from the parietal pleura to the parasternal and para-aortic chains. There are unidirectional channels through the diaphragm from the abdomen which facilitate the spread of fluid and infection from the abdomen to the pleural space but not in the reverse direction.

Lymph from the parietal pleura and chest wall drains into the nodes of the internal mammary, axillary and posterior mediastinal chains. The thoracic duct enters the thorax through the aortic orifice and runs up in the posterior mediastinum between the aorta and azygos vein. The thoracic duct continues on the anterior aspect of the vertebrae to the level of the seventh thoracic vertebra where the duct crosses obliquely behind the oesophagus then proceeds along the left oesophageal border into the neck where it joins the venous system.

Pleura

The lungs and chest wall are covered by the visceral and parietal pleura. A single layer of mesothelial cells line the pleura, their microvilli enmesh hyaluronic acid and glycoproteins to form a smooth frictionless surface.

There is a negative pressure within the pleural space of 3–4 cmH_2O. During inspiration the chest wall and diaphragm move to increase the intrathoracic volume. A traction tension between the layers of the pleura pulls on the visceral surface of the lung, so the lung expands, such is inspiration. During quiet expiration the elastic recoil of the lung pulls the visceral pleura inwards and the parietal pleura and the chest wall follow. Therefore intrapleural pressure is always negative other than in forced expiration.

There is a differential in the intrapleural pressure between the apical and basal pleural space. At the apex it is -10 cmH_2O and at the base -2 cmH_2O. This difference is due the weight of the lungs being supported by the diaphragm and the rib cage. Combined with gravity these are the reasons for differential ventilation and perfusion of the lung.

A hydrostatic pressure difference of 6 mmHg between the capillary beds of the parietal pleura and the pleural space is responsible for the formation of pleural fluid, while a difference of 13 mmHg between the pleural space and the capillaries of the visceral pleura encourages reabsorption of fluid. If this balance is disrupted for any reason, e.g. congestive cardiac failure or infection, fluid will collect within the pleural space forming an effusion with a greatly enhanced turnover of fluid. The pleura is a semipermeable membrane where proteins and cells are only absorbed through stomata in the parietal pleura which coalesce to form the lymphatics.

During quiet breathing, the lungs do not completely fill the costophrenic recess, the two layers of parietal pleura being in apposition for up to 7.5 cm in the mid-axillary line. Thus a liver biopsy through the right ninth and tenth intercostal spaces should be performed at full expiration to prevent lung damage. The standard chest X-ray is taken with postero-anterior exposure at full inspiration.

Section 49.2 • Surfactant

Pulmonary surfactant is a complex phospho lipid (dipalmitoyl phosphatidyl choline, DPPC). It is secreted by type 2 pneumocytes from the latter part of pregnancy at around 32 weeks of gestation. DPPC is synthesized from fatty acid. Electron microscopy shows surfactant to be stored as lamellar bodies which are excreted into the alveoli, where the surfactant unfolds to coat the air liquid interface with a lipid protein film. The synthesis is fast and turnover rapid.

The main function of surfactant is to reduce the surface tension of the alveoli and prevent collapse. The mechanism of action of surfactant is through DPPC, whose molecules are hydrophilic at one end and hydrophobic at the other. The molecules align themselves at the air liquid interface repelling each other in all directions against the attracting forces of the liquid surface molecules, thus reducing the surface tension.

Laplace's principle states that pressure within a bubble is equal to twice the surface tension ($2T$) divided by the radius (R), i.e. $P = 2T/R$. Therefore, the smaller the bubble the greater the tendency to collapse. One can imagine the alveoli as bubbles connected together by interalveolar ducts. Those alveoli that are small do not collapse and this is where surfactant plays its important role. The concentration of DPPC increases as the surface area of the alveoli decreases and the alveoli are kept open (Figure 49.2).

The physiological advantages of surfactant are that it decreases surface tension of the alveoli, increasing lung

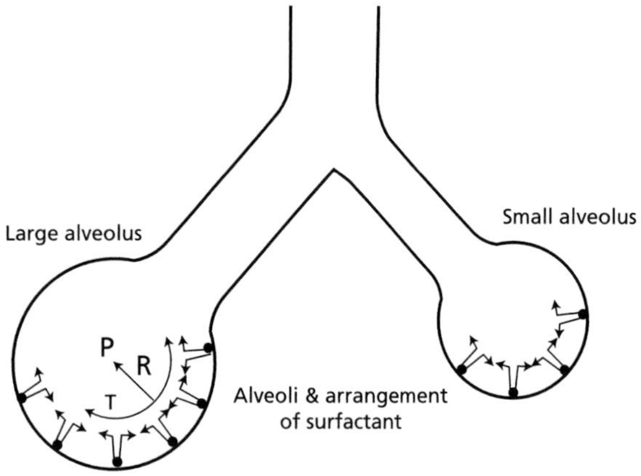

Figure 49.2 Laplace's law states that the pressure is proportional to wall tension and inversely proportional to the radius for a sphere. The figure shows that alveolar patency is maintained by the presence of surfactant: relatively more surfactant is in the smaller alveolus as it contracts, thus denying collapse in spite of Laplace's law.

compliance, thus reducing the work of breathing and maintaining alveolar stability. Surfactant's further function is to prevent alveolar flooding; by merely reducing the surface tension alveolar collapse is prevented.

Surfactant is also important in the pressure volume curve (compliance). If the lung is inflated in steps of increasing pressure, the lungs expand to total lung capacity (TLC). As the lung deflates, the deflation curve is not the same as the inflation curve. The difference between the inflation and deflation curves is called hysteresis. This is mainly the result of surfactant but other structures within the lung contribute: smooth muscles of blood vessels and connective tissues.

Consequences of surfactant deficiency are:

- atelectasis
- stiff lungs and increased work of breathing
- alveolar flooding, e.g. infant respiratory distress syndrome which is now treated by surfactant directly.

Section 49.3 • Functions of the lung

The main function of the lung is ventilation, the transfer of oxygen to the tissues and carbon dioxide excretion. The lung does have other functions.

Defence function of the lungs

The lungs have a large surface area for gas exchange, but present a small barrier to diffusion between air and the blood flowing through. The lungs possess the largest surface area of the body in contact with the external environment and are most susceptible to damage by foreign materials. The surface area of the lung is about 85 m^2, equivalent to a tennis court. Both lungs have about 300 million alveoli and yet their volume is only about 4 litres. They are susceptible to a variety of toxic damage by dust particles, bacteria, viruses and other airborne pollutants. Therefore defence mechanism are needed to prevent infection and reduce the damage from inhaled particles. The lungs are protected by physical barriers and immunological responses.

Physical barriers

Nose and nasopharynx

This acts as a filter and as a first line of defence against inhaled particles. The nose can filter particles above 5 μm in size. It can certainly trap all particles above 10 μm in size. The nose and the nasopharynx warm and humidify inspired air and also absorb soluble and reactive gases.

Swallowing mechanism

This acts to prevent aspiration into the upper airways. There are irritant fibres situated here.

Lower respiratory tract

The lower respiratory tract has a number of defence mechanisms: the cough reflex, the mucociliary escalator with its enzyme components and the alveolar macrophages.

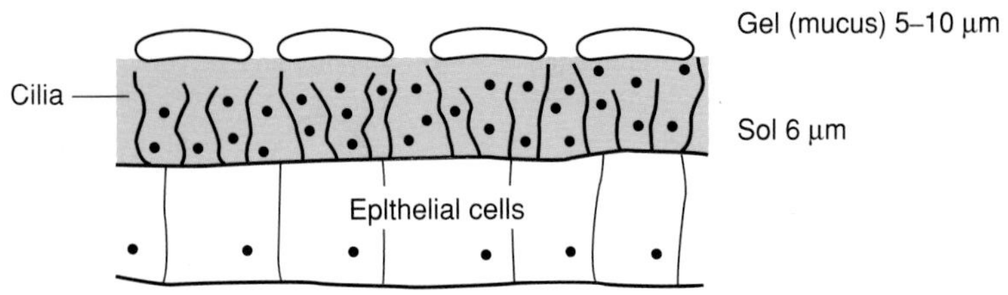

Figure 49.3 The mucous layer, sol and the cilia of the epithelial layer.

To initiate the cough reflex, there are many irritant receptors, cough receptors, in the trachea and the proximal bronchi. These protect the upper airways from foreign bodies and aspiration.

The main defence mechanism in the lower airway is the mucociliary barrier. This mechanism is facilitated by mucociliary transport. A mucous layer lies upon a low viscosity periciliary fluid called sol (Figure 49.3). The epithelial cells in the lower airways are covered by cilia. There are about 200 cilia per cell. Sol facilitates ciliary beating to propel the upper mucous gel. The length of the cilia is 6 μm reaching into the mucous gel. The mucous layer has a thickness of about 5–10 μm and contrary to the periciliary fluid, has high viscosity, it is very sticky, and captures the bacteria in the lower airways and other particles. The mucous gel unlike surfactant is not a continuous layer. The cilia beat rhythmically at about 20 beats/s, moving the mucous blanket proximally into the nasopharynx. The cilia beat and move the mucous blanket about 2.5 mm/min, but this may increase to 20 mm/min in some areas of the respiratory tract. The trachea and proximal airways have a faster clearance rate. The ciliary function is inhibited by cigarette smoking, viruses and drugs. The cells responsible for the secretion of this mucociliary layer are Clara cells in the proximal airways and goblet cells in the smaller airways. Eosinophils, polymorphs and macrphages as well as airborne particles move proximally on this mucociliary escalator into the trachea then to the nasopharynx where it is swallowed.

The mucous secretion consists of 95% water, 3% protein, 1% lipid and 1% minerals. It also contains albumin, protease inhibitors and immunoglobulins. IgA is the major bronchial antibody, but IgG and IgM are also present. These proteins are involved in agglutination and opsonization of antigens as well as in complement fixation.

Lysozymes are secreted in large quantities into the airways. Lysozymes are cationic enzymes that catalyse the hydrolysis of bacterial cell walls and fungi. Lysozymes also inhibit chemotaxis and the production of oxygen radicals by polymorphs, so reducing the tissue damage of inflammation. Lysozymes are expressed in a variety of tissues, e.g. salivary glands and lacrimal glands.

Lactoferrin is an iron chelator that inhibits iron dependent growth of micro-organisms.

Peroxidases catalyse the reduction of hydrogen peroxide to produce free oxygen radicals. Peroxidases are found in the secretary granules of goblet cells.

The airway epithelium has a barrier function whereby it separates the airway lumen and interstitium. This epithelium consists of sheets of cells joined by tight junctions to inhibit solute and water movement across the epithelium.

Alveolar macrophages

Since the alveolar cells have no cilia, the airways are protected by a different immune mechanism. This is fulfilled by the alveolar macrophages which are derived from blood monocytes and are situated above the alveolar cells in continuity with the surfactant (Figure 49.4). Alveolar macrophages are resident in the alveoli and very mobile. Their main functions are phagocytosis and digestion of bacteria and debris and secreting destructive enzymes: proteases, lysozymes, superoxides and oxygen radicals. Macrophages phagocytose micro-organisms and debris and then are transported proximally to the bronchi where they are removed by mucociliary clearance or pass directly into the interstitium to be removed by the lymphatics. Besides antimicrobial activity, phagocytosis and digestion of micro-organisms, macrophages respond to chemotactic factors especially C5a of complement.

Alveolar macrophages generate a weak cellular immune response, compared with the interstitial macrophages. Alveolar macrophages have an armament of enzymes that include peroxidases, proteases and nitrous oxide and can produce cytokines (leukotrienes, platelet activating factor and C5a) in inflammation.

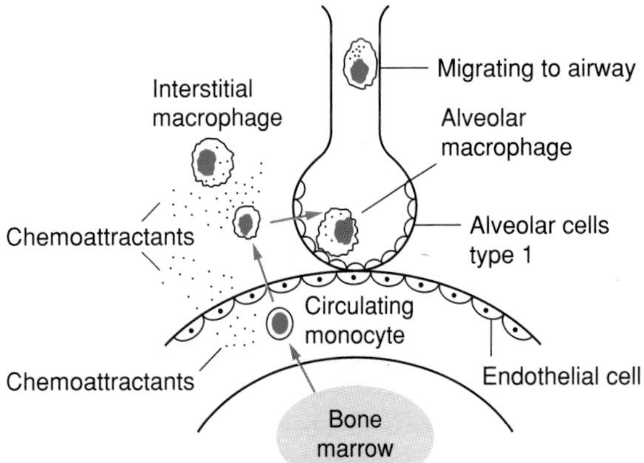

Figure 49.4 The origin of the alveolar macrophage from the blood-borne monocyte from the marrow to its maturation in the alveolus and its subsequent transport.

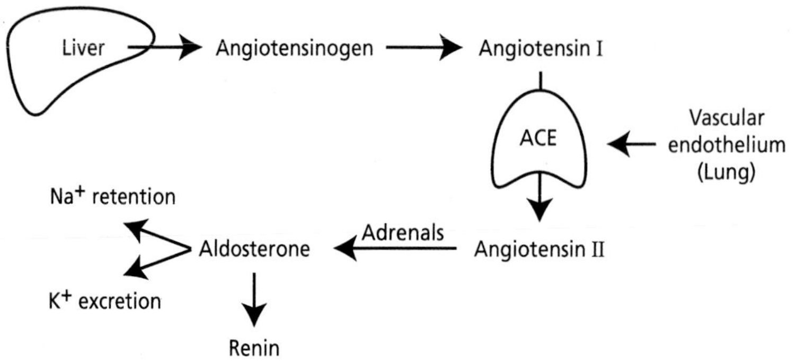

Figure 49.5 The renin–angiotension system.

Alveolar macophages are also essential in lung homoeostasis especially in inflammation when a number of cytokines are produced leading to cell death and remodelling. Macrophages have been found to produce cytokines responsible for cell death and proliferation of certain cells such as fibroblasts with resultant production of fibrous tissue.

One enzyme produced by macrophages and neutrophils is alpha-1-antitrypsin. Alpha-1-antitrypsin is involved in emphysema. Cigarette smoking increases the number of pulmonary macrophages that release chemicals to attract leucocytes that produce proteases which attack the elastic tissue of the lung. This is inhibited by alpha-1-antitrypsin. The imbalance between protease and antiprotease leads to the destruction of the lung tissue and the development of emphysema. The inherited deficiency of alpha-1-antitrypsin leads to lung destruction and emphysema by itself and smoking has a devastating effect.

Aggregates of lymphoid tissue are present in the mucosa of the bronchi. These are called mucosa associated lymphoid tissue (MALT). MALT is present in the upper airways and the gastrointestinal tract. They are aggregates of B-cells and drain into the regional lymphatics. These lymphoid tissues provide protection as the site of lymphocytic activation.

Metabolic function of the lungs

A number of metabolic functions are carried out in the lungs. Angiotensin-converting enzyme (ACE) is produced by the vascular endothelial cells of the lung and facilitates the conversion of angiotensin I to angiotensin II (Figure 49.5), which is a potent vasoconstrictor. The lung is also responsible for deactivation of vasoactive substances, like bradykinin. This is also facilitated by ACE. ACE inhibitors are drugs that prevent the conversion of angiotensin I to angiotensin II, and are used in patients with hypertension and congestive cardiac failure.

The lung makes a number of important products from arachidonic acid, itself derived from phospholipids in the cell walls, and generates two main metabolites. One, through lipo-oxygenase, produces leukotrienes which are responsible for asthma; recently a few leukotriene inhibitors have been developed for the management of asthma. Montelukast and Zafirlukast are examples. The other pathway is through cyclo-oxygenase and leads to the production of prostaglandins and thromboxane A_2 (Figure 49.6). All these compounds are produced and removed by the lungs. The lung also produces the phospholipid DPPC. The lung conducts protein synthesis for collagen and elastin from the lung parenchyma and their synthesis and breakdown are important to the normal function of the lung. This is controlled by protease and anti-protease activity.

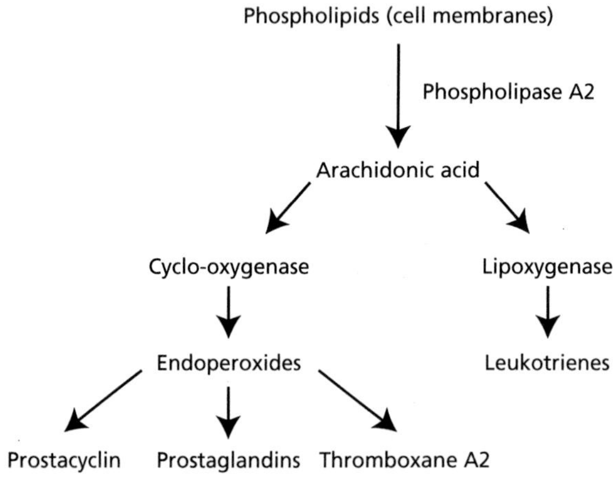

Figure 49.6 The metabolism of arachidonic acid with its end products and leukotriene production pathway.

Respiratory functions of the lungs

Ventilation is the transport of oxygen and carbon dioxide and the factors influencing gas exchange. Lung mechanics and neural control are an integrated system for breathing.

Ventilation, the main function of the lung, is the uptake of oxygen and the excretion of CO_2. This requires a rapid and efficient exchange of gases. Lung volumes are key to this process.

Measurements of lung volumes

The main method of measuring static lung volumes is by spirometry which measures tidal volume (V_t), total lung capacity (TLC) and forced vital capacity (FVC) (Figure

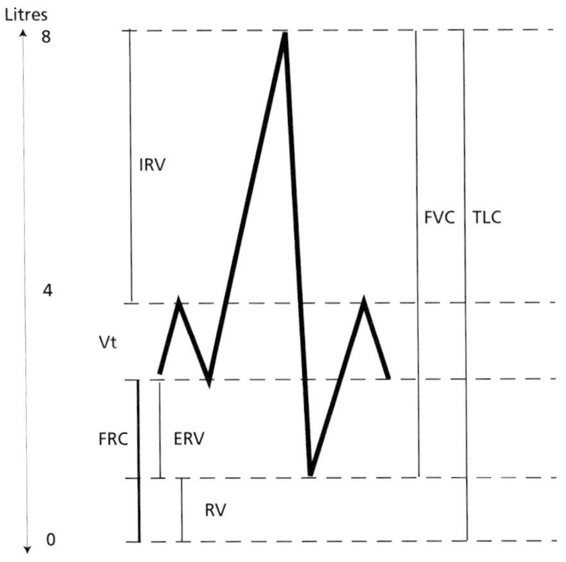

Figure 49.7 An ideal spirometry trace showing the estimation points and the measurements derived.

49.7). The spirometer is not able to measure functional residual capacity (FRC), which is the resting lung volume at the end of expiration, or residual volume (RV), which is the volume of air remaining after maximum expiration. FRC and RV are measured by helium dilution. This method relies on helium's being inert and not absorbed. The subject is connected to a spirometer containing a known concentration of helium. After taking several breaths in a closed system the concentrations in the spirometer and the lung equalize. Since no helium has been lost, then the amount of helium present before equilibrium equals the amount of helium present after equilibrium. This is represented in the following equation: $C_1V_1 = C_2(V_1 + V_2)$ (Figure 49.8).

Plethysmography is used to measure the FRC; it depends on the process of recording changes in pressure within a sealed box (Figure 49.9). This applies Boyle's law, which states that at a constant temperature, the volume of a gas varies inversely with the pressure. The box measures changes in lung volumes as pressure changes in the box, whilst the patient breaths through a spirometer. The whole body plethysmograph measures the volume of gas in the lung, including residual volume, i.e. the air that is trapped behind closed airways. By contrast, helium dilution measures only communicating gases or ventilated lung volume. Normally, these measurements are the same in healthy lungs but in patients with lung disease such measurements may be different, especially in patients with air trapping as in chronic obstructive pulmonary disease (COPD).

Ventilation

Ventilation is the flow of air in and out of the respiratory system during breathing. Not all the air inspired reaches the alveoli. Some of the air stays in the trachea and conducting airways and is not involved with gas transfer. There are two aspects of ventilation: minute ventilation (MV) and alveolar ventilation.

MV is the total amount of air entering the respiratory tract through the nose in 1 min. This is calculated as tidal volume (V_t) × respiratory rate (RR). Tidal volume is around 500 ml and breathing rate about 12 per minute. We can write this equation, MV= $V_t \times$ RR. This will amount to 6000 ml/min. This is the total minute ventilation. However, not all the air that passes the lips reaches the alveolar gas compartment for gas exchange. Of the 500 ml, 150 ml remain in the conducting airways from the mouth to the bronchi, including terminal bronchioles and are not involved in gas transfer. This is called the anatomical dead space.

Alveolar ventilation is the actual amount of air that reaches the alveoli in 1 min. The anatomical dead space is usually about 150 ml and therefore the alveolar minute ventilation amounts to 350 × 12. We can summarize this conveniently with symbols: MV = $V_d + V_a$, where MV is minute ventilation, V_d is dead space ventilation and V_a is alveolar ventilation (Figure 49.10).

Physiological dead space

Physiological dead space is the volume of gas in the lung that does not exchange with the capillary blood

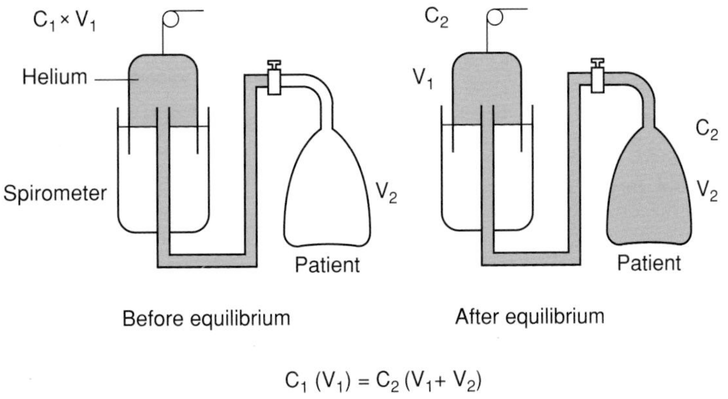

Figure 49.8 The measurement of the functional residual capacity by helium dilution.

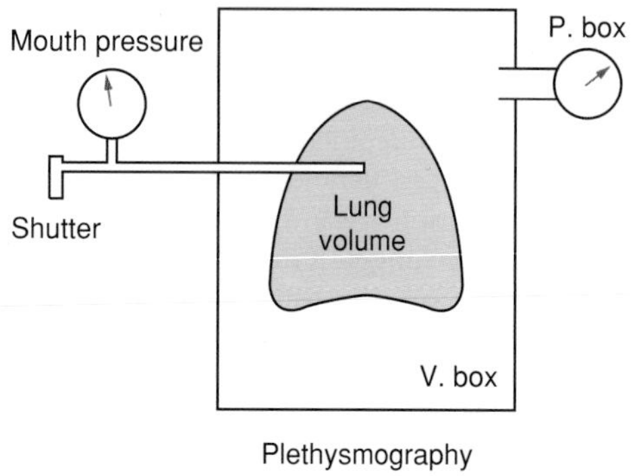

Figure 49.9 The volume measurement by the whole body box (plethysmography).

and includes anatomical and alveolar dead space. This can be measured by Bohr's method which depends on measuring CO_2 at the mouth. CO_2 comes totally through diffusion from the capillaries into the alveoli, therefore it can be used to measure alveolar ventilation. The mechanism behind physiological dead space is ventilation–perfusion mismatch, as some alveoli may be ventilated but not perfused, when ventilation is said to be wasted. In normal healthy people, the anatomical and physiological dead space are almost equal.

Regional differences in ventilation

Ventilation per unit volume is greatest near the bottom of the lung and becomes progressively smaller towards the apex of the lung, and perfusion follows the same pattern. This is seen in isotope studies.

Laws of diffusion

Diffusion is the transfer of gas across the blood gas barrier. Diffusion occurs from an area of high concentration to an area of low concentration, hence the driving force is the concentration gradient. Diffusion will continue until the concentration gradient equalizes in both compartments. Diffusion through tissues is described by Fick's law, which states that the rate of diffusion of a substance is proportional to the surface area of the membrane, solubility of this substance in the membrane and the difference in partial pressure of the gas between the two sides. Diffusion is inversely proportional to thickness of the membrane and the square root of the molecular weight:

$$V_g \propto AK(P_1 - P_2)T^{-1} \quad K = \text{Sol. MW}^{-2}$$

where V_g is volume of gas, A is area, K is the diffusion constant, P is partial pressure, Sol is solubility, MW molecular weight and T is thickness.

Therefore, the rate of diffusion across alveoli is directly dependent upon the partial pressure difference between the alveolar and the arterial gas.

Perfusion and diffusion limitation

At the alveolar capillary surface, gas transfer depends on two mechanisms: diffusion across the alveolar capillary membrane, and perfusion of the blood through the pulmonary capillaries (Figure 49.11). The uptake of gas into the blood depends on the solubility of the gas and the affinity of the gas to haemoglobin. Carbon monoxide has a high affinity to haemoglobin, so a large amount of carbon monoxide combines with haemoglobin even at low partial pressure, hence the amount of carbon monoxide that crosses the alveolar capillary membrane is limited only by the properties of the membrane and not by the pulmonary blood flow. Hence the transfer of the carbon monoxide is diffusion limited and it measures the function of the alveolar capillary membrane.

Nitrous oxide and oxygen are poorly soluble, hence the rate of transfer of the gas into the soluble phase is slow with a slow rise of the partial pressure in the blood. This limits the power of partial pressure difference between the alveoli and the blood as the driving force for diffusion. Therefore, nitrous oxide and oxygen

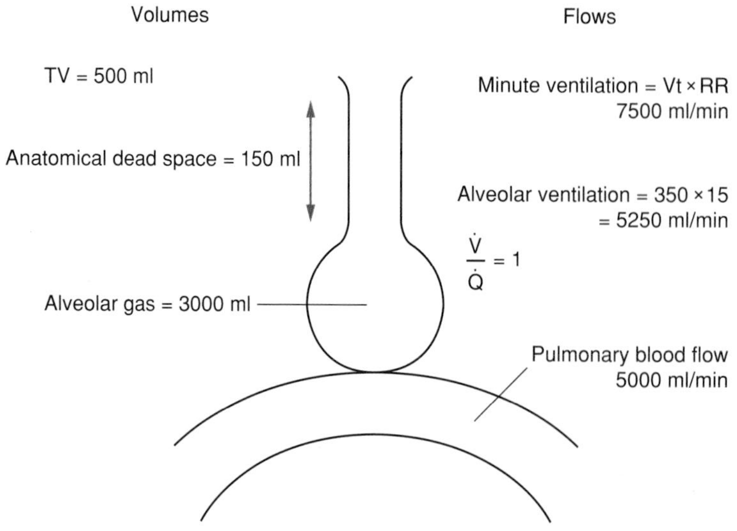

Figure 49.10 Demonstration of the minute volume and the dead space estimations.

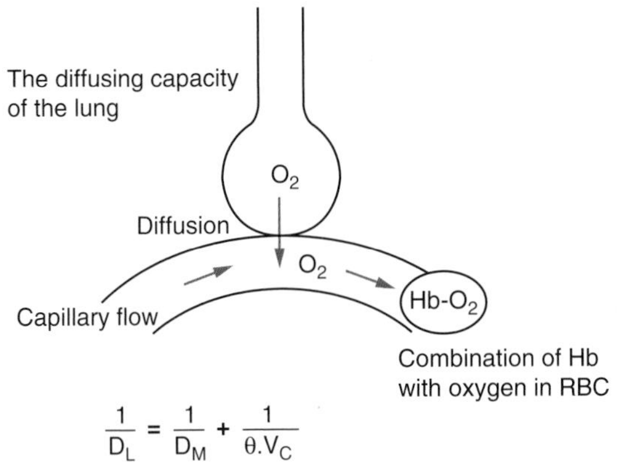

Figure 49.11 The diffusion across from the alveolus into the blood and the subsequent combination with haemoglobin of oxygen.

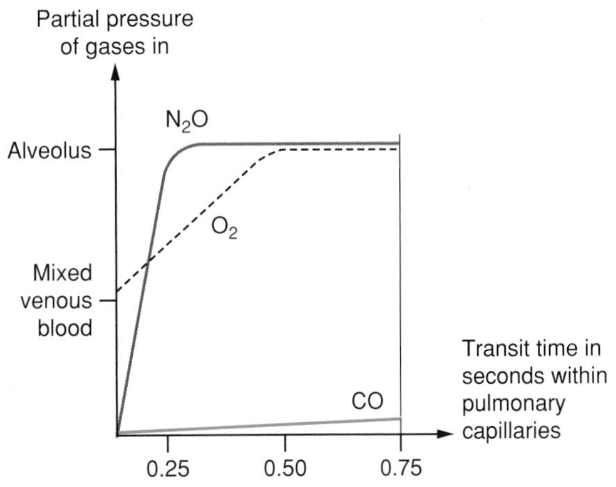

Figure 49.12 The plot of the rates of uptake of different gases diffusing from the alveolus into the lung capillaries.

are said to be perfusion limited as the amount of N_2O taken up by the blood depends on the blood flow (Figure 49.11).

The transfer of oxygen is perfusion limited and the partial pressure of the oxygen reaches equilibrium by about one-third of the transit time in the pulmonary capillary. No further driving force for diffusion exists after this point.

Oxygen uptake in the capillaries

The time taken for the partial pressure of oxygen to reach its plateau is 0.25 s. The pulmonary capillary volume is about 75 ml under resting conditions which is approximately equal to the stroke volume of the right ventricle. Thus the oxygen uptake is optimal (Figure 49.12). During exercise the cardiac output increases and the pulmonary capillary flow increases. The lungs cope with increased cardiac output by vasodilatation and recruitment of new capillaries, thus optimizing diffusion of oxygen. This mechanism allows the lung to cope with the whole cardiac output after pneumonectomy.

Measuring diffusion

This can be done by a single breath test. A single breath of a mixture of carbon monoxide and helium is taken. The breath is held for approximately 10 s. The difference between inspiratory and expiratory concentration of carbon monoxide is measured. This is the transfer factor. It is corrected to the alveolar volume, V_a, This is the transfer coefficient, TLCO.

Partial pressures of respiratory gases in the alveoli are demonstrated in Figure 49.13.

Reaction rate with haemoglobin

There is a further resistance to gas transfer caused by the finite rate of reaction of oxygen or carbon monoxide with haemoglobin inside the red blood cell (RBC). When CO is added to blood it combines with haemoglobin very quickly. The reaction has two phases: diffusion through the alveolar capillary membrane barrier, and the reaction of CO with haemoglobin. The sum of the resistances will produce the overall resistance. This can be written as $1/D_L = 1/D_M + 1/\theta.V_c$, where $1/D_L$ is total resistance of the lung, $1/D_M$ is the resistance of the membrane, θ is the rate of chemical combination of the gas, and V_c is the pulmonary capillary blood volume.

Oxygen transport

Oxygen is carried in the blood in two forms, dissolved and combined with haemoglobin. The dissolved form obeys Henry's law, which states that the amount dissolved is proportional to the partial pressure of the gas above the surface of the liquid, and normally amounts to 0.3/100 ml blood.

Haemoglobin has four polypeptide chains, two alpha and two beta. Associated with each polypeptide chain is a haem group that acts as a binding site for oxygen. This contains iron within its structure. This iron is normally in ferrous form and therefore it can bind to oxygen. Haemoglobin is capable of binding to four oxygen molecules and its main function is to take up oxygen in the

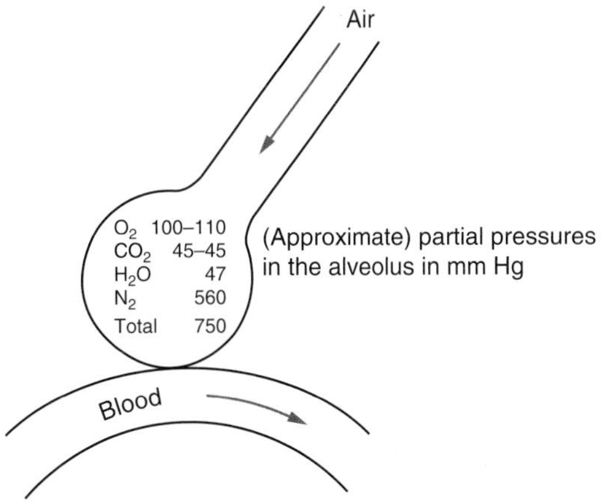

Figure 49.13 Partial pressure of different gases in the alveolus.

blood at the alveolar capillary membrane and transport and release oxygen into the tissues.

Haemoglobin also acts as a buffer for hydrogen ions and transports CO_2 as carbamino compounds.

Haemoglobin has four combining sites for oxygen and if all these binding sites are completely saturated, then every gram of haemoglobin carries 1.34 ml of oxygen. Since the blood has 15 g of haemoglobin per 100 ml, then the oxygen capacity is about 20.1 ml oxygen per 100 ml of blood (1.34 × 15). The oxygen saturation (SaO_2) of the blood is defined as the amount of oxygen carried in the blood expressed as a percentage of oxygen capacity. The oxygen saturation of arterial blood is about 97.5%, while that of mixed venous blood is about 75%.

Oxygen dissociation curve

The plot of the pO_2 and the oxygen saturation is sigmoid (Figure 49.14). The flatness of the curve in the arterial range is an advantage because a decrease in the arterial pO_2,as might be expected in lung disease, will still allow for a relatively normal oxygen content. As the reduction of the pO_2 approaches 50 mmHg there is a steep reduction in the oxygen content. This is important in the peripheral tissues as a large amount of oxygen for only a small drop in the capillary pO_2 is released. The maintenance of pO_2 assists the diffusion of oxygen into the tissues. Reduced haemoglobin is purple and therefore low oxygen saturation causes cyanosis. There are many factors that affect the oxygen dissociation curve. The curve is shifted to the right by increasing hydrogen ion concentration, pCO_2, temperature and concentration of 2,3-DPG (diphosphoglycerate) in the red cell. This means more unloading of haemoglobin at a given pO_2 in tissue capillary. A simple way to remember is that exercise produces acid, high CO_2 and heat load and benefits from unloading oxygen at the capillaries. 2,3-DPG is an end product of RBC metabolism and can shift the curve to the right. Increased 2,3-DPG occurs in hypoxia. Carbon monoxide interferes with the oxygen dissociation curve by combining with haemoglobin firmly. CO has an affinity 240 times greater than O_2 to combine with haemoglobin. Carbon monoxide shifts the oxygen dissociation curve to the left and thus interferes with unloading of oxygen, causing hypoxia.

Carbon dioxide transport

Carbon dioxide is carried in the blood in three ways: dissolved in the plasma, as bicarbonate ions and as carbamino compounds (Figure 49.15).

Dissolved carbon dioxide: carbon dioxide is 20 times more soluble than oxygen in the blood, and therefore a

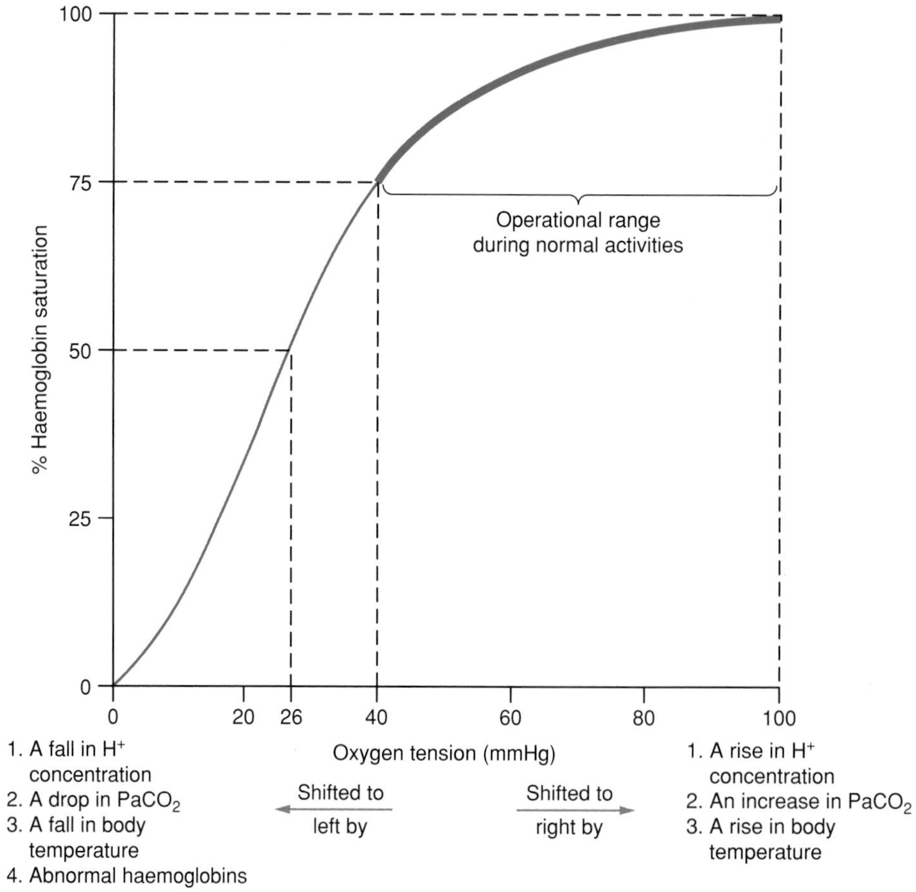

Figure 49.14 The oxygen haemoglobin dissociation curve.

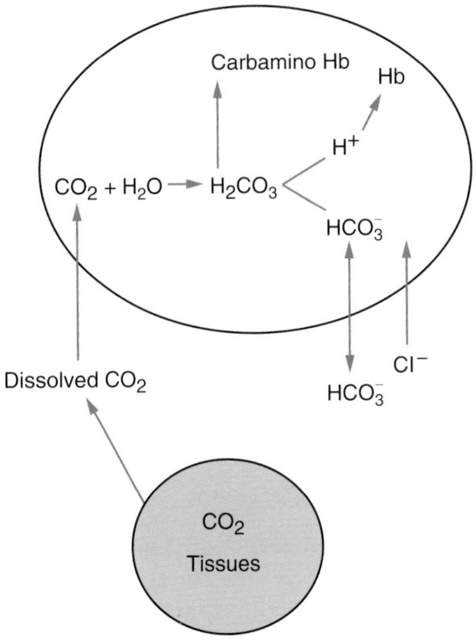

Figure 49.15 Carbon dioxide uptake from the tissues. The reverse occurs in the lung capillaries.

significant amount, 10%, of carbon dioxide is carried in solution. Solubility of carbon dioxide is 5.2 ml/kPa/l.

Bicarbonate ion: approximately 60% of CO_2 is transported as carbonic acid, which dissociates quickly into hydrogen and bicarbonate ions. The first reaction is slow in the plasma, but in the red cell it is dramatically speeded up by the presence of carbonic anhydrase. The reaction sequence is: $CO_2 + H_2O = H_2CO_3 = H^+ \; HCO_3^-$.

Haemoglobin in turn can take up the hydrogen ion produced, acting as a buffer, allowing the reaction to proceed rapidly. The bicarbonate produced in the red cell diffuses down the concentration gradient into the plasma in exchange for chloride. This is called chloride shift.

Carbamino compounds: CO_2 can react with proteins in the RBC to form carbamino compounds. This interaction of CO_2 with the haemoglobin is rapid and there is no enzyme involved. Approximately 30% of carbon dioxide is carried in this way. The presence of reduced haemoglobin in the peripheral blood helps with the loading of CO_2 while oxygenation in the pulmonary capillaries assists in unloading. Deoxygenation of the blood increasing its ability to carry CO_2 is known as the Haldane effect. The uptake of CO_2 in the peripheral blood increases the osmolar content of the red cell and consequently water enters the cell, increasing its volume.

Section 49.4 • Mechanics of breathing

General concept

During inspiration the chest wall expands and the diaphragm contracts, producing negative pressure in the pleura, thus drawing air into the lungs. Expiration occurs as the lungs return to their normal size by elastic recoil.

Intrapleural pressure during quiet breathing is always negative. There is a difference in intrapleural pressure between the apex and the base of the lung. From the apex to the base of the lung there is a rise in the intrapleural pressure from −10 cmH_2O to −2 cmH_2O.

Muscles of respiration

The main muscle of respiration, the diaphragm, is attached to the costal margin anteriorly and laterally, and to the lumbar vertebrae posteriorly. The motor nerve supply is via the phrenic nerve at C3, 4 and 5.

Intercostal muscles

External intercostal muscles originate from the anterior part of the upper rib and are inserted into the superior border of the rib below.

Internal intercostal muscles originate from the subcostal groove of the rib above and attach to the superior border of the rib below.

The internal intercostal muscles pull the ribs downwards and inwards while the external intercostal muscles pull the rib downwards and forwards. The muscles are supplied segmentally by the appropriate intercostal nerve.

Accessory muscles of inspiration include the scalene muscles and sternomastoids, which do not contribute to quiet breathing but during exercise may contract vigorously.

Elastic properties of the lung

Compliance is the slope of the pressure–volume curve or the volume change per unit pressure change. Normally the expanding pressure varies between −3 and −10 cmH_2O. The lung is remarkably tensile and compliant. The compliance of the human lung is about 200 ml/cmH_2O.

Elastance is the reciprocal of compliance, that is the resistance to the stretch of the lung. There are two types of compliance: lung compliance and chest wall compliance; the combination is total lung compliance. Compliance is expressed as dV/dP.

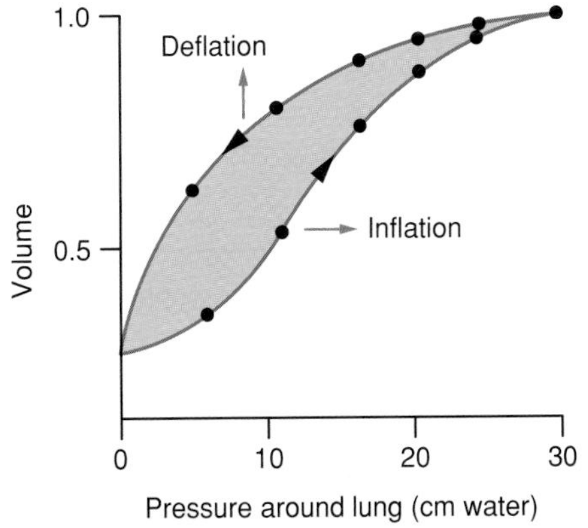

Figure 49.16 Compliance curve showing hysteresis.

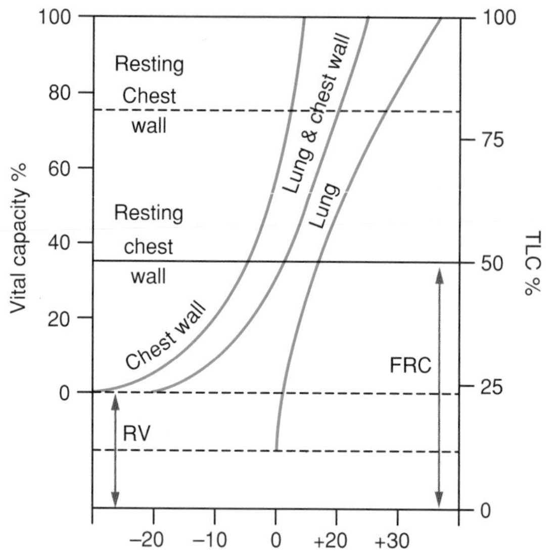

Figure 49.17 The balanced compliance of the chest wall and lung.

The dynamic lung compliance is a measure of the changing volume of the lung during breathing. This includes the work required to overcome airway resistance. The static lung compliance, measured *in vitro*, involves the inflation of the isolated lung in steps recording the volume at each step in inflation pressure, up to the TLC. Measurements are also taken during deflation. These measurements constitute the inflation deflation curve. The difference between the curves is called hysteresis (Figure 49.16). The lung volume at the base is less relative to the apex because it is compressed. Thus the base of the lung has greater initial compliance than the apex, and as both are submitted to the same intrapleural pressure during inspiration the base expands to a greater extent than the apex.

Chest wall compliance: the chest wall has elastic properties antagonistic to the lung. The chest wall tends to expand; if air is introduced into the pleural space at operation or pneumothorax, then the chest wall tends to spring open. The balance between the lung compliance and chest wall compliance is the total compliance of the lung (Figure 49.17).

Compliance is reduced in the following conditions:

- alveolar oedema
- pulmonary fibrosis
- pulmonary venous congestion
- pleural effusion and ascites
- obesity.

It is increased with age and in emphysema.

Patterns of air flow

The pattern of fluid flowing through a tube varies with the velocity, viscous properties of the fluid and the geometry of the tube. Laminar flow is stable flow, whereas turbulent flow is unstable. For any fixed geometry and viscosity, the velocity is the determinant.

The Reynolds number $Re = 2RVD/N$ determines the character of flow, where R is the radius, V is velocity, D is density and N is the viscosity of the fluid. If the Reynolds number is over 2000 it usually indicates turbulent flow. In any system there is an upper limit for the Reynolds number where flow is always turbulent and a lower limit where flow is always laminar.

Airways resistance

This can be defined as a resistance to the flow of the air within the airways of the lung. Resistance occurs only when there is flow. Resistance equals pressure divided by flow: $R = P/Q$. For laminar flow conditions the flow is directly related to the change in the pressure: $R = 8NL/(\pi r^4)$, where R is resistance, N is viscosity, L is the length, and r is the radius.

Determinants of airways resistance

The main site of airways resistance is the upper respiratory tract, i.e. large and medium airways to the seventh generation of the bronchial tree. The small airways, less than 2 mm, contribute 20% of the resistance; this is called the silent zone. Determinants of airways resistance include:

- lung volume: increased volume of the lung leads to decreased resistance from radial traction on the bronchi of the smooth muscles
- density and viscosity of the inspired gas.

Dynamic compression of the airways

This is the pressure difference between the airways and the pleura. During inspiration the pleural pressure is negative and the alveolar pressure is greater than the intrapleural pressure, which keeps the airways open. Alveolar pressure remains positive with respect to intrapleural pressure during expiration, and again the alveoli stay open. The transmural pressure depends on expiratory flow rate and intrapleural pressure (Figure 49.18). However, during

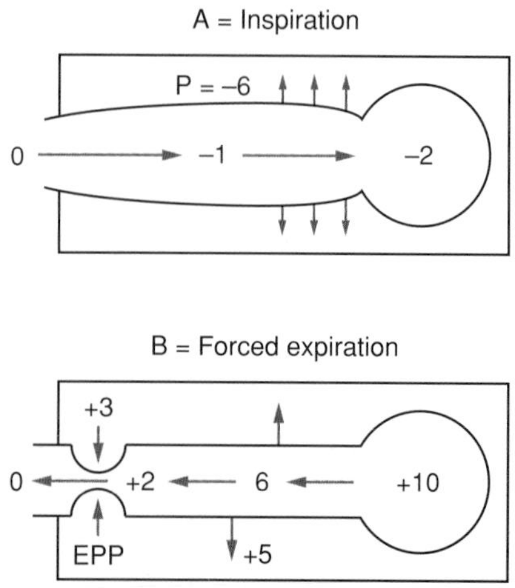

Figure 49.18 The change in pulmonary pressures during (a) inspiration and (b) expiration. Equal pressure points (EPP) are indicated.

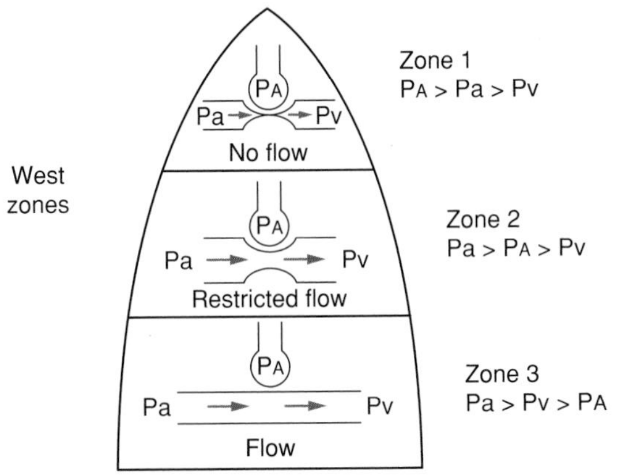

Figure 49.19 West zones illustrating the variation of blood flow in the lung in the upright position.

forced expiration there is positive intrapleural pressure which is transmitted through the lungs to the external walls of the airways. There is also a dynamic pressure drop from the alveoli to the airways caused by airways resistance. Hence the pressure at some point equalizes between the pleura and the airway leading to collapse of the airways. This point is called the equal pressure point. The harder the subject exhales forcibly, the more the airways are compressed. The pressure gradient will reduce the calibre of the airways during forceful expiration due to positive pressure inside the pleura exceeding the airway pressure inside the airway. This phenomenon is known as dynamic compression of the airways.

Distribution of blood within the lungs

The blood flow within the normal healthy lung is uniform. Blood flow at the base of the lung is greater than at the apex, and ventilation follows the same pattern. Because the lungs are vertical in the upright position they are under the influence of gravity and therefore lung bases have greater hydrostatic pressure than at the apex. Hence pressures at the lung base are higher so the lung will distend easily. As mentioned earlier, ventilation also increases from the apex to the base following blood flow.

The pattern of the blood flow in the lung in the upright position can be described in three zones, the West zones (Figure 49.19):

- Zone 1: At the apex where the alveolar pressure is higher than the arterial and capillary pressure, therefore the capillaries collapse and no flow occurs.
- Zone 2: Arterial pressure is greater than alveolar and venous pressure; hence there is flow from the arterial to the venous side. This is determined by the arterial alveolar pressure gradient.
- Zone 3: At the base of the lungs, where arterial is greater than venous pressure and greater than alveolar pressure, but flow is determined by the arterial venous pressure gradient.

Section 49.5 • Control of ventilation (Figure 49.20)

Homoeostasis of blood pH and blood gas tension requires proper matching of ventilation to oxygen consumption and CO_2 production. CO_2 and oxygen are the control variables that need to be kept within strict normal physiological limits. The control of ventilation is achieved through several components:

- the controller is that collection of brain nuclei that control the automatic function of breathing
- the effectors include the inspiratory and expiratory muscles, the power component of ventilation
- variables that can be physiologically detected; these include pCO_2, pO_2 and pH
- sensors which feed back to the central controller.

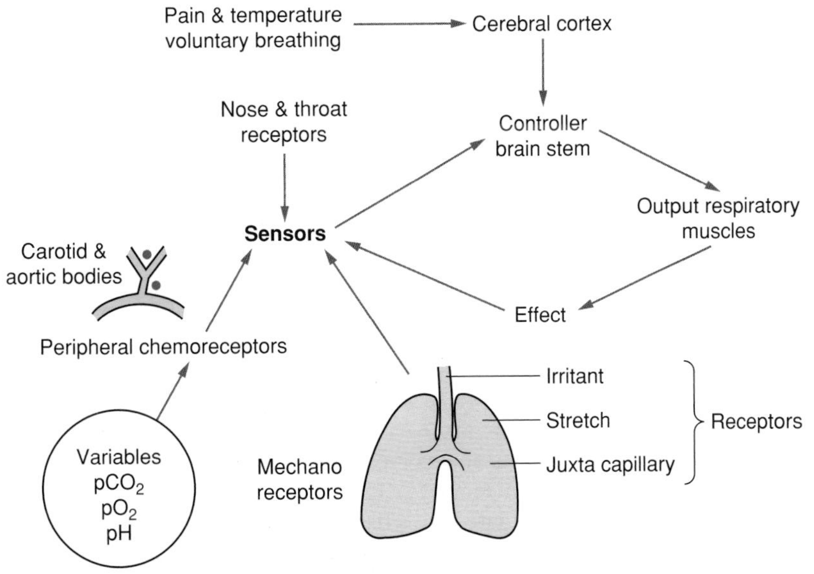

Figure 49.20 The neurological control of breathing.

The controller consists of two collections of neurones: the dorsal and ventral respiratory groups. The dorsal respiratory group has the property of intrinsic periodic firing and is responsible for the rhythm of ventilation. These nuclei have a second function of inhibiting the expiratory neurones in the ventral respiratory group. Thus they modulate the rate and depth of inspiration.

The ventral respiratory group of neurones is located in the nucleus ambiguus. These respiratory neurones supply the intercostal muscles, diaphragm and accessory muscles of respiration. The Botzinger complex is part of the ventral respiratory group and inhibits the neurones of the dorsal and ventral respiratory groups and may stimulate the expiratory neurones in the ventral respiratory group. The medulla is responsible for the respiratory rhythm and the dorsal respiratory group of neurones act like a pacemaker and discharge in a rhythmic manner, inhibiting expiratory neurones.

Effectors include the diaphragm, internal and external intercostal muscles and abdominal muscles. The effectors respond to control the rate and the strength of the contraction set by the central controller.

Variables, pH, pO_2 and pCO_2, are the end product of ventilation. These variables are kept within physiological range through the chemoreceptors. The chemoreceptors are responsible for 80% of the drive of respiration. There are two types of chemoreceptors: the central chemoreceptors situated in the medulla and those in the periphery. The medullary receptors are sensitive to carbon dioxide which crosses passively through the blood brain barrier and is converted to hydrogen ions, therefore stimulating ventilation. Peripheral chemoreceptors are situated in the carotid and aortic bodies and respond to changes in pO_2 and pH mainly, and to a lesser extent, to changes in pCO_2.

As well as chemoreceptors there are mechanoreceptors. These are joint stretch receptors, muscle spindles and Golgi apparati. Such receptors send stimuli and sensation from the chest wall directly to the dorsal group of nuclei in the medulla.

There are several receptors in the lungs:

- pulmonary stretch receptors situated in the airway smooth muscles
- irritant receptors situated between the epithelial cells, stimulated by noxious gases
- receptors situated in the alveolar walls close to the capillaries, called bronchial C fibre receptors
- all lung receptor responses are carried through the vagus nerve centrally to the dorsal respiratory group of neurones.

Other influences on the controller exist. Nose and upper airway receptors are irritant receptors; stimuli are carried by the glossopharyngeal and vagus nerves centrally to the dorsal respiratory group of neurones. Arterial baroreceptors sense changes in pressure. Their real pathway is unknown. Other receptors for pain and temperature, with emotion and volition are integrated through the cerebral cortex and influence the rate and depth of breathing.

The cerebral cortex has an influence on the breathing pattern as breathing is within voluntary control and the cerebral cortex can override the brain stem within limits. The controller always tends to reassert itself: witness the limits of the Valsalva manoeuvre, and those of voluntary hyperventilation, which can reduce pCO_2 leading to alkalosis which is always short lived.

Co-ordinated responses of the respiratory systems

Response to CO_2 is most important in control of ventilation. CO_2 is held within very tight limits and the ventilatory response is very sensitive to small changes in pCO_2. An increase in pCO_2 causes a significant increase in ventilation. Ventilatory response to pCO_2 is decreased during sleep and old age. Reduced response to CO_2 is caused by drugs such as morphine and genetic predisposition, and is modified by training in athletes.

Response to oxygen is only to low levels. Hypoxia stimulates peripheral chemoreceptors but this only becomes significant if the PO_2 is lower than 50 mmHg, i.e. 6.6 kPa. The response of the chemoreceptors to hypoxia varies at different levels of pCO_2. The higher the pCO_2 the earlier the response to low oxygen tension. Under normal conditions, pO_2 does not fall to values below 6.6 kPa, hence daily control of ventilation does not rely on hypoxic drive. The hypoxic drive becomes significant in severe lung diseases and becomes the main drive for ventilation. Patients with chronic lung disease rely entirely on the hypoxic drive, having lost the CO_2 drive. As the central chemoreceptors become less responsive to carbon dioxide, administration of high levels of oxygen may abolish hypoxic drive, depressing ventilation and worsening the patient's condition.

Hydrogen ions do not cross the blood brain barrier. Any change in pH above 7.46 may be compensated in the long term by the kidneys, as in high altitude living. Metabolic acidosis, most commonly caused by hypoperfusion of tissue, is a potent cause of hyperventilation as the respiratory alkalosis is compensatory. The falling pH below 7.34 acts on the peripheral chemoreceptors to drive the hyperventilation.

Human beings can increase ventilation in response to exercise to a much higher minute ventilation. This is achieved by increasing the respiratory rate and tidal volumes. During exercise pH, pO_2 and pCO_2 change very little. The real stimulus for increasing ventilation during exercise is not as well understood as the normal pattern of breathing.

Cheyne–Stokes respiration is the cyclical breathing pattern of apnoea followed by progressive deep breathing. This occurs in hypoxic patients and during sleep; however, it can also occur in patients with congestive heart failure and in patients with brain damage.

Communication

The larynx and bellows action of the lungs are essential for speech and communication. Voice changes resulting from involvement of the recurrent laryngeal nerves may be the first indication of pulmonary pathology. The development of speech has increased the proprioception in the chest wall. This increased sensory supply explains the severity of pain associated with chest injuries and why chest wall incisions are so painful.

Section 49.6 • Pulmonary function tests

The main indication for pulmonary function tests (PFTs) is the evaluation of pulmonary complaints, quantifying the impairment of different respiratory diseases and disability evaluation. PFTs can be useful in pre-operative assessment and assessing the risk for post-operative complications in non-thoracic operations and tolerance for lung resection.

Spirometry

PFTs can be measured with a volume displacement spirometer. It is now more common for flow to be the primary measurement with integration of flow over time to obtain volume. Spirometry includes measure of forced vital capacity (FVC), forced expiratory volume in 1 second (FEV1) and the ratio of FEV1 to FVC. Usually the best of three tests is accepted as the curve should be smooth and continuous and should have a reasonable duration of about 6 s. The FEV1 and FVC are reported as the largest value from any acceptable test (Figure 49.7).

Lung volume measurement

This usually relates to residual volume (RV), expiratory reserve volume (ERV), tidal volume (V_t) and inspiratory reserve volume (IRV). Lung volumes calculated from two volume addition are referred to as capacities.

Functional residual capacity (FRC) is the volume of air that is left in the lung at the end of expiration and equals RV + ERV.

- Inspiratory capacity (IC) equals tidal volume V_t + IRV.
- TLC (total lung capacity) equals vital capacity (VC) + RV.
- Lung volumes are measured by plethysmography and helium dilution.

The interpretation of PFTs

The most widely used prediction equations come from white populations of northern European ancestry. Studies of other groups find lower predicted values standardized against height. The normal range is ±20% of predicted, for sex and height.

An obstructive pattern is recognized when FEV1 is reduced, with a reduced ratio of FEV1/FVC below 80%.

The distinction between obstructive and restrictive patterns is based on the FEV1 to FVC ratio. In an obstructive pattern, FEV1 is reduced far more than FVC. COPD and asthma show an obstructive pattern with a reduced FEV1 and FEV1/FVC ratio with evidence of air trapping in the form of increased residual volume.

In asthma the bronchodilator response to beta-agonists is evidenced by increased FEV1, while patients with COPD usually elicit no or minimal reversibility. Significant reversibility is a 20% increase in FEV1 or an absolute increase of 200 ml in severe COPD with markedly reduced flows. The severity of obstruction can be measured according to the FEV1%. Severe obstruction is usually less than 50% of the predicted value.

A restrictive pattern is usually shown as reduced volumes of FVC, TLC and RV. Full lung volumes are required to confirm the restrictive pattern.

Flow–volume loops are generated using the spirometer to plot flow against volume.

Forced expiratory flow (FEF 25–75) is a measure of expiratory flow at 25 and 75% of FVC. FEF is usually a good marker of obstructive airways disease and particularly a marker for small airway disease.

Diffusing capacity has been discussed earlier. This may be reduced in obstructive airway disease (emphysema), in restrictive lung disease such as interstitial lung disease and in pulmonary vascular disease.

Role of PFTs in pre-operative assessment

PFTs should be used to assess the risk for post-operative complications. FEV1 less than 1 litre is a powerful predictor for mortality for life-threatening events. Consequently FEV1 is a necessary test in any patient who might have impaired lung function from whatever cause. Comorbidity assessments for peri-operative risk for morbidity and mortality all use FEV1 < 1 litre as an important marker.

The frequency of pulmonary complications is operation site dependent and is less likely if the operation is away from the diaphragm. Hence, thoracic and upper abdominal operations carry higher risk than lower abdominal and orthopaedic operations.

PFTs are vital if the patient has severe lung disease, when a conservative non-operative approach might be indicated. PFTs are necessary where a significant respiratory impairment is to be identified for the first time, especially when a tobacco related history is identified. Aggressive peri-operative therapy for COPD may be helpful. PFTs are always performed prior to coronary bypass grafting or upper abdominal operations. If there is a history of dyspnoea or tobacco use patients need pre-operative respiratory assessment and care but should not be excluded from these operations if at all possible. They are mandatory in all patients undergoing lung resection. The role of PFT's in lung resection surgery is discussed in Module 52.

Section 49.7 • Respiratory failure

The main function of the lung is the transfer of oxygen to the tissues and carbon dioxide out of the tissues, i.e. ventilatory function. When this system fails, then respiratory failure ensues. Acute respiratory failure is classified into two major categories:

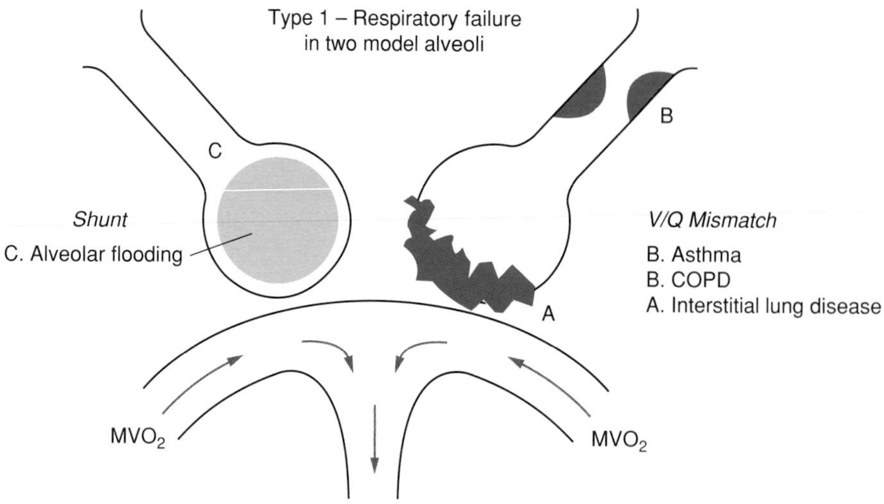

Figure 49.21 Type 1 respiratory failure demonstrating ventilation/perfusion mismatch leading to hypoxia. MVO_2 = mixed venous oxygen, COPD = chronic obstructive pulmonary disease.

- hypoxic respiratory failure, type 1
- hypercapnic respiratory failure, type 2.

However, there are two further categories which are a combination of types 1 and 2 failure:

- peri-operative respiratory failure
- hypoperfusion or shock related respiratory failure.

Type 1 – Hypoxic respiratory failure

Type 1 acute respiratory failure i.e. hypoxic respiratory failure (Figure 49.21), occurs when the gas exchange is impaired seriously, resulting in hypoxaemia with a paO_2 of less than 60 mmHg or SaO_2 less than 90%. Pathophysiology and the causes of hypoxic respiratory failure (HRF) are:

- Ventilation perfusion mismatch. This is caused by COPD, asthma and interstitial lung diseases or vascular obstruction due to pulmonary embolism. These conditions produce an abnormal ventilation to perfusion relationship. This type of hypoxaemia responds to increased inspired oxygen (FiO_2).
- Shunt. This refers to the fraction of mixed venous blood that passes into the arterial circulation bypassing the alveoli. This also occurs when the alveoli are filled with pus as in pneumonia, with blood as in pulmonary haemorrhage or fluid as in pulmonary oedema from either left ventricular failure or acute respiratory distress syndrome (ARDS). Shunt can occur in pulmonary embolism as well. These patients do not respond to oxygen. Shunts are associated with a wide $p(A\text{-}a)O_2$ gradient, i.e alveolar to arterial partial pressure of oxygen difference resulting in hypoxaemia. When a shunt is greater than 30% there is usually resistance to the correction of hypoxaemia.
- Alveolar hypoventilation. This is usually associated with high pCO_2 and the resultant hypoxaemia is due to increased alveolar CO_2 which displaces oxygen. Oxygen therapy will improve this type of hypoxaemia; however, it can worsen hypo-ventilation in some in patients with COPD or obesity hypoventilation syndrome. Primary treatment in this condition is correction of the cause of hypoventilation.
- Low inspired oxygen due to high altitude or inhalation of toxic gases.
- Diffusion impairment is seen in interstitial lung disease. Hypoxaemia is due to ventilation–perfusion abnormality.
- Low mixed venous oxygen returning to the lung capillary bed can lower the pO_2 significantly when either intrapulmonary shunting or ventilation–perfusion mismatch is present. Normally the lungs fully oxygenate pulmonary arterial blood. Low mixed venous oxygen can occur in anaemia, severe hypoxaemia, low cardiac output and with increased oxygen consumption.

Management of hypoxic respiratory failure (type 1)

Oxygen therapy

The main goal of oxygen administration is to facilitate oxygen uptake by the blood to meet the demands of the peripheral tissues. Oxygen can be delivered by nasal prongs or Venturi masks if variable percentages of oxygen need be delivered. One has to be careful in patients with COPD and hypercapnia. Non-rebreathing masks will achieve higher oxygen concentrations up to 80%. A one-way valve prevents exhaled gases from re-entering the reservoir in non-rebreathing systems to maximize the FiO_2.

Continuous positive airway pressure (CPAP) is delivered by a close fitting facemask and an expiratory resistance valve. This can be used if the pO_2 is less than 60 mmHg. The patient should be conscious and cooperative and should be able to protect his upper airways as well as able to initiate breathing. He or she should also be haemodynamically stable.

Bilevel positive airway pressure (BIPAP) is another mode of non-invasive ventilation whereby inspiratory and expiratory supplementary pressures can be applied via a close fitting mask to a patient's face when breathing spontaneously. Indications are similar to the CPAP but this mode has a back-up rate in case the patient has a low respiratory rate.

Type 2 – Hypercapnic respiratory failure

Hypercapnia occurs when CO_2 production increases without a corresponding increase in alveolar ventilation.

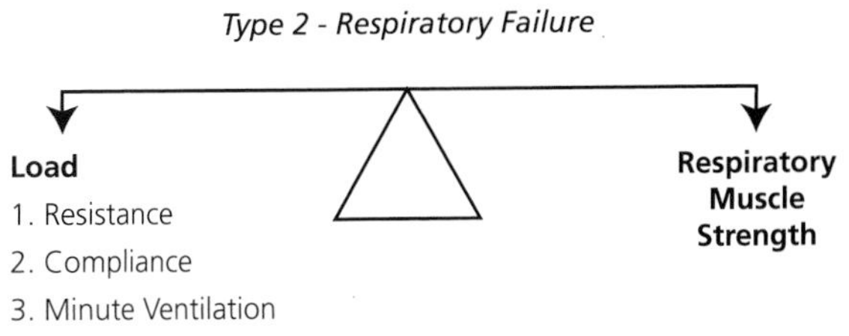

Figure 49.22 Type 2 respiratory failure illustrating the balance between the respiratory muscle strength and the breathing load.

CO_2 production is related to metabolic rate and the lung is responsible for clearing the CO_2 from the circulation. Therefore primary failure of alveolar ventilation is one major cause of hypercapnic respiratory failure. This may be due to weakness of the respiratory muscles. The diaphragm is the main muscle of respiration and it is innervated by the phrenic nerve at C3, 4 and 5.

Muscle weakness can be caused by:

- Depressed CNS drive. The brain stem and cerebral cortical region involved in respiratory control may be damaged or influenced by stroke, drug overdose such as morphine or alcohol intoxication and hypothyroidism.
- Motor neurone disorder. This is caused by spinal cord disease and motor neurone disease.
- Peripheral nerve dysfunction such as peripheral neuropathy, Guillain–Barré syndrome and critical illness neuropathy.
- Neuromuscular junction dysfunction such as myasthenia gravis, botulism and after neuromuscular blockade during relaxation anaesthesia and in patients on mechanical ventilation in intensive care units.
- Myopathy such as polymyositis and endocrine abnormalities (hyperthyroidism).
- Myocyte dysfunction due to electrolyte abnormalities: hypokalaemia, hypomagnesaemia, hypophosphataemia and hypocalcaemia.

Excessive load on the respiratory muscles

- Increased airways resistance. This occurs in bronchospasm, airway oedema and excessive secretions or upper airways obstruction. Obstructive sleep apnoea is a functional intermittent form.
- Decreased airway compliance. Lung compliance can be reduced when there is atelectasis, infection or pulmonary oedema. Chest wall compliance can be reduced in pleural effusion, pneumothorax or rib fractures, obesity and ascites.
- Increased minute ventilation will increase the load on the respiratory system. Ventilation is a product of respiratory rate and tidal volume. An increase in respiratory rate occurs in fever, acidosis, hypovolaemia, sepsis and pulmonary embolus.

Management approach to hypercapnic respiratory failure (type 2)

Conservative management is mainly to pre-empt mechanical ventilation dose inhaler or nebulizers. Ipratropium bromide (Atrovent), an anticholinergic agent, is also a bronchodilator and can be used especially in patients with COPD. Aminophylline is an effective bronchodilator in patients with COPD and may be given synergistically with other bronchodilators. Aminophylline has an added effect on the diaphragm as it increases the strength of contraction. Steroids can be given orally or intravenously especially in patients with COPD or asthma. Antibiotics should be given if there is evidence of bacterial infection.

CPAP and BIPAP via facemask should be capable of reducing the work of breathing in patients with impending type 2 respiratory failure. Arrhythmias are not common but may limit the dosage of bronchodilating drugs. The most common arrhythmias in these situations are the supraventricular tachyarrhythmias caused by a combination of hypoxia and metabolic derangement. If this fails then the patient will need intubation and mechanical ventilation.

Intubation and mechanical ventilation will correct hypoxaemia and reduce the CO_2 level. During mechanical ventilation the specific cause of type 2 respiratory failure is treated effectively, after which liberation from mechanical ventilation should be swift.

Type 3 – Peri-operative respiratory failure

Peri-operative respiratory failure is a combination of types 1 and 2 respiratory failure which occurs as a result of a reduction in the functional residual capacity below the closing volume leading to hypoventilation and hypoxaemia from progressive collapse of dependent parts of the lung. Causes of peri-operative respiratory failure include atelectasis, the supine position, excessive secretions and major tranquillizers. Splinting of the diaphragm is a result of major operations which cause excessive pain. These are particularly thoracic and upper abdominal procedures. Obesity and ascites also contribute to peri-operative respiratory failure.

The management of these patients should include monitoring of pain and effective analgesia with anti-atelectasis protocols such as physiotherapy, positioning the patient in an upright position and early mobilization.

Type 4 – Shock-related respiratory failure

The mechanism is shared between types 1 and 2 respiratory failure. Hypoperfusion states lead to increased work of breathing and in shock the proportion of oxygen consumption increases from 5 to 18% for the work of breathing. There are three major types of shock: cardiogenic shock due to myocardial infarction or left ventricular failure, hypovolaemic shock from acute haemorrhage and septic shock from endotoxaemia. The management of shock should be supportive, including oxygen, mechanical ventilation and specific treatment of the cause of shock.

Section 49.8 • Disorders of sleep and breathing

Obstructive sleep apnoea (OSA)

The muscles of the upper airways and thoracic muscles play major roles in maintaining adequate ventilation and oxygenation during sleep. Some patients, during sleep, have been shown to have elevated airways resistance with episodes of apnoea and or hypopnoea leading to cyclical hypoxaemia and hypercapnia with profound destruction of sleep architecture. Such patients commonly complain of excessive daytime sleepiness as a result of sleep fragmentation from upper airway narrowing and/or closure. This is called OSA. In physiology, apnoea is defined as absence of airflow at the nose or the mouth for over 10 s. Hypopnoea can be defined as a reduction in the airflow below 50% from the previous baseline flow, lasting more than 10 s. Apnoea during sleep is classified by character: central, obstructive and mixed. Central apnoea is characterized by absence of airflow and respiratory effort while obstructive apnoea is characterized by persistent respiratory effort during an apnoeic period. Apnoea that commences with central component followed by an obstructive component is called mixed apnoea.

The presence of apnoea during sleep may not be pathological. In normal younger adults up to five apnoeas per hour of sleep is considered physiological. However, an apnoea frequency of over 20 per hour of sleep is associated with increased morbidity. Physiological apnoeas are not associated with significant oxygen desaturation of less than 85%.

Epidemiology of OSA

OSA has a strong male predominance – the male to female ratio is 5:1 – and a mean age between 40 and 50 years. OSA has been described in children and adolescents. Sleep disordered breathing has been shown to increase with age. The true incidence is not known.

The main symptoms are disruptive snoring during sleep with sleep difficulties and daytime sleepiness, mood and psychiatric disturbances and cardiopulmonary complications. Some of these patients would have had road traffic accidents.

The main risk factors are male gender, obesity, hypertension and advancing age. Craniofacial and anatomical abnormalities that reduce upper airway size have been shown to be risk factors for OSA as well as familial factors. Smoking, excessive alcohol consumption and sedatives may also be risk factors.

Epidemiological studies have shown associations between snoring, obstructive sleep apnoea and hypertension. Correction of sleep apnoea has a modest effect on hypertension. Obstructive sleep apnoea is associated with ischaemic heart disease; snoring increases the odds for myocardial infarction approximately four-fold. A self-reported history of myocardial infarction is recorded more frequently in snorers than non-snorers. Cerebro-vascular disease and the risk of stroke is increased two-fold in OSA. Pulmonary hypertension is reported in between 10 and 30% of patients with OSA.

Cerebrovascular and cardiovascular diseases, road traffic accidents and work related accidents are more frequent causes of mortality in these patients. An apnoea index above 20 is the threshold for increased risk of mortality.

Polysomnography is used to diagnose sleep disordered breathing including obstructive sleep apnoea. This is an overnight study that measures respiratory flow, abdominal and thoracic movements with muscle tone, eye movements, electroencephalography, oximetry and electrocardiographic changes during sleep. Some centres titrate CPAP in the same setting and adjust the CPAP pressure accordingly for long-term management.

Management of OSA

General measures include weight reduction: all patients should be encouraged to lose weight. Opiates and excessive alcohol consumption tend to depress the upper airway motor tone during sleep and increase the apnoea threshold. These drugs should be avoided. Positive airway pressure, nasal CPAP, is the most effective non-surgical therapy for obstructive sleep apnoea. The effects are felt immediately after a single night of sleep. Nasal CPAP acts by elevating the pressure in the oropharynx and maintaining positive airway pressure throughout the respiratory cycle. It requires variable adjustment of the pressure; however, there are now new nasal CPAP systems that can adjust to the optimum pressures automatically.

The main problem with nasal CPAP is long-term compliance. This is known to be poor in spite of the immediate benefits to the patient. Only 46% of patients use the device for over 4 hours on 70% of nights.

As well as CPAP, BIPAP can also treat obstructive sleep apnoea but the device is more expensive. Antidepressants can be useful.

Surgical techniques

Uvulo-palatal pharyngeoplasty (UPPP) has received the greatest attention in medical and surgical investigations. It can reduce the apnoea hypopnea index by approximately 50%. However, normalization of breathing in these patients rarely occurs. The major problem is the functional area of obstruction in these patients. Somnaplasty is the reduction of tissue volume at the uvular soft palate area and at the base of the tongue and may prove to be efficacious but proper data are lacking.

Maxillomandibular advancement using mouth splints at night is useful in the majority (80%) of these patients. Tracheostomy is sometimes used in life threatening obstructive sleep apnoea or when there is failure of nasal CPAP or intolerance to the CPAP.

Further reading

CME Unlimited. Pulmonary Board Review (1996–2000). In: Seaton, A., Seaton, D. and Gordon Leitch, A., eds. *Crofton and Douglas's Respiratory Diseases*, 5th edn. Oxford: Blackwell Science.

Hall, J. B. and Wood, L. (1998) *Principles of Critical Care*, 2nd edn. New York: McGraw-Hill.

Scadding, J. G. and Cumming, G. (1981). *Scientific Foundations of Respiratory Medicine*. London: Heinemann.

West, J. B. (1999). *Respiratory Physiology. The Essentials*, 5th edn. Baltimore, MD: Lippincott, Williams and Wilkins.

MODULE 50

Pulmonary infections

Section 50.1 • Bronchiectasis

Bronchiectasis is defined as chronic irreversible dilatation and destruction of the large- or medium-sized bronchi (fourth to ninth generations) demonstrable at bronchography or high-resolution computed tomography (HRCT) and may be confirmed by examination of resected or post-mortem lung specimens. There are several causal mechanisms with differing clinical and radiological presentations. While the details of each pathological process are not fully understood, two factors are common:

1. The outward tension applied to the exterior of the bronchial walls may develop in several ways:
   (a) During acute respiratory infections in infancy the smaller bronchi may become blocked by mucopus with collapse of the lung parenchyma distally, so that tension is applied to the outside of the bronchial walls which, if damaged, will become dilated.
   (b) Chronic suppurative pneumonias, including some adenoviral and influenzal infections in childhood, may grumble on with the progressive destruction of the smaller bronchi and lung parenchyma. Such loss of lung volume increases the tension and stretch across the bronchial walls in the absence of any significant bronchial obstruction.
   (c) The obstruction of a major bronchus initially causes segmental or lobar collapse, followed by the accumulation of fluid in the affected bronchi and alveoli. If the obstruction is not relieved quickly, suppuration invariably supervenes with considerable tissue destruction and healing by fibrosis, both of which increase the destruction of the bronchial walls in the affected areas.
2. Weakening of the bronchial wall results from inflammatory damage to bronchial muscle or elastic tissue. The usual cause is infection which invades the wall with destruction of both elements, often occurring as part of the same process. In some bronchiectatic cysts there may be little evidence of any normal bronchial architecture, but damage is usually less severe.

Pathogenesis

Factors important in the pathogenesis include infectious insult, impaired drainage, airway obstruction and defects in host-defence mechanisms.

Classification

Traditionally, bronchiectasis has been classified according to the type of bronchial dilatation seen on bronchography, e.g. cylindrical, saccular or cystic (Figures 50.1–50.6). Recently bronchography has fallen into disuse. With increased experience it may prove possible to group bronchiectasis according to CT scanning appearances (Figure 50.7).

Although attempts at a classification based on clinical and pathological findings are incomplete, this causal classification is possible:

1. Post-infective bronchiectasis
   (a) follicular
   (b) saccular.
2. Post-collapse bronchiectasis
   (a) proximal obstruction
   (b) distal obstruction.
3. Post-tuberculous bronchiectasis.
4. Allergic bronchiectasis.
5. Congenital bronchiectasis
   (a) arrested development
   (b) cilial dysfunction.
6. Defective host-defence mechanisms.
7. Rheumatic diseases.
8. Cystic fibrosis.

Post-infective follicular bronchiectasis

This invariably develops in children under the age of 7 years with symptoms occurring before puberty.

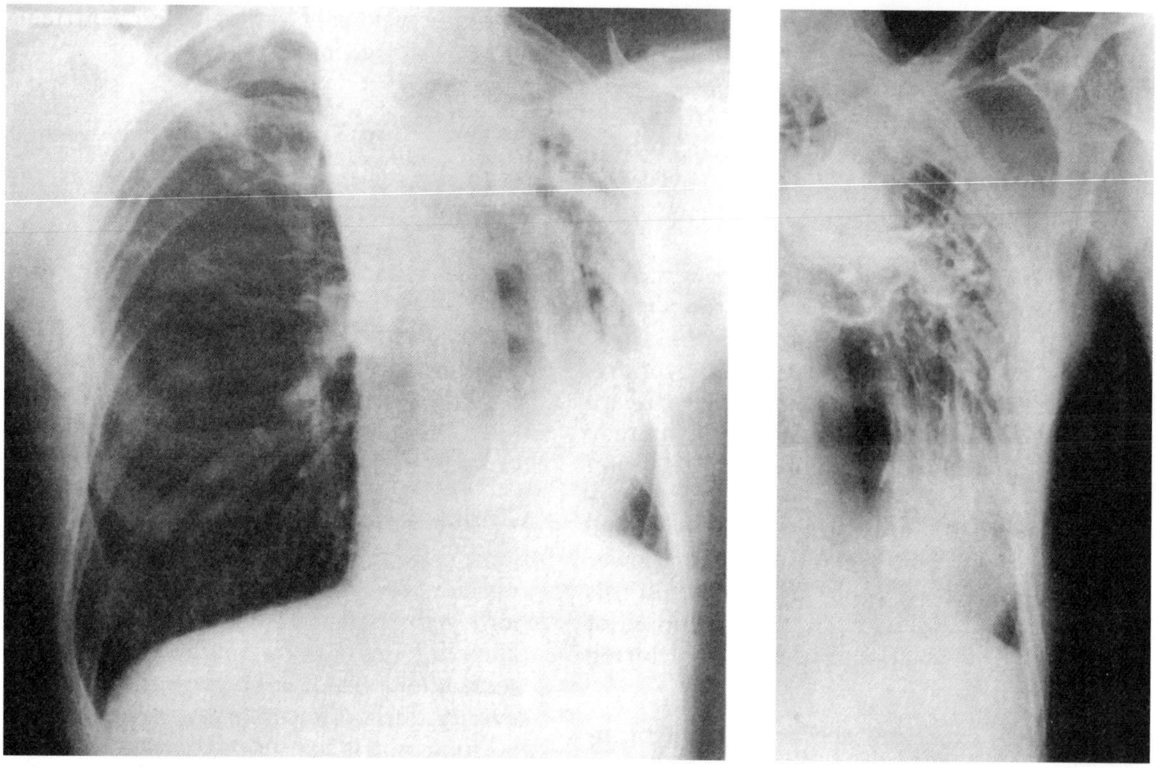

Figure 50.1 Contracted fibrotic left lung with bronchiectatic change from previous tuberculosis.

Two-thirds of cases follow measles or whooping cough, while grumbling adenoviral or influenzal infections account for many others.

Post-infective saccular bronchiectasis

In this there is often a history of severe bronchopneumonia in childhood although the symptoms develop much later. Bronchiectatic and normal bronchi are interspersed within the same lobe and although the smaller bronchi of the involved segments are destroyed collateral ventilation between normal and diseased areas leads to compensatory emphysema in the affected alveoli so that there is little loss of lung volume. There are numerous, pus-filled, saccular dilatations in continuity with medium-sized bronchi. The bronchial architecture of these cysts is completely disrupted, their walls consisting of fibrous granulation tissue with an ulcerated squamous epithelium.

Post-collapse bronchiectasis

The obstruction of a segmental or lobar bronchus by a bronchial neoplasm, foreign body, adenoma or hilar gland enlargement (usually tuberculous), if not relieved quickly, is followed by suppuration, abscess formation, fibrosis and collapse within the affected area. The larger bronchi lying distal to the obstruction become bronchiectatic presenting as dilated, pus-filled, 'finger-like' swellings. Even if the obstruction is relieved and the lobe or segment re-expands, e.g. following the removal of a foreign body, or the resolution of tuberculous glands, bronchiectasis may still develop as a

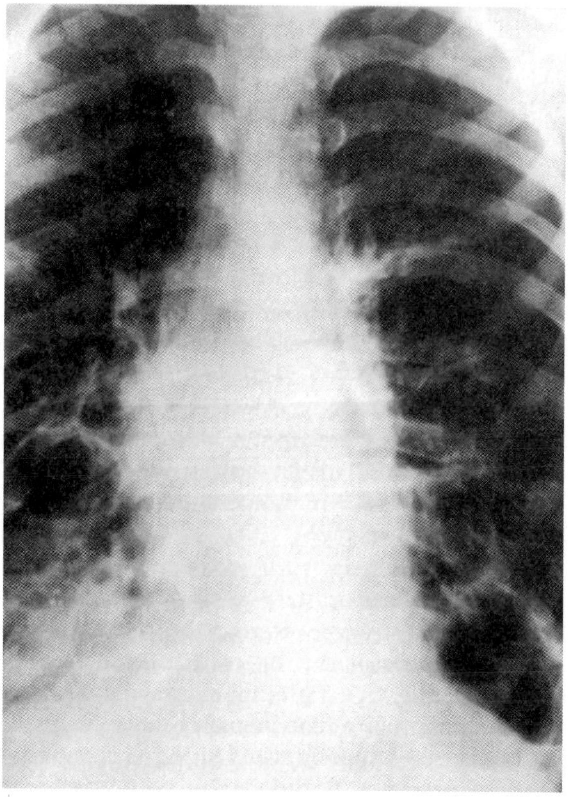

Figure 50.2 PA chest film showing extensive ring shadows throughout both lower lobes; several of the ring shadows show fluid levels representing saccular bronchiectasis. (Courtesy of Paul Grech.)

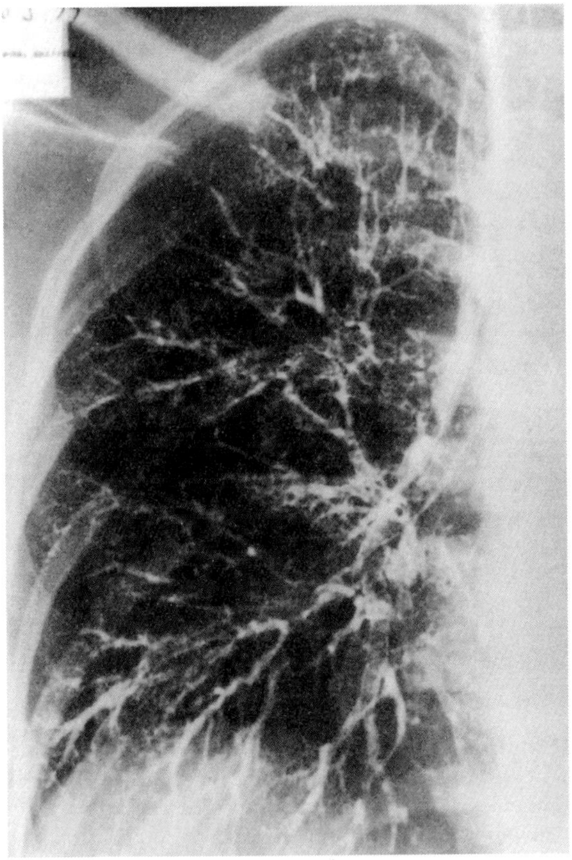

Figure 50.3 PA view of a normal right bronchogram performed via an intratracheal catheter positioned in the right main bronchus. (Courtesy of Paul Grech.)

result of parenchymal and bronchial damage which occurred during the obstruction (middle lobe syndrome).

Rarely, bronchiectasis develops after a viral or atypical pneumonia in adults if there has been peripheral collapse due to diffuse obstruction of the smaller bronchi by thick mucopus with coincidental damage to the walls of the proximal bronchi.

Post-tuberculosis bronchiectasis

Lung destruction and fibrosis are characteristic features of pulmonary tuberculosis resulting in contraction of a lobe or segment with distortion of the proximal bronchi (Figure 50.1). When the tuberculous process involves the bronchial walls (tuberculous endobronchitis) the resultant suppuration, caseation and fibrosis weaken the bronchi, predisposing them to bronchiectasis. These changes are most frequently seen in the upper lobes where they are often asymptomatic.

Allergic bronchopulmonary aspergillosis (ABPA)

In allergic bronchopulmonary aspergillosis, damage occurs at the sites of impaction of mucous plugs. These plugs may contain small quantities of the fungus *Aspergillus fumigatus*, which provokes a destructive allergic reaction within the bronchial walls. There is an associated collapse of the distal lung. ABPA represents a hyperimmune reaction to the fungus with features of a peripheral eosinophilia, high IgE and precipitating antibodies to the fungus. CT scan of the chest reveals central bronchiectasis which is characteristic of ABPA. Corticosteroids have a dramatic effect. Future episodes occurring in different segments result in bronchiectasis scattered throughout the medium-sized bronchi of both lungs.

Congenital bronchietasis

Congenital bronchiectasis resulting from the **arrested development** of the smaller bronchi and alveoli undoubtedly occurs but its frequency is disputed. Symptoms begin in early childhood. The affected lobe

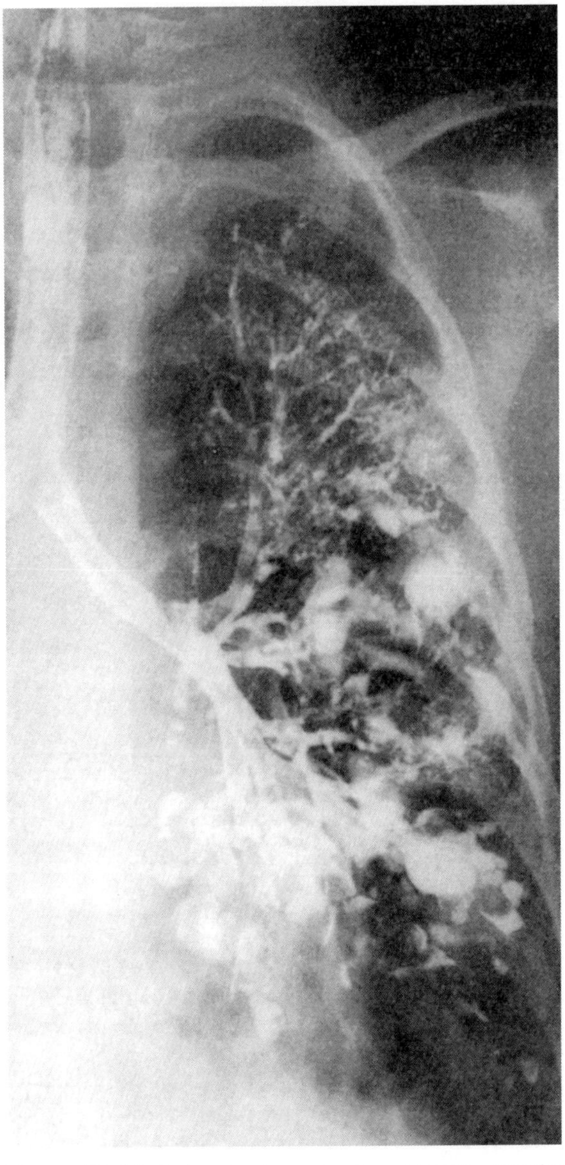

Figure 50.4 Left bronchogram showing extensive saccular bronchiectasis of the lingular and left lower lobe bronchi. (Courtesy of Paul Grech.)

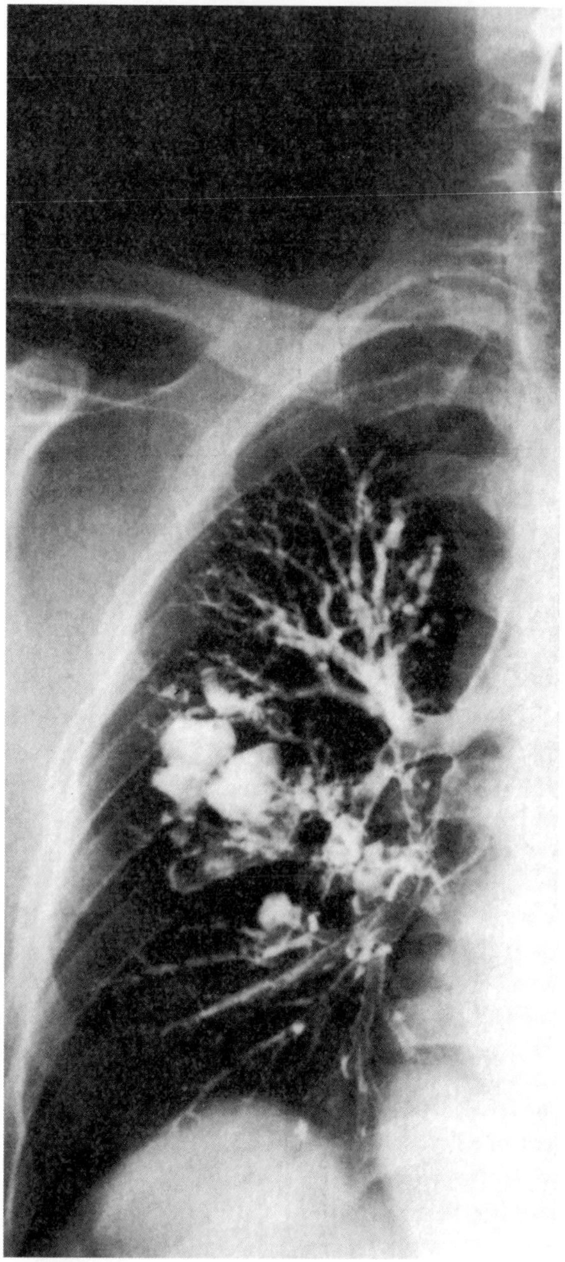

Figure 50.5 PA view of a right bronchogram performed through the cricothyroid route (note needle at the cricothyroid membrane). The anterior branch of the upper lobe bronchus is affected with cystic bronchiectasis. (Courtesy of Paul Grech.)

or lung is small, adherent to the chest wall and supplied by hypoplastic pulmonary arteries. The proximal bronchi while containing their normal complement of elastic tissue, muscle and cartilage are present as tubular structures. There is little recognizable parenchymal tissue.

In a sequestrated lung segment the bronchi are ectatic. Arrested parenchymal development between birth and 8 years may produce unilateral emphysema (MacLeod's syndrome) in which bronchiectasis features prominently.

Primary cilial dysfunction

A rare hereditary defect of cilial ultrastructure has been found in patients with Kartagener's syndrome (bronchiectasis, sinusitis, male infertility and transposition of the viscera). Dysfunction of cilia interferes with the activity of the respiratory ciliated epithelium and mucous escalator (mucociliary clearance), predisposing to recurrent infections and diffuse bronchiectasis. Incidence is from 1/20 000 to 1/60 000 of the population. Diagnosis is confirmed by nasal or bronchial epithelial brushings showing absence of the dynein arm at electron microscopy.

Defective host-defence mechanisms

Any condition which leads to a reduction in immunity may be a cause of bronchiectasis. Hypogammaglobulinaemia leaves the patient open to recurrent respiratory infection of varying severity, the overall result of which is to cause a loss of peripheral lung tissue and a weakening of the bronchial walls. Some patients have primary IgG subclass deficiencies. It is important to diagnose IgG deficiencies in view of effective treatment with immunoglobulins and reduction of lung destruction.

Rheumatic diseases

Rheumatoid arthritis is now considered a cause of bronchiectasis. Bronchiectasis can precede joint disease. Ankylosing spondylitis is another associated arthropathy.

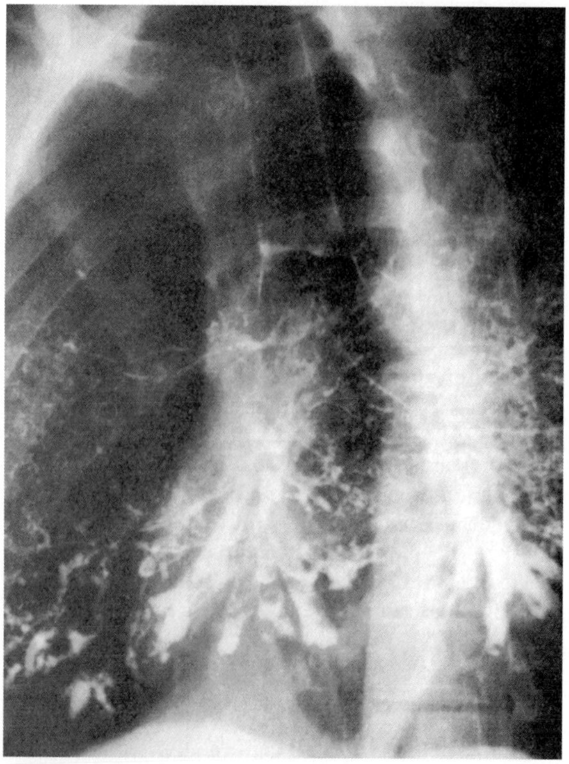

Figure 50.6 Inhalation bronchogram showing cylindrical bronchiectasis of all the bronchi of both lower lobes. (Courtesy of Paul Grech.)

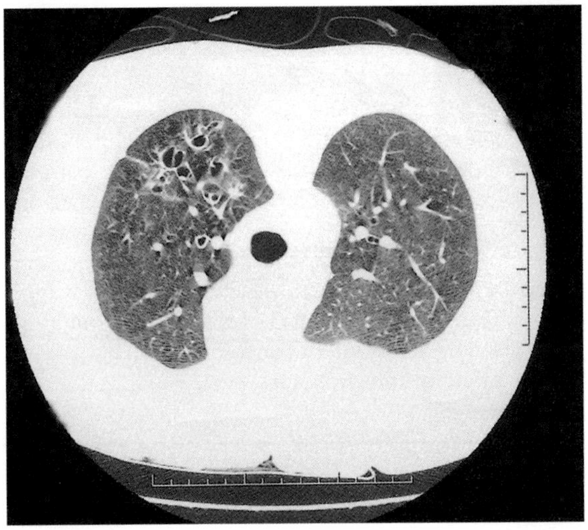

Figure 50.7 CT scan of patient with bronchiectasis affecting predominantly the right middle lobe; there are minor ectatic lesions widely distributed.

Cystic fibrosis

Cystic fibrosis is characterized by sinusitis and bronchiectasis and increased sweat chloride ions, >55 meq/l. Recurrent infections and inspissated mucus plugs predispose to bronchiectasis.

Bronchiectasis is multilobular in 70% of cases and often involves both lungs. The posterior basal segment of the left lower lobe is most frequently affected while the anterior and apical segments of that lobe are often spared. When the lingula is involved there is usually concomitant disease in the left lower lobe. In the presence of chronic inflammation the bronchial arteries hypertrophy and the blood flow through them is greatly increased. The arteries arise directly from the aorta at systemic pressure. Thus, haemoptysis of varying degree is common. Ventilation and perfusion are reduced in the affected areas.

Clinical features

The classic manifestations are cough and daily production of mucopurulent sputum.

Cough is present in 90% of cases and sputum production in >75%. Haemoptysis is another complaint present in about 50% of patients. Recurrent localized pneumonitis should alert the physician to the diagnosis of bronchiectasis. There may be pain and dyspnoea with wheeziness but these are less frequent. Patients may give a past history of pneumonia or tuberculosis earlier.

Physical findings include coarse crackles of the affected side, with occasional rhonchi and occasionally pleural rub. Clubbing occurs. Chronic sinusitis is often associated with bronchiectasis, being particularly troublesome in advanced cases. Brain abscess, although a classic complication, is now uncommon. In severe cases amyloidosis may develop and periodic checks for proteinuria and hepatosplenomegaly backed up by rectal biopsy are advisable.

Investigations

Chest X-ray

Linear atelectasis, dilated and thickened bronchi and tramline or ring shadows may be seen on a chest X-ray. Mucous plugging may be seen as irregular peripheral opacities or lobar collapse (Figure 50.2).

HRCT

HRCT of the thorax has now taken over from bronchography as the investigation of choice in: (1) establishing the diagnosis, (2) identifying the sites, and (3) defining the extent of bronchiectatic areas and the presence of confounding diseases. This is necessary when planning resection or postural drainage. HRCT in bronchiectasis has a sensitivity of 97%. HRCT demonstrates airway dilatation, and bronchial wall thickening with or without the presence of obstruction. Small cysts may also be seen. Central bronchiectasis is suggestive of ABPA. Upper lobe bronchiectasis is present in cystic fibrosis and tuberculosis. Pulmonary fibrosis may be seen on HRCT and traction bronchiectasis may be the result.

Pulmonary function tests allow functional assessment. Obstructive impairment with reduced forced expiratory volume in 1 second (FEV1) and FEV1/ forced vital capacity (FVC) is common.

Management

Although the incidence of bronchiectasis appears to be falling preventive measures continue to be essential. Vaccines against whooping cough and measles, improved management of neonatal and infantile bronchiolitis and the early treatment of childhood infections have all contributed. Effective treatment of tuberculosis, prophylactic chemotherapy in tuberculin-positive and BCG vaccination in tuberculin-negative children remain important. An awareness of the possibility of foreign body inhalation, particularly in children, with prompt investigation, removal and intensive physiotherapy to promote early re-expansion of any segmental or lobar collapse are important factors.

Medical measures may control but not eradicate the disease and secondary bronchitis, emphysema or asthma may often develop. Unfortunately, the cases which respond least well to conservative measures usually have extensive involvement which prevents resection. Resection may be curative in selected cases, provided all the diseased areas can be excised, leaving reasonable pulmonary function. However, careful case selection allows the benefit of reduced sputum load and recurrent infection to be the major contribution of resection.

Successful medical management depends on effective postural drainage backed up by appropriate antibiotic therapy. Good drainage clears the secretions, controls infection and reduces the chance of secondary damage. As co-operation is essential, it is important to educate the patient as to the nature of his or her disease and the rationale behind drainage which is often best achieved by a spell in hospital during which correct positioning can be demonstrated, breathing exercises taught and a close relative instructed in basic physiotherapy. A bronchodilator taken 10–15 min before drainage may relieve bronchospasm and improve the results

Broad spectrum antibiotics are required in acute exacerbations and should be given in high doses,e.g. amoxycillin 3 g daily. In complicated bronchiectasis antibiotics need be given intravenously to cover Gram-negative micro-organisms: *Klebsiella*, *Pseudomonas* or *Proteus*.

Surgical resection should be considered at an early stage in cases of severe or recurrent haemoptysis, recurrent disabling pneumonia, persistent cough with significant sputum production or lobar collapse due to bronchial obstruction, provided that the patient is young, otherwise fit, with a reasonable respiratory reserve and the disease is restricted to one lobe or lung.

In cases where the disease is multilobular but not extensive, careful assessment is required before considering operative intervention. The response to medical treatment, the age and general condition of the patient, the degree of respiratory reserve and the extent of upper respiratory tract involvement are important factors. Distorted but not obviously bronchiectatic segments may become frankly diseased after resection of other areas. Bilateral disease is not an absolute contraindication to resection, provided selective segmental resection leaves adequate functioning lung. Occasionally it may be justified to remove a badly damaged lobe even in the presence of significant disease elsewhere. Saccular bronchiectasis with lobar collapse responds better than cylindrical disease with compensatory emphysema.

Careful pre-operative preparation is essential, including sputum checks for tuberculosis, a full otolaryngological assessment and intensive physiotherapy, postural drainage and antibiotic therapy leading up to resection. Operative mortality is low (1%) as good pain relief, minitracheostomy and intensive physiotherapy have dramatically improved post-operative care. Cough and sputum production persist in up to 40% of cases but is usually less severe. Several factors may be responsible including: (1) failure to remove all the diseased areas; (2) post-operative collapse with fresh damage; (3) associated bronchitis and emphysema; and (4) re-infection from chronic sinusitis.

The place of resection requires careful evaluation. Results in children suggest 50–75% are cured or improved but 10–40% later develop bronchitis. A comparison of medical and surgical treatment over 16–25 years showed that one-third of each group were symptom free with a few deaths from severe disease in the medical group. Resection undoubtedly benefits selected cases but the criteria for referral have become increasingly stringent with improvements in medical control.

Section 50.2 • Lung abscess

Any process which causes lung suppuration may produce an abscess although the definition is usually restricted to necrotic cavitating lesions caused by pyogenic organisms, excluding tuberculosis, fungal infections and cavitating tumours. Following the introduction of antibiotics the incidence has fallen but a chronic abscess causing emaciation, cerebral sepsis or amyloidosis may still be encountered in developing countries. Suppuration and necrosis develop and spread circumferentially destroying most tissue, including blood vessels, which lie in its path. An abscess may rupture into a bronchus with the expectoration of pus, or into the pleura causing an empyema which may be associated with a persistent bronchopleural fistula. With treatment most abscesses heal leaving a fibrotic scar. Some debilitating abscess may be multilocular, spreading across interlobar fissures.

The mode of infection varies considerably, the chief causes being:

- **Aspiration** of infected material from the oropharynx or nasal cavity.
- **Bronchial obstruction** to a major bronchus by tumour; foreign body or glands predisposing to distal suppuration.
- **Suppurative pneumonias**, particularly staphylococcal, klebsiella and pseudomonas infections.
- **Infected infarcts** either resulting from septic emboli or due to secondary infection of a pulmonary infarct.
- **Transdiaphragmatic spread** from hepatic or subphrenic sepsis.
- **Lung cysts or bullae** which become secondarily infected.

Aspiration

Aspiration used to be the commonest cause but now bronchial obstruction due to carcinoma predominates (Figure 50.8). For aspiration to produce an abscess three conditions predispose to impairment of defence mechanisms:

- depression of the cough or gag reflexes by drugs, anaesthesia, alcohol, epileptic fits or electroconvulsive therapy
- disruption of the action of the ciliated epithelium and mucous blanket by smoking or anaesthetics
- ineffective coughing following thoracic or abdominal surgery or due to general debility.

The source of infected material is usually the mouth;

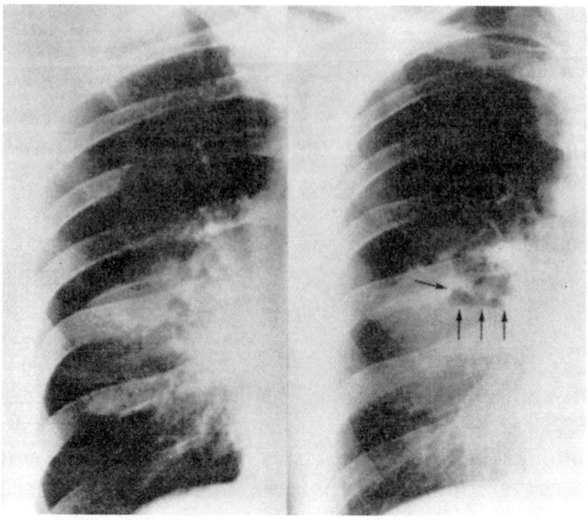

Figure 50.8 Aspiration lung abscess in the apical segment of the right lower lobe.

80% have dental sepsis causing pyorrhoea or tartar masses. Tonsillectomy and dental extraction were formerly responsible for 25% of cases but improved techniques have reduced their importance.

Bronchial obstruction

Obstruction of a major bronchus by tumour, foreign body or glandular enlargement, unless relieved quickly, invariably leads to segmental or lobar suppuration. The symptoms, signs and radiographic appearances suggest an unresolving pneumonia. Bronchoscopy will indicate the nature of the obstruction and will permit removal of a foreign body. It may be difficult to distinguish between a cavitating tumour and a proximal neoplasm with a distal abscess but, if feasible, both should be resected.

Suppurative pneumonias

Lung abscesses most frequently complicate staphylococcal or *Klebsiella* infections although any pneumonia may cause suppuration given suitable conditions.

The incidence of staphylococcal lung abscesses is highest at the extremes of life. In the elderly they usually occur as part of a staphylococcal bronchopneumonia, often a mixed infection with *Haemophilus influenzae*. The mortality is high. There are multiple small peribronchial abscesses from which the inflammation rapidly spreads causing considerable lung destruction. If the process is arrested there may be extensive residual fibrosis.

Children tend to develop a staphylococcal lobar pneumonia which is less severe than the bronchopneumonia of the elderly. Abscesses form and during coughing and crying they may become inflated through a check-valve mechanism producing tension pneumatoceles (Figure 50.9). These may: (a) compress the lung causing respiratory embarrassment, or (b) rupture into the pleural space forming a pyopneumothorax. The former usually respond to conservative measures; open procedures are rarely indicated. Effective antibiotics are needed.

Suppurative *Klebsiella* pneumonia occurs in patients over the age of 40 years, and is common in alcoholics and diabetics and those with chronic obstructive pulmonary disease (COPD). It usually affects the right upper lobe producing extensive oedema, destruction and multiple abscess formation. Chest X-ray shows typical cavitating pneumonia with expansion of the consolidated lobe.

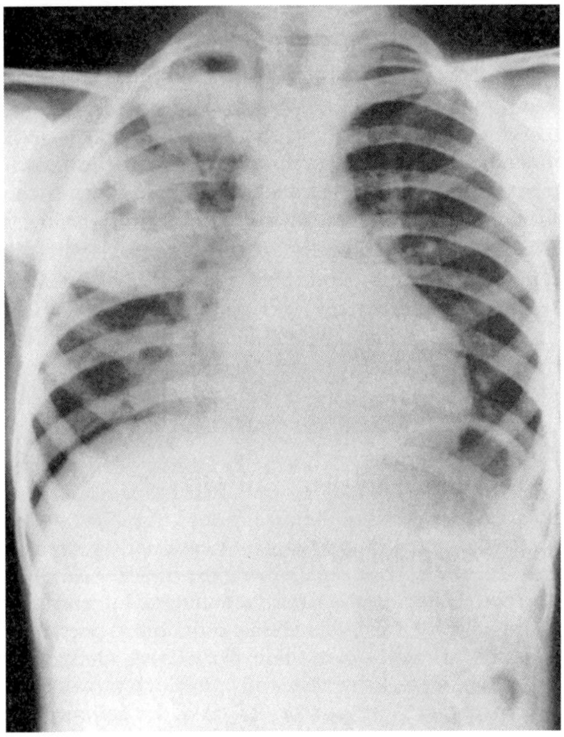

Figure 50.9 Multiple staphylococcal abscesses of the right lung in a child.

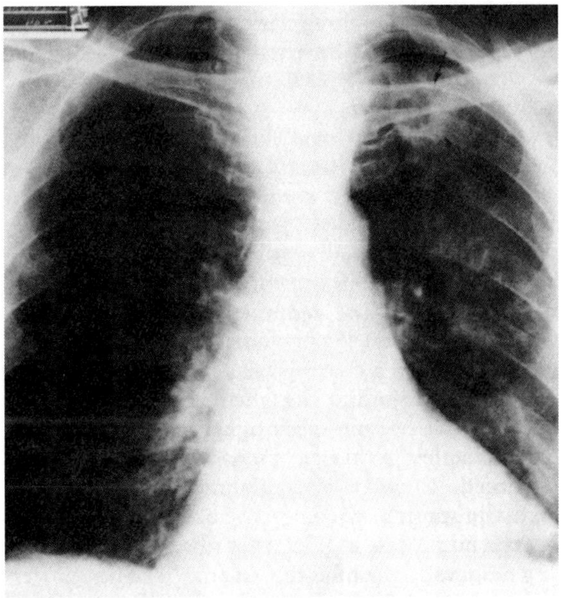

Figure 50.10 Abscess in the left upper lobe resulting from an infected cavitating pulmonary infarct.

Infected infarcts

Septic emboli most frequently arise from an infected venous cannula and less commonly from thrombophlebitis of the pelvis or lower limb veins or infective endocarditis involving the right side of the heart or a ductus arteriosus. The result is usually numerous small bilateral peripheral abscesses but occasionally a larger artery is involved with segmental suppuration (Figure 50.10).

Transdiaphragmatic spread

A subphrenic abscess invariably produces fixation and elevation of the hemidiaphragm with basal atelectasis and a 'sympathetic' pleural effusion. Infection may spread to the effusion (empyema) or the lung (suppurative pneumonia) or the abscess may rupture through the diaphragm into the lower lobe with expectoration of pus. Initial treatment is directed towards the subphrenic infection, but an empyema will need draining and the lung abscess may require resection.

When amoebiasis affects the right lobe of the liver inflammation may spread through the diaphragm often producing pleural adhesions which may prevent the formation of an effusion or empyema. The right lower lobe may become infected by direct spread or by the transdiaphragmatic rupture of a hepatic abscess. The resultant lung abscess eventually ruptures into a bronchus with the expectoration of a thick reddish-brown liquid ('anchovy' or 'chocolate' sauce). A fistula may connect the biliary and pulmonary systems with the expectoration of bile. The amoebiasis should be treated medically [see Module 5, Vol. I] before any hepatic or pulmonary surgery is undertaken.

Lung cysts or bullae

Infected bullae or cysts may resemble a lung abscess radiologically and present diagnostic difficulties. The patient is usually less severely ill although the radiological appearances are slower to resolve due to poorer drainage. The bulla may resolve as the inflammatory process obstructs the bronchiolar connection. Resection is rarely indicated.

Clinical picture

The initial symptoms, fever, rigor and malaise, are non-specific and may be modified by antibiotic therapy. Later, cough, haemoptysis, deep-seated pain and pleurisy may develop. Intrabronchial rupture is followed by the expectoration of large quantities of foul-smelling pus. When a lung abscess follows oral, otolaryngeal or abdominal surgery there has usually been a stormy post-operative period with respiratory symptoms beginning within a few days of the operation. There may be a history of excessive alcohol ingestion or altered conscious level or vomiting. There may be a recent history of a choking event.

Examination of the chest may be normal and any findings will be non-specific. The patient is usually quite toxic, with evidence of sepsis. Investigations show neutrophil leucocytosis. Sputum culture may show mixed organisms including anaerobes. Blood cultures may be positive.

The chest X-ray early in the disease process often suggests a segmental or lobar pneumonia, but later a fluid level usually develops within the opacity. The abscess cavity may have an irregular outline with variable surrounding infiltration and no fluid levels.

CT scanning may show evidence of consolidation with or without empyema, cavitation or occaisionally there may be an underlying tumour.

Bronchoscopy may be helpful to exclude bronchial obstruction due to tumour, foreign bodies or glands, or to clear secretions from the bronchial tree.

Treatment

The majority of aspiration lung abscesses respond to postural drainage, physiotherapy and large doses of intra-muscular benzylpenicillin but antibiotic treatment may have to be modified in the light of the organisms isolated and their sensitivities. Anaerobes are commonly present; metronidazole is valuable in lung abscess. Antibiotics should be tailored to culture and sensitivity advice. Broad spectrum antibiotics are usually indicated. Healing usually occurs leaving a fibrous scar although treatment may need to be continued for 2–3 months. Very occasionally surgical drainage may be required in severely ill patients failing to respond to medical treatment. A chronic cavity or a fibrotic lobe may need to be resected and if there is any doubt about a possible underlying neoplasm, exploratory thoracotomy should be undertaken.

Improved dental hygiene, post-operative treatment of respiratory infections, advances in oral and otolaryngeal surgery, better anaesthesia and improved post-operative care have all contributed to the falling incidence.

Rare complications of lung abscesses – severe haemoptysis, cerebral abscess, cachexia, weight loss and amyloid – are not seen in Western countries.

Section 50.3 • Pulmonary hydatid disease

Of the hydatid onchospheres (embryos) which gain entry to the portal circulation [see Module 5, Vol. I] about 25% pass through the liver to lodge in the pulmonary circulation. These onchospheres develop into classic hydatid cysts with an outer laminated ectocyst and inner germinal layer from which the primitive adult worms are formed. Apart from a thin rim of fibrous tissue (pericyst or adventitia) little host response is provoked.

The lower lobes are most frequently involved (55%) and in 20% the pulmonary lesions are bilateral. Some reports have suggested concomitant liver involvement in up to 70% of cases. The pulmonary hydatid cysts are usually round or oval but may be indented by any rigid structure they encounter during their slow growth. Occasionally the cyst fills a hemithorax. The cysts appear as white, pearly-grey patches just beneath the pleural surface.

Clinical features

Pulmonary hydatid cysts are often symptomless, presenting on routine chest radiography. Pleural pain and cough are the commonest symptoms although compression may produce dyspnoea or dysphagia. Occasionally severe dyspnoea occurs with a small cyst, but the mechanism is uncertain. Haemoptysis usually precedes intrabronchial rupture when clear salty fluid, containing portions of membrane or pearly cysts, is expectorated. Occasionally a large fragment of the cyst wall can block a main bronchus causing acute respiratory distress. Intrapleural rupture is accompanied by severe pleuritic pain. Allergic reactions (itch, urticaria and wheeze) often precede while anaphylactic shock may follow either bronchial or pleural rupture. A lung abscess invariably follows intrabronchial rupture with continuing cough and sputum production. Hepatic or diaphragmatic pain with associated hepatic tenderness and fever may precede transdiaphragmatic rupture or spread of infection from a liver cyst.

A dense, round or oval, clearly demarcated shadow, which if small may resemble a neoplasm or if large fill the hemithorax, is the commonest radiological finding (Figure 50.11); when multiple and small they may resemble cannonballs. A small leak prior to rupture may produce an 'air halo' between the cyst wall and pericyst (adventitia). Following intrabronchial rupture with partial expectoration, the redundant laminated layer may curl up and float on the surface of the fluid (the 'water-lily' sign). Rarely a cyst calcifies (Figure 50.12). An abscess with surrounding lung collapse or consolidation usually follows rupture although occasionally resolution occurs. Diaphragmatic paralysis or a pleural effusion may precede or follow intrapleural rupture or transdiaphragmatic spread. CT scanning of the thorax shows sharply delineated cysts with multiple daughter cysts within; less distinct masses with a necrotic centre and calcification may be seen.

In endemic areas, a dense cyst on chest radiography is highly suggestive while the 'air halo' and 'water-lily' signs are diagnostic. If clear, salty fluid is expectorated it should be examined for parts of the laminated layer, brood capsules and small worms. Details of the Casoni, complement fixation and the newer immunological tests are given in [see Module 5, Vol. I]

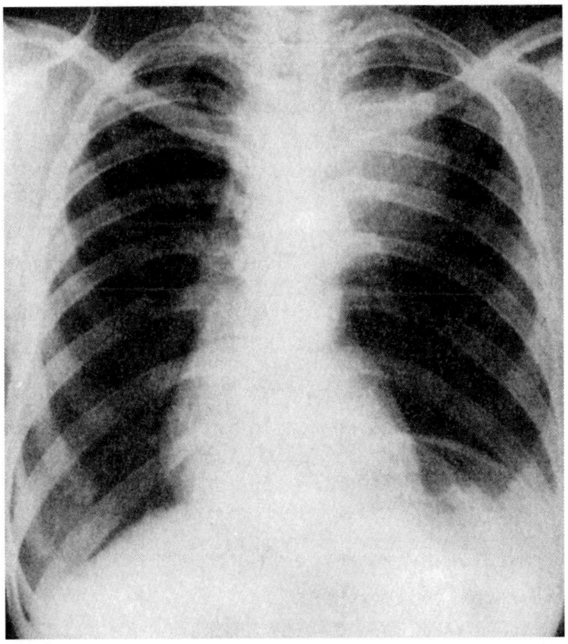

Figure 50.11 Hydatid cyst in the left upper lobe. The shadow is homogeneous and presents a clear-cut outline. (Courtesy of Paul Grech.)

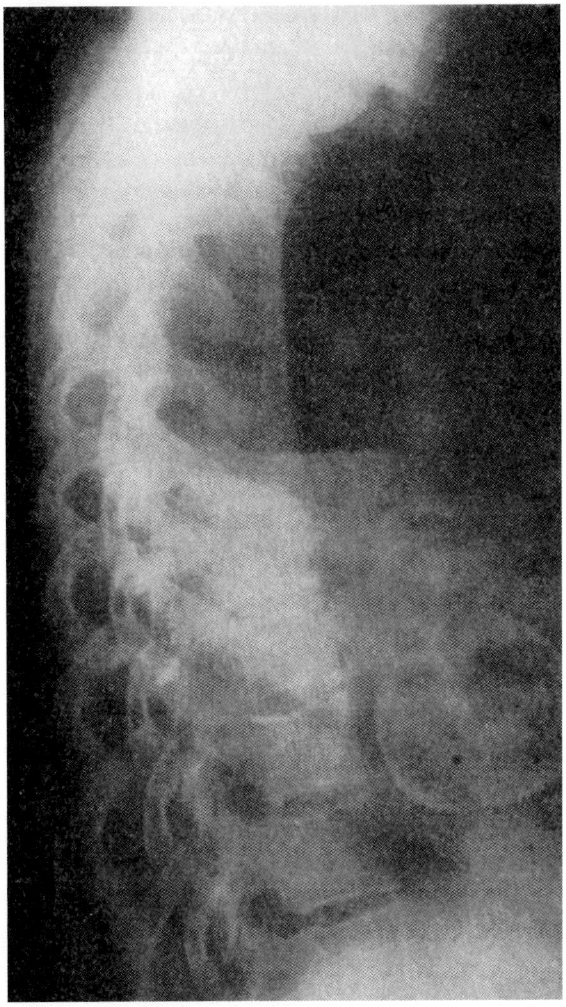

Figure 50.12 Left lateral chest film showing two calcified hydatid cysts in the left lung. There is also a fluid level posteriorly indicating secondary infection in one of the cysts. (Courtesy of Paul Grech.)

Diagnosis

A history of travel to or living in an endemic area with radiological evidence is suggestive of hydatid disease. An ultrasound scan of the liver is best for identifying liver cysts. Complementation test and the Casoni test are sensitive in 60–90% of cases. Eosinophilia is found in 30% of cases.

Treatment

Initially treatment is with albendazole and mebendazole [see Module 5, Vol. I]. Surgery is advisable if there is no response to medical therapy as rupture may cause anaphylaxis, dissemination or chronic pulmonary sepsis. Where possible the cyst should be removed intact. Three procedures are available: (1) resection of the cyst after careful aspiration of a little fluid and instillation of either 20% sodium chloride, 10% formalin or 0.5% silver nitrate to kill the parasite; (2) following exposure of the superficial wall the proximal intrabronchial pressure is raised sufficiently to extrude the cyst *in toto*; or (3) lobectomy for a ruptured cyst with secondary infection. An empyema or a trans-diaphragmatic fistula may require excision.

Section 50.4 • Pulmonary tuberculosis

Pulmonary tuberculosis must be considered in its world context where it remains a major problem with a high mortality. Effective chemotherapy, BCG vaccination and environmental improvements have drastically reduced the incidence in Western countries. However, inadequate treatment has produced strains of *Mycobacterium tuberculosis* resistant to some of the first-line drugs in several developing countries. The incidence in children and adolescents has reached low levels in the Western world in contrast to the situation in developing countries. A major source of new cases in Europe is the breakdown of quiescent primary foci or healed lesions inadequately treated in the past in patients whose immune response has decreased either as a result of the ageing process or because they have developed a debilitating disease, e.g. diabetes, chronic alcoholism. The speed of modern travel, the increased mobility of the population and long incubation period mean that immigrants (or tourists) contracting the disease in endemic areas may present many months later in their new environment, the second major source of new cases in Britain.

Epidemics of pulmonary tuberculosis are occurring in areas with a sizeable population of patients with the acquired immunodeficiency syndrome (AIDS). In this group the presentation and radiographic appearances of pulmonary tuberculosis are often atypical with a consequent delay in diagnosis. This now presents a significant epidemiological problem and vigilance is essential in this situation.

Pulmonary tuberculosis usually results from airborne spread of human *M. tuberculosis* from open cases of the disease. The initial reaction, the primary complex, may heal with calcification, lead on to the various forms of post-primary pulmonary disease, or involve other organs by haematogenous spread.

The primary complex consists of a localized area of pneumonitis, and regional gland involvement may follow inhalation of mycobacteria. Any part of the lung may be involved although the upper lobes are preferred in adults. After the initial acute reaction the bacilli are engulfed by alveolar macrophages. There is early spread to the lymph nodes where most bacilli are arrested, only a few gaining entry to the general circulation. After 3–8 weeks the patient develops hypersensitivity to the tubercular protein, the tuberculin test becomes positive and the macrophages release their contained bacilli. Classical granulomatous lesions develop containing epithelial cells, Langhans' giant cells, lymphocytes and fibroblasts with caseation (cheesy necrosis which results from hypersensitivity to the tubercular protein). The reaction usually subsides over several months with fibrosis and calcification, but the scar may continue to contain viable organisms capable of reactivation under suitable conditions. Most primary infections are asymptomatic or associated with a mild respiratory illness. Occasionally malaise, weight loss, fever, erythema nodosum or phlyctenular conjunctivitis may occur. The radiological appearances are variable; the pneumonitis may predominate with little glandular involvement but in children and African–Asians the glandular component often overshadows any lung lesion (Figure 50.13).

Lobar collapse or occasionally obstructive emphysema may result from pressure by the enlarged hilar nodes while localized tuberculous endobronchitis, in the vicinity of a node, may lead to bronchial stenosis. The intrabronchial rupture of a gland with aspiration of tuberculous material may result in an acute exudative lesion (epituberculosis) which is the result of either a hypersensitivity reaction to the tubercular protein or less commonly a caseous pneumonia. These complications may be symptomless although cough and wheeze are commonly found. Chemotherapy, corticosteroids and postural drainage usually produce slow resolution and bronchoscopy is rarely indicated. Thoracotomy may be necessary to relieve obstructive emphysema or stridor and if the damage has caused bronchiectasis surgical resection may be required at a later date (Figure 50.14).

A change in the tuberculin status from negative to positive while under observation is diagnostic of primary tuberculosis. With an extensive primary lesion, tubercle bacilli may be identified on smears or cultures of sputum or gastric washing but this is unusual.

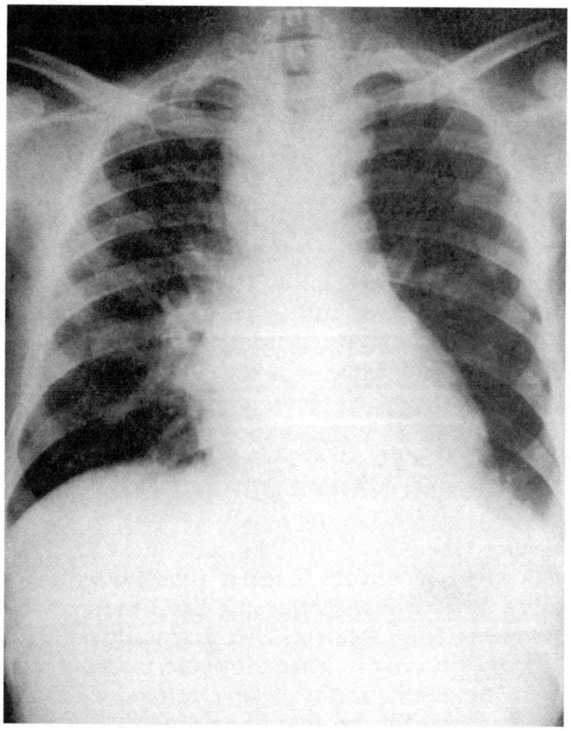

Figure 50.13 Mediastinal glandular involvement and a small left-sided basal effusion due to primary tuberculosis in a 20-year-old African. Note that there is little radiological evidence of parenchymal involvement.

When hilar or paratracheal glandular enlargement predominates, whether unilateral or bilateral, gland biopsy may be necessary to exclude a lymphoma. Mediastinoscopy may be helpful, otherwise left anterior mediastinotomy or thoracoscopy should be considered.

Infants and young children developing a primary lesion or who react strongly to a tuberculin test should be prescribed prophylactic antituberculous chemotherapy to prevent progression to the potentially lethal miliary or meningeal forms of the disease.

Occasionally the primary lesion merges into post-primary pulmonary tuberculosis. More commonly, haematogenous spread leads to: (1) miliary tuberculous with widespread organ involvement; (2) pleural involvement producing an effusion; (3) the apical lesions of classic post-primary tuberculosis; or (4) focal infection of other organs, e.g. bones or kidney, which may present as active disease only after the lapse of several years.

Post-primary pulmonary tuberculosis is the most important source of continuing infection in any community. It may arise from direct extension of a primary lesion, reactivation of a healed primary lesion, or haematogenous spread to the apices from a primary lesion (commonest cause). In an active case the following pathological stages are occurring side by side: **pre-exudative** with vasodilatation, interstitial oedema and swollen macrophages; **exudative** with varying degrees of oedema, fibrinous exudation, histiocytic, lymphocytic and leucocytic infiltration; **caseation** where necrosis occurs with the formation of a cheesy debris; **productive** when epithelioid, histiocytic and Langhans' giant cells encircle a caseous area and early fibrotic containment begins; **fibrotic** during which fibrosis, often commencing peripherally, invades the tubercles; and **cavitating** when liquefaction and expectoration of caseous material leads to cavity formation; the walls of the cavities are lined by soft, caseous material.

Clincal picture

There are no specific clinical features, the presentation depending on the nature and extent of the disease. Mild debility may pass unnoticed, the patient being picked up on routine radiography. The insidious progression of malaise, anorexia and weight loss over several months suggests tuberculosis. The development

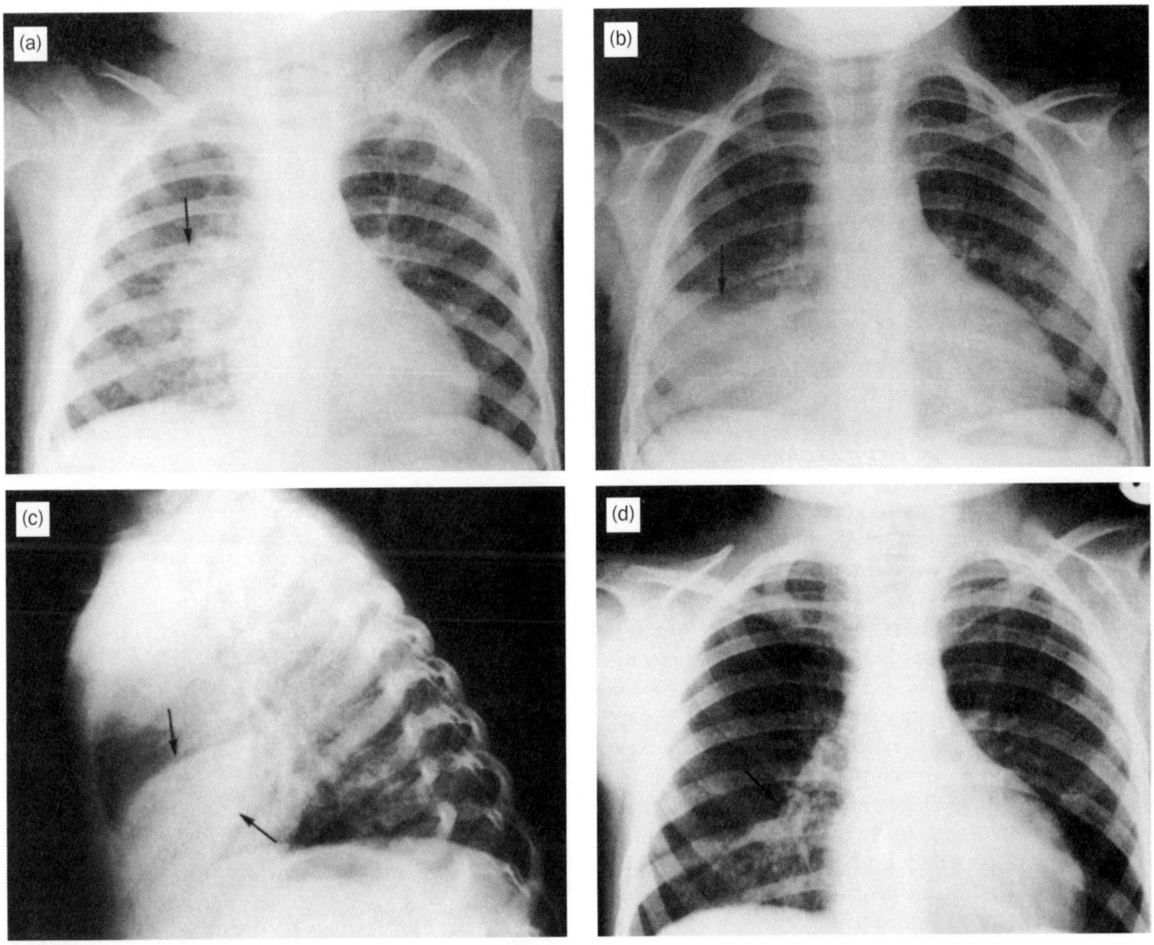

Figure 50.14 (a) Primary pulmonary tuberculosis with glandular involvement in a child aged 3 years. (b) Three months later: poor response to treatment resulting in progression of the disease with middle lobe collapse/consolidation. (c) Lateral view of the collapse/consolidation. (d) One year after (b) and (c) following successful chemotherapy: there is considerable improvement but increased striation is visible in the right lower zone suggesting early bronchiectatic change.

or worsening of a cough, which does not respond quickly to antibiotics warrants a chest X-ray. The sputum may be mucoid, purulent or bloodstained and occasionally severe haemoptysis follows involvement of a major vessel. Nagging chest pain is common. In advanced disease dyspnoea and wheeze may occur. Recurrent colds with intervening malaise or pneumonia which fails to respond to treatment are frequent presentations. The classic night sweats and fever are encountered often. Many patients complain of dyspepsia and a routine chest radiograph is always advisable in such cases.

The patient's general condition may be good in minimal disease but in the advanced stages they are pale, cachetic, flushed and pyrexial. The most characteristic signs are post-tussive crepitations at the apices, but these may be absent or replaced by the features of pneumonic consolidation. In chronic fibrocaseous disease the trachea and mediastinum may be drawn to the affected side.

The earliest radiological signs are usually unilateral or bilateral soft apical shadows which gradually extend and become confluent and which may cavitate. In fibrocaseous disease there are large thick-walled cavities with extensive fibrosis. Residual fibrosis may shrink the upper lobes with shift of the upper mediastinum and elevation of the hilar shadows (Figure 50.15–50.17).

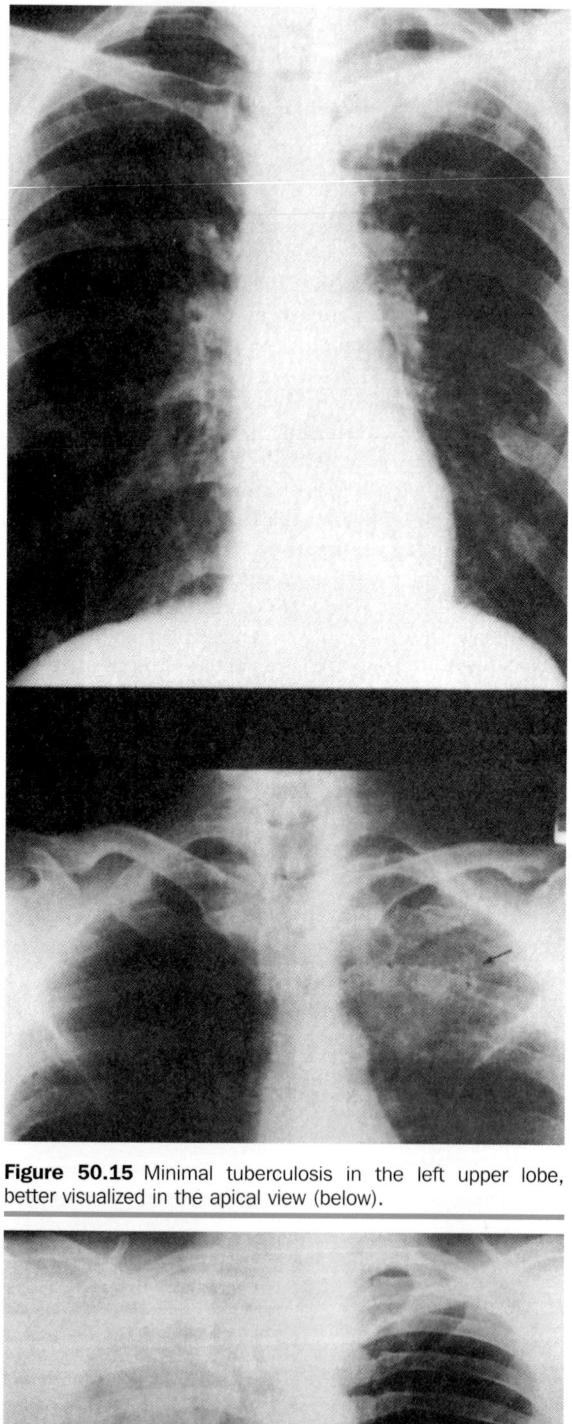

Figure 50.15 Minimal tuberculosis in the left upper lobe, better visualized in the apical view (below).

Diagnosis

The history, physical findings and radiological appearance often suggests the diagnosis which may be confirmed from direct smears or culture of sputum; today bronchoscopy with bronchial washings has a much higher sensitivity and is commonly used. The tuberculin test is usually strongly positive but may be negative in advanced disease or in patients with immunosuppression from whatever cause. A therapeutic trial of antituberculous chemotherapy may be justified on the clinical findings and tuberculin reaction in the absence of sputum confirmation.

The majority of cases respond well to antituberculous chemotherapy although considerable pulmonary fibrosis may still follow treatment. In Western countries sputum-positive cases are treated as outpatients. As treatment is commenced most patients soon cease to be infectious; most patients are no longer infectious within 2 weeks.

The scope for operative intervention varies considerably. In Western countries operation is restricted to cases with resistant organisms, persistent infection in a badly damaged lung. Segmental or lobar resections are preferred. Resections (including pneumonectomies) and thoracoplasties still have a place in developing countries in the treatment of progressive or persistent infections due to inadequate chemotherapy or resistant organism. Usually 3 months' chemotherapy should be given before any surgical intervention, to lessen the risks of dissemination or empyema, and continued for the appropriate time post-operatively.

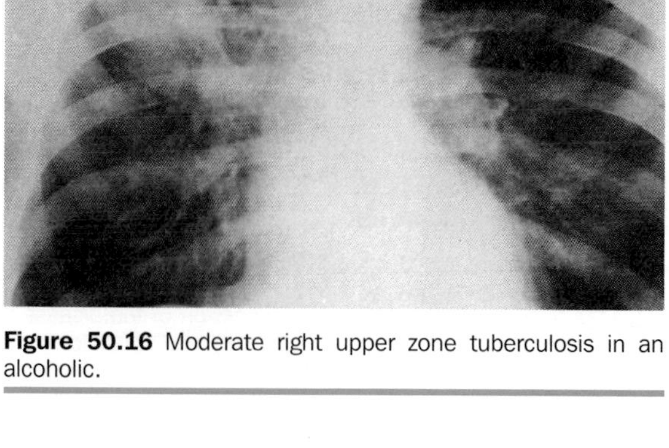

Figure 50.16 Moderate right upper zone tuberculosis in an alcoholic.

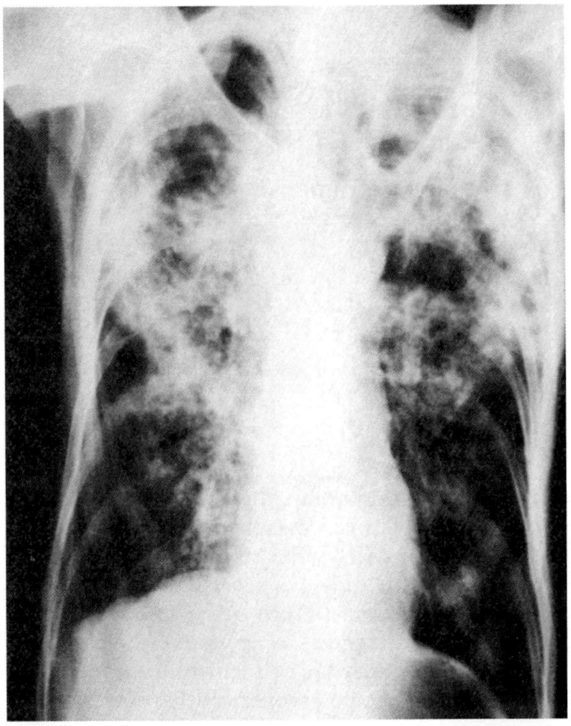

Figure 50.17 Advanced bilateral cavitating tuberculosis. The patient was an alcoholic and weighed 32 kg at the time of death.

A **tuberculoma** is a dense, slowly growing, peripheral tuberculous granuloma usually 1–3 cm in diameter which is often asymptomatic, being picked up on routine radiography. It must be differentiated from benign or malignant neoplasms. Radiologically its outline is poorly defined and its density variable. CT of the thorax may reveal calcification or small adjacent satellite lesions. The lesion may have been present in a radiograph taken months or years earlier. Therefore previous X-rays are of paramount importance. The tuberculin test is usually positive but may be negative. Tubercle bacilli are rarely obtained from sputum smear or culture. In a fit patient where the diagnosis is in doubt thoracotomy is indicated followed by a wedge or segmental resection of the tuberculoma. If operation is contraindicated the diagnosis may be established by percutaneous aspiration needle biopsy or antituberculous chemotherapy may be given and the response assessed.

Chest wall tuberculosis

A cold abscess or tuberculous sinus of the chest wall usually arises as a result of pus tracking from caseous lymph nodes in the anterior or posterior intercostal or mediastinal chains or from tuberculous osteitis of a vertebra. It may also follow reactivation of pulmonary disease previously treated with recurrent artificial pneumothoraces in the days before adequate chemotherapy was available and where pleural involvement had occurred. The ribs and cartilage may be infected as part of the spread. Response to chemotherapy is usually good and operation should be avoided if possible. Unfortunately inadvertant exploration of a chest wall swelling is not uncommon. If the disease is properly identified the antituberculous chemotherapy usually facilitates healing without consequence. Unfortunately if unrecognized it proceeds to scrofula and local tuberculous abscess of skin.

The late effects of pulmonary tuberculosis

Tuberculosis often leads to considerable fibrosis, destruction and bronchiectasis in a segment, lobe or lung and if this gives rise to persistent symptoms, resection should be considered provided the function of the remaining lung is satisfactory. Severe or recurrent haemoptysis from an area of 'dry' bronchiectasis or following the erosion of a broncholith may warrant resection. An aspergilloma resulting from fungal superinfection of a persistent cavity is best resected although residual lung function often prevents this. Pleural fibrosis or calcification may require decortication to allow full re-expansion (Figure 50.18). Patients are still encountered with a fixed, fibrotic, calcified hemithorax following previous artificial pneumothoraces although there is usually little that can be done to improve the situation. Thoracoplasty is compatible with normal life, particularly in non-smokers, although underlying bronchiectasis may aggravate any associated bronchitis. Rarely infection around a thoracoplasty or plumbage material may require further operative intervention.

Antituberculous chemotherapy

The introduction of effective drug regimens has revolutionized the management of tuberculosis. It is important that any regimen uses the combination of drugs which takes into account the resistance patterns of the local organisms, and modified in the light of the sensitivity tests when these become available. The initial regimens should include at least four drugs to which the organism is likely to be sensitive. Failure to adhere to these principles may lead to the emergence of resistant strains.

To be effective a regimen must be taken regularly and continued for sufficient time. Regular treatments should be either daily or intermittent regimens taken two to three times weekly. With the falling incidence of tuberculosis it is becoming increasingly difficult to persuade patients to continue treatment for sufficient time once the initial improvement has been achieved. Failure to take regular treatment for sufficient time may lead to relapse.

Directly observed therapy (DoT) can be used in non-compliant patients, and has been shown to be successful.

Several drugs have been developed possessing varying antituberculous activity.

First-line drugs

Bactericidal:

- isoniazid
- rifampicin
- streptomycin (in an alkaline pH)
- pyrazinamide (in an acid pH).

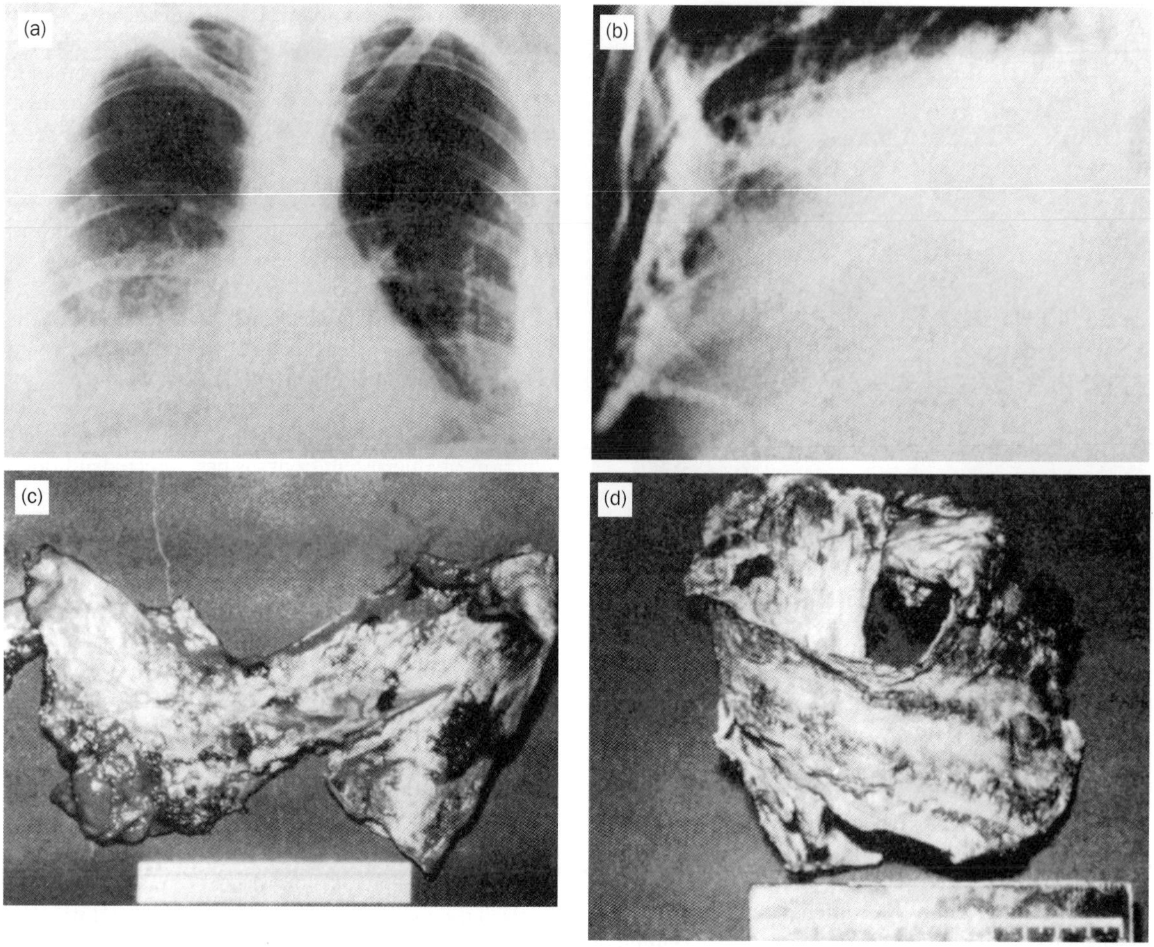

Figure 50.18 This 32-year-old male presented 10 years after a full course of antituberculous therapy for pulmonary tuberculosis. (a) PA chest film showing bilateral calcified pleural reactions. (b) Tomogram of the right lower zone showing extensive calcification. (c) Resected calcified pleura immediately after decortication. (d) Fixed specimen 24 hours later showing rib indentations.

Bacteriostatic:

- ethambutol
- thioacetazone.

Second-line drugs include ethionamide, prothionamide, capreomycin, ciprofloxacin, vibramycin and cycloserine.

First-line drugs are those in common usage while second-line drugs are reserved for resistant cases. In principle, bactericidal drugs (those which destroy the organism *in situ*) are preferred to bacteriostatic (those that interfere with the organism's reproduction allowing the body's defence mechanisms to deal with the infection).

In consequence various regimens (similar to that shown below) have been built around the combination of isoniazid and rifampicin daily for 6 months: rifampicin: 450 mg (under 50 kg) or 600 mg (over 50 kg) and isoniazid: 300 mg. Plus: pyrazinamide: 30 mg/kg to a maximum of 2 g daily and ethambutol: 15 mg/kg daily for the first 2 months. (It is advisable to give pyridoxine 10 mg daily with these regimens.)

In general, these regimens have few side-effects, are well tolerated giving 100% cure in 6 months and have become standard therapy in Western countries. A major disadvantage is their cost.

Ethambutol can cause retrobulbar neuritis (RBN) if used in high doses (>15 mg/kg) or for longer than 3 months. Visual acuity should be checked at the start of treatment. RBN usually recovers once the drug is stopped. As the drug is excreted by the kidney renal function should also be evaluated before initiating therapy.

Isoniazid can cause peripheral neuritis and hepatitis.

Rifampicin is an enzyme inducer and can interfere with the action of other drugs and cause liver function abnormalities. Discoloration of the urine occurs and the orange colour should be anticipated.

Pyrazinamide may cause arthralgia and hyperuricaemia.

The British Thoracic Society (BTS) recommend prior to initiation of therapy, liver function tests (LFTs), visual acuity test by Snellen chart and renal function tests if ethambutol and/or streptomycin are to be used. Further LFTs are to be checked after 3 weeks.

In many developing countries intermittent regimens using various combinations of isoniazid, streptomycin, rifampicin, ethambutol and thioacetazone have been introduced in an attempt to treat widespread disease within a limited budget. Such regimens have the advantage of administration two or three times weekly under supervision (DoT). Similar regimens may be used in the West to treat patients who have defaulted from previous follow-up or who are considered unreliable.

Section 50.5 • Pulmonary actinomycosis

The two bacteria *Actinomyces israelii* and *Nocardia asteroides* both cause actinomycosis, producing similar chronic respiratory infections. *Nocardia asteroides* accounts for only 10% of cases of pulmonary actinomycosis.

Actinomyces israelii lung infections usually result from the inhalation of infected material from the oropharynx but are occasionally due to the spread of actinomycosis from the abdomen or cervicofacial region. Nocardia gains entry by the inhalation of spores from the soil.

Pulmonary actinomycosis starts insidiously as a peripheral focus in a lower lobe. The advancing lesion crosses fascial planes to involve other lobes or extends to the pleura where it forms either an empyema or pleural adhesions with the subsequent invasion of the chest wall and the formation of chronic sinuses. The involved lung is densely fibrotic and honeycombed with small abscesses. Fever, toxaemia, malaise, weight loss, cough with bloodstained sputum and pleuritic pain develop and become progressively worse. Not only is tuberculosis mimicked but it may co-exist. Radiologically there are varying-sized cavitating pneumonic lesions, effusion or rib periostitis (Figure 50.19).

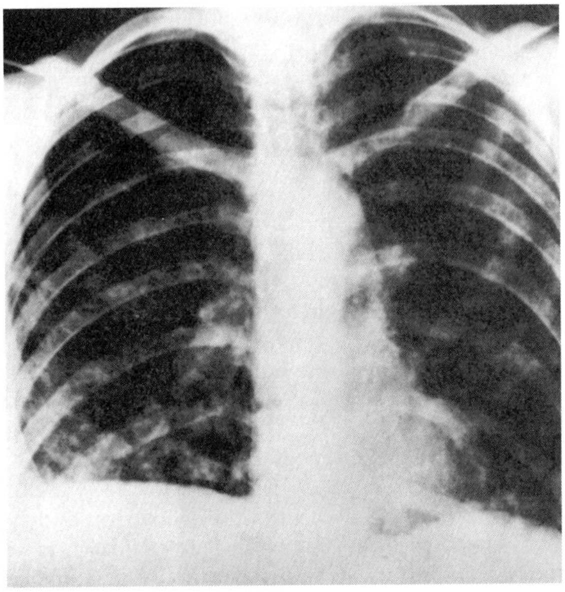

Figure 50.19 This 16-year-old male developed ileocaecal actinomycosis a few weeks after an appendicectomy. A month later he developed a cough and a chest film showed diffuse patchy consolidation throughout both lung fields. There is also a right pneumothorax. The more common radiological appearance of pulmonary actinomycosis is massive consolidation. (Courtesy of Paul Grech.)

Actinomyces israelii infections may be diagnosed by the presence of sulfur granules in either the sputum or pus from a sinus, or the organism may be cultured using anaerobic or micro-aerophilic techniques. *Nocardia asteroides* has to be grown using aerobic cultures.

High doses of penicillin for several months cure *A. israelii* infections. *Nocardia asteroides* usually responds to high dose sulfonamides or trimethoprim-sulfamethoxazole combinations. Failing this, imipenem, minocycline, amikacin or one of the third-generation cephalosporins may be tried. Sensitivity tests are important. It may be necessary to drain an empyema or resect damaged lungs after the completion of medical treatment.

Section 50.6 • Pulmonary fungal disease

Recent therapeutic changes have increased the importance of the respiratory fungal diseases while improved investigative techniques have advanced our understanding of them. The introduction of new drugs has had two effects: prolonged usage of broad spectrum antibiotics affects the bacterial flora of the respiratory tract allowing colonization by fungi which may later invade the lung parenchyma with subsequent widespread dissemination; and corticosteroids and cancer chemotherapy impair both cellular and humoral immunity permitting growth of organisms normally rejected.

Suppression of the immune response, either induced intentionally in order to prevent tissue rejection following organ transplantation or occurring as part of AIDS, has been a further factor in the increasing incidence of fungal infections of the lung.

Only a few fungi cause respiratory disease in humans. The majority are inhaled as spores from their natural habitat: the soil. Some being ubiquitous are found world-wide, e.g. *Aspergillus*, others require specialized soil conditions, e.g. *Coccidioides*, while others prefer soil rich in bird or bat excreta, e.g. *Histoplasmosis*. *Candida* lives symbiotically with man, requiring altered immunity before producing disease. Person-to-person spread is rare.

The resultant infection may be:

- **Opportunistic,** where impaired defence mechanisms or lung fibrosis permit the growth of otherwise harmless organisms. Such infections occur world-wide, e.g. moniliasis.
- **Parasitic,** where the fungus invades normal lung tissue usually producing a subclinical primary infection which occasionally progresses to chronic disease, e.g. coccidiodomycosis. Most of these fungi are endemic in specific regions but the speed of modern travel means they may present anywhere. These organisms are highly infectious and present problems to laboratory workers handling specimens.

The nature of the lesions produced by fungi varies from necrosis and fibrosis resembling fibrocaseous tuberculosis, e.g. coccidioidomycosis, through bronchitis and pneumonia, e.g. moniliasis, to the allergic manifestations of aspergillosis.

The diagnosis may be difficult, particularly in opportunistic infections where, with the exception of an aspergilloma, there are no distinctive clinical or radiological features, and is usually based on exclusion in the presence of repeated heavy cultures of the fungus. Post-mortem diagnoses require special histological staining. Most of the parasitic fungi have a specific delayed skin test although in acute cases it may be necessary to make the diagnosis from smears, cultures or animal inoculations.

In opportunistic infections antibiotic, steroid or cytotoxic therapy should be modified to allow recovery of the host's defence mechanisms. Amphotericin B is a good broad spectrum antifungal agent for inhalation or intravenous use but side-effects (nephrotoxicity) limit its usefulness. Less toxic drugs, 5-fluorocytosine and the imidazoles (itraconazole and miconazole) are now the drugs of choice. With limited disease or for residual lung fibrosis surgical resection may be indicated.

The incidence of each disease varies considerably. In endemic areas, the parasitic fungi may infect 80–90% of the population, e.g. coccidioides, of which 20–25% have mild symptoms but only 0.1–0.2% progress to serious disease.

At present it is not possible to produce a complete classification of the respiratory fungal infections but Table 50.1 serves as a framework for discussion.

Moniliasis (candidiasis)

Although oropharyngeal and laryngeal candidiasis are fairly common, bronchopulmonary involvement is unusual even in chronically debilitated patients or those receiving long-term antibiotics, high-dose steroids or cytotoxic therapy. *Candida albicans* is usually responsible although other species may be involved. Three types of pulmonary moniliasis have been described.

- **Monilial bronchitis** occurs in infancy, fibrocystic lung disease or debilitated elderly patients. The bronchial walls are studded with greyish-yellow plaques containing fibrin, hyphae and spores. Clinically there is an irritating cough productive of scanty 'milky' sputum with basal striations or normal appearances on radiography. Diagnosis depends on repeated culture of the fungus from the sputum.
- **Monilial pneumonia.** Rarely a necrotic pneumonia develops in severely debilitated patients giving patchy ill-defined shadows radiologically. The patient has a fever with tachycardia, dyspnoea and a cough productive of bloodstained sputum. The fungus is repeatedly obtained on sputum cultures.
- **Generalized moniliasis.** Occasionally following aggressive antibiotic, steroid or cytotoxic therapy, particularly in the presence of an indwelling venous cannula, a severe generalized candidal infection develops. Monilial pyaemia occurs with septic infarcts and abscesses developing in many organs including the lungs. The prognosis is poor, the diagnosis often being made at post-mortem.

Cryptococcosis (torulosis)

Cryptococcus neoformans is a yeast found world-wide. It has a diameter of 4–8 μm and has a capsule. While most infections occur in patients suffering from chronic diseases, e.g. diabetes, alcoholism, occasionally healthy subjects are infected. The inhaled fungus sets up a symptomless subpleural focus with hilar gland enlargement (resembling primary tuberculosis) which is often self-limiting with complete resolution. The lesion may:

- form a localized granuloma in immunocompetent patients, with a well-defined fibrous capsule and central caseation. This is usually symptomless, being mistaken for a neoplasm on routine radiography; or
- spread by progressive infiltration to produce cavitating consolidation. If the pleura is involved an empyema may develop. The clinical picture resembles tuberculosis with malaise, cough, sputum, chest pain and soft cavitating opacities on radiography.

Haematogenous spread can occur at any stage, especially in immunosuppressed patients: those with the human immunodeficiency virus (HIV), Hodgkin's disease and organ transplant recipients. They may develop a chronic meningitis (resembling tuberculous meningitis) or lesions in other organs. The meningitis is often the presenting feature and in any case of pulmonary cryptococcosis lumbar puncture is essential before commencing treatment.

Special stains are required to identify the organism in smears of sputum or cerebrospinal fluid (CSF). Latex agglutination test is positive in 95% of cases. CSF shows mononuclear cytosis. Sputum examination should be cautiously interpreted as there are many non-pathogenic organisms.

Table 50.1 Fungal infections of the respiratory tract

Organism	*Distribution*	*Infection*
Candida albicans	World-wide	Opportunistic
Cryptococcus neoformans	World-wide	Opportunistic
Aspergillus fumigatus (and other species)	World-wide	Opportunistic
Mucor (several species)	World-wide	Opportunistic
Coccidiodes immitis	South-western USA	Parasitic
Histoplasma capsulatum	World-wide (rare in Britain)	Parasitic
Blastomyces dermatitis	Eastern USA, Africa	Parasitic
Paracoccidioides brasiliensis	South and Central America	Parasitic
Sporotrichum schenckii	South Africa, France, USA	Parasitic

Fluconazole is standard therapy along with intravenous amphoteracin. Flucytocine can be used with other drugs for 6 weeks. Fluconazole can be tried in progressive lung lesions as an alternative to or in combination with intravenous amphotericin B.

Aspergillosis

The inhalation of spores of *Aspergillus fumigatus*, which reach their peak in the damp winter months, is the usual cause of aspergillosis but other species may be involved. *Aspergillus fumigatus* is a common laboratory contaminant and several sputum cultures may be necessary to confirm the diagnosis. Immediate and delayed skin tests and serum precipitins can be useful in distinguishing between the different disease entities. The clinical, radiological, immunological and mycological findings are all important when diagnosing aspergillosis. Several disease entities are encountered.

Hypersensitivity reactions

Allergic bronchopulmonary aspergillosis

This may take the form of acute type I allergic asthma following exposure to large concentrations of spores when the immediate skin test is usually strongly positive. The principal features are recurrent asthmatic attacks associated with malaise, cough productive of bronchial casts, sputum and blood eosinophilia, and fleeting shadows more common in the upper lobe at radiography (Figure 50.20). Permanent proximal bronchial damage (bronchiectasis) occurs at the site of the impaction of the casts. The immediate and delayed skin tests are positive in 40% and precipitins in 10%. The natural history of the disease is remission and exacerbation. The diagnosis is confirmed by skin test, high IgE and increased specific antibody to aspergillus. Long-term corticosteroids may be required to control the symptoms. Antifungal agents have little place in therapy.

Aspergilloma

Any chronic cavity, e.g. tuberculous, may become secondarily infected with *A. fumigatus* which grows on necrotic debris to form a mycelial mass. There is little surrounding reaction, the mass gradually filling and distending the cavity. There is usually a small crescentic halo of air above the mass, best seen on tomography (Figure 50.21). Cough, intermittent haemoptysis and expectoration of brown sputum containing the fungus is the usual presentation. The haemoptysis is occasionally severe. Systemic upset, fever, malaise and weight loss may occur. The fungus can be grown from the sputum and precipitin tests are invariably strongly positive. Although resection is desirable when the disease is symptomatic, this is uncommon and the symptomless patient should be observed. Furthermore, the disease which produced the cavity has often compromised lung function making operation impracticable.

Invasive pulmonary aspergillosis

Diffuse pneumonic shadowing or lobar consolidation develops invariably in immunosuppressed and myelosupressed subjects. The infection may be fulminating with rapid haematogenous spread to many organs and generalized toxaemia. Alternatively, there may be a good tissue response with the formation of multiple small abscesses when cough, sputum, malaise and fever

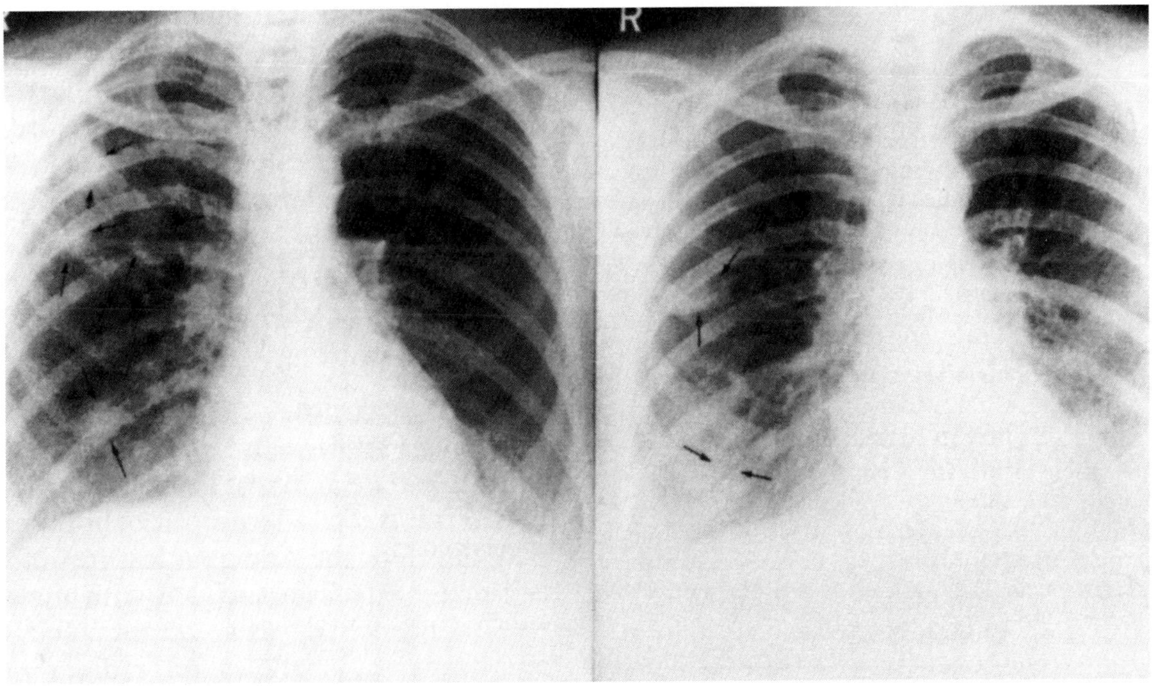

Figure 50.20 Chest films of the same patient demonstrating the changing pattern of pulmonary infiltrates in bronchopulmonary aspergillosis.

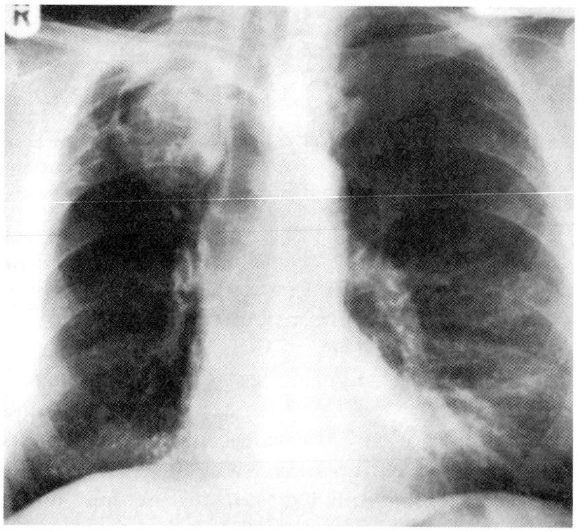

Figure 50.21 Chest film showing a large mass lying loose inside an old cavity in the right apex. The mass is outlined by air inside the cavity and it can be shown to move when the patient changes position. Diagnosis: aspergilloma.

predominate. The fungus may be cultured from sputum, bronchial washings obtained at bronchoscopy or material obtained from lung biopsy. Precipitating antibodies are often present and a rising titre is diagnostic. Intravenous amphotericin B is the treatment of choice. Alternatively itraconazole has proved effective in some trials. The resection of an infected lobe may be considered although the risk of developing a bronchopleural fistula is high.

Mucormycosis

Mucormycosis usually causes destructive skin lesions with involvement of the upper respiratory tract and meninges. Rhinocerebral disease occurs in patients with diabetic ketoacidosis and immunocompromised patients. Occasionally the lungs are involved, usually in drug addicts or following splenectomy for malignancy. Pneumonia or localized bronchial invasion followed by erosion into the pulmonary vessels may occur. Clinically there is cough, haemoptysis and pleurisy with ill-defined diffuse shadowing on radiography. The organism can be obtained from smears or culture of sputum. Prognosis is poor but intravenous and inhaled amphotericin B or surgical resection should be considered.

Coccidioidomycosis

Inhalation of the arthrospores of *Coccidioides immitis* produces a primary infection in up to 84% of the population in endemic areas, Argentina and south-western USA. Occasionally the primary lesions spread directly or break down later to give progressive lung disease.

Primary infection

Within 3 weeks the arthrospores release spherules which produce localized subpleural inflammation. This is usually asymptomatic resolving within 2 months to leave a small scar which may later calcify. Occasionally mild respiratory symptoms (pyrexia, cough with blood-stained sputum, pleurisy, malaise and headache), the so-called Valley fever or Desert rheumatism, may develop and rarely erythema nodosum or erythema multiforme occurs. Scattered soft shadows with hilar adenopathy are seen radiologically. A single dense lesion resembling a tumour or tuberculum may persist requiring resection for diagnosis.

Progressive pulmonary coccidioidomycosis

This may be acute or chronic with an overall mortality of 60% within 2 years. The **acute** form is associated with rapid intrapulmonary dissemination causing acute bronchopneumonia, necrosis and oedema. The systemic effects predominate with anorexia, weight loss, fever, malaise and the signs of a bronchopneumonia. There are diffuse patchy or confluent shadows radiologically. Should healing occur it produces extensive fibrosis, bronchiectasis and cavity formation. Haematogenous spread, particularly in infants or the elderly, produces miliary foci (resembling tuberculosis) in many organs and is usually rapidly fatal.

More frequently a **chronic** infection occurs with the formation of granulomas, which are surrounded by fibrous walls and contain a mass of caseating material. Satellite lesions are common. Rupture into a bronchus may produce a chronic cavity. Similar granulomas are found in skin, bone, lymph nodes and brain. There is progressive malaise, cough and sputum with radiological evidence of solid or cavitating lesions.

Coccidioidomycosis has to be distinguished from tuberculosis and tumour. Histologically, spherules are present but may be difficult to identify in chronic lesions. Sputum culture is hazardous. Risk factors are native Americans, African-Caribbeans, males, diabetics and pregnant women in the third trimester. Diagnosis is confirmed by skin test to coccidioidin skin test and serological tests, which include coccidioido diffusion test for IgM detection and complement fixation test, IgG. This last test is positive after 2 months of infection. IgM precipitin test is also valuable. In endemic areas a calcified primary complex on radiography with negative tuberculin but positive coccidioidin test is diagnostic.

Most patients need no treatment. In progressive disease intravenous and inhaled amphotericin B, ketoconazole or itraconazole may be helpful. Surgical resection of local pulmonary or bone lesions or drainage of an empyema may be necessary.

Histoplasmosis

The incidence of histoplasmosis shows considerable variation, being 85% in some areas of central USA, 10–15% in river valleys in India and Malaysia with only sporadic cases occurring in the UK and then usually as a result of previous travel or exposure to imported material, e.g. cotton. *Histoplasma capsulatum* prefers soil rich in bird or bat excreta and has been responsible for several minor epidemics of respiratory illness in cavers and poultry workers, e.g. cave sickness. Most infections follow the inhalation of spores causing severe respiratory disease especially in children with miliary mottling on the chest X-ray.

A **primary lesion** consisting of parenchymal and glandular components (resembling a primary tuberculous focus) follows inhalation of the fungus. The organism is taken up by and then destroys the macrophages causing a local reaction and caseation. The enlargement and necrosis of the regional glands is milder than in tuberculosis but may still lead to right middle lobe collapse or subsequent erosion of a phlebolith through the bronchial wall with haemoptysis. Most primary lesions heal rapidly with fibrosis and calcification but in older patients resolution may take up to 2 years with the production of a solid primary lesion consisting of layers of fibrosis and necrosis which may be mistaken for a tumour. Blood-borne dissemination may occur at any stage and is believed to account for characteristic disseminated calcified opacities seen on chest radiography (Figure 50.22). The majority of primary foci are asymptomatic although there may be mild influenzal symptoms which settle rapidly. Rarely, fever, malaise, weight loss, chest pain, cough and haemoptysis may develop and last for several months. Radiologically, localized or diffuse pneumonic shadowing with hilar adenopathy which heal with fibrosis and later calcification may be seen.

Rarely (0.2%) either acute or chronic **progressive pulmonary histoplasmosis** follows the primary lesion. The **acute** form consisting of a progressive caseating pneumonia with extensive lung destruction and severe systemic upset has a high mortality and must be distinguished from tuberculosis. This form of the disease is seen in patients with AIDS.

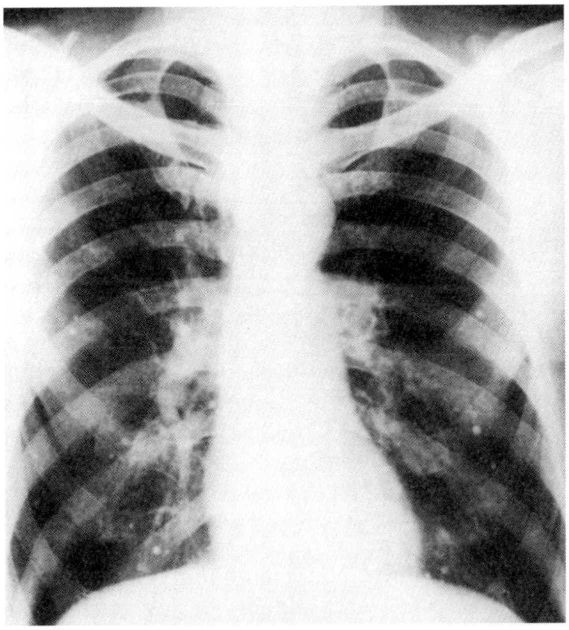

Figure 50.22 Chest film showing small round opacities in the lower parts of both lungs. The calcification is dense and appears homogeneous although with magnification some of the nodules consist of a central core surrounded by a halo of decreased density which is characteristic of histoplasmosis. (Courtesy of Paul Grech.)

The commoner **chronic** form affects the upper lobes with progressive caseation, fibrosis and cavity formation resembling tuberculosis with mediastinal involvement leading to extensive mediastinal fibrosis which may go on to superior vena cava obstruction and pulmonary hypertension. Blood-borne dissemination leads to chronic granulomata in other organs. The clinical features include increasing debility, weight loss, dyspnoea, a chronic productive cough, intermittent haemoptysis, the signs of pneumonia or cavitation over the upper lobes and a radiological picture suggesting fibrocaseous tuberculosis.

The organism may be identified from smears and culture using silver or periodic acid–Schiff (PAS) staining. The histoplasmin test becomes positive within 8 weeks but may be negative in severe cases. Complement fixation, agglutination or immunodiffusion precipitating antibody to H or M antigen may be helpful. Radioimmuno assay is the best for detecting fungal antigen. Treatment with oral ketoconazole, itraconazole or intravenous amphotericin B is required for progressive symptomatic disease. Isolated granulomas may need surgical resection.

North American blastomycosis

This disease, which principally affects forestry and agricultural workers, was first isolated along the eastern seaboard of the USA, but subsequently found in Africa and is thought to have reached America at the time of the slave trade. The spores of *Blastomyces dermatitis* produce a granulomatous caseating lesion in the lower lobes with regional gland enlargement. Haematogenous spread may involve other organs. The initial infection may be asymptomatic or produce acute respiratory symptoms of varying severity. The primary lesion may heal with calcification or extend producing either an acute fulminating pneumonia or chronic fibrocaseous disease with progressive disability clinically resembling tuberculosis. An empyema or a chronic chest wall sinus may develop. The radiological findings include pneumonic shadowing, fibrocaseous destruction with cavitation, miliary mottling and hilar gland enlargement. Tuberculosis frequently co-exists. Accessible lesions, e.g. skin, should be biopsied and sputum sent for culture. The intradermal blastomycin test produces a delayed reaction but may be negative in severe cases. Serological tests are unreliable. Oral ketoconazole, itraconazole or intravenous amphotericin B are the drugs of choice.

Paracoccidioidomycosis

Infection with *Paracoccidioides brasiliensis* is largely restricted to southern and central America. Primary infections principally involve the mucocutaneous junctions with considerable disfiguration. Inhalation may lead to lung involvement with small granulomas, extensive pneumonia or chronic suppuration, cavitation and fibrosis. Rarely blood-borne spread produces miliary lung lesions.

The diagnosis may be obtained by biopsying an accessible lesion, sputum culture or immunofluorescent studies. An intradermal skin test is available and the complement fixation test may be positive in acute cases. Oral ketoconazole, itraconazole or intravenous amphotericin B may effectively control the infection although reactivation may occur several years later. Reports using miconazole are encouraging.

Sporotrichosis

In South Africa, France and southern USA sporotrichosis is endemic. *Sporotrichum schenckii* lives in soil and usually enters the body through skin abrasions causing a subcutaneous granulomatous nodule with local lymphatic spread and blood-borne dissemination. Only rarely are the lungs involved either by haemoatogenous spread or by direct inhalation, with the production of chronic thin-walled cavities and satellite granuloma. Skin biopsy, sputum culture, mice inoculation or the sporotrichin skin test may be helpful in diagnosis. The skin lesion responds to high doses of potassium iodide while pulmonary sporotrichosis may be arrested by itraconazole or intravenous amphotericin B permitting later surgical resection of the damaged lung.

Further reading

American College of Chest Physicians. *Pulmonary Board Review*, 2000.

British Thoracic Society 2000. Guidelines: control and prevention of tuberculosis in the United Kingdom: Code of Practice. *Thorax* **55**: 887–901.

Citron, K. M. and Thomas, G. O. (1986). Occular toxicity from ethambutol. *Thorax* **41**: 737–9.

Murray, J. F. (2000). *Textbook of Respiratory Medicine*, 3rd edn. Philadelphia, PA: W.B. Saunders.

Pinching, A. (1987). The acquired immunodeficiency syndrome: with special reference to tuberculosis! *Tubercle* **68**: 6.

Richardson, M. D. and Warnock, D. W. (1993). *Fungal Infections – Diagnosis and Management*. Oxford: Blackwell.

Sanderson, J. M., Kennedy, M. C. S., Johnson, M. F. *et al.* (1974). Bronchiectasis – the results of surgical and conservative management. *Thorax* **29**: 407.

Thurlbeck, W. M. (1988). *Pathology of the Lung*. New York: Thieme.

MODULE 51

Diseases of the pleura, pneumothorax and emphysema

Section 51.1 • Pleural effusion

A pleural effusion exists when there is an abnormal amount of fluid within the pleural space detectable on clinical or radiological examination. The pleurae are normally kept moist by a thin layer of fluid (up to 15 ml), which is constantly being formed and reabsorbed (with a daily turnover of up to 400 ml), the flow is from the parietal to the visceral membranes. A collection of 100–300 ml is necessary for radiological and at least 500 ml for clinical detection.

A pleural effusion will develop when the equilibrium between formation and absorption is disturbed. The Starling forces govern the exchange of fluid as at any other capillary/tissue interface.

The capillary hydrostatic pressure is dependent on the venous pressure. An increase in systemic venous pressure, e.g. congestive cardiac failure or constrictive pericarditis, is an important factor in the formation of an effusion. If there is a concomitant rise in the pulmonary venous pressure, e.g. left ventricular failure, then the effects are additive.

The colloidal osmotic pressure is proportional to the molar concentrations of the proteins such that the lower molecular weight proteins, e.g. albumin, have the greatest effect. Any cause of hypoproteinaemia, for example, the nephrotic syndrome or liver disease, will reduce the plasma colloid pressure and encourage the formation of an effusion. Proteins from the pleural space drain solely into the lymphatic system principally through the mediastinal pleura via stomata. Although the turnover of protein is slower than water and electrolytes, 1 g of albumin may be exchanged in 24 hours. In normal subjects the pleural fluid contains 10–20 g/l of protein. Decreased reabsorption may be as important as increased output in the formation of some effusions.

The capillary permeability is increased in pleural inflammation, i.e. pneumonia or pulmonary infarction, allowing more fluid and protein to enter the pleural space.

Lymphatic drainage. Cells and protein leave the pleural space via stomata in the parietal pleura directly into the lymphatic system and any impairment of lymphatic drainage, i.e. lymph node infiltration by tumour, a maldeveloped lymphatic system (yellow nail syndrome) or increased venous pressure, will encourage the formation of an effusion.

A pleural effusion is always a manifestation of local or systemic disease. Its size may vary from just sufficient to blunt the costophrenic angle to sufficient to fill a hemithorax with displacement of the heart and mediastinum to the contralateral side. The effusion may lie free within the pleural space when it will gravitate to the most dependent part; or be loculated within an interlobar fissure; or may become encapsulated by adhesions in the pleural spaces.

An asymptomatic effusion may be picked up on routine radiography. The symptomatic presentation is of progressive dyspnoea which may be associated with pleuritic pain or a dull ache. There may be fever and toxaemia which settles after aspiration. Cough and haemoptysis usually indicate an underlying pulmonary cause.

The physical findings in a moderate or large effusion lying free in the pleural space are diminished expansion, stony dullness on percussion, diminished or absent breath sounds and reduced vocal fremitus and resonance over the affected side. A pleural friction rub may be audible at the top of an effusion with an area of bronchial breathing below. If large, there may be a shift of the heart and mediastinum to the contralateral side. A subpulmonary effusion presents with the features of an elevated hemi-

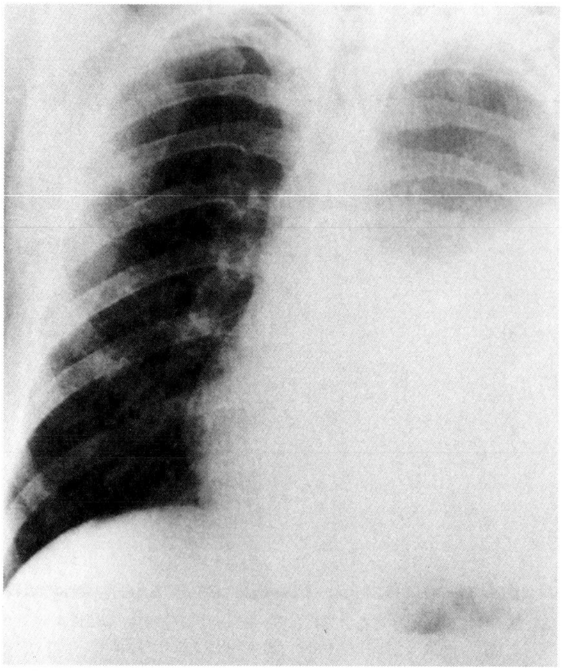

Figure 51.1 Large left pleural effusion with mediastinal shift to the right.

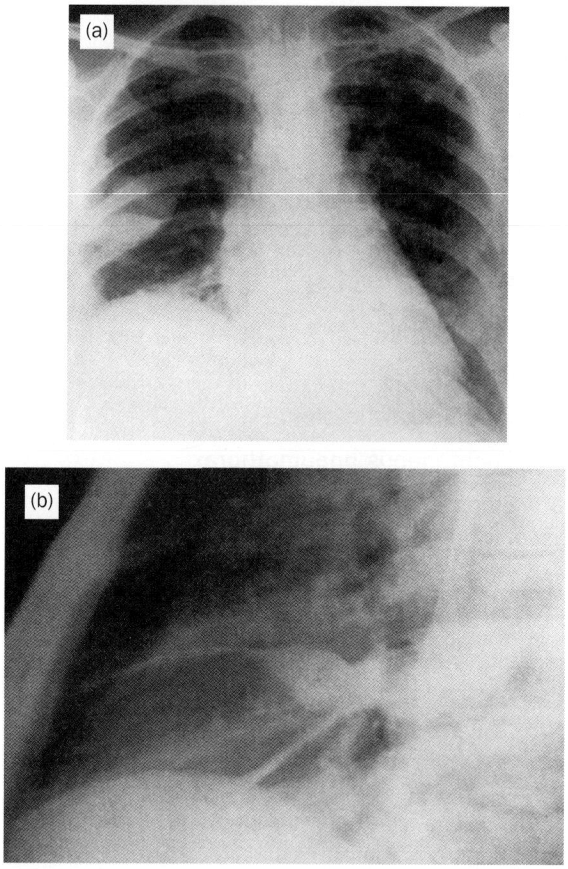

Figure 51.2 Interlobar pleural effusion. An opacity seen in the right midzone (a) is better visualized in the lateral projection (b), where it proved to be due to shadows along the lines of the transverse and oblique fissures. (Courtesy of Paul Grech.)

diaphragm. If the effusion lies within an interlobar fissure there may be no abnormal clinical findings.

Radiologically, blunting of the costophrenic angle may be the only finding. A small effusion may be distinguished from pleural thickening and its size by a lateral decubitis film when the fluid will collect as a puddle in the most dependent area of the thorax. Large effusions show the characteristic axillary tail with a concave upper border (the upper margin is at the same level right round the effusion but in the PA chest film the fluid in the axilla is seen end on and appears as a dense concave shadow). In a large effusion the hemithorax may appear opaque with the mediastinum shifted to the opposite side (Figure 51.1).

It may be difficult to distinguish an infrapulmonary effusion from an elevated hemidiaphragm. Such effusions will be displaced in a decubitus film. If loculation has occurred a small artificial pneumoperitoneum, the gastric air bubble or ultrasound scanning will help delineate the lower margin from the diaphragm. Interlobar effusions may present bizarre appearances on the PA radiograph but a lateral film usually shows the characteristic round or oval shadow in the line of a fissure (Table 51.2).

Computed tomography (CT) of the thorax is now routine for the assessment of pleural effusions with the added advantage of information on lung pathology.

While the causes of a pleural effusion are numerous, the patient's age and environmental circumstances will influence the likely aetiology. Thus tuberculosis would be more likely in an adolescent from a developing country than in an elderly Western male. Similarly the size of the effusion and whether it is unilateral or bilateral will be of diagnostic significance. The major causes for each group are set out in Tables 51.1 and 51.2.

These usually suggest a systemic cause (Table 51.2).

An indication as to the aetiology may be obtained from the history. Pleuritic pain suggests inflammation prior to the effusion, i.e. pneumonia or pulmonary infarction, while a dull ache may accompany malignant infiltration. Dyspnoea out of keeping with the size of the effusion may indicate underlying cardiac or pulmonary disease and haemoptysis suggests carcinoma, pulmonary infarction or pneumonia. Peripheral oedema might indicate cardiac failure or hypoproteinaemia. In difficult cases, some help may be obtained from the mode of onset and duration (the more rapid the more acute), any abdominal symptoms (pancreatitis or perforated bowel), recent abdominal surgery (subphrenic abscess, pneumonia or infarction), previous mastectomy (secondary malignancy), occupation (including exposure to asbestos many years previously), travel (amoebiasis), contact with tuberculosis or drug history (remembering that an effusion may develop after drug withdrawal).

A chest radiograph taken after aspiration or in the lateral decubitus position may indicate an underlying pulmonary lesion while a previous film may give a valuable lead (Figure 51.3).

Table 51.1 Unilateral effusions

	Small to moderate effusions	*Large effusions occupying most of a hemithorax*
Frequent causes	Secondary malignancy Bacterial pneumonia Cardiac failure Pulmonary infarction Tuberculosis Connective-tissue disorders Pneumothorax	Secondary malignancy Tuberculosis Cardiac failure Empyema Haemothorax
Less frequent	Lymphoma Subphrenic abscess Pancreatitis Primary pleural tumours Fungal infection Viral infection Post-myocardial infarction	
Rare	Drug induced (methyseride, practolol, nitrofurantoin) Lung abscesses Bronchiectasis Amoebiasis Yellow nail syndrome	

Smear, culture, tuberculin or fungal skin tests, bronchoscopy, electro- and echocardiography, ventilation and perfusion lung scans, and immunological tests (rheumatoid factor, antinuclear factor and LE cells) may give valuable diagnostic leads.

Aspiration of a little fluid (20–30 ml) from an area of maximum dullness confirms the diagnosis and its appearance may be diagnostically valuable.

- **Transudates**. Usually clear, light straw-coloured fluid which fails to clot. Protein less than 30 g/l. Systemic cause, e.g. congestive cardiac failure or hypoproteinaemia.
- **Exudates**. Clear but darker yellow, clotting on standing. Protein greater than 30 g/l. Local cause, e.g. tumour, infection.
- **Bloodstained**. Traumatic pleural taps will cause fresh bleeding. Continuous aspiration of old, dark red blood is characteristic of malignancy but may also occur in tuberculosis, infarction and pancreatitis.
- **Frank blood** (haemothorax). Pure blood usually follows chest trauma, usually from fractured ribs. Haemothorax passes through the same breakdown processes as blood in other tissues, therefore its colour will reflect the time since its accumulation.
- **Turbid**. Indicative of a high cell count as found in parapneumonic effusions.
- **Frank pus** (empyema). Frankly purulent fluid of varying viscosity, pH < 7 indicates empyema, i.e. it needs operative intervention.
- **Opalescent effusions.** Shimmering whitish, semi-translucent due to a high cholesterol content. A rare feature of longstanding effusions of whatever cause, i.e. malignancy, tuberculosis or nephrotic syndrome.
- **Chyle** (chylothorax). White and oily due to the collection of lymph secondary to involvement of the main lymphatic canals (e.g. damage or involvement of thoracic duct).

Table 51.2 Bilateral effusions

Transudates	Most commonly occur in congestive cardiac failure, hypoproteinaemia in nephrotic syndrome or liver disease and constrictive pericarditis. Rarer causes are Meigs's syndrome and myxoedema
Exudates	Seen in multiple pulmonary infarcts, connective-tissue disorders, secondary malignancy and rarely, tuberculosis

A large volume of fluid may be aspirated either for diagnostic purposes or to relieve symptoms (dyspnoea, fever). The needle is usually inserted in the posterior axillary line just below the upper level of dullness with the patient leaning forward. For loculated effusions the site may be determined from posteroanterior and lateral films or thoracic ultrasound scanning or the procedure done at thoracic CT scan. The needle size will depend on the nature of the fluid. Failure to obtain sufficient fluid usually results from either aspiration at too low a level due to an elevated diaphragm secondary to pulmonary collapse or loculation with adhesions. The initial aspiration should be limited to 1 litre in adults

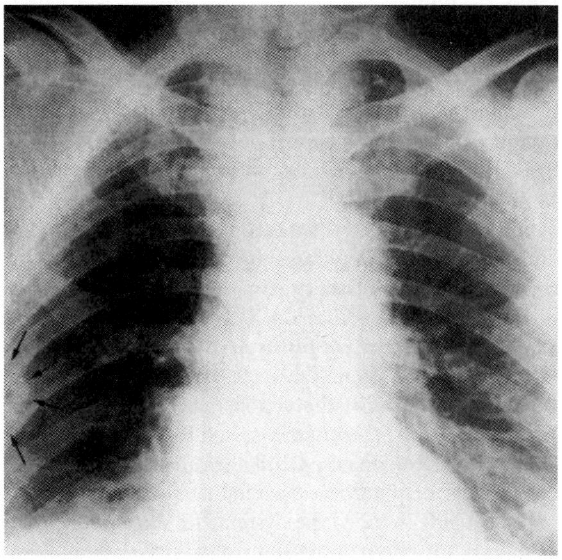

Figure 51.3 Peripheral right lower lobe shadow discovered after tapping of right pleural effusion. The lesion was a carcinoma.

(less in children) as too rapid or too large an aspiration may precipitate: (1) unilateral pulmonary oedema (the exact mechanism being uncertain); (2) respiratory distress and pain; (3) tachycardia; or (4) hypotension. Other less acute complications include pneumothorax, haemorrhage or infection. Aseptic technique is vital; the risk of iatrogenic infection is high if repeated aspiration is performed.

Aliquots of the aspirate should be sent for cytological, biochemical and bacteriological examination.

Cytology

While the total cell count is of little value, differential cell counts may provide useful information. Malignant cells may be identified. While a high lymphocyte count is common to both tuberculosis and secondary malignancy, mesothelial cells are frequently found in the latter but not in the former. Neutrophilia is found in parapneumonic effusions. Some effusions have a high eosinophil count which has little diagnostic significance.

Bacteriological examination

This may be by direct smear of sulphur granules or pus (fungi or actinomycosis), or culture for anaerobes, aerobes, fungi or tuberculosis (positive in only 25% of tuberculous effusions).

Pleural biopsy

Pleural effusions are always the manifestation of disease and should never be considered idiopathic. The introduction of a closed pleural biopsy technique using the Abrams' needle did prove a simple, safe and effective means of diagnosing pleural effusions of tuberculous (80%) or malignant (60–70%) origin, particularly if three or four biopsies were taken each time and the procedure repeated if necessary. The Abrams' needle biopsy should only be attempted in the presence of fluid. Complications of pneumothorax and slight bleeding are rare.

Increasingly, with the spread of thoracoscopic skills, direct inspection and open biopsy under vision are practised with aspiration to dryness and assessment of trapped lung. Such an approach to pleural biopsy in the presence or absence of effusion is safe and effective and highly specific (>95%).

A diagnosis may be made on clinical grounds, e.g. congestive cardiac failure, but if the effusion fails to respond to appropriate treatment, i.e. diuretics, then further investigation may reveal a different aetiology.

Congestive cardiac failure is the commonest cause of a transudate (Figure 51.4). It may develop with 24 hours of elevation of the venous pressure and is more likely to occur if both the systemic and pulmonary venous pressures are raised. Initially unilateral, usually on the right, it may become bilateral if the failure remains uncontrolled. Provided the dyspnoea is not severe, a trial of diuretics without aspiration is usually justified.

Most **pulmonary infarcts** involve the pleural surface with subsequent inflammation and the formation of a small to moderate effusion which is usually clear, yellow fluid but may be bloodstained. Most effusions are self-limiting and rarely require aspiration. The diagnosis depends on identifying the underlying infarction by lung scans or contrast CT.

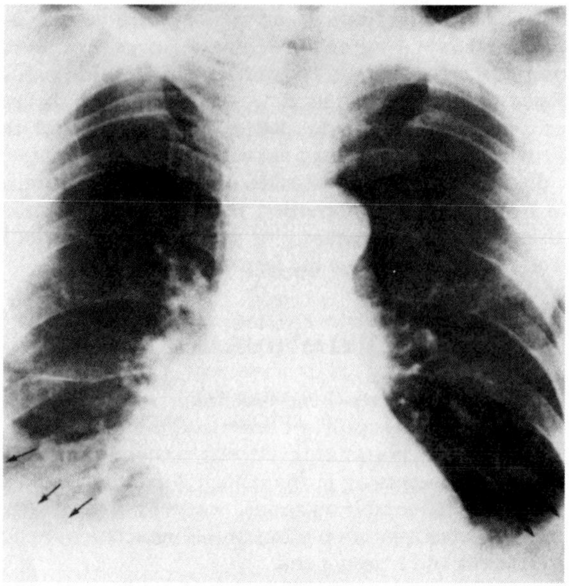

Figure 51.4 Bilateral basal pleural effusions and a prominent horizontal fissure due to cardiac failure.

Eighty per cent of **subphrenic abscesses** develop a 'sympathetic effusion' which contains polymorphs but no organisms. The effusion should be aspirated, the abscess drained, and antibiotics given to lessen the risk of an empyema.

Hepatic amoebiasis may cause a 'sympathetic effusion' but more often the infection spreads directly to the right lower lobe.

A pleural effusion, usually on the left, may complicate up to 10% of cases of **severe acute pancreatitis,** the fluid often being bloodstained with a high amylase content.

Ascites secondary to cirrhosis is often associated with bilateral effusion which arises from a combination of hypoproteinaemia and the direct passage of fluid through the diaphragm via the lymphatics or diaphragmatic defects. Rarely an ovarian tumour is associated with ascites and bilateral pleural effusions which resolve after resection of the tumour (**Meig's syndrome**).

Peritoneal dialysis may be complicated by bilateral effusions.

Ten per cent of patients with **acute rheumatic fever** develop a small or moderate, transient pleural effusion, at times bilateral, which usually requires no treatment.

A protracted unilateral effusion requiring repeated aspiration may be the first manifestation of **rheumatoid arthritis**. The fluid, which may be opalescent, has a low glucose content and is usually positive for the rheumatoid factor. Pleural rheumatoid nodules may be visible on thoracoscopy. At post-mortem pleural adhesions are common in rheumatoid arthritis and are believed to result from recurrent pleurisy or effusions. Bilateral effusions occasionally complicate **systemic lupus erythematosus** and may be the presenting feature.

Pleural involvement in a **bacterial pneumonia** may progress to the formation of a serous effusion called a parapneumonic effusion. The frequency with which an effusion develops depends on the causal organism, i.e. 10% with pneumococcal, 35% with anaerobic and 50% with staphyloccoccal pneumonias. The turbid fluid is rich in neutrophils but an organism is rarely cultured from it. The effusion may either remain serous, resolving without complications, or develop into an empyema. In view of the latter possibility such effusions should be aspirated to dryness, when the fever invariably settles. pH > 7 indicates that the diffusion gradient for oxygen is effective and antibiotics are still likely to enter the pleural space.

Pleural effusions are infrequent in **viral infections** and when they occur they are usually small and only detected radiologically. The diagnosis depends on showing a rising viral antibody titre.

Pleurisy and pleural effusions occur early in actinomycosis as a prelude to an empyema and chest wall involvement. Sulphur granules in pus or sputum are diagnostic of *Actinomyces israelii* infections.

Pleural effusion may complicate primary coccidioidomycosis, blastomycosis, histoplasmosis or cryptococcosis and if suspected special culture media will be required.

Tuberculous pleural effusions may arise: (1) during the course of the primary complex in children (7%) when the effusion is often small and self-limiting, resolving over 3–4 months without residual fibrosis or calcification; (2) as the main post-primary tuberculous manifestation in adolescents; or (3) as a complication of post-primary pulmonary tuberculosis. The pleura are usually studded with small tubercles, the effusion resulting from the combination of an inflammatory exudate and a hypersensitive reaction to the tubercular protein.

Classic adolescent tuberculous effusions which develop within a year of the primary complex are still frequently encountered in the developing countries but have become uncommon in Western countries. Several weeks of vague ill-health, pleural pain and fever are usual but progressive dyspnoea may be the presenting feature. A pleural rub may be heard, particularly if the effusion is small. The effusion is the principal radiological abnormality, the lung fields and hilar shadows often appearing normal. The tuberculin test is strongly positive. The pleural fluid is rich in lymphocytes, but smears of centrifuged debris are rarely positive and culture of the organism is difficult. Closed pleural biopsy using the Abrams' needle is positive in 70–80% of cases and thoracoscopic biopsy in almost all cases. Treatment with chemotherapy, pleural aspiration (repeated as necessary), and breathing exercises, usually ensures rapid and complete recovery. Inadequate treatment or delayed diagnosis can lead to tuberculous empyema which requires decortication.

If a post-primary tuberculous cavity ruptures into the pleural space, a pneumothorax and effusion results but this has become rare with good chemotherapy. The chest radiograph shows a hydropneumothorax. If inadequately treated there is the danger of developing a tuberculous empyema with progressive contraction and fibrosis of the hemithorax. A similar situation resulting from previous artificial pneumothorax treatment may still be encountered. When treating a tuberculous empyema, resection of the affected lobe or a pleuropneumonectomy may be necessary.

Most **malignant pleural effusions** result from the secondary involvement of the pleura from primary tumours arising in other organs. The effusion is an exudate which is formed as a result of obstruction to the lymphatic drainage in the mediastinum. The pleurae are often studded with metastatic deposits. Bronchial and breast primaries are the commonest followed by pancreatic, gastric and uterine. The effusion may be the first indication of malignancy with little evidence of the primary site, or result from the extension of a previously diagnosed lesion. It may herald the end of many symptom-free years in breast carcinoma. At autopsy a third of patients dying of Hodgkin's disease have a pleural effusion but the cause may be other than metastatic spread, i.e. infection. Effusions may complicate lymphoma. With lymphomas and some extrathoracic primaries, e.g. breast, the effusions may be bilateral. When associated with lymphangitis carcinomatosa the effusions are often bilateral and add to the patient's distress.

There may be few symptoms if the effusion is small or develops slowly. A careful history and examination may reveal the site of a primary lesion. A post-aspiration chest radiograph may show metastatic pleural deposits or enlarged mediastinal nodes. Occasionally the fluid is a clear, yellow exudate but more often it is uniformly bloodstained. Cytology may show malignant cells or lymphocytes but normal cytology does not exclude tumour. Closed pleural biopsy (Abrams' needle) may confirm the diagnosis and give some indication of histological type, but today thoracoscopy is used to better effect.

Most malignant pleural effusions cause considerable distress, i.e. dyspnoea and chest pain, but are difficult to control as they often reaccumulate rapidly following aspiration in spite of the variety of therapies on offer. A few cases respond to hormone therapy (some breast tumours), systemic cytotoxic chemotherapy (some breast, ovarian and small cell bronchial carcinomas or lymphoma) and radiotherapy (some lymphomas). Parietal pleural resection is an effective palliation. Repeated aspiration only depletes the patient's proteins and increases the risk of empyema.

Life expectancy determines the level of palliation. Aspiration followed by installation of sclerosing agents, of which talc is more effective than tetracycline. Cytotoxic agents are not sufficiently consistent in their effect to be recommended. Such pleurodesis must only be attempted if the two surfaces of the pleura are approximated after drainage of the effusion. When there is trapped lung a Denver shunt may be inserted. This drains the pleural effusion into either a great vein or the subphrenic space. Parietal pleurectomy in patients with a life expectancy greater than 6 months is invaluable.

Section 51.2 • Chylothorax

The collection of chyle within the pleural space following rupture or trauma to the thoracic duct or the right bronchomediastinal trunk, although comparatively rare, is increasing in frequency. The fluid is rich in protein, fat, fat-soluble vitamins, lymphocytes, water and electrolytes and its repeated aspiration often causes emaciation, hypoproteinaemia and lymphopenia.

The major causes are as follows:

- **Surgical trauma.** The technical advances in thoracic and oesophageal surgery have increased the chance of trauma to the lymphatic ducts. The incidence is 1–2% after oesophagectomy. The risks are greatest with surgery in the vicinity of the left subclavian artery. Block dissection of neck glands or scalene node biopsy has also been implicated. If the injury is recognized at the time of surgery and the duct ligated, chylothorax does not develop. With the development of total thoracic oesophagectomy as an *en bloc* excision it is routine to tie the duct on the anterior aspect of the eighth thoracic vertebrae.
- **Trauma.** Sudden hyperextension of the spine may lead to rupture of the thoracic duct just above the diaphragm. Chylothorax may also complicate falls, compression injuries or blows to the trunk, stab or gunshot wounds and severe episodes of coughing or vomiting.
- **Obstruction** to the thoracic duct from enlarged lymph nodes usually secondary to malignancy, but occasionally from tuberculosis or filariasis, may cause a chylothorax. Rarely, thrombosis of the left subclavian vein, aortic aneurysm or benign lymphangioma has been implicated.
- **Miscellaneous.** Congenital fistulas and birth injury are rare causes.

Two to 10 days may elapse between the damage and the formation of a chylothorax. Chyle collects initially in the posterior mediastinum then leaks into the hemithorax. Up to 2.5 litres of chyle may be produced daily. In patients who present with the chylous effusion late after injury an initial conservative approach may be successful. If the fluid losses are high an early a direct operative approach is needed.

The sudden onset of dyspnoea and pyrexia without toxaemia is the usual presentation. The clinical and radiological features are those of an effusion. The aspirate is characteristically white and oily with a high fat content, and can usually be easily distinguished from an opalescent effusion. Occasionally the ingestion of a lipophilic dye, which when absorbed rapidly passes into the chyle, may be used to establish the diagnosis. The effusion rapidly reaccumulates and repeated aspirations may lead to cachexia and death. Do not procrastinate, operate.

Table 51.3 Causes of empyema

Pulmonary infections	Pneumonia	Staphylococcal Pneumococcal Streptococcal
	Lung abscess Bronchiectasis Fungal infections Tuberculosis	
Trauma	Chest injuries – including implanted foreign bodies Post-thoracotomy Ruptured oesophagus/leaking anastomosis	
Transdiaphragmatic spread	Subphrenic abscess Hepatic amoebiasis	
Iatrogenic	Multiple aspirations for effusion	
Osteomyelitis	Ribs or vertebrae	
Septicaemia	Multiple small lung abscesses	

Section 51.3 • Empyema

The incidence of empyema has fallen since the introduction of antibiotics for the treatment of pulmonary infections. Early diagnosis and effective therapy are essential. The late complications of untreated empyema with a fixed fibrotic chest cavity should only remain in the history books. Of the sources of infection in Table 51.3, pulmonary infections remain the most important, with iatrogenic causes increasing because people now live so long with cardiac failure, rheumatic disorder and breast cancer.

'Dry pleurisy' may be the first indication of pleural inflammation although this is quickly followed by the outpouring of fluid rich in protein and polymorphs. Although frank purulence should develop before an effusion is referred to as an empyema, a pH< 7 is the best marker for the need for operative intervention, and therefore is probably the discrimminator for empyema. Continued accumulation of pus compresses the lung with shift of the mediastinum to the opposite side. Fibrin is continually deposited on the pleural surfaces producing a thickening rind, the deeper layers of which become fibrotic and avascular. The established empyema is walled off and the space is fixed. This allows for open drainage or easy stripping during surgical decortication. Such decortication at this stage will produce full re-expansion of the lung with gradual resolution of the pleural inflammation and no functional impairment. It is this fibrin deposition which limits the diffusion of oxygen that leads to anaerobic respiration and the fall in pH within the empyema. If the oxygen cannot diffuse neither can antibiotics.

If the pus is not drained effectively or the empyema excised, the continual formation and fibrosis of the pleural rind progressively restricts chest wall and diaphragmatic movement, eventually producing a shrunken, flattened, immobile hemithorax with overlapping ribs and scoliosis to the affected side.

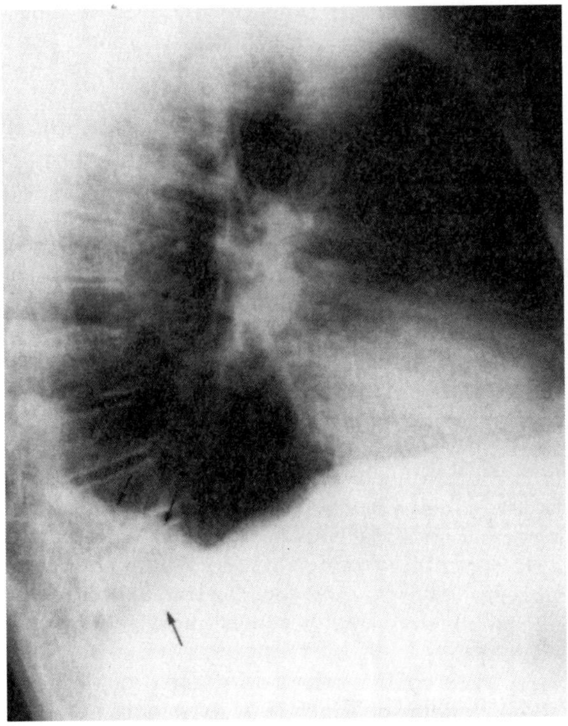

Figure 51.5 Empyema right base posteriorly. Triangular outline.

Occasionally an empyema pushes through the chest wall at one of the perforating pathways of the neurovascular bundle, forming a collar-stud abscess which may break down giving a discharging fistula in continuity with the empyema cavity (empyema necessitatis).

The term 'pyopneumothorax' refers to the situation where there is air and pus within the pleural space. This may occur: (1) if the empyema discharges into a bronchus forming a bronchopleural fistula; (2) if the empyema results from the rupture of a lung abscess or cyst (hydatid), again with the formation of a bronchopleural fistula; (3) following pleural aspiration if the lung is bound down by fibrotic rind and unable to re-expand; or (4) if the empyema contains gas-forming organisms usually associated with aspiration and is often present in the right paravertebral area. The right apical lower lobe bronchus is dependent in the supine position and the commonest site of aspiration damage.

The pathological process is modified by the infecting organism. Streptococcal infections produce thin pus with few adhesions and considerable toxaemia while a pneumococcal empyema becomes rapidly encapsulated with less systemic upset. Empyema secondary to lung abscesses often contain mixed anaerobic, microaerophilic and aerobic organisms capable of producing putrefaction with foul-smelling pus. An empyema associated with spreading infection distal to a bronchial carcinoma may go unnoticed in the patient's general deterioration.

In a hierarchy of systemic effect subphrenic abscess is worst, then pelvic abscess, followed by empyema. This relates to the access to the lymphatics of toxic materials. This also explains why empyema may remain occult for some time before diagnosis.

Clinical presentation

The patient may present with pyrexia from a respiratory infection which has failed to respond or had relapsed during or after treatment. There may be a history of recent thoracic or abdominal surgery, trauma or liver disease. A sudden deterioration in a child with staphylococcal pneumonia or severe pleurisy in hydatid disease may herald the development of an empyema.

Fever, rigors, a swinging temperature, malaise, anorexia, weight loss and pleurisy, followed by a gnawing chest pain, are common but may be modified by antibiotic therapy, i.e. into a low-grade grumbling pyrexia. Cough is unusual except with a bronchopleural fistula when large quantities of pus may be expectorated. Dyspnoea may arise if there is lung compression. These signs may be quite indolent.

The signs of an empyema lying free within the pleural space are those of a pleural effusion, but encapsulated lesions in the interlobar fissures, mediastinum or subpulmonary area may produce no abnormal signs. Finger clubbing can develop within 2–3 weeks but this is uncommon. Occasionally a collar-stud abscess (empyema necessitatis) develops usually in relation to an area of penetration of the chest wall by the neurovascular supply.

A leucocytosis of 15 000–30 000 is common. The C-reactive protein (CRP) is usually >200. Pus, aspirated through a wide-bore needle, should be cultured for anaerobic, microaerophilic and aerobic organisms, including fungi and tuberculosis. Previous antibiotic therapy may affect the results. Unfortunately positive culture is not possible in 40% of cases.

Radiologically, empyema resembles a pleural effusion and, if large, the entire hemithorax may be opaque. PA and lateral films or thoracic ultrasound scanning are necessary to localize an encapsulated lesion. The fluid level of a pyopneumothorax (Figure 51.6) may simulate a lung abscess but an empyema has a sharper outline and lacks a segmental or lobar distribution. Increasingly CT scanning is routine and aspiration at CT or ultrasound control is reducing false negative test aspiration.

Late empyema most frequently follows inadequate treatment or failure to recognize that empyema is extant. Generalized toxaemia, malaise, anorexia, weight loss, grumbling pyrexia, gnawing chest pain and cutaneous fistulas may develop particularly in the immunocompromised and with fungal infections. A persistent cough productive of sputum, particularly when lying on the contralateral side, or an aspiration pneumonia in the 'good lung' are features of a persistent bronchopleural fistula.

Progressive pleural fibrosis produces a shrunken, immobile hemithorax with scoliosis to the affected side. Finger clubbing is common. When bronchopleural and cutaneous fistulas co-exist, air is expelled through the skin sinus on coughing. A normochromic,

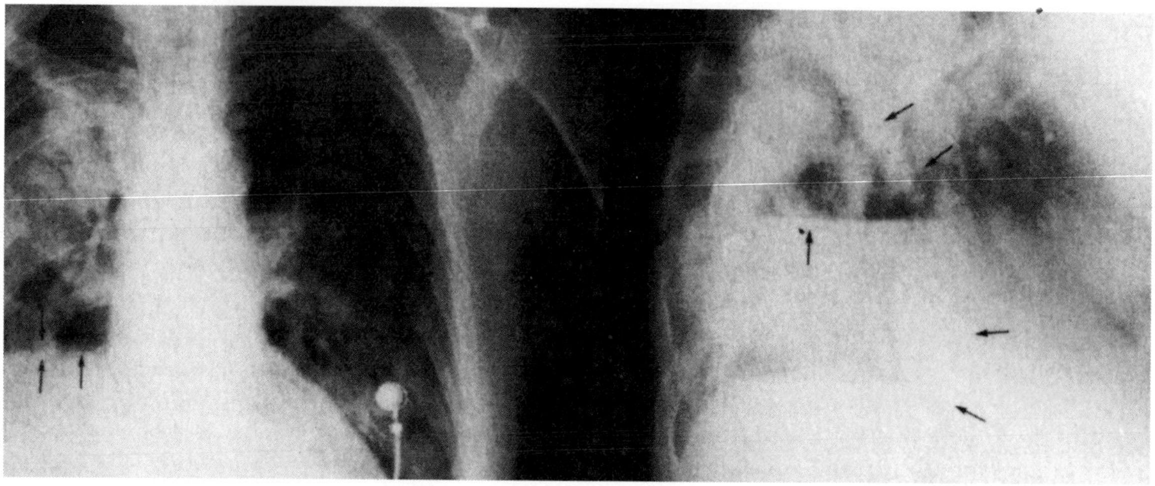

Figure 51.6 Right-sided pneumonia with pyopneumothorax. The limits of the empyema are outlined by the arrows in the lateral film.

normocytic anaemia and leucopenia are common. There is a risk of amyloidosis if this chronic purulent state is not controlled. Today in the Western world such conditions are rare.

Radiologically, there is dense pleural opacification, elevation of the hemidiaphragm, crowding of the ribs (some of which may show periostitis) and a shift of the mediastinum to the affected side. Fluid levels, which may be multiple within a loculated empyema, occur with bronchopleural or cutaneous fistulas or after aspiration. Pleural calcification may complicate an old tuberculous or post-traumatic empyema (Figures 51.6 and 51.7).

Pleural aspiration is often difficult but any pus or sputum should be sent for bacteriological examination, including cultures for tuberculosis and fungi.

Treatment

The principles of treatment are drainage of pus and obliteration of space, which leads to eradication of infection. When this is not possible marsupialization with an operculum is an effective control.

When planning treatment the state of the underlying lung is important and bronchoscopy necessary to exclude bronchial obstruction. Thoracic CT delineates the empyema and gives good evidence of underlying lung pathology. If the pH is > 7 it should be treated as a parapneumonic effusion and the pleural space should be aspirated to dryness through a wide-bore needle and an appropriate antibiotic given systemically. Regular aspirations should be continued until the pus ceases to re-collect. Vigorous physiotherapy, including breathing exercises, will aid lung re-expansion and encourage good chest wall movement. If repeated aspirations are difficult, a wide-bore intercostal tube with drainage to an underwater seal system may be considered.

If the pH is < 7 active intervention is indicated. There are three options: antibiotic irrigation for 5–7 days, rib resection with empyema drain or decortication. There is a further option – fenestration, called a Claggett window or Eloesser flap used in late empyema with a fixed lung or patients with poor general condition.

Empyema space irrigation

The cavity is intubated usually at its dependent part and a y-tube fitting attached. This allows repeated cavity irrigation with antibiotic or antiseptic solutions. Betadine in saline is the usual choice. At least 5 days of irrigation is needed.

Rib resection

A generous segment of a rib which lies just above the bottom of the cavity is resected and the cavity fully explored with the removal of all the pus and fibrin deposits. Biopsies from the cavity wall should be sent for pathological and bacteriological examination. The resulting cavity is drained initially as a closed system in which a wide-bore tube is left in the space and connected to an underwater seal drainage bottle. After 2 or 3 days conversion to an open system with a short length of wide-bore tubing draining to a stoma bag allows outpatient management.

Most parenchymal lung leaks close spontaneously with adequate treatment. A wide-bore tube draining to a stoma bag keeps the patient active and often in work. Closure of the fistula, checked if necessary by sinograms, is essential before removal of the tube.

The empyema drains are changed every 3 weeks and drain into a stoma bag. The cavity is studied 10–12 weekly with sinograms. As the cavity contracts to the size of the tube keep the tube a maximal diameter. When the cavity is reduced to the size of the tube then is the time to shorten but do not reduce the diameter too quickly.

Thoracotomy and decortication

If the patient is fit and there is no significant bronchopleural fistula open operation is the best choice for the larger empyema or when the empyema is loculated. Apical and basal drains connected to underwater

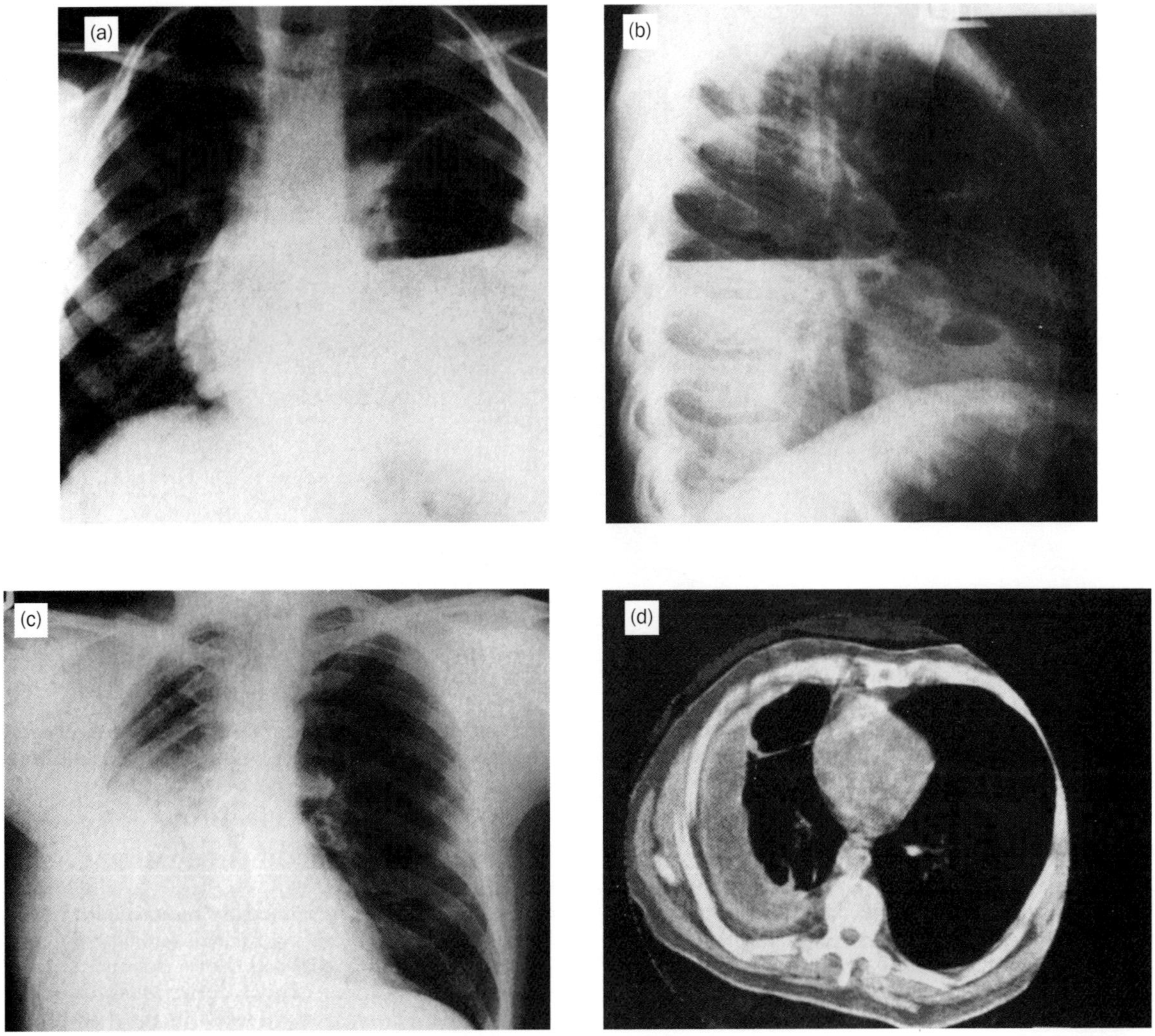

Figure 51.7 Chronic empyema. (a) PA and lateral views of a chest showing a large cavity containing pus. Note the fluid level and the thickness of the cavity wall. (Courtesy of Paul Grech.) (c) PA radiographs and (d) CT scan of a patient with a fully established empyema with some contraction of the hemithorax.

seal systems ensure adequate drainage and lung re-expansion. Appropriate antibiotic therapy and vigorous physiotherapy are essential. If effective the chest drains will be removed within a week.

In late empyema with a fixed lung or a large space in a patient with poor general condition fenestration is a simple procedure (*vide infra*).

When considering thoracotomy the patient's physical state and the condition of the underlying lung are important. If these are good then decortication and excision of the empyema and any cutaneous sinuses followed by free drainage usually ensures full re-expansion, although there may be permanent functional impairment if there has been alveolar destruction and fibrosis.

If there is underlying bronchiectasis, pulmonary fibrosis, a lung abscess or bronchial obstruction due to a resectable tumour or foreign body, then lobectomy plus decortication or pleuropneumonectomy should be considered provided the overall lung function permits.

Occasionally a limited thoracoplasty, a muscle flap or an omental patch or plug may be used to obliterate the residual cavity.

When the lesion is extensive, the lung function impaired or the patient's general condition poor, it may be impossible to eradicate an empyema and fenestration is indicated. The Claggett window or Eloessor flap is usually made in the axilla where two or three rib segments are removed with overlying muscle and skin. A large defect is left in the chest wall for open drainage. Modern fenestrated stoma bags cope well with these defects.

Post-pneumonectomy empyema

The development of a leak in the bronchial stump left after pneumonectomy invariably leads to infection in the space (Figure 51.8). If the leak is at an early post-operative stage then it may be closed using a muscle flap then with adequate toilet and 7 days' antibiotic

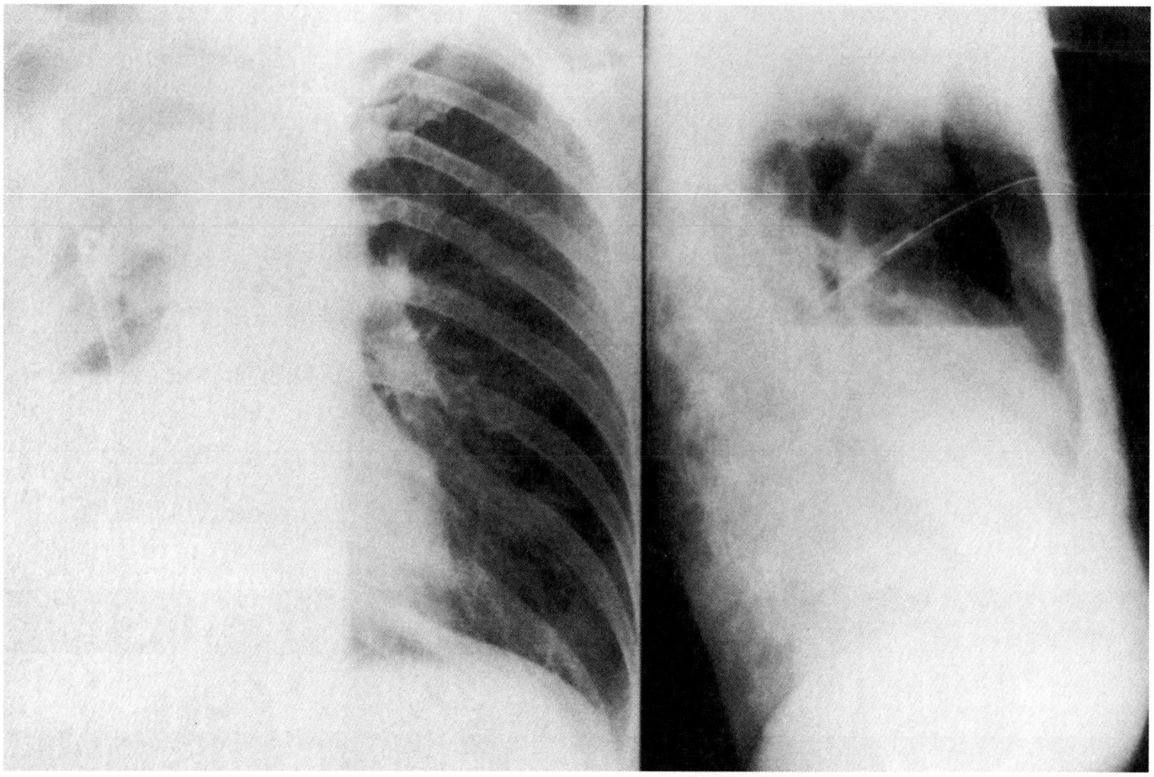

Figure 51.8 A right persistent post-pneumonectomy empyema.

irrigation control should be effected in 80% of cases. However, once infection is established in the hemithorax, treatment is by open drainage with a wide-bore tube for some months then eight rib thoracoplasty.

Section 51.4 • Tumours of the pleura

The pleural cavities are lined by mesothelial tissue containing both mesothelial and connective tissue elements. Tumour may arise from both. Histologically, epithelial and fibrous elements may co-exist in the same tumour, suggesting perhaps a common mesothelial origin.

Pleural tumours may be classified in various ways, but a useful clinical division is between:

- localized pleural lesions
- diffuse malignant mesothelioma
- secondary malignant spread.

Localized pleural lesions (Figure 51.9) microscopically, are usually firm well encapsulated lesions of either the parietal or visceral pleura, but they may occasionally be nodular or pedunculated. Commonly they have the histological appearance of a fibroma, but they can resemble a lipoma, haemangioma or a pericytoma. In some instances there is marked cellularity and pleomorphism suggesting a fibrosarcoma or a liposarcoma while in most instances they are benign. In time or a lesion recurring after previous local resection they may become locally invasive. They vary in size from 1 cm to a large mass filling most of the hemithorax. Occasionally there is an associated arthropathy.

Diffuse malignant mesothelioma

Currently mesothelioma is increasing and will continue to rise in incidence to 2025. This is the product of exposure to asbestos, usually in the working environment. These patients are already exposed and with increasing life expectancy will live long enough post-exposure so that it will be the cause of death in more than 10%. Asbestos exposure has also been associated with the development of localized fibrous pleural plaques, but there is no evidence that malignant mesotheliomas develop from these lesions. Malignant mesotheliomas occur with an incidence of 1750 per million per annum in the asbestos exposed population and one per million per annum in the unexposed.

The tumour gradually spreads out as a thick yellow-grey fibrotic sheet to encase the lung. It may have a multi-nodular appearance or grow as a local mass. Usually it is contained in the pleural membrane for some years and then breaks out and begins to directly invade local structures. This is the common time for presentation, the disease is advanced and most patients are dead within 12 months. The pericardium, chest wall and diaphragm may become involved by direct extension. The contralateral pleura and peritoneum may also be involved by direct spread. Presentation with large blood-stained pleural effusions is not uncommon, but as the

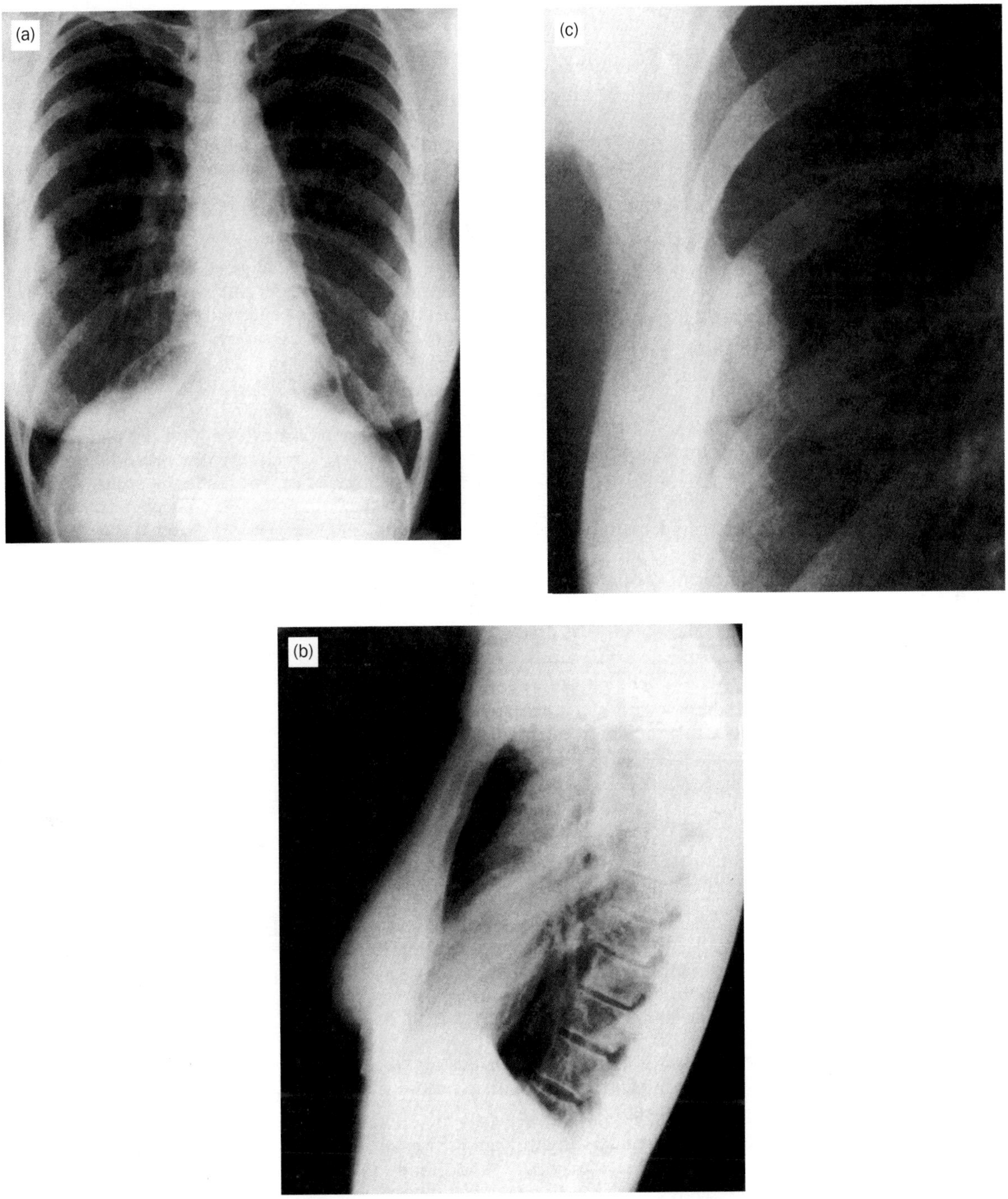

Figure 51.9 PA (a) and lateral (b) radiographs of a benign pleural tumour. (c) Close-up radiograph of a benign pleural tumour.

tumour advances the fluid tends to be replaced by tumour tissue. Mediastinal and hilar gland involvement occurs but is not clinically important although often found at post-mortem, as is other blood-borne spread to liver, contralateral lung, bone, adrenals and meninges.

Histological features fall into four patterns: epithelial, sarcomatous, mixed and desmoplastic. The histological type allows for survival estimates using median life expectancy: sarcomatous 6 months, mixed 11 months, epithelial 14 months and desmoplastic 18 months. The major modifier is the stage of the disease at presentation.

Clinical features

Localized pleural lesions rarely produce symptoms and are often diagnosed by chance on a routine chest radiograph. The commonest symptoms are dyspnoea, chest pain and cough, although occasionally they may be associated with joint pains, chills, pyrexia and finger clubbing. Pleural effusions rarely occur with this type of tumour. Localized pleural lesions are commonly peripherally situated, forming a D-shaped homogeneous opacity against the inner aspect of the chest wall. Oblique views and CT may improve the pre-operative diagnostic understanding for planned treatment.

There are no characteristic features associated with a diffuse malignant mesothelioma although a history of exposure to asbestos demands a high index of suspicion. Chest discomfiture and fatigue are the commonest symptoms often associated with a large pleural effusion. Cough and weight loss are not uncommon presenting features. Pain may be a very severe persistent symptom indicating advanced disease at presentation. Abdominal distension with palpable hard masses may occur if the peritoneum is involved. The disease progresses relentlessly with a prognosis of 6–18 months. The diagnosis may be suspected from the chest radiological appearance: a fixed mediastinum in the midline with loss of volume on the affected side and obvious pleural thickening onto the mediastinum.

The tumour may eventually spread to involve the lung parenchyma, mediastinum and diaphragm. CT gives a good picture of the extent of pleural involvement and will also indicate the presence of an effusion even in an extensive mesothelioma (Figure 51.10). Any effusion should be aspirated and its cellular content examined. The diagnosis of mesothelioma can be difficult unless histological proof is obtained. Thoracoscopy and open biopsy with aspiration of effusion to dryness and inspection of trapped lung confirm the diagnosis and allow for palliation judgements.

Management

In the UK, diffuse malignant mesothelioma is a proscribed industrial disease, and patients suspected of suffering from it should be referred to the Benefits Agency. If the patient is in receipt of a disability pension his or her death needs be reported to the coroner.

Treatment

The appropriate treatment for localized pleural lesions is excision, which usually presents no difficulty although recurrence can occasionally occur.

Diffuse malignant mesothelioma management is essentially that of accurate diagnosis and palliation with terminal care. Radical pleuropneumonectomy may be an attempt at cure in a few less aggressive cases diagnosed at an early stage but there are few survivors after 3 years. Responses to cytotoxic drugs are under intense investigation. Methotrexate is most effective with a response rate over 35% but again long-term survival is not improved. Multi-modal therapy is under review with resection, cytotoxic agents and radiotherapy but as yet no improvement in survival is extant.

Large pleural effusions should be drained at thoracoscopy and trapped lung identified. There should be no rush to pleurodesis as the effusions recur slowly. The space may fill with tumour and further drainage may be unnecessary. If the lung is mobile and expands to fill the hemithorax after drainage of the effusion, parietal decortication or talc pleurodesis is effective if the recurrent effusion requires control. The Denver shunt may be useful in persistent recurrent effusion with trapped lung.

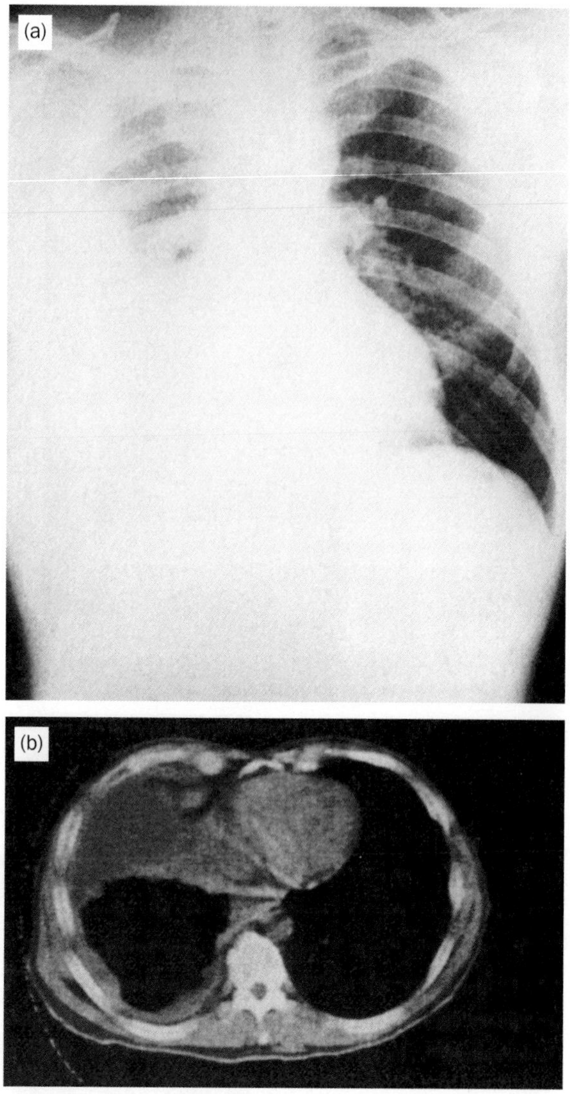

Figure 51.10 PA chest radiograph (a) and CT scan (b) of a patient with a diffuse malignant mesothelioma.

Currently the vogue is to treat the biopsy site with local radiotherapy to control recurrence in the track. Adequate analgesia for relief of chest wall pain is essential together with appropriate supportive measures for terminal care.

Section 51.5 • Spontaneous pneumothorax

Pneumothorax (air in the pleural space) was recognized in the nineteenth century usually as a complication of pulmonary tuberculosis. With the advent of chest radiography the frequent occurrence of spontaneous pneumothorax not associated with active tuberculosis was recognized. A pneumothorax may be limited when the volume of air and amount of lung collapse is prevented by pleural adhesions. Otherwise the whole lung recoils towards the hilum with the air lying free in the pleural space, the collapse being limited by the closure of the leak.

A **tension pneumothorax** develops when a valve-like mechanism comes into play. Air enters the space on inspiration repeatedly and the mediastinum is displaced and the hemidiaphragm depressed. If the tension continues to develop the venous return and oxygenation are impaired and cardiovascular collapse is imminent.

Several factors may predispose to the development of a spontaneous pneumothorax, of which the following are the most important:

- The formation of **subpleural blebs** containing air which has leaked through minor injuries in the alveolar walls and tracked up to collect at the apices, often bilaterally. Minor scars and subpleural blebs are common and are thought to be gravitational stresses from the upright position.
- The development of a **bulla** as part of generalized emphysema, in α_1-antitrypsin deficiency or in paraseptal or postfibrotic emphysema (Figure 51.11).
- Following diffuse **air trapping** in generalized emphysema or severe asthma when there may be leakage of air from the rupture of alveoli in different areas.
- **Hyperinflation** of alveoli during intermittent positive pressure ventilation.
- **Progressive dilatation and rupture** of congenital cysts (Figure 51.12), the pneumatoceles of childhood staphylococcal pneumonias or occasionally of the cysts which may develop in tuberculosis, carcinoma, honeycomb lung or pneumoconiosis and cystic fibrosis.

Clinical features

Spontaneous pneumothoraces are most common in association with apical gravitational stress, occurring from the age of 14 to 45 years. They are more common in men and tend to occur in taller individuals, supporting the gravitational stress thesis. Patients with chronic bronchitis and emphysema are usually over 50 years old, more frequently over 70. In this group of patients with poor respiratory reserve it is often associated with the final stage of the disease and contributes to the death.

The sudden onset of unilateral pleuritic chest pain and dyspnoea is the commonest presentation. These symptoms are only rarely associated with exercise. In an otherwise healthy adult the dyspnoea may soon abate although there may be no radiological change. Alternatively, worsening dyspnoea is indicative of progressive lung collapse and may be the first sign of a tension pneumothorax, other features of which are increasing anxiety, restlessness, cyanosis, hypotension, tachycardia, clammy extremities and shock. In a severe asthma attack or during assisted ventilation a deterioration in the patient's condition should alert the clinician to the possibility of a pneumothorax, the signs of which may be masked and a radiograph is often required to establish the diagnosis. Between 3 and 5% of patients sustaining a pneumothorax also suffer significant intrapleural haemorrhage which may be associated with systemic effects, i.e. malaise, hypotension, pronounced tachycardia and poor peripheral perfusion.

The physical signs of air in the pleural space are a hyper-resonant percussion note, diminished movement and faint or absent breath sounds on the affected side. Occasionally, in a small pneumothorax, there may be a clicking sound in time with the heart beat. In a tension pneumothorax the chest wall may be distended on the affected side, with shift of the trachea and apex beat to the opposite side made worse by expiration (Figure 51.12).

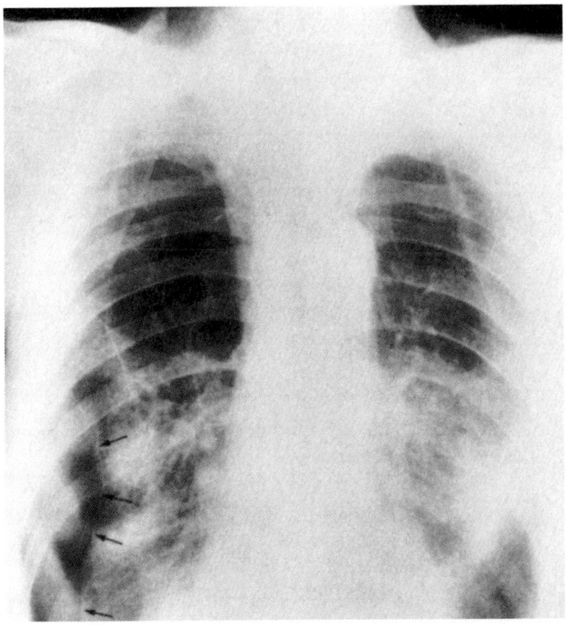

Figure 51.11 Right localized pneumothorax in a chronic bronchitic.

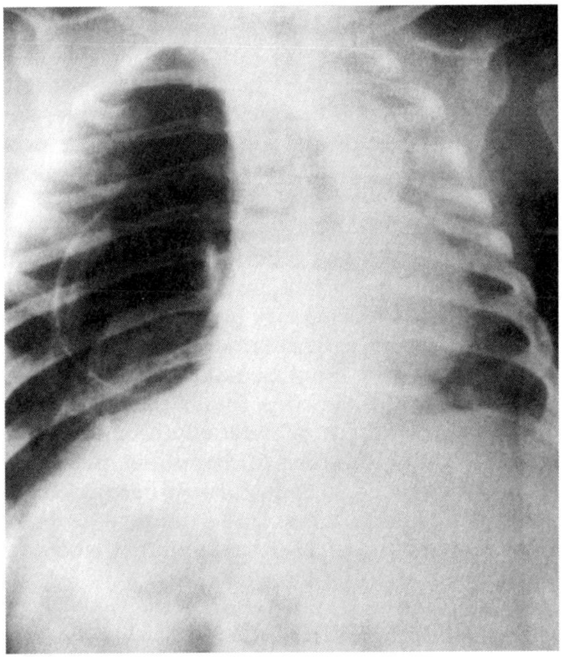

Figure 51.12 Tension cyst in a child with an associated tension pneumothorax causing mediastinal shift to the left side.

Occasionally a subpleural bleb ruptures but the visceral pleura remains intact. After tracking to the hilum, air enters the mediastinum from where it may spread to the neck producing the distinctive crepitus of subcutaneous (surgical) emphysema.

Investigations

A standard chest radiograph is the only relevant investigation. If the patient is not severely distressed, erect posteroanterior films taken on inspiration and expiration will demonstrate the extent of the pneumothorax (Figure 51.13).

Treatment

There are several methods of treatment, the choice being dictated by the clinical and radiological findings. However, even a small pneumothorax may show rapid progression or develop into a tension pneumothorax and needs a period of observation.

Conservative management

A fit patient with a pneumothorax of 30–40% may safely be observed. Once it has been established that the pneumothorax is static or resolving the patient may safely be allowed home without further treatment. A chest X-ray as an outpatient a week later should confirm progress to resolution. At least one-quarter of patients treated in this way will present later with a recurrent pneumothorax.

Needling

In patients distressed from, or in whom there is a rapidly developing tension pneumothorax, the insertion of a large-bore needle, cannula or tube into the affected hemithorax may be life-saving, relieving the situation until a more formal chest drain can be inserted.

Aspiration

With a spontaneous pneumothorax > 40% simple aspiration of the air using a wide-bore needle is successful in two-thirds of patients. If it fails it suggests that a persisting air leak and a chest drain is indicated.

Intercostal drain

Intercostal drainage is indicated if the above methods fail, in tension pneumothorax and in those with significant underlying lung pathology. It is a simple, safe technique when carried out properly and usually produces a rapid re-expansion of the lung. The pitfall is inadvertant intubation of a large lung cyst or bulla.

There are several points of importance regarding technique which should be stressed.

Site of insertion

The midaxillary line in the 4th or 5th space and the second intercostal space anteriorly in the midclavicular line are the safest sites for insertion. In a loculated or localized basal pneumothorax drainage tubes should be appropriately sited, preferably with CT scanning guidance.

Anaesthesia

A local anaesthetic is required and the chest wall should be anaesthetized in layers down to and including the pleura. The infiltrating needle should be inserted into the pleural cavity to check that the space contains air at the chosen site. Use a large volume of low concentration lignocaine (20 ml 0.5%). Maximize the effect by supplementary subcostal blocks posteriorly at 4, 5, 6 and 7 ribs.

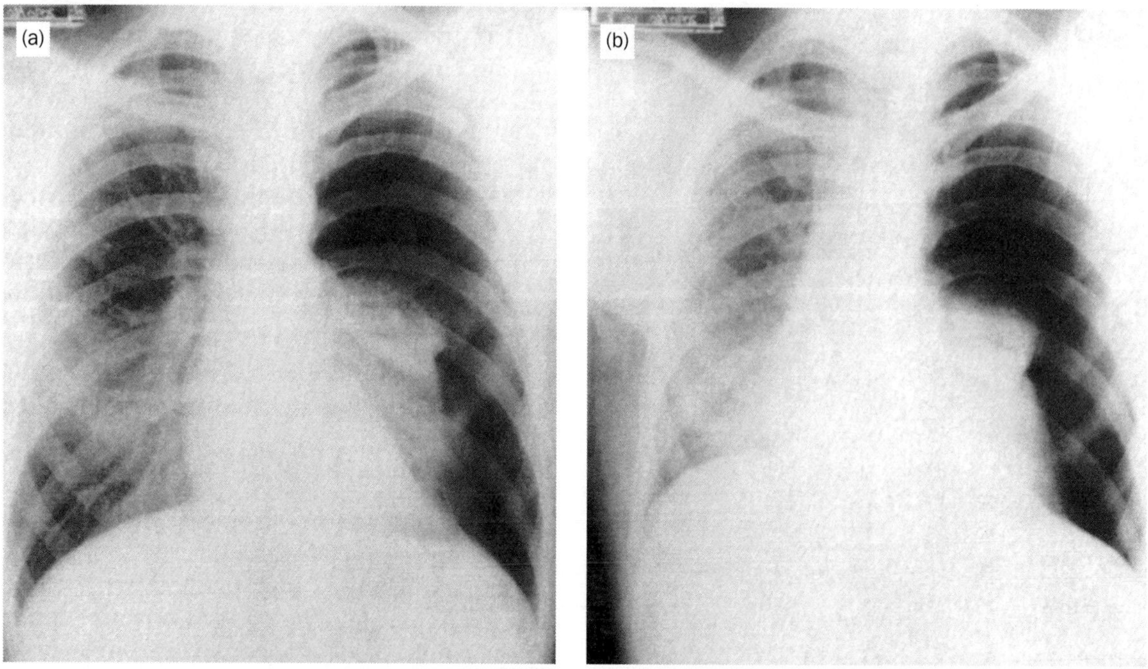

Figure 51.13 Large left pneumothorax (a) with mediastinal shift during expiration (b).

Choice of drain
The majority of clinicians now use a sterile polythene tube with a radio-opaque marker and several side holes. A size 24 Fr or larger is preferable.

Insertion of drain
The principles of Advanced Trauma Life Support now govern the insertion of chest drains. After anaesthetizing the site of insertion, under sterile conditions an incision is made in the skin and through into deeper tissues. Then with a dissecting instrument and a finger a track is developed over the upper border of the rib. The finger is inserted into the pleura to identify the pleural space and the drain inserted.

Management
When the drain is connected to the underwater seal system there should be an immediate stream of bubbles as the lung inflates. This will continue until full inflation is obtained at which point the patient may experience some pleuritic chest discomfort. Thereafter the air leak usually diminishes although some patients continue to leak large quantities of air even with the lung inflated. If clinical examination suggests the lung has fully inflated, observation and a chest X-ray before drain removal after 24 hours without an air leak is sufficient. If there is a persistent and continuing air leak beyond 7–10 days then closure at thoracoscopy with pleurodesis as necessary is indicated.

A second episode of spontaneous pneumothorax on the same side may be managed in the same way. If three or more pneumothoraces have occurred then some form of pleurodesis is required. Today this is executed at thoracoscopy, when apical bullectomy and/or pleurodesis with talc or tetracycline can be done.

Installation of talc slurry or tetracycline into the pleural space through the intercostal tube when the lung is fully expanded, with or without a small air leak is also an effective way of producing pleurodesis. This is often practised in the more fragile patient when general anaesthesia is high risk. But a word of caution: it is very painful and the patient may develop respiratory problems. Good pain control without respiratory depression is needed.

Section 51.6 • Emphysema

In emphysema the air spaces distal to the terminal bronchioles are irreversibly increased in size above the normally accepted limits as a result of either dilatation or destruction of their walls. This definition embraces a number of distinct entities, the pathogenesis of the majority being incompletely understood.

Centrilobular (centriacinar), panacinar and periacinar describe specific types of dilatation of the airspaces related to the acinus or lobule in emphysema. The centre of the lobules is principally involved in the centrilobular form while the emphysema is diffusely spread throughout the affected segment in the panacinar type. The periacinar distribution tends to occur in the subpleural region and is often associated with pneumothorax. Air spaces of more than 1 cm in diameter are referred to as bullae or cysts, the terms often being interchangeable. Emphysema may be unilateral or bilateral, segmental, lobar or generalized.

There is impairment of both ventilation and perfusion in any emphysematous area.

Impaired ventilation

The transference of gas through the distal air spaces occurs by diffusion, a process which becomes less efficient the larger the space. When the bronchus to an emphysematous area is obstructed ventilation occurs by diffusion from neighbouring alveoli via the pores of Kohn, further increasing the inefficiency of gas exchange.

Impaired perfusion

Three mechanisms – (1) attenuation and destruction of the capillary bed; (2) distension of the wall not accompanied by any increase in the capillary bed, thus the capillary alveolar interface is less efficient; and (3) hypoxia in the emphysematous space causing reflex vasoconstriction of the feeding arterioles – acting individually or in concert have been suggested as causes for the reduction in blood flow seen in emphysematous areas.

The major aspects of emphysema are categorized by cause and character. This list is neither exhaustive nor original.

Types of emphysema
Causal mechanism and type of emphysema:

- Overinflation
  - Senile
  - Fibrotic scarring
  - Compensatory
- Atrophy or hypoplasia
  - Paraseptal
  - MacLeod's syndrome
  - Lung agenesis
- Destructive process
  - α_1-antitrypsin deficiency
  - Primary emphysema
  - Associated with chronic bronchitis
- Check valve mechanism
  - Obstructive emphysema
  - Tension cysts
  - Bullae

Senile emphysema
With age the elasticity of the lungs declines, predisposing to a generalized dilatation of the air sacs which has little functional significance.

Fibrotic scarring
The alveoli around small areas of fibrosis, e.g. tuberculous scars, become distended and cysts can form, which, if lying subpleurally, may rupture causing a

spontaneous pneumothorax. The apical scarring that occurs in the lung is thought to be a maladaptation to the upright position. This is thought to be the underlying pathology in spontaneous pneumothorax.

Compensatory emphysema

This refers to the hyperinflation of a segment, lobe or lung, which follows collapse, fibrotic contraction or resection in another area. If the cause of the collapse, e.g. a foreign body, can be removed and the lung re-expands the emphysema resolves.

Compensatory emphysema is important in two contexts:

- Diagnosis: As a collapsed left lower lobe lies behind the heart it may be missed on routine radiography but an increased hypertransradiancy in the left upper zone from compensatory emphysema is an important sign.
- Post-operative function: The success of any lung resection is dependent upon the state of the remaining lung. In a healthy child requiring lobectomy for obstructive emphysema the residual lung will expand to fill the void without significant alteration in function.
- In lung resection for carcinoma careful lung function assessment may allow benefit for some patients from a volume reduction effect (*vide infra*).

Paraseptal emphysema

This occurs along connective-tissue septa, particularly-down the anterior lung margin, and is thought to result from atrophy in the surrounding lung tissue lessening support and allowing the alveoli to distend. This is again part of the gravity induced pathology of the upright position. Clinically it has significance as a cause of spontaneous pneumothorax or giant bullae.

Macleod's syndrome

MacLeod's syndrome is a condition in which there is unilateral panacinar emphysema resulting from arrested development of a lung occurring between birth and 8 years of age, the other lung being unaffected. Few patients recall any childhood illnesses although the syndrome has been shown to follow measles and tuberculosis. Most patients are asymptomatic, being diagnosed on routine chest radiography. Occasionally the affected lung may be the site of persistent or recurrent infection when pneumonectomy may be considered. Alternatively, pneumonia in the unaffected lung may cause sufficient additional functional impairment to bring the disorder to light. Clinically the percussion note is hyper-resonant and the air entry diminished over the affected lung.

Radiologically there is unilateral hypertransradiancy with a decrease in hilar and peripheral vascular markings and a shift of the mediastinum to the unaffected side on expiratory films. Contrast thoracic CT confirms the small pulmonary artery and bronchiectatic bronchial tree. There is reduced ventilation, the affected lung accounting for less than 10% of the oxygen uptake. Other causes of unilateral hypertransradiancy, e.g. congenitally absent pectoral muscles and mastectomy, must be excluded. If the remaining lung is healthy there are usually few problems but any respiratory infection should be promptly treated.

Lung agenesis

Agenesis of one lung leads to considerable enlargement of the other, the disorder presenting as progressive emphysema in the third or fourth decade.

α_1-Antitrypsin deficiency

The lung contains high concentrations of the proteolytic enzyme trypsin, which is thought to play an important role in the removal of foreign and damaged proteins from the circulation. In congenital α_1-antitrypsin deficiency the levels of this enzyme may be insufficient to deactivate the available trypsin. Following an insult to the lung, e.g. by smoking, a process of autodigestion begins with the progressive destruction of alveolar tissue and the formation of large bullae initially in the lower lobes (Figure 51.14). Patients usually present between the ages of 30 and 50 with progressive dyspnoea and a chest X-ray showing basal bullous emphysema. Resection of the affected lobes may produce temporary improvement but the process inevitably recurs in the remaining lung. As α_1-antitrypsin levels and phenotype measurements are readily available, family studies are recommended with genetic counselling and advice to affected youngsters regarding smoking.

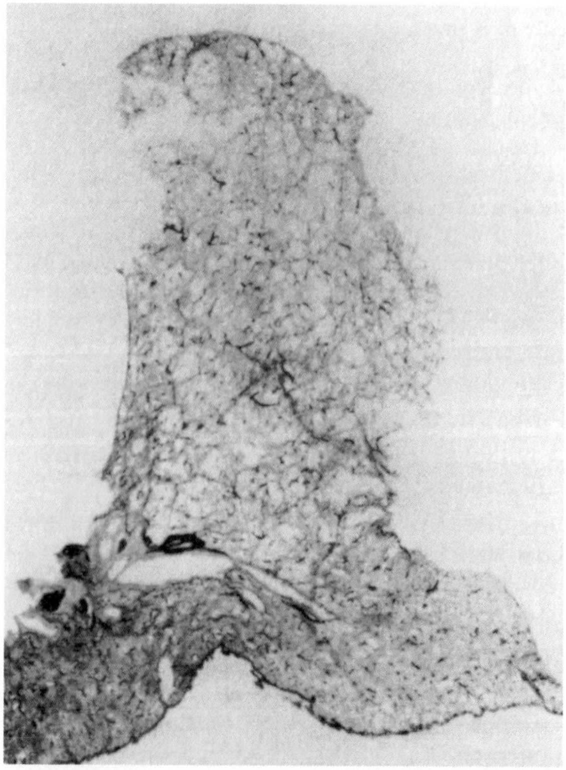

Figure 51.14 Slice through the right lower lobe in a patient with α_1-antitrypsin deficiency showing diffuse emphysematous change.

Primary emphysema (vanishing lung)

In this condition generalized involvement arises from widespread destruction of the alveolar walls producing varying sized air sacs. There may be pathological evidence of associated chronic bronchitis. The disease progresses remorselessly to early death from respiratory failure (Figure 51.15).

Primary emphysema is believed to develop as a result of autodigestion although the mechanism is not fully understood. The constituents of cigarette smoke or inhaled irritants are believed to induce an inflammatory reaction at the level of the terminal bronchioles and alveolar sacs, which leads to an accumulation of alveolar macrophages and white blood cells in the affected area. Both types of cell are rich in proteolytic enzymes which normally destroy ingested foreign proteins and bacteria. Other constituents of cigarette smoke damage both the alveolar macrophages and the white blood cells leading to the local release of high concentrations of these proteolytic enzymes. Under normal circumstances the blood contains antiproteolytic enzymes which deactivate any proteolytic enzymes that are released in the lungs.

Unfortunately, cigarette smoke contains agents which inactivate the antiproteolytic enzymes, undermining this defence mechanism. Thus the released proteolytic enzymes embark on a process of progressive autodigestion of terminal bronchi and alveolar spaces replacing them by emphysematous cysts.

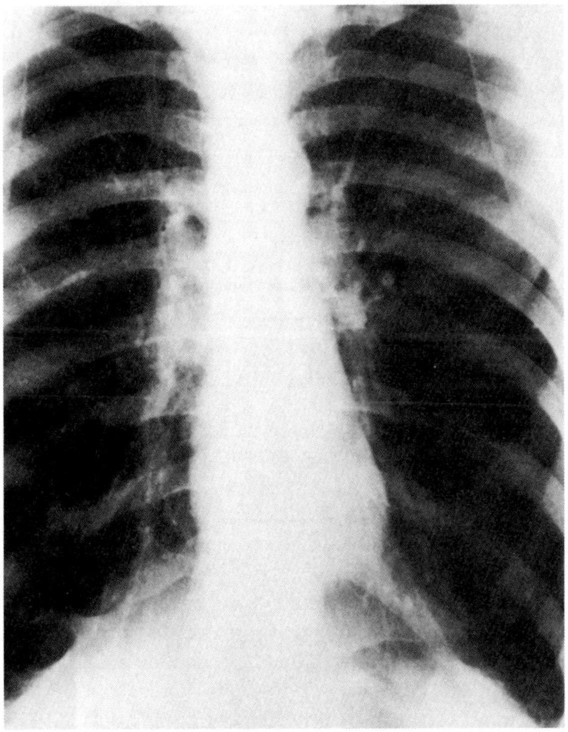

Figure 51.15 PA film showing loss of lung architecture (vanishing lung), depression of the diaphragm revealing 11th and 12th ribs, and widening of the rib spaces. This is typical of advanced primary emphysema.

Obstructive emphysema

Partial obstruction of a bronchus may lead to segmental or lobar emphysema through a check-valve mechanism, i.e. the air entering during inspiration cannot fully escape on expiration causing 'air trapping'. It may be the earliest sign of an inhaled foreign body (particularly in children) and rarely of bronchial carcinoma. Radiologically there is an area of hypertransradiancy which fails to deflate on expiration, causing a shift of the mediastinum to the contralateral side. Xenon slowly enters the zone during a ventilation scan. The obstructive emphysema progresses with compression of normal lung tissue and dyspnoea which may require surgical relief. Rarely, unilateral or bilateral obstructive emphysema arises from obstruction in the mediastinum, e.g. enlarged bronchogenic cyst or tuberculous glands, when exploration may be necessary.

This condition in a previously well child is a surgical emergency and is caused by an inhaled foreign body. If any child is thought to have inhaled a foreign body bronchoscopy is mandatory. Asphyxia remains the commonest cause of death in children aged 1–5 years in the Western world.

Tension cyst

In infancy the partial obstruction of a bronchus feeding a congenital cyst may lead to its progressive enlargement with compression of the surrounding lung causing acute dyspnoea, when resection of the cyst may be life-saving. These tension cysts of congenital origin may present in young adults who benefit greatly from resection of such lesions.

Emphysematous bullae

Many apical bullae result from paraseptal or postfibrotic emphysema. Basal bullae may complicate α_1-antitrypsin deficiency. Of greater clinical importance are the giant bullae which occur most frequently in association with primary emphysema.

A bulla may protrude from the lung being attached by a narrow pedicle, when resection and obliteration of the stem can be readily achieved or, alternatively, it may be broadly based lying either superficially where it is covered by pleura or deep within the lung when much of a lobe or segment may be involved.

A bulla arises as a result of the destructive process causing emphysema where a differential dilatation occurs. Although check-valve mechanisms have been postulated nothing has ever been demonstrated pathologically. The laws of physics would suggest La Place's law applies and once a differential in radius develops, larger diameter bullae will tend to expand as the wall tension/interalveolar pressure relationships dictate. As a bulla enlarges local compression of the surrounding lung occurs. The re-inflation of compressed potentially functioning lung underlies the operative management in all types of emphysema.

Most apical bullae are asymptomatic, being picked up at routine radiography (Figure 51.16) and need only periodic review. They may cause spontaneous

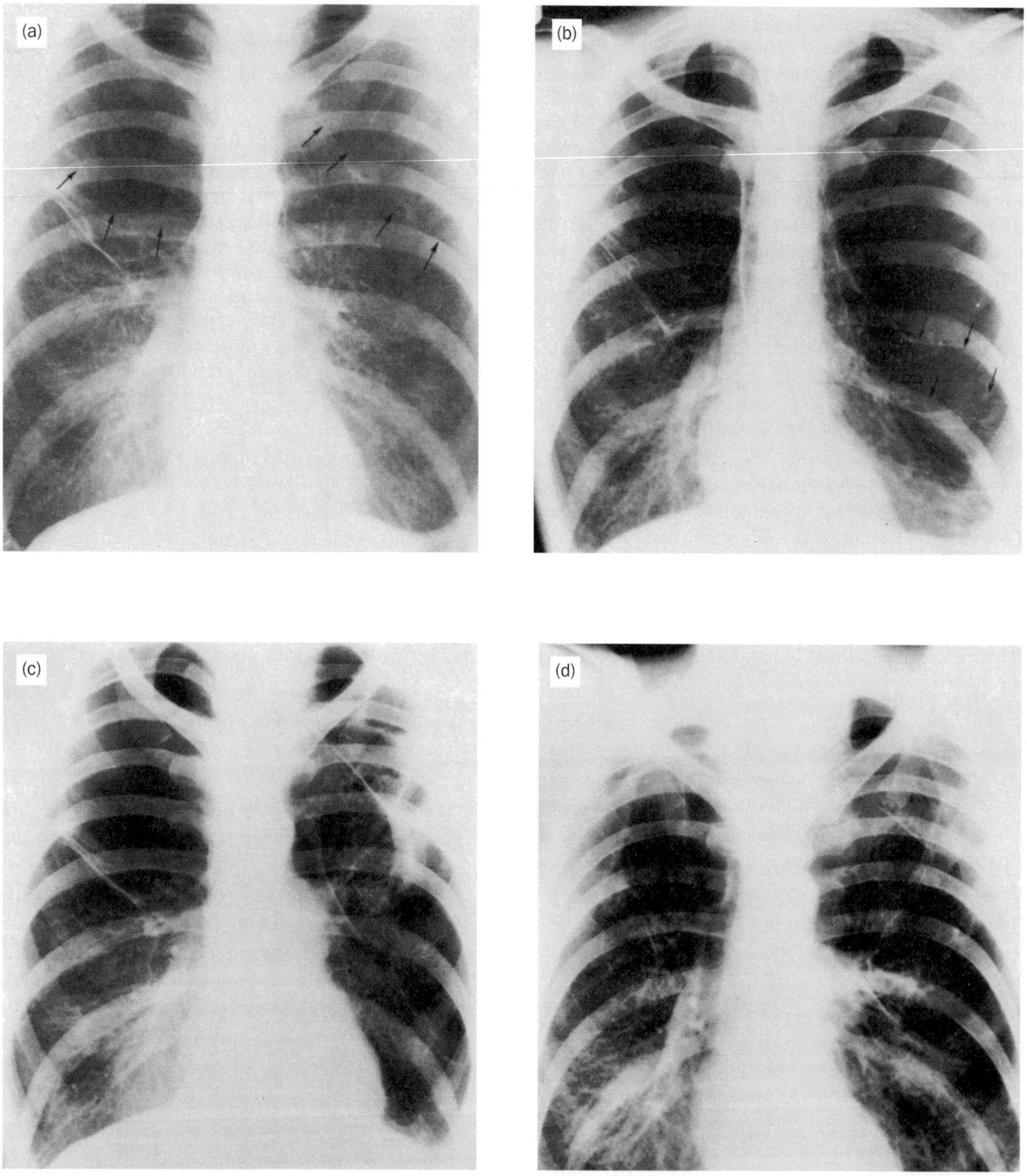

Figure 51.16 (a) Large emphysematous bullae in both apices. Chest film taken in 1971. (b) Follow-up film in 1974 demonstrating compression of the left lower lobe by the expanding bullae. (c) 1975, marked radiological improvement after a Monaldi procedure on the left side. The procedure improved the patient's breathlessness considerably. (d) Follow-up film in 1979 after a Monaldi procedure on the right side. The patient was active and mobile for some years afterwards.

pneumothorax and if this is recurrent, obliteration may be indicated. Rarely a large bulla causes chest discomfort, when resection may be helpful.

Management of emphysema

As the emphysema worsens the patient expends considerable energy in hyperventilating to maintain his arterial oxygen tension. The chest remains hyperinflated throughout respiration and during inspiration there may be paradoxical indrawing of the lower ribs resulting from the action of the flattened diaphragm. Air entry is poor but there may be a few added sounds. The liver may be palpable from the downward displacement of the diaphragm.

Treatment is mainly supportive using bronchodilators and oxygen. Patients with primary emphysema and some cases of α_1-antitrypsin deficiency have undergone single lung transplantation. Single lung transplant is very effective but the availability of organs is poor. Rationing in Great Britain is to 60 year olds and younger.

The majority of giant bullae occur in patients with long-standing chronic obstructive airways disease. In many patients with large bullae the underlying lung has multiple further bullae as a manifestation of bullous emphysema. Their appearance may lead to a worsening in the patient's condition although it is often difficult to assess their contribution to the overall functional impairment. If the respiratory function is reasonable, a period of observation and full medical treatment for the underlying obstructive airways disease, i.e. bronchodilators, antibiotics, oxygen and occasionally corticosteroids should be encouraged. Pulmonary rehabilitation is an increasingly valuable therapy and will improve many patients' coping strategies. Pulmonary rehabilitation is a valuable pre-operative tool for volume reduction and lung transplantation procedures. This often produces a significant clinical improvement but should the patient's condition continue to deteriorate or if the initial impairment is severe, operative treatment for the bullae should be considered. The development of volume reduction procedures followed the evaluation of excision of bullae. The principle of removal of non-functional expanded areas of lung, i.e. bullae, to improve the recruitment of compressed functional lung for ventilation is now extended to heterogeneous emphysema. Apical poorly functioning lung can be excised with modern techniques minimizing the air leaks.

Careful evaluation of patients is necessary prior to operation and includes:

- detailed respiratory function tests with transfer function
- HRCT of the lung to define the extent of a bulla and determine the state of the remaining lung particularly heterogeneity and other bullae
- bronchoscopy
- ventilation and perfusion scanning for functional assessment
- shuttle walk test.

Various operative procedures are available depending on the patient's condition and the extent of the disease for the management of bullae, although open procedures are very similar to volume reduction for emphysema.

If the patient is severely disabled with a large superficial bulla, a one-stage Monaldi procedure with the introduction of a catheter into the space to allow gradual deflations over several weeks should be considered. Operative mortality is low and significant functional improvement may be obtained even though symptoms are likely to recur at a later date (Figure 51.16).

Thoracotomy or thoracoscopy with stapling excision and use of tissue sealants is effective although a bilateral approach via a median sternotomy is popular.

Following thoracotomy the post-operative course may be stormy depending on the underlying obstructive airways disease. Adequate analgesia and aggressive physiotherapy are essential. If respiratory failure ensues controlled oxygen therapy will be required, because of the character of the lung operation positive pressure is avoided if at all possible. The operative and immediate post-thoracotomy mortality for severe cases has been as high as 10–15%; but improved control of persistent air leak and peri-operative care, improving case selection and earlier intervention are steadily improving outcomes.

With careful selection considerable subjective improvement can be obtained which may be reflected in improved respiratory function tests. The underlying disease process is usually progressive and respiratory failure from recurrence of bullae or emphysema may develop in time, but if the quality of life has been improved in the intervening period intervention will have been justified. Such operative management is now used for staged management prior to lung transplantation.

Further reading

Antony, V. B. (1998). Clinics in chest medicine. *Diseases of the Pleura*, Vol. 19. Philadelphia, PA: W.B. Saunders.

Seaton, A., Seaton, D. and Leitch, A. G. (2000). *Crofton and Douglas's Respiratory Diseases*, 5th edn. Oxford: Blackwell Science.

MODULE 52

Tumours of the lung

1 • Bronchogenic carcinoma
2 • Small cell lung cancer
3 • Metastatic pulmonary tumours
4 • Rare lung tumours

The most common pulmonary tumours are metastases. These can occur with any malignancy but typically arise from breast, gastrointestinal, renal, melanoma and osteogenic primaries although intrapulmonary metastatic spread from a primary bronchogenic carcinoma is not uncommon. Primary pulmonary tumours can be divided into benign and malignant types and further stratified according to histological characteristics identified by light microscopy which relate to the presence of characteristic features of different cell types such as keratin production in squamous tumours (Table 52.1). This chapter will be predominantly concerned with bronchogenic carcinoma as this is the most frequent lung neoplasm and, indeed, the commonest cause of cancer death for both men and women in the UK. Unfortunately, bronchogenic carcinoma is a generic term that includes all carcinomatous lesions. This is somewhat unhelpful as it includes a range of tumours in which there are significant differences regarding pathological features and clinical management. For this reason it is customary to differentiate between small cell lung cancer (SCLC) and other carcinomas, with the latter frequently being referred to as non-small cell lung cancer (NSCLC).

Section 52.1 • Bronchogenic carcinoma

Epidemiology

Bronchogenic carcinoma affects approximately 36 000 people each year in the UK. It can arise without any obvious predisposing cause but the risk of developing this disease is known to be increased by several factors (Table 52.2).

Cigarette smoking

The association with cigarette smoking was first demonstrated in case controlled studies nearly 50 years ago. These demonstrated a 10–20-fold increase in risk compared with non-smokers and a progressive yearly decrease in risk after cessation of smoking. Despite the strength of the evidence regarding the adverse effects of smoking and widespread dissemination of this information, smoking still remains the most important causative factor. Cigarette tar contains many potentially carcinogenic agents, notably the *N*-nitrosamines of which there are various tobacco specific types, of which NNK [4-(methylnitrosamine)-1-(3-pyridyl)-1-butanone] appears to be the most important with regard to lung cancer and is known to induce DNA mutations. Others have been implicated in carcinoma of the oesophagus, bladder, pancreas, mouth and upper airway, all of which are more frequent in smokers.

Table 52.1 Pathological groupings of primary lung tumours

Tissue element	*Benign*	*Malignant*
Epithelial	Adenoma	Adenocarcinoma Squamous carcinoma Large cell carcinoma Adenosquamous
Epithelial of salivary gland type		Adenoid cystic carcinoma Mucoepidermoid carcinoma
Epithelial with neuroendocrine features		Small cell carcinoma Carcinoid: Typical Atypical
Lymphoid		Lymphoma
Mesenchymal	Adenochondroma	Sarcoma

Table 52.2 Factors associated with the development of bronchogenic carcinoma

- Cigarette smoking
- Exposure to: arsenic, abestos, heavy metals (beryllium, cadmium, chromium, nickel), radon, silica, chloromethyl ethers, vinyl chloride, polycyclic aromatic compounds
- Gender
- Diet

Although cigarette smoking is strongly associated with bronchogenic carcinoma, less than 20% of smokers develop lung cancer, suggesting that individual susceptibility is an important component. This may be influenced by genetic factors which determine how carcinogens are absorbed and metabolized within the lung tissue and how susceptible the individual is to mutagens.

Interestingly, attempts to reduce the nicotine and tar content of cigarettes have been temporally associated with an increase in peripheral adenocarcinomas. One hypothesis advanced to explain this phenomenon is that the smoker is then driven by nicotine need to inhale more deeply and more frequently thereby subjecting more peripheral parts of the bronchial tree to carcinogens. Secondary smoking has been calculated to increase the risk to non-smokers by about 30%.

Industrial exposure

Most exposure to the chemicals and minerals listed in Table 52.2 occurs within an industrial setting. Although health awareness has been greatly increased in this area there is a legacy of exposure that will still be reflected in new cases of bronchogenic carcinoma for years to come. This is particularly relevant to asbestos exposure as fibres remain within the thorax permanently. Asbestos is thought to increased the risk of developing bronchogenic carcinoma in existing smokers by 1.5–5-fold yielding a very significant overall risk approaching 30 times that of non-smokers. It should also be noted that while radon, which damages lung tissue by alpha particle release, is normally associated with uranium mines, it can also be found in domestic buildings from ground release.

Gender

Although bronchogenic carcinoma remains more frequent in males, the rate in females has increased whilst that in males has decreased (Figure 52.1). This can partly be explained by the post-war increase in cigarette use among women. It is interesting to note that bronchogenic carcinoma is more common in non-smoking women than men (odds ratio 1.2–1.7) but, as with secondary smoking, this effect has to be seen within the context of the very low basic risk of developing bronchogenic carcinoma for non-smokers.

Diet

A carotene intake in the lowest quartile has been shown to be associated with a 50–100% increase in bronchogenic carcinoma risk suggesting that vitamin A and beta-carotene may have a protective value. Studies of dietary supplementation have, however, shown either no benefit or, paradoxically, have been stopped due to increased mortality in the supplementation group. Diet may be a surrogate for other issues or only a relevant consideration in those with a deficient intake.

Molecular biological aspects of bronchogenic carcinoma

One possible mechanism for the evolution of malignancy including bronchogenic carcinoma is the occur-

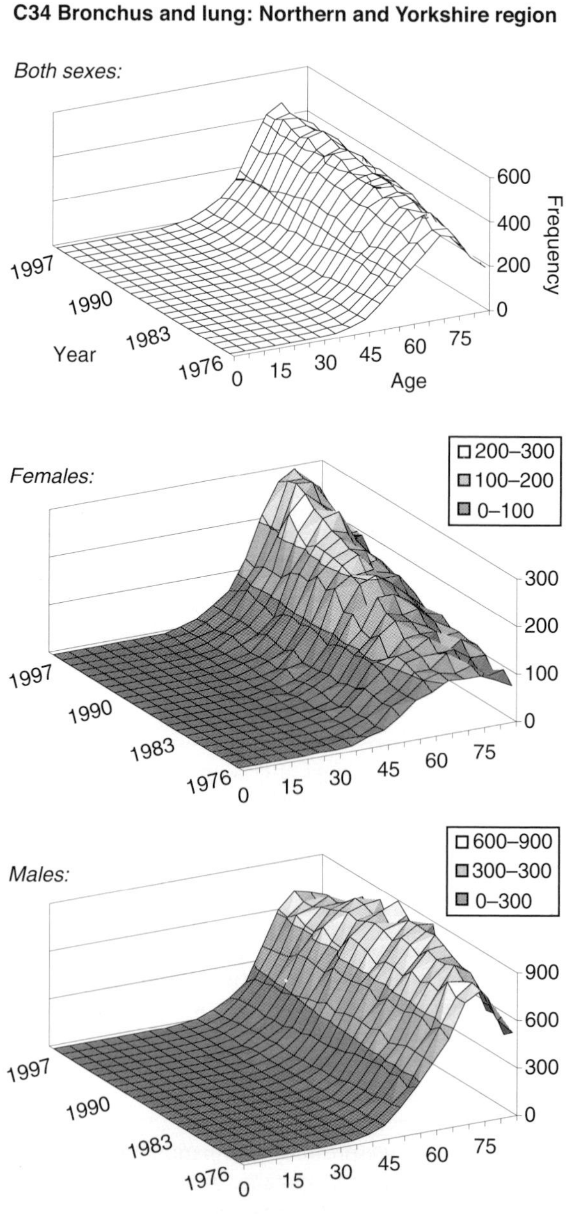

Figure 52.1 Change in incidence of male and female bronchogenic carcinoma between 1976 and 1997. Note the large increase in female and small decrease in male incidence. (Source – Yorkshire Cancer Registry Data.)

rence of DNA errors either as a sporadic phenomenon or as a result of a mutagenic stimulus. These errors give rise to abnormalities in cancer-related genes which are involved in regulation of cell proliferation or cell death, facilitating neoplastic growth. From a functional perspective, these cancer-related genes may be categorized as oncogenes where the oncogenic effect results from overactivity of the genes that enhance cell growth (proto-oncogenes) or as onco-suppressor genes where loss or inactivation of the gene causes malignant transformation. In general, oncogenes exert their actions via:

- signal transduction proteins
- nuclear proteins
- growth factors
- growth factor receptors.

The end result is to promote cell proliferation and to interrupt the normal processes that cause abnormal cells to die through apoptosis.

These molecular mechanisms may prove useful in facilitating diagnosis and identifying poor prognosis subgroups and as the basis for potential new treatment strategies.

Oncogenes

Proto-oncogenes

Activation of a number of proto-oncogenes has been implicated in bronchogenic carcinoma. Well-established examples (Table 52.3) include:

myc. This family of genes codes for nuclear phosphoproteins which appear to be important mediators of proliferation, differentiation and apoptosis. They have been described particularly in SCLC but also in NSCLC.

K-ras. This oncogene codes for a protein, K-ras, which is a membrane-associated G-protein linking tyrosine-kinase growth factor receptors to the cytoplasmic signal transduction cascade. Normally, this protein has GTPase activity and is activated by binding GTP and inactivated by binding GDP. K-ras mutation occurs in bronchogenic adenocarcinoma causing loss of GTPase activity. This leaves the protein persistently bound to GTP and hence activated, leading to unregulated cellular proliferation. The NNK *N*-nitrosamine found in tobacco smoke is associated with DNA mutations resulting in the activation of k-ras oncogenes in animal adenocarcinoma models.

Her2/neu. This oncogene codes for $p185^{HER2}$, a tyrosine-kinase associated membrane growth factor receptor. Overexpression of Her2/neu is found in 30–60% of NSCLC but not in SCLC.

bcl-2. Apoptosis is a process of programmed cell death in which the dead cells do not lyse thereby inducing an inflammatory response but are phagocytosed by macrophages. The protein coded for by this gene is a major inhibitor of apoptosis. Overexpression of bcl-2 is reported in 15–40% of primary bronchogenic carcinoma.

Tumour suppressor genes

These genes are negative regulators of the cell cycle so that loss or inactivation may result in cell proliferation. The best known example of this type of gene is p52. Loss of p53 activity is the most common genetic abnormality identified in lung cancer and is found in 90% of SCLC and 60% of NSCLC. This defect does not seem to affect long-term survival but it may decrease the effectiveness of chemotherapy as p53 is involved in the regulation of apoptosis due to DNA damage. Other examples include the genes coding for RBI, p16 and cyclin D1, all of which are concerned with control of the cell cycle. Abnormalities within these three genes collectively are found in over 90% of bronchogenic carcinoma.

Promoting tumour survival

In a teleological sense it is in the interest of malignant cells to promote their own survival. There are several examples of this phenomenon in bronchogenic carcinoma:

- As noted above, malignant cells may escape apoptosis due to the actions of oncogenes. They may also extend self-protection by secretory functions. For example, Fas-ligand (Fas-L) secreted by malignant cells will bind to receptors on T-lymphocytes and cause them to die thus interfering with an important component of cellular immunity. Fas-L production is described in 80–90% of bronchogenic carcinomas.
- Many bronchogenic carcinoma cancers express telomerase. This enables them to maintain telomere length which otherwise shortens with each cell reproduction until inadequate length is left for further reproduction.
- Growth factors secreted by malignant cells influence their own (autocrine) growth and that of other cells (paracrine). Some are exclusive to NSCLC, some to SCLC and some are common to both.
- Growing tissue requires a blood supply. This is stimulated via a variety of tumour derived cytokine products such as vascular endothelial growth factor, interleukin-8 (IL-8), platelet derived endothelial growth factor, and basic fibroblast growth factor, all of which promote angiogenesis.

Table 52.3 Examples of proto-oncogenes in bronchogenic carcinoma

Area of effect	*Oncogenes*	*Mechanism*
Nuclear transcription factors	c-myc, L-myc	Amplification/overexpression
Membrane-associated G protein	K-ras	Mutation/loss of GTPase activity
Growth factor receptor kinases	Her2/neu	Amplification/overexpression
Cytoplasmic kinases	c-src	Inappropriate expression
Apoptosis inhibitor	bcl-2	Inappropriate expression

Adapted from Kalemkerian, G. P., Pass, H. I. Present concepts in the molecular biology of lung cancer. In: Shields, T. W., LoCicero, J., Ponn, R. B. eds. *General Thoracic Surgery*, 5th edn. Philadelphia, PA: Lippincott Williams and Wilkins, 2000.

Pathological features of carcinoma of the lung

Initial development

It was formerly thought that malignancy may develop in bronchial mucosa through a sequence which proceeds from hyperplasia through metaplasia and dysplasia before culminating in carcinoma *in situ*. This sequence follows a logical process of deterioration such as might be expected with continued exposure to carcinogens in tobacco smoke. Unfortunately, while molecular biological abnormalities (p53, K-ras, etc.) can be found in these abnormal mucosae, the sequence of events may not follow this pathway. It is not even clear whether these changes are necessarily pre-malignant as regression has often been observed and tumours may arise at sites separate from an area of change under surveillance. Ultimately, these features may be best regarded as indicative of a bronchial tree with potentially unstable mucosa at risk of malignant change.

From a cellular perspective, it is also unclear whether all lung tumours arise from differentiation of a pluripotential stem cell (currently the favoured concept) or whether different tumours may have come from different originating cells. Although cellular heterogeneity is common in lung tumours, this could argue for either situation.

Specific cell types

Epithelial

Squamous carcinoma

This histological group is the most common found in the UK where it accounts for about 35% of bronchogenic carcinoma. Interestingly, this is not the case in North America or Japan where adenocarcinoma is now more frequent. It is more likely to develop in the central areas of the lung and tends to spread in a step-wise manner with late blood borne dissemination and a relatively slow doubling time. Peripheral squamous carcinomas may develop central necrosis and cavitate. Cavitation is more likely with squamous carcinoma but it is not a diagnostic feature as it can be seen with any cell type.

Microscopically, the tumour consists of groups of polygonal cells which exhibit stratification and intercellular bridge formation. Keratin may be produced and can form epithelial pearls. Histological variants include clear cell, papillary and basaloid types. A small cell variant is described which has a different chromatin pattern and different immunohistochemical profile to neuroendocrine small cell carcinoma. Spindle cell patterns occur which can cause confusion with sarcoma.

Adenocarcinoma

Approximately 30% of UK and European bronchogenic carcinoma exhibit this form of histology. Adenocarcinoma may be more common in the pulmonary periphery. It often grows more rapidly than squamous carcinoma but some peripheral lesions may progress very slowly. Peripheral adenocarcinomas may arise in association with pulmonary scars and areas of fibrosis. Bronchoalveolar carcinoma is a variant which accounts for about 5% of all lung carcinoma and may present as an incidentally detected small peripheral pulmonary opacity or with a pneumonic picture due to tumorous lobar consolidation. In general, adenocarcinomas tend to metastasize early to regional lymph nodes and are more likely to present with systemic metastases when the primary lesion is still relatively small.

Light microscopy typically shows cuboidal or columnar cells with uniform nuclei and pink or vacuolated cytoplasm. The cells may be arranged in acinar or glandular patterns becoming clumped, haphazard and variably sized as differentiation becomes poorer. Bronchoalveolar tumours have a tendency to grow along alveolar septae.

Large cell carcinoma

These are tumours which appear undifferentiated at the light microscopic level. Immunohistochemistry, mucin stains and other special investigations show that this group is not a distinct entity but is rather a collection of very poorly differentiated epithelial tumours. They make up about 5–10% of bronchogenic carcinoma and tend to exhibit the aggressivity that would be anticipated with an anaplastic type of lesion.

Adenosquamous carcinoma

Approximately 5% of bronchogenic carcinoma exhibit this mixed pattern. Generally, the adeno element is more significant but the ratios differ. Earlier dissemination and poorer prognosis are described.

Epithelial of salivary gland type

These uncommon tumours arise in the submucosal glands of the tracheobronchial tree and have similarities to salivary gland growths. These are slow growing, typically affect patients in middle age and account for only 1% of all pulmonary tumours.

Adenoid cystic carcinoma

This growth usually involves the trachea and main bronchi where it accounts for about one-quarter of tumours in this location. The degree of cellular differentiation varies from a cribiform or cylindromatous type where cuboidal cells are arranged around spaces through a cord-like morphology to sheets of layered cells with high mitotic activity. The cells show duct and myoepithelial characteristics on electron microscopy with the latter being reflected in the immunohistochemical staining characteristics (keratin, vimentin, actin, S100).

This tumour characteristically grows in the submucosal layers and outside the airway particularly along the perineural tissues. Luminal encroachment is usually a late feature. Complete resection is potentially curative. When clinically detected, however, the tumour has often extended to a degree that precludes resection and when undertaken resection is not infrequently associated with positive resection margins. Long-term palliation is feasible using radiotherapy and bronchoscopic debulking.

Mucoepidermoid carcinoma

Mucoepidermoid carcinoma is one-tenth as frequent as adenoid cystic carcinoma and tends to affect the more peripheral bronchial tree. In the low-grade type clear columnar cells and goblet cells are arranged into glandular formations and the tumour grows as an endoluminal polyp with a narrow stalk and little deep invasion High-grade lesions exhibit higher mitotic rates and are more invasive. Wide local resection usually by some form of bronchoplastic procedure is curative for low-grade lesions but often impossible for high-grade lesions due to central structure invasion.

Epithelial with neuroendocrine features

Small cell carcinoma

Small cell carcinoma comprises about 25% of all bronchogenic carcinoma but a minute proportion of operated cases as it is not generally considered to be an operable condition. It is frequently (80%) central in origin and is characterized clinically by very rapid growth (doubling time 20 days) with early lymphatic and systemic metastatic spread such that it is often regarded as being metastatic at presentation. It is not uncommon to see a small peripheral small cell lesion associated with gross mediastinal lymphadenopathy.

Microscopy reveals small, round, oval or spindle shaped cells with little cytoplasm and small dark nuclei showing a finely granular chromatin pattern. Extensive necrosis is frequent.

Small cell carcinoma appear to be very active metabolically and may produce a wide range of peptides and hormones as might be expected from their neuroendocrine differentiation.

Carcinoid

Carcinoid tumours constitute about 1% of all lung tumours but a greater proportion of surgical cases as most are resectable. These tumours are divided into typical and atypical types according to the histological appearance. Most (90%) are typical carcinoids that exhibit clusters or cords of round or polygonal cells with smooth oval nuclei and few mitoses. Osseous metaplasia with calcification can occur in the tumour stroma. Atypical lesions have the same pattern but exhibit greater pleomorphism with a higher mitotic rate and show vascular invasion, necrosis and palisading. Unlike SCLC carcinoids are not associated with smoking.

The clinical progress of these lesions is often quite indolent. Peripheral lesions are usually detected as incidental radiographic findings. Central lesions may cause bronchial obstruction mimicking asthma or bronchitis and can cause haemoptysis. Typical carcinoids tend to be located centrally while atypical lesions have a more peripheral distribution. Carcinoid lesions can bleed heavily when biopsied and may require adrenaline application or a more circumspect approach including needle biopsy or even excision without biopsy.

Surgical resection is curative for most typical lesions. Atypical lesions can metastasize to lymph nodes and may recur up to 15 years after resection.

Pathological determination of cellular type

Diagnosis and classification of lung carcinoma is dependent upon good haematoxylin and eosin stained sections from formalin fixed, paraffin embedded tissue. From these, characteristic morphological appearances augmented by chemical stains such as alcian blue and mucicarmine, which may be used to highlight mucin and demonstrate glandular differentiation, may provide sufficient material to allow a diagnosis of cell type. Subclassification may, however, be difficult from small bronchoscopic biopsies where crush artefact may be a problem for the pathologist or in specimens without adequately specific features.

The main role of immunohistochemistry in the diagnosis of lung carcinoma is to differentiate small cell from non-small cell carcinoma. To this end a panel of antibodies including anti-CD56, CAM5.2 and anti-CD45 are frequently used. CD56 (N-CAM) is expressed by most neuroendocrine tumours including small cell carcinoma but very rarely and focally in non-small cell lesions. Small cell carcinomas frequently show dot-like positivity with CAM 5.2 unlike the diffuse strong staining seen in other carcinomas with this anti-cytokeratin antibody. CD45 (leucocyte common antigen) expression helps differentiate small cell carcinoma from reactive and neoplastic lymphoid infiltrates. Immunohistochemistry may also augment diagnosis of cell type in NSCLC. For example, cytokeratin 14 is specific to squamous cell carcinoma and antibodies to surfactants, and membrane-associated glycoprotein may be useful in distinguishing poorly differentiated adenocarcinoma.

Patterns of spread of bronchogenic carcinoma

As with all malignant tumours bronchogenic carcinoma will extend locally and eventually disseminate.

Local spread

The local effects of a tumour tend to depend on whether the tumour develops in a central position, i.e. in the perihilar area, or in a more peripheral location.

Central tumours often cause airway obstruction and distal pneumonia. The obstruction may be due to tumour within the lumen of the bronchus but is more commonly due to extrinsic compression. Invasion of central structures is usually a relatively late feature of locally advanced tumours and is a significant cause of inoperability. Large vessel invasion within the lung or hilum usually leads to occlusion or thrombosis rather than bronchovascular fistula and massive haemoptysis which is very uncommon. Tumour may, however, extend along the pulmonary veins into the left atrium with subsequent thrombus or tumour embolism. Dysphagia may result from oesophageal compression and progression to an oesophago-bronchial fistula is, unfortunately, well recognized. Aortic involvement occurs with advanced left sided lesions and these may also injure the left recurrent laryngeal nerve producing hoarseness. Right upper hilar lesions may involve or compress the superior vena cava (SVC) producing upper body venous hypertension (superior vena cava syndrome). Pericardial and left atrial direct invasion are well recognized and may be associated with the onset of atrial fibrillation, pericardial effusion and phrenic nerve paresis. Ventricular invasion is rare and has only been seen once by this author.

Peripheral tumours can occlude airways but these are small in the periphery of the lung so that the volume of associated collapse is correspondingly modest. Direct invasion effects from these tumours usually concern the chest wall. Initially invasion is restrained by the parietal pleura but once this is breached the tumour can extend either between the ribs or by destruction of the ribs, eventually presenting as an external mass. Invasion of the apical thoracic cage may produce a 'Pancoast' syndrome. In this condition the first rib, vertebra and lower elements of the brachial plexus are involved resulting in intractable arm pain and often a Horner's syndrome due to interruption of the sympathetic chain on the neck of the first rib. The phrenic nerve may occasionally be involved by a peripheral tumour invading the lower left pericardium. Diaphragm invasion can occur with lower lobe tumours but is uncommon.

All tumours can invade the local microstructure. Thus small blood vessel invasion is frequent and is an adverse indicator of long-term survival. Direct invasion of lymph nodes seems to be less significant prognostically than conventional spread to these nodes but lymphatic permeation particularly around the bronchus is a negative feature.

Lymphatic spread

Lymphatic spread occurs first to intrapulmonary nodes, then to the node groups at the hilum and finally to the mediastinum. In some instances the intrapulmonary and hilar nodes are bypassed so that the first involved node station is at mediastinal level. This can occur with tumours in any location but is particularly associated with left upper lobe tumours. The overall frequency of this effect varies between lobes and tumour types but is between 5 and 15%. Similarly, although upper lobe lesions tend to spread to the upper mediastinal nodes and lower lobe lesions to the lower mediastinum, any variation is possible. These findings merely underline the fact that cancer spread does not necessarily follow a set sequence. From the mediastinum, nodal spread passes to the scalene and lower cervical glands. In advanced cases gross mediastinal lymphadenopathy can cause oesophageal compression and dysphagia or SVC obstruction.

As noted above, bronchogenic carcinoma can travel along the bronchus for some distance within lymphatic vessels and/or within the submucosal layers so that a 1.5–2 cm macroscopically clean stump length is required to avoid leaving disease at the resection margin.

The question of lymph node status is extremely important in the staging of lung cancer as one part of the stratification process and as an essential element in determining operability.

Metastatic spread

Post-mortem data demonstrate that systemic spread occurs principally to liver (35%), adrenal (25%), lung (23%), brain (17%), bone (15%) and kidney (15%) and often multiple sites are involved. It does seem that the metastatic potential of a tumour is related to histological type, degree of cellular differentiation, presence of blood vessel invasion and the molecular biological processes outlined above. Interestingly, immunoassays for malignant cells can often be positive in peripheral blood samples when no clinically detectable metastatic disease is present. The importance of this finding is unclear as it may either confirm the effectiveness of anti-tumour responses to continued cell shedding or, more likely, these assays may simply be detecting portions of cell membrane debris or non-viable cells.

Initial clinical assessment of patients with bronchogenic carcinoma

The initial clinical assessment of the potential lung cancer patient is the first step in a continual filtration process designed to determine the diagnosis, extent of disease and optimal treatment for that patient. This process begins with the initial interview during which the history, examination and simple chest X-ray will enable a working diagnosis and basic management plan to be formulated. The point at issue at this stage is whether or not the patient has potentially operable disease. If not, attention will be directed towards confirming diagnosis and determining the extent of disease with a view to best non-surgical management which may include curative or palliative chemo-radiotherapy and supportive care. If surgical intervention does appear to be at least conceivable, arrangements are made to proceed with detailed surgical assessment and staging.

Many patients, particularly those seen as referrals to a surgical clinic, have no symptoms but have an abnormality on the chest film. Common presenting symptoms include:

- cough
- weight loss
- haemoptysis
- lassitude.

Specific symptoms of advanced disease include:

- chest wall pain
- headache and suffusion of the head and neck
- hoarseness
- severe weight loss
- jaundice
- bone pain.

Although non-specific, degree of weight loss is the presenting feature which has the best correlation with adverse outcome.

Examination is frequently negative in early stage tumours. Occasionally, chest findings consistent with pulmonary collapse/consolidation or effusion may be encountered. Many patients exhibit clubbing but this is

Table 52.4 Non-metastatic syndromes in bronchial carcinoma

Endocrine
Gynaecomastia
Hormone secretion: ADH, ACTH, parathormone, insulin, TSH
Neurological
Cerebellar degeneration
Myasthenic syndrome
Neuropathy
Musculoskeletal
Myopathy
Finger clubbing
Hypertropic osteoarthropathy
Cutaneous
Dermatomyositis
Scleroderma
Acanthosis nigricans
Circulatory
Non-bacterial endocarditis
Gammaglobulin abnormality
Purpura
Thrombophlebitis migrans

not universal and features of other non-metastatic syndromes occur in 10% of patients (Table 52.4). The presence of scalene lymphadenopathy, SVC obstruction, Horner's syndrome, vocal cord paresis and any features of metastatic disease such as hepatomegaly, skin deposits (5% of metastatic cases) and bony tenderness should be excluded.

Perusal of the initial chest and CT films should confirm the presence, location and nature of the lesion (Figure 52.2a–d) and may indicate areas of potential concern such as chest wall involvement (Figure 52.3), elevation of a diaphragm (Figure 52.4) and the presence of any associated pleural effusion. Modern high resolution spiral computed tomography (CT) scanning is helpful in excluding other intrapulmonary lesions which may not be evident on the initial chest film (Figure 52.5) and will demonstrate the presence and size of mediastinal nodes (Figure 52.6). The upper abdominal phase provides a useful initial screen for liver and adrenal metastases (Figure 52.7).

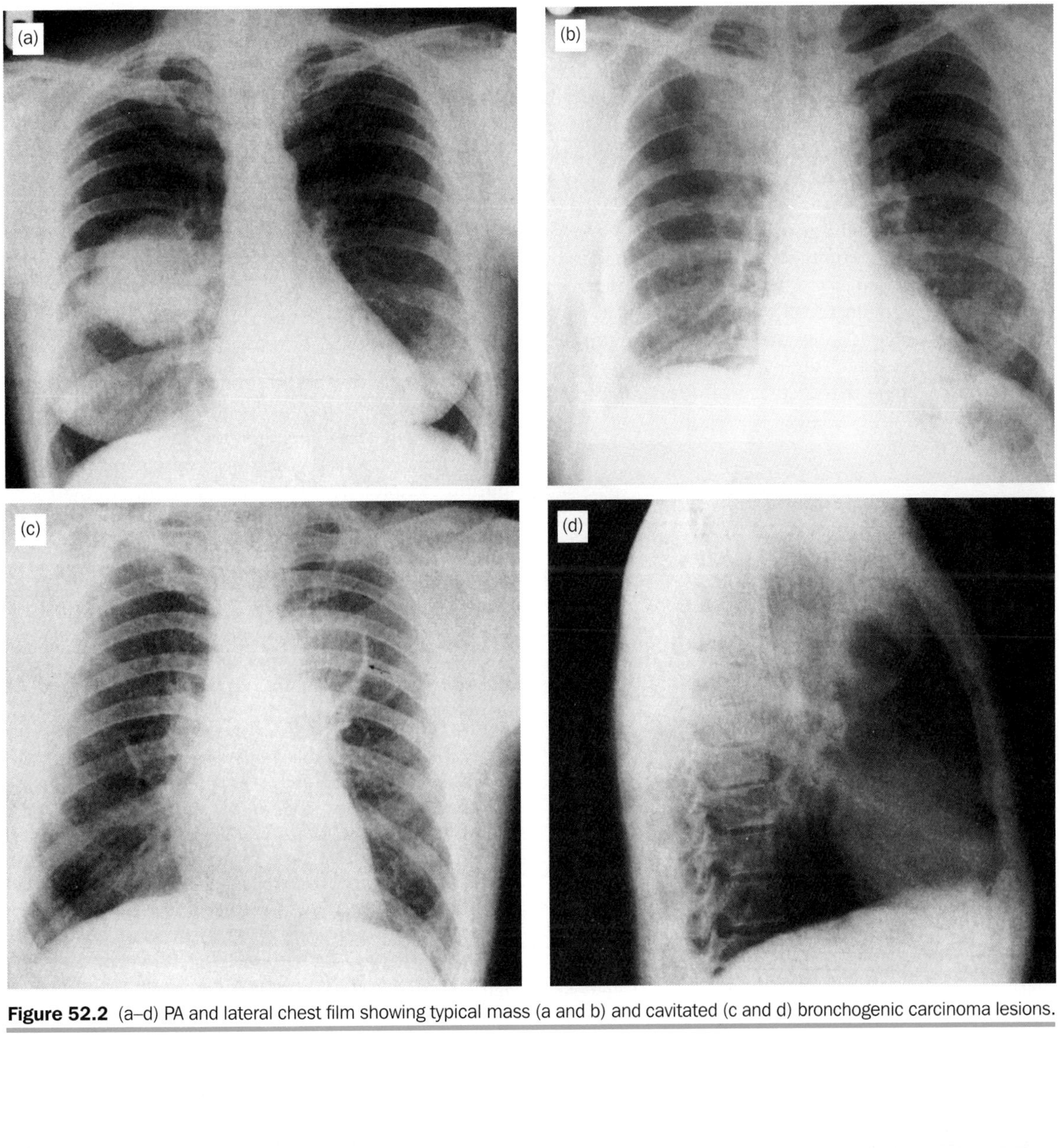

Figure 52.2 (a–d) PA and lateral chest film showing typical mass (a and b) and cavitated (c and d) bronchogenic carcinoma lesions.

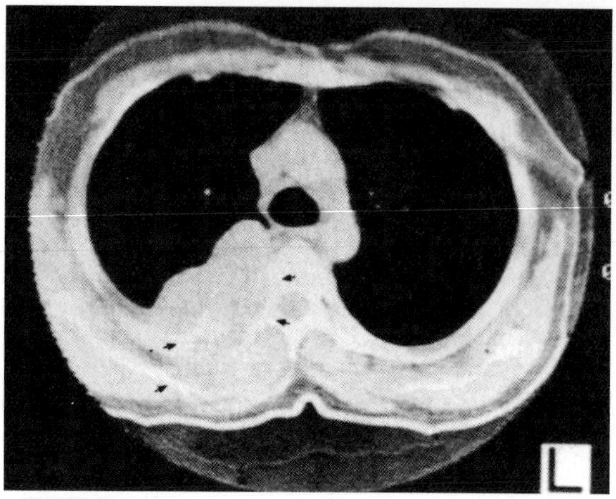

Figure 52.3 CT scan showing extensive chest wall invasion. If this occurs lateral to the posterior rib angle, resection with prosthetic replacement of the excised portion of chest wall may be possible. Medial involvement as in this case is inoperable as it is not practicably feasible to excise the tumour with a clear margin due to vertebral invasion.

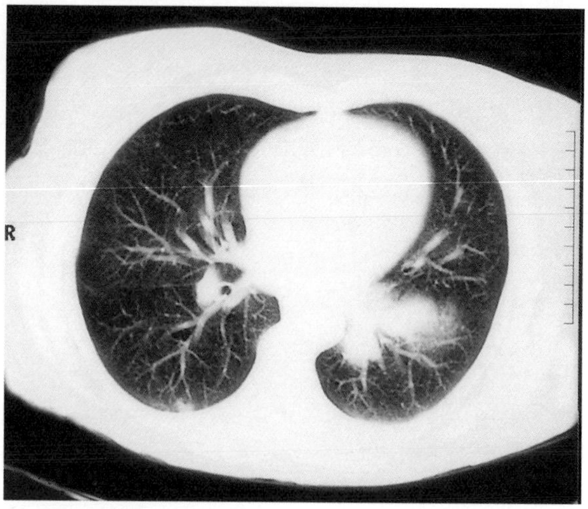

Figure 52.5 CT scan showing a large left sided hilar mass and small right apical lower segment lesion which was not evident on the initial chest film.

Diagnosis and staging

Histological diagnosis and staging determine the therapeutic options. These processes may be interlinked. Thus, for example, a staging procedure that confirms metastatic disease may also prove to be the simplest method of obtaining the histological diagnosis.

Achieving a tissue diagnosis

A tissue diagnosis is required to confirm that the lesion is a bronchogenic carcinoma and to distinguish between small cell and non-small cell types. Intrathoracic sampling options include attempts to sample the tumour directly and those which are part of the staging process and are intended to detect spread of disease. Clearly, a good sample derived from the primary tumour will always generate a histological answer whereas a staging sample will only do so in the presence of disseminated disease. Direct sampling of the primary lesion is, therefore, of particular relevance to surgical candidates who have negative staging samples and for those patients who are generally unfit and would not be suitable for invasive staging procedures.

Direct sampling options include, in order of increasing invasiveness:

- sputum cytology
- bronchoscopy
- transthoracic needle biopsy
- thoracoscopy
- thoracotomy.

Sputum cytology has high specificity but the sensitivity of this test depends upon the degree of main airway involvement by tumour. Consequently, positive sputum samples may be obtained from over 80% of central tumours but less than 40% of those in a peripheral location. It should also be observed that these

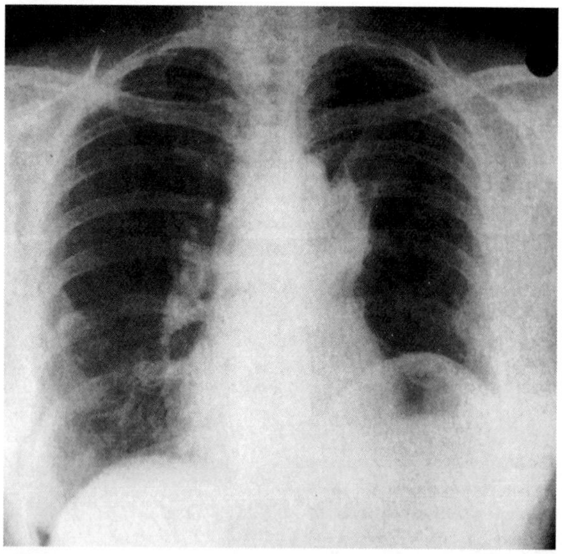

Figure 52.4 PA chest radiograph showing a left hilar tumour with marked elevation of the left diaphragm implying paralysis of the left phrenic nerve due to central tumour involvement.

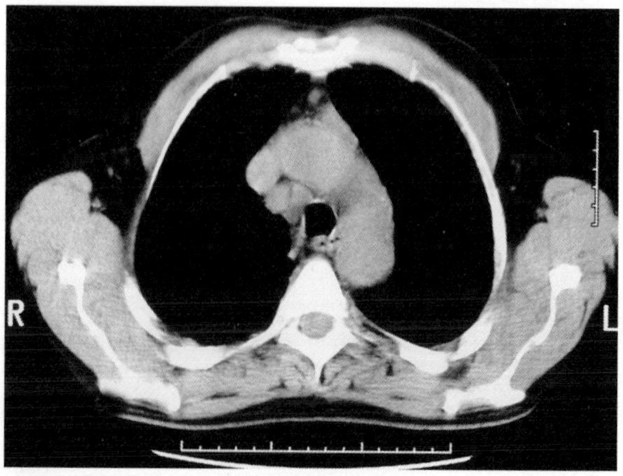

Figure 52.6 CT image of enlarged mediastinal nodes immediately to the right of the trachea.

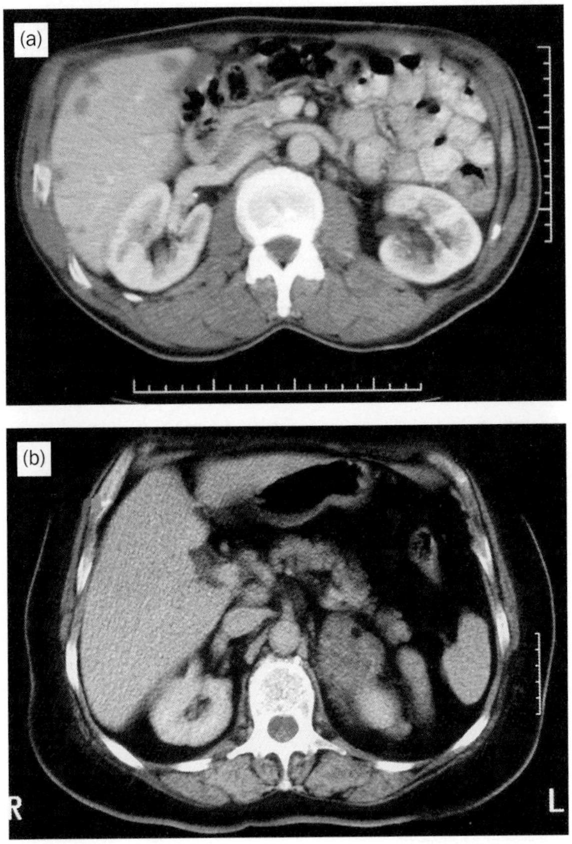

Figure 52.7 CT images of (a) hepatic metastases; (b) adrenal mass lesion.

data relate to adequate sputum samples. Many patients may not have a productive cough and others find it difficult to comply so that a useless salivary sample is obtained.

Bronchoscopy is mandatory for all potentially operable lung cancer. Fibre-optic examination may be performed under sedation and naso-laryngeal topical anaesthesia but rigid bronchoscopy will require a general anaesthetic. These are largely complementary investigations. Either will allow biopsy of central endobronchial tumours. Fibre-optic examination has a higher probability of direct access to tumours in the smaller airways and is a better way of obtaining cytological brushing samples. These are particularly helpful in achieving proof of malignancy with peripheral carcinomas which may be inaccessible to direct biopsy but may be diagnosed from shed cells brushed from the nearby bronchi. Rigid bronchoscopy also has specific advantages. The operator can take a much deeper bite and may obtain a positive result by detecting submucosal tumour which has evaded fibre-optic biopsy. Endobronchial suction is superior making it more effective when large quantities of mucus or pus are present. It is safer to biopsy tumours which appear vascular via the rigid bronchoscope as post-biopsy bleeding can be controlled by pressure from pledglets soaked in dilute adrenaline and the airways suctioned clear of blood and clot. It is also said that hilar fixity can be assessed by the tactile feedback gained while manoeuvring the rigid bronchoscope but this is largely of historic interest as other less subjective assessments of the extent of hilar tumour are now utilized. Transbronchial needle biopsy can be undertaken with either system but is most relevant to subcarinal lymphadenopathy and even in experienced hands has a less than 50% sensitivity with known enlarged glands.

CT guided transthoracic needle biopsy is a highly effective method of obtaining a tissue diagnosis with a sensitivity of about 80%. It is not practical for lesions much below 1 cm in diameter and a negative result does not exclude malignancy as the sampling volume is small. Pneumothorax occurs in about 30% of cases. It is more likely in emphysematous patients or those with central tumours and about half require a chest drain. Bleeding occurs in about 5% of cases. Implantation of malignant cells into the chest wall appears to be rare (<0.1%) and it is not considered to alter long-term survival following resection.

A histological diagnosis may not be available in up to one third of candidates for surgical resection because the primary lesion cannot be sampled and staging is negative. In these cases management will depend upon the location of the tumour. A relatively peripheral lesion may be suitable for either core or excision wedge biopsy using videothoracoscopic techniques (Figure 52.8). However, it may be impracticable or dangerous to biopsy a lesion seated deep within a lobe and in this circumstance many surgeons take the view that lobectomy is indicated because of the high (>85%) probability of bronchogenic carcinoma. In these cases definitive diagnosis must await the outcome of formal histology.

A central tumour will usually require resection by pneumonectomy which most surgeons would be reluctant to undertake without histological proof of appropriate malignancy. Videothoracoscopy may be used to obtain samples from central tumours (Figure 52.9) but if the lesion is not accessible to this approach open thoracotomy and frozen section histology are required.

Staging

Staging addresses three issues: the primary tumour, the status of the mediastinal and intrapulmonary lymph nodes, and detection of distant spread. The results of this process generate the clinical TNM grading (Table 52.5) which may be further refined with pathological data if resection is undertaken. This process is pursued to the maximum required extent in patients with potentially operable disease who may therefore undergo a variety of invasive assessments. For those with obviously inoperable disease, investigation is often restricted to confirmation of advanced disease status using imaging techniques with invasive biopsy being used only to confirm histological type by the simplest means possible.

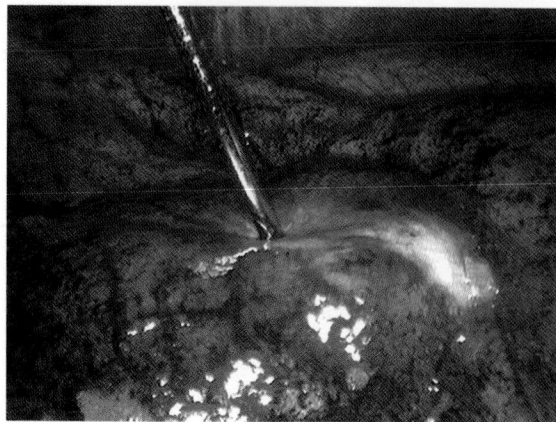

Figure 52.8 Operative view obtained during videothoracoscopic core biopsy of an undiagnosed peripheral pulmonary mass.

Evaluation of the primary tumour (T status)

Operability is questionable in most T3 and virtually all T4 lesions. The proximity of tumour to the carina is assessed by bronchoscopy. Tumour size can be reasonably accurately evaluated by CT imaging for lesions which are neither central nor adjacent to the chest wall but size is not of itself important in determining operability. The presence of chest wall or mediastinal invasion is important but unless gross invasion is present, the CT scan is not particularly accurate in differentiating contiguity from invasion. MRI is no better than CT in this respect and may be more difficult for clinicians to interpret. Magnetic resonance imaging (MRI) does have a specific role in assessing neural involvement in Pancoast lesions with possible involvement of the brachial plexus. The presence of a pleural effusion can indicate pleural dissemination of malignant disease but may also simply represent an inflammatory reaction to pneumonia or consolidation secondary to bronchial obstruction by tumour. The combination of pleural fluid cytology and pleural biopsy has a 70% chance of detecting pleural dissemination of bronchogenic carcinoma. If significant doubt persists despite negative samples, thoracoscopic evaluation is indicated in otherwise operable candidates.

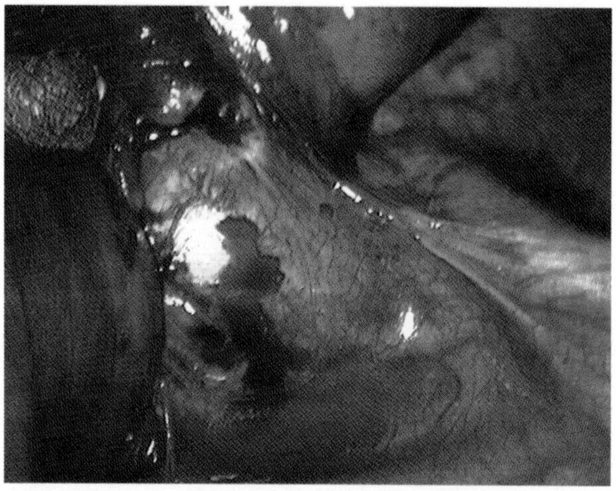

Figure 52.9 Operative view obtained during videothoracoscopy of a central hilar tumour abutting the left pulmonary artery. Videothoracoscopic evaluation is useful as a final screening measure prior to performing open thoracotomy in order to prevent open and shut thoracotomy in patients with irresectable disease or who would require too large a resection for their level of lung function. In this case pneumonectomy will be required. If the patient has poor lung function and could only tolerate a lobectomy, the surgeon could withdraw at this stage.

Evaluation of the intrathoracic lymph nodes (N status)

The topography of the pulmonary and mediastinal nodes and the relationship between involved node stations and long-term survival has been studied in detail. These are described in a 'lymph node map' (Figure 52.10) which has evolved through several iterations to reach the current form. It is not practicable to stage the intrapulmonary nodes by direct sampling prior to surgery and this is anyway not necessary as N0/N1 status does not affect suitability for surgery or curative radiotherapy. Mediastinal node (N2/3) status is, however, regarded by most surgeons as pivotal to surgical selection.

The available options to assess the mediastinal nodes include:

- CT
- PET
- trans-oesophageal biopsy
- mediastinoscopy
- mediastinotomy
- thoracoscopy
- thoracotomy.

The CT scan interrogated at mediastinal settings demonstrates mediastinal nodes very effectively. Unfortunately, there is considerable controversy about what to do with the information it provides. One extreme view is simply that it indicates the presence of nodes which should be removed at surgery by a 'radical' mediastinal lymphadenectomy. The other view is based on the observation that patients with pre-operatively diagnosed mediastinal node disease have no significant 5 year survival following surgery. It, therefore, holds that the status of these nodes should be determined prior to proceeding with resection. Even within this group there is not uniform practice as the decision regarding lymph nodes status may be based on CT size, positron emission tomographic (PET) scanning or biopsy.

Using a size criterion relies upon nodes larger than a specified value – typically 1 cm in long axis – being likely to be malignant and those beneath this threshold benign. There is, indeed, an association between size and the probability of malignant involvement but this is sufficiently inaccurate to mean that at least 10% of patients with glands less than 1 cm on CT will yield positive samples on mediastinoscopic sampling. The reverse is also true as a significant proportion of patients have enlarged mediastinal nodes which exhibit only reactive changes or other histology such as sarcoidosis when biopsied. Taken overall CT scanning has a sensi-

Table 52.5 TNM grading and stage distribution

Tumour status
T1 = peripheral tumour < 3 cm and not involving pleura
T2 = tumour > 3 cm or involves main bronchus beyond 2 cm from carina or parietal pleura
T3 = tumour involves: chest wall/mediastinal pleura/pericardium/diaphragm or main bronchus within 2 cm of carina
T4 = tumour involves: mediastinal structures/vertebral column/carina; tumour is associated with pericardial or pleural malignant effusion; satellite tumour deposits are present within lobe containing primary tumour

Node status
N0 = no lymph nodes involved by tumour
N1 = ipsilateral peribronchial or intrapulmonary nodes involved
N2 = ipsilateral mediastinal or subcarinal nodes involved
N3 = contralateral mediastinal nodes involved; involvement of scalene nodes on either side

Metastatic status
M0 = no distant metastases
M1 = distant metastases present

Stage category	*TNM classification*		
0	Carcinoma *in situ* (Tis)		
IA	T1	N0	M0
IB	T2	N0	M0
IIA	T1	N1	M0
IIB	T3	N0	M0
	T2	N1	M0
IIIA	T3	N1	M0
	T1/T2/T3	N2	M0
IIIB	Any T4,	Any N3,	M0
IV	Any M1		

Abbreviated descriptions derived from: Mountain, C. F. and Dressler, C. M. Regional lymph node classification for lung cancer staging. *Chest* 1997; **111**: 1718–23.

tivity of about 70% and a specificity of about 80% using the 1 cm size criterion discussed.

PET scanning detects photons resulting from positron emissions produced by the radiotracer [^{18}F] fluoro-2-deoxy-D-glucose (FDG). This is taken up by cells according to their rate of glucose metabolism and as this is increased in cancer cells, PET scanning can be used to identify possible areas of malignant tissue. It is more sensitive (80%) and more specific (90%) than CT but the scan images are anatomically imprecise (see Module 57) and benefit from superimposition on a CT image in order to provide accurate anatomical location of areas of increased uptake. This prevents adjacent hilar tumour or positive intrapulmonary nodes being misinterpreted as positive mediastinal nodes. PET is not 100% specific as positive scans can be generated in nodes with an inflammatory component including, in some instances, the enlarged nodes seen in industrial workers with significant dust exposure. The major advance offered by PET is that it provides almost no false negative results.

Mediastinal node sampling provides the definitive information on node status. It is usually achieved by three different approaches either singly or in combination. All require general anaesthesia and are often combined with rigid bronchoscopy. Mediastinoscopy is performed through a 4 cm low anterior cervical incision which is used to introduce the mediastinoscope into the peritracheal region. This technique allows the subcarinal (station 7) and both ipsilateral and contralateral (station 2 and 4) paratracheal nodes to be sampled. Thus both N2 (ipsilateral) and N3 (contralateral) node stations can be assessed. As will be evident from the lymph node map, there are other stations. Those situated around the aortic arch (stations 5 and 6) can be accessed via a mediastinotomy procedure. This utilizes a 5 cm paramediastinal approach in the second or third left interspace anteriorly and either an extrapleural or a transpleural route. These techniques are described in further detail in Module 57. Videothoracoscopic techniques are used to achieve a video assisted thoracic surgery (VATS) procedure (Figure 52.11). This allows the surgeon not only to access stations 5 and 6 but also to sample nodes lateral to the superior vena cava (station 3) and the lower para-oesophageal nodes (station 8) and pulmonary ligament nodes (station 9) (Figure 52.12). The invasiveness tariff does progressively increase with these different node biopsy procedures so that a judgement regarding the likely value of mediastinoscopy and VATS is required in each case. One further sampling option is the use of endoscopic ultrasound guided trans-oesophageal biopsy. This is confined to the para-oesophageal and subcarinal regions and is highly operator dependent but can be a useful method for obtaining a tissue sample in undiagnosed poor-risk patients with locally advanced bronchogenic carcinoma.

A rational solution to mediastinal node assessment would be to undertake routine CT and PET scanning

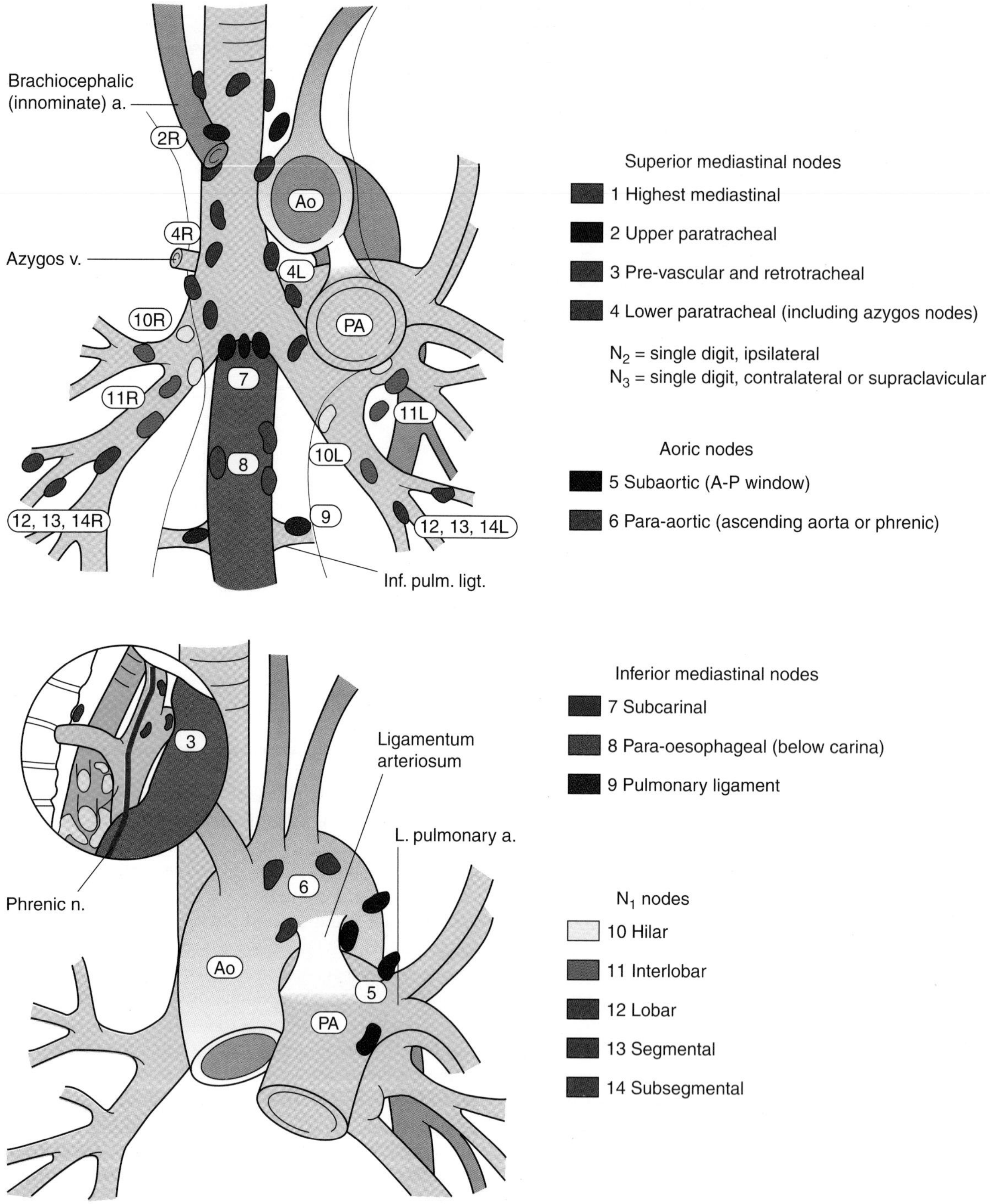

Figure 52.10 Diagrammatic representation of the thoracic lymph node stations. (Adapted from Mountain, C. F. and Dressler, C. M. Regional lymph node classification for lung cancer staging. *Chest* 1997; **111**: 1718–23.)

utilizing invasive surgical biopsy procedures for positive areas on the PET scan. At present, however, PET scanners are in limited supply and the thoracic surgical community is entirely divided between those who undertake routine mediastinoscopy on all patients, those who reserve it for patients with enlarged mediastinal nodes and those who would appear to have limited belief in mediastinal staging. To some extent this issue is the reciprocal of attitudes to intra-operative management as is discussed below.

Determination of the presence of metastatic spread (M status)

Detection of extrathoracic disease is provided by biopsy of palpable deposits such as cutaneous lesions or scalene lymph nodes, and scanning techniques. As

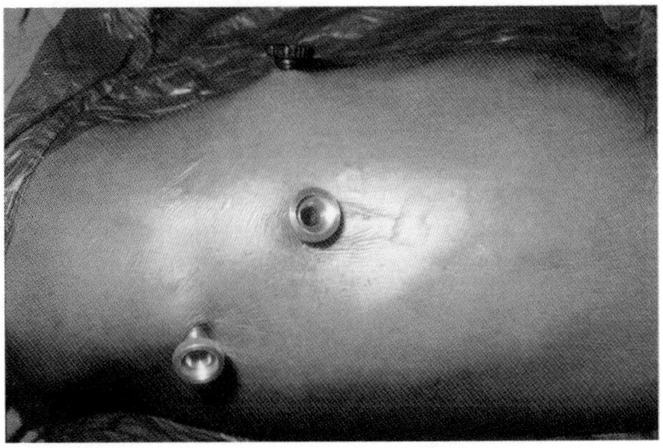

Figure 52.11 Access ports for VATS biospy procedures.

noted above CT imaging routinely should include the liver and adrenals in order to provide a first estimate of the presence of any lesions in these structures. Occasionally, ultrasound may be required to differentiate hepatic cyst(s) from metastatic disease and CT guided biopsy may be useful to determine whether an adrenal lesion is a metastasis or a simple primary adrenal adenoma. Isotope bone scanning is reserved for patients with abnormal biochemistry or specific bone pain. Similarly, the yield from CT or MRI brain scanning in asymptomatic operable patients is less than 3 % and this investigation is not usually performed in surgical candidates unless there are specific clinical signs or symptoms consistent with cranial involvement. Brain scans are indicated in SCLC as part of primary assessment as these cases often have intracerebral disease at presentation. They are also indicated in locally advanced NSCLC adenocarcinoma cases who may be on the borderline of surgical acceptance as these patients frequently relapse with a cerebral secondary.

Depending on the availability of scanners, PET imaging may ultimately prove to be an excellent 'one stop' body scan assessment which could detect metastases anywhere in the body except the brain where the intrinsic glucose metabolic rate is high. The available studies confirm that it is more effective at identifying metastases than conventional scans, with a 15% higher detection rate. It also offers the additional advantage of generating fewer false positives than bone scans and can distinguish between adrenal metastases and benign adenoma.

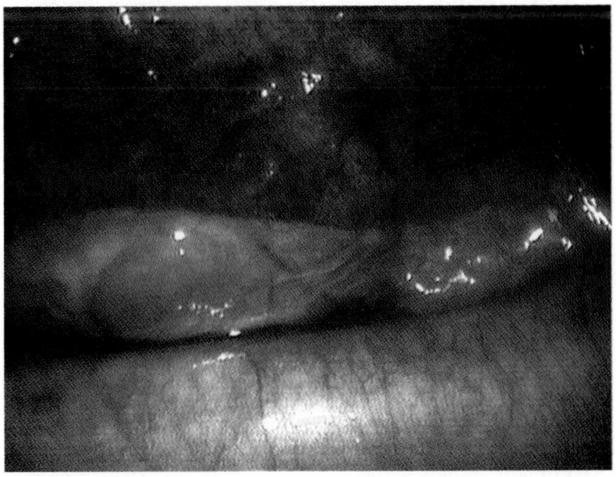

Figure 52.12 Examples of the view obtained at videothoracoscopic nodal assessment: Station 8, para-oesophageal nodes.

Surgical management

Resection is generally regarded as the optimum treatment strategy for all patients with pre-operative T1 or T2 and N0 or N1 disease. Selected T3 cases may also be suitable for resection where there is confidence that all intrathoracic disease can be excised. There is no role for 'palliative' resection as survival is not enhanced while the patient must bear the not inconsiderable morbidity of a thoracotomy. Patients identified as having N2 disease are not normally considered suitable candidates for resection unless it is undertaken within the context of a trial of neoadjuvant therapy as discussed below.

Assessment of fitness

A candidate for pulmonary resection must have adequate pulmonary reserve and should not have critical cardiac disease. From a pulmonary perspective the factors to consider are the:

- underlying pulmonary function
- extent of lung to be resected
- functionality of the lung to be resected.

Underlying pulmonary function

The most commonly used measure of pulmonary function is the forced expiratory volume in 1 second (FEV1). It is often stated that patients undergoing pulmonary resection should have an FEV1 that is above a certain value, typically 1.5 l. This is a crude oversimplification as the FEV1 value should be interpreted in the context of the patient. For example, an FEV1 of 1.5 l would be almost normal for a 75-year-old woman of small stature but it would be a very low value for a 50-year-old male of normal height. It is therefore better to consider the relationship between the predicted and actual FEV1. Using this measure, patients with a FEV1 of less than 40% of predicted are considered to be at increased risk of respiratory compromise following resection. FEV1 is a measure of air movement and does not assess the functionality of the alveolar air/blood exchange. This can be partly evaluated by measuring the carbon monoxide (CO) transfer factor and arterial blood gas levels. CO transfer assesses the ease with which CO can diffuse across the alveolar membrane and compares the value obtained with a predicted value for that patient. This test becomes less meaningful in patients with marked bullous emphysema because of air trapping effects but within a wide range of FEV1 it provides a useful further insight into underlying lung function. The third particularly useful assessment is a resting arterial blood gas sample taken while the patient is breathing room air. Mild depression in arterial oxygen tension is not important but an elevated pCO_2 is an absolute contraindication to surgical intervention.

Extent of lung to be resected
Standard pulmonary resection for cancer involves a pneumonectomy, lobectomy or bilobectomy. Right pneumonectomy is a significantly greater intervention than left pneumonectomy since it removes about 55% of the lung tissue as opposed to 45% with a left pneumonectomy, leaving less residual function. This is reflected in a greater operative mortality for right pneumonectomy particularly in patients over 70 years. Lobectomy involves the loss of a variable number of segments (Figure 52.13) and these can be used to calculate from the observed pre-operative FEV1 the predicted post-operative FEV1 which should be greater than 35% of the predicted pre-operative value. In practical terms, this calculation is more relevant to pneumonectomy patients as most will tolerate a lobectomy. Those with very poor pulmonary function and who are not thought likely to sustain a lobectomy will often cope with a limited sublobar resection of either a bronchopulmonary segment or small wedge (typically, 7 × 7 × 7 cm) of lung tissue. Sublobar resection provides a possible surgical option for the resection of a suitably placed small peripheral carcinoma in poor-risk cases.

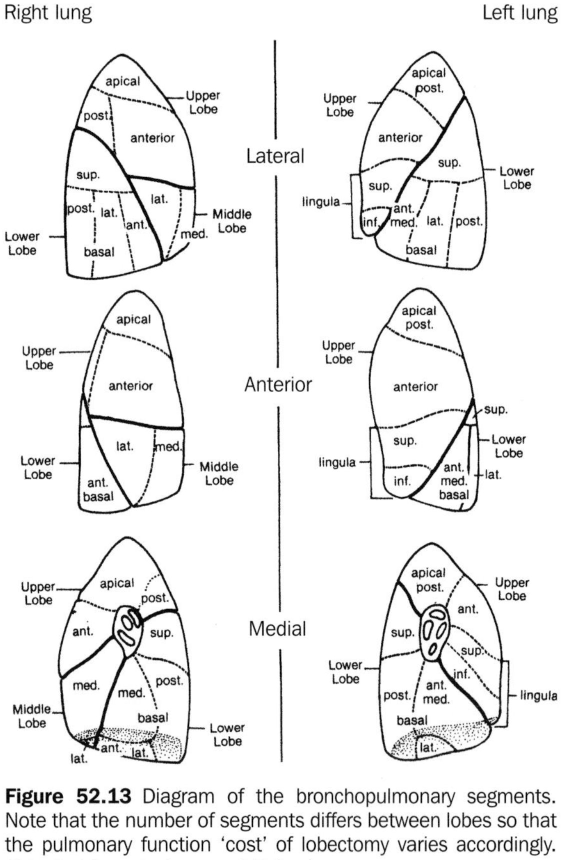

Figure 52.13 Diagram of the bronchopulmonary segments. Note that the number of segments differs between lobes so that the pulmonary function 'cost' of lobectomy varies accordingly. (Adapted from Jackson and Huber.)

Functionality of the lung to be resected
This is a crucial consideration which is frequently ignored. If the lung to be resected is non-functional as with proximal bronchial occlusion (Figure 52.14a, b) or destruction of an upper lobe by bullous disease, surgery will not affect residual lung function. This then becomes somewhat irrelevant although the patient must have sufficient reserve to tolerate surgery.

Principles of pulmonary resection

Routine surgery proceeds through a standard series of steps which may be summarized as: gaining access, assessment, selection of procedure and resection, lymph node staging and closure.

Positioning and aspects of anaesthesia
Patients undergoing pulmonary resection must be placed in the lateral decubitus position with a bridge or pillows under the lower chest until sufficient lateral flexion is produced to make the upper, operated side convex. This opens the interspaces and improves the access gained by rib retraction. Modern pulmonary surgery utilizes double lumen split lung ventilation. This is not essential but greatly facilitates surgery by improving access to the chest, safeguarding the contralateral dependent lung from spillage of infected material from the operated lung and by maintaining ventilation to the contralateral lung in the event of a major air leak on the operated side. Frequent bronchial toilet is necessary to minimize the risk of post-operative infection in the dependent lung.

Access
Pulmonary resection is usually undertaken via a posterolateral thoracotomy (Figure 52.15). This involves complete division of the latissimus and serratus anterior muscles and division of portions of the trapezius and rhomboid muscles. It provides exemplary access to the chest but is highly destructive and, consequently, is associated with impaired respiratory function and considerable post-operative pain. While this approach is optimal for large and central tumours, smaller lesions can be resected using less traumatic incisions. These fall into two groups. The muscle sparing approaches use a similar skin and intercostal incision but divide either less or no muscle relying instead on retraction to allow access through to the chest cavity. Muscle mobility is gained by elevating skin flaps. These approaches have the advantage of maintaining the general open style of surgery but the disadvantages of restricted access and of wound seroma formation which can occur in up to 12% of cases when a fully muscle sparing incision is used. The second option is the use of a VATS approach with minimal access techniques. This is suitable for early stage tumours but remains controversial and is used in relatively few centres despite significant advantages regarding pain and post-operative mobility.

Assessment
It is often possible to predict prior to operation whether a lobectomy or pneumonectomy will be required but,

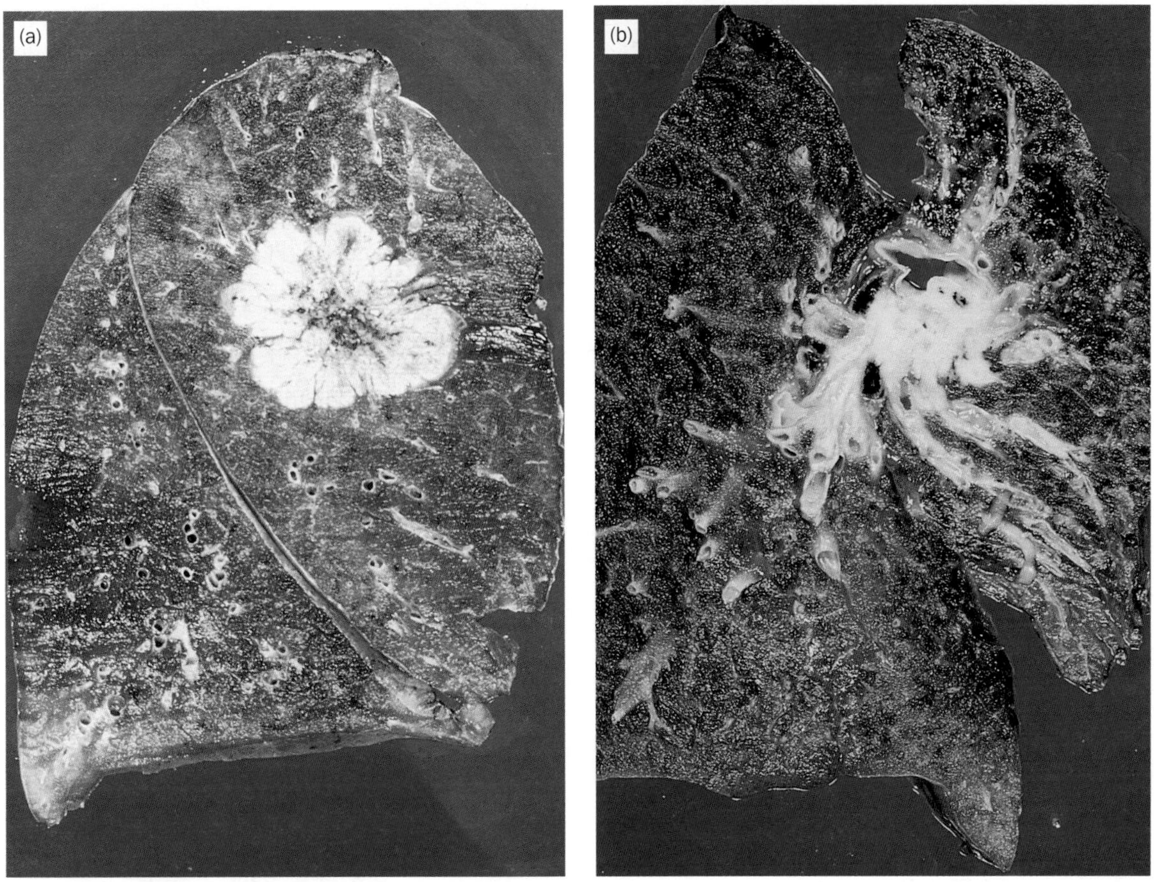

Figure 52.14 (a) Slice section through a lung with a peripheral pulmonary lesion. (b) Slice section through a lung with a carcinoma causing occlusion of a lobar bonchus. The degree of functional tissue lost with resection in patient (a) is significantly greater than that lost in patient (b).

as with all surgery, the final decision is made after full exploration of the thoracic cavity. Regrettably, despite full pre-operative staging, the operative findings may indicate that resection is not possible. This may reflect locally advanced disease or disease which exceeds the level of procedure that the patient was considered able to tolerate. At present the incidence of 'open and shut' thoracotomy in the UK is over 10%, which must be regarded as unacceptable. The risk of this outcome would be greatly reduced by routine pre-operative VATS assessment of the chest immediately prior to proceeding with an open approach. This enables the surgeon to detect unanticipated disease and consequently allows the patient to proceed quickly and relatively unscathed to alternative therapy.

Selection of procedure and resection

In general, the basic cancer principles of achieving adequate clearance apply so that the options tend to be between lobectomy for intralobar lesions which do not cross a fissure and pneumonectomy otherwise. In patients with impaired lung function, however, intra-operative evaluation may show that it is possible to perform a lung sparing bronchoplastic resection procedure. This technique is applicable to small tumours which are located at the origin of a lobar bronchus which is a situation which often results in a pneumonectomy. It may be possible to resect a sleeve of main bronchus around the orifice of the affected lobe and then reconstruct the airway by anastomosing the main bronchus to the stump of the residual lobe (Figure 52.16).

The sequence of division of the hilar structures may be dictated by circumstances but it is usually possible to follow a routine such as: arterial supply, venous drainage and bronchus. This will vary according to surgical preference. Some surgeons, for example, prefer to divide the pulmonary vein(s) as a first step in the belief that this may reduce the risk of tumour cell shedding with handling of the lung, while others prefer to interrupt the arterial supply first in order to reduce congestion within the lung. The pulmonary fissures are frequently poorly developed and are therefore separated at lobectomy using either a linear stapler or suture oversewing of the cut edges.

In advanced central tumours it may be necessary to resect a portion of pericardium and then secure the pulmonary veins adjacent to, or even including a cuff of, the left atrium. This is referred to as an intrapericardial pneumonectomy.

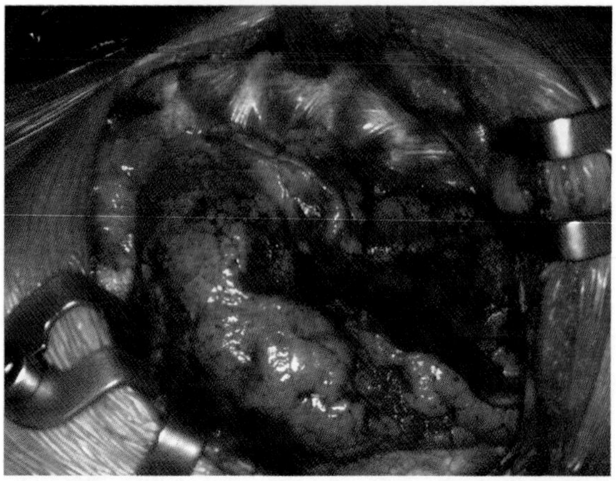

Figure 52.15 Incisional arrangement for left side open major pulmonary surgery.

Lymph node staging

At the end of the resection further mediastinal lymph node staging is carried out. This leads to a debate regarding intra-operative management of mediastinal lymphatics which is largely the reciprocal of the aforementioned arguments over pre-operative staging. Practice therefore varies between those who advocate sampling and those who undertake a radical mediastinal lymphadenectomy.

Closure

Closure involves coaption of the ribs with pericostal sutures, reconstruction of the divided muscles and insertion of one (pneumonectomy) or two (lobectomy) chest drains. It is also a phase during which a paravertebral catheter can be inserted by the surgeon to reduce post-operative pain (see Module 58).

Post-operative complications and peri-operative outcomes

Lobectomy carries a peri-operative mortality of 2–3% and pneumonectomy of 6%. Common causes of morbidity and death are pneumonia, adult respiratory distress syndrome (ARDS) (which may be associated with pneumonia) and peri-operative myocardial infarction. Bronchopleural fistula is uncommon (circa 3%) and occurs about 10 days following surgery due to breakdown of the bronchial suture line usually after pneumonectomy. It is almost always due to ischaemic necrosis of the bronchial stump and is more likely with radical lymphadenectomy. This is a dangerous complication which exposes the remaining bronchial tree to aspiration of pleural fluid and inevitably results in an empyema. Urgent tube drainage of the operated side is required. Revisional surgery is possible but most patients are treated by a permanent rib resection with open tube drainage. Unless an empyema has occurred, wound infection is remarkably uncommon. Pain is a major problem following thoracic surgery. Apart from the severe immediate wound pain, long-term neuralgic pain from intercostal nerve or root injury is experienced by 12% of patients, with 3–5% having sufficient pain to significantly interfere with their quality of life and require permanent medication. (This subject is discussed in further detail in Module 54). Operative trauma as measured by cytokine production and pain are reduced by a VATS approach.

Long-term survival

Survival following complete resection for NSCLC is largely stage dependent (Figure 52.17) although, as noted above, various histological and immunohistochemical features may be associated with an adverse outcome within any stage group. Approximately two-thirds of patients relapse at a distant site and one-third relapse locally within the thorax. The local relapse rate is higher in patients with positive mediastinal nodes. N2 positive patients benefit from adjuvant mediastinal irradiation which does not improve survival but does reduce the risk of local mediastinal recurrence. This is valuable as local recurrence produces distressing side-effects such as dysphagia and SVC obstruction.

This is one further area where the dispute regarding mediastinal lymph node management resurfaces.

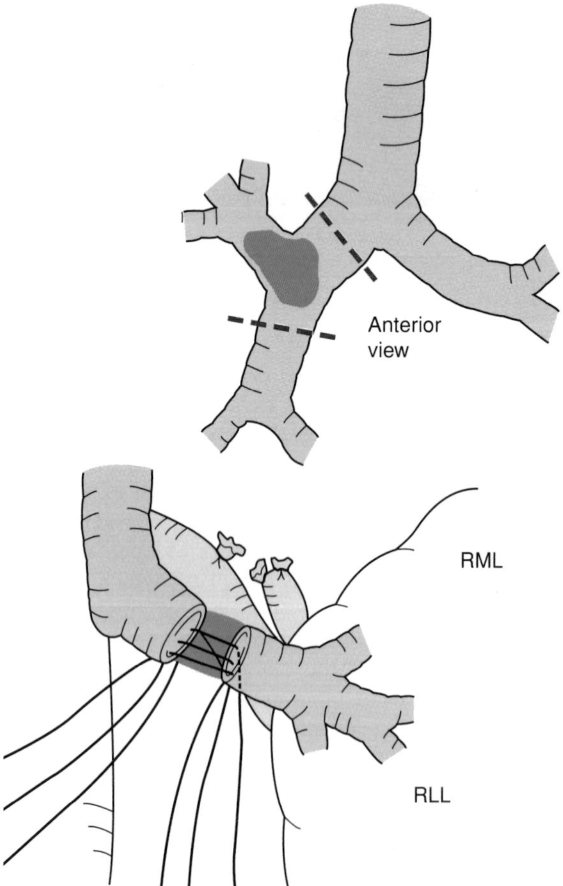

Figure 52.16 Diagram of the principle of sleeve lobar resection. In this case a tumour exists within the right upper lobe bronchus origin precluding standard lobectomy. Excision of the lobe together with a cuff of main and intermediate bronchus allows adequate tumour clearance and conservation of the lower and middle lobes.

Advocates of mediastinal gland clearance argue that their approach offers better survival and cite excellent 5 year survival data for stage I and II (i.e. mediastinal node negative disease). Those who do not subscribe to the mediastinal gland clearance concept point out that clearance of the mediastinum in stage I and II could hardly affect prognosis and argue that the apparently enhanced results achieved by the clearance group are simply the result of more accurate stage allocation. This improves the appearance of population curves but makes no difference to survival of the individual patient.

Arguments as to the merit of mediastinal gland clearance when the nodes turn out to be positive follow similar lines. The cleared group are accurately staged and even subdivided into the number of involved nodes. In contrast, some of the patients in the sampling group with minimal involvement of mediastinal nodes may be missed and are therefore understaged. This worsens the survival in sampled stage I and II cases and leaves only the more severe cases in the stage III group which accordingly acquires a correspondingly worse survival. To date, there has only been one randomized trial comparing node sampling with dissection and that showed no difference between the two groups in overall survival.

Improving surgical resection rates and outcomes

There is no dispute that surgical resection is associated with better survival than any other form of treatment but relatively few patients are suitable for surgery. Resection rates expressed as a percentage of presenting cases range from as low as 10% in the UK to 16–18% in the USA and parts of northern Europe.

These differences may have many causes. The general fitness of the aged population in different countries varies. While it is easy to determine the number of resections in a country, the accuracy of the denominator value is sometimes questionable. Notwithstanding these issues, however, the most important factor is that many patients have metastatic disease at presentation and 50% of NSCLC cases have involved mediastinal nodes. Ultimately, an increase in the resection rate requires either that more patients are referred to the surgeon while still resectable by conventional critera or that currently irresectable cases are brought back into the surgical arena.

Earlier stage tumours might be seen by reducing the time taken to reach surgical attention or by detecting tumours at an earlier stage in their development. Delay between initial presentation and surgery has been cited as a possible adverse factor and has recently been addressed in the UK by Department of Health guidelines detailing the acceptable delay between the decision to operate and surgery. These guidelines do not, however, deal with the more important delays in which the patient is reluctant to attend a general practitioner and the time then taken for referral through the medical system until a surgical referral is made. Earlier diagnosis implies a screening programme. These have not been shown to alter survival when carried out using plain chest films but interest has been rekindled by a US study using high resolution CT imaging in at-risk individuals. This is currently the subject of a multicentre UK MRC trial but it will take 10 years to know whether this project is of functional value and there are other concerns regarding screening in this way. Detection of small lesions of uncertain origin which then require observation and/or biopsy may generate significant and unnecessary worry for patients and will certainly constitute an additional demand on existing resources.

Neoadjuvant treatment, i.e. the administration of pre-operative chemotherapy (induction chemotherapy) or radiotherapy, has been suggested to 'down-stage'

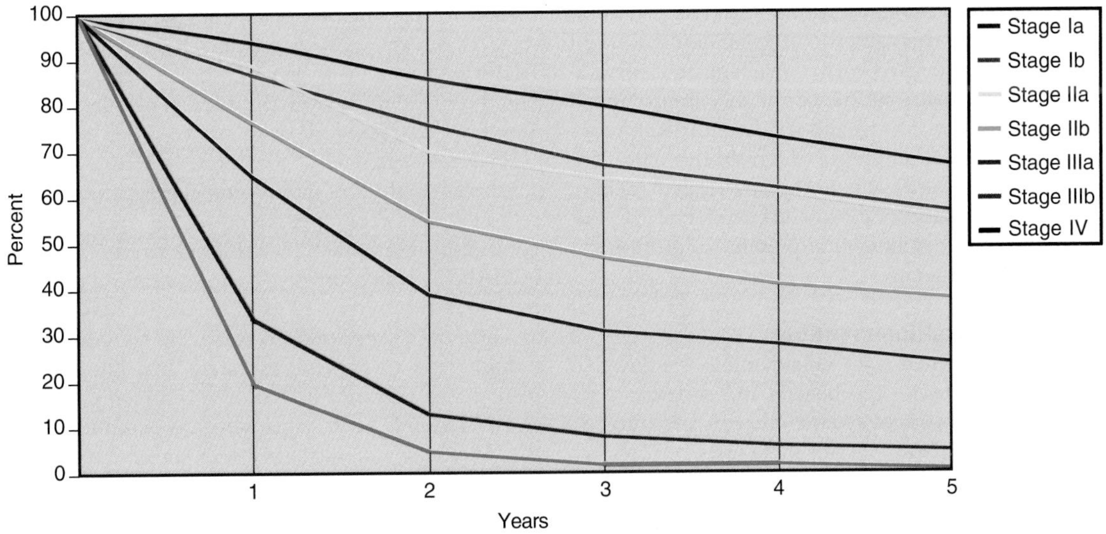

Figure 52.17 Survival in NSCLC following resection (Ia–IIIa) or non-surgical treatment (IIIb, IV).

lung tumours so that resection is possible. Two small randomized studies have compared induction chemotherapy + surgery with surgery alone and suggested a benefit with the induction chemotherapy arm in terms of resectability rates and survival. Both are open to major criticism, however, on the basis that the results in the surgery arm were below expected and the distribution of adverse markers was notably worse in the surgery group. This approach may prove useful for selected advanced tumours but it presents important difficulties including an increase in the surgical complication rate. The incidence of post-operative pulmonary dysfunction is increased and combined radiotherapy and chemotherapy produces more difficult operating conditions with a much increased risk of bronchopleural fistula presumably related to impaired peritracheal and bronchial blood supply.

Neoadjuvant therapy has also been advocated for early stage disease on the assumption that pre-treatment with induction chemotherapy will eliminate micrometastatic disease and therefore improve the results with resection. There is no evidence for this assertion which is currently being tested in Europe under the auspices of a clinical trial (LU22) but it is apparent that the pulmonary toxicity of current agents may significantly compromise the post-operative course of operated patients. The treatment also delays access to surgery, is expensive and carries both mortality and morbidity.

Adjuvant treatment

Evidence is available concerning the value of post-operative radiotherapy and chemotherapy from two large meta-analyses. The PORT meta-analysis trialist group report (1998) actually demonstrated worse survival with adjuvant radiotherapy for N0 and N1 cases. They did, however, confirm a reduced rate of local mediastinal recurrence in N2 disease and, as noted above, this is consequently the only indication for post-operative radiotherapy in completely resected NSCLC. The NSCLC Collaborative Group reported (1995) on 16 chemotherapy trials and showed that cisplatin based regimens were associated with a small apparent survival benefit (5% at 5 years) but the confidence limits ranged from −1 to +10% at 5 years and we therefore lack proof of a true survival advantage. Conversely, there are obvious problems with chemotherapy related toxicity such that some patients cannot even tolerate the full course required. It is difficult at present to justify post-operative chemotherapy.

Palliative surgical interventions

These are concerned with maintaining the luminal patency of the airway, oesophagus and superior vena cava, managing recurrent pleural effusion and mitigating the consequences of distant metastases.

Airway patency can be maintained by several techniques including stent insertion and physical dis-obliteration by reducing the endobronchial tumour mass using forceps, laser, cautery or cryotherapy. Oesophageal compression or invasion may be controlled by dilatation and stenting with a self expanding mesh stent or a plastic tube prosthesis; airway fistulation is a particularly difficult problem to manage but may be relieved by the use of a plastic oesophageal tube prosthesis with a surrounding balloon cuff. Superior caval compression is best managed with an endovascular stent inserted under radiological guidance. If this cannot be achieved it is possible to utilize both saphenous veins as bypass grafts. These are mobilized up to the sapheno-femoral junction and then tunnelled subcutaneously into the neck where sapheno-jugular anastomoses are constructed.

Recurrent pleural effusion will usually respond to pleurodesis using kaolin (calcium silicate) powder to generate a chemical pleurisy. The kaolin is administered after draining the effusion and can be insufflated under general anaesthesia or introduced through the intercostal drain catheter as a marcaine and kaolin slurry.

Metastatic NSCLC is very rarely relevant to surgical practice but occasionally a pathological fracture may require to be plated and an isolated cranial or intraspinal metastasis is worth excising on palliative grounds.

Non-surgical treatment

An extensive review of non-surgical treatment of NSCLC is outside the remit of this chapter but these therapies are numerically far more significant that surgical treatment and it is appropriate to briefly consider the available modalities. Although cure is described with non-surgical treatment these therapies are best thought of as palliative with occasional cure and the survival data usually quoted: median survival, response rates and recurrence intervals are compatible with this view.

Radiotherapy

Radiotherapy can be curative in stage I and possibly stage II disease with occasional good results in stage IIIa. It is delivered in divided doses to reduce toxicity but there is debate over the ideal schedule. Recently, attention has focused on a move from once daily 3–4 week regimens to more intense treatment schedules with the intention of preventing tumour regrowth between treatments. One such regimen, continuous hyperfractionated accelerated radiotherapy (CHART) which involves administration of 54 Gy in 36 fractions over 12 days, is of particular interest as survival is reported to superior to conventional radiotherapy for squamous carcinoma. The treatment plan poses significant resource problems, however, as it requires that treatment is continued over the weekend and may therefore prove impossible to implement.

Palliative treatment with up to 20 Gy is used for poor-risk candidates with a view to treating or reducing the risk of mediastinal complications such as SVC obstruction and tumour induced dysphagia and may also be used to control metastatic deposits elsewhere, notably bone and brain.

Apart from general fatigue, the side-effects of thoracic radiotherapy relate to the organs affected. Oesophagitis is frequent but usually mild and transient although stricturing can occur. Neural problems include spinal myelopathy with lower limb weakness and sensory disturbance and aggravation of neuralgic pain in post-thoracotomy cases. Cardiac irradiation can cause radiation pericarditis and ventricular dysfunction. These potential complications may have to be taken into account when planning irradiation fields and dosages.

Chemotherapy

The best results have been achieved with cisplatin based regimens which are associated with a modest (10%) survival improvement at 1 year equating to a gain of about 1.5 months in median survival. Newer agents including taxels, vinorelbine and gemcitabine in combination with chemosensitizing agents and alternative schedules with fewer agents in higher dosage are under investigation and seem likely to produce further modest gains. Chemotherapy is associated with well-known side-effects including nausea and vomiting, marrow suppression, pulmonary, renal, neural and cardiac toxicity and hair loss. There is, therefore, a judgement to be made in discussion with the patient regarding the value of these therapies in relation to pre-existing health status and anticipated quality of life.

Combination treatment with chemotherapy and thoracic radiation increases effectiveness by a further few percentage points.

Section 52.2 • Small cell lung cancer

SCLC is not normally considered to be a surgical condition. Conventional management of SCLC utilizes combinations of: cyclophosphamide, doxorubicin, vincristine, etoposide and cisplatin or their more recent derivatives and analogues. Concurrent mediastinal irradiation, with dosages in the order of 45 Gy, has been shown to improve survival in meta-analysis and prophylactic cranial irradiation is of further benefit in reducing the incidence of cerebral relapse in younger patients with a complete response to chemotherapy. Cure is anecdotal. Median survival is of the order of 15 months for limited disease and 9 months for those with advanced disease.

Resection of SCLC usually occurs as a pathological finding after resection of a previously undiagnosed peripheral pulmonary opacity. In this instance the patient is then referred to an oncologist and further treatment with standard chemotherapy is often given with a view to treating presumed micrometastatic disease. Rarely, resection may be undertaken for histologically proven SCLC in what is effectively a neoadjuvant context when a small cell lesion has failed to progress over a significant interval following chemotherapy. In either case, surgical evaluation and operative management are the same as that used for NSCLC. Several small surgical series describe 30% 5 year survival rates with surgically managed stage I SCLC but these results apply to a very small, non-representative and highly selected subset of these tumours.

Section 52.3 • Metastatic pulmonary tumours

Most metastatic pulmonary disease is not suitable for surgical intervention because it is widespread within the lung and/or there is further disease elsewhere. Pulmonary metastases are resected under two circumstances: inadvertent resection of a nodule which proves to be a metastatic deposit on histology and as a planned intervention in patients with limited metastatic disease confined to the lung.

Planned resection of metastatic disease (pulmonary metastasectomy) is infrequent and is normally undertaken for metastases from primary renal, colonic, testicular, melanoma and sarcomatous (notably osteogenic) primaries. Detailed scanning is essential to exclude disease elsewhere as it is clearly undesirable to inflict major thoracic surgery and potentially reduce quality of life by removing lung tissue without good evidence that this is a reasonable course of action. In the author's opinion, it is wise to keep an apparently solitary pulmonary metastasis under review for several months so that other occult deposits can declare their presence. Resection of multiple deposits is particularly relevant to persistent or recurrent osteogenic sarcoma deposits following resection of the primary and full chemotherapy. With this lesion the problem is that CT scanning underestimates the number of deposits so that direct palpation of both lungs is essential to ensure that all deposits are detected.

Resection is usually performed with a view to conserving as much functional lung tissue as is consistent with adequate local clearance. For a solitary lesion, a lateral thoracotomy approach can be utilized and wedge resection performed if possible but a central deposit may require a lobectomy or even a pneumonectomy. In some cases, it may be possible to perform the procedure using a VATS approach with obvious advantages regarding preservation of quality of life. Multiple deposits can, realistically, only be excised locally and these are usually approached via a median sternotomy. Osteogenic sarcoma metastases can be enucleated but with other soft tissue lesions the best option is to utilize a laser to vaporize the tissue around each deposit allowing local removal without leaving residual cells.

The results of metastasectomy vary with tumour type but taken overall a useful 5 year survival of approximately 25% can be obtained. Rarely repeat surgery is undertaken for further deposits.

Section 52.4 • Rare lung tumours

These tumours are all uncommon and collectively account for less than 4% of all lung tumours. With the exception of hamartomas, most would be seen in single figure numbers by any practising surgeon within a working lifetime.

Benign

Benign lesions can originate from all pulmonary tissue elements. Except for hamartoma, itself an uncommon lesion, these tumours are very rare and are usually diagnosed following excision of a peripheral lesion or of a tumour causing chronic bronchial obstruction.

Hamartoma

A hamartoma is a neoplasm of bronchial fibrous connective tissue. It often contains cartilage and fat and may be referred to as an adenochondroma. This tumour frequently presents as an asymptomatic, incidentally detected and slow growing peripheral lesion often with some calcification but it may arise in a central bronchus causing airway obstruction. The presence of fat on CT imaging implies the diagnosis but this can be confirmed by transthoracic needle biopsy or endobronchial biopsy of a central lesion. Resection is only required for a peripheral lesion where doubt as to diagnosis persists. These tumours are often mobile within the lung tissue when they can be enucleated quite easily. Central lesions may require resection together with the distal lung as a lobectomy procedure because chronic obstruction has usually caused lung destruction with bronchiectasis.

Malignant

Primary pulmonary lymphoma

Non-Hogkin's lymphoma and, less frequently, Hogkin's lymphoma can originate in the lung. These tumours arise in lymphoid tissue in the bronchial mucosa or intrapulmonary glands and are generally only of surgical interest to the extent that biopsy material may be required or inadvertent resection of a lymphomatous mass lesion is undertaken when the diagnosis is not known prior to surgery.

Sarcoma

Primary pulmonary sarcoma is very rare and affects patients of all ages. These lesions arise from primitive mesenchymal cells and only rarely breach the bronchial walls although they may cause external compression. Sarcomas up to 15 cm in diameter have been reported and dissemination tends to occur by haematogenous rather than lymphatic dissemination. They are subgrouped according to the stucture of origin into: parenchyma and bronchial, large vessel and small vessel types, with cellular classifications that reflect the differentiation of the proliferating sarcomatous cells: fibrosarcoma, leiomyosarcoma, angiosarcoma, etc. Those arising in central vessels may extend into the main pulmonary artery or left atrium. Treatment involves radical resection where that is possible with poor overall prognosis. Adjuvant chemo-radiotherapy may be given on an inferential rather than evidential basis.

Carcinosarcoma

As the name implies a carcinosarcoma is a malignancy of both epithelial and mesenchymal origin. It occurs in more elderly patients and is reputed to account for 0.3% of primary lung tumours. Extensive intrabronchial growth can occur. Progress is slow but prognosis is generally poor despite surgical excision due to both lymphatic and haematogenous dissemination.

Pulmonary blastoma

This lesion is of similar frequency to carcinosarcoma. It affects all ages with a preponderence of males. Histologically, columnar epithelium arranged in patterns similar to fetal lung exists within either a malignant mesenchymal stroma (pulmonary blastoma) or a benign appearing stroma (well differentiated fetal adenoma). A further variant (pleuropulmonary blastoma) is described in children. These tumours are treated by resection possibly with chemo-radiotherapy and have a prognosis which reflects the grade of mesenchymal malignancy, i.e. those with low-grade mesenchymal change do well, but those with high-grade changes exhibit a high tendency to recur.

Others

Other extremely rare malignant lesions have been reported at case report level and merely serve to illustrate that the lung is a fertile bed of multipotential cells capable of malignant transformation in virtually any direction. These include primary malignant melanoma of the bronchus, a lymphoepithelioma-like carcinoma and even tumours of germ cell origin such as pulmonary choriocarcinoma and teratoma.

Summary points

This chapter has presented a large amount of clinical information in a highly compressed form. The key surgical issues, concepts and controversies may be summarized as follows.

- Bronchogenic carcinoma is the most common cause of cancer death in males and females
- Smoking is strongly associated with risk of developing bronchogenic carcinoma
- The resectability rate is low at 10–18% of presenting cases due mainly to advanced disease at presentation
- Bronchogenic carcinoma is subdivided into small cell and non-small cell types
- Surgery is reserved for non-small cell lesions
- Detailed pre-operative staging is essential to determine suitability for surgery
- CT of thorax and upper abdomen and PET scanning, mediastinoscopy and VATS assessment are valuable and mutually complementary staging modalities
- Adequacy of lung function for surgery depends on: (a) baseline function which is assessed by FEV1 (> 40% predicted), CO transfer (> 60% predicted) and arterial blood gas (no evidence of CO_2 retention), and (b) the functionality of the lung to be resected

- The preferred operative options are lobectomy or pneumonectomy but lesser resection by wedge or segment is acceptable in poor-risk cases. Bronchoplastic lung conserving operations are relevant to localized and slow growing tumours, patients with poor lung function and lesions involving the main carinal area
- Surgical management of mediastinal nodes is controversial; opinion is divided between sampling and clearance and the degree of nodal dissection tends to be inversely related to the extent of mediastinal node assessment undertaken prior to surgery
- Standard post-operative mortality is 3% for lobectomy and 6% for pneumonectomy; complications include: pneumonia, ARDS, bronchopleural fistula, pulmonary embolism, myocardial infarction and atrial fibrillation
- Operative mortality rises to 20% for surgery involving the main carina and in poor-risk cases
- 5 year survival for resected NSCLC is of the order of 65% for stage I, 40% for stage II and 20% for stage IIIa
- Adjuvant radiotherapy is indicated in mediastinal node positive (N2) cases
- Adjuvant chemotherapy may yield a 5% survival benefit but this is uncertain
- Neoadjuvant chemo-radiotherapy and screening may increase the number of patients eligible for resection
- Resection of pulmonary metastases is indicated in solitary metastases which are usually from kidney and colon and for multiple metastases in osteogenic sarcoma cases.

Further reading

Hood, R. M. (1993). *Techniques in General Thoracic Surgery*, 2nd edition, Philadelphia, PA: Lea and Febiger.

Shields, T. W., LoCicero J., Ponn, R. B., eds (2000). *General Thoracic Surgery*, 5th edn. Philadelphia, PA: Lippincott William and Wilkins.

MODULE 53

Diseases of the mediastinum

Section 53.1 • Anatomy and clinical features

The mediastinum is defined as that part of the thorax contained between the two pleural sacs and divided somewhat arbitrarily into four areas as indicated in Figure 53.1. The superior mediastinum is the area bounded anteriorly by the manubrium and posteriorly by the first four thoracic vertebrae. The superior boundary is the thoracic outlet formed by the first thoracic vertebra, the first ribs and the superior margin of the manubrium. The inferior boundary is an artificial plane drawn from the manubriosternal angle to the lower border of the fourth thoracic vertebra. Through the superior mediastinum pass the arch of the aorta and its three branches, the brachiocephalic veins, the superior vena cava and vena azygos, the trachea and oesophagus, the thoracic duct, vagus, phrenic, recurrent laryngeal and sympathetic nerves. It also contains part of the thymus gland and several lymph nodes.

The anterior mediastinum lies between the body of the sternum and the pericardium. Its main contents are the lower part of the thymus gland, lymph nodes and fat.

The middle mediastinum is occupied by the heart, the intrapericardial portion of the great vessels, the pericardium itself, the phrenic nerves and their accompanying pericardiacophrenic vessels.

The posterior mediastinum is the remaining volume bounded anteriorly by the pericardium, above by the line from the manubriosternal angle to the fourth vertebra, and the diaphragm below. It contains the descending thoracic aorta and its branches, the azygos and hemiazygos veins, the thoracic duct, various lymph nodes, the oesophagus, the vagus and sympathetic nerve trunks.

The arbitrary anatomical divisions of the mediastinum are not of major clinical import, but have their greatest value in defining the exact situation of any mediastinal opacity on the chest X-ray when considering the differential diagnosis. The location of the more common mediastinal lesions is indicated in Figure 53.2.

In the superior mediastinum the commonest tumour is a retrosternal extension of an enlarged thyroid gland; occasionally ectopic thyroid tissue is found in the mediastinum. The latter is entirely detached from the cervical thyroid gland and has a separate mediastinal blood supply. Arterial aneurysms and oesophageal tumours occur in the superior mediastinum but are considered in detail in the appropriate modules. The most common mass lying posteriorly in the superior mediastinum is a neurogenic tumour. Radiological opacities around the trachea are most often due to lymph node enlargement from a wide variety of pathological processes the commonest being tuberculosis, sarcoidosis, lymphoma and bronchial carcinoma. Such lymph node involvement, particularly lymphoma, may also extend into the anterior compartment. The common anterior mediastinal lesions, i.e. thymic tumours and teratomas, may also extend into the superior mediastinum behind the manubrium.

The range of differential diagnoses in anterior mediastinal lesions is small, there being few structures in this area. Thymic cysts and tumours are the commonest abnormalities encountered with the germ cell tumours as the other major group of solid tumours occurring here. When the mass lies anteriorly at the level of the diaphragm two other possibilities must be considered, namely pleuropericardial cyst and a hernia through the foramen of Morgagni. Lymphoid tumours, lymph node enlargement, cystic hygroma and ectopic thyroid may occur in this space.

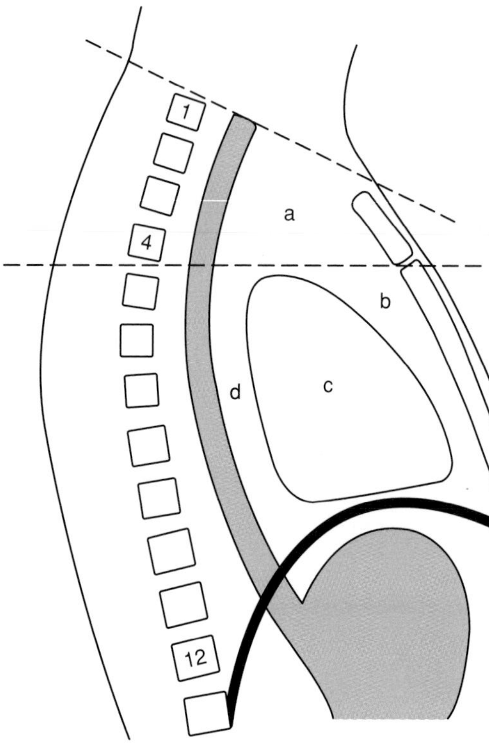

Figure 53.1 Anatomy of the mediastinal compartments. (a) Superior; (b) anterior; (c) middle; (d) posterior.

Most abnormalities arising in the middle mediastinum originate in the heart and great vessels and have to be distinguished from the enlargement of one or other of the cardiac chambers. Primary tumours of the pericardium are rare. Foregut duplications and thymic tumours may overlie the middle mediastinum on the straight X-ray.

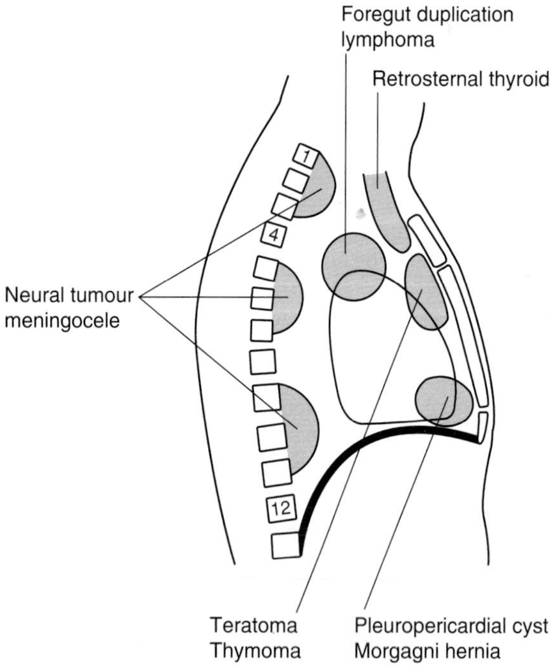

Figure 53.2 Pathological anatomy of the mediastinum.

Oesophageal pathology and aneurysms of the descending thoracic aorta are amongst the most common abnormalities in the posterior mediastinum but are not described further in this module. Of those lesions considered to be of posterior mediastinal origin, neural tumours are the most frequent and are typically situated in the paravertebral area. Cystic lesions related to the trachea or oesophagus may represent one or other variety of duplication in the mediastinum, the majority are relatively benign cysts and tumours. There are many abnormalities of developmental origin as a product of the complexity of the embryology of this area; witness the complexities of cardiovascular development and the migration of the thyroid and thymus glands during development.

Pulmonary, spinal, chest wall and metastatic tumours occasionally invade the mediastinum directly.

Clinical features

The clinical effect produced by a mediastinal mass depends on its site, size and rate of growth. Cysts and benign tumours usually enlarge slowly and may be completely asymptomatic even when large. Eventually this type of growth will compress adjacent structures, but interference with function is a late phenomenon. In contrast, malignant tumours, aneurysms and infections tend to produce more dramatic symptoms and signs. The mediastinum contains structures vital to several different systems of the body, all of which may be affected by an enlarging mediastial mass.

Respiratory

It is common for a retrosternal goitre to cause both tracheal compression and displacement at the level of the thoracic outlet (Figure 53.3); but symptoms of tracheal air flow obstruction, i.e. stridor and breathlessness occur late. The narrowing needs to reach the critical diameter of the trachea to generate the Reynolds number* for the system. The critical diameter is 4 mm, but longer stenoses may cause stridor at slightly larger diameters. These conditions cause turbulent air flow. Thus stridor is present and the work of breathing is increased. Direct invasion of the tracheal lumen in malignant thyroid disease causes such physical signs much earlier in the trachea and main bronchi producing stridor and dyspnoea. The trachea may occasionally be compressed by a neurogenic or other solid tumour enlarging within the thoracic oulet.

Cough is a symptom when there is tracheal or bronchial invasion or compression. Haemoptysis is not commonly associated with mediastinal tumours unless there is malignant invasion of the tracheobronchial tree. Aortic and brachiocephalic aneurysms may distort

*Reynolds number (*Re*) is a dimensionless number: $Re = VDr/n$, where V is velocity, D is the diameter, r is the density and n is the viscosity.

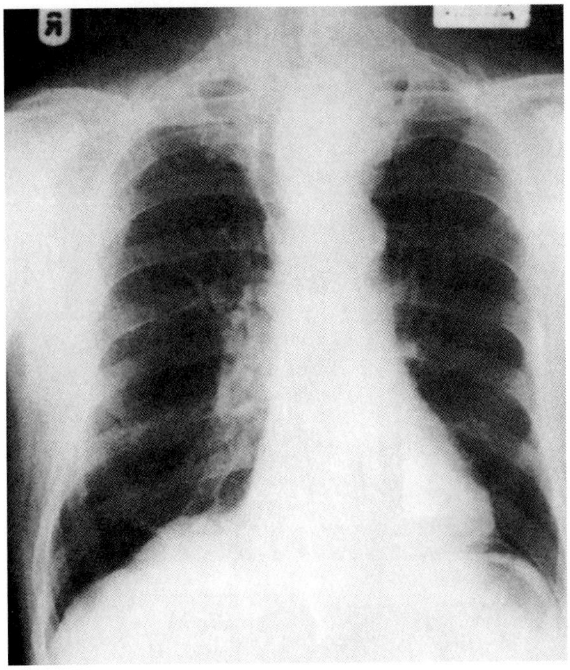

Figure 53.3 PA chest radiograph demonstrating a large retrosternal goitre with displacement of the trachea.

and compress the trachea and thus produce a more dramatic form of haemoptysis on rare occasions. Large mediastinal tumours may also cause stridor and dyspnoea.

Cardiovascular
Compression, displacement or invasion of the heart or great vessels may cause various cardiac symptoms and signs including tachycardia and arrhythmias. Obstruction of the superior vena cava with typical venous congestion in head, neck and upper limbs is most often due to metastatic bronchial carcinoma but may also occur with other solid superior mediastinal tumours such as lymphoma and thymoma. Anterior mediastinal masses press upon the right ventricular outflow and pulmonary artery to produce a systolic murmur in inspiration.

Alimentary
Herniation through the foramen of Morgagni is usually omentum and is asymptomatic. If stomach, small bowel or colon enters the hernia obstructive symptoms may be produced. Dysphagia is the most common alimentary symptom of mediastinal tumours, but is more often due to primary oesophageal disease or extrinsic compression of the oesophagus by metastatic mediastinal glands. Large benign posterior mediastinal tumours often displace the oesophagus but dysphagia is a late symptom.

Neurological
The phrenic, vagus and recurrent laryngeal nerves may be invaded directly by malignant mediastinal tumours or by metastatic tumour from bronchial carcinoma. Horner's syndrome is seen occasionally with neural tumours at the thoracic outlet. Posterior mediastinal neural tumours are usually benign and although they may involve one or more intercostal nerves, they do not often produce pain in the distribution of that particular nerve. About 10% of neural tumours have a dumb-bell like extension through the intervertebral foramina and this may cause spinal cord compression.

Section 53.2 • Investigations

Radiological imaging

The standard postero-anterior chest radiograph has limited value for the mediastinum. A normal mediastinal outline radiographically can conceal an opacity of considerable size. It is therefore, common for mediastinal anormalities not to be observed until they are of sufficient size to change the outline of the mediastinum on the posteroanterior chest film. A good lateral film is essential in the assessment of any suspected mediastinal opacity. Contrast computed tomography (CT) scanning will delineate the various mediastinal structures. Recent advances in imaging techniques have dramatically changed the accuracy of non-invasive diagnosis and the staging process. Contrast CT, magnetic resonance imaging (MRI), positron emission tomography (PET) and oesophageal ultrasound are now established in mediastinal disease assessment.

Barium swallow
Barium swallow is indicated in any patient presenting with dysphagia but may also be useful in patients with a superior or posterior mediastinal mass to demonstrate whether there is any oesophageal displacement, compression or invasion.

Computed tomography
This technique is particularly suitable for the localization and identification of mediastinal abnormalities. It can indicate the exact site, size, shape and density of a mediastinal cyst or tumour and can often detect invasion of surrounding structures. CT scanning may also be used to identify vertebral abnormalities and the presence of relatively small gland masses in the mediastinum. In a patient with a suspected thyroid mass it will demonstrate whether or not there is continuity with the cervical thyroid. Lymph node sizing can be critical: nodes greater than 1 cm in diameter are likely to be pathologically affected. Contrast CT scanning is now commonplace and helps identify all the significant vessels clearly.

Aortography
Suspicion of an aneurysm of the great vessels was the indication for aortography but is now rarely indicated.

Contrast enhancement of CT scanning and digital subtraction arteriography (DSA) have replaced formal catheterization in many centres. Transoesophageal ultrasound is now used for the oesophagus, the heart and for the aorta as the definitive investigation for many conditions.

Venography

Venography of the superior cava is not usually necessary to confirm the presence of caval obstruction as the clinical picture is typical. Where the clinical features are less obvious, or where a good collateral circulation has developed, it is relatively easy to inject dye into the great veins to confirm the diagnosis. More often venography is part of the palliative process when stenting the superior vena cava from the groin. Occasionally individual veins may be selectively cannulated and dye injected to demonstrate a tumour circulation – this may be done in patients with myasthenia gravis who are suspected of having thymic tumours and in pursuit of occult parathyroid tumours.

Magnetic resonance imaging (MRI)

This technique is increasingly available world-wide. Its value for neurological disorders is well established. The ability to identify anatomical planes improves staging information in the chest and particularly the mediastinum. Mediastinal lymphadenopathy is well imaged (Figure 53.4). Thymic tumours are easily identified and their invasive character is demonstrated.

Positron emission tomography (PET) scanning

PET scanning is increasingly available as the equipment becomes cheaper and more readily available. The usual agent is 18-fluorodeoxyglucose. An isotope of fluorine which emits two positrons at 180° is attached to glucose. The glucose is taken up differentially according to glucose metabolism. In the resting non-speaking patient malignant cells take up glucose more avidly than other cells. This activity is detected and images are produced. This is increasingly used to stage lung cancer and mediastinal involvement is clearly shown when present (Figure 53.5).

Other imaging techniques

Radiological screening of the patient may assist in the diagnosis of some cardiovascular abnormalities and should also be done to confirm the presence of paradoxical movement of the diaphragm when phrenic nerve paralysis is suspected. Pulmonary arteriography will confirm extrinsic compression of the pulmonary artery as a cause of a systolic murmur. Doppler ultrasound scanning now allows turbulent flow to be detected non-invasively. The indications for invasive angiography continue to fall as the non-invasive techniques become more widely available.

Artificial pneumomediastinum at one time gained some popularity as a method of delineating mediastinal lymphadenopathy but is rarely used today. Lymphangiography may occasionally be helpful and is still used to identify tumour invasion of nodes as the resolution of CT scanning is not adequate for this task. It is likely that PET scanning will be used instead in the future.

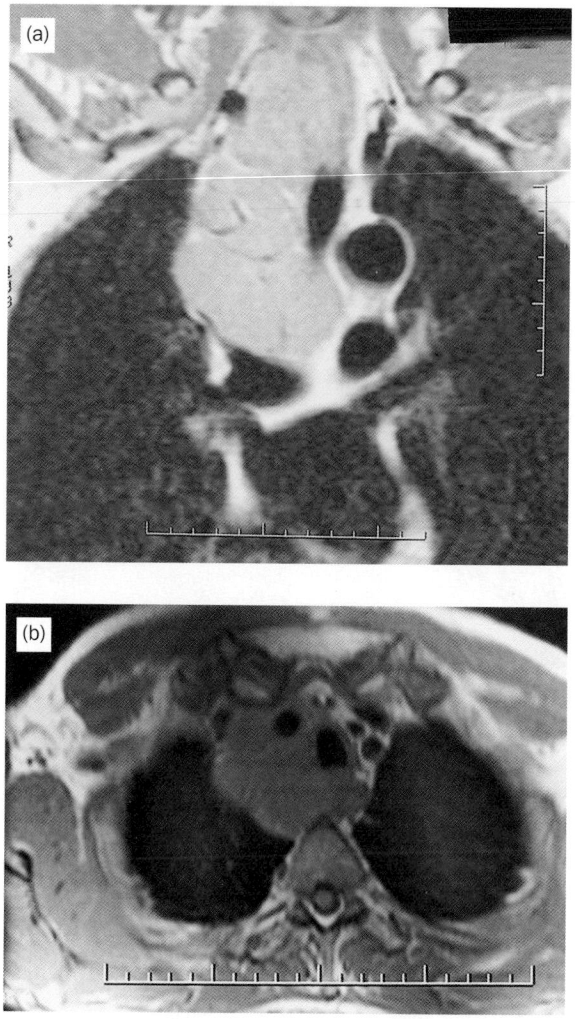

Figure 53.4 Magnetic resonance imaging in a patient with lymphoma in the mediastinum. (a) Coronal, (b) axial views.

Other investigations

Bronchoscopy

This is of value in mediastinal disease to confirm suspected tracheal or bronchial compression, and exclude primary tracheobronchial pathology.

Mediastinoscopy

This is an invasive investigation which carries with it a low morbidity and is extremely useful in making a histological diagnosis without resorting to thoracotomy. The mediastinoscope is inserted in the pretracheal plane and a limited area of the mediastinum is accessible in this way. Anterior mediastinoscopy, to inspect the retrosternal space, has been replaced by anterior mediastinotomy (*vide infra*).

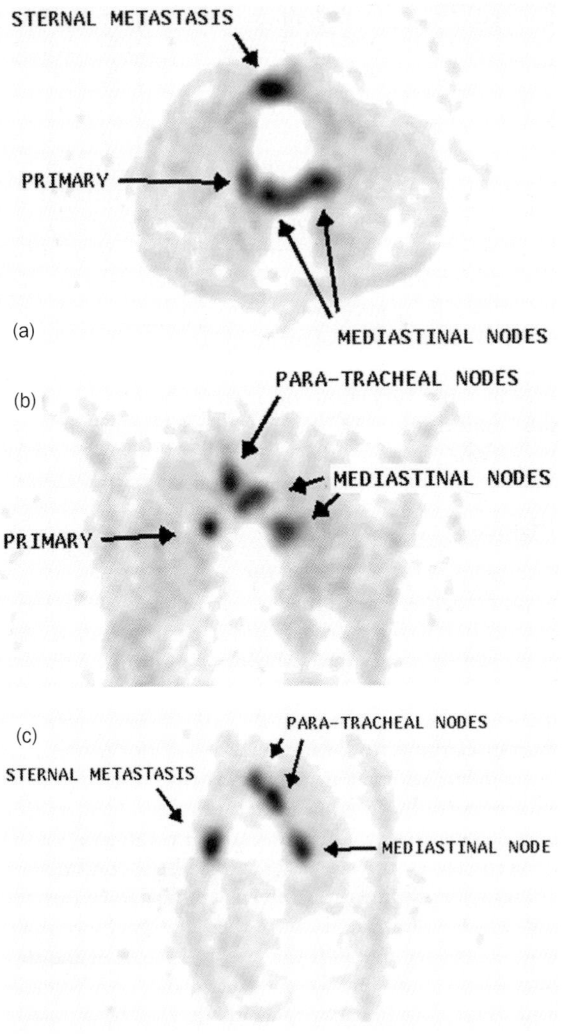

Figure 53.5 PET scanning in a patient with carcinoma of lung showing left hilar primary, mediastinal nodes and a sternal metastasis. The sternal metastasis did not show on a bone scan, illustrating the greater sensitivity of PET scanning. (a) Coronal, (b) sagittal, (c) axial views.

Mediastinoscopy has great value when there is a suspicion of the following problems as mediastinoscopy allows access for biopsy to paratracheal, tracheobronchial and even carinal lymph nodes:

- lymphadenopathy due to sarcoidosis, tuberculosis and bronchial carcinoma
- mediastinal lymphoma
- idiopathic mediastinal fibrosis
- occasionally a bronchogenic cyst may accidentally be drained. They do not recur afterwards.

Anterior mediastinotomy

This involves a small incision to either side of the sternum directly over the costal cartilage which is removed to create a window for extra- and intrapleural inspection, palpation and biopsy. Commonly the left second costal cartilage is excised for access to the anterior mediastinum and left hilar area in staging of carcinoma of bronchus. It is also of great value for the histological identification of all accessible lesions of the anterior mediastinum to confirm the diagnosis before planned resection. Access is via either right or left second to fifth costal cartilage excision.

Section 53.3 • Tumours and cysts of the mediastinum

Tracheal and oesophageal disease, and aneurysms of the heart and great vessels are discussed elsewhere. Lymphadenopathy associated with tuberculosis and sarcoidosis commonly occur and the diagnosis is established at mediastinoscopy or mediastinotomy. Tuberculosis is treated effectively by modern chemotherapy. Sarcoidosis is a self-limiting disease which may require steroids to contain the more severe symptoms and to minimize the end stage fibrotic problems.

Thyroid

Mediastinal thyroid tissue is most commonly found as the retrosternal extension of a multinodular goitre. Ectopic thyroid tissue is rare, but presents usually as an anterior mediastinal opacity which has no continuity with the cervical thyroid tissue and often derives its blood supply from the mediastinum. The siting of this ectopic thyroid tissue is related to the complicated developmental migration of the thyroid, islands of which may be found anywhere from the base of the tongue to the pericardium. Clinically, ectopic thyroid is usually asymptomatic and is a chance radiological finding. A retrosternal extension of a multinodular goitre will displace the structures in the superior mediastinum, particularly the trachea and oesophagus, which may eventually be compressed. Thus dyspnoea can occur, but dysphagia is a late symptom and is associated more often with malignant thyroid tumours. Ectopic thyroid tissue must always be suspected of being well-differentiated malignant disease of the thyroid.

Investigations

In the postero-anterior chest film a rounded mediastinal opacity will be seen (Figure 53.6) which is situated anteriorly in the lateral film. There may occasionally be calcification within thyroid cysts and tumours. Barium swallow should be carried out if there is dysphagia. A radioisotope thyroid scan may indicate functioning thyroid tissue within the thorax. A negative scan excludes neither retrosternal extension of a cervical goitre nor ectopic thyroid tissue. CT scanning of the neck and mediastinum is the standard imaging process for the thyroid with any retrosternal extension.

Management

Retrosternal extensions of multinodular goitres derive their blood supply from the neck and can almost always be safely enucleated through a standard low cervical

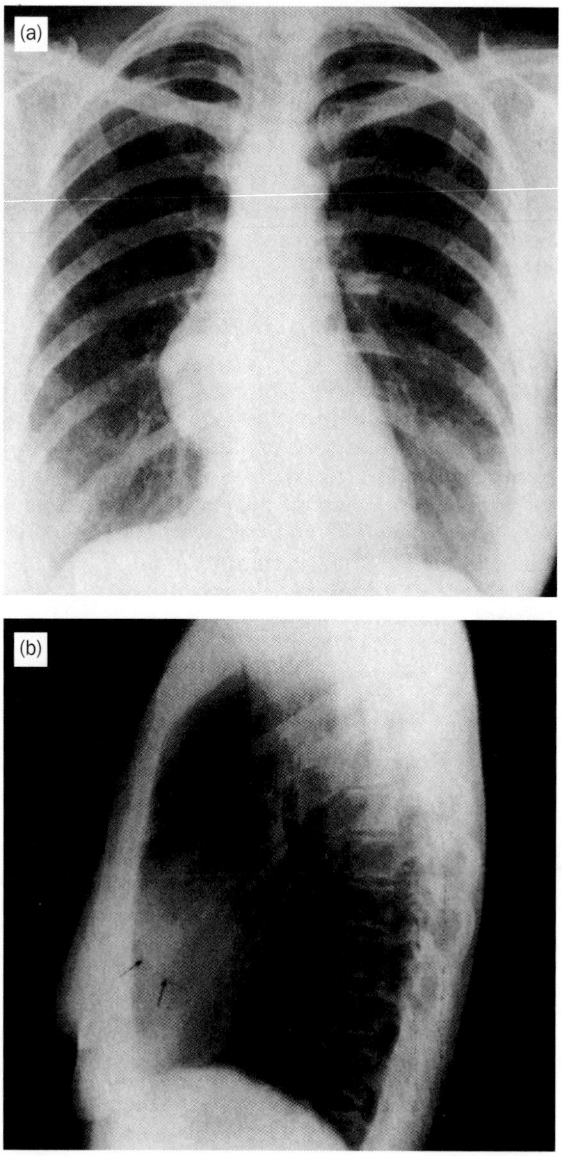

Figure 53.6 (a) PA and (b) lateral chest radiographs showing an anterior mediastinal thymic cyst.

incision. Occasionally the retrosternal element may be so large that it cannot be delivered through the thoracic outlet without splitting part or all of the sternum. The diagnosis of a retrosternal thyroid should certainly be made pre-operatively and it is very helpful to the surgeon to know whether or not a retrosternal extension is in continuity with the main thyroid mass. When an anterior mediastinal mass is not in continuity with the cervical thyroid tissue it should be approached by either median sternotomy or later lateral thoracotomy.

Parathyroid

Parathyroid adenomas occurring within the mediastinum are rare, being found in less than 5% of patients with hyperparathyroidism. The explanation of this ectopic parathyroid tissue is related to the fairly complicated developmental migration of the parathyroid tissue. As with parathyroid adenomas in the neck, the diagnosis is suspected on clinical and biochemical grounds and these tumours are very rarely visible on routine radiography. It is occasionally possible to demonstrate a tumour circulation by selective angiography, but multiple sampling from the veins of the neck and mediastinum for estimation of parathormone levels may give a more accurate indication of the site of the parathyroid adenoma. DSA has value as an imaging technique for parathyroid tissue. Surgical exploration involves complete examination of the neck before the sternum is split and the mediastinum explored. Pre-operative injection of methylene blue may aid the identification of the parathyroid gland at open operation.

Thymus

The thymus gland has right and left lobes closely bound together which may overlap each other to some extent. It lies anteriorly in the superior mediastinum and extends both superiorly into the front of the left brachiocephalic vein and inferiorly into the anterior mediastinum. The lower poles are closely related to the pericardium. Its relative size is greatest in the full-term infant when it is as large as the heart itself, but after puberty the thymus undergoes fatty degeneration to a varying extent. This process of involution is said to be complete by the age of 28 years. The thymus derives a blood supply from the internal thoracic arteries and the venous drainage is into the left brachiocephalic vein. In the young child the size and shape of the thymus varies considerably and the gland is subdivided into lobules by fibrous septa. In the elderly, it may be represented by just two stands of rather unimpressive fatty tissue. In the child, the thymus can be recognized to have a cortex and a medulla, the former contains predominantly lymphocytes, whereas the latter has epithelial cells and Hassall's corpuscles. Some aspects of thymic function are of considerable relevance to surgeons. Thymic agenesis is characterized by an absence of T-cells and a failure of cell mediated antibody response.

The part played by the thymus in myasthenia gravis is still not fully understood but thymectomy appears to reduce the production of the motor end-plate antibodies which block the response to acetylcholine. Thymectomy has also been demonstrated on occasions to influence the course of other diseases, such as polymyositis and subacute sclerosing panencephalitis. Pathological abnormalities in the thymus gland have been recorded in many diseases – in particular thyrotoxicosis, systemic lupus erythematosus, acquired haemolytic anaemia and hypogammaglobulinaemia. Thymic involution in the young is in general associated with immunological deficiency states and thymic hyperactivity, both hyperpalsia and neoplasia, with disease processes such as myasthenia, myocarditis and polymyositis.

Thymic cysts

These are usually relatively small, asymptomatic, benign lesions which occur anteriorly in the mediastinum. In adults thymic cysts are often small but may be multiple and have an attachment to the thymus gland. Small cysts are lined by ciliated epithelium or by columnar cells, larger ones by flattened epithelial or cuboidal cells. It remains unclear whether these cysts are derived from branchial pouch remnants or whether they differentiate from the thymic tissue. The majority of patients are asymptomatic but children with large thymic cysts may develop respiratory distress. Chest radiography shows a well-defined rounded opacity lying within the anterior mediastinum of anterior portion of the superior medastinum (Figure 53.6). On occasions the mass may be closely related to the pericardium. Contrast CT scanning should demonstrate a well-defined fluid-containing opacity and may assist considerably with the diagnosis (Figure 53.7). Even though most of these thymic cysts are asymptomatic surgical excision is recommended. The reasons for this are several – doubt about the diagnosis, the possibility of malignancy and the likelihood of enlargement. The latter may occur with considerable rapidity if there is haemorrhage into the cyst. Median sternotomy gives excellent access to these thymic lesions and is now the preferred incision. They can also be excised with little difficulty through a lateral thoracotomy. Surgical excision establishes the diagnosis and thymic cysts do not recur.

Thymic tumours

These are the most common anteriorly situated tumours in the mediastinum but have also been reported around the hila and even within the lung. There is considerable difference of opinion regarding the correct pathological classification. Some can confidently be called benign and others malignant but a considerable number are on the borderline between the two. Similarly, some tumours are clearly of epithelial origin whereas others consist almost entirely of lymphoid tissue. The most common appearance is a mixture of the two varieties with one or other element predominating. A clinical subdivision is also possible on the basis of whether or not myasthenia gravis is present. Another peculiar aspect of thymic tumours is that their clinical behaviour may bear little relationship to the pathological appearance. A small encapsulated and apparently benign tumour may recur locally or even on a more widespread basis. In contrast, apparently infiltrative malignant tumours even when incompletely resected may be compatible with prolonged survival. In general, local invasion at the time of surgery is a poor prognostic factor associated with local recurrence, though distant metastases are quite unusual. Classification as malignant or benign for thymoma is therefore best used descriptively about the behaviour of the individual lesion.

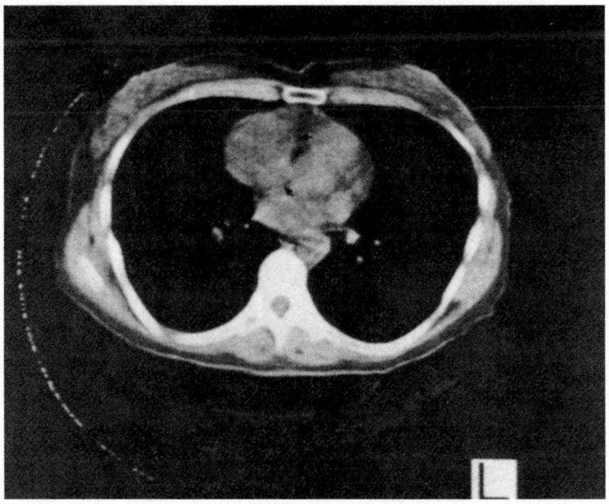

Figure 53.7 CT scan of the same patient as in Figure 53.6.

Thymomas (without myasthenia)

The majority of such patients are asymptomatic. Even when symptoms occur, they are often non-specific – chest pain, cough and occasionally breathlessness. Superior vena caval obstruction is a poor prognostic sign and hiccup has been reported. Radiologically a thymoma does not have a characteristic appearance and the presence of any anterior mediastinal mass should suggest this diagnostic possibility. Today initial assessment is by CT scanning and operability and staging identified by MRI.

Treatment

Any opacity suspected of being a thymoma should be surgically excised. The contraindication is clear cut evidence of invasion of the great vessels demonstrated either by the presence of caval obstruction with a cavogram supporting invasion rather than compression, or by an arteriogram indicating invasion of the aorta or its branches. Contrast CT scanning and MRI have now replaced arteriography. Superior vena caval obstruction is now palliated by endoluminal stenting. The most suitable incision is a median sternotomy, though such tumours can also be removed without difficulty through a thoracotomy. Even benign thymic tumours may be adherent to surrounding structures and because of the possibility of local recurrence excision *en bloc* with adjacent pericardium and pleura may be needed. Radiotherapy is an important adjunct to the management of patient who have thymic tumours which are towards the lymphomatous end of the spectrum and it is certainly indicated in irresectable tumours or those which have been incompletely resected. Combination chemotherapy has also been tried, but the response is unpredictable and presently no clear cut recommendations are apparent.

The thymus and myasthenia gravis

The pathogenesis of myasthenia is still not fully understood but it is probable that part of the disease process is related to the production of an antibody which blocks the effect of acetylcholine at the motor end-plate. These antibodies are not produced within the thymus but it has been recognized for over 80 years that patients with myasthenia gravis have abnormalities of the thymus gland.

The diagnosis, clinical features and medical management of myasthenia are outside the scope of this book. Some 75–80% of patients with myasthenia may derive some benefit from thymectomy; about half have a satisfactory remission. The pathological appearance of the thymic gland in the majority of myasthenics shows some degree of hyperplasia particularly of the lymphoid elements but between 10 and 30% of myasthenics are reported to have thymomas. These are usually small – under 2 cm – and may not be visible on routine chest radiography. CT scanning may pick up quite small thymic tumours and they may also be identified by selective cannulation and angiography through the thymic vein. An important development has been the demonstration that patients with myasthenia gravis benefit temporarily by plasmapheresis reducing the motor end-plate antibodies, levels of which in the blood can now be measured by radioimmuno-assay. After plasmapheresis the benefit may last for several weeks and includes significant improvement in respiratory function.

Access for operative excision of the thymus is the subject of some debate. For simple excision of the thymus the cervical approach is recommended by some authorities, as the more major procedure of sternotomy is thought to be unnecessary. Median sternotomy gives excellent access and is the incision of choice in a patient with suspected thymic tumour. It is, however, an incision which does have a certain morbidity, including the unpleasant, but uncommon, complication of mediastinal infection with sternal dehiscence. Division of the upper half of the sternum, extending to the second or third intercostal space, has never gained much popularity although access is adequate. A wide excision of the thymus is the best approach and if there is a tumour present, a block of mediastinal tissue including both pleura and pericardium should be removed. These measures are justified because the principal problem with thymic tumours is their propensity to local recurrence. The mortality from elective thymectomy should now be nil as long as the post-operative care is appropriate. The benefit from thymectomy is not immediate and patients will usually still require their anticholinesterase drugs in the early post-operative period. Steroid therapy and even immunosuppression may be of assistance to the patient, combined with thymectomy and plasmapheresis, in inducing remission. The best results are obtained in young females in whom the disease has been diagnosed relatively recently and who do not have a thymic tumour.

Thymic tumours may be carcinoids, 35% of which secrete inappropriate adrenocorticotrophic hormone (ACTH). Hydrocortisone support will be required post-operatively. The condition should be recognized pre-operatively as some features of Cushing's syndrome are usually apparent.

Teratoma and extragonadal germ cell tumours

By definition teratoma contains tissue from all three germinal layers though the degree of representation of each layer may vary considerably. The most common mediastinal teratoma is the dermoid, which derives principally from the ectodermal layer and is usually cystic. Its development in this situation is thought to be related to the complexity of the embryology of the mediastinum. These lesions are rarely found anywhere other than anteriorly in the mediastinum and probably arise from cells originating in the area of the third branchial pouch and cleft. The solid tumours may contain an odd mixture of adult and embryonic tissue, with varying degrees of maturity.

Presentation

Most mediastinal teratomas are symptomless and are found on routine chest radiography. Infection occasionally occurs in the cystic variety of tumour but malignant change is much the most important complication. About one-third of dermoid cysts and two-thirds of solid teratomas may undergo malignant change. Occasionally pathognomonic symptoms do occur, such as the coughing up of hair or sebaceous material; but in general when symptoms arise they are due to compression of surrounding mediastinal structures.

Investigations

Most of these tumours are symptomless and are chance radiographic findings. They are rounded homogeneous shadows which have a well-defined margin and lie anteriorly in the mediastinum (Figure 53.8). They may

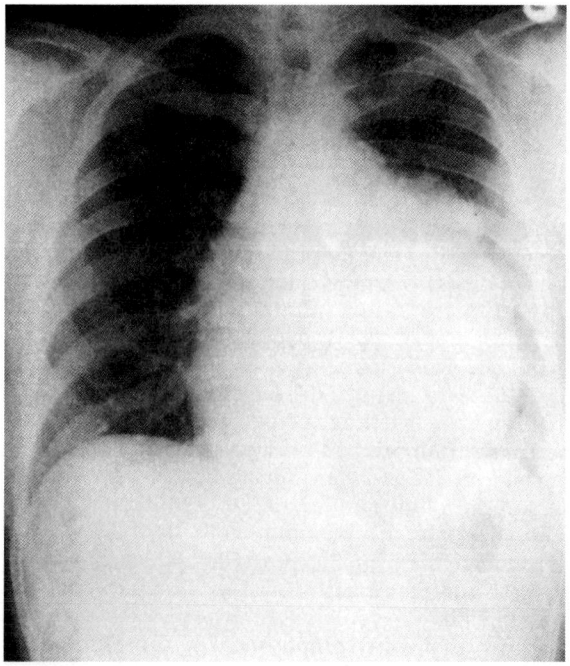

Figure 53.8 AP chest radiograph of an adult with a large benign teratoma.

extend very considerably laterally to displace the lung, particularly in infants. Calcification is present in about one-third of these tumours and recognizable teeth may occasionally be seen. The presence of a fluid level is an indication of a fistulous communication with the lung or tracheobronchial tree. It is not usually necessary to undertake further sophisticated investigation but CT scans will delineate the opacity accurately and may give more information about the nature of its contents.

Management

Surgical exploration and removal of the lesion is always the treatment of choice. There are several reasons for this – up to 30% of the relatively benign dermoid cysts become malignant whereas the proportion is very much higher for the solid teratomas, particularly in men. Although teratomas tend to enlarge gradually, they occasionally enlarge quite rapidly and produce pressure effects. The other problem is simply doubt about the diagnosis and it is very important in patients with mediastinal tumours that an accurate pathological diagnosis is made in order that all appropriate therapy may be given. Surgical access to the anterior mediastinum is best obtained by median sternotomy, particularly when it is suspected that an anterior mediastinal tumour is malignant. Benign teratomas usually project to one or other side of the mediastinum and can easily be removed at lateral thoracotomy. Patients in whom the teratoma has apparently involved the pericardium have also been recorded and it is not unusual for portions of the pericardium and pleura to need to be resected in order to be sure of mediastinal clearance. The surgical removal of a teratoma is a simple procedure which involves little dissection unless either infection or malignant change has occurred. If a benign teratoma is excised completely then local recurrence is unusual, but there is a much higher incidence of this complication and even of more distant metastasis if the lesion is malignant.

Previously teratoma as a classification embraced a rarer group of primary mediastinal tumours now identified as of germ cell origin. Earlier opinion that these tumours might be metastatic from primary tumours of the gonads no longer pertains; their primary mediastinal origin is now widely accepted. They are consequently categorized as germ cell tumours of the mediastinum. The category includes seminoma, embryonal cell tumour and choriocarcinoma; less commonly teratocarcinoma, endodermal sinus/yolk sac tumours and germ cell tumours of mixed histology occur.

Although they may present in much the same way as an anterior mediastinal tumour, their behaviour tends to be more aggressive with invasion of surrounding structures and early distant metastases, particularly to the lungs. As with chorionepitheliomas elsewhere, chorionic gonadotrophin may be secreted and occasionally gives rise to gynaecomastia and testicular atrophy.

Complete surgical excision offers the best chance of survival, and may be followed by radiotherapy and chemotherapy. In patients with mediastinal seminoma good results have been obtained by irradiation and chemotherapy without surgical resection. However, the patient requires an initial histological diagnosis. The usual approach is that of effective excision as the investigative and therapeutic singular event, initial anterior mediastinotomy may often have produced the histological information if the diagnosis of germ cell tumour was not suspected.

Modern solid tumour chemotherapy often involves an operative debulking procedure, so that modern management of malignant teratoma and germ cell tumours of the mediastinum usually involves a major operative excision.

Neurogenic tumours (Table 53.1)

Approximately 75% of tumours of the posterior mediastinum are of neurogenic origin. Benign tumours arising from the nerve sheath take two forms, the neurofibroma and neurilemmoma. Neurofibroma is non-encapsulated and shows a tangle of neurofibrils of Schwannian origin. Neurolemmoma is encapsulated and consists of Antoni type A and B tissue with collections of foamy macrophages. It is not unusual to see elements of neurofibroma and neurilemmoma within the same specimen. Malignant change may occur in the neurofibroma to fibrosarcoma of neural origin. Sarcomatous change in neurolemmoma is very rare, although occasional local recurrence may occur after

Table 53.1 Neurogenic tumours of the mediastinum

Benign	*Malignant*
Nerve sheath origin	
Neurolemmoma	Malignant Schwannoma – neurogenic sarcoma
Neurofibroma	
Autonomic ganglia	
Ganglioneuroma	Neuroblastoma – sympathetico-blastoma
	Ganglioneuroblastoma – partially differentiated neuroblastoma
Paraganglion system	
Phaeochromocytoma	Malignant phaeochromocytoma
True paraganglionoma	Malignant praraganglionoma
Non-chromaffinoma – chemodectoma	

resection. Tumours of the sympathetic nervous system demonstrate variable differentiation between individual tumours and often within the same tumour. Neuroblastoma is more common in children, it tends to occur in the upper posterior mediastinum, is unencapsulated and often infiltrative at presentation. There is a more differentiated form of tumour of the sympathetic nervous system called a ganglioneuroblastoma or a differentiating neuroblastoma; this is to identify the less aggressive aspect of the tumour which is encapsulated, appears lobular and is usually not infiltrative at presentation. The benign form occurs in adults as a ganglioneuroma. This is the most common form of tumour of the sympathetic nervous system. Grossly the presentation is of a smooth well-encapsulated mass in the posterior mediastinum which on cross-section usually has a fibrous yellow/grey appearance. Survival is directly proportional to the differentiation at microscopy. Effective resection will cure ganglioneuroma. Solid tumour chemotherapy is developing apace for the neuroblastomas of childhood and cure rates are rising.

Presentation

Most patients with neural tumours are entirely asymptomatic and the diagnosis is made as a chance radiographic finding. Very large neural tumours may produce pressure symptoms, such as dyspnoea, cough or dysphagia. Root pain in the distribution of the involved nerve is uncommon but Horner's syndrome may be produced by involvement of the cervical sympathetic chain at the thoracic oulet. Extension of neural tumours through the intervertebral foramina may press upon the spinal cord. Patients with multiple neurofibromatosis, Von Recklinghausen's disease, may have intrathoracic and mediastinal manifestations of their disease. A recent major population survey in multiple neurofibromatosis has suggested that previous estimates of rates of malignant change have been exaggerated.

Investigations

Mediastinal neural tumours are posteriorly situated, have a 'D' shaped outline on chest X-ray and are of uniform density (Figure 53.9). Up to 20% of patients have associated rib and vertebral abnormalities, apart from the local effect of a large tumour pressing on the posterior end of the ribs. Barium swallow examination may demonstrate oesophageal displacement in those patients with large tumours but bronchoscopy is unhelpful. A CT scan is the initial investigation after discovery on chest radiograph. It is usual to try fine needle aspiration in this investigation. MRI should be used to assess any spinal involvement or anomaly and any tumour extending into the vertebral foramina.

Neuroblastomas of the mediastinum are somewhat less aggressive than those in the retroperitoneum, but they do secrete catecholamines which can be estimated in a urine sample. Recently a new biochemical test has been evaluated. Neurone specific enolase is an enzyme present in the serum in patients with neural tumours. It is most valuable to have a high probability of diagnosis before thoracotomy so that the operation is properly executed. Both these tests should be done in children with posterior mediastinal masses. It is also wise to use these estimates if the adult disease is thought to be progressive.

Management

In general the policy with patients suspected of having mediastinal neurogenic tumours has been to advise thoracotomy and resection of the tumour because of doubt about the diagnosis and the possibility of malignancy. Increasingly VATS is the routine approach. Certainly if a tumour is enlarging, it should be excised as it will produce pressure effects on surrounding structures. Of patients who have neurogenic tumours, particularly ganglioneuromas, 1–15% have direct

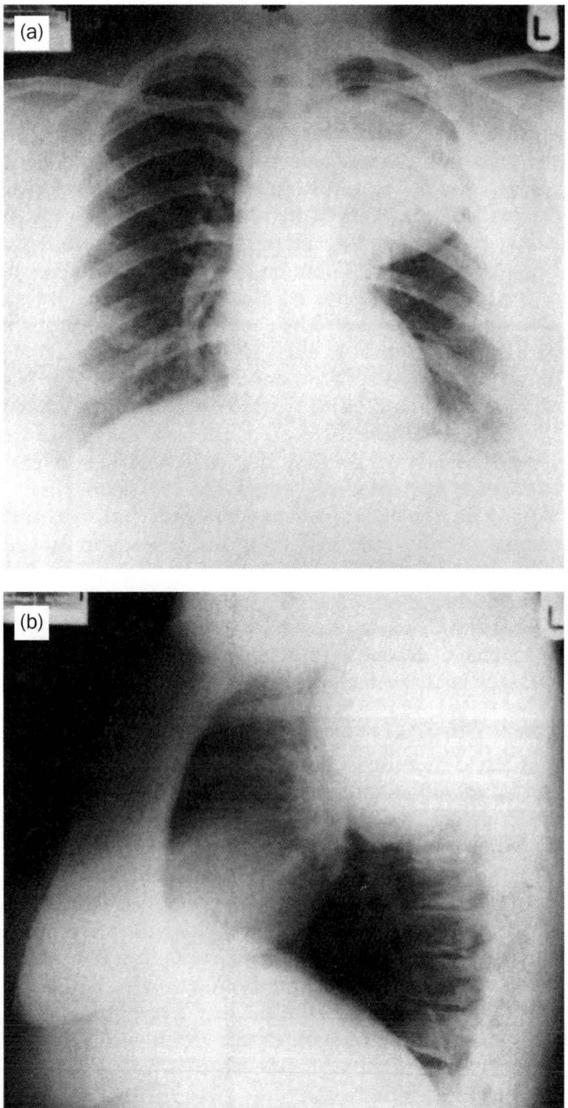

Figure 53.9 (a) PA and (b) lateral chest radiographs in a patient with a benign ganglioneuroma.

extension of their tumour into intervertebral foramina. Such patients should have the initial thoracotomy with excision of the intrathoracic mass and a careful attempt to remove the intraforaminal aspect. Should this not remove all of the tumour a seond stage planned procedure, a laminectomy or fenestration with extradural exploration, should follow immediately. Excellent results follow such a combined procedure. In patients who have generalized neurofibromatosis the presence of a typical posterior mediastinal opacity is not sufficient indication for exploratory surgery but resection is required if the lesion is enlarging.

Operation is carried out through a posterolateral thoracotomy at a level appropriate to the site of the tumour although video assisted thoracoscopic operations are effective in this situation. Immediate complications of surgery are few and consist principally of incomplete resection and the consequences of division of the sympathetic nerves near the thoracic outlet. Recurrence after apparently complete resection of a benign lesion is quite unusual. Other than rapid growth, there are no features which distinguish a malignant from a benign tumour. If the latter type of tumour is excised completely, no further treatment is required. Neuroblastoma is often large at presentation, although the use of radiotherapy is declining it is still used to reduce tumour mass before operation. Postoperatively pulsed chemotherapy is used. Cis-platinum based regimens are given at monthly intervals for six pulses in neuroblastoma. Presently the 5 year survival proportion in neuroblastoma is 60–70% with operative removal and chemotherapy. Spontaneous regression and maturation phenomena have been described in neuroblastoma. The mechanisms are ill understood but when the phenomenon occurs the prognosis is markedly improved.

Tumours of the paraganglion system

Chemically active and inactive tumours occur. Phaeochromocytoma is rare in the mediastinum, and if symptoms are present various manifestations of hypertension, hypermetabolism and diabetes may occur. Such symptoms associated with a mediastinal mass suggest an active phaeochromocytoma. Either or both adrenaline (epinephrine) and nor-adrenaline (norepinephrine) may be produced. Urinary and serum catechol amine estimation is now the preferred confirmatory test as it has a postive test probability of disease presence of >90%. One per cent of phaeochromocytomas present in the thorax, usually in the paravertebral gutter. The approach at removal is the routine for paravertebral tumours associated with the precautions for removal of phaeochromocytomas below the diaphragm, i.e. the use of alpha and beta-blockade. The tumour is usually highly vascular and bleeding is common. The tumour is a reddish brown soft glandular structure. Effective removal of the benign lesion is curative, but the malignant lesion carries a very poor prognosis.

Chemodectomas are rare, they may be found in the posterior mediastinum or associated with the viscera. This soft tumour is richly vascular, uncommonly malignant, and should be removed *en bloc* if possible. Occasionally, excision of the tumour is not feasible, but a biopsy must be done. Radiotherapy is given when malignancy is confirmed.

Thoracic meningocele

The thoracic meningocele is a cystic lesion arising from the spinal meninges protruding through an intervertebral defect. It extends beneath the pleura and presents a radiological appearance very similar to a neurogenic tumour though rather more translucent. The anatomy is clearly demonstrable at MRI. Two-thirds of patients with intrathoracic meningoceles also have multiple neurofibromatosis and almost all have vertebral or rib abnormalities adjacent to the opacity. These are usually in the form of kyphosis, scoliosis or bone defects. The treatment of choice is surgical excision, though if the lesion is large, it may be complicated by a spinal fluid fistula.

Pleuropericardial cysts

Thin-walled cysts containing clear fluid are occasionally found in the anterior cardiophrenic angle. They are closely related to the pericardium and are probably due to a developmental abnormality when a lacunar cavity fails to fuse with the main pericardial sac. They have been given various names including pericardial coelomic cysts and springwater cysts. They are seen more often on the right side of the chest than on the left and are usually asymptomatic.

Presentation

The great majority are detected as a chance radiography finding. Symptoms are few, chest discomfort is commonest, then dyspnoea and cough. Clinical signs are rare, but when the cyst is very large dullness to percussion over the anterior chest wall and diminished air entry at the base anteriorly may be noted.

Investigations

Radiographically they present as smooth, round opacities usually at the right cardiophrenic angle. The lateral film demonstrates that they occupy the anterior angle between the sternum and the diaphragm. The principal differential diagnosis is from a hernia through the foramen of Morgagni. Barium enema and CT scans may be helpful in resolving the diagnosis. At CT scanning the density estimate is diagnostic, i.e. Hounsfield number for water.

Management

It may be difficult to make a firm diagnosis without surgical intervention. If an irrefutable diagnosis could be made without thoracotomy, there would be no justification for removal of the cysts. Resection presents no technical difficulty and no patient should come to harm from this procedure. Occasionally a communication exists between the cyst and the pericardium but no problems arise because of this. If previous films are available which show that the opacity has been present, unchanged in size, for several years, then operation is probably not justifiable. In this situation the diagnosis may be confirmed by aspiration of the cyst, with the removal of the typical clear fluid. Malignant change does not occur.

Cystic duplications of the foregut

There are two principal varieties of foregut duplications, which between them account for 10% of all mediastinal cysts and tumours. The first arises from a relatively localized abnormality at the stage of development when the tracheobronchial tree is growing from the primitive foregut wall. The resulting duplication may be either in the wall of the oesophagus – a gastroenteric or enterogenous cyst – or in the wall of the tracheobronchial tree – a bronchogenic cyst. These cysts develop within the muscle of the foregut canal and are almost always lined by ciliated columnar epithelium. The second variety develops much earlier in fetal life as part of a more diffuse congenital lesion called the split notochord syndrome, and is commonly associated with vertebral and sometimes with spinal cord abnormalities. Is is thought that these defects are the result of varying degrees of adhesions between endoderm and ectoderm so that the ectodermal cells from which the notochord develops are split into two separate centres. In this way cystic lesions develop in association with congenital scoliosis or hemivertebrae. The duplication may occasionally lie low in the posterior mediastinum and be associated with thoracoabdominal abnormalities, such as mesenteric duplications. Such a lesion is called a neuroenteric cyst.

Bronchogenic cysts

These may also be called bronchial cysts and arise as a result of abnormal budding of the bronchial pathways during development. They are thin-walled and often merely have some connective tissue and a little smooth muscle in the wall. They may also contain cartilage and glandular elements. Cysts which have not been infected are filled with clear, yellow or milky fluid and they may be classified according to their location: (1) paratracheal – attached to the tracheal wall just above the bifurcation; (2) carinal – the attachment is at the level of the carina and the cyst is often adherent to the anterior oesophageal wall; (3) hilar – the cyst is attached to one or other main bronchus. Occasionally bronchogenic cysts are also found attached to lobar bronchi.

Presentation

The majority of these cysts are asymptomatic and the abnormality is diagnosed on routine radiography or an incidental film. As the cysts enlarge they may cause pressure symptoms, in particular respiratory distress, cough and dysphagia. Occasionally infection occurs and there may be a fistula between the cyst and the tracheobronchial tree. This complication may produce systemic disturbance with haemoptysis and purulent sputum.

Investigations

Standard postero-anterior and lateral chest radiographs demonstrate a smooth, rounded, homogeneous mediastinal opacity, usually situated just anterior to the vertebral column. The presence of a fluid level indicates a fistula into the tracheobronchial tree. A barium swallow may be helpful in demonstrating that the cyst is anterior to the oesophagus and may in fact displace it. Bronchoscopy is usually carried out but demonstrates little more than tracheobronchial compression on occasions.

Management

Pre-operatively the diagnosis can rarely be made with complete certainty. When doubt exists thoracotomy with excision is indicated. Any cyst that is producing pressure symptoms should obviously be removed.

Enterogenous cysts

Developmentally these are segments of the alimentary tract which have separated off completely or partially. They tend to be lined by mucosa similar to that of the foregut – usually columnar but occasionally squamous.

Two types are recognized:

- **Oesophageal cysts:** these lie either within or very close to the wall of the oesophagus and are lined by ciliated columnar epithelium. They probably represent true duplication and share a common blood supply with the oesophagus. Their usual site is at the middle third of the oesophagus more frequently on the right than on the left.
- **Neuroenteric cysts:** these are cystic structures lying in the posterior mediastinum separate from the oesophagus. They have a variable epithelium and a muscular wall resembling that of the intestine. They have a fibrous posterior attachment to the spine and are commonly associated with vertebral abnormalities.

These are the cystic derivatives of the split notochord syndrome. Because the vertebral column and the foregut elongate at different rates, the final position of the cyst is often caudal to that of the vertebral defect. Accordingly radiographs of the cervical and upper thoracic spine may be required to demonstrate the vertebral abnormalities. These cysts also tend to present as a chance radiological finding and are usually asymptomatic. The complications of infection and tracheobronchial obstruction are seen occasionally as with bronchogenic cysts. One additional complication is that mediastinal cysts lined by gastric-type mucosa are prone to all the complications of peptic ulceration. Because of these potentially serious complications and the difficulty of making an unequivocal diagnosis, surgical excision at thoracotomy remains the treatment of choice.

Section 53.4 • Lymphoma

Mediastinal involvement occurs in up to 50% of patients with Hodgkin's disease and in 10–20% of patients with non-Hodgkin's lymphoma. The mediastinal abnormality is part of the generalized lymphomatous disease and involves particularly the superior and anterior mediastinum.

Presentation

A proportion of these patients present with lymphoma elsewhere and the mediastinal abnormality is noted on routine chest radiography. Where the mediastinal masses reach a considerable size pressure effects may be noted, particularly cough, dyspnoea and stridor. Sometimes the mediastinal mass is large enough to produce superior vena caval (SVC) obstruction.

Investigations

Chest radiography initially, then contrast high-resolution CT (HRCT) will demonstrate whether the mass is paratracheal, hilar or anterior mediastinal. Staging in lymphoma is increasingly by non-invasive techniques: MRI and PET scanning are now in common use. Further investigation is directed principally towards making a histological diagnosis and determining the extent of the disease elsewhere in the body. Bronchoscopy is relatively unhelpful in most cases other than when assessing tracheobronchial compression. Mediastinoscopy or left anterior mediastinotomy will usually provide a histological diagnosis and will also serve to distinguish lymphoma from other causes of multiple lymph gland enlargement in the mediastinum, particularly sarcoidosis, metastatic carcinoma and primary pulmonary tuberculosis. Giant cell hyperplasia of the lymph gland may occur and is an important differential diagnosis as it is a self-limiting condition requiring no treatment. After treatment for lymphoma recurrence is not uncommon as is post-radiation fibrosis and repeat mediastinal staging operative procedures are often necessary.

Management

The details of management of lymphoma are discussed in Module 11. The majority of patients will respond to a greater or lesser extent to intermittent combination chemotherapy with or without radiotherapy. Surgical treatment has little to offer in that the disease is generalized though it is thought by some that reduction in tumour bulk may improve the efficacy of the chemotherapy. Dramatic pressure symptoms such as caval obstruction or stridor are usually taken as an indication for urgent chemotherapy and radiotherapy. SVC obstruction is not a contraindication to mediastinoscopy. SVC obstruction is often relieved by endoluminal stenting prior to mediastinoscopy. Because lymphoma does have an effective response to chemotherapy some authorities would not stent and proceed to chemotherapy as soon as the histology was established.

Section 53.5 • Rare mediastinal tumours

Mediastinal cysts and tumours present a particularly interesting diagnostic challenge, as they are rare and because of the difficulty of being certain of the pre-operative diagnosis even when apparently typical clinical and radiological appearances are present. Many of the conditions already discussed in this module are uncommon but the differential diagnosis is further lengthened by the occurrence of several more groups of even rarer mediastinal tumours (Figure 53.10). As expected, any area of the body that contains fat and fibrous tissue may occasionally produce lipomas, fibromas and their malignant counterparts, the liposarcoma and fibrosarcoma. Similarly, there is a wide variety of vascular and lymphatic tissue in the thorax which does produce many unusual tumours, classified according to their cellular composition. Thus a vascular tumour consisting of capillaries alone is called a capillary haemangioma except where the vessels are widely dilated when it becomes a cavernous haemangioma. If one or other cell group within the vessel wall predominates then the tumour may be called a haemangio-endothelioma. These are relatively benign tumours. However, the malignant angiosarcoma and haemangiopericytoma have been reported. They can occur in any age group and in any part of the mediasinum. If they involve the posterior mediastinum then extension on to the vertebral bodies and into the spinal canal can cause insuperable problems.

Contrast CT scanning and MRI are standard investigations, inevitably pre-operative as there is little alternative management. Excision is the treatment of choice but is a high-risk procedure in the more extensive tumour.

A slightly more common and rather different tumour is the lymphangioma or cystic hygroma which is seen particularly in children. As the name suggests they are benign cystic tumours which occur in the anterior mediastinum and have a good prognosis. The aetiology is not fully understood – they may arise from lymphoid tissue normally present in the area or may grow from mesodermal rests which produce abnormal lymphoid channels. The cystic hygroma is a particular variety of lymphangioma developing in relations to the lymph vessels of the jugular or iliac region; such a mediastinal lesion is usually associated with a cervical hygroma. They consist of a number of cysts of varying size, lined with epithelium, and the walls may contain smooth muscle and lymphocytes. The contents are clear or straw-coloured fluid. Standard chest radiographs may show a mass extending from the hilar area well up into the neck, and cystic spaces may be visible in it. Occasionally there is involvement of the pericardium with the production of chylopericardium. Early surgical removal is the treatment of choice.

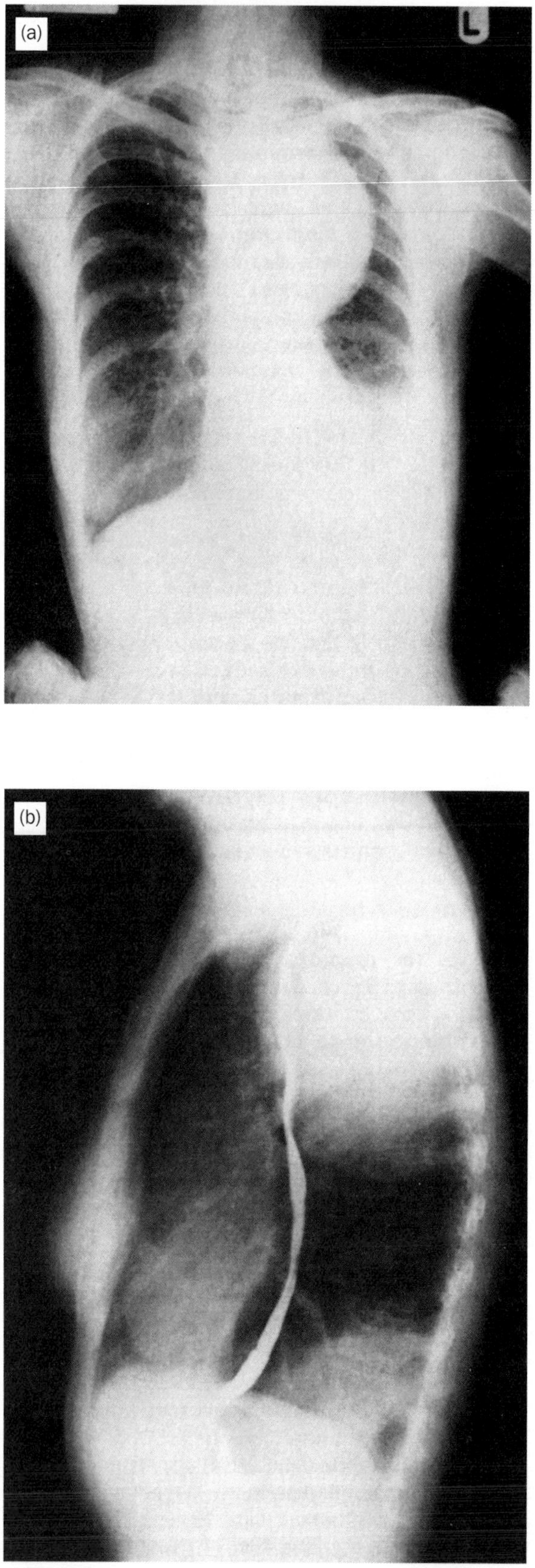

Figure 53.10 (a) PA and (b) lateral barium radiographs of a patient with a malignant mediastinal sarcoma and left pleural effusion.

The thoracic duct has occasionally been the site of cystic change. This may be suspected on CT scan and confirmed at MRI.

There are two varieties:

- **Degenerative:** these are usually found incidentally in the elderly at the time of autopsy. They may be multiple and the presence of atherosclerosis and calcification may be found in the walls of the cysts.
- **Lymphangiomatous:** there may be single or multiple cyst-like spaces filled with chyle.

Thoracic duct cysts occasionally rupture into the pleura to cause spontaneous chylothorax. Enhanced CT scanning and MRI may assist in the diagnosis if other dilated lymphatic channels can be identified. Lymphangiography is diagnostic and is indicated if doubt still exists after MRI.

Section 53.6 • Mediastinitis

Mediastinitis is rarely a primary disease entity. It is most frequently caused by perforation of the oesophagus which may be either spontaneous or traumatic and this is dealt with in Module 7. The formation of pus within mediastinal lymph nodes secondary to infection of the lungs or oesophagus may lead to acute mediastinitis as can vertebral tuberculosis or osteomyelitis. The clinical features are those of severe systemic upset with chest pain, rigors, pyrexia, dyspnoea and sometimes cyanosis and dysphagia. The mediastinal pleura is inflamed and a pleural effusion develops. This may proceed to a pyopneumothorax and mediastinal emphysema may also be seen. The management consists of treatment of the primary condition, antibiotics and surgical drainage of any abscess or pyopneumothorax.

Deep cervical infection extends into the mediastinum down the fascial planes and may even spread directly into the pericardium via the perivascular spaces.

Section 53.7 • Idiopathic mediastinal fibrosis

This condition is sometimes called cryptogenic fibrosing mediastinitis and its aetiology is still not understood. Mediastinal fibrosis may be related to retroperitoneal fibrosis and perhaps even to other fibrosing diseases, such as Riedel's thyroiditis, Dupuytren's contracture and possibly sclerosing cholangitis. The term mid-line fibroses has been suggested as a group description. The co-existence of two or more of these conditions has now been recorded more than once and the term multifocal fibrosclerosis has been suggested. An immunological mechanism for this process has been postulated but has not yet conclusively been demonstrated, nor has there been any consistent evidence of an infective basis although histoplasma has been isolated in a few cases. The drug methysergide which has been used in the treatment of migraine is associated with the production of retroperitoneal but not mediastinal fibrosis. The condition is characterized by the appearance of masses of hard white tissue infiltrating diffusely throughout the mediastinum but not invading the heart or lung. It is seen most frequently in the superior mediastinum in men, and obstruction and compression of the tracheobronchial tree, great veins, oesophagus and pulmonary vessels may occur.

Presentation

The clinical features are insidious and are mainly due to compression of the superior vena cava and innominate veins. The veins of the head, neck and upper limbs become distended and the face and neck swell, particularly when the patient is lying flat. There may be swelling of the eyelids, subconjuntive oedema, headache, breathlessness and epistaxis. With the passage of time venous collateral channels develop, some of which are clearly visible over the anterior chest wall; some of the clinical features resolve as this occurs.

Complications

Extensive fibrosis around the trachea or bronchi may produce increasing dyspnoea, stridor and eventually death. The pulmonary arteries and veins may be involved in the disease process usually as a separate entity which is identified as pulmonary hilar fibrosis and is usually unilateral.

Investigation

Chest radiography may be relatively unimpressive, showing merely some broadening of the superior mediastinum. Bronchoscopy may show evidence of compression of the tracheobraonchial tree. Contrast CT scanning is necessary to image the vessels. Venography of the superior vena cava will confirm the extent of the obstruction and the collateral circulation. Barium swallow may demonstrate oesophageal involvement.

Management

The principal problem is the differentiation from malignant mediastinal infiltration and this can usually only be made at either mediastinoscopy, mediastinotomy or thoracotomy. Steroid therapy and immunosuppression have been exhibited without impressive clinical results. Surgical treatment has little to offer in that the fibrosis is widely infiltrating and cannot usually be resected. Caval obstruction has been treated by a venous bypass from the left brachiocephalic vein to the right atrial appendage. Patency rates are low in this condition because the disease progresses. An adequate collateral circulation will normally develop in time. Sapheno-jugular bypass has been used effectively but is a recent innovation without long-term evaluation. Occasionally there is a localized area of mediastinal fibrosis which can be removed surgically. The disease is not necessarily progressive and some patients undergo slow improvement as collateral venous channels develop. If stricture of the tracheobronchial tree, oesophagus or pulmonary vessels occurs, then the outlook is not good.

Section 53.8 • Mediastinal emphysema

This is a condition produced by rupture of an air-containing viscus either within the mediastinum or in a position where the air may track into the mediastinum. It is seen following rupture of the oesophagus, either spontaneously or following instrumentation. It is more often produced by the spontaneous rupture of a subpleural pulmonary cyst or bulla. If the overlying pleura remains intact then air may track in the subpleural plain to the hilum and thence into the mediastinum. The clinical features depend on the aetiology but the classic physical finding is of crepitus in the tissues of the neck as the air tracks upwards out of the mediastinum. Chest radiography demonstrates a translucency produced by the air between the pleura and the mediastinum and between the mediastinal structures. If the source is an oesophageal injury there will be a toxic response and the patient will be ill.

Management

All patients with spontaneous mediastinal emphysema should have a period of observation. If there develop any signs of sepsis, injury to the oesophagus should be suspected and a water soluble contrast swallow carried out.

Further reading

Economous J. S., Trump, D. L., Holmes, E.C. and Eggleston, J. E. (1982). Management of primary germ cell tumors of the mediastinum. *J Thorac Cardiovasc Surg* **83**: 643–9.

Glenn, W. L., Liebow, A. A. and Lindskog, G. E. (eds) (1976). The mediastinum and mediastinal tumours. In *Thoracic and Cardiovascular Surgery with Related Pathology*, 3rd edn. Englewood Cliffs, NJ: Prentice-Hall, 405–53.

Holmes Sellors, T., Thackray, A. C. and Thomson, A. D. (1976). Tumours of the thymus. *Thorax* **22**: 193–220.

Le Roux, B. T. (1960). Mediastinal teratoma. *Thorax* **15**: 338–8.

Sabiston, D. C. Jr, Duke, J. B., Spencer, F. C. and Stewart, D. G. (1995). *Surgery of the Chest*, 6th edn. Philadelphia, PA: Harcourt Publishing.

Shields, T. W. and Reynolds, M. (1988). Neurogenic tumours of the thorax. *Surg Clin North Am* **68**: 645.

MODULE 54

Disorders of the chest wall

Section 54.1 • Congenital anomalies of the chest wall

Congenital abnormalities of the bony thorax are often incidental findings on routine chest radiography; for example, a midthoracic rib with a bifurcated anterior end which may be fused with the rib above or below (Figure 54.1a). There may be complete absence of one or more ribs, but an accessory or cervical rib is more common (Figure 54.1b). When such costal anomalies occur they are sometimes associated with defects of the vertebral bodies, such as hemivertebrae, and with thoracic and neurological defects. The majority of rib abnormalities are of little significance and only if extensive do they present a clinical problem. (Cervical rib, *vide infra*.)

Pectus excavatum

This is a deformity of the anterior chest wall characterized by depression of the sternum (Figure 54.2). It may be localized to the lower sternum but most often begins at the manubriosternal junction. The rib growth is thought to to be uncontrolled such that the ribs are too long. Accommodations occur in other structures within the chest wall and the area of the rib ends at the costal cartilages becomes prominent.

Pectus carinatum

This is also known as 'pigeon' or 'keel' chest deformity and is much less common than pectus excavatum. It may be associated with vertebral abnormalities. Two main varieties are seen: at manubrial level, in which case the manubrium and the body of sternum are almost at right-angles to one another; and at a much lower level near the xiphisternum (Figure 54.3). The deformity may be either symmetrical or asymmetrical – in the latter the sternum lies obliquely with depression of the costal cartilages on one side and elevation on the other. Again it seems likely that disordered asymmetrical growth of of the ribs at the costal cartilages is responsible.

Symptoms directly due to such physical abnormality are rare. Patients may be very conscious of the unusual shape of their chest wall and be unwilling to participate in activities such as swimming and sunbathing. Limitation of peak cardiac output may occur in severe pectus excavatum as maximal venous return is impaired. Most patients with moderate to severe degrees of depression, even with displacement of their heart to the left, have no clinical disability whatsoever. An ejection systolic murmur may be audible at the left sternal edge, which is from the pulmonary artery flow in a distorted vessel. Routine pulmonary function tests usually show that lung volumes and dynamic function are within normal limits. The degree of abnormality may be assessed clinically and radiologically – the latter by measuring the distance between the body of the sternum and the vertebral column in the lateral chest radiograph.

Treatment

These conditions so rarely cause symptoms that the indications for treatment are usually cosmetic. There is no general agreement with regard to the optimum timing for surgical correction; some surgeons operate in early childhood, but there is always the possibility of asymmetrical growth of costal cartilage continuing. There will not be further growth after the mid-teens. As the decision to operate is almost always cosmetic, it should be made by the individual and not the parents. The case for masterful inactivity is strong in the growing years. Breast development in the pubescent girl often modifies her attitude to minor deformity which may no longer be so obvious.

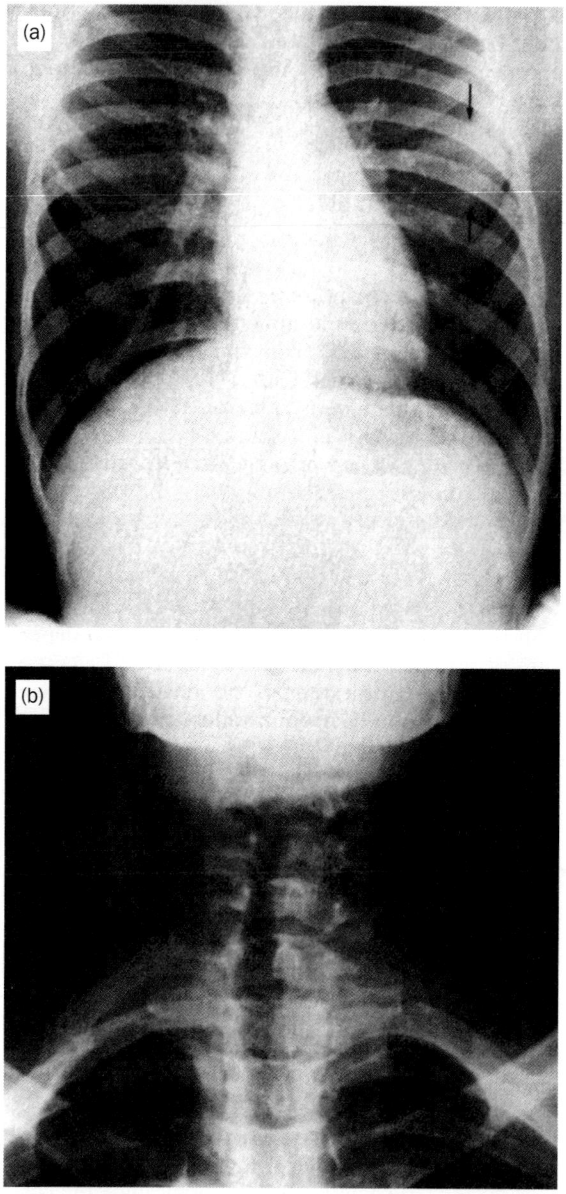

Figure 54.1 (a) Bifid fourth left rib anteriorly – congenital noted on a routine PA chest X-ray. (b) AP X-ray of thoracic outlet showing a cervical rib articulating with the first rib on the right side.

The potential hazards of major reconstructive surgery – anaesthesia, infection, pulmonary embolism, etc. – must always be borne in mind when considering such cosmetic surgery. The operation under general anaesthesia consists of two parts. **Mobilization** – a bilateral submammary incision gives excellent access from the sternal notch to ninth costal cartilages. The involved costal cartilages, usually the third to the seventh or eighth, are resected subperichondrially. A sternal osteotomy is done at about the manubriosternal junction and the body of the sternum elevated as far as is required. **Fixation** – the sternum needs to be stabilized in its new position. Wiring at the site of the osteotomy should be sufficient. External fixation is no longer practised, as with modern implant materials so few complications occur. Most methods of internal fixation rely on retrosternal struts, plates or steel wires resting on the rib ends at either side. These internal fixation devices are removed after the anterior chest wall

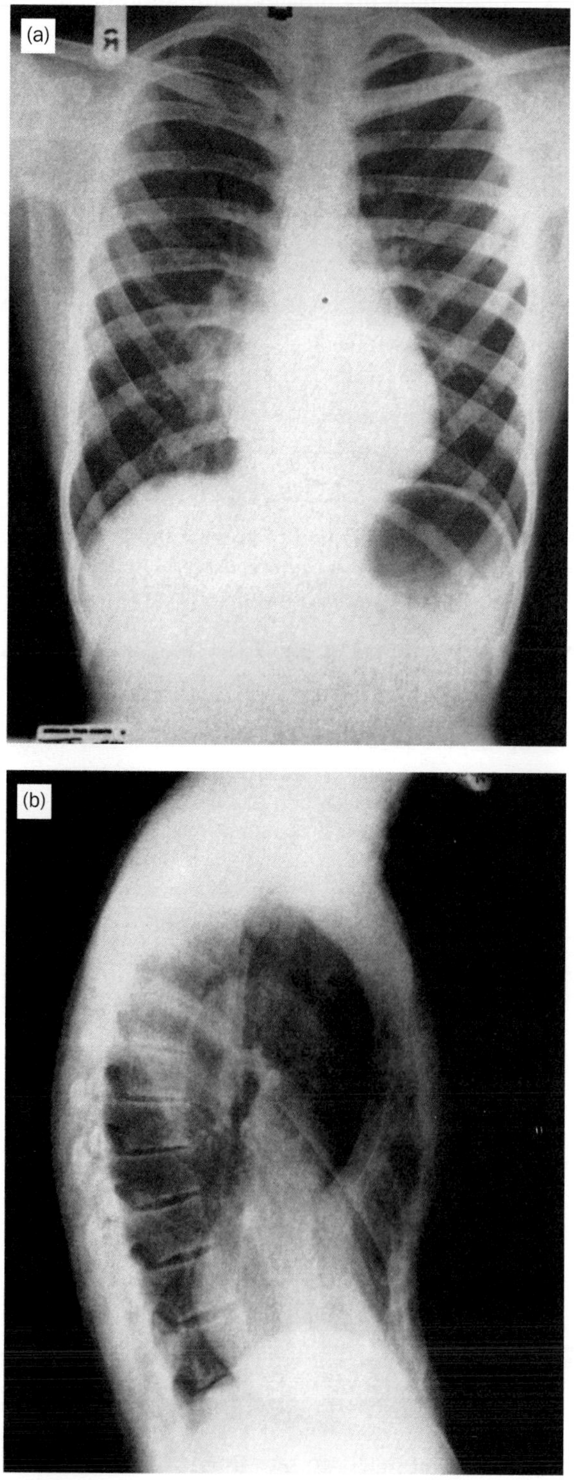

Figure 54.2 (a) PA and (b) lateral chest X-rays showing the typical bony deformity associated with pectus excavatum.

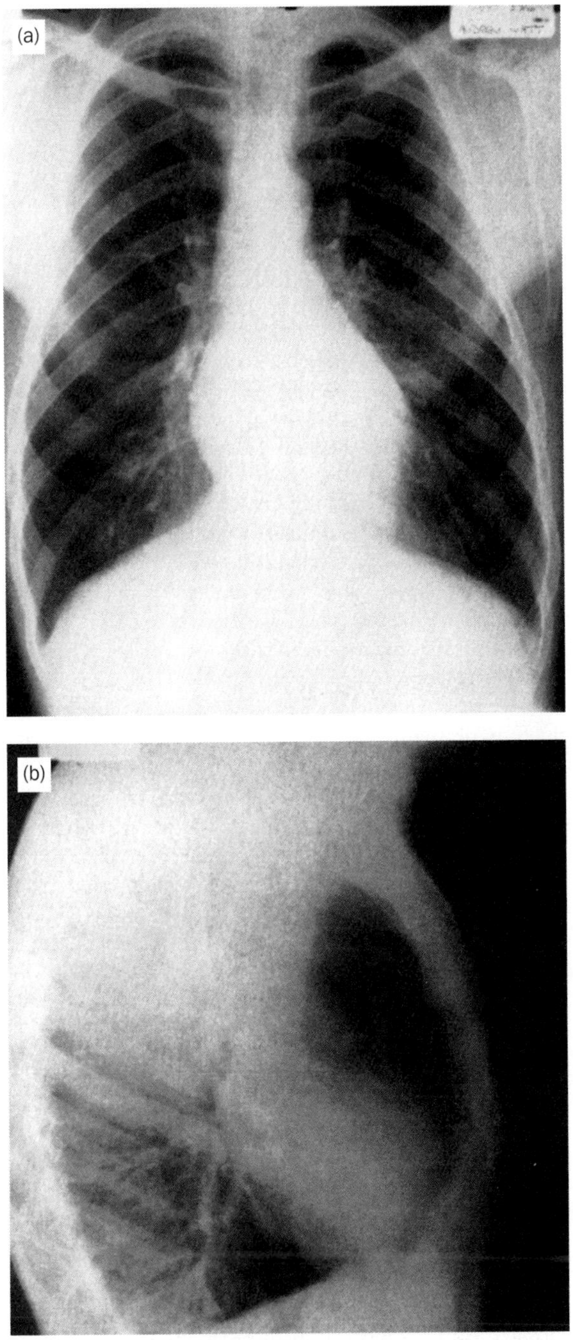

Figure 54.3 (a) PA and (b) lateral chest X-rays showing the thoracic deformity of pectus carinatum.

has united. Patients with lesser abnormalities may only require the reduction of prominent costal cartilages. Patients are usually discharged on the fourth day. The strut is removed electively at day surgery after 18 months. Many surgeons only remove the support if it is causing trouble.

Cleft sternum

Embryologically the sternum is a paired mesenchymal structure which becomes cartilaginous and migrates towards the midline. There are three major components, the manubrium, the body and the xiphoid, which each have a separate centre of ossification.

Failure of fusion of the sternum may lead to a cleft in the midline and there maybe associated defects of the diaphragm, pericardium and abdominal wall. If the heart is exposed then the condition is termed 'ectopia cordis'. Such patients usually have other congenital heart defects in the form of septal defects, valvular abnormalities, or even the tetralogy of Fallot. If sternal closure is carried out in infancy, satisfactory closure of the defect in the sternum can be obtained, but in later life much more complex surgical procedures may be required.

Thoracic outlet syndrome

The thoracic outlet is the space bounded anteriorly by the manubrium sterni, the first ribs laterally and the first thoracic vertebra. This is a narrow channel through which pass various important structures. These structures may be adversely affected by congenital abnormality as well as degenerative processes, tumours and trauma. The various conditions which produce symptoms and signs of compression in this area may be grouped together under the term 'thoracic outlet syndrome'. This includes accessory cervical ribs, the scalenus anterior syndrome and may also include symptoms due to hyperabduction or thrombosis of the subclavian vein.

Section 54.2 • Infection of the chest wall

Osteomyelitis

Primary osteomyelitis of the ribs or sternum occurring through haematogenous spread from a soft-tissue infection elsewhere in the body is now unusual. A destructive osteomyelitis of the sternum can occur as a complication of median sternotomy, the most common organisms responsible being staphylococci. Tuberculosis and fungal infections may involve the chest wall by direct extension from underlying infection of the lungs, pleura or lymph nodes. Treatment consists principally of the institution of appropriate antibiotic therapy and, on occasion, surgical resection of the involved segment of rib or cartilage. Occasionally chronic infections of the sternum fail to respond to simple measures and radical chest wall resection may then be required to eliminate the infection.

Infections of the soft tissues

The skin and subcutaneous tissues of the chest wall are subject to all the common infections which occur anywhere in the body. More serious are the deeper chest wall infections which are now uncommon. Subpectoral and subscapular abscesses, usually due to streptococci or staphylococci, originate in the ribs or the scapula. They require appropriate antibiotic therapy and surgical drainage. If an empyema within the pleural space is not treated appropriately then it may track along the perforating neurovascular bundles, into the subcutaneous tissues and present as an empyema necessitatis. Cold abscess of the chest wall may present similarly as a collar stud abscess. Deep cervical infection will spread on to Sibson's fascia and may present below the clavicle as a fluctuant swelling.

Section 54.3 • Tumours of the chest wall

Bone and cartilage

The most common primary chest wall tumours are the chondromata and chondrosarcomata which originate in the costal cartilages. They often occur close to the costochondral junction and present as visible and palpable swelling in this area. Radiologically a chondroma usually shows expansion of the rib but the cortex remains intact. Chondrosarcoma, by contrast, has a more destructive effect on the surrounding bone. Surgical treatment consists of resection of a block of chest wall – this may be a relatively limited resection when benign. Chondrosarcomata are very prone to local recurrence therefore radical resection with wide clearance is indicated. Large areas of chest wall may be resected and replaced with a prosthesis with little loss of breathing capacity.

Other tumours do occur in the bony thorax but are less frequent – osteogenic sarcoma probably accounts for about 10% of malignant chest wall tumours. The radiographic appearance is fairly typical with a dense cortex and the radiating subperiosteal calcification so often seen with this type of tumour in other sites. Osteogenic sarcoma is best dealt with by a combination of wide resection, radiotherapy and chemotherapy.

Myeloma is occasionally seen as an apparently solitary lesion in a vertebra or rib but is more commonly encountered as multiple lytic lesions. Solitary plasmacytoma is the commonest tumour of the sternum. Radical resection gives good results. The patient must be followed up for the development of systemic myeloma. Other lesions occasionally encountered are neuroectodermal tumours (pNET; Askin's and Ewing's sarcoma), eosinophilic granuloma and monostotic fibrous dysplasia.

Primary pulmonary and pleural tumours may invade the chest wall and cause bone destruction. The majority of tumours in ribs and thoracic vertebrae are not primary but metastatic, arising from primary tumours in other viscera – particularly breast, lung, thyroid and prostate. The majority of these metastases, with the exception of those from the prostate, produce bone destruction, and a pathological fracture is quite often the presentation. Radiotherapy or chemotherapy may offer effective palliation.

Tumours of soft tissues

These tumours may arise in any of the soft tissues of the chest wall – skin, subcutaneous fat, breast, connective tissue or muscle. Lipomas of the chest wall do not usually present a major diagnostic problem as they have typical clinical features, particularly on palpation. They occasionally arise in the deeper planes of the chest wall and a diagnosis may not be clear until they are explored surgically. The malignant tumour of fat, the liposarcoma, is also seen in the chest wall – it is slow-growing and should be excised widely as local recurrence is the main problem. Fibromas occur in the chest wall as well as in the pleura and multiple thoracic neurofibromas may be found as part of the syndrome of von Recklinghausen's disease. Other tumours are found including haemangiomas, haemangiopericytomas, desmoid tumours, rhabomyomas and rhabdomyosarcomas. These are all rare and the diagnosis is often unclear until biopsy or surgical excision.

The best investigatory approach is to optimize the imaging information, then decide on excision biopsy for smaller lesions, and incision biopsy for large lesions. Planned resection and reconstruction with excision of biopsy site then follows. With all such tumours a relatively wide margin of normal rib and intercostal muscles, including the underlying pleura, thymus or pericardium is best resected. The excision should be extended to include an apparently normal rib above and below and 4 cm laterally whenever possible. Large areas of the chest wall may require excision and the resulting defects of ribs or sternum may be reconstructed with rib grafts, Marlex mesh or an acrylic plate. Myocutaneous flaps are often used to fill in the defects after excision or to cover the prosthesis.

Section 54.4 • Miscellaneous chest wall disorders

Lung hernia

A lung hernia or pneumatocele is the protrusion of pulmonary tissue outside the normal pleural boundaries. (Figure 54.4). This may occur through the chest wall via an intercostal space, at the apex through the thoracic outlet, or through the diaphragm. These hernias are seen following trauma and surgery, and may also occur spontaneously. The most common variety other than following surgery is the intercostal lung hernia which is usually either alongside the sternum or the vertebral column where the intercostal muscles are relatively incomplete. A congenital deficiency of Sibson's fascia, the aponeurosis overlying the apex of the lung, may allow herniation of the lung into the neck. This usually develops in adults, particularly those with bronchitis and emphysema, and is occasionally seen in people whose occupation involves maintaining high expiratory pressures, such as trumpeters and glass blowers. These hernias are usually asymptomatic but may require surgical repair.

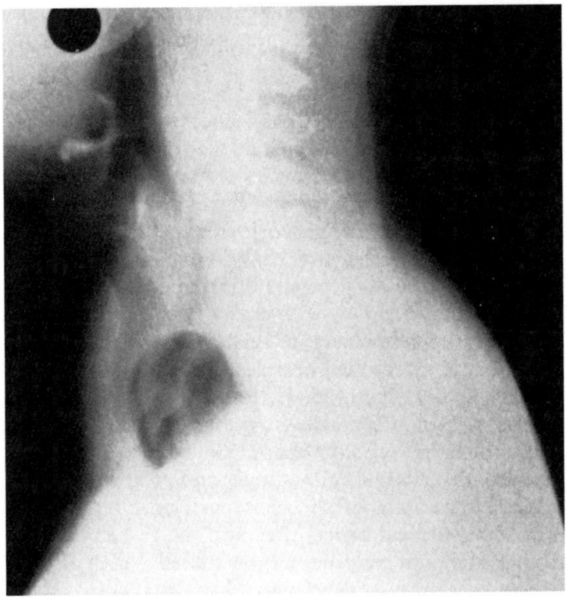

Figure 54.4 Lateral X-ray of of the neck showing a cervical lung hernia displacing the trachea.

Costochondritis

In 1921 Tietze described a syndrome of painful swelling in the area of the second or third costochondral junction. There is tenderness and some swelling over the costal cartilages but no inflammatory change in the skin. Radiography of the area is unhelpful and no treatment is required. It has been reported that surgical resection provides complete relief but it is very unusual for the symptoms to be sufficiently severe to warrant such interference. Local anaesthetics and long-acting steroids are often used for symptomatic improvement but the condition is self-limiting and treatment is poorly evaluated.

Section 54.5 • Tracheostomy

The operation of tracheostomy has been known and practised for hundreds of years but had an unenviable reputation in its earlier days, being performed almost entirely for high respiratory obstruction due to foreign bodies, 'croup' or one of the 'quinsies'. The operation made a major contribution to the management of laryngeal diphtheria in the nineteenth century but as diphtheria antitoxin became available it was used less and less. With the epidemic of poliomyelitis in the 1950s the value of intermittent positive pressure ventilation on a long-term basis was appreciated and the interest in tracheostomy changed from use in relieving upper airway obstruction to providing access for mechanical ventilation. Experience confirmed the use of routine tracheostomy for the control of bronchial secretions. In patients who are deeply unconscious or uncooperative following some intracranial incident or particularly following recoverable head injuries, control of the airway and bronchial secretions is vital.

Tracheostomy through the second and third ring of the trachea was increasingly preferred over the cricothyroid membrane incision as the problems of late laryngeal dysfunction were recognized after the latter. The standard tracheostomy tube was too large and caused disturbance of the function of the glottis, and quite obvious speech abnormalities were commonly present after the use of cricothyroidotomy for intubation. Consequently cricothyroid membrane intubation for ventilation access to the trachea has been abandoned. However, more recently the use of a simple catheter at the level of the cricothyroid membrane for the aspiration of secretions and the delivery of oxygen has been further developed as minitracheostomy. Minitracheostomy at the level of the cricothyroid membrane should now be the treatment of choice for simple control of bronchial secretions.

Indications

The majority of patients may be ventilated quite easily in the short term by the passage of an endotracheal tube through the mouth. If weaning from mechanical ventilation is expected to take any length of time, early tracheostomy is indicated by the Seldinger technique. The earlier practice of formal passage of a nasotracheal tube and ventilation for 2 weeks has been abandoned as it produced severe pharyngeal functional problems after extubation, and the patients were slow to eat properly. Tracheostomies are still required for long-term ventilation, and access for secretion control for the unstable larynx, when there is supraglottic stenosis, or as a final pathway as a tracheostome for laryngectomy or pharyngolaryngectomy. Occasionally it is necessary to perform a tracheostomy and use a cuffed tube to prevent the soiling of the bronchi from pharyngeal overspill to the trachea.

Technique

Percutaneous tracheostomy

Modern materials and transfer of principle have brought about changes in tracheostomy: the Seldinger technique of initial needle insertion followed by progressive dilatation then insertion of the tubular instrument or prosthesis over the introduced guidewire, is now the established method and standard kits are available. The commonest indication now for tracheostomy is mechanical ventilation. The anaesthetists have now become expert at Seldinger technique and as they make the decision for tracheostomy they tend to do it themselves. This now leaves the surgeon with little experience in training and only the very difficult tracheostomies to do. These are in the overweight patient with a short neck or patients on halo traction for cervical spine injuries. Experience with mediastinoscopy is now vital as the training competence for surgeons.

Standard tracheostomy

The formal tracheostomy operation should be carried out electively and be performed in an operating theatre under local or general anaesthesia with all facilities available. Unless the patient has supratracheal obstruction, an endotracheal tube will usually be *in situ* at the time of tracheostomy. Occasionally elective tracheostomy may be necessary before proceeding to an operative procedure and this may be carried out under local anaesthetic with no prior general anaesthesia.

The patient should be supine with a support under the shoulders, allowing maximum extension of the head and neck. The standard approach is a 2–3 cm transverse incision 2 cm above the sternal notch. The deep fascia is divided in the midline and the infrahyoid muscles are separated. The thyroid isthmus is exposed and the pretracheal fascia divided to display the trachea down to about the fourth ring. The thyroid isthmus normally covers the second and third tracheal rings and may have to be mobilized and retracted upwards. If the isthmus is bulky or the access is poor, it should be clamped and divided in the midline and the two halves secured by suture. Access may be considerably improved by traction with a sharp hook in an upwards direction on the first tracheal ring. Before any incision is made in the trachea, the surgeon must check that the correct sizes of tracheostomy tube are available, that the cuff inflates properly and that the correct catheter mounts and connections are available. Complete haemostasis is advisable before making the tracheal incision.

Although various tracheal incisions have been described over time and there was previously an enthusiasm for a 'U' shaped flap in the tracheal wall (Bjork flap), long-term experience has demonstrated that such flap types of tracheostomy have been associated with a higher incidence of late tracheal stenosis. The theoretical short-term advantage of ease of access when the need for reinsertion arises during the first 48 hours after tracheostomy is outweighed by the problems of late tracheal stricture. Therefore, the present recommendation is for a short vertical incision adequate for the insertion of the tracheostomy tube having gauged the size necessary. Adult males usually take a 39 or 42 Fr gauge, while the female trachea accepts 33 or 36 Fr.

Structures at risk during standard tracheostomy are few, but, if necessary, the thyroid isthmus can be tied without difficulty. However, in small children before the angle of descent of the ribs is fully established, the inominate vein lies high on the trachea and is at risk. Similarly, the apical pleura may be breached.

Minitracheostomy

Minitracheostomy is performed with the patient supine with the head extended on a flexed neck. It is unusual for the patient to require general anaesthesia, but elective minitracheostomy for post-operative bronchial toilet in patients with a secretion load is routine. The minitracheostomy would be inserted at the end of the elective procedure prior to extubation.

With the head extended on a flexed neck the cricothyroid membrane is palpated and a small amount of local anaesthetic introduced. The surgeon stands immediately behind the patient's head or to the side and the guarded knife, held with the cutting edge pointing caudally, is used to make a vertical incision straight through the cricothyroid membrane. The introducer is then passed into the trachea and the minitracheostomy tube – usually a 4 mm paediatric tube with a flange – is passed over the introducer into the trachea. The introducer is removed and the flange fixed, either by direct suturing or with tapes (Figure 54.5). Once the minitracheostomy tube is *in situ* a 12 Fr gauge catheter can be passed and secretions aspirated. A 14 Fr catheter can be wedged in the tracheostomy tube and humidified oxygen delivered more accurately than has previously been possible.

Management

The management of the minitracheostomy is simple and demands minimal care.

The standard tracheostomy is indicated for the patient who requires long-term ventilation. This is executed with the cuffed standard tracheostomy tube. The development of the low pressure high volume cuff has virtually eliminated the late endotracheal stenosis and tracheomalacia from necrosis of tracheal cartilage. Occasionally the end of the tube may be driven into the wall causing local necrosis and even fistulous involvement of the innominate artery. Careful attention paid to the ventilatory attachment to the tracheostomy tube and the swinging arm control which takes the weight of the ventilator attachments, holding the tracheostomy tube in the unstressed midline position, should eliminate such problems.

Bronchial toilet is executed via both tracheostomy and minitracheostomy tubes without difficulty using sterile soft catheters of the appropriate size. Catheter design has developed to stop the use of the endhole catheter which tends to engage against the bronchial walls as suction is applied. Venturi-flow catheters and side-aspirating catheters are available for use with

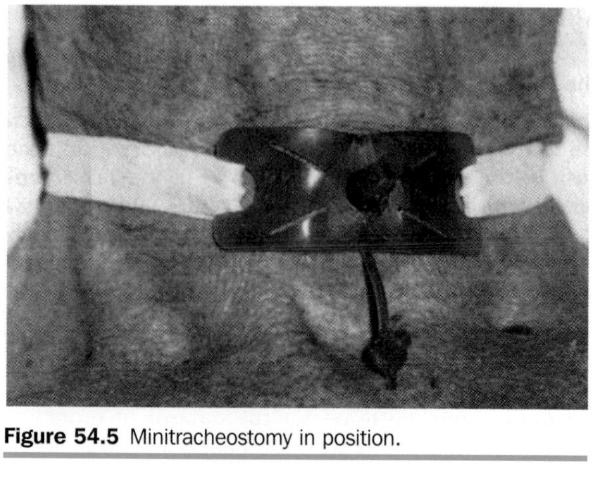

Figure 54.5 Minitracheostomy in position.

suction down endotracheal, tracheal and tracheostomy tubes. Catheters should be introduced disconnected from the suction or with the suction side-vented and the catheter occluded until withdrawal starts. Aspiration suction must only be applied as the catheter is withdrawn.

Any standard tracheostomy tube must be presented with well-humidified air or oxygen for both spontaneous breathing or assisted ventilation. When the minitracheostomy is being used to introduce oxygen into the trachea, this oxygen must be adequately humidified. The use of the open minitracheostomy tube purely for access for secretions does not require humidification because the flow characteristics dictate that the major air flow will be through the larynx rather than through the long narrow minitracheostomy tube. Removal of the tube is simple and a dry dressing is all that is needed. The wound heals in 72 hours. Occasionally a weaning period is necessary and a whole range of devices is available for maintaining access to the trachea and to allow the patient to speak.

Complications of tracheostomy

The complications of tracheostomy are very occasionally fatal and are nearly always caused by avoidable technical error. There is a small mortality associated with the operation itself because of the difficult circumstances under which it is sometimes executed. The problem of anoxia associated with trying to establish an airway in very difficult circumstances generates anxiety in all participants. Occasionally bleeding may present problems, particularly in small infants when the higher position of the innominate vein is not appreciated.

Displacement of the tube

For 48 hours after standard tracheostomy the track between the skin and the tracheostome is not fully established and should the tracheostomy tube be displaced in this early period reinsertion of the tube can be difficult. It should be a strict rule that no tracheostomy tube is formally changed within 72 hours. The tracheostomy should be checked for position and function immediately on insertion and sutured or tied firmly in position at this time. Incorrect reinsertion of the tube is life-threatening if the initial indications for tracheostomy still pertain. Any attempt to ventilate in a misplaced tube will meet high resistance and the ventilator pressures will rise. Under these circumstances ventilated air can be forced into the tissues and surgical emphysema develop. Tracheostomies in the first 48 hours must be in the care of skilled and aware attendants. It is inevitable that patients on ventilators will be in intensive care wards and that nurses will be in constant attendance. Good training and understanding is vital for the bedside staff. In the acute situation during this early period, reintubation by the endotracheal method to re-establish the airway is best as the tracheostomy tube can be reintroduced at leisure. It was this complication that led to the Bjork flap type of procedure which makes the early period much safer should the tube be displaced. However, with increased bedside skills in the management of tracheostomy, the late complication of the Bjork flap procedure – tracheal stenosis – is presently a more significant risk than the problem of early dislodgement of the tracheostomy tube.

Pneumothorax

Pneumothorax is a complication of any ventilated patient. It can complicate tracheostomy in small children when the apical pleura is closer to the tracheostomy site, and thus may be opened at operation because of the late descent of the ribs. The ribs are horizontal in the infant and the angle of descent, i.e. the angle between the upper border of the first thoracic vertebrae and the first rib in full expiration, is undeveloped. Although descent begins at 6 months of age the angle is not complete, i.e. 60 degrees, until the child is 7 years old.

Haemorrhage

Haemorrhage occurring during the operative procedure should be completely controlled before the tracheal incision is made. Late haemorrhage causes more tracheostomy-related deaths than any other complication. Classically the haemorrhage is from the brachiocephalic artery or the origin of the right common carotid artery. It occurs because of pressure necrosis by the tracheostomy tube through the anterior tracheal wall into the major artery which is its immediate relation. This is due to angulation of the tracheostomy tube and is wholly avoidable. This complication is usually fatal within a few minutes, death more often being due to drowning rather than to exsanguination. Sometimes there is a significant but brief spontaneous arterial haemorrhage which may be taken as a warning of impending disaster. There are occasional reports of this complication being temporarily controlled by insertion of a finger into the stoma and digital compression of the relevant artery against the sternum, or judicious endotracheal intubation by using the cuff for control of haemorrhage. Survival is rare.

Tracheal stricture

Stricture of the trachea related to tracheostomy occurs at three sites: the level of the stoma, the level of the cuff and at the tube tip. It is hoped that with intelligent use of low pressure cuffs, at least one of these sites will be relatively rare. The reported incidence of tracheal stenosis varies considerably but is probably at least 10%, though few of these constrictions have clinical significance. Severe strictures require excision.

Tracheo-oesophageal fistula

The incidence of this complication is fortunately low. Previous estimates of about 1 in 200 were related to prolonged assisted ventilation, over-inflation of the earlier narrow cuff and the presence of a nasogastric tube in the oesophagus. It is a complication which in itself carried a high mortality but nevertheless could be surgically repaired. The incidence of this complication has fallen dramatically with the use of low pressure high volume cuffs and fine bore enteral feeding tubes.

The way forward

Minitracheostomy is a routine procedure to be expected as a technical skill from junior doctors under local anaesthesia in the wards. Bronchoscopy for bronchial secretion should be a thing of the past. The Seldinger technique type tracheostomy will remain the norm on intensive care units, usually performed by anaesthetists.

Section 54.6 • Respiratory mechanics and post-operative pain

Clinically significant alterations in post-operative ventilatory mechanics and pulmonary gas exchange occur in all patients following anaesthesia, operation or trauma. These changes are most exaggerated in the elderly, the obese, in smokers and in those with pre-existing cardiopulmonary disease. Following operations on the abdominal and thoracic cavities, these inevitable post-operative changes are marked, with recovery of function delayed for days or weeks,. These changes are not clinically apparent in many patients, but set the stage for pulmonary complications in some normal and in many high-risk patients.

Decreased functional residual capacity (FRC) is the most important functional abnormality with its expected effects on pulmonary mechanics and gas exchange. This reduction in FRC is not accompanied by any significant alteration in the closing volume (CV)★★. When the CV becomes greater than the FRC, atelectasis in the dependent lung segments is inevitable. This leads to hypoxaemia from regional ventilation perfusion mismatching. Mucous plugs and infection are secondary to airway closure and alveolar collapse. Intra-operative and post-operative changes in pulmonary mechanics have different causes but pulmonary complications appear to be a progression of universal changes in pulmonary function after anaesthesia and operation.

Pre-operative risk factors

Age

As ageing occurs, the elastic recoil of the lung is diminished, resulting in airway closure at higher residual volumes. The effect of body position is such that changing from supine to the sitting position increases the closing volume only slightly, while the accompanying FRC increases by 20%. In the lateral position, reduction in FRC occurs which is most marked in the dependent lung. Closing volume begins to exceed FRC in a normal 44-year-old in the supine position, with airway closure in the dependent lung regions during resting tidal breathing. This condition exists in an upright 65 year old. The closing volume increases at a considerably greater rate with age than FRC, so that in elderly subjects CV is greater than FRC.

Smoking

Smoking has the same effect on closing volume as adding 10 years of age. In addition, smoking impairs small airway function, impairs the mucociliary transport mechanism and is associated with excess sputum production.

Obesity

Obesity causes a restrictive defect with changes in chest wall compliance from adipose tissue encasing the chest and abdomen. The chest wall and abdomen at end expiration are less deformable and CV encroaches on FRC and expiratory reserve volume (ERV). The CV is often greater than FRC and the resulting airway closure is responsible for arterial hypoxaemia even in young non-smoking subjects. These changes are most marked in the supine position.

COPD

Patients with chronic obstructive pulmonary disease (COPD) have significantly abnormal mechanical lung function, ventilation distribution and gas mixing. Non-uniform mechanical function produces a substantial decrease in dynamic pulmonary compliance. Airway resistance is increased and is only partly reversible with a bronchodilator. Because of the primary disease, the residual volume and FRC are abnormally expanded and hence protected to a small degree from alveolar collapse secondary to shallow breathing. As a result of the abnormally large dead space together with the significant ventilation–perfusion mismatch, hyperventilation is required to achieve adequate gas exchange. The effect of the post-operatively decreased ventilatory response in these patients is not atelectasis as would occur in normal lung, but rather CO_2 retention and hypoxaemia, i.e. type II respiratory failure. Atelectasis nevertheless does occur as the tidal volume is distributed non-uniformly.

Malnutrition

Malnutrition reduces both respiratory muscle strength and maximal voluntary ventilation thus impairing respiratory muscle capacity to handle increased ventilatory loads. Malnourished patients have reduced muscle mass of the diaphragm.

Lung function changes induced by anaesthesia and surgery

General anaesthesia causes reduction of FRC and impairment of gas exchange in all patients. The FRC is reduced by approximately 18% soon after induction of anaesthesia, but the reduction is not progressive with time. This holds true irrespective of anaesthetic agents used or whether the patient is breathing spontaneously or on positive pressure ventilation. The mechanisms causing the reduction in FRC remain controversial and

Table 54.1 Anaesthetic causes of reduction in FRC

- Cephalad displacement of the diaphragm
- Reduced transverse cross-sectional area of the thorax from muscle paralysis
- In lateral position gravitational effects of the mediastinum
- Absorption atelectasis due to increased FiO_2 up to 100%
- Changes in the activity of the inspiratory and expiratory muscles

are summarized in Table 54.1. The reduction in respiratory muscle tone is a fundamental change. Changes in vascular tone play a secondary role. The reduction of FRC is promptly followed by the development of atelectasis in dependent lung regions.

Post-operative period

Post-operative abnormalities in pulmonary mechanics and gas exchange may present early or late.

Early

Immediate post-operative period (recovery phase). Arterial hypoxaemia immediately following anaesthesia and operations lasting up to 2 hours is related to the preceding anaesthetic causes of hypoxaemia and is rapidly reversible in patients who have had extremity or superficial surgery, e.g. inguinal herniorraphy. Treatment consists of O_2 administration until the effects of anaesthesia have dissipated.

Late

Late post-operative period (delayed phase). Persistent abnormalities in gas exchange characterized by arterial hypoxaemia without hypercarbia modified by pre-existing cardiac and pulmonary dysfunction, may occur following operations on the abdominal and thoracic cavities. Mechanical factors are the cause and are not immediately reversible.

Persisting post-operative decrease in FRC (Table 54.2)

Post-operative hypoxaemia in the presence of hypoventilation is inevitable and most marked following thoracic and upper abdominal surgery. Pain after operation is the most important factor responsible for ineffective ventilation, ineffectual cough and impaired ability to breathe deeply and sigh. Such functional disturbances lead to atelectasis, hypoxaemia, infection and respiratory distress. One of the earliest changes in post-operative ventilatory mechanics is the substantial reduction in effort dependent lung measurements (forced expiratory volume in 1 second (FEV1), forced vital capacity (FVC), peak expiratory flow rate (PEFR)). This occurs before any change in FRC can be detected. By 24 hours following upper abdominal and thoracic surgery, FRC decreases to about 70% of the pre-operative levels, and remains depressed for several days, then gradually returns to normal by days 7–10. Most importantly, the reduction in FRC is not accompanied by any significant alteration in the CV during tidal breathing.

Table 54.2 Causes of post-operative decrease in FRC

Major:	Pain
Aggravated by:	Altered pattern of breathing Narcotic analgesia Bed rest in the supine position Diaphragmatic dysfunction particularly after upper abdominal operations Abdominal distension Electrolyte disturbances involving Ca^{2+}, K^+, Mg^{2+} and PO_4^-

The pattern of ventilation after operation is monotonous shallow breathing without spontaneous deep breaths. Impaired lung volumes, particularly FRC, ventilatory mechanics and oxygenation in the post-operative period are the consequences of such a breathing pattern. Sighing reverses these changes. A decrease in FRC results in a shift of the pressure volume curve to the right and the lesser gradient of this curve indicates a condition of decreased compliance. Increased work of breathing is necessary for adequate gas exchange because of altered compliance and increased dead space to tidal volume ratio. Elderly, malnourished patients and those in poor physical condition will be adversely affected by the increased muscular effort of breathing.

The diaphragm's contribution to quiet tidal breathing after upper abdominal surgery is reduced. This is secondary to impairment of diaphragmatic mechanics related to an increase in abdominal wall tone and/or a reflex decrease of phrenic nerve activity by inhibitory afferents arising from the abdominal compartment. Aminophylline and epidural analgesia have been shown to reverse diaphragmatic failure and to increase phrenic nerve activity.

Age, smoking, pre-operative respiratory disorders, obesity and intra- and post-operative surgical complications correlate positively with the development of pulmonary complications through airway closure during tidal breathing. Decreased FEV1 correlates inversely with the incidence of pulmonary complications.

Prevention and treatment of pulmonary complications

The main therapeutic goal remains maintenance or restoration of FRC. Although some patients with compromised pulmonary function must be managed initially with controlled ventilation, it is imperative that spontaneous breathing is re-established as quickly as possible. Prophylactic measures must be implemented early if they are to be effective.

Prophylactic measures

Pre-operative

Pre-existing pulmonary disease, FEV1 < 1 litre, smoking, sepsis, old age and obesity increase the risk of post-operative pulmonary complications. Detection and correction of these factors are important in order to reduce post-operative morbidity and mortality. Pre-operative physiotherapy will improve pulmonary function and thus decrease post-operative pulmonary complications in patients with chronic lung diseases such as bronchitis, bronchiectasis and emphysema. Sustaining muscular strength through adequate nutrition and maximal physical activity is an important but often neglected aspect of pulmonary care.

Intra-operative

- Decreased time under anaesthetic
- Use of PEEP (positive end-expiratory pressure) during anaesthesia
- Respiratory function less impaired by transverse rather than a median vertical laparotomy incision.

Post-operative

- Adequate analgesia
- Adequate humidification and low FiO_2 of inspired gas
- Sat up in bed and/or seated in a chair as soon as possible
- Encouraged to walk on the first post-operative day
- Use of incentive spirometer
- Adequate nutrition.

Pain management

Inadequate analgesia results in needless suffering, prevents early ambulation, limits deep breathing and prolongs hospital stay. Effective analgesia minimizes impairment of pulmonary function, aids in its recovery and prevents post-operative pulmonary complications. An ideal post-operative analgesic regimen has to be simple, effective and have the least number of complications. There is increasing evidence for the pain pathways to be the mediators and initiators of the metabolic response to trauma, often called the stress response. The effective use of pain prevention techniques peri-operatively limits the stress response.

Post-operative analgesia

Narcotic analgesia

Systemic opioid analgesics given on demand are not effective and should no longer be used. Patient controlled analgesia (PCA) systems are more effective. Opioids cause respiratory depression and obtund the periodic sigh response. The unilateral nature of most thoracic surgical procedures makes pain control by regional analgesic techniques more appropriate.

Non-steroidal anti-inflammatory drugs (NSAIDs)

The severity of pain in the immediate post-operative period makes the use of simple analgesics inappropriate. NSAIDS used alone are usually insufficient to control pain after major surgery, but have a significant complementary role when used with other analgesic techniques. Their peripheral action, anti-inflammatory activity and the convenience of administration by suppository are notable advantages.

Significant disadvantages associated with NSAIDs include gastric ulceration, impairment of renal function and impaired blood clotting by inhibition of platelet aggregation and fluid retention. Renal complications are related to inhibition of prostaglandin synthesis. Consequently, the use of NSAIDs post-operatively may be contraindicated in patients with congestive cardiac failure, renal disease or hepatic cirrhosis with ascites.

Epidural analgesia

Thoracic or lumbar epidural analgesia using either narcotic or local anaesthetic agents, or a combination of the same, provide post-operative analgesia and improve respiratory mechanics. Despite these advantages the use of epidural analgesia for post-thoracotomy pain is limited by associated problems and side-effects. Epidural analgesia, particularly with bupivacaine, is associated with bilateral sympathetic blockade in the upper thoracic region causing hypotension in many patients. Patients who are old or have had previous myocardial infarction or those after lung resections are at a greater risk of hypotension. Correction of hypotension by the administration of fluid load is particularly contraindicated in those who have had a pneumonectomy. Epidural morphine is also associated with a high incidence of respiratory depression (10%), which is subtle, insidious and unpredictable in duration. Other complications associated with epidural analgesics are muscle weakness with bupivacaine, while pruritus (15–30%), nausea, vomiting (12%) and disturbances of micturition are associated with morphine.

Intercostal and paravertebral blocks

Intercostal nerve and paravertebral blocks are found to be as effective an analgesic as epidural blocks using either morphine or bupivacaine without the associated complications and demand on personnel. A major component of the post-operative pain after thoracotomy is strained ligaments of the costovertebral and costotransverse joints as well as the posterior spinal muscles from rib retraction. Pain from these sources is mediated by the posterior penetrating branch of the intercostal nerve. Pain from a thoracotomy also comes from visceral pleura and organs conducted via afferent fibres in sympathetic nerves. Paravertebral block effectively interrupts such pathways and would be more effective than more distal blocks from local anaesthetic agents or cryoprobe neurolysis (Figure 54.6).

Continuous extrapleural intercostal nerve block

Repeated multiple intercostal or paravertebral blocks performed post-operatively are painful and time consuming. Continuous infusion techniques are more appropriate. Continuous extrapleural intercostal nerve block is a paravertebral localized eqivalent epidural block with complete local sympathetic block. Continuous extrapleural intercostal nerve block provides safe, effective analgesia after thoracotomy and reduces the early loss of post-operative pulmonary

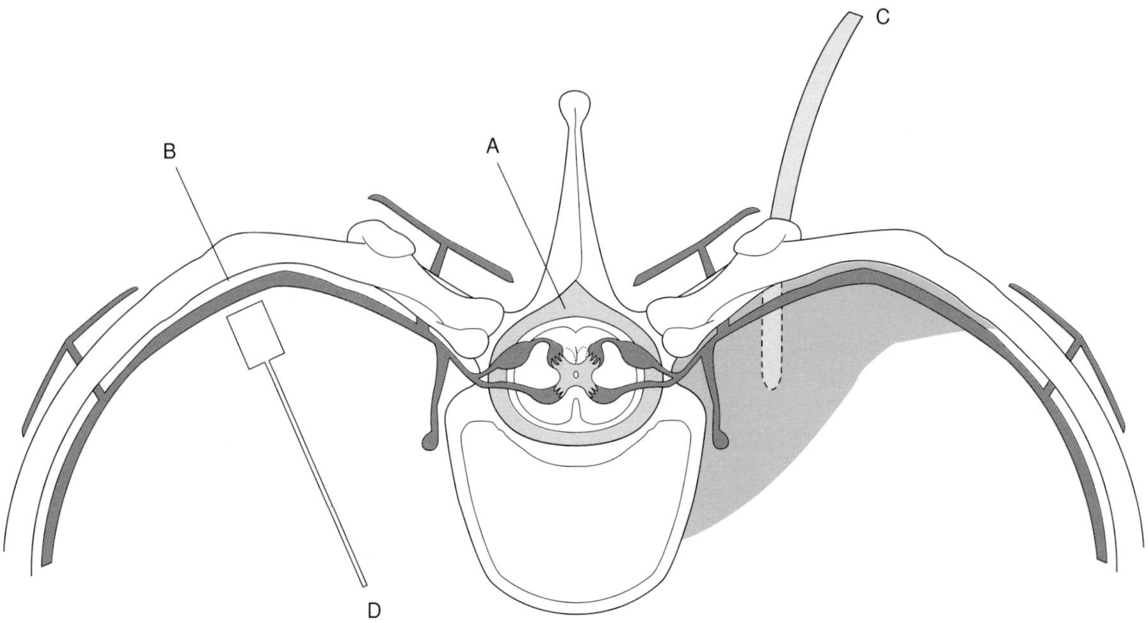

Figure 54.6 Methods of pain control in the thorax. A – Epidural. B – Subcostal block. C – Paravertebral catheter infusion. D – Cryoprobe. The epidural and paravertebral infusions block the posterior penetrating branch of the intercostal nerve. The paravertebral infusion blocks the sympathetic chain as well.

function significantly at 24 hours. It rapidly restores respiratory mechanics and minimizes post-operative pulmonary complications after thoracotomy.

Technique

Open paravertebral

The posterior parietal pleura at the posterior end of the thoracotomy wound is raised as far as the vertebral bodies to expose the paravertebral space. A small defect is then made in the extrapleural fascia using Lahey's forceps into the paravertebral space. A percutaneously inserted epidural cannula is passed into the extrapleural pocket under direct vision to infuse the paravertebral space.

Percutaneous paravertebral

With the patient in the lateral position the line of the rib for thoracotomy is identified. The rib two spaces higher is found and a Tuohy needle passed onto the transverse process. The needle is then walked off the upper border of the transverse process into the paravertebral space. Bupivacaine is injected and the space developed by hydrostatic pressure. An epidural catheter is passed into the paravertebral space and an infusion is now possible. The effective paravertebral block is immediately apparent. There is no change in pulse rate or blood pressure at incision, but there is much more subcutaneous bleeding as there will be a sympathetic blockade.

The paravertebral space is infused with 0.5% bupivacaine at a rate of 0.1 ml/kg body weight per hour for the first 48 hours and then 0.25% bupivacaine subseqently. The infusion runs for 4 or 5 days. The determinant for metabolism of bupivacaine is lean muscle mass, therefore a correction estimate for fat mass should be made to avoid a toxic dose.

Cryoprobe neurolysis

Cryoprobe neurolysis of intercostal nerves does not include posterior primary rami or the sympathetic chain. Severe discomfort may still be experienced by patients after cryoanalgesia as back pain in many cases. Deafferentation symptoms are not uncommon late post-operatively as part of the post-thoracotomy pain syndrome.

Intrapleural analgesia

As originally described, intrapleural analgesia is given through an epidural catheter placed in the pleural space. Post-operatively, the technique is most effective after cholecystectomy and renal surgery, but seems unsatisfactory in controlling pain after thoracotomy. This is primarily due to loss of the local anaesthetic via the chest tube, but dilution by irrigation fluid or blood, binding to blood proteins and rapid absorption by damaged lung are all likely to reduce effectiveness.

Lung expansion techniques

Decreased FRC is the product of inadequate pulmonary inflation; prevention and treatment are aimed at maximal inflation. Improvement in FRC can be achieved by moving the surgical patient from the bed to a chair as soon as possible following operation. Walking is even more effective than sitting, as it further increases FRC and requires the patient to breathe deeply as a result of exertion. Retained secretions are only partly responsible for post-operative atelectasis;

attention to circulating blood volume and adequate humidification of inspired gases with low levels of inspired oxygen concentration will minimize the influence of secretions in deranged pulmonary function.

Physiotherapy should be mandatory to clear tracheobronchial secretions and to encourage the patient to inspire deeply and cough. Incentive spirometry encourages sustained maximal inspiration and reduces post-operative pulmonary complications. Any manoeuvre that causes the patient to expire below FRC is undesirable.

Non-invasive ward-based ventilation techniques are increasingly used pre-emptively to assist patients with post-operative breathing problems. These techniques are especially valuable in the tiring patient and restore the patients' well being and keep them out of intensive care wards. Continuous positive airways pressure equipment is now simplified, nursing skills are easily developed and the respiratory care physiotherapists are eager to take up this challenge.

Further reading

Tracheostomy

Matthews, H. R. and Hopkinson, R. B. (1984). Treatment of sputum retention by minitracheotomy. *Br J Surg* **71:** 147–50.

Shields, T. W. and Locicero J. P. eds (2000). *General Thoracic Surgery*, 5th edn. Baltimore, MD: Lippincott, Williams and Wilkins.

Respiratory mechanics and post-operative pain

Richardson, J., Sabanathan, S., Jones, J. *et al.* (1999). A prospective, randomized comparison of preoperative and continuous balanced epidural or paravertebral bupivacaine on post-thoracotomy pain, pulmonary function and stress responses. *Br J Anaesth* **83**: 387–92.

Sabanathan, S., Eng, J. and Mearns, A. J. (1990). Alteration in respiratory mechanics following thoracotomy. *J R Coll Surg Edin* **35**: 144–50.

Sabanathan, S., Mearns, A. J., Bickford-Smith, P. J. *et al.* (1990). Efficacy of continuous extrapleural intercostal nerve block on post-thoracotomy pain and pulmonary mechanics. *Br J Surg* **77**: 221–5.

MODULE 55

Urological investigations

1 • Urine
2 • Blood
3 • Radionuclide (isotope) studies
4 • Imaging
5 • Endoscopy
6 • Investigation of bladder function

The clinician should start with what is simple, cheap, safe and least disturbing to the patient. More complex and invasive investigations are determined by the results of the initial tests and the clinical circumstances. Clinicians have a duty to use the resources of laboratories and imaging departments in a responsible way, avoiding unnecessary investigation and unjustified exposure of the patient to radiation or other risks.

This account is not comprehensive. It is a brief guide with emphasis on some practical points which have been found useful.

Section 55.1 • Urine

Urine can be obtained and tested simply, cheaply and safely. No patient should be seen for consultation without having at least a full urinalysis. Many men with impotence or urinary frequency have had their diabetes first diagnosed by a urologist.

Inspection

- Crystal clear urine is not infected; it is a waste to send it for routine culture.

Frank blood is obvious; lesser degrees of haematuria give a smokey pale brown colour.

'Stix' testing

A wide choice of testing strips is available, from those testing for a single substance such as protein or glucose, to strips with up to ten separate indicators. The following are of most relevance to urology.

Blood. The reagents react to haemoglobin (and myoglobin) so will detect this in its free form or in red cells. Differentiating a small amount of blood (+) from greater amounts (++, etc.) is of no value.

- All patients with haematuria need investigation.

The exception is the finding of a 'non-haemolysed trace', i.e. a few spots representing very small numbers of red cells. This is so common that a single such finding is often of no significance.

Protein. Moderate levels of proteinuria are found in infections and are sometimes associated with stones and tumours but should also raise the possibility of 'nephritis'. A result greater than 'trace' should be checked by 24 hour urine protein measurement.

Nitrites. Many urinary Gram-negative bacteria convert nitrates (normally found in the urine) to nitrites. A positive result indicates infection: a negative one does not exclude it.

Leucocytes. A positive result indicates the presence of white cells and suggests inflammation, most commonly caused by infection. White cells may also be found in patients with interstitial cystitis and papillary necrosis, and after surgery on the urinary tract.

- If blood, protein, nitrites and leucocytes are all absent, the urine is not infected and should not be sent for culture.

pH. Urine is normally acidic. Alkaline urine may be found in patients with Proteus infection and those taking alkalizing agents to reduce dysuria. Patients with renal tubular acidosis, which is associated with calcium phosphate stones, have urine which is alkaline or at least has a pH greater than 6.1.

Urine culture

- Obtaining reliable information from culture requires correct collection and transportation. The laboratory must be given appropriate information.

The results need to be interpreted with care and if necessary discussed with the laboratory. These conditions apply especially when infection is clinically suspected but routine culture is 'negative'.

Mid-stream urine (MSU). The patient must be given adequate instructions to avoid contamination. This is especially important in elderly women. Preparation of the introitus/vulva should be with normal saline. The sample should either be transported to the laboratory immediately or refrigerated and transported within an hour (although overnight refrigeration is acceptable) or a 'dipslide' should be used to sample the urine onto a culture medium which can be sent to the laboratory at room temperature, or incubated immediately.

There has been a significant change in the interpretation of MSU results. For 40 years the classical criterion was the presence of 100 000 (10^5) organisms/ml. Lower numbers indicated 'no significant growth on culture'. It is now realized that this applies to *asymptomatic* patients.

- When symptoms are present as few as 10^3 or even 10^2 organisms/ml together with leucocytes in the urine may be diagnostic of infection.

Catheter specimen of urine (CSU). A sample obtained by 'in and out' catheterization can be useful when there is doubt about the validity of MSU culture, and in elderly women where vulval contamination is difficult to avoid. Wash the peri-meatal area with saline, and avoid lubricating the catheter with jelly containing an antiseptic. Tell the laboratory that this is a CSU because the significant level of organisms is much lower than for a MSU.

- Urine should not *routinely* be cultured from indwelling catheters, which are always colonized with organisms, mostly of no clinical significance.

Suprapubic aspiration. This is usually done on children but may be used in adults where other specimens are equivocal. Any growth of organisms (except skin pathogens) is significant.

Urostomy specimens of urine

- Samples collected from the drainage bag are useless; 'clean catch' specimens of urine dripping from the stoma are little better. Specimens should be taken by catheter after washing the stoma with saline.

Samples should be obtained only if there are clinical signs of infection and the results then interpreted with caution.

'Negative' culture when infection is clinically likely. There are several reasons why culture may be 'negative' when symptomatic infection is present. Antibiotics excreted in the urine will inhibit bacterial growth in culture. Many patients with recurrent urinary infection learn to begin copious drinking when symptoms begin. The resulting repeated washing out of the bladder and dilution of the urine may reduce the concentration of organisms below that considered abnormal. Such patients, and those who self-administer antibiotics at the first sign of infection, should be given a 'dipslide' to take a sample at home before these measures begin.

- The classical cause of 'negative' culture in the presence of urinary leucocytes is tuberculosis. Such 'sterile pyuria' also occurs with papillary necrosis, interstitial cystitis and after surgery on the urinary tract.

Fastidious organisms not found by routine overnight culture in air may cause urethral and bladder symptoms. The clinician should liaise with the laboratory about the special requirements for detecting a range of these organisms.

Urine cytology

- Positive cytology is diagnostic of malignancy: negative cytology does not exclude it. Results may be equivocal in the presence of stones or infection, and after instrumentation.

Section 55.2 • Blood

A detailed account of all relevant blood tests is not appropriate here. The following points have practical clinical importance.

Creatinine and urea. Creatinine is a more useful variable than urea, which is more dependent on the level of hydration.

- Creatinine concentration does not rise until almost two-thirds of glomerular function have been lost: a normal creatinine concentration does not necessarily indicate normal renal function.

Creatinine clearance (as an estimation of glomerular filtration rate, GFR) may be measured by blood and urine collection using the standard formula, but GFR is now more commonly measured by isotope renography (see below). Each method has its potential inaccuracies.

Electrolytes. The most important electrolyte level in urological practice is potassium, which may rise to potentially fatal levels in acute renal failure. A very high creatinine concentration with a normal potassium concentration indicates that renal failure is chronic. This distinction may be important in the immediate management of patients admitted with obstructive uropathy.

Patients with some forms of urinary diversion are at risk of developing hypernatraemic hyperchloraemic acidosis.

In the 'TUR syndrome' (essentially water intoxication) sodium may fall to dangerous concentrations: recovery is rare if sodium concentration falls below 120 mmol/l.

Prostate specific antigen (PSA) is covered in Module 59.

Tests for causes of stone formation are covered in Module 60.

Section 55.3 • Radionuclide (isotope) studies

These have made two major contributions to urological investigations. First, the evaluation of upper tract function; second, the detection of bone metastases, especially from carcinoma of the prostate. The latter is dealt with in Module 59. Here we concentrate on the use of these studies for upper tract evaluation.

Radionuclide studies produce images by gamma-radiation detected on a sensitive film, in a similar manner to the production of a radiograph by the action of X-rays on sensitized film. These images are less anatomically precise than those of an X-ray, but as the 'gamma camera' can quantify gamma-radiation, functional information is obtained. Thus, one can measure the uptake of radionuclides from the blood into the kidney, their excretion from the parenchyma into the pelvi-calyceal system, their transit from the pelvi-calyceal system into the ureter and bladder and, in cases of vesico-ureteric reflux, their return up the ureter from the bladder to the kidney. The radiation dose from these studies is much less than that from X-ray studies such as intravenous urography (IVU), so serial studies can safely be used to monitor changes in function or the results of surgery.

'Static' isotope renography

Dimercaptosuccinic acid (DMSA) can be labelled with ^{99m}Tc, an isotope which emits gamma-radiation. After intravenous injection the labelled compound is taken up by the kidneys and 95% is retained in the proximal tubules. By counting over each kidney 3 hours after injection, the relative function of each kidney is measured and expressed as a percentage of total function. Such 'split function' studies can be helpful when there is bilateral renal pathology and one needs to operate on the 'better' side first, as well as in deciding whether a damaged kidney is worth attempted salvage or is better removed. The images produced, while anatomically imprecise, can show areas with no uptake of isotope caused by scarring, cysts or tumours.

GFR measurement

Diethylenetriamine penta-acetic acid (DTPA) labelled with ^{99m}Tc (or ^{51}Cr-labelled ethylenediamine tetra-acetic acid – EDTA), when injected intravenously, is taken up from the blood by the glomeruli but is not taken up by the tubules: it is all excreted into the collecting system. By sequential venous sampling over 4 hours its rate of disappearance from the blood, as a result of uptake by the kidneys (after correcting for decay), can be measured. From this, GFR can be calculated (see Figure 55.1).

Dynamic isotope renography

DTPA, or mercaptoacetyl triglycine (MAG3), labelled with ^{99m}Tc can be used to assess several aspects of renal function. Information obtained by counting over each kidney for 20–40 min will produce a plot of counts against time – a renogram, and a series of semi-anatomical images. The normal renogram has three phases (Figure 55.1). The short, rapidly rising first phase corresponds to arrival of isotope-containing blood in the kidney. The second phase lasts about 4 min and indicates extraction of the isotope by the kidney from the blood at a faster rate than its passage from the parenchyma into the pelvi-calyceal system. After about 4 min the curve normally falls from a peak, indicating loss of the isotope (= urine) from the kidney (phase 3).

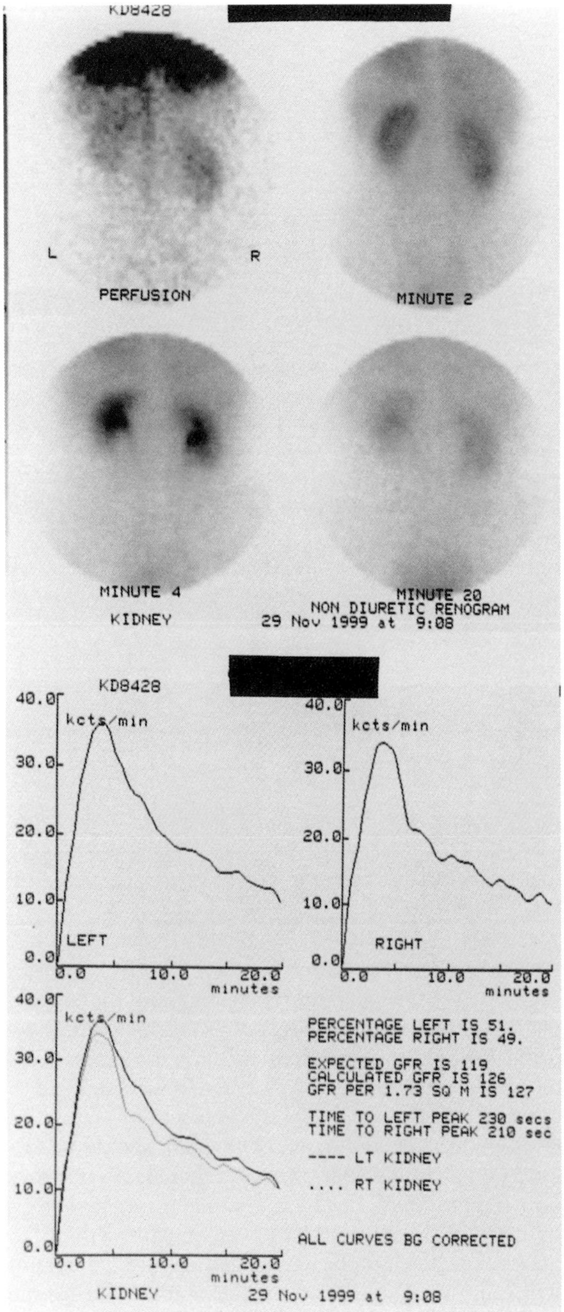

Figure 55.1 A normal DTPA isotope renogram. The 'films' in the upper half give some (imprecise) anatomical information. The plots of counts over each kidney, in the lower half, give a measure of function. Each kidney shows the accumulation of isotope (second phase) followed by its excretion (third phase). Sequential sampling continued beyond this phase allow calculation of the GFR.

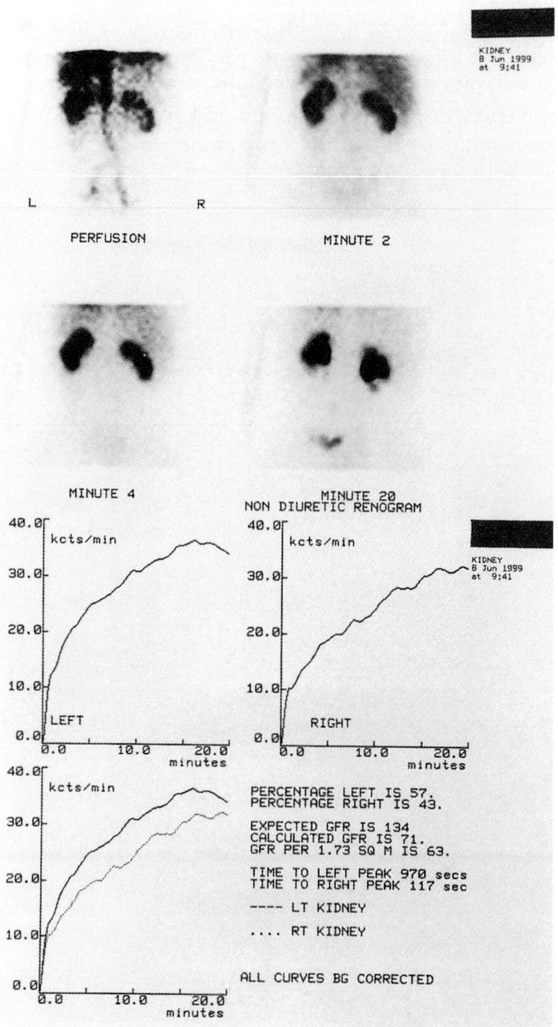

Figure 55.2 A DTPA renogram showing continued accumulation of isotope in the kidneys, i.e. a rising phase 3. This suggests obstruction, but may be due to slow flow through a dilated but non-obstructed system (see Figure 55.3).

In cases of renal outflow obstruction the second phase continues to rise. This may also happen with slow urine flow due to impaired function or more commonly to a 'baggy' dilated, but non-obstructed, pelvicalyceal system (Figure 55.2). The administration of furosemide at 20 min (F +20 renogram) should be followed by a rapidly falling curve if there is no obstruction (Figure 55.3), but by a continued rise if there is obstruction. In equivocal cases giving furosemide 15 min before the isotope is injected (F −15 renogram) will cause maximum load on the outflow during the study and may give an unequivocal result.

Section 55.4 • Imaging

Uroradiology benefits from the use of all of the diagnostic and therapeutic imaging modalities. The evaluation of specific urological problems also benefits from the use of a specific order of imaging techniques. The use of relatively simple, cheap and readily available techniques may answer a clinical problem as efficiently as a more expensive and less available modality.

A plain abdominal radiograph

Typically performed in inspiration, this covers the kidneys, ureters and bladder. Depending on patient size, a separate bladder film may be required. A second film of the renal areas in expiration is taken if there is a suspicion of renal calcification. Intra-renal calcifications will maintain a constant position relative to the renal outline. Oblique and tomographic views may be helpful.

A baseline plain film should always precede contrast administration. Renal size may be estimated. The presence or absence of a psoas outline is occasionally useful but neither excludes nor confirms the presence of retroperitoneal pathology. The spine may show evidence of spinal dysraphism, renal osteodystrophy or metastatic disease.

Intravenous urography

Intravenous urography provides a relatively quick screening evaluation for intra-renal pathology and function. Bowel preparation will improve the quality of the examination but is often omitted in the acute set-

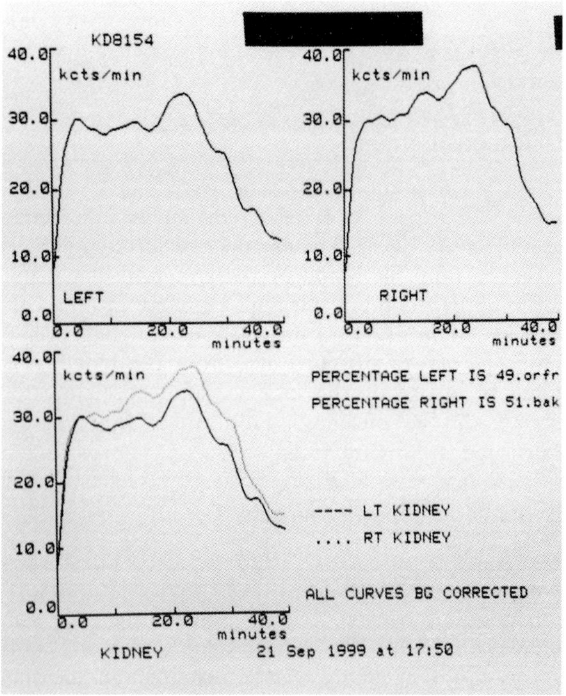

Figure 55.3 Diuretic renogram. After giving furosemide at 20 min the counts rapidly fall, ruling out obstruction.

ting. Fluid restriction is no longer used; it does not increase pyelographic density. Patients with renal impairment and diabetes should be well hydrated to decrease the risk of exacerbating or causing renal impairment. While low-osmolar non-ionic contrast agents are safer, they are expensive. Their benefits for patients with cardiac or renal disease or a history of allergies justify their use in these, if not in all, patients. After control films, contrast is administered and films of the renal areas are taken at 1 and 5 min. Compression is applied to distend the pelvicalyceal systems and a renal area film taken at 10 min. Compression is then released and a full-length film taken at 15 min. If ureteric filling is inadequate this can be improved by repeating the film with the patient prone. Additional films required may include: tomography of the renal areas, post-micturition films to assess drainage of upper tracts and bladder residual volume, erect films if there is doubt regarding a potential obstruction and post-micturition oblique views for assessment of the distal ureter and vesico-ureteric junction. In the absence of a nephrogram or pyelogram in the renal area at 5 min, a full-length film should be taken to check for a pelvic kidney. Oblique views will help evaluate posterior renal calyces and the relationship of calcifications to the ureter.

Retrograde ureteropyelography is occasionally needed to better define the collecting systems and ureters. Its use has been reduced by ureterorenoscopy (see Section 55.5).

Urethrography (Figure 55.4)

Urethography provides excellent anatomical definition of the urethra. Using a Knutsson clamp or a small Foley catheter inflated in the navicular fossa, the urethra is distended with contrast, and images are taken with the patient at an oblique angle. This provides anatomical detail to the level of the distal sphincter mechanism. If required, contrast can be instilled into the bladder and the catheter removed. The patient is then asked to void and a descending urethrogram is performed to visualize the bladder neck and posterior urethra.

Micturating cystourethrography

This is the most accurate technique for demonstrating vesicoureteric reflux. The bladder is catheterized and filled to maximal comfort with dilute contrast, using intermittent screening to identify reflux. The catheter is removed and images are taken during and after bladder emptying to detect reflux, with additional oblique views of the posterior urethra as required.

Ultrasound

This is a quick, cheap and non-invasive technique for evaluating the kidneys, bladder, testes and prostate.

Renal ultrasound is useful for assessing renal size, collecting system dilatation, differentiating solid from cystic masses and for guiding intervention. Using liver echogenicity as a reference, parenchymal changes can

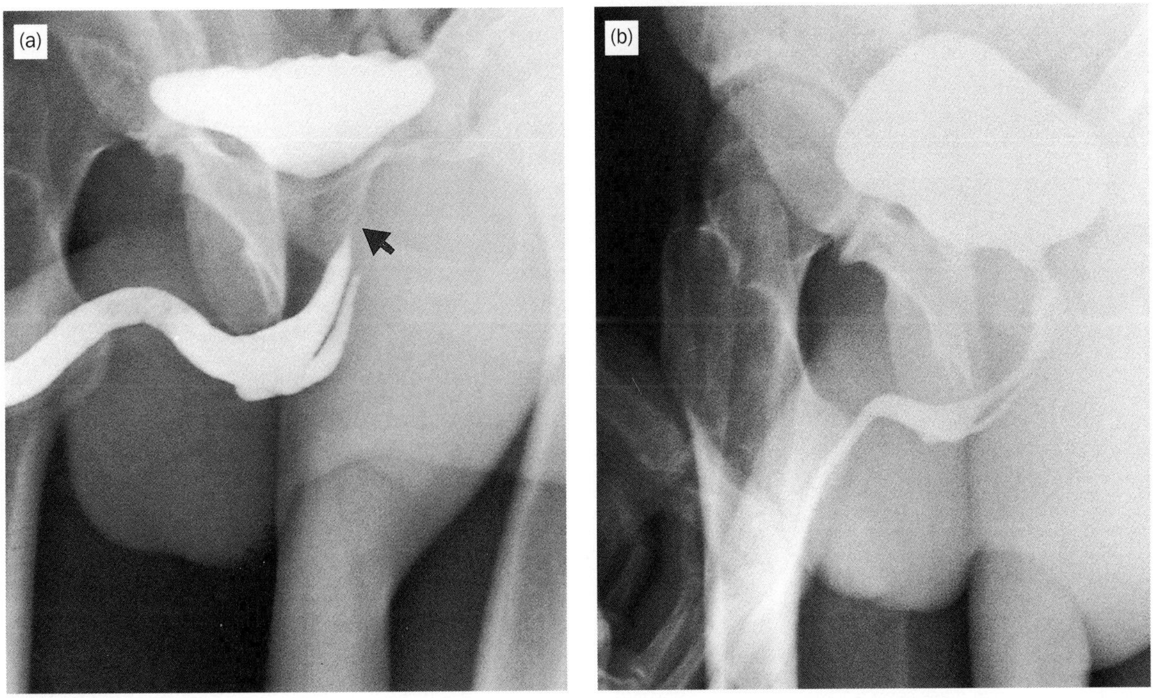

Figure 55.4 Ascending urethrogram. (This patient had the rare condition of partial duplication of the urethra.) Retrograde injection of contrast material (a) fills the main urethral channel to the level of the external sphincter (arrow), beyond which contrast passes in a fine stream through the prostatic urethra to enter the bladder. After the bladder is filled, micturition (b) outlines the normal bladder neck and prostatic urethra.

be evaluated in native and transplanted kidneys. Renal calcification can often be identified but should be correlated with plain radiographs.

Transabdominal scanning will often detect bladder tumours but is no substitute for cystoscopy.

Transrectal ultrasound (TRUS), best demonstrates prostatic volume and the internal morphology of the prostate gland. Ultrasound-guided sextant and lesion-focused biopsies are increasingly important in the evaluation of suspected prostate cancer.

Testicular ultrasound is a reliable technique for evaluating intra-testicular or epididymal pathology, hydroceles, male infertility and searching for undescended testes. Colour and spectral Doppler techniques can be used for evaluating testicular trauma, torsion and pain.

Doppler ultrasound is useful in distinguishing tumour from haematoma (Figure 55.5) and in monitoring for arterial and venous complications in transplant kidneys. The role of Doppler ultrasound as a screening test for renal artery stenosis is hampered by technical problems, particularly the non-visualization of accessory renal vessels. Future developments in urological ultrasound will involve the use of harmonic imaging and intravascular ultrasound contrast agents.

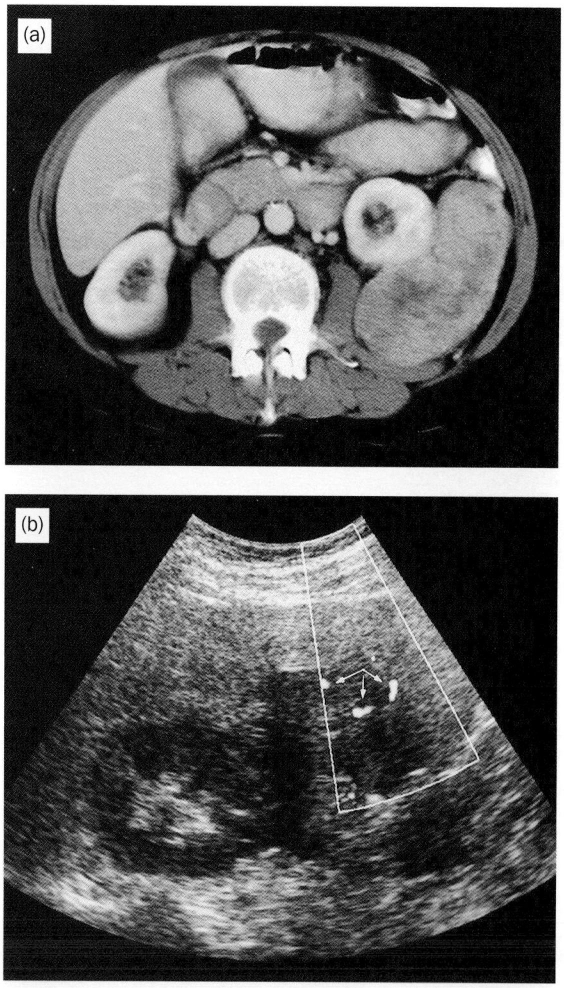

Figure 55.5 A large mass seen on axial CT (a) arising from the left kidney, following a blow to the flank in an anticoagulated patient. Doppler ultrasound (b) showed blood flow in the mass (arrows), excluding the diagnosis of haematoma. The lesion was an oncocytoma.

The appropriate use of more advanced imaging techniques, such as CT or MRI, requires consideration of factors such as cost, availability and the effect on proposed patient management.

Computed tomography (CT)

CT has applications in evaluating complex renal cysts and masses, particularly lesions containing fat and calcification. Multiphasic pre- and post-contrast enhanced scanning allows for accurate local staging of renal cell carcinoma (Figure 55.6a), the exclusion of a second tumour in the contralateral kidney, the local staging of transitional cell carcinoma of the kidney and, when MRI is not available, the staging of tumours of the bladder and prostate. CT allows for evaluation of retroperitoneal pathology affecting the ureter and the assessment of pelvic masses (Figure 55.7). CT is more accurate than urography and angiography in the assessment of renal trauma and other abdominal injuries (see Module 56).

CT has improved significantly with the advent of helical technology. With earlier technology, each slice was acquired and the patient was then moved to the next slice location. Helical CT slip-ring technology allows the X-ray tube and detectors to rotate continuously. A sliding table moves the patient through the scanner resulting in helical rather than axial acquisition of data. This technique is fast, 60 slices taking approximately 60 s. Because a volume of tissue, rather than individual axial slices, has been scanned the images can be reconstructed using different slice intervals and different planes. Varying the table speed alters the pitch and speed of the examination. With additional improvements in scanning and reconstruction speeds this technology will in the future be even faster, with 60 slices being acquired in 10–20 s. There is increasing interest in the use pre- and post-contrast enhanced-helical CT in the evaluation of renal and ureteric stones.

Magnetic resonance imaging (MRI)

MRI technology has advanced significantly with more rapid imaging sequences, improved coil design and contrast enhancement techniques.

MRI is unequivocally better than CT for the local staging of bladder cancer (Module 58) and prostate cancer (Module 59) and for the identification of undescended testes (Module 62).

The inability of MRI reliably to detect calcification in the kidney is a problem, but in all other respects the results for evaluating solid and cystic renal masses are comparable with CT. MRI offers certain advantages when assessing venous involvement and patency (Figure 55.6b). The higher resolution possible with MRI also offers advantages for pre-surgical

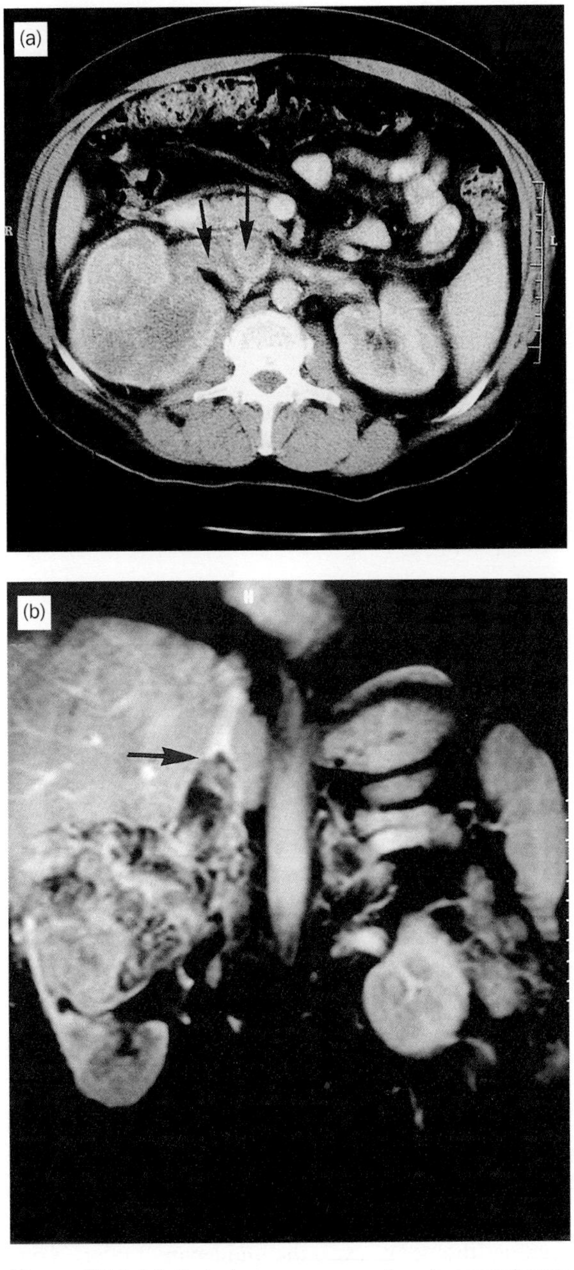

Figure 55.6 (a) Typical appearances of a hypernephroma on axial CT. The patient presented with a painful right varicocele. The tumour is invading the renal vein and vena cava (arrow), but the extent of caval involvement is not easily determined. (b) MRI of the same patient. The upper extent of caval involvement is clearly shown (arrow), allowing pre-operative planning.

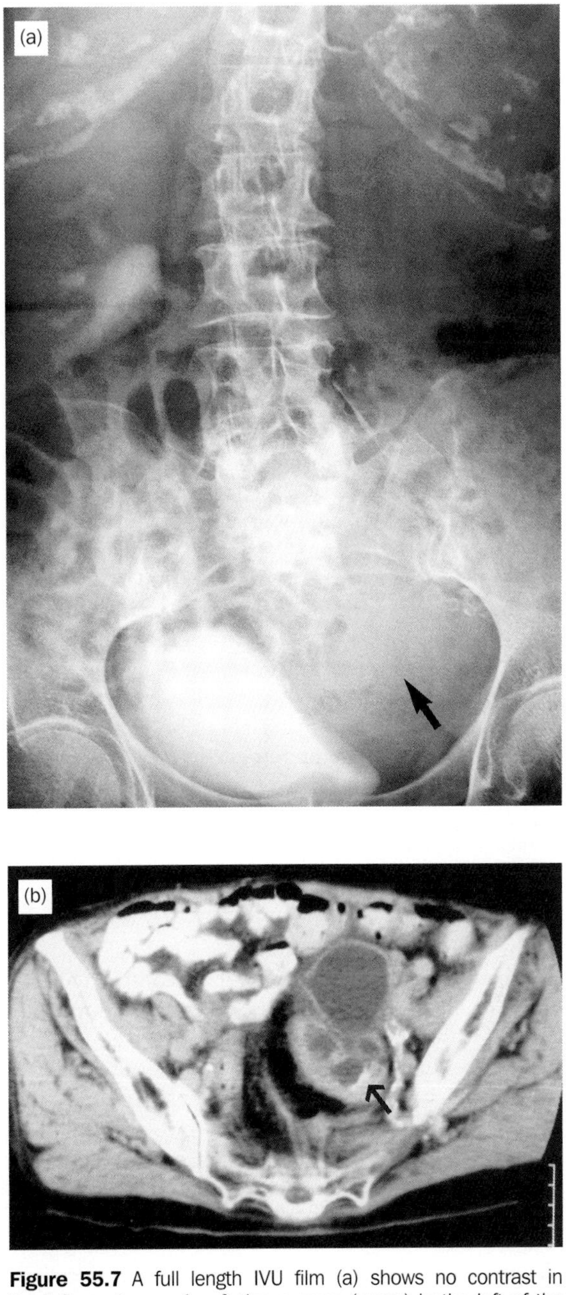

Figure 55.7 A full length IVU film (a) shows no contrast in the left renal area. A soft tissue mass (arrow) in the left of the pelvis pushes the bladder to the right. A post-contrast axial CT scan (b) shows the mass to be an obstructed left pelvic kidney (arrow).

planning prior to partial nephrectomy. Future developments will include the use of MRI urography and contrast enhanced MRI measurements of renal function.

Ultrasound, CT and MRI have virtually replaced angiography for the evaluation of renal masses.

Recent developments in CT and MR angiography are replacing standard angiography for the assessment of unexplained haematuria, renovascular hypertension and the assessment of potential renal transplant donors.

Section 55.5 • Endoscopy

Changes in endoscope technology, including fibre-optic illumination, the rod-lens system and, more recently, fibre-optic viewing systems, have transformed urological endoscopy. Another major development has been the routine use of small, light, endoscopic CCTV cameras which reduce risk and fatigue to the operator, allow other theatre staff to see what is being done and assist training.

Cystourethroscopy

Using rigid instruments

The inspection technique is essentially unchanged since the early days of the twentieth century. A standard rigid cystoscope (Figure 55.8) of 17–21 Fr calibre can be passed in a female or stoical male under topical analgesia, but general or regional anaesthesia is standard in males to avoid pain (largely caused by negotiating the bends in the urethra and by traction on the perineal membrane) and in females to avoid embarrassment.

- Inspection of the male urethra using a 0° to 30° telescope (i.e. a telescope whose axis of view is directly or almost directly ahead) is an essential first part of the examination.

The interior of the bladder is then inspected using a 70° telescope in a systematic fashion in 'strips' at each of the eight equidistant points of a circle (i.e. 12 o'clock, half past one, 3 o'clock, half past four, etc.). In males the area inside the bladder neck may be hidden by intravesical prostatic enlargement, in which case a retrograde viewing (120°) telescope is needed. Intravesical manoeuvres such as biopsy, diathermy, removal of stents, small stones or foreign bodies and injection of material can be done. Ureteric stenting and retrograde ureterography are best done via a rigid cystoscope.

- After emptying the bladder and withdrawing the cystoscope, bimanual examination of the pelvic organs is an essential part of the examination in both males and females.

Using flexible instruments

Flexible cystoscopes (Figure 55.9) are constructed similarly to flexible gastroscopes, with an illumination bundle, viewing bundle, irrigating and operating channel in an outer sheath of about 16 Fr calibre. These instruments have had a significant impact on urological practice.

- More than 95% of diagnostic and check cystoscopies are done using a flexible instrument.

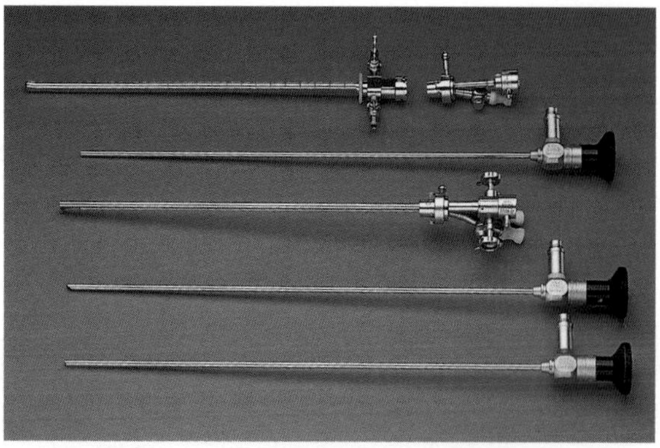

Figure 55.8 A modern version of the traditional rigid cystoscope, with directing insert for ureteric catheters, diathermy or injection devices, etc., and telescopes with differing viewing angles. (Illustration courtesy of Karl Storz Endoscopie.)

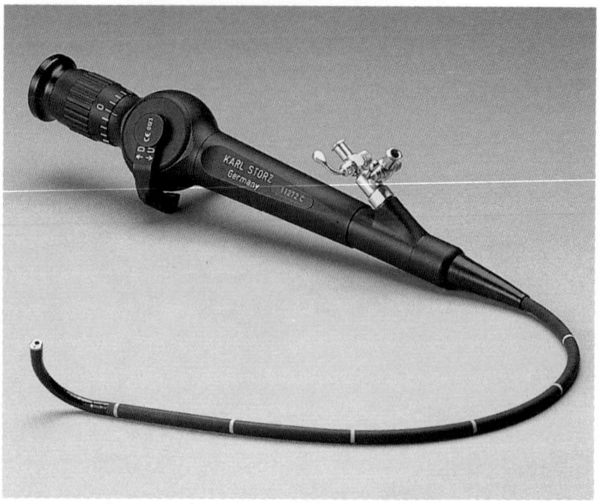

Figure 55.9 A flexible cystoscope. (Illustration courtesy of Karl Storz Endoscopie.)

The instrument is passed along the urethra after topical anaesthesia with gel. Men have some discomfort when the external sphincter is passed. Discomfort at the sphincter/prostatic urethra/bladder neck areamakes these the least well-inspected parts of the lower urinary tract: when it is essential to have a leisurely and detailed look at these areas a rigid endoscopy under general anaesthetic may still be preferred. Once the bladder is entered it is examined in strips around the clock as for rigid cystoscopy. The area inside the bladder neck is easily examined using the 'J manoeuvre' in which the tip of the instrument is angled through almost a 'hairpin bend' to look back on itself and the area around the internal meatus. Minor intravesical procedures such as biopsy using fine forceps, tumour destruction using a laser fibre and retrieval of ureteric stents, are easily done.

In patients not fit for general anaesthesia, ureteric stenting can be done by first passing a guidewire up the ureter via a flexible cystoscope, removing the cystoscope (through which a stent will not pass), then feeding the stent over the guidewire under X-ray control.

Ureteroscopy and ureterorenoscopy

- Upper tract endoscopy for diagnosis and treatment has been a major advance. It is possible to inspect the whole ureter and the pelvi-calyceal system, to take biopsies and to destroy calculi *in situ*.

Ureteroscopes are passed under general or regional anaesthesia via the urethra, bladder and ureteric orifice.

Rigid and semi-rigid ureteroscopes

Ten years ago the available ureteroscopes were essentially long thin cystoscopes of at least 12 Fr calibre. Dilatation of the intramural ureter was needed, with a risk of splitting and stricture formation. Flexion of the instrument (e.g. to negotiate the pelvic brim) caused a 'crescent moon' loss of part of the view. Recent improvements have provided instruments of about 7.5 Fr calibre (Figure 55.10a) containing an illuminating bundle, a viewing system, an irrigating channel and an operating channel of just over 3 Fr which will take fine biopsy forceps, stone disintegrating probes and retrieval baskets. Such an instrument about 45 cm long can be passed up most ureters into the pelvi-calyceal system. The instrument may be passed over or alongside a guidewire and in skilled hands without a guidewire. A fibre-optic viewing system allows a significant amount of bending without loss of field. Such fine instruments inevitably have limited irrigation and working channels, so for stones in the lower third of the ureter most urologists use a more robust (10.5 Fr) shorter (35 cm) instrument to make stone disintegration and fragment removal easier and safer.

Flexible ureteroscopes

These are essentially long (70 cm), thin (7.5 Fr) flexible cystoscopes which are passed (usually over a guidewire) as far as the pelvi-calyceal system, which can be inspected by the deflectable tip (Figure 55.10b).

The irrigation/instrument channels are necessarily very small so these instruments are mainly used for inspection and biopsy of urothelial lesions, but they can accommodate a fine laser fibre for stone disintegration.

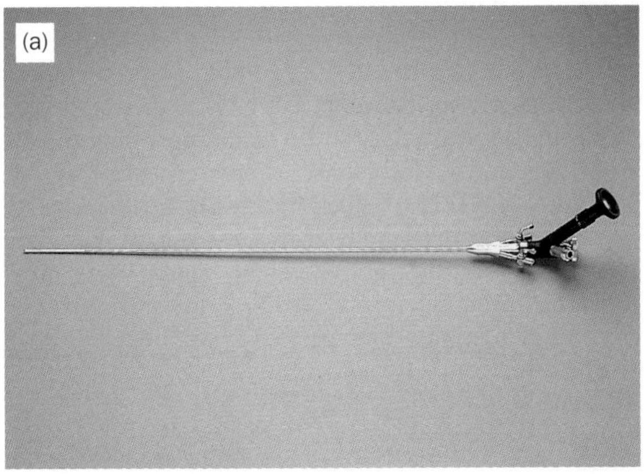

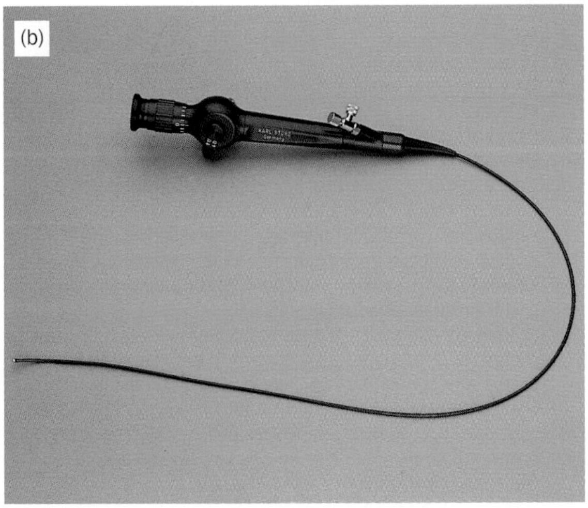

Figure 55.10 (a) A semi-rigid ureteroscope with irrigation and instrument channels. (Illustration courtesy of Karl Storz Endoscopie.) (b) A flexible ureteroscope with common irrigation/instrument channel. (Illustration courtesy of Karl Storz Endoscopie.)

Section 55.6 • Investigation of bladder function

Tests of bladder function are collectively known as 'urodynamic studies'. They involve a range of measurements, some simple and some very complex, which need to be tailored to suit the clinical problem and may need to be modified as they proceed in the light of the information obtained.

The simplest and commonest urodynamic measurements are estimation of residual urine volume and uroflowmetry.

Residual urine volume measurement

This measurement is important in the assessment of suspected bladder outflow obstruction and of patients with urinary tract infection. Residual urine following micturition is at risk of infection and eventually causes upper tract damage. The normal residual urine volume is a few millilitres at most.

There is no agreed level considered abnormal and many asymptomatic healthy people have residual urine volumes of 50 ml, or even up to 100 ml at first measurement in the clinic. Repeated volumes of over 100 ml are definitely abnormal. Rising sequential levels are more significant than a single modestly elevated level.

- Measurement is usually done by ultrasound to avoid the risks of catheterization. There is error in the measurement which is insignificant for clinical purposes.

Simple, relatively inexpensive portable bladder scanners are widely used in clinics and wards, or the more sophisticated equipment used for abdominal imaging in the radiology department may be used.

Residual urine volume must be measured after a voluntary void in privacy. Unreliable results are obtained when the patient is instructed to void to order before the bladder feels full or if the patient fears interruption or is intimidated by the clinical surroundings. No treatment decision should be based on a single estimation.

Uroflowmetry

- The rate of urine flow depends on two factors: the strength of bladder contraction and the resistance of the bladder outflow. In clinical practice a reduced flow rate is most commonly caused by increased outflow resistance, e.g. due to prostatic enlargement or urethral stricture; but weak bladder contraction will have the same effect.

Common causes of impaired contraction are diabetes mellitus with impairment of the autonomic supply to the bladder, detrusor decompensation due to chronic overdistension of the bladder from long-standing obstruction, or detrusor failure of the elderly.

- The patient must feel comfortably full before being asked to void. Reliable results require a voided volume of at least 150, preferably 200 ml, in the absence of fear of interruption. No treatment decision should be based on a single measurement.

Figure 55.11 shows a normal uroflow trace. The most important variable is the peak flow rate (Q_{max}). Interpretation is given in Table 55.1.

Table 55.1 Interpretation of peak urine flow rate (Q_{max})

Peak urine flow rate	*Interpretation*
>25 ml/s	Definitely normal
20–25 ml/s	Almost certainly excludes obstruction (except minor degrees of obstruction in young men with powerful detrusors)
15–20 ml/s	Equivocal. May be significant obstruction partially compensated by increased detrusor contraction, or mild obstruction
10–15 ml/s	Definitely abnormal, usually indicates obstruction
<10 ml/s	Grossly abnormal. Seen with severe obstruction or detrusor failure

Pressure–flow studies

These are most used in the specialized investigation of incontinence and may be valuable in investigating lower urinary tract symptoms when bladder outflow obstruction is suspected (see Module 61).

Pressure–flow studies involve artificial filling of the bladder and the continuous measurement of bladder pressure, relating this to bladder volume and urine flow rate in a continuous graphical representation. Thus the study has two phases: the filling phase and the voiding phase.

The bladder is filled with normal saline at room temperature infused at a fixed rate (usually 50 ml/min). This allows the bladder volume to be measured indirectly as a function of time. Filling is done through a fine (4 Fr) catheter (usually an infant feeding tube) inserted along the urethra. A second fine catheter (maximum 6 Fr) is similarly inserted and connected to a pressure transducer. It continuously measures vesical pressure (P_{ves}). As the vesical pressure is the sum of the detrusor pressure plus abdominal pressure (P_{abd}), subtraction of abdominal pressure (measured in the rectum) from the measured bladder pressure gives the true detrusor pressure (P_{det}) which is the important variable. The sequence of events in a typical urodynamic study is given in Table 55.2. This sequence may be modified in response to findings as they are obtained during the study. The filling phase of such a study is shown in Figure 55.12.

Urodynamic studies can be made more sophisticated by including radiological screening using contrast medium to fill the bladder, by measuring the closure pressure along the length of the urethra, by including sphincter electromyography or by 'ambulatory urodynamics' using telemetry. These modifications may be needed in complex unexplained incontinence and in neuropathic bladder disorders.

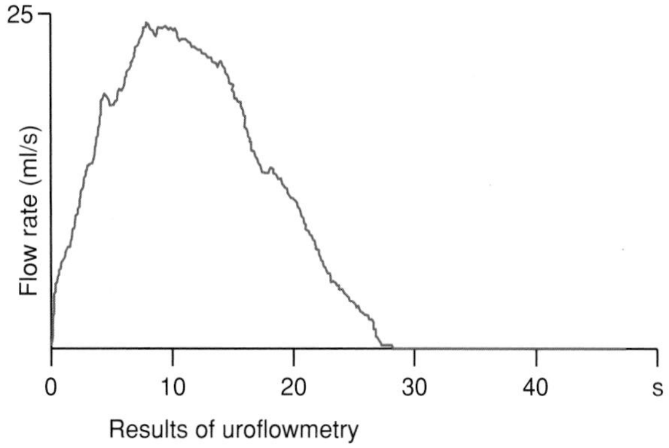

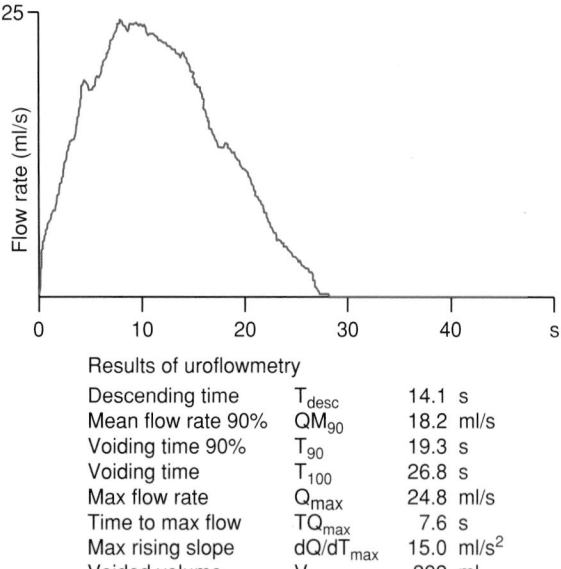

Results of uroflowmetry

Descending time	T_{desc}	14.1 s
Mean flow rate 90%	QM_{90}	18.2 ml/s
Voiding time 90%	T_{90}	19.3 s
Voiding time	T_{100}	26.8 s
Max flow rate	Q_{max}	24.8 ml/s
Time to max flow	TQ_{max}	7.6 s
Max rising slope	dQ/dT_{max}	15.0 ml/s^2
Voided volume	V_{comp}	392 ml

Figure 55.11 A normal uroflow trace. The most important variable is the peak flow rate: Q_{max}.

Table 55.2 Sequence of events in a typical pressure–flow study

1. Patient voids from a full bladder into a flow meter to obtain uroflow trace.
2. Residual urine volume is measured by bladder ultrasound.
3. Fine catheters for filling and pressure measurement are passed into the bladder.
4. A fine catheter is passed into the rectal ampulla to measure rectal (abdominal) pressure.
5. Bladder and rectal catheters are connected to the appropriate transducers and all air is flushed out by water, leaving a continuous fluid column between tip of catheter and transducer.
6. Patient sits (female) or stands (male) over a urine flow meter which detects urine escape during the filling phase and measures flow rate during voiding.
7. The filling pump is switched on and the patient is asked to report: first sensation of bladder fullness; sensation of normal desire to void ('when you would normally go to the toilet') and maximal desire to void ('when you feel you can't hold on any longer'). During the filling phase detrusor pressure is continually monitored.
8. When maximal comfortable capacity is reached the patient is asked to void. Detrusor pressure is continuously monitored during voiding.

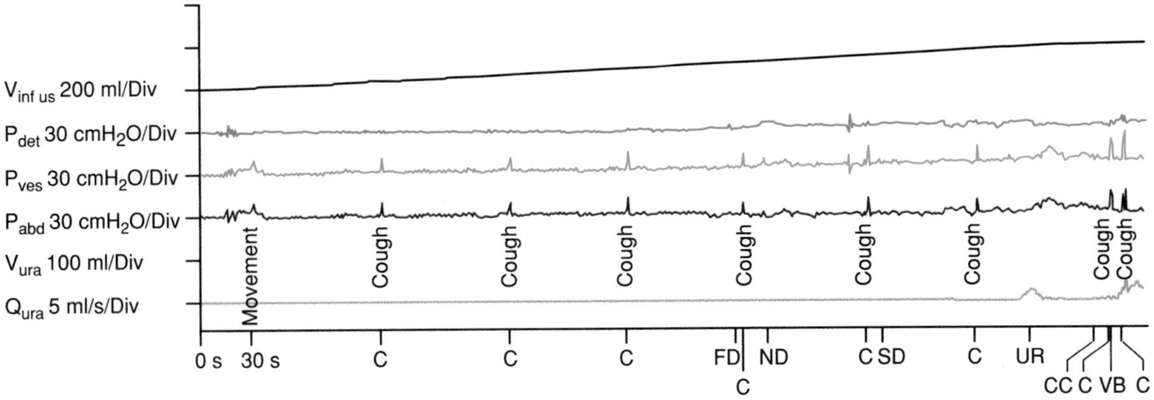

Figure 55.12 The filling phase of a pressure–flow study (cystometrogram). Half way through this phase the measured bladder pressure (P_{ves} – blue line) begins to rise. The abdominal pressure (P_{abd} – red line, measured from the rectum) remains at baseline, indicating that this is a true detrusor pressure rise (P_{det} – green line). Towards the end of this phase urine flows (Q_{ura} – yellow line) after coughing.

Further reading

Urology in general

Walsh, P.C., Retik, A.B., Vaughan, E.D. and Wein, A.J., eds (1998). *Campbell's Urology*, 7th edn. Philadelphia, PA: W.B. Saunders.

Whitfield, H. N., Hendry, W. F., Kirby, R. S. and Duckett, J. W., eds (1998). *Textbook of Genitourinary Surgery*, 2nd edn. Oxford: Blackwell Science.

Urological investigations

Anderson, R. U. (1999). Management of lower urinary tract infections. *Urol Clin North Am* **26**: 729–735.

Whitfield, H. N., Hendry, W. F., Kirby, R. S. and Duckett, J. W., eds (1998). Principles of urological investigations, Chapter 1. In *Textbook of Genitourinary Surgery*, 2nd edn. Oxford: Blackwell Science.

Uroradiology

Becker, J. (1998). A commentary on the past and a look at the future of genitourinary imaging. *Radiology* **207**: 7–8.

Whitfield, H. N., Hendry, W. F., Kirby, R. S. and Duckett, J. W., eds (1998). Basic uroradiological investigations, Chapter 2. In: *Textbook of Genitourinary Surgery*, 2nd edn. Oxford: Blackwell Science.

Zagoria, R. J., ed. (1997). *Urol Clin North Ame* **24**: 471–702.

Pressure–flow studies

Chapple, C. R, Christmas, T. J. and MacDiarmid, S., eds (1999). *Urodynamics Made Easy*. Edinburgh: Churchill Livingstone.

MODULE 56

Urogenital trauma

Most renal injuries are treated conservatively unless there are clear indications for intervention. If renal injury is suspected clinically, imaging must be used to assess the extent.

Section 56.1 • Renal trauma

Epidemiology

Blunt renal trauma is becoming more common because of the increase in motor vehicle accidents (MVAs) and the increasing number of people participating in contact sports.

Penetrating renal trauma is also on the increase because of injury caused by firearms in civilian assaults and in wars.

Mechanism of injury

The kidney is relatively protected by:

- its retroperitoneal position, protected by the abdominal wall posteriorly and the abdominal viscera anteriorly
- the rib cage
- the perinephric fat and fascia.

Because considerable force is required to damage a normal kidney, always consider an underlying pathology (hydronephrosis, tumour, cyst or stone) when trauma has been minor, or in children where hydronephrosis is the commonest underlying abnormality.

Most cases of **blunt** renal trauma are related to a direct blow to the loin. Renal artery thrombosis is rare, but is classically associated with an acceleration/deceleration injury, such as a fall from a height onto the feet.

Blunt renal trauma (especially if associated with a MVA) may be associated with other major intra-abdominal injuries.

The aetiology of **penetrating** renal trauma is outlined in Table 56.1.

Classification of renal trauma

After clinical and radiological assessment of the patient with renal trauma, an attempt must be made to classify the **extent** of the renal injury. A suggested classification is given in Figure 56.1.

Contusion and minor lacerations are regarded as **minor injuries** (80%): major laceration, vascular injury and injury to the renal pelvis are regarded as major injuries.

Contusion is a subcapsular haematoma due to blunt trauma or to penetrating trauma without caliceal penetration (i.e. no extravasation on radiological studies).

Minor laceration is a single tear through the capsule and renal parenchyma communicating with a calix. There is no major tear in the perinephric fascia so haemorrhage is contained. Extravasation is demonstrable radiologically but the kidney usually functions well.

Major laceration involves multiple parenchmal lacerations into calices. There are major tears in the perirenal fascia with loss of the containing effect, allowing extensive bleeding.

Radiologically, there is extensive extravasation with parts of the kidney functioning poorly.

Table 56.1 Aetiology of penetrating renal trauma

Traumatic	*Iatrogenic*
1. Stab wounds – often associated with trauma to other viscera 2. Gunshot wounds Low velocity – similar effect to stab wounds High velocity – enormous damage due to hydraulic shock	1. Percutaneous nephrolithotomy (PCNL) 2. Renal biopsy Either may cause primary bleeding, or secondary haemorrhage due to a false aneurysm

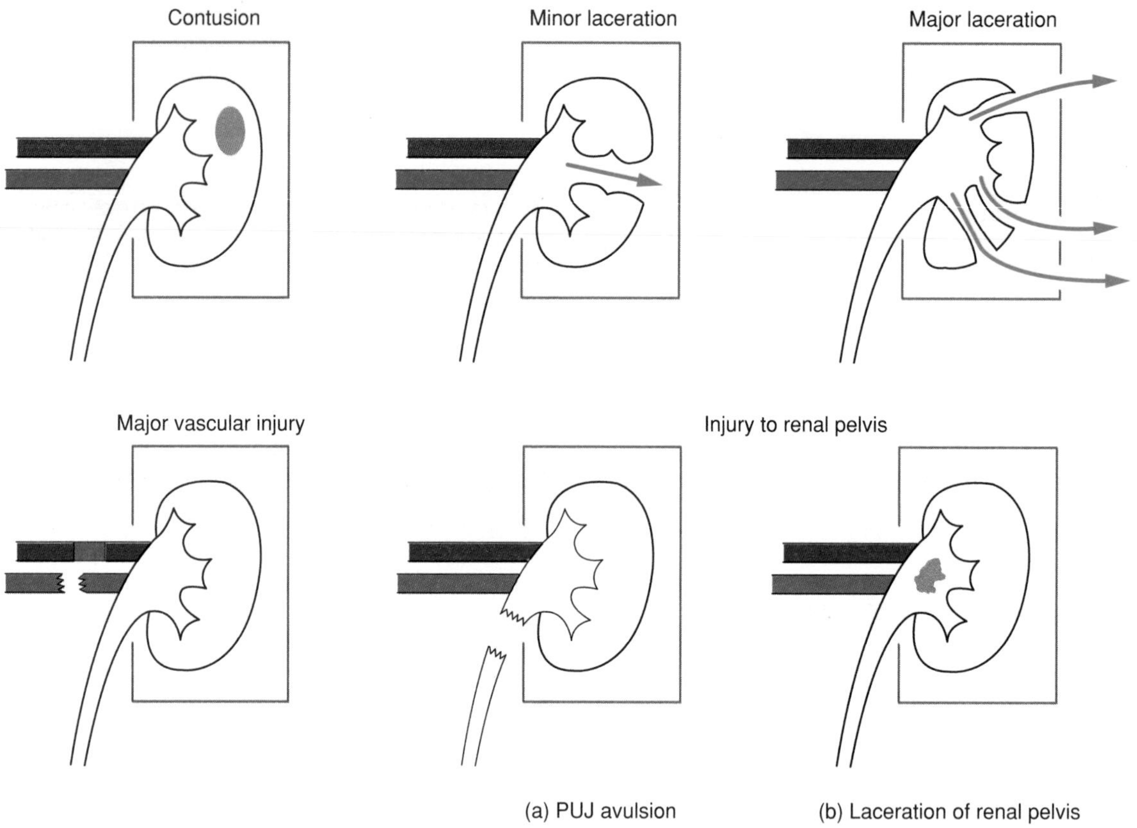

Figure 56.1 Classification of renal trauma.

Major vascular injury

- The classical vascular injury after blunt renal trauma is an intimal tear causing renal artery thrombosis. Renal artery avulsion is rare following blunt trauma.
- Penetrating renal trauma may cause injury to the renal artery and/or vein.

Injury to the renal pelvis

- Avulsion of the pelvis from the upper ureter.
- Penetrating renal trauma may perforate the renal pelvis directly (without going through renal parenchyma).

Complications of renal trauma

These are shown in Table 56.2.

Clinical presentation

Renal trauma usually presents in one of two ways:

- The patient sustains a blunt or penetrating injury to the loin, upper abdomen or lower chest and subsequently has macroscopic haematuria.
- The patient is involved in a MVA, has abdominal tenderness, and is subsequently found to have macroscopic haematuria (usually on catheterization).

The patient must be assessed for evidence of hypovolaemic shock. In patients with blunt trauma flank bruising, seatbelt marks and loin tenderness should be looked for. In patients with stab wounds the site is very important, as stab wounds posterior to the anterior axillary line have a much lower incidence of intra-abdominal injury than anterior stab wounds. In renal gunshot wounds it is useful to know the type and calibre of the weapon. Entrance and exit wounds should be looked for. In penetrating trauma, the degree of haemorrhage from the wound should be noted, because occasionally it may be severe.

Table 56.2 Complications of renal trauma

1. **Haemorrhage**
   - persistent primary haemorrhage
   - secondary (delayed) haemorrhage 10–14 days post-injury
2. **Urinary extravasation**
   - urinary fistula
   - urinoma/pseudocyst
   - hydronephrosis (secondary to pelviureteric junction (PUJ) obstruction) due to fibrosis or to pressure from a urinoma
3. **Infection**
   - pyelonephritis
   - infected perinephric haematoma/urinoma
   - septicaemia
4. **Infarction (segmental or total)**
5. **Hypertension: following infarction or scarring**
6. **Death: usually from associated injuries**

A renal mass on abdominal examination suggests a major injury associated with a perinephric haematoma or urinoma. After penetrating trauma, a bruit suggests a traumatic arteriovenous fistula; signs of peritonitis suggest an associated intra-abdominal injury. The possibility of chest involvement must not be forgotten.

All patients with suspected renal injury and haematuria (macroscopic or microscopic) must be investigated radiologically, as the degree of haematuria does not correlate with the severity of the injury. There is an exception following blunt trauma in an adult. Microscopic haematuria, but no history of rapid deceleration, no shock, no loin bruising or tenderness and no evidence of intra-abdominal injury does not need radiological investigation. In such patients the incidence of major renal injury is less than 1%. Some minor renal injuries will be missed but they would in any case be treated conservatively and have a low complication rate. This exception does not apply to paediatric patients. Any degree of haematuria in a child following blunt trauma must be investigated fully because:

- Kidneys are less protected in children (greater relative size, less muscle and perinephric fat).
- Pre-existing renal abnormalities occur in up to 23% of children sustaining blunt renal trauma.
- Children are able to maintain normal blood pressure despite significant blood loss.

Radiological diagnosis

Intravenous pyelography

A high-dose intravenous pyelogram (IVU) is the time-honoured way of assessing renal trauma, but tends to understage renal injury (see Figures 56.7 and 56.8).

On the control film, fractured lower ribs and/or fractured transverse processes of L1 or L2 suggest possible renal injury. An absent psoas shadow may be due to a retroperitoneal haematoma. A soft tissue mass with bowel displacement may be seen if there is a major laceration. Absence of a nephrogram on the injured side needs investigation to exclude renal artery thrombosis (Figures 56.2 and 56.3). Is the function good, as found in a contusion, or are there areas of non-function due to poor perfusion as found in a major laceration (Figure 56.4). Next, look for evidence of extravasation, which tends to increase with time. Extravasation is associated with lacerations (Figure 56.5) or rarely with a pelviureteric junction (PUJ) avulsion or direct pelvic injury. Pelvic injury is suggested when extravasation is medial (as opposed to lateral with caliceal injury) and when the ureter is not seen. This is important as pelvic injury needs exploration.

Confirmation of the presence of a normal contralateral kidney is important, particularly if the traumatized kidney has sustained major injury.

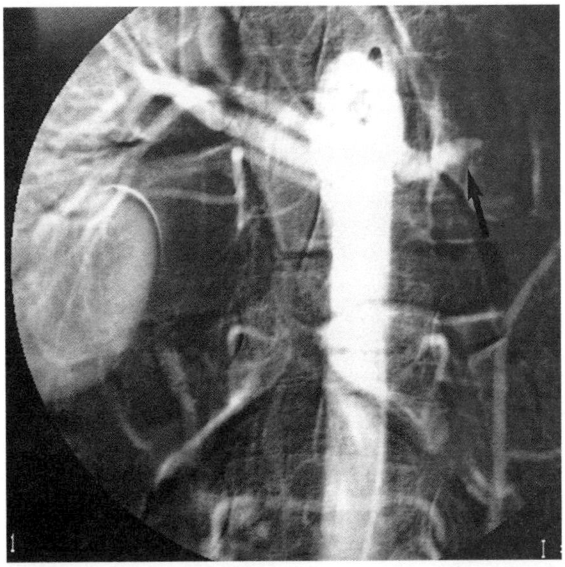

Figure 56.3 Aortogram in the same patient as Figure 56.2 shows renal artery thrombosis (arrow).

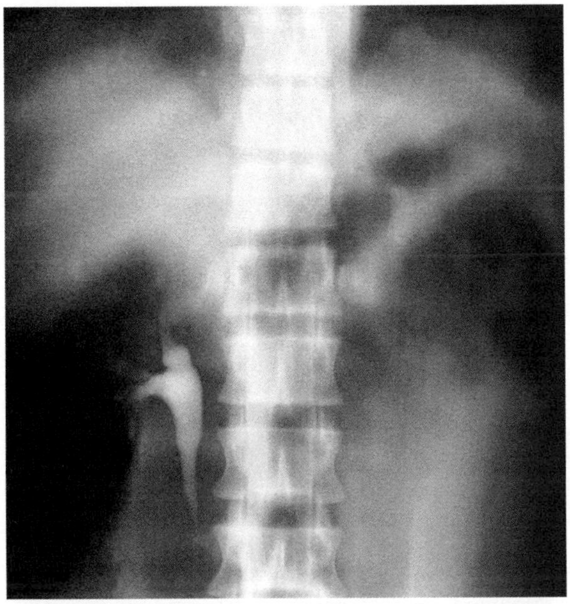

Figure 56.2 Blunt abdominal trauma and microscopic haematuria. IVU reveals no nephrogram on left.

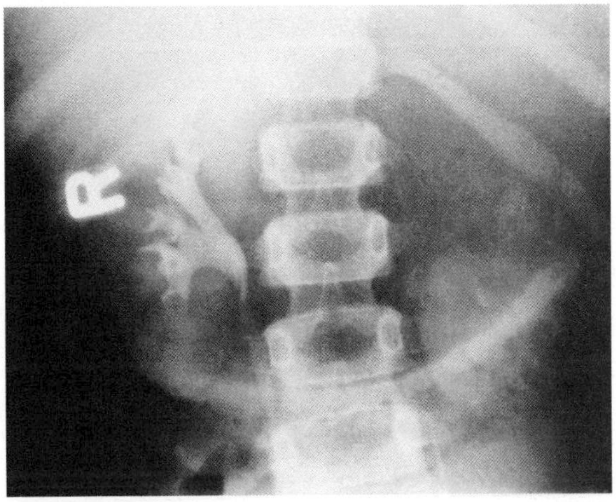

Figure 56.4 Major injury to left kidney – perfusion of lower pole only.

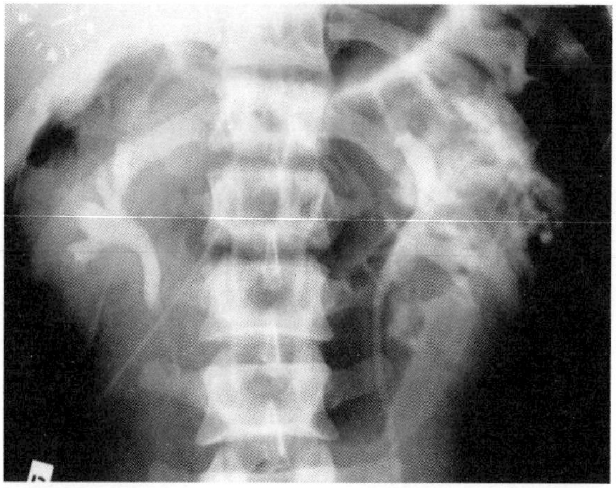

Figure 56.5 Minor laceration involving left kidney – good function but obvious contrast extravasation.

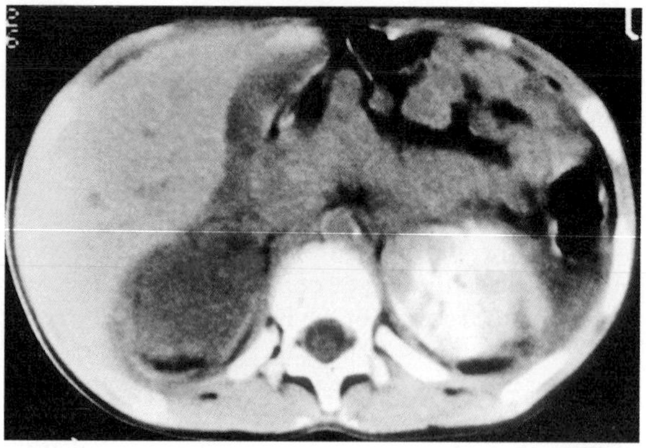

Figure 56.8 Computed tomography (same patient as in Figure 56.7) – non-perfusion of right kidney due to traumatic renal artery thrombosis, and laceration of left kidney with contrast extravasation, not seen on IVU.

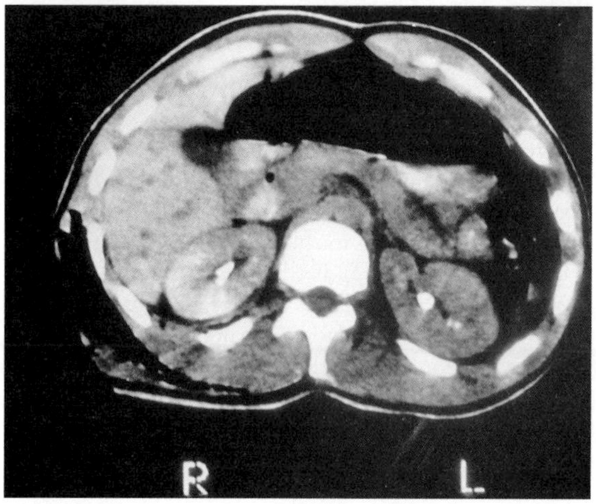

Figure 56.6 The patient presented with blunt abdominal trauma and haematuria. IVU normal. Computed tomography showed subcapsular extravasation involving right kidney.

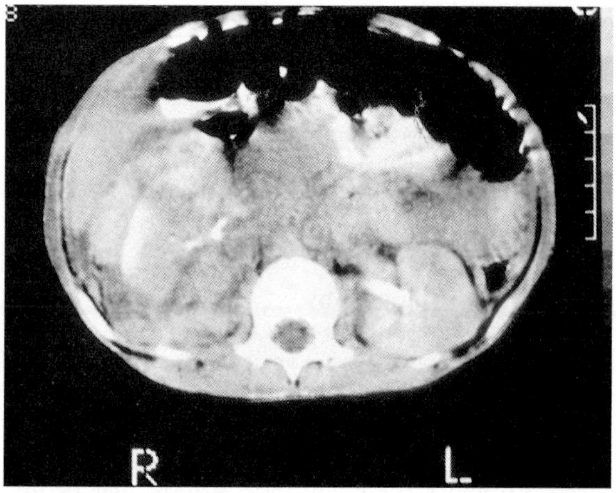

Figure 56.9 Computed tomographic appearance of major laceration of the right kidney.

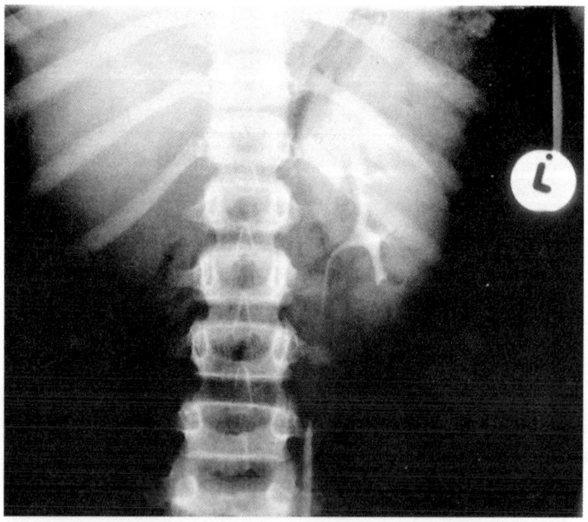

Figure 56.7 This patient had macroscopic haematuria after a MVA. IVU – left kidney 'normal', no nephrogram seen on right side.

Computed tomography

The advantages of computed tomography (CT) are demonstrated by the two cases shown in Figures 56.6–56.8. Figure 56.9 shows a major laceration of a right kidney.

Renal angiography

Angiography has largely been replaced by CT, but it still has an important role in the management of secondary haemorrhage by demonstrating a false aneurysm before embolization of the feeding vessel (Figures 56.10 and 56.11).

Angiography is also useful in interval exploration for a major laceration, where partial nephrectomy is contemplated (Figure 56.12).

Renal ultrasound

Ultrasound shows parenchymal lacerations and perinephric collections well and is a useful complement to IVP if CT is unavailable.

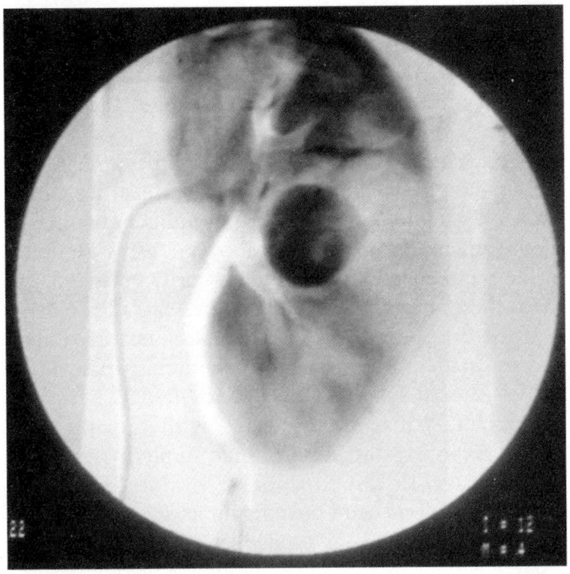

Figure 56.10 Renal angiogram showing large false aneurysm in midpole of left kidney.

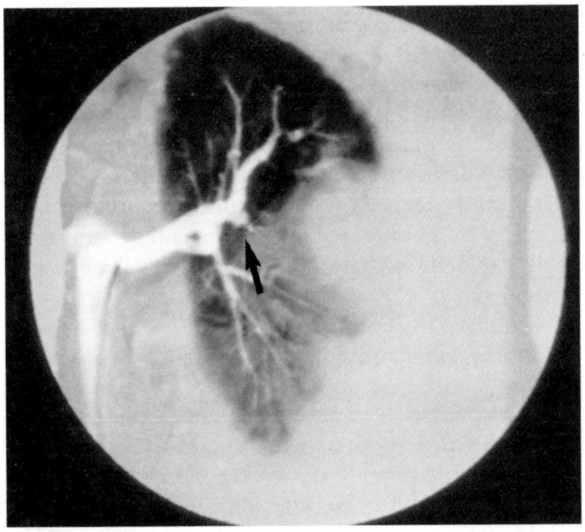

Figure 56.11 Post-embolization angiogram showing obstructed feeding vessel (arrow) and area of infarction peripherally.

Management of renal trauma

The initial management of renal trauma (blunt or penetrating) is usually conservative. The principles of conservative management are outlined in Table 56.3.

The patient being treated conservatively must be closely watched for the development of complications, such as an infected perinephric haematoma/urinoma (swinging pyrexia and tender mass) or the development of abdominal signs secondary to initially unsuspected intra-abdominal visceral damage.

The indications for acute renal exploration are outlined in Table 56.4. Haemodynamic instability due to haemorrhage (either internal, external or both) is the most important indication, as this can be life-threatening.

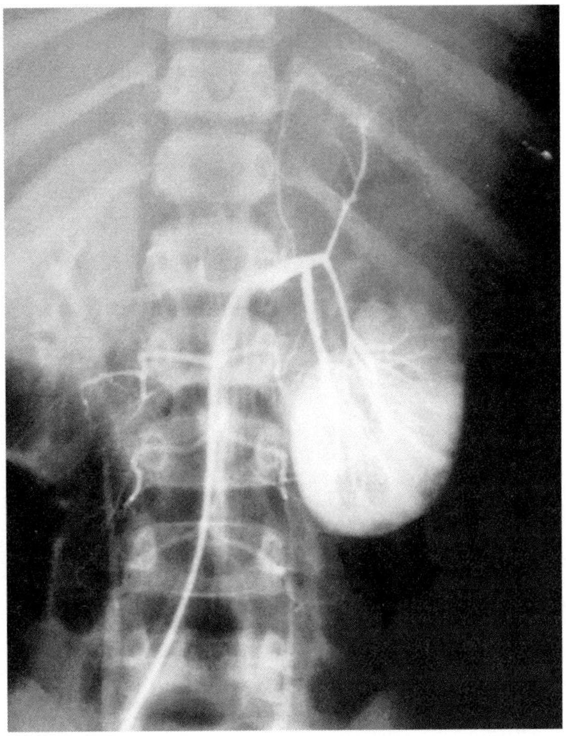

Figure 56.12 Left renal angiogram showing a normal lower pole. Upper pole poorly perfused because of a major injury.

Renal reconstruction

The aim is to preserve 30% or more function in the kidney. Operative options are renorraphy (kidney repair), partial nephrectomy or (as a last resort) total nephrectomy.

The principles of renal reconstruction are outlined in Table 56.5.

Renal pedicle injuries

Renal artery thrombosis is managed by vascular control, renal cooling, thrombectomy, renal perfusion with cold solution and segmental excision of the involved renal artery. Vascular continuity is re-established by end to end anastomosis; vein, artery or synthetic graft interposition; or autotransplantation. The results of surgery for renal artery thrombosis, even when treated early, are poor.

Table 56.3 Conservative management of renal trauma

1. Admit
2. Strict bed rest
3. Intravenous fluids
4. Monitor vital signs
   - temperature
   - blood pressure
   - pulse rate
   - haemoglobin
5. Repeated, frequent abdominal examination
   - renal mass
   - renal bruit
   - signs of peritonitis
6. Monitor macroscopic haematuria
7. Antibiotics for penetrating trauma

Table 56.4 Indications for acute surgery in renal trauma

1. Haemodynamic instability due to haemorrhage: obtain pre-operative imaging if at all possible
2. Renal artery thrombosis: requires immediate exploration if diagnosed within 12 hours
3. Laparotomy for suspected intraperitoneal visceral damage
4. High-velocity gunshot wounds: always need exploration due to extent of damage
5. Suspected renal pelvis injury
6. Non-function of a major part of the kidney

Table 56.5 Principles of renal reconstruction

1. Adequate exposure (midline laparotomy)
2. Control renal vessels
3. Inspect kidney, hilar vessels, renal pelvis
4. Debride devitalized tissue
5. Preserve renal capsule if possible
6. Control haemorrhage
7. Repair defects in collecting system
8. Cover parenchymal defect with:
   - capsule
   - synthetic mesh
   - omentum
9. Drain

Lacerations of the renal artery and vein can be repaired with 5/0 vascular sutures after vascular control. If necessary the left renal vein can be tied off because of the existence of a collateral circulation.

Renal pelvis injuries

A renal pelvis injury secondary to penetrating trauma requires debridement before closure and drainage. PUJ avulsion is managed with a spatulated end to end anastomosis over a stent with covering nephrostomy and perirenal drain. These repairs can be covered with omentum.

Unexpected retroperitoneal haematoma at laparotomy

The finding of an unexpected retroperitoneal haematoma at laparotomy for suspected intra-abdominal injury is managed according to the algorithm in Figure 56.13.

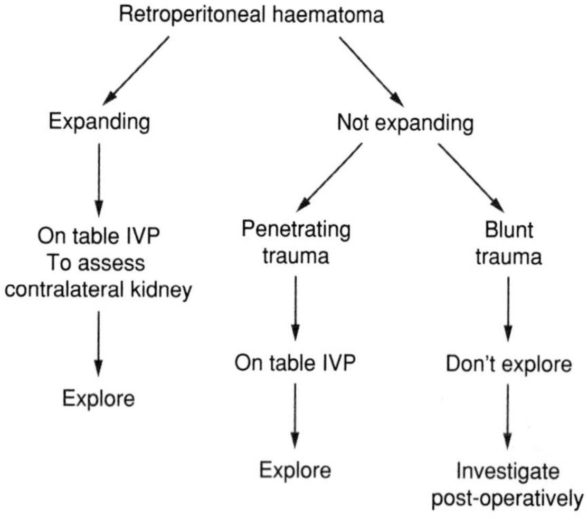

Figure 56.13 Management of unexpected retroperitoneal haematoma at laparotomy.

An **expanding** retroperitoneal haematoma suggests a serious renal injury or involvement of the great vessels, and must be explored. First establish that a contralateral kidney is present and functioning by a single on-table film 10 min after contrast injection. If on-table radiology facilities are not available, a dye that is excreted by the kidney (such as indigo carmine or methylene blue) can be given intravenously. The ureter of the traumatized kidney is temporarily occluded, and the catheter bag checked for the presence of the dye.

If the retroperitoneal haematoma is not expanding and the patient has sustained penetrating trauma, the kidney should be exposed and repaired if necessary. Blunt trauma may be associated with a major renal injury. Exposing the kidney may result in torrential haemorrhage. In this situation, it is more prudent to 'leave well alone' and investigate post-operatively. If surgery to the kidney is needed later it can be done on a stable patient in a relatively bloodless field.

Management of complications

Secondary haemorrhage presents acutely with gross haematuria. A bruit may be heard over the kidney. Initial management consists of resuscitation, transfusion and bladder washout if necessary. Renal angiography usually demonstrates a false aneurysm (Figure 56.10), which is embolized (Figure 56.11). If embolization facilities are not available, or if haemorrhage recurs post-embolization (rare) surgical exploration is needed.

Infected perinephric haematoma/urinoma is suggested by a swinging temperature and a loin mass. It needs exploration, drainage of the collection and repair of the kidney.

Secondary PUJ obstruction is due to fibrosis round a urinoma and is treated by pyeloplasty.

Section 56.2 • Ureteric injuries

The possibility of a ureteric injury should always be considered in a patient who has sustained a gunshot wound to the abdomen or who has had difficult pelvic surgery.

Early diagnosis leads to a good result. Delayed diagnosis increases the complication rate.

Epidemiology

Penetrating ureteric injuries occur with gunshot wounds, during difficult pelvic surgery and at ureteroscopy.

Aetiology

The causes of ureteric injury are shown in Table 56.6.

Complications of ureteric injuries

A missed ureteric injury is often silent at first. Urine in the peritoneal cavity may produce an ileus. A urinoma may become infected, presenting as an abscess, or may cause a urinary fistula – for example a post-hysterecto-

Table 56.6 Aetiology of ureteric trauma

Traumatic	*Iatrogenic*
1. Penetrating trauma • gunshot wounds – low velocity – high velocity • Stab wounds (rarely involve the ureter) 2. Blunt trauma (rare – usually involves PUJ avulsion – see section on renal trauma)	1. Open surgery – gynaecological – colorectal – vascular – urological 2. Ureteroscopy (risk much reduced with latest small calibre or flexible instruments – see Module 55)

my ureterovaginal fistula. Healing by fibrosis produces a ureteric stricture and the patient may present later with loin pain.

Clinical presentation

1. Penetrating ureteric injuries

Ninety-two per cent of penetrating ureteric injuries are associated with injury to other intra-abdominal viscera, thus most patients will have a laparotomy.

(a) Ureteric injury suspected pre-operatively
Haematuria (usually microscopic) is present in 90% of patients with penetrating ureteric injuries. Imaging is needed, as below.

(b) Ureteric injury suspected intra-operatively
A ureteric injury may be suspected because of the trajectory of the bullet or stab wound or excessive clear fluid accumulation intra-abdominally. Urine leak can be confirmed by intravenous injection of a dye excreted by the kidney (indigo carmine or methylene blue).

(c) Post-operative diagnosis of ureteric injury
When a ureteric injury is missed it presents post-operatively as:

- ileus with raised serum creatinine due to reabsorption
- urinary fistula through drain site
- intra-abdominal abscess
- loin pain due to ureteric stricture.

2. Iatrogenic ureteric injuries associated with abdominal surgery

(a) Prevention
If difficult surgery is anticipated, do an intravenous pyelography (IVP) pre-operatively and consider ureteric catheterization to help identify the ureters.

(b) Ureteric injury suspected intra-operatively
The ureter may have been crushed, divided or included in a ligature or suture. Most injuries involve the distal ureter, thus the ureter can be exposed proximally and followed distally to the suspect area. If in doubt catheterize the ureters via open cystotomy or cystoscopy. Avoid a proximal ureterotomy and distal passage of a ureteric catheter as it may cause a ureteric stricture, whereas open cystotomy has negligible morbidity.

(c) Post-operative diagnosis of ureteric injury
A missed ureteric injury will present as described in 1(c).

3. Ureteroscopic ureteric injuries

The ureter is usually damaged by perforation. Avulsion is (fortunately) rare.

A missed injury may present later as a ureteric stricture.

Radiological diagnosis

In a patient with penetrating abdominal trauma, an IVU will show extravasation in up to 90% of cases (Figure 56.14). CT is often done for patients with penetrating abdominal trauma. It will show extravasation and lack of distal ureteric filling.

If iatrogenic ureteric injury is suspected post-operatively, IVU is again very useful as extravasation and/or obstruction is seen in most cases of ureteric damage (Figure 56.15). A retrograde pyelogram is useful to delineate the site and extent of the injury prior to definitive treatment. If a percutaneous nephrostomy has already been inserted, an antegrade nephrostogram will give the same information.

Treatment

There are four considerations in deciding on treatment for a ureteric injury:

Site of the injury

This determines the incision used for open repair.

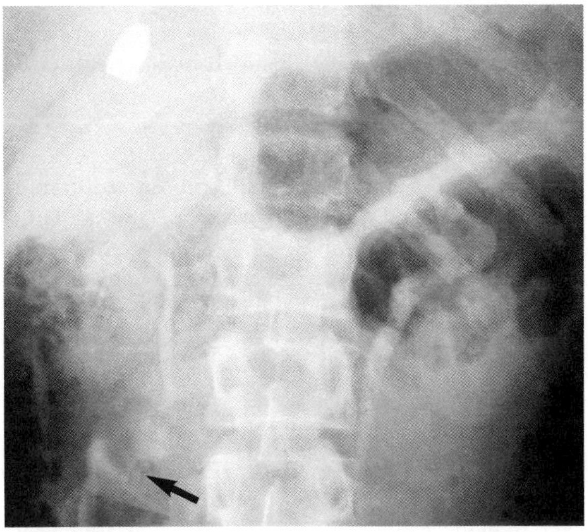

Figure 56.14 Gunshot wound to abdomen (bullet visible in right upper quadrant). Extravasation of contrast from right upper ureter (arrow).

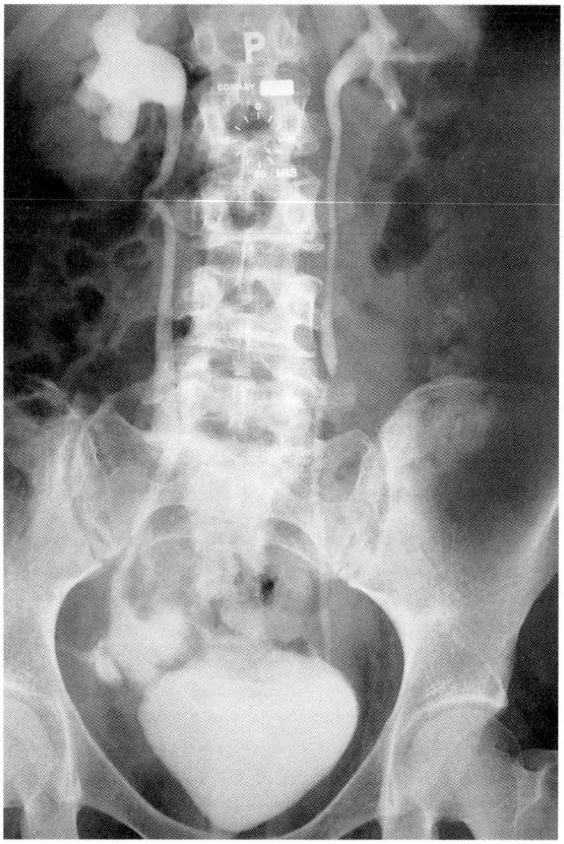

Figure 56.15 Post-hysterectomy injury to right ureter. IVU shows hydronephrosis and hydroureter down to the point of injury, and adjacent extravasation.

Cause of the injury

Low-velocity gunshot wounds and stab wounds require minimal debridement before anastomosis. High-velocity gunshot wounds need extensive debridement and often 're-look surgery' at 48–72 hours to check viability.

Time to recognition of injury

The earlier the diagnosis, the better the results. Late diagnosis is associated with a much higher nephrectomy rate.

Associated injuries

Ureteric injuries due to penetrating abdominal trauma are often associated with damage to other viscera. Duodenal and pancreatic injuries are especially important and require a watertight ureteric closure with omental interposition. Colonic injuries, even if there is significant soiling, do not appear to affect ureteric healing.

The ureter should be stented regardless of the type of repair. (It has been suggested that patients with adjacent ureteric and vascular injuries should have nephrostomy drainage rather than stenting due to the danger of fistula formation.) A double J stent works very well, but if the latter is not available an 8 Fr feeding tube (with the connector cut off) works well. For example, if the upper ureter has been repaired, one end of the 'stent' can be passed through the anastomosis into the kidney and the other end brought out of the ureter distal to the anastomosis and then through the skin – ureterostomy *in situ* (Figure 56.16). Similarly a ureteroneocystostomy can be stented by a tube brought out through the bladder (Figure 56.17).

Treatment options for ureteric injuries

For a ureteric injury **below** the pelvic brim, the treatment of choice is a **ureteroneocystostomy**, while for injuries **above** the pelvic brim the treatment of choice is **ureteroureterostomy**.

The different surgical options are well covered in operative urology textbooks and will not be described in detail here.

Temporary percutaneous nephrostomy (PCN)

This is very useful in two situations:

1. Late presentation of ureteric injury with obstruction (e.g. post-hysterectomy), where insertion of a PCN allows the kidney to recover, pending definitive repair.
2. At laparotomy for penetrating trauma where the patient is unstable and there is large segment ureteric loss, the proximal ureter may be tied off (and the distal ureter marked with a suture) and a PCN inserted in the early post-operative period. This allows good renal drainage while the other problems are addressed. The ureteric injury can be repaired electively.

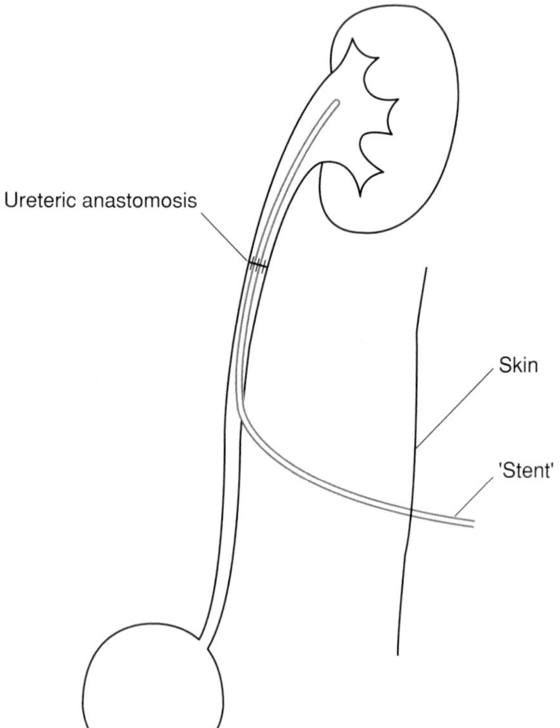

Figure 56.16 When a double J stent is not available, an 8 Fr infant feeding tube can be used to splint the anatamosis, by ureterostomy *in situ* draining through the skin.

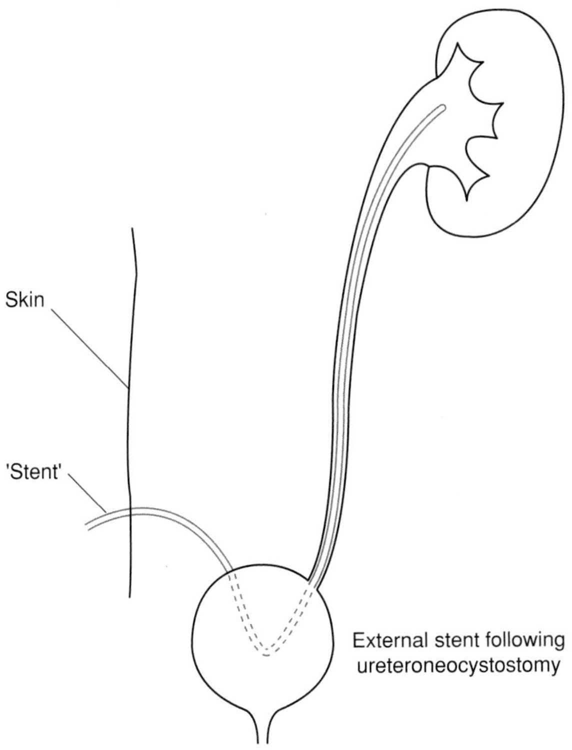

Figure 56.17 An infant feeding tube can also be used to splint a ureteroneocystostomy.

Ureteric stent
As well as in ureteric repair as above, stents are useful for partial or suspected ureteric injury The stent is passed through the area retrogradely via a cystoscope or a cystotomy, or antegradely via a PCN.

When PCN facilities are not available, the proximal ureter can be intubated with a feeding tube which is tied in place and brought out on the skin as a ureterostomy *in situ*, pending definitive repair.

Simple suture
This can be done (over a stent) where the ureter is still in continuity (i.e. a partial injury). Care must be taken not to produce narrowing.

Ureteroureterostomy (end-to-end repair)
Mobilization of the proximal and distal ureters (taking care to preserve ureteric blood supply) and complete mobilization of the kidney within Gerota's fascia will give 2–3 cm of 'length', ensuring a tension-free anastomosis (see Table 56.7).

Table 56.7 Principles of ureteric repair

1. Adequate debridement of damaged ureter
2. Spatulated water-tight tension-free anastomosis (if end to end), using fine (e.g. 4/0) polyglycolic acid or monofilament absorbable interrupted sutures
3. Isolation of anastomosis from associated injuries or contamination, by wrapping with omentum, which also brings a blood supply
4. Adequate drainage to avoid urinoma leading to fibrosis and obstruction
5. Ureteric stenting

Ureteroneocystostomy
An anti-reflux anastomosis is preferable but not essential, as obstruction and tension must be avoided. Hitching the ipsilateral part of the bladder up onto the psoas muscle with non-absorbable sutures helps to give a tension-free anastomosis.

Boari flap
When there has been 'large segment' ureteric loss of the distal ureter (or even the mid ureter if bladder capacity is good) then the Boari flap is a very useful manoeuvre. It is usually combined with a psoas hitch (Figure 56.18).

Transureteroureterostomy
This is especially useful for injuries to the distal third of the ureter where reimplantation is not possible or is contraindicated (e.g. previous pelvic irradiation with a frozen pelvis), or where an anti-reflux vesico-ureteric junction is important (e.g. in children).

Autotransplantation into the iliac fossa
This can be used where most of the ureter has been destroyed. It is an interval elective procedure done in a major centre with renal transplant experience.

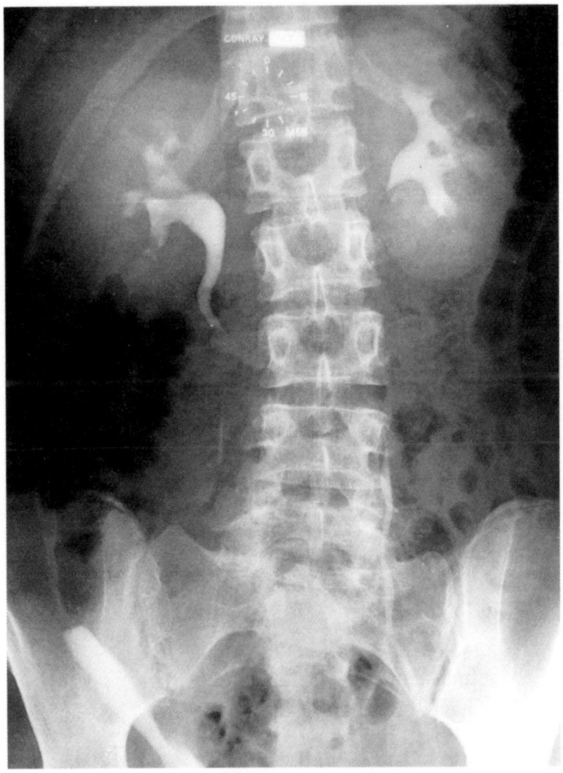

Figure 56.18 Right distal ureteric injury treated with a Boari flap and ureteric reimplantation. Note undilated right upper urinary tract.

Ileal replacement of the ureter

This is another way of managing massive loss of the ureter. It is an interval procedure and should not be undertaken lightly. Incorporating bowel into the urinary tract brings its own problems, including recurrent urinary tract infection and the long-term risk of malignancy.

Nephrectomy

This is the **last** resort, but may be considered if there is large segment ureteric loss and multiple other visceral damage (especially pancreatic and duodenal injuries).

Management of ureteroscopic ureteric injury

Perforation is managed by a double J stent left in place for 6 weeks, or a percutaneous nephrostomy if stenting is not possible. These injuries usually heal without stricture formation.

Avulsion of the ureter needs immediate exploration. The ureter is repaired if possible, but if the whole ureter is involved autotransplantation, ileal replacement or nephrectomy may be needed.

Late presentation

A ureteric stricture after missed ureteric injury is managed initially with balloon dilatation, and by open surgery if this fails.

Section 56.3 • Bladder injuries

A bladder injury diagnosed and treated early leads to a good result. Late diagnosis increases morbidity.

Epidemiology

MVAs are an important cause of bladder injury. In some parts of the world gunshot wounds are the second most common cause, in others iatrogenic injury takes second place.

Aetiology

The causes of bladder injury are shown in Table 56.8.

Blunt trauma

The bony pelvis is a rigid ring joined at the sacroiliac joints posteriorly so it is not possible to break the pelvis at one point without fracture, dislocation or diastasis at another point. The pubovesical ligaments extend from the bladder to the back of the symphysis pubis. The dome has the least support and is the weakest part of the bladder.

Extraperitoneal bladder rupture is almost always associated with a fractured pelvis and an empty bladder at the time of injury. 10% of patients with a pelvic fracture have an associated bladder rupture. The mechanism is direct penetration of the bladder wall by a bone fragment or tearing of the bladder anteriorly related to the attachments of the pubovesical ligaments. The latter is a serious injury as it may extend into the bladder neck. Intraperitoneal bladder rupture occurs when a patient with a full bladder receives a blow to the lower abdomen, causing a horizontal tear in the dome of the bladder.

Penetrating trauma

Gunshot wounds to the abdomen or perineum have become an important cause of penetrating bladder injury. In 80% of cases there is associated intra-abdominal injury, particularly rectal injury. Stab wounds are a rare cause of bladder injury.

Iatrogenic injury

Bladder injury can occur during pelvic operations such as abdominal hysterectomy, caesarean section or rectal surgery; or inguinal hernia repair, where part of the bladder has prolapsed into the sac. Rarely, bladder injury has been associated with hip surgery. The bladder can be injured during lower tract endoscopic procedures, such as tumour resection and litholapaxy.

Complications of bladder injuries

Urinary ascites may follow an undiagnosed intraperitoneal bladder rupture. Sequelae of this may be peritonitis, intra-abdominal abscess or even respiratory difficulty.

Urinary fistula occurs particularly after missed iatrogenic injuries, for example vesicovaginal fistula following missed bladder injury at hysterectomy.

Pelvic abscess may occur as a complication of extraperitoneal bladder rupture.

Table 56.8 Aetiology of bladder injuries

Traumatic	*Iatrogenic*
1. Blunt trauma • Extraperitoneal bladder rupture • Intraperitoneal bladder rupture • Combined extra- and intraperitoneal bladder rupture	1. Open surgery
2. Penetrating trauma • Gunshot wounds – low velocity – high velocity • Stab wounds	2. Endoscopic surgery

Clinical presentation

Traumatic bladder injury

The classical acute presentation of traumatic bladder injury is a patient who is unable to void, has no sign of urethral injury (i.e. urethral bleeding) and has an impalpable bladder. Urethral catheterization reveals macroscopic haematuria. Local examination may reveal bruising over the lower abdomen, entrance and exit wounds (in the case of gunshot wounds) or clinical features of a fractured pelvis. Abdominal examination may reveal lower abdominal tenderness or features of peritonitis. The latter is usually due to associated intra-abdominal injury as the presence of uninfected urine in the peritoneal cavity elicits a minimal inflammatory response. Rectal and vaginal examination are very important to exclude injury to those structures (particularly following gunshot wounds).

The diagnosis of delayed presentation of an intraperitoneal bladder rupture can be very difficult. It usually follows an assault on an intoxicated patient, who presents 2–3 days later. By this time the bladder laceration may have been 'plugged' by omentum and the patient may be voiding urethrally, often with clear urine. Abdominal examination typically reveals features of an ileus with ascites, and there is uraemia due to reabsorption.

Patients with a fractured pelvis may rarely have a combined intra- and extraperitoneal bladder rupture.

Iatrogenic bladder injury

Iatrogenic bladder injury at open surgery or endoscopy is usually evident. A missed bladder injury will present with complications as above.

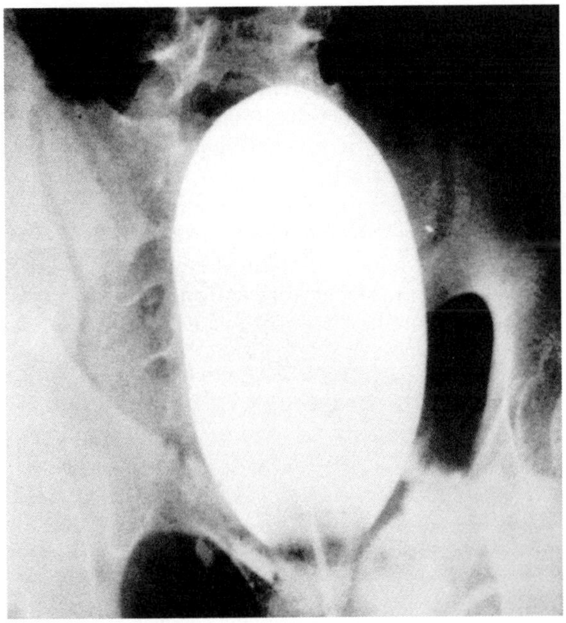

Figure 56.19 Extraperitoneal bladder rupture. Note fracture of the right superior pubic ramus, lateral compression of the bladder by pelvic haematoma and contrast extravasation around the bladder base.

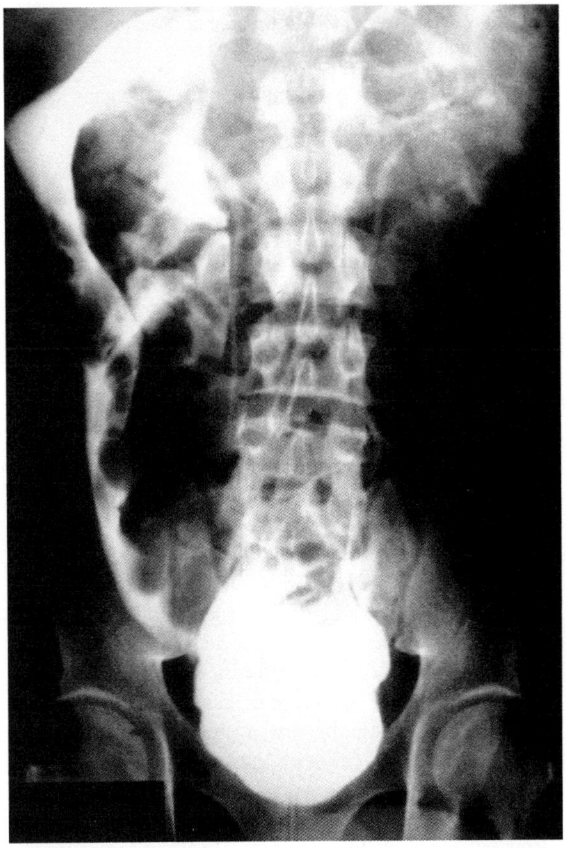

Figure 56.20 Intraperitoneal bladder rupture. Note extensive extravasation of contrast from bladder dome and accumulation in right paracolic gutter. Upper urinary tract contrast due to IVU done simultaneously.

Radiological diagnosis

The definitive investigation for the diagnosis of the bladder injury is an ascending cystogram.

The bladder is filled via a urethral catheter with a water soluble contrast agent under gravity until flow stops (usually 300–500 ml). Radiological screening should be used because an intraperitoneal bladder rupture is often quickly obvious, and the procedure can then stop. A post-drainage film is very important as extravasation may be minimal in extraperitoneal bladder ruptures, and may be seen only on this film.

Extraperitoneal bladder rupture is characterized by extravasation of contrast confined to the pelvis, particularly around the bladder base (Figure 56.19). Intraperitoneal bladder rupture is characterized by extravasation of contrast from the bladder dome and diffusely throughout the peritoneal cavity, particularly in the paracolic gutters (Figure 56.20).

If urethral catheterization is contraindicated (as in a patient with a fractured pelvis and suspected membranous urethral injury), the cystogram phase of an IVU may show contrast extravasation. If additional renal or ureteric injury is suspected clinically, a CT scan or IVU must be performed.

Table 56.9 Indications for surgical repair of extraperitoneal bladder rupture

1. During laparotomy for trauma to abdominal organs
2. Presence of associated injury to:
   - bladder neck
   - membranous urethra
   - rectum
   - vagina
3. Severe haematuria

Management of bladder injuries

Extraperitoneal bladder rupture

Most extraperitoneal bladder ruptures can be treated non-operatively by a urethral catheter and broad spectrum antibiotics. A cystogram at 10 days post-injury confirms healing. The indications for surgical repair of extraperitoneal bladder rupture are given in Table 56.9. Open the dome of the bladder, check bladder neck integrity (bladder neck injury requires repair over a urethral catheter), look for clear urine from both ureteric orifices and repair bladder lacerations transvesically with absorbable sutures. Avoid opening the pelvic haematoma, which will cause severe haemorrhage. Leave a suprapubic and a urethral catheter, and a perivesical drain.

Intraperitoneal bladder rupture

Intraperitoneal bladder rupture always needs surgery. Evacuate urine from the peritoneal cavity, repair the defect in the bladder in two layers, insert a drain and a urethral and a suprapubic catheter.

Penetrating bladder trauma

Surgery is always indicated because of the possibility of bladder neck or utereric injury and the high incidence of associated intra-abdominal visceral damage. After laparotomy, repair the bladder as above. Rectal injury may require end colostomy and omental interposition between bladder and rectal repairs. Vaginal injury also needs separate repair of bladder and vagina with interposition of omentum.

Iatrogenic bladder injury at open surgery

The possibility of bladder injury must always be considered when doing difficult pelvic surgery. If the injury is recognized and repaired, and adequate catheter drainage instituted, there is seldom any further problem.

A missed injury presents later with complications, e.g. vesicovaginal fistula after hysterectomy. This usually requires delayed repair. Omental interposition is useful to bring in blood supply.

Iatrogenic bladder injury at endoscopic surgery

Most of these injuries occur in the extraperitoneal part of the bladder, and are treated conservatively with an indwelling catheter for a week.

An intraperitoneal injury (on the dome of the bladder) needs exploration and repair.

Section 56.4 • Urethral injuries

Injuries to the male urethra only are discussed here. The female urethra, because of its short length and protected position under the symphysis pubis, is very rarely injured.

Epidemiology

Pelvic fractures from road accidents cause most posterior urethral injuries, some of the most serious injuries seen in urological practice.

The increased incidence of gunshot injuries has caused an increase in the incidence of penetrating urethral trauma, although this is still an uncommon injury.

Aetiology

The causes of urethral injuries are shown in Table 56.10.

Classification of urethral injuries

Urethral injuries may be classified as in Figure 56.21. In a **urethral mucosal tear** the urethra is intact. An example is urethral bleeding following intercourse, or the clinical picture of a urethral injury following blunt trauma, with a normal urethrogram. A **partial rupture** has a laceration in the wall of the urethra but there is still continuity. Radiologically, contrast will pass through the area into the urethra beyond, but there will be extravasation. **Major distraction** injuries are seen in posterior urethral trauma, where the bladder and

Table 56.10 Aetiology of urethral injuries

Traumatic	*Iatrogenic*
1. Blunt trauma • Membranous urethral injury (associated with fractured pelvis) • Bulbar urethral injury (fall astride or blow to perineum) • Penile urethral injury	1. Open surgery • Pelvic rectal operations • Anorectal surgery • Perineal debridement for necrotizing fasciitis
2. Penetrating trauma • Gunshot wounds – low velocity – high velocity • Stab wounds	2. Traumatic catheterization/inadvertent inflation of balloon in urethra 3. Endoscopes, especially resectoscopes

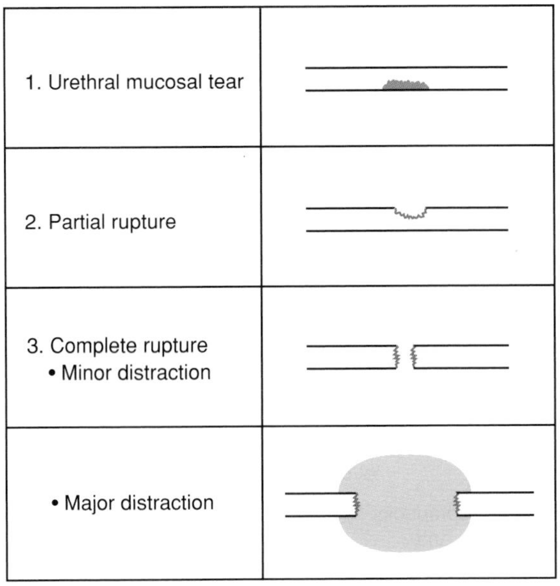

Figure 56.21 Classification of urethral injury.

prostate are displaced upwards, and the ends are separated by a pelvic haematoma. The degree of distraction is shown by simultaneous ascending and descending (via a suprapubic cystostomy) urethrography.

Complications of urethral injuries

The complications of urethral injury are shown in Table 56.11.

Clinical presentation

Any patient who sustains blunt or penetrating trauma to the lower abdomen, perineum or external genitalia is at risk of sustaining a urethral injury. This is particularly relevant if he has a fractured pelvis (10% will have a posterior urethral injury).

The hallmark of urethral injury is urethral bleeding. Classically, the patient is unable to void, although occasionally patients with a partial injury may void small volumes. In patients who have sustained a bulbar urethral injury, a scrotal haematoma may be found. The patient is usually in acute urinary retention with a palpable bladder. In a patient with a fractured pelvis and suspected urethral injury, failure to palpate a bladder after adequate resuscitation should alert one to the possibility of an associated bladder rupture which occurs in 15% of patients with a posterior urethral injury.

In patients with a fractured pelvis, rectal examination is important to exclude rectal injury and to palpate the prostate. A prostate in the normal position indicates a partial injury or a complete injury with only minor distraction. If the prostate is impalpable, and one can only feel a boggy mass (the pelvic haematoma) this suggests a complete injury with major distraction.

Patients with a fractured pelvis and posterior urethral injury often have multiple other injuries and the diagnosis of a urethral injury may be overlooked without a high index of suspicion.

Table 56.11 Complications of urethral injury

Stricture – the most important complication
- partial rupture heals either without stricture or with a short soft stricture easily managed endoscopically
- complete rupture always forms a stricture

Erectile dysfunction
Usually due to damage to nerves posterolateral to apex of prostate

Incontinence
Injury damages external sphincter. Associated bladder neck injury or previous surgery, e.g. prostatectomy, leaves patient with no competent sphincter mechanism

Fistula
- urethrorectal – due to original injury or attempted endoscopy of an impassable stricture
- urethrocutaneous

Peri-urethral complications
- urine extravasation
- peri-urethral abscess
- necrotizing fasciitis of perineum
- pelvic abscess
- chronic peri-urethral cavity – may cause urethrocutaneous fistula

Radiological diagnosis

If a urethral injury is suspected clinically following blunt trauma, most surgeons would recommend a urethrogram. The authors disagree, for two reasons. First, the danger of introducing infection to the area of rupture when exploration, repair and drainage is not contemplated in the acute phase. Second, the findings on urethrogram will not change the initial management (i.e. suprapubic cystostomy) in most cases.

However, there are indications for a urethrogram in the acute phase:

- penetrating trauma with a suspected urethral injury, where immediate exploration is contemplated, to help plan surgery
- where a patient with a fractured pelvis has not passed urine and has no urethral bleeding. If a catheter is passed but no urine drains a urethrogram must be done to exclude urethral injury.

If a urethrogram is done, it should be done carefully with a sterile technique and using a water-soluble contrast medium. Fluoroscopy should be used to minimize extravasation by halting the examination as soon as the diagnosis is made.

An IVU is useful in patients with a fractured pelvis and suspected posterior urethral injury. It excludes significant renal trauma and gives important information about the bladder. If the bladder is in the pelvis and has an 'inverted teardrop' shape (due to lateral compression by pelvic haematoma) this suggests a partial injury or a complete injury with only minor distraction (Figure 56.22). If the bladder is displaced out of the pelvis and has a relatively normal shape this suggests a complete injury with a major distraction (Figure 56.23). The cystogram phase of the IVU may show a ruptured

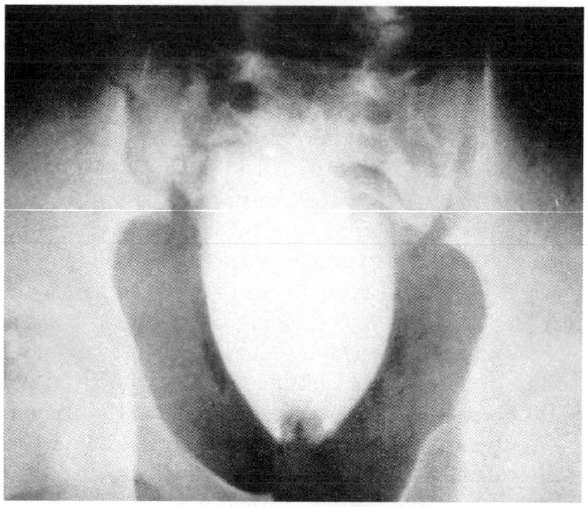

Figure 56.22 Patient with fractured pelvis and suspected posterior urethral injury. Cystogram phase of the IVU: note 'inverted teardrop' shape to bladder situated in the pelvis.

bladder. If a 'push-in' suprapubic cystostomy is done for a suspected posterior urethral injury, and blood stained urine is obtained, a cystogram must be done to exclude a bladder rupture, particularly an extraperitoneal rupture which involves the bladder neck.

Management

Bulbar urethral injury due to blunt trauma

The management is summarized in Figure 56.24. As these patients do not usually have other injuries, a

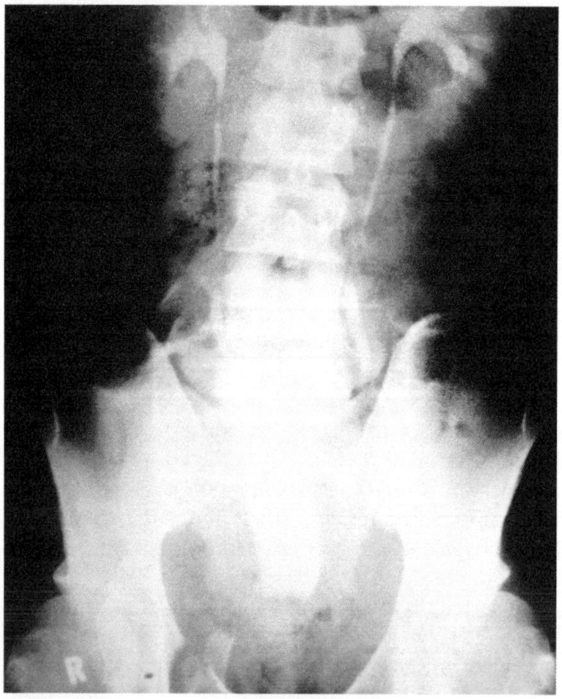

Figure 56.23 Patient with fractured pelvis and suspected posterior urethral injury. IVU: normal upper urinary tracts, bladder 'high riding'.

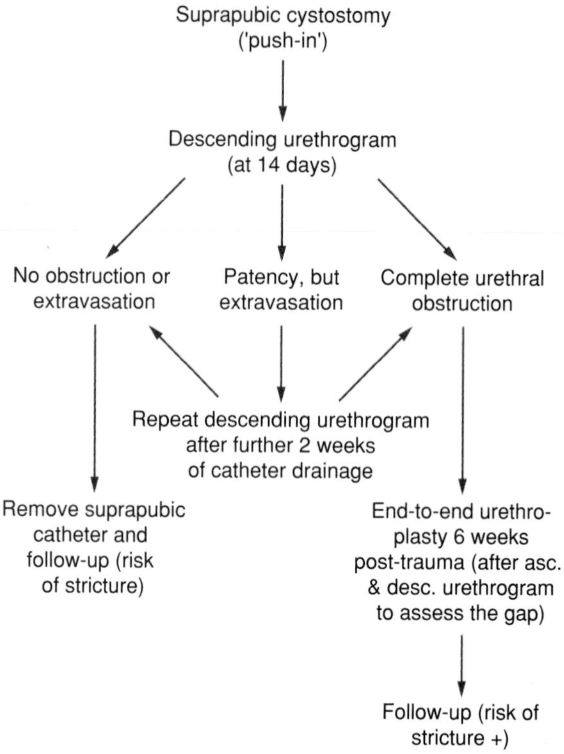

Figure 56.24 Management of bulbar urethral injury (blunt trauma).

'push-in' suprapubic cystostomy works well. Patients with a partial injury need to be followed up because a small percentage develop a urethral stricture later. Such strictures are usually easily managed with optical urethrotomy or urethral dilatation.

Membranous urethral injury due to blunt trauma

The management is summarized in Figure 56.25. The standard initial urological management is suprapubic cystostomy, unless there are indications for urethral realignment ('railroading'), which will be discussed later.

A 'push-in' suprapubic cystostomy may be technically difficult because of the fractured pelvis and pelvic haematoma. The alternative is a formal suprapubic cystostomy which, in any case, would be done if the patient required a laparotomy for intra-abdominal injury or a ruptured bladder. Avoid the pelvic haematoma, as entering it may cause severe haemorrhage. Examine the bladder carefully for lacerations and particularly for a bladder neck injury. The catheter should be brought out through the dome of the bladder and through the wound high and in the midline. This facilitates posterior urethral instrumentation during the subsequent urethroplasty.

Following suprapubic cystostomy, endoscopic re-establishment of urethral continuity can be achieved within the first few weeks after injury by a combined urethral and suprapubic approach. Although this

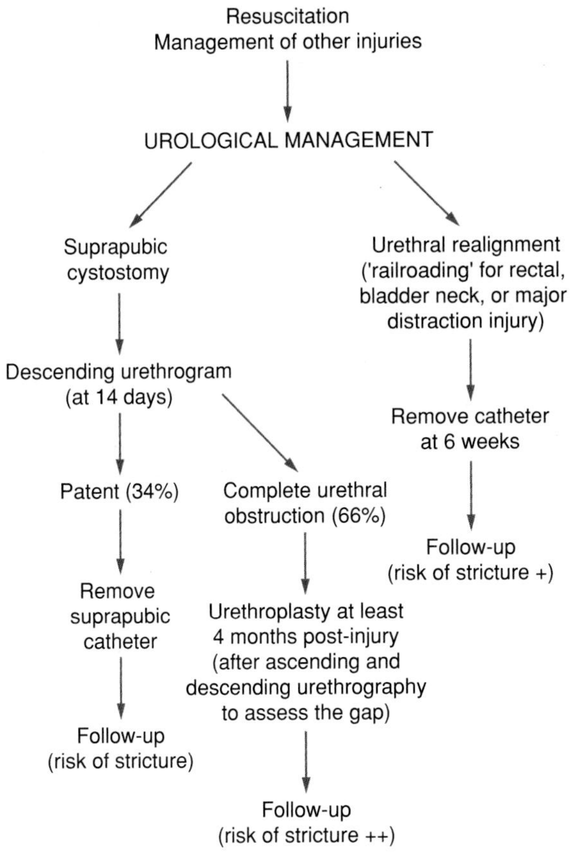

Figure 56.25 Management of membranous urethral injury (blunt trauma).

achieves urethral continuity, stricture formation is inevitable and this treatment is not the 'gold standard' for the treatment of posterior urethral injuries. Recently Professor Mundy of Guy's Hospital has advocated delayed primary repair, i.e. exploration at 7–10 days after injury with evacuation of pelvic haematoma and urethral anastomosis. Numbers are small and the follow-up is short. In most centres the preferred definitive treatment is formal urethroplasty at least 4 months after injury. The principles of such surgery are shown in Table 56.12.

Urethral realignment ('railroading')

There are three indications for urethral realignment as a primary procedure.

Table 56.12 Principles of end-to-end urethroplasty

- Adequate perineal exposure
- Freeing of corpus spongiosum proximal and distal to injury for tension-free anastomosis
- Excision back to normal urethra
- Spatulation of urethral ends
- Anastomosis with interrupted sutures (e.g. 4/0 polyglycolic acid)
- Transanastomotic silastic catheter plus suprapubic cystostomy
- Perineal drain

Rectal injury

When exploration is required to evacuate the contaminated haematoma. Do a colostomy and drain the area adequately.

Bladder neck injury

Repair must be done over a urethral catheter, thus 'railroading' is required.

Major distraction injury

Where the bladder and prostate are displaced superiorly. Treating these cases with initial suprapubic cystostomy only may leave one with a very difficult urethroplasty, especially if the eventual 'gap' is more than 7 cm.

The disadvantages of 'railroading' are:

- Difficult surgery, with bleeding from the pelvic haematoma.
- An increased incidence of erectile dysfunction and incontinence post-operatively, compared to patients treated by suprapubic cystostomy and subsequent urethroplasty.
- A stricture rate of approximately 45%.

A suggested protocol for 'railroading' is:

- Open the bladder formally.
- Pass a catheter up the urethra – the tip will appear in the retropubic space.
- Pass a catheter down through the bladder neck – its tip will also appear in retropubic space.
- Tie the tips of the catheters together and 'railroad' the urethral catheter into the bladder.
- Tie a silk suture to the tip of the urethral catheter and bring the suture out on to the skin with the suprapubic catheter (to facilitate changing the urethral catheter).
- Remove the urethral catheter at 6 weeks. Monitor the patient for development of a urethral stricture, for at least 2 years. Strictures may present many years later.

Penetrating urethral injury

All penetrating urethral injuries should have a pre-operative urethrogram followed by immediate exploration, repair of the urethra, drainage of the area and a suprapubic cystostomy.

An exception to this would be a penetrating injury to the posterior urethra, where immediate surgery would be technically very difficult. After placement of a suprapubic cystostomy, delayed repair is done.

Iatrogenic urethral injuries

Iatrogenic urethral injury found at open pelvic surgery should be repaired over a urethral catheter. Interposition of omentum is useful. Drain the area and insert a suprapubic cystostomy. Monitor the patient for development of a urethral stricture. Urethral injury at endoscopy is managed by placement of a urethral catheter for a week.

Iatrogenic urethral injury due to inadvertent inflation of the balloon of the Foley catheter in the urethra is relatively common. Initially, a gentle urethral catheterization should be attempted. If successful leave the catheter for 1 week. If not, insert a percutaneous suprapubic catheter. The subsequent descending urethrogram will determine future management.

Section 56.5 • Injuries to the male external genitalia

Epidemiology and aetiology

There are many causes of injuries to the male external genitalia (Table 56.13). Penetrating injuries are usually due to gunshot wounds while blunt trauma is due to accident or assault. Genital skin loss is associated with MVAs or industrial accidents. Penile amputation occurs as a result of self-mutilation, assault or accident. Neonatal or ritual circumcision may have very serious complications.

Penetrating trauma to male external genitalia

Penetrating trauma may be due to gunshot wounds (low or high velocity), stab wounds or occasionally 'blow-out' injuries due to power driven machinery.

Low-velocity gunshot wounds or stab wounds are not usually associated with life-threatening injuries. The clinical picture will depend on the site and the trajectory of the wounds. Urethral bleeding would suggest a urethral injury, and a pre-operative urethrogram should be done. Clinical features of scrotal injury, such as a haematocele, would make scrotal exploration mandatory. Penile involvement will require repairing defects in the corpora cavernosa (Figures 56.26 and 56.27) and urethral injuries should be repaired primarily over a urethral catheter, with a covering 'push-in' suprapubic cystostomy. If a testicular rupture (disruption of the tunica albuginea and extrusion of seminiferous tubules) is found at exploration, foreign material must be removed, necrotic tubules debrided and the tunica albuginea closed. Drain the scrotum and give antibiotics.

Table 56.13 Classification of injuries to male external genitalia

Penetrating trauma
- Penis
  - glans
  - corpora cavernosa
  - urethra
- Scrotal contents
  - testis
  - epididymis
  - spermatic cord

Blunt trauma
- Fractured penis
- Testicular trauma

Genital skin loss
- Penis
- Scrotum

Amputation
- Penis
- Testis

Complications of circumcision
- Neonatal
- Ritual

Miscellaneous
- Genital burns
- Bites – human or animal
- Penile strangulation

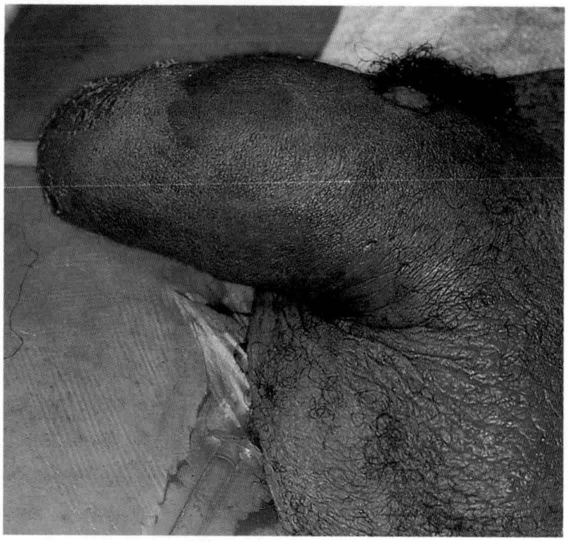

Figure 56.26 Low-velocity wound to the penis – entrance wound on the dorsum.

High-velocity gunshot wounds and 'blow-out' injuries may cause enormous damage. Primary repair of structures is not indicated, but haemostasis and debridement is needed, with suprapubic diversion (urethral injury will need to be treated later). Rectal injury must be carefully excluded. Scrotal exploration may be required, and if the testis is involved an orchidectomy is usually needed.

Fractured penis

Traumatic rupture of the corpus cavernosum (fractured penis) is an uncommon injury. It is usually caused by bending of the erect penis against the perineum or symphysis during coitus. Thirty per cent of cases have an associated penile urethral injury.

Typically, the patient hears a 'cracking' sound, feels immediate pain and the penis undergoes rapid detumescence. On examination there is a haematoma at the site

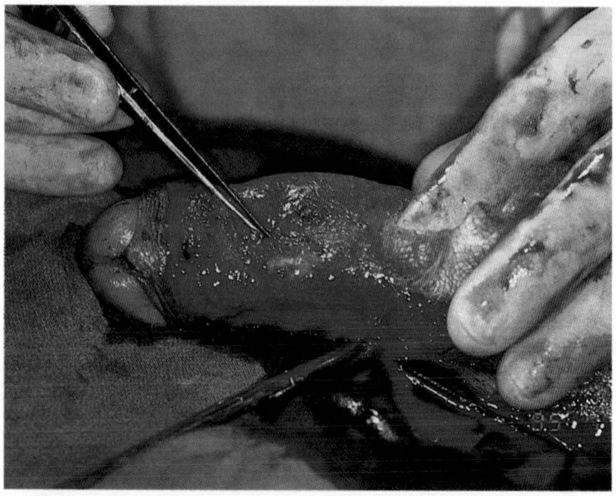

Figure 56.27 Same patient as in Figure 56.26 at operation. The defect in the corpus cavernosum is shown.

of the injury (usually confined to the penis, unless Buck's fascia has been torn). If a urethral injury is suspected, a urethrogram is indicated, prior to exploration. The management is urgent surgical exploration. Make a subcoronal circumferential incision, degloving the skin back to the area of injury. Evacuate the haematoma and repair the defect in the tunica albuginea with interrupted absorbable sutures. If the defect is very large, a patch graft (from tunica vaginalis or using synthetic material) may be needed. If there is a urethral injury, repair it primarily over a urethral catheter and insert a suprapubic cystostomy. Antibiotics are not needed.

Testicular trauma

A very large force to the scrotum is needed to cause testicular injury. When a patient presents following minor trauma, a testicular tumour must be excluded. If the testis is easily palpable, serious injury is unlikely. Scrotal ultrasound is very accurate in detecting testicular rupture. A large haematocele may conceal a testicular rupture.

The indications for exploration following blunt scrotal trauma are: suspected testicular rupture, and a large haematocele. The testis is explored through a scrotal incision, or an inguinal incision if a tumour is suspected. The haematocele is drained and the testis repaired. Antibiotics are not necessary.

A haematoma in the scrotal wall, with a normal testis, is best managed conservatively by bed rest and scrotal elevation.

Genital skin loss

Genital skin loss may be due to traumatic avulsion, but an important cause is extensive skin debridement in patients with necrotizing fasciitis of the perineum.

If skin is avulsed from the shaft of the penis it must be debrided up to the coronal sulcus to prevent subsequent distal lymphoedema. Small areas of skin loss over the penis and scrotum can be managed by primary closure if not infected. Loss of penile shaft skin can be managed by split-skin graft later, but if the patient is potent, a full thickness graft should be considered as split skin on the shaft interferes with erection.

When there has been extensive loss of scrotal skin, the testes can be 'stored' in subcutaneous thigh pouches. Later, the testes should be removed from the thigh and covered with a split skin graft or a perineal flap.

Amputation injuries

Penile amputation is rare: the commonest cause is self-mutilation in psychotic individuals. It has also been performed as an act of revenge by a jealous partner. The part should be cleaned and packed in ice in a sterile saline solution. Bleeding from the stump should be controlled by a tourniquet, and the patient transferred within 8 hours to a hospital with microsurgical facilities.

Testis amputation is an even rarer occurrence than penile loss, and is almost always associated with self-mutilation. Autotransplantation is possible, but is not usually indicated.

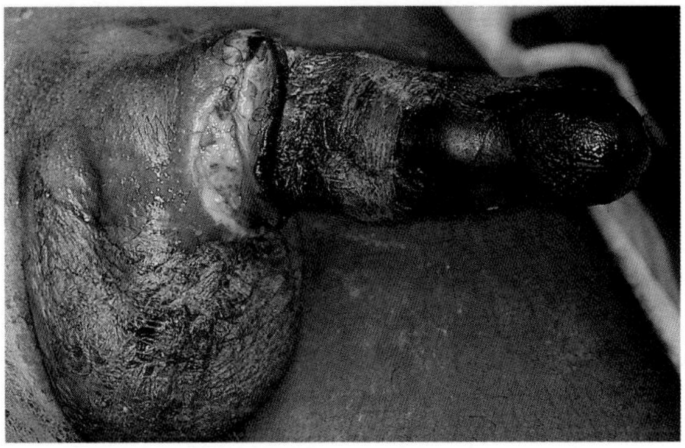

Figure 56.28 Necrotic penis as a complication of ritual circumcision. The patient required penectomy.

Complications of circumcision

Neonatal circumcision may be associated with complications because of the small size of the penis and often inadequate anaesthesia or analgesia. Skin complications (too much excised) and glandular injury (with possible meatal stenosis) are the most common. Necrosis of part or all of the penis has been described.

Ritual circumcision is practised among some African tribes, as part of an adolescent's initiation into manhood. The procedure is performed with a spear, and leaves are applied as a tight dressing. Devastating complications may be seen: septicaemia (with loss of life), extensive skin loss, urethral fistulas and necrosis of part or all of the penis (Figure 56.28). Initially the patient needs antibiotics and topical dressings. Skin grafting and urethroplasty may be needed later.

Genital burns are managed in the same way as burns elsewhere but a urethral catheter may be needed initially to facilitate dressings.

Human and animal bites to the external genitalia have a high incidence of sepsis. Wounds should never be closed primarily and liberal debridement should be done under antibiotic cover.

Incarceration or strangulation of the penis by an encircling object (often used to heighten sexual excitement) is occasionally seen. Innovative ways of removing the offending object have been described. In most cases, no permanent damage to the penis is done, but occasionally debridement and skin grafting are needed.

Further reading

Blunt urologic trauma (1995) *Seminars in Urology* **13**(1). *Trauma and Emergency Medicine* (1995), **12**: 169–96.

Urogenital trauma (1989). *Urol Clin North Am* **16**(2).

Whitfield, H. N., Hendry, W., Kirby, R. S. and Duckett, J. W. eds (1998). Injury to the genitourinary tract. *Textbook of Genitourinary Surgery*, 2nd edn. Oxford: Blackwell Science, 989–1054.

MODULE 57

Tumours of the upper urinary tract

1 • Childhood tumours

2 • Adult tumours

Primary kidney tumours account for 3–4% of adult malignancies. They are important because the mainstay of management in adults is still surgical removal. Advances in our knowledge of genetic events involved in their development have led to a greater understanding of carcinogenesis and will guide the design of future treatments, but as yet have no effect on routine clinical practice.

Upper tract tumours (Table 57.1) can be divided into:

- childhood tumours, of which Wilms' tumour is the most common
- adult tumours, of which renal cell carcinoma is the most common.

This chapter will describe the characteristics of the common tumours, give details of current treatment and briefly discuss controversies and new developments in their management.

Section 57.1 • Childhood tumours

Renal cancers are rare in childhood but represent a success story in co-operative cancer management derived from the participation of multiple centres in co-ordinated randomized controlled trials.

Wilms' tumour

Epidemiology

The annual incidence of Wilms' tumour is approximately 1 case per 100 000. There is little variation in prevalence across the world suggesting that environmental factors are not of major importance. Boys and girls are equally affected. The tumour usually presents before the age of 6 (median 3.5) years. Bilateral or multicentric tumours tend to present at a younger age (median 2 years) and are more likely to be associated with congenital syndromes including **WAGR** syndrome (**W**ilms' tumour, **a**niridia, **g**enitourinary malformations and mental **r**etardation); Beckwith–Wiedemann (overgrowth) syndrome and Denys–Drash syndrome (nephropathy and pseudohermaphroditism). Children with congenital anomalies account for 10% of those with Wilms' tumour.

Table 57.1 Classification of renal tumours

Childhood tumours
Wilms' tumour (nephroblastoma)
Clear cell sarcoma
Rhabdoid sarcoma
Congenital mesoblastic nephroma
Adult tumours
Renal cell carcinoma
Oncocytoma
Angiomyolipoma (hamartoma)
Secondary tumour
Transitional cell carcinoma of renal pelvis

Genetics

Knudson and Strong formulated a 'two-hit' hypothesis of familial cancer development in 1971 following statistical study of retinoblastoma. They hypothesized that the absence of both copies or alleles of a single gene (tumour suppressor) within a particular cell could result in the development of a cancer. In familial cancer syndromes the first allele is lost through a germ line deletion or mutation; the first 'hit'. The second 'hit' occurs in a clone of cells within a particular organ during development, again by mutation or deletion. Clonal expansion can then occur in the absence of the tumour suppressor gene, leading to a clinically apparent cancer. Tumours that form in this way occur at a younger age than sporadic cases, may be bilateral and are associated with familial cancer syndromes. Using genetic and molecular techniques, detailed study of a number of families with a predisposition to Wilms' tumour has led to the identification of two tumour suppressor genes that may be involved in the development of Wilms' tumour.

Pathology

Wilms' tumour is derived from embryonic metanephric blastema, so a wide spectrum of histological patterns is seen. The gross appearance is of a large multi-lobulated mass that compresses surrounding tissue into a pseudocapsule. The cut surface is usually homogeneous but can be altered by haemorrhage, necrosis or cyst formation. Histologically the tumour

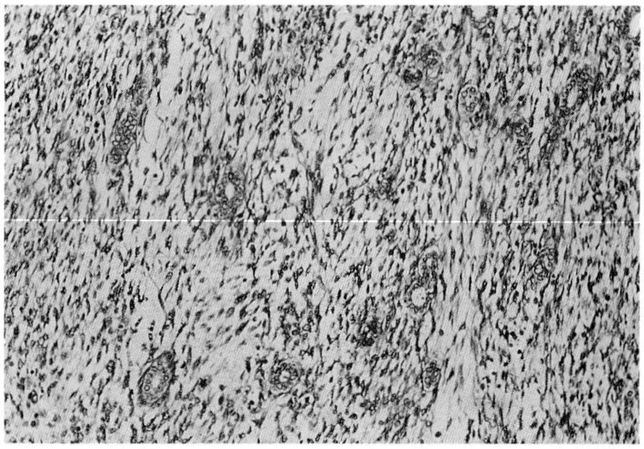

Figure 57.1 Photomicrograph showing the triad of histological features (haemoxylin and eosin stain) typical of Wilms' tumour. Sheets of immature blastemal cells are set in a fibromuscular stroma interspersed with primitive renal tubules.

consists of varying proportions of three elements: persistent blastema, dysplastic tubules and stroma (Figure 57.1). Unfavourable histology, including anaplastic nuclear appearance such as large size, hyperchromatism and abnormal mitoses, is found in 13% of patients and implies a worse prognosis (see Table 57.2).

Normal renal tissue in patients with Wilms' tumour often has groups of persistent embryonal cells, termed nephrogenic rests or nephroblastomatosis. These are thought to represent pre-malignant lesions and indicate more careful follow-up to detect further tumour development in remaining renal tissue.

Clinical presentation

Tumours are often large and asymptomatic. Most children (75%) present with an abdominal mass (Figure 57.2) noted by a parent or relative. Others present with abdominal pain, loss of appetite, failure to thrive or a paraneoplastic syndrome such as hypercalcaemia or erythrocytosis. Metastatic disease is present at diagnosis in 15% and is almost always confined to the lung (92%) and/or liver (18%).

Investigation

Ultrasound can locate the mass, differentiate between solid and cystic components and assess lymph node and liver masses. Further clinical staging is by computed tomography (CT) scanning, with intravenous contrast, of the abdomen and chest under sedation or anaesthesia. Most children are entered into co-operative trials of treatment regimens so accurate initial imaging is essential for later measurement of response. Clinical, radiological, operative and pathological findings are combined to establish the stage of the disease (Table 57.2).

Table 57.2 Clinicopathological staging for Wilms' tumour

Stage definition		*Four year survival*
Stage I	Confined to the kidney and completely excised	97%
Stage II	Tumour outside kidney but completely excised	92%
Stage III	Incomplete excision without haematogenous metastases	84%
Stage IV	Distant (haematogenous) metastases	83%
Stage V	Bilateral disease	Variable
Stage I–III	With unfavourable histology	68%
Stage IV	With unfavourable histology	55%

Treatment

Surgical excision is essential for cure, but the great improvement in survival has been due to the development of effective adjuvant chemotherapeutic regimens.

Surgery

In North America laparotomy and radical nephrectomy is the initial treatment for all cases except when the primary tumour is unresectable or bilateral. European centres are studying the effectiveness of neoadjuvant chemotherapy given prior to nephrectomy for all children. The operation is performed through a generous transverse, transperitoneal incision. It is important to detect and fully excise extension of tumour into the renal artery or vein and to perform lymph node sampling to detect lymph node involvement that is present in 15–20% of cases. Radical node dissection does not improve outcome. In North America and Europe, patients with bilateral disease or unresectable lesions receive neoadjuvant chemotherapy, allowing subsequent surgery using nephron-sparing techniques if required.

Chemotherapy

When bowel function has returned, children with stage I and II disease receive 18 or 24 week cyclical chemotherapy using a combination of actinomycin and vincristine. Stage III, IV and V disease and the presence of unfavourable histology need the addition of doxyrubicin and increased duration and intensity of treatment. Cyclophosphamide, ifosfamide, etoposide and cisplatin are under trial for high-risk and relapsed patients.

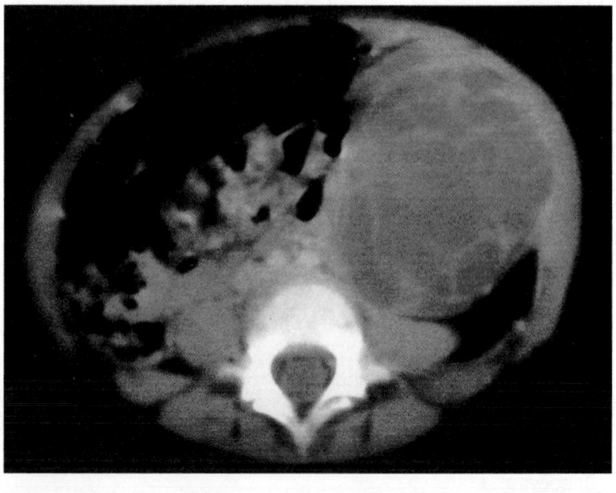

Figure 57.2 CT of abdomen of a 4-year-old girl presenting with a right loin mass. A large, partly solid, partly cystic mass with patchy enhancement is seen arising from the left kidney. This was a Wilms' tumour.

Radiotherapy

When bowel function has returned children with stage III disease or greater, and those with unfavourable histology, receive radiotherapy to the flank, abdomen and liver or lung as appropriate.

Prognosis

Prognosis is related to stage and the presence of anaplastic elements (Table 57.2).

With the latest combined treatment protocols the overall relapse rate is less than 25%. Relapse usually occurs within 2 years of nephrectomy. Survival in children with recurrent disease can approach 40% with second line chemotherapy and targeted radiation treatment.

Specific long-term adverse effects of treatment include bone necrosis, liver damage, cardiomyopathy, second tumour development and female infertility. Improved, reduced dose chemotherapy and radiation therapy may lessen these problems in the future.

Future prospects

Further study of genetic changes in Wilms' tumour will inform our knowledge of tumour development, allow design of gene therapeutic approaches and improve genetic counselling. The investigation of substances secreted by these tumours, particularly hyaluronic acid, may lead to a useful tumour marker. Current therapeutic trials are designed to minimize dosage and duration of treatment whilst maintaining survival rates. This includes the use of neoadjuvant chemotherapy and nephrectomy alone for low-risk stage I disease. The use of newer chemotherapeutic agents may improve survival in poor prognosis groups.

Other childhood tumours

Clear cell sarcoma

Clear cell sarcoma has a similar presentation to Wilms' tumour but a higher rate of metastasis to bone and brain. Histology shows abundant fibrovascular stroma and an alveolar growth pattern distinct from Wilms' tumour. The previous poor prognosis associated with this tumour has been improved with combined surgery, chemotherapy and radiotherapy.

Rhabdoid sarcoma

Rhabdoid sarcoma is again similar to Wilms' tumour from a clinical viewpoint. Histology however shows a characteristic pattern of large cells with eosinophilic cytoplasm. It presents in the first 2 years of life and has a high relapse rate and mortality despite combined aggressive treatment.

Congenital mesoblastic nephroma

Congenital mesoblastic nephroma generally presents under 3 months of age. The pathological appearance is of a rubbery dense white tumour consisting mainly of spindle cells. Complete cure is usual following radical surgery.

Section 57.2 • Adult tumours

This section will review the characteristics and treatment of renal cell carcinoma together with the presentation and treatment of transitional cell carcinoma of the renal pelvis and ureter.

Despite many therapeutic trials, effective adjuvant treatment is still lacking and since surgery can cure only localized disease, overall survival rates have changed little over the past 40 years.

Renal cell carcinoma

Epidemiology

- Renal cell carcinoma (RCC) accounts for 2–3% of adult cancers and has a male:female ratio of 2:1. Most tumours present between the ages of 60 and 75 years.

Prevalence is highest amongst Scandinavians and lowest in Chinese, Japanese and Indians living in their home countries. Intermediate levels are found in the UK with an annual incidence of 4 per 100 000. The incidence has risen over the past 20 years with an improvement in survival suggesting a trend towards earlier diagnosis.

The risk of developing RCC is doubled by smoking and is increased in the obese. Other risk factors include exposure to petroleum products, heavy metals and asbestos and the presence of acquired cystic renal disease in patients on dialysis. A family history of RCC in a first degree relative gives a four-fold risk of tumour.

A number of familial cancer syndromes include RCC, notable for their multifocal nature and young age at diagnosis. The commonest such syndrome is Von Hippel–Lindau (VHL) disease which has an autosomal dominant inheritance and is characterized by varying combinations of retinal angiomas, central nervous system haemangioblastomas, cysts in solid organs, multiple renal tumours and phaeochromocytomas. The lifetime risk of developing RCC in VHL disease is 50–70%.

Genetics

Current theories concerning the aetiology of cancer suggest a sequence of genetic events that result in genetic instability and loss of growth control within a single cell leading to uncontrolled clonal expansion. These genetic changes arise through a combination of inheritance, spontaneous mutation, action of chemical or physical carcinogens and viral infection. The overexpression of dominant oncogenes, the deletion/mutation of recessive tumour suppressor genes and loss of function of DNA repair genes are thought to be key events.

In the case of the common clear cell variant of RCC the key event is thought to be mutation or loss of both alleles of the VHL gene and hence its tumour suppressor function. Such changes are found in 95% of clear cell RCCs. The cause of the mutation is unknown. The

Table 57.3 Pathological classification of renal cell carcinoma

Histological type	*Genetic defect*	*Percentage of total*
Conventional (clear cell) renal carcinoma	3p25 (VHL)	75–85%
Papillary (chromophilic) renal cell carcinoma	Trisomy 7, 17; loss of Y	14%
Chromophobe renal cell carcinoma	Chromsome loss (hypodiploid)	5%
Collecting duct carcinoma	Monosomy 1,6,14,15,22	1%
Renal cell carcinoma unclassified	Undetermined	3%

VHL gene encodes for a protein that inhibits products of a variety of target genes, including those responsible for the production of erythropoietin and vascular endothelial growth factor. Loss of the VHL gene results in the uncontrolled and inappropriate expression of these polypeptides. The less common variants of RCC have different genetic defects with normal VHL function (Table 57.3). The relevance of other mechanisms thought to be important in cancer development (including changes in the expression of proteins such as p53 that control the cell cycle, or over-expression of oncogenes) is unclear.

A common feature of RCC is metastasis. The process of metastasis and its possible relation to over- or under-expression of polypeptides that would normally maintain tissue integrity in RCC have been investigated. It is hoped that therapeutic inhibition of these processes may prevent the development of metastases.

Pathology

Renal cell carcinomas are typically rounded masses that can arise anywhere within the kidney. They vary in size from 1 cm in diameter to huge masses occupying large areas of the abdominal cavity. Initially the tumour is confined within the renal capsule but local extension will involve the perinephric fat and pelvicalyceal system, although invasion of neighbouring organs is unusual. The cut surface is nodular, yellow and shows areas of necrosis and cyst formation (see Figure 57.3c). Extension into the renal vein may represent direct invasion (see Figure 57.3d) or tumour thrombus.

The tumour probably originates from proximal tubular cells. The cells are classically lipid-laden. The lipid material dissolves in processing, leaving the classical 'clear cell' appearance (Figure 57.4). Previously, tumours were classified according to cell type or growth pattern: this was unrelated to clinical findings and has been abandoned. Current classification is based on recently discovered genetic changes and is now generally accepted (Table 57.3).

Staging of RCC combines clinical, imaging, operative and pathological findings and provides useful prognostic information (Table 57.4). The diameter indicating division between T1 and T2 remains controversial with opinions varying between 3 and 10 cm. Nuclear grading systems are commonly used but show poor reproducibility and do not correlate with outcome.

Clinical presentation

The commonest symptoms are caused by locally advanced disease and include haematuria (50%), loin pain (30%) and a palpable mass (30%). Fewer than 10% of patients present with all three. An increasing number (up to 40%) of locally confined tumours are discovered incidentally by imaging for unrelated symptoms.

Non-specific systemic symptoms such as weight loss, nausea, night sweats and bowel disturbance, or those related to paraneoplastic syndromes such as fever, neurological symptoms or muscle pains are present in approximately 20% of cases. Some cases present as pathological fracture, hypercalcaemia due to metastases or secretion of a parathormone-like substance, or with erythrocytosis from uncontrolled erythropoietin production. Rarely the gonadal vein may be obstructed, particularly on the left, causing a varicocele. Non-specific changes in liver enzymes are also seen: they resolve on removing the primary tumour and are not a sign of metastatic disease (Stauffer's syndrome).

- Despite earlier diagnosis up to 30% of patients will have metastases at presentation.
- Metastases are mostly in lung (50–60%), bone (30–40%) (Figure 57.5), liver (30–40%) or brain (5%). Unusual sites include thyroid and skin.

Investigation

The purpose of investigation is to stage the tumour as accurately as possible in order to determine the likely prognosis, decide therapeutic options and plan the surgical approach. This is a achieved using a combination of imaging modalities, as below.

Simple blood tests including full blood count, liver function, calcium and erythrocyte sedimentation rate (ESR) or plasma viscocity may detect paraneoplastic manifestations.

Imaging

A plain chest X-ray is mandatory to detect gross pulmonary metastatic disease but further investigation with chest CT and radionuclide bone scan is only performed if indicated by clinical suspicion. Intravenous urography is only useful to exclude upper tract transitional cell carcinoma and angiography is only used if nephron-sparing surgery is planned

Ultrasound

This gives 80% accuracy in local and regional staging and can also distinguish simple cysts from complex cystic RCC. No functional information is obtained. The renal vein and interior vena cava (IVC) can be examined to detect invasion and tumour thrombus (Figure 57.6).

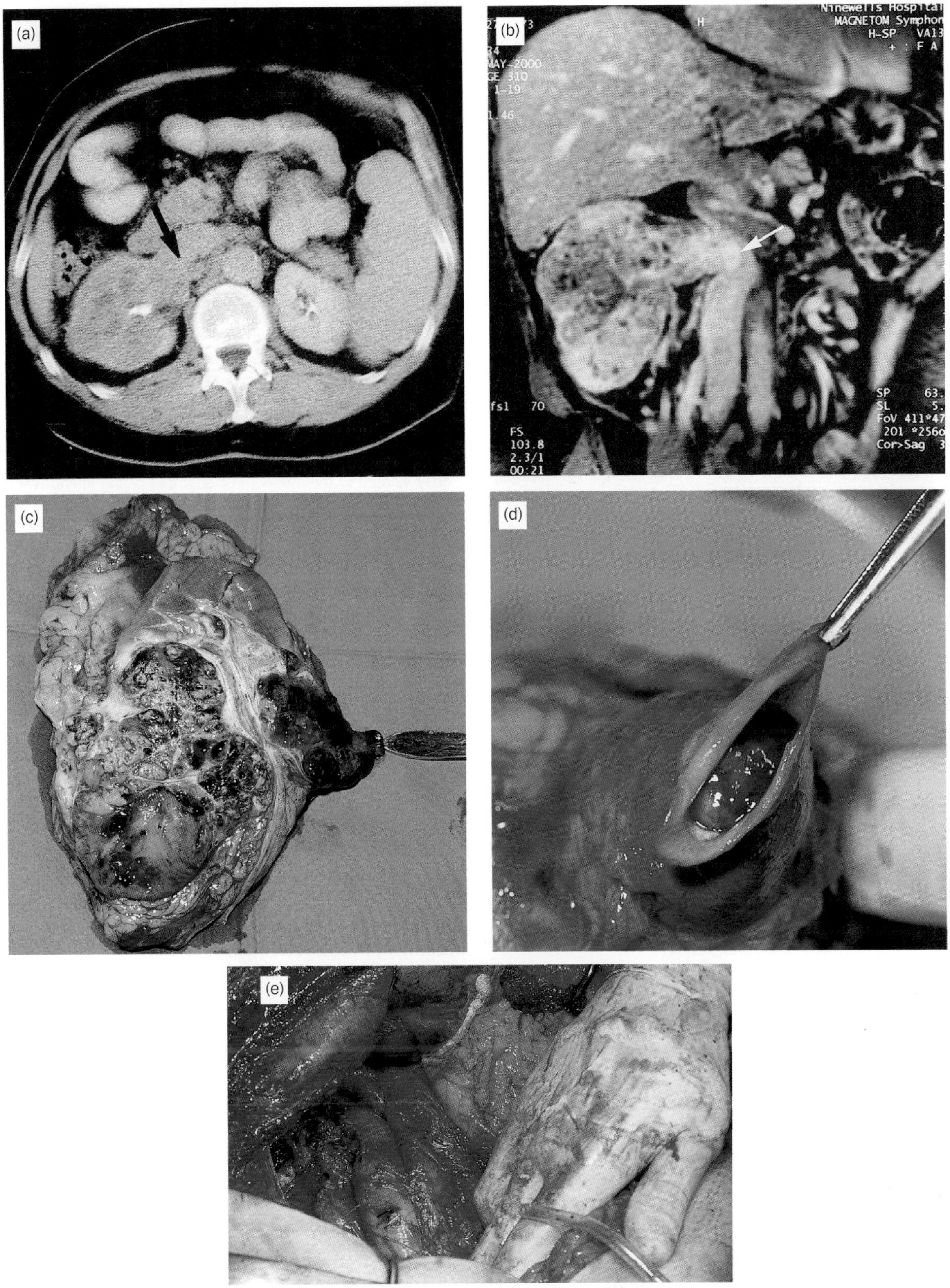

Figure 57.3 (a) CT scan showing large renal cell carcinoma involving most of right kidney, spreading into renal vein and vena cava (arrow). The extent of caval involvement is difficult to assess. Contrast excretion by the left kidney is sufficient indication of function. The patient presented with frank haematuria and a painful right varicocele. (b) Reconstructed MRI image showing that tumour extends into vena cava at level of right renal vein (arrow) but some lumen remains patent and intracaval tumour does not extend into intrahepatic cava. (c) Operative specimen showing classical nodular yellow cut surface of tumour with areas of necrosis and cyst formation. (d) Operative specimen showing direct invasion into renal vein with free edge projecting into vena cava. (e) Operative photograph showing closure of cava after resection of kidney, renal vein and cuff of cava to obtain tumour clearance.

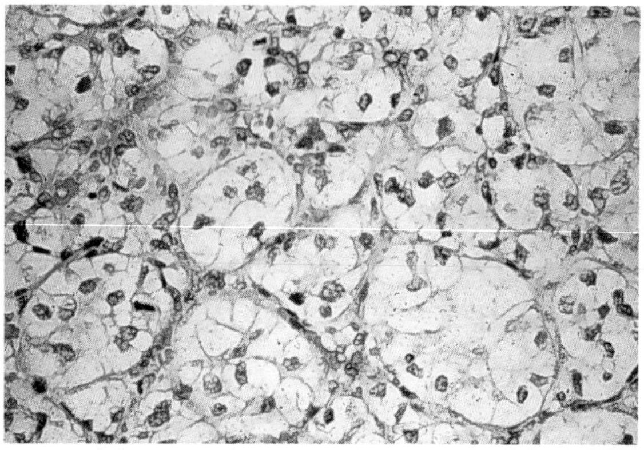

Figure 57.4 The histological features of a conventional (clear cell) renal cell carcinoma. Note the abundant non-staining (clear) cystoplasm. (Courtesy of Dr Marie O'Donnell, Freeman Hospital, Newcastle upon Tyne, England.)

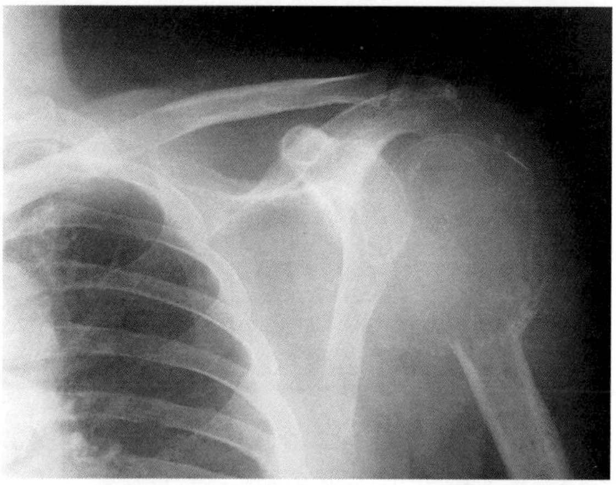

Figure 57.5 Destruction of humeral head by metastatic RCC, presenting 19 years after nephrectomy.

CT scanning

This allows local and lymph node staging with 94% accuracy. Lymph nodes greater that 2 cm are considered malignant: smaller ones may be reactive and should not preclude surgery. Due to flow artefacts CT is less sensitive than ultrasound for detecting venous invasion.

For most patients assessment of function of the contralateral kidney by CT following intravenous

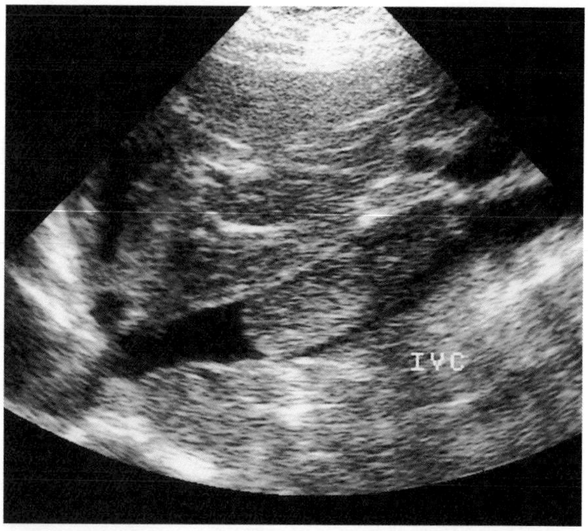

Figure 57.6 Ultrasound image of a tumour thrombus arising from a locally advanced renal cell carcinoma of right kidney located in the intrahepatic segment of the inferior vena cava.

contrast is sufficient (Figure 57.4a). (Radionuclide renography best determines function of the contralateral kidney but is unnecessary for patients with normal creatinine levels.) The chest can be scanned if a thorough search for metastases is required. Small renal masses (<1.5 cm) can be examined in more detail for diagnosis, and for follow-up if conservative management is chosen. This is best done with helical CT or standard CT using thin (5 mm) sections. Synchronous ipsilateral or contralateral tumours are found in up to 5%.

Magnetic resonance imaging

MRI gives staging accuracy similar to that of CT, with the added advantage of avoiding radiation and iodine-containing contrast agents. MRI gives more accurate imaging of IVC involvement (Figures 57.4a and 57.4b) and can survey the axial skeleton for metastases.

Treatment

Surgical removal of the tumour by radical (or occasionally partial) nephrectomy remains the only curative option and is effective for localized disease (T1–3, N0,

Table 57.4 Clinicopathological staging and prognosis of renal cell carcinoma

TNM	*Robson (1969)*	*% Survival at 5 years*
T1 Tumour ≤ 7 cm confined to kidney	1	80–95%
T2 Tumour > 7 cm confined to kidney	1	60–80%
T3a Tumour invades adrenal or perinephric fat	2	47–80%
T3b Tumour extends into renal vein or IVC below diaphragm	3A	38–70%
T3c Tumour in IVC above diaphragm	3A	38–70%
T4 Tumour invades beyond Gerota's fascia	4A	3%
N1 Metastasis in single lymph node	3B	10–40%
N2 Metastases in more than one lymph node	3B	10–40%
T3b/c and N1/2	3C	10–30%
M1 Distant metastasis	4B	3%

M0). An aggressive surgical approach is justified in the fit patient with locally advanced but non-metastatic disease (T3/4). As yet no effective systemic treatment is available for the 30% of patients who present with metastatic disease and the 30% who develop metastases after nephrectomy.

Surgery for localized disease

Radical nephrectomy

Radical nephrectomy through an anterior transperitoneal approach with early ligation of the renal artery and vein remains the standard treatment of renal cancer localized to the kidney (T1–3, N0, M0). The operation involves the excision of the kidney, ipsilateral adrenal gland and perinephric fat within Gerota's fascia. Radical para-aortic lymph node dissection has been abandoned by most surgeons as any small improvement in outcome is offset by greater operative morbidity. Limited sampling of lymphatic tissue from the midline of the IVC and from the midline of the aorta, for tumours of the right and left kidney respectively, is done instead. The small incidence of adrenal metastases (<2%) suggests the ipsilateral adrenal gland can be preserved unless the tumour margin is compromised.

Removal of tumour thrombus contained in the renal vein or sub-hepatic IVC must be done in the absence of metastases (Figure 57.3). When feasible it is worthwhile even if cure is unlikely, to prevent massive tumour embolus or distressing caval obstuction. It needs control of the IVC above and below the renal veins, and of the contralateral renal vein.

The presence of tumour thrombus in the proximal IVC and right atrium does not worsen prognosis for T3 tumours provided there is no nodal or distant metastatic disease. Thrombus above the porta hepatis requires more extensive mobilization of the liver, or cardiac bypass with hypothermia and mechanical perfusion.

Peri-operative adjuvant systemic treatment is not helpful.

Nephron-sparing surgery

A range of surgical techniques is available for localized removal of renal tumours. These include partial nephrectomy suitable for polar tumours, wedge excision and enucleation. Accepted indications for such surgery include bilateral tumours and tumour in a solitary kidney. Controversial situations are: tumours presenting as part of a familial cancer syndrome such as VHL (when further tumours are likely), and small (<5 cm) asymptomatic RCCs. The main concern following such surgery is the local recurrence rate of 2–7%, higher than that seen with radical nephrectomy for T1 disease. Such surgery should be confined to specialist centres within a randomized study.

Management by surveillance of asymptomatic, incidentally found renal masses has been advocated for tumours < 1.5 cm. This remains controversial. In the elderly, tumours grow slowly and small ones may be best managed by surveillance, especially when there is comorbidity.

Surgery for metastatic disease

Lymph nodes

- Survival of patients with macroscopic lymph node involvement is not improved by lymphadenectomy.

A small subgroup of patients with microscopic nodal disease without distant metastases might benefit from radical lymph node dissection, but few groups practise this extended surgery.

Distant metastases

- The often-quoted spontaneous regression of metastases following nephrectomy occurs in less than 1%. In the absence of symptoms nephrectomy is not routinely advised for patients with established N1/2 or M1 disease. However, nephrectomy may be needed to control bleeding or pain, and removal of a large haemorrhagic and partly necrotic mass produces a non-specific temporary improvement in well-being.

Resection of a solitary synchronous or metachronous metastasis (usually pulmonary) may result in unexpected long survival, but the disease may have a prolonged natural history resulting in lead-time bias.

Systemic treatment for metastatic disease

Radiotherapy

- Radiotherapy has no effect on the primary tumour and is virtually never indicated for soft tissue metastases.

Targeted radiotherapy relieves pain from skeletal metastases (Figure 57.5) in 70% of cases and aids stabilization of pathological fractures.

Chemotherapy

- Complete or partial responses occur in less than 10%, whatever the regimen.

Clinical trials have shown no treatment advantage of progestogens over other non-specific steroids.

Immunotherapy

Interferon-α (IFNα) in high dose systemic treatment was too toxic but low dose treatment given by sub-cutaneous injection showed a response rate of 12% and a slight increase in survival from 6 to 8 months.

Interleukin-2 (IL-2), usually combined with an infusion of lymphokine-activated killer (LAK) cells, has a response rate of 19% which is more durable than that of IFNα. The latest trials involve a combination of IL-2, IFNα and 5-fluorouracil. One group obtained a 48% response rate using this regimen but this has yet to be reproduced by others.

- Immunotherapy remains the best hope of developing systemic treatment that will improve survival for those with metastatic disease. Patients with good performance status, long disease-free interval and metastases confined to the lung will benefit most.

Outcome

Prognosis is good following nephrectomy in those with T1 and T2 disease (Table 57.4). Intermediate survival rates are seen in those with advanced localized disease, due to later relapse with distant metastases. Prolonged survival with established metastatic disease is rare.

- Follow-up after nephrectomy is controversial: advice ranges from none at all to regular chest X-ray and CT scan. The surgeon has to steer a course between giving the impression that no interest is being taken in the patient's future, and frequent investigations (with attendant anxiety) to detect early but probably untreatable recurrence.

A pragmatic approach, in the present context of lack of benefit of systemic therapy for metastatic disease, would be to individualize the follow-up protocol according to tumour stage, patient age and personal preference.

Future developments

Case-finding of asymptomatic tumours by imaging for unrelated complaints will continue but formal screening programmes are not practical due to the low prevalence of RCC. It is likely that surveillance or nephron-sparing surgery will be more widely used for small localized tumours. Novel immunotherapeutic approaches include the use of adoptive immunity generated by the harvesting, activation *in vitro* and re-infusion of immune-competent cells. Tumour vaccination (using cancer cells from the tumour that are transfected with cytokine genes, attenuated by radiation and re-infused with an adjuvant such as bacille-Calmette-Guérin (BCG)) is under assessment.

Other renal parenchymal tumours

Oncocytoma

Oncocytoma is a benign tumour which can only be differentiated from RCC on histological examination. It is found in 3% of radical nephrectomy specimens (Figure 56.5a, b).

Angiomyolipomas

Angiomyolipomas are hamartomas that give a diagnostic appearance on ultrasound and CT. They are benign developmental abnormalities that can cause local symptoms by haemorrhage or expansion. Most cases are sporadic but multiple lesions are found in tuberose sclerosis. Management is based on size at presentation. Lesions less than 4 cm can be ignored; larger ones have a 50% chance of developing complications due to growth or bleeding and should be monitored.

Secondary tumours

Secondary tumours are often found at post-mortem examination in people dying from metastatic non-renal tumour. Lymphoma is the commonest secondary kidney tumour to present in life.

Transitional cell carcinoma of the renal pelvis and ureter

Transitional cell carcinoma (TCC) of the upper urinary tract shares the aetiological, genetic and pathological features described for TCC of the bladder (see Module 58). The major differences are a worse prognosis for comparable stage and a poor response to systemic chemotherapy and external beam radiotherapy. Surgery remains the main curative option.

Epidemiology

- Only 5% of TCC occurs in the upper urinary tract.

Patients with bladder cancer have a 5% risk of developing a metachronous upper tract tumour. This is more common in those with invasive, multiple or high-grade superficial tumours (including carcinoma *in situ*). Conversely patients with an upper tract TCC have up to a 50% chance of developing a bladder tumour on follow-up and a 5% chance of developing TCC in the contralateral upper tract, both more common with high tumour grade. Aetiological factors in common with TCC of the bladder include male sex, tobacco smoke and exposure to industrial carcinogens. Balkan nephropathy and abuse of phenacetin are particularly associated with the development of upper tract TCC.

Pathology

The majority of tumours are typical papillary or solid TCCs (see Module 58) that invade through the lamina propria into the renal substance or wall of the ureter. Local lymph node metastasis and distant spread to lungs, liver and bone will occur. The staging and grading systems are in common with bladder TCC (see Module 58).

Clinical presentation

Ninety per cent will be detected by investigation of gross or microscopic haematuria. Others will be found during routine upper tract monitoring of patients with bladder cancer (Figure 58.8), and a few by urography or ultrasound performed for loin pain or other reasons.

Investigation

Ultrasound usually gives non-specific indication of a tumour because of dilatation of the affected upper tract. Upper tract TCC can reliably be imaged by contrast examination achieved by intravenous urography (IVU) or retrograde pyelography. CT is useful to differentiate a radiolucent stone from a renal cell carcinoma (Figure 57.7) and more accurately to stage locally advanced disease. A chest film is usually obtained to exclude gross metastatic disease.

Cytological examination of urine will detect malignant cells in 20–50% of cases of low-grade carcinoma, 50–80% of cases of high-grade carcinoma and >90% of those with carcinoma *in situ*. It is possible to localize the tumour site by obtaining separate urine samples or washings from the bladder and from each renal pelvis.

Ureteroscopy (Module 55 and Figure 55.10) allows inspection and biopsy of upper tract TCC and is essential if conservative surgery is contemplated (see below).

Treatment

Radical surgery

The standard treatment for TCC of the upper tract is nephroureterectomy: resecting the kidney, ureter and a cuff of bladder through an extended anterolateral incision, or through separate loin (or subcostal extraperitoneal) and suprapubic incisions.

Endoscopic resection of the intramural ureter followed by nephrectomy and finger dissection (plucking) of the lower ureter through a single incision gives equivalent results for tumours in the upper ureter and renal pelvis.

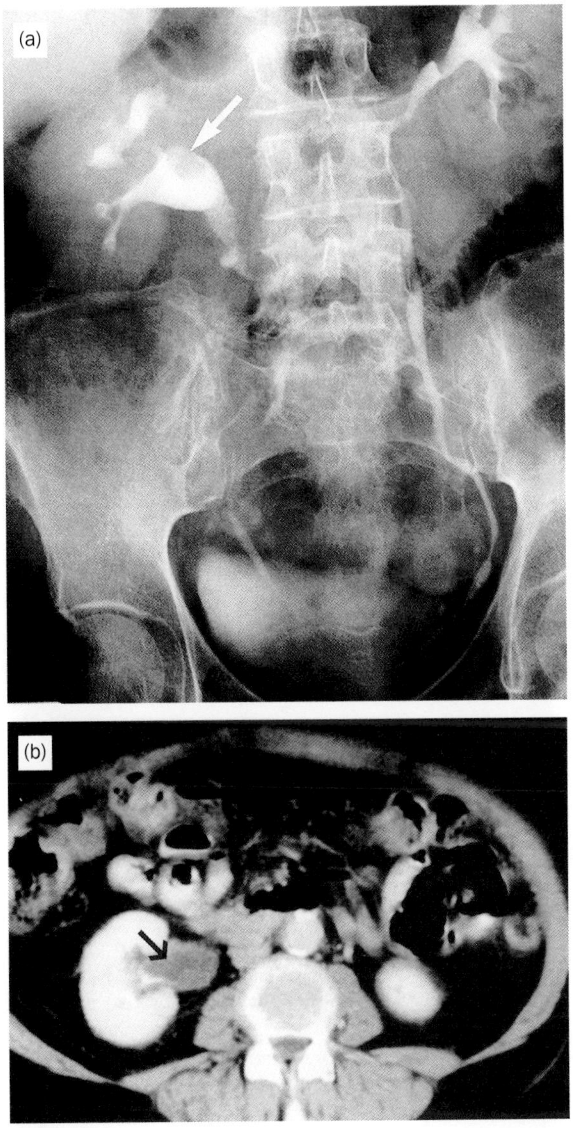

Figure 57.7 (a) Intravenous urogram shows a radiolucent filling defect (arrow) in the right renal pelvis. (b) CT shows the lesion to be a soft tissue mass, not a stone. It proved to be a TCC.

Conservative surgery

Low-grade superficial tumours (G1/2 Ta) of the lower ureter can be excised by segmental ureterectomy and reimplantation into the bladder using a psoas hitch and/or Boari flap (Figure 56.18), which are described in textbooks of operative urology. Superficial tumours of any part of the ureter and of the renal pelvis can be treated by retrograde endoscopic ablation using electrocautery or laser energy. Percutaneous resection has also been tried, although tumour seeding along the access track remains a worrying potential complication. These techniques are unproven and require time-consuming subsequent ureteroscopic surveillance. They are best limited at present to specific indications where renal preservation is important such as in the solitary kidney and in patients with Balkan nephropathy.

- Radical and conservative surgical techniques give equivalent results for low-grade and stage tumours, radical surgery is superior for medium risk tumours and the results for both forms of surgery are disappointing for high-grade and locally advanced tumours.

Chemotherapy

Chemotherapy by retrograde instillation of chemotherapeutic substances such as epirubicin or mitomycin has been tried together with the use of instillation of BCG as immunotherapy. Systemic chemotherapy using cisplatin-based regimens can be offered for locally advanced or metastatic disease on the basis of the 20–30% response rates seen in bladder TCC.

Radiotherapy

Radiotherapy by external beam may improve local control for invasive tumours but does not improve survival.

Outcome

In common with TCC of the bladder, stage and grade are prime prognostic factors. Low grade and stage (G1/2 Ta/1) tumours show 80–100% survival at 5 years. This is reduced to 30–40% for locally confined muscle invasive tumours (G1/2 T2) and falls to 0–10% in high-grade or deeply invasive tumours (G3 T1/2/3). Most cases progress with lymph node and distant metastatic disease. Follow-up should consist of regular surveillance cystoscopy as for bladder TCC and IVU every 2 years to image the contralateral upper tract.

Future developments

These currently seem limited to an increased use of endoscopic or conservative open surgery with endoscopic follow-up, and local or systemic chemotherapy.

Further reading

Wilms' tumour

Wiener, J. S., Coppes, M. J. and Ritchey, M. L. (1998). Current concepts in the biology and management of Wilms' tumour. *J Urol* **159**: 1316–25.

Renal cell carcinoma

Bower, M., Roylance, R. and Waxman, J. (1998). Immunotherapy for renal cell cancer. *Q J Med* **91**: 597–602.

Clifford, S. C. and Maher, E. R. (1999) The molecular genetics of renal cell carcinoma. In: Mundy, A. R., Fitzpatrick, J. M., Neal, D. E. and George, N. J. R., eds (1999). *The Scientific Basis of Urology*. Oxford: Isis Medical Media: 319–41.

Fleming, S. (1997). Genetics of renal tumours. *Cancer Metastasis Rev* **16**: 127–40.

Motzer, R. J., Bander, N. H. and Nanus, D. M. (1996). Renal cell carcinoma. *N Engl J Med* **335**: 865875.

Transitional cell carcinoma of the upper urinary tract

Tawfiek, E. R. and Bagley, D. H. (1997). Upper tract transitional cell carcinoma. *Urology* **50**: 321–329.

MODULE 58

Carcinoma of the bladder

Bladder cancer is one of the commonest and most important diseases treated by urologists. Most bladder tumours are transitional cell carcinomas: squamous cell and adenocarcinoma are less common. Bladder tumours can display the complete spectrum of behaviour from benign to very aggressive disease. In practice, the disease exists mostly in two forms: superficial, well to moderately differentiated tumours; and poorly differentiated, invasive tumours with metastatic potential.

In spite of abundant clinical experience there is much debate about how best to treat many of the stages and grades of this common malignancy.

Both the superficial and poorly differentiated types of bladder cancer are areas of current clinical and research interest. There is increasing interest in chemotherapy or immunotherapy to reduce the recurrence rate of superficial disease, and uncertainty as to how we should best manage invasive disease. Should this initially be by radiotherapy, with or without adjuvant chemotherapy or should one proceed directly to radical cystectomy with orthotopic bladder substitution or the more traditional ileal conduit?

Section 58.1 • Epidemiology

Bladder carcinoma presents in 18 people per 100 000 per year in the UK. It is three times more common in men than in women and is the fourth most common cancer in men after lung, prostate and colorectal cancers. The incidence of the disease is increasing, at least in the USA. It causes 2.6% of all cancer deaths in men and 1.4% in women.

Although bladder cancer can occur at any age (even in children) it is very much a disease of the elderly. The median age at diagnosis is 70 years.

Section 58.2 • Aetiology

Bladder carcinoma is much more common in the UK and the USA than in Japan and Finland, stongly suggesting that environmental or genetic factors are involved.

- The most significant associated factor is cigarette smoking. Bladder cancer is four times more common in smokers than in non-smokers. There is a direct relationship between the prevalence of the disease and the number of cigarettes smoked, the duration of smoking and whether or not smoke is inhaled.

Aromatic amines are present in tobacco smoke and are known to cause tumours in both animals and humans. Exposure to aromatic amines has occurred in some occupations, including dye manufacture and the rubber industry, both associated with bladder carcinoma. The disease has also been associated with coffee and tea drinking, analgesic abuse, artificial sweeteners (at least in rodents) and treatment with cyclophosphamide.

- Other patients at risk include those with chronic cystitis due to indwelling catheters, calculi or large residual urine volumes. These patients often produce squamous cell carcinoma. Up to 10% of paraplegics with long-term catheters develop squamous bladder carcinoma.

Schistosoma haematobium, endemic in the Middle East and parts of Africa, can cause both squamous cell and transitional cell carcinomas. Patients who have undergone pelvic irradiation, usually for carcinoma of the cervix, are at a slightly higher risk for carcinoma of the bladder. Familial or hereditary bladder carcinoma is extremely rare.

Section 58.3 • Molecular biology of bladder carcinoma

All neoplastic diseases reflect disordered cell growth and therefore have a genetic basis. Our understanding of the derangement is limited, but a number of tumour-associated phenomena have been described: oncogenes, tumour suppressor genes and receptor expression.

Oncogenes

Oncogenes are genes which are normally active only during embryological development at times of differential cell growth. In the adult, these genes can become inappropriately active, often because of damage to the genes' flanking or promoting regions. Several oncogenes appear to be associated with the development of bladder carcinoma although they are present in only a small proportion of tumours. The p21 ras gene and c-myc appear to correlate with tumour grade and tumour progression, respectively.

At present knowledge and demonstration of oncogenes is of research interest only, although it is possible that they will be used for molecular staging and to predict prognosis of equivocal superficial tumours in the future.

Tumour suppressor genes

Tumour suppressor genes occur normally within the cell and regulate cell growth. If they are damaged the result may be unregulated cell growth or failure to direct DNA-damaged cells to programmed cell death (apoptosis). These effects result in uncontrolled proliferation of cloned cells with nuclear damage, possibly resulting in neoplasia.

A number of tumour suppressor genes have been described in different malignant diseases. The commonest damaged gene in bladder carcinoma is p53. It normally suppresses cell proliferation and directs DNA-damaged cells towards apoptosis prior to cell replication. Damage to p53 causes unsuppressed division of genetically damaged cells leading to further genetic instability. Bladder carcinomas with p53 abnormalities behave more aggressively than those with normal p53.

The retinoblastoma gene has also been implicated in bladder carcinomas as have other cell cycle regulators.

Receptor expression

Epidermal growth factor (EGF) is an important regulator of cell division. Increased expression of the EGF receptor within bladder tumour cells has been associated with aggressive tumour behaviour. EGF receptor expression may be the first molecular marker to achieve clinically useful status.

Section 58.4 • Pathology

The bladder urothelium consists of a basal cell layer, several layers of intermediate cells and a superficial coat of umbrella cells. Hyperplasia and metaplasia can occur in benign lesions, and squamous metaplasia is often observed over the trigone in women. Various benign changes can occur in the urothelium including von Brunn's nests, cystitis cystica and glandular metaplasia.

Some benign lesions can undergo malignant transformation, though this is very rare. An inverted papilloma is a benign lesion occurring in the base of the bladder, consisting of papillary fronds of normal epithelium projecting into the fibrovascular stroma.

Nephrogenic adenoma is a benign, solid, mucosal lesion occurring predominantly in men which may be associated with dysuria and frequency.

Leucoplakia is a form of squamous metaplasia with marked keratinization, often found in older women with a residual urine and chronic infection. Leucoplakia is generally considered to be the most common premalignant 'benign' lesion; up to 20% of patients develop invasive carcinoma, often of squamous cell type.

- Epithelial dysplasia is common. Mild or moderate dysplasia is of little clinical significance, but severe or grade 3 epithelial dysplasia is equivalent to carcinoma *in situ* (CIS – Figure 58.1). In the bladder this is an important and potentially serious condition. CIS is characterized by poorly differentiated carcinoma cells, which are confined to the urothelium. It has great potential to proceed directly to poorly differentiated, invasive tumours without going through an exophytic papillary stage. Progression to invasion and metastasis can be very rapid. CIS needs aggressive intravesical treatment, careful cystoscopic monitoring and radical treatment at the first sign of progression.

Section 58.5 • Transitional cell carcinoma

- More than 90% of bladder cancers are transitional cell carcinomas (TCC). TCC is characterized by an increased number of epithelial cell layers with papillary folding of the mucosa, abnormal cell maturation, giant cells, an increased nuclear-to-cytoplasmic ratio, prominent nucleoli, clumping of chromosomes and an increased number of mitoses.

The gross appearance can vary from the papillary, exophytic tumour (see Figure 58.5), usually well differentiated, to a solid, nodular invasive tumour (usually poorly differentiated). Both growth patterns may be seen in one tumour or in different tumours in the same bladder.

Grading of TCC

- Tumour grading is based on the architecture of the tumour and the cytological features. It is very important as a predictor of future behaviour. In particular, grade 3 tumours (see below) even at an early, non-invasive, stage can be dangerous and need careful management.

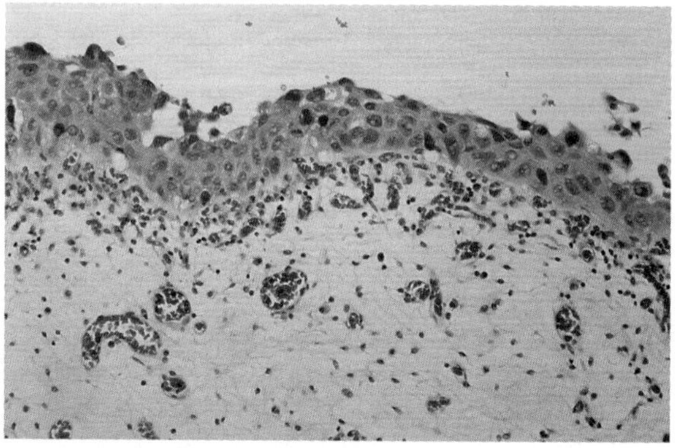

Figure 58.1 CIS of the bladder, showing severe cytological atypia in a flat mucosa with no invasion of basement membrane. (Courtesy of Dr S. Lang, Department of Pathology, Ninewells Hospital, Dundee, Scotland.)

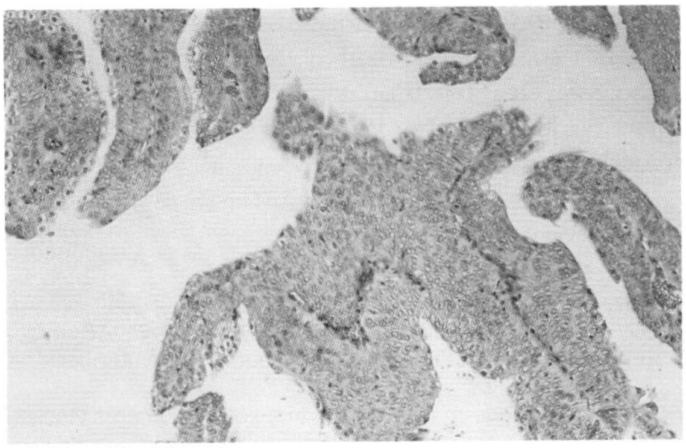

Figure 58.2 Papillary transitional cell carcinoma: G1 pTa. (Courtesy of Dr S. Lang, Department of Pathology, Ninewells Hospital, Dundee, Scotland.)

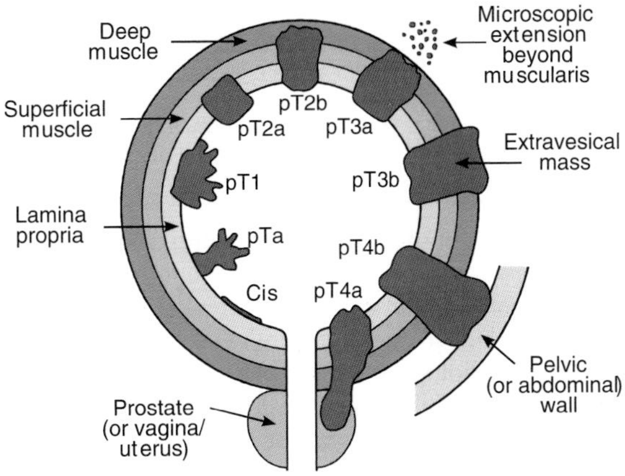

Figure 58.4 The common system of staging for carcinoma of the bladder.

Well-differentiated, grade 1 tumours consist of papillary fronds (Figure 58.2) with a thin fibrovascular stalk and a thickened urothelium containing more than seven layers with little cytological abnormality.

Moderately differentiated, grade 2 tumours have a wider fibrovascular core with disturbed cellular maturation, increased nuclear-to-cytoplasm ratio and increased mitotic figures.

Poorly differentiated, grade 3 tumours (Figure 58.3) have cells which do not differentiate as they progess from the basement membrane and have a high nuclear-to-cytoplasm ratio, with frequent mitotic figures.

Different grades of differentiation may be found within the same bladder, or even within the same tumour. Squamous cell carcinoma and adenocarcinoma can occur as metaplastic elements within a predominantly TCC. The presence of these changes does not alter the classification of the tumour, or its biological behaviour. Pure squamous cell carcinoma and adenocarcinoma behave differently.

Staging of TCC

Staging is initially done clinically, by bimanual examination of the empty bladder under anaesthesia, and may later be supplemented by imaging. Definitive staging is by histological examination (p stage).

- The currently accepted standard is the TNM classification as illustrated in Figure 58.4. The key distinction is between superficial (pTa, pT1) disease and invasive tumours (pT2, pT3, pT4). It is important to note that CIS is a distinct disease from pTa transitional carcinoma.

Metastatic spread occurs in 5% of patients with moderately differentiated tumours, and 20% of those with high-grade, *superficial* disease (G3, pT1). Metastatic spread is even more common in patients with *invasive* disease, particularly poorly differentiated (G3) disease.

Lymphatic spread can occur to the pelvic, iliac and aortic lymph nodes. Vascular spread is most commonly to bone, particularly the axial skeleton although liver and lung metastases do occur, usually at a very late stage.

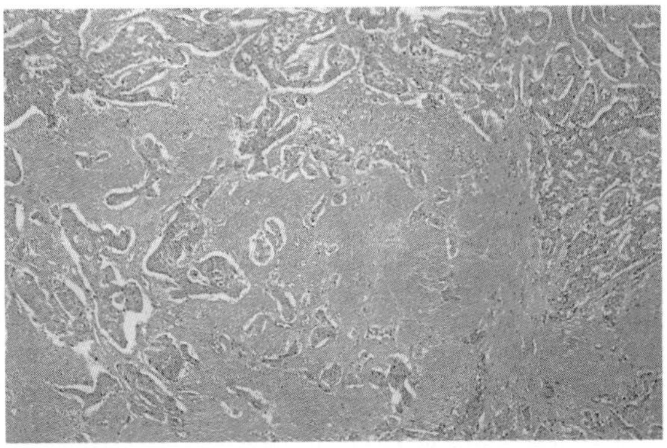

Figure 58.3 G3 transitional cell carcinoma of the bladder invading detrusor muscle (pT2). (Courtesy of Dr S. Lang, Department of Pathology, Ninewells Hospital, Dundee, Scotland.)

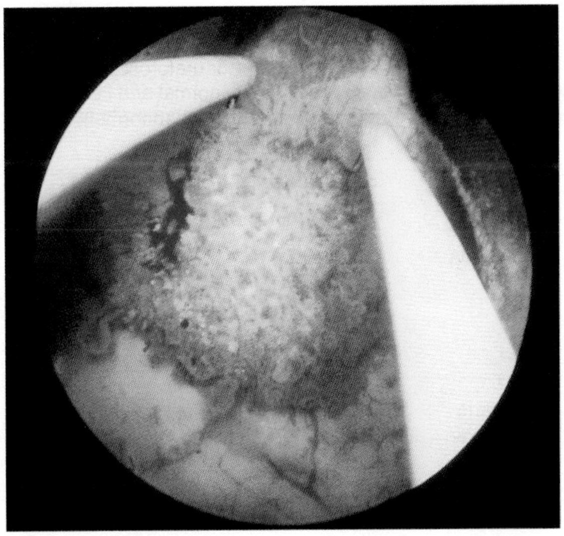

Figure 58.5 Endoscopic view of the start of resection of a papillary tumour (G1 pT1). The yellow, insulated arms of the resecting loop end in the bare wire loop itself which is hidden by the tumour 'chip' being resected.

Natural history of TCC

- More than one-half of tumours are superficial and non-aggressive. Tumour recurrence tends to mimic the original tumour staging and grade but about 20% recur at higher grade and 10% of patients with superficial disease develop metastases.

Forty per cent of patients present initially with high-grade muscle invasive lesions with a high likelihood of distant disease or subsequent recurrence. Patients with metastatic bladder carcinoma are nearly all dead within 2 years, so radiological staging of patients with invasive disease is important when considering radical extirpative surgery with curative intent.

Clinical presentation of TCC

Bladder carcinoma almost invariably presents with haematuria, frank or so-called 'microscopic' (usually detected by dipstick examination of the urine). Figure 58.6 is a suggested algorithm for the investigation of haematuria. It is based on a 'cystoscopy first' approach, since bladder carcinoma is the commonest serious underlying cause in the Western world.

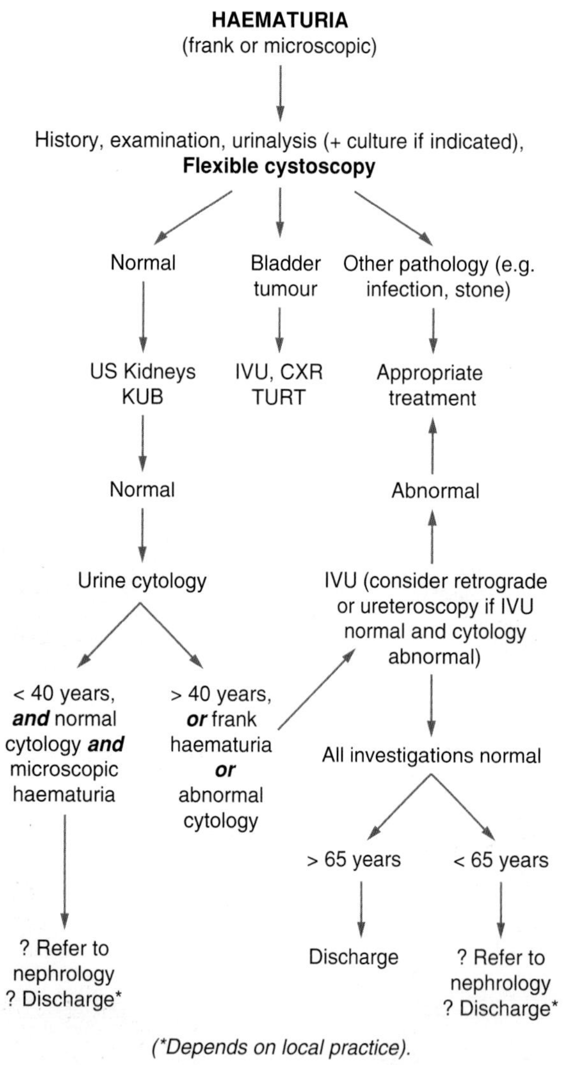

Figure 58.6 A suggested algorithm for the investigation of haematuria, based on a 'cystoscopy first' approach. US, ultrasound; KUB, kidneys, ureter, bladder; IVU, intravenous pylogram; CXR, chest X-ray; TURT, transurethral resection of tumour.

Patients with haematuria must have a cystoscopy **and** upper urinary tract imaging.

The few exceptions to this rule are:

- children with haematuria, who are best first investigated by a paediatrician as glomerular causes greatly outnumber urological causes
- the **first** episode of haematuria in a young woman associated with a **proven** urinary tract infection which responds clinically and bacteriologically to antibiotics and where the post-treatment urinalysis is normal
- in areas where schistosomiasis is endemic, the first episode of haematuria, which responds to treatment and does not recur.

There is an argument that in adults under 40 years (others say 50) with asymptomatic **microscopic** haematuria the incidence of bladder tumour is so low that nephrological investigation is the better first option, whether or not proteinuria is present. The counter-argument is that flexible cystoscopy with topical analgesia has such a low morbidity, and the consequences of overlooking a bladder tumour are so serious, that this investigation (and at least renal ultrasound) is always justified.

Unusually, bladder carcinoma can present with symptoms of advanced local disease, such as bilateral ureteric obstruction causing renal failure; or as a pelvic mass, bone pain, etc. It is an occasional incidental finding during transurethral resection of the prostate. Rarely, the papillary fronds become necrotic and act as a nidus of recurrent urinary infection.

Investigations

Once a bladder carcinoma is found an intravenous pyelogram (IVU) must be done to exclude synchronous urothelial tumour in the upper tract. Chest X-ray is only indicated in patients with invasive or poorly differentiated disease. Normal urine cytology does not exclude a tumour as it is relatively insensitive for TCC generally, but it is invaluable in the diagnosis (and monitoring) of carcinoma *in situ*.

If radical surgery is planned, staging investigations are needed. Cystoscopy, bimanual examination and histological examination of the resected biopsy are essential. Further staging is by magentic resonanace imaging (MRI) of the pelvis, abdomen and chest, and by isotope bone scanning. MRI (Figure 58.7) is more sensitive than computed tomography in detecting invasion of adjacent structures, especially after radiotherapy.

Endoscopic management

- Transurethral resection of the bladder tumour (Figure 58.5) is the mainstay of treatment. It prevents further haematuria, provides material for histological examination and allows local staging of the tumour endoscopically and on bimanual examination of the anaesthetized, relaxed patient.

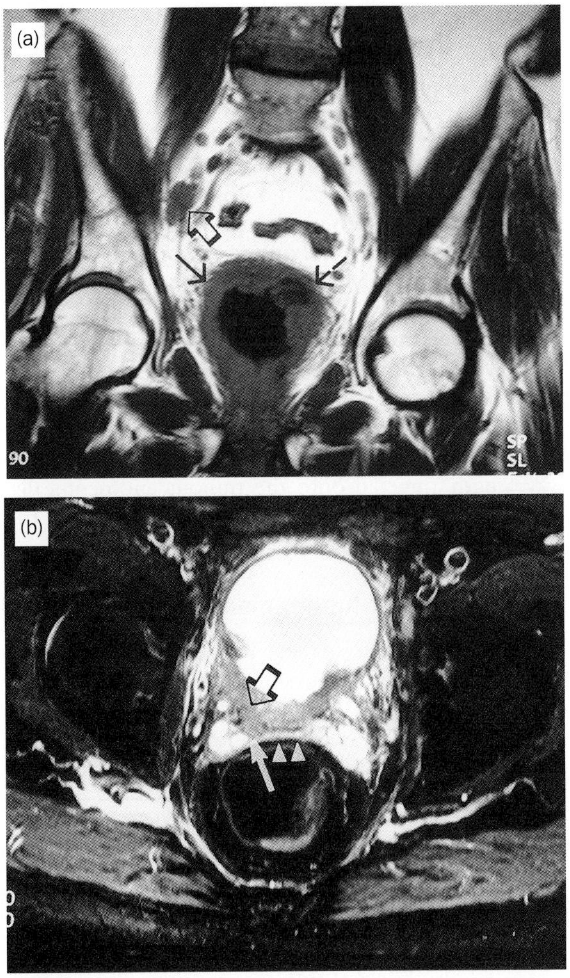

Figure 58.7 Magnetic resonance imaging staging of carcinoma of the bladder. Image (a) demonstrates bladder wall thickening (closed arrows) consistent with the known bladder tumour and previous radiotherapy. Also demonstrated is right iliac adenopathy (open arrow). Image (b) is an axial sequence which better demonstrates the tumour invasion posterolaterally on the right (open arrow). There is no evidence for rectal involvement (arrow heads) but the right seminal vesicle (closed arrow) was involved. Cystectomy was unlikely to be curative but was indicated after failure of radiotherapy and to prevent distressing strangury. (Courtesy of Dr D. Sheppard, Department of Imaging, Ninewells Hospital, Dundee, Scotland.)

The tumour should be carefully and systematically resected down to the level of the bladder mucosa. Resection is continued into the muscle underlying the tumour base to ensure complete clearance of the tumour and to allow the pathologist to identify or exclude muscle invasion. To detect invasion, take a second resection sample from the base of the tumour after having washed out the initial chips, and send this as a separate specimen.

Surrounding irregular areas, and other secondary smaller satellite lesions should be diathermied. Care is needed when resecting or diathermying the vault of the bladder to avoid perforating the peritoneal aspect of the bladder. In this area, 'spray' coagulation diathermy should not be used as it can cause electrical injury to the adjacent bowel without perforation of the bladder wall.

Resection to perivesical fat is appropriate for tumours in the base and side wall of the bladder and may be important to complete tumour clearance and ensure that muscle is included in the specimen. It is important to resect more cautiously in the bladder vault, where deep resection may cause intraperitoneal perforation, requiring open exploration to establish the integrity of adjacent small bowel and close any perforation. Care is needed when resecting lateral to the trigone: electrical stimulation of the obturator nerve may cause intense and sudden adduction of the legs. This may cause perforation of the bladder (into the pelvic rather than peritoneal space) and will alarm a patient under spinal anaesthetic. Obturator spasm can be reduced by using coagulating rather than cutting diathermy when resecting in this area.

An irrigating catheter is inserted at the end of this procedure and removed when haematuria has settled. The catheter is left in for 5 days if perforation of the bladder wall has occurred. Although bladder carcinoma tends to recur within the bladder because of widespread field changes throughout the urothelium, a number of 'recurrent' tumours occur because of implanation at the time of initial tumour resection. This is the rationale for the use of single dose, intravesical chemotherapy to reduce implantation of viable cells in the surrounding mucosa. Tumour recurrence is less likely if a single dose of adriamycin or mitomycin C is instilled into the bladder just before catheter removal.

Superficial disease: further management

Check cystoscopy

If histological examination confirms that the tumour is well or moderately differentiated and not invading muscle (G1, G2, pTa, pT1) no further treatment is done at this stage. The patient is placed on a check cystoscopy programme.

- Traditionally, check cystoscopy is perfomed at 3 monthly intervals for 1 year, 6 monthly intervals for a further 2 years and yearly thereafter. Any recurrence returns the patient to the start of the programme. The patient may be discharged after 10 years without recurrence.

It is now possible to predict the probability of further tumour recurrence and tailor check cystoscopy intervals to a given patient. Frequent recurrence is more likely in patients with large tumours, multiple tumours or recurrent disease at the first check cystoscopy. Caution is needed in interpretation of the first check cystoscopy as persistent rather than recurrent disease may be present, especially when the original tumour was large or multiple. A patient with GI, pTa disease with no recurrence at 3 months can then have only annual follow-up. Large or multiple tumours or G2, pT1 disease require more frequent follow-up for the first year, then annual follow-up if no recurrence occurs.

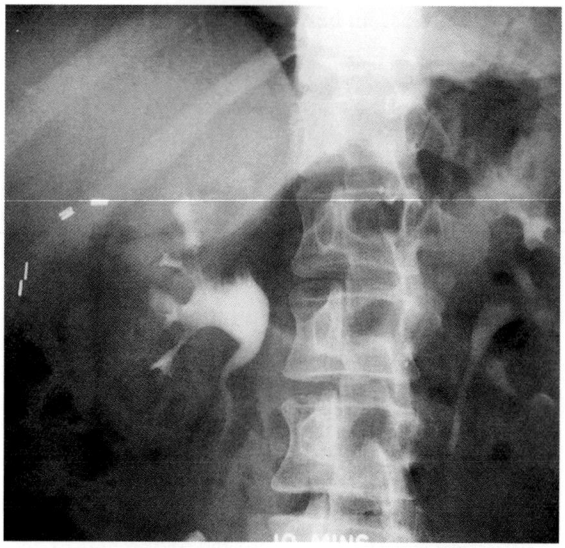

Figure 58.8 Asymptomatic TCC of the right renal pelvis found on routine IVU as part of follow-up after treatment of carcinoma of the bladder. (Courtesy of Mr R. Pickard, Department of Urology, Freeman Hospital, Newcastle upon Tyne, England.)

- Because of the significant risk of urothelial tumours in the upper tracts, an IVU should be done during cystoscopic follow-up; every 2 years if bladder recurrences are frequent, otherwise every 3 years (see Figure 58.8).

Chemotherapy

Although there is no defined role for *systemic* chemotherapy in patients with bladder carcinoma, *intravesical* schemes have improved the management of recurrent superficial disease. Adriamycin and mitomycin C given either as a single post-operative dose (as above), or as six doses at weekly intervals, can reduce the risk of recurrence at subsequent check cystoscopy. A 6 week course can also reduce the frequency and number of recurrences, and increase the time to recurrence, in patients who have frequent crops of small superficial tumours. Intravesical bacille-Calmette-Guérin (BCG) treatment (to stimulate a local immune response) is even more effective and offers improved resolution of bladder tumours and protection from progression in patients with carcinoma *in situ*. The morbidity of BCG is significantly greater than that of mitomycin with an increased incidence of cystitis and occasional systemic 'BCG-osis', a tuberculosis-like syndrome. BCG treatment may be ineffective when the patient is taking some antibiotics or anti-inflammatory drugs.

Although endoscopic follow-up is adequate for patients with well or moderately differentiated, non-invasive disease, it may not be so for patients with poorly differentiated disease invading the lamina propria (G3, pT1 disease). Such disease has a higher recurrence rate than truly superficial disease and may progress rapidly to muscle invasive disease with the risk of metastasis. It is not appropriate to regard G3, pT1 disease in the same way as G1 or G2, pTa or pT1 disease. Management is controversial and partly determined by age, general fitness and personal preferences. A full course (6 weeks) of intravesical BCG treatment is very useful in G3, pT1 disease to minimize tumour recurrence and progression. A minority of surgeons advocate primary cystectomy. Others perform a further resection of the tumour base after 2 months: if residual tumour is present, radical treatment is recommended. Radical radiotherapy may have a role in the treatment of this disease in the elderly patient.

Future developments

Photodynamic therapy is an experimental technique. It involves systemic administration of a 'dye' which is selectively taken up by the tumour and which absorbs a specific wavelength of light. Laser light of this wavelength, directed onto the tumour endoscopically, converts the 'dye' to toxic substances which kill the tumour cells.

Invasive disease: further management

It is not acceptable to manage invasive bladder carcinoma with endoscopic treatment alone(except in the very elderly or unfit). Invasive disease needs radical treatment completely to clear the tumour deep to, and surrounding, the resected area. The choice is between:

- radical ablative surgery, i.e. primary cystectomy
- bladder-conserving treatment, i.e. radiotherapy, reserving 'salvage' cystectomy for residual or recurrent invasive tumour
- an initial subtotal course of radiotherapy followed 4–6 weeks later by planned cystectomy.

There is no consensus and there are strong arguments for and against each option. Primary cystectomy inflicts major surgery on some patients who would have been cured by radiotherapy and on others who have occult metastases and are incurable. Radiotherapy has significant side-effects; it makes salvage cystectomy difficult, with significantly increased morbidity and mortality. Radiotherapy and planned cystectomy might combine the best or the worst of the two options.

Primary chemotherapy is not a current option: complete regression is uncommon and the morbidity of treatment significant.

Radical radiotherapy

This usually consists of 50 Gy in 20 fractions over 4 weeks. Morbidity consists of radiation cystitis, proctitis and occasional small bowel problems. Morbidity can be reduced with accurate planning and by keeping treatment volumes to a minimum. This regimen will not treat malignant tissue outside the bladder but it is unlikely that lymph node positive disease is curable by any means. Malignant pelvic lymph nodes may respond to chemotherapy, although this is probably best reserved for younger patients.

After radiotherapy the check cystoscopy programme (above) begins, but the first check should be delayed for at least 4 months after the completion of radiotherapy as 'residual disease' seen within this time may be non-viable. True residual disease, or recurrent invasive disease, is treated by salvage cystectomy. Staging investigations should be done before contemplating this, as distant disease may already exist, but cystectomy may still be appropriate when metastases are present, to give relief from distressing bladder symptoms, including intractable haematuria (see Figure 58.7).

Cystectomy

- This operation should remove the entire bladder, perivesical fat and nodes and prostate (and the urethra if there is TCC in, or distal to, the prostatic urethra) and is curative if the tumour has not spread to pelvic lymph glands, lung or bone. It is a major procedure in older patients with significant comorbidity.

Cystectomy gives improved local control and *possibly* improved tumour specific survival compared to radiotherapy, but its impact on the the patient's quality of life and overall survival is not necessarily better.

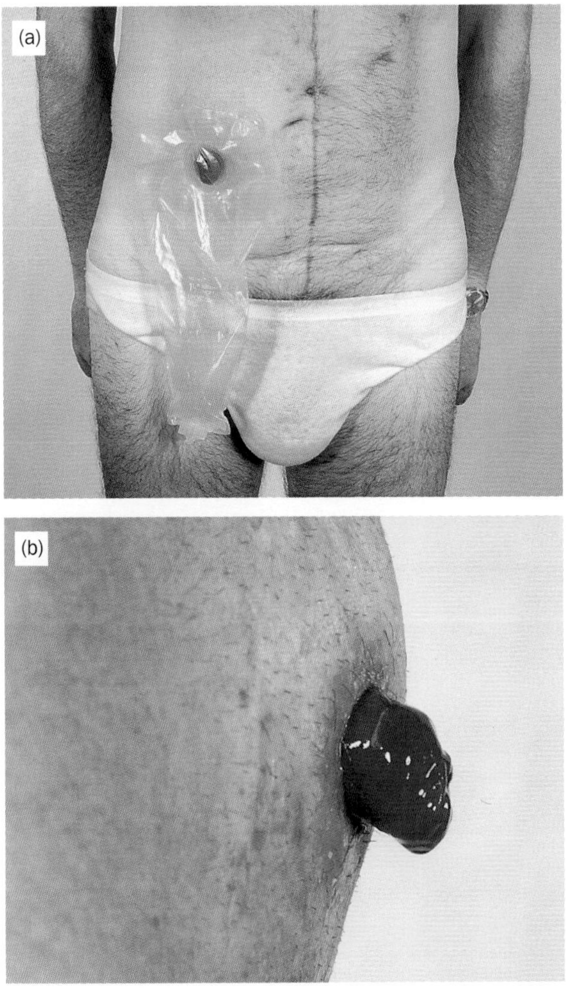

Figure 58.9 Standard urinary diversion by 'incontinent' ileal conduit. Although this is the simplest, safest and best-tried form of urinary diversion, orthotopic bladder substitution and continent urinary diversion are gaining acceptance.

Having removed the bladder the surgeon has a number of options for urinary diversion. The simplest, safest and most tested is to make an ileal conduit, in which the distal ends of the ureters are anastomosed to the proximal end of a 6 inch length of isolated ileum, the distal end of which is brought out to the skin of the iliac fossa as an everted stoma (Figure 58.9). An alternative is to do an orthotopic bladder substitution using detubularized right colon or distal ileum. Detubularizing the bowel, rather than using it intact, reduces the pressures in the neo-bladder, enhancing continence and preserving renal function. After the appropriate segment is isolated and bowel continuity restored, the isolated intestinal segment is divided along its anti-mesenteric border and a neo-bladder fashioned using one of several techniques. The ureters are usually anastomosed into the back of the neo-bladder. It is unclear whether an anti-reflux technique is essential. The neo-bladder is then anastomosed to the proximal cut end of the urethra. To preserve sphincter function it is essential that the cystectomy is done using a nerve-sparing technique, akin to radical prostatectomy.

- After radiotherapy or radical surgery, the upper tract needs monitoring by IVU, as for superficial disease.

Future developments

Radiotherapy and primary cystectomy remain the standard treatments for invasive bladder carcinoma. There is increasing interest in the use of chemotherapy, either in the adjuvant or neo-adjuvant role, before or after radical cystectomy. The commonest regimen is MVAC but newer agents are being evaluated.

There is also interest in these agents as chemosensitizers for patients undergoing primary radical radiotherapy, as a number of agents seem to enhance tumour susceptibility to radiation.

Chemotherapy would be useful for younger patients who present with locally advanced or distant disease and who are not amenable to simple resection but where the morbidity of radical extirpative surgery is not warranted.

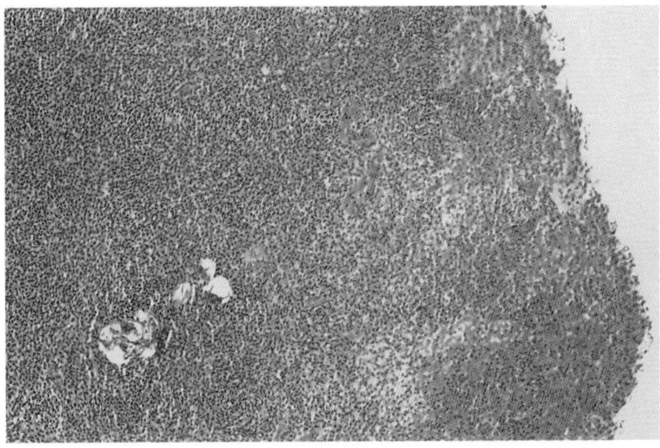

Figure 58.10 Intense eosinophilic reaction to ova of *Schistosoma haematobium*. This condition predisposes to squamous (and to transitional cell) carcinoma of the bladder.

Section 58.6 • Squamous carcinoma of the bladder

In Africa and the Middle East squamous carcinoma is common as a late complication of bilharziasis (infection with *Schistosoma haematobium* – Figure 58.10). Squamous carcinoma is not radiosensitive. Primary cystectomy is usually advocated, as many of these patients are young and need curative rather than palliative treatment.

In non-bilharzia areas, squamous metaplasia of TCC is more common than primary squamous carcinoma and is radiosensitive. Primary squamous carcinoma is almost confined to elderly women (often associated with residual urine, chronic urinary tract infection or bladder stones) and to patients with long-term catheters.

Section 58.7 • Adenocarcinoma of the bladder

Primary adenocarcinoma of the bladder is rare. Tumour markers on histological examination may be helpful in diagnosis. Cystectomy is the treatment of choice. Adenocarcinoma can also arise in the urachal remnant in the bladder vault. This disease carries a very poor prognosis and seems to metastasize early. If the disease appears to be confined to the bladder then total excision of the bladder, urachal remnant and median umbilical ligament is necessary to achieve tumour clearance.

Adenocarcinoma in the bladder is more often due to local invasion from carcinoma of the colon or ovary. It can also be metastatic from the ovary or, less commonly, colon, stomach or breast, so it is important to look for other sites of the disease.

Further reading

Hall, R. R., ed. (1999). *Clinical Management of Bladder Carcinoma.* London: Arnold.

Khadra, M. H., Pickard, R. S., Charleton, M. *et al.* (2000). A prospective analysis of 1,930 patients with haematuria to evaluate current diagnostic practice. *J Urol* **163**: 524–7.

Loughlin, K. R. ed. (2000). Superficial bladder cancer: new strategies in diagnosis and management. *Urol Clin North Am* **27**(1).

Montie, J. E., ed. (1997). Bladder surgery. *Atlas of the Urologic Clinics of North America* **2**(5).

Sultana, S. R., Goodman, C. M., Byrne, D. J. and Baxby, K. (1996). Microscopic haematuria: investigation using a standard protocol. *Br J Urol* **78**: 691–8.

Van der Meijden, A. P. M. (1998). Fortnightly review: bladder cancer. *BMJ* **317**: 1366–9.

Whittlestone, T. H. and Persad, R. (2000). Radical cystectomy and bladder substitution. *Hosp Med* **62**(1): 336–40.

MODULE 59

Carcinoma of the prostate

1 • Epidemiology
2 • Aetiology
3 • Pathology
4 • Screening for prostate cancer
5 • Diagnosis of prostate cancer
6 • Clinical presentations of prostate cancer
7 • Treatment of prostate cancer

Prostate cancer is the second most common cause of death from malignant disease in Western European and North American men. As the prevalence of lung cancer decreases following the decline of male cigarette smoking, prostate cancer may soon be the commonest cause of male cancer-related death. Two of the most controversial issues in urology are: should we screen for early prostate cancer, and what should we do when we find it?

The clinical management of carcinoma of the prostate presents several challenges:

- Should we screen asymptomatic men for cancer of the prostate?
- How do we deal with cancer found incidentally after surgery for 'benign' disease?
- What is the natural history of the condition in the individual patient and in men in general?
- Whom do we treat surgically, whom medically, and who is better with 'watchful waiting'?
- What are the roles of radical surgery, hormonal manipulation and radiotherapy?
- How can we best control advanced disease?
- How can we best manage hormone-escaped disease?
- What is the best management of bone pain and of spinal cord compression?

Section 59.1 • Epidemiology

The incidence is highest in black American men, intermediate in white men and lowest in Chinese and other Asian men. The black population in the USA has an incidence of 100 in 100 000 per year, compared to the incidence of 1 in 100 000 per year in some parts of Asia and North Africa. In the USA, the incidence in African-Americans is 1.7 times higher than in Caucasians. Migrant men acquire the level of incidence of their new home.

There appears to have been a 6% decrease in mortality rate from prostate cancer from 1991 to 1995 in the USA. There has been a similar decline in mortality from other cancers during this time so it is not clear whether the decline in prostate cancer is due to early detection and treatment.

Brothers of men with prostate cancer have a three-fold risk of developing the disease at an early age. In some cases there is a pattern of autosomal dominant inheritance, accounting for 9% of all cases and 45% of cases in men under 55. Male carriers of the BRCA1 gene (associated with breast cancer) are at three-fold risk.

Section 59.2 • Aetiology

Prostate cancer, at least in its early stages, is androgen dependent. Testosterone is converted into dihydrotestosterone (DHT) by 5-alpha-reductase within the prostate cells. DHT is essential for growth and development of the prostate.

Dietary, environmental and lifestyle factors may influence the prevalence of prostate cancer in different populations, but no aetiological factor has been conclusively implicated so far. A high-calorie diet rich in saturated fat, red meat and vitamin A has been associated with a high prevalence of prostate cancer. Vitamin E may be protective. Phyto-oestrogens, such as lignans and isoflavonoids, may protect against the development of prostate cancer.

Other lifestyle factors, sexual activity, alcohol and smoking have no known role in the promotion of, or protection from, prostate cancer.

Section 59.3 • Pathology

Pathological anatomy

The prostate is composed of four anatomically and pathologically distinct zones: peripheral, central, transitional and anterior.

The peripheral zone constitutes 70% of the normal young prostate: it is the commonest site of prostatic intra-epithelial neoplasia (PIN) and 70% of clinically apparent cancers occur here. This is the zone accessible by digital rectal examination (DRE). It is divided into right and left lobes by the median sulcus.

The central zone is a cone-shaped area at the base of the gland and around the ejaculatory ducts. Five per cent of cancers arise here.

The transitional zone comprises two lateral zones and the periurethral glands. This zone is the site of almost all benign prostatic hyperplasia and 25% of cancers. The anterior zone contains no glandular elements.

Histopathology

- Ninety-eight per cent of prostate cancers are adenocarcinomas, from glandular elements.

PIN is considered to be a precursor of invasive adenocarcinoma. PIN shows abnormal cytological features (large hyperchromatic nuclei with multilayering and nucleolar enlargement) with a normal basal cell layer. Low-grade PIN on biopsy is not associated with frank histological malignancy elsewhere in the gland.

High-grade PIN is associated with concomitant cancer in 50% of cases (detected by re-biopsy). In autopsy studies, the prevalence of high-grade PIN increases with increasing age.

- Adenocarcinoma has similar cytological features, but lacks a basal cell layer.
- Perineural invasion is a common feature of progressive disease.
- Prostate cancer dedifferentiates with time.
- Testosterone withdrawal causes squamous metaplasia in the glandular cells.

The Gleason system of grading is based on architectural features and is described below.

Section 59.4 • Screening for prostate cancer

Prostate specific antigen (PSA, see below) and DRE can be used to screen the population of men at risk of developing prostate cancer (those over 40 or 50 years, depending on the protagonists' views). Detection rates in men aged 50–79 will be 3–6%. Whether or not screening is helpful, many men ask for it after reading the lay press and doctors find it hard to resist taking blood for PSA testing if the patient wants it as part of a general health check. Major private health insurers offer PSA measurement as part of a 'well man' check.

PSA and DRE are far from being perfect screening tools.

- An elevated PSA in the intermediate range (4–10 ng/ml) predicts cancer on biopsy in 25–35%.
- Serum PSA over 10 ng/ml predicts cancer on biopsy in 50–60% of men.
- DRE abnormality alone is a poor predictor of cancer on biopsy.
- The strongest predictor is a combination of a PSA concentration greater than 10 ng/ml and a hard prostate (positive predictive value 80%).

When considering screening asymptomatic men the following points are relevant:

- In an unscreened population the majority of men are incurable at diagnosis. Cancer detected by screening is more likely to be at an early stage. More men are reaching old age with increasing life expectancy and the numbers of men who will die from prostate cancer will increase. There is a strong case for trying to eliminate prostate cancer as a major cause of morbidity and death in these men.
- Screening for early prostate cancer by serum PSA and DRE does not meet many of the accepted criteria for a valid screening programme.
- A single PSA measurement lacks the required sensitivity and specificity to be the main screening tool.
- Men with 'positive' PSA results will need further investigation by prostate biopsy.
- Prostate biopsy has a morbidity, and even a mortality. Biopsy is uncomfortable for all, painful for some and often causes bleeding. The most serious risk is sepsis. Five per cent of patients have significant complications needing medical attention.
- A negative biopsy does not exclude carcinoma (because of sampling error). This may lead to a false sense of security in patient and doctor and may have medico-legal implications.
- Sampling error is inversely proportional to the number of biopsies taken; but the greater the number of biopsies, the greater the risk of bleeding and sepsis.
- There is no consensus on the best management for early, subclinical, microscopic disease.
- It seems reasonable to assume that radical treatment of early disease is both necessary and beneficial, but this has not been proved in a randomized, controlled trial.
- There is a significant risk of over-treatment of early disease. Several men whose disease would never have harmed them may need to have radical treatment to give benefit to one who would have come to harm if untreated.
- There are serious financial implications for health services in terms of the resources needed for biopsies, radical treatment and their complications. There is as yet no evidence that these costs will be offset by benefit to patients.

Early diagnosis may lead to lead-time and length-time bias, which may be especially difficult to detect in a disease with such a prolonged natural history.

- An 'abnormal' PSA level followed by a 'negative' biopsy may serve only to worry the patient. Some urologists consider PSA to be only a 'Promoter of Stress and Anxiety'.
- Asymptomatic men requesting 'screening' by PSA estimation should be made aware of these considerations.

The above reservations do not apply to men with a first degree relative with prostate cancer. Such men have a significantly increased risk of developing the disease at a young age. They should be screened annually from the age of 40 years. Some urologists would apply this to African-Caribbean men.

A European prospective, randomized, controlled trial to determine whether screening reduces mortality is in progress. About 300 000 men will take part, and an answer is expected by the year 2015.

Section 59.5 • Diagnosis of prostate cancer

The diagnostic tools are:

- DRE
- PSA
- imaging
- biopsy.

Digital rectal examination

DRE is an essential part of a good physical examination and is mandatory in men with lower urinary tract symptoms and in those over 40 years with back pain. A normal DRE (obviously) does not exclude prostate cancer. At least one-third of prostate cancers diagnosed on biopsy or incidentally found in transurethral prostatic resection (TURP) specimens are not palpable.

The benign prostate has a smooth contour, with a distinct midline sulcus and lateral borders. Palpable cancers feel hard often with bulging and irregularity of the contour of the gland.

A prostate can be described as suspect if there is one (or more) of the following:

- obliteration of the median sulcus
- induration or extension of a lobe
- obliteration of the lateral borders
- asymetry of the gland or excessive firmness.

Experienced examiners will disagree about these criteria in up to 40% of examinations.

DRE (preferably by bimanual examination under anaesthesia) is used clinically to stage prostate cancer using the TNM staging system:

- T1: not palpable ('incidental carcinoma' found on subsequent histology)
- T2: nodule palpable within the prostate, not deforming the contour
- T3: hard nodule deforming contour, invading capsule of gland
- T4: fixed mass involving and extending from the prostate, fixed to the pelvic side wall or rectal wall.

Prostate specific antigen

A glycoprotein of prostatic epithelial origin, PSA was originally used for forensic purposes in the detection of semen.

Measurement of PSA in circulating blood is now important in the diagnosis and management of prostate cancer. In general, PSA is a good marker of prostate cancer activity (though cancer often expresses PSA histochemically less well than does benign tissue). For clinical trials of treatment it is a surrogate for disease activity. It is less precise as a screening or diagnostic tool.

PSA enters peripheral blood by leakage from the prostate and its concentration is proportional to the bulk of the prostate and to its 'leakiness', which is increased by malignant and inflammatory changes. The half-life in serum is 3.5 days.

Healthy men may not have detectable PSA: 0–4 ng/ml is accepted as the normal range. Kits for PSA testing vary in their methodology and range of 'normal'. When comparing results between centres, the assay used must be given.

Interpretation of laboratory results should take account of the patient's age, as follows (based on surveys of men in the community).

Population PSA (ng/ml)

- All men: 0–4.
- Age 40–49: 0–2.5.
- Age 50–59: 0–3.5.
- Age 60–69: 0–4.5.
- Age 70–79: 0–6.5.
- Age >80: up to 10 ng/ml.

Thus a man of 45 years with a PSA of 3.5 ng/ml is at increased risk of prostate cancer in spite of a PSA in the 'normal range'.

Because of the significant overlap of values for benign and early malignant disease, attempts have been made to refine the interpretation of PSA as follows.

- **PSA density**. Men with larger benign prostate glands tend to have elevated PSA concentrations approximately proportional to the size of the gland. Serum PSA (ng/ml) divided by the weight of the prostate in grams should be below 0.15.
- **PSA velocity**. Increase of PSA over time (normally up to 0.75 ng/ml/year).
- **PSA doubling time.** A doubling of PSA concentration in 2 years suggests cancer.
- **Free/total PSA.** Most of the PSA circulates bound to serum proteins. The ratio is often lower than 0.2 in cancer patients and higher in men with BPH.

Up to 5% of men with advanced prostate cancer do not express serum PSA at levels in keeping with the disease, which in these cases is usually very poorly differentiated.

Urinary infection, acute retention and instrumentation may raise PSA concentrations to over 100 ng/ml. If a high concentration is found during such an episode, repeat measurement should be delayed for 3 weeks. PSA is not much affected by digital rectal examination.

Imaging

Plain radiography

Metastases from the prostate are typically osteosclerotic (Figure 59.1). Bone metastases are present in about 20% of men at first presentation. They are commonly painless and found on routine imaging, but they may be the presenting feature.

In advanced disease the chest may show lymphangitis carcinomatosa or pleural effusion.

Transrectal ultrasound (TRUS)

Seventy per cent of cancers arise in the peripheral zone of the prostate, the part nearest the examining finger and the transrectal ultrasound probe. If the peripheral zone contains a hypo-echoic area corresponding to a nodule felt on DRE there is a 90% chance of cancer on biopsy of this area. Many cancers show more subtle changes on TRUS. These include loss of differentiation between the transitional zone (the benign prostatic hypertrophy area) and the peripheral zone, and asymmetry and expansion of the peripheral zone. TRUS helps systematic sampling of the prostate, the most likely sites for cancer detection being the lateral peripheral zone and towards the apex. Other than as a guide to biopsy, TRUS has a role in the measurement of prostate volume for calculation of PSA density (and as a guide to treatment in benign disease, see Module 61).

Isotope bone scanning

Technetium phosphate is taken up by the skeleton (and excreted by the kidneys). Bony metastases show increased uptake on bone scan. Areas often affected include the pelvis, spine, ribs and skull and long bones

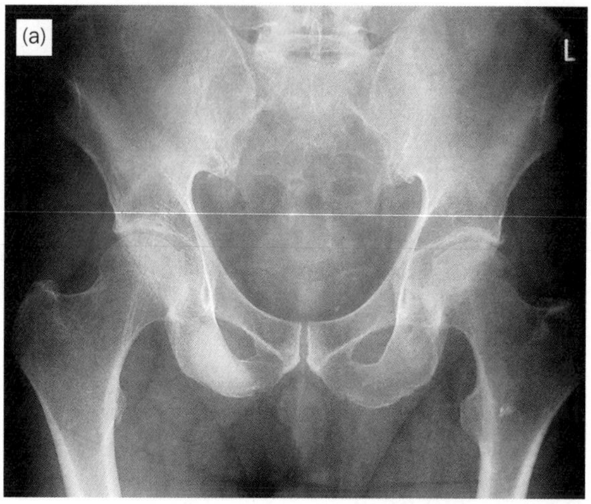

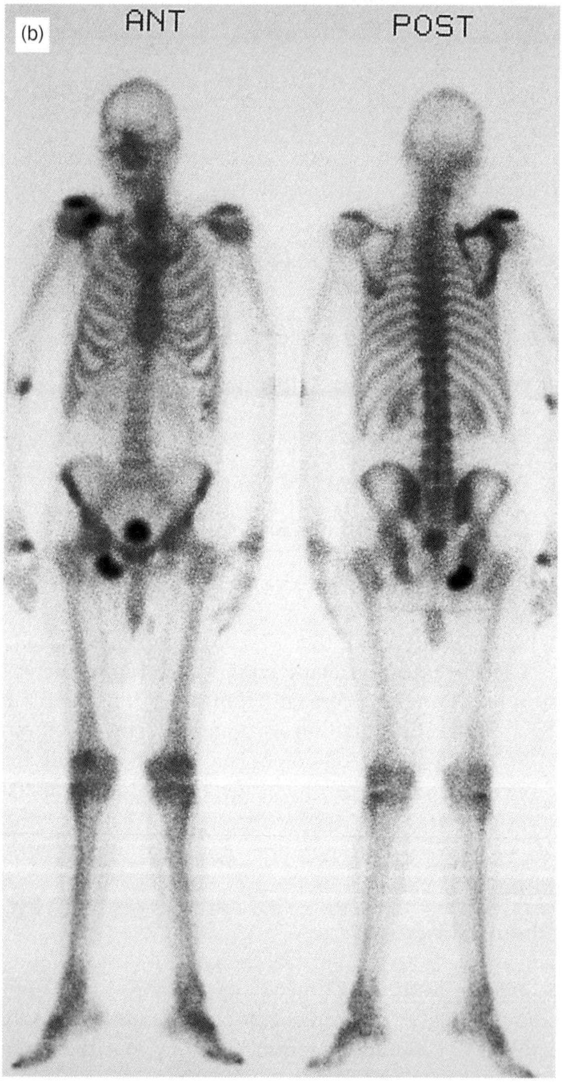

Figure 59.1 (a) Typical sclerotic metastasis in right ischium. (b) Isotope bone scan of the same patient showing a localized 'hot spot' corresponding to a sclerotic lesion. The kidneys can be seen, as they take up the isotope, which is also in the bladder. (The 'hot spot' in the right shoulder is a result of degenerative change and the two 'hot spots' in the right hand and elbow are caused by extravasated isotope at the sites of difficult injections.)

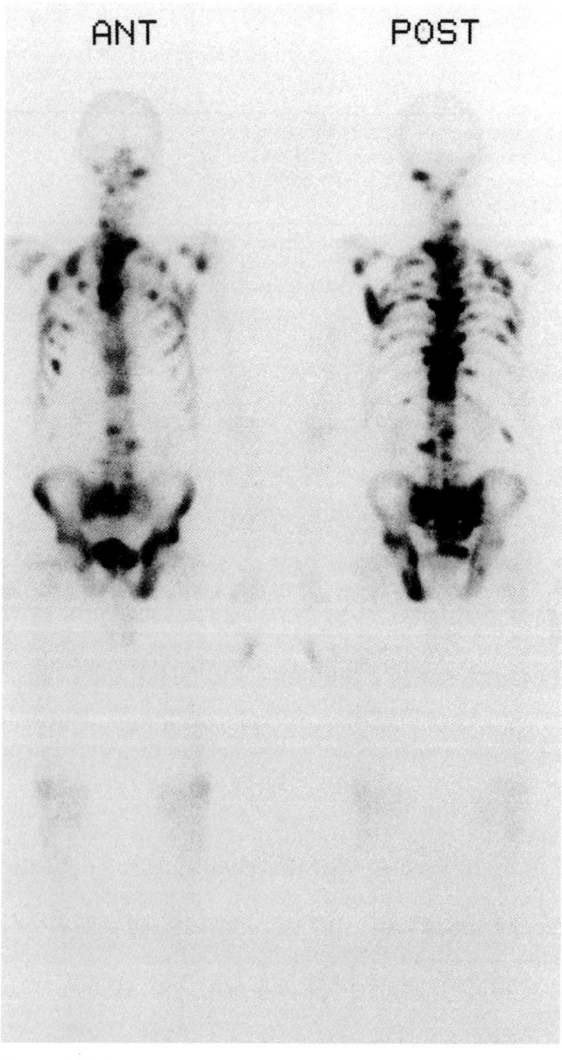

Figure 59.2 Multiple bony metastases from prostate cancer, typically in the spine, ribs and pelvis, as well as other sites.

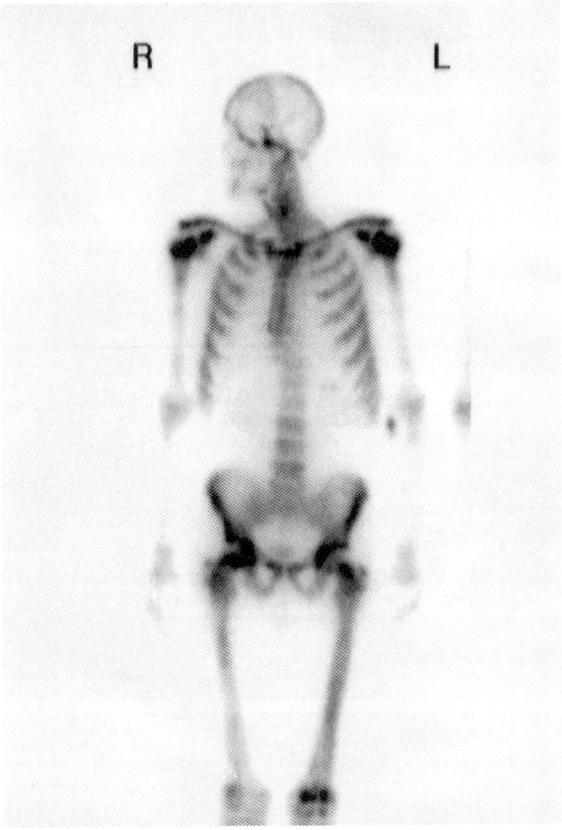

Figure 59.3 'Superscan' showing intense uptake of isotope by virtually the whole skeleton as a result of widespread metastases, with no excretion by the kidneys.

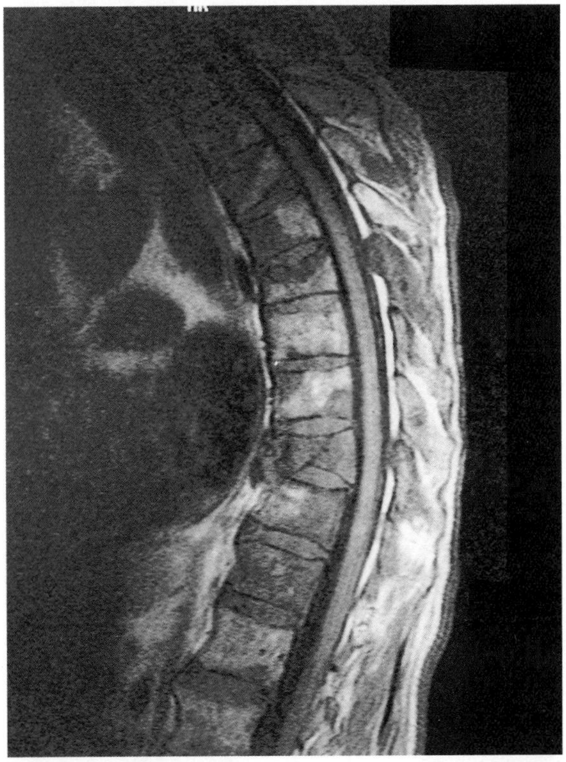

Figure 59.4 MRI of the spine showing multiple metastases from prostate cancer, with collapse of at least two thoracic vertebrae.

(Figure 59.2). A 'superscan' shows intense uptake by the entire skeleton and no excretion by the kidneys (Figure 59.3). This represents an extensive disease burden. Abnormal uptake is found in arthritis, degenerative spinal disease, healing fractures and Paget's disease. These conditions may be distinguished from metastases by PSA concentration and plain radiography. Unless radical local treatment is being considered, bone scanning is not justified if the PSA is less than 10 and the Gleason score (see below) less than 8.

Computed tomography and magnetic resonance imaging

Computed tomography (CT) will differentiate bone metastases from degenerative and other lesions, but magnetic resonance imaging (MRI) is better for this (Figure 59.4) and is far superior to CT for assessing local spread, especially capsular penetration and invasion of the seminal vesicles (Figures 59.5–59.7).

- Lymph node metastases may be difficult to image by either method.

Biopsy

Before treatment is planned, histological proof is needed. Except in patients in whom the diagnosis has been made on examination of operative specimens, this will require needle biopsy. Accurate systematic biopsy and specific targeting of suspicious areas are done using transrectal ultrasound. 'Blind biopsy' is no longer justified, other than to obtain histological confirmation in a large gland which is diffusely and obviously malignant.

By convention, four to six or more biopsies are taken. The number of positive tissue cores and the proportion of the core infiltrated by cancer correlate well with disease stage and the presence of positive margins at subsequent radical prostatectomy. The cores are about 22 mm long and 2 mm wide and are not always easy to assess by histology. There is often only a small area of cancer and it may be impossible accurately to provide Gleason grade (see below) on needle biopsy. The pathologist will usually be able to say how much of the specimen is malignant and whether this is well or poorly differentiated. The value of the report to the clinician is enhanced by dialogue with the pathologist.

Biopsy can, rarely, be omitted when the patient presents with an extensive craggy prostate, sclerotic lesions on plain radiographs and a very high PSA concentration, when treatment needs to start urgently (e.g. because of imminent spinal cord compression or ureteric obstruction with renal impairment). Treatment without histological proof is not otherwise justified: multiple prostatic calculi and granulomatous prostatitis can simulate carcinoma.

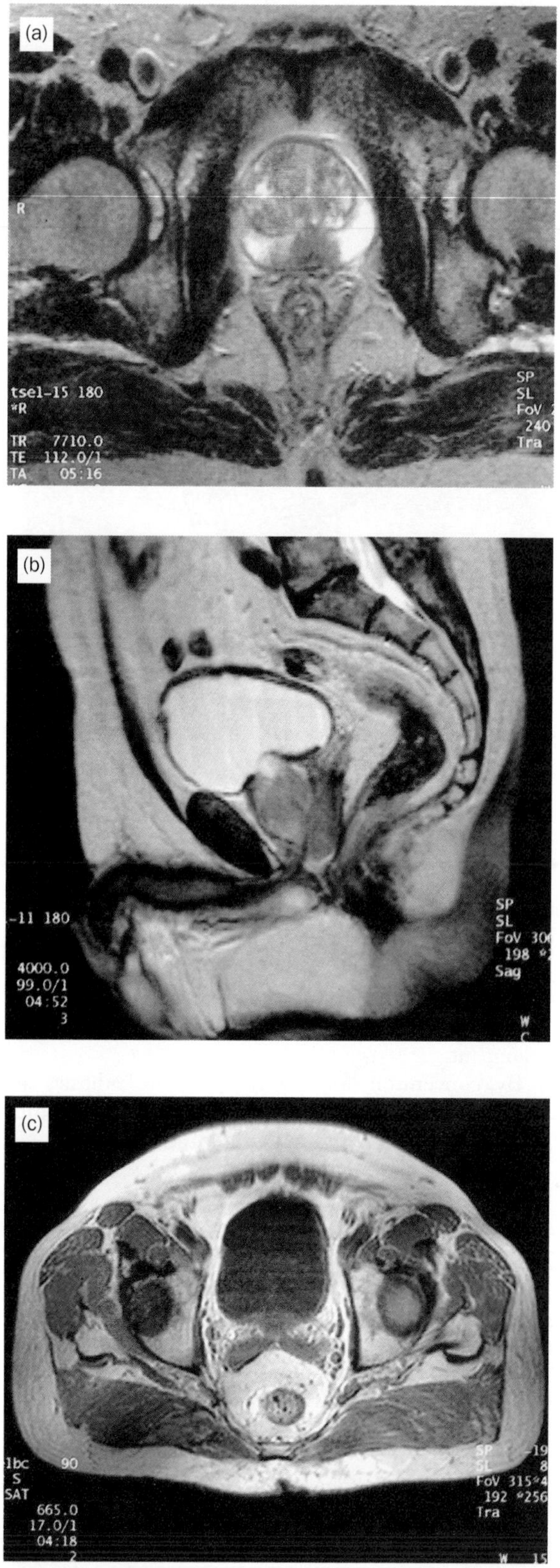

Figure 59.5 MRI (T2-weighted) images. (a) Large tumour in peripheral zone within true capsule. Axial view. (b) Sagittal image. (c) Further axial view. The seminal vesicles are uninvolved – 'bow-tie' appearance. (Courtesy of Drs Barry, Russell and McDermott, Department of Radiology, Stirling Royal Infirmary, Stirling, Scotland.)

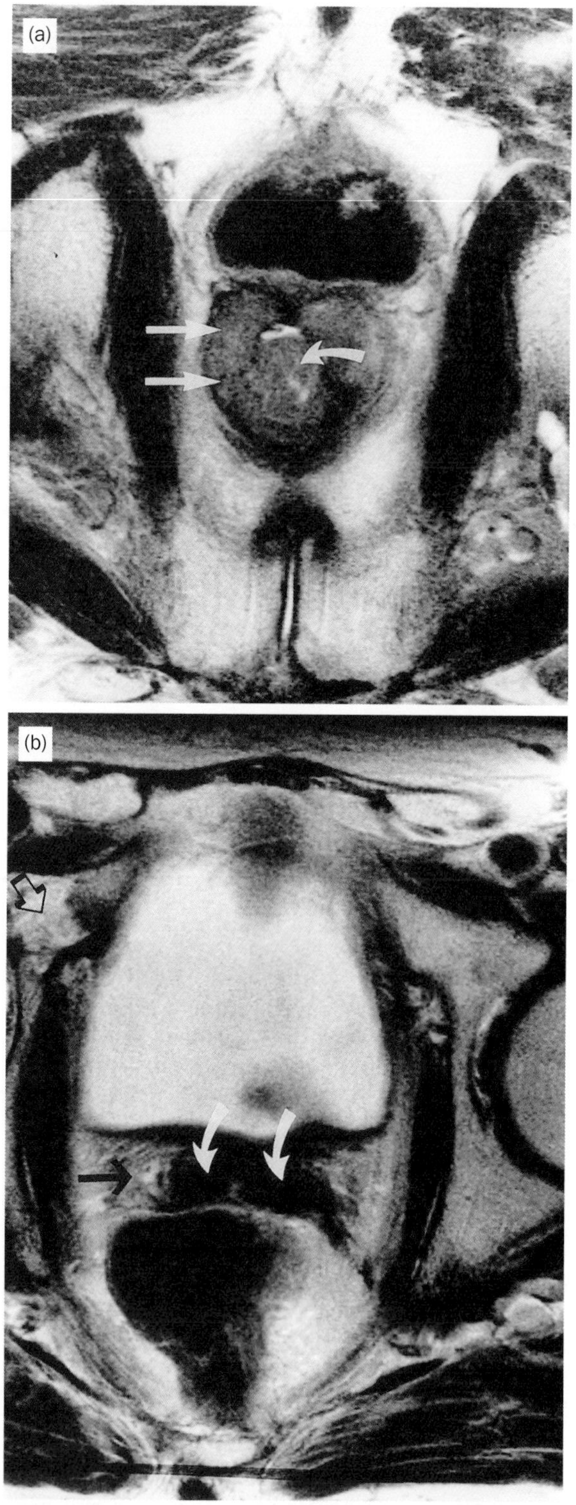

Figure 59.6 MRI (T2-weighted) images in a patient with prostatic carcinoma after previous TURP. On an axial sequence (a) tumour mass is shown in the TURP defect (curved arrow) and replacing the normal hyperintense peripheral zone (straight arrows). A further axial image (b) shows extensive involvement of the seminal vesicles (curved arrows) with a small residual area of normal seminal vesicle on the right (closed black arrow). Metastatic bone disease near the right acetabulum is also shown (open arrow). (Courtesy of Dr D. Sheppard, Department of Imaging, Ninewells Hospital, Dundee, Scotland.)

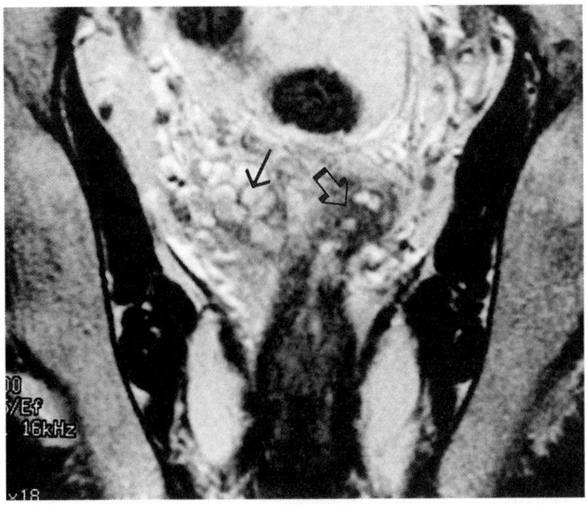

Figure 59.7 A coronal T2-weighted MRI image shows a normal right seminal vesicle (closed arrow) and partial replacement of the left seminal vesicle by tumour (open arrow). (Courtesy of Dr D. Sheppard, Department of Imaging, Ninewells Hospital, Dundee, Scotland.)

Staging prostate cancer

Staging is mostly by the TNM system. In North America the Jewett–Whitmore staging system is still popular (see Table 59.1).

For practical prognostic and therapeutic purposes staging can be grouped into:

- organ-confined disease
- locally advanced disease without metastases
- metastatic disease

as in Table 59.2.

Grading prostate cancer

It is said that men do not develop prostate cancer, they develop prostate cancers. Cancers are typically multiple and are heterogeneous in morphology, in aggressiveness and in genetic profile. Biopsy specimens can underestimate the grade of disease because of sampling error: a single area of high-grade tumour may be missed, yet the prognosis is determined by the highest grade.

The Gleason grading system is in general use. Five grades are described (1–5). The Gleason score is the sum of the scores of the predominant grade and of the second most common grade (which should be present in at least 5% of the biopsy) giving a total score between 2 and 10.

- The Gleason score is a good indicator of prognosis and the likelihood of spread.

The Gleason grading system correlates with histological features as follows:

- Well differentiated: Gleason sum 2–4.
- Moderately differentiated: Gleason sum 5–7.
- Poorly differentiated: Gleason sum 8–10.

Grade is important in locally confined disease because it relates directly to prognosis. Locally advanced and metastatic disease tend to be of high grade. Very poorly differentiated disease may be less hormone responsive and can cause clinical difficulties as it is often associated with *relatively* little rise in serum PSA concentration.

Section 59.6 • Clinical presentations of prostate cancer

Early local (organ-confined) disease

In areas where routine PSA measurement is prevalent, men are identified who have elevated PSA concentrations with minimal or no symptoms and early disease.

TUR for clinically benign disease is a common source of diagnosis of prostate cancer in stages T1a and T1b.

Locally advanced disease

This may present as lower urinary tract symptoms (LUTS) or haematuria and uraemia due to bladder outflow obstruction or ureteric obstruction by local extension or rarely, venous or lymphatic congestion of the leg(s) by direct mechanical pressure.

Table 59.1 Staging of prostate cancer

TNM (1997)	*Jewett–Whitmore*
• Tx: Primary tumour stage cannot be assessed	
• T1: Primary tumour not palpable, nor visible by imaging	
T1a: involving 5% or less of TUR chips	A1: Foci in <3 chips A2: Diffuse >3 chips
T1b: More than 5% TUR chips	
T1c: Cancer on needle biopsy	
• T2: Tumour palpable or visible confined within prostate	B1: One lobe, <2 cm
T2a: One lobe involved	B2: One lobe, >2 cm
T2b: Both lobes involved	B3: Both lobes, inside capsule
• T3: Tumour extends through prostate capsule	C1: Sulcus or sulci involved
T3a: Extracapsular extension, one or both lobes	C2: Invading base of seminal vesicles
T3b: Invasion of seminal vesicle(s)	C3: Seminal vesicles ± other local organs
• T4: Tumour fixed or invading bladder, urethra, rectum, pelvic wall	
• N1: Regional lymph nodes involved	D1: Lymph node disease
• M1: Distant metastases	D2: Distant metastases D3: Metastases resistant to hormonal treatment

Table 59.2 Clinically useful grouping of stages

Grouping		*10 year disease-specific survival*
Organ-confined disease (T1, T2, N0, M0)	May be curable	93–80% (depending on grade)
Locally advanced, non-metastatic disease (T3, T4, Nx, M0)	Not curable	50%
Bone metastases (T1–4, Nx–1, M1)	Not curable	10%

Metastatic disease

This can cause:

- bone pain
- renal failure
- anaemia – from renal failure or bone marrow infiltration
- leg swelling due to lymphatic or venous compression
- paraplegia
- pathological fracture
- proptosis.

Section 59.7 • Treatment of prostate cancer

Dr Willet F. Whitmore, a urologist who himself died of prostate cancer, posed two important questions.

- Is cure possible when it is necessary?
- Is cure necessary when it is possible?

Early local (organ-confined) disease

We know of the high prevalence of prostate cancer on post-mortem histology in elderly men who have had no sign of the disease in life. There is therefore debate about the need to treat men with asymptomatic localized disease. Many such men will live out their lives with no clinical evidence of prostate cancer. Some will develop overt disease but not die from it. Others will develop progressive disease which will kill them. We have no means of predicting at an early stage which course the disease will follow in a given patient. Men with T1 and T2 low-grade cancer have a good prognosis without treatment (85% 10 year survival). However, there is some evidence to support the treatment of men with higher grade disease, who have a 10 year survival of 33%. Fit patients with significant volume, higher grade tumours are most likely to benefit from treatment.

Locally advanced disease

Once disease is beyond the prostatic capsule it can be suppressed for a time but is no longer curable and prognosis is poor. However, treatment can be deferred if the patient does not have significant symptoms and is not at immediate health risk from the tumour, especially if age and comorbidity play a major part in his prognosis.

Metastatic disease

Virtually all patients with metastases should have treatment. Hormone manipulation is the mainstay of treatment. There is evidence that early intervention is better than waiting until symptoms occur. Those who respond will have a survival benefit and a lower risk of serious complications such as ureteric obstruction, spinal cord compression and other causes of hospitalization for their disease.

Treatment options

Radical prostatectomy

In 1903 total removal of the prostate was first used to treat early stage cancer with the aim of curing the disease. A huge increase of numbers occurred the 1980s and 1990s in the USA, where in some urology departments this has become the most common operation on the prostate, outnumbering TURP for benign disease. This trend is spreading to Europe. Patient selection is important. A man has to be fit, with a 10–15 year life expectancy. The disease must pose a threat to his health and to his life. Dr Whitmore's conundrum applies. Most candidates for radical surgery are under 70, lack serious comorbidity, and have stage T1 or T2 disease, occasionally early T3. Usually the cancer will be medium or high grade (Gleason score 5–9).

High-grade PIN is not an indication for radical prostatectomy, nor is the finding on biopsy of one or two microscopic foci of frank malignancy, because of the risk of over-treatment of a non-significant cancer.

The technique of radical prostatectomy has been refined by Professor Patrick Walsh at Johns Hopkins University. A suprapubic incision is made and the retropubic space is developed. The obturator lymph nodes are taken for staging. Frozen section may be useful as there is no point in proceeding with radical surgery if the disease is extra-prostatic. The prostate is mobilized, opening the endopelvic fascia, securing and dividing the deep dorsal vein of the penis. A nerve-sparing and sphincter-saving procedure is preferred, provided this does not compromise tumour clearance. The nerves to the corpora cavernosa of the penis run immediately outside the postero-lateral angles of the prostate in the neurovascular bundles and can easily be damaged while mobilizing the prostate. The external urinary sphincter is closely applied and inserted into the apex of the prostate, making a degree of sphincter injury inevitable. The bladder neck is anastomosed end-to-end to the urethra to allow healing and a catheter is left *in situ* for 2–3 weeks.

Radical prostatectomy can also be done by the perineal route. This is not as popular as the retropubic operation and it is not possible to sample lymph nodes by this route.

Microscopic involvement of the margins of resection is common (Figure 59.8), but does not always predict disease relapse. Lymph node or seminal vesicle involvement predicts disease relapse in nearly every case. Extensive margin involvement can be managed by adjuvant radiotherapy and lymph node disease by hormonal manipulation or by observation.

The main post-operative complications are incontinence of urine and impotence.

Incontinence affects 70% of men initially. With supportive care this can be tolerated and up to 90% of men have good control at 1 year, but 30% will need a pad in their underpants for daily activity.

Impotence occurs in 50% of men who were potent before. Treatments such as sildenafil and injectable or intra-urethral prostaglandins are usually effective, and function may recover with time.

Radiotherapy

Radical radiotherapy

Prostate cancer is radiosensitive and radical radiotherapy has been used for many years in an effort to cure it. The same 'curability' criteria must apply as with surgery. Usually hormonal therapy is used with radiotherapy to shrink the prostate and give a smaller area for treatment, making treatment more effective and less toxic. Radiotherapy is sometimes seen as second-best to surgery and only patients unfit for surgery or with disease too advanced to be excised are then referred for radiotherapy. This should not be the case. Results following radiotherapy are comparable to those of surgery, although there seems to be a tendency for radiation treatment to fail at 5–7 years in poorly differentiated cancer. Radiotherapy provides good local control for many men for the duration of their life expectancy, but may not be as effective as surgery for men with high-grade, organ-confined disease and good life expectancy.

Radiotherapy is useful as an adjunct to surgery where surgery leaves residual disease or if there is local relapse. The converse does not as easily apply: salvage surgery after failure of irradiation is not an easy procedure.

Radical radiotherapy is given 5 days a week in fractions over 4–6 weeks to a total dose of 60 Gy. The side-effects are proctitis, cystitis, stricture, impotence and incontinence. The last two complications may be no less common after irradiation than after surgery. Alternatives currently in vogue include brachytherapy by the placement of radioactive iodine seeds in the prostate under ultrasound control.

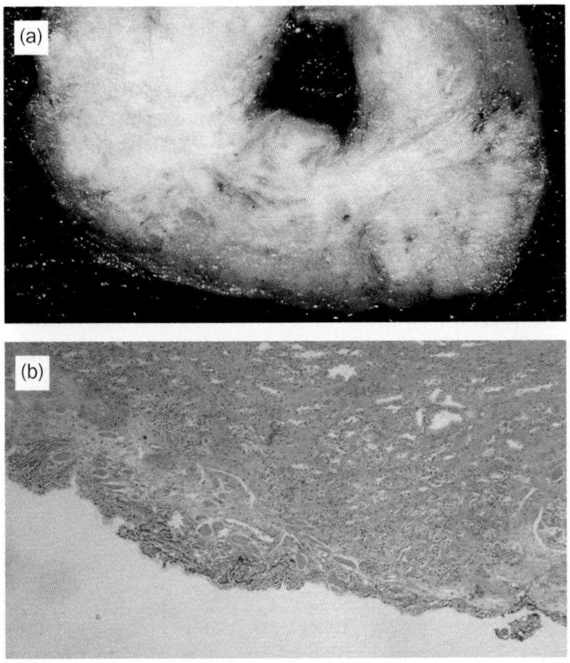

Figure 59.8 Radical prostatectomy specimen. (a) Macroscopic appearance showing area of tumour (yellowish area at lower margin). The margins are inked. (b) Microscopic appearances of this area show that the tumour extends to the margin of the specimen. In this situation some urologists would advise adjuvant radiotherapy post-operatively. Others would monitor PSA concentrations and advise adjuvant treatment only if these suggested progression.

Adjuvant and palliative radiotherapy

Radiotherapy as an adjuvant to surgery, for local recurrence, is helpful in managing local disease. Metastases are usually treated by hormonal methods. If hormone therapy has failed radiation to bony lesions gives fast relief. For multiple bony lesions hemibody radiation can be given. Palliative therapy is usually given over 1–2 days and can be repeated as needed.

Radionucleotide treatment

Strontium-89 and other radionucleotides can be used for palliation of bony pain. After they are are injected the radiation is emitted into the bony lesion from the isotope taken up by the metastasis. There is a danger of marrow suppression.

Hormone manipulation

In 1941 Dr Huggins produced the pioneering work showing that prostate cancer was hormone sensitive. Castration or oestrogen therapy produced shrinkage of the cancer.

Early local disease

This is rarely treated by hormone manipulation, which has significant side-effects and can never cure the disease but can only suppress it for about 3 years. If it is decided that a fit, relatively young man does need treatment for early local disease, he should have potentially curative treatment by radical surgery or radiotherapy. Older, less fit men with such asymptomatic disease are often best spared the side-effects of hormone therapy until symptoms develop.

Advanced local disease and metastatic disease

Orchidectomy is still the easiest, simplest and cheapest method of androgen ablation.

Luteinizing hormone releasing hormone (LHRH) agonists were introduced in the 1980s and are preferred to surgical orchidectomy by many men. A chemical castration results. For about 3 weeks after the first dose there is stimulation of luteinizing hormone (LH) and the serum testosterone can increase, risking a flare of disease activity. This period is usually covered by anti-androgen therapy.

Anti-androgens block androgen activity at the cellular level. Cyproterone acetate is a steroidal anti-androgen. Bicalutamide, flutamide and nilutamide are non-steroidal. Anti-androgens used alone are a helpful option in men who wish to preserve potency. There are a number of important side-effects. Liver toxicity can rarely be fatal and liver function should be monitored. Gynaecomastia and breast pain are a problem for many men.

Complete androgen blockade involves the use of anti-androgens with orchidectomy or LHRH agonists. There may be an advantage in survival and disease-free interval for a small subset of younger men with low volume metastases, although a meta-analysis has not shown this.

The main side-effects of orchidectomy and LHRH agonists are loss of masculinity, hot flushes and increase in body mass. The flushes will usually respond to cyproterone acetate and will diminish with time.

There is some evidence that intermittent hormone therapy can be as effective as continuous treatment, with reduced severity of side-effects.

About 80% of patients respond to hormone therapy. Rapidity and completeness of PSA response is a predictor of prognosis. Poorly differentiated tumours often respond incompletely, for a short period only, or not at all.

Relapse on hormone therapy

A population of hormone insensitive cells eventually emerges in most men on hormone therapy. The anti-androgens mentioned above will produce a temporary response in 25% of men after relapse following primary treatment.

In men who have shown a durable initial response to an anti-androgen used alone as first line treatment or in complete androgen blockade it is worth withdrawing the drug for a trial period as there may be a response (rare, but well documented).

Estramustine phosphate is a cytotoxic agent linked to an oestrogen. The principle of its use is that the oestrogen attaches to tumour receptors and the cytotoxic agent is released locally, giving a useful second-line treatment without the systemic cytotoxicity.

Ketoconazole, megestrol acetate, aminoglutethamide, prednisolone and dexamethasone have all shown secondary hormonal effects. Dexamethasone and prednisolone are most commonly used. As well as a direct effect on tumour tissue, they have a non-specific effect in increasing appetite and weight and producing a sense of well-being.

Chemotherapy

The response to non-hormonal chemotherapy has been disappointing. Such treatment is currently used only in clinical trials.

Palliative interventions

Transurethral resection (TUR) can relieve bladder outflow obstruction caused by the malignant prostate. Repeat TUR can fail due to encasement of the prostate area by rigid tumour and extension of the tumour to the external sphincter where resection would cause incontinence. Hormone manipulation may give as good a result over time in the patient presenting with obstruction.

Stenting of an obstructed ureter can help preserve kidney function in late stage disease when quality of life is good. Stenting from below by cystoscopy may not be possible. Antegrade stenting via percutaneous nephrostomy (Module 60 and Figure 60.11) is an alternative and usually more successful approach. Occasionally it may be justified to transpose the ureters into the dome of the bladder at open surgery.

Palliative radiotherapy is very useful for recurrent haemorrhage from a malignant prostate as well as for painful bony metastases as described above.

Medical palliation by steroid therapy and morphine with the help of palliative care physicians and nurses, blood transfusion for anaemia, catheter care and management of incontinence, family support, etc. are needed for the declining patient when specific therapy has failed. Quality of life is important and the patient should be looked after at home surrounded by his caring family wherever possible. Pointless interventions and hospital treatments should be avoided.

Paraplegia

This emergency, due to intradural extension of spinal metastases, can result in a paralysed dying patient, but if correctly managed can restore the ability to walk. It is occasionally the mode of presentation of prostate cancer. Immediate referral with a view to spinal decompression, radiotherapy and hormone therapy is essential and can give dramatic relief.

Future developments

Changes in attitudes, increased awareness and the trend towards screening will lead to more men presenting with earlier stage disease. The impact this may have on deaths from disease or on the burden of disease for society is unknown.

Gene therapy is already being used in studies on humans with prostate cancer. Adenovirus, vaccinia and dendritic cell therapy are among the exciting areas being studied.

Surgery will increasingly be in the hands of specialists. Laparoscopic radical prostatectomy, with lower morbidity and shorter hospital stay, is gaining popularity.

Hormone therapy will be the mainstay of treatment for advanced and metastatic disease. Novel agents such as LHRH antagonists are being developed but orchidectomy is likely to remain popular, as it has been for half a century.

Novel, less toxic chemotherapy may be used in earlier disease stages aiming to enhance the response to conventional therapies such as radiation and hormone therapy.

Further reading

Klein, E. A., ed. (2000). *Management of Prostate Cancer.* Totowa, NJ: Humana Press.

Lu Yao, G. L. and Yao, S. L. (1997). Population based study of long term survival in patients with clinically localised prostate cancer. *Lancet* **349**: 906–10.

Nixon, R. G. and Brawer, M. K. (1998). Refinements in serum prostate-specific antigen testing for the diagnosis of prostate cancer. In: Kirby, R. S. and O'Leary, M. P., eds. *Recent Advances in Urology*. Edinburgh: Churchill Livingstone.

Peeling, W. B., ed. (1996). *Questions and Uncertainties About Prostate Cancer*. Oxford: Blackwell Science.

Pienta, K. J., ed. (1999). Hormone refractory prostate cancer. *Urol Clin North Am* **26**(2).

Schroder, F. H. and Bangma, C. H. (1997). The European Randomised Study of Screening for Prostate Cancer. *Br J Urol* **79**(Suppl 1): 68–71.

Taneja, S. S. and Belldegrun, A. (1998). Prospects for the application of gene therapy to urologic malignancy. In: Kirby, R. S., O'Leary, M. P., eds. *Recent Advances in Urology*. Edinburgh: Churchill Livingstone.

MODULE 60

Urinary stone disease: upper urinary tract obstruction

The pathophysiology of upper tract obstruction is discussed in Section 12.1 of Volume I. Obstruction leads first to increased peristalsis in an attempt to overcome the obstruction. Later, muscle activity is reduced leading to stasis, dilatation and an increased risk of infection and stone formation.

Stones are the commonest cause of obstruction. Pelvi-ureteric junction obstruction and extrinsic ureteric obstruction account for almost all other cases. Urothelial tumours of the ureter are a rare cause of obstruction.

Stones in the urinary tract have been recorded as early as 4800 BC in Egyptian mummies. Despite advances in detection and treatment, the aetiology of most stones remains obscure. There have been several milestones in the treatment of stones, most notably extracorporeal shockwave lithotripsy (SWL). Endoscopic techniques and SWL have made the treatment of stone disease almost entirely minimally invasive. Open surgery is almost obsolete. The next challenge is to find simple and reliable ways to reduce stone recurrence rates, which can be as high as 75% at 10 years.

Section 60.1 • Epidemiology of stone disease

Urolithiasis in technologically developed countries principally occurs in the upper urinary tract, while bladder stones are common in less developed areas. The incidence of urinary calculi peaks between the ages of 30 and 50 years. The male-to-female ratio is about 3:1, and the prevalence 2–3%. Prevalence is related to geographic location: USA, UK, Scandinavian countries, northern India, Pakistan and China have particularly high levels. Climatic factors play a role: there is a relationship between high environmental temperatures and stone disease and a seasonal incidence of stone presentation. High fluid intake (hence high urine output) lowers the incidence of urinary calculi. There have been a few reports to suggest that urinary calculi are more likely in affluent people and those with sedentary occupations. The incidence of urolithiasis appears to be increasing, perhaps because of dietary changes.

Section 60.2 • Chemistry and pathophysiology of stone formation

Stone formation requires supersaturated urine. The point at which saturation is reached and crystallization occurs is known as the thermodynamic solubility product. High concentrations of calcium, oxalate, phosphate and urate, low concentrations of citrate and magnesium and low urinary volume increase the calcium/oxalate supersaturation, which may then exceed its thermodynamic solubility product. Even under these conditions, however, crystallization does not occur as urine contains inhibitors, which allow higher concentrations to be held in solution. Thus, urine is said to be metastable with respect to calcium oxalate. As concentration increases further, crystallization occurs. Concentration at this point is known as the formation product. These events are summarized in Figure 60.1.

Stasis

Stasis is an important factor in stone formation: it causes crystal retention, promoting stone growth. Anatomical abnormalities causing stasis or increased crystal adherence to the epithelium can predispose to stone formation. Most stones have a layered structure, suggesting intermittent growth during periods of supersaturation and/or stasis.

Modifiers of crystal formation

Urine contains many substances which alter or modify crystal formation, including inhibitors, complexers and

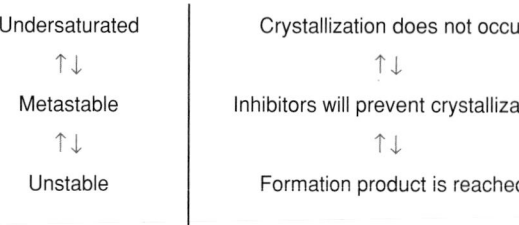

Undersaturated	Crystallization does not occur
↑↓	↑↓
Metastable	Inhibitors will prevent crystallization
↑↓	↑↓
Unstable	Formation product is reached

Figure 60.1 Chemistry of stone formation.

promoters. The potent inhibitors are Tamm–Horsfall protein, nephrocalcin and uropontin. In stone formers the concentration of these inhibitors has been shown to be lower than in non-stone formers. Citrate and magnesium are complexers and also inhibit crystallization. The promoters include certain glycosaminoglycans and Tamm-Horsfall protein (which may act as an inhibitor or promoter).

Nucleation

Nucleation occurs when calcium oxalate supersaturation is seven to 11 times its solubility. Crystal nuclei usually form on epithelial cell debris, urinary casts, other crystals and red blood cells. This is known as heterogeneous nucleation. Further crystals aggregate on these nuclei.

Epitaxy

The theory of epitaxy attempts to explain the formation of mixed stones. If the lattice structure of one crystal is similar to that of a different crystal, the second crystal may be able to nucleate and grow on the first. The most well-described example of this is the growth of calcium oxalate crystals on sodium urate crystals, which helps to explain the increased incidence of calcium oxalate stones in patients with elevated urinary concentrations of uric acid.

Matrix

Calculi usually contain organic material called matrix. The exact role of matrix in stone formation is unknown. It may act as a nidus for crystal aggregation or as a naturally occurring glue to adhere crystal components.

Section 60.3 • Aetiology of urolithiasis

- **Idiopathic urolithiasis** is said to account for 70–80% of stone disease, but some investigators report that meticulous investigation shows a cause in up to 90%.
- **Hypercalciuria** is the most common abnormality found in standard investigation. It may be idiopathic or due to increased intestinal absorption, renal leak or bone demineralization.
- **Hyperparathyroidism** causes 5%.
- **Inherited enzyme disorders** such as cystinuria or renal tubular syndromes cause 1%.
- **Hyperoxaluria** can be either primary (a rare genetic disorder), or enteric in patients with short bowel syndrome or fat malabsorption (due to increased binding of calcium in the bowel).
- **Hyperuricosuria** can be due to increased dietary purine intake, defective renal tubular handling of uric acid or rare hereditary enzyme deficiency.

An extensive list of causes is given in Table 60.1.

Section 60.4 • Types of urinary stones

- **Calcium oxalate**: 70% of stones.
- **Calcium phosphate**: 10% of stones. Pure calcium phosphate stones are rare and usually seen in renal tubular acidosis.
- **Struvite** (infective or triple phosphate stones): about 15% of stones. They are composed of calcium, magnesium, ammonium and phosphate. Infection with urease-producing bacteria, usually Proteus, is needed for struvite stone formation.
- **Uric acid**: 5% of stones. They form in acidic, concentrated urine.
- **Cystine**: 1% of stones. They occur in cystinuria, an autosomal recessive disorder.

Xanthine, silicate, triamterene and indinavir are contituents of rare stones.

Table 60.1 Causes of urolithiasis

Renal tubular syndromes
Renal tubular acidosis
Cystinuria
Hypercalcaemic disorders
Primary hyperparathyroidism
Immobilization
Milk-alkali syndrome
Sarcoidosis
Hypervitaminosis D
Neoplastic diseases
Cushing's syndrome
Hyperthyroidism
Uric acid lithiasis
Idiopathic
Gout
Low urine output states
Myeloproliferative disorders
Enzyme disorders
Primary hyperoxaluria
Xanthinuria
2,8-Dihydroxyadeninuria
Secondary urolithiasis
Enteric hyperoxaluria
Infection
Obstruction
Medullary sponge kidney
Urinary diversion
Drugs (e.g. indinavir)
Idiopathic calcium urolithiasis
Hypercalciuria
Normocalciuria

Adapted from Gillenwater, J. Y., Grayhack, J. T., Howard, S. S. and Duckett, J. W., eds. *Adult and Paediatric Urology*, 3rd edn. St Louis, MO: Mosby, 1996.

Section 60.5 • Clinical presentation

Renal stone disease most commonly presents as an acute episode of renal or ureteric colic as a result of the stone causing complete or partial obstruction.

The commonest area of impaction of a stone is at the vesico-ureteric junction, the narrowest part of the upper urinary tract.

Other common sites of impaction are:

- where the ureter crosses the iliac blood vessels, at the pelvic brim
- the pelvi-ureteric junction
- in the necks of the calices.

A typical episode of renal or ureteric colic is abrupt in onset; the patient is in very severe pain and cannot lie still. The pain usually starts in the loin and radiates anteriorly to the groin, scrotum or labia and sometimes to the tip of the urethra, depending on the site of the stone. A stone at the vesico-ureteric junction may cause urgency, frequency and pain referrred along the urethra as a result of irritation of the trigone.

Nausea and vomiting are commonly associated with renal colic and may raise the possibility of other acute abdominal pathology.

The differential diagnosis of renal colic includes:

- On either side:
  - **gonadal pathology** (the gonad has the same autonomic nerve supply as the kidney)
    - torsion of the testis
    - twisted ovarian cyst
    - tubo-ovarian abscess
  - **musculo-skeletal pain**, especially tearing of the insertion of quadratus lumborum at the lower border of the twelfth rib
  - **basal pneumonia**.
- On the right side:
  - **biliary disease**
  - **appendicitis**
  - inflammation of Meckel's diverticulum.
- On the left side:
  - **leaking abdominal aortic aneurysm**
  - **sigmoid diverticulitis.**

Other presentations of renal calculi include haematuria, recurrent urinary tract infections, pyonephrosis or septicaemia. Occasionally, the patient may be asymptomatic and calculous disease may be an incidental finding. Rarely the patient may present in end stage renal failure secondary to bilateral disease.

Section 60.6 • Investigations

Baseline tests

In any stone presentation evidence of sepsis should be sought on physical examination. Temperature, pulse, blood pressure and urine analysis are mandatory. In about 85% of cases, there is evidence of microscopic or gross haematuria on urinalysis. Pyuria and crystalluria may provide evidence of underlying calculous disease. A midstream urine for culture and sensitivity, full blood count and creatinine, urea and electrolytes are mandatory.

Imaging

Plain abdominal radiograph

Ninety per cent of stones in the urinary tract are radio-opaque. They should be seen on plain abdominal films (Figure 60.2a) but are notoriously easy to miss if overlying the sacro-iliac joint. A small ureteric calculus may be difficult to see due to gas and faeces or to confusion with other opacities such as phleboliths and arterial calcification. Renal tomography without contrast is occasionally helpful.

Ultrasound

Up to 25% of patients with ureteric stones have normal ultrasound appearances, because in severe obstruction renal shutdown may prevent hydronephrosis developing. Ureteric calculi are often difficult to see.

Intravenous urography

This will usually confirm the diagnosis by demonstrating a delay in function and dilatation down to the stone or filling defect (Figure 60.2b). It is essential to ensure that renal function is not significantly impaired (by serum creatinine concentration) before the urogram. Delayed films can be taken up to 24 hours after the injection of contrast if necessary.

Spiral computed tomography

This is rapidly emerging as the investigation of choice for the detection of ureteric calculi in an acute situation. The drawbacks are its availability and cost implications.

Retrograde studies

These are not usually done for diagnosis due to their invasive nature and the fact that the diagnosis can almost always be made by other means. They are occasionally needed when there is no function in the affected kidney.

Section 60.7 • Treatment

Treatment can be divided into:

- treatment of the acute episode
- interval treatment
- prevention of recurrences or new stone formation.

Treatment of the acute episode

Expectant treatment

If the greatest diameter of the stone is <4 mm, spontaneous passage is very likely, but surface characteristics of the stone may be as important as size.

The first priority is to relieve pain. This is best done by non-steroidal anti-inflammatory drugs. Diclofenac is the most commonly used. It is contraindicated in pregnancy, in asthmatic patients and in peptic ulcer disease, in which situations morphine is the drug of choice. The common measure of forced diuresis in the

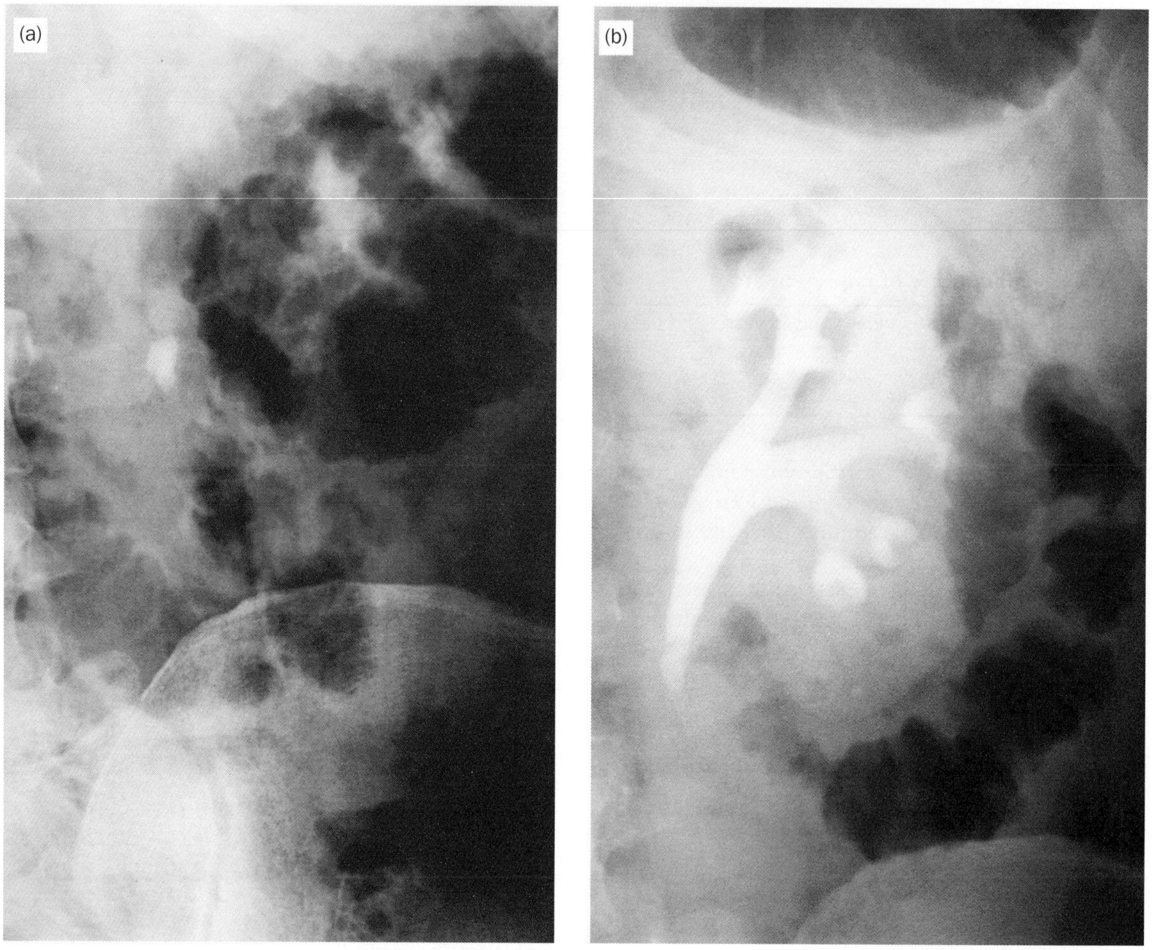

Figure 60.2 (a) Plain radiograph and (b) IVU showing obstructing upper ureteric calculus.

acute situation may be unhelpful, as an increase in diuresis may decrease ureteric peristalsis and hinder the passage of stones. Antibiotics must be given if there is any clinical suspicion of infection.

Expectant treatment can continue as long as pain is under control, there are no signs of infection, serum creatinine is normal and the patient is prepared to wait. The indications for emergency treatment are given below. Early elective treatment is indicated if the stone is of a size which is unlikely to pass (>7 mm) or if the stone fails to move after a 'reasonable period' (which is largely determined by the patient's preferences).

Intervention

The indications for emergency intervention are:

- significant obstruction with infection
- intractable pain
- progressive renal deterioration
- anuria due to obstruction in a solitary kidney
- pyelonephitis (without significant obstruction) not responding to antibiotic treatment.

The options for emergency treatment are:

- nephrostomy
- stenting
- ureteroscopic extraction
- SWL (see below) if on site.

The management of acute upper urinary tract obstruction is summarized in Figure 60.3. The advantages and disadvantages of stenting and nephrostomy are shown in Table 60.2.

Interval treatment

Surgical treatment

Surgery forms the mainstay of treatment of calculous disease of the urinary tract both in the acute presentation as described above and as interval treatment after an acute episode or in patients presenting to the outpatient clinic. There have been marked changes in the treatment of urinary stone disease with the increasing use of minimally invasive therapies. Percutaneous nephrolithotomy, extracorporeal shock wave lithotripsy and ureterorenoscopy have transformed treatment. Open surgery is virtually obsolete.

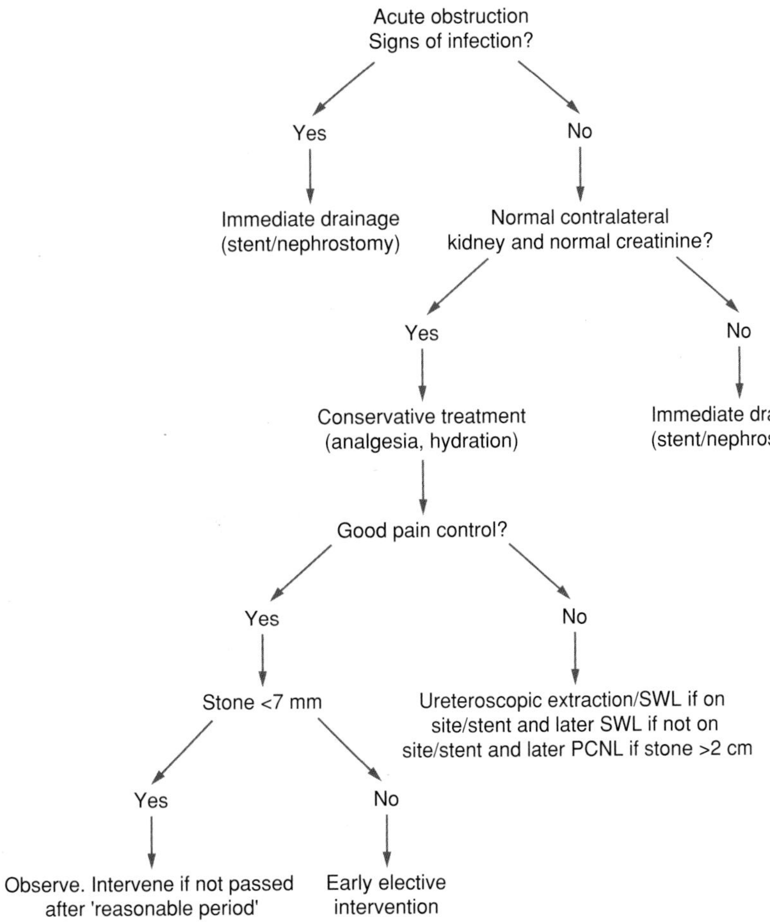

Figure 60.3 Management of acute upper urinary obstruction.

Shockwave lithotripsy

Since its initial use in 1982, shockwave lithotripsy (SWL) has become widely accepted as first-line treatment for the majority of urinary calculi. There are many different types of lithotriptors available, which are usually characterized by the type of shockwave generator: electrohydraulic, electromagnetic or piezoelectric. The shockwaves are focused on the stone by an ellipsoid reflector: imaging is by fluoroscopy and/or ultrasound (Figures 60.4 and 60.5).

Mechanism of action of SWL:

- As the shockwave strikes the anterior surface of the stone, it splits into two components. One is reflected back towards the source, the other enters the stone. These opposing forces create a pressure gradient, producing fragmentation and erosion.
- A similar phenomenon occurs as the shockwave strikes the posterior surface.
- Cavitation is an acoustic phenomenon in which pressure changes cause the rapid expansion of gas bubbles in a liquid medium. These unstable bubbles collapse explosively forming microjets, which strike the stone at high velocities, causing erosions and microscopic fractures.

Table 60.2 Advantages and disadvantages of stenting and nephrostomy

Stent	*Nephrostomy*
Usually needs general anaestheic for insertion and change	Usually placed and changed with local anaesthesia
Increases pressure in renal pelvis	Drains collecting system at low pressure
May not drain pyonephrosis	Drain pus well
Cannot be flushed after placement	Can be flushed if blocked
May irritate bladder	No bladder or trigone irritation
Vesico-renal reflux – may cause pain and ascending infection	No vesico-renal reflux
Cannot be dislodged by external force	Sometimes 'falls out'
May not resist external compression (e.g. by malignancy)	Drains kidney even when ureter totally obstructed
May be suitable for indefinite drainage (with changes every 3–6 months)	Not suitable for long-term drainage
May be 'lost to follow-up'	Unlikely to be 'lost to follow-up'

Indications for SWL:

- **Renal calculi** – stones less than 2 cm in diameter have up to a 90% chance of fragmentation and clearance. Stones in the lower pole or in caliceal diverticula give lower success rates.
- **Ureteric calculi** – SWL is recommended as first line treatment for most patients with stones 1 cm or less in the proximal ureter (Figure 60.6). SWL and ureteroscopy are equally acceptable choices for stones of this size in the distal ureter. Stones in the mid-ureter are often inaccessible to SWL because the sacro-iliac joint obscures them.
- **Bladder calculi** – can be treated with the patient prone.

Stone size is a very important factor. Renal calculi 2 cm or less and ureteric calculi 1 cm or less in diameter are the ideal stone sizes for SWL. Renal calculi between 2 and 3 cm in diameter may be treated after placement of a ureteric stent, but stone-free rates are poor and the risk of complications increases. Larger stones are best treated by PCNL (see below). Treatment of staghorn calculi is indicated only in rare cases with a normal collecting system and a relatively low stone burden.

Stone composition is relevant to the success of SWL. Calcium oxalate monohydrate, calcium phosphate and cystine stones are more difficult to fragment. The contraindications to SWL are given in Table 60.3, and the complications in Table 60.4.

Special cases and limitations:

Children usually require general anaesthesia. Treatment of stones over the sacro-iliac joint may damage the epiphyseal plates and cause skeletal growth disturbances.

Anomalous kidneys can safely be treated with SWL. The prone position is recommended in pelvic kidneys; in horseshoe kidneys stone visualization can be a problem because of the overlying bony skeleton. In solitary kidneys stent placement is recommended for stones >7 mm in diameter.

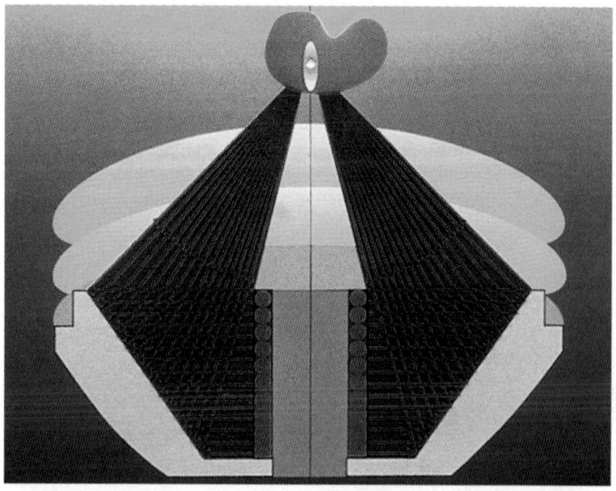

Figure 60.4 Principle of shockwave lithotripsy (SWL). Shockwaves produced by the generator (electrohydraulic, electromagnetic or piezoelectric) are focused by an ellipsoid reflector. (Courtesy of Karl Storz Medical.)

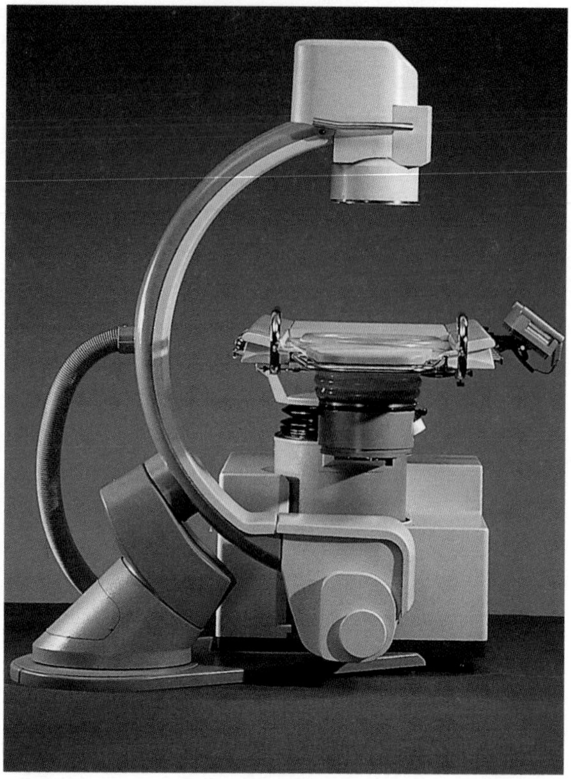

Figure 60.5 A modern lithotriptor. A fluid 'cushion' transmits the shockwaves from the generator/reflector to the skin surface, from where they travel through the tissues to the stone. (Courtesy of Karl Storz Medical.)

Aneurysms of the abdominal aorta and renal artery need caution, using intensive haemodynamic monitoring.

Cardiac pacemakers are not disturbed by SWL.

Obesity can make imaging difficult. Most machines have weight limits.

Uterorenoscopy

Advances in instrumentation (Module 55) allow access to the entire urinary tract. Devices such as the electrohydraulic, ultrasonic and ballistic lithotriptors and the holmium:YAG laser have made the treatment of refractory stones easier. Ureteroscopy may be the first option in centres with high a degree of expertise or where availability of SWL is limited.

Table 60.3 Contraindications to SWL

Absolute:	Pregnancy Uncontrolled coagulopathy Uncontrolled hypertension Urinary tract obstruction distal to the stone Urinary tract infection with fever
Relative:	Urinary tract infection Distal ureteric calculi in women of child-bearing age

Table 60.4 Complications of SWL

Steinstrasse ('stone street'): A column of fragments in the ureter
- may be prevented by stent placement
- nephrostomy is needed if there is infection, obstruction or intractable pain; this measure alone can clear the fragments in 70%
- the leading fragment can be treated by more SWL
- ureteroscopy may be required to clear remaining fragments

Bleeding
This is common and is usually self-limiting

Gastrointestinal side-effects
- pancreatitis
- elevation of hepatic enzymes
- incidental fragmentation of gallbladder calculi causing biliary colic
- mucosal erosions and submucosal haematomas of the colon

Mortality
There is a reported mortality rate of 0.02%

Hypertension
Some long-term studies show an 8.2% prevalence of new onset hypertension after SWL. This is controversial

The indications for ureteroscopy are:

- Ureteric calculi that cannot be visualized for SWL or which have not responded to SWL.
- Renal calculi not responding to SWL, or residual stones after percutaneous treatment.
- Radiolucent stones or filling defects which need to be inspected.

Stenting with a double pigtail stent is generally recommended after ureteroscopic treatment, but may not be needed after the use of small diameter ureteroscopes. Reported stone free rates following ureteroscopy vary from 62% to 100%. Clearing all fragments at the time of ureteroscopy gives better stone-free rates at 3 months than leaving even a few small fragments which are expected to pass. Complications such as perforation, false passage and avulsion of the ureter have been reported in up to 9% of cases. The placement of a safety guidewire and the use of grasping forceps instead of baskets can reduce the risk of avulsion. Injuries from the use of *in situ* lithotriptor devices are a potential problem. The risk of stricture formation is much reduced with careful instrumentation, use of small diameter ureteroscopes, use of flexible instruments, increasing experience and sound judgement.

Percutaneous nephrolithotomy

Percutaneous nephrolithotomy (PCNL) was the first 'keyhole surgery'. The pelvicaliceal system is punctured

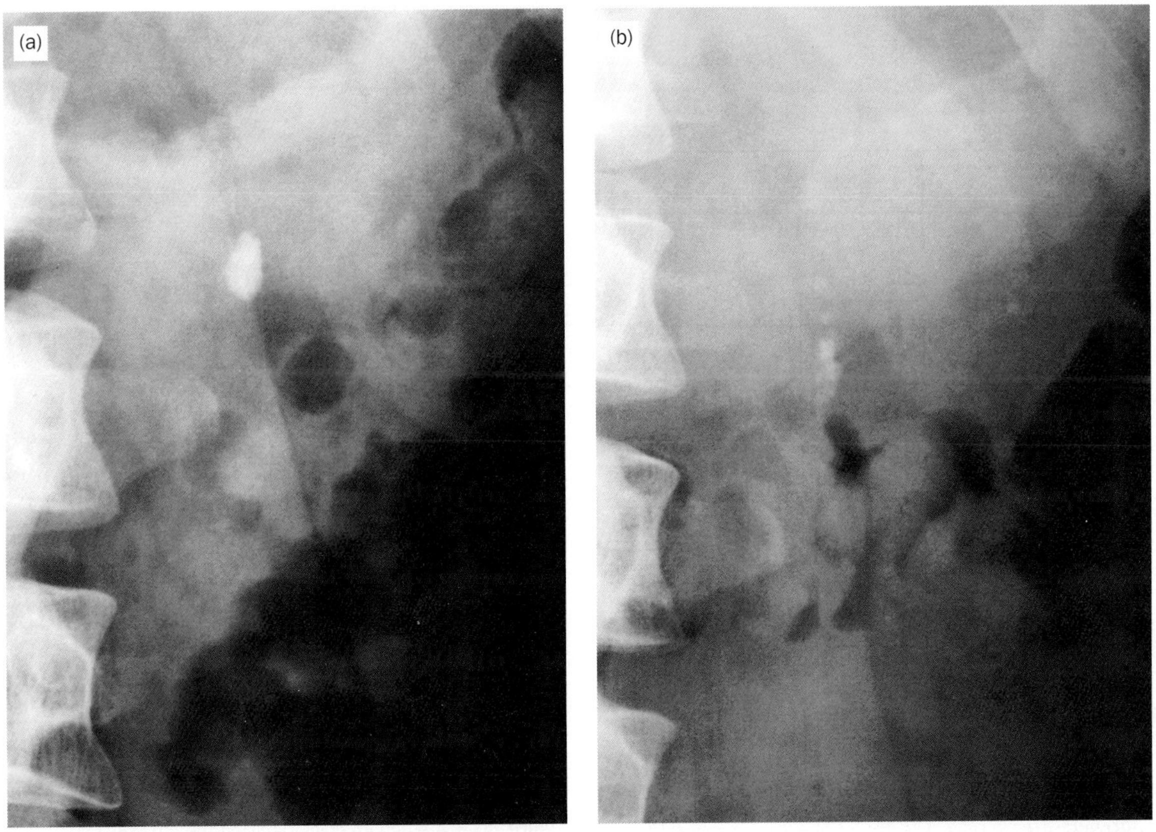

Figure 60.6 Plain radiographs showing an upper ureteric stone (a) before and (b) after SWL.

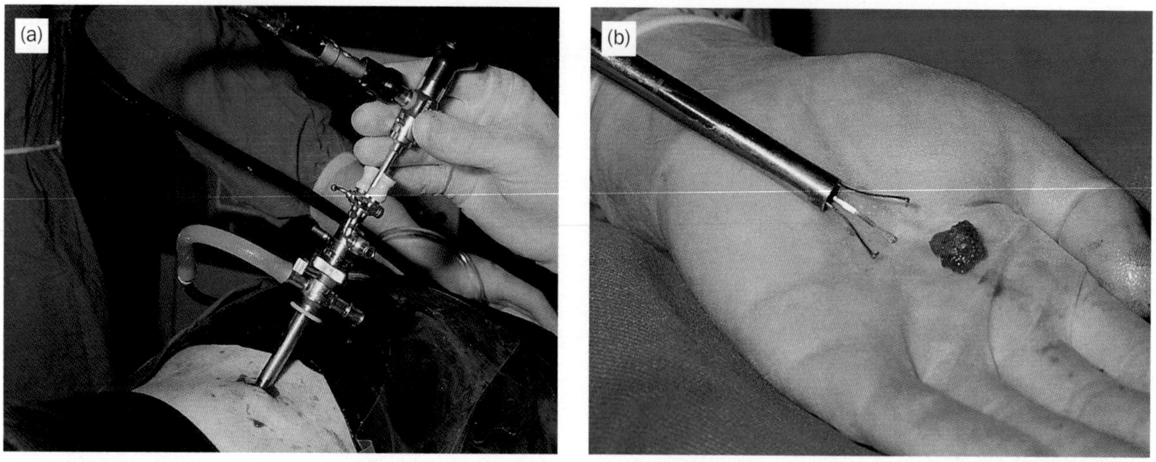

Figure 60.7 Percutaneous nephrolithotomy (PCNL). (a) A nephroscope is passed down the track from skin to pelvicaliceal system. (b) The stone is removed entire if <1 cm in diameter. Larger stones are fragmented by devices (ultrasonic, kinetic or laser) passed via the nephroscope.

under fluoroscopic control. A guidewire is inserted through the puncturing needle. A series of dilators is passed over the guidewire until a track 1 cm wide (30 Fr) is made through the skin, fat, muscle, perinephric fascia, renal capsule and cortex into the pelvicaliceal system. Instruments for stone removal and disintegration can be passed down this track (Figure 60.7).

The absolute indications for PCNL are:

- Staghorn calculi (Figure 60.8) and large (>3 cm) renal calculi.
- Failed SWL for stones < 3 cm.
- Cystine stones refractory to SWL.
- An infected obstructed system – PCNL is done in two stages: insertion of a nephrostomy followed by lithotomy after the patient has been stabilized (usually 1–3 days later).

The relative indications for PCNL are:

- Upper and mid-ureteric calculi (with a dilated system above the stone) can be approached in an antegrade fashion via a percutaneous nephrostomy. The patient becomes stone free, but general anaesthesia is needed.
- A single kidney, or patients with renal impairment, where PCNL may cause less renal damage than SWL.
- Horseshoe kidneys, where imaging the stone on the lithotriptor can be difficult due to the lumbar spine.
- Morbidly obese patients where stone imaging and the weight of the patient may be problems on the lithotriptor (but such patients are poor anaesthetic risks).
- First-line treatment for stones in a lower pole calix with unfavourable anatomy, such as a very dependent position or a narrow neck, making fragment clearance a problem.

Results of PCNL. Overall stone-free rates after percutaneous nephrolithotomy range from 90% to 100% for stones in all situations. Rates for staghorn calculi are lower at 60– 90%. The 'sandwich technique' has improved results for large staghorn calculi. This consists of PCNL to fragment and debulk the stone, followed after 1 or 2 days by SWL, then further PCNL if necessary to remove significant fragments.

Complications of PCNL. Complications can be caused by the formation of the PCNL track (access) or by surgical stone manipulation.

Complications of access include haemorrhage, pneumothorax, hydrothorax and injury to neighbouring viscera.

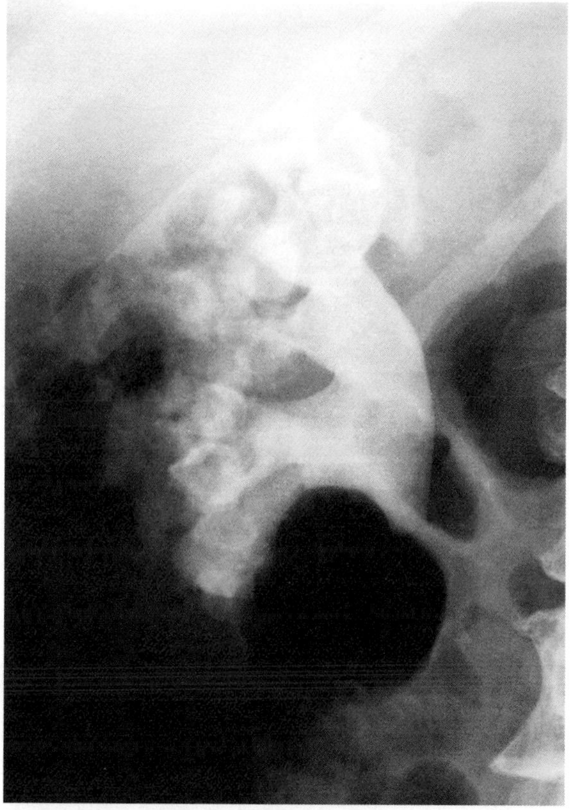

Figure 60.8 A staghorn calculus filling the intrarenal collecting system. Percutaneous debulking is needed before SWL.

Complications of stone manipulation include haemorrhage obscuring vision, irrigant absorption with fluid overload, perforation of the collecting system and extravasation of fluid, sepsis, residual and lost fragments, and delayed haemorrhage. If bleeding persists, percutaneous embolization of the bleeding vessel may be required. Operative time should be limited to 1 hour, as the risk of fluid absorption and sepsis increases after this.

The mortality rate following PCNL is 0.1–0.7%. Transfusion rates up to 10% are reported.

Open stone surgery

The prevalence of open stone surgery in specialist urology departments is well under 2%, but in some developing countries open stone surgery still has a significant role. In tertiary referral centres open surgery is reserved for a selected group of patients with complex stone burden, and for treatment failures. The procedures performed are pyelolithotomy, anatrophic and radial nephrolithotomy and partial nephrectomy. In these few, selected cases open surgery is a reasonable treatment alternative with a high success rate.

Laparoscopic ureterolithotomy

Laparoscopic procedures are performed in some centres for impacted stones that have failed SWL or ureteroscopic methods of management. Their role depends on the local availability of laparoscopic and ureteroscopic expertise and equipment.

Non-surgical treatment

Uric acid stones can be dissolved by a high fluid intake and alkalization of the urine with sodium bicarbonate or potassium citrate. Cystine and struvite stones can also be dissolved, although less successfully. Cystine stones can be dissolved by oral hydration, alkalization and cystine complexing agents, such as D-penicillamine and α-mercaptopropionylglycine (MPG). Struvite stones may undergo partial or complete dissolution after antimicrobial therapy. A list of pharmacological treatments for prevention or dissolution of stones is given in Table 60.5.

Metabolic investigations

All stones should be analysed if recovered. If the stone cannot be recovered a urine cystine screen should be performed. Patients most likely to have a detectable metabolic abnormality, such as those with multiple stones, recurrent stones (>1 per year), nephrocalcinosis, radiolucent stones or age <30 years at first presentation should undergo a complete evaluation. This consists of a detailed history including diet, fluid loss, medications and evidence of any underlying abnormalities or recurrent urinary tract infections. Laboratory tests include measurement of serum calcium, phosphate and urate. Serum parathormone concentration should be measured if the patient is hypercalcaemic. A 24 hour urine collection to measure urine pH, total volume, and concentrations of calcium, oxalate, magnesium, phosphate, sodium, citrate and uric acid is often the most useful test.

Table 60.5 Drugs used and their indications in the prevention of stone recurrence

Thiazides	Calcium oxalate stones, idiopathic hypercalciuria
Citrate	Hypocitraturic calcium stone formers; uric acid and cystine stones (by raising urine pH)
Allopurinol	Uric acid stones with high serum urate
Phosphate	Absorptive and renal hypercalciuria
Sodium cellulose phosphate	Absorptive hypercalciuria
Magnesium	Decreases calcium oxalate and phosphate crystal formation
Pyridoxine	Primary hyperoxaluria
α-Mercaptopropionylglycine	Cystine stones
D-penicillamine	Cystine stones

Prevention of recurrences

- Fifty to seventy-five per cent of patients have recurrences within 10 years of the first episode. Ideally, prevention requires analysis of the chemical composition of the stone and diagnosis of the cause.

There is controversy over which patients should undergo extensive metabolic investigation and, when appropriate, medical treatment. Patients with cystine and struvite stones, who have the highest risk of recurrence, require preventative treatment after surgical clearance of their stones. The majority of patients with calcium oxalate stones are best managed simply by sound dietary advice and regular follow-up. Compliance with strict medical regimens is notoriously poor, especially for a condition which is not usually life-threatening. The clinician must take into consideration the motivation of the patient, which generally increases with each subsequent episode of stone passage or treatment. There will be cases where the frequency of stone recurrence is such that pharmacotherapy is justified. Hyperuricaemia needs treatment with allopurinol. The drugs used, and their respective indications, in the attempted prevention of stone recurrence are shown in Table 60.5.

Dietary factors

Fluid intake

Increase in the fluid intake leads to dilute urine and decreases the risk of stone formation. A fluid intake to produce at least 2 litres of urine output a day is adequate. The simple advice 'drink enough always to keep your urine the colour of white wine' is easier for the patient than measuring urine output.

Calcium intake

Contrary to popular belief, restriction of calcium is not advised as it increases oxalate absorption and has minimal effect on the degree of supersaturation with calcium oxalate.

High levels of dietary protein and sodium increase the risk of calcium oxalate and uric acid stone recurrence. Citric acid (the highest concentrations are found in lemon juice) and dietary fibre reduce the risk.

Section 60.8 • Future developments in stone disease

Treatment

Current techniques allow for successful minimally invasive treatment of almost all stones in specialized units. There will inevitably be advances in instrumentation, but in the next 10 years advances will more likely be as a result of dissemination of effective techniques from specialist centres to general hospitals.

Prevention

There has been little progress here. Complex metabolic evaluations and unpalatable medications have made compliance a major issue. Simplified testing for specific disorders, such as the presence of abnormal Tamm–Horsfall protein, may allow more specific targeting of patients at highest risk of recurrence.

Section 60.9 • Pelvi-ureteric junction obstruction

Pelvi-ureteric junction (PUJ) obstruction restricts urine flow from the pelvis to the ureter, producing hydronephrosis. The natural history is varied: it may progress to complete loss of renal function on the affected side or remain stable or even improve without treatment. Patients may present at any age from the pre-natal period to the eighth decade. The increasing detection of hydronephrosis as a result of pre-natal ultrasound has brought into question traditional attitudes to the aggressive treatment of this disorder. Most newborns with PUJ obstruction need only observation.

PUJ obstruction may be primary or secondary. **Primary** PUJ obstruction presenting in childhood is thought to result from incomplete recanalization of the ureter during fetal development. Longitudinal and circular muscle fibres are dysfunctional, producing an adynamic segment of ureter. PUJ obstruction presenting in adults is associated with a lower pole crossing vessel in up to one half of cases: by contrast, PUJ obstruction detected in the neonatal period is generally not associated with crossing vessels. This suggests that PUJ obstruction associated with a crossing vessel may have a distinct aetiology.

Secondary PUJ obstruction is typically the result of stone disease or previous surgery.

Clinical presentation

This largely depends on the age of the patient. Adults typically present with loin pain, classically after drinking large volumes of fluids. Children may present with an abdominal mass or non-specific abdominal pain. The pain often simulates gastrointestinal disease, with episodes of nausea and vomiting. Occasionally, patients present with signs and symptoms of pyelonephritis or pyonephrosis.

Investigations

The diagnosis is often suggested by the finding of hydronephrosis on ultrasound (Figure 60.9). The diagnosis can be confirmed by intravenous urography (IVU), which typically demonstrates contrast filling an enlarged renal pelvis with little or no contrast reaching the ureter. Hydrocalicosis may or may not be present depending on whether the pelvis is intra- or extrarenal. A diuretic renogram is useful to determine relative renal function and to quantify the response of the collecting system to a diuretic load. Typically, the curve does not show the expected fall after diuretic administration (Figures 55.2 and 55.3) and remains horizontal or rises. False negative studies can occur in patients with intermittent obstruction.

A retrograde ureteropyelogram is essential to check the ureter prior to definitive treatment. In some cases of *lower* ureteric obstruction, delayed function allows filling of the pelvis but not of the ureter during the normal time span of an IVU. This may give a false impression of PUJ obstruction.

Management

Observation by renal ultrasound at 6 monthly intervals, with isotope renography if necessary, is appropriate for hydronephrosis with good cortical thickness diagnosed on routine pre-natal ultrasound. The onset of cortical thinning or deterioration in renal function indicates intervention.

Older children and adults present because of symptoms, so intervention is virtually always appropriate.

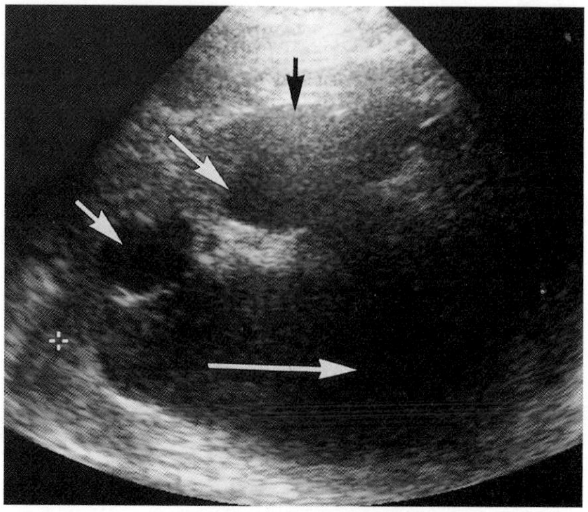

Figure 60.9 Ultrasound examination of the kidney in a young man presenting with loin pain after drinking beer. The pelvis and calices (white arrows) are dilated and the cortex (black arrow) is thinned.

Open surgery

The PUJ is exposed and may be excised and anastomosed over a stent ('dismembered pyeloplasty') or incised longitudinally (Davis procedure) or similarly incised with the insertion of a rotated flap of redundant pelvis (Culp–de Weerd pyeloplasty). A reduction pyeloplasty is often carried out with these procedures to reduce the volume of the pelvis; it improves the appearances on imaging and may well improve the urine transit time through the pelvis, reducing the risk of infection.

Laparoscopic surgery

Any of the above procedures can be carried out laparoscopically.

Endourological procedures

Modern endourological techniques are challenging open pyeloplasty as the 'gold standard' of treatment.

Endourological techniques include:

- endopyelotomy (pyelolysis)
  - antegrade, via a percutaneous nephrostomy track
  - retrograde, by ureteroscopic endopyelotomy
- balloon dilatation of the PUJ
- balloon dilatation with additional endopyelotomy by diathermy wire on balloon surface.

The main risk of these procedures is from cutting a vessel crossing in front of or behind the PUJ. Imaging studies such as endoluminal ultrasound and spiral CT (Figure 60.10) to detect crossing vessels prior to endopyelotomy improve the safety and success rate.

Results of surgery

Success rates are about 90% for open pyeloplasty, 80% for endopyelotomy and lower still for balloon dilatation with or without diathermy incision. Failure is more likely if there is poor function (<20%) on the affected side, or severe hydronephrosis.

Section 60.10 • Extrinsic ureteric obstruction

Extrinsic ureteric obstruction is unilateral in most cases. Any disease process affecting the retroperitoneal structures close to the ureter in the abdomen, or the retroperitoneal and intraperitoneal structures of the pelvis, can cause extrinsic compression. Urgent treatment is needed if obstruction is bilateral or if there is evidence of infection or uraemia. The causes of extrinsic ureteric obstruction are given in Table 60.6.

Clinical features and diagnosis

Ureteric obstruction may be an incidental finding in patients presenting with features of the underlying condition. It may occasionally present as uraemia, flank pain or sepsis. Although ultrasound may confirm dilatation, computed tomography (CT) scan with contrast is the investigation of choice. Magnetic resonance imaging (MRI) may be able to differentiate malignant disease from retroperitoneal fibrosis.

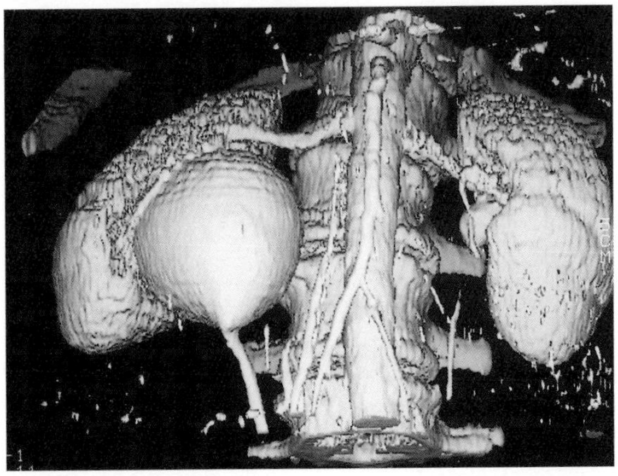

Figure 60.10 Three-dimensional reconstruction of computed tomography angiography in a case of right PUJ obstruction. In this case there are no crossing vessels.

Treatment

In an acute situation decompression is a priority. Decompression can be achieved by percutaneous nephrostomy or by retrograde stent insertion. Long-term stents, although well placed, may not relieve extrinsic obstruction as they may themselves be compressed. Specialized metallic coil stents are available. They may develop encrustation and be extremely difficult to replace, but in most cases where they are used (i.e. obstruction from extrinsic malignancy) the patient may not survive long enough for these problems to develop.

In general, acute decompression is appropriate in patients with obstruction from an unknown cause or a treatable cause. The development of bilateral ureteric obstruction secondary to pelvic malignancy raises ethical issues regarding quality of life. A frank discussion of the prognosis may be needed, especially when the underlying cause is recurrent malignancy with no effective treatment.

Percutaneous nephrostomy (Figure 60.11a) is the simplest method of acute decompression and allows for rapid restoration of renal function. It is less acceptable as a long-term solution. Antegrade stenting via a nephrostomy is often successful where a retrograde approach from the bladder has failed. If both techniques fail there is the possibility of tunnelling a stent subcutaneously from the nephrostomy puncture wound around the flank to the anterior abdominal wall and then into the bladder.

Other operative techniques such as a transuretero-ureterostomy, uretero-neocystostomy, ileal interposition or urinary diversion (e.g. by ileal conduit) are rarely appropriate. Again, the underlying disease process, prognosis and quality of life play a significant role in the decision-making process.

Retroperitoneal fibrosis

Retroperitoneal fibrosis (RPF) is characterized by encasement of retroperitoneal structures by inflammatory proliferation of fibrous tissue.

Table 60.6 Causes of extrinsic ureteric obstruction

Benign gynaecological disorders
Endometriosis
Benign pelvic masses
Uterine prolapse
Malignancies
Cervical
Bladder
Prostatic
Colorectal
Iatrogenic
Following surgery or radiotherapy
Retroperitoneal diseases
Retroperitoneal fibrosis
Retroperitoneal tumours, including lymph node disease
Retroperitoneal infections and haemorrhage
Vascular causes
Abdominal aortic aneurysm
Iliac aneurysm
After reconstructive vascular surgery
Retrocaval ureter
Ovarian vein syndrome
Post-partum ovarian vein thrombophlebitis
Gastrointestinal causes
Inflammatory bowel disease
Diverticular disease
Pancreatic lesions

Aetiology

There is no known cause in 70% of cases. The known causes and associations of RPF are given in Table 60.7.

Clinical features of RPF

- Predominantly a disease of the fifth and sixth decades
- male-to-female ratio is 2:1
- insidious onset with non-specific symptoms
- anorexia
- weight loss
- general malaise
- pyrexia of unknown origin
- non-specific gastrointestinal symptoms
- two-thirds present with uraemia due to bilateral ureteric obstruction
- flank or loin pain is common.

Diagnosis

- Raised erthrocyte sedimentation rate (ESR)
- anaemia
- uraemia
- IVU shows medial deviation of the ureter which:
  - is usually in the middle third
  - is usually bilateral
  - involves long segments of ureter
- CT scan:
  - usually shows dense fibrous tissue encasing retroperitoneal structures
  - involvement is commonly from renal pedicles to iliac bifurcation and out to lateral borders of psoas.

Definitive diagnosis depends on biopsy.

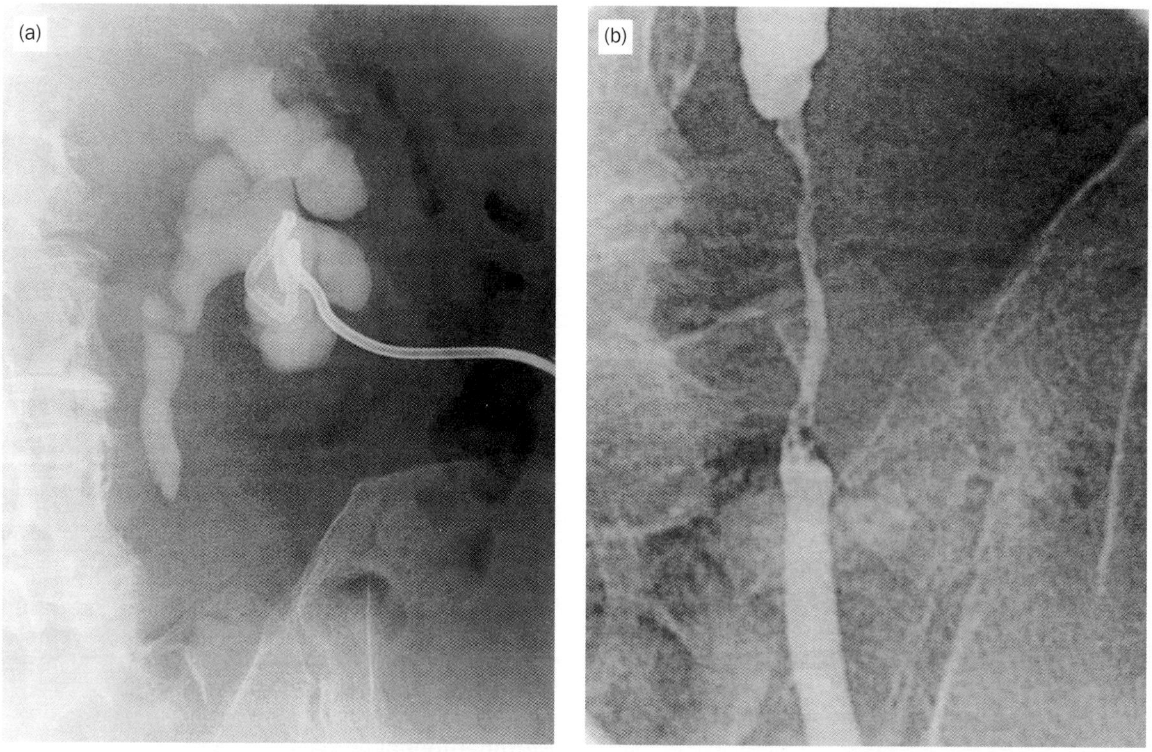

Figure 60.11 (a) Percutaneous nephrostomy as emergency treatment for mid-ureteric obstruction caused by retroperitoneal lymph nodes containing metastatic breast cancer. The patient presented with bacteraemia due to pyonephrosis. (b) A subsequent retrograde study confirms a long, tight rigid section. Retrograde stenting was impossible. Antegrade stenting via the nephrostomy succeeded.

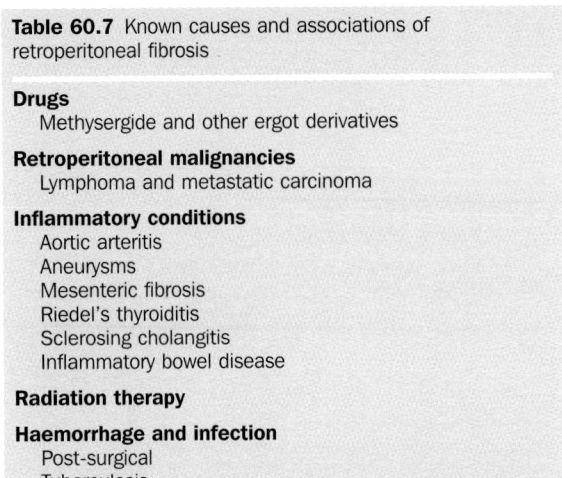

Table 60.7 Known causes and associations of retroperitoneal fibrosis

Drugs
Methysergide and other ergot derivatives
Retroperitoneal malignancies
Lymphoma and metastatic carcinoma
Inflammatory conditions
Aortic arteritis
Aneurysms
Mesenteric fibrosis
Riedel's thyroiditis
Sclerosing cholangitis
Inflammatory bowel disease
Radiation therapy
Haemorrhage and infection
Post-surgical
Tuberculosis
Schistosomiasis

Management

The principles of management are shown in Figure 60.12. Corticosteriods are effective, especially if the ESR is very high. Failure to respond in 3 weeks indicates surgery. Surgical treatment involves exploration, biopsy and ureterolysis. The ureters can be placed intraperitoneally or wrapped in omentum in an attempt to prevent recurrence.

Prognosis

This generally depends on the underlying cause and the degree of renal impairment at presentation. Recurrence is common and patients should be followed indefinitely.

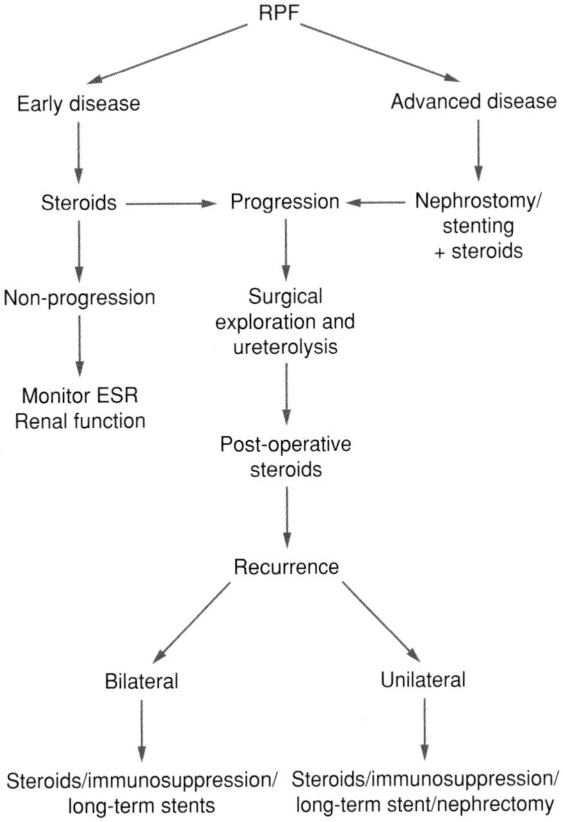

Figure 60.12 The management of retroperitoneal fibrosis.

Further reading

Gnanapragasam, V., Ramsden, P., Murthy, L. and Thomas, D. (1999). Primary in situ extracorporeal shock-wave lithotripsy in the management of ureteric calculi: results with a third-generation lithotripter. *Br J Urol* **84**: 770–4.

Jenkins, A. D. (1996). Calculus formation. In: Gillenwater, J.Y., Grayhack, J. T., Howard, S. S., Duckett, J. W., eds. *Adult and Paediatric Urology*, 3rd edn. St Louis, MO: Mosby, 461–505.

Martin, T.V. and Sosa, R. E. (1998). *Shock-wave Lithotripsy.* In: Walsh, P .C., Retik, A. B., Vaughan, E. D. Jr and Wein, A. J., eds. *Campbell's Urology*, 7th edn. Philadelphia, PA: W.B. Saunders, 2735–52.

Menon, M., Parulkar, B. G. and Drach, G. W. (1998). Urinary lithiasis: etiology, diagnosis and medical management. In: Walsh, P. C., Retik, A. B., Vaughan, E. D. Jr and Wein, A. J., eds. *Campbell's Urology*, 7th edn. Philadelphia, PA: W.B. Saunders, 2661–733.

Parivar, F., Low, R. K. and Stoller, M. L. (1996). The influence of diet on urinary stone disease. *J Urol* **155**: 432–40.

Peschel, R., Janetschek, G. and Bartsh, G. (1999). Extracorporeal shock wave lithotripsy versus ureteroscopy for distal ureteral calculi: a prospective randomised study. *J Urol* **162**: 1909–12.

Segura, J. W., Preminger, G. M., Assimos, D. G. *et al.* (1994). Nephrolithiasis clinical guidelines panel summary report on the management of staghorn calculi. The American Urological Association Nephrolithiasis Clinical Guidelines Panel. *J Urol* **151**: 1648–51.

Segura, J. W., Preminger, G. M., Assimos, D. G. *et al.* (1997). Ureteral stones clinical guidelines panel summary report on the management of ureteral calculi. *J Urol* **158**: 1915–21.

MODULE 61

Lower urinary tract symptoms: bladder outflow obstruction

1 • Lower urinary tract symptoms
2 • Bladder outflow obstruction
3 • Benign prostatic enlargement
4 • Bladder neck hypertrophy
5 • Urethral stricture
6 • Detrusor–sphincter dyssynergia
7 • Miscellaneous disorders causing bladder outflow obstruction
8 • 'Prostatitis'

Until recently this module would have been entitled 'prostatism' or 'BPH'. The title has been chosen to emphasize an important change in urological practice: in at least 30% of men with 'prostatism', the prostate is not the cause of the symptoms. Only 60% of men with classical 'prostatism' have significant symptomatic improvement after surgery. In good urological practice men are selected for medical or surgical treatment only after analysis of symptoms, and appropriate investigations to confirm prostatic obstruction as the cause of those symptoms. Management is then tailored to the individual patient's needs, wishes and circumstances. With this approach the proportion of patients who have good symptomatic outcomes after surgery should be at least 80% and can be as high as 93%.

The terms *prostatism*, *BPH* (benign prostatic hypertrophy) and *bladder outflow obstruction* are often used freely and inaccurately. 'Prostatism' is often used to refer to abnormalities of urine flow (hesitancy, poor flow and terminal dribbling) and of bladder storage function (frequency, nocturia and urgency) that have many causes and which, as a group, occur as commonly in elderly women as in elderly men.

- **'Prostatism'** makes an assumption about causation: it has been replaced by **LUTS** – lower urinary tract symptoms.
- **BPH** is a histological diagnosis which should not be used as a clinical descriptor. It should be replaced by **BPE** (benign prostatic enlargement) – the presence of an enlarged gland on clinical and ultrasonic examination, without suspicion of carcinoma.
- **Bladder outflow obstruction (BOO)** is properly defined as a relationship between bladder pressure and urine flow, in which bladder pressure is abnormally high for the flow rate. In clinical practice it is usually diagnosed on flow rate and residual urine volume.

LUTS, BPE and proven obstruction do not necessarily exist together in the individual patient. This has been succinctly expressed by Professor Hald of Copenhagen in a classic diagram showing three overlapping rings, reproduced in modified form in Figure 61.1. It is seen that there are several possible combinations, e.g. BPE with neither symptoms nor obstruction, symptoms with BPE but no obstruction, etc. Only when all three conditions overlap (i.e. in the minority of patients) is there a high chance of success from prostatic surgery.

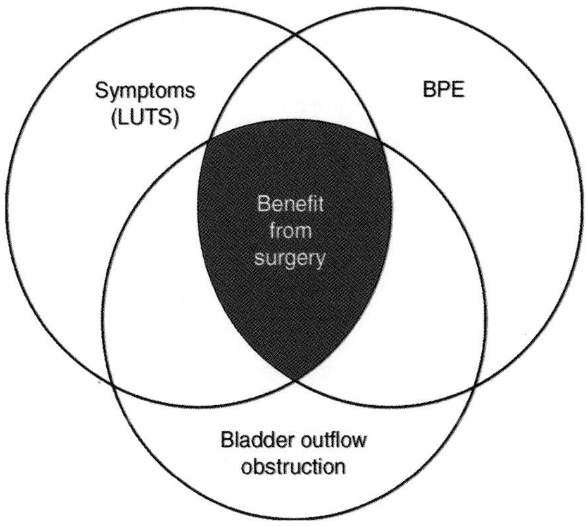

Figure 61.1 Only when benign prostatic enlargement, bladder outflow obstruction and symptoms coincide is there likely to be a good result from surgery on the prostate.

Section 61.1 • Lower urinary tract symptoms

One-half of all men over 65 years of age have some urinary symptoms. Many symptoms are caused by age-related changes in the bladder unrelated to prostatic disease or to outflow obstruction.

The symptoms discussed here will be frequency, nocturia, urgency, urge incontinence, dysuria, hesitancy, poor flow, intermittent stream, terminal dribbling, after-dribbling and a feeling of incomplete emptying. They will be discussed individually with particular reference to their relationship to bladder outflow obstruction. Urinary incontinence as a separate entity is not discussed here.

Anatomy of LUTS

- The bladder and urethra cannot be considered separately from each other.
- The lower urinary tract cannot be considered in isolation from its nerve supply.

Most of the bladder wall consists of a three-dimensional interlacing network of bundles of smooth muscle (the detrusor muscle) with small amounts of collagenous tissue around groups of muscle bundles. Its main motor (efferent) nerve supply is parasympathetic. In man acetylcholine is the main transmitter.

Around the bladder neck (internal urethral meatus) the smooth muscle is condensed in a circular fashion to form the internal (pre-prostatic) urinary sphincter. It has a rich sympathetic (norepinephric) nerve supply. Although the pre-prostatic sphincter can and does act as a urinary sphincter it has an important function in closing off the bladder neck during ejaculation so that emitted seminal fluid can pass only distally. Its almost inevitable involvement in prostatectomy is important in the after-effects of that operation (see Table 61.6). The prostatic stroma and the proximal urethra are also rich in norepinephric receptors.

Immediately distal to the prostate is the rhabdosphincter, composed of striated muscle. After prostatectomy it is the only structure preventing urinary leakage. The older term *external urethral sphincter* is no longer appropriate. It was used before the rhabdosphincter was described to denote those extrinsic perineal muscles which can compress the urethra for short periods.

Physiology: the micturition cycle

What follows is an outline to allow understanding of LUTS. It is necessarily an oversimplified account of a complex and not entirely understood series of events which depend for their successful completion on nerve pathways within the bladder wall, between the bladder and urethra, and at spinal, pontine and cortical levels.

As urine enters the bladder, stretch receptors in the bladder wall are stimulated but the impulses produced do not reach conscious level. During the filling phase the bladder pressure remains low (by definition less than 15 cmH_2O but usually much less). At about 300 ml filling volume the impulses are appreciated at cortical level. The desire to void they produce can be suppressed at cortical level if circumstances require it ('the postponement phase'). Detrusor contraction is suppressed and sphincter tone increased. At about 400 ml the desire to void becomes more urgent. It can still be suppressed if required, up to twice this volume, with increasing difficulty and discomfort. A socially acceptable site is reached and micturition begins.

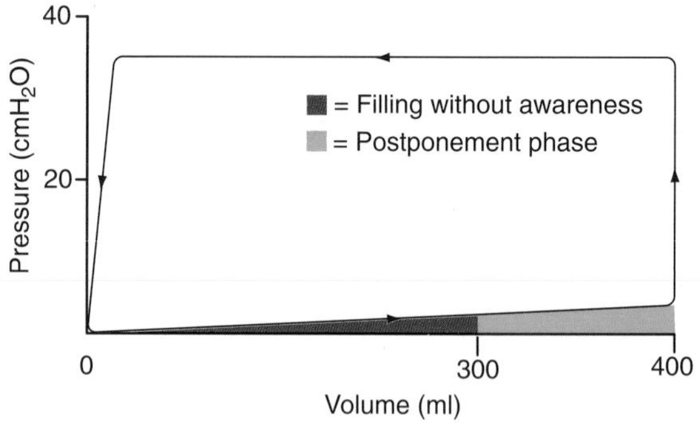

Figure 61.2 The micturition cycle in a normal bladder. During the filling phase (red area) the bladder volume increases but pressure remains low and there is no awareness of bladder filling. At about 300 ml the desire to void is felt. Micturition can be postponed (blue area) until a socially acceptable site is reached. Detrusor contraction continues until the bladder volume is effectively zero.

The urethral sphincters relax and cortical inhibition of detrusor activity is switched off. Detrusor contraction under parasympathetic stimulation causes a pressure rise typically 20–40 cmH_2O until the bladder is virtually empty, when the pressure falls to zero. These events are summarized in Figure 61.2. The rhabdosphincter closes, urine in the proximal urethra is milked back into the bladder and the bladder neck closes. The cycle begins again. Thus there are two phases: filling and voiding. Symptoms may occur in either phase.

- A common abnormality in the filling phase is development of unstable bladder contractions which, by definition, exceed 15 cmH_20 pressure. They often produce a desire to void, a feeling of urgency or urine loss (see Figure 61.3).

Analysis of LUTS

Symptoms in the filling phase

Frequency

- Frequency is determined by the urinary output divided by the functional bladder capacity (i.e. the capacity at normal desire to void). Frequency will increase if the urine output increases or if the functional bladder capacity decreases.

The commonest causes of an increase in urine output are diabetes, excessive drinking and the early stages of renal failure where concentrating power is impaired. Having excluded these, the urologist is mostly concerned with reduced functional bladder capacity. In the absence of infection, a reduced functional bladder capacity is due either to unstable detrusor contractions (Figure 61.3) or to reduced bladder compliance. Reduced compliance may be due to age-related changes in the bladder wall or to an increase in collagen in response to obstruction (see below).

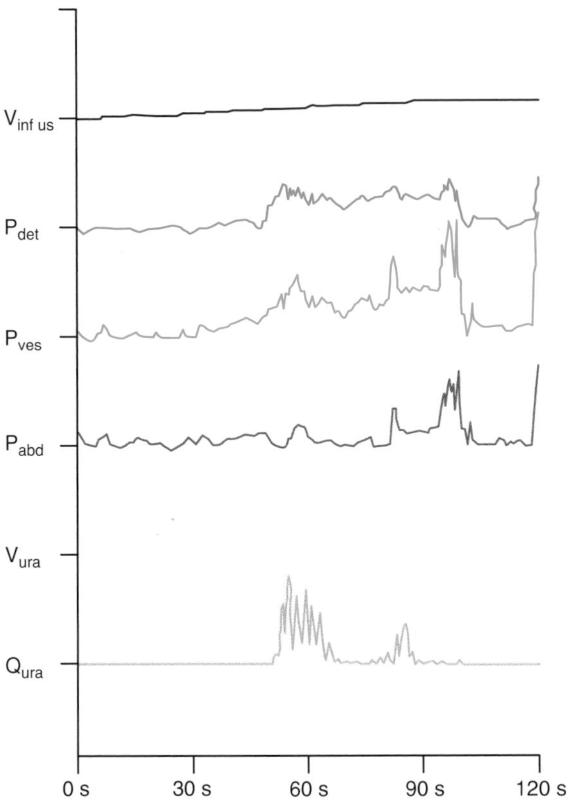

Figure 61.3 Cystometry showing detrusor pressure rise (green line) of up to 30 cmH_2O beginning after 30 s of artificial bladder filling (25 ml). Such 'unstable contractions' produce a desire to avoid, a feeling of urgency or, as in this case, urine loss (yellow line). This patient was referred with 'prostatism'. His urgency and urge incontinence were due to a cerebrovascular accident preventing cortical inhibition of bladder activity. Prostatic surgery will not improve this problem and may make it worse.

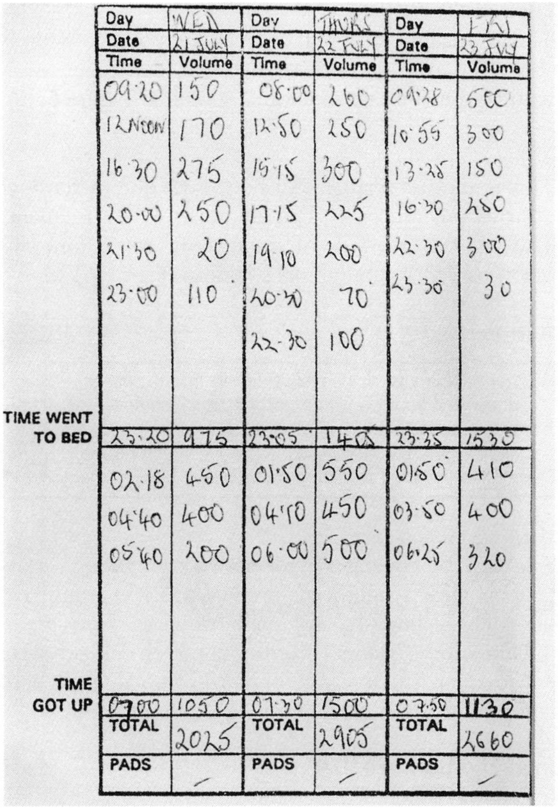

	Day WED		Day THURS		Day FRI	
	Date 21 JULY		Date 22 JULY		Date 23 JULY	
	Time	Volume	Time	Volume	Time	Volume
	09·20	150	08·00	260	09·28	500
	12 NOON	170	12·50	250	10·55	300
	16·30	275	15·15	300	13·25	150
	20·00	250	17·15	225	16·30	250
	21·30	20	19·10	200	22·30	300
	23·00	110	20·30	70	23·30	30
			22·30	100		
TIME WENT TO BED	23·20	975	23·05	1405	23·35	1530
	02·18	450	01·50	550	01·50	410
	04·40	400	04·10	450	03·50	400
	05·40	200	06·00	500	06·25	320
TIME GOT UP	07·00	1050	07·30	1500	07·50	1130
	TOTAL	2025	TOTAL	2905	TOTAL	2660
	PADS	/	PADS	/	PADS	/

Figure 61.4 Three day extract from a frequency/voiding chart. The patient was referred with 'prostatism' because of nocturia × 3. The chart shows good voided volumes with half of the 24 hour output occurring at night. His 'prostatism' was cured by treatment of his congestive cardiac failure. This simple, painless 'investigation' may save much unnecessary investigation and treatment.

Nocturia

The factors causing nocturia are the same as those causing diurnal frequency with the addition that nocturnal output may be increased in old age due to the loss of circadian rhythm in water and sodium excretion, and by reabsorption of oedema fluid which has accumulated during the day (see Figure 61.4).

- Untreated heart failure is a common cause of nocturia in the elderly.

Urgency

This symptom is not fully understood but is at least in part due to unstable bladder contractions causing an overwhelming desire to void which can be postponed for only a short time.

Urge incontinence

- The progression from urgency to urge incontinence depends on a balance between the severity of the urgency and the patient's ability to reach a socially acceptable site for micturition. It can often be solved without urological attention: a urinal bottle at the side of the bed may be more effective than urosurgical manoeuvres!

Symptoms in the voiding phase

Dysuria

By common usage this means painful micturition. In the absence of infection it is not a feature of bladder outflow obstruction.

Hesitancy

This is commonly found in outflow obstruction due to benign prostatic enlargement and is a marked feature of detrusor sphincter dyssynergia.

Poor flow

- Poor flow is the classic sign of 'prostatism' and correlates well with obstruction
- **but**: flow depends on the power of detrusor contraction as well as on outflow resistance; in both sexes the power of detrusor contraction reduces with age
- **and**: poor flow may be secondary to a low voided volume. If a patient's frequency and/or urgency are so severe that he can hold only 100 ml, the flow will never be good. This is a major source of misinterpretation and should be obvious from the frequency voiding chart.

Measurement of urine flow rate is discussed in Module 55.

Intermittent stream

This is usually a manifestation of very poor flow but is also seen in patients with detrusor decompensation who void mainly by abdominal straining (Figure 61.5).

Terminal dribbling

This is another feature of a poor flow due to outflow obstruction, especially benign prostatic enlargement. The last few seconds of micturition are commonly accompanied by abdominal straining (Figure 61.6).

After-dribbling

- After-dribbling must be distinguished from terminal dribbling. It is not a symptom of bladder outflow obstruction (except occasionally with a urethral stricture). It is due to failure of the bulbospongiosus muscle which normally empties the urethra, and is not relieved by prostatectomy.

A feeling of incomplete emptying

This may be associated with obstruction, though most patients with a significant residual urine volume have no such feeling. It may arise from the low-grade inflammatory changes commonly seen in prostatic enlargement. It is a feature of detrusor instability where 'after-contractions' may produce a desire to void.

Investigation of LUTS

History

Correct analysis of symptoms depends on care in listening to the patient. Time spent on this may prevent mistakes in investigation or treatment and will establish rapport with the patient which will be useful when one comes to discuss treatment options.

- Always take a drug history: many drugs, not only tricyclic antidepressants, affect bladder function.

Frequency voiding chart

- The simple, cheap, painless 'investigation' of a frequency voiding chart may save much inappropriate investigation and treatment.

The patient should note the time and volume of each void by day and by night. A three-day extract from such a chart is shown in Figure 61.4. This patient complained only of nocturia. His 'prostatism' was relieved by treating his congestive cardiac failure.

Symptom score

This is another cheap and painless 'investigation'. At least seven scoring methods are in use. One of the commonest is the IPSS (International Prostate Symptom Score). Its name is unfortunate because it presupposes that the prostate is the cause of the symptoms – the very practice this module aims to discourage! Symptom scores are widely used and the WHO has recommended their routine use in the evaluation of LUTS.

Symptom scores are:

- reproducible in a given patient
- used to monitor progress in untreated patients
- useful in comparing symptoms before and after surgery
- used in statistical comparison of treatment groups in trials
- without an absolute criterion against which they can be validated
- varied in the weighting they give to some symptoms.

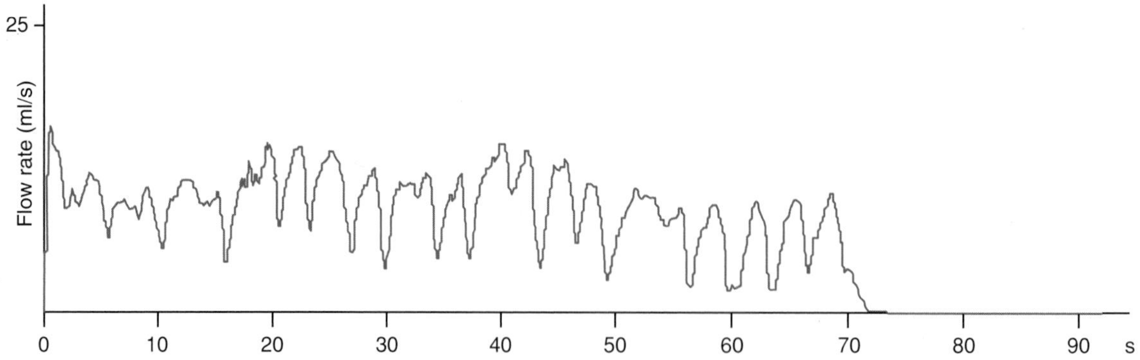

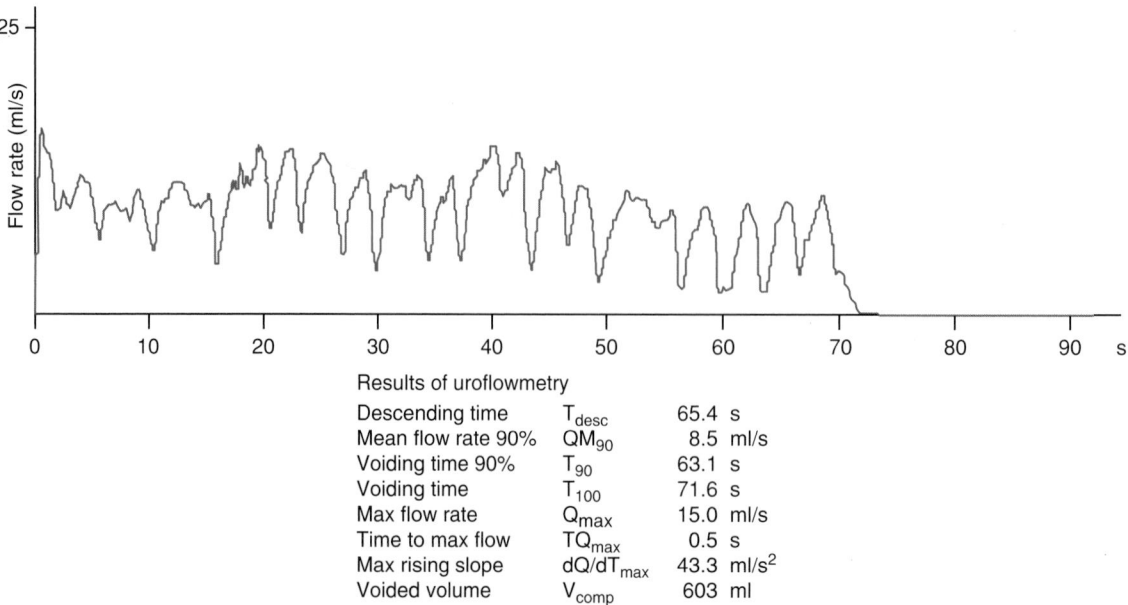

Results of uroflowmetry

Descending time	T_{desc}	65.4	s
Mean flow rate 90%	QM_{90}	8.5	ml/s
Voiding time 90%	T_{90}	63.1	s
Voiding time	T_{100}	71.6	s
Max flow rate	Q_{max}	15.0	ml/s
Time to max flow	TQ_{max}	0.5	s
Max rising slope	dQ/dT_{max}	43.3	ml/s^2
Voided volume	V_{comp}	603	ml

Figure 61.5 Uroflow trace from a patient with detrusor decompensation due to a combination of long-standing obstruction and diabetic neuropathy. Voiding is mostly by abdominal straining. He originally presented with chronic retention of urine (1.7 litres). After prostatectomy he voided to completion, but was doing so by using his abdominal muscles. In the absence of obstruction abdominal straining can produce a reasonable peak flow rate (in this case 15 ml/s).

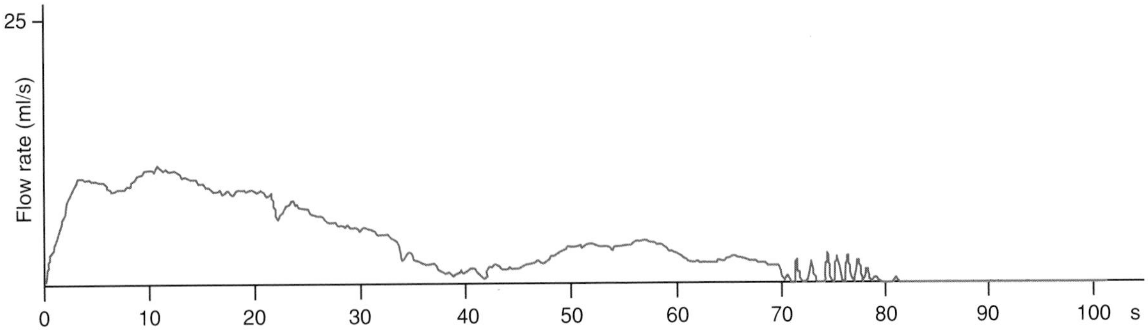

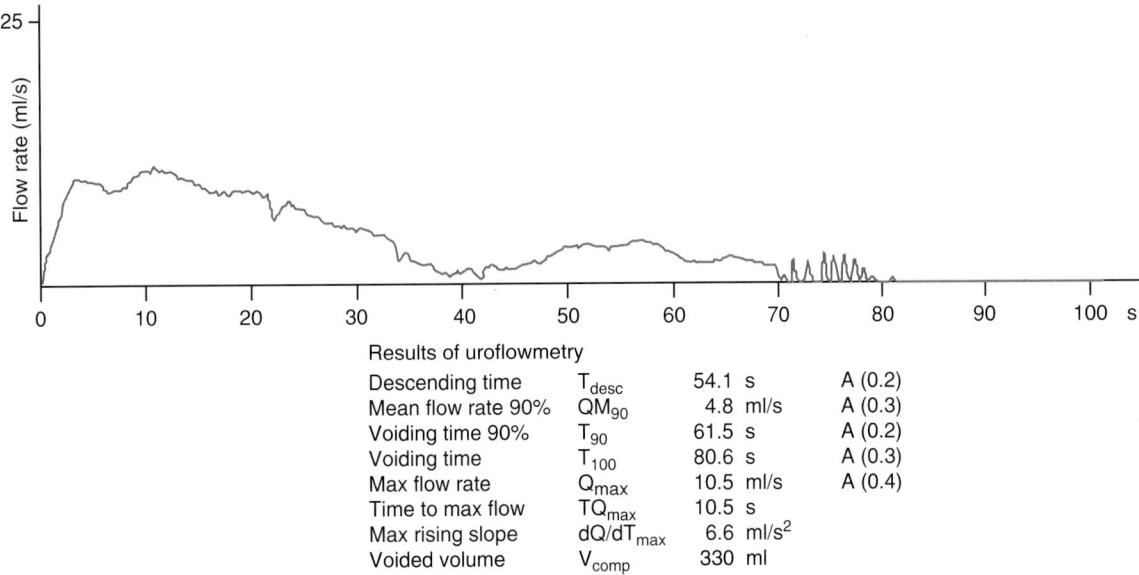

Results of uroflowmetry

Descending time	T_{desc}	54.1 s	A (0.2)
Mean flow rate 90%	QM_{90}	4.8 ml/s	A (0.3)
Voiding time 90%	T_{90}	61.5 s	A (0.2)
Voiding time	T_{100}	80.6 s	A (0.3)
Max flow rate	Q_{max}	10.5 ml/s	A (0.4)
Time to max flow	TQ_{max}	10.5 s	
Max rising slope	dQ/dT_{max}	6.6 ml/s^2	
Voided volume	V_{comp}	330 ml	

Figure 61.6 Typical uroflow trace from a man with bladder outflow obstruction due to benign prostatic enlargement, showing a slow rise to peak, low peak flow, prolonged flow and terminal dribbling. The end of the stream is augmented by abdominal straining. Note that in the presence of outflow obstruction abdominal straining has little effect (in contrast to Figure 61.5).

Clinical examination

This is often of little help but must include examination of the lower limb reflexes, anal tone and peri-anal sensation to detect obvious neuropathy. Digital rectal examination (DRE) is used to detect impacted faeces (a common cause of LUTS in the elderly), to assess anal sphincter tone and to judge the texture and consistency of the prostate. Estimating prostate size by DRE is difficult as the finger feels only a small part of the surface of a spheroid. Transrectal ultrasound, when available, is a more reliable indicator of size. A firm nodule, loss of the median sulcus and a hard or craggy surface raise the possibility of carcinoma and require appropriate investigations (see Module 59).

Urinalysis

Urinalysis is essential to exclude diabetes, proteinuria indicating renal disease and infection (see Module 55). The finding of red cells requires investigation as for any patient with haematuria (Module 58 and Figure 58.6).

Urine cytology

Frequency and urgency of recent onset are occasional presenting features of the dangerous condition of carcinoma *in situ* (Module 58). Most patients with this will have red cells in their urine and so will have a cystoscopy, but cytology is a useful back-up.

Plasma creatinine, urea and electrolytes

It is good practice to check these, with the proviso that a normal creatinine level does not necessarily confirm normal renal function.

Prostate specific antigen concentration

The controversy about prostate specific antigen (PSA) measurement to screen **asymptomatic** men for prostate cancer is covered elsewhere (Module 59).

- Patients with a family history (i.e. a first degree male relative with prostate cancer), or from ethnic groups with a high incidence of prostate cancer (see Module 59) should have their PSA concentration measured. Otherwise, there is no consensus on its routine use in the evaluation of LUTS.

The potential consequences for the patient of PSA estimation need to be considered. A raised concentration may set the patient off on a course of investigation ending in biopsy which has significant morbidity and even mortality. A negative biopsy does not exclude prostate cancer (although probably excludes it as a cause for the presenting symptoms). The recommendation is that PSA testing should be done only after counselling the patient about the implications of an abnormal result. This may not be appropriate at first consultation. However, many patients expect PSA testing and some present because of fear of cancer.

- Although routine use of PSA estimation in the evaluation of LUTS may not be supported by the evidence available so far, it is becoming standard practice, which raises medico-legal issues. On balance, it is probably wise to do it, except in patients over 75 years with normal-feeling prostates in whom the diagnosis of a small carcinoma, unrelated to the symptoms, would not lead to active treatment.

Urine flow rate and residual urine volume estimation

These simple investigations are those which most commonly lead to the diagnosis of BOO, which is classically associated with a peak flow rate of less than 15 ml/s and a residual urine volume of over 100 ml.

Uroflowmetry and its interpretation are discussed in Module 55 (and Table 55.1).

Transrectal ultrasound

Transrectal ultrasound (TRUS) should be used to measure prostate volume. There is little correlation between obstruction and prostate size at lower prostate volumes (below 30 cm^3) but better correlation at higher volumes.

Pressure–flow studies ('urodynamics')

Pressure–flow studies (Module 55) may be used in two situations: (1) when symptoms of frequency, nocturia, urgency and urge incontinence are predominant, suggesting instability, and (2) as the only certain indicator of BOO, which can only be defined in terms of a relationship between the pressure generated by the detrusor and the rate of urine flow. They will also identify patients whose poor flow is due to low detrusor pressure (rather than obstruction) and who will not do well with surgery. In spite of this, urodynamic studies are not used in the routine assessment of LUTS and it is impractical to suggest or expect that they should be so.

Lower tract endoscopy and upper tract imaging are not routinely needed in the investigation of LUTS when urinalysis is normal.

Section 61.2 • Bladder outflow obstruction

Bladder outflow obstruction (BOO) is clinically important for two reasons. First, it can cause symptoms which bother patients. Second, it may interfere with renal function and ultimately lead to renal failure which may occur 'silently'.

The indicators that LUTS are due to bladder outflow obstruction are:

- history of a diminishing urine flow over time
- an intermittent urine flow (90% positive predictive value for BOO)
- DRE: size estimation is difficult but gross enlargement makes BOO more likely
- TRUS volume (especially volume of the transition zone) correlates well with BOO
- uroflowmetry: peak flow below 10 ml/s – 79% positive predictive value at first void, rising to 93% at fourth void
- residual urine volume over 100 ml on repeat estimation suggests BOO, or detrusor decompensation.

Although it is standard practice to proceed with management decisions on the above basis, outflow obstruction is properly defined only in terms of the relationship between flow rate at any instant and the detrusor pressure required to produce that flow rate. Some authorities argue that bladder outflow obstruction *should* be diagnosed by urodynamic studies before any treatment is considered and *must* be so before surgery is chosen. This view is supported by outcome figures for prostatic surgery: good symptom relief is achieved in only 60% of men when decisions are made on symptoms and rectal examination, in 80% when symptoms are considered more critically and the results of uroflowmetry and residual volume measurement are taken into account, and in 93% with urodynamically proven 'high pressure/low flow' obstruction. This is a compelling argument for routine urodynamic studies but such a policy is very difficult to implement other than in large, well staffed specialist units. Medico-legal considerations may drive an increasing use of urodynamics in this situation.

In most urology departments urodynamic studies will be used in patients with high scores for instability symptoms (frequency, nocturia, urgency and urge incontinence) and in patients where hesitancy and high residual urine volumes suggest obstruction but flow rates are satisfactory. Such patients may have 'high pressure/high flow' obstruction and will be helped by surgery.

Cystoscopy is not generally helpful in diagnosing bladder outflow obstruction. It will diagnose a stricture, and a large, long prostate with lateral lobes obscuring the internal meatus and making it difficult to enter the bladder probably is causing obstruction. Except in such extreme cases cystoscopic appearances are a poor guide.

Upper tract studies are not indicated in suspected bladder outflow obstruction when urinalysis is normal, but many urologists ask for renal ultrasound as it is safe, painless and may identify a few patients with upper tract dilatation but normal creatinine concentrations. There is no statistical association between BOO and upper tract tumours or stones.

Consequences of bladder outflow obstruction

The first consequence of increasing bladder outflow resistance is that the detrusor must work harder to expel urine. It responds by hypertrophy. This process is accompanied by an increase in connective tissue (collagen). These two effects – hypertrophy of muscle cells and increasing collagen around them – result in enlargement of the muscle bundles giving the appearance we call trabeculation.

- Trabeculation is not a sign of obstruction. It is a sign of increased detrusor activity, of which obstruction is only one cause.

Increased muscle activity initially maintains urine flow and complete bladder emptying. Eventually the muscle is unable to compensate, flow is diminished and emptying incomplete. This is a late stage in the overall process. The end stage, unrelieved, is bladder failure with more collagen than muscle in the bladder wall. This is the stage of chronic retention, which may impair renal function as pressure in the lower urinary tract causes ureteric dilatation and hold-up at a higher pressure than the glomerular filtration pressure. Renal impairment may be made worse by vesico-ureteric reflux of urine, which may be infected.

Between the stage of compensated obstruction and decompensation with chronic retention, something else may happen: the development of detrusor instability (Figure 61.3). Detrusor instability is present in 50% of men with bladder outflow obstruction. The symptoms it causes (frequency, nocturia, urgency) are more troublesome than the obstructive symptoms of hesitancy and a poor flow.

Benign causes of bladder outflow obstruction

These include: benign prostatic enlargement; bladder neck hypertrophy; urethral stricture; detrusor-sphincter dyssynergia and other rare causes.

In clinical practice most BOO is caused by benign prostatic enlargement. Carcinoma of the prostate is also a cause and covered in Module 59.

Section 61.3 • Benign prostatic enlargement

In practice a diagnosis of benign prostatic enlargement (BPE) is made clinically by the presence of obstructive symptoms, the objective findings of a reduced urine flow and increased residual urine volume and the finding on rectal examination, or (preferably) transrectal ultrasound, of prostatic enlargement without evidence of malignancy. There is no agreed criterion for 'prostatic enlargement' but a prostate of more than 20 cm^3 is generally accepted as significantly enlarged.

Epidemiology

Benign prostatic disease is a large consumer of health service resources and is likely to become a massive potential problem with increasing life expectancy producing a large rise in the number of men at risk. Benign prostatic hyperplasia as a histological condition begins about age 35 years and occurs in 60% of men over 60 years. It does not necessarily cause obstruction or symptoms.

Community studies have shown a clinical incidence of *symptomatic* benign prostatic enlargement with reduced urine flow rate in 40% of men in their sixties, of whom one-half had significant impairment of daily living.

There are racial differences in incidence, but environmental factors appear to be more important. The disease is associated with a Western diet, hypertension and diabetes mellitus. It has even been suggested that it is part of the 'metabolic syndrome' characterized by insulin resistance. Sympathetic overactivity is another characteristic of this syndrome and it is interesting that alpha-blocking drugs, when effective, maintain their effect for at least 4 years, suggesting that reduction in alpha-adrenergic stimulation may slow prostatic growth.

Pathophysiology and pathological anatomy

Prostatic growth requires testosterone. Unlike most androgen-dependent tissues, the prostate converts testosterone to dihydrotestosterone (DHT), which is the active metabolite in the gland. This conversion depends on the enzyme 5-alpha-reductase. The cause of the fibro-epithelial hyperplasia which characterizes BPH is unknown. Suggestions include an increase in the amount of 5-alpha-reductase, an increase in the number of androgen receptors and alterations in the ratios of androgens to oestrogenic substances at the 'male menopause'.

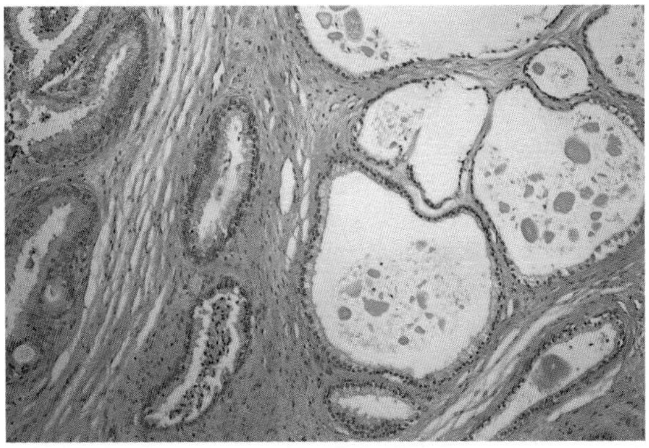

Figure 61.7 Haemoxylin and eosin stained section from a prostate showing benign hyperplasia. There is hyperplasia of both glandular and stromal elements. In this section glandular elements predominate. The glandular (epithelial) component predominates in larger prostates, and may respond to drugs which block the enzyme 5-alpha-reductase. Smaller glands, where stromal elements tend to predominate, may be better managed by alpha-adrenergic blocking drugs.

Histologically the process is characterized by an increase of both glandular and stromal elements, the glandular elements usually predominating (Figure 61.7). These changes take place mainly in the tissue around the urethra (properly called the transition zone). In young men this constitutes less than 20% of the gland (Figure 61.8a). As this portion enlarges it compresses the urethra centripetally and the rest of the prostate centrifugally (Figure 61.8b).

Eventually there is severe compression of the urethra, and the newly enlarged periurethral tissue makes up 80% of the gland, compressing the rest of it into a thin 'surgical capsule'(Figure 61.8c). There is little correlation between the overall size of the gland and the degree of obstruction, or the severity of symptoms. The degree of obstruction, due to pressure on the urethra, depends on the tension within the prostatic capsule which in turn depends of the ratio of smooth muscle and fibrous tissue to glandular elements, and on sympathetic tone.

The pathophysiological effects of obstruction have been described earlier.

Clinical presentations of benign prostatic enlargement

- The most common presentations are: in the outpatient clinic with urinary symptoms, as acute retention of urine and as chronic retention of urine. Occasionally patients present in unusual ways, such as with haematuria or infection and are found on investigation to have BPE as an underlying cause.

(a) (b) (c)

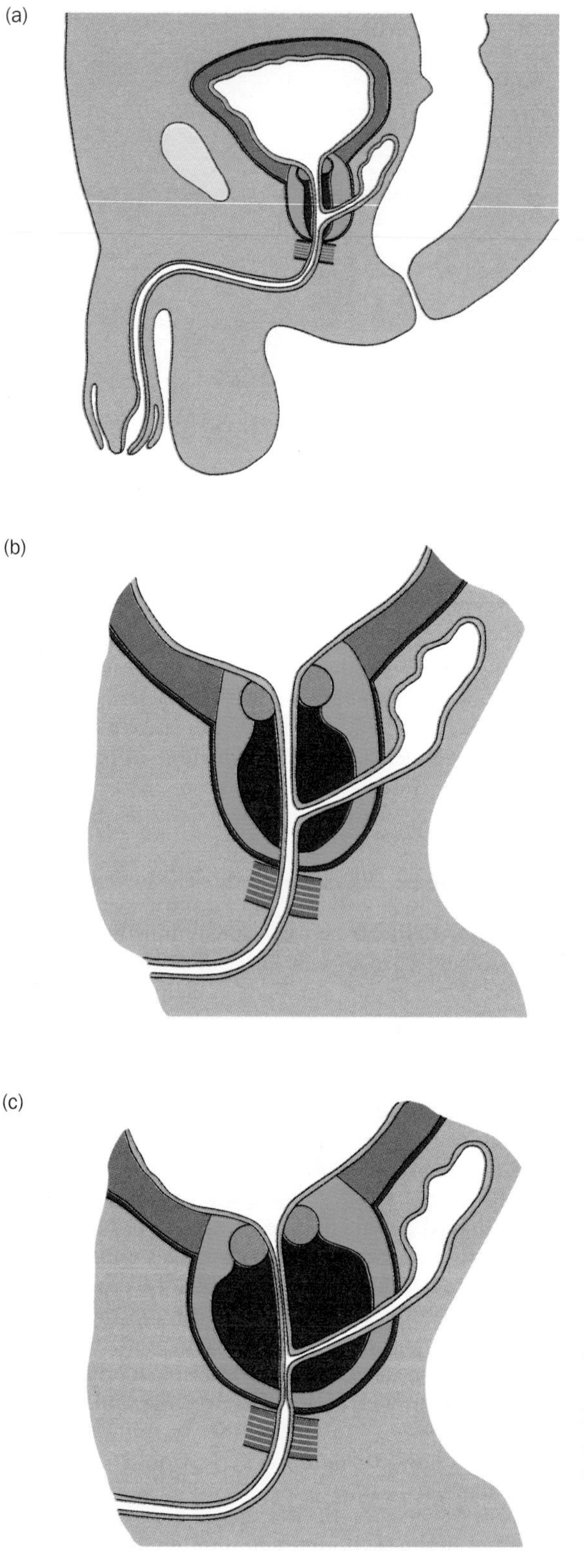

Figure 61.8 (a) Simplified diagramatic sagittal section of a young male pelvis. The periurethral/transition zone tissue (red) in a young man constitutes less than 20% of the gland. (b) Hyperplasia of this tissue begins to compress the urethra and the surrounding normal prostate. (c) At a late stage the adenomatous tissue is producing marked compression of the urethra, and has compressed the normal prostate into a thin 'surgical capsule'.

Routine presentation with symptoms

The classical symptoms occurring during the filling phase ('irritative' symptoms – frequency, nocturia, urgency and urge incontinence) and during the voiding phase ('obstructive' symptoms – hesitancy, poor flow and terminal dribbling) have been described in detail above. The 'irritative' symptoms cause more trouble than the 'obstructive' ones. Nocturia is especially troublesome, and some men present only because their partners are disturbed by this problem.

It is unfortunate that the 'irritative symptoms', particularly nocturia, have many causes other than BPE and even if due to it are least likely to be relieved by surgical treatment.

Patients vary in their tolerance of symptoms: many elderly men regard hesitancy, a poor flow and nocturia as an inevitable part of ageing, not something requiring medical attention; younger men still active in business may present at the first indication of hesitancy and perhaps the need to get up at night only once. Many men present because of publicity about prostatic disease, some of them requiring only reassurance of the absence of malignancy.

Acute retention of urine

This may happen with little or no warning, or after a long period of troublesome symptoms. It is commonly precipitated by an additional factor superimposed on obstruction. Such factors include drugs which reduce detrusor contraction (especially tricyclic antidepressants), drugs which increase tone in the prostatic urethra (alpha-stimulants, including some in proprietary cough and cold medication), surgical operation, immobilization and constipation. Men in their seventies with moderate to severe prostatic symptoms have a 3% per year risk of developing acute retention.

Chronic retention of urine

Gradually increasing, painless overdistension of the bladder may reach an advanced stage before presentation, especially in elderly men. It may present as urinary infection, as renal failure with its many manifestations, as overflow incontinence especially at night, or simply as increasing abdominal girth (Figure 61.9).

Investigations

There is consensus on the requirement for some investigations, consensus on some investigations which are not required, and less agreement on others, as indicated in Table 61.1.

Management of benign prostatic enlargement

Management of patients presenting to the clinic with symptoms

- Does the patient need treatment; and if so, which treatment?
- Many men with BPE do not need medical or surgical treatment.

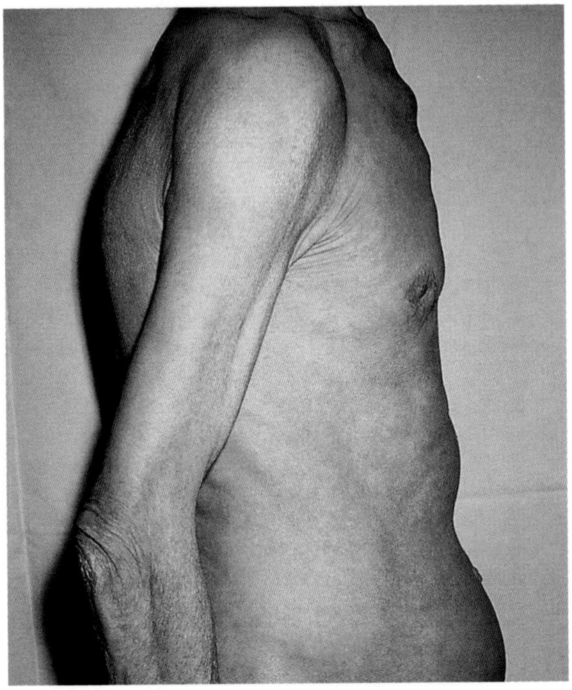

Figure 61.9 Chronic retention of urine. This man presented with shortness of breath due to anaemia, due to renal failure, due to chronic retention of urine. His only other complaint was of 'putting on weight'. He denied urinary symptoms. His peak flow rate was 2 ml/s – about one-tenth of normal, but he regarded this as 'good for my age'.

Table 61.1 Investigation of bladder outflow obstruction

Investigation	*Comment*
Urinalysis	Essential; for glucose, blood, protein, nitrites and leucocytes
Urine culture	Indicated only if analysis suggests infection
Plasma creatinine	Essential to rule out significant renal impairment which would alter management plan
Digital rectal examination	Essential to exclude obvious carcinoma and give estimate of prostate size
Uroflowmetry	Essential
Residual urine volume	Essential
Symptom score	Recommended by WHO
Transrectal ultrasound	Strongly advised. Gives accurate indication of prostate size
Prostate specific antigen	Commonly measured. Controversial (see text)
Urine cytology	Not indicated except in presence of haematuria or irritative symptoms of sudden onset, raising possibility of malignancy
Cystoscopy	Not indicated except in presence of haematuria or irritative symptoms of rapid onset
Renal ultrasound	Not routinely indicated. Often done because safe and cheap
Intravenous urogram	Contraindicated (in absence of haematuria)

Symptoms may progress very slowly or remain unchanged for years. Some seek only reassurance of the absence of malignancy or of the need for surgery. Others fear that benign prostatic disease, if not treated, will lead to malignancy: they can be told this is not so. Others have minimal symptoms (e.g. nocturia once or twice) which may be unrelated to prostatic disease.

- If the flow rate is above 15 ml/min, the residual volume is virtually zero, the symptom score low and the prostate less than 20 cm^3 in volume, the patient can be discharged.

Flow rates below 15 ml/s, significant residual volumes (say, 100 ml or more on repeated measurement) or prostate size over 20 cm^3 are more likely to be associated with progression and need more active management (though this may be 'watchful waiting').

- The options are: 'watchful waiting', pharmacotherapy and surgery. There are very few absolute indications for any of these. Within wide limits patient preference is paramount.

How would the patient feel if he had to spend the rest of his life with the condition as it has been in the month before the consultation? How much do the symptoms interfere with his work, leisure and sleep? Is he bothered enough to want to take pills every day? Is he bothered enough to want an operation?

'Watchful waiting'

Almost any out patient can be managed in this way, at least initially. Flow rates less than 10 ml/s, residual volumes over 200 ml and prostates over 40 ml are relative indications that this course may **not** be appropriate, but many patients wish to avoid drugs or surgery and will better accept them if symptoms and clinical findings deteriorate during the period of observation. Patients are seen every 6 months for symptom score, flow rate and residual urine volume. If there is no significant change after 2 years the intervals can be increased to 1 year.

- Watchful waiting is safe and can be abandoned at any time, but for men with moderate symptoms it has twice the rate of failure (acute retention or need for surgery) of pharmacological or surgical treatment.

Pharmacological treatment

- The options are: phytotherapy, 5-alpha-reductase inhibitors, and alpha-blocking agents.

The results of pharmacotherapy are difficult to assess because of the conflicting evidence from clinical trials and the common placebo effect (up to 30%) of any medication for urinary symptoms.

Phytotherapy

Plant extracts may reduce prostatic congestion and inflammation and affect enzyme activity. Controlled trials are scarce.

5-Alpha-reductase inhibitors

These inhibit the enzyme converting testosterone to its active metabolite, reducing cell proliferation whilst increasing cell atrophy and apoptosis. At the time of writing the only such drug available is finasteride. Others are under trial.

- Sixty per cent of patients respond to finasteride, with a mean reduction in prostate volume of 20%.
- The effect is not apparent for 3 months and is maximal at 6 months.
- Symptom scores and flow rates significantly improve and urodynamic studies show reduced voiding pressures.
- The effects are maintained for at least 4 years.
- Low libido, ejaculatory problems and impotence occur in about 3%.
- Finasteride is most useful in glands over 40 cm^3, where epithelial elements predominate.

Finasteride reduces the risk of acute retention and need for surgery by 50%, but about 40 patients need to be treated to prevent one such episode. It may be most usefully prescribed for older men with larger glands and high symptom scores, who are known to have the highest risk of developing retention.

Alpha-blocking agents

These drugs block alpha-1-adrenergic receptors in the prostate and proximal urethra.

- Alpha-blocking agents reduce resistance in the prostatic urethra, improving flow, reducing symptoms of bladder irritability and improving symptom scores.
- The effect is apparent within a few days.
- There are several available: prazosin, indoramin, doxazosin, alfuzosin, terazosin and tamsulosin.
- All may produce postural hypotension, especially in men already taking anti-hypertensive drugs.
- They are equally effective but newer ones have reduced incidence and severity of side-effects.
- The effects are maintained for at least 4 years.

If there is no response to an alpha blocker after 1 month or to finasteride after 6 months, the drug should be withdrawn. Drugs are not a cheap alternative to surgery. There is concern that they may merely delay the need for surgery by a few years, by which time the patient may be less fit. Patients whose symptoms and clinical findings warrant drug treatment should have formal follow-up as for watchful waiting.

Surgical treatment

Other than chronic retention and repeated acute retention there are few strong indications for surgery. They include renal deterioration, bladder stone formation, a large bladder diverticulum, repeated infection with high residuals and persistent bleeding from the prostate. Otherwise, all indications are relative and patient preference is paramount.

Older men with large glands (more than 40 cm^3), high symptom scores and flow rates below 10 ml/s are most likely to have a progressive clinical course or develop retention and are often best advised to consider surgery before their health deteriorates. For all others the benefits of surgery (Table 61.2) must be weighed against the risks (Table 61.3) and complications (Tables 61.4–61.6).

The surgical options are:

- open prostatectomy
- transurethral resection of the prostate (TURP)
- transurethral incision of the prostate (TUIP)
- alternative surgical and 'parasurgical' treatments.

Open prostatectomy. The principles of prostatectomy (open or transurethral) are shown in Figure 61.10. Less than 2% of operations for BPE are now done by the open route (Figure 61.11). Indications include the presence of a large bladder stone or a diverticulum needing removal, and a prostate too large for safe transurethral removal (more than 60–80 g). The threshold may be lower for patients with chronic retention where the surgeon wants to be sure that all obstructing tissue has been removed and that any post-operative voiding difficulties are due to detrusor failure. The morbidity and mortality of open prostatectomy are higher than for TURP but published figures may not reflect this as less fit patients will not have open surgery. The short- and long-term sequelae are as for TURP, except that prostatic re-growth tends to occur later as more tissue has been removed.

Transurethral resection of the prostate. The adenomatous tissue is removed piecemeal (in 'chips' – Figure 61.12). In theory, the tissue removed is the same as that in open prostatectomy (Figure 61.10b). Although TURP is described as 'the gold standard' treatment for BPE, radiological studies have shown that even in the most expert hands, adenoma removal by TURP is incomplete.

Pre-operative preparation is as for any other major surgery with the additional consideration that there is often significant bleeding, so that prophylactic low-dose heparin is avoided by most urologists, and many recommend that patients on low-dose aspirin should stop the medication for 2 weeks before surgery, starting

Table 61.2 Benefits of surgery for BPE

- Proven best option for symptom relief
- Proven best option for improvement in objective indicators of obstruction (flow rate, residual volume, voiding pressure)
- effects apparent within days
- Provides permanent solution for most men
- Avoids long-term medication and follow-up
- Provides material for histological examination (but see Table 61.3)

Table 61.3 Disadvantages of surgery for BPE

- Mortality and morbidity of surgery (Tables 61.4 and 61.5)
- Long-term sequelae (Table 61.6)
- Does not remove the periphery of the gland where carcinoma is most common
- Material removed cannot all be examined histologically. Overlooking an 'incidental' carcinoma may lead to false impression that future symptoms cannot be due to prostatic disease
- Adenoma will re-grow if patient lives long enough (most have significant re-growth at 15 years)

Table 61.4 Peri-operative complications of TURP

Complication	*Comment*
1. Severe intra-operative bleeding	Usually controlled by halting the resection and using tamponade with an overinflated catheter balloon (50 ml if necessary) pulled **onto** (not into) the prostatic cavity by external traction. Occasionally requires open surgery and packing of prostatic cavity
2. 'TUR syndrome'	Irrigant inevitably enters veins in the prostatic bed. When water was used as the irrigant this produced haemolysis, as well as dilutional hyponatraemia and cerebral oedema. The syndrome occurs less commonly using glycine, usually after proloned resection of large glands or after capsular perforation. Treatment is with furosemide. Mortality is high
3. Sepsis	Patients with indwelling catheters at the time of surgery must have prophylaxis (usually gentamycin plus a broad spectrum penicillin or cephalosporin unless pre-operative culture indicates otherwise). In the absence of a catheter and in the presence of sterile urine many patients become bacteraemic as urethral organisms enter the blood stream. It is therefore common to give all patients prophylaxis
4. Excessive immediate post-operative bleeding	Treated by transfusion and if necessary return to theatre for evacuation of clots and diathermy of discrete bleeding points. Further measures as for operative bleeding. Antifibrinolytic agents (e.g. tranexamic acid) may be helpful

Table 61.5 Early post-operative complications of TURP

Complication	*Comment*
1. Secondary haemorrhage	Classically occurs on tenth to twelfth day; can be as early as third day and as late as 6 weeks. Usually associated with infection. Treated by recatheterization, bladder washout, antibiotics and transfusion if necessary
2. Epididymo-orchitis	Said to be due to spread of organisms from prostatic bed along vas. At first indication of scrotal pain or swelling use bed rest and antibiotics
3. Deep vein thrombosis	Significant risk because of position on table and avoidance of prophylactic low-dose heparin Reduce risk by graduated compression stockings, and by intermittent calf compression during surgery. Management may be difficult because anticoagulation within 3 weeks of surgery may cause serious haemorrhage from the prostatic bed
4. Incontinence	Minor stress incontinence due to temporary external sphincter dysfunction rapidly subsides and needs only reassurance. Urgency and urge incontinence due to unstable bladder contractions may take weeks or months to settle and often require anticholinergic treatment. Long-term incontinence due to surgical damage to the sphincter is rare (less than 1%)

Table 61.6 Late complications of TURP

Complication	*Comment*
1. Retrograde ejaculation	Almost inevitable consequence of destruction of internal sphincter. Patients **must** be warned of this. Not reliable contraception. Some complain that quality of orgasm is impaired
2. Impotence	Controversial. Probably a small (<5%) incidence due to damage to neurovascular bundles posterolaterally on prostatic capsule. Medico-legal situation not clear but probably best to warn patients of 'very small risk'
3. Stricture formation	Occurs in about 3%. Presents as diminished flow weeks, months or years after surgery Most respond to dilatation or urethrotomy followed by intermittent self-dilatation
4. Bladder neck stenosis	Occurs in about 3%. Excess scar tissue produces a 'camera shutter diaphragm' effect. Most respond to single incision or resection but some recur whatever is done and may even require open Y-V plasty
5. Re-growth of prostate	Almost inevitable if patient lives long enough (10–15 years). Should be explained before surgery
6. Malignancy	Not a consequence of surgery, but patients should be told that no form of surgery for benign disease prevents cancer
7. Stress incontinence	Significant damage to external sphincter at time of surgery may result in permanent stress incontinence. May require treatment by intra-urethral bulking injections or insertion of artificial sphincter
8. Detrusor instability	If present before surgery may persist, or may be 'unmasked' by surgery. May need long-term anticholinergic treatment. Patients with symptoms of instability before surgery must be warned that these may persist after surgery

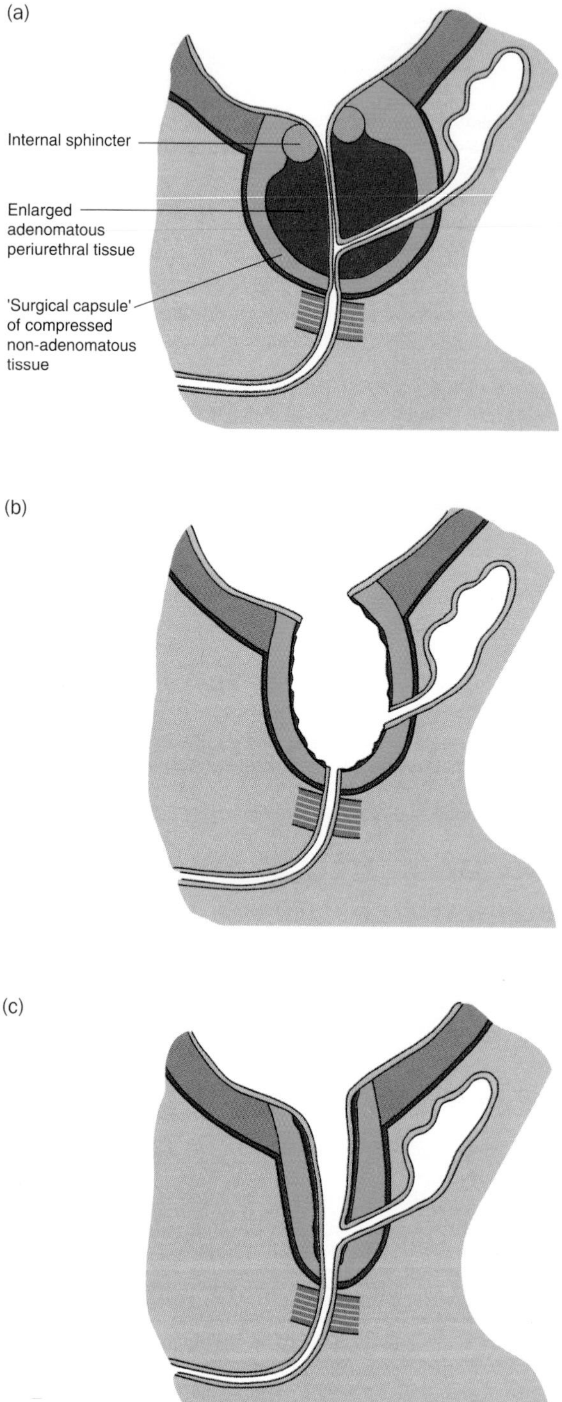

Figure 61.10 The principles of prostatectomy. (a) The enlarged adenomatous tissue, now comprising most of the gland, will be removed. The internal sphincter is inevitably removed with it. (b) Immediately after removal of the adenoma. The capsule will contract down very quickly. The plane between adenoma and surgical capsule is not 100% clean and some potentially adenomatous tissue remains. If the patient lives long enough this may re-grow, requiring further surgery. (c) The end result. The capsule has contracted down and re-epithelialization has occurred. The bladder neck can no longer close, resulting in retrograde ejaculation. Continence depends on the rhabdosphincter. Most of the prostate present in a young man (Figure 61.8a) remains. This is where malignant change occurs.

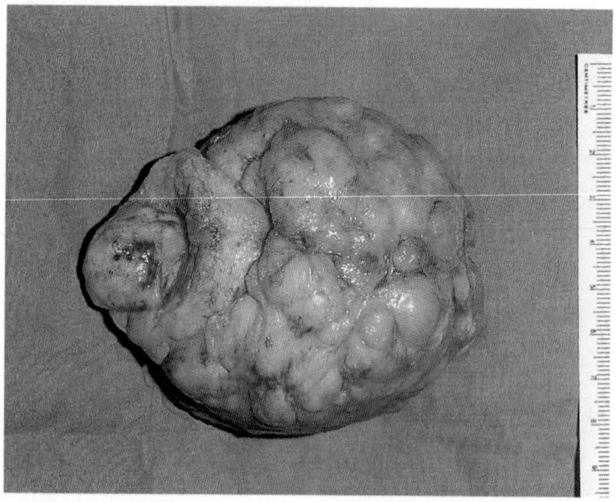

Figure 61.11 A benign (250 g) 'prostate gland', i.e. prostatic adenoma, enucleated at open surgery, now a rare operation.

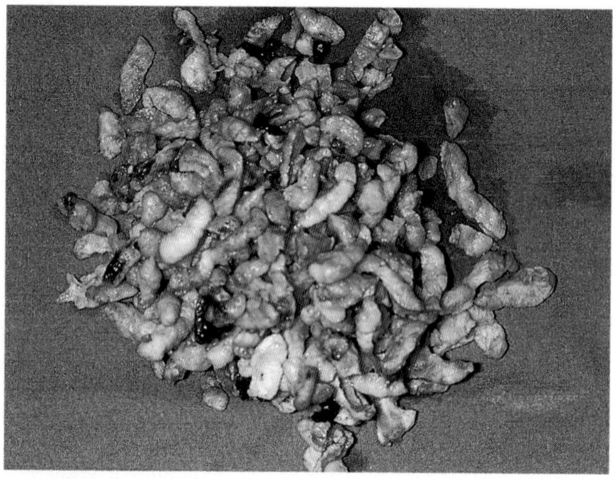

Figure 61.12 Prostate 'chips' removed by TURP.

it again only after the main risk of secondary haemorrhage has passed (about 12 days). Others feel that the risks of stopping aspirin in patients taking it for secondary prophylaxis outweigh any benefits from reduced bleeding. The complications specific to TURP can be divided into peri-operative, early post-operative and late, as in Tables 61.4–61.6.

Despite the formidable list of potential problems, with proper selection at least 80% of patients should have good symptomatic relief after surgery and be 'satisfied or very satisfied' with the results.

As shown in Figure 61.10, in open or transurethral surgery for benign disease only the adenoma is removed. Most of the prostate present in youth remains. This tissue is where cancer occurs. The term 'prostatectomy' is inaccurate and may lead to dissatisfaction if the patient develops recurrent BPE or carcinoma. The term 'adenomectomy' is coming into use in some parts of the world.

Transurethral incision of the prostate. This can give good results when obstruction is due to a small gland ('the small fibrous prostate'). The prostate is deeply incised, from midway between the ureteric orifice and bladder neck, down to the level of the verumontanum (i.e. just proximal to the rhabdosphincter). The incision is made at 5 or 7 o'clock (or both) and must be deepened into prostatic capsule or periprostatic fat. In appropriate cases this has good results with a lower incidence of retrograde ejaculation and urethral stricture, and a shorter hospital stay, than TURP. It is much underused.

Alternatives to standard surgery for BPE. The high incidence of side-effects from traditional surgery has prompted a search for alternatives to TURP. Several have appeared over the past 10 years. Many have had only brief popularity; others show promise. They should all be regarded as semi-experimental, to be evaluated against the 'gold standard' of TURP in specialist units. An indication of some of these alternatives is given in Table 61.7. They are mentioned here because they often feature in the lay press and patients expect their surgeons to know about them.

Management of acute retention of urine

This requires immediate relief by catheterization. The urethral route is traditional. The suprapubic route has advantages (if there has been no previous lower abdominal surgery). Suprapubic catheterization allows trial clamping and unclamping rather than trial removal and insertion, and leaves the urethra clean for surgery.

- All patients who have been catheterized for acute retention should have a trial removal of the catheter. The morbidity and mortality of prostatectomy in catheterized patients are significantly higher than in those without catheters.
- Some may have a reversible precipitating cause (e.g. constipation, medication). Even when there is a history of symptoms before this episode, and interval surgery is required, operating on a non-catheterized patient has advantages. An alpha-blocking drug started 24 hours before trial removal/clamping significantly increases the chances of success.

Management of chronic retention of urine

After catheterization for chronic retention there may be significant diuresis with loss of sodium and potassium which can be dangerous. Catheterization for chronic retention should always be done on an in-patient basis. 'Gradual decompression' by releasing the catheter for a few minutes every hour is unnecessary and unhelpful.

Patients with bladder volumes over 1 litre, especially if elderly, are unlikely to void well after prostatectomy. Where surgery would carry a high risk, bladder pressure studies are indicated to measure detrusor power and hence estimate the chances of success after surgery.

- An elderly man with a painless retention of more than 1 litre may well be better served by avoiding surgery. In such cases (or after failed surgery) the choice is between clean intermittent self-catheterization or an indwelling catheter, preferably suprapubic. Once all hope of regaining detrusor power is lost, continuous drainage has no merit. Such patients may be happier with a valved spigot rather than a leg bag.

Table 61.7 Surgical and 'parasurgical' alternatives to TURP

Technique	*Comment*
Balloon dilatation of prostate	Very short-term relief. Minimal bleeding. Needs regional or general anaesthesia. Virtually abandoned
Prostatic stents ('internal catheter')	Can be inserted under local anaesthesia. Avoids catheter in those unfit for surgery. Not always well tolerated. Removal can be very difficult. Newer expanding titanium stents may have wider use
Laser coagulation	Using side-firing Nd:YAG laser. Virtually abandoned due to prolonged catheterization and pain
Transurethral microwave therapy (thermotherapy)	Prostate heated to around 45°C under local analgesia. May have good subjective improvement but little objective evidence of it. Easily repeated. No tissue for histology
Transurethral needle ablation (TUNA)	Radiofrequency ablation under general or regional anaesthesia. Creates cavity within prostate without breaching mucosa. Cavity collapses to reduce overall size. The effects may be delayed while shrinkage occurs. Some early promising results. Capital cost high. No tissue for histology
Interstitial laser ablation	Similar effects to TUNA. Same remarks apply
Laser resection of prostate	Using Ho:YAG laser to resect tissue as in TURP. Immediate result, minimal bleeding. Early results promising. Capital cost high
Transurethral vaporization of prostate (TUVP)	Similar effect to TURP using rolling electrode at high setting instead of resection loop, to vaporize tissue. Immediate effect. Short catheter time. May be as good as laser but without capital cost. No tissue for histology.
Focused high-intensity ultrasound/ extracorporeal pyrotherapy/prostatic Necrosis by prostatic ethanol injection	All experimental. No large series. No significant follow-up.

Future developments in the management of BPE

Prevention by 'prophylactic' finasteride or an alpha-blocker starting at age 40 years is not a realistic suggestion. Treatment will become more refined, with improved patient selection and, perhaps, an increased use of laser, radiofrequency or other forms of prostatic ablation less invasive than TURP.

Section 61.4 • Bladder neck hypertrophy

This is caused by hypertrophy of the smooth muscle at the bladder neck. It causes the same symptoms as BPE but tends to affect younger men. Irritative symptoms are common and the muscle hypertrophy may be part of general detrusor hypertrophy associated with overactivity – i.e. the bladder neck hypertrophy may not be the primary problem. A trial of alpha-blocking drugs is the first line of treatment. A deep bladder neck incision is the surgical solution, following which persisting irritative symptoms are treated by anticholinergic drugs. The contrasting appearances of BPE and bladder neck hypertrophy are shown in Figure 61.13.

Section 61.5 • Urethral stricture

Epidemiology and aetiology

- In developed countries the commonest cause is iatrogenic trauma, usually following TURP or other urethral instrumentation. The second commonest cause is trauma of other causes, e.g. a fall astride crushing the bulb of the urethra against the pubic arch, or disruption of the membranous urethra associated with a fractured pelvis (see Module 56).

In countries where access to medical care is difficult gonorrhoea is a very common cause of strictures which may be multiple and associated with fistulas from the urethra to penile or scrotal skin.

Pathophysiology

The bladder responds to obstruction as already described. The scar tissue which forms the stricture usually involves the full thickness of the urethral wall and may involve the surrounding corporeal tissue. Hence the results of stricture surgery, whilst initially good, are almost uniformly poor with prolonged follow-up.

Presentation

This is usually as a poor flow or other symptoms of bladder outflow obstruction, sometimes with urinary tract infection and occasionally with acute retention. The latter is initially managed by suprapubic catheterization.

Investigations

Uroflowmetry classically shows a prolonged very flat trace with a very poor peak flow.

Urethrography is described in Module 55. It is essential to define both ends of the stricture, which requires descending as well as ascending urethrography.

Management

- Virtually all strictures recur after initial treatment, unless further measures are taken.

Most respond to initial dilatation or urethrotomy under vision, followed by intermittent self-dilatation which the patient must do initially at intervals of a few days, then weekly, most patients eventually continuing with a once-a-month regimen. Self-dilatation is done using a disposable catheter with a hydrophilic coating, usually size 16 Fr. The aim is to 'calibrate' the urethra to prevent stricture recurrence, rather than to dilate a recurring stricture.

- Strictures which recur very rapidly or complex strictures in the proximal urethra need open urethroplasty, often in two stages, using pedicle grafts of scrotal or perineal skin, or free grafts of buccal mucosa. The natural history of strictures is measured in decades rather than in years and the very long-term results of open urethroplasty are not good. Open surgery should therefore be followed by self-'dilatation' as above.

Section 61.6 • Detrusor–sphincter dyssynergia

This is caused by lack of co-ordination between detrusor contraction and relaxation of the rhabdosphincter. There is often a long history of hesitancy of micturition, especially in unfamiliar surroundings. Uroflow-

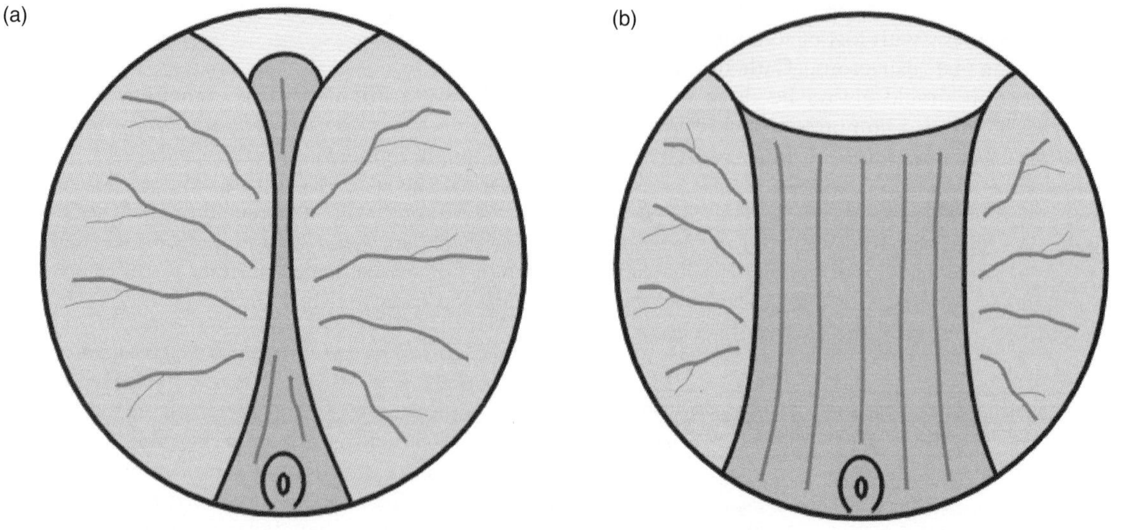

Figure 61.13 (a) The typical endoscopic appearance of trilobar prostatic enlargement, with convex projections into the lumen. (b) Bladder neck hypertrophy has a concave border to the 'middle lobe'.

metry shows a reduced peak flow and a rapid 'fluttering' due to opening and closing of the rhabdosphincter. There is no generally successful treatment and an explanation of the problem and reassurance of the absence of serious consequences is usually sufficient. Some patient develop prostatic pain due to urine reflux into the prostatic ducts.

Section 61.7 • Miscellaneous disorders causing bladder outflow obstruction

Obstruction due to sphincter spasm is seen in neurological diseases, especially multiple sclerosis, and is managed by intermittent self-catheterization.

A stone impacted in the urethra may rarely cause obstruction.

Young women may develop retention associated with excess rhabdosphincter activity (Fowler's syndrome). They were often formerly described as cases of 'hysterical retention'.

Section 61.8 • 'Prostatitis'

Although this condition causes bladder outflow obstruction only in the rare cases of acute bacterial prostatitis with abscess formation, 'prostatitis' as a group of symptoms causes distress and dismay to men and their urologists world-wide and is appropriately discussed here.

Clinical types of 'prostatitis' are:

- acute bacterial prostatitis
- recurrent subacute/chronic bacterial prostatitis
- chronic non-bacterial prostatitis
- prostatodynia.

Acute bacterial prostatitis

This causes severe constitutional upset, a high fever and an exquisitely tender prostate. Treatment is by bed rest, copious fluids and antibiotics appropriate to urinary pathogens. Failure to show improvement within 24 hours suggests abscess formation which may be detected by digital or ultrasonic rectal examination (which may need general anaesthesia). An abscess is drained by transurethral resection. Because of the architecture of the prostate gland and the difficulty of eradicating infection, antibiotics should be continued for at least 4 weeks after the initial episode.

Recurrent subacute/chronic bacterial prostatitis

This may or may not follow an acute episode. Patients may be disabled by chronic pain in the perineum radiating along the urethra, to the sacral area and scrotum, and in a sciatic distribution. The pain is often worse after ejaculation. The gland contains fibrous tissue and small calculi and may feel malignant on digital examination. Expressed prostatic secretion contains an excess of leucocytes.

The mainstays of treatment are antibiotics and alpha-blocking drugs. Culture of expressed prostatic secretion often grows organisms such as diphtheroids and staphylococci which are irrelevant. Antibiotics normally given for urinary tract infections, such as trimethoprim, may be helpful but the characteristics of the prostate indicate that quinolone antibiotics, especially ofloxacin, are the most suitable in most cases. A minimum of 1 month's treatment should be given. Recently the older treatment of frequent prostatic massage has been shown to help but needs to be done two or three times a week. Transurethral resection should not be done. It may produce initial improvement, followed by worsening as fibrosis occurs.

Chronic non-bacterial prostatitis

This is not always distinct from the preceding category, since specific organisms are often absent in both conditions. Some cases may be due to chlamydia or other fastidious organisms. The prostate is tender and there are excess leucocytes in the expressed prostatic secretion. Treatment with quinolone antibiotics and alpha-blocking drugs for prolonged periods is again the mainstay of treatment. A few patients are helped by finasteride. Many of these men have prolonged misery with frequent relapses at times of stress over a clinical course of 10 years or more, although eventually the condition does tend to 'burn itself out'.

Prostatodynia

This is the most difficult of all to treat. There is prostatic pain but no sign of inflammation. Alpha-blocking drugs and non-steroidal anti-inflammatory drugs may help. Depression, neurosis and introspection are common. One theory is that these patients do not have prostatic pain as such but may have dysfunction in the parts of the levator ani closest to the prostate and rectum and may be helped by drugs which reduce skeletal muscle spasm.

Further reading

Abrams, P. (1994). New words for old: lower urinary tract symptoms for 'prostatism'. *BMJ* **308**: 929–30.

Abrams P. (1995). Managing lower urinary tract symptoms in older men. *BMJ* **310**: 1113–1117.

Blandy, J. and Notley, R. (1998). *Transurethral Resection*, 4th edn. Oxford: Isis Medical Media.

Hald, T. (1989). Urodynamics in benign prostatic hyperplasia: a survey. *Prostate* **2**(Suppl): 69–77.

Lepor, H., Williford, W. O., Barry, M. J. *et al.* (1996). The efficacy of terazosin, finasteride, or both in benign prostatic hyperplasia. *N Engl J Med* **335**: 533–9.

McConnell, J. D., Bruskewitz, R., Walsh, P. *et al.* (1998). The effect of finasteride on the risk of acute urinary retention and the need for surgical treatment among men with benign prostatic hyperplasia. *N Engl J Med* **338**: 557–63.

Nickel, J. C., ed. (1999). *Textbook of Prostatitis*. Oxford: Isis Medical Media.

MODULE 62

The male external genitalia

1 • The testis, epididymis and vas

2 • The penis

3 • The scrotum

Section 62.1 • The testis, epididymis and vas

The main functions of the testis are to produce spermatozoa and to secrete testosterone.

Surgical anatomy

The undifferentiated gonad gives rise, during the sixth week of intrauterine life, to a group of cells (blastema) which will form the testis. The gubernaculum is a band of connective tissue, which joins the caudal end of the developing gonad to the genital swelling. Growth in length of the fetus, and failure of the gubernaculum to elongate, results in a relative caudal migration of the gonad. The testis lies behind a pouch of peritoneum (the processus vaginalis) as it traverses the inguinal canal to reach the scrotal sac by the eighth month. The lower part of the processus vaginalis becomes the tunica vaginalis. Its persistence results in the infantile type of hernia.

The epididymis is formed from part of the mesonephric duct, the closed proximal portion of which remains as the appendix of the epididymis. The remainder of the mesonephric duct becomes the vas deferens and the seminal vesicles

The arterial supply of the testis is by vessels from the aorta which follow the descent of the testis. Further blood supply follows the course of the vas deferens and cremaster muscle and may be sufficient to maintain testicular viability if the testicular artery is divided above the level of the inguinal canal.

Venous drainage of the testis is through multiple veins of the pampiniform plexus to the spermatic vein(s), usually double, emerging from the upper end of the cord before passing retroperitoneally. On the right side the testicular vein empties into the inferior vena cava and on the left into the renal vein.

The lymphatic drainage of the testis is to the common iliac and para-aortic nodes. The latter communicate across the midline at the level of the kidneys and also communicate with the mediastinal and supraclavicular chains, hence the classical finding of enlarged supraclavicular nodes in disseminated testicular malignancy.

Testicular nerves are derived from the aortic and renal plexuses, which in turn communicate with the solar plexus. Thus testicular pathology may produce abdominal and not scrotal pain. This may lead to misdiagnosis of testicular pathology, especially torsion.

The epididymis is a single coiled tubule about 5 m long. Spermatozoa undergo maturation during passage along the epididymis, which also acts as a storage reservoir.

The vas deferens transports spermatozoa from the epididymis via the spermatic cord through the inguinal canal and extraperitoneally to the ampulla of the vas and the seminal vesicles.

The maldescended testis

Faced with a problem of testicular descent there are basic questions to be answered which help to categorize the problem and thus decide on the correct management.

- Is the problem unilateral or bilateral?
- Is the testis palpable, impalpable or intermittently palpable?
- If the testis is palpable, is it retractile or ectopic?
- If the testis is not palpable, is it present at all ?
- If the testis is present, where is it?

The palpable testis

Retractile testis. This condition is common and requires careful assessment by accurate examination in a relaxed atmosphere, with warm hands.

Under these circumstances it should be possible to coax the testis into the scrotum where it can be held without tension. The retractile testis is usually bilateral and does not need surgery.

Ectopic testis. The ectopic positions include: superficial inguinal (most common), femoral, perineal and pubopenile.

An undescended testis may be intermittently palpable due to its movement into and out of the inguinal canal. This may be difficult to differentiate from an ectopic testis in the superficial inguinal pouch.

The impalpable testis

The impalpable testis constitutes 20% of all problems related to descent.

Anorchism (bilateral absence of testes) is very rare. Monorchism occurs in 3% of maldescended testes. The testis is impalpable when it is absent, atrophic, intra-abdominal or in the inguinal canal.

The testis should be descended in the full-term infant and since the cremasteric reflex is poorly developed at birth, confusion with a retractile testis should not occur if early examination has been performed.

The impalpable testis is associated with a higher incidence of hernia, malignant transformation, spermatogenic failure, incomplete orchidopexy and a smaller adult testis than a palpable maldescended one. Torsion of an impalpable testis is more difficult to diagnose and results in a higher incidence of ischaemic damage.

Investigation of a child with bilateral impalpable testes requires:

- a search for Müllerian structures
- karyotyping
- endocrine tests to identify functioning testicular tissue.

A rise in serum testosterone after administration of human chorionic gonadotrophin (hCG) indicates functioning testicular tissue: surgical exploration is appropriate. (This method of investigation is unreliable in the adult male as the intra-abdominal gonad may have undergone premature failure of endocrine function.)

Investigations to locate the impalpable testis before surgical exploration include:

- ultrasound
- computed tomography (CT) or magentic resonance imaging (MRI) (Figure 62.1)
- laparoscopy
- selective testicular arteriography or selective testicular venography.

Results aid accurate planning of the surgical approach. In practice, most impalpable testes are in the inguinal canal or close to the deep ring.

Endocrine therapy for undescended testes

Failure of descent may be due to a failure of the hypothalamic-pituitary-gonadal axis. Some authors suggest that hCG or luteinizing hormone releasing hormone (LHRH) treatment may be tried first in patients up to 5 years with a success rate between 10 and 50%. Others report the development of irreversible histological lesions in both the undescended and the contralateral normal testis by the age of 2 years, leading to infertility and possible testicular carcinoma. They recommend that failure of hormonal treatment by 2 years requires surgical intervention.

Orchidopexy

The purposes of orchidopexy are:

- to improve spermatogenesis
- to prevent malignant change, trauma and torsion
- to remove any psychological ill-effects.

The aims of orchidopexy are:

- to locate the testis
- to secure a viable organ in the scrotum without tension
- to remove an associated hernial sac.

Psychological problems can be minimized by day case surgery in suitable patients.

Orchidopexy may be best performed before 24 months of age, and must be done before the child is 5. Before 24 months the operation is technically more difficult but future spermatogenesis is more likely to be improved.

The operation should be performed through a skin crease incision in the groin. After identification of the testis and dissection of any associated hernial sac, careful dissection of the vas and vessels is performed to provide sufficient length for the testis to be placed in the scrotum without tension. Various methods have been described to maintain the position of the testis in the scrotum; the subdartos pouch is most popular.

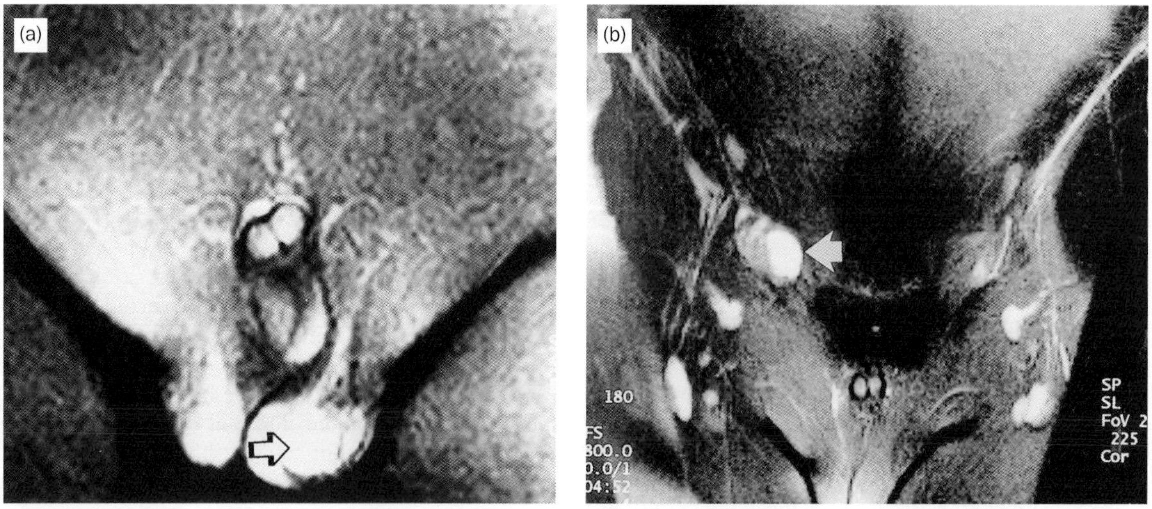

Figure 62.1 Use of magnetic resonance imaging to locate an impalpable testis before surgery. Coronal T2-weighted fat-suppressed images demonstrate a normally positioned left testis [(a) – open arrow] and an ectopic right testis in the inguinal canal [(b) – closed arrow].

If sufficient length of the vessels cannot be achieved, the options are:

- extension of the dissection to the retroperitoneum to provide a straighter (shorter) course
- fixation of the testis in the best position obtainable and re-exploration 1 year later
- division of the intra-abdominal spermatic vessels, or preliminary laparoscopic clipping and mobilization of the testis months later on a pedicle of peritoneum and the artery of the vas
- auto-transplantation using microvascular anastomosis to the inferior epigastric vessels.

Testicular tumours

Testicular tumours are uncommon but are increasing in incidence. Effective chemotherapy means that early stage and low bulk disease are almost always curable, so early diagnosis and accurate staging are important.

Epidemiology

The incidence is highest in Scandinavia at nine cases per 100 000 per year, a three-fold increase in 50 years. Black men in the USA have the lowest incidence of one per 100 000 per year with no evidence of an increase.

Aetiology of testicular tumours

There are several risk factors for testicular tumours. The most obvious is young age. It is well known that maldescent is a strong risk factor; however a wide range of urogenital congenital abnormalities including hypospadias, inguinal hernia and the 'bell clapper' deformity have a similar risk association. The common pathway seems to be the disruption of normal germ cell development leading to carcinoma *in situ* then overt cancer. The case for a single common pathway is supported by the finding of an increased risk of carcinoma in the anatomically normal contralateral testes in unilateral maldescent. Other risk factors include:

- fetal exposure to maternal oestrogens
- race – Caucasians have a higher risk than blacks
- there may be some human leucocyte antigen (HLA) associations
- trauma and viral (mumps) orchitis
- professional or agricultural occupation.

The hypothesis is that the above risk factors exert their influences via a common effect: failure of germ cell differentiation. This could be the initiating step of malignant change promoted by hormonal stimulation in puberty, resulting in a peak incidence in the next 15–20 years.

Pathology

Tumours may arise from all the tissue types represented within the testis. The common tumours are: seminoma, arising from the seminiferous tubular epithelium; and the non-seminomatous germ cell tumours (teratomas).

Seminoma (Figure 62.2) is the commonest tumour and occurs predominantly in the 35–40 years age group. Teratomas occur at an earlier age (peak age 25–30 years) and may also occur in childhood.

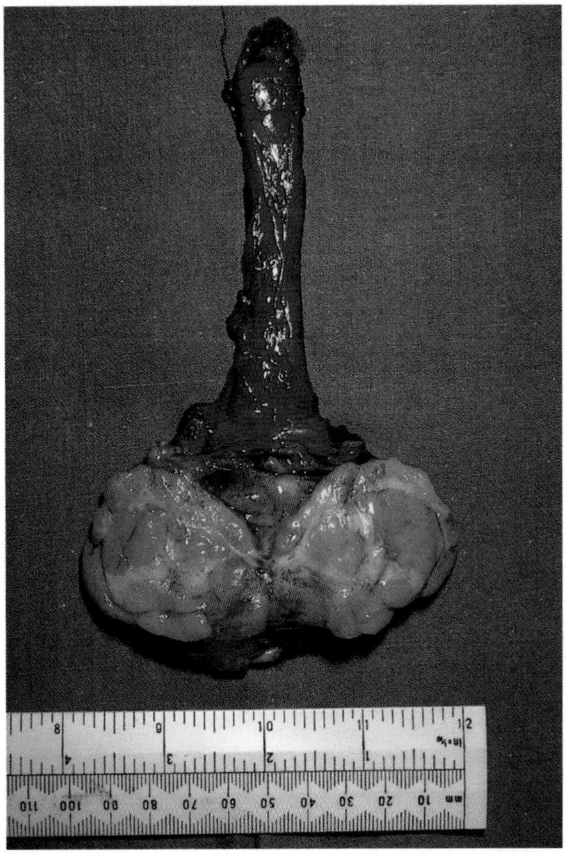

Figure 62.2 A seminoma of the testis with pearly, bulging surface on cutting. The 40-year-old patient presented with a swollen testis noticed after a collision with a large dog. One-third of testicular tumours present in 'atypical' ways.

The differentiated teratoma of childhood can be regarded as a benign lesion but this is not so in adults. In men over 60 the commonest tumour is malignant lymphoma.

Carcinoma in situ

Carcinoma *in situ* (CIS) has been found in men with testicular cancer, elsewhere in the removed testis and in the contralateral one. It is usually asymptomatic although it may produce slight tenderness and very poor semen quality. It is not associated with an increased plasma alpha-fetoprotein (AFP), hCG or placental alkaline phophatase (PLAP). There is a 50% risk of developing invasive germ cell cancer in 5 years. Diagnosis is currently by testicular biopsy but semen analysis may reveal malignant germ cells. Treatment depends on the age and testicular status of the patient. For unilateral CIS, orchidectomy should be performed but in unitesticular men or bilateral CIS, radiotherapy should be considered.

Presentation

Every testicular swelling must be assessed with the possibility of tumour in mind. The classical presentation is with a painless enlargement of the testicle. One-third of testicular tumours are misdiagnosed on the first clinical assessment. The common errors in diagnosis result from the presence of pain (which may result from haemorrhage into the tumour), hydrocele (a not uncommon accompaniment of tumour) and a history of 'trauma' which may merely bring the swelling to attention (Figure 62.2).

Preliminary ultrasound examination of the scrotum may be helpful, especially where the testis cannot be palpated because of the presence of a large hydrocele. The differential diagnosis includes epididymo-orchitis, torsion, a syphilitic gumma, granulomatous orchitis and tuberculosis. If there is doubt about the diagnosis surgical exploration should be undertaken.

Surgical exploration

Exploration should be undertaken through an inguinal approach with early dissection and soft clamping of the cord prior to delivery of the testis. Frozen section histology is not necessary in every case and can be reserved for those in whom there is doubt about the diagnosis after inspection of the testis, or before removal of a solitary testis.

Staging

Staging investigations should not postpone the orchidectomy.

The essential pre-operative investigations are a chest radiograph and preferably two separate measurements of AFP and beta-hCG

Post-operative staging requires:

- histological analysis of the extent of the primary tumour, with particular reference to invasion of the cord structures and the histological type
- CT scan of abdomen
- plain chest radiograph, and chest CT if negative
- full blood count, liver function tests, urea, electrolytes, calcium, AFP, beta-hCG (and creatinine clearance before chemotherapy).

The patient can then be placed in one of the stages shown in Table 62.1. The TNM classification has been altered (fifth edition) to incorporate the prognostic information from serum markers. The 'S categories' are shown in Table 62.2a, and the stage groupings incorporating these are shown in Table 62.2b.

Tumour markers

Measurement of markers is of some prognostic guide in assessing response to orchidectomy but their main value is in follow-up. Rising concentrations indicate active metastases, often long before disease becomes obvious on clinical or radiological examination.

The two commonly used markers are AFP and beta-hCG. Significant concentrations of one or other marker are found in the serum of up to 90% of patients with non-seminomatous germ cell tumours. Both markers will be raised in 40% of patients. The half-life of AFP is 4-6 days, and of hCG 24–36 hours. hCG levels are occasionally raised in seminomas, but AFP elevation indicates the presence of a teratomatous element, even if this has not been detected histologically.

Table 62.1 Staging of testicular cancer

pTX	Primary tumour cannot be assessed. If radical orchiectomy has not been performed then TX is used
pT0	No evidence of primary tumour
pTis	Carcinoma *in situ* (intra-tubular germ cell neoplasia)
pT1	Tumour limited to testis and epididymis without vascular or lymphatic invasion
pT2	Tumour limited to testis and epididymis with vascular or lymphatic invasion or tumour extends through tunica albuginea with involvement of tunica vaginalis
pT3	Tumour invades spermatic cord
pT4	Tumour invades scrotum
NX	Regional lymph nodes cannot be assessed
N0	No regional lymph node metastases
N1	Metastasis with a lymph node mass ≤ 2 cm or multiple nodes none >2 cm in greatest dimension
N2	Metastasis with a lymph node mass >2 cm ≤ 5 cm or multiple nodes >2 cm but ≤ 5 cm in greatest dimension
N3	Metastasis with a lymph node mass >5 cm
MX	Distant metastasis cannot be assessed
M0	No distant metastasis
M1	Distant metastasis
M1a	Non-regional lymph nodes or pulmonary metastases
M1b	Distant metastases other than non-regional lymph nodes or pulmonary metastases

Table 62.2a S (Serum tumour marker) categories and stage groupings for testis cancer

SX Serum markers not available

S0 Serum marker study levels within normal limits

	LDH		*HCG (U/ml)*		*AFP (ng/ml)*
S1	<1.5 × N	and	<5000	and	<1000
S2	1.5 – 10 × N	or	5000–50 000	or	1000–10 000
S3	>10 × N	or	>50 000	or	>10 000

N: indicates the upper limit or normal for the LDH assay.

Table 62.2b Stage groupings for testis cancer

Stage 0	pTis	N0	M0	S0, SX
Stage I	pT1–4	N0	M0	SX
Stage IA	pT1	N0	M0	S0
Stage IB	pT2–4	N0	M0	S0
Stage IS	Any pT/TX	N0	M0	S1–3
Stage II	Any pT/TX	N1–3	M0	SX
Stage IIA	Any pT/TX	N1	M0	S0, S1
Stage IIB	Any pT/TX	N2	M0	S0, S1
Stage IIC	Any pT/TX	N3	M0	S0, S1
Stage III	Any pT/TX	Any N	M1, M1a	SX
Stage IIIA	Any pT/TX	Any N	M1, M1a	S0, S1
Stage IIIB	Any pT/TX	N1–3	M0	S2
	Any pT/TX	Any N	M1, M1a	S2
Stage IIIC	Any pT/TX	N1–3	M0	S3
Stage IV	Any pT/TX	Any N	M1, M1a	S3
	Any pT/TX	Any N	M1b	Any S

Management

Testicular tumours are relatively rare. Management requires expertise in chemotherapy, radiotherapy and surgery, in addition to active surveillance with easy access to CT scanning. Referral to a centre with a special interest is strongly advised.

Semen banking should be offered when appropriate, before further treatment begins, but should not cause significant delay.

Seminoma

This tumour is usually diagnosed in the early stages as it is relatively slow growing. A careful search of all pathological material should be made to exclude a small teratomatous element. If the tumour markers are elevated there is a teratomatous element, which affects management of the patient.

Seminomas are very sensitive to radiotherapy, which forms the main treatment of stage I disease and is used in selected patients in other stages, with or without chemotherapy.

Stage I disease is managed by radiotherapy to the para-aortic and ipsilateral pelvic nodes. The scrotum need not be irradiated unless there has been violation of the scrotal skin. In stage I patients the relapse rate should be less than 1%. Surveillance alone for stage I seminoma has shown it to be a safe alternative but relapse may occur late and when it does occur, treatment becomes more intense than might otherwise be necessary.

Low volume stage II disease can treated by a similar regimen. Relapse rates are 9% for radiotherapy and 18% for surveillance. For patients with large stage II tumour volume, the relapse rate after radiotherapy alone is unacceptably high and these patients are best treated with cisplatin-based chemotherapy.

Stage III and IV disease is managed by cisplatin-based chemotherapy, with radiation for residual disease.

Non-seminomatous tumours

The management of teratomas has undergone a dramatic change in recent years. The conventional management with orchidectomy and radiotherapy or retroperitoneal node dissection has been altered by the development of potent chemotherapy. After adequate chemotherapy patients are restaged and persistent bulky disease is resected.

Stage I patients with negative markers can be treated by orchidectomy then intensive surveillance to identify those with progressive disease, which is then treated by chemotherapy. In some centres such patients (with progressive disease) may be offered the alternative of retroperitoneal lymph node dissection. Patients with definite metastatic disease or positive markers are treated with chemotherapy until the markers become negative.

Stage II and III patients receive four to six cycles of chemotherapy and if the markers return to normal but a mass persists then surgical excision of the residual disease is performed. Persistent marker-positive disease may require further chemotherapy.

Chemotherapy

Testicular tumours have a unique sensitivity to a broad range of anti-neoplastic agents. A major advance occurred with the discovery that cisplatin was effective with single agent response rates of approximately 70%. Cisplatin was found to work in synergy with vinblastine and bleomycin. This drug combination has formed the basis of modern chemotherapy for non-seminomatous tumours. For patients with favourable prognostic factors the long-term survival rates are over 90%.

Chemotherapy is toxic and considerable expertise is required to prevent unnecessary renal toxicity.

In spite of treatment with four to six cycles of combination chemotherapy, some patients cannot be salvaged, or relapse early. Large tumour volume, very high levels of tumour markers (especially hCG), the presence of undifferentiated tumour in the primary and involvement of liver, bone or central nervous system are all important factors. These factors indicate 'unfavourable prognosis' disease with a 60% cure rate. For these patients trials are in progress assessing the role of more intensive chemotherapy and new drugs.

Surgery for residual disease after chemotherapy

Accurate planning (from spiral CT or MRI images) of residual disease is the key to success in this important facet of therapy. Although the majority of residual masses are in the retro-peritoneum, combined thoraco-abdominal procedures may be required.

Mixed tumours

Prognosis for these tumours relates to the non-seminomatous elements and they are therefore managed along the lines for teratomas.

Follow-up of testicular tumours

There is a risk (up to 3%) of tumour developing in the remaining testis after orchidectomy for tumour. This risk is much higher (up to 45%) if the testis was originally undescended.

Infections and inflammations of the testis and epididymis

Epididymitis

For descriptive purposes epididymitis, its aetiology and treatment, will be separated from orchitis. Epididymitis presents as pain, felt locally or referred along the spermatic cord, with swelling and tenderness. It may occur in association with inflammation of the adjoining testis to give the clinical picture of epididymo-orchitis.

Patients with epididymitis can usefully be divided into three groups: children, adults up to the age of 35, and older men.

In children and men over 35 years, epididymitis is usually related to bacterial infection of the urinary tract. In the middle group of sexually active young men, epididymitis usually follows urethritis caused by sexually acquired infection. The common organisms in this group are the chlamydial organisms and *Neisseria gonorrhoeae*.

In all age groups epididymitis may be related to a systemic infectious or inflammatory disease, e.g. tuberculosis, brucella, sarcoid and cryptococcus. These disorders usually cause chronic rather than acute epididymitis.

Diagnosis
The differential diagnosis of acute epididymitis includes testicular torsion and tumour. Differentiation from torsion depends on the history of preceding urinary or urethral irritation, the examination findings and the finding of pus cells and bacteria on urine microscopy. Radionuclide studies and Doppler ultrasound of the testicular vessels have been reported as helpful but may not be available in the emergency situation and are not 100% accurate. If doubt exists, prompt surgical exploration should be undertaken.

Chronic epididymitis needs investigation to exclude the systemic disorders mentioned above.

Complications
These include abscess formation, testicular infarction, chronicity and inflammatory obstruction of sperm transport with resultant subfertility.

Abscess formation should be suspected if pain, swelling and fever show no response to bed rest and adequate antibiotic therapy within 24 hours. Ultrasound will diagnose this complication, which is treated by surgical drainage. If abscess formation has produced extensive tissue destruction epididymectomy (and often orchidectomy) is needed.

Management
Ideally, treatment of epididymitis should be directed at a specific organism. In practice, 'best guess' therapy has to be started in advance of bacteriological culture results.

For young men in whom the infection is likely to be associated with urethritis, a Gram stain of urethral secretion should be followed by special culture. If cultures are not helpful serological tests may be so. Treatment is with oral oxytetracycline (or a derivative) for 14–21 days in uncomplicated cases. Erythromycin and 4-quinolones are alternatives. Treatment of patient and consort should proceed simultaneously.

Epididymitis in children and older men should be managed by culture of the urine, followed by administration of an antibiotic active against the common urinary pathogens according to local sensitivities, changed if necessary when the culture results are available. Subsequent evaluation of the urinary tract should be done to exclude obstruction and other abnormalities predisposing to infection.

Non-specific measures for all patients include bed rest, analgesia and scrotal elevation to improve lymphatic drainage.

Orchitis
Infection may reach the testis by direct extension from the vas and epididymis, via the lymphatics or by blood spread. The common causes of orchitis are those associated with epididymitis. A focus of pyogenic orchitis may also occur after an episode of septicaemia. The clinical picture of epididymo-orchitis is treated in the same way as epididymitis. Orchitis alone is relatively rare. Non-bacterial causes include viruses, chemicals, parasites and trauma. Syphilitic and filarial orchitis occur where these diseases are endemic.

Viral orchitis
The best-known form of orchitis is that associated with mumps. It occurs in one in five post-pubertal mumps patients, about 5 days after the parotitis. Other causes are influenza and coxsackie viruses. Testicular swelling is prominent and there is often a reactive hydrocele. Treatment is directed to relief of symptoms. No significant benefit from adrenocorticotrophic hormone (ACTH) or steroids has been demonstrated. Aspirating a tense hydrocele may relieve pain.

Granulomatous orchitis
Non-specific inflammation may occur in the testis, epididymis and spermatic cord following infection, trauma, exposure to chemicals, and occasionally after vasectomy. The testis is usually enlarged and tender. The aetiology is often not clear. Biopsy may be required to exclude specific pathology such as tuberculosis, sarcoid, and other rare conditions.

Testicular torsion

The pathological event is torsion of the spermatic cord. Torsion can occur in the extravaginal or intravaginal cord. Compression of the testicular veins, then the arterial supply, causes pain: within 6 hours cells in the testis suffer ischaemic damage.

Neonatal torsion
Extra-vaginal torsion of the testis may occur in the neonatal or even pre-natal period. There is often no apparent pain or systemic upset but the testis is swollen. Commonly the testis is completely infarcted by the time of surgical exploration. Fixation of the other testis must be done.

Torsion in young adults
The underlying defect that allows an intra-vaginal torsion of the cord to occur is a high insertion of the tunica vaginalis ('bell clapper' deformity – Figure 62.3), leaving a length of cord free within the tunica. This anomaly is usually bilateral and the testis may take up a horizontal lie. Torsion of the testis alone may occur with the congenital anomaly of a long mesorchium (Figure 62.4).

Clinical features
Torsion is most common around the time of puberty. There are often preceding attacks of pain probably representing episodes of torsion, which resolve spontaneously.

There is a sudden onset of pain, which may be felt in the scrotum, groin or in the lower abdomen, often associated with nausea and vomiting.

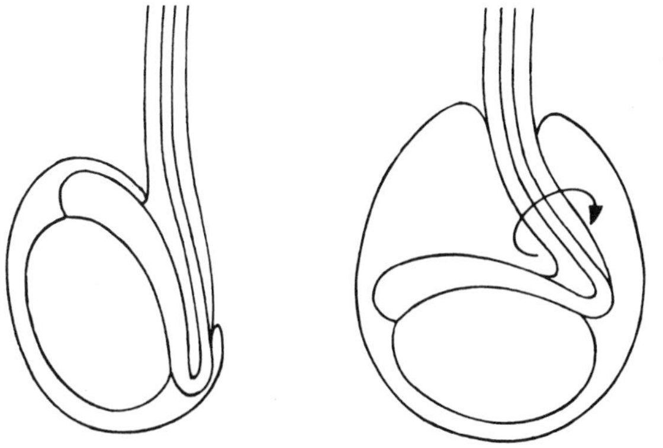

Figure 62.3 The high insertion of the tunical vaginalis allows an intravaginal torsion to occur.

Examination often shows the relevant testis sitting high in the scrotum, often with a horizontal lie. The testis and cord are tender and swollen.

Differential diagnosis

Infection and tumour are the main differential diagnoses. The common mistake is to treat a painful testis as infection without making a definite diagnosis (Figure 62.5). If the urine has no pus cells or bacteria infection is unlikely and surgical exploration is needed.

Treatment

Prompt surgical exploration should be undertaken through a scrotal incision. The twist in the cord is reduced and the testis observed. If the testis is viable it should be fixed by suturing the tunica albuginea to the dartos at three points using non-absorbable sutures. If the testis is not viable it should be removed. The other testis should be fixed at the same time.

Although the time limit of 6 hours after the onset of pain is classically associated with non-viability, it is worth performing exploration even after this time as the vascular occlusion is not always complete and the testis may be salvageable.

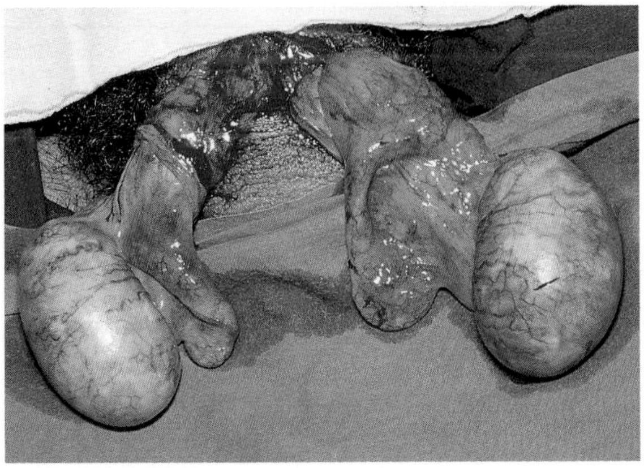

Figure 62.4 This 23-year-old patient had recurrent testicular pain and swelling for 5 years. The long mesorchium allows torsion of the testis alone, which easily corrects itself. Bilateral orchidopexy cured his pain.

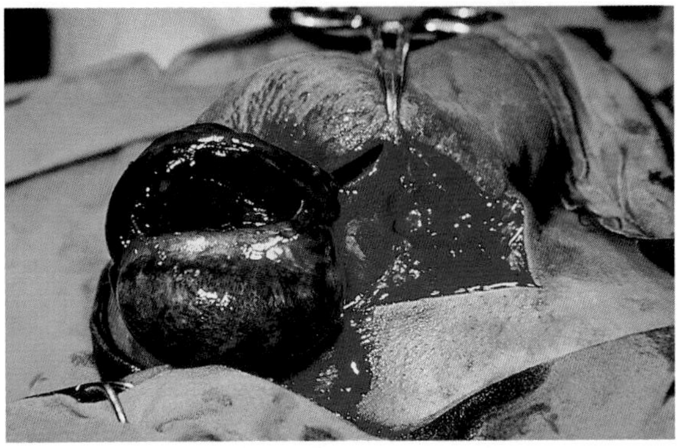

Figure 62.5 The late effects of torsion. The testis, appendages and intravaginal cord are necrotic. This 18-year-old man was treated for 48 hours with antibiotics for 'epididymitis' despite normal urinalysis and the absence of urinary symptoms.

Torsion of testicular or epididymal appendages

Embryonic remnants form cysts attached to the upper pole of the testis or epididymis. They may undergo torsion and produce pain and swelling out of all proportion to their size. Careful examination may demonstrate localized tenderness and the rotated cyst may be seen by transillumination of the associated small hydrocele ('blue spot sign'). If the diagnosis is certain, surgical exploration is not essential, but may be needed to exclude testicular torsion (Figure 62.6).

Testicular trauma

Testicular trauma is dealt with in Module 57.

Chronic testicular pain

Chronic testicular pain is a difficult problem which seems to be increasingly common.

Patients require careful assessment. A thorough history should include an attempt to identify events associated with the onset of the pain and the patient's theories of the cause. Examination and scrotal ultrasound will identify local pathology. If the testis and cord are normal, referred pain from intra-abdominal, retroperitoneal or musculoskeletal causes should be

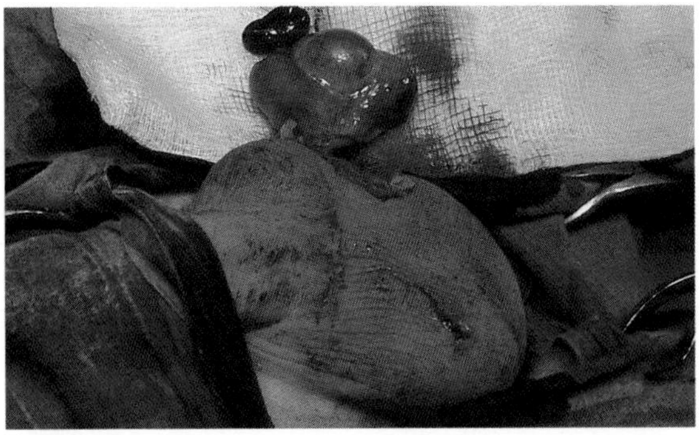

Figure 62.6 Torsion of the appendix of the epididymis. Exploration was needed because testicular torsion could not be excluded.

sought. Commonly, no formal diagnosis can be made or the problem may be one manifestation of 'visceral hyperalgesia'. Assessment in the pain clinic is recommended. Surgery virtually never helps and commonly results in transference of the pain to the incision or opposite testis.

Section 62.2 • The penis

Surgical anatomy

The penis consists of two dorso-laterally situated parallel erectile compartments, the corpora cavernosa, and the corpus spongiosum which surrounds the urethra ventrally and terminates distally in the erectile glans penis. Each is surrounded by fascial sheaths. The three corpora are surrounded by the dense fibrous Buck's fascia.

The arterial supply to the penis comes from the internal iliac artery via the internal pudenal artery. The internal pudendal artery becomes the penile artery and divides into the dorsal, bulbo-urethral and cavernous arteries. The cavernous arteries in turn give off the helicine arteries, which supply the erectile tissue. The helicine arteries become dilated and straight during erection.

The venous drainage of the penis consists of emissary veins, which drain the sinusoidal spaces beneath the tunica albuginea into deep dorsal, circumflex and peri-urethral veins.

The main motor nerve supply to the penis is from the sacral parasympathetic nerves. These delicate nerves run in the lateral pelvic fascia between the rectum and prostate. At the apex of the prostate they course anteriorly to reach the lateral aspect of the membranous urethra (Figure 62.7). An understanding of this anatomical pathway has allowed development of techniques to avoid their division in the course of radical pelvic surgery. The thoracolumbar sympathetic nerves form an additional nerve supply to the corpora and may be the pathway for psychologically mediated erection.

Lymphatic drainage from the corpora cavernosa and the skin passes through the superficial and deep inguinal nodes to the iliac nodes.

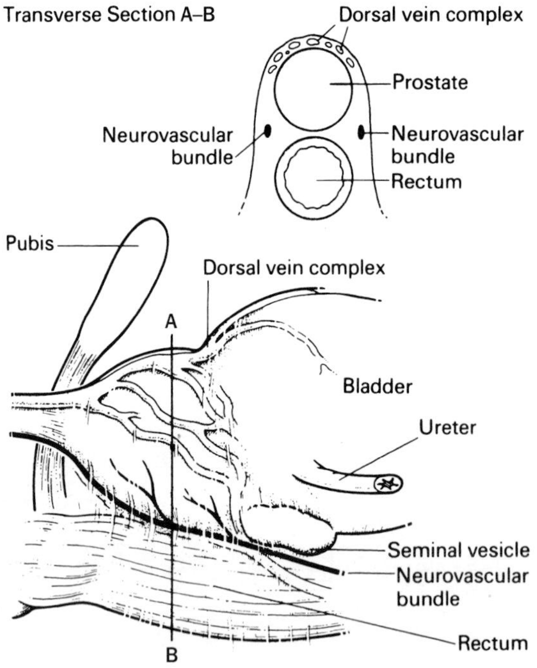

Figure 62.7 Course of the nerve supply of the corpora cavernosa.

Congenital lesions of the penis

Hypospadias

Hypospadias is a common developmental abnormality in which the urethra opens in an abnormal position on the underside of the penis. The most common associated abnormalities are undescended testes and inguinal herniae.

Hypospadias can be classified according to the site of urethral opening:

- glandular
- coronal
- penile
- penoscrotal
- scrotal
- perineal.

Severe hypospadias raises the possibility of an intersex state; chromosome studies are needed.

The associated hooded prepuce must be preserved for future repair of the hypospadias. When religious practice requires early circumcision, a dispensation to avoid this may be obtained. Hypospadias is commonly associated with chordee and correction of this is an important component of any repair.

The choice of surgical procedure depends on the severity of the hypospadias. Not all cases require surgery.

The aims of surgery are to:

- correct the cosmetic defect
- produce a meatus situated at the tip of the glans
- produce a forward projected urinary stream
- allow erection without ventral curvature.

Techniques are advancing and the trend is towards one-stage procedures. These are best performed by surgeons with experience and training in this exacting area.

Epispadias

Dorsal opening of the urethral meatus may occur alone or in conjunction with bladder exstrophy. In the glandular or penile variety the bladder neck is intact and continence is preserved. In the more posterior penopubic or sub-symphyseal variety (Figure 62.8) the bladder neck is incompetent and dribbling incontinence is present. The trigone of the bladder is often poorly developed and there is a high incidence of vesico-ureteric reflux. The corpora cavernosa are poorly developed giving rise to erectile abnormalities.

Surgical reconstruction aims to restore continence, reposition the urethral opening and correct penile deformity. It is a major reconstructive undertaking needing referral to a specialist centre.

Phimosis and paraphimosis

The prepuce is normally closely applied to the glans penis until the age of 2–3 years. Separation of the prepuce or circumcision before this age are not recommended as exposure of the glans to urine may result in ammoniacal dermatitis.

Phimosis describes a condition where the opening of the prepuce is narrowed and retraction is prevented. Separation of adhesions between glans and prepuce may be all that is needed in the younger child, and can be done under local anaesthesia, followed by daily retraction of the prepuce by a parent. Circumcision may be indicated in the older child if the phimosis is associated with scarring, recurrent balanoposthitis (Figure 62.9) or severe ballooning during voiding.

Paraphimosis results from trapping of a tight phimotic ring behind the glans to produce vascular congestion and oedema. A vicious cycle of increasing oedema and vascular insufficiency is created and may result in ischaemia of the glans.

The management of paraphimosis involves anaesthesia (a ring block of plain lignocaine around the base of the penis is usually satisfactory) and gentle, persistent manual compression of the glans. This compression reduces the oedema and allows reduction of the constriction ring. Early elective circumcision is recommended. Emergency dorsal slit, or circumcision, is rarely required and often leaves a poor cosmetic result.

Trauma to the penis and urethra

Trauma to the penis and urethra is dealt with in Module 56.

Disorders of erection

Mechanism of erection

The neurovascular events involved in erection are mediated by the cavernous nerves, which contain sympathetic and parasympathetic fibres. The smooth muscle of the corporeal erectile tissue is the key to understanding the mechanism of penile erection. In the flaccid state this smooth muscle is tonically contracted. Sexual stimulation results in release of neurotransmitters (including nitric oxide), which lead to relaxation of the cavernous smooth muscle. This relaxation results in arteriolar dilatation, pooling of blood in the expanding sinusoids and compression of the venous outflow, leading to penile enlargement and rigidity.

Nitric oxide produces vasodilatation by stimulating the production of cyclic guanosine monophosphate (cGMP). cGMP is normally broken down in the corporeal tissues by phosphodiesterase type 5. Sildenafil (Viagra) is a phosphodiesterase type 5 inhibitor and therefore promotes and prolongs the erectile response.

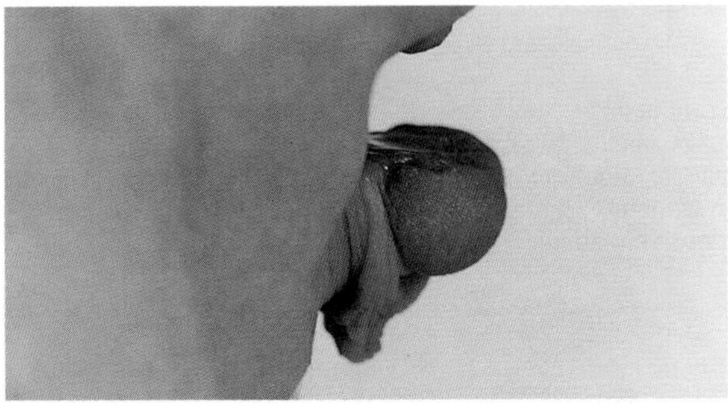

Figure 62.8 Severe epispadias with a dorsal urethral plate, severe penile shortening and bladder neck incompetence.

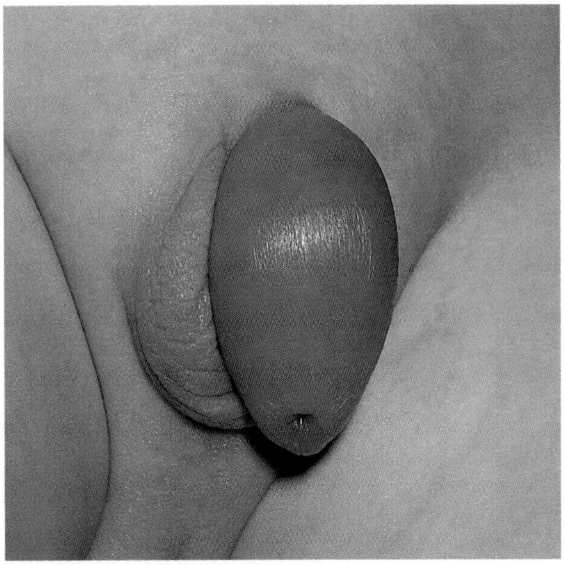

Figure 62.9 Severe balanoposthitis in a child aged 18 months. Recurrent attacks are one of the few indications for circumcision at this age.

Priapism

Priapism is an abnormally prolonged erection without sexual stimulation or desire.

- The erection is confined to the corpora cavernosa so the glans is not erect.
- Detumescence does not occur following ejaculation.
- Most cases are idiopathic.
- Some cases are associated with:
  - sickle-cell disease
  - leukaemia
  - drug therapy (systemic and intra-corporeal)
  - alcohol abuse
  - perineal trauma
  - dialysis
  - inflammatory disorders of the urinary tract.

Priapism can be classified as 'low flow' or 'high flow'. 'Low flow' priapism is usually painful and there is venous occlusion: blood gas analysis will reveal readings similar to venous (deoxygenated) blood. Untreated low flow priapism leads to fibrosis and erectile dysfunction.

'High flow' priapism usually follows trauma to the corpora and is associated with increased inflow of arterial blood – a form of AV fistula.

Management is summarized in Figure 62.10. Extreme care must be taken in giving metaraminol, as life-threatening hypertension can occur when it reaches the systemic circulation.

Peyronie's disease

This idiopathic disorder causes fibrotic changes in the elastic tissue of the tunica of the corpora cavernosa. The fibrotic plaque may cause pain and/or curvature of the penis. In a minority of cases an asymptomatic lump appears in the penis. The disease may progress slowly over a period of years or may follow a rapid course producing marked angulation of the erect penis preventing intercourse. The plaque may be dorsal (Figure 62.11), lateral or ventral.

About 10% of patients with Peyronie's disease also have Dupuytren's contracture and there are familial associations. The aetiology is unknown. Some cases follow trauma to the corpora. Spontaneous remission is common.

Impotence may result from pain, psychological effects or mechanical progress of the disease.

Management

No non-surgical treatment has been proved effective in randomized, controlled trials, but oral vitamin E, oral or locally injected steroids, oral sodium para-amino benzoate and ultrasound applied to the plaque are still commonly used. The pain experienced by some patients is usually self-limiting.

Angulation interfering with satisfactory intercourse makes some patients opt for surgery. Operative techniques are based on: (1) surgical excision of the fibrotic plaque with replacement of the defect with dermal or synthetic grafts; or (2) plication or resection of the corpus cavernosum opposite the site of maximum concavity. The former have been disappointing; the latter may cause an 'hour-glass ' appearance with impairment of distal blood flow.

Impotence in association with Peyronie's disease merits full investigation to exclude other causes but may require combined treatment of the plaque with insertion of a penile prosthesis (see below).

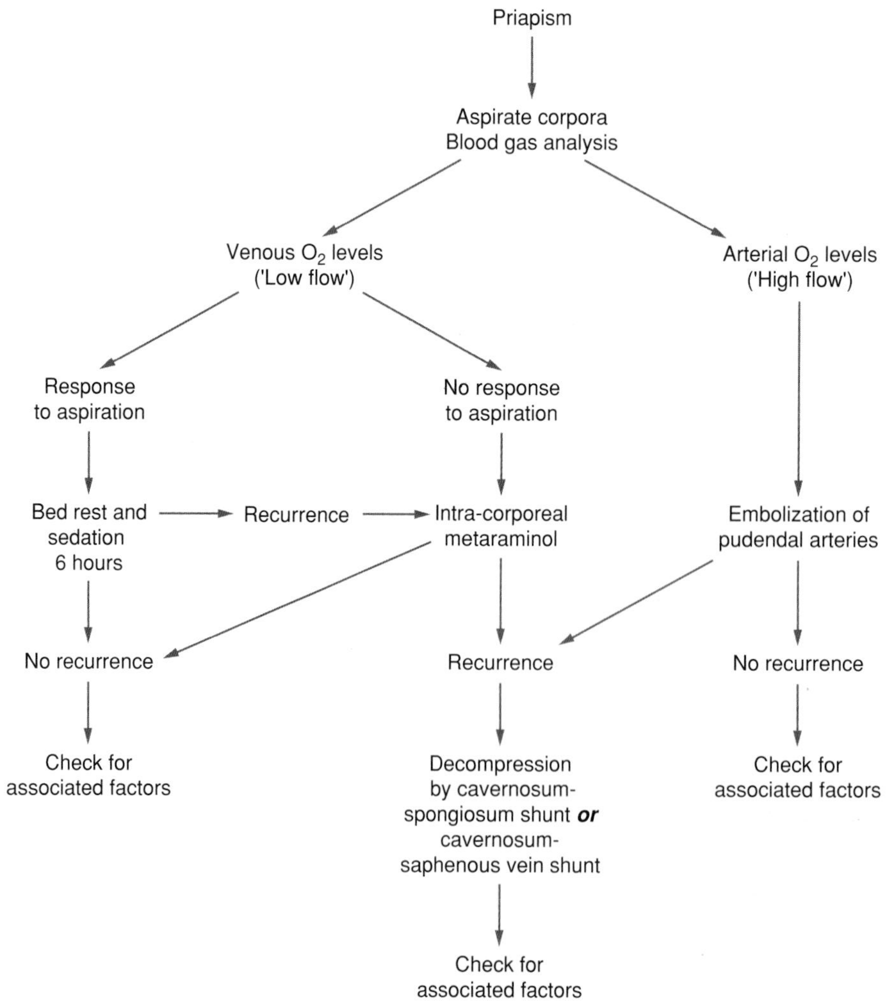

Figure 62.10 The management of priapism.

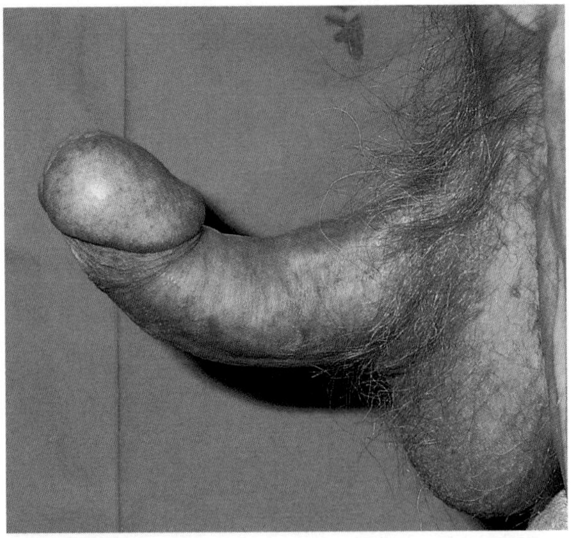

Figure 62.11 Peyronie's 'disease' causing severe angulation, in this case dorsally.

Erectile dysfunction ('impotence')

Assessment

A full history, including a complete drug history, should be taken. The drugs known to affect erectile function are shown in Table 62.3. Physical examination and urinalysis should include a search for peripheral vascular disease and diabetes. A history suggesting psychogenic factors may lead to more detailed investigation by a psychologist or psychiatrist with an interest in erectile dysfunction. Plasma testosterone should be measured. The concentration of free testosterone may be more important than the total. Many patients expect that hormone supplements will be used: they are contraindicated unless these measurements are low. It is now known that most secondary erectile dysfunction in middle-aged or older men is due to insufficient arterial inflow to the corpora. This may or may not be associated with generalized arterial disease which accompanies a Western lifestyle, a diet high in saturated fat, smoking and sympathetic overactivity.

Intra-cavernosal injection of prostaglandin E1 or a papaverine/phentolamine mixture is a useful test of overall cavernosal function. More detailed investigation may require Doppler flow studies, electromyography, selective penile angiography and assessment of penile rigidity after psycho-sexual stimulation in specialist laboratories.

Table 62.3 Drugs implicated in erectile dysfunction

Drug class	*Drug example*
Anti-hypertensives	Beta-blocking drugs
Anti-depressants	Tricyclic anti-depressants
Tranquillizers	Diazepam
CNS depressants	Ethanol, opiates
Anti-androgens	Cyproterone acetate
Anti-cholinergics	Probanthine

Management

Management should be directed by the findings obtained from the history, physical examination and special investigations. Many patients accept reassurance that their problem is shared by many men of the same age and is not a sign of serious disease.

The development of effective oral therapy has changed management and led to a significant reduction in the use of intra-cavernosal injection therapy.

Sildenafil (Viagra). Sildenafil (Viagra) is an effective oral agent, which is well tolerated. The main side-effects are of facial flushing, headaches and distortion of colour vision. Cardiovascular events are due to unaccustomed physical activity in unfit people rather than to the drug itself. The drug takes effect within 2 hours of oral ingestion and is not associated with a risk of prolonged erections or priapism. Sildenafil is contraindicated in patients on nitrate therapy. Other oral agents such as vasodilators, and the centrally acting apomorphine, are under investigation.

Vacuum devices. Vacuum devices fit over the penis and draw blood into the cavernosal tissues. Some patients find the use of an external mechanical device inhibiting.

Intra-cavernosal injection therapy. Intra-cavernosal injection therapy using papaverine, phentolamine or prostaglandin E1 has been used extensively for treatment of erectile dysfunction. The treatment is limited by its invasive nature and complications, which include prolonged erection, pain at the injection sites and the development of fibrosis in the corpus cavernosa.

The medicated urethral system for erection (MUSE). MUSE was developed as an alternative to intra-cavernosal injection. With this system prostaglandin is introduced as a pellet into the distal urethra and absorbed into the erectile tissue.

A very few selected patients benefit from surgery to insert a malleable (Figure 62.12a) or inflatable (Figure 62.12b) penile prosthesis, or from surgery to reduce venous outflow or augment the arterial inflow.

Disorders of ejaculation

The process of ejaculation has three main phases: bladder neck closure, seminal emission into the posterior urethra and propulsion of semen along the urethra. The efferent limb for the reflex is the anterior lateral column of the spinal cord and the thoracolumbar sympathetic outflow. This latter is particularly vulnerable during surgical dissection around the distal aorta.

The important disorders of ejaculation are: haemospermia; retrograde ejaculation; premature ejaculation and failure of ejaculation due to failure of orgasm.

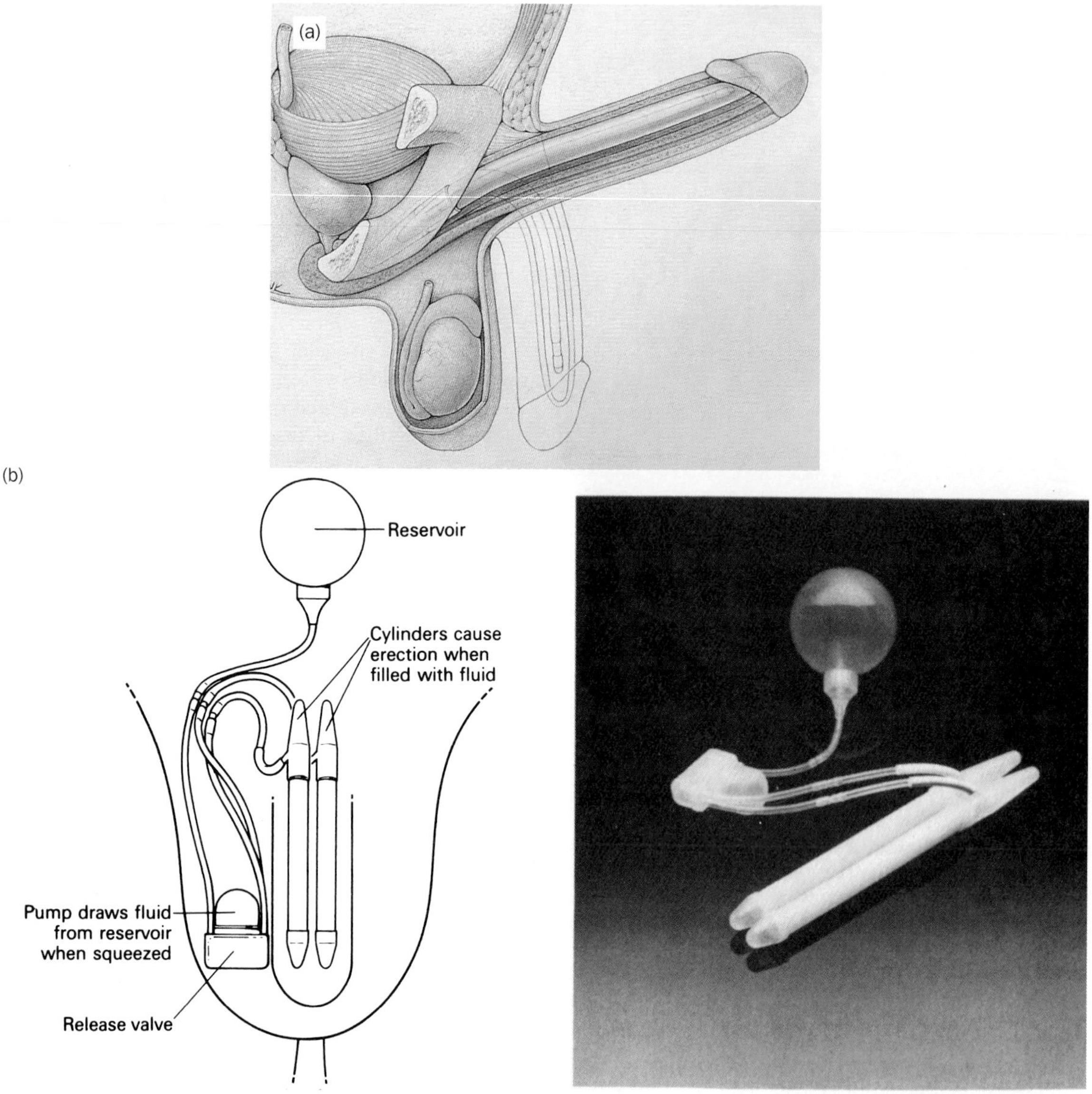

Figure 62.12 (a) A malleable penile prosthesis. The shaft of the penis is permanently elongated and thickened and is made 'erect' simply by bending. Surgery is straightforward and there are few complications. (b) An inflatable prosthesis. This gives a natural resting appearance. The device is more expensive, surgery is more complex and complications are more frequent than with a malleable prosthesis. (Illustrations courtesy of American Medical Systems.)

Haemospermia

Haemospermia is common and alarming to the patient, but rarely indicates serious disease. In patients under 40 years, if clinical examination of the prostate and external genitalia is normal, only explanation and reassurance are indicated. It is reasonable to do transrectal ultrasound and even cystoscopy if the patient will not be reassured without them, but they are not otherwise needed. In patients over 40 years, prostate-specific antigen (PSA) measurement and transrectal ultrasound are advisable. Most cases are self-limiting, but persistence may indicate prostatic infection: trimethoprim, a tetracycline derivative or a 4-quinolone antibiotic may help.

Retrograde ejaculation

Retrograde ejaculation is caused by failure of closure of the bladder neck, causing reflux of the ejaculate into the bladder. Prostatic surgery or alpha-blocking drugs (Module 61), diabetic autonomic neuropathy and surgical damage to the thoracolumbar outflow can cause retrograde ejaculation.

Premature ejaculation

Premature ejaculation is common, is virtually never due to urogenital disease and is treated by psychosexual counselling (Masters and Johnson technique) and clomipramine or selective serotonin re-uptake inhibitors.

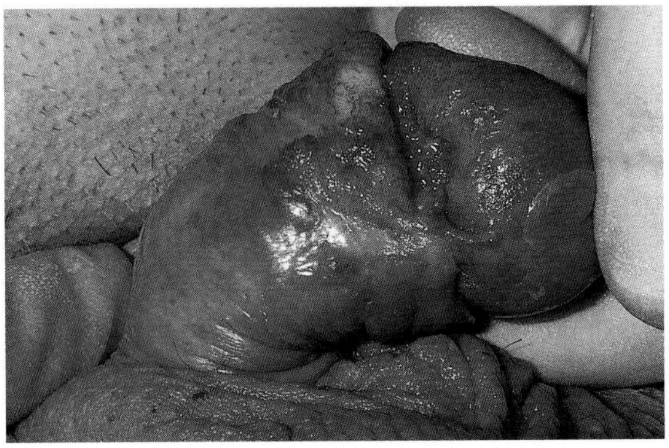

Figure 62.13 Ulcerating carcinoma of the penis. The patient was a 53-year-old doctor who had noticed a discharge from under his prepuce for 1 year.

Failure of orgasm

Failure of orgasm (hence failure of ejaculation) is rare and usually psychogenic. Organic causes include autonomic neuropathy, some psychotrophic drugs and surgical division of the thoracolumbar sympathetic outflow.

Carcinoma of the penis

Aetiology

Circumcision in infancy gives complete protection from developing carcinoma of the penis. Circumcision performed after infancy but before puberty greatly decreases the risk. A non-retractile foreskin and poor hygiene are clearly associated with the development of carcinoma of the penis but there is no clear association with venereal or herpetic infection.

Table 62.4a TNM classification of carcinoma of the penis

TX	Primary tumour cannot be assessed
T0	No evidence of primary tumour
Tis	Carcinoma *in situ*
Ta	Non-invasive verrucous carcinoma
T1	Tumour invades subepithelial connective tissue
T2	Tumour invades corpus spongiosum or cavernosum
T3	Tumour invades urethra or prostate
T4	Tumour invades other adjacent structure
NX	Regional lymph nodes cannot be assessed
N0	No regional lymph node metastases
N1	Metastasis in a single superficial inguinal node
N2	Metastases in multiple or bilateral superficial inguinal lymph nodes
N3	Metastases in deep inguinal or pelvic lymph node(s), unilateral or bilateral
MX	Distant metastasis cannot be assessed
M0	No distant metastasis
M1	Distant metastasis

Table 62.4b Stage groupings for carcinoma of the penis

Stage 0	Tis	N0	M0
	Ta	N0	M0
Stage I	T1	N0	M0
Stage II	T1	N0, N1	M0
	T2	N0, N1	M0
Stage III	T1	N2	M0
	T2	N2	M0
	T3	N0, N1, N2	M0
Stage IV	T4	Any N	M0
	Any T	N3	M0
	Any T	Any N	M1

Pathology

The lesion is usually a squamous cell carcinoma. Very rarely a basal cell carcinoma, malignant melanoma, sarcoma or secondary carcinoma occurs. Carcinoma *in situ* of the penis shows the typical cytological features of malignancy.

Clinical features

Invasive penile cancer usually presents in elderly men but may occur in patients as young as 30 years. The tumours are proliferative or ulcerating (Figure 62.13). Secondary infection is common. The inguinal lymph nodes are enlarged in two-thirds of cases but in one-half the lymphadenopathy is the result of secondary infection, not metastases.

Carcinoma *in situ* (erythroplasia of Queyrat – indistinguishable from Bowen's disease at other epidermal sites) appears as moist, velvety red or dry, scaly patches or even as a warty lesion. Progression to invasive cancer is probably rare but the condition is certainly potentially malignant.

TNM classification and staging

These are summarized in Table 62.4.

Management

Diagnosis is established by biopsy, which may require a dorsal slit or circumcision. The large infected and fungating tumour is best dealt with by partial or radical amputation.

Stage I and II lesions can be treated with radiotherapy with a good cosmetic and functional result and survival at least as good as for surgery (70–90% 3 year survival).

Palpable lymph nodes should be treated with antibiotics and carefully watched while the primary tumour is treated. If the lymphadenopathy increases, or does not resolve after 1 month, a biopsy should be taken to look for metastatic involvement. Bilateral inguinal node dissection may be complicated by lymphoedema and delayed wound healing, and may not cure the disease. An alternative is to irradiate the nodal area. When the disease is extensive with iliac nodes involved, the prognosis is dismal. So far the best chemotherapeutic agent for advanced disease is bleomycin.

Carcinoma *in situ* may be treated with either radiotherapy or topical 5-fluorouracil cream.

Infections and inflammations of the penis

Balanitis and balanoposthitis. The presence of the prepuce creates a warm moist atmosphere for the growth of organisms. Regular hygiene normally prevents abnormal growth and may be used to manage minor infections. Persistent balanitis unresponsive to local hygiene and antibiotics, guided by culture results, should be investigated to exclude other specific pathology. Not all balanitis is caused by infection and the differential diagnosis includes pre-cancerous lesions, drug eruptions, psoriasis, scabies, dermatitis and lichen planus. If phimosis co-exists then a dorsal slit may be required to expose underlying lesions of the glans penis. If doubt exists about the pathology, biopsy should be performed.

Gangrenous balanitis may result from combined infection by spirochaetes and vibrio organisms and untreated may result in extensive destruction of the glans and shaft of the penis.

Balanitis xerotica obliterans is lichen sclerosus et atrophicus of the prepuce, of unknown cause. The typical white firm prepuce bleeds easily and causes a dense phimosis. The process may extend to the glans and cause meatal stenosis. The lesion is not pre-malignant but may require circumcision and meatotomy or meatoplasty.

Genital warts are caused by papilloma viruses and do not usually cause diagnostic difficulty. Warts on the genitalia outside the urethra can be treated by application of podophyllin, diathermy or cryotherapy. Warts in the urethra can be treated by local instillation of thiotepa or 5-fluorouracil.

Section 62.3 • The scrotum

Necrotizing fasciitis of the scrotum (Fournier's gangrene)

This is usually caused by infection with more than one organism, particularly haemolytic streptococci in association with coliforms, bacteroides, diphtheroids or pseudomonas. The onset is sudden and constitutional upset severe. Pain and inflammation are marked and patchy necrosis of the scrotal skin occurs which may be followed by extensive sloughing. Treatment is with appropriate antibiotics (including metronidazole) and **wide** surgical debridement. Despite the severe clinical signs recovery is usually complete.

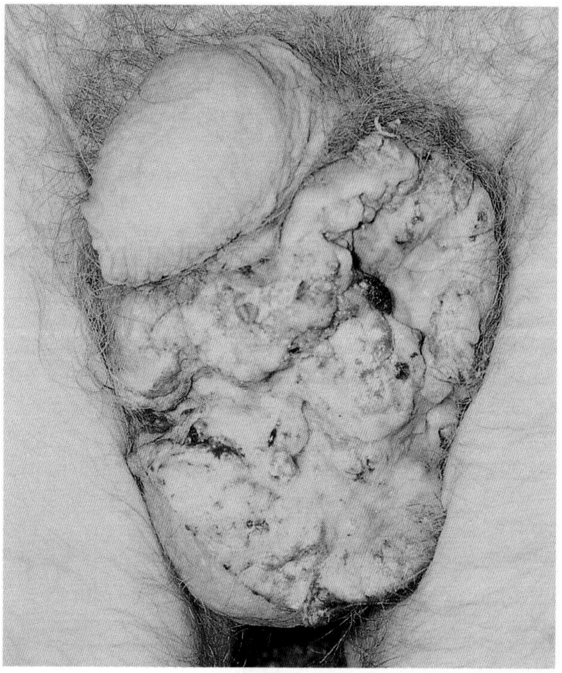

Figure 62.14 Carcinoma of the scrotum in a former jute mill worker.

Carcinoma of the scrotum (Figure 62.14)

An occupational aetiology has been known for this condition since it was first described in chimney sweeps and later in cotton spinners. Even today it is still likely to have resulted from occupational exposure to carcinogens so a full occupational history should be taken. Treatment is by a wide local excision with later dissection of the inguinal nodes if involved.

Genital filariasis

Wüchereria bancrofti is the common lymphatic filarial parasite to infect the genitalia. The diagnosis can be confirmed from microscopic examination of smears of blood or hydrocele fluid. Complement-fixation and skin tests are also useful. Management includes treatment with diethylcarbamazine. Plastic surgery may be required to remove oedematous tissue and reconstruct the scrotum.

Scrotal swellings

Diagnosis

The diagnosis of a scrotal swelling depends on a careful history and examination, scrotal ultrasound and a minimum of other investigations.

There are three important issues in the examination of a scrotal swelling:

- Does the swelling arise in the scrotum or has it come down from above through the inguinal canal (is its upper limit palpable)?
- Is it cystic or solid (does it transilluminate)?
- Is the swelling in the body of the testis or not?

Hydrocele

Infantile hydroceles

Infantile hydroceles are due to continued patency of the processus vaginalis and may be associated with an inguinal hernia. Ligation of the processus vaginalis will resolve the problem. The sac is fenestrated to drain the fluid but need not be removed.

Adult hydroceles

Adult hydroceles may be primary (idiopathic) or secondary to trauma, tumour or infection. Primary hydroceles are common in the elderly. The basic defect is a delay in the absorption of fluid, presumably due to lymphatic obstruction. In all cases the body of the testis should be carefully palpated and it may be necessary to aspirate a tense hydrocele before this can be done. In 5% of cases the testis lies anteriorly in the hydrocele sac so its position should be demonstrated by transillumination before aspiration. If ultrasound examination is needed, it can easily be done through the fluid 'window'. Treatment is surgical (subtotal excision or plication of the sac) unless the patient is unfit or unwilling to undergo surgery. Repeated aspirations may keep the patient comfortable but risk causing bleeding or infection. Aspiration with injection of sclerosant (tetracycline or STD) sometimes prevents recurrence.

Epididymal cysts and spermatoceles

Cysts arising in the region of the head of the epididymis may contain either clear fluid (epididymal cysts) or 'barley water' containing spermatozoa (spermatoceles). They may be multiple or multi-locular. Aspiration is followed by recurrence and if they are large, uncomfortable or causing undue anxiety they should be excised. Excision risks interrupting the single coiled tubule which forms the epididymis, interfering with ipsilateral sperm transport. This should be considered when advising young men.

Varicocele

Sixteen per cent of normal adult men have abnormal dilatation of the pampiniform plexus of veins. Most varicoceles cause no symptoms but a dull ache is sometimes complained of. The left side is nearly always affected with only 2% of cases affecting the right side. A cough impulse is present and there is retrograde flow of blood down the testicular vein. There is an increase in scrotal temperature which affects both sides of the scrotum. The relationship of a varicocele to subfertility is controversial. Treatment, if needed, is by transvenous embolization under radiological control; or by resection of a segment of the spermatic vein extraperitoneally above the internal inguinal ring. Ligation in the scrotum carries a high risk of testicular infarction. The appearance of a left varicocele in a middle-aged or older man is classically associated with a renal tumour occluding the left renal vein. A varicocele can also occur with occlusion of the spermatic vein on the right (Module 57, Figure 57.4).

Idiopathic scrotal oedema

This is a benign self-limiting condition of unkown cause, occuring in young children. The oedema and erythema are painless and may affect both sides and extend onto the groin and penis. Spontaneous resolution occurs in a few days.

Vasectomy

Vasectomy (more correctly vasotomy and occlusion, as there is no medical or medico-legal need to remove a segment of vas) is a safe and effective method of contraception. The procedure is normally performed under local anaesthesia as an outpatient and has few complications.

Pre-operative counselling should include a description of the procedure and the need for follow-up semen analyses (beginning at 3 and 4 months) until two consecutive samples have shown azoospermia. Most important from a medico-legal point of view is that even after two such samples there is a chance of 1 in 2600 that sperms will appear in the semen, temporarily or permanently, at some time during the next 20 years. The incidence of pregnancy is very much less than this, as temporary reappearance may not coincide with intercourse or the partner's fertile time. This must be explained and recorded.

The procedure involves division of the vasa (usually at the neck of the scrotum) and occlusion of the ends with ligatures, clips or diathermy. Fascial interposition reduces the risk of re-canalization.

The complications of vasectomy are usually related to the technique. A haematoma occuring within 24 hours of surgery must be drained to avoid discomfort and disability which otherwise may last many weeks. Swelling presenting later than 10 days is often misdiagnosed as infection. It is usually due to a sperm granuloma, an exquisitely tender immune reaction to extravasated sperms. Some respond to a short course of oral steroids: others require removal of the epididymis and vas up to the vasotomy site. Long-term scrotal pain is a difficult problem in a very few men, and is said to be less likely if the fascia around the vasotomy site is infiltrated with local anaesthetic (without epinephrine) at the end of the procedure.

Reversal of vasectomy

Vasectomy can be reversed by vaso-vasostomy or vaso-epididymostomy. The best results (>95% vas patency) follow microsurgical anastomosis in two layers. Failure to achieve patency may result from technical failure or unrecognized secondary obstruction elsewhere in the vas or epididymis Late stenosis, following initial patency, may occur.

Further reading

Bianchi, A. (1995).The impalpable testis. *Ann R Coll Surg Engl* **77**: 3–6.

Hendry, W. H. and Horwich, A. (1998). Testicular tumours. In: Whitfield, H. N., Hendry, W. F., Kirby, R. S. and Duckett, J. W., eds. *Textbook of Genitourinary Surgery*. Oxford: Blackwell Science.

Parkinson, M. C. and Harland, S. J. (2000). Testis cancer. In: Mundy, A. R., Fitzpatrick, J. M., Neal, D. E. and George, J. R., eds. *The Scientific Basis of Urology*. Oxford: Isis Medical Media, 375–93.

Sobin, L.H. and Wittekind, C., eds (1997). *TNM Classification of Malignant Tumours*, 5th edn. New York: John Wiley.

Soomro, N. A. and Neal, D. E. (1998). Treatment of hypospadias: an update of current practice. *Hosp Med* **57**: 553–6.

United Kingdom Testicular Cancer Study Group (1994). Aetiology of testicular cancer: association with congenital abnormalities, age at puberty, infertility, and exercise. *BMJ* **308**: 1393–9.

MODULE 63

Management of the surgical neonate

Section 63.1 • Neonatal surgery

The term neonatal surgery originally described the surgery of children up to 28 days after birth. In practice it has come to describe specialized neonatal surgical care, frequently commencing during the newborn period, of children born with congenital malformations and other conditions specific to this age group. Thus the child suffering from necrotizing enterocolitis or the premature infant with a large inguinal hernia will require neonatal surgical expertise even if the condition arises well outside the 28th day of life.

The neonatal surgical unit

Antenatal diagnosis has provided the opportunity for better planning of the pregnancy and delivery. It is evidently in the best interest of the mother and her child that the neonatal surgical unit is situated within easy distance from the obstetric and antenatal services and particularly the delivery suite. This facilitates the neonatal surgeon's involvement in antenatal counselling and in fetal investigation and therapy. In particular it allows and encourages parental (particularly maternal) access to the child, enhancing the bonding process and the acceptance of the child within the family. Clearly, neonatal surgery forms an integral part of perinatal services and is essential to them.

Most surgical neonates are cared for primarily by neonatologists with the assistance of neonatal surgeons. Others are managed by a team of neonatal surgeons and a neonatal anaesthetic-intensivist, with consultation and backup from the neonatologists. Thus the neonatal anaesthetic-intensivist has become a key member who is involved not only in the operating theatre but also in the day to day management of the surgical neonate. Successful management depends entirely on the availability of specialized neonatal surgical nursing staff, integral to whom are the neonatal operating room staff and the outreach family care sisters who will support the family once the child is discharged from the unit.

The spectrum of conditions managed by a neonatal surgical unit largely depends on the expertise available within the team at all levels. In the UK most units accept a wide range of congenital anomalies, but exclude cardiac and occasionally neurological conditions, which are managed in dedicated centres by specialized personnel.

The neonatal/fetal surgeon

Much of the surgery of congenital malformations is of a reconstructive nature. The paediatric surgeon aspiring to the specialized field of neonatal surgery should have a broad training incorporating the principles and practice of general and reconstructive surgery with the specialized fields of fetal medicine, antenatal care, neonatology and paediatric intensive care, genetics and paediatrics. Expertise in psychological management and counselling are integral to the skills of the modern neonatal surgeon. The neonatal surgeon is often faced with complex moral and ethical dilemmas and should therefore educate himself in these fields.

Refinements in antenatal ultrasound and consequently accurate evaluation of congenital malformations at an early stage in pregnancy, has involved the neonatal surgeon in the joint management of the mother, the fetus and its family. Close co-operation with colleagues from diverse specialties, e.g. ultrasound, obstetrics, genetics, neonatology, pathology, has led to the evolution of the 'fetal management team' of which the neonatal surgeon is a key member. His involvement immediately after birth and his knowledge of the long-term prognosis of congenital malformations is particularly relevant to the management of the pregnancy and the fetus. The neonatal surgeon has come to play a vital role in antenatal counselling of prospective parents, as well as in the dissemination of accurate information to colleagues in other specialties. He must be familiar with the developments in fetal physiology and advances in other specialties, e.g. neonatology, genetics, plastic surgery and organ transplantation. He is already involved in interventional fetal investigation and therapy and must look towards his possible role in antenatal fetal surgery. Equally his unique experience in the management of congenital malformations is invaluable in stimulating, as well as curbing, enthusiasm in the new and developing field of antenatal fetal surgery and the ethical issues arising from it.

Aesthetics and neonatal surgery

The goal of neonatal surgical management is a normal long-term survivor with a fully functional body and a healthy mind. It is precisely the surviving child for whom body image and self-acceptance are of major relevance to the development of personality. The surgeon, in planning his operation, must be constantly conscious of normal physiological development, and of the psychological needs of the growing child through adolescence to adulthood. The needs and feelings of the parents in relation to their abnormal child are also matters for consideration. Thus at the time of first, often serious life-saving surgery, scars should be carefully planned and placed within natural skin creases where they will be least conspicuous in later life.

To the growing child, who naturally seeks to conform to his peers, 'function' and 'aesthetics' are of equal relevance, and are as important as 'survival'. Thus survival at the expense of a significantly scarred and embarrassing body is no longer acceptable to the adolescent and his family. The neonatal surgeon therefore works to the concept of 'a healthy mind in a functional aesthetic body'.

Aetiology

Despite major advances the causes of most (65%) congenital malformations remain unclear. Some 7.5% are said to have a known genetic base, e.g. cystic fibrosis, congenital adrenal hyperplasia, and approximately 6% are chromosomal in origin, e.g. Down's syndrome, trisomy 13. Others relate to environmental factors such as maternal infection with rubella, cytomegalovirus and toxoplasma, or maternal exposure to teratogens such as thalidomide, mercury, alcohol and radiation. Congenital malformations may be of multifactorial origin, the result of an interaction of genetic and environmental factors, e.g. Hirschsprung's disease, spina bifida, cleft lip and palate. The majority of such insults act during the first trimester at a time of early embryogenesis. Others arise later, having a more obvious cause as is exemplified by intestinal atresia which is due to interference with the bowel blood supply, and club foot and Potter's syndrome which are thought to be due to direct uterine pressure on the fetus. The study of these aetiological factors is of obvious relevance to the understanding and future incidence of congenital malformations, and underpins genetic counselling for 'at-risk' individuals and families.

Table 63.1 Consideration prior to transfer of a neonate

Transport of the neonate
Airway
Temperature (prevent loss, provide heat)
Blood glucose (monitor, provide sugar)
Cardiovascular support
Metabolic problems
Render the child stable and safe

The neonate

The newborn child is not a 'small adult', and an understanding of the basic physiological differences from the adult is crucial to a successful outcome. Babies with congenital anomalies are best delivered close to the neonatal services. Antenatal transfer of the pregnant mother is the best and indeed the cheapest way of transporting the child. Post-natal transfer is rather more stressful. Before embarking on a journey, however short, it is absolutely essential that the child should be 'stable and safe'. Vain attempts at crash transfer of an ill and unstable child will often end in tragedy. Stable neonates travel well over considerable distances, as long as attention is given to basic physiology (Table 63.1). Thus the airway must be stable. This may involve muscle paralysis and ventilation through an endotracheal tube. Active measures should be in place to prevent heat loss and to maintain body temperature. Hypovolaemia and acidosis must be corrected and blood glucose levels stabilized. A period of relative stability prior to transfer will greatly enhance the child's chances of safe travel. During this time the advice and services of the Neonatal Flying Squad are a great asset.

Airway

Immediately at birth the pharynx should be cleared of all secretions. Since the baby is unable to lift its head and to clear its pharynx, it should always lie flat and on its side, for gravity to assist in clearing the airway of secretions. The anatomy of the pharynx and the higher position of the larynx in the newborn are reflected in the predominance of nasal breathing, such that occlusion of the nasal passages (choanal atresia, nasogastric tubes) may rapidly cause respiratory distress. The newborn child uses its diaphragm as the main muscle of respiration, so that impaired diaphragmatic movement, e.g. raised intra-abdominal pressure, diaphragmatic paralysis, is likely to compromise ventilation. Similarly, situations causing an increased respiratory effort or rate (normal 30 breaths per minute) rapidly lead to exhaustion and metabolic acidosis. Anticipation of such situations, e.g. post-operatively, is essential to appropriate elective preventive measures. The newborn child's central respiratory control is relatively immature and somewhat erratic. Apnoeic spells are a frequent and significant problem in the premature child and the ill or stressed child particularly after anaesthesia. Monitoring for apnoea therefore forms a routine part of neonatal care. Central stimulation with an intravenous aminophylline infusion is often effective in alleviating the situation. Persistent apnoeic episodes are an indication for mechanical ventilatory support. Clearly the surgical neonate, premature and otherwise, requires respiratory support much more frequently than an adult. Such a possibility should be anticipated and should form part of the overall management plan, rather than a response to a crisis. It is therefore relevant for all neonatal medical and nursing staff to acquire skills for endotracheal intubation and for ventilation of the newborn.

Temperature

In relation to its body weight the neonate has a much larger surface area than the adult. Its skin is thinner and capillary beds are closer to the surface such that heat loss to the environment is much more marked and rapid. The temperature regulating centres in the brain are relatively immature. Mechanisms for heat conservation such as vasoconstriction in the skin, and for heat production by shivering and muscular activity, are absent or much reduced so that the child is unable to compensate for heat loss. The development of sclerema or cold injury, a rare event in recent times, is a preventable life threatening complication.

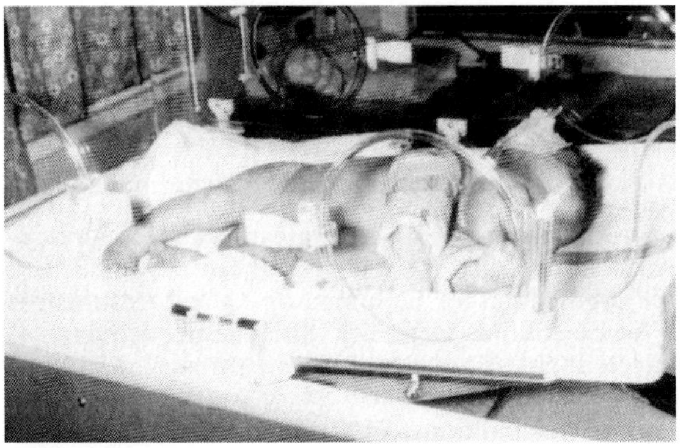

Figure 63.1 A stable child in a controlled environment in an incubator.

In planning management, heat loss should be anticipated and preventive measures instituted. The child should be kept in a draught-free, warm environment and unnecessary exposure avoided. Covering the baby with foil can reduce heat lost by radiation. In view of the neonate's reduced ability to produce heat, prevention of heat loss and active measures to provide heat, e.g. incubator (Figure 63.1), warming blanket, hot air blower are axiomatic to proper management of all surgical neonates.

Blood glucose

The normal term neonate lays down sufficient glycogen and brown fat body stores during the third trimester of a normal pregnancy, to avoid hypoglycaemia until maternal breast milk becomes available. Such stores are much reduced in the premature and the growth-retarded newborn. Blood sugar control is markedly disrupted by severe illness, so that hypoglycaemia is a common and dangerous complication. It may occur in specific situations because of high insulin levels as in the child of a diabetic mother, in association with the EMG (Beckwith–Wiedemann) syndrome, and nesideoblastosis. Symptoms of hypoglycaemia are hypotonia and lethargy, jittering, convulsions and apnoeic spells. All are an index of the brain's dependence on blood glucose for its nutrition, and indicate cerebral cell dysfunction and eventual injury. Babies at risk from hypoglycaemia should have their blood sugar monitored at least every 2–4 hours until they are stable. Intragastric or intravenous glucose supplements are required to maintain blood sugar levels. Reactive hypoglycaemia may follow infusions of concentrated glucose solutions. In difficult situations it should be remembered that an intraperitoneal or even subcutaneous infusion of glucose would rapidly reach the blood stream. However, high concentrations beneath the skin will cause sloughing and should be avoided.

Cardiovascular system

The transition from a fetal to an adult type of circulation involves major alterations in the pattern of blood flow. Lung expansion is associated with a marked reduction in pulmonary vascular resistance and pulmonary artery pressure. Blood flow through the pulmonary vascular bed rises from 7% of the blood volume during fetal life to virtually 100% following closure of the foramen ovale and the ductus arteriosus. During this period the cardiovascular system is relatively unstable. Adverse factors such as acidosis, hypoxia and hypercapnia may cause pulmonary vasoconstriction. There is a consequent rise in pulmonary vascular resistance and reversion to a fetal type of circulation with deoxygenated blood shunting from right to left across the foramen ovale and the patent ductus arteriosus.

Blood volume

The full-term neonate has been calculated to have a blood volume of 85 ml/kg. Loss of a relatively small volume of blood is therefore significant, and represents a major percentage of the total blood volume, the more so since compensatory mechanisms are relatively immature or absent. A loss of over 10% of the blood volume will induce signs of hypovolaemia, e.g. a rapid thready pulse, a drop in blood pressure and in central venous pressure, poor peripheral perfusion and a metabolic acidosis which may rapidly progress to circulatory collapse and cardiac arrest. It is evident that techniques which limit blood loss during surgery, e.g. dissection within tissue planes, bipolar diathermy are essential surgical practice. A careful ongoing estimate of blood loss is undertaken during surgery, and blood transfusion given for losses over 10% of the blood volume. In the event of circulatory collapse, e.g. septic shock, hypovolaemic shock, an intravenous bolus dose of 20 ml/kg of whole blood, plasma or colloid is a safe initial volume for resuscitation. The child's general condition and peripheral perfusion, his pulse and blood pressure and his central venous pressure determine further transfusion. Metabolic acidosis develops rapidly during hypovolaemic shock and should correct spontaneously once a normal circulation is restored. In the acute phase correction with 8.4% sodium bicarbonate (1/3 of base deficit × body weight in kg) may be helpful. Infusions of platelets and clotting factors are often required, e.g. septic shock from necrotizing enterocoloitis, large haemangiomas and liver dysfunction. It cannot be overemphasized that prevention of hypovolaemia constitutes best practice and that blood volume monitoring and rapid correction are crucial to successful neonatal surgery.

Red cell mass

Most neonates are polycythaemic at birth. Over subsequent weeks there is a steady reduction in the red cell mass so that the breast-fed child at 3 months of age has a haemoglobin level of around 11 g%. Introduction of a weaning diet and possibly haematinics is usually the only treatment required. Blood transfusion is occasionally necessary. The volume to be transfused is calculated from the Hb deficit (g%) × body weight (kg) × 3 for packed cells and × 6 for whole blood. Blood transfusion should be given slowly over several hours to allow for circulatory adjustment and to avoid cardiac embarrassment. The blood sugar should be constantly monitored to avoid hypoglycaemia during transfusion.

Hypocalcaemia

The symptoms are somewhat similar to those of a low blood sugar. The child is jittery in response to minimal stimuli, and increased muscle tone and twitching may progress to convulsions. Premature babies, stressed and ill infants are most at risk from hypocalcaemia. Most episodes are temporary and occur in the course of a specific illness. Persistent hypocalcaemia requires full investigation. Extensive blood transfusion with citrated blood may also induce hypocalcaemia and interfere with clotting. Treatment consists of a bolus intravenous injection of 30 mg/kg (0.3 ml/kg) of 10% calcium gluconate. Serum calcium levels can be sustained by constant intravenous calcium infusion (4 ml of 10% calcium gluconate added to each 100 ml of the daily maintenance fluids).

Jaundice

A mild jaundice is a normal occurrence in virtually all babies during the first 3–7 days of life. This unconjugated (fat-soluble) hyperbilirubinaemia is due to a temporary enzyme deficiency in hepatic handling of bilirubin. Premature babies are at greater risk of kernicterus (the effect of deposition of fat-soluble bilirubin in the basal ganglia of the brain) from the rapidly rising levels of unconjugated bilirubin. Treatment consists of adequate hydration and phototherapy with artificial light of wavelength 400–500 nm, to induce bilirubin conversion in the skin. If unsuccessful, repeated exchange blood transfusion will be required to keep the bilirubin level down. Persistent jaundice, particularly of a mixed variety, is always pathological and requires urgent investigation. Common surgical causes include sepsis and biliary atresia.

Feeding

The act of feeding, commencing immediately after birth, links nutrition with the essential stimulus (food in the mouth) for brain learning. Appropriate corticoneural connections develop during this critical postnatal phase of brain plasticity, which subserve the functions of recognition and appreciation of different foods, of taste and texture, of bolus formation and of swallowing. The neonate is born with a strong 'rooting reflex', responding avidly to the stimulus of a nipple close to the mouth. This reflex is rapidly reduced and lost within a few days if not sustained by the satisfaction of feeding and the presence of food in the mouth. Thus neonates who are not offered food orally, e.g. fed by nasogastric tube or gastrostomy, will fail to learn bolus formation, taste and texture, and will lose the will to feed. If oral diversion is sustained, they will never develop food appreciation and will eventually reject all foods placed in the mouth. The surgical neonate, because of bowel related problems, often faces lengthy periods of food denial. Such children should not be deprived of the food stimulus and should be 'sham fed' to a normal feeding pattern. The stomach should be aspirated during and after sham feeding until absorptive capability becomes established. Sham feeding teaches and comforts the child and assists parent bonding. It is relevant to the child with an oesophagostomy, to the premature infant being supplemented by nasogastric tube and to the child awaiting establishment of absorptive function, e.g. post-laparotomy, gastroschisis.

The best possible feed for the human infant is fresh warm maternal breast milk preferably direct from the mother. In addition to its nutrient value, it transfers immunity from the mother to the child such that there is a reduced incidence of enterocolitis and gut-related infections. The act of breast-feeding assists the bonding process between the child, the mother and the family. It is unfortunate that breast-feeding may be contraindicated in the event of possible transmission of the human immunodeficiency virus (HIV) virus or of acquired immunodeficiency syndrome (AIDS). Breast milk contains reduced levels of vitamin K rendering the child liable to haemorrhagic disease of the newborn. Prolonged unsupplemented breast-feeding is associated with iron deficiency anaemia. Although not ideal, cow's milk formulae are a reasonable substitute. However, many differences exist such that lactose intolerance and cow's milk protein allergy are not uncommon. Soya based preparations can be used in such circumstances. Early and rapidly increased feeding of premature infants with cow's milk preparation renders them more liable to necrotizing enterocolitis. In special circumstances, e.g. short bowel syndrome, predigested milk preparations or elemental diets may be necessary.

Nutrition is an essential consideration in the management of the surgical neonate. There is evidence to suggest that insufficient early nutrition may have a lasting effect on cerebral development and body growth. When enteral nutrition is not possible then calorie and fluid requirements must be met parenterally.

- **Maintenance of fluids and electrolytes** – For practical purposes relatively simple formulae are used for estimating daily maintenance fluids. The normal term neonate requires 60 ml/kg/day on the first day of life, increasing to 120–150 ml/kg/day by the fourth day. Older infants and children require less fluid at 100 ml/kg/day for the first 10 kg body weight, 50 ml/kg/day for the next 10 kg body weight, and 25 ml/kg/day thereafter. Thus a 21 kg child requires 1525 ml/day. Maintenance sodium requirements are calculated at 3 mmol/kg/day and potassium at 2–3 mmol/kg/day. Intravenous maintenance fluids and electrolytes are given as isotonic solutions made up to isotonicity with dextrose. The basic solution contains 0.18% sodium chloride in 4% dextrose with 10 mmol potassium chloride added to a 500 ml volume. Substituting to a 10% dextrose solution can provide additional sugar (Table 63.2).
- **Fluid and electrolyte deficits** – Deficits already incurred will require correction. Thus a mild deficit is calculated at 2.5% of body weight (wt in kg × 25), a moderate deficit at 5% of body weight (wt in kg × 50) and a severe deficit at 8% of body weight (wt in kg × 80). The difference between the present weight and the weight prior to the onset of the acute illness is a good indicator of the extent of a fluid deficit. The electrolytic content of the replacement fluid is tailored to the type and extent of the disease (Table 63.3).
- **Ongoing losses** – Nasogastric aspirates, peritoneal or pleural drainage require 'ongoing' correction. Replacement should be undertaken with fluids similar to those being lost, e.g. exudates are replaced with plasma.
- **Other special conditions** – Fluid losses for other reasons, e.g. burns, must also be included in the replacement plan.

Table 63.2 Fluid balance regimen

- Planning a fluid balance chart
- Maintenance fluids
- Correction of deficits
- Correction of on-going losses
- Special considerations – phototherapy

Table 63.3 A practical estimate for replacement of a fluid deficit

Fluid deficits

- Mild deficit: 2.5% body weight (weight in kg × 25)
- Moderate deficit: 5% body weight (weight in kg × 50)
- Severe deficit: 8% body weight (weight in kg × 80)

Having established the total fluid requirement under each heading, replacement must be undertaken slowly at least over a 24 hour period, to allow fluid and electrolyte equilibrium between the various body compartments to establish gradually. In severe cases an initial resuscitative fluid bolus at 10–20 ml/kg should be given rapidly to stabilize the blood pressure and central venous pressure. The fluid regimen is adjusted frequently in line with decreasing losses and deficit reduction. Since all replacement formulae are simply guidelines, fluid management effectively relies on frequent and careful clinical assessment and judgement. Thus the child's general condition and activity, the fontanel tension, skin turgor, central venous pressure, peripheral perfusion, liver size and urine output are all relevant. Twice daily weight is a useful indicator and helps prevent fluid overload (1 ml of fluid = 1 g). Biochemical parameters such as serum and urinary electrolytes and osmolarity are helpful.

Vascular access

Small calibre atraumatic cannulae have allowed stable venous access in the neonate. Peripheral and central venous and arterial cannulation for monitoring and for treatment is now basic, routine practice. Short-term parenteral fluids are usually given through peripheral limb veins using 22–26 Fr gauge cannulae. Accurate delivery of small volumes is essential and is achieved through sophisticated infusion pumps. Because of vein rupture and fluid extravasation, all cannula sites should be visible and constantly monitored. Serious rises in tissue pressure can lead to tissue sloughing and even loss of a limb.

Venous access for parenteral nutrition or for central venous pressure monitoring can be achieved by percutaneous subclavian or internal jugular puncture, or alternatively by open access onto the external or internal jugular veins or the sapheno-femoral junctions. Non-reactive silastic or polyurethane catheters are positioned in the superior or inferior vena cava and catheter position is confirmed radiologically. It is relevant to avoid positioning the catheter in the atrium since even the softest and finest catheters can erode through the heart muscle into the pericardium, causing cardiac tamponade. At the time of catheter insertion there should be free blood withdrawal and easy infusion before the catheter position is accepted. The catheters should be monitored by blood culture for infection and by ultrasound for 'vegetations'. Arterial access is established for monitoring of arterial oxygen levels and blood pressure. The right or left radial arteries are most commonly used, but should be avoided if a congenital hand anomaly exists, e.g. absent or hypoplastic thumb, since loss of the artery may jeopardize hand reconstruction. The anterior and posterior tibial arteries, the femoral and axillary arteries are all available, the larger vessels being particularly useful for haemodialysis. Umbilical artery cannulae are best avoided since they carry a high incidence of aortic thrombosis and embolism, and are associated with an increased risk of necrotizing enterocolitis.

Parenteral nutrition

Parenteral nutrition may be total or may be a supplement to enteral nutrition. This is a specialized and complex management and should be undertaken in, or under guidance from specialist centres. Solutions of amino acids (Vamin), fats (10–20% Intralipid) and carbohydrates (10–12% Dextrose) are combined with electrolytes, vitamins and trace elements to provide a comprehensive balanced daily nutrition. The neonate requires around 85 kcal/kg/day for daily maintenance and for growth. Higher levels of calorie intake particularly in the form of lipid solutions, constitute hyperalimentation and may induce liver dysfunction (cholestasis). Parenteral nutrition is often spread over the full 24 hours, but may be used cyclically over 10–16 hours to allow freedom and a family life, thereby enhancing the quality of life. For children with chronic intestinal failure, e.g. short bowel state and food intolerance, home parenteral nutrition should be considered. The commitment to parenteral nutrition, particularly long-term, should not be taken lightly. Apart from the major financial burden, complications such as severe septicaemia, loss of venous access and liver dysfunction are a constant source of anxiety. Social and economic factors should be considered since the impact on the family is considerable.

Venous access is most commonly established through the neck veins. Meticulous care is necessary at all times since venous accessibility is the child's 'life-line'. Modern silastic (Broviac, Hickman) and polyurethane catheters are available in various sizes and are provided with Teflon cuffs for subcutaneous fixation. Catheter blockage and infection will require catheter replacement, which should be undertaken through the same venous access site as often as is possible. Gram positive (*Staphylococcus aureus* or *albus*) and Gram negative (*Escherichia coli*) sepsis accounts for the majority of catheter-related sepsis. Prophylactic antibiotics are not advised since they may lead to superinfection with resistant strains, with pseudomonas or with *Candida albicans*. Management is preventive and there is no substitute for meticulous technique when handling central venous feeding catheters. Established catheter infection is first controlled with antibiotics until the catheter is changed through the same venous port within 24–48 hours. Parenteral nutrition constitutes a major breakthrough in management of the surgical neonate. It remains however a serious and high-risk therapy, even in the best of units.

Section 63.2 • Anomalies of the gastrointestinal tract

Intestinal obstruction arising antenatally may affect any part of the gastrointestinal tract. It may be mechanical because of interruption of bowel continuity (atresia), narrowing of the lumen (stenosis) or intraluminal obstruction as in meconium ileus. Alternatively obstruction may be functional or adynamic because of absent neurones (Hirschsprung's disease), abnormal neural networks (neuronal intestinal dysplasia), abnormal smooth muscle (megacystis microcolon syndrome) or of unknown aetiology (chronic idiopathic intestinal pseudo-obstruction).

Bowel atresia, other than oesophagus, duodenum and rectum constitutes the end point following an intrauterine vascular insult. The commonest causes are segmental small bowel volvulus, midgut volvulus, intussusception, and bowel strangulation from an internal hernia, an adhesion (vitello-intestinal band) or herniation at the umbilicus as in gastroschisis. The majority of bowel atresias are therefore secondary phenomena occurring later in pregnancy, and carrying no known genetic implications. In a sterile intra-uterine environment devitalized bowel is resorbed. The end result is a spectrum of lesions from a simple stenosis to an intraluminal membrane causing partial or complete obstruction, through to the more common complete bowel atresia with a missing segment of bowel and a V-shaped defect in the attendant mesentery. The bowel immediately proximal to the atresia is grossly dilated and the distal bowel is narrow and unused, containing only pellets of shed mucosal cells. However, when lesions occur later in pregnancy, meconium may be present in the bowel distal to the atresia.

Oesophageal atresia and tracheo-oesophageal fistula

Oesophageal atresia (OA) was first described in 1670 by William Durston, and the associated tracheo-oesophageal fistula (TOF) by Thomas Gibson (1697). It has an incidence of 1:3500 live births, but is commoner if aborted fetuses are included. There is a definite association with chromosomal anomalies, e.g. trisomy 13 and 18. Despite evidence of a genetic link – it occurs in twins and in parents of affected children – the majority are said to follow on some major insult during the fourth week of gestation. Vogt (1929) classified the various anatomical types of oesophageal atresia (Figure 63.2). In the most commonly encountered form (86.5%), there is a markedly dilated blind upper oesophageal pouch, a missing oesophageal segment of variable length, and a lower pouch terminating as a fistulous communication to the posterior wall of the trachea. Other anatomical variations are pure OA with no TOF, TOF from the upper oesophageal pouch only, multiple TOFs to one or both pouches, and TOF with intact oesophagus (H-type). The high incidence of associated anomalies has been characterized as the **VACCTERL**

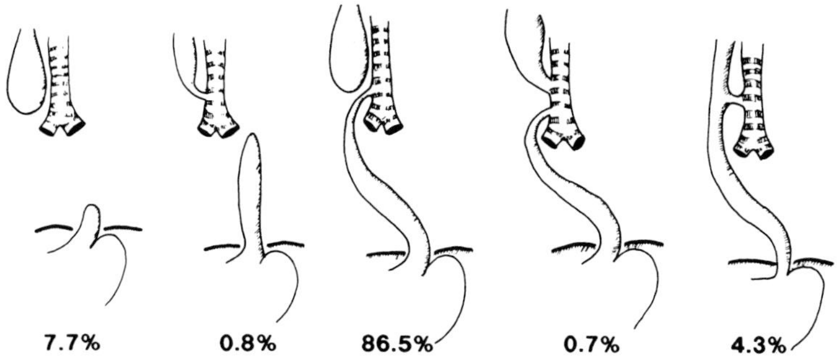

Figure 63.2 Varieties of oesophageal atresia.

Association which is an acronym for **V**ertebral (fused or hemivertebrae), **A**norectal (imperforate anus), **C**ardiac (ventricular and atrial septal defects), **C**hromosomal (trisomy 13,18), **T**racheal (TOF, tracheomalacia), (o)**E**sophageal (atresia), **R**enal (single kidney, vesicoureteric reflux) and **L**imb anomalies (absent thumb, radial aplasia).

The diagnosis of oesophageal atresia is now often made in mid-pregnancy, by which time a suspicion may have already arisen because of hydramnios, a consequence of the child's inability to swallow liquor. Antenatal ultrasound may delineate the dilated blind upper pouch, but more often it is the absence of a fluid filled stomach, which raises the possibility of oesophageal atresia. The VACCTERL association demands a detailed fetal scan, which is particularly relevant to antenatal counselling. Chromosomal anomalies can be excluded on a choriovillus biopsy or fetal cordocentesis, in a much shorter time than amniocentesis. At birth the child presents as a 'mucousy' baby in respiratory difficulty, which is relieved by pharyngeal suction of accumulated saliva and air. The passage of a firm nasogastric tube (8–10 Fr) is held up at T2–4 level and cannot be advanced to reach the stomach. A plain X-ray of the whole baby (babygram) is indicated to confirm the position of the tube, to outline any pneumonic changes from aspiration of pharyngeal secretions or from gastric acid reflux, and to assess the size and shape of the heart. Air in the bowel confirms the presence of a TOF to the distal oesophagus. Costal, vertebral and sacral anomalies can also be identified. Cerebral, cardiac and renal abnormalities are confirmed on ultrasound examination and appropriate specialist review is sought. Chromosomal analysis and post-natal counselling should be undertaken jointly with the geneticists.

The child is nursed flat and turned on its side to avoid pharyngeal accumulation of secretions. A sump-suction Replogyle (double lumen) tube is passed into the blind upper oesophagus, which is kept free of secretions by constant low-grade suction (10 cm water) to avoid tracheal aspiration of saliva. Operation is planned semi-urgently during the first 24–36 hours after birth, the actual timing being determined by the child's condition. Evidence of respiratory distress syndrome requiring a high ventilatory pressure is an indication for urgent division of the TOF to facilitate ventilation and to avoid gastric rupture from transmitted pressure. Tracheoscopy allows for an 'informed thoracotomy' and is always indicated pre-operatively in all varieties of oesophageal atresia. It is performed under general anaesthesia but with the child breathing spontaneously. The site and number of fistulas, the structure of the trachea (tracheomalacia), the condition of the mucosa (reflux tracheitis), the laryngeal anatomy (laryngo-tracheo-oesophageal cleft) and the position of the aortic arch in relation to the trachea can be assessed. A left-sided pulsatile indentation of the trachea suggests a normal left aortic arch. Surgery is undertaken through a right thoracotomy to avoid the aortic arch and the segmental aortic branches. Access is through an aesthetic high right axillary skin crease incision or through the more conventional vertical mid-axillary line incision. The pectoralis major, latissimus dorsi and serratus anterior are retracted, protecting the long thoracic nerve of Bell. The thorax is entered through the fouth and fifth intercostal space (no ribs are resected) and the dissection carried bluntly extrapleurally, pushing the right lung and mediastinum medially and forwards. The azygos vein is divided and the lower oesophagus located. Mobilization of the lower pouch and of the TOF should attempt to preserve the oesophageal segmental blood supply and the nerve branches from the vagus nerve. The fistula is followed to its insertion into the posterior wall of the trachea or at the carina. It is transected allowing the mucosa to retract towards the tracheal lumen, and is then oversewn with fine absorbable sutures to eliminate air leak. TOF ligation alone is insufficient and carries a high risk of recurrence. The upper oesophageal pouch is then identified, and a wide oblique tension-free anastomosis is constructed turning down a vascularized pedicle flap of oesophageal tissue from the upper pouch and insetting it into the circumference of the lower pouch. This procedure achieves a wider, more uniform oesophagus and is associated with fewer swallowing difficulties than the conventional funnel-shaped end-to-end anastomosis. The chest is closed with extrapleural low-grade (10 cm water) suction drainage. Post-operative recovery is usually unremarkable and most will heal primarily, commencing feeding at 3–5 days. Potential early complications include anastomotic breakdown and leakage with subsequent stricture formation and recurrence of the TOF.

Long-term swallowing problems may be due to oesophageal stenosis or to functional dysmotility. Significant gastro-oesophageal reflux may coexist. Respiratory infections are more frequent and require aggressive management. The increased incidence relates to the co-existent tracheomalacia, which accounts also for the characteristic barking cough which these children virtually always demonstrate. Uncomplicated oesophageal atresia and tracheo-oesophageal fistula should not carry any mortality, and death is due to the associated severe anomalies, particularly cardiac and chromosomal. With modern management the long-term prognosis and quality of life are excellent, with a steady improvement in respiratory symptoms and in the ability to swallow all foods. Mental and physical development should be normal.

Less common forms of oesophageal atresia

Treatment for the other varieties of oesophageal atresia follows the same principles. Multiple fistulas are all identified at pre-operative tracheoscopy and must all be divided at surgery. The H- or N-type fistula with intact oesophagus is situated at the thoracic inlet and can be reached through a low cervical incision such that a thoracotomy is not indicated. The child with a long gap between oesophageal pouches where direct anastomosis is not possible is best managed by temporary oesophagostomy and gastrostomy, and eventual oesophageal replacement with stomach or colon. This allows a full sham feeding programme to ensure that the child learns to eat. Various complex procedures have been described in attempts to mobilize or elongate the upper and lower pouches to allow for a delayed anastomosis. Although of value they have a greater incidence of complications. Given appropriate and skilled management the long-term life expectancy for such children is excellent with potential for a full and good quality life.

Duodenal atresia

Atresia or stenosis typically occurs in the second part of the duodenum at the level of the ampulla of Vater. The duodenum proximal to the obstruction becomes massively dilated. Immediately below the atresia the duodenum is deficient such that the pancreas occupies the space between the proximal and distal duodenal segments giving the impression of an annular pancreas. The distal duodenum is essentially normal but appears narrow relative to the large proximal segment. Duodenal atresia is not often associated with other bowel atresias except for those affecting the oesophagus and the anus. The ampulla of Vater commonly drains into the proximal dilated segment accounting for the typical bile stained vomiting. Uncommonly an accessory or additional duct may straddle the atretic zone and drain also into the distal segment. In some 10% of cases the ampulla discharges into the distal bowel beyond the atresia so that bile stained vomiting is not a presenting feature. Some 30% of cases are associated with Down's syndrome, suggesting a genetic aetiology for duodenal atresia. The diagnosis can be made on antenatal ultrasound at 16–20 weeks of gestation by detection of the large fluid filled proximal duodenal loop. Hydramnios may be present and there may be the obvious features of Down's syndrome, e.g. globular head, nuchal fat pad, short fingers and square pelvis. The diagnosis should be confirmed by chromosome analysis. Delivery is usually vaginal and complicated only by bile stained liquor. Within a few hours of birth 90% of cases present with bile stained vomiting. Because of the high obstruction no air passes to the distal bowel and the abdomen remains flat. An abdominal X-ray reveals only the typical 'double bubble' appearance (Figure 63.3) that is formed by the gastric air bubble and an additional air–fluid level in the dilated proximal duodenum. Air within the bowel distal to the duodenum suggests a partial obstruction from a perforated mucosal diaphragm, or a duodenal stenosis. Treatment is operative and consists of a wide diamond shaped duodeno-duodenostomy with tailoring of the dilated proximal duodenum when relevant. Enteral feeding will often become established within 5–10 days, and the long-term prognosis for uncomplicated duodenal atresia or stenosis is excellent.

Small bowel atresia

Atresia of the small bowel may be single or multiple, occurring anywhere from the duodeno-jejunal flexure

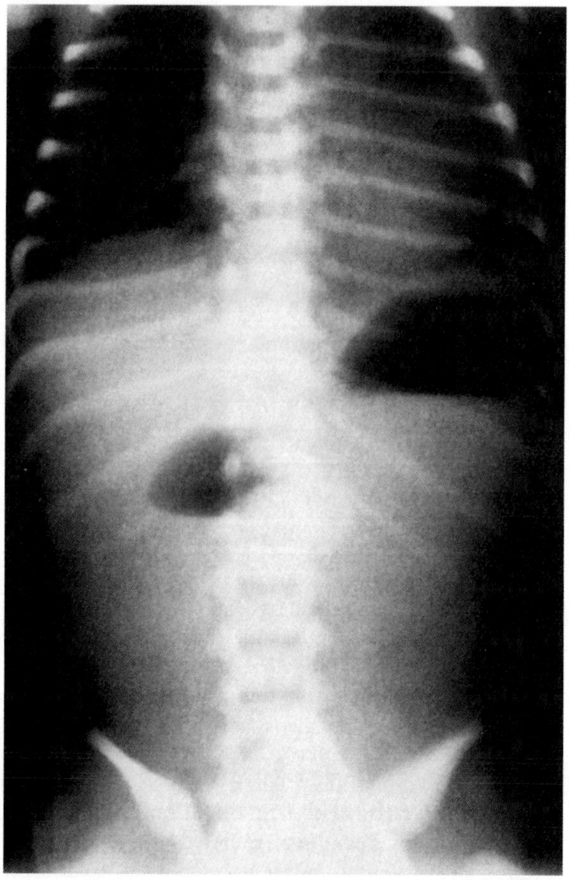

Figure 63.3 'Double bubble' appearance typical of congenital duodenal obstruction.

to the ileo-caecal valve. Small bowel atresia encompasses a spectrum of lesions from a simple stenosis, an intraluminal membrane causing partial or complete obstruction, to the more common complete bowel atresia with a missing segment of bowel and an obvious V-shaped mesenteric defect. The bowel proximal to the atresia is massively dilated and thickened relative to the narrow 'unused' distal bowel (Figure 63.4). Since these lesions are 'acquired', arising later in pregnancy, meconium may be present in the distal bowel and colon. In 1957 Lowe and Barnard, in experimental work in puppies, established the vascular origin of these lesions. Interruption to the blood supply, because of segmental or midgut volvulus, intussusception or bowel infarction, e.g. internal hernia, leads to loss of varying lengths of small bowel. Long-term survival will depend on the adaptability of the residual absorptive mucosa. In this context the possibility of cystic fibrosis (meconium ileus) as the underlying cause should always be considered. It is often possible to make a diagnosis of small bowel atresia at antenatal ultrasound when dilated loops of fluid filled bowel can be seen in the fetal abdomen. At delivery the liquor is bile stained and the child soon presents with varying abdominal distension and bile stained vomiting. The degree of abdominal distension varies according to the level of the lesion. Air contrast radiography reveals dilated loops of small bowel containing air–fluid levels with one large air–fluid level in the dilated loop at the site of the atresia. Operative treatment is always indicated, with resection of the massively dilated non-propulsive proximal segment and a wide bowel anastomosis. It is axiomatic that further distal atresias should have been excluded by injection of saline and air through to the anus prior to anastomosis. In the event of the 'short bowel state' all available bowel is valuable and resection should not be performed. A tube drain may be placed in the dilated bowel and the abdomen closed. The child should be referred to a specialist centre for further management.

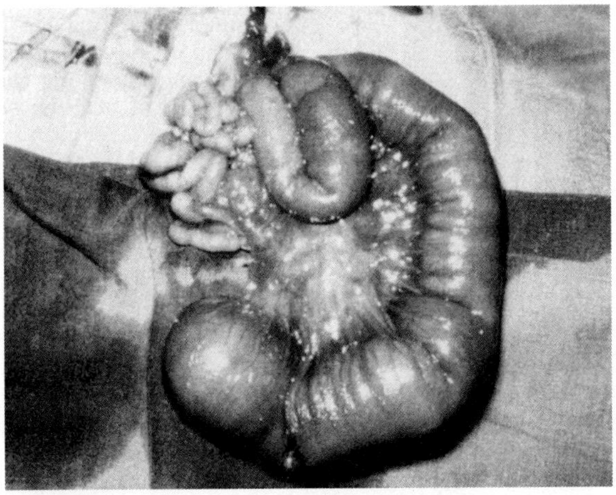

Figure 63.4 Small bowel atresia showing the dilated proximal segment, the V-shaped mesenteric defect and missing bowel, and the collapsed distal bowel.

The short bowel state

Loss of long segments of absorptive small bowel becomes increasingly serious when the residual small bowel length is less than 60 cm, and particularly if the ileo-caecal valve and the right colon are not present. The dilated bowel just proximal to the atresia should not be resected and all available bowel should be preserved since it constitutes a significant proportion of the absorptive mucosa on which the child's survival and future will depend. Preferably no bowel surgery should be performed or at best a tube drain inserted to relieve distension in the dilated bowel, and the child referred to an 'intestinal failure service'. If the problem is significant the child will require support with parenteral nutrition while awaiting bowel adaptation and improved absorption from the residual bowel. Various dietary, pharmacological and surgical techniques are available to enhance bowel adaptation which may require a period of several months or years, but is most progressive during the first year. Surgical techniques have attempted to increase mucosal contact time to allow for a greater absorption. Most successful amongst these have been tissue expansion followed by bowel tailoring and lengthening procedures, also combined with reversed antiperistaltic segments. Children with persistent intestinal failure from inadequate mucosal surface area can achieve a good quality life and growth on home-based parenteral nutrition despite the risk of feeding-catheter related sepsis, loss of venous access and hepatic dysfunction. Advances in bowel transplantation have allowed consideration of an isolated small bowel or a combined liver and small bowel transplant when all else has failed or in the event of life threatening circumstances. Post-transplant management is complex and 3 year survival is around 40–50%, such that transplantation should not presently be regarded as the first line of management.

Non-fixation and malrotation of the midgut

Around the sixth to tenth week of gestation the bowel migrates from the physiological umbilical hernia into the peritoneal space. It undergoes a 270° counterclockwise rotation, which creates a G-shaped duodenal configuration, with the duodenum and duodenojejunal flexure passing beneath the superior mesenteric vascular pedicle. The colon continues its rotation, passing over these vessels such that the caecum and appendix eventually come to lie in the right iliac fossa. Bowel fixation in this wide normal configuration is associated with a stable mesenteric base running from the duodenojejunal flexure to the left of the spine towards the right iliac fossa. Failure, arrest or abnormal rotation results in a narrow mesenteric pedicle with a significant risk of midgut volvulus. An upper gastrointestinal contrast study will demonstrate the typical S-shaped duodenum with absence of a duodeno-jejunal flexure and passage of the small bowel towards the right side of the abdomen (Figure 63.5). The colon lies towards the left side with the caecum and appendix in the left hypochondrium. At operation peritoneal bands (Ladd's bands) will be seen to run across the duodenum from the subhepatic space towards the left-sided caecum. Incomplete rotation or lesser degrees of non-rotation and non-fixation account for a high caecum lying beneath the liver. Reverse rotation leads to the duodenum passing in front of the transverse colon and interferes with mesenteric fixation thus also carrying a risk of midgut volvulus.

Failure of appropriate rotation and fixation is associated with a narrow mesenteric base through which passes the superior mesenteric vascular pedicle – the only blood supply to the midgut. The situation is unstable and midgut volvulus with loss of the major portion of the absorptive small bowel is an ever-present danger and may occur at any time. Antenatal midgut volvulus is followed by resorption of the sterile dead bowel, so that the child presents with features of a high small bowel atresia and the 'short bowel state'. Post-natal volvulus typically presents with sudden onset of features suggestive of duodenal obstruction in a previously well child. There is copious bile stained vomiting and a flat, relatively featureless non-tender abdomen except for left hypochondrial stomach distension. Serial abdominal X-rays will reveal the distended stomach and the reducing volume of gas distal to the second part of the duodenum. A suspicion of malrotation and midgut volvulus constitutes the most acute diagnostic and surgical emergency. No time should be lost since midgut strangulation may be imminent. Rectal bleeding is a late and ominous sign. If the child and the abdomen are in good condition then an urgent upper gastrointestinal contrast study will demonstrate the typical S-shaped duodenum with variable obstruction at the second part below the bile duct. Contrast enema is unnecessary but will reveal the high caecum possibly lying over to the left side. Treatment is by urgent operation with derotation of the midgut and release of Ladd's peritoneal bands. The mesentery should be laid open widely and the bowel replaced such that the duodenojejunal junction and the small bowel pass towards the right of the abdomen and the caecum towards the left hypochondrium. An appendicectomy is best performed. Every measure should be taken to ensure a widely splayed mesentery and to induce fixation by adhesion formation.

Midgut volvulus constitutes the most acute diagnostic and surgical emergency for which immediate simple action is rewarded by complete success, whereas delay can be catastrophic, frequently resulting in death. In the absence of small bowel loss the long-term prognosis is excellent.

Meconium ileus (cystic fibrosis)

Some 15% of children with cystic fibrosis present to the neonatal surgeon with meconium ileus. Cystic fibrosis is a genetically determined condition inherited as an autosomal recessive. The genetic coding for the condition has been identified and some 85% of mutations occur at the Delta F508 locus. The diagnosis can thus be rapidly established within the first week of life but should be further confirmed by a sweat test after the sixth week. High values for sodium and chloride (>80 mmol/l) will be found in the sweat. Cystic fibrosis is associated with the production of abnormal tenacious

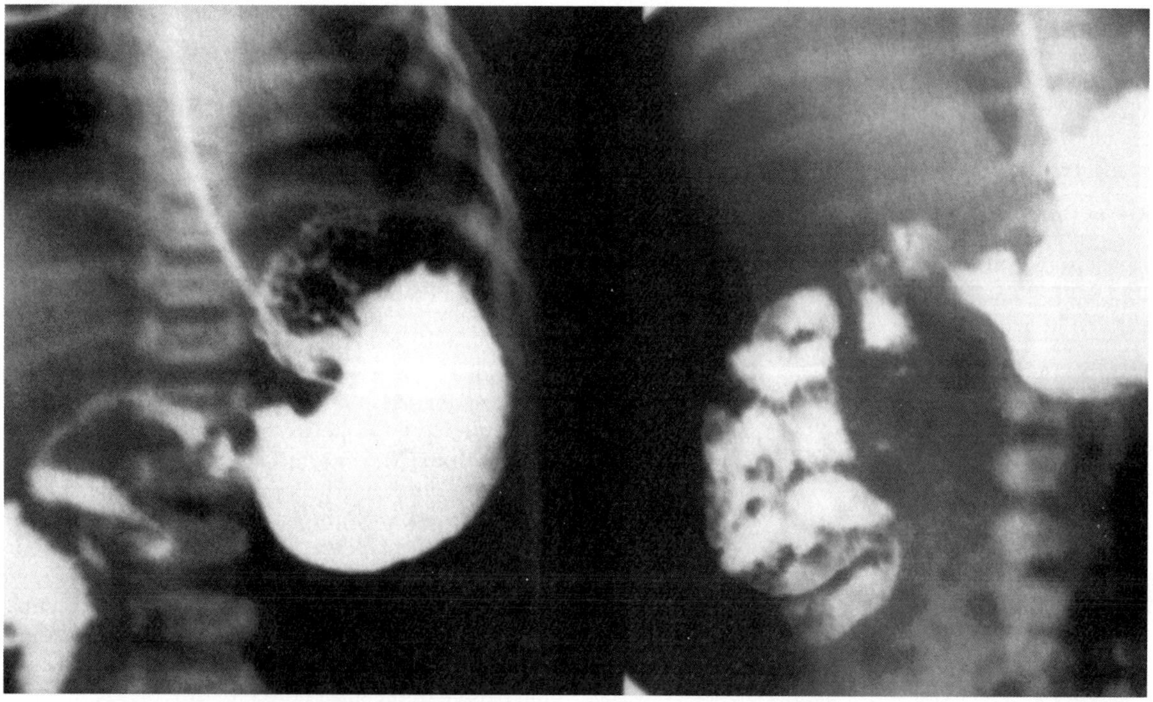

Figure 63.5 Barium meal showing the non-rotated duodenum and the small bowel passing to the right side of the abdomen in midgut malrotation.

mucus of high salt content. The pancreas undergoes marked fibrocystic dysplasia. Loss of pancreatic enzymes and abnormal mucus leads to the formation of a thick and tacky meconium, which obstructs the lower ileum. Affected bowel loops become thickened, dilated and heavy with tacky meconium so that they are prone to segmental volvulus. The ileum and colon distal to the obstructive meconium are of narrow calibre (microcolon) and filled with amorphous pellets of desquamated cells and other detritus containing no bile.

In view of the genetic basis to cystic fibrosis, it is relevant to assess all siblings and to provide counselling for the parents. In known families, an affected fetus can be detected by DNA probing at the time of *in vitro* fertilization and prior to implantation. During early pregnancy, fetal cells can be obtained by placental choriovillus biopsy. Subsequently antenatal ultrasound scans may reveal abdominal distension and the presence of large loops of meconium filled bowel. At birth the child presents a distended abdomen with visible and palpable loops of bowel. Segmental volvulus and bowel loss present as small bowel atresia. Alternatively a meconium cyst containing sterile meconium and dead bowel may form. A plain abdominal X-ray shows variably dilated bowel loops of granular appearance, and no fluid levels. Eventually features of intestinal obstruction become apparent above the obstructed segment. Contrast enema shows a microcolon filled with pellets (Figure 63.6). In some 50% of non-complicated cases, a dilute gastrograffin enema (a high osmolality contrast medium) may dislodge the meconium sufficiently to overcome the obstruction. Persistent obstruction or the development of complications is an indication for surgery. At laparotomy an attempt can be made to liquefy and detach the meconium by bowel massage and intraluminal injection of warm saline or dilute gastrograffin. It is frequently necessary to resect the dilated thickened meconium filled loops. Bowel continuity is restored by end-to-end anastomosis and a stoma is not usually necessary.

Children born with meconium ileus require careful long-term medical supervision for the management of the underlying cystic fibrosis. Pancreatic enzyme supplements are provided with each feed and are regulated to ensure sufficient food absorption and growth. Care of the respiratory tract (daily intensive physiotherapy, antibiotics) is crucial to long-term survival and is best managed by dedicated specialists. Recent advances suggest the possibility of 'gene therapy' using a live virus vector delivered by inhalation, to carry a normal replacement gene into the lungs. In the longer term these children are prone to meconium ileus equivalent, constipation, intussusception and to rectal prolapse, and may require further surgery. Respiratory failure is common and may lead to consideration of lung or heart–lung transplantation in the second or third decade of life.

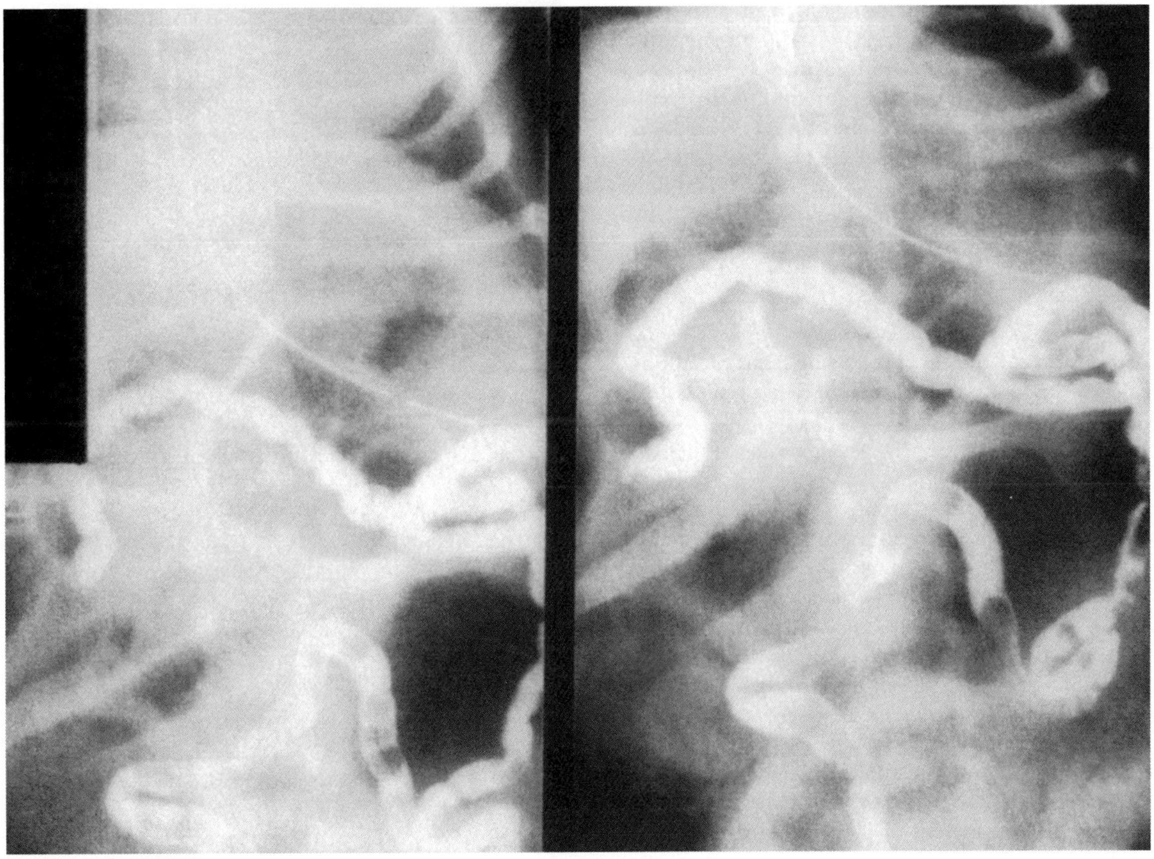

Figure 63.6 Microcolon containing 'pellets' in meconium ileus.

Section 63.3 • Anterior abdominal wall anomalies

Over the last 20 years there has been a definite increase in anterior abdominal wall anomalies world-wide, such that they now form a greater proportion of referrals for antenatal counselling and eventual admission to the neonatal surgical service. The term is used to denote a variety of conditions from the relatively minor herniation into the umbilical cord (exomphalos minor) to the more spectacular exomphalos major and gastroschisis.

Exomphalos minor and major

Exomphalos minor presents as an intact hernial sac passing into the umbilical cord through an expanded umbilical port. The hernial sac lies to the right with the cord vessels passing along its left side. The sac frequently contains loops of terminal ileum and a patent vitellointestinal duct opening at its apex. The presence of an exomphalos or even simply an umbilical hernia should alert the clinician to the possibility of associated cardiac, syndromic or bowel anomalies. Exomphalos in association with macroglossia and gigantism constitutes the EMG or Beckwith–Wiedemann syndrome, which is of special concern because of the accompanying large pancreas and hyperinsulinaemia. Severe hypoglycaemia may develop rapidly after birth such that the blood sugar should be constantly monitored to avoid cerebral injury. The situation stabilizes within hours or days leaving no long-term morbidity. Exomphalos minor requires relatively minor surgery, aesthetically performed, to resect the vitellointestinal duct and to achieve appropriate umbilical cicatriztion. The umbilical cord should never be excised since loss of the normal umbilical scar is psychologically detrimental to the growing child.

Exomphalos major presents as a supraumbilical midline hernia of at least 5 cm diameter. There is a wide divarication of the recti extending from the umbilical port to the splayed costal margin. The divarication also affects the anterior fibres of the diaphragm. The umbilical cord attaches along the undersurface of the sac and may appear to be opening into it. The hernial sac may be intact or may have ruptured at the time of delivery. The sac contains a large proportion of the small and large bowel, the stomach and the spleen. The liver in whole or in part, herniates out of the abdomen and is attached to the sac at its dome. It is of an abnormal globular shape and often appears to hang on a 'mesentery'. There is non-fixation of the midgut and failure of formation of the mesenteric base so that the midgut is attached by a narrow based pedicle and is at risk of volvulus. Despite this, antenatal midgut volvulus is uncommon. The bowel is of normal texture but the ileum may be adherent to the inner surface of the sac at the level of the Meckel's diverticulum. Other anomalies, particularly cardiac and chromosomal, must be excluded. Unruptured exomphalos major (Figure 63.7) does not pose immediate problems to the child. However, accommodation of all the extruded viscera in the underdeveloped abdominal cavity can be difficult so that primary abdominal wall closure may not be possible. Manipulation of the liver and abdominal wall closure under excessive tension can seriously interfere with venous return to the heart and may also compromise respiration by splinting the diaphragm. Conservative management, consisting of attempts to dry out the sac by painting with cicatrizing agents until creeping epithelialization occurs, is a prolonged procedure often punctuated by septic episodes. It has the advantage of avoiding difficult early surgery. If successful the resultant large ventral hernia will need eventual repair. The surgical alternatives are primary, staged or delayed closure. Primary closure is always under some tension and requires experienced judgement to avoid serious circulatory, respiratory and renal compromise. If fascial closure is not possible, then midline skin closure alone is acceptable. Skin flaps or other 'plasty' procedures are contraindicated since they lead to unnecessary abdominal wall scarring. Muscle paralysis and ventilatory support are a routine part of post-operative management until the abdomen becomes more supple and accommodating. Should it prove impossible to

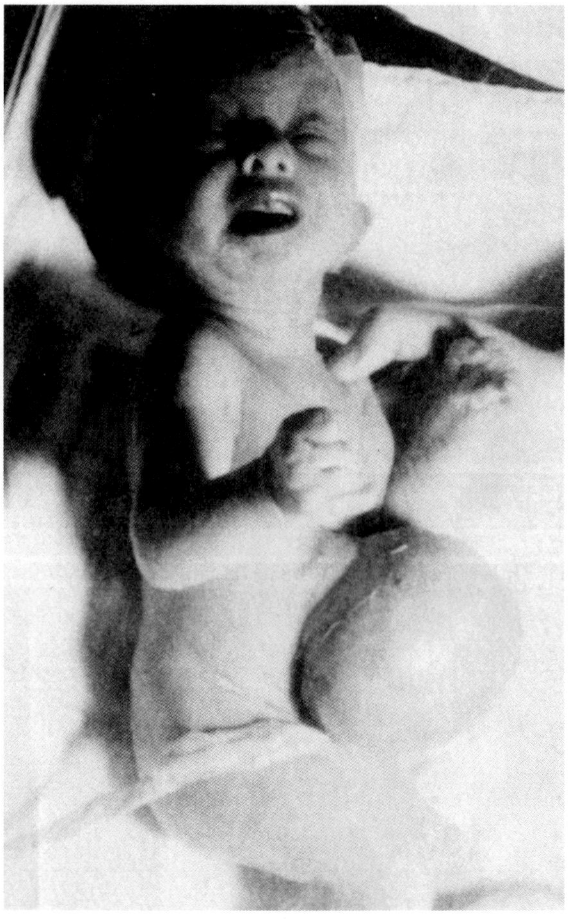

Figure 63.7 Unruptured exomphalos major.

achieve primary closure, then a staged technique is adopted. Any remaining extruded viscera are enclosed within a silastic pouch, which is sutured to the edges of the abdominal wall (Figure 63.8). The child is kept paralysed and the contents of the pouch are gradually returned to the abdomen over some days, by a combination of gravity and pouch plication. The midline abdominal divarication is then closed by direct fascial and skin apposition. More recently the concept of delayed surgery has become more attractive. The child is electively paraysed and ventilated, and the sac contents are gradually accommodated in the abdomen by a process of gravity and sac plication over several days. Surgical repair is only undertaken when abdominal wall closure without tension can be assured.

Ruptured exomphalos (Figure 63.9) imposes a degree of urgency in management. Sac rupture may occur at or around the time of delivery. The unprotected sac contents are exposed and the peritoneal cavity is open. There is a marked risk of heat and fluid loss, which is reduced by placing the extruded organs in a clean plastic bag. Further resuscitation consists of cardiovascular support with plasma or colloid, and correction of body temperature. Primary or staged surgical closure is only undertaken once the child's condition is stable. Since the bowel is relatively unaffected, enteral nutrition establishes rapidly post-operatively.

The long-term prognosis for exomphalos minor and major is excellent with full prospects of a normal life. Mortality relates to the associated cardiac or chromosomal anomalies.

Gastroschisis

The increased incidence of gastroschisis (Figure 63.10) in recent years remains unexplained. Although anatomically similar to a ruptured exomphalos minor, several differences exist. Children born with gastroschisis are usually smaller and of lower weight, not infrequently delivering prematurely. The umbilical port is expanded to the right of the umbilical cord such that the cord vessels are situated on its left margin. Port expansion to the left of the cord has been described, but is very rare. A hernial sac is never present. The whole of the midgut is extruded together with the sigmoid colon. Occasionally the fundus of the bladder, the ovaries or testes may lie outside the peritoneal space, however the liver and spleen are always retained at their normal location within the abdomen. The expanded umbilical port may be of any diameter with the narrower defects more frequently associated with loss of the midgut and intestinal atresia. The presence of dilated fluid-filled loops of bowel on antenatal ultrasound is an indication of bowel loss and intestinal atresia. Since the reason for bowel loss is usually a midgut volvulus, the situation is serious because of the short bowel state. Bowel exposed to amniotic fluid during the third trimester of pregnancy becomes thickened and covered over with a grey, friable, vascular 'peel' consisting of granulation tissue. Other associated anomalies are uncommon. Management is similar to that for ruptured exomphalos, with reduction of the extruded viscera into the peritoneal space. The procedure is undertaken electively when the child is in the best condition. Since reduction is not painful, it may also be performed on the conscious child without general anaesthesia. The condition of the bowel following prolonged exposure to

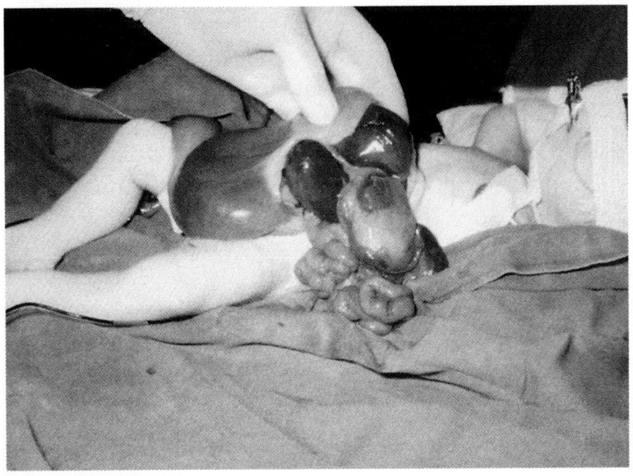

Figure 63.9 Ruptured exomphalos major. Extruded contents include liver and spleen.

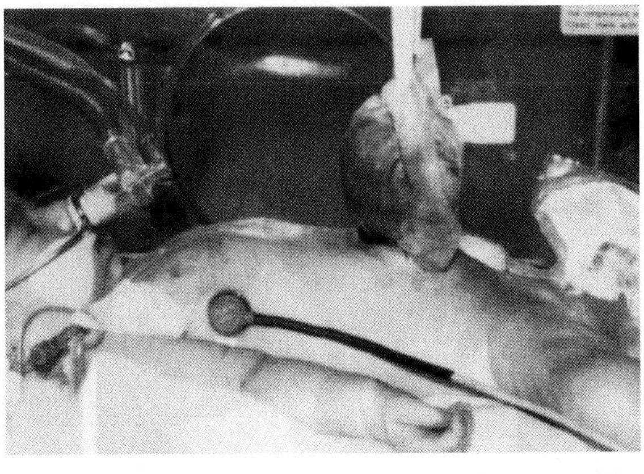

Figure 63.8 Temporary silastic pouch or 'Silo', containing bowel during staged midgut reduction and abdominal wall closure. The child is kept paralysed and ventilated.

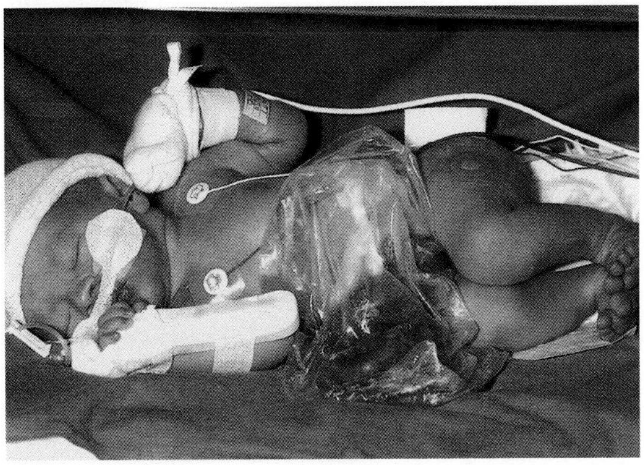

Figure 63.10 Gastroschisis.

the amniotic fluid often precludes early function and parenteral nutrition may be required for a brief period. Meanwhile oral 'sham feeding' should be commenced to maintain the rooting reflex and to allow the child to learn the nature of food. Unless complicated by midgut volvulus and short bowel, or food intolerance from mucosal injury, the long-term prognosis for these children is excellent.

Section 63.4 • Teratoma

Teratomas arise from totipotential cells and may occur anywhere in the body. Girls are more frequently affected than boys, with a ratio of 4:1. They are most commonly found in the sacrococcygeal area, the neck, the mediastinum, the ovary and the testes. The majority are benign, however some, e.g. sacrococcygeal, show a significant tendency to malignancy within months of birth. The lesions are multilocular, consisting of cystic and solid structures showing varying degrees of differentiation of diverse tissues. They do not infiltrate but rather compress and stretch surrounding normal tissues as they increase in size (Figure 63.11). Thus in the cervical area structures such as the trachea and the oesophagus may be grossly elongated and displaced. The sacrococcygeal teratoma displaces the rectum, pushing the anus and perineum anteriorly as it expands outwards (Figure 63.12). Sacrococcygeal lesions may grow

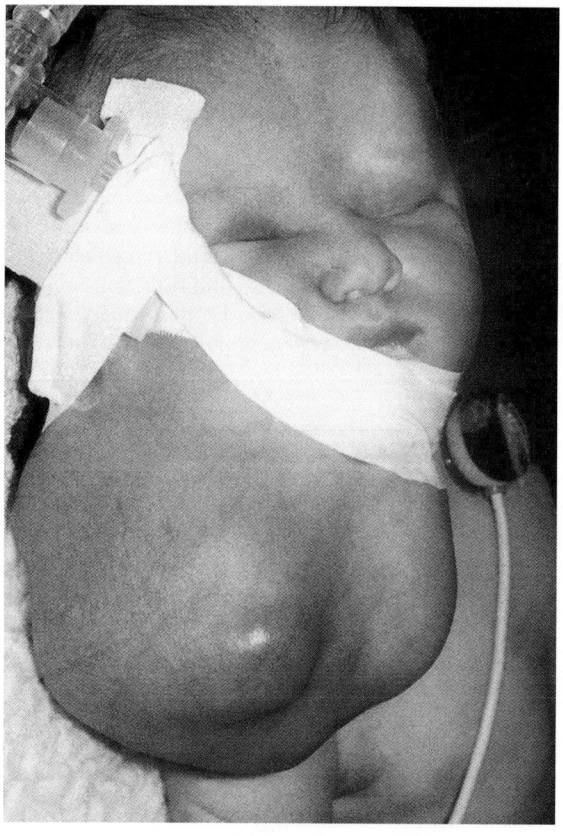

Figure 63.11 Cervical teratoma markedly displacing trachea.

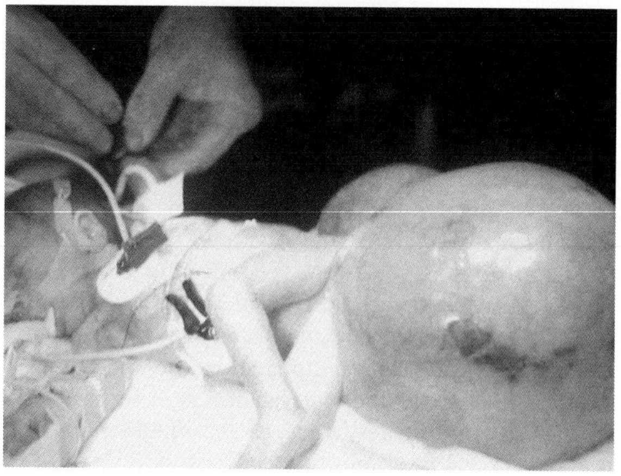

Figure 63.12 Sacrococcygeal teratoma.

entirely intrapelvically so that they are not obvious at birth and may only come to light later because of malignant transformation. They can be detected easily on digital rectal examination, lying in the presacral space behind the rectum. Ultrasound scans will confirm the presence of the lesion and a rising serum alpha-fetoprotein levels suggest malignancy.

Most teratomas are now diagnosed antenatally on ultrasound scan. Appropriate counselling and planning for delivery, commonly by Caesarean section, is offered. Although impressive and daunting because of their size and position, teratomas are eminently resectable. Surgical dissection must respect the natural tissue plane between the tumour capsule and the overstretched normal tissues, which must be preserved for functional and aesthetic reconstruction. Complete tumour excision and aesthetic reconstruction are associated with an excellent long-term prognosis. Psychological problems arising from major residual deformity and unsightly scars can be markedly reduced by appropriately planned surgery. Pelvic nerve injury should be minimal, so that normal bladder and bowel continence and sexual function is to be expected.

Section 63.5 • Necrotizing enterocolitis

This is a serious bowel inflammatory condition of unknown aetiology, which arises during the first few weeks of life. Premature and 'stressed' babies are most vulnerable. Other predisposing factors include intrauterine growth retardation, difficult delivery, congenital heart disease and maternal diabetes. Children requiring exchange transfusion and those with indwelling umbilical artery or venous catheters may be prone to necrotizing enterocolitis (NEC). Of particular relevance is the association with early and high volume feeding of cow's milk formulae to premature babies. Necrotizing enterocolitis is less common in breast-fed babies, suggesting the possibility of an immunological basis for the condition. The disease only occurs post-natally and predominantly affects the terminal ileum and the proximal two-thirds of the colon. In severe cases all of the small bowel may be involved. The underlying lesion appears to be an ischaemic mucosal injury with ulceration and sloughing of the mucosa and possible eventual destruction of the full thickness of the bowel wall. Secondary bacterial invasion, frequently with colonic organisms (*E. coli, Clostridium difficile*), rapidly occurs with severe septicaemia and endotoxic shock. Disseminated intravascular coagulation further complicates the situation and presents as a severe haemorrhagic state with low clotting factors and marked thrombocytopenia. Bone marrow depression with inability to mount an effective response is a serious and frequent complication. In mild cases of NEC the clinical picture is that of an unwell child with a distended tender abdomen. There is bilious vomiting and eventually the passage of loose stools containing blood and mucus. Severe cases may be fulminant with circulatory collapse and endotoxic shock. The abdomen is acutely tender, and inflamed oedematous loops of bowel may be palpable. Bowel perforation with peritonitis may follow rapidly. Abdominal X-ray may show dilated loops of bowel with thickened oedematous walls. Mucosal ulceration and sloughing gives a ground glass appearance, with bubbles of gas in the bowel wall (pneumatosis intestinalis) being typical of advanced disease (Figure 63.13). Gas within the portal tracts in the liver is of serious prognosis.

Management is preventive in the first instance. Susceptible children should be carefully watched and known predisposing factors avoided. Suspicious and early cases are treated conservatively with antibiotics and prolonged 'bowel rest' for some 15–21 days during which the child should not be fed enterally. Parenteral nutrition will be required to support the child during this phase. Early surgical consultation and appropriately timed surgery is particularly relevant to avoid deterioration. Localized disease is best managed by limited bowel resection and end-to-end anastomosis or a temporary stoma. Other indications for surgery include local or generalized bowel perforation and intra-abdominal abscess formation. More severe states require aggressive resuscitation with correction of hypovolaemia and blood, platelet and clotting factor deficits. The peritoneal cavity should be drained with a large catheter and peritoneal washout performed with a dialysate solution Pre-operative peritoneal dialysis may be necessary to optimize the child's condition and as a prelude to surgery. Drainage alone can occasionally be successful but is not recommended. Once the child's condition is optimal, bowel-conserving surgery is undertaken. Only obviously dead bowel is resected, and all potentially viable bowel is retained. The bowel lumen is extensively washed out from mouth to anus. Multiple anastomoses may be necessary in an attempt to conserve bowel and to avoid the short bowel state. A temporary stoma above the anastomoses may be useful. The abdomen is only very loosely closed over extensive free drainage. Further elective 'peritoneal cleansing' at 48–72 hours may benefit the child by preventing

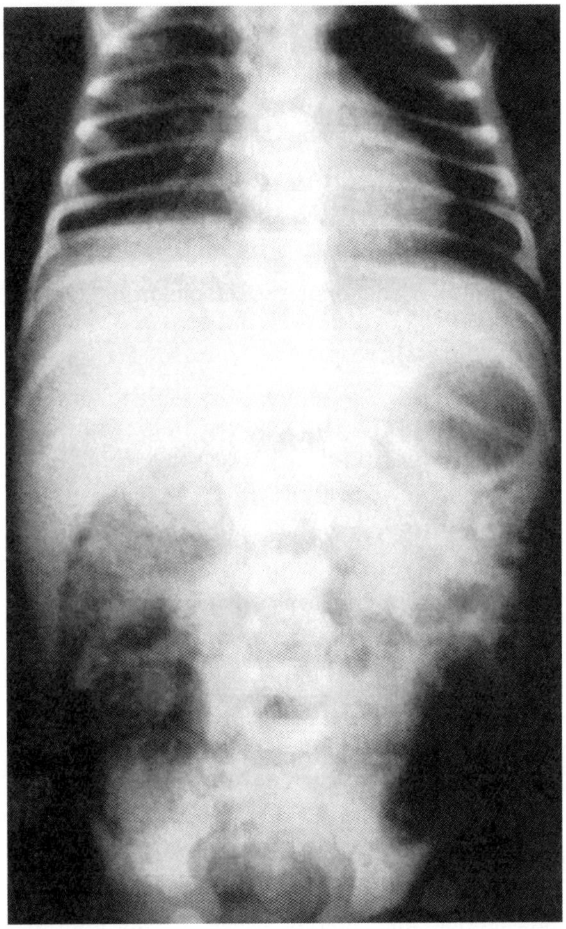

Figure 63.13 Necrotizing enterocolitis showing pneumatosis intestinalis.

the development of septic collections. Second-look laparotomy with a view to bowel resection is best avoided, and fistulas are allowed to develop along the drain tracks as natural repair occurs. Residual fistulas or strictures will require resection at a later date in a well survivor with a quiescent abdomen. NEC may lead to extensive loss of the small and large bowel, leaving the surviving child with a short bowel state. Given an avid programme of 'prevention – early diagnosis – aggressive but conservative surgery' the majority will avoid this fate and will survive to an excellent long-term prognosis without residual disability.

Colonic atresia

Atresia of the colon is far less common than that affecting the small bowel. Any variety of atresia may occur in any part of the colon, and the features are similar to atresias elsewhere, with a proximal dilated segment and a collapsed atrophic distal bowel. Within a few days of birth the child presents features of low intestinal obstruction with a distended abdomen and late onset of bilious vomiting. The presence of a competent ileocaecal valve may cause rapid massive distension and perforation of the grossly distended colon. Since these lesions arise late in pregnancy, meconium may be present in the distal colon. Abdominal radiographs confirm intestinal obstruction and show the massively dilated air–fluid filled colon proximal to the atresia. Treatment consists of surgical resection of the atretic bowel and end-to-end anastomosis, with tailoring of the dilated proximal segment to propulsive proportions. The long-term prognosis is excellent.

Congenital aganglionosis – Hirschsprung's disease

Hirschsprung's disease (congenital aganglionosis) most frequently (75%) involves the rectosigmoid portion of the large bowel. However, any length of intestine may be affected so that 'total colonic aganglionosis' and 'very long segment' Hirschsprung's disease affecting varying lengths of the small bowel are well recognized. The condition has an incidence of 1:4500 live births and is of multifactorial inheritance. The incidence is higher and the hereditary influence more manifest in long segment cases if there has been a previously affected sibling, or if the mother has been a sufferer as well. In view of the genetic influence, siblings of affected infants should be screened after birth. The genetic influence is also manifest in the increased association with other genetic conditions such as Down's syndrome and Wardenburg's syndrome. Genetic counselling for parents and affected families is always relevant.

Congenital aganglionosis is the result of a failure of intra-uterine migration of ganglion cells from the neural crest. Embryologically these cells travel distally along the vagus nerve pathways within the bowel wall, eventually reaching the anus. Arrest of migration will result in aganglionosis of all bowel distal to this point. 'Skip' lesions are extremely uncommon and difficult to explain. Within the aganglionic segment there is a proliferation of nerve fibrils, some of which are hypertrophic, demonstrating an increased acetylcholinesterase activity. Other ganglion anomalies, in particular neuronal intestinal dysplasia (NID), are considered to coexist with Hirschsprung's disease in some 15% of cases and may account for persistent problems after treatment. Failure of development of local autonomic innervation leads to absence of peristalsis within the affected bowel and consequent adynamic obstruction. The bowel immediately proximal to the congenital obstruction becomes markedly dilated and hypertrophic, eventually tapering into the aganglionic segment (Figure 63.14). This tapered 'transition zone' accounts for the 'cone effect' which is diagnostic on contrast enema and at operation.

The pregnancy is usually uncomplicated and the condition does not show any distinctive features antenatally. Commonly the child is born at full term, is of normal birth weight, and feeds and behaves normally, except for a failure to pass meconium during the first 24 hours of life, and despite a normal anus. Presentation is commonly at 2–4 days of age (80%) with abdominal

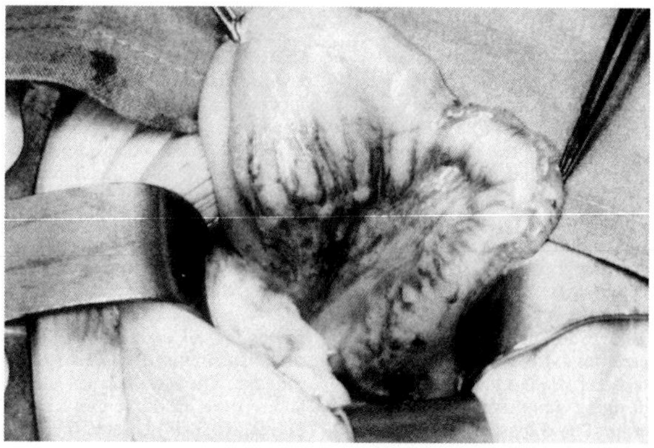

Figure 63.14 Hirschsprung's disease demonstrating the dilated bowel proximal to the 'transition zone' or 'cone', and the spastic aganglionic distal bowel.

distension, bile stained vomiting and passage of meconium only after stimulation. Digital rectal examination is followed by immediate explosive evacuation or a steady passage of flatus and meconium over several hours. Serious enterocolitis and life threatening septicaemia may complicate delayed diagnosis. The condition may sometimes be missed, the children eventually presenting at an older age group because of failure to thrive and constipation. The diagnosis of Hirschsprung's disease depends on a high index of suspicion. Failure to pass meconium within the first 24 hours after birth is always an indication for investigation. Definitive diagnosis depends on histological demonstration on a rectal biopsy, of an absence of ganglia, hypertrophy and proliferation of nerve fibrils and an increased acetylcholinesterase content in Auerbach's and Meissner's neural plexi. Mucosal and submucosal specimens are obtained by rectal suction biopsy or at formal operation. Other investigations such as contrast radiography and manometry are helpful in confirming and possibly demonstrating the level of the lesion, but are not as conclusive as histology.

At first presentation, management is that of intestinal obstruction, with nasogastric aspiration and intravenous fluid and electrolyte replacement. Because of the possibility of enterocolitis, antibiotics should also be given. The most important aspect to treatment is evacuation of the obstructed bowel. This can be achieved by 4–6 hourly digital rectal dilatation of the adynamic segment. Evacuation may not be immediate, and may occur gradually over several hours. Bowel washouts could be hazardous and should only be undertaken with measured volumes of isotonic solutions, ascertaining that all is returned. Once the child's condition has improved and the diagnosis confirmed on rectal biopsy, elective curative surgical resection is undertaken. Conventional management consists of a temporary transverse or left iliac fossa colostomy in normal ganglionic bowel. This is followed some months later by more definitive resection of the aganglionic segment and a reconstructive pullthrough. Intra-operative frozen section histology on serial seromuscular biopsies is essential to determine the level of resection. The three most commonly performed operations are those of Swenson, Soave and Duhamel. All follow the same aim of resecting the aganglionic bowel and transferring normal ganglionic bowel to the anus, as far down as the dentate line. The colostomy may be closed at the time of pullthrough (two-stage reconstruction) or at a third procedure once the anastomosis has healed and is widely patent. Improved neonatal anaesthesia, monitoring and intensive care has made possible a single-stage neonatal resection and pullthrough without a covering colostomy. More recently the open abdominal phase of the operation has been undertaken laparoscopically. A further advance has been the introduction of a completely transanal Soave or Swenson pullthrough. These single stage approaches do not carry any mortality, and morbidity is minimal such that they have become the treatment of choice in specialized centres. They have the advantage of one operation at the time of neonatal admission, no stoma and rapid return of a relatively normal child to the family. The long-term prognosis and quality of life for the large majority of children with Hirschsprung's disease is excellent with only a very low incidence of residual constipation or incontinence. Some 15% of affected children continue to suffer from bouts of abdominal distension, constipation and enterocolitis, suggestive of a dysfunctional residual colon despite apparent histological normality. There is still much controversy regarding the possible association between Hirschsprung's disease and NID or other anomalies of the ganglia, which has been suggested as the cause of the residual bowel dysfunction.

Long segment disease affecting the whole of the colon may be treated by colonic resection and ileo-anal anastomosis. The Lester Martin procedure, which sought to preserve colonic mucosa by side-to-side anastomosis of aganglionic colon to ganglionic ileum, is associated with an increased incidence of enterocolitis and has largely been abandoned. Extensive involvement of the small bowel is a serious issue, and is a cause of the short bowel state. Because of intestinal failure there is a total dependence on parenteral nutrition. Extensive aganglionosis is a possible indication for isolated small bowel transplantation.

Imperforate anus

The term imperforate anus covers a wide spectrum of associated anomalies with an incidence of approximately 1:3500. This condition is considered to be due to abnormal differentiation and not to have genetic implications. Imperforate anus may occur in association with other abnormalities, e.g. oesophageal atresia, cloacal extrophy. There is a high incidence of other abnormalities affecting the urinary tract (neurogenic bladder, vesico-ureteric reflux), the lumbosacral spine (sacral hypoplasia) and its associated nerves.

Imperforate anus is relevant to the development of anorectal continence, which is a highly complex learned activity. Continence involves the development of an ano-cortico-neural circuitry, which depends on sensory stimuli from the anorectum to the brain. Brain learning and patterning is particularly active during the early days and weeks of life at a time of maximal 'brain plasticity', which then matures during the first years of life. Basic management eventually transfers to the subconscious, such that nocturnal as well as diurnal continence is achieved. Continence therefore depends not only on intact and delicate sphincter muscle complexes and nerves (sensory and motor), but also on a highly sophisticated, stimulus-dependent ano-cortico-neural network which is continuously active at subconscious level, but which can be voluntarily overridden.

The anatomy of the sphincter muscle complex has been well clarified by Pena and de Vries and it is now well established that all of the muscles of continence are present in all cases of imperforate anus. The quality and function of these muscles is variable and depends on the degree of innervation. The external sphincter muscle complex is an integral but specialized section of the pelvic floor (diaphragm). The most superficial parasagittal fibres run in an anteroposterior direction from the coccyx towards the perineum just beneath the perianal skin. Other fibres criss-cross anteriorly and posteriorly to form a specialized concentric muscle ring surrounding the anal orifice. The major portion of the external sphincter complex is situated just beneath the highly sensitive perianal skin which lines the anal canal. The sphincter complex is in constant tone and acts with the levator ani to constrict, elevate and angulate the anorectum. The muscle is of the striated variety and possesses both a voluntary and an autonomic nerve supply. The internal rectal sphincter is an integral part of the rectal muscle wall and is found at the lowermost part of the rectum just above the dentate line. Though essentially separate structures, the internal and external sphincters are normally in anatomical continuity and each complements the other, such that they function as a single motor unit. At rest the anus is normally held closed, with the sphincter muscles in constant resting tone, but can be activated to relax or retain by conscious voluntary override. The internal sphincter responds to stretch reflexes originating in the rectal wall and relaxes in response to rectal distension.

The wide spectrum of pathology in imperforate anus has been extensively described and classified by Douglas Stephens and revised by Pena. At the better end of the scale lie anal stenosis and covered anus where the anorectum is well developed and continence is not likely to be a problem. Even in these cases the rectum shows the marked dilatation associated with bowel atresias. Poor propulsion in this segment causes faecal retention and overflow incontinence. Next along the spectrum are various forms where the anal canal is absent, but there is an anal dimple covered over by highly sensitive perianal skin. Anterior to the anal dimple the dilated rectum opens in the midline of the perineum through a fistulous track which is surrounded by the internal sphincter. The perineum is well-featured, indicative of good muscle tone and appropriate innervation such that continence is highly likely (Figure 63.15). The more severe varieties of imperforate anus have a poorly formed anal dimple and a featureless perineum with poor muscle tone and little sphincteric activity (Figure 63.16). The fistula from the dilated rectum communicates with the posterior urethra at bulbar or prostatic level in the male, and at the vulva or vagina in the female, lying well away from the external sphincter complex. There is a high incidence of sacral nerve abnormality with a neurogenic perineum and incontinence. Associated abnormalities of the renal tract and the sacrum are particularly common.

Imperforate anus can be readily diagnosed at the first routine post-natal examination by simple inspection of the perineum. The anus is stenotic or imperforate and the perineum is of variable tone. There is often a failure to pass meconium, however this may still appear on the perineum, in the vulva or through the urethra because of a fistulous communication from the rectum. Should evacuation through the fistula be unsatisfactory, then signs of intestinal obstruction develop (distended abdomen, bilious vomiting). The high incidence of associated urological, sacral and pelvic nerve abnormalities calls for a full study to include a cystogram. Relief of intestinal obstruction is the most urgent priority. It may be possible to deflate the bowel through the fistulous track on the perineum or in the vulva, in preparation for full reconstruction. Excessive dilatation or injudicious surgery to widen the fistulous orifice is contraindicated and may cause injury. In all other circumstances, it has traditionally been considered safer to perform a colostomy at the transverse colon or at the descending colon-sigmoid junction, leaving reconstruction to a later date. The nature of the fistulous communication can be evaluated by contrast enema down the distal limb of the colostomy. It is now becoming commoner practice for primary reconstruction to be undertaken in the neonatal phase and without a stoma. Whichever policy is preferred, the goal in reconstruction of the anorectum is to achieve full continence and voluntary control for flatus, and for liquid and solid faeces by day and night. The reconstructive plan should recognize the relevance to continence of the anorectal sensory receptors, intact neural pathways, brain patterning and learning at the normal physiological age, a functional sphincter muscle complex and a propulsive rectum. It is evident that the anomalous rectal fistula must be closed. The reconstructive plan therefore includes:

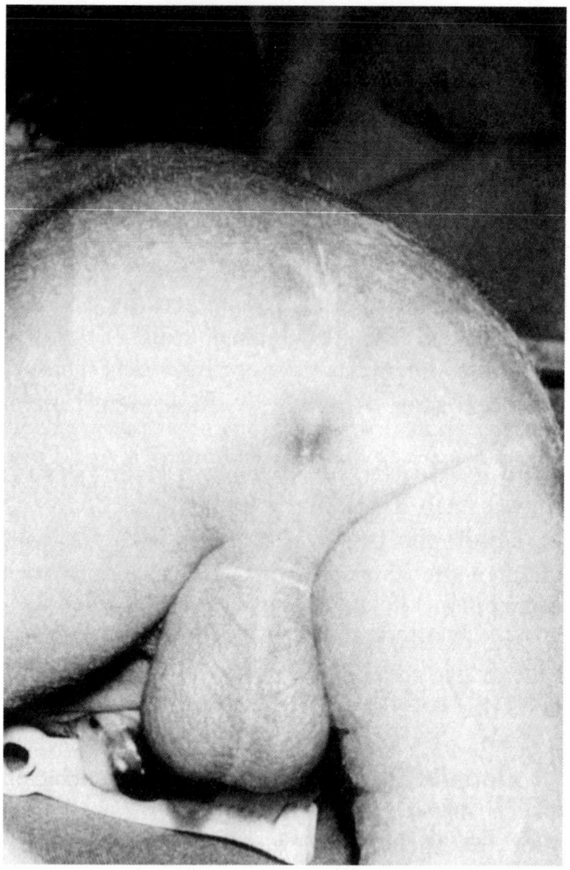

Figure 63.16 Imperforate anus without a visible fistula, but a probable recto-urethral fistula.

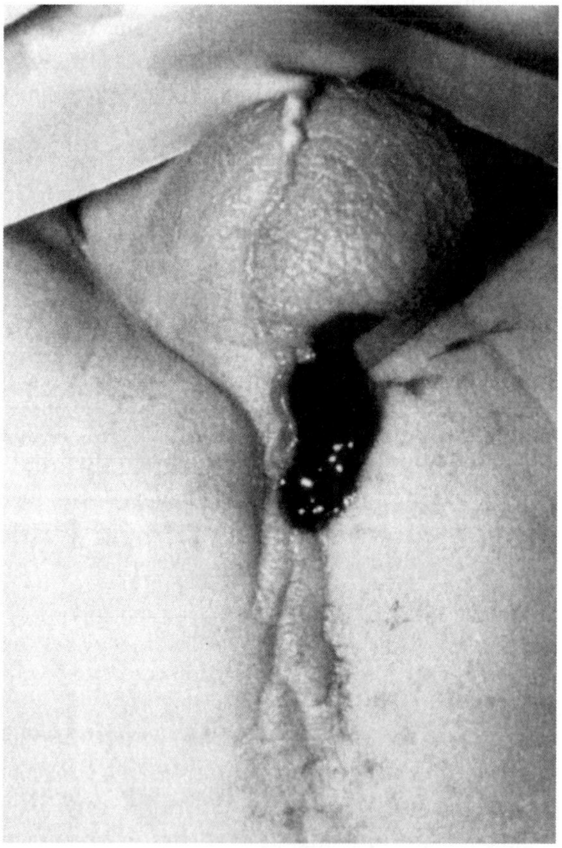

Figure 63.15 Imperforate anus with recto-perineal fistula.

- Construction of a patent anus with an anal canal of normal dimensions lined with sensitive perianal skin. No perianal tissue should be excised
- Identification of the external sphincter muscle complex with the Pena muscle stimulator
- Identification of the rectum through an anterior perineal, a posterior sagittal or an open or laparoscopic abdominal approach. Division of the rectal fistula at its lowermost point preserves the internal sphincter around the lower end of the rectum
- Re-routing of the rectum and its internal sphincter, to anastomose with the previously prepared anal canal at the dentate line
- Reconstruction of the disrupted vulva and perineum towards normal.

When a colostomy has been performed, reconstructive procedures are usually undertaken at 3–12 months of age. In some centres in well-experienced hands, full primary reconstruction without a stoma is undertaken as the definitive procedure during the first 48 hours after birth. This approach recognizes the relevance to long-term continence of sensory input from the anus for the development of normal ano-cortico-neural pathways at the physiological time of 'brain plasticity'. Clearly reconstruction for imperforate anus is a difficult and delicate undertaking which is best performed in specialized neonatal and paediatric centres.

Biliary atresia

Persistent jaundice during the neonatal period should always raise the suspicion of biliary atresia. The histological features suggest an ongoing destructive process affecting the biliary tree, however the aetiology remains unclear. Some 85% of cases are of the intrahepatic variety involving the intrahepatic and frequently the extrahepatic bile ducts as well, whereas 15% affect the extrahepatic bile ducts alone. It is particularly important to differentiate between biliary atresia and neonatal hepatitis, since the latter requires only a conservative approach, whereas biliary atresia requires relatively urgent surgery, preferably within the first 6 weeks of life. Routine biochemical investigations are equivocal and isotope scanning is unsatisfactory. Diagnosis may eventually depend on expert histological evaluation of liver biopsy specimens and may ultimately only become clear at surgical exploration of the porta hepatis. Despite biochemical evidence of obstructive jaundice, ultrasound scans never demonstrate bile duct distension even in cases of extrahepatic biliary atresia. An inability to outline the gallbladder and the extrahepatic bile ducts is highly suspicious. In pure extrahepatic biliary atresia the extrahepatic ductular system is fibrosed, but the intrahepatic ducts are patent. At surgery the blind-ending hepatic ducts can be found at some level below the porta hepatis. Intrahepatic biliary atresia is more sinister in that no obvious intrahepatic drainage system can be found. The gallbladder and extrahepatic bile ducts are often fibrosed and no lumen can be found. Occasionally sections of the extrahepatic system may remain patent and may communicate with the duodenum. Treatment attempts to provide biliary drainage for the liver. A Roux-en-Y jejunal loop hepatic portoenterostomy, as described by Kasai, is the treatment of choice. Successful surgery is followed by relatively rapid clearance of jaundice, so that in extrahepatic biliary atresia the long-term prognosis may be good. Children with intrahepatic biliary atresia in whom drainage has been achieved will enjoy a marked improvement in their growth and quality of life. However, the process of intrahepatic fibrosis and eventual cirrhosis progresses unrelentingly towards portal hypertension and liver failure, commonly between 3 and 5 years of age. Although the Kasai portoenterostomy may not offer a permanent cure, it provides an opportunity for improved growth and well being towards an eventual elective liver transplant.

Choledochal cyst

This lesion presents with jaundice and occasionally with cholangitis. Ultrasound scan reveals a variable cystic dilatation of the extrahepatic ductular system. The lesion may be associated with abnormalities at the junction of the pancreatic and common bile ducts. Treatment is by resection of the dilated ducts and replacement by Roux-en-Y choledochojejunostomy. Reconstruction of the extrahepatic ducts using available ductular tissue from the cyst is not recommended since it does not deal with the anomaly at the junction with the pancreatic duct. In other situations the friability and vascularity of the cyst wall makes such reconstruction difficult. It is relevant that such tissue has been associated with an increased risk of malignancy.

Section 63.6 • Infantile hypertrophic pyloric stenosis

Pyloric stenosis is characterized by marked hypertrophy of the pyloric musculature. It is a common condition carrying an incidence of 1:400. Both sexes are affected with a male to female ratio of 4:1, with a particular bias towards first born males. The aetiology of the condition remains unknown. Pyloric stenosis develops some 4–6 weeks after birth, regardless of whether the child was born prematurely or at term, and has never been reported in stillbirths. There is a definite genetic predisposition, since a mother who had pyloric stenosis has a 1:5 chance of an affected child. Pyloric stenosis also has a racial bias, occurring more commonly in Caucasians. Presentation is with vomiting of a few days' duration, in a previously well and thriving child. Typically the child is constantly hungry, demonstrating a desperate wish to feed. The vomitus is initially of small amount, but steadily increases in volume, force and frequency until virtually all of the feed is returned. It is rarely bile stained, and consists of curdled milk and altered blood because of inflammatory gastritis from food stasis. The strongly contracting stomach is often visible as waves of painful peristalsis passing from left to right across the left hypochondrium. Features of dehydration eventually become evident, and the initially alert child becomes lethargic and hypotonic. The fontanelles are depressed, skin turgor is lost and the child is sunken eyed. Weight loss, largely an index of dehydration, is rapid and significant. The blood chemistry reflects the fluid and electrolyte losses, particularly for sodium, potassium and chloride. Compensatory buffer mechanisms result in an intracellular acidosis and an extracellular alkalosis. Only small amounts of concentrated urine are passed and the stools are small, firm and green. The diagnosis is suggested by the typical history and is determined by definite palpation of the hypertrophied muscle mass. Ultrasound scan and contrast radiology is helpful in the difficult case, but is not a substitute for careful clinical examination. The hypertrophic pylorus is easier to palpate when the baby is pain free and relaxed. The stomach is emptied and then constantly aspirated with a large (8 Fr gauge) nasogastric tube and the baby is offered a milk or dextrose feed. With the child thus comforted and relaxed it is possible to palpate deeply in the upper abdomen. Examination is undertaken from the left side with the operator's left hand. The position of the pylorus is variable and somewhat dependent on the size of the stomach. The palpating index and middle fingers search beneath the right edge of the liver in the paraspinal gutter and moving towards the midline and above the umbilicus. The hypertrophied pylorus is palpable as a moderately mobile firm swelling about the size of a small walnut. It can be localized against the spine and tends to be slightly uncomfortable, eliciting a reaction from the child. Accuracy in diagnosis depends on operator experience.

Early management is conservative with correction of the fluid and electrolyte losses. Reduction in the metabolic alkalosis is a good index of correction of the severe intracellular potassium deficit. Meanwhile the child is allowed to sham feed to maintain his sucking reflex and for comfort. Surgery is only entertained once all deficits are corrected and the serum biochemistry has returned to normal. The mainstay of surgery is Ramstedt's pyloromyotomy, which splits and widely separates the hypertrophic muscle at the submucosal plane, from stomach to duodenum. Every attempt is made to avoid a mucosal perforation, however if this occurs it is patched over with omentum and the stomach is kept empty for some 3 days post-operatively to allow adequate healing prior to feeding. The vertical midline epigastric incision has largely been abandoned in favour of the transverse right hypochondrial approach. This in its own right is now being replaced by the more aesthetic circum-supraumbilical incision which lies in a skin crease just above the umbilicus (Figure 63.17). Pyloromyotomy can also be undertaken laparoscopically, however considering the risks and additional skills required the indication for this is questionable. Normal milk feeds are started once the child recovers from anaesthesia, but are delayed in the event of a mucosal perforation. No 'special' regimens are necessary and full feeding, a contented mother and child and home discharge are usually achieved within 24–72 hours after surgery. The long-term prognosis is excellent.

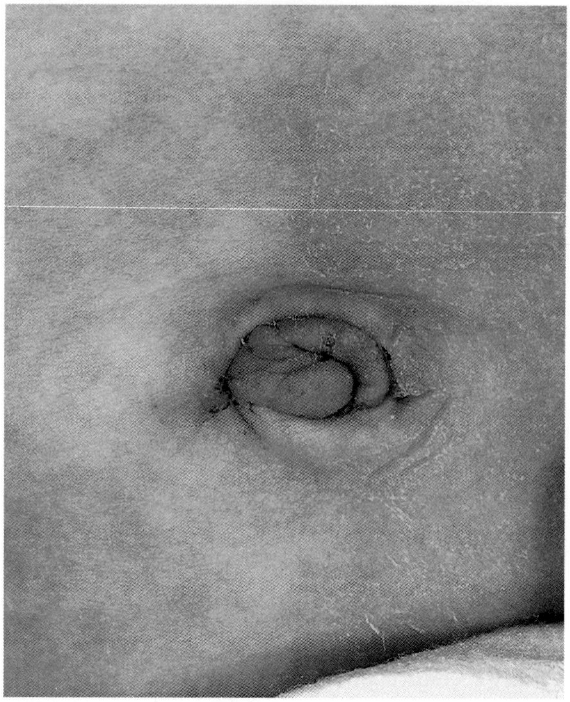

Figure 63.17 Circum-supraumbilical incision.

Section 63.7 • Intussusception

The term describes an invagination of the bowel into itself. As it progresses more and more bowel is drawn in, such that the intussusception becomes progressively more bulky. Compression of the mesentery within the intussusception leads to increasing vascular congestion and bowel strangulation. Intussusception may occur antenatally when it is followed by resorption of the sterile infarcted mass of bowel and the typical features of intestinal atresia.

The condition occurs most commonly in a previously well child of 9–18 months of age. There is a seasonal incidence with increased frequency in the spring and autumn, which coincides with epidemics of upper respiratory (largely viral) infections. The most frequent lesion forming the apex of the intussusception is a hyperplasia of lymphoid tissue in a Peyer's patch within the antimesenteric wall of the ileum. As the intussusceptum progresses, it passes through the ileo-caecal valve and along the colon, and may even reach the anus. Other causes include a Meckel's diverticulum, mucosal polyps, Peutz–Jegher syndrome, Henoch–Schönlein purpura, cystic fibrosis and foreign bodies. There are spasms of severe abdominal colic causing the child to scream and to draw its legs up towards the abdomen. Major autonomic upset causes marked pallor, sweating and retching such that the child looks ill and is often described by the mother as 'white as a sheet'. Initial reflex vomiting of gastric content is followed by reflux vomiting of bile and small bowel content as intestinal obstruction establishes. Frequent episodes of severe colic and vomiting eventually lead to exhaustion and lethargy as the condition progresses. Vascular congestion within the intussusception causes oozing of mucus and blood, which is then passed rectally as the typical 'redcurrant jelly' stools. This is a late and ominous sign suggesting vascular compromise in the affected bowel. Sequestration of blood within the intussusception reduces the circulating blood volume and leads to hypovolaemic shock. Abdominal examination during an early quiescent phase reveals a soft relatively non-tender abdomen with a sausage shaped mass in the right hypochondrium just above the umbilicus. As the intussusceptum passes down the left colon, the mass is drawn beneath the umbilicus towards the left side. The apex may even present at the anus. In late cases signs of peritonitis suggest severely compromised or necrotic bowel.

The diagnosis is suggested by the typical history, an abdominal mass and the passage of redcurrant jelly stools. A plain abdominal X-ray shows an emptiness in the right iliac fossa, an opacity over the intussusception and features of small bowel obstruction. Following resuscitation and blood volume replacement, the diagnosis can be confirmed on ultrasound scan or by contrast enema (air or fluid). Positive backward pressure during the enema is used to 'push back' the intussusceptum, and is maintained until contrast is seen to pass freely into the small bowel, confirming complete reduction. As long as the child is stable and the abdomen does not show signs of peritonitis, the length of the history is not a contraindication to contrast enema reduction. It is not infrequent for reduction to be incomplete at the first attempt, with the intussusceptum held up at the ileo-caecal valve. A second or third attempt may prove successful. Deterioration in the child's general condition or the state of the abdomen, repeated failed reduction or uncertainty as to completeness are indications for surgical intervention. In older children intussusception is more likely to be due to lesions other than hypertrophic Peyer's patches, such that the indication for surgery is stronger. Reduction may be undertaken at open surgery or laparoscopically. The abdomen is opened through a transverse incision placed aesthetically in a skin crease in the right iliac fossa. The intussusception is delivered through the wound and the reduction completed by gentle push back. Hypertrophic Peyer's patches do not require excision. Severely compromised or gangrenous bowel is resected and continuity established by end-to-end anastomosis. There is a 7% incidence of recurrence of the intussusception, when reduction by contrast enema is again indicated. Repeated recurrence should raise the suspicion of other lesions and is a definite indication for surgery.

Section 63.8 • Hydrocele, inguinal and femoral hernias

The processus vaginalis develops as a peritoneal sac ahead of the descending testis as it passes from the abdomen to the scrotum. Once the testicle reaches its most caudal position in the scrotum, the processus fuses and is represented by the tunica vaginalis around the testis. A similar peritoneal sac develops alongside the round ligament in the female. Patency of the processus vaginalis is a normal occurrence in the full-term neonate, but is pathological after the sixth month. Sac distension with fluid constitutes a hydrocele. A sac with a neck wide enough to allow passage of viscera classifies as a hernia. Since the left testis is the first to descend and the left processus the first to fuse, a right-sided hernia or hydrocele is commoner. Equally, continuing left patency carries a higher incidence of an associated right hernia. Bilateral patent processi are particularly common in premature male babies and in girls.

Hydrocele

These are rarely seen in the female, but are very common in the male. Typically there is a non-tender bluish swelling of varying size in the inguinal area and in the scrotum, which becomes large and tense following straining or physical activity. The clear peritoneal fluid within the sac will transilluminate and the cord and testicle will be seen to lie posteromedial to the sac. Unless the hydrocele is excessively tense, it is usually possible to palpate the cord structures between the upper limit of the sac and the inguinal ring. The processus may remain patent only in its mid-section such that an 'encysted cord hydrocele' results. Hydroceles are not associated with complications and initial management is conservative, awaiting spontaneous fusion of the processus vaginalis during the first 6 months after birth. Persistent patency or discomfort due to size and weight is an indication for surgery. The operation is the same as for inguinal hernia, and the processus is ligated and divided at the internal inguinal ring. Recurrence is unlikely.

Inguinal hernia

Inguinal hernia affects both sexes but is commoner in the male. Almost all inguinal hernias are of the indirect variety. The hernial sac (processus vaginalis) passes through the inguinal canal alongside the vas deferens and the testicular vessels, lying within the cremasteric sheath. A variety of intra-abdominal organs can find their way into the sac. Unlike the adult the child's omentum is poorly formed, and it is often the ileum which herniates into the sac. Other organs include the appendix, the ovary and fallopian tube and even the uterus and bladder. The presence of a gonad in the groin in a child with normal female genitalia should raise the possibility of 'testicular feminization' (androgen insensitivity syndrome).

The hernia, of the indirect variety, usually presents as a non-tender swelling passing down the inguinal canal and into the scrotum. The bowel within the sac does not transilluminate and no upper limit can be found. Spontaneous reduction may occur when the child is quiet or asleep. However, excessive tension within the inguinal canal will lead to incarceration and irreducibility, with eventual possible bowel strangulation. Compression of the testicular vessels and the vas at the inguinal ring may lead to testicular infarction or vasal occlusion. The diagnosis of inguinal hernia may have to rely on the history since an uncomplicated hernia may not always be easy to demonstrate. Examination may reveal only a thickened cord. Treatment is surgical and is best undertaken electively. Irreducibility demands urgent attention to avoid strangulation and injury to the testicle and vas. It is relevant to warn the parents of possible testicular atrophy following incarceration of an inguinal hernia. Reduction is achieved by steady massage over the cord and inguinal ring with appropriate taxies at the fundus in order to push back the hernial contents. Failed or incomplete reduction is an indication for immediate surgery. Operation consists of high ligation and division of the processus vaginalis at or above the internal ring. The procedure can be performed through a skin crease groin incision exposing the spermatic cord and opening the inguinal canal when necessary. Alternatively the more aesthetic high scrotal incision (Figure 63.18) or a 'groin crease' incision in the female (Figure 63.19) will provide excellent access. Since the underlying lesion is a congenital patency of the processus vaginalis, a simple herniotomy is usually sufficient. However, excessively large hernias, which are commoner in premature babies, cause major disruption of the inguinal canal such that a herniorrhaphy is relevant to avoid recurrence. There is really no indication for laparoscopic hernia repair in the child.

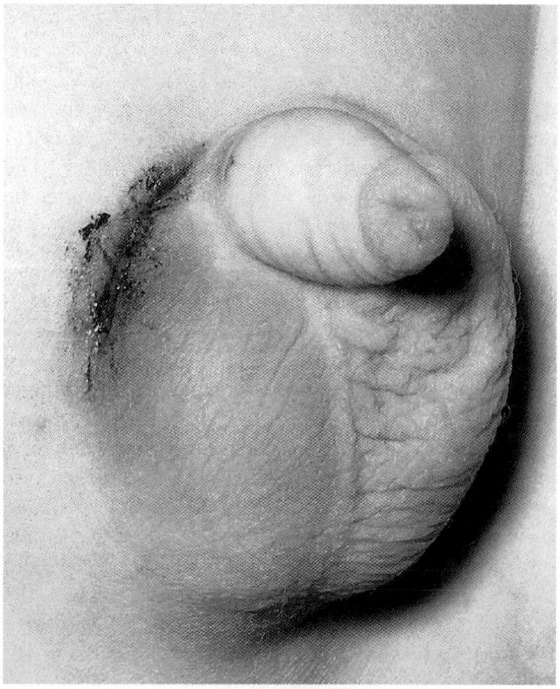

Figure 63.18 Scrotal skin crease incision for hydrocele and hernia repair, and for orchidopexy.

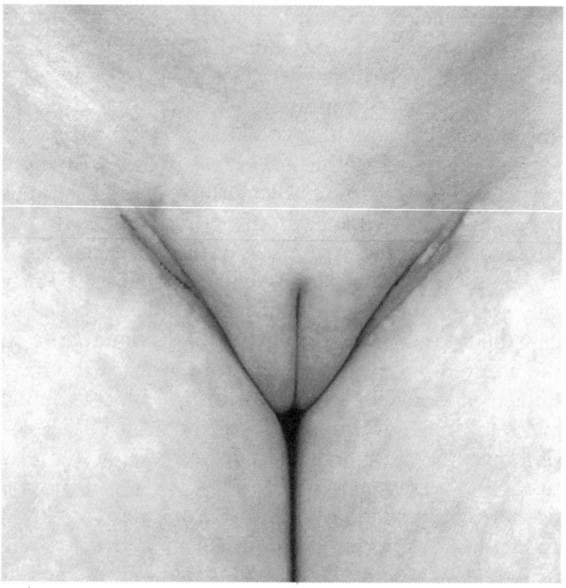

Figure 63.19 Aesthetic skin crease groin incisions for hernia repair in girls.

Femoral hernia

This uncommon hernia occurs more often in girls and presents as a tender swelling below the inguinal ligament and medial to the femoral vein. It usually contains fat, and bowel herniation is infrequent. The femoral hernia is distinguished from an inguinal hernia or an enlarged femoral lymph node by its position and its consistency. Treatment consists of a herniotomy and a herniorrhaphy, either from below the inguinal ligament or through a McEvedy approach from above. Recurrence is uncommon and the long-term prognosis is excellent.

Section 63.9 • Undescended testis

The testis develops from the genital ridge just below the mesonephrogenic ridge on the posterior abdominal wall. By an as yet unclear process of fetal unfolding and hormonal influences (including Müllerian inhibiting substance), the testis reaches the internal inguinal ring. At around the second to ninth month of gestation, under the influence of chorionic gonadotrophin and testosterone, it passes through the inguinal canal to lie in the scrotum at the time of birth. Testosterone (androgen) exerts its effect through the anterior spinal nucleus and the genital branch of the genitofemoral nerve, utilizing the neurotransmitter calcitonin gene related peptide (CGRP). Despite increasing knowledge the exact cause(s) for testicular undescent remains unclear. Some testes are primarily abnormal and fail to respond to normal stimuli. However, most recent studies suggest that around 80% of undescended testes are intrinsically normal at birth. However, if continually exposed to body heat in the undescended position, the testis shows a marked loss of spermatogonia and tubular degeneration, particularly after the second year of life.

The incidence of testicular undescent in the full-term normal male is around 4%. There is a much higher incidence in the premature infant, which relates to gestational age. Spontaneous descent continues during the first 6 months after birth, so that the incidence at 1 year is around 1.4%. At this time and subsequently residual undescent is pathological and demands surgical referral. The true undescended testis must be distinguished from the normal retractile gonad, which often lies in the superficial inguinal pouch. The examining left hand, in a sliding movement from the anterior superior iliac spine to the scrotal neck, overcomes the cremasteric retraction, such that the normal testis on long vessels and vas deferens passes into the well developed scrotum effortlessly and without discomfort or pain.

Testicular descent may be unilateral or bilateral, with the right side being more commonly affected, possibly because of the later descent of the right testis. The scrotum on the undescended side is hypoplastic, giving a flat unfilled appearance. Some 80% of true undescended testes are palpable in the groin. They may be 'incompletely' descended lying along the normal pathway of descent, or they may be 'ectopic' lying laterally in the groin crease, overlying the femoral vessels, at the base of the penis or even in the perineum between the scrotum and the anus. The ectopic testis is frequently of normal volume (1–1.5 ml in the neonate) and of normal histology, demonstrating also a fused processus vaginalis. By comparison the incompletely descended testis is associated with a patent processus vaginalis which is short, and together with a variably fibrotic cremaster muscle, acts to retain the testis in an undescended state. It is commonly of smaller volume and is frequently histologically abnormal, with a higher content of potentially neoplastic dysgenetic tissue. By far the majority of palpable undescended testes have a normal vas deferens and testicular vessels of normal length, neither of which hinder passage to the most caudal scrotal position. Some 15–20% of undescended testes are impalpable. Most will be found to lie high in the inguinal canal or intraperitoneally close to the internal inguinal ring. Some 10% will be absent, either because of failure of development or more commonly because of loss secondary to intra-uterine testicular torsion. It follows that it is always important to determine the presence and location of an impalpable testis. These testes are always smaller and contain a considerable amount of potentially neoplastic dysgenetic tissue such that they carry the highest incidence of malignancy. Thus it follows that the clinical prognostic indicators of normality for all testes are testicular volume and the most caudal position to which the testis can be brought into the scrotum without any discomfort or pain to the child. In assessing testicular undescent these parameters should be clearly recorded in the case notes.

Testicular undescent is associated with several potential complications. Since the testis has failed to reach the most caudal scrotal position, the processus vaginalis remains patent and constitutes a hernial sac (hydrocele or hernia). The testis has an unstable lie and is prone to torsion. Constant exposure to a higher body temperature has a detrimental effect leading to loss of spermatogonia and failure of tubular development such that fertility is steadily reduced. Sterility may be due to the higher incidence of epididymo-testicular dissociation and other epididymal anomalies (atresias, stenoses). The undescended testis is at greater risk of malignancy because of the higher content of dysgenetic tissue. Some 60% of tumours are seminomas and are more frequent around 35–45 years of age. Finally and of major relevance, the psychological impact of abnormal genitalia on the adolescent and his family should not be underestimated. The main indications for treatment are the preservation of spermatogenesis and hence fertility, and the removal of the psychological concerns of the cryptorchid child and family. Since there is no further spontaneous descent after 6 months of age, referral and treatment should be instituted as soon as possible after this time. Hormonal stimulation with human chorionic gonadotrophin or LHRH (luteinizing hormone releasing hormone), or combinations of both, is only effective in the small number of very low lying testes already at the scrotal neck. Treatment is essentially surgical. The operation of orchidopexy as described by Schuller (1881) and Bevan (1899, 1903) has been conventionally performed through a groin incision. The testis is isolated on its vas and vessels, and the short processus vaginalis is ligated and divided above the internal inguinal ring. Tension-free descent of some 1.5–3.5 cm is usually achieved. Through a separate scrotal incision the testis, attached solely by the vas and the testicular vessels, is brought through into an ipsilateral subdartos scrotal pouch as described by Schoemaker (1932). More recently orchidopexy through a single transscrotal skin crease incision (previously described for inguinal hernia and hydrocele) (Figure 63.18) has been proposed for the palpable testis. This single incision provides good access for mobilization of the testis in the inguinal area and for formation of the ipsilateral subdartos pouch. It involves less dissection and is more comfortable for the 'day-case' child, also leaving an aesthetically superior, skin crease scrotal scar. Complications of orchidopexy are few. Damage to the vas and testicular vessels from rough handling or excessive tension may lead to testicular atrophy or vasal occlusion. Recurrence of undescent is usually due to insufficient mobilization of the testicular vascular pedicle such that the testis is brought to the scrotum under tension. Adhesion of the cord structures to the external inguinal ring will occasionally result in an 'ascending' testis with slow recurrence of undescent as the child grows.

Impalpable testes should be located at laparoscopy, this being the single definitive and informative investigation. Surgical groin exploration should be avoided since it disrupts tissue planes and adds to the difficulty of definitive surgery. The high inguinal and intra-abdominal testis has a short vascular pedicle and will rarely reach the scrotum by conventional orchidopexy. Multistage orchidopexy is frequently unsuccessful. Division of the main testicular vessels (Fowler-Stephens technique) allows the testis to reach the scrotum, but relies for testicular survival on the collateral circulation from the flimsy vasal vessels. There is a prolonged period of relative ischaemia and venous congestion which results in a 30–50% risk of testicular infarction and atrophy. The two-stage Fowler-Stephens technique, with initial ligation of the vascular pedicle at open operation or laparoscopically, and subsequent testicular transfer to the scrotum is said to have a greater success in terms of testicular survival. Immediate return of a full arterial supply and venous drainage recommends microvascular orchidopexy as the treatment of choice for the high inguinal and intra-abdominal testis on a short vascular pedicle. Through an extended groin incision the testis is mobilized extensively on its vas and vessels, also preserving the collateral circulation from the vasal vessels. The testicular vessels are divided above the confluence of the pampiniform plexus to form a single testicular vein, and the testis with intact vas is placed in a subdartos pouch. A full blood supply is restored within some 90 min, by anastomosis of the testicular artery (0.5 mm diameter) to the inferior epigastric artery (1.2 mm diameter) and the testicular vein (1 mm diameter) to an inferior epigastric vein (0.8 mm diameter). Microvascular anastomosis requires the use of the operating microscope and a technically perfect technique to avoid anastomotic thrombosis. When undertaken in a specialized centre regularly offering microsurgical expertise, microvascular orchidopexy has a 92% testicular survival rate with a well placed psychologically and aesthetically acceptable scrotal testis. The long-term effect on spermatogenesis and on malignancy following the Fowler–Stephens technique and microvascular orchidopexy at <2 years of age remains to be determined. In view of the higher risk of neoplasia, patients who have undergone scrotal transfer of a high testis should be taught careful self-examination.

Section 63.10 • Intersex disorders

During early embryological development, the external genitalia for both male and female are essentially similar, and of female configuration. The Y-chromosome determines the development of the primordial non-committed gonad towards a testis, which becomes hormonally active. Increasing levels of testosterone are converted by 5-alpha-reductase to the active dihydrotestosterone, which is picked up by cell membrane androgen receptors and transferred to the nucleus. This induces the external genitalia to undergo virilization and primes the brain and spinal cord towards a male orientation. The Sertoli cells in the testis produce Müllerian inhibiting substance (MIS), a locally acting hormone that induces regression of the Müllerian ducts from which the upper two-thirds of the vagina, the uterus and fallopian tubes are derived. The virilization process involves a marked growth in the size of the phallus and an alteration in its structure and direction to form the normal penis. The developing urethral tube on the ventral surface of the shaft closes over from a proximal to distal direction, eventually passing through a subglanular tunnel. The scrotum, the ventral shaft skin and the prepuce unite at a midline raphe. Fusion of the labioscrotal folds initially forms a bifid scrotum, and is followed by development of the central partition to give a normal scrotal shape. Concomitant with this process there is a regression of the lower one-third of the vagina, which originates from the external genital structures.

Inappropriate virilization will lead to the various forms of intersex. Thus the 'male pseudohermaphrodite', chromosomally XY, who only undergoes partial virilization, will present with hypospadias of varying severity. Treatment is surgical and is designed to complete the virilization process. Total inability to respond to androgens because of absence of cell membrane receptors leads to 'testicular feminization' with a total failure of masculinization. The external genitalia retain a female form, however the secretion of MIS by the otherwise normal testes causes regression of the Müllerian ducts leading to an absence of the upper vagina, the uterus and the fallopian tubes. Not infrequently the gonads remain undescended and present in a hernial sac at the external inguinal ring. Thus the presence of a gonad in an inguinal hernia in a child with a normal female vulva, should always stimulate consideration of XY testicular feminization. Since these chromosomally male (XY) children are unable to respond to androgens and therefore cannot virilize, they are in effect functionally female and should be reared as such. The testes will require removal and female hormones given at puberty and subsequently. Vaginal elongation is usually necessary to allow intercourse. Since these girls have no ovaries and no uterus they are of necessity sterile and cannot bear children. Both the children and their parents require counselling at all stages of management.

The 'female pseudohermaphrodite', chromosomally XX, who has virilized because of exposure to androgenic substances in early pregnancy (congenital adrenal hyperplasia (CAH), androgen producing tumour, maternal progestogen ingestion), will present with ambiguous genitalia tending towards male. Such children may be mistaken for males with severe hypospadias. However, the gonads are ovaries and there has been no exposure to MIS such that the internal female organs are all present. Treatment is directed towards medical control of excessive androgen production, e.g. hydrocortisone in CAH, and surgery is designed to return the overvirilized external genitalia towards normal female.

Varying combinations of gonadal structures (ovotestes, primordial gonad) classify as 'mixed gonadal dysgenesis'. The sex of rearing and future function will depend on the configuration of the internal and external genitalia, which in turn depend on the presence of active testicular tissue and the end organ response to therapy with androgens. Chromosomal mosaicism is a frequent association.

The final form of intersex is the 'true hermaphrodite' with a normal testis and male internal genitalia on one side, and a normal ovary with female internal structures on the other. The genitalia may be ambiguous but tend towards male. The presence of androgens will have primed the brain and spinal cord towards a male orientation. Chromosomal mosaicism is not uncommon. Management depends on the extent of development of the external genitalia and the response to hormones.

Intersex disorders should be referred to specialist centres for investigation by an expert multidisciplinary team. The child should not be allocated a sex until full determination of the anatomy and the response to hormonal therapy. The psychological impact on these children and their families should not be underestimated, and they require early and ongoing counselling.

Section 63.11 • Hypospadias

Undervirilization of an otherwise normal male child may result in varying degrees of hypospadias. This is a common condition occurring in 1:150 liveborn boys. A genetic influence is evident in some families. Hypospadias also occurs in association with other chromosomally determined conditions. The anatomy of the genitalia will depend on the timing of the interference with the virilization process. For the majority this occurs late and virilization will be well advanced but incomplete (Figure 63.20). The phallus will have achieved a good size and will be relatively free and well positioned. Failure of glanular development leads to a splayed and ventrally flexed appearance (glanular flexion) similar to that of the clitoris. The meatus is represented at the normal glanular site but ends as a blind pit. The prepuce does not unite ventrally and is collected on the dorsal aspect of the glans. The urethral meatus opens proximally in the midline on the ventral penile shaft, and the urethra distal to the meatus is represented as an open urethral plate extending onto the glans. The spongiosal tissue is divided with each half lying lateral to the urethral plate on either side. In severe cases development is poor, with a severe lack of urethral plate and marked ventral shaft tethering (chordee) particularly during erection (Figure 63.21). The testes are often normally descended in the scrotum. Disrupted virilization at a very early stage will result in perineal or penoscrotal hypospadias with limited penile and scrotal development. The phallus is small and tethered and the scrotum is often bifid and extending up around the penile base in 'shawl' fashion. The urethral meatus is very proximal and may even be perineal. The testes may not have descended. Indeed ambiguous genitalia and impalpable testes should raise the possibility of a virilized female.

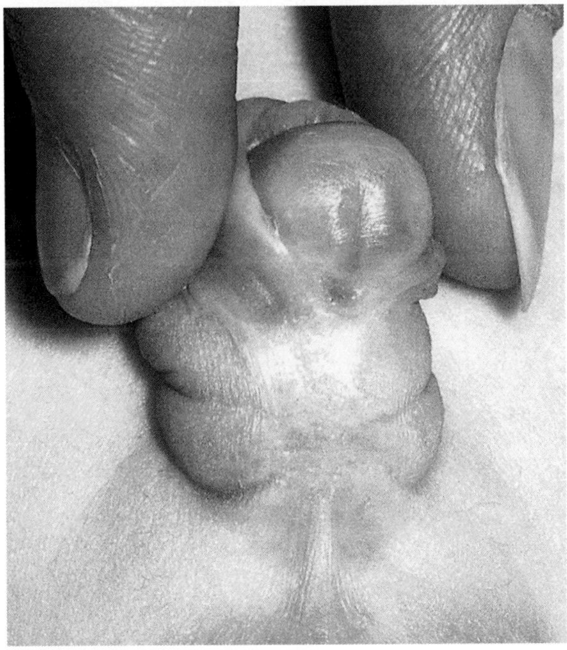

Figure 63.20 Hypospadias showing glanular flexion and splayed glans, distal shaft urethral meatus, ventral shaft skin deficit and split prepuce collected dorsally.

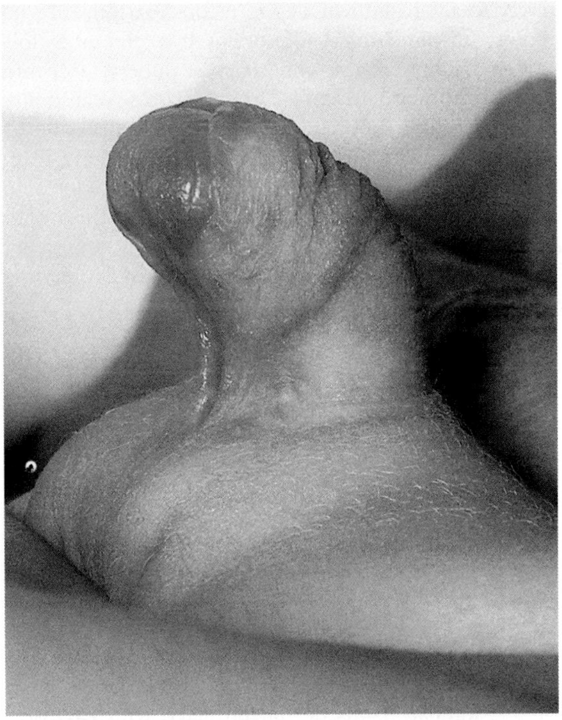

Figure 63.21 Penoscrotal hypospadias with marked chordee in erection.

The degree of hypospadias is classified according to the position of the urethral meatus and the presence of chordee. However, the full extent of the defect and therefore the real classification can only be ascertained at operation once full correction has been achieved. The reasons for surgery in hypospadias relate to the psychological impact of ambiguous genitalia and to eventual sexual performance. Meatal stenosis and ability to micturate as a male are further indications. Treatment is entirely surgical and is designed along embryological lines, to complete the virilization process. When possible all surgery should be complete by the second to fourth year of life. Operative techniques, which achieve complete correction in a single stage, are now available and should be the norm. It is essential that the penis is fully released and able to rise freely in erection. The urethra is constructed from the urethral plate; alternatively a neourethra is fashioned from ventral shaft skin or from the transposed prepuce. A bladder or buccal mucosal graft may occasionally be relevant if local tissues are insufficient. Whenever possible the hemispongiosal tissue is united in the midline to support the urethral reconstruction. The glans is rotated ventrally and the glanular flexion corrected to give a well-directed glanular meatus and urinary stream. It is very important to preserve the meatal lips and the 'vertical slit' meatal configuration since this concentrates the urinary steam and avoids spraying during micturition. Temporary urinary diversion can be achieved with a through-repair catheter or by suprapubic catheterization. Present day techniques carry a 7% complication rate, mainly related to ventral glanular disruption, meatal stenosis, fistula formation and rarely total breakdown of the reconstruction. All will require further surgical adjustment. It is relevant to follow and support these children past puberty and into young adulthood to ensure appropriate sexual ability and counselling. Aesthetic functional reconstruction by the early age of 2–4 years has an excellent long-term prognosis with little residual psychological upset in later life. It is evident that children and families with severe forms of hypospadias require expert evaluation, skilled surgical management and long-term counselling and support, which can only be provided by a specialized multidisciplinary team.

Section 63.12 • Congenital adrenal hyperplasia

This autosomal recessive condition (1:4 inheritance), the result of a gene defect at CyP21B (the active 21 hydroxylase gene) on chromosome 6, occurs more frequently in females. It is due to an enzyme deficiency, commonly 21-hydroxylase, along the pathway to hydrocortisone production in the adrenal gland. The lack of hydrocortisone leads to uninhibited stimulation of the adrenal glands by the pituitary, with excessive production of androgens. At the sixth to ninteenth week of gestation, the critical stage of external genital development, high androgen levels induce virilization of the female external genitalia and male brain priming in an otherwise normal XX female. The associated mineralocorticoid deficiency presents as a salt-losing state. At birth these girls have ambiguous genitalia and may be mistaken for severely hypospadiac males. The clitoris is large, resembling a penis protruding from the vulva. The labia are fused at the midline beneath the phallus, with the single orifice of the urogenital sinus opening on the ventral shaft at the penile base (Figure 63.22). The distal one-third of the vagina regresses and is stenotic. However, the absence of testicular MIS preserves the internal genital structures as those of a normal female.

Presentation is usually because of ambiguous genitalia at birth. The severe mineralocorticoid deficiency and the inability to mount a normal stress response lead to 'crises' with vomiting, abdominal distension, lethargy, dehydration and circulatory collapse. Low serum levels of sodium and chloride and raised potassium levels may cause cardiac arrhythmias. In the long-term inadequately treated children with sustained high androgen levels will demonstrate rapid and excessive somatic growth and early fusion of bony epiphyses. Male children have macrogenitosomia and a well-developed physique, and have been likened to an infant Hercules. The diagnosis can be confirmed by the presence of a high serum and salivary 17-OH progesterone level. Genetic counselling is essential for the family and the child. Transplacental fetal therapy by maternal treatment with dexamethasone, commencing before or

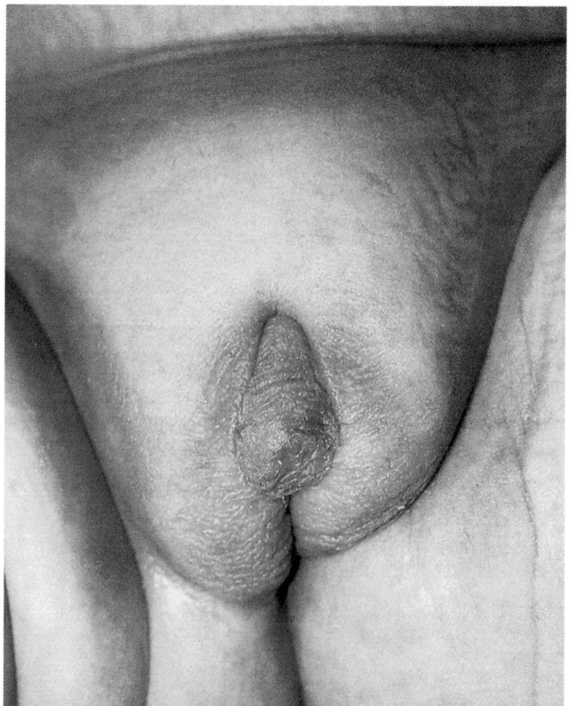

Figure 63.22 Ambiguous genitalia. A virilized female with congenital adrenal hyperplasia.

during early pregnancy, has been effective in preventing or limiting virilization of the female fetus. CAH children require life-long replacement therapy with hydrocortisone and a mineralocorticoid (fludrocortisone). Patient compliance with therapy and expert supervision are essential to ensure a normal somatic growth rate and to avoid early epiphyseal fusion. Affected females require reconstructive surgery. A reduction cliteroplasty and vulvovaginoplasty should be undertaken at a few weeks or months of age, but only when the baby is hormonally stable. The urogenital sinus is laid open to expose the urethra and the vagina. The corpora cavernosa and glans are reduced in size and repositioned within the vulva. It is important to preserve the neurovascular bundles to ensure normal glanular blood supply and sensation. The prepuce and redundant shaft skin are preserved and used to fashion labia minora and to line the vestibular area in the vulva. Additional surgery may be required in adolescence or young adulthood to release cicatricial stenosis at the vaginal orifice or to reconstruct an inadequate or small vagina. Since these girls have ovaries and retain normal female internal genitalia, they are able to conceive and carry a pregnancy. Long-term supervision and patient compliance with therapy are essential to satisfactory somatic growth and outcome. Counselling (personal and genetic) is a major component of good management.

Section 63.13 • Urinary tract anomalies in the fetus and the neonate

Abnormalities affecting the kidneys may take the form of anomalies of rotation, number (single), position (ectopic, pelvic), form (horseshoe, duplex) or development (agenesis, multicystic, cystic dysplasia). Even more common are anomalies of the pelvicalyceal system (pelvi-ureteric junction obstruction), the ureter (vesico-ureteric obstruction, vesico-ureteric reflux, duplex, ureterocele), the bladder (neurogenic bladder, diverticulum), and the urethra (posterior urethral valves). Antenatal scanning allows diagnosis of urinary tract anomalies at an early stage in pregnancy. Obstructive uropathy at the urethra or bladder neck presents with a large dilated bladder and bilateral hydroureteronephrosis. Rupture of one kidney into the peritoneal space leads to urinary ascites but also helps to relieve pressure on the parenchyma and to preserve additional renal tissue. Significant obstruction in early pregnancy interferes markedly with renal parenchymal development and leads to severe dysplasia and impaired function. Oligohydramnios is an ominous sign suggesting a failure of micturition by the fetus. Urinary tract anomalies are not uncommon in association with other congenital malformations and particularly those affecting the anorectum (imperforate anus, cloaca), the oesophagus (atresia) and the sacrum (hypoplasia, spina bifida). So great is the incidence of such association that investigation of the urinary tract is mandatory at the time of first admission. Enthusiasm for antenatal assessment of fetal renal function by fetal bladder aspiration, and therapeutic bladder drainage by transuterine insertion of a pigtail vesico-amniotic shunt has waned markedly since it was realized that such procedures did not lead to significant improvement or protection of renal parenchyma. Indeed the long-term prognosis was no different, and there is now little indication for such management.

Immediate post-natal investigation consists of serialized assessment of renal function (urea, creatinine clearance, osmolality) over the first weeks of life, and evaluation of the anatomy of the urinary tract by ultrasound studies and micturating cystourethrography. Transurethral bladder catheterization in the newborn should never be traumatic, and should only be undertaken for the clearest indications. Antibiotic cover is essential to avoid potential urinary infection and potentially fatal sepsis. Intravenous urography and isotope scanning are best delayed for about 6 weeks until renal function has stablized. It is usually possible to delay cystoscopy to a later age, thus avoiding trauma to the neonatal urethra. Meanwhile, temporary urinary tract drainage can be established by vesicostomy or ureterostomy to bypass obstructive lesions.

The management of children with urinary tract anomalies commences antenatally at first contact with the fetal management team, which includes a nephrologist and a neonatal urologist who will oversee the child's post-natal care. An action plan is drawn up with the parents, which provides appropriate counselling, genetic advice, investigation and management at all stages, and covers all relevant scenarios from termination of the pregnancy to dialysis and potential renal transplantation.

MODULE 64

Organ transplantation

Over the past 100 years, advances in surgical techniques and immunobiology have resulted in the successful clinical application of organ transplantation. Presently, transplantation of the liver, kidney and pancreas is considered standard treatment for failure of these organs. In 1998 there were 4487 liver, 131 392 kidney and 1221 pancreas (with or without combined kidney) transplants performed in the USA. The continued success of transplantation is likely to depend on a number of factors including technical refinement and the development of new immunosuppressive strategies, along with increases in the organ donor pool.

Section 64.1 • Introduction

The modern era of transplantation began at the beginning of the twentieth century with the development of successful suturing techniques. Payr, Murphy and Jaboulay refined existing suturing methods and, in 1905, Alexis Carrel working with Guthrie developed a successful means of vascular anastomosis. This allowed for the revascularization of a variety of organs. Using this technique, Carrel transplanted kidneys, hearts, parathyroids and vessels.

Ullman performed the first experimental kidney transplantation in 1902. Using a prosthesis technique for the anastomosis, he transplanted kidneys to the necks of dogs. A few years later, in 1906, Jaboulay performed the first experimental human kidney transplants. Kidneys from goats and pigs were grafted to the extremities. It was not until 1933 that a Ukrainian surgeon, Voronoy, carried out the first kidney transplant from a human donor. There was a mismatch for blood groups and the graft never worked. By 1949, Voronoy had performed six similar transplants, but these were also unsuccessful. In 1947 transient function of a kidney allograft was obtained by Hoofnagle, Hume and Landsteiner at the Peter Bent Brigham Hospital in Boston. This patient was suffering from acute renal failure and this transient function may have helped her recovery. This event, along with the development of dialysis machines, renewed interest in kidney transplantation. In the early 1950s, two separate groups in Boston and Paris developed successful heterotopic techniques. However, long-term survival was not achieved because of immunological barriers. The first successful kidney transplant occurred in 1954 between identical twins carried out by Murray at the Brighman hospital. His surgical technique is the basis for the kidney transplant procedure performed today.

Encouraged by the technical progress in kidney transplantation, experimental liver transplantation developed also using a heterotopic technique. Welch performed a liver transplant in the lower abdomen of a dog. Portal flow was established by an anastomosis between the portal vein and the iliac artery, venous drainage was into the inferior vena cava and a cholecystoduodenostomy provided biliary drainage.

Orthotopic procedures were described by Moore in 1959 and by Starzl in 1960 independently. Several concerns made the heterotopic position less desirable, including a loss of hepatotrophic factors from the gut, which Starzl demonstrated to be important for normal physiology and the concern that an extra organ in the abdomen often resulted in respiratory compromise. Orthotopic liver transplantation, however, also presented a challenge. It was clear that cross-clamping of the portal vein and inferior vena cava was not tolerated well by dogs. This prompted development of the technique of veno-venous bypass. The first attempt at liver transplantation was in 1963 by Starzl but was unsuccessful. The patient, who had biliary atresia, died as a result of haemorrhage. Starzl was later successful in 1967. He transplanted an 18-month-old child with hepatoma at the University of Colorado Health Sciences Center in Denver, Colorado.

Experimental pancreatic transplantation began with Hedon in 1913. He transplanted a portion of the pancreas to the neck of a dog. In 1966, Kelley, Lillehei and Merkel performed the first human pancreas transplant. This was a segmental pancreas transplant in diabetic woman who became insulin independent but unfortunately suffered from rejection and later died. Zollinger, Corry, Starzl and other investigators popularized pancreas transplantation in the early 1980s, which led to the modern era of pancreas transplantation.

Section 64.2 • Immunological development

Around the beginning of the twentieth century, several theories attempted to explain the mechanism of rejection. Peter Medawar, in a series of skin grafts experiments in rabbits in the 1940s, documented the immunological nature of rejection and tolerance. The initial attempt in the control of rejection was with the use of total body irradiation in Boston and Paris. However, long-term survival was infrequent due to graft rejection and bone marrow suppression. Pharmacological immunosuppression began with the introduction of an antiproliferative drug, 6-mercaptopurine (6-MP), by Schwartz and Dameshek. They demonstrated that 6-MP could inhibit the clonal proliferation of rabbit lymphocytes when given a foreign protein as an antigenic stimulus. A derivative of this compound, azathioprine, was then shown by Calne to prolong canine renal allograft survival. Azathioprine interferes with purine synthesis and suppresses both B- and T-cell activity.

The anti-inflammatory effect of corticosteroids has been known since the early twentieth century. In 1960 Goodwin demonstrated that they could reverse a rejection episode. The mechanism of action is complex but they inhibit T-cell activation by blocking the activation of the interleukin-2 (IL-2) gene.

In 1978, Calne introduced cyclosporine, a fungal metabolite that has a profound immunosuppressive effect. Cyclosporine binds to cyclophilin in the cytoplasm and blocks the enzymatic function of the calcium-activated calcineurin. This results in prevention of IL-2 synthesis and a significant improvement in graft survival.

Tacrolimus, a macrolide derived from *Streptomyces tsukubaensis*, was recognized to have immunosuppressive properties in 1984. In 1989 it was shown to reverse liver allograft rejection. Its ability to control ongoing steroid or orthoclone (OKT3) or muromonab-CD3-resistant acute rejection and prevent the progression of chronic rejection (or even reverse chronic rejection in some cases) was unprecedented and was the impetus for subsequent primary liver transplantation trials.

Mycophenolate mofetil is a semisynthetic derivative of mycophenolic acid and inhibits the *de novo* purine nucleotide synthesis in lymphocytes which are unable to use alternative salvage pathways. It has replaced azathioprine, the use of which is associated with bone marrow toxicity.

Rapamycin is a macrolide produced by *Streptomyces hygroscopicus*. It prevents the action of IL-2 on T-cells and thymocyte proliferation and B-cell activation. The site of action is late in the G1 phase of the cell cycle. When used with cyclosporin A it has a synergistic effect with a lower incidence of rejection in renal transplant recipients.

IL-2 receptor (IL-2R) antibodies, anti-TAC or HAT

These novel agents have been used in clinical trials on both sides of the Atlantic in combination with conventional immunosuppressive agents and preliminary studies have shown promising results in renal transplantation. T-cell activation is initiated when appropriately processed and presented antigen interacts with the 90 kDa polymorphic heterodimeric T-cell surface receptor for the specific antigen. This is characterized by the expression of IL-2 and high-affinity IL-2R by the T-cell. IL-2 exerts its effects on T-lymphocytes by binding to the IL-2R. The IL-2R is composed of three distinct membrane components: the 'α' chain (IL-2Ra, T-cell activation antigen or Tac), the 'β' chain (IL-2Rb) and the 'γ' chain (IL-2Rg). The genes encoding these receptors have been cloned and characterized.

A hyperchimeric humanized anti-IL-2Ra antibody Daclizumab (HAT, humanized anti-Tac, Zenapax®) was constructed resulting in the total retained mouse segments to account for less than 10% of the protein mass, making HAT more than 90% human. Vincenti *et al.* recently reported the results of multicentre clinical trials using five doses of Daclizumab (1 mg/kg of body weight, maximum of 100 mg; first dose within 24 hours before transplantation, with subsequent doses given 2, 4, 6 and 8 weeks after transplantation) in 126 renal transplant recipients and concluded that it reduced the frequency of acute rejection in kidney-transplant recipients. Baseline immunosuppression was CyA, azathioprine and prednisone based in all patients.

Basiliximab (Simulect®), another form of IL-2Ra humanized chimeric antibody, is produced *in vitro* by continuous culture fermentation of a murine-myeloma cell-line transfected with plasmid-borne recombinant gene constructs coding for murine variable regions and human constant regions. It has been shown to reduce the incidence of biopsy proven acute rejection after renal transplantation.

The combination of a calcineurin inhibitor, purine antagonist and corticosteroids has served as the basis of conventional maintenance immunosuppression since 1978. Antilymphocyte preparations are generally used for induction in some high-risk patients and for the treatment of steroid-resistant rejection.

Section 64.3 • Organ donation

There has been a progressively increasing discrepancy between the number of available cadaver donors and potential recipients. This is a result of the relative static number of donors over the past few years and the increasing number of recipients. It is estimated that there could potentially be between 50 and 55 potential donors per million in USA. However, the national organ retrieval rate is only 19 donors per million. In 1988 there were 16 026 patients on the United Network for Organ Sharing (UNOS) waiting list for organs and 4080 cadaver donors. In 1998 the number waiting has increased to 64 423 while the number of donors has only increased to 5799. This increasing discrepancy has resulted in longer waiting times for patients on the list and an increase in the number of patients dying while waiting for an organ.

Several strategies have been used to address this issue, including national education campaigns and legislation aimed at closing poorly performing organ procurement organizations (OPOs). Many centres have expanded their use of marginal and non-heart-beating donors which would have been discarded in the past. An important and successful strategy has been to utilize living donors, either related or unrelated. The general public is aware of the organ shortage and has accepted the application of brain death criteria for patients who are on life support in most parts of the world. Educational programmes are available in many large cities to address the issues of organ shortage and answer issues of equity and utility.

Recently, UNOS has issued a notice that it will require OPOs to meet minimum performance criteria to maintain federal designation. OPOs unable to achieve these requirements will be recognized. Subsidization of the burial costs of cadaver organ donors seems attractive without eliminating the altruistic nature of the gift and avoiding the issue of organ commerce. This is currently practised in many areas. Several studies have investigated the use of marginal donors for organ donation. Current data indicate that older donors are acceptable for organ donation provided that a critical evaluation has been performed, including a pre-transplant biopsy and an assessment for vascular disease. Organs from paediatric donors can be successfully placed in adults; however, when possible, paediatric organs should go into children.

A few centres are recovering organs for transplantation from non-heart-beating cadaver donors. The technique, which was developed in Europe, differs from the standard in that the flush occurs after the heart has stopped. The organs are cooled and removed in a similar fashion to the standard technique.

Presumed consent assumes that every 'brain dead' patient is an organ donor without family consent. This has been practised successfully in some countries; however in many regions it is unlikely that donor physicians will agree to remove organs without obtaining permission from the next of kin.

The use of living donors can be traced to the early years of renal transplantation. At present, living donors provide 42% of the organs for transplantation. This represents an increase of 10% over the past 10 years. Living-related transplants are attractive for several reasons, including improved initial and long-term function and shorter waiting times for recipients. Major complications occur in less than 5% of kidney and liver donors for paediatric recipients and are usually related to deep vein thrombosis, pulmonary embolus and infection. The morbidity and mortality of adult to adult liver donation is currently being established. Over the past few years there has been renewed interest in living unrelated donors (spouses, distant relatives, friends with close emotional bonds to the recipients and anonymous). There are several complex ethical issues involved in living non-related donation, but this should be encouraged when medically and ethically appropriate. The buying and selling of human organs and tissue for transplantation are unacceptable.

With the introduction of new immunosuppressive agents and transgenic animals the field of xeno-transplantation is making important progress. The risk of viral transmission to the recipient and their contacts remains a critically unresolved issue. Again there are significant ethical issues and it remains to be seen how the general public will respond. This is especially true for kidney recipients since renal failure is not a life-threatening emergency. There will probably be no single solution to the donor shortage and a combination of strategies will be necessary to solve this major obstacle.

Section 64.4 • Renal transplantation

Renal transplantation is the treatment of choice for the vast majority of patients with end-stage renal disease (ESRD). The incidence of renal failure continues to grow as the population ages. Unfortunately, the supply of organs to transplant has not been meeting the demand for many years. Currently, more than 20 000 new patients are added to the waiting list for kidney transplantation each year in the USA alone while only about 12 000 kidney transplants are performed each year in America. In fact, there are now nearly 45 000 ESRD patients waiting to be transplanted in the U.S. and the list is growing by about 4000 new patients per year. Increasing the number of living donors has been the most effective way to address this discrepancy. The donor operation, which traditionally was done through a flank approach, can now be done laparoscopically, resulting in a faster recovery and hopefully a more desirable option.

The causes of ESRD are numerous and listed in Table 64.1. Type I diabetes is the most common cause of renal failure at this time. While some of the causes of native renal failure such as IgA nephropathy may recur in the renal allograft, these recurrences usually occur late and, therefore, are not contraindications to transplantation. Many type I diabetics may be candidates for combination kidney and pancreas transplantation, which, if successful, will eliminate the recurrence of diabetic nephropathy in the allografted kidney. On occasion patients will require one or both of the native kidneys to be removed prior to transplantation. Patients with severe nephrotic syndrome or difficult to control hypertension may necessitate bilateral nephrectomy.

Table 64.1 Causes of end-stage disease

Glomerulonephritis
Idiopathic
Focal glomerulosclerosis
Membranous
Mesangiocapillary (type I)
Mesangiocapillary (type II)
IgA nephropathy
Infectious
Chronic pyelonephritis
Hereditary
Alport's syndrome
Polycystic kidney disease
Medullary cystic disease
Congenital
Aplasia
Hypoplasia
Horseshoe kidney
Metabolic disorders
Hyperoxaluria
Nephrocalcinosis
Diabetes mellitus
Gout
Fabry's disease
Amyloidosis
Obstructive uropathy
Acquired
Congenital
Toxic
Lead
Analgesic nephropathy
Opiate abuse
Tumours
Renal cell carcinoma
Wilms' tumour
Myeloma
Irreversible acute renal failure
Cortical necrosis
Acute tubular necrosis
Haemolytic uraemic syndrome
Trauma
Other
Systemic lupus erythematosis
Scleroderma

Chronic pyelonephritis or nephrolithiasis may also make unilateral or bilateral nephrectomy necessary. Additionally it may be necessary to remove a very large polycystic kidney in order to make room for the new kidney.

There are relatively few contraindications to renal transplantation. Physiological age is more important than chronological age and, as a result, there is no specific age limitation. Of course, increasing age (generally men >50 and women >55 years) is associated with occult cardiovascular disease which should be evaluated as part of their work-up prior to undergoing kidney transplantation. This also true for all patients with diabetes, long-standing hypertension, hyperlipidaemia, a strong family history, or a long-standing history of smoking. Ongoing infections, human immunodeficiency virus (HIV) positivity, incurable malignancies, debilitating cardiorespiratory diseases that preclude safely operating on the patient, ongoing substance abuse and incapacitating mental illnesses are usually considered absolute contraindications to renal transplantation.

The work-up of the potential candidate for renal transplantation includes a complete history and physical examination, serological testing for venereal disease, HIV, cytomegalovirus (CMV), Epstein–Barr virus (EBV), and hepatitis B and C. The patient should also be evaluated for psychosocial issues including compliance with dialysis, diet and drug regimens pre-transplant, support from family or friends at home, ability to obtain the necessary medications post-transplantation, and transportation to and from the transplant clinic. If the candidate appears to be acceptable for transplantation, blood is drawn for ABO testing, tissue typing and assessment for sensitization against human leucocyte anigens (HLA). Patients with risk factors for cardiovascular disease as noted above should undergo a non-invasive cardiac stress test. If the stress test is positive, cardiac catheterization should be performed and any significant coronary artery lesions should be treated with either angioplasty or bypass surgery if feasible. Patients who are overweight are asked to undergo a weight reduction programme prior to being transplanted. Patients with a substance abuse problem or a history of non-compliance are asked to demonstrate their ability to abstain from alcohol or drugs for a 6 month period or prove compliance during a similar time period before being accepted for kidney transplantation. They should be monitored for behavioural changes closely by the dialysis social worker.

Once a patient has met all the criteria for acceptance as a kidney transplant candidate, (s)he is placed on the UNOS waiting list for an available cadaver kidney or a living kidney donor is sought. Risks and benefits of kidney transplantation are explained to the recipient including the side-effects of immunosuppression. Cadaver kidney allocation is based upon waiting time, HLA matching, degree of sensitization to HLA antigens or age. (Patients < 10 years of age are given more points.) The national UNOS waiting list was established to provide recipients with the opportunity to receive organs from cadaver donors who are zero antigen mismatches. Long-term graft survival is significantly improved when there are no HLA mismatches between the donor and recipient. For this reason, if there are multiple siblings who are able to donate a kidney, the sibling found with the closest match by HLA tissue typing should be the first choice as a donor.

Donor selection

It is incumbent upon the transplant surgeon to establish suitability of the cadaver donor. This includes reasonable and stable renal function, or at least recoverable renal function (a young donor with ATN may be perfectly acceptable as a donor). In uncertain cases a biopsy of the kidney can be helpful to assess the degree of nephrosclerosis or fibrosis especially in older donors or donors with long-standing hypertension.

There is evidence that kidneys with greater than 20% nephrosclerosis are at higher risk for primary non-function. An abbreviated urine creatinine clearance test may be useful to identify donors whose kidneys may be suboptimal for transplantation. In addition, the risk for transmission of diseases such as HIV or hepatitis should be minimal as assessed by history and serological testing. Donors with a history of cancer with metastatic potential should be avoided. Those who have died as a result of central nervous system malignancies are usually acceptable as organ donors if they have not undergone a ventriculo-peritoneal shunt or recent resection/biopsy. Kidneys from infants may be used in adults when kept attached to the donor aorta and vena cava. This allows for an *en bloc* transplant into the same recipient and reduces technical problems.

Living kidney donors should be healthy and willing to donate for truly altruistic reasons only. A psychological evaluation may be warranted to establish altruistic motives when the transplant personnel suspect otherwise. Donors should be free of systemic diseases such as diabetes and hypertension, however these criteria might be relaxed if the donor is highly motivated (such as a parent to child donation) and there is no evidence of injury to the donor's renal function. If the prospective donor is ABO blood type compatible, the work-up should proceed and include a urinalysis, urine culture, 12 hour urine collection for protein and creatinine clearance, serological testing to rule out transmissable diseases, CBC and chemistry panel, chest X-ray, and electrocardiogram (ECG). If the donor remains a suitable candidate to donate after these tests, (s)he must have an anatomical evaluation of his or her kidneys.

This may include an aortogram, magnetic resonance angiogram, or a spiral computed tomography (CT). The latter test offers ease of performance, lower cost, and provision of both the venous and arterial anatomy. Knowledge of the venous anatomy has become more important with the use of laparoscopic techniques to remove a kidney from a living donor.

Recipient operation

The recipient is evaluated for volume overload, hyperkalaemia and acidosis just prior to transplantation. Dialysis may be required to correct these before going to the operating room. The recipient is placed supine on the table and, after induction of anaesthesia, a central venous catheter is placed to monitor volume status, and a Foley catheter is inserted into the bladder. A three-way connector is attached to the Foley in order to distend the bladder with GU irrigant to facilitate the ureteral anastomosis later.

The kidney is placed extraperitoneally in either the right or left iliac fossa. The right side is preferred because of the more superficial position of the iliac vein and the decreased incidence of deep venous thrombosis. Upon entering the retroperitoneal space, the inferior epigastric vessels are identified, ligated and divided. In males, the spermatic cord is encircled with a Penrose drain and retracted. In females, the round ligament is ligated and divided. The peritoneal sac is retracted medially and superiorly to expose the iliac vessels. The peri-vascular lymphatic vessels are meticulously ligated with fine silk ligatures before division while dissecting out the iliac artery and vein.

The renal vein is sewn end-to-side to the external iliac vein. If there is a cuff of aorta on the renal artery, it is usually sewn end-to-end anastomosis to the external iliac artery. If there is no aortic cuff, such as with a living donor kidney, an end-to-side to the internal iliac artery is usually performed. Care must be taken that there is no significant stenosis at the origin of the internal iliac artery and that the contralateral internal iliac artery has not been used for a previous kidney transplant. Mannitol 1 g/kg is administered intravenously to the recipient prior to revascularizing the kidney and steroids are given shortly after reperfusion.

The ureter is anastomosed to the bladder with either an extravesical (modified Lich) or intravesical (Politano-Leadbetter) technique. In either case, the ureteral mucosa is sewn directly to the bladder mucosa. Some centres perform donor to native uretero-ureterostomies as a matter of routine, but, in general, this technique is reserved for cases where the donor ureter will not reach the bladder or when the bladder is excessively contracted and difficult to distend. It is usually safe to divide the native ureter and ligate the proximal end. The bladder is kept decompressed by Foley drainage until post-operative day 4 to allow healing of the ureteroneocystostomy.

Technical complications of renal transplantation include renal artery stenosis, renal artery or vein thrombosis, urine leak, bleeding, ureteral obstruction or lymphocele formation. Patients with a urinoma present with significant pain and tenderness as well as a rising creatinine and decreased urine output. Urine leaks most commonly occur at the bladder anastomosis. Lymphoceles are more insidious as they are usually painless until the lymphocele becomes tense. Also, renal function is usually not affected by a lymphocele until late in its course when the ureter may become compressed or kinked. Ureteral obstruction is also usually painless and may be first manifested by a rising creatinine. Ultrasonography is very effective at detecting peri-nephric fluid collections or hydronephrosis as well as evaluating blood flow into the kidney.

Immunosuppression post-kidney transplantation

Many transplant centres routinely 'induce' all kidney transplant patients with immunosuppressive antibody preparations. While episodes of acute rejection can be reduced or at least delayed, antibody induction is expensive, can increase the risk of opportunistic infections and post-transplant lymphoproliferative disorders, and has not been shown to significantly improve overall short- or long-term graft survival. Today, traditional horse or rabbit-derived polyclonal anti-lymphocyte preparations and the murine anti-CD3 monoclonal antibody are being replaced by genetically engineered humanized or chimeric mouse/human monoclonal antibodies directed against the IL-2 receptor protein (anti-CD25) for purposes of induction. These new antibodies, basiliximab and daclizumab, have been shown to be better tolerated and are longer lasting than the older preparations mentioned above. Because they are not eliminated as rapidly as non-humanized antibodies, fewer doses are required and thus the cost is reduced somewhat. Thus, the cost:benefit ratio of antibody induction is improved. Nevertheless, induction for all kidney transplant recipients remains controversial and not all centres routinely employ it. Most centres induce recipients who are at higher immunological risk, including recipients of second or more kidneys, those with prior sensitization to HLA antibodies (high PRA) or recipients of multiple organs such as a kidney and pancreas simultaneously.

Maintenance immunosuppression consists of tacrolimus or cyclosporin A, together with steroids and mycophenolate mofetil. Tacrolimus is associated with a dose-dependent incidence of diabetes among recipients. Cyclosporine associated diabetes is distinctly uncommon and idiosyncratic in nature.

The latest addition to the immunosuppressive armamentarium is sirolimus which was approved for use in the USA in late 1999. Clinical trials demonstrated acute rejection episodes of 10–15% after primary kidney transplantation when sirolimus was used with varying doses of cyclosporine. There is interest to eliminate the use of prednisone because of its long-term side-effects or to eliminate calcineurin inhibitors because of their nephrotoxicity and other side-effects. As chronic rejection is the greatest cause of graft loss after kidney transplantation, there is keen interest in finding the agent or combination of agents that will best reduce the risk for chronic rejection.

Results of kidney transplantation

During the past decade both cadaveric and living donor graft survivals have steadily improved to 88.3% and 94.2% respectively as reported by UNOS for the year 1997. The overall 1 year graft survival for 1998 was 89.3%, almost as good as that for living related kidney transplants alone reported only 8 years earlier. Some centres are now reporting 1 year cadaveric graft survival of 95% or better. There is little doubt that new agents used for immunosuppression have improved the graft survival rates, since the technique of kidney transplantation has changed little since it was first successfully performed in 1954 by Murray.

Section 64.5 • Pancreas transplantation

Type I diabetes mellitus is characterized by beta cell destruction, which usually leads to absolute insulin deficiency. This beta cell destruction could be immune mediated or idiopathic. In 1997 the Expert Committee on the diagnosis and classification of diabetes mellitus defined type I (DCCT) diabetes mellitus as random plasma glucose greater than or equal to 200 mg/l (11.1 mmol/l) associated with symptoms, or a fasting plasma glucose greater than or equal to 126 mg/l (7.0 mmol/l), or a 2 hour glucose greater than or equal to 200 mg/l (11.1 mmol/l) after a 75 g glucose load.

The diagnosis of type I diabetes mellitus is made by the findings of one of the above and the presence of detectable antibodies to cytoplasm of islet cells, gluconic acid decarboxylase or insulin or phosphatase-like protein. Typically this is characterized by low plasma C-peptide level.

Diabetes mellitus affects all organs causing microvascular changes leading to diabetic retinopathy and blindness, ischaemic heart disease, cardiovascular disease, diabetic nephropathy leading to renal failure, neuropathy, sexual dysfunction, autonomic disorders like postural hypotension and gastroparesis and keto-acidosis. The management essentially consists of insulin replacement therapy in addition to dietary regulation and periodic monitoring of haemoglobin A_{Ic} levels. Medical management does not prevent long-term complications and is dependent upon exogenously administered insulin.

The number of pancreas transplants performed in the USA has increased from 79 in 1988 to 1221 in 1998, as reported by UNOS. Each year, 50 individuals per million population develop insulin-dependent diabetes. The disease reduces life expectancy by about one-third, primarily due to chronic renal failure, cardiovascular disease and infection. Patients with insulin-dependent diabetes are 25 times more likely to develop blindness and it is the most common cause of blindness in Western societies. It is responsible for approximately one-third of patients with renal failure, and increases the susceptibility to peripheral gangrene and coronary atherosclerosis by a factor of 5 and 2, respectively.

Vascularized pancreatic allografts allow for euglycaemia and an insulin-independent state in almost all recipients. The number of diabetic patients treated with pancreatic transplantation has increased rapidly, and in 1991 765 procedures were carried out world-wide. One-year graft and patient survival is 69% and 88%, respectively.

The total number of registrants waiting for pancreas transplantation also has increased from 189 in 1988 to 455 in 1998 (pancreas alone), and 923 candidates in 1993 to 1841 candidates in 1998 (kidney/pancreas waiting list). In addition, the number of donors for pancreas transplantation has increased from 577 donors in 1988 to 1312 in 1997 (UNOS OPTN registry data, 21 September 1998).

Surgical options for treating type I diabetes mellitus are as follows:

- pancreas transplantation which includes:
  - simultaneous kidney/pancreas transplantation (SKP)
  - pancreas-after-kidney transplantation (PAK)
  - pancreas transplantation alone (PTA)
- islet cell transplantation.

Pancreas transplantation is the most efficacious method of returning glucose and haemoglobin A_{1c} levels to normal in type I diabetes mellitus. Simultaneous kidney/pancreas transplantation (SKP) is the most common procedure performed. This is done in patients with end-stage renal disease resulting from the effects of diabetes who have already been on a form of dialysis, or who have a creatinine clearance of less of 30 ml/minute with impending dialysis. Pancreas transplantation in these patients protects the newly transplanted kidney from hypoglycaemia and effects of diabetes. It has also been shown to protect from or slow down the secondary complications of diabetes and frees the patients from exogenous insulin, resulting in overall improvement in the quality of life.

Pancreas-after-kidney transplantation (PAK) is performed for type I diabetics who have had a previous kidney transplantation, or in patients who have a history of graft pancreatectomy following a SKP procedure. The most common indication for graft pancreatectomy after SKP is venous thrombosis of the graft. This almost always necessitates removal of the transplanted pancreas.

Pancreas transplantation alone (PTA) is indicated for patients with severe metabolic disability, severe autonomic dysfunction, and those who have a creatinine clearance of greater than 30 ml/min. The operation aims to improve the quality of life and overall it tends to forestall or prevent the complications related to diabetes.

Donor selection

Donors for patients for pancreas transplantation are cadaveric donors with no history of pancreatitis or heavy alcohol intake. Criteria for donors include haemodynamic stability and/or minimal use of pressors, normal or near-normal serum amylase and lipids levels, and the presence of minimal fat around the pancreas. In general, donors less than 50 years of age are preferred. Accepting organs from donors who have been on high doses of pressors is an important factor in graft loss following pancreas transplantation.

Living donors

Recently kidney and pancreas transplantation from live donors has been performed with success; however, this method has not gained too much popularity due to concerns over early and late risks associated with distal pancreatectomy on the living donor.

Recipient selection

Diabetes predisposes patients to development of multi-organ disease resulting from arteriosclerosis. In order to ensure maximum success from this procedure, this operation is avoided in patients with severe debilitating cardiovascular disease. In general, the listing criteria for patients for simultaneous kidney/pancreas transplantation include:

- type I diabetes with end-stage renal disease
- absence of debilitating cardiovascular disease
- absence of ongoing infection
- history of good compliance
- age up to 50–55 years in general
- no ongoing substance abuse
- no active malignancy
- negative HIV test.

Adherence to these criteria avoids or limits the technical complications and the incidence of any operative complications related to coronary arteriosclerosis.

Donor operation

The donor operation is usually done in conjunction with multi-organ retrieval. The aim is to procure the pancreas in conjunction with the duodenum, the superior mesenteric artery and the portal vein. The abdomen is opened with a long midline incision. A preliminary inspection of the pancreas is done by lifting the colon, thus stretching the transverse mesocolon which gives a reasonably good view of the body of the pancreas, the lesser sac is entered and the organ in the supracolic compartment is assessed. The presence of excessive fat, haemorrhage and saponification indicating pancreatitis contraindicates the use of this organ.

The next step consists of isolating the origin of the superior mesenteric artery followed by isolation of the portal vein. The mode of procurement depends on the choice of the donor surgeon. If it is decided the pancreas has to be procured separately from the liver, more dissection is necessary, and this includes dissecting and ligating the gastroduodenal artery, dissection of the common hepatic artery and isolation of the splenic artery. The portal vein is then isolated. The transverse colon is mobilized and retracted caudally and the stomach and the gastrosplenic ligaments are mobilized and divided.

The spleen–pancreas complex is then mobilized and lifted off the left renal bed. The infrarenal aorta is exposed and made ready for cannulation.

Some donor surgeons prefer to procure the liver and pancreas together *en bloc*, in which case extensive dissection is not necessary. After the heparin is administered, the inferior mesenteric vein is cannulated with a small size portal vein cannula, and the tip of this catheter is located and palpated in the portal vein at the hepatic hilum. 2–0 silk ties are encircled around the portal vein and this is tied off to vent the portal vein below the tie thus selectively perfusing the liver with cold University of Wisconsin (UW) solution.

After the donor is heparinized, the aorta is cannulated and flushed with cold UW solution, the small bowel mesentery is stapled off and the suprahepatic portion of the inferior vena cava is then transected to remove the liver. The organs are thus rapidly cooled and perfused with the UW solution, which acts as a preservative. The pancreas is procured with the spleen, which serves as a handle to manipulate the organ. The organs are inspected for any procurement-related injury. The liver and the pancreas are then separated. The remnant of the small bowel distal to the fourth portion of the duodenum and the pylorus are excised and the proximal and distal ends of the duodenum are oversewn in two layers. The common bile duct is ligated in addition to the gastroduodenal artery and inferior mesenteric vein. The small bowel mesentery is then individually isolated and ligated.

The donor common iliac artery is used to reconstruct the inflow for the graft. This is done by creating an anastomosis between external and internal iliac arteries to splenic and superior mesenteric artery, respectively. The portal vein can be lengthened by using the external iliac vein of the donor.

Recipient operation

The operative approach for SKP, PAK and PTA are similar and, therefore, the simultaneous SKP procedure will be described here. The operation is done under general anaesthetic and the presence of an arterial line and a central venous catheter is mandatory.

The SKP procedure can be performed by a midline incision which allows access to both the common and external arteries and veins. The vessels on each side can also be exposed by two separate incisions in the right and left iliac fossae. The right iliac fossa is prepared for the abdominal placement of the pancreas and the left iliac fossa for the extraperitoneal placement for the kidney. As a rule, the pancreas is always transplanted in the abdomen. In general, the pancreas is put in the right iliac fossa as it needs more room and the caecum can be easily mobilized to accommodate the pancreas.

The common iliac and the external iliac vessels are exposed and encircled with a vessel loop. Venous anastomosis is carried out first by clamping the proximal and distal common external iliac vein, and making a venotomy to match the size of the portal vein of the donor, then suturing the donor portal vein to the external iliac vein using 6–0 Prolene. This is followed by the end-to-side anastomosis of the reconstructed common iliac artery of the donor to the external iliac artery of the recipient. Following this the organ is reperfused. Any bleeders are then ligated. The pancreas is transplanted with the spleen. Following reperfusion the spleen is excised after ligating the splenic artery and vein. The anaesthesiologist measures the blood sugar post-reperfusion and subsequently at hourly intervals. Rapid spontaneous correction of euglycaemia confirms satisfactory organ function.

Several options have been used in the past to drain the exocrine pancreatic secretions. These include ligating of the pancreatic duct or injecting it with neoprene. The two current and most popular options are anastomosing the donor duodenum to the bladder or to the loop of the small bowel. The advantages of bladder technique include the availability of monitoring of urine to diagnose rejection, and the feasibility of doing a transcystoscopic biopsy of the pancreas to establish this diagnosis. However, this technique is prone to several disadvantages which include episodes of urinary tract infection, haematuria, rapid electrolyte loss and imbalance (patients lose a lot of bicarbonate as a result of exocrine pancreatic secretion and hence have to receive replacement of electrolytes). Other complications include transitional cell dysplasia, urethritis and stricture formation.

The authors' preferred technique is enteric drainage. It is more physiological and almost totally eliminates the side-effects associated with bladder drainage. Disadvantages of this procedure include diarrhoea, which is almost always self-limiting, and the possibility of generalized peritonitis if the anastomosis were to leak. Anastomotic bleed is also a known complication of enteric drainage. The single greatest disadvantage of this procedure is that there is a lack of urinary amylase estimation for the diagnosis of rejection. The success of enteric anastomosis depends on paying attention to technical details with a careful two-layer closure. If undue tension is to be expected, a Roux-en-Y technique is preferred to the usual side-to-side anastomosis.

The choice of venous drainage in pancreas transplantation is between systemic drainage and portal drainage. In systemic drainage, the donor portal vein drains into the recipient's iliac or vena cava. The disadvantage of this is that it is prone to cause hyperinsulinaemia and hyperlipidaemia. Recently some surgeons have resorted to a portal venous drainage of the portal vein, which is a physiologically more correct option. In these situations, the donor portal vein drains into the recipient superior mesenteric vein or the portal vein.

Complications

Complications of pancreas transplantation include graft thrombosis (5–10%), haemorrhage, infections and abcesses formation and pancreatitis. Other complications which can occur during the post-operative period include acute rejection, anastomotic leak and anastomotic bleeding. Late complications include CMV pancreatitis, graft thrombosis, autoimmune destruction and malignancies related to post-transplantation immunosuppression.

Immunosuppression

Immunosuppression, in the authors' practice at UCSD, consists of tacrolimus, mycophenolate mofetil, steroids and IL-2R antibodies. Some surgeons prefer to induce these patients with anti-IL-2 antibodies and these include daclizumab and basilxumab (Table 64.2).

The diagnosis of pancreas transplant rejection is based on presence of hyperglycaemia, increased lipase activity in serum, and the presence of graft tenderness.

Table 64.2 Immunosuppression for pancreas transplantation

At induction of anaesthesia	*At reperfusion of graft*	*Post-operatively*
Basilixumab 20 mg iv	Solumedrol 10 mg/kg i.v.	Basilixumab 20 mg i.v. Tacrolimus 0.5–0.1 mg/kg p.o. Mycophenolate 10–30 mg/kg divided Solumedrol taper

Fine needle biopsy

This technique, which has recently been popularized, is performed under ultrasound scan guidance using a 23-gauge needle. The presence of activated lymphocytes in the aspirate confirms the presence of rejection. Treatment of rejection consists of optimizing the tacrolimus levels to therapeutic levels and bolus treatment of steroids using 10 mg/kg Solu-Medrol i.v., tapering it down to 2 mg/kg i.v.

Clinical outcomes

Guzner and colleagues in 1999 reported the results of the international pancreas transplantation registry, and reported a greater than 93% patient survival at 1 and 3 years after transplantation with PTA, SPK and PAK. Mortality in most cases was associated with complications of diabetes, especially cardiovascular disease. The graft survival at 2 years for PTA, SPK and PTA respectively is 52%, 79% and 79%.

The indicators of a successful pancreas transplantation include normalization of fasting plasma sugar, haemoglobin A_{1c} levels, glucose induced insulin secretion and improved responses to hyperglycaemia. Successful pancreas transplantation results in partial reversal of renal lesions and established neuropathy. Patients report tremendous improvement in quality of life, sexual performance, return to employment, successful pregnancies, and independence from insulin and unpredictable hypo- and hyperglycaemia.

Improvement in motor and sensory conduction has been documented in patients after pancreas transplantation. However, this procedure does not have any beneficial effect on established retinopathy.

Pancreas transplantation: the future

Some centres have resorted to pancreas transplantation with the transfusion of donor bone marrow. This is reported to increase chimerism or presence of donor drive cells in the recipient's serum and blood. It has been postulated that it would cause organ tolerance and reduce the need for immunosuppression.

Islet cell transplantation

Islet cell transplantation is indicated for patients who have had a total pancreatectomy for chronic pancreatitis (islet autograft transplantation) or in patients with type I diabetes (islet allograft).

Islet cell transplantation is associated with a 2 year success rate of about 80%. Islet allograft transplantation has had very limited success. Islet cells can be obtained from donor pancreases after pancreas dissection and isolation in aseptic conditions. These islets are then infused into the recipient intrahepatically via the portal vein. These patients need immunosuppression post-infusion.

Alejando and colleagues in 1997 reported successful euglycaemia for 6 years after islet transplantation. However, the problems associated with this include difficulties with islet isolation, islet encapsulation and islet immune cell destruction in the pancreas. Hence, this procedure is still thought of as experimental.

Tremendous research efforts are being devoted to improvements in islet retrieval and encapsulation technique, thereby limiting the immune destruction of the number of islets after infusion.

Type I diabetes is, therefore, considered curable with pancreas transplantation which offers insulin independence and prevention of complications related to diabetes. Improved immunosuppression management leads to rejection-free survival.

Section 64.6 • Liver transplantation

Since its introduction by Starzl, liver transplantation has influenced the management of many aspects of liver disease. Selected patients with unresectable malignancy can be offered transplantation when in the past they would have received palliative therapy. Potential or actual candidates for liver transplant who develop variceal bleeding unresponsive to pharmacological or endoscopic therapy are now first offered a transjugular intrahepatic shunt or an operative shunt outside the hilum before considering a portacaval shunt. This approach is taken to minimize the impact on survival following transplant.

The introduction of cyclosporine by Calne and the development of other immunsuppressive agents dramatically reduced the incidence of rejection and improved results. Currently rejection rates are between 10 and 20%. As a result the procedure has gained wide clinical application. Another significant advance has been a better understanding of organ selection and preservation. High-risk donors on large doses of pressors or with significant steatosis are avoided due to the risk of primary non-function, the incidence of which is approximately 5%.

Indications

In 1983 the National Institutes of Health consensus conference recognized orthotopic liver transplantation as the procedure of choice in the treatment of end-stage liver disease which prompted an increase in the number of procedures. In 1991, 2946 liver transplants were performed and by 1998 this increased to 4450 in the USA. The options for liver transplantation are shown in Table 64.3. In the USA, the most common indication in adults is hepatitis C and in children it is biliary atresia.

Although irreversible hepatic failure is the unequivocal indication for liver transplantation, the timing of this procedure is often difficult and should be based on the expected natural history of the various kinds of liver disease and associated medical problems. In general all patients should be referred early for evaluation for liver transplantation so that developing complications can be managed to optimize outcome. Patients with fulminant hepatic failure or primary non-function require an emergency transplant. This requires prioritization on the list and widespread sharing. Patients with chronic disease should be referred before the complications of end-stage liver disease develop, resulting in a decrease in survival.

When severe complications develop, such as refractory ascites, severe encephalopathy, persistent variceal haemorrhage or hepatorenal syndrome, an urgent transplant should be done to reduce mortality while waiting. Unfortunately, the survival of these patients is not as good as those transplanted before the development of complications.

Patients with primary biliary cirrhosis, primary sclerosing cholangitis, inborn errors of metabolism and trauma have the best results following liver transplantation, with survival rates of 80% at 5 years and no recurrence of their original disease. Patients transplanted for alcoholic cirrhosis and hepatitis C have good results. Patients with active hepatitis B can be successfully transplanted with the use of post-operative antiviral treatment. With improved operative and post-operative management, many traditional contraindications to transplantation are disappearing. There is no absolute chronological age limit for liver transplant candidates: neonates and patients in their eighth decade have been successfully transplanted. The physiological status of the patient is more important than the actual age.

Table 64.3 Liver transplantation – options

Cadaveric
Whole organ
Split:
in situ
ex vivo
Living
Related
Unrelated

Advanced cardiopulmonary disease, active alcohol or drug abuse, active sepsis outside the hepatobiliary system, metastatic maglignancy and inability of the patient and/or family to understand the implications of liver transplantation are absolute contraindications. Relative contraindications include certain non-metastatic hepatobiliary malignancies, splanchnic and portal vein thrombosis, extensive previous abdominal surgery and severe hypoxaemia.

The pre-operative assessment of candidates for liver transplantation requires the establishment of a firm diagnosis and an evaluation of the patient's physiological reserve. This will allow for a rational decision as to the prognosis with and without transplantation.

Recipient operation

A bilateral subcostal incision, longer on the right, with a midline extension to the xiphoid is used to enter the abdomen. The recipient hepatectomy is the most difficult portion of the recipient operation and care must be taken to achieve excellent haemostasis. The hilar dissection is preformed first with division of the bile duct and hepatic artery as close to the liver as possible. The portal vein is isolated and can be cannulated along with the femoral and axillary veins if bypass is to be used. The sub- and suprahepatic vena cava can then be encircled and clamped and the liver removed. Alternatively, by using the piggyback technique, the vena cava can be left intact and the hepatic veins ligated and divided. The bare area is a source of bleeding which should be controlled with the use of the argon beam coagulator. If the vena cava is removed then the remaining cuffs should be fashioned and end-to-end anastomoses are performed to the donor vena cava. A 3–0 or 4–0 Prolene suture is used. If the cava is left intact this anastomosis is done in a side-to-side fashion. With either technique a vent should be created to allow for air debris and the cold perfusate to flush out.

Upon completion of the vena cava anastomosis the portal vein is sewn in an end-to-end fashion to the donor portal vein using a 6–0 Prolene suture. Care must be taken to avoid twisting the vessels or leaving excessive vessel length, which results in kinking. Pursestring constriction is avoided by leaving a 'growth factor', that is, the first knot is tied down snugly, but the second and remaining knots are tied 2–4 mm away from the first. This allows the suture line to expand once the clamp is removed. When this anastomosis is completed, the clamps are removed and the liver is revascularized. The arterial anastomosis is performed next. The authors most commonly use a patch of aorta to provide a cuff for an end-to-side anastomosis to the recipient's common hepatic gastroduodenal circuit. The anastomosis is performed using 7/0 Prolene. Following completion of the vascular anastomoses the gallbladder is removed. In adults with a normal common bile duct an end-to-end choledochocholedochostomy is performed using an interrupted 5–0 absorbable synthetic monofilament suture. The placement of a T-tube is optional (at the authors' institution) and is dependent on concerns about size discrepancy. In adults with sclerosing cholangitis or with an inadequate recipient bile duct, a Roux-en-Y choledochojejunostomy is required.

Immunosuppression

Our current immunosuppressive protocol consists of tacrolimus with levels of 10 ng/ml during the first 30 days, mycophenolate mofetil 1 g twice per day and tapering doses of prednisone. Pulse steroids are used to treat rejection and antilymphocyte preparations are rarely used to treat steroid-resistant rejection.

Results

Survival following liver transplant has improved significantly over the past 10 years. In 1997 UNOS reported 1 year patient and graft survival at 86.2% and 78.4% respectively.

Paediatric liver transplantation

The field of paediatric hepatology has seen many advances over the last few years as the aetiological factors and pathology of paediatric liver diseases have been brought to light. The number of paediatric patients less than 17 years of age on the waiting list has increased from 252 patients in 1989 to 854 patients in 1998 (UNOS OPTN Report). The mortality of paediatric patients less than 17 years of age on the waiting has increased from 41 in 1989 to 115 reported deaths in 1998.

Liver transplantation is indicated for a variety of paediatric liver diseases, listed in Table 64.4. The clincial presentations of patients with end-stage liver disease include malnournishment, delayed growth, ascites, jaundice, bleeding related to portal hypertension, coagulopathy and hepatic encephalopathy. Children who have an obstructive biliary tract also can present with multiple episodes of sepsis and/or cholangitis. Paediatric patients who have metabolic diseases commonly present with hepatic encephalopathy, acidosis and/or coma. Patients with a tumour often present with abdominal swelling and palpable liver mass. Patients with acute fulminant hepatic failure can present with encephalopathy of rapid onset, coagulopathy and/or multi-organ system failure.

During the last decade, liver transplantation has evolved into an accepted therapy for patients with end-stage liver disease. Due to improvement in operative techniques, introduction of more specific and better immunosuppressions, and better diagnostic tests being introduced to detect post-transplantation diseases, the overall 5 year patient survival has improved tremendously to 90%. Immunosuppressants with limited toxicity have gained widespread usage. Due to scientific advancements and improved abilities to monitor the patients post-operatively and diagnose rejection an increasing number of patients have been either taken completely off immunosuppression or taken off prednisone following liver transplantation. This has been particularly useful in paediatric patients in whom steroid related growth inhibition is a major concern.

Table 64.4 Indications for orthotopic liver transplantation

Adults
Chronic active hepatitis
Primary biliary cirrhosis
Sclerosing cholangitis
Cirrhosis post-viral hepatitis
Neoplasms
Metabolic errors
Autoimmune hepatitis
Budd-Chiari
Trauma
Children
Obstructive and cholestatic diseases
Biliary atresia
Sclerosing cholangitis
Familial intrahepatic cholestasis (Byler disease)
Alagille syndrome (syndromic bile duct paucity)
Metabolic diseases
α_1-Anti-trypsin deficiency
Tyrosinaemia
Urea cycle defect
Glycogen storage diseases
Wilson's disease
Fulminant hepatic failure
Acute viral hepatitis
Drug induced chronic hepatitis
Post-viral
Autoimmune
Tumours
Hepatoblastoma
Hepatocellular carcinoma
Haemangioendothelioma
Miscellaneous
Cryptogenic cirrhosis
Congenital hepatic fibrosis
Caroli's disease
Hyperalimentation-induced cirrhosis

Pre-operative evaluation

Pre-operative evaluation of the paediatric liver candidate starts at the outpatient setting when the patients are referred by either the paediatric hepatologist, paediatric surgeon or primary care physician. The evaluation process consists of a good history and physical examination, a family history, recognition of any obvious anomalies, for example hyperteleorism in patients who have Alagille syndrome and presence of any cardiac murmur in patients who can have congenital anomalies related to biliary atresia. Blood tests are sent for liver function, haematology and screening for hepatitis A, B, C and D. Serologies are also performed for CMV, EBV and HIV. If cardiac anomaly is suspected, the patient undergoes an echocardiogram. Other blood tests include determination of the patient's blood type and blood cultures to rule out sepsis. An ultrasound scan of the abdomen is done to assess the patency of liver vessels including hepatic artery, portal vein and hepatic veins.

In addition to diagnostic tests, social worker evaluation, nutritional assessment and an anaesthesiologist assessment are carried out. A dedicated paediatric liver transplant co-ordinator can play a key role in getting the work-up completed. The patient is then presented to the liver transplantation selection committee, which comprises surgeons, hepatologists, social worker, nutritionist and anaesthesiologist. If felt appropriate, the patient is listed on the UNOS waiting list for a liver transplantation.

Contraindications to liver transplantation, as with other organs, include HIV positivity, presence of systemic infections and involvement of extrahepatic organs with tumours. Transplantation is also contraindicated in patients with fulminant hepatic failure who have compromised cerebral blood flow as evidenced on a flow scan or magnetic resonance imaging (MRI) of the head. Presence of severe multisystem organ failure is a relative contraindication to liver transplantation.

Prior to proceeding with liver transplantation, the patient's medical condition is optimized with medical management, which is geared towards correction of hepatic encephalopathy, coagulopathy and controlling infection. Various surgical options include cadaveric liver transplantation, which includes cadaveric whole liver, whereby the donor organ comes from an age or size matched donor and the entire liver is used for the recipient. The second option is a cadaveric split liver transplantation whereby the donor is an adult and the liver divided to obtain a portion of the liver, which is usually the left lateral segment, for the paediatric recipient. The split liver transplantation can be split *in situ*, which is the more common or preferred method of splitting, as it reduces the ischaemic damage to the liver. The lateral segment of the liver or the left lobe of the liver is used for the paediatric recipient, whereas the right lobe is used for an adult recipient. *Ex vivo* split is also performed in some situations whereby the removed donor organ is split on the back table to provide two separate segments to be implanted into two different recipients.

Another option is a living related transplantation. This procedure was introduced due to increased organ shortage and has gained popularity in the last 5 years. The amount of liver necessary for the recipient has to be a minimum of 1% of the recipient's body weight. Living-related transplantation for paediatric patients is becoming increasingly popular. In this procedure the lateral segment of the liver of one of the parents or a living related donor is removed and implanted in the child.

Donor operations

For cadaveric liver procurement, the principles include laparotomy to rule out any intra-abdominal problems or presence of tumour. This is followed by mobilization of both the left and right lobes of the liver, and exploration of the liver hilum to isolate and divide the common bile duct, and determine any hepatic artery anomaly. The portal vein is then identified and skeletonized followed by the hepatic artery. The gallbladder is flushed of bile and heparin is administered to the donor. The infrarenal aorta is cannulated and the portal vein is cannulated. The aorta is cross-clamped and the abdominal viseral are rapidly cooled. The suprahepatic vena cava is then divided to vent the perfusate and blood. The organs are perfused with UW solution which acts as a preservative. For adult donors in whom an *in situ* split is contemplated, the donor surgery is usually prolonged by about 2 hours. The principles of *in situ* splitting include identification of any vascular anomaly, and mobilization of the left and right triangular ligaments, and left lateral segment (segments 2 and 3 of the left lobe of the liver).

The left branch of the hepatic artery, the left portal vein and the left bile duct draining segments 2 and 3 are identified and encircled. The left hepatic vein is also identified and encircled with a vessel loop. The left branch of the hepatic artery and left portal vein is ligated and transected followed by ligation and transection of the left hepatic vein. The left lateral segment having been previously mobilized is then taken out and put in ice and the hepatic artery and the portal vein is flushed with cold UW solution containing 1000 units of heparin. The right lobe procurement goes ahead while the lateral segment of the liver is being prepared by a separate team.

Absolute contraindications to procurement of the organs for transplantation include HIV positivity of the donor, high pressor requirement and presence of traumatic damage to the liver.

Orthotopic liver transplantation in the paediatric patient

The approach to this is similar to the adult procedure with some technical modifications if a reduced sized graft is used.

After the recipient hepatectomy, the suprahepatic cava (whole liver) or the left hepatic vein is anastomosed to the suprahepatic cava or inferior vena cava of the recipient. This is followed by an anastomosis of the donor portal vein to recipient portal vein. The liver is then flushed by opening the portal vein clamp and the suprahepatic clamp. This is followed by restoration by arterial inflow to the liver by anastomosing the donor left hepatic artery to the recipient artery. If the vessels are very small, the microvascular surgeons can be of immense help in anastomosing the donor and recipient hepatic artery. In paediatric patients, biliary construction is always performed by doing biliary-enteric anastomosis. The abdomen is then closed after placement of closed-suction drains (Jackson-Pratt type) into the abdominal cavity.

Post-operative immunosuppression

The regimen which is most commonly used is shown in Table 64.5.

Table 64.5 Immunosuppression for hepatic transplantation

Tacrolimus	0.1 mg/kg p.o.q. day
or	
Cyclosporin	10 mg/kg p.o.q. day
Prednisone	20 mg/kg Solu-Medrol intra-operative followed by steroid
Mycophenolate mofetil	10–30 mg/kg p.o.q. day

Post-operative complications

The immediate post-operative complications include haemorrhage and primary non-function of the liver graft. The latter requires liver re-transplantation. Other immediate post-operative complications include pulmonary problems and diminution of urine output. These complications are usually seen within the first few days after liver transplantation. A week after transplantation acute rejection of the allograft is the most common complication feared. Luckily with the introduction of newer immunosuppressants this complication is being seen less and less (Table 64.6).

Acute rejection is diagnosed by the presence of acute elevation in liver enzymes including alanine aminotransferase (ALT), aspartate aminotransferase (AST), gamma-glutamyltransferase (GGT) and alkaline phosphatase. A liver biopsy is confirmatory and this shows evidence of lymphocytes around the central veins (central venulitis) and the presence of inflammatory cells around the portal tract (portal triaditis). Treatment essentially consists of a steroid bolus of 10 mg/kg i.v., Solu-Medrol followed by gradually tapering doses of steroids. Tacrolimus levels are kept between 10 and 12 ng/ml.

The nursing staff and transplant co-ordinator educate the parents on administration of immunosuppressive and post-transplant medications, which include immunosuppressive drugs and prophylactic antibiotics. These include septran to control pneumocystis pneumonia, acyclovir to avoid viral infections and fluconazole to avoid fungal infections. Normal liver function is confirmed by the improving liver function tests (AST, ALT, GGT and bilirubin), weaning off the ventilator, normalization of other systems, namely improvement in oxygenation and an overall improvement of neurological status. With increasing expertise the overall 5 year patient survival has been about 90%.

A late complication is stricture of biliary anastomosis. This can be treated with external drainage, stent placement or balloon dilatation. Other complications include post-transplant lymphoproliferative diseases as a consequence of immunosuppression. Increasing EBV PCR titres or the presence of obvious lymphoid lesions in the digestive tract are diagnostic. Biopsy confirms the diagnosis. The treatment essentially consists of reducing the immunosuppressive drug doses. In some centres, lymphokine activated cells have been used to treat these lesions. Reduction in growth or absence of growth is another long-term complication following immunosuppressive therapy. The aim is to reduce the steroid dose as soon as and by as much as possible following liver transplantation.

Another post-operative complication is hepatic artery thrombosis. This usually presents as an acute elevation in the liver numbers during the post-operative period. The diagnosis is confirmed by ultrasound examination. In most children this can be prevented by introduction of aspirin or heparin during the immediate post-transplant period. If diagnosed, immediate exploration and revascularization of the hepatic graft is the treatment of choice. However, if this entity is diagnosed late, collaterals develop and these patients develop bile duct problems, especially related to stricturing and cholangitis. This is because the biliary system has the hepatic artery branches as the sole blood supply. Some patients later on require liver re-transplantation if this continues to be a problem.

Section 64.7 • Conclusions

The overall outcome of transplantation in adults and children has improved tremendously with the advancement of surgical techniques and immunosuppression. The rate of primary graft non-function has significantly decreased as there has been a better understanding of donor management and organ preservation. Overall patient and graft survival for most abdominal grafts is in excess of 90% at 1 year. These procedures, however, are specialized and to achieve optimal results should be conducted in centres dedicated to the management of these patients.

Table 64.6 Post-operative complications after liver transplantation

Immediate	*Early post-op < 1 week*	*Late post-op > 1 week*
Haemorrhage	Pulmonary	Acute rejection
Primary non-function	Renal	Bile leak
	Haemorrhage	Wound infection
	Hepatic artery thrombosis	Chronic rejection
		Sepsis
		Lymphoproliferative diseases
		Hepatic artery thrombosis

Further reading

Alejandro, R., Lehmann, R., Ricordi, C. *et al.* (1997). Long-term function (6 years) of islet allografts in type 1 diabetes. *Diabetes* **46**: 1983–9.

Billingham, R. E., Brent, L. and Medawar, P B. (1953). Actively acquired tolerance of foreign cells. *Nature* **172**: 603.

Diabetes Control and Complications Trial Research Group (1993). The effect of intensive treatment of diabetes on the development and progression of long-term complications in insulin-dependent diabetes mellitus. *N Engl J Med* **329**: 977.

Griffith, B. P., Shaw, B. W. Jr, Hardesty, R. L. *et al.* (1987). Veno-venous bypass without systemic anticoagulation for transplantation of the human liver. *Surg Gynecol Obstet* **165**: 343–8.

Hume, D. M., Merrill, J. P., Miller, B. F. *et al.* (1955). Experiences with renal homotransplantation in the human: report of nine cases. *J Clin Invest* **34**: 327.

Iwatsuki, S., Starzl, T. E., Todo, S. *et al.* (1988). Experience in 1000 liver transplants under cyclosporin-steroid: a survival report. *Transplant Proc* **20**: 498–504.

Jain, A. B., Khanna, A., Molmenti, E. P. *et al*: (1949). Immunosuppressive therapy, new concepts. *Surg Clin North Am* **79**: 59–76.

Khanna, A., Jain A. B. and Bonham, A. (1999). Principles of immunosuppression. In: Ayer, S. M., Grenvik, A., Holbrook, P. R., Shoemaker, W. C., eds. *Textbook of Critical Care*, 4th edn. Philadelphia, PA: W.B. Saunders.

Makowka, L., Gordon, R. D., Todo, S. *et al.* (1990). Early trials with FK 506 as primary treatment in liver transplantation. *Transplant Proc* **22**: 13–16.

Medawar, P. B. (1944). The behaviour and fate of skin autografts and skin homograft in rabbits. *J Anat* **78**: 176.

Morris, P. J., ed. (1988). *Kidney Transplantation. Principles and Practice*, 3rd edn, Philadelphia, PA: W.B. Saunders.

Report of the Expert Committee on the Diagnosis and Classification of Diabetes Mellitus (1997). *Diabetes Care* **20**: 1183.

Reyes, J. and Mazariegos, G. V. (1999). Pediatric transplantation. *Surg Clin North Am* **79**:163–89.

Sutherland, D. E., Cecka, M. and Gruessner, A. C. (1999). Report from the International Pancreas Transplant Registry – 1998. *Transplantation Proc* **31**: 597–601.

Sutherland, D. E., Gruessner, A. C. and Gruessner, R. W. (1998). Pancreas transplantation: a review. *Transplantation Proc* **50**: 1940–3.

Vincenti, F., Kirkman, R. Light, *et al.* (1988). Interleukin-2-receptor blockade with daclizumab to prevent actue rejection in renal transplantation. Daclizumab Triple Therapy Study Group. *N Engl J Med* **338**: 161–5.

MODULE 65

Plastic and reconstructive surgery

Plastic and reconstructive surgery is one of the most rapidly expanding faculties of the surgical subspecialties. It encompasses such varied *foci* as cosmetic surgery, burn and reconstructive surgery, peripheral neurosurgery, hand and microsurgery, congenital deformity, oncological, transplant and post-traumatic reconstruction.

The term *plastic surgery* is thought to be derived from the Greek *plastickos*, meaning to mould, shape or form. The efforts of the plastic surgeon are directed at restoring function, form and appearance by incorporating the concepts of physiology, function and anatomy with those of balance, symmetry and aesthetics. The practice of plastic and reconstructive surgery has a perceived origin in 1600 BC when the Susruta described the reconstruction of the nose using forehead and cheek flaps in the *Hindu Book of Revelation*. At that time in India the nose was amputated as a punitive measure for criminal acts.[1]

[1]*First the leaf of creeper, long and broad enough to fully cover the hole of the severed or clipped off part should be gathered; and a patch of living flesh equal in dimension of the preceding leaf, should be sliced off from down upward from the region of the cheek and, after scarifying it with a knife, swiftly adhered to the severed nose. Then the cool-headed physician should steadily tie it up with a bandage decent to look at and perfectly suited to the end for which it has been employed. The physician should make sure that the adhesion of the severed parts has been fully effected and then insert two small pipes into the nostrils to facilitate respiration and to prevent the adhesioned flesh from hanging down. After that the adhesion part should be dusted with the powders of sappanwood, licorice-root and bayberry pulverized together; and the nose should be enveloped in cotton and several times sprinkled over with a refined oil of pure sesamum … As soon as the skin has grown together with the nose, he cuts through the connection with the cheek.*

Section 65.1 • Wound healing

Wound healing historically and today remains one of the most fundamental concerns for the surgeon and the patient. It has evolved into a rapidly developing specialty of its own. An understanding of the pathophysiology is essential to all physicians. Wounds that in the past would not or could not be closed in a timely fashion often led to deformed, poorly functional and scarred sequelae. By applying an understanding of the fundamentals of wound healing, the surgeon can improve function, aesthetics and quality of life.

Numerous ancient Egyptian, Greek, Hebrew, Indian and European texts all detail the importance of proper wound handling, foreign body removal, cleanliness and closure. Ancient Hindu texts describe the use of insect mandibles for closure in a fashion similar to modern day stapling techniques.

During the gunpowder era historical concepts of wound care began to change. Boiling oils and salves were often employed. Atraumatic wound and tissue handling techniques were neglected and the results proved disastrous. It was not until the mid-1500s AD when Ambroise Pare, a surgeon at the Battle of Villaine, noted that when his supply of boiling oil ran out wound healing improved. The modern era of wound healing began with Lister's work on sepsis and Alex Carrel's work on transplantation rapidly expanded and evolved the field.

The physiological process of wound healing is usually divided into three phases. These phases overlap each other are probably best thought of as a continuum. Immediately after the body first suffers an injury or wounding whether by trauma, accident or surgical incision the first and life saving response is to stop the bleeding.

The *inflammatory phase* begins at the time of wounding with platelet deposition and vasoactive contraction. In a surgical wound, this phase continues over the next 3–4 days. During this phase, platelet derived factors are released and act as chemoattractants for neutrophils and macrophages. Histamine and prostaglandin release results in vasodilatation and increase in vascular permeability. Monocytes promote fibroblasts; fibronectin derived from the early granulation tissue promotes adhesion and migration of polymorphonuclear cells, monocytes, fibroblasts and epithelial cells. Proteolytic and collagenolytic enzymes are released. The complement cascade is activated. In this manner, bacteria and devitalized debris are removed from the wound. This wound characteristically appears red and swollen and may easily be disrupted.

The second phase of wound healing starts around day 3 post-injury and continues for 2–4 weeks. This phase is usually called the *proliferative* or *fibroblastic phase.* During this phase fibroblasts lay down the extracellular matrix and calcium dependent collagen synthesis provides scaffolding and structure to the wound defect. Growth factors released from macrophages promote angiogenesis. New capillaries are formed in a process termed neovascularization. During this second phase the collagen content and tensile strength of the wound rapidly increases.

The third phase of wound healing is termed the *maturation* or *remodelling phase.* The collagen, which at first appears to be randomly laid down begins to be reorientated and reorganized, and undergoes cross-linking. Collagen synthesis begins to equal collagen degradation. Embryonic type III collagen is replaced by mature type I collagen until the normal 4:1 ratio (depending on the type of tissue) is achieved. These processes significantly increase the overall strength of the wound, attaining approximately 70–80% of the original pre-wound strength. The remodelling phase usually lasts approximately 1 year but may last up to 2 years in young children with burns (Figures 65.1 and 65.2).

We know that prolongation of the phases of wound healing whether due to infection, inadequate debridement, steroids, radiation, etc., results in impaired wound healing. When wounds are not closed surgically but rather are left open to heal by secondary intention, i.e. dressing changes, the inflammatory phase continues until the wound is completely closed.

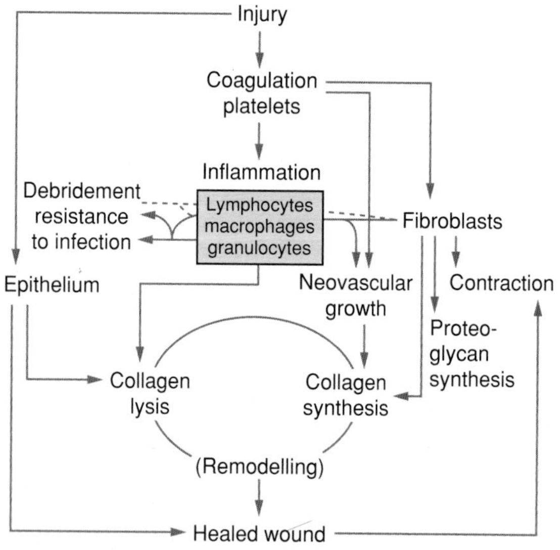

Figure 65.1 Schematic representation of key events in wound healing. (From Barbul, A. (1990). *Clinics in Plastic Surgery*, **17:** 434, with permission.)

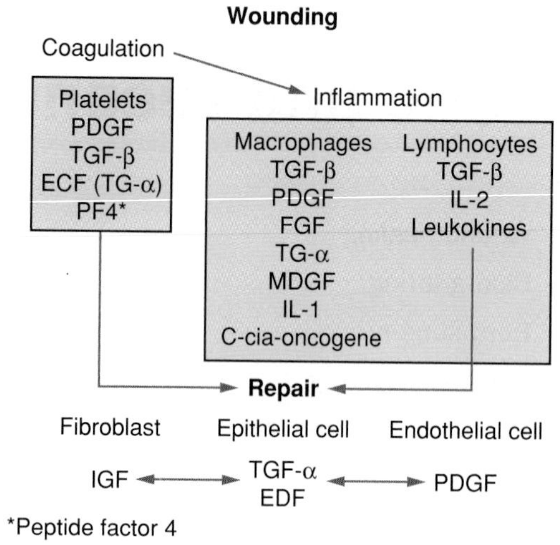

Figure 65.2 Peptide growth factors released by the cells recruited into the injured area. (From McGrath, H. (1990). *Clinics in Plastic Surgery* **17:** 424, with permission.)

The physician can create a more favourable wound-healing environment by careful attention to atraumatic wound handling and meticulous debridement of all devitalized tissue. The nutritional state of many patients can often be optimized as can the control of many comorbid factors like that of blood sugar in the diabetic patient and blood pressure in the hypotensive patient. Medicines like non-steroidal anti-inflammatories, steroids and chemotherapeutic agents all directly affect wound healing. Supplementation of vitamin A in the steroid dependent patient and platelet derived growth factors in the treatments of diabetic lower extremity wounds may all directly aid in wound healing.

Contractile forces also contribute to the closure of the open wound. Contraction is the normal centripetal force of closure thought to result from contractile myofibroblastic cells. Contracture, on the other hand is a resultant abnormal, shortened and scarred deformity.

The surface of a wound defect closes by the concurrent mechanisms of epithelialization and contraction. A linear scar may only need epithelium to advance a few cell lengths but a large open wound will require extensive epithelial migration. A granulating wound bed covered gradually with advancing epithelium is usually one of poor quality and durability. Epithelialization involves the mobilization and migration of epithelial cells across the wound. They enlarge, flatten and detach from neighbouring cells and the basement membrane. Migration is thought to be due to the loss of contact inhibition and continues until another cell is met. The fixed basal cells undergo mitosis replacing peripherally migrating cells. These cells then divide and multiply thickening the new epithelial layer. Keratinocytes differentiate and re-establish the stratum. Advancing cells from the perimeter then bridge the gap. Normal cell differentiation from basal to surface re-establishes the height of the wound.

Simultaneously, the wound's surface area will decrease as specialized fibroblasts induce intracellular actin and myosin frameworks for the purpose of contracting the wound. Finally, after the wound is closed, the fibroblasts continue to deposit collagen, which matures through cross-linking, yielding a wound of greater tensile strength (Figure 65.3).

Many defects in the phases of epithelialization and contraction are recognized. Patients with Ehlers-Danlos syndrome cannot generate an appropriate collagen subtype for stable and mature wound healing. Whenever wounds fail to self-regulate, collagen deposition proceeds in excess of collagen degeneration. This leads to either a hypertrophic or a keloid scar, both examples of 'excessive healing'. Only by unravelling the physiology of wound healing through basic research may we better affect the clinical condition to the patient's benefit.

Local tissue and free microvascular transfer of flaps provide healthy vascularized muscle and/or soft tissue to areas of deficit such as poorly vascularized or non-healing wounds. In doing so we can often facilitate wound healing, control local chronic infection and aid in bony union.

Abnormal scars

There are two major classes of abnormal scars that most clinicians routinely face, hypertrophic scars and keloids. Hypertrophic scars are raised, pruritic and do not extend beyond the original borders of the wound. Keloids on the other hand tend to enlarge beyond the borders of the wound and tend to be progressive, irritating, deforming and prone to recurrence. Keloid scars appear to demonstrate some degree of genetic transmission. They occur more commonly in darker skinned individuals. Unfortunately, to date there is no reliable cure for these problematic scars. There are however numerous treatments available. Intralesional injections of steroids, calcium channel blockers and chemotherapeutic agents have all been described. The use of pulse dye lasers, pressure therapy, excisional therapies and radiation treatments has also been shown to help (Figures 65.4 and 65.5).

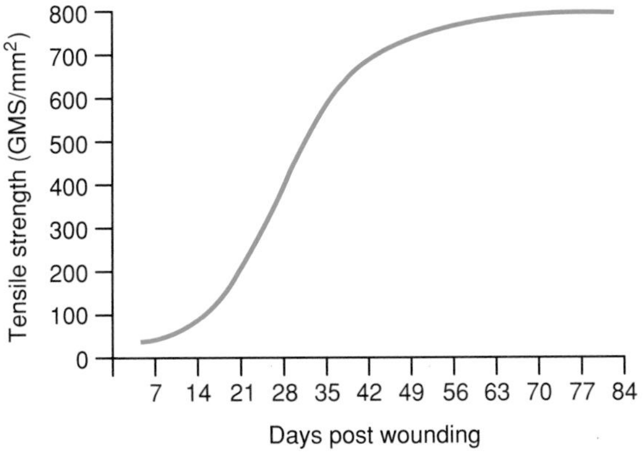

Figure 65.3 Tensile strength graph.

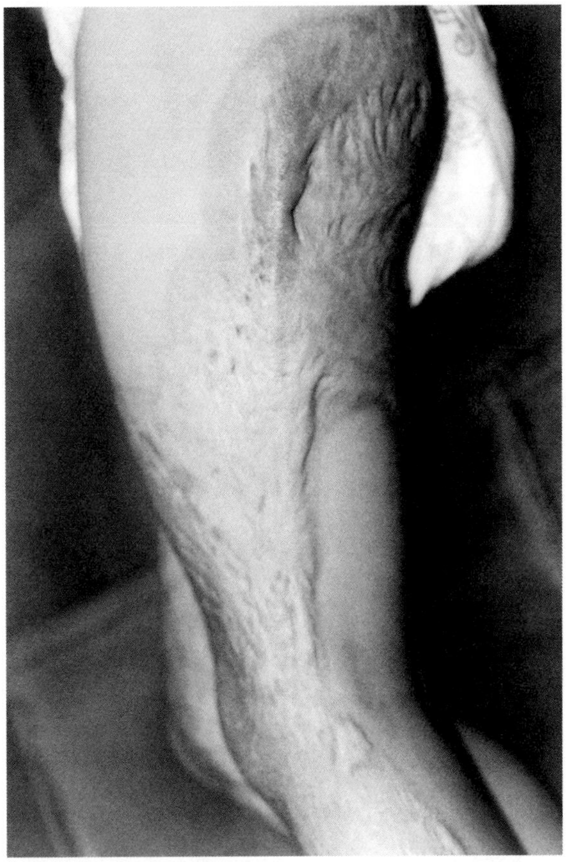

Figure 65.4 Keloid scar.

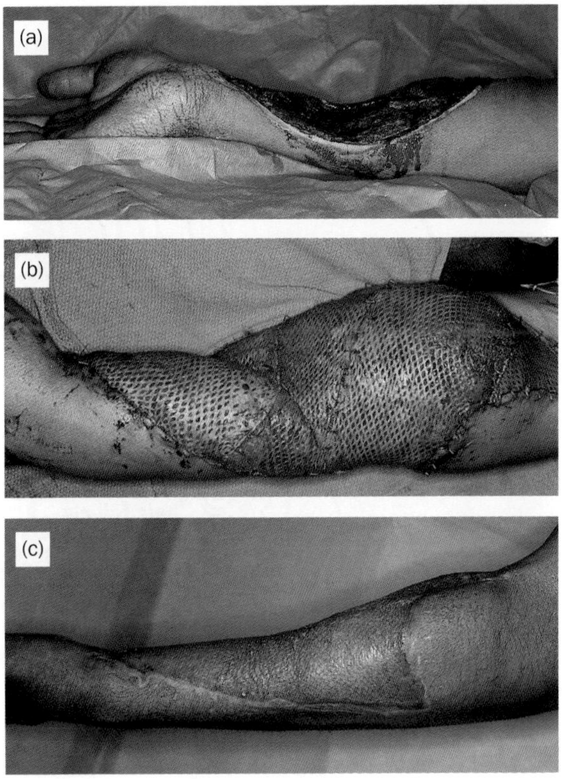

Figure 65.5 Treatment of hypertropic scarring.

Section 65.2 • Skin grafting

In 1822 Bunger and again in 1830 Warren first successfully grafted autologous skin to a nasal defect. This humble application proved to become one of the greatest advances in reconstructive surgery.

A skin graft can be thought of as a portion of skin that is transferred without its own blood supply. Skin grafts are categorized by the amount of dermis included in the graft (Figure 65.6).

A split thickness skin graft includes the epidermis and a portion of the dermis. A thick split thickness graft has proportionately more dermis included than a thin split thickness graft. In retaining some dermis in the donor site, the donor site may then heal by the re-epithelialization from adnexal elements like hair follicles and sebaceous glands, as well as contraction. Full thickness skin grafts include all of the epidermis and all of the dermis. The donor site, devoid of adnexae, will only heal if closed primarily or itself skin grafted.

The presence and extent of expansion further categorize skin grafts. By meshing a skin graft, the graft may be expanded many times much like a woven stocking might be stretched to cover greater areas. The interstices allow transudates and exudates to drain, and facilitate contouring over irregular surfaces.

Thinner skin grafts take more reliably but tend to contract more. Thicker skin grafts look better, contract less but have a less reliable take and require donor site closure.

Skin grafts initially adhere via a fibrin to collagen interaction and survive by *inhibition* or diffusion of plasma from the recipient bed. Over the ensuing 2–5 days a miscrovascular supply is established. This process is called *inosculation*.

Skin grafts may be taken from almost any place in the body. One tries to match the quality, thickness and colour of the recipient site to that of the donor site while minimizing donor site morbidity.

Flaps

A flap, as opposed to a graft, is simply tissue that is transferred with its own blood supply. The orientation of the blood supply, the pattern of transfer and the elements contained in the transfer all further differentiate the types of available flaps.

When we look at the particular vascular supply of the flap, we can divide flaps into axial and random patterns. Random flaps rely on the underlying dermal and subdermal vascular plexi for their vascularity. Axial flaps on the other hand have a well-defined artery and vein contained. As a result axial flaps may be constructed of a considerably greater length to width ratio.

One can also classify flaps based on their composition. Flaps that only contain muscle are called muscle flaps, those that contain muscle and the overlying skin are called myocutaneous flaps, those that contain fascia alone are called fascial flaps and those that contain fascia as well as the overlying skin are called fasciocutaneous flaps.

Flaps can also be defined based on their pattern of transfer. By capitalizing on the elastic nature of most biological tissues and employing fundamental geometric rules we can often fill defects by rotating, transposing or advancing tissues into adjoining defects (Figure 65.7).

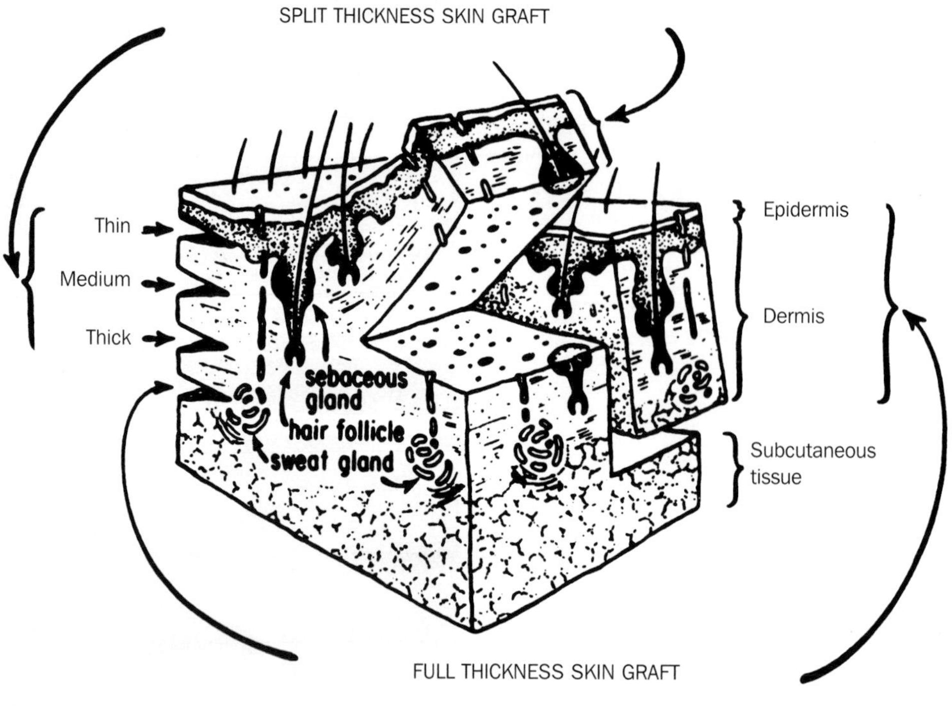

Figure 65.6 Split thickness skin graft.

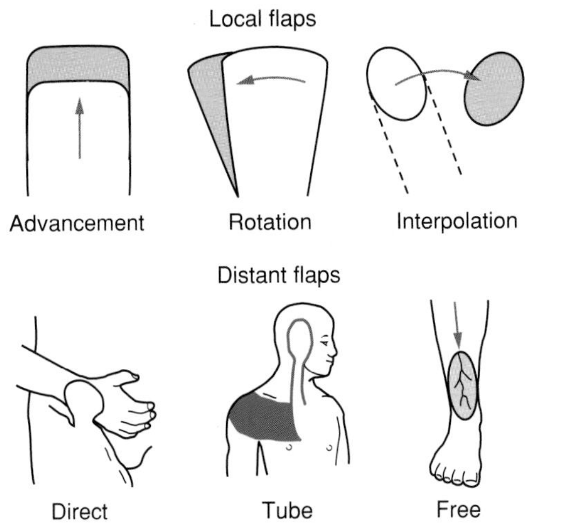

Figure 65.7 Classification of skin flaps by method of movement. (From McCarthy, J. G. (1990). *Plastic Surgery*. Philadelphia, PA: W.B. Saunders, 1990, p. 277, with permission.)

Flaps may also be transferred with greater bulk, to further distances and with improved vascularity by microvascular techniques. Muscle or myocutaneous, fascia or fasciocutaneous or even composite flaps containing vascularized bone or necrotized functional tissue may be procured with their vascular supply and re-anastomosed at the recipient site under the microscope to a new vascular supply (Figures 65.8–65.10).

Section 65.3 • Burn surgery

In the USA alone, burn injuries account for over 100 000 hospital admissions and approximately 12 000 deaths/year.

Prior to the 1970s most patients succumbed to wound sepsis. Zora Janzekovich promoted early aggressive excision and closure within days of the injury. This as well as the establishment of dedicated burn centres, improved surgical and critical care techniques have all resulted in significantly decreased mortality. The most frequent cause of death in the burn patient today is pulmonary, usually inhalation injury or pneumonia.

Plastic surgeons are involved in both the acute and late reconstruction of burn injuries. This requires a close co-ordinated effort among intensivists, paediatricians, rehabilitative specialists, nutritionists, opthalmologists, psychiatrists, pain specialists and others as needed, all of whom together constitute the multidisciplinary burn care team.

Burns are categorized by depth of involvement. Superficial burns like sunburns often heal without significant sequelae. Superficial and deep partial thickness burns include injury to the dermis. These wounds appear blistered and are very painful. Full thickness injuries involve all layers of the epidermis and full thickness involvement of the dermis. These are usually leather-like in appearance and often painless due to the destruction of the cutaneous sensory nerves. These wounds will not heal and should be excised early and covered.

Acutely the burn wound is debrided and treated with either antimicrobials or biological dressing. Burn patients who have suffered significant total body surface involvement are aggressively fluid resuscitated using formulae specifically derived for this. Most commonly these are based on variations of the Parkland formula. In adults, fluids for the first 24 hours = (3–4 cm^3) × (patient weight in kg) × (percentage total body surface area involved in second or third degree burn). One half of this fluid is administered in the first 8 hours from the onset of the burn injury; the residual is administered over the next 16 hours and titrated to the patient's pulmonary and haemodynamic status. Escarotomies and fasciotomies are performed for circumferential limb threatening distributions. Extremities and critical joints are often splinted and ranged early.

Deep facial burns are best excised and grafted within a week to 10 days to improve the overall quality of the final result as well as to decrease the chance of hypertrophic scar development. Major joints and functional areas are usually covered with thicker and non-expanded grafts when possible to decrease the likelihood of future contracture deformities. Periorbital burns are often difficult to manage due to the very thin multilaminate nature of the eyelids as well as the critical functional importance in ocular protection. Combined reconstructions are often performed in concert with the ophthalmic surgeons to protect the eye. Full thickness grafts and a variety of local flaps are well described for periorbital coverage. Grafts to the face are usually best taken from areas above the clavicles for optimal colour and textural match. Pre- and post-auricular grafts as well as uninvolved contralateral eyelid skin or even upper inner arm skin may be used.

Pressure ulcers manifest when sufficient pressures develop locally to overcome the microcirculation (32 mmHg). These are usually areas over bony prominences, and result in local ischaemia and soft tissue loss.

The most common sites for the development of pressure ulcers are ischial, trochanteric and sacral. Other areas like the heel and occiput are also seen quite frequently. The location of the pressure ulcer is dependent on the patient's habitus and position. Patients who spend prolonged periods sitting up, e.g. the patient in a wheelchair, will more commonly develop ischial pressure ulcers while patients who are bed ridden tend to develop ulcers, in the sacral, occipital and heel distributions.

Significant risk factors in the development of a pressure ulcer include immobility, spasticity, impaired nutritional status, altered levels of consciousness and incontinence. Like burns, pressure ulcers are staged based on depth of involvement (Table 65.1).

Certainly not all pressure ulcers require surgical intervention and the best treatment plan is usually prophylactic and includes the optimization of comorbid

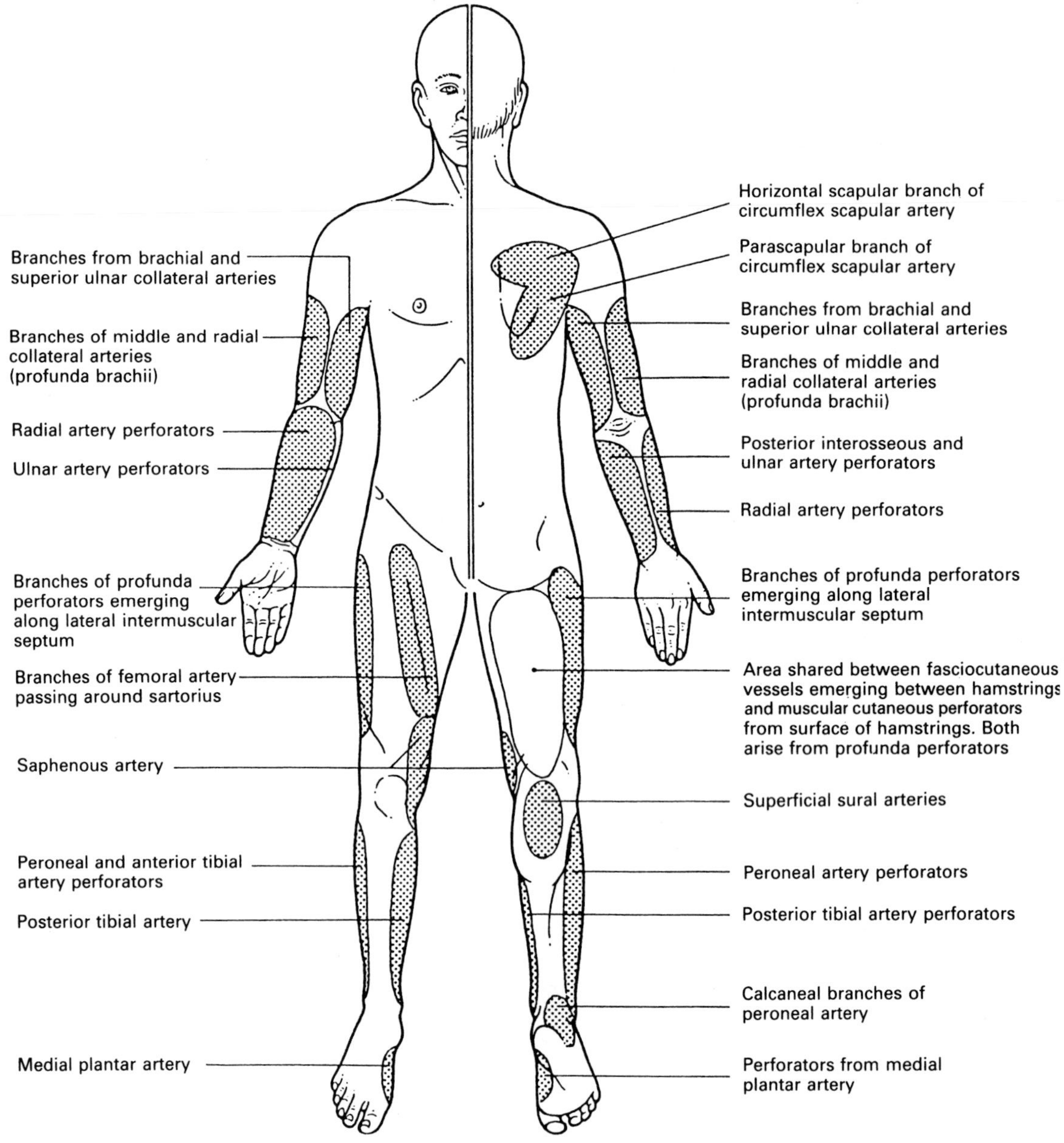

Figure 65.8 Areas suitable for the raising of fasciocutaneous flaps. Proportions of actual flaps will differ from the above. (From Cormack, G. C. and Lamberty, B. G. H. (1986). *The Arterial Anatomy of Skin Flaps*. Edinburgh: Churchill Livingstone: 92, with permission.)

risk factors. Spasticity is often managed medically with drugs like baclofen and diazepam; occasionally surgical neuroablative techniques are required. Frequent positional changes, appropriate cushioning and supportive measures all help to decrease local pressure effects. These are co-ordinated with the patient's carer, prosthetist or therapist. Nutrition is optimized and local wound care helps to heal the more superficial ulcers.

The surgical principles involved in the treatment of pressure ulcers include drainage of any collections with wide surgical debridement of all devitalized tissues. Pseudobursae are excised and judicious local ostectomy is performed to resect involved bone and smooth the remaining contour of irregularities. Bone cultures are often taken to evaluate for osteomyelitis. When the wound is clean, the patient optimized and found to be a suitable candidate for reconstruction, local fasciocutaneous and muscle flaps are usually required for coverage.

Section 65.4 • Aesthetic surgery

In this era of lengthier and more active lifespans, significant solar exposure as well as the increasingly competitive nature of the workplace environment there is little surprise that more and more individuals are seeking

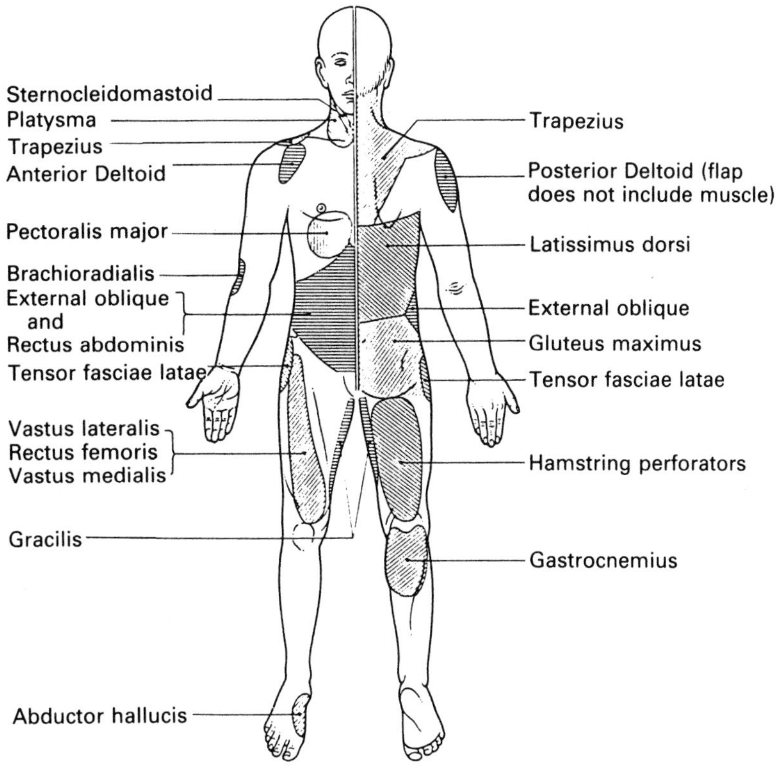

Figure 65.9 Areas suitable for the raising of musculocutaneous flaps. Proportions of actual musculocutaneous flaps will vary from the above. (From Cormack, G. C. and Lamberty, B. G. H. (1986). *The Arterial Anatomy of Skin Flaps*. Edinburgh: Churchill Livingstone: 76, with permission.)

aesthetic and rejuvenative procedures. These techniques have evolved significantly with the improved appreciation for the changes that occur during ageing. The skin undergoes atrophic changes with loss of elasticity, subcutaneous atrophy to the normal fatty layers and bony skeleton. Retaining ligaments that once held the skin and soft tissues of the face attenuate and the characteristic jowling, malar and brow descent become evident. Folds are accentuated and wrinkles develop, creating a tired and often angry appearance.

Laser resurfacing, mechanical dermabrasion and chemical peels all remove the superficial layers of the skin. New collagen is deposited; the skin is tightened and re-epithelialized in a more regular pattern. Facelifts are designed to excise excess skin of the neck and face. Numerous suspensory techniques are employed to raise the midfacial elements, neck and improve the cheek

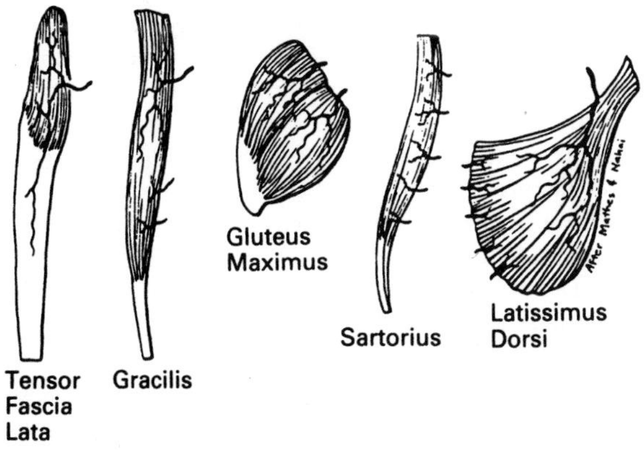

Figure 65.10 Classification of muscles by the type of blood supply (after Mathes and Nahai). Areas suitable for the raising of musculocutaneous flaps. Proportions of actual musculocutaneous flaps will vary from the above. (From McCarthy (1990), Vol. 1, p. 283, with permission.)

Table 65.1 Pressure sore staging system

Stage I	Non-blanchable erythema of intact skin (heralding lesion of skin ulceration)
Stage II	Partial thickness skin loss involving epidermis or dermis. The ulcer is superficial and presents clinically as an abrasion, blister or shallow crater
Stage III	Full thickness skin loss involving damage to or necrosis of subcutaneous tissue that may extend down to, but not through, underlying fascia. The sore presents clinically as a deep crater with or without undermining of adjacent tissue
Stage IV	Full thickness skin loss with extensive destruction, tissue necrosis, or damage in muscle, bone or supporting structures (e.g. tendon or joint capsule)

From US Department of Health and Human Services: Pressure Ulcers in Adults: Prediction and Prevention. *Clinical Practice Guideline No. 3*, Publication 97-004, 1992.

and malar regions. Reorientating vectors of pull create a more youthful appearance. Blepharoplasty is the excision of excess skin and often muscle of the eyelids to crate a fresher and less baggy appearance. Occasionally ptotic or bulging fat may be concomitantly excised or repositioned.

Liposuction involves the removal subcutaneous fatty collections with vacuum and suction catheters. These fatty accumulations often do not go away with routine weight loss and exercise. As a result they are termed lipodystrophic. Liposculpture techniques include not only aspirating fatty collections but also reinjecting fat to areas of depletion and atrophy in an attempt to improve contours and rejuvenate. Ultrasonic and laser techniques are also utilized adjunctively by some surgeons in areas of denser and more fibrous fat as is seen in gynaecomastia.

As with all surgical procedures it is important to remember that aesthetic surgery is *real* surgery with very *real* risks and complications. Proper patient education and selection is imperative.

Tissue expansion

Neumann first described the expansion of peri-auricular skin using a subcutaneously placed air-filled balloon in 1956. Since that time the technique of tissue expansion has lent itself to almost routine use in burn surgery, post-mastectomy breast reconstruction and scalp reconstruction.

Tissue expanders are usually placed with the goal of expanding and advancing healthy local tissues or flaps so that they may be advanced to augment or supplant defects and deformities. In this way, like or similar tissue, i.e. matched for colour, thickness, hair distribution and texture, may augment or replace the lost tissue while minimizing the donor defect.

The expanding balloon is thought to force interstitial fluid out of the overlying tissues allowing for early extension. Later viscoelastic change and recruitment of adjacent tissue results in a net gain of available tissue. Histologically, there is an increase in the vascularity and collagen content of the expanded tissue with thinning of the dermis and epidermal thickening.

Section 65.5 • Peripheral neurosurgery

Significant improvements have been made in our ability to identify, understand and repair peripheral nerve injuries, particularly over the past decades. Seddon in 1943 classified three types of nerve injury; Sutherland in 1968 and finally Mackinnon in the 1980s further expanded this classification to include six degrees of injury to the internal structure of a peripheral nerve.

First degree injuries involve an interruption of the conduction in the axon with *preservation* of the anatomical continuity of all the components of the nerve. This is termed *neuropraxia*. These injuries usually recover completely in a period of days to 12 weeks.

Second degree injuries involve axonal damage; as a result there is Wallerian degeneration occurring distal to the site of injury. This is termed *axonotmesis*. These injuries usually recover completely without surgical intervention at a rate of approximately 2-3 cm per month.

Third degree injuries involve transection and interruption of the continuity of the nerve. This constitutes *neurotmesis*. This degree of injury requires surgical intervention including nerve repair, nerve grafting and neurolysis. The rate of recovery usually requires approximately 1 month to cross the repair site and another month or so per 3 cm distal. To put this into perspective, an injury to a nerve that is repaired at the level of the axilla may take over 2 years to restore sensation to the hand.

Open peripheral nerve injuries (stab wound, laceration, etc.) are best repaired early by microscopic re-anastomosis. Gaps of less than 3 cm or so can be reconstructed by using conduits such as vein or with nerve grafts. Gaps of greater than 3 cm or so require the use of nerve grafts; these are often procured from the arm, i.e. antebrachial nerve, or leg, i.e. sural nerve.

Blunt or closed peripheral nerve injuries are usually watched clinically for 6 weeks or so. If no recovery is seen then electromyographic and nerve conduction studies are undertaken and followed for several months. If little or no improvement is noted then surgical renervation techniques are undertaken. Occupational and rehabilitative therapies are used in the intervening periods to maintain length, position, range of motion, tone and fluidity.

Section 65.6 • Major trauma

The plastic and reconstructive surgeon is often involved in the evaluation and treatment of wounds and injuries in almost any part of the body. It is impossible within the scope of this chapter to fully detail the management of this complicated issue. We will concentrate mainly on facial and lower extremity injuries.

Facial injuries may span the gamut from the management of the simple laceration or abrasion to complex craniofacial fractures. When one evaluates a patient with a facial or head injury attention to the ABC of trauma must take priority. Trauma to the face may include significant airway, neck or intracranial injury. Jaw fractures may posteriorly displace and with the resultant oedema, result in airway obstruction. Obtundation, whether due to drug or neurological injury may facilitate aspiration. Haemorrhage, from the well-vascularized head and neck, is often profuse. Nasal bleeding is often controlled by pressure. If external pressure does not suffice, careful anterior and posterior packing may be required. Occasionally, angiographic and surgical interruption is required. Ophthalmological evaluation is always warranted with injuries to the periorbital regions.

As with all wounds and lacerations, facial injuries should be copiously irrigated. Sterile saline is usually preferred, as it is quite forgiving to the eyes and local tissues. All foreign bodies should be debrided and edges freshened up while maintaining as much healthy, native tissue as possible. The wounds are closed as meticulously as possible for the initial efforts lay the foundation for future revision and reconstruction.

The observer's eye tends to view the face as an inverted triangle. The nose and mouth constitute the apex and the eyebrow and eyes make up the base. By realigning key anatomical landmarks like the vermilion border, eyebrow and nostril sill, aesthetic symmetry and continuity is re-established.

As opposed to wounds in many other locations, those of the face are often closed even after significant delay on presentation. The face is very well perfused with numerous adnexal structures and significant cross-innervation. As a result, the majority of superficial injuries to the face often result in a favourable outcome.

Puncture wounds should always raise the suspicion for retained foreign body and deep underlying injury. Domestic cat and dog bite wounds can usually be gently re-approximated if the wound is uncomplicated, the animal is clean with vaccines up to date and the patient presents early. Thorough debridement and antimicrobial therapy is employed. The patient must be instructed on meticulous wound care and follow-up. Human bites, contaminated wounds, and wounds that have resulted from high energy mechanisms like military injuries or significant crush injuries pose special problems and are often treated with aggressive local wound care and delayed closure techniques. Road crash debris is best treated with early and meticulous debridement of all foreign body impregnation. Saline pulse lavage, gentle cleansing with surgical scrub sponges and even loupe magnified hand debridement in the operating theatre may be necessary to help minimize the post-traumatic scarring and tattooing that often results.

The ear with its delicate invested cartilaginous framework is prone to injury, infection and permanent deformity resulting in the 'cauliflower ear'. Lacerations should be repaired in a layered anatomical fashion realigning the cartilage. Hematomas should be evacuated early; bolsters, moulded dressings and drains are often employed.

The lower extremity is usually divided into thirds when considering reconstructive options. Defects of the proximal two-thirds of the lower leg are readily covered by the gastrocnemius and soleus muscles. The medial gastrocnemius tends to be larger than the lateral gastrocnemius muscle and is easier to mobilize with the fibula and peroneal nerve located laterally. The distal third of the lower extremity poses more difficult reconstructive options. There is a smaller muscle mass to tendon ratio here and as a result larger defects often require free tissue transfer with microvascular anastomosis outside the zone of injury (Figure 65.11).

Basic principles of post-traumatic wound care are thorough irrigation and debridement of all contaminants and devitalized tissue, atraumatic handling and protection of remaining viable soft tissues as well as the accurate reduction and stabilization of bony elements and length.

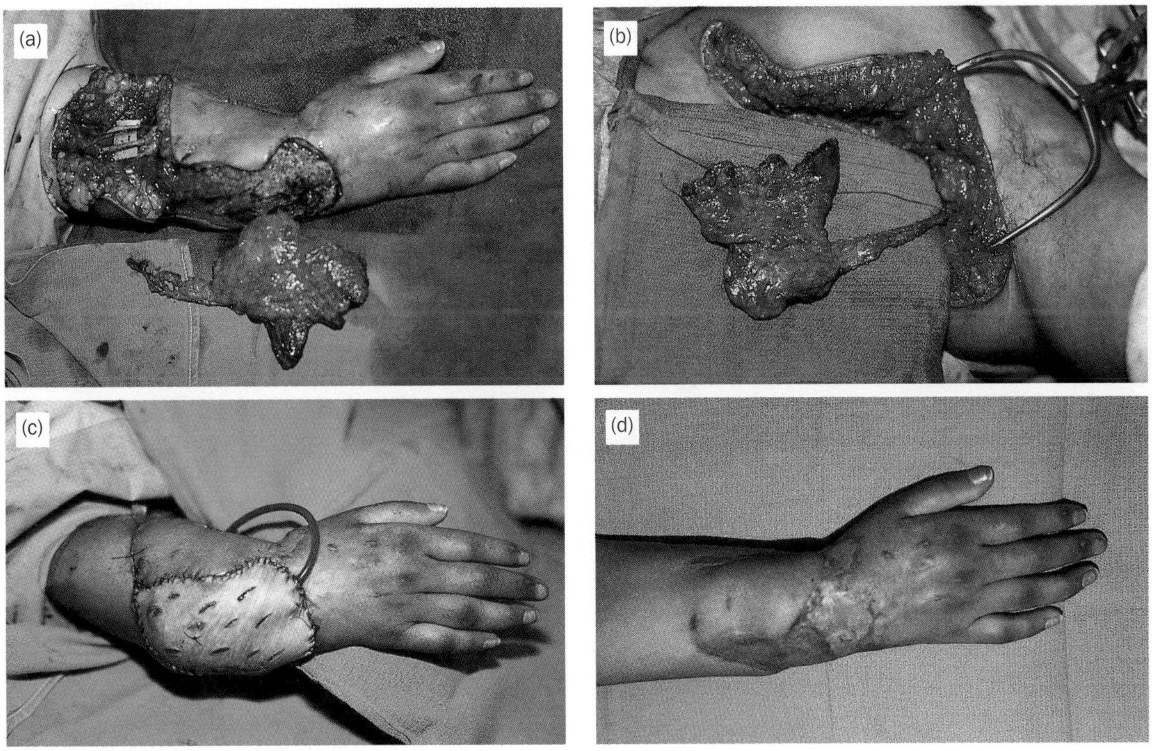

Figure 65.11 Lower external reconstruction and free flap.

Amputation is often best reserved for extremities that have suffered significant non-reconstructable injuries such as severe crush injuries and injuries that have resulted in prolonged ischaemia times. Occasionally, due to significant comorbid factors or concomitant injury amputation may be life saving.

Several studies over the past decade have demonstrated that when *all* costs to the patient, hospital and society are factored in, free flap reconstruction of lower extremity injuries is cost effective.

Burn reconstruction

The ideal timing for burn reconstruction is of great debate. Time often has a dramatic effect on the quality of the burn scar deformity. These improvements continue for up to several years post-burn, particularly in the paediatric burn population. In an ideal situation one might try to spare and plan reconstructive options and donor locations during the initial burn treatment. Often the acute life saving requirements preclude such strategies.

Preventive measures such as early rehabilitative exercises, massage, range of motion activities, moisturization and splinting can certainly diminish future reconstructive needs. These modalities also tend to motivate and include the patient in his or her own rehabilitation. The early use of compression garments, silicone sheeting and laser therapies all attempt to control the hypertrophic stages of burn scar and donor site deformities that so often complicate the burn injury and recovery (Figure 65.12).

Acute reconstructive efforts are usually directed towards protection of critical functions. Injuries to the eyelids and cheeks often produce progressive scarring, traction and contracture with resultant exposure, which may lead to keratopathy infection or blindness. Contracture of major joints like the axilla, antecubital region or knees often requires early release with soft tissue augmentation to prevent frozen joints, shortening of critical muscle and tendon units which significantly limit rehabilitative progress and potential.

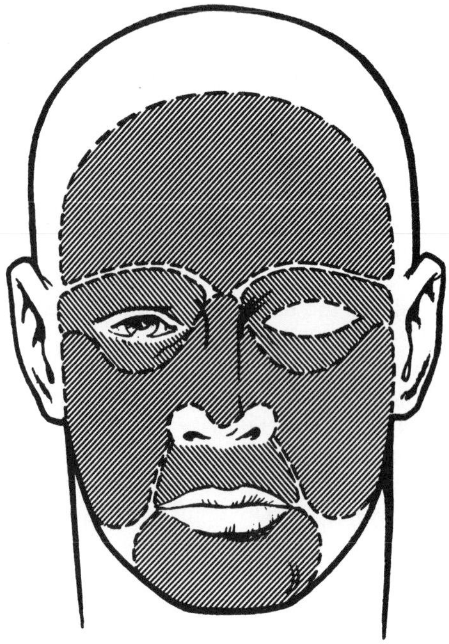

Figure 65.13 Aesthetic units.

Most burn reconstruction surgeons acutely try to prevent untoward sequelae and may occasionally plan future reconstructive options during the initial presentation.

General reconstructive principles are to try and replace like tissue with like tissue (Figure 65.13). Replacing and recontouring deformities respecting aesthetic unit guidelines often allows for the most natural end result.

Later burn reconstructive measures often involve the use of tissue expanders and free flap reconstructions to recruit and reintroduce healthy and aesthetic tissue to areas of contracture and deformity (Figure 65.14).

While attempts at biosynthetic development continue, these technologies remain prohibitively expensive for most applications.

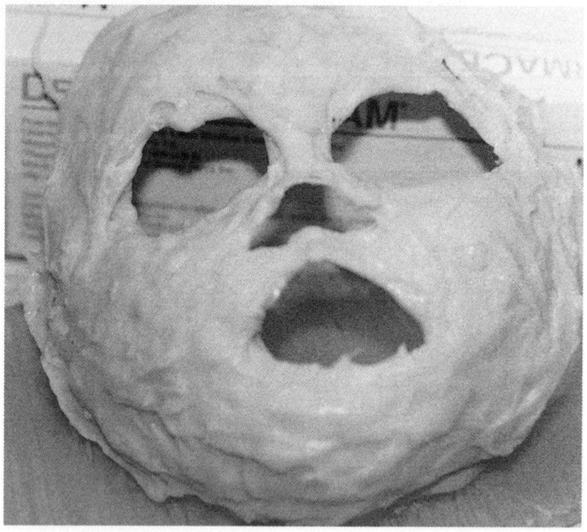

Figure 65.12 Silicone face mask.

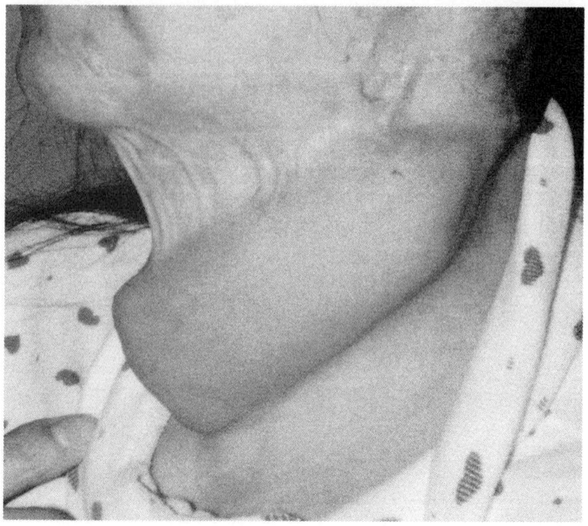

Figure 65.14 Tissue expander to the neck.

Section 65.7 • Congenital malformations

Birth defects are usually categorized on the basis of both morphology and pathogenesis. The dysmorphologist recognizes three different subtypes of birth defects:

- **Malformation** – At the earliest phase of development, a defect in migration, proliferation or differentiation of tissue occurs. As a result the organism is not formed correctly in the first place.
- **Deformation** – The child is initially formed correctly but, later, an external force alters that form. This might be related to fetal position *in utero*, twinning, uterine pathology, etc. Usually, but not every time, a deformation will self-correct, presumably because the message for normal growth is inherent in the genetic code.
- **Disruption** – Normal formation of tissues has occurred, but some time during gestation a disrupting event takes place, e.g. premature rupture of the amniotic membranes or injury to an embryonic artery.

While the frequency of birth defects has remained relatively unchanged throughout the twentieth century, more and more children are benefiting from the skills of the plastic surgeon. We better appreciate the negative impact a deformity tends to have on the psychological development and social integration of an affected child.

Prior to undertaking the surgical reconstruction of a child's birth defect, the mechanism of the deformity should be defined and categorized. Associated defects must also be catalogued and the sequence of the entire defect understood so that a safe reconstructive plan can be undertaken and prioritized. Valid genetic counselling, which is so important for both the affected child and family, requires accurate definition of a birth defect's mechanism.

Developmental malformations

As a child develops, abnormalities may become apparent that were never recognized early in life. Certain vascular anomalies are not visible at birth; they may evolve weeks, months or even years afterwards.

At the time of puberty, a sudden change in hormone secretion can produce unwanted deformity. Gynaecomastia in an adolescent boy or mammary hypoplasia in a teenage girl can be emotionally devastating events. The nose, one of the last facial structures to complete its growth, may undergo a significant growth spurt, which is disproportionate to overall facial form. In each case, a plastic surgeon is often able to influence a patient's self-esteem favourably.

Cleft lip and palate

For many plastic and reconstructive surgeons, cleft lip and palate reconstruction remains one of the most gratifying surgeries for the physician, family and patient. Cleft lip and palatal deformities occur during the first trimester. Embryologically there are five facial elements which come together to create the developing face and jaw. Genetic, viral and nutritional causes have all been implicated as causes for this deformity.

The basic surgical principles involved in the correction of these deformities traditionally involve a recreation of the normal lip contours, reorientation and alignment of the underlying musculature without significantly compromising maxillary growth centres, and closing the palatal to nasal communication to facilitate feeding and speech. The operations are usually performed when the child is stable enough to tolerate the surgery. Many use the rule of 10s to help determine surgical timing: 10 weeks of age, 10 pounds, 10 g haemoglobin.

Debates continue as to the optimal timing for the repair of the associated nasal and occlusal deformities. Some opt for very early intervention and others prefer later reconstructions (Figure 65.15).

The early use of maxillary orthopaedic devices is advocated by several large centres in an attempt to mould the bony shelves and teeth into alignment and decrease the overall width of the defect, facilitating the repair.

Genetic counselling, nutritionists, speech and hearing therapists co-ordinate in a multidisciplinary fashion the progress of the affected child and assist the parents and physicians.

Section 65.8 • Craniofacial surgery

As a result of the work of pioneers like Paul Tessier and Joseph G. McCarthy, the field of craniofacial surgery has evolved rapidly since the 1920s. In combination with well-established orthognathic (jaw corrective) techniques, exposure of the craniofacial skeleton is obtained through a combination of scalp, periorbital, intraoral and base of skull approaches. As a result, the appearance of the abnormal appearing child can be dramatically improved.

Patients likely to benefit from this new subdiscipline are those born with one of the craniofacial dysostoses (Apert, Crouzon, Pfeiffer syndromes) or mandibulofacial dyostosis (Treacher–Collins), hypertelorism (lateral displaced orbits) or one of the major facial clefts.

As craniofacial surgery becomes a safer and more refined practice, its principles are being applied to younger children and eventually to newborns. Premature cranial suture closure (craniosynostosis) has been recognized as a common precursor or accompaniment to the severest craniofacial deformities. We do not yet fully understand the pathogenesis of the various craniosynostoses. However, surgeons are recognizing a need to release joined sutures early, not just to prevent development of hydrocephaly, but also to advance a restrained forehead and to encourage maxillary growth.

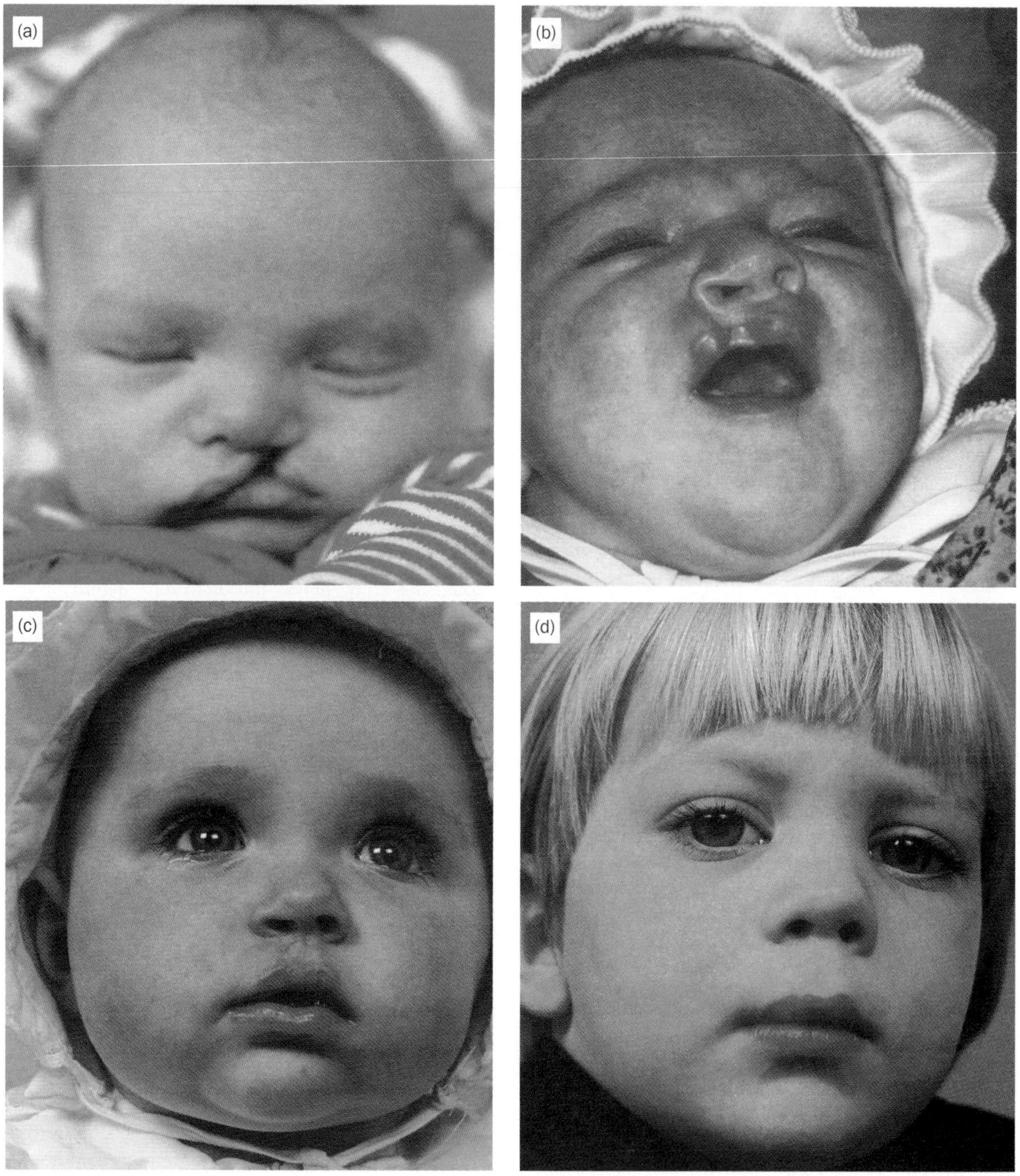

Figure 65.15 Cleft lip and palate repair.

The technical achievements of craniofacial surgery are now being applied to victims of the severest facial trauma, and also to aesthetic surgery patients who can benefit from facial bone contouring.

Section 65.9 • Hand surgery

As with all reconstructive surgery a multidisciplinary approach is often employed for optimal recovery of form and function in hand surgery. Plastic surgeons, orthopaedic surgeons, occupational, rehabilitative and pain specialists all play an important role in the care and management of the hand injured patient.

A thorough discussion of hand reconstruction is beyond the scope of this brief chapter. The hand is a source of fascination for any surgeon who respects its anatomical efficiency. Yet, the inherent biology of the inflammatory and repair processes often gets in the way of reversing the effects of trauma or degenerative disease on hand function.

Hands suffer predictable patterns of accidental injury: skin avulsion, lacerated tendons, burns and even amputation. The principles of resurfacing a hand wound are not very different from other deficit wounds. The challenge of tendon repair is maintenance of gliding function. The trend has been in the direction of early repair and motion.

Replantation of amputated parts has become quite commonplace in microsurgical practice. However, the biological limitations of incomplete nerve regeneration compromise the final functional result, despite a technically perfect procedure. Replantations in the upper arm have not reliably provided return of ulnar function to the intrinsic muscles of the hand. The decision to undergo replantation must weigh the factors of the patient's general health, the degree of local trauma and contamination, and realistic prediction of the functional outcome. In recent years transplantation of the upper extremity has been performed by several centres. It is too early to predict the long-term cost, benefits and results.

Degenerative disease can severely impact hand function. Compression of the median nerve as it courses through the carpal tunnel may result in a weakened grasp, altered sensation and eventually atrophy to the thenar musculature. The diagnosis is usually established clinically often with the help of nerve conduction and electromyographic studies. If conservative management fails, surgical release of the carpal tunnel is indicated. Open and endoscopic techniques have been devised for median nerve release.

Dupuytren's disease leads to contraction and thickening of the palmar fascia and overlying skin, and flexor contraction of digits. It is most common among those of Celtic descent. The time of intervention varies, but once 30° of flexion exists at the metacarpo-phalangeal joint, release is indicated. Early release of digital contractures is indicated because these deficits can be more difficult to correct once advanced. Surgical management varies from limited fasciotomy to complete fascia/skin excision of the palm with grafting. The minor procedures have high recurrence rates and low morbidity. Conversely, major resection has lower recurrence, but increased complication rates.

Countless neoplasms, mostly benign, appear on the hand. Some are stable and insensitive and can be ignored. Others are progressive and painful. The common ganglion cyst appears most frequently on the extensor surface of the wrist, sometimes also on the flexor side. These should be excised rather than purposefully ruptured by force. The glomus tumour derived from thermoregulatory and neurovascular tissue is characteristically painful. Rarely, a skin carcinoma will appear on the dorsal skin, or a melanosarcoma within a nailbed.

Young hands can suffer developmental errors: duplications, inappropriate union of digits (syndactyly), angulation (clinodactyly), absence of parts or misshapen parts such as short fingers (brachydactyly). Many congenital hand deformities are surgically correctable. The trend today is towards earlier repair.

Section 65.10 • Breast reconstructive surgery

Breast cancer is the most common form of cancer in women. In the USA, there is a one in eight general lifetime risk for the disease with approximately 140 000 new cases expected in 1 year alone. The mainstay of treatment remains surgical. Breast reconstructive surgery does not affect disease free survival and for many patients the restoration of normal body contours significantly improves physical and psychosocial recovery. As a result, reconstruction of the breast has become a very important part in the treatment of breast cancer (Figure 61.16).

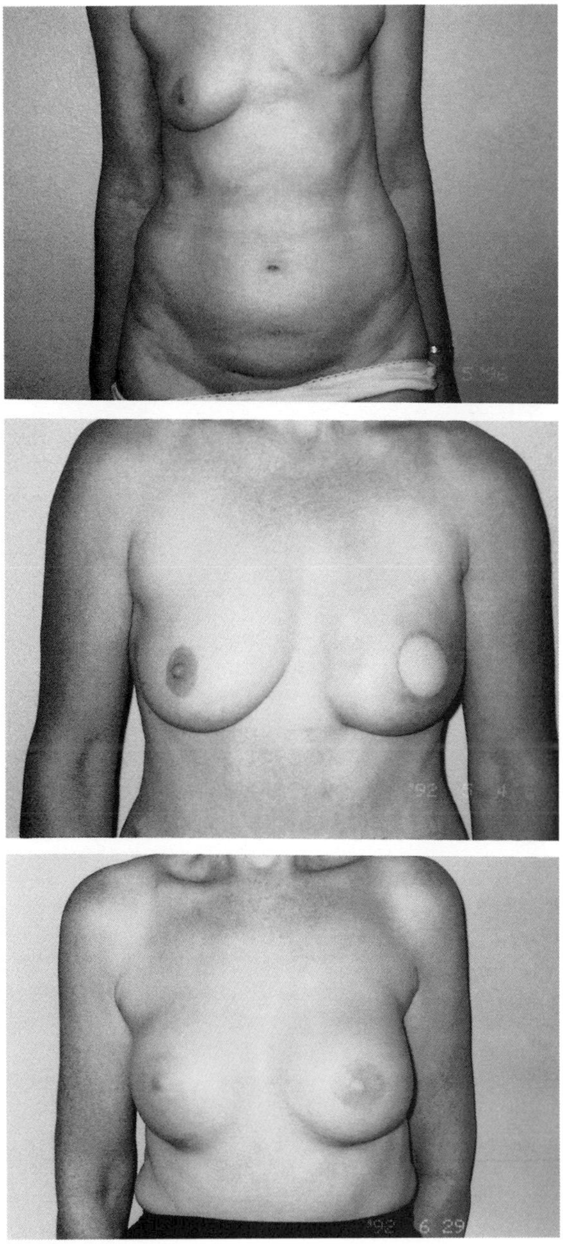

Figure 65.17 Breast reconstruction.

In the appropriate candidate, options include the use of autologous and non-autologous tissues in the reconstruction of the breast. The TRAM (transverse rectus abdominis myocutaneous) flap employs the abdominal pannus either as a pedicled flap or alternatively as a free microvascular transfer. Latissimus muscle based flaps as well as gluteal and peri-iliac fat pad flaps are also commonly used. Non-autologous options include the placement of tissue expanders followed by the placement of permanent prostheses under the remaining muscle and soft tissue.

Candidates for breast reconstruction must first of all desire breast reconstruction surgery. They must be healthy enough to tolerate the added surgical procedures; usually several stages are involved. The cancer must be controlled.

Section 65.11 • The future

This is a very exciting time in the field of plastic and reconstructive surgery. The development of new and expanding techniques in medicine, surgery and rehabilitation pose ever increasing challenges to the reconstructive surgeon. Neonates are operated on *in utero*, people are living longer and experiencing more active lives. Our understanding of the anatomical and pathophysiological processes involved in tumours, wounds, flaps and ageing along with the technological advances in biosynthesis and biotechnology hold great promise for the future.

Further reading

Bhisragratna, K. K. (1907). *The Sushruta Sanhita*. An English translation base on the original Sanscrit text. Calcutta.

Janzekovic Z. A. (1970). New concept in the early excision and immediate grafting of burns. *J Trauma* **10**: 1103–8.

Index

Visual glossary: Leaves

Structure of a leaf

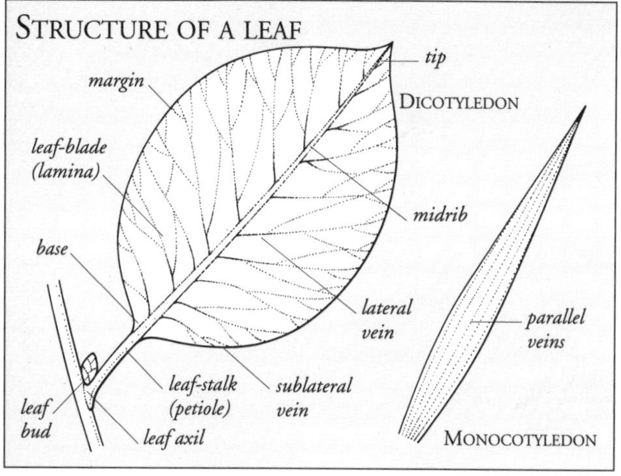

Arrangements

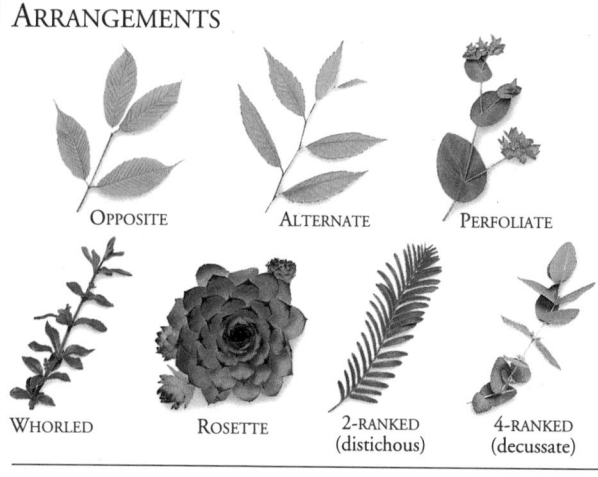

Coniferous leaves

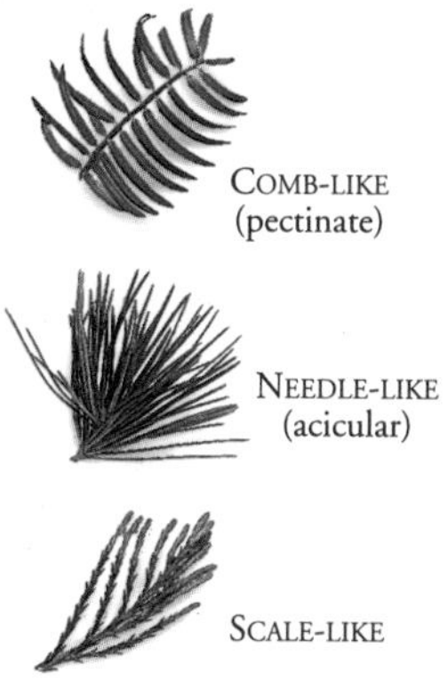

Lobing and division

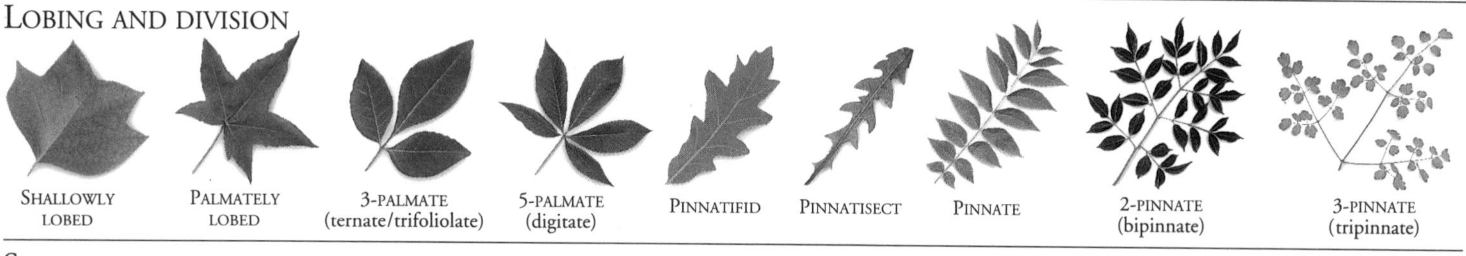

Shapes

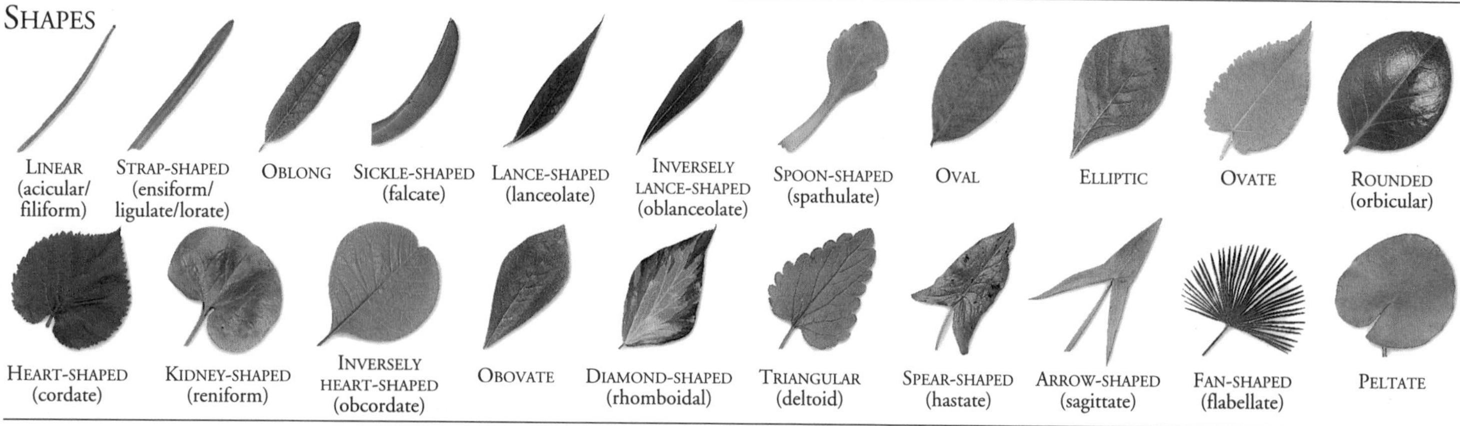

Margins

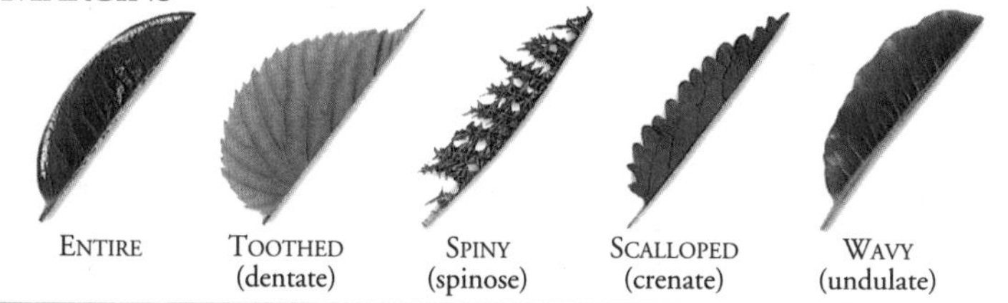

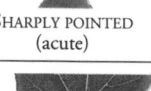

Tips

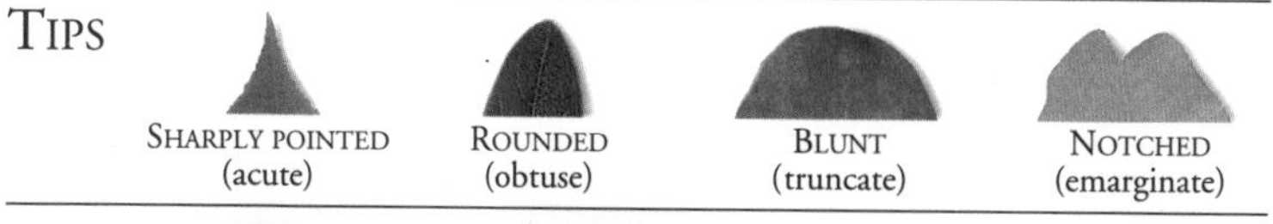

Bases

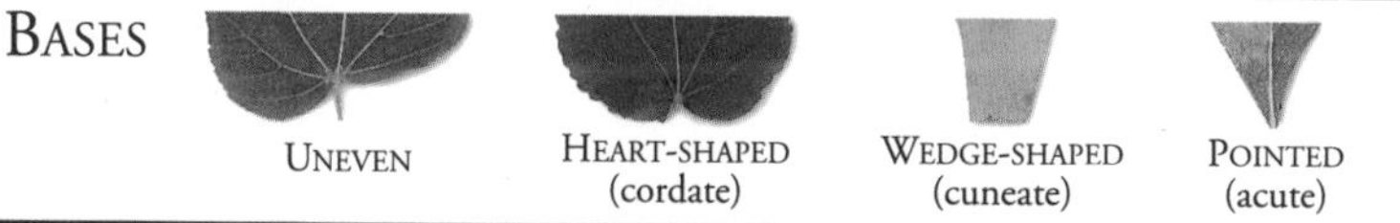

Key to symbols

Miscellaneous	Plant dimensions	Tree shapes		
Cross-reference	Typical height	Rounded to broadly spreading	Broadly conical	Small weeping
Plant is pictured (on same page as entry or facing page)	Typical spread	Rounded to broadly columnar	Narrowly conical	Single-stemmed palm, cycad, or similar tree
Plant has received the RHS Award of Garden Merit	Typical height and spread (if the same)	Broadly columnar	Narrowly conical (flame-shaped)	Multi-stemmed palm, cycad, or similar tree
		Narrowly columnar	Large weeping	

Hardiness ratings

Frost tender: plant may be damaged by temperatures below 5°C (41°F)	Half hardy: plant can withstand temperatures down to 0°C (32°F)	Frost hardy: plant can withstand temperatures down to -5°C (23°F)	Fully hardy: plant can withstand temperatures down to -15°C (5°F)

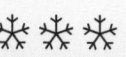

THE ROYAL HORTICULTURAL SOCIETY

A-Z ENCYCLOPEDIA of GARDEN PLANTS

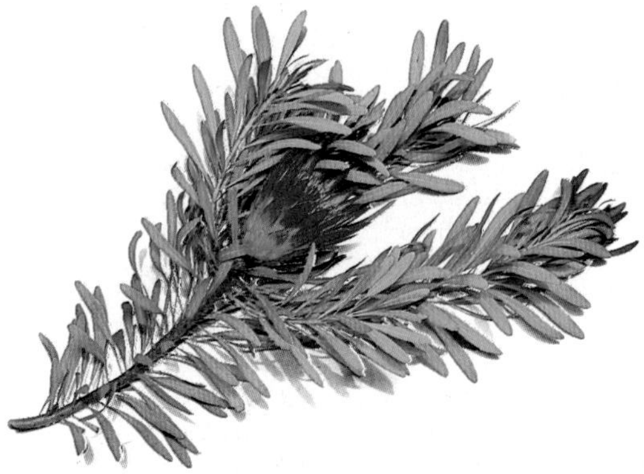

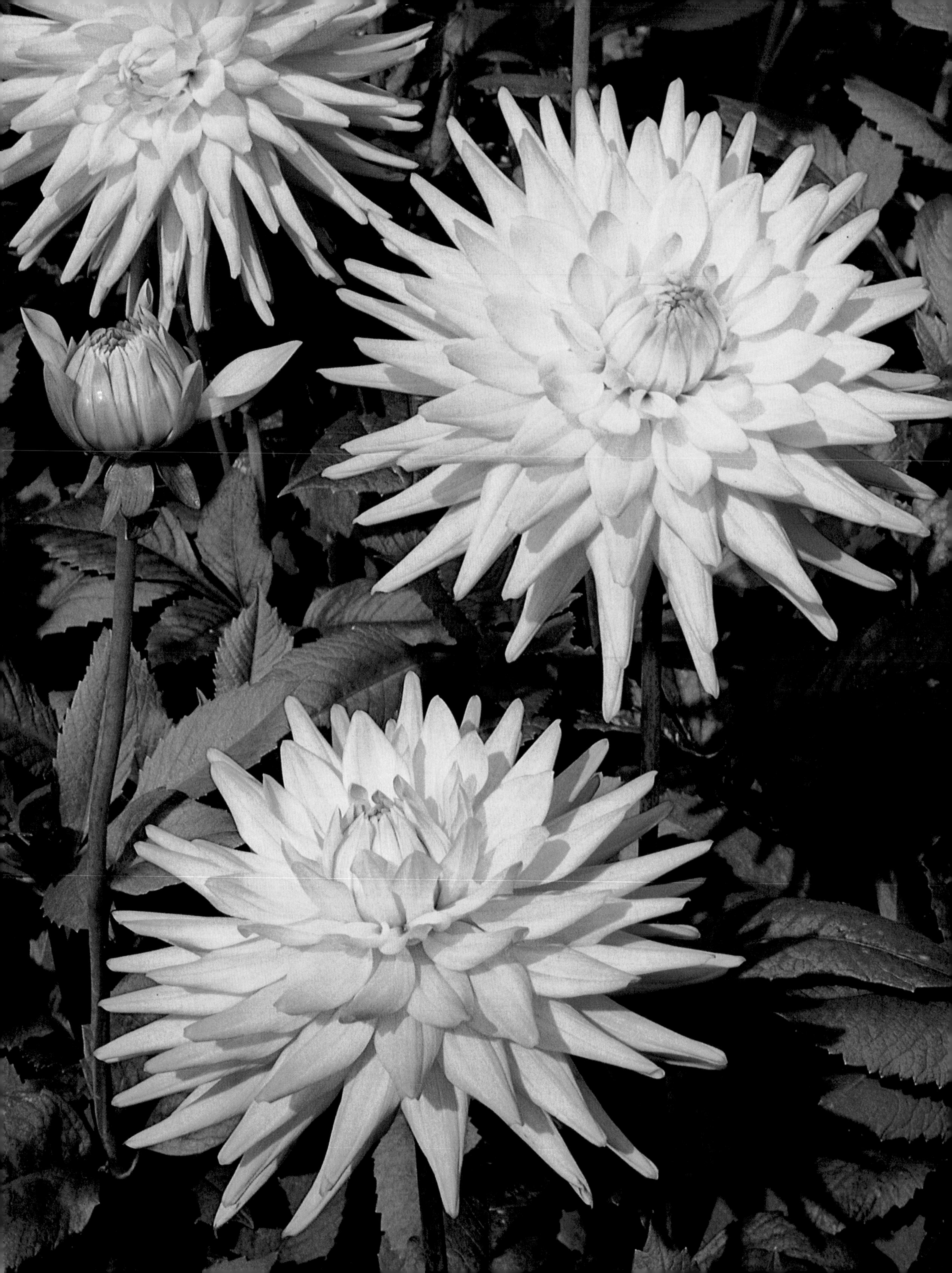

THE ROYAL HORTICULTURAL SOCIETY

A-Z ENCYCLOPEDIA of GARDEN PLANTS

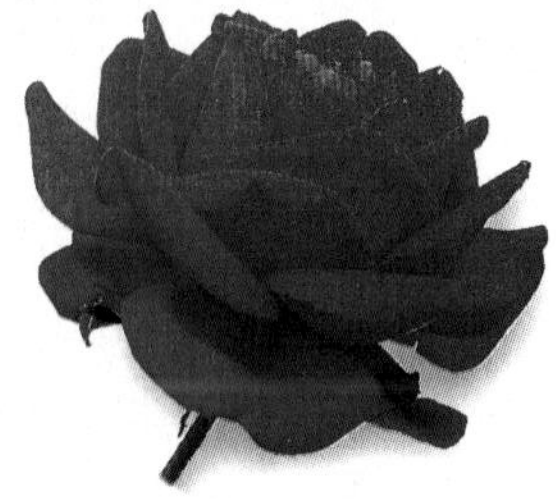

CHRISTOPHER BRICKELL
Editor-in-Chief

DORLING KINDERSLEY
London • New York • Stuttgart • Moscow

A DORLING KINDERSLEY BOOK

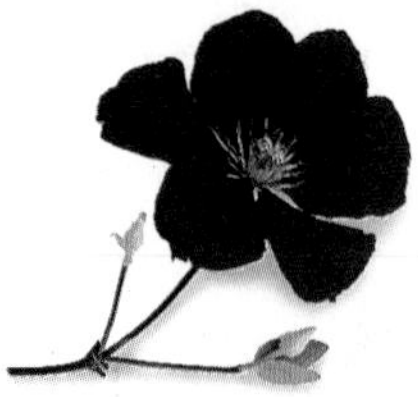

IMPORTANT NOTICE

This encyclopedia follows Royal Horticultural Society guidelines on potentially hazardous plants, although the properties of many garden plants have yet to be fully evaluated. Where a plant is known to have potentially harmful properties, a warning has been included in the appropriate alphabetical entry. However, any plant substance has the potential to cause an allergic reaction in some people, so due caution should be exercised when handling plants.

MANAGING EDITOR Jonathan Metcalf
SENIOR ART EDITORS Peter Cross, Ina Stradins

EDITORS Polly Boyd, Monica Byles, Anna Cheifetz, Joanna Chisholm, Alison Copland, Clare Double, Peter Frances, Angeles Gavira, Richard Hammond, Maggie O'Hanlon, Lin Hawthorne, Sally Paxton, Lesley Riley, Harriet Stewart-Jones, Jo Weeks, Tony Whitehorn, Sarah Widdicombe, Fiona Wild
ART EDITORS Pauline Clarke, Elaine Hewson, Kate Poole, Helen Robson, Helen Taylor

PROOFREADING AND INDEXING Marion Dent, Ilse Gray, Jane Parker
DESIGN ASSISTANTS Robert Campbell, Murdo Culver
ADMINISTRATIVE SUPPORT Susila Baybars, Ian Hambleton, Paula Hardy, Simon Maughan, Paul Rundle

PRODUCTION CONTROLLER Michelle Thomas
PRODUCTION ASSISTANT Hélène Lamassoure
DTP MANAGER Mark Bracey

CULTIVATION EDITORS Cathy Buchanan, Lin Hawthorne, Andrew Mikolajski
HORTICULTURAL ADVISORS Peter Barnes, Sabina Knees, Nigel Rowland
PICTURE RESEARCHERS Denise Greig, Emily Hedges, Dr Alan Hemsley
ILLUSTRATORS Karen Cochrane, Martine Collings, Gill Tomblin

SENIOR MANAGING EDITOR Mary-Clare Jerram
MANAGING ART EDITOR Amanda Lunn

EDITORIAL DIRECTOR Jackie Douglas
ART DIRECTOR Peter Luff

First edition published in Great Britain in 1996 by
Dorling Kindersley Limited, 9 Henrietta Street, London WC2 8PS

Visit us on the World Wide Web at http://www.dk.com

A CIP catalogue record for this book is available from the British Library

ISBN 0-7513-0303-8

Text film output by The R & B Group, Isleworth, Middx., UK
Colour reproduction by G.R.B. Editrice, Verona, Italy
Printed and bound in Germany by Mohndruck GmbH, Gütersloh

Frontispiece: *Dahlia* 'Wootton Impact'

CONTENTS

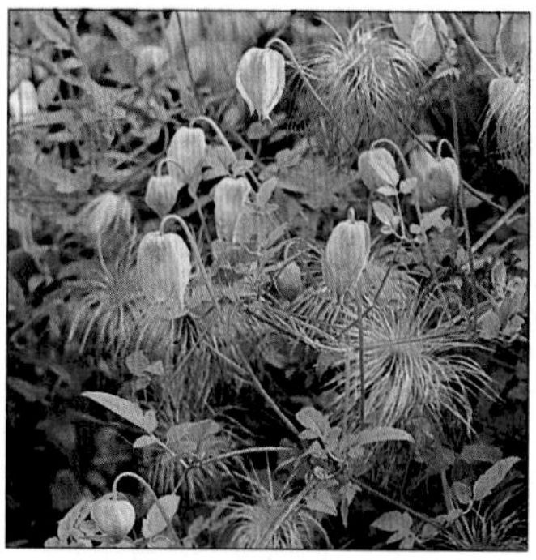

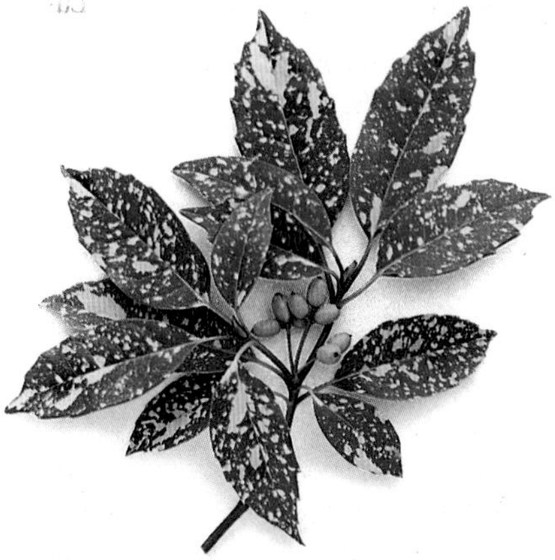

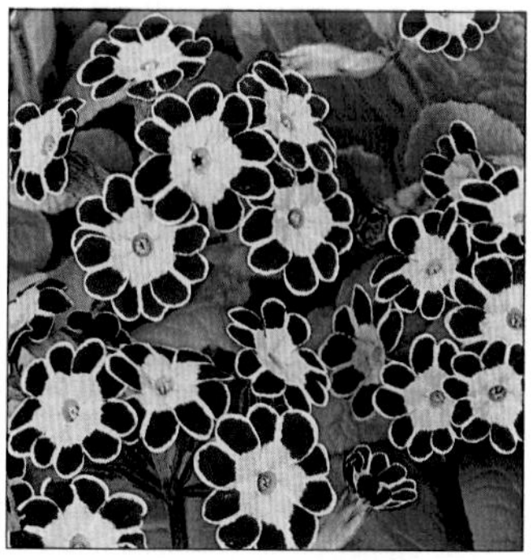

Editor-in-Chief

Christopher Brickell

CBE, BSc (Hort), FInstHort, VMH

Former Director General, The Royal Horticultural Society
Chairman, International Commission for the Nomenclature of Cultivated Plants

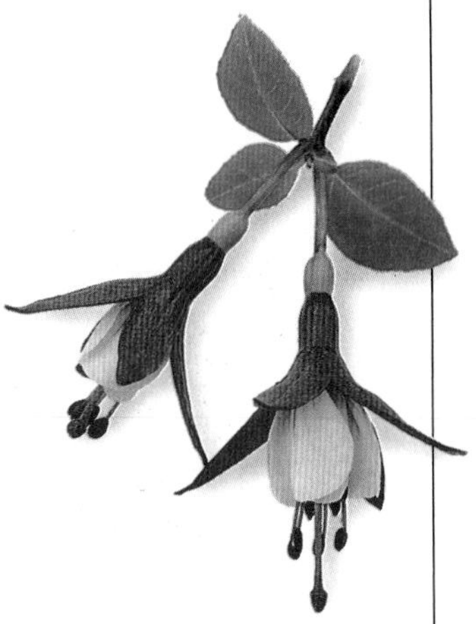

Contributors and Consultants

Susyn Andrews

George Argent

Roger S. Aylett
FIHort

David G. Barker
BSc

Larry Barlow

Peter Barnes

George Bartlett

Kenneth A. Beckett
VMM

Jeffrey Brande

Cathy Buchanan
MA, DipHort (Kew), MIHort

David Burnie

Brian Burrow

Eric Catterall

Roy Cheek
MHort (RHS), FIHort

Ian Cooke
MHort (RHS)

Allen J. Coombes

Jack Elliott
VMH

Raymond J. Evison
VMH

John & Eileen Galbally

Richard W. Gilbert

Pippa Greenwood
BSc, MSc

Diana Grenfell

Dr Christopher Grey-Wilson
BSc (Hort)

Dr Patricia Griggs

Peter Harkness
DHM

Lin Hawthorne

Tony Hender

Peter Hovenkamp

Clive Innes
VMH

Clive Jermy

Hazel Key

Sabina G. Knees
BSc, MSc

W.A. Lord

Brian Mathew
VMH

Peter R. Maynard

Margaret E. McKendrick

Tim Miles
MIHort

Jim Pearce

Martin Rickard
BSc (Botany)

Wilma Rittershausen

Peter Robinson
MHort (RHS), FIHort, DipHort (Edin)

Peter Q. Rose
MHort, FLS, MIHort

Keith Rushforth

Tony Schilling
MArb, FIHort, FLS, VMH

Christine Skelmersdale

David Small

Arthur Smith

Joyce Stewart
MSc, FIHort, FLS

Nigel Taylor

David Trehane
BSc (Hort)

Ray Waite

Dr Trevor G. Walker
DSc

Photographers

Clive Boursnell

Deni Bown

Jonathan Buckley

Andrew Butler

Eric Crichton

Christine M. Douglas

John Fielding

Neil Fletcher

John Glover

Jerry Harpur

Sunniva Harte

C. Andrew Henley

Andrew Lawson

Andrew de Lory

Howard Rice

Bob Rundle

Juliette Wade

Matthew Ward

Dave Watts

Steven Wooster

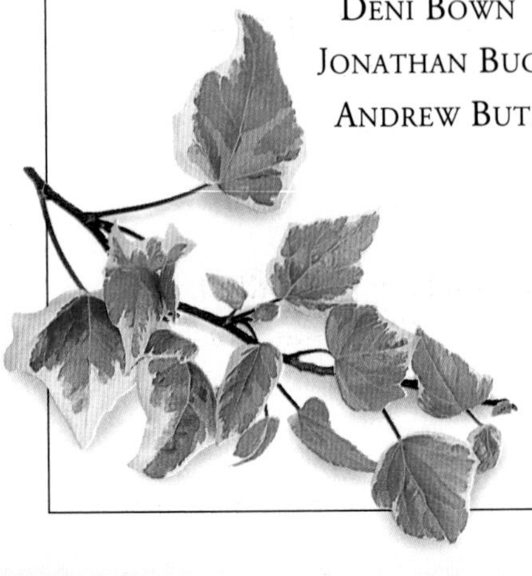

FOREWORD

THE FOURTH IN A SERIES of encyclopedias published by Dorling Kindersley in association with the Royal Horticultural Society, *The RHS A–Z Encyclopedia of Garden Plants* is the third on which I have acted as Editor-in-Chief. It is, I believe, a unique work, being extremely comprehensive in its coverage and authoritative in its approach, but nonetheless accessible to all gardeners. Complementary to the remarkably successful *RHS Gardeners' Encyclopedia of Plants & Flowers*, in which some 8,000 plants are arranged by plant type, this new encyclopedia provides detailed descriptions of over 15,000 ornamental garden plants in alphabetical order, using the most up-to-date botanical names, and with thousands of synonyms and common names exhaustively cross-referenced throughout. With more than 6,000 colour photographs closely integrated with the text profiles, it is undoubtedly a landmark in contemporary garden reference.

Great care has been taken in the preparation of this encyclopedia to include as broad a range of ornamental plants as possible, satisfying not only traditional tastes but also inspiring new ideas and approaches. To that end, many half-hardy and tender plants are featured, from delicate orchids to exotic palms and tree ferns, together with some of the most outstanding recent introductions – many bearing the Royal Horticultural Society's own Award of Garden Merit. The selection of species and cultivars in each category, from annuals to garden trees, was made in each case by a gardener or horticulturist with current and direct experience of those plants. In short, therefore, all of the plants presented here, although very varied in origin, type, and habit, and with a wide range of cultivation requirements, are fully deserving of their place in any garden, greenhouse, conservatory, or home.

Equally as important as the range of plants covered is the depth, consistency, and accuracy with which they are described. Drawing on the combined contributions of over 40 of the most distinguished plantsmen and plantswomen worldwide, every plant is described in clear and precise terms, with information necessary for identification and comparison, including diagnostic measurements where appropriate, uniformly presented. Concise introductions to each genus provide background detail on native habitat, hardiness, ornamental features, and where to grow in the garden, and offer unambiguous advice on cultivation, pruning, propagation, and pests and diseases. The entire text has been painstakingly formatted and verified by a dedicated team at both Dorling Kindersley and the Royal Horticultural Society, and its accessibility and authority are further enhanced by the thorough introduction and glossary, the illustrated plant anatomy key on the inside front cover, and of course by the superb pictures, the work of some of our finest gardening photographers.

Immense patience and meticulous attention to detail have been required from all involved, and I am very grateful for the untiring efforts of Jonathan Metcalf, the Managing Editor, and his team, without whom a work of this magnitude and complexity could not have been achieved.

The RHS A–Z Encyclopedia of Garden Plants continues the very long tradition of the Royal Horticultural Society in producing publications of excellence to help, advise, and instruct gardeners, not only in the UK but also in many other parts of the world. It will, I hope, inspire new generations to cultivate some of the vast range of ornamental plants now available to us, and serve as a reliable and comprehensive source of reference to those already practised in this most fascinating of arts, gardening.

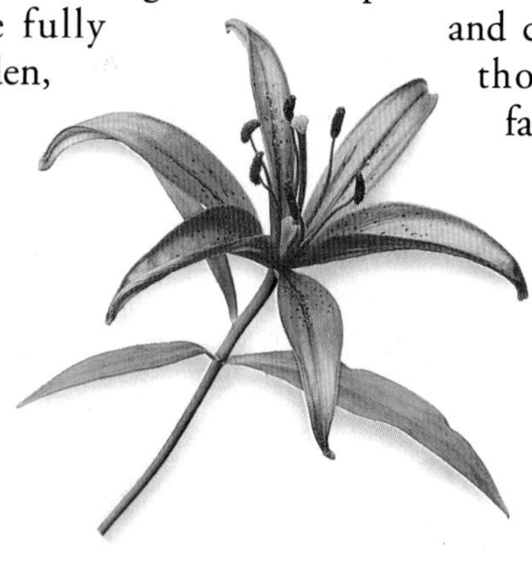

CHRISTOPHER BRICKELL
Editor-in-Chief

How to use the encyclopedia

The encyclopedia is arranged in three main sections: an introduction to gardening; the A–Z plant directory itself, in which over 15,000 garden plants are listed by their current botanical names, within genus entries; and a full glossary. An index of topics found in the introduction appears on p.1080, and both endpapers feature a visual key to terms and concepts used in the plant entries. Common names and synonyms are cross-referenced in alphabetical order throughout the plant directory. Many plants listed have received the Royal Horticultural Society's prestigious Award of Garden Merit (AGM), which recognizes plants of outstanding quality, both in appearance and all-round garden performance, whether grown outdoors or under glass.

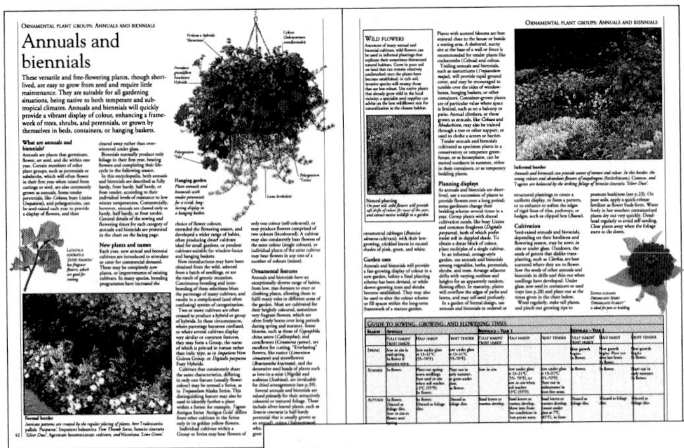

Introduction

Illustrated features outline the key elements of gardening, including plant classification and anatomy, outdoor and under-glass cultivation, propagation, and pruning, and provide a concise introduction to each of the major ornamental plant categories, from trees to tender ferns.

PAGE HEADINGS

Left-hand headings name the first genus described on the page (either continued from the previous page or a new entry); right-hand headings name the last genus on the page.

PHOTOGRAPHS

Plant portraits appear in alphabetical order within the genus text, and illustrate different growth habits and ornamental features, as appropriate.

ARTWORKS

Distinctive or complex features of larger genera, such as variations in flower and leaf form, are illustrated and labelled for clearer understanding.

CLOSE-UP DETAIL

Inset photographs show ornamental features with greater clarity.

MARGINAL MARKERS

Coloured tabs move down the margin with the alphabet, for quick location of the letter required.

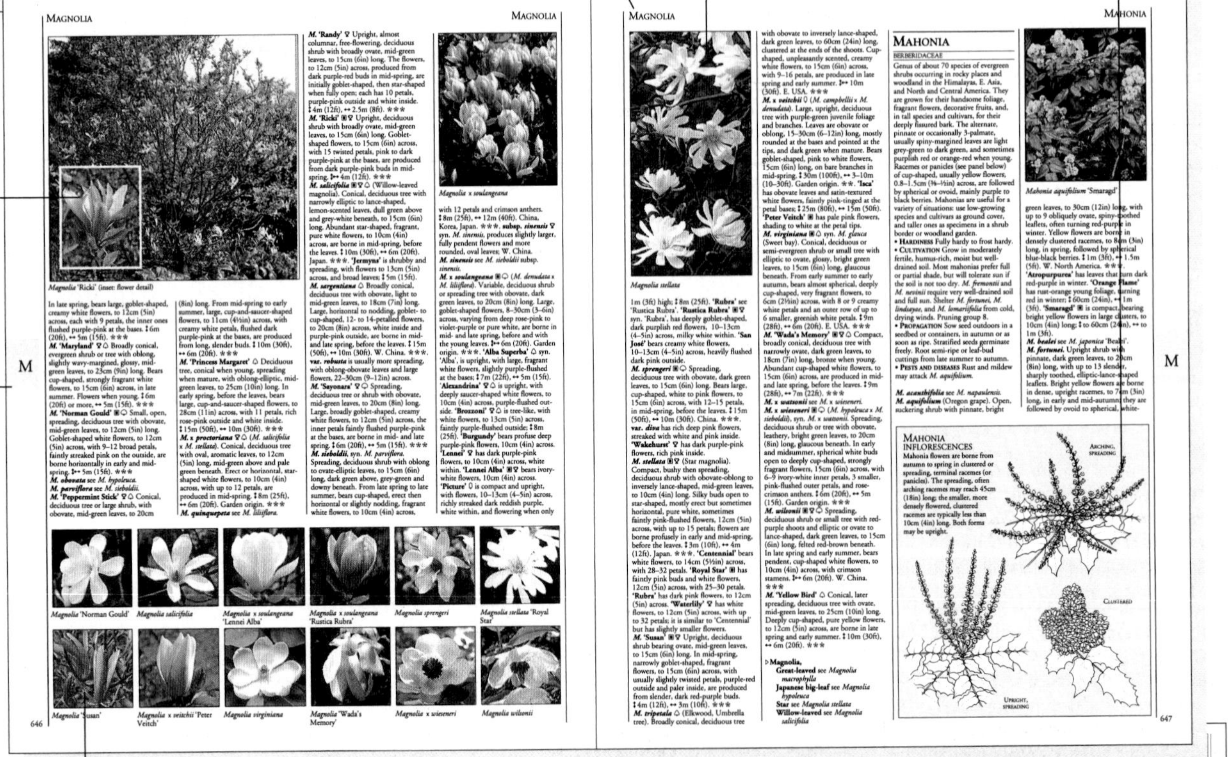

A–Z plant directory

All plants are arranged in alphabetical order within a genus entry, which consists of a short introduction followed by individual plant descriptions. Pictures appear within their relevant text; common names and synonyms are cross-referenced.

FEATURE PANELS

Close-up views of leaves or flowers may be grouped within major genera, allowing differences in form, colour, or markings to be seen clearly. Panels read alphabetically from left to right.

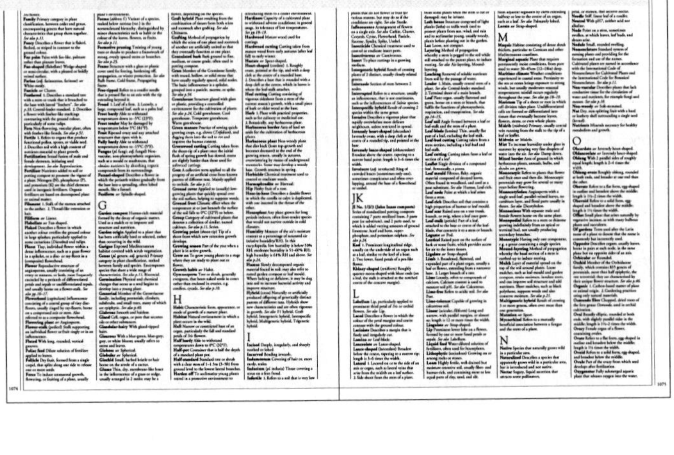

Glossary

All horticultural and botanical terms used in the encyclopedia, as well as other terms used in gardening, are defined here. Some are cross-referenced to related topics in the glossary and the introduction.

Endpapers

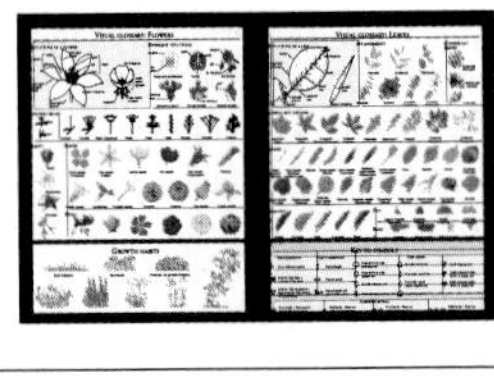

Quick-reference, visual glossaries to terms and concepts used in the plant entries appear on both front and back endpapers.

THE GENUS ENTRY

All plants in the A–Z directory are described within a genus entry, the genus being a grouping of one or more species with similar characteristics (see p.11). Each entry includes an introduction to the entire genus, outlining its composition and extent, and the salient features of plants within it. Where information is common to all plants in the genus, it may be presented here but omitted from each individual plant entry. Sections on hardiness, cultivation, propagation, and pests and diseases appear after the introduction, the advice given being applicable to all cultivated plants in the genus. Individual plant entries follow, under their own bold headings. Variants and cultivars of a species are presented under the main plant entry; only characteristics that distinguish them from the species are described. In all entries, perennials are assumed to be deciduous, and leaves simple and mid-green, unless otherwise stated. All measurements are rounded, for ease of use.

CROSS-REFERENCES
Common names are cross-referenced in alphabetical order, between genus entries; they are prefaced by the ▷ symbol. Many are inverted (e.g. Mulberry, Red) for more logical access. Synonyms may be cross-referenced between genera, as for common names, or within a genus entry. Cross-references to synonyms of variants and cultivars within a species are included where appropriate.

GARDEN USE
Suitable sites for planting are suggested, either in the garden or, where applicable, under glass (see p.24 for definitions of the various greenhouse categories). Additional information on subjects such as attractiveness to wildlife, herbal uses, or potentially harmful qualities may also be included.

HARDINESS
The resistance to cold of all cultivated plants in the genus is defined here, sometimes as a range (see also pp.18–19).

PROPAGATION
Precise details of propagation techniques set out the most appropriate ways of increasing stock, including any special requirements.

SYMBOLS
Located after the plant name, symbols indicate that the plant is pictured on that page or the facing page (■), or that it has received the RHS Award of Garden Merit (🏆). A range of symbols, such as △, are used to indicate the habits of trees, palms, cycads, and tree-like shrubs (see key right).

INDIVIDUAL PLANT ENTRY
Each entry begins with the botanical name, in bold type, with the genus name abbreviated. Most entries include a description of habit, leaf and flower characteristics, and other ornamental features, such as fruits, as appropriate.

GEOGRAPHICAL ORIGIN
The country or region from which the plant originates appears after the plant dimensions. "Garden origin" indicates that an interspecific hybrid has been artificially selected, rather than occurring naturally in the wild.

VARIANTS AND CULTIVARS
Subspecies, forma, varietas, and cultivar descriptions follow on from the main plant entry. Their names appear in bold type, without the generic name or species epithet, and with "subsp.", "f.", and "var." disregarded for purposes of alphabetization. Only those characteristics that distinguish them from the species are described, including height and spread, hardiness, and geographical origin.

PICTURE CAPTION
Plants are identified by their full botanical names.

▷**Hyssop** see *Hyssopus, H. officinalis*
Anise see *Agastache foeniculum*

HYSSOPUS
Hyssop
LABIATAE/LAMIACEAE

Genus of about 5 often variable species of aromatic herbaceous perennials and evergreen or semi-evergreen shrubs, occurring in dry, sandy, and rocky sites from the Mediterranean to C. Asia. The linear to lance-shaped, ovate, or oblong leaves are mid- or blue-green. Tubular, violet-blue to pink flowers are borne in whorls on narrow, spike-like, terminal inflorescences. *H. officinalis* and its cultivars are grown for their aromatic foliage and flowers, and are excellent for a rock garden or herb garden. They are also suitable for low hedging, and for growing at the base of a warm, sunny wall or in containers. The flowers are attractive to bees and butterflies; the foliage has culinary and medicinal uses.
• **HARDINESS** Fully hardy.
• **CULTIVATION** Grow in fertile, well-drained, neutral to alkaline soil in full sun. Pruning group 10, in mid-spring.
• **PROPAGATION** Sow seed in containers in a cold frame in autumn. Root softwood cuttings in summer.
• **PESTS AND DISEASES** Trouble free.

H. officinalis ■ (Hyssop). Dwarf, semi-evergreen, aromatic shrub with erect shoots and linear to narrowly lance-shaped, or oblong, mid-green leaves, to 5cm (2in) long. Slender spikes of whorled, funnel-shaped, 2-lipped, dark blue flowers, 1.5cm (½in) long, are produced from midsummer to early autumn. ↕60cm (24in), ↔1m (3ft). S. Europe. ❄❄❄. **f. *albus*** has white flowers. **subsp. *aristatus*** has a dense, upright habit, and produces bright green leaves. **f. *roseus*** has pink flowers.

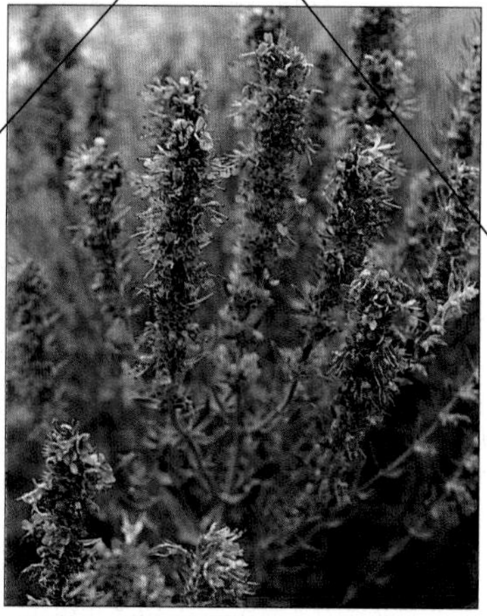
Hyssopus officinalis

GENUS HEADING
The botanical genus name is followed by any common names or synonyms for the genus. Synonyms only apply where one genus has been completely "sunk" into another.

FAMILY NAME
The botanical family to which the genus belongs appears after the genus heading. Where opinion differs, more than one name may be listed, in alphabetical order.

GENUS INTRODUCTION
A broad description of the genus includes the number of species, plant categories, native habitat, geographical origin, and main characteristics of plants in the genus.

CULTIVATION
Care requirements are given for all cultivated plants in the genus. Pruning advice (for woody plants) refers to one of the 13 groups described on pp.26–27. For tender plants, suggestions for growing both outdoors and "under glass" (which may be in a greenhouse, alpine house, conservatory, or indoors) are included.

PESTS AND DISEASES
The pests, diseases, and disorders most likely to afflict plants in the genus are listed. "Trouble free" means the genus has no specific problems.

ALTERNATIVE NAMES
Common names and synonyms are listed directly after the plant name and any symbols. Parents of hybrids, where known, appear in parentheses. Synonyms are prefaced by "syn.".

HEIGHT AND SPREAD
Unless otherwise specified, height (↕) and spread (↔) are for typical mature plants, cultivated in an appropriate site. Where height and spread are the same, only one measurement is given, after the combined symbol (↕↔). Where appropriate, height is of the plant in flower. Container-grown plants may be smaller than the dimensions given. For bulbous plants, ↔ can be used as a guide to planting distance. Height is not given for floating or submerged aquatic plants; spread is not given for climbers.

HARDINESS RATING
Each full plant description is accompanied by a hardiness rating (see key right). A minimum temperature for successful cultivation is also given for tender plants; individual plants may be able to withstand night temperatures slightly lower than this, depending on local conditions and the maturity and health of the plant. Entries for tender orchids include both a minimum and a maximum temperature that will be tolerated. See also pp.18–19.

HAZARDOUS PLANTS

The majority of garden plants are safe to grow and handle. However, any plant substance is capable of causing an allergic reaction in some people, either through contact or ingestion, so care should always be taken. Warnings are included in the encyclopedia for plants known to have potentially harmful properties, but many plants have yet to be scientifically screened.

Children and animals are most at risk, as they are often attracted to brightly coloured fruits and seed pods, which may cause stomach upset if ingested. Gardeners may also come into contact with plants whose foliage or sap may irritate skin, aggravate allergies, or cause photodermatitis (severe sensitivity to sunlight). The reaction is not always immediate, and may include itching, redness, or blistering.

If an adverse reaction to a plant occurs, seek immediate medical help, and take a sample of the plant for examination. Do not force the affected person to vomit.

KEY TO SYMBOLS

▷ Cross-reference
🏆 Plant has received the RHS Award of Garden Merit
■ Plant is pictured (on same page as entry or facing page)

HARDINESS RATINGS

Frost tender: plant may be damaged by temperatures below 5°C (41°F). The minimum temperature (min.) for cultivation appears after the symbol
❄ Half hardy: plant can withstand temperatures down to 0°C (32°F)
❄❄ Frost hardy: plant can withstand temperatures down to -5°C (23°F)
❄❄❄ Fully hardy: plant can withstand temperatures down to -15°C (5°F)

PLANT DIMENSIONS

↕ Typical height
↔ Typical spread
↕↔ Typical height and spread (if the same)

TREE SHAPES

Rounded to broadly spreading
Rounded to broadly columnar
Broadly columnar
Narrowly columnar
Broadly conical
Narrowly conical
Narrowly conical (flame-shaped)
Large weeping
Small weeping
Single-stemmed palm, cycad, or similar tree
Multi-stemmed palm, cycad, or similar tree

The plant kingdom

Plants constitute one of the five kingdoms that are used to classify all living organisms. The plant kingdom, Plantae, is divided into progressively smaller groups according to shared botanical characteristics, usually represented as a family tree. The first, most basic division is between vascular and non-vascular plants. It is the vascular plants that are of interest to gardeners.

Non-vascular and vascular

Primitive, non-vascular plants, such as fungi, liverworts, and mosses, lack conductive tissue for the circulation of water and nutrients, and are thus confined to a moist environment. Widespread in the wild, their small size and relatively dull appearance render them of limited value in gardens. Vascular plants, on the other hand, which include both flowering and non-flowering plants, are very diverse, the adaptability of their root and shoot systems (see pp.12–13) having enabled them to thrive in many habitats. Although some, such as ferns, reproduce by means of spores, like non-vascular plants, the vast majority (over 250,000 species) reproduce by means of seeds.

Seed-bearing plants

Vascular plants that bear seed are divided into gymnosperms (literally "naked seed") and angiosperms ("covered seed"). Gymnosperms produce seed that is only partly enclosed by tissues from the parent plant. Conifers, which normally bear seed on the scales of cones, form the largest family, containing some 550 species. Many, such as cedars (*Cedrus*) and yews (*Taxus*), are very tolerant of heat, cold, or drought, and are therefore of great horticultural importance. Other gymnosperms in cultivation include cycads and ginkgos.

Angiosperms (usually referred to as flowering plants) produce seed in an ovary – a protective chamber that forms part of the fruit when seeds ripen, and often aids in their dispersal (see pp.13, 16). Flowering plants consist of 300 families, containing some 250,000 species. They are further defined as monocotyledons or dicotyledons, according to their seed-leaves (cotyledons) and other differences in their anatomy and growth patterns (see panel below).

Life-span

Flowering plants can also be categorized by life-span as annuals, biennials, or perennials. Annuals complete their life-cycle within a single season of growth. Biennials live for two seasons, most producing only foliage and amassing food reserves in the first year, then flowering, fruiting, and dying in the next. Perennials thrive for several or many seasons, most flowering annually, once established.

In cultivation, some perennials that bloom most vigorously in their first year are treated as annuals or biennials, and are uprooted after flowering. Tender perennials may also be grown for a season, then discarded in autumn in frost-prone climates. Herbaceous, or soft-stemmed perennials die back to ground level each autumn, then become dormant before producing new shoots in spring. Woody perennials, largely trees and shrubs, may also lose their foliage and become dormant, but they retain their stems, which resume growth with the new season.

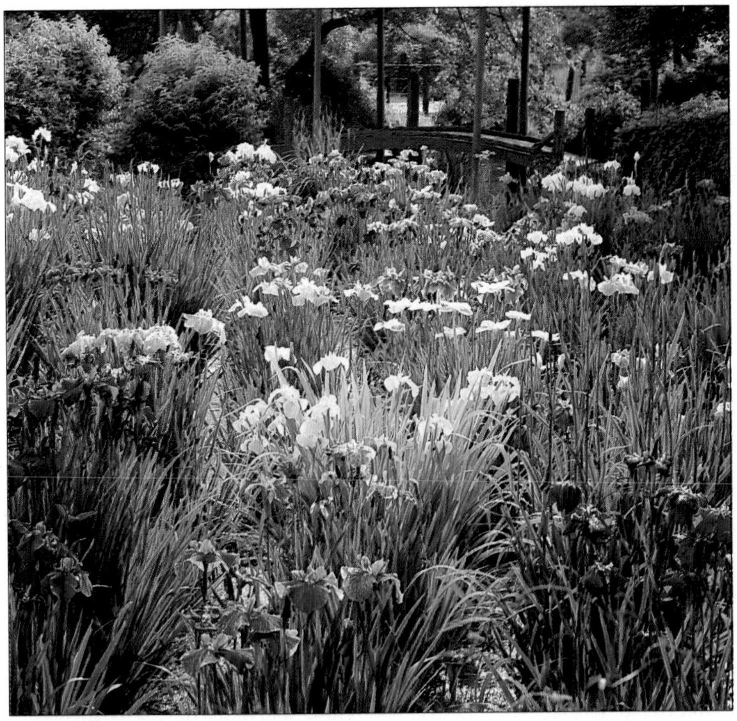

Natural diversity, artificial selection
The ability of vascular plants to adapt to different habitats has brought about a vast range of flowering plants. In this water garden, naturally occurring iris species grow alongside cultivars artificially selected by plant breeders.

MONOCOTS AND DICOTS

All flowering plants are classified either as monocotyledons or dicotyledons (known as monocots and dicots). Monocots have a single seed-leaf (cotyledon), leaves with veins that run parallel to their length, slender, non-woody stems (except in palms), and flower parts arranged in threes. Their modified sepals resemble petals. Dicots have 2 seed-leaves, a network of veins on their foliage, thick or woody stems, and flower parts (enclosed in leaf-like sepals) arranged in multiples of 4, 5, 7, or more. See also pp.14–16.

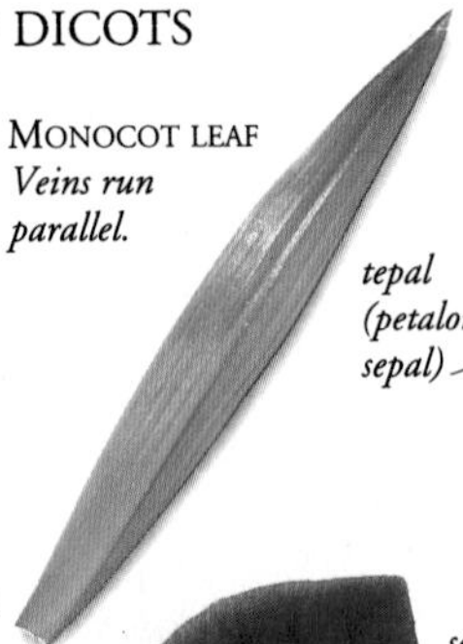

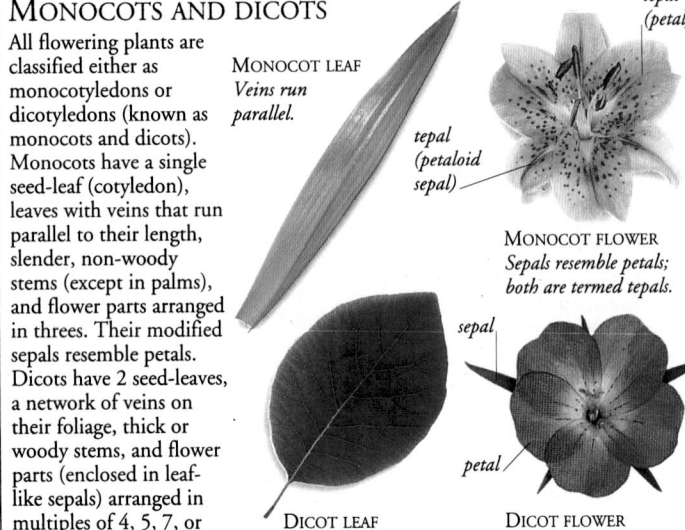

MONOCOT LEAF
Veins run parallel.

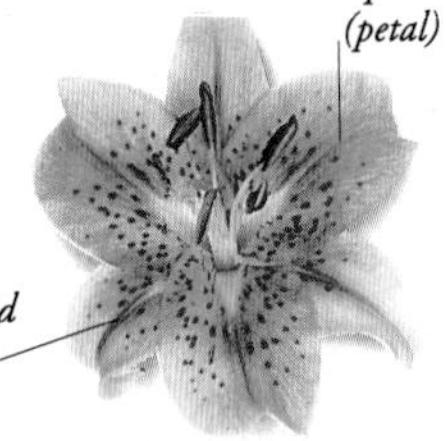

MONOCOT FLOWER
Sepals resemble petals; both are termed tepals.

DICOT LEAF
Veins form a network.

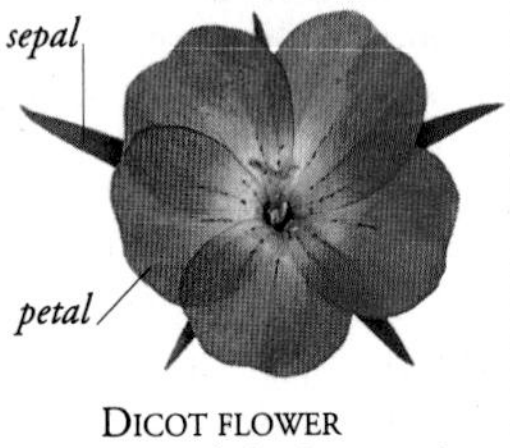

DICOT FLOWER
Petals differ from sepals.

Species, hybrids, and cultivars

In the wild, species are more or less uniform in habit, foliage, flowers, and fruit. Any variation is part of an evolutionary process, and botanists apply subdivisions within a species (subspecies, varietas, and forma) to recognize such differences. A subspecies is a "mini-species" with distinct morphological or genetic variation, and sometimes distinct geographical distribution; a varietas is a wild variety, and its differences from the species are less clear cut; forma is used for colour variants or similar minor differences. All remain more or less stable in the wild, but when grown together in cultivation they may hybridize and the distinctions become blurred.

This variation is exploited by gardeners who select (recognize and name) an individual plant, and

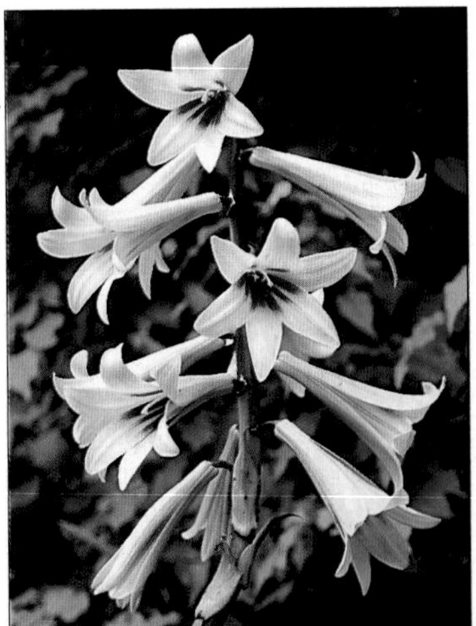

Monocarpic plants
Monocarpic plants, like Cardiocrinum giganteum *var.* yunnanense, *grow for a number of years, flower once, then die.*

PLANT CLASSIFICATION AND NOMENCLATURE

In this encyclopedia, all plants are listed by their up-to-date botanical names (except for a few genera, such as *Chrysanthemum*, where an older name has been preserved for the benefit of gardeners). Botanical names are preferred to common names, as they are recognized internationally and apply to one plant only. They may refer to the person who first collected the plant or to a salient characteristic (e.g. *Gilia tricolor*, named after Felipe Gil, a Spanish botanist, and the Latin for 3-coloured, referring to the flowers).

The basic unit of plant classification is the species, denoted by a binomial (see right). Naturally occurring variants of a species – subspecies, varietas, or forma – are given an additional epithet prefixed by "subsp", "var", or "f". Artificially selected cultivars of a species are given a vernacular name, often by the grower, which appears in single quotation marks after the species name, for example *Calluna vulgaris* 'Firefly'. Some cultivars are also registered with trademark names, which are often used commercially instead of the true cultivar names. Sexual hybrids are denoted by a multiplication sign (for example, *Rosa* x *odorata*), and graft hybrids by a plus sign (+ *Laburnocytisus adamii*). In this encyclopedia, parents of hybrids, where known, are given in brackets after the plant name.

Botanical names do occasionally change, mainly when research reveals a misidentification or an older name that takes precedence, or when plant groups are reclassified. When this occurs, the superseded names become synonyms. In this encyclopedia, these are given directly after the plant name and are cross-referenced. A name appended with "of gardens" indicates that the name is commonly used but misapplied.

Family
Group of one or more genera that share a set of underlying features. Family names usually end in -aceae. The limits of families are often controversial and unclear.

Genus (*pl.* **genera)**
Group of one or more plants that share a wide range of characteristics. Names are printed in italic type with an initial capital letter. Hybrid genera are denoted by a multiplication sign before the genus.

Species
Group of plants that are capable of breeding together to produce offspring similar to themselves. Species are given a two-part name, or binomial, printed in italic type: the first part, with an initial capital letter, is the genus; the second part is the species epithet, which distinguishes it from other species in the genus.

Subspecies
Naturally occurring, distinct variant of a species, often an isolated population. Indicated by "subsp." *in roman type, followed by the subspecific epithet in italic type.*

Varietas (variety) and forma (form)
Minor subdivisions of a species, differing slightly in their botanical structure. Indicated by "var." *or* "f." *in roman type, followed by the variety or form epithets in italic type.*

Cultivars
Selected or artificially raised, distinct variants of species, subspecies, varietas, forma, or hybrids. Denoted by a vernacular name in roman type within single quotation marks, e.g. Calluna vulgaris 'Firefly'. *If the parentage is obscure or complex, the vernacular name may directly follow the generic name, e.g. Rosa* 'Goldfinch'.

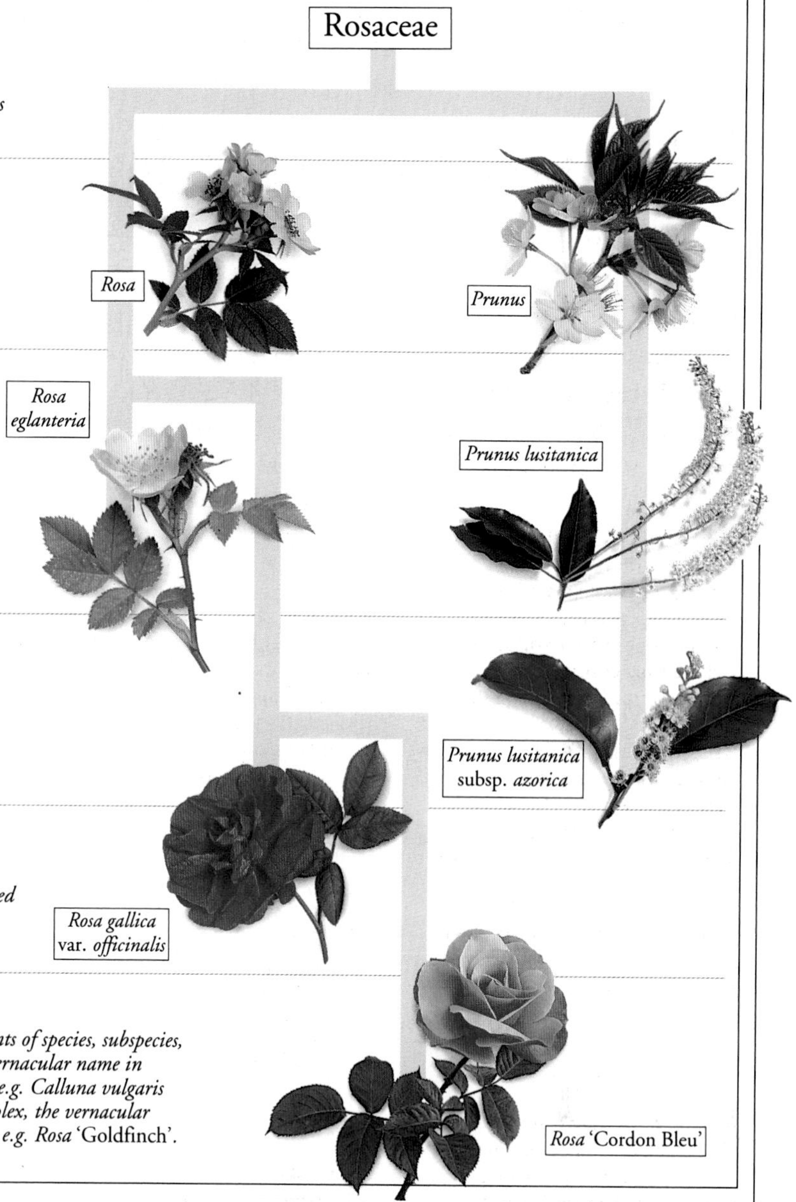

propagate it to maintain it. If several species of one genus are cultivated together, they may hybridize, giving rise to offspring sharing characters of both parents, for example *Camellia* x *williamsii* (*C. japonica* x *C. saluenensis*). Seedlings from these crosses may vary, and may be selected and given cultivar names, such as *C.* x *williamsii* 'Mary Christian'. If the resulting hybrids are fertile, several generations of plants may be produced. In time, the parentage of the offspring becomes obscured, reflected in the style of name chosen, for example *C.* 'Leonard Messel'. Although most are the result of hybridizing in cultivation, interspecific hybrids may also occur in the wild.

Closely related genera can also hybridize in cultivation; for example, *Cupressus* and *Chamaecyparis* have crossed to produce the intergeneric hybrid x *Cupressocyparis*. This name applies to all hybrids between the two genera, and individual cultivars may be selected, propagated, and named. A further category is the graft hybrid, which involves two or more genera or species being grafted together to produce a plant composed of the tissue of the parent plants. Only a few examples are known, such as + *Laburnocytisus adamii*.

A cultivar is any artificially raised or selected plant (the name being a contraction of cultivated variety) that is clearly distinct, uniform, and stable in its characteristics, and able to be maintained by propagation. Some cultivars are increased vegetatively (asexually, also referred to as cloning) from an individual plant, and are maintained by this method. Other cultivars are raised from seed (normally sexually); these are usually annuals, but may also be herbaceous perennials, and their characteristics can only be maintained by removing all plants not true to type. If rigorous selection is not carried out, plants sold under those cultivar names may not have the expected characteristics.

Sports are mutations resulting from genetic change, which produce shoots or flowers differing from those of the parent plant. If a mutation is propagated vegetatively, it may be named as a cultivar and maintained – many variegated plants occur in this way. Not all sports are stable; some often revert to the parent's characteristics.

Groups, Grexes, and Series

Hybridization and subsequent selection has produced many cultivars with similar characteristics. For convenience, these are often classified in named cultivar Groups that denote their similarities, for example *Tulipa* Lily-flowered Group. Some Groups may at first not contain any named cultivars; these may be included at a later date once selected. In orchid nomenclature, the term Grex is used as an equivalent of Group but is based on known parentage, whereas the parentage in Groups may not be certain. Commercially, the terms Series and Group are used interchangeably. Series are often based on breeding lines that give a high degree of consistency in their offspring, often coming almost true. A Series usually includes a number of cultivars differing only in one characteristic, such as flower colour. In some cases a Series may be deliberately constituted as a mixture of cultivars, so that it provides a range of flowers of different colours but of the same character – often for use in bedding schemes.

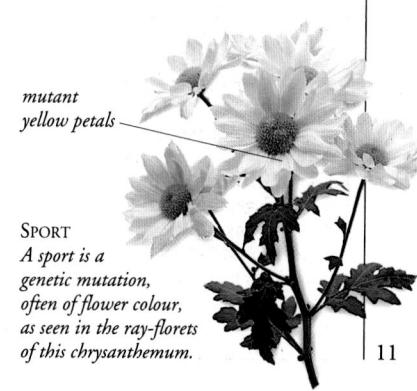

SPORT
A sport is a genetic mutation, often of flower colour, as seen in the ray-florets of this chrysanthemum.

The life of a plant

Flowering plants have evolved a range of strategies and structures that enable them to survive and reproduce in diverse habitats. Knowing how plants function and understanding their life-cycle are a vital part of raising and maintaining healthy specimens, and successfully increasing stocks, whether from seed or by other means.

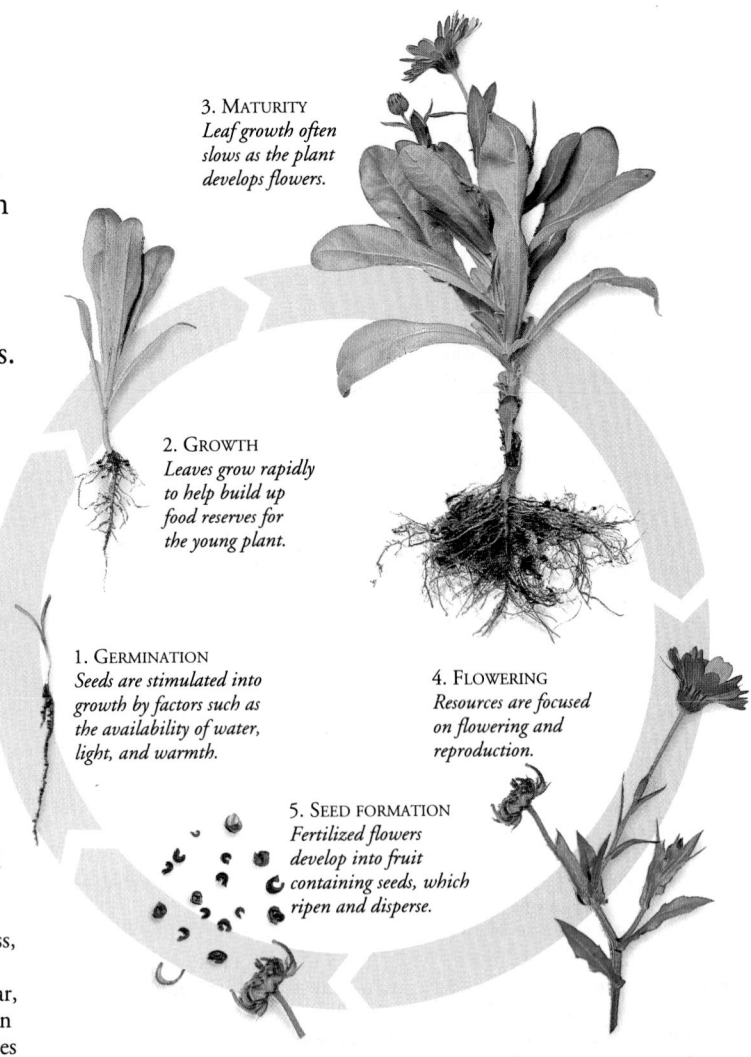

3. MATURITY
Leaf growth often slows as the plant develops flowers.

Leaves grow rapidly to help build up food reserves for the young plant.

5. SEED FORMATION
Fertilized flowers develop into fruit containing seeds, which ripen and disperse.

Seeds, shoots, and roots

Seeds are a plant's essential agent of reproduction. Each seed contains the embryo of a new plant, and is genetically programmed to start into growth only when conditions are absolutely right. In temperate climates, for example, the soft growth of many flowering plants is unable to withstand severe winter cold. The seeds of plants from such areas remain dormant in the soil until spring, when they germinate, triggered mainly by water intake, but also by factors such as rising temperatures of air and soil, higher levels of light and humidity, and increasing day length.

Some seeds, such as those of many alpine plants, must experience a period of cold before they will germinate. In cultivation, dormancy may be broken by stratification, which involves the intake of water by the seed, followed by a period of cold: the seeds must be sown outdoors in autumn, then exposed to winter frost; or kept warm and moist for a few days and then placed in a refrigerator for 3–18 weeks. For tough-coated seeds, dormancy may be broken by scarification: nicking or abrading the outer casing to encourage the seed to absorb water (see also p.28).

Successful germination is usually indicated by the emergence of seed-leaves (cotyledons) – a single leaf in monocotyledons, a pair of leaves in dicotyledons. These first leaves and a stem rapidly develop into the mature shoot system. Its initial function is to gather energy from sunlight, which is essential for photosynthesis. During this process, the plant uses a complex series of chemical reactions to produce sugar, in the form of glucose, from carbon dioxide and water. Glucose provides the plant with energy for growth, but it is also a component in the manufacture of more complex substances. One of these is cellulose, a tough, fibrous material that gives strength and flexibility to cell walls. Another is starch, which is stored in the cells to provide a supply of energy later on. Once a plant has reached maturity, the resources of the shoot system are concentrated on forming the structures involved in reproduction: flowers, followed by fruits, which contain seeds for regeneration (see pp.16–17).

Life-cycle of a flowering plant
The life-cycle of an angiosperm has several phases, often regulated by seasonal variations such as water availability, air temperature, and day length. Germination is followed by a period of growth. The mature plant then flowers and sets seed. With annuals and biennials, this cycle occurs once; with most perennials, growth and flowering recurs for many years.

Hidden below ground, the root system also makes an essential contribution to a plant's health and vigour, not only anchoring the plant but also absorbing a constant supply of moisture and nutrients from the soil. Some plants develop a tap root system with one main root; others form a widespreading, fibrous root system in which there is no main, or tap root. Microscopic root hairs fan out from the root tips, vastly increasing the surface area of each root, and therefore the amount of water and nutrients it can take up.

For a healthy root system, always prepare the ground thoroughly before sowing or planting: loose, well-aerated soil allows roots to spread widely in their search for food and water.

After it has entered through the roots, water is drawn up through the plant in a process known as transpiration, carrying minerals to the leaves where oxygen and water evaporate through stomata (microscopic pores) in the leaf surface. Most moisture leaves the plant in this manner, although some is used

GROWTH HABITS

As with other organisms, the way a plant grows – whether it is stemless, or climbing, or clump-forming, for example – is genetically determined, laid down in a blueprint carried in every cell. How well individual plants grow varies with availability of light, exposure to wind, and competition for food and space with other plants.

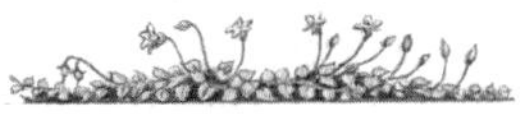

MAT-FORMING
Stems densely cover the ground; flowers extend above.

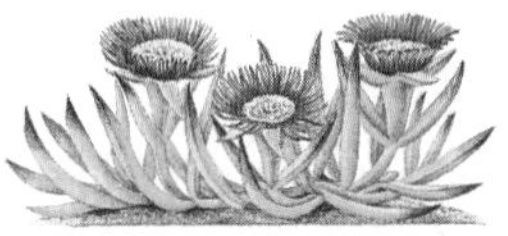

PROSTRATE AND TRAILING
Stems spread out on the ground; flowers are borne close to foliage.

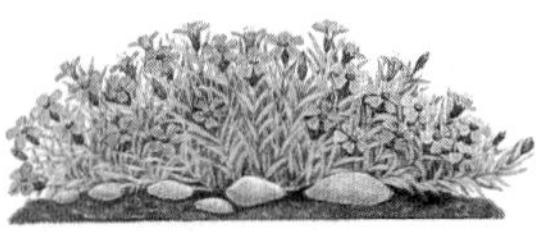

CUSHION- OR MOUND-FORMING
Tightly packed stems form a low clump; flowers are close to foliage.

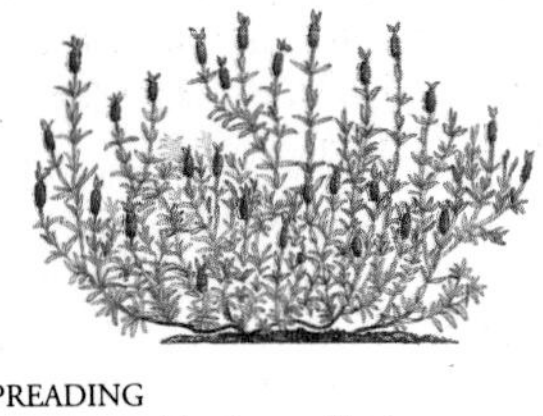

SPREADING
Stems extend horizontally then ascend, forming a densely packed mass.

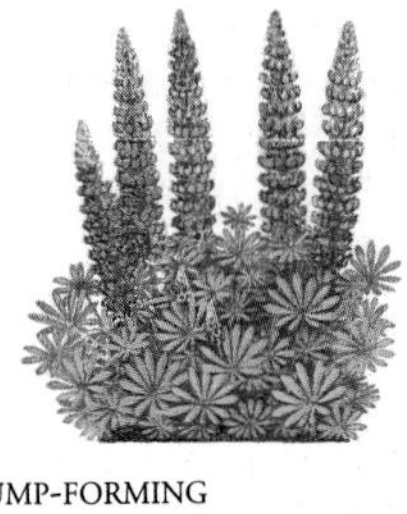

CLUMP-FORMING
Flower stems and leaf-stalks arise at ground level to form a dense mass.

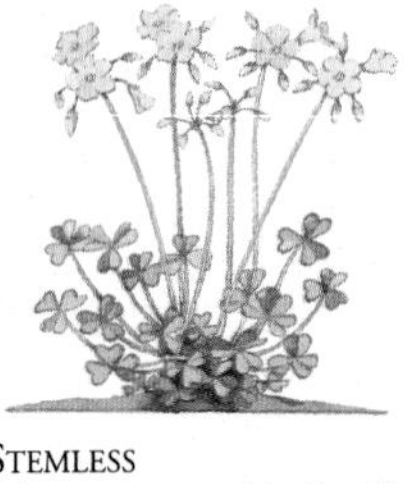

STEMLESS
Flower stems and leaf-stalks arise at ground level.

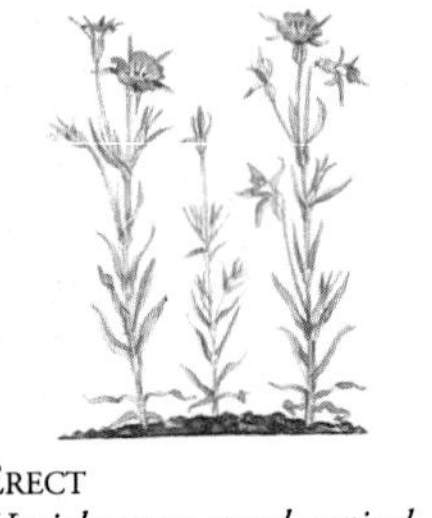

ERECT
Upright stems stand vertical, supporting leaves and flowers.

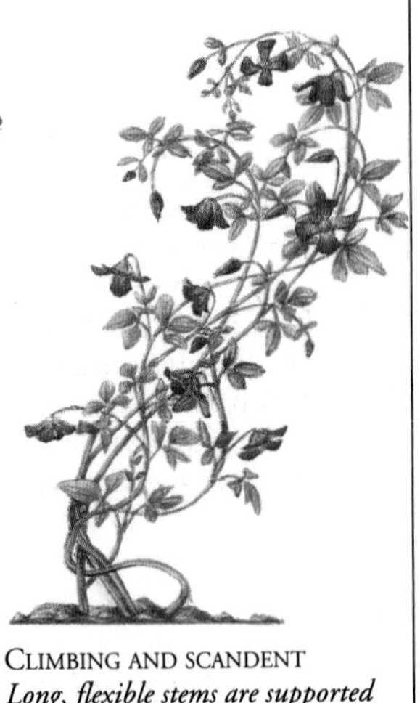

CLIMBING AND SCANDENT
Long, flexible stems are supported by other plants or structures.

MALE AND FEMALE

Most plants have bisexual (hermaphrodite) flowers, containing both male and female reproductive organs. These may pollinate themselves or be pollinated by another plant of the same species. Other plants produce unisexual flowers: on a monoecious plant, male and female flowers are borne separately; on a dioecious plant, the flowers are either all male or all female, so both male and female plants must be grown to produce fruit. A few species are polygamous, with both bisexual and unisexual flowers.

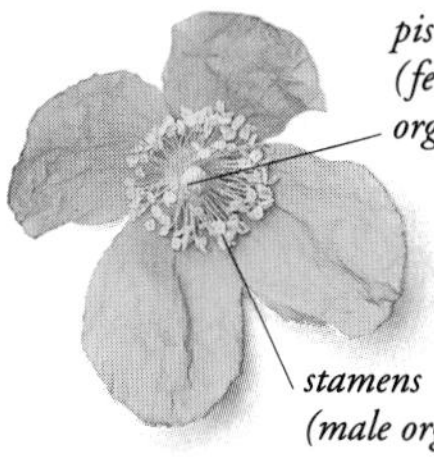

BISEXUAL (HERMAPHRODITE) PLANTS
Each flower contains both male and female organs. It may pollinate itself, or be pollinated by another plant of the species.

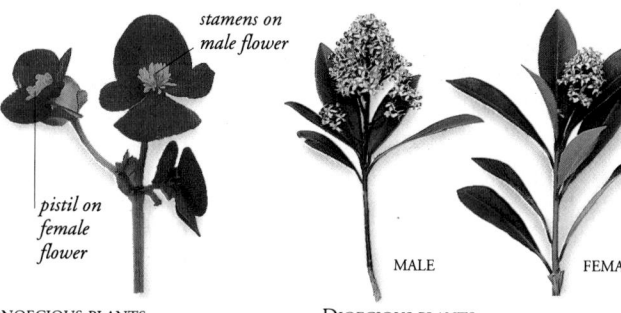

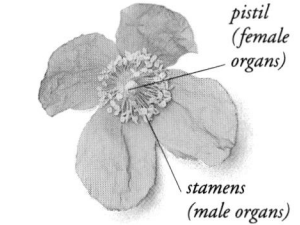

MONOECIOUS PLANTS
Flowers are either male or female, but are borne on the same plant.

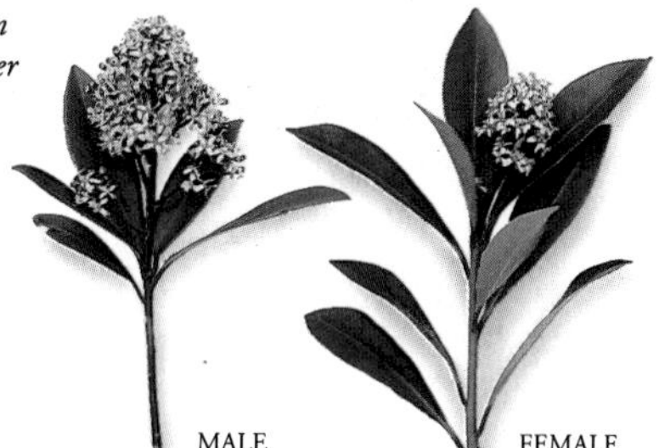

DIOECIOUS PLANTS
Male and female flowers form on separate plants; both are needed for fertilization.

FRUITS

Fruits are formed from the ovaries of flowering plants. They protect the seeds, and often aid their dispersal. Soft, fleshy fruits are eaten by animals and birds, which disperse the seeds in the process; dry pods or capsules split open when ripe to scatter the seeds.

The cones of many conifers and other gymnosperms are not true fruits, as they are not formed by the ovaries. However, conifers such as yews (*Taxus*) do produce soft, berry-like structures, but the flesh (the aril) is produced on the seed itself, rather than by the ovary of the parent plant.

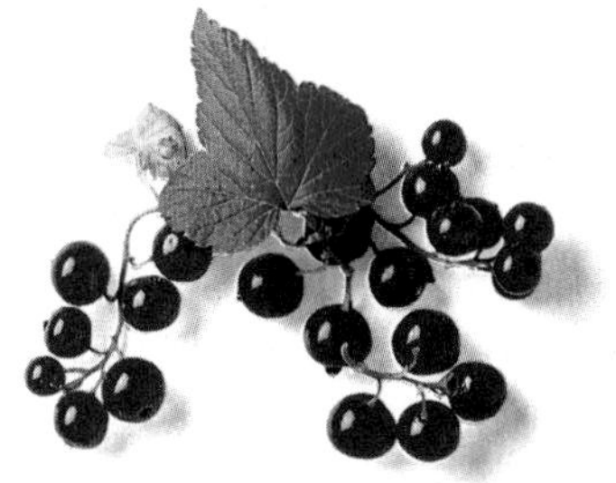

BERRY
Non-splitting fruit with one to numerous seeds surrounded by soft flesh. Many soft, fleshy fruits are loosely referred to as berries.

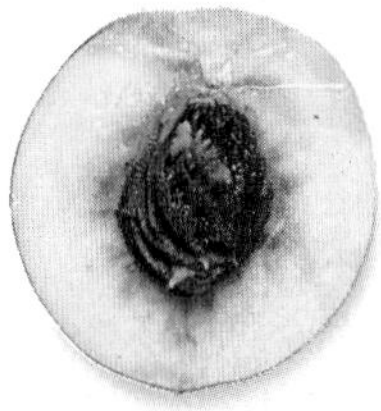

STONE FRUIT (drupe)
Non-splitting fruit with soft flesh surrounding one or several hard seeds (stones).

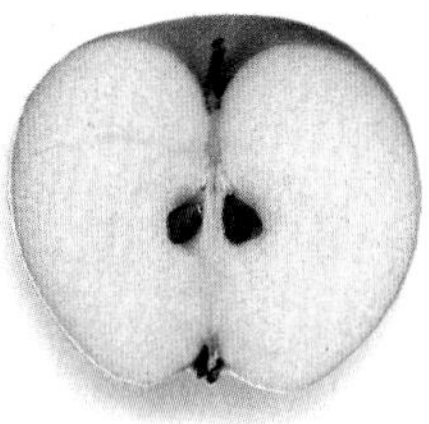

POME
Non-splitting fruit with firm flesh surrounding chambers containing seeds.

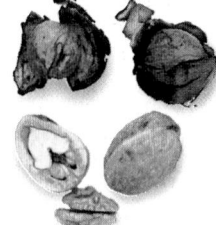

NUT
Non-splitting fruit with a hard casing surrounding a softer seed (kernel).

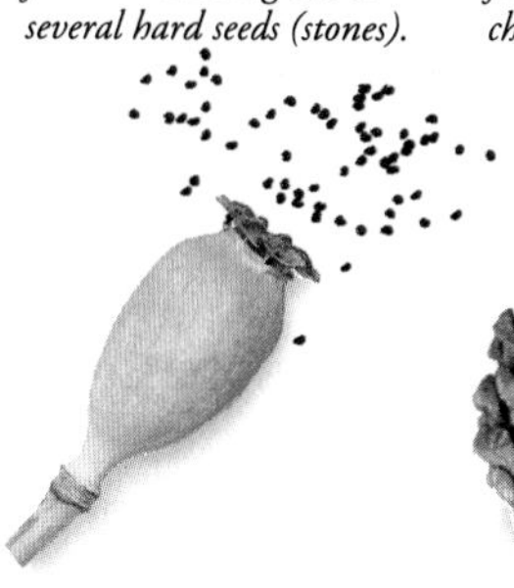

CAPSULE
Dry fruit that normally splits open when ripe to disperse seeds.

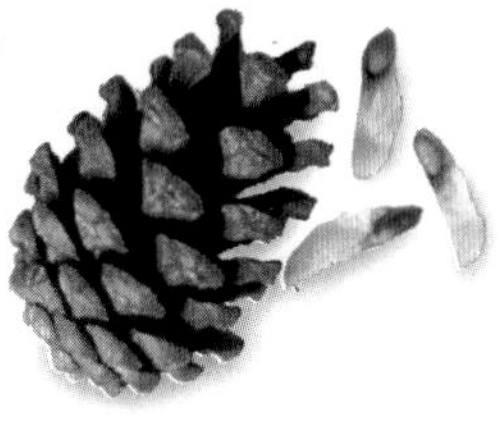

CONE
Not a true fruit. Woody scales part to release seeds when conditions are favourable.

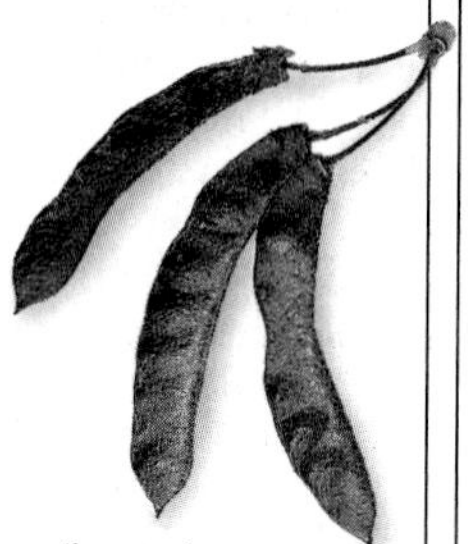

POD (legume)
Usually firm or dry fruit that splits along 2 sides when ripe to release seeds.

as a raw material in photosynthesis. The movement of water through a plant also keeps its cells turgid (swollen), enabling the stem to stay upright. When water is in short supply, the stem quickly loses its rigidity (wilts) and the plant may die, particularly if transpiration is increased by hot, dry, frosty, or windy weather. In cultivation, therefore, provide plants – especially those that are grown under glass or in containers outdoors – with a regular supply of water, and food in the form of fertilizers. Too much water, however, may inhibit growth by waterlogging the soil or compost, so that oxygen intake is impossible and the roots die or rot. On the other hand, an excess of nutrients, mainly nitrogen, may encourage the strong growth of lush foliage at the expense of flower production.

Modified shoots

Many plants have evolved modified shoot and root systems in response to the conditions in their native environments. Above ground, the winding tendrils of climbing plants are stems or leaves that have become adapted for grasping a support in the upward quest for light. Thorns are modified branches that deter plant-eating animals. In plants that live in arid conditions, such as cacti, leaves are often reduced to spines to minimize water loss, while the swollen, succulent stems perform photosynthesis and store water. Similarly, the trunk of the tropical baobab tree (*Adansonia digitata*) swells with water-filled tissue, permitting vital functions and growth to continue even during long periods of sparse rainfall.

In some plants, a significant part of the shoot system develops below ground. Subterranean stems include swollen structures such as bulbs, corms, tubers, and rhizomes, which act as food stores. They also increase in number, by producing offsets or bulbils for example. Such plants offer a simple means of propagation, since when dormant they may be lifted, divided, and replanted.

Unlike other swollen stems, rhizomes grow horizontally, often close to or at the surface of the soil. Adventitious roots arise at the nodes along the length of the rhizome, rather than from its base as with a conventional stem. The rhizomes of some perennials, such as certain irises, have a relatively slow growth rate. In others, however, such as the bamboo *Yushania anceps*, the rhizomes spread very vigorously, rapidly defeating more delicate competitors for available space, light, moisture, and nutrients. A knowledge of such growth habits is indispensable for gardeners, to avoid any one plant becoming dominant or invasive.

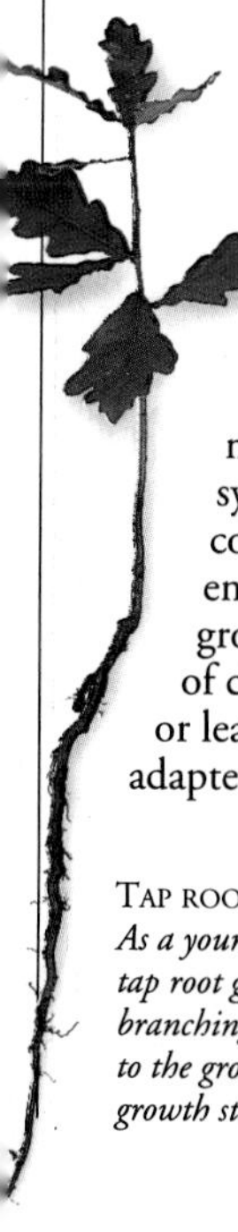

TAP ROOTS
As a young plant develops, its tap root grows downwards before branching, anchoring the plant to the ground and holding top-growth stable against wind-rock.

Alternative root systems

In the same way that shoots may sometimes develop below ground, so roots may grow above it. Climbing plants such as ivies (*Hedera*) have adventitious, aerial roots arising from their stems. These roots cling to any surface, and penetrate the smallest cracks and crevices, where they expand until the plant is securely attached to its support. Many low-growing plants of spreading habit, such as periwinkles (*Vinca*), produce adventitious roots from nodes on the stems. In cultivation, this is encouraged by layering (pinning stems down to root in the soil) for the purposes of propagation.

Aerial roots are also produced by epiphytic plants, which lodge on other plants and derive moisture and nutrients from the atmosphere, rather than from the soil. In tropical rainforest, epiphytes are often found in the higher branches of trees, where they benefit from increased levels of light near the upper canopy. In such plants, the root system is highly specialized for a permanent existence above ground. The plant is held secure by a network of generally thickened roots, which wrap themselves around twigs and branches in similar fashion to tendrils, and are able to take up rainwater.

A number of trees, such as screw pines (*Pandanus*) and banyans (*Ficus microcarpa, F. benghalensis*), develop additional roots above ground to support them when mature. Stilt roots, for example, are adventitious roots that arise from the trunk, whereas wide-spreading buttress roots are either outgrowths of the trunk or fused, adventitious, aerial roots, forming flanges that provide the tree with extra support; both are commonly found on trees in tropical rainforest, where the soil is relatively shallow, or may be heavily saturated.

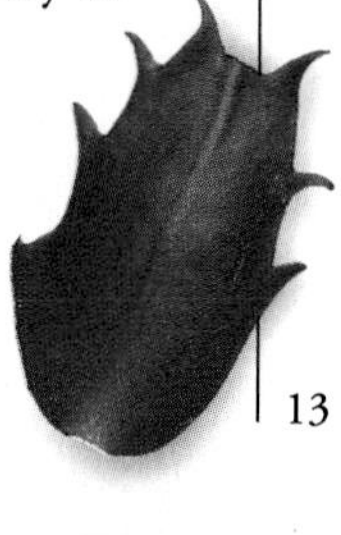

PHYLLOCLADE
The modified stems of some succulents, known as phylloclades, perform similar functions to leaves.

Leaves

Leaves fuel the growth of a plant by utilizing solar energy to manufacture food. They also control the passage of water through the plant, which gives it rigidity. The enormous diversity of leaf shapes, sizes, forms, and arrangements, as illustrated here, is the result of plants adapting to conditions in a vast range of habitats.

Structure and function

The basic component of a leaf is the blade (lamina). Simple leaves consist of one continuous blade, while compound leaves are divided into separate leaflets (see Lobing and division, right). Most leaves are attached to the stem by a slender stalk (petiole), but some, as in the case of many monocotyledons, are stalkless (sessile). The leaves (fronds) of ferns often have numerous divisions, and uncurl as they grow. Reproductive, spore-bearing structures usually form on their undersides (see p.51). Some flowering plants have modified leaves, such as the tendrils of climbers (see p.13).

The veins on a leaf are extensions of the food and watering tissue (xylem and phloem) of the stem. The leaves of dicotyledons usually have a primary vein (midrib), with a subsidiary network of veins fanning out from it. In monocotyledons, the veins run parallel to the length of the leaf and there is often no distinct midrib (see p.10).

The greatest division within leaf types lies between deciduous and evergreen foliage in trees and shrubs. Evergreen leaves are shed and replaced throughout the year, while deciduous leaves are all replaced annually, mostly falling in autumn to minimize moisture loss in winter.

A leaf's main functions are photosynthesis and transpiration (see pp.12–13). The first relies heavily on the presence of chlorophyll (the pigment that makes most leaves green), and the second on stomata (minute pores) on the leaf surface.

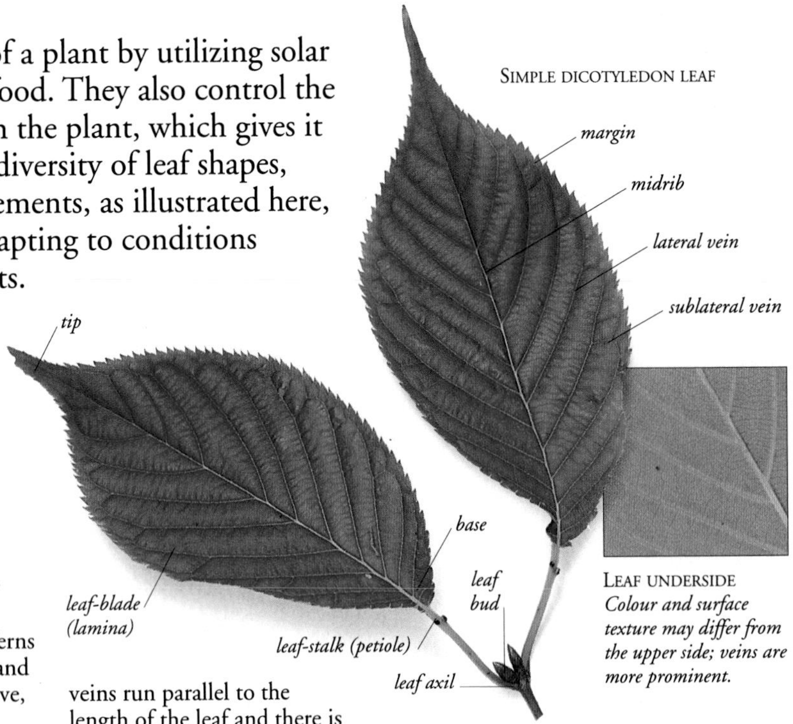

LEAF UNDERSIDE
Colour and surface texture may differ from the upper side; veins are more prominent.

Leaf structure
Although some are divided into separate leaflets, the leaves of most dicotyledons and virtually all monocotyledons consist of a single, flat leaf-blade.

CONIFER LEAVES

Most coniferous trees and shrubs have linear leaves, which are often needle-like or scale-like, and covered in a thick, waxy outer layer. These factors help to reduce moisture loss, especially useful in winter when roots cannot take up water from frozen soil. Leaves may be arranged singly, in pairs on either side of the stem (pectinate), or in whorls.

COMB-LIKE (pectinate)

NEEDLE-LIKE (acicular)

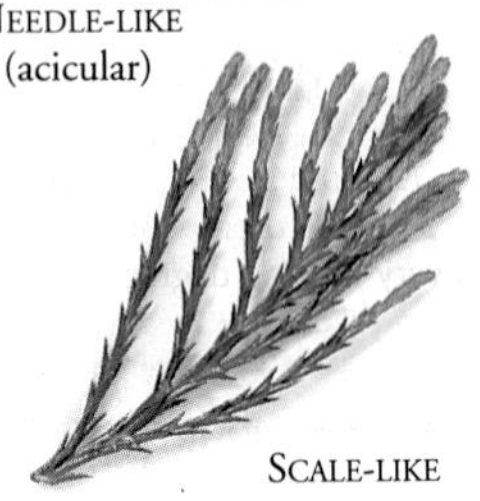

SCALE-LIKE

COLOUR AND TEXTURE

Leaf colour, which may be affected by surface texture, normally changes in deciduous plants as the leaf ages, due to the breakdown of pigments, especially chlorophyll. In variegated leaves, pigments are unevenly dispersed, usually due to a mutation.

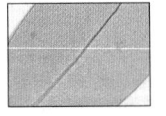

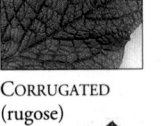

GLAUCOUS

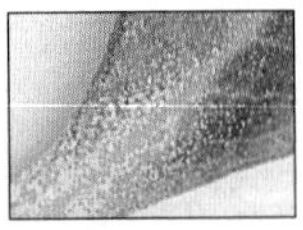

WHITE-MEALY (farinose)

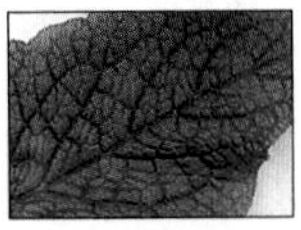

CORRUGATED (rugose)

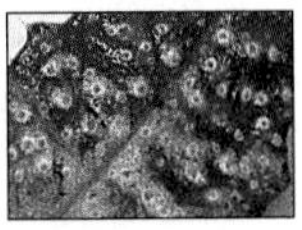

WARTY (pustulate)

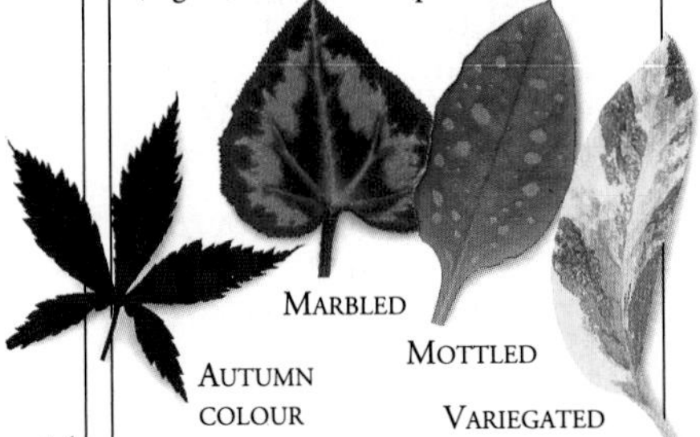

MARBLED

AUTUMN COLOUR

MOTTLED

VARIEGATED

LEAF ARRANGEMENTS

The leaves of plants are arranged in a variety of ways to ensure maximum exposure to sunlight in different environments. In some cases, the leaf arrangement may help collect rain-water. Members of a genus or family often have a common arrangement.

In some species, leaves are densely packed at each leaf node (joint with the stem), forming a rosette or whorl. In others, leaves are borne individually or in pairs, separated by a length of bare stem (internode), as in opposite, alternate, and perfoliate arrangements. Some leaves are spirally arranged around the stem.

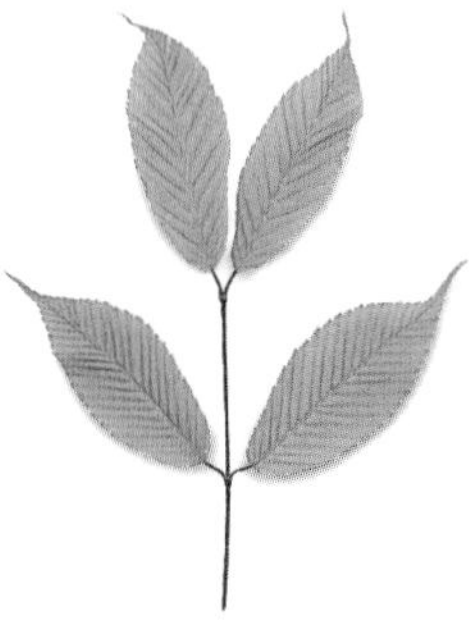

OPPOSITE
Leaves arranged in pairs on the same plane.

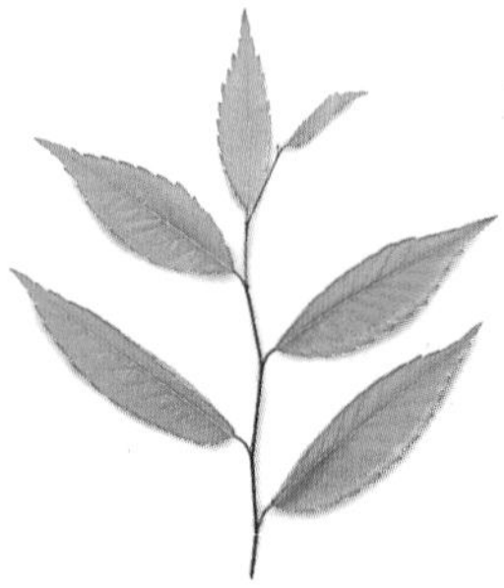

ALTERNATE
Leaves arranged singly on alternate sides of stem.

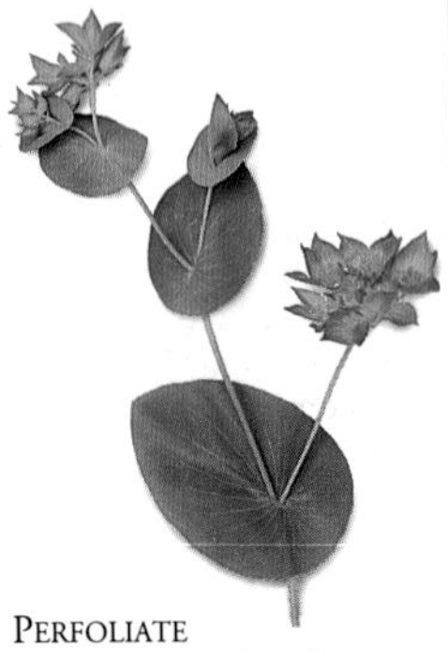

PERFOLIATE
Leaves arranged singly or in pairs, bases surrounding stem.

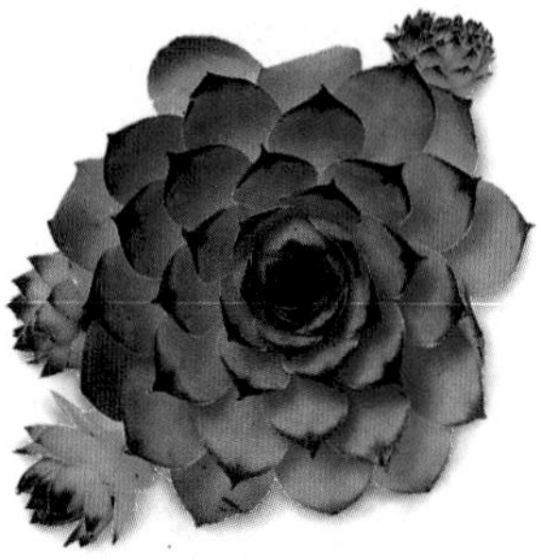

ROSETTE
Leaves densely packed, radiating from single point on stem or from base of plant.

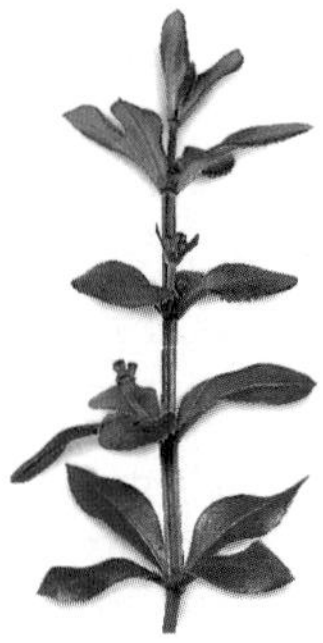

WHORLED
Leaves in groups of 3 or more around stem.

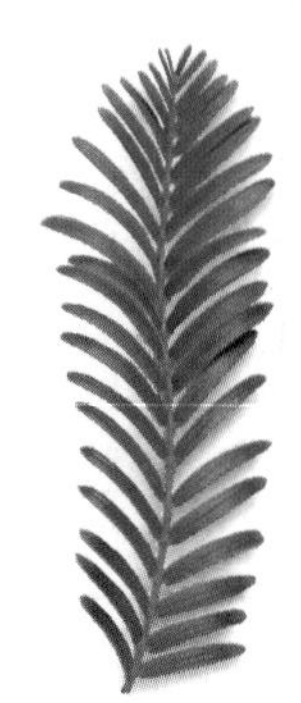

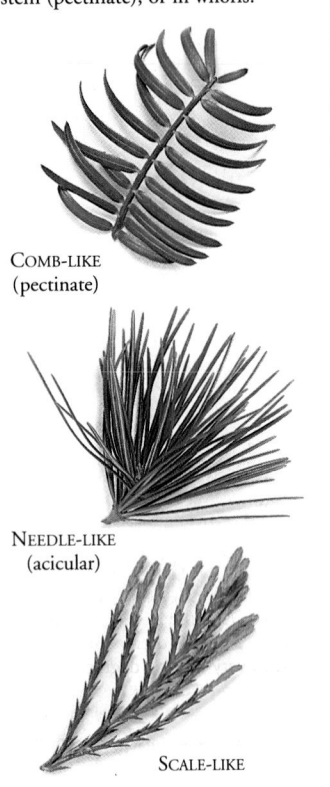

2-RANKED (distichous)
Leaves arranged on stem in 2 flattened, opposite ranks.

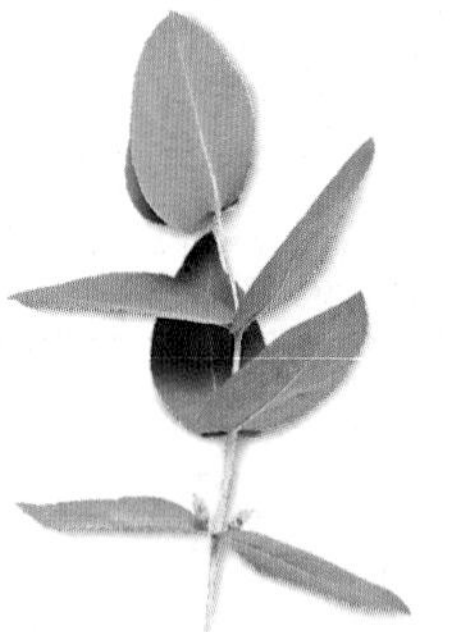

4-RANKED (decussate)
Leaves arranged in pairs at alternate right-angles.

SHAPE

Leaf shape may not be consistent within a species: in some, it depends on a leaf's position on the stem; in others, on whether plants are juvenile or adult. Certain aquatic plants produce one type of leaf under water, another type above the surface. This panel illustrates leaf shapes and terms, and characteristic length to width ratios.

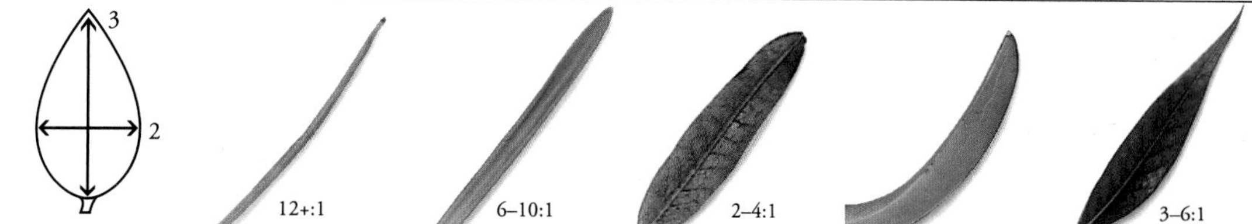

RATIO EXAMPLE *Length:width here is 3:2.*

LINEAR (acicular/filiform)

STRAP-SHAPED (ensiform/ligulate/lorate)

OBLONG

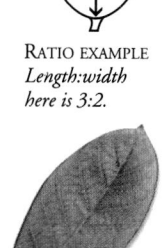

SICKLE-SHAPED (falcate)

LANCE-SHAPED (lanceolate)

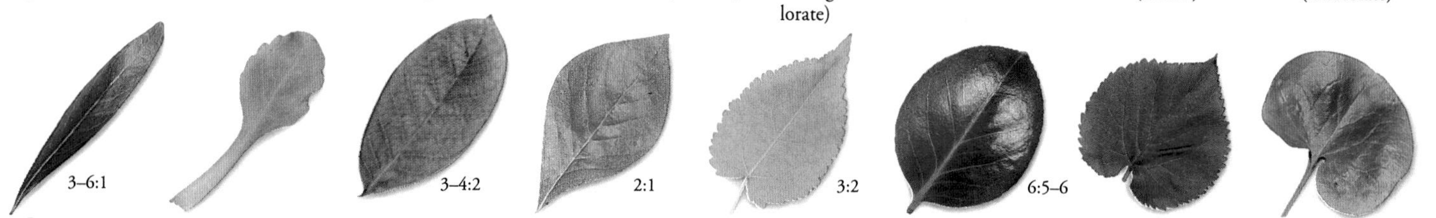

INVERSELY LANCE-SHAPED (oblanceolate)

SPOON-SHAPED (spathulate)

OVAL

ELLIPTIC

OVATE

ROUNDED (orbicular)

HEART-SHAPED (cordate)

KIDNEY-SHAPED (reniform)

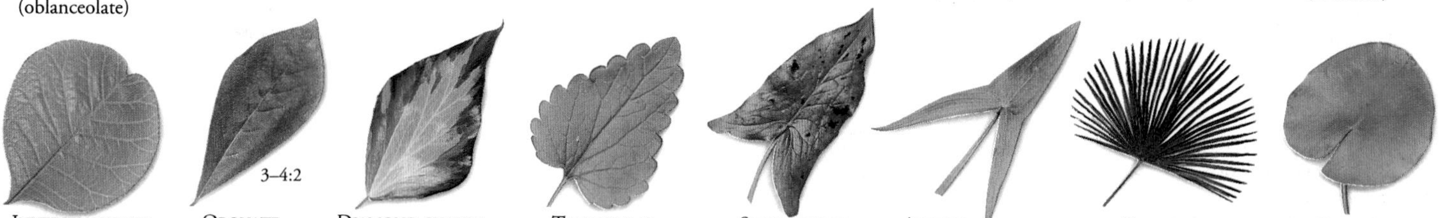

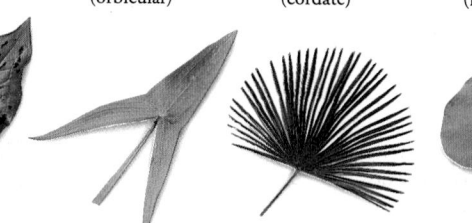

INVERSELY HEART-SHAPED (obcordate)

OBOVATE

DIAMOND-SHAPED (rhomboidal)

TRIANGULAR (deltoid)

SPEAR-SHAPED (hastate)

ARROW-SHAPED (sagittate)

FAN-SHAPED (flabellate)

PELTATE

LOBING AND DIVISION

Simple leaves consist of one blade with a continuous surface. This, however, does not preclude them from being lobed to very varying degrees. Shallowly lobed and pinnatifid leaves have lobes cut no deeper than halfway to the midrib. Palmately lobed and pinnatisect leaves have deeper, more distinct lobes.

Compound leaves have blades that are fully divided into leaflets. In palmate leaves, leaflets arise from a single point at the top of the leaf-stalk. In pinnate leaves, the leaflets arise on both sides of a main axis. The leaflets may be stalkless, and may themselves be subdivided. Two features can help to show that compound leaves are single entities, whatever their size or complexity: in many cases, they are shed as a single unit, and while buds form in the axil of a compound leaf, they do not occur in the axils of individual leaflets.

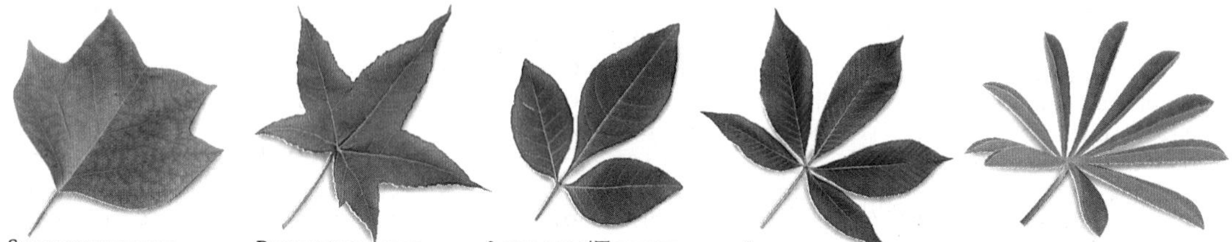

SHALLOWLY LOBED *With shallowly cut lobes.*

PALMATELY LOBED *With deeply cut lobes.*

3-PALMATE/TERNATE (trifoliolate) *With 3 leaflets.*

5-PALMATE (digitate) *With 5 leaflets.*

9-PALMATE *With 9 leaflets.*

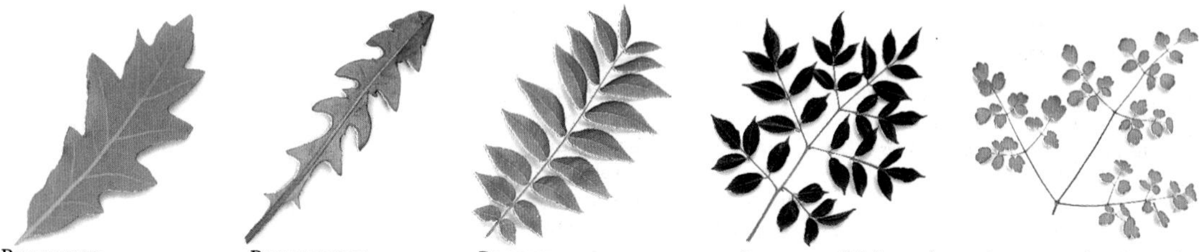

PINNATIFID *Pairs of shallowly cut lobes on each side of midrib.*

PINNATISECT *Pairs of deeply cut lobes on each side of midrib.*

PINNATE *Fully divided into leaflets along a single axis.*

2-PINNATE (bipinnate) *Each division divided along 2 axes.*

3-PINNATE (tripinnate) *Each division divided along 3 axes.*

TIPS AND BASES

The tips and bases of leaves vary greatly. The leaves of monocotyledons are often linear, with rounded or pointed tips. Leaves of dicotyledons display greater diversity of tip and base shapes, including lobed bases that meet the leaf-stalk, and narrow "drip tips", which channel rainwater away from the plant. In a decurrent leaf, the leaf-stalk, and sometimes the base of the leaf-blade, is joined to the stem below the node. Some leaf bases partly sheathe the stem.

TIPS

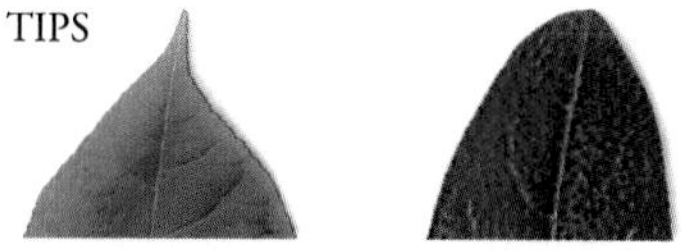

SHARPLY POINTED (acute)

ROUNDED (obtuse)

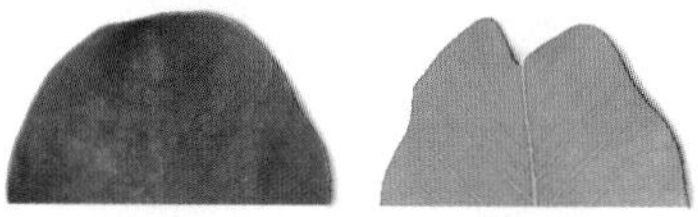

BLUNT (truncate)

NOTCHED (emarginate)

BASES

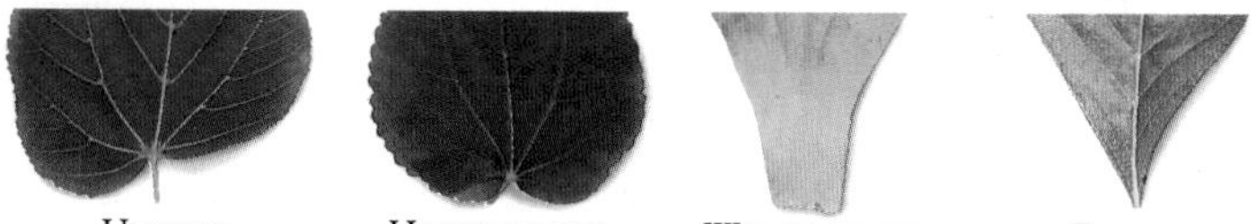

UNEVEN

HEART-SHAPED (cordate)

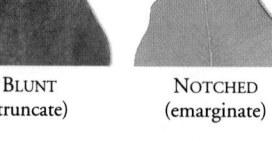

WEDGE-SHAPED (cuneate)

POINTED (acute)

MARGINS

Most monocotyledons have leaves with smooth margins, without indentations (entire). Many dicotyledons have more complex leaf margins: they may have sharply pointed teeth, or be scalloped, lobed, or deeply incised, as if cut or torn. Most leaves have flat blades, but in some the margins are wavy, or tightly rolled inwards or outwards. Ciliate leaves have marginal hairs.

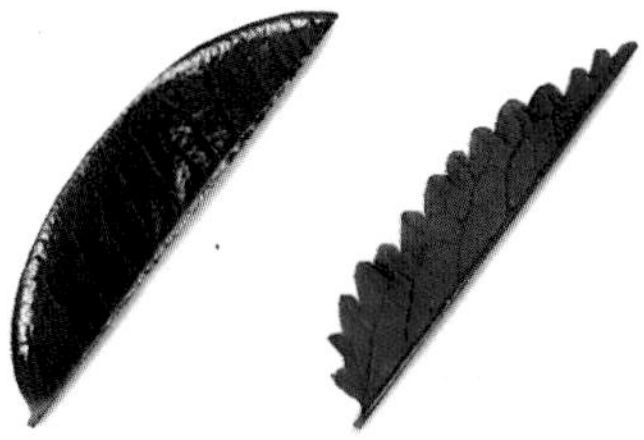

ENTIRE

SCALLOPED (crenate)

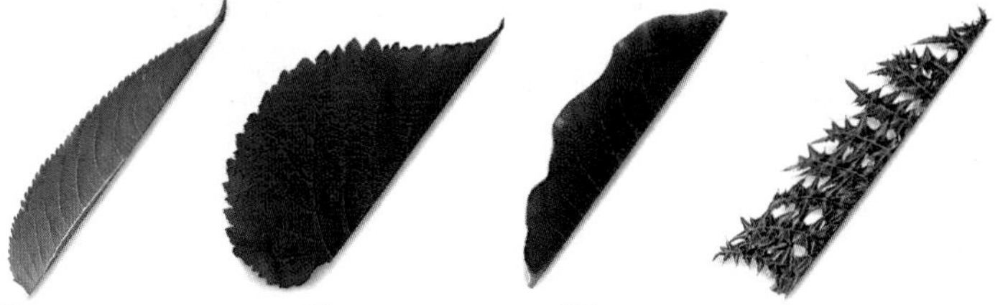

FINELY TOOTHED (serrate)

TOOTHED (dentate)

WAVY (undulate)

SPINY (spinose)

Flowers

Flowers are unique structures that house the reproductive organs of angiosperm plants. Although all flowers share similar underlying features, which enable them to produce seed, they have evolved an enormous variety of shapes, sizes, colours, and fragrances. In cultivation, this diversity has been further enhanced by selective breeding.

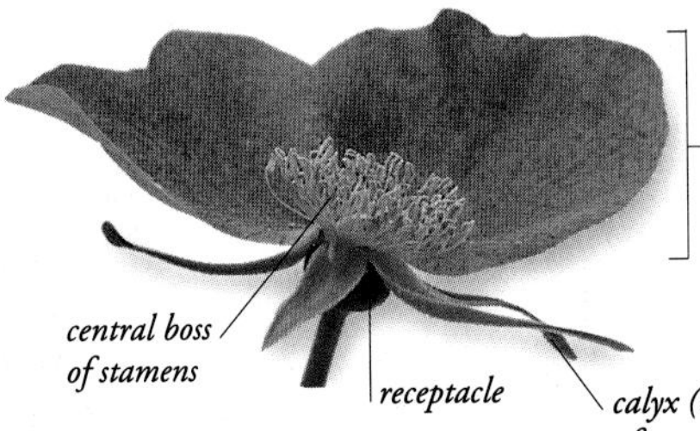

DICOTYLEDON

The parts of a flower
Ringed by whorls of petals and sepals, the male stamens surround the female carpels at the centre of the flower. The ovary or ovaries of the carpel or carpels contain ovules awaiting fertilization.

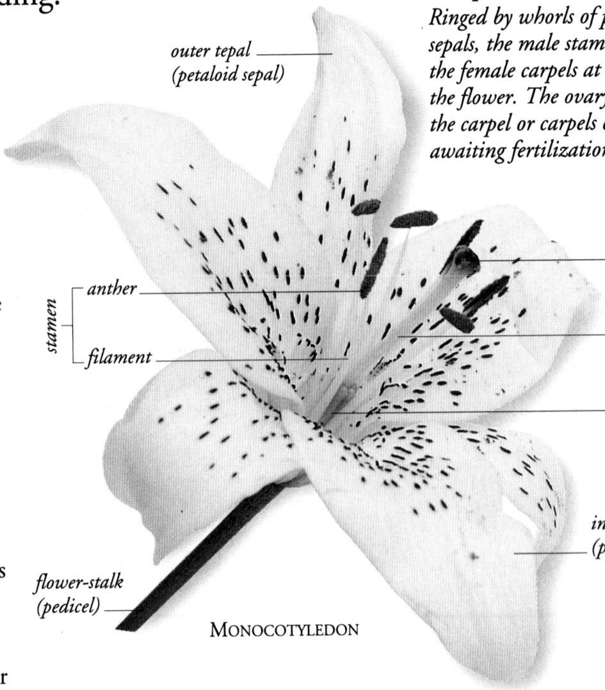

MONOCOTYLEDON

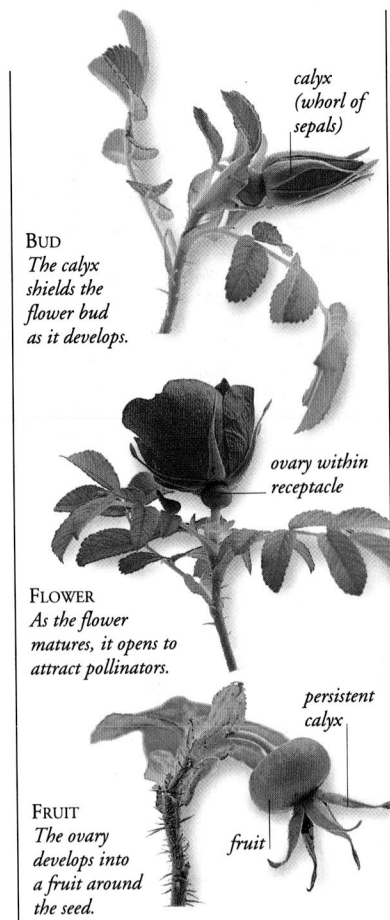

BUD
The calyx shields the flower bud as it develops.

FLOWER
As the flower matures, it opens to attract pollinators.

FRUIT
The ovary develops into a fruit around the seed.

Life-cycle of a flower
The calyx protects the developing flower bud, which eventually matures to reveal its reproductive organs. Once ovules are fertilized by pollen, the ovary develops into a fruit containing one or more seeds capable of germination into new plants.

Structure and function

All parts of a flower arise from the enlarged or elongated tip of a stem (the receptacle). Most flowers consist of a whorl of colourful petals (the corolla), surrounded by an outer whorl of leaf-like, often green sepals (the calyx). In most monocotyledons, the sepals look like the petals, and the two alternate around the rim of the flower; both are then known as tepals (or perianth segments in some genera).

At the centre of a bisexual flower, male reproductive organs (stamens) surround the female part or parts (carpels – collectively known as pistils). Each stamen consists of a pollen-producing anther at the end of a slender stalk (filament). Flowers may have one or more carpels: each carpel has a stigma, which receives the pollen, connected by a stalk (style) to an ovary containing one or more ovules. Once the ovules have been fertilized by pollen, they develop into seeds, which contain food to sustain the embryo plant until its shoot and root systems can fuel growth.

Although many plants are able to pollinate themselves, most have mechanisms that encourage cross-pollination – the transfer of pollen from one plant to another. This increases the genetic diversity of the seeds, improving seedlings' chances of survival. In cultivation, cross-pollination is used to produce plants with new or improved traits (see p.11).

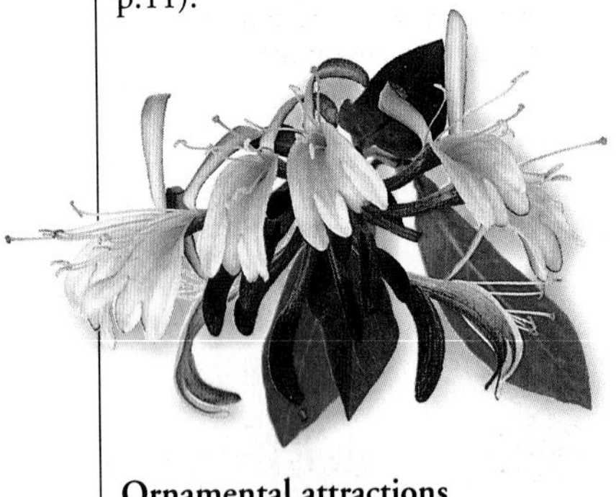

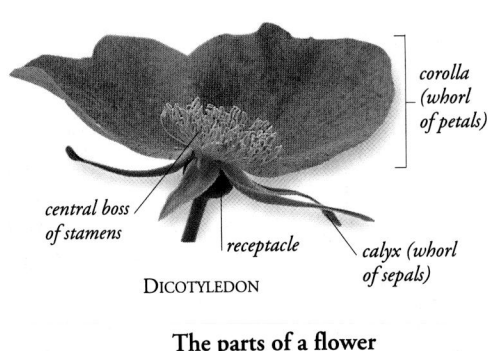

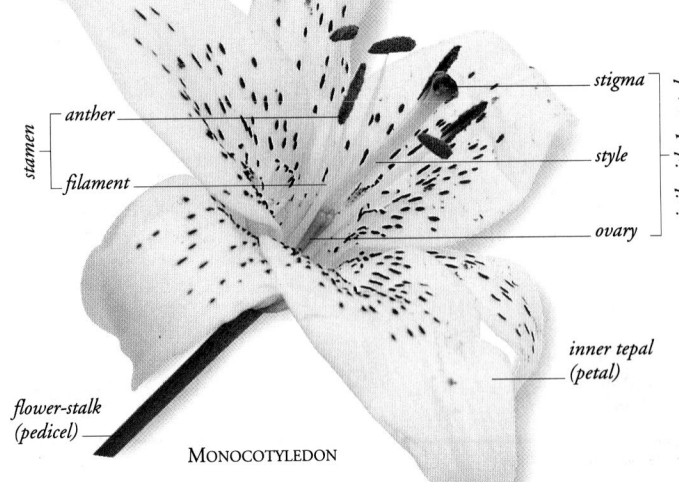

Ornamental attractions
Many insect-pollinated flowers, such as Lonicera periclymenum *'Serotina', have a sweet fragrance and attractive form that make them a popular choice among gardeners.*

DIFFERENT STRUCTURES

Flowers have evolved innumerable forms in order to facilitate pollination – by insects and other animals, wind, and, more rarely, by water. Flowers that are pollinated by insects or other animals are typically brightly coloured and sweetly scented, often containing sugar-rich nectar. Some have specialized forms to encourage a particular pollinator; the flowers of certain orchids, for example, resemble female insects, which attract the males. Wind-pollinated flowers tend to be smaller and less conspicuous, although in plants such as grasses, they are often crowded into attractive inflorescences.

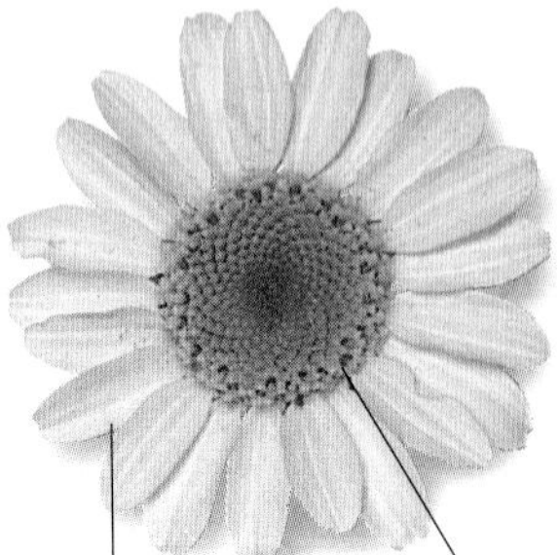

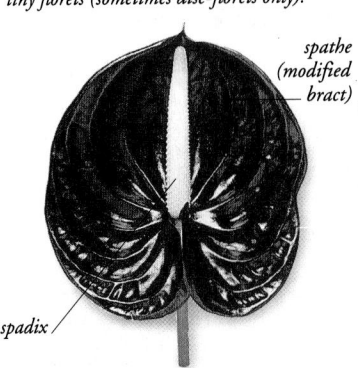

FLOWERHEAD (composite flower)
Inflorescence made up of usually 2 types of tiny florets (sometimes disc-florets only).

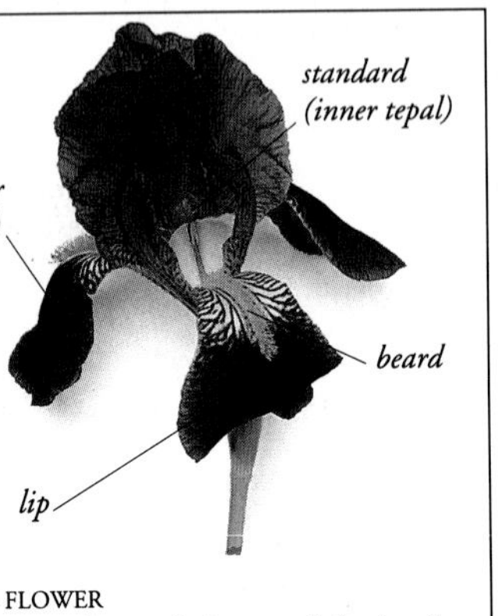

IRIS FLOWER
Flower with very distinct tepals (perianth segments) and parts in threes.

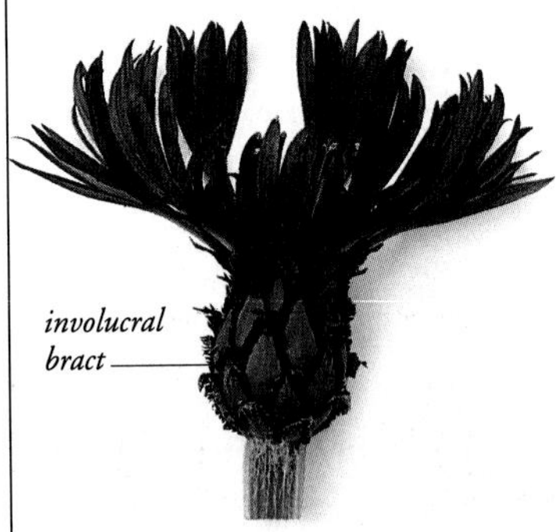

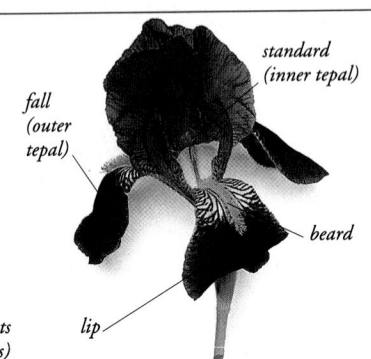

BRACTS
Modified leaves forming an involucre that surrounds the base of a flower or flowerhead.

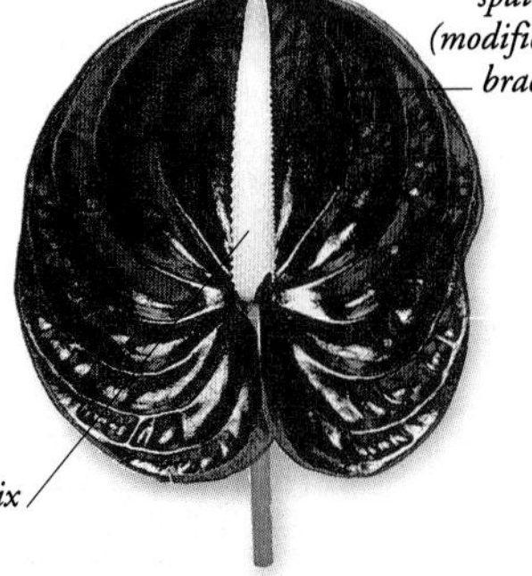

SPATHE
Modified, hood-like bract surrounding a spike of tiny flowers (spadix).

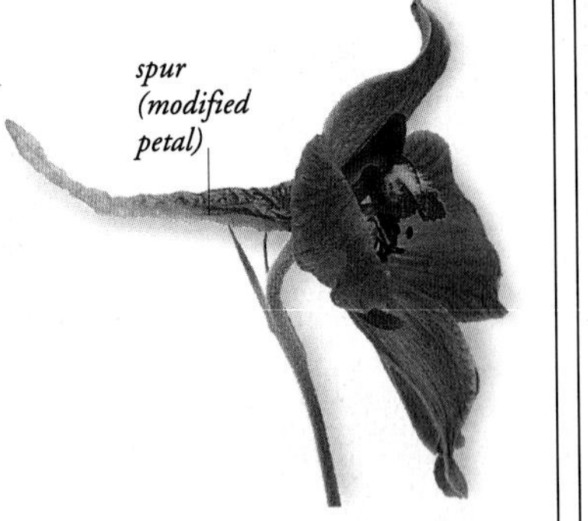

SPURRED FLOWER
Flower with a petal modified to form a hollow projection, often containing nectar.

INFLORESCENCES

Some plants bear solitary flowers, each on its own stem. In many others, flowers are grouped into inflorescences. The type of inflorescence may be identified by the way the flowers are arranged on the stem (the arrows in the diagrams indicate that the main axis may extend further). Some compound flowerheads resemble a single flower.

TERMINAL
Borne at the end of a stem.

AXILLARY
Borne from a leaf axil.

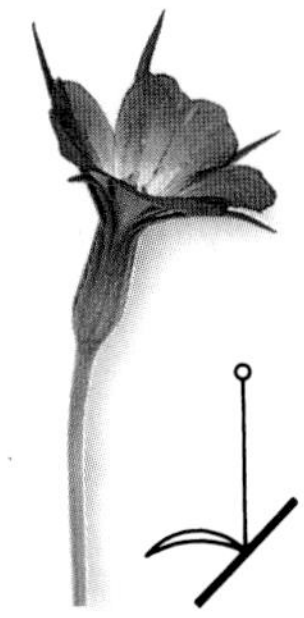

SOLITARY
Flowers are borne singly on a stem.

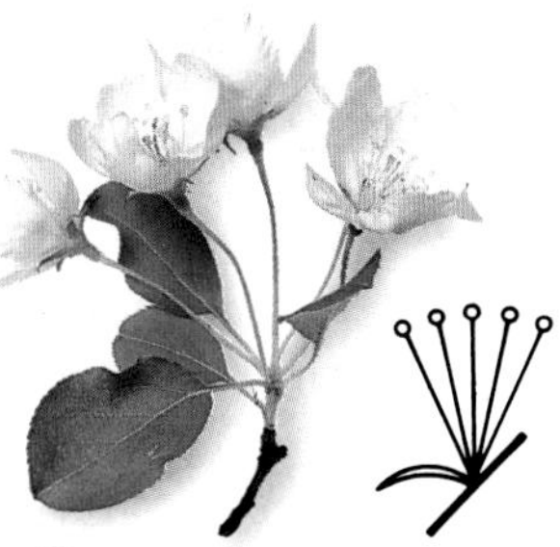

CLUSTER
Several stalked flowers arise from a single point on a stem.

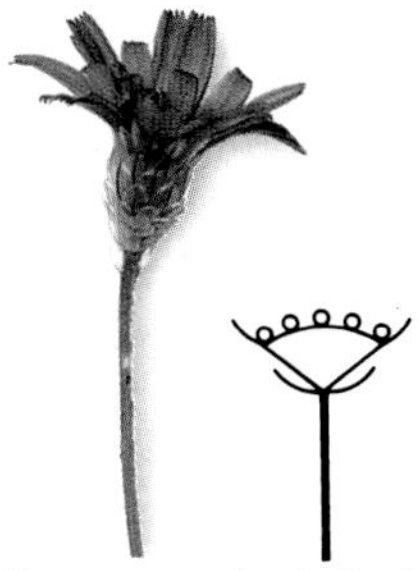

FLOWERHEAD (capitulum)
Stalkless florets are densely packed on a disc-like pad.

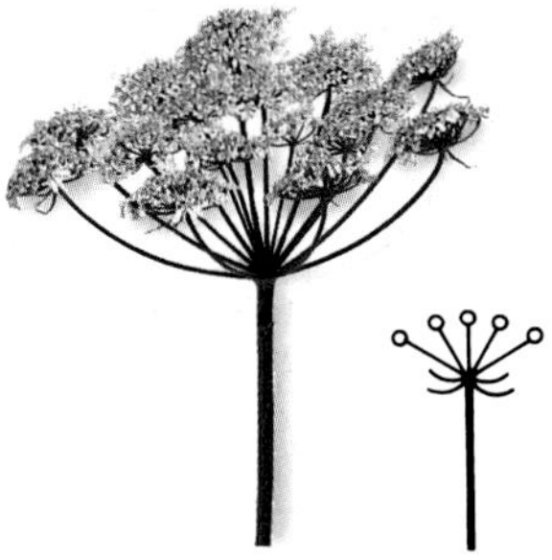

UMBEL
Stalked flowers radiate from a single point at the top of a stem.

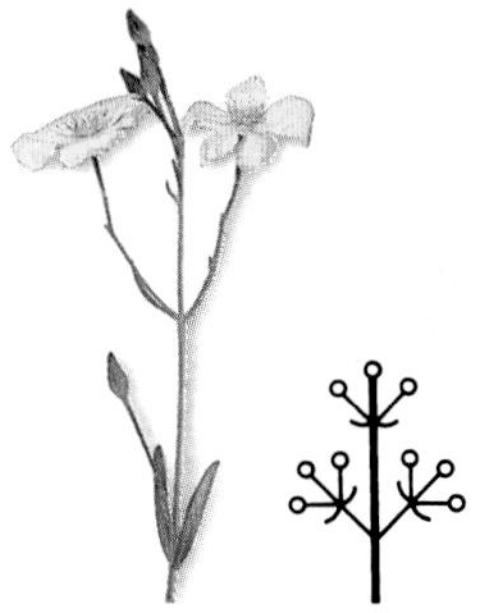

CYME
A flower terminates each branch, the oldest in the centre.

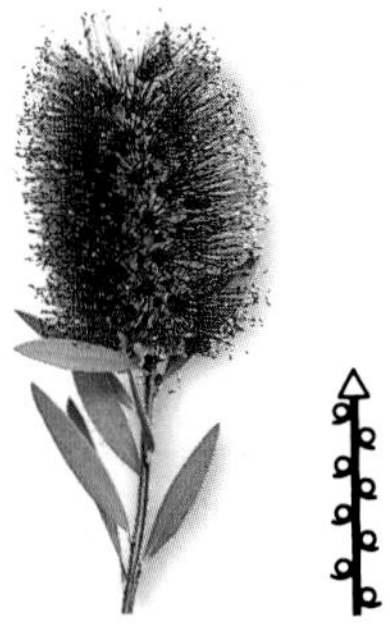

SPIKE
Stalkless flowers radiate from an unbranched stem.

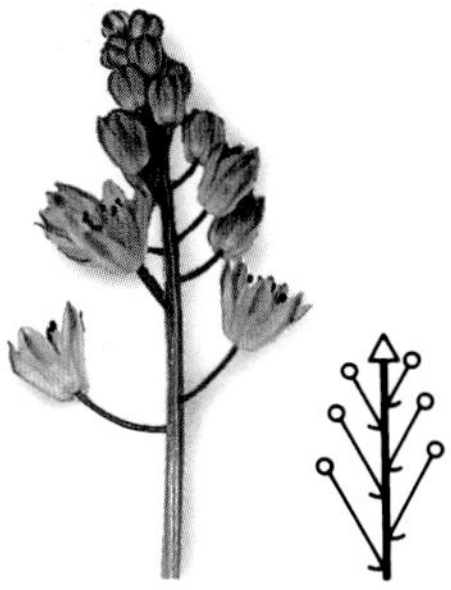

RACEME
Stalked flowers radiate from an unbranched stem.

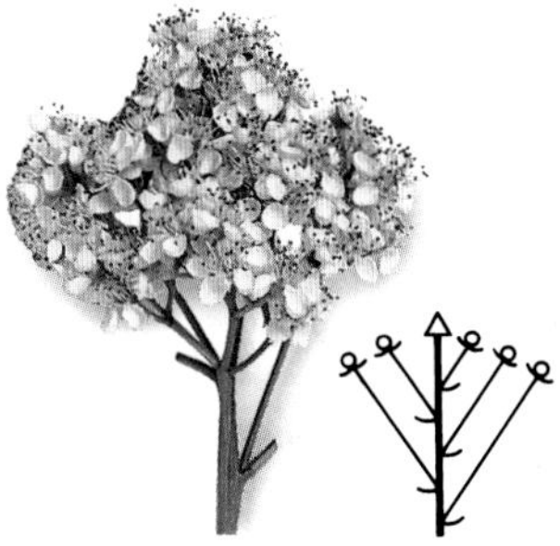

CORYMB
Flat-topped or domed, the stalked flowers alternating on the stem.

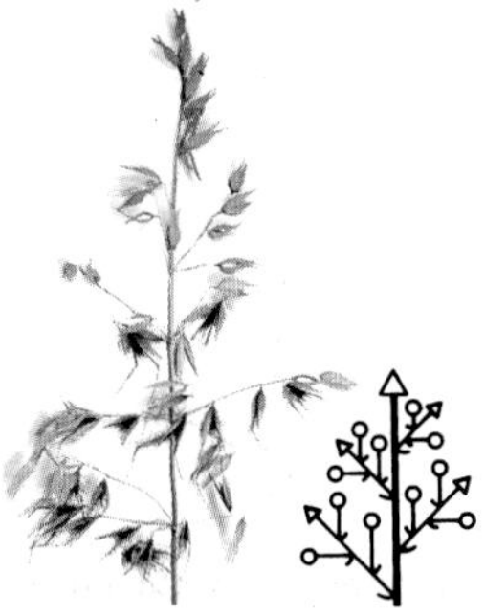

PANICLE
Branched raceme (or sometimes cyme or corymb) of stalked flowers.

SHAPE

Flower shapes are divided into 2 types: either regular or radially symmetrical and rounded in outline; or long, and irregular or symmetrical along one axis only. Petals may be separate (free) or partly fused, forming a funnel-shaped or tubular flower. In composite flowers, the florets may be elongated, but the flowerhead is usually rounded.

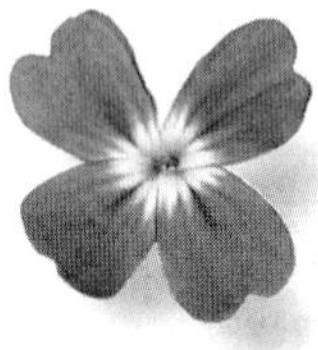

CROSS-SHAPED (cruciform)

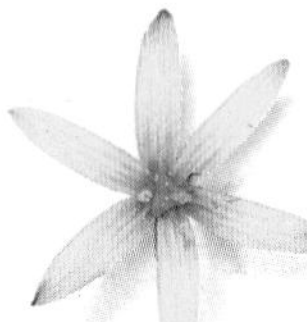

STAR-SHAPED (stellate)

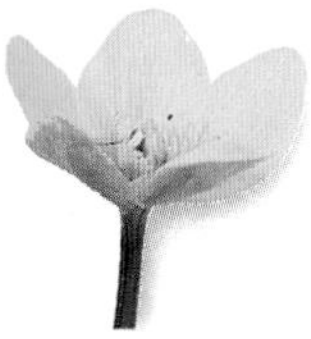

SAUCER-SHAPED

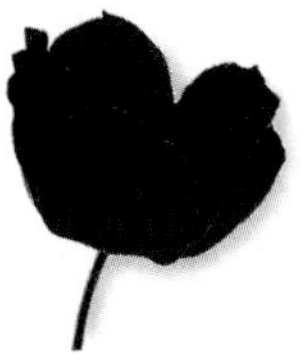

CUP-SHAPED

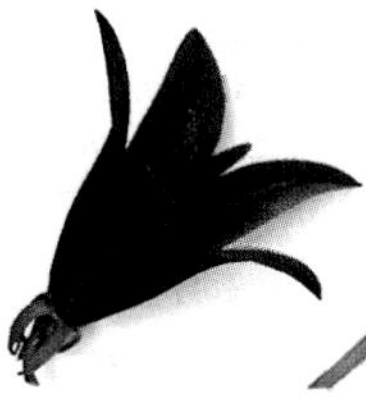

BELL-SHAPED (campanulate)

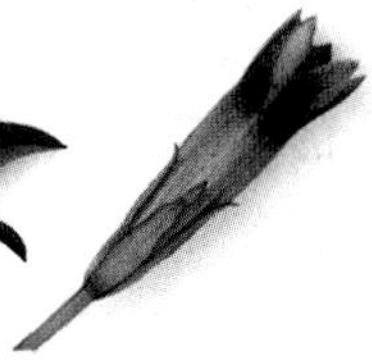

TUBULAR

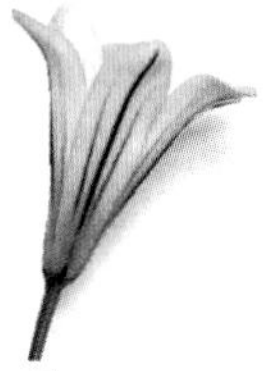

FUNNEL-SHAPED

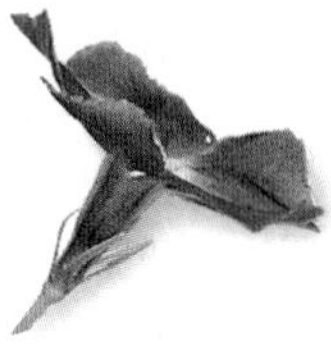

SALVERFORM

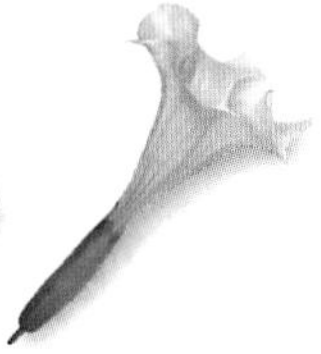

TRUMPET-SHAPED

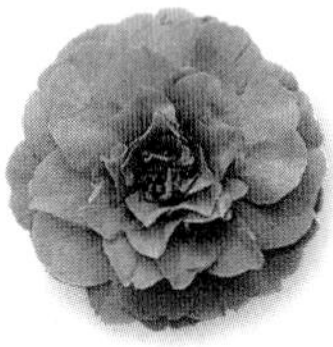

ROSETTE

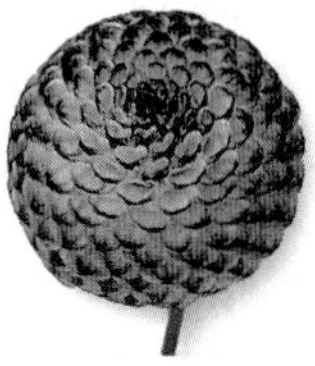

POMPON

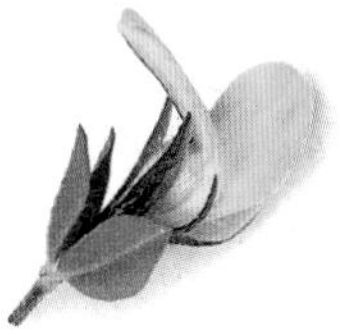

PEA-LIKE

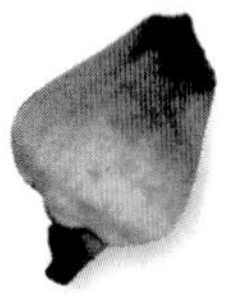

PITCHER-SHAPED

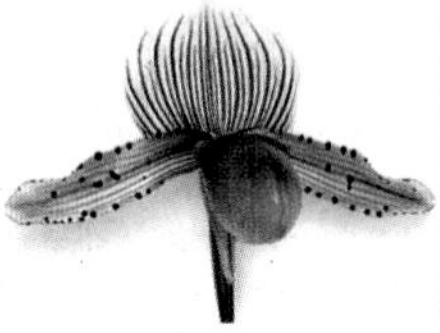

SLIPPER-SHAPED

PETAL ARRANGEMENTS

Virtually all flowers in the wild have a single whorl of petals. A few may have more, but this is much more common in cultivation. Semi-double flowers have 2 or 3 rows of petals; double flowers have many rows and few or no stamens; fully double flowers have a dense dome of petals and few or no stamens.

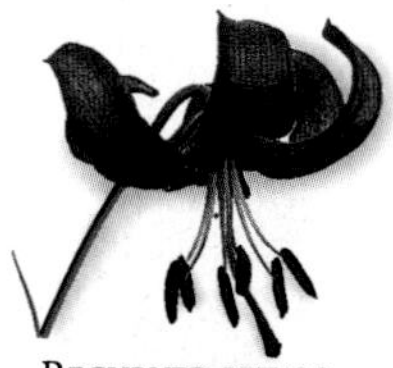

RECURVED PETALS

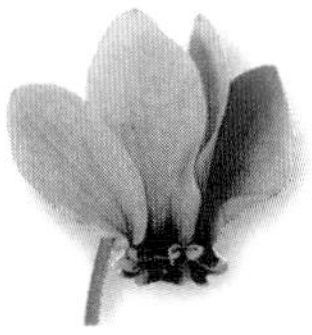

REFLEXED PETALS

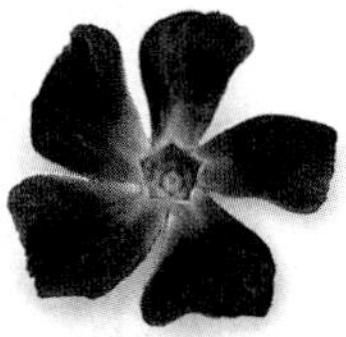

SINGLE

SEMI-DOUBLE

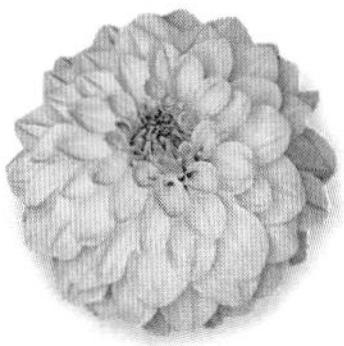

DOUBLE

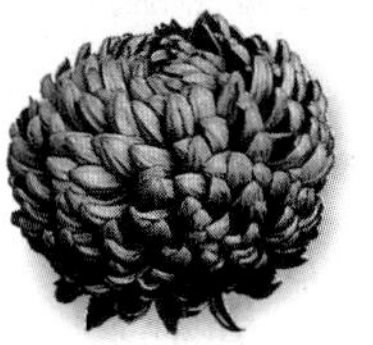

FULLY DOUBLE

HABITS

The habit of a flower or inflorescence describes its orientation on its stalk when mature. In some plants, this changes as the flower develops.

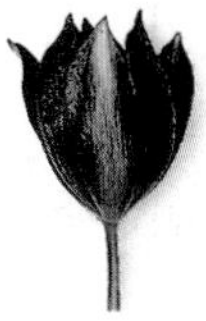

ERECT

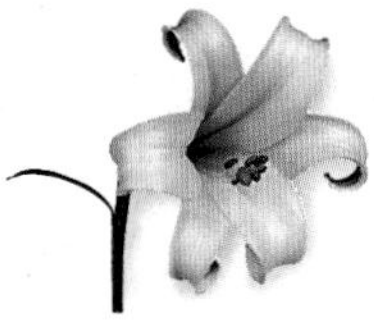

HORIZONTAL

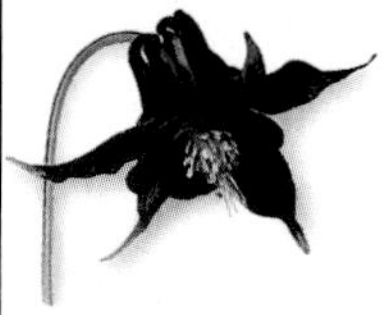

NODDING

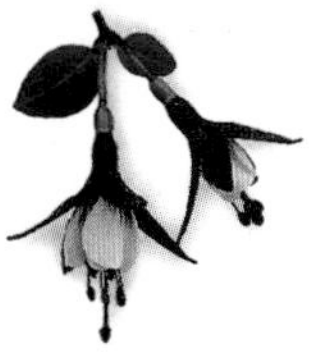

PENDENT

FLOWER COLOUR

The colours and markings of flowers originally evolved to attract pollinators; in cultivation, many have been modified to extend their decorative value.

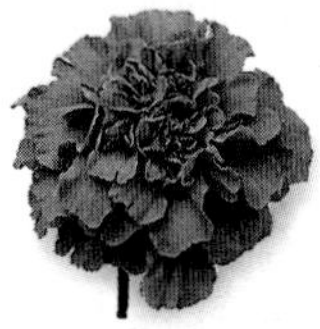

SELF-COLOURED

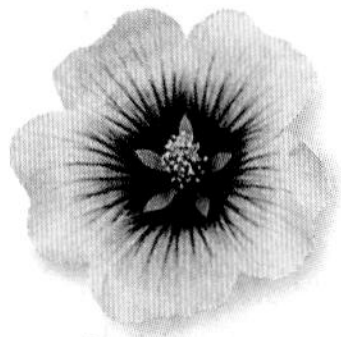

BICOLOURED

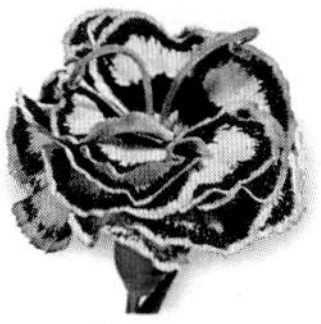

PICOTEE

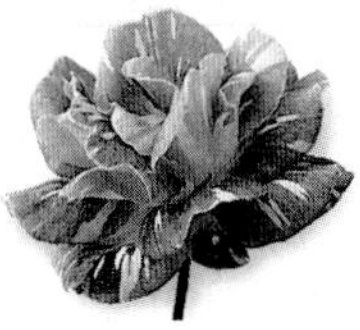

STRIPED

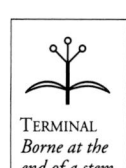

Hardiness

Every plant is hardy in its natural habitat, since it has adapted to the distinctive conditions that exist there. The concept of hardiness therefore applies only to cultivated plants, which almost invariably live in an alien environment. In simple terms, hardiness is the capacity of a plant to withstand prevailing climatic conditions all year round. In cold areas, it is generally used to refer to tolerance of low temperatures; in hot climates, it is sometimes used to describe resistance to such stresses as drought and extreme heat.

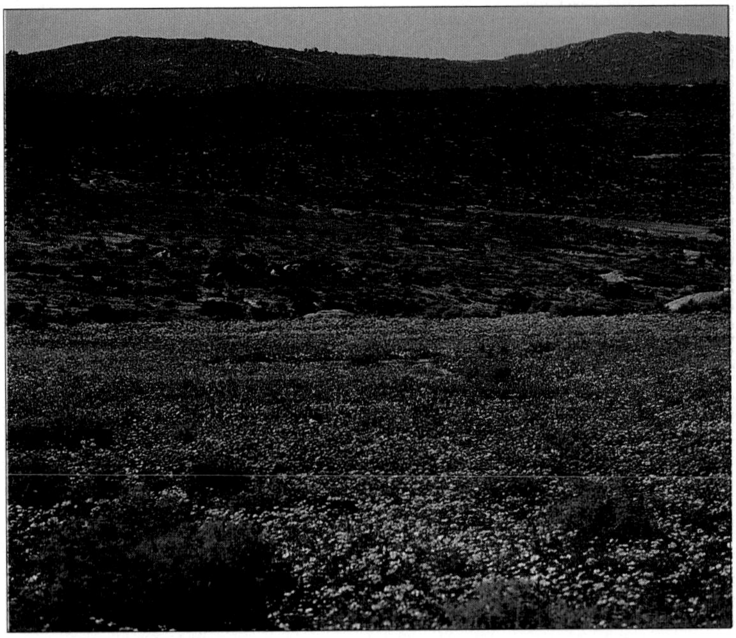

Hardiness and exposure
The plateau grasslands of South Africa (including Namaqualand, above) are divided into low veldt, middle veldt, and high veldt. Plants occurring at different altitudes are adapted to withstand different degrees of cold and exposure to wind.

Factors affecting hardiness

The ability of an individual plant to withstand severe conditions depends on a number of factors. In general, plants become increasingly hardy as they mature. The chief determinant of hardiness, however, is the degree of similarity between conditions in the garden and those in the plant's natural habitat, especially soil type and fertility, drainage, soil and air temperature, and levels of humidity, light, and rainfall. It is best, therefore, to select the right plant for the site, rather than to try to tailor the site to the plant's needs. Fortunately for gardeners, most plants readily acclimatize to new circumstances, although some will only thrive in their indigenous surroundings.

Adaptations for survival

Plants in the wild have developed a number of strategies to enable them to survive severe conditions. Many hardy plants become dormant in winter, restricting their growing period to those seasons when conditions of light, moisture, and temperature are favourable. Annuals complete their life-cycle in a single season, leaving dormant seed to germinate the following spring. The top-growth of many perennials dies down in autumn; the roots, safely insulated below ground, store food in order to permit rapid growth when favourable conditions return. Woody, deciduous plants protect themselves by shedding their leaves, the parts most vulnerable to winter cold, in autumn; their buds remain dormant until triggered into growth by increasing warmth and light in spring. Many hardy evergreens produce small leaves with a reduced surface area, which is often leathery or covered with an insulating layer of hairs to minimize the drying effects of strong winds. These plants often root deeply to levels where the soil will not freeze. They may also adopt a ground-hugging habit, or produce aromatic oils that help to conserve water and act in a similar way to antifreeze.

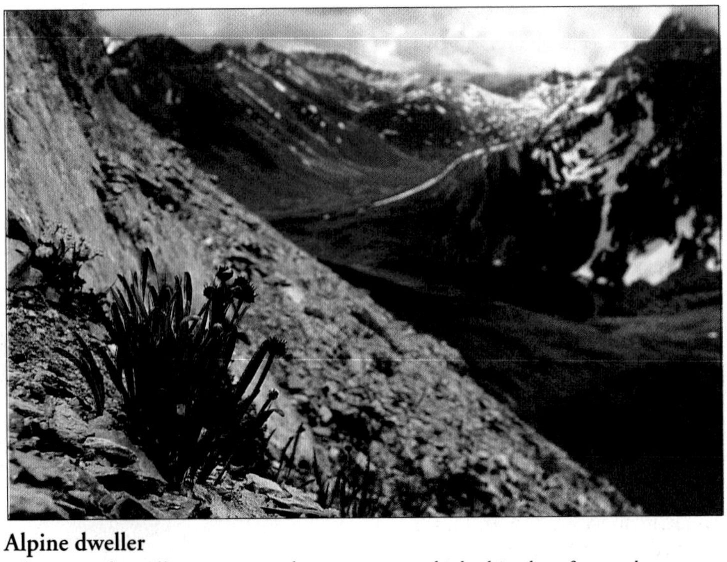

Alpine dweller
Alpines, such as Allium campanulatum, *occur at high altitudes, often under snow in winter; they are usually hardy, but seldom tolerate high winter rainfall.*

The effects of habitat

An understanding of a plant's natural habitat provides valuable clues to its needs in cultivation. For example, alpine plants that live in scree and rock crevices develop deep root systems that extend widely to take up moisture and the available nutrients. Beneath the rocks, the roots are insulated from extremes of both cold and heat. During winter, the top-growth is maintained at temperatures near freezing point by a blanket of dry snow. Snow melt in spring triggers a short but intense period of growth; many alpines bloom early so that they may set seed and become dormant before the snows return. In cultivation, therefore, alpine plants need a very free-draining, low-nutrient soil, a cool, deep root run, and shelter from high winter rainfall.

At another extreme, plants native to hot, desert-like areas are adapted to store moisture in succulent tissue, safeguarded against desiccation and the sun's heat by spines, hairs, or tough, waxy skin. In the dry season, succulents may lose up to 70 per cent of their water content, and may even experience severe cold. After the rains, plants swell and burst into bloom. When cultivated in a cool, wet climate, most succulents need the warmth of a heated greenhouse or must be grown as houseplants, with little or no watering outside their natural period of growth.

The effects of climate

The difference between continental and maritime (coastal) climates is a significant factor affecting plant hardiness. In continental interiors, most rainfall occurs in summer, and winters are relatively dry and often extremely cold. Seasonal differences are clearly defined: a large, sustained rise in temperature in spring is followed by a long, hot summer. These conditions are ideal for plant growth, maturing of flower buds, and ripening of woody growth.

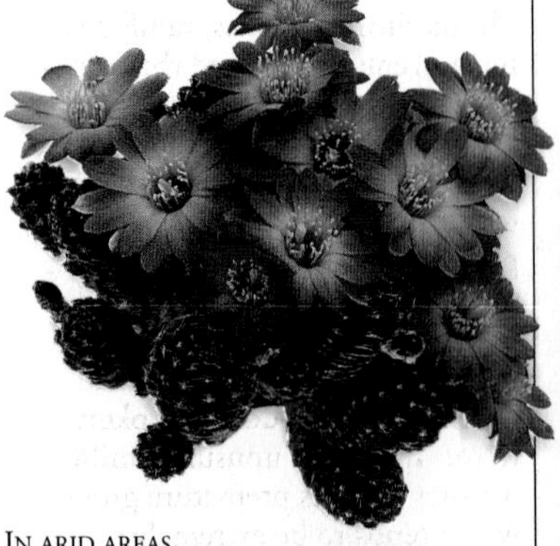

IN ARID AREAS, *cacti such as* Rebutia pygmaea *are resistant to cold, but may require frost protection in wetter climates.*

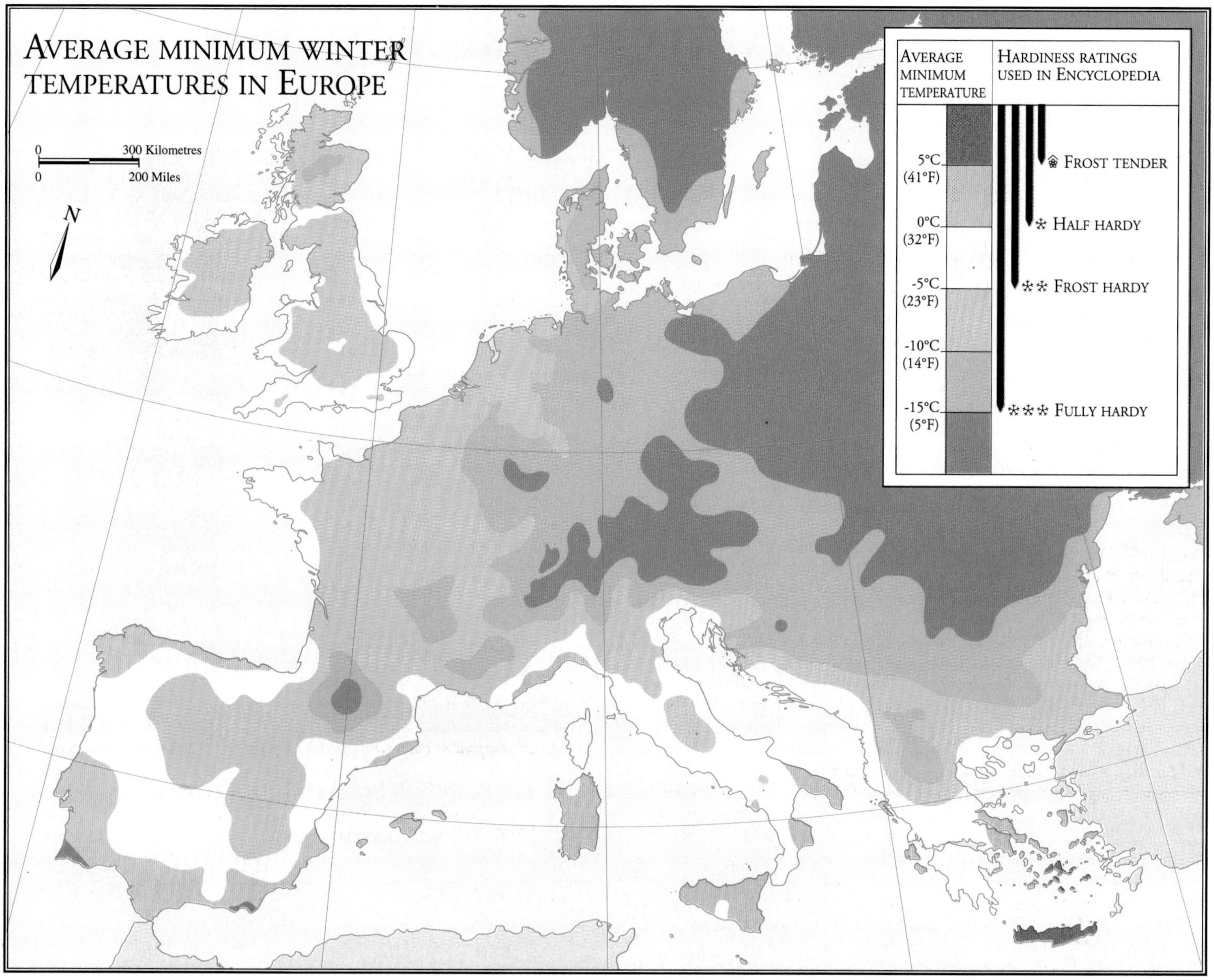

Using the temperature map to determine plant hardiness
The coloured bands on the map of Europe above indicate average minimum winter temperatures. To establish whether a plant in this encyclopedia will be hardy in a chosen region (and therefore whether it may safely be grown outdoors all year round), compare its hardiness rating with the prevailing minimum winter temperature.

Ripening encourages internal cell walls to become firm and tough, yet flexible, ensuring that the plant is better able to withstand severe winter cold and periods of freezing that follow.

In maritime climates, rainfall is more evenly distributed throughout the year, and temperature extremes are modified by the presence of vast bodies of water. The fluctuation of temperatures in summer may prevent adequate ripening, leaving growth soft and more susceptible to cold damage. Persistent rainfall in winter may cause the roots of dormant or semi-dormant plants to rot. In spring, unusually mild weather induces premature growth, which tends to be extremely vulnerable to damage, even in light frost. For this reason, in a maritime climate, plants that are fully hardy in the extremes of a continental winter may not grow to their full stature, or may fail to thrive at all.

Hardiness in cultivation

Plants exposed to temperatures below their normal tolerances may experience impairment of their physiological processes. In severe cases, this can lead to injuries, such as damage to shoots, stems, and leaves, or even to plant death. Some of these injuries may be avoided by identifying and improving those conditions that cause stress to plants grown beyond their prescribed limits of hardiness.

Perhaps the most vital factor, certainly for evergreen plants, is protection against cold, drying winds; these increase the rate of transpiration from leaf surfaces, causing moisture to be lost more quickly than it can be replaced from the soil, especially in a dry or frosty spell. Protect plants, especially young specimens, with a wind-filtering hedge or belt of trees, or more locally with fine-grade netting.

Frost damage to roots may often be avoided by growing plants in deep, crumbly, easily worked, well-drained soil, into which roots may penetrate easily, and by applying a thick, dry winter mulch, which will also protect dormant roots from excessive moisture in winter.

Promote ripening of wood by positioning plants in a warm, sunny site (providing they are tolerant of full sun). A warm wall retains and reflects the sun's heat in summer, and so enhances ripening. In winter, the few added degrees of warmth may make the difference between success and failure.

Hardiness ratings

All plants in this encyclopedia are assigned one of 4 hardiness ratings, according to the lowest temperature they are likely to withstand (see key to map above). For example, a plant that is rated as frost hardy will withstand temperatures to -5°C (23°F). For plants rated as frost tender, a minimum temperature for successful cultivation is also given. In some cases, a hardiness rating is qualified by the word "borderline", which means that the plant requires conditions 2–3°C (4–5°F) warmer than the minimum for the given category. Bear in mind, however, that the hardiness ratings are guidelines only, and, as discussed above, many other factors affect a plant's overall hardiness.

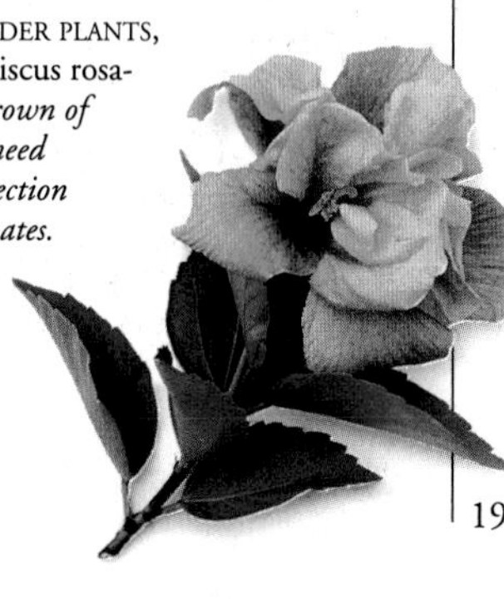

FROST-TENDER PLANTS, *such as* Hibiscus rosa-sinensis *'Crown of Bohemia', need winter protection in cold climates.*

The garden environment

All gardens contain a unique combination of light levels, exposure to wind and cold, soil type, and drainage. Understanding the prevailing conditions in a region and their small-scale variations in the garden is an important first step in devising a planting scheme, as plants from similar natural habitats can then be used. By combining the advice presented here with good design practice, it is possible to develop an attractive garden using plants that will thrive in the sites chosen.

WATER IN THE SOIL

Rainfall is the main source of water for plants grown outdoors, and is vital for plant growth. Rain drains through the soil, where it is absorbed by plant root hairs, along with essential minerals. In order to be able to take up water and nutrients readily, most plants require an aerated soil that is moist but nonetheless well-drained. Waterlogged soil lacks oxygen, and is normally fatal to plants, as the roots will rot if deprived of oxygen. These conditions are, however, ideal for cultivating plants that thrive in the saturated soil of such habitats as bogs, marshland, streambanks, and riversides.

SUNLIGHT AND GROWTH

All plants need light. It is the source of energy for photosynthesis, which fuels their growth. Heat from sunlight also warms the air and soil, and increases humidity through the evaporation of water. The rate of plant growth is largely dependent on the amount of light received, and therefore on day length and the extent of the growing season (determined, in turn, by latitude and altitude).

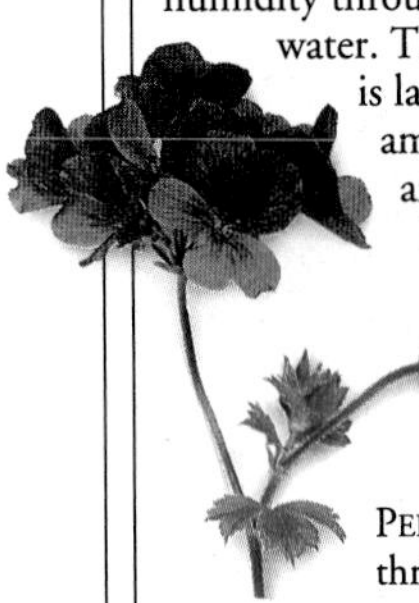

PELARGONIUM *'POLKA'* thrives in sunny sites.

Individual plants vary in their need for and response to sunlight. Those that need full sun grow pale and elongated (etiolated) in poor light. Conversely, the foliage of plants that are adapted to shaded conditions in their natural habitat will often scorch in strong sunlight.

In cold areas, plants from warm climates require a site in full sun, such as the base of a sunny wall. Summer warmth helps to increase a plant's food store, and ripens the shoots of woody plants, as well as roots, corms, bulbs, and tubers below ground. Plants with fully ripened tissue are also better able to withstand winter cold.

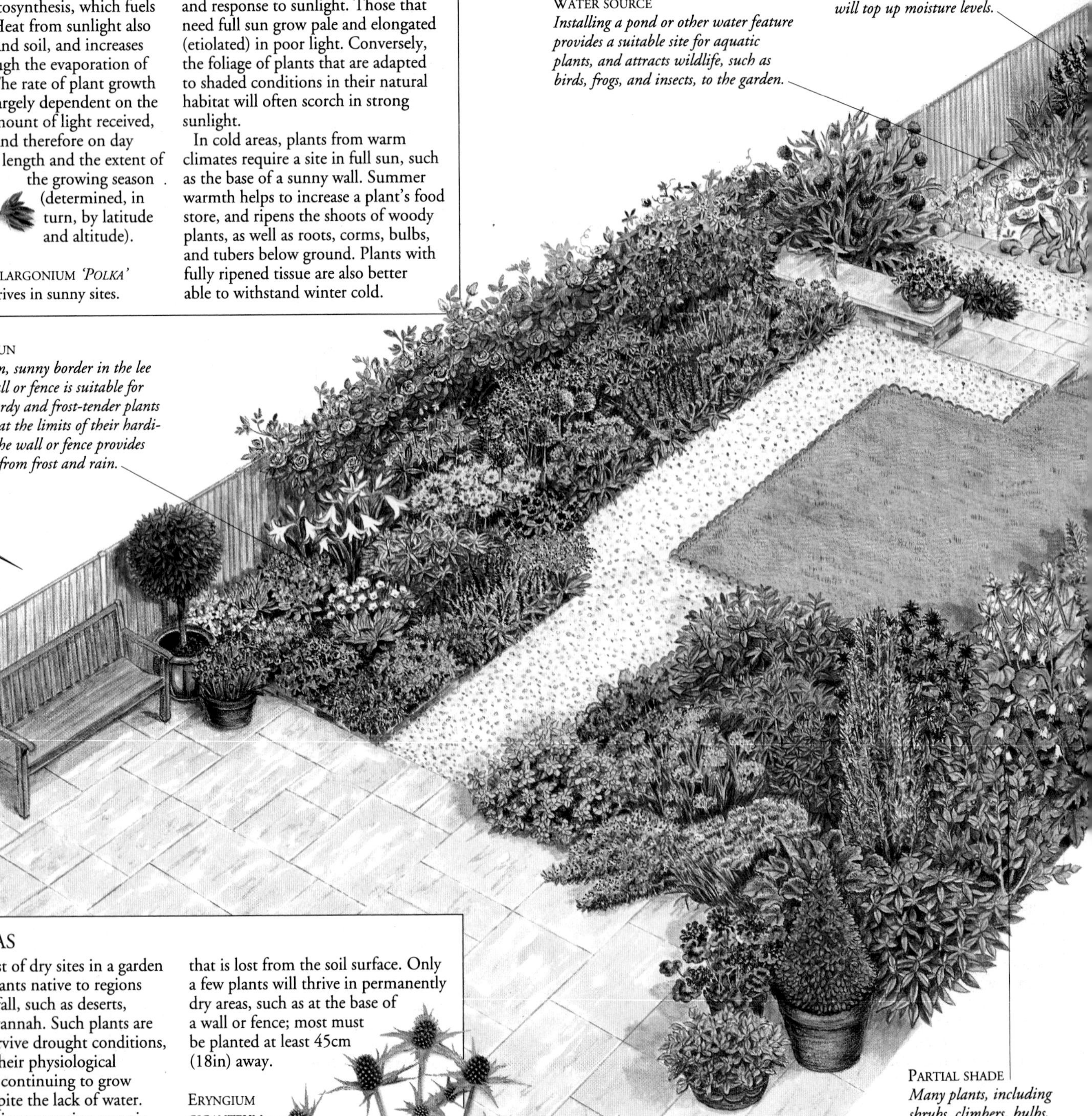

DAMP SOIL
Low-lying, damp soil is ideal for a bog garden; the overflow from an adjacent pond will top up moisture levels.

WATER SOURCE
Installing a pond or other water feature provides a suitable site for aquatic plants, and attracts wildlife, such as birds, frogs, and insects, to the garden.

FULL SUN
A warm, sunny border in the lee of a wall or fence is suitable for half-hardy and frost-tender plants grown at the limits of their hardiness. The wall or fence provides shelter from frost and rain.

PARTIAL SHADE
Many plants, including shrubs, climbers, bulbs, and ground-cover plants, either tolerate or prefer partial shade.

DRY AREAS

Make the most of dry sites in a garden by growing plants native to regions with low rainfall, such as deserts, scrub, and savannah. Such plants are adapted to survive drought conditions, maintaining their physiological processes and continuing to grow normally, despite the lack of water. Alternatively, incorporating organic matter into the soil will improve its ability to hold moisture. Mulching will help to reduce the amount of water that is lost from the soil surface. Only a few plants will thrive in permanently dry areas, such as at the base of a wall or fence; most must be planted at least 45cm (18in) away.

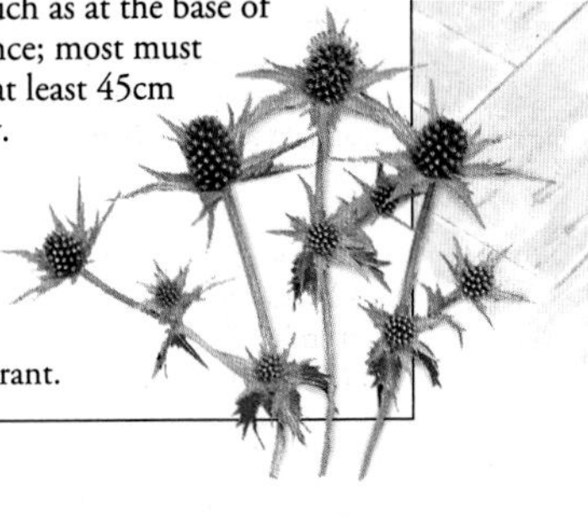

ERYNGIUM GIGANTEUM *'SILVER GHOST'* is drought-tolerant.

SHELTER FROM THE WIND

The movement of air over leaf surfaces increases the rate of transpiration and flow of water through a plant. If water loss is greater than uptake, however, the plant suffers leaf scorch and desiccation and, in extreme cases, will die. These effects are most severe in winter, particularly with evergreens, as water lost from the leaves cannot be replaced when the soil is frozen.

In coastal or exposed areas, strong, persistent winds may stunt the top-growth of woody plants, making them lop-sided. Windbreaks, ideally using trees or hedges from maritime areas, provide shelter for a distance equal to up to 5 times their own height.

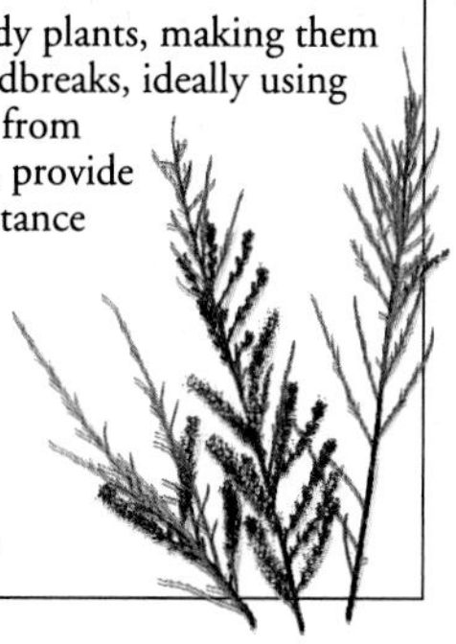

TAMARIX TETRANDRA *is wind-resistant.*

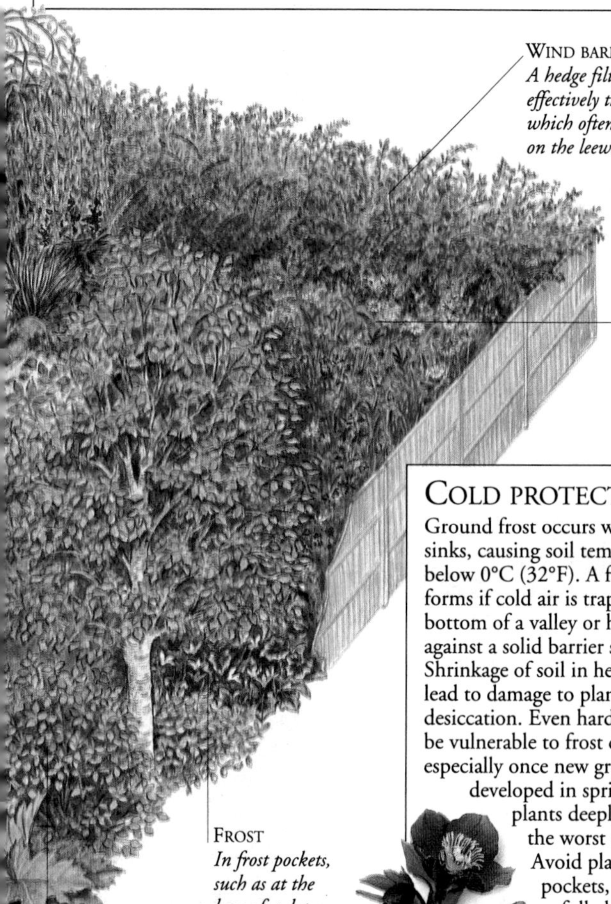

WIND BARRIER *A hedge filters wind more effectively than a solid wall, which often creates turbulence on the leeward side.*

POOR SOIL *Soil that is low in nutrients is ideal for a patch of wild-flower meadow.*

FROST *In frost pockets, such as at the base of a slope, provide protection or use only fully hardy plants.*

DAPPLED SHADE *Woodland plants and many spring-flowering bulbs are excellent for growing in the shade of a tree.*

COLD PROTECTION

Ground frost occurs when cold air sinks, causing soil temperature to fall below 0°C (32°F). A frost pocket forms if cold air is trapped at the bottom of a valley or hollow, or against a solid barrier such as a wall. Shrinkage of soil in heavy frosts may lead to damage to plant roots from desiccation. Even hardy plants may be vulnerable to frost damage, especially once new growth has developed in spring. Mulch plants deeply to combat the worst effects of frost. Avoid planting in frost pockets, or use only fully hardy plants, ideally with top-growth emerging in late spring, when the risk of severe frosts has passed.

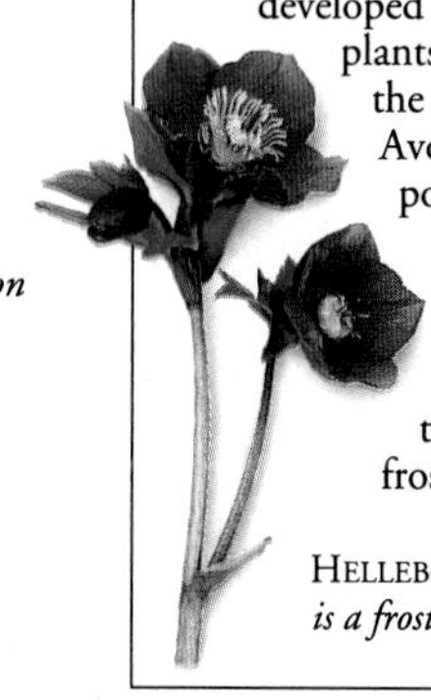

HELLEBORUS ORIENTALIS *is a frost-tolerant perennial.*

SHADY SITES

Shaded areas of the garden are often regarded as problematic, since many plants thrive only in full sun. These sites are, however, ideal for plants that occur naturally in shaded habitats, such as woodland, the bases of cliffs, or the bottoms of ravines, and which are tolerant of lower light levels. There are several different degrees of shade. Light dappled shade is similar to that found in hedgerows and green woodland, where patterns of shade and sunlight shift over the course of a day; plants may receive direct sunlight, but for short periods only. Partial shade describes a site where shade is more or less constant throughout the day, as found beneath a canopy of deciduous trees. A deeply shaded site, such as beneath evergreen trees and shrubs, or between cliffs or buildings, never receives direct sunlight.

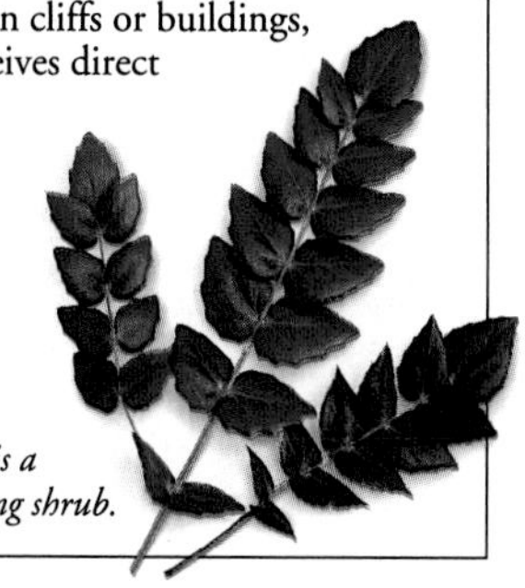

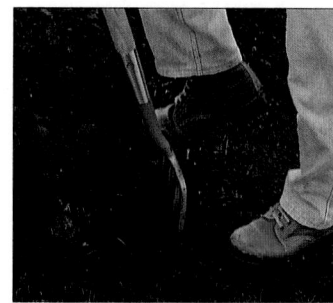

MAHONIA NERVOSA *is a shade-loving shrub.*

SOIL TYPES

Soils may be divided into mineral and organic types (although all have both mineral and organic components). Mineral soils, derived from weathered rock, are classified according to the size and composition of their particles.

Clay soils have tiny particles, and are often very fertile. They are also heavy to dig, may become waterlogged after rainfall, and warm up slowly in spring. They are easily compacted when wet, and prone to surface-capping (baking hard), reducing the amount of air available to roots and seeds.

Silty soils are moderately fertile and hold less water than clay soils, but are also prone to compaction and capping.

Calcareous (chalky) soils are shallow, free-draining, moderately fertile, and alkaline (see panel below).

Sandy soils contain particles up to 1,000 times larger than those of clay soils. They are light, free-draining, and easily worked, and warm up rapidly in spring, but are often of low fertility because nutrients are quickly leached away as water drains through the soil.

Loam soils are the best mineral soils for most purposes, as they have a balanced mix of particle sizes, and combine good drainage and moisture-retention with high fertility.

Organic soils, particularly those that contain peat, are formed by the decay of organic matter, and are low in nutrients. They are suitable for plants from acid habitats. A number of peat substitutes are available, based on such materials as leaf mould or coconut fibre, rather than natural peat.

Identifying soil type
The easiest way to identify the soil type in a garden is to examine its colour and texture. Soil pH (see panel below) may be measured using an electronic meter or a soil testing kit. The local geology, and the kind of weeds and other plants growing in a garden, will also provide further information on soil type.

SANDY SOIL *Light and free-draining, but often of low fertility.*

PEATY SOIL *Acid, of low fertility, moist, but often poorly drained.*

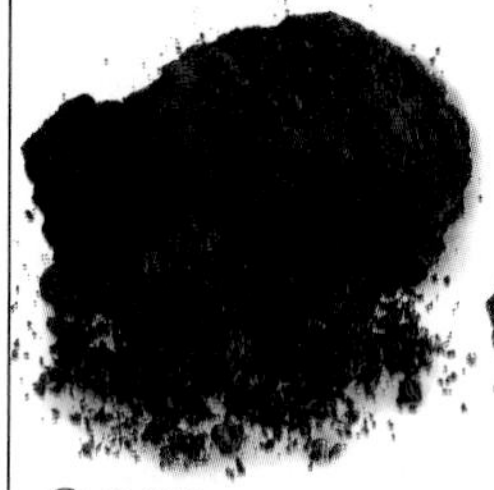

CLAY SOIL *Fertile, but heavy and prone to waterlogging.*

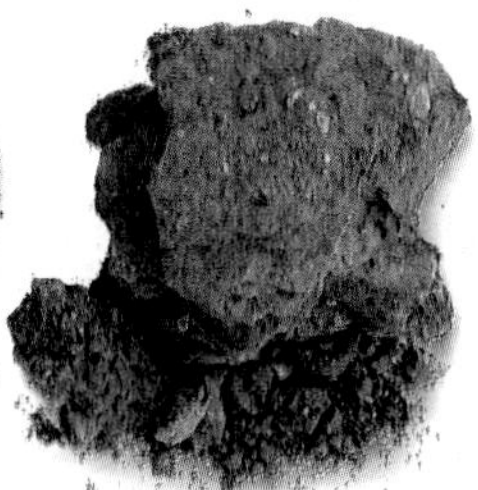

CALCAREOUS SOIL *Alkaline, well-drained, and usually moderately fertile.*

SILTY SOIL *Moderately fertile, but prone to compaction.*

IMPROVING THE SOIL

Few gardens have the fertile, well-drained, loamy soil that is ideal for most plants, but there are several ways in which soil can be improved. Incorporating organic matter, such as garden compost or manure, increases the humus content of soil, improving its structure. The addition of humus to clay and silty soils draws the fine particles together into larger, crumb-like structures, and improves the flow of air and water between them. If the soil is usually waterlogged, it may be necessary to install drainage pipes. Adding humus to sandy soils increases their ability to hold both moisture and nutrients.

Soil fertility may be improved by applying fertilizer, either in liquid form, or as solid slow-release pellets or concentrated granules.

The acidity or alkalinity of the soil is also important when considering what plants to grow. It is measured on the pH scale, which is numbered 1 to 14: acid soils have a pH value below 7, and alkaline soils a pH value above 7; neutral soils are pH7. Adding lime will reduce acidity; incorporating organic matter will lower alkalinity to some extent. In the long term, however, it is better to select plants that thrive in a given soil type, rather than trying to change its pH radically. Many plants prefer neutral to slightly acid soil. Others, such as heathers (*Calluna* and *Erica*), prefer acid conditions, and will thrive in peaty soil; those needing alkaline conditions flourish in limestone-rich, chalk soils.

Forking in organic matter
Improve soil structure by adding liberal quantities of organic matter, such as well-rotted manure or garden compost.

Outdoor cultivation

For successful outdoor cultivation, preparation is as important as routine maintenance. Wherever possible, select plants whose natural habitats are similar to the proposed planting site (see pp.20–21). Next, choose robust specimens that are free of pests and diseases. Finally, prepare the site carefully and plant out at the most favourable time of year.

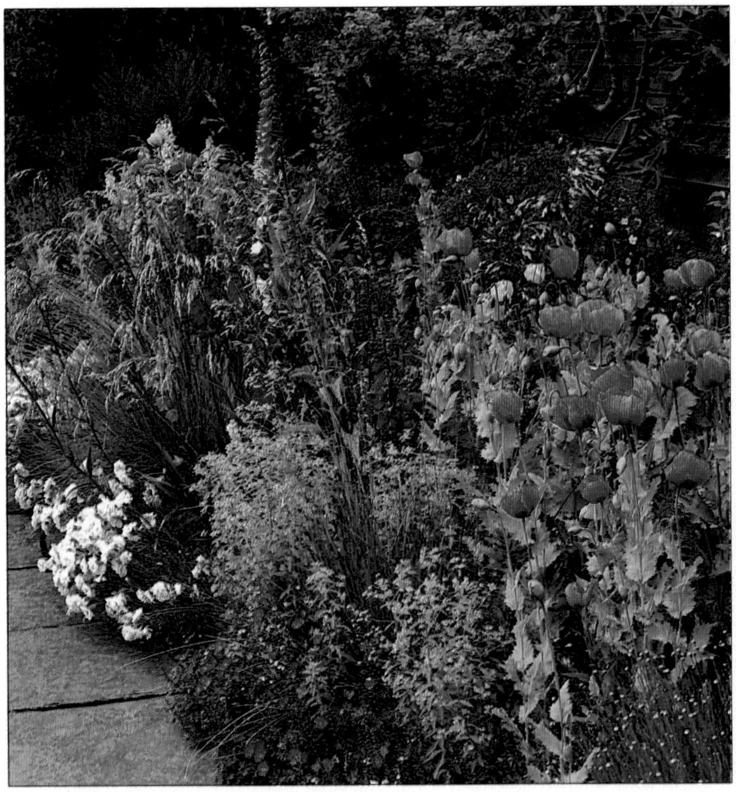

A well-maintained and healthy border
For flourishing, vigorous growth, provide plants with well-cultivated soil and good drainage. Allow plenty of space for each plant to develop, and keep free from weeds. Many plants will flower freely over a long period if they are regularly dead-headed.

Choosing the right plant

When planning a garden, bear in mind the characteristics of the site. Try to find a plant from a similar habitat, although the match need not be exact, since most plants will tolerate a range of conditions. Information on natural habitats is contained in the introduction to each genus in this encyclopedia.

It is important to acquire robust, well-grown plants. When buying plants, inspect for signs of pests or diseases, such as discoloured foliage or dieback (see pp.30–31). Take particular care over selecting plants that will have a long lifetime in the garden. With herbaceous perennials, look for vigorous top-growth, with strong, emergent shoots or plump, healthy buds, and an even network of established roots. Ensure that the potting compost is moist; a layer of moss or liverwort suggests a plant has been in its container for some time and may suffer from nutrient deficiency and waterlogging.

When buying a tree or shrub, make sure that it has a balanced framework of top-growth in proportion to the size of its root ball. Shrubs and trees are available either bare-rooted or root-balled (with a ball of soil around the roots, wrapped in netting or hessian) in the dormant season, or in containers at any time of year. Select bare-rooted plants with well-developed, fibrous roots that show no signs of desiccation. With root-balled plants, check that the root ball is firm and evenly moist, with the wrapping intact. As with perennials, when buying container-grown shrubs or trees, avoid plants with roots that are tightly coiled or that protrude from the base of the container. Plants with restricted roots will probably have suffered nutrient deficiency, and will establish poorly and slowly at best.

Soil preparation and planting

Careful preparation of the planting site is critical for vigorous, healthy growth. First clear the site of all weeds. Next, prepare the site by digging deeply or using a powered cultivator, and incorporating well-rotted organic matter to improve soil structure and fertility (see p.21). If possible, prepare the ground a season before planting.

Autumn or spring is the best time to plant herbaceous perennials. An autumn planting enables roots to become established while the soil is still warm. Those herbaceous plants, including certain *Kniphofia* species and cultivars, that are intolerant of cold and wet when not established, are better planted in spring.

Bare-rooted and root-balled trees and shrubs should be planted as soon as possible after purchase, in mild winter weather; do not plant in wet or frozen soil, as roots will not become established, and are likely to suffer frost damage.

Although container-grown plants may be planted at any time of year, spring and summer plantings need extra care, especially with watering; growth will be checked and the plant may die if the soil is allowed to dry out. Most trees and shrubs are best planted in autumn, at the start of the dormant season. Some, including certain evergreens, will establish better if planted in spring, although they should be watered well, particularly in dry weather.

Watering

An adequate supply of water is essential for plant growth. For most plants grown in the open, rainfall is the main source of water. However, due to the unreliability of rainfall in most areas, some form of artificial watering is usually required. The amount needed varies between plants, and also between sites, depending in part on soil type and structure (see p.21). Bear in mind that too much water can cause as much damage to plants as too little.

Most plants require more water when in active growth than at other times of the year. Plants that have a dormant period (such as some bulbs) should be kept moist, but no more, when dormant. Newly planted or transplanted plants should be watered until they have become established, unless rainfall has been sufficient.

Always water thoroughly, so that water is available deep in the soil; it is better to water infrequently in large quantities than to apply a little often. Try to deliver water directly to individual plants at ground level, and to avoid forming puddles at the soil surface. Water in the early morning or evening to reduce loss by evaporation.

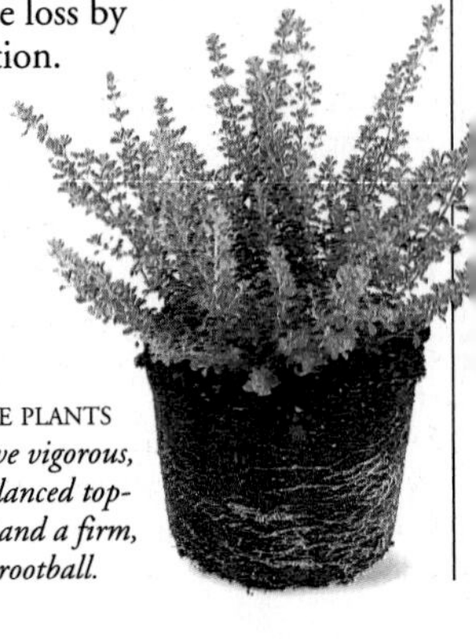

CHOOSE PLANTS *that have vigorous, well-balanced top-growth and a firm, fibrous rootball.*

CONTAINER GARDENING

Use plants grown in containers to decorate paved areas such as patios and courtyards, or as focal points in other areas of a garden. In frost-prone areas, many tender plants can be displayed in containers outdoors in summer, and moved under glass in winter.

In mixed plantings, it is important to group plants that grow at a similar rate and require similar conditions. Set containers in position before planting up, as they may be too heavy to move afterwards. Plants may need watering twice daily in hot spells. If grown in a container for more than one season, plants should be top-dressed in spring by replacing the upper layer of compost with new compost.

For permanent plantings, use fertile, loam-based potting compost, such as JI No.2 or No.3. Loamless composts, lightweight in structure as well as being clean to use, are most suitable for short-term plantings, especially for hanging baskets. Most loamless composts now contain slow-release fertilizer; if not, apply fertilizer regularly in the growing season. Do not allow the compost to dry out.

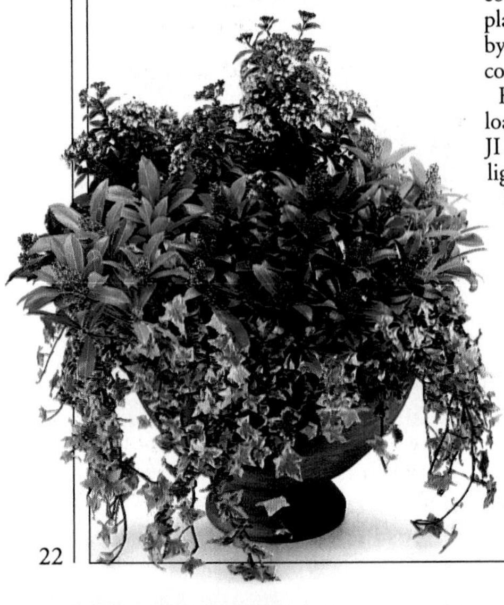

MIXED CONTAINER PLANTINGS *can provide a succession of ornamental features, with evergreen leaves providing prolonged interest, and acting as a foil to the flowers.*

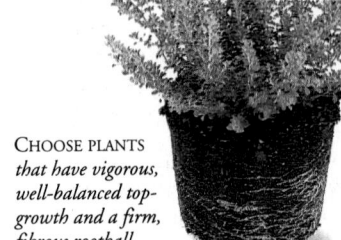

Staking

After planting, young trees usually require support for 1 or 2 years, until strong, anchoring roots are established. For most, a short stake is best, as it permits movement of the trunk, encouraging root establishment and stem growth. Stake trees with slender or flexible stems, or ones over 4m (12ft) tall, as high as the crown in the first year; reduce the height of the stake in the second year; remove it in the third.

Some perennials also need staking to prevent lax stems from over-hanging other plants, as well as to protect them from wind damage.

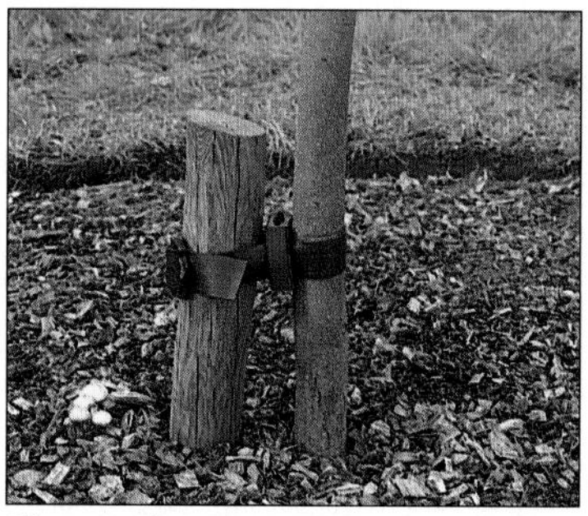

Short stake

Insert the stake before planting, with 60cm (24in) below ground and 50cm (20in) above. Secure stem with a tie and spacer, to avoid stem constriction.

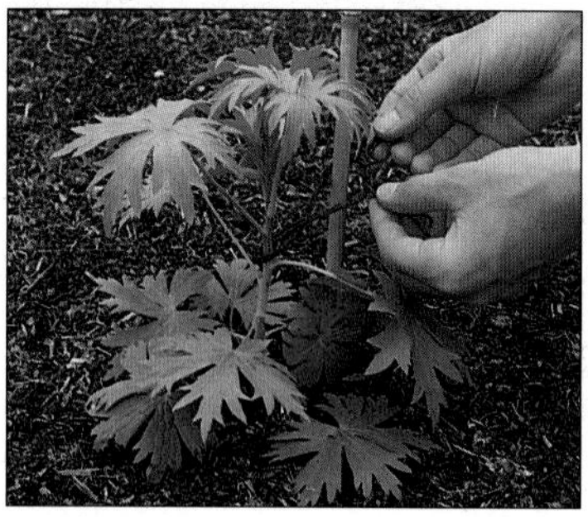

Single stake

Insert a single cane to two-thirds of the mature height of a tall, single-stemmed plant, when it is 20cm (8in) high. Tie the stem to the stake using soft twine.

Ring stake

Use ring stakes for clump-forming plants of medium size; link stakes together for taller plants. Set stakes in place early in the season, and raise as the plants grow.

Mulching

Mulching soil has three purposes. It helps to prevent the germination of weed seeds, minimizes evaporation of water from the soil surface, and keeps plant roots cooler in summer and warmer in winter. Organic mulches, such as garden compost or well-rotted farmyard manure, also improve soil structure and fertility.

There are 2 main types of mulch: continuous sheet mulches and loose mulches consisting of material such as garden compost or farmyard manure, bark chips, cocoa shells, coarse grit, or gravel. In areas with severe winter cold, apply a deep, dry mulch of bracken litter, leaf mould, ash, or straw to protect roots and dormant buds from freezing.

Mulches should be applied annually in spring or autumn, to soil that is moist but not water-logged; never mulch very cold or frozen soil. For effective control of weeds, lay the mulch at least 5–8cm (2–3in) deep. To provide adequate winter protection for the roots of plants growing at the limits of their hardiness, the mulch should be 10–15cm (4–6in) deep. A mulch should not be applied too close to the crown of a plant, since this will encourage rot and attract pests that damage new top-growth.

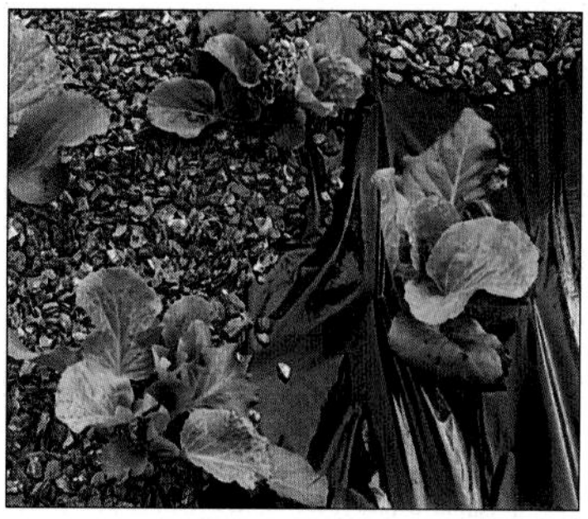

Sheet mulches

Black plastic or woven-fibre sheeting, disguised with a material such as bark chips, controls weeds over a large area and may raise soil temperature slightly.

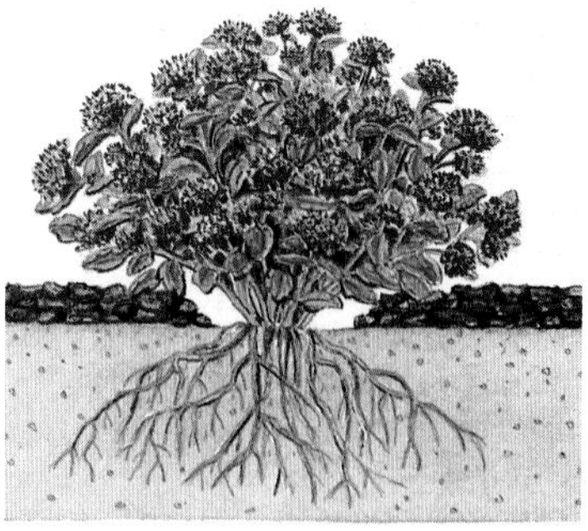

Loose mulches

Applying a loose mulch to soil regulates its temperature, improves moisture-retention, and discourages the growth of weeds.

Routine garden maintenance

A number of routine operations should be carried out during the growing season. For some plants, both thinning (cutting out weak shoots early in the year in order to encourage healthy development of the rest) and stopping increase the number and quality of flowers in certain perennials. Dead-heading prolongs flowering and prevents self-seeding. Cutting back dead, diseased, damaged, and flowered shoots and clearing residual weed growth in autumn help to maintain good hygiene, reduce risk of disease, and prevent rotting in winter, when plants are most vulnerable.

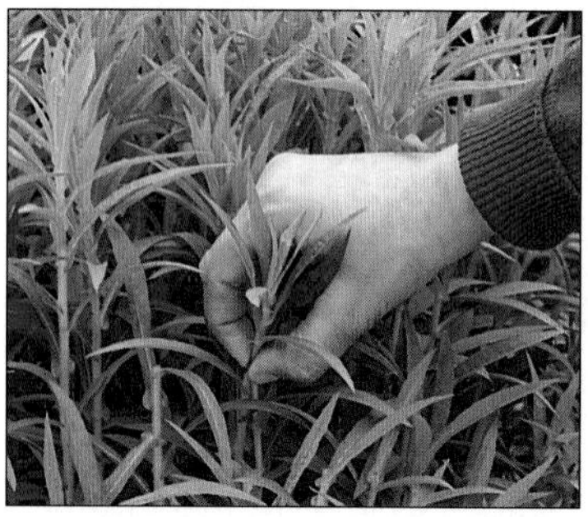

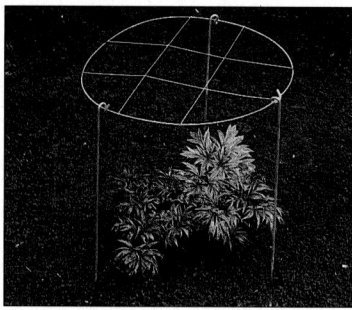

Stopping

As plants reach one-third of their final height, pinch out 2.5–5cm (1–2in) from the stem tip, to encourage shorter, sturdier stems and formation of flower buds in the upper leaf axils.

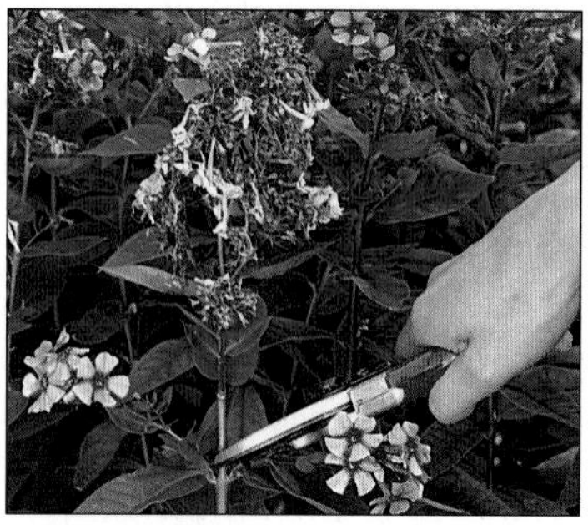

Dead-heading

Removing dead or fading flowers diverts energy into growth, improving flowering potential for the following season. Break stems cleanly using finger and thumb, or use secateurs for tougher stems.

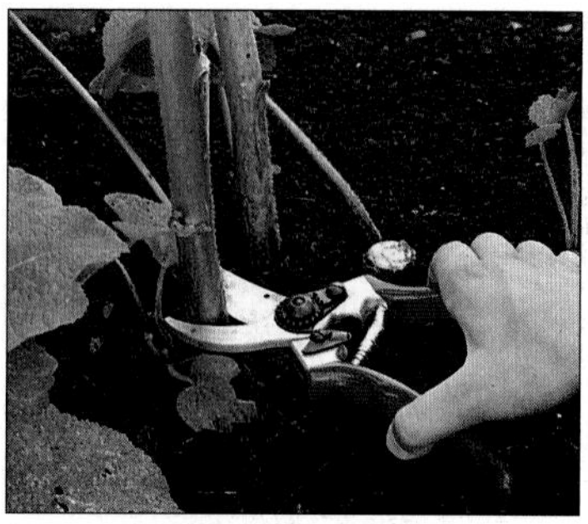

Preventing seed formation

Remove flowered stems, especially of short-lived perennials, before they set seed. As well as helping to prolong the plant's life, this also reduces the nuisance of unwanted, self-sown seedlings.

Winter protection

Small plants, particularly immature ones, should be protected from excessive winter rain, frost, or snow in a cold or heated frame. Cloches or, where practical, propped panes of glass may be used to shelter mature plants.

Protect larger shrubs growing at the limits of their climatic tolerance by packing them with straw and wrapping them loosely in hessian or horticultural fleece. Frost-tender, wall-trained shrubs and climbers are best covered with screens of fleece or fine netting, stretched over a framework of laths or canes. See also Mulching, above.

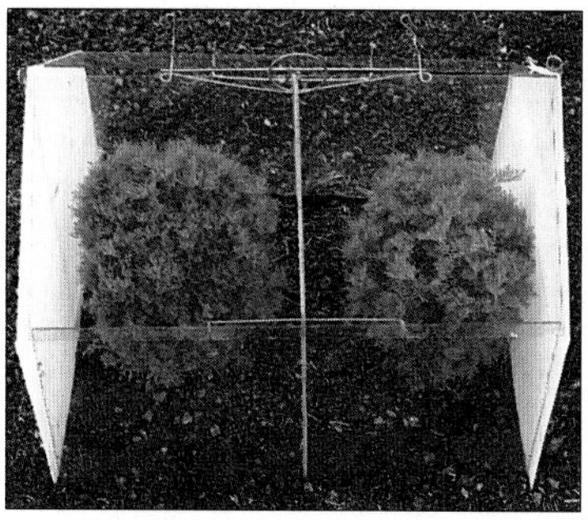

Barn cloche

A barn cloche is useful for protecting young seedlings, frost-tender to frost-hardy perennials, and small shrubs. Close the ends with sheets of glass or plastic to protect plants from cold winds.

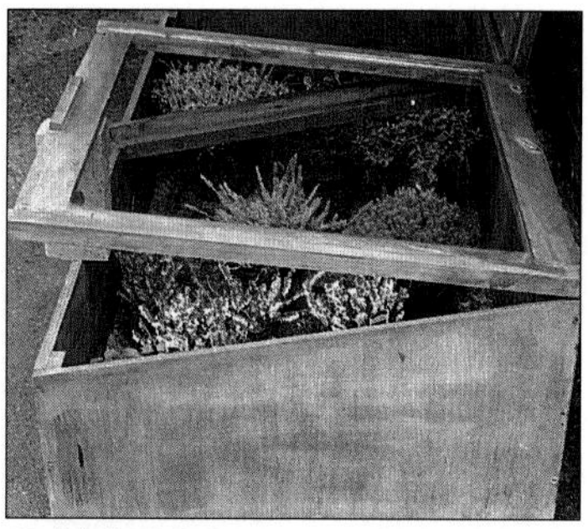

Cold frame

Use a cold frame to overwinter autumn-sown seedlings, and to protect alpines and other plants from excess moisture in winter and summer. It is also ideal for hardening off young plants in spring.

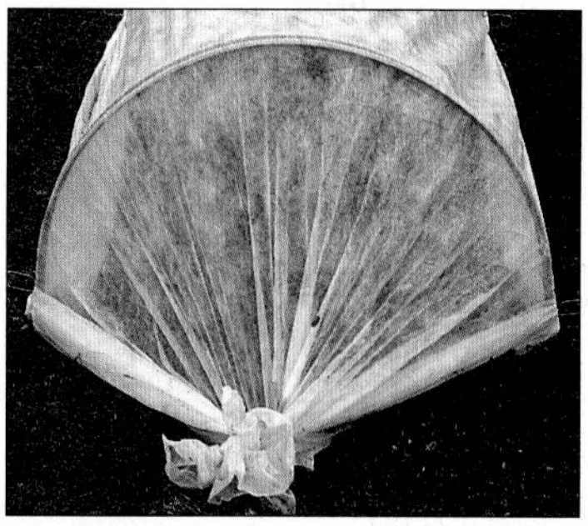

Tunnel cloche

A tunnel cloche made of horticultural fleece protects autumn-sown annuals and biennials from severe frosts. It will also allow air to circulate and water to penetrate.

Care under glass

Cultivation under glass, whether in a greenhouse or conservatory, or as houseplants, greatly extends the range of plants that can be grown, especially in cool climates. In greenhouses in particular, the environment should be regulated to suit specific plants, using one of four distinct regimes (see panel below right).

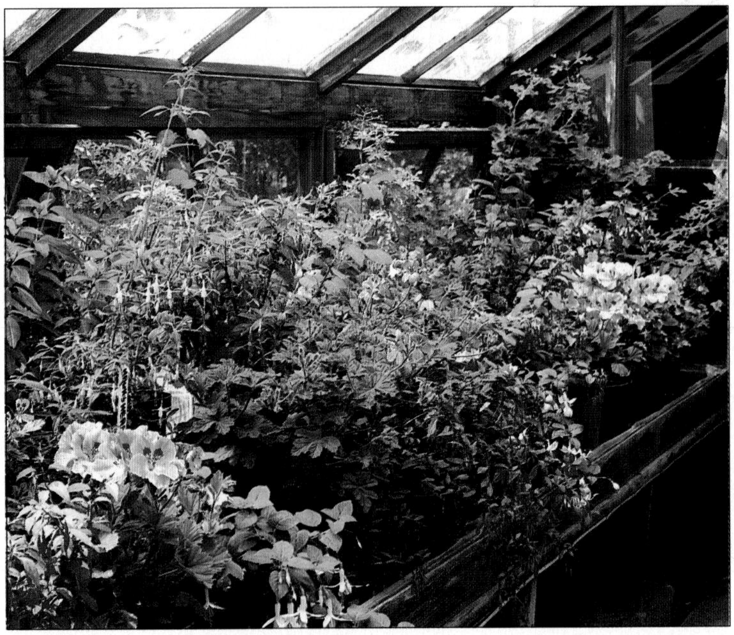

Regulating the greenhouse environment
A greenhouse offers the most versatile means of maintaining a controlled growing environment, especially with regard to temperature, ventilation, and humidity. Areas may also be sectioned off to enable a range of regimes to be set up.

Environments under glass

As a rule, plants that are grown as houseplants must be able to tolerate less than ideal light levels, as well as the dry air associated with central heating. Conservatories provide good levels of light but may become too hot and dry in summer for some plants, as they often lack good ventilation or any means of shading or increasing humidity, and may be too cold in winter if unheated.

Conditions in a greenhouse are easier to control. Ventilation and temperature can be adjusted in most, and humidity increased by damping down or using a hand-held sprayer. Shade may be provided with green shade netting or a shade wash. Alpine plants are best grown in a type of unheated greenhouse known as an alpine house, which is designed to provide a level of ventilation 2 or 3 times greater than in a standard greenhouse (see p.41).

With all plants grown under glass, the need for light, moisture, and nutrients varies from season to season, according to whether the plant is in growth or dormant.

In this encyclopedia, it is assumed that plants grown under glass are in containers, unless otherwise stated.

Light levels

A number of different light levels may be provided under glass. Plants described as needing full light must have the maximum possible level of light all day; for those needing full light with shade from hot sun, use screens or blinds to protect them from scorching in midday summer sun. Bright filtered light is achieved using screens, blinds, or a shade wash. Bright indirect light, such as that found near a well-lit window, is suitable for plants that require good light but not direct sun. Place plants that prefer low light beneath staging or green shade netting in a greenhouse; as houseplants, they should be sited away from windows.

Watering and feeding

When in growth, some plants need to be watered freely, which means that the potting compost should be kept evenly moist but not waterlogged. Others need only moderate watering: allow the compost to dry out partially before watering again. To water sparingly, allow the compost to dry almost completely between applications. When plants cease active growth, they need less water; most should be kept moist so the compost has just enough water to avoid desiccation. Some plants, such as many cacti, must be kept totally dry in winter, or when dormant; resume watering as growth restarts.

Plants in containers are restricted in their quest for nutrients, and usually need fertilizer in the growing season. Most conveniently applied in liquid form, a proprietary balanced fertilizer contains the nutrients needed for plant growth – nitrogen, phosphate, and potassium (NPK) – and a full range of trace elements.

Ventilation and humidity

Good ventilation serves to control temperature, maintains a flow of fresh air, and moderates levels of atmospheric humidity. Ventilation is particularly necessary with high humidity, to avoid stagnant air in which fungal diseases thrive. In this encyclopedia, low humidity is defined as less than 50% relative humidity (RH) – a percentage of saturation of the air. Moderate humidity is 51–60% RH, and high humidity 61% RH and above. If damping down is impractical, humidity may be increased locally by grouping plants on trays of moist gravel or expanded clay granules.

POTTING COMPOSTS

Container plants require potting compost that is moist but well drained, with good aeration, and a structure that will withstand heavy watering. In the long-term, most plants are best grown in loam-based composts, which are less prone to saturation than loamless mediums, do not dry out as rapidly, and are easier to re-wet if they become dry. John Innes loam-based composts are standardized mixes, each one suitable for a specific range of plants.

JOHN INNES NO.1 (JI NO.1)
Suitable for seedlings, short-term, and annual houseplants. Ingredients (by volume): 7 parts sterilized loam; 3 parts peat (or substitute); 2 parts sand. To each cubic metre (or cubic yard) is added 600g (1lb) ground limestone; 1.2kg (2lb) hoof and horn; 1.2kg (2lb) superphosphate; and 600g (1lb) potassium sulphate.
JOHN INNES NO.2 (JI NO.2)
Suitable for larger, established plants. Ingredients as for No.1, but with double the quantity of fertilizer.
JOHN INNES NO.3 (JI NO.3)
Suitable for long-term, established plants. Ingredients as for No.1, but with triple the quantity of fertilizer.
LOAMLESS POTTING COMPOST
Suitable for most short-term plants. Contains 1 part sand; 3 parts coarse peat or substitute; variable nutrients.
ERICACEOUS POTTING COMPOST
Suitable for plants that dislike alkaline soil; lime-free with pH6.5 or below.

GREENHOUSE ENVIRONMENTS

TEMPERATURE REGIME	VENTILATION	HUMIDITY	SHADING
COLD Unheated; no min. temp.	Ventilate in summer to lower temperature, and in winter to prevent damp, stagnant conditions.	Natural levels of humidity are adequate.	Admit full light in winter; shade vulnerable plants in summer.
COOL Day: 5–10°C (41–50°F) Night: 2°C (36°F)	Ventilate in summer to lower temperature, and in winter to disperse heater fumes and water vapour.	Damp down in summer to keep cool, with low humidity.	Admit full light in winter; shade vulnerable plants in summer.
TEMPERATE Day: 10–13°C (50–55°F) Night: 7°C (45°F)	Ventilate in summer to lower temperature, and in winter to disperse heater fumes and water vapour.	Damp down in summer to keep cool, with moderate humidity.	Admit full light in winter; shade vulnerable plants in summer.
WARM Day: 13–18°C (55–64°F) or above Night: 13°C (55°F)	Ventilate in summer and as needed in winter to lower temperature and prevent stagnant conditions.	Provide high humidity in summer; reduce in winter.	Admit full light in winter; shade vulnerable plants in summer.

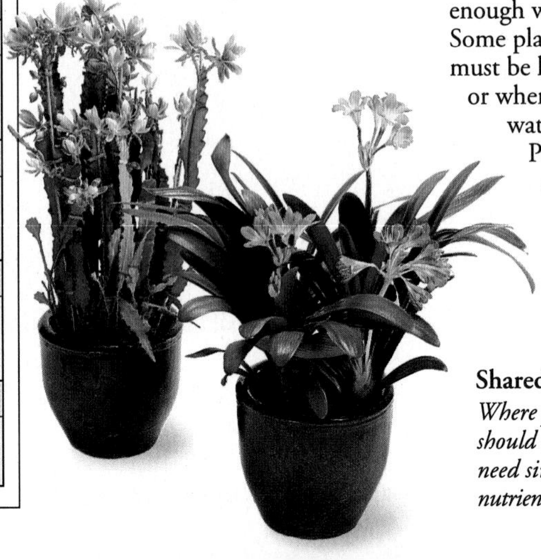

Shared needs
Where possible, plants under glass should be grouped with others that need similar levels of warmth, light, nutrients, water, and humidity.

Pruning

Woody plants are pruned for a number of reasons: to maintain good health, by removing dead, diseased or damaged wood; to encourage the formation of vigorous and bushy growth; to produce plants that have a sound structure when mature; and to shape and direct growth so that plants display their decorative features to optimum effect. Regular pruning also improves the supply of strong, young growth, which normally produces flowers and fruit in greater abundance and of better quality than does old or moribund wood.

Principles of pruning

Before making any cuts, assess the overall shape of the plant. Never cut indiscriminately. Begin by removing any wood that is dead, diseased, or damaged, as this helps to promote plant hygiene and good health. The timing and nature of subsequent pruning depend on the age and type of flowering wood, and also on an individual species' vigour and ability to produce new growth in response to pruning. Follow one of the 13 regimes set out on pp.26–27, as recommended in the introduction to each genus of woody plants.

Provided that a plant is healthy, has adequate nutrients, and tolerates drastic pruning, the harder a shoot is pruned, the more vigorously it will grow. Conversely, light pruning results in limited regrowth.

Woody plants that flower before midsummer usually bloom on the previous year's growth. They are therefore normally pruned after flowering, so that new growth has a full season in which to ripen before blooming the following year. Most plants that bloom after midsummer flower on the current season's growth; these are pruned in winter or spring, then flower later in the season on new growth. However, pruning in spring (when the sap is rising) should be avoided for plants that "bleed" (leak sap) when cut. Pruning of evergreens is best carried out in mid-spring, so that resultant young shoots will develop after the danger of hard frosts has passed.

Formative pruning

The aim of formative pruning is to produce a balanced framework of sturdy, well-spaced branches that permits maximum light and air to reach the entire plant. Most evergreen trees and shrubs require little formative pruning, but may need light shaping after planting in spring, to ensure balanced growth. Formative pruning of deciduous species should be carried out in the dormant season, either at or soon after planting. For the vast majority of woody plants, formative pruning follows the procedure illustrated (centre right). If a young shrub does not have a balanced framework, cut it back hard, then select 4 or 5 of the strongest, most evenly spaced branches from the resulting growth to form the new framework, and cut out the rest. Some plants (mainly those assigned pruning group 1) need only minimal pruning; these include slow-growing shrubs with an intricate, ornamental branch structure whose appearance is easily spoiled by cutting back.

Restrictive pruning

It is best to select plants whose natural size suits an allotted area in a garden, rather than to prune to restrict size. Under glass, however, such pruning is often unavoidable. Follow the principles outlined above with regard to timing, referring also to the pruning group. However, the pruning should be more severe than usual, and in many cases needs to be performed every year. Aim to reduce the previous season's growth by one- to two-thirds of its length after flowering, retaining only the strongest shoots to maintain a well-spaced and open framework.

Renovation (renewal) pruning

Some old or overgrown shrubs – such as those that produce new shoots from the base or from old wood – may be rejuvenated by hard pruning. Renovate deciduous shrubs after flowering or when dormant, and evergreen shrubs in mid-spring. For drastic renovation in a single operation, cut back all main stems to 30–45cm (12–18in) above the ground. Select the strongest 3 or 4 shoots that then sprout from each stem to produce a new framework and cut out the rest. However, for all but the most resilient shrubs, it is best to stagger pruning over 2 or 3 years, as illustrated (bottom right). After both types, mulch the soil to a depth of 5–10cm (2–4in), apply a slow-release, balanced fertilizer, and keep the plant well watered.

PRUNING CUTS

Different techniques are used to prune plants depending on whether buds are alternately or oppositely arranged (see right). Keep tools clean and blades sharp so that they do not produce a ragged cut that is slow to heal. Use secateurs to sever small branches up to about 1cm (½in) in diameter. For larger branches, use loppers or a pruning saw to avoid crushing plant tissue.

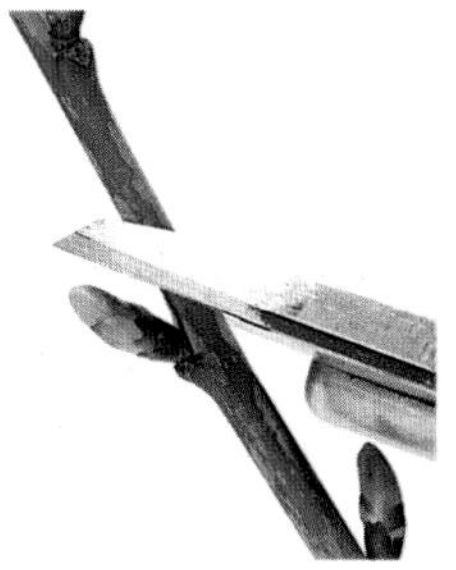

Alternate buds
For plants with alternate buds, angle the cut away from and just above an outward-facing bud.

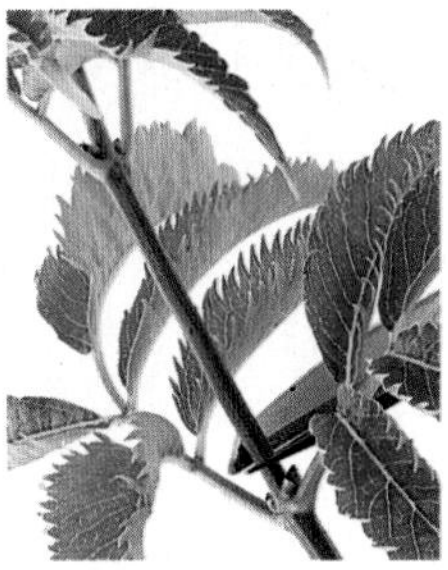

Opposite buds
For plants with opposite buds, cut straight across immediately above a strong pair of buds.

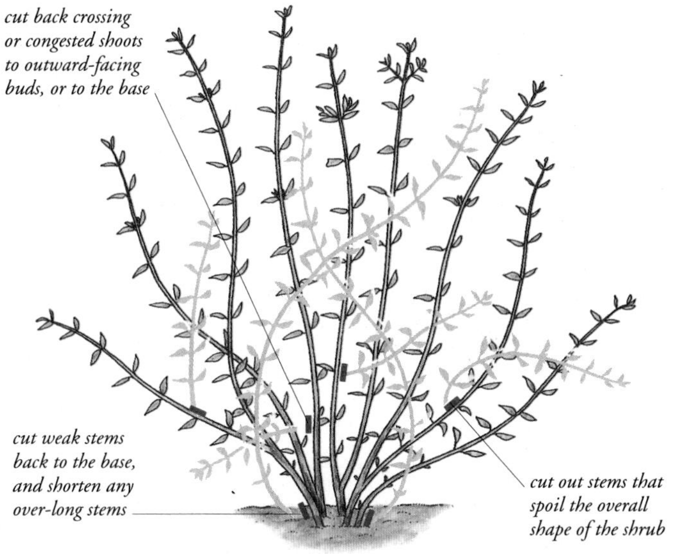

cut weak stems back to the base, and shorten any over-long stems

Formative pruning
Formative pruning aims to produce a balanced framework of strong, evenly spaced stems. After planting, remove dead, diseased, and damaged wood. Cut out or shorten crossing, rubbing, or congested stems, and cut all weak growth back to the base.

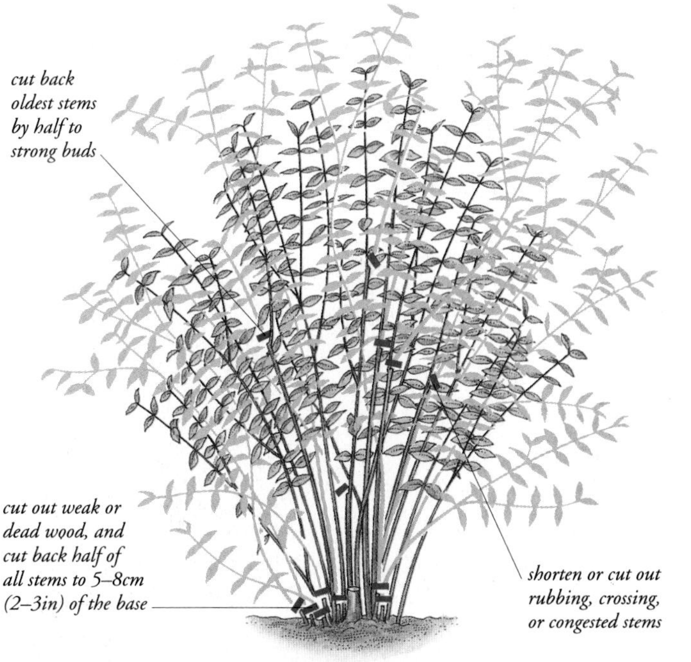
cut back oldest stems by half to strong buds
cut out weak or dead wood, and cut back half of all stems to 5–8cm (2–3in) of the base
shorten or cut out rubbing, crossing, or congested stems

Gradual renovation
To renovate a woody plant, remove dead wood and cut back up to one-third of the oldest stems close to the base. Of those that then remain, shorten the oldest. Repeat the following year, cutting back the remaining old main stems.

Pruning groups

In this encyclopedia, all woody plants that require pruning are assigned one of the groups outlined here (see relevant genus cultivation notes). An individual species may be assigned a different group to the genus as a whole, or may be assigned more than one group if it can be grown in a variety of ways. As all woody plants require routine removal of dead, diseased, and damaged wood, this is not stated for each group. In groups 10–13, the correct time to prune depends on the type of flowering wood: plants that flower on the previous year's growth usually bloom between early spring and early summer; those that bloom on the current year's growth usually flower after midsummer. In the illustrations below, red cut marks show where to prune.

GROUP 1 e.g. *Acer palmatum, Hamamelis,* some *Magnolia* species

TYPE Evergreen and deciduous trees and some deciduous shrubs that flower on previous or current year's growth and need minimal pruning.

ACTION Remove wayward or crossing shoots to maintain permanent, healthy framework.

WHEN In late winter or early spring, when dormant; some in late summer or early autumn to prevent bleeding of sap.

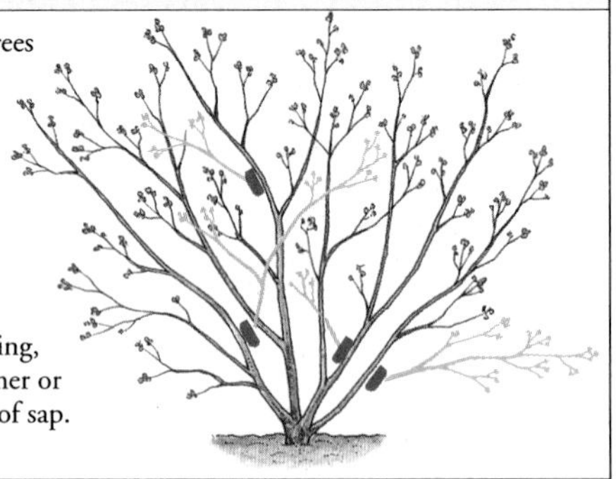

GROUP 2 e.g. *Buddleja alternifolia, Deutzia, Forsythia, Philadelphus*

TYPE Deciduous shrubs (and a few trees) that flower in spring or early summer on previous year's growth.

ACTION Cut back flowered shoots to strong buds or young lower or basal growth. On established plants, cut back about one-quarter to one-fifth of old shoots to the base, to promote replacement growth.

WHEN Annually, after flowering.

GROUP 3 e.g. *Cytisus scoparius* and hybrids, *Kerria*

TYPE Deciduous shrubs that flower in spring or early summer on previous year's growth, and produce new growth at or near ground level.

ACTION Cut back flowered shoots to young sideshoots or to strong buds low down on branch framework, to encourage strong new growth.

WHEN Annually, after flowering.

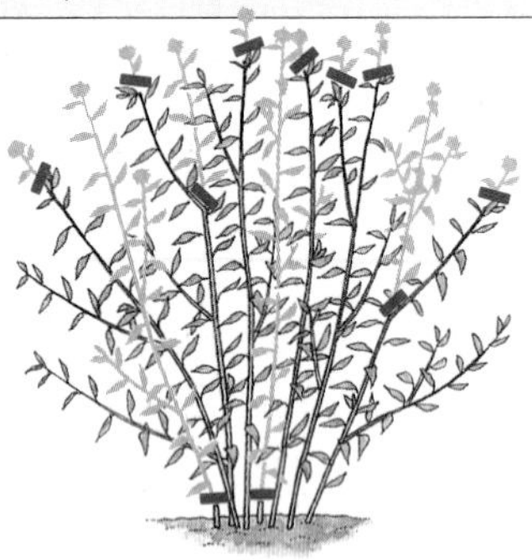

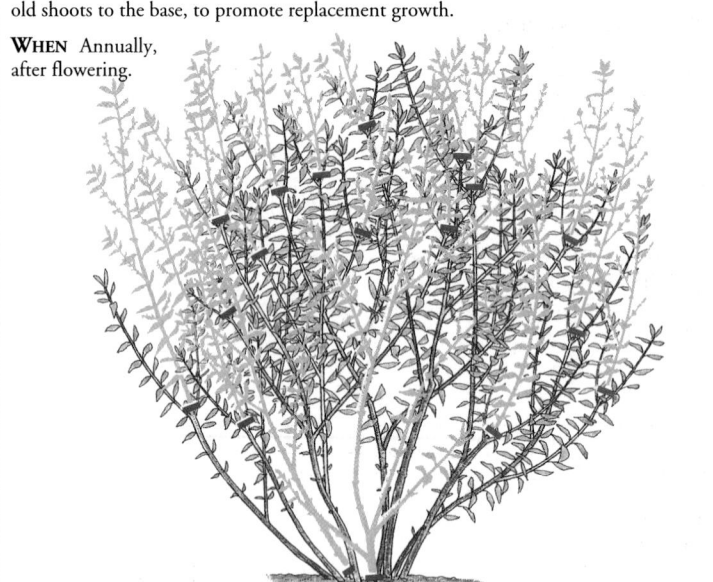

GROUP 4 e.g. *Hydrangea macrophylla*

TYPE Deciduous shrubs that flower in mid- to late summer or autumn on previous year's growth.

ACTION Trim off last season's flowerheads to the first bud or pair of buds beneath each flowerhead. With established plants, cut back about one-third to one-quarter of the oldest flowered shoots to the base, to promote replacement growth.

WHEN Annually, from early to mid-spring.

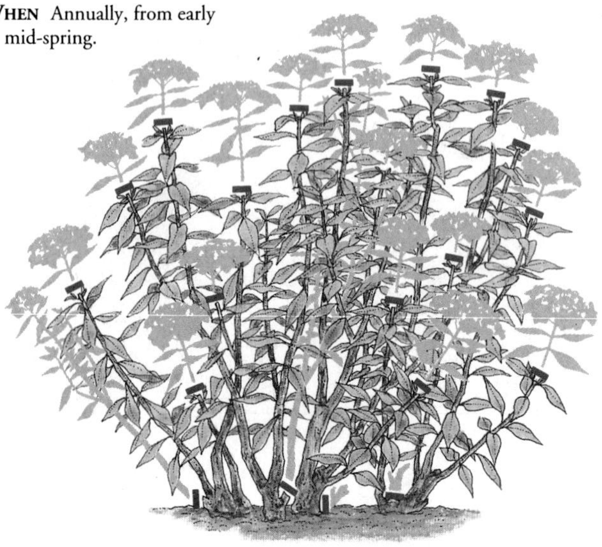

GROUP 5 e.g. *Prunus triloba*

TYPE Deciduous shrubs that flower between late winter and early spring on previous year's growth.

ACTION Cut back all stems to strong buds or to developing shoots close to the base of the plant, to promote replacement growth.

WHEN Annually, after flowering.

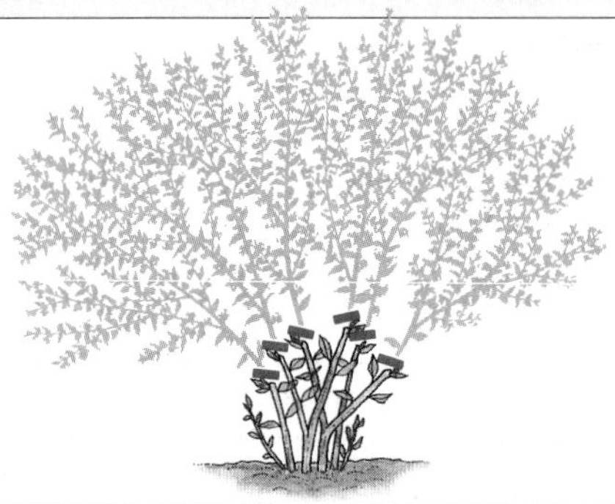

GROUP 6 e.g. *Buddleja davidii, Caryopteris, Perovskia*

TYPE Deciduous shrubs that flower in mid- to late summer or autumn on current year's growth.

ACTION Cut back to low permanent framework. For subshrubs, and for drastic renovation, cut back all flowered stems close to the base.

WHEN Annually, as buds begin to swell in early spring.

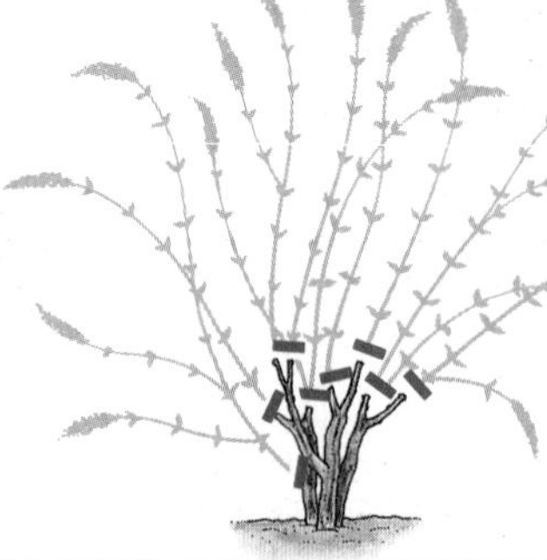

GROUP 7 e.g. *Cornus alba, Cotinus,* some *Eucalyptus* species, *Sambucus*

TYPE Deciduous trees and shrubs that, when pruned hard, produce colourful winter stems, or large or brightly hued foliage, as ornamental features. Plants that flower on previous year's wood do not bloom if pruned this way.

ACTION Cut back stems to within 2 or 3 buds of the base (suckering species close to base), or to permanent framework. Feed or apply well-rotted farmyard manure, and mulch to compensate for loss of vigorous wood.

WHEN Annually, in early spring.

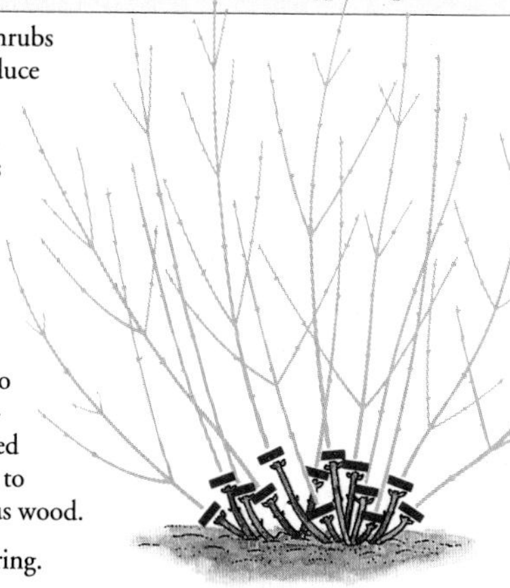

GROUP 8 e.g. *Camellia, Rhododendron*

TYPE Evergreen shrubs that flower between winter and early summer on previous or current year's growth, and need minimal pruning.

ACTION Trim or lightly cut back shoots that spoil symmetry. Dead-head regularly if practical (unless fruit are required).

WHEN Annually, after flowering. Remove dead and damaged growth in mid-spring.

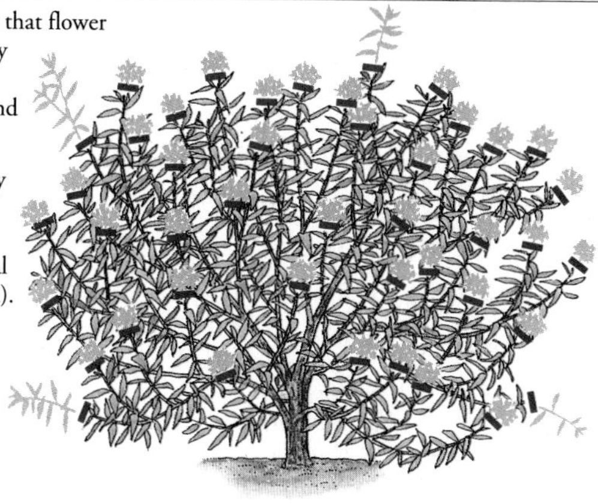

GROUP 9 e.g. *Eucryphia, Prunus laurocerasus, P. lusitanica*

TYPE Evergreen shrubs that flower between midsummer and late autumn on previous or current year's growth, or that bear insignificant flowers, and that need minimal pruning.

ACTION Trim or lightly cut back shoots that spoil symmetry. Shrubs grown for foliage often tolerate harder pruning. Dead-head regularly if practical (unless fruit are required).

WHEN Annually, or as necessary, from mid- to late spring.

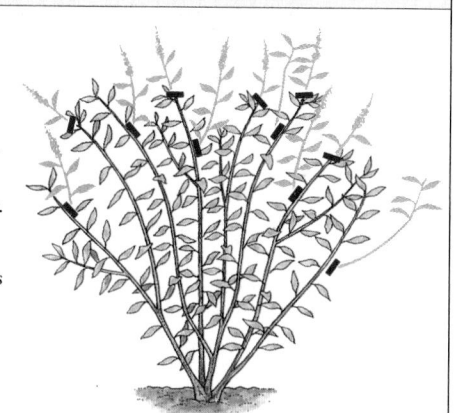

GROUP 10 e.g. *Bouvardia, Calluna, Erica, Lavandula*

TYPE Evergreen shrubs that flower on previous year's growth in spring or early summer, or on current year's growth in late summer or autumn. (Tree heathers require only minimal pruning.)

ACTION Cut back flowered shoots to within 1.5–2.5cm (½–1in) of previous year's growth.

WHEN Annually:
- after flowering, if flowering on previous year's growth.
- in early or mid-spring, if flowering on current year's growth.

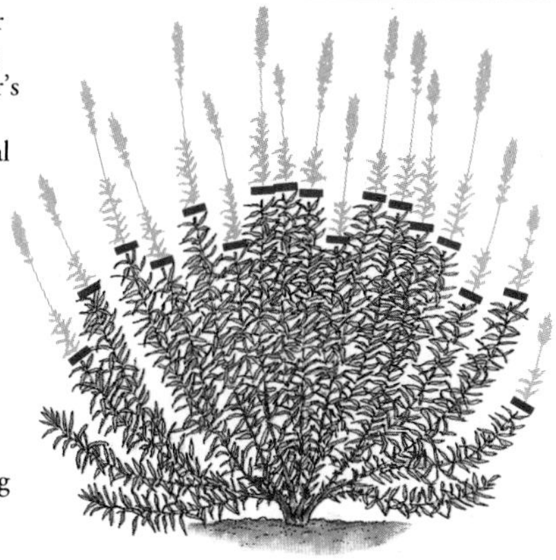

GROUP 11 e.g. *Akebia, Clematis montana, Fallopia baldschuanica*

TYPE Vigorous, deciduous and evergreen climbers that flower on previous or current year's growth, and need no regular pruning.

ACTION Trim to fit available space; carry out renovation pruning as needed (see p.25).

WHEN Annually, or as needed:
- after flowering, if flowering on previous year's growth.
- in late winter or spring, if flowering on current year's growth.

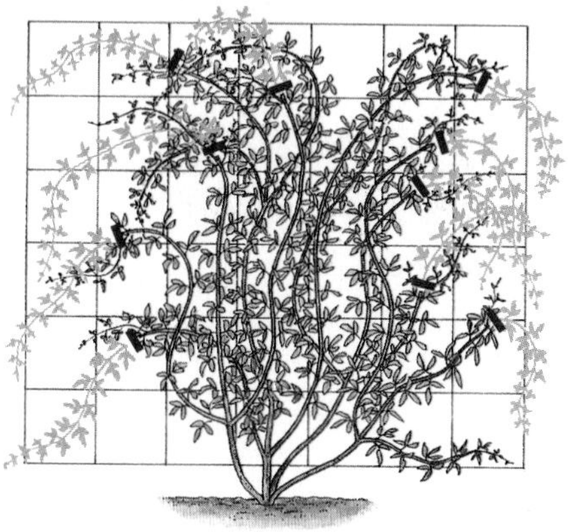

GROUP 12 e.g. *Bougainvillea, Solanum crispum*

TYPE Less vigorous, deciduous and evergreen climbers that flower on previous or current year's growth. (For *Wisteria*, see cultivation notes in genus introduction.)

ACTION "Spur prune" by cutting back side-shoots to within 3 or 4 buds of permanent framework. Thin out overcrowded shoots.

WHEN Annually:
- after flowering, if flowering on previous year's growth.
- in late winter or early spring, if flowering on current year's growth.

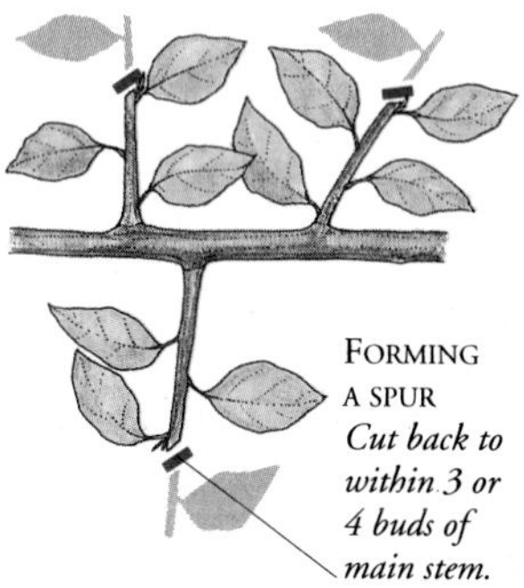

FORMING A SPUR *Cut back to within 3 or 4 buds of main stem.*

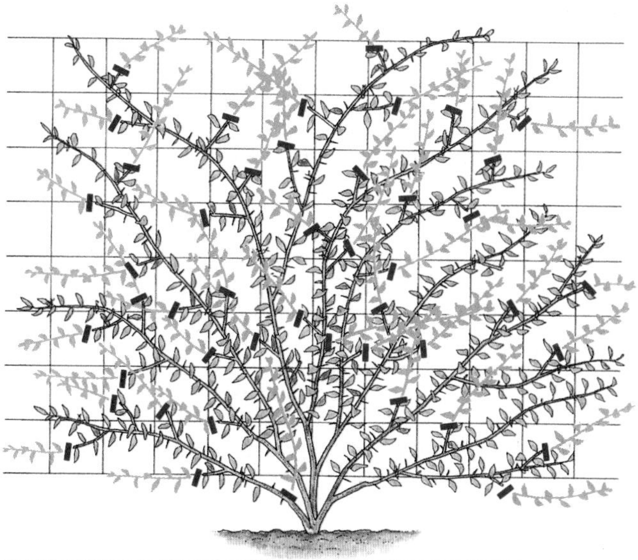

GROUP 13 e.g. *Ceanothus, Chaenomeles*

TYPE Wall-trained, deciduous and evergreen shrubs that flower on previous or current year's growth. (For *Cotoneaster* and *Pyracantha*, see cultivation notes in each genus introduction.)

ACTION Cut back flowered shoots to within 2–4 buds of permanent framework. Trim outward-facing shoots and those growing towards the wall.

WHEN Annually:
- after flowering, if flowering on previous year's growth.
- in late winter or early spring, if flowering on current year's growth.

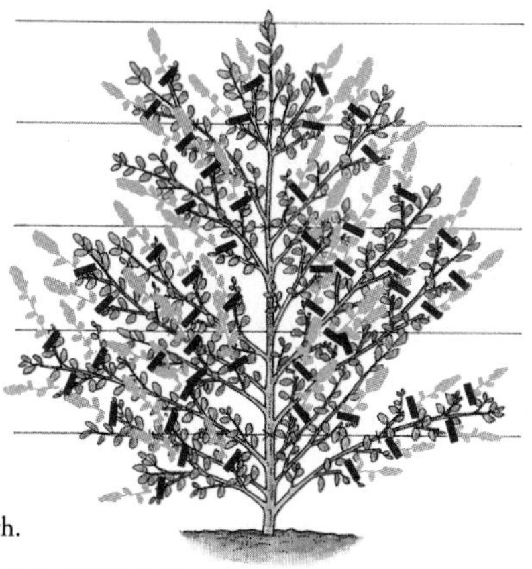

Propagation

Plants propagate naturally in ways that can be exploited by gardeners to increase stocks or preserve the distinct characteristics of individual plants. The cultivation notes for each genus described in this encyclopedia specify the methods that may be used. Techniques fall into two categories: propagation by seed or by vegetative means. Raising plants from seed is relatively simple, although variants of garden origin are unlikely to breed true from garden-collected seed (see p.11). Such plants should instead be increased by asexual, vegetative means, such as from suckers, by division, grafting, or layering, or by taking cuttings.

Propagation from seed

Most seed is best sown as soon as ripe. If necessary, soak fruits in water first, then extract seeds by rubbing the flesh, and leave to dry. Hard-coated seeds may need soaking or scarification before germination. Soak in recently boiled water for between 10 minutes and 72 hours, depending on the species; viable seeds will swell, and should then be sown immediately. To scarify small seeds, abrade with emery paper; with large seeds, file the coats or chip (nick) with a knife. Some seeds need cold stratification to break dormancy: sow in a cold frame or open frame for exposure to winter cold. Alternatively, place in moist peat inside a plastic bag, and keep warm for 3 or 4 days, then place in a refrigerator at 1–5°C (34–41°F). Sow on germination – after 3–18 weeks, depending on the species.

Seed may be sown *in situ*, or in a tray or seedbed; sow thinly to avoid damping off, and, except tiny seeds or seeds that need light, cover with soil or compost. Most will germinate at 5°C (41°F) above the minimum temperature prescribed for each plant. As a rule, maintain seeds of plants from the tropics at 19–24°C (66–75°F); from warm-temperate and subtropical areas at 13–18°C (55–64°F); from cool-temperate areas at 6–12°C (43–54°F).

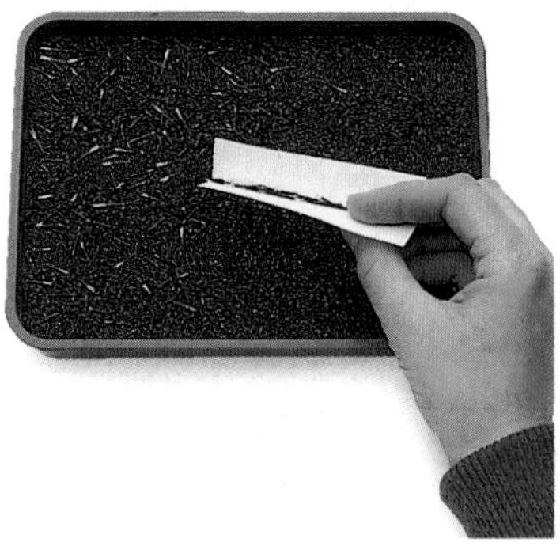

Sowing in a seed tray
Sow seed thinly and evenly on to moist seed compost and cover, if required, to its own depth in sieved compost. Cover with glass, shade from hot sun, and keep at an appropriate temperature.

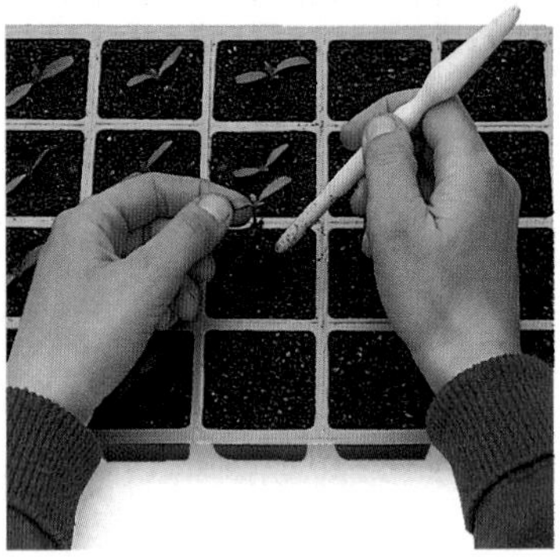

Pricking out
When seed leaves are strong enough to be handled, prick out singly into modular trays or small containers. Pot on when large enough, or harden off, then plant out in open ground.

Division

Division is the most rapid means of increasing perennials that have a spreading rootstock and produce new shoots annually from the crown, as well as rhizomatous plants and some tuberous ones. The term is also loosely used to describe the separation of offsets from clump-forming bulbous plants (see p.45).

Division is best carried out when the plant is dormant, normally between late autumn and early spring, but never in very wet or frosty weather. However, fleshy-rooted plants, or those that are not fully hardy, are best divided in early spring, when young plants are less likely to suffer damage from cold.

Lift the parent plant and shake off excess soil from the roots. Separate the plant into sections, using forks, a spade, or a sharp knife, so that each part has a good root system and several new shoots or growth buds. Discard old, damaged, or unproductive pieces, and replant vigorous material immediately, at the original depth of soil. Small divisions may be potted up and grown on in a cold frame until established. For plants with thick rhizomes, cut the rhizomes into sections; retain at least two growing points on each section. Dust cut surfaces with fungicide before replanting at the original depth.

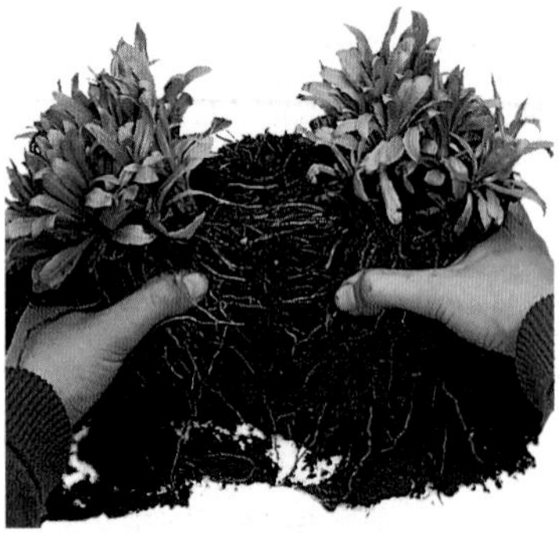

Loose, fleshy roots
Lift the parent plant and shake off surplus soil. Separate the plant into sections by hand. Replant vigorous, healthy sections, each with several new shoots, at their previous depth of soil.

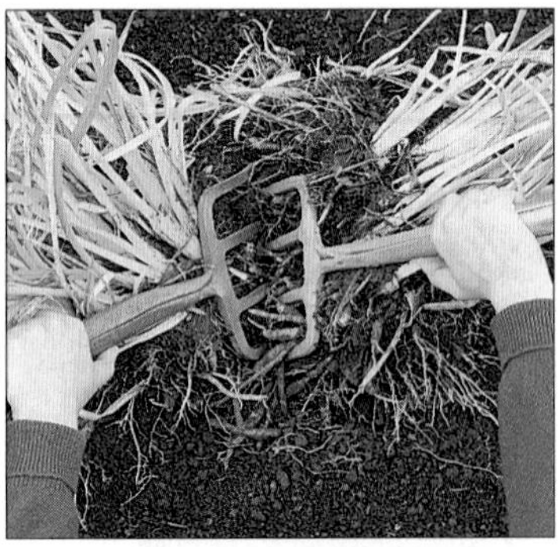

Fibrous roots and woody crowns
Lever apart fibrous-rooted plants using two forks set back-to-back. To section plants with tough, woody crowns, use a spade or knife to cut through the roots, avoiding growth buds.

Layering, suckers, and grafting

Layering is a simple technique for increasing plants whose stems will produce roots if wounded: the stem is pegged to the ground and left to form roots, while still attached to the parent plant.

Suckering plants, such as *Cornus alba* and kerrias, naturally produce suckers that may be detached and inserted as ready-rooted plants.

Several trees, shrubs, and house- or greenhouse plants may be increased by air layering. Cut a slit in an aerial stem, pack the resulting tongue with a wad of damp sphagnum moss, and enclose it in a plastic sleeve. Once roots have grown into the moss, which may take up to 2 years, separate the layered stem from the parent plant and pot up.

Grafting involves taking the stem of one plant and uniting it with the rootstock of a closely related plant. It is used to increase stocks of newly bred woody cultivars, and to improve the rate of development or flowering of slow-growing plants by joining them to more vigorous ones. The union is achieved by making a close-fitting join between woody parts of the rootstock (the plant with roots and stem) and the scion (the plant with top-growth). Budding is a form of grafting, in which a vegetative bud of one plant is grafted on to another plant.

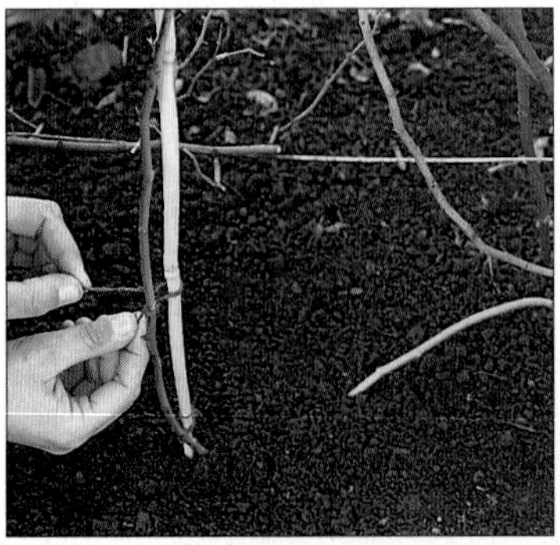

Simple layering
Wound the underside of a pliable young stem. Apply rooting hormone, peg the wounded section down, and cover with soil. Bend the stem tip upright and tie to a cane. Sever when roots have formed.

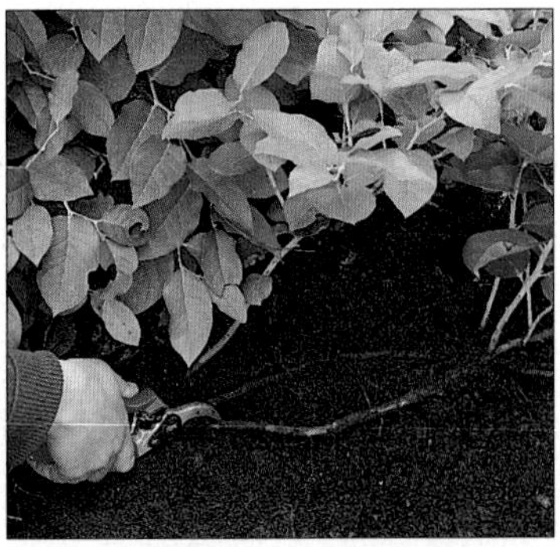

Suckers
To detach a sucker, uncover its long suckering root and sever this close to the parent plant. Dig up the sucker with its own fibrous roots, replant, then cut back top-growth by half.

Taking cuttings

Raising plants from cuttings is one of the most common methods of vegetative propagation. In general, the technique involves taking a small piece of material from a living plant. After insertion in a rooting medium (usually in a propagating case to maintain humidity), this develops new roots, and may then be grown on until large enough to be planted out. There are 3 main types of cutting: stem, leaf, and root. Several types of stem cutting are used, differentiated by the ripeness of the wood. Instructions for propagation from each of the main types are given in the table below.

Two other types of cutting (not listed below) are also used. Semi-ripe leaf-bud cuttings are trimmed just above an axillary leaf bud, and 2cm (¾in) below it. Wound 5mm (¼in) of the base, and insert in cutting compost with the leaf axil just above the surface. Heel cuttings are taken as other stem cuttings, using sideshoots with a heel (sliver) of old wood at the base.

Simple propagating case
Use a clear plastic bag, inflated and supported by canes or wire hoops, as an alternative to a propagating case.

Cuttings from conifers
For most conifers, propagate from semi-ripe cuttings, choosing leaders or sideshoots typical of the parent plant.

GUIDE TO TAKING CUTTINGS

	TYPE OF CUTTING	WHEN TO CUT	CUTTING MATERIAL	PREPARATION	ROOTING MEDIUM	ROOTING ENVIRONMENT
TREES, SHRUBS, AND CLIMBERS (WOODY PLANTS)	SOFTWOOD AND GREENWOOD CUTTINGS 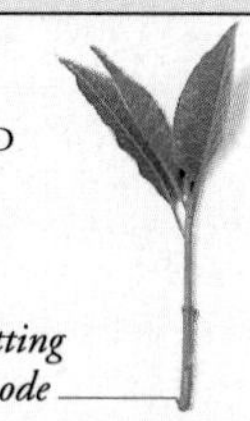	Spring to early summer.	Soft, pliable tips of fast-growing, non-flowering shoots of current season's growth, with 3–5 pairs of leaves. Greenwood is slightly firmer.	Take early in morning, and seal in an opaque plastic bag to conserve moisture. Do not allow to wilt. Trim to 8–10cm (3–4in) long, with a straight cut just below a node. Remove leaves on lower third of cutting.	Insert into standard cutting compost, or equal parts peat (or substitute) and perlite or sharp sand. Ensure that leaves do not touch. Water with fungicide solution.	Place in a mist unit or propagating case at 18–24°C (64–75°F). Remove fallen leaves daily. Apply fungicidal spray weekly.
	SEMI-RIPE AND RIPEWOOD CUTTINGS 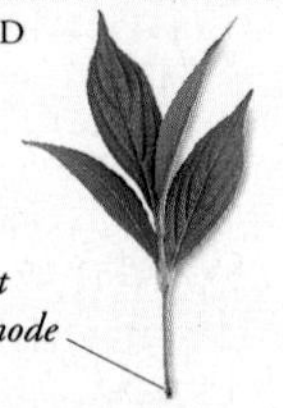	Semi-ripe: mid- or late summer, occasionally early autumn. Ripewood: early autumn to early winter.	Soft-tipped shoots of current season's growth, firm and woody at the base. Cut just below a node for nodal cuttings, or with a heel of older wood at the base.	Remove sideshoots. Trim nodal cuttings to 8–10cm (3–4in) long; heel cuttings to 5–7cm (2–3in) long; trim heel. Remove leaves on lower third, and for semi-ripes also soft tips. Reduce large leaves by half. Wound 2.5–4cm (1–1½in) of the stem base.	Dip base of cutting in rooting hormone. Insert into standard cutting compost, or equal parts peat (or substitute) and perlite or sharp sand. Ensure that leaves do not touch. Water with fungicide solution.	Place in a mist unit or propagating case at 21°C (70°F), if bottom heat is needed, or use an insulated cold frame (vital for ripe-wood). Shade from hot sun. Remove fallen leaves daily. Once rooted, apply liquid fertilizer every 2 weeks.
	HARDWOOD CUTTINGS 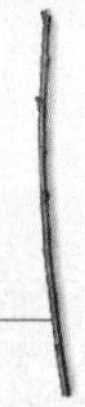 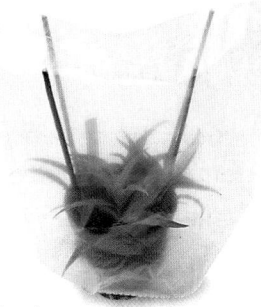	Early autumn (after leaf fall) to early winter.	Leafless shoots of fully ripe current year's growth, cut at join with previous year's growth. On pithy stems, take with a heel of older wood at the base.	Trim to 15–23cm (6–9in) long, with the top cut just above a bud or pair of buds, and the bottom cut just below a bud or pair of buds. Make a wound in the stem base up to 1.5cm (½in) long, if difficult to root.	Dip base in rooting hormone. Insert in a trench in a prepared bed; line the bottom with coarse sand (vital in heavy soil) and cover with soil. Alternatively, insert in containers in a cold frame; use equal parts peat (or substitute) and fine grit.	Firm into the trench with the top 2.5–5cm (1–2in) of the cutting visible above soil level; check and re-firm after frost. If slow-rooting, place in bundles in a sand bed in a cold frame; move to the trench in spring.
	BASAL STEM CUTTINGS 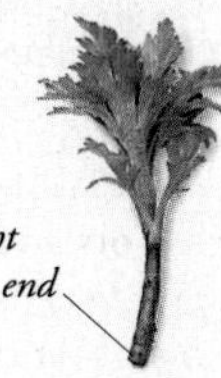	Early or mid-spring.	New shoots, when about 3.5–5cm (1½–2in) high, as first leaves unfurl, taken from close to the base or crown, with a heel of older, woody tissue at the base.	Trim to 3.5–5cm (1½–2in) long, with a straight cut at the base, and with a heel of basal tissue. Remove leaves on lower third of cutting.	Dip base in rooting hormone. Insert singly or severally into standard cutting compost, or equal parts peat (or substitute) and perlite or sharp sand. Ensure that leaves do not touch. Water with fungicide solution.	Place in a propagating case or cold frame, or cover with a clear plastic bag supported by canes or wire hoops.
PERENNIALS (NON-WOODY PLANTS)	STEM-TIP (SOFT-TIP) CUTTINGS 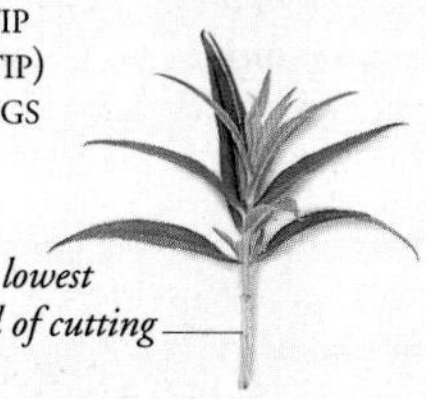	Spring to autumn, or any time in growing season when suitable shoots are available.	Soft, pliable tips of fast-growing, non-flowering shoots, 7–12cm (3–5in) long, cut just above leaf nodes.	Take early in morning, and seal in an opaque plastic bag to conserve moisture. Do not allow to wilt. Trim to 5–7cm (2–3in) long, with a straight cut just below a node. Remove leaves on lower third of cutting.	Insert into standard cutting compost, or equal parts peat (or substitute) and perlite or sharp sand. Ensure that leaves do not touch. Water with fungicide solution.	Place in a mist unit or propagating case, or cover with a clear plastic bag supported by canes or wire hoops. Shade from hot sun. Remove fallen leaves daily.
	ROOT CUTTINGS 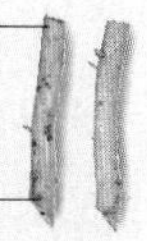	In dormant period, usually late winter.	Vigorous young roots, preferably at least 5mm (¼in) in diameter, taken from close to the crown of the parent plant.	Trim thick roots to 5–10cm (2–4in) long; thin roots to 7–12cm (3–5in) long. Make a straight cut at the proximal end (nearest to crown), and a slanted cut at the distal (opposite) end to ensure correct orientation. Remove fibrous roots. Dust with fungicide powder.	Insert thick roots upright in containers of moist standard cutting compost, the proximal end flush with the surface. Lay thin roots flat in trays; cover with compost. Top-dress with fine grit or sand.	Place in a cold frame or propagating case. Do not water until rooted.
	LEAF CUTTINGS 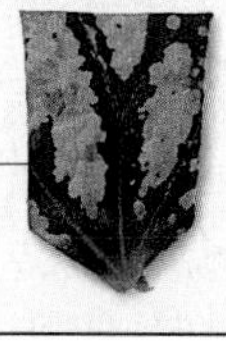 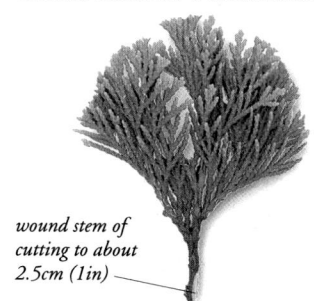	Any time of year.	Mature, healthy, undamaged leaves, cut off close to the bases of the leaf-stalks.	Whole leaves, e.g. *Saintpaulia*: cut leaf-stalk straight across, 3cm (1¼in) below leaf-blade. Half-leaf sections, e.g. *Streptocarpus*: cut in half, removing the midrib. Scored leaf/leaf squares, e.g. Rex begonias: make 1cm (½in) cuts across undersides of main veins.	Use equal parts fine sand and peat (or substitute). Insert whole leaves upright, with leaf-blades touching compost. Pin scored leaves or leaf squares flat on compost, cut side down. Insert half-leaf sections cut edge down. Water with fungicide solution.	Place in a propagating case at 18–24°C (64–75°F). Keep in bright indirect light; always shade from hot sun.

Plant problems

These pages list the most common pests, groups of diseases, and disorders that can afflict garden plants. In general, pests are creatures that feed on plants or cause abnormal growth. Diseases are brought about by the presence of fungi, bacteria, viruses, or similar organisms. Disorders usually result from unsatisfactory growing conditions. Fortunately, many problems can be prevented before they arise.

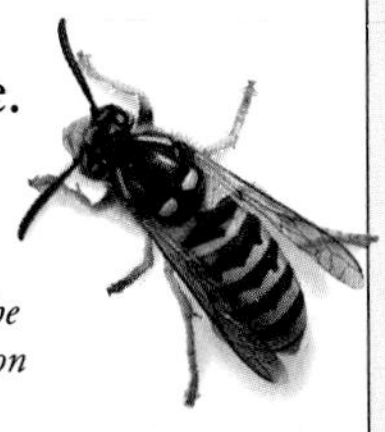

WASPS FEED ON *fruit, but also help the gardener by preying on other pests.*

Preventing problems

Good cultivation practices and simple garden hygiene considerably reduce the risk of plant problems. Buy only vigorous, healthy plants with sound, uncongested root systems (see p.22), and try to find pest- and disease-resistant cultivars wherever possible. To help prevent physiological disorders, select plants for sites in the garden where conditions match their specific needs (see pp.20–21). Thereafter, provide the correct amount of water (see p.22), and maintain adequate levels of nutrients in the soil (see p.21). Avoid over-watering and over-fertilizing; both can kill plants. Mulch beds and borders annually to suppress weeds (see p.23), and clear away all withered or damaged plant material, composting only healthy plant waste. Where feasible, grow annuals, vegetables, and bulbs in different sites each year to prevent the build-up of pests and diseases.

Methods of control

Once a problem occurs, it is always important to tackle it quickly. Two common strategies are chemical and biological control. Chemical control refers to the destruction of pests by applying a synthetic compound, such as a fungicide, insecticide, or weedkiller, to plants or to the soil. Biological control involves the deliberate introduction of insects, bacteria, or fungi that attack specific pests (see panel below); for example, to attract hoverflies, which feed on aphids, grow French marigolds (*Tagetes patula*). This approach is referred to as companion planting.

Alternatively, remove larger pests by hand and destroy them. Either incinerate infected plant material, if permitted locally, or dispose of it along with other household waste.

Using chemicals

To use chemical controls safely, always follow the manufacturer's instructions exactly. In general, observe the following precautions. Avoid contact with skin and eyes, and do not inhale dust, smoke, or spray. Never eat, drink, or smoke when applying a chemical. It is best to spray when the weather is dry and dull with no breeze, preferably in the evening, when pollinating insects are less active. Always keep chemicals well away from children, pets, ponds, and wildlife.

Store chemicals in their original, labelled containers, together with explanatory notes, out of reach of children and animals. Rinse all equipment thoroughly before and after use, keeping each item solely for applying either pesticides or weedkillers. Ideally, use a dribble bar when applying weedkiller. Never flush excess chemicals into the sewage system. Instead, excess of any type should be applied to gravel paths or waste ground, avoiding drains and watercourses.

BIOLOGICAL PEST CONTROL

Many pests, especially under glass, can be curbed by biological control. The list below shows pests (in bold type), and suggested control organisms.

Aphids Fly larvae parasite (*Aphidius*) and predators (*Aphidoletes aphidimyza*)
Caterpillars Bacterial disease (*Bacillus thuringiensis*)
Mealybugs Predatory ladybird (*Cryptolaemus montrouzieri*)
Red spider mite Predatory greenhouse mite (*Phytoseiulus persimilis*)
Slugs Slug nematode (*Steinernema capense*)
Soft scale insects Parasitic wasp (*Metaphycus helvolus*)
Thrips Predatory mites (*Amblyseius*)
Vine weevil larvae Eelworm (*Heterorhabditis, Steinernema*)
Whiteflies Parasitic wasp (*Encarsia formosa*)

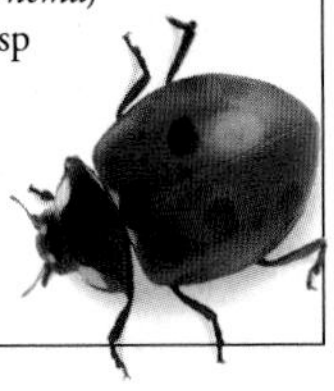

LADYBIRDS *feed on mealybugs.*

PESTS, DISEASES, AND DISORDERS

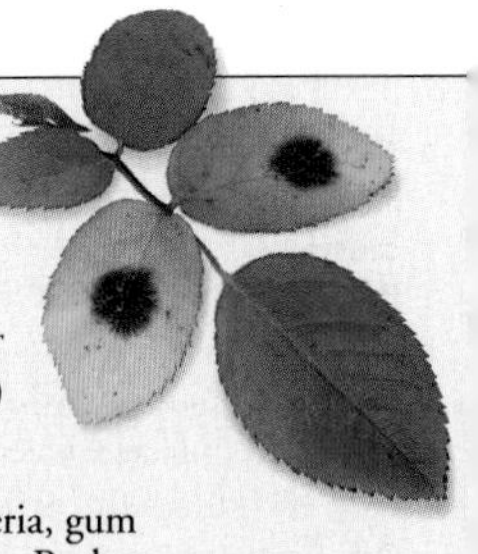

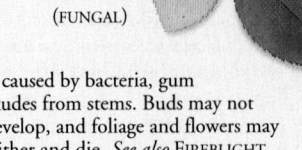

LEAF SPOT (FUNGAL)

Key to entries

Each entry indicates what part of the plant is affected (see symbols below), briefly describes the nature of the pest, disease, or disorder, then suggests appropriate action.

☘ Leaves
✿ Flowers and inflorescences
❍ Fruit
♢ Underground structures
✱ Stems, trunks, whole plant
➪ Action for prevention or cure

ADELGIDS ☘✱ Small, greyish black, sap-sucking insects, similar to aphids, that weaken leaves and stems, produce white waxy fibres, and excrete honeydew. ➪ *Apply insecticide.*

ANTHRACNOSE ☘❍✱ Fungus causing spots on leaves, which then wither; shoots and fruit are infected; plant may die. ➪ *Destroy affected parts; apply fungicide; improve ventilation; maintain hygiene.*

ANTS ♢✱ Insects whose nest-building disturbs roots, causing growth to be stunted; plant wilts. ➪ *Apply ant-killer.*

APHIDS ☘✿✱ Sap-sucking insects (also known as blackflies and greenflies) that excrete honeydew, cause galls, and transmit viruses. They may also cause leaf distortion. Woolly aphids suck sap from bark in spring and secrete white waxy fibres. ➪ *Apply insecticide; use biological control.*

BACTERIA ☘✿❍✱ Micro-organisms that cause distortion and discoloration of leaves or flowers, dieback, or death. ➪ *Prune out affected areas or remove plant if necessary; control insects that spread infection; select resistant plants; maintain hygiene.*

BEETLES ☘✿❍✱ Insects that create holes or pits in various parts of plants, depending on the species. ➪ *Destroy pests; apply insecticide to seedlings; maintain hygiene.*

BLACKFLIES *see* APHIDS

BLOSSOM WILT ☘✿♢✱ Symptom of fungus that attacks trees, entering through flowers, which wither but remain on the tree. Leaves may discolour; pustules appear. Infection spreads, causing dieback. ➪ *Cut back to well below affected parts; apply fungicide.*

BOTRYTIS *see* GREY MOULD

BUD BLAST ✿ Fungus that causes buds to turn brown; they may have a silvery grey sheen and be covered in black bristles. Buds remain on the plant but do not develop. ➪ *Destroy affected parts; control insects that spread spores (leafhoppers).*

BUGS ☘✿❍ Sap-sucking insects that make holes in leaves, flowers, and fruit. ➪ *Destroy affected parts; apply insecticide.*

BULB SCALE MITES ☘✱ Tiny pests that tunnel into bulbs. ➪ *Destroy affected bulbs; immerse bulbs in hot water before planting.*

CANKER ✱ Root or stem lesion. If caused by fungi, raised rings of bark, sometimes oozing gum, may lie close to a wound or bud, with pustules nearby; plant may die. If caused by bacteria, gum exudes from stems. Buds may not develop, and foliage and flowers may wither and die. *See also* FIREBLIGHT, SHOTHOLE. ➪ *Destroy affected parts; apply fungicide.*

CATERPILLARS ☘✿❍ Larvae of moth and butterfly species that feed on leaves, flowers, or fruit, leaving powdery excreta. ➪ *Crush eggs; destroy pests; use biological control; apply insecticide.*

CHAFERS *see* BEETLES

CHLOROSIS (*adj.* chlorotic) ☘ Virus or mineral deficiency that causes leaves to turn pale green, yellow, or white. *See also* MAGNESIUM DEFICIENCY, MANGANESE OR IRON DEFICIENCY. ➪ *Correct mineral imbalance; if caused by virus, destroy plant.*

CLUBROOT ☘♢✱ Distortion or swelling of roots and discoloration of foliage, caused by slime mould. Growth is stunted and plant wilts. ➪ *Destroy affected plants; improve drainage; add lime to soil; select resistant plants; apply fungicide before planting; maintain hygiene.*

CUCKOO SPIT *see* FROGHOPPERS

CUTWORMS ☘♢✱ Caterpillars of moth species that gnaw tap roots, stem bases, and lower leaves. Plant wilts and dies. ➪ *Destroy pests; apply insecticide to plant or soil.*

DAMPING OFF ♢✱ Blackening and decay of stem bases and roots, caused by fungi; seedlings collapse. *See also* RHIZOCTONIA, ROTS. ➪ *Apply fungicide to seedlings; maintain hygiene.*

DIEBACK ☘✱ Death of shoots of trees and shrubs, caused by poor growing conditions, frost damage, or fungal disease. Whole plant often dies. ➪ *Cut back beyond affected parts; treat cause; improve conditions.*

DOWNY MILDEW *see* MILDEWS

EARWIGS ☘✿ Insects whose larvae and adults feed on leaves and flowers. ➪ *Destroy pests; apply insecticide; set traps; maintain hygiene.*

EELWORMS ☘✱ Microscopic, worm-like invertebrates (also known as nematodes) that infest plant tissues, causing distortion and discoloration of leaves and flowers. Plant usually dies. ➪ *Destroy affected plants; use crop rotation; in some cases, immerse dormant rootstock in hot water.*

FIRE ☘♢ Fungus that attacks bulbs, usually daffodils and tulips, causing leaves to turn brown. ➪ *Destroy infected bulbs; apply fungicide; change soil; use crop rotation.*

FIREBLIGHT ☘✱ Bacterial disease that attacks certain trees in the Rosaceae family, mainly entering through flowers. Infection spreads to branches; cankers form at base of diseased tissues. Where spread is extensive, plant usually dies. ➪ *Cut back to well below affected parts, or destroy whole plant.*

FROGHOPPERS ☘✱ Young, sap-sucking insects that produce froth (cuckoo spit) on stems and leaves, causing distortion of growth. ➪ *Destroy pests; apply insecticide.*

GALL MIDGES Small flies, whose adults and larvae feed on plant tissues, causing galls to form on stems, leaves, and flowers. Growth may be stunted. *Destroy affected parts; apply insecticide.*

GALL MITES Small pests that feed on or within plant tissues, causing galls to form on foliage and buds. *Destroy affected parts.*

GALLS Irregular swellings, usually on woody plants, caused by bacteria, fungi, insects, or mites. *Destroy affected parts; improve drainage; avoid injury to plant.*

GREENFLIES *see* APHIDS

GREY MOULD (*Botrytis*) Fungi that cause patches of rot on leaves, stems, flowers, and fruit; mould may spread to rest of plant. *Destroy affected plants; apply fungicide; improve ventilation; avoid injury to plant; maintain hygiene.*

GRUBS Plump insect larvae that are often found in soil, where they feed on underground structures. *Apply insecticide to soil.*

GUMMING Leakage of clear, amber-coloured gum from trunk and branches of conifers and other trees; trees with stone fruits also exude gum around stone inside fruit. Caused by poor growing conditions. *Improve conditions.*

HONEYDEW Sticky excreta of various pests that encourages growth of moulds on leaves and stems. *See also* ADELGIDS, APHIDS, MEALYBUGS, SCALE INSECTS, WHITEFLIES. *Destroy pests.*

HONEY FUNGUS Fungus that causes mycelium and black fungal strands; fruiting bodies appear in autumn. Conifers may exude gum or resin. Growth is stunted; plant often dies. *Destroy affected plants including roots; select resistant plants.*

LEAF BLOTCHES *see* SPOTS

LEAF-CUTTER BEES Small, hairy bees that cut semi-circular pieces from leaves. *No treatment necessary.*

LEAFHOPPERS Sap-sucking insects, related to aphids, that may transmit viruses and spread fungal spores. When disturbed, they leap away. Larvae feed on undersides of leaves, causing mottling on upper surfaces. *Apply insecticide.*

LEAF MINERS Larvae of flies, moths, beetles, and sawflies that tunnel into leaves, producing usually white or brown, linear, blotched, or irregular discoloration. *Destroy pests and affected leaves; apply insecticide.*

LEAF SPOT *see* SPOTS

LEATHERJACKETS Cranefly larvae that cause brown patches on grass in midsummer. *Water grass, and cover with black plastic sheets to bring larvae to surface, then destroy pests; apply insecticide.*

MAGGOTS Legless larvae, especially of flies, that feed on fruit and underground structures; plant may die. *Destroy affected parts; apply insecticide.*

MAGNESIUM DEFICIENCY Disorder that often occurs in acid soils, causing foliage to discolour (magnesium is one of the main constituents of chlorophyll). *See also* CHLOROSIS. *Apply Epsom salts (hydrated magnesium sulphate) to plants or soil.*

MANGANESE OR IRON DEFICIENCY Disorder that often occurs in alkaline soils, manifested as chlorosis on mature leaves, or as disorders specific to certain genera. *Match plant to soil type; clear any builder's debris; add trace elements and chelated iron to soil; apply acid mulch; irrigate with rainwater.*

MEALYBUGS Sap-sucking insects, whose adults and young produce tufts of waxy wool and excrete honeydew on leaves and stems. Under glass, root mealybugs infest underground structures; plant may die. *Use biological control; apply insecticide.*

MILDEWS Mouldy growth. Downy mildew (white tufts or down, usually on the undersides of leaves) and powdery mildews (dusty white coatings) are both caused by fungi. *Destroy affected parts; apply fungicide; keep roots moist; avoid overhead watering; improve ventilation; select resistant plants.*

MILLIPEDES Small, dark brown pests, with 2 legs to each body segment, that feed on underground structures, extending injuries caused by other pests. *Apply inorganic fertilizer and insecticide; maintain hygiene; cultivate soil regularly.*

MOSAIC VIRUSES *see* VIRUSES

MOTHS Insects whose larvae (caterpillars) bite holes in leaves, flowers, and fruit. *Apply insecticide; use biological controls.*

MOTTLES *see* VIRUSES

NECROSIS Death of plant cells, caused by fungal infection. *Apply fungicide.*

NEEDLE CAST Discoloration and shedding of coniferous foliage, caused by fungal infection. *Apply fungicide; maintain hygiene.*

NEMATODES *see* EELWORMS

OEDEMA Formation on leaves of warty patches, which later turn brown; caused by excess moisture in soil or air. *Do not remove affected foliage; improve ventilation and drainage.*

PEACH LEAF CURL Fungus that shows as white spores on surfaces of blistered red leaves, usually of peach trees; overwintered spores enter developing leaf buds. *Destroy affected leaves; apply fungicide.*

PEAR LEAF BLISTER MITE Small pest that causes formation of pale green, raised markings (later turning brown) on the undersides of leaves, corresponding to brown areas on the upper surfaces; leaves may become distorted. Particularly affects *Pyrus* and *Sorbus* species. *Destroy affected leaves.*

PHYLLOXERIDS Small yellow, sap-sucking insects, related to aphids, that infest undersides of leaves, causing discoloration and withering. *Apply insecticide.*

POTASSIUM DEFICIENCY Disorder that causes leaves to turn dull blue-green with brown areas; broad-leaved foliage curls down at margins. Growth is stunted. *Improve soil; apply high-potash fertilizer.*

POWDERY MILDEWS *see* MILDEWS

PSYLLIDS *see* SUCKERS

RED SPIDER MITES Tiny, sap-sucking insects that appear mainly under glass, or outdoors in warm climates. Fine webbing may appear over plant, which may die. *Under glass, use biological control. Apply insecticide.*

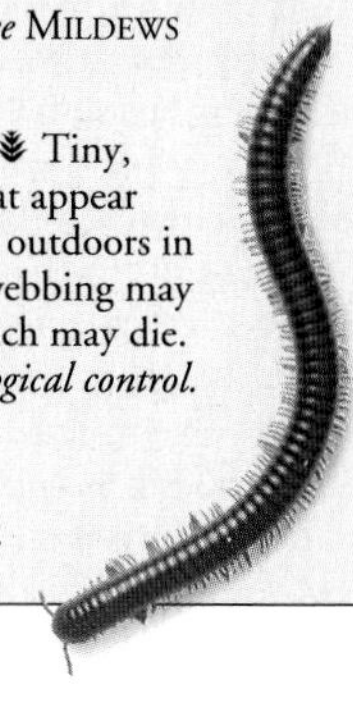

MILLIPEDE

REPLANT DISEASE Loss of vigour, dieback, and discoloration or stunting of roots, caused by eelworms, nutrient depletion, soil-borne fungi, or viruses. Particularly affects roses. *Change soil; improve conditions; plant trees, shrubs, and perennials in fresh soil.*

RHIZOCTONIA Fungus that causes damping off in seedlings. In mature plants, it encourages root rots and causes discoloration of foliage; plant may die. *Destroy affected parts; apply fungicide; improve conditions; maintain hygiene.*

ROOT FLIES Insects whose larvae tunnel into roots, causing wilting and sometimes death. *Destroy affected parts; apply insecticide; cover soil around plant; dress seed.*

ROOT MEALYBUGS *see* MEALYBUGS

ROTS Decay caused by water-logging, fungi, or bacteria. Leads to root damage, and wilting, discoloration, and dieback of leaves and stems; plant dies. *Destroy affected plants; improve drainage; use crop rotation; maintain hygiene.*

RUSTS Fungal disease that causes raised, brown, orange, or buff pustules or spores to appear, usually on stems or on undersides of leaves, with corresponding discoloration on upper surfaces; leaves may drop. If stem is affected, growth may be stunted and plant may die. *Destroy affected leaves; apply fungicide; improve ventilation; reduce humidity.*

SAWFLIES Insects whose larvae feed on leaf surfaces or on the insides of plant tissues and galls. *Destroy affected parts; apply insecticide.*

SCAB Dark lesions on fruit surfaces, caused by fungi. Fruit may become distorted or discoloured; leaves may blister and drop. *Destroy affected parts; apply fungicide; improve soil; use resistant plants.*

SCALE INSECTS Insects resembling small raised scales on stems and undersides of leaves; they excrete honeydew on leaves. *Use biological control; apply insecticide.*

SHOTHOLE Holes in leaves, resulting from death of tissue due to cankers or leaf spots. *Apply fungicide; improve conditions; fertilize annually; mulch and irrigate in spring.*

SILVER LEAF Fungal disease that causes foliage to turn silver, later brown. Wood is stained; shoots or branches suffer dieback; fruiting bodies form on dead wood. Particularly affects trees with stone fruits. *Cut back beyond affected parts; prune susceptible trees in summer only.*

SLUGS Soft-bodied pests that feed on underground structures and low-growing leaves, which may be stripped. Slime trails may be visible. *Use biological control; apply pellets or liquid; cultivate soil regularly; maintain hygiene.*

SLUGWORMS Black, slime-covered sawfly larvae, similar to small slugs, that feed on upper leaf surfaces, causing opaque patches. *Spray with insecticide.*

SMUTS Fungal diseases that cause pale swellings, later releasing black spores, on stems and foliage. Parts affected may wither and die. *Destroy affected parts or plants; disinfect greenhouse; apply fungicide.*

SNAILS Hard-shelled pests that feed on leaves; plant may be stripped. Slime trails may be visible. *Apply pellets or liquid; cultivate soil regularly; maintain hygiene.*

SOFT SCALE INSECTS *see* SCALE INSECTS

SPOTS Bacterial or fungal diseases that affect leaves. Bacterial spots may be angular with a yellow rim; fungal spots have concentric zones and an area of fruiting bodies. *See also* ANTHRACNOSE, SHOTHOLE. *Destroy affected parts; apply fungicide; improve conditions; sow seed thinly; fertilize annually; mulch and water in spring.*

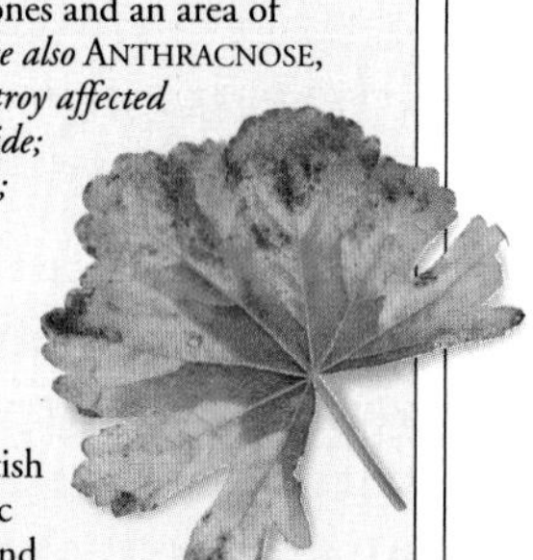

POTASSIUM DEFICIENCY

SPRINGTAILS Tiny, whitish pests, often prolific on roots, that extend damage caused by other pests. When disturbed, some leap using rear of body. *Apply insecticide to soil; maintain hygiene.*

SUCKERS Sap-sucking insects, related to aphids but with flattened bodies and prominent eyes and wing buds. Larvae and adults excrete honeydew on leaves and stems, causing distortion of young growth. *Destroy affected parts; apply insecticide.*

THRIPS Insects whose juveniles and adults cause pale white flecks on petals and leaves; buds may fail to turn green. *Use biological control; apply insecticide; water regularly; improve ventilation.*

VINE WEEVIL LARVAE *see* WEEVILS

VIRUSES Diseases that cause distortion and discolouring of leaves and flowers. Growth is stunted; plant may die. *Destroy affected plants; control insects that spread infection; select resistant plants; maintain hygiene.*

WASPS Insects that feed on fruit, but also prey on other pests. *Destroy nests at dusk if treatment is required.*

WEEVILS Small, dark-coloured insects that feed on plants. Grubs gnaw cuttings, underground structures, and seedlings. Plant or seedlings wilt, discolour, and die. *Destroy pests; use biological control; apply insecticide.*

WHIPTAIL Molybdenum deficiency in brassicas, often in acid soils, that causes development of narrow, ribbon-like leaves. *Add lime to soil; add molybdenum to soil before sowing or planting out.*

WHITE BLISTER Fungal diseases that cause unsightly, gleaming white patches on foliage. *Destroy affected leaves.*

WHITEFLIES Insects, related to aphids, whose juveniles and tiny white, moth-like adults suck sap on leaf undersides and excrete honeydew, causing distortion of young growth. *Apply insecticide outdoors; use biological control under glass.*

WILT Fungal disease that enters via roots or is carried on secateurs. Plant wilts and usually dies. *Destroy affected plants; use crop rotation; maintain hygiene.*

WIREWORMS Small, orange-yellow click beetle larvae that feed on underground structures and bases of seedlings. Plant or seedlings may die. Most common on newly cultivated former grassland. *Destroy pests and affected plants; apply insecticide to plants or soil; cultivate soil regularly.*

WOODLICE Pests that feed on young or damaged roots, stems, and leaves. *Maintain hygiene.*

WOOLLY APHIDS *see* APHIDS

Trees

As the largest and most prominent of all garden plants, trees establish the basic, long-term framework of a garden, and their forms and colours influence the selection of other plants. Since they originate from most regions of the world, there is an immense variety of ornamental trees suitable for almost any garden site.

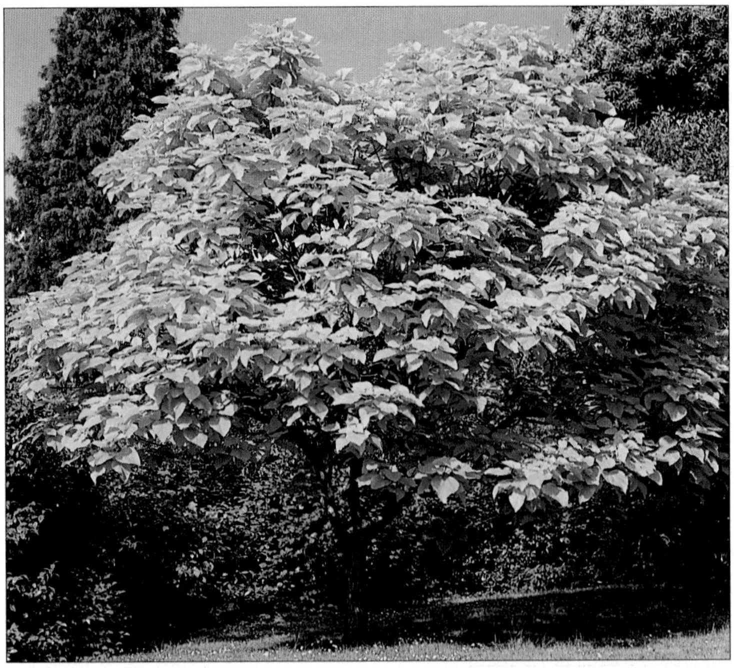

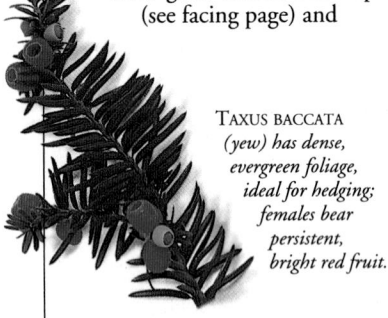

An ideal specimen
The best specimen trees display a succession of ornamental features. Catalpa bignonioides *'Aurea' has bronze young foliage in mid-spring, soon turning bright yellow, and bears bell-shaped flowers in summer, followed by bean-like pods.*

What are trees?

Trees may be broadly defined as long-lived, woody perennial plants, deciduous or evergreen, each usually with a single stem, although some, such as birches (*Betula*), may have 2 or 3 stems and still be regarded as trees. They are generally quite distinct from shrubs, which produce several or many stems that branch from or near soil level. As a group, trees are larger than shrubs, but show great variation in shape (see facing page) and height, ranging from dwarf cultivars only 1m (3ft) high to specimens of 90m (300ft). In horticulture, a grafted shrub that is grown as a standard, even if only 2m (6ft) or so high, is often referred to as tree-like.

TAXUS BACCATA *(yew) has dense, evergreen foliage, ideal for hedging; females bear persistent, bright red fruit.*

Most trees are angiosperms (see p.10). Exceptions include conifers, which reproduce by means of naked ovules borne on the scales of cones. Conifers can withstand extreme climatic conditions, and have distinctive, regular branching, often conical crowns, and linear, needle-like leaves. They are popular as specimen trees, and for hedging and screening. Dwarf conifers are ideal in beds and containers.

Shape and size

A tree's shape and size have a strong impact on the style of a garden. Tall, narrow trees can lend a formal air; trees that are open and spreading seem more informal. Weeping trees are graceful, whereas conical trees are strong and sculptural.

When choosing a tree, take note of its size at maturity and the proximity of other plants to ensure that it will be appropriate for the size and style of the garden. A weeping willow (*Salix* x *sepulcralis* 'Chrysocoma'), for example, would overwhelm a small garden and cause problems for other plants growing nearby, whereas the same tree would look magnificent in a larger area.

Ornamental features

The leaves of trees are often highly decorative, and vary greatly in size, shape, surface texture, and colour. Occurring in all shades of green, as well as yellow, purple, and other hues, their dense mass of colour can complement other plants throughout the year. Leaf textures, whether smooth and glossy, or hairy or woolly, add further interest. Some trees bear aromatic foliage.

Many trees are also cultivated for their attractive, often scented flowers, which range from the small, clustered flowers of hawthorn (*Crataegus*) to the large single blooms of *Magnolia*. The berries, pods, or other fruits that follow the flowers, with their bold shapes and colours, often persist throughout autumn or winter. Some species bear fruit only in maturity, while dioecious trees, such as most hollies (*Ilex*), must be cross-pollinated by a second plant of the opposite sex before setting fruit. Bisexual and monoecious trees can usually set their own fruit (see p.13).

Bark can also provide fascinating patterns, textures, and colours (see panel, left). Some species may need to be pruned to the base annually to stimulate vividly coloured new growth.

Garden uses

Trees are most commonly grown in an open site as specimen plants, visible from all angles, generally on a lawn or underplanted with ground cover, or they may be grown in a large shrub border as a focal point. Single trees can also be used to mark an entrance or change of levels in a garden. Ideally, a specimen tree will display one or more features at different times during the year.

In larger gardens, trees can be planted in groups. Year-round interest is ensured if both evergreen and deciduous trees are included, since the branches of deciduous trees may be bare for up to half of the year in cool climates.

Trees may also be used as hedging, as wind or sound barriers, to screen eyesores, to frame a view, or to line a pathway. They can give shelter from sun or rain, as well as provide a home for wildlife.

DECORATIVE BARK

Bark performs the essential function of protecting the sensitive growth tissue of the tree stem or branches beneath. As their girth expands with age, the bark may fissure or peel, sometimes resulting in patterns, textures, and hues with ornamental interest. Brightly coloured bark is also produced on the young branches of some trees. Bark may be conspicuously marked with lenticels (pores), which provide access for air to the inner tissues.

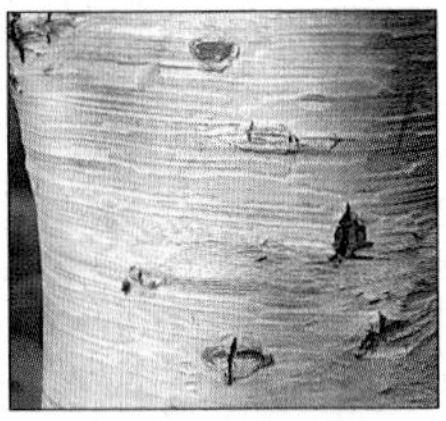

ATTRACTIVELY COLOURED
Betula ermanii

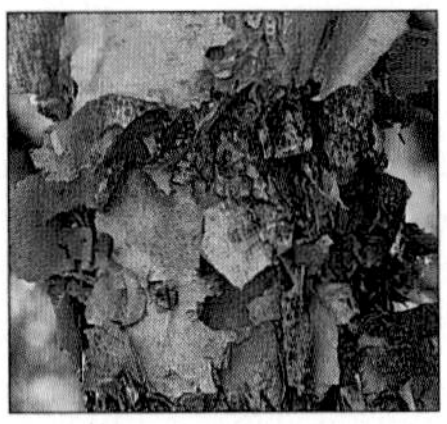

PEELING IN FLAKES
Betula nigra

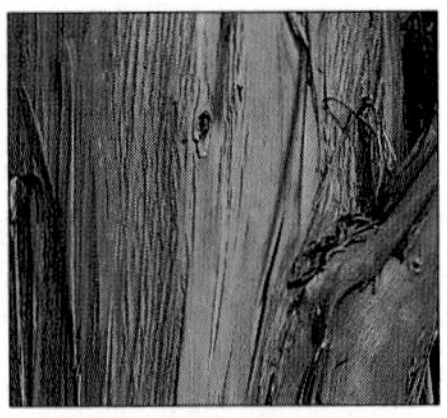

PEELING VERTICALLY
Eucalyptus johnstonii

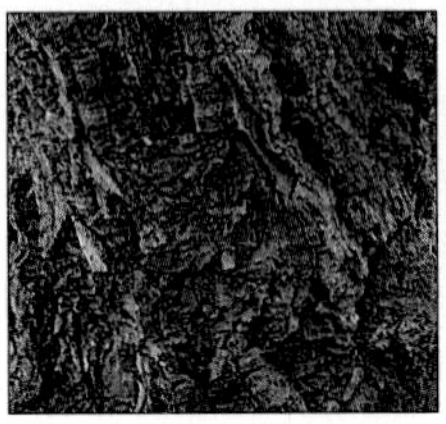

FISSURED
Quercus suber

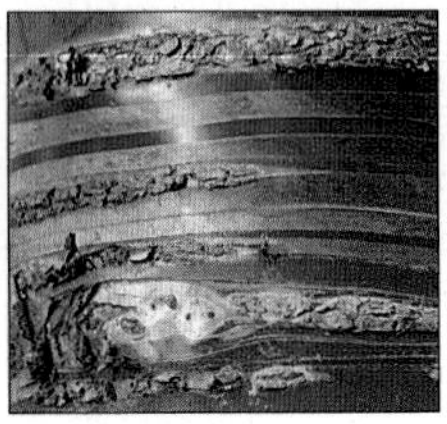

PEELING HORIZONTALLY
Prunus serrula

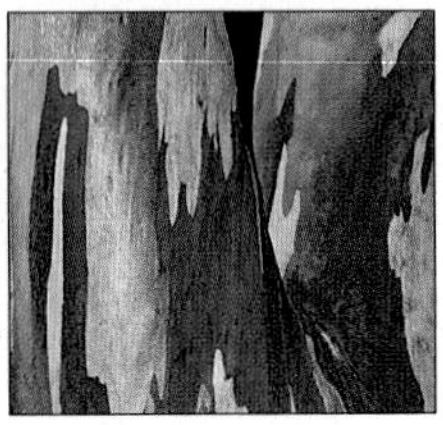

PEELING IN PATCHES
Eucalyptus pauciflora

FORMATIVE PRUNING

A young tree, particularly if deciduous, requires formative pruning in order to develop even growth. A "feathered" tree, with a stem branched to the base, can be trained either as a central-leader standard, with a clear stem and lateral branches tapering towards the bottom third of the trunk, or as a branched-head standard, with a clear stem and a more fully developed crown. Mature trees require little pruning, except to maintain their vigour and shape (see pp.26–27). More drastic pruning, such as for renewal, is described on p.25.

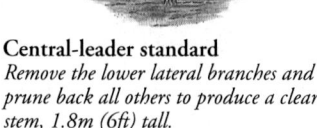

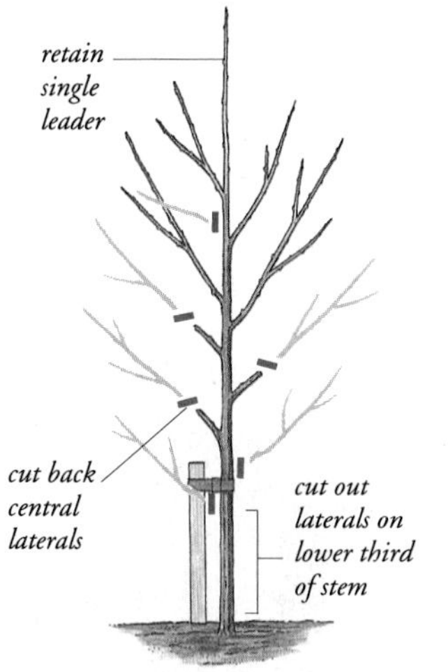

Central-leader standard
Remove the lower lateral branches and prune back all others to produce a clear stem, 1.8m (6ft) tall.

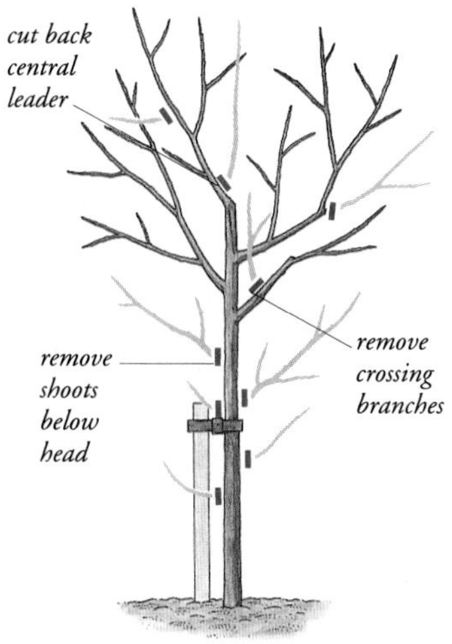

Branched-head standard
Train as a central-leader standard with a clear stem, 1.8m (6ft) tall, then cut back the leader to open the crown.

TREE SHAPES

The basic shape of every tree in this encyclopedia is represented by one of the stylized shape symbols shown below (for palms and cycads, see p.50). The symbols appear within the plant entry, directly after the botanical name, and indicate the general outline of each tree, regardless of its internal branch structure (see right) and the differences that naturally occur from one specimen to another. When choosing a tree, consider the impact of its overall shape on the planting site.

Branch structure
Each of these 3 trees is classified as ⚲ *(rounded to broadly spreading), despite their different branch structures.*

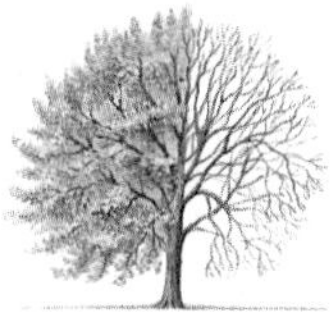
Fagus sylvatica

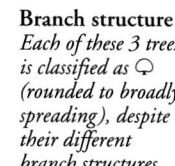

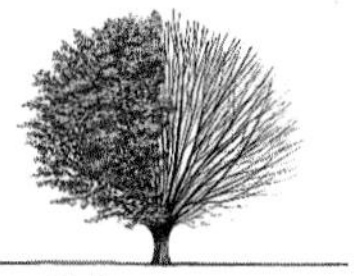
Zelkova serrata

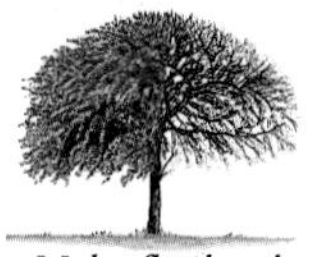
Malus floribunda

SHAPES AND SYMBOLS

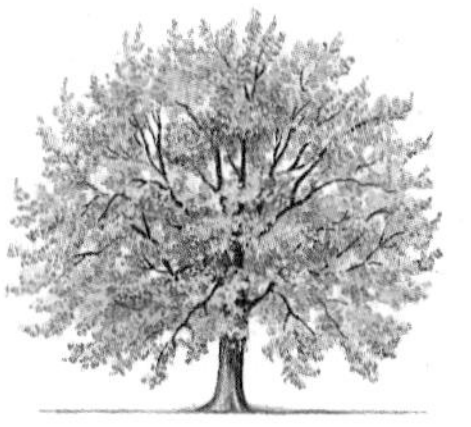
ROUNDED TO BROADLY SPREADING
e.g. *Fagus sylvatica*

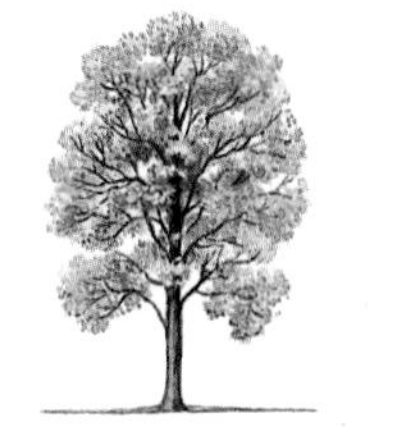
ROUNDED TO BROADLY COLUMNAR
e.g. *Populus szechuanica*

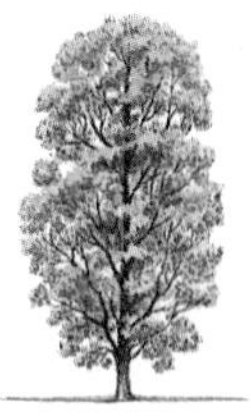
BROADLY COLUMNAR
e.g. *Quercus pontica*

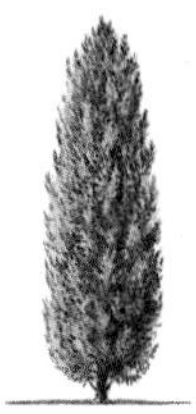
NARROWLY COLUMNAR
e.g. *Juniperus chinensis* 'Obelisk'

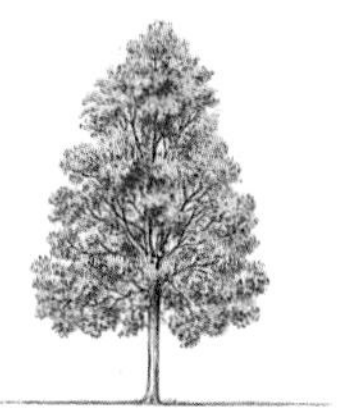
BROADLY CONICAL
e.g. *Betula papyrifera*

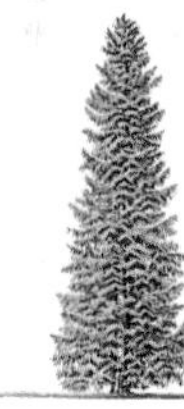
NARROWLY CONICAL
e.g. *Thuja koraiensis*

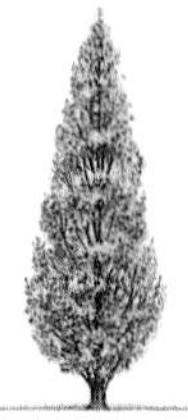
NARROWLY CONICAL (FLAME-SHAPED)
e.g. *Cupressus sempervirens*

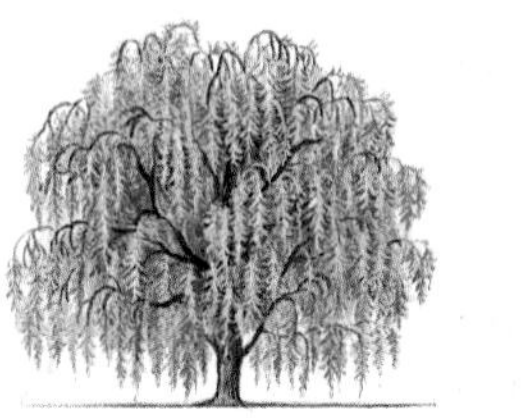
LARGE WEEPING
e.g. *Salix babylonica*

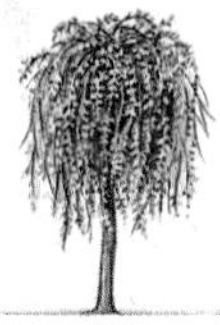
SMALL WEEPING
e.g. *Salix caprea* 'Kilmarnock'

A woodland garden provides a naturalistic, shady, and sheltered environment in which to nurture shrubs, perennials, and bulbs that grow best in dappled shade. Larger birches or oaks (*Quercus*) can provide an excellent canopy above smaller trees, such as some magnolias and maples (*Acer*).

Many trees are also tolerant of cultivation in containers. As it is possible to move them around, they can be used in varied displays in areas such as patios and courtyard or roof-top gardens, or to flank steps or doorways. Container-grown trees can also be underplanted with annuals and trailing plants for colour and variety. In cold climates, ensure that containers are frost-proof; tender trees can be moved under glass for protection in winter.

Cultivation

Trees can thrive for decades, some even for centuries, if they are grown in the right soil and climate, and have adequate shelter, levels of light, and rainfall. Plant away from pipes, drains, cables, and usually walls and buildings, although some tender trees are best grown against a sunny wall. On slopes, plant trees halfway down, where it is warmer and less windy. In coastal zones, select trees that tolerate salt winds and spray.

Plant bare-root, usually deciduous trees between mid-autumn and mid-spring, but not in frosty weather; evergreen trees are best planted in autumn or mid-spring. Plant hardy trees with fleshy roots, whether evergreen or deciduous, in mid-autumn or in mid- or late spring; in cold areas, half-hardy and evergreen trees should be planted only in mid-spring. Plant root-balled trees in early or mid-autumn, or in early or mid-spring; deciduous root-balled trees may be planted in winter when the weather is mild. Plant out container-grown trees at any time, except in frost or drought.

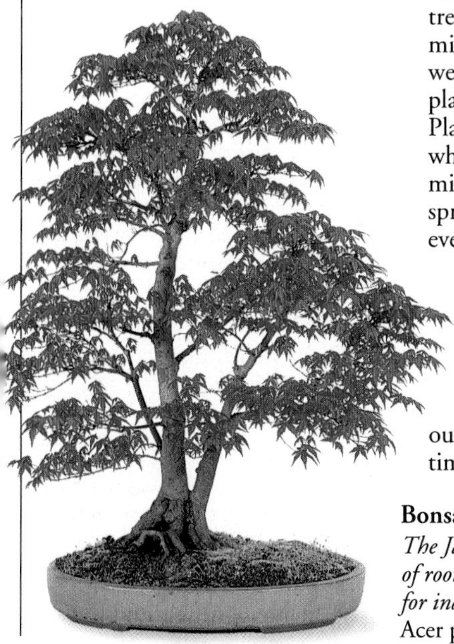

Bonsai tree
The Japanese art of restrictive pruning of roots and branches produces tiny trees for indoor and outdoor use, such as this Acer palmatum *'Schindeshojo'.*

Dig the planting hole 2 to 4 times as wide as the root ball, and 1½ times as deep, working organic matter into the base. If necessary, drive a stake off-centre into the hole (see p.23). Plant the tree, backfill with soil mixed with organic matter, tread it in firmly, and water well, mulching thickly or top-dressing with bark chips or a similar organic mulch. Secure the tree to the stake and protect it with a stem guard. Until established, water young trees regularly, especially those on light, sandy soils; keep them free of weeds to a diameter of 1m (3ft) around the trunk. Provide a winter mulch. Remove suckers as they appear.

Feed and water trees grown in containers regularly, watering freely in hot, dry weather. In spring, replace the top 5cm (2in) of compost with fresh compost and apply a slow-release fertilizer. Pot on every 3 to 5 years.

Trees may be propagated by seed, cuttings, layering, or grafting (rarely used by amateur gardeners). Species are often grown from seed, although they take a long time to establish. Hybrids and cultivars rarely come true from seed, and must be increased by vegetative means, usually from cuttings.

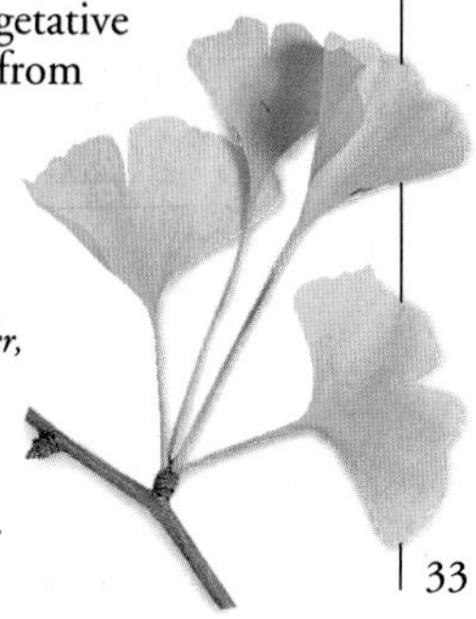

GINKGO BILOBA, *a deciduous conifer, has fan-shaped, mid-green leaves that turn golden yellow in autumn.*

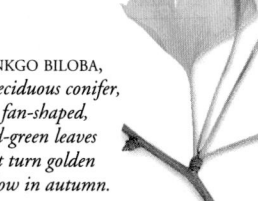

Shrubs

Both deciduous and evergreen shrubs are prized as essential elements in most garden designs. The diversity of their ornamental features – architectural habits, fragrant flowers, striking fruits, or attractive foliage – and the year-round presence of their woody, often decorative stems, offers an almost infinite choice for gardeners. Like trees, they occur in the wild in a broad spectrum of habitats, ensuring there is a wide range of shrubs suitable for every soil and aspect.

What are shrubs?

Shrubs are woody-stemmed plants, usually freely branching from the base. Whereas a tree usually has a single stem (see p.32), a shrub has several or many stems arising from or near ground level. Most shrubs reach no more than 5–6m (15–20ft) in height, the majority of species and cultivars attaining considerably smaller stature.

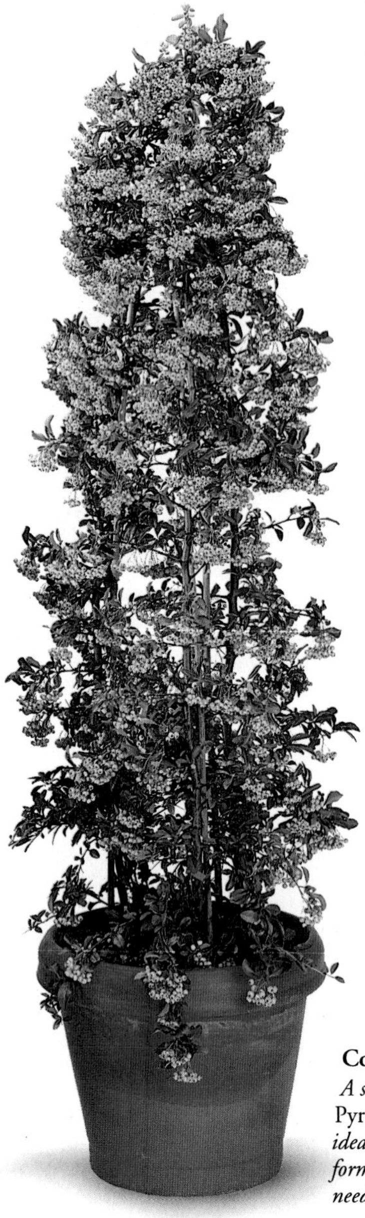

Container display
A shrub grown in a pot, such as this Pyracantha *'Golden Charmer', is ideal for a small, paved garden or formal area. Container-grown shrubs need careful watering and pruning.*

However, a degree of overlap occurs between shrubs and other plant groups. Larger shrubs, such as lilac (*Syringa*), that grow on a single stem, can also be considered trees, although this depends on their size at maturity. Subshrubs (shrubs that are woody only at the base), such as *Perovskia*, and shrubs that die back annually as a result of winter frosts, such as *Fuchsia*, are often cultivated as herbaceous perennials.

Essential framework

In every size and style of garden, shrubs are invaluable for their structural forms and their woody stems, which provide the garden with a long-term framework. They offer a variety of shapes and sizes, from prostrate, mat-, or clump-forming subshrubs, such as dwarf cultivars of *Erica carnea*, only 15cm (6in) high, to erect, tree-like shrubs like *Buddleja colvilei*, 6m (20ft) tall.

Ornamental features

Shrubs display an immense range of decorative features. They are often cultivated for their foliage, occurring in many shades of green, yellow, red, purple, silver, or grey. Some are especially favoured for their brilliant autumn coloration: Japanese maples (*Acer palmatum*) include numerous cultivars that turn from yellow through orange to shades of red, while the purple leaves of some *Cotinus* cultivars turn red between autumn and early winter. The notable autumn colour of witch hazels (*Hamamelis*) ranges from yellow to orange-red or purple.

The flowers of shrubs vary enormously in shape, size, and scent, and occur in almost every colour. At one end of the spectrum are the abundant, tiny flowers of

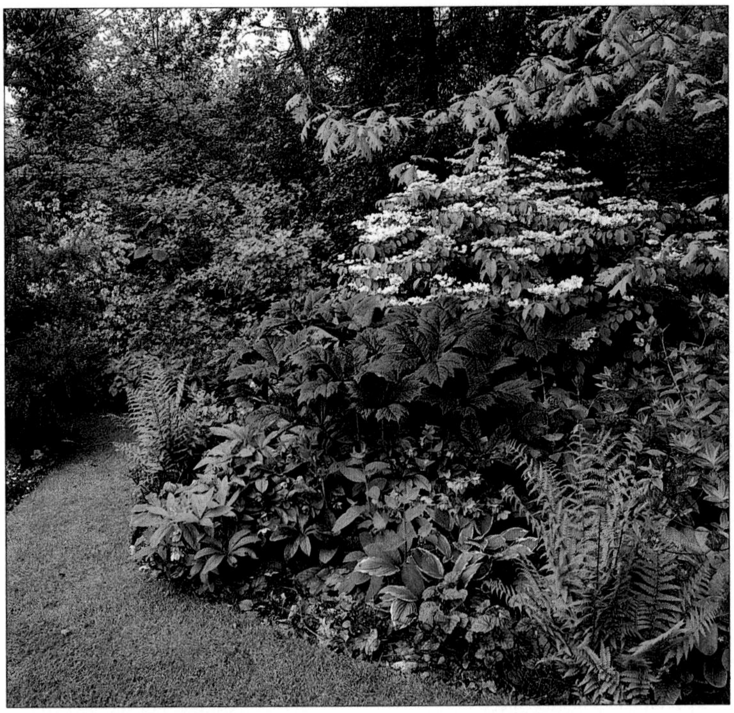

Designing for a mature border
Positioned too close together, larger plants may compete for space, light, moisture, and nutrients. Here, Viburnum plicatum *'Mariesii' is centrally placed at the back of the border, with ample room for its spreading growth. Its magnificent white flowerheads cascade towards the bronze foliage of the perennial* Rodgersia podophylla.

Ceanothus; at the other are the giant blooms of tree peonies (*Paeonia*). While numerous shrubs bloom for only a few weeks each year, others, including *Hypericum* and *Potentilla*, flower reliably over several months; shrubs of the latter type are valuable during periods when little else is in bloom. Some shrubs, such as Mexican orange blossom (*Choisya ternata*) are remontant, regularly flowering twice in a year. Winter-flowering shrubs, such as *Viburnum* x *bodnantense*, often bear scented blooms over a long period.

Many popular shrubs, including *Cotoneaster*, *Gaultheria*, holly (*Ilex*), and *Pyracantha*, bear vividly coloured berries in autumn, which persist into winter. Other types of fruit range from those of *Dipelta*, which are covered by papery bracts, to the pendent, bean-like, deep blue pods of *Decaisnea fargesii*.

Some shrubs display brightly coloured winter stems. In dogwoods (*Cornus*), the stems can be blazing red through to bright greenish yellow. A special pruning regime may be required to stimulate new growth for the best display of colour (see pruning group 7, p.27).

Garden uses

Most shrubs are grown in a shrub border, or in a mixed border among annuals or perennials. When designing a border, it is advisable first to establish a theme. Consider whether the border is to display a selection of favourite species, to provide interest in a particular season or throughout the year, and whether plants should feature ornamental or scented flowers, decorative foliage, or fruit, or various combinations of all of these.

For a dedicated shrub border, select larger shrubs that will flower in different seasons: for example, choose *Viburnum tinus* to flower from late winter to spring, lilacs (*Syringa*) or *Philadelphus* for flowers in summer, and *Garrya elliptica* or witch hazel (*Hamamelis*) for winter blooms. For year-round foliage interest, include both deciduous and evergreen shrubs.

Shrub borders are usually designed with larger shrubs planted at the back of the border, and dwarf or ground-cover shrubs, such as *Chaenomeles japonica*, at the front, although other arrangements can also be successful. It is particularly important to provide sufficient space for each shrub; as plants become established, they should not crowd one another. If necessary, any bare patches can be filled in with small, fast-growing shrubs, such as *Cistus*, fuchsias, or hebes, which can

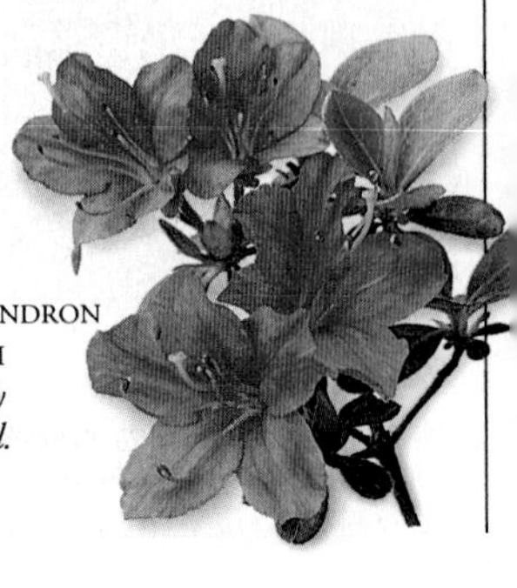

RHODODENDRON KIUSIANUM *thrives only on acid soil.*

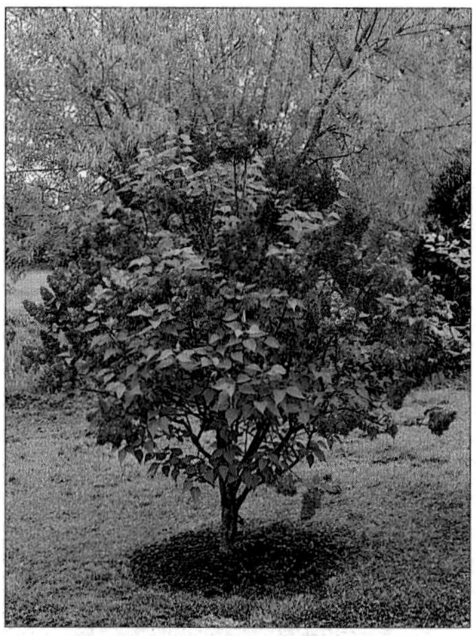

Scented specimen
Syringa vulgaris *'Congo' is ideal for use as a lawn specimen. Tree-like in habit, it also has fragrant flowers, which are particularly attractive to butterflies.*

be removed when shrubs with a slower growth rate have reached maturity. Some shrubs are best trained against a warm, sunny wall, particularly tender shrubs, which may not thrive elsewhere in the garden; a few, such as *Ceanothus*, may grow to twice their usual height in this situation.

In a mixed border, cultivate shrubs alongside annuals, biennials, bulbs, or herbaceous perennials, seeking associations of colour and texture of flowers and foliage, and contrasts in form and habit. When dividing (see p.28) or transplanting perennials within a mixed border, take care not to damage the roots of plants growing nearby.

Shrubs that exhibit a variety of ornamental features make excellent specimen plants, and are ideally sited where they may be viewed from different angles. A specimen shrub should be appealing in habit and branch structure, particularly if it is deciduous, as well as in its foliage, flowers, or fruit. In a small garden, where a single specimen serves as a focal point throughout the year, versatility is essential; it is less important in a large garden that can accommodate a selection of shrubs of different sizes and features.

Growing in containers

Many shrubs thrive in containers, and are excellent for a small garden, patio, or roof terrace. Use an isolated specimen in a decorative container as an arresting focal point, or group containers in different arrangements for variety.

Container growing also enables cultivation of shrubs that may not survive in the open garden due to the acidity or alkalinity of the local soil, poor drainage, or an unsuitable climate. Tender plants can be displayed outdoors in summer, and then moved under glass before the first frosts. Ensure that hardy plants kept outside in frost-prone areas are grown in frost-proof containers.

Cultivation

Shrubs will thrive for many years, given the right growing conditions. The majority will grow in any type of garden soil, but generally prefer a fertile, well-drained but moisture-retentive loam. Plant bare-root and root-balled shrubs from autumn to spring, although planting should be delayed if the ground is frozen. Container-grown plants can be planted at any time, except in frost or drought, but usually establish best if planted in autumn or spring.

For root-balled or container-grown plants, make the planting hole 2 or 3 times the width of the root ball and deep enough for the roots to be buried to their original depth of soil. For bare-root plants, allow room for the roots to fan out fully around the shrub.

Plant the shrub, backfilling with a mixture of soil and organic matter, and firm in. In sandy soils, leave a depression around the shrub to retain moisture; in clay soils, plant the shrub slightly higher than the surrounding soil level so that water will readily drain off. Water and mulch well with garden compost or bark chips. Protect newly planted shrubs from cold, drying winds. Plant wall-trained shrubs about 45cm (18in) from the wall; lean the plant against the wall and support it with canes tied into wires. Young plants require regular watering until established. Apply fertilizer in early spring, and mulch thickly with bark chips or garden compost in spring or autumn.

From early spring to midsummer, water shrubs in containers freely and apply a quick-release fertilizer 2 or 3 times. In spring, replace the top 5–10cm (2–4in) of compost with fresh compost, mixed with a slow-release, balanced fertilizer. Pot on in late summer or autumn, when the root growth appears congested.

For all shrubs, remove suckers and cut out reverted (plain) shoots from variegated plants as soon as they appear. Dead-head regularly to encourage stronger growth.

General pruning advice and details of the pruning groups for each shrub genus in this encyclopedia are given on pp.25–27. Unless otherwise stated, coniferous shrubs do not require pruning.

Shrubs can be propagated by seed (for species), from cuttings, or by layering, division, or grafting (not usually used by amateur gardeners). Hybrids and cultivars must be propagated by vegetative means as they do not come true from seed.

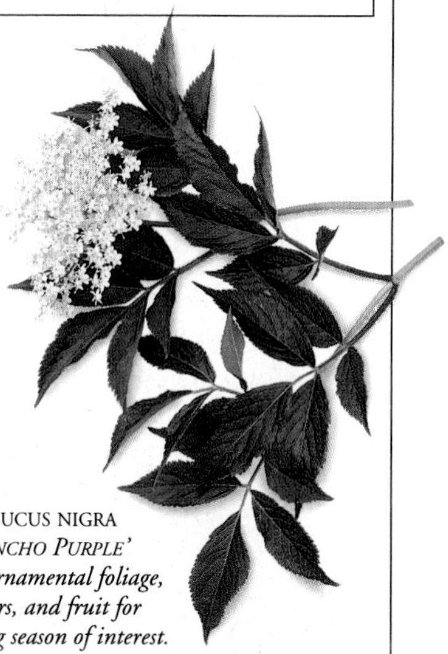

SAMBUCUS NIGRA *'GUINCHO PURPLE' has ornamental foliage, flowers, and fruit for a long season of interest.*

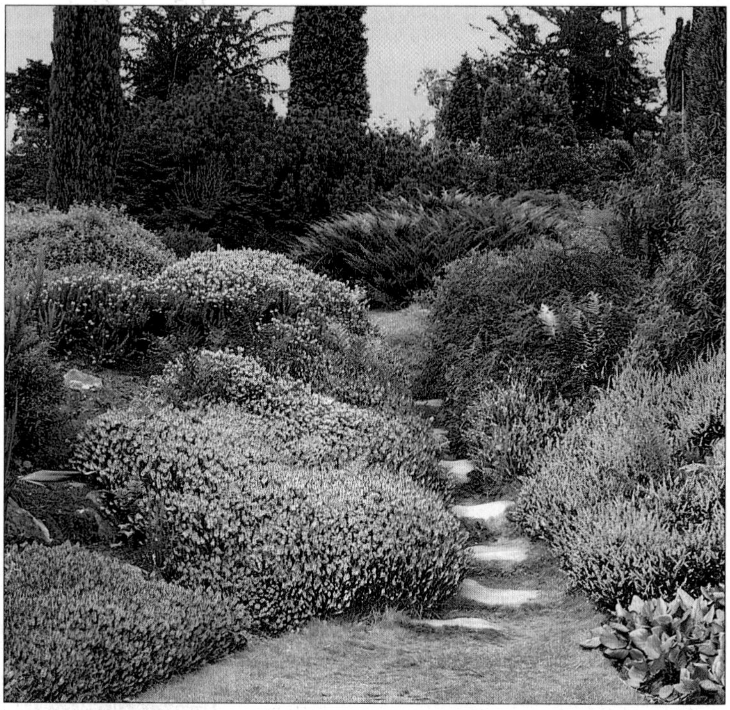

Heather border
In this border, the low, rounded form of the heathers, interspersed with ferns and bergenias, is accented by the columnar habit of Chamaecyparis lawsoniana *and other conifers in a pleasing combination of shape, habit, texture, and colour.*

HEDGES AND SCREENS

Many shrubs can be used as boundary markers or screens, as low edging, or to divide areas within a garden. Those most suitable are robust, dense, and erect in habit, and tolerate clipping.

Spiny-leaved or thorny shrubs, such as cultivars of *Berberis thunbergii, Ilex aquifolium,* and roses, as well as shrubs with dense growth, including *Taxus baccata* 'Adpressa', are excellent for creating an impenetrable hedge. Dwarf shrubs, such as *Buxus sempervirens* 'Suffruticosa', are good for low edging. Herbs, such as lavender (*Lavandula*) and rosemary (*Rosmarinus*), make fragrant low hedges. In coastal areas, select plants resistant to wind and salt, such as *Elaeagnus* or *Griselinia.*

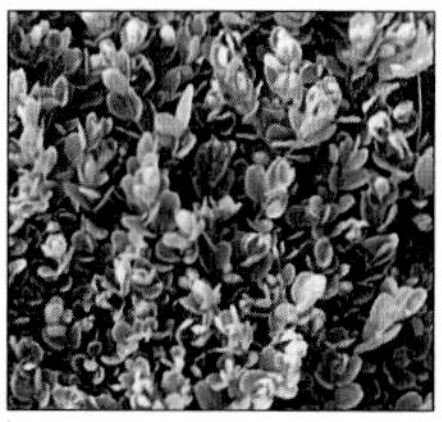

Buxus sempervirens 'Suffruticosa'

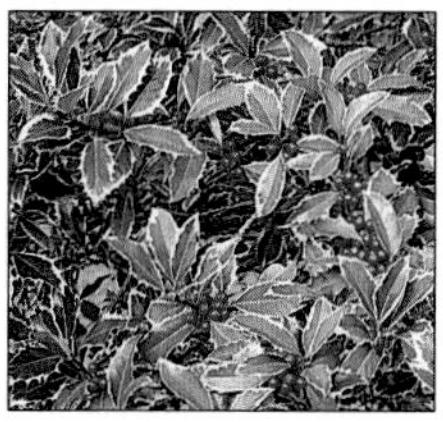

Ilex aquifolium 'Handsworth New Silver'

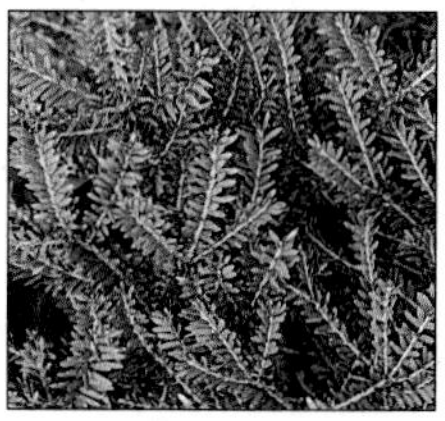

Taxus baccata 'Adpressa'

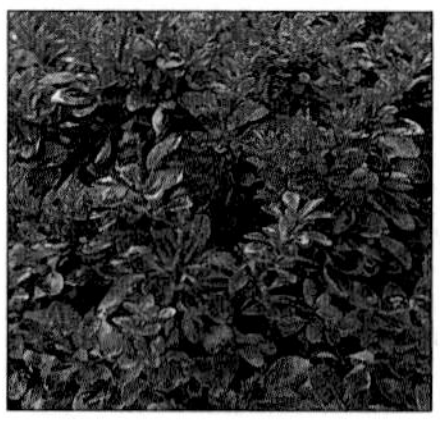

Berberis thunbergii 'Dart's Red Lady'

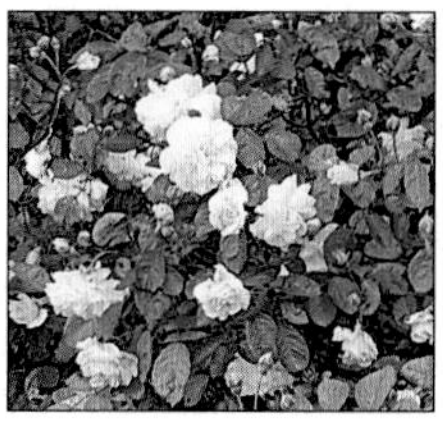

Rosa 'Buff Beauty'

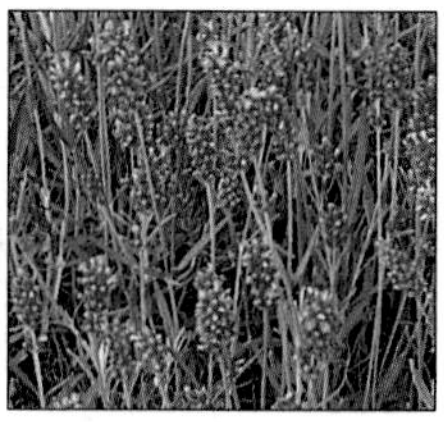

Lavandula angustifolia 'Hidcote'

Climbers

Gardeners value evergreen and deciduous climbing plants for their ability to cover walls, tree stumps, or buildings, or to grow through the branches of robust trees or shrubs. Many can be used as ground cover or as living ornamental screens. Climbers provide diverse attractions of flowers, fruits, and foliage, and there is an ample choice of woody or herbaceous perennials, or annuals.

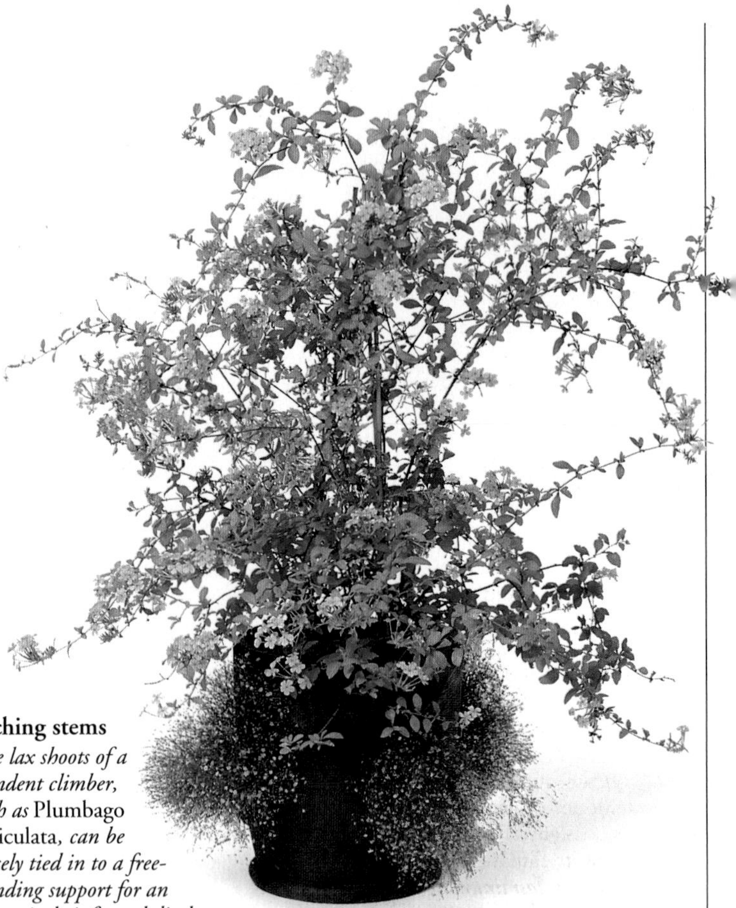

Arching stems
The lax shoots of a scandent climber, such as Plumbago auriculata, *can be loosely tied in to a free-standing support for an attractively informal display.*

What are climbers?

Climbing plants may be self-clinging or twining, or scandent, scrambling, or trailing. Self-clinging plants use aerial roots or terminal adhesive pads to attach themselves to any surface that offers purchase, for example rock faces, tree trunks, or walls, and need only initial guidance. Twining climbers twine their stems, coil their tendrils, or use modified leaf-stalks to wind through trees, shrubs, or trellis. They will thread their way through shrubs and trees without additional support, but require wires or trellis if wall-trained. If used as ground cover, they need to be pinned down so that they root at the nodes. Scandent, scrambling, and trailing plants have long stems that attach themselves loosely, if at all, to their support. To climb, they must be tied in to their support, or they can be allowed to tumble over walls or banks.

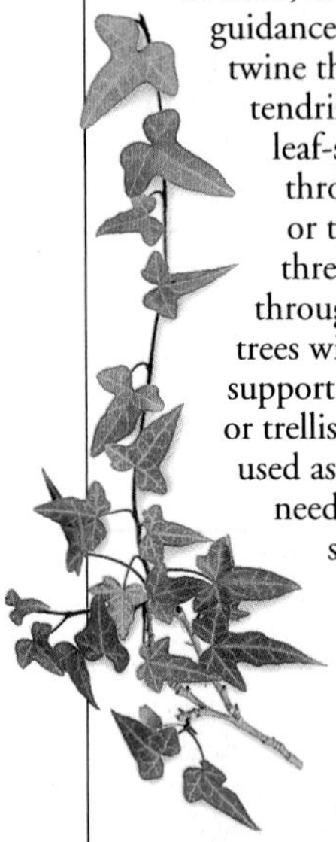

HEDERA NEPALENSIS *'SUZANNE' is excellent for clothing a sheltered, shady wall.*

Garden uses

Evergreens, such as *Hedera colchica* and its variegated cultivars, provide handsome foliage all year round. Deciduous climbers can display attractive foliage from their first bright new spring growth through to autumn, when many, such as *Parthenocissus tricuspidata*, provide brilliant autumn colour. *Actinidia kolomikta* has decorative green foliage splashed pink and white.

Many climbers, including clematis, honeysuckle (*Lonicera*), and jasmine (*Jasminum*), are cultivated for their colourful or fragrant flowers. Some produce ornamental fruits: the silky seed heads of clematis often remain decorative for some time after the flowers have gone; many honeysuckles follow their blooms with red berries. Climbers grown mainly for their fruits include *Celastrus*, whose fruits split open in autumn, revealing brightly coloured seeds.

Vigorous climbers, such as *Fallopia baldschuanica* or *Wisteria*, can be used to hide unsightly outbuildings. To cover low objects, such as old tree stumps, and for use as ground cover, choose self-clinging plants, such as ivies (*Hedera*), *Hydrangea petiolaris*, and Virginia creeper (*Parthenocissus*), which require no training or support. Climbers can also be trained to form attractive screening between various parts of a garden. For example, a trellis can be used to support a screen of fragrant annuals, or can be smothered with both climbing roses and honeysuckle.

Many climbers will easily twine through the branches of a tree, complementing the host tree's own features and extending its period of interest. Self-clinging climbers planted at the base of a tree will establish themselves against the trunk; twining or tendril climbers will need to be trained into the lower branches. *Clematis montana* and *C. armandii*, as well as honeysuckles, *Hydrangea petiolaris*, ivies, *Vitis coignetiae*, and *Wisteria* can all be grown this way. Shade-loving honeysuckles flower beneath the foliage of the tree, while sun-loving clematis will flower only at the sunlit top of the canopy.

Pergolas and pillars are ideal for supporting climbers, as they can be admired from all sides. These structures also provide strong vertical elements in garden design.

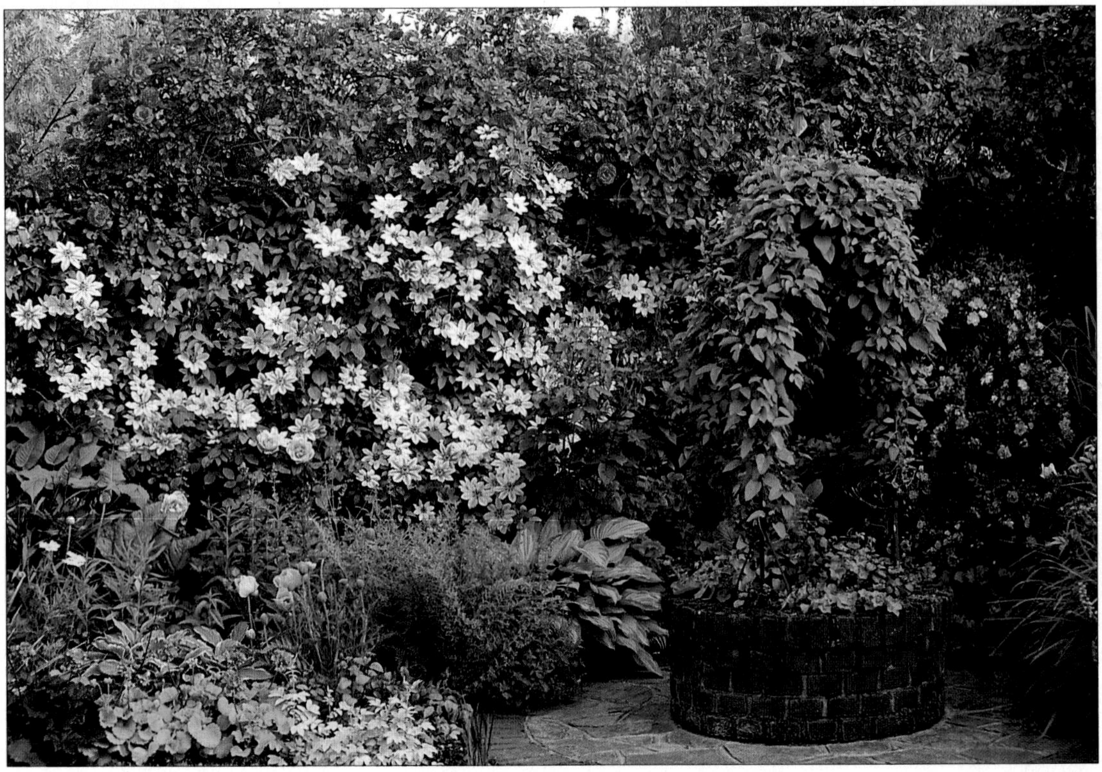

Visual counterpoint
Here, climbers are used as the focus of a raised bed improvised from a well-head. The lush foliage of Humulus lupulus *and a clematis, trained over a wire loop, are offset by abundantly flowering roses, honeysuckle (*Lonicera*),* Clematis *'Nelly Moser', and* C. *'William Kennett'.*

Short-term climbers

Climbing annuals, and perennials grown as annuals (such as *Eccremocarpus scaber*), are useful for providing temporary screens, for short-term cover on arches or trellis until permanent plantings are established, or for providing shade during summer. The fragrant sweet pea (*Lathyrus odoratus*) is ideal for a cottage-style garden, with attractive flowers suitable for cutting. Slender perennial climbers, such as species of *Codonopsis*, can be used to twine through subshrubs. Herbaceous species, for example *Tropaeolum speciosum*, *Lathyrus grandiflorus*, and *L. latifolius*, will scramble through robust shrubs. All die back in autumn, thereby avoiding problems with pruning among the host plants.

HOW CLIMBERS ATTACH

Twining plants use tendrils or leaf-stalks to coil their stems in spirals around a support; guide them into the branches of a tree or shrub, or train them on to a wire framework or wooden trellis against a wall. Self-clinging plants climb by using aerial roots or adhesive pads on their tendrils until they have become established against the trunk of a tree or a wall. Scandent and scrambling climbers need to be tied in to a support in order to climb, or they can be left to trail. All types can be used as ground cover.

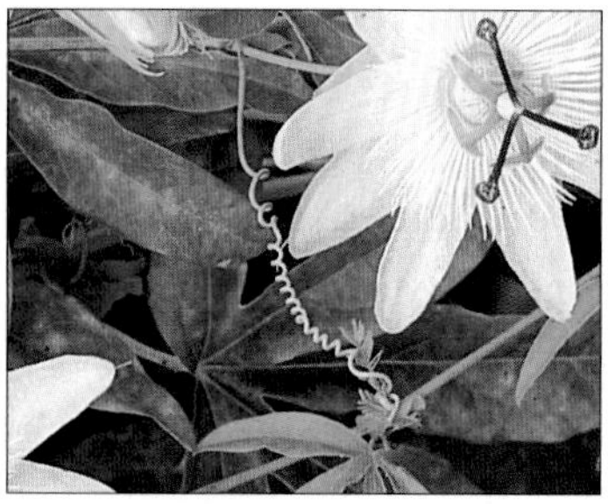

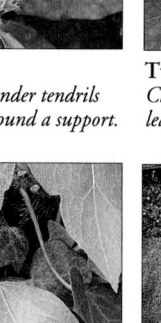

Twining tendrils
Passion flowers send out slender tendrils (modified stems) to curl around a support.

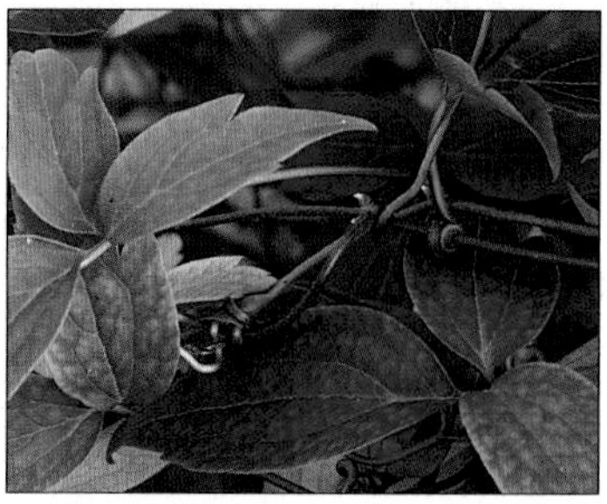

Twining leaf-stalks
Clematis climb by spiralling modified leaf-stalks around an appropriate support.

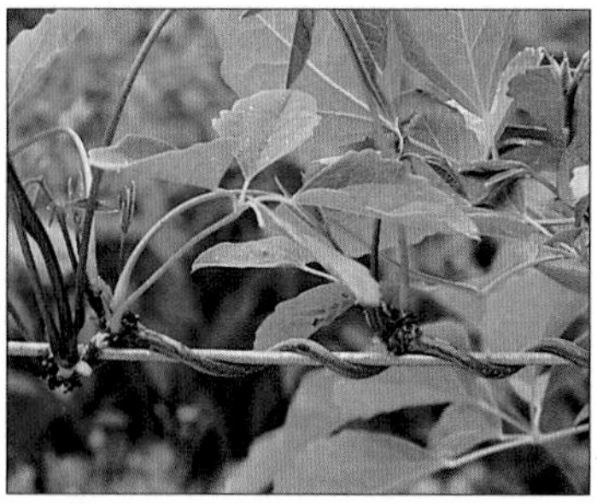

Twining stems
The flexible stems of Akebia *curl and extend around the support as they grow.*

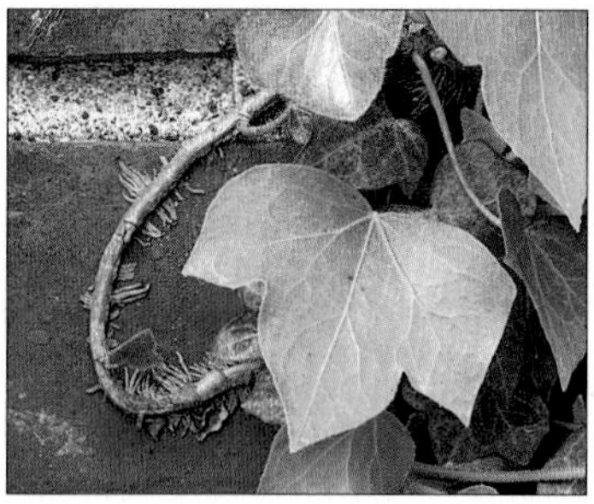

Self-clinging aerial roots
Ivies fasten to a surface by means of their aerial roots (adventitious rootlets).

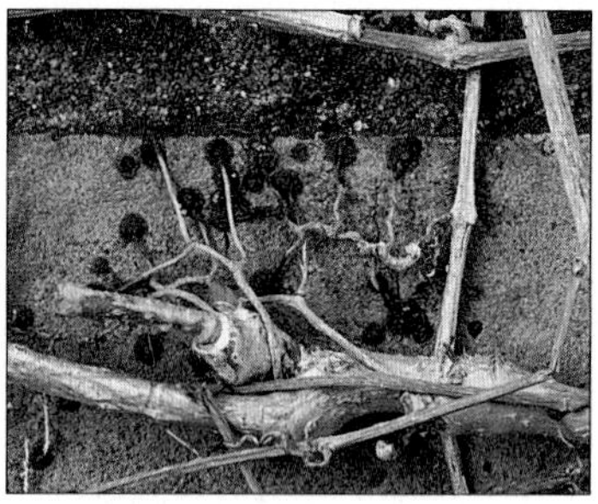

Self-clinging adhesive pads
Virginia creepers cling to a surface using adhesive pads at the end of their tendrils.

Choosing a climber

Consider the aspect of the intended site before choosing a climber. Many climbers, including *Actinidia*, *Clerodendrum*, and passion flowers (*Passiflora*), need a sunny wall to thrive, as does any climber grown at the limits of its climatic tolerance. *Akebia quinata*, *Jasminum officinale*, *Stauntonia hexaphylla*, and *Wisteria* tolerate a shaded wall, but flower and fruit more reliably in full sun. A few, like *Hydrangea petiolaris* and Virginia creeper, thrive in sun or shade. *Parthenocissus henryana* will colour better in shade. For shaded walls, use a robust ivy, or *Pileostegia viburnoides*, *Schizophragma hydrangeoides*, or *S. integrifolium*.

Take care to match the vigour of the chosen climber to the size and strength of the host tree or the scale of the building to be covered. Very vigorous climbers, such as *Fallopia baldschuanica*, or rampant ramblers, such as *Rosa wichurana* and *R. filipes* 'Kiftsgate', may cause an elderly or small tree to topple, or may rapidly overwhelm a small structure.

Types of support

Choose a support that will accommodate the eventual height, spread, and vigour of the chosen climber. The main types are wooden or plastic trellis panels, wire or plastic mesh, and wires (usually plastic-covered) stretched between vine eyes. Trellis is the most reliable support for twining climbers; use wire or mesh for tendril climbers, and trellis or wire framework for scandent or scrambling climbers.

Purpose-built structures, such as pergolas and pillars, must be strong and durable to support plants throughout their life-span.

Cultivation

When planting climbers against a wall or fence, position the plant at least 45cm (18in) from the base of the support. This allows the roots to receive sufficient rainwater, once established. After planting, water and apply mulch 5–7cm (2–3in) deep to a radius of about 60cm (24in) around the plant. Top-dress climbers in spring during their first two seasons, using 50–85g (2–3oz) of a balanced fertilizer, and apply a mulch each spring. Apply a slow-release fertilizer annually.

In hot, dry periods, water weekly. Dead-head plants regularly, unless fruits are desired. Tie in new shoots, and cut back overgrown plants (see p.25). Protect tender climbers grown outdoors in cold weather.

In frost-prone areas, climbers that are not reliably hardy, such as the spectacular, tropical *Bougainvillea*, *Hoya*, *Mandevilla*, and *Pandorea*, may be grown in a greenhouse or conservatory; some are suitable as houseplants. Climbers grown permanently under glass will outgrow their allotted space, so early restrictive pruning is essential (see p.25). Small climbers grown in containers with free-standing supports, such as cane tripods or trellis panels, can be moved outside during summer and returned under glass before autumn frosts. Plant vigorous species in large containers or in a greenhouse border. If they are allowed to grow very large, they may need to be replaced, since few respond to hard renovation pruning. Climbers in containers need to be repotted and fed regularly.

Climbing plants can be propagated by seed, by stem or root cuttings, or by layering. For species, seed is the most practical method, particularly for annuals and herbaceous species, although woody plants take some time to establish. Cultivars and hybrids do not come true from seed; take cuttings or layer.

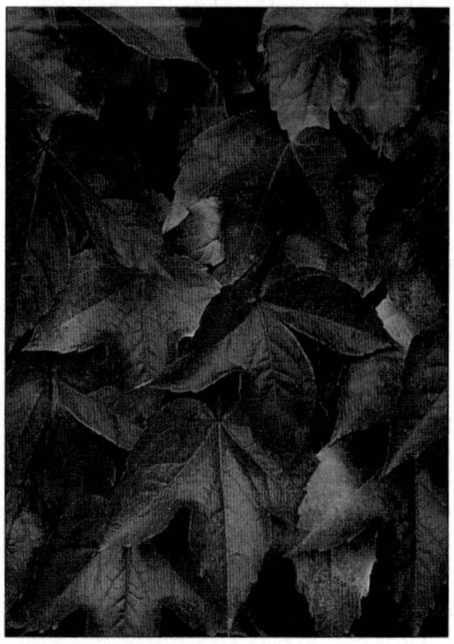

Instant colour
Parthenocissus tricuspidata *offers a spectacular display of autumn colour, and is one of the best climbers for covering a bare wall rapidly.*

ESTABLISHING A CLIMBER

It is important that climbers become well established against their support early on. Plants with aerial roots or adhesive pads are best planted at the base of a wall without support and allowed to establish themselves.

To grow a climber that requires support against a wall, fix a wooden trellis or wire support 30cm (12in) above the soil, slightly away from the wall. Dig a hole 45cm (18in) from the foot of the wall, deep enough so that the top of the root ball, when planted, will be level with the surrounding soil. Drench the root ball, then place it at an angle of 45° to the support. Fan the roots out away from the wall. Fill in the hole with soil, firm in, and water well. Remove the stake that comes with the plant, and fasten each main shoot to a new stake, fixing them to the lower rungs of the support. As new shoots appear, tie in to the support; do not damage the stems by tying too tightly. Cut out any weak or wayward shoots. Water freely until established.

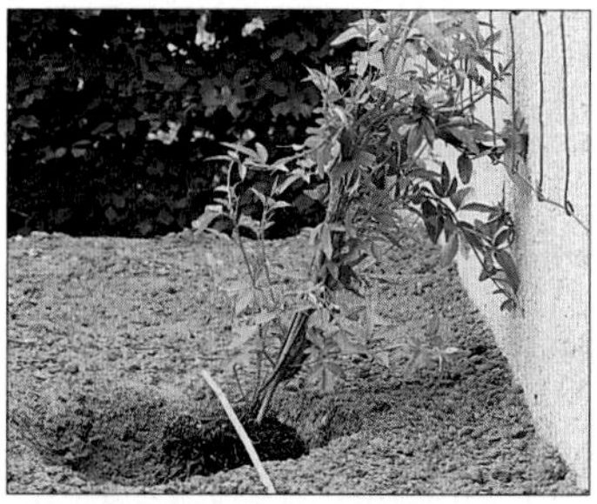

Check the level of the root ball.

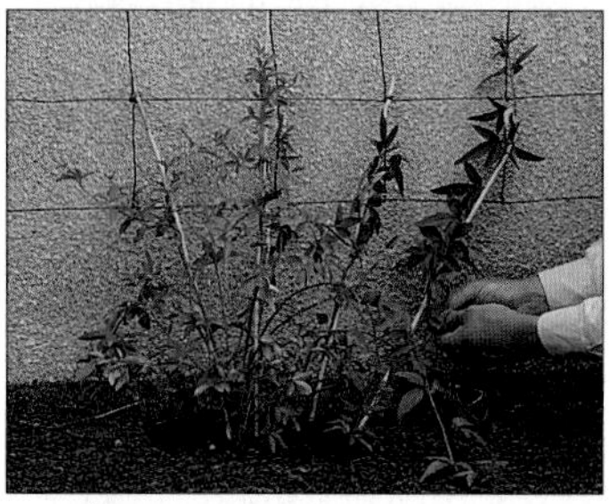

Tie shoots to stakes, fixed to the support.

Perennials

Perennials reach maturity in as little as two seasons. A well-chosen selection rapidly forms a fine tableau of textures and colours, both foliage and flowers providing visual interest for months. They can be featured as specimen plants, massed in a traditional herbaceous border, or interspersed with shrubs, annuals, and biennials in a mixed border. For variety, they can be cultivated in containers or window boxes, or grown among fruit and vegetables in a kitchen garden.

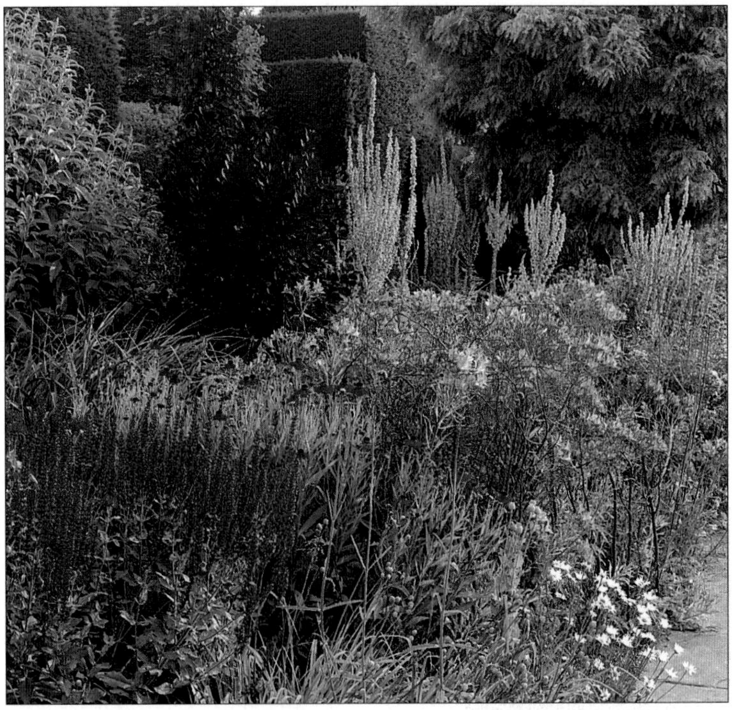

Mixed border
Shrubs and perennials have been planted here in a series of groupings, some of them providing colour harmonies, others striking contrasts. Heights are unevenly arranged with taller plants such as alstroemerias, heleniums, salvias, and verbascums brought to the front, surrounding smaller plants such as Argyranthemum frutescens.

What are perennials?

Precisely defined, perennials are plants that live for 2 years or longer and, once mature, flower annually. In gardens, however, the term perennial is commonly applied to herbaceous plants that form flowering stems each year before seeding, then die back in autumn to ground level, sending up new growth in spring. The term is also used to describe some non-woody, evergreen plants, such as *Bergenia* and *Yucca*, as well as subshrubs like *Artemisia* and *Penstemon.*

Ornamental features

Perennials are probably the most diverse plant group, providing a huge variety of shape, form, colour, texture, and scent with which to design a planting. They range in height from low, creeping plants, useful for ground cover, to feature plants, such as *Rheum palmatum,* which is 2.5m (8ft) or more high.

Colourful foliage plants can add contrast to a predominantly mid-green backdrop, accentuating each plant's structural form. Possible choices include the glossy, dark green leaves of *Acanthus,* the purple foliage of some *Canna* species, the variegated leaves of *Hosta* cultivars, or the silvery foliage of *Onopordum.*

Perennials with unusual shapes, arrangements, or textures of leaf can also produce eye-catching effects, especially when used as dot plants (usually taller feature plants used to accentuate contrasts).

Flowers of perennials are extremely varied in colour, size, and form, presenting the gardener with endless possibilities for contrasting, complementary, and single-colour plantings. Well-chosen groupings can also provide form and structure, for example the flat corymbs of *Achillea,* the tall spikes of lupins (*Lupinus*), or the tiered whorls of *Phlomis russeliana.* Popular fragrant perennials, attractive to bees and butterflies, include species of clematis, *Hemerocallis, Nicotiana,* phlox, and verbenas.

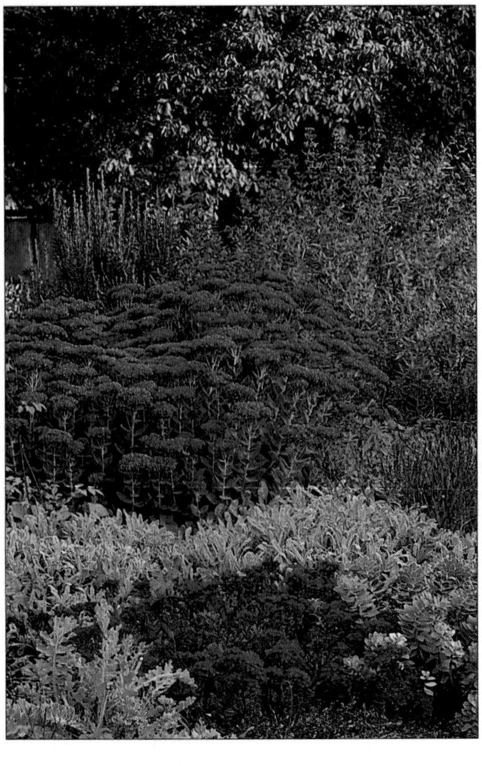

Late-season interest
*Many perennials provide interest throughout autumn and winter. A fine clump of ice plant (*Sedum spectabile*), whose stems and seed heads remain attractive in winter, dominates the centre of this planting, with salvia and rosemary (*Rosmarinus*) at the rear. At the front, the deep red flowers of* Sedum *'Ruby Glow' contrast with the cool, silvery green foliage of various species of* Stachys *and* Senecio.

Borders

The traditional herbaceous border dates back to the nineteenth century and earlier. It was usually a large rectangular plot, set into a lawn or against a hedge or wall, filled with summer- and autumn-flowering perennials, banked according to height. Today, herbaceous borders are frequently more modest in scale, often incorporating a carefully planned colour scheme, and using foliage as well as flowers for colour, texture, and structure. Some gardeners still prefer a banked effect. Others choose to arrange plant heights unevenly.

Borders can be planned as a series of incidents (groupings of 3 or more plants) or as a progression of subtle associations along the border. Swathes of massed plants, at an oblique angle to the front of the border, have strong visual impact. Experiment with merging informal drifts of several different species and cultivars, or create intricate patterns using regularly spaced groups of a more limited number of plants.

For ground cover, choose low, mat-forming, or creeping perennials displaying attractive foliage, such as *Lamium,* or flowering, clump-forming plants, such as geraniums; evergreens, such as *Bergenia* and some hellebores, can soften stark winter borders in cold areas. (See also panel, far right.)

SPECIALIST GROWING

The cultivation and exhibition of prodigious and flawless blooms can be a source of immense satisfaction to many gardeners. Popular hobby plants, such as carnations, chrysanthemums, dahlias, delphiniums, and gladioli, can all be grown with other plants in garden beds and borders. Specialist growers, however, will often set aside a designated area for such plants, such as a kitchen garden or in a greenhouse, to provide them with extra space, careful tending, and to protect them from any damage from pests or diseases, or from adverse weather conditions. Specialist societies have been established to distribute information to enthusiasts about species, hybrids, and cultivars of their favoured plants, and to give advice on sources, cultivation, and the exhibition of blooms.

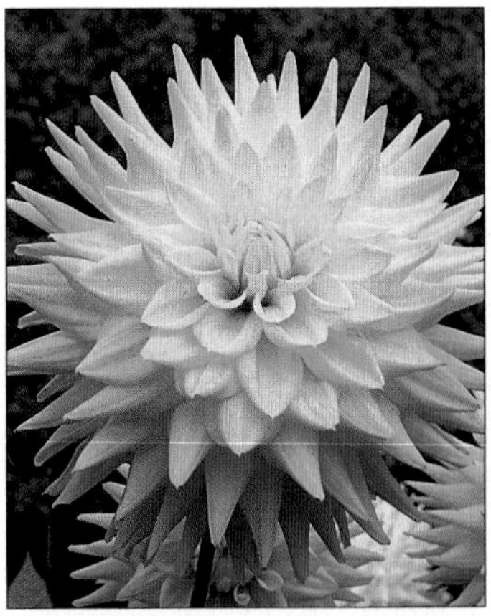

Show bloom
This Dahlia *'Hamari Accord' flower is ready for exhibition, demonstrating perfect petals and ideal proportions.*

CULTIVATING HERBS

In gardens, herbs are simply perennials grown for culinary or medicinal use, although many are also popular for their ornamental qualities. Most are of Mediterranean origin, preferring full sun and sharply drained soil, although mint (*Mentha*) thrives in moist soil and tolerates partial shade. A few, such as lavender (*Lavandula*) and chives (*Allium schoenoprasum*), bear showy flowers, and many have attractively coloured or variegated leaves. Sow annual or biennial herbs in succession against a framework of perennials to provide a continuous supply and to avoid gaps in the herb garden in late summer. Some medicinal herbs are of benefit only if prescribed by a qualified herbalist; unsupervised use may have harmful consequences.

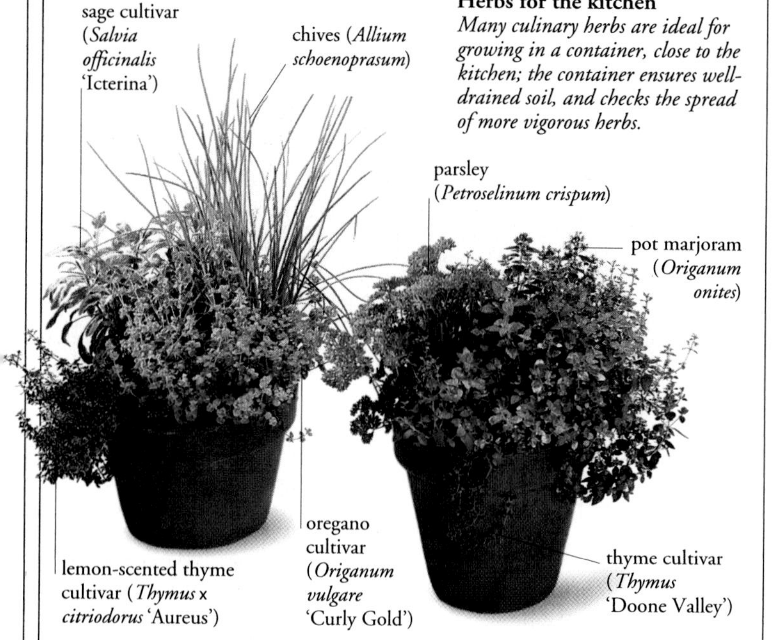
sage cultivar (*Salvia officinalis* 'Icterina')
chives (*Allium schoenoprasum*)
parsley (*Petroselinum crispum*)
pot marjoram (*Origanum onites*)
lemon-scented thyme cultivar (*Thymus* x *citriodorus* 'Aureus')
oregano cultivar (*Origanum vulgare* 'Curly Gold')
thyme cultivar (*Thymus* 'Doone Valley')

Herbs for the kitchen
Many culinary herbs are ideal for growing in a container, close to the kitchen; the container ensures well-drained soil, and checks the spread of more vigorous herbs.

Mixed borders of herbaceous perennials, shrubs, bulbs, climbers, annuals, and biennials are excellent for providing year-round interest. A careful selection of perennials and deciduous and evergreen shrubs that fill up to a third of the border will provide a balanced planting. Fill out the border with annuals until the perennials and shrubs mature. For extra interest in spring, many perennials, particularly those coming into growth in mid- to late spring, such as hostas, can be underplanted with bulbs or other early-flowering plants, such as tulips, anemones, and scillas. Tender perennials, such as dahlias, can be added to enhance a late-summer and autumn display.

Container ideas

Some hardy perennials are ideal for use in containers; ornamental grasses, for example, offer excellent choices of shape, structure, and colour. Less hardy plants, such as *Agave, Cordyline, Melianthus major*, and variegated *Phormium* cultivars, are also attractive, but may need overwintering under glass. Perennial subshrubs in decorative containers, for example *Argyranthemum* and lavender (*Lavandula*), can serve as focal points in paved areas. For a long floral display, choose summer- and autumn-flowering perennials, such as *Felicia* and pelargoniums.

Cutting and drying

Perennials include some of the best garden plants for cutting. Blooms often last well if they are cut early in the morning. Remove leaves from the bases of the stalks. To encourage them to take up water, bruise or slit the base of each stem, or plunge stems briefly in boiling water, before immersing them in cool water to the necks (where the flowers begin).

The flowers and seed heads of some perennials are also good for drying, particularly those that hold their shape and colour well, such as *Achillea* and *Eryngium.* Some less rigid flowers with a higher water content may be air-dried if this is done quickly, by suspending small bunches in a dark and airy place. Flowers with papery petals can be dried in a proprietary desiccant. Pick blooms as they begin to open. If picked too soon, the stems will not be sufficiently stiff; if picked too late, the colour of the flowers will have deteriorated or the petals (or seed, in the case of grasses) will fall.

Cultivation

When planning a herbaceous or mixed border, match the needs of plants to the aspect and conditions of the chosen site. Plant in carefully prepared ground, usually in spring or autumn. Keep the surrounding area free of weeds, and water young plants regularly until established. Mature perennials require little watering except during prolonged dry periods. Apply an annual top-dressing of bone meal or a balanced, slow-release fertilizer, preferably in early spring after rain.

Most herbaceous plants produce vigorous shoots in spring, but some may be spindly. When the plant is one-quarter to one-third of its final height, pinch out or cut back weak shoots; the remaining sturdy shoots will usually bear larger flowers. This particularly benefits plants such as Michaelmas daisies (*Aster*), delphiniums, and phlox. Plants that require support should be staked when young to ensure that lax stems remain upright (see p.23). Dead-head regularly to prolong flowering.

In autumn, cut shoots down to the base, and remove dead and faded growth and weeds, leaving the border tidy in winter. In spring, when the ground is moist, apply a mulch of organic matter, such as mushroom compost or bark chips. Where practical, perennials grown in a border should be divided not only for propagation, but also to maintain vigour, ideally every 3 to 5 years. Take care when lifting and replanting not to damage the roots of surrounding trees and shrubs.

To appreciate grasses and other plants throughout the winter months, delay cutting and mulching until spring. In very cold areas, leaving top-growth in place during winter will also offer some frost protection to the crown of a plant.

For container-grown perennials, use loam-based compost, or lighter soilless compost mixed with a slow-release, balanced fertilizer. Although the extra weight of the loam adds stability, use soilless composts in plastic containers for roof gardens or balconies where heavy containers may be too great a load; lighter containers are also easier to move.

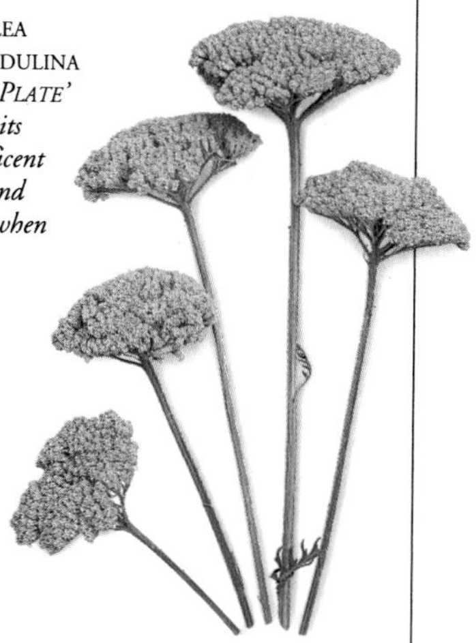

ACHILLEA FILIPENDULINA *'GOLD PLATE' retains its magnificent shape and colour when dried.*

Ensure that compost in containers does not dry out when plants are in growth; water daily in hot, dry weather. Plants in larger containers require less frequent watering, especially if moisture-retentive polymer granules have been mixed in with the compost. Mulching also helps to retain moisture; replace this when dividing or repotting plants.

Perennials can be propagated by seed, division, cuttings, or grafting (rarely used by amateur gardeners). Sowing seed is preferable for species where large numbers of plants are required. Hybrids and cultivars do not come true from seed; divide or take cuttings.

GROUND COVER

A wide variety of perennials can be used as decorative, low-maintenance ground cover, with the added benefit of reducing the labour of weeding. Geraniums are often chosen for their abundant flowers, while others, such as hostas, are grown mainly for their attractive foliage. Cerastiums prefer full sun, but many perennials, such as geraniums, hostas, *Lamium*, and *Persicaria*, also thrive in partial shade. Tiarellas prefer partial to deep shade.

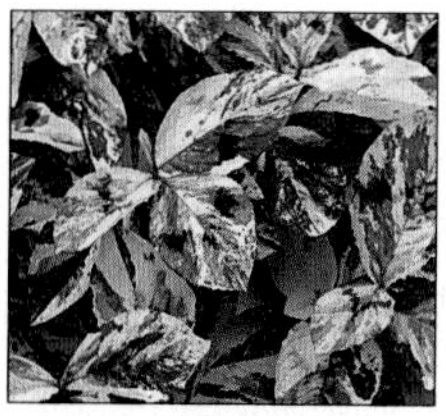

Persicaria virginiana 'Painter's Palette'

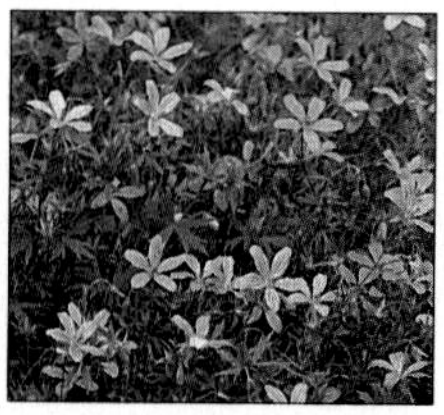

Geranium asphodeloides

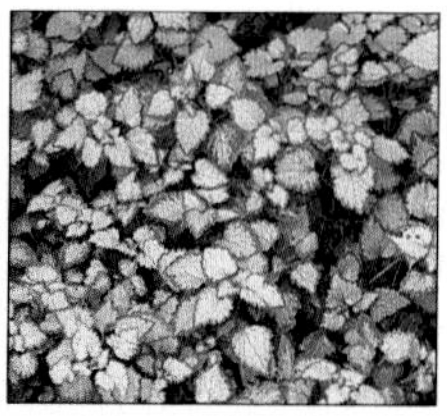

Lamium maculatum 'Beacon Silver'

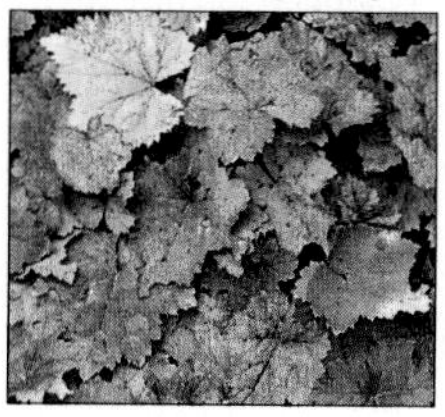

Tiarella cordifolia

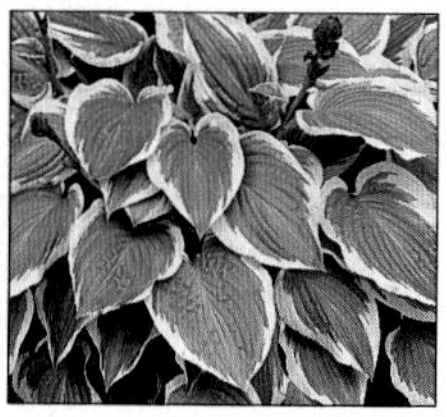

Hosta 'Shade Fanfare'

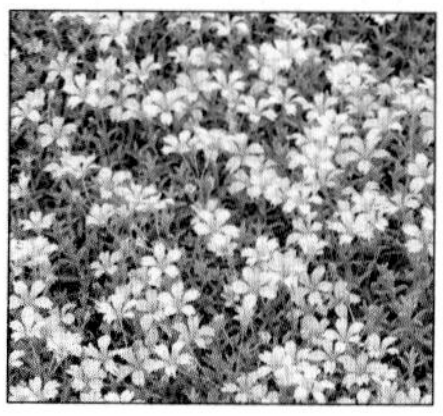

Cerastium tomentosum

Rock plants

As a group, rock plants represent an extensive range of hardy perennials, shrubs, and bulbous plants, many of which originate in mountain ranges. Many rock plants will flourish in a suitably well-drained site with an appropriate aspect; some require special conditions in the garden or in an alpine house. Delicate, simple, clear-coloured flowers are often prolifically borne in spring and early summer.

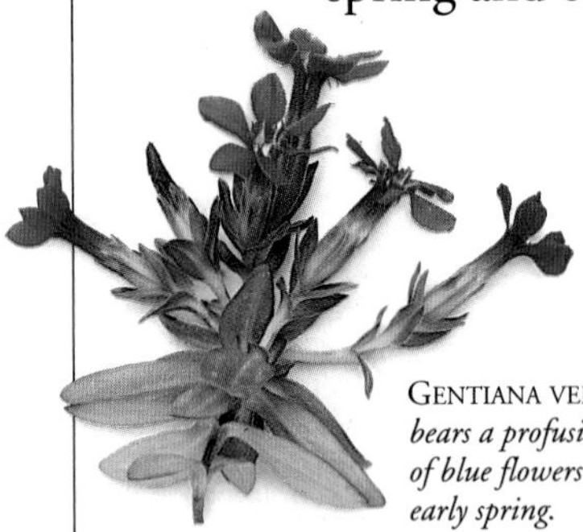
GENTIANA VERNA *bears a profusion of blue flowers in early spring.*

What are rock plants?

The term rock plant is often used more or less interchangeably with alpine. In fact, true alpines are native to mountains in temperate, subtropical, and tropical regions, where they grow above the tree-line in screes, rocky crevices, and turf. Subalpines occur just below the tree-line. Most alpines are compact in habit, and rarely over 15cm (6in) tall. This minimizes wind resistance and water loss at high altitudes.

When more broadly defined, a rock plant is any plant sufficiently dwarf in its habit to associate well with true alpines. Many rock plants are found in mountain pasture and woodland, or on dry hillsides. A few occur on coastal cliffs and shores.

Adapted to growth in thin, rapidly draining soil, often at high altitudes, most alpines and rock plants will survive extremes of temperature but not excessive wet. In cultivation, many prefer an artificial environment that reproduces the aspect, light level, exposure to the elements, and soil conditions of their natural habitat. Rock gardens, raised beds, scree beds, and alpine houses (see panel opposite) will all provide suitable growing conditions. Other less specialized plants, like aubretias (*Aubrieta*), will thrive in any well-drained site with a suitable aspect.

Ornamental features and uses

Rock plants in the broadest sense encompass a diverse mixture of mat- or cushion-forming plants, dwarf shrubs and trees, and bulbous plants. Dwarf coniferous shrubs and trees, such as *Juniperus communis* 'Compressa', can provide height and structure in a planting, contrasting with specimens of more open or rounded habit like hebes. Lower-growing, tufted, or mat-forming plants, like sandworts (*Arenaria*), are useful as ground cover or edging.

Some rock plants, like houseleeks (*Sempervivum*), have fleshy, water-storing leaves. Others, like edelweiss (*Leontopodium*), have small, closely arranged, sometimes hairy leaves, which minimize water loss through transpiration. These provide a varied choice of foliage textures for garden plantings. Specimens like *Celmisia semicordata*, with its sword-shaped, silvery leaves, will offset rosette-forming, fleshy plants like stonecrops (*Sedum*), or those with feathery leaves, such as pulsatillas.

Many rock plants are evergreen and will provide year-round interest in the open garden. Spaces within a framework of miniature shrubs can be filled with rock plants; their tufts, clumps, or cushions of foliage are often as interesting as their blooms.

Rock plants flower mainly over a relatively short period in spring and early summer, but often produce a profusion of tiny, clear-coloured blooms. Autumn- and late winter-flowering bulbs, such as some cyclamen or crocuses, may be used to extend the flowering season.

Rock gardens

The most popularly constructed environment for rock plants is a rock garden. This is best located in an open, sunny site on a slope, clear from the shade cast by trees, and sheltered from cold, drying winds. Where possible, include a source of water, such as a pond or stream, to enhance the basic design.

Construct the rock garden on a bed of coarse rubble, covered with standard rock garden soil (see right). Set rocks into the soil in a natural formation. Pockets between the rocks will accommodate the rock plants and provide them with a deep, cool root run. Top-dress the surface after planting with grit, gravel, or stone chippings.

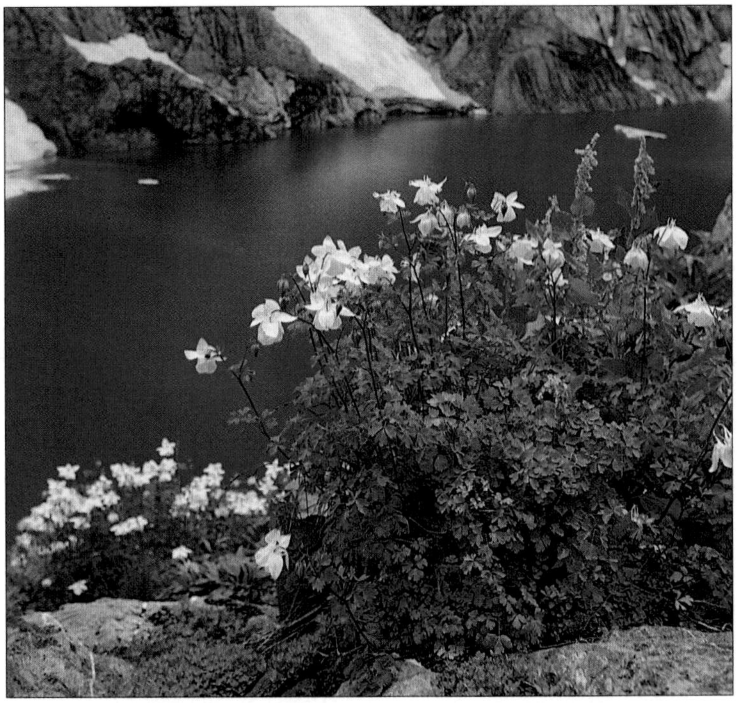
Mountain dwellers
True alpines, like this Aquilegia fragrans, *grow above the tree-line in mountain ranges to over 3,000m (10,000ft) high. In the garden, such plants require conditions that replicate their high-altitude habitats: well-drained soil and a cool root run.*

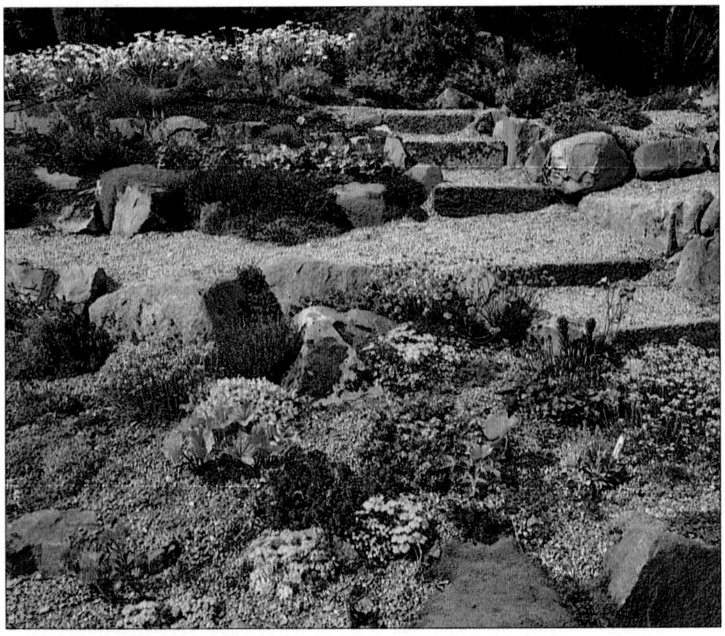
Establishing a rock garden
Alpines and other rock plants, such as Antennaria, Armeria, *hebes, saxifrages, stonecrops, and houseleeks, will rapidly establish themselves on the gentle slopes of a sunny, well-planned rock garden.*

GESNERIADS

A plant family of about 2,500 species, the Gesneriaceae are mainly evergreen perennials (some epiphytic) or shrubs, and a few trees. Most are native to tropical or subtropical regions, with a few from temperate zones. Of the latter group, rock plants such as *Ramonda* and *Haberlea* are ideal for growing in the niches of a cool, shady wall or rock, or in a scree bed, where their rosettes will remain free of excess moisture. Often grown in an alpine house, *Jancaea heldreichii* will also thrive outdoors in tufa, in a shady site.

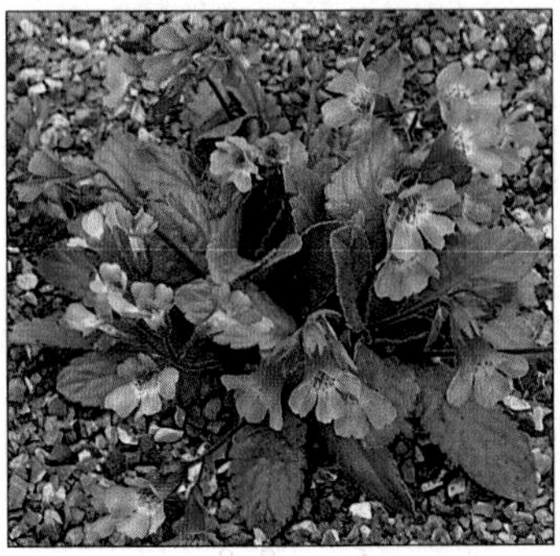
Haberlea ferdinandi-coburgii

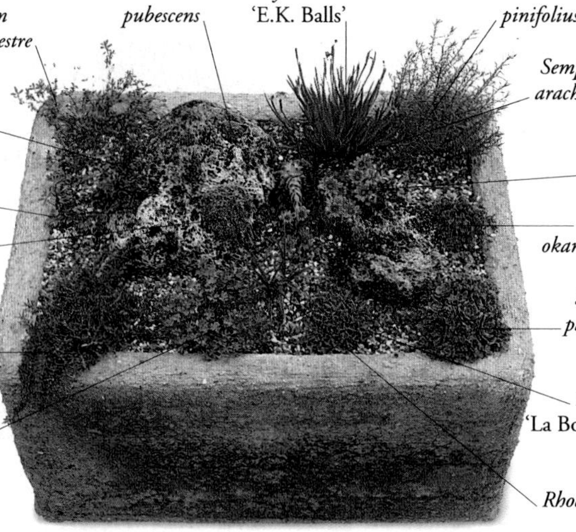
Helianthemum oelandicum subsp. *alpestre*
Androsace pubescens
Sisyrinchium 'E.K. Balls'
Penstemon pinifolius
Saxifraga cotyledon
Sempervivum arachnoideum
Draba aizoides
Oxalis 'Ione Hecker'
Talinum okanoganense
Saxifraga cochlearis 'Minor'
Saxifraga paniculata
Phlox douglasii
Dianthus 'La Bourboule'
Oxalis enneaphylla 'Minutifolia'
Rhodohypoxis baurii

Planting a trough
As with raised beds, carefully placed rocks can enhance the natural effect of a trough or sink planting. If using tufa, bore holes in them to fill with compost and appropriate small plants.

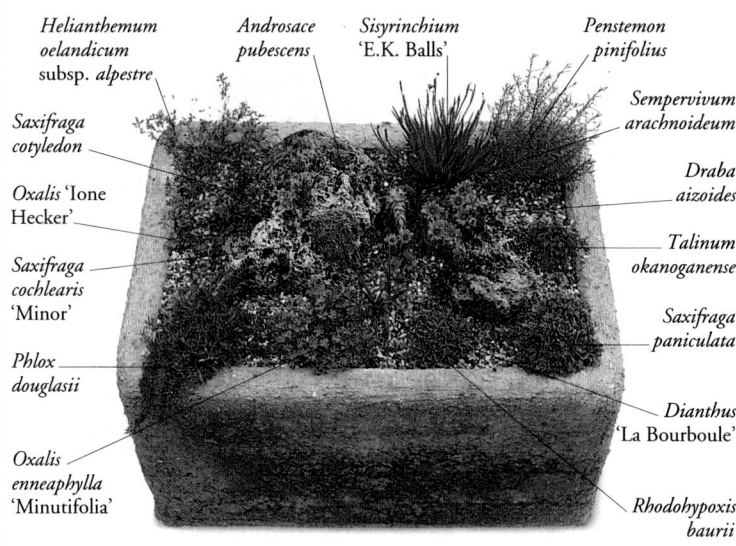

Niches or crevices in a wall, or between paving, can provide similar growing conditions to a rock garden. Some rosette-forming plants, such as *Lewisia* and *Ramonda*, are best planted on their sides in cracks in a wall, so that water drains away quickly from their collars.

Grow mat-forming plants like *Sedum acre* or *Dianthus deltoides* in pockets of soil on the top of a wall, or in vertical cracks, to produce a cascade of colour. Use trailing or spreading plants, such as *Saponaria ocymoides* or *Saxifraga* 'Tumbling Waters', to soften the lines of a boundary wall or the retaining wall of a bank or raised bed.

Beds and containers

Raised beds and scree beds are ideal for growing plants on a level site. Rock plants that prefer very gritty soil and a well-drained root run, like alpine forget-me-nots (*Myosotis alpestris*), will grow best in a scree bed. If the bed is designed to be a free-standing feature, it should be slightly raised to assist drainage. A scree bed may also be constructed as part of a larger rock garden.

A raised bed can be constructed in a garden of any size, and is useful where garden soil is heavy or slow-draining. Its added height improves drainage and brings the attractions of low-growing plants closer to eye-level. Grow species and cultivars that prefer acid soil, such as *Cassiope* or *Arctostaphylos*, in a peat bed or peat bank, which may be top-dressed with bark chips.

The retaining walls of a raised or scree bed can be constructed from natural or artificial stone, bricks, wooden logs, or railway sleepers. As with a rock garden, all beds should have a rubble base, covered with a suitable soil mix and top-dressed with grit, stone chippings, or gravel.

Rock plants will also flourish in containers such as sinks, troughs, and tubs. Provide a generous top-dressing of grit around the bases of the plants to improve drainage and reduce the evaporation of moisture from the compost.

Cultivation

In general, alpines and other rock plants prefer an open site in full sun, with moderately fertile soil, a cool, deep root run, and sharp drainage.

With some cushion-forming plants, like *Dionysia* or *Androsace*, the rotting of one or two rosettes may rapidly lead to the death of the whole plant. Such species and their cultivars are best grown within the controlled environment of an alpine house or cold frame. Some bulbous plants, like *Calochortus*, also benefit from a controlled environment as they require protection from moisture when dormant in summer.

In the open garden, shelter susceptible plants from damp by providing very well-drained soil and a thick dressing of grit around the collar of each plant. Panes of glass or clear plastic can also be propped up over the plants, or they can be covered with an open-ended cloche of glass or transparent plastic.

At planting, incorporate a slow-release, balanced fertilizer into the soil or compost. Thereafter, apply a general-purpose fertilizer in spring, if vigorous growth is required. Plants grown in a free-draining scree bed may require watering until established. Rock plants grown in an alpine house, in raised beds, or in containers should be watered regularly. In an alpine house, soak the medium in which plants are plunged, as well as the individual plants. For species and cultivars that resent moisture from above, soak the plunging medium only.

Dead-head rock plants, where practical, to encourage further flowering, and remove withered or damaged growth immediately. Trim plants as required to maintain their neat, compact form and, where necessary, to restrict their spread.

Various propagation methods are used for rock plants; consult individual genus entries for the most appropriate method in each case.

ALPINE HOUSES

The needs of moisture-sensitive rock plants are best met in an alpine house – an unheated greenhouse with maximum levels of ventilation, usually provided by a door at each end, and extra windows or louvred panels set into the sides, along the roof ridge, and below the staging. Some growers heat an alpine house just sufficiently to prevent hard-freezing of soil and compost, enabling the cultivation of frost-hardy to half-hardy plants.

Most plants are grown in clay pots, plunged to the rims in sand on staging; this reduces the need for watering and offers some frost protection. Plants in plastic containers do not require plunging, but they risk dehydration if the growing medium freezes hard in winter. A raised bed allows for landscaping and provides a deep root run, but plants cannot then be moved.

To keep plants cool in summer, shade an alpine house (see p.24) from late spring to early autumn and, where possible, move containerized plants that have finished flowering to an open plunge bed or cold frame outdoors.

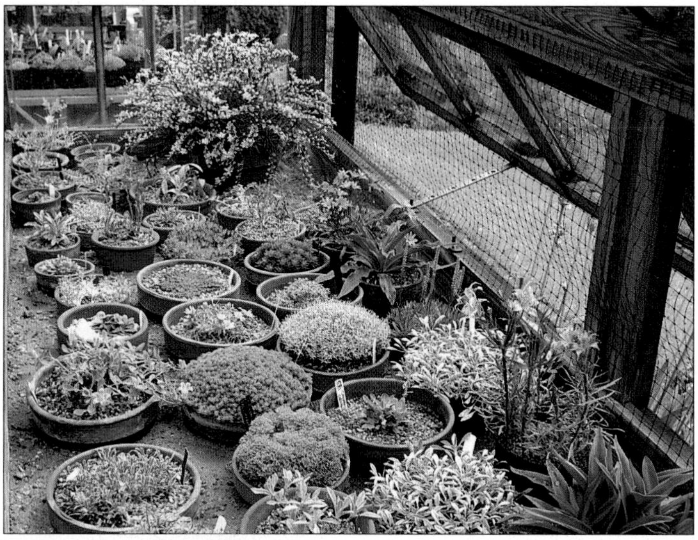

Maintaining healthy plants
In an alpine house, most rock plants are grown in clay pots, plunged to the rims in a layer of sand upon staging. In summer, maximum levels of ventilation reduce the risk of disease, while green shade netting protects foliage and flowers from scorching.

COMPOSTS

Special soil mixes aim to reproduce the mediums in which alpines and other rock plants grow in the wild. For acid-loving plants, use lime-free loam and grit, supplemented with granitic or sandstone chippings; for alkaline-loving plants, use limestone chippings. Peat substitutes include decomposed bark, bracken litter, garden compost, and leaf mould.

ROCK GARDEN (STANDARD MIX)
2 parts JI No.2 or 3 (or 1 part sterilized loam; 1 part peat or peat substitute); 1 part sharp sand or grit.
SCREE BED
1 part sterilized loam; 1 part peat or substitute; 3 parts grit or stone chippings (in dry areas, 2 parts grit or chippings). Or 2 parts sterilized loam; 2 parts leaf mould; 1 part sharp sand; 4 parts grit or chippings.
RAISED BED
3 parts sterilized loam; 2 parts peat or substitute; 1–2 parts sharp sand or coarse grit.
PEAT BED (< pH6.5)
1 part peat or substitute; 1 part acid leaf mould; 1 part fibrous acid loam; 1 part lime-free sharp sand or coarse grit. Add a slow-release, balanced fertilizer.
WALLS
3 parts sterilized loam; 2 parts peat or substitute; 1–2 parts sharp sand or coarse grit. Add extra sand, grit, or stone chippings to improve drainage in crevices.
FOR ACID-LOVING PLANTS (< pH6.5)
4 parts acid leaf mould, or peat or substitute (such as decomposed bark, or bracken litter); 1 part sharp sand.
FOR HIGH-ALTITUDE ALPINES
1 part JI No.3; 1 part gravel or stone chippings. Or 1 part sterilized loam; 1 part leaf mould, or peat or substitute (such as decomposed bark); 2–3 parts gravel or stone chippings.
FOR CONTAINERS
3 parts JI No.1; 1 part coarse grit. Add a slow-release, balanced fertilizer.

Annuals and biennials

These versatile and free-flowering plants, though short-lived, are easy to grow from seed and require little maintenance. They are suitable for all gardening situations, being native to both temperate and sub-tropical climates. Annuals and biennials will quickly provide a vibrant display of colour, enhancing a framework of trees, shrubs, and perennials, or grown by themselves in beds, containers, or hanging baskets.

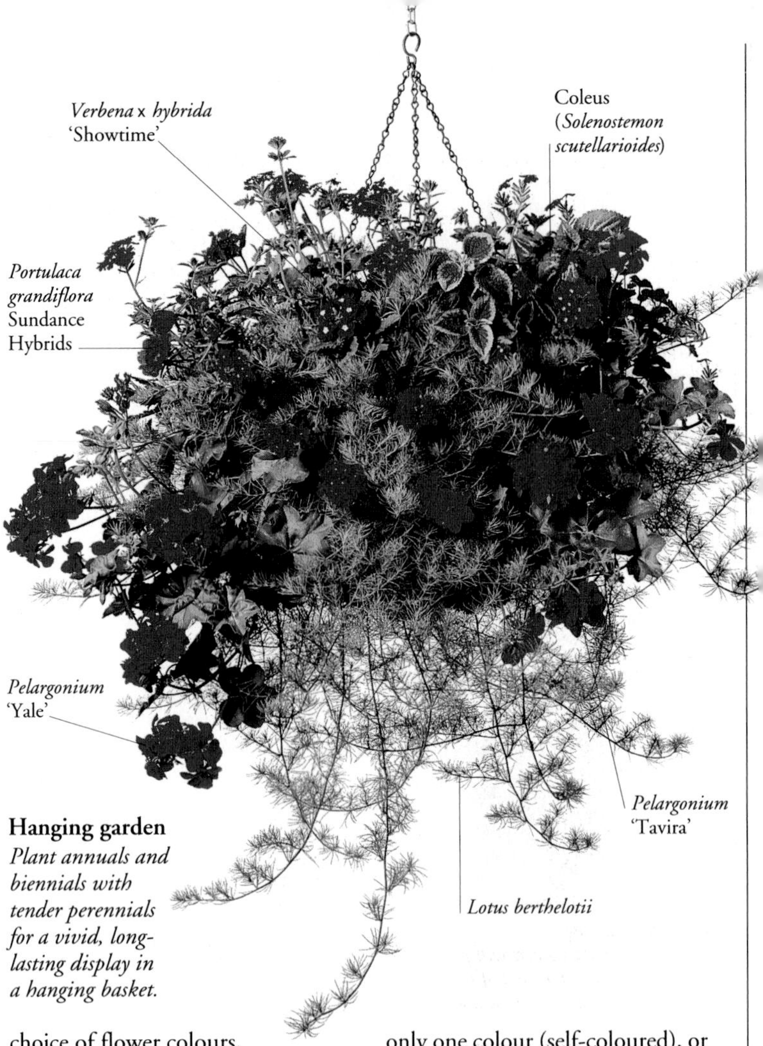

Hanging garden
Plant annuals and biennials with tender perennials for a vivid, long-lasting display in a hanging basket.

What are annuals and biennials?

Annuals are plants that germinate, flower, set seed, and die within one year. Certain members of other plant groups, such as perennials or subshrubs, which will often flower in their first year when raised from cuttings or seed, are also commonly grown as annuals. Some tender perennials, like *Cobaea*, busy Lizzies (*Impatiens*), and pelargoniums, can be seed-raised each year to provide a display of flowers, and then cleared away rather than over-wintered under glass.

Biennials normally produce only foliage in their first year, bearing flowers and completing their life-cycle in the following season.

In this encyclopedia, both annuals and biennials are described as fully hardy, frost hardy, half hardy, or frost tender, according to their individual levels of resistance to low winter temperatures. Commercially, however, annuals are classed only as hardy, half hardy, or frost tender. General details of the sowing and flowering times for each category of annuals and biennials are presented in the chart on the facing page.

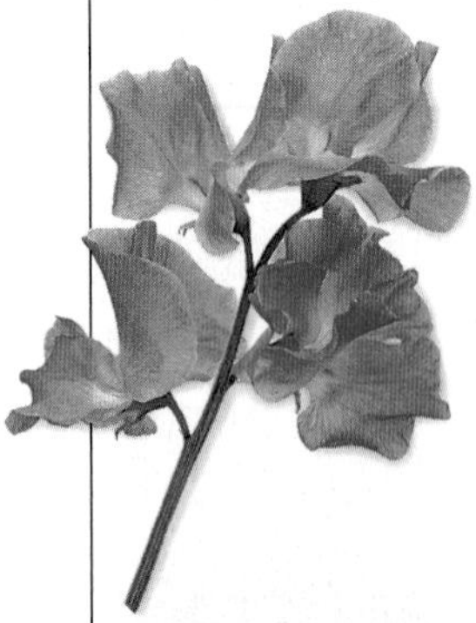

LATHYRUS ODORATUS *'JAYNE AMANDA' has fragrant flowers, which are good for cutting.*

New plants and names

Each year, new annual and biennial cultivars are introduced to stimulate or cater for commercial demand. These may be completely new plants, or improvements of existing cultivars. In many species, breeding programmes have increased the choice of flower colours, extended the flowering season, and developed a wider range of habits, often producing dwarf cultivars ideal for small gardens, or pendent cultivars suitable for window-boxes and hanging baskets.

New introductions may have been obtained from the wild, selected from a batch of seedlings, or are the result of genetic mutation. Continuous breeding and inter-breeding of these selections blurs the parentage of many cultivars, and results in a complicated (and often confusing) system of categorization.

Two or more cultivars are often crossed to produce a hybrid or group of hybrids. In these circumstances, where parentage becomes confused, or where several cultivars display very similar or common features, they may form a Group, the name of which is printed in roman rather than italic type, as in *Impatiens* New Guinea Group, or *Digitalis purpurea* Foxy Hybrids.

Cultivars that consistently share the same characteristics, differing in only one feature (usually flower colour) may be termed a Series, as in *Tropaeolum* Alaska Series. This distinguishing feature may also be used to identify further a plant within a Series: for example, *Tagetes* Antigua Series 'Antigua Gold' differs from other cultivars in the Series only in its golden yellow flowers.

Individual cultivars within a Group or Series may bear flowers of only one colour (self-coloured), or may produce flowers comprised of two colours (bicoloured). A cultivar may also consistently bear flowers of the same colour (single colours), or individual plants of the same cultivar may bear flowers in any one of a number of colours (mixes).

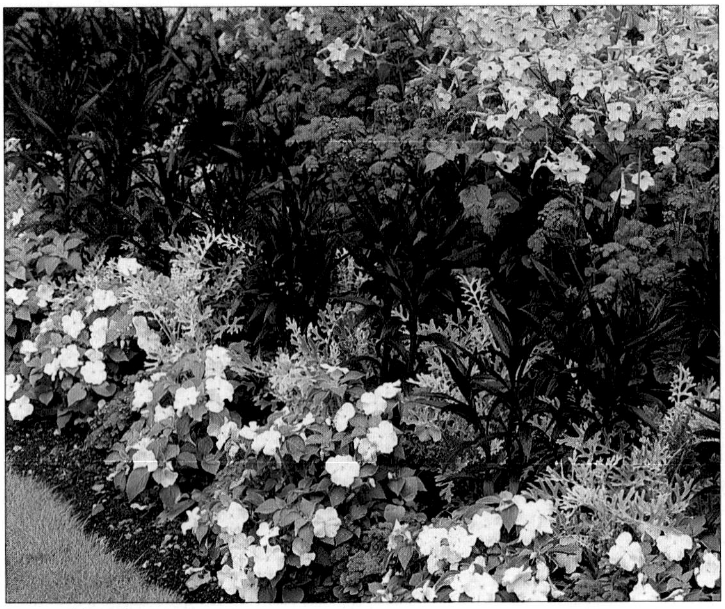

Formal border
Intricate patterns are created by the regular placing of plants, here Tradescantia pallida *'Purpurea',* Impatiens balsamina *Tom Thumb Series,* Senecio cineraria *'Silver Dust',* Ageratum houstonianum *cultivars, and* Nicotiana *'Lime Green'.*

Ornamental features

Annuals and biennials have an exceptionally diverse range of habits, from low, mat-formers to erect or climbing plants, allowing them to fulfil many roles in different areas of the garden. Most are cultivated for their brightly coloured, sometimes very fragrant flowers, which are often freely borne over long periods during spring and summer. Some blooms, such as those of *Gypsophila*, china asters (*Callistephus*), and cornflowers (*Centaurea cyanus*), are excellent for cutting. "Everlasting" flowers, like statice (*Limonium sinuatum*) and strawflowers (*Bracteantha bracteata*), and the decorative seed heads of plants such as love-in-a-mist (*Nigella*) and scabious (*Scabiosa*), are invaluable for dried arrangements (see p.39).

Several annuals and biennials are valued primarily for their attractively coloured or textured foliage. These include silver-leaved plants, such as *Senecio cineraria* (a half-hardy perennial that is usually grown as an annual), coleus (*Solenostemon*), which have foliage in yellows and greens to reds and purples, and

WILD FLOWERS

Ancestors of many annual and biennial cultivars, wild flowers can be used in informal plantings that replicate their sometimes threatened natural habitats. Grow in poor soil on land that can remain relatively undisturbed once the plants have become established; in rich soil, invasive species will swamp those that are less robust. Use native plants that already grow wild in the local vicinity; a specialist seed supplier can advise on the best wildflower mix for naturalization in the chosen habitat.

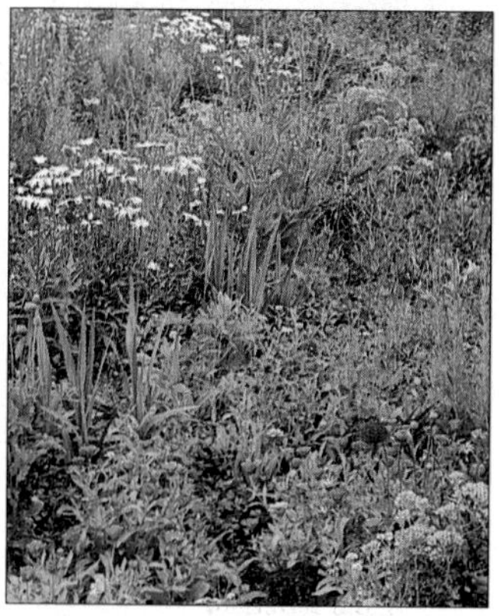

Natural planting
On poor soil, wild flowers will provide soft drifts of colour for most of the year, and attract native wildlife to a garden.

ornamental cabbages (*Brassica oleracea* cultivars), with their low-growing, crinkled leaves in muted shades of pink, green, and white.

Garden uses

Annuals and biennials will provide a fast-growing display of colour in a new garden, before a final planting scheme has been devised, or while slower-growing trees and shrubs become established. They may also be used to alter the colour scheme or fill spaces within the long-term framework of a mature garden.

Plants with scented blooms are best enjoyed close to the house or beside a seating area. A sheltered, sunny site at the base of a wall or fence is recommended for tender plants like cockscombs (*Celosia*) and coleus.

Trailing annuals and biennials, such as nasturtiums (*Tropaeolum majus*), will provide rapid ground cover, and may be encouraged to tumble over the sides of window-boxes, hanging baskets, or other containers. Container-grown plants are of particular value where space is limited, such as on a balcony or patio. Annual climbers, or those grown as annuals, like *Cobaea* and *Rhodochiton*, may also be trained through a tree or other support, or used to clothe a screen or barrier.

Tender annuals and biennials cultivated as specimen plants in a conservatory or temperate greenhouse, or as houseplants, can be moved outdoors in summer, either in their containers, or as temporary bedding plants.

Planning displays

As annuals and biennials are short-lived, use a succession of plants to provide flowers over a long period; some gardeners change their bedding scheme several times in a year. Group plants with shared cultivation needs, like busy Lizzies and common foxgloves (*Digitalis purpurea*), both of which prefer moist soil in dappled shade. To obtain a dense block of colour, plant multiples of a single cultivar.

In an informal, cottage-style garden, use annuals and biennials among vegetables, herbs, perennials, shrubs, and trees. Arrange adjacent drifts with varying outlines and heights for an apparently random, flowing effect. In maturity, plants will overflow the edges of paths and lawns, and may self-seed profusely.

In a garden of formal design, use annuals and biennials in ordered or structured plantings to create a uniform display, to form a pattern, or to enhance or soften the edges of rigid lines of tiles, pathways, or hedges, such as clipped box (*Buxus*).

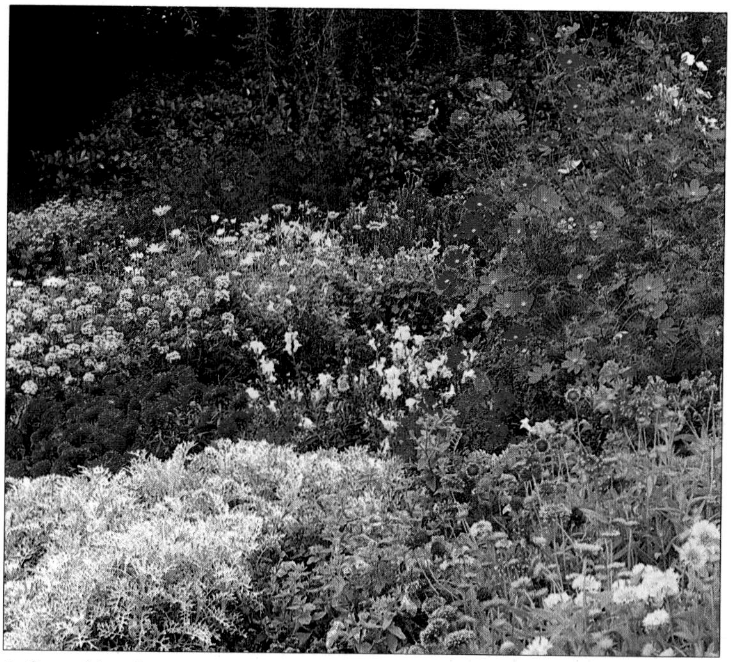

Informal border
Annuals and biennials can provide waves of texture and colour. In this border, the strong colours and abundant flowers of snapdragons (Antirrhinum), Cosmos, *and* Tagetes *are balanced by the striking foliage of* Senecio cineraria *'Silver Dust'.*

Cultivation

Seed-raised annuals and biennials, depending on their hardiness and flowering season, may be sown *in situ* or under glass. Outdoors, the seeds of genera that dislike transplanting, such as *Clarkia*, are best scattered where they are to flower. Sow the seeds of other annuals and biennials in drills and thin out when seedlings have developed. Under glass, sow seed in containers or seed trays (see p.28) and plant out at the times given in the chart below.

Weed regularly, stake tall plants, and pinch out growing tips to promote bushiness (see p.23). On poor soils, apply a quick-release fertilizer as flower buds form. Water freely in hot weather; containerized plants dry out very quickly. Deadhead regularly to avoid self-seeding. Clear plants away when the foliage starts to die down.

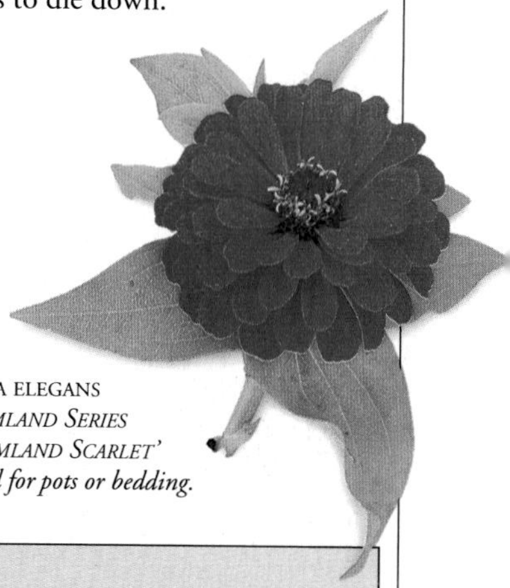

ZINNIA ELEGANS *DREAMLAND SERIES 'DREAMLAND SCARLET'* *is ideal for pots or bedding.*

GUIDE TO SOWING, GROWING, AND FLOWERING TIMES

SEASON	ANNUALS			BIENNIALS – YEAR 1			BIENNIALS – YEAR 2		
	FULLY HARDY/ FROST HARDY	HALF HARDY	FROST TENDER	FULLY HARDY/ FROST HARDY	HALF HARDY	FROST TENDER	FULLY HARDY/ FROST HARDY	HALF HARDY	FROST TENDER
SPRING	Sow *in situ* in mid-spring. In flower if autumn-sown.	Sow under glass at 13–21°C (55–70°F).	Sow under glass at 13–21°C (55–70°F).				New growth begins. In flower.	New growth begins. Plant out after last frosts. In flower.	New growth begins. In flower.
SUMMER	In flower.	Plant out spring-sown seedlings. Sow seed *in situ* when soil reaches 13°C (55°F). In flower.	Plant out in early summer, or grow under glass. In flower.	Sow *in situ.*	Sow under glass at 13–21°C (55– 70°F), or sow *in situ* when soil reaches 13°C (55°F).	Sow under glass at 13–21°C (55–70°F). Plant out in midsummer in frost-free areas.	In flower.	In flower.	Plant out in early summer. In flower.
AUTUMN	In flower. Discard as foliage dies. Sow *in situ* to flower next spring.	In flower. Discard as foliage dies.	Discard as foliage dies.	Basal leaves or rosettes develop.	Basal leaves or rosettes develop. Move into frost-free conditions in frost-prone areas.	Basal leaves or rosettes develop. Ensure under glass at 7°C (45°F), in frost-prone areas.	Discard as foliage dies.	Discard as foliage dies.	Discard as foliage dies.
WINTER	Autumn-sown seed overwintering.			Overwintering.	Overwintering.	Overwintering.			

Bulbous plants

Bulbous plants occur worldwide in habitats from scrub, meadows, and woodland to mountains and streamsides. Sometimes evergreen, bulbs are valued mainly for the beauty of their flowers, which can provide welcome colour in early spring. Summer-flowering bulbs, like lilies or gladioli, are splendid in borders or integrated into a bedding scheme; their tall, showy blooms often last well when cut. Excellent in containers, bulbs can also be used to brighten the home or garden in winter.

What are bulbous plants?

The term bulb is generally used to describe a range of different structures including true bulbs, corms, tubers, and rhizomes. These fleshy storage organs enable bulbous plants to survive a long dormant period, often spent underground.

True bulbs have fleshy scales (swollen leaves or leaf bases), sometimes tightly overlapping, attached to a small basal plate. In plants such as daffodils (*Narcissus*), each bulb is encased in a thin, papery tunic; others, like lilies (*Lilium*), have loosely arranged, unclothed scales.

Corms are enlarged, compressed stems, often marked with leaf scars. The majority, including those of crocuses and gladioli, are sheathed in a papery or fibrous tunic. Each corm usually lasts for one year, and is then replaced by a new one.

Tubers are swollen sections of stem or root, modified to store food. They are solid in form, like those of dahlias and cyclamen, and usually lack scales or tunics.

Rhizomes are stems that usually creep at or below ground level, often dividing as they spread. Ridged with leaf scars, rhizomes may be thin and wiry, as with lily-of-the-valley (*Convallaria*), or thick and fleshy, as with bearded irises.

A bulbous structure that has died down out of sight is often described as being dormant. Far from a state of low activity, however, this period represents a significant time in the plant's life-cycle, when the bulb ripens and flower buds form, ready for the new season of active growth.

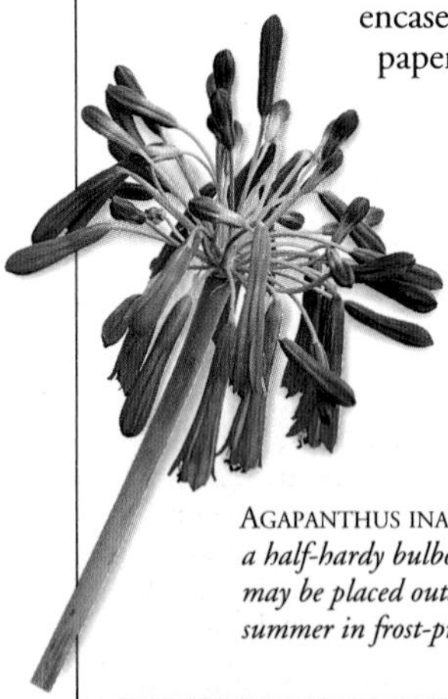

AGAPANTHUS INAPERTUS, *a half-hardy bulbous plant, may be placed outdoors in summer in frost-prone areas.*

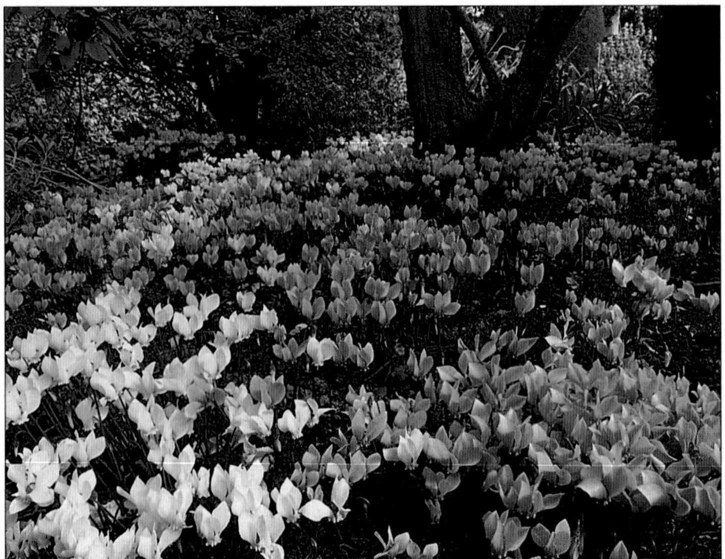

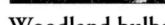

Woodland bulbs

Bulbous plants native to woodland soon naturalize when planted in the dappled shade of a tree. Here, Cyclamen hederifolium *has colonized a shady bank to form a carpet of colour with its vivid autumn blooms.*

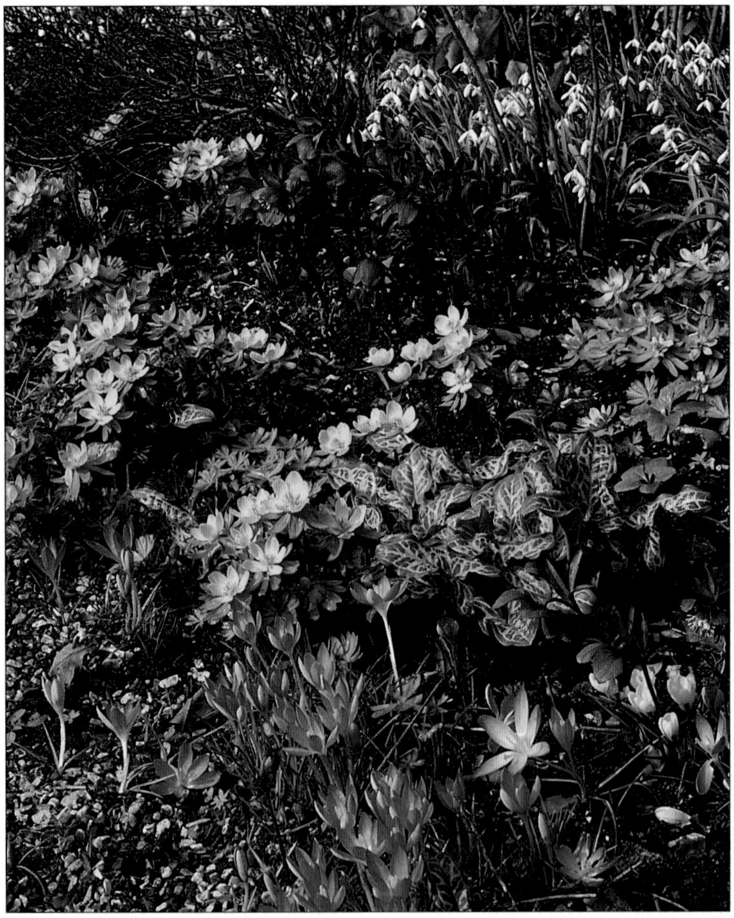

Spring border

A burst of early spring colour is produced here by Crocus tommasinianus, *winter aconites (*Eranthis*),* Arum italicum *'Marmoratum', hellebores, and snowdrops.*

Ornamental features

Bulbous plants are grown mainly for their decorative and sometimes fragrant flowers. These can have the delicate appeal of tiny snowdrops (*Galanthus*) or the imposing effect of tall gladiolus spikes. Many, like those of irises and lilies, are good for cutting. Their floral parts are usually arranged in multiples of 3.

Most bulbous plants are monocotyledons (see p.10), having long, narrow to fairly broad, strap-shaped leaves with near-parallel veins along their length. Some, like cannas, are particularly valued for their foliage, which is erect or semi-erect, sometimes attractively coloured, and forms striking clumps.

Year-round interest

A spectacular array of flowering bulbs, from snowdrops and crocuses to daffodils, provides some of the first blooms of spring. Different species and cultivars may be interplanted with each other to create a rich display that will last for several months until perennials and shrubs come fully into flower.

Later-flowering bulbs can be used to provide highlights of seasonal colour, extending interest throughout the year. Summer-flowering bulbs are often tall, robust plants, bearing flowers in vivid colours, such as the brilliant red or yellow of montbretias (*Crocosmia*) or the purple globes of *Allium aflatunense*. Autumn-blooming bulbs, including colchicums and some crocuses, are dormant during summer, but provide a late flush of colour with the onset of autumn rains.

STORAGE ORGANS

Gardeners commonly refer to any swollen, underground, food-storage organ as a bulb. True bulbs consist of fleshy scales attached to a basal plate, often within a papery tunic. Corms are swollen stem bases. Tubers are unevenly swollen stems or roots. Rhizomes are horizontal, swollen stems.

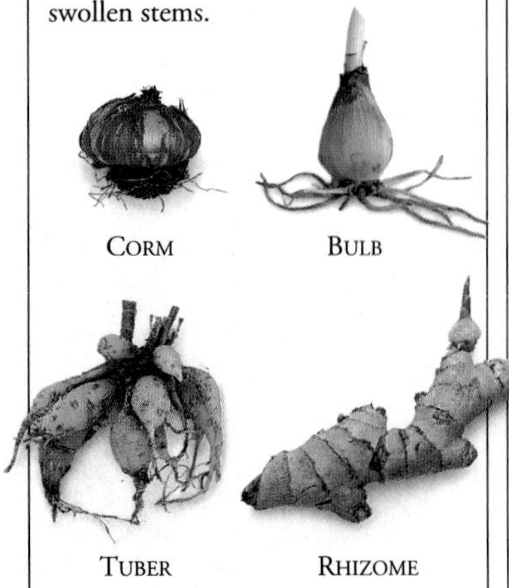

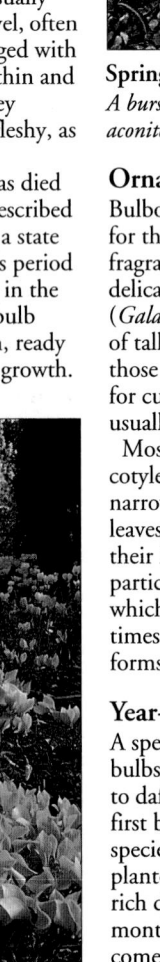

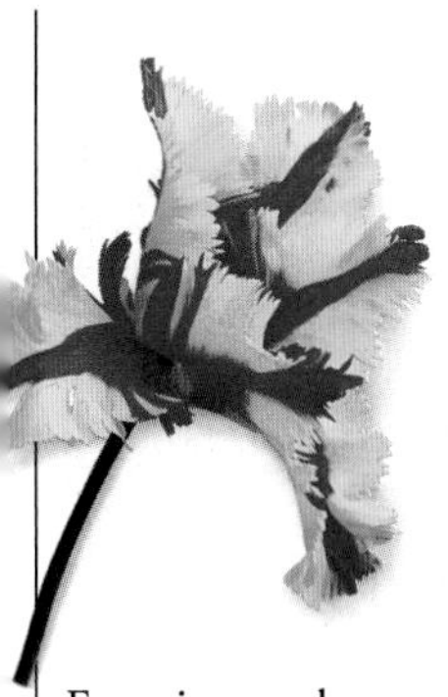

TULIPA *'FLAMING PARROT' bears showy, vibrantly striped blooms in late spring.*

For winter colour, grow bulbous plants such as *Chionodoxa*, grape hyacinths (*Muscari*), snowdrops, or scillas. Several species can be successfully forced indoors.

Where to grow

Interesting contrasts can be achieved by associating bulbs with other plants. Small bulbs, like autumn daffodils (*Sternbergia*), are ideal for growing among rock plants. Those with larger leaves and flowers, like lilies and *Crinum*, are good for infilling or naturalizing in a mixed or shrub border. After flowering, bulbs may be lifted to make room for new plantings, or left in place to increase and flower the next year.

To encourage an abundant crop of flowers, plant bulbs originating from Mediterranean climates in a site where they will receive maximum sun. *Amaryllis*, nerines, and autumn daffodils can be planted at the base of a warm wall or fence.

Bulbs native to woodland habitats, such as some cyclamen, *Eranthis*, erythroniums, snowdrops, and many lilies, will thrive in the light shade of deciduous trees or large shrubs.

Some bulbs, including daffodils, scillas, and crocuses, can be planted in quantity in grass. Cease mowing when the noses of the bulbs appear in late summer or early autumn, and recommence only when the foliage has died down in late spring.

Bulbs are excellent for providing a display of flowers in window-boxes or in containers on a patio. Plant species with differing flowering times to extend the show.

Cultivation

Many bulbs thrive outdoors without protection, even in areas of severe frost. Their main requirement is a near-neutral, well-drained soil in full sun, although bulbs of woodland origin prefer partial shade.

Improve the texture of heavy, wet soil by digging in grit, coarse sand, and organic matter. On poor soil, incorporate a balanced fertilizer on planting. Supplement very light soil with decomposed organic matter to assist moisture retention.

After flowering, allow the foliage to die down naturally; do not knot leaves together, as this reduces their ability to photosynthesize and thus store food in the bulb.

Bulbs from dry summer habitats may rot if subjected to summer rainfall. They are best grown in a raised bed to provide sharp drainage, or in a bulb frame (a raised bed with a protective shelter). Small, rare bulbs with specialized needs are best grown in an alpine house (see p.41) or in a cool greenhouse (see p.24).

In frost-prone areas, plant summer-flowering, half-hardy and frost-tender bulbs in late spring; lift them in autumn and store in frost-free conditions. They may also be grown in a conservatory or warm greenhouse, or indoors. Keep tender bulbs that are dormant in summer, like some nerines and *Hippeastrum*, in a cool, dry site; in early autumn, move them to a frost-free place, such as a sunny window-sill, to flower.

The atmosphere in a home may not be sufficiently humid to support bulbs for long periods. They can be brought indoors when in bud, but returned under glass for their foliage to mature and for their dormant period. When in growth, apply a potash-rich (tomato-type) liquid fertilizer each month to bulbs grown in containers for more than one year. Water freely when in flower. When the leaves die back after flowering, allow bulbs to dry off, and keep warm and dry while dormant. At the end of this period, repot and water to stimulate growth.

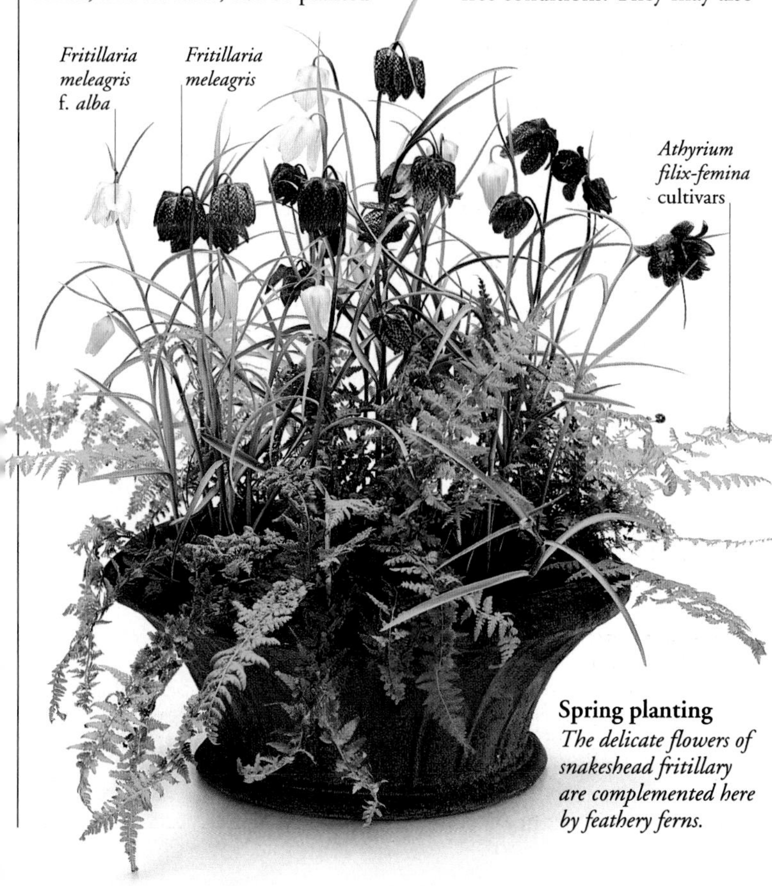

Spring planting
The delicate flowers of snakeshead fritillary are complemented here by feathery ferns.

PLANTING BULBS

Bulbs must be planted at the correct depth (see below) and distance apart. In the individual plant entries in this encyclopedia, the ideal planting distance between single bulbous plants of the same species is given against the symbol (↔) normally used for spread.

Once planted, protect bulbs from extremes of temperature. Those prone to rotting are best laid on a layer of sharp sand to improve drainage. Place bulbs with a hollow top, such as crown imperials (*Fritillaria imperialis*), on their side, to prevent water from lying in the crown.

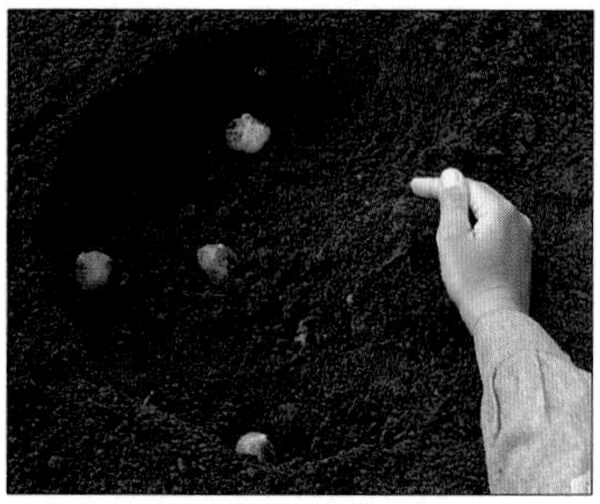

Planting bulbs in the open
Plant bulbs randomly at the correct depth with growing points uppermost, at least their own width apart.

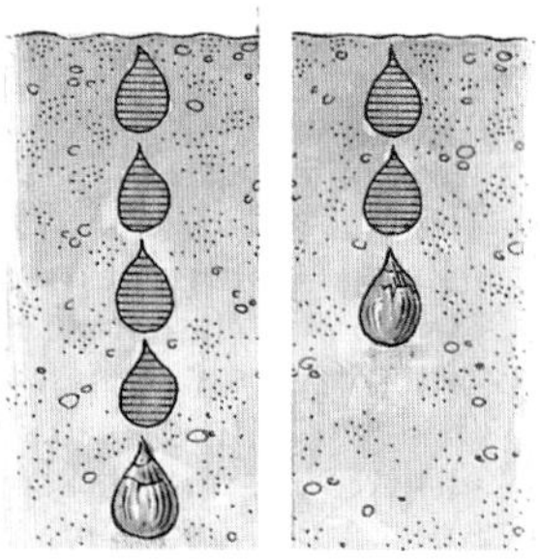

Planting depths
In frost-prone areas and sandy soil, plant at 4–5 times bulb depth (left). Elsewhere, plant at 2–3 times bulb depth (right).

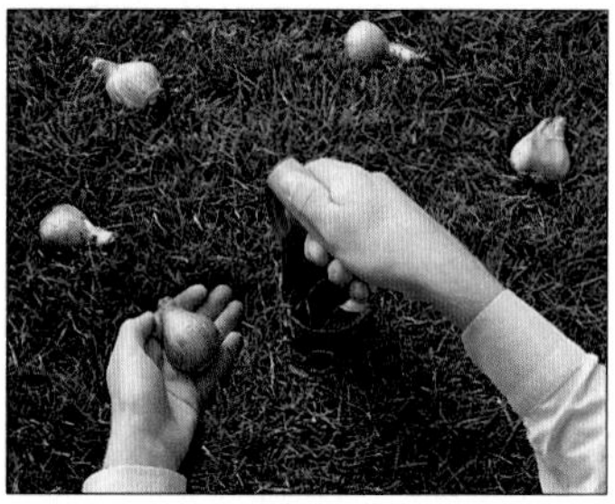

Planting bulbs singly or in grass
Remove a core of soil for each bulb. Place bulb on a little bone meal, and replace soil. If in grass, cover with a lid of turf.

Forcing

To induce unseasonal flowering (forcing), pot up bulbs such as hyacinths in early autumn; keep them in the dark for 8–10 weeks, either plunged outdoors or in a cool place indoors, until flower buds show. Then keep indoors at about 10–15°C (50–59°F), gradually increasing to 20–23°C (68–73°F) as the flower buds develop. Kept too warm or dry, flowers may not open. Once the flowers have died back, return the bulbs to a bulb frame and plant them outdoors in spring.

"Prepared" bulbs are also available; these are specially treated to bear flowers earlier than forced bulbs.

INCREASING STOCKS

Bulbous plants can be raised from seed, but may take several years to flower. In true bulbs, like daffodils, scales or the offsets that form on mature bulbs can be removed for propagation. Plants like lilies form bulbils in the flowerheads and stem and leaf axils. Other plants produce bulblets at the stem bases. Place offsets, scales, bulbils, and bulblets in trays of loam-based compost; when rooted, grow them on in deep boxes of moist compost in a cold frame.

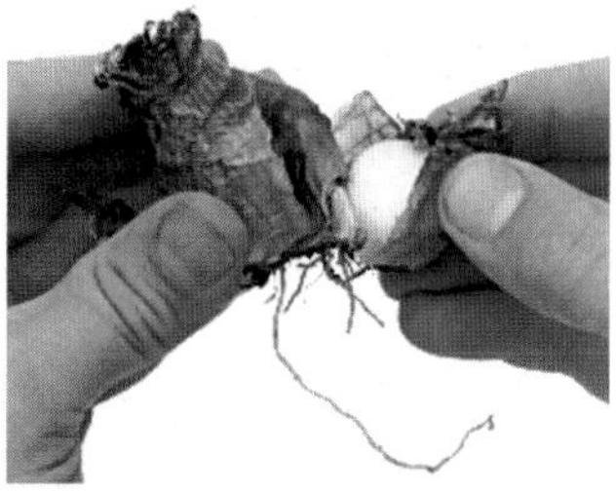

Offsets
Detach large offsets and plant them in trays of loam-based potting compost.

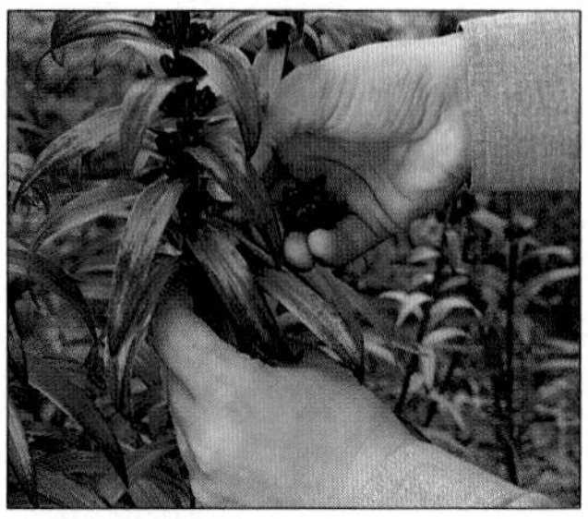

Stem bulbils
Collect ripe bulbils in late summer. Press them gently into soil or compost.

Orchids

All orchids belong to the huge Orchidaceae family, which contains 25,000 species and 100,000 hybrids in some 835 genera. They are evergreen or deciduous perennials, epiphytic, lithophytic (rock-dwelling), or terrestrial in habit, and distinguished by a unique flower structure that has diversified into numerous shapes and spectacular colour combinations.

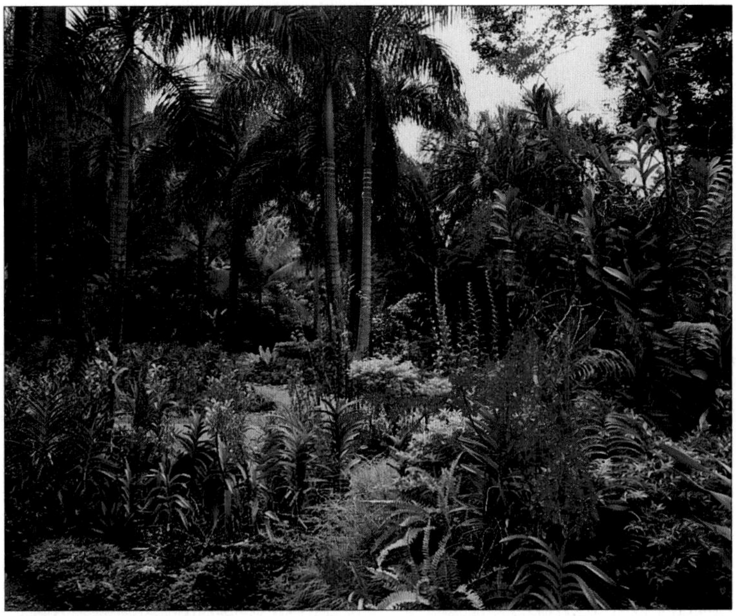

Orchids outdoors
In tropical climates, orchids thrive outdoors if shaded from strong sun by trees or a lath house. In cool areas, use the vivid colour and unusual shape of orchid flowers for an exotic effect under glass, or grow hardier orchids from temperate zones outdoors.

What are orchids?

Most orchid species are rhizomatous epiphytes from tropical rainforest. They often bear fleshy, aerial roots, which are fully or partially attached to the host tree, and which absorb atmospheric moisture; some species are lithophytic. Most cultivated orchids are complex hybrids. The majority are grexes, denoted by a vernacular name in roman type, as in *Lycaste* Wyldfire (see also p.11).

Epiphytic orchids have 2 distinct patterns of growth. Sympodial epiphytes, mainly from rainforest at sea level or at low altitudes, arise from horizontal rhizomes. Each season, growing points (buds) on the rhizomes produce new pseudobulbs – erect, swollen stems that store water and food, and bear leaves and flowers. Active buds usually cease growth by flowering time, and any new growth occurs from lateral buds on older rhizomes. Backbulbs (pseudobulbs that no longer bear leaves) may be used for propagation (see panel); their removal reactivates dormant buds on the bulbs.

Monopodial epiphytes are usually native to dense, steamy rainforest at higher altitudes. Instead of pseudobulbs, they have extended stems that produce new growth from the shoot tips and growing points.

Terrestrial orchids, mainly native to temperate regions, are distinct from epiphytes in that they have underground tubers or rhizomes. These bear a rosette of leaves from which flower stems arise.

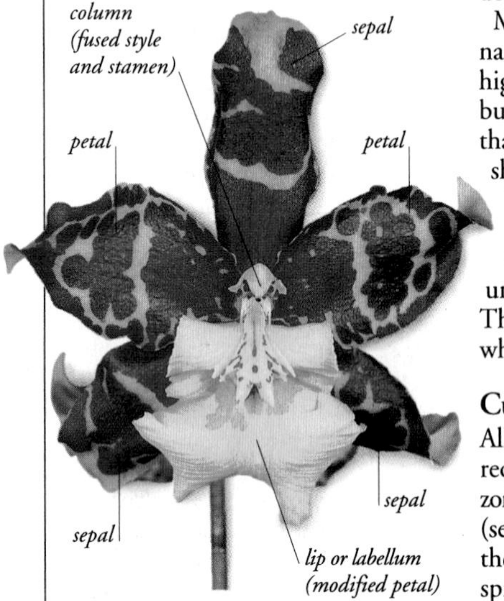

Flower structure
x Odontocidium *Tiger Hambühren clearly displays the typical anatomy and brilliant coloration of an orchid flower.*

Cultivation

All epiphytes, and a few terrestrials, require 1 of 3 controlled temperature zones – cool, intermediate, or warm (see panel below) – depending upon their native origins. Use shading in spring and summer to regulate temperatures and protect foliage from scorching (see p.24).

In hot climates, orchids of tropical origin provide a spectacular and colourful outdoor display. Epiphytes that need moist, shaded conditions, such as moth orchids (*Phalaenopsis*), are best grown in a lath house to protect them from strong sunlight.

In cool regions, terrestrial orchids from northern temperate zones, like lady's slipper orchids (*Cypripedium*), can be cultivated outdoors in a rock garden, in woodland, or on a peat bank. Most die back after flowering and undergo a dormant period.

Some epiphytic orchids may be mounted on slabs of bark, others on branches anchored to form an orchid "tree". Genera with pendent or semi-pendent flowers, such as *Stanhopea*, are best grown in open-slatted hanging baskets.

Both epiphytic and terrestrial orchids are suitable for growing in a conservatory, greenhouse, or, in certain cases, as houseplants. Grow those kept as houseplants in half-pots or wooden baskets, in humid but well-ventilated conditions. When the roots of a plant overfill its container, repot at the onset of the growing season into a container that has room for 2 years' new growth.

Orchids are not easily propagated from seed; in the wild, the tiny seeds usually germinate only with the help of a mycorrhizal fungus, which must be replicated in cultivation. Alternative methods of propagation are given below.

As illegal collecting is depleting orchid species in the wild, it is vital that gardeners obtain only plants that have been raised in cultivation.

Cultivation requirements

Temperature regime	Growing medium	Light	Humidity	Watering	Fertilizer
COOL Min. 10–13°C (50–55°F). Max. 21–24°C (70–75°F). INTERMEDIATE Min. 14–19°C (57–66°F). Max. 30–33°C (86–91°F). WARM Min. 20–24°C (68–75°F). Max. 30–33°C (86–91°F).	STANDARD EPIPHYTIC COMPOST 3 parts bark chippings (use fine-grade granulated bark for fine-rooted orchids); 1 part perlite; 1 part fine charcoal. STANDARD TERRESTRIAL COMPOST 3 parts fibrous peat; 3 parts coarse grit; 1 part perlite; 1 part fine charcoal.	IN SUMMER Most need shade from direct sunlight: shade the greenhouse from late spring until early autumn. IN WINTER Provide full light.	IN SUMMER Damp down daily in early morning (tropical species also in late afternoon). Also mist foliage to reduce leaf temperature. Ventilate well. IN WINTER Do not damp down in cold, clammy conditions, except to counteract drying effects of heating in very cold weather.	IN GROWTH When new growth appears, water regularly in the early morning. Use rainwater or soft water at ambient temperature; compost should remain moist. Mist foliage. WHEN DORMANT Water species that retain leaves sufficiently to prevent dehydration; allow compost to dry out between applications. Keep orchids that lose their leaves dry.	IN GROWTH Apply proprietary orchid fertilizer or ¼- to ½-strength balanced liquid fertilizer every 2–3 weeks, when watering. (Some growers use a high-nitrogen fertilizer for leaf growth, followed by a high-potash fertilizer for better flowering.) WHEN DORMANT Do not feed.

Orchid propagation

Increase stocks by division, removal of backbulbs, or from stem cuttings. Professional growers also raise plants from seed or by meristem culture.

For division, select a plant that has outgrown its container, and split the rhizome so that each part retains at least 3 healthy pseudobulbs; cut out any dead roots, then pot up with the oldest pseudobulb against the rim. With backbulbs, detach from the rhizome, and pot up singly in a 6cm (2½in) container, the cut surface against the rim. For stem cuttings, use sections 7cm (3in) long, with at least 1 dormant bud. Store on moist moss in indirect light until rooted.

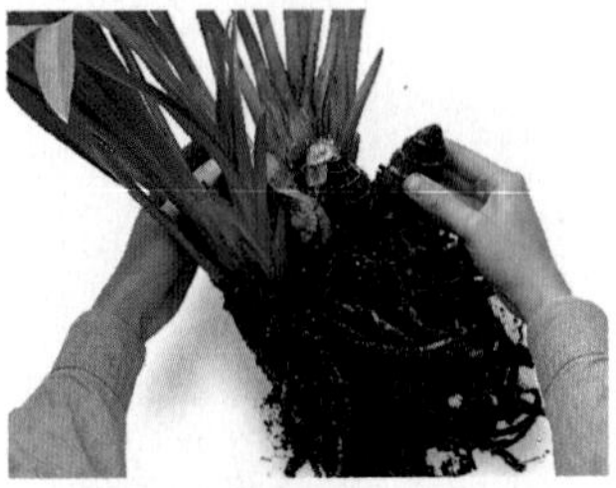

Selecting backbulbs
Choose firm backbulbs, such as the examples on this Cymbidium.

Bromeliads

Members of the Bromeliaceae family, bromeliads number over 2,000 species, most of which grow wild from the southern states of the USA through to Central and South America, and in the West Indies. Producing striking inflorescences and colourful, often variegated leaves, they are easy to cultivate in a greenhouse, as houseplants, or even outdoors in warm regions.

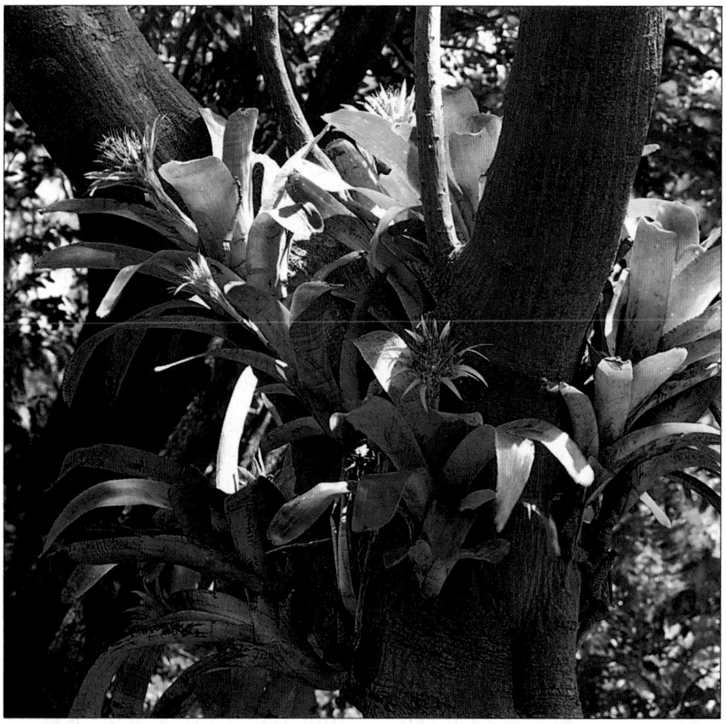

Rainforest epiphytes
In the wild, many epiphytes (here, Aechmea fasciata*) cling to the highest branches of trees to obtain maximum levels of moisture and light. In cultivation, such plants may be displayed on bare branches, secured with adhesive or wedged into notches.*

What are bromeliads?

Bromeliads are mainly rainforest plants, although some are found in mountainous or semi-desert areas, with a few in marshes and on sea-shores. Most are tropical epiphytes, thriving in humid conditions, lodged in trees or on rocks with little soil around their roots. Others are terrestrial.

Most bromeliads are rosette-forming. They range greatly in size, from low-growing plants that form dense colonies, like *Bromelia balansae*, through to tree-like species up to 5m (15ft) tall, such as *Puya berteroniana*. The erect or semi-prostrate rosettes comprise brightly coloured or variegated, sometimes toothed or spiny-margined leaves, which are often adapted to absorb or conserve moisture. Some bromeliads, including air plants (*Tillandsia*), have leaves covered in tiny scales that enable them to retain and absorb moisture and nutrients from the atmosphere, often from mists and low, moisture-laden cloud. In other bromeliads, like *Guzmania*, *Vriesea*, and *Aechmea*, the centre of the rosette forms a "cup" or "vase" that retains water and nutrients.

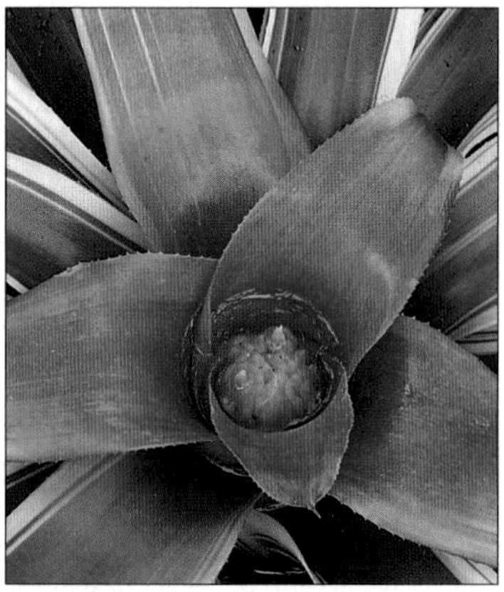

Water-retaining cup
The leaves of some bromeliads, such as Neoregelia*, form a cup, which should be wiped clean and refilled regularly.*

Brightly coloured inflorescences of bracts and flowers are borne in the centre of the rosettes, or are set low in the central cup in certain bromeliads. As monocotyledons (see p.10), bromeliads have flower parts in groups of 3. After flowering, the rosettes begin to die, although new offsets are borne from dormant buds in the basal leaf axils, or on the rhizomes or roots. These offsets can be used for propagation (see below).

Cultivation

Bromeliads are best cultivated by simulating the conditions of their natural habitat (see panel below). Given the right growing environment, they require relatively little maintenance.

In cool areas, most rock-dwelling and terrestrial bromeliads will thrive in a greenhouse or conservatory, or as houseplants. In warmer climates, cultivate bromeliads outdoors, with protection from extremes of heat, sunlight, and rain. Most epiphytes require partial shade, both outdoors and under glass, as bright light may fade their foliage. In many terrestrial species, however, full light improves the coloration of their rigid leaves.

Epiphytes may be attached to a tree or branch, which can be secured in a container, or to a metal or wire framework covered in bark.

To propagate bromeliads, detach offsets from the base or leaf axils of mature plants. Pot up each offset individually into a mix of equal parts shredded peat (or substitute), leaf mould, and granitic grit. Water sparingly until new growth develops.

Sow seed as soon as ripe in a mix of 1 part each leaf mould and shredded peat (or substitute), and 3 parts sharp sand or fine granitic grit. Sow winged seeds (like those of air plants) on slabs of moistened wood or bark; place these at regular intervals on a tray containing a mix of equal parts sharp sand and moist, chopped sphagnum moss.

Apply a proprietary fungicide to prevent damping-off, then place the containers or tray in a propagator with bottom heat at about 21°C (70°F). The slow-growing seedlings will be large enough to prick out and grow on after a few months.

CULTIVATION REQUIREMENTS

TYPE		TEMPERATURE REGIME	GROWING MEDIUM	LIGHT	HUMIDITY AND VENTILATION	WATERING	FERTILIZER
UNDER GLASS	EPIPHYTES	RAINFOREST SPECIES Min. 13–15°C (55–59°F). MOST OTHER SPECIES Min. 10°C (50°F); some hardy, alpine species can tolerate lower temperatures.	IN CONTAINERS Equal parts shredded peat or granulated bark; leaf mould; and granitic grit. GROWN EPIPHYTICALLY Wrap roots in moist sphagnum moss.	Most need bright filtered light.	Rainforest species need high humidity; all others need moderate humidity. Damp down daily in growth, less often when dormant. Ventilate well.	Mist daily, using rain-water or soft water; also mist moss around roots of epiphytes. Watering is not generally necessary.	IN GROWTH Apply ¼-strength proprietary orchid foliar fertilizer every 4–5 weeks when misting. WHEN DORMANT Do not feed.
	TERRESTRIALS AND ROCK-DWELLERS		1 part peat or coconut fibre (coir); 1 part leaf mould; 3 parts granitic grit.	Most need full light.	Maintain low to moderate humidity. Ventilate well.	Water freely; allow compost to dry partially between applications. Where appropriate, regularly replenish cup with fresh rainwater.	IN GROWTH Apply ½-strength low-nitrogen liquid feed every 3–4 weeks when watering. WHEN DORMANT Do not feed.
OUTDOORS	EPIPHYTES, TERRESTRIALS, AND ROCK-DWELLERS	Minimum temperatures as above.	Most prefer sharply drained, humus-rich soil.	Most epiphytes need partial shade; most terrestrials and rock-dwellers need full sun.	Rainforest epiphytes need high humidity. Terrestrials need low to moderate humidity.	Watering is generally not necessary, although light misting is advisable in extremely hot weather.	Feeding is not necessary.

Cacti and other succulents

The fascinating shapes of cacti and other succulents are the result of the adverse conditions they endure in their natural habitats. They vary in habit from small cushions of rosetted leaves to the tall, branching columns of desert cacti. Their unusual textures include smooth, waxy, hairy, or spiny surfaces. Many produce subtly or brightly coloured flowers, enhancing their appeal in desert gardens, and as greenhouse and houseplants.

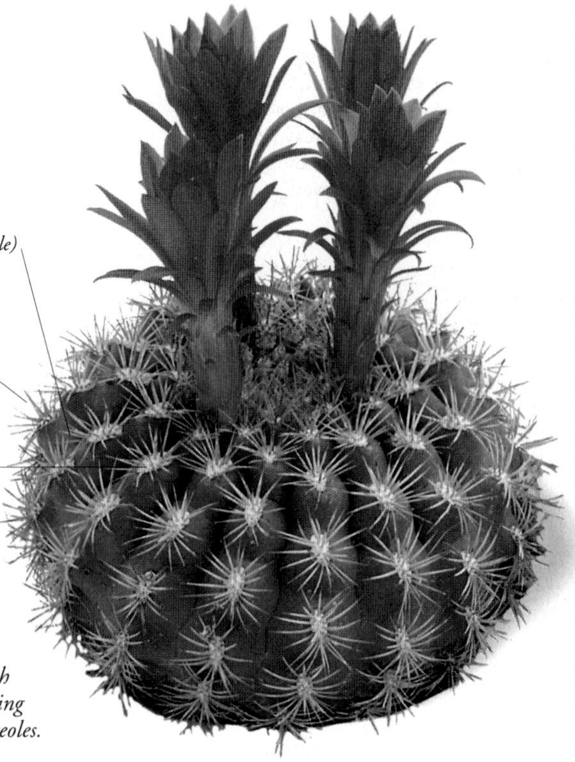

Spiny cactus
Cacti like Oreocereus intertexta *(syn.* Matucana intertexta*) are stem succulents with characteristic growing points known as areoles.*

What are succulents?

Succulents are plants that have adapted to extreme conditions, particularly frequent periods of drought. Typical adaptations include reduced leaf size and the presence of fleshy, water-storing tissue in the stems, leaves, or roots. They are native to a range of habitats, from cold alpine climates, and semi-desert areas in temperate and subtropical zones, to moist rainforest; many may undergo a dormant period in either summer or winter. Succulents may be loosely grouped as stem succulents (including cacti), leaf succulents, root succulents, and caudiciform succulents.

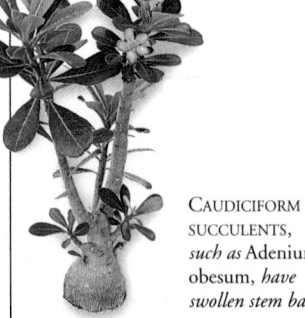

CAUDICIFORM SUCCULENTS, *such as* Adenium obesum, *have swollen stem bases.*

Stem succulents

Stem succulents (most of which are cacti) have swollen, moisture-retaining stems, usually slender, oval, columnar, or spherical in shape. They may be climbing, pendent, or tree-like in habit; some resemble flat, leaf-like pads. Epiphytic succulents native to dry regions often produce aerial roots on their stems that absorb moisture from the atmosphere.

Cacti, which originate in North, Central, or South America (except for *Rhipsalis baccifera*), are distinguished from other stem succulents by their unique growing points, known as areoles. Although a few, such as *Pereskia*, have semi-succulent leaves, most lack foliage, thereby minimizing water loss through transpiration in very dry conditions; chlorophyll for photosynthesis is contained in the stems.

Most cacti have ribs arranged longitudinally on the stems, which expand or contract according to their water content. Along the ribs are the areoles, from which arise flowers, new growth, and spines. Cactus spines are modified leaves, borne as radials (around the edge of an areole) or as centrals (in the centre of an areole). These condense moisture which drips on to the soil around the plant's roots. Epiphytic cacti from humid rainforests have flattened stems with broad surface areas to absorb as much of the limited available light as possible.

Some cacti, such as *Melocactus*, produce a terminal, head-like, almost woody structure, the cephalium, which produces a mass of woolly spines and flowers, and stops further vegetative growth. In other genera, the cephalium is lateral, allowing growth in height to continue. It is then often referred to as a pseudocephalium.

Leaf succulents

The foliage of leaf succulents is usually fleshy, very variable in shape, and downy, felted, glaucous, powdery, waxy, or glossy in texture. Many species have opaque areas at the leaf tips to diffuse the sun's rays. To lessen the rate of transpiration in a dry climate, leaves have a limited number of stomata (pores), which remain closed in the heat of the day.

Water-storage tissues inside the leaves enable the plants to survive in arid conditions. Leaves swell and shrink according to their water content, and usually drop away during periods of severe drought. In many species, the leaves form tight rosettes, which are borne on short stems. This minimizes evaporation both from the plant itself and from the soil beneath.

Root succulents

These succulents are usually found in places where the climate is harsh, or the soil thin and poor. They have swollen roots, hidden below ground, which lose moisture relatively slowly. Most root succulents develop from

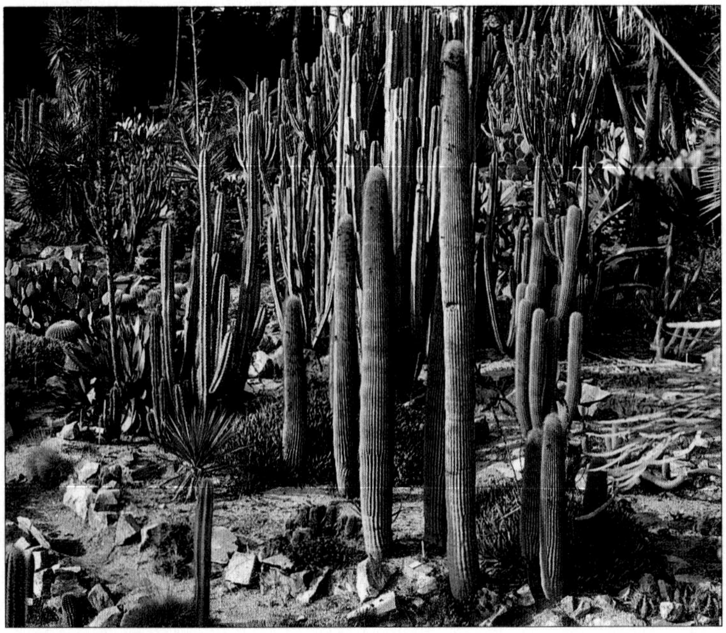

A desert garden
In warm, dry climates, dramatic effects can be achieved by contrasting the columnar habits of Cereus, Cleistocactus, *and* Haageocereus *species with the more complex outlines of such plants as* Agave, Aloe, *or* Opuntia *species.*

LEAF AND STEM SUCCULENTS

Leaf succulents have foliage but often lack a stem, whereas cacti and other stem succulents have a swollen stem but mostly lack leaves. In both types, stems or foliage expand when water is plentiful and contract or, in the case of foliage, drop away, in a drought. The fibrous root system of leaf and stem succulents extends over a wide area just below the surface level to maximize the collection of water. New root hairs are quickly formed to take up any available moisture from dew and passing rain showers.

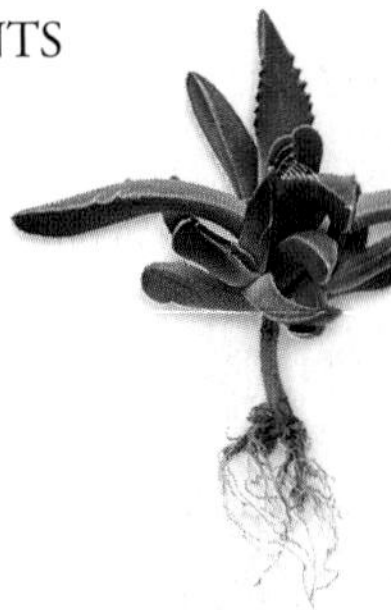

LEAF SUCCULENT
Thick, fleshy leaves retain water.

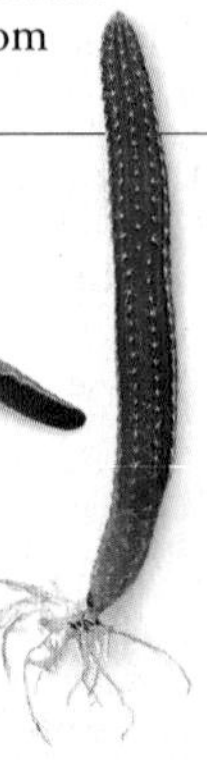

STEM SUCCULENT
Stem contains water-storage tissue.

a normal root system, but some have a specialized rootstock, usually in the form of a tuber. Many also have deciduous succulent leaves or stems, which regenerate when good conditions for growth prevail.

Caudiciform succulents

Some succulents, such as certain species of *Adenium, Dioscorea, Euphorbia,* and *Pachypodium,* have a rootstock that may develop to large proportions, and gradually emerge above ground to form a rounded, sometimes slightly flattened, bottle-shaped or tree-like growth, known as a caudex. The caudex is defined botanically as a swollen base formed at the junction of root and stem. More generally, any succulent with a swollen stem or root above ground is described as caudiciform.

PROPAGATION

Increase succulents by the following methods, or by offsets or grafts.

Divide clump-forming species and cultivars as soon as new growth appears, so that each part has a healthy bud or shoot and roots.

Take stem cuttings from early to mid-spring: trim a leaf-bearing stem to 1cm (½in), or cut sections of leaf-like or columnar cacti into lengths of 5–10cm (2–4in). Take leaf cuttings in spring or early summer, each with a sliver of stem at the base. Allow all cuttings to callus, then insert upright into equal parts peat (or substitute) and sharp grit or sand. Top-dress with grit or gravel and place in bright indirect light at 21°C (70°F). Spray with tepid water until rooted.

Sow seed as soon as ripe from late winter to late spring; cover with twice their depth of standard seed compost, top-dressed with fine grit. Keep moist and place in a propagator in indirect light. On germination, gradually admit more light and air. Apply fungicide to minimize damping-off. Maintain half-hardy and tender species at 21°C (70°F). Plunge containers of seed of hardy species in a cold frame. After pricking out, grow on at 15°C (59°F).

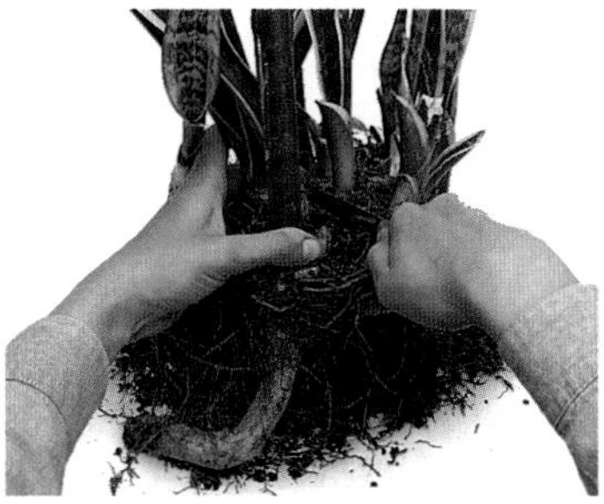

Division of rootstock
Split rootstock into sections; discard old or damaged material; repot each section.

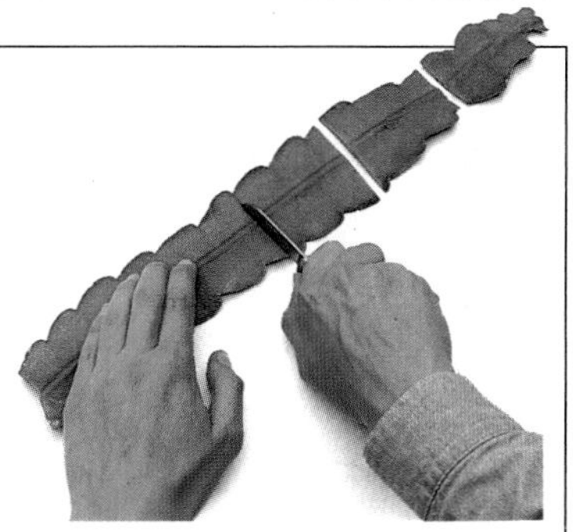

Stem cuttings
Cut leaf-like stems laterally into sections about 5–10cm (2–4in) long.

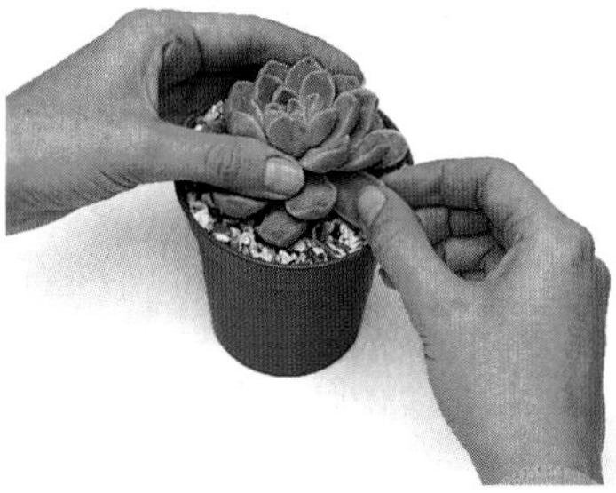

Leaf cuttings
Detach a healthy leaf with a small piece of stem attached to the base.

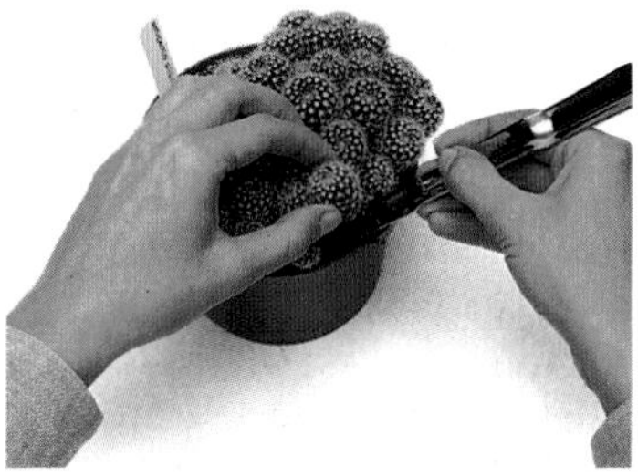

Cacti seedlings
Prick out seedlings as soon as they can be handled (several months after sowing).

Garden and indoor displays

Where climate allows, cacti and other succulents can provide an impressive outdoor display. Planted out or grouped in containers, their foliage, flowers, and unusual forms create an eye-catching feature on a sunny patio or terrace. Even in frost-prone areas, plants may be moved outdoors to a sheltered site during the hottest summer months. Some succulents from mountainous regions are hardy, particularly when protected from moisture in winter, and are ideal for cultivating outdoors in a raised bed. Those originating from cooler areas are best shaded from full sun.

Cacti and other succulents are very popular as houseplants, individually or grouped in bowl gardens. They are often also grown in a temperate or warm greenhouse, where they may be displayed in containers, in landscaped indoor borders, or in raised beds.

Epiphytic succulents, such as *Epiphyllum* and *Schlumbergera,* require partial or dappled shade. They are particularly effective when used in plantings with epiphytic bromeliads (see p.47), which have similar cultivation requirements. Many epiphytic species can be wedged into the crevices of a wall or between roof tiles; those with pendent or trailing habits are suitable for hanging baskets. Some can be lodged in the branches of a tree, with moistened sphagnum moss wrapped around their roots, and held in place with fine wire or garden twine; the roots will eventually anchor themselves.

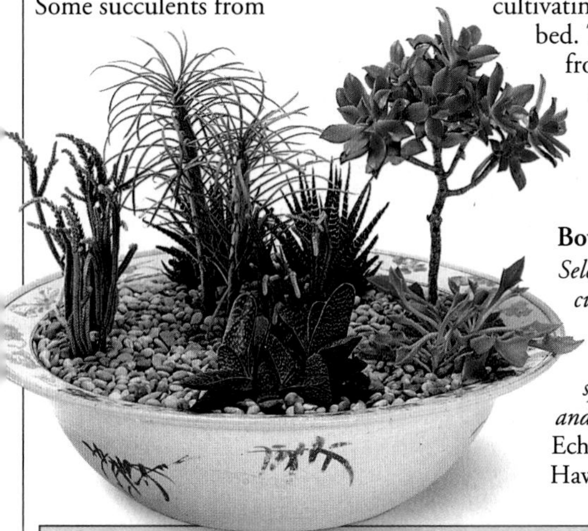

Bowl display
Select plants with similar cultivation requirements that are unlikely to outgrow their allotted space, such as dwarf species and cultivars of Crassula, Echeveria, Gasteria, Haworthia, *and* Senecio.

Cultivation

The panel below gives details of the general growing requirements of cacti and other succulents.

Suitable containers for growing succulents include shallow pans or half-pots, which should contain a layer of crocks at the base to ensure sharp drainage. Plants should also be top-dressed with grit or stone chippings to protect their collars from excess moisture, which tends to lead to fatal rotting.

CULTIVATION REQUIREMENTS

	TEMPERATURE REGIME	GROWING MEDIUM	LIGHT	HUMIDITY	WATERING	FERTILIZER
UNDER GLASS	MOST SPECIES Optimum day temp: 15–30°C (59–86°F). Min. night temp: 10–15°C (50–59°F). When dormant: 7–10°C (45–50°F). TROPICAL AND EQUATORIAL SPECIES Optimum day temp: 21–32°C (70–90°F). Min. night temp: 13–20°C (55–68°F). When dormant: 10–15°C (50–59°F).	Most need pH 6–7.5 and sharply drained soil. STANDARD CACTUS COMPOST 3 parts loam-based compost (JI No.2) or 2 parts loamless compost; 1 part 6mm (¼in) grit. Top-dress with grit, or apply limestone chippings for species that require alkaline conditions. EPIPHYTIC CACTUS COMPOST 3 parts loam-based compost (JI No.2) or loamless compost; 2 parts 6mm (¼in) grit; 1 part leaf mould.	SUMMER Most species require full light with shade from hot sun. Epiphytes and trailing/climbing members of the Asclepiadaceae family require partial shade or bright filtered light. WINTER Provide full light in winter. Supplement light for winter-growing species, if possible.	Most require low humidity and good ventilation. Damp down in very hot weather. Many rainforest epiphytes require high humidity (*Rhipsalis* species need 80% humidity); mist on warm days. Shelter all from draughts.	IN GROWTH Soak thoroughly, using rain-water or soft water; allow compost to dry between applications; avoid wetting the foliage. Keep compost of tropical and epiphytic species just moist. WHEN DORMANT Keep most species dry; mist with tepid water at noon on warm days to prevent dessication. Keep compost of tropical species and epiphytes just moist.	Add slow-release balanced fertilizer to compost. IN GROWTH Apply proprietary cactus fertilizer or ½-strength balanced liquid fertilizer every 4–5 weeks when watering. WHEN DORMANT Do not feed when dormant or when compost is dry.
OUTDOORS	Min. temp. 10°C (50°F) for most. In frost-prone areas, move plants outdoors only in warm summer months (except for fully hardy species).	CONTAINERS AND RAISED BEDS 2 parts loamless compost, coconut fibre, or granulated bark; 1 part 6mm (¼in) grit. Apply slow-release balanced fertilizer.	Most require full sun. Very succulent, smooth-skinned species require full sun with some midday shade.	Most require low humidity. Many rainforest epiphytes need high humidity.	Watering is not necessary. Many rainforest epiphytes require light misting on warm days.	Apply slow-release balanced fertilizer to soil.

Palms and cycads

These evergreen trees or shrubs, with arching, divided leaves, are similar in appearance, yet botanically unrelated. Mainly from tropical and subtropical regions, palms and cycads can be grown outdoors as specimen plants in warm climates. In frost-prone areas, most are best cultivated as short-term young plants, either under glass or as houseplants.

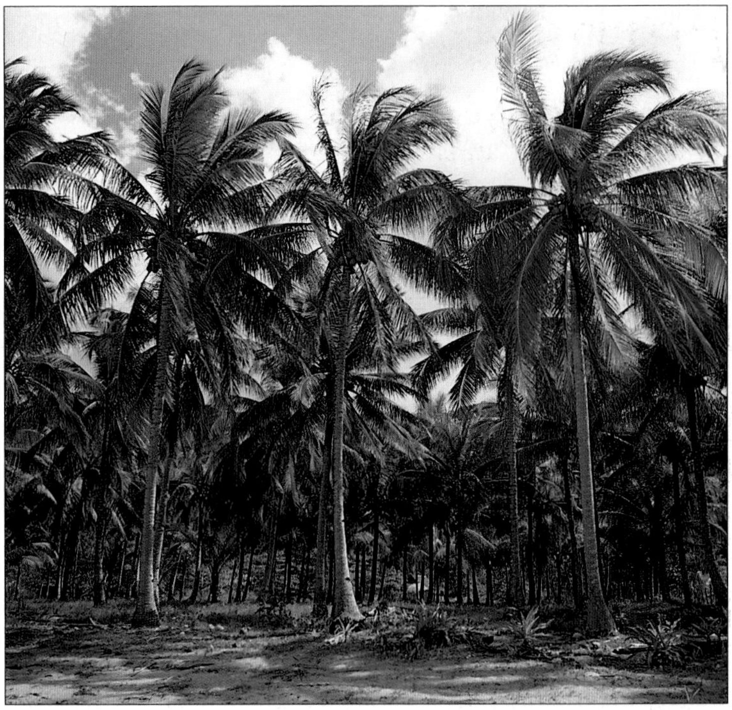

Coconut palms
Cocos nucifera *(coconut palm) thrives in tropical climates as a specimen or avenue tree, reaching a height of 20–30m (70–100ft). Young specimens are impressive as houseplants or grown under glass, and will last until they outgrow their site.*

What are palms?

Palms range from usually unbranched large trees to dwarf shrubs that grow on the rainforest floor or in open, rocky sites. Some appear stemless; most have an upright trunk. Many have a distinctive crownshaft (a usually green, slightly swollen extension of the stem tip) formed from tightly rolled, flattened leaf-stalks.

The leaves may be pinnate, palmately lobed, or semi-palmate. Palms with pinnate foliage, such as the coconut palm (*Cocos nucifera*), are known as feather palms. The leaflets may be lobed or cut, forming a 2-pinnate leaf, as in fish-tail palms (*Caryota*). The palmately lobed leaves of fan palms, such as *Trachycarpus*, are basically hand-shaped, sometimes with radiating lobes. Semi-palmate leaves, such as those of some species of *Livistona*, appear palmate, but have a short extension of the leaf-stalks between each pair of leaflets.

Palm trees produce panicles of small flowers among the leaves or just beneath the lowest leaf. They are monocotyledons (see p.10), their floral parts occurring in multiples of 3. The variably sized fruits have moist flesh, as in the date palm (*Phoenix dactylifera*), or dry flesh, as in the coconut palm.

Cultivating palms

In warm climates, grow palms in moist but well-drained, neutral to slightly acid soil in full sun to deep shade, depending on the species. Many require shelter from strong winds, although some, such as the coconut palm and *Trachycarpus*, are wind-tolerant.

Indoors or under glass, grow palms as dwarf or young specimens in loamless potting compost. Place them in bright, indirect light to minimize leaf scorch: those native to rainforests are particularly sensitive to harsh light. From late spring to late summer, water moderately and apply a balanced liquid fertilizer monthly. At other times water sparingly. Repot in spring. Palms do not usually require pruning.

Most palms are grown from seed, although some species may be divided, and a few produce suckers that may be transplanted. Sow fresh seed singly, as soon as ripe, in standard seed compost in containers 7–9cm (3–3½in) in diameter. Cover each seed with its own depth in compost, although very large seeds should be only half-buried. Sow seed of tropical species at 22–30°C (72–86°F), and seed of temperate species at 13–18°C (55–64°F). Germination often occurs within 2 or 3 months, but may take from 10 days to 2 years. Grow seedlings in partial shade with moderate humidity.

What are cycads?

Cycads are primitive seed plants. Most have short, sometimes branched, occasionally tuber-like trunks, either fully or partly below ground. Some produce suckers. The foliage is pinnate or 2-pinnate, usually tough, leathery, and often rigid; the leaflets may be tipped or margined with spines.

The majority of cycads reproduce by means of primitive, unisexual, cone-like structures, which bear either ovules or pollen sacs. *Cycas* species differ in bearing large, naked ovules along the margins of structures similar to reduced leaves. The ovules develop into nut-like seeds up to 8cm (3in) long, with a tough, woody casing, covered by a thin, sometimes bright red or orange pulp.

Cultivating cycads

Cycads, with their slow growth and elegant habit, are popular house-plants. They are becoming scarce in their native habitats, so always ensure that plants purchased have not been collected in the wild.

In warm climates, grow cycads outdoors in well-drained, neutral to acid soil in full sun or partial shade. Indoors or under glass, grow them in bright but indirect light, in a mix of 2 parts well-drained, loam-based potting compost, such as JI No.1, and 1 part grit or washed sand. Water plants sparingly, and keep dry in cooler temperatures. Apply a half-strength balanced liquid fertilizer monthly to container-grown plants when in growth. Repot in spring. Cycads do not usually require pruning.

PROPAGATING CYCADS

Cycads can be increased from seed or by transplanting suckers. Sow seed singly in small, deep containers. Use a standard, loam-based potting compost or a mix of equal parts gritty sand and peat (or substitute). Seeds should protrude slightly above the surface of the soil. Maintain at a temperature of 16–30°C (61–86°F). Germination, if successful, may take from 3 months to 2 years. The subsequent growth rate will also be slow, with each plantlet producing 1–3 leaves per year. To propagate from suckers, detach the suckers produced by mature plants in spring and pot them up separately.

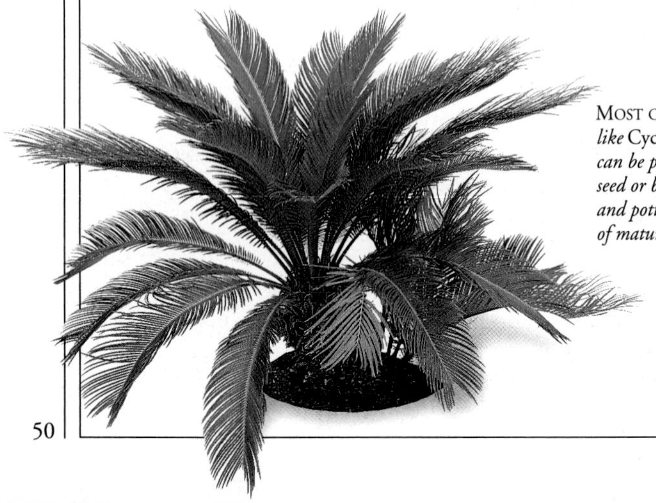

MOST CYCADS, *like* Cycas revoluta, *can be propagated from seed or by detaching and potting up suckers of mature plants.*

SHAPE SYMBOLS

Each palm, cycad, or other tree of similar appearance described in this encyclopedia is assigned a shape symbol. This identifies it either as a single-stemmed tree, or as a multi-stemmed tree that spreads outwards from its base, near ground level.

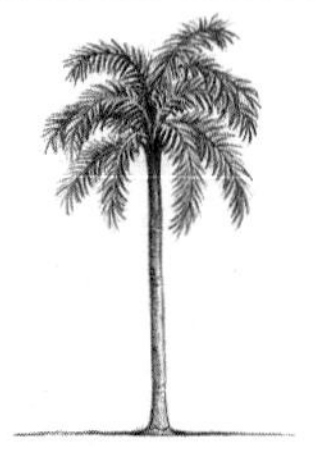

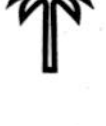

SINGLE-STEMMED
e.g. *Roystonea regia*

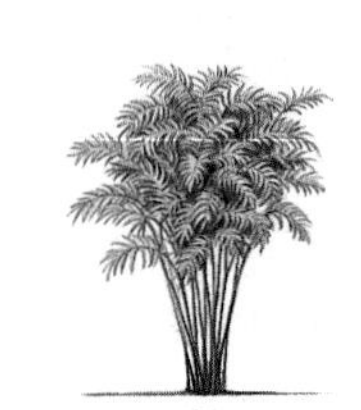

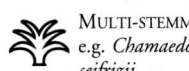

MULTI-STEMMED
e.g. *Chamaedorea seifrizii*

Ferns

Attractive foliage, year-round interest, and a preference for damp, shaded areas where many flowering plants are unable to survive make ferns deservedly popular as houseplants, or for growing outdoors or under glass. Hardy ferns are especially effective in streamside and woodland settings, and frost-tender, tropical ferns are handsome plants for greenhouses or conservatories.

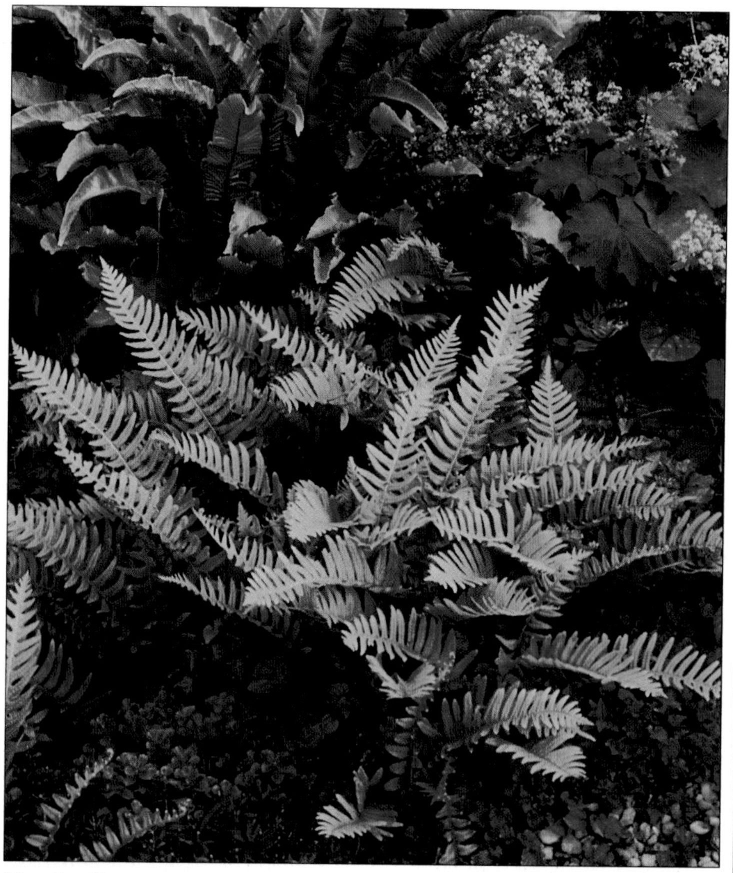

Planting for contrasts
Successful plantings of ferns often contrast textures, habits, and colours of foliage. Here, the glossy, strap-shaped leaves of Asplenium scolopendrium *arch over the feathery fronds of* Polypodium vulgare.

What are ferns?

Ferns are primitive plants that produce evergreen or deciduous leaf-like structures, known as fronds. Together with club mosses and horsetails, they belong to the Pteridophytes, a group of plants that lack flowers and reproduce by spores rather than seeds. Ferns are epiphytic (lodging on trees or rocks), or terrestrial (rooted in soil). Their reproductive spores are sometimes borne in sporangia, usually clustered within indusia (covers of epidermal tissue) on the underside of their fronds. After germination, spores form a flap of green tissue (the prothallus), where the male and female reproductive organs are both sited. Fertilization occurs on the underside of the prothallus.

Ornamental features

Ferns are highly valued for the elegant symmetry of their fronds, and the textural contrasts of their lush, usually green foliage, varied in some species with displays of red, yellow, or grey. Fronds may also have brown scales at their bases, or have silvery undersides.

Their diversity of habit presents a wide choice for the gardener. Shuttlecock ferns like *Matteuccia* have erect rhizomes, each bearing a crown of fronds. Creeping ferns, such as *Phlebodium*, are prostrate, and provide good ground cover, producing single fronds at intervals along each rhizome. Tree ferns, such as *Dicksonia,* have erect, trunk-like rhizomes, ridged with scars left by the stalks of old fronds. Staghorn ferns (*Platycerium*) are tender epiphytes with some clasping fronds produced from the base of each plant, and some erect fronds, slightly arching outwards.

If carefully chosen, ferns provide year-round garden interest. Most uncurl bright foliage in spring, the fronds of deciduous plants starting to fade by late summer and dying back after the first frosts. Evergreen ferns often remain attractive throughout autumn and winter.

Cultivation

Once established, ferns usually require little maintenance. The majority prefer conditions ranging from partial to deep shade. Some, such *Matteuccia*, *Onoclea*, and *Osmunda* require damp soil. Others, such as *Asplenium*, *Polypodium*, and *Polystichum*, tolerate relatively dry sites. Dwarf species of *Asplenium* and ferns from desert areas, such as *Cheilanthes*, prefer full sun, and are ideal in rock crevices. Most other hardy species will thrive outdoors in well-aerated, humus-rich soil.

Many ferns, particularly half-hardy and frost-tender species, may be grown in a conservatory or greenhouse, or as houseplants. They are best grown in bright indirect light. Species native to desert habitats, such as *Cheilanthes* and *Pellaea*, will thrive in full light in an alpine house (see p.41).

Water ferns only when compost is barely moist to the touch, as they are intolerant of excessive water. As a rule, they should be watered more freely in summer than in winter. Do not allow ferns in containers to remain standing in water.

Most ferns prefer high levels of humidity, which can be achieved indoors by standing containers on a tray of moistened, expanded clay granules or gravel. In winter, the humidity level may be reduced by the drying effects of central heating. This can be offset by keeping ferns in a cool room or hallway.

Grow terrestrial ferns in a mix of 1 part each of loam, medium-grade granulated bark, and charcoal, 2 parts sharp sand, and 3 parts coarse leaf mould; add 1 part limestone chippings for species that require alkaline conditions. Include a slow-release, balanced fertilizer in the mixture; alternatively apply a half-strength, general-purpose or tomato-type liquid fertilizer every 3–4 weeks during growth. Grow epiphytic ferns in a mix of equal parts fine-grade granulated bark, perlite, and charcoal.

Repot all container-grown ferns in spring or summer when their roots overfill the containers.

To propagate ferns, cut rhizomes into sections, or divide crowns, in spring, or use bulbils or spores (see panel).

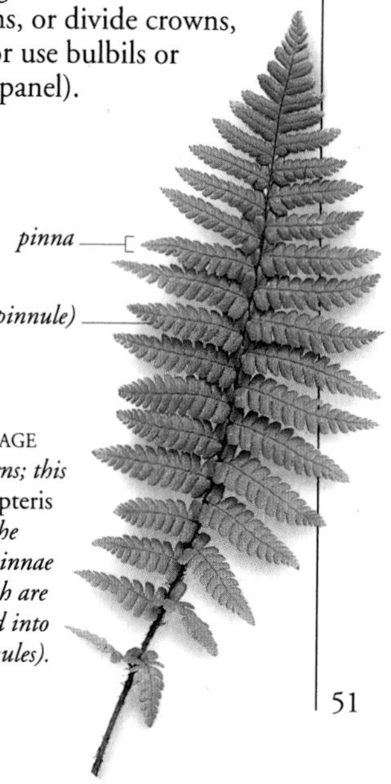

PINNATE FOLIAGE *is typical of ferns; this frond of* Dryopteris affinis *shows the division into pinnae (leaflets), which are further divided into segments (pinnules).*

PROPAGATION BY BULBILS OR SPORES

To propagate from bulbils, sever a frond full of bulbils at the base. Peg it flat on to seed or cutting compost in a tray, water, label, and seal in an inflated plastic bag, and leave in a warm, light place until the bulbils have rooted. Grow on singly in 6cm (3in) containers of moist, soilless compost. To propagate from spores, place a frond with plump sporangia on clean paper to collect the spores. As soon as possible, sow them thinly on to moist, sterilized seed compost, place in a propagator, and mist twice weekly until prothalli appear. Firm small clumps on to compost, spray, and return to propagator. Grow sporelings on until fronds develop; pot up singly.

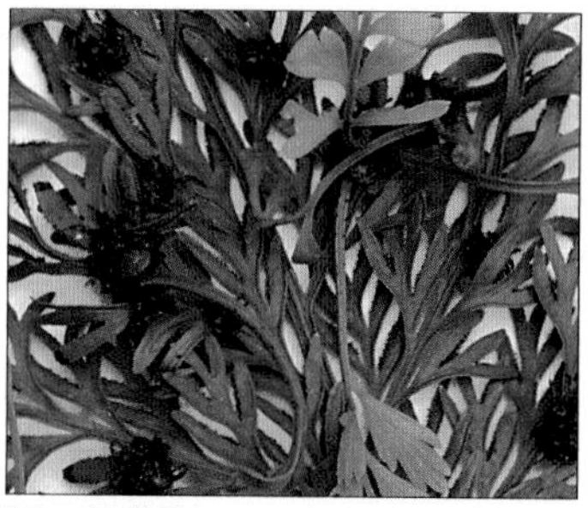

Ripe bulbils
Select a frond that is drooping under the weight of bulbils, which may have tiny green fronds emerging from them.

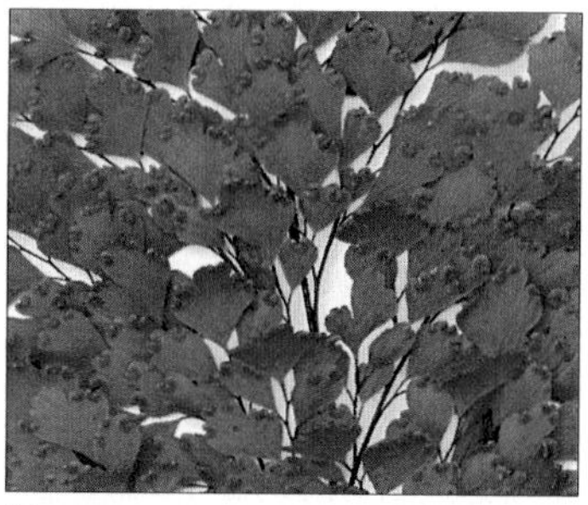

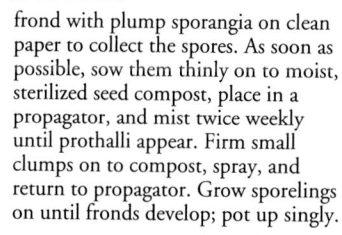

Ripe spores
Select fronds with sporangia that are neither rough (too old) nor still tightly wrapped in the indusium (too young).

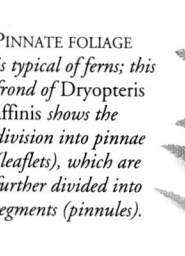

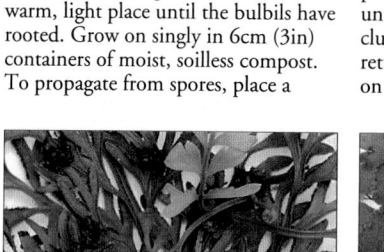

Aquatic plants

Many aquatic plants, prized over the centuries for their beauty, can be cultivated in artificial or natural water features in the garden. Large and small ponds, formal or informal pools, streams, bog gardens, and even small barrel ponds all present different conditions and varying water depths that will support an exciting diversity of aquatic plant, insect, and animal life.

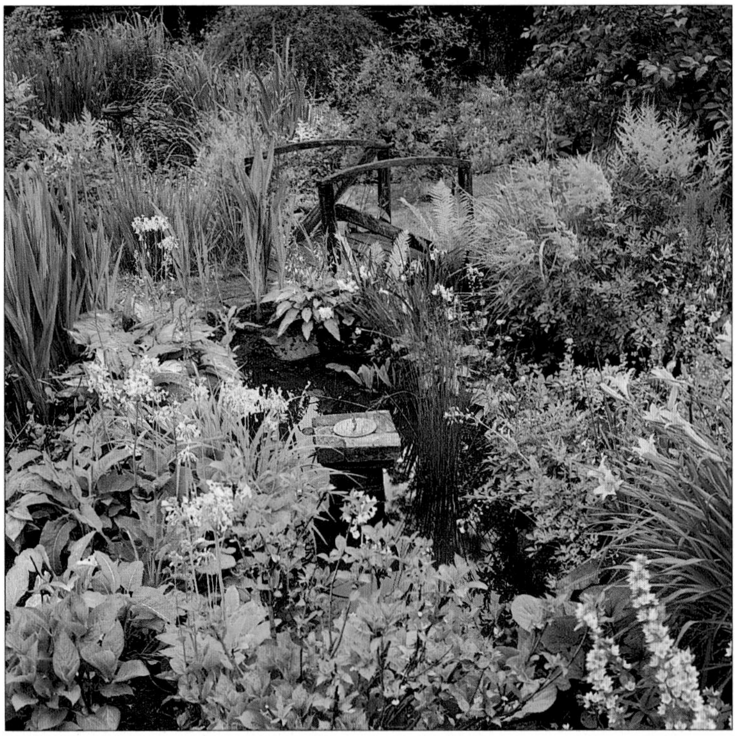

An emphasis on marginals
Marginals, bog plants, and moisture-loving plants link a pond with the rest of the garden and provide a habitat for wildlife. They are also useful in smaller ponds, leaving the water surface clear to reflect the colours and forms of the planting.

What are aquatic plants?

All plants that grow rooted, floating, or submerged in water are broadly termed aquatic plants. They are categorized as submerged, deep-water, surface-floating, marginal, bog, or moisture-loving plants, according to the depth of water in which they grow best. Depth is measured from the surface of the soil around a plant's roots to the surface of the water.

Most aquatic plants are both ornamental and functional. They produce attractive foliage and flowers but also play a vital role in the ecosystem of water features, by providing a habitat for myriad micro-organisms, insects, and wildlife, and by helping to suppress algal growth and maintain the clarity of water. A healthy balance of animal and plant life can be achieved only if a pond is stocked with an appropriate range of plant species.

Submerged and floating plants

Certain plants, such as *Lagarosiphon major* and milfoils (*Myriophyllum*), remain totally submerged below water. They are fast-growing, and usually produce slender stems and leaves. Submerged plants are grown mainly for their ability to reduce algae by competing with them for mineral salts (released by the breakdown of organic matter, such as dead leaves) dissolved in the water. They are often called oxygenators, because they release oxygen into the water as a by-product of photosynthesis – an asset if fish are to be kept in a pool. The fine strands of submerged plant foliage also provide valuable shelter for fish fry.

Deep-water plants, like water lilies (*Nymphaea*), grow with their root systems at depths of 30–90cm (12–36in), and with their foliage and flowers floating at surface level. The shade cast by their leaves reduces underwater light levels, which helps to control algal growth.

Surface-floating plants, such as *Azolla filiculoides*, usually have tiny leaves and spreading roots that absorb nutrients from the water. They multiply rapidly during summer, forming dense colonies.

Ideally, 50–70 per cent of a pool's surface should be covered with the foliage of deep-water and floating plants to keep the water clear. In a new pond this allows other aquatics to become established. If coverage is greater than 70 per cent, insufficient light will filter through the water for submerged plants to survive.

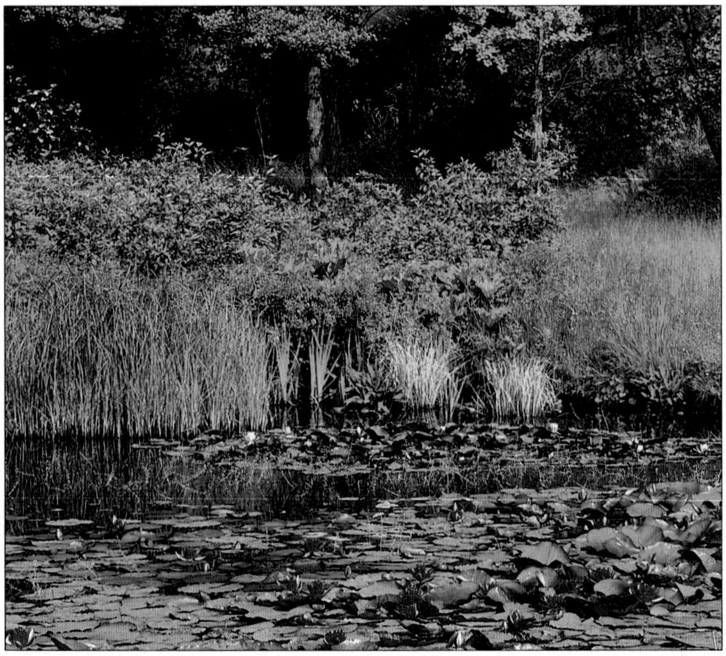

Water lily pond
*Deep-water plants, such as these water lilies (*Nymphaea *'Escarboucle'), are ideal for larger ponds; they are complemented here by marginal clumps of sedges and rushes.*

Shallow-water and bog plants

Marginal plants tolerate conditions ranging from pure mud to water 30–45cm (12–18in) deep over their roots, and are perhaps the most diverse of all aquatic plants. They are best used to conceal the artificial outline of an informal water feature, such as a wildlife pond or watercourse, but also provide cover for birds and other wild creatures.

Bog plants are also marginal plants but prefer a site in shallower water. However, the term is commonly used to describe any plant that grows in saturated soil just beyond the water's edge, normally without a covering of water. Such plants represent the transition between true aquatics and plants that are simply moisture-loving. In nursery catalogues, the latter are sometimes referred to as bog plants, despite their intolerance of waterlogged ground and need for oxygen around their roots.

Planning a water feature

Formal and informal water features and their associated aquatic plants have been used throughout history as major elements of garden design. As with all plantings, water gardens should be designed to take advantage of the contrasts and similarities between plants, and provide a long succession of flowers and seed heads or decorative foliage throughout the year. In selecting aquatic plants, it is worth bearing in mind that many die back after frost, reducing winter interest in cold regions. Native plants provide food for insect life, such as dragonflies, which in turn fall prey to other creatures.

Always choose a water feature that is appropriate for the size and style of the garden, and take great care when deciding on its position. A pond is best sited in full sun, away from overhanging trees, and should not be constructed in an exposed site or frost pocket. Since most gardens lack a brook or natural spring, a pond should lie near an accessible water source so that moisture lost through evaporation can be replaced easily.

A formal pond of any dimensions provides an impressive focal point

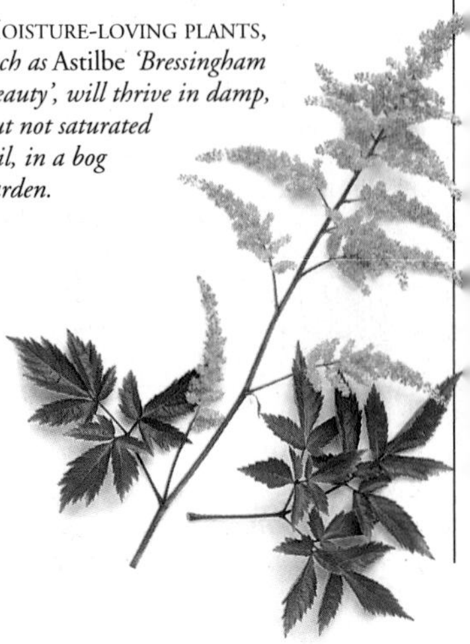

MOISTURE-LOVING PLANTS, *such as* Astilbe *'Bressingham Beauty', will thrive in damp, but not saturated soil, in a bog garden.*

PLANTING A POND

Aquatic plants are best introduced into a pond from late spring to midsummer. Slide surface-floaters on to the water with roots trailing downwards. Plant deep-water, submerged, and marginal plants in an underwater bed, or in containers, using heavy loam or a proprietary aquatic compost that will not cloud the water. Containers will curb invasive species and allow easier relocation and division of plants.

Aquatic containers have a broad, flat base with open-meshed sides to prevent stagnation of the growing medium: unless the mesh is fine, line pots with polypropylene or hessian. Firm plants into the soil and top-dress with grit or pea shingle for ballast and to prevent fish disturbing the roots. Apply a slow-release aquatic fertilizer in summer.

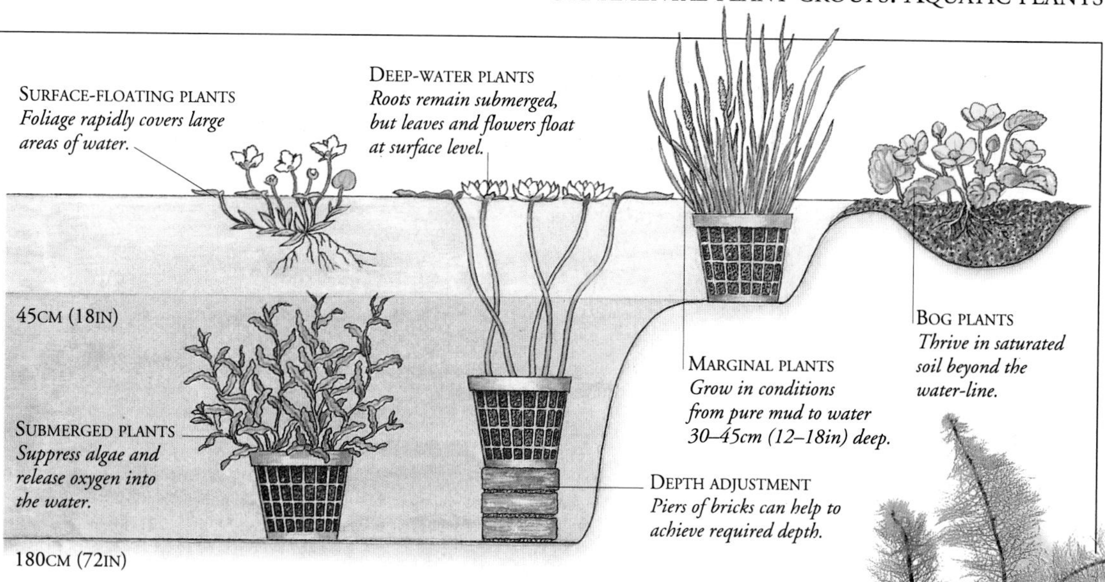
SURFACE-FLOATING PLANTS
Foliage rapidly covers large areas of water.
DEEP-WATER PLANTS
Roots remain submerged, but leaves and flowers float at surface level.
45CM (18IN)
SUBMERGED PLANTS
Suppress algae and release oxygen into the water.
180CM (72IN)
MARGINAL PLANTS
Grow in conditions from pure mud to water 30–45cm (12–18in) deep.
BOG PLANTS
Thrive in saturated soil beyond the water-line.
DEPTH ADJUSTMENT
Piers of bricks can help to achieve required depth.

within a garden. It may be sunken or raised, made from concrete or stone, and is usually geometric in shape, with straight sides. Use ornamental materials to decorate its perimeter, either as paving, or in the form of a raised edge or seat.

A small formal pond will support a limited but choice range of species and cultivars. These are often best selected for their architectural interest. Ideal examples are water lilies, with their spreading, rounded foliage and exquisite flowers, or water irises, like *Iris pseudacorus*, which have upright blooms on strongly erect stems.

Informal pools are mostly sunken and irregular in outline, often designed to attract native wildlife to a garden. To suit amphibians, the pool should ideally have a muddy bottom and gently sloping sides, dotted with large, flat stones. Birds and other wild creatures, such as hedgehogs, will be attracted to the bathing and drinking facilities provided by an area of shallow beach. Soften or disguise the edges of an informal pool with natural materials, like rocks or turves, partially concealed by clumps of marginal and bog plants.

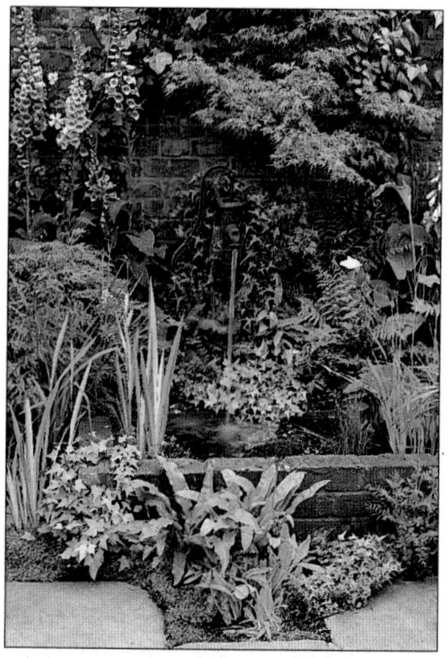

Corner feature
Even small gardens may be enlivened by a small pool and fountain, ringed with ferns and other moisture-loving plants.

A bog garden is an attractive way of using waterlogged ground, and also provides good conditions for local wildlife. To create an artificial bog garden, place a perforated synthetic liner under soil next to a pool; this will retain sufficient moisture for bog plants.

Almost any water-tight container may be used to grow oxygenators, dwarf water lilies, and marginal plants. Metal containers must be sealed inside with rubber paint or a synthetic liner to avoid poisoning either fish or plants. In cold regions, containers also enable frost-tender plants to be grown outdoors in summer, then overwintered indoors.

Maintenance

Synthetic liners, plastic modules, and electric pumps for filtering water have all simplified pond maintenance. Ensure that drainage is adequate for occasions when the pond may overflow. On sloping ground, a tumbling or split-level watercourse or waterfall may be constructed. If fish are kept, install a fountain or similar device to aerate the water during still summer nights, when oxygenating plants are unable to photosynthesize. Most aquatic plants are intolerant of splashing water, so they are best sited in more tranquil parts of the pond. In areas with cold winters, move fish that are normally kept in a container pond, such as a barrel, to a sunken pool, where they are more likely to survive.

Aquatic plants require little regular care, although submerged plants grown in a soil-bottomed pond need regular thinning and cutting back. In autumn, cut back any leaves or stems that would rot in the water, together with damaged or diseased marginals and bog plants. With wildlife ponds, however, foliage is best left until spring to provide winter cover for birds and animals.

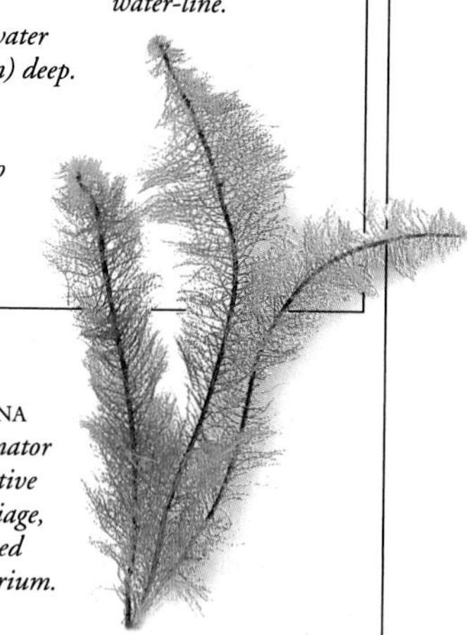

CABOMBA CAROLINIANA
is an oxygenator with attractive feathery foliage, best displayed in an aquarium.

Aquarium plants

An indoor aquarium enables year-round cultivation of tender plants, and also displays the foliage of submerged plants and the feathery roots of surface-floaters to good effect. Grow aquatic plants from temperate regions in a cold water aquarium. Tropical plants and fish must have a heated aquarium.

Line the base of the aquarium with an inert medium, such as grit, sand, or gravel. Maintain the balance of the water chemistry by growing a suitable range of oxygenating plants, and provide a good filtration system and correct temperature. Ensure that lighting is adequate but not too bright (excess light will encourage algal growth). Trim foliage as necessary, and occasionally apply proprietary slow-release fertilizer tablets to the growing medium.

PROPAGATION

Aquatic plants can be propagated by seed, division, cuttings, turions (see below), offsets, and runners. Most are increased by division of the rootstock in summer; divide every 1–2 years, as roots soon become thickly enmeshed.

Moisture-loving and some aquatic plants can be grown from ripe seed in summer or autumn. Sow on an inert medium and top-dress with fine grit. Keep submerged under glass in bright indirect light at 18°C (64°F). Prick out plantlets, retain under glass, and plant out in spring of the second year.

With submerged plants, take stem-tip cuttings in spring or summer. Trim to 10–15cm (4–6in) long, and insert singly or in bunches of 3–6 into submerged pots of loam; transplant when rooted. Alternatively, float weighted bunches on the water to root in the bottom of a soil-based pond.

Certain aquatic species bear turions – swollen buds that overwinter at the bottom of a pond. When they surface in spring, pot up singly as new plants.

Many surface-floating plants of tropical origin may be increased from offsets or runners, which form on long, adventitious shoots. If detached from the parent, these plantlets will multiply rapidly on the water's surface.

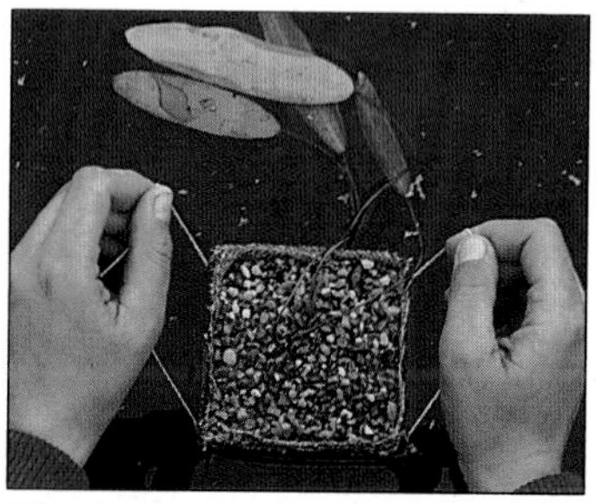

Planting cuttings in containers
Insert cuttings singly or in bunches in a container that is sufficiently large to accommodate the adult plant.

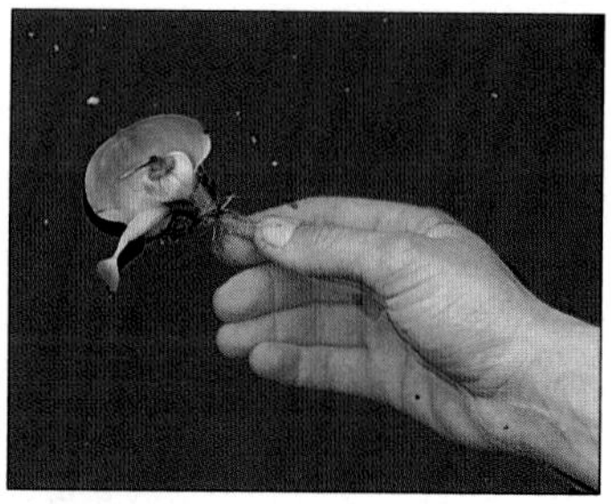

Offsets
Place offsets of floating plants directly on the surface of the water, supporting each one until it floats upright.

Grasses and bamboos

True grasses, including bamboos, are members of a vast family of plants that grow wild throughout the world. A few are very commonly grown as lawns, but many ornamental grasses are valued for their stately habit, feathery inflorescences, and slender, sometimes unusually coloured leaves. Some bear decorative seed heads, and many are suitable for indoor displays.

What are grasses?

Grasses are evergreen or deciduous annuals or perennials belonging to the Gramineae family. Their erect or arching stems are usually round and hollow, with regularly spaced nodes, very clearly seen in the jointed canes of bamboos. The foliage is borne in 2 ranks from sheaths, which may be split or peeled back. Colours include yellow, silvery blue, and red, as well as shades of green; numerous cultivated grasses have attractively variegated leaves, with longitudinal stripes or cross-bands.

The delicate inflorescences, in the form of spikes, panicles, or racemes of tiny spikelets, are usually light and feathery, and subtle in colour. Many are suitable for cutting and displaying indoors, either fresh or dried (see p.39).

In the garden, grasses have a variety of uses. Those of imposing habit, like pampas grass (*Cortaderia selloana*), are splendid as specimen plants, while some lower-growing grasses, such as hair grass (*Aira elegantissima*), provide excellent ground cover. Many grasses can also be used in a mixed border, where their soft curves and vertical lines contrast well with more rounded, broader-leaved plants.

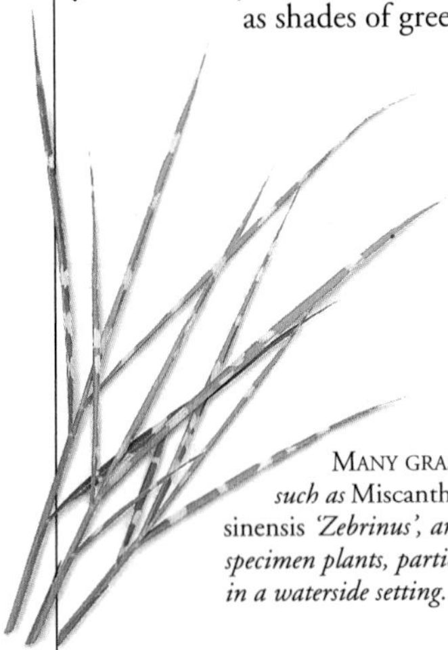

MANY GRASSES, *such as* Miscanthus sinensis *'Zebrinus', are fine specimen plants, particularly in a waterside setting.*

Cultivation

Once established, grasses need little maintenance. Most prefer full sun and moist but well-drained soil, not too rich in nutrients. Feeding is rarely required. Grow grasses that prefer damp soil near a water feature.

Plant hardy, container-grown grasses in any season. Half-hardy and tender grasses are best planted in spring; in areas with high rainfall, use sharply drained, gritty soil, and top-dress with stone chippings in winter. Bamboos should be watered freely until established.

Restrain vigorous and invasive grasses by growing in containers, or place a barrier, such as thick plastic sheeting, in the soil around them. Alternatively, cut back invasive roots with a spade when new growth appears in spring, and again in mid- or late summer. Cut perennials to ground-level in autumn or early winter, but leave attractive foliage and seed heads until late winter. Cut back tender grasses in spring.

Propagate grasses by seed, sown as soon as ripe, or divide rhizomatous and clump-forming grasses in late spring or early summer. Divisions are often best potted up and established before planting out; use moist but well-drained compost and keep cool in bright indirect light.

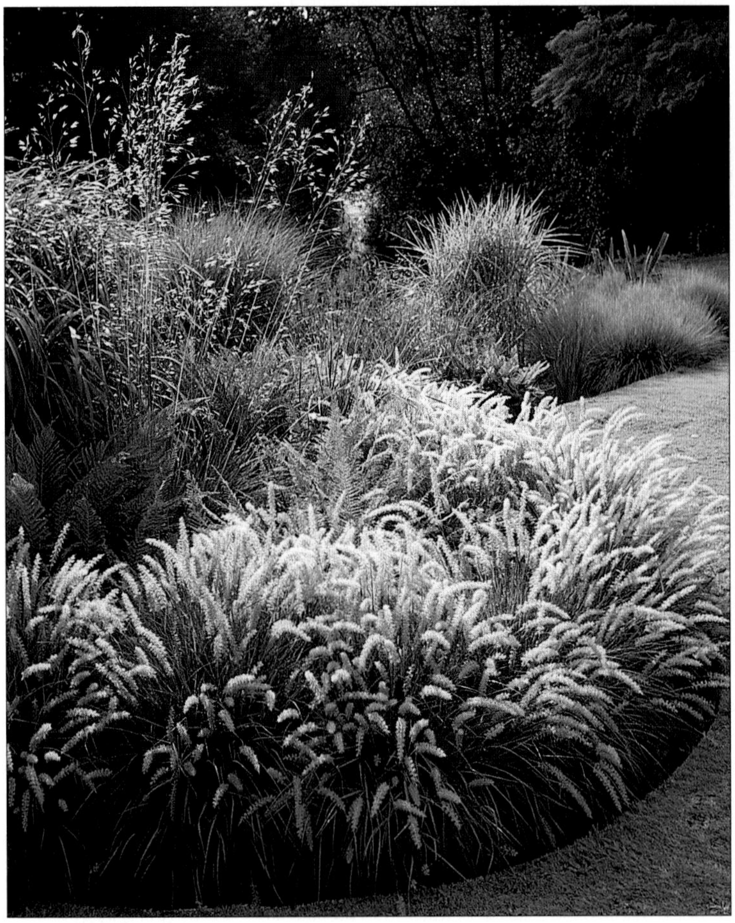

Grass border
Use grasses to give a border strong visual impact. Select species that contrast in height and habit, as well as in the shape and texture of their inflorescences. Here, the tall panicles of Stipa gigantea *are offset by the soft mounds of* Pennisetum orientale.

BAMBOOS

Most of these woody-caned, perennial grasses originate in tropical and subtropical regions, particularly E. Asia. The majority are frost tender and evergreen; the few that are fully hardy are from temperate zones. Bamboos range in habit from low-growing plants like *Pleioblastus pygmaeus* var. *distichus* to those with a tall, almost tree-like habit, such as *Phyllostachys aureosulcata* 'Spectabilis'. Popularly grown as specimen or accent plants, for screening and hedging, or as decorative ground cover, bamboos have elegant, ornamental foliage, which is sometimes variegated with green, cream, or yellow.

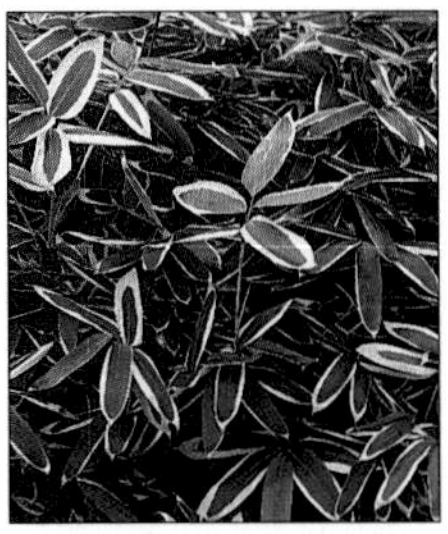

Sasa veitchii

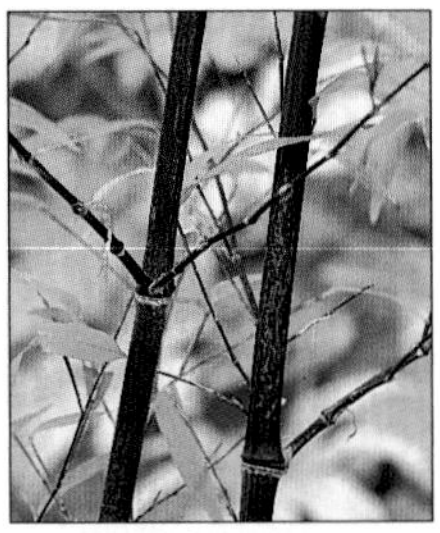

Phyllostachys nigra

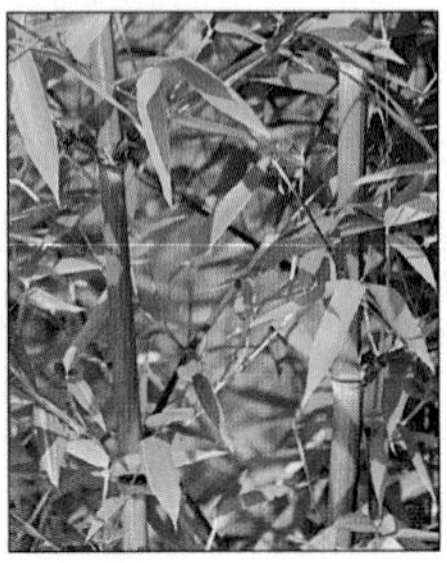

Phyllostachys aureosulcata 'Spectabilis'

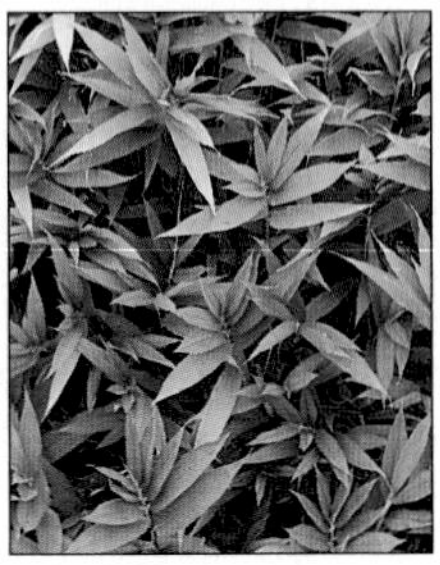

Pleioblastus pygmaeus var. *distichus*

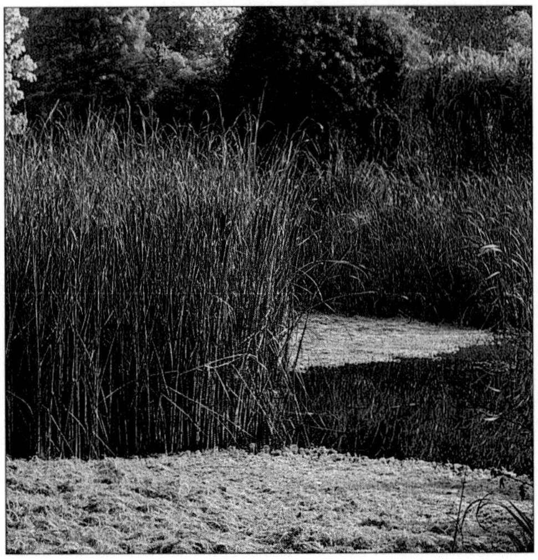

Sedges and rushes
Sedges (Cyperaceae) and rushes (Juncaceae) are large families of perennials from temperate and arctic regions. Grown for their attractive foliage and inflorescences, they are similar to grasses in appearance and garden use, but differ botanically. Many, such as the Carex *species shown here, thrive in or close to water. Some rushes also flourish in damp or dry shade.*

THE A-Z PLANT DIRECTORY

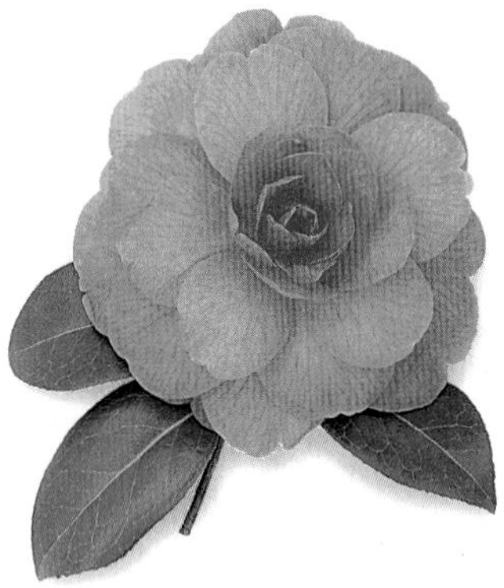

A

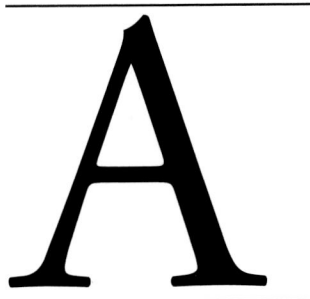

▷ **Aaron's beard** see *Hypericum calycinum*
▷ **Aaron's rod** see *Solidago, Verbascum thapsus*
▷ **Abele** see *Populus alba*

ABELIA

CAPRIFOLIACEAE

Genus of about 30 species of deciduous and evergreen shrubs found on hillsides and in open woodland from the Himalayas to E. Asia, and in Mexico. They are cultivated for their attractive foliage and profusion of flowers. The ovate to rounded leaves are opposite or occasionally in whorls of 3 or 4. Funnel-shaped or tubular flowers are borne in axillary cymes or terminal panicles on the current year's growth in summer and autumn; they have persistent calyces which, in several species, remain attractive after the flowering period. Abelias are ideal for a sunny border. In frost-prone climates, grow less hardy species against a warm, sunny wall.

- **HARDINESS** Frost hardy to half hardy.
- **CULTIVATION** Grow in fertile, well-drained soil in full sun, sheltered from cold, dry winds. Pruning group 1 for deciduous shrubs (group 6, if very vigorous); group 8 for evergreen shrubs.
- **PROPAGATION** Root greenwood cuttings in early summer, or semi-ripe cuttings in late summer.
- **PESTS AND DISEASES** Trouble free.

A. chinensis, syn. *A. rupestris*. Spreading, deciduous shrub with ovate, glossy, dark green leaves, to 4cm (1½in) long. From summer to autumn, bears terminal panicles of fragrant, funnel-shaped, pink-tinged white flowers, 5mm (¼in) long, with 5-lobed pink calyces. ↕ 1.5m (5ft), ↔ 2.5m (8ft). China. ✻✻
***A.* 'Edward Goucher'** 🏆 Semi-evergreen shrub with arching branches and ovate, glossy, dark green leaves, to 5cm (2in) long, bronze when young. Trumpet-shaped, lilac-pink flowers, 2cm (¾in) long, with 2-lobed pink calyces, are borne singly or in small axillary cymes from summer to autumn. ↕ 1.5m (5ft), ↔ 2m (6ft). ✻✻
A. floribunda ■ 🏆 Evergreen shrub with arching shoots and ovate, glossy, dark green leaves, to 5cm (2in) long. Pendent, tubular, bright cerise flowers, 3–5cm (1¼–2in) long, with 5-lobed green calyces, are borne in profuse terminal panicles in early summer. ↕ 3m (10ft), ↔ 4m (12ft) (more if against a wall). Mexico. ✻
A.* x *grandiflora ■ 🏆 (*A. chinensis* x *A. uniflora*), syn. *A. rupestris* of gardens. Vigorous, rounded, evergreen or semi-evergreen shrub with arching branches which produce ovate, glossy, dark green leaves, to 5cm (2in) long. Axillary cymes and terminal panicles of funnel-shaped, fragrant, pink-tinged white flowers, 2cm (¾in) long, with 2- to 5-lobed pink calyces, are borne from midsummer to autumn. ↕ 3m (10ft), ↔ 4m (12ft). Garden origin. ✻✻ (borderline).
'Francis Mason' 🏆 is less vigorous, and has yellow leaves marked with dark green; ↕ 1.5m (5ft), ↔ 2m (6ft).
'Goldsport', syn. 'Gold Strike', has all-yellow foliage.
A. rupestris see *A. chinensis.*
***A. rupestris* of gardens** see *A.* x *grandiflora.*
A. schumannii ■ Deciduous shrub with arching shoots and ovate, mid-green leaves, bronze when young, to 3cm (1¼in) long. Funnel-shaped, slightly scented, orange-marked, lilac-pink flowers, 2.5cm (1in) long, with 2-lobed, pinkish green calyces, are produced singly or in axillary cymes, from late summer to autumn. ↕ 2m (6ft), ↔ 3m (10ft). C. China. ✻✻
A. triflora ■ Large shrub or tree, vigorous and erect in habit, with deeply ridged bark and deciduous, ovate, dark green leaves, to 8cm (3in) long. Small, very fragrant, pink-tinged white flowers, 1.5cm (½in) long, with 5-lobed, bronze-red, narrowly segmented calyces, are produced in threes from the upper leaf axils, in clusters to 5cm (2in) across, in summer. ↕ 5m (15ft) or more, ↔ 3m (10ft). N.W. Himalayas. ✻✻

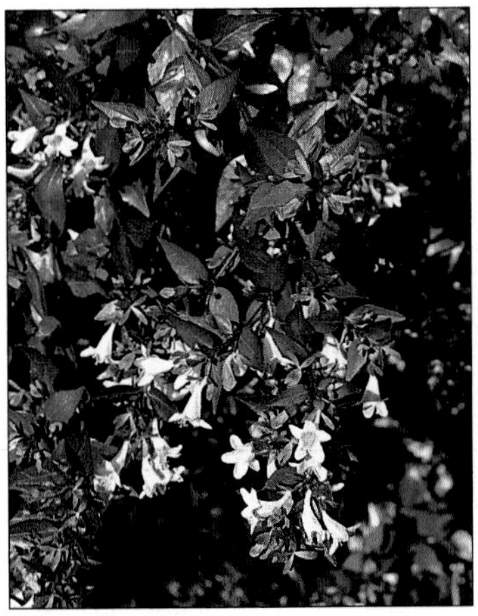
Abelia x *grandiflora*

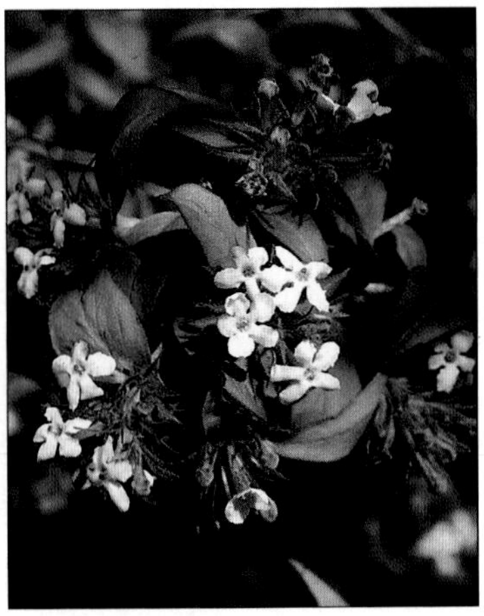
Abelia triflora

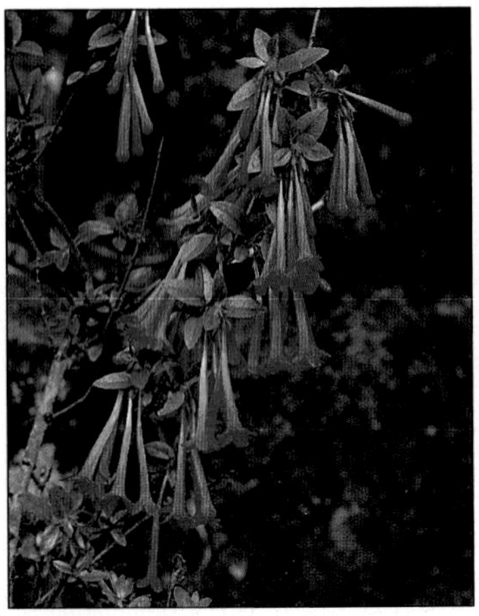
Abelia floribunda

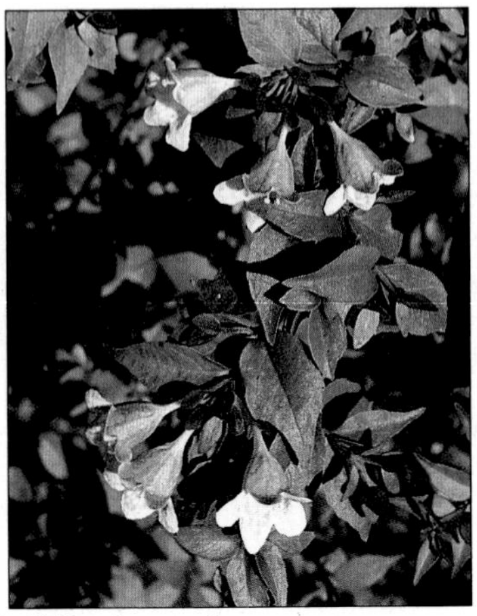
Abelia schumannii

ABELIOPHYLLUM

White forsythia

OLEACEAE

Genus of one species of deciduous shrub occurring on open hillsides in Korea. Related to *Forsythia*, it is cultivated for its fragrant flowers, borne in late winter or spring on the previous year's growth. Grow *A. distichum* in a sunny border or train against a warm wall.

- **HARDINESS** Fully hardy, if wood has adequately ripened in summer. Early flowers may be damaged by late frosts.
- **CULTIVATION** Grow in fertile, well-drained soil in full sun. Pruning group 5, or group 13 if wall-trained.
- **PROPAGATION** Root greenwood or semi-ripe cuttings, or layer, in summer.
- **PESTS AND DISEASES** Trouble free.

A. distichum ■ Open, spreading shrub with opposite, ovate, matt, dark green leaves, to 8cm (3in) long, often turning purple in autumn. Long, axillary racemes of small, cross-shaped, 4-petalled, fragrant white, sometimes pink-tinged flowers, with purple-tinged calyces and stalks, are produced in late winter or early spring. ↕↔ 1.5m (5ft) (taller if against a wall). Korea. ✻✻✻

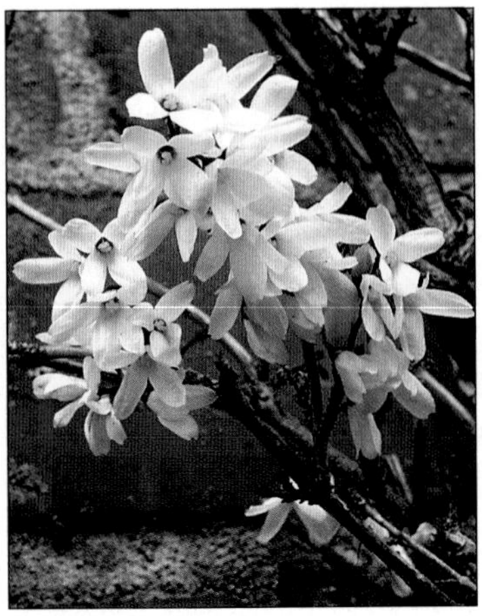
Abeliophyllum distichum

ABELMOSCHUS

MALVACEAE

Genus of 15 species of hairy annuals and perennials from meadows and waste-land in tropical Asia. They are grown mostly for their flowers, although some are tropical crops, grown for their edible pods (okra and gumbo) and leaves. They have large, palmately lobed, toothed leaves, and 5-petalled flowers, usually yellow with purple centres, borne in terminal racemes or singly from the leaf axils. Grow *A. moschatus* as an annual in a mixed border, or in summer bedding.

- **HARDINESS** Frost tender.
- **CULTIVATION** Under glass, grow in loam-based potting compost (JI No.1), in full light. In the growing season, water freely and apply a balanced liquid fertilizer monthly; water more sparingly in winter. Outdoors, grow in fertile, well-drained soil in full sun.
- **PROPAGATION** Sow seed at 10–13°C (50–55°F) in late winter or early spring, or sow *in situ* in mid- or late spring, after any danger of frost has passed.
- **PESTS AND DISEASES** Susceptible to slugs and fungal diseases, including powdery mildew and possibly rust. Red spider mites and whiteflies may be a problem under glass.

A. moschatus, syn. *Hibiscus abelmoschus* (Musk mallow). Bushy perennial, often grown as an annual, with broadly ovate, 3- to 7-lobed, coarsely hairy leaves, to 45cm (18in) long. Hibiscus-like flowers, to 10cm (4in) across, usually yellow with purple centres, sometimes pink or red with white centres, are borne singly or in terminal racemes from midsummer to autumn, followed by musk-scented seeds. ↕ 1.5m (5ft), ↔ 45cm (18in). Tropical Asia. ❀ (min. 5°C/41°F)

ABIES

Silver fir

PINACEAE

Genus of about 50 species of evergreen conifers from Europe, N. Africa, Asia, and North America, dominating northern and mountainous regions. The whorled branches bear linear, flattened, sometimes glossy, mid- to dark green leaves, often with 2 longitudinal silver bands beneath. The female cones are often purplish blue, erect, with occasionally protruding bracts, and are produced on the upper branches in late spring and early summer. After ripening in autumn, they break up to release the seeds, leaving the central stalk on the shoot. Male cones are pendent, green when young, usually purple, purplish blue, or brown when mature, and are borne throughout the crown. In the descriptions below, all the cones are female. Silver firs provide good shelter and screening, and also make fine specimen trees.

- **HARDINESS** Fully hardy, although frost may damage new foliage.
- **CULTIVATION** Grow in fertile, moist but well-drained, neutral to slightly acid

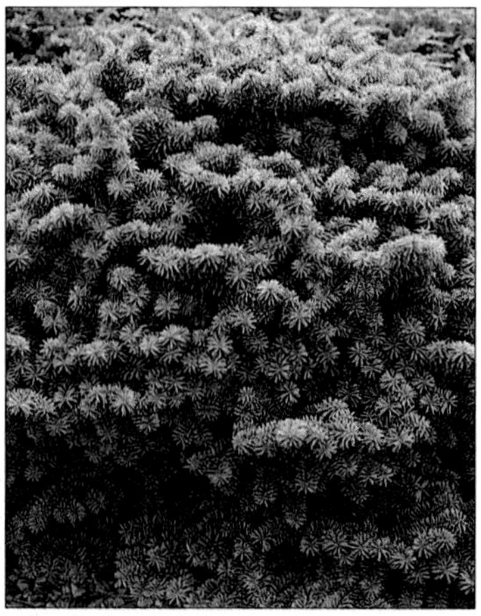
Abies balsamea 'Nana'

soil in full sun, with some shelter from cold winds. Most are shade tolerant, especially when young. *A. amabilis* prefers acid soil; *A. pinsapo* and *A. vejarii* tolerate alkaline and drier soils.
• **PROPAGATION** Sow seed in containers in a cold frame as soon as ripe or in late winter; stratify for 21 days to aid germination. Graft cultivars in winter.
• **PESTS AND DISEASES** Prone to adelgids and honey fungus.

A. alba ◊ syn. *A. pectinata* (European silver fir, Silver fir). Columnar tree with dark green leaves, silver beneath, to 2.5cm (1in) long, arranged on the shoots in a V-shape. Cylindrical cones are yellow-green ripening to brown, 10–15cm (4–6in) long, with protruding bracts. ↕ 25–45m (80–150ft), ↔ 4–6m (12–20ft). Mountains of C. and S.E. Europe. ❄❄❄
A. amabilis ◊ (Beautiful fir, Pacific fir). Conical tree with shoots covered in pale hairs, and with small, spherical, resinous buds. Square-tipped, dark green leaves, silvery white beneath, 2–3cm (¾–1¼in) long, are densely borne on the upper surface of each shoot in neat, forward-pointing rows. Ovoid-cylindrical purple cones, 9–15cm (3½–6in) long, have hidden bracts. Grows best in cool, moist climates in acid soil. ↕ 20–30m (70–100ft), ↔ 4–6m (12–20ft). USA (S. Alaska to N. California). ❄❄❄
A. balsamea ◊ (Balsam fir). Conical tree with smooth grey bark interspersed with fragrant resin blisters. Dark green leaves, whitish green beneath, and 1.5–2.5cm (½–1in) long, are semi-erect, forward pointing, and densely arranged on the shoots in a V-shape. Oblong-cylindrical, purplish blue cones, 5–8cm (2–3in) long, have hidden bracts. Needs a moist site. ↕ to 15m (50ft), ↔ to 5m (15ft). C. and E. Canada, N.E. USA. ❄❄❄. **f. *hudsonia*** 🏆◊ is a dwarf, irregularly rounded variant, with leaves to 1.5cm (½in) long, and no cones; ↕ to 60cm (24in), ↔ 1m (3ft). **'Nana'** ▣◊ is rounded, with short leaves, 4–10mm (⅛–½in) long, arranged radially around the shoots; ↕↔ 1m (3ft).
A. bracteata ◊ syn. *A. venusta* (Bristle-cone fir, Santa Lucia fir). Columnar tree with distinctive spindle-shaped, pointed, non-resinous buds. Sharp-pointed, glossy, dark green leaves, silvery green beneath, to 5cm (2in) long, spread either side of each shoot in 3 or 4 ranks. Ovoid, golden brown cones, 8cm (3in) long, have large, protruding bracts, with long, narrow, reflexed points, and often exude resin. ↕ 25m (80ft), ↔ to 6m (20ft). USA (Santa Lucia Mountains, California). ❄❄❄
A. cephalonica ◊ (Greek fir). Conical tree with a spreading crown in old age. Stiff, glossy, dark green leaves, greenish white beneath, 2–3cm (¾–1¼in) long, are arranged radially around each shoot, with a rounded, sucker-like pad at each leaf base. Cylindrical, tapering, resinous, green-brown cones, 10–16cm (4–6in) long, have protruding, reflexed bracts, and nipple-like apexes. ↕ to 30m (100ft), ↔ 5–8m (15–25ft). C. and S. Greece. ❄❄❄. **'Meyer's Dwarf'** ▣◊ syn. 'Nana', produces short leaves, 0.8–1.5cm (⅜–½in) long, and forms a low, spreading mound; ↕ 50cm (20in), ↔ 1–3m (3–10ft).

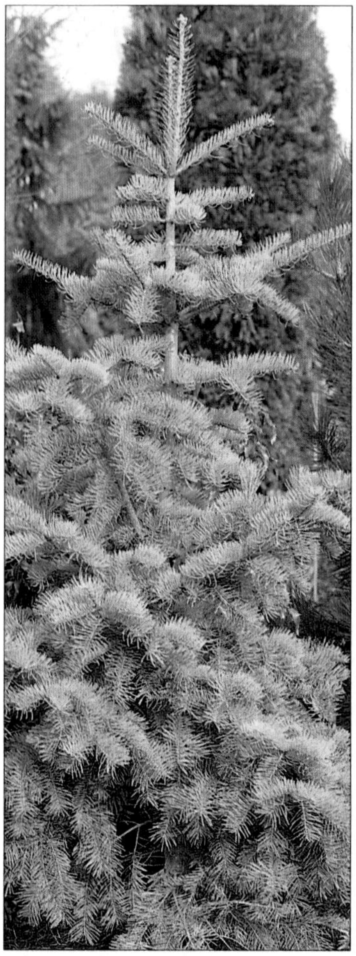
Abies concolor 'Argentea'

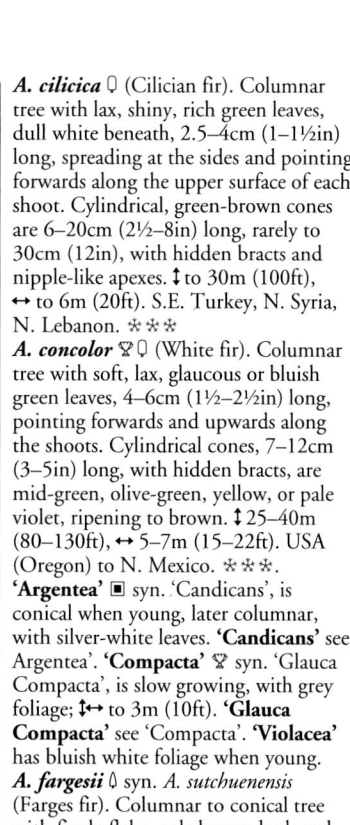

A. cilicica ◊ (Cilician fir). Columnar tree with lax, shiny, rich green leaves, dull white beneath, 2.5–4cm (1–1½in) long, spreading at the sides and pointing forwards along the upper surface of each shoot. Cylindrical, green-brown cones are 6–20cm (2½–8in) long, rarely to 30cm (12in), with hidden bracts and nipple-like apexes. ↕ to 30m (100ft), ↔ to 6m (20ft). S.E. Turkey, N. Syria, N. Lebanon. ❄❄❄
A. concolor 🏆◊ (White fir). Columnar tree with soft, lax, glaucous or bluish green leaves, 4–6cm (1½–2½in) long, pointing forwards and upwards along the shoots. Cylindrical cones, 7–12cm (3–5in) long, with hidden bracts, are mid-green, olive-green, yellow, or pale violet, ripening to brown. ↕ 25–40m (80–130ft), ↔ 5–7m (15–22ft). USA (Oregon) to N. Mexico. ❄❄❄. **'Argentea'** ▣ syn. 'Candicans', is conical when young, later columnar, with silver-white leaves. **'Candicans'** see Argentea'. **'Compacta'** 🏆 syn. 'Glauca Compacta', is slow growing, with grey foliage; ↕↔ to 3m (10ft). **'Glauca Compacta'** see 'Compacta'. **'Violacea'** has bluish white foliage when young.
A. fargesii ◊ syn. *A. sutchuenensis* (Farges fir). Columnar to conical tree with finely flaky, pale brown bark and deep purple, year-old shoots with conical, resinous purple buds. Shiny, dark green leaves, banded with silver beneath, to 2.5cm (1in) long, spread below and point forwards above each shoot. Ovoid, slightly resinous cones, 5–8cm (2–3in) long, are violet-purple with protruding bracts. ↕ 10–15m (30–50ft), ↔ 3–4m (10–12ft). China (Gansu, Sichuan, Hubei). ❄❄❄
A. forrestii ▣◊ (Forrest fir). Conical tree with an open, whorled habit, becoming denser when old, and smooth, silvery grey bark. Shoots are red-brown, with spherical, resinous white buds. Dark green leaves, silvery white beneath, 2–4cm (¾–1½in) long, are arranged densely and radially around each shoot. Ovoid-cylindrical, violet-blue cones, 8–15cm (3–6in) long, have protruding bracts. ↕ 10–20m (30–70ft), ↔ 3–6m (10–20ft). China (Yunnan). ❄❄❄
A. grandis ▣🏆◊ (Giant fir, Grand fir). Very fast-growing, conical to columnar tree with smooth grey bark, cracked into squares on old trees, and small, conical, resinous buds. Produces soft, shiny, dark green leaves, 3–5cm (1¼–2in) long, with whitish green bands on the reverse, arranged like the teeth of a 2-sided

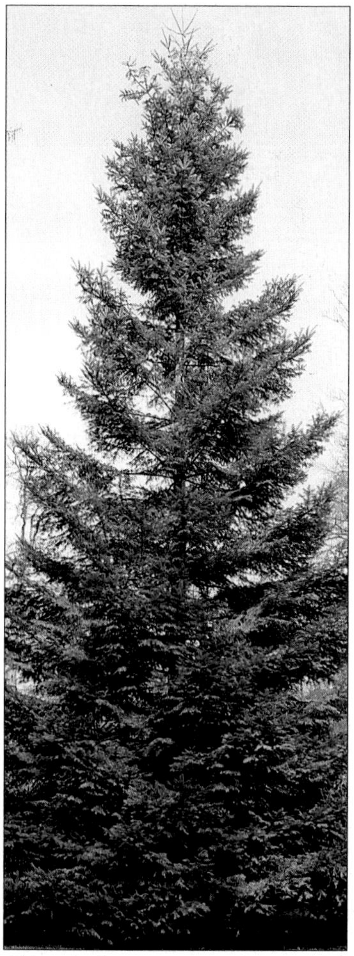
Abies grandis

comb. Cylindrical cones, 5–11cm (2–4½in) long, with hidden bracts, are green, ripening to brown. ↕ 25–60m (80–200ft), ↔ 5–8m (15–25ft). W. North America (British Columbia, Oregon to Idaho). ❄❄❄
A. homolepis ◊ (Nikko fir). Conical tree with tiered branches and deeply ridged shoots. Glaucous green leaves, 1.5–3cm (½–1¼in) long, with silver bands beneath, are arranged on the shoots like the teeth of a 2-sided comb. Cylindrical, violet-blue cones, 7–12cm (3–5in) long, have hidden bracts. ↕ to 25m (80ft), ↔ 5–8m (15–25ft). S. Japan. ❄❄❄
A. koreana ▣◊ (Korean fir). Small, conical tree with shiny, dark green leaves, silver beneath, 1–2cm (½–¾in) long, arranged radially but mainly on the upper surface of each shoot. From

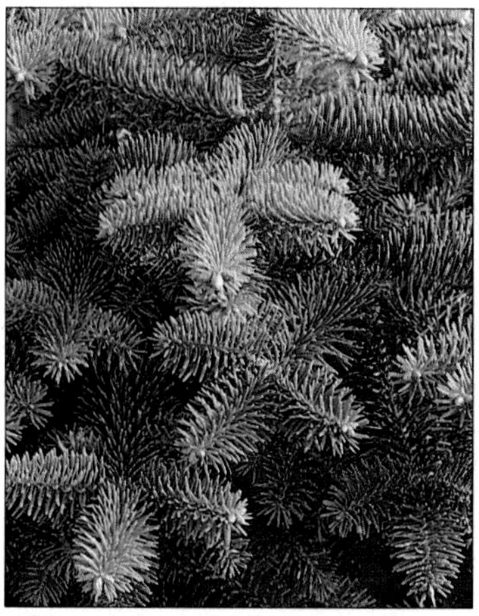
Abies cephalonica 'Meyer's Dwarf'

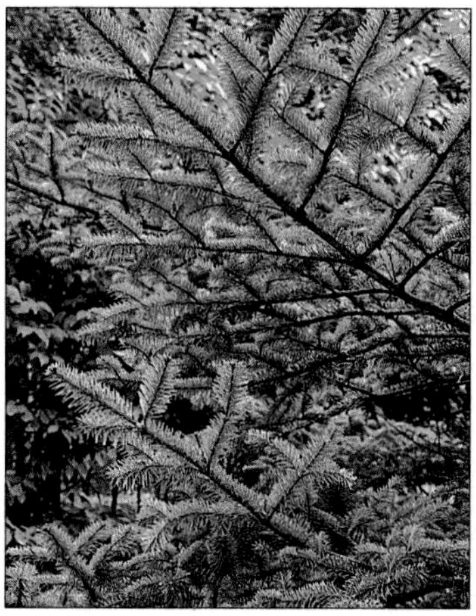
Abies forrestii

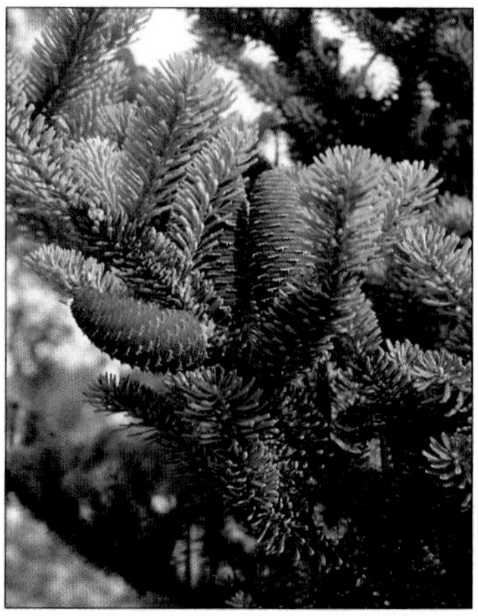
Abies koreana

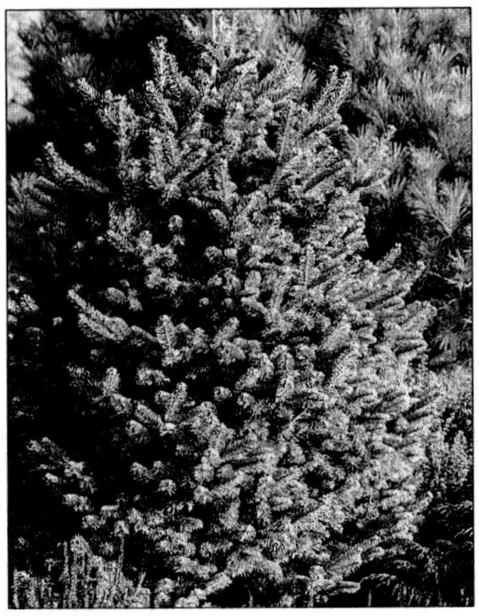

Abies lasiocarpa var. *arizonica* 'Compacta'

a young age, produces cylindrical, violet-blue cones, 5–7cm (2–3in) long, with either hidden or protruding bracts. ↕ 10m (30ft), ↔ to 6m (20ft). S. Korea. ✻✻✻. **'Silberlocke'** 🏆 has leaves that twist above the fawn-coloured shoots to reveal the silver undersides.

A. lasiocarpa ◊ Small, narrowly pyramidal tree with corky bark. Densely arranged but spreading, 2-ranked, grey-green leaves, 1.5–3.5cm (½–1½in) long, have a waxy coating. Oblong-cylindrical cones, 8–10cm (3–4in) long, with hidden bracts, are dark purple, ripening to brown. ↕ to 10m (30ft), ↔ 3–4m (10–12ft). North America (Alaska to Oregon, Wyoming to N. Colorado). ✻✻✻. **var. *arizonica*** (Corkbark fir) has thicker, soft bark, silvery grey leaves,

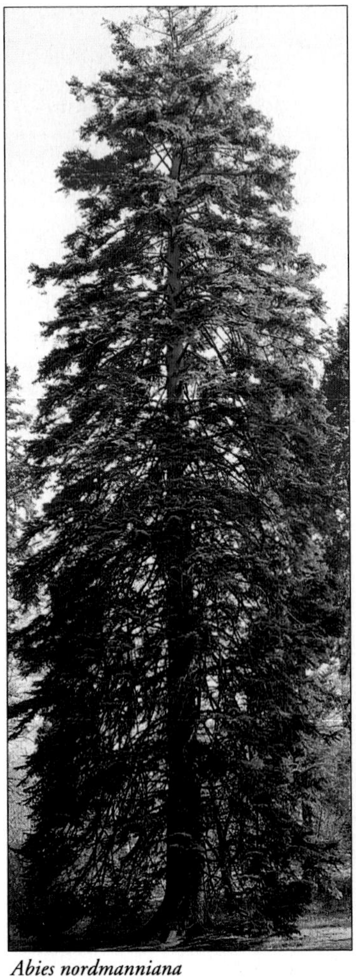

Abies nordmanniana

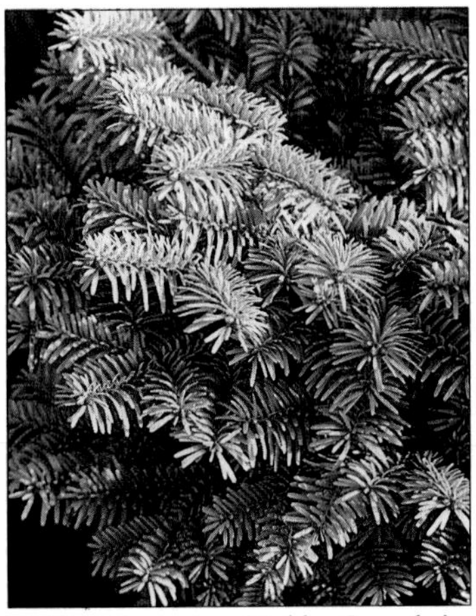

Abies nordmanniana 'Golden Spreader'

2.5–3.5cm (1–1½in) long, and cones 6–8cm (2½–3in) long; USA (Arizona, New Mexico). **var. *arizonica* 'Compacta'** ▣ 🏆 is slow growing, forming a conical to oval tree with blue-grey leaves; ↕ 3–5m (10–15ft), ↔ 2–3m (6–10ft). **'Roger Watson'** is a slow-growing dwarf cultivar, with grey-green leaves, reaching its full height after about 10 years; ↕↔ to 90cm (36in).

A. magnifica ◊ (California red fir). Columnar tree with a narrow crown and stout trunk. Leaves, 4–5cm (1½–2in) long, grey-green to bright blue-grey above, inconspicuously grey-banded beneath, lie flat along the upper surfaces of the shoots and are arranged like the teeth of a comb beneath. Barrel-shaped, golden green cones, 18–25cm (7–10in)

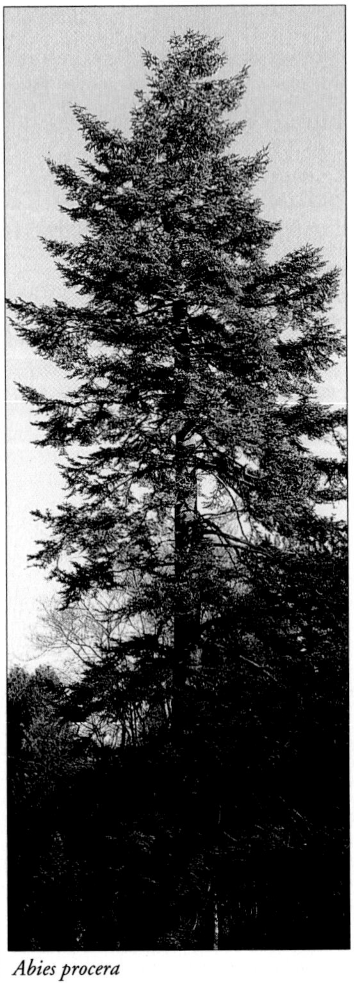

Abies procera

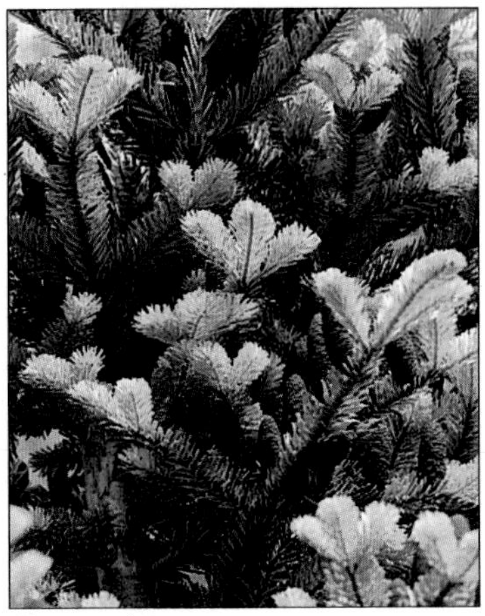

Abies veitchii

long, have concealed bracts. ↕ 25–35m (80–120ft), ↔ 5–6m (15–20ft). USA (S. Oregon to N. California). ✻✻✻

A. nobilis see *A. procera.*

A. nordmanniana ▣ 🏆 ◊–◊ (Caucasian fir, Nordmann fir). Columnar tree with tiered branches. Densely arranged, glossy, rich green leaves, dull white beneath, 2–3cm (¾–1¼in) long, point forwards and overlap above on each shoot. Ovoid-cylindrical, greenish brown cones, to 15cm (6in) long, have protruding bracts. ↕ to 40m (130ft), ↔ to 6m (20ft). Caucasus, N. Turkey. ✻✻✻. **'Golden Spreader'** ▣ 🏆 ◊ is slow-growing, and usually dwarf, with spreading branches and bright golden yellow leaves, pale yellowish white beneath; ↕ to 1m (3ft), ↔ to 1.5m (5ft), but occasionally forms a small tree.

A. pectinata see *A. alba.*

A. pinsapo ◊ (Hedgehog fir, Spanish fir). Tree with a conical crown, later becoming untidy. Rigid, dark green to glaucous, grey-blue leaves, 1–2cm (½–¾in) long, are arranged radially around each shoot. Cylindrical cones, 10–15cm (4–6in) long, with hidden bracts, are green, ripening to brown. ↕ to 25m (80ft), ↔ 5–8m (15–25ft). S. Spain. ✻✻✻. **'Glauca'** 🏆 has striking, glaucous, grey-blue leaves.

A. procera ▣ 🏆 ◊ syn. *A. nobilis* (Noble fir). Conical tree, later becoming broad and columnar, with whorled branches when young, and silvery grey bark. Grey-green to bright blue-grey leaves, 1–3.5cm (½–1½in) long, with narrow grey bands beneath, lie flat along the upper surfaces of the shoots, and are 2-ranked and slightly downward-curving below. Cylindrical, green and brown cones, 15–25cm (6–10in) long, with protruding, reflexed bracts, are borne on the uppermost branches when the tree is 6m (20ft) or more tall. ↕ 25–45m (80–150ft), ↔ 6–9m (20–28ft). USA (Oregon, Washington). ✻✻✻. **'Glauca'** has glaucous, bright blue foliage and forms a tall tree or, if no leader develops, a spreading shrub.

A. sutchuenensis see *A. fargesii.*

A. veitchii ▣ 🏆 ◊ (Veitch fir). Fast-growing, conical tree with soft, densely arranged, glossy, dark green leaves, to 3cm (1¼in) long, which curve upwards and are silver on the reverse. Cylindrical, bright grey-blue cones, 5–7cm (2–3in) long, bear either protruding or hidden bracts. ↕ 15–20m (50–70ft), ↔ 4–6m (12–20ft). Japan. ✻✻✻

A. vejarii ◊ (Vejar fir). Conical tree with olive-green shoots and forward- and upward-pointing, grey-green or glaucous leaves, grey-banded on the reverse, 2–2.5cm (¾–1in) long. Produces cylindrical or ovoid violet cones, 6–15cm (2½–6in) long, which have protruding bracts. Very drought tolerant. ↕ 10–20m (30–70ft), ↔ 3–5m (10–15ft). N.E. Mexico. ✻✻✻

A. venusta see *A. bracteata.*

ABROMEITIELLA

BROMELIACEAE

Genus of 2 or 3 species of low, mound-forming, terrestrial, evergreen perennials (bromeliads) occurring in dry, rocky sites in the Andes of Bolivia and Argentina. They form large mats or cushions of numerous small, dense rosettes of triangular, succulent, greyish green leaves, with spiny margins and tips. Short-branched inflorescences, made up of groups of 3 greenish yellow or green flowers with twisted petals, develop from the centres of the rosettes in summer, and are followed by dull, greyish green berries. Where temperatures fall below 5°C (41°F), grow in a cool or temperate greenhouse, or as houseplants; in warmer areas, they are excellent for a border.

- **HARDINESS** Frost tender.
- **CULTIVATION** Under glass, grow in terrestrial bromeliad compost in full light. Keep almost dry in winter; water moderately at all other times of the year. Excess water may cause rotting at temperatures below 5°C (41°F). Apply a low-nitrogen liquid fertilizer every 3–4 weeks from mid-spring to late autumn. Outdoors, grow in moderately fertile, lime-free, well-drained soil in full sun. See also p.47.
- **PROPAGATION** Sow seed at 27°C (81°F) in spring. Detach and root rosettes in spring and summer.
- **PESTS AND DISEASES** Mealybugs may be a problem at flowering time.

A. brevifolia ▣ 🏆 syn. *A. chlorantha.* Terrestrial bromeliad with narrowly triangular, densely arranged leaves, 2cm (¾in) long, toothed only at the bases, and with sharp-pointed tips. Cylindrical green flowers, 3cm (1¼in) long, with a white basal scale to each petal, are produced in summer. ↕ 15cm (6in) or more, ↔ indefinite. S.W. Bolivia, N.W. Argentina. ❀ (min. 5°C/41°F)

A. chlorantha see *A. brevifolia.*

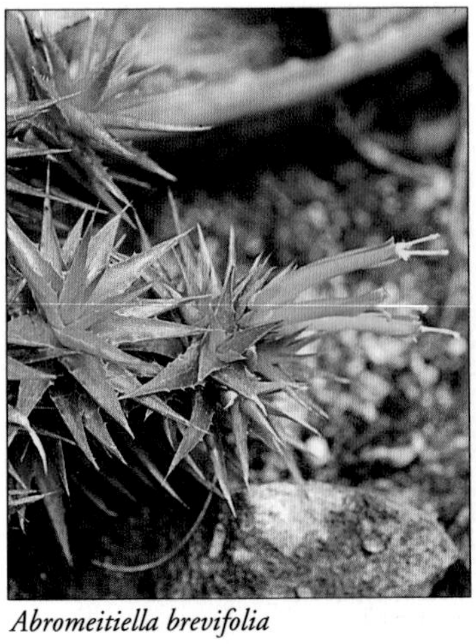

Abromeitiella brevifolia

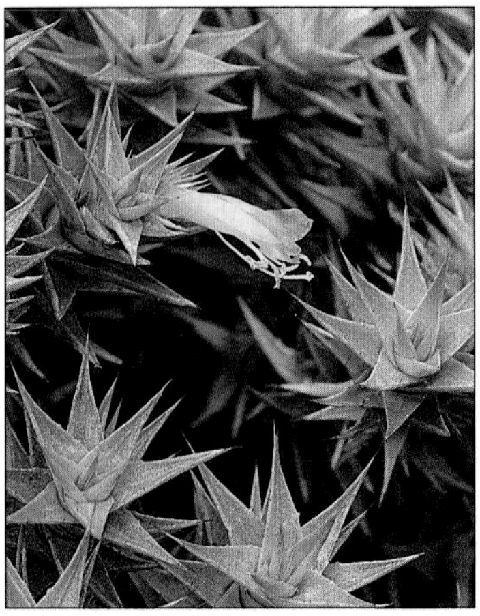

Abromeitiella lorentziana

A. lorentziana ▣ Terrestrial bromeliad with triangular, spine-tipped, greyish green leaves, 4–15cm (1½–6in) long. In summer, bears long-tubed yellow, green-tipped flowers, to 3.5cm (1½in long). Very similar to *A. brevifolia*, but with leaves that are more spiny, and with a white-fringed basal scale to each petal. ↕24cm (10in) or more, ↔ indefinite. N.W. Argentina. ⊛ (min. 5°C/41°F)

▷**Absinth** see *Artemisia absinthium*

ABUTILON

Flowering maple, Indian mallow, Parlour maple

MALVACEAE

Genus of about 150 species of evergreen and deciduous shrubs, small trees, perennials, and annuals from tropical and subtropical regions of Africa, Asia, Australia, and North and South America. The leaves vary from simple to palmately 3- to 7-lobed. Abutilons are cultivated for their showy, mostly bell-, cup-, or bowl-shaped axillary flowers, some with highly coloured calyces and stamens. The flowers are usually solitary and pendent, occasionally borne in racemes or panicles, and often produced continuously from spring to autumn. Some abutilons also have attractive variegated foliage. In frost-prone areas, grow tender and half-hardy abutilons in a conservatory or cool or temperate greenhouse, or as houseplants; half-hardy species are also suitable for bedding in a sunny, sheltered border; train frost-hardy species of arching habit against a warm wall. In frost-free areas, grow abutilons in a shrub border.

• **HARDINESS** Frost hardy to frost tender.

• **CULTIVATION** Under glass, grow in loam-based potting compost (JI No.2) in full light. In the growing season, water freely and apply a balanced liquid fertilizer monthly; water sparingly in winter. Outdoors, grow in moderately fertile, well-drained soil in full sun. Pruning group 1 or 6, as required, for deciduous shrubs; group 9 for evergreens. Pruning group 13 for wall-trained abutilons.

• **PROPAGATION** Sow seed at 15–18°C (59–64°F) in spring. Root softwood cuttings in spring, or greenwood cuttings in summer.

• **PESTS AND DISEASES** Whiteflies, red spider mites, mealybugs, and scale insects may be a problem, particularly under glass.

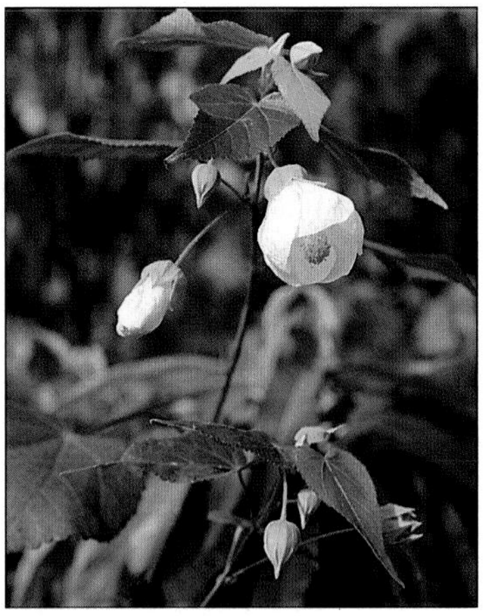

Abutilon 'Boule de Neige'

***A.* 'Ashford Red'** ♀ ⚲ Erect to spreading, evergreen shrub or small tree with broadly ovate to rounded, 3- to 5-lobed, pale to mid-green leaves, 10–20cm (4–8in) long. Bears nodding to pendent, bell-shaped red flowers, 6–8cm (2½–3in) long, from spring to autumn. ↕↔ to 3m (10ft). ❄

***A.* 'Boule de Neige'** ▣ ⚲ Vigorous, evergreen shrub or small tree, of erect to spreading habit, with broadly ovate to rounded, 3- to 5-lobed, mid-green leaves, 10–20cm (4–8in) long. From spring to autumn, bears pendent, bell-shaped white flowers, 6–8cm (2½–3in) long. ↕ to 4m (12ft), ↔ to 3m (10ft). ❄

***A.* 'Canary Bird'** ♀ ⚲ Erect to spreading, evergreen shrub or small tree with broadly ovate to rounded, 3- to 5-lobed, mid-green leaves, 10–20cm (4–8in) long. From spring to autumn, produces pendent, bell-shaped, lemon-yellow flowers, 6–8cm (2½–3in) long. ↕↔ to 3m (10ft). ❄

***A. globosum* of gardens** see *A.* x *hybridum.*

A.* x *hybridum ⚲ (*A. darwinii* x *A. pictum* and other species) syn. *A. globosum* of gardens. Erect to spreading, evergreen shrub or small tree with ovate to rounded, 3- to 5-lobed, pale to mid-green leaves, 10–20cm (4–8in) long, which may be variegated. Bears pendent, bowl- or bell-shaped, white, yellow, red, or orange flowers, 5–8cm (2–3in) long, from spring to autumn. ↕ to 5m (15ft), ↔ 2–5m (6–15ft). Garden origin. ❄

***A.* 'Kentish Belle'** ▣ ♀ Evergreen or semi-evergreen shrub with slender, arching, dark purple-brown shoots and narrowly ovate, shallowly lobed, dark green leaves, to 4cm (1½in) long. Pendent, bell-shaped flowers, 6–8cm (2½–3in) long, with apricot-yellow petals and purple stamens, protruding from red calyces, are produced along the young shoots from summer to autumn. ↕↔ to 2.5m (8ft). ❄❄

***A.* 'Louis Marignac'** ⚲ syn. *A.* 'Louise de Marignac'. Evergreen shrub or small tree, of erect to spreading habit, with ovate to rounded, 3- to 5-lobed, pale to mid-green leaves, 10–20cm (4–8in) long. Distinctive, pendent, bell-shaped, pale pink flowers, 6–8cm (2½–3in) long, are borne from spring to autumn. ↕↔ to 3m (10ft). ❄

***A.* 'Louise de Marignac'** see *A.* 'Louis Marignac'.

A. megapotamicum ▣ ♀ (Trailing abutilon). Evergreen or semi-evergreen shrub with slender, arching shoots and

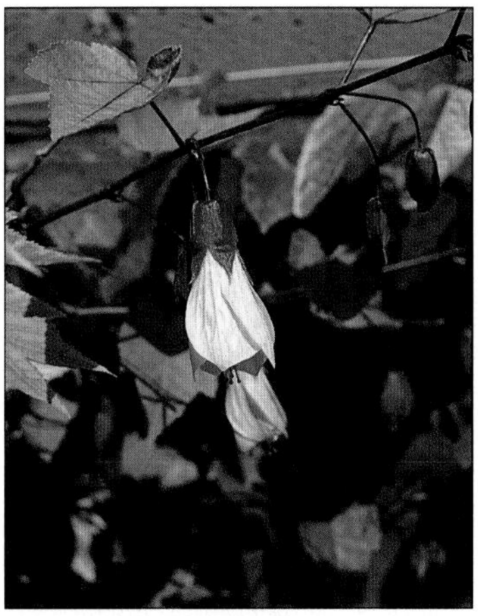

Abutilon 'Kentish Belle'

lance-shaped to ovate, bright green leaves, to 12cm (5in) long, sometimes shallowly lobed, and heart-shaped at the bases. Pendent, bell-shaped flowers, to 4cm (1½in) long, with yellow petals and purple stamens, protruding from red calyces, are borne along the young shoots from summer to autumn. ↕↔ 2m (6ft). Brazil. ❄❄. **'Variegatum'** has leaves heavily mottled yellow.

A.* x *milleri ♀ (*A. megapotamicum* x *A. pictum*). Evergreen shrub with thin, arching shoots and narrowly ovate, bright green leaves, to 12cm (5in) long, with 3 long-pointed lobes. Pendent, bell-shaped flowers, to 4cm (1½in) long, with dusky pink calyces surrounding petals of dark apricot, flushed dark red inside the bases, are borne along the young shoots from summer to autumn. ↕↔ 2.5m (8ft). Garden origin. ❄❄

***A.* 'Nabob'** ♀ ⚲ Erect to spreading, evergreen shrub or small tree. Leaves are ovate to rounded, 3- to 5-lobed, 10–20cm (4–8in) long, and rich green in colour. From spring to autumn, bears large, nodding to pendent, open bowl-shaped, deep crimson flowers, to 7cm (3in) across. ↕↔ to 3m (10ft). ❄

A. ochsenii. Fast-growing, upright, deciduous shrub, sometimes tree-like, with stout, grey-felted shoots and ovate, 3- to 5-lobed, dark green leaves, to 15cm (6in) long. Pendent, cup-shaped, violet-blue flowers, to 6cm (2½in) across, are borne on long stalks in late spring and early summer. ↕3m (10ft), ↔ 2.5m (8ft). Chile. ❄❄

***A.* 'Patrick Synge'** ⚲ Very vigorous, evergreen shrub or small tree, of erect to spreading habit, bearing ovate to rounded, 3- to 5-lobed, pale to mid-green leaves, 10–20cm (4–8in) long. Bears pendent, open bowl-shaped flowers, to 7cm (3in) across, with slightly reflexed, flame-red petals, from spring to autumn. ↕↔ to 3m (10ft). ❄

A. pictum ⚲ syn. *A. striatum* of gardens. Evergreen shrub or small tree, erect at first, then spreading, with ovate to rounded, 3- to 5-lobed, mid- to deep green leaves, to 15cm (6in) long. From spring to autumn, bears pendent, bell-shaped, yellow to orange flowers, 6cm (2½in) long, with dark red veins. ↕5m (15ft), ↔ 2–5m (6–15ft). Brazil. ❄. **'Thompsonii'** ▣ ⚲ is erect, with 5- to 9-lobed leaves, mottled with yellow, and orange-flushed, salmon-pink flowers.

***A.* 'Souvenir de Bonn'** ▣ ♀ ⚲ Vigorous, erect, evergreen shrub or small tree with ovate to rounded, 3- to 5-lobed, pale to mid-green leaves, 10–20cm (4–8in) long, margined and occasionally mottled creamy white. From spring to autumn, bears pendent, bowl-shaped flowers, to 7cm (3in) across, soft orange with darker veins. ↕ to 3m (10ft), ↔ 2–3m (6–10ft). ❄

***A. striatum* of gardens** see *A. pictum.*

A.* x *suntense (*A. ochsenii* x *A. vitifolium*). Fast-growing, upright, deciduous shrub with stout, grey-felted shoots and narrowly ovate, 3- to 5-lobed, grey-green leaves, to 12cm (5in) long, with toothed margins. In late spring and early summer, bears long-stalked, pendent, saucer-shaped, white to dark violet-blue flowers, to 6cm (2½in) across. ↕4m (12ft), ↔ 2.5m (8ft). Garden origin. ❄❄. **'Geoffrey Gorer'** has sprays of purple-blue flowers.

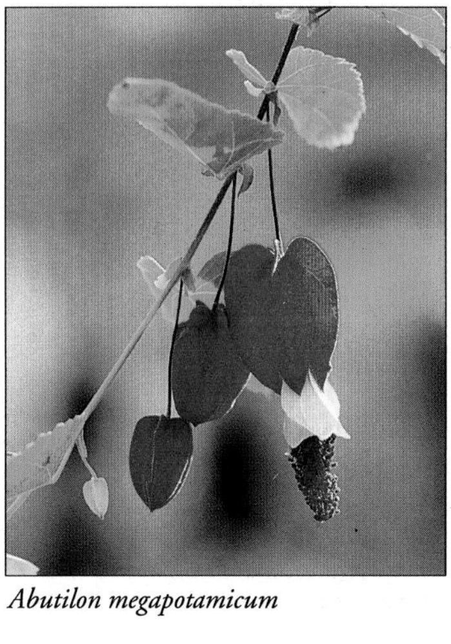

Abutilon megapotamicum

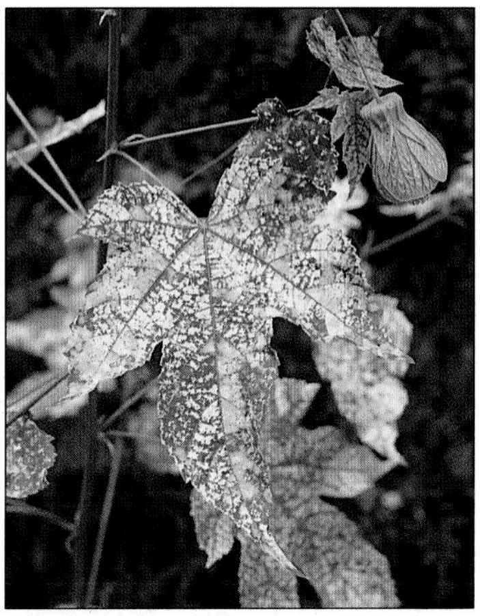

Abutilon pictum 'Thompsonii'

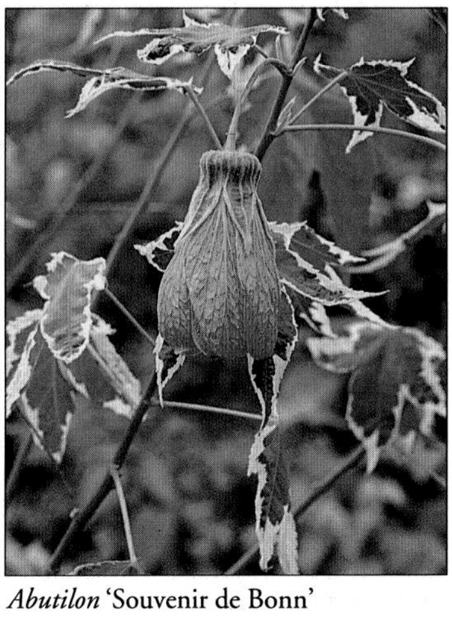

Abutilon 'Souvenir de Bonn'

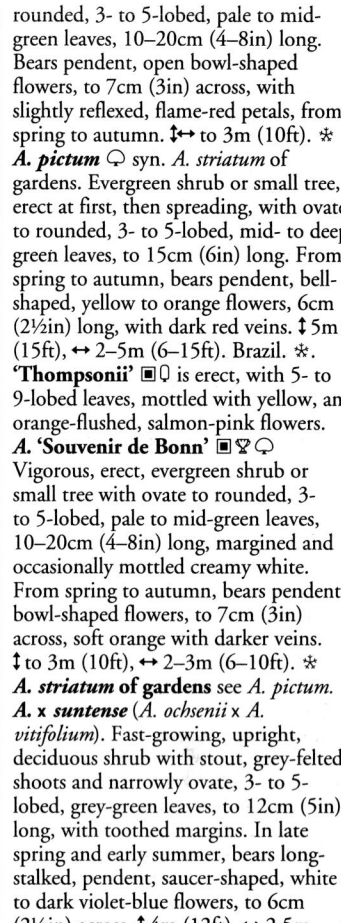

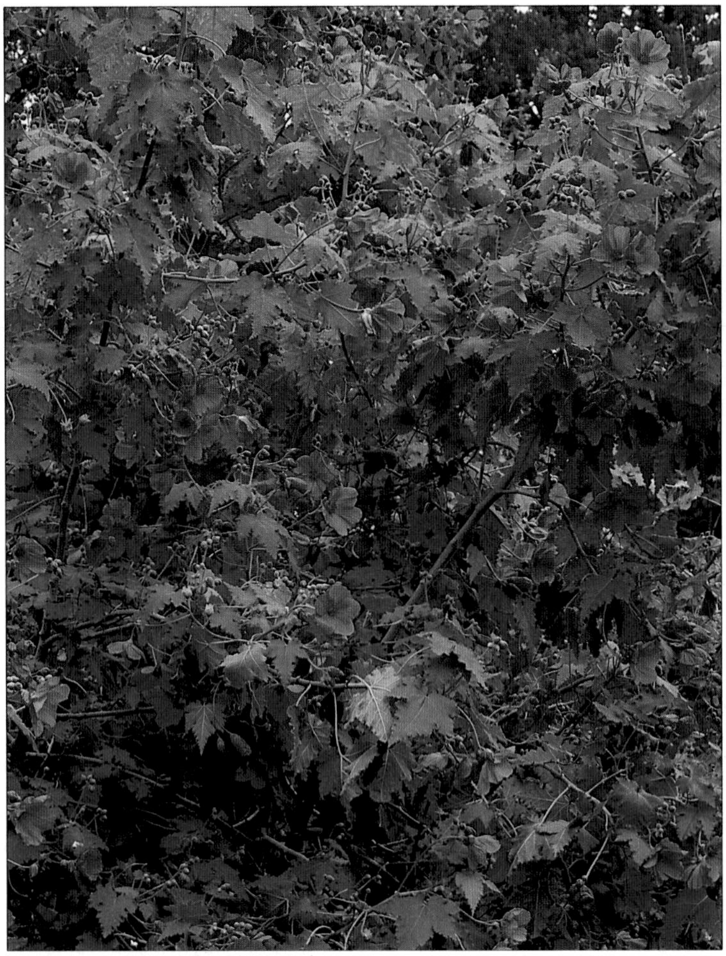
Abutilon x *suntense* 'Ralph Gould'

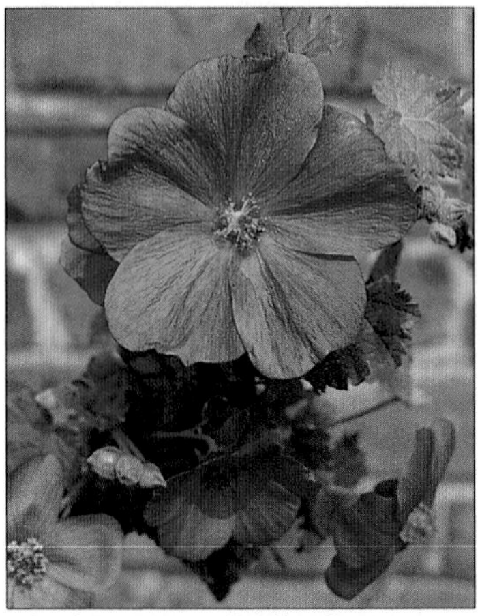
Abutilon x *suntense* 'Violetta'

'Gorer's White' has pure white flowers. **'Ralph Gould'** ▣ bears larger, flatter flowers, to 8cm (3in) wide. **'Violetta'** ▣ bears abundant dark violet-blue flowers.
A. vitifolium. Fast-growing, upright, deciduous shrub, sometimes tree-like, with stout, grey-felted shoots, and ovate, shallowly 3- to 5-lobed, toothed, softly grey-hairy leaves, to 15cm (6in) long. Bears long-stalked, pendent, saucer-shaped, white to purple-blue flowers, to 8cm (3in) across, with long stamens, in early summer. ↕5m (15ft), ↔ 2.5m (8ft). Chile. ✻✻. **var. *album*** ▣ has white flowers. **'Veronica Tennant'** ▣ 𝕐 bears profuse, mauve flowers, to 9cm (3½in) across.

▷**Abutilon, Trailing** see *Abutilon megapotamicum*

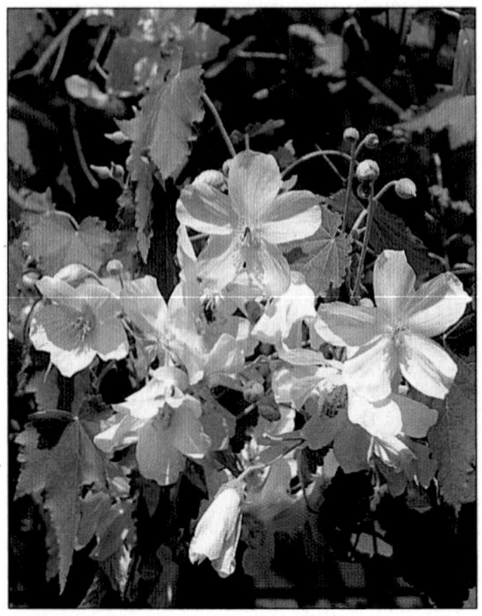
Abutilon vitifolium var. *album*

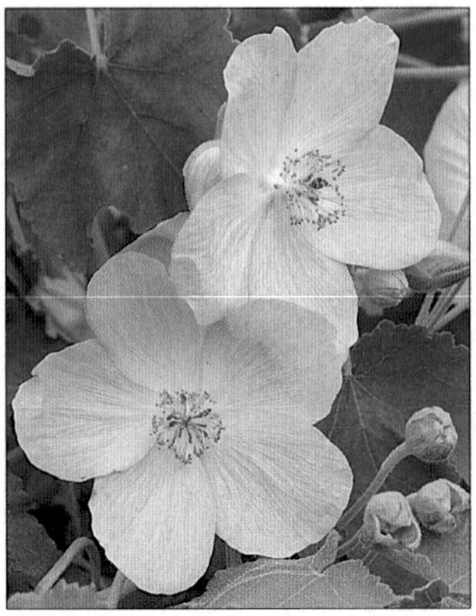
Abutilon vitifolium 'Veronica Tennant'

ACACIA

Wattle

LEGUMINOSAE / MIMOSACEAE

Genus of at least 1,100 species of deciduous and evergreen trees, shrubs, and climbers, cultivated mainly for their flowers, and sometimes foliage. Acacias are found in tropical to warm-temperate regions of Central and South America, Kenya, southern Africa, Polynesia, and Australia. Leaves are alternate and 1- or 2-pinnate, or may be reduced to flattened leaf-stalks known as phyllodes, mostly lance-shaped to ovate and entire. Tiny flowers, often sweetly scented, with 4 or 5 minute petals and long stamens, form either spherical heads, 5–10mm (¼–½in) across, in racemes or panicles, or are borne in short, cylindrical spikes, 1–8cm (½–3in) long. They are usually produced in winter or spring. These are followed by varyingly shaped seed pods, mostly green, sometimes flushed with red or purple. In frost-prone areas, grow tender species in a cool or cold greenhouse and half-hardy species against a warm wall outdoors; in frost-free areas, grow in a border, or as specimen plants.

• **HARDINESS** Half hardy to frost tender.

• **CULTIVATION** Under glass, grow in loam-based potting compost (JI No.2) in full light. In the growing season, water freely and apply a balanced liquid fertilizer monthly; water sparingly in winter. Outdoors, grow in moderately fertile, neutral to acid soil in a sheltered site in full sun. Pruning group 1 for deciduous acacias; group 8 for evergreen acacias; and group 13 for wall-trained plants. Most acacias resent hard pruning.

• **PROPAGATION** Sow seed in spring at not less than 18°C (64°F), after soaking in warm water until swollen. Root semi-ripe cuttings in summer.

• **PESTS AND DISEASES** Red spider mites may be a problem under glass.

A. armata see *A. paradoxa.*
A. baileyana ▣ 𝕐 ⚲ (Cootamundra wattle). Small tree or large shrub with spreading, dense branches and fern-like, 2-pinnate, evergreen, silvery grey leaves, to 5cm (2in) long, composed of 16–40 tiny, linear leaflets. Spherical, bright yellow flowerheads, 5mm (¼in) across, open in dense axillary racemes, 7–10cm (3–4in) long, from winter to spring. ↕5–8m (15–25ft), ↔ 3–6m (10–20ft). Australia (New South Wales). ✻

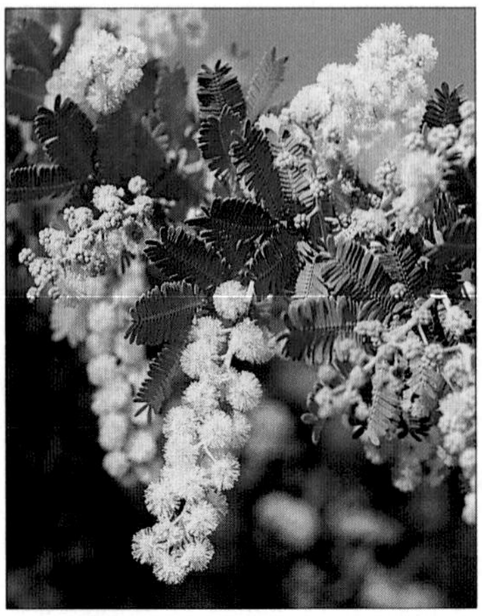
Acacia baileyana

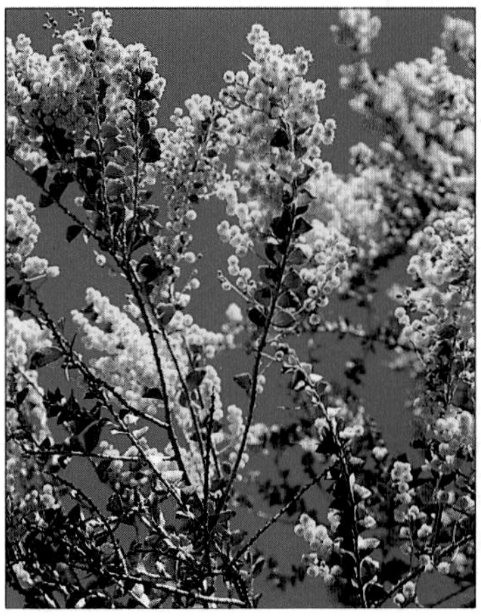
Acacia cultriformis

A. cultriformis ▣ (Knife-leaf wattle). Erect, evergreen shrub, becoming bushy and spreading with age. Bluish green phyllodes are 1–2.5cm (½–1in) long, and lopsidedly oval to triangular. In spring, bears spherical, bright yellow flowerheads, 5mm (¼in) across, in axillary racemes, 4–8cm (1½–3in) long, which are crowded towards the tips of the stems. ↕↔ 2–4m (6–12ft). Australia (Queensland to New South Wales). ✻
A. dealbata ▣ 𝕐 ⚲ (Mimosa, Silver wattle). Open, evergreen tree with fern-like, 2-pinnate, hairy leaves, 12cm (5in) long, each with 40–80 linear, glaucous to silvery leaflets. Terminal racemes, 10–20cm (4–8in) long, of spherical, fragrant yellow flowerheads, 5mm (¼in) across, are borne from winter to spring. ↕15–30m (50–100ft), ↔ 6–10m (20–30ft). Australia (New South Wales to Tasmania). ✻
A. decurrens ⚲ (Early black wattle, Green wattle). Spreading, evergreen large shrub or medium-sized tree with 2-pinnate, fern-like, dark green leaves, to 8cm (3in) long, composed of 60–80 linear leaflets. In spring, bears spherical, rich yellow flowerheads, 5mm (¼in) across, in profuse axillary racemes and panicles, 10–15cm (4–6in) long. ↕5–15m (15–50ft), ↔ 3–8m (10–25ft). Australia (New South Wales). ✻
A. drummondii (Drummond's wattle). Open, spreading, evergreen shrub producing sparse, 1- or 2-pinnate leaves, 2–3cm (¾–1¼in) long, with up to 12 oblong, mid-green or slightly glaucous leaflets. During late winter and spring, bright to rich yellow flowerheads, in the form of cylindrical spikes, 1–3cm (½–1¼in) long and 8–10mm (⅜–½in) across, are produced at the tips of short side branches. ↕0.6–1.8m (2–6ft), ↔ 0.9–1.5m (3–5ft). Australia (Western Australia). ✻

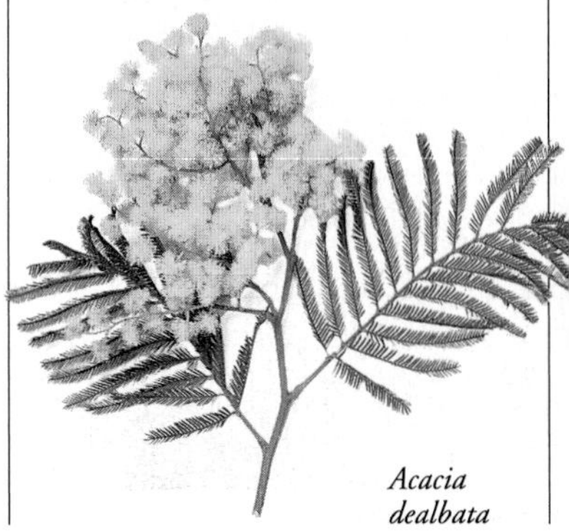
Acacia dealbata

A. floribunda ♀ (White sallow wattle). Tall shrub or small tree, usually open in habit, but sometimes bushy. Evergreen, mid-green phyllodes, 5–12cm (2–5in) long, are linear to lance-shaped with slender, curved tips. Produces 1–3 spikes of loosely cylindrical, fragrant, pale yellow flowerheads, 2.5–6cm (1–2½in) long and 7–10mm (¼–½in) across, from each upper phyllode axil, in spring. ↕4–8m (12–25ft), ↔3–6m (10–20ft). Australia (Queensland to Victoria). ✲

A. mearnsii ♀ (Black wattle). Spreading, evergreen tree producing 2-pinnate, fern-like leaves, 8–15cm (3–6in) long, with 18–40 tiny, linear, grey-green leaflets. Many spherical, richly fragrant, pale yellow flowerheads, 5mm (¼in) across, are borne in axillary racemes and panicles, 8–15cm (3–6in) long, in spring. ↕8–20m (25–70ft), ↔5–10m (15–30ft). Australia (New South Wales, Victoria). ✲

A. melanoxylon ♀ (Blackwood). Evergreen tree or shrub with an erect to spreading habit and freely branching, angular stems. Tapered, deep matt to greyish green phyllodes, to 15cm (6in) long, are oblong to lance-shaped. From late winter to late spring, bears branched axillary racemes, 5–10cm (2–4in) long, of spherical, cream to pale yellow flowerheads, 1cm (½in) across. ↕5–25m (15–80ft), ↔4–12m (12–40ft). Australia (South Australia, Queensland to Tasmania). ✲

A. paradoxa ■ syn. *A. armata* (Hedge wattle, Kangaroo thorn). Evergreen shrub with erect, spiny stems and lance-shaped to oblong, deep green phyllodes, 1–3cm (½–1¼in) long, often with strongly waved margins. Solitary, long-stalked, spherical, golden yellow flowerheads, 1cm (½in) across, are produced from the phyllode axils in spring. ↕↔2–4m (6–12ft). Australia (New South Wales). ✲

A. pendula ♀ (Weeping myall). Bushy, broad-headed, evergreen tree with pendent branches. Bears lance- or slightly sickle-shaped, greyish green to glaucous phyllodes, to 10cm (4in) long. Short, branching racemes, 2–5cm (¾–2in) long, of spherical, pale yellow flowerheads, 1cm (½in) across, are borne from the phyllode axils in winter. ↕6–10m (20–30ft), ↔6–7m (20–22ft). Australia (Queensland to Victoria). ✲

A. podalyriifolia (Queensland silver wattle). Erect, loosely branched, evergreen, hairy shrub, often grown for its attractive foliage. Downy, white to blue-white phyllodes are ovate to oblong and 2–4cm (¾–1½in) long. Produces spherical, fragrant, rich yellow flowerheads, 1cm (½in) across, in terminal and axillary racemes, 7–15cm (3–6in) long, in spring. ↕3–5m (10–15ft), ↔3–4m (10–12ft). Australia (Queensland to New South Wales). ✲

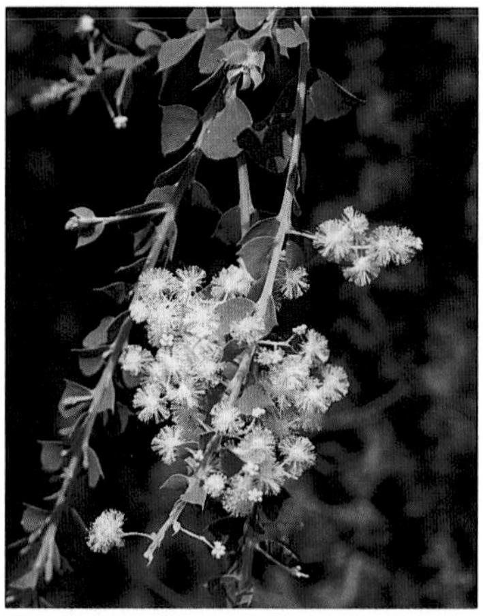
Acacia pravissima

A. pravissima ■♀ (Ovens wattle). Large shrub or small tree, open to dense in habit, with short, pendent branches, crowded with lopsidedly triangular, evergreen, grey-green phyllodes, 0.5–2cm (¼–¾in) long. Spherical, fragrant, bright yellow flowerheads, 5mm (¼in) across, are profusely borne in axillary racemes, 5–10cm (2–4in) long, in late winter and spring. ↕3–8m (10–25ft), ↔3–7m (10–22ft). Australia (New South Wales, Victoria). ✲

A. pulchella (Western prickly Moses). Bushy, evergreen, prickly shrub with 2-pinnate leaves, 1–2cm (½–¾in) long, composed of 4–22 narrowly oblong, deep green leaflets. Solitary, spherical, golden yellow flowerheads, to 1cm (½in) across, are produced from the phyllode axils in winter and spring. ↕0.6–1.5m (2–5ft), ↔1–2m (3–6ft). Australia (Western Australia). ✲

A. retinodes ■♀♀ (Silver wattle, Swamp wattle). Spreading, large shrub or small tree with slender, angular, often pendent stems, and linear to narrowly lance-shaped, evergreen, bluish green phyllodes, 10–20cm (4–8in) long. Short axillary racemes, 2–4cm (¾–1½in) long, of spherical, lemon-yellow flowerheads, 5mm (¼in) across, are produced periodically throughout the year. ↕4–8m (12–25ft), ↔3–7m (10–22ft). Australia (South Australia, Victoria, Tasmania). ❀ (min. 3–5°C/37–41°F)

A. verticillata ♀ (Prickly Moses). Tall, bushy, evergreen shrub or sometimes small tree, bearing linear, spine-tipped, dark green phyllodes, 2cm (¾in) long, usually in whorls, or scattered. Bears panicles, to 1.5cm (½in) long, of 1–3 ovoid to rod-shaped, lemon-yellow flowerheads, 3cm (1¼in) long, in spring. ↕2–8m (6–25ft), ↔3–8m (10–25ft). Australia (South Australia, New South Wales to Tasmania). ✲

▷**Acacia,**
False see *Robinia pseudoacacia*
Mop-head see *Robinia pseudoacacia* 'Umbraculifera'
Rose see *Robinia hispida*

ACAENA

Bidi-bidi, New Zealand burr

ROSACEAE

Genus of about 100 species of mainly evergreen, creeping, mat-forming perennials and semi-prostrate subshrubs, widely distributed over the S. hemisphere, most from open habitats at high altitudes. Acaenas are cultivated for their variously coloured, narrowly oblong-ovate, pinnate leaves, and petalless flowers. These are produced in stalked spikes or dense, ovoid or spherical heads, which develop into colourful, spiny burrs in mid- or late summer. The prostrate stems root where they touch the ground and rapidly form dense mats of foliage. The burrs may be a nuisance to pets. *A. microphylla* 'Kupferteppich' is an effective and restrained rock garden plant. Other acaenas are good – although invasive – ground-cover plants.

• **HARDINESS** Fully hardy.
• **CULTIVATION** Grow in moderately fertile, well-drained soil in sun or partial shade. Pull out rooted stems to restrict growth.
• **PROPAGATION** Sow seed in containers in an open frame in autumn. Separate rooted stems from the parent plant in autumn or early spring, or take softwood cuttings in late spring.
• **PESTS AND DISEASES** Trouble free.

***A. anserinifolia* of gardens** see *A. novae-zelandiae.*

***A.* 'Blue Haze'** ■ syn. *A.* 'Pewter'. Creeping, vigorous, evergreen perennial producing pinnate leaves, to 8cm (3in) long, grey-blue, shaded bronze at the margins, with 9–13 oval leaflets.

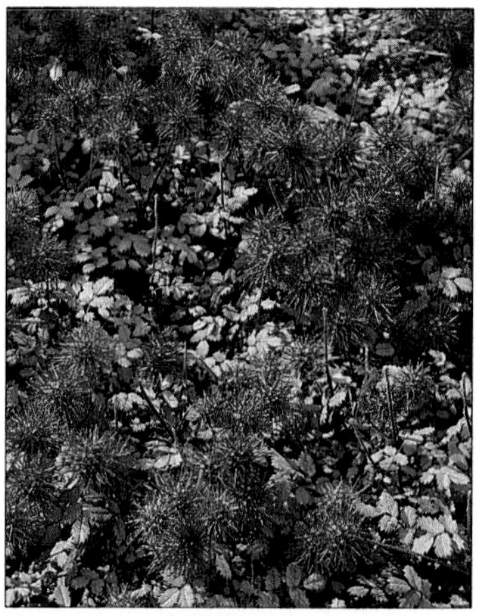
Acaena microphylla 'Kupferteppich'

Spherical flowerheads are followed by dark red burrs, to 2cm (¾in) across, with pinkish red spines, in midsummer. ↕10–15cm (4–6in), ↔1m (3ft). ✲✲✲

A. caerulea see *A. caesiiglauca.*

A. caesiiglauca, syn. *A. caerulea.* Creeping, usually evergreen perennial with pinnate, glaucous blue leaves, to 10cm (4in) long, divided into 7–13 obovate leaflets. Spherical flowerheads are followed by reddish brown burrs, to 2cm (¾in) across, in late summer. ↕8–12cm (3–5in), ↔to 1m (3ft). New Zealand. ✲✲✲

***A. microphylla* 'Copper Carpet'** see *A. microphylla* 'Kupferteppich'.

***A. microphylla* 'Kupferteppich'** ■ syn. *A. microphylla* 'Copper Carpet'. Compact, creeping, usually evergreen perennial with pinnate bronze leaves, to 3cm (1¼in) long, with 9–15 rounded leaflets. Small, spherical flowerheads are followed by bright red burrs, 2.5–3cm (1–1¼in) across, in late summer. ↕3cm (1¼in), ↔to 60cm (24in). ✲✲✲

A. novae-zelandiae, syn. *A. anserinifolia* of gardens. Vigorous, creeping, evergreen perennial producing pinnate, grey-green or rich green leaves, to 10cm (4in) long, with 9–15 oblong leaflets. Small, ovoid to spherical flowerheads are followed by red burrs, 1.5cm (½in) across, in late summer. ↕to 15cm (6in), ↔1m (3ft) or more. New Zealand. ✲✲✲

***A.* 'Pewter'** see *A.* 'Blue Haze'.

ACALYPHA

EUPHORBIACEAE

Genus of about 430 species of evergreen shrubs and trees, and annuals, grown for their foliage and flowers. They are found in tropical and subtropical regions, from tropical woodland to open savannah. Their alternate leaves are oval to ovate, simple, and toothed. Tiny, petalless flowers are borne in terminal or axillary, catkin-like racemes, either small and insignificant, or large and brightly coloured. Where temperatures fall below 10–13°C (50–55°F), grow in a warm greenhouse or as a houseplant. In warmer areas, grow in a border, or use for hedging or as specimen plants.

• **HARDINESS** Frost tender.
• **CULTIVATION** Under glass, grow in loamless potting compost in full or filtered light. Water freely in the growing season, applying a balanced liquid fertilizer monthly during summer; water moderately in winter. Pot on or

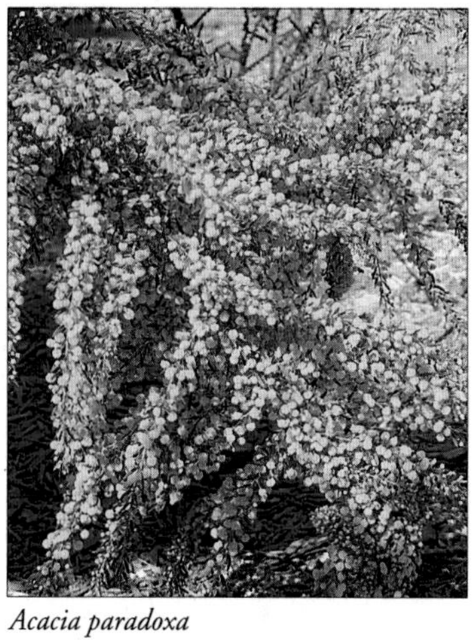
Acacia paradoxa

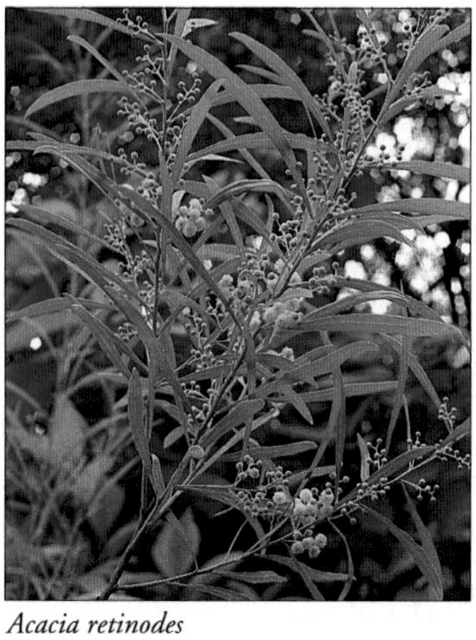
Acacia retinodes

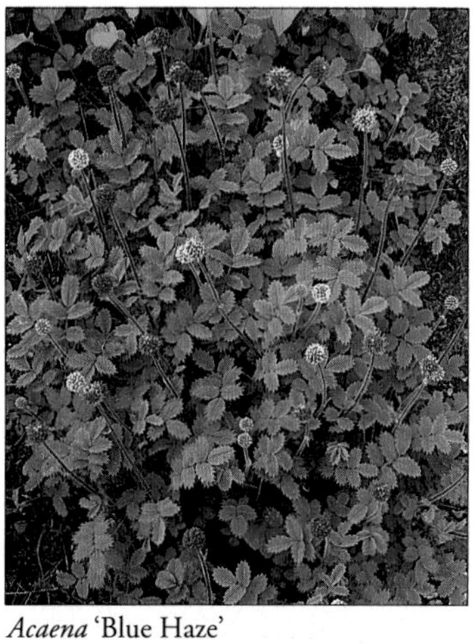
Acaena 'Blue Haze'

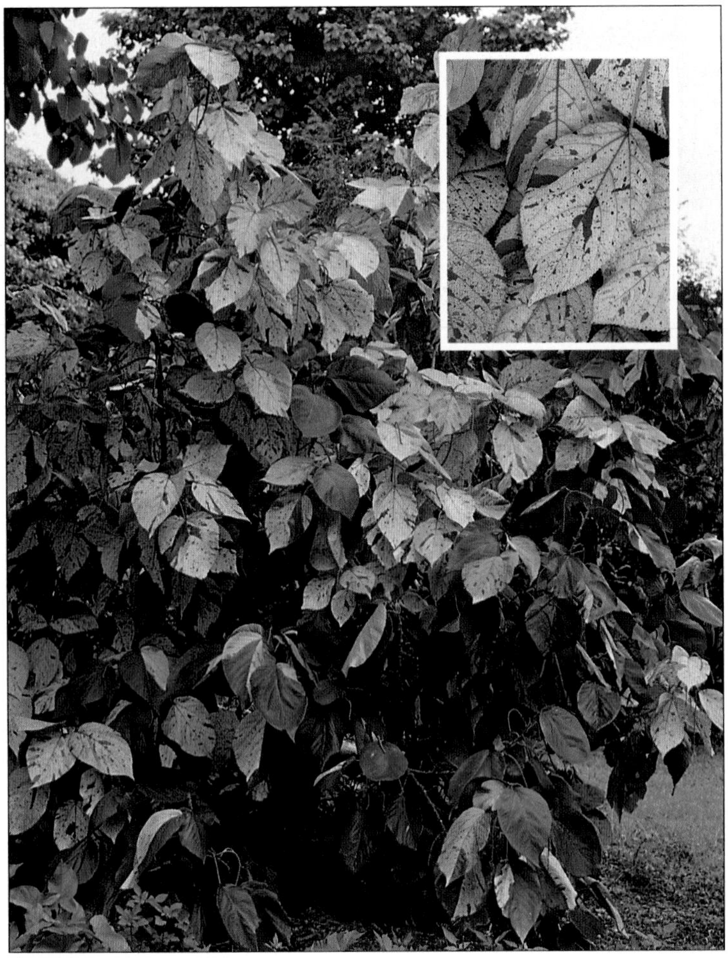

Acalypha wilkesiana (inset: leaf colour variation)

top-dress in early spring or autumn. Outdoors, grow in fertile, humus-rich, moist but well-drained soil in sun or partial shade. Pruning group 9.
• **PROPAGATION** Divide rhizomatous or clump-forming species in spring. Root softwood cuttings in early spring, or semi-ripe cuttings in late summer, with bottom heat.
• **PESTS AND DISEASES** Scale insects, mealybugs, whiteflies, and red spider mites may be a problem under glass.

A. hispida 🏆 (Red-hot cat's tail). Erect shrub, usually sparsely branched, with oval, rich green leaves, 10–25cm (4–10in) long. Bears thick, fluffy, deep crimson or bright red catkins, 25–50cm (10–20in) long, periodically during the year. ↕ 2–3m (6–10ft), ↔ 1–2m (3–6ft). Malaysia, New Guinea. ❀ (min. 13°C/55°F). **'Alba'** has off-white catkins.
A. wilkesiana ■ (Copperleaf). Spreading shrub, with oval, multi-coloured, mottled, and often variegated leaves, 10–20cm (4–8in) long. Bears catkin-like racemes, 10–20cm (4–8in) long, usually green- or copper-tinted, and often hidden among the leaves, periodically during the year. ↕ to 2m (6ft), ↔ 1–2m (3–6ft). Pacific islands. ❀ (min. 10°C/50°F). **'Marginata'** has leaves with crimson to white margins. **'Musaica'** has foliage heavily mottled red and orange.

▷***Acanthocalycium aurantiacum*** see *Echinopsis thionantha*
▷***Acanthocalycium violaceum*** see *Echinopsis spiniflora*
▷***Acanthocalyx*** see *Morina*

ACANTHOLIMON

PLUMBAGINACEAE

Genus of about 120 species of evergreen, mat-forming perennials, found in open, rocky areas at high altitudes, from the E. Mediterranean to C. Asia. They are grown for their dense, spiny rosettes of needle-like leaves, 1–7cm (½–3in) long, and short spikes or panicles of shallowly funnel-shaped flowers, borne in early and midsummer. Suitable for a scree bed, or a wall, although in cold climates with high winter rainfall, most species are best grown in an alpine house.
• **HARDINESS** Fully hardy.
• **CULTIVATION** Outdoors, grow in moderately fertile, very well-drained soil in full sun; only *A. glumaceum* tolerates winter wet. Under glass, grow in a mix of equal parts loam-based potting compost (JI No.1) and sharp grit, with additional limestone chippings; top-dress with grit. Established plants resent disturbance.
• **PROPAGATION** Sow seed as soon as ripe in containers in an open frame. Root softwood cuttings in spring. Layer shoot tips in sandy potting compost in spring.
• **PESTS AND DISEASES** Red spider mites may be a problem under glass.

A. glumaceum ■ Slow-growing perennial with crowded rosettes of stiff, linear-lance-shaped, spiny, dark green leaves, to 2.5cm (1in) long. In summer, dense spikes of 3–8 deep rose-pink flowers are produced on stems 2.5cm (1in) long. ↕ 5–8cm (2–3in),

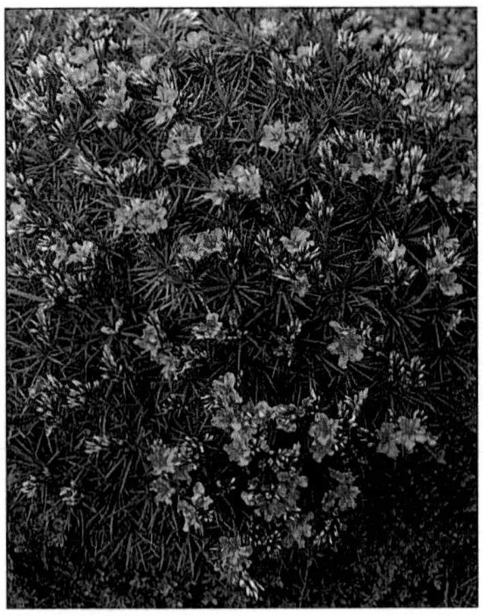

Acantholimon glumaceum

↔ 20–30cm (8–12in). Caucasus, Armenia, Turkey. ❄❄❄
A. venustum. Slow-growing perennial with rosettes of linear-lance-shaped, spiny, silver-margined, blue-grey leaves, 1.5–4cm (½–1½in) long. Bears spikes of up to 20 pink flowers on stems to 3cm (1¼in) long, in midsummer. ↕ 5–8cm (2–3in), ↔ 15–20cm (6–8in). Turkey, Syria, Iraq, Iran. ❄❄❄

▷***Acanthopanax*** see *Eleutherococcus*
A. ricinifolius see *Kalopanax septemlobus*
A. sieboldianus see *Eleutherococcus sieboldianus*

ACANTHOPHOENIX

Barbel palm

ARECACEAE/PALMAE

Genus of one very variable species of single-stemmed palm from coastal woodland in the Mascarene Islands in the Indian Ocean. Pinnate leaves are produced in a terminal tuft on the stem, and small, separate male and female flowers are borne in panicles just beneath them. In cool climates, grow young specimens as foliage plants in a conservatory or warm greenhouse. In warmer regions, barbel palms are fine specimen trees for growing outdoors.
• **HARDINESS** Frost tender.
• **CULTIVATION** Under glass, grow in loam-based potting compost (JI No.3), with additional sharp sand, in full light. In the growing season, water freely and apply a balanced liquid fertilizer monthly; water moderately in winter. Pot on or top-dress in spring. Outdoors, they are best grown in fertile, sandy soil in full sun.
• **PROPAGATION** Sow seed at 27°C (81°F) in spring.
• **PESTS AND DISEASES** Red spider mites may be a problem under glass.

A. crinita see *A. rubra.*
A. rubra 🏆 syn. *A. crinita.* Elegant palm with a slender trunk, swollen at the base and topped by a prominent crownshaft. The pinnate leaves, 2–4m (6–12ft) long, have prickly stalks and midribs, and are divided into many crowded, linear, rich green leaflets with cleft tips. Small, inconspicuous, dull white, yellow, pink, red, or purple flowers are produced in panicles, to 45cm (18in) long, during summer. ↕ to 18m (60ft), ↔ 4–8m (12–25ft). Mascarene Islands. ❀ (min. 10–13°C/50–55°F)

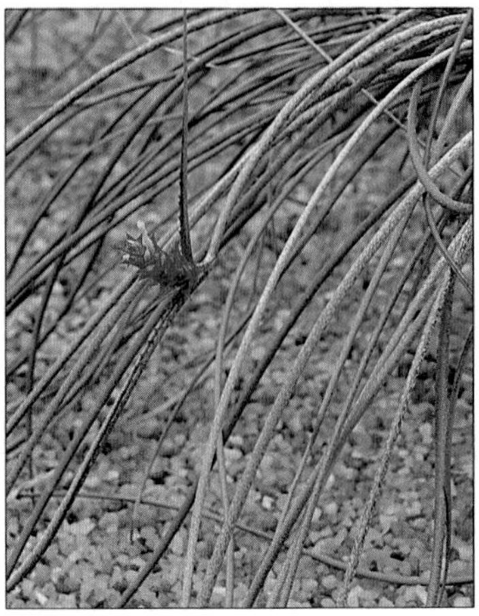

Acanthostachys strobilacea

ACANTHOSTACHYS

Prickle ear

BROMELIACEAE

Genus of one species of stemless, evergreen, epiphytic or rock-dwelling perennial (bromeliad) occurring at altitudes above 800m (2,600ft) in Brazil, Paraguay, and N. Argentina. Cone-shaped inflorescences are borne from the centre of loose rosettes of arching, slender leaves, and develop into edible, sweet-tasting fruit resembling small pineapples. Where temperatures fall below 10°C (50°F), grow in a warm greenhouse or as a houseplant; in warmer areas, grow *A. strobilacea* in a border or epiphytically.
• **HARDINESS** Frost tender.
• **CULTIVATION** Under glass, grow epiphytically or in standard epiphytic bromeliad compost, in full light. Water moderately from spring to autumn; keep moist in winter. Apply a low-nitrogen granular fertilizer 3 or 4 times when in growth. Outdoors, grow in well-drained, fertile, humus-rich soil in an open, sunny site. See also p.47.
• **PROPAGATION** Sow seed at 27°C (81°F) as soon as ripe. Sever offsets in early spring; grow on new plantlets *in situ* or pot up separately.
• **PESTS AND DISEASES** Vulnerable to scale insects, especially before flowering.

A. strobilacea ■ Epiphytic bromeliad with short rhizomes and open rosettes of a few linear, spiny, white-scaly, bright green leaves, to 1m (3ft) long. In summer, tubular yellow flowers, 1cm (½in) long, are borne in dense, cone-shaped inflorescences, on erect, leafless stems, 50cm (20in) long, just above 2 leaf-like, widely spreading, reddish orange bracts. ↕↔ to 1m (3ft). Brazil, Paraguay, Argentina. ❀ (min. 10°C/50°F)

ACANTHUS

Bear's breeches

ACANTHACEAE

Genus of about 30 species of perennials from dry, rocky sites, mostly in the Mediterranean. They are vigorous, architectural plants, with striking foliage and flowers. The dark green, oblong-lance-shaped to broadly ovate, usually basal leaves, up to 90cm (36in) long, are variously lobed and toothed, sometimes spiny. The tubular, 2-lipped flowers are generally 3.5–5cm (1½–2in) long, usually with spiny bracts and sepals in combinations of white, green, yellow, pink, or purple. They are borne, sometimes in ranks of 4, in erect, terminal racemes, to 1.2m (4ft) tall. Grow acanthus in a spacious border; they are also good for cutting or drying. In frost-prone areas, grow *A. montanus* in a cool or temperate greenhouse or conservatory.

• **HARDINESS** Fully hardy to frost tender. *A. montanus* will withstand short periods at 0°C (32°F).

• **CULTIVATION** Under glass, grow in loam-based potting compost (JI No.2) in full or filtered light. In the growing season, water moderately and apply a balanced liquid fertilizer monthly; keep just moist in winter. Outdoors, grow in any soil in sun or partial shade, although they thrive in deep, fertile, well-drained loam.

• **PROPAGATION** Sow seed in containers in a cold frame in spring. Divide in spring or autumn. Take root cuttings in winter.

• **PESTS AND DISEASES** Powdery mildew may be a problem.

A. balcanicus see *A. hungaricus.*

A. dioscoridis. Variable perennial with a fleshy, running rootstock which produces rosettes of narrowly lance-shaped, lobed, spiny, dark green leaves, 8–20cm (3–8in) long. Racemes, 20–25cm (8–10in) long, of purplish pink or rich pink flowers, with green bracts, are borne from late spring to late summer. ↕ 20–40cm (8–16in), ↔ 90cm (36in). Turkey, Lebanon, W. Iraq, W. Iran. ✻✻✻. **var. *perringii*** has pinnatifid, spiny, grey-green leaves; ↕ 30–40cm (12–16in), ↔ 60cm (24in); Turkey (S. Anatolia).

A. hirsutus ▣ Clump-forming perennial with slender, semi-erect, lance-shaped, pinnatifid, weakly spiny, dark green leaves, 25–35cm (10–14in) long. Racemes, 15cm (6in) long, of pale yellow or greenish white flowers with hairy, weakly spiny, yellowish green bracts, are produced from late spring to midsummer. ↕ 15–35cm (6–14in), ↔ 30cm (12in). Turkey. ✻✻✻

A. hirsutus* var. *syriacus see *A. syriacus.*

A. hungaricus ▣ syn. *A. balcanicus, A. longifolius.* Clump-forming perennial with oblong-ovate, dark green leaves, 60–90cm (24–36in) long, with deep lobes narrowed at the bases, and wide, winged midribs between the main lobes.

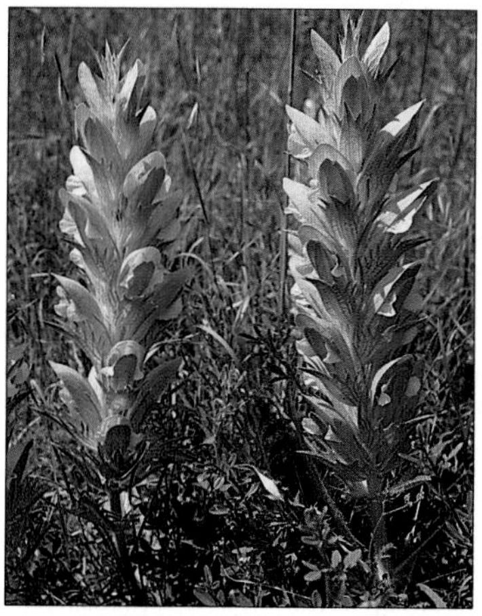

Acanthus hirsutus

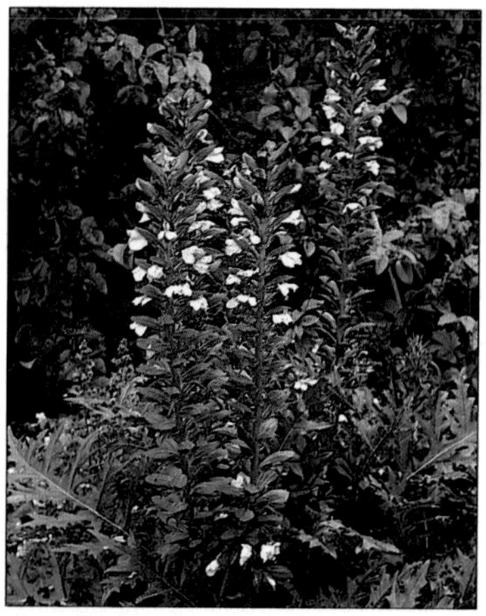

Acanthus hungaricus

Racemes, 65–70cm (24–28in) long, of white or pale pink flowers with purple-shaded bracts, are produced in early and midsummer. ↕ 60–120cm (2–4ft), ↔ 60–90cm (24–36in). Balkans. ✻✻✻

A. longifolius see *A. hungaricus.*

A. mollis ▣ Clump-forming perennial with obovate, deeply lobed, dark green leaves, shiny above, to 1m (3ft) long. In late summer, white flowers with purple-shaded bracts are borne in 1m- (3ft-) long racemes, often with purple-tinted stems. ↕ 1.5m (5ft), ↔ 90cm (36in). S.W. Europe, N.W. Africa. ✻✻✻. **Latifolius Group** includes variants with broad, shallowly lobed, conspicuously veined, shiny, rich green leaves, to 1.2m (4ft) long.

A. montanus (Mountain thistle). Shrubby perennial with few branches and oblong-lance-shaped, pinnatifid, spiny, leathery leaves, 30cm (12in) long, that are glossy, dark green, with silver markings and wavy margins. Bears racemes, 23–30cm (9–12in) long, of rose-pink or pale mauve flowers with spiny calyces in late summer and early autumn. ↕ 2m (6ft), ↔ 60cm (24in). W. Africa. ✻

A. spinosissimus see *A. spinosus* Spinosissimus Group.

A. spinosus ▣ 🏆 Variable, clump-forming perennial producing narrowly oblong-ovate, arching, dark green leaves, to 1m (3ft) long, often deeply cut to the midribs, with spiny margins. Tall racemes, to 1m (3ft) long, of pure white flowers with purple bracts are borne from late spring to midsummer. ↕ 1.5m (5ft), ↔ 60–90cm (24–36in). Italy to W. Turkey. ✻✻✻. **Spinosissimus Group**, syn. *A. spinosissimus*, includes variants with deep greyish green leaves, 50cm (20in) long, deeply cut to the bold white midribs, and with white-spiny margins; ↕ 1.2m (4ft), ↔ 60cm (24in).

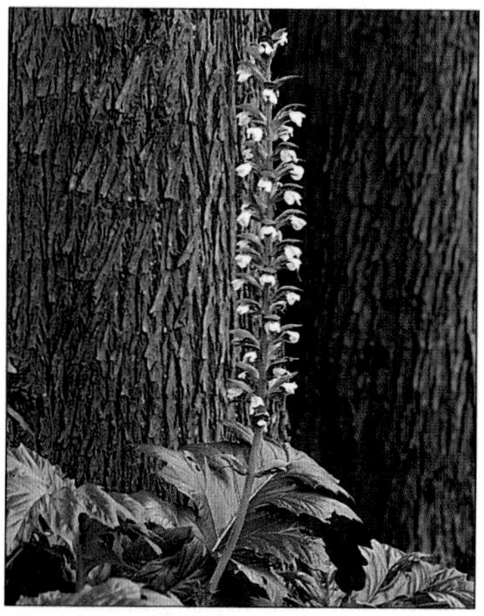

Acanthus mollis

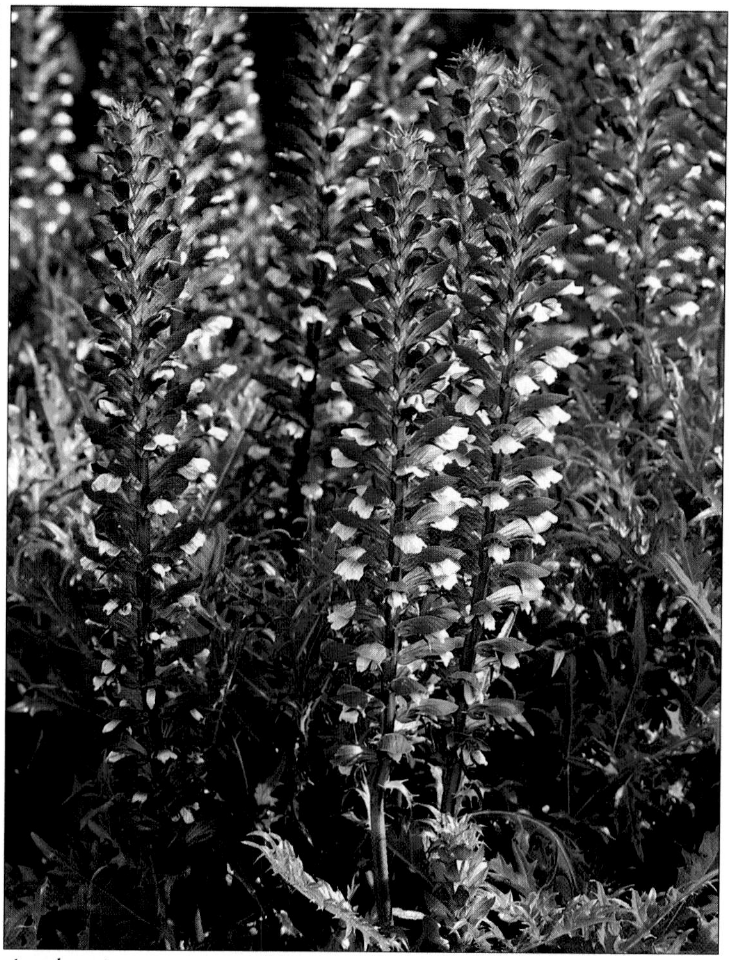

Acanthus spinosus

A. syriacus, syn. *A. hirsutus* var. *syriacus.* Clump-forming perennial with clusters of long-stalked, pinnatifid, lance-shaped, spiny, hairy, dark green leaves, to 20cm (8in) long. Racemes, 15–23cm (6–9in) long, of greenish white flowers with purple-shaded bracts, are borne from late spring to midsummer. ↕↔ 60cm (24in). Turkey, Syria, Jordan, Israel, Lebanon. ✻✻✻

ACCA *syn.* FEIJOA

MYRTACEAE

Genus of 2 or 3 species of evergreen, opposite-leaved shrubs occurring in dry upland slopes, scrub, and open woodland in subtropical South America. They are cultivated for their attractive, shallowly cup-shaped flowers, which are produced singly from the upper leaf axils in midsummer. In hot climates, edible fruits may also be produced. To obtain fruit in areas where temperatures fall below 5°C (41°F), grow in a cool greenhouse. *A. sellowiana* is tolerant of salt and drought, and may be used as hedging in mild coastal areas.

• **HARDINESS** Frost hardy.

• **CULTIVATION** Under glass, grow in loam-based potting compost (JI No.3) in full light. During the growing season, water freely and apply a balanced liquid fertilizer every 4 weeks; water plants more sparingly in winter. Outdoors, grow in light, well-drained soil in full sun in a sheltered site.

• **PROPAGATION** Sow seed at 13–16°C (55–61°F) as soon as ripe. Take semi-ripe cuttings in summer.

• **PESTS AND DISEASES** Trouble free.

A. sellowiana ▣ (Pineapple guava). Bushy shrub with elliptic-oblong, grey-green leaves, to 7cm (3in) long, white-woolly beneath. Flowers, 4cm (1½in) across, with long red stamens, purple-red petals, white on the margins and reverse, are produced singly from the upper leaf axils in midsummer, followed in warm climates by ovoid, red-tinged, green berries, 5cm (2in) long. ↕ 2m (6ft), ↔ 2.5m (8ft). Brazil, Uruguay. ✻✻. **'Variegata'** has leaves that are margined creamy white.

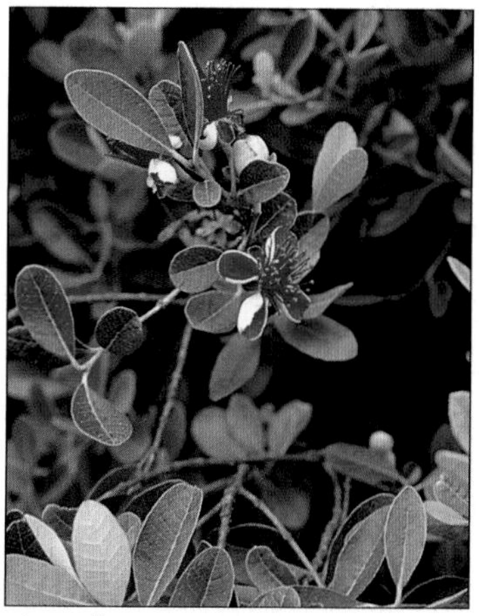

Acca sellowiana

ACER
Maple
ACERACEAE

Genus of about 150 species of evergreen and deciduous trees and shrubs from Europe, N. Africa, Asia, and North and Central America. Mainly woodland plants, they either form large trees or grow as part of the understorey. The opposite leaves are usually shallowly to deeply palmately lobed, but in some species and cultivars are unlobed or, more rarely, 3-palmate or pinnate. The small, often greenish yellow flowers are borne in generally pendent, occasionally upright racemes, panicles, or umbels, in early or mid-spring, and are followed by usually brown, occasionally colourful, winged fruits, joined in pairs. Maples are valued for their foliage, which may be variegated or have good autumn colour; some also have attractive bark. Grow large maples as specimen trees; smaller trees and those of shrubby habit are excellent for gardens of any size. Maples are also suitable for growing in large containers, although doing so will restrict their growth.

• **HARDINESS** Most are fully hardy; some are frost hardy.

• **CULTIVATION** Grow in fertile, moist but well-drained soil, in sun or partial shade. Shelter cultivars of *A. palmatum* from cold winds and from late frosts, which may kill the young leaves. Where temperatures fall below -10°C (14°F), mulch the roots of *A. palmatum* and *A. japonicum* and their cultivars in autumn. Pruning group 1, but prune only from late autumn to midwinter. Train large species as central leader standards.

• **PROPAGATION** Sow seed *in situ* or in containers outdoors as soon as ripe. Graft in late winter; bud in late summer.

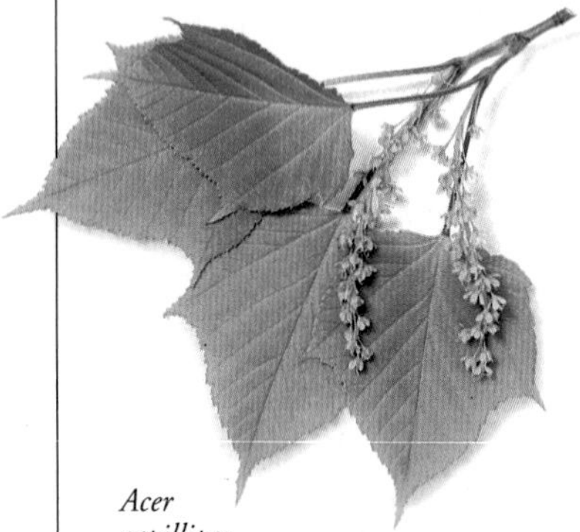
Acer capillipes

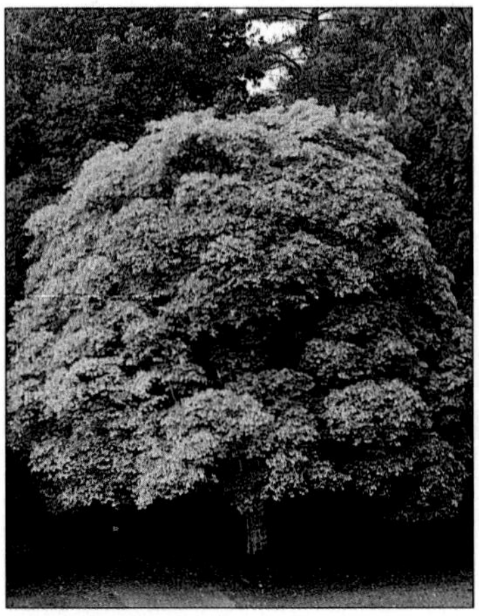
Acer cappadocicum

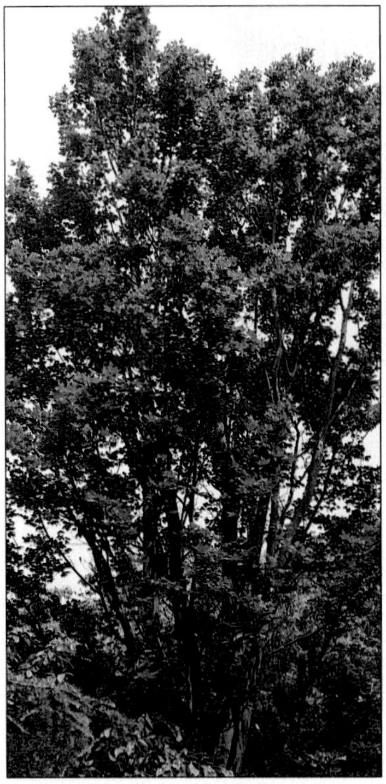
Acer cappadocicum subsp. *lobelii*

• **PESTS AND DISEASES** Prone to aphids, mites, scale insects, caterpillars, tar spot, *Verticillium* wilt, leaf scorch, and honey fungus. In several species, mites may cause the production of galls.

A. buergerianum ♀ (Three-toothed maple, Trident maple). Spreading, deciduous tree with obovate, 3-lobed, glossy leaves, to 9cm (3½in) long, dark green above, blue-green beneath, turning orange and red in late autumn and early winter. Bears erect racemes of pale yellow flowers. Ideal in a small garden or large containers; also popular for bonsai work. ↕10m (30ft), ↔ 8m (25ft). E. China, Korea, Japan. ***
A. caesium* subsp. *giraldii see *A. giraldii.*
***A. campestre* 'Schwerinii'** ▯ Broadly upright, narrow-crowned, deciduous tree with ovate to rounded, 5-lobed leaves, to 6cm (2½in) long, reddish purple when young, dark green by late summer. Bears erect umbels of green flowers, followed by spreading fruit wings, which ripen to red. ↕8m (25ft), ↔ 4m (12ft). ***
A. capillipes ■ ♈ ♀ (Snake-bark maple). Deciduous tree with spreading,

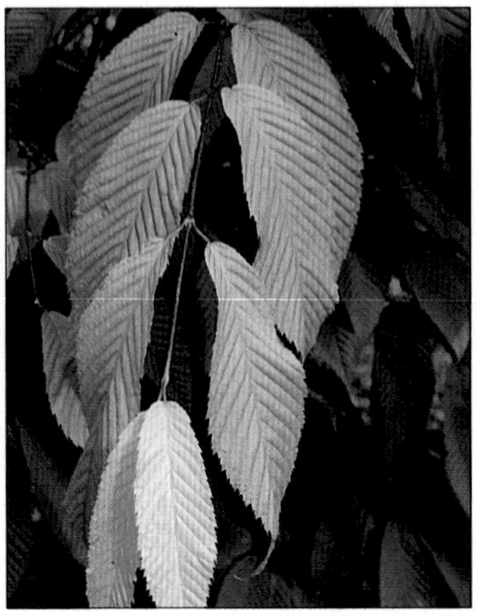
Acer carpinifolium

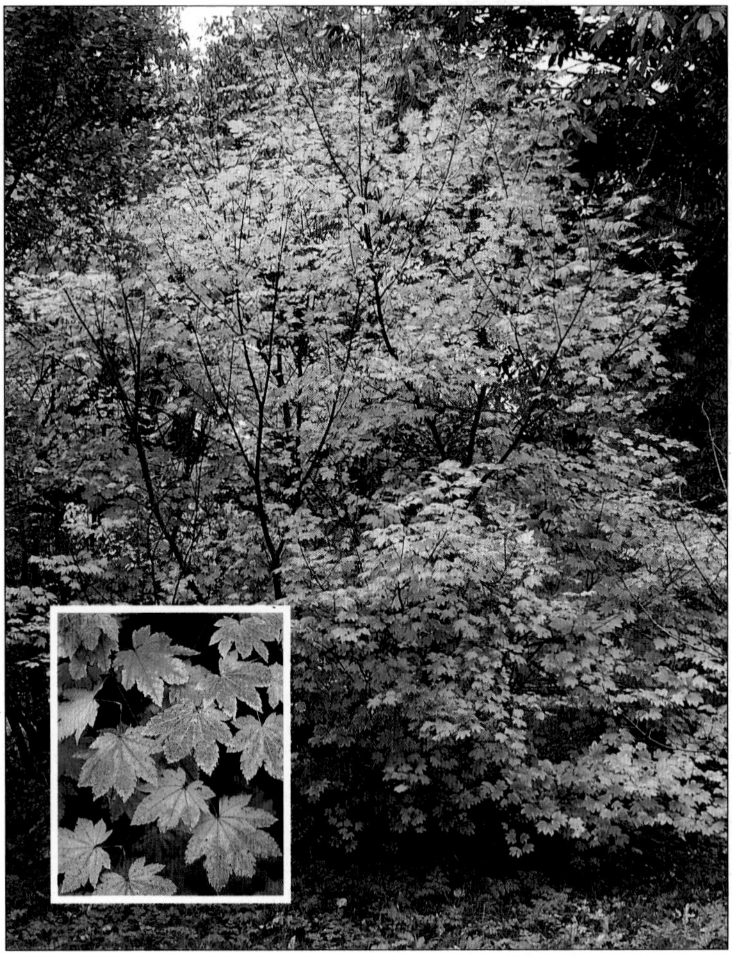
Acer circinatum (inset: autumn leaf colour)

arching branches, streaked green and white, and with red young shoots. Broadly ovate, mid- to dark green leaves, to 12cm (5in) long, with 3 pointed lobes, turn bright red in autumn. Bears pendent racemes of greenish white flowers. ↕↔ 10m (30ft). Japan. ***
A. cappadocicum ■ ♀ (Cappadocian maple, Caucasian maple). Spreading, deciduous tree with broadly ovate, bright green leaves, to 10cm (4in) long, with 5–7 tapered lobes, which turn yellow in autumn. Bears erect umbels of pale yellow flowers. ↕20m (70ft), ↔ 15m (50ft). Caucasus, N. Turkey, Iran, Himalayas, China. ***. **'Aureum'** ♈ has bright yellow young leaves, which turn green in summer, and yellow again in autumn; ↕15m (50ft), ↔ 10m (30ft). **subsp. *lobelii*** ■ ▯–♀ syn. *A. lobelii* (Lobel's maple), is narrow, with upright branches and dark green leaves, 8–13cm (3–5in) long, each with 3–5 wavy-margined lobes, on glaucous shoots; ↕20m (70ft), ↔ 6m (20ft); Italy. **var. *mono*** see *A. mono.* **'Rubrum'** ♈ produces dark red young leaves on red shoots.
A. carpinifolium ■ ♀ (Hornbeam maple). Bushy, spreading, deciduous tree with upright branches and simple, ovate to ovate-oblong, tapered, sharply toothed, prominently veined, mid-green leaves, to 15cm (6in) long, which turn golden brown in autumn. Green flowers are borne in short, pendent racemes. ↕↔ 10m (30ft). Japan. ***
A. circinatum ■ ♈ ♀ (Vine maple). Spreading, bushy, sometimes shrubby, deciduous tree with rounded, deeply 7- to 9-lobed, light green leaves, to 13cm (5in) long, which turn orange and red in autumn. Bears pendent umbels of small, purple and white flowers. ↕5m (15ft), ↔ 6m (20ft). W. North America. ***
A. cissifolium ♀ Spreading, deciduous tree with deeply toothed, 3-palmate, dark green leaves, with oval or obovate leaflets, each to 8cm (3in) long, that open bronze, become dark green, then turn brilliant red in early autumn. Bears upright racemes of pale yellow flowers. Acid or neutral soils give the best autumn colour. ↕8m (25ft), ↔ 10m (30ft). Japan. ***. **subsp. *henryi*** see *A. henryi.*
A. crataegifolium ♀ (Hawthorn maple). Spreading, deciduous tree with green- and white-streaked bark and arching branches. Ovate, shallowly 3-lobed, dark green leaves, to 8cm (3in)

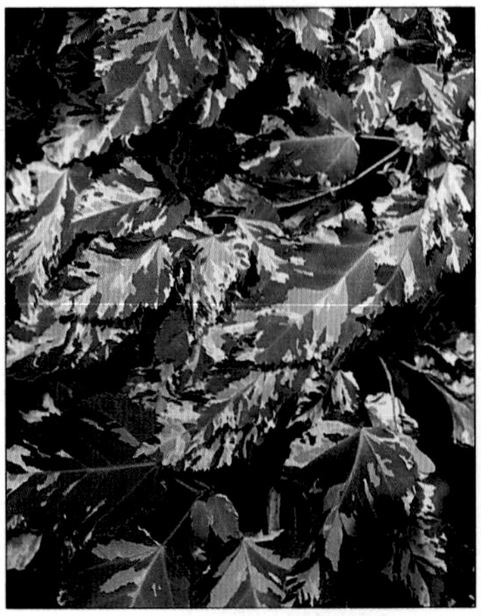
Acer crataegifolium 'Veitchii'

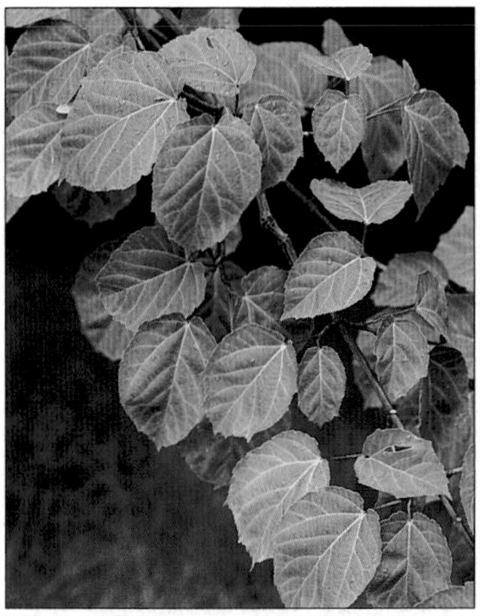
Acer davidii 'George Forrest'

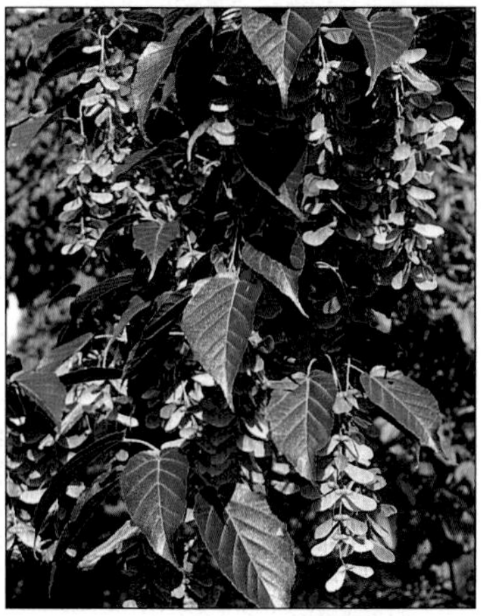
Acer davidii 'Madeline Spitta'

long, with toothed margins, turn orange in autumn. Produces pale yellow flowers in upright racemes. ↕↔ 10m (30ft). Japan. ❄❄❄. **'Veitchii'** ▣ has white-mottled leaves, sometimes also pink-mottled, which turn pink and purple in autumn; ↕↔ 6m (20ft).
A. dasycarpum see *A. saccharinum.*
A. davidii ○ (Père David's maple, Snake-bark maple). Variable, deciduous tree with arching branches and green- and white-streaked bark. The ovate, unlobed or shallowly lobed, mid-green leaves, to 15cm (6in) long, turn orange to yellow in autumn, when pink-brown fruit are also borne. Bears pendent racemes of pale yellow flowers. ↕↔ 15m (50ft). China. ❄❄❄. **'Ernest Wilson'** has pale green leaves that turn bright orange in autumn; ↕ 8m (25ft), ↔ 10m

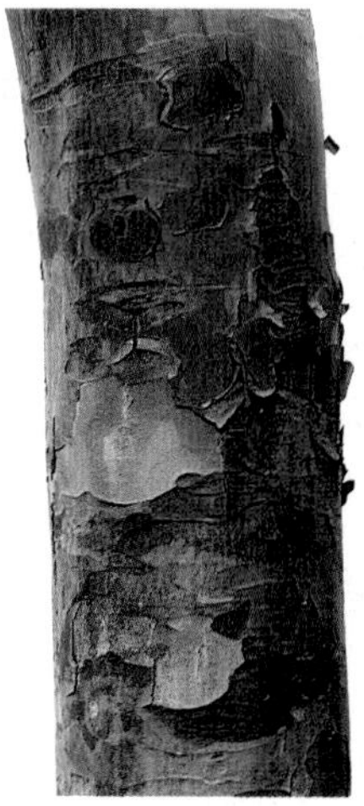
Acer griseum

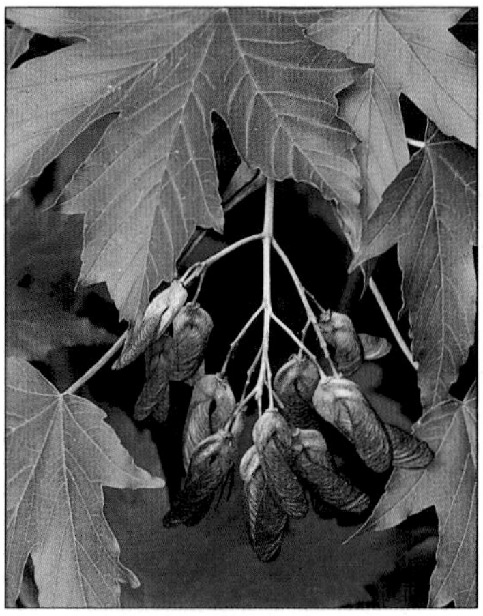
Acer heldreichii subsp. *trautvetteri*

(30ft). **'George Forrest'** ▣ ♀ ○ is broadly upright, with large, mid- to dark green leaves, to 20cm (8in) long, but with poor autumn colour. **subsp. *grosseri*** ♀ syn. *A. grosseri, A. grosseri* var. *hersii, A. hersii,* has boldly streaked bark and triangular-ovate leaves, each with 3 shallow side lobes, which turn orange or yellow in autumn; N. China. **'Madeline Spitta'** ▣ ▯ is narrowly erect, with glossy, dark green leaves, orange-red in late autumn; ↕ 12m (40ft), ↔ 5m (15ft). **'Serpentine'** ♀ has leaves to 10cm (4in) long and dark purple shoots.
***A.* 'Dissectum'** see *A. palmatum* var. *dissectum.*
A. forrestii see *A. pectinatum* subsp. *forrestii.*
A. ginnala see *A. tataricum* subsp. *ginnala.*
A. giraldii ○ syn. *A. caesium* subsp. *giraldii.* Spreading, deciduous tree with glaucous young shoots and broadly ovate, 3-lobed, glossy, dark green leaves, 13cm (5in) long, glaucous beneath, borne on stout red leaf-stalks. Produces greenish white flowers in upright umbels. ↕↔ 15m (50ft). C. China. ❄❄
A. grandidentatum see *A. saccharum* subsp. *grandidentatum.*
A. griseum ▣ ♀ ○ (Paper-bark maple). Slow-growing, spreading, deciduous tree with peeling, orange-brown bark. Dark green, 3-palmate leaves, to 10cm (4in) long, have ovate leaflets, and turn orange to red and scarlet in autumn. Bears yellow flowers in pendent racemes. ↕↔ 10m (30ft). C. China. ❄❄❄
A. grosseri see *A. davidii* subsp. *grosseri.*
A. grosseri* var. *hersii see *A. davidii* subsp. *grosseri.*

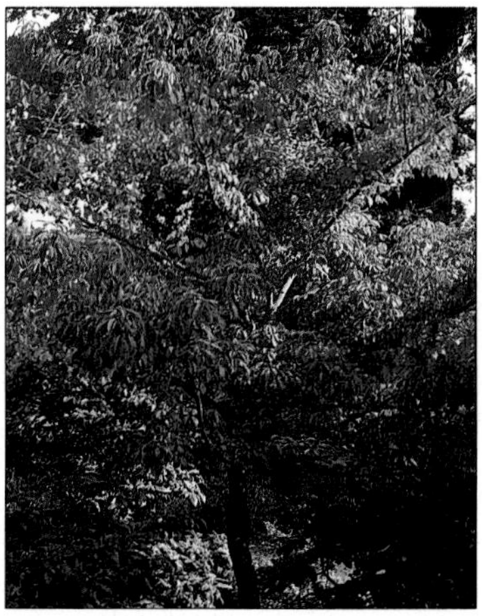
Acer henryi

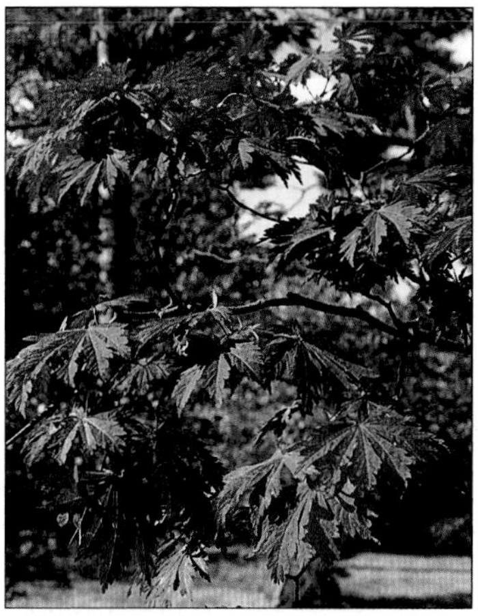
Acer japonicum 'Aconitifolium'

A. heldreichii* subsp. *trautvetteri ▣ ▯ (Greek maple, Red bud maple). Upright, deciduous tree with heart-shaped, deeply 5-lobed, dark green leaves, 10–15cm (4–6in) long, which open from red buds and turn dark yellow in autumn. Erect umbels of yellow flowers are followed by fruit wings that ripen to red. ↕↔ 15m (50ft). Caucasus, N. Turkey. ❄❄❄
A. henryi ▣ ○ syn. *A. cissifolium* subsp. *henryi.* Spreading, deciduous tree producing 3-palmate, dark green leaves, to 10cm (4in) long, with entire or nearly entire, elliptic leaflets, which open bronze and turn brilliant red in early autumn. Produces green flowers in slender, pendent racemes. ↕ 8m (25ft), ↔ 10m (30ft). C. China. ❄❄❄
A. hersii see *A. davidii* subsp. *grosseri.*
***A.* x *hillieri* 'West Hill'** ○ Rounded, deciduous tree with deeply heart-shaped leaves, 10–20cm (4–8in) long, with 5–7 tapered lobes, slightly glossy, mid-green, turning yellow in autumn. Bears upright umbels of yellow-green flowers. ↕↔ 10m (30ft). ❄❄❄
A. japonicum ○ (Full-moon maple, Japanese maple). Spreading, bushy, deciduous tree or shrub with rounded, 7- to 11-lobed, toothed, mid-green leaves, 15–20cm (6–8in) long, turning red in autumn. Bears upright umbels of conspicuous, small, red-purple flowers. ↕↔ 10m (30ft). Japan. ❄❄❄. **'Aconitifolium'** ▣ ♀ syn. 'Filicifolium', 'Laciniatum', has deeply lobed leaves and is very free flowering; ↕ 5m (15ft), ↔ 6m (20ft). **'Aureum'** see *A. shirasawanum* 'Aureum'. **'Filicifolium'** see 'Aconitifolium'. **'Laciniatum'** see 'Aconitifolium'. **'Vitifolium'** ▣ ♀ has large, shallowly lobed leaves, 5–25cm (2–10in) long, with coarsely toothed margins, turning dark red in autumn.
A. laxiflorum ○ syn. *A. pectinatum* subsp. *laxiflorum.* Rounded, deciduous tree with arching branches and green- and white-streaked bark. Simple, ovate, leathery, glossy, mid-green leaves, to 8cm (3in) long, on red leaf-stalks, turn orange in autumn. Bears brownish green flowers in slender, pendent racemes. ↕↔ 10m (30ft). W. China. ❄❄❄
A. lobelii see *A. cappadocicum* subsp. *lobelii.*
A. macrophyllum ▣ ○ (Big-leaf maple, Oregon maple). Vigorous, deciduous tree with broadly ovate, deeply 5-lobed, glossy, dark green leaves, 20–30cm (8–12in) long, which turn orange-brown in autumn. Yellow-green flowers, in long, pendent racemes, are followed by large, bristly, winged fruit. ↕↔ 20m (70ft). W. North America. ❄❄❄
A. maximowiczianum ○ syn. *A. nikoense* (Nikko maple). Rounded, deciduous tree producing 3-palmate leaves, to 10cm (4in) long, with oval, entire or nearly entire leaflets, dark green above, glaucous and softly hairy beneath, which turn red in autumn. Bears yellow flowers in small umbels. ↕↔ 12m (40ft). Japan, China. ❄❄❄
A. micranthum ♀ ○ Deciduous tree or shrub with upright, arching branches and red young shoots. Ovate, deeply 5-lobed, mid-green leaves, 5–7cm (2–3in) long, with lobes tapered and sharply toothed, turn yellow and red in autumn. Produces pendent racemes of greenish white flowers. ↕ 10m (30ft), ↔ 8m (25ft). Japan. ❄❄❄
A. mono ▣ ○ syn. *A. cappadocicum* var. *mono, A. pictum.* Rounded, deciduous tree with almost heart-shaped leaves, 8–15cm (3–6in) long, each with 5–7 tapered lobes, bright green, turning yellow in autumn. Bears erect umbels of greenish yellow flowers. ↕↔ 12m (40ft). China, Korea, Japan. ❄❄❄

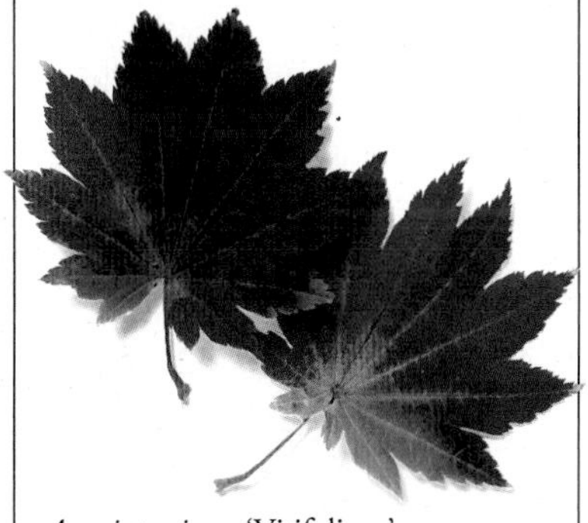
Acer japonicum 'Vitifolium'

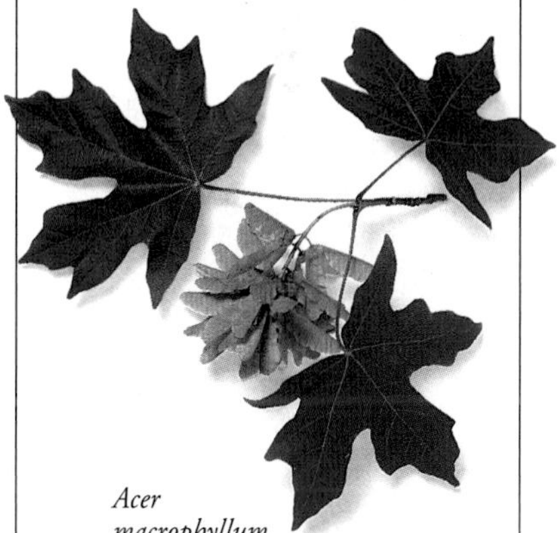
Acer macrophyllum

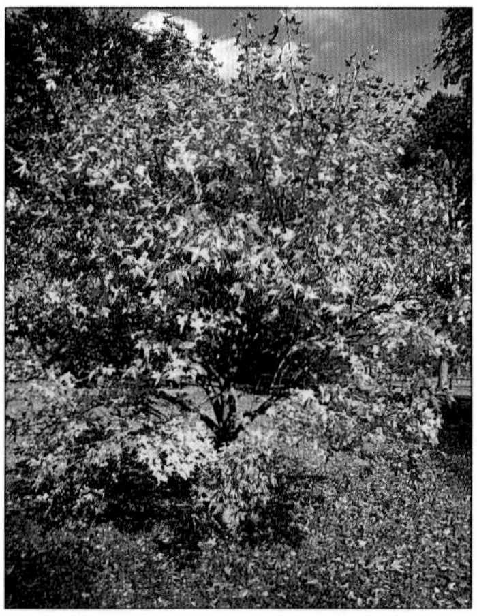
Acer mono

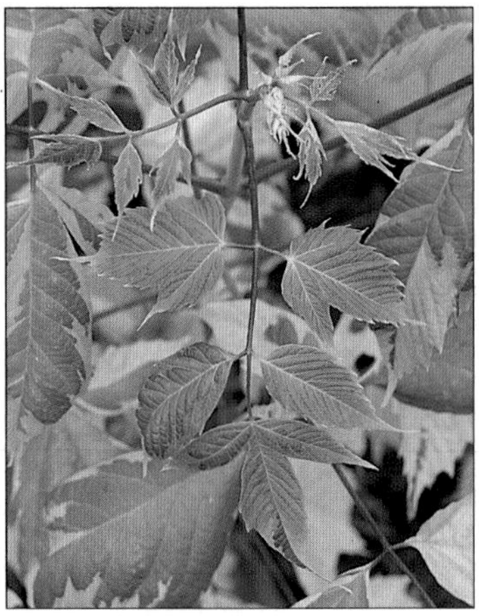

Acer negundo 'Flamingo'

A. monspessulanum ⚲ (Montpellier maple). Variable, bushy, deciduous shrub or small, rounded tree bearing leathery, ovate, glossy, dark green leaves, 3–5cm (1¼–2in) long, with 3 rounded lobes. Bears a profusion of yellow-green flowers in pendent racemes, followed by red-winged fruit in midsummer. ↕↔ 8m (25ft). Mediterranean. ❄❄❄
A. negundo ♀ (Ash-leaved maple, Box elder). Fast-growing, upright, deciduous tree, mostly cultivated in the variants described below. Pinnate leaves, 20cm (8in) or more long, have 3–7 (sometimes 9) ovate, light green leaflets, to 10cm (4in) long, turning yellow in autumn. Greenish yellow flowers are borne in pendent racemes, males and females on separate plants. ↕ 15m (50ft), ↔ 10m (30ft). North America. ❄❄❄.

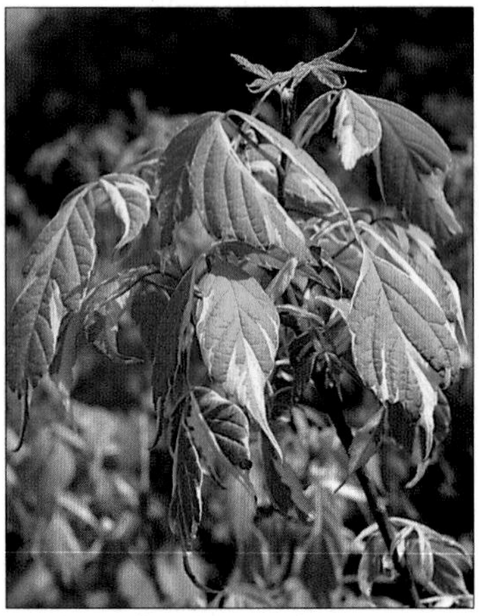

Acer negundo 'Variegatum'

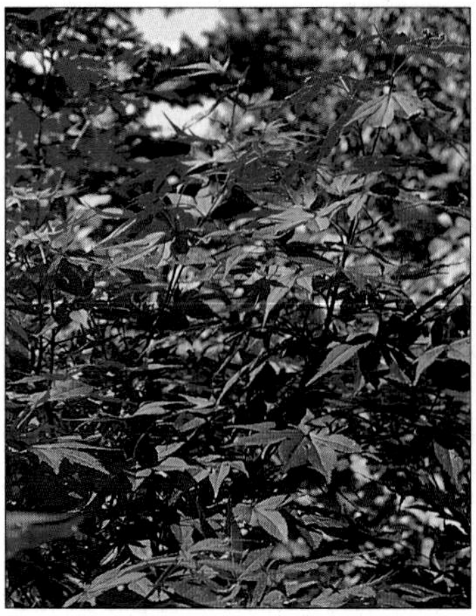

Acer palmatum f. *atropurpureum*

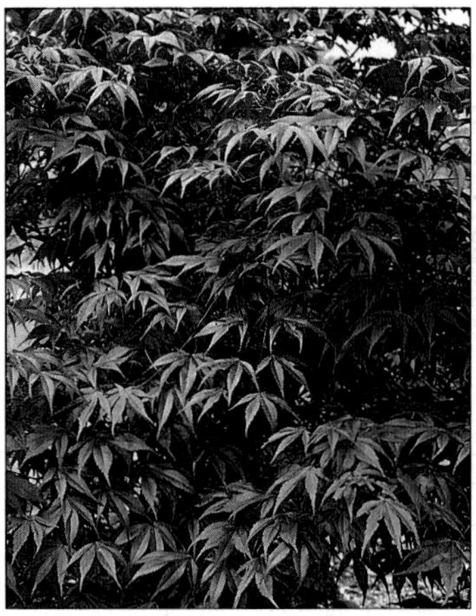

Acer palmatum 'Bloodgood'

'Argenteovariegatum' see 'Variegatum'. **'Auratum'** ⚲ is slow growing, with bright yellow leaves in spring, becoming paler in summer; ↕↔ 8m (25ft). **'Flamingo'** ▣ 🏆 ⚲ has glaucous shoots and leaves with broad pink margins that turn white in summer. **'Variegatum'** ▣ ⚲ syn. 'Argenteovariegatum', has leaves broadly margined with white. **var. *violaceum*** 🏆 has very glaucous shoots and long, hanging tassels of tiny, purple-violet flowers.
A. nikoense see *A. maximowiczianum*.
A. oliverianum ⚲ Graceful, deciduous tree with spreading, arching branches. Ovate, shallowly lobed, mid-green leaves, 5–12cm (2–5in) long, each with 5 tapered and finely toothed lobes, turn orange, red, and purple in autumn. Bears pale yellow flowers in long-

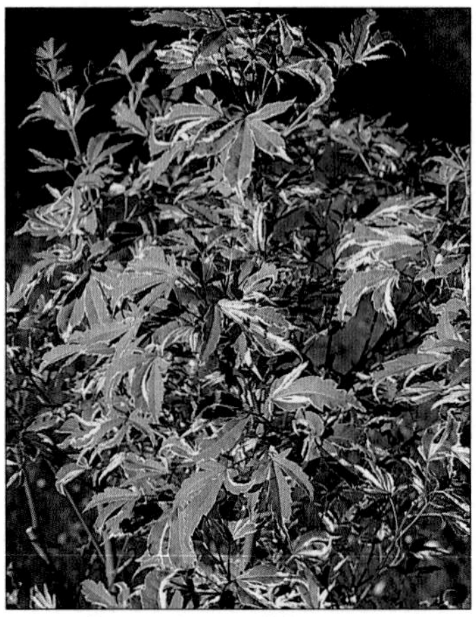

Acer palmatum 'Butterfly'

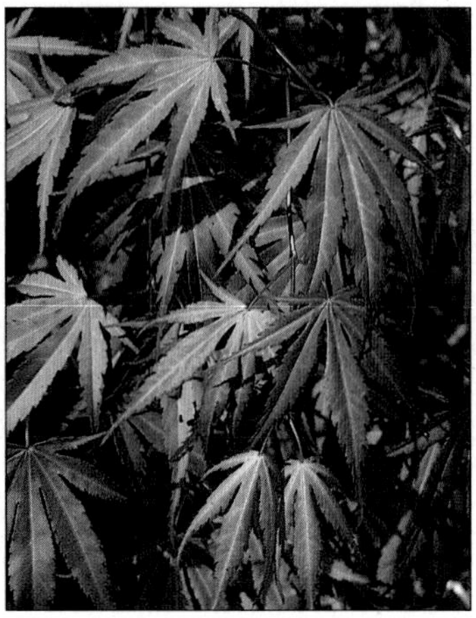

Acer palmatum 'Chitoseyama'

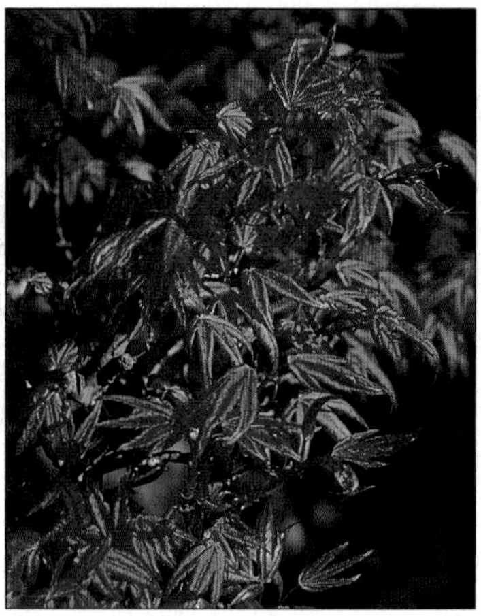

Acer palmatum 'Corallinum'

stalked, upright, corymb-like umbels. ↕ 8m (25ft), ↔ 10m (30ft). China. ❄❄❄
A. opalus ⚲ (Italian maple). Round-headed, deciduous tree with ovate to obovate, 5-lobed, dark green leaves, 6–15cm (2½–6in) long, turning yellow in autumn. Bears showy, pendent corymb-like umbels of yellow flowers. ↕↔ 15m (50ft). S. Europe. ❄❄❄
A. palmatum ⚲ (Japanese maple). Round-headed, deciduous tree with rounded, shallowly to deeply 5- to 9-lobed, mid-green leaves, 5–12cm (2–5in) long, which turn orange to yellow or red in autumn. Tiny, purple-red flowers, borne in small, pendent corymbs, are followed by red-winged fruit in late summer. ↕ 8m (25ft), ↔ 10m (30ft). China, Korea, Japan. ❄❄❄. Most cultivars are low growing and shrubby; taller ones form trees or large shrubs. Several, particularly var. *dissectum* and similar mound-forming cultivars with arching shoots, may be top-grafted to make miniature trees. **'Atrolineare'** see 'Linearilobum Atropurpureum'. **f. *atropurpureum*** ▣ syn. 'Atropurpureum', has deeply lobed, red-purple leaves, turning brilliant red in autumn. **'Beni-kagami'** has pendent branches and very deeply cut, 5-lobed, red-purple leaves; ↕↔ 8m (25ft). **'Bloodgood'** ▣ 🏆 has deeply cut, 5-lobed, dark red-purple leaves, turning bright red in autumn, and red fruit; ↕↔ 5m (15ft). **'Burgundy Lace'** 🏆 has very deeply cut, 5-lobed, dark red-purple leaves; ↕ 4m (12ft) ↔ 5m (15ft). **'Butterfly'** ▣ 🏆 ♀ is upright with small, shallowly 5-lobed, grey-green leaves,

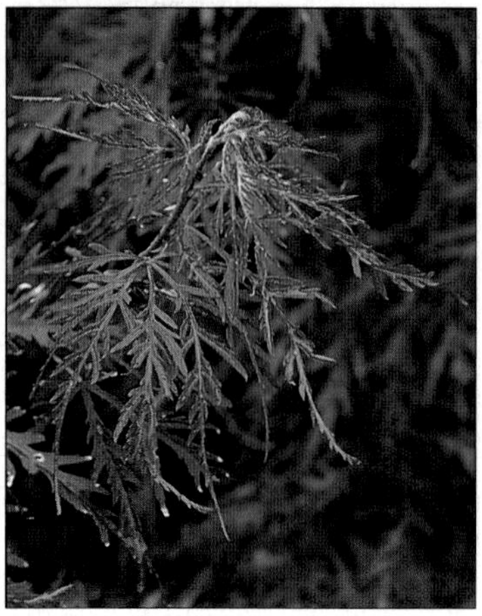

Acer palmatum 'Garnet'

3–5cm (1¼–2in) long, margined white and pink; ↕ 3m (10ft), ↔ 1.5m (5ft). **'Chishio'** see 'Shishio'. **'Chitoseyama'** ▣ 🏆 ⚲ is mound-forming, with deeply 7-lobed, pale crimson-green leaves, which turn rich purple-red in autumn; ↕ 2m (6ft), ↔ 3m (10ft). **'Corallinum'** ▣ is slow growing, with small, deeply lobed, pale green leaves, 3–8cm (1¼–3in) long, opening brilliant pink in spring; ↕ 1.2m (4ft), ↔ 1m (3ft). **'Crimson Queen'** 🏆 has arching shoots and red-purple leaves divided into finely cut, deeply toothed lobes; ↕ 3m (10ft), ↔ 4m (12ft). **var. *dissectum*** 🏆 syn. *A.* 'Dissectum', is mound-forming, with arching shoots, and has 7- to 11-lobed leaves, each deeply and finely cut, turning gold in autumn; ↕ 2m (6ft), ↔ 3m (10ft). **'Dissectum Atropurpureum'** ▣ is similar to var. *dissectum*, but has red-purple leaves. **'Dissectum Nigrum'**, syn. 'Ever Red', is similar to 'Dissectum Atropurpureum', but has dark red-purple leaves, silvery-hairy beneath when young. **'Dissectum Ornatum Variegatum'** is similar to var. *dissectum*, but has leaves with white markings. **'Ever Red'** see 'Dissectum Nigrum'. **'Filigree'** is similar to var. *dissectum*, but has very finely cut leaves, opening pale green mottled with cream, turning gold in autumn. **'Garnet'** ▣ 🏆 is similar to 'Dissectum Atropurpureum', but with leaves remaining red-purple into autumn. **var. *heptalobum*** ▣ has leaves with 7–9 broad lobes, turning orange to red in autumn; ↕ 5m (15ft), ↔ 6m (20ft). **var. *heptalobum* 'Lutescens'** is similar to var. *heptalobum*, but has

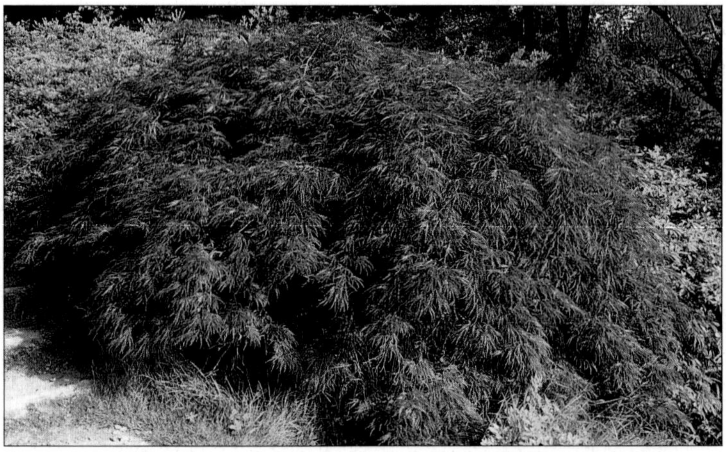

Acer palmatum 'Dissectum Atropurpureum'

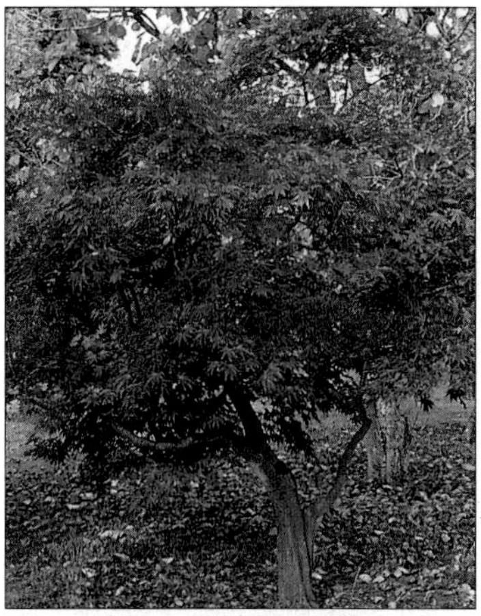

Acer palmatum var. *heptalobum*

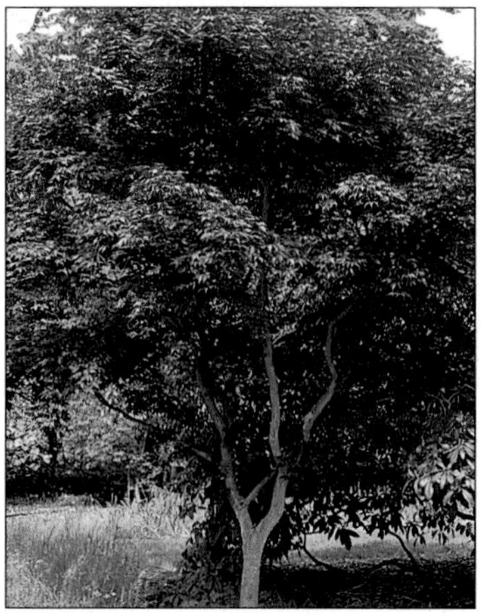

Acer palmatum var. *heptalobum* 'Rubrum'

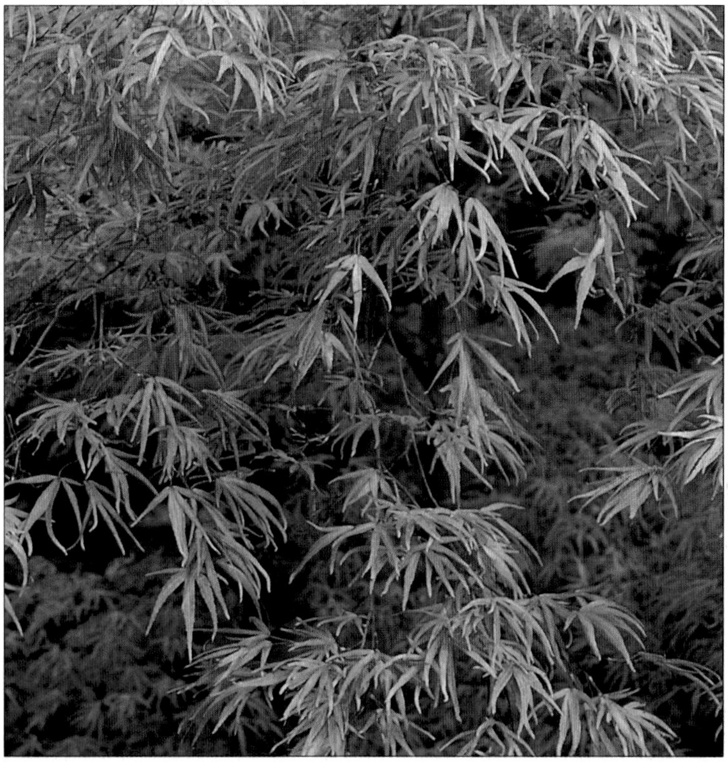

Acer palmatum 'Linearilobum'

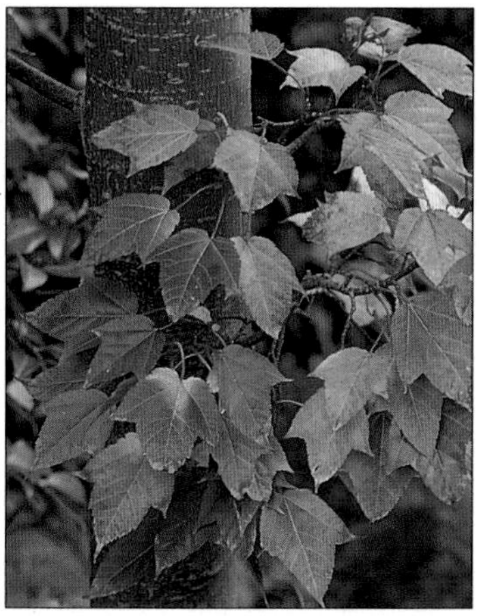

Acer pectinatum subsp. *forrestii*

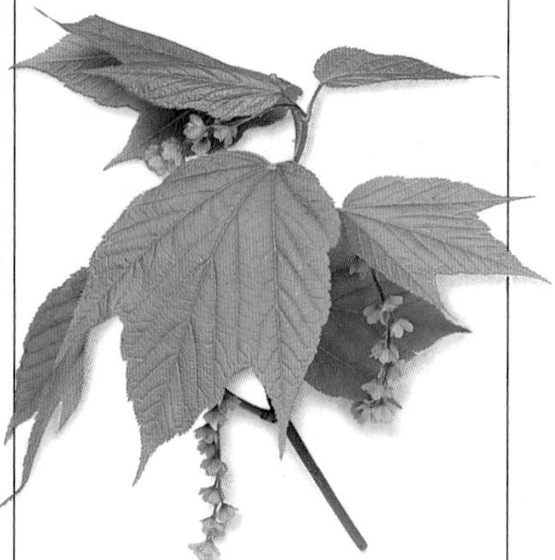

Acer pensylvanicum

yellow-green leaves in spring, turning bright gold in autumn. **var. *heptalobum* 'Rubrum'** ■ is similar to var. *heptalobum*, but with dark red-purple leaves, turning red in autumn. **'Higasayama'** has small leaves, 5–8cm (2–3in) long, margined white and pink, turning yellow to red in autumn; ↕↔ 5m (15ft). **'Kagiri-nishiki'**, syn. 'Roseomarginatum', has blue-green leaves with deeply cut, often curved lobes, margined white and pink, and turning pink and red in autumn; ↕↔ 3m (10ft). **'Linearilobum'** ■ ♀ syn. 'Scolopendrifolum', has deeply cut, bright green leaves with 7 long, slender lobes, turning yellow in autumn; ↕ 5m (15ft), ↔ 4m (12ft). **'Linearilobum Atropurpureum'**, syn. 'Atrolineare', is similar to 'Linearilobum', but with red-purple foliage. **'Osakazuki'** ■ ♀ produces large, deeply 7-lobed leaves, 10–12cm (4–5in) long, which turn brilliant red in autumn; ↕↔ 6m (20ft). **'Red Pygmy'** ♀ ◊ is vase-shaped, with linear leaves that are dark red in spring, turning gold in autumn; ↕↔ 1.5m (5ft). **'Ribesifolium'** see 'Shishigashira'. **'Roseomarginatum'** see 'Kagiri-nishiki'. **'Sango-kaku'** ■ ♀ syn. 'Senkaki', has bright coral-red shoots in winter and deeply 5-lobed leaves, 3–7cm (1¼–3in) long, opening orange-yellow, turning soft yellow in autumn; ↕ 6m (20ft), ↔ 5m (15ft). **'Scolopendrifolum'** see 'Linearilobum'. **'Senkaki'** see 'Sango-kaku'. **'Shindeshojo'** has 5- to 7-lobed leaves, that are brilliant red when young, white- and pink-speckled green in summer, and orange and red in autumn; ↕↔ 2m (6ft). **'Shishigashira'** ◊ syn. 'Ribesifolium', is upright, with densely clustered leaves; ↕ 4m (12ft), ↔ 3m (10ft). **'Shishio'**, syn. 'Chishio', has 5-lobed leaves, bright red when young, green in summer, and red in autumn; ↕↔ 2.5m (8ft). **'Ukigumo'** ◊ has small, deeply cut, 5-lobed leaves, 3–7cm (1¼–3in) long, irregularly mottled white and pink; ↕↔ 2m (6ft). **'Waterfall'** is similar to var. *dissectum*, but has slightly deeper cut, semi-pendent leaves.

A. pectinatum* subsp. *forrestii ■ ○ syn. *A. forrestii*. Spreading, deciduous tree with arching branches, red when young, later becoming green-and-white-striped. Broadly ovate leaves, to 12cm (5in) long, each with 3, sometimes 5 lobes, open red-tinged green, turn dark green in summer, and orange-red in autumn. Produces pendent racemes of brownish green flowers. ↕↔ 10m (30ft). W. China. ❄❄❄

A. pectinatum* subsp. *laxiflorum see *A. laxiflorum*.

A. pensylvanicum ■ ♀ ◊ (Moosewood, Striped maple). Broadly upright, deciduous tree with green-and-white-striped bark. Obovate, bright green leaves, to 20cm (8in) long, have 3 forward-pointing lobes, and turn clear yellow in autumn. Bears pendent panicles, 10–15cm (4–6in) long, of greenish yellow flowers. ↕ 12m (40ft), ↔ 10m (30ft). E. North America. ❄❄❄. **'Erythrocladum'** ♀ has brilliant pink young shoots, striking in winter, which become orange-red with white stripes as they mature.

A. pentaphyllum ○ Spreading, deciduous tree with slender shoots. The 5- to 7-palmate leaves, to 7cm (3in) long, with long red leaf-stalks, are divided into narrow, oblong to lance-shaped, entire or nearly entire leaflets, which are glossy, light green above, and blue-green beneath. Bears upright corymbs of yellow-green flowers. ↕ 10m (30ft), ↔ 8m (25ft). S.W. China. ❄❄

A. pictum see *A. mono.*

A. platanoides ♀ ○ (Norway maple). Vigorous, spreading, deciduous tree with large, broadly ovate, dark green leaves, 8–15cm (3–6in) long, each with 3–5 lobes, ending in slender-pointed teeth. The leaves turn clear yellow or sometimes red in autumn. Bears small but conspicuous, upright corymbs of yellow flowers. ↕ 25m (80ft), ↔ 15m (50ft). Europe. ❄❄❄. **'Chas. F. Irish'** has an open, rounded crown with upswept branches; ↕ 15m (50ft) or more. **'Columnarbroad'** ◊ syn. 'Parkway', is compact and broadly upright, with an oval crown and bright yellow autumn colour; ↕ 12m (40ft), ↔ 8m (25ft). **'Columnare'** ◊ is similar to 'Columnarbroad', but is taller and has a narrower spread; ↕ 20m (70ft), ↔ 6m (20ft). **'Crimson King'** ■ ♀ has dark red-purple foliage, maturing dark purple, and red-tinged yellow flowers. **'Crimson Sentry'** ◊ is narrowly upright, and has red-purple foliage; ↕ 12m (40ft), ↔ 5m (15ft). **'Deborah'** produces wavy-

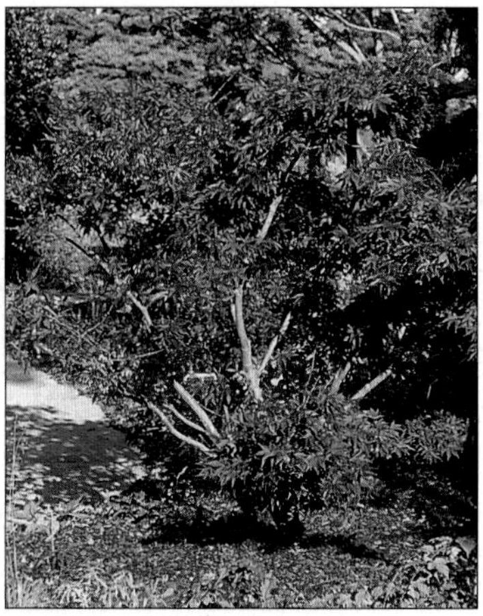

Acer palmatum 'Osakazuki'

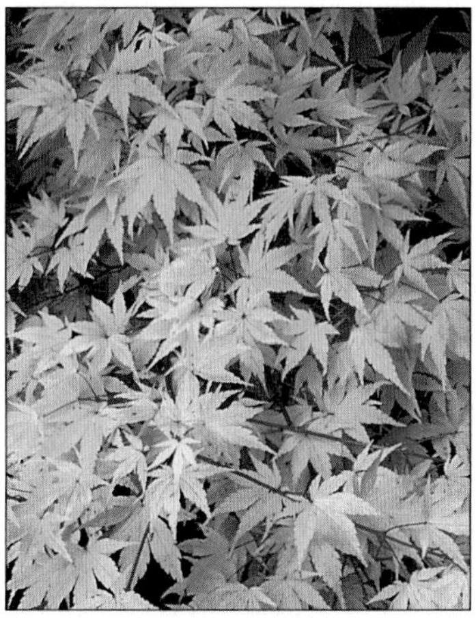

Acer palmatum 'Sango-kaku'

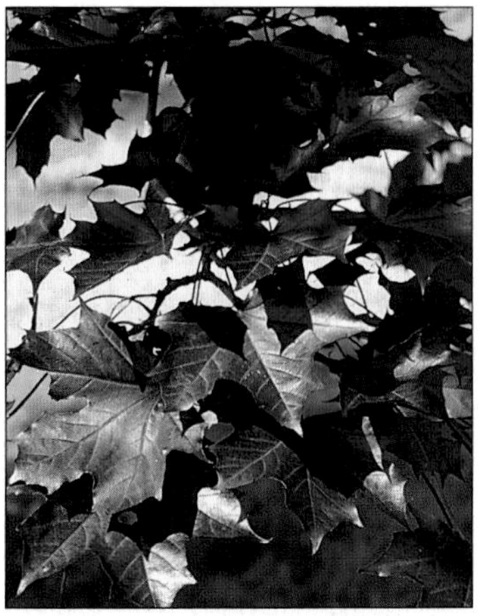

Acer platanoides 'Crimson King'

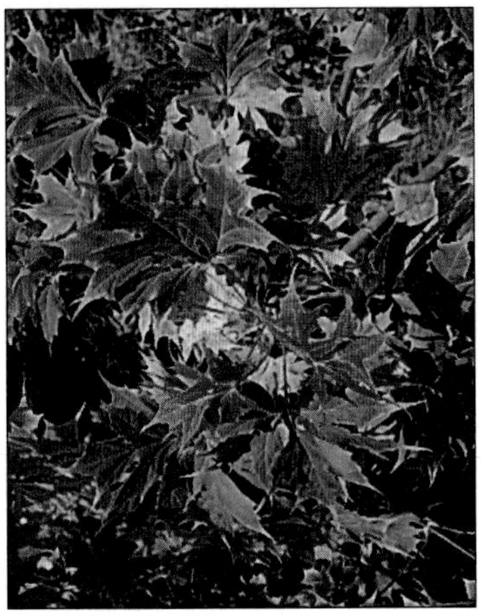
Acer platanoides 'Palmatifidum'

margined leaves, which open brilliant red, turn dark green in summer, and become orange-yellow in autumn. **'Drummondii'** ♀ has leaves broadly margined creamy white; ↕↔ 10–12m (30–40ft). **'Faassen's Black'** is similar to 'Crimson King', but has duller and darker, red-purple leaves, turned up at the margins, becoming bright red in autumn. **'Fairview'** has leaves opening dark red, then turning dark green in summer. **'Globosum'** has a dense, rounded head; ↕ 6m (20ft), ↔ 8m (25ft). **'Goldsworth Purple'** is similar to 'Crimson King', but has lighter red-purple leaves, wrinkled when young. **'Jade Glen'** is fast growing, with an open head. **'Laciniatum'** ⬮ (Eagle's claw maple) is upright, and has fan-shaped, deeply lobed leaves with claw-like lobes;

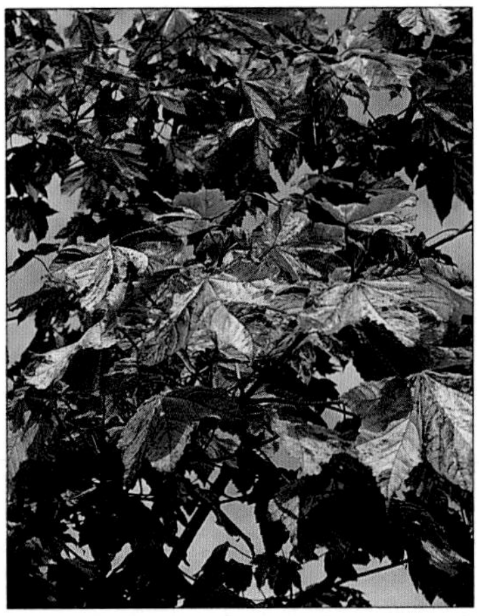
Acer pseudoplatanus 'Simon Louis Frères'

↕ 20m (70ft), ↔ 10m (30ft). **'Lorbergii'** see 'Palmatifidum'. **'Olmsted'** ⬮ is dense and upright; ↕ 10m (30ft), ↔ 5m (15ft). **'Oregon Pride'** is fast growing, with shallowly lobed leaves that turn golden bronze in autumn. **'Palmatifidum'** ■ syn. 'Lorbergii', has shallowly to deeply lobed leaves, the lobes ending in long, slender teeth. **'Parkway'** see 'Columnarbroad'. **'Schwedleri'** ♀ bears conspicuous, purplish yellow flowers before the leaves. The leaves open red at first, then turn dark purple-green in summer.

A. pseudoplatanus ⚲ (Sycamore). Fast-growing, spreading, rounded, deciduous tree producing ovate, 5-lobed, dark green leaves, 10–20cm (4–8in) long. Yellow-green flowers are borne in pendent panicles, to 12cm (5in) long, followed by green, sometimes red, winged fruit. ↕ 30m (100ft), ↔ 25m (80ft). Europe, S.W. Asia. ❄❄❄. **'Atropurpureum'** has dark green leaves, dark red-purple beneath, with red leaf-stalks; it bears clusters of red-winged fruit in late summer; ↕ 25m (80ft), ↔ 20m (70ft). **'Brilliantissimum'** ■ ♀ is slow growing, with a dense head, and bright pink leaves that turn yellow, then green in summer; ↕ 6m (20ft), ↔ 8m (25ft). **f. *erythrocarpum*** ■ produces fruit with bright red wings. **'Leopoldii'** ♀ has leaves that open pink, later turning yellow, then green speckled with yellow and pink; ↕↔ 10m (30ft). **'Nizetii'** produces leaves splashed and streaked with pale green and white above, red-purple beneath; ↕↔ 12m (40ft). **'Prinz Handjery'** is similar to 'Brilliantissimum', but with leaves that are red-purple beneath. **'Simon Louis Frères'** ■ is slow-growing, with leaves opening pink, then turning creamy green speckled with white in summer; ↕↔ 10m (30ft). **'Worley'** ♀ syn. 'Worlei', 'Worleei', has leaves that open yellow, then turn green in summer, with red leaf-stalks.

A. pseudosieboldianum ⚲ (Korean maple). Small, rounded, deciduous tree with a bushy head and rounded, glossy, mid-green leaves, to 12cm (5in) long, with 9–11 finely toothed lobes. The leaves turn red, orange, or purple in autumn. Red-purple flowers are borne in erect corymbs. ↕↔ 6m (20ft). N.E. China, Korea. ❄❄❄

A. rubrum ⚲ (Red maple, Scarlet maple, Swamp maple). Round-headed to open-crowned, deciduous tree with 3- or 5-lobed, ovate, dark green leaves, to 10cm (4in) long, blue-white beneath, turning bright red in autumn. Produces erect clusters of tiny red flowers. Grow in acid soil for best autumn colour. ↕ 20m (70ft), ↔ 10m (30ft). E. North America. ❄❄❄. **'Armstrong'** ⬮ is erect; ↔ to 6m (20ft). **'Autumn Flame'** ⬮ has foliage that turns brilliant red in early autumn. **'Columnare'** ■ ⬮ is narrow, with red-orange autumn colour; ↔ 3m (10ft). **'Gerling'** is conical when young; ↕ 8m (25ft), ↔ 10m (30ft). **'Indian Summer'** see 'Morgan'. **'Morgan'**, syn. 'Indian Summer', is vigorous and extremely hardy, with leaves that turn brilliant orange-red in autumn. **'October Glory'** ■ ♀ ⬮ has glossy foliage, which turns brilliant red in early autumn. **'Red Sunset'** has bright red colour very early in autumn. **'Scanlon'** ■ ♀ ⬮ is dense and columnar, and has foliage that turns red-orange in autumn; ↕ 15m (50ft), ↔ 5m (15ft). **'Scarlet Sentinel'** ⬮ syn. 'Scarsen', is vigorous and columnar, with leaves that turn orange-red in autumn; ↕ 12m (40ft). **'Scarsen'** see 'Scarlet Sentinel'. **'Schlesingeri'** ■ has leaves that turn dark red very early in autumn.

A. rufinerve ■ ♀ ⚲ (Snake-bark maple). Arching, deciduous tree with glaucous young shoots, green-and-white-striped branches, and ovate, 3-lobed leaves, to 12cm (5in) long, which turn red in autumn. Greenish yellow flowers are borne in erect racemes, followed by red-winged fruit. ↕↔ 10m (30ft). Japan. ❄❄❄. **'Hatsuyuki'**, syn. f. *albolimbatum*, has leaves that are boldly mottled white.

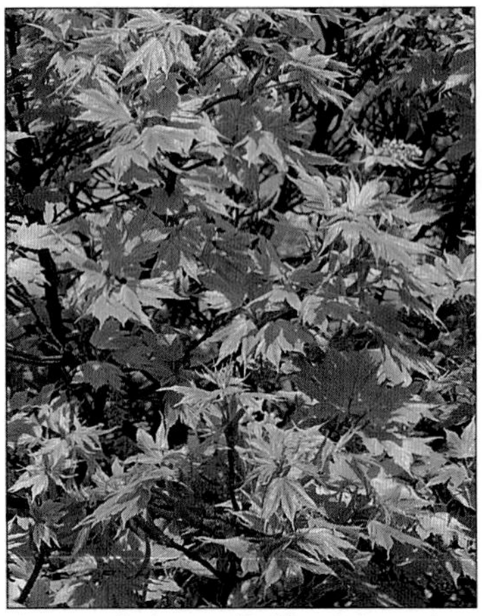
Acer pseudoplatanus 'Brilliantissimum'

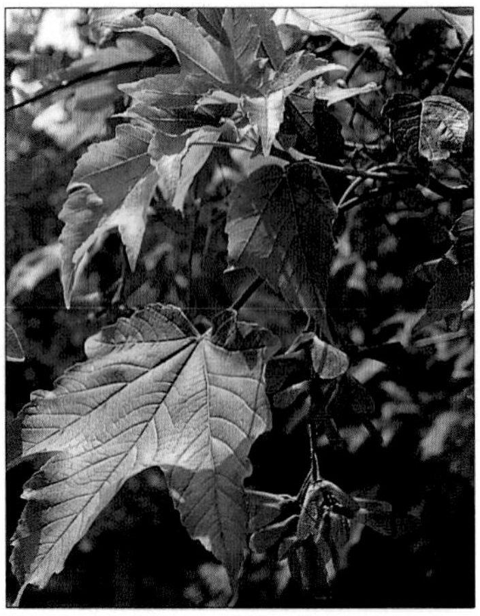
Acer pseudoplatanus f. *erythrocarpum*

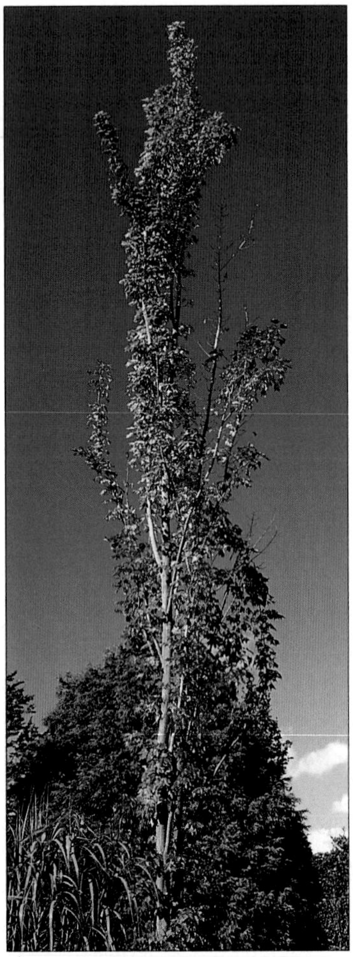
Acer rubrum 'Columnare'

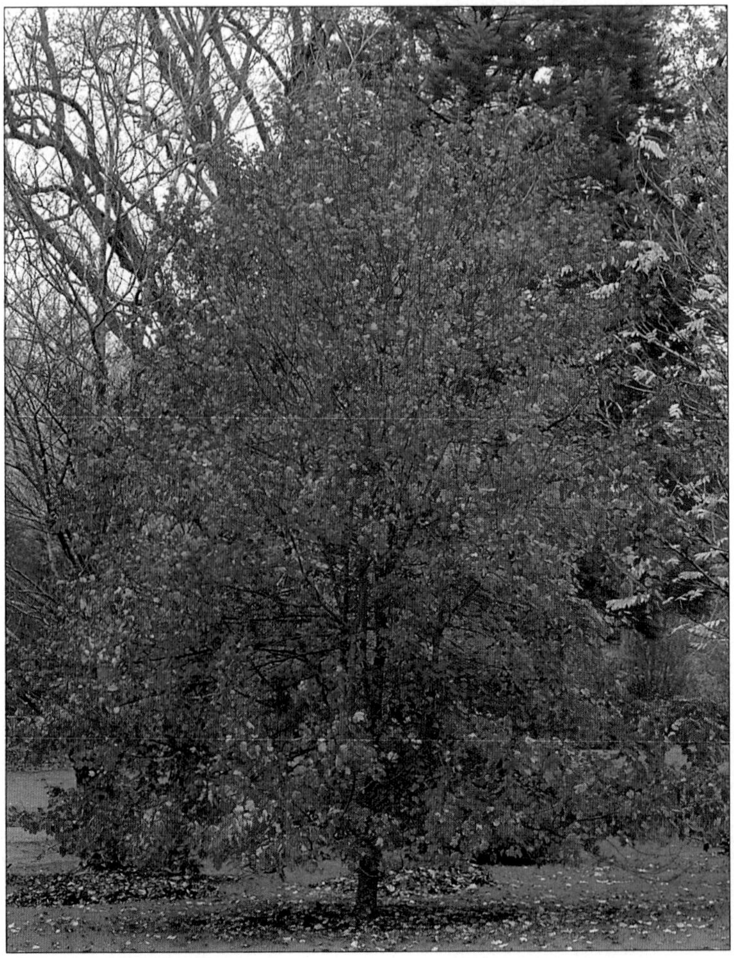
Acer rubrum 'October Glory'

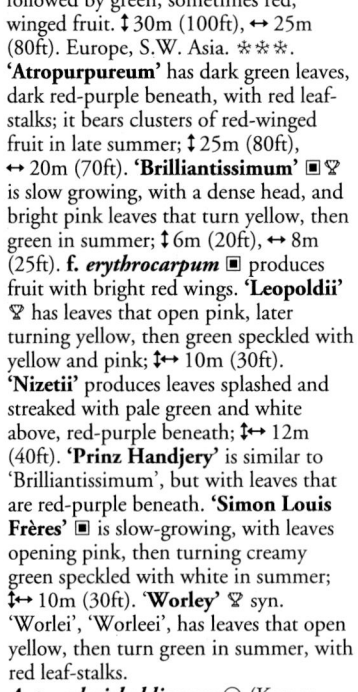

A. saccharinum ■ syn. *A. dasycarpum* (Silver maple). Spreading, fast-growing, deciduous tree, often with pendent branches. Sharply toothed, shallowly to deeply 5-lobed leaves, 10–20cm (4–8in) long, are light green above, silvery white beneath, and turn yellow to orange or red in autumn. Greenish yellow flowers are borne in small, erect corymbs. ↕25m (80ft), ↔ 15m (50ft). E. North America. ✻✻✻. **'Laciniatum Wieri'** syn. 'Wieri' has pendent lower branches and very deeply cut leaves. **'Lutescens'** has yellow-green leaves that turn yellow in autumn. **'Pyramidale'** is broadly upright, with deeply cut leaves. **'Silver Queen'** is broadly upright, with bright green leaves turning yellow in autumn, and produces few fruit. **'Wieri'** see 'Laciniatum Wieri'.

A. saccharum (Rock maple, Sugar maple). Deciduous tree with a dense, oval to rounded crown and large, broadly ovate, dull, mid-green leaves, 8–18cm (3–7in) long, with 3–5 blunt lobes, which turn brilliant orange to red and yellow in autumn. Greenish yellow flowers are borne in upright corymbs. ↕20m (70ft), ↔ 12m (40ft). E. North America. ✻✻✻. **'Bonfire'** is vigorous, with glossy, mid-green leaves, turning bright red and orange in autumn. **'Columnare'** see 'Newton Sentry'. **'Goldspire'** is columnar, with leaves that turn bright yellow-orange in autumn. **subsp. *grandidentatum*** syn. *A. grandidentatum* (Canyon maple), is much smaller than *A. saccharum*, and has glossy, mid-green leaves, 6–12cm (2½–5in) long, which turn brilliant scarlet, orange, or yellow in autumn; ↕↔ 10m (30ft); W. USA. **'Green Mountain'** is upright, and ideal for growing in hot, dry areas. **'Monumentale'** see 'Temple's Upright'. **'Newton Sentry'** syn. 'Columnare', has upright branches, which have short, spur-like shoots, and lacks a central leader; ↕10m (30ft), ↔ 2.5m (8ft). **subsp. *nigrum* 'Green Column'** ■ is broadly columnar, with leaves that turn bright yellow in autumn; ↕12m (40ft), ↔ 8m (25ft). **'Sweet Shadow'** has deeply lobed leaves, turning orange in autumn. **'Temple's Upright'** ■ syn. 'Monumentale', is narrowly upright, and has ascending branches; ↕20m (70ft), ↔ 5m (15ft).

***A. shirasawanum* 'Aureum'** ■ syn. *A. japonicum* 'Aureum'. Rounded, bushy, deciduous tree or shrub producing rounded, 7- to 11-lobed, bright yellow leaves, 7–10cm (3–4in) long, which turn red in autumn. Tiny, red-purple flowers are borne in upright corymbs. ↕↔ 6m (20ft). ✻✻✻

A. sieboldianum Rounded, bushy, deciduous tree with rounded, 7- to 11-lobed, mid-green leaves, 6–9cm (2½–3½in) long, which turn orange-yellow to red in autumn. Bears small, nodding corymbs of tiny yellow flowers. ↕↔ 6m (20ft). Japan. ✻✻✻

A. spicatum (Mountain maple). Deciduous tree or shrub with upright shoots, red-tinged when young, and ovate, shallowly 3-lobed, toothed, bright green leaves, to 12cm (5in) long, turning red in autumn. Creamy white flowers are borne in slender, upright panicles. ↕8m (25ft), ↔ 5m (15ft). E. North America. ✻✻✻

A. tataricum (Tatarian maple). Bushy, deciduous tree with a rounded crown. Produces broadly ovate, glossy, bright green leaves, to 10cm (4in) long, entire or with up to 3 lobes, and with toothed margins; the leaves turn red or yellow in autumn. Upright panicles of creamy white flowers are followed by red-winged fruit. ↕10m (30ft), ↔ 8m (25ft). S.E. Europe, S.W. Asia. ✻✻✻.

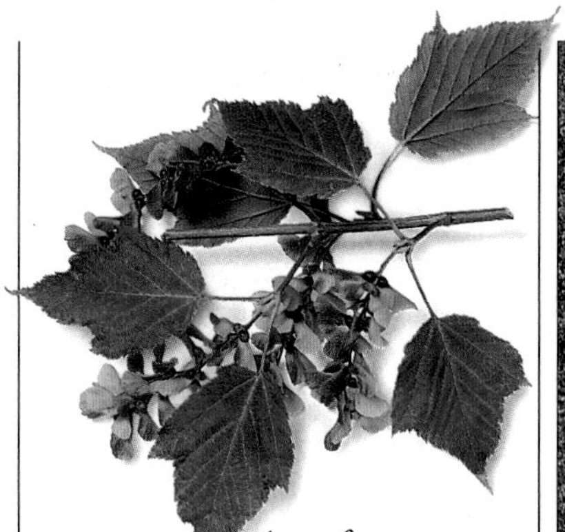

Acer rufinerve

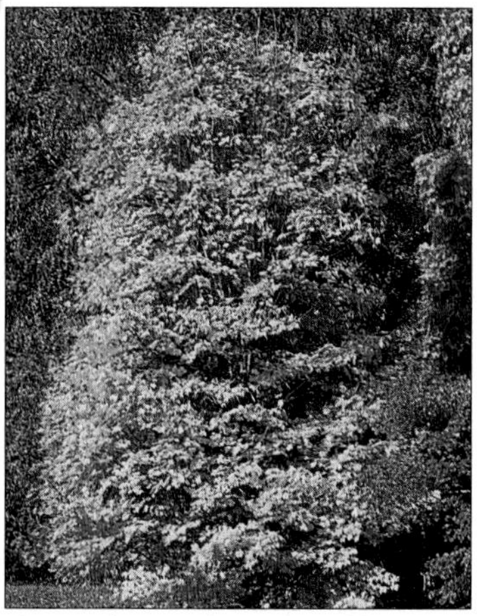

Acer saccharum subsp. *nigrum* 'Green Column'

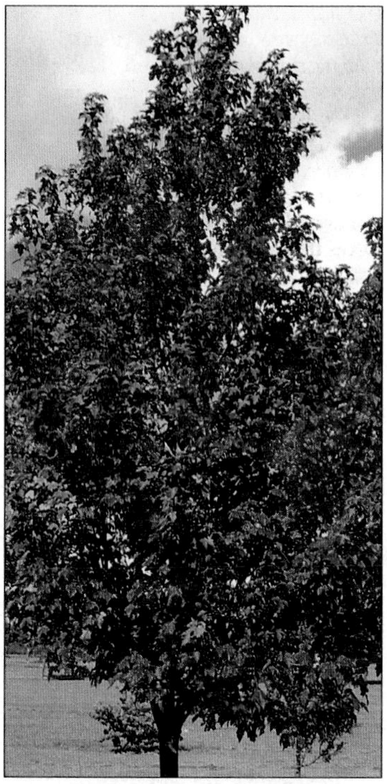

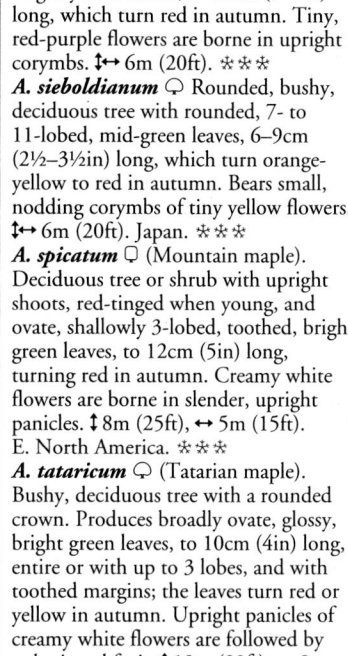

Acer rubrum 'Scanlon'

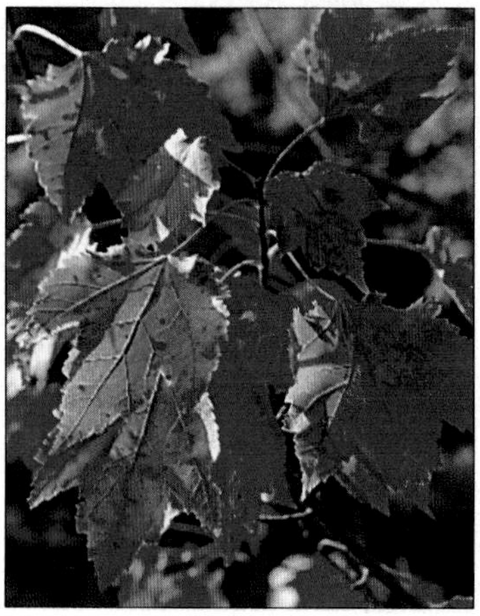

Acer rubrum 'Schlesingeri'

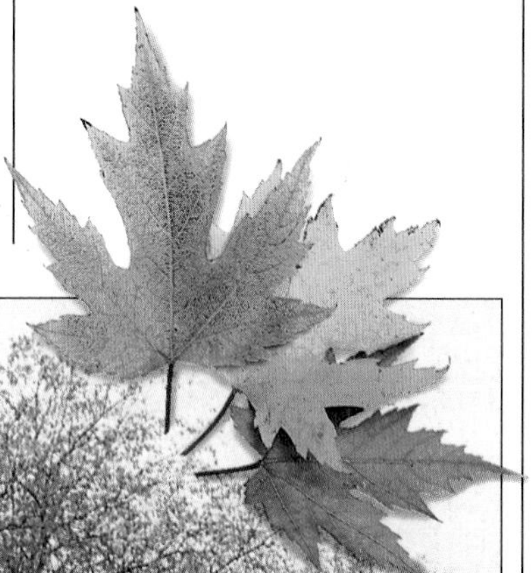

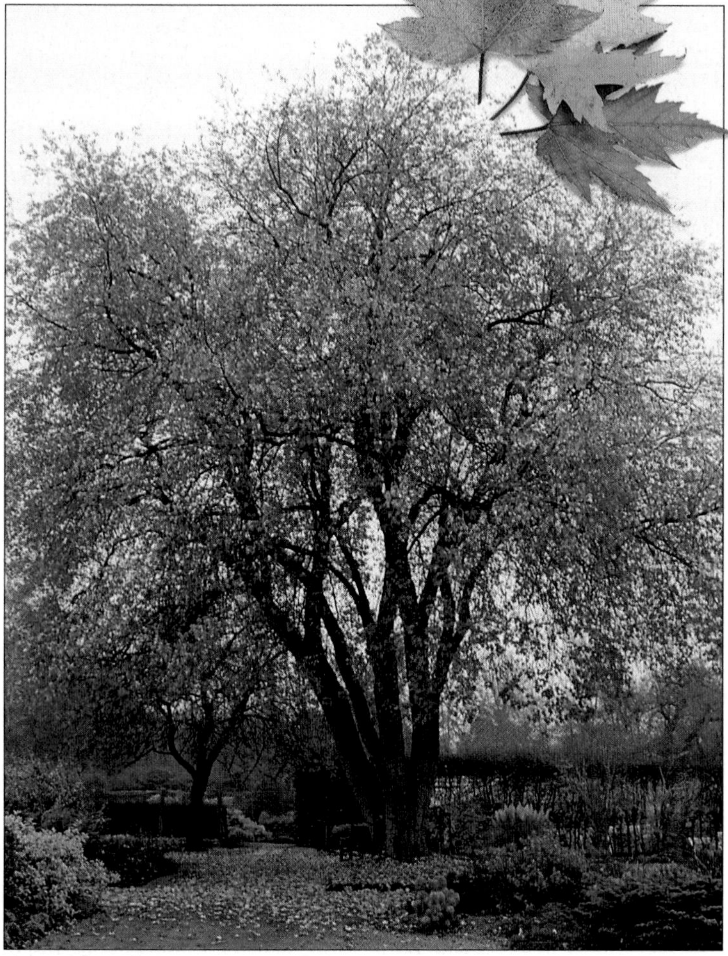

Acer saccharinum (inset: autumn leaf colour)

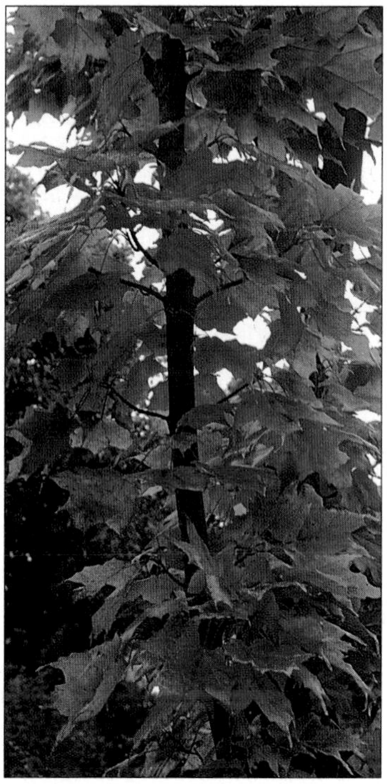

Acer saccharum 'Temple's Upright'

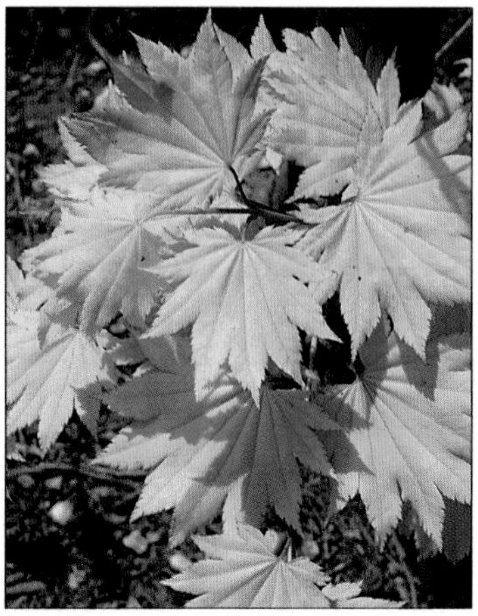

Acer shirasawanum 'Aureum'

A

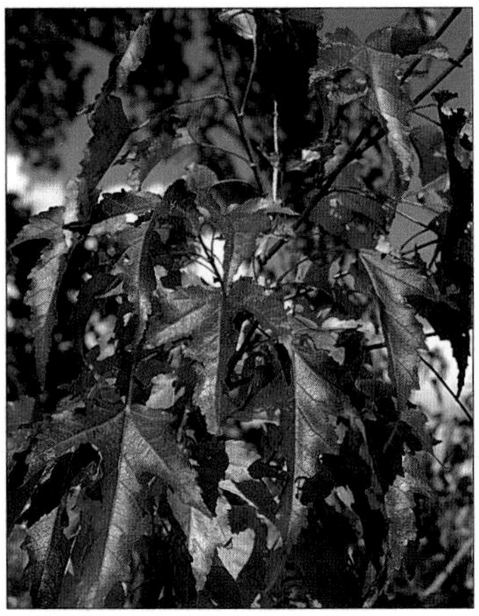

Acer tataricum subsp. *ginnala*

subsp. *ginnala* ▣ 🏆 syn. *A. ginnala* (Amur maple), has slender, arching branches and deeply 3-lobed leaves, which turn deep red in autumn. **subsp. *ginnala* 'Durand Dwarf'** is dense and shrubby, and has leaves, to 4–8cm (1½–3in) long, which turn light to dark red in early autumn; ↕ 1.5m (5ft), ↔ 2m (6ft). **subsp. *ginnala* 'Flame'** has red leaves and fruit in autumn.
A. tegmentosum ♀ Spreading, deciduous tree with green-and-white-striped branches, and ovate, shallowly 3-lobed, bright green leaves, to 15cm (6in) long, yellow in autumn. Bears yellowish green flowers in pendent racemes. ↕ 8m (25ft), ↔ 10m (30ft). N.E. Asia. ❄❄❄
A. triflorum ▣ ♀ Broadly columnar to spreading, deciduous tree with peeling, grey-brown bark and unevenly toothed, 3-palmate, mid-green leaves, to 8cm (3in) long, with obovate to lance-shaped leaflets, orange in autumn. Bears clusters of yellow-green flowers. ↕ 10m (30ft), ↔ 8m (25ft). N.E. Asia. ❄❄❄
A. truncatum ♀ (Shantung maple). Compact, rounded, deciduous tree with a spreading head and glossy, mid-green, broadly ovate leaves, 8–12cm (3–5in) long, usually with 5 tapered lobes, turning yellow in autumn. Yellowish green flowers are produced in upright corymbs. ↕ 8m (25ft), ↔ 10m (30ft). N. China, Korea. ❄❄❄
A. velutinum ▣ ♀ Vigorous, spreading, deciduous tree with ovate, 5-lobed, dark green leaves, 15–25cm (6–10in) long, downy on the reverse, on red leaf-stalks. Bears upright corymb-like panicles of yellow-green flowers. ↕ 20m (70ft), ↔ 15m (50ft). Caucasus, N. Iran.

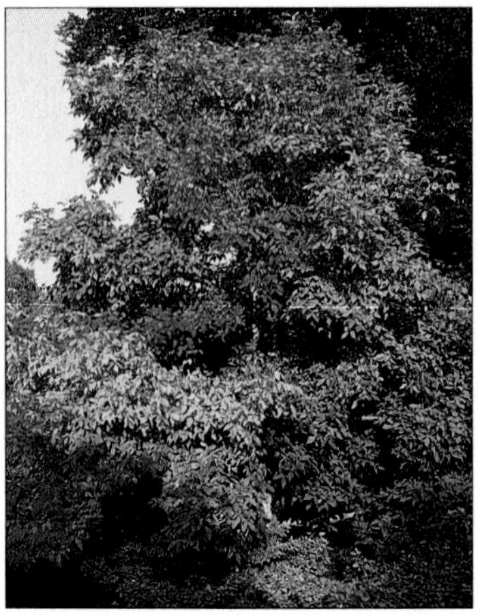

Acer triflorum

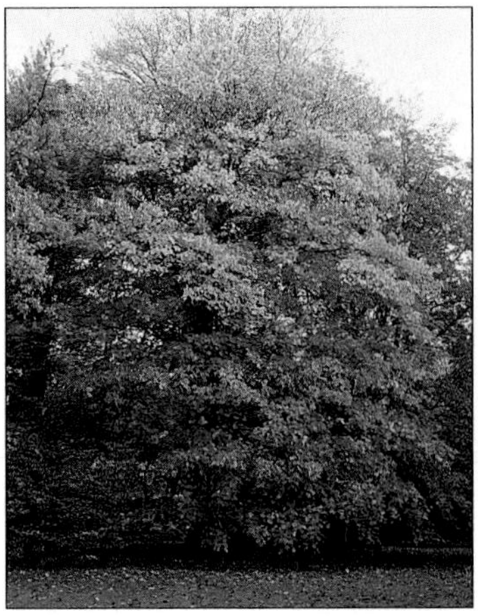

Acer velutinum

❄❄❄. **var. *vanvolxemii*** has large leaves, 20–30cm (8–12in) long, blue-green beneath.
A.* x *zoeschense ♀ (*A. campestre* x *A. cappadocicum* subsp. *lobelii*). Rounded, deciduous tree with broadly ovate leaves, deeply heart-shaped at the bases, and 7–12cm (3–5in) long. The leaves usually have 5 tapered, shallowly toothed lobes, and are glossy, dark green, turning yellow in autumn. Bears yellowish green flowers in upright, softly hairy corymbs. ↕↔ 15m (50ft). Garden origin. ❄❄❄. **'Annae'** has red-purple leaves that turn dark green in summer.

▷ ***Aceriphyllum*** see *Mukdenia*
A. rossii see *M. rossii*

ACHILLEA

Yarrow

ASTERACEAE/COMPOSITAE

Genus of about 85 species of mainly deciduous perennials from temperate regions of the N. hemisphere. Some, from mountainous regions, are low growing and mat-forming; other species, from grassland or dry wasteground, are taller and herbaceous. The grey or green, often aromatic leaves are mostly 1- to 3-pinnate or pinnatifid, and fern-like, although some are entire. They are elliptic to lance-shaped, toothed, and 15–30cm (6–12in) long in most species, 5–12cm (2–5in) long in smaller-growing achilleas. The basal leaves are usually larger than the stem leaves. Most achilleas produce daisy-like flowerheads, 3–15mm (⅛–½in) across, in corymbs, 7–12cm (3–5in) across, in summer and autumn; the disc- and ray-florets are usually both white or both yellow. Newer cultivars and hybrids, including the Galaxy Hybrids (*A. millefolium* x *A.* 'Taygetea'), offer a wide colour range, and produce flowerheads in compound corymbs, 15–20cm (6–8in) across. Grow achilleas in a wildflower or rock garden; the taller ones are excellent for a mixed or herbaceous border, and for cutting and drying. Contact with foliage may aggravate skin allergies.
• **HARDINESS** Fully hardy.
• **CULTIVATION** Grow in moist but well-drained soil in an open site in full sun, although most will tolerate a wide range of soils and conditions. *A. ageratum* 'W.B. Childs' and *A. ptarmica* cultivars require more moisture than other achilleas, but not waterlogged soils, and partial shade. *A. clavennae* and *A.* x

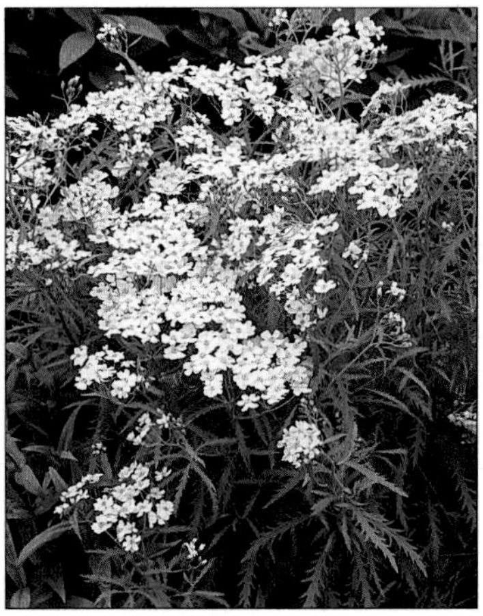

Achillea ageratum 'W.B. Childs'

kellereri will not tolerate winter wet in poorly drained soils. Dwarf species and silver- and hairy-leaved alpine species must have sharp drainage.
• **PROPAGATION** Sow seed *in situ* or divide in spring. *A. clypeolata* is short-lived, so divide annually to maintain stocks. Divide *A.* 'Moonshine' regularly to maintain vigour.
• **PESTS AND DISEASES** Aphids may be a problem; powdery mildew is common, especially on *A. ptarmica* cultivars.

***A. aegyptica* of gardens** see *A.* 'Taygetea'.
A. ageratum, syn. *A. decolorans.* Spreading perennial producing linear, pinnatifid, sharply toothed, grey-white leaves. Yellowish white flowerheads are borne in loose corymbs, 8cm (3in) wide, from midsummer to early autumn. ↕↔ 60cm (24in). Portugal, W. Mediterranean. ❄❄❄. **'W.B. Childs'** ▣ bears many attractive white flowerheads with creamy white disc-florets; ↕ 60–70cm (24–28in).
A. argentea see *Tanacetum argenteum.*
***A. argentea* of gardens** see *A. clavennae.*
A. chrysocoma. Mat-forming, spreading perennial with ovate, 2- or 3-pinnate, mid-green leaves. In early summer, produces corymbs, 1–2cm (½–¾in) across, of golden yellow flowerheads. ↕ 5–8cm (2–3in), ↔ 30cm (12in). Greece, Turkey (Anatolia). ❄❄❄
A. clavennae ▣ syn. *A. argentea* of gardens. Mat-forming perennial with semi-evergreen, narrowly obovate, pinnatifid or pinnate, light grey-green, silver-hairy leaves. Bears clusters of up to 25 white flowerheads, in corymbs

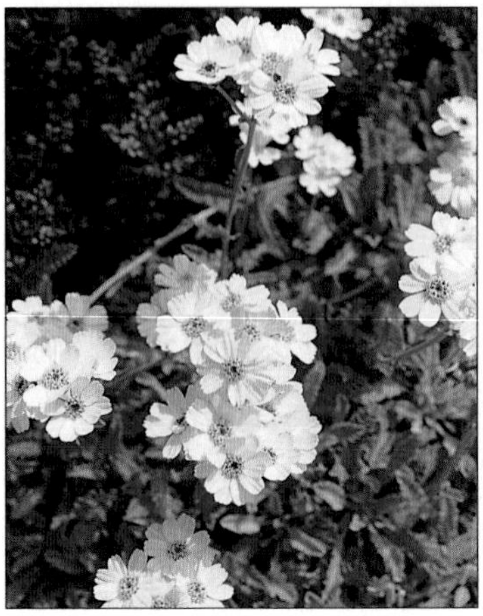

Achillea clavennae

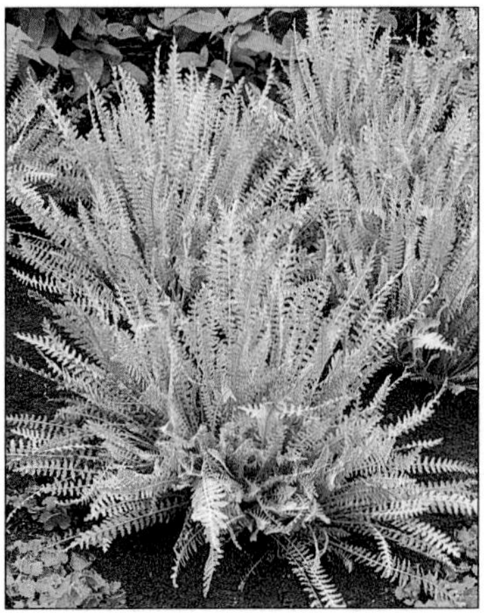

Achillea clypeolata

4–5cm (1½–2in) across, in summer and early autumn. ↕ 15–20cm (6–8in), ↔ 30cm (12in) or more. E. European Alps. ❄❄❄
A. clypeolata ▣ Mat-forming perennial with ovate to lance-shaped, pinnatifid, silvery green leaves. Corymbs, 5–7cm (2–3in) across, of tiny, golden yellow flowerheads are produced from early to late summer. ↕ 45–60cm (18–24in), ↔ 30cm (12in). Balkans. ❄❄❄
***A.* 'Coronation Gold'** ▣ 🏆 Clump-forming perennial with evergreen, oblong, pinnatifid, silvery grey leaves. Bears tiny, golden yellow flowerheads in corymbs, 10cm (4in) across, from mid-summer to early autumn. ↕ 75–90cm (30–36in), ↔ 45cm (18in). ❄❄❄
A. decolorans see *A. ageratum.*
A. eupatorium see *A. filipendulina.*

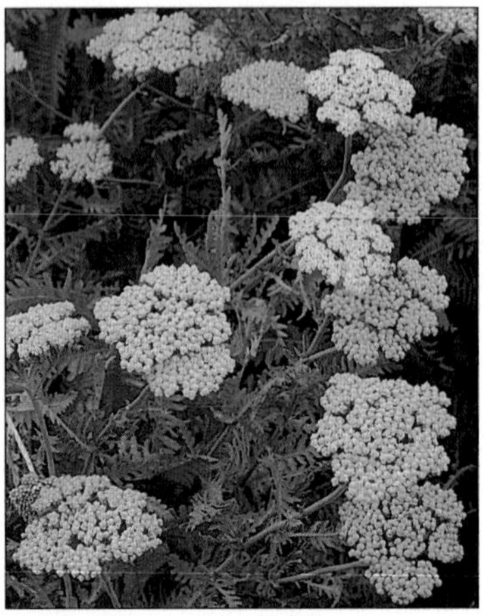

Achillea 'Coronation Gold'

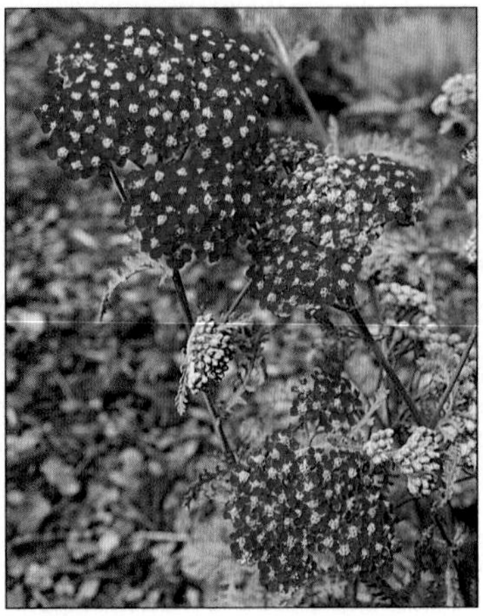

Achillea 'Fanal'

ACHILLEA

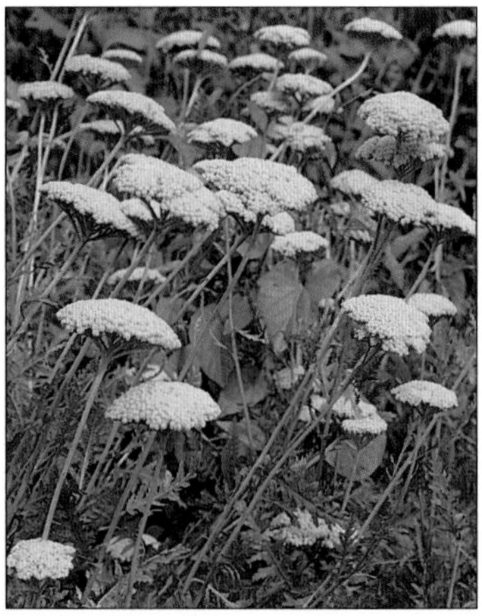

Achillea filipendulina 'Gold Plate'

***A.* 'Fanal'** ■ syn. *A.* 'The Beacon'. Mat-forming Galaxy Hybrid with broadly linear, 2-pinnate, slightly greyish green leaves. In early summer, bears corymbs, to 15cm (6in) across, of bright red flowerheads with yellow disc-florets that fade with age. ↕75cm (30in), ↔60cm (24in). ❄❄❄
***A. filipendulina*,** syn. *A. eupatorium.* Clump-forming, evergreen perennial with rosettes of oblong, 1- or 2-pinnate, mid- to grey-green leaves. Strong, leafy stems bear golden yellow flowerheads in flat corymbs, 12cm (5in) across, from early summer to early autumn. ↕1.2m (4ft), ↔45cm (18in). Caucasus. ❄❄❄. **'Altgold'** has grey-green leaves and corymbs of copper-tinged yellow flowerheads; ↕60cm (24in). **'Cloth of Gold'** has light green leaves and corymbs of deep golden yellow flowerheads; ↕1.5m (5ft). **'Gold Plate'** ■🏆 has bright golden yellow flowerheads in slightly convex corymbs, 15cm (6in) across.
***A.* 'Flowers of Sulphur'** see *A.* 'Schwefelblüte'.
***A.* 'Forncett Candy'** ■ Clump-forming, evergreen perennial producing rosettes of fern-like, broadly linear, pinnatifid, grey-green leaves. During summer, freely branching stems bear a profusion of pale pink flowerheads in corymbs to 15cm (6in) across; the ray-florets fade almost to white with age; ↕85cm (34in), ↔45cm (18in). ❄❄❄
***A.* 'Forncett Ivory'.** Clump-forming perennial with rosettes of evergreen, broadly linear, fern-like, pinnatifid, mid-green to grey-green leaves. In summer, bears corymbs, to 15cm (6in) across, of ivory flowerheads, the disc-florets tinged reddish brown. ↕85cm (34in), ↔45cm (18in). ❄❄❄
A. grandifolia. Clump-forming perennial with ovate, coarsely pinnate, greyish green leaves. Stout stems bear white flowerheads, in corymbs to 12cm (5in) across, from early summer to autumn. ↕90cm (36in), ↔60cm (24in). C. Balkans. ❄❄❄
***A.* 'Great Expectations'** see *A.* 'Hoffnung'.
***A.* 'Hartington White'.** Spreading perennial with linear, finely divided, pinnatifid, sharply toothed, greyish green leaves. White flowerheads are borne in corymbs, 10–15cm (4–6in) across, in early summer. ↕↔60cm (24in). ❄❄❄
***A.* 'Hoffnung'**, syn. *A.* 'Great Expectations'. Compact, clump-forming Galaxy Hybrid with broadly linear, 2-pinnate, mid-green leaves. In summer, freely bears corymbs, 10–15cm (4–6in) across, of creamy, sand-coloured flowerheads with disc-florets that darken with age. ↕75cm (30in), ↔60cm (24in). ❄❄❄
A.* x *kellereri (*A. ageratifolia* x *A. clypeolata*). Semi-evergreen perennial with lance-shaped, pinnatifid, grey-green leaves. Loose clusters of 6–8 cream flowerheads, each 2cm (¾in) across, with darker disc-florets, are produced in summer. ↕15–20cm (6–8in), ↔30cm (12in) or more. Garden origin. ❄❄❄
***A.* x *kolbiana* 'Weston'**, syn. *A. umbellata* 'Weston'. Mat-forming perennial with semi-evergreen, linear, pinnate, silver-grey leaves. Short-stemmed white flowerheads, 1–2cm (½–¾in) across, are borne in corymbs 3–10cm (1¼–4in) wide, in summer and early autumn. ↕10–15cm (4–6in), ↔ to 30cm (12in). ❄❄❄
***A.* 'Lachsschönheit'** ■ syn. *A.* 'Salmon Beauty'. Clump-forming Galaxy Hybrid with broadly linear, pinnatifid, dark green leaves. In summer, many-branched stems bear a profusion of light salmon-pink flowerheads, fading to pink-flushed, creamy white, in corymbs 14cm (5½in) across. ↕75–90cm (30–36in), ↔60cm (24in). ❄❄❄
***A.* x *lewisii* 'King Edward'** ■🏆 Woody-based, mat- to low-mound-forming perennial with semi-evergreen, linear, fern-like, pinnatifid, sharply toothed, soft grey-green leaves. Pale yellow flowerheads are borne in dense corymbs, to 10cm (4in) across, in early and midsummer. ↕8–12cm (3–5in) or more, ↔23cm (9in) or more. ❄❄❄

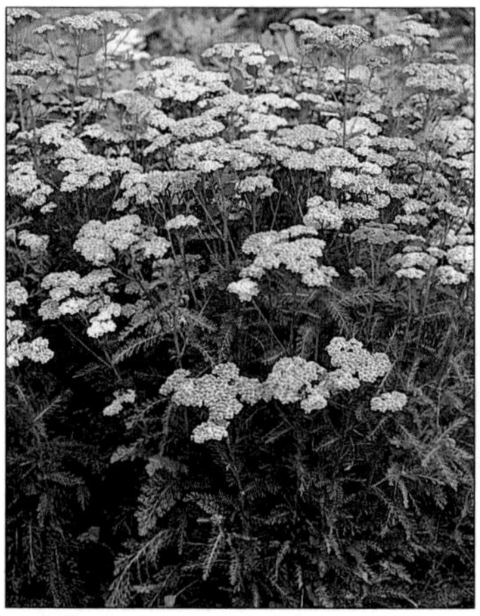

Achillea 'Forncett Candy'

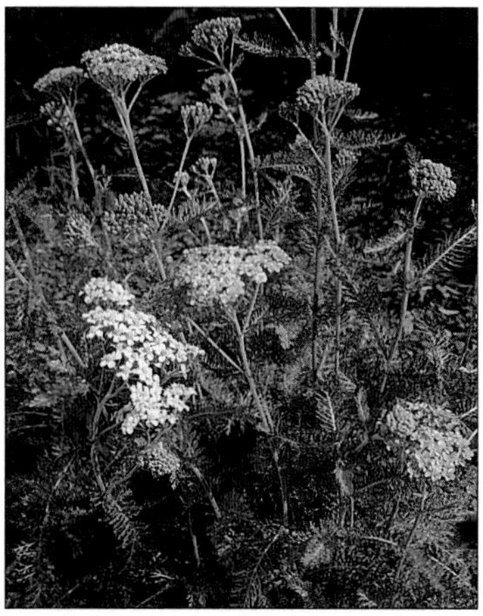

Achillea 'Lachsschönheit'

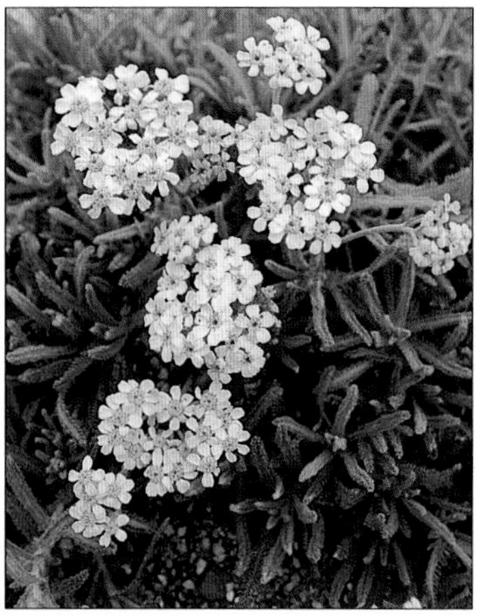

Achillea x *lewisii* 'King Edward'

***A. millefolium* cultivars.** Selections from this rhizomatous, mat-forming and invasive perennial have linear to lance-shaped, pinnatisect, mid-green leaves. Flowerheads are borne in flat corymbs, 7–10cm (3–4in) across, from early to late summer. ↕↔60cm (24in). ❄❄❄. **'Burgundy'** bears deep red flowerheads. **'Cerise Queen'** ■ is very vigorous and forms a mat of dark green leaves; the bright magenta-pink flowerheads have white disc-florets, fading with age. **'Fire King'** is vigorous and upright, with richer red flowerheads than 'Cerise Queen'. **'Lavender Beauty'** see 'Lilac Beauty'. **'Lilac Beauty'**, syn. 'Lavender Beauty', is very free-flowering, with lilac flowerheads fading with age; ↕80cm (32in). **'Paprika'** bears orange-red flowerheads that fade with age. **'Sammetriese'** has dark green leaves and heavy, dark red flowerheads, in corymbs 20cm (8in) across, slightly darker and brighter than those of 'Cerise Queen', and fading to bright magenta; ↕80cm (32in).
***A.* 'Moonshine'** ■🏆 Clump-forming perennial producing evergreen, linear to lance-shaped, pinnatifid, grey-green leaves. Light yellow flowerheads with slightly darker disc-florets are borne in corymbs, to 15cm (6in) across, from early summer to early autumn. ↕↔60cm (24in). ❄❄❄
***A.* 'Moonwalker'.** Clump-forming, aromatic perennial with linear to lance-shaped, pinnatifid, dark green leaves. In summer, bears flat corymbs, 10–15cm (4–6in) across, of scented, golden yellow, copper-tinged flowerheads that fade with age. ↕↔60cm (24in). ❄❄❄
A. ptarmica (Sneezewort). Strong, rhizomatous perennial with simple, linear-lance-shaped, finely toothed, dark green leaves. From early to late summer, bears loose corymbs, 2–10cm (¾–4in) across, of usually off-white flowerheads, 1.5–2cm (½–¾in) across. ↕30–90cm (12–36in), ↔60cm (24in). Europe, W. Asia. ❄❄❄. **'Ballerina'** bears small, double white flowerheads, which open to show disc-florets that fade to grey; ↕ to 60cm (24in), ↔30cm (12in). **'Boule de Neige'** ■ syn. 'Schneeball', has double, pure white flowerheads; ↕45–60cm (18–24in). **'Perry's White'** has larger, double white flowerheads; ↕80–100cm (32–39in). **'Schneeball'** see 'Boule de Neige'. **'The Pearl'** has tight, button-like, double white flowerheads; the flowers may be variable when seed-raised. ↕75cm (30in).
***A.* 'Salmon Beauty'** see *A.* 'Lachsschönheit'.
***A.* 'Schwefelblüte',** syn. *A.* 'Flowers of Sulphur', *A.* 'Sulphur Flowers'. Clump-forming perennial with broadly linear, pinnatifid, greyish green leaves. In early and midsummer, bears corymbs, to 10cm (4in) across, of sulphur-yellow flowerheads, that fade to a paler shade of

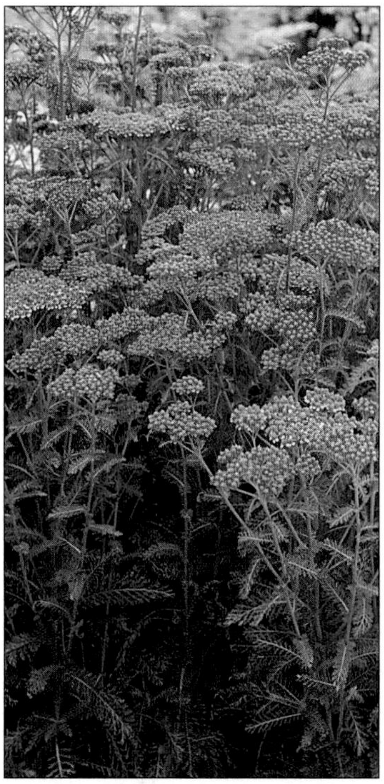

Achillea millefolium 'Cerise Queen'

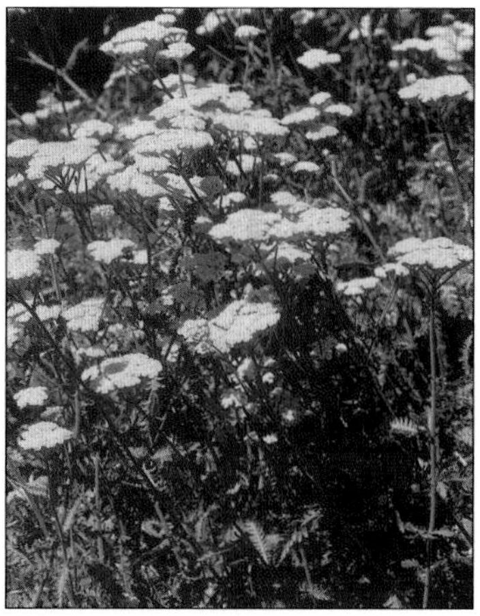

Achillea 'Moonshine'

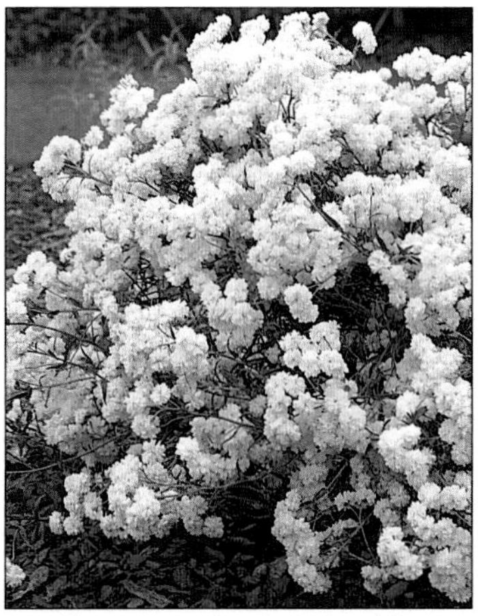

Achillea ptarmica 'Boule de Neige'

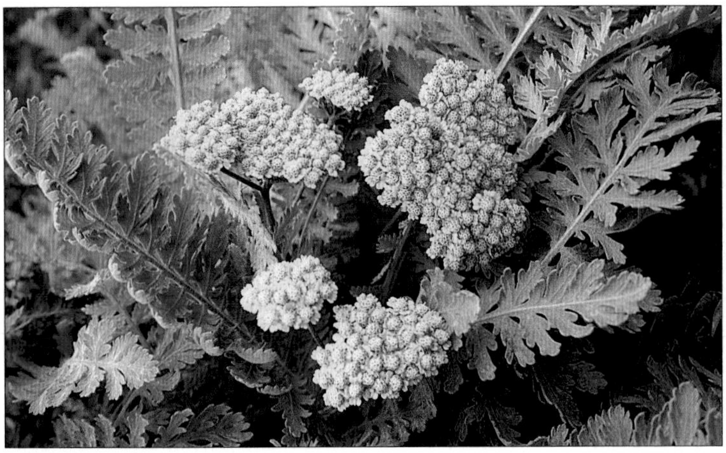

Achillea 'Schwellenburg'

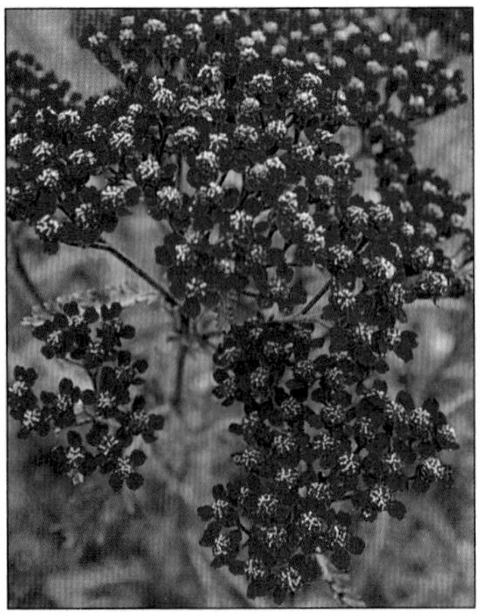

Achillea 'Summerwine'

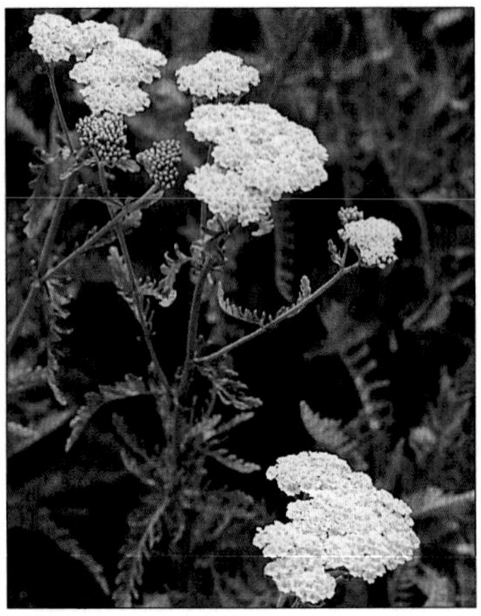

Achillea 'Taygetea'

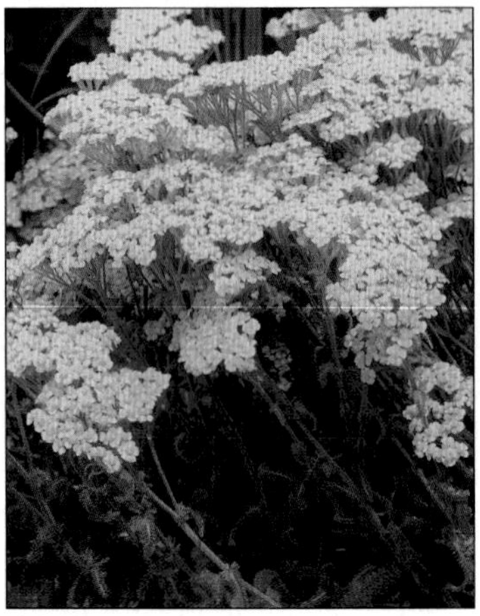

Achillea tomentosa

yellow with age. ↕ 60cm (24in), ↔ 45cm (18in). ❄❄❄

***A.* 'Schwellenburg'** ■ Low-growing, spreading perennial producing oblong-ovate, pinnatifid, grey-green leaves. From early summer to early autumn, branched stems bear corymbs, 10–20cm (4–8in) across, of lemon-yellow flowerheads, opening from silvery buds. ↕ 45cm (18in), ↔ 60cm (24in). ❄❄❄

***A.* 'Sulphur Flowers'** see *A.* 'Schwefelblüte'.

***A.* 'Summerwine'** ■ Upright Galaxy Hybrid with linear, pinnatifid, dark green leaves. Dark red flowerheads, 2cm (¾in) across, with white disc-florets, are produced in corymbs, to 7cm (3in) across, in mid- and late summer. ❄❄❄

***A.* 'Taygetea'** ■ syn. *A. aegyptica* of gardens. Clump-forming perennial with evergreen, linear, pinnatifid, greyish green leaves. In mid- and late summer, bears pale, creamy yellow flowerheads in corymbs, 5–10cm (2–4in) across. ↕ 60cm (24in), ↔ 45cm (18in). ❄❄❄

***A.* 'The Beacon'** see *A.* 'Fanal'.

A. tomentosa ■ 🏆 Mat-forming perennial with linear, pinnatifid, woolly, grey-green leaves. Bears dense corymbs, to 7cm (3in) across, of lemon-yellow flowerheads from early summer to early autumn. ↕ to 35cm (14in), ↔ 45cm (18in). S. Europe to W. Asia. ❄❄❄. **'Aurea'**, syn. 'Maynard's Gold', is more compact, with brighter (but fewer) flowerheads in early summer; ↕ 20cm (8in). **'Maynard's Gold'** see 'Aurea'.

A. umbellata. Clump-forming, semi-evergreen perennial with ovate, pinnate, silver-grey, white-hairy leaves. Hairy stems bear umbels, 3cm (1¼in) across, of 3–6 white flowerheads, to 1.5cm (½in) across, in summer. ↕ to 20cm (8in), ↔ to 30cm (12in). Greece. ❄❄❄.

'Weston' see *A.* x *kolbiana* 'Weston'.

***A.* 'Wesersandstein'** ■ Mat-forming, many-branched Galaxy Hybrid with linear to lance-shaped, pinnatifid, mid-green leaves. In summer, bears corymbs, to 15cm (6in) across, of pinkish red flowerheads, fading to a creamy sand colour. ↕ 45–60cm (18–24in), ↔ 60cm (24in). ❄❄❄

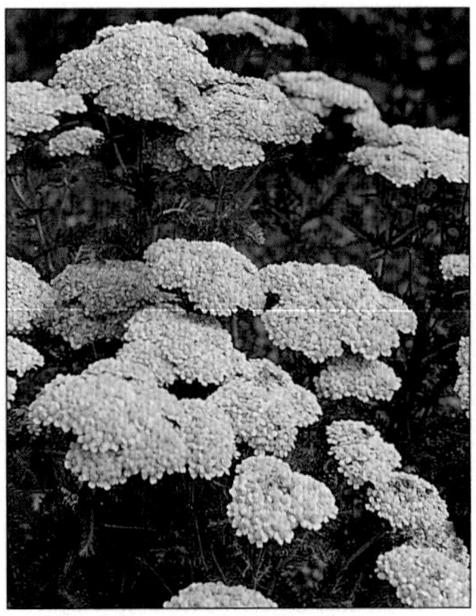

Achillea 'Wesersandstein'

x ACHIMENANTHA

GESNERIACEAE

Hybrid genus, a cross between *Achimenes* and *Smithiantha*, of upright, rhizomatous, herbaceous perennials, cultivated for their brightly coloured flowers. The ovate to oval leaves are opposite and usually hairy. The axillary clusters of tubular flowers vary greatly in colour. In frost-prone areas, grow in a warm greenhouse; in warmer regions, grow in a border.

- **HARDINESS** Frost tender.
- **CULTIVATION** Under glass, grow in loamless or loam-based potting compost (JI No.2) in bright filtered light and moderate humidity. Water sparingly in spring; in summer, water moderately and apply a quarter-strength balanced liquid fertilizer at each watering. After flowering, reduce water until growth has withered; remove any dead growth. Overwinter dormant rhizomes in dry, frost-free conditions. Outdoors, grow in fertile, humus-rich, moist but well-drained soil in partial shade.
- **PROPAGATION** Divide rhizomes or plant individual scales in containers in spring. The latter will produce flowering plants only after several years.
- **PESTS AND DISEASES** Greenfly, red spider mites, and particularly western flower thrips may be a problem.

x *A. naegelioides.* Upright, rhizomatous perennial with hairy, ovate to oval, mid-green leaves, to 12cm (5in) long. In summer, bears tubular, slightly nodding, red to white flowers, to 5cm (2in) long, often marked yellow, maroon, or purple. ↕ 35cm (14in), ↔ 23cm (9in). Garden origin. ❀ (min. 10°C/50°F). **'Ginger Peachy'** is compact, with peach-pink flowers; ↕ 20cm (8in), ↔ 15cm (6in). **'Inferno'** has bright red, yellow-centred, red-veined flowers. **'Rose Bouquet'** has small leaves, to 7cm (3in) long, and double magenta flowers.

ACHIMENES

Cupid's bower, Hot water plant

GESNERIACEAE

Genus of about 25 species of winter-dormant, rhizomatous perennials, grown for their flowers, occurring mainly in subtropical forest in Mexico and Central America. Each of the small, scaly rhizomes produces a single upright, spreading, or trailing stem, which may be either branched or unbranched. The simple, ovate, dark green leaves are opposite (sometimes in unequal pairs) or in whorls, have toothed margins, and are fleshy and usually hairy; the undersides are often red and less hairy. From summer to autumn, salverform flowers are borne singly, in pairs, or in cymes from the leaf axils. There are many cultivars, with flowers in a wide range of colours. In frost-prone areas, grow in containers or hanging baskets in a temperate greenhouse, or as houseplants. In frost-free areas, grow in a border.

- **HARDINESS** Frost tender.
- **CULTIVATION** Under glass, grow in loamless or loam-based potting compost (JI No.2) in bright filtered light and moderate humidity. Bring into growth at 16–18°C (61–64°F) in spring, and water sparingly. In summer, water freely and apply a quarter-strength balanced liquid fertilizer at each watering. In autumn, remove dead top growth, and store in containers at 10°C (50°F) in dry conditions until spring. Outdoors, grow in fertile, humus-rich, moist but well-drained soil in full sun; needs partial shade in very hot areas.
- **PROPAGATION** Divide rhizomes or take stem cuttings in spring.
- **PESTS AND DISEASES** Aphids, thrips, and red spider mites may be a problem.

A. antirrhina. Erect perennial with unequal pairs of ovate, toothed, downy, dark green leaves, 10cm (4in) long, red beneath. Solitary, cream or yellow flowers, to 2.5cm (1in) across, striped purple and spotted red in the throats, are borne from summer to autumn. ↕ 30cm (12in), ↔ 15cm (6in). Mexico, Guatemala. ❀ (min. 10–15°C/50–59°F)

A. coccinea see *A. erecta.*

A. erecta, syn. *A. coccinea, A. pulchella.* Long-stemmed perennial, trailing to 45cm (18in), with whorls of 3 ovate to elliptic, toothed, dark green leaves, 6cm (2½in) long, often red-flushed beneath. Bears numerous solitary, long-tubed, bright red, occasionally rose-pink flowers, 1cm (½in) across, from summer to autumn. ↕ 45cm (18in), ↔ 30cm (12in). Mexico to Panama. ❀ (min. 10–15°C/50–59°F)

A. grandiflora. Erect perennial bearing pairs of ovate, pointed, toothed, dark green leaves, 15–18cm (6–7in) long, hairy and dark green above, red-flushed beneath. From summer to autumn, produces solitary or paired, reddish purple flowers, to 5cm (2in) across, each with a white eye and a purple-dotted throat. ↕↔ 60cm (24in). Mexico to Honduras. ❀ (min. 10–15°C/50–59°F)

***A.* 'Little Beauty'** ■ Bushy perennial with 3-whorled, ovate, pointed, dark green leaves, 15–18cm (6–7in) long, with toothed margins. Solitary, deep pink flowers, 3cm (1¼in) across, with yellow eyes, are produced from summer

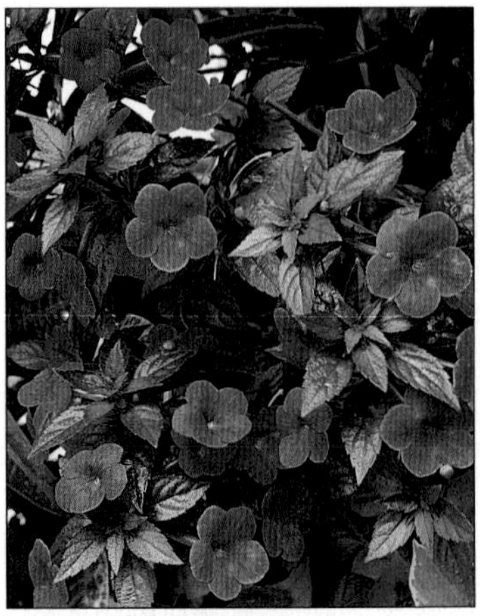

Achimenes 'Little Beauty'

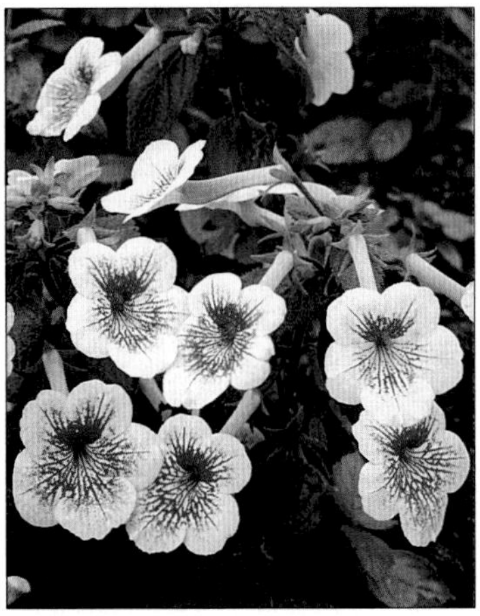

Achimenes longiflora 'Ambroise Verschaffelt'

to autumn. ↕ 25cm (10in), ↔ 30cm (12in). ❄ (min. 10–15°C/50–59°F)
A. *longiflora* 'Ambroise Verschaffelt' ▣ Free-flowering perennial, trailing to 30cm (12in). Dark green leaves, usually in whorls of 3 or 4, sometimes opposite, are ovate to oblong, 5cm (2in) long, coarsely toothed, and sometimes red-tinted on the reverse. From summer to autumn, bears numerous solitary white flowers, 5cm (2in) across, with purple-red veins and dots in the yellowish throats. ↕ 24cm (10in), ↔ 35–40cm (14–16in). ❄ (min. 10–15°C/50–59°F)
A. 'Paul Arnold' ▣ Erect, compact perennial with whorls of 3 or 4 ovate, toothed, dark green leaves, 6cm (2½in) long, red-purple beneath. Attractive, solitary, deep purple-blue flowers, 5cm (2in) across, with white throats suffused with yellow and purple, are borne from summer to autumn. ↕↔ 40cm (16in). ❄ (min. 10–15°C/50–59°F)
A. 'Peach Blossom'. Trailing perennial with whorls of usually 3 ovate, pointed, toothed, dark green leaves, 6cm (2½in) long. Solitary, magenta-pink flowers, 5cm (2cm) across, each with a darker ring around the eye, are borne from summer to autumn. ↕↔ 20cm (8in). ❄ (min. 10–15°C/50–59°F)
A. pulchella see *A. erecta.*
A. 'Purple King'. Vigorous, upright or spreading perennial, trailing to 40cm (16in), with whorls of 3 ovate, toothed, dark green leaves, red beneath. Solitary, ruffle-margined, reddish purple flowers, 5cm (2in) across, open from summer to autumn. ↕ 35–40cm (14–16in), ↔ 30cm (12in). ❄ (min. 10–15°C/50–59°F)

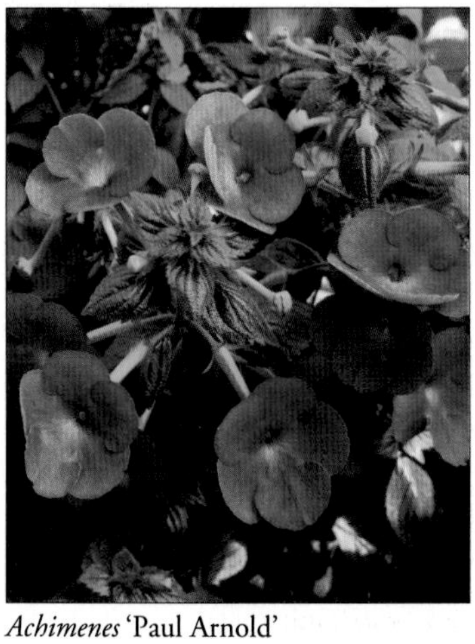

Achimenes 'Paul Arnold'

A. 'Yellow Beauty'. Erect perennial with pairs of ovate, toothed, slightly hairy, dark green leaves, 5cm (2in) long. Solitary, primrose-yellow flowers, 5cm (2in) across, are produced from summer to autumn. ↕ 24cm (10in), ↔ 30cm (12in). ❄ (min. 10–15°C/50–59°F)

▷**Achiote** see *Bixa orellana*
▷***Achnatherum*** see *Stipa*
▷***Acidanthera*** see *Gladiolus*
A. bicolor* var. *murieliae see *G. callianthus*
A. murieliae see *G. callianthus*

ACINOS
Calamint

LABIATAE/LAMIACEAE

Genus of 10 species of annuals and evergreen or semi-evergreen, spreading, woody-stemmed perennials found in mountainous areas and open sites from C. and S. Europe to Asia. They have small, aromatic, usually mid-green, opposite leaves, and tubular, 2-lipped flowers, borne in erect, spike-like whorls in midsummer. Grow in a rock garden or at the front of a border.
• **HARDINESS** Fully hardy to frost hardy.
• **CULTIVATION** Grow in poor to moderately fertile, well-drained soil in full sun; they resent wet conditions.
• **PROPAGATION** Sow seed in containers in a cold frame in autumn or spring. Separate rooted stems, or root basal softwood cuttings, in late spring or summer.
• **PESTS AND DISEASES** Prone to aphids and red spider mites under glass.

A. alpinus, syn. *Calamintha alpina* (Alpine calamint). Woody-based, low-growing, evergreen perennial with entire or slightly toothed, elliptic to rounded leaves, to 2cm (¾in) long, with pointed or blunt tips. In midsummer, produces spike-like whorls of 3–8 purple flowers, 1–2cm (½–¾in) long, marked white on the lower lips, from the upper leaf axils. ↕ 10–20cm (4–8in), ↔ 8–16cm (3–6in). S. and C. Europe. ❄❄❄
A. arvensis ▣ syn. *Clinopodium acinos* (Basil thyme, Mother of thyme). Spreading, short-lived perennial or annual with ovate to elliptic leaves, to 1.5cm (½in) long, on erect, branching stems. In mid- and late summer, produces loose, axillary whorls of 3–8 violet flowers, 7–10mm (¼–½in) long, marked white on the lower lips. ↕ 20cm (8in), ↔ to 30cm (12in). N. Europe, Mediterranean, W. Asia. ❄❄❄

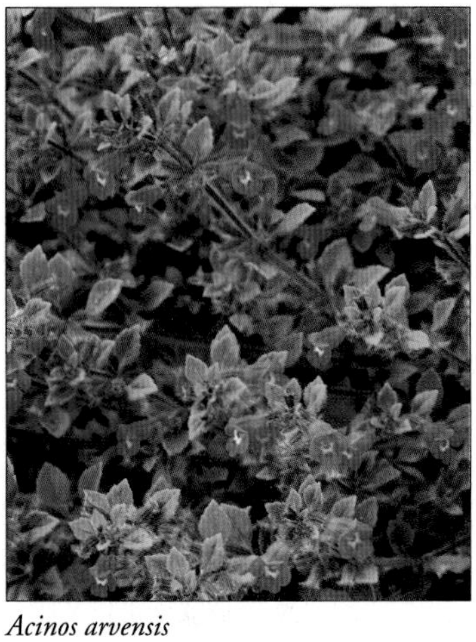

Acinos arvensis

A. corsicus, syn. *Calamintha corsica, Micromeria corsica.* Low, mat-forming, semi-evergreen perennial with obovate to spoon-shaped leaves, 4–10mm (⅛–½in) long, blunt at the tips. Short, spike-like whorls of 2–4 violet flowers, to 1.5cm (½in) long, are borne in midsummer. ↕ to 10cm (4in), ↔ 20–30cm (8–12in). Corsica. ❄❄❄

ACIPHYLLA
Bayonet plant, Speargrass

APIACEAE/UMBELLIFERAE

Genus of about 40 species of evergreen, mostly dioecious perennials, mainly from New Zealand and a few from Australia. Most species are from sparse mountain grassland or alpine regions, but some are from lower altitudes. They form stiff, grassy clumps, the rosettes of flattened, linear, leathery leaves having divided, much-reduced leaf-blades, large terminal spines, and usually conspicuous stipules, also spined. Aciphyllas bear terminal panicles of numerous compound umbels, 2–4cm (¾–1½in) across, of tiny, star-shaped, white or yellow-green flowers, to 2mm (1/16in) long, which are protected by spiny bracts, usually larger and more colourful than the flowers themselves. Most species seldom flower in cool climates. Both male and female plants are needed to produce fruit. Grow larger species in a mixed border and smaller species in a rock garden.
• **HARDINESS** Fully hardy to frost hardy.
• **CULTIVATION** Grow in moist but well-drained, fertile, humus-rich, gritty soil in an open site in full sun.
• **PROPAGATION** Sow seed in containers in a cold frame as soon as ripe, although it may remain viable for up to one year. Plant out seedlings *in situ* as soon as possible, because the deep roots resent disturbance. Divide rhizomatous species, such as *A. pinnatifida*, in spring.
• **PESTS AND DISEASES** Slugs may damage young plants.

A. aurea ▣ Rosette-forming perennial with narrowly strap-shaped, pinnate or 2-pinnate, spine-tipped, grey-green leaves, to 60cm (24in) long, with bold yellow margins and midribs. From early to late summer, bears numerous golden brown flowers. ↕↔ 1m (3ft). New Zealand. ❄❄❄
A. colensoi (Speargrass, Wild Spaniard). Rosette-forming perennial with strap-shaped, pinnate or 2-pinnate, stiff,

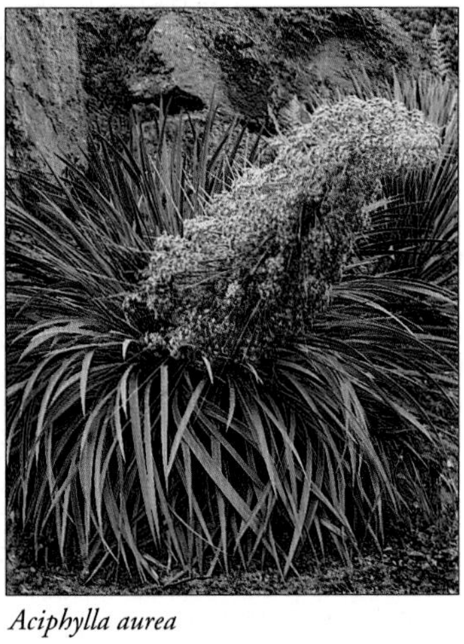

Aciphylla aurea

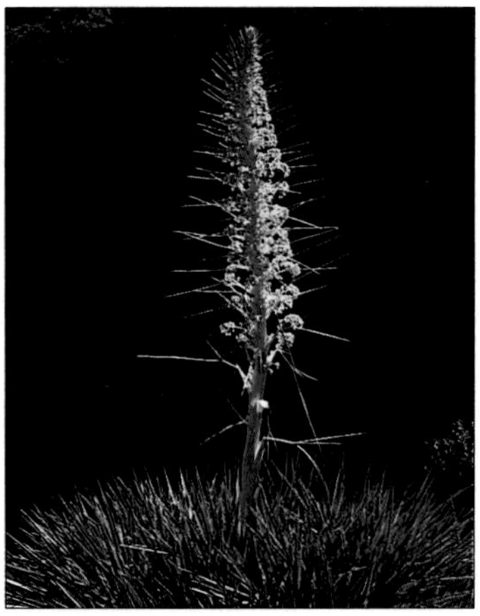

Aciphylla scott-thomsonii

spiny, bluish green leaves, 30–50cm (12–20in) long, with toothed margins and red or reddish brown main veins. In summer, bears small, yellowish green flowers on prickly stems. ↕ to 2.5m (8ft), ↔ 1.5–2m (5–6ft). New Zealand. ❄❄❄
A. glaucescens. Rosette-forming perennial producing very narrow, strap-shaped, 3-pinnate, spine-tipped, silvery grey leaves, to 1m (3ft) long; they have prominent, almost white midribs, toothed margins, and stipules divided into 3 unequal lengths. Yellow-green flowers are borne from early to late summer. ↕↔ 1m (3ft). New Zealand. ❄❄❄
A. hectoris. Dwarf, rosette-forming, perennial producing flat, lance-shaped, dark green leaves, 20–25cm (8–10in) long, deeply divided into 3 slender segments; they have toothed, almost spineless, narrow, red-gold margins and shiny stipules. Pale yellow-green flowers are borne in midsummer. ↕↔ 15cm (6in). New Zealand. ❄❄❄
A. latifolia see *Anisotome latifolia.*
A. pinnatifida. Low-growing, fern-like, rhizomatous perennial producing linear, deeply pinnatifid, spine-tipped, bronzed, dark green leaves, 15–20cm (6–8in) long, with yellow midribs and shiny stipules. Bears off-white flowers in summer. ↕ 10–15cm (4–6in), ↔ 30cm (12in). New Zealand. ❄❄❄
A. scott-thomsonii ▣ (Giant Spaniard). Rosette-forming perennial with linear, pinnate or 2-pinnate, sharply spined, glaucous, blue-green leaves, to 1.5m (5ft) long, with green or pale yellow midribs and finely toothed margins. Yellowish green flowers are produced from early to late summer. ↕ 3m (10ft) or more, ↔ 2m (6ft). New Zealand. ❄❄❄

ACMENA

MYRTACEAE

Genus of 7 species of evergreen trees, occurring in rainforest and moist woodland from Australia to New Guinea. The opposite leaves are oval to lance-shaped, simple, and entire. Small, 5-petalled flowers are borne in axillary racemes or terminal panicles, followed by colourful, succulent berries. In frost-prone regions, grow in a temperate greenhouse; in frost-free areas, grow as specimen trees.
• **HARDINESS** Frost tender, although *A. smithii* may survive short periods at just above 0°C (32°F).

• **CULTIVATION** Under glass, grow in loam-based potting compost (JI No.3) in full light (they will also tolerate filtered light). Pot on or top-dress in early spring or autumn. In the growing season, water freely and apply a balanced liquid fertilizer monthly; water sparingly in winter. Outdoors, grow in moist but well-drained, moderately fertile soil in full sun. Pruning group 8, or 13 if wall-trained.
• **PROPAGATION** Sow seed at 13–18°C (55–64°F) as soon as ripe, or in spring. Root semi-ripe cuttings with bottom heat in late summer.
• **PESTS AND DISEASES** Whiteflies, scale insects, and aphids may be a problem.

A. smithii ♀ syn. *Eugenia smithii* (Lillypilly). Rounded, bushy tree producing ovate to lance-shaped, glossy, dark green leaves, 4–10cm (1½–4in) long, with long, slender tips. Terminal panicles, 2–5cm (¾–2in) long, of greenish white flowers are borne in late spring and early summer. Edible, white, pink, or red-purple berries, 1cm (½in) across, ripen in autumn. In cool areas, only established container plants will bear fruit. ↕8–15m (25–50ft), ↔6–10m (20–30ft). Australia (Northern Territory, Queensland to Victoria). ❀ (min. 5°C/41°F)

ACOELORRAPHE

Saw palm

ARECACEAE/PALMAE

Genus of one species of cluster-stemmed palm from moist forest and swampland in S. Florida in the USA, and from Mexico to Central America and the West Indies. Panicles of bowl-shaped, hermaphrodite flowers are borne among fan-shaped leaves, which are produced in terminal tufts. In frost-prone areas, grow young saw palms in a temperate or warm greenhouse; in frost-free areas, grow outdoors as specimen trees.
• **HARDINESS** Frost tender.
• **CULTIVATION** Under glass, grow in loamless or loam-based potting compost (JI No.3) in full light. In the growing season, water freely and apply a balanced liquid fertilizer monthly; water sparingly in winter. Pot on or top-dress in spring. Outdoors, grow in fertile, well-drained soil in full sun.
• **PROPAGATION** Sow seed at 27°C (81°F) in spring.
• **PESTS AND DISEASES** Red spider mites may be a problem under glass.

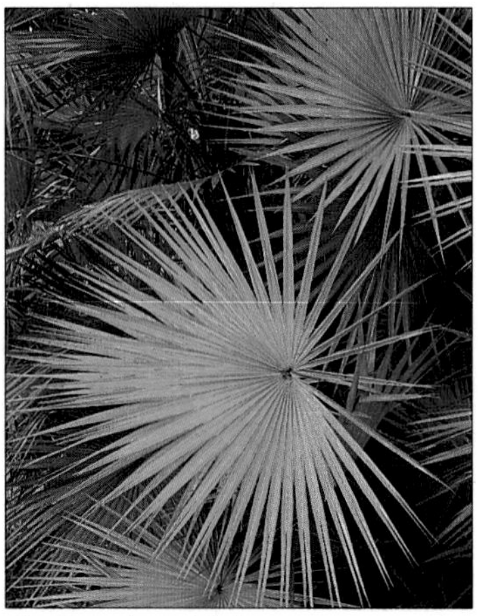

Acoelorraphe wrightii

A. wrightii ■ ✲ syn. *Paurotis wrightii* (Everglades palm, Saw cabbage palm, Silver saw palm). Compact-crowned palm with no crownshaft and 3–10 slender stems clothed with brown fibres and old leaf bases. Rounded, deeply cut, fan-like leaves, with spiny stalks, are glossy, mid-green above, light green to silvery beneath, and to 1m (3ft) long. In summer, bears small white flowers in slender panicles, to 1m (3ft) long, partly hidden by the leaves, followed by black fruit. ↕5–8m (15–25ft), ↔2.5–6m (8–20ft). Mexico to Central America, West Indies. ❀ (min. 10°C/50°F)

ACOKANTHERA

APOCYNACEAE

Genus of 5 species of evergreen trees and shrubs from arid to seasonally moist scrub in tropical to subtropical regions, from southern and eastern Africa to the Arabian Peninsula. They are cultivated mainly for their clusters of long-tubed, 5-petalled flowers, which are borne on the previous year's growth, and for their simple, leathery leaves, produced in opposite pairs. In frost-prone climates, grow in a temperate greenhouse; in frost-free areas, grow in a border. The sap and small, plum-like fruits that follow the flowers are highly toxic if ingested.
• **HARDINESS** Frost tender, although *A. oblongifolia* will survive short periods down to 2°C (36°F).
• **CULTIVATION** Under glass, grow in loam-based potting compost (JI No.3) in full light; top-dress or pot on in autumn. From late spring to autumn, water freely and apply a balanced liquid fertilizer monthly; water sparingly in winter. Outdoors, grow in moderately fertile, well-drained soil in full sun. Pruning group 9; plants under glass may need restrictive pruning.
• **PROPAGATION** Sow seed at 19–24°C (66–75°F) in spring. Root semi-ripe cuttings with bottom heat in summer.
• **PESTS AND DISEASES** Trouble free.

A. oblongifolia ■ ♀ syn. *A. spectabilis, Carissa spectabilis* (Poison arrow plant, Wintersweet). Bushy shrub or small tree producing elliptic, glossy, dark green leaves, to 12cm (5in) long. Fragrant white flowers, 1.5–2cm (½–¾in) long, are borne in axillary clusters, 5–10cm (2–4in) long, from winter to spring. The flowers are followed by ellipsoid, purple-black fruit, to 2.5cm (1in) long. ↕3–6m (10–20ft), ↔1.5–4m (5–12ft). Mozambique, South Africa (KwaZulu/Natal, Northern Cape). ❀ (min. 5°C/41°F)
A. spectabilis see *A. oblongifolia.*

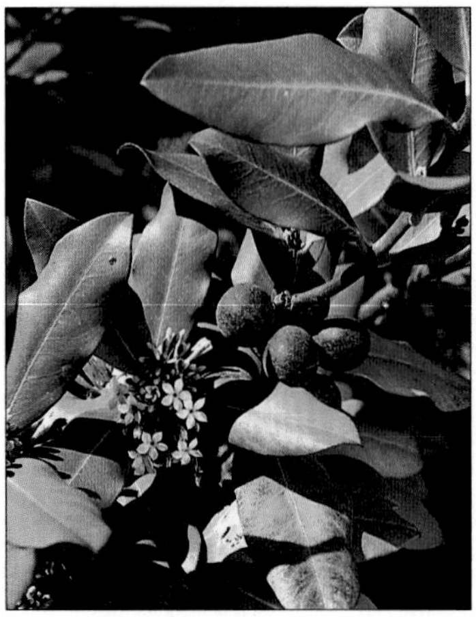

Acokanthera oblongifolia

▷**Aconite** see *Aconitum*
Winter see *Eranthis, E. hyemalis*

ACONITUM

Aconite, Monkshood

RANUNCULACEAE

Genus of 100 species of perennials and biennials, mainly from mountainous grassland or scrub in the N. hemisphere. Most have tuberous or occasionally fibrous roots and erect, sometimes twining stems. The stems bear shallowly to palmately lobed, kidney-shaped to rounded or ovate, usually rich green leaves, mostly 5–10cm (2–4in) long. The curious, hooded flowers, usually 2.5–5cm (1–2in) long, are borne in racemes or panicles, 30–60cm (12–24in) long, well above the leaves. Flower shape and colour are provided by the sepals, because the petals are converted to nectaries under the "hood" of sepals. Ideal for a woodland garden and for borders; grow twining species through shrubs for support. Aconites are good for cutting, but contact with the foliage may irritate skin; all parts are highly toxic if ingested.
• **HARDINESS** Fully hardy.
• **CULTIVATION** Best grown in cool, moist, fertile soil in partial shade, but will tolerate most soils and full sun. Taller aconites require staking.
• **PROPAGATION** Sow seed in containers in a cold frame in spring. Divide every third year in autumn or late winter to maintain vigour, although plants are sometimes slow to re-establish.
• **PESTS AND DISEASES** Fungal stem rot, aphids, and *Verticillium* wilt may be a problem.

A. anthora ■ Upright, usually hairy perennial with rounded, deeply lobed, dark green leaves. In mid- and late summer, bears compact racemes of pale yellow, sometimes blue-violet flowers. ↕60–75cm (24–30in), ↔30cm (12in). C., S., and E. Europe. ✻✻✻
A. 'Blue Sceptre'. Erect perennial with rounded, 3- to 5-lobed, glossy, dark green leaves. From midsummer to early autumn, bears bicoloured, violet and white flowers in tapering racemes. ↕60cm (24in), ↔30cm (12in). ✻✻✻

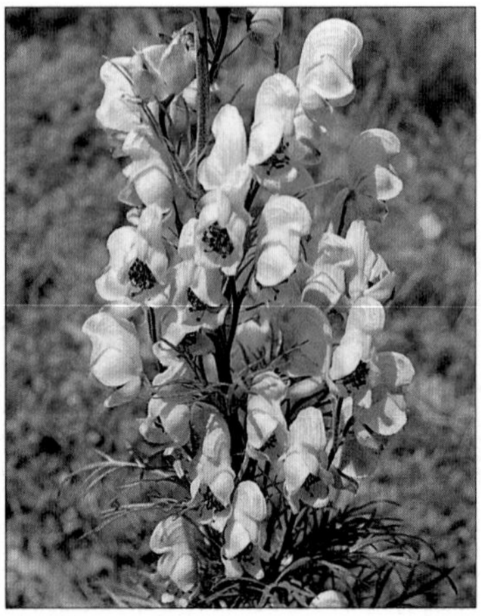

Aconitum anthora

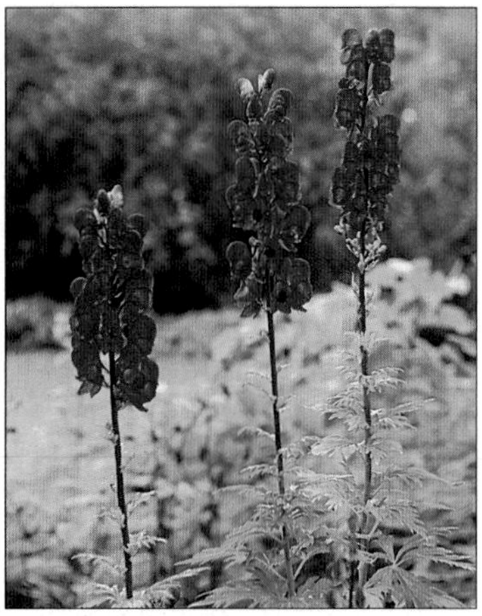

Aconitum 'Bressingham Spire'

A. 'Bressingham Spire' ■ 🏆 Upright perennial with rounded, 3- to 5-lobed, glossy, dark green leaves. Bears tapering racemes of deep violet flowers from midsummer to early autumn. ↕0.9–1m (36–39in), ↔30cm (12in). ✻✻✻
***A. x cammarum* cultivars.** Selections from *A. x cammarum* are erect with ovate to rounded, deeply 3- to 7-lobed, glossy, dark green leaves. They bear panicles or racemes of purple to white, sometimes bicoloured flowers in mid- and late summer. ↕1.2–1.5m (4–5ft), ↔30cm (12in). ✻✻✻. **'Bicolor'** ■ 🏆 bears loose panicles of blue-and-white flowers on arching branches; ↕to 1.2m (4ft). **'Grandiflorum Album'** has white flowers, evenly spaced in long racemes. **'Nachthimmel'** bears loose racemes of deep violet flowers on arching branches.
A. carmichaelii, syn. *A. fischeri* of gardens. Erect perennial with ovate, 3- to 5-lobed, leathery, dark green leaves. In early autumn, bears dense panicles of large, violet or blue flowers. ↕1.5–1.8m (5–6ft), ↔30–40cm (12–16in). Russia to China. ✻✻✻. **'Arendsii'** ■ syn. 'Arends', has sturdy stems and rich blue flowers in branched panicles in early and mid-autumn; ↕to 1.2m (4ft), ↔30cm (12in). **'Barker's Variety'** bears deep violet flowers. **'Kelmscott'** 🏆 has tall panicles of lavender-blue flowers in early and mid-autumn.
***A. compactum* 'Carneum'** see *A. napellus* 'Carneum'.
***A. fischeri* of gardens** see *A. carmichaelii.*
A. hemsleyanum ■ syn. *A. volubile* of gardens. Perennial, twining climber with ovate, 3- to 5-lobed leaves. Racemes of

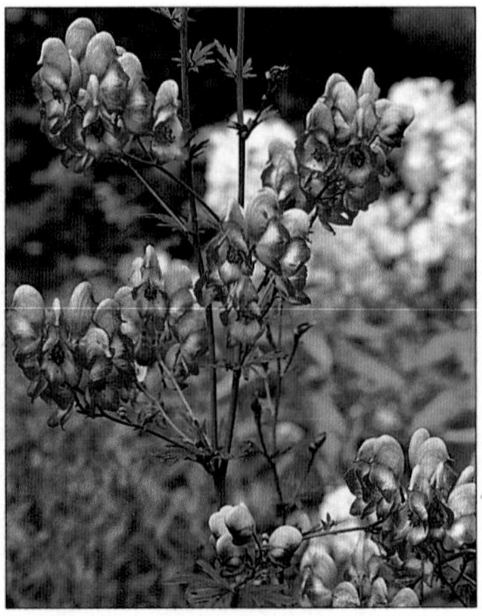

Aconitum x *cammarum* 'Bicolor'

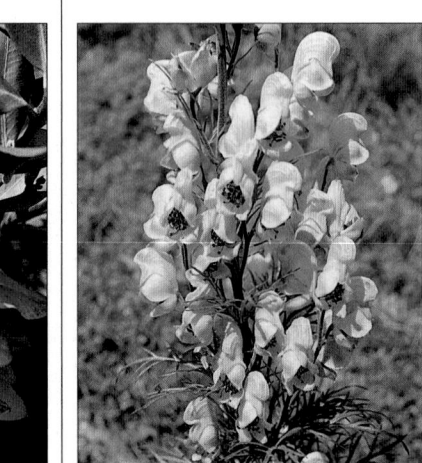

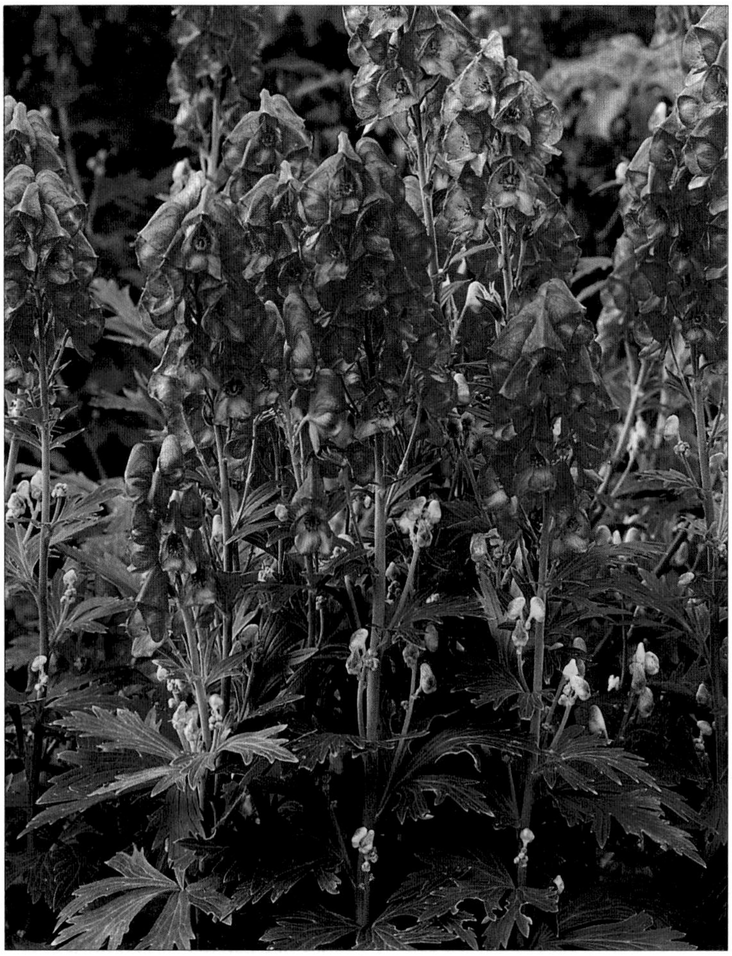
Aconitum carmichaelii 'Arendsii'

large violet flowers are borne from midsummer to early autumn. ↕ 2–3m (6–10ft). W. and C. China. ❄❄❄
***A.* 'Ivorine'** ▣ syn. *A. septentrionale* 'Ivorine'. Upright, bushy perennial with rounded, deeply 3- to 7-lobed leaves. Dense racemes of ivory flowers are borne in late spring and early summer. The flowers are larger and clearer in colour in cool, moist climates. ↕ 90cm (36in), ↔ 45cm (18in). ❄❄❄
A. lamarckii see *A. lycoctonum* subsp. *neapolitanum*.
A. lycoctonum (Wolf's bane). Erect perennial with rounded, 5- to 7-lobed, dark green leaves and panicles of usually yellow, sometimes purple flowers borne in mid- and late summer. ↕ 1–1.5m (3–5ft), ↔ 30cm (12in). C. and S. Europe. ❄❄❄. **subsp. *lycoctonum***, syn. *A. septentrionale*, has deeply lobed leaves and often scandent stems, bearing erect racemes of tall, narrowly hooded, pale yellow, cream, or purple flowers; W. Europe to Romania. **subsp. *neapolitanum***, syn. *A. lamarckii*, *A. neapolitanum*, *A. pyrenaicum*, has 7- or 8-lobed leaves and bears yellow flowers in large racemes or panicles; ↕ 1–1.2m (3–4ft); Pyrenees to Balkans. **subsp. *vulparia*** ▣ syn. *A. orientale* of gardens, *A. vulparia*, has 5- to 9-lobed leaves and pale yellow flowers; C. and S. Europe.
A. napellus (Monkshood). Variable, erect perennial with rounded, deeply 5- to 7-lobed, dark green leaves, the lobes toothed or further divided. Bears dense racemes of indigo-blue flowers in mid- and late summer. ↕ 1.5m (5ft), ↔ 30cm (12in). N. and C. Europe. ❄❄❄.

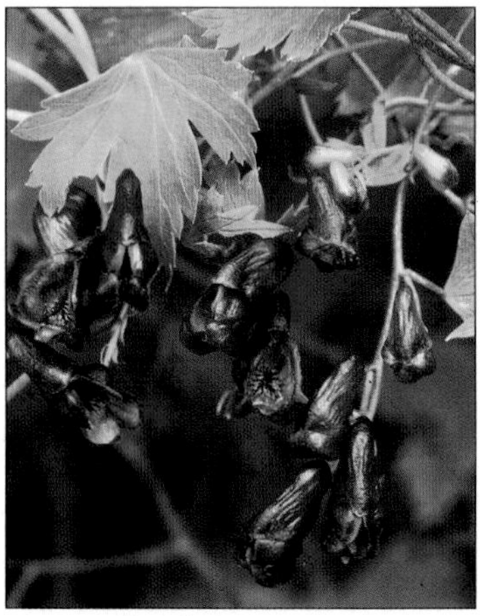
Aconitum hemsleyanum

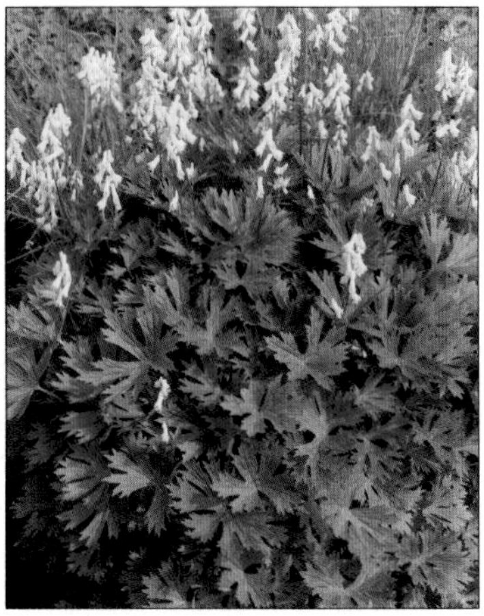
Aconitum 'Ivorine'

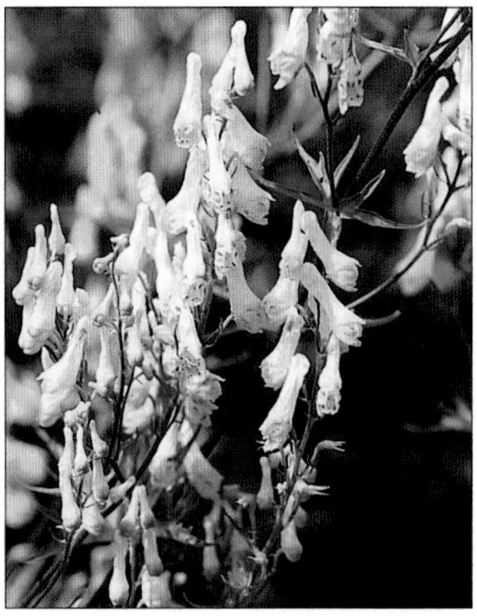
Aconitum lycoctonum subsp. *vulparia*

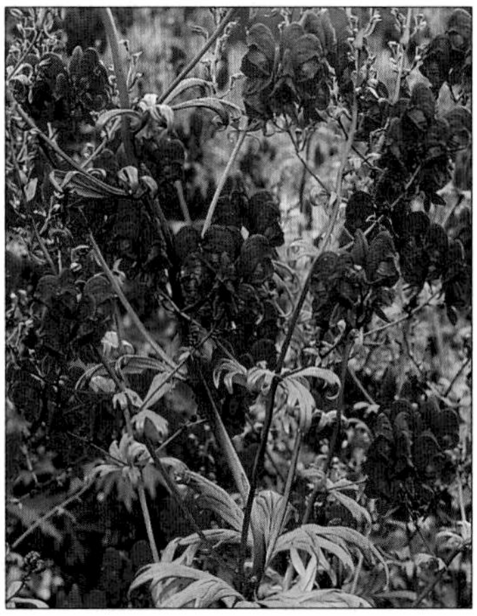
Aconitum 'Spark's Variety'

'Albidum' bears grey-white flowers. **'Carneum'**, syn. *A. compactum* 'Carneum', has leaves with deep, narrow lobes and dusty pink flowers, which are a clearer colour in cool, moist climates.
A. neapolitanum see *A. lycoctonum* subsp. *neapolitanum*.
***A.* 'Newry Blue'.** Erect perennial with rounded, 5- to 7-lobed, dark green leaves, and many-branched, dense racemes of mid-blue flowers produced in mid- and late summer. ↕ to 1.5m (5ft), ↔ 30cm (12in). ❄❄❄
***A. orientale* of gardens** see *A. lycoctonum* subsp. *vulparia*.
A. pyrenaicum see *A. lycoctonum* subsp. *neapolitanum*.
A. septentrionale see *A. lycoctonum* subsp. *lycoctonum*.
***A. septentrionale* 'Ivorine'** see *A.* 'Ivorine'.
***A.* 'Spark's Variety'** ▣ ♀ Upright perennial with rounded, deeply 5- to 7-lobed leaves on thin stems. Large, widely branched panicles of deep violet flowers are produced in mid- and late summer. ↕ 1.2–1.5m (4–5ft), ↔ 45cm (18in). ❄❄❄
A. volubile. Perennial climber, often confused with *A. hemsleyanum*, with small, rounded, 3-lobed leaves. Racemes of lilac or greenish blue flowers are produced in mid- and late summer. ↕ to 2m (6ft) or more. E. Siberia, China (Manchuria), Japan. ❄❄❄
***A. volubile* of gardens** see *A. hemsleyanum*.
A. vulparia see *A. lycoctonum* subsp. *vulparia*.

▷ ***Aconogonon*** see *Persicaria*

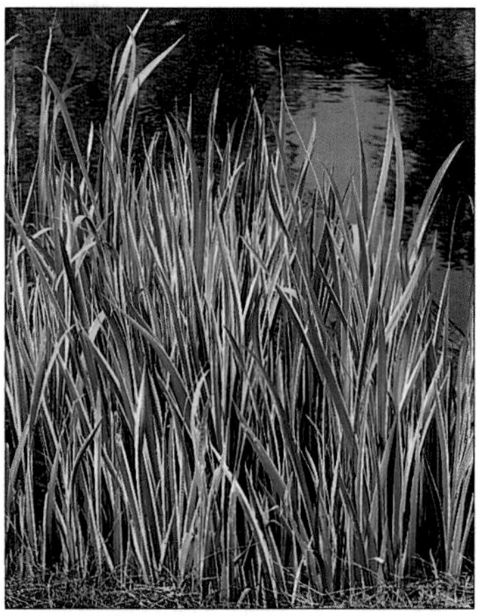
Acorus calamus 'Variegatus'

ACORUS

ARACEAE

Genus of 2 species of rhizomatous, marginal aquatic perennials, one semi-evergreen and one deciduous, found in shallow water by streams and lakes throughout the N. hemisphere, particularly E. Asia. They have sheathed, radical, linear or strap-shaped leaves, which die off in autumn leaving a small basal tuft of foliage that develops the following year. In midsummer, insignificant flowers, resembling small horns, 5–7cm (2–3in) long, are produced laterally just below the tips of central, leaf-like flower stems. They are excellent foliage plants for the shallow margins of a pool, for a bog garden or sink garden, or for marshy areas. Some cultivars of *A. gramineus* are useful aquarium plants.
• **HARDINESS** Fully hardy to half hardy. *Acorus* species are short-lived in an aquarium if the water temperature exceeds 22°C (72°F) for long periods.
• **CULTIVATION** Grow at pool margins in wet or very moist soil in full sun; use aquatic planting baskets for *A. gramineus* and its cultivars, which thrive in shallow water, to 10cm (4in) deep. In an aquarium, grow *A. gramineus* and its cultivars in containers to avoid disturbing the roots. See also pp.52–53.
• **PROPAGATION** Divide rhizomes at the beginning of the growing season and pot up, planting out only when established; repeat every 3–4 years to prevent congestion.
• **PESTS AND DISEASES** Trouble free.

***A. calamus* 'Variegatus'** ▣ Spreading, deciduous, aquatic perennial with strap-shaped, aromatic, bright green leaves, 1.5m (5ft) long, longitudinally striped white and cream, and with distinct midribs and occasionally wrinkled margins. Grows best in water no deeper than 22cm (9in). ↕ 60–90cm (24–36in), ↔ 60cm (24in). ❄❄❄
A. gramineus (Japanese rush). Semi-evergreen, aquatic perennial with fans of 2-ranked, linear, glossy, rich green leaves, 8–35cm (3–14in) long. ↕ 8–35cm (3–14in), ↔ 10–15cm (4–6in). E. Asia. ❄. **'Ogon'**, syn. 'Wogon', bears glossy, variegated leaves, striped with pale green and cream; ↕ to 25cm (10in), ↔ 10–15cm (4–6in). **'Pusillus'** (Dwarf Japanese rush) is compact, with stiff, dark green leaves, 4–16cm (1½–6in)

long; ↕ 10cm (4in), ↔ 10–15cm (4–6in); ❄. **'Variegatus'** (Variegated Japanese rush) has leaves 8–30cm (3–12in) long, striped cream and yellow; ↕ 25cm (10in), ↔ 15cm (6in); ❄❄. **'Wogon'** see 'Ogon'.

ACRADENIA

RUTACEAE

Genus of 2 species of evergreen shrubs or trees native to riverbanks in Australia (Tasmania). *A. frankliniae* is not often cultivated, yet is attractive both for its aromatic, opposite, 3-palmate leaves and for its panicles of 5-petalled flowers, which are borne in late spring on the previous year's growth. In frost-prone areas, grow in a cool greenhouse; in frost-free areas, grow in a shrub border.

• **HARDINESS** Frost hardy.

• **CULTIVATION** Under glass, grow in lime-free (ericaceous) potting compost in filtered light. In the growing season, water freely and apply a balanced liquid fertilizer monthly; water sparingly in winter. Outdoors, grow in moist but well-drained, fertile soil in partial shade, sheltered from cold, dry winds. Pruning group 8; plants under glass may need restrictive pruning.

• **PROPAGATION** Take semi-ripe cuttings in summer.

• **PESTS AND DISEASES** Trouble free.

A. frankliniae 🏆 (Whitey wood). Erect shrub, or occasionally small tree, producing glossy, dark green leaves, to 7cm (3in) long, with 3 narrowly oval leaflets, aromatic when crushed. Star-shaped white flowers open in terminal corymbs, to 5cm (2in) across, in late spring. ↕ 3m (10ft), ↔ 1.5m (5ft). Australia (Tasmania). ❄❄

▷ ***Acroclinium*** see *Rhodanthe*
A. roseum see *R. chlorocephala* subsp. *rosea*

ACTAEA

Baneberry

RANUNCULACEAE

Genus of 8 species of rhizomatous woodland perennials from temperate regions of the N. hemisphere. Grown mainly for their foliage and fruit, they have 2-, 3-, or 5-ternate, toothed leaves and usually terminal, compact, fluffy, spherical to ovoid racemes of small white flowers with prominent stamens, followed by longer clusters of colourful berries. Grow in a woodland garden, or in a shady mixed or herbaceous border. The berries are highly toxic if ingested.

• **HARDINESS** Fully hardy.

• **CULTIVATION** Grow in cool, moist, moderately fertile soil, enriched with leaf mould, in partial shade. Water thoroughly in very dry weather. *A. spicata* will thrive even in full shade and beneath conifers.

• **PROPAGATION** Sow seed in containers in a cold frame in autumn. Divide in early spring.

• **PESTS AND DISEASES** Trouble free.

A. alba ▣ 🏆 syn. *A. pachypoda* (Doll's eyes, White baneberry). Clump-forming perennial with irregularly pinnate leaves, to 60cm (24in) long, composed of 3–12 ovate leaflets. White flowers are borne in spherical racemes, 2–5cm (¾–2in) long,

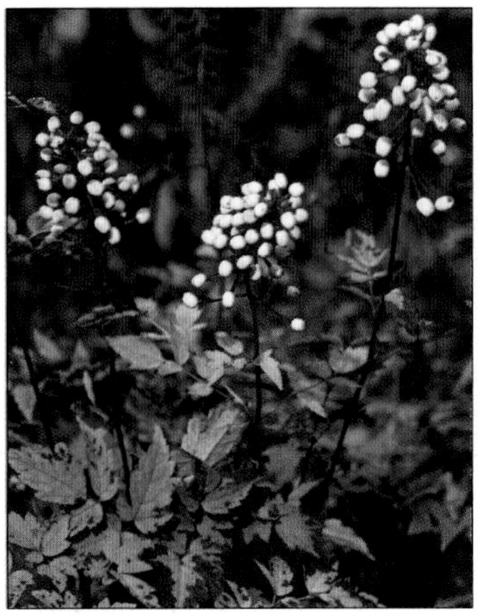

Actaea alba

in late spring and early summer, followed by spherical white berries, 8mm (⅜in) across, each with a black eye, on stalks that elongate, thicken, and turn red. ↕ 90cm (36in), ↔ 45–60cm (18–24in). E. North America. ❄❄❄

A. erythrocarpa, syn. *A. spicata* var. *rubra*. Clump-forming perennial with pinnate leaves, to 40cm (16in) long, composed of 3–12 ovate to lance-shaped leaflets. White flowers in ovoid racemes, 3–5cm (1¼–2in) long, are borne in late spring and early summer; they are followed by spherical maroon berries, 7–9mm (¼–⅜in) across, on arching red stalks. ↕ 60cm (24in), ↔ 45cm (18in). N. Europe to E. Asia. ❄❄❄

***A. erythrocarpa* of gardens** see *A. rubra*.

A. nigra see *A. spicata*.

A. pachypoda see *A. alba*.

A. rubra ▣ 🏆 syn. A. *erythrocarpa* of gardens (Red baneberry). Clump-forming perennial with 2- or 3-pinnate leaves, to 40cm (16in) long, composed of 3–15 ovate leaflets. From mid-spring to early summer, bears white flowers in ovoid racemes, 3–5cm (1¼–2in) long, followed by spikes of shiny red, spherical or ellipsoid berries, 5–10mm (¼–½in) across, on slender green stalks. ↕ 45cm (18in), ↔ 30cm (12in). C. and E. North America. ❄❄❄. **subsp. *arguta*** is smaller than the species and has almost spherical red berries; ↕ 45cm (18in), ↔ 30cm (12in). **f. *neglecta*** has white berries to 1.5cm (½in) long; W. USA.

A. spicata, syn. *A. nigra* (Herb Christopher). Clump-forming perennial with usually 2-ternate leaves, to 60cm (24in) long, with 9–15 ovate leaflets. From mid-spring to early summer, bears

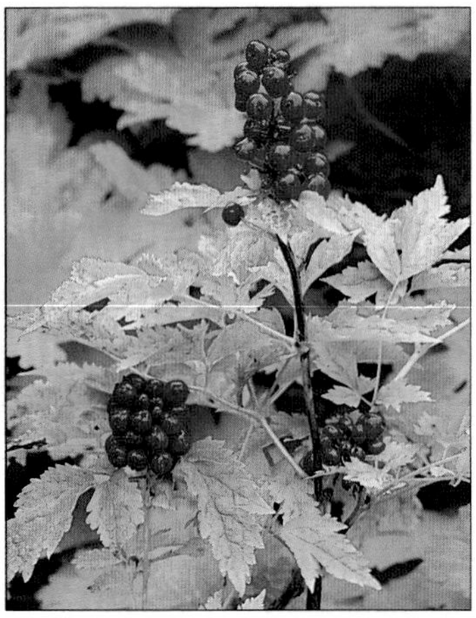

Actaea rubra

white flowers in ovoid racemes, 2–6cm (¾–2½in) long, followed by ovoid black berries, to 1cm (½in) across, on slender green stalks. ↕↔ 45cm (18in). N. Europe, Asia. ❄❄❄. **var. *rubra*** see *A. erythrocarpa*.

ACTINIDIA

ACTINIDIACEAE

Genus of about 40 species of mainly deciduous, twining climbers with alternate, simple leaves, found among shrubs in areas of light forest in E. Asia. They are valued for their ornamental, sometimes variegated foliage, their cup-shaped, occasionally scented flowers, produced singly or in axillary cymes in summer, and their edible fruits, which ripen in autumn. Train against a wall or into a tree. Both male and female plants are usually needed to obtain fruit, although some self-fertile cultivars are available for commercial fruit production. In frost-prone areas, *A. deliciosa* will produce fruit if grown in a sheltered garden or cool greenhouse.

• **HARDINESS** Frost hardy to fully hardy; *A. deliciosa* is frost hardy unless the wood has been well ripened in summer.

• **CULTIVATION** Under glass, grow in loam-based potting compost (JI No.3) in full light. In the growing season, water freely and apply a balanced liquid fertilizer monthly; keep moist in winter. Outdoors, grow in fertile, well-drained soil in sun, with shelter from strong winds. Grow in full sun to maximize fruiting. Prune in late winter: if grown for fruit, pruning group 12; otherwise, pruning group 11.

• **PROPAGATION** Sow seed in containers in a cold frame in autumn or spring. Root semi-ripe cuttings, or graft cultivars, in late summer.

• **PESTS AND DISEASES** Trouble free.

A. arguta (Tara vine). Deciduous climber with ovate to ovate-oblong, bristle-toothed, dark green leaves, to 12cm (5in) long. In early summer, bears clusters of 3 fragrant white flowers, each 2cm (¾in) wide. Female plants produce smooth-skinned, oblong, yellow-green fruit, 2.5cm (1in) long. ↕ 7m (22ft). E. Asia. ❄❄❄. **'Issai'** is self-fertile and fruits without cross-pollination.

***A. chinensis* of gardens** see *A. deliciosa*.

A. deliciosa ▣ syn. *A. chinensis* of gardens (Chinese gooseberry, Kiwi fruit). Vigorous, deciduous climber with stout shoots covered in red-brown hairs and

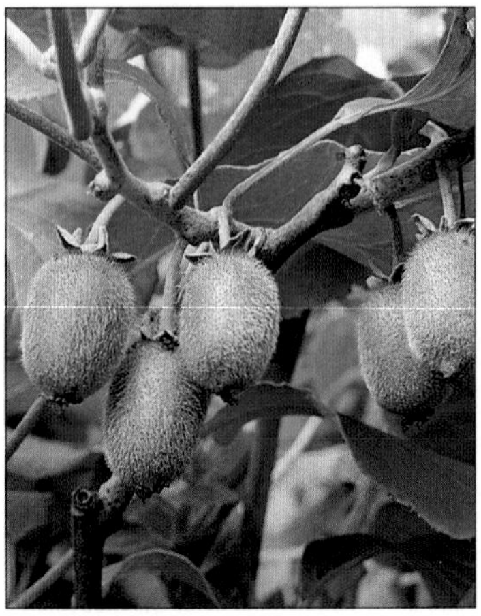

Actinidia deliciosa

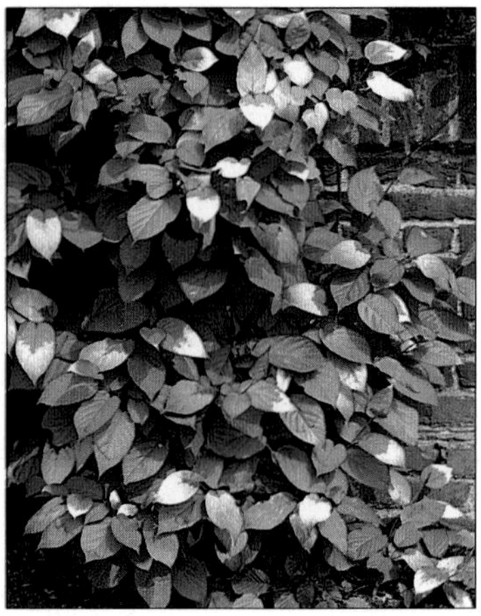

Actinidia kolomikta

broadly ovate, heart-shaped, mid-green leaves, to 20cm (8in) long. In early summer, bears clusters of 2 or 3 (occasionally more) creamy white, later yellow flowers, 4cm (1½in) across. Female plants produce ovoid-oblong bristly-skinned, greenish brown fruit, to 7cm (3in) long. ↕ 10m (30ft). China. ❄❄. Several female cultivars, including **'Blake'** (which is self-fertile), **'Bruno'**, and **'Hayward'**, and several males, such as **'Matua'** and **'Tomuri'**, are grown.

A. kolomikta ▣ 🏆 Deciduous climber with ovate-oblong, dark green leaves, to 15cm (6in) long, purple-tinged when young, becoming variegated with white and pink in the top half. Bears clusters of 3 fragrant white flowers, 2cm (¾in) across, in early summer. Female plants produce smooth, ovoid-oblong, yellow-green fruit, 2.5cm (1in) long. ↕ 5m (15ft) or more. E. Asia. ❄❄❄

A. polygama (Silver vine). Deciduous climber with elliptic or ovate-oblong leaves, to 15cm (6in) long, dark green with silver-white tips, or silvery white in the top half. Clusters of 3 fragrant white flowers, 2cm (¾in) across, open in early summer. Female plants bear smooth, ovoid, yellow-green fruit, 2.5cm (1in) long. ↕ 5m (15ft). Japan. ❄❄❄

ADA

ORCHIDACEAE

Genus of about 20 species of evergreen, epiphytic orchids, growing at an altitude of 2,500m (8,000ft) in Central and South America. They have short rhizomes and small, oblong pseudobulbs with 2 narrowly oval leaves at the tips. In spring or summer, arching racemes of bell-shaped flowers are borne from the bases of the pseudobulbs. Grow in containers or epiphytically.

• **HARDINESS** Frost tender.

• **CULTIVATION** Cool-growing orchids. Grow epiphytically or in epiphytic orchid compost in the smallest possible containers. Supply high humidity and good ventilation. Provide bright filtered light in summer; in winter, remove shading. Water freely when in growth, more sparingly in winter. In summer, apply a half-strength liquid fertilizer at every third watering. See also p.46.

• **PROPAGATION** Divide when the plant overgrows its container, or pot up back-bulbs separately.

• **PESTS AND DISEASES** Aphids, red spider mites, mealybugs, and whiteflies may be a problem.

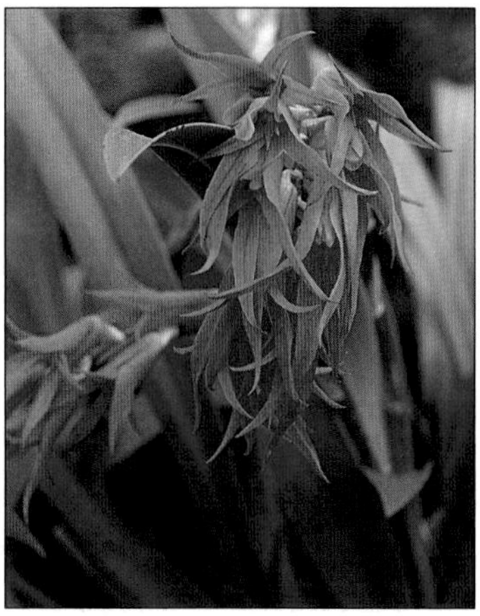

Ada aurantiaca

A. aurantiaca ■ Evergreen, epiphytic orchid with oblong pseudobulbs and 2 narrowly oval, mid-green leaves, 10cm (4in) long. Bears basal racemes of bright orange flowers, 2.5cm (1in) long, in spring. ↕ 23cm (9in), ↔ 15–23cm (6–9in). Colombia, Venezuela. ❅ (min. 10°C/50°F; max. 24°C/75°F)

▷**Adam's needle** see *Yucca filamentosa*

ADANSONIA

BOMBACACEAE

Genus of 9 or 10 species of mostly deciduous trees from tropical, semi-arid regions of Africa, the Comoros Islands, Madagascar, and N. and N.W. Australia. They have succulent, often swollen trunks and short, branched crowns. The simple to palmate (sometimes only palmately lobed) leaves are borne only on mature plants, in summer. The large, solitary, pendent flowers are usually creamy white with 5 crinkled, waxy petals and "powder puffs" of numerous stamens; they are followed by spherical to oblong-obovoid, fleshy, often woody-coated, edible, velvety, pale brown fruits. Where temperatures fall below 16°C (61°F), grow in a warm greenhouse; in warmer climates, grow in a desert garden.

• **HARDINESS** Frost tender.

• **CULTIVATION** Under glass, grow in loam-based potting compost (JI No.2), with added grit or sharp sand, in full light. Water sparingly in spring and autumn, moderately in summer; keep dry in winter. In the growing season, apply a low-phosphate liquid fertilizer monthly. Outdoors, grow in well-drained, sandy, moderately fertile soil in full sun.

• **PROPAGATION** Sow seed as soon as ripe at 19–24°C (66–75°F).

• **PESTS AND DISEASES** Aphids may infest young leaves and flower buds.

A. digitata ♆ (Baobab tree). Deciduous tree with a thick, swollen, succulent trunk and short branches. These bear rounded, usually 5- to 9-palmate, occasionally only lobed leaves, to 17cm (7in) long. Pendent flowers, 10–12cm (4–5in) across, with partially reflexed white petals and extended, central "balls" of purple-anthered stamens, are borne on long stalks, with or just before the leaves, in summer. Woody, ovoid fruit, 25cm (10in) long, contain large black seeds. ↕ to 18m (60ft), ↔ 30m (100ft). S.W. Africa, N.E. South Africa, Comoros Islands, W. Madagascar. ❅ (min. 16°C/61°F)

▷**Adder's tongue,**
Footed see *Scoliopus bigelovii*
Yellow see *Erythronium americanum*

ADENIA

PASSIFLORACEAE

Genus of over 90 species of deciduous, perennial succulents, sometimes semi-evergreen, with caudiciform rootstocks and vine-like climbers with thin, thorny, tendril-bearing stems; they are found in scrub or desert in Africa, Madagascar, and Burma. All have alternate, palmate or simple leaves. The axillary cymes of tiny, sometimes scented flowers, to 1cm (½in) across, are followed by conical to obovoid, capsular, yellow, green, or red fruits, 2–4cm (¾–1½in) long. Where temperatures fall below 15°C (59°F), grow in a warm greenhouse; in warmer regions, grow in a desert garden.

• **HARDINESS** Frost tender.

• **CULTIVATION** Under glass, grow in standard cactus compost in full light in dry, airy conditions. Water sparingly in spring and autumn, freely in summer; keep dry in winter. In the growing season, apply a balanced liquid fertilizer every 4–6 weeks. Outdoors, grow in well-drained soil in full sun. See also pp.48–49.

• **PROPAGATION** Sow seed at 19–24°C (66–75°F) as soon as ripe. Take cuttings from non-flowering stems in summer; small tubers develop about 3 months from rooting.

• **PESTS AND DISEASES** Vulnerable to mealybugs during the growing season.

A. buchananii see *A. digitata.*
A. digitata, syn. *A. buchananii, Modecca digitata.* Perennial succulent with a cylindrical grey caudex, to 30cm (12in) or more across, which tapers into an erect, slender stem, crowned by a cluster of 3- to 5-palmate, sometimes semi-evergreen, dark green leaves, 10cm (4in) or more long. Small, star-shaped yellow flowers open with the leaves in summer, followed by obovoid, yellow to red fruit. The sap may cause severe discomfort if ingested. ↕ 1.5m (5ft), ↔ to 1m (3ft). Mozambique, N.E. South Africa. ❅ (min. 15–16°C/59–61°F)
A. globosa ■ Perennial succulent with a spherical, greyish green caudex, to 1m (3ft) across. Interlaced, stiff, spiny, thick, greyish green branches have lance-shaped, warty, mid-green, deciduous leaves, 7–10mm (¼–½in) long. Small, star-shaped, scented, bright red flowers open in spring, followed by ovoid, green then orange fruit. ↕ to 1.5m (5ft), ↔ 1m (3ft). Kenya, Tanzania. ❅ (min. 15–16°C/59–61°F)
A. spinosa. Perennial succulent with a swollen, grey-green caudex, to 2m (6ft) wide, and stiff, sharply spiny branches with ovate to elliptic, mid-green, deciduous leaves, 3cm (1¼in) long. Small, tubular, creamy white flowers open in summer with the leaves; they are followed by obovoid yellow fruit. ↕ 3m (10ft), ↔ 1m (3ft). N.E. South Africa. ❅ (min. 15–16°C/59–61°F)

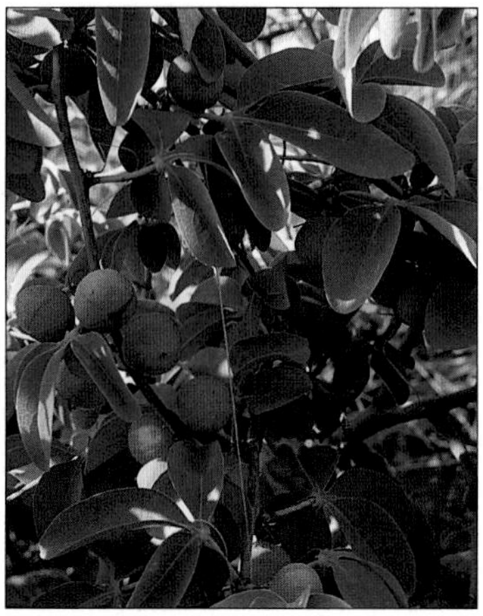

Adenia globosa

ADENIUM

Desert rose, Impala lily

APOCYNACEAE

Genus of one very variable species (sometimes considered to be 5 or 6 species) of perennial succulents found in semi-arid regions of the Arabian Peninsula and E. to S.W. Africa. The swollen caudex may be very low, with its base partly underground, or may grow taller and be widely bottle-shaped. The irregular, spineless branches bear glossy leaves in spiral, terminal clusters, with salverform flowers varying in colour from rich red to pink or white. Where temperatures fall below 15°C (59°F), grow in a warm greenhouse or as house-plants; in warmer areas, grow in a desert garden. The milky sap that exudes from broken stems may irritate skin and cause severe discomfort if ingested.

• **HARDINESS** Frost tender.

• **CULTIVATION** Under glass, grow in loam-based potting compost (JI No.2) with added sharp sand, in full light with shade from hot sun. When in growth, water moderately and apply a balanced liquid fertilizer 2 or 3 times; water more sparingly in winter. Outdoors, grow in well-drained, slightly alkaline, humus-rich soil in full sun with some midday shade. See also pp.48–49.

• **PROPAGATION** Sow seed as soon as ripe at 21°C (70°F). Root cuttings from non-flowering shoots in summer with bottom heat.

• **PESTS AND DISEASES** Prone to aphids.

A. arabicum see *A. obesum.*
A. micranthum see *A. obesum.*
A. obesum ■ syn. *A. arabicum, A. micranthum, A. speciosum, Nerium obesum.* Variable, perennial succulent with a thick, usually bottle-shaped, twisted, greyish brown caudex, often more than 1m (3ft) long, and tapering to a many-branched tip. Upright, succulent brown branches produce ovate, grey-green leaves, to 10cm (4in) long. Red, pink, or white flowers, to 4–6cm (1½–2½in) across, are borne in small terminal corymbs throughout summer, sometimes before the leaves. ↕ 1.5m (5ft), ↔ 1m (3ft). E. to S.W. Africa, Arabian Peninsula. ❅ (min. 15°C/59°F; optimum 21°C/70°F).
subsp. *oleifolium* has an almost spherical or ovoid caudex, and produces 1–5 slender branches with lance-shaped, grey-green leaves, to 15cm (6in) long, arranged in loose rosettes; ↕ 45cm (18in), ↔ 30cm (12in); S.W. Africa.
A. speciosum see *A. obesum.*

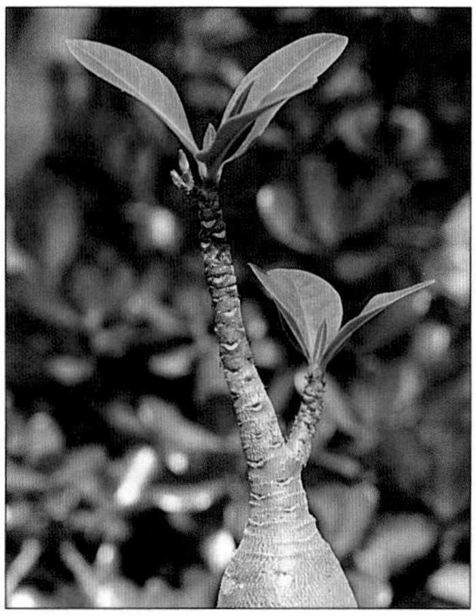

Adenium obesum

ADENOCARPUS

LEGUMINOSAE/PAPILIONACEAE

Genus of about 15 species of deciduous and evergreen, sometimes semi-evergreen shrubs, occasionally trees, found in scrub or light woodland in S. W. Europe, the Mediterranean, Canary Islands, and N. Africa. They have alternate, 3-palmate leaves and are valued for their broom-like yellow flowers, which are borne in terminal, sometimes congested racemes on the previous year's growth in spring or summer. Grow in a sunny shrub border in frost-free climates, or against a warm, sunny wall in frost-prone areas.

• **HARDINESS** Frost hardy.

• **CULTIVATION** Grow in light, moderately fertile, very well-drained soil in full sun; in frost-prone areas, protect from winter wet and wind. Pruning group 8, or 13 if wall-trained.

• **PROPAGATION** Sow seed in containers in a cold frame in autumn or spring. Root semi-ripe cuttings in summer.

• **PESTS AND DISEASES** Trouble free.

A. complicatus. Variable, upright or spreading, deciduous shrub producing 3-palmate leaves with inversely lance-shaped leaflets, to 2.5cm (1in) long. In summer, bears dark yellow flowers, occasionally red-tinged, to 1.5cm (½in) long, in dense, arching terminal racemes, to 10–15cm (4–6in) long. ↕↔ 4m (12ft). Mediterranean, S.W. Europe. ✻✻
A. decorticans ■ Stiff, horizontally branching, deciduous shrub with flaky

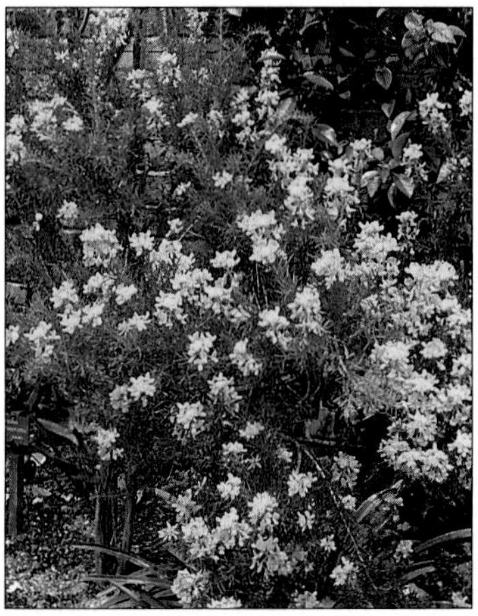

Adenocarpus decorticans

grey to white bark and dense clusters of small, silver-hairy leaves with 3 narrowly elliptic leaflets, 0.5–1.5cm (¼–½in) long, with inrolled margins. Bright yellow flowers, to 1.5cm (½in) long, are borne in short, erect racemes, to 6cm (2½in) long, in late spring and early summer. ↕↔ 2.2m (7ft). Spain. ❄❄
A. viscosus. Semi-evergreen shrub with erect, then spreading branches covered with 3-palmate, stalkless, grey-green leaves with narrowly elliptic leaflets, to 1cm (½in) long. In late spring, bears dark golden yellow to orange flowers, 1.5–2cm (½–¾in) long, in dense terminal racemes, to 6cm (2½in) long. ↕ 1m (3ft), ↔ 1.5m (5ft). Canary Islands (Tenerife and La Palma). ❄❄

ADENOPHORA

CAMPANULACEAE

Genus of more than 40 species of fleshy-rooted perennials, similar to campanulas (differing in having discs at the bases of the styles). They are found in temperate woodland and grassland, sometimes at high altitudes, in Europe and Asia. They produce rounded basal leaves (dying back before flowering in some species) and small, lance-shaped to ovate, entire or toothed stem leaves, arranged alternately or, occasionally, in whorls. The pendent or semi-pendent, bell- or funnel-shaped flowers, 0.5–2cm (¼–¾in) long, with protruding styles, are pale to dark lavender-blue and are mostly produced in terminal racemes or panicles. Grow in a border or in open woodland; smaller species are suitable for a rock garden.

• **HARDINESS** Fully hardy.

• **CULTIVATION** Grow in light, humus-rich, moist but well-drained soil in sun or partial shade. Plant seedlings when young, then avoid disturbing the deep roots.

• **PROPAGATION** Sow seed thinly in containers outdoors as soon as ripe or in late winter; plant out potfuls of seedlings to avoid disturbing the roots. Root cuttings of basal shoots in late spring. Seldom tolerates division.

• **PESTS AND DISEASES** Vine weevils may attack the fleshy roots. Slugs and snails will eat young growth.

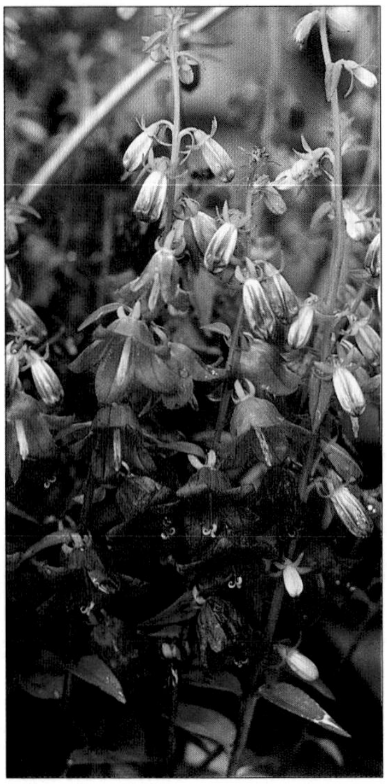

Adenophora bulleyana

A. bulleyana ■ Erect perennial with alternate, lance-shaped, toothed stem leaves, to 8cm (3in) long. In late summer, bears spike-like racemes of nodding, narrowly funnel-shaped, pale to mid-blue flowers, 1cm (½in) long, often in groups of 3. ↕ 1.2m (4ft), ↔ 30cm (12in). W. China. ❄❄❄
A. liliiflora see *A. liliifolia.*
A. liliifolia, syn. *A. liliiflora.* Erect perennial with alternate, lance-shaped, stalkless, toothed, hairy stem leaves, 5–8cm (2–3in) long; the basal leaves die back before flowering. Produces panicles of pendent, widely bell-shaped, fragrant, pale blue flowers, to 2cm (¾in) long, in midsummer. ↕ 45cm (18in), ↔ 30cm (12in). C. Europe to Siberia. ❄❄❄
A. polymorpha* var. *tashiroi see *A. tashiroi.*
A. potaninii. Upright perennial with alternate, ovate to lance-shaped, toothed stem leaves, to 5cm (2in) long. Racemes of pendent, open bell-shaped violet flowers, to 2cm (¾in) long, are borne in mid- and late summer. ↕ 60–90cm (24–36in), ↔ 30cm (12in). W. China. ❄❄❄
A. tashiroi, syn. *A. polymorpha* var. *tashiroi.* Semi-decumbent perennial producing small, alternate, ovate to elliptic, coarsely toothed stem leaves, 1.5–3cm (½–1¼in) long. Pendent, bell-shaped violet flowers, to 2cm (¾in) long, are borne in few-flowered racemes on branching stems in midsummer. ↕ 10–50cm (4–20in), ↔ 15cm (6in). Korea, Japan. ❄❄❄
A. triphylla. Erect perennial with ovate to elliptic, toothed stem leaves, 4–8cm (1½–3in) long, borne in whorls of 4. In early summer, bears dense, short-branched, lax panicles of bell-shaped violet flowers, to 1cm (½in) long. ↕ 60–100cm (24–39in), ↔ 15cm (6in). Japan (particularly Hokkaido). ❄❄❄. **var. *hakusanensis*** has a tighter, less lax inflorescence; ↕ 30–50cm (12–20in).

▷ ***Adhatoda duvernoia*** see *Justicia adhatoda*

ADIANTUM

Maidenhair fern

ADIANTACEAE / PTERIDACEAE

Genus of 200–250 species of evergreen, semi-evergreen, and deciduous ferns, many from tropical and subtropical areas of North and South America, but a few from temperate regions of Europe, Asia, Australasia, and North America. Most grow at woodland margins, in shady crevices in rocks, or at stream-sides; some prefer deeper forest shade. The fronds are 1- to 5-pinnate, with oblong or diamond-shaped to rounded segments and usually long, shiny black or deep purple-red stalks; these are produced from often many-branched, long- to short-creeping, sometimes erect rhizomes. Rounded or oblong sori form on the margins of the frond divisions and are covered by kidney-shaped or semi-circular indusia. Adiantums are grown for their elegant foliage and, in many species, the purplish pink colour

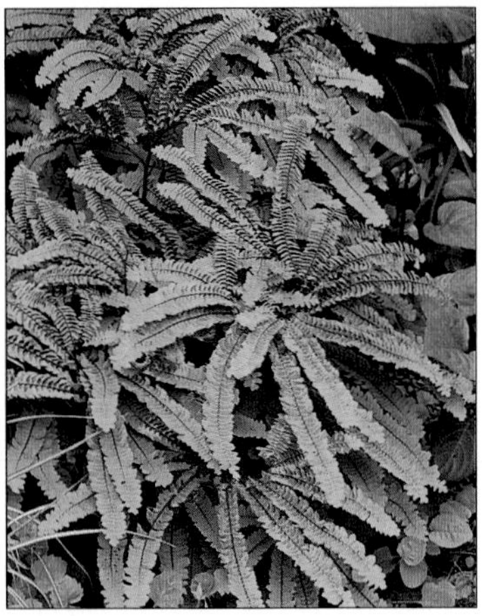

Adiantum aleuticum

of the croziers and young fronds. Where temperatures fall below 10°C (50°F), grow tender species in a temperate or warm greenhouse (*A. formosum* in a cool greenhouse). Grow hardy species, or tender species in warmer regions, in woodland, or in a shady border.

• **HARDINESS** *A. aleuticum, A. capillus-veneris, A. pedatum,* and *A. venustum* are fully hardy or frost hardy. In mild areas, *A. formosum* will survive short periods of frost if given protection and a sheltered site. The remaining species and cultivars are frost tender.

• **CULTIVATION** Under glass, grow in 1 part each of loam, medium-grade bark, charcoal, and limestone chippings; 2 parts sharp sand; 3 parts leaf mould. Provide bright indirect light in summer, bright filtered light in winter, and medium to high humidity with good ventilation; water less if air flow is poor, and sparingly in winter. When in growth, apply a half-strength balanced liquid fertilizer monthly. Remove old, damaged fronds in spring. If moving plants from a humid to a drier environment, do so gradually to avoid wilting. Outdoors, grow hardy species in moist but well-drained, moderately fertile soil in partial shade; *A. capillus-veneris* prefers moist, alkaline soil. Grow tender species in humus-rich, well-drained soil in a partially shaded, open site.

• **PROPAGATION** Sow spores as soon as ripe, at minimum 15°C (59°F) for hardy species and 21°C (70°F) for tender ones. Divide rhizomes in early spring. Root plantlets from *A. caudatum* and others that root at the frond tips. See also p.51.

• **PESTS AND DISEASES** Scale insects may be a problem under glass.

A. aleuticum ■ syn. *A. pedatum* subsp. *aleuticum* (Aleutian maidenhair fern, Northern maidenhair fern). Deciduous or semi-evergreen fern with short rhizomes and broadly ovate to kidney-shaped, pedate, pale to mid-green fronds, 20–30cm (8–12in) long, with oblong segments, and black stalks and midribs. New fronds may be tinged pink when very young. Closely allied to *A. pedatum* but with shorter rhizome internodes. ↕↔ to 75cm (30in). W. North America, E. Asia. ❄❄❄. **'Japonicum'** has golden red new fronds, maturing to green. **var. *subpumilum,*** syn. subsp. *subpumilum* (Dwarf maiden-hair fern), has fronds 10–12cm (4–5in) long; ↕ to 15cm (6in), ↔ 30cm (12in).
A. capillus-veneris (True maidenhair fern). Evergreen fern, deciduous at around -2°C (28°F), with short-creeping rhizomes. Triangular, 2- or 3-pinnate, light green fronds, 70cm (28in) long, with fan-shaped pinnae, are produced on glossy black stalks. ↕ 30cm (12in), ↔ 40cm (16in). Temperate and tropical regions worldwide. ❄❄
A. caudatum (Trailing maidenhair fern, Walking maidenhair fern). Evergreen fern, with short-creeping rhizomes, bearing ladder-like, linear, pinnate fronds, to 60cm (24in) long, with entire to shallowly lobed, sometimes deeply cut pinnae. Young fronds are pale green to pale pink with red-brown stalks that darken with age, and prominent veins. Plantlets are produced on the elongated frond tips. Ideal for hanging baskets.

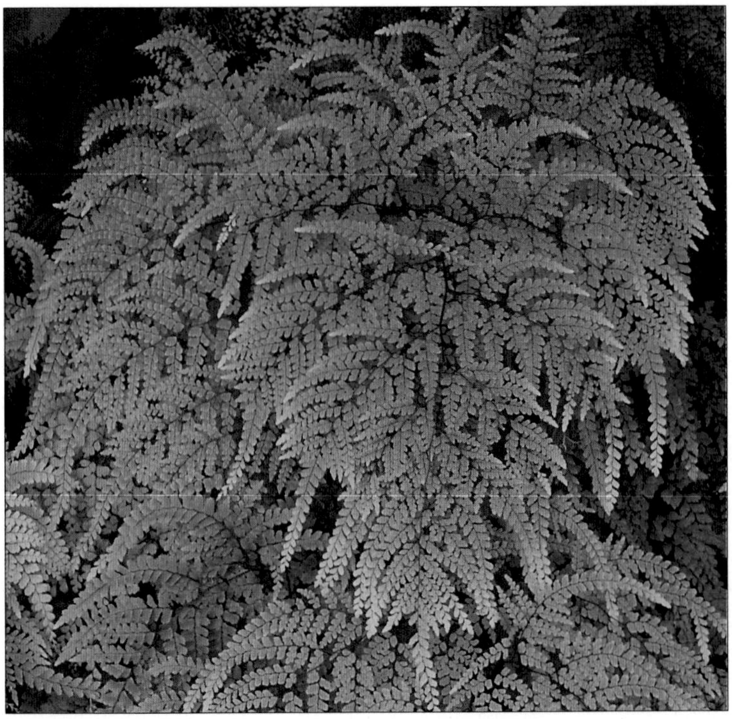

Adiantum formosum

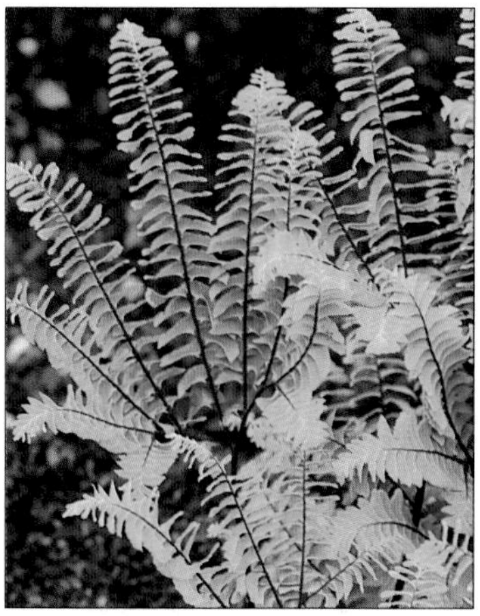
Adiantum pedatum

↕ 10–40cm (4–16in), ↔ 60cm (24in). India to Philippines, New Guinea, Taiwan, China. ❀ (min. 10°C/50°F)
A. cuneatum see *A. raddianum.*
A. formosum ■ (Australian maidenhair fern, Giant maidenhair fern). Evergreen fern with erect, roughly triangular, 2- to 4-pinnate fronds, to 1m (3ft) long, on long purple-black stalks, arising from long-creeping rhizomes. Segments are triangular to diamond-shaped and deeply cut. Fronds are pale green when young, darkening with age. Grow in a cool greenhouse in cold climates. ↕ to 1m (3ft), ↔ 2m (6ft) or more. E. Australia, New Zealand. *
A. pedatum ■ ♀ Deciduous fern with stout, creeping rhizomes, producing lance-shaped, broadly ovate to kidney-shaped, pinnate, mid-green fronds, to 35cm (14in) long, on glossy, dark brown or black stalks. The segments are oblong or obliquely triangular, and lobed or toothed on their upper margins. ↕↔ 30–40cm (12–16in). E. North America. ***.
subsp. *aleuticum* see *A. aleuticum.*
A. peruvianum (Silver dollar maidenhair fern). Evergreen fern with short-creeping rhizomes, producing triangular, 1- to 3-pinnate, dark green fronds, to 1m (3ft) long, on black-purple stalks. Diamond-shaped to ovate-rhomboid segments are to 5cm (2in) long. Young fronds are pale pink with a silky sheen. ↕ 1m (3ft), ↔ 1.5m (5ft). Ecuador, Peru, Bolivia. ❀ (min. 14°C/57°F)
A. raddianum, syn. *A. cuneatum* (Delta maidenhair fern). Evergreen fern with short rhizomes and roughly triangular, 3- or 4-pinnate, black-stalked fronds, to 60cm (24in) long, with rounded to triangular, variably lobed segments. Fronds are pale green, darkening with age. ↕ to 60cm (24in), ↔ 80cm (32in). Tropical North and South America, West Indies, W. South America. ❀ (min. 7°C/45°F). **'Elegans'** has fronds to 25cm (10in) long, with small, narrowly wedge-shaped segments, 1cm (½in) long, tapered at the bases and often curved towards the centres of the fronds. **'Fragrantissimum'**, syn. 'Fragrans', has dense fronds with deeply lobed, often overlapping, segments; ↕ to 75cm (30in). **'Fritz Luth'** has light green fronds with segments that are held almost horizontally or arch downwards. **'Gracillimum'** ■ syn. 'Gracilis', has pendent, broadly triangular, much-dissected fronds, with oblong segments, tapered at the bases. Some variants are

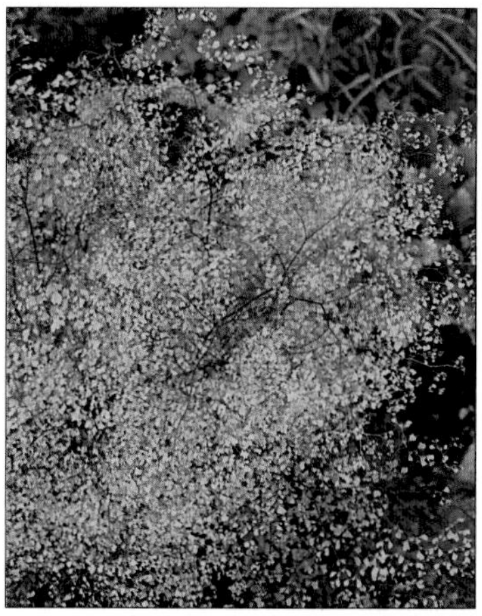
Adiantum raddianum 'Gracillimum'

crested; young foliage may be pale pink; ↕ 80cm (32in). **'Grandiceps'** (Tassel maidenhair fern) is crested, with each frond tip forming a dissected fan. Use in a hanging basket. **'Victoria's Elegans'** is often confused with 'Elegans', but has fronds with broad, wedge-shaped, more rounded segments. **'Weigandii'** is compact, and has dense, erect fronds with broadly fan- to diamond-shaped, deeply cut segments; ↕ to 40cm (16in). **'White Fritz Luth'** has fronds that unfold pure white and turn pale green.
A. tenerum ■ (Brittle maidenhair fern). Evergreen fern with broadly triangular, 1- to 3-pinnate, mid-green fronds, to 1m (3ft) long, borne on dark purple-brown to black stalks, arising from short rhizomes. Superficially similar to *A. raddianum*, but the segments are ovate and deeply cut, with jointed stalks, and softly hairy when young. Some cultivars will overwinter in a cool garden if given a dry mulch. ↕ to 60cm (24in), ↔ to 90cm (36in). S. USA, Central America, N. South America. ❀ (min. 5°C/41°F). **'Farleyense'** (Barbados maidenhair fern, Glory fern) is a variable complex of large ferns with broadly fan-shaped, deeply cut segments, tinged bronze-pink when young and becoming light green with age; many of its selections are infertile; ↕ to 90cm (36in). **'Lady Moxham'** has pendent fronds with broad, fan-shaped segments. **'Pacific May'** has broadly fan-shaped segments with many narrow, deeply cut divisions; ↕ to 75cm (30in). **'Scutum Roseum'** has erect, 3-pinnate fronds with crowded, rhomboidal segments. Young fronds are rose-pink; ↕ 50cm (20in).

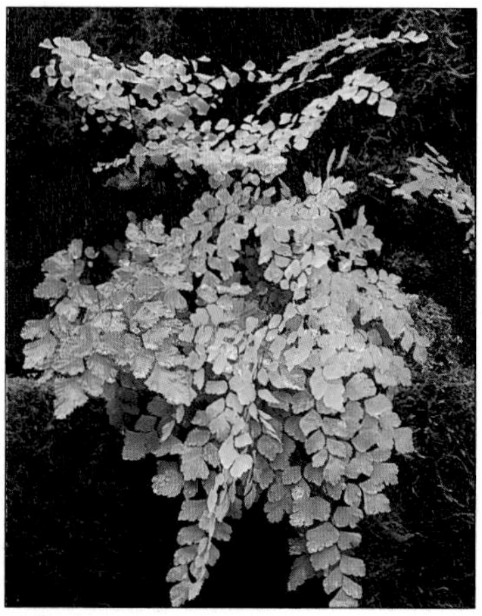
Adiantum tenerum

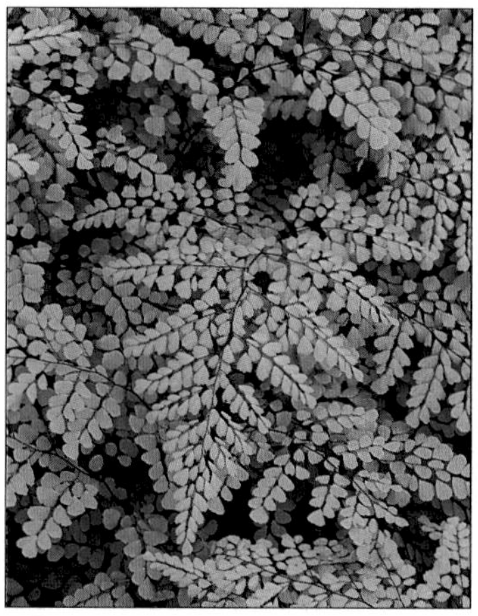
Adiantum venustum

A. trapeziforme (Diamond maidenhair fern, Giant maidenhair fern). Evergreen fern with short rhizomes, producing erect to spreading, broadly triangular, 3-pinnate fronds, to 2m (6ft) or more long, on black stalks. Segments, to 6cm (2½in) long, vary from ovate-diamond-shaped to rhomboidal, and are mid-green, sometimes glaucous beneath. ↕ to 2m (6ft) or more, ↔ 2.5m (8ft) or more. Tropical North and South America, West Indies, Cuba. ❀ (min. 14°C/57°F)
A. venustum ■ ♀ (Himalayan maidenhair fern). Evergreen fern, deciduous below -10°C (14°F), with creeping rhizomes. Narrowly triangular, usually 3-pinnate, mid-green fronds, 15–30cm (6–12in) long, with narrowly fan-shaped segments, are produced on black stalks. New fronds emerge bright bronze-pink in late winter and early spring. Hardy to -30°C (-22°F). ↕ 15cm (6in), ↔ indefinite. China, Himalayas. ***

ADLUMIA

FUMARIACEAE

Genus of one species of biennial climber found at the edges of moist woodland in temperate areas of Korea and E. North America, grown for its delicate foliage and nodding to pendent flower panicles. The leaves are 2- to 4-pinnate, and form a basal rosette on the plant when young, becoming alternate as the flowering stem elongates in the second year. The flowers, borne in axillary, nodding to pendent panicles, each have 2 pairs of petals, the outer pair with basal pouches. *A. fungosa* is effective grown over an arch, pergola, or through a large shrub.
• **HARDINESS** Fully hardy.
• **CULTIVATION** Grow in any fertile, humus-rich, moist but well-drained soil in sun or partial shade, with shelter from strong winds.
• **PROPAGATION** Sow seed as soon as ripe or in spring, either in containers in a cold frame or *in situ.* May self-seed.
• **PESTS AND DISEASES** Prone to aphids.

A. cirrhosa see *A. fungosa.*
A. fungosa, syn. *A. cirrhosa* (Allegheny vine, Climbing fumitory, Mountain fringe). Slender biennial climber with leaf-stalk tendrils and 2- to 4-pinnate, light green, fern-like leaves, 10–25cm (4–10in) long. Green- or purple-tinted, pale pink or white flowers, 1.5cm (½in) long, are borne in panicles, 5–10cm (2–4in) long, from summer to autumn. As the flowers fade, the persistent petals enclose the developing seed pods. ↕ 3–5m (10–15ft), occasionally more. Korea, E. North America. ***

▷***Adonidia merrillii*** see *Veitchia merrillii*

ADONIS

RANUNCULACEAE

Genus of about 20 species of annuals and perennials from Europe and Asia, mainly from alpine habitats. The fern-like foliage dies back by midsummer in some species. The solitary, terminal, anemone-like flowers are usually yellow in perennials and red in annuals; double-flowered cultivars have up to 30 petals. The Asiatic species are best grown in shady woodland and the European species in an open, rocky site.
• **HARDINESS** Fully hardy.
• **CULTIVATION** *Adonis* species have varying cultivation requirements. For ease of reference, these have been divided into the following groups:
1. Humus-rich, cool, moist, light, acid soil in full shade.
2. Moist but well-drained, humus-rich soil in partial shade.
3. Well-drained, moderately fertile, alkaline soil in full sun.
• **PROPAGATION** Sow seed of perennials in containers in a cold frame as soon as ripe; germination in spring is slow and erratic, and seedling growth slow. Sow seed of annuals *in situ* in autumn or spring. Perennial species resent division, but if required, divide after flowering.
• **PESTS AND DISEASES** Susceptible to slug damage, especially *A. vernalis.*

A. aestivalis. Erect annual with 1- to 3-pinnate leaves, 3–5cm (1¼–2in) long, with linear to thread-like leaflets. In midsummer, bears cup-shaped, dark-centred red flowers, 1.5–2.5cm (½–1in) wide, with 5 spreading petals, and sepals pressed to the petal backs. Cultivation group 3. ↕ 40cm (16in), ↔ 15–30cm (6–12in). C. and S. Europe. ***
A. amurensis ■ Clump-forming perennial producing triangular to ovate, 3-pinnate leaves, to 10cm (4in) long, with many linear leaflets with pointed lobes. Bowl-shaped yellow, sometimes bronze-backed flowers, 3–5cm (1¼–2in) across, with 20–30 petals, are borne in late winter and early spring, before the leaves emerge, on short stems that gradually lengthen. Cultivation group 1.

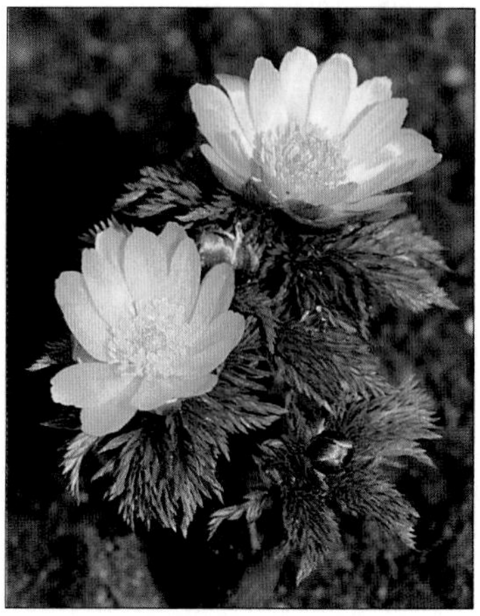
Adonis amurensis

↕ 20–40cm (8–16in), ↔ 30cm (12in). China (Manchuria), Korea, Japan. ❄❄❄. **'Flore Pleno'** ■ has double, green-tinged yellow flowers. **'Fukujukai'** has semi-double, sterile, bright yellow flowers, 5cm (2in) across. **'Hinomoto'** has orange-red, green-tinted flowers. **'Pleniflora'**, syn. 'Plena', produces neat, double yellow flowers, each with a prominent green eye.

A. annua (Pheasant's eye). Erect annual producing finely divided, 3-pinnate leaves, 3–5cm (1¼–2in) long, with linear leaflets. Cup-shaped, dark-centred scarlet flowers, 1.5–2.5cm (½–1in) across, are borne in early summer. The 5 almost erect petals are clearly separated from the sepals. Cultivation group 3. ↕ 45cm (18in), ↔ 15–30cm (6–12in). S. Europe to S.W. Asia. ❄❄❄

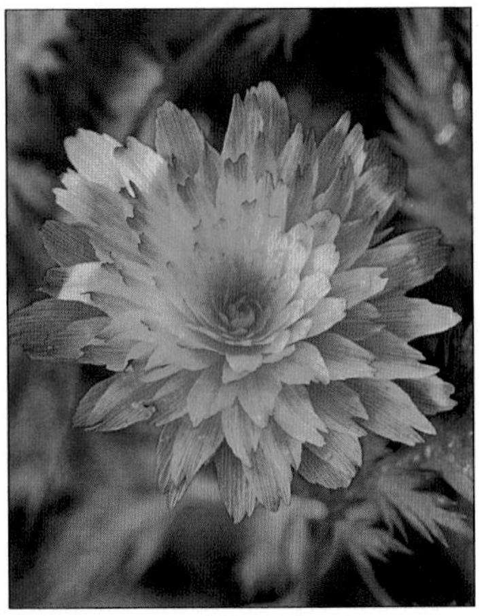

Adonis amurensis 'Flore Pleno'

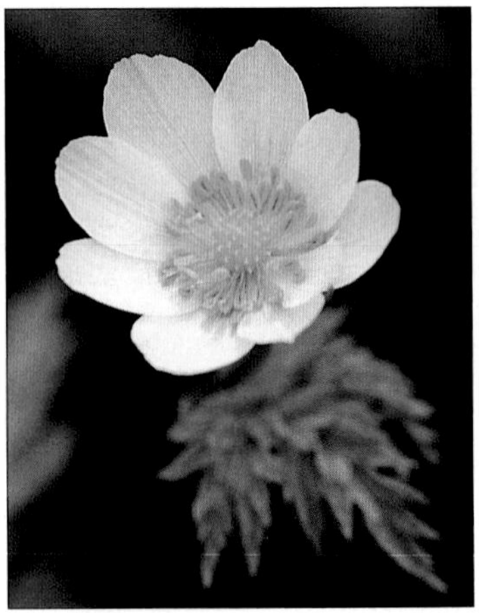

Adonis brevistyla

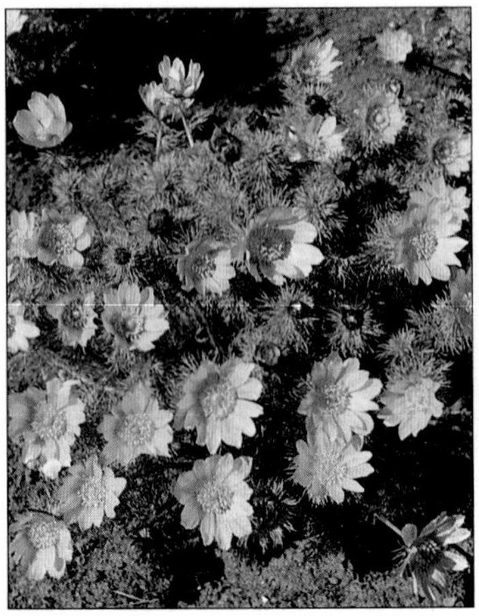

Adonis vernalis

A. brevistyla ■ Clump-forming perennial with narrowly ovate, 1- or 2-pinnate leaves, 5–12cm (2–5in) long, the leaflets with pointed lobes. Shallowly cup-shaped flowers, to 5cm (2in) across, with 20 or more petals, usually white with blue on the outside, open in late spring. Cultivation group 1. ↕ 20–40cm (8–16in), ↔ 20cm (8in). China (Yunnan), S. Tibet, Bhutan. ❄❄❄

A. chrysocyathus. Clump-forming perennial with triangular, 3-pinnate leaves, to 16cm (6in) long, the leaflets with long, flat, sharp-pointed lobes. Many cup-shaped, bright yellow flowers, to 5cm (2in) across, with 20–25 petals, are produced from early summer to early autumn. Cultivation group 2. ↕ 15–40cm (6–16in), ↔ 30cm (12in). W. Himalayas, Tibet. ❄❄❄

A. vernalis ■ Clump-forming perennial producing 2- or 3-pinnate, bright green leaves, 3–5cm (1¼–2in) long, with linear leaflets, the lower ones scale-like. Shallowly cup-shaped, bright golden yellow flowers, to 8cm (3in) across, with up to 20 elliptic petals, open in mid- and late spring. Cultivation group 3. ↕ to 38cm (15in), ↔ 45cm (18in). Finland to Italy, E. Europe to the Urals. ❄❄❄

ADROMISCHUS

CRASSULACEAE

Genus of about 30 species of stemless or short-stemmed perennial succulents, closely related to *Cotyledon*, from semi-arid areas of southern Africa. The thick, fleshy leaves are clustered or spirally arranged, and the small, tubular flowers, with spreading lobes, are borne in spike-like cymes, mainly in summer. Where temperatures fall below 7°C (45°F), grow in a temperate greenhouse or as houseplants; in warmer areas, grow in a raised bed.

- **HARDINESS** Frost tender.
- **CULTIVATION** Under glass, grow in sharply drained standard cactus compost in full light with good ventilation. In summer, water only when the soil has become dry; at other times, water only in warm weather; excess watering may encourage root rot. Apply a low-nitrogen fertilizer 2 or 3 times in the growing season. Outdoors, grow in well-drained, fertile soil, enriched with leaf mould, in full sun. See also pp.48–49.
- **PROPAGATION** Sow seed at 19–24°C (66–75°F) in spring. Take stem or leaf cuttings in summer.
- **PESTS AND DISEASES** Susceptible to mealybugs and greenfly.

A. clavifolius see *A. cooperi*.

A. cooperi, syn. *A. clavifolius, Cotyledon cooperi, Echeveria cooperi.* Freely branching succulent with greyish brown stems and inversely lance-shaped, glossy, grey-green leaves, to 5cm (2in) long, often purple-marked above. Tubular, green-and-red flowers, to 1.5cm (½in) long, with white-margined, pink or purple lobes, are borne in spike-like cymes, 25cm (10in) or more long, in summer. ↕ 10cm (4in), ↔ to 15cm (6in). South Africa (Eastern Cape, Western Cape). ❁ (min. 7°C/45°F)

A. cristatus* var. *zeyheri, syn. *Cotyledon zeyheri.* Perennial succulent with semi-erect stems and many aerial roots. Inversely lance-shaped to obovate, hairy, grey-green leaves, to 4cm (1½ in) long, spotted purple-red, are fan-like and wavy near the tips. In summer, bears tubular, greenish red flowers, to 1.5cm (½in) long, with white and pink lobes, in spike-like cymes, to 12cm (5in) long. ↕ 10cm (4in), ↔ indefinite. South Africa (Eastern Cape). ❁ (min. 7°C/45°F)

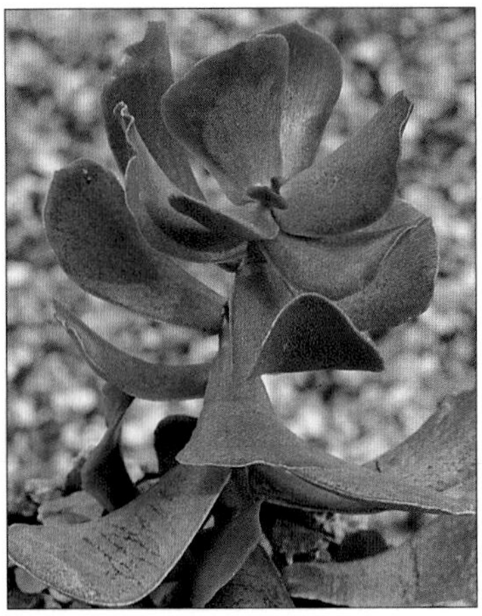

Adromischus maculatus

A. maculatus ■ syn. *Cotyledon alternans, Cotyledon maculata, Crassula maculata* of gardens. Perennial succulent with a sparsely branched brown caudex. Inversely lance-shaped, glossy, bright green leaves, to 5cm (2in) long, are mottled dark purplish red, and often have horny margins. Spike-like cymes, 25–30cm (10–12in) long, of tubular green flowers, to 1.5cm (½in) long, with pinkish white or pale purple lobes, are borne in summer. ↕ 15cm (6in), ↔ to 15cm (6in). South Africa (Eastern Cape, Western Cape). ❁ (min. 7°C/45°F)

AECHMEA

BROMELIACEAE

Genus of nearly 200 species of rosette-forming, often rhizomatous, mostly epiphytic, evergreen perennials (bromeliads), mainly from rainforest in S. Mexico, Central America, South America, and the West Indies. Their arching leaves are narrowly strap-shaped to triangular. Terminal, simple or compound, spike-like inflorescences with long-lasting, brightly coloured, tubular flowers and triangular bracts are produced in summer, and are often followed by persistent, fleshy, colourful fruits. Where temperatures fall below 10°C (50°F), grow in a warm greenhouse or as houseplants; in warmer areas, grow epiphytically in a moist site.

- **HARDINESS** Frost tender.
- **CULTIVATION** Under glass, grow either epiphytically or in epiphytic bromeliad compost in bright filtered light with low humidity. In the growing season, water freely and apply a low-nitrogen fertilizer monthly. Keep the central "cup" filled with soft water. Outdoors, grow epiphytically or in moist, gritty, humus-rich soil. See also p.47.
- **PROPAGATION** Root offsets in early summer.
- **PESTS AND DISEASES** Scale insects and mealybugs may be a problem.

A. candida. Epiphytic perennial with wide funnel-shaped rosettes of strap-shaped, stiff, grey-scaly, mid-green leaves, to 45cm (18in) long, with spiny margins. In summer, bears pyramidal, floury-white inflorescences, to 20cm (8in) long, of 4- to 9-flowered spikes, 1cm (½in) long, with woolly, pink and white bracts, pale yellow sepals, and white petals. These are followed by spherical, woolly, yellowish white fruit. ↕ 70cm (28in), ↔ 60cm (24in). S. Brazil. ❁ (min. 10°C/50°F)

A. caudata. Epiphytic perennial with funnel-shaped rosettes of strap-shaped, grey-scaly, dark green leaves, to 1m (3ft) long, with finely sharp-toothed brown margins. In summer, bears panicle-like inflorescences, to 25cm (10in) long, of spreading spikes of 4–7 lilac-pink-bracted yellow flowers, 2.5cm (1in) long, followed by ovoid, woolly white fruit. ↕ 1.2m (4ft), ↔ 80cm (32in). S.E. Brazil. ❁ (min. 10°C/50°F)

A. chantinii ■ ♀ Epiphytic perennial with wide-spreading rosettes of strap-shaped, mid-green leaves, to 40cm (16in) long, margined with short brown spines and cross-banded in greyish white. Lax pyramidal inflorescences, 15cm (6in) long, with short spikes of up to 8 bright yellow to orange flowers, 3cm (1¼in) long, are borne on erect, white-scaly, red-bracted stems in summer. They are followed by ovoid, greenish red fruit. ↕ to 1m (3ft), ↔ to 80cm (32in). S.E. Colombia, N.E. Peru, N. Brazil. ❁ (min. 10°C/50°F)

A. cylindrata. Rhizomatous, epiphytic or terrestrial perennial with dense, flat, open rosettes of strap-shaped, grey-scaly, mid-green leaves, to 50cm (20in) long, with red tips and lilac-grey stripes. In summer, bears simple, cylindrical inflorescences, to 20cm (8in) long, composed of many rows of red-bracted flowers, 2cm (¾in) long, with blue petals and rose-red sepals. They are followed by ovoid, woolly white fruit. ↕ 60cm (24in), ↔ to 35cm (14in). S.E. Brazil. ❁ (min. 10°C/50°F)

A. distichantha ■ Variable, epiphytic or terrestrial perennial with funnel-shaped rosettes of narrowly triangular to strap-shaped, grey-scaly, dull, mid-green leaves, 1m (3ft) long, with pointed tips and brown marginal spines. Pyramidal or ovoid inflorescences composed of erect to spreading spikes of 2–12 white-felted, pink-bracted, purple, blue, or white flowers, to 3cm (1¼in) long, are borne on white-woolly stems in summer. These are followed by cylindrical, woolly white fruit. ↕↔ 1m (3ft) or more. S. Brazil, Bolivia, N.E. Argentina, Paraguay, Uruguay. ❁ (min. 10°C/50°F)

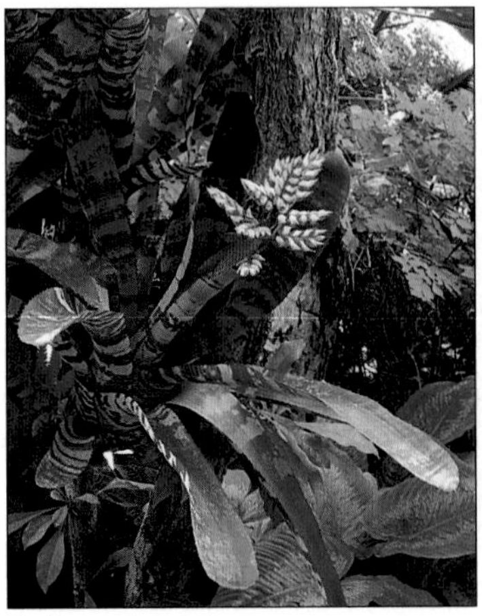

Aechmea chantinii

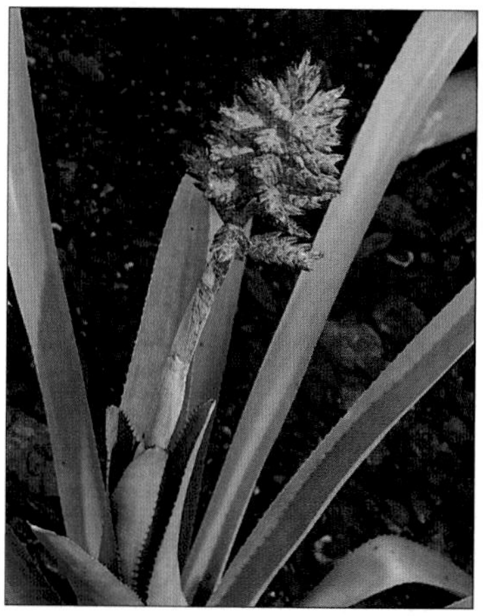
Aechmea distichantha

A. fasciata ■ ♀ syn. *Billbergia rhodocyanea* (Vase plant). Rhizomatous, epiphytic perennial with funnel-shaped rosettes of strap-shaped, lilac-grey leaves, to 60cm (24in) long, cross-banded with grey scales, and with tiny brown marginal spines. In summer, densely white-woolly stems bear wide pyramidal inflorescences, 8cm (3in) long, consisting of dense clusters of flowers, 3.5cm (1½in) long, with blue petals, rose-pink bracts, and white-scaly, rose-pink sepals. These are followed by spherical, woolly white fruit. ↕ 40cm (16in) or more, ↔ to 50cm (20in). S.E. Brazil. ❁ (min. 10°C/50°F)
***A.* Foster's Favorite Group** ■ ♀ Terrestrial perennial with erect rosettes of strap-shaped, wine-red leaves, 45cm (18in) long, with tiny marginal spines. Semi-pendent inflorescences, to 50cm (20in) long, of pink-tipped, red-bracted blue flowers, 2cm (¾in) long, are borne in summer, followed by pear-shaped red fruit. ↕↔ 30–60cm (12–24in). ❁ (min. 10°C/50°F)
A. fulgens ■ Epiphytic perennial with funnel-shaped rosettes of broadly strap-shaped, bright green leaves, 40cm (16in) long, grey-waxy beneath, with marginal spines. In summer, red stems bear branched inflorescences, 20cm (8in) long, consisting of spikes of 2–5 flowers, 2cm (¾in) long, with red sepals and violet petals, fading to red; the bracts are absent or reduced to scales. The red fruit are spherical and stalked. ↕ to 50cm (20in), ↔ 40cm (16in). E. Brazil. ❁ (min. 10°C/50°F). **var. *discolor*** ♀ produces leaves purplish or brownish red beneath.

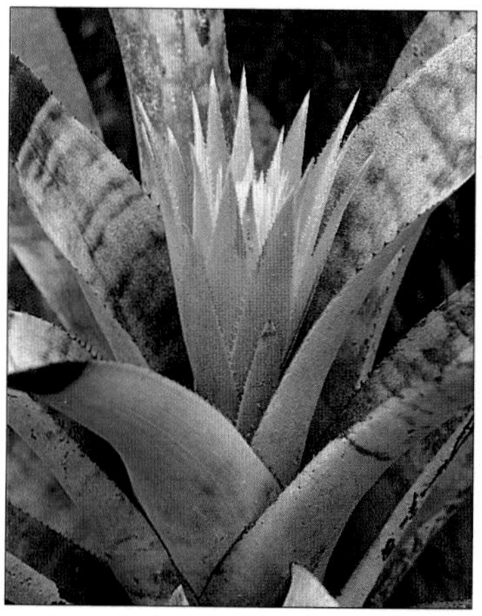
Aechmea fasciata

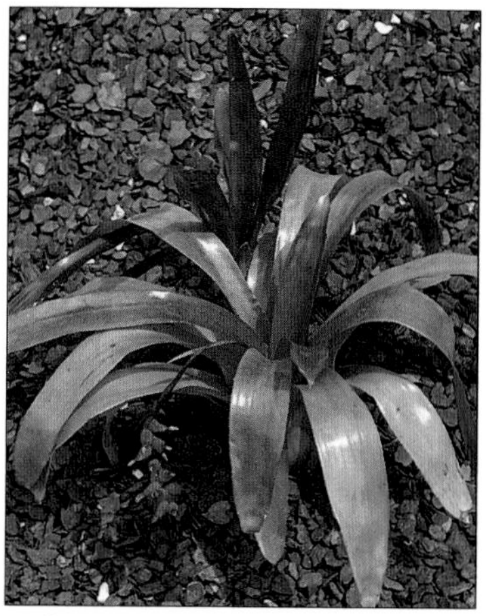
Aechmea Foster's Favorite Group

A. gamosepala ■ Epiphytic or terrestrial perennial with erect, funnel-shaped rosettes of broadly strap-shaped, bright green leaves, 25–55cm (10–22in) long, grey-scaly beneath, with rounded, spiny tips. In summer, bears cylindrical inflorescences, to 25cm (10in) long, of flowers, 1.5cm (½in) long, with pale blue or purple petals, red or pink sepals, and reddish brown bracts. These are followed by spherical, rose-pink fruit. ↕ 50cm (20in), ↔ to 60cm (24in). S.E. Brazil. ❁ (min. 10°C/50°F)
A. marmorata see *Quesnelia marmorata.*
A. mertensii. Variable, epiphytic perennial with funnel-shaped rosettes of strap-shaped, lilac-grey, white-scaly leaves, to 70cm (28in) long, with black marginal spines. In summer, spikes of 2–8 red-bracted, red or yellow flowers, 2cm (¾in) long, are borne in cylindrical inflorescences, 30cm (12in) long, followed by ovoid pink fruit. ↕ to 70cm (28in), ↔ 35–40cm (14–16in). Venezuela, Colombia, Ecuador, Peru, Brazil, Guyana, Trinidad. ❁ (min. 10°C/50°F)
A. mexicana. Epiphytic or terrestrial perennial with wide funnel-shaped rosettes of broadly strap-shaped, spiny-margined, mid-green leaves, 1m (3ft) or more long, irregularly marked with darker green patches. In summer, bears pyramidal or cylindrical, branched inflorescences, to 70cm (28in) long, on grey-scaly stems; they consist of spikes of 5–10 red, lilac, or violet flowers, 1.5cm (½in) long, with rose-pink bracts, and are followed by spherical white fruit. ↕↔ 1m (3ft) or more. Mexico. ❁ (min. 10°C/50°F)

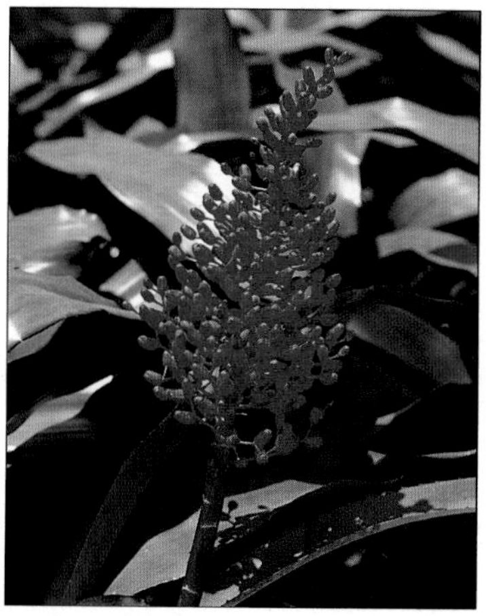
Aechmea fulgens

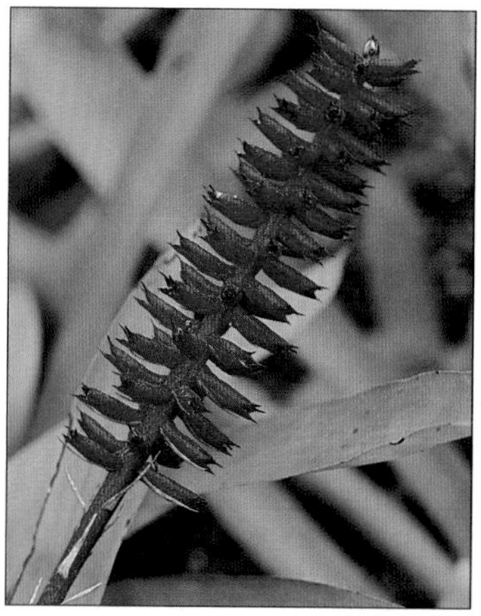
Aechmea gamosepala

A. nudicaulis ■ ♀ Variable, epiphytic or terrestrial perennial with rosettes of strap-shaped, grey-green leaves, 30–90cm (12–36in) long, cross-banded with darker grey-green beneath, and with black marginal spines. In summer, bears simple, cylindrical inflorescences, 5–25cm (2–10in) long, of 15–20 red-bracted yellow flowers, 2cm (¾in) long, followed by cylindrical, scaly green fruit. ↕ to 70cm (28in), ↔ 25cm (10in). Central America, N. and N.E. South America, West Indies. ❁ (min. 10°C/50°F). **var. *cuspidata*** has triangular yellow bracts; ↕ to 50cm (20in); Brazil.
A. orlandiana ■ ♀ Epiphytic perennial with funnel-shaped rosettes of strap-shaped, mid-green, grey-scaly leaves, 30cm (12in) long, spotted and banded dark purple with purple marginal spines. In summer, red stems bear pyramidal inflorescences, to 10cm (4in) long, with spikes of 4–6 red-bracted, yellow-white flowers, 2–3cm (¾–1¼in) long; they are followed by ovoid, pale green fruit. ↕ to 50cm (20in), ↔ 40–50cm (16–20in). S.E. Brazil. ❁ (min. 10°C/50°F)
A. pineliana. Variable, mainly epiphytic perennial with funnel-shaped rosettes of strap-shaped, silvery grey-scaly, dark green leaves, to 70cm (28in) long, often cross-banded with silver-grey beneath, and with dark reddish brown marginal spines. In summer, slender, white-woolly stems bear cylindrical inflorescences, 7cm (3in) long, with clusters of brown bristles, and long-bracted yellow flowers, 1.5cm (½in) long, which gradually turn black. The white fruit is spherical and woolly. ↕ to 80cm (32in), ↔ 50cm (20in) or more. S.E. Brazil. ❁ (min. 10°C/50°F)
A. pubescens. Epiphytic perennial with wide-spreading rosettes of strap-shaped, mid-green leaves, 1m (3ft) long, which have spiny, sometimes grey margins. In summer, white-woolly, red-bracted stems bear pyramidal inflorescences, 35cm (14in) long, composed of spikes of 8–16 pale violet flowers, 1.5cm (½in) long. These are followed by ellipsoid blue fruit. ↕ 1m (3ft), ↔ to 40cm (16in). Central America, Colombia, Venezuela. ❁ (min. 10°C/50°F)
A. recurvata ■ Variable, terrestrial perennial with dense, tubular rosettes of narrowly triangular, channelled, often strongly recurved, dark or mid-green leaves, 40cm (16in) long, with curved marginal spines; the central leaves turn red at flowering time and in strong sun. Ovoid inflorescences, 6cm (2½in) long,

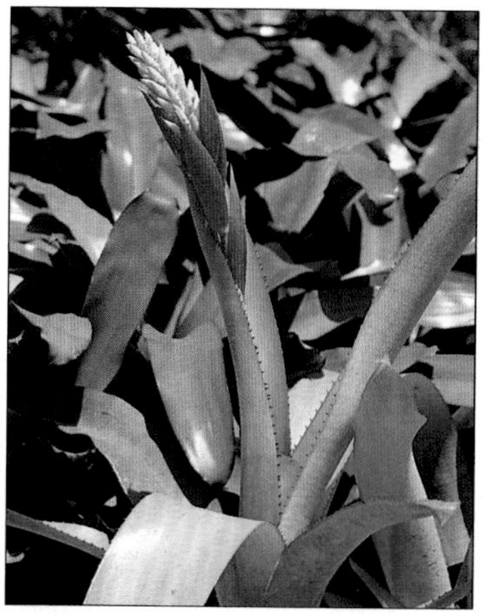
Aechmea nudicaulis

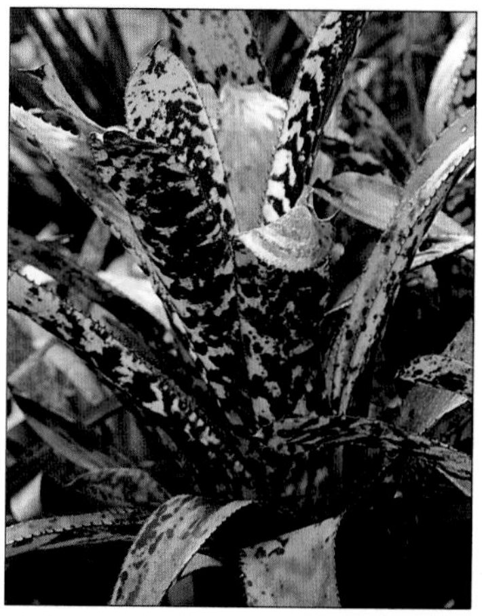
Aechmea orlandiana

have red bracts almost hiding the pinkish white or purple flowers, 3.5cm (1½in) long; they are followed by ovoid white fruit. ↕ to 20cm (8in), ↔ to 50cm (20in). Brazil, Paraguay, Argentina, Uruguay. ❁ (min. 10°C/50°F)
A. weilbachii. Epiphytic perennial with funnel-shaped rosettes of strap-shaped, almost smooth-margined, dark green leaves, to 60cm (24in) long, often tinged purple. In summer, red-bracted pink stems bear slender inflorescences, 15cm (6in) long, composed of spikes of 5–10 red-bracted, bluish purple flowers, 1.5cm (½in) long. They are followed by ellipsoid, rough, lilac-red fruit. ↕ to 70cm (28in), ↔ 30cm (12in). S.E. Brazil. ❁ (min. 10°C/50°F)

▷ ***Aegle*** see *Poncirus*

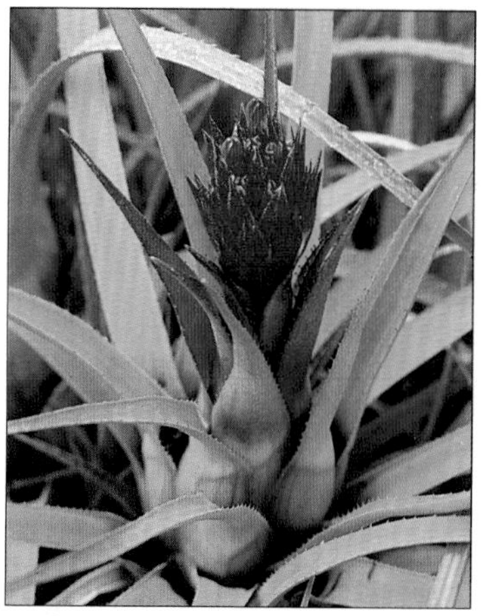
Aechmea recurvata

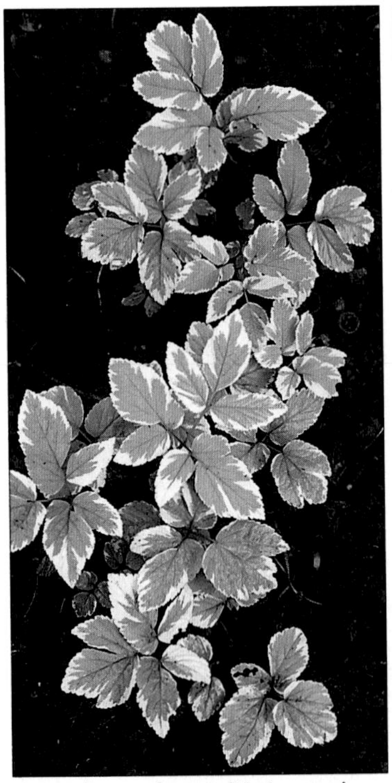

Aegopodium podagraria 'Variegatum'

AEGOPODIUM

Ground elder

APIACEAE/UMBELLIFERAE

Genus of about 5 species of perennials, with invasive rhizomes and deep roots, occurring in woodland in N. and C. Europe, Siberia, and W. Asia. The alternate, deep green leaves have 3 ovate leaflets, and the many-rayed umbels of white flowers are borne on branching, hairless stems. Only the variegated cultivars are suitable for a garden; plant either in containers or as ground cover in poor soil in a shady site, where little else flourishes and where they cannot spread into other plants.

- **HARDINESS** Fully hardy.
- **CULTIVATION** Grow in any soil in full or partial shade. Dead-head before the flowers set seed.
- **PROPAGATION** Separate rhizomes in autumn or spring.
- **PESTS AND DISEASES** Trouble free.

***A. podagraria* 'Variegatum'** ■ (Variegated goutweed, Variegated ground elder). Ground-covering perennial with ternate or 2-ternate, toothed, deep green leaves, 10–20cm (4–8in) long, margined and splashed creamy white. Bears flat umbels, 2–6cm (¾–2½in) across, of tiny, creamy white flowers in early summer. ↕30–60cm (12–24in), ↔ indefinite. ✻✻✻

AEONIUM syn. MEGALONIUM

CRASSULACEAE

Genus of about 30 species of evergreen, perennial, occasionally biennial succulents, often subshrubby, mainly found on hillsides in Madeira, the Canary Islands, Cape Verde Islands, N. Africa, and the Mediterranean. Neat rosettes of fleshy leaves are produced at the ends of clustered basal shoots. Terminal cymes, panicles, or racemes of numerous star-shaped, many-petalled flowers, 8–15mm (⅜–½in) across, develop from the centres of the rosettes from spring to summer. In some species, the flowering branches die once the seeds have ripened. Where temperatures fall below 10°C (50°C), grow in a cool or temperate greenhouse or as houseplants; elsewhere, grow in a border.

- **HARDINESS** Frost tender; they may withstand occasional short periods of frost in dry conditions.
- **CULTIVATION** Under glass, grow in standard cactus compost in filtered light.Water freely and apply a balanced liquid fertilizer 2 or 3 times during the growing season; allow the compost to dry out almost completely between waterings. Keep dry when dormant. Outdoors, grow in moderately fertile, well-drained soil in partial shade. See also pp.48–49.
- **PROPAGATION** Sow seed at 19–24°C (66–75°F) in spring. Take rosette cuttings in early summer, wait until calluses have formed, then insert in sandy cactus cutting compost in moderate light, at 18°C (64°F), and keep barely moist until rooted.
- **PESTS AND DISEASES** Prone to greenfly, especially while flowering, and to mealybugs in autumn and winter.

A. arboreum ♀ syn. *Sempervivum arboreum.* Erect, succulent subshrub with few branches, each bearing a tightly packed rosette, 20cm (8in) across, of spoon-shaped, light green leaves, to 15cm (6in) long, margined with fine hairs and sometimes mottled purplish green. Bears large, pyramidal panicles, to 30cm (12in) long, of many bright yellow flowers in late spring. ↕↔ to 2m (6ft). Morocco, but naturalized in other frost-free areas. ❀ (min. 10°C/50°F).
'Zwartkop' ■♀ syn. 'Schwarzkopf', has rich, almost black-purple leaves.
A. balsamiferum, syn. *Sempervivum balsamiferum.* Shrubby, balsam-scented, perennial succulent with thick branches, each crowned by a saucer-shaped rosette, 20cm (8in) across, of spoon-shaped, sticky, pale green leaves, 7cm (3in) long, with pointed tips. Bears pyramidal panicles, 15cm (6in) or more long, of many pale yellow flowers in late spring. An unusual species needing dry conditions. ↕1.2–1.5m (4–5ft), ↔ 60cm (24in). Canary Islands (Lanzarote). ❀ (min. 10°C/50°F)
A. bertoletianum see *A. tabuliforme.*
A. canariense, syn. *A. exsul.* Short-stemmed, perennial succulent, often branching at the base. Produces rosettes, to 40cm (16in) across, of broadly spoon-shaped, dark green leaves, to 25cm (10in) long, with glandular, sticky white hairs. In spring, bears pale green and white flowers in pyramidal, leafy racemes, 50–70cm (20–28in) long. ↕ to 20cm (8in), ↔ 50cm (20in). Canary Islands (Tenerife). ❀ (min. 10°C/50°F)
***A. domesticum* 'Variegatum'** see *Aichryson* x *domesticum* 'Variegatum'.
A. exsul see *A. canariense.*
A. haworthii ■♀ syn. *Sempervivum haworthii.* Succulent subshrub with slender branches, each crowned by a rosette, 6–15cm (2½–6in) across, of spoon-shaped, pointed, toothed, bluish green leaves, to 8cm (3in) long, keeled beneath, and with red margins. Bears lax panicles, 10–15cm (4–6in) long, of pale yellow to pinkish white flowers in spring. ↕↔ 60cm (24in). Canary Islands (Tenerife). ❀ (min. 10°C/50°F)

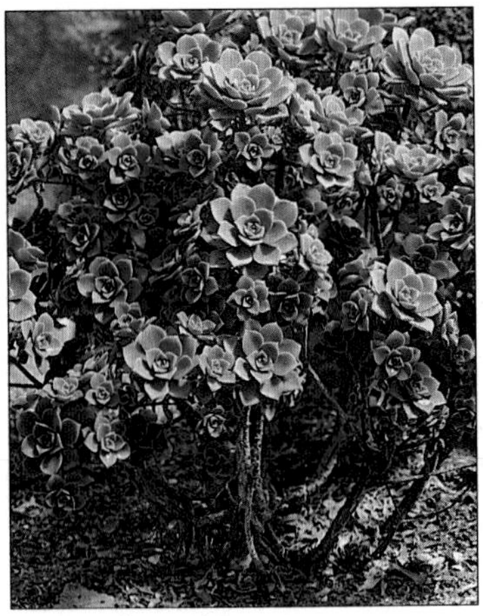

Aeonium haworthii

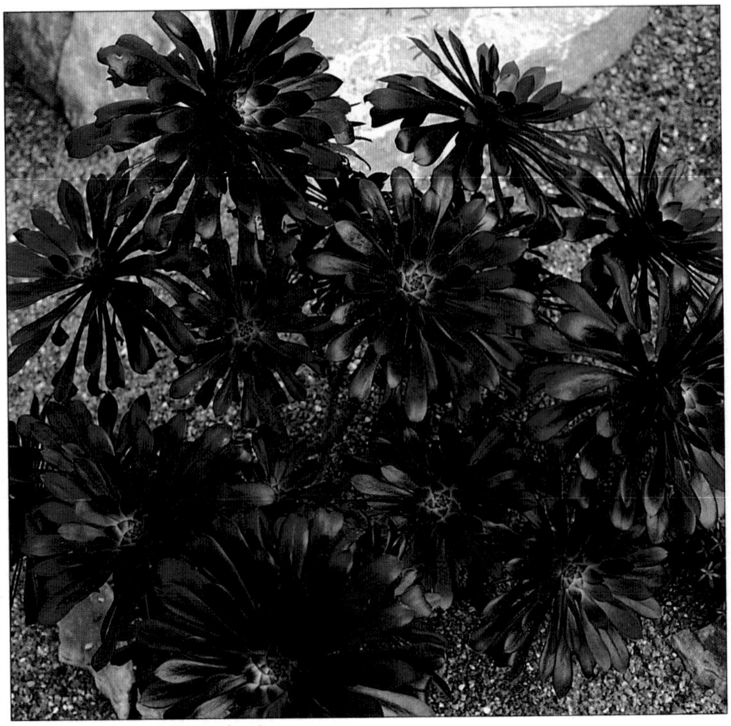

Aeonium arboreum 'Zwartkop'

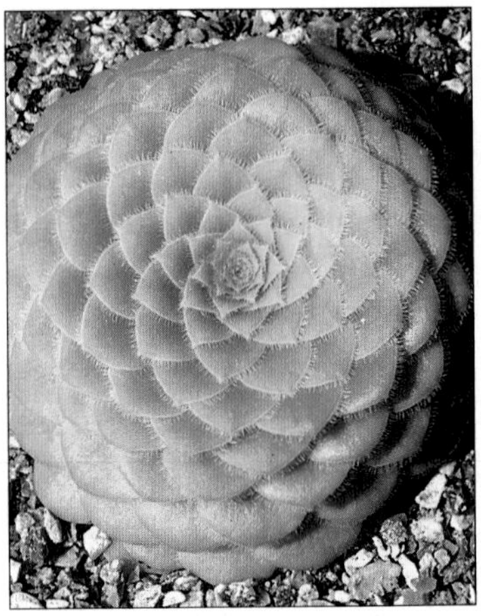

Aeonium tabuliforme

A. nobile, syn. *Megalonium nobile, Sempervivum nobile.* Subshrubby, usually unbranched, short-stemmed succulent. Produces rosettes, 50cm (20in) across, of broadly obovate to rounded, very fleshy, often red-tinged, olive-green leaves, to 30cm (12in) long, with incurved margins. Bears large, pyramidal, flat-topped cymes, 20–40cm (8–16in) long, of copper-red or yellow flowers, lined with red, in late spring. The rosettes often die soon after flowering. ↕60cm (24in), ↔ 50cm (20in). Canary Islands (La Palma). ❀ (min. 10°C/50°F)
A. sedifolium, syn. *Aichryson sedifolium, Sempervivum masferreri.* Dense, succulent subshrub with slender, erect branches that later become pendent. Club-shaped, sticky, fleshy, mid-green to yellowish green, red-lined leaves, to 1.5cm (½in) long, are borne in rosettes, 6cm (2½in) across. Bears large, golden yellow flowers, in racemes, 2–7cm (¾–3in) long, in spring. ↕15–40cm (6–16in), ↔ 13cm (5in). Canary Islands (Tenerife). ❀ (min. 10°C/50°F)
A. tabuliforme ■♀ syn. *A. bertoletianum, Sempervivum complanatum.* Biennial or perennial succulent with very short, unbranched stems bearing plate-like rosettes, to 50cm (20in) across, of many spoon-shaped, bright green leaves, to 25cm (10in) long, margined with fine hairs. Yellow flowers are produced in large panicles, 30cm (12in) or more long, in spring. ↕8–10cm (3–4in), ↔ to 50cm (20in). Canary Islands (Tenerife). ❀ (min. 10°C/50°F)

AERANGIS

ORCHIDACEAE

Genus of about 35 species of evergreen, epiphytic, monopodial orchids, mostly from lowland forest and savannah or woodland in tropical Africa and Madagascar. The fleshy or leathery leaves are generally oval, obovate, or inversely lance-shaped, occasionally narrowly linear-oblong, and are arranged in 2 ranks. Racemes of white, sometimes red- or yellow-tinted, usually star-shaped, long-spurred flowers, in most cases night-scented, are borne at various times of the year, but mostly in winter or spring.

- **HARDINESS** Frost tender.

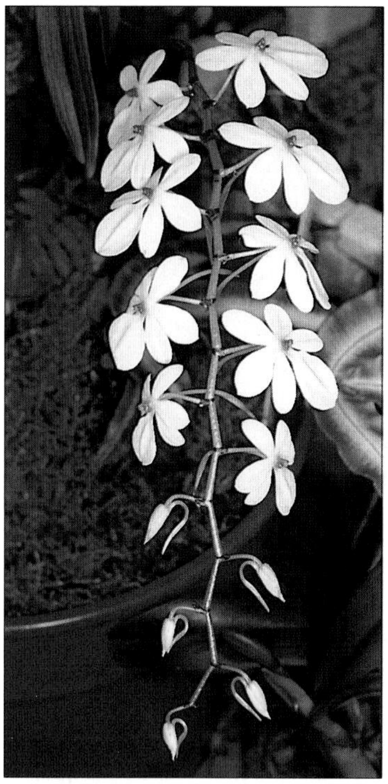

Aerangis luteoalba var. *rhodosticta*

• **CULTIVATION** Intermediate- to warm-growing orchids. Grow epiphytically on an orchid raft or cork slab; provide shade in summer and high humidity. Water freely throughout the year, more sparingly in winter. In spring and summer, apply a half-strength, balanced foliar fertilizer at every third watering. Spray aerial roots with water once or twice daily in summer. See also p.46.
• **PROPAGATION** Not suitable for division, although cuttings or offshoots may be rooted successfully.
• **PESTS AND DISEASES** Aphids, red spider mites, and mealybugs may be a problem.

A. ellisii* var. *grandiflora. Epiphytic orchid with oblong-obovate leaves, 20–25cm (8–10in) long. Pendent racemes, to 60cm (24in) long, of star-shaped, fragrant, pure white flowers, 5cm (2in) across, with curved spurs, 18–27cm (7–11in) long, and tinted pale orange, are borne from summer to autumn. ↕25cm (10in), ↔30cm (12in). Madagascar. ❀ (min. 13–18°C/55–64°F; max. 30°C/86°F)
A. luteoalba* var. *rhodosticta ■ Epiphytic orchid with oblong-obovate leaves, to 15cm (6in) long. Star-shaped, fragrant white to creamy white flowers, 3cm (1¼in) across, with a striking bright red column and spurs, 2–4cm (¾–1½in) long, are borne in arching racemes, 10–30cm (4–12in) long, in winter. ↕↔15cm (6in). Cameroon, Ethiopia, Kenya, Tanzania. ❀ (min. 13–18°C/55–64°F; max. 30°C/86°F)

AERIDES

ORCHIDACEAE

Genus of about 40 species of evergreen, monopodial, epiphytic orchids from India, the Himalayas, and S.E. Asia, mostly found at low altitudes in tropical forest. Strap-shaped to linear, leathery leaves are borne alternately in 2 ranks, with moth-like, often fragrant flowers produced in dense, arching racemes from the leaf axils in summer. They develop numerous aerial roots, sometimes up to 1m (3ft) long.
• **HARDINESS** Frost tender.
• **CULTIVATION** Cool- to intermediate-growing orchids. Grow in epiphytic orchid compost in an orchid basket or epiphytically on slabs of bark. Provide high humidity and filtered light. Water freely throughout the year, watering more sparingly in winter. Apply a half-strength, balanced foliar fertilizer at every third watering in spring and summer. They will bloom in spring and summer if grown suspended in a position with good light. See also p.46.
• **PROPAGATION** Not suitable for division, although cuttings or offshoots may be rooted successfully.
• **PESTS AND DISEASES** Aphids, white-flies, red spider mites, and mealybugs may be a problem.

A. japonica see *Sedirea japonica.*
A. odorata. Epiphytic orchid with linear leaves, to 25cm (10in) long. In summer, produces arching racemes, to 25cm (10in) long, of fragrant, white-tinted, rose-pink to purple, often spotted flowers, 4cm (1½in) long, with incurved green- or yellow-tipped spurs. ↕45cm (18in), ↔30cm (12in). India to Philippines. ❀ (min. 11–13°C/52–55°F; max. 30°C/86°F)
A. rosea. Epiphytic orchid with linear leaves, to 25cm (10in) long. Many fragrant, white-spotted amethyst flowers, 2.5cm (1in) across, with white spurs, are produced in pendent racemes, to 60cm (24in) long, in early summer. ↕↔30cm (12in). Himalayas. ❀ (min. 11–13°C/52–55°F; max. 30°C/86°F)

AESCHYNANTHUS

GESNERIACEAE

Genus of about 100 species of evergreen subshrubs, climbers, and trailing and semi-trailing perennials, some of which are epiphytic, from subtropical forest in the Himalayas, S. China, Malaysia, Indonesia, and New Guinea. They have ovate to lance-shaped, leathery, fleshy leaves in opposite pairs or whorls. From summer to winter, vividly coloured flowers are produced in pairs from the leaf axils near the stem tips, or in terminal corymbs or clusters. The flowers often have prominent calyces, sometimes in a contrasting colour, and long, tubular, often curved, sometimes hooded corollas, with protruding stamens and styles. In frost-prone areas, grow in hanging baskets in a warm conservatory or greenhouse; compact species are good houseplants. In tropical or subtropical areas, grow outdoors in a shady site.
• **HARDINESS** Frost tender.
• **CULTIVATION** Under glass, grow in a mix of 3 parts fibrous peat and 1 part sphagnum moss, with high humidity. Grow in filtered light to encourage flowering. Water freely with soft water during the growing season, more sparingly in winter; when established, apply a half-strength, balanced liquid fertilizer monthly. Outdoors, grow in humus-rich, well-drained soil in partial shade; they will tolerate a more sunny position if humidity is high.
• **PROPAGATION** Take cuttings of young shoots, 3–5cm (1¼–2in) long, in spring, or semi-ripe cuttings in summer; root in gritty compost at 15–19°C (59–66°F).
• **PESTS AND DISEASES** Aphids may infest young growth.

***A.* 'Black Pagoda'** ■ Semi-trailing perennial producing elliptic leaves, to 10cm (4in) long, pale green with dark brown marbling above, and purple beneath. Terminal clusters of 3 or 4 deep burnt-orange flowers, to 5cm (2in) long, with green calyces, are borne from summer to winter. ↕60cm (24in), ↔ to 45cm (18in). ❀ (min. 15–18°C/59–64°F)
A. bracteatus. Scrambling epiphyte, often growing on rocks in the wild, with elliptic to ovate, sharply pointed, dark green leaves, 10cm (4in) long. Produces terminal clusters of 4 or 5 scarlet flowers, to 5cm (2in) long, with dark purple calyces, from summer to winter. ↕15cm (6in), ↔60cm (24in). E. Himalayas. ❀ (min. 15–18°C/59–64°F)
A. hildebrandii, syn. *A.* 'Hillbrandii'. Small subshrub with ovate, dark green leaves, to 2.5cm (1in) long, tinged red at the margins. From summer to autumn, bears terminal clusters of 2 or 3 orange-red flowers, 5cm (2in) long, with green calyces. ↕20cm (8in), ↔30cm (12in) or more. Burma. ❀ (min. 15–18°C/59–64°F)
***A.* 'Hillbrandii'** see *A. hildebrandii.*
A. lobbianus ■ syn. *A. radicans* var. *lobbianus* (Lipstick vine). Spreading, trailing perennial with elliptic, dark green leaves, 4.5cm (1¾in) long, tinged purple at the margins. Bears terminal clusters of 2 or 3 red flowers, 5cm (2in) long, with purple calyces, from summer to winter. ↕20cm (8in), ↔ to 90cm (36in). Indonesia (Java). ❀ (min. 15–18°C/59–64°F)
A. longicaulis 🏆 Semi-trailing perennial with lance-shaped, dark green leaves, 8cm (3in) long. Orange-red flowers, 5cm (2in) long, with green calyces, are produced in axillary and terminal clusters of 1–3 from summer to winter. ↕60cm (24in), ↔ to 90cm (36in). Malaysia. ❀ (min. 15–18°C/59–64°F)
A. marmoratus, syn. *A. zebrinus.* Semi-trailing perennial producing oval leaves, 8–10cm (3–4in) long, light green with dark marbling above and red beneath. Solitary, axillary, greenish yellow flowers, 3.5cm (1½in) long, with maroon- or brown-tinged throats and deeply cut green calyces, are produced from summer to winter. Often confused with *A. longicaulis.* ↕60cm (24in), ↔90cm (36in). Burma, Thailand, Malaysia. ❀ (min. 15–18°C/59–64°F)

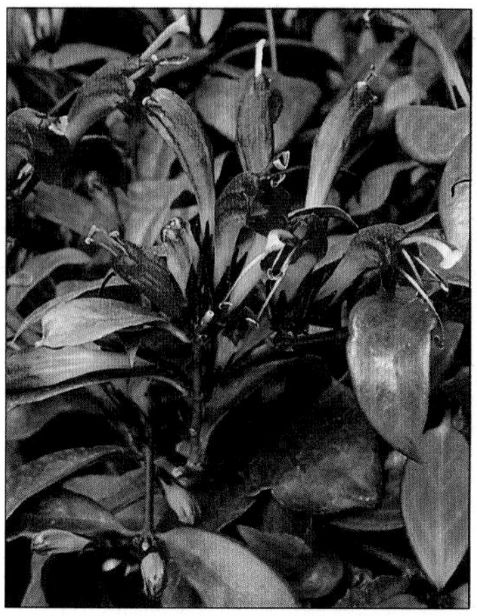

Aeschynanthus 'Black Pagoda'

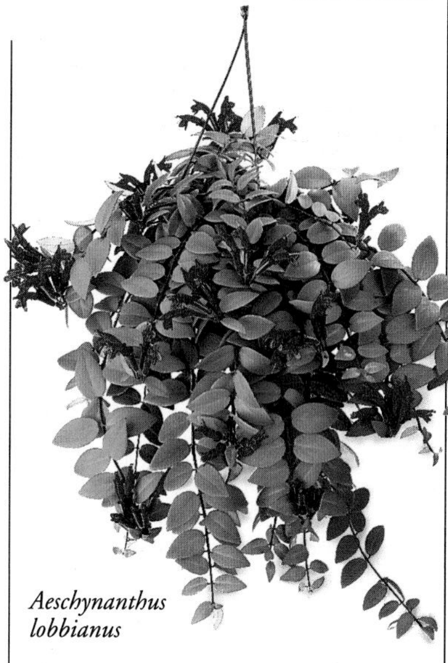

Aeschynanthus lobbianus

A. pulcher 🏆 (Lipstick plant). Epiphytic climber with thin, rooting branches and oval, slightly toothed, dark green leaves, 4.5cm (1¾in) long. From summer to winter, bears terminal corymbs of 6–8 hooded, bright red flowers, 6cm (2½in) long, with green calyces and yellow throats. ↕75cm (30in). Indonesia (Java). ❀ (min. 15–18°C/59–64°F)
A. radicans* var. *lobbianus see *A. lobbianus.*
A. speciosus 🏆 Trailing perennial with lance-shaped, pale green leaves, to 10cm (4in) long. From summer to winter, bright orange flowers, 10cm (4in) long, marked red across the lower lobes and with green calyces, are borne in terminal clusters of 6–20. ↕↔80cm (32in). Malaysia. ❀ (min. 15–18°C/59–64°F)
A. zebrinus see *A. marmoratus.*

AESCULUS

Buckeye, Horse chestnut

HIPPOCASTANACEAE

Genus of about 15 species of deciduous trees and shrubs, mainly from woodland in S.E. Europe, the Himalayas, E. Asia, and North America. They have opposite, palmate leaves, mostly mid- to dark green, some turning deep yellow or red in autumn. Large, upright, conical to cylindrical panicles of 4- or 5-petalled flowers, each 1.5–3cm (½–1¼in) across, with prominent stamens, are borne usually in late spring and early summer. The spiny or smooth-skinned, rounded to pear-shaped fruits contain 1 or 2 large, usually brown or blackish brown seeds. Most horse chestnuts are suitable only for large gardens, where they are best planted as specimen trees, although *A.* x *mutabilis* 'Induta' and *A. parviflora* may be grown in a medium-sized garden. All parts may cause mild stomach upset if ingested.
• **HARDINESS** Most are fully hardy. *A. californica* and *A. indica* will be damaged below -15°C (5°F).
• **CULTIVATION** Grow in deep, fertile, moist but well-drained soil in sun or partial shade. Grow *A. californica* and *A. chinensis* in a hot, but not dry, sunny site for best results. Pruning group 1, when dormant; train trees as central leader standards.
• **PROPAGATION** Sow seed in a seedbed as soon as ripe. *A.* x *carnea* comes true

A

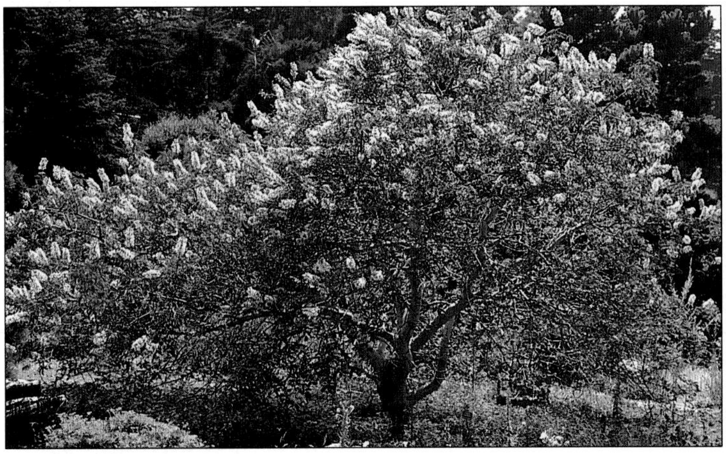
Aesculus californica

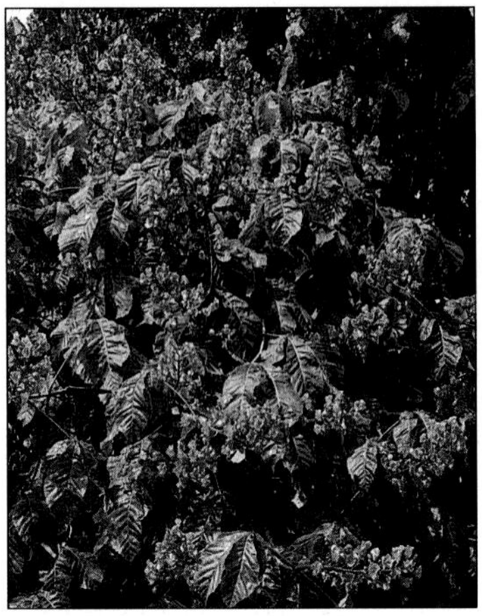
Aesculus x *carnea* 'Briotii'

from seed. Graft in late winter or bud in summer. Propagate *A. parviflora* from suckers.

• **PESTS AND DISEASES** Prone to canker, coral spot, leaf blotch, and scale insects.

A. californica ▣ 🌳 (California buckeye). Spreading, rounded, short-trunked tree with 5- to 7-palmate, mid-green leaves divided into narrowly ovate leaflets, 10cm (4in) or more long. Bears fragrant, white or pink-tinged white flowers, with long, protruding stamens, in dense, cylindrical panicles, to 20cm (8in) tall, in early summer, followed by rough-skinned fruit, 5–7cm (2–3in) long. Grow in full sun. ↕8m (25ft), ↔10m (30ft). USA (California). ❄❄❄

A.* x *carnea 🌳 (*A. hippocastanum* x *A. pavia*) (Red horse chestnut). Spreading tree with 5- to 7-palmate, dark green leaves composed of stalkless or short-stalked, often slightly twisted, obovate leaflets, 25cm (10in) long. Bears dark red or rose-red flowers with yellow centres in conical panicles, 20–30cm (8–12in) tall, in early and midsummer, followed by spiny fruit. ↕20m (70ft), ↔15m (50ft). Garden origin. ❄❄❄. **'Briotii'** ▣ 🏆 has glossy leaves and larger panicles of dark rose-red flowers. **'Plantierensis'** has pale pink flowers and does not develop mature fruit.

A. chinensis ▣ 🌳 (Chinese horse chestnut). Slow-growing, spreading tree with 5-palmate (occasionally 7-palmate), glossy, mid-green leaves composed of narrowly oblong, finely pointed leaflets, 20cm (8in) or more long. White flowers with protruding stamens are produced in slender, cylindrical panicles, to 30cm (12in) tall, in midsummer, followed by rough-skinned fruit. ↕15m (50ft), ↔10m (30ft). N. China. ❄❄❄

A. flava ▣ 🏆 △ syn. *A. octandra* (Yellow buckeye). Broadly conical tree with 5- to 7-palmate, glossy, dark green leaves with obovate or ovate leaflets, 8cm (3in) or more long. Bears yellow flowers in conical panicles, to 18cm (7in) tall, in late spring and early summer, followed by smooth-skinned fruit. ↕15–25m (50–80ft), ↔10–15m (30–50ft). E. USA. ❄❄❄

A. glabra △ (Ohio buckeye). Broadly conical tree with rough, fissured bark, bearing 5-palmate, glossy, light green leaves with obovate to ovate, long-pointed leaflets, 15cm (6in) or more long. In late spring and early summer, bears yellow-green flowers in conical

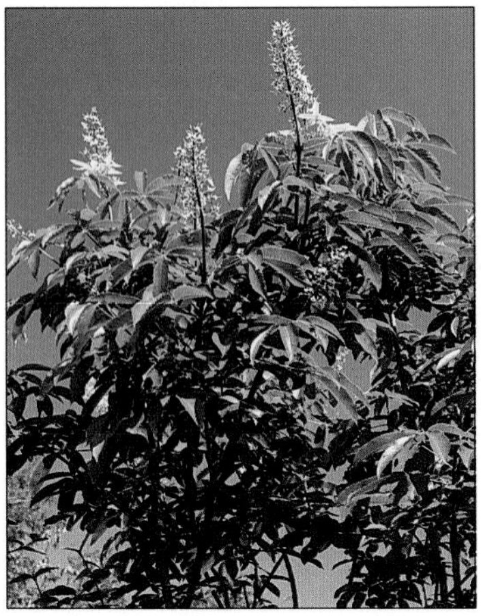
Aesculus chinensis

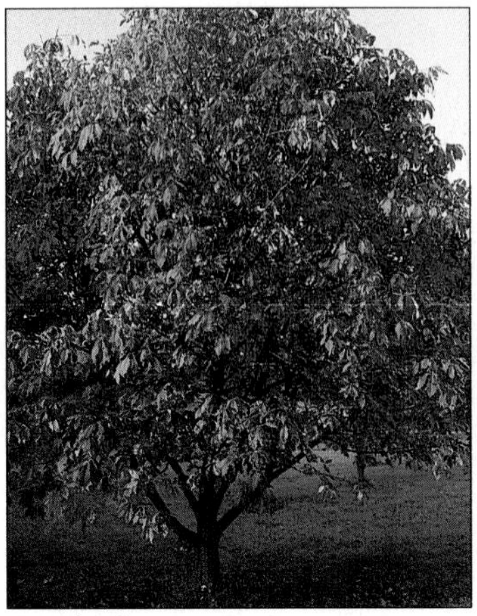
Aesculus flava

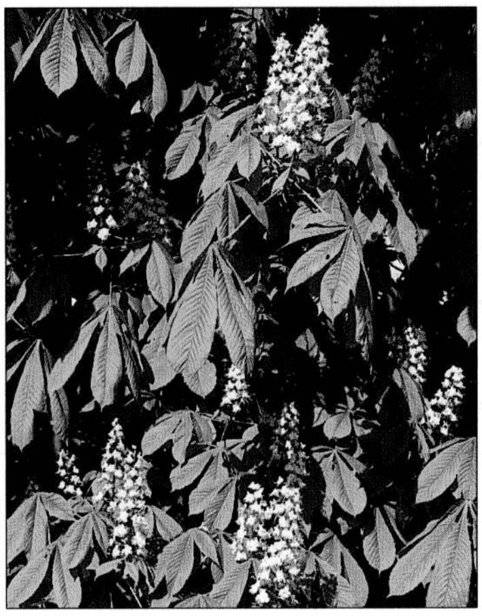
Aesculus hippocastanum

panicles, to 15cm (6in) tall, followed by sparsely prickly fruit. ↕15m (50ft), ↔10m (30ft). C. and E. USA. ❄❄❄

A. hippocastanum ▣ 🏆 🌳 (Horse chestnut). Vigorous, spreading, rounded tree with 5- to 7-palmate, mid-green leaves comprising obovate leaflets, 30cm (12in) or more long. White flowers, with yellow, later pink marks, open in conical panicles, to 30cm (12in) tall, in late spring and early summer; flowers are followed by the well-known, spiny "horse chestnut" fruit. ↕25m (80ft), ↔20m (70ft). S.E. Europe. ❄❄❄. **'Baumannii'** 🏆 syn. 'Flore Pleno', has double flowers and does not bear fruit.

A. indica 🏆 🌳 (Indian horse chestnut). Spreading, rounded tree with usually 7-palmate leaves composed of obovate to lance-shaped leaflets, 30cm (12in) or

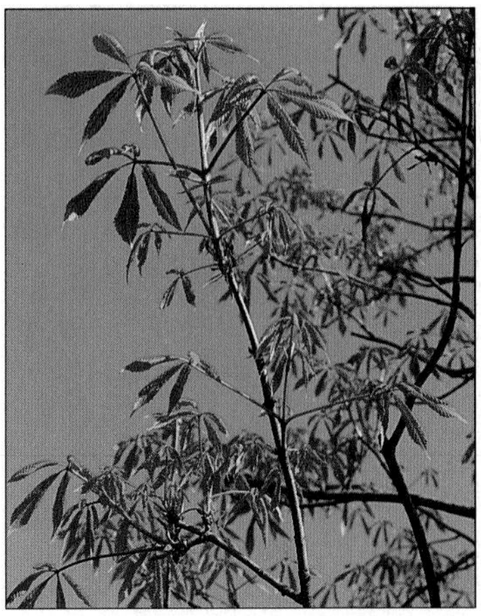
Aesculus x *neglecta* 'Erythroblastos'

more long, opening bronze and turning glossy, mid-green. White or pink flowers, with central red and yellow marks, are borne in cylindrical panicles, 30–40cm (12–16in) tall, in summer, followed by smooth-skinned fruit. ↕↔15m (50ft). N.W. Himalayas. ❄❄❄. **'Sydney Pearce'** ▣ is vigorous, with freely produced panicles of deep pink, yellow-centred flowers.

***A.* x *mutabilis* 'Induta'** 🌳 Small tree, sometimes shrubby in habit, producing 5- to 7-palmate, mid-green leaves with ovate leaflets, 20cm (8in) or more long. Profuse yellow-flushed pink flowers are borne in panicles, to 20cm (8in) tall, in late spring and early summer. Does not bear fruit. ↕↔5m (15ft). ❄❄❄

A.* x *neglecta △ (*A. flava* x *A. sylvatica*). Conical tree with 5-palmate, mid-green

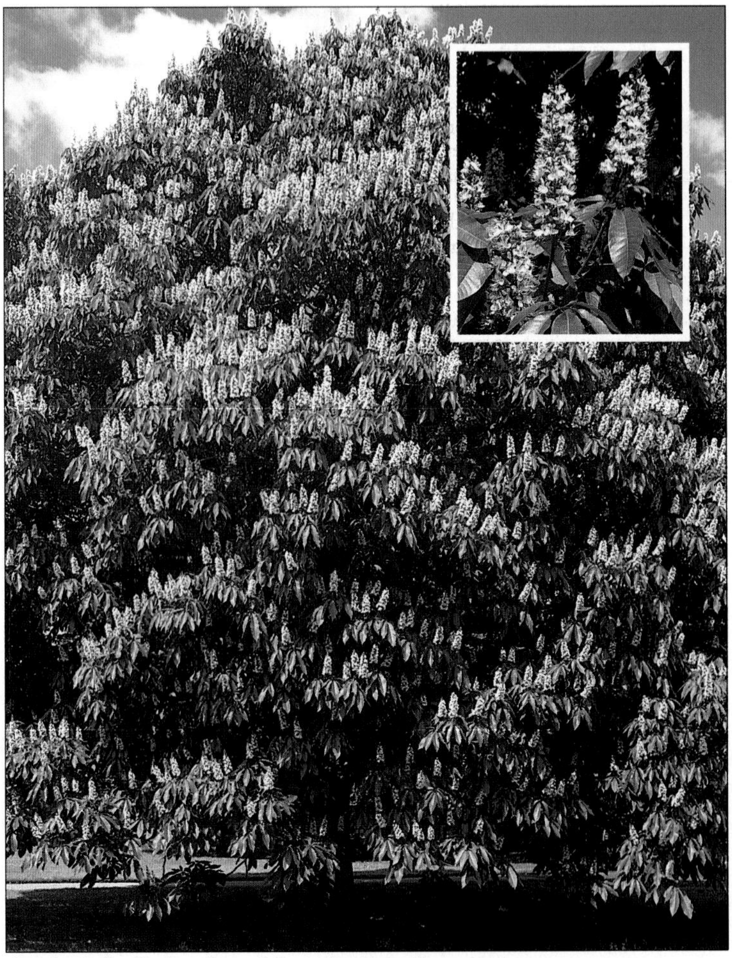
Aesculus indica 'Sydney Pearce' (inset: flower detail)

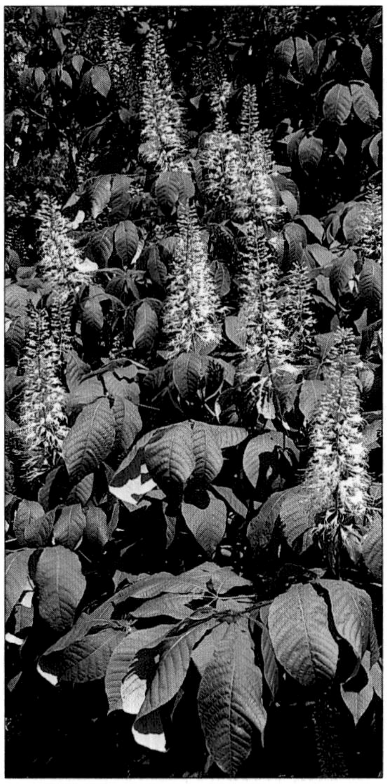
Aesculus parviflora

leaves composed of obovate to ovate leaflets, 15cm (6in) or more long. Bears yellow or yellow-flushed red flowers in conical panicles, to 15cm (6in) tall, in midsummer, followed by smooth-skinned fruit. ↕ 10m (30ft) or more, ↔ 8m (25ft). S.E. USA. ❄❄❄.
'Erythroblastos' ■ ♀ (Sunrise horse chestnut) has red leaf-stalks and leaves that unfold cream, bright pink, become yellow, then turn green by midsummer.
A. octandra see *A. flava.*
A. parviflora ■ ♀ (Bottlebrush buckeye). Suckering shrub with 5- to 7-palmate, mid-green leaves divided into ovate leaflets, 23cm (9in) or more long, bronze when young. Bears spidery white flowers, with protruding stamens, in conical panicles, to 30cm (12in) tall, in midsummer, followed by smooth-skinned fruit. Tolerant of all but very poorly drained sites. ↕ 3m (10ft), ↔ 5m (15ft). S.E. USA. ❄❄❄
A. pavia ♀ ⌂ syn. *A. splendens* (Red buckeye). Conical shrub or small tree, producing 5- to 7-palmate, mid-green leaves with obovate to oblong to lance-shaped leaflets, 13cm (5in) or more long. Red, sometimes yellow-marked flowers are borne in conical panicles, to 15cm (6in) tall, in early summer, followed by smooth-skinned fruit. ↕ 5m (15ft), ↔ 3m (10ft). E. USA. ❄❄❄.
'Atrosanguinea' ■ has dark red flowers.
A. splendens see *A. pavia.*
A. turbinata ♣ (Japanese horse chestnut). Vigorous, spreading tree producing 5- to 7-palmate, mid-green leaves with obovate leaflets, 40cm (16in) or more long. White flowers, each with a yellow, later pink mark, are borne in cylindrical panicles, to 30cm (12in) tall, in early and midsummer, followed by smooth-skinned fruit. ↕ 20m (70ft), ↔ 12m (40ft). Japan. ❄❄❄

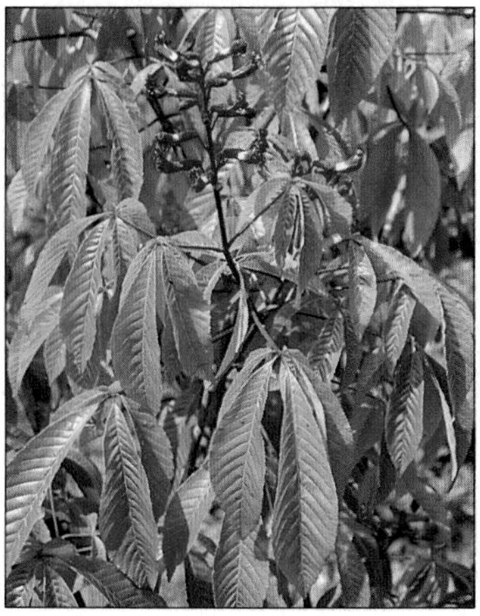
Aesculus pavia 'Atrosanguinea'

AETHIONEMA

syn. EUNOMIA
Stone cress
BRASSICACEAE/CRUCIFERAE

Genus of more than 40 species of evergreen or semi-evergreen, dwarf subshrubs, woody-based perennials, and annuals from sunny, open sites, on limestone, in the mountains of Europe and W. Asia, particularly Turkey. They are grown for their dense to loose, terminal racemes of small, 4-petalled, cross-shaped, sometimes fragrant flowers, in red, pink, or creamy to pure white, profusely borne on stems 2–4cm (¾–1½in) long, usually from spring to early summer. The leaves are small, usually stalkless, fleshy, and arranged alternately, or sometimes in opposite pairs. Grow in a rock garden or wall crevice; *A. oppositifolium* prefers a scree bed or alpine house.

- **HARDINESS** Fully hardy, given good drainage.
- **CULTIVATION** Grows best in fertile, well-drained, alkaline soil in full sun, but will tolerate poor, acid soils.
- **PROPAGATION** Sow seed of perennials in containers in a cold frame in spring. Sow seed of annuals *in situ* as soon as ripe or in autumn. Seedlings grown from garden seed often prove to be hybrids. Root softwood cuttings in late spring or early summer.
- **PESTS AND DISEASES** Aphids and red spider mites may be a problem.

A. armenum ■ Short-lived, compact, evergreen or semi-evergreen subshrub with linear-oblong, blue- to grey-green leaves, 0.5–1.5cm (¼–½in) long. Dense racemes of small, pale pink flowers, 5mm (¼in) across, are borne in late spring. ↕↔ 15–20cm (6–8in). Caucasus, Turkey. ❄❄❄

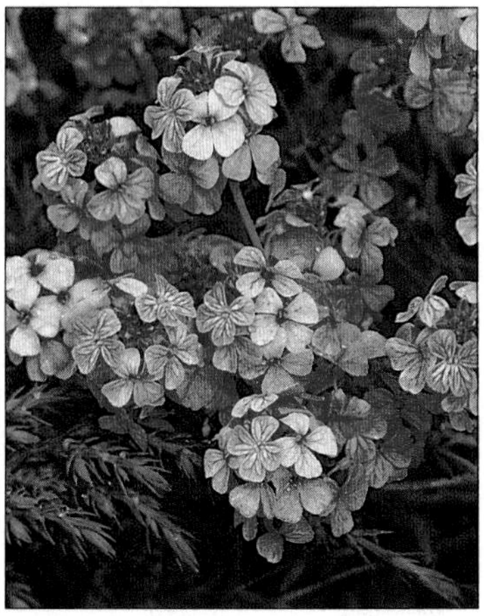
Aethionema armenum

A. grandiflorum ■ ♀ syn. *A. pulchellum.* Short-lived, evergreen or semi-evergreen, loosely branched sub-shrub or woody-based perennial with blunt-tipped, linear-oblong, blue-green leaves, to 1cm (½in) long. Bears pale to deep rose-pink flowers, to 7mm (¼in) wide, in loose racemes in late spring and early summer. ↕↔ 20–30cm (8–12in). Caucasus, Turkey, Iraq, Iran. ❄❄❄
A. oppositifolium, syn. *Eunomia oppositifolia.* Mat- or cushion-forming, evergreen or semi-evergreen perennial with opposite, obovate, blue-grey leaves, 1cm (½in) long. Bears small racemes of lavender-pink flowers, 6–8mm (¼–⅜in) across, in late spring. ↕ to 5cm (2in), ↔ 10–15cm (4–6in). Caucasus, Turkey, Syria, Lebanon. ❄❄❄
A. pulchellum see *A. grandiflorum.*
***A.* 'Warley Rose'** ■ ♀ Short-lived, evergreen or semi-evergreen, compact subshrub with linear, blue-grey leaves, 1cm (½in) long. Profuse racemes of rich pink flowers, to 7mm (¼in) across, are borne in late spring and early summer. ↕↔ 15–20cm (6–8in). ❄❄❄

▷**African daisy** see *Arctotis*
Blue-eyed see *A. venusta*
▷**African violet** see *Saintpaulia*

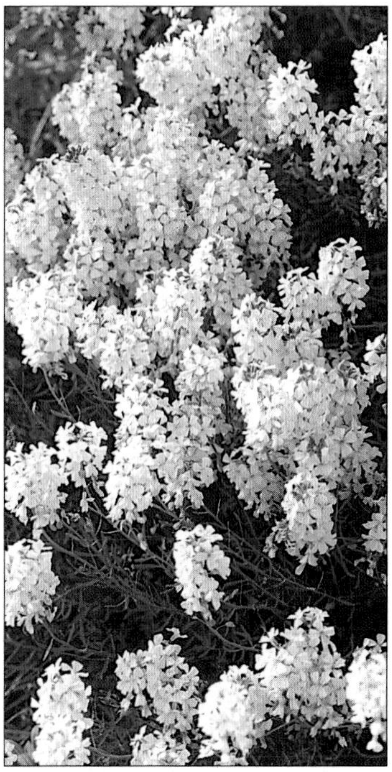
Aethionema grandiflorum

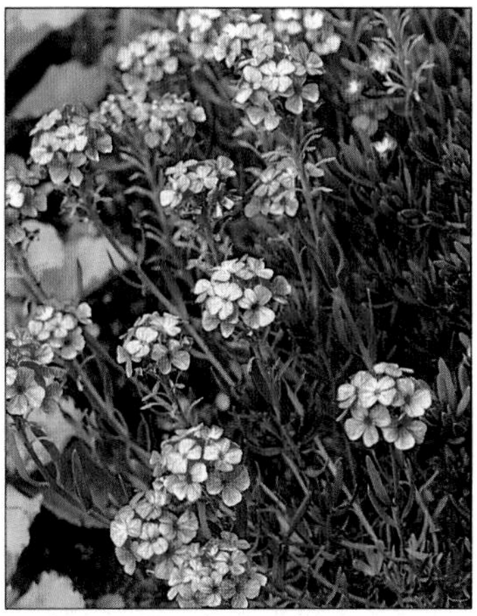
Aethionema 'Warley Rose'

AGAPANTHUS

African blue lily
ALLIACEAE/LILIACEAE

Genus of about 10 species of vigorous perennials, some of them evergreen, from southern Africa. The evergreen species occur in coastal areas, the deciduous ones in moister, mountain grassland in inland regions. They form bold clumps of large, strap-shaped, usually arching, often deep green leaves, and bear rounded, intermediate, or pendent umbels of many tubular, bell- or trumpet-shaped, blue or white flowers. The inflorescences are good for cutting, and are followed by decorative seed heads. Grow in a border or in large containers. Most hybrids are deciduous and usually hardier than the species, with dense, rounded umbels, to 20cm (8in) across, of 3cm (1¼in) long flowers, and with leaves to 45cm (18in) long. The name Headbourne Hybrids, originally referring to selected seedlings raised by the Hon. Lewis Palmer, is now misapplied to cover a range of mixed seedlings that vary greatly in flower colour, size, and quality, and so is not included here.

AGAPANTHUS INFLORESCENCES

Agapanthus flowers are borne in 3 main inflorescence types: rounded umbels of bell- to trumpet-shaped flowers; intermediate umbels of usually trumpet-shaped flowers; and pendent umbels of tubular flowers.

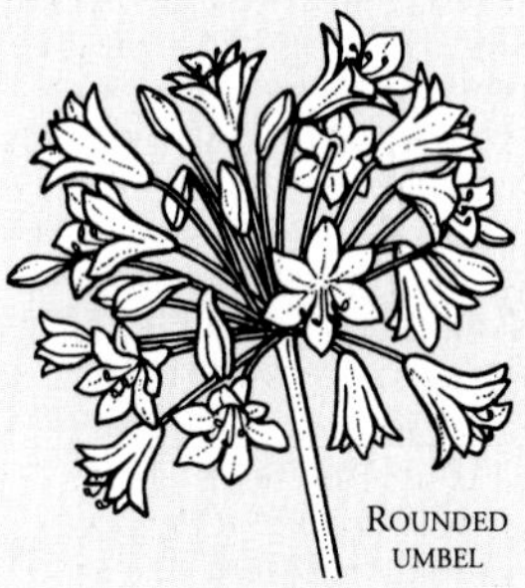
ROUNDED UMBEL

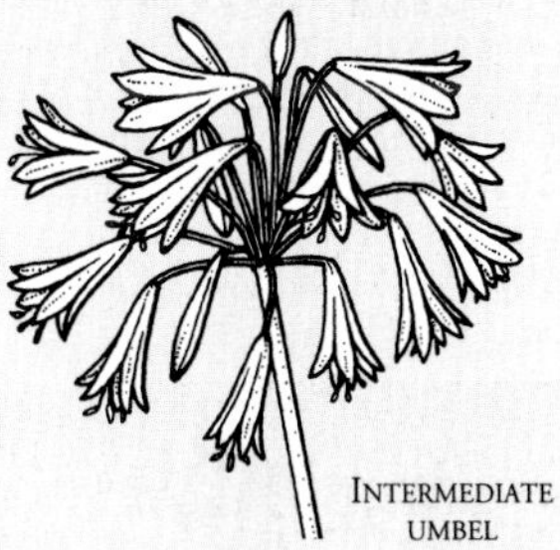
INTERMEDIATE UMBEL

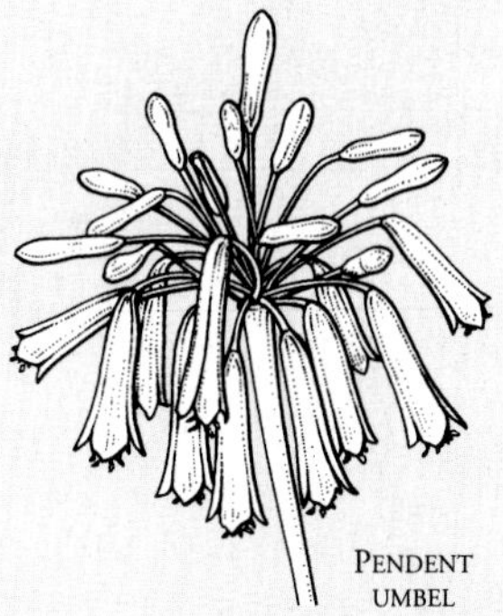
PENDENT UMBEL

A

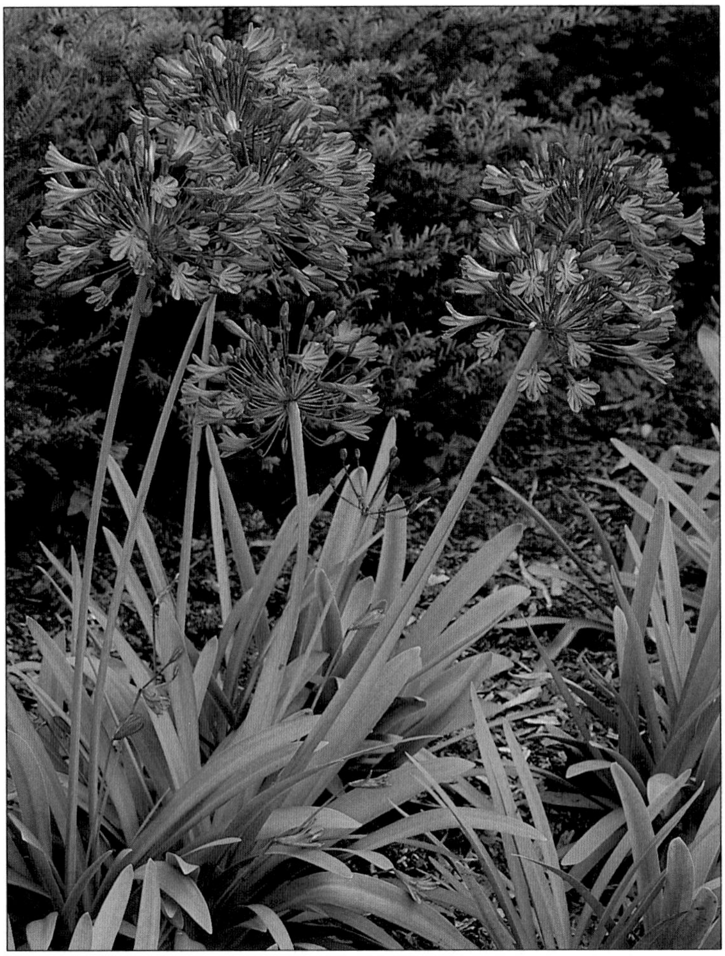

Agapanthus 'Blue Giant'

- **HARDINESS** Fully hardy to half hardy.
- **CULTIVATION** Grow in fertile, moist but well-drained soil in full sun. In cold areas, mulch hardy hybrids in winter. In containers, grow in loam-based compost (JI No.3). Water freely when in growth, sparingly in winter. Apply a balanced liquid fertilizer monthly from spring until flowering. Overwinter *A. africanus*, *A. campanulatus* 'Albovittatus', and *A. praecox* subsp. *orientalis* under cover, except in the warmest areas.
- **PROPAGATION** Sow seed at 13–15°C (55–59°F) when ripe or in spring; keep the seedlings in a frame for the first winter in frost-prone climates. They will flower in 2–3 years. Most seedlings grown from garden seed do not come true. Divide in spring.
- **PESTS AND DISEASES** Slugs, snails, and viruses may be a problem.

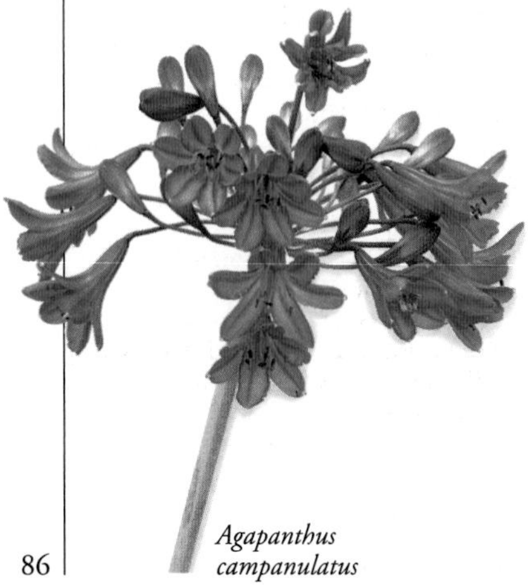

Agapanthus campanulatus

A. africanus 🏆 Clump-forming, evergreen perennial with strap-shaped leaves, to 30cm (12in) or more long. In late summer, bears trumpet-shaped, deep blue flowers, 2.5–5cm (1–2in) long, in rounded umbels, 15–30cm (6–12in) across. ↕60–90cm (24–36in), ↔45cm (18in). South Africa (Northern Cape, Western Cape, Eastern Cape). ✻
***A.* 'Alice Gloucester'.** Clump-forming perennial that produces intermediate umbels of trumpet-shaped white flowers, the buds and pedicels tinged lilac, in mid- and late summer. ↕90cm (36in), ↔45cm (18in). ✻✻✻
***A.* 'Ben Hope'.** Clump-forming perennial bearing rounded umbels of trumpet-shaped, dark blue flowers in mid- and late summer. ↕to 1.2m (4ft), ↔60cm (24in). ✻✻✻
***A.* 'Blue Giant'** ▣ Clump-forming perennial producing rounded umbels of open bell-shaped, rich blue flowers in mid- and late summer. ↕1.2m (4ft), ↔60cm (24in). ✻✻✻
***A.* 'Blue Moon'.** Clump-forming perennial bearing large, rounded umbels of open bell-shaped, pale blue flowers in late summer and early autumn. ↕60cm (24in), ↔45cm (18in). ✻✻✻
***A.* 'Blue Triumphator'.** Clump-forming perennial producing rounded to intermediate umbels of open bell-shaped, clear blue flowers in mid- and late summer. ↕90cm (36in), ↔45cm (18in). ✻✻✻
***A.* 'Bressingham White'.** Clump-forming perennial bearing intermediate umbels of trumpet-shaped, pure white flowers in mid- and late summer. ↕90cm (36in), ↔60cm (24in). ✻✻✻

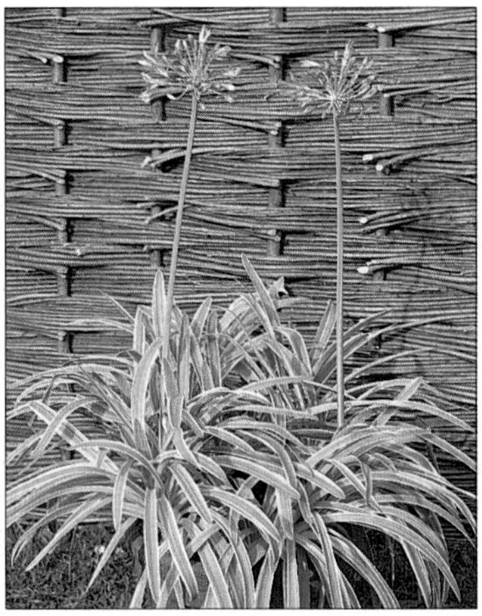

Agapanthus campanulatus 'Albovittatus'

A. campanulatus ▣ Vigorous, clump-forming perennial producing narrow, strap-shaped, deciduous, greyish green leaves, 15–40cm (6–16in) long. Rounded umbels, 10–20cm (4–8in) across, of bell-shaped, pale to dark blue, sometimes white flowers, 2–3.5cm (¾–1½in) long, are borne on strong stems in mid- and late summer. ↕60–120cm (24–48in), ↔45cm (18in). South Africa (KwaZulu/Natal, Northern Cape). ✻✻✻. **'Albovittatus'** ▣ is less vigorous and has broad leaves, boldly striped white; ✻✻. **'Isis'** produces dark blue flowers; ↕75cm (30in), ↔30cm (12in); ✻✻✻ (borderline). **subsp. *patens*** 🏆 bears light blue flowers, with shorter tubes and more open mouths than the species, in late summer and early autumn; ↕to 45cm (18in), ↔30cm (12in); South Africa (Drakensberg mountains to Northern Transvaal); ✻✻✻ (borderline)
***A.* 'Castle of Mey'.** Clump-forming perennial bearing rounded to intermediate umbels of broadly trumpet-shaped, deep blue flowers in mid- and late summer. ↕60cm (24in), ↔45cm (18in). ✻✻✻
A. caulescens 🏆 Clump-forming perennial with a leek-like stem, bearing deciduous, narrowly strap-shaped lower leaves, to 15cm (6in) long, and broader upper leaves, to 60cm (24in) long. From midsummer to early autumn, produces open, rounded umbels, 15–24cm (6–10in) across, of bell-shaped violet-blue flowers, 3–5cm (1¼–2in) long, with tepals spreading at the mouths, and long, projecting stamens. ↕90–120cm (3–4ft), ↔60cm (24in). Swaziland. ✻✻

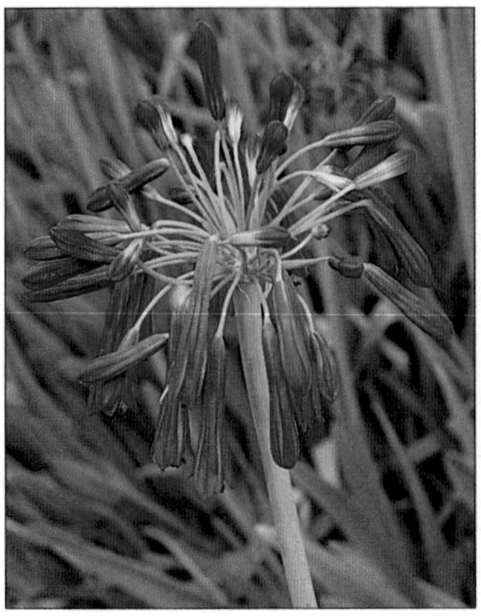

Agapanthus inapertus

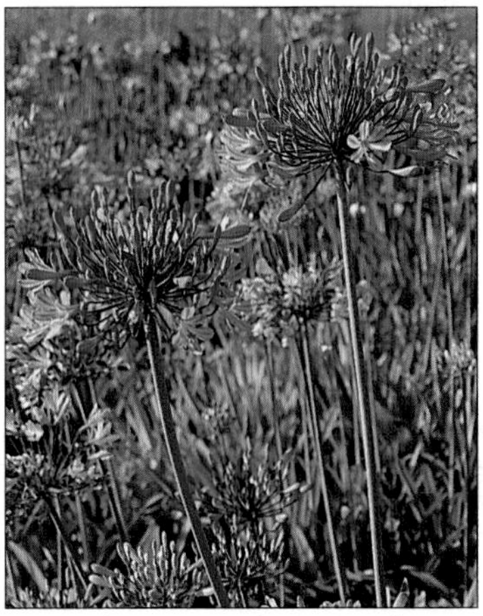

Agapanthus praecox subsp. *orientalis*

***A.* 'Cherry Holley'.** Clump-forming perennial bearing intermediate umbels of open, trumpet-shaped, dark blue flowers in midsummer. Often flowers again in early autumn. ↕75cm (30in), ↔60cm (24in). ✻✻✻
***A.* 'Dorothy Palmer'.** Clump-forming perennial bearing intermediate umbels of open trumpet-shaped, rich blue flowers, fading to reddish mauve, in mid- and late summer. ↕90cm (36in), ↔60cm (24in). ✻✻✻
***A.* 'Golden Rule'.** Slow-growing, clump-forming perennial with small, narrow, yellow-margined leaves. Bears rounded to intermediate umbels of bell-shaped, light blue flowers in mid- and late summer. ↕40–60cm (16–24in), ↔30–40cm (12–16in). ✻✻✻ (borderline)
A. inapertus ▣ Clump-forming perennial with erect, strap-shaped leaves, to 70cm (28in) long. In late summer and early autumn, stiff, upright stems bear pendent umbels, 10–15cm (4–6in) across, of pendent, tubular blue flowers, narrowed at the mouths, and 2.5–4.5cm (1–1¾in) long. ↕90–150cm (3–5ft), ↔60cm (24in). South Africa (Northern Transvaal, Eastern Transvaal). ✻✻

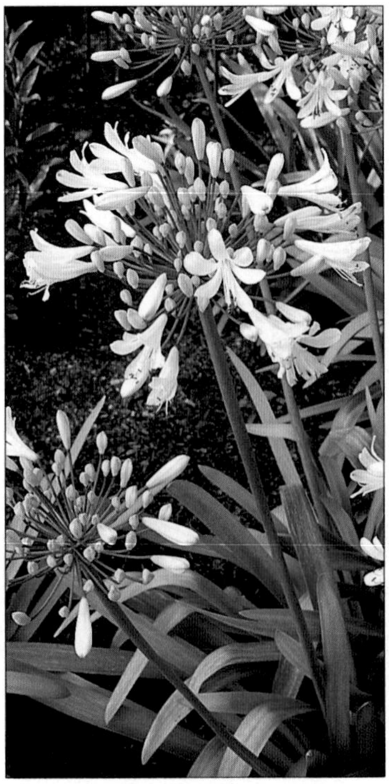

Agapanthus 'Snowy Owl'

***A.* 'Lilliput'.** Clump-forming perennial bearing rounded to intermediate umbels of trumpet-shaped, deep blue flowers in mid- and late summer. ↕↔ 40cm (16in). ✲✲✲
***A.* 'Loch Hope'** 🏆 Clump-forming perennial with rounded to intermediate umbels of broadly trumpet-shaped, deep blue flowers in late summer and early autumn. ↕ to 1.5m (5ft), ↔ 60cm (24in). ✲✲✲
***A.* 'Midnight Blue'.** Clump-forming perennial with intermediate umbels of broadly trumpet-shaped, very dark blue flowers in mid- and late summer. ↕ 45cm (18in), ↔ 30cm (12in). ✲✲✲
A. orientalis see *A. praecox* subsp. *orientalis.*
A. praecox* subsp. *orientalis ■ syn. *A. orientalis.* Clump-forming, evergreen perennial with broad, strap-shaped, dark green leaves, 30–70cm (12–28in) long. Bears large, rounded umbels, 15–30cm (6–12in) across, of trumpet-shaped, rich mid-blue flowers, 4–6cm (1½–2½in) long, in late summer and early autumn. ↕ 60–90cm (24–36in), ↔ 60cm (24in). South Africa. ✲
***A.* 'Snowy Owl'** ■ Clump-forming perennial with rounded umbels of bell-shaped white flowers in late summer. ↕ 1.2m (4ft), ↔ 60cm (24in). ✲✲✲

AGAPETES

ERICACEAE

Genus of about 95 species of spreading to erect or scandent shrubs, sometimes epiphytic in the wild, found in scrub and forest from warm-temperate regions of E. Asia to the western Pacific, including Australia. The evergreen, occasionally briefly deciduous leaves are simple, usually entire, and leathery, and are borne in opposite pairs. They are cultivated mainly for their solitary or clustered, pendent flowers, which are tubular, or bell- or urn-shaped, with 5 short petal lobes. In frost-prone areas, grow in a cool or temperate greenhouse; in frost-free areas, grow in a border or against a wall or arbour.

• **HARDINESS** Frost tender, although *A. serpens* and *A.* 'Ludgvan Cross' will survive temperatures to 0°C (32°F).

• **CULTIVATION** Under glass, grow in well-drained, lime-free (ericaceous) potting compost in bright filtered light. In the growing season, water freely and apply a balanced liquid fertilizer monthly; water sparingly in winter. Pot on or top-dress in late winter or spring.

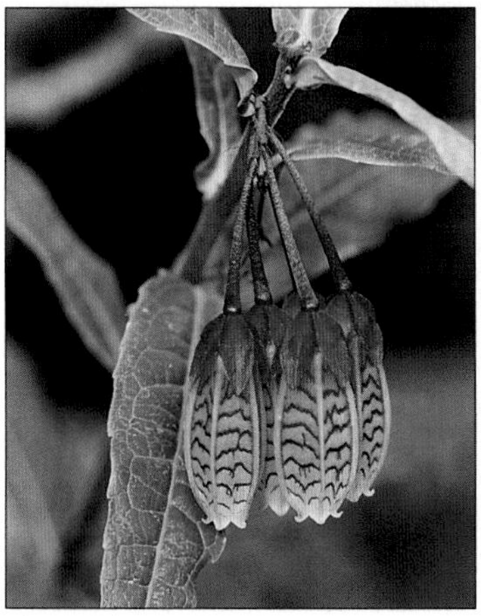

Agapetes incurvata

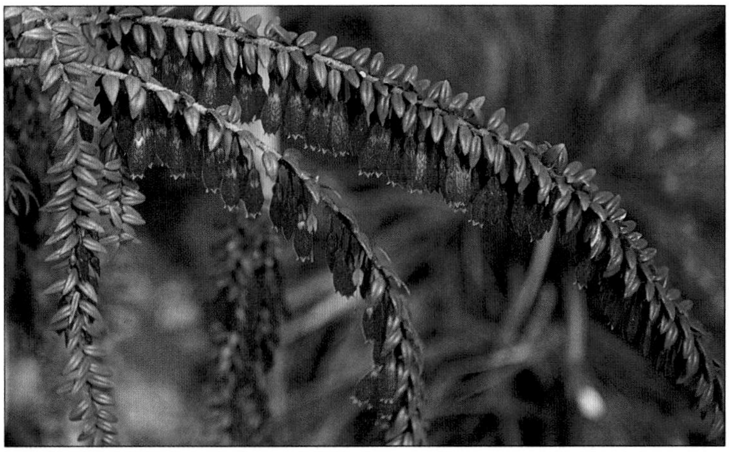

Agapetes serpens

Outdoors, grow in moist but well-drained, neutral to acid, moderately fertile soil, enriched with composted bark. They prefer partial shade, but tolerate some sun. Mulch in spring every other year. Pruning group 11, but pruning is best kept to a minimum.

• **PROPAGATION** Root semi-ripe cuttings with bottom heat in late summer, or layer in spring.

• **PESTS AND DISEASES** Scale insects may be a problem.

A. incurvata ■ syn. *A. rugosa.* Sparsely branched shrub, which may be trained as a climber, with flexible, arching to pendent stems. Dark green leaves, to 10cm (4in) long, are broadly lance-shaped to ovate, shallowly toothed, and conspicuously veined. In summer, bears pendent clusters of up to 5 angular, narrowly urn-shaped, white to pink, purple-veined flowers, 2cm (¾in) long, with prominent, ovate calyx lobes. ↕ to 1m (3ft), ↔ 1–2m (3–6ft) as a shrub; ↕ 2–3m (6–10ft) as a climber. E. Nepal to India (Arunachal Pradesh). ❄ (min. 5–7°C/41–45°F). **var. *hookeri*** has yellow flowers.
***A.* 'Ludgvan Cross'** (*A. incurvata* x *A. serpens*). Pendent shrub with lance-shaped, mid- to dark green leaves, to 5cm (2in) long. From spring to summer, bears pendent clusters of up to 6 urn-shaped pink flowers, 2–3cm (¾–1¼in) long, with dark crimson veins. ↕↔ 1.2–1.5m (4–5ft). ✲
A. macrantha see *A. variegata* var. *macrantha.*
A. rugosa see *A. incurvata.*
A. serpens ■ 🏆 Initially erect, then arching shrub, which may be trained as a climber. Small, crowded, lance-shaped leaves, to 2cm (¾in) long, are rich green and glossy. From late winter to spring, usually solitary, narrowly urn-shaped red flowers, 2cm (¾in) long, with V-shaped, darker red markings, are produced from the leaf axils. ↕ 60–90cm (24–36in), ↔ 2–3m (6–10ft); ↕ 2–3m (6–10ft) if grown as a climber. Nepal, Bhutan, India (Assam). ✲
***A. variegata* var. *macrantha*,** syn. *A. macrantha.* Spreading, arching shrub with lance-shaped-elliptic, mid- to deep green leaves, 8–12cm (3–5in) long. From winter to spring, older stems bear clusters of up to 5 urn-shaped, white to pink flowers, 4–5cm (1½–2in) long, patterned with V-shaped red lines. ↕↔ 1–2m (3–6ft). N.E. India. ❄ (min. 7–10°C/45–50°F)

AGASTACHE

syn. BRITTONASTRUM

LABIATAE/LAMIACEAE

Genus of about 30 species of aromatic perennials from dry, often hilly habitats in China, Japan, USA, and Mexico. Most are stiffly erect, bushy plants, with lance-shaped to ovate, greyish green leaves, borne in opposite pairs. Spikes of long-lasting, small, 2-lipped, tubular flowers are produced in whorls from midsummer to autumn. They are suitable for a mixed border; *A. barberi* and *A. mexicana* may also be grown as annuals in frost-prone areas.

• **HARDINESS** Fully hardy to half hardy.

• **CULTIVATION** Grow in well-drained, fertile soil in full sun. In warmer areas, less hardy species will overwinter in a sheltered site.

• **PROPAGATION** Sow seed at 13–18°C (55–64°F) in early spring. Divide in spring. Root semi-ripe cuttings in late summer; overwinter young plants under cover in frost-prone areas. Root semi-ripe cuttings of *A. mexicana* in early summer to maintain stocks.

• **PESTS AND DISEASES** Powdery mildew may affect the leaves in dry summers.

A. anethiodora see *A. foeniculum.*
A. anisata see *A. foeniculum.*
A. barberi. Upright, bushy perennial with aromatic, ovate leaves, 3–5cm (1¼–2in) long. Loose spikes, to 30cm (12in) long, of red-purple flowers are produced from midsummer to late autumn. ↕ 60cm (24in), ↔ 30cm (12in). S. USA to N. Mexico. ✲. **'Firebird'** has copper flowers. **'Tutti-Frutti'** ■ has strongly aromatic foliage and pinkish red flowers.

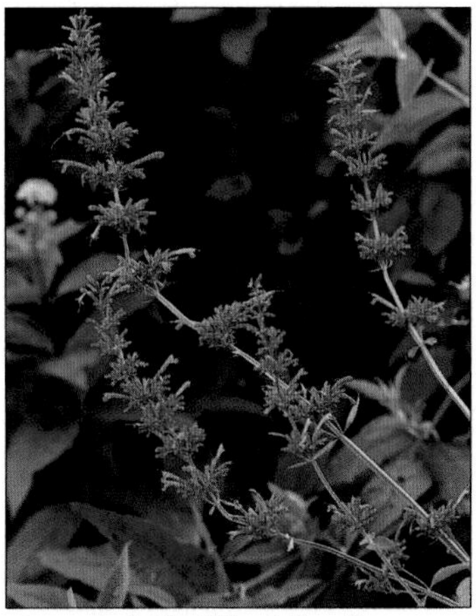

Agastache barberi 'Tutti-Frutti'

***A. foeniculum*,** syn. *A. anethiodora, A. anisata* (Anise hyssop). Erect, leafy, aniseed-scented perennial with ovate-lance-shaped, veined leaves, 5–8cm (2–3in) long, downy and whitish green beneath. Dense spikes, 4–8cm (1½–3in) long, of blue flowers, with violet bracts and calyces, are borne from midsummer to early autumn. ↕ 90–150cm (3–5ft), ↔ 30cm (12in). North America. ✲✲. **'Alabaster'** has white flowers.
***A. mexicana*,** syn. *Brittonastrum mexicanum, Cedronella mexicana.* Bushy, aromatic, short-lived perennial with ovate to lance-shaped leaves, 4–6cm (1½–2½in) long. Rose-red flowers are produced in spikes, to 30cm (12in) long, in mid- and late summer. ↕ 60–90cm (24–36in), ↔ 30cm (12in). Mexico. ✲

▷ ***Agathaea*** see *Felicia*

AGATHIS syn. DAMMARA

Kauri pine

ARAUCARIACEAE

Genus of 13 species of evergreen, coniferous trees with broad, flat leaves, from tropical areas without a dry season, from Malaysia and the Philippines to New Guinea, Australia (Queensland), Fiji, and New Zealand. The male cones are cylindrical, the females spherical. They are monoecious, but may be dioecious when young. In frost-prone areas, grow young plants for their foliage in a cool greenhouse or conservatory. In frost-free areas, grow as specimen trees.

• **HARDINESS** Half hardy to frost tender.

• **CULTIVATION** Under glass, grow in loam-based potting compost (JI No.3) in full light, with ample ventilation. When in growth, water freely and apply a balanced liquid fertilizer monthly; water sparingly in winter. Outdoors, grow in any moist but well-drained soil in full sun, sheltered from cold winds.

• **PROPAGATION** Sow seed at 10–13°C (50–55°F) in early spring.

• **PESTS AND DISEASES** Trouble free.

A. australis ♤ (Kauri pine). Coniferous tree, conical when young, with a massive spreading crown on a stout trunk when mature. Leathery leaves are opposite, lance-shaped, to 8cm (3in) long, and bright green when young, maturing to grey-green. Female cones, 5–7cm (2–3in) long, are woody and green; male cones are 3–4cm (1¼–1½in) long. ↕ 40m (130ft), ↔ to 15m (50ft). New Zealand (North Island). ✲ (borderline)

AGATHOSMA

RUTACEAE

Genus of 135 species of heather-like, evergreen shrubs and subshrubs from open, sandy savannah in South Africa. They are grown for their small, 5-petalled flowers, borne singly or in axillary clusters. The crowded leaves are small, often narrow, and aromatic. In frost-prone areas, grow in containers in a cool greenhouse, and place outside in summer; in frost-free areas, grow in a border or against a wall.

• **HARDINESS** Frost tender; *A. pulchella* may survive short spells at 0°C (32°F).

A

• **CULTIVATION** Under glass, grow in lime-free (ericaceous) potting compost in full light, with good ventilation. During the growing season, water moderately and apply a balanced liquid fertilizer monthly; water sparingly in winter. Outdoors, grow in moist but well-drained, neutral to acid, preferably sandy soil in full sun. Pruning group 8.
• **PROPAGATION** Sow seed in spring, or root semi-ripe cuttings in summer, both at 13–18°C (55–64°F).
• **PESTS AND DISEASES** Trouble free.

A. pulchella, syn. *Barosma pulchella*. Wiry-stemmed, branching shrub with crowded, alternate, ovate to lance-shaped leaves, 6mm (¼in) long. From spring to summer, purplish pink, mauve, or white flowers, 5mm (¼in) across, are produced singly or in pairs from the upper leaf axils. ↕↔ 1m (3ft) or more. South Africa. ✲ (borderline)

AGAVE

AGAVACEAE

Genus of more than 200 species of rosette-forming, perennial or monocarpic succulents from desert and mountain regions of North, Central, and South America, and the West Indies. The leaves are often rigid and fleshy, usually having sharp terminal spines and toothed margins. The funnel-shaped, short-tubed flowers, each with 6 tepals, are borne in umbel-like clusters, racemes or panicles on leafless stems from the centres of the rosettes. The ovoid or spherical, capsular fruits contain numerous flat black seeds. In

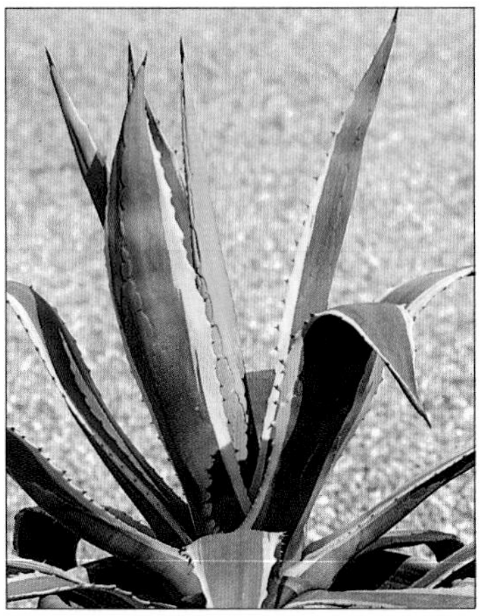
Agave americana 'Marginata'

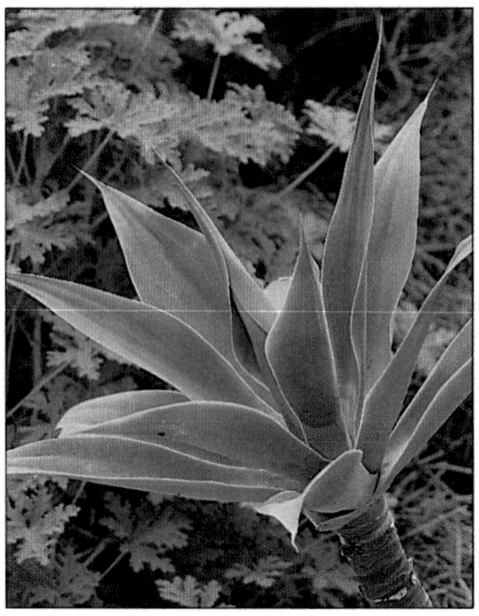
Agave attenuata

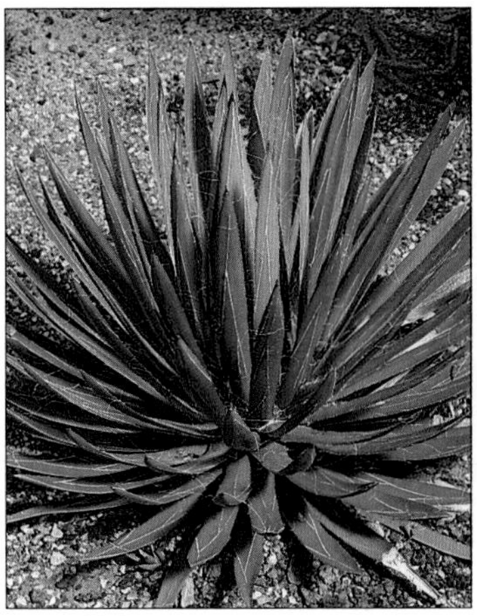
Agave filifera

most species, the rosettes die after flowering and fruiting, leaving offsets to mature and flower in subsequent years. In frost-prone areas, grow in a cool or temperate greenhouse; in frost-free areas, grow as specimen plants.
• **HARDINESS** Half hardy to frost tender.
• **CULTIVATION** Under glass, grow in standard cactus compost in full light. In summer, water freely and apply a low-nitrogen fertilizer 3 or 4 times; reduce water in autumn; keep dry in winter. Outdoors, grow in slightly acid, moderately fertile, sharply drained soil in full sun. See also pp.48–49.
• **PROPAGATION** Sow seed at 21°C (70°F) in early spring. Remove offsets in spring or autumn; if already rooted, treat as mature plants. Insert unrooted offsets, or plantlets of *A. americana* and other species in a mix of equal parts peat and sharp sand until rooted.
• **PESTS AND DISEASES** Prone to scale insects, particularly on young growth.

A. altissima see *A. americana*.
A. americana 🏆 syn. *A. altissima*. Monocarpic succulent producing basal rosettes of spreading, lance-shaped, spine-tipped and spiny-margined, grey-green leaves, often to 2m (6ft) long. In summer, bears clusters of yellowish green flowers, 9–10cm (3½–4in) long, in spreading panicles, to 8m (25ft) long. ↕ to 2m (6ft), ↔ to 3m (10ft). Mexico. ❁ (min. 5°C/41°F). **'Marginata'** ■ has pale yellow-margined leaves that often become white with age. **'Mediopicta'** 🏆 has a broad, pale yellow central band along each leaf. **'Striata'** produces leaves vertically striped yellow or white.

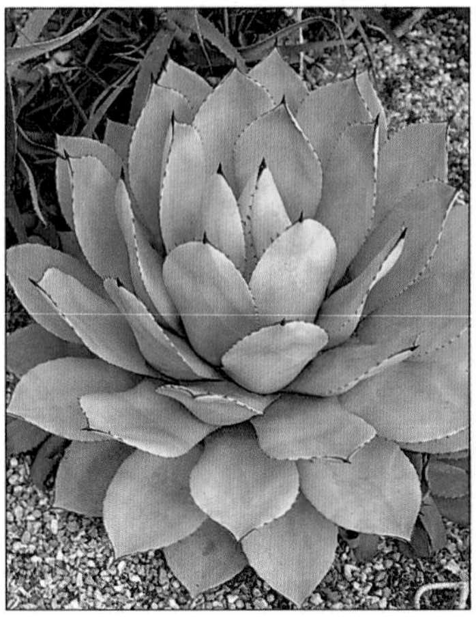
Agave parryi

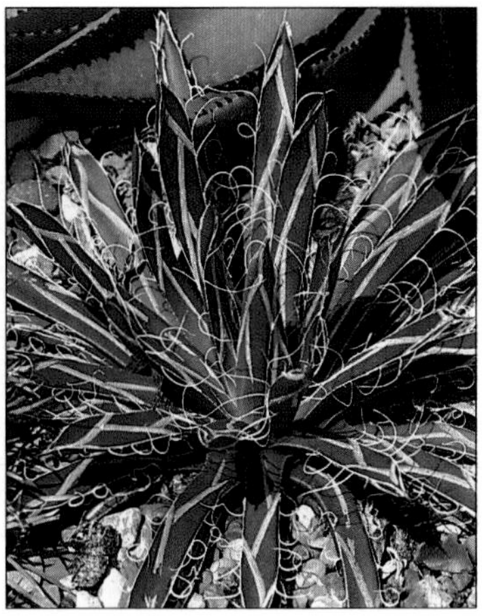
Agave parviflora

A. attenuata ■ syn. *A. cernua*, *A. glaucescens*. Perennial succulent with a thick trunk, often branching at the base. The branches are crowned by rosettes of ovate, sometimes finely toothed, pale yellowish green or greyish green leaves, 50–70cm (20–28in) long, with no terminal spines. Recurving racemes, to 3.5m (11ft) or more long, bear greenish white flowers, 6cm (2½in) long, in summer. ↕ to 1m (3ft), ↔ to 2m (6ft). C. Mexico. ❁ (min. 10°C/50°F)
A. cernua see *A. attenuata*.
A. consideranti see *A. victoriae-reginae*.
A. cupreata. Basal-rosetted or short-stemmed, perennial succulent. Pointed, pale green leaves are ovate to obovate, 75cm (30in) long, with twisted, spiny, reddish brown marginal teeth, and brown terminal spines. Yellow flowers, 3.5–7cm (1½–3in) long, are produced in erect panicles, 60cm (24in) or more long, in summer. ↕ to 1m (3ft), ↔ 1.5m (5ft). W. Mexico. ❁ (min. 10°C/50°F)
A. dentiens see *A. deserti*.
A. deserti, syn. *A. dentiens*, *A. nelsonii*, *A. pringlei*. Variable, perennial succulent with basal rosettes of thick, sharp-tipped, greyish green leaves, 15–40cm (6–16in) long. The concave to flat leaves are triangular to linear to lance-shaped, channelled above, sometimes banded, usually with spiny margins, occasionally entire. In summer, bears erect panicles, 2–7m (6–22ft) long, of silvery yellow flowers, to 5cm (2in) long. ↕ to 50cm (20in), ↔ to 1m (3ft). USA (California, Arizona), N. Mexico. ❁ (min. 10°C/50°F)
A. ferox. Rosetted, perennial succulent with a stout stem. Oblong to spoon-shaped, rigid, fleshy, sharp-tipped, dark green leaves, 1m (3ft) long, have marginal hooked teeth, to 2cm (¾in) long, and terminal spines, to 8cm (3in) long. In summer, bears greenish yellow flowers, 8cm (3in) long, in erect then spreading panicles, to 10m (30ft) long. ↕ to 4–5m (12–15ft), ↔ to 2m (6ft). Mexico. ❁ (min. 10°C/50°F)
A. filifera ■ 🏆 Stoloniferous, perennial succulent with basal rosettes of slender, lance-shaped, dark green leaves, to 25cm (10in) long, margined with white threads, and each with a brown terminal spine. Erect, spike-like inflorescences, to 2.5m (8ft) long, with dense clusters of greenish yellow flowers, 5cm (2in) long, are borne in late summer and early autumn. ↕ 30–50cm (12–20in), ↔ 1m (3ft). C. Mexico. ❁ (min. 10°C/50°F)

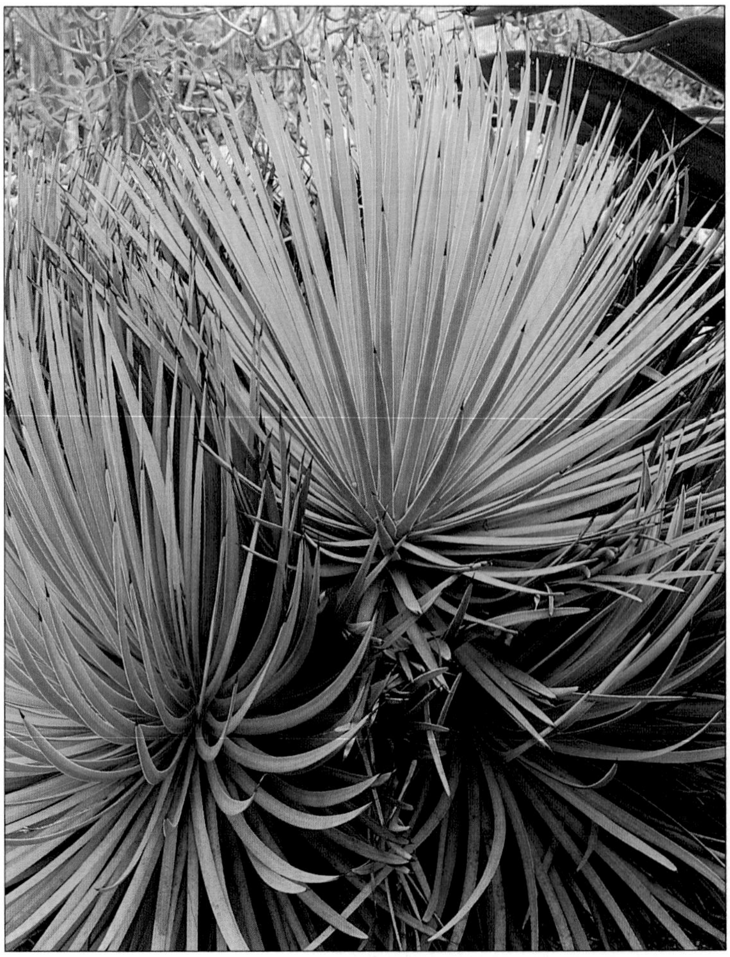
Agave stricta

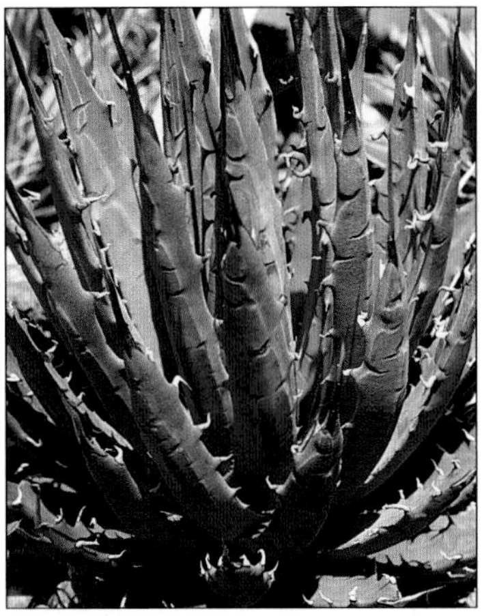

Agave utahensis

A. glaucescens see *A. attenuata.*
A. hartmanii see *A. parviflora.*
A. huachucensis see *A. parryi* var. *huachucensis.*
A. hystrix see *A. stricta.*
A. nelsonii see *A. deserti.*
A. neomexicana see *A. parryi.*
A. parryi ■ syn. *A. neomexicana.* Perennial succulent producing a dense, compact, basal rosette of broadly oblong, spiny, grey-blue leaves, to 30cm (12in) long. Numerous creamy yellow flowers, pink- or red-tinged in bud, and 6cm (2½in) long, open in erect panicles, to 5m (15ft) long, in summer. ↕ 50cm (20in), ↔ to 1m (3ft). Mountains of USA (Arizona) to N. Mexico. ❁ (min. 5°C/41°F). **var. *huachucensis*,** syn. *A. huachucensis,* has broadly oblong leaves to 65cm (26in) long, and flowers 7cm (3in) long; USA (S. Arizona).
A. parviflora ■ 🏆 syn. *A. hartmanii.* Basal-rosetted, perennial succulent with narrowly lance-shaped, white-marked, dark green leaves, 4–10cm (1½–4in) long, margined with white threads, and each with a greenish brown terminal spine. Erect racemes, 1–1.8m (3–6ft) or more long, with clusters of pale yellow flowers, 1.5cm (½in) long, are borne in summer. ↕ 15cm (6in), ↔ 50cm (20in). USA (S. Arizona) to N. Mexico. ❁ (min. 10°C/50°F)
A. pringlei see *A. deserti.*
A. scaphoidea see *A. utahensis.*
***A. schidigera*,** syn. *A. vestita.* Basal-rosetted or short-stemmed, perennial succulent with lance-shaped, shiny, dark green or purplish green leaves, to 50cm (20in) long, margined with coiled white threads, and each with a brown terminal spine. Produces erect, spike-like inflorescences, 2–2.5m (6–8ft) long, with yellow-green or reddish brown flowers, 5cm (2in) long, in summer. ↕ to 50cm (20in), ↔ to 75cm (30in). C. Mexico. ❁ (min. 10°C/50°F)
A. stricta ■ 🏆 syn. *A. hystrix.* Short-stemmed, perennial succulent with rosettes of linear-lance-shaped, sharply tapered, mid-green leaves, to 35cm (14in) long, with red-brown terminal spines. In summer, bears red to purple-red flowers, 2cm (¾in) long, in dense, erect, spike-like racemes, 2–2.5m (6–8ft) long. ↕↔ 25–50cm (10–20in). S.E. Mexico. ❁ (min. 10°C/50°F)
A. utahensis ■ syn. *A. scaphoidea.* Variable, basal-rosetted, clump-forming, perennial succulent with linear to lance-shaped, grey-green leaves, to 30cm (12in) long, each with a long terminal spine; indented, wavy margins have hooked spines. In summer, bears yellow flowers, 3cm (1¼in) long, in erect panicles or racemes, 1.5–4m (5–12ft) long. ↕ 30cm (12in), ↔ indefinite. USA (Utah). ❁ (min. 10°C/50°F)
A. vestita see *A. schidigera.*
A. victoriae-reginae ■ 🏆 syn. *A. consideranti.* Variable, perennial succulent with basal rosettes of straight or incurved, triangular-oblong, white-marked, dark green leaves, 15–30cm (6–12in) long, with thick, rounded tips, and each with a brown terminal spine. The horny leaf margins are usually entire, but may have small white spines. In summer, bears erect or curved, spike-like racemes, 4–5m (12–15ft) long, of creamy white flowers, to 5cm (2in) long, sometimes tinged purple. ↕↔ to 50cm (20in). USA (California), N. and W. Mexico. ❁ (min. 10°C/50°F)

▷ ***Ageratina altissima*** see *Eupatorium rugosum*
▷ ***Ageratina ligustrina*** see *Eupatorium ligustrinum*

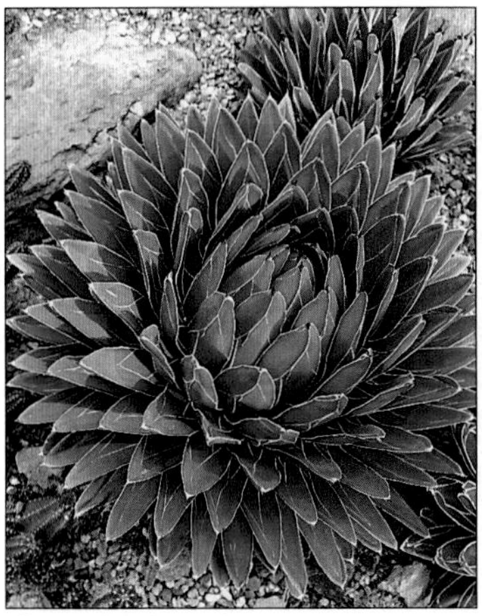

Agave victoriae-reginae

AGERATUM

Floss flower

ASTERACEAE/COMPOSITAE

Genus of about 40 species of annuals, perennials, and shrubs from diverse habitats in tropical and warm-temperate North and South America, some of which have become naturalized in many tropical and subtropical countries. They may be erect, spreading, or mound-forming in habit, and have oval to lance-shaped, mid-green leaves. In summer and early autumn, panicles of 30–50 small flowerheads form soft, rounded, brush-like clusters, varying in colour from bright blue or grey-blue to pink or white; they are attractive to butterflies. Ageratums are usually grown as annuals; use *A. houstonianum* and its cultivars for bedding or as edging in borders. They may also be grown in containers.

• **HARDINESS** Half hardy.
• **CULTIVATION** Grow in fertile, moist but well-drained soil in full sun, in a sheltered site. Water freely in mid-summer to prolong flowering. Dead-head to encourage a second flowering.
• **PROPAGATION** Sow seed at 16–18°C (61–64°F) in early spring, or sow in autumn and overwinter at 10°C (50°F).
• **PESTS AND DISEASES** Prone to root rot.

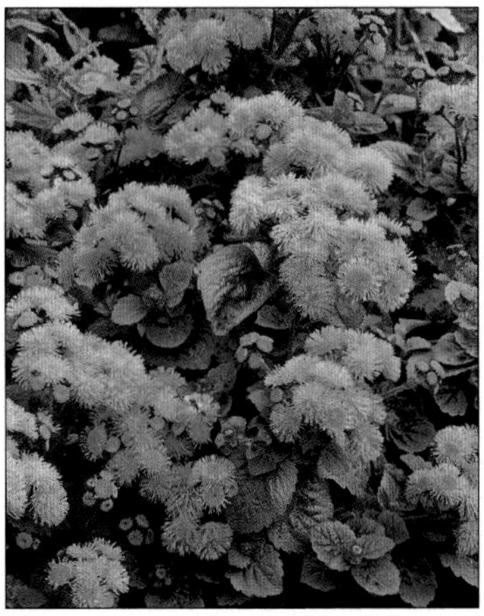

Ageratum houstonianum 'Adriatic'

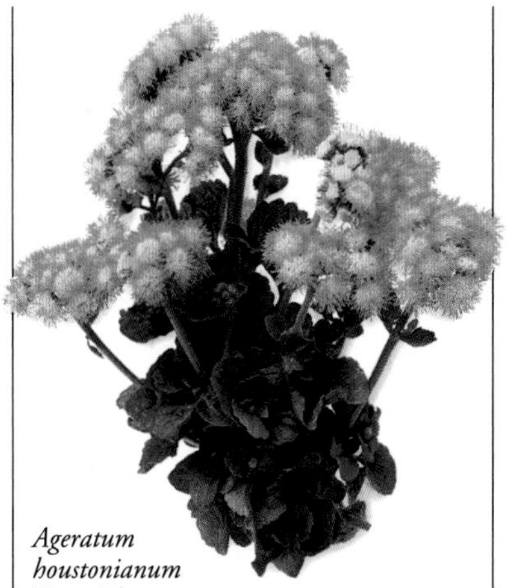

Ageratum houstonianum 'Bavaria'

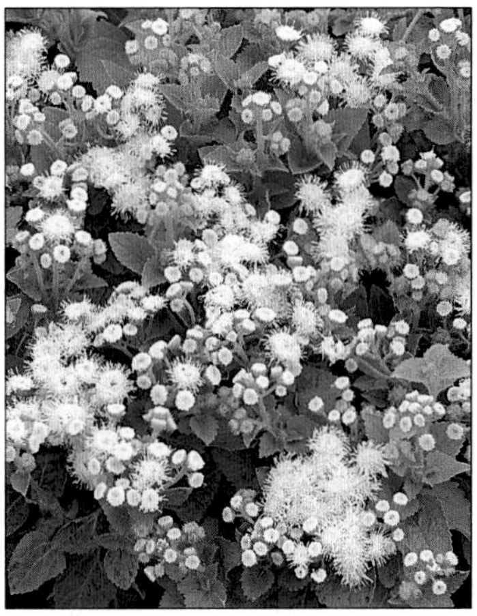

Ageratum houstonianum Hawaii Series 'Hawaii White'

***A. houstonianum* cultivars.** Selections from the fast-growing, Mexican annual *A. houstonianum* are mostly compact, mound-forming, and of uniform habit. They have oval, downy leaves, 5–7cm (2–3in) long, heart-shaped at the bases. Rounded panicles, 5–10cm (2–4in) across, of 40 or more small flowerheads are borne just above the foliage from midsummer until the first frosts. ↕↔ 15–30cm (6–12in). ❄. **'Adriatic'** ■ is bushy, with clear, mid-blue flower-heads; ↕ 15–20cm (6–8in). **'Atlantic Plus'** has deep blue flowerheads; ↕ 15–20cm (6–8in). **'Bavaria'** ■ has blue-and-white flowerheads; ↕ 25cm (10in). **'Blue Danube'** bears many small, weather-resistant, lavender-blue flowerheads while plants are still young; ↕ 15–18cm (6–7in). **'Blue Horizon'** produces purple-blue, weather-resistant flowerheads on long, sturdy stems, good for cutting; ↕ 45cm (18in). **'Blue Mink'** is vigorous and of relatively open habit, with powder-blue flowerheads; ↕ 20–30cm (8–12in). **Hawaii Series** includes uniform, compact plants, with deep to pale blue and white flowerheads; **'Hawaii White'** ■ has fluffy white flowerheads; ↕ to 15cm (6in). **'Pacific'** 🏆 is neat, with tight clusters of deep violet-blue flowerheads; ↕ 20cm (8in). **'Swing Pink'** ■ is dwarf, with attractive pink flowerheads; ↕ 15–20cm (6–8in).

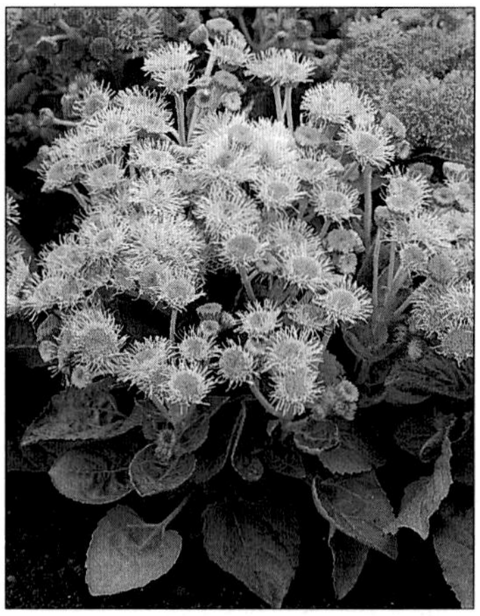

Ageratum houstonianum 'Swing Pink'

AGLAOMORPHA

POLYPODIACEAE

Genus of 10 or more species of evergreen, mostly epiphytic ferns, usually with thick, creeping rhizomes, found on tree trunks, rocks, and cliff faces in rainforest and scrub in tropical S.E. Asia. The large, pinnate fronds are erect, then often arching or pendent, with thin, leathery leaflets. In most species, organic matter accumulates in the closely overlapping bases of the fronds. Sori are dispersed over the undersides of the fronds, or are arranged serially between the veins. Aglaomorphas are attractive specimen plants, and their foliage forms a good backdrop for other ferns. In frost-prone areas, grow in a warm greenhouse.

• **HARDINESS** Frost tender.
• **CULTIVATION** Under glass, grow in an orchid basket, shallow container, or hanging basket, in equal parts fine-grade bark, perlite, and charcoal in filtered light with high humidity. When in growth, water freely and apply a half-strength, balanced liquid fertilizer monthly; water sparingly in winter. Pot on annually in early spring to prevent the rhizomes covering the outside of the container. Outdoors, grow epiphytically, or in moist, coarse, moderately fertile, humus-rich soil in a shady, humid site.
• **PROPAGATION** Sow spores at 21°C (70°F) as soon as ripe. Divide rhizomes as growth begins in spring, making sure that each division has a growing tip. See also p.51.
• **PESTS AND DISEASES** Susceptible to scale insects under glass.

***A. coronans*,** syn. *Pseudodrynaria coronans.* Epiphytic or terrestrial, rhizomatous fern producing arching, overlapping, triangular to lance-shaped, dark green fronds, strongly waved or

A

shallowly lobed at the bases, and deeply pinnatifid or pinnatisect with lance-shaped to oblong segments. ‡↔ to 2m (6ft). India to Taiwan. ❁ (min. 10°C/50°F)
A. meyeniana (Bear's paw fern). Epiphytic, rhizomatous fern with overlapping, triangular to lance-shaped, deep green fronds, 80cm (32in) long, almost entire at the bases, and pinnate in the middle and at the top; the upper segments on fertile fronds are very short. ‡↔ to 1m (3ft). Taiwan, Philippines. ❁ (min. 10°C/50°F)

AGLAONEMA

ARACEAE

Genus of about 20 species of usually rhizomatous, evergreen perennials from tropical forest in Asia. The leaf-blades are borne on long, sheathing leaf-stalks from a central growing point, and are variegated in many species. The stems are erect and cane-like, or short, decumbent, and creeping. Insignificant flowering spadices, enclosed in cream or greenish white spathes, are borne sporadically. In frost-prone areas, grow in a temperate or warm greenhouse or conservatory, or as houseplants; in frost-free areas, grow in a shady border.
• **HARDINESS** Frost tender.
• **CULTIVATION** Under glass, grow in well-drained, loamless or loam-based potting compost (JI No.2 or 3), in filtered light, with high humidity. Water moderately; allow some drying out between applications in winter; excess watering may encourage stem or root rot. Apply a balanced liquid fertilizer monthly in the growing season. Pot on every 2–3 years. Outdoors, grow in well-drained, moderately fertile, humus-rich soil in partial shade.
• **PROPAGATION** Separate basal shoots with 3 or 4 leaves, ideally with roots attached, or divide in spring.
• **PESTS AND DISEASES** Mealybugs may infest the leaf axils.

A. commutatum ■ Erect perennial, becoming decumbent with age. Leaf-stalks, to 15cm (6in) long, bear oblong-elliptic, dark green leaf-blades, feathered and barred grey, and 30cm (12in) long. ‡↔ 50cm (20in). Philippines, Indonesia (Sulawesi). ❁ (min. 13°C/55°F). **'Malay Beauty'**, syn. 'Pewter', has green-marbled white stems and yellow- and green-mottled leaf-blades, 30cm (12in) long, with white veins. **'Pewter'** see

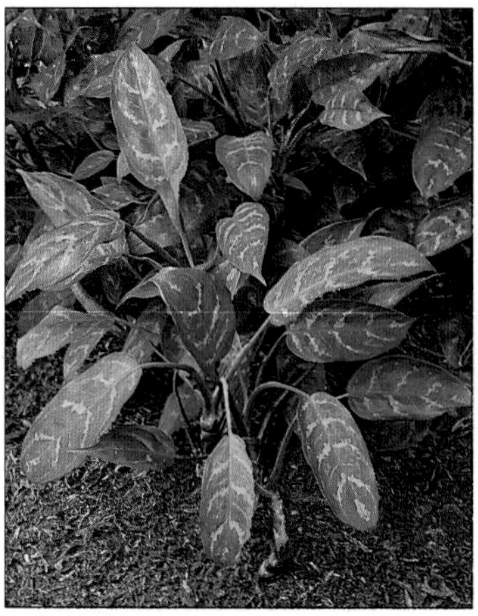

Aglaonema commutatum

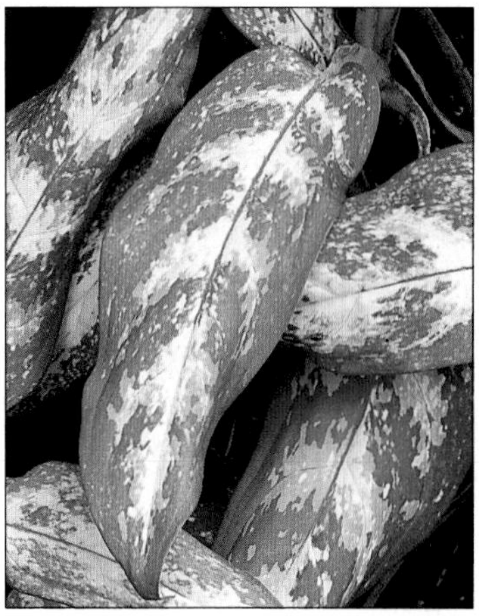

Aglaonema commutatum 'Pseudobracteatum'

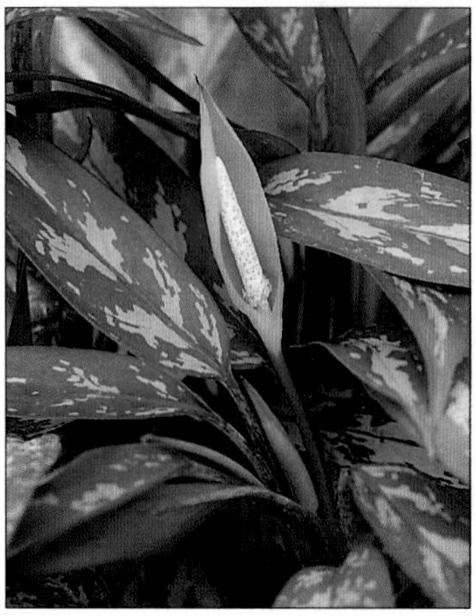

Aglaonema commutatum 'Treubii'

'Malay Beauty'. **'Pseudobracteatum'** ■ produces narrowly elliptic leaf-blades, 20cm (8in) long, which are mid- to dark green, with irregular white and pale green markings radiating from the leaf veins; ‡↔ 60cm (24in). **'Treubii'** ■ is compact, with narrowly lance-shaped, pointed, grey-green leaf-blades, 25cm (10in) long, irregularly marked with silver or pale green; ‡↔ 40cm (16in).
A. costatum. Rhizomatous, creeping perennial with leaf-stalks to 12cm (5in) long, bearing ovate to lance-shaped, dark green leaf-blades, 20cm (8in) long, with broad white midribs, and spotted white on both surfaces. ‡↔ 75cm (30in). Malaysia. ❁ (min. 13°C/55°F)
A. crispum, syn. *A. roebelinii* (Painted drop-tongue). Erect perennial with lance-shaped to elliptic, leathery, silvery

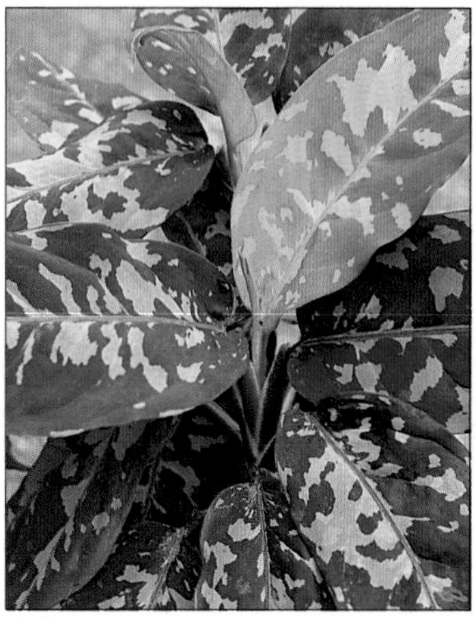

Aglaonema pictum

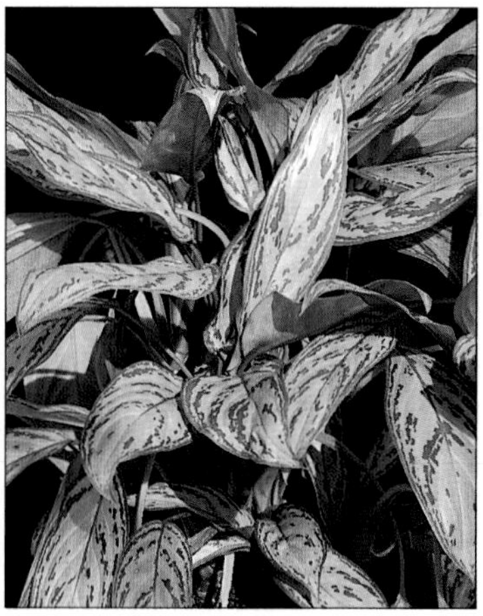

Aglaonema 'Silver King'

grey-green leaf-blades, 20cm (8in) long, with dark green margins, on leaf-stalks to 25cm (10in) long. ‡↔ 1.2m (4ft). Philippines. ❁ (min. 13°C/55°F)
A. modestum ♀ Erect perennial bearing lance-shaped to ovate, waxy, glossy, dark green leaf-blades, 20cm (8in) long, with wavy margins, on leaf-stalks 10–20cm (4–8in) long. ‡↔ 60cm (24in). S. China to N. Thailand. ❁ (min. 7°C/45°F)
A. pictum ■ Erect perennial producing narrowly elliptic to oval, wavy-margined leaf-blades, 20cm (8in) long, lustrous bluish green in colour, and irregularly marked with pale green and silvery grey, on leaf-stalks 5–6cm (2–2½in) long. ‡↔ 60cm (24in). Indonesia (Sumatra). ❁ (min. 13°C/55°F)
A. roebelinii see *A. crispum.*
***A.* 'Silver King'** ■ Upright perennial bearing lance-shaped leaf-blades, 30cm (12in) long, light to dark green, strongly suffused silver, and with short-pointed tips, on leaf-stalks to 10cm (4in) long. ‡↔ 60cm (24in). ❁ (min. 13°C/55°F)

AGONIS

MYRTACEAE

Genus of 10–12 species of evergreen shrubs and small trees from dry to seasonally moist scrub, often near the sea, in Western Australia. They are grown mainly for their small, 5-petalled, fragrant flowers, which are produced in clusters from the upper leaf axils. The alternate leaves vary from ovate to lance-shaped. In frost-prone climates, over-winter in a cool greenhouse. In frost-free areas, grow *A. flexuosa* as an elegant specimen tree; smaller species are effective in a border or against a wall.
• **HARDINESS** Frost tender, but *A. flexuosa* may tolerate temperatures around 0°C (32°F) for short periods.
• **CULTIVATION** Under glass, grow in well-drained, lime-free (ericaceous) potting compost in full light, with good ventilation. In the growing season, water moderately and apply a balanced liquid fertilizer monthly; water more sparingly in winter. Outdoors, grow in moist but well-drained, moderately fertile, neutral to slightly acid soil in full sun; established plants will tolerate partial shade and dry spells. Pruning group 8, but pruning is best kept to a minimum.
• **PROPAGATION** Sow seed at 16°C (61°F) in spring. Root semi-ripe cuttings with bottom heat in summer.
• **PESTS AND DISEASES** Prone to scale insects and red spider mites under glass.

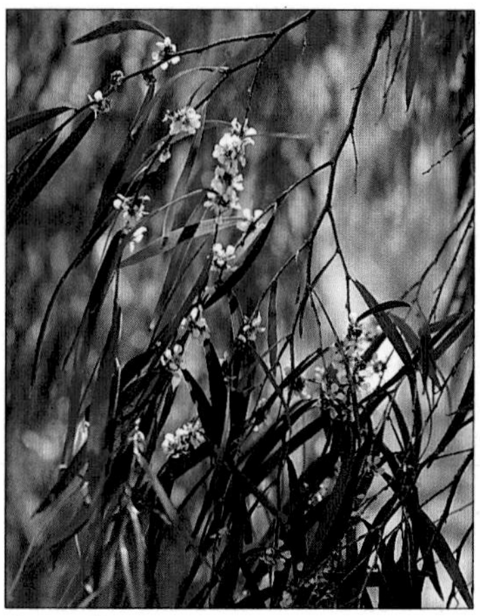

Agonis flexuosa

A. flexuosa ■ ◌ Bushy tree, willow-like in growth, with pendent branches and lance-shaped, bright green leaves, 5–15cm (2–6in) long. Numerous axillary clusters of 2 or 3 white flowers, 1cm (½in) across, are produced in summer. ‡ 6–12m (20–40ft), ↔ 5–10m (15–30ft). Australia (S.W. Western Australia). ✲ (borderline)

AGROSTEMMA

Corn cockle

CARYOPHYLLACEAE

Genus of 2–4 species of erect, branching annuals from scrub, stony slopes, and cultivated fields in S. Europe, the Mediterranean, and W. Asia. They have linear, opposite leaves and, in summer, bear usually solitary, 5-petalled, open trumpet-shaped flowers with long-toothed calyces. The stems are slender and covered with a soft down. Grow in a wildflower or cottage garden, or in containers. The flowers are suitable for cutting and are attractive to bees. Seeds may cause severe discomfort if ingested.
• **HARDINESS** Fully hardy.
• **CULTIVATION** Grow in preferably poor, well-drained soil in full sun. The lax growth needs staking. Dead-head to prolong flowering, but allow last seed crop to self-sow.
• **PROPAGATION** Sow seed *in situ* as soon as ripe, or in early spring; thin seedlings to 23–30cm (9–12in) apart. For summer-flowering container plants, sow seed in autumn, overwinter in a cold frame, and then pot on the following spring.
• **PESTS AND DISEASES** Trouble free.

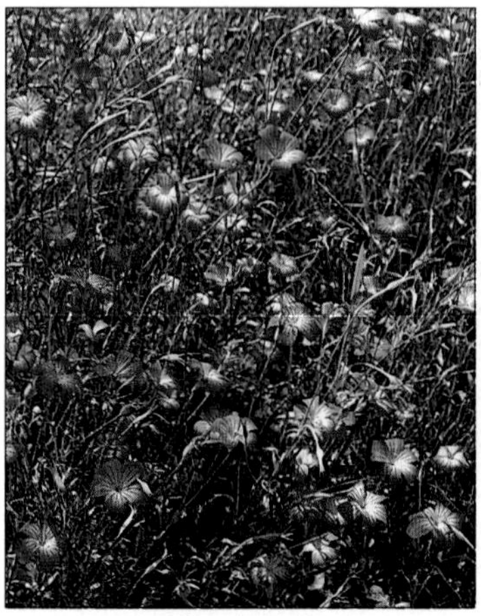

Agrostemma githago 'Milas'

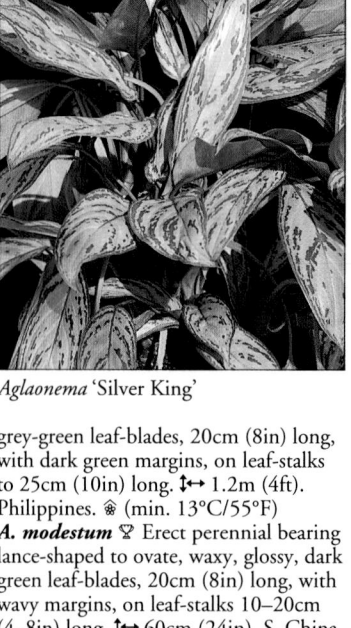

A. coeli-rosa see *Silene coeli-rosa.*
A. githago. Summer-flowering annual with linear to lance-shaped, grey-green leaves, to 8cm (3in) long. Produces magenta-purple, sometimes white-eyed, or white flowers, to 5cm (2in) across, with ribbed, hairy calyces. ↕60–90cm (24–36in), ↔ 30cm (12in). Mediterranean. ❄❄❄. **'Milas'** ■ syn. 'Rose Queen', has deep plum-pink flowers. **'Milas Cerise'**, syn. 'Purple Queen', has cerise-pink flowers, darker than those of 'Milas'. **'Purple Queen'** see 'Milas Cerise'. **'Rose Queen'** see 'Milas'.

AGROSTIS

GRAMINEAE/POACEAE

Genus of 120–150 species of annual and perennial grasses found at high altitudes in tropical regions and temperate zones; some species are important fodder grasses, while others are used in fine lawn seed mixtures. A few annual species with light, airy panicles are suitable for a border and for cutting and drying. The perennial species are more commonly cultivated and are useful for the front of a border or a wildflower meadow.
• **HARDINESS** Fully hardy.
• **CULTIVATION** Grow in well-drained soil in full sun. *A. canina* thrives in all but very dry soils in sun or partial shade. Dead-head before seed is set.
• **PROPAGATION** Divide between mid-spring and early summer.
• **PESTS AND DISEASES** Trouble free.

A. canina (Velvet bent). Mat-forming, evergreen perennial with short stolons and erect, rounded stems bearing flat, slightly rough, linear, mid-green leaves, 6cm (2½in) long. From early to late summer, bears slender panicles, to 11cm (4½in) long, of shiny, reddish brown spikelets. ↕6cm (2½in), ↔ 30cm (12in) or more. Europe, Asia, N.E. USA. ❄❄❄. **'Silver Needles'** has leaf-blades with silvery white margins.

AICHRYSON

CRASSULACEAE

Genus of about 10 annual or perennial succulents, mostly from hilly areas of the Azores, Madeira, and the Canary Islands. They have erect, often forked stems and rosettes of mid- to dark green, mainly alternate, hairy leaves, produced close to the stem tips. Panicles or cymes of star-shaped yellow or red flowers are borne from late spring to summer. In frost-prone areas, grow in a temperate greenhouse or as houseplants. In frost-free areas, grow in a desert garden.
• **HARDINESS** Frost tender.
• **CULTIVATION** Under glass, grow in standard cactus compost or loam-based potting compost (JI No.2), with additional grit, in full or bright filtered light. Water moderately at all times, and apply a balanced liquid fertilizer 3 or 4 times when in growth. Outdoors, grow in an open site in poor to moderately fertile, well-drained soil in full sun. See also pp.48–49.
• **PROPAGATION** Sow seed at 19–24°C (66–75°F) in spring; flowers are usually borne after 2 years. Root cuttings of rosettes in spring or early summer.
• **PESTS AND DISEASES** Susceptible to mealybugs and aphids.

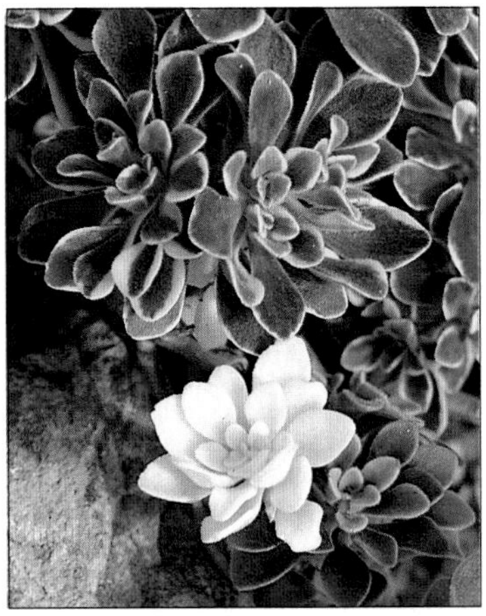
Aichryson x *domesticum* 'Variegatum'

A. x domesticum 'Variegatum' ■ ♀ syn. *Aeonium domesticum* 'Variegatum'. Shrubby, branching, perennial succulent with rosettes of diamond-shaped, or obovate to ovate, finely hairy, dark green leaves, 2–5cm (¾–2in) long, margined and marbled white or creamy white. Occasionally produces shoots with only creamy white or white leaves. In early summer, bears panicles of bright yellow flowers, 1.5–2cm (½–¾in) wide. ↕15cm (6in) or more, ↔ 40cm (16in). ❀ (min. 7°C/45°F; optimum 13–26°C/55–79°F)
A. sedifolium see *Aeonium sedifolium.*
A. villosum. Densely branched, annual or short-lived perennial succulent with sticky, usually rough, white-hairy stems and diamond-shaped, mid-green leaves, to 3cm (1¼in) long, densely covered with long hairs. Cymes of golden yellow flowers, to 1.5cm (½in) wide, are borne in late spring. ↕20cm (8in), ↔ to 40cm (16in). Azores, Madeira. ❀ (min. 7°C/45°F; optimum 13–26°C/55–79°F)

AILANTHUS

SIMAROUBACEAE

Genus of 5 species of deciduous trees and shrubs occurring in woodland in China and from S.E. Asia to Australia, with large, alternate, pinnate leaves. *A. altissima*, the most commonly cultivated species, is grown as a specimen tree, mainly for its striking foliage and colourful, winged fruit. It is suitable for a large garden. Individual plants usually have either male or female flowers; both are needed to produce fruit. Male flowers are unpleasantly scented; the pollen may cause an allergic reaction.

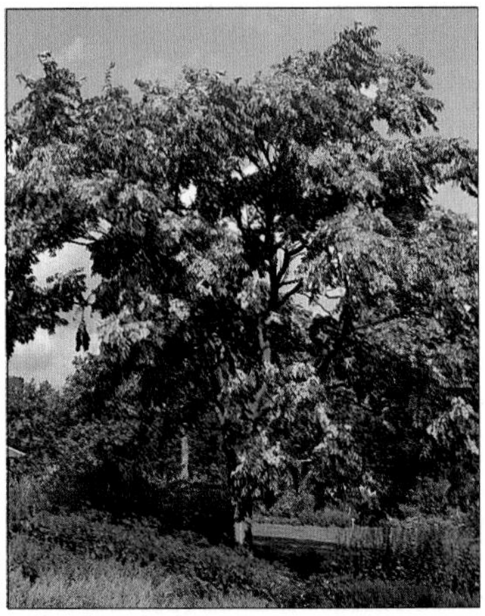
Ailanthus altissima

Flowering and fruiting are most profuse in areas with hot summers.
• **HARDINESS** Fully hardy.
• **CULTIVATION** Grow in deep, fertile, well-drained soil in sun or partial shade. Suckers may be a problem with *A. altissima.* Pruning group 1; train as a central leader standard or prune hard annually to grow as a large-leaved shrub.
• **PROPAGATION** Sow seed in containers in a cold frame as soon as ripe, or in spring. Remove and pot up suckers or take root cuttings in winter.
• **PESTS AND DISEASES** Trouble free.

A. altissima ■ ♀ ○ (Tree of heaven). Spreading tree with large, oblong-elliptic, pinnate leaves, to 60cm (24in) long, composed of up to 30 ovate to lance-shaped leaflets, which open reddish green and later turn mid-green. Bears terminal panicles, to 30cm (12in) across, of small green flowers in summer, followed by red-brown fruit, similar to those of ash (*Fraxinus*). ↕25m (80ft), ↔ 15m (50ft). China. ❄❄❄

AIPHANES

Ruffle palm

ARECACEAE/PALMAE

Genus of about 40 species of single-stemmed, spiny, monoecious palms from dry forest in the West Indies and Central and South America. The pinnate leaves are arranged in terminal tufts, and small, cup-shaped flowers are borne in panicles among them. In frost-prone areas, grow young plants as foliage specimens in a temperate or warm greenhouse. In frost-free areas, grow as specimen trees.
• **HARDINESS** Frost tender.
• **CULTIVATION** Under glass, grow in loam-based potting compost (JI No.3), with additional leaf mould, in full light. In the growing season, water freely and apply a balanced liquid fertilizer monthly; water more sparingly in winter. Outdoors, grow in fertile, moist but well-drained soil in full sun.

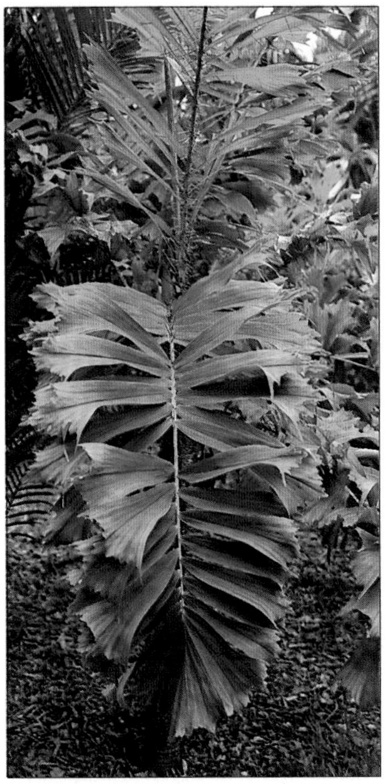
Aiphanes caryotifolia

• **PROPAGATION** Sow seed at 25–30°C (77–86°F) in spring.
• **PESTS AND DISEASES** Red spider mites may be a problem under glass.

A. caryotifolia ■ ♈ (Spine palm). Slender-stemmed palm, ringed with spines, and producing pinnate leaves, 1–3m (3–10ft) long, with prickly stalks and 4–10 strap-shaped, light to mid-green leaflets. In summer, bears yellow flowers in panicles, to 1.5m (5ft) long, followed by spherical red or yellow fruit. ↕6–12m (20–40ft), ↔ 2.5–3m (8–10ft). N. South America. ❀ (min. 7°C/45°F)

AIRA

Hair grass

GRAMINEAE/POACEAE

Genus of 8 or 9 species of annual, sometimes biennial grasses from dry, open areas in Europe, the Mediterranean, N. Africa, and mountainous regions of tropical Africa, the Middle East, and N. and W. Asia. They have linear, often inrolled leaves. Several species are cultivated for their delicate, lax, finely branched flower panicles, and provide good cut or dried flowers. Grow at the front of a border.
• **HARDINESS** Fully hardy.
• **CULTIVATION** Grow in any well-drained soil in sun or partial shade.
• **PROPAGATION** Sow seed *in situ* in spring.
• **PESTS AND DISEASES** Trouble free.

A. elegantissima (Hair grass). Tufted annual grass with linear, inrolled, mid-green leaves, to 5cm (2in) long. Open, diffuse panicles, to 10cm (4in) long, of small silvery or purple spikelets, 2–3mm (1/16–⅛in) long, are borne on hair-fine branches in late spring and early summer. ↕30cm (12in), ↔ 25cm (10in). Mediterranean. ❄❄❄
A. flexuosa see *Deschampsia flexuosa.*

▷**Air plant** see *Tillandsia*

AJANIA

ASTERACEAE/COMPOSITAE

Genus of 30 species of low-mound-forming perennials, subshrubs, or shrubs from exposed, rocky hillsides in C. and E. Asia. The leaves are shallowly lobed to pinnatifid, and often white-woolly. They bear attractive racemes or branched corymbs of button-like yellow flowers in summer and autumn, and are suitable for a sunny rock garden or herbaceous border.
• **HARDINESS** Fully hardy.
• **CULTIVATION** Grow in poor, well-drained soil in full sun.
• **PROPAGATION** Sow seed in containers in a cold frame in spring. Divide runners in spring, or take basal cuttings in spring or summer.
• **PESTS AND DISEASES** Trouble free.

A. pacifica, syn. *Chrysanthemum pacificum, Dendranthema pacificum.* Low, mound-forming perennial or subshrub with short runners and lobed, ovate, silky-white, silver-margined, mid-green leaves, to 5cm (2in) long. Small yellow flowerheads, to 2cm (¾in) across, are borne in branched corymbs, to 10cm (4in) across, in autumn. ↕30cm (12in), ↔ 90cm (36in). C. and E. Asia. ❄❄❄

AJUGA

Bugle

LABIATAE/LAMIACEAE

Genus of about 40 species of annuals and clump-forming or spreading, evergreen or semi-evergreen, usually rhizomatous perennials found in shady habitats throughout temperate Europe and Asia. The attractive leaves are opposite and entire, or occasionally toothed, and the 2-lipped, tubular, usually blue flowers are produced in whorls from the axils of leaf-like bracts from spring to early summer. Bugles are excellent for ground cover, spreading freely from rhizomes or stolons, especially in moist conditions.

• **HARDINESS** Fully hardy.

• **CULTIVATION** Grow in any moist soil in partial shade or part-day sun, as the foliage may scorch in full sun. *A. reptans* and its cultivars will tolerate poor soils, even in full shade.

• **PROPAGATION** Separate rooted stems, or root softwood cuttings, in early summer. Divide *A. pyramidalis* 'Metallica Crispa' every 2–3 years to maintain vigour.

• **PESTS AND DISEASES** Susceptible to powdery mildew.

A. genevensis ▣ (Blue bugle, Upright bugle). Clump-forming, densely hairy to almost hairless, evergreen perennial, rhizomatous but without stolons, and with upright stems to 40cm (16in) long. Long-stalked, mid- or light green, obovate, basal leaves, to 12cm (5in) long, are shallowly lobed or toothed. In spring, bears spike-like whorls, to 10cm (4in) tall, of bright deep blue (sometimes pink or white) flowers, 2cm (¾in) long. ↕ 20–40cm (8–16in), ↔ 45cm (18in). S. Europe, S.W. Asia. ❄❄❄

A. metallica see *A. pyramidalis.*

A. pyramidalis, syn. *A. metallica* (Pyramidal bugle). Clump-forming, evergreen or semi-evergreen, rhizomatous perennial, without stolons,

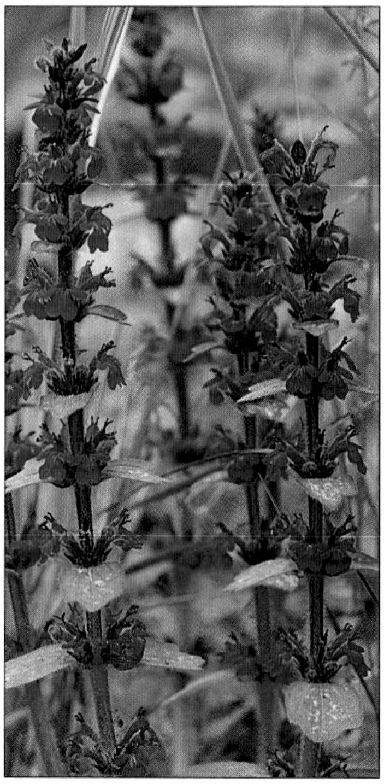

Ajuga genevensis

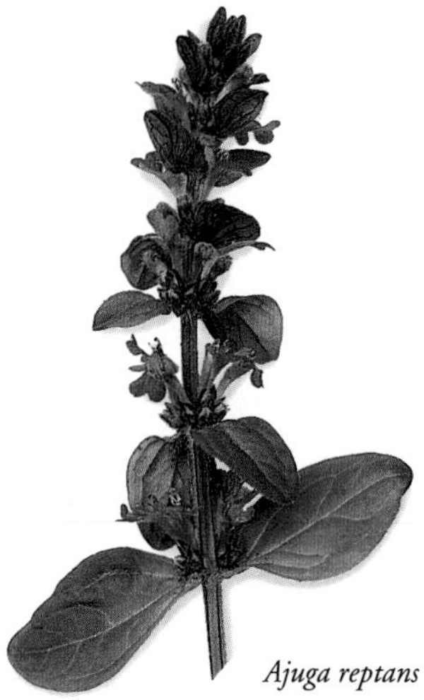

Ajuga reptans

producing basal rosettes of obovate, slightly toothed, softly hairy, dark green leaves, to 11cm (4½in) long. Deep blue or pale violet-blue (sometimes pink or white) flowers, 2cm (¾in) long, are borne in dense, pyramidal, spike-like whorls, to 10cm (4in) tall, among purple-tinged bracts, from spring to early summer. ↕ 15–25cm (6–10in), sometimes to 30cm (12in), ↔ 45–60cm (18–24in). N. and C. Europe, Alps. ❄❄❄. **'Metallica Crispa'** forms tight cushions of crinkled and curled, metallic green-purple leaves; ↕ 15cm (6in), ↔ 30–40cm (12–16in).

A. reptans ▣ Creeping, evergreen, rhizomatous perennial, spreading rapidly by stolons, with partly hairy stems producing ovate to oblong-spoon-shaped, dark green leaves, 9cm (3½in) long. Dark blue flowers, 1.5cm (½in) long, are borne in spike-like whorls, to 15cm (6in) tall, in late spring and early summer. ↕ 15cm (6in), ↔ 60–90cm (24–36in) or more. Europe, Caucasus, Iran. ❄❄❄. The wild species is invasive, but selected cultivars, varying in flower and foliage, are excellent ground-cover plants. **'Burgundy Glow'** ♀ has silvery green leaves suffused deep wine-red. **'Catlin's Giant'** ♀ has very large, dark bronze-purple leaves, to 15cm (6in) long, and produces inflorescences to 20cm (8in) long. **'Multicolor'** ▣ syn. 'Rainbow', is mat-forming, with dark bronze-green leaves marked with cream and pink. **'Pink Elf'** is compact, with deep pink flowers on stems 5cm (2in) long. **'Rainbow'** see 'Multicolor'. **'Variegata'** is dense and slow-spreading, with grey-green leaves margined and splashed cream.

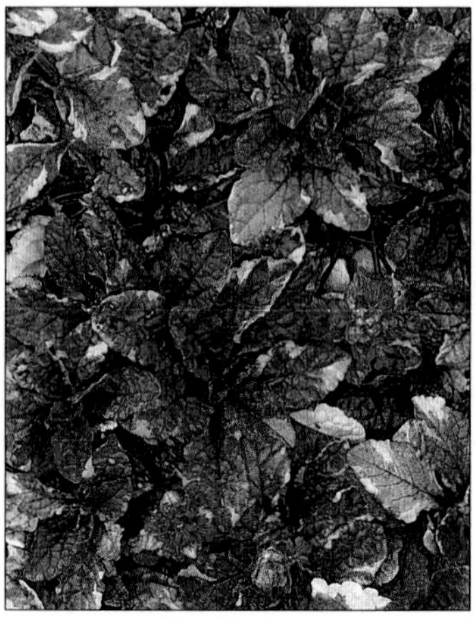

Ajuga reptans 'Multicolor'

AKEBIA

Chocolate vine

LARDIZABALACEAE

Genus of about 5 species of deciduous or semi-evergreen, twining climbers from forest margins in E. Asia, grown for their flowers and foliage. They have alternate, 3- to 5-, occasionally 7-palmate, mid-green leaves, often bronze-tinted when young. Racemes of self-sterile, shallowly cup-shaped flowers, with both sexes borne in each raceme, and with the larger, deeper-coloured female flowers at the base, are produced in spring, followed by unusual, sausage-shaped, fleshy purple fruits. To ensure cross-pollination, grow 2 plants from the same species (not of the same clone); they need warm springs and long, hot summers to fruit well. Grow against a wall or train into a tree or on a pergola.

• **HARDINESS** Fully hardy, but late frosts may damage the flowers.

• **CULTIVATION** Grow in moist but well-drained, fertile soil, in sun or partial shade. Pruning group 11, after flowering.

• **PROPAGATION** Sow seed in containers in a cold frame as soon as ripe. Root semi-ripe cuttings in summer. Layer in winter.

• **PESTS AND DISEASES** Trouble free.

A. lobata see *A. trifoliata.*

A. quinata ▣ Semi-evergreen climber with rounded leaves, 4–8cm (1½–3in) long, composed of usually 5 oblong to obovate, entire leaflets, notched at the tips, dark green above, blue-green below, tinged purple in winter. Spicily fragrant, brownish purple flowers are borne in pendent racemes, to 12cm (5in) long, in early spring, followed by fruit to 10cm (4in) long. ↕ 10m (30ft). China, Korea, Japan. ❄❄❄

A. trifoliata, syn. *A. lobata.* Deciduous climber with rounded leaves, 10cm (4in) long, composed of 3 broadly ovate, shallowly lobed leaflets, opening bronze, then turning glossy, dark green. Purple flowers are produced in pendent racemes, to 12cm (5in) long, in spring, and are followed by fruit, to 12cm (5in) long. ↕ 10m (30ft). China, Japan. ❄❄❄

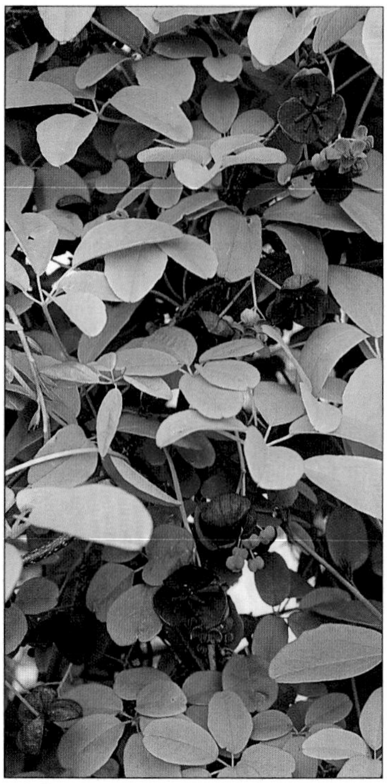

Akebia quinata

ALANGIUM

ALANGIACEAE

Genus of about 17 species of deciduous and evergreen trees, shrubs, and climbers from open scrub in tropical Africa and warm-temperate to tropical regions from E. Asia to E. Australia. *A. platanifolium*, the most commonly grown species, has attractive, alternate leaves and axillary cymes of unusual, tubular flowers. They are best grown in a shrub border.

• **HARDINESS** Frost hardy to frost tender; unripened wood may be damaged by frost.

• **CULTIVATION** Grow in fertile, well-drained soil in sun or partial shade. In frost-prone areas, grow against a wall or among other plants for protection. Pruning group 1.

• **PROPAGATION** Sow seed in containers in a cold frame in autumn or early spring. Root semi-ripe cuttings in summer.

• **PESTS AND DISEASES** Trouble free.

A. platanifolium. Upright, deciduous shrub with rounded, maple-like, shallowly 3- to 7-lobed leaves, to 20cm (8in) long, dark green above and mid-green beneath. In summer, produces clusters of 4 (sometimes up to 7) tubular, fragrant white flowers, to 4cm (1½in) wide, with recurving petal lobes. ↕ 3m (10ft), ↔ 2m (6ft). Korea, Japan. ❄❄

ALBIZIA

syn. PARASERIANTHES

LEGUMINOSAE/MIMOSACEAE

Genus of about 150 species of deciduous trees, shrubs, and climbers, often found in poor soils, in tropical and subtropical regions from Africa and Asia to Australia. They are grown for their filigree foliage and attractive flowerheads of small florets with long stamens, which may be borne on plants only a few years old. The alternate, 2-pinnate leaves have numerous oblong-ovate to sickle-shaped leaflets. In frost-prone areas, overwinter container-grown plants in a cool greenhouse; elsewhere, grow as specimen plants.

• **HARDINESS** Frost hardy to frost tender; *A. julibrissin* may survive to -20°C (-4°F) if growth has been ripened in summer. Alternating mild and cold spells may damage top-growth.

• **CULTIVATION** Under glass, grow in loam-based potting compost (JI No.2) in full light, with shade from hot sun. When in growth, water freely and apply a balanced liquid fertilizer monthly; water sparingly in winter. Pot on or top-dress in late winter. Outdoors, grow in poor to moderately fertile, well-drained soil in full sun. Pruning group 1, or 13 if wall-trained; plants under glass may need restrictive pruning in early spring.

• **PROPAGATION** Sow seed in spring, at not less than 15°C (59°F), after soaking for 24 hours in warm water. Root semi-ripe cuttings with bottom heat in summer. Take root cuttings in winter.

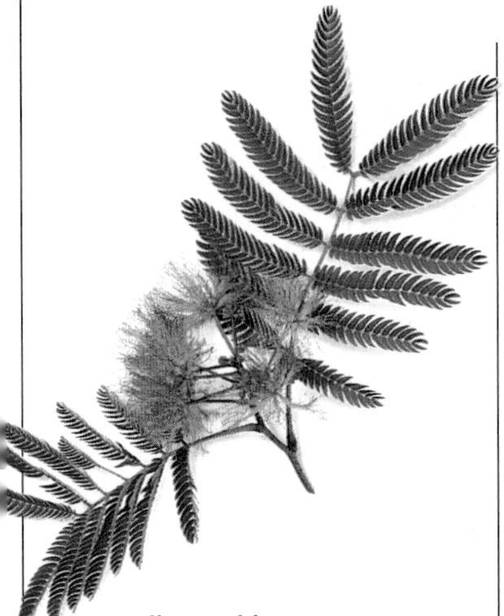

Albizia julibrissin var. *rosea*

• **PESTS AND DISEASES** Red spider mites and whiteflies may be a problem under glass. Outdoors, prone to vascular wilt.

A. distachya see *A. lophantha.*
A. julibrissin ♀ (Silk tree). Large shrub or small tree with a domed crown when mature. Fern-like, light to mid-green leaves, 30–45cm (12–18in) long, have many small, sickle-shaped leaflets. Bears terminal clusters, 7–15cm (3–6in) wide, of spherical, yellow-green flowerheads, 3.5cm (1½in) across, in summer. ↕ 6m (20ft), ↔ 4–6m (12–20ft). Iran to Japan. ✲✲. **var. *alba*** has white flowerheads. **var. *rosea*** ■ ♀ has pink flowerheads.
A. lophantha ♀♀ syn. *A. distachya, Paraserianthes lophantha* (Cape wattle, Swamp wattle). Erect to spreading, large shrub or small tree with fern-like, bright green leaves, 30cm (12in) long, with numerous small, oblong-ovate, lop-sidedly pointed leaflets. In spring, bears tiny, yellow-green or gold flowerheads in cylindrical, axillary spikes, 3–6cm (1¼–2½in) long. ↕ 2–10m (6–30ft), ↔ 1–3m (3–10ft). Australia (Western Australia). ❀ (min. 4–5°C/39–41°F)

ALBUCA

LILIACEAE

Genus of 30 species of bulbous perennials from grassland in the Middle East and Africa. Most of those cultivated come from South Africa, and have open tubular flowers and long, strap-shaped to lance-shaped or narrowly linear, deep green to grey-green, basal leaves. The narrowly bell-shaped or tubular flowers, 2–4cm (¾in–1½in) across, are borne in

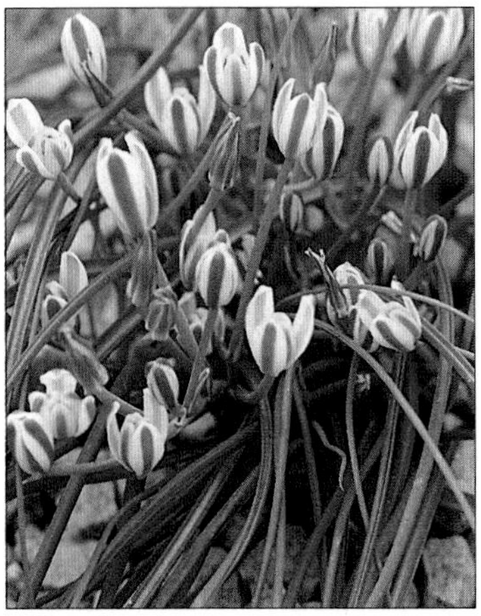

Albuca humilis

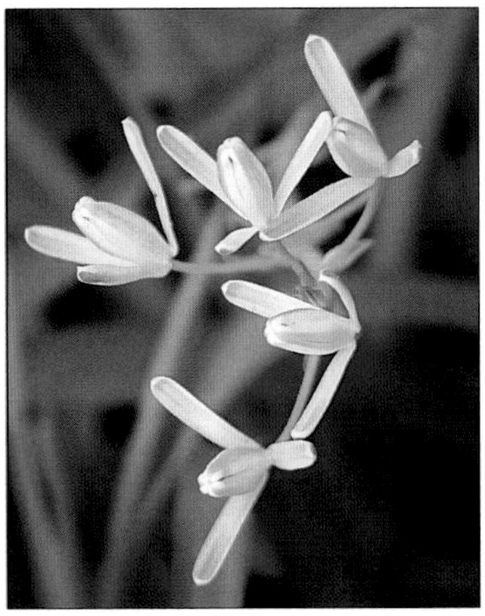

Albuca nelsonii

loose racemes, and are usually white or yellow with a green or dull red central stripe on each tepal. In frost-prone areas, grow in a temperate greenhouse; in warmer areas, use in an open, sunny site.
• **HARDINESS** Half hardy to frost tender; *A. canadensis* may survive brief spells at around -5°C (23°F). *A. humilis* is half hardy; in mild areas, it will survive in a sheltered site, mulched in winter.
• **CULTIVATION** Plant bulbs 5cm (2in) deep in spring. Under glass, grow in sandy, loam-based potting compost (JI No.2) in full light. In the growing season, apply a balanced liquid fertilizer monthly. Water freely when flowering, more sparingly in spring and autumn; keep dry in winter. Pot on in spring, if required. Outdoors, grow in moderately fertile, well-drained soil in full sun.
• **PROPAGATION** Sow seed at 13–18°C (55–64°F) as soon as ripe, or remove offsets in autumn.
• **PESTS AND DISEASES** Trouble free.

A. canadensis, syn. *A. minor.* Bulbous perennial with 3–6 lance-shaped leaves, 15cm (6in) long. In late spring and early summer, produces up to 7 nodding, narrowly bell-shaped, pale yellow flowers, the tepals each with a wide green central stripe. ↕ 50cm (20in), ↔ 21cm (8in). South Africa. ✲
A. humilis ■ Bulbous perennial with 1–3 narrowly linear leaves, 7–15cm (3–6in) long. Produces 1–3 narrowly bell-shaped white flowers in late spring and early summer. Outer tepals are green-striped; inner ones have yellow tips. ↕ 10cm (4in), ↔ 5cm (2in). South Africa. ✲
A. minor see *A. canadensis.*
A. nelsonii ■ Tall, bulbous perennial with 4–6 lance-shaped leaves, 90–120cm (3–4ft) long. Bears dense racemes of many, almost erect, tubular white flowers, the tepals each with a green, or occasionally dull red central stripe, in late spring and early summer. Good for cutting. ↕ 1.5m (5ft), ↔ 21cm (8in). South Africa. ❀ (min. 7°C/45°F)

ALCEA

Hollyhock

MALVACEAE

Genus of about 60 species of biennials and short-lived perennials found in temperate regions of Europe and Asia, usually in rocky sites and on dry, grassy wasteland. They are cultivated for their tall, slender inflorescences of large,

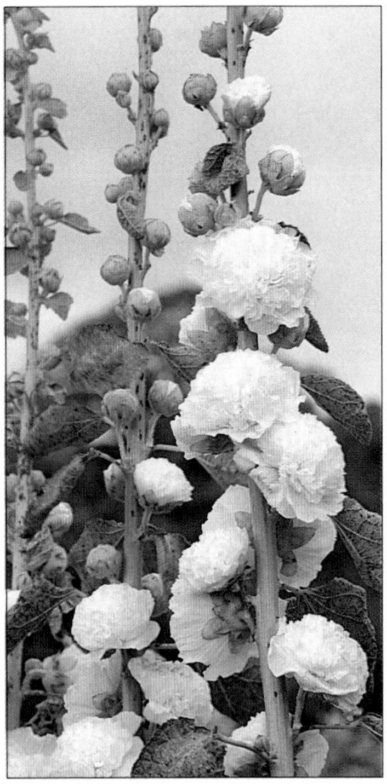

Alcea rosea 'Chater's Double'

stalkless or short-stalked, funnel-shaped, 5-petalled, brightly coloured flowers, often double in cultivars, which are borne in summer. Suitable for a mixed border, or for growing along a wall; they are attractive to butterflies and bees.
• **HARDINESS** Fully hardy.
• **CULTIVATION** Grow in moderately fertile, well-drained soil in full sun. May require staking in exposed sites. Grow as annuals or biennials to limit the spread of hollyhock rust.
• **PROPAGATION** To grow as annuals, sow seed at 13°C (55°F) in late winter, or *in situ* in mid-spring. For biennials and perennials, sow seed *in situ* in midsummer. If required, transplant in early autumn, when 2 or 3 true leaves have developed.
• **PESTS AND DISEASES** Susceptible to hollyhock rust. Cutworms and slugs may damage young growth. Mallow flea beetles, aphids, and capsid bugs may be a problem in dry conditions.

A. ficifolia. Erect biennial or short-lived perennial with rounded, 5- to 7-lobed, conspicuously veined, rough, mid-green leaves, to 18cm (7in) long. Terminal spikes of single, sometimes double yellow flowers, 5–8cm (2–3in) across, are produced in early summer. ↕ to 2.5m (8ft), ↔ 90cm (36in). Siberia. ✲✲✲
A. rosea, syn. *Althaea rosea* (Hollyhock). Vigorous, upright perennial producing rounded, roughly hairy, light green leaves, to 3.5cm (1½in) long, cut into 3–7 shallow lobes. Long, terminal racemes of single, purple, pink, white, or yellow flowers, 5–10cm (2–4in) across, are borne in early and midsummer. ↕ 1.5–2.5m (5–8ft), ↔ to 60cm (24in). Probably W. Asia. ✲✲✲. **'Chater's Double'** ■ bears peony-form, double flowers in a range of bright colours and paler shades, including pink, apricot, red, white, lavender-blue, yellow, and purple; ↕ 2–2.5m (6–8ft). **'Indian Spring'** bears single, white, pink, or yellow flowers. **'Majorette'** is dwarf and bushy, bearing rosette-like, fringed,

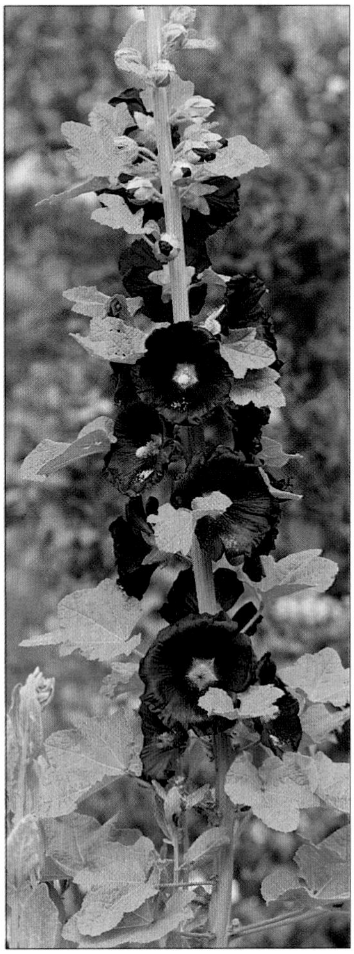

Alcea rosea 'Nigra'

semi-double flowers in pale shades, including yellow, carmine-red, and apricot, in early summer; ↕ 1m (3ft), ↔ to 30cm (12in). **'Nigra'** ■ has single, deep chocolate-maroon flowers with yellow throats; ↕ to 2m (6ft). **'Summer Carnival'**, bred for annual cultivation, bears double flowers in colours such as pale yellow and red, in early summer. Flowers are produced lower on the flowering stems than in other cultivars.

ALCHEMILLA

Lady's mantle

ROSACEAE

Genus of about 250 species of perennials from meadows and light woodland, some from rocky habitats, in N. temperate and arctic zones, and from mountain regions in tropical Africa, India, Sri Lanka, and Indonesia (Java). Alchemillas are valued for both their attractive foliage and their frothy sprays of flowers. Most have woody rhizomes, and shallowly to palmately lobed, rounded or kidney-shaped, often silky-haired leaves. The many-branched cymes of tiny, green or yellowish green flowers, 2–3mm (1/16–⅛in) across, are good for cutting. Alchemillas are suitable for a wildflower or large rock garden, or for a border.
• **HARDINESS** Fully hardy to frost hardy; *A. ellenbeckii* is hardy to -8°C (18°F).
• **CULTIVATION** Grow in any moist, humus-rich soil in sun or partial shade. Dead-head *A. mollis* soon after flowering, as it self-seeds very freely.
• **PROPAGATION** Sow seed in containers in a cold frame in spring. Transplant

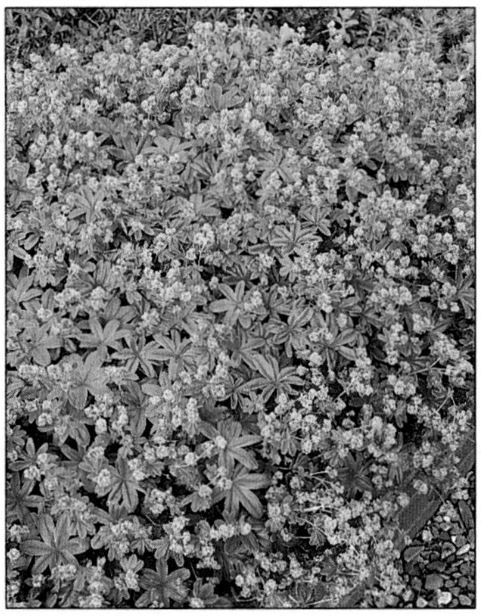

Alchemilla alpina

seedlings while small. Divide in early spring or autumn.

• **PESTS AND DISEASES** Slugs and snails may damage young foliage.

A. alpina ■ (Alpine lady's mantle). Mat-forming perennial with a creeping, woody rootstock and rounded or kidney-shaped, very deeply 5- to 7-lobed leaves, to 3.5cm (1½in) long, deep green and smooth above, silver-hairy beneath, with toothed tips. Loose cymes of tiny, yellow-green flowers are borne on stems 8–12cm (3–5in) long, in summer. Often confused with *A. conjuncta.* ↕8–12cm (3–5in), ↔ to 50cm (20in). N. Europe, mountains of W. and C. Europe, Greenland. ❄❄❄

A. conjuncta ■ Clump-forming, spreading perennial producing rounded, very deeply 7- to 9-lobed leaves, 3.5–4.5cm (1½–1¾in) long, blue-green above and silver-hairy beneath. Cymes of tiny, greenish yellow flowers are borne from early summer to early autumn. ↕40cm (16in), ↔ 30cm (12in). Jura mountains, S.W. Alps. ❄❄❄

A. ellenbeckii. Evergreen, mat-forming perennial with wiry red stems and small, kidney-shaped, deeply 5-lobed, pale green leaves, to 2cm (¾in) long. Bears tiny, yellow-green flowers in loose cymes in summer. Flowers resemble those of *A. alpina*, but are fewer, on shorter stems, and almost hidden by the foliage. Thrives in moist but well-drained soil. ↕2.5–5cm (1–2in), ↔ 30cm (12in) or more. Mountains of E. Africa. ❄❄

A. erythropoda ♀ Clump-forming perennial with rounded, shallowly 7- to 9-lobed, sharp-toothed, hairy, bluish

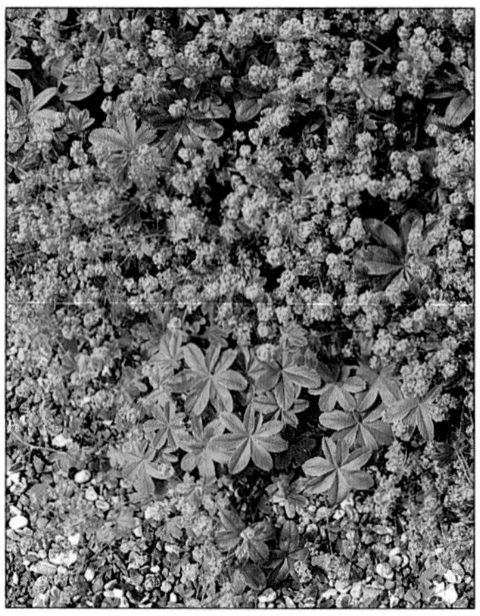

Alchemilla conjuncta

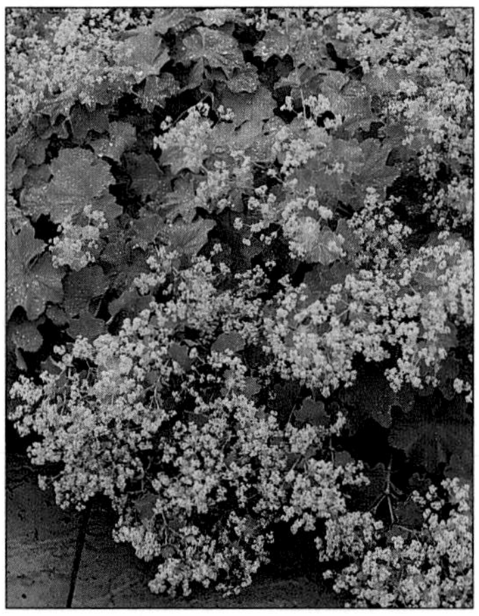

Alchemilla mollis

green leaves, 3–5cm (1¼–2in) long. Cymes of yellowish green flowers are produced from late spring to late summer. ↕20–30cm (8–12in), ↔ 20cm (8in). Carpathian and Balkan mountains, Caucasus, Turkey. ❄❄❄

A. faeroensis. Clump-forming perennial with kidney-shaped, deeply 7- to 9-lobed leaves, 3.5–4.5cm (1½–1¾in) long, blue-green above and silver-hairy beneath. Bears cymes of tiny, greenish yellow flowers from early summer to early autumn. ↕40cm (16in), ↔ 30cm (12in). E. Iceland. ❄❄❄

A. fulgens, syn. *A. splendens* of gardens. Spreading, rhizomatous perennial with rounded, shallowly 7- to 9-lobed, toothed, hairy leaves, 4.5–5cm (1¾–2in) long, blue-green above and silvery green beneath. Cymes of greenish yellow flowers are borne from early to late summer. ↕30cm (12in), ↔ 25cm (10in). Pyrenees. ❄❄❄

A. mollis ■♀ Clump-forming perennial with rounded, shallowly 9- to 11-lobed, toothed, densely softly hairy, pale green leaves, to 15cm (6in) long. Bears loose cymes of many tiny, greenish yellow flowers from early summer to early autumn. Drought-tolerant. Excellent for ground cover and for providing cut flowers. ↕60cm (24in), ↔ 75cm (30in). E. Carpathians, Caucasus, Turkey. ❄❄❄

***A. splendens* of gardens** see *A. fulgens.*

A. xanthochlora. Clump-forming perennial producing kidney-shaped, shallowly 9- to 11-lobed, often yellowish green leaves, 5cm (2in) long, hairless above and hairy beneath, with hairy leaf-stalks. Cymes of tiny, yellow-green flowers are borne in profusion from early to late summer. ↕50cm (20in), ↔ 60cm (24in). N.W. and C. Europe, Greece. ❄❄❄

▷**Alder** see *Alnus*
African red see *Cunonia capensis*
Black see *Ilex verticillata*
Common see *Alnus glutinosa*
Green see *Alnus viridis*
Grey see *Alnus incana*
Italian see *Alnus cordata*
Japanese see *Alnus japonica*
Mountain see *Alnus tenuifolia*
Oregon see *Alnus rubra*
Red see *Alnus rubra*
Sitka see *Alnus sinuata*
Thinleaf see *Alnus tenuifolia*
White see *Alnus rhombifolia, Clethra*
Witch see *Fothergilla gardenii*
▷**Alecost** see *Tanacetum balsamita*

ALEURITES

EUPHORBIACEAE

Genus of 6 species of evergreen trees from tropical to subtropical rainforest and moist woodland in China, Indonesia, and W. Pacific islands. The usually alternate leaves are shallowly lobed or entire. The small, 5-petalled white flowers are borne in terminal, panicle-like cymes, followed by fruits containing oil-bearing seeds. Where temperatures fall below 7°C (45°F), grow in a cool greenhouse. In warmer areas, grow as shade or specimen trees.

• **HARDINESS** Frost tender; *A. fordii* may tolerate short spells around 0°C (32°F).

• **CULTIVATION** Under glass, grow in lime-free (ericaceous) potting compost in full light. In the growing season, water freely and apply a balanced liquid fertilizer monthly; water sparingly in winter. Outdoors, grow in fertile, moist but well-drained, neutral to acid soil in full sun; they will tolerate partial shade. Pruning group 1; plants under glass may need restrictive pruning.

• **PROPAGATION** Sow seed at 13–18°C (55–64°F) as soon as ripe or in spring. Root semi-ripe cuttings in late summer.

• **PESTS AND DISEASES** Prone to red spider mites and whiteflies under glass.

A. fordii ♀ Erect to spreading tree with ovate, pointed, 3-lobed, light green leaves, to 25cm (10in) long, mostly arranged in whorls. Red-tinted white flowers are borne in panicle-like cymes, 10–15cm (4–6in) long, in summer, followed by spherical, greenish brown fruit, 6–7cm (2½–3in) across. ↕5–7m (15–22ft), ↔ 3–6m (10–20ft). W. and C. China. ❀ (min. 5°C/41°F).

▷**Alexanders, Perfoliate** see *Smyrnium perfoliatum*
▷**Alfalfa** see *Medicago sativa*

x ALICEARA

ORCHIDACEAE

Hybrid genus of evergreen, epiphytic orchids that are crosses between *Brassia*, *Miltonia*, and *Oncidium.* Basal rhizomes produce groups of oval pseudobulbs, each pseudobulb bearing 2 narrowly oval, mid-green leaves with pointed tips. Up to 12 long-lasting flowers, varying in size and colour, are borne in racemes from the bases of the pseudobulbs at various times during the year.

• **HARDINESS** Frost tender.

• **CULTIVATION** Cool-growing orchids. Grow in epiphytic orchid compost in the smallest possible containers. Provide shady, well-ventilated conditions and high humidity in summer; remove shading in winter. Water moderately throughout the year, more sparingly in winter. In summer, spray the foliage lightly with water once or twice a day; apply a half-strength fertilizer at every third watering. See also p.46.

• **PROPAGATION** Divide when the plant overgrows its container.

• **PESTS AND DISEASES** Susceptible to aphids, red spider mites, and mealybugs.

x *A.* 'Dark Warrior' ■ Evergreen hybrid orchid with oval pseudobulbs and oval leaves, 23cm (9in) long. Racemes of up to 12 flowers, each 4cm

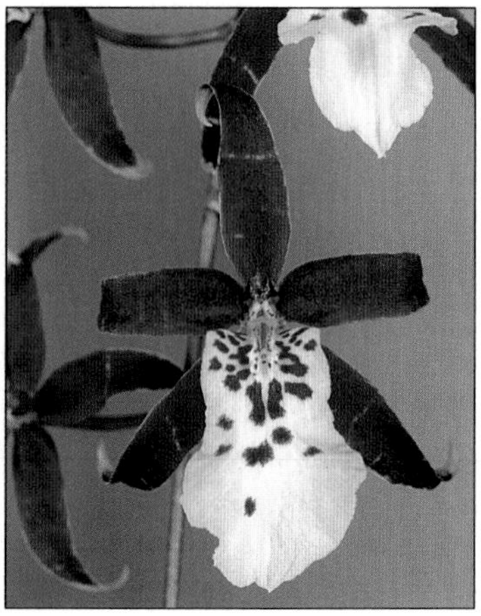

x *Aliceara* 'Dark Warrior'

(1½in) across, typically brown with cream lips, are borne throughout the year. ↕25cm (10in), ↔ 30cm (12in). ❀ (min. 11–13°C/52–55°F; max. 24°C/75°F)

ALISMA

Water plantain

ALISMATACEAE

Genus of 9 species of rhizomatous, deciduous, marginal aquatic perennials from temperate regions of the N. hemisphere, southern Africa, and from Australia. Basal rosettes of plantain-like leaves, with long leaf-stalks and elliptic to lance-shaped leaf-blades, are held above the water surface in spring. Whorled, umbel-like panicles of 3-petalled, saucer-shaped, white or pink flowers are borne above the foliage in mid- and late summer. Grow in large groups or drifts at pool margins. *A. plantago-aquatica* is ideal for a large pond and for naturalizing in a lake.

• **HARDINESS** Fully hardy.

• **CULTIVATION** Flowering is most profuse in water 15cm (6in) deep; they will tolerate water up to 30cm (12in) deep. *A. plantago-aquatica* self-seeds freely; dead-head regularly, once established. See also pp.52–53.

• **PROPAGATION** Sow seed as soon as ripe in seed trays or pots half submerged in shallow trays of water. Divide tuber-like rhizomes in late spring.

• **PESTS AND DISEASES** Trouble free.

A. gramineum. Aquatic perennial with growth above the water surface, or submerged to a depth of 23cm (9in). Above water, the dark green leaves are elliptic to lance-shaped, and 10cm (4in) long; submerged, they are linear, and to 45cm (18in) long. White or pinkish white flowers, to 6mm (¼in) across, are borne in dense panicles, 12–15cm (5–6in) tall. ↕↔ 15–20cm (6–8in). Europe, N. Africa, W. Asia, North America. ❄❄❄

A. lanceolatum. Aquatic perennial that thrives in water 20–23cm (8–9in) deep. Lance-shaped, bluish green leaves, to 30cm (12in) long, often smaller, grow above water. Bears panicles, 20–70cm (8–28in) tall, of purplish pink flowers, to 1.5cm (½in) across. ↕50–70cm (20–28in), ↔ 23cm (9in). Europe, Africa, C. and S.W. Asia. ❄❄❄

A. plantago-aquatica ■ Aquatic perennial with rosettes of elliptic to lance-shaped, greyish green leaves, to 30cm (12in) long, heart-shaped at the

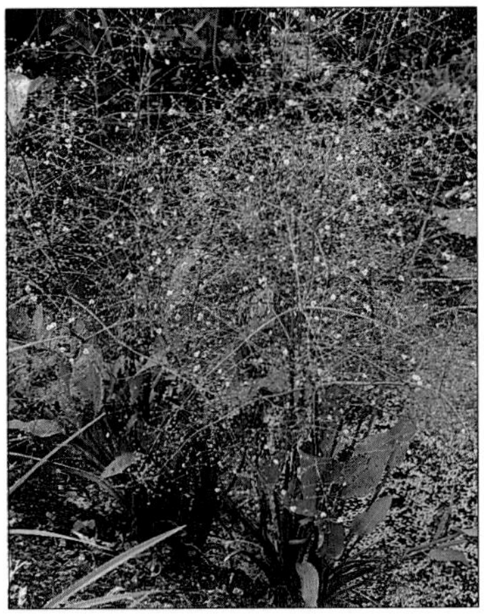

Alisma plantago-aquatica

bases, with pointed tips, borne on long stalks above the water. Bears white or pinkish white flowers, to 1.5cm (½in) wide, in panicles, 20–75cm (8–30in) tall. ↕60–75cm (24–30in), ↔45cm (18in). Europe, N. and southern Africa, E. Asia, North America. ❄❄❄

▷**Alison, Sweet** see *Lobularia*
▷**Alkanet** see *Anchusa*
Green see *Pentaglottis, P. sempervirens*

ALKANNA

BORAGINACEAE

Genus of 30–40 species of annuals or evergreen, clump-forming perennials, mostly found in scree and rock crevices from S. Europe to Iran. Few species are cultivated. They have basal tufts of alternate leaves, 8–15cm (3–6in) long, which are usually entire and hairy. They are grown for their funnel-shaped or salverform, bright blue flowers, borne in erect, terminal cymes on leafy stems in early summer. Grow in a raised scree bed or alpine house.

• **HARDINESS** Fully hardy.
• **CULTIVATION** Outdoors, grow in sharply drained soil in a raised scree bed, protected from winter wet; alternatively, grow in an alpine house in very gritty potting compost. Water moderately in the growing season; keep just moist in winter; avoid wetting the foliage.
• **PROPAGATION** Sow seed in containers in a cold frame in autumn, or root softwood cuttings in summer.
• **PESTS AND DISEASES** Prone to aphids and red spider mites under glass.

A. incana. Low, mound-forming, evergreen perennial with linear to lance-shaped, very hairy, grey-green leaves, to 15cm (6in) long, and salverform, bright blue flowers, 1cm (½in) across, on stiff stems, to 4–5cm (1½–2in) long. Needs good drainage. ↕5–15cm (2–6in), ↔5–10cm (2–4in). Turkey. ❄❄❄

ALLAMANDA

syn. ALLEMANDA

APOCYNACEAE

Genus of 12 species of evergreen shrubs and scandent climbers from scrub and forest in tropical North, Central, and South America. They have simple leaves, which may be alternate, opposite, or whorled, and are grown for their showy, usually terminal cymes of large, funnel- or trumpet-shaped flowers, each with 5 broad petal lobes. These are followed by spiny seed capsules. Where temperatures fall to 7°C (45°F), grow in a temperate or warm greenhouse. In warmer areas, grow in a border or on a wall. Contact with sap may irritate skin; all parts may cause mild stomach upset if ingested.

• **HARDINESS** Frost tender; *A. blanchetii* and *A. cathartica* may survive very short spells at about 0°C (32°F).
• **CULTIVATION** Under glass, grow in loam-based potting compost (JI No.3) in full light. Water freely in growth, applying a balanced liquid fertilizer every 2–3 weeks; water sparingly in winter. Outdoors, grow in moist, fertile soil in full sun. Pruning group 11 or 12 in late winter or early spring.
• **PROPAGATION** Sow seed at 18–20°C (64–68°F) in spring. Root greenwood cuttings in late spring or early summer.
• **PESTS AND DISEASES** Red spider mites and whiteflies may be a problem.

A. blanchetii, syn. *A. violacea.* Erect shrub or semi-scandent climber, with whorls of 4 oblong-obovate leaves, 8–12cm (3–5in) long. From summer to autumn, produces axillary and terminal cymes of broadly trumpet-shaped flowers, 6–9cm (2½–3½in) long, which are purplish pink, deeper toned inside. ↕↔2–3m (6–10ft). South America. ❀ (min. 7–10°C/45–50°F)
A. cathartica (Golden trumpet). Strong-growing climber with whorls of 3 or 4 lance-shaped to obovate leaves, 10–15cm (4–6in) long. Axillary and terminal cymes of yellow flowers, 12cm (5in) or more long, are borne from summer to autumn. ↕8–16m (25–52ft). Central and South America. ❀ (min. 7–10°C/45–50°F). **'Hendersonii'** ▣🏆 has bronze-tinted buds that open to bright yellow flowers, sometimes white-flecked in the throats.
A. violacea see *A. blanchetii.*

▷***Allemanda*** see *Allamanda*
▷**All heal** see *Valeriana officinalis*

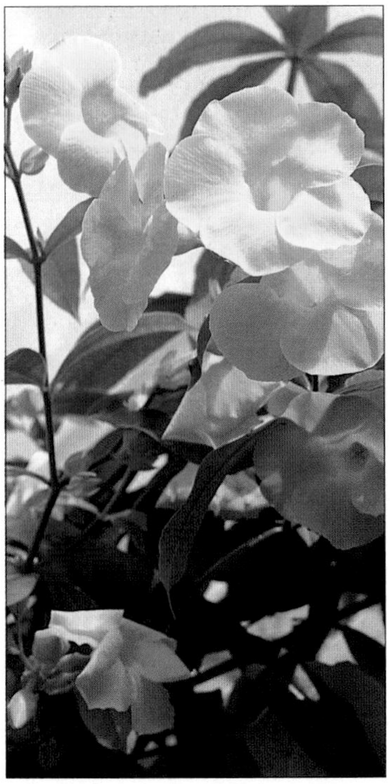

Allamanda cathartica 'Hendersonii'

ALLIUM

Onion

LILIACEAE

Genus of about 700 species of spring-, summer-, and autumn-flowering, bulbous and rhizomatous perennials, mainly from dry and mountainous areas of the N. hemisphere. In most species, a single bulb produces clusters of offset bulbs around it, which gradually form clumps. A few species have elongated bulbs, which develop on short, fleshy rhizomes; some produce bulbils in the flowerheads. The upright to spreading, sometimes cylindrical, linear to strap-shaped, basal or stem-clasping leaves have a pungent aroma when crushed; they are often withered by flowering time. The tubular-based flowers are bell-, star-, or cup-shaped; they are borne, few to many, in usually spherical, sometimes hemispherical or ovoid, occasionally pendent umbels, mostly 1–10cm (½–4in) across, sometimes to 30cm (12in) across. Grow taller species in groups in a border; some have flowerheads that dry well. Grow shorter species at the front of a border or in a rock garden. Contact with the bulbs may irritate skin or aggravate some skin allergies. Several species have culinary uses, including *A. sativum* (garlic), *A. schoenoprasum* (chives), and *A. tuberosum* (Chinese chives).

• **HARDINESS** Fully hardy to frost hardy.
• **CULTIVATION** Grow in fertile, well-drained soil in full sun. Plant bulbs 5–10cm (2–4in) deep in autumn; plant clump-forming species with rhizomes at, or just below, the soil surface in spring. Grow alliums from areas with hot, dry summers in sandy, loam-based potting compost (JI No.1) in an alpine house; keep dry when dormant in summer.
• **PROPAGATION** Sow seed in containers in a cold frame, when ripe or in spring; sow seed of *A. schoenoprasum* in drills *in situ.* Remove offsets of bulbous species in autumn. Divide clump-forming, rhizomatous species in spring.
• **PESTS AND DISEASES** Susceptible to white rot, downy mildew, and onion fly.

A. acuminatum ▣ Bulbous perennial with linear, channelled, mid-green basal and stem-clasping leaves, 10–20cm (4–8in) long. Hemispherical umbels, 4–6cm (1½–2½in) across, of 10–30 star-shaped, pinkish purple, occasionally white or pale pink flowers are produced in early summer. ↕10–30cm (4–12in), ↔5cm (2in). W. North America. ❄❄❄

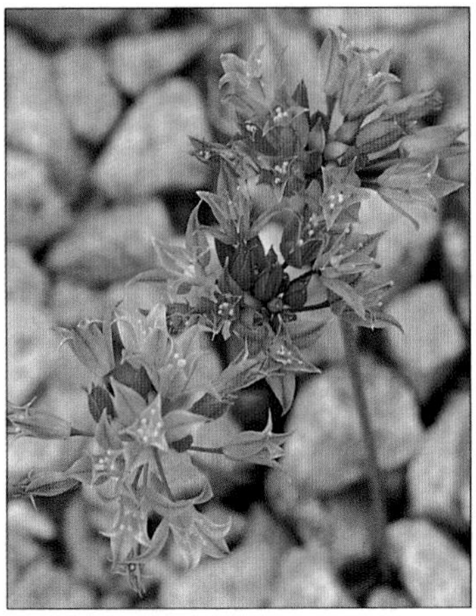

Allium acuminatum

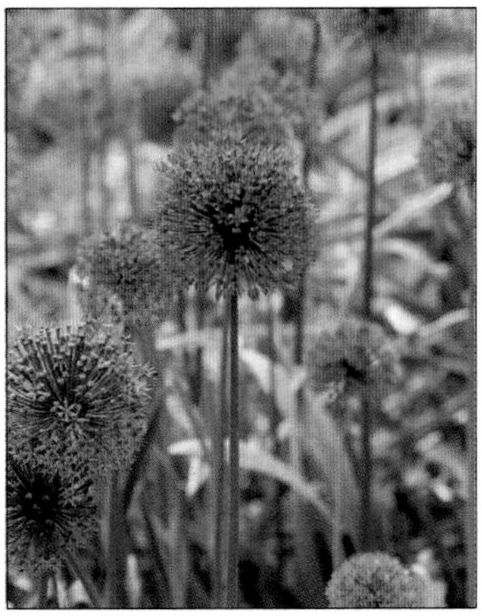

Allium aflatunense

A. aflatunense ▣ Bulbous perennial with slightly ribbed stems and linear, mid-green, basal leaves, 30–60cm (12–24in) long. Dense umbels, 10cm (4in) across, of many star-shaped, purplish pink flowers, are produced in summer. ↕1m (3ft), ↔10cm (4in). C. Asia. ❄❄❄
***A. aflatunense* of gardens** see *A.* x *hollandicum.*
A. akaka. Bulbous perennial with oblong-elliptic, grey-green, basal leaves, to 20cm (8in) long. Virtually stemless umbels, 6cm (2½in) across, of 30–40 small, star-shaped, lilac-pink flowers are produced in spring. ↕12cm (5in), ↔10cm (4in). Caucasus, Turkey, Iran. ❄❄❄
A. albopilosum see *A. cristophii.*
A. azureum see *A. caeruleum.*
A. beesianum 🏆 Bulbous perennial with linear, grey-green, basal leaves, 15–20cm (6–8in) long, and umbels, 2.5cm (1in) across, of 6–12 pendent, bell-shaped, blue or white flowers, with short stamens, from late summer to autumn. ↕15–20cm (6–8in), ↔5cm (2in). W. China. ❄❄❄
A. bulgaricum see *Nectaroscordum siculum* subsp. *bulgaricum.*
A. caeruleum ▣🏆 syn. *A. azureum.* Bulbous perennial with linear, mid-green, stem-clasping leaves, 7cm (3in) long, which die back before flowering. Dense umbels, 2.5cm (1in) across, of 30–50 small, star-shaped, bright blue flowers are borne on stiff stems in early summer. ↕60cm (24in), ↔2.5cm (1in). N. and C. Asia. ❄❄

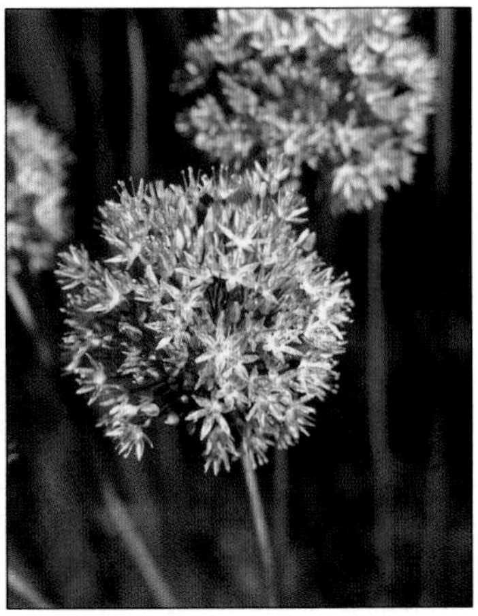

Allium caeruleum

A

A. callimischon. Bulbous perennial with grass-like, linear, mid-green, stem-clasping leaves, to 30cm (12in) long. Wiry stems bear loose umbels, 2.5cm (1in) across, of 8–25 cup-shaped, white or pale pink flowers in autumn. ↕ 9–35cm (3½–14in), ↔ 5cm (2in). Greece, W. Turkey. ❄❄. **subsp. *haemostictum*** has white or pale pink flowers with maroon spots; Crete.
A. campanulatum. Bulbous perennial with linear, mid-green, stem-clasping leaves, to 30cm (12in) long, which die back at flowering time. Bears dense umbels, 3–6cm (1¼–2½in) across, of up to 20 cup-shaped, rose-pink flowers in summer. ↕ 10–30cm (4–12in), ↔ 5cm (2in). USA (California, Nevada). ❄❄
A. carinatum. Bulbous perennial with linear, mid-green basal and stem-clasping leaves, to 20cm (8in) long. Bears loose umbels, 5cm (2in) across, of up to 30 bell-shaped purple flowers in midsummer, usually accompanied by bulbils; the outer flowers are pendent. Spreads rapidly, so best in informal plantings. ↕ 30–60cm (12–24in), ↔ 5cm (2in). C. and S. Europe, Turkey, former USSR. ❄❄❄. **subsp. *pulchellum*** 🏆 syn. *A. pulchellum*, has rich purple flowers in dense, elongated umbels, 6cm (2½in) across, with no bulbils. Virtually evergreen, since new leaves are produced with the flowers. Rapidly forms clumps, but is not invasive. ↕ 30–45cm (12–18in), ↔ 5cm (2in). S. Europe. **subsp. *pulchellum* f. *album*** has white flowers.
A. cernuum ■ 🏆 (Nodding onion, Wild onion). Vigorous, bulbous perennial with narrowly strap-shaped, dark green, basal leaves, 10–20cm (4–8in) long. In summer, stiff stems, curving over sharply at the tips, bear pendent umbels, 6cm (2½in) across, of 25–40 bell-shaped, mid- to deep pink flowers. ↕ 30–60cm (12–24in), ↔ 5cm (2in). North America. ❄❄❄
A. christophii see *A. cristophii.*
A. cowanii see *A. neapolitanum.*
A. cristophii ■ 🏆 syn. *A. albopilosum, A. christophii.* Bulbous perennial with ribbed stems and strap-shaped, grey-green, basal leaves, 15–40cm (6–16in) long, with stiff marginal hairs. The leaves wither before large umbels, 20cm (8in) across, of up to 50 star-shaped, pinkish purple flowers with a metallic sheen are produced in early summer. The flowerheads dry well. ↕ 30–60cm (12–24in), ↔ 15–19cm (6–7in). Turkey, C. Asia. ❄❄

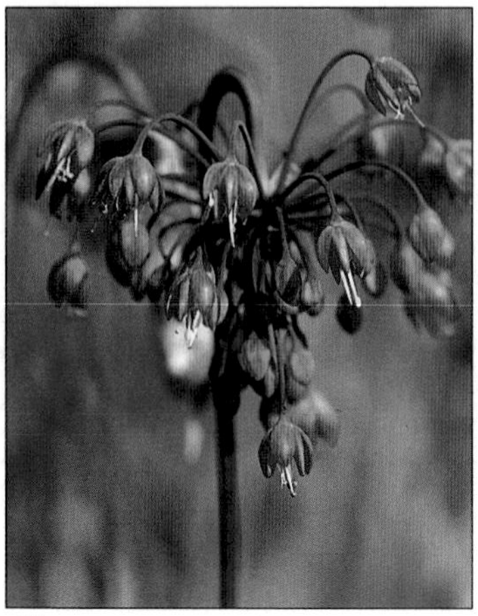

Allium cernuum

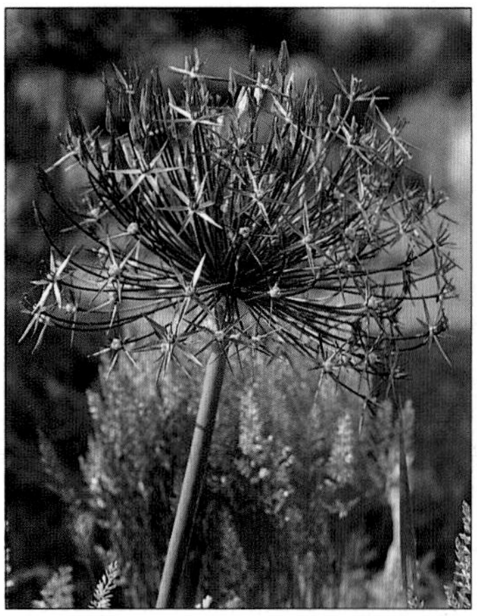

Allium cristophii

A. cyaneum 🏆 Bulbous perennial with short rhizomes and thread-like, dark green, basal leaves, to 15cm (6in) long. Produces small umbels, 2cm (¾in) across, of 6–8 bell-shaped blue flowers in summer. ↕ 10–25cm (4–10in), ↔ 8cm (3in). China. ❄❄❄
A. cyathophorum* var. *farreri ■ syn. *A. farreri.* Vigorous, bulbous perennial with narrowly strap-shaped, mid-green, basal leaves, 18–24cm (7–10in) long. In summer, bears loose umbels, 1.5cm (½in) across, of 6–30 small, pendent, bell-shaped, deep violet-purple flowers. ↕ 15–30cm (6–12in), ↔ 5cm (2in). China. ❄❄❄
A. dichlamydeum. Bulbous perennial with narrowly strap-shaped, short, mid-green, basal leaves, 10–20cm (4–8in) long. Bears thick-stemmed, compact umbels, 4cm (1½in) across, of up to 20 large, bell-shaped, bright pinkish purple flowers in early summer. ↕ 10–24cm (4–10in), ↔ 5cm (2in). USA (California). ❄❄
A. elatum see *A. macleanii.*
A. farreri see *A. cyathophorum* var. *farreri.*
A. flavum ■ 🏆 Very variable, bulbous perennial with cylindrical, narrowly strap-shaped, glaucous, stem-clasping leaves, to 20cm (8in) long. In summer, produces loose umbels, 1.5cm (½in) across, of up to 60 bell-shaped, bright yellow flowers with prominent stamens. The flowers bend downwards as they open. ↕ 10–35cm (4–14in), ↔ 5cm (2in). Europe, W. Asia. ❄❄❄
A. giganteum ■ Bulbous perennial with large, strap-shaped, pale green, basal leaves, 30–100cm (12–39in) long,

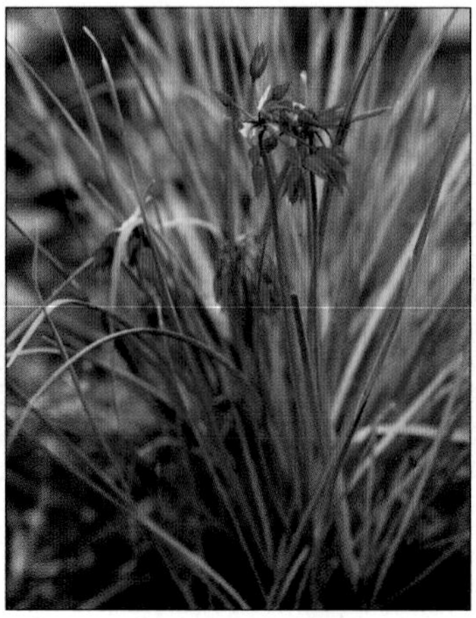

Allium cyathophorum var. *farreri*

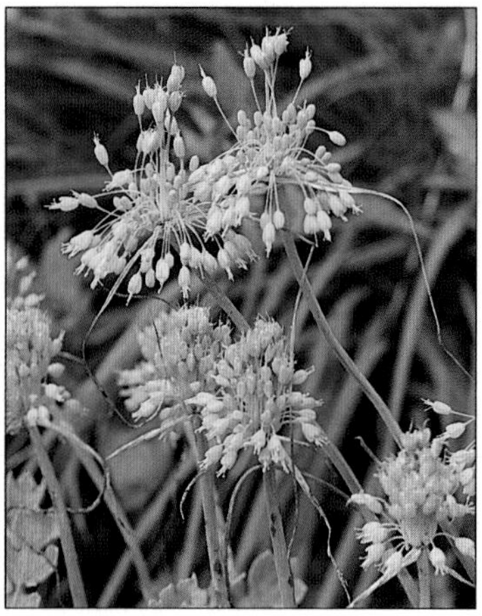

Allium flavum

which wither before flowering. In summer, bears dense umbels, 10cm (4in) across, of 50 or more star-shaped, lilac-pink flowers with prominent stamens. ↕ 1.5–2m (5–6ft), ↔ 15cm (6in). C. Asia. ❄❄❄
***A.* 'Globemaster'** ■ Bulbous perennial with strap-shaped, grey-green, basal leaves, 40–100cm (16–39in) long. Bears large umbels, 15–20cm (6–8in) across, of numerous star-shaped, deep violet flowers in summer. ↕ 80cm (32in), ↔ 20cm (8in). ❄❄❄
A. x hollandicum, syn. *A. aflatunense* of gardens. Bulbous perennial with unribbed stems and strap-shaped, mid-green, basal leaves, 30–60cm (12–24in) long, dying back at flowering time. Numerous star-shaped, purplish pink flowers are borne in dense umbels, 10cm (4in) across, in summer. Excellent for drying. ↕ 1m (3ft), ↔ 10cm (4in). Garden origin. ❄❄❄
A. insubricum 🏆 Bulbous perennial with short rhizomes and narrowly strap-shaped, mid-green, stem-sheathing leaves, 12–20cm (5–8in) long. Umbels, 2.5cm (1in) across, of 3–5 pendent, bell-shaped, pink-purple flowers are produced in summer, and are followed by pendent seed heads. Often confused with *A. narcissiflorum*, which has more flowers and erect seed heads. ↕ 15–25cm (6–10in), ↔ 5cm (2in). N. Italy. ❄❄❄
A. kansuense see *A. sikkimense.*
A. karataviense ■ 🏆 Bulbous perennial grown for its pairs of elliptic, almost horizontal, red-margined, grey-green or greyish purple, basal leaves, 15–23cm (6–9in) long. In summer, bears umbels, 5–8cm (2–3in) across, of 50 or more

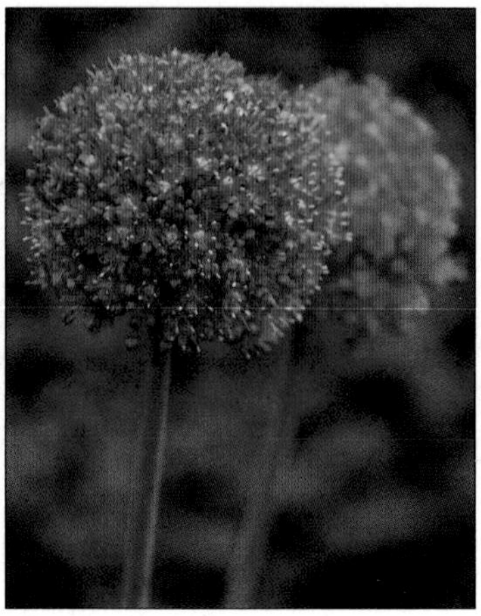

Allium giganteum

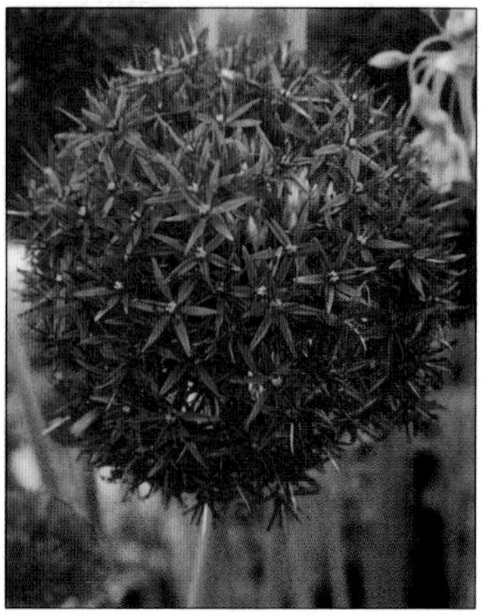

Allium 'Globemaster'

star-shaped, pale pink flowers with purple midribs. ↕ 10–25cm (4–10in), ↔ 10cm (4in). C. Asia. ❄❄❄
A. lemmonii. Bulbous perennial with sickle-shaped, grass-like, mid-green, basal leaves, 10–20cm (4–8in) long. In early summer, bears numerous tiny, star-shaped, white to pink flowers in umbels, 4cm (1½in) across. ↕ 10–15cm (4–6in), ↔ 5cm (2in). USA (California). ❄❄
***A.* 'Lucy Ball'.** Robust, bulbous perennial with strap-shaped, pale green, basal leaves, to 1m (3ft) long. In early summer, bears 50 or more star-shaped, dark lilac flowers in tight umbels, 5–8cm (2–3in) across. ↕ 1m (3ft), ↔ 15cm (6in). ❄❄❄
A. macleanii, syn. *A. elatum.* Bulbous perennial with deeply ridged stems and strap-shaped, glossy, mid-green, basal leaves, to 30cm (12in) long. In summer, bears umbels, 5–8cm (2–3in) across, of 50 or more star-shaped violet flowers, fading to rose-pink. ↕ 60–110cm (24–42in), ↔ 15cm (6in). C. and S.E. Asia. ❄❄
A. macranthum, syn. *A. oviflorum.* Bulbous perennial with short rhizomes and channelled, linear, mid-green, basal leaves, 15–45cm (6–18in) long. Loose umbels, 7–10cm (3–4in) across, of up to 20 pendent, bell-shaped, deep plum-purple flowers are borne in summer. ↕ 20–30cm (8–12in), ↔ 5cm (2in). India (Sikkim), W. China. ❄❄❄
A. mairei. Slender, bulbous perennial with short rhizomes and linear, grass-like, mid-green, basal leaves, to 25cm (10in) long. In late summer, bears loose umbels, 2.5cm (1in) across, of up to 10 bell-shaped, pale to bright pink flowers

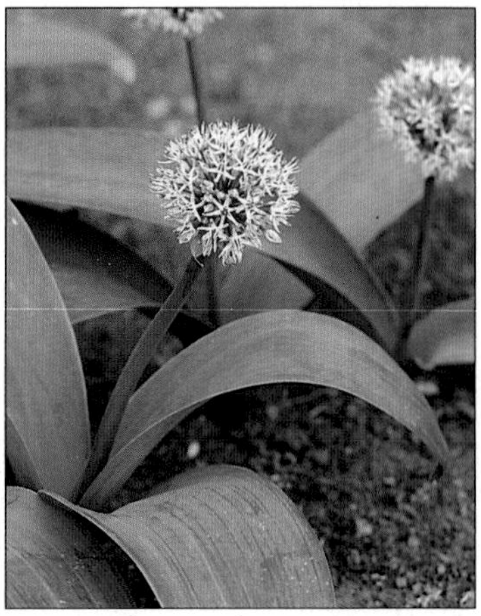

Allium karataviense

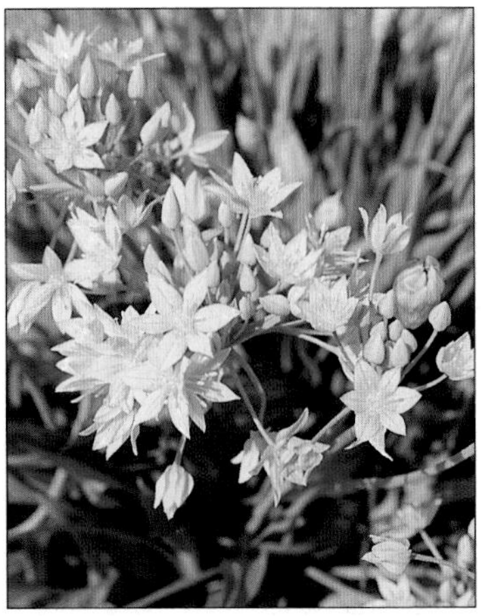

Allium moly

with red spots. ↕ 15–25cm (6–10in), ↔ 5cm (2in). S.W. China. ❄❄❄
A. moly ■ 🏆 (Golden garlic). Bulbous perennial with lance-shaped, grey-green, basal leaves, 20–30cm (8–12in) long, usually produced in pairs. In summer, bears dense umbels, 5cm (2in) across, of up to 30 star-shaped, bright golden yellow flowers. Increases rapidly and is ideal for naturalizing in light woodland or around shrubs. ↕ 15–25cm (6–10in), ↔ 5cm (2in). S.W. and S. Europe. ❄❄❄. **'Jeannine'** 🏆 flowers in early summer and has larger umbels, 8cm (3in) across, on stiff stems; ↕ 30–40cm (12–16in), ↔ 7cm (3in); Pyrenees.
A. multibulbosum see *A. nigrum.*
A. murrayanum see *A. unifolium.*
A. narcissiflorum, syn. *A. pedemontanum* of gardens. Bulbous perennial with short rhizomes and strap-shaped, grey-green, stem-sheathing leaves, 9–18cm (3½–7in) long. Pendent umbels, 2.5cm (1in) across, of up to 10 relatively large, bell-shaped, pink-purple flowers are borne in summer, followed by erect seed heads. Often confused with *A. insubricum*, which has fewer flowers and pendent seed heads. ↕ 15–35cm (6–14in), ↔ 5cm (2in). Portugal, France, N. Italy. ❄❄❄
A. neapolitanum ■ syn. *A. cowanii.* Bulbous perennial with linear-lance-shaped, mid-green, stem-sheathing leaves, 8–35cm (3–14in) long, which wither before flowering time. Umbels, 5cm (2in) across, of up to 30 star-shaped, pure white flowers are produced in summer. Excellent for cut flowers. ↕ 20–40cm (8–16in), ↔ 5cm (2in). S. Europe, N. Africa. ❄❄
A. neriniflorum see *Caloscordum neriniflorum.*
A. nigrum, syn. *A. multibulbosum.* Bulbous perennial with lance-shaped, grey-green, basal leaves, to 50cm (20in) long. In summer, bears flattish umbels, 7cm (3in) across, of 20–35 large, open cup-shaped flowers, usually creamy white, sometimes pale lilac, each with a prominent dark green ovary. ↕ 35cm (14in), ↔ 8cm (3in). Mediterranean. ❄❄
A. obliquum. Bulbous perennial with short rhizomes and linear, grey-green, stem-clasping leaves, to 35cm (14in) long. In midsummer, stiff stems bear dense umbels, 2.5cm (1in) across, of up to 50 or more cup-shaped, pale yellow-green flowers, with protruding stamens. ↕ 60cm (24in), ↔ 5cm (2in). Romania, C. Asia, Siberia. ❄❄

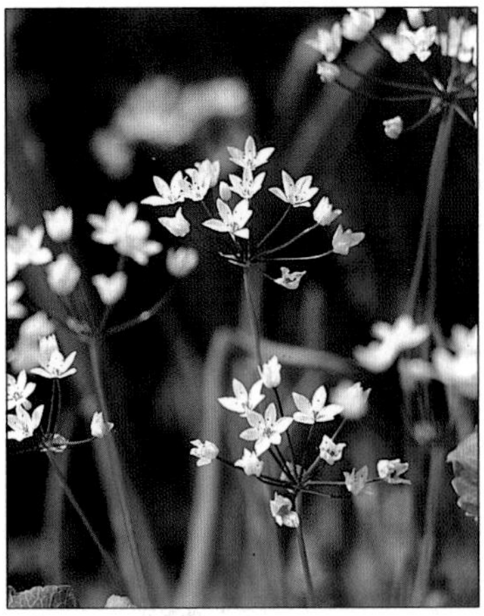

Allium neapolitanum

A. oreophilum ■ 🏆 syn. *A. ostrowskianum.* Bulbous perennial with linear, mid-green leaves, 10–15cm (4–6in) long, sheathing the lower part of the stems. In early summer, produces loose umbels, 4cm (1½in) across, of up to 15 long-lasting, bell-shaped, bright pinkish purple flowers. Each tepal has a darker midrib. ↕ 5–20cm (2–8in), ↔ 3cm (1¼in). Caucasus, C. Asia. ❄❄❄. **'Zwanenburg'** 🏆 has brighter, carmine-red flowers.
A. ostrowskianum see *A. oreophilum.*
A. oviflorum see *A. macranthum.*
A. paniculatum. Vigorous, bulbous perennial with linear, mid-green leaves, 25cm (10in) long, sheathing the lower part of the stems. In summer, bears ovoid umbels, 5cm (2in) across, of up to 40 bell-shaped, white, pink, or yellowish brown flowers, with prominent stamens; the flowers become pendent as they open. ↕ 30–70cm (12–28in), ↔ 5cm (2in). Europe, C. Asia. ❄❄❄
***A. pedemontanum* of gardens** see *A. narcissiflorum.*
A. pulchellum see *A. carinatum* subsp. *pulchellum.*
***A.* 'Purple Sensation'** 🏆 Bulbous perennial with long, strap-shaped, grey-green, basal leaves, 30–60cm (12–24in) long. In summer, bears umbels, 8cm (3in) across, of 50 or more star-shaped, deep violet flowers. Remove immature seed heads to prevent paler-flowered, self-sown seedlings. ↕ 1m (3ft), ↔ 7cm (3in). ❄❄❄
A. rosenbachianum ■ Bulbous perennial with ridged stems and long, strap-shaped, glaucous-green, basal leaves, 30–60cm (12–24in) long. In

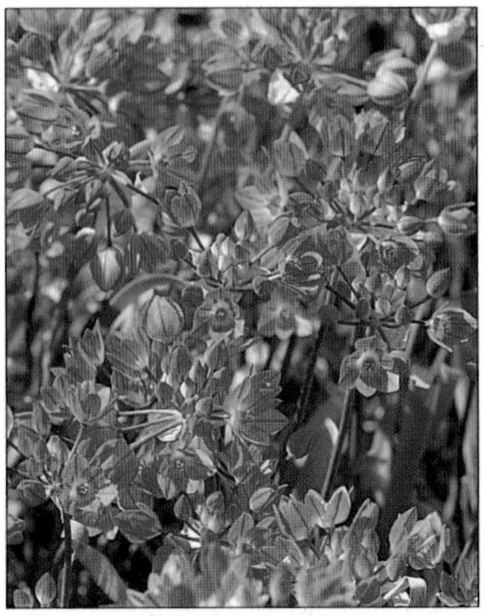

Allium oreophilum

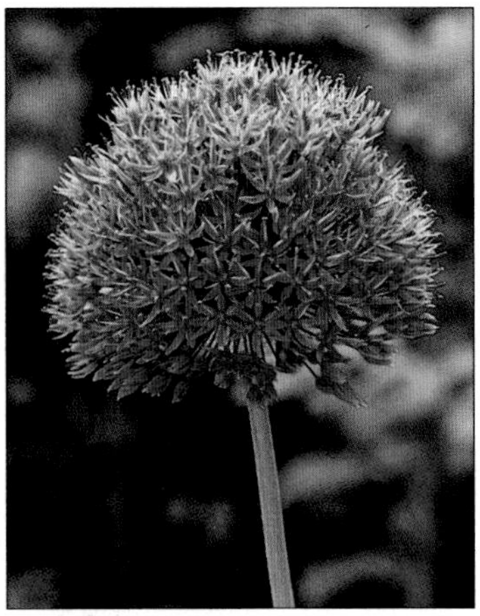

Allium rosenbachianum

summer, bears umbels, 10cm (4in) across, of 50 or more star-shaped, deep purple flowers with protruding violet stamens. Often confused with *A. stipitatum.* ↕ 1m (3ft), ↔ 10cm (4in). C. Asia. ❄❄
A. roseum (Rosy garlic). Very variable, bulbous perennial with linear, mid-green, basal leaves, 12–35cm (5–14in) long. In summer, bears small, loose umbels, 1cm (½in) across, of 5–25 cup-shaped, pale pink flowers, often with bulbils present. Few-flowered plants with many bulbils may be invasive and are best removed. ↕ 10–65cm (4–26in), ↔ 5cm (2in). S. Europe, N. Africa, Turkey. ❄❄❄
A. sativum (Garlic). Aromatic perennial grown for its ovoid bulbs, each comprising 5–18 bulblets enclosed by a papery tunic, and producing linear, grey-green leaves, to 60cm (24in) long, sheathing the lower part of the stems. In summer, hollow stems bear umbels, 2.5–5cm (1–2in) across, of 5–10 bell-shaped white flowers and many bulbils, and sometimes no flowers and only bulbils. ↕ to 1m (3ft), ↔ 23–30cm (9–12in). Probably C. Asia. ❄❄❄
A. schoenoprasum ■ (Chives). Bulbous perennial with short rhizomes, usually grown for its edible, cylindrical, hollow, dark green leaves, to 35cm (14in) long. Bears dense umbels, 2.5cm (1in) across, of up to 30 bell-shaped, pale purple, sometimes pure white flowers in summer. ↕ 30–60cm (12–24in), ↔ 5cm (2in). Europe, Asia, North America. ❄❄❄. **'Forescate'** ■ is vigorous, with deep bright purplish pink flowers; ↕ 60cm (24in), ↔ 7cm (3in).

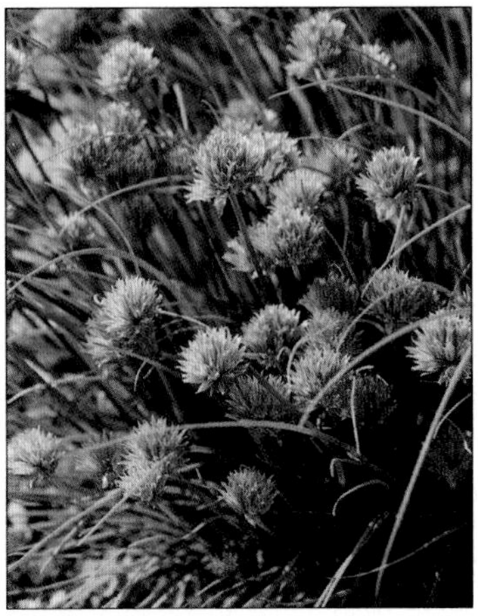

Allium schoenoprasum

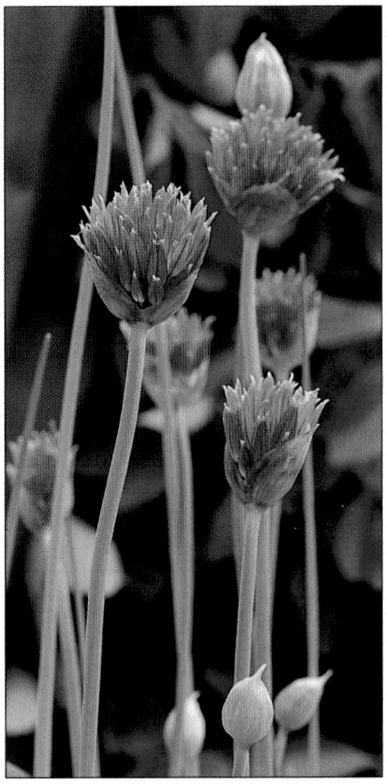

Allium schoenoprasum 'Forescate'

A. schubertii. Bulbous perennial with strap-shaped, bright green, basal leaves, 20–40cm (8–16in) long, which die back before flowering. Umbels, to 30cm (12in) across, of up to 50 star-shaped, pale purple flowers are borne on stalks of differing lengths in early summer. ↕ 30–60cm (12–24in), ↔ 20cm (8in). E. Mediterranean to C. Asia. ❄❄
A. senescens. Vigorous, bulbous perennial with short rhizomes and short strap-shaped, mid-green, basal leaves, 4–30cm (1½–12in) long. In mid- and late summer, bears dense umbels, 2cm (¾in) across, of up to 30 long-lasting, cup-shaped, pale to mid-purple-pink flowers. ↕ 8–60cm (3–24in), ↔ 5cm (2in). Europe, N. Asia. ❄❄❄. **var. *calcareum*** see subsp. *montanum.* **subsp. *montanum*** ■ syn. var. *calcareum*, has grey-green, often twisted leaves, and pink flowers; ↕ 45cm (18in). **subsp. *montanum* var. *glaucum***, syn. *A. spiralis*, a variant of the subspecies, has twisted grey leaves and bears bright pink flowers; ↕ 15cm (6in).
A. siculum see *Nectaroscordum siculum.*
A. sikkimense, syn. *A. kansuense*, *A. tibeticum.* Slender, bulbous perennial with short rhizomes and linear, mid-

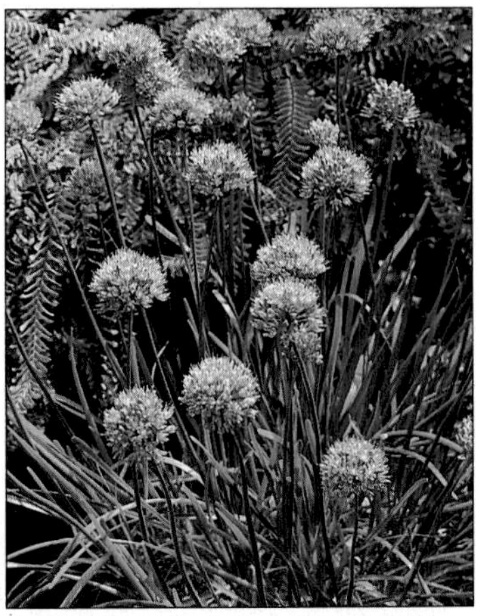

Allium senescens subsp. *montanum*

green, basal leaves, 30cm (12in) long. In early summer, bears nodding umbels, 2.5cm (1in) across, of up to 10 small, bell-shaped, bright blue, sometimes white flowers. ↕15–25cm (6–10in), ↔10cm (4in). W. China, Tibet, Nepal, India (Sikkim). ❄❄❄

A. sphaerocephalon (Round-headed leek). Bulbous perennial with linear, mid-green, basal leaves, to 35cm (14in) long. Ovoid umbels, 2.5cm (1in) across, of up to 40 tightly packed, bell-shaped flowers, varying from pink to dark red-brown, are produced in summer, and are sometimes accompanied by bulbils. ↕50–90cm (20–36in), ↔8cm (3in). Europe, N. Africa, W. Asia. ❄❄❄

A. spiralis see *A. senescens* subsp. *montanum* var. *glaucum.*

A. stipitatum. Bulbous perennial with ribbed stems and broadly strap-shaped, grey-green, basal leaves, 30–45cm (12–18in) long, hairy beneath. In early summer, bears tightly packed umbels, 10cm (4in) across, of 50 or more star-shaped, pale lilac flowers. Excellent for drying. Often confused with *A. rosenbachianum.* ↕1.4m (4½ft), ↔10cm (4in). C. Asia. ❄❄. **'Album'** has smaller heads of white flowers.

A. tibeticum see *A. sikkimense.*

A. tuberosum (Chinese chives). Fast-growing, bulbous perennial with short rhizomes and solid, linear, keeled, edible, mid-green basal and stem-sheathing leaves, to 35cm (14in) long. From late summer to autumn, bears many star-shaped, fragrant white flowers in umbels, 5cm (2in) across. ↕25–50cm (10–20in), ↔5cm (2in). S.E. Asia. ❄❄

A. unifolium ▣ syn. *A. murrayanum.* Bulbous perennial with short, linear, grey-green, basal leaves, 15–20cm (6–8in) long, that wither by flowering time. In spring, each stem produces a hemispherical umbel, 6cm (2½in) across, of up to 20 large, open bell-shaped, clear purple-pink flowers. ↕30cm (12in), ↔5cm (2in). USA (Oregon, California). ❄❄

A. wallichii. Bulbous perennial with short rhizomes and linear, keeled, mid-green basal and stem-clasping leaves, 60–90cm (24–36in) long. Many star-shaped purple flowers are borne in loose umbels, 5–7cm (2–3in) across, in late summer and early autumn. Bulbs are slender and poorly developed. ↕30–90cm (12–36in), ↔8cm (3in). Nepal to W. China. ❄❄❄

A. zebdanense. Bulbous perennial producing strap-shaped, mid-green, basal leaves, 10–30cm (4–12in) long. In spring, bears umbels, 3cm (1¼in) across, of 6–10 large, bell-shaped, lightly scented white flowers. ↕25–40cm (10–16in), ↔5cm (2in). Lebanon. ❄❄

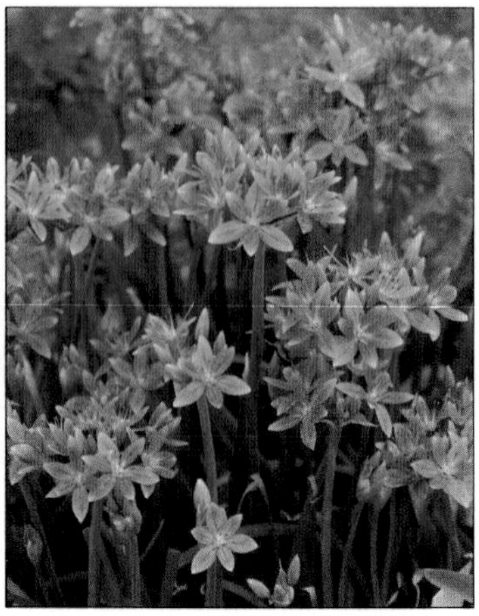

Allium unifolium

▷**Allspice** see *Calycanthus*
Californian see *C. occidentalis*
Carolina see *C. floridus*

ALLUAUDIA

DIDIEREACEAE

Genus of about 6 species of tree-like, perennial succulents from dry regions of S.W. and S. Madagascar. They have mainly thick, fleshy trunks and often thorny stems. The fleshy leaves are shed in dry periods and are apparent only during the growing season. The unisexual flowers are borne in umbel-like cymes. Where temperatures fall below 15°C (59°F), grow in a temperate or warm greenhouse. In warmer climates, grow in a desert garden.

- **HARDINESS** Frost tender.
- **CULTIVATION** Under glass, grow in loam-based potting compost (JI No.2), with up to 10 per cent each of added leaf mould and sharp sand, in full light. Water moderately in summer; keep almost dry at other times. Apply a balanced liquid fertilizer 2 or 3 times in the growing season. Outdoors, grow in sharply drained, humus-rich, slightly alkaline soil, with additional sharp sand, in partial shade. See also pp.48–49.
- **PROPAGATION** Sow seed at 19–24°C (66–75°F) as soon as ripe. Take stem cuttings in spring, and place in partial shade until rooted.
- **PESTS AND DISEASES** Trouble free.

A. comosa. Perennial succulent with 4 or 5 erect main branches and slender, twiggy, long-thorned stems bearing obovate to rounded, mid-green leaves, to 2cm (¾in) long, sometimes indented at the tips. Minute white flowers in small cymes, 4–8cm (1½–3in) across, are produced directly from branches, below a thorn, in summer. ↕to 20m (70ft), ↔1m (3ft). S.W. and S. Madagascar. ❀ (min. 15°C/59°F)

A. dumosa. Erect, freely branching succulent producing twig-like stems, with short, isolated thorns and cylindrical, mid-green leaves, 0.8–2cm (⅜–¾in) long, which soon fall. Cymes, 2cm (¾in) across, of tiny, pale pinkish white flowers are borne directly from branches in summer. ↕2–8m (6–25ft), ↔1.5m (5ft). S. Madagascar. ❀ (min. 15°C/59°F)

▷**Almond,**
Common see *Prunus dulcis*
Dwarf Russian see *Prunus tenella*
Flowering see *Prunus triloba*
Indian see *Terminalia catappa*

ALNUS

Alder

BETULACEAE

Genus of about 35 species of deciduous trees and shrubs from all parts of the N. hemisphere, usually found on poor or wet soils. Alders have alternate, simple, toothed leaves, and bear male and female flowers in separate catkins on the same tree. The male catkins are conspicuous; the females are smaller,

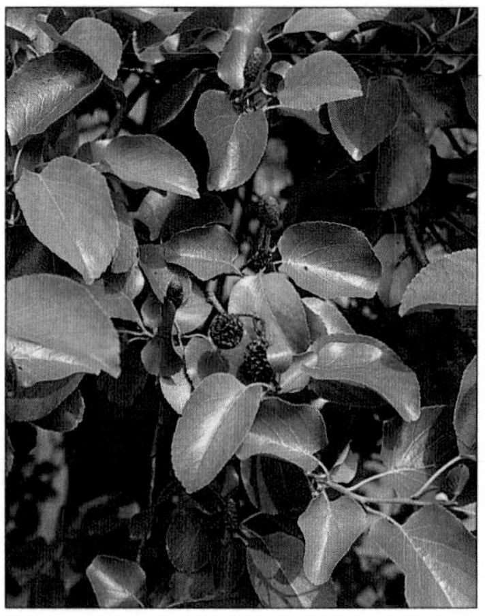

Alnus cordata

and after pollination develop into persistent, woody, cone-like green fruits, which turn brown in autumn. Some alders, such as *A. rubra* and selected forms of *A. cordata*, *A. glutinosa*, and *A. incana*, are grown for their ornamental foliage, and are particularly effective planted close to water. Most, however, are notable for their ability to thrive on poor, wet soils, and are widely used in land reclamation. *A. cordata*, *A. incana*, and *A. rubra* are fast-growing and valuable as windbreaks.

- **HARDINESS** Fully hardy.
- **CULTIVATION** Alders will thrive in moderately fertile, moist but well-drained soil in full sun; *A. cordata* and *A. incana* tolerate dry soils. Pruning group 1, between leaf fall and midwinter.
- **PROPAGATION** Sow seed in a seedbed as soon as ripe. Root hardwood cuttings in winter. Bud in late summer.
- **PESTS AND DISEASES** Prone to *Phytophthora* root rot.

A. cordata ▣ ♀ ♢ (Italian alder). Conical tree with broadly ovate, glossy, dark green leaves, heart-shaped at the bases, and to 10cm (4in) long. Groups of 3–6 pendent, yellow-brown male catkins, to 8cm (3in) long, open before the leaves, in late winter or early spring. Bears ovoid fruit, 2–3cm (¾–1¼in) long, in summer. ↕25m (80ft), ↔6m (20ft). Corsica, S. Italy. ❄❄❄

A. crispa see *A. viridis* subsp. *crispa.*

A. glutinosa ♢ (Common alder). Broadly conical tree with ovate, dark green leaves, to 10cm (4in) long, sticky when young. Groups of 3–5 pendent, yellow-brown male catkins, 10cm (4in) long, are produced in late winter or early spring. Bears ovoid fruit, 1–2cm (½–¾in) long, in summer. ↕25m (80ft), ↔10m (30ft). Europe, N. Africa, W. Asia. ❄❄❄. **'Aurea'** has yellow leaves that mature to light green; ↕12m (40ft), ↔5m (15ft). **'Imperialis'** ▣ ♀ has mid-green leaves with deeply cut lobes. **'Laciniata'** resembles 'Imperialis', but the leaves are more shallowly cut. **'Pyramidalis'** ⇑ is stiffly erect, with upright branches and dark green leaves; ↕15m (50ft), ↔5m (15ft).

A. incana ▣ ♢ (Grey alder). Conical tree with ovate, dark green leaves, to 10cm (4in) long, grey-white and hairy beneath. Clusters of 3 or 4 pendent, yellow-brown male catkins, to 10cm (4in) long, are borne in late winter and

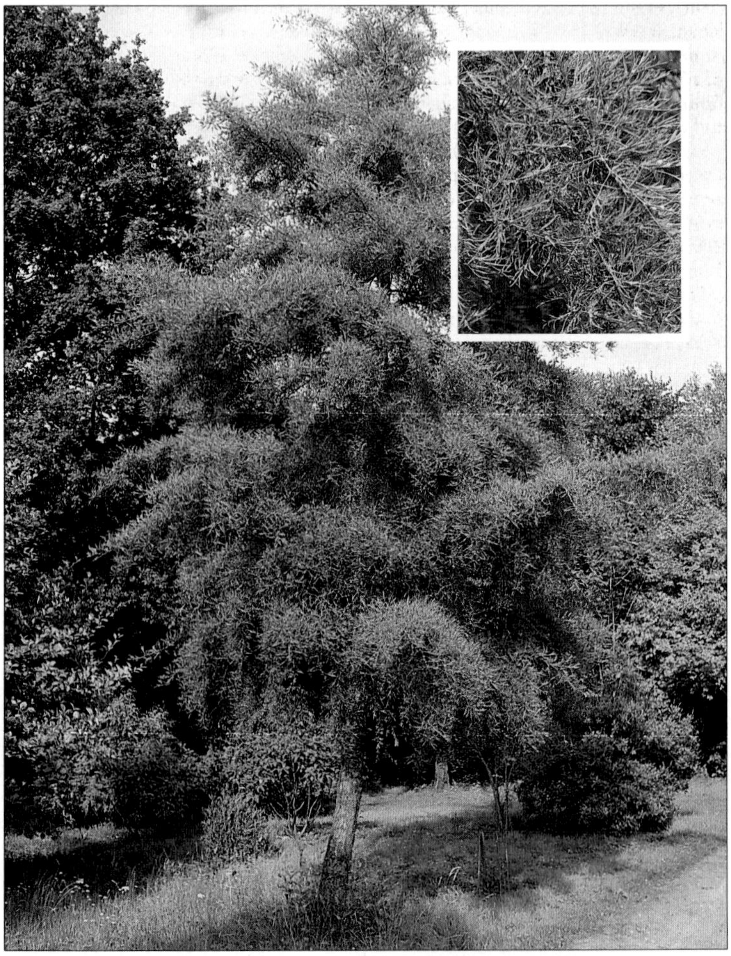

Alnus glutinosa 'Imperialis' (inset: leaf detail)

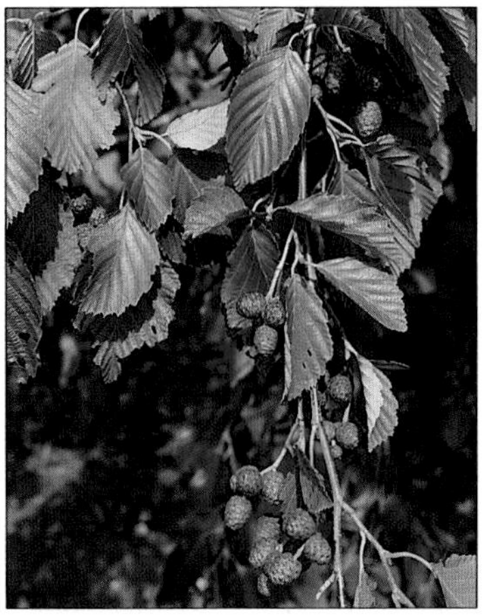
Alnus incana

early spring, before the leaves. Produces ovoid fruit, 1.5cm (½in) long, in summer. ↕20m (70ft), ↔10m (30ft). Europe, Caucasus. ❄❄❄. **'Aurea'** ■ ◊ has yellow leaves, pale green in summer, and orange shoots and catkins in winter; ↕10m (30ft), ↔5m (15ft). **'Laciniata'** ◊ has narrow-lobed leaves. **'Pendula'** ◊ has weeping branches; ↕10m (30ft), ↔6m (20ft). **'Ramulis Coccineis'** ◊ has yellow leaves in spring, red shoots and buds in winter, and orange catkins; ↕10m (30ft), ↔5m (15ft).
A. japonica ♤ (Japanese alder). Conical tree with narrowly ovate, glossy, dark green leaves, paler beneath, to 10cm (4in) long. Clusters of 4–8 pendent, yellow-brown male catkins, to 8cm (3in) long, open before the leaves in early spring. Ovoid fruit, 1.5–2.5cm (½–1in) long, are borne in summer. ↕20m (70ft), ↔8m (25ft). N. China, Korea, Japan. ❄❄❄
A. oregona see *A. rubra*.
A. rhombifolia ♀ (White alder). Rounded tree with spreading branches and arching shoot-tips. Ovate, glossy, dark green leaves, to 10cm (4in) long, are yellow-green beneath. Groups of 2–7 pendent, yellowish brown male catkins, to 10cm (4in) long, open before the leaves in early spring. Bears ovoid fruit, 1.5cm (½in) long, in summer. ↕25m (80ft), ↔20m (70ft). W. USA. ❄❄❄
A. rubra ♤ syn. *A. oregona* (Oregon alder, Red alder). Very vigorous, conical tree with semi-pendent shoots and ovate, red-veined, glossy, dark green leaves, to 10cm (4in) or more long. Clusters of 2–5 pendent yellow male catkins, to 15cm (6in) long, open in

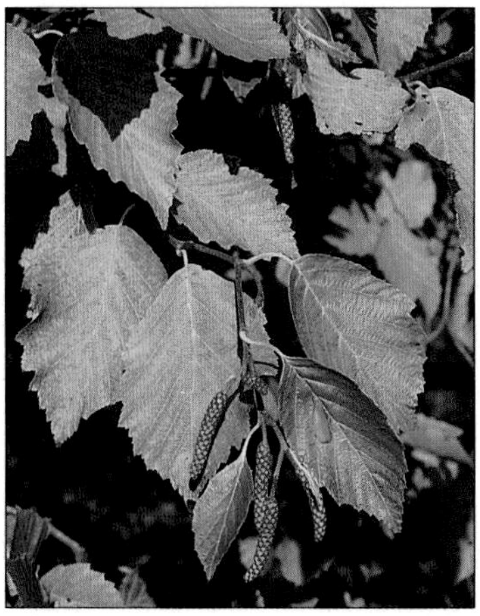
Alnus incana 'Aurea'

early spring, followed by ovoid-oblong fruit, 3cm (1¼in) long, in summer. ↕25m (80ft), ↔10m (30ft). W. North America. ❄❄❄
A. sinuata ◊ (Sitka alder). Narrowly conical tree, sometimes shrubby, with ovate, light green leaves, to 15cm (6in) long, glossy beneath and sticky when young. Bears clusters of 3–6 pendent yellow male catkins, to 12cm (5in) long, in spring, after the leaves; they are followed in summer by ellipsoid fruit, 1.5cm (½in) long. ↕10m (30ft), ↔4m (12ft). N.W. North America. ❄❄❄
A. tenuifolia ♀ (Mountain alder, Thinleaf alder). Spreading tree with a rounded head and red buds. Ovate leaves, to 10cm (4in) long, are dark green above and paler beneath. Pendent clusters of 3 or 4 small, yellow-brown male catkins, to 6cm (2½in) long, open in early spring, before the leaves. Produces narrowly ovoid fruit, 2cm (¾in) long, in summer. ↕↔8m (25ft). W. North America. ❄❄❄
A. viridis (Green alder). Upright shrub with ovate leaves, to 9cm (3½in) long, matt, mid-green above, glossy, yellow-green beneath. Groups of up to 10 stout, yellow-brown male catkins, to 8cm (3in) long, open in spring – erect at first, later pendent. In summer, bears ovoid fruit, to 1.5cm (½in) long. ↕3m (10ft), ↔2m (6ft). Europe. ❄❄❄. **subsp. *crispa***, syn. *A. crispa*, has slightly larger, fine-toothed, bright green leaves, to 8cm (3in) long; Canada, N.E. USA.

ALOCASIA

Elephant's ear plant

ARACEAE

Genus of about 70 species of large, evergreen, mainly rhizomatous, sometimes tuberous-rooted perennials, found in tropical forest and sunny, open or shaded, usually damp sites by streams and marshes in S. and S.E. Asia. They are cultivated for their large, usually peltate, heavily veined, oblong to ovate, arrow-shaped leaves, which are often marked in black, dark violet, or bronze, and have cylindrical leaf-stalks. The relatively insignificant spathes, borne at any time of year, are followed by clusters of red or orange fruits. In frost-prone areas, grow in a warm greenhouse; some species are suitable as houseplants. In frost-free areas, grow in a shady border. Contact with sap may irritate skin; all parts may cause mild stomach upset if ingested.

- **HARDINESS** Frost tender.
- **CULTIVATION** Under glass, grow in a mix of equal parts composted bark, loam, and sand, in filtered light. In the growing season, provide high humidity, water freely, and apply a balanced liquid fertilizer every 2–3 weeks; water moderately in winter. Outdoors, grow in moderately fertile, humus-rich, moist but well-drained soil in partial shade.
- **PROPAGATION** Sow seed at 23°C (73°F) as soon as ripe. Divide the rhizomes, or separate offsets, in spring or summer. Root stem cuttings in early spring.
- **PESTS AND DISEASES** Mealybugs may be a problem.

A. cuprea ■ Rhizomatous perennial with oblong-ovate leaf-blades, 45cm (18in) long, and leaf-stalks 60cm (24in)

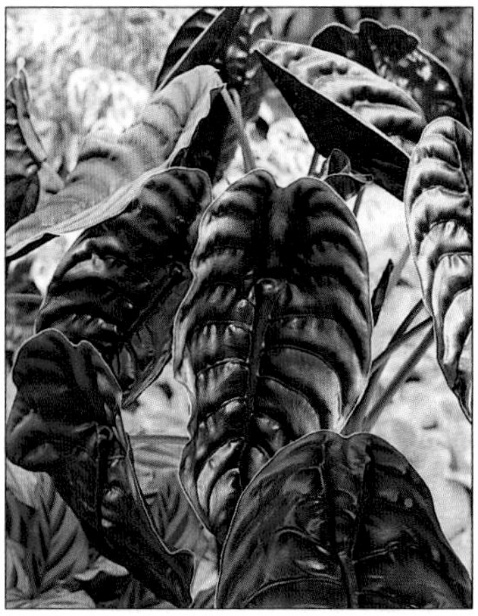
Alocasia cuprea

long. Upper leaf surfaces have dark green zones and midribs with copper-coloured areas in between; the undersides are reddish violet. Produces purple spathes, to 15cm (6in) long. ↕1m (3ft), ↔75cm (30in). Malaysia, Borneo. ❀ (min. 15–18°C/ 59–64°F)
***A. indica* var. *metallica* of gardens** see *A. plumbea*.
A. lowii* var. *veitchii see *A. veitchii*.
A. macrorrhiza ■ (Giant taro). Imposing, rhizomatous perennial with large, ovate, glossy, mid- to dark green leaves, arrow-shaped at the bases, with pale green veins, borne on "false stems" to 2m (6ft) long. Each leaf-blade is 1–1.2m (3–4ft) long, and each leaf-stalk 1.2m (4ft) long. Produces yellow-green spathes, to 20cm (8in) long. Widely cultivated in tropical areas for its edible rhizomes and shoots. ↕4–5m (12–15ft), ↔2–2.5m (6–8ft). India, Sri Lanka, Malaysia. ❀ (min. 15–18°C/59–64°F)
A. picta see *A. veitchii*.
A. plumbea, syn. *A. indica* var. *metallica* of gardens. Rhizomatous perennial producing purple or dark olive-green stems, and similarly coloured, ovate leaves that are arrow-shaped at the bases, with wavy margins, purple veins, and silvery purple beneath. Each leaf-blade is 1–1.2 (3–4ft) long, and each leaf-stalk 1.2 (4ft) long. Produces white spathes, 15–17cm (6–7in) long. ↕4–5m (12–15ft), ↔2–2.5m (6–8ft). Indonesia (Java). ❀ (min. 15–18°C/59–64°F)
A. sanderiana ■ (Kris plant). Rhizomatous perennial with arrow-shaped, dark green leaves, sometimes purple beneath, with wavy or deeply lobed silver margins, a metallic sheen,

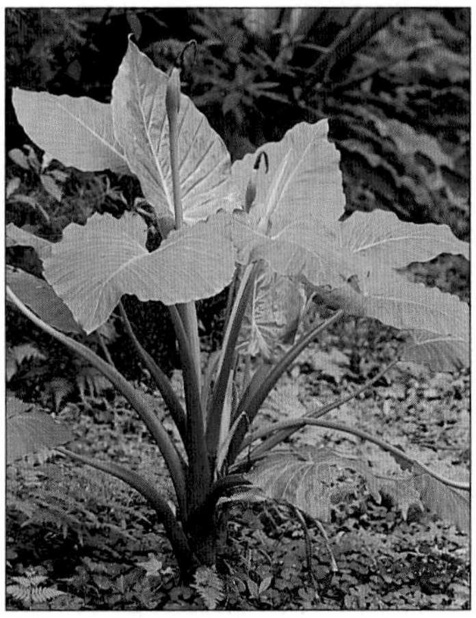
Alocasia macrorrhiza

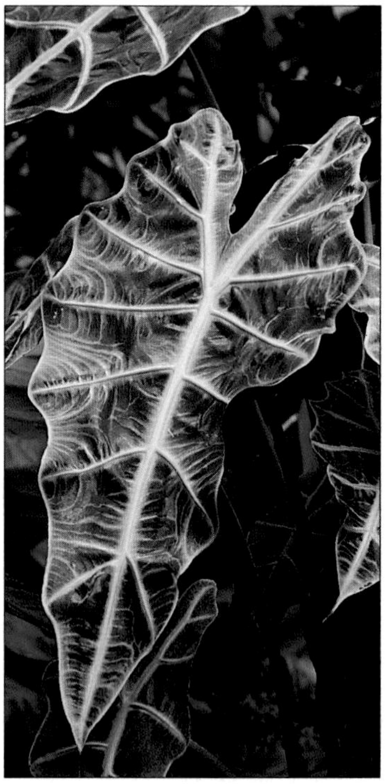
Alocasia sanderiana

and silver veins. Each leaf-blade is 30–40cm (12–16in) long, the leaf-stalk to 60cm (24in) long. The creamy white spathes are 12cm (5in) long. ↕2m (6ft), ↔ to 2m (6ft). Philippines (Mindanao). ❀ (min. 15–18°C/59–64°F)
A. veitchii, syn. *A. lowii* var. *veitchii*, *A. picta*. Rhizomatous perennial with very dark green, pointed, narrowly ovate-triangular leaves, arrow-shaped at the bases, with grey margins and veins, and red-purple beneath. Each leaf-blade is to 75cm (30in) long, the leaf-stalk 1.3m (4½ft) long. Produces yellowish green spathes, 11–12cm (4½–5in) long. ↕2–2.2m (6–7ft), ↔1.2m (4ft). Borneo. ❀ (min. 15–18°C/59–64°F)

ALOE

ALOEACEAE / LILIACEAE

Genus of about 300 species of small to large, rosetted, evergreen perennials. Some are shrub-like or climbing, a few tree-like. They are found at various altitudes in the Cape Verde Islands, tropical and southern Africa, Madagascar, and the Arabian Peninsula. Most have succulent leaves and axillary or terminal racemes or panicles of cylindrical to 3-angled, tubular, or bell-shaped flowers. The leaves of many *Aloe* species become suffused red in poor soils and dry conditions. The cylindrical or spherical fruits are papery or woody, and contain flat or angular seeds. Where temperatures fall below 10°C (50°F), grow in a cool or temperate greenhouse or as houseplants. In warmer climates, grow in a desert garden or in a border.

- **HARDINESS** Frost tender.
- **CULTIVATION** Under glass, grow in loam-based potting compost (JI No.2), with added sharp sand or perlite, in full light with good ventilation. Water moderately throughout the year, but sparingly when dormant. In the growing season, apply a balanced liquid fertilizer 2 or 3 times. Outdoors, grow in fertile, well-drained soil in full sun. See also pp.48–49.

• **PROPAGATION** Sow seed at 21°C (70°F) as soon as ripe. Separate offsets late spring or early summer. Insert unrooted offsets in standard cactus potting compost.
• **PESTS AND DISEASES** Prone to scale insects and mealybugs.

A. albiflora, syn. *Guillauminia albiflora.* Basal-rosetted, clump-forming succulent producing spirally arranged, linear, tapering, fleshy, dark green leaves, 12–15cm (5–6in) long, slightly grooved and rough, white-warty above and with small white marginal teeth. Terminal racemes, 60cm (24in) tall, of bell-shaped white flowers, to 1.5cm (½in) long, are borne in early summer. ↕ 15cm (6in), ↔ indefinite. Madagascar. ❄ (min. 10°C/50°F)
A. arabica see *A. vera.*
A. arborescens, syn. *A. perfoliata* var. *arborescens.* Tree-like, many-branched succulent with rosettes of sword-shaped, very fleshy, bright green leaves, to 60cm (24in) long, partly concave above, with wavy, toothed margins. Each rosette produces terminal racemes, to 30cm (12in) long, of cylindrical red flowers, to 4cm (1½in) long, in late spring and early summer. ↕ 2–4m (6–12ft), ↔ 2m (6ft). Malawi, Mozambique, Zimbabwe, South Africa. ❄ (min. 10°C/50°F). **'Variegata'** ▣ has yellow-striped leaves.
A. aristata ▣ syn. *A. ellenbergeri.* Stemless, clump-forming succulent with a dense rosette of lance-shaped, minutely toothed, white-margined, dark green leaves, 8–10cm (3–4in) long, cross-banded with very small white spots and soft white spines, particularly on the undersides. Terminal panicles, to 50cm (20in) long, and usually 2- to 6-branched, bear cylindrical, orange-red flowers, to 4cm (1½in) long, in autumn. ↕ to 12cm (5in), ↔ indefinite. E. and S. South Africa. ❄ (min. 10°C/50°F)
A. atherstonei see *A. pluridens.*
A. ausana see *A. variegata.*
A. bakeri ♀ Mat-forming succulent with clustered rosettes of very slender, linear, fleshy, white-mottled, greenish or reddish brown leaves, to 10cm (4in) long, sometimes partially banded red or pink, with softly toothed margins. In summer, bears tubular, green-tipped scarlet or yellowish orange flowers, 2cm (¾in) long, in axillary racemes, 30cm (12in) long. ↕ 10–20cm (4–8in), ↔ 40cm (16in). Madagascar. ❄ (min. 10°C/50°F)
A. barbadensis see *A. vera.*

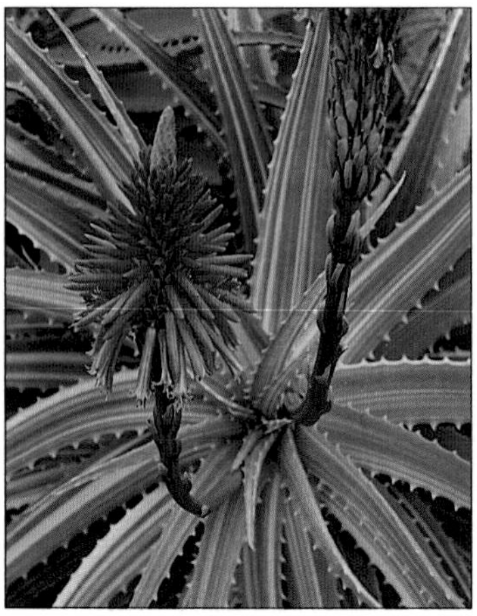

Aloe arborescens 'Variegata'

A. bellatula. Stemless, suckering succulent forming dense, rosetted clumps of linear to lance-shaped, grooved, warty, fleshy, dark green leaves, to 13cm (5in) long, spotted with pale green; the leaf margins are horny and minutely toothed. Terminal racemes, to 60cm (24in) long, with bell-shaped, coral-red flowers, to 1.5cm (½in) long, are produced throughout the summer. ↕ 15cm (6in), ↔ indefinite. Madagascar. ❄ (min. 10°C/50°F)
A. brevifolia, syn. *A. prolifera.* Stemless or short-stemmed succulent producing groups of compact rosettes with erect to spreading, triangular-lance-shaped, fleshy, glaucous leaves, 7–18cm (3–7in) long, with toothed margins. Each rosette bears an axillary raceme, 40–50cm (16–20in) long, of cylindrical red flowers, 4cm (1½in) long, in autumn. ↕ 10cm (4in), ↔ indefinite. South Africa (Western Cape). ❄ (min. 10°C/50°F)
A. ciliaris ▣ Scrambling or climbing succulent with freely branching, warty stems bearing narrowly lance-shaped, fleshy, dull green leaves, 10–15cm (4–6in) long, with white marginal teeth. Broadly cylindrical, axillary racemes, 15cm (6in) or more long, of tubular, curving, scarlet and greenish yellow flowers, 3cm (1¼in) long, are produced in summer. ↕ 5m (15ft). South Africa (Eastern Cape). ❄ (min. 10°C/50°F)
A. comptonii. Stemless or short-stemmed succulent with large, compact rosettes of upright, lance-shaped, fleshy, toothed, bluish green leaves, to 30cm (12in) long, concave above, keeled and spiny below. Terminal panicles, 80cm (32in) long, with 3–5 branches, bear

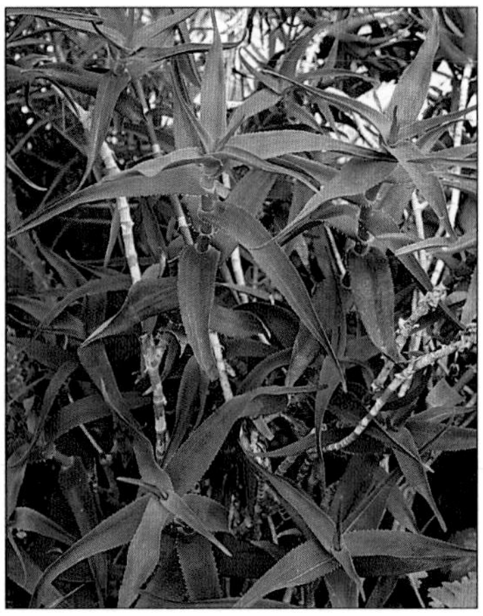

Aloe ciliaris

pendent, cylindrical scarlet flowers, 4cm (1½in) long, in autumn. ↕ 40cm (16in), ↔ indefinite. South Africa (Eastern and Western Cape). ❄ (min. 10°C/50°F)
A. descoingsii. Stemless, clump-forming succulent with rosettes of ovate, tapered, dull green leaves, 3–4cm (1¼–1½in) long, with small white tubercles on both surfaces, and incurved, toothed margins. Flattened racemes, to 15cm (6in) long, terminate in cylindrical to bell-shaped, deep red and yellowish orange flowers, 8mm (⅜in) long, in summer. ↕ 4–5cm (1½–2in), ↔ indefinite. Madagascar. ❄ (min. 10°C/50°F)
A. distans ▣ Trailing succulent with stems often 2–3m (6–10ft) long, and rooting at the nodes. Lance-shaped to broadly ovate, fleshy, white-spotted, bluish green leaves, 8cm (3in) long, are

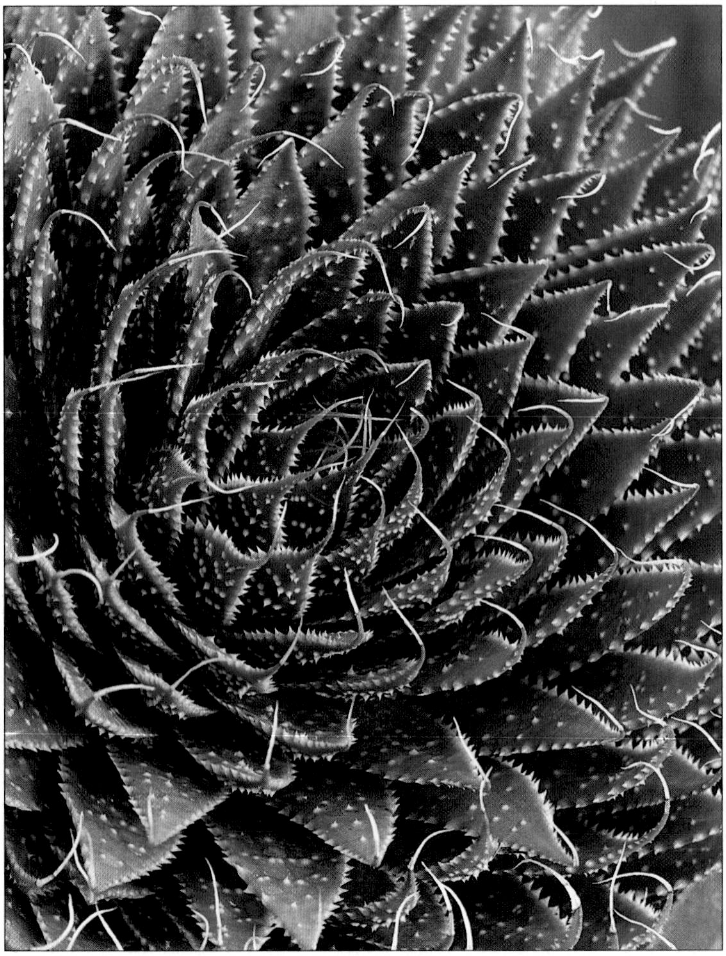

Aloe aristata

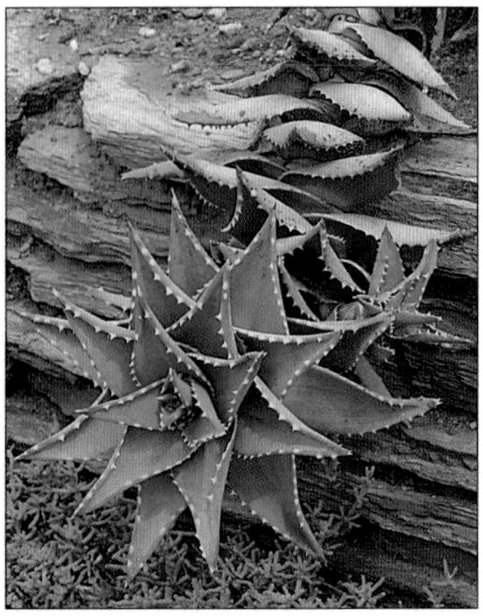

Aloe distans

sharply pointed and have horny yellow marginal teeth. In winter, panicles, 40–60cm (16–24in) long, with 3 or 4 branches, bear cylindrical, red and yellow flowers, 4cm (1½in) long, in terminal clusters. ↕ 50cm (20in), ↔ indefinite. South Africa (Western Cape). ❄ (min. 10°C/50°F)
A. ellenbergeri see *A. aristata.*
A. excelsa. Tree-like succulent with very thick stems bearing dense rosettes of lance-shaped, fleshy, dull green leaves, 60–65cm (24–26in) long, with toothed margins and undersides. Each rosette has 1 or 2 many-branched panicles, to 1.3m (4½ft) tall, bearing terminal clusters of cylindrical, orange-red to rich scarlet flowers, to 3cm (1¼in) long, in summer. ↕ 6–9m (20–28ft), ↔ 75cm (30in). Zimbabwe. ❄ (min. 10°C/50°F)
A. ferox ▣ syn. *A. galpinii, A. socotrina, A. supralaevis.* Single-stemmed, tree-like succulent crowned by a rosette of narrowly to broadly lance-shaped, fleshy, sometimes red-tinged, dull green leaves, to 1m (3ft) long, hairless or spiny above, spiny beneath, and with red marginal teeth. Erect, terminal panicles with 5–10 branches, 30–80cm (12–32in) long, covered with tubular, scarlet-orange flowers, 2–3cm (¾–1¼in) long, are produced in summer. ↕ 2–3m (6–10ft), ↔ 1.5m (5ft). South Africa (Northern Cape, Eastern Cape, Western Cape). ❄ (min. 10°C/50°F)
A. galpinii see *A. ferox.*
A. haemanthifolia. Stemless, suckering succulent with 2-ranked, broadly strap-shaped, round-tipped, fleshy, grey-green to bluish green leaves, to 20cm (8in) long, which are concave above and have

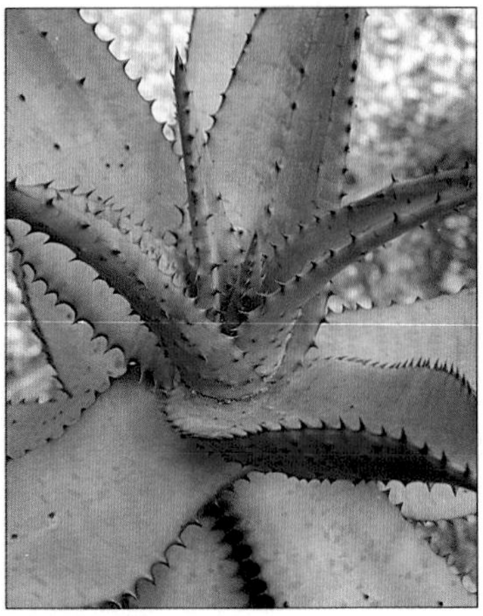

Aloe ferox

red margins. The flattened, terminal racemes, 30–45cm (12–18in) long, produce clusters of tubular, stiffly pendent scarlet flowers, 4cm (1½in) long, in autumn. ↕ 20cm (8in), ↔ to 50cm (20in). South Africa (Eastern and Western Cape). ❄ (min. 10°C/50°F)
A. haworthioides ■ syn. *Aloinella haworthioides.* Stemless, suckering succulent with dense rosettes of lance-shaped, fleshy, white-warty, grey-green leaves, 3–6cm (1¼–2½in) long, suffused red in dry conditions; each has a terminal spine and white marginal teeth. Bears terminal racemes, to 30cm (12in) long, of tubular orange flowers, 8mm (⅜in) long, with projecting stamens, in summer. ↕ 6cm (2½in), ↔ 10cm (4in). Madagascar. ❄ (min. 10°C/50°F)
A. indica see *A. vera.*
A. jucunda. Stemless or short-stemmed, clump-forming succulent with rosettes of ovate, recurved, fleshy, deep green leaves, 4cm (1½in) long. These are brown-tinged towards the tips and have pale green and white spots, and reddish brown marginal teeth. In summer, bears sublateral racemes, to 30cm (12in) long, of cylindrical, pale pink flowers, 2cm (¾in) long. ↕ to 5cm (2in), ↔ indefinite. Somalia. ❄ (min. 10°C/50°F)
A. marlothii. Tree-like succulent with persistent old leaves, on a thick stem crowned with a dense rosette of semi-erect, broadly lance-shaped, fleshy, mid-green or glaucous, grey-green leaves, 1m (3ft) long; both upper and lower surfaces and margins are spiny. Many-branched, dense, terminal panicles, to 80cm (32in) or more long, of cylindrical, yellowish orange flowers, to 3cm (1¼in) long, are borne in summer. ↕ to 4m (12ft), ↔ 1.5m (5ft). Botswana, E. South Africa. ❄ (min. 10°C/50°F)
A. mitriformis ■ syn. *A. xanthocantha.* Variable, clump-forming succulent with thick, nearly erect or horizontal stems bearing terminal rosettes of ovate-lance-shaped, fleshy, bluish green leaves, 45cm (18in) long, keeled beneath, and suffused red in poor soil conditions.

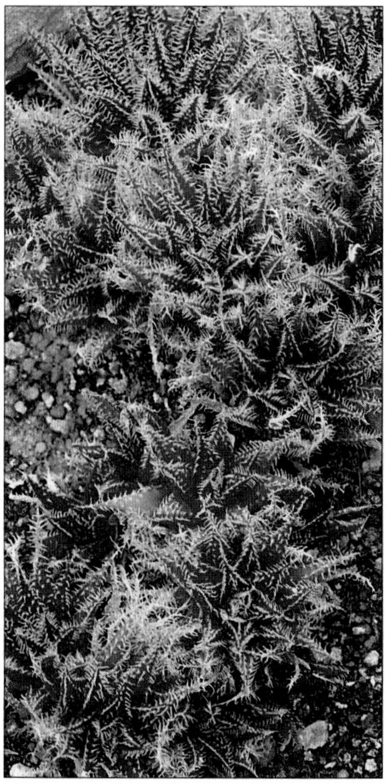

Aloe haworthioides

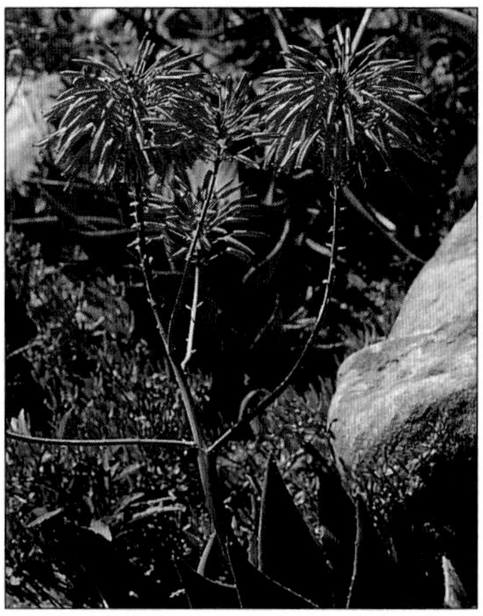

Aloe mitriformis

Both keel and leaf margins are yellow-toothed. In winter, broadly conical, occasionally branched, axillary racemes, 40–60cm (16–24in) long, of tubular, dull scarlet flowers, 4–5cm (1½–2in) long, are borne on branched stems. ↕ to 2m (6ft), ↔ indefinite. South Africa (Western Cape). ❄ (min. 10°C/50°F)
A. niebuhriana. Stemless, suckering, semi-prostrate succulent with rosettes of lance-shaped, fleshy, grey-green leaves, 45–60cm (18–24in) long, purple-flushed above, with close-set marginal teeth. In summer, bears dense, broadly conical, occasionally branched, axillary racemes, 1m (3ft) tall, of slightly pendent, tubular, scarlet or greenish yellow flowers, to 3cm (1¼in) long. ↕ to 60cm (24in), ↔ 80cm (32in). S.W. Arabian Peninsula. ❄ (min. 10°C/50°F)
A. paniculata see *A. striata.*
A. perfoliata* var. *arborescens see *A. arborescens.*
A. platyphylla see *A. zebrina.*
A. pluridens ■ syn. *A. atherstonei.* Tree-like succulent with simple or branching stems, each crowned by a dense rosette of strap-shaped, recurved, fleshy, pale green or yellowish green leaves, 70–80cm (28–32in) long, with horny, grooved white marginal teeth. Conical, axillary racemes, to 80cm (32in) long, of cylindrical, rose-pink to scarlet flowers, 3.5–4.5cm (1½–1¾in) long, are borne in spring. ↕ 2–3m (6–10ft), ↔ 1m (3ft). South Africa (Eastern Cape). ❄ (min. 10°C/50°F)
A. prolifera see *A. brevifolia.*
A. punctata see *A. variegata.*
A. rauhii 🏆 Stemless, clump-forming succulent with rosettes of spreading,

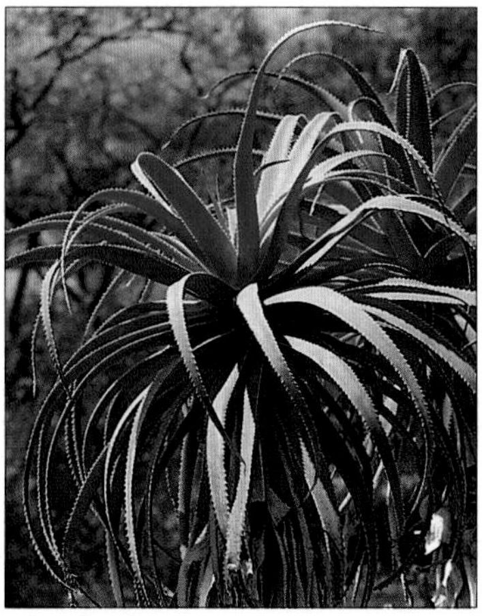

Aloe pluridens

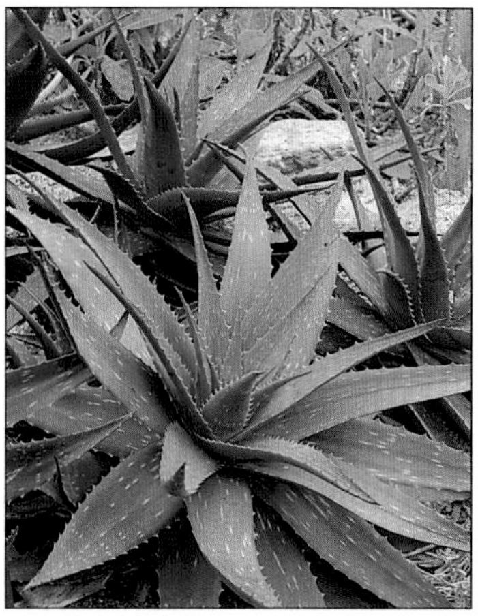

Aloe saponaria

lance-shaped, fleshy, grey-green leaves, to 10cm (4in) long. They are sometimes tinged brown, with H-shaped markings and minute white marginal teeth. In summer, produces tubular, rose-scarlet flowers, 2.5cm (1in) long, in cylindrical, terminal racemes, to 30cm (12in) long. ↕ 10–15cm (4–6in), ↔ indefinite. Madagascar. ❄ (min. 10°C/50°F)
A. saponaria ■ Stemless or short-stemmed, suckering succulent with solitary or multiple rosettes of toothed, lance-shaped, pale to dark green leaves, 20cm (8in) or more long, with oblong white marks. In summer, bears terminal panicles, 40–60cm (16–24in) long, with up to 3 branches, of cylindrical red to yellow flowers, 3.5–4.5cm (1½–1¾in) long. ↕ 70cm (28in), ↔ indefinite. E. South Africa. ❄ (min. 10°C/50°F)
A. socotrina see *A. ferox.*
A. striata ■ syn. *A. paniculata.* Almost stemless succulent with a dense rosette of lance-shaped, fleshy, white-margined leaves, 45cm (18in) or more long. They are often reddish green, indistinctly spotted and striped, and with a waxy white bloom. Corymb-like, many-branched, terminal panicles, to 1m (3ft) long, of tubular, orange-red flowers, 2.5cm (1in) long, are borne in summer. ↕ 1m (3ft), ↔ 85cm (34in). S.W. to southern Africa. ❄ (min. 10°C/50°F)
A. supralaevis see *A. ferox.*
A. variegata ■ 🏆 syn. *A. ausana, A. punctata* (Partridge-breasted aloe). Stemless, stoloniferous succulent, forming dense clumps, with rosettes of semi-erect, overlapping, lance-shaped, fleshy, dark green leaves, 12cm (5in) long. They are V-shaped in cross-

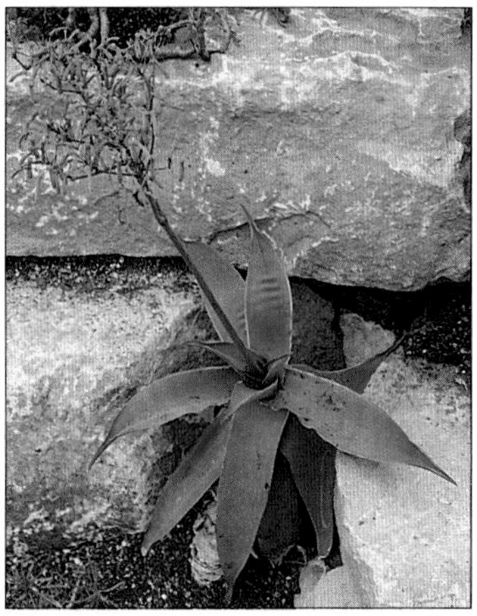

Aloe striata

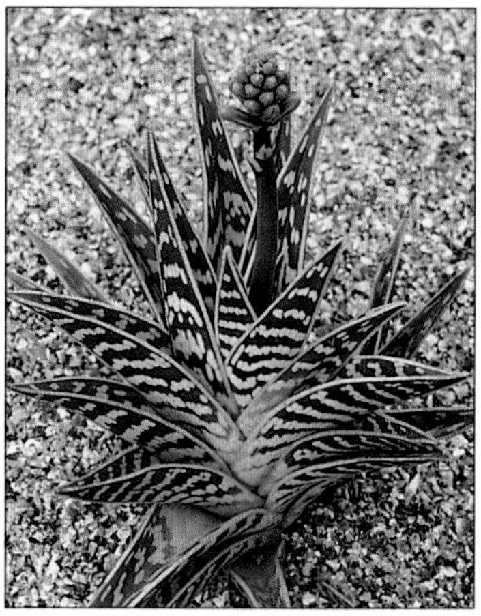

Aloe variegata

section, with irregular white cross-bands and small white marginal teeth. Each rosette produces axillary racemes, 30cm (12in) long, sometimes branched, of pendent, tubular, pink or scarlet flowers, 3–4.5cm (1¼–1¾in) long, in summer. ↕ 20cm (8in), ↔ indefinite. South Africa. ❄ (min. 10°C/50°F)
A. vera ■ 🏆 syn. *A. arabica, A. barbadensis, A. indica.* Clump-forming, suckering succulent producing basal rosettes of lance-shaped, fleshy, grey-green leaves, 45cm (18in) long, slightly grooved above, with toothed pink margins. In summer, bears tubular yellow flowers, to 3cm (1¼in) long, in terminal racemes, 90cm (36in) or more long, sometimes with up to 4 branches. ↕ 60cm (24in), ↔ indefinite. Origin unknown, but widespread in tropical and subtropical regions. ❄ (min. 10°C/50°F)
A. xanthocantha see *A. mitriformis.*
A. zebrina, syn. *A. platyphylla.* Usually stemless succulent with rosettes of linear-lance-shaped, fleshy, powdery glaucous, sometimes red-flushed, dark green leaves, to 30cm (12in) long, with stout brown marginal teeth and white-spotted cross-banding. Many-branched, erect, terminal panicles, 1–1.5m (3–5ft) long, of cylindrical, deep red or orange-red flowers, 3–3.5cm (1¼–1½in) long, are produced in spring. ↕ 30cm (12in), ↔ 80cm (32in). S.W. to southern Africa. ❄ (min. 10°C/50°F)

▷**Aloe, Partridge-breasted** see *Aloe variegata*
▷***Aloinella haworthioides*** see *Aloe haworthioides*

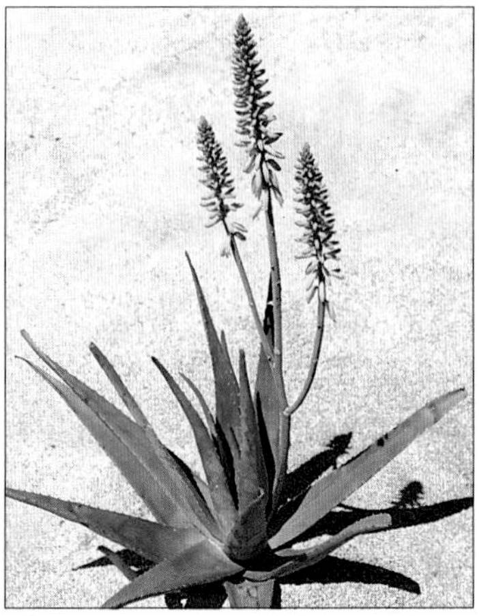

Aloe vera

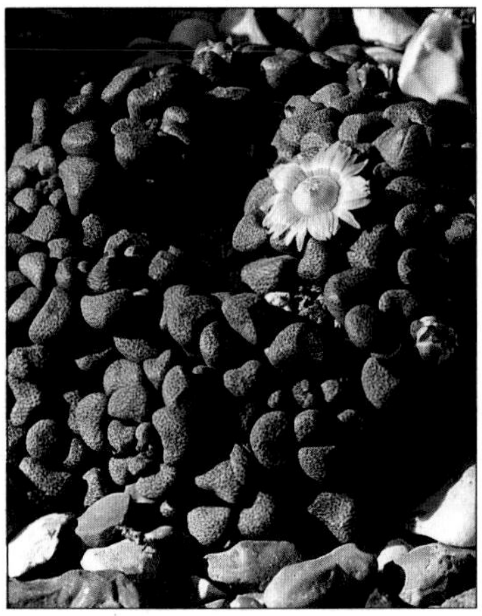

Aloinopsis schooneesii

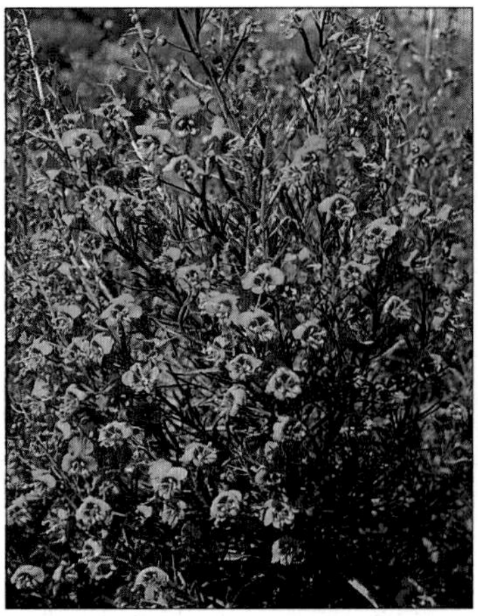

Alonsoa linearis

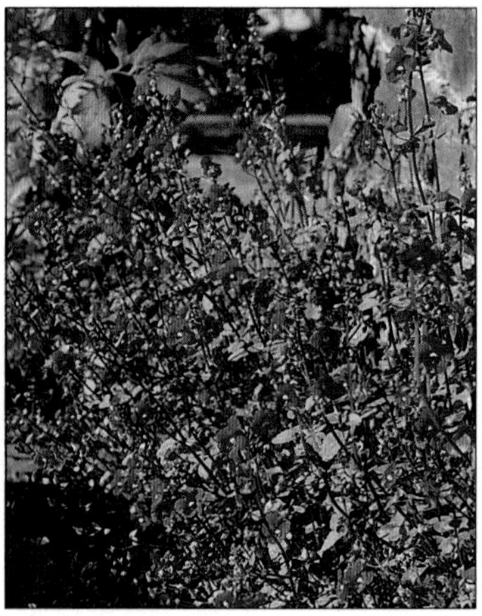

Alonsoa warscewiczii

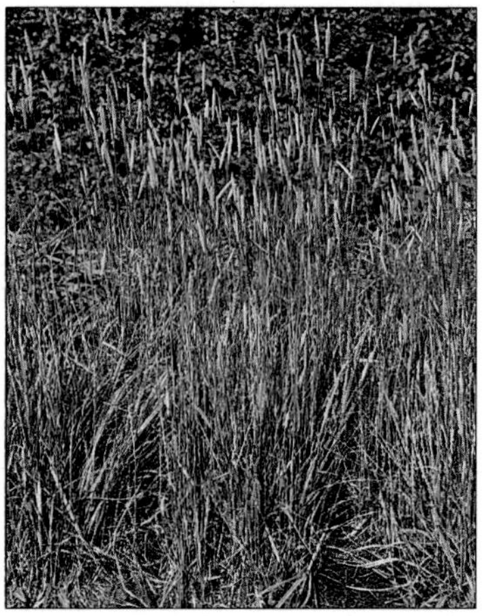

Alopecurus pratensis 'Aureovariegatus'

ALOINOPSIS

AIZOACEAE

Genus of 10–15 species of dwarf, fleshy- or tuberous-rooted, tufted, perennial succulents, closely related to *Nananthus* and *Titanopsis*, from low, hilly areas of South Africa. Most species have loose, basal rosettes of warty leaves and bear usually solitary, stalked, 2-bracted, many-petalled flowers in late autumn; the flowers open in late afternoon or early evening. Below 10°C (50°F), grow in a temperate greenhouse; in warm, dry areas, grow in a raised bed or border.
• **HARDINESS** Frost tender.
• **CULTIVATION** Under glass, grow in standard cactus compost in full light. In the growing season, water moderately and apply a half-strength, balanced liquid fertilizer 2 or 3 times; keep almost dry in winter. Outdoors, grow in sharply drained soil in full sun. See also pp.48–49.
• **PROPAGATION** Sow seed at 21°C (70°F) in early spring. Take stem or leaf cuttings in late spring or early summer; root in equal parts fine peat and sand in partial shade.
• **PESTS AND DISEASES** Vulnerable to mealybugs and root mealybugs.

A. rubrolineata, syn. *Nananthus rubrolineata.* Fleshy-rooted succulent producing rosettes of 4–6 ovate, slightly recurved, dull, mid-green leaves, 2.5cm (1in) long. Bears daisy-like yellow flowers, 2.5cm (1in) across, with a central red stripe along each petal. ↕ 3cm (1¼in), ↔ to 25cm (10in). South Africa. ⚘ (min. 10°C/50°F)
A. schooneesii, syn. *Nananthus schooneesii* ■ Tuberous-rooted succulent with irregular rosettes of 8–10 roughly diamond-shaped, dark green leaves, to 1.5cm (½in) long. Yellowish red flowers, 1cm (½in) across, are silky and daisy-like. ↕ 2cm (¾in), ↔ 30cm (12in). South Africa. ⚘ (min. 10°C/50°F)

ALONSOA

Mask flower

SCROPHULARIACEAE

Genus of about 12 species of evergreen shrubs, subshrubs, and perennials from stony slopes and scrub in tropical and subtropical W. South America. The leaves are arranged in opposite pairs or in whorls of 3, on 4-angled, branching, slender shoots, and often alternately on the flowering shoots. Delicate, spurred, unequally 2-lipped, orange or red, sometimes white flowers are borne in spring and autumn in lax, terminal racemes. Use as colourful winter-flowering container plants in a temperate greenhouse or conservatory, as summer bedding, or in a mixed border. They also provide good cut flowers. Modern, compact-growing seed selections for bedding are now available. The species described are usually grown as annuals.
• **HARDINESS** Half hardy.
• **CULTIVATION** Under glass, grow in loam-based potting compost (JI No.2) in full light with a minimum of 10°C (50°F). Water moderately. Outdoors, grow in any fertile, well-drained soil in full sun.
• **PROPAGATION** Sow seed at 15–18°C (59–64°F) in early spring; plant out in late spring. Sow seed in late summer for winter-flowering container plants. Root semi-ripe cuttings in late summer.
• **PESTS AND DISEASES** Aphids may be a problem, particularly under glass.

A. acutifolia, syn. *A. myrtifolia.* Erect, spreading subshrub with lance-shaped, pointed, toothed, downy, dark green leaves, 2–3cm (¾–1¼in) long. Lax racemes of spurred, orange or deep red flowers, 2–2.5cm (¾–1in) across, are produced continuously throughout summer. ↕ 50–90cm (20–36in), ↔ 15–23cm (6–9in). Andes in Peru and Bolivia. ✻. **var. *candida***, syn. *A. albiflora* of gardens, has white flowers.
***A. albiflora* of gardens** see *A. acutifolia* var. *candida.*
A. caulialata see *A. meridionalis.*
A. grandiflora see *A. warscewiczii.*
A. linearis ■ syn. *A. linifolia.* Erect, moderately compact subshrub with linear to ovate to lance-shaped, pointed, entire or minutely toothed, dark green leaves, to 4cm (1½in) long. Lax racemes of spurred, brick-red flowers, 2–2.5cm (¾–1in) across, with black-spotted throats, are borne for much of the summer. Useful for cutting. ↕ to 1m (3ft), ↔ 30cm (12in). Peru, Chile. ✻
A. linifolia see *A. linearis.*
A. meridionalis, syn. *A. caulialata.* Bushy, red-stemmed perennial or subshrub with ovate to lance-shaped, pointed, toothed, mid-green leaves, to 3.5cm (1½in) long. Lax racemes of spurred, orange or deep red flowers, to 2cm (¾in) across, are borne in summer. Useful for cut flowers. ↕ 30–90cm (12–36in), ↔ 30cm (12in). Colombia, Peru. ✻. Cultivars in **Firestone Jewels Series** produce scarlet, orange, salmon-pink, pink, or white flowers, with red shades predominating; selected cultivars are also available from seed.
A. myrtifolia see *A. acutifolia.*
A. warscewiczii ■ 🏆 syn. *A. grandiflora.* Bushy, compact, red-stemmed perennial or subshrub with ovate to lance-shaped, toothed, dark green leaves, to 4cm (1½in) long, heart-shaped at the bases. From summer to autumn, bears lax racemes of spurred, scarlet, sometimes white flowers, 1.5–2cm (½–¾in) wide. ↕ 45–60cm (18–24in), ↔ 30cm (12in). Peru. ✻

ALOPECURUS

Foxtail grass

GRAMINEAE/POACEAE

Genus of 25–40 species of annual and perennial grasses from meadows and pastures, occasionally scree and rocky sites, in N. temperate regions. They produce tufts of usually flat, sometimes channelled leaves and dense, terminal panicles of cylindrical, single-flowered spikelets. Some are important fodder crops; several have ornamental foliage and are suitable for a rock garden or mixed border.
• **HARDINESS** Fully hardy.
• **CULTIVATION** Grow in gritty soil in a sunny scree bed or trough with a top-dressing of grit, or in a mix of equal parts loam, leaf mould, and grit in an alpine house. *A. lanatus* does not tolerate wet conditions in winter. *A. pratensis* 'Aureovariegatus' thrives in fertile, well-drained soil in sun or partial shade. Clip back in spring for best foliage effect.
• **PROPAGATION** Sow seed in containers in a cold frame when ripe, or in spring. Divide with care in spring or early summer.
• **PESTS AND DISEASES** Trouble free.

A. lanatus (Woolly foxtail grass). Densely tufted perennial producing linear, often channelled, white-woolly, blue-green leaves, to 5cm (2in) long, appearing silvery grey overall. Bears ovoid-spherical, densely hairy, light green panicles, to 2cm (¾in) long by 1.5cm (½in) wide, from mid-spring to midsummer. ↕ to 10cm (4in), ↔ 12cm (5in). E. Mediterranean, Turkey. ✻✻✻
***A. pratensis* 'Aureovariegatus'** ■ Spreading, but not invasive perennial with striped, rich yellow and green, linear leaves, 5–6cm (2–2½in) long, arranged in basal tufts. Produces dense, cylindrical, pale green to purple panicles, to 10cm (4in) long by 1cm (½in) across, from mid-spring to mid-summer. ↕ to 1.2m (4ft), ↔ 40cm (16in) or more. ✻✻✻

▷ ***Alophia lahue*** see *Herbertia lahue*

ALOYSIA

VERBENACEAE

Genus of 37 species of deciduous or evergreen shrubs from warm areas of North and South America, favouring dry, rocky soils. The simple leaves are aromatic, and opposite or whorled, and small, salverform flowers are borne in slender, spike-like panicles or racemes. *A. triphylla* (Lemon verbena) is cultivated for its strongly lemon-scented foliage, which is used for culinary purposes or in pot-pourri. In frost-prone areas, grow in a cool greenhouse or at the base of a warm, sheltered wall. In frost-free areas, grow in a sunny border.
• **HARDINESS** Frost hardy to frost tender.
• **CULTIVATION** Under glass, grow in loam-based potting compost (JI No.2) in full light. In the growing season, water moderately and apply a balanced liquid fertilizer monthly; keep just moist in winter. Outdoors, grow in well-drained, poor, dry soil in full sun. Mulch in autumn to protect the roots. Pick and dry leaves in summer before flowering. Pruning group 6, or 13 if wall-trained.
• **PROPAGATION** Root softwood or greenwood cuttings in summer.
• **PESTS AND DISEASES** Trouble free.

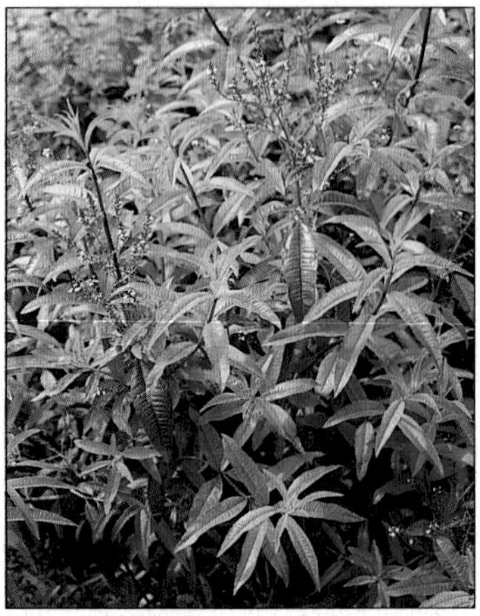

Aloysia triphylla

A. citriodora see *A. triphylla.*
A. triphylla ■ ♀ syn. *A. citriodora, Lippia citriodora* (Lemon verbena). Bushy, upright, deciduous shrub with whorled, narrow, lance-shaped, lemon-scented, rough, bright green leaves, to 10cm (4in) long. Bears tiny, pale lilac to white flowers in slender panicles, to 12cm (5in) long, in late summer. ↕↔ 3m (10ft). Chile, Argentina. ❄❄

▷ **Alpenrose** see *Rhododendron ferrugineum*
▷ **Alpine chrysanthemum** see *Leucanthemopsis alpina*

ALPINIA
Ginger lily

ZINGIBERACEAE

Genus of about 200 species of rhizomatous, evergreen, clump-forming perennials from open forest and forest margins in moist tropical areas of India, China, S.E. Asia, and Australia. The ginger-scented rhizomes give rise to slender but strong, reed-like stems, to 3m (10ft) high, which bear 2-ranked, lance-shaped leaves and a panicle or raceme of showy, narrowly bell-shaped, slightly hooded flowers; these each have a 3-lobed calyx and a 3-petalled corolla, with a 2-lobed lip, enclosed in prominent bracts. The fruits are ovoid or spherical capsules. In frost-prone areas, grow smaller species in a warm greenhouse or conservatory, preferably in a border, so their growth is not restricted; they may be difficult to grow in containers. In frost-free areas, they are best grown in a shady border.

• **HARDINESS** Frost tender.
• **CULTIVATION** Under glass, grow in loam-based potting compost (JI No.3), with up to 25 per cent each added leaf mould and composted bark, in bright filtered light. In the growing season, water freely and apply a balanced liquid fertilizer every month; water moderately in winter. Pot on container-grown plants, and cut out flowered stems in spring. Outdoors, grow in moist, fertile, humus-rich soil in partial shade.
• **PROPAGATION** Sow seed as soon as ripe at 20°C (68°F), or divide in spring. Treat plantlets produced in the inflorescence of *A. purpurata* as offsets.
• **PESTS AND DISEASES** Trouble free.

A. calcarata (Indian ginger). Slender, upright perennial with narrowly lance-shaped, stalkless, glossy, mid-green leaves, 30cm (12in) long, with minute, well-spaced bristles on the margins. Yellow flowers, 4–5cm (1½–2in) long, with lower petals veined dark red or maroon, are usually borne in pairs in spreading or more or less erect panicles, 10–13cm (4–5in) long, in summer. ↕ 1m (3ft), ↔ 30–60cm (12–24in). India, China. ❀ (min. 16°C/61°F)
A. nutans **of gardens** see *A. zerumbet.*
A. purpurata ■ (Red ginger). Robust, upright perennial with stalked, hairless, lance-shaped, mid-green leaves, 80cm (32in) long. In summer, pendent to semi-erect racemes, to 90cm (36in) long, of many small white flowers, to 2.5cm (1in) long, are produced from the axils of persistent red bracts. ↕ 3–4m (10–12ft), ↔ 60–90cm (24–36in). S. Pacific islands. ❀ (min. 16°C/61°F)
A. sanderae **of gardens** see *A. vittata.*
A. speciosa see *A. zerumbet.*
A. vittata, syn. *A. sanderae* of gardens (Variegated ginger). Robust, upright perennial with almost stalkless, lance-shaped, mid-green leaves, 15cm (6in) long, striped with white and cream, and with bristly hairy margins. In summer, pale green flowers, 2cm (¾in) long, are borne in pendent racemes, 15cm (6in) long, from the axils of green, pink-tinged bracts. ↕ 1.5m (5ft), ↔ 60–90cm (24–36in). Solomon Islands. ❀ (min. 16°C/61°F)
A. zerumbet ■ syn. *A. nutans* of gardens, *A. speciosa* (Pink porcelain lily, Shell ginger). Robust, upright perennial with stalkless, oblong-lance-shaped, mid-green leaves, to 60cm (24in) long. Fragrant white, purple-tinged flowers, to 5–6cm (2–2½in) long, with yellow lips striped red and brown, are borne mostly in pairs, in pendent racemes, to 40cm (16cm) long, in summer. ↕ 3m (10ft), ↔ 1–1.2m (3–4ft). E. Asia. ❀ (min. 7°C/45°F). **'Variegata'** has dark green foliage, banded or striped pale yellow.

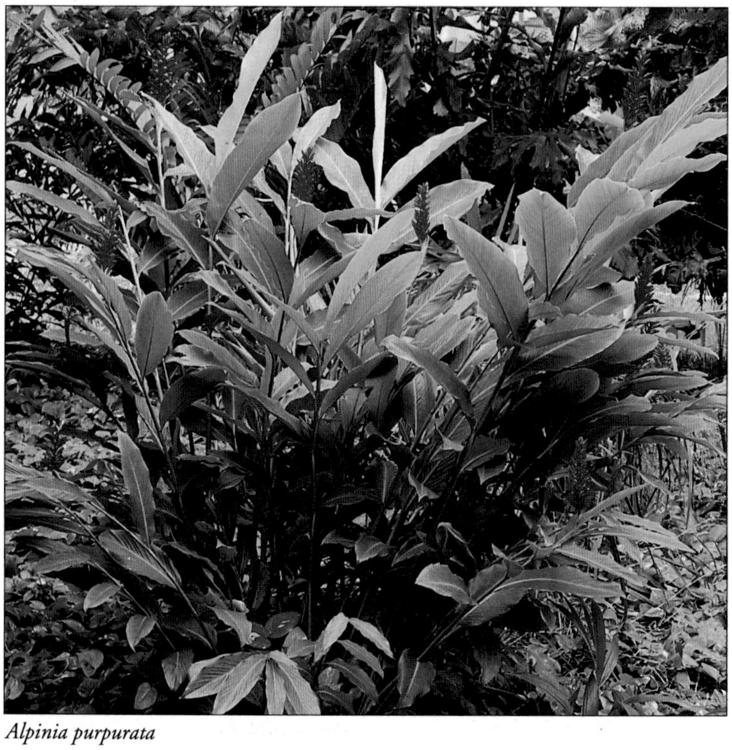

Alpinia purpurata

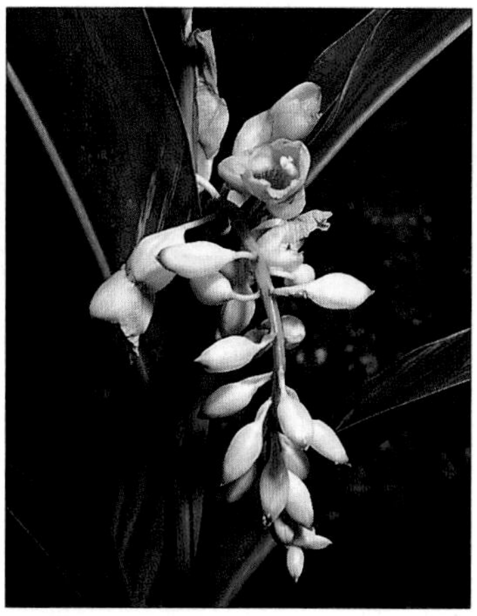

Alpinia zerumbet

▷ ***Alsobia*** see *Episcia*
A. **'Cygnet'** see *E.* 'Cygnet'
A. dianthiflora see *E. dianthiflora*
▷ ***Alsophila*** see *Cyathea*
A. australis see *C. australis*
A. australis **of gardens** see *C. cooperi*

ALSTROEMERIA
Peruvian lily

ALSTROEMERIACEAE

Genus of about 50 species of perennials from open mountain screes and grassland in South America. The fleshy, sometimes rhizome-like tubers spread to form clumps, 30–60cm (12–24in) across. They produce erect stems with alternate or scattered, linear to lance-shaped, mid- to grey-green leaves, usually 7–12cm (3–5in) long, with twisted leaf-stalks. Showy, funnel-shaped, 6-tepalled flowers, 3.5–10cm (1½–4in) long (smaller in the dwarf species), are borne in summer; they are produced in loose, often compound, few- to many-rayed, terminal umbels, 7–12cm (3–5in) across. They are ideal for a mixed or herbaceous border, although *A. pygmaea* and *A. hookeri* are best grown in an alpine house. Many species are good for cut flowers. Contact with foliage may aggravate skin allergies.

• **HARDINESS** Hardy to -10°C (14°F), although *A. aurea* and *A. ligtu* and their hybrids will tolerate brief falls in temperature to -15°C (5°F).
• **CULTIVATION** Plant tubers 20cm (8in) deep in late summer or early autumn. Take care when handling. In an alpine house, grow in a mix of loam, leaf mould, and sharp sand. In the growing season, water freely and apply a balanced liquid fertilizer monthly; water sparingly in winter. Outdoors, grow in moist but well-drained, fertile soil in sun or partial shade. Mulch for the first 2 years; in frost-prone areas, protect with a dry mulch in winter. Leave undisturbed to form clumps.
• **PROPAGATION** Sow seed in containers in a cold frame as soon as ripe. Plant out seedlings by the potful to avoid damaging the tubers. Divide established clumps in autumn or very early spring.

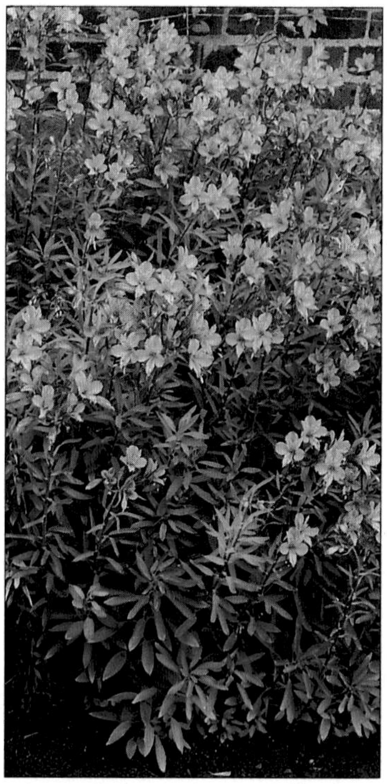

Alstroemeria aurea

• **PESTS AND DISEASES** Susceptible to slug damage and viruses; red spider mites may be a problem under glass.

A. aurantiaca see *A. aurea.*
A. aurea ■ syn. *A. aurantiaca.* Tuberous perennial bearing 3- to 7-rayed umbels, each ray with 1–3 bright orange or yellow flowers, the inner tepals streaked dark red, in summer. ↕ 1m (3ft), ↔ 45cm (18in). Chile. ❄❄. **'Dover Orange'** has deep orange flowers with paler orange inner tepals, streaked red. **'Lutea'** has bright yellow flowers with brown-spotted inner tepals.
A. **'Ballerina'.** Tuberous perennial producing 3- to 7-rayed umbels, each ray with 1–3 rose-pink flowers, with bronze-green tips and purple stripes, in summer. ↕ 1m (3ft), ↔ 75cm (30in). ❄❄
A. **'Beatrix'**, syn. *A.* 'Stadoran'. Tuberous perennial bearing 3- to 8-rayed umbels of vivid orange flowers, 2 or 3 per ray, in summer. ↕ 1m (3ft), ↔ 75cm (30in). ❄❄
A. gayana see *A. pelegrina.*
A. hookeri ■ Dwarf, tuberous perennial with grey-green leaves to 2.5cm (1in) long, and stems to 15cm (6in) long,

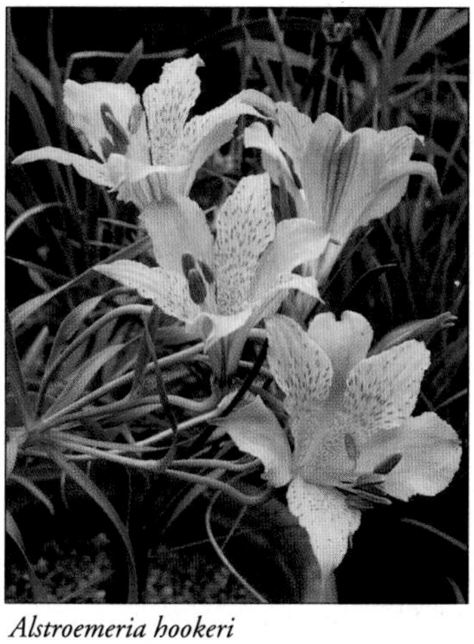

Alstroemeria hookeri

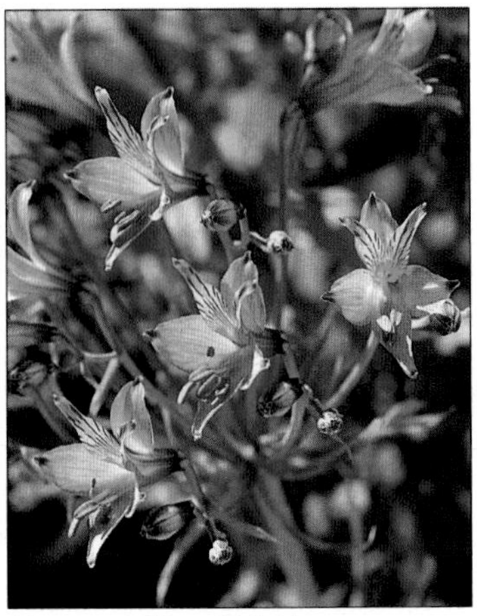

Alstroemeria Ligtu Hybrids

bearing up to 6-rayed umbels, each ray with 1–3 pink flowers, in summer. The inner tepals have yellow flashes and are streaked with purple. ↕ 30–60cm (12–24in), ↔ to 60cm (24in). Peru. ❄❄

A. ligtu. Tuberous perennial producing 3- to 8-rayed umbels, each ray with 2 or 3 flowers, varying in colour from white to pale lilac or pinkish red, in summer. The obovate inner tepals are usually yellow with white, yellow, red, or purple markings; the stamens are shorter than the tepals. ↕ 50cm (20in), ↔ 75cm (30in). Chile, Argentina. ❄❄. **Ligtu Hybrids** ■ 🏆 is a collective name given to seedlings derived mainly from crosses between *A. ligtu* and *A. haemantha.* Flower colour varies considerably.

***A.* 'Margaret'** ■ syn. *A.* 'Stacova'. Tuberous perennial bearing 3- to 8-rayed umbels, each ray with 2 or 3 deep red flowers, in summer. ↕ 1.1m (3½ft), ↔ 75cm (30in). ❄❄

***A.* 'Orchid'** see *A.* 'Walter Fleming'.

***A.* 'Parigo Charm'** ■ Tuberous perennial with 3- to 8-rayed umbels, each ray bearing 2 or 3 salmon-pink flowers, in summer. The inner tepals are primrose-yellow, marked carmine-red. ↕ 1m (3ft), ↔ 60cm (24in). ❄❄

A. paupercula, syn. *A. violacea.* Tuberous perennial with 3- to 6-rayed umbels, each ray with 3–5 violet flowers, in summer; the inner tepals have white centres, spotted purple. ↕ 50–90cm (20–36in), ↔ 45cm (18in). Chile. ❄❄

A. pelegrina ■ syn. *A. gayana.* Tuberous perennial, similar to *A. hookeri*, producing white flowers, flushed pink or purple and with a darker

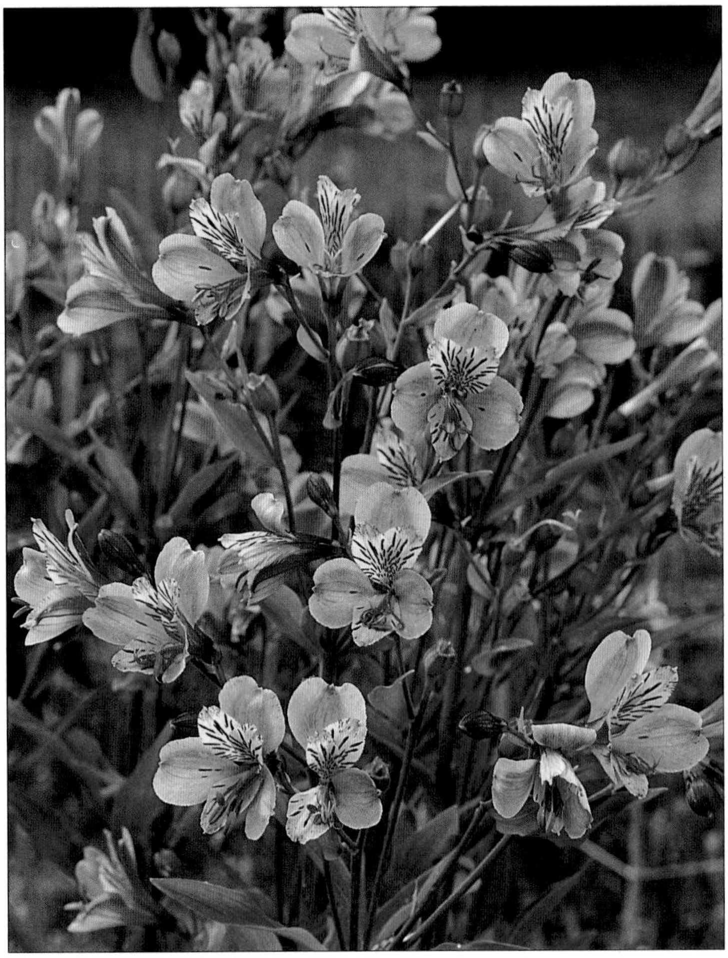

Alstroemeria 'Parigo Charm'

central area, in summer. The inner tepals are yellow at the bases, with maroon flecks. Blooms are solitary or borne in 2- or 3-rayed umbels, with 1–3 flowers per ray. ↕ 30–60cm (12–24in), ↔ to 60cm (24in). Peru. ❄❄. **'Alba'** produces green-flushed white flowers, the inner tepals with yellow or green markings.

A. psittacina, syn. *A. pulchella.* Tuberous perennial with mauve-spotted stems bearing 4- to 6-rayed umbels, each ray with 1–3 green flowers, heavily overlaid with deep red, in summer. ↕ 1m (3ft), ↔ 45cm (18in). Brazil. ❄❄

A. pulchella see *A. psittacina.*

A. pygmaea ■ Dwarf, fleshy-rooted perennial producing grey-green leaves to 2.5cm (1in) long, and stems to 15cm (6in) long. In summer, solitary, deep yellow flowers, 5cm (2in) long, the inner tepals spotted with red, are borne in single-rayed umbels. Attractive species for a scree bed or cold greenhouse. ↕↔ 15–20cm (6–8in). Andes of Argentina, Bolivia, and Peru. ❄❄

***A.* 'Regina'** see *A.* 'Victoria'.

***A.* 'Rosy Wings'.** Tuberous perennial producing 3- to 8-rayed umbels, each ray with 2 or 3 flowers, in summer. The outer tepals are red with green-marked tips, the inner ones are pink, marked with yellow and red. ↕ 1m (3ft), ↔ 50cm (20in). ❄❄

***A.* 'Sonata'.** Tuberous perennial producing 3- to 8-rayed umbels of red flowers, with 2 or 3 blooms per ray, in summer; the tepals have green margins and yellow and purple markings. ↕ 1m (3ft), ↔ 1m (3ft). ❄❄

***A.* 'Stacova'** see *A.* 'Margaret'.

***A.* 'Stadoran'** see *A.* 'Beatrix'.

***A.* 'Sweetheart'.** Tuberous perennial bearing 3- to 8-rayed umbels, each ray with 2 or 3 flowers, in summer. The outer tepals are pink, each with a darker central mark; the inner ones are paler, with red, yellow, and brown markings. ↕ 1m (3ft), ↔ 50cm (20in). ❄❄

***A.* 'Victoria'**, syn. *A.* 'Regina'. Tuberous perennial bearing 3- to 6-rayed umbels, each ray with 2 or 3 pale pink flowers with bright yellow and red markings, in summer. ↕ 1m (3ft), ↔ 60cm (24in). ❄❄

A. violacea see *A. paupercula.*

***A.* 'Walter Fleming'**, syn. *A.* 'Orchid'. Tuberous perennial producing 3- to 8-rayed umbels of yellow- and purple-marked cream flowers in summer. Each ray bears 2 or 3 blooms. ↕ 60cm (24in), ↔ 20cm (8in). ❄❄

ALTERNANTHERA

AMARANTHACEAE

Genus of about 200 species of bushy annuals and perennials from moist, open forest areas in tropical and subtropical Central and South America. They are grown for their colourful leaves, which are opposite, linear to obovate, often toothed, and variable in size. They bear insignificant flowers in terminal or axillary spikes. In frost-prone areas, use as annuals in summer bedding, or grow in a cool or temperate greenhouse or conservatory; they are excellent for hanging baskets. In frost-free climates, use for bedding or as ground cover.

- **HARDINESS** Frost tender.
- **CULTIVATION** Under glass, grow in loam-based potting compost (JI No.2) in full light. In the growing season, water freely and apply a balanced liquid fertilizer monthly; in winter, water sparingly and keep well ventilated. Outdoors, plant out after any risk of frost has passed; grow in moist but well-drained soil, in full sun for best leaf colour, or in partial shade. Clip over to maintain compactness.
- **PROPAGATION** Sow seed at 13–18°C (55–64°F) as soon as ripe, or in spring; seedlings will vary in leaf colour, making the plants less suitable for a uniform display. Divide in spring. Take softwood or greenwood cuttings in late summer. Overwinter young plants under glass.
- **PESTS AND DISEASES** Red spider mites may be a problem.

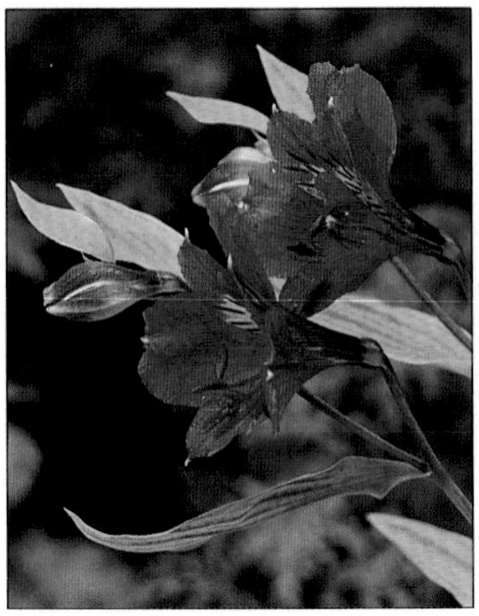

Alstroemeria 'Margaret'

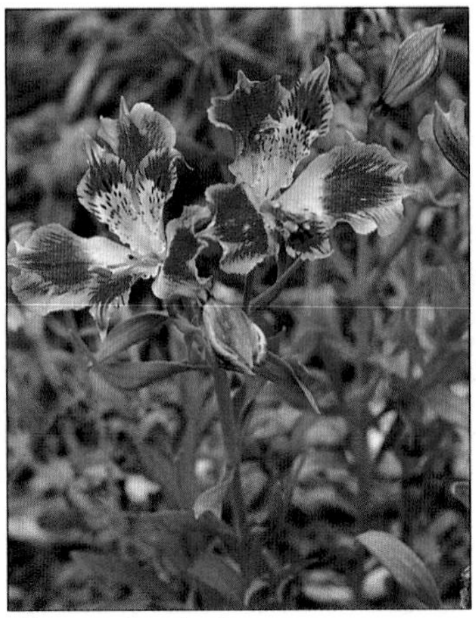

Alstroemeria pelegrina

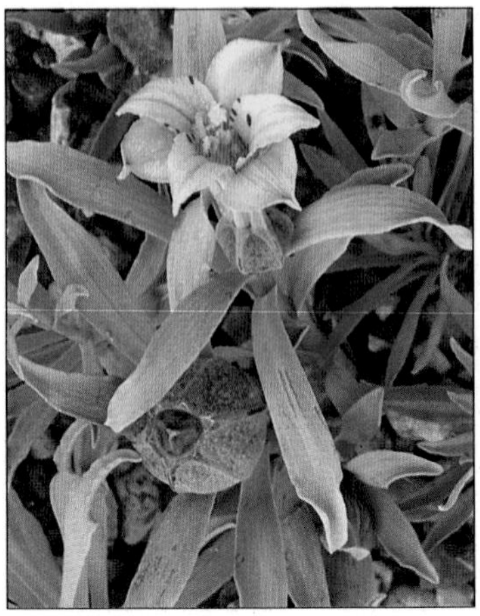

Alstroemeria pygmaea

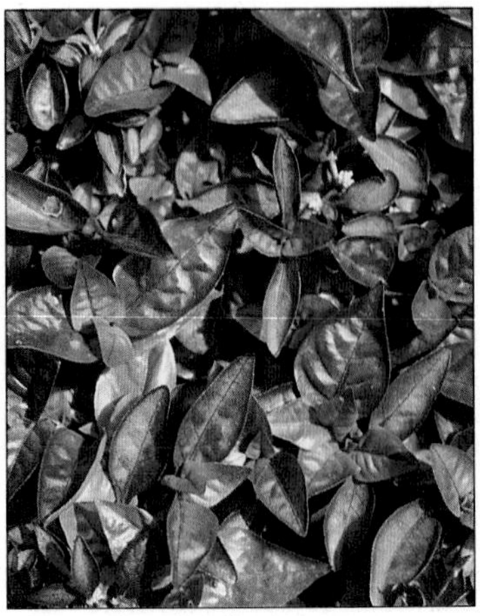

Alternanthera ficoidea var. *amoena*

A. amoena see *A. ficoidea* var. *amoena*.
A. bettzichiana (Calico plant). Mat-forming to erect annual or short-lived perennial with narrow, spoon-shaped, olive-green to yellow leaves, to 2.5cm (1in) long, mottled in combinations of red, purple, and bronze. Insignificant white flowers are borne in axillary spikes, 5–10mm (¼–½in) long, and are similar to those of *A. ficoidea*, of which this species is sometimes considered a variety. ↕ 5–20cm (2–8in), ↔ indefinite. Brazil. ❀ (min. 5°C/41°F)
A. ficoidea (Parrot leaf). Mat-forming to erect perennial with elliptic to obovate, pointed, mid-green leaves, 2.5cm (1in) long, which are marked with combinations of red, orange, purple, and yellow. Insignificant white flowers are produced in spherical to ovoid, axillary spikes, 3–10mm (⅛–½in) long. ↕ 20–30cm (8–12in), ↔ indefinite. Mexico, South America. ❀ (min. 5°C/41°F). **var. *amoena*** ■ syn. *A. amoena*, is dwarf, with lance-shaped to elliptic, mid-green leaves, heavily mottled and veined brown-red, orange, and purple; ↕ to 5cm (2in). **'Versicolor'**, syn. *A. versicolor*, is erect with bluntly spoon-shaped, copper or blood-red to maroon leaves; ↕↔ 30cm (12in).
A. versicolor see *A. ficoidea* 'Versicolor'.

ALTHAEA

MALVACEAE

Genus of about 12 species of annuals and perennials, similar to *Alcea* but bearing smaller, usually stalked flowers, found mainly in moist, sometimes brackish coastal habitats from W. Europe to C. Asia. They have strong, wiry stems that seldom need support, and broadly ovate, shallowly to deeply lobed, dark green leaves. Racemes or panicles of small, pink to bluish purple, 5-petalled flowers are produced from summer to autumn. They are suitable for a mixed or herbaceous border or wildflower garden.
• **HARDINESS** Fully hardy.

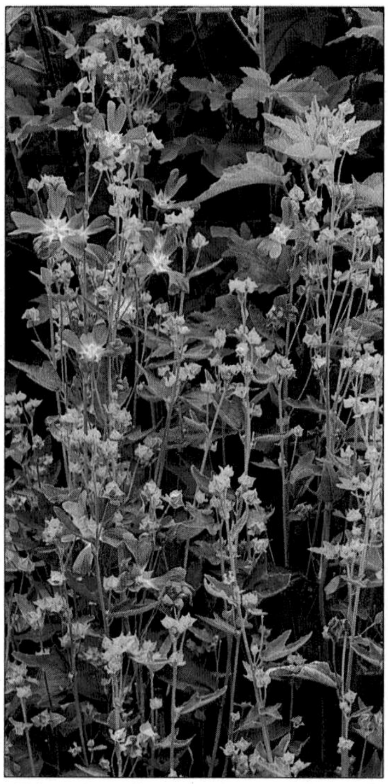

Althaea cannabina

• **CULTIVATION** They will tolerate a wide range of situations, but for best results grow in fertile, moist but well-drained soil in full sun.
• **PROPAGATION** Sow seed of annuals at 13°C (55°F) in late winter, or *in situ* in mid-spring. For perennials, sow seed in drills in midsummer; transplant in early autumn, when 2 or 3 true leaves have developed.
• **PEST AND DISEASES** Rust and flea beetles may be a problem.

A. armeniaca. Erect, woody-based perennial with triangular-ovate, toothed or deeply 3- to 5-lobed leaves, to 15cm (6in) long, dark green above, paler beneath, and densely softly hairy. From midsummer to early autumn, produces leafy racemes of open funnel-shaped, deep rose-pink flowers, to 5cm (2in) across, on short stalks from the leaf axils. ↕ 1.2m (4ft), ↔ 30cm (12in). C. and S.W. Asia, S.E. Russia. ✻✻✻
A. cannabina ■ Erect, woody-based perennial with rounded, hairy leaves, to 35cm (14in) long, each with 3–5 lobes, which are themselves lobed or toothed, and dark green above, paler beneath. Axillary clusters of small, cupped, lilac to deep pink flowers, 3–5cm (1¼–2in) across, sometimes with darker eyes, open from midsummer to early autumn. ↕ 2m (6ft), ↔ 60cm (24in). C., S., and E. Europe. ✻✻✻
A. officinalis (Marsh mallow). Erect perennial producing softly hairy leaves with 3–5 shallow, toothed lobes. From midsummer to early autumn, bears pale lilac-pink flowers, 1.5–2cm (½–¾in) across, singly or in short axillary or terminal clusters. Sometimes grown for culinary or medicinal purposes. ↕ 2m (6ft), ↔ to 1.5m (5ft). C., S., and E. Europe. ✻✻✻
A. rosea see *Alcea rosea*.

▷**Aluminium plant** see *Pilea cadierei*

ALYOGYNE

MALVACEAE

Genus of 4 species of evergreen shrubs, formerly included in *Hibiscus*, growing wild in dry scrub in Australia (Northern Territory, Southern Australia, Western Australia). The leaves are alternate and entire to deeply lobed. They are valued for their large, attractive, hibiscus-like flowers, which are produced singly from the upper leaf axils from late spring to autumn. In frost-prone areas, grow in a cool greenhouse and stand plants outdoors in summer. In frost-free areas, grow in a border or at the base of a wall. Established plants will tolerate short periods of drought.
• **HARDINESS** Half hardy to frost tender.
• **CULTIVATION** Under glass, grow in loamless or loam-based potting compost (JI No.3) in full light. Pot on or top-dress in spring. In the growing season, water moderately and apply a balanced liquid fertilizer every 2–3 weeks; water sparingly in winter. Outdoors, grow in any well-drained soil in full sun. Pruning group 9, or 13 if wall-trained.
• **PROPAGATION** Sow seed in spring, at not less than 16°C (61°F). Root semi-ripe cuttings in late summer.
• **PESTS AND DISEASES** Aphids, whiteflies, and red spider mites may be a problem.

A. huegelii, syn. *Hibiscus huegelii*. Erect, fast-growing shrub, spreading with age, bearing palmate, hairy, bright green leaves, 3–8cm (1¼–3in) long, each with 5 irregularly toothed lobes. Solitary, funnel-shaped, satiny, lilac, mauve, or purple flowers, to 10cm (4in) across, are produced from the leaf axils of young shoots from late spring to autumn. ↕↔ 1–2m (3–6ft). Australia (Western Australia). ✻. **'Santa Cruz'** is a free-flowering, mauve-purple cultivar.

ALYSSUM

BRASSICACEAE/CRUCIFERAE

Genus of over 150 tufted, mat- or hummock-forming, sometimes erect annuals, and evergreen perennials and subshrubs, mostly found in open, rocky sites in C. and S. Europe, N. Africa, and S.W. and C. Asia. They have simple, alternate leaves, 0.4–2.5cm (⅛–1in) long, and are cultivated mainly for their corymb-like racemes of cross-shaped, 4-petalled, yellow or white flowers, produced in early summer. They are suitable for growing in a rock garden, at the front of a mixed border, or in wall crevices.
• **HARDINESS** Fully hardy.
• **CULTIVATION** Grow in well-drained, moderately fertile, preferably gritty, loamy soil in full sun. Trim lightly after flowering to maintain compactness.
• **PROPAGATION** Sow seed in containers in a cold frame in autumn or spring. Root greenwood cuttings in early summer.
• **PESTS AND DISEASES** Aphids, flea beetles, white blister, and downy mildew may be a problem.

A. maritimum see *Lobularia maritima*.
***A. montanum* 'Berggold'**, syn. *A. montanum* 'Mountain Gold'. Evergreen, mat-forming perennial with prostrate stems and rosettes of small, oblong to obovate grey leaves. Racemes of many fragrant, golden yellow flowers, each to 5mm (¼in) across, are borne in early summer. ↕ 10–15cm (4–6in), ↔ to 50cm (20in) or more. ✻✻✻
***A. montanum* 'Mountain Gold'** see *A. montanum* 'Berggold'.
A. saxatile see *Aurinia saxatilis*.
A. spinosum, syn. *Ptilotrichum spinosum*. Compact, mounded, evergreen subshrub with densely branching, spine-tipped stems. Dense, corymb-like racemes of white flowers, each to 7mm (¼in) across, are borne in early summer above tiny, obovate, silvery grey leaves. ↕↔ 30–50cm (12–20in). S.E. France, S. Spain. ✻✻✻. **var. *roseum*** ♀ has pale to deep rose-pink flowers.
A. vesicaria see *Coluteocarpus vesicarius*.
A. wulfenianum ■ Erect or prostrate, tufted, evergreen perennial producing rosettes of small, oblong-obovate, grey- or white-hairy leaves. Corymbs of tiny pale yellow flowers, each to 6mm (¼in) across, are borne in early summer. ↕ 10–15cm (4–6in), ↔ to 50cm (20in). S.E. Alps. ✻✻✻

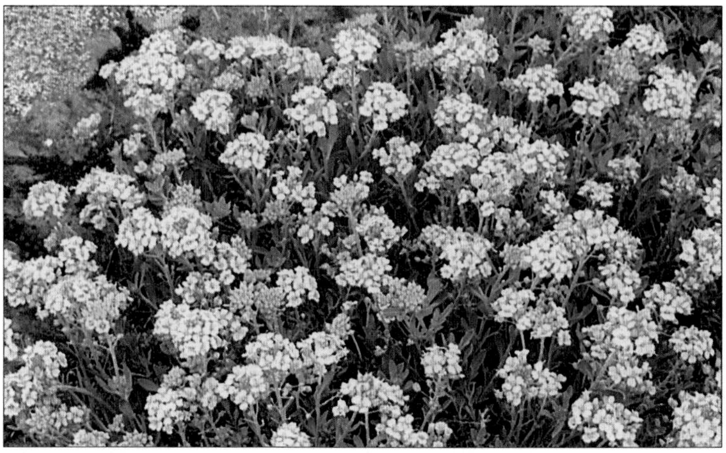

Alyssum wulfenianum

▷**Alyssum, Sweet** see *Lobularia*
▷***Amana*** see *Tulipa*
A. edulis see *T. edulis*
▷**Amaranth,**
Globe see *Gomphrena globosa*
Purple see *Amaranthus cruentus*
Red see *Amaranthus cruentus*

AMARANTHUS

AMARANTHACEAE

Genus of about 60 species of erect, spreading, or prostrate annuals or short-lived perennials, often invasive, from a range of habitats, including wasteland and fields, in temperate and tropical regions worldwide. They have alternate, entire leaves, and bear large, upright or pendent, catkin-like cymes of numerous densely packed, small, red or green flowers in summer and early autumn. The flowers are followed by variously coloured seed heads. In frost-prone areas, use as summer bedding, or grow in containers or hanging baskets; they may also be grown as short-lived house-plants or in a temperate greenhouse. *A. tricolor* cultivars are best grown under glass in cool climates. In frost-free areas, use for summer bedding. *A. caudatus* and *A. hypochondriacus* cultivars are good for cut or dried flowers.
• **HARDINESS** Half hardy.
• **CULTIVATION** Under glass, grow in loam-based potting compost (JI No.2) in full light. Water freely in summer, and provide high humidity. Outdoors, grow in moderately fertile, humus-rich, moist soil in full sun in a sheltered site. *A. caudatus* will tolerate poor soil. Water freely during dry periods in summer to prolong flowering.
• **PROPAGATION** Sow seed at 20°C (68°F) in mid-spring. *A. caudatus* may also be sown *in situ* in mid-spring; thin to 60cm (24in) apart.
• **PESTS AND DISEASES** Aphids and viruses may be a problem.

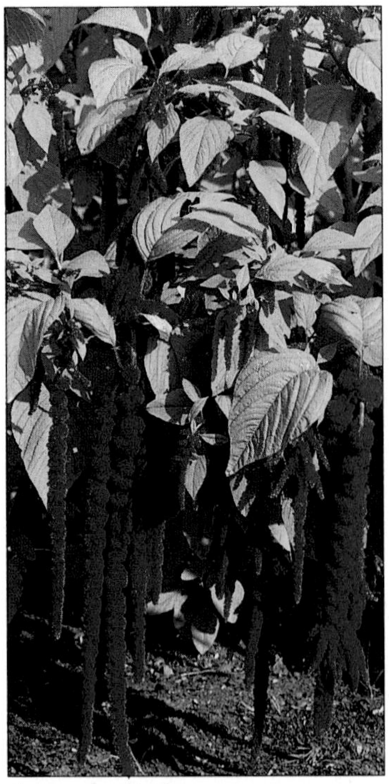
Amaranthus caudatus

A. caudatus ■ (Love-lies-bleeding, Tassel flower). Bushy, erect annual or short-lived perennial with red, purple, or green stems, and ovate to ovate-oblong, light green leaves, to 15cm (6in) long. Some cultivars have red or purple-green leaves. Tassel-like, pendent, terminal and axillary panicles, 45–60cm (18–24in) long, of crimson-purple flowers are borne freely from summer to early autumn. ↕ 1–1.5m (3–5ft), ↔ 45–75cm (18–30in). Africa, India, Peru. ❄. **'Viridis'** ■ has tassels of vivid green flowers, fading to cream.
A. cruentus (Prince's feather, Purple amaranth, Red amaranth). Coarsely hairy, erect annual with ovate to lance-shaped, purplish green leaves, to 15cm (6in) long. Bears pendent, cylindrical, terminal cymes, to 60cm (24in) long, of tightly packed, red-suffused green flowers from summer to early autumn, followed by red-brown or purple, sometimes yellow seed heads. ↕ to 2m (6ft), ↔ 45cm (18in). Tropical North and South America. ❄. **'Golden Giant'** has prominent golden seed heads.
***A. hypochondriacus* cultivars.** Erect, bushy annuals with oblong-lance-shaped, dark purple-green leaves, 15cm

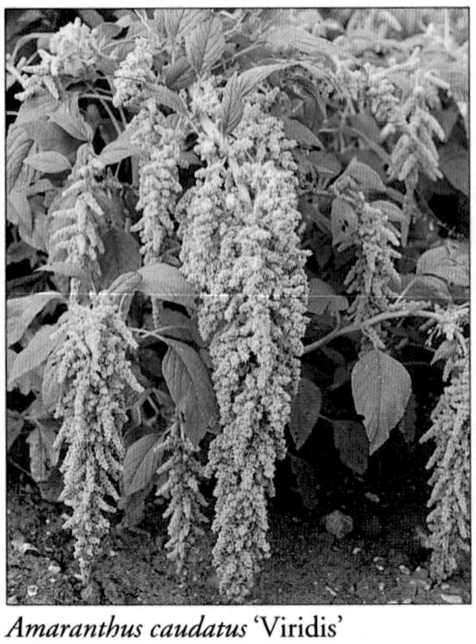
Amaranthus caudatus 'Viridis'

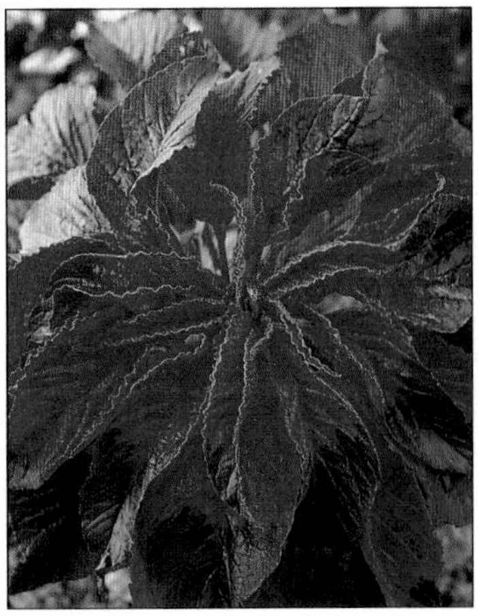
Amaranthus tricolor 'Illumination'

(6in) long. From summer to early autumn, bears tiny crimson flowers in erect, plume-like, sometimes flattened, terminal cymes, to 15cm (6in) or more long. ↕ 0.9–1.2m (3–4ft), ↔ 30–45cm (12–18in). ❄. **'Green Thumb'** 🏆 has much-divided cymes of brilliant yellow-green flowers; ↕ to 60cm (24in), ↔ 30cm (12in). **'Pygmy Torch'** 🏆 is dwarf, with erect cymes of maroon flowers; ↕ 30–45cm (12–18in), ↔ 30cm (12in).
***A. tricolor* cultivars** (Chinese spinach, Tampala). Erect, bushy annuals, grown for their ovate or elliptic, sometimes lance-shaped, multi-coloured leaves, to 20cm (8in) or more long, which vary in colour from green or purple to brilliant crimson or maroon, often suffused with gold, rose-pink, and bronze in the different cultivars. Insignificant green or red flowers are borne in often thickened and flattened, terminal or axillary cymes, from summer to early autumn. ↕ 1.3m (4½ft), ↔ 30–45cm (12–18in). ❄. **'Flaming Fountains'** has willow-like, lance-shaped leaves in carmine-red, crimson, and bronze. **'Illumination'** ■ has ovate to elliptic, bright rose-red upper leaves topped with gold, and lower leaves in copper-brown; ↕ to 45cm (18in). **'Joseph's Coat'** has ovate to elliptic, gold and crimson upper leaves, and a mix of green, yellow, and chocolate-brown lower leaves.

x AMARCRINUM

syn. x CRINODONNA

AMARYLLIDACEAE

Hybrid genus of a single summer-flowering, evergreen, bulbous perennial, a cross between *Amaryllis* and *Crinum*. x *A. memoria-corsii* is similar to *Crinum* in both its growth and showy, funnel-shaped flowers. Where temperatures do not fall below -5°C (23°F), grow in a mixed or herbaceous border or at the base of a sheltered wall. In colder climates, grow in a cool greenhouse or conservatory.
• **HARDINESS** Frost hardy.
• **CULTIVATION** Plant in late summer or spring, with the nose of the bulb just below soil level. Under glass, grow in well-drained, loam-based potting compost (JI No.2), with additional leaf mould and sharp sand, in full light. In the growing season, water moderately and apply a balanced liquid fertilizer monthly; reduce water after flowering and keep almost dry in winter. Outdoors, grow in moderately fertile,

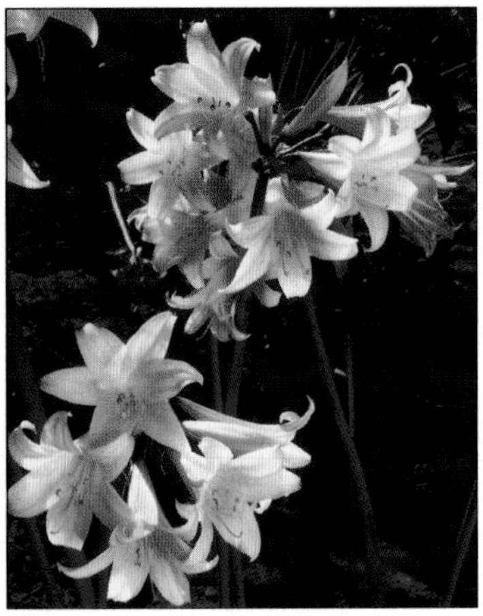
x *Amarcrinum memoria-corsii*

dry, well-drained soil in full sun. Protect foliage from prolonged frost.
• **PROPAGATION** Remove offsets from established plants in early spring; grow on under glass for 1–2 years before planting outside in spring.
• **PESTS AND DISEASES** Susceptible to slug damage; aphids and red spider mites may be a problem under glass.

x *A. howardii* see x *A. memoria-corsii.*
x *A. memoria-corsii* ■ syn. x *A. howardii*, x *Crinodonna corsii.* Robust, bulbous perennial with semi-erect, wide, strap-shaped, basal leaves, to 60cm (24in) long. In late summer, stout stems bear loose umbels of up to 10 funnel-shaped, fragrant, rose-pink flowers, 6–10cm (2½–4in) long. ↕ 1m (3ft), ↔ 60cm (24in). Garden origin. ❄❄

x AMARYGIA

syn. x BRUNSDONNA

AMARYLLIDACEAE

Hybrid genus of a single bulbous perennial, a cross between *Amaryllis belladonna* and *Brunsvigia*, cultivated for its umbels of showy flowers, which are borne before the leaves from summer to autumn. In areas where temperatures do not fall below -5°C (23°F), grow in a mixed or herbaceous border, or at the base of a warm, sheltered wall. In cooler areas, grow in a cool greenhouse or conservatory.
• **HARDINESS** Frost hardy.
• **CULTIVATION** Plant from early to late summer with the neck of the bulb just above soil level. Under glass, grow in loam-based potting compost (JI No.2)

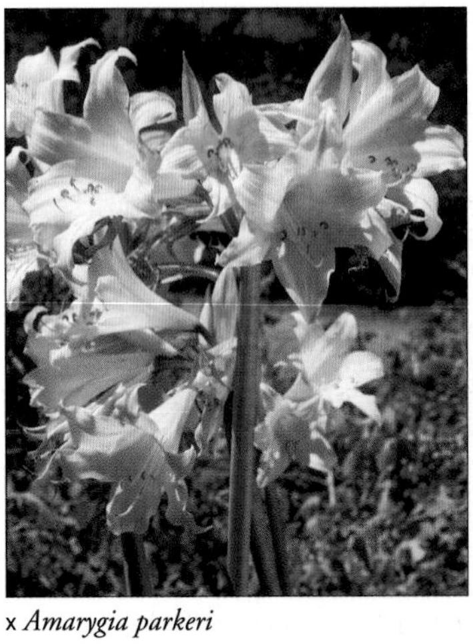
x *Amarygia parkeri*

with additional leaf mould and sharp sand. Provide full light, but shade when flowering to prevent scorching. Water moderately during the growing season, more sparingly when the leaves fade; keep dry while dormant. Allow the bulbs to become congested before potting on. Outdoors, grow in humus-rich, sandy, well-drained soil in full sun; protect foliage from prolonged frost.
• **PROPAGATION** Remove offsets from congested plants only, just before the plant comes into growth in summer.
• **PESTS AND DISEASES** Prone to leaf scorch. Narcissus eelworm, narcissus bulb fly, aphids, mealybugs, whiteflies, and red spider mites may be a problem.

x *A. parkeri* ■ syn. x *Brunsdonna parkeri.* Robust, bulbous perennial bearing loose umbels of up to 12 large, funnel-shaped, frilled pink flowers, 6–10cm (2½–4in) long, on stout stems in summer. Semi-erect, strap-shaped, basal leaves, 30–45cm (12–18in) long, are borne after flowering. ↕ 1m (3ft), ↔ 30cm (12in). Garden origin. ❄❄

AMARYLLIS

AMARYLLIDACEAE

Genus of one species of deciduous, autumn-flowering, bulbous perennial from coastal hills and streambanks in S. Western Cape, South Africa. It is cultivated for its showy flowers. Where temperatures fall below -5°C (23°F), grow in a cool greenhouse; in warmer areas, grow against a sheltered wall.
• **HARDINESS** Frost hardy.
• **CULTIVATION** Plant bulbs just below the soil or compost surface when dormant in late summer, or in spring. Under glass, grow in loam-based potting compost (JI No.2), with additional leaf mould and sharp sand, in full light. In the growing season, water moderately and apply a balanced liquid fertilizer monthly; keep dry when dormant. Outdoors, grow in moderately fertile, well-drained soil in full sun. Protect foliage from frost.
• **PROPAGATION** Sow seed thinly in containers at 16°C (61°F) as soon as ripe; grow on under glass. Remove offsets in spring, and grow on under glass for 1 or 2 seasons, before planting outdoors.
• **PESTS AND DISEASES** Prone to slug damage and narcissus bulb fly; aphids and red spider mites may be a problem under glass.

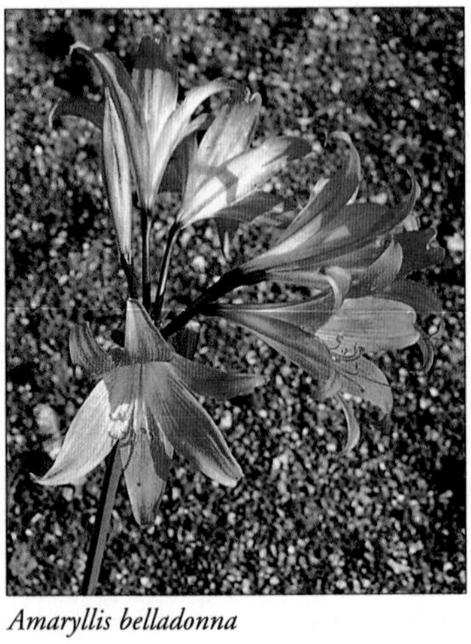
Amaryllis belladonna

A

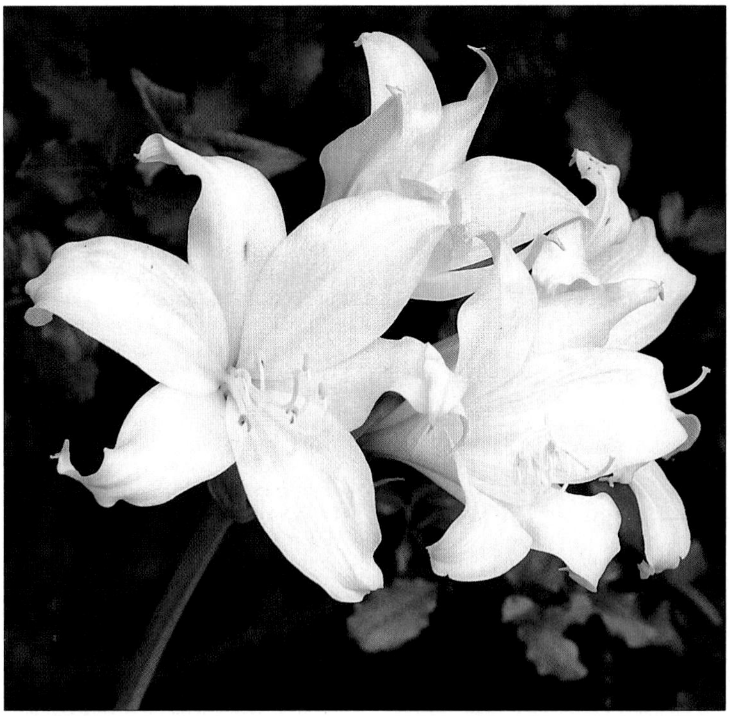

Amaryllis belladonna 'Hathor'

A. belladonna ▣ Bulbous perennial producing stout, purple or purple-green stems with umbels of 6 or more funnel-shaped, scented pink flowers, 6–10cm (2½–4in) long, in autumn. Strap-shaped, fleshy leaves, 22–40cm (9–16in) long, are produced after flowering. ↕60cm (24in), ↔10cm (4in). South Africa. ❄❄. **'Barberton'** produces dark rose-pink flowers. **'Cape Town'** bears deep rose-red flowers. **'Hathor'** ▣ has white flowers, which are pink in bud. **'Johannesburg'** is free flowering, with pale pink flowers. **'Kimberley'** bears deep carmine-pink flowers with white centres.

▷**Amaryllis, Blue** see *Worsleya*

AMBERBOA

Sweet sultan

ASTERACEAE/COMPOSITAE

Genus of about 6 species of upright annuals or biennials found in gravelly and sandy soils from the Mediterranean to W. and C. Asia, with alternate, entire to deeply divided, pinnatifid, grey-green leaves. Attractive, solitary flowerheads, each with a thistle-like centre of disc-florets and soft, fringed rings of long, outer ray-florets, are borne from spring to autumn. Grow sweet sultans in a border or cottage garden, or in containers. Good for cutting.

- **HARDINESS** Fully hardy.
- **CULTIVATION** Grow in any moderately fertile, well-drained, neutral to alkaline soil in full sun. Provide plants with light, twiggy support when they reach 7–10cm (3–4in) high. Dead-head to prolong flowering.
- **PROPAGATION** Sow seed thinly in containers in a cold frame or *in situ* in early spring; plant out *A. moschata* seedlings in potfuls to avoid root disturbance. Alternatively, sow seed in autumn; in very cold areas, overwinter young plants under glass.
- **PESTS AND DISEASES** Powdery mildew may be a problem in dry summers.

A. moschata, syn. *Centaurea moschata* (Sweet sultan). Strongly branched annual with grey-green leaves, the basal leaves entire, to 10cm (4in) long, the stem leaves lobed or pinnatifid. Bears scented, fringed flowerheads, to 5cm (2in) across, resembling large corn-flowers, in white, yellow, pink, or purple, on erect stems, from spring to summer. ↕to 60cm (24in), ↔23cm (9in). Turkey, Caucasus. ❄❄❄

▷***Amblyopetalum caeruleum*** see *Tweedia caerulea*

AMELANCHIER

Juneberry, Shadbush, Snowy Mespilus

ROSACEAE

Genus of about 25 species of deciduous trees and shrubs, often suckering, mostly from moist woodland and streambanks in Europe, Asia, and North America. Amelanchiers are cultivated for their racemes of 5-petalled, star-shaped, flat to very shallowly saucer-shaped, usually white or pink-flushed flowers, 1–2cm (½–¾in) across, borne from spring to early summer, and for their fine autumn colour and fruit. The alternate, ovate to oblong leaves are often bronze when young, and open with the flowers. Grow in a shrub border or as specimen plants. The spherical or pear-shaped, purple to maroon fruits, attractive to birds, ripen in summer and are edible when cooked.

- **HARDINESS** Fully hardy.
- **CULTIVATION** Grow in lime-free (acid), fertile, moist but well-drained soil in sun or partial shade. *A. asiatica* is lime-tolerant. Pruning group 1.
- **PROPAGATION** Sow seed in a seedbed as soon as ripe; the species hybridize freely. Root greenwood or semi-ripe cuttings in summer. Remove suckers of stoloniferous species in winter.
- **PESTS AND DISEASES** Susceptible to fireblight.

A. asiatica ▣ ○ Spreading tree with arching branches and ovate leaves,

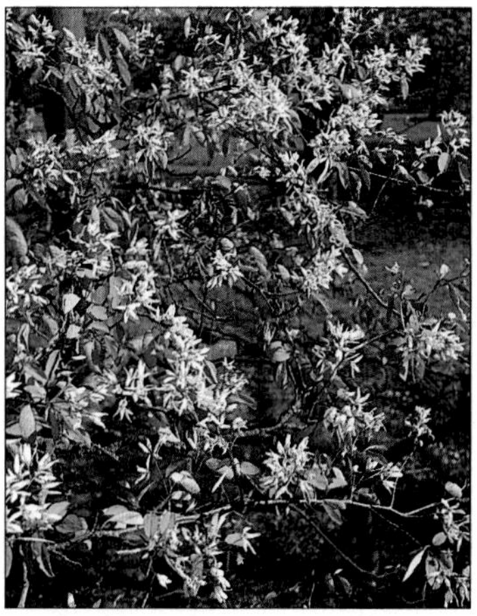

Amelanchier asiatica

4–7cm (1½–3in) long, white-hairy beneath when young, mid-green in summer, then orange to red in autumn. Bears scented white flowers in upright racemes, 3–6cm (1¼–2½in) long, in late spring, followed by insipid-tasting, blue-black fruit, 5–10mm (¼–½in) across. ↕8m (25ft), ↔10m (30ft). China, Korea, Japan. ❄❄❄

***A.* 'Ballerina'** ▣ ♀ ○ Spreading, shrubby tree with broadly elliptic, glossy leaves, 5–8cm (2–3in) long, bronze-tinted when young, becoming mid-green in summer, and red and purple in autumn. White flowers are borne in arching racemes, 15cm (6in) long, in mid-spring. Sweet, juicy fruit, to 1.5cm (½in) across, are red at first, ripening to purplish black. Free-flowering hybrid of *A. laevis*. ↕6m (20ft), ↔8m (25ft). ❄❄❄

A. canadensis (Shadbush). Dense, erect, suckering shrub with oblong-elliptic to obovate leaves, 3.5–5cm (1½–2in) long, white-hairy when young, becoming almost hairless when mature, and mid-green in summer, yellow to orange and red in autumn. Erect racemes, 2.5–6cm (1–2½in) long, of white flowers open in spring, followed by sweet, blue-black fruit, 7–10mm (¼–½in) across. Often confused in European gardens with *A. arborea*, *A. laevis*, and *A. lamarckii*. ↕6m (20ft), ↔3m (10ft). E. North America. ❄❄❄

A. confusa. Upright shrub with ovate leaves, 2–3.5cm (¾–1½in) long, light green above, glaucous beneath, turning red and yellow in autumn. White flowers are borne in erect racemes, 3–8cm (1¼–3in) long, in late spring

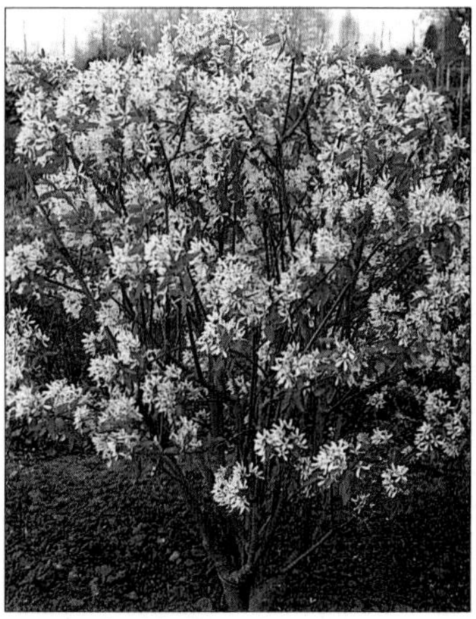

Amelanchier 'Ballerina'

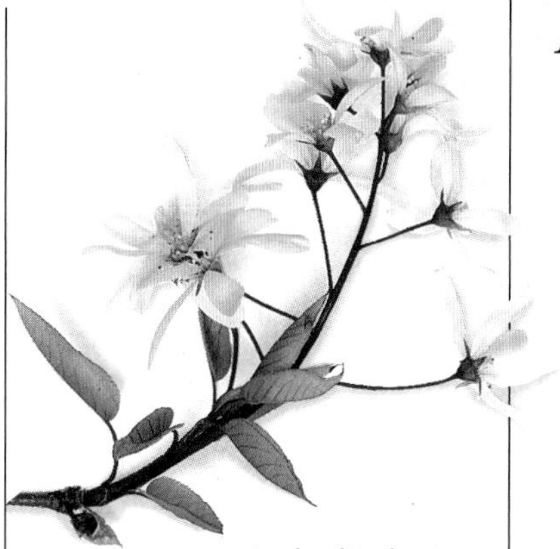

Amelanchier laevis

and early summer, followed by insipid-tasting, blue-black fruit, 7–9mm (¼–⅜in) across. Often confused with *A. lamarckii*. ↕3m (10ft), ↔2m (6ft). Sweden. ❄❄❄

A. x grandiflora ○ (*A. arborea* x *A. laevis*). Spreading, sometimes shrubby tree producing ovate leaves, 4.5–8cm (1¾–3in) long, bronze with hairy undersides, turning green in late spring, orange and red in autumn. Bears pendent racemes, 6–8cm (2½–3in) long, of white flowers in mid-spring, followed by sweet, juicy, blue-black fruit, 7–10mm (¼–½in) across. ↕8m (25ft), ↔10m (30ft). Garden origin. ❄❄❄. **'Autumn Brilliance'** is vigorous, with brilliant red autumn colour. **'Robin Hill'** ○ is compact and broadly upright, with white flowers and pink-tinged buds; ↕8m (25ft), ↔5m (15ft). **'Rubescens'** syn. *A. lamarckii* 'Rubescens', has dark pink buds and paler pink flowers.

A. laevis ▣ ○ (Allegheny serviceberry). Spreading, sometimes shrubby tree with ovate leaves, 4–6cm (1½–2½in) long, bronze and hairless when young (unlike *A. lamarckii*), turning mid-green in summer, then orange or red in autumn. Pendent racemes, 4–12cm (1½–5in) long, of white flowers are borne in mid-spring, followed by sweet, blue-black fruit, to 1.5cm (½in) long. Often confused with *A. lamarckii*. ↕↔8m (25ft). North America. ❄❄❄

A. lamarckii ▣ ♀ ○ Upright-stemmed shrub or small tree with white-haired young shoots and leaves, soon becoming hairless. Elliptic to oblong bronze leaves, to 8cm (3in) long, turn dark green, then orange and red in autumn. In mid-spring, bears pendent racemes, 6–12cm

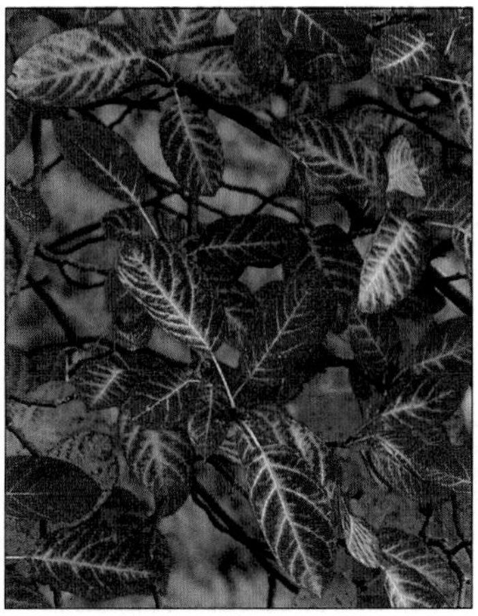

Amelanchier lamarckii

(2½–5in) long, of white flowers, followed by sweet, juicy, purple-black fruit, 7–10mm (¼–½in) across. Often confused with *A. canadensis* or *A. laevis.* ↕ 10m (30ft), ↔ 12m (40ft). Uncertain origin; naturalized in Europe. ❄❄❄.
'Rubescens' see *A.* x *grandiflora* 'Rubescens'.
A. stolonifera. Dense, erect, thicket-forming, suckering shrub with oval to rounded leaves, 1–3cm (½–1¼in) long, white-hairy beneath when young, mid-green, turning yellow to orange and red in autumn. Bears erect, compact racemes, to 4cm (1½in) long, of 4–10 white flowers in mid- and late spring, followed by sweet, blue-black fruit, 6–8mm (¼–⅜in) across. ↕ 2m (6ft), ↔ 1.5m (5ft). E. North America. ❄❄❄

AMESIELLA

ORCHIDACEAE

Genus of one species of evergreen, epiphytic, monopodial orchid from the Philippines, where it grows in mountain forest at an altitude of 800m (2,600ft). Short stems, 3–6cm (1¼–2½in) long, bear 2-ranked leaves (usually no more than 4) and produce racemes of spurred, almost spherical flowers, mostly in autumn.
- **HARDINESS** Frost tender.
- **CULTIVATION** Intermediate-growing orchid. Grow in small pots or slatted baskets of epiphytic orchid compost in filtered light and humid conditions. Water moderately throughout the year, applying a fertilizer at every third watering in summer. See also p.46.
- **PROPAGATION** Not suitable for division, although cuttings or offshoots may be rooted successfully.
- **PESTS AND DISEASES** Prone to red spider mites, aphids, and mealybugs.

A. philippinensis. Miniature, evergreen, epiphytic orchid with elliptic-oblong, fleshy leaves, to 5cm (2in) long. Short, axillary racemes of 1–3 almost spherical white flowers, 3cm (1¼in) across, each with a yellow stain on the lip, and spurs 4cm (1½in) long, are produced in autumn. ↕ 6cm (2½in), ↔ 10cm (4in). Philippines. ⌂ (min. 16°C/61°F; max. 30°C/86°F)

AMHERSTIA

CAESALPINIACEAE/LEGUMINOSAE

Genus of one species of evergreen tree, found on riverbanks in tropical forest in Burma. It has alternate, large, pinnate leaves, and long racemes of 5-petalled, orchid-like flowers. Where temperatures fall below 16°C (61°F), grow *A. nobilis* in a warm greenhouse, although it rarely flowers in a container. In tropical areas, it is a spectacular specimen tree.
- **HARDINESS** Frost tender.
- **CULTIVATION** Under glass, grow in loam-based potting compost (JI No.3) in bright filtered light and high humidity. In the growing season, water freely and apply a balanced liquid fertilizer monthly; water sparingly in winter. Outdoors, grow in moist, fertile soil in a sheltered, reasonably sunny site. Pruning group 1; plants under glass may need restrictive pruning in late winter or after flowering.
- **PROPAGATION** Sow seed in spring at a minimum temperature of 21–24°C (70–75°F); the seedlings are delicate and must be handled with care.
- **PESTS AND DISEASES** Red spider mites may be a problem under glass.

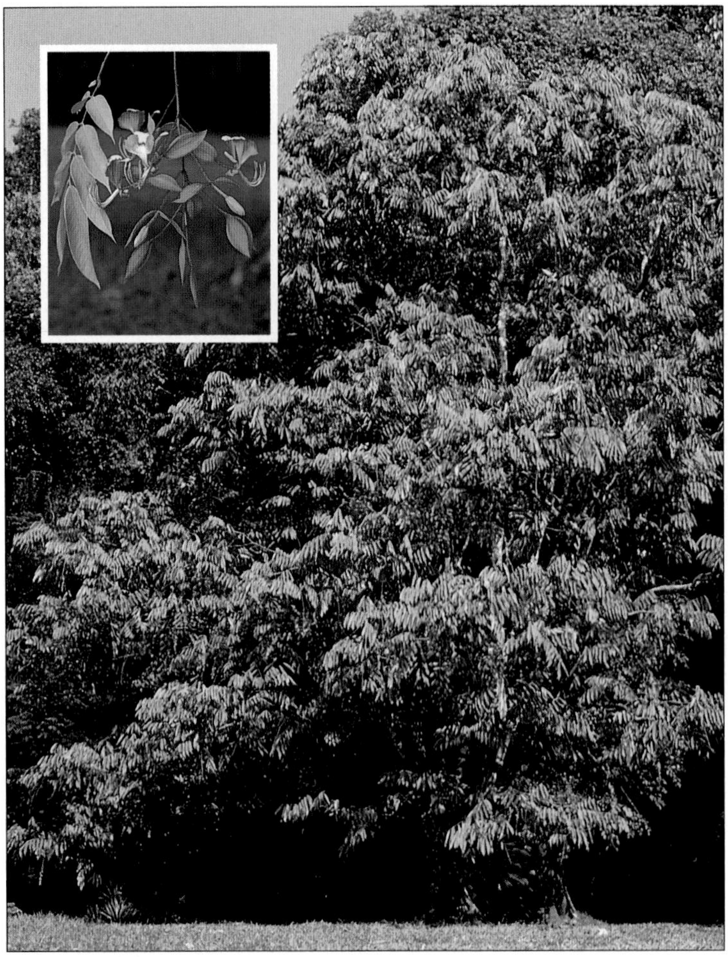

Amherstia nobilis (inset: flower detail)

A. nobilis ▣ ♀ (Orchid tree, Pride of Burma). Erect, open-branched tree producing pinnate leaves, 60–90cm (24–36in) long, divided into 8–18 copper-pink leaflets, which turn deep green with age. The orchid-like flowers, 6–10cm (2½–4in) across, are bright red, suffused pink and white, with yellow tips and protruding stamens, and are borne in pendent racemes, 40–90cm (16–36in) long, in early summer. ↕ 10m (30ft), ↔ 15m (50ft). Burma. ⌂ (min. 16°C/61°F)

AMICIA

LEGUMINOSAE/PAPILIONACEAE

Genus of 7 species of upright, woody-based perennials found on riverbanks and in woodland in the mountains of Mexico and in the Andes. They are grown mainly for their alternate leaves, each with 2 pairs of leaflets and, when young, large, pale green stipules with purple veins. The pea-like autumn flowers may be damaged by early frosts, except in mild areas. Where temperatures fall below -10°C (14°F), grow in containers in a cool greenhouse and move outdoors in summer. Elsewhere, grow in a mixed or herbaceous border.
- **HARDINESS** Half hardy to frost hardy; *A. zygomeris* will tolerate temperatures down to -10°C (14°F), and will regenerate from the woody base if cut back by frost.
- **CULTIVATION** Under glass, grow in loam-based potting compost (JI No.2) in full light. In the growing season, water freely and apply a balanced liquid fertilizer monthly; keep just moist in winter. Outdoors, grow in well-drained, fertile soil in full sun; mulch in winter in frost-prone sites.
- **PROPAGATION** Sow seed at 13–18°C (55–64°F) in spring. Root basal cuttings in late spring, or semi-ripe cuttings in summer.
- **PESTS AND DISEASES** Slugs and snails may be a problem.

A. zygomeris ▣ Woody-based perennial with mid-green leaves, 15–20cm (6–8in) long. Each leaf has 2 pairs of inversely heart-shaped leaflets with rounded, pale green stipules, to 4cm (1½in) across, veined purple and diffused reddish purple. Racemes of 3–10 pea-like yellow flowers, to 3cm (1¼in) across, with purple keels, are borne in early and mid-autumn. ↕ 2.2m (7ft), ↔ 1.2m (4ft). Mexico. ❄❄

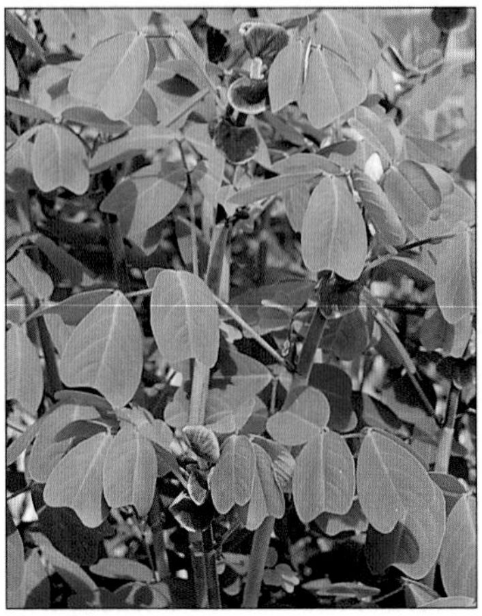

Amicia zygomeris

AMMI

APIACEAE/UMBELLIFERAE

Genus of about 10 species of slender, upright to spreading, summer-flowering annuals and biennials occurring in scrub in Europe, N. Africa, and W. Asia. They have pinnate to 3-pinnate or ternate to 3-ternate, fern-like leaves, and white or creamy white, lace-like flowers borne in large, rounded, branched umbels in summer. Suitable for a border or a cottage garden.
- **HARDINESS** Fully hardy.
- **CULTIVATION** Grow in any moist but well-drained, fertile soil in sun or partial shade. Provide support when seedlings are 7–10cm (3–4in) high.
- **PROPAGATION** Sow seed *in situ* in spring.
- **PESTS AND DISEASES** Trouble free.

A. majus. Slender, upright, branched annual producing 2- or 3-pinnate, light green leaves, 15–20cm (6–8in) long, divided into many finely toothed, ovate to lance-shaped leaflets. Compound umbels with 30 or more rays, each with 10 or more small white flowers, resembling delicate lacework, are borne in summer. ↕ 30–90cm (12–36in), ↔ 30cm (12in). S. Europe, Turkey, N. Africa. ❄❄❄

AMMOBIUM

Winged everlasting

ASTERACEAE/COMPOSITAE

Genus of 2 or 3 upright, branched or unbranched perennials occurring in grassland and open forest in E. Australia. The white-woolly, lance-shaped leaves are produced in broad, basal rosettes. Bright green flowering stems, winged and flattened, and usually branched, bear loose clusters of papery flowerheads, each to 2.5cm (1in) across. Suitable for an annual border; *A. alatum* is excellent for dried flower arrangements.
- **HARDINESS** Half hardy, but may tolerate temperatures to -5°C (23°F) in well-drained soil.
- **CULTIVATION** Grow in any light, well-drained soil, preferably low in nutrients, in full sun. Cut flowerheads for drying before fully open.
- **PROPAGATION** Sow seed at 13–16°C (55–61°F) in early spring, or *in situ* in mid-spring.
- **PESTS AND DISEASES** Trouble free.

A. alatum (Winged everlasting). Rosette-forming perennial, grown as an annual, with lance-shaped, white-woolly leaves, to 18cm (7in) long. In summer, winged, bright green stems bear clusters of "everlasting" flowerheads, to 2.5cm (1in) across, with orange or yellow disc-florets and reflexed, papery, silvery outer bracts and scales. ↕ 50–90cm (20–36in), ↔ 45cm (18in). Australia (Queensland, New South Wales). ❄

▷ ***Amomyrtus luma*** see *Myrtus lechleriana*

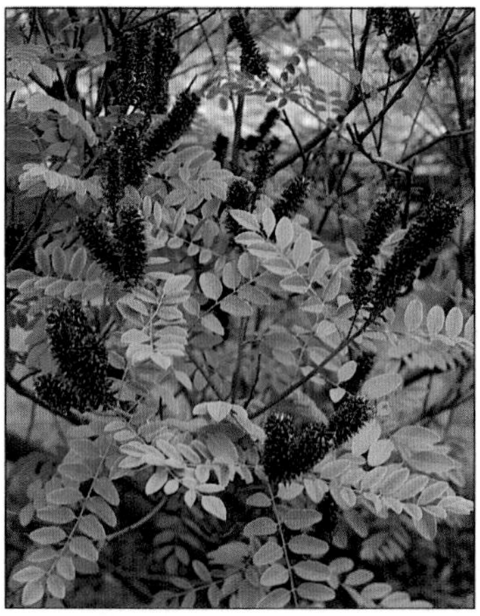
Amorpha fruticosa

AMORPHA

LEGUMINOSAE/PAPILIONACEAE

Genus of 15 species of deciduous shrubs from North America, found in dry, often sandy areas, such as prairies, scrub, and hills, and sometimes in woodland and on riverbanks. They are grown for their aromatic leaves, which are alternate and pinnate, comprising 7–45 leaflets, and their dense, erect racemes of small flowers, which have only a single petal (the standard). They are also valued for their ability to thrive on very poor, dry soils, particularly where temperatures fall to -30°C (-22°F) or below. Grow in a mixed or shrub border.
• **HARDINESS** Fully hardy.
• **CULTIVATION** Grow in light, sandy, well-drained soil in sun or partial shade. Pruning group 6.
• **PROPAGATION** Sow pre-soaked or scarified seed in autumn in containers in an open frame. Separate rooted suckers of *A. fruticosa* in autumn or winter.
• **PESTS AND DISEASES** Vulnerable to rust and mildew.

A. fruticosa ▣ (Bastard indigo). Fast-growing, spreading shrub with pinnate leaves, to 30cm (12in) long, composed of 13–33 oval or oblong leaflets. Orange- or yellow-anthered, purple-blue flowers, 2cm (¾in) long, are produced in narrow racemes, to 15cm (6in) long, in summer. ↕↔ to 5m (15ft). E. USA. ✻✻✻

AMORPHOPHALLUS

Devil's tongue, Snake palm

ARACEAE

Genus of 90–100 species of perennials, with corm-like rhizomes, from moist, shaded habitats in tropical Africa and Asia, grown for their magnificent, deeply lobed leaves. The large, purple-red to greenish white spathes, produced in summer, are usually unpleasantly scented. Outside tropical regions, grow in a warm greenhouse, although they may be moved outdoors in summer after any danger of frost has passed.
• **HARDINESS** Frost tender.
• **CULTIVATION** Plant dormant tubers 10cm (4in) deep in late winter or early spring. Under glass, grow in loam-based potting compost (JI No.3) in containers 60–90cm (24–36in) wide, in filtered light. In the growing season, water freely and apply a balanced liquid fertilizer

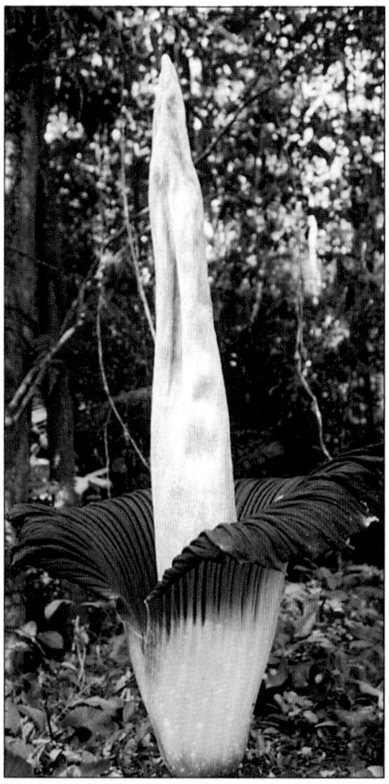
Amorphophallus titanum

monthly. Reduce water as the foliage dies down; overwinter tubers in warm, barely moist conditions. Outdoors, grow in moist, humus-rich soil in partial shade.
• **PROPAGATION** Sow seed at 19–24°C (66–75°F) in autumn or early spring. Separate offsets when dormant.
• **PESTS AND DISEASES** Trouble free.

A. konjac, syn. *A. rivieri* (Devil's tongue, Snake palm, Umbrella arum). Perennial with corm-like rhizomes, to 25cm (10in) across. Reddish purple spathes, to 40cm (16in) long, each with a protruding, dark brown spadix, are borne on stalks 60cm (24in) long, in summer. Each spathe is followed by a solitary, 2-pinnate leaf, to 1.3m (4½ft) long, with oblong-elliptic leaflets or lobes, on a brownish green, white-mottled leaf-stalk, 1–1.3m (3–4½ft) long. ↕ 1–1.3m (3–4½ft), ↔ 1m (3ft). S.E. Asia. ❀ (min. 13–16°C/55–61°F)
A. rivieri see *A. konjac.*
A. titanum ▣ Perennial with huge, corm-like rhizomes, to 50cm (20in) across, and weighing up to 7kg (15lb) each. In summer, produces reddish purple spathes, 1.5m (5ft) long, each with a protruding white spadix, on stalks 1m (3ft) long. The spathes are followed by solitary, 3-parted, deeply lobed leaves, to 4m (12ft) across, borne on leaf-stalks 4.5m (14ft) long. ↕ 5m (15ft), ↔ 4m (12ft). Indonesia (Sumatra). ❀ (min. 13–16°C/55–61°F)

AMPELOPSIS

VITACEAE

Genus of about 25 species of woody, deciduous climbers and a few shrubs from woodland in Asia and North America. They are cultivated for their attractive foliage, which often colours well, turning red and yellow in autumn; the leaves are alternate, simple, palmate or pinnate, often lobed or toothed, with clinging tendrils on the stems opposite the leaves. They are also valued for their sometimes ornamental, spherical or top-shaped berries, which develop from insignificant cymes of small green flowers. The climbers are excellent for covering a wall, fence, pergola, old tree stump, or tree. If grown on house walls, keep clear of gutters and roof tiles. *A. brevipedunculata* 'Elegans' may also be grown as a houseplant.
• **HARDINESS** Fully hardy to frost hardy.
• **CULTIVATION** Under glass, grow in loam-based potting compost (JI No.2) in bright filtered light. During the growing season, water freely and apply a balanced liquid fertilizer monthly; water sparingly in winter. Outdoors, grow in any moist but well-drained, fertile soil in sun or partial shade. Fruiting will be most reliable in a sunny site, especially where root growth can be restricted. *A. brevipedunculata* 'Elegans' grows best against a warm, sheltered, partially shaded wall. Pruning group 11, in spring.
• **PROPAGATION** Sow seed in containers in an open frame in autumn, or stratify and sow in containers in a cold frame in spring. Root softwood cuttings in summer.
• **PESTS AND DISEASES** Trouble free.

A. aconitifolia, syn. *Vitis aconitifolia.* Vigorous, slender-stemmed climber with 3- or 5-palmate, glossy, dark green leaves, to 12cm (5in) long, composed of lance- to diamond-shaped, deeply lobed leaflets. In late summer, bears axillary cymes of small green flowers, followed by spherical orange fruit, to 6mm (¼in) across. ↕ 12m (40ft). Mongolia, N. China. ✻✻✻
A. brevipedunculata ▣ Vigorous climber producing palmately 3-lobed, occasionally 5-lobed, dark green leaves, hairy beneath, and 5–15cm (2–6in) long. Branched, axillary cymes of small green flowers are borne in summer, followed by attractive, spherical, pinkish purple, later clear blue fruit, 5–8mm (¼–⅜in) across. ↕ 5m (15ft). N.E. Asia. ✻✻✻. **'Elegans'** is less vigorous, and has dark green leaves, heavily mottled white and pink. **var. *maximowiczii***, syn. *A. heterophylla, Vitis heterophylla,* has very variable, slightly longer leaves than the species, sometimes broadly heart-shaped at the bases and shallowly lobed, or deeply cut into 3–5 lobes.
A. heterophylla see *A. brevipedunculata* var. *maximowiczii.*
A. megalophylla. Vigorous climber with glaucous shoots and large, 2-pinnate, occasionally pinnate leaves, to 60cm (24in) long, composed of 7–9 ovate to ovate-oblong, dark green leaflets, glaucous on the reverse. Few-flowered, axillary cymes of green flowers are borne in late summer, followed by top-shaped black fruit, 6mm (¼in) across. ↕ 10m (30ft). W. China. ✻✻✻
A. sempervirens see *Cissus striata.*
A. veitchii see *Parthenocissus tricuspidata* 'Veitchii'.

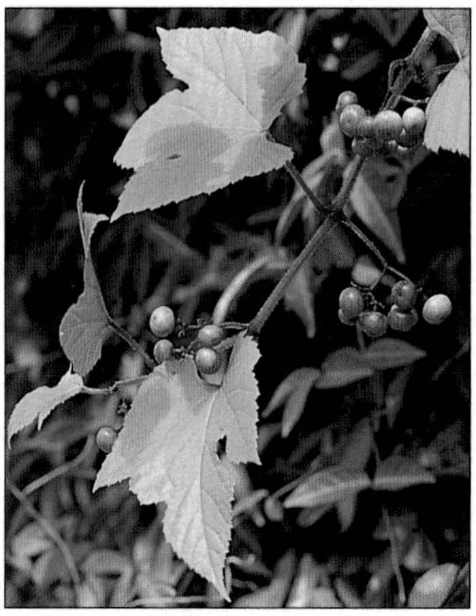
Ampelopsis brevipedunculata

▷***Amphicome*** see *Incarvillea*

AMSONIA syn. RHAZYA

APOCYNACEAE

Genus of about 20 species of clump-forming perennials from light woodland or grassland in moist, stony or heavy soils in S.E. Europe, Turkey, Japan, and N.E. and C. USA. They have alternate, lance-shaped or ovate to elliptic, entire leaves. Long-lasting cymes or panicles of narrowly funnel-shaped blue flowers, with 5 spreading petal lobes, are borne from spring to summer. They are suitable for a mixed or herbaceous border. Contact with the milky sap may irritate skin.
• **HARDINESS** Fully hardy.
• **CULTIVATION** Grow in any moist but well-drained soil in full sun. Will tolerate some drought.
• **PROPAGATION** Sow seed in containers in a cold frame in autumn or spring. Divide in spring. Root softwood or basal cuttings in early summer.
• **PESTS AND DISEASES** Trouble free.

A. illustris. Clump-forming perennial with broadly ovate to lance-shaped or elliptic, glossy, bright green leaves, 3–7cm (1¼–3in) long. Open panicles of light blue flowers, to 1.5cm (½in) across, are produced on erect stems, in late spring and early summer. ↕ 1.2m (4ft), ↔ 45cm (18in). C. and S. USA. ✻✻✻
A. orientalis ▣ 🏆 syn. *Rhazya orientalis.* Clump-forming perennial with many erect stems rising from a woody rootstock, and with narrowly ovate to lance-shaped, willow-like, greyish green leaves, 3–7cm (1¼–3in) long. Short, compact or loose panicles of violet-blue flowers, 1–2cm (½–¾in) across, are produced in early and midsummer. ↕ 50cm (20in), ↔ 30cm (12in). N.E. Greece, N.W. Turkey. ✻✻✻
A. salicifolia see *A. tabernaemontana* var. *salicifolia.*

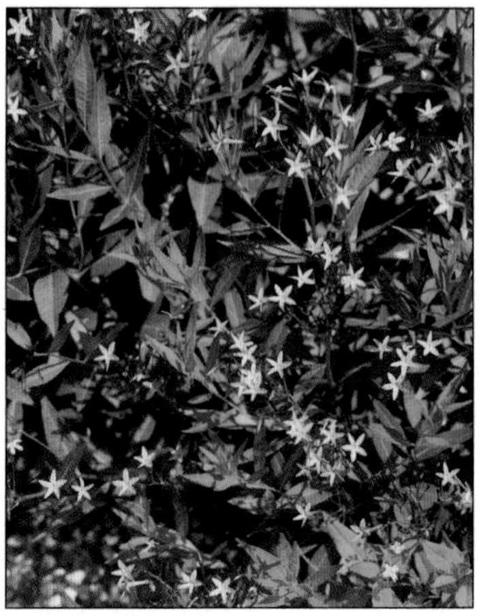
Amsonia orientalis

A

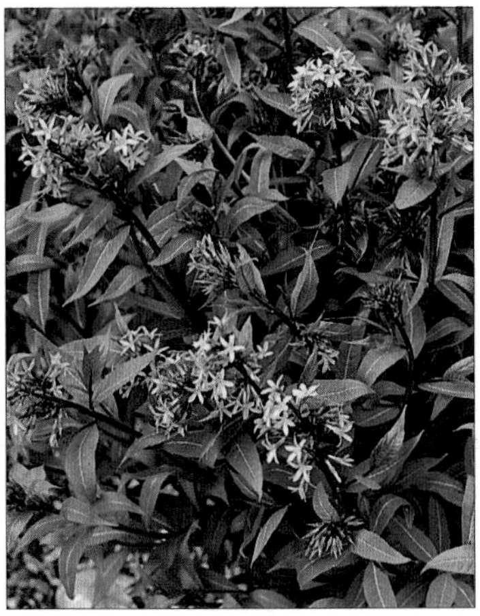

Amsonia tabernaemontana

A. tabernaemontana ■ Clump-forming perennial with many stems and small, ovate to elliptic or lance-shaped, matt, dark green leaves, 3–7cm (1¼–3in) long. Dense, rounded, cyme-like panicles of pale blue flowers, 1–2cm (½–¾in) across, are borne from late spring to midsummer. ↕60cm (24in), ↔45cm (18in). E. USA. ❄❄❄. **var. *salicifolia***, syn. *A. salicifolia*, has much narrower leaves, glaucous beneath, and produces flowers in more open panicles.

▷***Amygdalus*** see *Prunus*

ANACAMPSEROS

PORTULACACEAE

Genus of about 50 species of perennial succulents, mainly from the most arid regions of Africa and Australia, with either minute leaves, often covered by hairs or hidden by stipules, or fleshy, ovoid to spherical, conspicuous leaves. In summer, the 5-petalled, white, pink, or red flowers, produced singly or in racemes, open only for a brief period, in full sun. In frost-prone areas, grow in a temperate greenhouse; in frost-free areas, grow in a desert garden.

• **HARDINESS** Frost tender.

• **CULTIVATION** Under glass, grow in standard cactus compost in full light with good ventilation. In the growing season, water moderately and apply a dilute liquid fertilizer monthly; keep almost dry when dormant in winter. Outdoors, grow in poor to moderately fertile, sharply drained soil in full sun. See also pp.48–49.

• **PROPAGATION** Sow seed as soon as ripe at 18°C (64°F), or take stem cuttings in spring and root at the same temperature.

• **PESTS AND DISEASES** Prone to aphids.

A. alstonii. Tufted, many-branched succulent with a tuberous rootstock, which, when exposed, is caudex-like. Tiny leaves are arranged in rows along the branches and are hidden by small, overlapping, triangular silver stipules, 2mm (1/16in) long. Solitary, open white flowers, 3cm (1¼in) across, are borne in summer. ↕3cm (1¼in), ↔8cm (3in). South Africa (Northern Cape). ❁ (min. 7°C/45°F)

A. comptonii. Succulent with a short, thick stem, much of which is buried, becoming swollen and caudex-like. The aerial stems produce spherical, olive-green or bronzed leaves, 3–5cm (1¼–2in) long, tapered at the tips, grooved above, and covered with white hairs. Solitary, open, red-purple, pink, or white flowers, 6mm (¼in) across, are borne in summer. ↕↔2.5cm (1in). Namibia, South Africa. ❁ (min. 7°C/45°F)

A. intermedia see *A. telephiastrum*.

A. telephiastrum, syn. *A. intermedia*, *A. varians*. Mat-forming succulent, becoming tufted when mature, with ovoid, short-pointed, fleshy, brownish green leaves, 2cm (¾in) long. Racemes of 1–4 deep pink flowers, 3cm (1¼in) or more across, open in summer. ↕5cm (2in), ↔10cm (4in). South Africa (Western Cape). ❁ (min. 7°C/45°F)

A. varians see *A. telephiastrum*.

▷***Anacharis densa*** see *Egeria densa*

ANACYCLUS

ASTERACEAE/COMPOSITAE

Genus of 9 species of annuals and herbaceous perennials from stony slopes and sandy and disturbed ground in the Mediterranean. The 2- or 3-pinnatisect leaves, with finely cut lobes, are produced on creeping stems radiating from a central rootstock. Solitary or paired, daisy-like flowerheads are borne on short stems in summer. Grow in an alpine house or a rock garden.

• **HARDINESS** Frost hardy, but may tolerate temperatures below -5°C (23°F) with protection from winter wet.

• **CULTIVATION** Under glass, grow in a mix of equal parts loam, leaf mould, and sharp sand or grit, in full light. Outdoors, grow in gritty, sharply drained, poor to moderately fertile soil in full sun, protected from winter wet.

• **PROPAGATION** Sow seed in containers in an open frame in autumn. Root softwood cuttings in spring or early summer.

• **PESTS AND DISEASES** Aphids may be a problem under glass.

A. depressus see *A. pyrethrum* var. *depressus*.

A. pyrethrum* var. *depressus ■ syn. *A. depressus*. Prostrate, mat-forming perennial with rosettes of 2- or 3-pinnatisect, grey-green leaves, 10–14cm (4–5½in) long. Bears numerous solitary flowerheads, 2.5–5cm (1–2in) across, with white ray-florets; the ray-florets are red on the reverse, each with a white stripe. ↕2.5–5cm (1–2in) or more, ↔10cm (4in). Atlas Mountains in Morocco, Algeria, and Tunisia. ❄❄

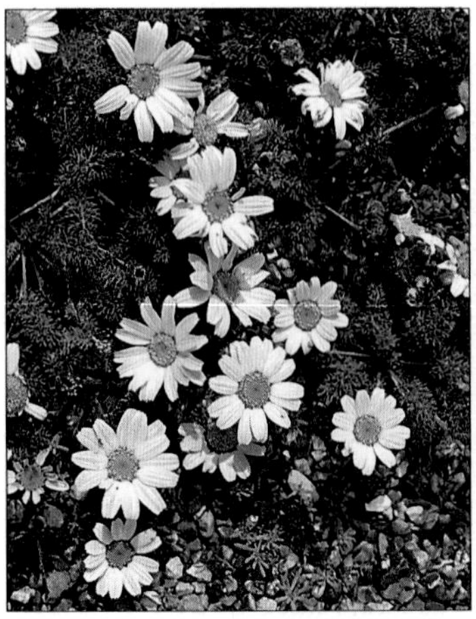

Anacyclus pyrethrum var. *depressus*

ANAGALLIS

Pimpernel

PRIMULACEAE

Genus of about 20 species of low-growing or creeping annuals and evergreen perennials, occurring in open meadows, bogs, and dry sites in the Mediterranean and W. Europe. The opposite or alternate leaves (occasionally borne in threes) are entire and smooth, with very short or no leaf-stalks. The solitary, bell-shaped to open saucer-shaped flowers, each with 5 petals, are produced from the leaf axils. Easily cultivated, pimpernels provide colourful ground cover for a rock garden or the front of a border. *A. tenella* 'Studland' is also an excellent specimen for growing in pans in an alpine house.

• **HARDINESS** Fully hardy to frost hardy.

• **CULTIVATION** Under glass, grow *A. tenella* 'Studland' in gritty, loam-based potting compost (JI No.1) in full light. Outdoors, grow pimpernels in fertile, moist but well-drained soil in full sun; *A. monellii* needs moderately fertile, well-drained soil in full sun. Overwinter young plants in a cool greenhouse and plant out after danger of frost has passed. Pimpernels are often short-lived, so propagate regularly.

• **PROPAGATION** Sow seed in containers in a cold frame in spring, or divide in spring. Increase *A. tenella* 'Studland' and cultivars of *A. monellii* by soft tip cuttings in spring or early summer.

• **PESTS AND DISEASES** Prone to aphids.

A. collina see *A. monellii*.

A. linifolia see *A. monellii*.

A. monellii ♀ syn. *A. collina*, *A. linifolia* (Blue pimpernel). Low-growing perennial with branching stems bearing stalkless, lance-shaped to elliptic, mid-green leaves, to 2.5cm (1in) long, in opposite pairs or in threes. Open saucer-shaped flowers, to 1.5cm (½in) or more across, usually deep blue, sometimes reddish at the bases, are produced on long stalks in summer. Red- and pink-flowered variants are also available. ↕10–20cm (4–8in), ↔ to 40cm (16in). Mediterranean. ❄❄. **'Phillipii'**, syn. *A. phillipii* of gardens, has deep blue flowers; ↕ to 25cm (10in).

***A. phillipii* of gardens** see *A. monellii* 'Phillipii'.

***A. tenella* 'Studland'** ■♀ Mat-forming perennial with alternate or opposite, stalkless, elliptic to rounded, bright green leaves, 4–9mm (⅛–⅜in) long. In late spring and early summer, the leaves are almost hidden by upright, bell-shaped, scented, deep pink flowers, 6–10mm (¼–½in) across. ↕5–10cm (2–4in), ↔ to 40cm (16in). ❄❄❄

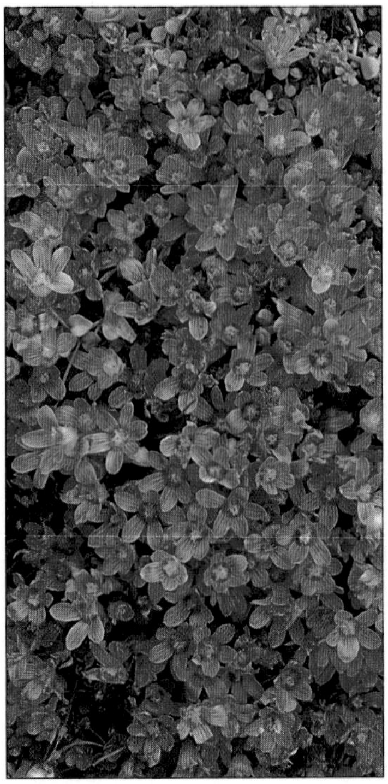

Anagallis tenella 'Studland'

ANANAS

Pineapple

BROMELIACEAE

Genus of 5 or 6 species of evergreen, terrestrial perennials (bromeliads) from South America, occurring in habitats ranging from fairly dry to extremely humid, and from low terrain to mountains over 1,000m (3,000ft). They form rosettes of lance-shaped, spiny leaves and, in summer, produce showy flowers in dense, terminal, cone-like inflorescences on stout stems, giving rise to fleshy, swollen, edible fruits. In areas where temperatures fall below 15°C (59°F), grow pineapples as houseplants or in a warm greenhouse. In tropical climates, grow in a border.

• **HARDINESS** Frost tender.

• **CULTIVATION** Under glass, grow in terrestrial bromeliad compost in full light with low to moderate humidity and in draught-free conditions. Water freely during the growing and flowering season; reduce water slightly and apply a balanced liquid fertilizer weekly as the fruits begin to swell. Keep barely moist at other times of the year. Outside, grow in well-drained, fertile, humus-rich soil in full sun. See also p.47.

• **PROPAGATION** Root basal offsets in early summer; or carefully sever the leafy rosette at the top of the fruit, allow it a day or two to callus, then root it in a barely moist mix of peat and sand, in indirect light at 21°C (70°F).

• **PESTS AND DISEASES** Scale insects may be a problem under glass.

A. bracteatus (Red pineapple, Wild pineapple). Terrestrial bromeliad with green-brown, coarsely spiny leaves, 45cm (18in) or more long, the spines

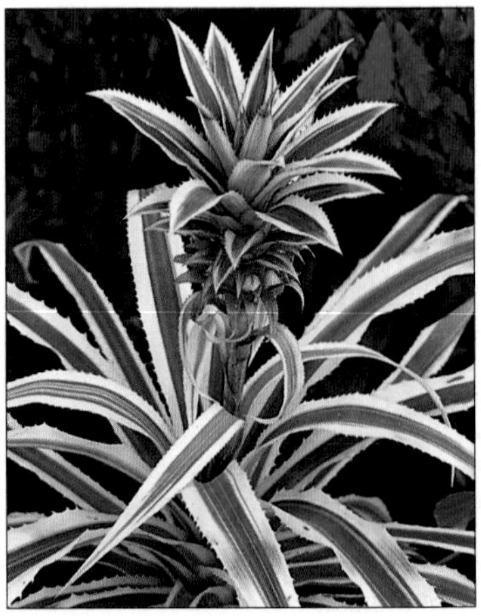

Ananas bracteatus 'Tricolor'

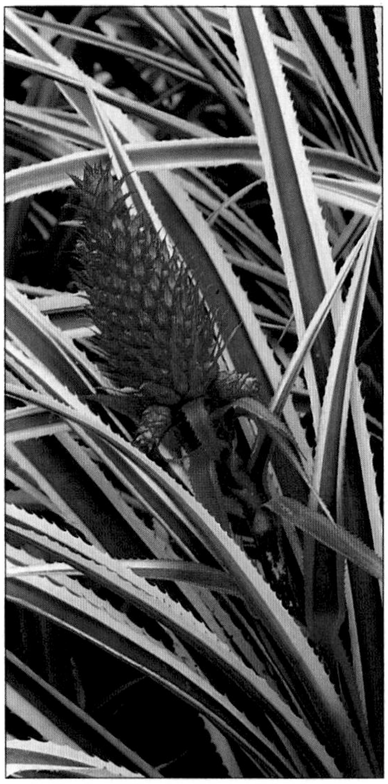

Ananas comosus 'Variegatus'

upward-pointing. In summer, bears red-bracted, yellowish red flowers in almost cylindrical inflorescences, to 15cm (6in) long, followed by edible but not very fleshy, greenish brown fruit, 15cm (6in) long. ↕ to 70cm (28in), ↔ 50cm (20in). Brazil, Paraguay, Argentina. ❁ (min. 15°C/59°F). **'Tricolor'** ▣ ♀ syn. 'Striatus', var. *tricolor*, has deep green, yellow-striped leaves.
A. comosus. Variable, terrestrial bromeliad with dense rosettes of slightly recurved, spiny-margined, dark green leaves, to 1m (3ft) long. In summer, produces oblong-ovoid inflorescences, 30cm (12in) or more long, of small, reddish yellow bracts and violet-purple or violet-blue flowers. They are followed by bright red fruit, to 30cm (12in) long. These are the pineapples grown commercially. ↕ 1m (3ft), ↔ 50cm (20in). Presumed to have originated in Brazil. ❁ (min. 15°C/59°F).
'Variegatus' ▣ syn. var. *variegatus*, has leaves longitudinally striped yellowish white, occasionally also with red stripes.
A. nanus. Terrestrial bromeliad resembling a miniature *A. comosus.* Slightly recurved, dark green leaves, to 60cm (24in) long, have upward-pointing marginal spines. Cone-shaped inflorescences, 10cm (4in) long, comprising lilac-purple or red flowers with small yellow bracts, are produced in summer. They are followed by fruit to 10cm (4in) long, with a large crown. ↕ 45cm (18in), ↔ 60cm (24in). Surinam, Brazil. ❁ (min. 15°C/59°F)

ANAPHALIS

Pearl everlasting

ASTERACEAE/COMPOSITAE

Genus of about 100 species of spreading to upright perennials, some evergreen, from dry slopes, dry forests, sunny riverbanks, or moist woodland in the N. hemisphere. They have woolly grey foliage and produce corymbs of papery "everlasting" white flowerheads, 0.6–2.5cm (¼–1in) across, which are good for cutting and drying. The larger species provide pale foliage contrast in borders too moist for most sun-loving, grey-leaved plants, while the smaller species are excellent, long-lasting rock-garden plants.

- **HARDINESS** Fully hardy.
- **CULTIVATION** Grow in full sun in moderately fertile, reasonably well-drained soil that does not dry out in summer (very important for *A. nepalensis* and its variants). Most will also grow in partial shade.
- **PROPAGATION** Sow seed in containers in a cold frame in spring. Divide in early spring, or take basal or stem tip cuttings in spring or early summer.
- **PESTS AND DISEASES** Trouble free.

A. cinnamomea see *A. margaritacea* var. *cinnamomea.*
A. margaritacea ▣ Clump-forming, rhizomatous perennial with erect, leafy stems and lance-shaped, mid-green leaves, 7–14cm (3–5½in) long, white-woolly beneath. From midsummer to early autumn, bears dense corymbs, to 15cm (6in) across, of yellow flowerheads surrounded by white bracts. ↕↔ 60cm (24in). N.E. Asia, North America. ✽✽✽. **var. *cinnamomea*,** syn. *A. cinnamomea*, has broader leaves, white or cinnamon-coloured beneath, with 3 main veins, and flowerheads in tighter, rounder, many-branched corymbs; ↔ 45–50cm (18–20in). Mountains of India and Burma. **var. *yedoensis*** ♀ syn. *A. yedoensis*, has shorter, narrow, single-veined, white-woolly leaves, 6cm (2½in) long; Japan.
A. nepalensis ▣ syn. *A. triplinervis* var. *intermedia.* Clump-forming perennial with lance-shaped, pale grey-green leaves, 3–10cm (1½–4in) long, white-woolly beneath, with 3 main veins, on short, silvery green stems. In late summer and early autumn, produces solitary to several yellow flowerheads, surrounded by pointed white bracts, in rounded corymbs, 2cm (¾in) across. ↕ 30cm (12in), ↔ 15cm (6in) or more. Himalayas, W. China. ✽✽✽. **var. *monocephala*,** syn. *A. nubigena*, has short, densely leafy, white-woolly stems, and inversely lance-shaped to linear-lance-shaped leaves, light grey-green above, white-woolly beneath, to 2.5cm (1in) long. Solitary to several, white or yellow flowerheads in corymbs, 1.5cm (½in) across, are borne in midsummer; ↕ 10–20cm (4–8in), ↔ 30cm (12in). China (Yunnan) to Tibet.

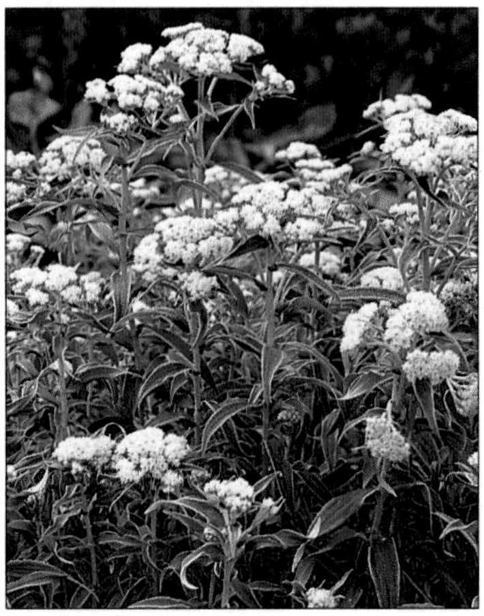

Anaphalis margaritacea

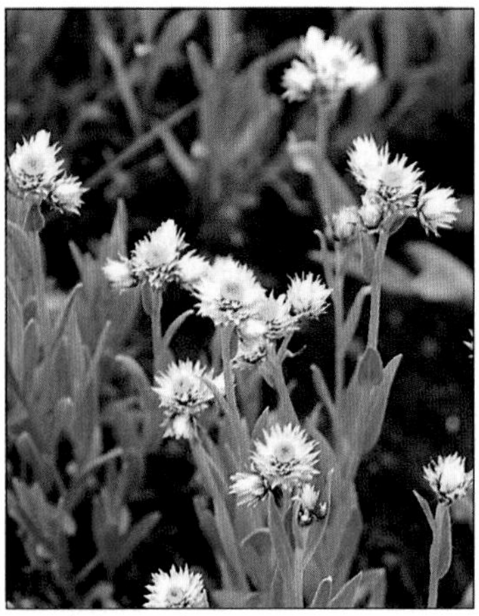

Anaphalis nepalensis

A. nubigena see *A. nepalensis* var. *monocephala.*
A. sinica* subsp. *morii. Upright, evergreen, silvery grey, downy perennial, which is a dwarf variant of *A. sinica*, with linear-lance-shaped leaves, to 2cm (¾in) long. In late summer and early autumn, bears spherical corymbs, 3–7cm (1¼–3in) across, of white flowerheads surrounded by pointed white bracts. Tolerates heavy soils and partial shade. ↕ to 20cm (8in), ↔ to 60cm (24in). Mountainous areas of China, Korea, Japan (Kyushu). ✽✽✽
A. triplinervis ♀ Clump-forming perennial with spoon-shaped to obovate-elliptic, pale grey-green, white-woolly leaves, 3–10cm (1¼in–4in) long, with 3–5 main veins. Domed corymbs, 4–5cm (1½–2in) across, of white-bracted, yellow-centred flowerheads, are produced in mid- and late summer. ↕ 80–90cm (32–36in), ↔ 45–60cm (18–24in). Himalayas to S.W. China. ✽✽✽. **var. *intermedia*** see *A. nepalensis.* **'Sommerschnee'** ♀ syn. 'Summer Snow', has brilliant white bracts.
A. yedoensis see *A. margaritacea* var. *yedoensis.*

ANCHUSA

Alkanet

BORAGINACEAE

Genus of about 35 species of erect to spreading or mound-forming annuals, biennials, and perennials, often short-lived, occurring in sunny, dry sites, including roadsides, stony hills, cliffs, and grassland, in temperate regions of Europe, Africa, and W. Asia. They have alternate, linear-lance-shaped to elliptic leaves, sometimes with a covering of bristly hairs, and are grown for their tubular, usually blue flowers with 5 spreading lobes, borne in terminal and axillary cymes. Grow dwarf species, such as *A. cespitosa*, in tufa or in a rock garden, raised bed, or trough. Taller species are ideal for a herbaceous border. The flowers are attractive to bees.

- **HARDINESS** Fully hardy to frost hardy.
- **CULTIVATION** Grow in any moist but well-drained, moderately fertile soil in full sun. Tall species and cultivars may need staking when in flower. Cut back top-growth after flowering to encourage the development of overwintering basal rosettes. Dead-head after the first flush of flowers to encourage a second flush. Most species resent excessive winter wet.
- **PROPAGATION** Sow seed of annuals at 13–16°C (55–61°F) in late winter or early spring. Sow seed of perennials in containers in a cold frame in spring. Root basal cuttings in spring, or insert root cuttings in winter.
- **PESTS AND DISEASES** Prone to mildew.

A. angustissima see *A. leptophylla* subsp. *incana.*
A. azurea, syn. *A. italica.* Erect, clump-forming perennial with mainly basal leaves, 10–40cm (4–16in) long, which are linear-elliptic to lance-shaped, mid- to dark green, and stiffly hairy. Branching panicles of gentian-blue flowers, to 1.5cm (½in) across, turning blue-purple with age, are borne in early summer. ↕ 90–150cm (3–5ft), ↔ 60cm (24in). S. Europe, N. Africa, W. Asia. ✽✽✽. **'Feltham Pride'** is compact, with clear, bright blue flowers. Although perennial, it is often grown as a seed-raised biennial; ↕ to 90cm (36in). **'Little John'** is long-lived and dwarf, with deep blue flowers. It is ideal for the front of a border or a rock garden; ↕ 45cm (18in), ↔ 30cm (12in). **'Loddon Royalist'** ▣ ♀ is sturdy, so seldom needs staking, and has bright, deep blue flowers; ↕ 90cm (36in). **'Morning Glory'** has flowers in a bright shade of deep blue; ↕ 1m (3ft). **'Opal'** has paler blue flowers than the other cultivars; ↕ 90cm (36in).
A. barrelieri. Erect, clump-forming perennial with elliptic or lance-shaped to oblong-spoon-shaped, wavy-margined or sometimes toothed, mid-green leaves, 5–7cm (2–3in) long. Panicles of white-eyed blue flowers, 6–8mm (¼–⅜in) across, similar to forget-me-nots, are borne in early summer. ↕ 60cm (24in), ↔ 30cm (12in). N. Balkans to Ukraine, Turkey. ✽✽✽
A. caespitosa see *A. cespitosa.*
A. capensis. Erect biennial, often grown as an annual, with rough, narrowly lance-shaped, mid-green leaves, to 12cm (5in) long, covered in bristly hairs. Bears a mass of terminal, open panicles of saucer-shaped, bright blue, white-

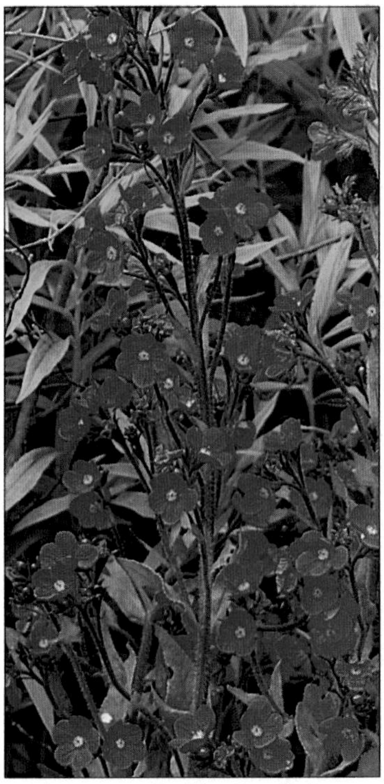

Anchusa azurea 'Loddon Royalist'

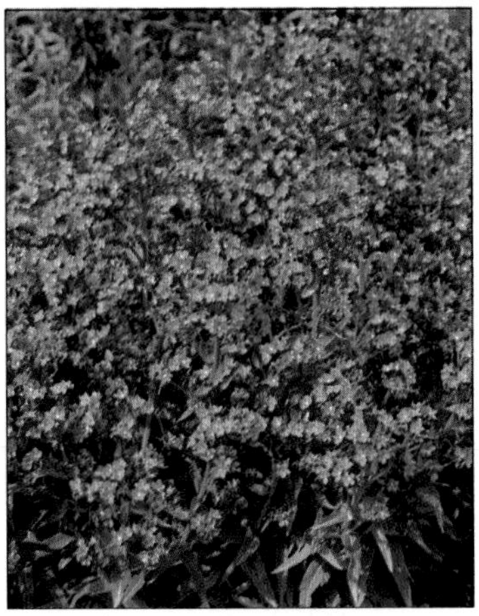

Anchusa capensis 'Blue Angel'

throated flowers, 4–8mm (1/8–3/8in) across, in summer. ↕ 12–18cm (5–7in), ↔ 9–12cm (3½–5in). South Africa. ❄❄. **'Blue Angel'** ■ is upright and compact with ultramarine-blue flowers; ↕ 20cm (8in), ↔ 15cm (6in). **'Blue Bird'** bears indigo-blue flowers; ↕ 45cm (18in), ↔ 15–23cm (6–9in). **'Dawn'** has blue, pink, or white flowers; ↕ 45cm (18in), ↔ 15–23cm (6–9in).

A. cespitosa ■ ♀ syn. *A. caespitosa*. Dense, mound-forming perennial with rosettes of narrowly linear, hairy, dark green leaves, to 6cm (2½in) long. Bears clusters of stemless, white-eyed, vivid blue flowers, to 1.2cm (½in) across, in spring. Needs sharp drainage. ↕ 5–10cm (2–4in), ↔ 15–20cm (6–8in). Mountain rocks in Greece (Crete). ❄❄❄

A. italica see *A. azurea*.

A. leptophylla* subsp. *incana, syn. *A. angustissima*. Upright, tufted, many-branched perennial with loose rosettes of narrowly lance-shaped, dark green leaves, 6–11cm (2½–4½in) long. Bears one-sided cymes of bright azure-blue, white-eyed flowers, 4–6mm (1/8–¼in) across, throughout the summer. ↕ to 30cm (12in), occasionally more, ↔ 20cm (8in). Turkey. ❄❄❄

A. myosotidiflora see *Brunnera macrophylla*.

A. sempervirens see *Pentaglottis sempervirens*.

▷***Ancistrocactus*** see *Sclerocactus*
A. crassihamatus see *S. uncinatus* var. *crassihamatus*
A. megarhizus see *S. scheeri*
A. scheeri see *S. scheeri*
A. uncinatus see *S. uncinatus*

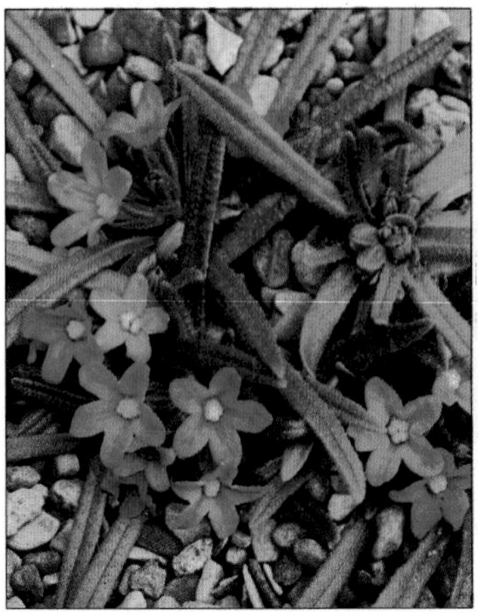

Anchusa cespitosa

ANDROMEDA

Bog rosemary

ERICACEAE

Genus of 2 species of low-growing, wiry-stemmed, evergreen shrubs, found in acid peat bogs in the arctic and cool-temperate regions of the N. hemisphere. The leaves are simple, alternate, and linear-lance-shaped to oblong; the small, urn-shaped flowers, produced in terminal umbels from spring to early summer, are white or pink. Grow with woodland plants in a peat bed; they are also suitable for a shady rock garden, or a damp border in acid soil.

- **HARDINESS** Fully hardy.
- **CULTIVATION** Grow in moist, acid, humus-rich soil, in partial shade or full sun. Mulch annually in spring with leaf mould in dry sites.
- **PROPAGATION** Root softwood cuttings in early to midsummer; pot up suckers or rooted layers in autumn or spring.
- **PESTS AND DISEASES** Trouble free.

A. polifolia ■ syn. *A. rosmarinifolia* (Common bog rosemary, Marsh andromeda). Variable, erect or semi-prostrate shrub producing pointed, linear-oblong, leathery, dark green leaves, 1.5–3.5cm (½–1½in) long. White or pale pink flowers are borne on slender flower-stalks, in 2- to 5-flowered umbels, to 3cm (1¼in) across, from spring to early summer. ↕ to 40cm (16in), ↔ to 60cm (24in). N. Europe. ❄❄❄. **'Alba'** ■ syn. 'Compacta Alba', is semi-prostrate and freely produces pure white flowers; ↕ 15cm (6in),

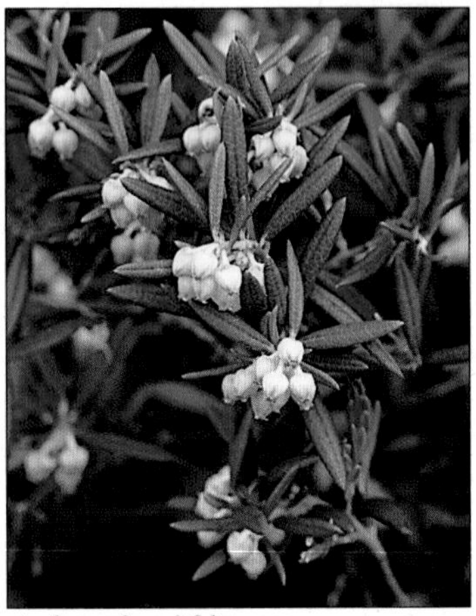

Andromeda polifolia

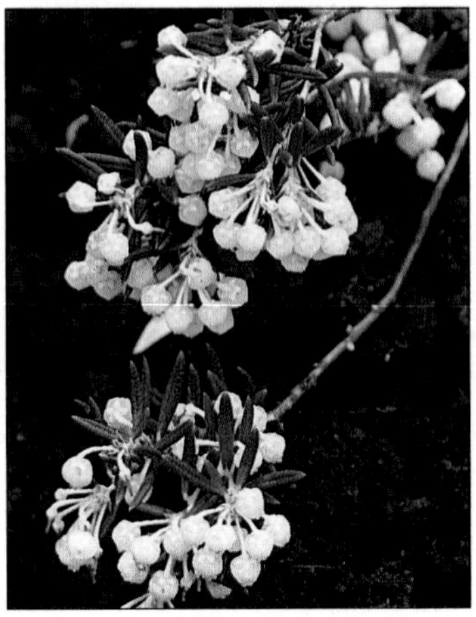

Andromeda polifolia 'Alba'

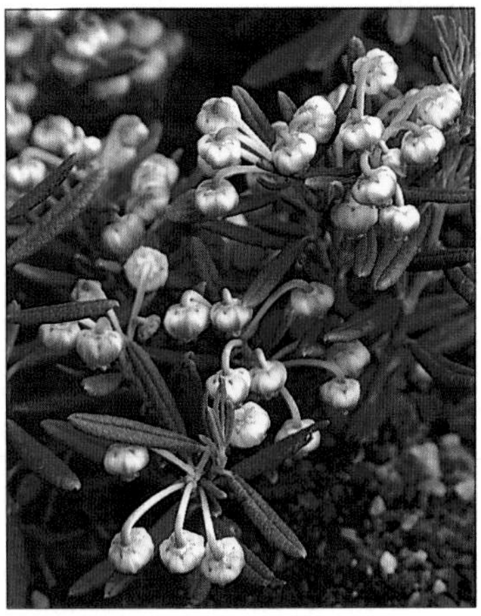

Andromeda polifolia 'Compacta'

↔ 20cm (8in). **'Compacta'** ■ ♀ is a densely twiggy shrub, with broad, glaucous leaves and pink flowers; ↕ to 30cm (12in), ↔ to 20cm (8in). **'Compacta Alba'** see 'Alba'. **'Macrophylla'** ♀ is low-growing, with broad, ovate, dark green leaves, to 3cm (1¼in) long. It produces numerous deep pink and white flowers, which are slightly larger and more rounded than the species; ↕ 5–15cm (2–6in), ↔ 25cm (10in). **'Nikko'** is a vigorous, compact, rounded shrub. It has grey-green leaves, to 2.5cm (1in) long, and bears umbels of clear pink flowers; ↕↔ 20–25cm (8–10in).

A. rosmarinifolia see *A. polifolia*.

▷**Andromeda, Marsh** see *Andromeda polifolia*

ANDROPOGON

GRAMINEAE/POACEAE

Genus of over 100 species of annual or perennial, rhizomatous and clump-forming grasses, mostly from grassland in tropical regions, but also from the temperate zones of both hemispheres. They have flat, sheathed, linear leaves and produce racemes of small spikelets, on erect, sometimes branching stems in summer or autumn. Only *A. gerardii*, which has colourful foliage and flower-heads, is of ornamental value; it is suitable for growing at the back of a herbaceous border.

- **HARDINESS** Fully hardy.
- **CULTIVATION** Grow in light, fertile, well-drained, and preferably sandy soil, in full sun. *A. gerardii* does not tolerate excessive winter wet. Cut back old stems to the ground in early spring before growth begins.
- **PROPAGATION** Divide from mid-spring to early summer. Sow seed in containers in a cold frame in spring.
- **PESTS AND DISEASES** Trouble free.

A. gerardii (Big bluestem). Densely tufted perennial, with short rhizomes, producing erect clumps of arching, linear, blue-green leaves, to 30cm (12in) long, which turn purple in autumn. Strong, erect stems, to 2m (6ft) tall, bear 3–6 terminal, finger-like, deep red-purple racemes, to 10cm (4in) long, in early and mid-autumn. ↕ to 2m (6ft), ↔ 60cm (24in). Canada to Mexico. ❄❄❄

A. scoparius see *Schizachyrium scoparium*.

ANDROSACE

syn. DOUGLASIA

Rock jasmine

PRIMULACEAE

Genus of about 100 species of annuals, biennials, and predominantly evergreen, mat- or cushion-forming perennials. They have small rosettes of hairy leaves and produce stemless or short-stemmed, tubular-based flowers, with flat or cup-shaped lobes, singly or in umbels from late spring to late summer. Most occur in the mountains of the N. hemisphere, growing in rock crevices, scree, or turf. The high-alpine (Aretian), cushion-forming species are superb for a well-ventilated alpine house; most of the remainder are ideal for a rock garden, scree bed, or trough.

- **HARDINESS** Fully hardy, but the Aretian species need protection from excessive wet, especially in winter.
- **CULTIVATION** Under glass, grow in pans in full light with good ventilation. Grow Aretian species in a very sharply drained mix of equal parts loam-based potting compost (JI No.2) and grit, with a collar of grit around the neck of the plant. They are best watered from below to keep the plant neck and foliage dry; do not allow the compost to dry out. Outdoors, grow other species in a scree bed, in vertical crevices in rock-work, or in moist but gritty, well-drained soil in a trough in full sun. The smallest cushion-forming species also grow well in tufa.
- **PROPAGATION** Sow seed in containers in an open frame as soon as ripe or in autumn. Root single rosettes as cuttings in early to midsummer. Keep moist, but water from below to avoid wetting the rosettes.
- **PESTS AND DISEASES** Prone to aphids under glass, and to fungal diseases in damp conditions. Remove dead rosettes to reduce the risk of infection.

A. carnea ■ Tufted perennial with loose rosettes, 1–2cm (½–¾in) wide, of evergreen, hairy-margined, linear, fleshy, mid-green leaves, to 2cm (¾in) long. In late spring, bears umbels of 3–8 pink, yellow-eyed flowers, 5–8mm (¼–3/8in) across, on stems 2.5–5cm (1–2in) tall. ↕ 5cm (2in), ↔ 8–15cm (3–6in). Pyrenees, Alps, Tyrol. ❄❄❄. **subsp. *laggeri*** ■ ♀ syn. *A. laggeri*, is more densely tufted with smaller rosettes, 7–10mm (¼–½in) across, and flowers that are a deeper pink; E. Pyrenees.

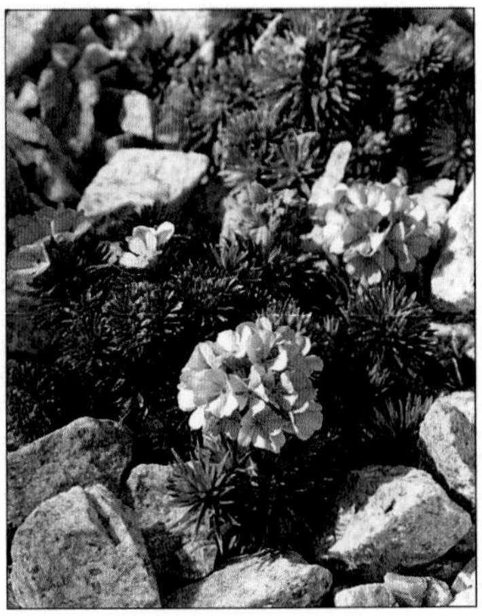

Androsace carnea

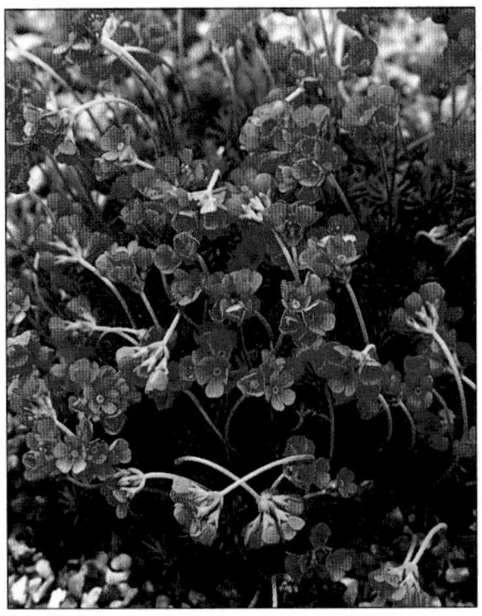
Androsace carnea subsp. *laggeri*

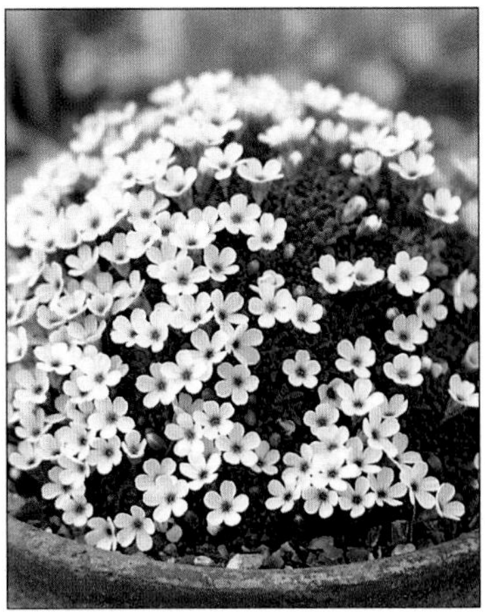
Androsace pyrenaica

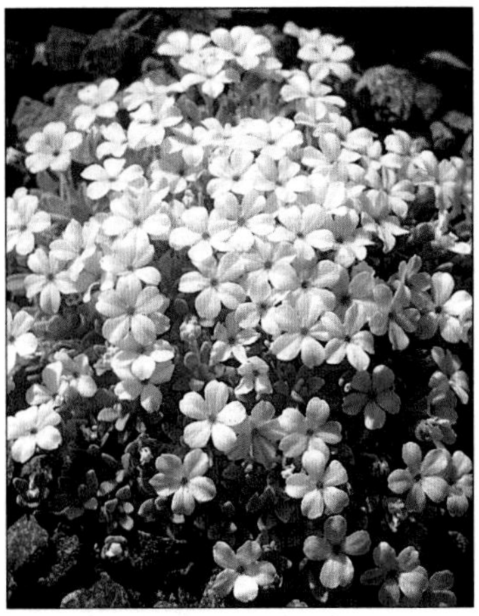
Androsace vandellii

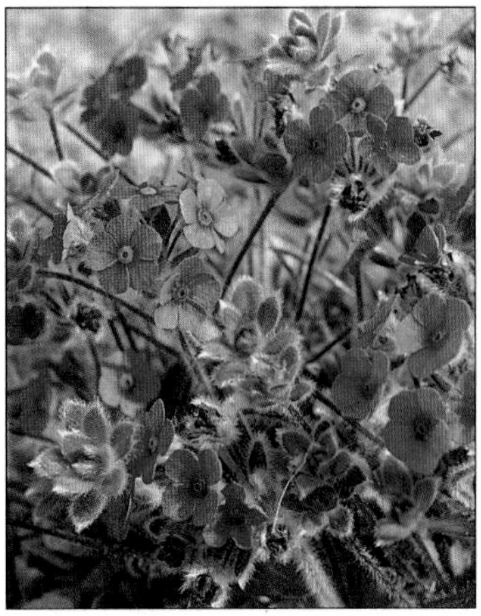
Androsace villosa var. *jacquemontii*

A. chamaejasme. Mat-forming, evergreen perennial with short stolons and open rosettes, 1–2cm (½–¾in) across, of oblong-lance-shaped to elliptic, silky-hairy, mid-green leaves, to 1.5cm (½in) long. In late spring, bears umbels of 2–8 pink or white, yellow-eyed flowers, to 8mm (⅜in) across, sometimes turning pink- or red-eyed with age, on stems to 6cm (2½in) tall. ↕ 3–6cm (1¼–2½in), occasionally to 12cm (5in), ↔ to 15–20cm (6–8in). Europe to North America. ❄❄❄
A. ciliata. Cushion-forming Aretian with loose, evergreen rosettes, 1.5–2.5cm (½–1in) across, of inversely lance-shaped to ovate, hairy, glossy, mid-green leaves, to 1.5cm (½in) long. In late spring and early summer, pale to deep pink, yellow- to orange-eyed flowers, 8–15mm (⅜–½in) across, are borne singly above the cushions, on stems 1.5cm (½in) long. ↕ 2.5cm (1in), ↔ 5–8cm (2–3in). Pyrenees. ❄❄❄
A. cylindrica. Compact, cushion-forming, evergreen Aretian with rosettes, 1.5–2cm (½–¾in) wide, of linear-elliptic, hairy-margined, grey-green leaves, to 1cm (½in) long. In mid- and late spring, white flowers, 1cm (½in) across, with greenish yellow eyes, are borne singly on stems, to 1.5cm (½in) high. ↕ 1–2cm (½–¾in), ↔ 10–15cm (4–6in). Pyrenees. ❄❄❄
A. imbricata see *A. vandellii.*
A. jacquemontii see *A. villosa* var. *jacquemontii.*
A. laevigata, syn. *Douglasia laevigata.* Densely tufted, evergreen perennial with rosettes, 1–4cm (½–1½in) across, of oblong-lance-shaped, glossy, dark grey-green leaves, 1–2cm (½–¾in) long. Compact umbels of 2–10 deep rose-pink flowers, 1–2cm (½–¾in) across, are borne on stems 2–7cm (¾–3in) long, in early summer. ↕ 5cm (2in), ↔ to 20cm (8in). N.W. USA. ❄❄❄
A. laggeri see *A. carnea* subsp. *laggeri.*
A. lanuginosa ■ ♀ Prostrate, evergreen, mat-forming perennial with trailing, reddish green stems and alternate, elliptic, silky-hairy, grey-green leaves, to 1.5cm (½in) long. Produces compact umbels of 10–15 pale pink flowers, 8–12mm (⅜–½in) across, with greenish yellow eyes, on stems 8–10cm (3–4in) long, in mid- and late summer. ↕ to 5cm (2in), sometimes to 10cm (4in), ↔ to 30cm (12in). Himalayas. ❄❄❄
A. pubescens. Cushion-forming, evergreen perennial with dense rosettes, 9–15mm (⅜–½in) across, of elliptic to spoon-shaped, hairy, mid-green leaves, to 1cm (½in) long. Solitary white flowers, 6–10mm (¼–½in) across, with green or yellow eyes, are borne on stems to 5mm (¼in) long, in spring and early summer. ↕ to 6cm (2½in), ↔ to 10cm (4in). Pyrenees. ❄❄❄
A. pyrenaica ■ Compact, cushion-forming, evergreen perennial with dense rosettes, 4–5mm (⅛–¼in) across, of elliptic, hairy, grey-green leaves, to 4mm (⅛in) long. Solitary, almost stemless white flowers, 5mm (¼in) across, with yellow eyes, are borne in mid- and late spring. ↕ 4–5cm (1½–2in), ↔ 7–12cm (3–5in). Pyrenees. ❄❄❄
A. sarmentosa ♀ Mat-forming, stoloniferous, evergreen perennial, with rosettes, 1.5–3cm (½–1¼in) across, of narrowly to broadly elliptic, white-hairy, light green leaves, 1.5–3cm (½–1¼in) long. In late spring and early summer, stems to 10cm (4in) long, bear compact umbels of 3–8 pale to deep rose-pink flowers, 7–9mm (¼–⅜in) across, with greenish yellow eyes. Vigorous species for a rock garden. ↕ 5–10cm (2–4in), ↔ to 30cm (12in). Himalayas to W. China (Sichuan). ❄❄❄
A. sempervivoides ■ ♀ Mat-forming, stoloniferous, evergreen perennial with open rosettes, 1–2.5cm (½–1in) across, of oblong to spoon-shaped, leathery, hairy-margined, mid-green leaves, 5mm (¼in) long. In mid- and late spring, umbels of 4–10 pink to mauve-pink, yellow-eyed, scented flowers, 8–10mm (⅜–½in) across, their eyes turning red with age, open on stems 2–8cm (¾–3in) long. ↕ 2.5–5cm (1–2in), ↔ 15–20cm (6–8in). N.W. Himalayas. ❄❄❄
A. strigillosa. Vigorous, stoloniferous, evergreen perennial with loosely clustered rosettes, to 8cm (3in) across, of broadly elliptic, mid-green, downy leaves, to 6cm (2½in) long. In early and midsummer, bears open umbels of 5–15 usually white, purplish red-backed, yellow-eyed flowers, 5mm (¼in) across, on stems to 25cm (10in) tall. Variants with white or pink flowers are also grown. ↕ to 25cm (10in), ↔ to 15cm (6in). C. Himalayas. ❄❄❄
A. vandellii ■ syn. *A. imbricata.* Evergreen, cushion-forming Aretian with dense rosettes, 5–10mm (¼–½in) wide, of linear to elliptic, silvery grey-hairy leaves, to 6mm (¼in) long. Produces attractive white, yellow-eyed flowers, 4–8mm (⅛–⅜in) across, singly from the leaf axils on short stems, 1–5mm (¹⁄₁₆–¼in) long, in early and mid-spring. ↕ 4–5cm (1½–2in), ↔ 7–12cm (3–5in). Sierra Nevada, Pyrenees, Alps. ❄❄❄
A. villosa ■ Mat- or cushion-forming, evergreen perennial with densely silky-hairy rosettes, to 1.5cm (½in) across, of linear to broadly elliptic leaves, 5–7mm (¼in) long, mid-green above and covered in long, silky hairs beneath. In spring, bears tight umbels of 3–7 white flowers, 6–10mm (¼–½in) across, with yellow eyes, sometimes turning pink- and red-eyed with age, on stems 2–3cm (¾–1¼in) long. ↕ to 4cm (1½in), ↔ to 20cm (8in). W. Europe to W. Asia. ❄❄❄. **var. *jacquemontii*** ■ syn. *A. jacquemontii*, is stoloniferous, with deep pink-purple, yellow- to green-eyed flowers; Himalayas.
A. vitaliana see *Vitaliana primuliflora.*

ANDRYALA

ASTERACEAE/COMPOSITAE

Genus of about 25 species of drought-resistant annuals and perennials from rocky sites, including scree and cliffs, in the Mediterranean. They have milky sap and alternate leaves, which are simple or deeply pinnatisect, sometimes with deep, wavy margins. The yellow, daisy-like flowerheads may be borne singly or in many-flowered panicles, the outer-most florets often having red stripes on the undersides. They are useful for dry wall crevices or for a raised bed in a rock garden. Grow in an alpine house for protection against winter wet.

- **HARDINESS** Fully hardy to half hardy. *A. agardhii* is hardy to -10°C (14°F), except in very wet winters.
- **CULTIVATION** Under glass, grow in deep pots in a mix of equal parts loam, leaf mould, and sharp sand, with a top-dressing of grit, in full light. Water freely when in growth, more sparingly in winter. Outdoors, grow in sharply drained, poor, gravelly soil in full sun.
- **PROPAGATION** Sow seed in containers in a cold frame when ripe, or in spring. Root heel cuttings in summer.
- **PESTS AND DISEASES** Trouble free.

A. agardhii. Woody-based perennial forming a densely tufted mound of lance-shaped to spoon-shaped, entire, softly white-hairy, mid-green leaves, 3–4cm (1¼–1½in) long, which taper to long leaf-stalks. Bears solitary, clear yellow flowerheads, 2.5cm (1in) across, from early to late summer. ↕↔ 15cm (6in). S. Spain. ❄❄

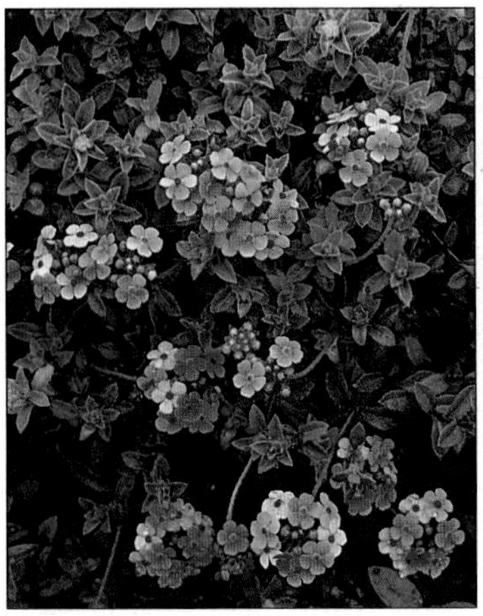
Androsace lanuginosa

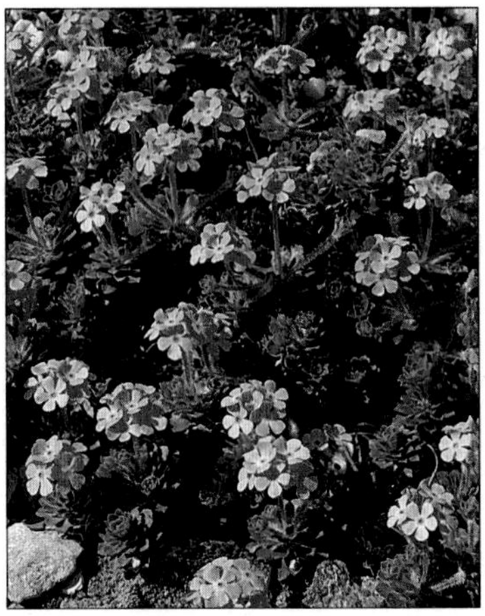
Androsace sempervivoides

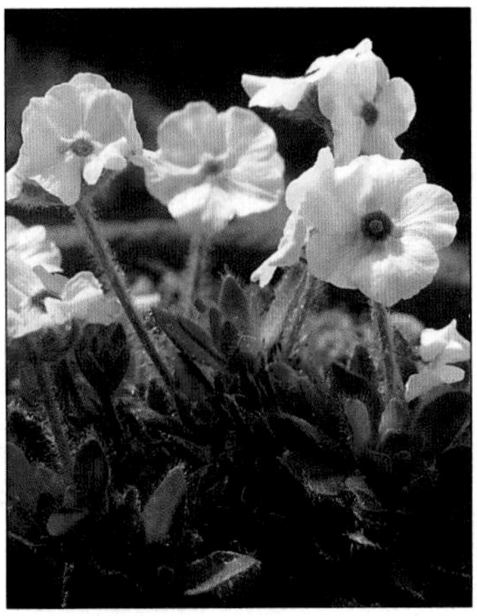
Androsace villosa

ANEMONE

Windflower

RANUNCULACEAE

Genus of about 120 species of variable perennials from a wide range of habitats in temperate regions, mainly of the N. but also of the S. hemisphere. Anemones have rhizomatous, tuberous, fleshy, or fibrous rootstocks. They may be divided into 3 main groups: spring-flowering species, some with tubers or rhizomes, which are found in woodland and alpine pastures; tuberous Mediterranean and C. Asian species from areas with hot, dry summers, flowering in spring or early summer; and larger, mainly tall, herbaceous species with fibrous roots, occurring in moist, open woodland and grassy sites, and flowering from late summer to autumn. Most anemones produce both basal and stem leaves. The basal leaves are rounded to oval in outline, 3- to 7-palmate or palmately lobed, rarely entire, and mid- to dark green. The leaflets and lobes are often shallowly to deeply dissected or toothed, and may be either hairless or hairy. Smaller, stalkless or short-stalked stem leaves are often produced in a whorl beneath the flowers.

Anemones are grown for their open saucer-shaped to shallowly cup-shaped flowers, each with a central boss of stamens. The flowers are solitary or borne in cymes or umbels, on branched or unbranched stems. Larger species are ideal for a border, smaller species for a woodland or rock garden. Some anemones, such as *A. blanda* and *A.* *apennina*, are excellent for naturalizing in a variety of sites. Contact with the sap may irritate skin.

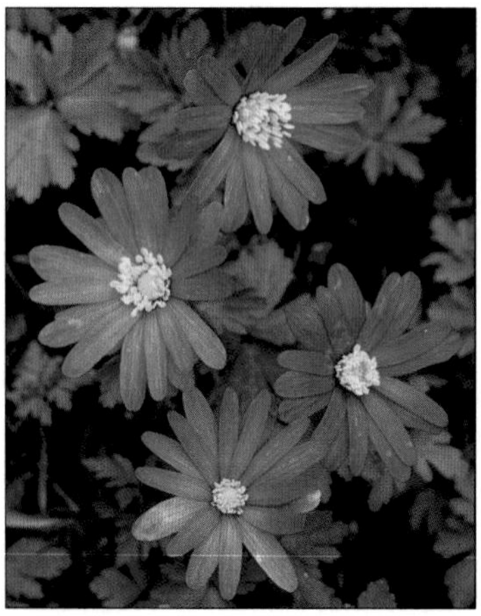

Anemone blanda 'Atrocaerulea'

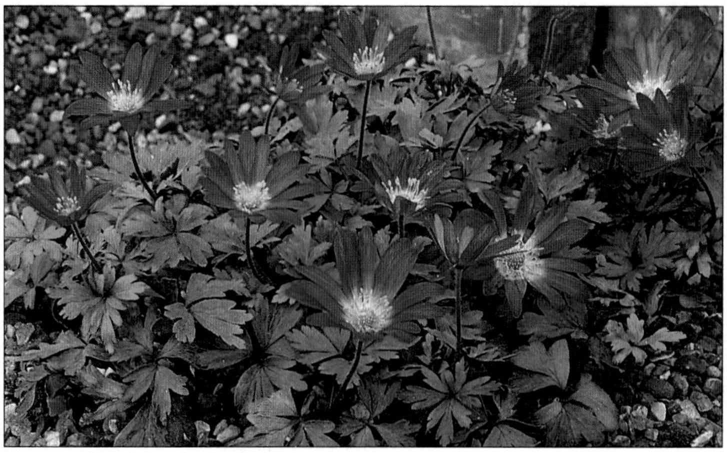

Anemone blanda 'Violet Star'

• **HARDINESS** Fully hardy to half hardy.
• **CULTIVATION** Anemones have varying cultivation requirements. For ease of reference, these are grouped as follows:
1. Moist but well-drained, humus-rich soil in partial shade, although drier conditions are tolerated when dormant in summer.
2. Well-drained, humus-rich soil in sun or partial shade.
3. Light, sandy soil in full sun. Ensure a dry dormancy after flowering. Mulch for winter protection, or lift and overwinter in sand in a frost-free place.
4. Moist, fertile, humus-rich soil in sun or partial shade. Some species may be invasive once established. They will not tolerate excessive winter wet. Mulch in spring and late autumn in cold areas.

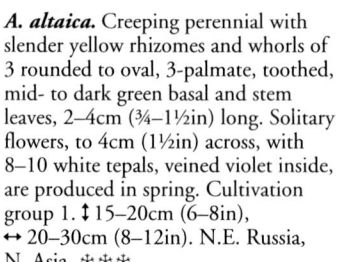

Most species are best planted in autumn, but plant *A. coronaria* De Caen Group and St. Brigid Group in spring. Plant anemones with tubers 5–8cm (2–3in) below the surface of the soil.
• **PROPAGATION** Sow seed in containers in a cold frame as soon as ripe (use dry sand to rub hairs off the woolly-coated seeds); germination may be slow and erratic. Divide autumn-flowering anemones in early spring or autumn, growing on in containers for a year before planting out in spring. Separate the rhizomes of rhizomatous species in spring, or after the leaves have died down. Separate the tubers of tuberous species in summer, when dormant.
• **PESTS AND DISEASES** Susceptible to leaf eelworms and, occasionally, anemone smut. All species are prone to leaf spot and powdery mildew, and to damage from caterpillars and slugs.

A. altaica. Creeping perennial with slender yellow rhizomes and whorls of 3 rounded to oval, 3-palmate, toothed, mid- to dark green basal and stem leaves, 2–4cm (¾–1½in) long. Solitary flowers, to 4cm (1½in) across, with 8–10 white tepals, veined violet inside, are produced in spring. Cultivation group 1. ↕ 15–20cm (6–8in), ↔ 20–30cm (8–12in). N.E. Russia, N. Asia. ❄❄❄
A. apennina 🏆 Perennial with short, creeping rhizomes and rounded to oval, 3-palmate, dark green, basal and stem leaves, 3–8cm (1¼–3in) long, with hairy undersides, and toothed and lobed leaflets. Solitary, usually blue flowers, 2.5–3cm (1–1¼in) across, with 8–14 tepals, are borne in spring; white flowers, sometimes pink-flushed, also occur. Cultivation group 1 or 2. ↕ 20cm (8in), ↔ 30cm (12in). S. Europe. ❄❄❄
A. baldensis. Clump-forming, fibrous-rooted perennial producing rounded, 3-palmate, dark green basal and stem leaves, 3–8cm (1¼–3in) long, with 3-lobed leaflets. Slightly nodding, solitary white flowers, 2.5–4cm (1–1½in) across, with 8–10 tepals, often flushed blue on the reverse, open in mid- and late spring. Cultivation group 2. ↕ 20cm (8in), ↔ 10–15cm (4–6in). Mountains of N. Italy, rocky sites in former Yugoslavia. ❄❄❄
A. biflora. Tuberous perennial with rounded, 3-palmate, mid-green basal and stem leaves, 3–5cm (1¼–2in) long, with toothed and lobed leaflets. Red flowers, occasionally yellow or orange, 3–4cm (1¼–1½in) across, with 5 tepals, are borne in 2- or 3-flowered clusters in spring. Cultivation group 3. ↕ 12cm (5in), ↔ 10cm (4in). Iran. ❄❄

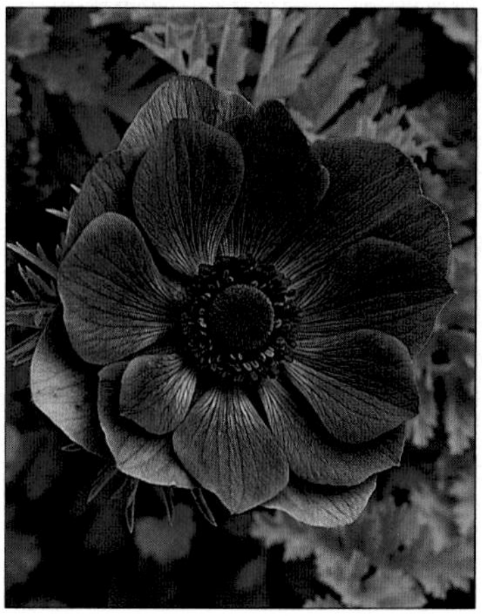

Anemone coronaria 'Lord Lieutenant'

A. blanda 🏆 Spreading perennial with knobbly tubers. Produces 1 or 2 broadly oval to triangular, 3-palmate, dark green basal and stem leaves, 3–10cm (1¼–4in) long, with irregularly lobed leaflets. In spring, solitary flowers, 2–4cm (¾–1½in) across, with 10–15 deep blue to white or pink tepals, are borne above the leaves. Quickly forms large clumps. Cultivation group 2 or 3. ↕↔ 15cm (6in). S.E. Europe, Turkey. ❄❄❄. **'Atrocaerulea'** ▣ has deep blue flowers. **'Blue Star'** produces pale blue flowers. **'Charmer'** has deep pink flowers. **'Ingramii'** 🏆 bears deep blue flowers with purple-backed tepals. **'Pink Star'** has bright pink flowers. **'Radar'** ▣🏆 bears magenta flowers with white centres. **'Violet Star'** ▣ bears large, amethyst flowers with white backs. **'White Splendour'** ▣🏆 produces large white flowers with pink-tinged backs.
***A.* 'Bressingham Glow'** see *A. hupehensis* var. *japonica* 'Bressingham Glow'.
A. bucharica. Clump-forming perennial with knobbly tubers and rounded, 3-palmate, light to dark green basal and stem leaves, 5–12cm (2–5in) long, with lobed and toothed leaflets. In spring, branched stems bear pairs of red or violet-red flowers, 3–4cm (1¼–1½in) across, with 5 tepals, hairy on the outside. Cultivation group 3. ↕ 20cm (8in), ↔ 10cm (4in). C. Asia. ❄❄❄

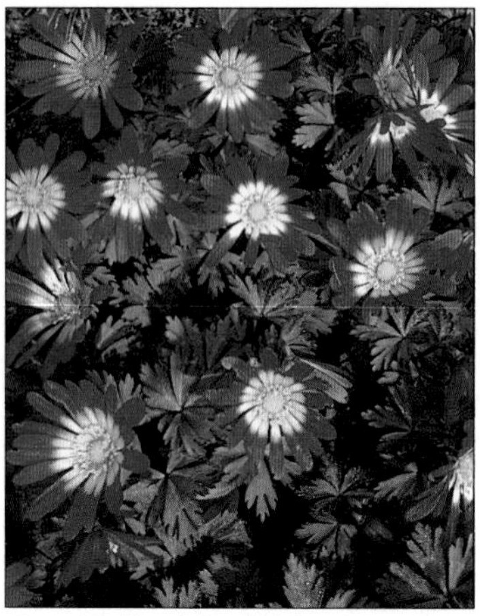

Anemone blanda 'Radar'

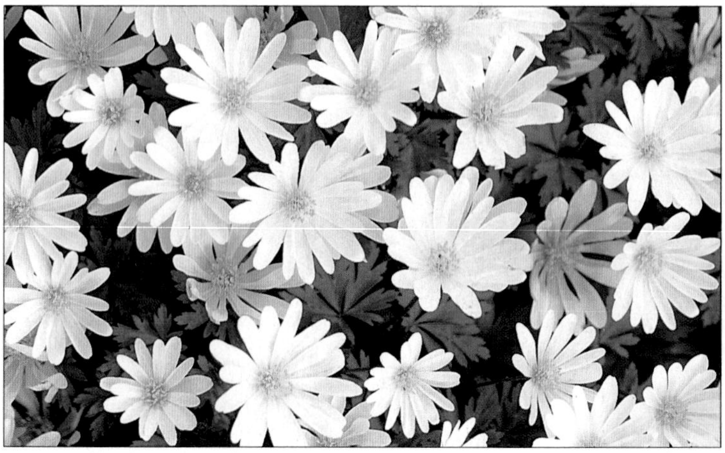

Anemone blanda 'White Splendour'

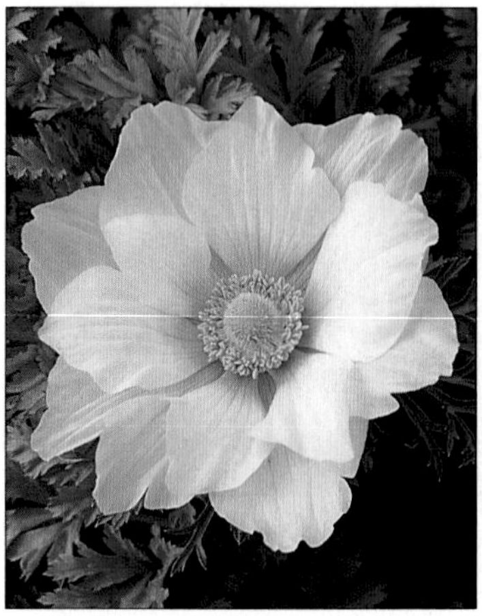

Anemone coronaria 'The Bride'

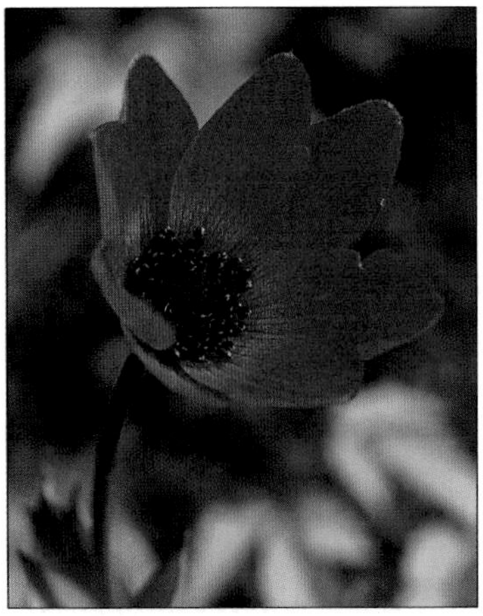

Anemone x *fulgens*

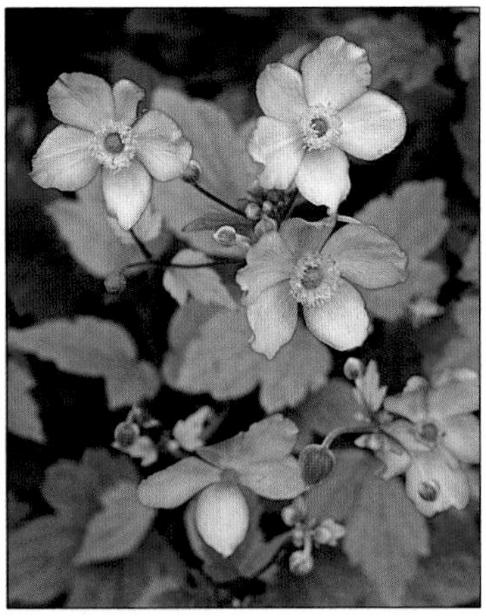

Anemone hupehensis

A. coronaria. Erect perennial with knobbly tubers, producing rounded to oval, 3-palmate, mid-green basal and stem leaves, 5–12cm (2–5in) long, with finely lobed leaflets. Solitary, showy, single flowers, 3–8cm (1¼–3in) across, with 5–8 tepals, in red, blue, or white, are borne in spring. Cultivation group 3. ↕ 30–45cm (12–18in), ↔ 15cm (6in). Mediterranean. ✻✻✻. There are many cultivars, both single- and double-flowered; all are useful as cut flowers. **De Caen Group** is a collective name for a race of single-flowered cultivars with 5–8 tepals. **'Lord Lieutenant'** ■ has semi-double, deep blue flowers. **'Mr. Fokker'** has single, violet-blue flowers. **St. Brigid Group** is a collective name for a race of double-flowered cultivars. **'The Admiral'** produces semi-double violet flowers. **'The Bride'** ■ has semi-double, pure white flowers.
A. demissa. Clump-forming perennial with a woody-based, fibrous rootstock, and rounded, deeply 5-lobed, sharply toothed, mid-green basal and stem leaves, 5–15cm (2–6in) long. Branched stems bear spreading umbels of 3–6 white, blue, or purple flowers, 2–4cm (¾–1½in) across, with 5–7 tepals and bold, golden yellow stamens, from early to late summer. Cultivation group 2. ↕ 15–40cm (6–16in), ↔ 15cm (6in). W. Himalayas to S.W. China. ✻✻✻
A. x elegans see *A.* x *hybrida.*
A. eranthoides. Erect, tuberous perennial with congested rhizomes and stalkless, rounded, 3- to 5-palmate, mid-green basal leaves, to 12cm (5in) long, the leaflets further 3-lobed and toothed; stem leaves are stalkless, 3-palmate and narrowly obovate. Flowers, 1–2.5cm (½–1in) across, with up to 8 tepals, yellow-green outside and golden yellow inside, are borne, usually in pairs, in spring. Cultivation group 3. ↕ to 12cm (5in), ↔ to 8cm (3in). C. Asia. ✻✻✻
A. flaccida. Erect, rhizomatous perennial forming mounds of oval, 3-palmate, fleshy basal and stem leaves, 3–10cm (1¼–4in) long, with lobed and toothed leaflets, bronze at first, later dark green with white-marked bases. In late spring, bears clusters of 1–3 creamy white, sometimes pink-flushed flowers, 1.5–3cm (½–1¼in) across, with 5–7 tepals. Cultivation group 1. ↕ to 20cm (8in), ↔ 15–20cm (6–8in). Mountain forests in Russia, China, Japan. ✻✻✻
A. x fulgens ■ (*A. hortensis* x *A. pavonina*). Tuberous perennial with rounded to oval, 3-palmate to deeply 3-lobed, mid-green basal and stem leaves, 3–12cm (1¼–5in) long, with lobed and toothed leaflets. In spring, bears solitary, narrow-petalled scarlet flowers, 5–7cm (2–3in) across, with 10–15 tepals. Cultivation group 3, but will tolerate summer rain without protection. ↕ 30cm (12in), ↔ 15cm (6in). Garden origin. ✻✻✻. **'Annulata Grandiflora'** has large red flowers with yellow centres.
A. globosa see *A. multifida.*
A. heldreichiana ■ syn. *A. stellata* var. *heldreichii.* Slow-growing perennial with a tuber-like, congested rhizome. Produces rounded, 3-palmate, light green basal leaves, 3–6cm (1¼–3½in) long, and small, rounded stem leaves, 5–10mm (¼–½in) long, with lobed leaflets. Solitary flowers, 2–4cm (¾–1½in) across, with 8–14 tepals, grey-blue on the outside and white inside, are borne in spring. Cultivation group 3. ↕ 10–15cm (4–6in), ↔ to 10cm (4in). Greece (Crete). ✻✻✻
A. hepatica see *Hepatica nobilis.*
A. hupehensis ■ Erect perennial with a woody-based, fibrous rootstock and suckering shoots. Long-stalked, rounded to oval, 3-palmate, dark green basal leaves, 10–20cm (4–8in) long, and smaller stem leaves, are sharply toothed, and sparsely hairy beneath. In mid- and late summer, branched stems bear umbels of up to 15 white or pink flowers, 5–6cm (2–2½in) across, with 5–6 tepals, the outer ones often deep pink outside. Cultivation group 4. ↕ 60–90cm (24–36in), ↔ 40cm (16in). W. and C. China. ✻✻✻. **'Hadspen Abundance'** ■🏆 has flowers with dark reddish pink outer tepals. **var. *japonica*** (Japanese anemone) is taller than the species and has creamy pink flowers with 10–20 narrow tepals; ↕ 60–120cm (2–4ft), ↔ 45cm (18in); S. China, Japan. **var. *japonica* 'Bressingham Glow'** ■ syn. *A.* 'Bressingham Glow', has slightly darker pink flowers and longer tepals than var. *japonica*, the silky hairs on the outer surfaces producing a white sheen. **var. *japonica* 'Prinz Heinrich'** 🏆 syn. *A.* x *hybrida* 'Prince Henry', is very similar to var. *japonica* 'Bressingham Glow', but more invasive. **'Pink Shell'** see 'Rosenschale'. **'Rosenschale'**, syn. 'Pink Shell', is vigorous and produces flowers with large, overlapping, broad-based, dark rose-pink outer tepals. **'September Charm'** 🏆 has uniform, pale pink flowers, 9cm (3½in) across.
A. x hybrida (*A. hupehensis* var. *japonica* x *A. vitifolia*) syn. *A.* x *elegans, A. japonica* of gardens (Japanese anemone). Vigorous, erect, woody-based perennial with suckering shoots and oval, usually 3-palmate, toothed, mid-green leaves, softly hairy beneath. Basal leaves are 10–20cm (4–8in) long; stem leaves are 5–12cm (2–5in) long. Branched stems bear umbels of 12–18 semi-double, pale pink flowers, to 9cm (3½in) across, with 6–11 (sometimes up to 15) tepals, from late summer to mid-autumn. Cultivation group 4. ↕ 1.2–1.5m (4–5ft), ↔ indefinite. Garden origin. ✻✻✻. **'Géante des Blanches'** 🏆 syn. 'White Giant', 'White Queen', is vigorous and has semi-double flowers with broad white tepals, shaded green on the reverse. **'Honorine Jobert'** ■🏆

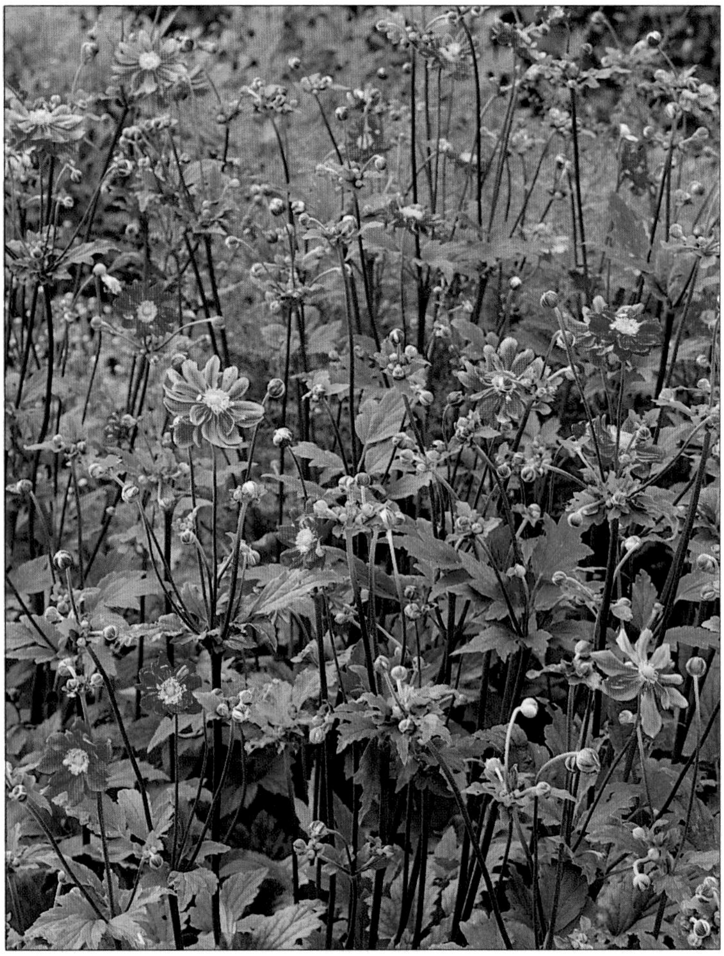

Anemone hupehensis var. *japonica* 'Bressingham Glow'

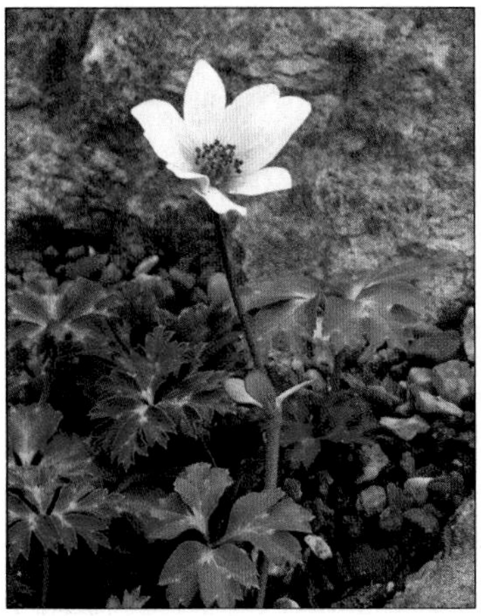

Anemone heldreichiana

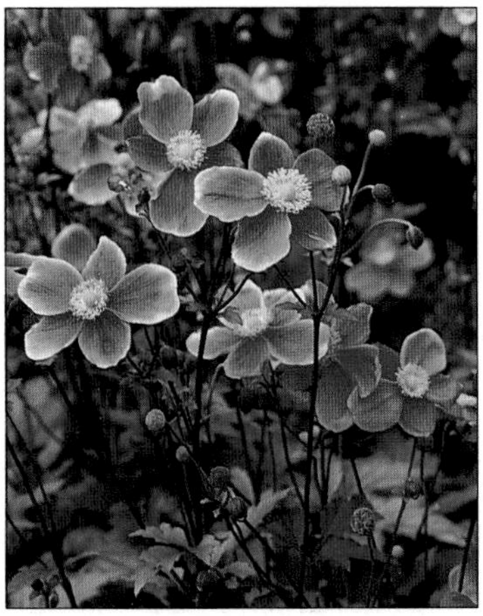

Anemone hupehensis 'Hadspen Abundance'

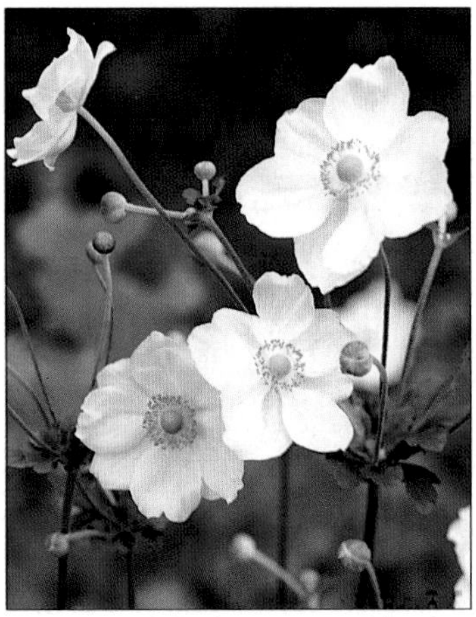

Anemone x *hybrida* 'Honorine Jobert'

ANEMONE

A

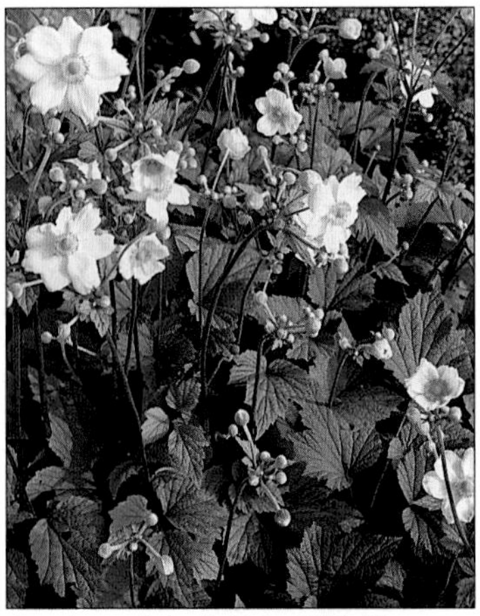

Anemone x *hybrida* 'Luise Uhink'

has single white flowers, pink-tinged on the reverse, with golden yellow stamens. **'Königin Charlotte'** ♀ syn. 'Queen Charlotte', is vigorous with large, semi-double pink flowers, 10cm (4in) across, shaded purple on the reverse of the outer tepals; ↕1.5m (5ft). **'Kriemhilde'** bears semi-double, pale purple-pink flowers, darker on the reverse of the tepals. **'Lady Gilmour'** see 'Margarete'. **'Luise Uhink'** ■ is vigorous with large, semi-double white flowers. **'Margarete'**, syn. 'Lady Gilmour', 'Margaret', bears almost double, pale pink flowers. **'Max Vogel'** ■ bears single, light pink flowers that become paler with age, the 3 or 4 outer tepals slightly darker than the 5 or 6 inner ones. **'Prince Henry'** see *A. hupehensis* var. *japonica* 'Prinz Heinrich'. **'Profusion'** is vigorous with semi-

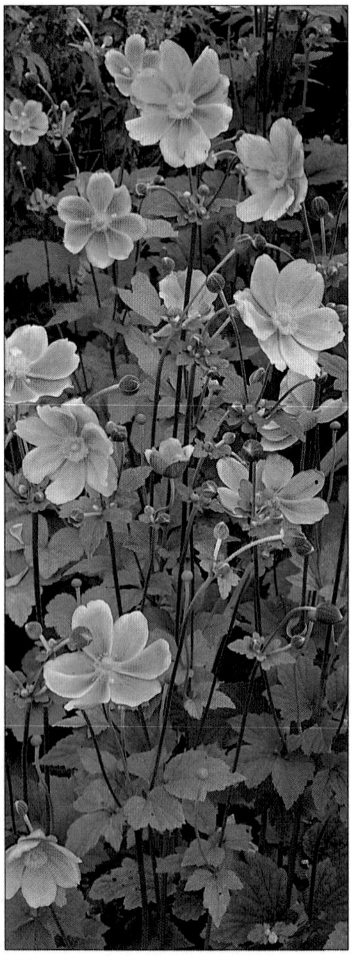

Anemone x *hybrida* 'Max Vogel'

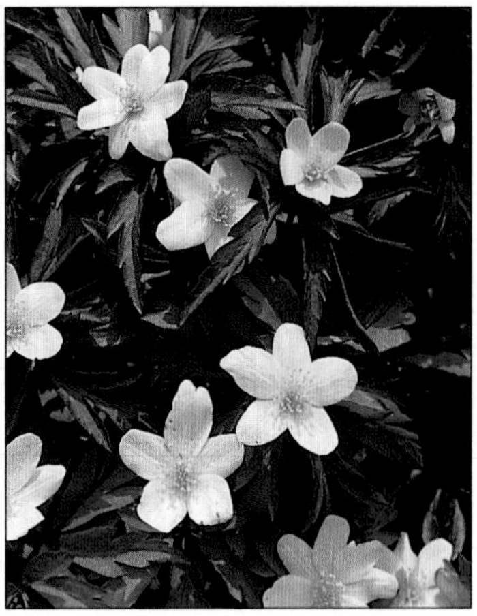

Anemone x *lipsiensis*

double, rose-pink flowers, 6–7cm (2½–3in) across. **'Queen Charlotte'** see 'Königin Charlotte'. **'Whirlwind'** has semi-double white flowers, often with twisted, greenish white tepals at the centres. **'White Giant'** see 'Géante des Blanches'. **'White Queen'** see 'Géante des Blanches'.

A.* x *intermedia see *A.* x *lipsiensis.*

***A. japonica* of gardens** see *A.* x *hybrida.*

A.* x *lesseri (*A. multifida* x *A. sylvestris*). Erect, fibrous-rooted perennial forming clumps of large, rounded, 3- to 5-palmate, hairy, mid-green basal and stem leaves, 5–12cm (2–5in) long, with very finely lobed and toothed leaflets. In summer, bears reddish pink flowers, to 3cm (1¼in) across, with 5–8 tepals, singly or in umbels of 2 or 3. There are also variants with purple, yellow, or white flowers. Cultivation group 2. ↕40cm (16in), ↔ to 30cm (12in). Garden origin. ❄❄❄

A.* x *lipsiensis ■ (*A. nemorosa* x *A. ranunculoides*) syn. *A.* x *intermedia, A.* x *seemannii.* Vigorous perennial with slender brown rhizomes and rounded, 3-palmate, mid-green basal and stem leaves, 5–8cm (2–3in) long, with deeply lobed leaflets. Similar to *A. nemorosa,* but bears solitary, pale creamy yellow flowers, 1.5–2cm (½–¾in) across, with 6–8 tepals, in spring. Cultivation group 1. ↕5–15cm (2–6in), ↔ to 45cm (18in). Europe. ❄❄❄

***A. magellanica* of gardens** see *A. multifida.*

A. multifida ■ syn. *A. globosa, A. magellanica* of gardens. Vigorous, rhizomatous perennial with rounded, 3- to 5-palmate, mid-green basal and stem leaves, 3–8cm (1¼–3in) long, with finely lobed leaflets. In summer, bears umbels of 2 or 3 creamy yellow flowers, to 2.5cm (1in) across, with 5–9 tepals. Cultivation group 2. ↕to 30cm (12in), ↔ to 15cm (6in). N. America. ❄❄❄

A. narcissiflora ■ Clump-forming perennial with a slightly woody rootstock. Rounded, 3- to 5-palmate, mid-green basal leaves, 8–15cm (3–6in) long, and smaller stem leaves have deeply lobed and toothed leaflets. In late spring and early summer, bears umbels of 3–8 (sometimes 9 or 10), white flowers, 2–4cm (¾–1½in) across, occasionally flushed pink on the reverse of the 5–7 tepals. Cultivation group 2. ↕40cm (16in), ↔ 45cm (18in). Mountains of C. and S. Europe to Turkey, Caucasus, Siberia, W. North America. ❄❄❄

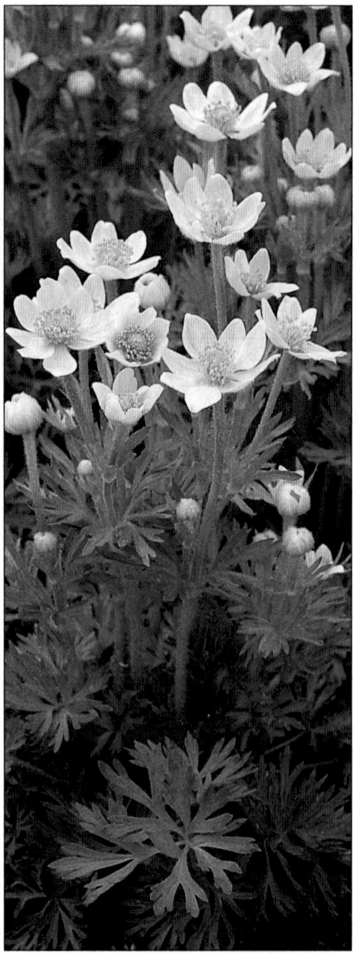

Anemone multifida

A. nemorosa ♀ (Windflower, Wood anemone). Vigorous, low-growing, creeping perennial with slender brown rhizomes and rounded, 3-palmate, mid-green basal and stem leaves, 5–12cm (2–5in) long, the narrow leaflets further lobed and toothed. From spring to early summer, bears solitary white, often pink-flushed flowers, 2–3cm (¾–1¼in) across, with 6–8 tepals. Cultivation group 1. ↕8–15cm (3–6in), ↔ 30cm (12in) or more. Woods and mountain pastures of Europe. ❄❄❄. **'Allenii'** ♀ produces deep lavender-blue flowers, 4cm (1½in) across, shaded paler blue on the outside of the tepals. **'Blue Bonnet'** is late-flowering, with deep blue flowers, 3–4cm (1¼–1½in) across. **'Bracteata Pleniflora'** ■ has semi-double flowers with a ruff of leaves below the narrow

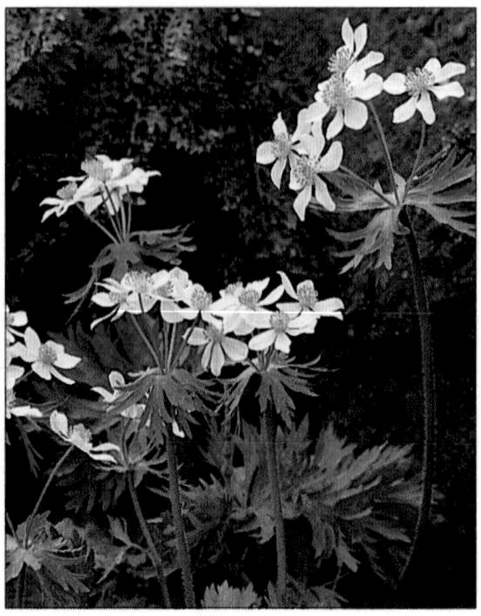

Anemone narcissiflora

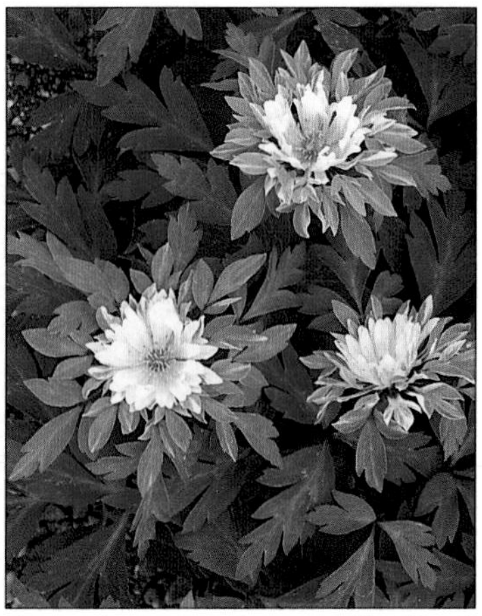

Anemone nemorosa 'Bracteata Pleniflora'

tepals, the inner tepals white or white with green tips and the outer ones green. **'Flore Pleno'**, syn. 'Plena', has small, double white flowers, 2–3cm (¾–1¼in) across. **'Plena'** see 'Flore Pleno'. **'Robinsoniana'** ■♀ produces large, pale lavender-blue flowers, 3–4cm (1¼–1½in) across, with creamy-grey backs. **'Vestal'** ♀ bears double white flowers, 2–2½cm (¾–1in) across, with central buttons of symmetrically arranged tepals. **'Wilk's Giant'** bears single white flowers, 4–5cm (1½–2in) across, the largest blooms of all *A. nemorosa* cultivars.

A. obtusiloba. Tufted, fibrous-rooted perennial with rounded, deeply lobed, mid-green basal and stem leaves, 5–12cm (2–5in) long, the 3 lobes subdivided and spreading. In late spring, produces umbels of 2 or 3 white, yellow, or deep blue flowers, 2–3cm (¾–1¼in) across, with 4–6 tepals. Cultivation group 2. ↕5cm (2in), ↔ to 25cm (10in). Himalayas, S.W. China. ❄❄❄

A. pavonina ■ Tuberous perennial with rounded, 3-palmate or deeply 3-lobed, dissected, sparsely toothed, mid- to dark green basal and stem leaves, 8–15cm (3–6in) long. In early spring, bears solitary, red, pink, or purple flowers, 3–10cm (1¼–4in) across, with 7–9 tepals, often with white tepal bases. Cultivation group 3. ↕25cm (10in), ↔ 15cm (6in). Mediterranean. ❄❄❄. **var. *ocellata*** bears scarlet flowers with white centres. **St. Bavo Group** has large flowers, 10cm (4in) across, in shades of purple, pink, and salmon-pink.

A. petiolulosa. Tuberous perennial, closely related to *A. biflora,* with

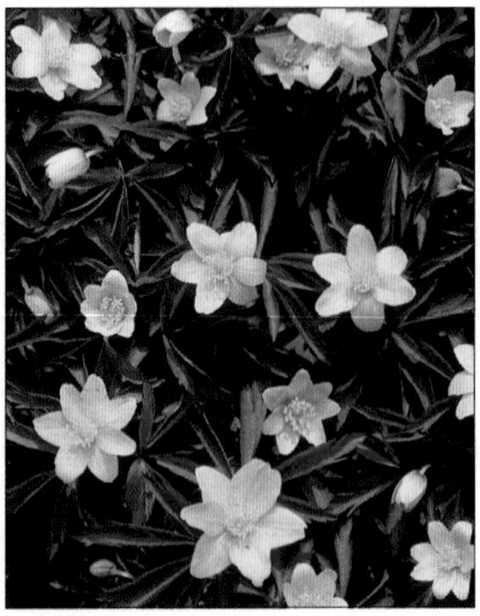

Anemone nemorosa 'Robinsoniana'

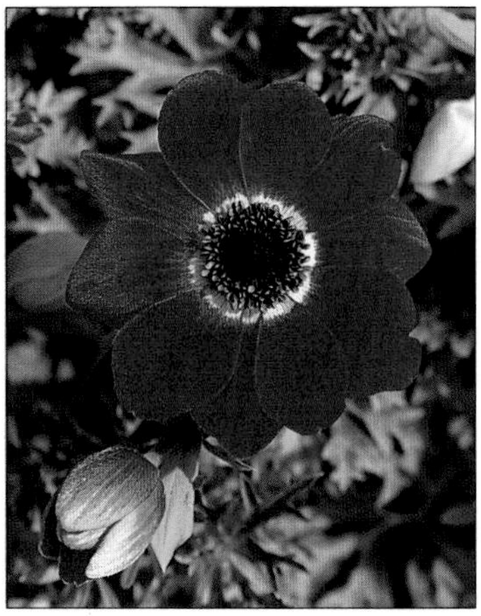
Anemone pavonina

rounded, 3-palmate, mid-green basal and stem leaves, 5–12cm (2–5in) long, with deeply lobed leaflets. In spring, bears clusters of up to 4 slightly pendent yellow, red-backed flowers, 2–4.5cm (¾–1¾in) across, with 5 tepals. Cultivation group 3; best in a bulb frame. ↕ 15cm (6in), ↔ 10cm (4in). C. Asia. ❄❄❄

A. polyanthes. Clump-forming perennial with a woody-based, fibrous rootstock. Rounded, hairy, dark green basal and stem leaves, 15–30cm (6–12in) long, are shallowly 5- to 7-lobed, with rounded teeth. Umbels of 5 or more white, purple-blue, or reddish purple flowers, to 3cm (1¼in) across, with 4–6 tepals, are produced in late spring or early summer. Cultivation group 2. ↕ 50cm (20in), ↔ 45cm (18in). Pakistan to Bhutan. ❄❄❄

A. ranunculoides ■ 🏆 Spreading perennial with yellow rhizomes and rounded, deeply 3-lobed, mid-green basal and stem leaves, 8–15cm (3–6in) long, each lobe also deeply divided. Solitary, deep yellow flowers, 2–3cm (¾–1¼in) across, with 5 or 6 tepals, open in spring. Cultivation group 1. ↕ 5–10cm (2–4in), ↔ to 45cm (18in) or more. Woodland in Europe. ❄❄❄. **'Pleniflora'**, syn. 'Flore Pleno', has double flowers.

A. rivularis ■ Variable, clump-forming perennial with a woody-based fibrous rootstock and long-stalked, rounded, 3-palmate to deeply 3-lobed, softly hairy, dark green leaves, the lobes or leaflets further divided and toothed. Basal leaves are 8–18cm (3–7in) long, stem leaves are slightly smaller. Umbels of 10–20

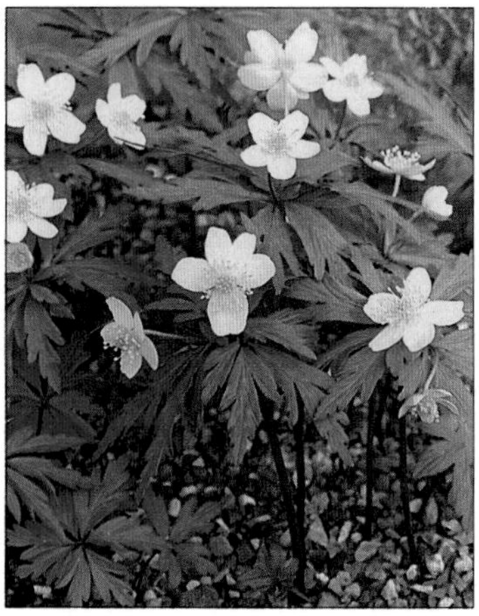
Anemone ranunculoides

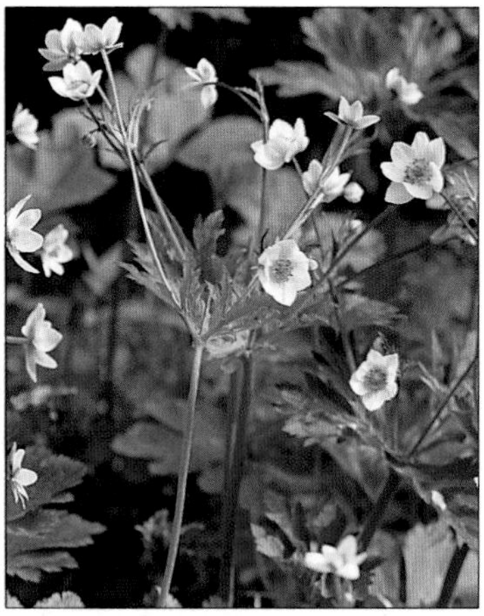
Anemone rivularis

or more white flowers, 4–7cm (1½–3in) across, with 5–8 tepals, often blue on the reverse, are borne on long, spreading stalks from the branching stems, in late spring and early summer, and sometimes again in autumn. Cultivation group 2. ↕ 60–90cm (24–36in), ↔ 30cm (12in). India, S.W. China. ❄❄❄

A. x seemannii see *A.* x *lipsiensis.*

A. stellata* var. *heldreichii see *A. heldreichiana.*

A. sylvestris ■ (Snowdrop anemone). Perennial with a woody-based, fibrous rootstock, spreading rapidly by root suckers. Long-stalked, mid-green basal and stem leaves, 5–15cm (2–6in) long, are rounded to oval, and deeply 5-lobed, the lobes also deeply divided. In late spring and early summer, bears solitary, single, semi-pendent white flowers, 2.5–8cm (1–3in) across, with 5 or more tepals and golden yellow stamens. Cultivation group 2. ↕↔ 30–50cm (12–20in). S. Sweden, N.E. France, C. and E. Europe, Caucasus. ❄❄❄. **'Flore Pleno'** bears double white flowers. **'Macrantha'** has large, single white flowers.

A. tomentosa, syn. *A. vitifolia* of gardens, *A. vitifolia* 'Robustissima'. Clump-forming perennial with a woody-based, fibrous rootstock, spreading by underground shoots. Oval, toothed, mid-green basal and stem leaves, 10–20cm (4–8in) long, are 3- to 7-palmate, conspicuously veined, and white-woolly on the reverse. In late summer and early autumn, branched stems bear clusters of 10 or more pale pink flowers, 5–8cm (2–3in) across, with 5 or 6 tepals. Cultivation group 4.

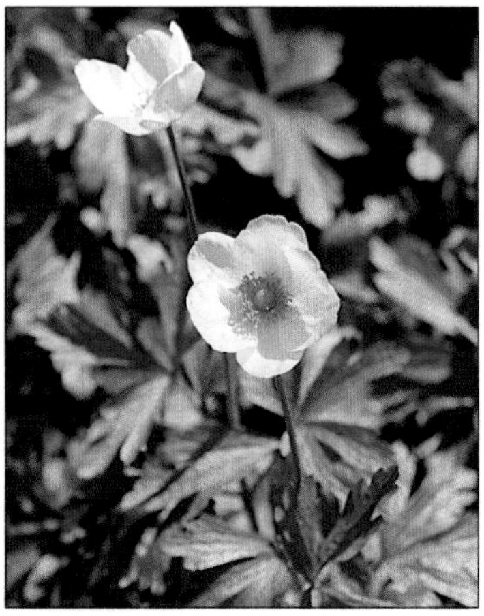
Anemone sylvestris

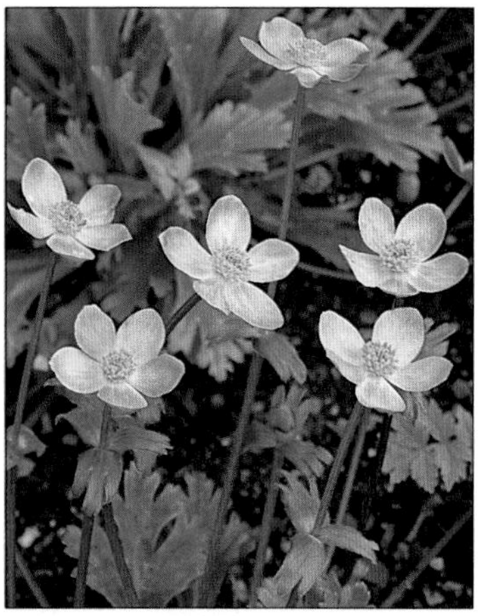
Anemone trullifolia

↕ 1–1.5m (3–5ft), ↔ 60cm (24in). N. and C. China. ❄❄❄

A. trifolia. Creeping perennial with slender brown rhizomes and long-stalked, rounded to oval, 3-palmate, toothed, light green basal and stem leaves, 5–12cm (2–5in) long, with narrow leaflets. In spring, leafy stems bear solitary white flowers, sometimes pink on the reverse, 2cm (¾in) across, with 5–8 tepals and a conspicuous boss of blue or white anthers. Cultivation group 1. ↕ to 15cm (6in), ↔ to 30cm (12in). Woodland in S. Europe. ❄❄❄

A. trullifolia ■ Compact, tufted, fibrous-rooted perennial, resembling *A. obtusiloba*, but producing wedge-shaped, deeply 3-lobed, mid-green basal and stem leaves, 5–12cm (2–5in) long, the lobes further divided and toothed. Solitary, blue, white, or yellow flowers, 2cm (¾in) across, with 4–6 tepals, are borne in late spring and early summer. Cultivation group 2. ↕ to 15cm (6in), ↔ to 20cm (8in). E. Himalayas, S.W. China. ❄❄❄

A. tschaernjaewii. Tuberous perennial producing oval, 3-palmate, mid-green basal and stem leaves, 3–8cm (1¼–3in) long, the leaflets shallowly 3-lobed. In

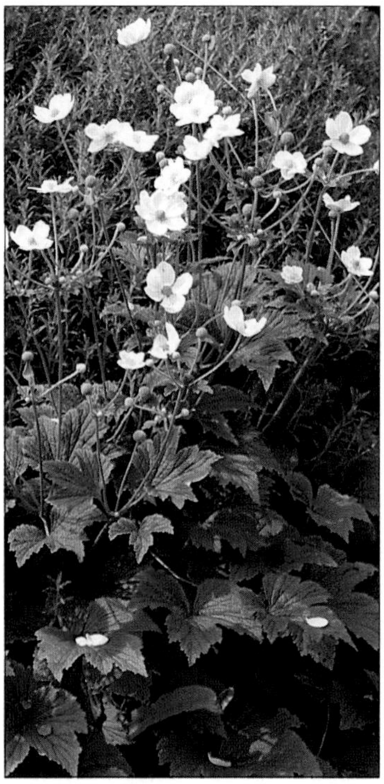
Anemone vitifolia

spring, each stem bears 1–3 white or pink flowers, 2–4.5cm (¾–1¾in) across, with purple centres and 5 tepals. Cultivation group 3; best grown in a bulb frame. ↕ 22cm (9in), ↔ 10cm (4in). C. Asia. ❄❄❄

A. vitifolia ■ Clump-forming perennial with a woody-based, fibrous rootstock and oval, shallowly 5-lobed, vine-like, dark green basal and stem leaves, 10–20cm (4–8in) long, the lobes conspicuously toothed and sparsely white-woolly beneath. Loose umbels of 3–7 white flowers, 3–6cm (1¼–3½in) across, with 5 or 6 tepals, are produced in late summer and early autumn. Cultivation group 4. ↕↔ 1m (3ft), ↔ indefinite. Afghanistan to W. China, Burma. ❄❄❄ (borderline).

'Robustissima' see *A. tomentosa.*

***A. vitifolia* of gardens** see *A. tomentosa.*

▷**Anemone,**
False rue see *Isopyrum*
Japanese see *Anemone* x *hybrida*, *A. hupehensis* var. *japonica*
Rue see *Anemonella thalictroides*
Snowdrop see *Anemone sylvestris*
Wood see *Anemone nemorosa*

ANEMONELLA

RANUNCULACEAE

Genus of one species of tuberous, clump-forming perennial occurring in woodland in E. North America. *A. thalictroides* is cultivated for its attractive flowers, and is suitable for growing in a woodland garden, or for underplanting in a shady shrub border or rock garden. Although slow to establish, it will eventually increase to form colonies to 30cm (12in) across.

- **HARDINESS** Fully hardy.
- **CULTIVATION** Grow in moist, moderately fertile, humus-rich soil in partial shade. Tubers may rot in very wet soils.
- **PROPAGATION** Sow seed in containers in a cold frame as soon as ripe, or divide young plants in early spring.
- **PESTS AND DISEASES** Susceptible to slug damage.

A. thalictroides ■ (Rue anemone). Tuberous perennial producing loose umbels of 2–4 fragile, cup-shaped, white or pale pink flowers, to 2cm (¾in) wide, on slender stems, from spring to early summer. Flowers are borne above 2- to 3-ternate, delicate, fern-like, dark bluish green leaves, 10–15cm (4–6in) long,

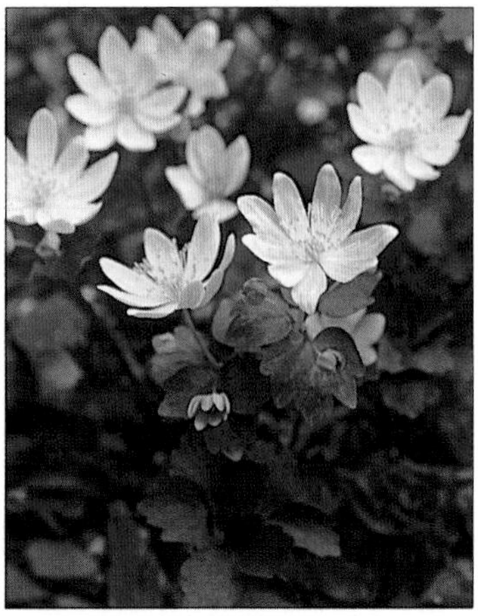
Anemonella thalictroides

A

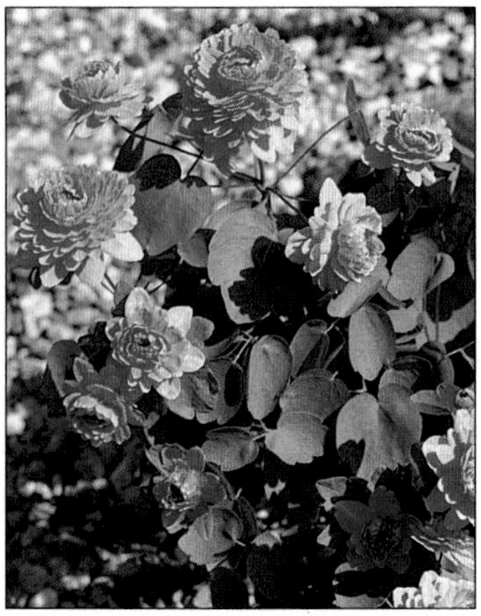

Anemonella thalictroides 'Oscar Schoaf'

with 5–9 ovate leaflets, arising from clusters of small tubers. ↕ 10cm (4in), ↔ 30cm (12in). E. North America. ❄❄❄. **'Oscar Schoaf'** ■ syn. 'Flore Pleno', 'Schoaf's Double', 'Schoaf's Pink', has double pink flowers.

ANEMONOPSIS

RANUNCULACEAE

Genus of a single species of clump-forming perennial from mountain woodland in Japan. It produces 2- or 3-ternate leaves with lobed or sharply toothed leaflets, and bears racemes or loose panicles of pendent, lilac and violet flowers. Grow *A. macrophylla* in a woodland garden or peat garden, or in a shady border.
• **HARDINESS** Fully hardy.
• **CULTIVATION** Grow in deep, cool, moist, moderately fertile, humus-rich, preferably acid soil, in partial shade. Protect from cold, drying winds, which will damage or kill the foliage.
• **PROPAGATION** Sow seed in containers in a cold frame as soon as ripe; germination is unreliable. Carefully divide the thick, fleshy roots in spring.
• **PESTS AND DISEASES** Trouble free.

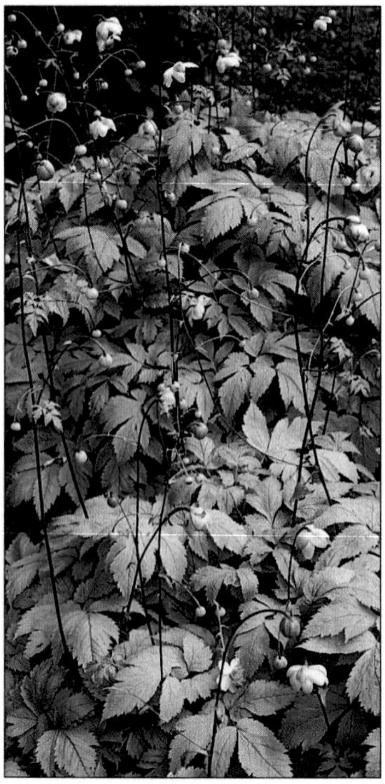

Anemonopsis macrophylla

A. macrophylla ■ Clump-forming perennial with 2- or 3-ternate, glossy, hairless, dark green leaves, 6–10cm (2½–4in) long, with diamond-shaped to ovate or oblong, sharply toothed, often 3-lobed leaflets. Racemes of cup-shaped, nodding flowers, to 3cm (1¼in) across, each with 3 waxy lilac sepals and several rows of 7–10 smaller violet petals, are borne in mid- and late summer. ↕ 75cm (30in), ↔ 45cm (18in). Japan. ❄❄❄

ANEMOPAEGMA

BIGNONIACEAE

Genus of over 40 species of evergreen, tendril climbers from moist forest in tropical North and South America. They are grown for their terminal or axillary racemes of showy, foxglove-like flowers. The leaves are opposite and 2- to 5-pinnate. In frost-prone areas, grow in a temperate or warm greenhouse. In warmer areas, they are ideal for growing on a house wall, pergola, arbour, or tree.
• **HARDINESS** Frost tender, but *A. chamberlaynii* may survive short periods down to 2°C (36°F).
• **CULTIVATION** Under glass, grow in loam-based potting compost (JI No.3) in full or bright filtered light. When in growth, water freely and apply a balanced liquid fertilizer monthly; water sparingly in winter. Outdoors, grow in fertile, moist but well-drained soil in sun or partial shade. Pruning group 11, or group 12 in a restricted site; prune in late winter or early spring.
• **PROPAGATION** Sow seed at minimum 16°C (61°F) in spring. Root cuttings of short-jointed, lateral shoots in summer.
• **PESTS AND DISEASES** Prone to red spider mites, whiteflies, and mealybugs.

A. chamberlaynii. Vigorous climber, supporting itself by claw-like tendrils at the leaf tips. Ovate-lance-shaped, pinnate leaves, 5–14cm (2–5½in) long, have 2 large, lance-shaped or ovate, glossy, mid-green leaflets with wavy margins. Bears axillary racemes of 2–8 trumpet-like, pale yellow flowers, 5–7cm (2–3in) long, with purple-and-white-striped throats, from summer to early autumn. ↕ 4–6m (12–20ft). Brazil. ❁ (min. 7°C/45°F)

ANETHUM

Dill

APIACEAE/UMBELLIFERAE

Genus of 2 species of aniseed-scented annuals or biennials with smooth, branching stems, feathery, blue-green foliage, and umbels of small yellow flowers in summer. They are probably native to S.W. Asia and India, but *A. graveolens* has become widely naturalized on roadsides and wasteland in Europe and N. USA. *A. graveolens* is grown in herb and vegetable gardens for its aromatic leaves and seeds, which have many culinary uses.
• **HARDINESS** Fully hardy.
• **CULTIVATION** Grow in fertile, well-drained soil in full sun with shelter from strong winds. Water freely during the growing season to inhibit bolting.
• **PROPAGATION** Sow seed *in situ* at monthly intervals from spring to midsummer to produce a succession of fresh foliage.
• **PESTS AND DISEASES** Trouble free.

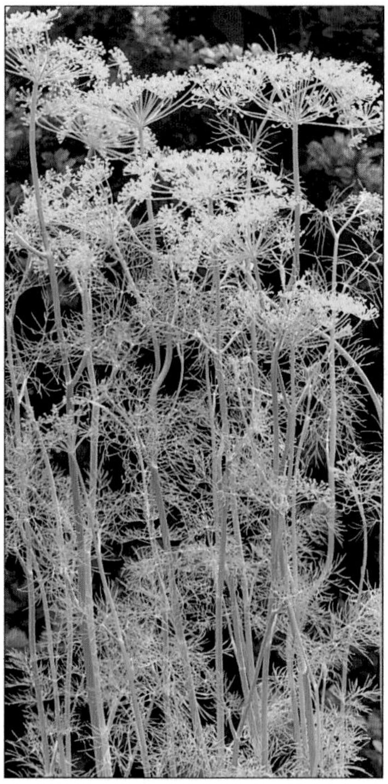

Anethum graveolens

A. graveolens ■ syn. *Peucedanum graveolens* (Dill). Aromatic annual with hollow, finely ridged stems. It has 3- or 4-pinnate, obovate to oblong leaves, to 35cm (14in) long, finely divided into numerous thread-like, blue-green leaflets. In midsummer, produces flattened umbels, 9cm (3½in) across, of tiny, deep yellow flowers. ↕ 60cm (24in) or more, ↔ 30cm (12in). Probably S.W. Asia and India. ❄❄❄

ANGELICA

APIACEAE/UMBELLIFERAE

Genus of 50 species of herbaceous perennials and biennials, some monocarpic, mainly from damp woodland, meadows, fens, and streambanks in the N. hemisphere. They are large, architectural plants producing alternate, 2- or 3-pinnate or 2- or 3-ternate, usually diamond-shaped leaves, 30–90cm (12–36in) long. They bear large umbels of small, white, greenish yellow, or purple flowers, followed by flat, ribbed brown fruit. Angelicas are excellent for a large border, as specimens in a woodland setting, or for growing by a pond or stream. *A. archangelica* also has culinary and medicinal uses, and is suitable for a herb garden.
• **HARDINESS** Fully hardy.
• **CULTIVATION** Grow in deep, moist, fertile, loamy soil in full or partial shade, although most species will tolerate drier conditions; *A. sylvestris* prefers full sun. *A. archangelica* dies after flowering, but if flowering is prevented, or the spent flowers are removed before setting seed, it will often flower a second year.
• **PROPAGATION** Sow seed in containers in a cold frame as soon as ripe; exposure to light is required for germination. Transplant the seedlings while small, as older plants resent disturbance. They normally flower within 2 or 3 years.
• **PESTS AND DISEASES** Powdery mildew may be a problem in dry summers. Susceptible to aphids, snails, slugs, and leaf miners.

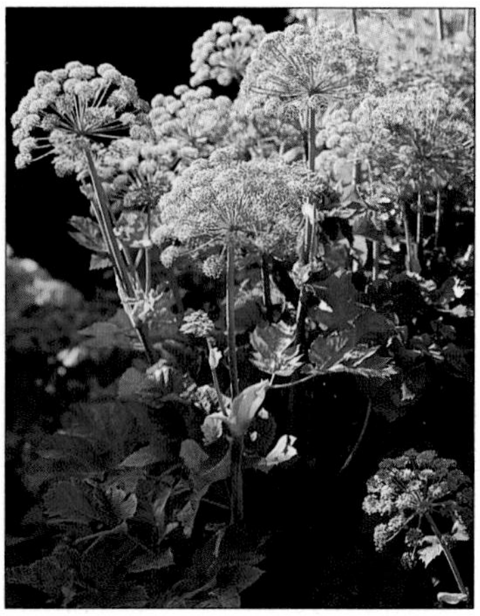

Angelica archangelica

A. archangelica ■ syn. *A. officinalis* (Archangel). Stout, upright, herbaceous or monocarpic perennial, often grown as a biennial, with 2- or 3-pinnate, mid-green leaves, to 60cm (24in) long, which have ovate-lance-shaped, toothed leaflets. Rounded umbels, to 25cm (10in) across, of greenish yellow flowers are borne on thick, ribbed stems in early and midsummer. ↕ 2m (6ft), ↔ 1.2m (4ft). N. Europe. ❄❄❄
A. gigas ■ Clump-forming biennial or short-lived herbaceous perennial with toothed, tripartite, mid-green leaves, 30–40cm (12–16in) long, composed of diamond-shaped to ovate, lobed leaflets. Produces conspicuous, inflated, red-purple leaf-sheaths and dense, purple-bracted umbels, 12cm (5in) across, of rich, dark purple flowers on dark red stems, in late summer and early autumn. ↕ 1–2m (3–6ft), ↔ 1.2m (4ft). N. China, Korea, Japan. ❄❄❄
A. montana see *A. sylvestris.*
A. officinalis see *A. archangelica.*
A. sylvestris, syn. *A. montana* (Wild angelica). Robust biennial or short-lived herbaceous perennial producing ridged, purple-flushed stems and 2- or 3-pinnate, light green leaves, to 60cm

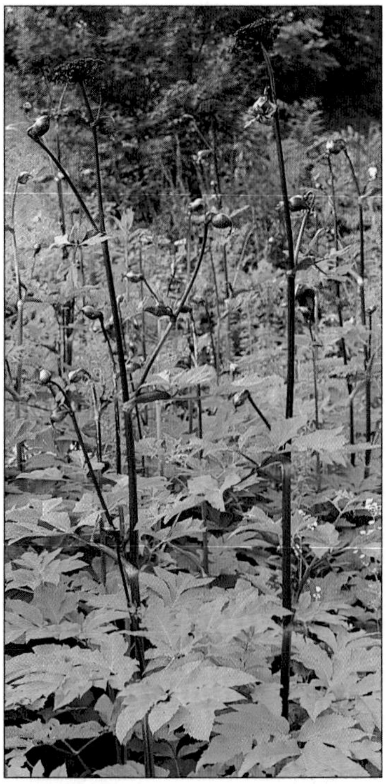

Angelica gigas

(24in) long, divided into sharply toothed, oblong-ovate leaflets. Bears many white or pale pink flowers in rounded, compound umbels, to 15cm (6in) across, in late summer and early autumn. Suitable for a wildflower garden. ↕ to 2.5m (8ft), ↔ 1m (3ft). Europe to C. Asia. ❄❄❄

▷ **Angelica, Wild** see *Angelica sylvestris*
▷ **Angelica tree,**
American see *Aralia spinosa*
Japanese see *Aralia elata*

ANGELONIA

SCROPHULARIACEAE

Genus of about 30 species of small subshrubs and evergreen, soft-stemmed perennials from damp savannah in tropical and subtropical Central and South America. They have opposite or alternate, broadly to narrowly lance-shaped leaves. The 2-lipped, shallowly cup-shaped, white, pink, mauve, or blue flowers, with spreading lobes, are borne in terminal racemes or singly from the leaf axils. In frost-prone areas, grow as summer bedding annuals or in a warm greenhouse; elsewhere, grow in a border.

• **HARDINESS** Frost tender.
• **CULTIVATION** Under glass, grow in loam-based potting compost (JI No.2) in full light, with filtered light in summer. Water freely and apply a balanced liquid fertilizer monthly. Containerized plants are best discarded after flowering. Outdoors, grow in moist but well-drained, fertile soil in full sun.
• **PROPAGATION** Sow seed in spring at 24°C (75°F). Divide or take softwood cuttings in spring in frost-prone areas, or at any time in frost-free areas.
• **PESTS AND DISEASES** Prone to aphids in spring and summer.

A. gardneri. Subshrubby perennial with stalkless, broadly lance-shaped, softly hairy leaves, 4–6cm (1½–2½in) long, with toothed margins. In summer, bears purple flowers, 2cm (¾in) across, with white disc-florets dotted red, in terminal racemes, to 15cm (6in) high. ↕ 1m (3ft), ↔ 60cm (24in). Brazil. ⌂ (min. 10°C/50°F)

▷ **Angel's fishing rod** see *Dierama*
▷ **Angel's tears** see *Narcissus triandrus*
▷ **Angels' trumpets** see *Brugmansia*
Common see *B. arborea*
Red see *B. sanguinea*
▷ **Angel wings** see *Caladium bicolor*

ANGOPHORA

MYRTACEAE

Genus of about 8 species of evergreen trees and shrubs, closely related to *Eucalyptus*, found in dry to moist, tropical to warm-temperate woodland and thickets in Australia. The leathery leaves are simple and entire, opposite on mature plants, but often alternate on immature ones. The 5-petalled, creamy white flowers have a prominent crown of stamens, and are borne in terminal, corymb-like cymes. *A. hispida*, the most commonly grown species, is valued for its foliage, although flowers may be borne once the plant is 2–3m (6–10ft) tall. In frost-prone climates, grow in a cool greenhouse; in frost-free regions, use as handsome specimen trees.

• **HARDINESS** Half hardy to frost tender.
• **CULTIVATION** Under glass, grow in loam-based potting compost (JI No.3), with additional sharp sand, in full light. In the growing season, water moderately and apply a balanced liquid fertilizer monthly; reduce water in winter. Outdoors, grow in fertile, well-drained soil in full sun. Pruning group 1; plants grown under glass need restrictive pruning.
• **PROPAGATION** Sow seed in spring at 19–24°C (66–75°F); pot on seedlings singly as soon as possible.
• **PESTS AND DISEASES** Trouble free.

A. cordifolia see *A. hispida.*
A. hispida ♀ syn. *A. cordifolia* (Dwarf apple). Erect to spreading shrub or small tree with peeling grey to grey-brown bark, orange-brown when young, and young branchlets with red-brown hairs. The opposite, short-stalked or stalkless, elliptic to ovate, grey-green leaves, to 10cm (4in) long, dark purple-red when young, are heart-shaped at the bases, and have wavy, scalloped margins. From early to late summer, bears corymb-like cymes of 3–7 creamy white flowers, each 2cm (¾in) across. ↕ 3–8m (10–25ft), ↔ 3–6m (10–20ft). E. Australia (New South Wales). ❄ (borderline)

ANGRAECUM

ORCHIDACEAE

Genus of about 200 species of mostly evergreen, epiphytic, monopodial orchids, found mainly in warm, humid regions at sea level or at low altitudes in Africa and Madagascar. They have semi-rigid, linear to oblong leaves, produced in 2 ranks, and bear white to green or yellowish green, spurred flowers, singly or in racemes from the leaf axils, at various times of the year.

• **HARDINESS** Frost tender.
• **CULTIVATION** Warm-growing orchids. Grow epiphytically or in baskets of epiphytic orchid compost; provide humid conditions and full shade. Water

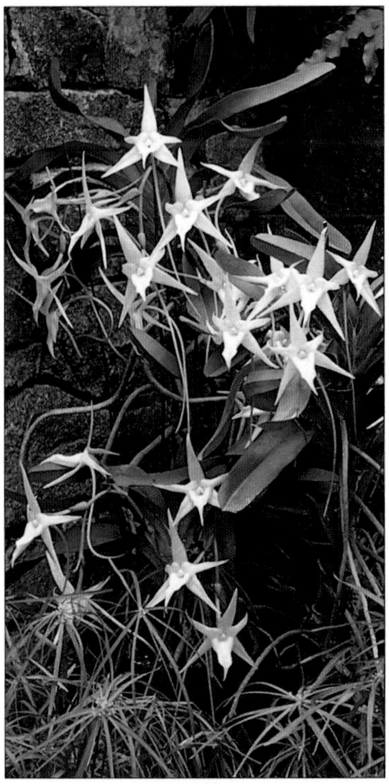

Angraecum sesquipedale

freely all year, more sparingly in winter. In summer, apply a half-strength liquid fertilizer at every third watering and spray foliage lightly with water once or twice daily. See also p.46.
• **PROPAGATION** Not suitable for division, although robust species sometimes produce offsets, which may be detached and rooted.
• **PESTS AND DISEASES** Susceptible to whiteflies, aphids, red spider mites, and mealybugs.

A. distichum. Miniature, evergreen, epiphytic orchid with broadly elliptic-oblong, curved, mid-green leaves, 8–12cm (3–5in) long. Many stalkless, night-scented white flowers, 1cm (½in) across, with spurs 8mm (⅜in) long, are produced singly from the leaf axils from summer to autumn. ↕↔ 15cm (6in). Tropical Africa, from Guinea to Uganda and Angola. ⌂ (min. 18°C/64°F; max. 30°C/86°F)
A. eburneum, syn. *A. superbum.* Variable, robust, evergreen epiphytic orchid with rigid, strap-shaped, leathery, mid- to dark green leaves, 30–50cm (12–20in) long. Night-scented, light green flowers, 8cm (3in) long, with white lips and spurs, to 10cm (4in) long, are borne in one-sided axillary racemes, to 60cm (24in) long, from autumn to winter. ↕ 1.2m (4ft), ↔ 60cm (24in). E. tropical Africa, Madagascar, islands of the Indian Ocean. ⌂ (min. 18°C/64°F; max. 30°C/86°F)
A. sesquipedale ▣ ♀ Robust, evergreen, epiphytic orchid with strap-shaped to oblong, dark green leaves, to 30cm (12in) long. In winter, produces axillary racemes, 25–30cm (10–12in) long, of 2–4 night-scented, waxy, ivory-white flowers, 17–22cm (7–9in) across, with spurs, 20–30cm (8–12in) long. ↕ 60cm (24in), ↔ 30cm (12in). Madagascar. ⌂ (min. 18°C/64°F; max. 30°C/86°F)
A. superbum see *A. eburneum*

ANGULOA

Cradle orchid, Tulip orchid

ORCHIDACEAE

Genus of about 10 species of deciduous, epiphytic or terrestrial orchids from South America, where they are found at high altitudes in the Andes. They have cylindrical to conical pseudobulbs, each of which produces 3 strongly ribbed and folded, broadly lance-shaped, soft-textured leaves. Cradle orchids are cultivated for their superb, tulip-like, solitary, fragrant flowers with waxy tepals, which are borne on basal stems in summer. They are closely related to, and hybridize readily with, the genus *Lycaste.*

• **HARDINESS** Frost tender.
• **CULTIVATION** Cool- to intermediate-growing orchids. Grow in containers of epiphytic or terrestrial orchid compost with high humidity and full shade in summer. In spring and summer, while the plants are in leaf, water freely and apply a half-strength liquid fertilizer at every third watering. In autumn, reduce water and temperature, and remove shading. Keep dry after the leaves have died away; resume watering and pot on when new growth develops. Avoid spraying the foliage, as this encourages fungal diseases. See also p.46.
• **PROPAGATION** Remove the oldest pseudobulbs and pot up separately, but

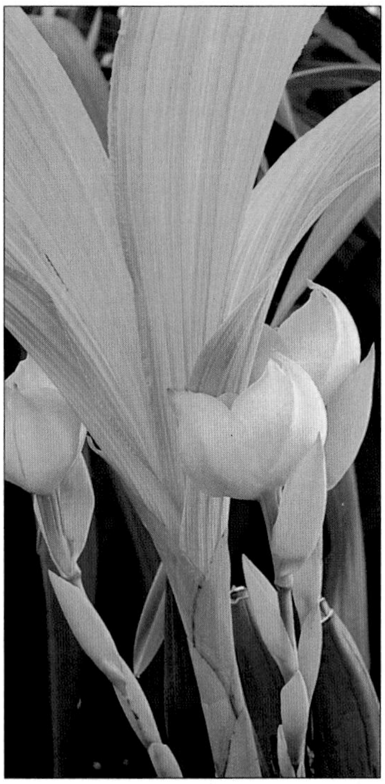

Anguloa clowesii

leave no fewer than 4 on the main plant.
• **PESTS AND DISEASES** Prone to red spider mites, aphids, and mealybugs.

A. clowesii ▣ Deciduous, terrestrial orchid with conical pseudobulbs and folded, deep green leaves, 45–80cm (18–32in) long. Solitary, bright lemon-yellow flowers, 10cm (4in) long, are chocolate- and wintergreen-scented, and are produced on stems to 23cm (9in) long from spring to summer. ↕↔ 60cm (24in). Colombia, Venezuela. ⌂ (min. 11°C/52°F; max. 30°C/86°F)
A. ruckeri. Deciduous, epiphytic or terrestrial orchid producing conical pseudobulbs and folded, deep green leaves, 45cm (18in) long. Solitary flowers, 9cm (3½in) long, are greenish brown on the outside and ochre, spotted red on the inside; they are borne on stems 23cm (9in) long in early summer. ↕↔ 60cm (24in). Colombia. ⌂ (min. 11°C/52°F; max. 30°C/86°F)

x ANGULOCASTE

ORCHIDACEAE

Bigeneric hybrid genus of deciduous orchids, a cross between *Anguloa* and *Lycaste,* with conical pseudobulbs and broadly lance-shaped, soft, folded leaves, to 60cm (24in) or more long. They are grown for their large, solitary, tulip-like, fragrant, often colourful flowers, which are borne in profusion in spring.

• **HARDINESS** Frost tender.
• **CULTIVATION** Cool- to intermediate-growing orchids. Grow in epiphytic orchid compost in humid conditions with full shade in summer. In spring and summer, water freely and apply a half-strength liquid fertilizer at every third watering. In autumn, when the pseudobulbs are fully formed, reduce water and temperature, and remove shading. Keep dry after the leaves have died; resume watering and pot on when new growth develops. Do not spray the foliage, as this encourages fungal diseases. See also p.46.

• **PROPAGATION** Remove oldest pseudobulbs and pot up separately, leaving at least 4 on the main plant, or divide when the plant overgrows its container.
• **PESTS AND DISEASES** Prone to red spider mites, aphids, and mealybugs.

x *A.* Apollo 'Goldcourt'. Deciduous hybrid orchid with conical pseudobulbs and folded, dark green leaves, to 60cm (24in) long. In spring, bears numerous solitary, fragrant, deep yellow, red-flecked flowers, to 10cm (4in) across. ↕↔ 60cm (24in). ❀ (min. 11°C/52°F; max. 30°C/86°F)
x *A.* Olympus 'Magnolia'. Deciduous hybrid orchid with conical pseudobulbs and folded, dark green leaves, to 60cm (24in) long. Bears many solitary, fragrant, creamy yellow flowers, 10cm (4in) across, in spring. ↕↔ 60cm (24in). ❀ (min. 11°C/52°F; max. 30°C/86°F)

▷ ***Anhalonium retusum*** see *Ariocarpus retusus*
▷ ***Anhalonium trigonum*** see *Ariocarpus trigonus*

ANIGOZANTHOS

Cat's paw, Kangaroo paw

HAEMODORACEAE

Genus of 11 species of evergreen, clump-forming perennials from a variety of habitats in S.W. Australia, including winter-wet swamps, sandy plains, open dry woodland, and coastal heathland. They have short rhizomes, fans of sheathing, lance- or strap-shaped, light to dark green leaves, and erect, slender, sometimes branched stems that bear terminal racemes or panicles of curious, 2-lipped, tubular flowers, thought to resemble a kangaroo's paws. These are densely covered with red, orange, yellow, or green woolly hairs. They flower from spring to midsummer outdoors, but under glass may flower at any time of year. They hybridize freely, both in the wild and in cultivation. In frost-prone areas, grow in a cool greenhouse or conservatory. In frost-free regions, use to add interest to a border. They are also excellent for cut flowers.
• **HARDINESS** Half hardy to frost tender.
• **CULTIVATION** Under glass, grow in 3 parts leaf mould and 1 part each loam and sharp sand in full light. Water freely in spring and summer, applying a balanced liquid fertilizer monthly; keep almost dry in winter. Outdoors, grow in moist but well-drained, humus-rich, sandy loam in full sun. Water freely during dry periods; mulch with straw or bark chips in autumn to protect the crowns.
• **PROPAGATION** Sow seed at 13–18°C (55–64°F) as soon as ripe; divide in spring.
• **PESTS AND DISEASES** Susceptible to leaf spot.

A. bicolor (Little kangaroo paw). Clump-forming perennial with mid-green leaves, 30–40cm (12–16in) long, usually with bristly margins. Racemes, 3–10cm (1¼–4in) long, of 4–10 olive-green flowers, 3.5–6cm (1½–2½in) long, blue-green inside with red- or yellow-felted ovaries and reflexed lobes, are borne from spring to summer. ↕70cm (28in), ↔ 40cm (16in). S.W. Australia. ✲

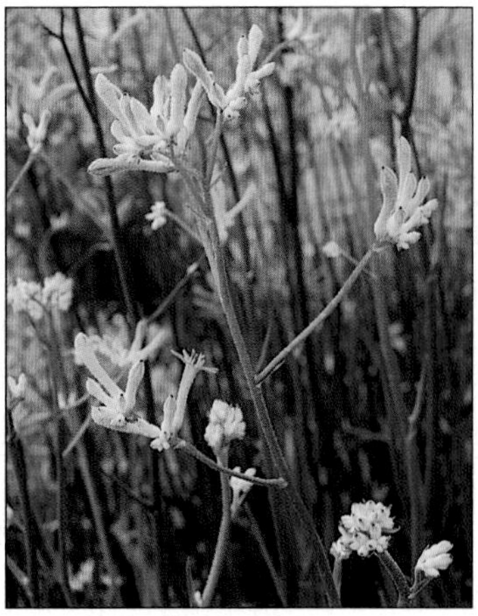

Anigozanthos flavidus

***A.* 'Bush Dawn'.** Clump-forming perennial with dark green leaves, 22–45cm (9–18in) long. From late spring to midsummer, bears racemes, 8–15cm (3–6in) long, of up to 100 yellow flowers, each 3–4cm (1¼–1½in) long, green inside and with reflexed lobes, on branched stems. ↕ 1–1.5m (3–5ft), ↔ 60cm (24in). ❀ (min. 5°C/41°F)
***A.* 'Bush Emerald'.** Clump-forming perennial with glaucous, blue-green leaves, to 35cm (14in) long. Red-purple, occasionally forked stems bear racemes, 5–12cm (2–5in) long, of 12–15 yellow-green flowers, 5cm (2in) long, from late spring to midsummer. ↕ 60–100cm (24–39in), ↔ 60cm (24in). ❀ (min. 5°C/41°F)
***A.* 'Dwarf Delight'.** Clump-forming perennial with bright green leaves, to 50cm (20in) long. From late spring to midsummer, erect stems bear panicles, 5–12cm (2–5in) long, of 5–15 greenish yellow flowers, 5–7cm (2–3in) long, covered with red hairs, appearing rich orange-red. ↕ 80cm (32in), ↔ 50cm (20in). ✲
A. flavidus ■ Clump-forming, evergreen perennial with olive to mid-green leaves, 35–100cm (14–39in) long. From late spring to midsummer, panicles, 4–7cm (1½–3in) long, of 9–10 yellow-green to brownish red flowers, to 5cm (2in) or more long, the lobes not reflexed, are borne on widely branched stems. ↕ 1–3m (3–10ft), ↔ 60–80cm (24–32in). S.W. Australia. ❀ (min. 5°C/41°F)
A. humilis ♀ (Common cat's paw). Clump-forming perennial with light to mid-green leaves, 15–20cm (6–8in) long, with hairy margins. In early and mid-spring, bears racemes, 5–12cm (2–5in) long, of up to 15 yellow-green, yellow, orange, or red flowers, 5cm (2in) long, with lobes not reflexed. ↕ to 50cm (20in), ↔ to 30cm (12in). S.W. Australia. ✲

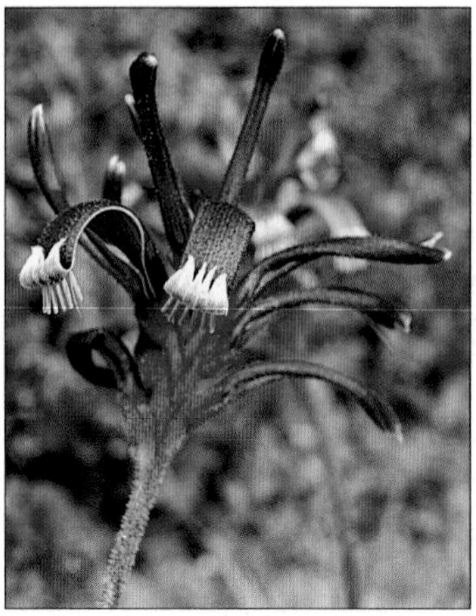

Anigozanthos manglesii

A. manglesii ■ ♀ (Mangles' kangaroo paw). Clump-forming perennial with erect, grey-green leaves, 10–40cm (4–16in) long. From mid-spring to early summer, red-hairy, rarely branched stems bear racemes, 5–14cm (2–5½in) long, of up to 7 yellow-green flowers, 6–10cm (2½–4in) long, with reflexed lobes, grading to dark green with lime-green hairs outside and red, sometimes yellow or apricot-yellow hairs at the bases. ↕ 30–120cm (1–4ft), ↔ 40–60cm (16–24in). S.W. Australia. ✲
A. pulcherrimus (Yellow kangaroo paw). Clump-forming perennial with grey-green, sometimes silky-haired leaves, 20–40cm (8–16in) long. From late spring to late summer, branched stems bear panicles, 3–8cm (1¼–3in) long, of 5–15 yellow flowers, 3.5–5cm (1½–2in) long, with spreading lobes and yellow hairs. ↕ to 1m (3ft), ↔ 40–60cm (16–24in). S.W. Australia. ✲
A. rufus. Clump-forming perennial producing mid-green leaves, 20–40cm (8–16in) long, with rough, hairy margins. Broad panicles, 3–9cm (1¼–3½in) long, of 5–15 or more red or deep claret, purple-woolly flowers, to 4.5cm (1¾in) or more long, with lobes not reflexed, are produced on branched stems from mid-spring to midsummer. ↕ to 1m (3ft), ↔ 40–60cm (16–24in). S.W. Australia. ❀ (min. 5°C/41°F)
A. viridis (Green kangaroo paw). Clump-forming perennial with narrow, grey-green leaves, 10–50cm (4–20in) long. Racemes, 5–14cm (2–5½in) long, of up to 15 yellow-green flowers, 5–8cm (2–3in) long, with reflexed lobes and covered with greenish yellow hairs, are produced from early spring to early summer. ↕ to 1m (3ft), ↔ 40–60cm (16–24in). S.W. Australia. ✲

▷ **Anise,**
Chinese see *Illicium anisatum, I. verum*
Purple see *Illicium floridanum*
Star see *Illicium verum*

ANISODONTEA

MALVACEAE

Genus of 19 species of woody-based perennials and shrubs from a variey of habitats in South Africa. The evergreen, alternate, usually toothed leaves vary from linear to elliptic or ovate and are sometimes lobed or 3-palmate. They are grown for their shallowly cup-shaped, 5-petalled flowers, borne singly or in racemes, corymbs, or cymes from spring to autumn. In frost-prone areas, grow in a cool greenhouse, standing plants outside or bedding them out in summer. In frost-free areas, grow in a border.
• **HARDINESS** Half hardy; *A. capensis* and *A.* x *hypomadarum* may withstand spells to -5°C (23°F) if wood is well-ripened.
• **CULTIVATION** Under glass, grow in loam-based potting compost (JI No.2) in full light. Pot on or top-dress in late winter. From spring to autumn, water freely and apply a balanced liquid fertilizer monthly; water sparingly in winter. Outdoors, grow in moderately fertile, well-drained soil in full sun. Tip prune young plants to encourage a bushy habit. Pruning group 9.
• **PROPAGATION** Sow seed at 13–18°C (55–64°F) in spring. Root semi-ripe cuttings with bottom heat in summer.
• **PESTS AND DISEASES** Susceptible to red spider mites, whiteflies, and aphids.

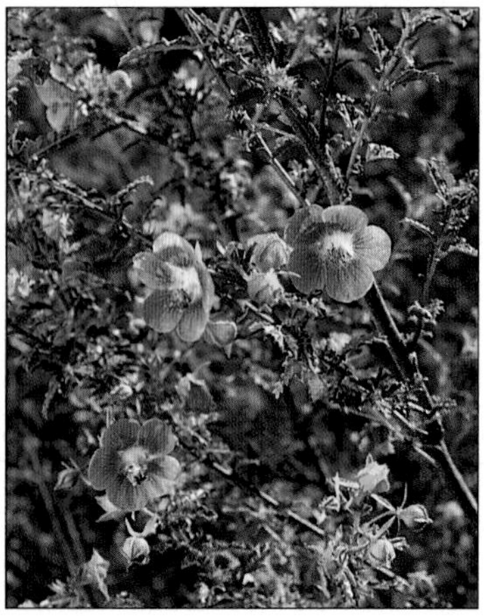

Anisodontea capensis

A. capensis ■ syn. *Malvastrum capensis.* Erect shrub with hairy stems and hairy, triangular to ovate, mid-green leaves, 2.5cm (1in) long, with 3–5 shallow to deep lobes, which may also be lobed and toothed. From summer to autumn, produces dark-veined, pale to deep red-purple flowers, 2.5cm (1in) wide, singly or in 2- or 3-flowered racemes from the leaf axils. ↕ 60–100cm (24–39in), ↔ 40–80cm (16–32in). South Africa. ✲
***A.* x *hypomadarum*,** syn. *A.* x *hypomandarum.* Bushy shrub or sub-shrub, with slender, erect, densely hairy stems, and obovate to oblong, 3-lobed, toothed, mid- to deep green leaves, to 3.5cm (1½in) long. From spring to autumn, produces purple-veined, pale pink flowers, 2.5–3cm (1–1¼in) wide, singly from the upper leaf axils. ↕ 1.5m (5ft), ↔ 1m (3ft). Garden origin. ✲
A.* x *hypomandarum see *A.* x *hypomadarum.*

ANISOTOME

APIACEAE/UMBELLIFERAE

Genus of 13 species of perennials, related to *Aciphylla,* from New Zealand (mainly South Island) and adjacent sub-antarctic islands. They occur mostly in shady sites in moist, rich soil in lowland areas or mountain grassland, and have large, pinnate leaves and broad umbels of small, white, red, or purple flowers. Grow in moist woodland. Alpine species are suitable for a rock garden or trough.
• **HARDINESS** Frost hardy; *A. latifolia* is hardy to -7°C (19°F).
• **CULTIVATION** Grow in deep, fertile, moist but well-drained soil in a cool site with partial shade.
• **PROPAGATION** Sow seed in containers in a cold frame in spring. Divide carefully as growth begins in spring.
• **PESTS AND DISEASES** Prone to blackfly.

A. latifolia, syn. *Aciphylla latifolia.* Clump-forming perennial with ovate, 2- or 3-pinnate, thick, leathery, glossy, mid-green leaves, 30–60cm (12–24in) long, with spiny tipped, ovate to lance-shaped leaflets. In summer, umbels, 4–10cm (1½–4in) wide, of small, white to reddish purple flowers, grouped into larger, compound umbels, over 20cm (8in) across, are borne on branched, furrowed stems. ↕ 1–2.2m (3–7ft), ↔ indefinite. New Zealand (Auckland Islands, Campbell Islands). ✻✻

▷**Annatto** see *Bixa orellana*
▷***Anneliesia candida*** see *Miltonia candida*
▷**Annuals** see pp.42–43

ANODA

MALVACEAE

Genus of about 10 species of upright to spreading annuals, perennials, and subshrubs, widespread in moist soils in meadows and near streams, some from woodland or rocky areas, from S.W. USA to Mexico, in the West Indies, and in N. South America. They have slightly hairy, unlobed, palmately lobed or palmate, lance-shaped to spear-shaped, mid-green leaves, and 5-petalled, mallow-like flowers borne singly or in racemes or panicles from summer to autumn. The short-lived perennials, usually grown as annuals, may survive mild winters with a mulch to protect the root system. They are suitable for a mixed or annual border.

• **HARDINESS** Half hardy.
• **CULTIVATION** Grow in any moist but well-drained soil, preferably low in nutrients, in full sun. Provide early support, when the seedlings are 7–10cm (3–4in) high. Dead-head to prolong flowering.
• **PROPAGATION** Sow seed at 13–15°C (55–59°F) in early spring, or *in situ* in mid-spring.
• **PESTS AND DISEASES** Trouble free.

A. cristata. Upright or spreading annual or short-lived perennial with ovate, unlobed to deeply 3- to 7-lobed, entire or toothed leaves, usually to 10cm (4in) long, but varying greatly in size and shape, even on the same plant. Saucer-shaped, white, lavender-blue, lilac, or purple-blue, veined flowers, 1.5–5cm (½–2in) across, are produced singly or in pairs from the upper leaf axils, from summer to autumn. ↕ to 1.5m (5ft), ↔ to 60cm (24in). S.W. USA to Mexico, West Indies, N. South America. ✻. **'Opal Cup'** ▣ produces silver-lilac flowers with darker veins, and leaves sometimes marked purple. **'Silver Cup'** has pure white flowers.

▷***Anoiganthus breviflorus*** see *Cyrtanthus breviflorus*
▷***Anoiganthus luteus*** see *Cyrtanthus breviflorus*

ANOMATHECA

IRIDACEAE

Genus, closely related to *Freesia*, of 6 species of cormous perennials from upland grassland in C. and southern Africa. They have flat, broadly lance-shaped leaves, and bear terminal racemes of small, trumpet- to funnel-shaped flowers in late spring and early summer. The flowers are followed in autumn by brown capsules containing bright red seeds. In frost-prone climates, they are effective grown in containers in a cool or cold greenhouse. In frost-free regions, they are suitable for a sunny border or terrace.

• **HARDINESS** Half hardy, but will withstand occasional falls to -5°C (23°F).
• **CULTIVATION** Plant corms in spring, 5cm (2in) deep. Under glass, grow in sandy, loam-based potting compost (JI No.2) in full light. In the growing season, water moderately and apply a balanced liquid fertilizer monthly; keep completely dry when dormant. Outdoors, grow in sandy, moderately fertile soil in full sun.
• **PROPAGATION** Sow seed at 13–16°C (55–61°F) in spring. Divide clumps in spring. Seedlings will flower in 2 years.
• **PESTS AND DISEASES** Trouble free.

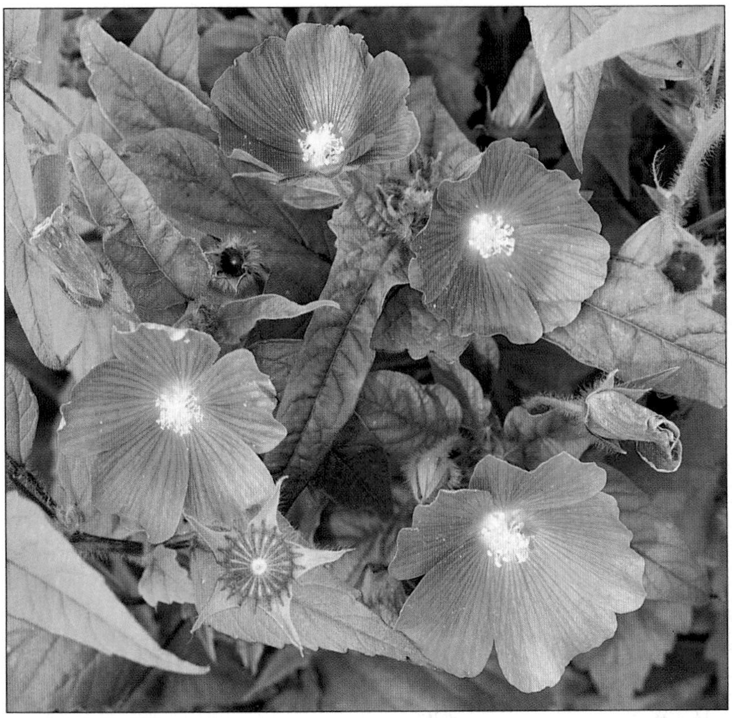

Anoda cristata 'Opal Cup'

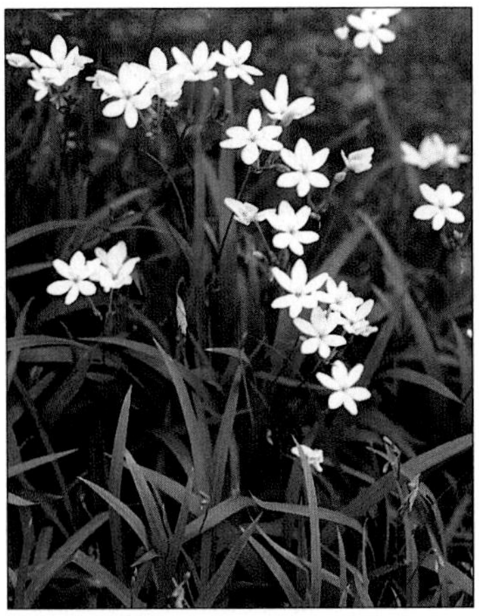

Anomatheca laxa var. *alba*

A. cruenta see *A. laxa*.
A. laxa, syn. *A. cruenta*, *Lapeirousia cruenta*, *L. laxa*. Cormous perennial with mid-green leaves, 10–35cm (4–14in) long. In early summer, bears stems of up to 6 open trumpet-shaped red flowers, 2cm (¾in) across, with darker red spots on the lower petals. ↕ 15–30cm (6–12in), ↔ 5cm (2in). Southern Africa, Mozambique. ✻. **var. *alba*** ▣ has pure white flowers.
A. viridis. Cormous perennial with mid-green leaves, 10–25cm (4–10in) long. In early summer, bears stems of 2–10 green flowers, to 2cm (¾in) across, shaped like curved funnels, with narrow, recurved petals. ↕ 30cm (12in), ↔ 5cm (2in). South Africa (Northern Cape, Eastern Cape, Western Cape). ✻.

ANOPTERUS

ESCALLONIACEAE

Genus of 2 species of evergreen shrubs from moist forest in E. Australia and Tasmania. They have simple, alternate leaves and are cultivated for their attractive, terminal racemes of flowers. They are effective when planted in light woodland. In frost-prone areas, grow in a cool greenhouse and move outdoors during the summer.

• **HARDINESS** Half hardy.
• **CULTIVATION** Under glass, grow in lime-free (ericaceous) potting compost in full or filtered light. In the growing season, water freely and apply a balanced liquid fertilizer monthly; water sparingly in winter. Outdoors, grow in cool, moist, lime-free, humus-rich soil in partial shade, ideally among trees and other shrubs for protection from hard frosts and cold winds. Pruning group 8.
• **PROPAGATION** Root semi-ripe cuttings in summer.
• **PESTS AND DISEASES** Trouble free.

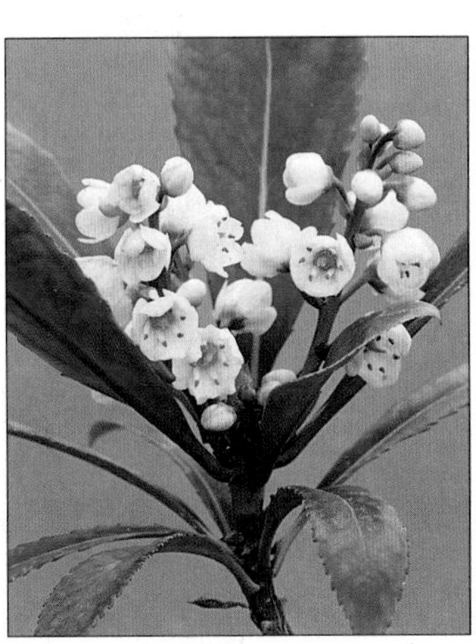

Anopterus glandulosus

A. glandulosus ▣ (Tasmanian laurel). Upright, evergreen shrub with narrowly obovate, toothed, leathery, glossy, dark green leaves, to 12cm (5in) long. In mid- and late spring, bears cup-shaped white, sometimes pink-tinged flowers in terminal racemes, to 12cm (5in) long. ↕ 10m (30ft), ↔ 8m (25ft). Tasmania. ✻

ANREDERA

syn. BOUSSINGAULTIA

BASELLACEAE

Genus of 10 species of tuberous-rooted, twining, evergreen climbers found in dry scrub and thickets in South America. The leaves are alternate, simple, and fleshy, often with bulbils produced in the leaf axils. Racemes of tiny, 5-petalled flowers are produced from the upper axils of long, young shoots. In frost-prone areas, grow *A. cordifolia* in a cool greenhouse. In frost-free areas, train over a support.

• **HARDINESS** Half hardy to frost tender; the rootstock of *A. cordifolia* often survives in frost-prone areas if planted deeply and protected with a mulch.
• **CULTIVATION** Under glass, grow in loam-based potting compost (JI No.3) in full light. Water freely when in growth, applying a balanced liquid fertilizer monthly; water sparingly in winter. Outdoors, grow in any well-drained soil in full sun. Pruning group 11; prune in late winter or early spring.
• **PROPAGATION** Divide the tuberous roots in early spring. Root softwood cuttings in early summer. Collect tubers and bulbils in autumn and store in frost-free conditions; plant in early spring.
• **PESTS AND DISEASES** Prone to aphids and red spider mites under glass.

A. cordifolia, syn. *Boussingaultia baselloides* of gardens (Madeira vine, Mignonette vine). Fast-growing twiner with reddish green stems and oblong, fleshy, bright green leaves, 3–10cm (1¼–4in) long, with heart-shaped bases. In autumn, bears numerous racemes, 30cm (12in) long, of sweetly scented white flowers. ↕ 4–6m (12–20ft). S. Brazil to N. Argentina. ✻ (borderline)

ANTENNARIA

Cat's ears, Pussy-toes

ASTERACEAE/COMPOSITAE

Genus of about 45 species of evergreen or semi-evergreen, dioecious, mat-forming perennials from open habitats in the N. hemisphere. They have basal rosettes of hairy leaves and solitary or corymb-like heads of small, "everlasting" flowerheads on short stems. Use in a rock garden, as low ground cover at the front of a border, and in crevices in walls or paving. The flowerheads may be dried for use in flower arrangements.

• **HARDINESS** Fully hardy.
• **CULTIVATION** Grow in any moderately fertile, well-drained soil in full sun.
• **PROPAGATION** Sow seed in containers in an open frame in spring or autumn. Separate rooted stems in spring.
• **PESTS AND DISEASES** Trouble free.

A

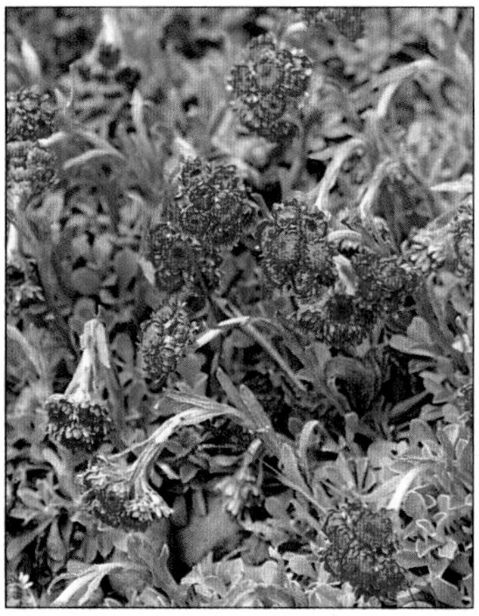

Antennaria dioica 'Rosea'

A. dioica. Semi-evergreen, mat-forming, stoloniferous perennial with grey-green, spoon-shaped leaves, to 4cm (1½in) long, densely white-hairy beneath. Bears corymbs of small, fluffy, white or pale pink flowerheads, on stems 2cm (¾in) long, in late spring and early summer. ↕5cm (2in), ↔ to 45cm (18in). Europe, N. Asia, North America. ❄❄❄. **'Nyewoods'** is compact, bearing deep pink flowerheads; ↔ to 20cm (8in). **'Rosea'** ■ 🏆 has rose-pink flowerheads.

ANTHEMIS

ASTERACEAE/COMPOSITAE

Genus of about 100 species of mat- or clump-forming, occasionally hummock-forming annuals and perennials from a wide range of well-drained, sunny habitats from Europe to N. Africa, Turkey, the Caucasus, and Iran. They are valued in a border or rock garden for their filigree foliage and extended flowering season, from late spring to late summer. They have usually pinnatisect to 3-pinnatisect, hairy, aromatic leaves and daisy-like, white or yellow flowerheads with yellow disc-florets; some species are good for cutting.

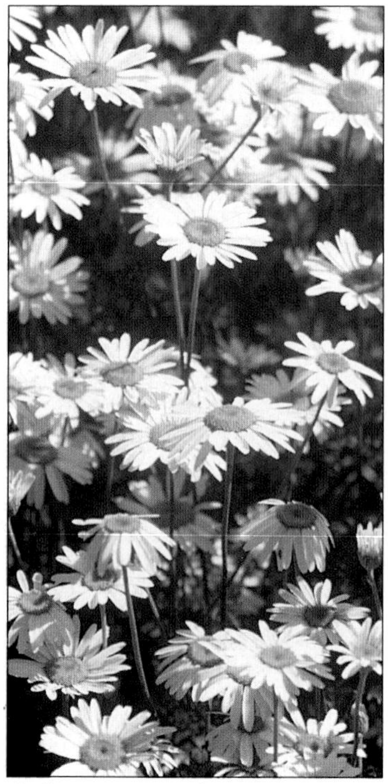

Anthemis punctata subsp. *cupaniana*

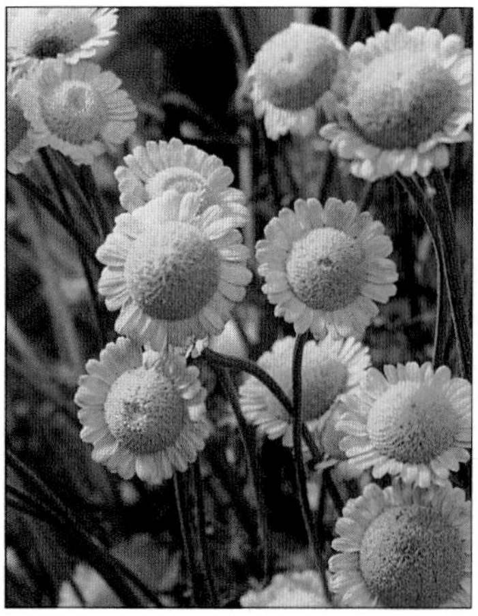

Anthemis sancti-johannis

- **HARDINESS** Fully hardy to frost hardy.
- **CULTIVATION** Grow in moderately fertile, well-drained, sandy or gravelly soil in full sun. *A. marschalliana* prefers partial shade with protection from winter wet. *A. sancti-johannis* and *A. tinctoria* are often short-lived; to increase their longevity, cut back hard after flowering to encourage the development of strong, overwintering, basal growth.
- **PROPAGATION** Sow seed in containers in a cold frame in spring. Divide in spring, or root basal cuttings in spring and late summer.
- **PESTS AND DISEASES** Prone to slug damage, aphids, and powdery mildew.

A. biebersteiniana see *A. marschalliana.*
A. marschalliana, syn. *A. biebersteiniana, A. rudolphiana.* Mat-forming perennial with obovate, 2-pinnatisect, silky-grey leaves, to 7cm (3in) long, densely arranged on the stems. Solitary yellow flowerheads, 1.5cm (½in) across, with white-woolly, black-margined involucral bracts, are borne in late spring and early summer. ↕20–45cm (8–18in), ↔ 45–60cm (18–24in). Caucasus, N. Turkey. ❄❄❄
A. nobilis see *Chamaemelum nobile.*
A. punctata* subsp. *cupaniana ■ 🏆 Mat-forming perennial with ovate to obovate, pinnatisect or 2-pinnatisect, silvery grey leaves, 7–12cm (3–5in) long, turning dull grey-green in winter. In early summer, bears long-lasting white flowerheads, to 6cm (2½in) wide, with fewer blooms later. ↕30cm (12in), ↔ 90cm (36in). Italy (Sicily). ❄❄
A. rudolphiana see *A. marschalliana.*
A. sancti-johannis ■ Clump-forming, short-lived perennial bearing oblong, pinnatisect, grey-hairy, white-tipped leaves, to 5cm (2in) long, and bright orange flowerheads, 3–5cm (1¼–2in) across, throughout summer. Hybridizes freely with *A. tinctoria*, and many plants offered under this name are hybrids. ↕60–90cm (24–36in), ↔ 60cm (24in). S.W. Bulgaria. ❄❄❄
A. tinctoria (Golden marguerite, Ox-eye chamomile). Clump-forming, free-flowering perennial with inversely lance-shaped to obovate, 2- or 3-pinnatisect basal leaves, 1–5cm (½–2in) long, and smaller stem leaves. Leaves are mid-green above and grey-downy beneath. In summer, branching stems bear solitary, golden yellow to cream flowerheads, 3cm (1¼in) across, with grey-woolly involucral bracts. ↕↔ 90cm (36in). Europe, Caucasus, Turkey, Iran. ❄❄❄. The cultivars are excellent in borders, flowering for many weeks, and are also good for cutting; ↕↔ 60–90cm (24–36in) for most cultivars. **'Beauty of Grallach'** has orange-gold flowerheads. **'E.C. Buxton'** ■ produces attractive lemon-yellow flowerheads; ↕45–70cm (18–28in). **'Grallach Gold'** bears vivid gold flowerheads. **'Kelwayi'** has clear mid-yellow flowerheads; ↕↔ 60cm (24in). **'Sauce Hollandaise'** has very pale cream, almost white flowerheads, and dark green foliage; ↕ to 60cm (24in), ↔ 40–60cm (16–24in). **'Wargrave'** has pale yellow flowerheads.

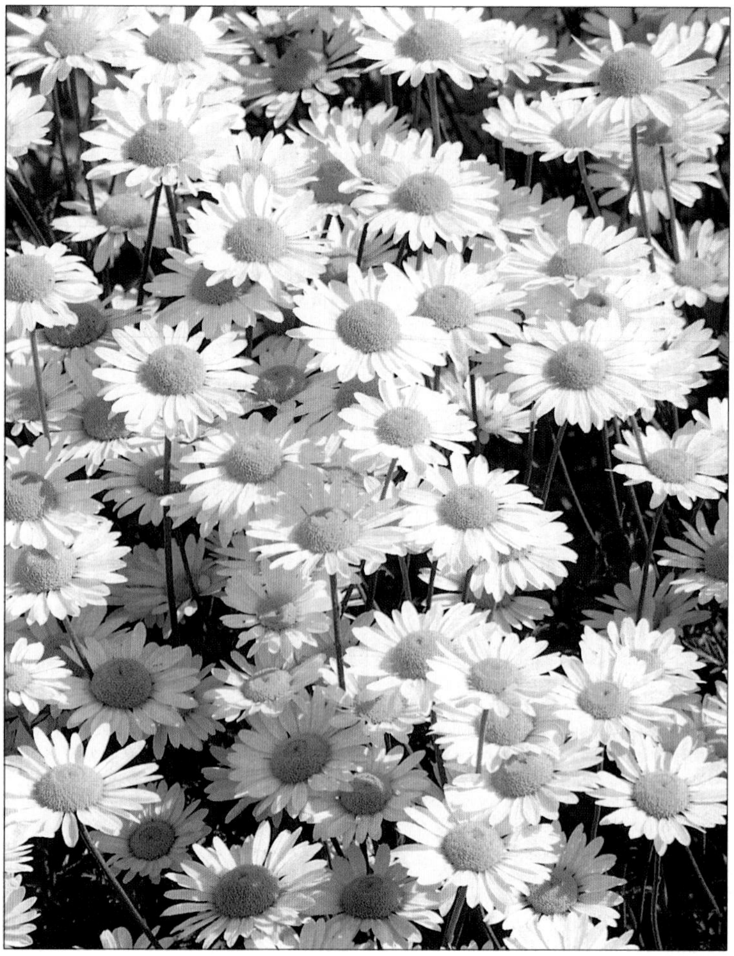

Anthemis tinctoria 'E.C. Buxton'

ANTHERICUM

ANTHERICACEAE/LILIACEAE

Genus of about 50 species of fleshy-rooted, rhizomatous perennials from grassy scrub on hillsides in Europe, Turkey, and Africa. They form clumps of narrow, linear, radical leaves and produce attractive, small, lily-like white flowers in racemes or panicles on slender stems, mainly in spring or summer, followed by decorative brown capsular fruits. They are ideal for a herbaceous border, or for naturalizing in grass; also excellent for cutting.

- **HARDINESS** Fully hardy to frost hardy.
- **CULTIVATION** Grow in any fertile, well-drained soil in full sun.
- **PROPAGATION** Sow seed in containers in a cold frame in autumn or spring (they may flower within 3 years) or divide as growth begins in spring.
- **PESTS AND DISEASES** Susceptible to damage from slugs and snails.

A. algeriense see *A. liliago* 'Major'.
A. graminifolium see *A. ramosum.*
A. liliago ■ 🏆 (St. Bernard's lily). Rhizomatous perennial with grass-like, linear, mid-green leaves, to 40cm (16in) long. Open trumpet-shaped, lily-like white flowers, 2–3cm (¾–1¼in) across, with tepals to 2cm (¾in) long, are borne in racemes in late spring and early

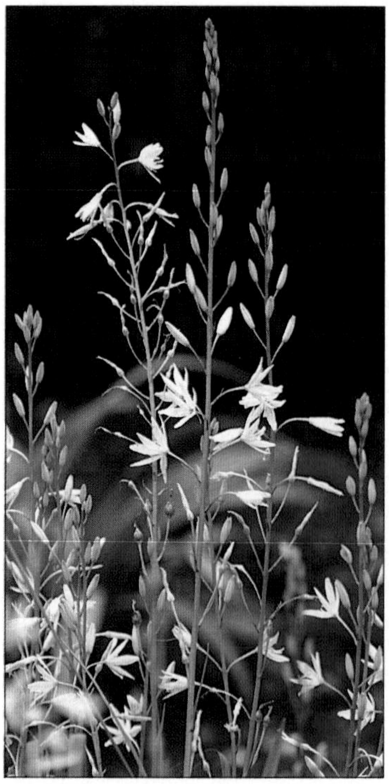

Anthericum liliago

summer. ↕60–90cm (24–36in), ↔30cm (12in). N., C., and S. Europe. ❄❄❄. **'Major'**, syn. *A. algeriense*, has large, wide-opening flowers, to 3cm (1¼in) across.

A. ramosum, syn. *A. graminifolium*. Rhizomatous perennial with linear, grey-green leaves, to 40cm (16in) long. During early and midsummer, bears branched, open panicles of star-shaped, lily-like white flowers, to 1.5cm (½in) across, with tepals 1–2cm (½–¾in) long. ↕90cm (36in), ↔30–60cm (12–24in). N. to S. Europe, Turkey, Crimea. ❄❄❄

▷***Antholyza*** see *Crocosmia*
A. paniculata see *C. paniculata*

ANTHRISCUS

APIACEAE/UMBELLIFERAE

Genus of about 12 species of annuals, biennials, and perennials from grassland, wasteland, and light woodland in temperate regions of the N. hemisphere. They have 2- or 3-pinnate, finely divided, light to mid-green leaves and tiny white flowers in umbels, 5–7cm (2–3in) across. Common chervil (*A. cerefolium*) has many culinary uses. Cow parsley (*A. sylvestris*) is attractive as a meadow plant. *A. sylvestris* 'Ravenswing' is good for providing dark foliage contrast in a herbaceous border.

• **HARDINESS** Fully hardy.
• **CULTIVATION** Grow in any well-drained soil in sun or partial shade. Water *A. cerefolium* in dry periods to inhibit bolting. *A. sylvestris* self-seeds prolifically if not dead-headed.
• **PROPAGATION** Sow *A. cerefolium* seed *in situ*, in succession from early spring to midsummer. Sow seed of perennials in containers in a cold frame in autumn or spring. Insert root cuttings in mid-winter. Grown in isolation, *A. sylvestris* 'Ravenswing' produces many dark-leaved seedlings, but take care to select stock with dark, purple-brown foliage.
• **PESTS AND DISEASES** Slugs, snails, and caterpillars may damage young growth; powdery mildew may also be a problem.

A. cerefolium (Common chervil). Erect annual with 2- or 3- pinnate, aniseed-flavoured leaves, 3–5cm (1¼–2in) long, and hairy beneath, composed of ovate, toothed or pinnatifid leaflets. In mid-summer, bears umbels of white flowers. ↕to 50cm (20in), ↔24cm (10in). Europe, W. Asia. ❄❄❄

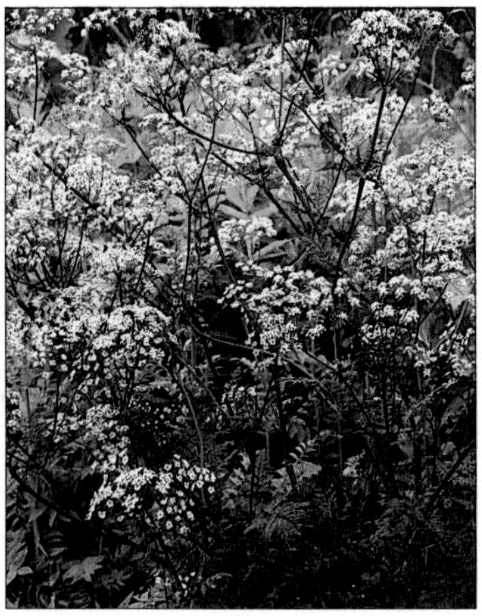

Anthriscus sylvestris 'Ravenswing'

A. sylvestris (Cow parsley, Queen Anne's lace). Clump-forming biennial or short-lived perennial with lacy, 3-pinnate leaves, 15–30cm (6–12in) long, composed of ovate, pinnatifid leaflets. Umbels of tiny white flowers open from mid-spring to early summer. ↕60–100cm (24–39in), ↔30cm (12in). Europe, Caucasus, Turkey, N.W. Africa. ❄❄❄. **'Ravenswing'** ▣ has purple-brown leaves, and bears umbels of tiny white flowers with small pink bracts from late spring to summer; ↕1m (3ft).

ANTHURIUM

Flamingo flower, Tail flower

ARACEAE

Large genus of 700–900 species of evergreen perennials, many epiphytic, with erect, sometimes climbing stems, from wet mountain forest in tropical and subtropical North and South America. They have large, entire or palmately lobed, often glossy leaves, and produce brightly coloured, flat or concave spathes and cylindrical spadices, to 45cm (18in) long. The spadices usually taper evenly upwards but may be pendent or contorted. The fruits are ovoid or spherical berries, which ripen to orange, red, or purple. In frost-prone areas, anthuriums may be grown in containers or epiphytically on false "trees" in a warm greenhouse; species that tolerate drier conditions, such as *A. scherzerianum*, are suitable for use as houseplants. All provide excellent, long-lasting cut flowers. In humid, tropical areas, grow outdoors as epiphytes or in a border. If ingested, all parts may cause mild stomach disorder; contact with sap may irritate skin.

• **HARDINESS** Frost tender.
• **CULTIVATION** Plant with the crowns just above the soil surface and cover with a layer of sphagnum moss to protect the uppermost roots from drying out. Under glass, grow epiphytically or in a mix of 1 part fibrous loam, 1 part coarse sand, and 2–3 parts leaf mould, with additional charcoal. Provide high humidity and a constant temperature, with filtered light in summer and full light in winter. In the growing season, water freely and apply a balanced liquid fertilizer every 2–3 weeks; reduce humidity and water sparingly in winter. Top-dress annually and pot on every 2 years. Outdoors, grow epiphytically or in coarse, moist, fertile, humus-rich soil, enriched with leaf mould, in full or partial shade.
• **PROPAGATION** Sow seed at 24–27°C (75–81°F) as soon as ripe; they may take several months to germinate. Divide rootstock in winter. Root stem cuttings or offsets at 24–27°C (75–81°F) in spring or summer.
• **PESTS AND DISEASES** Mealybugs and scale insects may be a problem. Leaf spotting may be caused by fungal attack.

A. andraeanum ▣ (Flamingo flower). Upright, epiphytic perennial with stems to 30cm (12in) tall, and ovate, reflexed, dark green leaves, which are arrow-shaped at the bases. Both leaf-blades and leaf-stalks are to 30cm (12in) long. Erect, ovate to heart-shaped red spathes, 10–12cm (4–5in) long, often puckered, with yellow spadices, are produced

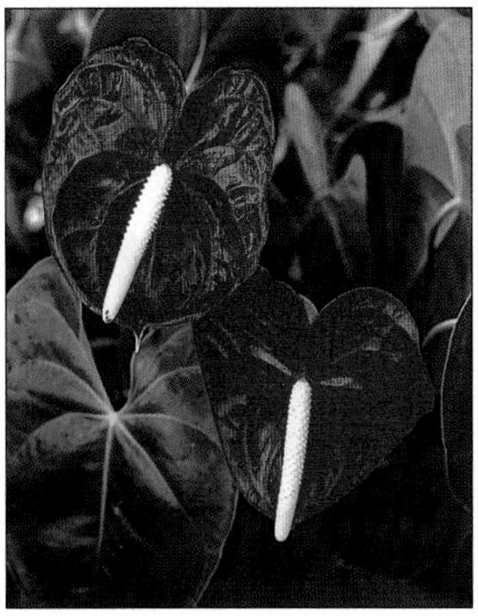

Anthurium andraeanum

throughout the year. Used extensively for hybridization. ↕60cm (24in), ↔20–30cm (8–12in). Colombia, Ecuador. ❀ (min. 16°C/61°F)

A. 'Aztec'. Upright, epiphytic perennial, similar to *A. andraeanum*, with ovate, reflexed, dark green leaves, arrow-shaped at the bases, on stems 30cm (12in) tall. Leaf-blades and leaf-stalks are to 30cm (12in) long. Erect, rounded-ovate scarlet spathes, 10–12cm (4–5in) long, often puckered, with prominent, golden yellow spadices, are borne throughout the year. ↕60cm (24in), ↔20–30cm (8–12in). ❀ (min. 16°C/61°F)

A. 'Brazilian Surprise'. Upright, epiphytic perennial with stems, 30cm (12in) tall, and ovate, reflexed, dark green leaves, arrow-shaped at the bases. Both leaf-blades and leaf-stalks are to 30cm (12in) long. Erect, rounded-ovate, orange to red spathes, often puckered, and 10–12cm (4–5in) long, have white spadices, turning yellow with age, and are borne periodically throughout the year ↕60cm (24in), ↔20–30cm (8–12in). ❀ (min. 16°C/61°F)

A. crystallinum ▣ Upright, epiphytic perennial with stems 25cm (10in) tall, cultivated for its large, broadly ovate to elliptic, velvety, deep green leaves, which are pink-bronze when young. The blades are sharply reflexed and 30–45cm (12–18in) long, with prominent white veins; the leaf-stalks are 21cm (8in) long. Erect and spreading, narrow green spathes, 8cm (3in) long, with greenish yellow spadices, are borne intermittently throughout the year. ↕↔60cm (24in). Colombia. ❀ (min. 16°C/61°F)

A. x cultorum see *A.* x *ferrierense*.

A. x ferrierense (*A. andraeanum* x *A. nymphaeifolium*), syn. *A.* x *cultorum*. Upright, epiphytic perennial with dense growth. Stems are to 30cm (12in) tall; leaves are ovate, reflexed, bright to mid-green, and arrow-shaped at the bases. The leaf-blades are 35–40cm (14–16in) long, the leaf-stalks 1m (3ft) long. Erect, fleshy, smooth, ovate to heart-shaped spathes, to 15cm (6in) long, varying in colour from dark red to pink and orange-white, with curving yellow spadices, are borne at any time of year. ↕1m (3ft), ↔75cm (30in). Guatemala. ❀ (min. 16°C/61°F). **'Guatemala'** has broad, thick, bright red spathes with yellow spadices. **'Reidii'** produces large pink spathes, 15–20cm (6–8in) long.

A. 'Flamingo'. Upright, epiphytic perennial, similar to *A. andraeanum*, with reflexed, ovate, dark green leaf-

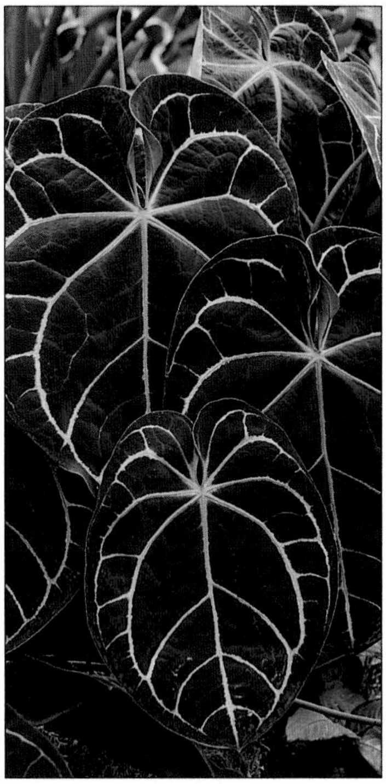

Anthurium crystallinum

blades, arrow-shaped at the bases. Leaf-blades and leaf-stalks are both 30cm (12in) long. Erect, rounded-ovate, puckered, bright pink spathes, 18cm (7in) long, with white spadices, which turn yellow with age, are produced sporadically throughout the year. ↕60cm (24in), ↔20–30cm (8–12in). ❀ (min. 16°C/61°F)

A. 'Negrito'. Erect, epiphytic perennial with ovate, reflexed, dark green leaf-blades, arrow-shaped at the bases; blades and leaf-stalks are 30cm (12in) long. Erect, rounded-ovate, deep copper spathes, 7–12cm (3–5in) long, with purple spadices, are borne throughout the year. ↕60cm (24in), ↔20–30cm (8–12in). ❀ (min. 16°C/61°F)

A. scherzerianum ▣ Variable, upright, epiphytic or terrestrial perennial with oblong-elliptic to lance-shaped, reflexed, leathery, dark green leaf-blades, 15–21cm (6–8in) long, on leaf-stalks to 25cm (10in) long. Broadly elliptic, reflexed, bright red spathes, 8–10cm (3–4in) long, with twisted, orange-red spadices, are borne intermittently throughout the year. ↕50–60cm (20–24in), ↔30cm (12in). Costa Rica, Guatemala. ❀ (min. 16°C/61°F).

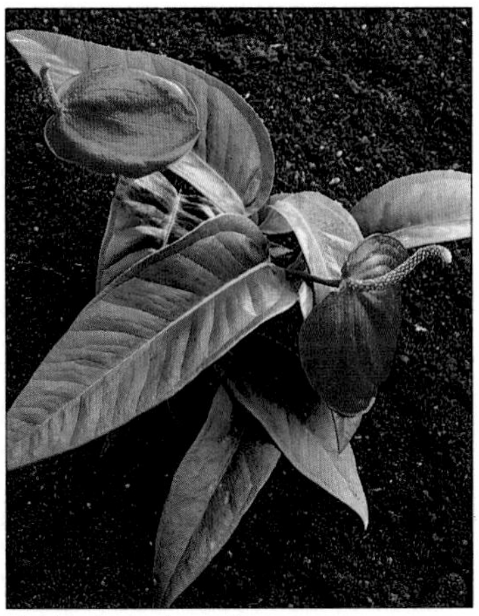

Anthurium scherzerianum

A

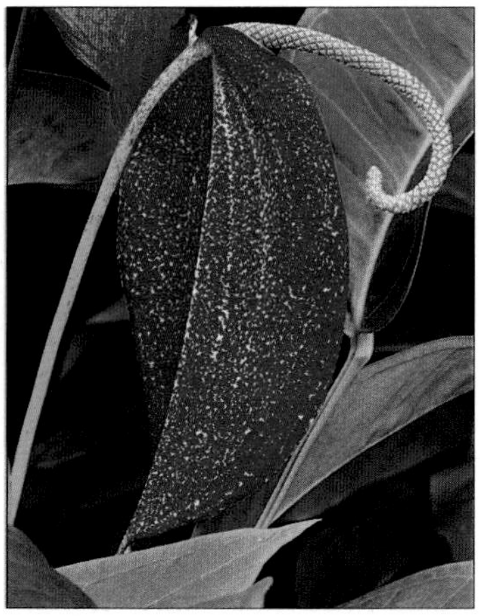

Anthurium scherzerianum 'Rothschildianum'

'Rothschildianum' ◼ has red spathes with white spots and yellow spadices. **'Wardii'** has red stems and large, dark red spathes with long red spadices.

A. veitchii. Upright, epiphytic perennial with oblong-ovate, corrugated, reflexed, glossy, dark green leaves, arrow-shaped at the bases, with pale green midribs. The leaf-blades are to 1.1m (3½ft) long, the leaf-stalks to 60cm (24in) long. Bears spreading, ovate to lance-shaped, recurved ivory spathes, 8–15cm (3–6in) long, with cream or rose-pink spadices, at any time of year. ↕ 1–1.2m (3–4ft), ↔ 60–90cm (2–3ft). Colombia. ❄ (min. 16°C/61°F)

A. warocqueanum. Climbing, epiphytic perennial with narrowly ovate to lance-shaped, reflexed, velvet-textured, glossy, emerald green leaf-blades, 50–90cm (20–36in) long; the leaf-stalks are 15–60cm (6–24in) long. Bears narrow, reflexed green spathes, to 10cm (4in) long, with yellow-green spadices, at any time of year. ↕ 1.2m (4ft), ↔ 60–90cm (2–3ft). Colombia. ❄ (min. 16°C/61°F)

ANTHYLLIS

LEGUMINOSAE/PAPILIONACEAE

Genus of about 20 species of annuals, perennials, and shrubs found on rocky cliffs or in open grassland, mainly in the Mediterranean. They have pinnate or 3-palmate leaves, and bear racemes of pea-like, mostly yellow, cream, or red flowers in dense heads, occasionally in clusters or singly from the leaf axils. They thrive in areas with long, hot summers and tolerate poor, dry soils. Some species are suitable for a rock garden or the front of a mixed border.

- **HARDINESS** Fully hardy.
- **CULTIVATION** Grow in well-drained, poor to moderately fertile soil in full sun. Trim untidy plants after flowering.
- **PROPAGATION** Sow seed in containers in a cold frame in autumn. Root semi-ripe cuttings in late summer.
- **PESTS AND DISEASES** Trouble free.

A. hermanniae. Compact, rounded shrub with spiny, tangled branches and tiny, 3-palmate leaves, to 1cm (½in) long, with oblong to lance-shaped, bright to grey-green leaflets, the 2 lateral leaflets sometimes very small. In early summer, bears a mass of bright golden yellow flowers, 5–10mm (¼–½in) long, in short, 2- to 8-flowered racemes, 2–3cm (¾–1¼in) long, with 2 large, leaf-like bracts. ↕ to 45cm (18in), ↔ to 60cm (24in) or more. Mediterranean, from Balearic Islands to Turkey. ✻✻✻ (borderline). **'Minor'**, syn. 'Compacta', is compact; ↕ 10cm (4in), sometimes more, ↔ 30cm (12in).

A. montana ◼ Clump-forming, woody-based perennial with pinnate leaves, to 6cm (2½in) long, comprising 8–15 or more pairs of narrowly elliptic to obovate-oblong, silky-haired, grey-green leaflets. During late spring and early summer, bears red, pink, or purple, white-tipped flowers, to 1.5cm (½in) long, in dense, spherical, clover-like heads, 2–3cm (¾–1¼in) across, above 2 deeply lobed, leaf-like bracts. Suitable for a rock garden or retaining wall. ↕ to 30cm (12in), ↔ to 60cm (24in). Alps and mountains of S. Europe. ✻✻✻. **'Rubra'** 🏆 produces bright crimson flowers.

A. vulneraria (Kidney vetch). Very variable, spreading, silky-hairy annual or short-lived perennial with erect or spreading stems and pinnate, mid-green leaves, to 14cm (5½in) long, consisting of oblong to elliptic leaflets with a larger terminal leaflet. In summer, bears rounded, umbel-like clusters, to 1.5cm (½in) across, of cream or yellow, often purple-tipped flowers, 1.5cm (½in) long, surrounded by palmately lobed, silky, leaf-like bracts. Colour variations from red, orange, and purple to white also occur. Suitable for a large rock garden or a wildflower meadow. ↕ 20–60cm (8–24in), ↔ to 80cm (32in). Europe and North Africa to W. Asia. ✻✻✻. **var. *coccinea*** is applied to variants bearing bright red flowers.

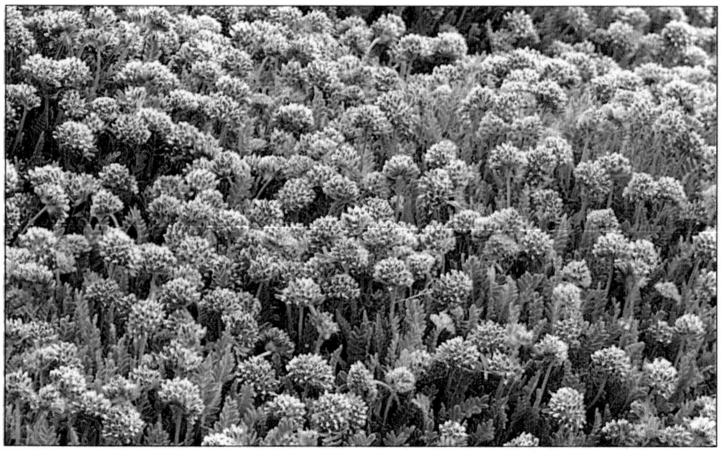

Anthyllis montana

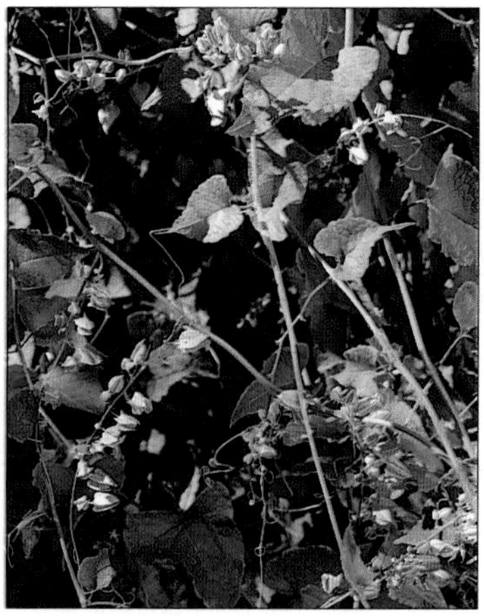

Antigonon leptopus

ANTIGONON

Corallita, Coral vine, Queen's wreath

POLYGONACEAE

Genus of 3 species of tendril climbers from Mexico and Central America, where they thrive in moist, tropical forest and scrub. They have tuberous roots, alternate, simple leaves, and are grown for their small, pink or white flowers, usually borne in panicles at the tips of the shoots. Where temperatures fall below 7°C (45°F), grow in a temperate greenhouse or conservatory. In warmer areas, train over a pergola, against a house wall, or through a tree.

- **HARDINESS** Half hardy to frost tender. The roots of *A. leptopus* may survive short spells of frost if protected with a mulch in autumn.
- **CULTIVATION** Under glass, grow in loam-based potting compost (JI No.2) in full light. From spring to autumn, water freely and apply a low-nitrogen liquid fertilizer monthly; keep just moist in winter. Outside, grow in moderately fertile, well-drained soil in full sun. Pruning group 11, in spring.
- **PROPAGATION** Sow seed at 13–16°C (55–61°F) in spring. Root semi-ripe cuttings with bottom heat in summer.
- **PESTS AND DISEASES** Aphids, red spider mites, and whiteflies may be a problem, especially under glass.

A. leptopus ◼ (Confederate vine, Mexican creeper). Fast-growing climber with heart-shaped to almost triangular, bright green leaves, 5–14cm (2–5½in) long. From summer to autumn, bears coral-pink to red, occasionally white flowers, 1.5–2cm (½–¾in) across, in airy racemes and panicles, to 15cm (6in) or more long. The tuberous roots are edible. ↕ 8–12m (25–40ft). Mexico. ✻

ANTIRRHINUM

Snapdragon

SCROPHULARIACEAE

Genus of about 30–40 species of annuals, perennials, and semi-evergreen subshrubs from mainly rocky sites in Europe, USA, and N. Africa. They are cultivated for their broadly tubular, 2-lipped flowers, with a characteristic hairy palate on the lower lip, which are produced from the leaf axils or in terminal racemes from early summer to autumn. The leaves, borne on branching stems, are linear-lance-shaped to ovate, and sometimes glandular. The common snapdragon, *A. majus*, is a short-lived perennial, usually grown as a bedding annual. Shrubby perennial species are ideal for growing in a rock garden or retaining wall.

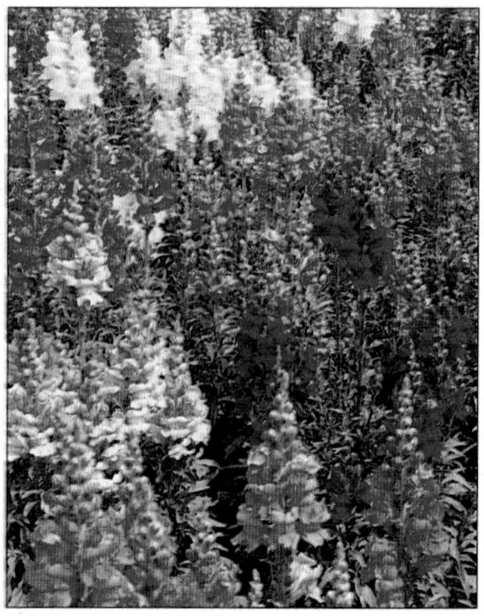

Antirrhinum majus Coronette Series

- **HARDINESS** Fully hardy to half hardy.
- **CULTIVATION** Grow *A. majus* cultivars in fertile, sharply drained soil in full sun. Dead-head to prolong flowering. Shrubby perennial species require very well-drained soil and shelter from wind; they are extremely brittle and sensitive to winter wet.
- **PROPAGATION** Sow seed of *A. majus* cultivars at 16–18°C (61–64°F) in late summer, early autumn, or early spring. Root softwood cuttings of shrubby species in summer, or sow seed in containers in a cold frame in autumn or spring; they may not come true. Overwinter young plants under glass.
- **PESTS AND DISEASES** Susceptible to antirrhinum rust; also prone to aphids and powdery mildew.

A. asarina see *Asarina procumbens.*

A. majus. Variable, strongly branched, short-lived perennial, often woody at the base, with mostly alternate, lance-shaped, glossy, deep green leaves, to 7cm (3in) long. Upright racemes of fragrant, 2-lipped flowers, 3–4.5cm (1¼–1¾in) across, with spreading, rounded, upper and lower lobes, vary in colour in cultivated selections from white, yellow, and bronze, to purple, pink, and red, often including bicolours; they are borne all summer and into autumn. ↕ 0.25–2m (¾–6ft), ↔ 15–60cm (6–24in). S.W. Europe, Mediterranean. ✻. Cultivars fall into 3 groups: tall, excellent for cut flowers and as "fillers" in a mixed border, ↕ 1m (3ft), ↔ to 45cm (18in) or more; intermediate, the most suitable for bedding, ↕ 30–60cm (12–24in), ↔ to 45cm (18in); and dwarf, for a small bedding scheme, edging, and containers, ↕ 20–30cm (8–12in), ↔ to 30cm (12in). **'Bells'** is dwarf and early-flowering, with long-lasting, open-faced or hyacinth-like flowers, in purple, purple and white, red, rose-pink, pink, bronze, yellow, or white. **'Chimes'** is exceptionally dwarf and compact, producing flowers in a wide colour range including several bicolours; ↕ to 15cm (6in). **Coronette Series** ◼ 🏆 cultivars are tall, weather- and rust-resistant bedding antirrhinums, good for cutting; they produce flowers in colours that include pale salmon-orange, scarlet, deep velvet-red, light

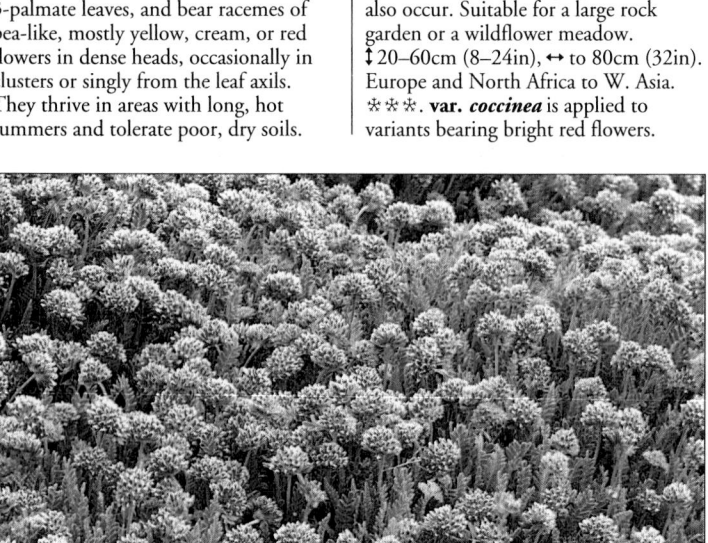

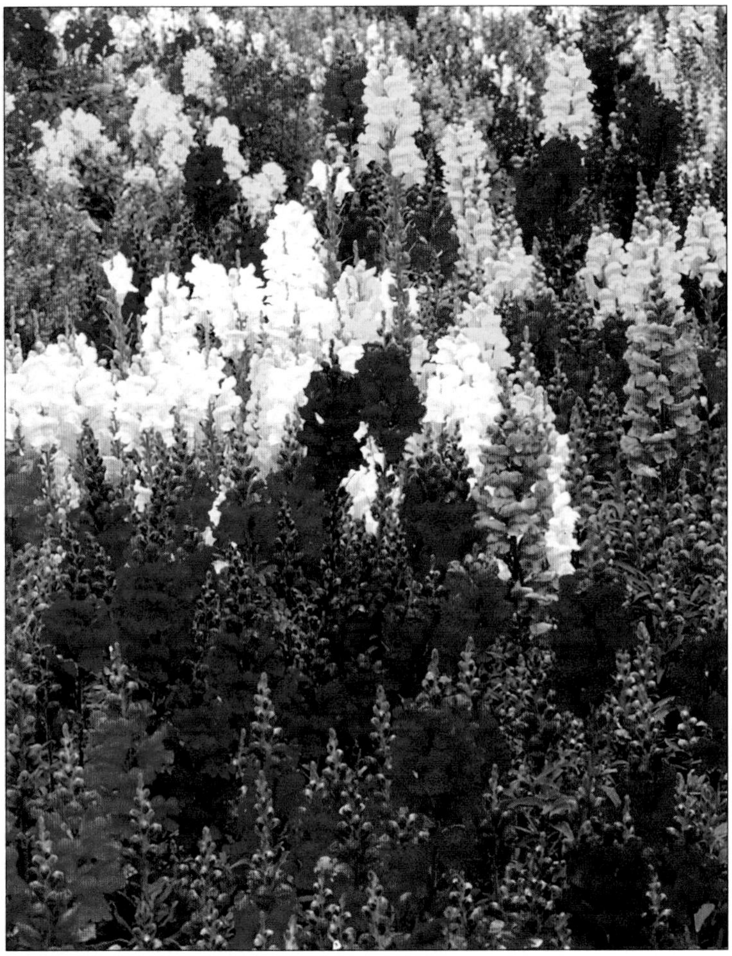

Antirrhinum majus Sonnet Series

pink, deep rose-pink, rich purple, lemon-yellow, and white; they are also available in single colours; ↕ to 65cm (26in). **'Floral Showers'** is dwarf and early-flowering, bearing flowers in up to 10 colours, including some bicolours. Tolerates wet weather; ↕ to 20cm (8in). **Rocket Series** cultivars are vigorous, tall antirrhinums, producing flowers in a broad colour range; they are excellent for cut flowers; ↕ to 1.2m (4ft). **Sonnet Series** ▣ ♀ cultivars are very early and free-flowering, intermediate antirrhinums. They are bushy in habit, with good wet-weather tolerance, and produce bronze, pink, carmine-red, crimson, burgundy, white, and yellow flowers. **Tahiti Series** ▣ cultivars are dwarf and rust-resistant, producing flowers in red, orange, rose-pink, and

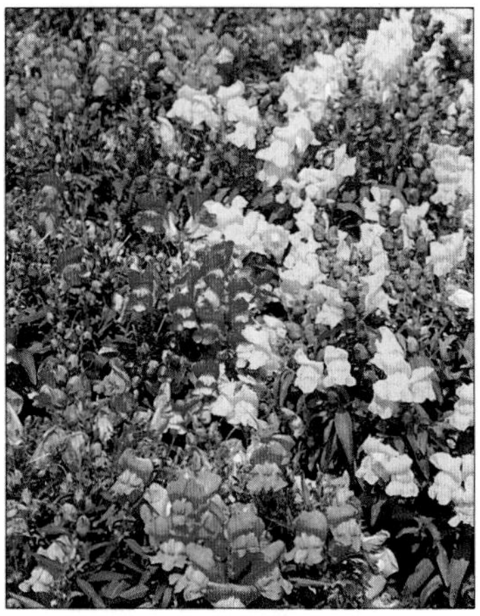

Antirrhinum majus Tahiti Series

bronze, with a pink and white bicolour; ↕ to 20cm (8in).

A. molle. Vigorous, dwarf subshrub with both procumbent and almost erect stems producing alternate, broadly ovate to elliptic, sticky-hairy, mid-green leaves, 1–2cm (½–¾in) long. White or pale pink flowers, 2.5–3cm (1–1¼in) long, with yellow palates, are produced from the upper leaf axils in early and midsummer. ↕ 15–20cm (6–8in), ↔ 20–30cm (8–12in). N.E. Spain, Portugal. ❄❄❄ (borderline)

A. pulverulentum ▣ Decumbent, dwarf shrub with opposite and alternate, ovate to elliptic, hairy, mid-green leaves, to 3cm (1¼in) long. Pale yellow flowers, 2–2.5cm (¾–1in) long, are produced from the upper leaf axils in early and midsummer. ↕ 15–20cm (6–8in),

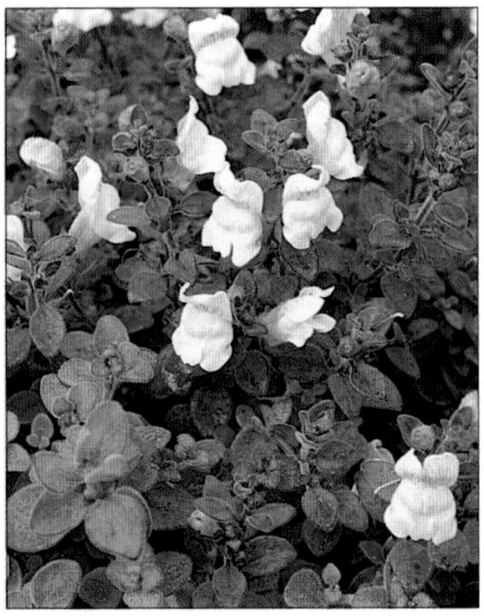

Antirrhinum pulverulentum

↔ 20–30cm (8–12in). Chalky, alkaline soils in E. Spain. ❄❄❄ (borderline)

A. sempervirens. Dwarf shrub, similar to *A. pulverulentum*, with trailing or erect, branching stems bearing opposite, oblong-ovate to elliptic, slightly sticky-hairy, mid-green leaves, 5–15mm (¼–½in) long. In early and midsummer, produces cream or white flowers, to 2.5cm (1in) long, with purple veins and yellow palates, from the upper leaf axils. ↕ 15–20cm (6–8in), ↔ 20–30cm (8–12in). Pyrenees, E. central Spain. ❄❄❄ (borderline)

APHELANDRA

ACANTHACEAE

Genus of about 170 species of evergreen shrubs and subshrubs from moist woodland in tropical North, Central, and South America. They are grown for their attractive flowerheads and opposite pairs of simple, fleshy, glossy leaves produced on stout or slender stems. Terminal, occasionally axillary, 4-sided spikes with long-lasting, overlapping, brightly coloured bracts and a succession of short-lived, tubular, red to yellow flowers are usually borne sporadically throughout the year. In frost-prone areas, grow in a temperate or warm greenhouse or as houseplants; elsewhere, use for bedding and for a border. Plants in containers grow to only about a third of the dimensions given below.

• **HARDINESS** Frost tender.

• **CULTIVATION** Under glass, grow in loam-based potting compost (JI No.2), with additional leaf mould, one-third by volume; grow in full light with filtered light in summer. Water freely with soft water when in growth, more sparingly in winter. Apply a balanced liquid fertilizer every 2 weeks in summer, and monthly in winter. Outdoors, grow in moderately fertile, humus-rich, well-drained soil in partial shade.

• **PROPAGATION** After flowering, cut back the main stems to a strong pair of leaves to encourage sideshoots. When these are 8–10cm (3–4in) long, detach them and root at 21°C (70°F). Propagate regularly, as older specimens deteriorate rapidly.

• **PESTS AND DISEASES** New growth is prone to infestation by aphids, scale insects, and mealybugs.

A. aurantiaca ▣ syn. *A. fascinator.* Erect shrub with slender stems and ovate to elliptic, deep green leaves, 10–15cm (4–6in) long, flushed or mottled with silver. In winter, bears dense, terminal spikes, to 45cm (18in) long, of overlapping bracts and protruding, orange-scarlet or vermilion flowers, 4–5cm (1½–2in) long. ↕ 0.75–1.3m (2½–4½ft) ↔ 0.6–1.2m (2–4ft). Mexico to Colombia. ❁ (min. 7°C/45°F). **'Roezlii'** has wavy and puckered, grey-green leaves with bold silver markings, and scarlet flowers.

A. fascinator see *A. aurantiaca.*

A. squarrosa (Saffron-spike, Zebra plant). Compact shrub with stout stems and ovate to elliptic, dark green leaves, to 30cm (12in) long, with white, silver, or yellow veins and mid-ribs. Produces terminal spikes, to 20cm (8in) long, of waxy yellow flowers, 2.5–3cm (1–1¼in) long, and maroon-tinged yellow bracts. ↕ 1.5–2m (5–6ft), ↔ 1.5m (5ft).

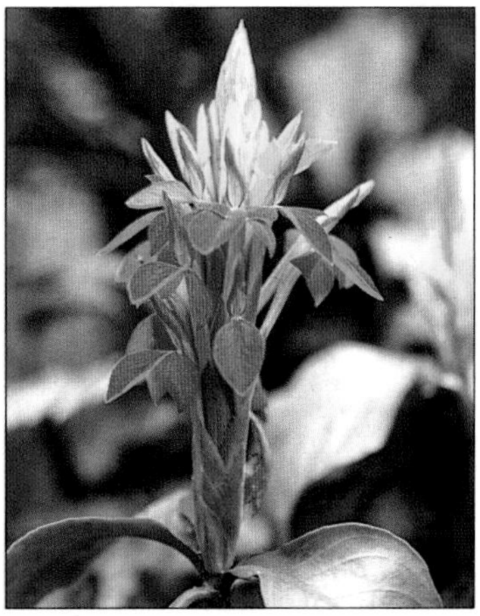

Aphelandra aurantiaca

Tropical and subtropical America. ❁ (min. 7–10°C/45–50°F; optimum 19°C/66°F). **'Dania'** has ovate to ovate-elliptic leaves with very prominent white veins that are feathered at the margins. Flowers, rarely produced, are yellow or orange-yellow, and 2.5cm (1in) long; ↕↔ 30cm (12in). **'Louisae'** ▣ ♀ has leaves with prominent white midribs and bold cross-bands of white around the veins. Bears spikes, 8–10cm (3–4in) long, of waxy, green-tipped, golden yellow flowers, resembling those of 'Dania'. Produces smaller flowerheads from the leaf axils just below the main spike; ↕ to 45cm (18in), ↔ 30cm (12in). **'Snow Queen'** is erect, with ovate, dark green leaves, which have silvery white veins. Flowers are pale lemon-yellow; ↕ to 45cm (18in), ↔ 30cm (12in).

A. tetragona. Spreading shrub with slender stems bearing broadly ovate, dark green leaves, 22cm (9in) long. Produces axillary and terminal spikes, 5–8cm (2–3in) long, of small orange bracts and hooded, bright red flowers, 3.5–8cm (1½–3in) long, with curved tubes. ↕↔ 1.2m (4ft). West Indies, Costa Rica, N. South America. ❁ (min. 7–10°C/45–50°F; optimum 19°C/66°F)

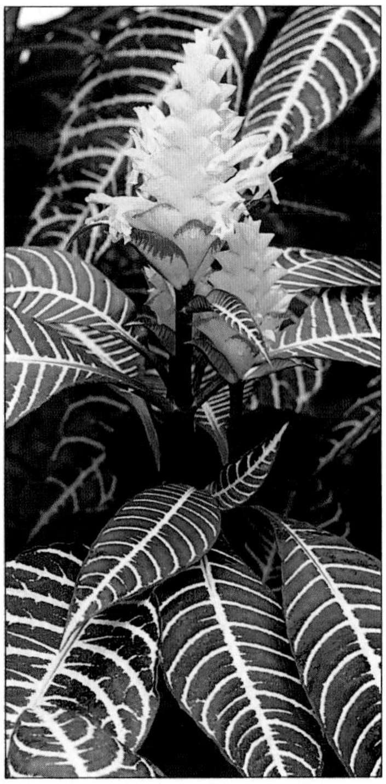

Aphelandra squarrosa 'Louisae'

APHYLLANTHES

APHYLLANTHACEAE / LILIACEAE

Genus of one species of densely tufted or clump-forming perennial occurring on hot, dry hillsides in S.W. Europe and Morocco. It has rush-like stems, and leaves that are reduced to membranous, basal sheaths. Attractive, saucer-shaped, deep to pale blue flowers are borne on slender stems in early summer. *A. monspeliensis* is suitable for a rock garden or an alpine house.

- **HARDINESS** Frost hardy.
- **CULTIVATION** Under glass, grow in a mix of 1 part each loam and grit with 2 parts leaf mould or peat. Water freely during the growing season; keep just moist when dormant. Outdoors, grow in sharply drained, sandy, peaty soil in full sun, with shelter from cold winds.
- **PROPAGATION** Sow seed in containers in a cold frame when ripe, or in spring; plant out seedlings as soon as possible, as young seedlings do not transplant well and larger plants resent disturbance. Divide with care in early spring.
- **PESTS AND DISEASES** Trouble free.

A. monspeliensis. Tufted or clump-forming, fibrous-rooted perennial with stiff, ribbed stems. In early summer, the stems bear deep blue to pale blue, dark-veined flowers, to 2.5cm (1in) across, singly or in groups of 2 or 3, above papery, reddish brown bracts. ↕ 10–25cm (4–10in), sometimes to 40cm (16in), ↔ 10–15cm (4–6in). S.W. Europe, Morocco. ❄❄

APONOGETON

APONOGETONACEAE

Genus of 44 species of rhizomatous, submerged aquatic perennials from temperate and tropical regions of Africa, S.E. Asia, and N. and E. Australia. The linear to elliptic or lance-shaped, floating leaves are produced from a tuber-like rhizome. Compound panicles or simple, forked racemes of tiny, often scented flowers, with 1–6 tepals and 6 or more stamens, are borne, mainly in summer, from a spathe-like bract just above the water surface. Some species will grow in water to 1m (3ft) deep. *A. distachyos* and *A. madagascariensis* are the most commonly cultivated species and are suitable for a pond outdoors, although in frost-prone areas *A. madagascariensis* is best in an aquarium.

- **HARDINESS** Frost hardy to frost tender.
- **CULTIVATION** Grow *A. distachyos* in soil at the bottom of a pond, or in aquatic planting baskets, at least 30cm (12in) across, in water 30–90cm (12–36in) deep. Prefers full sun, but will tolerate partial shade. Grow *A. madagascariensis* outdoors in a shady pool in frost-free regions or, in frost-prone areas, in an aquarium with filtered light, in water up to 50cm (20in) deep, at 23–28°C (73–82°F); the flowers last longer in the high humidity of a closed aquarium. Remove dying foliage after the growing season. See also pp.52–53.
- **PROPAGATION** Sow seed as soon as ripe, or seed that has been kept moist since collection, in small containers, covered by 5–7cm (2–3in) of water, at 13–16°C (55–61°F) for *A. distachyos* and 19–24°C (66–75°F) for *A. madagascariensis.* Divide rhizomes of large clumps when dormant.
- **PESTS AND DISEASES** Young leaves are often eaten by water snails and the larvae of the brown china-mark moth. Algae may easily smother the delicate leaves of *A. madagascariensis.*

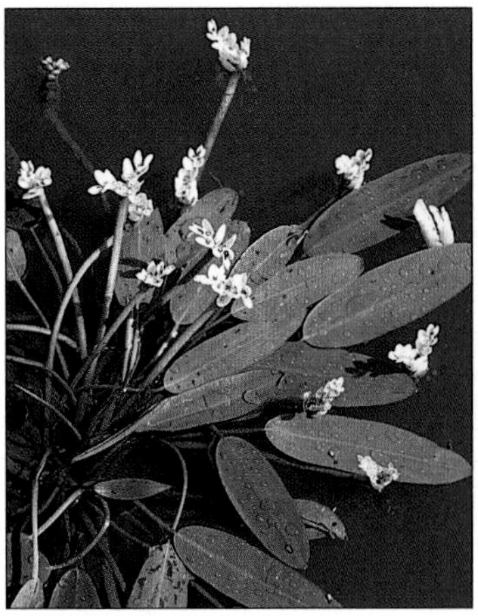

Aponogeton distachyos

A. distachyos ■ (Cape pondweed, Water hawthorn). Aquatic perennial with oblong-lance-shaped, bright green floating leaves, to 20cm (8in) long, which are almost evergreen in mild winters. Small, hawthorn-scented white flowers, 3cm (1¼in) across, with purplish brown anthers, are enclosed in white spathes, to 2cm (¾in) long, and borne in racemes with forked branches, 10cm (4in) long, above the water surface in spring and autumn. ↔ 1.2m (4ft). Southern Africa. ❄❄

A. madagascariensis (Lace plant, Lattice leaf plant). Aquatic perennial with unusual, skeletonized foliage reduced to a network of veins with no tissue in between. Leaves, to 55cm (22in) long, with very long leaf-stalks, are elliptic, light green, and submerged below the water surface. In summer, bears small white flowers, with white anthers, in compound panicles of white-spathed spikes, 2.5–5cm (1–2in) long. After fertilization, the flowers turn mauve. ↔ 30–35cm (12–14in). Madagascar. ⊛ (min. 15°C/59°F)

APOROCACTUS

Rat's tail cactus

CACTACEAE

Genus of 2 species of perennial, often epiphytic cacti found in sparsely wooded areas of S. Mexico and N. Central America. They are cultivated for their trailing stems, sometimes up to 2m (6ft) long, and colourful flowers. The pencil-like, pendent, fleshy stems have low ribs and closely arranged areoles bearing short, fine spines. The irregular, tubular to funnel-shaped, diurnal, bright red or purple flowers, with stamens longer than the petals, are borne singly, mainly on more mature growth. They are followed by spherical, soft-bristly red berries, containing numerous small, reddish brown seeds. In frost-prone areas, they are excellent for hanging baskets in a temperate greenhouse or conservatory. In frost-free areas, they are best grown outdoors in hanging baskets, epiphytically, or cascading over rocks.

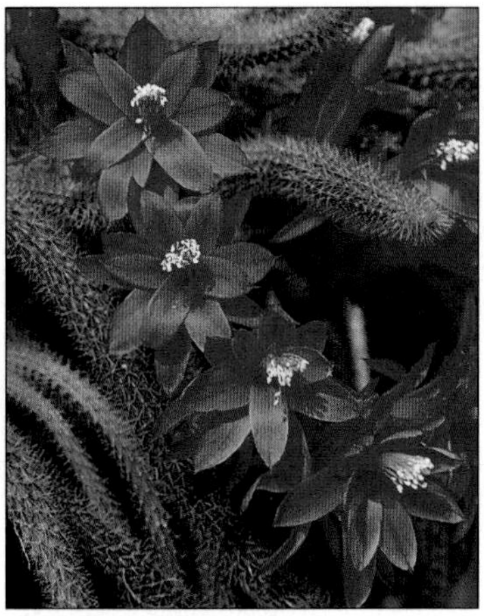

Aporocactus flagelliformis

- **HARDINESS** Frost tender.
- **CULTIVATION** Grow in epiphytic cactus compost in bright filtered light. During the growing season, water moderately and apply a high potash liquid fertilizer monthly; keep just moist at other times of the year. Outdoors, grow in sharply drained, gritty, humus-rich soil in a sheltered site in partial shade. See also pp.48–49.
- **PROPAGATION** Sow seed at 21°C (70°F) as soon as ripe; keep just moist and provide filtered light. Root stem cuttings in early summer.
- **PESTS AND DISEASES** Young or new growth is particularly vulnerable to mealybugs.

A. conzattii see *A. martianus.*
A. flagelliformis ■ syn. *Cereus flagelliformis.* Pendent, perennial cactus producing greyish green stems with 10–14 ribs, and areoles each bearing reddish brown spines (8–12 radials and 3 or 4 centrals). Narrowly tubular, funnel-shaped, purple-red flowers, 8cm (3in) long, with narrow, reflexed outer petals and wider, spreading inner ones, are borne in late spring and early summer. ↕ 10cm (4in), ↔ to 1.5m (5ft). S. Mexico, N. Central America. ⊛ (min. 7–10°C/45–50°F)
A. mallisonii see x *Aporoheliocereus smithii.*
A. martianus, syn. *A. conzattii, Eriocereus martianus.* Pendent or creeping, perennial cactus producing grey-green stems with 8 ribs and yellow-spiny areoles, each bearing 6–8 radial spines and 2 or more centrals. Funnel-shaped, bright scarlet flowers, 10cm (4in) long, are borne in early summer. ↕ 10–12cm (4–5in), ↔ to 1m (3ft). S. Mexico. ⊛ (min. 7–10°C/45–50°F)

x APOROHELIOCEREUS

CACTACEAE

Hybrid genus, a cross between *Aporocactus* and *Heliocereus*, of one creeping, pendent, perennial cactus, whose parents originate from wooded areas in Mexico. It has pencil-like, fleshy stems, often up to 2m (6ft) long, closely set, fine-spiny areoles, and solitary, large, funnel-shaped flowers that form mainly on mature growth. In frost-prone climates, x *A. smithii* is excellent in a hanging basket in a temperate greenhouse or conservatory. In frost-free regions, it is effective trailing over a wall.

- **HARDINESS** Frost tender.
- **CULTIVATION** Under glass, grow in epiphytic cactus compost in bright filtered light. When in growth, water moderately and apply a high potash liquid fertilizer monthly; keep just moist at other times. Outdoors, grow in sharply drained, gritty, humus-rich soil in a sheltered site in partial shade. See also pp.48–49.
- **PROPAGATION** Take stem cuttings in early summer.
- **PESTS AND DISEASES** Vulnerable to mealybugs.

x *A. mallisonii* see x *A. smithii.*
x *A. smithii*, syn. *Aporocactus mallisonii*, x *Aporoheliocereus mallisonii.* Pendent, perennial cactus with dark green stems with 6–8 prominent ribs, brown areoles, and radiating dark yellow spines. In summer, funnel-shaped, diurnal red flowers, to 7cm (3in) long, are produced mainly on the upper parts of the stems. ↕ 15cm (6in), ↔ to 75cm (30in). Garden origin. ⊛ (min. 7–10°C/45–50°F)

▷**Apple** see *Malus*
Balsam see *Clusia major*
Chinese may see *Podophyllum pleianthum*
Crab see *Malus*
Dwarf see *Angophora hispida*
Kangaroo see *Solanum aviculare, S. laciniatum*
Love see *Mandragora officinarum*
May see *Podophyllum peltatum*
▷**Apple berry,**
Common see *Billardiera scandens*
Purple see *Billardiera longiflora*
▷**Apple of Peru** see *Nicandra, N. physalodes*
▷***Aprica arachnoidea*** see *Haworthia arachnoidea*
▷**Apricot, Japanese** see *Prunus mume*

APTENIA

AIZOACEAE

Genus of 2 species of prostrate, perennial succulents from arid regions of South Africa. They have opposite, lance- or heart-shaped, fleshy and papillose leaves. In summer and autumn, small, daisy-like red flowers, solitary or borne in threes, are produced terminally or laterally from the leaf axils, and are followed by ovoid, 4-celled red fruits. In frost-prone areas, use in a hanging basket or as ground cover in a temperate greenhouse border; in warmer areas, grow in a desert garden.

- **HARDINESS** Frost tender.

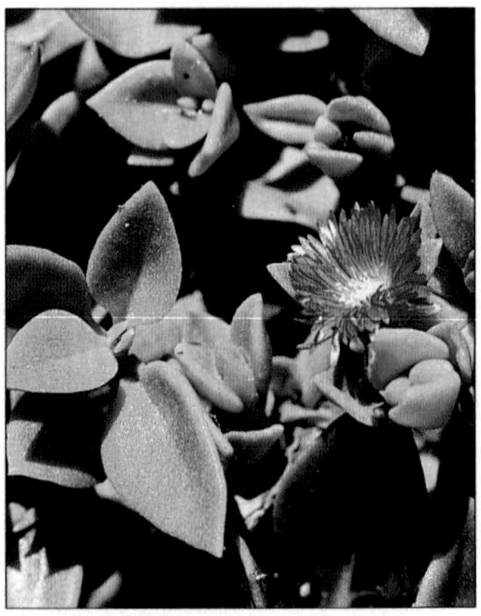

Aptenia cordifolia

• **CULTIVATION** Under glass, grow in standard cactus compost with added sharp sand in full light. Water moderately when flowering and in growth; keep completely dry in winter. Apply a low-nitrogen fertilizer in early spring. Outdoors, grow in any gritty, sharply drained soil in partial shade. Protect from excessive winter wet. See also pp.48–49.
• **PROPAGATION** Sow seed at 20–25°C (68–77°F) in early spring. Take stem cuttings in early spring.
• **PESTS AND DISEASES** Trouble free.

A. cordifolia ■ syn. *Litocarpus cordifolia, Mesembryanthemum cordifolium.* Freely branching, perennial succulent with cylindrical, greyish green stems, to 60cm (24in) long, and broadly ovate, fleshy, bright green leaves, 2.5cm (1in) long. Solitary, terminal or lateral, red-purple flowers, to 1.5cm (½in) across, are borne in summer or autumn. ↕ 5cm (2in), ↔ indefinite. E. South Africa. ❀ (min. 6–7°C/43–45°F). **'Variegata'** has leaves with creamy white margins.

▷**Aquatic plants** see pp.52–53

AQUILEGIA
Columbine
RANUNCULACEAE

Genus of about 70 species of clump-forming perennials from meadows, open woodland, and mountainous areas in the N. hemisphere. They produce basal rosettes of long-stalked, deeply 3-lobed or ternate to 3-ternate, often glaucous, blue-green leaves; the leaflets are mostly obovate or rounded, wedge-shaped at the bases, and often shallowly or deeply divided into 2 or 3 lobes. Distinctive, mainly bell-shaped flowers, usually 2.5–10cm (1–4in) long, with colourful tepals and spurred petals, are borne singly or in short panicles on branched, leafy stems.

Biedermeier Group, McKana Hybrids, and Mrs. Scott-Elliot Hybrids are all complex hybrids of *A. canadensis, A. longissima, A. vulgaris,* and possibly also other species. The larger species and cultivars, including *A. canadensis* and *A. vulgaris,* are effective in light woodland or in a herbaceous border. Most alpine species, such as *A. jonesii* and *A. saximontana,* require sharp drainage and will thrive in a scree bed or alpine house; they prefer cool conditions in summer. Contact with sap may irritate skin.
• **HARDINESS** Fully hardy.
• **CULTIVATION** Grow in fertile, preferably moist but well-drained soil in full sun or partial shade. Grow alpine species in gritty, humus-rich, moist but sharply drained soil in full sun.
• **PROPAGATION** Sow seed in containers in a cold frame as soon as ripe, or in spring. Seed of alpine species may take 2 years to germinate. All aquilegias self-seed profusely but also hybridize freely. Grown in isolation, *A. vulgaris* 'Nivea', 'Nora Barlow', and Vervaeneana Group cultivars produce a good proportion of true seedlings. Divide named cultivars in spring, although they are slow to recover as the rootstocks resent disturbance.
• **PESTS AND DISEASES** Susceptible to powdery mildew, aphids, leaf miners, sawflies, and caterpillars.

A. akitensis see *A. flabellata.*
A. alpina ■ syn. *A. montana* (Alpine columbine). Upright perennial with finely divided, ternate or 2-ternate, bluish green leaves divided into leaflets, 3cm (1¼in) long. Bears terminal, leafy racemes of 2 or 3 nodding blue flowers, sometimes with white petal tips, and with straight or curving spurs, to 2.5cm (1in) long, in late spring. Prefers rich soil in sun or partial shade. ↕ 45cm (18in), sometimes more, ↔ to 30cm (12in). Alps. ✻✻✻
A. bertolonii ♀ syn. *A. reuteri.* Delicate, upright perennial with finely divided, 2-ternate, smooth, dark green leaves with leaflets, to 2cm (¾in) long. From spring to early summer, each stem bears terminal, leafy racemes of 2–4 nodding, deep violet flowers, with incurved spurs, to 1.5cm (½in) long. ↕ to 30cm (12in), ↔ 10cm (4in). S. France, Italy. ✻✻✻
***A.* Biedermeier Group.** Short-stemmed perennials with 2-ternate, bluish green leaves divided into leaflets, 1–3cm (½–1¼in) long. From late spring to midsummer, they bear dense, terminal, leafy racemes of many almost upward-facing flowers, 3.5cm (1½in) long, with spurs to 3cm (1¼in) long, in colours that include white, deep pink, lilac, and shades of purple or blue. ↕ 50cm (20in), ↔ 30cm (12in). ✻✻✻
A. caerulea ♀ Upright perennial with 2-ternate, mid-green leaves with deeply lobed leaflets, 1–3cm (½–1¼in) long, usually hairy beneath. Terminal, leafy racemes of upright, bicoloured flowers with wide-spreading blue sepals and usually white petals with slender spurs, to 5cm (2in) long, are borne from late spring to midsummer. ↕ 60cm (24in), ↔ 30cm (12in). USA (mountains of S.W. Montana to N. Arizona, and N. New Mexico). ✻✻✻

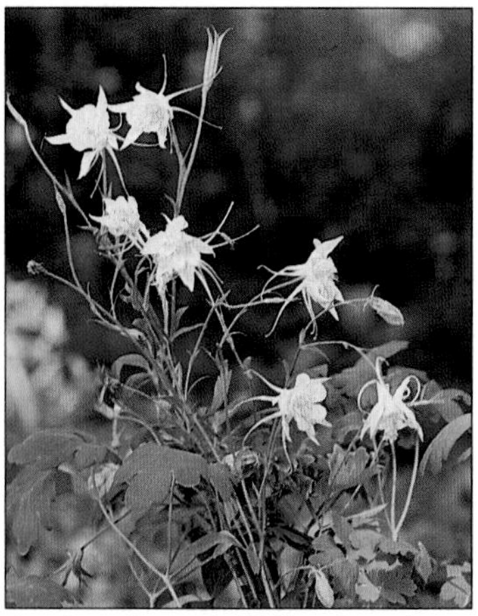
Aquilegia chrysantha 'Yellow Queen'

A. canadensis ♀ Airy perennial with 2-ternate, fern-like, dark green leaves divided into leaflets, 1–2cm (½–¾in) long. Bears terminal, leafy racemes of up to 20 nodding flowers from mid-spring to midsummer. The sepals are scarlet and forward-pointing; lemon-yellow petals taper into straight, erect red spurs, 1.5cm (½in) long; the stamens and styles extend outwards and downwards. ↕ 60–90cm (24–36in), ↔ 30cm (12in). E. Canada to S. USA (Florida, Texas, New Mexico). ✻✻✻
A. chrysantha. Vigorous, erect perennial with 3-ternate, fern-like, mid-green leaves divided into leaflets, 1–3cm (½–1¼in) long. Produces axillary and terminal, leafy racemes of 4–12 upward- or horizontal-facing flowers from late spring to late summer. Sepals are wide-spreading and light to golden yellow, sometimes tinged pink. Petals, paler than the sepals, have gently curving spurs, 4–7cm (1½–3in) long. ↕ 90cm (36in), ↔ 60cm (24in). S. USA to N. Mexico. ✻✻✻. **'Yellow Queen'** ■ has soft, golden yellow flowers.
***A.* 'Crimson Star'.** Upright perennial with 2-ternate, mid-green leaves comprising leaflets, 1–3cm (½–1¼in) long. Each stem bears 2 or 3 terminal, pendent flowers with red sepals and creamy white petals and spurs, to 5cm (2in) long, from late spring to mid-summer. Breeds almost true from seed. ↕ 60cm (24in), ↔ 30cm (12in). ✻✻✻
A. flabellata ♀ syn. *A. akitensis.* Strong-growing perennial with ternate or 2-ternate, bluish green leaves divided into leaflets, 1.5–4cm (½–1½in) long. In early summer, bears terminal, semi-erect to nodding, soft blue-purple flowers, 1 or 2 per stem, with white or cream petal tips and incurved spurs, to 2cm (¾in) long. Requires moist soil and partial shade. ↕ 10–30cm (4–12in), ↔ 10–15cm (4–6in). E. Asia, Japan. ✻✻✻. **var. *pumila* f. *alba*** ♀ syn. 'Nana Alba', is compact, with 1–3 white flowers per stem; ↕↔ to 10cm (4in).
A. formosa. Airy perennial producing 2-ternate, blue-green leaves with deeply divided leaflets, 2–4cm (¾–1½in) long. Axillary and terminal, leafy racemes of pendent flowers, produced in late spring and early summer, have wide-spreading orange sepals, and yellow petals with red lobes and upright, reddish orange spurs, 1–2cm (½–¾in) long. ↕ 60–90cm (24–36in), ↔ 45cm (18in). W. North America (Alaska to California, Montana, Utah). ✻✻✻
A. fragrans ■ syn. *A. glauca.* Upright perennial with 2-ternate, finely divided, glaucous, blue-green leaves with deeply lobed leaflets, 2–4cm (¾–1½in) long. Each stem bears 1–3 terminal, nodding, fragrant white or cream, sometimes blue-tinted flowers, with spurs to 2cm (¾in) long, in early summer. Needs rich soil, and will tolerate partial shade. ↕ 15–40cm (6–16in), ↔ 15–20cm (6–8in). W. Himalayas. ✻✻✻
A. glauca see *A. fragrans.*
***A.* 'Hensol Harebell'** ♀ Upright perennial with 2-ternate, mid-green leaves, purplish green when young, with deeply incised leaflets, 1–4cm (½–1½in)

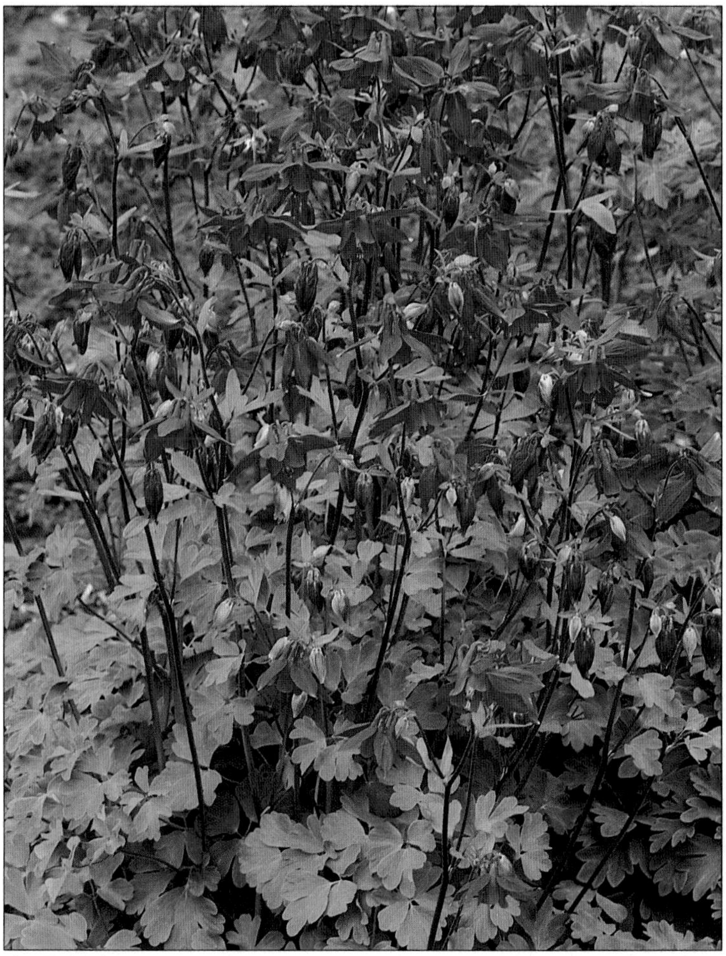
Aquilegia alpina

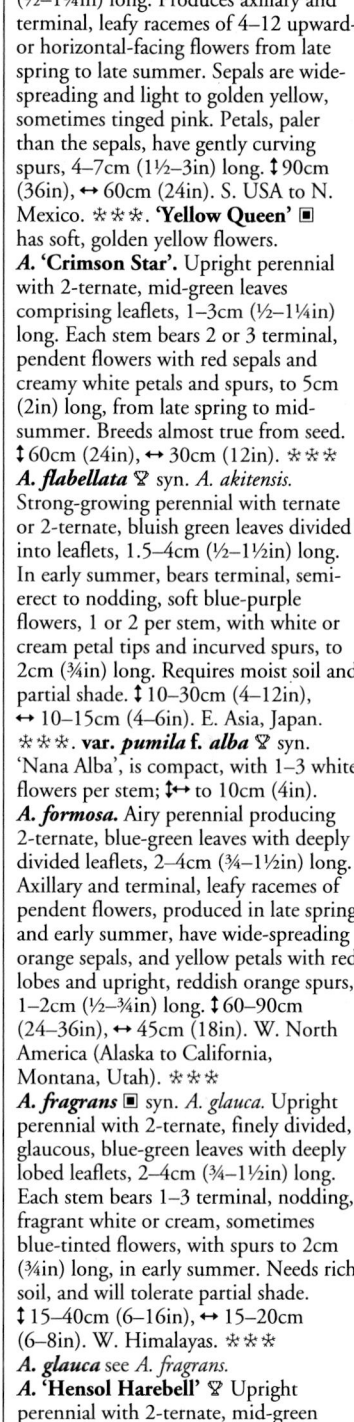

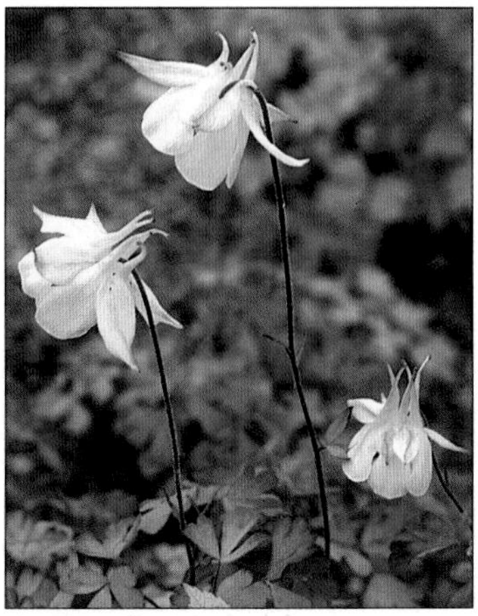
Aquilegia fragrans

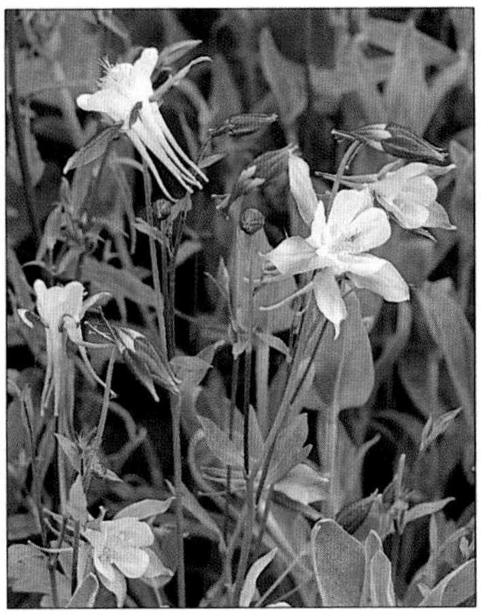

Aquilegia McKana Hybrids

long. Terminal, nodding, soft blue flowers, with spurs, 3.5cm (1½in) long, are borne, 2 or 3 per stem, from late spring to midsummer. Other colour variations are sometimes offered incorrectly under this name. ↕ 75cm (30in), ↔ 30cm (12in). ❄❄❄

A. jonesii. Densely tufted perennial with tight clusters of 2-ternate, softly hairy, blue-grey leaves with lobed leaflets, 1–2cm (½–¾in) long. Bears terminal, solitary, upturned, blue to violet flowers, with short spurs, to 1cm (½in) long, in early summer. Thrives in a scree or raised bed. Rarely flowers freely. ↕ 2–10cm (¾–4in), ↔ to 10cm (4in). USA (Rocky Mountains in Montana, Wyoming). ❄❄❄

A. longissima. Short-lived, upright perennial with fern-like, 3-ternate, mid-green leaves with deeply lobed leaflets, 2–4cm (¼–1½in) long. Produces terminal, leafy racemes of 4–12 semi-erect, scented flowers with slender, backward-pointing, bright yellow spurs, to 15cm (6in) long. Petals and spreading sepals are pale yellow. ↕ 60–90cm (24–36in), ↔ 45cm (18in). USA (mountains of S. Arizona and W. Texas), Mexico. ❄❄❄

***A.* McKana Hybrids** ■ Vigorous but short-lived, erect perennials with 3-ternate, mid-green leaves divided into leaflets, 1–4cm (½–1½in) long. From late spring to midsummer, they produce terminal, leafy racemes of 3–15 upright and pendent flowers with very long spurs, to 10cm (4in) long, self-coloured or bicoloured in shades of blue, yellow, and red. ↕ 75cm (30in), ↔ 60cm (24in). ❄❄❄

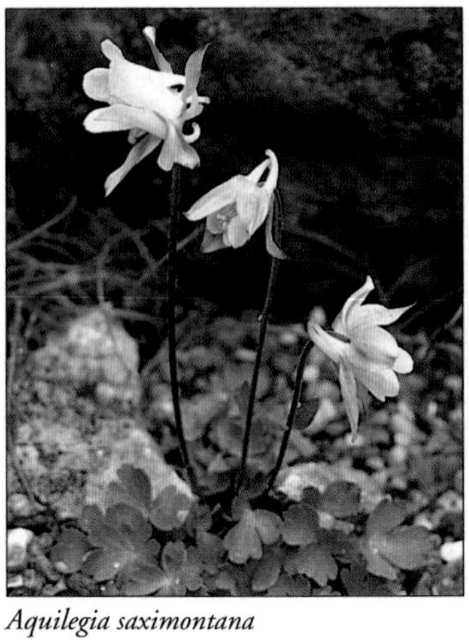

Aquilegia saximontana

A. montana see *A. alpina.*

***A.* 'Mrs. Scott-Elliot'** see *A.* Mrs. Scott-Elliot Hybrids.

***A.* Mrs. Scott-Elliot Hybrids** syn. *A.* 'Mrs. Scott-Elliot'. Vigorous perennials with 2-ternate, mid-green leaves divided into leaflets, 1–4cm (½–1½in) long. Bear nodding and upright flowers in a variety of shades, including red-yellow and blue-white bicolours, with spurs to 5cm (2in) long, in terminal, leafy racemes of 5–11 blooms, from late spring to midsummer. ↕ 90cm (36in), ↔ 60cm (24in). ❄❄❄

A. reuteri see *A. bertolonii.*

A. saximontana ■ (Rocky Mountain columbine). Densely tufted perennial with tight clusters of 2-ternate, slightly crinkled, bluish green leaves with leaflets, 1–2cm (½–¾in) long. In late spring and early summer, bears terminal, nodding, deep lavender-blue flowers, 1–2 per stem, with yellowish white petals and short, hooked spurs, to 7mm (¼in) long. Will tolerate partial shade. ↕ 10–15cm (4–6in), ↔ to 15cm (6in). USA (Rocky Mountains of Utah, Colorado). ❄❄❄

***A.* 'Schneekönigin'**, syn. *A.* 'Snow Queen'. Strong-growing, erect perennial bearing 2-ternate, glaucous, grey- or blue-green leaves with leaflets, 1–4cm (½–1½in) long. Produces terminal, leafy racemes of 5–15 nodding white flowers with long spurs, 5–8cm (2–3in) long, from late spring to midsummer. ↕ 75cm (30in), ↔ 30cm (12in). ❄❄❄

A. scopulorum. Tufted perennial with dense clusters of 2-ternate, blue-green leaves, with leaflets 0.5–1.5cm (¼–½in) long. Stems with 1–5 upright flowers, 3–4cm (1¼–1½in) across, with slender spurs, 2.5–3cm (1–1¼in) long, are borne in early summer. The flowers are usually lavender-blue to violet, but may vary from pale blue to deep blue, pink, or white, with white or cream petals. ↕ 8–15cm (3–6in), ↔ to 10cm (4in). W. USA. ❄❄❄

***A.* 'Snow Queen'** see *A.* 'Schneekönigin'.

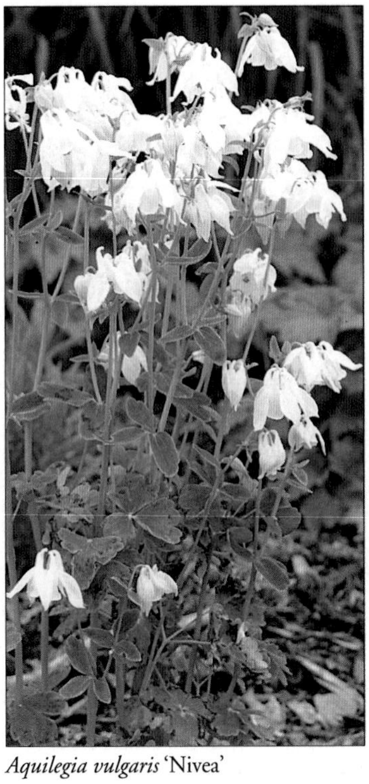

Aquilegia vulgaris 'Nivea'

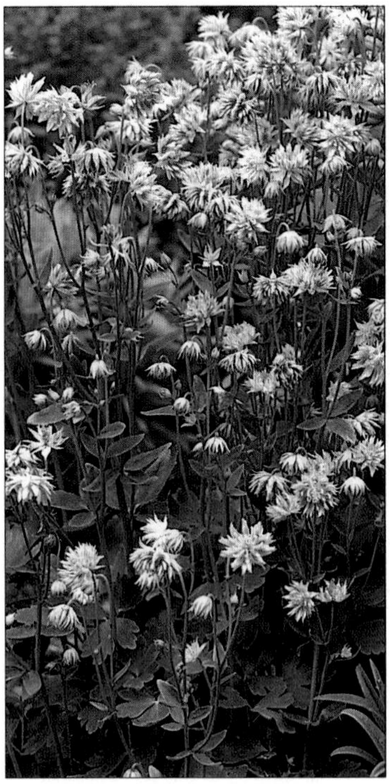

Aquilegia vulgaris 'Nora Barlow'

A. viridiflora. Upright, short-lived perennial with 2-ternate, mid-green leaves divided into leaflets, 1–3cm (½–1¼in) long. In late spring and early summer, bears stems of 2 or 3 terminal, nodding, fragrant flowers with dark green sepals and purplish brown petals with spurs, to 1.5cm (½in) long. ↕ 20–30cm (8–12in), ↔ 15–20cm (6–8in). Russia (E. Siberia), W. China. ❄❄❄

A. vulgaris (Granny's bonnet). Upright, reliable perennial with 2-ternate, mid-green leaves, glaucous beneath, divided into lobed leaflets, 1–4cm (½–1½in) long. In late spring and early summer, many-branched, stiff stems bear terminal, leafy racemes of 5–15 pendent to horizontal flowers with short, hooked spurs, to 2cm (¾in) long, in colours ranging from deep violet and blue to pink and white. ↕ 90cm (36in), ↔ 45cm (18in). Europe. ❄❄❄. **var. *clematiflora*** see var. *stellata.* **'Gisela Powell'** has yellow-orange flowers. **'Munstead White'** see 'Nivea'. **'Nivea'** ■🏆 syn. 'Munstead White', is vigorous, with greyish green foliage, pale green stems, and pure white flowers. **'Nora Barlow'** ■🏆 has double pompon flowers with numerous narrow, spurless, quilted tepals in pale green and red. **var. *stellata***, syn. var. *clematiflora*, has spurless flowers with spreading tepals, in white or shades of blue or pink. **Vervaeneana Group** cultivars have variegated leaves, mottled and streaked yellow, and bear white, reddish pink, and purple flowers.

ARABIS

Rock cress

BRASSICACEAE/CRUCIFERAE

Genus of some 120 species of annuals and mainly evergreen perennials, mostly from rocky, mountainous areas of Europe, Asia, and North America. They are erect or mat- or cushion-forming, with branching, often woody-based stems. The leaves are simple, toothed or

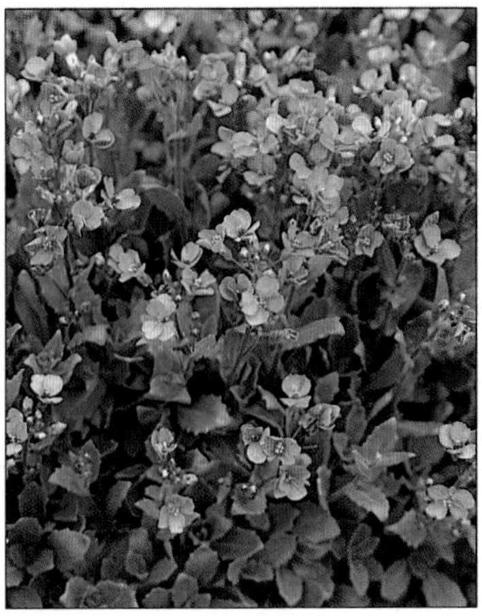

Arabis x *arendsii* 'Rosabella'

entire, and sometimes hairy. Small, cruciform, 4-petalled, white to purple flowers are borne in racemes, 3–8cm (1¼–3in) long. Rock cress are easily cultivated, and are useful for growing in a rock garden, dry bank, or at the edge of a border; they are also suitable for crevice plantings in a retaining wall. *A. caucasica* is effective ground cover.

- **HARDINESS** Fully hardy.
- **CULTIVATION** Grow in any well-drained soil in full sun. Will tolerate hot, dry conditions and poor, infertile soils. Protect *A. blepharophylla* 'Frühlingszauber' from winter wet, or grow in an alpine house in a mix of equal parts loam, leaf mould, and sharp sand; water freely when in growth, sparingly in winter. Vigorous species such as *A. caucasica* will swamp smaller plants, so site with care. Trim after flowering to maintain compactness.
- **PROPAGATION** Sow seed in containers in a cold frame in autumn. *A. blepharophylla* 'Frühlingszauber' is best raised from seed. Root softwood cuttings in summer.
- **PESTS AND DISEASES** Prone to downy mildew, aphids, and white blister. The arabis midge causes malformation of flowering shoots, which should be removed and burned if affected.

A. albida see *A. caucasica.*

A. alpina* subsp. *caucasica see *A. caucasica.*

***A.* x *arendsii* 'Rosabella'** ■ syn. *A. caucasica* 'Rosabella'. Compact, mat-forming, evergreen perennial with rosettes of elliptic to ovate, hairy, grey-green leaves, 3–5cm (1¼–2in) long.

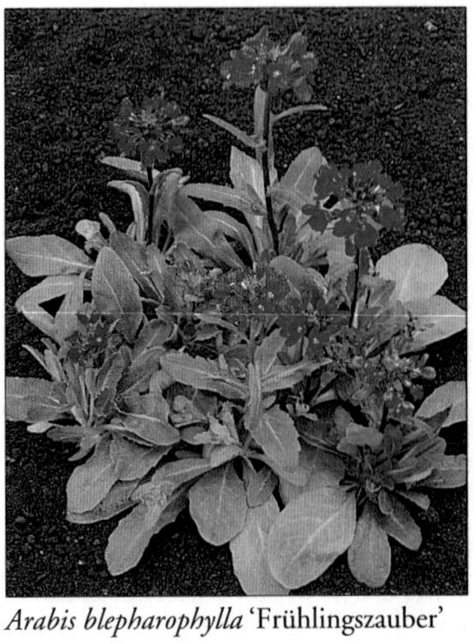

Arabis blepharophylla 'Frühlingszauber'

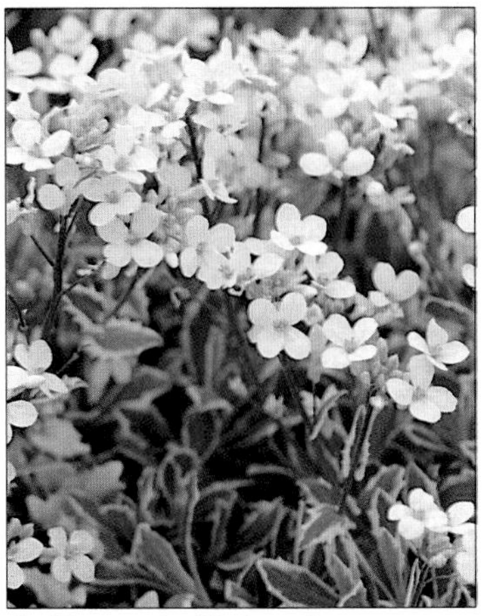

Arabis caucasica 'Variegata'

Bears short racemes of deep rose-pink flowers, to 1.5cm (½in) across, in late spring and early summer. ↕ 5–10cm (2–4in), ↔ 20–30cm (8–12in). ❄❄❄

A. billardieri see *A. caucasica.*

***A. blepharophylla* 'Frühlingszauber'** ■ 🏆 syn. *A. blepharophylla* 'Spring Charm'. Mat- or cushion-forming, evergreen, short-lived perennial with loose rosettes of obovate, toothed, dark green leaves, 3–5cm (1¼–2in) long, with grey-hairy margins. Compact racemes of fragrant, deep pink-purple flowers, to 1.5cm (½in) across, are produced in late spring and early summer. Dislikes winter wet. ↕ to 10cm (4in), ↔ to 20cm (8in). ❄❄❄

***A. blepharophylla* 'Spring Charm'** see *A. blepharophylla* 'Frühlingszauber'.

A. bryoides. Densely tufted, evergreen perennial with rosettes of elliptic-ovate, grey-green, white-hairy leaves, to 1.5cm (½in) long, and short, compact racemes of white flowers, to 1cm (½in) across, in late spring and early summer. ↕ 2–6cm (¾–2½in), ↔ to 8cm (3in). Greece, Balkan Peninsula. ❄❄❄

A. caucasica, syn. *A. albida, A. alpina* subsp. *caucasica, A. billardieri.* Vigorous, mat-forming, evergreen perennial with loose rosettes of obovate, toothed, grey-green leaves, 3–5cm (1¼–2in) long. Loose racemes of fragrant white flowers, to 1cm (½in) across, open in late spring. ↕ 15cm (6in), ↔ 50cm (20in) or more. S. Europe. ❄❄❄. **'Flore Pleno'** 🏆 syn. 'Plena', produces double, pure white flowers. **'Plena'** see 'Flore Pleno'. **'Rosabella'** see *A.* x *arendsii* 'Rosabella'. **'Variegata'** ■ has green leaves, boldly margined pale yellow.

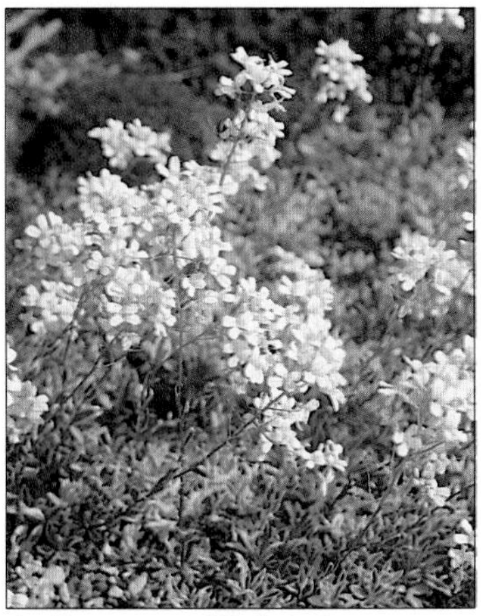

Arabis procurrens 'Variegata'

***A. ferdinandi-coburgi* 'Variegata'** see *A. procurrens* 'Variegata'.

***A. procurrens* 'Variegata'** ■ 🏆 syn. *A. ferdinandi-coburgi* 'Variegata'. Mat-forming, evergreen or semi-evergreen perennial with flattened rosettes of narrowly oblong to lance-shaped, glossy, mid-green, sometimes pink-tinged leaves, 2–3cm (¾–1¼in) long, with creamy white margins. Numerous loose racemes of white flowers, 8–10mm (⅜–½in) across, are produced in late spring. Remove any stems that revert to the green-leaved form. ↕ 5–8cm (2–3in), ↔ 30–40cm (12–16in). ❄❄❄

ARACHNIS

Scorpion orchid

ORCHIDACEAE

Genus of 6 or 7 species of evergreen, monopodial orchids, often initially terrestrial but becoming epiphytic, from S.E. Asia, New Guinea, and the Philippines, occurring mainly on trees or rocks in wet areas. They are robust plants with long, branching stems, 2-ranked, strap-shaped, thick, fleshy leaves, and axillary racemes of attractive, highly coloured, fragrant flowers. Cultivated mainly in a lath house in tropical regions, where they are grown for use as cut flowers, they require full, year-round sun to flower regularly. In frost-prone areas, grow scorpion orchids in a warm greenhouse. They seldom flower well outside their native areas.

• **HARDINESS** Frost tender.

• **CULTIVATION** Warm-growing orchids. Grow in terrestrial orchid compost, either in containers or in a greenhouse border. Provide full light, ample water, and high temperatures and humidity all year round. In summer, apply a balanced liquid fertilizer at every third watering. Outdoors, in humid, tropical areas, grow in coarse, moist, humus-rich soil. Grow in a lath house to shelter from wind, heavy rain, and the hottest sun. See also p.46.

• **PROPAGATION** Root stem cuttings, at least 60cm (24in) long, or divide when the plant outgrows its container.

• **PESTS AND DISEASES** Aphids, red spider mites, whiteflies, and mealybugs may be a problem.

A. flos-aeris. Evergreen, terrestrial orchid with dark green leaves, 18cm (7in) long. Fragrant, yellow-green flowers, horizontally striped or spotted maroon, to 10cm (4in) across, are borne in arching panicles or racemes, 1.2m (4ft) high, in late summer. ↕ 5m (15ft), ↔ 4m (12ft). Malaysia and Singapore to the Philippines. ⊛ (min. 18°C/64°F; max. 30°C/86°F)

ARAEOCOCCUS

BROMELIACEAE

Genus of 5 species of rosette-forming, evergreen, mostly epiphytic perennials (bromeliads). They occur in areas ranging from low foothills to terrain over 500m (1,500ft) and rainforest, in S. Central America, N. and E. South America, and the West Indies. The slender leaves have scales pressed close to one or both surfaces, and smooth or spiny margins. The inflorescence, borne in late summer, consists of few-flowered spikes of small, tubular flowers. Where temperatures fall below 19°C (66°F), grow in a warm greenhouse. In tropical regions, grow epiphytically outdoors.

• **HARDINESS** Frost tender.

• **CULTIVATION** Under glass, grow epiphytically or in epiphytic bromeliad compost. Keep moist, and provide shade and moderate humidity at all times. Apply a nitrogen-based fertilizer every month from early spring to late autumn. In tropical areas, grow epiphytically in a shady, humid site. See also p.47.

• **PROPAGATION** Root offsets in spring.

• **PESTS AND DISEASES** Susceptible to root mealybugs and scale insects.

A. flagellifolius. Epiphytic bromeliad with smooth, grass-like leaves, over 1m (3ft) long, the spiny sheaths forming a bulbous base to the few-leaved rosette. Produces pyramidal inflorescences, to 30cm (12in) long, of white or greenish white flowers in late summer. ↕ 1m (3ft), ↔ 15cm (6in) or more. S.E. Colombia, Amazonian Brazil. ⊛ (min. 19°C/66°F)

ARALIA

ARALIACEAE

Genus of about 40 species of vigorous, deciduous and evergreen trees and shrubs, and rhizomatous perennials, from S. and E. Asia, Malaysia, and North, Central, and South America, found mainly in mountain woodland. The striking, large leaves are simple or pinnate to 3-pinnate, and are sometimes covered in large bristles. Numerous white or greenish white flowers are borne in terminal panicles of spherical umbels or cymes, and are followed by spherical, usually black fruits. Aralias are suitable for a shady border in a large garden (to which they can lend an exotic air) or for woodland or a streambank.

• **HARDINESS** Fully hardy to frost hardy.

• **CULTIVATION** Grow in fertile, humus-rich, moist soil in an open or partially shaded site, sheltered from strong winds, which may damage the large leaves. In very fertile soil, they may produce vigorous but soft growth, which is vulnerable to frost damage. Pruning group 1 for trees and shrubs. Remove suckers at any time to control their spread; variegated forms may send out suckers with green foliage, which should be removed completely. Cut perennials to the ground after fruiting in autumn.

• **PROPAGATION** Sow seed in containers in a cold frame when ripe, or stratify and sow in spring. Divide rhizomatous perennials in spring. Insert root cuttings of woody species in winter. Transplant suckers of trees and shrubs in early spring or winter. Graft variegated cultivars of *A. elata* in winter.

• **PESTS AND DISEASES** Aphids may attack the relatively soft flower-stalks.

***A. chinensis* of gardens** see *A. elata.*

A. elata 🏆 ♤ syn. *A. chinensis* of gardens (Japanese angelica tree). Vigorous, suckering, upright then spreading, deciduous tree with stout, spiny stems. The large, 2-pinnate leaves, to 1.2m (4ft) long, have 80 or more ovate leaflets, dark green above, and paler beneath, turning yellow, orange, or purple in autumn. In late summer and early autumn, bears small white flowers, in large, spreading, panicle-like, compound umbels, to 60cm (24in) long, followed by spherical black fruit, to 6mm (¼in) across. ↕↔ 10m (30ft). E. Asia. ❄❄❄. **'Albomarginata'** see 'Variegata'. **'Aureovariegata'** ♤ is less vigorous, with leaflets broadly and irregularly margined yellow, becoming paler with age; ↕↔ 5m (15ft). **'Variegata'** ■ 🏆 ♤ syn. 'Albomarginata', is similar to 'Aureovariegata', but has leaflets irregularly margined with creamy white.

A. elegantissima see *Schefflera elegantissima.*

A. japonica see *Fatsia japonica.*

A. papyrifer see *Tetrapanax papyrifer.*

A. racemosa. Spreading, rhizomatous perennial with tall stems producing pinnate, mid-green leaves, to 75cm (30in) long, with 3–5 ovate leaflets, which are toothed but not bristly.

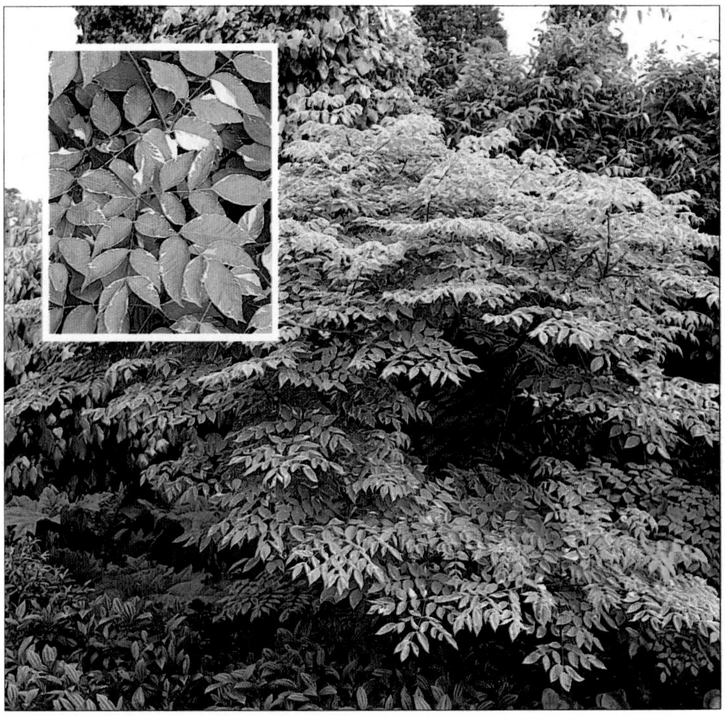

Aralia elata 'Variegata' (inset: leaf detail)

Umbels of small, greenish white flowers are borne in imposing spike-like inflorescences, 20–40cm (8–16in) long, in late spring and early summer, followed by spherical, dark purple fruit, 3mm (⅛in) across. ↕ to 3m (10ft), ↔ 1.2m (4ft). C., E., and S.W. North America. ✻✻✻

A. sieboldii see *Fatsia japonica.*

A. spinosa ◊ (American angelica tree, Devil's walking stick, Hercules' club). Upright, suckering, deciduous tree or shrub with stout, spiny stems. Large, 2-pinnate leaves, to 1.5m (5ft) long, with 80 or more ovate leaflets, are dark green above and glaucous beneath. Umbels of white flowers are borne in conical, terminal panicles, to 60cm (24in) long, in summer, followed by spherical black fruit, to 6mm (¼in) across. ↕ 10m (30ft), ↔ 5m (15ft). E. USA. ✻✻✻

▷**Aralia,**
False see *Schefflera elegantissima*
Fern-leaf see *Polyscias filicifolia*
Geranium see *Polyscias guilfoylei*
Japanese see *Fatsia japonica*
Lace see *Polyscias guilfoylei* 'Victoriae'

ARAUCARIA

ARAUCARIACEAE

Genus of 18 species of evergreen, coniferous trees from tropical rainforest with a pronounced dry season in New Guinea, Australia, New Hebrides, New Caledonia, Norfolk Island, and South America. The leaves are spirally arranged and usually broadly triangular to needle-like. Male and female cones are green, maturing to brown, and are normally borne on separate trees. The female cones are spherical, ovoid, or ellipsoid, with seeds fused to the bract scale; the male cones are conical or cylindrical. They are all elegant specimen trees and, except for *A. araucana*, require a warm, temperate climate. In colder areas, grow young plants in a cool conservatory or greenhouse. *A. heterophylla* may be grown as a houseplant.

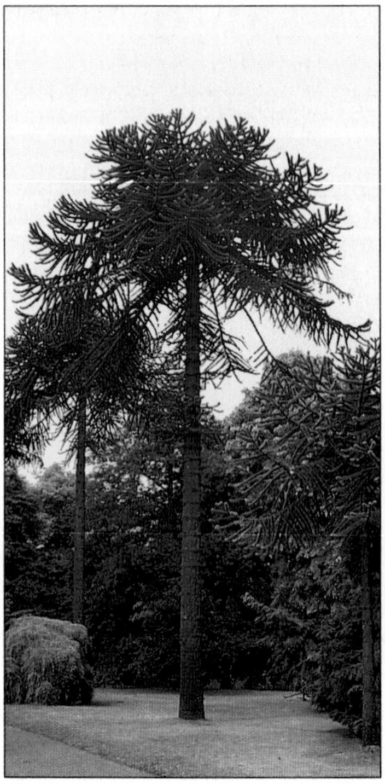
Araucaria araucana

• **HARDINESS** Half hardy to frost tender, except *A. araucana*, which is fully hardy.
• **CULTIVATION** Under glass, grow in loam-based potting compost (JI No.2) in full light with good ventilation. In the growing season, water freely and apply a balanced liquid fertilizer every 2 weeks; keep just moist in winter. Outdoors, grow in moderately fertile, moist but well-drained soil in an open site with shelter from cold, drying winds.
• **PROPAGATION** Sow seed in a seedbed as soon as ripe. Take cuttings, 7–10cm (3–4in) long, of vertical shoot tips in midsummer and root in a cold frame; cuttings of the horizontal side branches will never form an erect tree.
• **PESTS AND DISEASES** Honey fungus may be a problem.

A. araucana ▣ ◊–◌ syn. *A. imbricata* (Chilean pine, Monkey puzzle). Coniferous tree with whorled branches, conical when young, becoming rounded and losing its lower branches when old, with tough, horizontally ridged, dark grey-brown bark. The radially arranged, triangular-ovate, leathery, bright then dark green leaves are sharply pointed, 3–5cm (1¼–2in) long, and persist for up to 10 years. Female cones are ovoid, to 15cm (6in) long, and ripen over 2–3 years. Male cones are cylindrical to ovoid and to 15cm (6in) long. Seeds are edible. ↕ 15–25m (50–80ft), ↔ 7–10m (22–30ft). Volcanic slopes of Chilean Andes and into Argentina. ✻✻✻

A. bidwillii ▣ ◊–◌ (Bunya-bunya). Coniferous tree with whorled branches, conical when young, eventually becoming rounded and losing its lower branches. It has blackish brown bark and flattened, spreading, glossy, mid-green leaves, 2–5cm (¾–2in) long; these are oblong-lance-shaped and spirally arranged in 2 rows when young; leaves on mature trees are 2–3cm (¾–1¼in) long, lance-shaped, twisted, and overlapping. Female cones, to 27cm (11in) long, are spherical; male cones, 10–18cm (4–7in) long, are cylindrical.

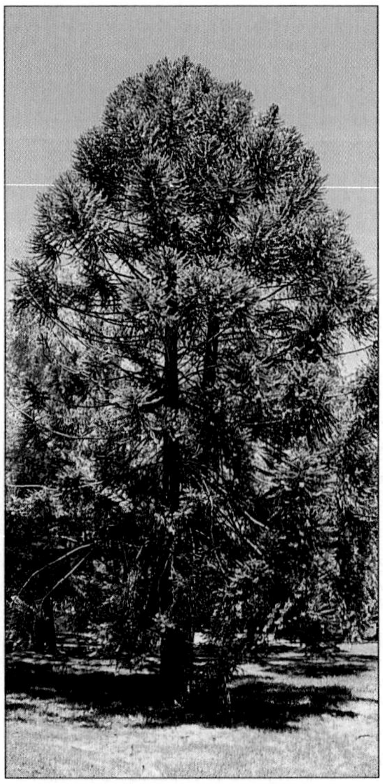
Araucaria bidwillii

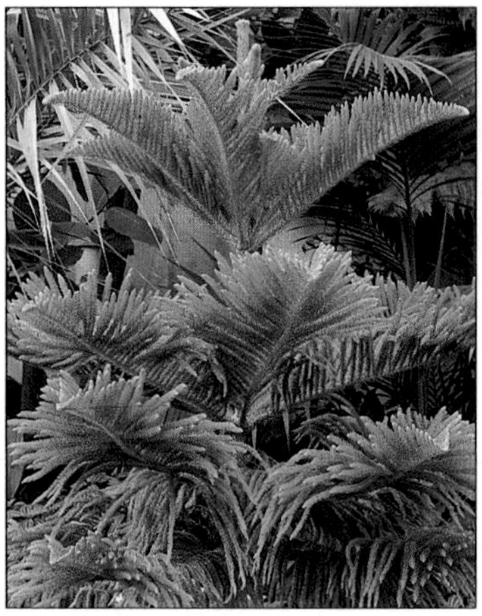
Araucaria heterophylla

↕ 30–45m (100–150ft), ↔ 6–10m (20–30ft). Australia (S.E. Queensland). ❀ (min. 5°C/41°F)

A. columnaris ◊ syn. *A. cookii* (Cook pine, New Caledonian pine). Conical to columnar, coniferous tree with whorled branches when young. Lateral branches are soon lost and replaced by short, epicormic shoots on the main stem, producing a narrow column of foliage. The alternate, ovate, light green leaves are to 1.5cm (½in) long on young trees; on mature trees, leaves are 6–8mm (¼–⅜in) long and closely overlapping. Female cones, to 15cm (6in) long, are ellipsoid; male cones, 2.5–6cm (1–2½in) long, are conical. ↕ 30–50m (100–160ft), ↔ 3–6m (10–20ft). New Caledonia. ❀ (min. 5°C/41°F)

A. cookii see *A. columnaris*

A. cunninghamii ◊ (Hoop pine, Moreton Bay pine). Columnar or conical, coniferous tree with red-brown, horizontally peeling bark, and whorled branches with tufts of young shoots at the tips, and rising either side of the branches. On young trees, the mid-green leaves are needle-like to ovate, flattened, spirally arranged, and to 1.5cm (½in) long; on mature trees, they are crowded and overlapping, incurved, scale-like, and to 6–8mm (¼–⅜in) long. Female cones, to 10cm (4in) long, are ovoid; male cones, 5–8cm (2–3in) long, are cylindrical. ↕ to 50m (160ft), ↔ to 6m (20ft). Australia (Queensland, N. New South Wales). ❀ (min. 5°C/41°F)

***A. excelsa* of gardens** see *A. heterophylla.*

A. heterophylla ▣ ♀ ◊ syn. *A. excelsa* of gardens (Norfolk Island pine). Conical, coniferous tree with distinctive, whorled branches of fan-like foliage. On young trees, leaves are narrowly wedge-shaped, light green, and to 1.5cm (½in) long; on mature trees, they are crowded, scale-like, incurved, and to 5mm (¼in) long. Spherical female cones are to 10cm (4in) long; cylindrical male cones are 4–7cm (1½–3in) long. ↕ 25–45m (80–150ft), ↔ 6–8m (20–25ft). Norfolk Island. ✻

A. imbricata see *A. araucana.*

ARAUJIA

ASCLEPIADACEAE

Genus of 4 species of evergreen, twining climbers, growing wild in scrub and at forest margins in dry, warm-temperate to tropical areas of South America, and cultivated for their flowers and foliage. The opposite leaves are simple. The

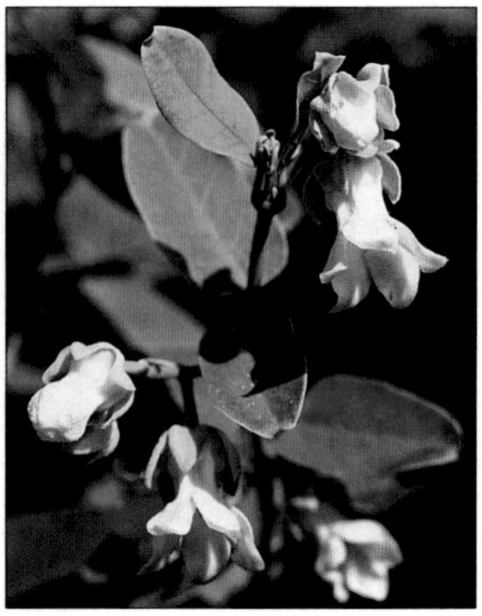
Araujia sericifera

tubular-based, 5-petalled flowers, borne in terminal racemes, may be either bell-shaped or salverform. The stems contain a white latex. In frost-prone areas, grow in a cool greenhouse; in frost-free areas, grow on a pergola, arbour, or wall, or through a strong-growing shrub.
• **HARDINESS** Most are frost tender, but *A. sericifera* may survive short spells down to 0°C (32°F).
• **CULTIVATION** Under glass, grow in coarse, loam-based potting compost (JI No.2) in full light. In growth, water moderately, and apply a balanced liquid fertilizer monthly; keep just moist in winter. Outdoors, grow in well-drained, moderately fertile soil in sun or partial shade. Pruning group 11, in early spring.
• **PROPAGATION** Sow seed in containers in a cold frame when ripe or in spring. Root semi-ripe cuttings of lateral shoots with bottom heat in late summer.
• **PESTS AND DISEASES** Red spider mites may be a problem.

A. sericifera ▣ (Cruel plant). Twining-stemmed climber with wavy, lance-shaped leaves, to 10cm (4in) long, mid- to pale green above, and thinly felted with hairs beneath. From late summer to autumn, bears racemes, 5–10cm (2–4in) long, of oblong-bell-shaped, fragrant, white or pale pink flowers, 2.5cm (1in) across, and swollen at the bases. Sticky pollen masses temporarily trap visiting moths, giving rise to the common name. ↕ 7–10m (22–30ft). South America. ✻ (borderline)

▷**Arborvitae** see *Thuja*

ARBUTUS

Manzanita, Strawberry tree

ERICACEAE

Genus of about 14 species of evergreen trees or shrubs, favouring rocky habitats, from Portugal to Turkey, Cyprus, and Lebanon, and from W. North America to Mexico and Guatemala. They have often attractive, peeling, red-brown bark, and simple, toothed or entire, leathery leaves, variable in length, and arranged alternately. The small, pitcher-shaped, white or pink flowers, 6–8mm (¼–⅜in) long, are borne in terminal panicles, followed by strawberry-like fruits, 1–3cm (½–1¼in) across. They are excellent for a large shrub border, for a woodland garden, or as specimen trees. In frost-prone climates, grow half-hardy species in a cool greenhouse.

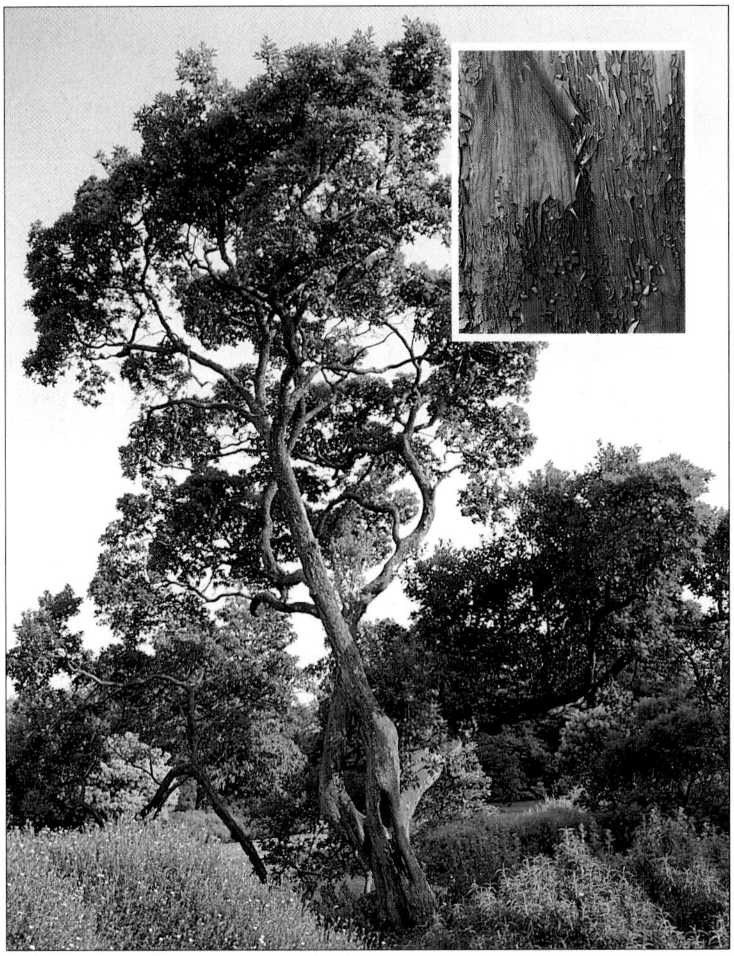

Arbutus x *andrachnoides* (inset: bark detail)

• **HARDINESS** Fully hardy when mature (young plants less so) to frost hardy; a few rare species are half hardy.
• **CULTIVATION** Grow in fertile, humus-rich, well-drained soil, in a sheltered site in full sun. Protect from cold winds, even when mature. *A. andrachne*, *A.* x *andrachnoides*, and *A. unedo* will tolerate alkaline soils. *A. menziesii* (and other species) need acid soils. Pruning group 1; but keep pruning to a minimum.
• **PROPAGATION** Sow seed in containers in a cold frame as soon as ripe. Root semi-ripe cuttings in late summer.
• **PESTS AND DISEASES** Leaf spot and aphids may be a problem.

A. andrachne ♀ (Grecian strawberry tree). Spreading, sometimes shrubby tree with smooth, peeling, red-brown bark. Ovate to ovate-oblong, glossy, dark green leaves, 5–10cm (2–4in) long, are usually entire, occasionally finely toothed. White flowers are produced in leafy, erect panicles, to 10cm (4in) long, in late spring, followed by spherical, warty, orange-red fruit, 1–2cm (½–¾in) across, which ripen in the autumn of the following year. ↕↔ 6m (20ft). S.E. Europe, Turkey, Lebanon. ❄❄
A.* x *andrachnoides ▣ ♀ ♀–♀ (*A. andrachne* x *A. unedo*). Broadly upright, then often spreading, sometimes shrubby tree with peeling, red-brown bark and ovate to lance-shaped, finely toothed, glossy, mid-green leaves, to 10cm (4in) long, and glaucous beneath. Semi-pendent panicles, to 8cm (3in) long, of small white flowers, sometimes pink-tinged, are borne from autumn to spring. Fruit are rarely produced. ↕↔ 8m (25ft). S.E. Europe, S.W. Asia. ❄❄❄
A. menziesii ▣ ♀ ♀ (Madroño). Spreading, sometimes shrubby tree with peeling, red-brown bark. Oval, toothed leaves, 5–15cm (2–6in) long, are glossy, dark green, glaucous beneath. White flowers in erect panicles, to 20cm (8in) tall, are borne freely in early summer, followed by spherical, warty, orange-red fruit, 1cm (½in) across, which ripen in autumn the following year. ↕↔ 15m (50ft). W. North America. ❄❄❄
A. unedo ▣ ♀ ♀ (Strawberry tree). Spreading, sometimes shrubby tree with rough, shredding, red-brown bark and oval to obovate, shallowly toothed, glossy, mid-green leaves, to 10cm (4in) long. Small white flowers, sometimes pink-tinged, open in pendent panicles, to 5cm (2in) long, in autumn; spherical, warty red fruit, 2cm (¾in) across, ripen in the following autumn. ↕↔ 8m (25ft). S.E. Europe, Turkey, Lebanon. ❄❄❄. **'Elfin King'** is compact, flowering and fruiting freely when small. ↕ 2m (6ft), ↔ 1.5m (5ft). **f. *rubra*** ♀ has dark pink flowers.

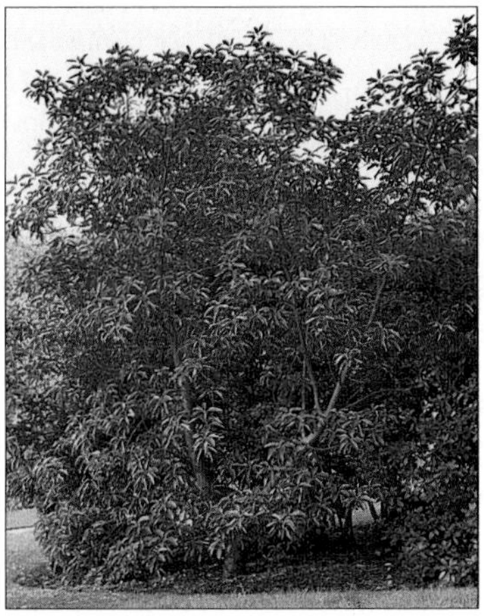

Arbutus menziesii

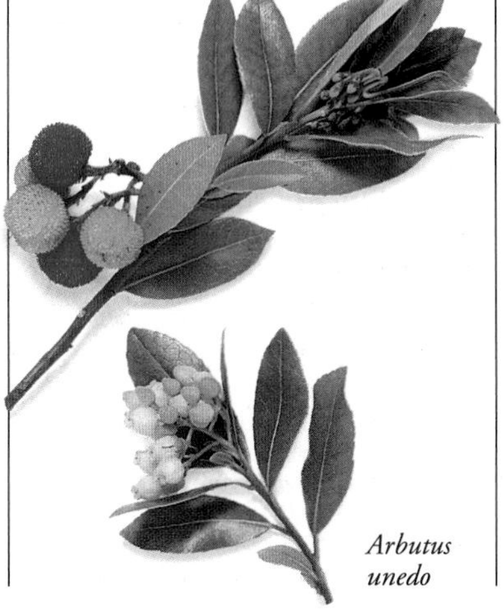

Arbutus unedo

▷**Arbutus, Trailing** see *Epigaea repens*
▷**Archangel** see *Angelica archangelica*

ARCHONTOPHOENIX
King palm
ARECACEAE/PALMAE

Genus of 2 species of single-stemmed palms from rainforest in E. Australia. Large, pinnate leaves are arranged in a terminal tuft above a prominent crown-shaft, and large panicles or racemes of monoecious, cup-shaped flowers are borne beneath them. Where temperatures fall below 10–13°C (50–55°F), grow young plants in a temperate greenhouse or conservatory; in warmer areas, grow as specimen trees.
• **HARDINESS** Frost tender.
• **CULTIVATION** Under glass, grow in loamless potting compost in bright, filtered light with moderate humidity. When in growth, water moderately and apply a balanced liquid fertilizer monthly; keep just moist in winter. Outdoors, grow in fertile, humus-rich, moist but well-drained soil in partial shade to prevent leaf scorch.
• **PROPAGATION** Sow seed in spring at 24–27°C (75–81°F).
• **PESTS AND DISEASES** Red spider mites may be a problem under glass.

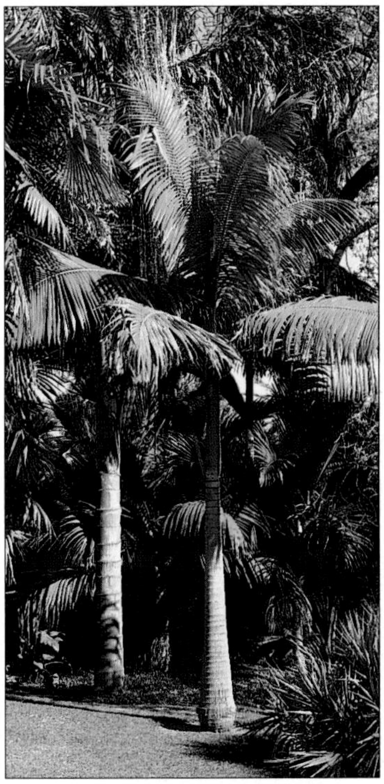

Archontophoenix alexandrae

A. alexandrae ▣ ⚘ syn. *Ptychosperma alexandrae* (Alexander palm, Northern bangalow palm). Tall, fast-growing palm with a slender trunk, swollen at the base and covered in ring-like leaf scars. Arching, pinnate leaves, 2–4m (6–12ft) long, have numerous narrowly lance-shaped leaflets, pale green or purple-flushed above, silver to grey beneath. In summer, cream to yellow flowers open in large panicles, to 80cm (32in) long, followed by ellipsoid to almost spherical, pinkish red fruit. ↕ to 25m (80ft), ↔ 5–7m (15–22ft). Australia (Queensland). ❀ (min. 10–13°C/50–55°F)
A. cunninghamiana ♀ ⚘ (Bangalow palm, Illawarra palm, Piccabeen palm). Slender-stemmed palm with a ringed trunk and arching, pinnate leaves, 2–4m (6–12ft) long, comprising many lance-shaped, grey-green or light green leaflets. When mature, produces small lilac flowers in large, pendent racemes, to 60–90cm (24–36in) long, in summer, followed by ovoid red fruit. ↕ 15–20m (50–70ft), ↔ 2–5m (6–15ft). Australia (Queensland). ❀ (min. 10–13°C/50–55°F)

▷***Arcterica nana*** see *Pieris nana*

ARCTOSTAPHYLOS
syn. COMAROSTAPHYLIS
Bearberry, Manzanita
ERICACEAE

Genus of about 50 species of prostrate or upright shrubs, or small trees, all evergreen except for *A. alpina*, mainly from W. North America, particularly California. They are found in a range of moist or dry habitats from coastal scrub to mountain slopes, pine forest, and high moors. They have alternate, simple, entire or toothed leaves, and terminal panicles or racemes of tiny, urn-shaped flowers, 4–7mm (⅛–¼in) long, followed by spherical fruits, 6–10mm (¼–½in) across. Use the prostrate and compact species as ground cover or in a rock garden. The more upright species, with their often attractive bark, are effective in open areas of a woodland garden. In frost-prone climates, grow half-hardy species in a cool greenhouse.
• **HARDINESS** Fully hardy to half hardy.
• **CULTIVATION** Under glass, grow in lime-free (ericaceous) potting compost in full light. When in growth, water freely and apply a balanced liquid fertilizer monthly; water sparingly in winter. Grow in moist but well-drained, moderately fertile, lime-free soil in full sun or partial shade. Shelter less hardy species from cold, drying winds.
• **PROPAGATION** Sow seed in containers in a cold frame in autumn (immerse seed in boiling water for 20 seconds before sowing), or root semi-ripe cuttings in summer. Layer in autumn. Prostrate species and hybrids often root

at the nodes, providing rooted pieces that may be removed and potted up.
• **PESTS AND DISEASES** Prone to leaf spot.

A. alpina, syn. *Arctous alpinus* (Alpine bearberry). Deciduous, creeping shrub with obovate to inversely lance-shaped, white-woolly, toothed leaves, 1.5–3cm (½–1¼in) long, bright green, turning red in autumn. In late spring, bears axillary racemes, 1–2cm (½–¾in) long, of pendent, pink-flushed white flowers, followed in autumn by small, spherical, red then purple-black fruit. ↕ 5cm (2in), ↔ to 20cm (8in). Mountain moors and heaths in N. circumpolar regions. ❄❄❄
***A. densiflora* 'Howard McMinn'.** Dense, mound-forming shrub with smooth, dark red bark and elliptic, glossy, mid-green leaves, 3cm (1¼in) long. Pink-tinged white flowers are borne in small racemes, to 4cm (1½in) long, in spring. ↕ 1.5m (5ft), ↔ 2m (6ft). ❄❄
A. diversifolia, syn. *Comarostaphylis diversifolia* (Summer holly). Upright shrub with peeling or shredding bark and oblong to elliptic, toothed, glossy, dark green leaves, to 8cm (3in) long. Small white flowers are borne in racemes, to 6cm (2½in) long, in spring, and are followed by small, spherical, warty red fruit in autumn. ↕ 5m (15ft), ↔ 3m (10ft). USA (California). ❄
A. glandulosa (Eastwood manzanita). Rounded shrub with smooth, red-brown bark. Ovate to lance-shaped, leathery, matt green leaves, to 5cm (2in) long, are covered with sticky hairs on both sides when young, becoming hairless when mature. Bears small white flowers in racemes, to 4cm (1½in) long, in late winter and early spring, followed by small, flattened-spherical, sticky, red-brown fruit in summer. ↕↔ 2m (6ft). USA (Oregon, California). ❄❄
A. glauca (Bigberry manzanita). Rounded shrub, sometimes tree-like, with smooth, red-brown bark and elliptic to ovate, leathery, glaucous leaves, to 4cm (1½in) long. White or pink flowers open in racemes, to 8cm (3in) long, from spring to early summer, followed in late summer by spherical, sticky brown fruit. ↕↔ 6m (20ft). USA (California). ❄
***A. hookeri* 'Monterey Carpet'.** Low-growing, sometimes mat-forming shrub with purple-tinged branches and ovate to elliptic, narrow-pointed, glossy, pale green leaves, 2–4cm (¾–1½in) long. In early summer, produces racemes, 7cm (3in) long, of pinkish white flowers, followed by spherical scarlet fruit. ↕ to 20cm (8in), ↔ to 1m (3ft) or more. ❄❄❄ (borderline)
A. manzanita 🏆 (Manzanita, Parry manzanita). Upright shrub or small tree with smooth, red-brown bark and ovate, leathery, bright green to grey-green leaves, to 5cm (2in) long, sometimes hairy on both sides. Dark pink, sometimes white flowers in racemes, to 4cm (1½in) long, are produced in late winter and early spring, followed by flattened-spherical white fruit, ripening to red, in autumn. ↕ 4m (12ft), ↔ 3m (10ft). USA (California). ❄❄
***A. x media* 'Snow Camp'**, syn. *A. uva-ursi* 'Snow Camp'. Mat-forming shrub, closely resembling *A. uva-ursi*, with prostrate branches, erect or ascending stems, and obovate, dark

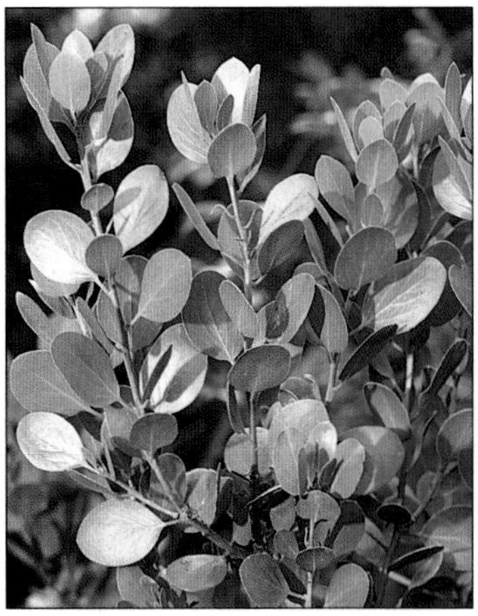

Arctostaphylos patula

green leaves, to 3cm (1¼in) long. In summer, bears a profusion of compact racemes, 5–10cm (2–4in) long, of pale pink flowers, followed by flattened-spherical red fruit. ↕ 10cm (4in), ↔ to 1m (3ft) or more. ❄❄❄
A. nevadensis (Pine-mat manzanita). Prostrate, mat-forming shrub with spreading branches, often rooting at the nodes, and narrowly lance-shaped to obovate, sharply tipped, glossy, bright green leaves, 2–3cm (¾–1¼in) long. In early summer, bears erect, raceme-like clusters, 4–8cm (1½–3in) long, of white, sometimes pink-tinged flowers, followed by flattened-spherical, reddish brown fruit in autumn. ↕ to 30cm (12in), ↔ to 1m (3ft). USA (California, W. Oregon). ❄❄❄ (borderline)
A. patula ■ (Greenleaf manzanita). Spreading shrub with smooth, red-brown bark and broadly ovate to rounded, leathery, hairless, bright green leaves, 2.5–4cm (1–1½in) long. Bears pink or white flowers in loose panicles, to 8cm (3in) long, from spring to early summer, followed by flattened-spherical, dark brown to black fruit in late summer. ↕↔ 2m (6ft). USA (California). ❄❄
A. pumila ■ (Dune manzanita). Trailing, dense, mat-forming shrub with upright branch tips and obovate to spoon-shaped, dark green leaves, 2cm (¾in) long, paler and sometimes white-downy beneath. Short, dense racemes, 4–8cm (1½–3in) long, of white flowers, sometimes pink-tinted, are borne in summer, followed by small, flattened-spherical, reddish brown fruit in autumn. ↕ 30cm (12in), ↔ 40cm (16in),

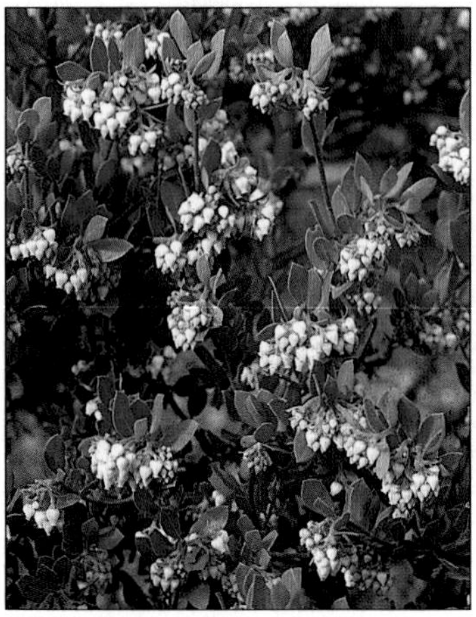

Arctostaphylos pumila

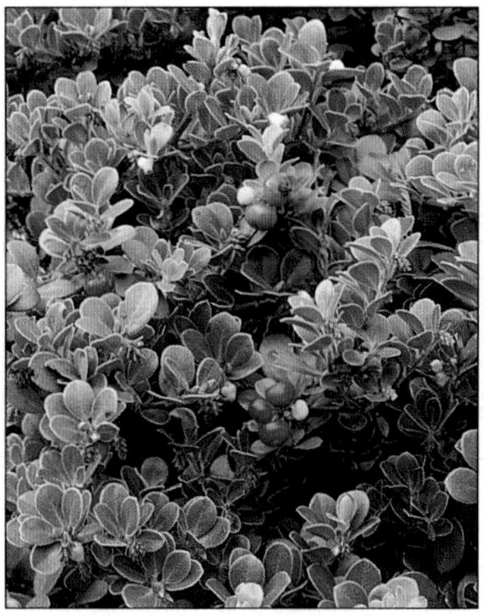

Arctostaphylos uva-ursi 'Wood's Red'

possibly reaching 75cm (30in) in cultivation. USA (California). ❄❄❄ (borderline)
A. stanfordiana (Stanford manzanita). Erect shrub with slender shoots and smooth, red-brown bark. Narrowly ovate, pointed, bright green leaves, to 6cm (2½in) long, held upright, are hairless and leathery. From spring to early summer, pink-flushed white flowers open in racemes, to 6cm (2½in) long, followed by flattened-spherical fruit, ripening to bright red in autumn. ↕↔ 2m (6ft). USA (California). ❄
A. uva-ursi (Common bearberry, Kinnikinnick). Low-growing, intricately branched, sometimes mat-forming shrub with small, obovate, leathery, dark green leaves, 2–4cm (¾–1½in) long. Small racemes, 2–3cm (¾–1¼in) long, of pink-tinted white flowers are borne in summer, followed by spherical, bright scarlet fruit in autumn. ↕ to 10cm (4in), ↔ to 50cm (20in). N. Eurasia, North America. ❄❄❄. **'Snow Camp'** see *A.* x *media* 'Snow Camp'. **'Vancouver Jade'** is a low, arching shrub with glossy leaves and small pink flowers; ↕ 15cm (6in), ↔ 45cm (18in). **'Wood's Red'** ■ is a dwarf cultivar with pink flowers and large, shiny red fruit.

ARCTOTHECA

ASTERACEAE/COMPOSITAE

Genus of 4 species of low-growing, usually rosette-forming perennials from open, sandy areas in South Africa; some species have become naturalized in Portugal, Spain, and Australia. The leaves, often white-woolly, are pinnatifid with prominent lobes, toothed, or sometimes entire. The yellow, daisy-like flowerheads, with purplish black disc-florets in some species, are often tinged with bronze or purple, especially on the undersides; they are mostly solitary, but sometimes borne in twos or threes, on long, slender stems. Use for covering banks or for edging; usually treated as annuals in frost-prone areas.
• **HARDINESS** Half hardy but will survive short periods to -5°C (23°F).
• **CULTIVATION** Grow in well-drained, moderately fertile soil in full sun.
• **PROPAGATION** Sow seed at 16–18°C (61–64°F), or divide in spring.
• **PESTS AND DISEASES** Trouble free.

A. calendula ■ syn. *Cryptostemma calendulaceum*. Low-growing, rhizomatous perennial with rosettes of

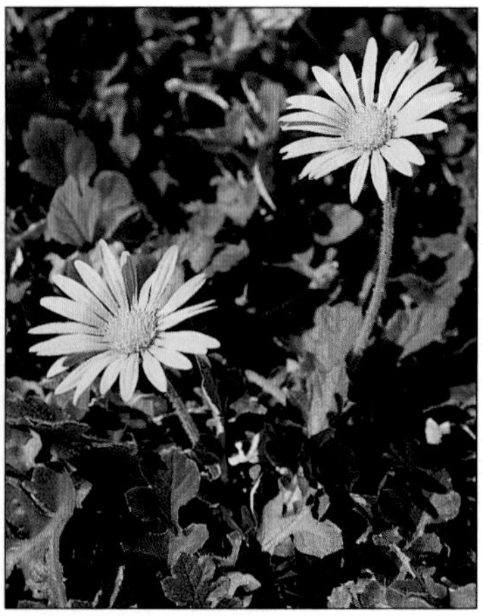

Arctotheca calendula

oblong-obovate, pinnatifid, occasionally entire leaves, 15cm (6in) long, and white-woolly beneath. Flowerheads, to 4cm (1½in) across, with yellow ray-florets, tinged purple on the undersides, and purplish black disc-florets with yellow anthers, are borne in spring or early summer. ↕ 50cm (20in), ↔ indefinite. South Africa. ❄
A. populifolia. Low-growing, rhizomatous perennial with alternate, elliptic to ovate, occasionally pinnatifid, mid-green leaves, 7cm (3in) long, and white-woolly beneath. From summer to autumn, bears flowerheads 1.5–2cm (½–¾in) across, with yellow ray-florets and yellow disc-florets. ↕ 30cm (12in), ↔ 60cm (24in). South Africa. ❄

ARCTOTIS

syn. x VENIDIOARCTOTIS, VENIDIUM
African daisy

ASTERACEAE/COMPOSITAE

Genus of about 50 species of erect to spreading annuals and perennials, occasionally subshrubs, found in dry stony soils in South Africa. They form basal rosettes of entire to lobed, lance-shaped to elliptic, grey-green to silvery green leaves. Solitary, daisy-like, brightly coloured flowerheads are borne on long, thick, ribbed stems from midsummer to early autumn. Grow as an annual in bedding schemes, a gravel garden, or containers. The flowerheads of modern cultivars, bred for bedding display, tend to stay open longer than those of the original species, which close in mid-afternoon and in dull weather. African daisies are attractive, if short-lived, cut flowers.
• **HARDINESS** Frost tender.
• **CULTIVATION** Grow in sharply drained but relatively moist, light soil in full sun.
• **PROPAGATION** Sow seed at 16–18°C (61–64°F) in early spring or autumn. Prick out individually into 9cm (3½in) containers to avoid further root disturbance. Root stem cuttings of good colour selections at any time.
• **PESTS AND DISEASES** Aphids and leaf miners may be a problem.

A. fastuosa ■ syn. *Venidium fastuosum* (Monarch of the veldt). Spreading perennial, usually cultivated as a half-hardy annual, with elliptic, deeply lobed, silvery white leaves, 12cm (5in) long, with a dense covering of woolly hairs. Rich orange flowerheads, to 10cm (4in) across, with deep purple or black

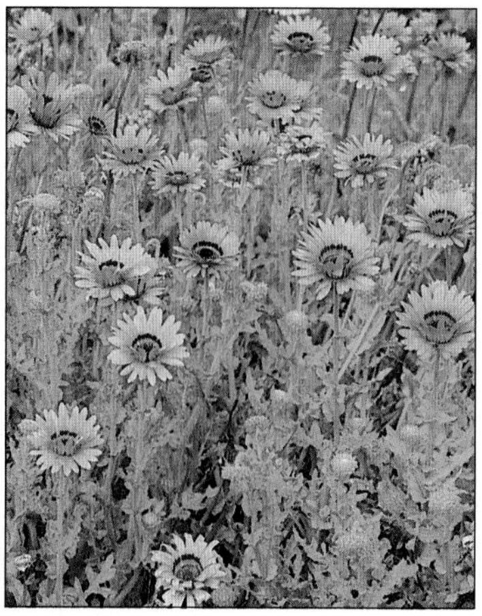

Arctotis fastuosa

disc-florets, are borne from midsummer to early autumn. ↕30–60cm (12–24in), ↔ 30cm (12in). South Africa. ❅ (min. 5°C/41°F). **'Zulu Prince'** ■ has intensely silvery white foliage and creamy yellow flowerheads, with a small black triangle with orange margins at the base of each ray-floret.

***A.* Harlequin Hybrids**, syn. *A.* x *hybrida*, x *Venidioarctotis*. Interspecific hybrids bred for cultivation as half-hardy annuals or perennials. They have elliptic, wavy-margined, lobed, felted, silvery green leaves, to 12cm (5in) long. From midsummer to early autumn, they bear pink, orange, white, carmine-red, or apricot-yellow flowerheads, 8–9cm (3–3½in) across, with dark disc-florets, sometimes with darker markings on the ray-florets. ↕45–50cm (18–20in), ↔ to 30cm (12in). ❅ (min. 5°C/41°F). A number of named cultivars, originally introduced under the name x *Venidioarctotis*, are very free-flowering and are propagated by cuttings; they include **'Bacchus'**, with reddish purple flowerheads, **'China Rose'**, with dusky pink flowerheads, and **'Flame'**, which has brilliant orange-red flowerheads.

A.* x *hybrida see *A.* Harlequin Hybrids.

A. stoechadifolia see *A. venusta*.

A. venusta, syn. *A. stoechadifolia* (Blue-eyed African daisy). Spreading perennial, often cultivated as a half-hardy annual, with elliptic-obovate, wavy-margined, lobed leaves, to 12cm (5in) long, dark green above, and silvery green beneath. Creamy white flowerheads, to 8cm (3in) across, with blue disc-florets, are borne from midsummer to early autumn. ↕60cm (24in), ↔ 40cm (16in). South Africa. ❅ (min. 5°C/41°F)

▷ ***Arctous alpinus*** see *Arctostaphylos alpina*

ARDISIA

MYRSINACEAE

Genus of about 250 species of evergreen trees and shrubs from moist woodland in tropical and warm-temperate areas of Asia, Australasia, and North and South America. They are grown for their whorled or spiralled, mid- to dark green leaves, their panicles or umbel-like corymbs of white or pink flowers, and their showy red fruits. In frost-free areas, grow in woodland; *A. japonica* is good ground cover where temperatures do not fall below -5°C (23°F). In frost-prone areas, grow *A. crispa* in a temperate greenhouse or as a houseplant.

- **HARDINESS** Frost hardy to frost tender.
- **CULTIVATION** Under glass, grow *A. crispa* in loam-based potting compost (JI No.3) in bright filtered light. When in growth, water freely and apply a balanced liquid fertilizer monthly; water moderately at all other times. Outdoors, grow in moist but well-drained, humus-rich soil in a shady site, sheltered from strong winds. Pruning group 9; plants under glass need restrictive pruning.
- **PROPAGATION** Sow seed at 13°C (55°F) in spring. Root semi-ripe cuttings in summer. Divide runners of *A. japonica* in spring.
- **PESTS AND DISEASES** Trouble free.

A. crispa ■ ♀ Erect shrub with spiralled or alternate, lance-shaped, leathery, mid- to dark green leaves, 5–14cm (2–5½in) long, with shallowly scalloped margins. In summer, bears terminal, umbel-like corymbs, to 10cm (4in) long, of star-shaped pink flowers, 9–12mm (⅜–½in) across, followed by spherical red berries, to 7mm (¼in) wide. ↕0.6–1.5m (2–5ft), ↔ 45–60cm (18–24in). S.E. Asia. ❄

A. japonica (Marlberry). Compact shrub with erect, clustered stems, underground runners, and whorls of toothed, ovate, glossy, mid- to dark green leaves, 4–9cm (1½–3½in) long. In summer, bears umbel-like corymbs, 3–8cm (1¼–3in) long, of pendent, star-shaped, white to pale pink flowers, 1.5cm (½in) across, followed by persistent, spherical red berries, 6mm (¼in) across. ↕45cm (18in), ↔ indefinite. China, Japan. ❄❄

ARECA

ARECACEAE/PALMAE

Genus of 50–60 species of single-stemmed, monoecious palms found in woodland from Malaysia and Indonesia to the Solomon Islands. Linear or lance-shaped, 2-pinnate leaves are produced in a terminal tuft above a distinct crown-shaft, with panicles of cup-shaped flowers borne beneath them. In frost-prone regions, grow young plants in a warm greenhouse. In frost-free climates, use arecas as specimen plants.

- **HARDINESS** Frost tender.
- **CULTIVATION** Under glass, grow in loamless potting compost in bright filtered light. During the growing season, water moderately and apply a balanced liquid fertilizer monthly; keep just moist in winter. Outdoors, grow in fertile, moist but well-drained soil in partial shade.
- **PROPAGATION** Sow seed at 24–27°C (75–81°F) in spring.
- **PESTS AND DISEASES** Red spider mites may be a problem under glass.

A. catechu ■ ♀ (Betel nut palm, Pinang). Slender palm with a trunk ringed with old leaf scars and topped by a crownshaft. Arching, pinnate leaves, 1–2m (3–6ft) long, have lance-shaped, soft-textured, truncate, mid-green leaflets. In summer, produces large panicles, to 60cm (24in) long, of pale yellow flowers, followed by orange to red fruit containing betel nuts, which are popular for chewing in some countries. ↕20–25m (70–80ft), ↔ 2–4m (6–12ft). Probably mainland Malaysia, Singapore. ❅ (min. 13–15°C/55–59°F)

A. lutescens see *Chrysalidocarpus lutescens*.

▷ ***Arecastrum*** see *Syagrus*
A. romanzoffianum see *S. romanzoffiana*

▷ ***Aregelia*** see *Neoregelia*
A. carolinae see *N. carolinae*

ARENARIA

Sandwort

CARYOPHYLLACEAE

Genus of about 160 species of annuals and mainly low-growing perennials, some of which are evergreen, mostly from mountainous, arctic, and temperate regions of the N. hemisphere. They have opposite pairs of small, linear to ovate leaves and bear solitary or few-flowered cymes of 5-petalled, usually white flowers. Several *Arenaria* species are attractive mat- or cushion-forming plants for a rock garden, alpine house, or scree bed, or for growing in the crevices of a wall or paving.

- **HARDINESS** Fully hardy.
- **CULTIVATION** Grow in moist but well-drained, sandy, poor soil in full sun. *A. tetraquetra* requires very sharp drainage. *A. balearica* thrives in partial shade.
- **PROPAGATION** Sow seed in containers in an open frame in autumn, divide in spring, or root basal cuttings in early summer.
- **PESTS AND DISEASES** Trouble free.

A. balearica ■ (Corsican sandwort). Prostrate, mat-forming, evergreen perennial with broadly ovate, shiny, light green leaves, 2–4mm (1/16–⅛in) long. From late spring to summer, it is studded with solitary, star-shaped white flowers, 6–10mm (¼–½in) across. ↕1cm (½in), ↔ 30cm (12in) or more. W. Mediterranean islands. ❄❄❄

A. montana ■ ♀ Vigorous, low-growing, evergreen perennial with wiry, prostrate stems and linear to lance-

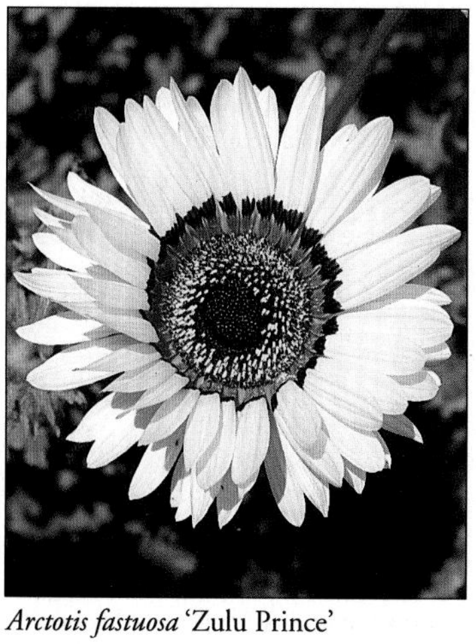

Arctotis fastuosa 'Zulu Prince'

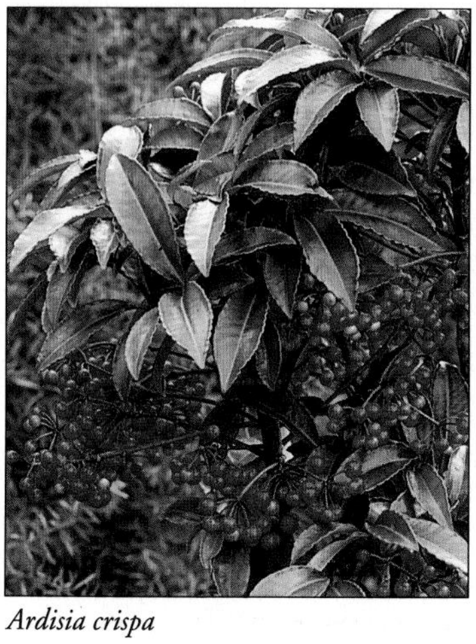

Ardisia crispa

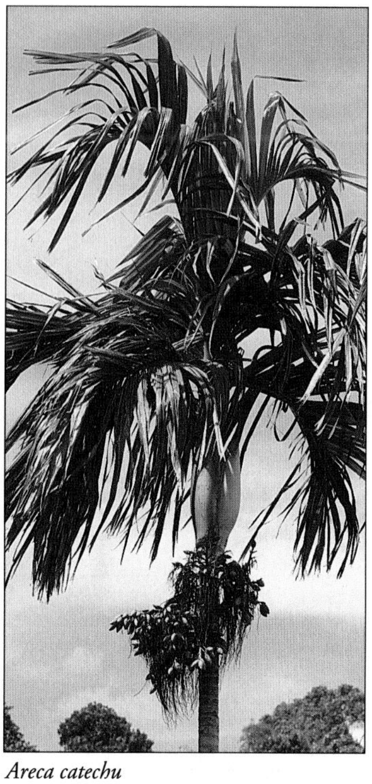

Areca catechu

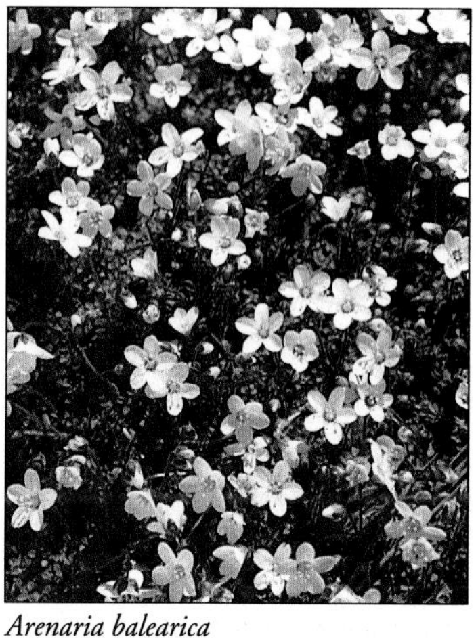

Arenaria balearica

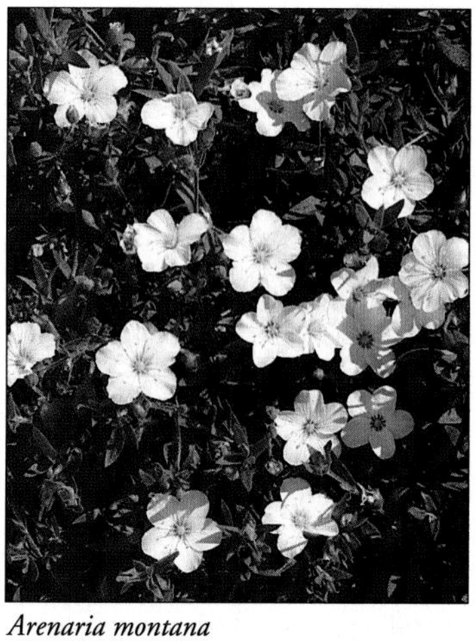

Arenaria montana

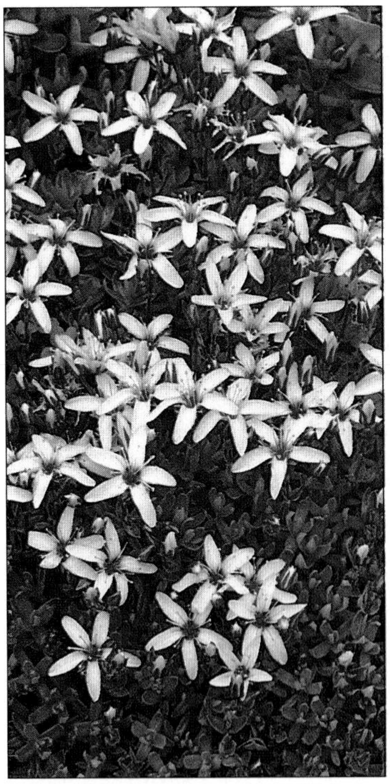
Arenaria purpurascens

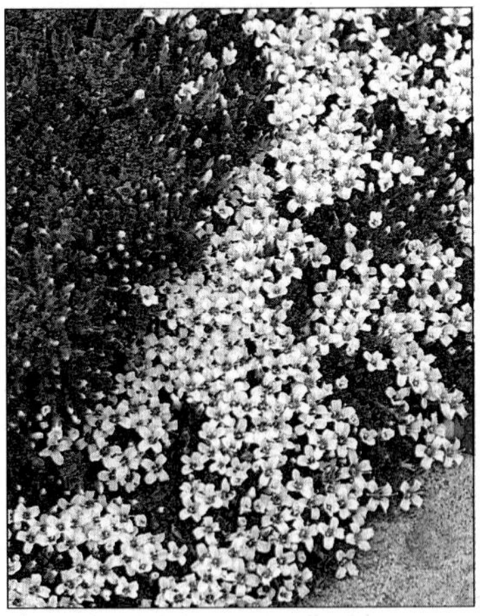
Arenaria tetraquetra

shaped, greyish green leaves, 1–2cm (½–¾in) long. Shallowly cup-shaped white flowers, 1.5–2cm (½–¾in) across, are freely borne, singly or in few-flowered cymes, in early summer. Easily grown in a rock garden, or in crevices in a wall or paving. ↕ 2–5cm (¾–2in), ↔ 30cm (12in). Mountains of S.W. Europe. ❄❄❄

A. purpurascens ▣ (Pink sandwort). Evergreen, mat- or cushion-forming perennial with elliptic to lance-shaped, sharp-pointed, glossy, dark green leaves, 6–9mm (¼–⅜in) long, with hairy margins. In midsummer, bears profuse cymes of 2–4 star-shaped, deep pink flowers, to 1.5cm (½in) across. ↕ 2–5cm (¾–2in), ↔ 20cm (8in). Pyrenees and mountains of N. Spain. ❄❄❄

A. tetraquetra ▣ Dense, cushion-forming, evergreen perennial with tiny, ovate, overlapping, grey-green leaves, 1–4mm (1/16–⅛in) long, smothered with solitary, very short-stemmed, star-shaped white flowers, 6–10mm (¼–½in) across, in spring. Suitable for a scree bed, a trough, or an alpine house. ↕ 2.5–5cm (1–2in), ↔ 15–20cm (6–8in). Pyrenees and mountains of N. Spain. ❄❄❄

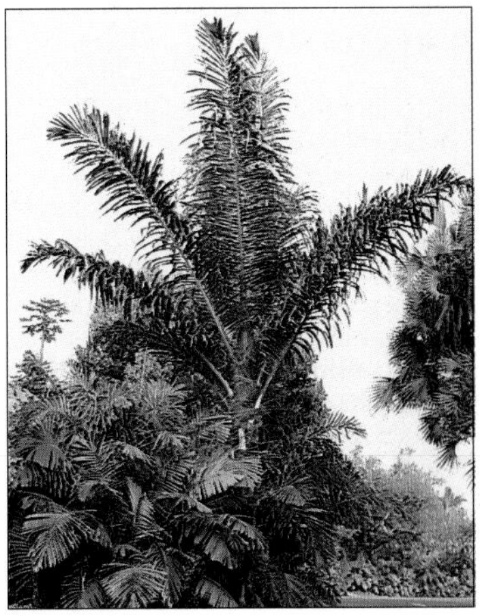
Arenga pinnata

ARENGA

ARECACEAE/PALMAE

Genus of 17 species of single- or cluster-stemmed palms from tropical lowland and hilly forest areas in S.E. Asia. Erect to arching, pinnate leaves are borne in a terminal tuft, with no crownshaft. The monoecious (rarely dioecious), cup-shaped flowers are produced only at the end of the tree's life, initially from the top leaf axils, then from all the lower ones. After fruiting, the tree usually dies. Where temperatures fall below 10–13°C (50–55°F), grow as a houseplant or in a temperate greenhouse. In tropical regions, grow as a specimen tree.

- **HARDINESS** Frost tender.
- **CULTIVATION** Under glass, grow in loamless potting compost in bright filtered light. In the growing season, water freely and apply a balanced liquid fertilizer monthly; keep just moist in winter. Outdoors, grow in fertile, moist but well-drained soil, ideally in partial shade when young.
- **PROPAGATION** Sow seed at 24–27°C (75–81°F) in spring.
- **PESTS AND DISEASES** Red spider mites may be a problem under glass.

A. pinnata ▣ 🌴 (Sugar palm). Tall, single-stemmed palm, the trunk clothed with leaf bases and the remains of fibrous black sheaths. Pinnate leaves, 6m (20ft) or more long, are composed of linear, rich green leaflets arranged in several ranks. Bears panicles, to 2m (6ft) long, of green to bronze flowers over a long period in summer, followed by black fruit. When tapped, the flowering stems yield a sweet sap, which is the basis of palm sugar. ↕ to 20m (70ft), ↔ to 12m (40ft) or more. Malaysian islands. ⌂ (min. 10–13°C/50–55°F)

▷ ***Arequipa hempeliana*** see *Oreocereus hempelianus*

ARGEMONE
Prickly poppy

PAPAVERACEAE

Genus of 28 species of vigorous, erect to spreading, usually prickly annuals, perennials, and one shrub, from scrub and wasteland in S. and S.E. USA, Central America, and the West Indies. The fleshy roots produce large clusters of mostly basal, entire to deeply lobed, smooth to prickly, glaucous leaves.

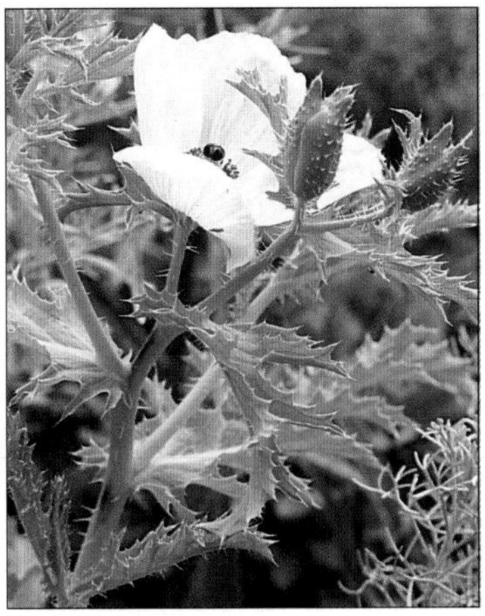
Argemone grandiflora

Paper-thin, poppy-like, white, yellow, or mauve flowers are borne singly or in corymbs in a long succession from summer to autumn. The flowers are followed by very prickly seed pods; the seeds may cause severe discomfort if ingested. The stems, when cut, exude a pale yellow to orange latex. Although some species are perennial, they are often cultivated as annuals. Grow in a gravel garden, or in a sunny mixed border. Prickly poppies self-seed freely.

- **HARDINESS** Half hardy.
- **CULTIVATION** Grow in very poor, gritty, or stony soil in full sun. Dead-head to prolong flowering.
- **PROPAGATION** Sow seed at 18°C (64°F) in early spring. Established plants resent disturbance.
- **PESTS AND DISEASES** Trouble free.

A. grandiflora ▣ Spreading, clump-forming annual or short-lived perennial with inversely lance-shaped to elliptic, deeply lobed, white-veined, blue-green leaves, to 12cm (5in) or more long; the leaves are often prickly beneath and have prickle-tipped margins. Showy, poppy-like, white or yellow flowers, to 10cm (4in) across, are borne singly or in few-flowered corymbs throughout the summer. ↕ to 1.5m (5ft), ↔ 30–40cm (12–16in). Mexico. ❄

A. mexicana ▣ (Devil's fig, Prickly poppy). Spreading, clump-forming annual with inversely lance-shaped to elliptic, deeply lobed, silver-veined, blue-green leaves, to 12cm (5in) long, with spine-tipped teeth. In late summer and early autumn, bears solitary, poppy-like, slightly scented, pale to deep yellow flowers, to 8cm (3in) across. ↕ to 1m (3ft), ↔ 30–40cm (12–16in). S. USA to Central America. ❄. **'White Lustre'** has pure white blooms. **'Yellow Lustre'** has yellowish orange flowers.

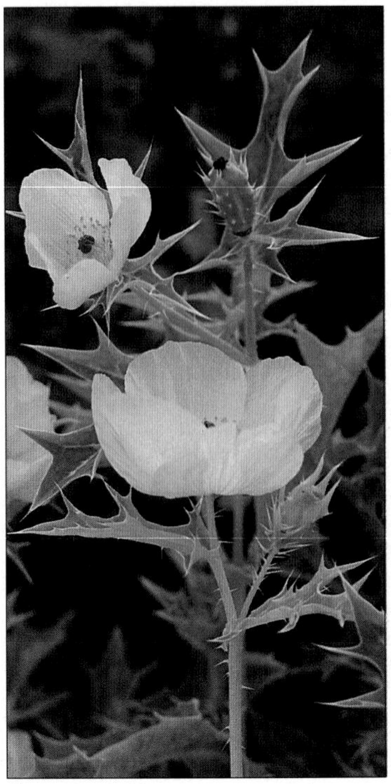
Argemone mexicana

ARGYRANTHEMUM

ASTERACEAE/COMPOSITAE

Genus of 23 species of procumbent or spreading to erect, evergreen subshrubs (sometimes offered as chrysanthemums) from the Canary Islands and Madeira. They occur in a wide range of habitats, from coastal beaches to light woodland and volcanic mountains, 2,300m (6,900ft) high. The opposite or alternate leaves are entire to finely dissected or coarsely lobed, usually 5–10cm (2–4in) long, and vary from green to intensely glaucous. Loose corymbs of daisy-like, single, sometimes anemone-centred or double flowerheads, in white, rose-pink, yellow, or apricot, are freely borne from late spring to early autumn. In frost-free areas, they are excellent for bedding or borders, as they may flower almost continuously. In frost-prone climates, grow as summer bedding or in containers.

- **HARDINESS** Frost hardy (in well-drained soil) to half hardy.
- **CULTIVATION** Grow in well-drained, moderately fertile soil in full sun. Most species will tolerate sea winds. Where temperatures fall below -5°C (23°F), apply a deep, dry winter mulch, and take cuttings as insurance against winter losses; even if top-growth is frosted, plants often regenerate from the base

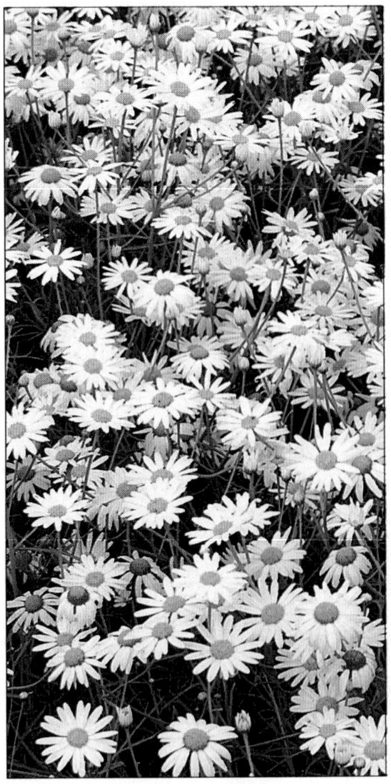
Argyranthemum foeniculaceum

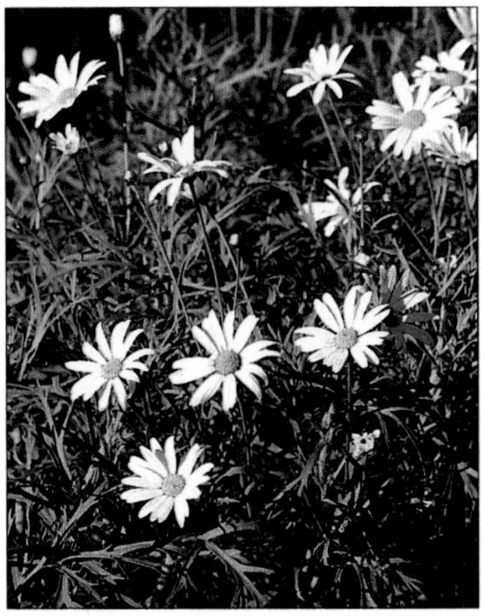

Argyranthemum frutescens

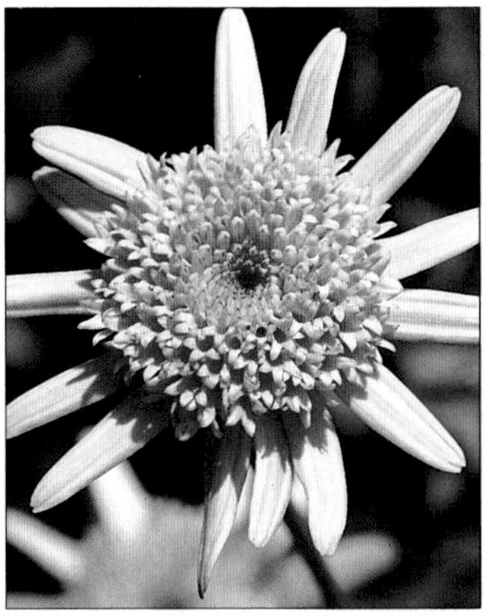

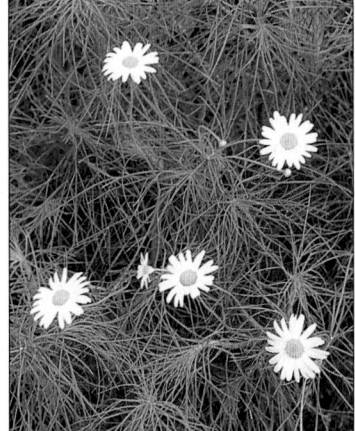

Argyranthemum 'Mary Wootton'

in spring. Pinch out the growing tips to encourage a compact habit. Pruning group 10, in early to mid-spring; may be trained as standards.
• **PROPAGATION** Root greenwood cuttings in spring, or semi-ripe cuttings of non-flowering shoots, 5–10cm (2–4in) long, in summer. Overwinter young plants in a cool greenhouse.
• **PESTS AND DISEASES** Coarse-leaved argyranthemums are prone to crown gall and chrysanthemum leaf miner.

***A.* 'Chelsea Girl'** see *A. gracile* 'Chelsea Girl'.
***A.* 'Cornish Gold'** 🏆 Compact subshrub producing pinnatisect, toothed, mid-green leaves and yellow flowerheads, 5cm (2in) across, with yellow disc-florets. ↕↔ 60cm (24in). ❄
A. foeniculaceum ■ Compact subshrub with 2- or 3-pinnatisect, finely dissected, blue-grey leaves. Bears white flowerheads, 3cm (1¼in) across, with yellow disc-florets. ↕↔ 80cm (32in). Canary Islands (N.W. Tenerife). ❄. **'Royal Haze'** 🏆 has intensely blue-grey foliage.
A. frutescens ■ Variable, rounded subshrub producing pinnatisect or 2-pinnatisect, coarsely dissected, bright green leaves and profuse white flowerheads, to 2cm (¾in) across, with yellow disc-florets. ↕↔ 70cm (28in). Canary Islands. ❄
***A. gracile* 'Chelsea Girl'** ■ 🏆 syn. *A.* 'Chelsea Girl'. Compact subshrub producing pinnatisect, grey-green leaves, with fine, hair-like lobes, and white flowerheads, 3cm (1¼in) across, with yellow disc-florets. ↕↔ 60cm (24in). ❄
***A.* 'Jamaica Primrose'** ■ 🏆 Open subshrub with pinnatisect, coarsely toothed, greyish green leaves. Long, branching stems bear primrose-yellow flowerheads, 6cm (2½in) across, with darker yellow disc-florets. Easily trained as a standard. ↕ 1.1m (3½ft), ↔ 1m (3ft). ❄
***A.* 'Jamaica Snowstorm'** see *A.* 'Snowstorm'.
A. maderense 🏆 syn. *A. ochroleucum*. Compact subshrub with pinnatisect, deeply toothed, greyish green leaves. Bears lemon-yellow flowerheads, 3cm (1¼in) across, with yellow disc-florets. ↕ 30cm (12in), ↔ 50cm (20in). Canary Islands (N. Lanzarote). ❄
***A.* 'Mary Cheek'** 🏆 Compact subshrub with pinnatisect, narrow-lobed, grey-green leaves. Produces double, hemi-spherical, light pink flowerheads, 3cm (1¼in) across, with pink disc-florets. ↕↔ 40cm (16in). ❄
***A.* 'Mary Wootton'** ■ Open subshrub with coarsely pinnatisect, greyish green leaves. Bears anemone-centred, light pink flowerheads, 5cm (2in) across, which fade almost to white, with pink disc-florets. Easily trained as a standard. ↕ 1.1m (3½ft), ↔ 1m (3ft). ❄
A. ochroleucum see *A. maderense*.
***A.* 'Petite Pink'** 🏆 syn. *A.* 'Pink Delight'. Neat, dome-shaped subshrub with finely pinnatisect, greyish green leaves and an abundance of light pink flowerheads, 2.5cm (1in) across, with yellow disc-florets. Excellent for bedding and containers. ↕↔ 30cm (12in). ❄
***A.* 'Pink Delight'** see *A.* 'Petite Pink'.
***A.* 'Snowstorm'** 🏆 syn. *A.* 'Jamaica Snowstorm'. Compact subshrub with pinnatisect, grey-green leaves and white flowerheads, 3cm (1¼in) across, with yellow disc-florets. ↕↔ 30cm (12in). ❄
***A.* 'Vancouver'** ■ 🏆 Compact subshrub producing coarsely pinnatisect, greyish green leaves. Double, anemone-centred flowerheads, 5cm (2in) across, have rose-pink disc-florets, and mid-pink outer ray-florets fading to buff pink. Easily trained as a standard. ↕ 90cm (36in), ↔ 80cm (32in). ❄

ARGYREIA

CONVOLVULACEAE

Genus of about 90 species of mainly woody-stemmed, evergreen climbers found in tropical rainforest and thickets from Asia to Queensland, Australia. The handsome, alternate leaves are large and usually broadly ovate; the funnel-shaped flowers are borne singly or in axillary cymes, followed by colourful berries. Where temperatures fall below 13°C (55°F), grow in a warm greenhouse. Elsewhere, grow on an arbour, pergola, or wall, or through a tree.
• **HARDINESS** Frost tender.
• **CULTIVATION** Under glass, grow in loam-based potting compost (JI No.3) in full light. From spring to autumn, water freely and apply a balanced liquid fertilizer monthly; reduce water in winter. Outdoors, grow in moderately fertile, moist but well-drained soil in full sun. Pruning group 11, in late winter.
• **PROPAGATION** Sow seed at 18–21°C (64–70°F) in spring. Root softwood cuttings with bottom heat in spring.
• **PESTS AND DISEASES** Prone to red spider mites, whiteflies, and aphids.

A. nervosa, syn. *A. speciosa* (Woolly morning glory). Twining climber with white-downy young shoots and broadly ovate, silver-backed leaves, 18–27cm (7–11in) long, with heart-shaped bases. From summer to autumn, bears axillary cymes, to 15cm (6in) long, of flowers 6–7cm (2½–3in) long, which are white-downy in bud, opening lavender-blue with darker bases, and flushed red-purple inside. Berries are rich brown. ↕ 8–10m (25–30ft). India (Assam), Bangladesh. ❀ (min. 13°C/55°F)
A. speciosa see *A. nervosa*.

▷ ***Argyrocytisus*** see *Cytisus*
A. battandieri see *C. battandieri*

ARGYRODERMA

AIZOACEAE

Genus of about 10 species of dwarf, stemless, sometimes clustered, perennial succulents occurring in arid regions of South Africa. They have finger-like or kidney-shaped, fleshy, evergreen leaves, arranged in pairs; some species are briefly deciduous, the new leaves forming quickly as the old leaves die away. Solitary, short-stalked or stalkless, daisy-like, yellow, purple, red, or white flowers are borne in late summer. In frost-prone areas, grow in a cool or temperate greenhouse; in dry, frost-free areas, use in a desert garden.
• **HARDINESS** Frost tender.
• **CULTIVATION** Under glass, grow in standard cactus compost in full light with low humidity. In summer, water moderately and apply a balanced liquid fertilizer monthly; water very sparingly in spring and autumn; keep dry in

Argyranthemum gracile 'Chelsea Girl'

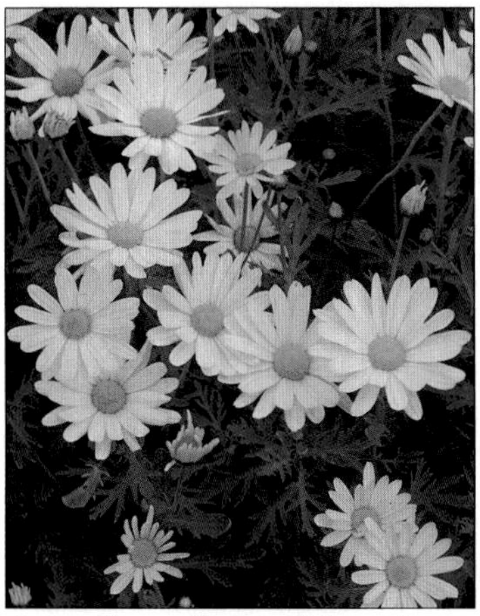

Argyranthemum 'Jamaica Primrose'

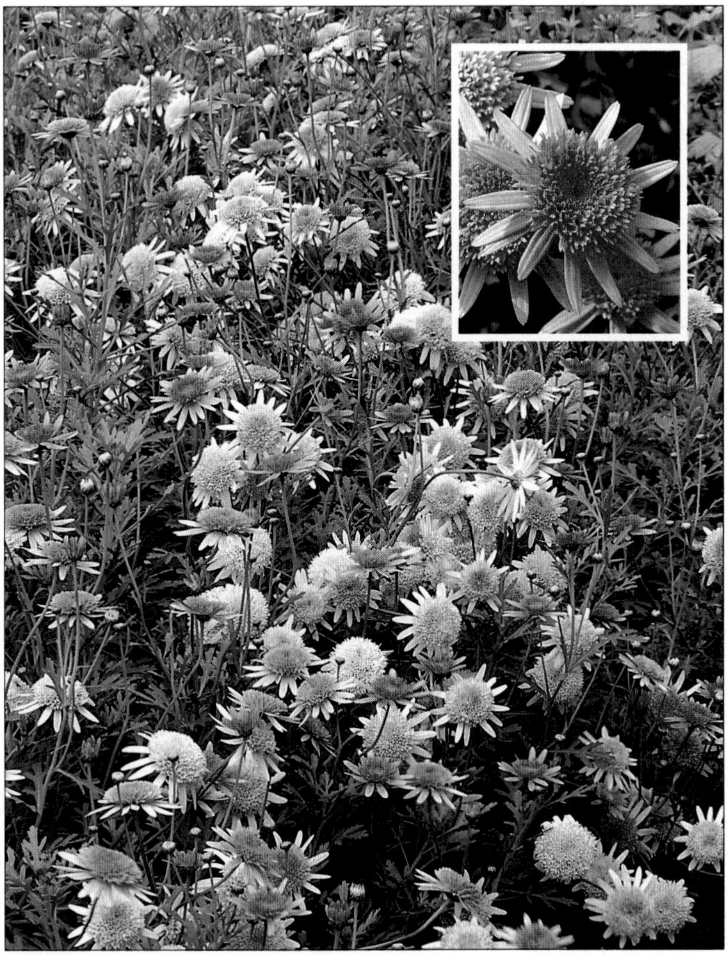

Argyranthemum 'Vancouver' (inset: flower detail)

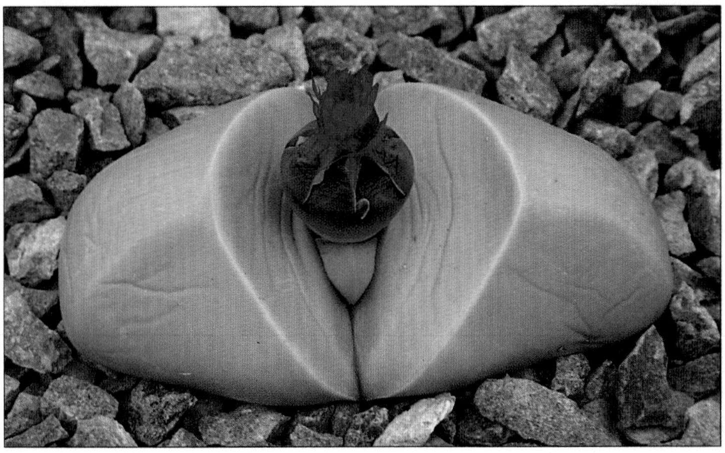

Argyroderma delaetii

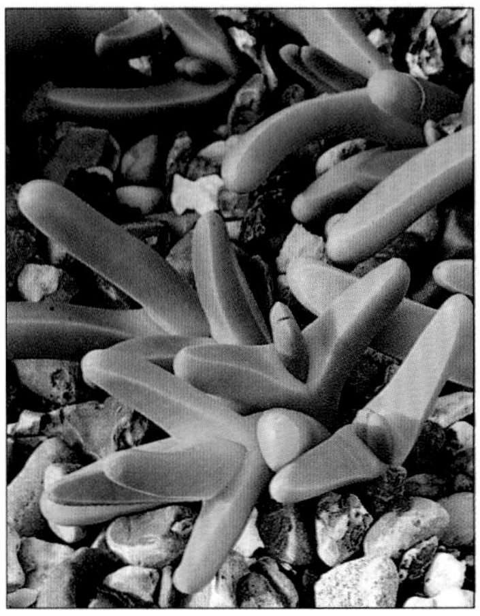

Argyroderma fissum

winter. Outdoors, grow in poor, sharply drained soil in full sun. See also pp.48–49.
• **PROPAGATION** Sow seed at 21°C (70°F) in early spring; provide partial shade until germinated, then give more light but maintain temperature.
• **PESTS AND DISEASES** Mealybugs and greenfly may be a problem.

A. aureum see *A. delaetii.*
A. blandum see *A. delaetii.*
A. brevipes see *A. fissum.*
A. delaetii ▣ syn. *A. aureum, A. blandum.* Usually unbranched succulent with a single pair of deciduous, kidney-shaped, silvery grey or bluish grey leaves, 2–5cm (¾–2in) long, united at the bases and partly sunken in the ground. The inner leaf surface is flat, and the outer one convex. In late summer, bears white, pink-purple, or yellow flowers, 5cm (2in) across. ↕ 3cm (1¼in), ↔ 5cm (2in). South Africa. ❅ (min. 7°C/45°F)
A. fissum ▣ syn. *A. brevipes.* Clump-forming succulent with pairs of finger-shaped, erect, deciduous, usually whitish green or grey-blue leaves, 5–10cm (2–4in) long, the upper surfaces rounded and smooth, and often red-tipped. Produces flowers 4cm (1½in) across, with white or yellow inner petals, and red or purple outer petals, in late summer. ↕ 12cm (5in), ↔ indefinite. South Africa. ❅ (min. 7°C/45°F)
A. pearsonii ▣ syn. *A. schlechteri.* Usually unbranched succulent with a single pair of kidney-shaped, deciduous, greenish or brownish grey leaves, 2cm (¾in) or more long, united near their bases, each with a flattish inner surface and a rounded and partly keeled outer one. In summer, produces flowers 3cm (1¼in) across, varying from violet or violet-white to yellow flushed with violet or orange. ↕ 3cm (1¼in), ↔ 5cm (2in). South Africa. ❅ (min. 7°C/45°F)
A. schlechteri see *A. pearsonii.*

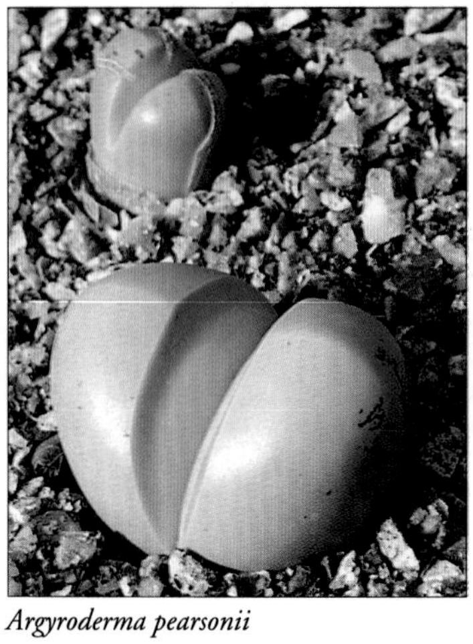

Argyroderma pearsonii

ARIOCARPUS

CACTACEAE

Genus of 5 or 6 species of slow-growing, spineless, perennial cacti from desert in Mexico. They have a long tap root, and a spherical, flat-topped stem, covered with lateral to semi-erect rosettes of triangular, rock-like tubercles. Solitary, funnel-shaped, diurnal, white, pink, yellow, or reddish purple flowers are borne in the centres of the crowns from autumn to winter, followed by ovoid green berries containing black seeds. Grow in a temperate greenhouse in frost-prone areas, or in a desert garden in frost-free areas.
• **HARDINESS** Frost tender.
• **CULTIVATION** Under glass, grow in standard cactus compost in full light. In the growing season, water moderately, and apply a balanced liquid fertilizer monthly; keep dry at other times. Outdoors, grow in poor, sharply drained soil in full sun. See also pp.48–49.
• **PROPAGATION** Sow seed at 24°C (75°F) in early spring.
• **PESTS AND DISEASES** Mealybugs may be a problem.

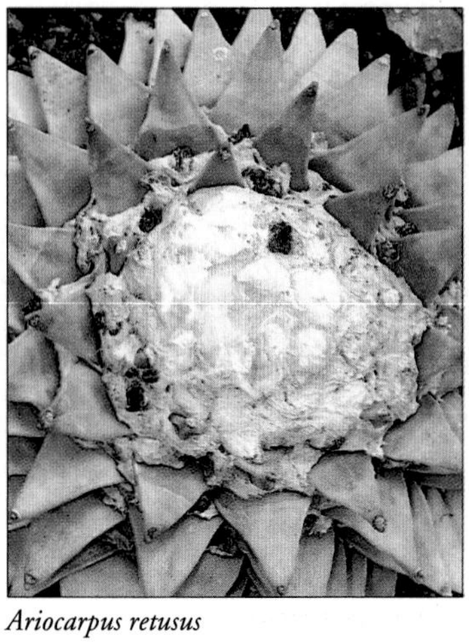

Ariocarpus retusus

A. fissuratus, syn. *Roseocactus fissuratus* (Living rock). Flat-topped cactus with blunt-tipped, grey-green tubercles, 2.5cm (1in) long and 2.5cm (1in) wide at the bases. In autumn, bears pink flowers to 4cm (1½in) across. ↕ 10cm (4in), ↔ to 15cm (6in). Mexico. ❅ (min. 10°C/50°F)
A. retusus ▣ syn. *Anhalonium retusum.* Flat-topped cactus with grey-green tubercles, 1.5–4cm (½–1½in) long and 1–3cm (½–1¼in) wide. White to pink flowers, 4–5cm (1½–2in) across, are produced in autumn. ↕ 9cm (3½in), ↔ to 25cm (10in). Mexico. ❅ (min. 10°C/50°F)
A. trigonus, syn. *Anhalonium trigonum.* Perennial cactus with flat-topped, grey-green tubercles, to 5cm (2in) long and 2.5cm (1in) wide at the bases. Bears yellow flowers, 5cm (2in) across, in autumn. ↕ 13cm (5in), ↔ to 25cm (10in). Mexico. ❅ (min. 10°C/50°F)

ARISAEMA

ARACEAE

Genus of about 150 species of spring- or summer-flowering, rhizomatous or tuberous perennials from moist woodland and rocky wasteland. The species in cultivation are mainly from the Himalayas, China, Japan, and North America. They are cultivated for their attractive, sometimes unusually shaped spathes and simple, palmately lobed or palmate, mid-green leaves. Insignificant flowers are borne at the bases of slender, sometimes striking spadices, and are followed by dense clusters of spherical to oblong red berries. They are best grown outdoors in partial shade, but are suitable for a cold greenhouse in frost-prone climates.

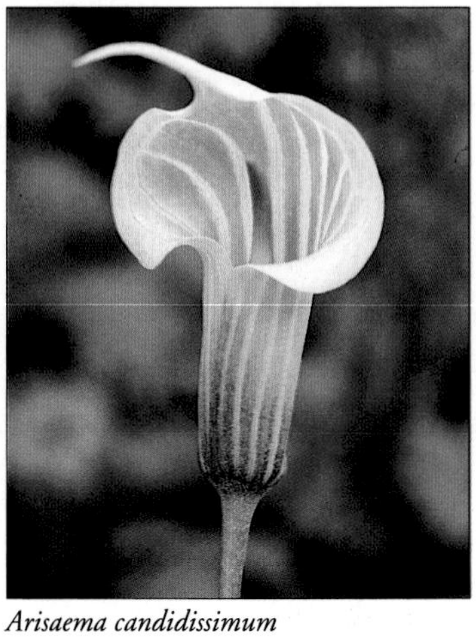

Arisaema candidissimum

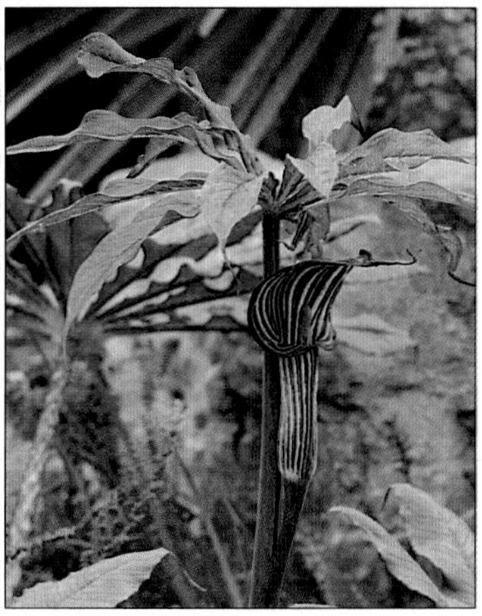

Arisaema consanguineum

• **HARDINESS** Fully hardy to half hardy.
• **CULTIVATION** Plant tubers or rhizomes 15–25cm (6–10in) deep in winter or spring. Under glass, grow in deep clay containers in equal parts loam, leaf mould, and grit in bright indirect light. Water freely when in growth, applying a balanced liquid fertilizer monthly; keep cool and moist in winter. Outdoors, grow in moist but well-drained, neutral to acid, humus-rich soil in a cool, partially shaded site. *A. candidissimum, A. consanguineum,* and *A. flavum* will tolerate more sun. Mulch in winter; protect the leaves of spring-flowering species from late frosts. Do not allow dormant tubers to dry out completely.
• **PROPAGATION** Sow seed in containers in a cold frame in autumn or spring. Most species produce offsets, which may be removed in late summer.
• **PESTS AND DISEASES** Vulnerable to slugs and vine weevils.

A. amurense. Tuberous perennial with a purple stem and usually a solitary leaf, divided into 5 radiating, oblong to linear-lance-shaped leaflets, 10–18cm (4–7in) long. In spring, bears hooded spathes, 8–12cm (3–5in) long, with dark purple and white stripes. ↕ 45cm (18in), ↔ 15cm (6in). N. Asia. ✻✻
A. atrorubens see *A. triphyllum.*
A. candidissimum ▣ ♡ Tuberous perennial bearing a conspicuous, sweetly scented, pink-striped white spathe, 8–15cm (3–6in) long, in summer, followed by a solitary, 3-palmate leaf with broadly ovate leaflets, 10–20cm (4–8in) long. ↕ 40cm (16in), ↔ 15cm (6in). W. China. ✻✻

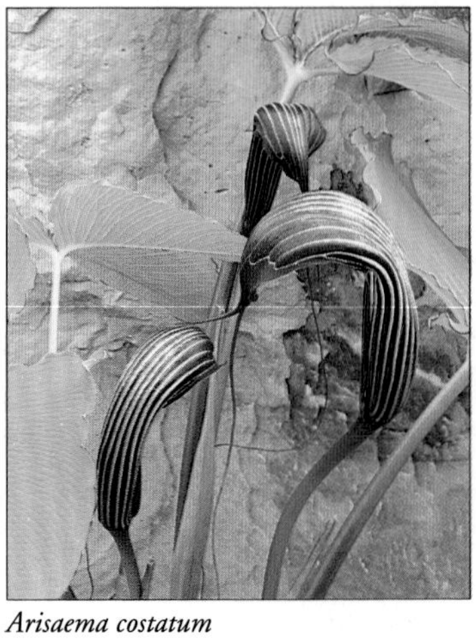

Arisaema costatum

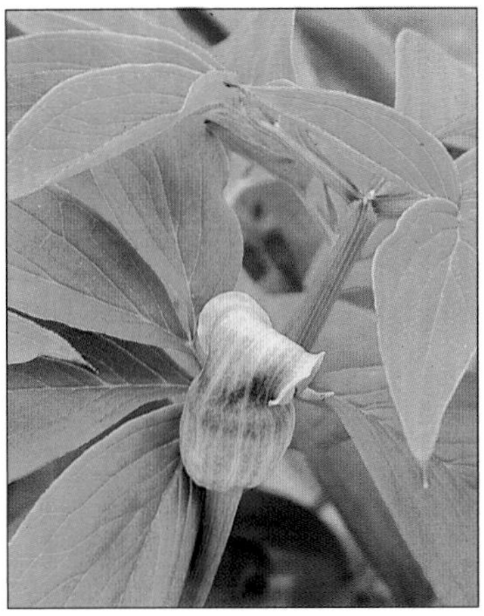

Arisaema flavum

A. consanguineum ■ Tuberous perennial producing a hooded, white-striped, brown-tinged green spathe, 10–20cm (4–8in) long, in summer, followed by a large cluster of red berries. The spathe forms below a solitary leaf with 11–20 broadly to narrowly ovate leaflets, to 20cm (8in) or more long. ↕ 1m (3ft), ↔ 15cm (6in). E. Himalayas to C. China. ❄❄
A. costatum ■ Tuberous perennial with a single, red-margined leaf divided into 3 ovate leaflets, to 40cm (16in) long. In early summer, produces a hooded, deep purple-brown spathe with white stripes, 10–15cm (4–6in) long, and a long, narrow, twisted spadix. ↕ 35–50cm (14–20in), ↔ 15cm (6in). Nepal. ❄❄
A. dracontium. Tuberous perennial bearing a single, pedate leaf, 10–20cm (4–8in) long, deeply divided into 7–15 lance-shaped lobes. Produces a narrow, hooded green spathe, 5–7cm (2–3in) long, in spring. ↕ 80cm (32in), ↔ 15cm (6in). E. North America. ❄❄❄
A. flavum ■ Tuberous perennial with 2 palmate leaves composed of 5–11 ovate to lance-shaped leaflets, 5–12cm (2–5in) long. Small but conspicuous, greenish yellow to bright yellow spathes, 2–4cm (¾–1½in) long, are borne in summer. ↕ 10–45cm (4–18in), ↔ 10cm (4in). Yemen to W. China. ❄❄❄
A. griffithii ■ Tuberous perennial with 2 large leaves, divided into 3 ovate to diamond-shaped leaflets, to 20cm (8in) long. In early summer, bears a spathe, 10–25cm (4–10in) long, just above the ground; it is purple or green, heavily veined, and hooded like a cobra. ↕ 60cm (24in), ↔ 15cm (6in). E. Himalayas. ❄

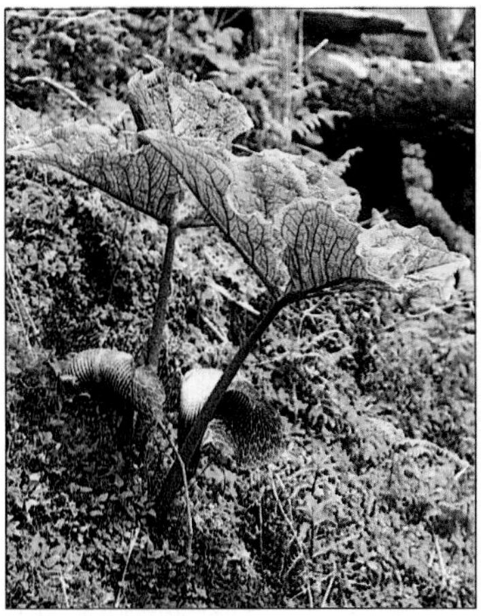

Arisaema griffithii

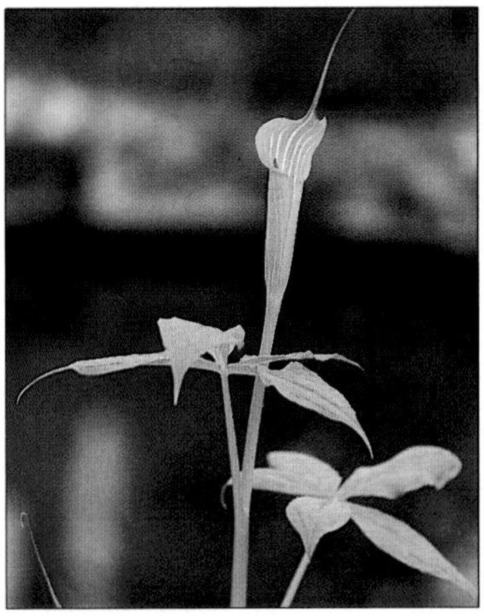

Arisaema jacquemontii

A. helleborifolium see *A. tortuosum.*
A. jacquemontii ■ Tuberous perennial producing a narrow, hooded, white-striped, light green spathe, 10–15cm (4–6in) long, in early summer. This is borne above the palmate or 2-palmate leaves, each divided into 3–9 ovate to inversely lance-shaped leaflets, 5–15cm (2–6in) long. ↕ 15–70cm (6–28in), ↔ 10cm (4in). Himalayas. ❄❄❄
A. japonicum see *A. serratum.*
A. ringens. Tuberous perennial with 2 glossy leaves, each composed of 3 elliptic to ovate leaflets, 15–20cm (6–8in) long, with long, tapering points. Bears a large, hooded and curled, green-and-purple-striped, purple-lipped spathe, 10–15cm (4–6in) long, below the leaves in early summer. ↕ 30cm (12in), ↔ 10cm (4in). China, Korea, Japan. ❄❄
A. serratum, syn. *A. japonicum.* Tall, tuberous perennial with 2 pedate leaves, each with 7–20 elliptic to lance-shaped lobes, 5–12cm (2–5in) long, on a mottled stem. In spring, bears a hooded spathe, 8–12cm (3–5in) long, varying from green to purple, and sometimes spotted or striped. ↕ 1m (3ft), ↔ 15cm (6in). China, Korea, Japan. ❄
A. sikokianum ■ Tuberous perennial with usually 2 pedate leaves, one 3- and one 5-lobed, the divisions broadly ovate and 5–15cm (2–6in) long. In spring, bears a large, deep purple spathe, 20cm (8in) long, which is open at the mouth, revealing the club-like white spadix. ↕ 30–50cm (12–20in), ↔ 15cm (6in). Japan. ❄❄
A. speciosum. Tuberous perennial with a hooded, trailing, white-striped purple spathe, 10–15cm (4–6in) long, borne in spring or early summer below a solitary 3-palmate leaf on a mottled stem. The leaf has ovate to lance-shaped leaflets, 20–45cm (8–18in) long. ↕ 60cm (24in), ↔ 15cm (6in). E. Himalayas. ❄

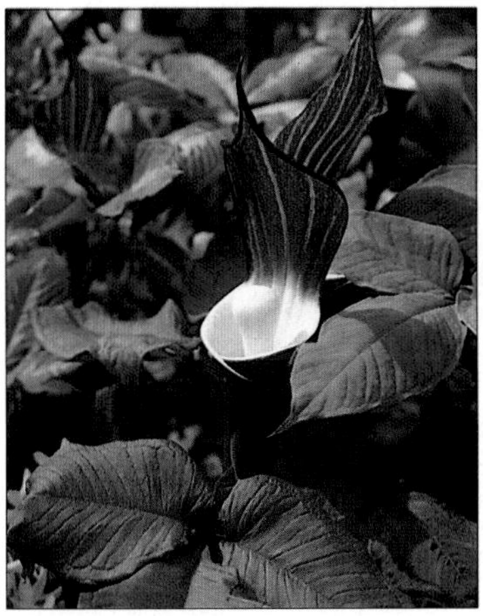

Arisaema sikokianum

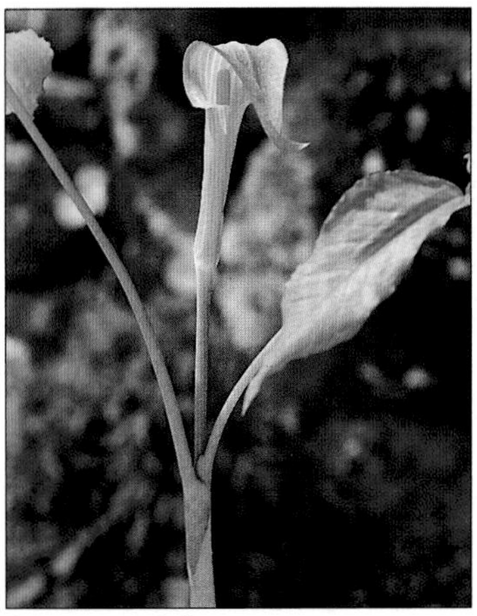

Arisaema triphyllum

A. tortuosum, syn. *A. helleborifolium.* Tuberous perennial with 2 or 3 pedate leaves, each divided into 5–17 elliptic leaflets, 15–20cm (6–8in) long. Hooded green spathes, 10–18cm (4–7in) long, with long, erect then outward-curving, purple or sometimes green spadices, are borne above the leaves in spring or early summer. ↕ to 1.5m (5ft), ↔ 20cm (8in). Himalayas. ❄
A. triphyllum ■ syn. *A. atrorubens* (Jack-in-the-pulpit). Tuberous perennial producing 1 or 2 leaves, each divided into 3 narrow, oblong to ovate leaflets, 8–15cm (3–6in) long. Bears hooded, green, sometimes purple-striped spathes, 10–15cm (4–6in) long, from spring to early summer, followed by clusters of red berries in autumn. ↕ 15–60cm (6–24in), ↔ 15cm (6in). E. USA. ❄❄❄

ARISARUM

ARACEAE

Genus of 3 species of rhizomatous or tuberous perennials from moist woodland or rocky ground and wasteland in Europe. They are grown for their small, hooded, tubular spathes, developing in winter or early to mid-spring, which enclose spadices that have minute flowers. The densely arranged, radical, ovate to arrow-shaped leaves, on long leaf-stalks, sometimes obscure the inflorescences. Ideal for an alpine house, or for a woodland or rock garden.

- **HARDINESS** Fully hardy to half hardy. *A. vulgare* will tolerate short spells to -5°C (23°F) if well mulched.
- **CULTIVATION** Plant tubers or rhizomes 8cm (3in) deep in autumn. Under glass, grow in gritty, humus-rich, loamless potting compost in filtered light. Outdoors, *A. proboscideum* requires humus-rich, moist soil in partial shade. *A. vulgare* needs a more open site in full sun, in well-drained soil that is dry in summer.
- **PROPAGATION** Sow seed in containers in a cold frame in spring, or divide in autumn or winter.
- **PESTS AND DISEASES** Trouble free.

A. proboscideum ■ (Mouse plant). Rhizomatous perennial with mats of arrow-shaped, glossy, dark green leaves, 6–15cm (2½–6in) long. In spring, bears hooded, dark brown-purple spathes, 3–5cm (1¼–2in) long, each with a long, thin, curled tip, to 15cm (6in) long, which looks like a mouse's tail; the spadices are insignificant. Often forms large colonies. ↕ 15cm (6in), ↔ to 25cm (10in) or more. Italy, Spain. ❄❄❄
A. vulgare. Tuberous perennial with arrow-shaped, mid- to yellowish green leaves, 5–12cm (2–5in) long, sometimes mottled with purple. In winter or early spring, produces small, hooded green spathes, 2.5–5cm (1–2in) long, striped brown or purple, with blackish brown spadices. Best grown in an alpine house. ↕ 15cm (6in), ↔ to 10cm (4in) or more. Mediterranean. ❄

ARISTEA

IRIDACEAE

Genus of 50 species of rhizomatous, evergreen, clump-forming, mainly spring- or summer-flowering perennials from coastal and mountain sites in W. and E. Africa, Madagascar, and South Africa. They have slender stems bearing spike-like, terminal panicles with lateral clusters of saucer-shaped flowers, each lasting only one day. The basal leaves, 10–70cm (4–28in) long, are erect and 2-ranked, and longer than the stem-clasping leaves. In frost-prone areas, grow in a cool greenhouse; in frost-free areas, grow in a border.

- **HARDINESS** Half hardy to frost tender.
- **CULTIVATION** Under glass, grow in loamless potting compost in bright filtered light. When in growth, water freely and apply a balanced liquid fertilizer monthly; keep moist at other

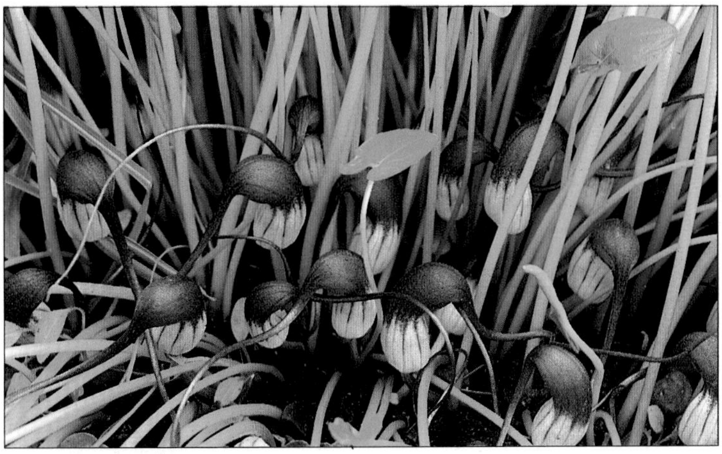

Arisarum proboscideum

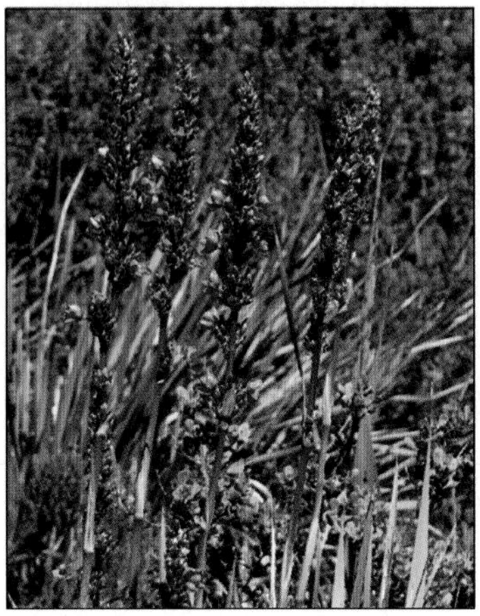

Aristea major

times. Outdoors, grow in well-drained, moderately fertile, humus-rich soil in full sun. They resent root disturbance.
• **PROPAGATION** Sow seed thinly at 13–16°C (55–61°F) in spring.
• **PESTS AND DISEASES** Trouble free.

A. ecklonii. Robust, clump-forming, evergreen, rhizomatous perennial with tufts of linear basal leaves, 30–45cm (12–18in) long, and smaller, linear stem-clasping leaves. Loose, spike-like panicles of saucer-shaped blue flowers, 2cm (¾in) across, are borne in summer. ↕1m (3ft), ↔45cm (18in). C. Africa, South Africa. ✲
A. major ■ syn. *A. thyrsiflora.* Clump-forming, evergreen, rhizomatous perennial with dense, spike-like panicles of saucer-shaped, blue or purple flowers, 3–4cm (1¼–1½in) across, in summer. Basal leaves are lance-shaped and 30–50cm (12–20in) long; stem leaves are linear and smaller. ↕1–1.5m (3–5ft), ↔45cm (18in). South Africa. ✲
A. thyrsiflora see *A. major.*

ARISTOLOCHIA

Dutchman's pipe

ARISTOLOCHIACEAE

Genus of about 300 species of evergreen and deciduous climbers, occasionally shrubs or scandent perennials, mostly from moist woodland in temperate and tropical regions of both hemispheres. The leaves are entire or lobed, and often heart-shaped. The petalless flowers, mostly in white, purple, liver-brown, or maroon, veined or mottled with darker hues, have a curved or S-shaped calyx with an inflated base, resembling the shape of a Dutch pipe. Aristolochias are unusual and useful climbing plants for screening, but some have unpleasantly scented flowers and are best grown away from the house. In frost-prone regions, grow tender species in a temperate or warm greenhouse. Some species were formerly included in the genus *Isotrema.*
• **HARDINESS** Fully hardy to frost tender.
• **CULTIVATION** Under glass, grow in loamless potting compost in bright filtered light. During the growing season, water freely and apply a balanced liquid fertilizer monthly; water more sparingly in winter. Outdoors, grow in fertile, well-drained soil in sun or partial shade. Hardy species overwinter most successfully in dry soils. Climbing species require strong support. Pruning group 11 or 12; prune after flowering.

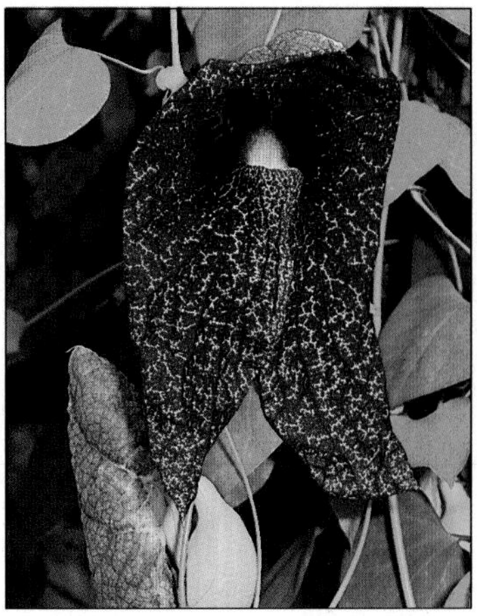

Aristolochia gigantea

• **PROPAGATION** Sow seed of hardy species at 13–16°C (55–61°F) and tender species at 21–24°C (70–75°F), as soon as ripe or in spring. Divide perennials in spring, or insert root cuttings in winter. Root softwood cuttings of climbing or scandent species grown under glass in early spring, and of hardy species in midsummer.
• **PESTS AND DISEASES** Trouble free.

A. clematitis (Birthwort). Deciduous perennial with creeping, branched rhizomes, and heart-shaped, mid- to dark green leaves, 6–15cm (2½–6in) long, on erect, then scandent stems. Axillary clusters of 3–8 narrow, tubular, pale yellow, brown, or yellowish brown flowers, 2–3cm (¾–1¼in) long, with pointed, curved upper lips, are borne from late spring to midsummer. Contact with sap may irritate skin. ↕90cm (36in), ↔60cm (24in). Europe. ✲✲✲
A. durior see *A. macrophylla.*
A. elegans see *A. littoralis.*
A. gigantea ■ Evergreen twiner with broadly triangular, dark green leaves, 5–10cm (2–4in) long. In summer, bears solitary, rounded, white, purple-veined flowers, white- or ivory-mottled maroon inside, to 16cm (6in) across. ↕10m (30ft). Panama. ❀ (min. 10°C/50°F)
A. gigas see *A. grandiflora.*
A. grandiflora, syn. *A. gigas.* Vigorous, evergreen twiner with heart-shaped, dark green leaves, 20–25cm (8–10in) long. Solitary, rounded, long-tailed white flowers, 15–18cm (6–7in) across, with brownish purple veins and dark purple eyes, are borne in summer. ↕to 10m (30ft) or more. Mexico to Panama, West Indies. ❀ (min. 10°C/50°F)
A. littoralis ■ ♀ syn. *A. elegans* (Calico flower). Evergreen twiner with kidney- to heart-shaped, glaucous, pale green leaves, 5–10cm (2–4in) long. Solitary, rounded, purple-brown flowers, 10cm (4in) across, with white markings and veins, are borne in summer. ↕5–8m (15–25ft). Brazil. ❀ (min. 7°C/45°F)
A. macrophylla, syn. *A. durior, A. sipho* (Dutchman's pipe). Strong-growing, deciduous twiner with broadly heart-shaped leaves, dark green above, lighter beneath, and 10–30cm (4–12in) long. In summer, bears solitary, rounded, mid-green flowers, 2.5cm (1in) across, mottled with yellow, purple, and brown, that are hidden among the leaves. ↕8–10m (25–30ft). S.E. USA. ✲✲
A. sipho see *A. macrophylla.*

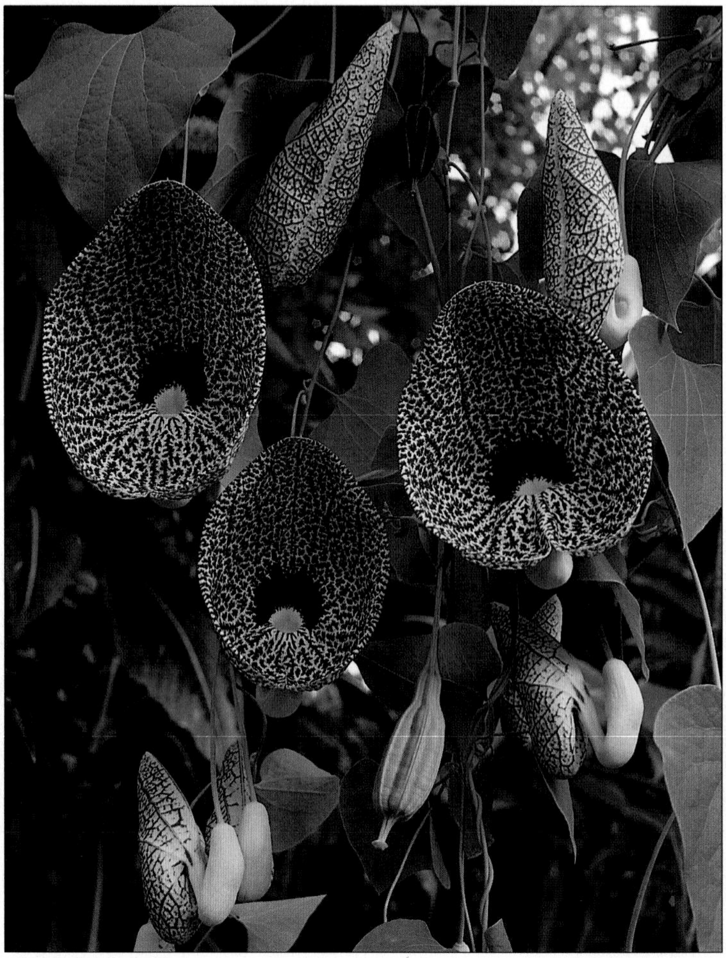

Aristolochia littoralis

ARISTOTELIA

ELAEOCARPACEAE

Genus of 5 species of deciduous and evergreen trees and shrubs often found in woodland and scrub in South America, Australia, and New Zealand. They are cultivated for their attractive, alternate or near-opposite, usually ovate leaves, their spreading cymes of tiny flowers, and their autumn fruits. Male and female flowers are borne on separate plants, so both sexes must be grown together to obtain fruit. They tolerate sea winds and are useful for a coastal garden or shrub border.
• **HARDINESS** Frost hardy.
• **CULTIVATION** Grow in fertile, well-drained soil in sun or partial shade in a warm site, sheltered from cold, drying winds. Pruning group 9.
• **PROPAGATION** Sow seed in containers in a cold frame in spring. Root semi-ripe cuttings in summer.
• **PESTS AND DISEASES** Trouble free.

A. chilensis, syn. *A. macqui* (Macqui). Evergreen shrub with near-opposite or alternate, ovate, glossy, dark green leaves, to 12cm (5in) long. Greenish white flowers, 5mm (¼in) across, are borne in axillary cymes in summer. Female plants produce small, spherical fruit, purple at first, ripening to black. ↕↔5m (15ft). Chile, Argentina. ✲✲
A. macqui see *A. chilensis.*

ARMERIA

Sea pink, Thrift

PLUMBAGINACEAE

Genus of about 80 species of tufted or hummock- or cushion-forming, evergreen perennials or subshrubs, distributed widely from sea cliffs to mountainous areas in Europe, Turkey, N. Africa, and the Pacific coast of North and South America. They produce dense rosettes of linear to strap-shaped leaves and compact, spherical heads of small,

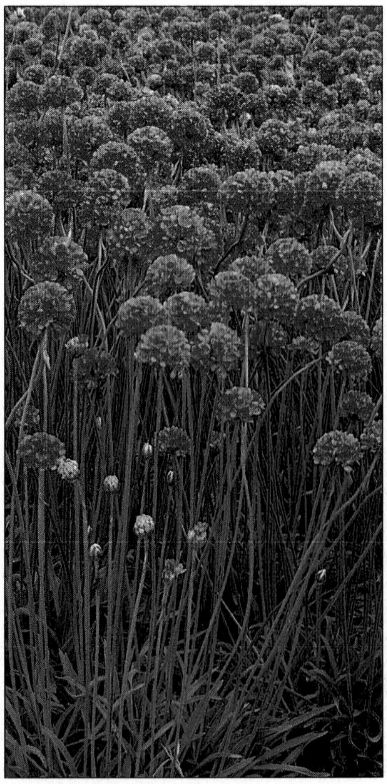

Armeria 'Bee's Ruby'

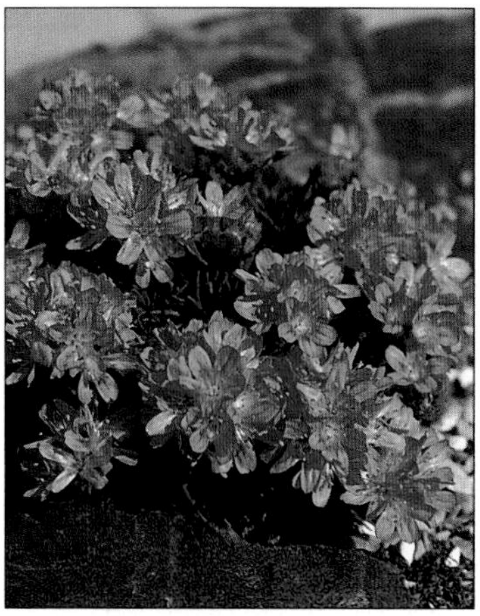
Armeria juniperifolia

saucer- or cup-shaped flowers on slender stems. They are ideal for a rock garden or trough, or for the front of a border.
• **HARDINESS** Fully hardy.
• **CULTIVATION** Grow in well-drained, poor to moderately fertile soil in an open situation in full sun.
• **PROPAGATION** Sow seed in containers in a cold frame in autumn or spring; the species cross freely and hybrids may result. Divide in early spring. Root semi-ripe, basal cuttings in summer.
• **PESTS AND DISEASES** Prone to red spider mites and aphids under glass.

A. alliacea, syn. *A. arenaria*, *A. plantaginea.* Robust, clump-forming perennial with narrow, inversely lance-shaped to linear, dark green leaves, to 15cm (6in) long. In summer, bears white to deep red-purple flowerheads, to 2cm (¾in) across, on wiry stems, 20–50cm (8–20in) long. ↕↔ to 50cm (20in). Mountains of W. Europe. ❄❄❄
A. arenaria see *A. alliacea.*
***A. atrosanguinea* of gardens** see *A. pseudarmeria.*
***A.* 'Bee's Ruby'** ■ ♀ Tufted, woody-based perennial with broadly strap-shaped, dark green leaves, to 15cm (6in) long. Deep, bright pink flowerheads, 3–4cm (1¼–1½in) across, are borne on strong stems, 20–30cm (8–12in) long, in early summer. ↕ 30cm (12in), ↔ 25cm (10in). ❄❄❄
A. caespitosa see *A. juniperifolia.*
A. juniperifolia ■ ♀ syn *A. caespitosa.* Hummock-forming subshrub with rosettes of linear, hairy, spine-tipped, grey-green leaves, to 1.5cm (½in) long. Purplish pink to white flowerheads, to

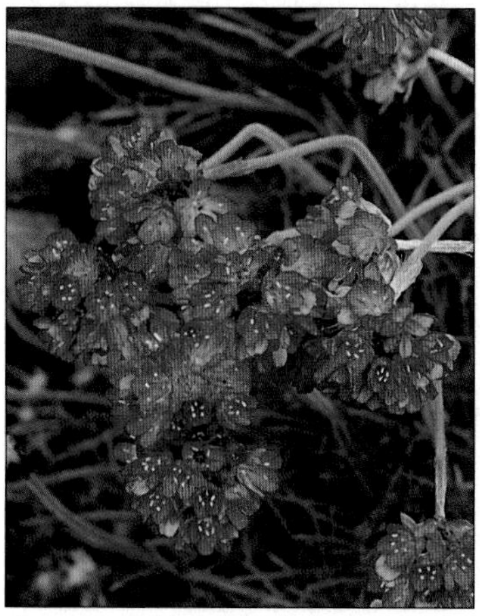
Armeria maritima 'Vindictive'

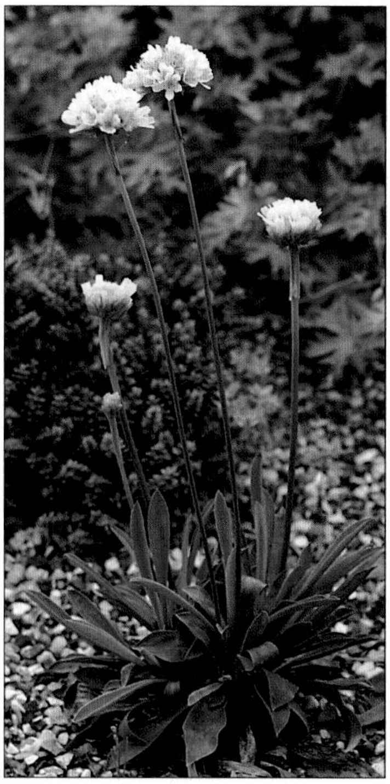
Armeria pseudarmeria

1.5cm (½in) across, are borne on stems, 1–2cm (½–¾in) long, in late spring. ↕ 5–8cm (2–3in), ↔ to 15cm (6in). Mountain pastures or rock crevices in C. Spain. ❄❄❄. **'Bevan's Variety'** ♀ is compact, with deep rose-pink flowers on very short stems; ↕ to 5cm (2in).
A. latifolia see *A. pseudarmeria.*
A. maritima (Sea thrift). Variable, clump-forming perennial with linear, dark green leaves, 4–12cm (1½–5in) long. Stiff stems, to 20cm (8in) long, bear profuse, white, pink, or red-purple flowerheads, to 2.5cm (1in) wide, from late spring to summer. ↕ to 20cm (8in), ↔ to 30cm (12in). Mountain and coastal areas in N. hemisphere. ❄❄❄. **'Bloodstone'** has dark, blood-red flowerheads. **'Vindictive'** ■ ♀ has stems to 15cm (6in) long, and rose-pink flowerheads to 2cm (¾in) wide.
A. plantaginea see *A. alliacea.*
A. pseudarmeria ■ syn. *A. atrosanguinea* of gardens, *A. latifolia.* Clump-forming subshrub with lance-shaped, mid-green leaves, to 20cm (8in) long. In summer, bears white or pale pink flowerheads, 3–4cm (1¼–1½in) across, on stems 25–50cm (10–20in) long. ↕ to 50cm (20in), ↔ 30cm (12in). Coastal pastures in W. Portugal. ❄❄❄

ARMORACIA

BRASSICACEAE/CRUCIFERAE

Genus of 3 species of erect perennials from a range of habitats at low altitudes, including wasteland, streamsides, and roadsides, in Eurasia and E. USA. They have simple or pinnatifid, dock-like, toothed, coarse, basal leaves arising from deep, woody or fleshy tap roots. Small, cruciform, 4-petalled white flowers are borne in large, terminal racemes or panicles on leafy, branching stems from late spring to late summer, and are followed by oblong to obovate fruits. *A. rusticana* (common horseradish) is widely grown for its pungent, fleshy roots, often used in sauces and relishes.
• **HARDINESS** Fully hardy.
• **CULTIVATION** Grow in full sun in light, fertile, moist but well-drained soil. Water freely during the growing season to prevent the roots becoming woody.
• **PROPAGATION** Divide or take root cuttings in winter. Roots left in place re-sprout vigorously and may be invasive.
• **PESTS AND DISEASES** Prone to black rot, clubroot, and turnip mosaic virus.

A. rusticana, syn. *Cochlearia armoracia* (Horseradish, Red cole). Clump-forming perennial with long-stalked, ovate-oblong, toothed, puckered, dark green leaves, 30–50cm (12–20in) long, arising from fleshy, branching, cream-coloured roots. Leafy, branched stems bear terminal panicles of white flowers, 5–8mm (¼–⅜in) across, from late spring to late summer. Contact with sap may irritate skin. ↕ 1m (3ft), ↔ 45cm (18in) or more. S.E. Europe, but naturalized in Europe, New Zealand, and North America. ❄❄❄

ARNEBIA

BORAGINACEAE

Genus of about 25 species of erect to spreading annuals and perennials found in woodland and dry, rocky areas, or on grassy slopes, from N. Africa to C. Asia. Simple or branching stems produce hairy leaves, 3–15cm (1¼–6in) long. Blue to purple or yellow to cream flowers are borne in short, coiled, usually terminal cymes. Ideal for a rock garden, a border, or a woodland glade.
• **HARDINESS** Fully hardy.
• **CULTIVATION** *A. pulchra* is best in partial shade in moist but well-drained soil; will tolerate full sun if kept moist. Most other species prefer more sharply drained soil in an open, sunny site.
• **PROPAGATION** Sow seed in containers in a cold frame as soon as ripe. Divide in spring or take root cuttings in winter.
• **PESTS AND DISEASES** Susceptible to aphids and red spider mites under glass.

A. echioides see *A. pulchra.*
A. pulchra ■ syn. *A. echioides*, *Echioides longiflorum*, *Macrotomia echioides* (Prophet flower). Clump-forming perennial with lance-shaped to oblong, stiffly hairy, light green leaves, to 15cm (6in) long. In summer, unbranched stems bear terminal cymes of trumpet-shaped yellow flowers, to 2.5cm (1in) across; each petal has a brown basal spot that fades with age. ↕↔ to 30cm (12in). Caucasus, Turkey, N. Iran. ❄❄❄

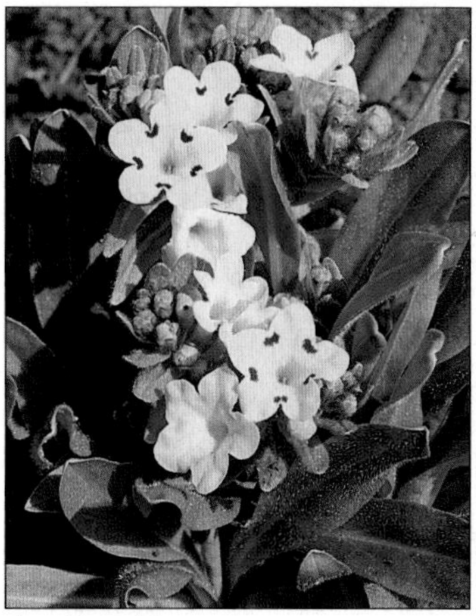
Arnebia pulchra

ARNICA

ASTERACEAE/COMPOSITAE

Genus of about 32 species of clump-forming and rhizomatous perennials from pasture and open woodland in N. temperate and arctic regions. They have mainly basal leaves, 11–20cm (4½–8in) long, and daisy-like flowerheads borne on unbranched stems. They are suitable for a herbaceous border or a large rock garden. All parts may cause severe discomfort if ingested, and contact with sap may aggravate skin allergies.
• **HARDINESS** Fully hardy.
• **CULTIVATION** Grow in moist but well-drained, humus-rich soil in full sun.
• **PROPAGATION** Sow seed in a cold frame in autumn, or divide in spring.
• **PESTS AND DISEASES** Caterpillars and slugs may be a problem.

A. montana. Clump-forming perennial with mainly basal, broadly obovate to inversely lance-shaped leaves, to 15cm (6in) long. In summer, produces solitary (occasionally 2 or 3), deep yellow or orange-yellow flowerheads, each 5–8cm (2–3in) across, on stems 25–50cm (10–20in) long. ↕ to 50cm (20in), ↔ 30cm (12in). Europe, W. Asia. ❄❄❄

ARONIA

Chokeberry

ROSACEAE

Genus of 2 species of deciduous, suckering shrubs, sometimes classified as *Photinia*, from woodland clearings, scrub, and swamps in E. North America. They are grown for their white, sometimes pink-tinged flowers, borne in late spring in corymbs, to 6cm (2½in) wide; for their colourful autumn leaves, which are alternate, simple, fine-toothed, and 8–10cm (3–4in) long; and for their spherical red or black fruits. Excellent for a shrub border or as specimen plants.
• **HARDINESS** Fully hardy.
• **CULTIVATION** Grow in any moist but well-drained soil (except shallow soil over chalk) in sun or partial shade. Pruning group 1 or 2.
• **PROPAGATION** Sow seed in a seedbed in autumn. Root softwood cuttings in early summer. Remove suckers when plants are dormant, and pot up.
• **PESTS AND DISEASES** Trouble free.

A. arbutifolia ■ (Red chokeberry). Erect shrub with narrowly ovate, matt,

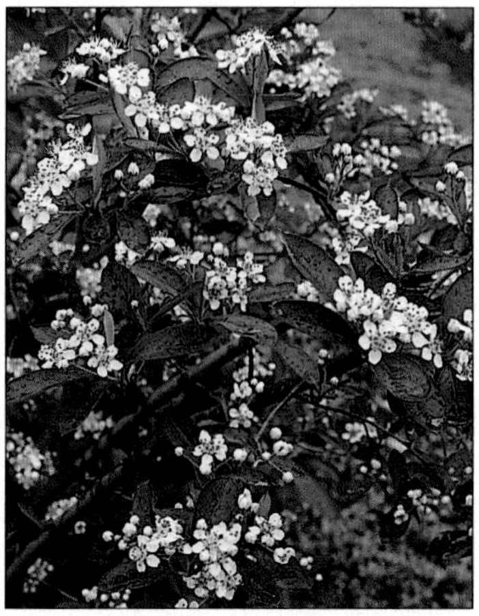
Aronia arbutifolia

A

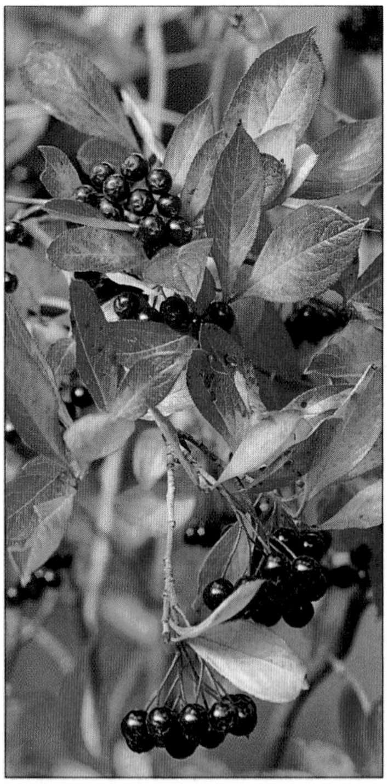

Aronia x *prunifolia*

dark green leaves, densely grey-hairy beneath, which turn orange, red, and yellow in autumn. Corymbs of white, occasionally pink-tinged flowers, to 1.5cm (½in) across, are borne in late spring, and are followed by persistent red berries, to 6mm (¼in) across. ↕3m (10ft), ↔1.5m (5ft). E. North America. ❄❄❄. **'Brilliant'** see *A.* x *prunifolia* 'Brilliant'.

A. melanocarpa (Black chokeberry). Upright shrub with obovate, hairless, glossy, mid-green leaves, which turn dark purple-red in autumn. Corymbs of white, occasionally pink-tinged flowers, to 1cm (½in) across, are borne in late spring and early summer, and are followed by black berries, to 1cm (½in) across. ↕2m (6ft), ↔3m (10ft). E. North America. ❄❄❄. **'Brilliant'** see *A.* x *prunifolia* 'Brilliant'.

A.* x *prunifolia ▣ (*A. arbutifolia* x *A. melanocarpa*) (Purple chokeberry). Variable, erect shrub producing obovate, matt, dark green leaves, grey-hairy beneath, which turn dark purple-red in autumn. Corymbs of white, sometimes pink-tinged flowers, to 1.5cm (½in) across, are borne in late spring, and are followed by purple-black berries, to 8mm (⅜in) across. ↕3m (10ft), ↔2.5m (8ft). E. North America. ❄❄❄. **'Brilliant'**, syn. *A. arbutifolia* 'Brilliant', *A. melanocarpa* 'Brilliant', has bright red leaves in autumn.

▷**Arorangi** see *Olearia macrodonta*

ARRABIDAEA

BIGNONIACEAE

Genus of about 50 species of evergreen, tendril climbers occurring in tropical and subtropical rainforest from Mexico to Argentina and the West Indies. They are cultivated mainly for their attractive flowers, which are salverform to bell-shaped, each with 5 petal lobes, often reddish purple or pink, and borne in terminal or axillary panicles. The opposite leaves are 3-palmate, or consist of a pair of leaflets with a tendril between them. Where temperatures fall below 10–13°C (50–55°F), grow in a temperate or warm greenhouse. In warmer climates, train on a pergola or wall, or through a tree.

• **HARDINESS** Frost tender.

• **CULTIVATION** Under glass, grow in loamless potting compost in full light. During the growing season, water freely and apply a balanced liquid fertilizer monthly; reduce water in winter. Outdoors, grow in moist but well-drained, reasonably fertile soil in sun or partial shade. Pruning group 11; prune in early spring or after flowering.

• **PROPAGATION** Sow seed in spring at not less than 16–18°C (61–64°F). Root semi-ripe cuttings in summer. Layer in spring.

• **PESTS AND DISEASES** Red spider mites may be a problem under glass.

A. corallina. Vigorous climber with mid-green leaves divided into 3 ovate leaflets, 3–11cm (1¼–4½in) long. In summer, produces terminal panicles, 10–30cm (4–12in) long, of bell-shaped, red-purple to lilac flowers, 5cm (2in) long, with spreading lobes and white throats. ↕5–8m (15–25ft). Mexico to Argentina. ❁ (min. 10°C/50°F)

A. magnifica see *Saritaea magnifica.*

ARRHENATHERUM

Oat grass

GRAMINEAE/POACEAE

Genus of 6 species of deciduous, loosely tufted, perennial grasses from meadows and grassland in Europe, N. Africa, and N. and W. Asia. While most species have unattractive, coarse foliage, and some are invasive, *A. elatius* subsp. *bulbosum* 'Variegatum' is useful for planting among dark-leaved ground cover at the front of a border, or in a rock garden.

• **HARDINESS** Fully hardy.

• **CULTIVATION** Grow in well-drained, fertile soil in full sun or partial shade. Cut to ground level in midsummer; in fertile soil, a second flush of leaves will follow.

• **PROPAGATION** Every third year, divide plants from mid-spring to early summer, to maintain stocks.

• **PESTS AND DISEASES** Prone to rust.

***A. elatius* subsp. *bulbosum* 'Variegatum'** (Bulbous oat grass, Onion couch). Loosely tufted perennial producing chains of small, usually pear-shaped "bulbs" (swollen stem bases), 1cm (½in) across, and erect, narrow, linear, grey-green leaves, to 25cm (10in) long, with bold, white-striped margins. Narrow, silvery green panicles, 20–30cm (8–12in) long, with open, oat-like spikelets, 1cm (½in) long, are borne from midsummer to early autumn. ↕↔ to 30cm (12in). ❄❄❄

▷**Arrow arum** see *Peltandra*
Green see *P. virginica*
White see *P. sagittifolia*

▷**Arrowhead** see *Sagittaria*
Japanese see *S. sagittifolia*

▷**Arrowroot,**
Florida see *Zamia pumila*
Japanese see *Pueraria lobata*

▷**Arrow-wood, Southern** see *Viburnum dentatum*

ARTEMISIA

Mugwort, Sagebrush, Wormwood

ASTERACEAE/COMPOSITAE

Genus of about 300 species of evergreen and deciduous shrubs, perennials, and annuals found in dry fields, prairies, and scrub in the N. hemisphere, with a few from South Africa and W. South America. Artemisias are cultivated for their alternate, variously shaped, often pinnatisect, usually aromatic, grey or silver leaves; the cylindrical flowerheads, 2–8mm (1⁄16–⅜in) across, occasionally solitary, but usually in terminal panicles or racemes, are generally of little interest. They are suitable for a rock garden or border; some have culinary uses and are grown in herb gardens.

• **HARDINESS** Fully hardy to frost hardy.

• **CULTIVATION** Grow in well-drained, fertile soil in full sun. A few, such as *A. lactiflora*, require fairly moist soil. Alpine species prefer sharp drainage; some, such as *A. glacialis*, are best grown in a scree or crevice. Most species die back in heavy, poorly drained soils and may be short-lived. Cut perennials to the bases in autumn; if necessary, cut shrubby species and cultivars back hard in spring to maintain a compact habit.

• **PROPAGATION** Sow seed in containers in a cold frame in autumn or spring. Divide in spring or autumn. Root greenwood cuttings or heel cuttings of side-shoots in early summer. *A.* 'Powis Castle' may not survive severe winters; maintain stocks by regular propagation from cuttings.

• **PESTS AND DISEASES** *A. absinthium*, its cultivars, and *A.* 'Powis Castle' are prone to aphids and gall. *A. lactiflora* is prone to powdery mildew in dry weather.

A. abrotanum ▣🏆 (Lad's love, Old man, Southernwood). Erect, deciduous to semi-evergreen shrub producing aromatic, pinnatisect to 3-pinnatisect, grey-green leaves, to 5cm (2in) long, with thread-like lobes, grey-hairy beneath. Yellowish grey flowerheads are borne in dense panicles, 10–30cm (4–12in) long, in late summer. ↕↔1m (3ft). S. Europe. ❄❄❄

A. absinthium (Absinth, Wormwood). Clump-forming, woody-based perennial producing 2- or 3-pinnatisect, aromatic, silky-hairy, silvery grey leaves, 6–10cm (2½–4in) long, with oblong lobes. Loose panicles, 5–12cm (2–5in) long, of greyish yellow flowerheads are borne

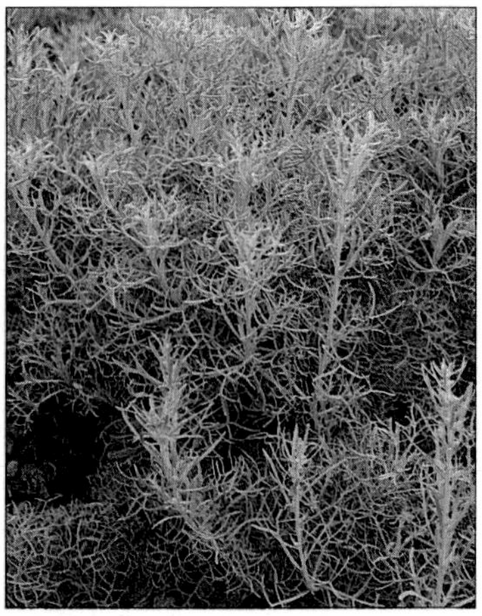

Artemisia alba 'Canescens'

in late summer. ↕90cm (36in), ↔60cm (24in). Europe, temperate Asia. ❄❄❄. **'Lambrook Silver'** 🏆 has deeply divided silver foliage; ↕to 75cm (30in).

***A. alba* 'Canescens'** ▣🏆 syn. *A. canescens, A. splendens, A. vulgaris* 'Canescens'. Clump-forming, semi-evergreen perennial producing pinnatisect to 3-pinnatisect silver leaves, 3–15mm (⅛–½in) long, with slender, curling lobes. Insignificant, brownish yellow flowerheads are borne in panicles, 5–20cm (2–8in) long, in late summer. ↕45cm (18in), ↔30cm (12in). ❄❄❄

A. arborescens ▣ Upright, evergreen shrub with pinnatisect or 2-pinnatisect, aromatic, fern-like, silvery white leaves, to 10cm (4in) long, with linear lobes. Small yellow flowerheads, borne in one-sided panicles, 30cm (12in) long, in summer and autumn, are initially semi-pendent and later erect. Grow against a warm wall in cold areas. ↕1m (3ft), ↔1.5m (5ft). Mediterranean. ❄❄❄. **'Brass Band'** see *A.* 'Powis Castle'.

A. assoana see *A. pedemontana.*

A. canescens see *A. alba* 'Canescens'.

A. discolor see *A. michauxiana.*

A. dracunculus (Tarragon). Clump-forming, subshrubby perennial with aromatic, lance-shaped, light to mid-green leaves, 10cm (4in) long. Insignificant, nodding, yellowish white flowerheads are borne in loose panicles, 5–35cm (2–14in) long, in late summer. The leaves are used for seasoning; European (French) tarragon has a finer flavour than the hardier and more vigorous Russian tarragon, but seldom sets seed. ↕1.2m (4ft), ↔30cm (12in). C. and E. Europe, S. Russia. ❄❄❄

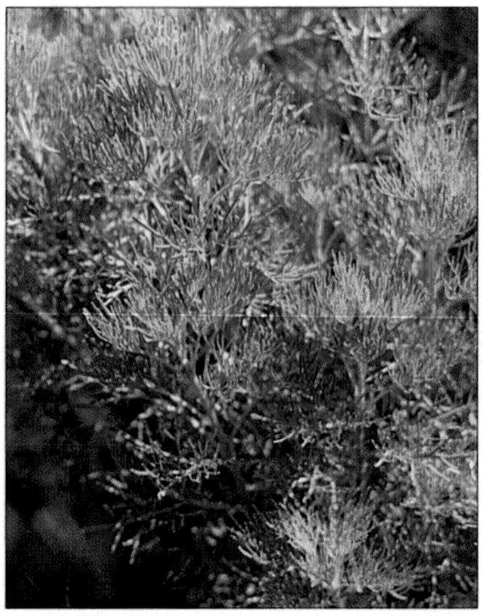

Artemisia abrotanum

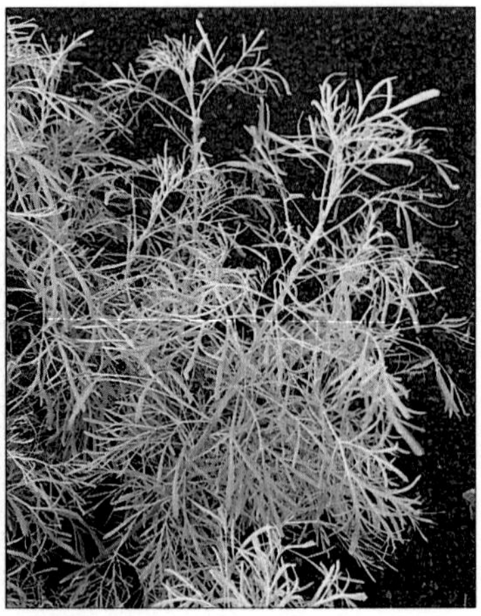

Artemisia arborescens

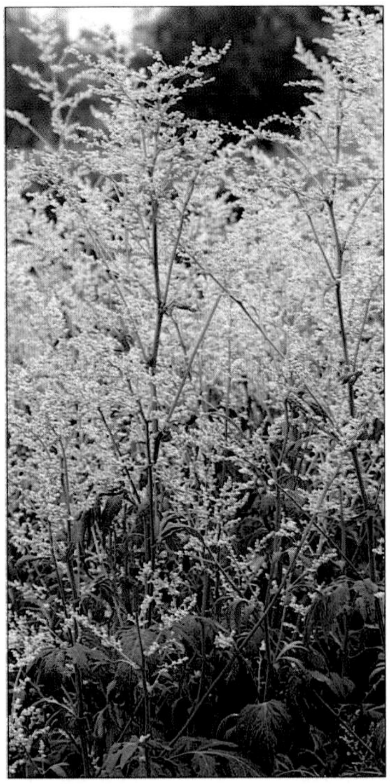

Artemisia lactiflora

A. glacialis. Low, densely tufted perennial with silver-hairy leaves, 1–3cm (½–1¼in) long, finely divided into 5 lobes, each 3-lobed. Bears insignificant yellow flowerheads in corymbs 0.5–2.5cm (¼–1in) across, in summer. Resents winter wet; best in an alpine house or scree bed. ↕ 5cm (2in), ↔ 15–20cm (6–8in). S.W. Alps. ❄❄❄
***A. kitadakensis* 'Guizhou'** see *A. lactiflora* 'Guizhou'.
A. lactiflora ■ ♀ (White mugwort). Clump-forming perennial producing jaggedly cut, pinnatisect, dark green leaves, 20–25cm (8–10in) long, with broadly lance-shaped segments. Spreading panicles, to 60cm (24in) long, of long-lasting, creamy white flowerheads are borne from late summer to mid-autumn. Excellent for a border and for cut or dried flowers. ↕ 1.5m (5ft), ↔ 60cm (24in). W. China. ❄❄❄. **'Guizhou'**, syn. *A. kitadakensis* 'Guizhou', often has purple-flushed stems and young leaves, and bears widely branched white flowerheads.
A. lanata see *A. pedemontana.*
A. ludoviciana, syn. *A. palmeri, A. purshiana* (Western mugwort). Rhizomatous, clump-forming perennial

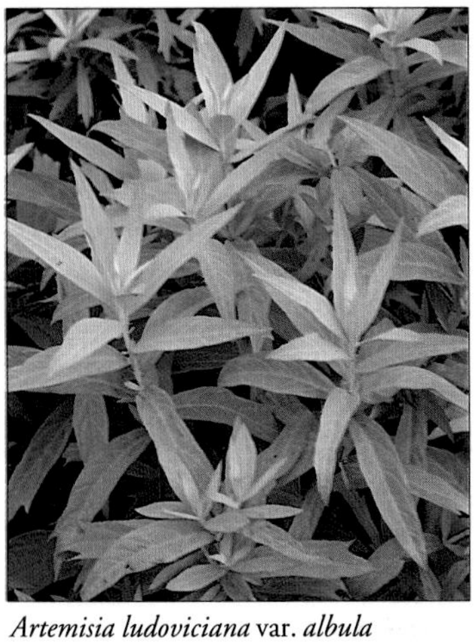

Artemisia ludoviciana var. *albula*

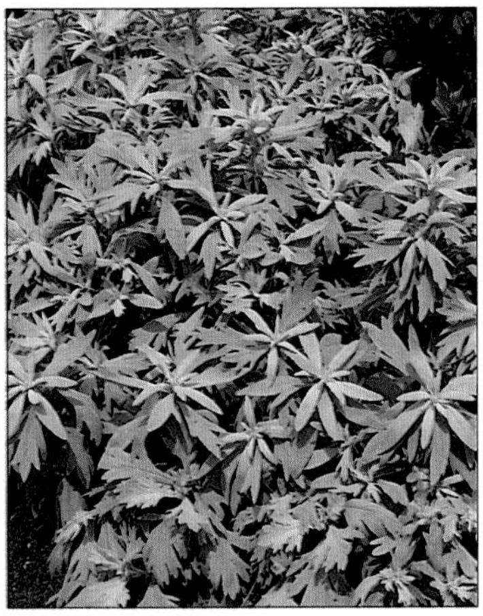

Artemisia ludoviciana 'Silver Queen'

with lance-shaped, downy, silvery white leaves, 10–12cm (4–5in) long, which become greener with age. Densely white-woolly panicles, to 20cm (8in) long, of brownish yellow flowerheads are produced from midsummer to autumn. ↕ 1.2m (4ft), ↔ 60cm (24in) or more. W. North America to Mexico. ❄❄❄. **var. *albula*** ■ has white-woolly leaves. **'Silver Queen'** ■ ♀ produces slightly larger leaves than *A. ludoviciana*, and flowers less freely; ↕ 75cm (30in). **'Valerie Finnis'** ♀ has silvery grey leaves, which have sharply cut margins; ↕ 60cm (24in); USA (California).
A. michauxiana, syn. *A. discolor.* Rhizomatous perennial, slightly woody at the base, producing pinnatisect or 2-pinnatisect leaves, to 3cm (1¼in) long, with slender, linear lobes, green above and white-hairy beneath. In summer, produces nodding yellowish flowerheads in narrow panicles, 5–25cm (2–10in) long. ↕ 45cm (18in), ↔ 60cm (24in). S.W. Canada, W. USA. ❄❄❄
A. nutans see *Seriphidium nutans.*
A. palmeri see *A. ludoviciana.*
A. pedemontana, syn. *A. assoana, A. lanata.* Evergreen or semi-evergreen, tufted, low-growing perennial producing silver-hairy, fern-like, pinnatifid leaves, 4–15mm (⅛–½in) long, with linear lobes. Racemes, 3–15cm (1¼–6in) long, of brownish yellow flowerheads are borne in summer. ↕ to 30cm (12in), ↔ to 45cm (18in). C. Spain to S.E. Ukraine. ❄❄❄
A. pontica ■ ♀ Vigorous, rhizomatous, aromatic, evergreen perennial forming a dense dome of erect, unbranched stems, with pinnatifid or 2-pinnatifid, woolly,

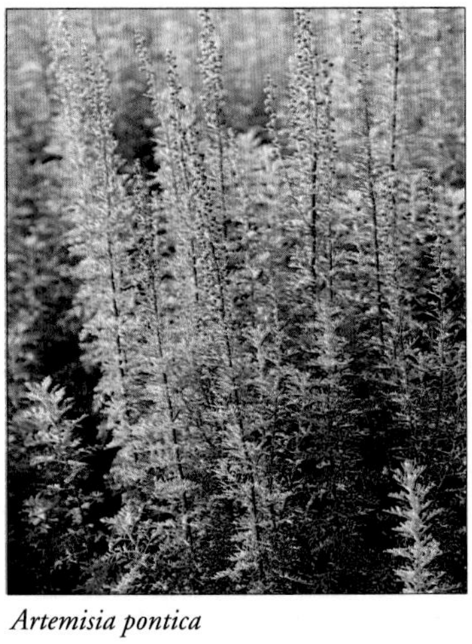

Artemisia pontica

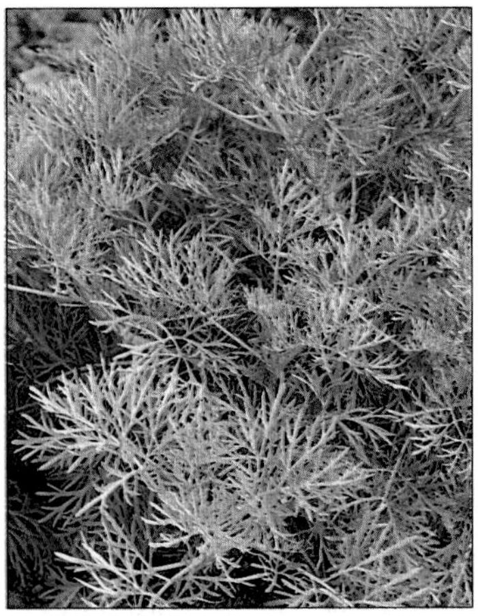

Artemisia 'Powis Castle'

greyish green leaves, 3–4cm (1¼–1½in) long, with narrow, linear lobes. In early summer, greyish yellow flowerheads are produced in panicles 5–20cm (2–8in) long. It is excellent as ground cover in poor soils in full sun. ↕ 40–80cm (16–32in), ↔ indefinite. C. and E. Europe. ❄❄❄
***A.* 'Powis Castle'** ■ ♀ syn. *A. arborescens* 'Brass Band'. Woody-based perennial forming a dense, billowing clump of pinnatisect or 2-pinnatisect, feathery, silver-grey leaves, 6cm (2½in) long, with linear lobes. Panicles, to 15cm (6in) long, of silver, yellow-tinged flowerheads are borne in late summer. ↕ 60cm (24in), ↔ 90cm (36in). ❄❄
A. purshiana see *A. ludoviciana.*
A. schmidtiana ♀ Low, rhizomatous, evergreen, tufted perennial, forming a silver carpet of 2-pinnatisect, silky-hairy leaves, 3–4.5cm (1¼–1¾in) long, with very fine linear lobes. Panicles, to 10cm (4in) long, of small yellow flowerheads are borne in summer. ↕ 30cm (12in), ↔ to 45cm (18in). Japan. ❄❄❄. **'Nana'** ■ ♀ is very similar, but smaller and more compact; ↕ 8cm (3in), ↔ 30cm (12in).
A. splendens see *A. alba* 'Canescens'.
***A. stelleriana* 'Boughton Silver'** ■ syn. *A. stelleriana* 'Mori', *A. stelleriana* 'Silver Brocade'. Compact, almost prostrate, rhizomatous, evergreen perennial with stalkless, deeply toothed or pinnatifid, white-hairy, silvery grey leaves, 5–10cm (2–4in) long. Panicles, 3–8cm (1¼–3in) long, of insignificant yellow flowerheads are borne on erect white stems in late summer and early autumn. ↕ to 15cm (6in), ↔ 30–45cm (12–18in). ❄❄❄

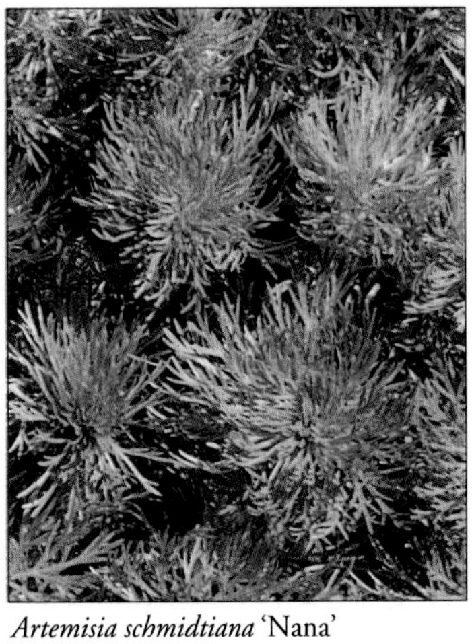

Artemisia schmidtiana 'Nana'

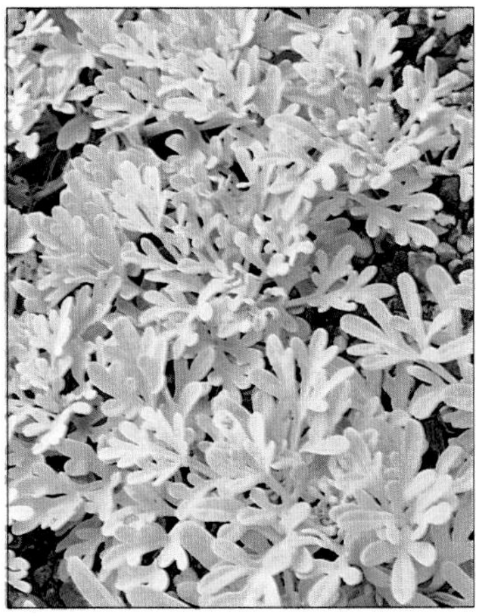

Artemisia stelleriana 'Boughton Silver'

***A. stelleriana* 'Mori'** see *A. stelleriana* 'Boughton Silver'.
***A. stelleriana* 'Silver Brocade'** see *A. stelleriana* 'Boughton Silver'.
A. tridentata see *Seriphidium tridentatum.*
***A. vulgaris* 'Canescens'** see *A. alba* 'Canescens'.

ARTHROPODIUM

ANTHERICACEAE/LILIACEAE

Genus of 12 species of evergreen or deciduous, rhizomatous, tufted perennials, found in a variety of open habitats, mainly in New Zealand and S. Australia. The radical, basally sheathing leaves are simple, entire, and linear to lance-shaped. Loose panicles or racemes of small flowers, with 6 spreading tepals and hairy anthers and filaments, are borne in summer. The hardier species, such as *A. candidum* and *A. milleflorum*, are excellent for a sunny rock garden. Grow half-hardy species, such as *A. cirratum*, in a cool greenhouse or conservatory in frost-prone areas.

• **HARDINESS** Most are frost hardy to half hardy; *A. candidum* and *A. milleflorum* are hardy to -10°C (14°F) with good drainage.

• **CULTIVATION** Under glass, grow in loam-based potting compost (JI No.2) with added sharp sand, in full light. Water moderately in growth, applying a balanced liquid fertilizer monthly; water sparingly in winter. Outdoors, grow in fertile, well-drained, gritty soil in full sun; grow at the base of a warm, sunny wall in frost-prone areas.

• **PROPAGATION** Sow seed in containers in a cold frame in autumn or early spring, or divide in spring. Overwinter young plants under glass.

• **PESTS AND DISEASES** New growth is particularly vulnerable to slugs.

A. candidum, syn. *A. reflexum.* Deciduous, tuberous-rooted perennial with linear, mid-green leaves, 15–20cm (6–8in) long. In early and midsummer, bears small, rounded white flowers, 8mm (⅜in) across, with white-hairy anthers and white filaments, in panicles or racemes, 5–10cm (2–4in) long. ↕ to 20cm (8in), ↔ to 10cm (4in). New Zealand. ❄❄. **'Maculatum'** and **'Purpureum'** are names applied to variants that produce bronze foliage when raised from seed.
A. cirratum, syn. *A. cirrhatum.* Tufted, evergreen perennial with short rhizomes

A

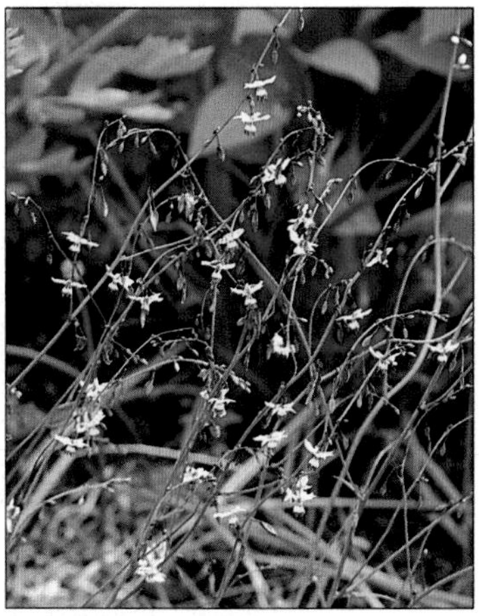

Arthropodium milleflorum

and linear to lance-shaped, channelled, grey-green leaves, 30–60cm (12–24in) long. Nodding, star-shaped white flowers, 2.5cm (1in) across, flecked purple and yellow, with white anthers and filaments are borne in lax panicles, 30cm (12in) long, in early summer. ↕ 90cm (36in), ↔ 30cm (12in). New Zealand. ❄❄
A. cirrhatum see *A. cirratum.*
A. milleflorum ■ syn. *A. millefoliatum, A. paniculatum.* Deciduous perennial with short rhizomes, fibrous roots, and lance-shaped, blue- or grey-green leaves, to 25cm (10in) or more long. In mid-summer, bears loose, branched panicles, 30–60cm (12–24in) long, of star-shaped, pale violet or blue flowers, 1.5cm (½in) across, with creamy white filaments and deep violet anthers. ↕ to 50cm (20in), ↔ to 20cm (8in). Australia (S.E. Australia, Tasmania). ❄❄
A. millefoliatum see *A. milleflorum.*
A. paniculatum see *A. milleflorum.*
A. reflexum see *A. candidum.*

▷**Artichoke, Globe** see *Cynara scolymus*
▷**Artillery plant** see *Pilea microphylla*

Arum

Lords and ladies

ARACEAE

Genus of 26 species of mainly spring-flowering, tuberous perennials found in a range of partially shaded habitats in S. Europe, N. Africa, and W. Asia to the W. Himalayas. They have often attractively marked leaves, which may be spear-, arrow-, or heart-shaped, and which are normally produced in late autumn or winter. Large spathes enclose thin spadices of tiny flowers, either sweetly or unpleasantly scented; these are followed by spikes of red or orange berries. All parts may cause severe discomfort if ingested, and the sap may irritate skin on contact. Some species are good foliage plants for growing with shrubs. The leaves of *A. italicum* 'Marmoratum' are often used in flower arrangements. In frost-prone areas, half-hardy species are best grown under glass.
• **Hardiness** Fully hardy to half hardy.
• **Cultivation** Plant tubers 10–15cm (4–6in) deep in autumn or spring. Under glass, grow in coarse, loamless potting compost with additional grit, in full or filtered light. In the growing season, water freely and apply a balanced liquid fertilizer monthly; reduce water as the leaves wither, and keep almost dry

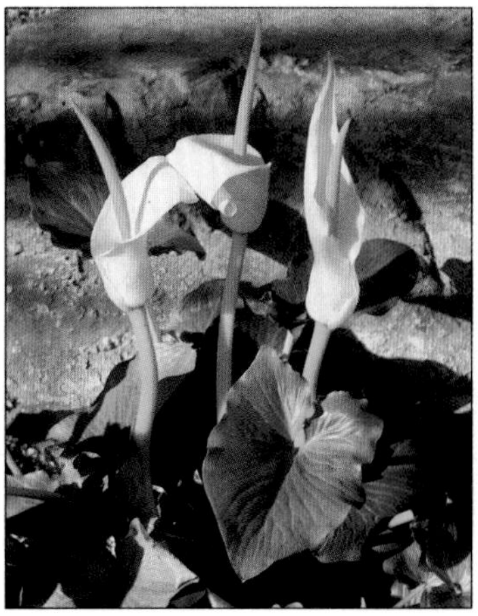

Arum creticum

when dormant. Outdoors, grow in well-drained, humus-rich soil in a sheltered site in sun or partial shade.
• **Propagation** Sow seed in autumn: remove the outer pulp from the berries (it may be caustic) and sow seed in containers in a cold frame. Divide clumps of tubers after flowering.
• **Pests and diseases** Trouble free.

A. creticum ■ Tuberous perennial bearing showy, creamy white or deep yellow spathes, 15–25cm (6–10in) long, in spring; they recurve at the tip to reveal stout, pale to deep yellow, sweetly scented spadices. The arrow-shaped leaves, 18–26cm (7–10in) long, are unmarked and dark green. Needs full sun. ↕ 30–50cm (12–20in), ↔ 15cm (6in). Greece (Crete). ❄❄

A. dioscoridis. Variable, tuberous perennial bearing large, deep purple or pale green spathes, 15–35cm (6–14in) long, in spring; they are stained or spotted dark maroon-purple and have unpleasantly scented spadices. Narrow, arrow- to spear-shaped leaves, 27–45cm (11–18in) long, are dark green. Requires full sun. ↕ 20–30cm (8–12in), ↔ 15cm (6in). E. Mediterranean. ❄❄
A. dracunculus see *Dracunculus vulgaris.*
A. hygrophilum. Tuberous perennial bearing green spathes, 5–13cm (2–5in) long, with purple-flushed margins and deep purple spadices, in late spring. The variable, spear-shaped leaves, 14–45cm (5½–18in) long, are light to mid-green. Best in a cool greenhouse in frost-prone areas. ↕ 15cm (6in), ↔ 15cm (6in). Morocco, Cyprus, Lebanon. ❄❄
A. italicum. Tuberous perennial with arrow- to spear-shaped, mid-green, white-veined leaves, to 35cm (14in) long, lasting from winter to late spring. In early summer, bears pale greenish white spathes, 15–40cm (6–16in) long, followed by spikes of bright orange-red berries, which may last until new leaves develop. Produces largest leaves in a partially shaded site; needs an open, sunny site to flower well. ↕ 30cm (12in), ↔ 15cm (6in). Europe, Turkey, N. Africa. ❄❄❄. **subsp. *albispathum*** has plain green leaves, to 20cm (8in) long, and white spathes; Crimea, Caucasus. **'Marmoratum'** ■ 🏆 syn. 'Pictum', has pale green or cream-veined leaves.
A. pictum. Tuberous perennial bearing blackish purple spathes, 15–25cm (6–10in) long, with short spadices, in autumn. Arrow- to heart-shaped leaves, 30cm (12in) long, are leathery, glossy, dark green, often with fine creamy white veins. Best grown in an alpine house in frost-prone areas. ↕ 15–25cm (6–10in), ↔ 15cm (6in). Balearic Islands, France (Corsica), W. central Italy, Sardinia. ❄

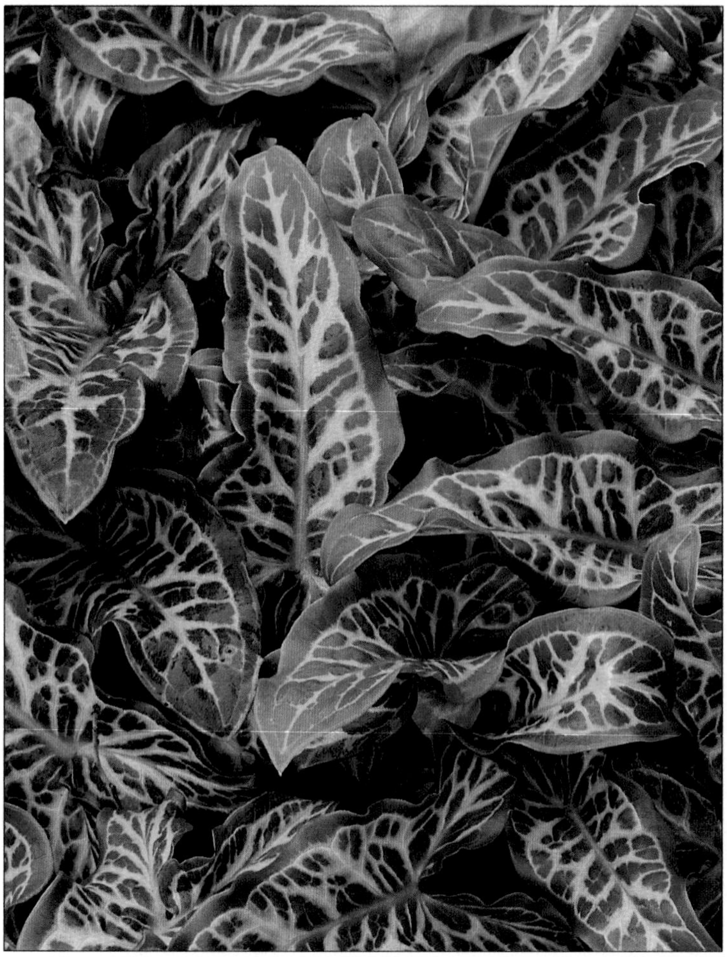

Arum italicum 'Marmoratum'

▷**Arum,**
Arrow see *Peltandra*
Bog see *Calla palustris*
Dragon see *Dracunculus vulgaris*
Golden see *Zantedeschia elliottiana*
Pink see *Zantedeschia rehmannii*
Umbrella see *Amorphophallus konjac*
▷**Arum lily** see *Zantedeschia, Z. aethiopica*

Aruncus

ROSACEAE

Genus of 2 or 3 species of clump-forming perennials with short rhizomes, closely related to *Filipendula* and *Spiraea*, from moist woodland, often in mountainous areas, in the N. hemisphere. They have alternate, pinnate leaves with long leaf-stalks and boldly veined, toothed leaflets. Tiny, unisexual (occasionally bisexual), white or creamy white flowers, to 5mm (¼in) across, are borne in terminal panicles above the leaves, and are useful for cutting. Grow in a moist border or woodland garden.
• **Hardiness** Fully hardy.
• **Cultivation** Grow in moist, fertile soil in full or partial shade. *A. dioicus* will tolerate drier conditions in full sun.
• **Propagation** Sow seed in containers in a cold frame in autumn or spring; will self-seed freely unless dead-headed. Divide in early spring or autumn.
• **Pests and diseases** Blackfly and sawfly larvae may be a problem.

A. aethusifolius. Compact perennial with 3- or 4-pinnate, mid-green leaves, to 25cm (10in) long, with ovate, deeply cut leaflets, turning yellow in autumn. Bears panicles, 5–15cm (2–6in) long, of numerous tiny, creamy white flowers in early and midsummer. ↕↔ 25–40cm (10–16in). Korea. ❄❄❄
A. dioicus ■ 🏆 syn. *A. sylvester, Spiraea aruncus* (Goatsbeard). Dioecious perennial producing 2-pinnate, toothed, hairless, fern-like, mid-green leaves, to 1m (3ft) long, with ovate leaflets. Flowers are borne in loose, pyramidal panicles, to 50cm (20in) long, in early and midsummer. The male inflorescences are creamy white; the females are more pendent and greenish

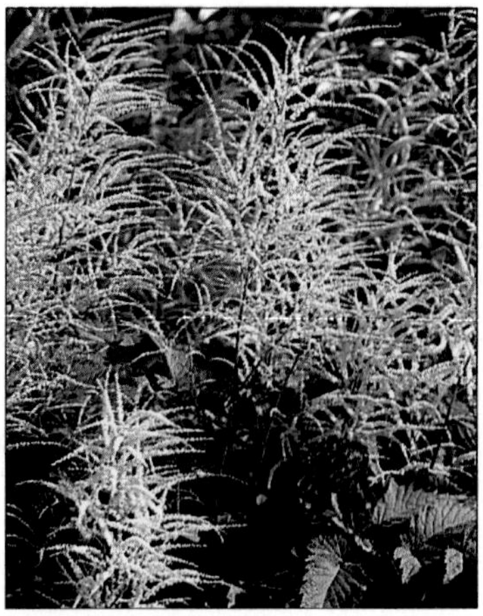

Aruncus dioicus

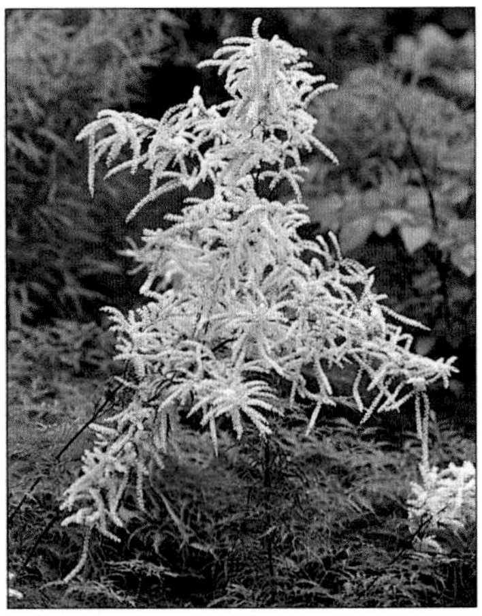

Aruncus dioicus 'Kneiffii'

white. ↕ to 2m (6ft), ↔ 1.2m (4ft). Europe to E. Siberia, E. North America. ❄❄❄. **'Kneiffii'** ■ has very finely divided, fern-like leaves, and bears tiny, nodding cream flowers on arching, wiry stems; ↕ 1.2m (4ft), ↔ 45cm (18in).
A. sylvester see *A. dioicus.*

ARUNDINARIA

GRAMINEAE/POACEAE

Genus of 1 or 2 species of bamboo from swampy areas in S.E. USA. They have spreading rhizomes and stout, rigid canes, 1.5–10m (5–30ft) high, which are simple in the first year, then branching in the second. The persistent cane sheaths produce 3–6 leafy branches from each node. Lateral panicles of 5–15 flower spikelets are borne among the branches at various times of the year. Grow as a dense hedge or screen.
• **HARDINESS** Hardy to -12°C (10°F), but needs warmer conditions to thrive.
• **CULTIVATION** Grow in moist, fertile, humus-rich soil in a sheltered position in sun or partial shade.
• **PROPAGATION** Divide in spring.
• **PESTS AND DISEASES** Prone to aphids.

A. anceps see *Yushania anceps.*
A. auricoma see *Pleioblastus auricomus.*
A. disticha see *Pleioblastus pygmaeus* var. *distichus.*
A. falconeri see *Himalayacalamus falconeri.*
A. fastuosa see *Semiarundinaria fastuosa.*
A. fortunei see *Pleioblastus variegatus.*
A. gigantea, syn. *A. macrosperma, A. tecta* (Canebrake). Rapidly spreading bamboo with yellow-green canes, lance-shaped leaves, to 20cm (8in) long, and lateral panicles of purple spikelets. Shorter plants that develop flowering panicles directly from the rhizomes are sometimes also sold as *A. tecta.* ↕ to 10m (30ft), ↔ indefinite. S.E. USA. ❄❄
A. humilis see *Pleioblastus humilis.*
A. jaunsarensis see *Yushania anceps.*
A. macrosperma see *A. gigantea.*
A. murieliae see *Fargesia murieliae.*
A. nitida see *Fargesia nitida.*
A. pygmaea see *Pleioblastus pygmaeus.*
A. quadrangularis see *Chimonobambusa quadrangularis.*
***A. simonii* 'Variegata'** see *Pleioblastus simonii* 'Variegatus'.
A. tecta see *A. gigantea.*
A. vagans see *Sasa ramosa.*
A. variegata see *Pleioblastus variegatus.*
A. viridistriata see *Pleioblastus auricomus.*

ARUNDO

GRAMINEAE/POACEAE

Genus of 2 or possibly 3 species of evergreen, rhizomatous, perennial grasses from riversides and ditches in warm-temperate regions of the N. hemisphere. They have alternate, broadly linear, flat leaves, borne on thick, reed-like stems, and terminal, feathery flower panicles. *A. donax* is grown for its attractive, bamboo-like foliage. In frost-prone areas, the variegated cultivars are ideal for a cool conservatory or greenhouse. In warmer areas, use as specimen plants or at the back of a large border.
• **HARDINESS** *A. donax* is hardy to about -12°C (10°F); variegated cultivars are half hardy.
• **CULTIVATION** Under glass, grow variegated cultivars in permanently moist, loamless potting compost in full light. Outdoors, *A. donax* grows well in any soil, but thrives in moist conditions in full sun, with protection from strong winds. For best foliage, cut back annually to the bases. To encourage flowering, cut down stems after their second year.
• **PROPAGATION** Sow seed of *A. donax* in containers in a cold frame in spring. Divide the rootstock from mid-spring to early summer. Root sections of stems in a water-filled tray from mid-spring to midsummer; pot up and keep moist.
• **PESTS AND DISEASES** Trouble free.

A. conspicua see *Chionochloa conspicua.*
A. donax (Giant reed). Clump-forming, rhizomatous perennial with stout stems and arching, broadly linear, mid-green, glaucous leaves, to 60cm (24in) long. In mid- and late autumn, produces terminal panicles of light green to purple spikelets, to 60cm (24in) long. ↕ 5m (15ft), ↔ 1.5m (5ft) or more. S. Europe. ❄❄❄ (borderline). **'Variegata'** see var. *versicolor.* **'Variegata Superba'** has wide leaves, 4–6cm (1½–2½in) across, and to 30cm (12in) long, striped and margined white; ↕ to 1m (3ft), ↔ indefinite; ❄. **var. *versicolor***, syn. 'Variegata', produces white-striped leaves; ↕ to 1.8m (6ft), more in mild climates, ↔ 60cm (24in); ❄

▷**Asarabacca** see *Asarum europaeum*

ASARINA

SCROPHULARIACEAE

Genus of one species of trailing, evergreen perennial, with softly sticky-hairy leaves, occurring among shaded rocks in the Pyrenees. *A. procumbens* is cultivated for its attractive, 2-lipped flowers, which resemble those of snapdragons (*Antirrhinum*). They are produced singly from the upper leaf axils over long periods in summer. It will trail effectively over shady walls or rocks, the side of a raised bed, or a shady bank.
• **HARDINESS** Hardy to -10°C (14°F).
• **CULTIVATION** Grow in fertile, well-drained, sandy soil in partial shade.
• **PROPAGATION** Sow seed at 16°C (61°F) in early spring, or root tip cuttings in summer.
• **PESTS AND DISEASES** Trouble free.

A. antirrhiniflora see *Maurandella antirrhiniflora.*

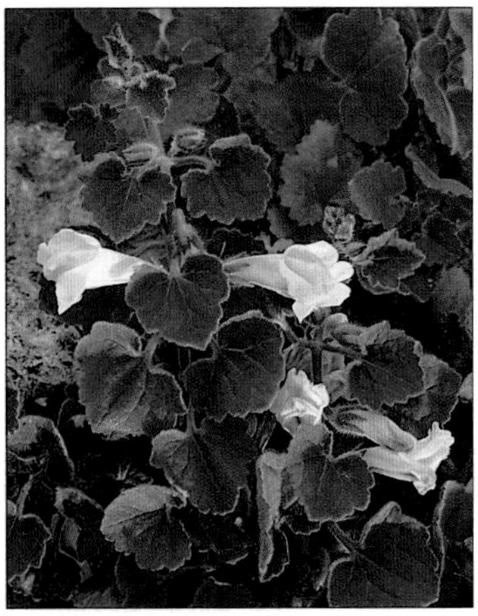

Asarina procumbens

A. barclayana see *Maurandya barclayana.*
A. erubescens see *Lophospermum erubescens.*
A. procumbens ■ syn. *Antirrhinum asarina.* Trailing, evergreen perennial with opposite pairs of shallowly lobed, kidney-shaped, hairy, grey-green leaves, to 6cm (2½in) long, on brittle stems. Pale yellow "snapdragon" flowers, to 3.5cm (1½in) long, with deep yellow throats and light purple veining, are produced in summer. Tolerates partial shade. ↕ 5cm (2in), ↔ to 60cm (24in). Pyrenees. ❄❄. **'Iberian Trail'** is a seed-raised cultivar of the species.
A. purpusii see *Maurandya purpusii.*

ASARUM

syn. HETEROTROPA, HEXASTYLIS
Wild ginger

ARISTOLOCHIACEAE

Genus of about 70 species of mainly evergreen, low-growing, rhizomatous perennials occurring in woodland in Europe, E. Asia, and North America. They have large, usually glossy, sometimes marbled leaves, concealing mildly malodorous, pitcher-shaped flowers, some with 3 slender, tail-like petal tips. Use as ground cover at the edge of a border or grow among shrubs. The rhizomes are aromatic, smelling rather like ginger.
• **HARDINESS** Fully hardy, but may shed leaves below -15°C (5°F).
• **CULTIVATION** Grow in partial to full shade in moderately fertile, humus-rich, moist but well-drained, preferably neutral to acid soil.
• **PROPAGATION** Sow seed in containers in a cold frame as soon as ripe. Some species self-seed freely. Divide in early spring.
• **PESTS AND DISEASES** Slugs and snails may be a problem, especially in spring.

A. europaeum ■ (Asarabacca). Evergreen, creeping, rhizomatous perennial, forming carpets of kidney-shaped, glossy, dark green leaves, 5–8cm (2–3in) long. These conceal small, narrowly bell-shaped, short-lobed, greenish purple then brown flowers, 1.5–2cm (½–¾in) long, borne in late spring. ↕ 8cm (3in), ↔ to 30cm (12in) or more. W. Europe. ❄❄❄
A. hartwegii, syn. *A. marmoratum.* Evergreen, prostrate, rhizomatous perennial with heart-shaped, pointed, dark green-bronze leaves, 6–12cm

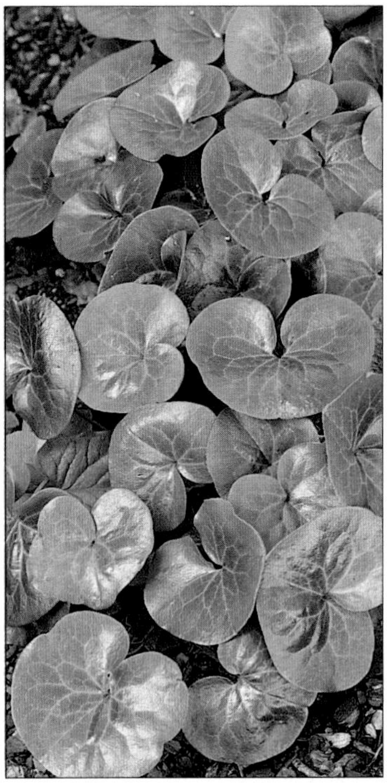

Asarum europaeum

(2½–5in) long, attractively marbled silvery green along the veins. Broadly tubular, brownish purple flowers, to 5cm (2in) or more long, with long, slender lobes, are produced in early summer. ↕ 8cm (3in), ↔ to 30cm (12in) or more. USA (California, Oregon). ❄❄❄
A. marmoratum see *A. hartwegii.*
A. shuttleworthii. Evergreen, prostrate, rhizomatous perennial with broadly heart-shaped, shiny, dark green, often silver-marbled leaves, 2.5–10cm (1–4in) long. Broadly tubular, purple-brown flowers, 1.5–4cm (½–1½in) long, with triangular lobes, patterned purple-red and cream within, are borne in early summer. ↕ 8cm (3in), ↔ to 30cm (12in) or more. S.E. USA. ❄❄❄

ASCLEPIAS

Milkweed, Silkweed

ASCLEPIADACEAE

Genus of about 110 species of evergreen or deciduous, clump-forming, sometimes spreading perennials, and a few subshrubs and shrubs, mainly from well-drained soils in scrub or grassland, some from marsh, wet scrub, and lakeside areas, in South Africa, temperate North America, and tropical North and South America. They have simple, narrowly elliptic to lance-shaped or ovate, opposite or alternate, sometimes spirally arranged leaves and umbel-like cymes of numerous small flowers, to 2.5cm (1in) across. The corolla lobes reflex to display the unusual, upright, horn-like, staminal appendages. The flowers are followed by pairs of spindle-shaped green fruits, variable in length, which ripen to yellowish brown, and split open to expose rows of seeds with long, silky white hairs, giving rise to the common name, silkweed. Asclepias are attractive to bees and are showy plants for a border or wildflower garden. In frost-prone areas, grow tender species in a cool or temperate greenhouse. Contact with the milky sap may irritate skin.

A

• **HARDINESS** Fully hardy to frost tender.
• **CULTIVATION** Under glass, grow in loam-based potting compost (JI No.2), with additional leaf mould, in full light. During the growing season, water freely and apply a balanced liquid fertilizer every 5–6 weeks; reduce water after flowering and keep almost dry in winter. Outdoors, grow in fertile, well-drained, loamy soil in full sun, although *A. incarnata* and *A. speciosa* prefer more moisture and will thrive near a pond or stream. Grow *A. hallii* and *A. syriaca* in a wildflower garden, because they spread by underground suckers and are unsuitable for a border.
• **PROPAGATION** Sow seed of tender species at 16–18°C (61–64°F) in late winter. Sow seed of perennials in containers in a cold frame in early spring, or divide in spring. Root basal cuttings in spring.
• **PESTS AND DISEASES** Whiteflies may be a problem under glass.

A. curassavica ▣ (Blood flower, Indian root, Swallow-wort). Evergreen subshrub, often grown as an annual, with upright branches and opposite, elliptic-lance-shaped, mid-green leaves, to 15cm (6in) long. Axillary or near-terminal, umbel-like cymes, 5–10cm (2–4in) across, of red or orange-red flowers, sometimes yellow or white, with orange-yellow hoods, are borne from summer to autumn. They are followed by erect fruit, to 8cm (3in) long. ↕ 1m (3ft), ↔ 60cm (24in). South America. ❁ (min. 7°C/45°F)
A. fruticosa see *Gomphocarpus fruticosus*.
A. hallii. Vigorous perennial with upright stems, spreading, fleshy roots, and alternate, lance-shaped, dark green leaves, 12cm (5in) long. Semi-pendent, terminal cymes, 5–8cm (2–3in) across, of deep pink flowers, are produced in mid- and late summer. The flowers are followed by erect fruit, to 15cm (6in) long. ↕ 90cm (36in), ↔ 60cm (24in). W. USA. ***
A. incarnata ▣ (Swamp milkweed). Thick-stemmed perennial with dense branches and opposite, narrowly elliptic to ovate, mid-green leaves, 7–15cm (3–6in) long. Clustered, umbel-like cymes, 5cm (2in) across, of pinkish purple flowers, with paler "horns", are produced from the upper leaf axils from midsummer to early autumn. The flowers are followed by erect fruit, to 7cm (3in) long. ↕ 1.2m (4ft), ↔ 60cm (24in). N.E. to S.E. USA. ***

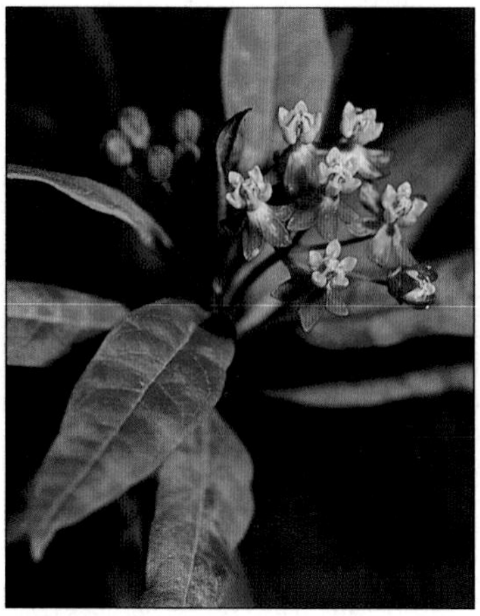

Asclepias curassavica

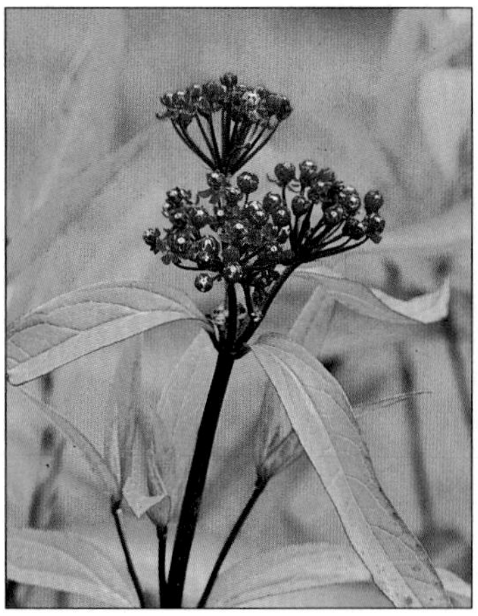

Asclepias incarnata

A. lanceolata. Erect, tuberous perennial with slender stems and opposite, lance-shaped, mid-green leaves, to 25cm (10in) long. Bears terminal, umbel-like cymes, 8–10cm (3–4in) across, of bright red flowers (orange or yellow in some garden cultivars) in mid- and late summer. They are followed by erect fruit, to 10cm (4in) across. ↕ 1.5m (5ft), ↔ 75cm (30in). S.W. USA. ***
A. physocarpa see *Gomphocarpus physocarpus*.
A. speciosa. Erect, softly hairy perennial with opposite, oblong-ovate, grey-white, woolly leaves, 8–20cm (3–8in) long. Numerous axillary, umbel-like cymes, 3–8cm (1¼–3in) across, of purple-pink flowers are borne in summer, and are followed by densely hairy, semi-pendent or pendent fruit, 6–10cm (2½–4in) long. ↕ 75cm (30in), ↔ 60cm (24in). W. and C. North America. ***
A. syriaca. Vigorous, softly hairy perennial with spreading, fleshy roots and upright stems with opposite, oblong-ovate leaves, 10–25cm (4–10in) long, mid-green above and blue-green beneath. In summer, bears scented, greenish purple and pink, occasionally white flowers in axillary, nodding, umbel-like cymes, 5cm (2in) across.

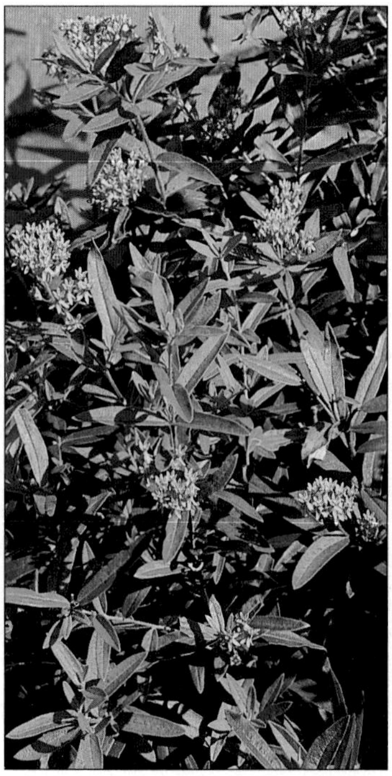

Asclepias tuberosa

These are followed by pendent, softly spiny fruit, to 12cm (5in) long. ↕ to 2m (6ft), ↔ indefinite. E. North America. ***
A. tuberosa ▣ (Butterfly weed). Tuberous, hairy perennial with stout, unbranched stems bearing numerous spirally arranged, lance-shaped to oblong-ovate, light to mid-green leaves, 10–14cm (4–5½in) long. Bears axillary and terminal, umbel-like cymes, 4–5cm (1½–2in) across, of orange-red, sometimes orange or yellow flowers, from midsummer to early autumn; they are followed by fruit 9–13cm (3½–5in) long, on nodding stalks. ↕ 90cm (36in), ↔ 30cm (12in). E. and S. North America. ***

x ASCOCENDA

ORCHIDACEAE

Bigeneric hybrid genus, a cross between *Ascocentrum* and *Vanda*, of several hundred compact, evergreen, epiphytic orchids, derived from species originally growing wild in Burma, India, and the Philippines. They have upright rhizomes producing semi-rigid, narrowly oval leaves, and axillary racemes of 6–8 delicate, open flowers, which are borne freely over long periods of the year, although mainly in winter. The flowers are often richly coloured and attractively overlaid with contrasting colours.
• **HARDINESS** Frost tender.
• **CULTIVATION** Warm-growing orchids. Grow in epiphytic orchid compost, ideally in slatted baskets. Provide full light and high humidity throughout the year, with shade from hot sun in spring and summer. In summer, water freely, mist twice daily, and apply a balanced liquid fertilizer at every third watering; water moderately in winter. See also p.46.
• **PROPAGATION** Plants occasionally produce basal shoots, which can be separated when rooted.
• **PESTS AND DISEASES** Aphids, red spider mites, and mealybugs may be a problem.

x *A.* Dong Tarn ▣ (x *A.* Eileen Beauty x x *A.* Medasand). Compact, evergreen, epiphytic orchid producing alternate, 2-ranked, mid-green leaves. Upright racemes of many bright red flowers, 6cm (2½in) across, flecked deep maroon and touched magenta and yellow, are borne in winter. ↕ 30cm (12in), ↔ 23cm (9in). ❁ (min. 18°C/64°F; max. 30°C/86°F)

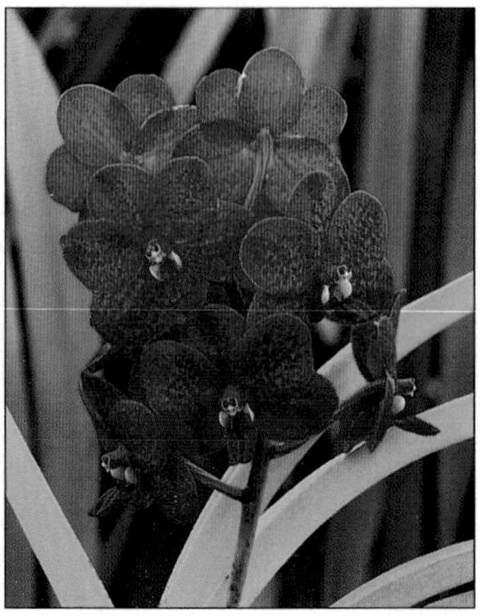

x *Ascocenda* Dong Tarn

ASCOCENTRUM

ORCHIDACEAE

Genus of 5 species of evergreen, epiphytic, monopodial orchids from the Himalayas to S.E. Asia and the Philippines. They have upright stems and 2-ranked, rigid, linear or strap-shaped leaves. They are grown for their axillary racemes of numerous brightly coloured flowers, 1–2cm (½–¾in) across, borne in spring and summer.
• **HARDINESS** Frost tender.
• **CULTIVATION** Warm-growing orchids. Grow in epiphytic orchid compost in containers or slatted baskets. Provide full light and high humidity all year, with shade from hot sun in spring and summer. In summer, water freely, mist twice daily, and apply a balanced liquid fertilizer at every third watering; water moderately in winter. See also p.46.
• **PROPAGATION** Plants occasionally produce basal shoots, which can be separated when rooted.
• **PESTS AND DISEASES** Prone to aphids, red spider mites, and mealybugs.

A. ampullaceum. Evergreen, epiphytic orchid with strap-shaped, dark green leaves, 10–12cm (4–5in) long. In early summer, bears bright rose-pink, spurred flowers, 1–2cm (½–¾in) across, in racemes 10cm (4in) long. ↕ 12cm (5in), ↔ 20cm (8in). Himalayas, Burma, Thailand. ❁ (min. 16–18°C/61–64°F; max. 30°C/86°F)

▷**Ash** see *Fraxinus*
American mountain see *Sorbus americana*
Arizona see *Fraxinus velutina*
Claret see *Fraxinus angustifolia* 'Raywood'
Common see *Fraxinus excelsior*
Green see *Fraxinus pennsylvanica*
Korean mountain see *Sorbus alnifolia*
Manna see *Fraxinus ornus*
Mountain see *Sorbus aucuparia*
Narrow-leaved see *Fraxinus angustifolia*
One-leaved see *Fraxinus excelsior* f. *diversifolia*
Oregon see *Fraxinus latifolia*
Red see *Fraxinus pennsylvanica*
Velvet see *Fraxinus velutina*
Weeping see *Fraxinus excelsior* 'Pendula'
White see *Fraxinus americana*

ASIMINA

ANNONACEAE

Genus of 8 species of deciduous and evergreen shrubs or small trees found in rich, moist soils in thickets and woodland, mainly in southern parts of E. North America. Their leaves are entire and alternate. *A. triloba*, the only species cultivated, has striking foliage, curious, solitary flowers, borne on the previous year's shoots, and edible fruit. Suitable for a shrub border or a sunny woodland clearing, it needs long, hot summers to achieve tree stature, and to flower and fruit freely. In cooler climates, it is grown as a multi-stemmed foliage shrub.
• **HARDINESS** Fully hardy.
• **CULTIVATION** Grow in moist but well-drained, fertile, humus-rich, neutral to acid soil, in full sun. Pruning group 1.

• **PROPAGATION** Sow seed in autumn in a seedbed, or stratify in moist sand at 5°C (41°F) for 90 days, and sow in spring. Alternatively, layer in autumn or insert root cuttings in winter.
• **PESTS AND DISEASES** Trouble free.

A. triloba ♀ (Pawpaw). Deciduous shrub or small tree with obovate, mid-green leaves, to 30cm (12in) long, turning yellow in autumn. Cup-shaped flowers, 3–5cm (1¼–2in) across, each with 3 large calyx lobes surrounding 6 purple-brown petals (3 large and 3 small), are borne singly or in small clusters in late spring. Ovoid, bottle-shaped, edible fruit, to 12cm (5in) long, are yellow-green, ripening to yellow-brown. ↕↔ 6m (20ft). E. USA. ✲✲✲

ASPARAGUS

ASPARAGACEAE/LILIACEAE

Genus of about 300 species of evergreen and deciduous perennials, climbers, and subshrubs from sandy and coastal sites in Europe, Asia, and Africa. They usually have spindle-shaped tubers or tuber-like rootstocks. Arching and spreading or climbing stems bear scale-like true leaves and more prominent leaf-like stems, which in some species have straight or curved spines. Slightly scented, white or pink flowers, borne singly or in racemes or small clusters, are followed by red, orange, or purple berries, 1cm (½in) across. In frost-prone regions, grow as houseplants or in a cool or temperate greenhouse. In frost-free climates, grow in a border, or train climbers on a trellis. The foliage is useful for floral arrangements.
• **HARDINESS** Fully hardy to frost tender.
• **CULTIVATION** Under glass, grow in loam-based potting compost (JI No.2) in bright filtered light, with shade from hot sun. Water freely from early spring to mid-autumn, applying a balanced liquid fertilizer monthly; water more sparingly in winter. Pot on in spring. Provide support for climbers. Outdoors, grow in fertile, moist but well-drained soil in a sheltered site in partial shade.
• **PROPAGATION** Sow seed at 16°C (61°F) in autumn or early spring. Divide clusters of tubers in early spring.
• **PESTS AND DISEASES** Red spider mites and scale insects may be a problem.

A. densiflorus (Asparagus fern). Evergreen, arching, tuberous perennial with feathery, linear, leaf-like, light green

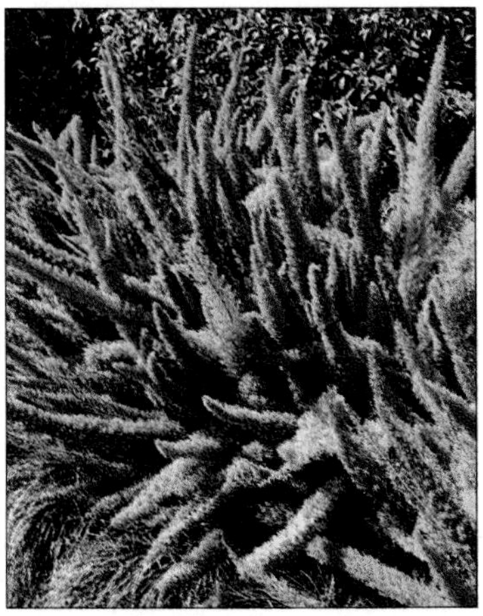

Asparagus densiflorus 'Myersii'

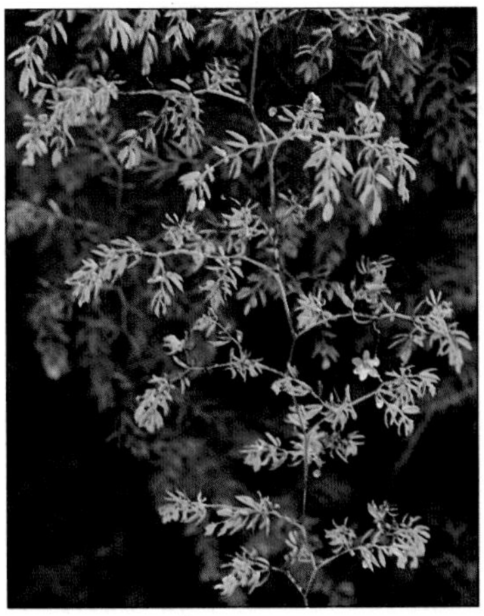

Asparagus scandens

stems, to 1.5cm (½in) long. In summer, bears axillary racemes of small white flowers followed by bright red berries. ↕ 60–90cm (24–36in), ↔ 1–1.2m (3–4ft). South Africa. ❀ (min. 7°C/45°F). **'Myersii'** ■ 🏆 syn. *A. meyeri*, *A.* 'Myers' (Foxtail fern), has dense, arching, foxtail-like fronds, 30–40cm (12–16in) long, of needle-like, leaf-like stems, each 2–2.5cm (¾–1in) long; ↕ 40cm (16in). **'Sprengeri'** 🏆 syn. *A. sprengeri* (Emerald feather, Emerald fern), has arching then pendent stems, giving an open, loose appearance, and needle-like, leaf-like stems, 5–15mm (¼–½in) long, borne in groups of 3.
A. meyeri see *A. densiflorus* 'Myersii'.
***A.* 'Myers'** see *A. densiflorus* 'Myersii'.
A. plumosus see *A. setaceus.*
A. scandens ■ Scrambling or climbing perennial producing fern-like foliage, with 2, or whorls of 3, lance- to sickle-shaped, light green, leaf-like stems, to 1.5cm (½in) long. Tiny, nodding, white, sometimes pink-flushed flowers are produced singly from the leaf axils in summer, and followed by red berries. ↕ 2m (6ft). South Africa. ✲
A. setaceus 🏆 syn. *A. plumosus* (Asparagus fern). Twining climber when mature (bushy at first), with feathery foliage, consisting of clusters of up to 20 bristle-like, leaf-like, deep green stems, 1cm (½in) long. Produces solitary, tiny, nodding white flowers from the leaf axils in summer, followed by purple-black berries. ↕ 3m (10ft). South Africa. ✲
A. sprengeri see *A. densiflorus* 'Sprengeri'.

▷**Asparagus, Bath** see *Ornithogalum pyrenaicum*
▷**Aspen** see *Populus*
American see *P. tremuloides*
Bigtooth see *P. grandidentata*
Common see *P. tremula*
Quaking see *P. tremuloides*
Weeping see *P. tremula* 'Pendula'

ASPERULA

Woodruff

RUBIACEAE

Genus of about 100 species of annuals, evergreen or deciduous perennials, and dwarf shrubs, from woodland and mountain sites, mainly in Europe and Asia. The stalkless leaves are opposite or whorled. Tubular or funnel-shaped flowers, with widely spreading lobes, are borne in branched, terminal or axillary panicles or cymes in spring or summer.

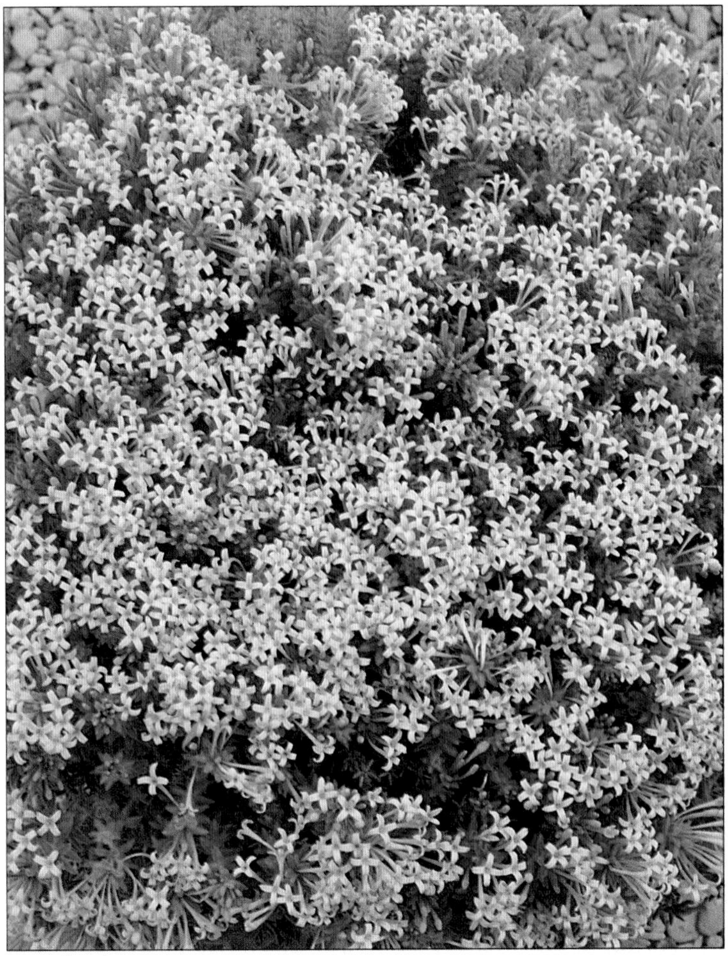

Asperula suberosa

Grow dwarf shrub or perennial species in an alpine house, or in a rock garden, a trough, tufa, or a scree bed. *A. orientalis* is useful for an annual border, and for cut flowers.
• **HARDINESS** Fully hardy, if protected from winter wet.
• **CULTIVATION** All are lime-tolerant. Under glass, grow perennials and dwarf shrubs in gritty, loam-based potting compost (JI No.1). Outdoors, grow in sharply drained, moderately fertile soil in sun or partial shade. Protect from excessive winter wet. Some perennials, especially *A. suberosa*, are very brittle.
• **PROPAGATION** Sow seed of perennials in an open frame in autumn; sow seed of annuals *in situ* in spring. Divide in spring or autumn, or root softwood cuttings in early summer.
• **PESTS AND DISEASES** Susceptible to aphids and red spider mites under glass.

A. aristata* subsp. *thessala see *A. sintenisii.*
***A. athoa* of gardens** see *A. suberosa.*
A. azurea see *A. orientalis.*
A. gussonii. Densely tufted, mat-forming, woody-based, evergreen perennial with whorls of narrowly ovate-oblong to linear, glaucous green leaves, 5–10mm (¼–½in) long. Bears clusters of tubular, deep pink flowers, to 5mm (¼in) long, in late spring and early summer. ↕ to 5cm (2in), ↔ to 15cm (6in). Italy (mountains in Sicily). ✲✲✲
A. nitida. Tufted, cushion-forming, evergreen perennial with rosettes of whorled, linear to lance-shaped, rich green leaves, to 1.5cm (½in) long. Few-flowered, terminal cymes of narrowly tubular pink flowers, to 8mm (⅜in) long, are produced in early summer. ↕ 10cm (4in), ↔ to 20cm (8in). Mountains of Greece and Turkey. ✲✲✲. **subsp. *hirtella***, syn. subsp. *puberula*, is very similar, but has leaves fringed with fine hairs. It is sometimes confused with *A. sintenisii.*
A. odorata see *Galium odoratum.*
A. orientalis, syn. *A. azurea.* Upright, then spreading annual with whorls of obovate to oblong-lance-shaped, bristly, mid-green leaves, to 2.5cm (1in) long. Powderpuff-like, flattened cymes of sweetly scented, tubular, bright blue, occasionally white flowers, 9mm (⅜in) long, are borne in summer. ↕ 30cm (12in), ↔ 8–10cm (3–4in). Caucasus, Syria, Iran, Iraq. ✲✲✲
A. sintenisii 🏆 syn. *A. aristata* subsp. *thessala.* Tufted, cushion-forming, evergreen perennial with rosettes of whorled, linear to oblong, glaucous, blue-green leaves, 4–8mm (⅛–⅜in) long. Bears paired or solitary, short-stemmed, narrowly tubular pink flowers, to 1cm (½in) long, in early summer. ↕ 10cm (4in), ↔ to 20cm (8in). Mountains of Turkey. ✲✲✲
A. suberosa ■ syn. *A. athoa* of gardens. Clump-forming, evergreen perennial with whorled, inversely lance-shaped, white-hairy, glaucous leaves, 4–10mm (⅛–½in) long. Bears profuse clusters of tubular, bright pink flowers, to 6mm (¼in) long, in early summer. ↕ to 8cm (3in), ↔ to 20cm (8in). Mountains of Greece, Bulgaria. ✲✲✲

▷**Asphodel** see *Asphodelus*
Yellow see *Asphodeline lutea*

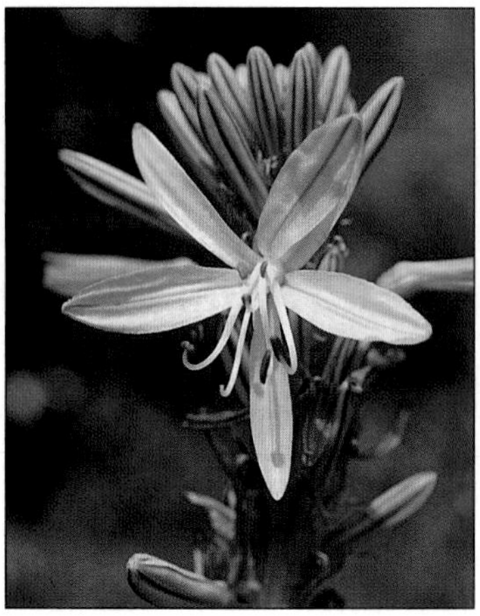

Asphodeline lutea

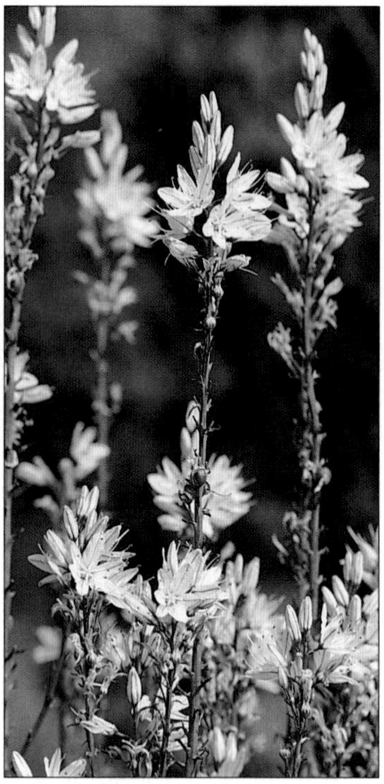

Asphodelus albus

Asphodeline

Jacob's rod

ASPHODELACEAE/LILIACEAE

Genus of up to 20 species of biennials and perennials from sunny, rocky meadows and scrub on dry slopes from the Mediterranean and Turkey to the Caucasus. They have clustered, fleshy or fibrous rhizomes, grass-like basal and stem leaves, and star-shaped, yellow or white flowers in erect, narrow racemes on erect, unbranched stems. Grow in a border or on a dry, sunny bank.

- **Hardiness** Fully hardy.
- **Cultivation** Grow in moderately fertile, well-drained, sandy, loamy, deep soil in full sun. Mulch in autumn in very cold areas.
- **Propagation** Sow seed in containers in a cold frame in spring. Divide in late summer and early autumn: tease apart the fleshy rhizomes, retaining 2 or 3 growing points on each piece.
- **Pests and diseases** Slugs, snails, and aphids may be a problem.

A. liburnica. Clump-forming perennial with narrowly triangular, blue-green leaves, to 25cm (10in) long, borne only on the lower part of the flower stems. In midsummer, bears slender racemes, 15–22cm (6–9in) long, of pale yellow flowers, 5cm (2in) wide, the backs of the tepals striped green, with narrowly ovate to lance-shaped bracts, 1.5cm (½in) long. ↕ 1m (3ft), ↔ 30cm (12in). S.E. Europe, E. Mediterranean. ❄❄❄
A. lutea ■ (King's spear, Yellow asphodel). Clump-forming perennial with furrowed, narrowly triangular, blue-green leaves, 35cm (14in) long, produced all along the flower stems. In late spring, bears dense racemes, to 20cm (8in) long, of fragrant, bright yellow flowers, 3cm (1¼in) wide, with large, ovate bracts, 2.5cm (1in) long. ↕ 1.5m (5ft), ↔ 30cm (12in). C. and E. Mediterranean, W. Turkey. ❄❄❄

Asphodelus

Asphodel

ASPHODELACEAE/LILIACEAE

Genus of 12 species of annuals and perennials found in open woodland, meadows, and scrub in well-drained, sometimes barren, rocky soils from C. Europe and the Mediterranean to the Himalayas. They have fleshy, congested rhizomes and dense tufts of radical, linear, flat or cylindrical, sometimes keeled, basal leaves, 15–60cm (6–24in) long. Leafless stems bear dense racemes or panicles of flowers, mostly 3–4cm (1¼–1½in) across, surrounded by persistent, scaly, white or brown bracts. The white or pink tepals have green or brown central veins. The taller perennial species are striking in a sunny border or wildflower garden; grow *A. acaulis* in a scree bed or in an alpine house.

- **Hardiness** Fully hardy.
- **Cultivation** Grow in deep, well-drained, moderately fertile, sandy loam in a warm, sunny, dry position. Under glass, grow *A. acaulis* in gritty, loam-based potting compost (JI No.1); outdoors, grow in a scree bed in full sun.
- **Propagation** Sow seed in containers in a cold frame in spring, or divide in early spring. Raise the short-lived *A. fistulosus* annually from seed.
- **Pests and diseases** Prone to aphids.

A. acaulis. Evergreen, rhizomatous, stemless perennial with rosettes of flat, linear, light green leaves, to 20cm (8in) long. In late winter and early spring, produces congested racemes of open funnel-shaped, pale pink or white, green-veined flowers, to 4cm (1½in) wide, with white bracts, on short stems in the centre of the leaf rosettes. ↕ to 15cm (6in), ↔ to 20cm (8in). Atlas Mountains. ❄❄❄
A. aestivus, syn. *A. microcarpus.* Clump-forming perennial with broad, linear, flat, thick and leathery, mid-green leaves, 20–40cm (8–16in) long. In mid- and late spring, bears star-shaped, white, sometimes pink-flushed flowers, 5–8cm (2–3in) across, with brown central veins and greenish white bracts, in branched panicles. ↕ 1m (3ft), ↔ 30cm (12in). Mediterranean, W. Turkey. ❄❄❄
A. albus ■ Clump-forming perennial with linear, flat but keeled, mid-green leaves, 30–60cm (12–24in) long, and leafless flowering stems. Star-shaped white flowers, 2–4cm (¾–1½in) across, with pink central veins and white or brown bracts (depending on the subspecies), are borne in occasionally branched racemes in mid- or late spring. ↕ 90cm (36in), ↔ 30cm (12in). C. and S. Europe, N. Africa. ❄❄❄
A. fistulosus, syn. *A. tenuifolius.* Annual or short-lived perennial with a dense, basal clump of narrow, cylindrical, keeled, mid-green leaves, to 35cm (14in) long. In mid- and late summer, hollow, usually branched stems bear panicles of star-shaped, pinkish white flowers, to 2.5cm (1in) across, with brown central veins, surrounded by white bracts. ↕ 45cm (18in), ↔ 20cm (8in). S.W. Europe to S.W. Asia. ❄❄❄
A. microcarpus see *A. aestivus.*
A. tenuifolius see *A. fistulosus.*

Aspidistra

CONVALLARIACEAE/LILIACEAE

Genus of 3 or more species of evergreen, rhizomatous perennials from woodland in the Himalayas, China, and Japan. The long-lasting, leathery, glossy, basal leaves are elliptic to lance-shaped, pointed at the tips, and narrowed at the bases into long, slightly winged leaf-stalks. Solitary, 6- to 8-lobed, purple or grey-white flowers with purple markings, borne on the rhizomes at soil level, are pollinated by snails or slugs and mostly hidden by the foliage. Aspidistras are valued for their tolerance of deep shade, fluctuating temperatures, and neglect. Although commonly grown as houseplants, they are also useful as ground cover in mild climates.

- **Hardiness** Frost hardy.
- **Cultivation** Under glass, grow in loam-based potting compost (JI No.2) in bright filtered light. Water moderately when in growth, sparingly in winter. Once established, apply a balanced liquid fertilizer monthly (variegated cultivars tend to revert if overfed). Grows best with a minimum of 7–10°C (45–50°F). Outdoors, grow in moist but well-drained, fertile, sandy loam with added leaf mould, in a sheltered site in full or partial shade.
- **Propagation** Divide in spring.
- **Pests and diseases** Mealybugs, red spider mites, scale insects, thrips, and vine weevil larvae may be a problem under glass.

A. elatior 🏆 (Cast-iron plant). Rhizomatous perennial, usually grown as a houseplant, with ovate to lance-shaped, glossy, dark green leaves, 30–50cm (12–20in) long, produced singly at short intervals along the rhizomes. Erect, fleshy, broadly bell-shaped, 8-lobed cream flowers, 2–3cm (¾–1¼in) across, and maroon inside, are borne singly along the rhizomes in early summer. ↕↔ to 60cm (24in). China. ❄❄. **'Milky Way'** has white-speckled foliage. **'Variegata'** ■ 🏆 has elliptic leaves, to 70cm (28in) long, with creamy white stripes or wider cream bands along the margins and down the leaf-stalks. Variegated areas on older leaves often turn brown in bright light.
***A. lurida* 'Irish Mist'.** Rhizomatous perennial producing stiff, lance-shaped leaves, 15–20cm (6–8in) long, with 2 or 3 leaves per node. Leaves are dark green and develop yellow markings when mature. Solitary, bell-shaped, 8-lobed, deep purple-red flowers, 2–3cm (¾–1¼in) across, are borne along the rhizomes in early summer. ↕↔ 15–20cm (6–8in). ❄❄

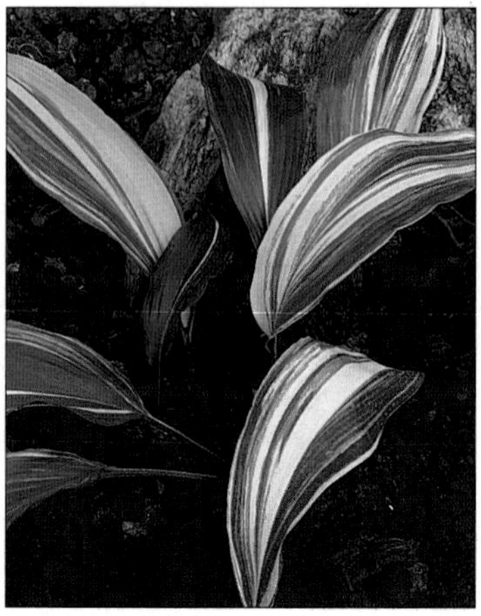

Aspidistra elatior 'Variegata'

Asplenium

syn. Ceterach, Phyllitis

Spleenwort

ASPLENIACEAE

Genus of over 700 species of evergreen or semi-evergreen, terrestrial and epiphytic ferns found in diverse habitats on all continents except Antarctica. Short, erect, occasionally creeping rhizomes produce tufts of fronds, which may be simple, or pinnate to 4-pinnate, or pinnatifid. Some aspleniums are "bird's-nest" ferns: striking epiphytes with long, entire fronds overlapping to form a "nest" in which organic matter collects. Sori are linear, and usually run parallel to each other from the midribs towards the margins of the fronds. Use smaller species in wall crevices, a rock garden, or an alpine trough. Grow larger species in woodland or among shrubs in a shady border. In frost-prone climates, grow tender species as houseplants or in a cool, temperate, or warm greenhouse.

- **Hardiness** Fully hardy to frost tender.

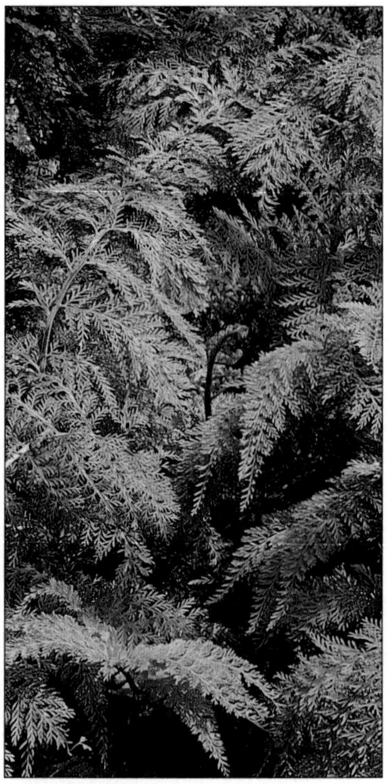

Asplenium bulbiferum

A. ceterach, *A. scolopendrium*, *A. trichomanes*, and their cultivars are hardy to -30°C (-22°F).

• **CULTIVATION** Under glass, grow in a mix of equal parts loam, coarse leaf mould or peat substitute (or peat), sharp sand, and charcoal. Provide bright filtered light and moderate humidity. When in growth, water moderately and apply a half-strength balanced liquid fertilizer monthly; water sparingly in winter. Outdoors, grow in humus-rich, moist but well-drained soil, with added grit, in partial shade. *A. rhizophyllum* needs alkaline soil; *A. ceterach*, *A. scolopendrium*, and *A. trichomanes* prefer alkaline conditions, but most other terrestrial species must be kept lime-free.

• **PROPAGATION** Sow spores as soon as ripe at 15°C (59°F) for hardy species, and at 21°C (70°F) for tender species. Divide hardy species in spring. Some species, such as *A. bulbiferum*, produce plantlets that may be potted up when 3 or 4 leaves have formed. See also p.51.

• **PESTS AND DISEASES** *A. scolopendrium* is prone to rust in wet winters. Bird's-nest ferns are vulnerable to scale insects.

A. australasicum (Bird's-nest fern). Evergreen, terrestrial or epiphytic fern with short, erect rhizomes, producing a "nest" of lance-shaped, entire to slightly wavy, bright green fronds, 2m (6ft) long. Sometimes confused with *A. nidus*. ↕ to 2m (6ft), ↔ 1.2m (4ft). Australia to Polynesia. ⌂ (min. 10°C/50°F)

A. bulbiferum ■ ♀ (Hen-and-chicken fern, Mother spleenwort). Evergreen or semi-evergreen, terrestrial or epiphytic fern with short, erect rhizomes and 2- or 3-pinnate, ovate, triangular, or lance-shaped to oblong, dark green fronds, 1.2m (4ft) long. The lance-shaped to oblong segments bear numerous plantlets. ↕↔ 1.2m (4ft). Australia, New Zealand. ❄❄ (borderline)

A. ceterach ■ syn. *Ceterach officinarum* (Rusty-back fern). Evergreen, terrestrial fern with short, erect rhizomes and tufts of narrowly lance-shaped, pinnate or deeply pinnatifid fronds, to 20cm (8in) long, with oblong to rounded pinnae, dark green above, covered with rusty brown scales beneath. Sori are intermixed with the scales. ↕ 15cm (6in), ↔ 20cm (8in). Widespread in much of Europe to Caucasus, W. Asia, Himalayas, N. Africa. ❄❄❄

A. dimorphum. Evergreen, terrestrial fern with 2- or 3-pinnate to pinnatifid, mid-green fronds, 90cm (36in) long, arising from short, erect rhizomes. Sterile and fertile pinnae may occur on the same frond. Sterile pinnae are coarsely divided into ovate segments; fertile pinnae are lacy and finely divided. ↕ to 80cm (32in), ↔ 60–80cm (24–32in). Australia (Norfolk Island). ⌂ (min. 10°C/50°F)

A. musifolium. Evergreen, epiphytic fern with short, erect rhizomes, producing "nests" of simple, broadly ovate to lance-shaped, glossy, bright green fronds, 1.2m (4ft) long, similar to those of *A. nidus*, but much wider. ↕ to 1.5m (5ft), ↔ 1m (3ft). Tropical S.E. Asia. ⌂ (min. 10°C/50°F)

A. nidus ■ ♀ (Bird's-nest fern). Slow-growing, evergreen, epiphytic fern with "nests" of ovate to lance-shaped, entire, glossy, bright green fronds, 1.5m (5ft) long, and short, erect rhizomes. Commonly cultivated, and has given rise to a number of cultivars. Several species have similar frond characteristics and may be confused with *A. nidus*. ↕ to 1.5m (5ft), ↔ 1m (3ft). Widespread in tropical areas. ⌂ (min. 10°C/50°F)

A. oblongifolium (Shining spleenwort). Evergreen, terrestrial or epiphytic fern with short, erect rhizomes and ovate to elliptic, pinnate, mid-green fronds, 60cm (24in) long, with elongated, ovate to elliptic pinnae, borne on purplish black stalks. ↕ to 1m (3ft), ↔ 80cm (32in). New Zealand. ❄

A. rhizophyllum, syn. *Camptosorus rhizophyllus* (Walking fern). Semi-evergreen or deciduous, terrestrial fern with short, erect rhizomes. Tapered, triangular-lance-shaped or linear, simple fronds, are 30cm (12in) long, heart-

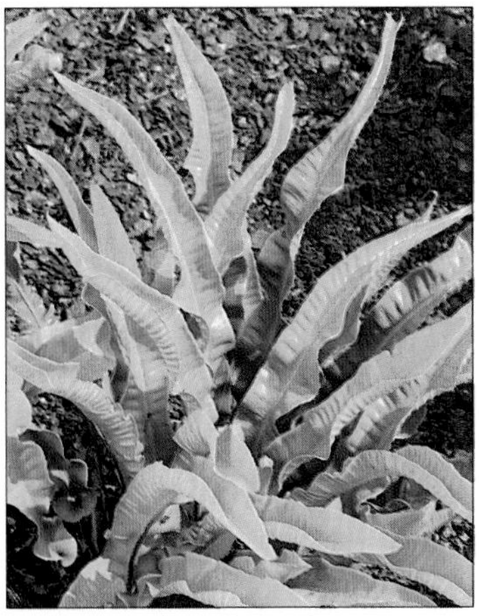

Asplenium scolopendrium

shaped, and sometimes pinnatifid at the bases, with short, reddish green stalks. The elongated frond tips curve over and root where they touch the ground, quickly producing new plantlets and forming large colonies. ↕ to 23cm (9in), ↔ indefinite. North America. ❄

A. scolopendrium ■ ♀ syn. *Phyllitis scolopendrium*, *Scolopendrium vulgare* (Hart's tongue fern). Terrestrial, evergreen fern with erect to shortly creeping rhizomes. It produces irregular, shuttlecock-like crowns of strap-shaped, leathery, glossy, bright green fronds, to 40cm (16in) or more long, which are heart-shaped at the bases and often have wavy margins. Sori are arranged in herringbone fashion. ↕ 45–70cm (18–28in), ↔ 60cm (24in). Europe, W. Asia, North America (as var.

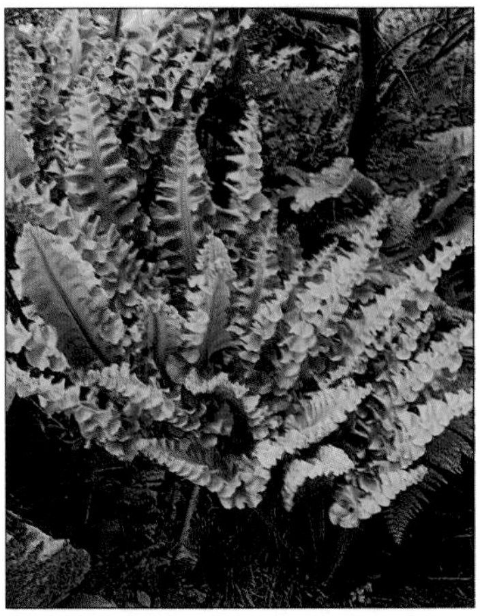

Asplenium scolopendrium 'Crispum'

americanum). ❄❄❄. **'Crispum'** ■ has mid-green fronds with strongly wavy margins, and is usually sterile. **Cristatum Group** cultivars have fronds that are fertile and crested at the tips; ↕ 60cm (24in), ↔ 80cm (32in). **Marginatum Group** contains variants that have fertile fronds with toothed or irregular margins and often fleshy ridges of tissue running along the undersides, close to the margins; ↕ 35cm (14in), ↔ 45cm (18in). **Ramocristatum Group** cultivars produce many-branched fronds, with each division lightly crested at the tip, eventually forming a ball of shining green foliage; ↕ 30cm (12in), ↔ 50cm (20in). **Ramomarginatum Group** cultivars have branched fronds with toothed or irregular margins, often with fleshy ridges running along the undersides, close to the margins; ↕ 30cm (12in), ↔ 50cm (20in). **'Undulatum'** has fertile fronds with wavy margins, the undulations less regular than those of 'Crispum'; ↕ 30cm (12in), ↔ 50cm (20in).

A. trichomanes ■ (Maidenhair spleenwort). Evergreen or semi-evergreen, terrestrial fern with erect, sometimes creeping rhizomes producing narrowly lance-shaped, pinnate, dark green fronds, usually 10–20cm (4–8in) long, on glossy black or dark brown stalks. Pinnae are distinctly stalked, elliptic or oblong, and rounded at the tips. ↕ 15cm (6in), ↔ 20cm (8in). Most temperate regions. ❄❄❄. **subsp. *quadrivalens*** is cultivated more frequently than *A. trichomanes*, and has fronds with short-stalked pinnae, which are squarer at the tips and closer together.

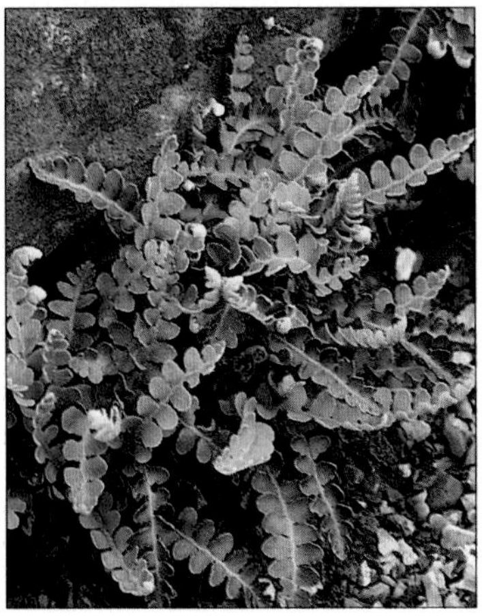

Asplenium ceterach

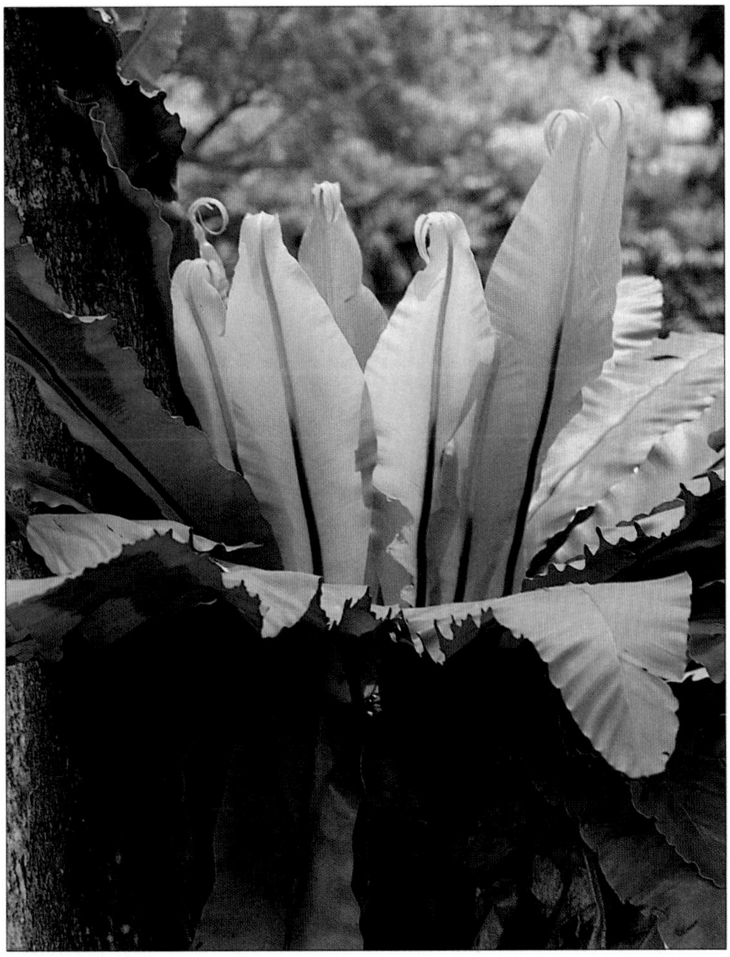

Asplenium nidus

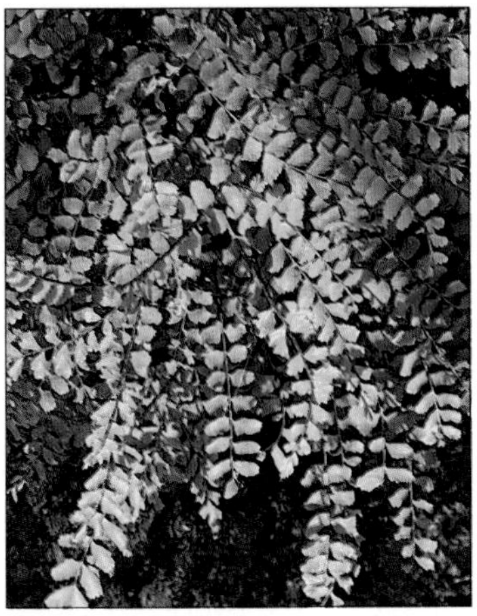

Asplenium trichomanes

A

ASTELIA

ASTELIACEAE/LILIACEAE

Genus of about 25 species of evergreen perennials with short rhizomes, mostly from subalpine or mountainous areas, in boggy, peaty soil, in New Guinea, Australasia, Hawaii, and southern areas of South America. They form large clumps of arching, usually keeled, linear leaves covered in silvery white scales, sometimes losing these at maturity. In spring or summer, they bear panicles of small, unisexual, pale-hued, often green, yellow, or brownish purple flowers. The 6 tepals may be spreading or reflexed, and often persist below the orange or red berries. *A. chathamica* and *A. nervosa* have particularly attractive foliage. In frost-free climates, grow in a peat bed or rock garden. In frost-prone regions, they are best grown in a cool greenhouse or conservatory.

- **HARDINESS** Frost hardy to half hardy.
- **CULTIVATION** Under glass, grow in loamless potting compost in full light with shade from hot sun and with good ventilation. Water freely during the growing season; keep just moist in winter. Outdoors, grow in moist, fertile, peaty soil in sun or partial shade.
- **PROPAGATION** Sow seed in containers in a cold frame as soon as ripe, or divide in spring.
- **PESTS AND DISEASES** Trouble free.

A. chathamica ■ ♀ syn. *A. nervosa* var. *chathamica*. Clump-forming perennial producing arching, leathery, silver-scaly leaves, to 1.5m (5ft) long. Long-stalked panicles of pale yellowish green flowers, 8mm (⅜in) across, with reflexed tepals, are borne in mid- and late spring. The flowers are followed by orange berries on female plants. ↕ 1.2m (4ft), ↔ to 2m (6ft). New Zealand (Chatham Islands). ❄❄

A. nervosa. Clump-forming perennial with tufts of arching foliage, green and silver-woolly above, bronze to white and scaly beneath, with green midribs. Leaves are usually 60cm (24in) long, sometimes to 2m (6ft). Long-stalked, open panicles of greenish yellow or brownish purple flowers, 7–8mm (¼–⅜in) across, with spreading tepals, are borne in summer; female plants produce orange or red berries. ↕ 60cm (24in), ↔ to 2m (6ft). New Zealand. ❄❄. **var. *chathamica*** see *A. chathamica*.

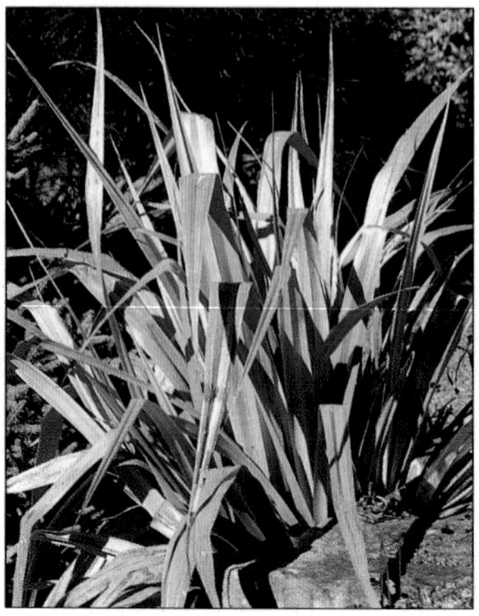

Astelia chathamica

ASTER

syn. CRINITARIA, MICROGLOSSA

ASTERACEAE/COMPOSITAE

Genus of about 250 species of annuals, biennials, perennials, and subshrubs from a variety of habitats, including well-drained, mountainous sites to moist woodland, in the N. hemisphere, particularly North America. The few shrubby species are mainly from South Africa. Most asters have alternate, entire, simple, lance-shaped leaves, some hairless, some softly hairy. The daisy-like flowerheads are either solitary or borne in terminal corymbs, racemes, or panicles on erect to spreading, usually branched stems; they have strap-shaped, female ray-florets in white, pink, blue, or purple, and tubular, hermaphrodite, usually yellow disc-florets. There are asters for almost all garden situations, including borders and rock gardens, streamsides, dry sites, and wildflower gardens. In frost-prone areas, grow the tender, shrubby species in a cool greenhouse.

- **HARDINESS** Fully hardy to frost tender.
- **CULTIVATION** Asters have varying cultivation requirements. For ease of reference, these are grouped as follows:

1. Well-cultivated, fertile, moist soil in sun or partial shade.
2. Well-drained, open, moderately fertile soil in full sun.
3. Moist, moderately fertile soil in partial shade.

Mulch all asters annually after cutting back in late autumn. Stake taller perennials, 75–90cm (30–36in) or more high, from early spring. To maintain vigour and flower quality, divide cultivars of *A. novae-angliae* and *A. novi-belgii* every third year.

- **PROPAGATION** Sow seed in containers in a cold frame in spring or autumn. Divide or separate runners, preferably in spring, otherwise in autumn; replant only vigorous, young shoots. Root basal cuttings of *A. amellus*, *A.* x *frikartii*, and *A. thomsonii* in spring.
- **PESTS AND DISEASES** Vulnerable to eelworms, aphids, slugs, snails, *Fusarium* wilt, leaf spot, and grey mould (*Botrytis*). *A. novi-belgii* cultivars are prone to powdery mildew and tarsonemid mites.

A. acris see *A. sedifolius*.
A. albescens, syn. *Microglossa albescens*. Open, spreading, deciduous subshrub with lance-shaped, tapered, toothed, aromatic, mid-green leaves, to 12cm (5in) long. In mid- and late summer, mauve-blue or white flowerheads, 9mm (⅜in) across, with yellow disc-florets, are borne in flattened corymbs, to 10cm (4in) across. Cultivation group 2. ↕ 1.2m (4ft), ↔ 2m (6ft). Himalayas. ❄❄❄
A. alpinus ■ ♀ Spreading, clump-forming perennial with short-stalked, spoon-shaped to narrowly lance-shaped, mid-green leaves, to 9cm (3½in) long. Bears solitary violet flowerheads, to 5cm (2in) across, with deep yellow disc-florets, on erect stems in early and mid-summer. Cultivation group 2. ↕ to 25cm (10in), ↔ 45cm (18in). Alps. ❄❄❄. Several outstanding cultivars are available, the ray-florets varying in colour, but all with deep yellow disc-florets. Suitable for the front of a border or a large rock garden. **'Dark Beauty'** see 'Dunkle Schöne'. **'Dunkle Schöne'**, syn. 'Dark Beauty', has deep purple flowerheads. **var. *himalaicus*** see *A. himalaicus*. **'Wargrave Variety'**, syn. 'Wargrave Park', has pale pink, purple-tinged flowerheads. **'White Beauty'** has white flowerheads.
A. amelloides see *Felicia amelloides*.
A. amellus. Clump-forming, erect or semi-decumbent, hairy perennial with lance-shaped, mid-green leaves, 3–5cm (1¼–2in) long. Loose corymbs, to 15cm (6in) across, of lilac-blue flowerheads, each 3–5cm (1¼–2in) wide, with yellow disc-florets, open from late summer to autumn. Cultivation group 2; thrives in alkaline soil. ↕ 30–60cm (12–24in), ↔ 45cm (18in). C. and E. Europe to W. Russia and Turkey. ❄❄❄. **'Brilliant'** has bright pink flowerheads; ↕ 75cm (30in). **'King George'** ■ ♀ has large violet-blue flowerheads; ↕ 45cm (18in). **'Mauve Beauty'** has large violet flowerheads; ↕ 60–90cm (24–36in). **'Nocturne'** ■ has deep lilac flowerheads; ↕ 75cm (30in). **'Peach Blossom'** is peach-pink; ↕ 70cm (28in). **'Pink Zenith'** see 'Rosa Erfüllung'. **'Rosa Erfüllung'**, syn. 'Pink Zenith', has soft pink flowerheads. **'Rudolph Goethe'** has deep lavender-blue flowerheads. **'Sonia'** ■ has light pink flowerheads. **'Veilchenkönigin'** ♀ syn. 'Violet Queen', has violet-purple flowerheads. **'Violet Queen'** see 'Veilchenkönigin'.

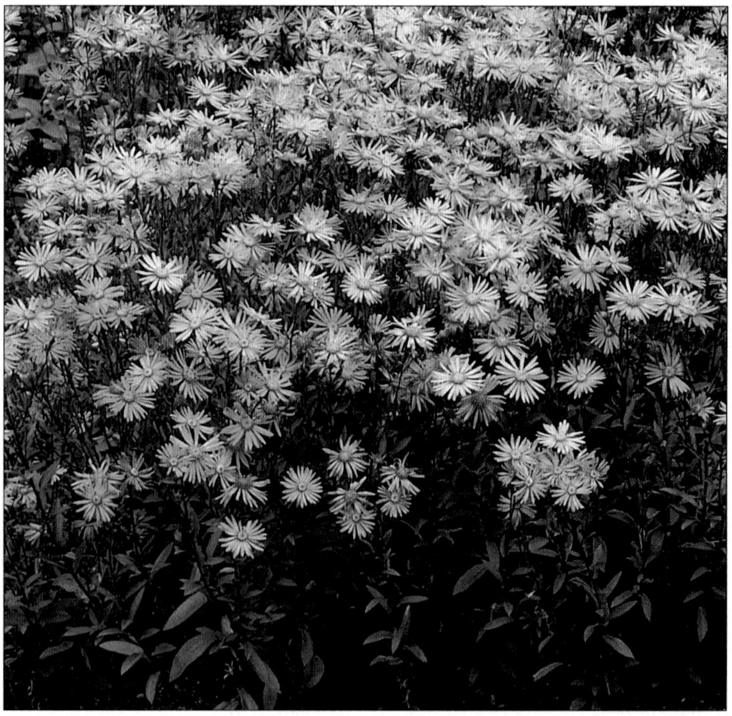

Aster amellus 'Sonia'

A. capensis see *Felicia amelloides*.
A. coelestis see *Felicia amelloides*.
A. 'Coombe Fishacre' ♀ Clump-forming, erect perennial, a hybrid of *A. lateriflorus*, with lance-shaped, finely toothed, dark green leaves, 6–10cm (2½–4in) long. From midsummer to mid-autumn, produces pink-flushed white flowerheads, 1.5cm (½in) across, with brownish yellow disc-florets, in corymbs to 20cm (8in) across. Cultivation group 3, but tolerates well-drained soil in full sun. ↕ 90cm (36in), ↔ 30cm (12in). ❄❄❄
A. cordifolius. Clump-forming, erect perennial with long-stalked, broadly ovate to heart-shaped, mid-green leaves, to 12cm (5in) long. From late summer to mid-autumn, produces loose panicles, 25cm (10in) across, of pale to deep blue flowerheads, to 2cm (¾in) across, with yellow disc-florets. Cultivation group 3. ↕ 0.6–1.5m (2–5ft), ↔ 45cm (18in). E. North America. ❄❄❄. **'Silver Spray'** ■ has pale pink, white-tinged flowerheads, to 3cm (1¼in) across; ↕ 1.2m (4ft). **'Sweet Lavender'** ♀ has arching sprays of lavender-blue flowerheads on lax stems; ↕ 1–1.2m (3–4ft).
A. corymbosus see *A. divaricatus*.
A. diffusus see *A. lateriflorus*.
A. divaricatus, syn. *A. corymbosus*. Clump-forming, rhizomatous perennial with arching, wiry, blackish purple stems bearing mid-green leaves, 6–12cm (2½–5in) long, the upper ones ovate-lance-shaped, the lower ones heart-shaped. Bears loose corymbs, 10cm (4in) across, of white flowerheads, to 1cm (½in) across, with brownish yellow disc-florets, from midsummer to mid-autumn. Cultivation group 3. ↕↔ 60cm (24in). E. North America. ❄❄❄
A. ericoides. Clump-forming, bushy perennial with slender, freely branched stems and small, linear-lance-shaped, mid-green leaves, to 7cm (3in) long. Bears white flowerheads, to 1cm (½in) across, sometimes shaded pink or blue, with yellow disc-florets, in loose panicles, 20cm (8in) across, from late summer to late autumn. Cultivation group 2. ↕ 1m (3ft), ↔ 30cm (12in). Canada, C. and E. USA. ❄❄❄. **'Brimstone'** ♀ has cream flowerheads with bold yellow disc-florets. **'Esther'** ■ is bushy, with small pink flowerheads; ↕ 70cm (28in). **'Golden Spray'** ■ ♀ is bushy, with pink-tinged white flowerheads and bold, golden yellow disc-florets. **'Pink Cloud'** ♀ bears a mass of small, pale pink flowerheads, each 1.5cm (½in) across. **'White Heather'** ■ is upright, with compact panicles of white flowerheads; ↕ 90cm (36in).
A.* x *frikartii (*A. amellus* x *A thomsonii*). Upright perennial with oblong-ovate,

rough, dark green leaves, 5–8cm (2–3in) long. In late summer and early autumn, bears loose corymbs, 20cm (8in) across, of light to dark violet-blue flowerheads, 5–8cm (2–3in) across, with orange disc-florets. Cultivation group 2. ↕70cm (28in), ↔ 45cm (18in). Garden origin. ✲✲✲. **'Flora's Delight'** has dense, bushy growth, greyish green foliage, and long-lasting lilac flowerheads; ↕50cm (20in), ↔ 30cm (12in). **'Mönch'** ■🏆 has long-lasting, clear lavender-blue flowerheads on stout stems; ↕70cm (28in), ↔ 35–40cm (14–16in). **'Wunder von Stäfa'** ■🏆 is similar to 'Mönch', with stout stems and long-lasting blue flowerheads; ↕70cm (28in), ↔ 35–40cm (14–16in).

A. himalaicus, syn. *A. alpinus* var. *himalaicus*. Rhizomatous, clump-forming perennial with obovate to spoon-shaped, mid-green leaves, to 5cm (2in) long. In early summer, bears erect, unbranched stems of solitary flowerheads, 3–8cm (1¼–3in) across, with lilac or purple-blue ray-florets and brownish yellow disc-florets. Cultivation group 2. ↕to 15cm (6in), ↔ to 30cm (12in). China to E. Himalayas. ✲✲✲

A. lateriflorus, syn. *A. diffusus*, *A. vimineus*. Clump-forming perennial with slender, hairy stems, spreading branches, and linear- or oblong-lance-shaped, mid-green leaves, to 15cm (6in) long. Corymbs, to 15cm (6in) across, of white to pale lilac flowerheads, to 1.5cm (½in) across, with rose-pink disc-florets, are produced from midsummer to mid-autumn. Cultivation group 3. ↕1.2m (4ft), ↔ 30cm (12in). North America. ✲✲✲. **'Delight'** has greyish green foliage and white flowerheads with pinkish brown disc-florets; ↕60cm (24in). **'Horizontalis'** ■🏆 has widely spreading branches and small leaves, to 8cm (3in) long. It bears white, sometimes pink-tinged flowerheads with pink-brown disc-florets; ↕60cm (24in).

A. linosyris ■ (Goldilocks). Clump-forming perennial with unbranched, erect stems and linear, mid-green leaves, 5–8cm (2–3in) long. In late summer or early autumn, bears tiny flowerheads, 2–4mm (1⁄16–⅛in) across, with golden yellow disc-florets and no ray-florets, in dense corymbs, 3–15cm (1¼–6in) across. Cultivation group 2. ↕70cm (28in), ↔ 30cm (12in). Europe. ✲✲✲

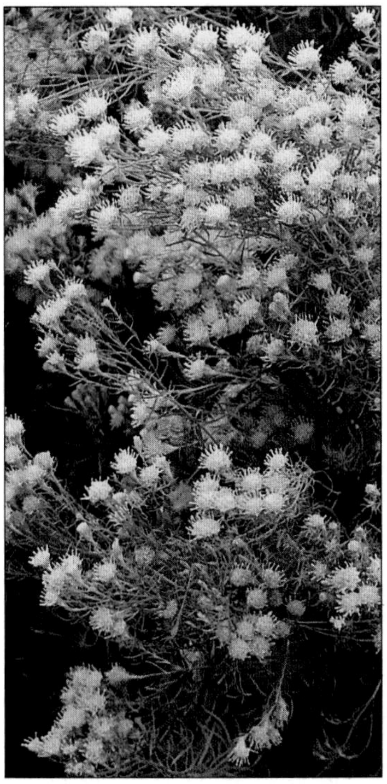
Aster linosyris

***A.* 'Little Carlow'** ■🏆 Clump-forming, erect perennial, a hybrid of *A. cordifolius*, with ovate to heart-shaped, toothed, dark green leaves, 10–12cm (4–5in) long. Produces loose panicles, 20cm (8in) across, of violet-blue flowers, to 2cm (¾in) across, with yellow disc-florets, in early and mid-autumn. Cultivation group 3, but tolerates well-drained soil in full sun. ↕90cm (36in), ↔ 45cm (18in). ✲✲✲

***A.* 'Little Dorrit'**. Clump-forming perennial, a hybrid of *A. cordifolius*, with erect stems bearing ovate to heart-shaped, toothed, dark green leaves, 10–12cm (4–5in) long. In early and mid-autumn, bears pink, sometimes mauve-shaded flowerheads, to 2cm (¾in) across, with yellow disc-florets, in loose panicles 20cm (8in) across. Cultivation group 3, but will tolerate well-drained soil in full sun. ↕1m (3ft), ↔ 45cm (18in). ✲✲✲

A. natalensis see *Felicia rosulata*.

A. novae-angliae (New England aster). Clump-forming, hairy perennial with short rhizomes and stout stems, densely covered with stalkless, stem-clasping, lance-shaped, mid-green leaves, to 12cm (5in) long. From late summer to mid-autumn, strong, almost woody stems bear terminal, corymb-like sprays, to 25cm (10in) across, of violet-purple flowerheads, to 5cm (2in) across, with yellow disc-florets. Cultivation group 1. ↕to 1.5m (5ft), ↔ 60cm (24in). E. North America. ✲✲✲. **'Andenken an Alma Pötschke'** ■🏆 syn. 'Alma Pötschke', has bright salmon-pink flowerheads; ↕1.2m (4ft). **'Andenken an Paul Gerber'** has dark red flowerheads in late summer and early autumn; ↕1.5m (5ft). **'Autumn Snow'** see 'Herbstschnee'. **'Barr's Pink'** ■ has semi-double, bright rose-pink flowerheads in early autumn; ↕1.3m (4½ft). **'Barr's Violet'** bears deep violet-blue flowerheads; ↕1.5m (5ft). **'Harrington's Pink'** ■🏆 has clear, light pink flowerheads; ↕1.2m (4ft). **'Herbstschnee'**, syn. 'Autumn Snow', bears large white flowerheads, to 7cm (3in) across; ↕1.2m (4ft). **'Lye End Beauty'** is lilac-pink; ↕1.7m (5½ft). **'Septemberrubin'**, syn. 'September Ruby', bears deep rose-pink flowerheads; ↕1.2m (4ft). **'September Ruby'** see 'Septemberrubin'.

A. novi-belgii (Michaelmas daisy, New York aster). Clump-forming, rhizomatous, hairless perennial with slender, branched stems and stalkless, lance-shaped, mid-green leaves, 5–10cm (2–4in) long. From late summer to mid-autumn, bears corymb-like panicles, 10–30cm (4–12in) across, of violet flowerheads, to 6cm (2½in) across, with yellow disc-florets. Cultivation group 1. ↕1.2m (4ft), ↔ 90cm (36in). North America. ✲✲✲. **'Ada Ballard'** bears large, lavender-blue flowerheads, 7cm (3in) across; ↕90cm (36in). **'Alice Haslam'** has rose-red flowerheads; ↕25cm (10in), ↔ 45cm (18in). **'Apple Blossom'** ■ has flowerheads in creamy pink; ↕90cm (36in). **'Audrey'** has lavender-blue flowerheads; ↕35cm

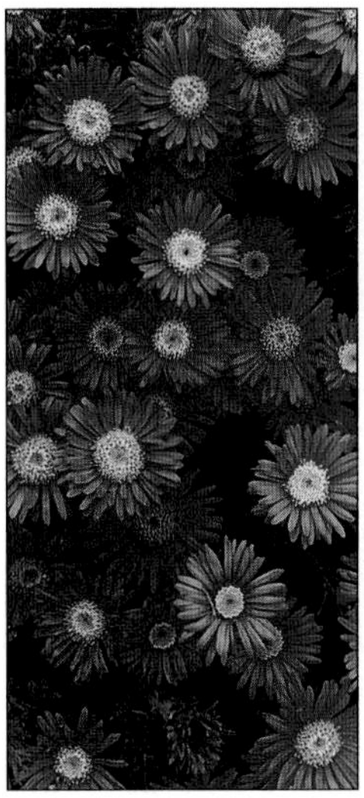
Aster alpinus

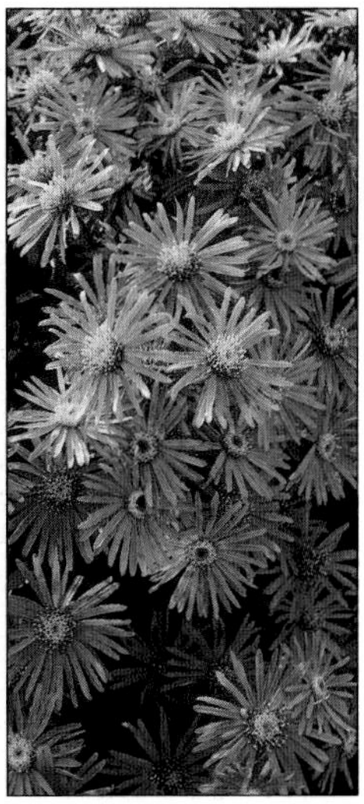
Aster amellus 'King George'

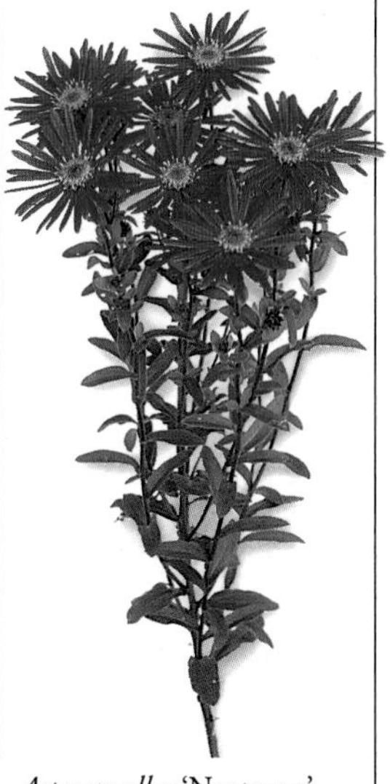
Aster amellus 'Nocturne'

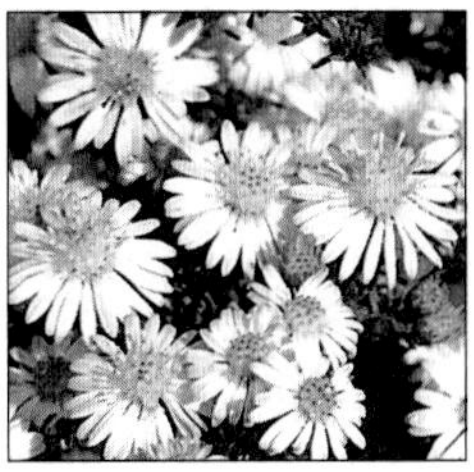
Aster cordifolius 'Silver Spray'

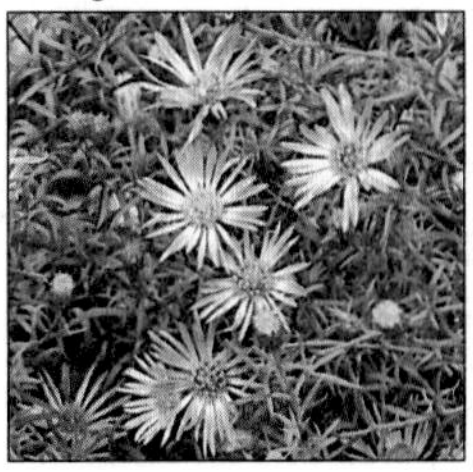
Aster ericoides 'Esther'

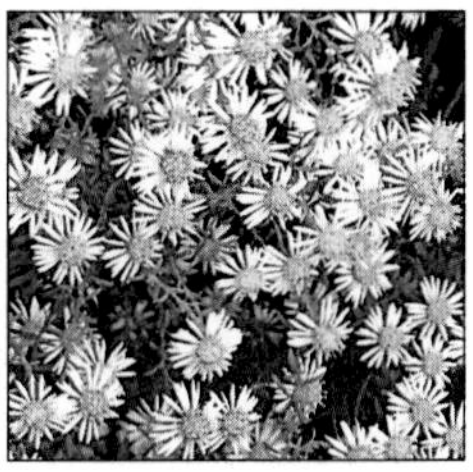
Aster ericoides 'Golden Spray'

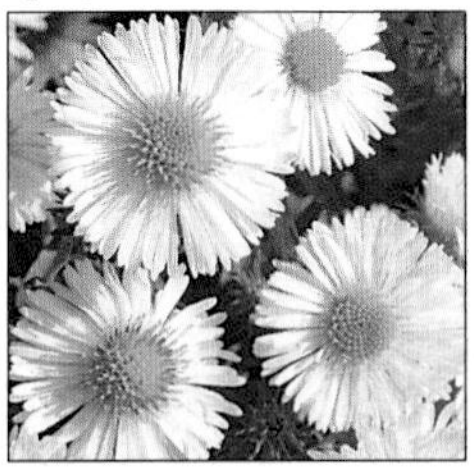
Aster ericoides 'White Heather'

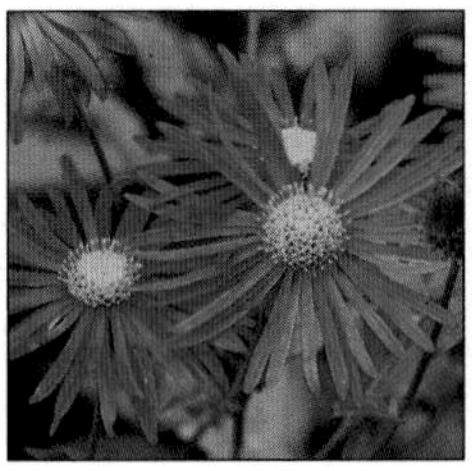
Aster x *frikartii* 'Mönch'

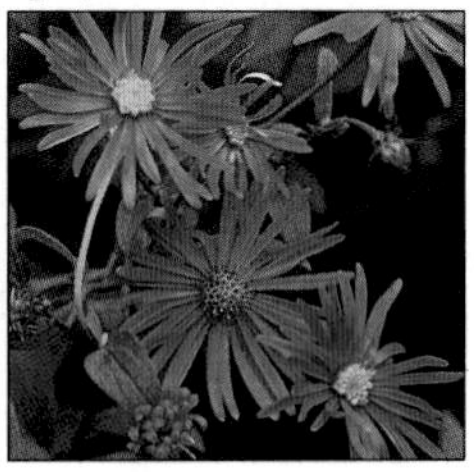
Aster x *frikartii* 'Wunder von Stäfa'

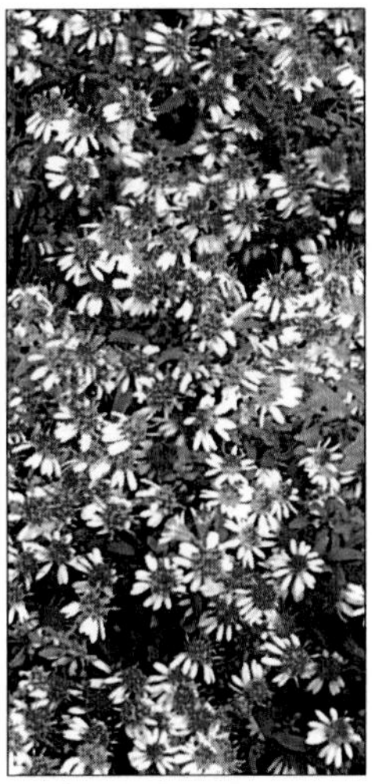
Aster lateriflorus 'Horizontalis'

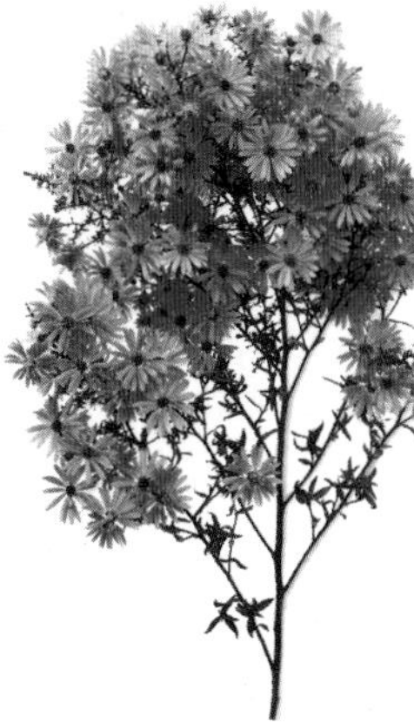
Aster 'Little Carlow'

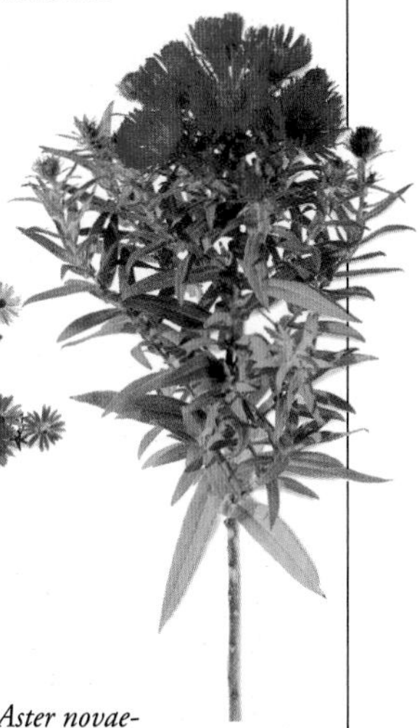
Aster novae-angliae 'Andenken an Alma Pötschke'

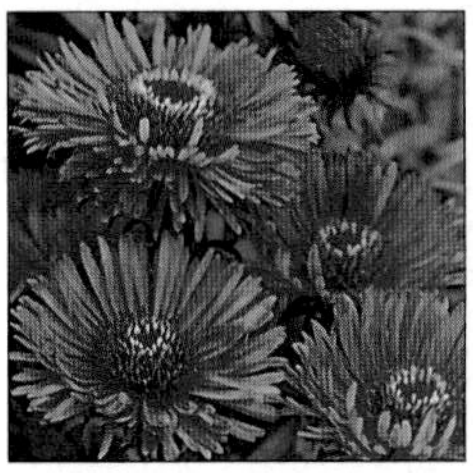
Aster novae-angliae 'Barr's Pink'

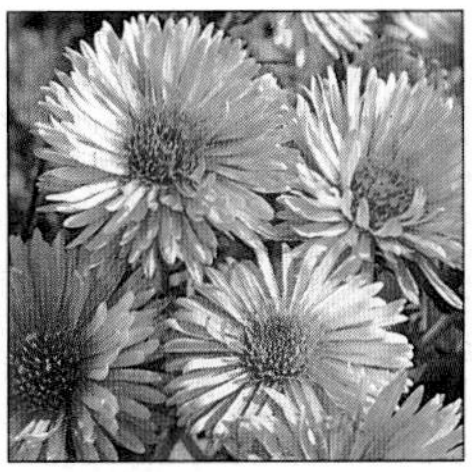
Aster novae-angliae 'Harrington's Pink'

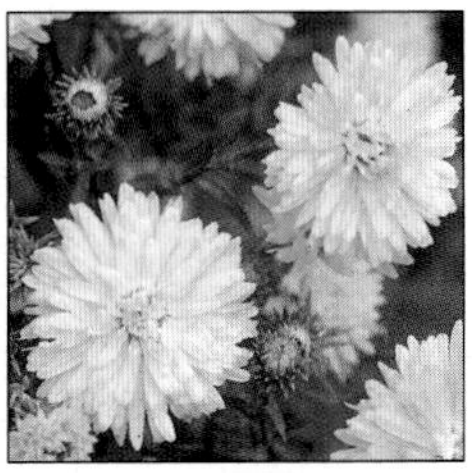
Aster novi-belgii 'Apple Blossom'

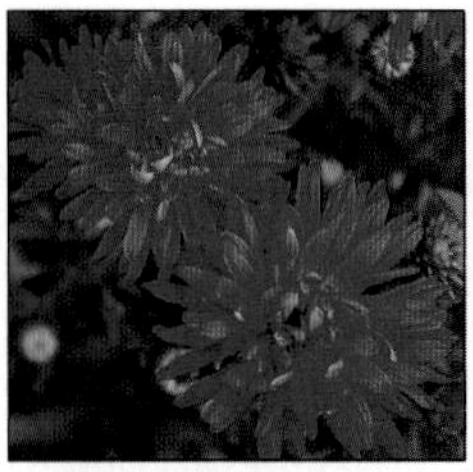
Aster novi-belgii 'Carnival'

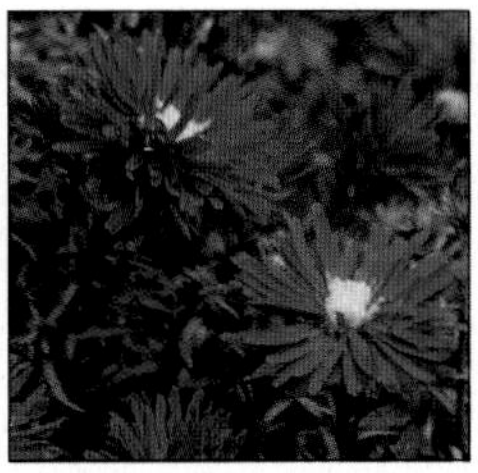
Aster novi-belgii 'Chequers'

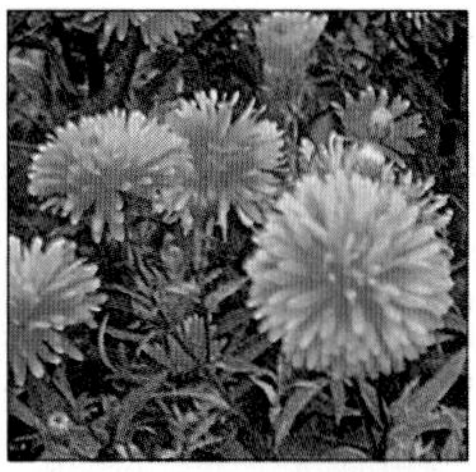
Aster novi-belgii 'Fellowship'

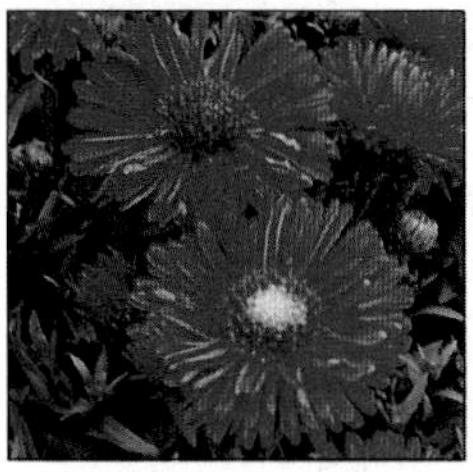
Aster novi-belgii 'Jenny'

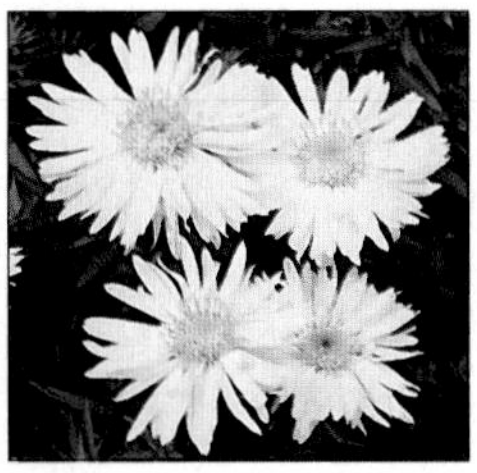
Aster novi-belgii 'Kristina'

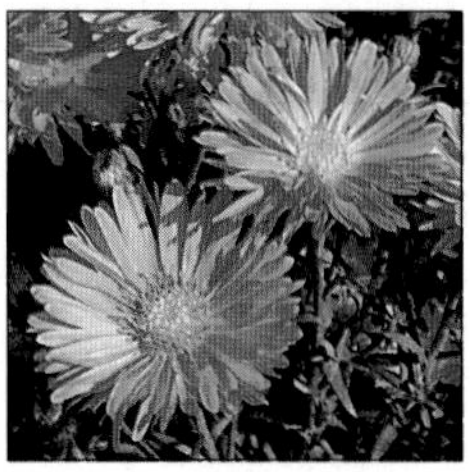
Aster novi-belgii 'Lassie'

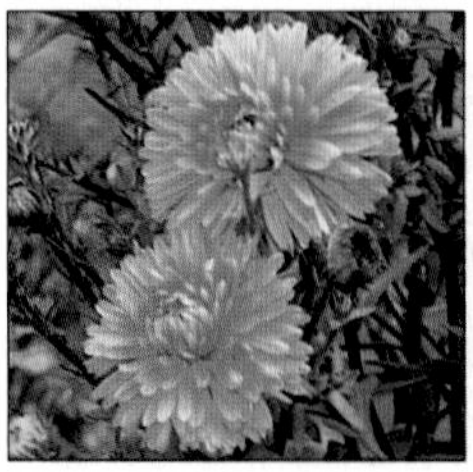
Aster novi-belgii 'Marie Ballard'

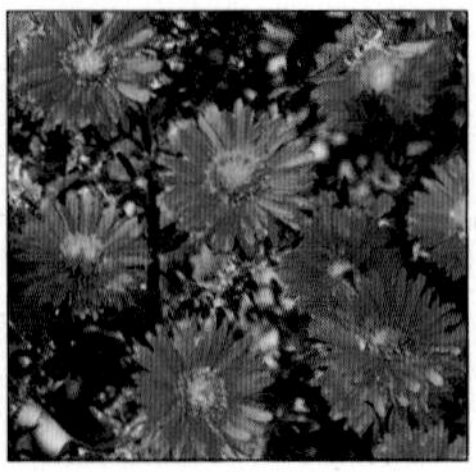
Aster novi-belgii 'Orlando'

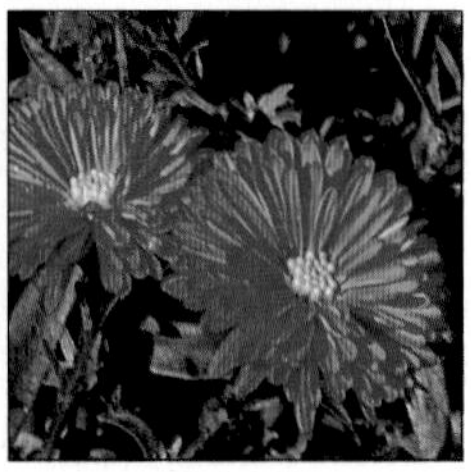
Aster novi-belgii 'Patricia Ballard'

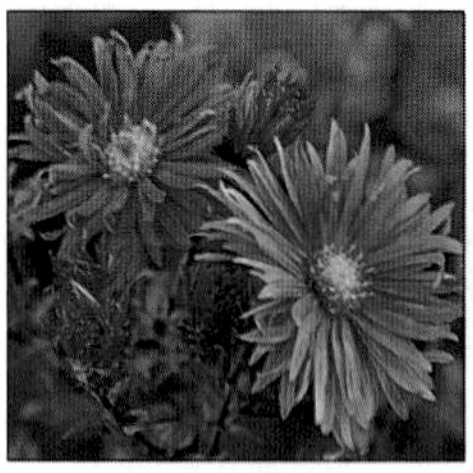
Aster novi-belgii 'Peace'

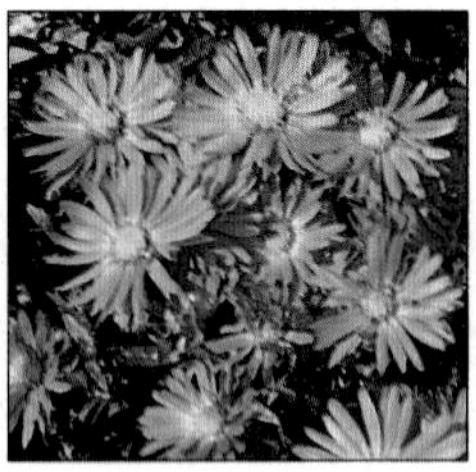
Aster novi-belgii 'Professor Anton Kippenberg'

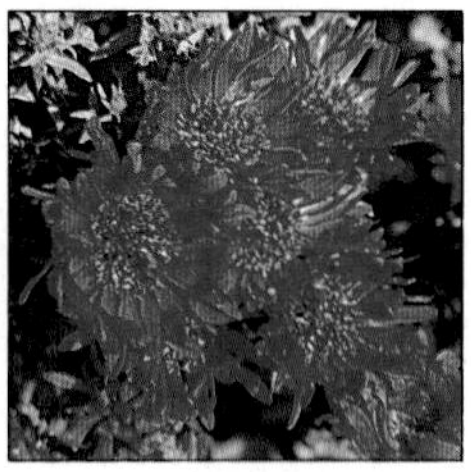
Aster novi-belgii 'Royal Ruby'

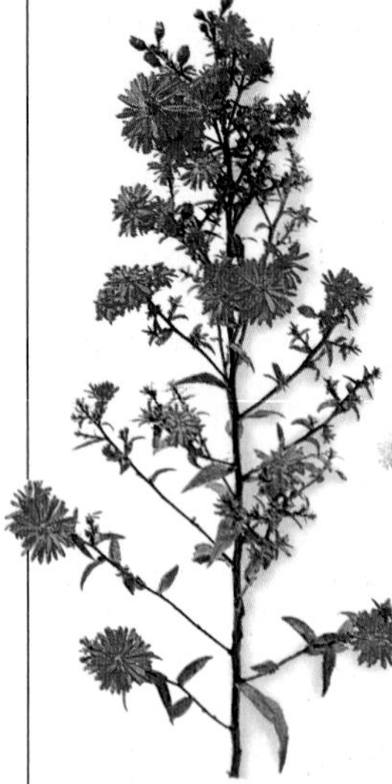
Aster novi-belgii 'Royal Velvet'

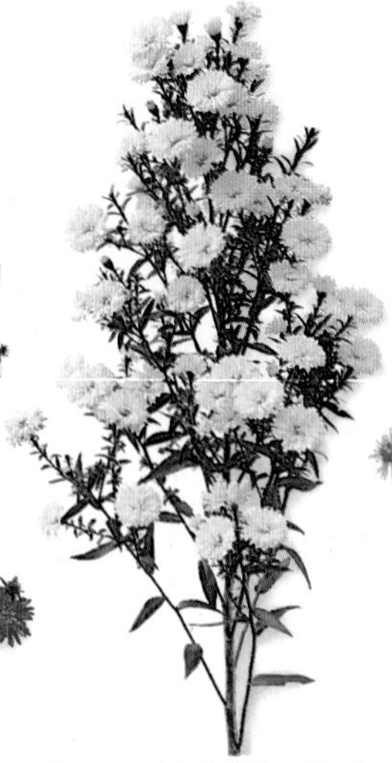
Aster novi-belgii 'Sandford White Swan'

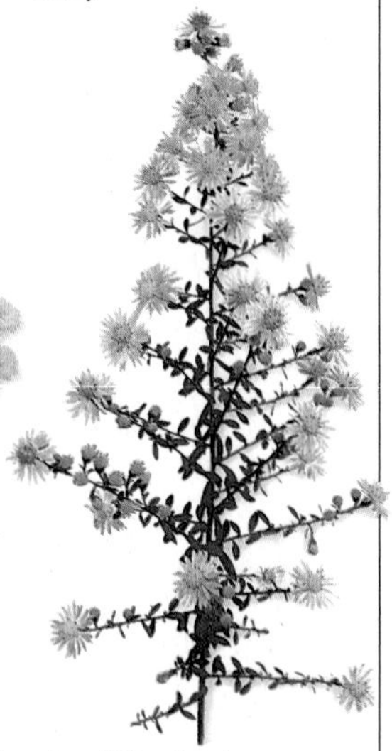
Aster 'Ringdove'

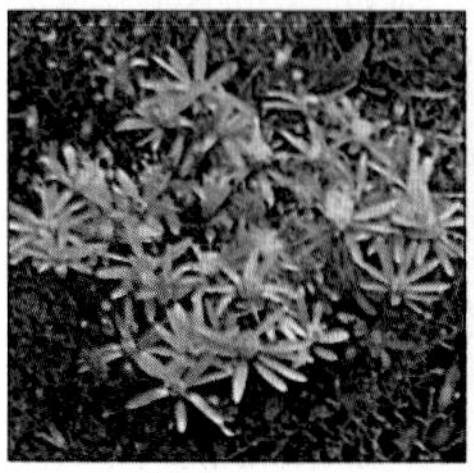
Aster sedifolius

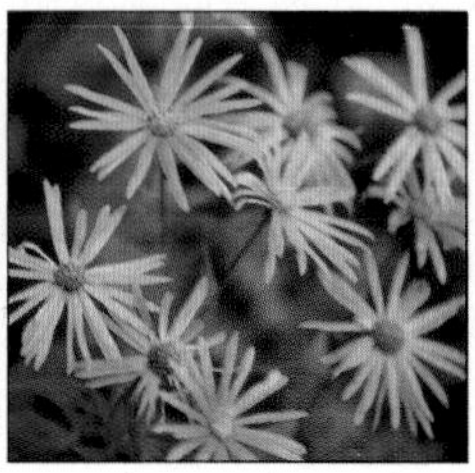
Aster thomsonii 'Nanus'

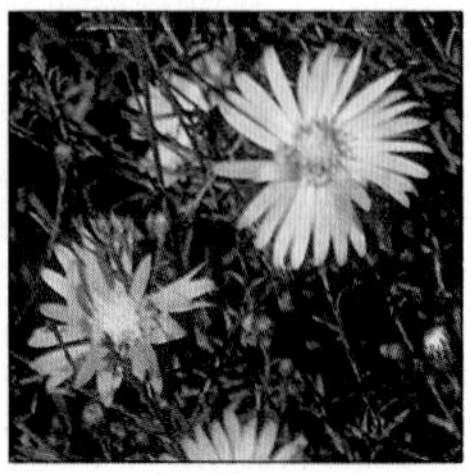
Aster turbinellus

(14in), ↔ 45cm (18in). **'Beechwood Challenger'** has crimson flowerheads; ↕ 90cm (36in). **'Blandie'** bears semi-double ivory flowerheads, becoming pink-tinged; ↕ 90cm (36in). **'Blue Gown'** bears mid-blue flowerheads. **'Carnival'** ■ bears bright cerise flowerheads; ↕ 60cm (24in). **'Chequers'** ■ has purple flowerheads; ↕ 60cm (24in). **'Climax'** has light lavender-blue flowerheads. **'Coombe Rosemary'** has double, violet-purple flowerheads; ↕ 90cm (36in). **'Crimson Brocade'** has semi-double crimson flowerheads; ↕ 90cm (36in). **'Ernest Ballard'** has large, carmine-red flowerheads; ↕ 90cm (36in). **'Fellowship'** ■ has large, double flowerheads, 7cm (3in) across, in deep pink; ↕ 90cm (36in). **'Freda Ballard'** bears semi-double, rich rose-red flowerheads; ↕ 90cm (36in). **'Gayborder Royal'** has bright crimson flowerheads; ↕ 90cm (36in). **'Harrison's Blue'** has violet-blue flowerheads; ↕ 90cm (36in). **'Heinz Richard'** has pink flowerheads, 7cm (3in) across; ↕ 30cm (12in), ↔ 45cm (18in). **'Helen Ballard'** bears dusky red flowerheads; ↕ 60cm (24in), ↔ 45cm (18in). **'Jean'** produces double, deep violet flowerheads; ↕↔ 45cm (18in). **'Jenny'** ■ bears double, red-purple flowerheads; ↕ 30cm (12in), ↔ 45cm (18in). **'Kristina'** ■ has large, semi-double white flowerheads; ↕ 30cm (12in), ↔ 45cm (18in). **'Lassie'** ■ has large flowerheads in clear pink; ↕ 90cm (36in), ↔ 45cm (18in). **'Little Pink Beauty'** has semi-double, soft pink flowerheads; ↕ 30cm (12in), ↔ 45cm (18in). **'Margaret Rose'** has light pink flowerheads; ↕ 30cm (12in), ↔ 45cm (18in). **'Marie Ballard'** ■ has double, pale blue flowerheads; ↕ 90cm (36in). **'Melbourne Belle'** bears bright pink flowerheads; ↕ 75cm (30in). **'Mount Everest'** has white flowerheads; ↕ 90cm (36in). **'Orlando'** ■ has deep pink flowerheads with golden yellow disc-florets; ↕ 1m (3ft). **'Patricia Ballard'** ■ has semi-double, dark pink flowerheads; ↕ 90cm (36in). **'Peace'** ■ has mauve flowerheads, 7cm (3in) across. **'Percy Thrower'** has double, deep violet-blue flowerheads; ↕ 90cm (36in). **'Professor Anton Kippenberg'** ■ bears mid-blue flowerheads; ↕ 35cm (14in), ↔ 45cm (18in). **'Prosperity'** has large, semi-double flowerheads, 7cm (3in) across, in rose-pink; ↕ 1.1m (3½ft). **'Raspberry Ripple'** has cerise flowerheads; ↕ 75cm (30in). **'Rosenwichtel'** has deep pink flowerheads; ↕ 20cm (8in), ↔ 35cm (14in). **'Royal Ruby'** ■ has semi-double, rich red flowerheads; ↕ 50cm (20in). **'Royal Velvet'** ■ has deep violet flowerheads. **'Sandford White Swan'** ■ has white flowerheads; ↕ 90cm (36in). **'Sarah Ballard'** has narrow, pointed violet flowerheads; ↕ 90cm (36in). **'Schneekissen'**, syn. 'Snow Cushion', has white flowerheads; ↕ 30cm (12in), ↔ 45cm (18in). **'Snow Cushion'** see 'Schneekissen'. **'Snowsprite'** ■ has pink buds opening white; ↕ 25–30cm (10–12in), ↔ 45cm (18in). **'The Cardinal'** bears deep rose-red flowerheads. **'Thundercloud'** has deep purple flowerheads; ↕ 90cm (36in). **'Winston S. Churchill'** has double, dark ruby-red flowerheads; ↕ 90cm (36in).

A. pappei see *Felicia amoena*.

***A. pringlei* 'Monte Cassino'** ■ 🏆 Clump-forming perennial with sparsely branched, upright stems and narrow oblong to lance-shaped, pale to mid-green leaves, to 7cm (3in) long. From late summer to late autumn, bears open sprays, to 10cm (4in) long, of white flowerheads, 8–10mm (3/8–½in) across, with yellow disc-florets. Cultivation group 1 or 3. ↕ to 1m (3ft), ↔ 30cm (12in). ❄❄❄

***A.* 'Ringdove'** ■ 🏆 Clump-forming, erect perennial, a hybrid of *A. ericoides*, with linear-lance-shaped, stalkless, mid-green leaves, to 7cm (3in) long. Bears numerous pale mauve flowerheads, to 1cm (½in) across, with yellowish brown disc-florets, in panicles, to 18cm (7in) long, in autumn. Cultivation group 2. ↕ 90cm (36in), ↔ 30cm (12in). ❄❄❄

A. sedifolius ■ syn. *A. acris*. Clump-forming perennial with weakly branched stems and stalkless, lance-shaped, mid-green leaves, 5–6cm (2–2½in) long. Terminal sprays, 5–15cm (2–6in) wide, of flowerheads to 4cm (1½in) across, are borne in late summer and early autumn. Ray-florets are widely spaced and blue-purple, lilac or lilac-pink, with yellow disc-florets. Cultivation group 2. ↕ to 1.2m (4ft), ↔ 60cm (24in). C., S., and E. Europe. ❄❄❄. **'Nanus'** is compact, bearing flowerheads with darker blue ray-florets; ↕ 45cm (18in).

A. thomsonii. Clump-forming perennial with erect, slender stems and ovate to elliptic, coarsely toothed, mid-green leaves, to 10cm (4in) long. Lilac-blue flowerheads, 4–5cm (1½–2in) across, with yellow disc-florets, are borne in terminal sprays, 5–15cm (2–6in) across, from midsummer to early autumn. Cultivation group 3. ↕ 60–75cm (24–30in), ↔ 50cm (20in). W. Himalayas. ❄❄❄. **'Nanus'** ■ has long-lasting, star-shaped, lilac-blue flowerheads; ↕ 45cm (18in), ↔ 25cm (10in).

A. tongolensis. Rhizomatous, mat-forming perennial with elliptic, softly hairy, mostly basal, dark green leaves, to 9cm (3½in) long. In early summer, erect, stout, almost leafless stems bear solitary flowerheads, to 6cm (2½in) across, with violet-blue ray-florets and orange-yellow disc-florets. Cultivation group 2, but will tolerate moister soil. ↕ 45cm (18in), ↔ 30cm (12in). W. China, Himalayas. ❄❄❄. The following cultivars bear profuse, large flowerheads, to 8cm (3in) across, which are useful for cutting. **'Berggarten'** has flowerheads with lavender-blue ray-florets and orange disc-florets; ↕ 40cm (16in). **'Napsbury'** has flowerheads with

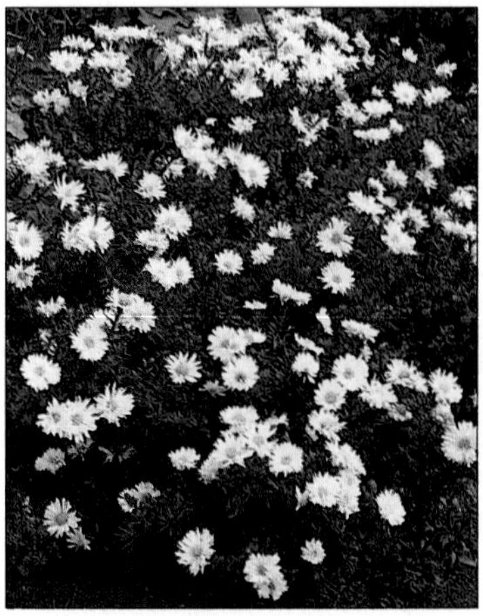
Aster novi-belgii 'Snowsprite'

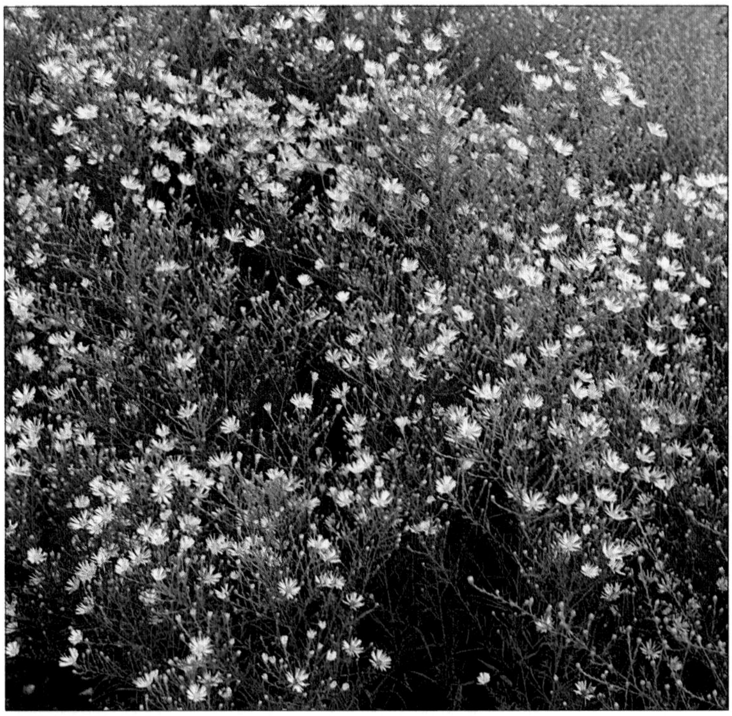

Aster pringlei 'Monte Cassino'

violet-blue ray-florets and bright orange disc-florets; ↕ 50cm (20in).
A. turbinellus ▣ 🏆 Clump-forming perennial with slender, erect, dark green stems and lance-shaped, mid-green leaves, 8–10cm (3–4in) long. In early and mid-autumn, bears airy panicles, to 15cm (6in) wide, of pale violet flowerheads, to 2cm (¾in) across, with yellow disc-florets. Cultivation group 2. ↕ 1.2m (4ft), ↔ 60cm (24in). C. and E. USA. ✻✻✻
A. vimineus see *A. lateriflorus.*

▷**Aster,**
Beach see *Erigeron glaucus*
China see *Callistephus*
Hairy golden see *Heterotheca villosa*
New England see *Aster novae-angliae*
New York see *Aster novi-belgii*
Stokes' see *Stokesia*

ASTERANTHERA

GESNERIACEAE

Genus of one species of evergreen, climbing or creeping shrub from humid, temperate forest in Chile and Argentina. Grown for its brightly coloured flowers, *A. ovata* is best trained against a shady wall, or grown in woodland against a tree trunk. In very cold areas, grow in a cool greenhouse or conservatory.
• **HARDINESS** Frost hardy, but thrives only in cool, humid climates.
• **CULTIVATION** Under glass, grow in lime-free (ericaceous) potting compost in full light, shaded from hot sun. Provide moderate humidity. When in growth, water freely and apply a balanced liquid fertilizer monthly; water sparingly in winter. Outdoors, grow in moist, lime-free, moderately fertile, humus-rich soil in partial shade; shelter from cold, drying winds.
• **PROPAGATION** Surface-sow seed in containers in a cold frame in autumn. Root semi-ripe cuttings in late summer. Detach and pot up rooted pieces in spring.
• **PESTS AND DISEASES** Trouble free.

A. ovata. Freely branching, evergreen, climbing or creeping shrub with opposite, ovate-rounded, toothed, bristly, deep green leaves, to 4cm (1½in) long, on white-hairy stems. Solitary, long-tubed, bright deep reddish pink flowers, to 6cm (2½in) long, each with 5 spreading lobes forming a 2-lipped mouth, are produced from the leaf axils in summer. ↕ 4m (12ft), ↔ 2m (6ft). Chile, Argentina. ✻✻

ASTILBE

SAXIFRAGACEAE

Genus of about 12 species of densely clump-forming, rhizomatous perennials from moist sites in mountain ravines, woodland, and streambanks in S.E. Asia and North America. Astilbes are grown for their striking, plume-like panicles, 18–35cm (7–14in) long, of tiny, red, pink, purple, or white flowers, borne mainly in summer. The dry flowerheads fade to decorative shades of brown in autumn, providing continued interest throughout the winter. They are attractive as cut flowers, but quickly fade. The handsome leaves, usually 23–75cm (9–30in) long, are 2- or 3-ternate, with each leaflet further divided into 3–5 toothed lobes. Grow in a damp border or a woodland garden, or use for waterside plantings.

Numerous *Astilbe* hybrids have been raised. They are the result of often complex crosses between *A.* x *arendsii, A. astilboides, A. chinensis, A. chinensis* var. *davidii, A. chinensis* var. *taquetii, A. japonica, A. simplicifolia,* and *A. thunbergii. A.* x *arendsii* hybrids are 50–120cm (20–47in) tall, with ovate to lance-shaped, 2- or 3-ternate leaves, 20–75cm (8–28in) long, and panicles to 45cm (18in) long in the largest cultivars. *A. chinensis* and *A. chinensis* var. *davidii* hybrids are either low-growing, 15–25cm (6–10in) high, or tall, growing to 80–130cm (32–54in) high. They have elliptic-ovate, 3-ternate leaves, 15–50cm (6–20in) long, and slender panicles, 10–20cm (4–8in) long. *A. japonica* hybrids are 50–100cm (20–39in) tall, with ovate to ovate-lance-shaped, 2- or 3-ternate leaves, 15–60cm (6–24in) long, and erect, branched panicles, 10–20cm (4–8in) long. *A. simplicifolia* hybrids are usually 30–50cm (12–20in) tall, occasionally dwarf, with ovate to narrowly ovate, 2-ternate leaves, 13–55cm (5–22in) long, and small, arched panicles, 10–20cm (4–8in) long. *A. thunbergii* hybrids are 50–80cm (20–32in) tall, with ovate to lance-shaped, 2-ternate leaves, 20–55cm (8–22in) long, and open panicles, 20–30cm (8–12in) long, of white or pink flowers.
• **HARDINESS** Fully hardy.
• **CULTIVATION** Grow in moist, humus-rich soil or boggy sites in full sun; in drier soils, grow in partial shade. Astilbes prefer fertile soil and will not thrive in chalky or clay soils that dry out in summer. Divide and replant every 3 or 4 years to maintain vigour and flower quality, discarding old, woody rhizomes. The flowers and young foliage may be damaged by late frosts.
• **PROPAGATION** Divide in winter or early spring when dormant; either replant the divisions immediately or pot them up to plant out in early summer when re-established.
• **PESTS AND DISEASES** Powdery mildew and leaf spot may be a problem.

***A.* 'Amethyst'.** Tall *A.* x *arendsii* hybrid with 3-ternate, mid-green leaves and open panicles of lilac-pink flowers in early summer. ↕ 80–100cm (32–39in), ↔ 60–90cm (24–36in). ✻✻✻
***A.* 'Aphrodite'** ▣ Clump-forming *A. simplicifolia* hybrid bearing panicles of red flowers above bronze foliage in midsummer. ↕ 40–60cm (16–24in), ↔ 60cm (24in). ✻✻✻
***A.* 'Brautschleier'** 🏆 syn. *A.* 'Bridal Veil'. Clump-forming *A.* x *arendsii* hybrid producing elegant sprays of nodding white flowers. They open in midsummer from bright green buds above bright green leaves, and fade to creamy yellow. ↕↔ 75cm (30in). ✻✻✻
***A.* 'Bressingham Beauty'.** Tall *A.* x *arendsii* hybrid with spreading, bronze-flushed, mid-green leaves and panicles of bright pink flowers in midsummer. ↕ 90cm (36in), ↔ 60cm (24in). ✻✻✻
***A.* 'Bridal Veil'** see *A.* 'Brautschleier'.
***A.* 'Bronce Elegans'** 🏆 syn. *A.* 'Bronze Elegance'. Clump-forming *A. simplicifolia* hybrid with dark green

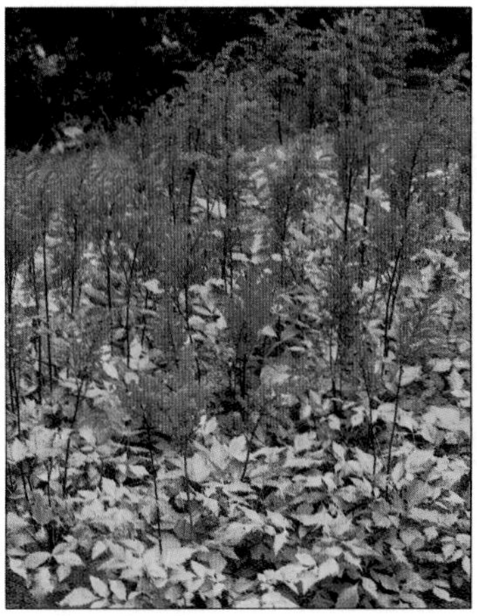

Astilbe 'Aphrodite'

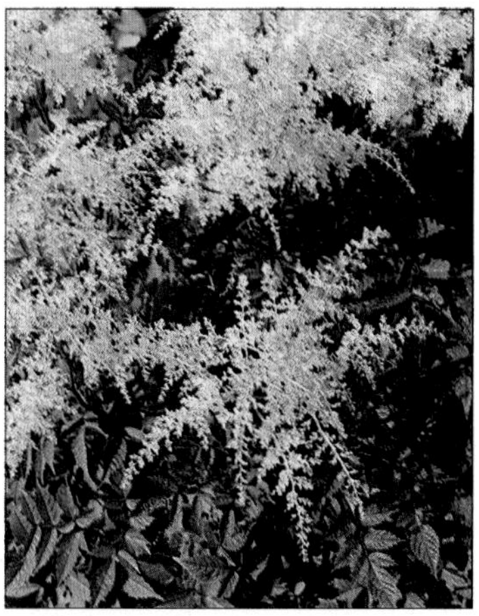

Astilbe 'Deutschland'

leaves. Panicles of pink-red flowers are produced on reddish green stems in late summer. ↕ 30cm (12in), ↔ 25cm (10in). ✻✻✻
***A.* 'Bronze Elegance'** see *A.* 'Bronce Elegans'.
A. chinensis. Vigorous perennial with 3-ternate, toothed, softly hairy, dark green leaves. In late summer, bears panicles of pinkish white flowers. ↕↔ to 60cm (24in). Siberia, China, Korea. ✻✻✻. **var. *davidii*,** syn. *A. davidii*, has bronze-tinted leaves and short, almost erect branches bearing slender panicles of purple-pink flowers. Thrives in sun or shade; ↕ to 2m (6ft), ↔ 60cm (24in); China. **var. *pumila*** 🏆 is dwarf, with red-green leaves and broad, dense, conical panicles of reddish pink flowers; ↕ to 25cm (10in), ↔ to 20cm (8in). **var. *taquetii* 'Purpurlanze'** see *A.* 'Purpurlanze'.
***A.* 'Cologne'** see *A.* 'Köln'.
***A.* x *crispa* 'Gnom'** see *A.* 'Gnom'.
***A.* x *crispa* 'Perkeo'** see *A.* 'Perkeo'.
A. davidii see *A. chinensis* var. *davidii.*
***A.* 'Deutschland'** ▣ Clump-forming *A. japonica* hybrid with erect panicles of pure white flowers above bright green foliage in late spring. ↕ 50cm (20in), ↔ 30cm (12in). ✻✻✻
***A.* 'Drayton Glory'** see *A.* 'Peach Blossom'.
***A.* 'Europa'.** Clump-forming *A. japonica* hybrid with mid-green leaves and dense panicles of light pink flowers in late spring and early summer. ↕ 60cm (24in), ↔ 45cm (18in). ✻✻✻
***A.* 'Fanal'** ▣ 🏆 Clump-forming *A.* x *arendsii* hybrid producing dark green foliage. Dense panicles of long-lasting,

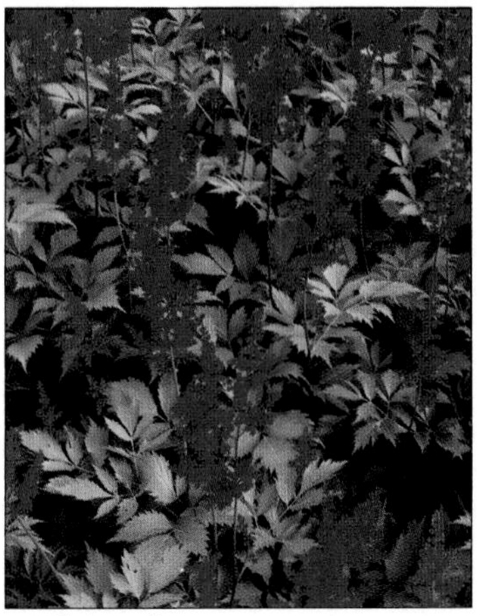

Astilbe 'Fanal'

A

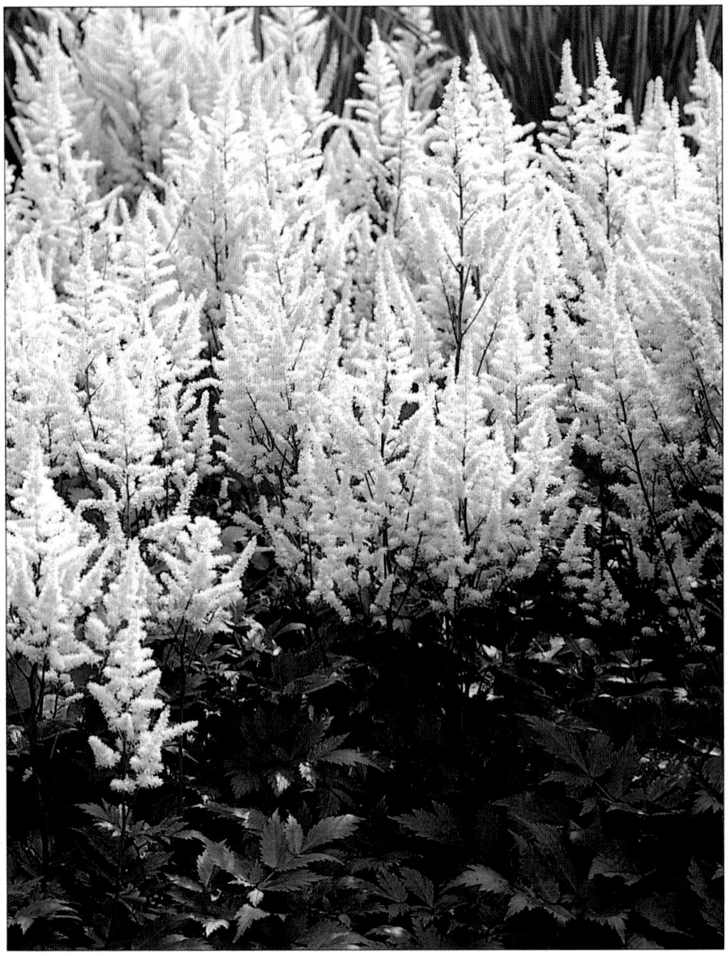
Astilbe 'Irrlicht'

dark crimson flowers are borne in early summer. ↕60cm (24in), ↔45cm (18in). ❄❄❄
A. 'Federsee'. Strong-growing *A.* x *arendsii* hybrid bearing dense, conical panicles of deep rose-pink flowers over mid-green foliage in mid- and late summer. ↕60cm (24in), ↔45cm (18in). ❄❄❄
A. 'Gertrud Brix'. Clump-forming *A.* x *arendsii* hybrid producing panicles of deep red flowers over mid-green foliage in early and midsummer. ↕60cm (24in), ↔45cm (18in). ❄❄❄
A. glaberrima* var. *saxatilis ♀ syn. *A. japonica* var. *terrestris.* Dwarf, clump-forming perennial with toothed, 2-ternate, deep green leaves, red-tinted beneath. Spikes, 8–10cm (3–4in) long, of white-tipped mauve flowers are borne in summer. Thrives in moist soil. ↕to 8cm (3in), ↔15cm (6in). Japan. ❄❄❄
A. 'Gnom', syn. *A.* x *crispa* 'Gnom', *A. simplicifolia* 'Gnome'. Arching, clump-forming *A. simplicifolia* hybrid with basal rosettes of deeply cut, reddish green leaves with wavy leaflets. Produces tiny pink flowers in dense spikes, 15cm (6in) long, in summer. ↕to 15cm (6in), ↔ to 20cm (8in). ❄❄❄
A. 'Granat'. *A.* x *arendsii* hybrid bearing pyramidal panicles of deep red flowers over dark green foliage in midsummer. ↕60cm (24in), ↔45cm (18in). ❄❄❄
A. 'Hyacinth' see *A.* 'Hyazinth'.
A. 'Hyazinth', syn. *A.* 'Hyacinth'. Tall *A.* x *arendsii* hybrid with compact panicles of lilac-pink flowers over bright green foliage in mid- and late summer. ↕1m (3ft), ↔45cm (18in). ❄❄❄

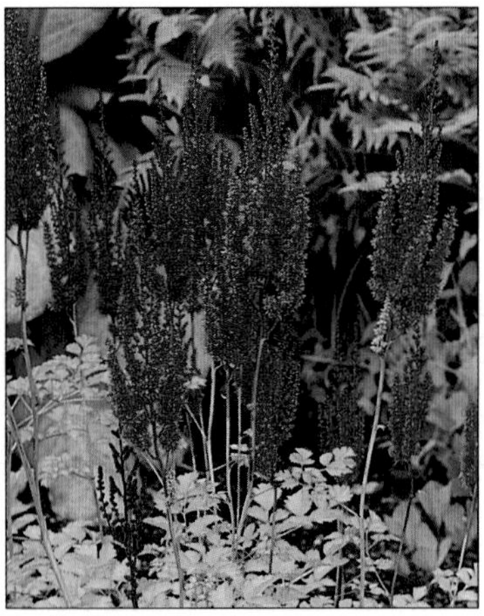
Astilbe 'Purpurlanze'

A. 'Irrlicht' ■ Clump-forming *A.* x *arendsii* hybrid bearing elegant panicles of white flowers over dark green foliage in late spring and early summer. ↕↔50cm (18in). ❄❄❄
A. japonica* var. *terrestris see *A. glaberrima* var. *saxatilis.*
A. 'Jo Ophorst'. Tall *A. chinensis* var. *davidii* hybrid producing dense, erect panicles of lilac-tinted pink flowers over mid-green foliage in late summer. ↕to 1.4m (4½ft), ↔60cm (24in). ❄❄❄
A. 'Koblenz'. Clump-forming *A. japonica* hybrid with bronze-tinted, dark green leaves and open panicles of deep salmon-pink flowers in midsummer. ↕60cm (24in), ↔50cm (20in). ❄❄❄
A. 'Köln', syn. *A.* 'Cologne'. Clump-forming *A. japonica* hybrid with bronze-suffused, dark green leaves and panicles of deep pink flowers in midsummer. ↕60cm (24in), ↔45cm (18in). ❄❄❄
A. 'Montgomery'. Clump-forming *A. japonica* hybrid bearing tapering panicles of deep red flowers over finely cut, dark red-bronze foliage in mid-summer. ↕60–70cm (24–28in), ↔45cm (18in). ❄❄❄
A. 'Ostrich Plume' see *A.* 'Straussenfeder'.
A. 'Peach Blossom', syn. *A.* 'Drayton Glory'. *A. japonica* hybrid producing peach-pink flower panicles over mid-green foliage in midsummer. ↕60cm (24in), ↔45cm (18in). ❄❄❄
A. 'Perkeo' ■♀ syn. *A.* x *crispa* 'Perkeo'. Compact, clump-forming perennial with finely cut, dark green leaves, bronze-tinted when young. Bears pyramidal spires, 15–20cm (6–8in) long, of small, deep pink flowers in

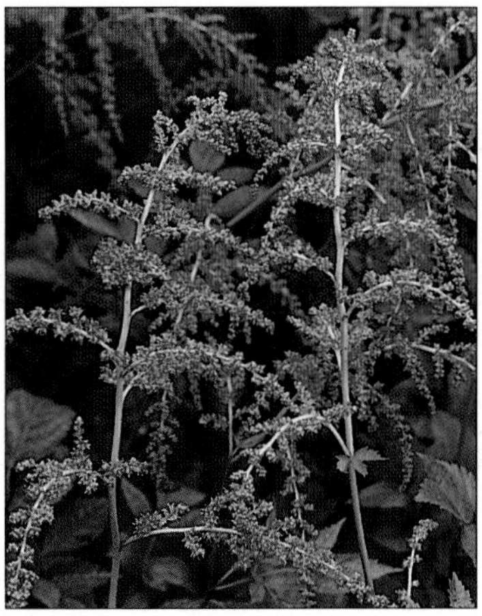
Astilbe 'Straussenfeder'

summer. Suitable for a border or a rock garden. ↕↔ to 20cm (8in). ❄❄❄
A. 'Professor van der Wielen' ■ Graceful *A. thunbergii* hybrid bearing open, arching plumes of white flowers over mid-green foliage in midsummer. ↕1.2m (4ft), ↔ to 100cm (39in). ❄❄❄
A. 'Purple Lance' see *A.* 'Purpurlanze'.
A. 'Purpurlanze' ■ syn. *A. chinensis* var. *taquetii* 'Purpurlanze', *A.* 'Purple Lance'. Tall, vigorous *A. chinensis* hybrid bearing panicles of purple-red flowers over mid-green foliage in late summer and early autumn. Will tolerate drier conditions than most cultivars. ↕1.2m (4ft), ↔90cm (36in). ❄❄❄
A. 'Red Sentinel'. Clump-forming *A. japonica* hybrid producing panicles of deep crimson-red flowers over dark green foliage in early summer. ↕1m (3ft), ↔50cm (20in). ❄❄❄
A. 'Rheinland' ♀ Clump-forming *A. japonica* hybrid with mid-green foliage, and compact, upright panicles of rich pink flowers throughout summer. ↕50cm (20in), ↔45cm (18in). ❄❄❄
***A. simplicifolia* 'Gnome'** see *A.* 'Gnom'.
A. 'Sprite' ■♀ Clump-forming *A. simplicifolia* hybrid with broad, mid-

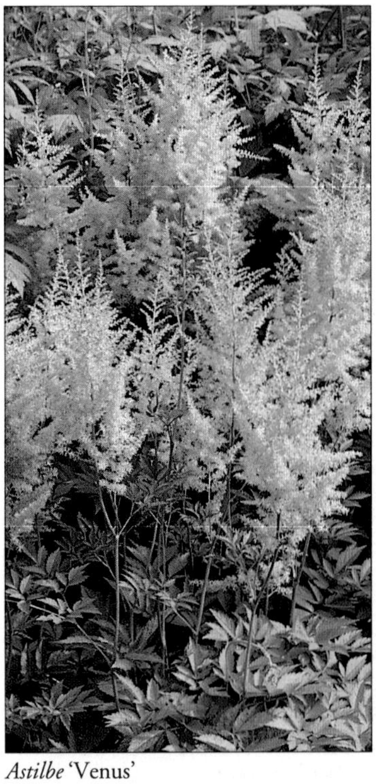
Astilbe 'Venus'

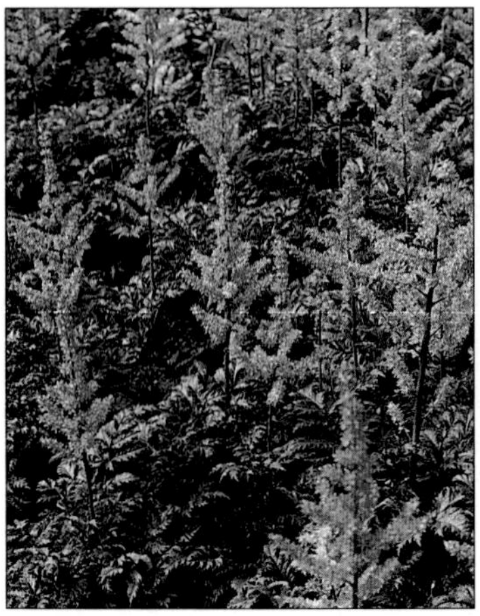
Astilbe 'Perkeo'

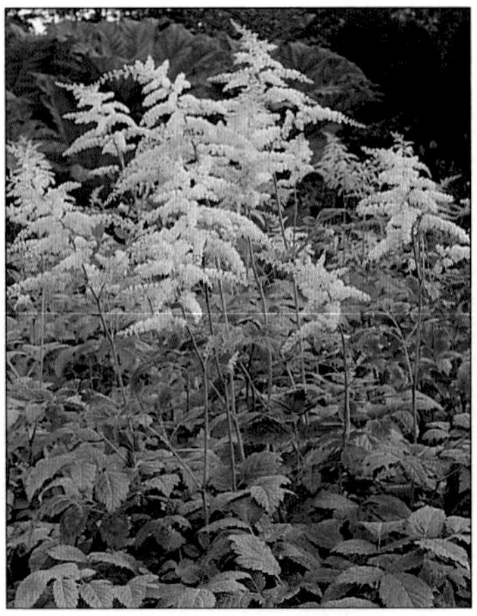
Astilbe 'Professor van der Wielen'

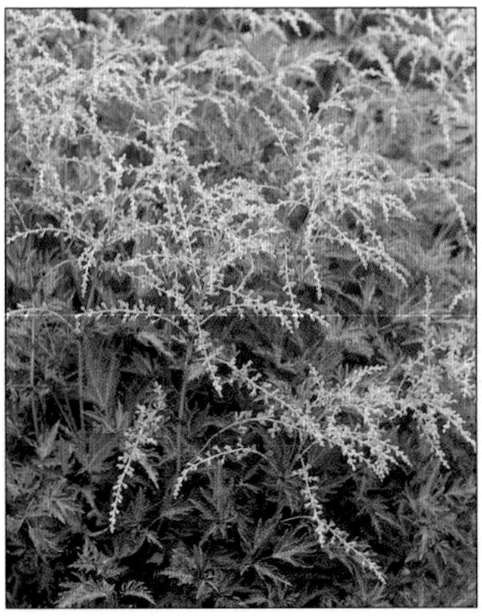
Astilbe 'Sprite'

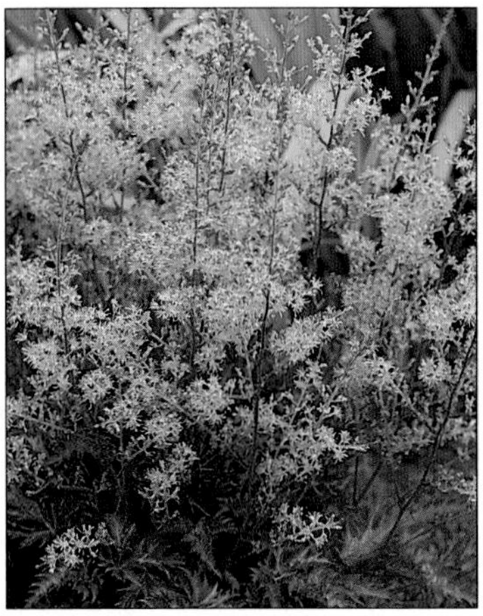

Astilbe 'William Buchanan'

green leaves composed of narrow leaflets. Bears feathery spikes of small, shell-pink flowers in summer. ↕ 50cm (20in), ↔ to 1m (3ft). ❄❄❄
A. 'Straussenfeder' ■ 🏆 syn. *A.* 'Ostrich Plume'. Vigorous *A. thunbergii* hybrid with bronze-tinted young foliage and open, arching sprays of rich coral-pink flowers in late summer and early autumn. Requires ample moisture in the growing season. ↕ 90cm (36in), ↔ 60cm (24in). ❄❄❄
A. 'Venus' ■ Tall *A.* x *arendsii* hybrid bearing tapering, feathery panicles of bright pink flowers over bright green foliage in early summer. ↕ 1m (3ft), ↔ 45cm (18in). ❄❄❄
A. 'Weisse Gloria', syn. *A.* 'White Glory'. Strong-growing *A.* x *arendsii* hybrid with mid-green leaves, and large panicles of white flowers in late summer and early autumn. ↕ 1m (3ft), ↔ 45cm (18in). ❄❄❄
A. 'White Glory' see *A.* 'Weisse Gloria'.
A. 'William Buchanan' ■ Dwarf *A. simplicifolia* hybrid producing red-tinted leaves and panicles of white flowers with red stamens, appearing pink overall, in mid- and late summer. ↕ 23–30cm (9–12in), ↔ 20cm (8in). ❄❄❄

ASTILBOIDES

SAXIFRAGACEAE

Genus of one species of perennial from moist woodland on the banks of lakes and streams in E. Asia. It produces panicles to 1.5m (5ft) tall, of numerous small, creamy white flowers above rounded clumps of large, lobed leaves. *A. tabularis* is an architectural plant, suitable for a woodland garden or for growing beside a pond or stream.

- **HARDINESS** Fully hardy.
- **CULTIVATION** Grow in cool, moist, humus-rich soil in partial shade. If grown beside water, plant with the roots above water level; it will not tolerate either waterlogging or drought.
- **PROPAGATION** Sow seed in containers in a cold frame in autumn, or divide in spring as growth begins.
- **PESTS AND DISEASES** Slugs may eat the large resting buds.

A. tabularis ■ syn. *Rodgersia tabularis.* Clump-forming perennial with long-stalked, rounded, peltate, shallowly but often sharply lobed, softly hairy, light green leaves, to 90cm (36in) long. In early and midsummer, bears plume-like panicles of numerous tiny, creamy white flowers. ↕ 1.5m (5ft), ↔ 1.2m (4ft). N.E. China, N. Korea. ❄❄❄

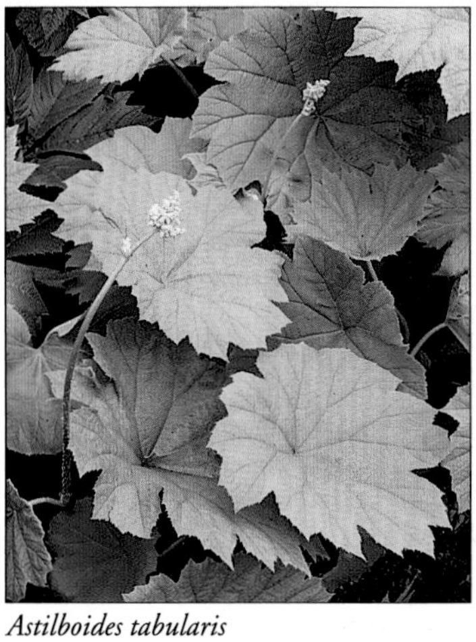

Astilboides tabularis

ASTRANTIA

Hattie's pincushion, Masterwort

APIACEAE / UMBELLIFERAE

Genus of about 10 species of clump-forming perennials found in alpine woods and meadows from Europe to W. Asia. They have loose, basal rosettes of palmately lobed or palmate leaves. Erect umbels of small, 5-petalled flowers, surrounded by ruff-like involucres of showy, papery bracts, are borne in sprays above the foliage. Astrantias will thrive in a woodland garden, on a streambank, or in a moist border. The flowerheads are useful for dried flower arrangements.

- **HARDINESS** Fully hardy.
- **CULTIVATION** Grow in moist, fertile, preferably humus-rich soil in sun or partial shade. Most variants of *A. major* will tolerate drier conditions; they also self-seed prolifically unless dead-headed before the seed is ripe. *A. major* 'Sunningdale Variegated' needs full sun to obtain the best leaf colour.
- **PROPAGATION** Sow seed in containers in a cold frame as soon as ripe. Divide in spring.
- **PESTS AND DISEASES** Slugs, aphids, and powdery mildew may be a problem.

A. major ■ Clump-forming, variable perennial with deeply 3- to 7-lobed, toothed, basal leaves, 8–15cm (3–6in) long. Green-veined white bracts, occasionally pink-tinted, surround the small, green or pink, occasionally deep purple-red flowers, which are borne in

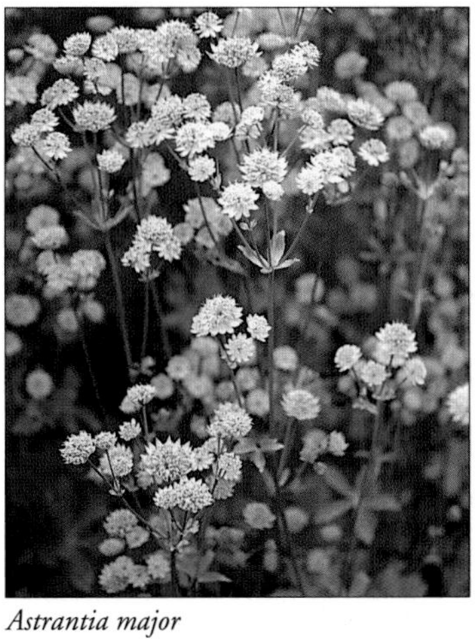

Astrantia major

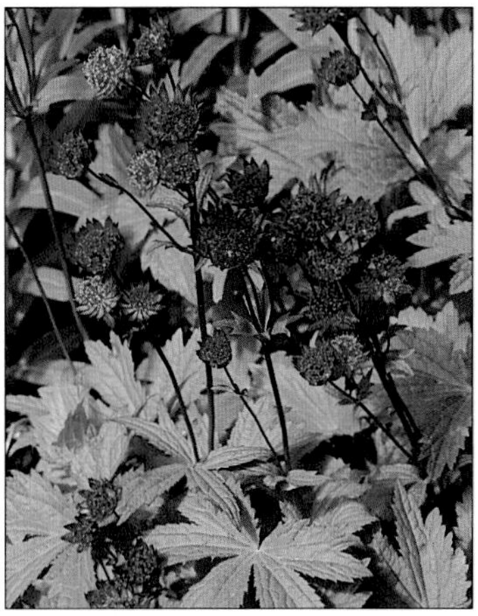

Astrantia major 'Hadspen Blood'

umbels, 2–3cm (¾–1¼in) or occasionally more across, in early and midsummer. ↕ 30–90cm (12–36in), ↔ 45cm (18in). C. and E. Europe. ❄❄❄. **subsp. *carinthiaca*** see subsp. *involucrata.* **'Hadspen Blood'** ■ has dark red bracts and flowers. **subsp. *involucrata*** ■ syn. subsp. *carinthiaca*, var. *involucrata*, has green and white bracteoles, twice as long as the umbel width. **'Margery Fish'** see 'Shaggy'. **'Rosensinfonie'** has rose-pink flowerheads. **'Shaggy'** 🏆 syn. 'Margery Fish', has very long bracts with prominent green tips, and deeply cut leaves. **'Sunningdale Variegated'** ■ 🏆 syn. 'Variegated', has pale pink bracts and attractive leaves unevenly margined creamy yellow. **'Variegated'** see 'Sunningdale Variegated'.

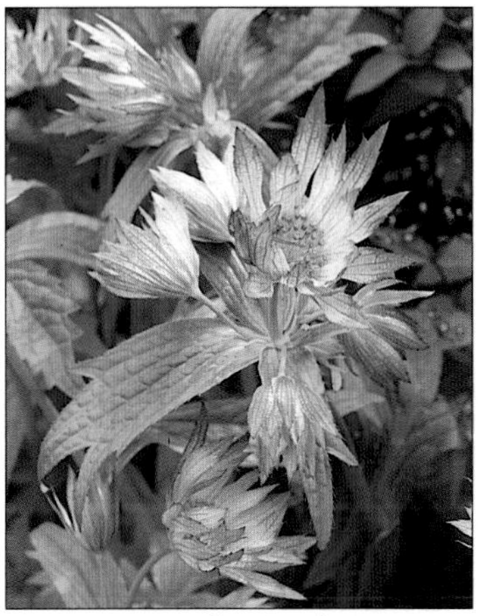

Astrantia major subsp. *involucrata*

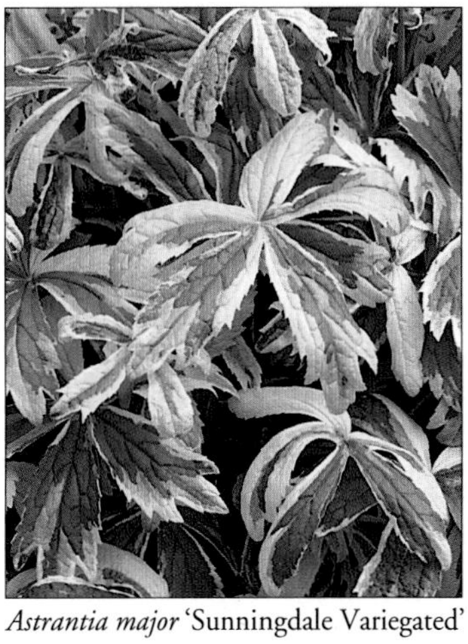

Astrantia major 'Sunningdale Variegated'

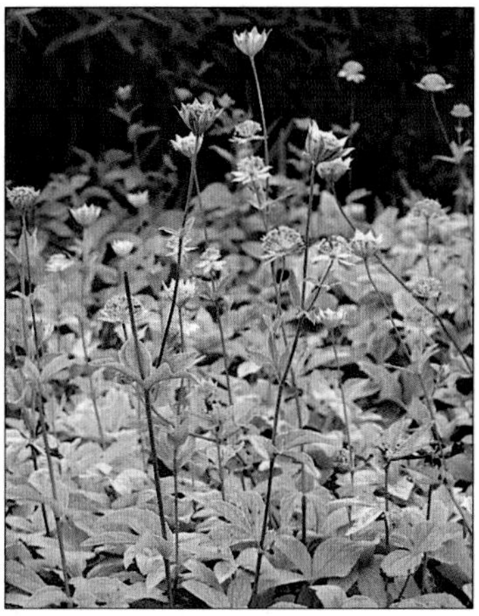

Astrantia maxima

A. maxima ■ Clump-forming perennial producing basal leaves, 3–10cm (1¼–4in) long, deeply divided into 3–5, occasionally almost separate lobes. Umbels, 4–6cm (1½–2½in) across, with sharp-pointed, broad pink bracts, each to 3cm (1¼in) long, surrounding tiny, soft pink flowers, are borne singly, or occasionally in twos or threes, in early and midsummer. ↕ 60cm (24in), ↔ 30cm (12in). Caucasus, Turkey, Iran. ❄❄❄

ASTROPHYTUM

CACTACEAE

Genus of 4–6 species of slow-growing, perennial cacti occurring in dry, arid areas of the USA (S. Texas), and N. and C. Mexico. They have spherical or hemispherical, ribbed stems, some becoming columnar when mature, with woolly, occasionally spiny areoles. Solitary, large, funnel-shaped, diurnal yellow flowers, some with red-tinted throats, are produced in summer. They are followed by ovoid, green or red berries containing boat-shaped, black or brown seeds. Where temperatures fall below 10°C (50°F), grow in a temperate greenhouse. In warmer climates, grow in a desert garden.

- **HARDINESS** Frost tender.
- **CULTIVATION** Under glass, grow in standard cactus compost, with added limestone chippings, in bright filtered light. Water moderately in the growing season; keep dry when dormant. Apply a low-nitrogen liquid fertilizer monthly from mid-spring to late summer. Outdoors, grow in sharply drained, poor, slightly alkaline soil in full sun. See also pp.48–49.
- **PROPAGATION** Sow seed at 21°C (70°F) in early spring.
- **PESTS AND DISEASES** Vulnerable to mealybugs.

A. asterias, syn. *Echinocactus asterias* (Sand dollar cactus, Sea-urchin cactus). Hemispherical cactus with 6–10 flat, purplish brown ribs with straight grooves between. Prominent, spineless white areoles are set along the ribs. Red-throated, bright yellow flowers, 3–7cm (1¼–3in) long, are borne in summer. ↕↔ 10cm (4in). USA (Texas), N.E. Mexico. ❀ (min. 10°C/50°F)
A. capricorne, syn. *Echinocactus capricornis* (Goat's horn cactus). Spherical to ovoid cactus with 7–9 white-flecked, pale green ribs, with deep

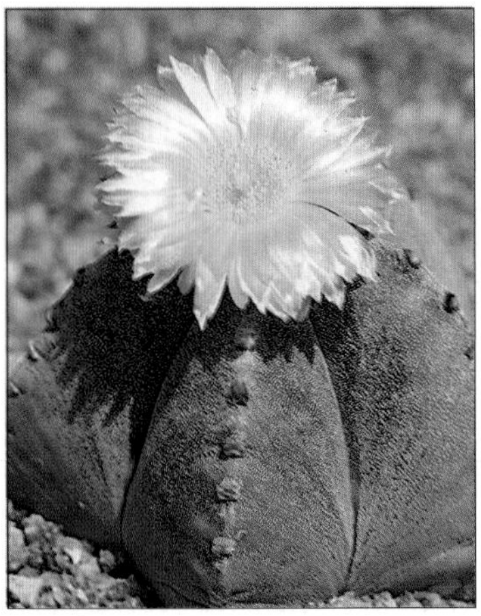

Astrophytum myriostigma

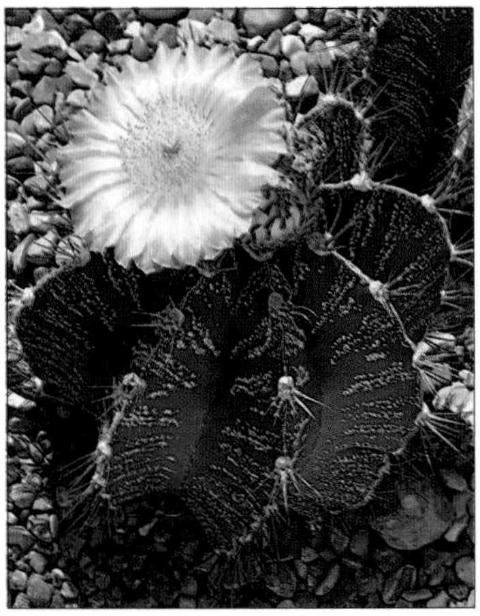

Astrophytum ornatum

grooves between. Areoles bear long, twisted, yellowish brown spines. Red-centred yellow flowers, 6–10cm (2½–4in) long, are produced in summer. ↕ 20–25cm (8–10in), ↔ 10cm (4in). N. Mexico. ❀ (min. 10°C/50°F)

A. myriostigma ■♀ syn. *Echinocactus myriostigma* (Bishop's cap). Spherical or occasionally columnar cactus with usually 4–8 ribs covered with minute, white-woolly scales. Areoles are brown and spineless. Yellow, often red-centred flowers, 4–6cm (1½–2½in) long, are produced in summer. ↕ 23cm (9in), ↔ 20–30cm (8–12in). N.E. Mexico. ❀ (min. 10°C/50°F)

A. ornatum ■ syn. *Echinocactus ornatus.* Spherical to columnar cactus with 6–8 ribs, straight or occasionally spiralled, and cross-banded with woolly scales. Close-set areoles bear brown or yellow spines. Yellow flowers, 7–10cm (3–4in) long, are produced in summer. ↕ 35cm (14in) or more, ↔ 15cm (6in). Central E. Mexico. ❀ (min. 10°C/50°F)

▷ ***Asystasia*** see *Mackaya*
A. bella see *M. bella*

ATHEROSPERMA

MONIMIACEAE

Genus of one species of evergreen tree occurring in woodland in S.E. Australia, including Tasmania. In its natural habitat, *A. moschatum* grows to 20–30m (70–100ft) tall, but it is much smaller in cultivation, when it is best grown in sheltered woodland. Both the opposite, simple, aromatic leaves and the white flowers produced in spring (the male and female blooms on different plants) are attractive. In very cold areas, grow in a cool greenhouse.

• **HARDINESS** Frost hardy.
• **CULTIVATION** Under glass, grow in lime-free (ericaceous) potting compost in full light, shaded from hot sun. Water freely when in growth, applying a balanced liquid fertilizer monthly; water more sparingly in winter. Outdoors, grow in moderately fertile, moist but well-drained, humus-rich, lime-free soil in sun or partial shade, sheltered from cold, drying winds. Pruning group 1.
• **PROPAGATION** Sow seed at 10–13°C (50–55°F) in spring. Root semi-ripe cuttings in summer.
• **PESTS AND DISEASES** Trouble free.

A. moschatum △ (Australian sassafras). Conical tree with lance-shaped, nutmeg-scented, dark green leaves, to 10cm (4in) long, glaucous on the reverse. Solitary, saucer-shaped, fragrant, creamy white flowers, 2.5cm (1in) across, are produced from the upper leaf axils in early spring. ↕ 6m (20ft), ↔ 3m (10ft) in cultivation. S.E. Australia, including Tasmania. ❄❄

ATHROTAXIS

Tasmanian cedar

TAXODIACEAE

Genus of 2 species and 1 natural hybrid of evergreen, coniferous trees, restricted to mountainous areas of W. Tasmania, Australia, where they grow in rocky gullies, on exposed ridges, or around lakes. They have fissured, red- to grey-brown bark, flaking in long shreds, and scale-like or ovate leaves, arranged in spirals, and lying flat to the shoots or spreading. Cones are spherical or ovoid, and green, ripening to brown at the end of the first year. The female cones have 10–16 scales. Useful as small specimen trees, these conifers thrive in areas with cool, humid summers.

• **HARDINESS** Fully hardy to frost hardy.
• **CULTIVATION** Grow in moist but well-drained, moderately fertile, humus-rich, preferably slightly acid soil in full sun, with shelter from cold, dry winds.
• **PROPAGATION** Sow seed in a seedbed or in containers in a cold frame in late winter or early spring. Root semi-ripe cuttings in late summer.
• **PESTS AND DISEASES** Trouble free.

A. x laxifolia ■◊–△ (*A. cupressoides* x *A. selaginoides*) (Tasmanian cedar). Coniferous, narrowly to broadly conical tree with an open crown and shaggy, fissured reddish brown bark. Glossy, dark green leaves, yellowish green when young, are ovate, 4–6mm (⅛–¼in) long, spreading and horizontally arranged along the shoots. Bright green, ovoid cones, 2–2.5cm (¾–1in) long, turn orange-yellow then brown as they ripen. ↕ 10–20m (30–70ft), ↔ 4–6m (12–20ft). Australia (W. Tasmania). ❄❄❄

A. selaginoides ◊ (King William pine). Conical, coniferous tree with an open crown and fissured, shredding, reddish brown bark. Similar to *A.* x *laxifolia*, except that the ovate leaves, to 1.5cm (½in) long, spread more widely, and are bright green with blue-white bands along their length; the bark is thicker and the spherical cones are larger, to

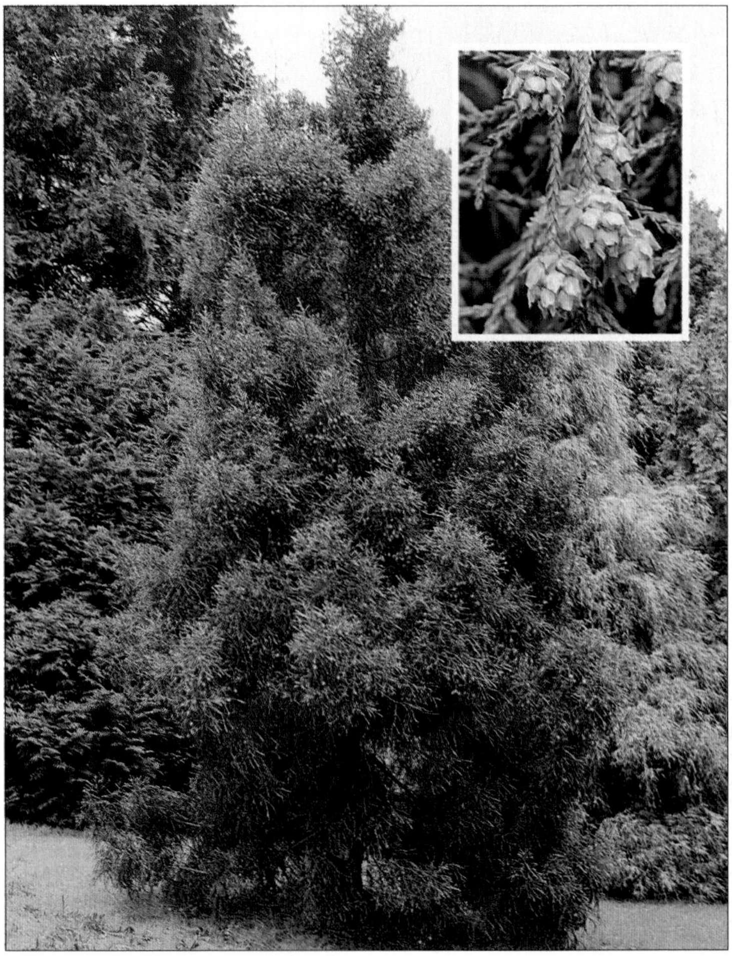

Athrotaxis x *laxifolia* (inset: cone detail)

3cm (1¼in) long, becoming orange-brown when ripe. It requires a moister site than *A.* x *laxifolia.* ↕ 15–30m (50–100ft), ↔ 4–8m (12–25ft). Australia (W. Tasmania). ❄❄

ATHYRIUM

Lady fern

ATHYRIACEAE/DRYOPTERIDACEAE/ WOODSIACEAE

Genus of 180 species of deciduous, terrestrial ferns found mainly in moist woodland or forest in temperate and tropical regions of the world. They have erect or creeping, sometimes branched rhizomes. Fronds are normally pinnate to 3-pinnate or pinnatifid, but in a few species are simple. Sori form in 2 rows and are usually covered by J-shaped indusia. Lady ferns tolerate all but dry conditions, and are useful for a range of sites, from a shady border to a woodland setting. In frost-prone areas, grow the tropical species as houseplants or in a warm greenhouse. *A. niponicum* is also suitable for a cool greenhouse or conservatory.

• **HARDINESS** Fully hardy to frost tender. *A. filix-femina* is hardy to -30°C (-22°F).
• **CULTIVATION** Under glass, grow in 1 part each of loam, medium-grade bark, and charcoal; 2 parts sharp sand; and 3 parts coarse leaf mould. Provide bright filtered light and high humidity. In growth, water freely and apply a half-strength fertilizer monthly; water sparingly in winter. Outdoors, grow in moist, fertile, neutral to acid soil, enriched with leaf mould or garden compost, in a shaded, sheltered site.
• **PROPAGATION** Sow spores as soon as ripe at 21°C (70°F) for tender species, and 15–16°C (59–61°F) for hardy ones. Divide in spring. See also p.51.
• **PESTS AND DISEASES** Trouble free.

A. filix-femina ♀ (Lady fern). Variable, deciduous fern with erect rhizomes and usually lance-shaped, 2- or 3-pinnate or pinnatifid, light green fronds, 1m (3ft) long, sometimes with red-brown stalks, borne like upright shuttlecocks and arching outwards with age. Pinnae are variably sized, but usually elliptic with long, pointed tips; segments are lance-shaped to oblong. ↕ to 1.2m (4ft), ↔ 60–90cm (24–36in). Widespread in temperate regions of N. hemisphere. ❄❄❄. **Cruciatum Group** cultivars have crested fronds, 30–50cm (12–20in)

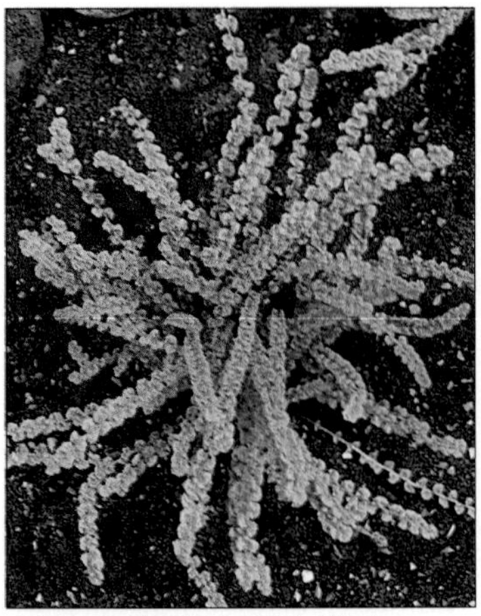

Athyrium filix-femina 'Frizelliae'

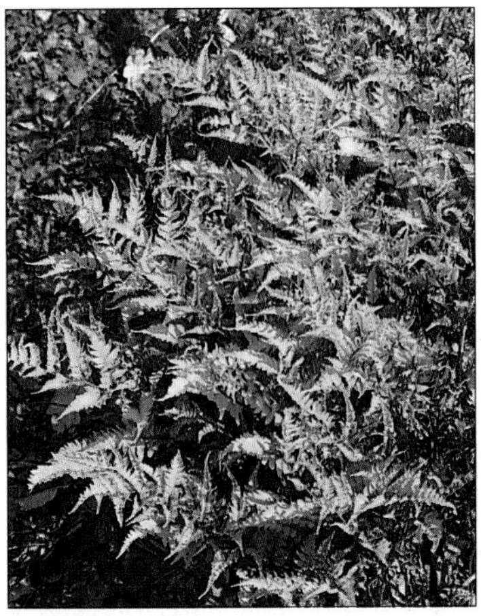

Athyrium niponicum

long, with each pinna branching at the midrib, producing the effect of a row of crosses; ↕90cm (36in); often sold incorrectly as 'Victoriae' (Queen Victoria's lady fern), a very rare cultivar with pinnae and segments branching to form crosses. **'Frizelliae'** ▣ (Mrs. Frizell's lady fern, Tatting fern) has fronds 10–20cm (4–8in) long, and pinnae reduced to rounded lobes along each side of the midribs, resembling tatting (handmade lace); ↕20cm (8in), ↔30cm (12in). **'Minutissimum'** is smaller than the species, and forms dense clumps; ↕30cm (12in), ↔40cm (16in). **Plumosum Cristatum Group** cultivars have finely cut fronds that are also crested; ↕↔90cm (36in). **Plumosum Group** cultivars have 3- or 4-pinnate fronds with finely cut segments; ↕1.2m (4ft), ↔90cm (36in). **'Vernoniae'** has narrowly triangular, crisped segments; ↕↔75cm (30in).
A. goeringianum see *A. niponicum*.
A. niponicum ▣ syn. *A. goeringianum*, *A. nipponicum* (Japanese painted fern). Deciduous fern with creeping red-brown rhizomes and 2- or 3-pinnate to pinnatifid, lance-shaped, silvery grey-green or mid-green fronds, to 35cm (14in) long, with red-purple midribs. Segments are lance-shaped to oblong or ovate, sometimes with notched or lobed margins. Frond colouring is variable; if growing from spores, select plants with the strongest silver markings. ↕20–30cm (8–12in), ↔ indefinite. Japan. ❄❄❄.
var. *pictum* ♀ syn. 'Pictum', f. *metallicum*, has fronds with purplish red stalks and silver-grey segments, sometimes flushed purple-red.
A. nipponicum see *A. niponicum*.

▷***Atragene*** see *Clematis*

ATRIPLEX

CHENOPODIACEAE

Genus of about 100 species of evergreen or semi-evergreen shrubs, subshrubs, annuals, and perennials, found on coasts and in saltmarshes, salt flats, and deserts worldwide. They have alternate or opposite, often grey or silver leaves and insignificant flowers. *A. halimus* is an attractive foliage shrub for a border, and also useful for hedging in coastal areas. Use the edible leaves of coloured variants of *A. hortensis* to provide contrast in summer bedding, or as a colourful addition to salads.
• **HARDINESS** Frost hardy to half hardy.
• **CULTIVATION** Grow shrubs in well-drained, dry, poor to moderately fertile soil in full sun, sheltered from cold, dry winds. Pruning group 1. Grow *A. hortensis* in moist but well-drained, fertile soil in full sun; water freely during dry periods to inhibit bolting.
• **PROPAGATION** Sow seed of *A. hortensis in situ* in succession from spring to early summer. Root softwood cuttings of shrubs in summer.
• **PESTS AND DISEASES** Trouble free.

A. halimus (Tree purslane). Dense, semi-evergreen shrub with alternate, ovate or diamond-shaped, sometimes toothed, leathery, silvery grey leaves, to 6cm (2½in) long. In late summer, bears tiny, greenish white flowers in terminal panicles, to 30cm (12in) long. Tolerates full exposure to sea winds. ↕2m (6ft), ↔2.5m (8ft). S. Europe. ❄❄
A. hortensis (Red mountain spinach, Red orache). Erect annual grown for its spinach-like, succulent, alternate or opposite, lance-shaped, green to purple-brown leaves, to 18cm (7in) long; they are slightly downy when young, and may be shallowly toothed or entire. Green or red-brown flowers are borne in tall, foxtail-like, terminal racemes, to 20cm (8in) long, in summer. ↕1.2m (4ft), ↔30cm (12in). Asia, also naturalized widely in Europe and North America. ❄. **Plume Series** contains variants selected for their yellow, green, or burgundy-red flowerheads and foliage. **var. *rubra*** has blood-red or purple-red foliage and flowering spikes.

▷**Aubretia** see *Aubrieta*

AUBRIETA

Aubretia

BRASSICACEAE/CRUCIFERAE

Genus of about 12 species of evergreen, mound- or carpet-forming perennials, occurring among rocks, in scree, and in coniferous woodland from Europe to C. Asia. They have small, obovate to oblong, entire or toothed, hairy, mid-green leaves, and few-flowered racemes of cross-shaped, 4-petalled, colourful flowers, usually borne in abundance in spring. Grow on walls, as ground cover on a sunny bank, or in a rock garden.
• **HARDINESS** Fully hardy.
• **CULTIVATION** Grow in moderately fertile, well-drained, preferably neutral or alkaline soil in full sun. Cut back after flowering to maintain compactness.

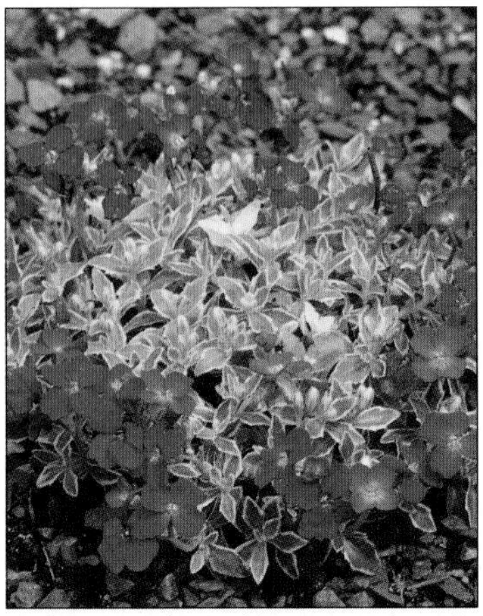

Aubrieta x *cultorum* 'Argenteovariegata'

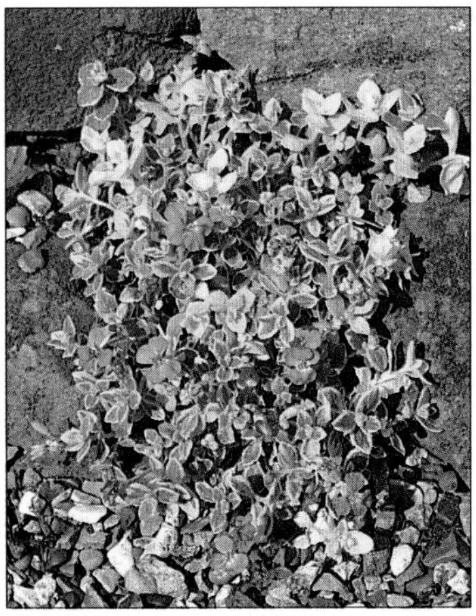

Aubrieta x *cultorum* 'Aureovariegata'

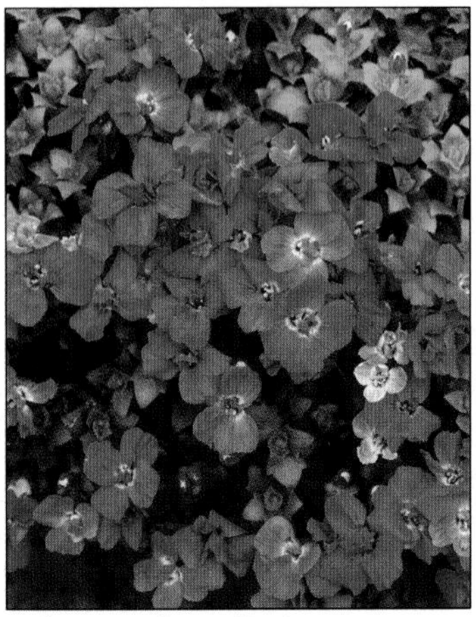

Aubrieta x *cultorum* 'Joy'

• **PROPAGATION** Sow seed in containers in a cold frame in autumn or spring; seed germinates freely, but rarely comes true from cultivated plants. Root softwood cuttings in early summer, or semi-ripe cuttings in midsummer. Division of clumps in autumn is less successful than taking cuttings.
• **PESTS AND DISEASES** Prone to aphids, eelworms, flea beetles, and white blister.

***A.* x *cultorum*.** Mat-forming perennials of complex hybrid origin, usually grown in preference to the species. They are available in a wide range of colours, with single or double flowers, to 1.5cm (½in) across, borne in profusion in spring. All are often listed under *A. deltoidea*. ↕5cm (2in), ↔ to 60cm (24in) or more. ❄❄❄.
'Albomarginata' see 'Argenteovariegata'. **'Argenteovariegata'** ▣ syn. 'Albomarginata', has soft, mid-green leaves, margined silvery white, and single, pinkish mauve flowers.
'Aureovariegata' ▣ is similar to 'Argenteovariegata', but has irregularly gold-margined leaves and single mauve-pink flowers. **'Barker's Double'** has double, pink-tinged purple flowers.
'Bressingham Pink' bears large heads of double pink flowers. **'Carnival'** see 'Hartswood Purple'. **'Greencourt Purple'** has single purple flowers.
'Hartswood Purple', syn. 'Carnival', has large, single violet flowers. **'Joy'** ▣ bears double mauve flowers on short stems. **'J.S. Baker'** ▣ produces single purple flowers with white eyes.

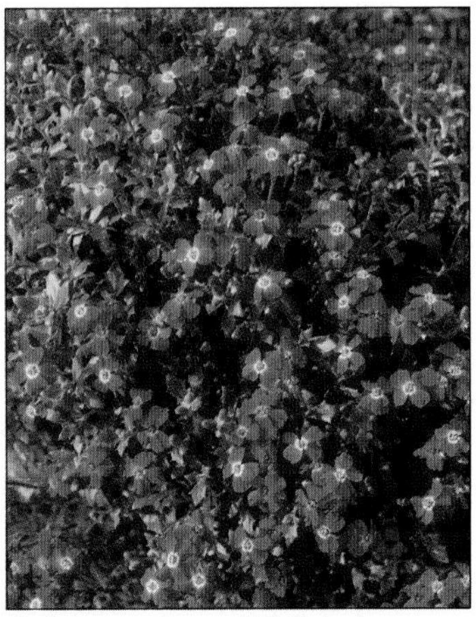

Aubrieta x *cultorum* 'J.S. Baker'

AUCUBA

CORNACEAE

Genus of 3 or 4 species of evergreen, dioecious shrubs from a wide variety of habitats from the Himalayas to E. Asia. While cultivated for their bold, alternate leaves and large fruits, aucubas are most valued for their tolerance of full shade, dry soils, pollution, and salt winds. Use as specimen plants, for hedges and screens, or to fill a dark corner where little else will flourish. They are also suitable for containers outdoors and as large houseplants.
• **HARDINESS** Fully hardy.
• **CULTIVATION** Grow in any but water-logged soil, in full sun or partial or full shade; variegated plants prefer partial shade. All are best in shade where summers are very hot. In containers, grow in loam-based potting compost (JI No.2). When in growth, water freely and apply a balanced liquid fertilizer monthly; water sparingly in winter. Pruning group 1. Trim hedges and cut back shrubs hard in spring.
• **PROPAGATION** Sow seed in containers in a cold frame in autumn or root semi-ripe cuttings in summer.
• **PESTS AND DISEASES** Trouble free.

A. japonica ▣ (Spotted laurel). Rounded, evergreen shrub with elliptic to ovate, glossy, mid-green leaves, to 20cm (8in) long, usually with a few marginal teeth. In mid-spring, bears small, red-purple flowers, the males with yellow anthers, in erect panicles to 10cm (4in) long. Female plants produce bright red berries, to 1cm (½in) across, in autumn. All parts may cause mild stomach upset if ingested. ↕↔3m (10ft).

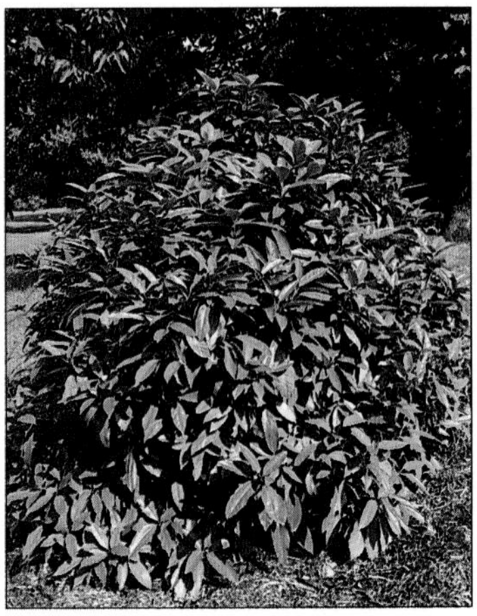

Aucuba japonica

A

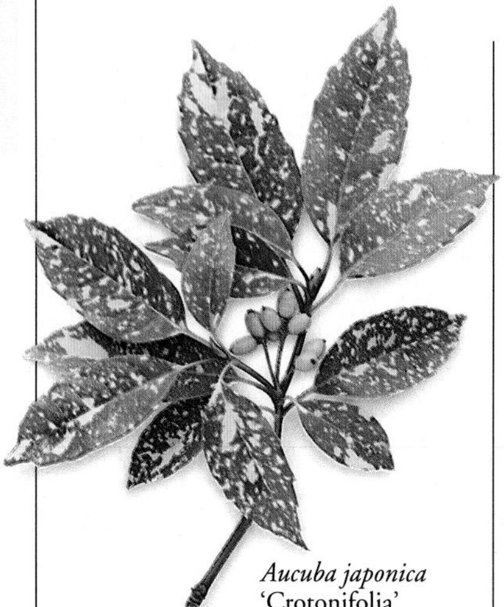

Aucuba japonica 'Crotonifolia'

Japan. ✻✻✻. **'Crassifolia'** is male, with large, leathery, dark green leaves, to 25cm (10in) long. **'Crotonifolia'** ▣ 🏆 is female, with yellow-speckled leaves. **'Gold Dust'** is female, with leaves heavily speckled golden yellow. **'Hillieri'** is female, with glossy, dark green leaves, to 25cm (10in) long. **'Lance Leaf'** is male, with lance-shaped, entire leaves. **'Picturata'** is female, and has leaves marked yellow in the centres; it often reverts. **'Rozannie'** is compact, with broadly elliptic, dark green leaves and bisexual flowers; ↕ 1m (3ft). **'Salicifolia'** is female, with slender leaves. **'Sulphurea Marginata'** is female, with yellow-margined leaves.

AURINIA

BRASSICACEAE/CRUCIFERAE

Genus, closely allied to *Alyssum*, of 7 species of clump-forming biennials or woody-based, evergreen perennials, found in rocky, mountainous areas from C. and S. Europe, eastwards to Russia and Turkey. They bear rosettes of hairy, usually inversely lance-shaped to spoon-shaped leaves, and racemes or panicles of 4-petalled, yellow or white flowers. They are robust plants for a rock garden, the front of a border, or a sunny bank.

- **HARDINESS** Fully hardy.
- **CULTIVATION** Grow in moderately fertile soil in full sun. Ensure good drainage. Cut back after flowering to maintain compactness.
- **PROPAGATION** Sow seed in containers in a cold frame in autumn, or root softwood cuttings in early summer.
- **PESTS AND DISEASES** Prone to aphids.

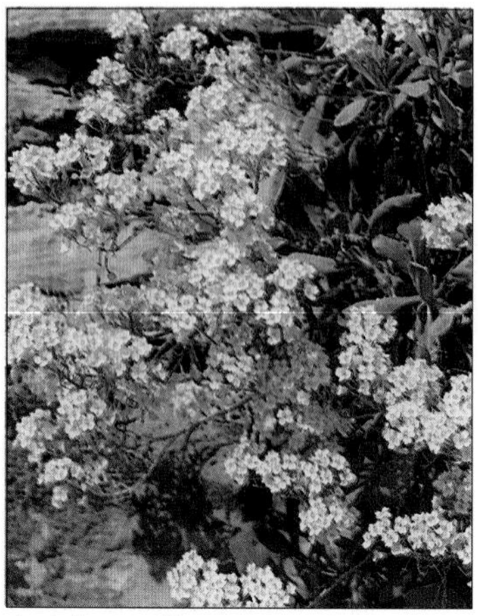

Aurinia saxatilis

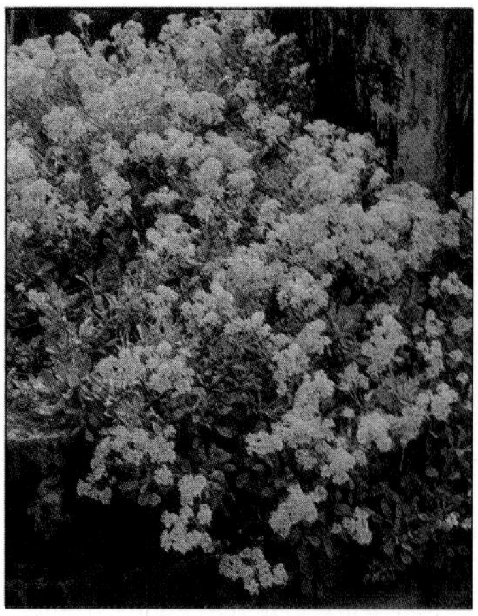

Aurinia saxatilis 'Dudley Nevill'

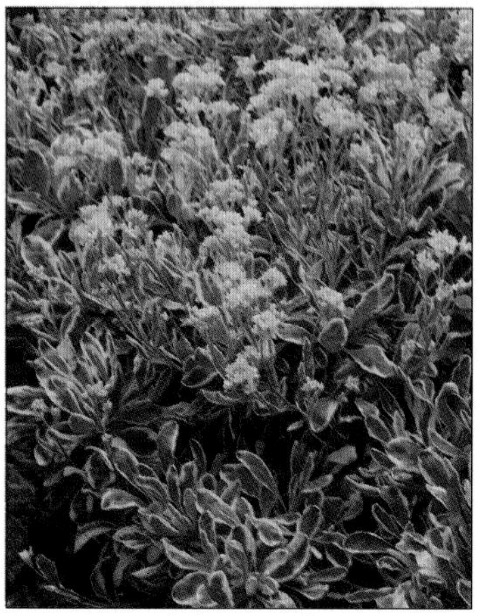

Aurinia saxatilis 'Variegata'

A. saxatilis ▣ 🏆 syn. *Alyssum saxatile* (Gold dust). Evergreen, mound-forming perennial with rosetted, obovate, occasionally pinnatifid, toothed, hairy, grey-green leaves, 3–7cm (1¼–3in) long, sometimes to 12cm (5in) long. Dense panicles of bright yellow flowers, to 1cm (½in) across, are borne in late spring and early summer. ↕ 20cm (8in), ↔ to 30cm (12in). C. and S.E. Europe. ✻✻✻. **'Citrina'** 🏆 bears abundant panicles of lemon-yellow flowers. **'Dudley Nevill'** ▣ bears soft yellowish buff flowers. **'Variegata'** ▣ has leaves with irregular creamy margins.

▷**Austrian briar** see *Rosa foetida*

AUSTROCEDRUS

CUPRESSACEAE

Genus of one species of evergreen, coniferous tree from the Andes of Chile and Argentina, where it grows on steep, dry mountain slopes with winter rain or snow and a prolonged dry season. *A. chilensis* forms a small, columnar tree, with flattened, moss- or fern-like sprays of foliage, similar to *Calocedrus*. The solitary cones each have 4 scales, hinged at the bases; only the central pair are fertile. Grow as a specimen tree.

- **HARDINESS** Fully hardy to frost hardy.
- **CULTIVATION** Grow in any moist but well-drained, moderately fertile soil in full sun. Shelter from cold, dry winds.
- **PROPAGATION** Sow seed in containers in a cold frame or in a seedbed in late winter or early spring. Root semi-ripe cuttings in late summer.
- **PESTS AND DISEASES** Trouble free.

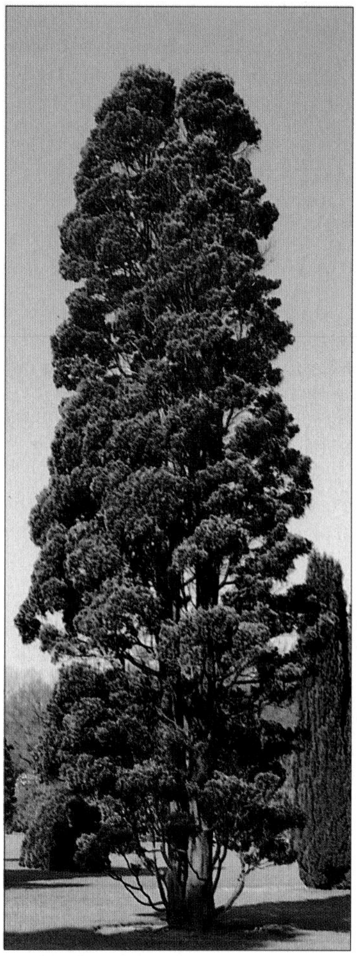

Austrocedrus chilensis

A. chilensis ▣ ▯ syn. *Libocedrus chilensis* (Chilean incense cedar). Narrowly columnar, densely branched tree with greyish green foliage and dark brown to orange-grey bark. Scale-like leaves are to 5mm (¼in) long, with long, decurrent bases, and are arranged in sets of 2 unequal pairs, often with glaucous bands on the reverse. Produces ovoid-oblong brown cones, to 1.5cm (½in) long. ↕ to 15m (50ft), ↔ to 4m (12ft). Andes of Chile and Argentina. ✻✻✻

▷**Autograph tree** see *Clusia major*
▷***Avena candida*** see *Helictotrichon sempervirens*
▷***Avena sempervirens*** see *Helictotrichon sempervirens*
▷**Avens** see *Geum*
Mountain see *Dryas, D. octopetala*
▷**Azalea** see *Rhododendron*
Alpine see *Loiseleuria*
Trailing see *Loiseleuria*

AZARA

FLACOURTIACEAE

Genus of 10 species of evergreen shrubs and small trees from South America, often found at woodland margins and lakesides. They have simple leaves, alternate or in unequal pairs, and usually glossy, entire or toothed. The fragrant flowers are small and petalless, but with showy stamens, and are borne in axillary spikes, clusters, or corymbs. They are followed in hot summers by pale mauve or white berries, to 6mm (¼in) across. Grow in a shrub border, in a sheltered, sunny site, or against a wall. In frost-prone areas, grow in a cool greenhouse.

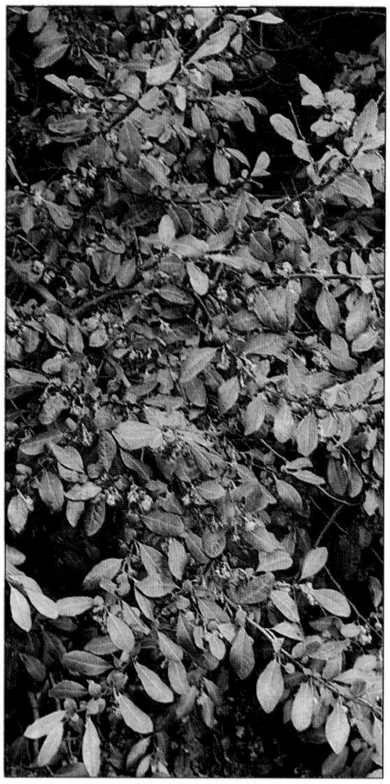

Azara integrifolia

- **HARDINESS** Fully hardy to half hardy.
- **CULTIVATION** Under glass, grow in loam-based potting compost (JI No.3) in full light with shade from hot sun. Water freely when in growth, applying a balanced liquid fertilizer monthly; water sparingly in winter. Outdoors, grow in moist, fertile, humus-rich soil, in sun or partial shade, sheltered from cold winds. Pruning group 8, or 13 if wall-trained.
- **PROPAGATION** Root semi-ripe cuttings in summer.
- **PESTS AND DISEASES** Trouble free.

A. dentata ⌓ Arching, evergreen shrub or small tree with ovate, toothed, glossy, dark green leaves, to 4cm (1½in) long, densely hairy beneath. In late spring, bears branching, dense corymbs, to 4cm (1½in) across, of fragrant, dark yellow flowers. ↕↔ 3m (10ft). Chile. ✻✻
A. integrifolia ▣ ▯ Upright, evergreen shrub or small tree with obovate or diamond-shaped, usually entire, hairless, glossy, dark green leaves, to 5cm (2in) long. From midwinter to early spring, fragrant yellow flowerheads are borne in mimosa-like clusters, 1cm (½in) wide. ↕ 5m (15ft), ↔ 3m (10ft) sometimes more. Chile, Argentina. ✻✻

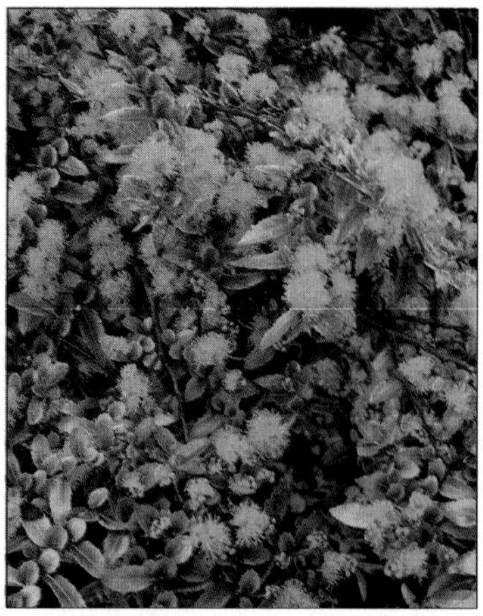

Azara lanceolata

A. lanceolata ■ Evergreen shrub with arching, fern-like branches and lance-shaped, sharply toothed, hairless, bright green leaves, to 6cm (2½in) long. Bears fragrant, bright yellow flowers in small, rounded, corymb-like clusters, to 2cm (¾in) across, in mid- and late spring. ↕↔ 5m (15ft). Chile, Argentina. ❄❄

A. microphylla ♀ Upright, evergreen tree or large shrub with semi-pendent shoots and small, obovate, entire or toothed, hairless, very dark green leaves, to 2.5cm (1in) long. In late winter and spring, produces tiny, vanilla-scented, greenish yellow flowers in clusters, to 1cm (½in) across, from leaf axils on the undersides of the shoots. Hardiest of the species, it tolerates full shade and grows well against a wall. ↕ 10m (30ft), ↔ 4m (12ft). Chile, Argentina. ❄❄❄

A. petiolaris Arching, evergreen shrub or sometimes small tree, bearing ovate, leathery, hairless, dark green leaves, to 8cm (3in) long, with a few large marginal teeth. In mid- and late spring, bears fragrant, pale creamy yellow flowers in nodding, catkin-like racemes, to 2.5cm (1in) long. ↕ 5m (15ft), ↔ 4m (12ft). Chile. ❄❄

A. serrata. Evergreen shrub with downy branches and oval, toothed, glossy, dark green leaves, hairless beneath, to 6cm (2½in) long. Fragrant, dark yellow flowers open in dense, spherical, umbel-like corymbs, to 2cm (¾in) across, in midsummer. ↕ 4m (12ft), ↔ 3m (10ft). Chile. ❄❄

AZOLLA

AZOLLACEAE

Genus of 8 species of floating, aquatic ferns found in lakes, ponds, and slow-flowing streams in both hemispheres. They have pinnately branched, floating rhizomes, with frail roots, producing 2-lobed, light green, scale-like fronds, which turn reddish brown in autumn. On a pool, they provide fast-growing surface cover, which partially suppresses algae and helps clear the water. In frost-prone areas, only *A. filiculoides* is suitable for outdoor pools; grow tender species in indoor pools in a cool or temperate conservatory or terrarium.

• **HARDINESS** Half hardy to frost tender.

• **CULTIVATION** Under glass, scatter plants on the water surface in spring and provide full light. Outdoors, scatter on the pool surface when any danger of frost has passed, in full sun or partial shade. Where temperatures do not fall below -5°C (23°F), plants overwinter as resting buds that sink to the pool bottom after the foliage is frosted, rising to the surface in spring. In frost-prone areas, remove before the first frosts and overwinter in frost-free conditions in a saucer of moist soil. See also pp.52–53.

• **PROPAGATION** Scatter small bunches of young plants on the water surface in early summer.

• **PESTS AND DISEASES** May be eaten by waterfowl.

A. caroliniana see *A. filiculoides.*

A. filiculoides ■ syn. *A. caroliniana* (Fairy moss, Mosquito plant). Aquatic perennial forming an attractive cover of soft foliage on the water surface. Pairs of delicate, lacy, light green fronds, 1mm (1/16in) long, are 2-ranked, and support single strands of fine roots, to 1.5cm (½in) long. ↔ indefinite. North and South America. ❄

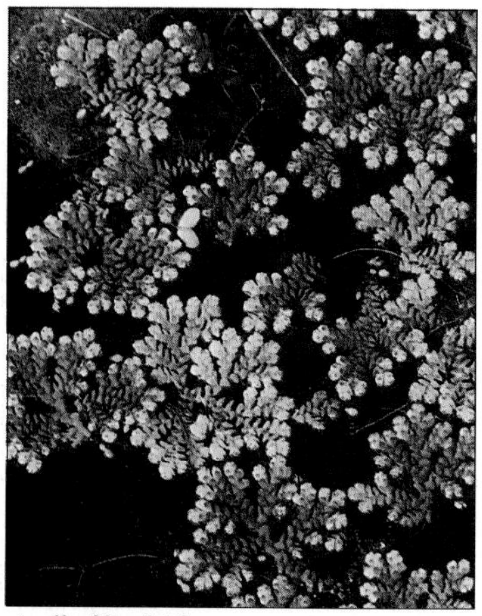

Azolla filiculoides

AZORELLA

APIACEAE/UMBELLIFERAE

Genus of about 70 species of evergreen, mat- or cushion-forming perennials from open, rocky areas in New Zealand and South America. They produce attractive mounds of foliage, comprising rosettes of toothed or lobed, leathery leaves, 0.5–1.5cm (¼–½in) long. Umbels of small flowers are borne in late spring or summer. Grow in a raised bed or scree bed, or in an alpine house. Often confused with the genus *Bolax.*

• **HARDINESS** Fully hardy, given good drainage.

• **CULTIVATION** Grow in gritty loam-based potting compost (JI No.1) in an alpine house in full light. Outdoors, grow in gritty, poor to moderately fertile, sharply drained soil in full sun.

• **PROPAGATION** Sow seed in containers in an open frame in autumn, or root rosettes as cuttings in spring.

• **PESTS AND DISEASES** Prone to aphids and red spider mites under glass.

A. glebaria see *Bolax gummifera.*

A. nivalis see *A. trifurcata.*

A. trifurcata ■ syn. *A. nivalis.* Dense, cushion-forming perennial with rosettes of overlapping, glossy, dark green leaves, to 1.5cm (½in) long, deeply cut into 3 (occasionally 5) sharp-tipped, triangular lobes. Inconspicuous umbels of tiny, creamy white flowers are borne in summer. ↕ to 10cm (4in) or more, ↔ to 20cm (8in). Chile, Argentina. ❄❄❄

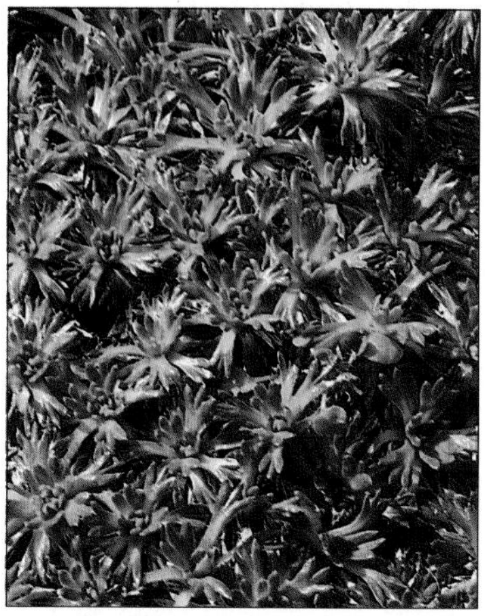

Azorella trifurcata

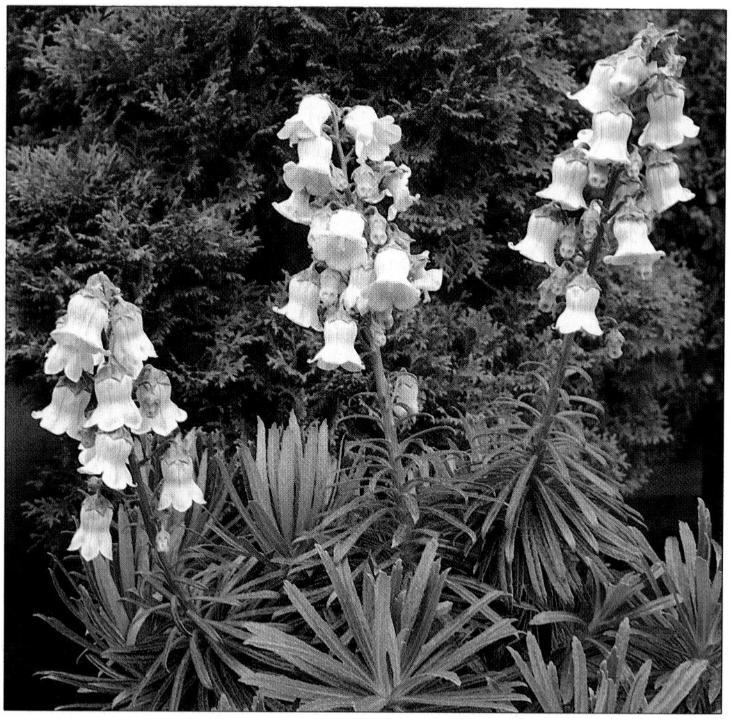

Azorina vidalii

AZORINA

CAMPANULACEAE

Genus of one species of erect, sparsely branched, evergreen shrub from volcanic cliffs or scree in the Azores. It has ridged stems and alternate, mid-green leaves, and bears racemes of bell-shaped flowers in late summer. In frost-prone areas, *A. vidalii* is an attractive plant for a cool conservatory or greenhouse. In frost-free climates, it is best grown among shrubs or in a border.

• **HARDINESS** Frost tender.

• **CULTIVATION** Under glass, grow in loam-based potting compost (JI No.2) in bright filtered light. Provide good ventilation. In the growing season, water freely and apply a balanced liquid fertilizer monthly; keep just moist in winter. Outdoors, grow in fertile, moist but well-drained soil in full sun with some midday shade.

• **PROPAGATION** Sow seed at 13–16°C (55–61°F) in spring, or root softwood or semi-ripe cuttings in summer.

• **PESTS AND DISEASES** Trouble free.

A. vidalii ■ syn. *Campanula vidalii.* Soft-stemmed, evergreen shrub with spoon-shaped, toothed, veined, glossy, mid-green leaves, 5–15cm (2–6in) long, crowded towards the stem tips. In late summer, bears loose racemes of up to 50 pendent, waisted, bell-shaped, white or pink flowers, 5cm (2in) long, with orange bases. ↕↔ 40–60cm (16–24in). Azores. ❀ (min. 5°C/41°F)

AZTEKIUM

CACTACEAE

Genus of one species of very slow-growing, tuberous-rooted, perennial cactus, occurring on scree slopes in N.E. Mexico. It has prominently ribbed stems and produces areoles in rows along the ribs. It occasionally forms compact colonies. In frost-prone regions, grow *A. ritteri* in a temperate greenhouse; in frost-free climates, it is suitable for a desert garden.

• **HARDINESS** Frost tender.

• **CULTIVATION** Under glass, grow in standard cactus compost in full light. Water moderately in growth; keep dry at all other times of the year. Outdoors, grow in sharply drained, gritty, poor soil in full sun. See also pp.48–49.

• **PROPAGATION** Sow seed at 13–16°C (55–61°F) in spring, or root semi-ripe cuttings in summer.

• **PESTS AND DISEASES** Mealybugs and root mealybugs may be a problem.

A. ritteri ■ syn. *Echinocactus ritteri.* Perennial cactus with a flattened-spherical, 8- to 11-ribbed, minutely furrowed, olive-green stem. Tiny areoles each bear 1–4 flat, papery, curved, yellow to grey spines, which fall once an areole produces flowers. Funnel-shaped, diurnal, white or pink flowers, 1cm (½in) long, are borne from new areoles at the centre of the stem from spring to autumn. ↕↔ 5cm (2in). N.E. Mexico. ❀ (min. 7–10°C/45–50°F)

▷***Azureocereus*** see *Browningia*
A. hertlingianus see *B. hertlingiana*

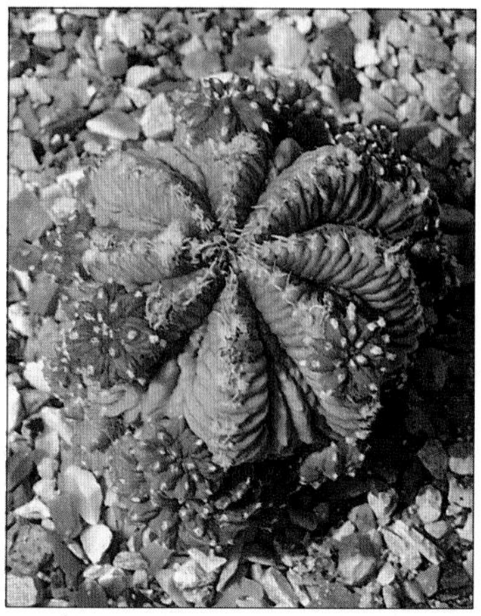

Aztekium ritteri

B

B

BABIANA
IRIDACEAE

Genus of 50–60 species of cormous perennials from open grassland and hill-sides in South Africa. They have ribbed or pleated, often hairy, lance-shaped, mid- to bright green leaves and spikes of funnel-shaped, often strongly scented flowers, 2–4cm (¾–1½in) across, borne mainly in spring. In frost-prone areas, grow in a cool greenhouse; in warmer climates, plant in a sunny border.
• **HARDINESS** Frost tender.
• **CULTIVATION** Under glass, plant corms in autumn in loam-based potting compost (JI No.2), and grow in full light. When in growth, water freely and apply a weak balanced liquid fertilizer every 3 weeks before flowering; dry off as the leaves die down in summer. Outdoors, plant 20cm (8in) deep, in light, rich, well-drained soil in full sun in autumn. Dormant corms are sometimes offered for spring planting in frost-prone areas to bloom in summer. If left in the soil, they revert to winter growing (if they survive).
• **PROPAGATION** Sow seed at 13–15°C (55–59°F) as soon as ripe. Remove offsets when dormant.
• **PESTS AND DISEASES** Red spider mites may be a problem.

B. disticha see *B. plicata.*
B. nana. Cormous perennial with hairy leaves, 3.5–6cm (1½–2½in) long. In spring, bears spikes of 2–6 scented, blue, lilac, or pink flowers, the lower lobes marked with white and mauve or with yellow. ↕ 12cm (5in), ↔ 5cm (2in). South Africa. ❁ (min. 5°C/41°F)
B. plicata, syn. *B. disticha.* Cormous perennial with hairy leaves, 8–12cm (3–5in) long. Spikes of 4–10 scented, pale lilac to violet flowers, often with a paler mark on the lower lobes, are borne in spring. ↕ 7–20cm (3–8in), ↔ 5cm (2in). South Africa. ❁ (min. 5°C/41°F)

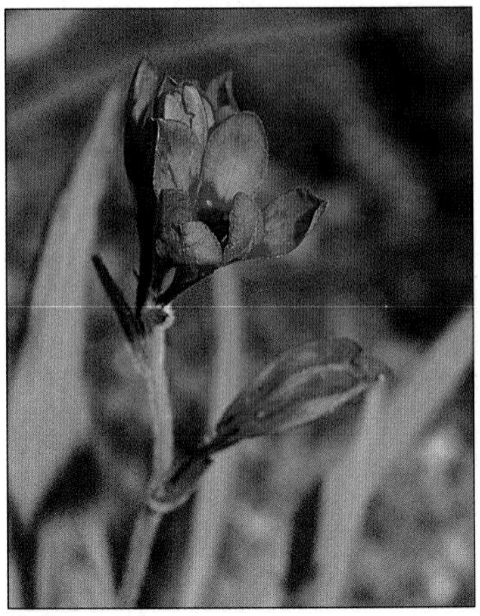
Babiana rubrocyanea

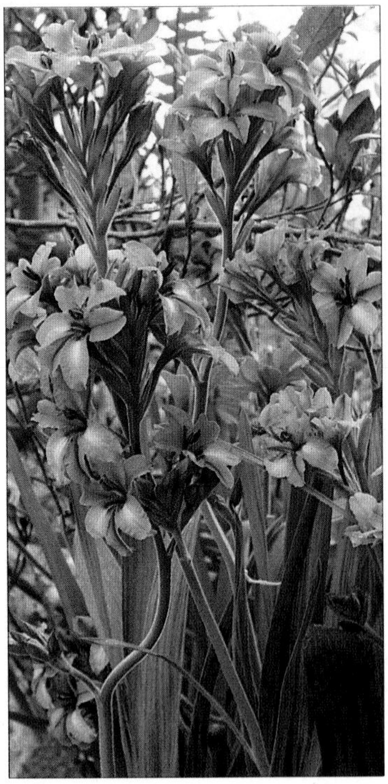
Babiana stricta

B. rubrocyanea ▣ Cormous perennial with hairy leaves, to 15cm (6in) long. Bears spikes of 5–10 scarlet and blue flowers in spring. ↕ 5–20cm (2–8in), ↔ 5cm (2in). South Africa. ❁ (min. 5°C/41°F)
B. stricta ▣ Variable, cormous perennial with hairy leaves, 4–12cm (1½–5in) long. In spring, bears spikes of 4–8 sometimes scented, purple, mauve, blue, or yellow flowers, occasionally with dark red centres. ↕ 10–30cm (4–12in), ↔ 5cm (2in). South Africa. ❁ (min. 5°C/41°F). **'Zwanenburg's Glory'** has alternate blue and white flower segments.
B. villosa. Cormous perennial with hairy leaves, 5–12cm (2–5in) long. In spring, bears spikes of 4–8 deep red flowers, with large, purple-black anthers. ↕ 12–20cm (5–8in), ↔ 5cm (2in). South Africa. ❁ (min. 5°C/41°F)

▷ **Baby blue-eyes** see *Nemophila menziesii*
▷ **Baby's breath** see *Gypsophila paniculata*
▷ **Baby's tears** see *Soleirolia soleirolii*

BACCHARIS
ASTERACEAE/COMPOSITAE

Genus of about 350 species of dioecious, deciduous or evergreen shrubs and herbaceous perennials from coasts, salt marshes, riverbanks, high mountains, and woodland margins in North, Central, and South America. Leaves are alternate or absent; flowerheads are borne in axillary panicles or corymbs. In frost-prone areas, grow tender species in a cool greenhouse. *B. halimifolia* is valued as a windbreak, especially near the sea, and for its silver seed heads.
• **HARDINESS** Fully hardy to frost tender.
• **CULTIVATION** Grow in fertile soil in full sun. Pruning group 1 or 4.
• **PROPAGATION** Sow seed in containers in a cold frame in spring. Root softwood cuttings in summer.
• **PESTS AND DISEASES** Trouble free.

B. halimifolia (Bush groundsel, Sea myrtle). Vigorous, upright, deciduous shrub with obovate to oval, grey-green leaves, to 8cm (3in) long, with large, marginal teeth. In autumn, bears axillary clusters of small white flowerheads in corymbs to 15cm (6in) across. Female plants produce thistle-like, silky white fruit. ↕↔ 4m (12ft). E. USA, S. central USA, Mexico, West Indies. ✻✻✻

▷ **Bachelor's buttons** see *Ranunculus aconitifolius, Craspedia, C. globosa, C. uniflora*
White see *Ranunculus aconitifolius* 'Flore Pleno'

BACKHOUSIA
MYRTACEAE

Genus of 7 species of evergreen shrubs and trees found mainly in subtropical and tropical rainforest in Australia. Ovate, elliptic, or lance-shaped, aromatic leaves are borne in opposite pairs. Small flowers, with 4 petals and conspicuous stamens, are borne in cymes, umbels, or panicles. In frost-prone areas, grow in a temperate greenhouse; elsewhere, grow in a border.
• **HARDINESS** Frost tender.
• **CULTIVATION** Under glass, grow in equal parts loam, peat, and sand in full light. Pot on or top-dress in spring. In growth, water freely and apply a balanced liquid fertilizer monthly; water sparingly in winter. Outdoors, grow in fertile, humus-rich, neutral to acid soil in full sun. Pruning group 9.
• **PROPAGATION** Surface-sow seed at 13–15°C (55–59°F) in spring. Root semi-ripe cuttings in summer.
• **PESTS AND DISEASES** Trouble free.

B. citriodora ⚲ (Lemon ironwood, Lemon-scented myrtle). Shrub or bushy tree with broadly lance-shaped, hairy, reddish green leaves, 5–12cm (2–5in) long, maturing to glossy, deep green. From summer to autumn, bears umbels, 10–15cm (4–6in) or more across, of creamy white flowers. ↕ 3–15m (10–50ft), ↔ 2–6m (6–20ft). Australia (Queensland). ❁ (min. 5–7°C/41–45°F)

BACTRIS
Spiny club palm
ARECACEAE/PALMAE

Genus of over 230 species of single- or cluster-stemmed, usually spiny palms from dry, open sites in Mexico, the West Indies, and South America. Pinnate or simple, cleft leaves are borne in terminal tufts, with no crownshafts, and 3-petalled flowers are produced in panicles among them. In frost-prone areas, grow in a warm greenhouse. In frost-free areas, use as specimen plants.
• **HARDINESS** Frost tender.
• **CULTIVATION** Under glass, grow in well-drained, loam-based potting compost (JI No.2) in bright filtered light. In growth, water moderately and apply a balanced liquid fertilizer monthly; water sparingly in winter. Pot on or top-dress in spring. Outdoors, grow in fertile, moist but well-drained soil with some midday shade.
• **PROPAGATION** Sow seed at 25–30°C (77–86°F) in spring.
• **PESTS AND DISEASES** Red spider mites may be troublesome under glass.

B. gasipaes 🌴 (Peach palm). Medium-sized or tall palm, usually single-stemmed, bearing rings of sharp spines. Pinnate, deep green leaves, to 3m (10ft) long, with many slender leaflets, are paler beneath. Bears light green flowers in upright then pendent panicles in summer, followed by edible, orange-red fruit. ↕ to 20m (70ft), ↔ to 6m (20ft). Possibly Peru. ❁ (min. 15°C/59°F)

BAECKEA
MYRTACEAE

Genus of about 70 species of evergreen shrubs and small trees occurring in scrub in subtropical to subalpine areas in China, Malaysia, Australia, and New Caledonia. Linear to narrowly lance-shaped, usually entire leaves are borne in opposite pairs. Saucer-shaped, 5-petalled flowers are produced singly or in umbels in summer. In frost-prone climates, grow in a cool greenhouse. In warmer climates, grow in a border, at the base of a warm, sunny wall, or as ground cover.
• **HARDINESS** Frost tender; but may tolerate short periods of light frost.
• **CULTIVATION** Under glass, grow in neutral to acid, loam-based potting compost in bright light, with some shade from hot sun. In the growing season, water freely and apply a balanced liquid fertilizer monthly; water sparingly in winter. Pot on or top-dress in late winter. Outdoors, grow in neutral to acid, well-drained soil in full sun. Pruning group 9.
• **PROPAGATION** Surface-sow seed at 13–15°C (55–59°F) in spring and keep moist. Root semi-ripe cuttings in a propagating case in late summer.
• **PESTS AND DISEASES** Trouble free.

B. virgata ⚲ (Twiggy baeckea). Prostrate to erect, bushy shrub or small tree with narrowly oblong to lance-shaped, dark green leaves, to 2.5cm (1in) long. In summer, numerous white flowers, to 6mm (¼in) across, are produced in umbels of 2–9 near the ends of the branchlets. ↕ 0.3–3m (1–10ft) or more, ↔ 1–3m (3–10ft). E. Australia. ❁ (min. 5°C/41°F)

▷ **Baeckea, Twiggy** see *Baeckea virgata*
▷ **Baldmoney** see *Meum athamanticum*
▷ **Balloon flower** see *Platycodon*

BALLOTA
LABIATAE/LAMIACEAE

Genus of 30–35 species of clump- or mat-forming perennials and evergreen subshrubs from rocky and waste ground in the Mediterranean, Europe, and W. Asia. The leaves are opposite, toothed to scalloped, and aromatic, sometimes unpleasantly so. Whorls of 2-lipped flowers, often with prominent, saucer- or funnel-shaped calyces, are produced from the leaf axils of terminal shoots. Grow in a sunny border.
• **HARDINESS** Fully hardy to frost hardy.
• **CULTIVATION** Grow in poor, dry, freely draining soil in full sun. Pruning group 10; cut back subshrubs in mid-spring to keep compact.
• **PROPAGATION** Divide perennials in spring. For subshrubs, root softwood cuttings in late spring or early summer, or semi-ripe cuttings in early summer.
• **PESTS AND DISEASES** Trouble free.

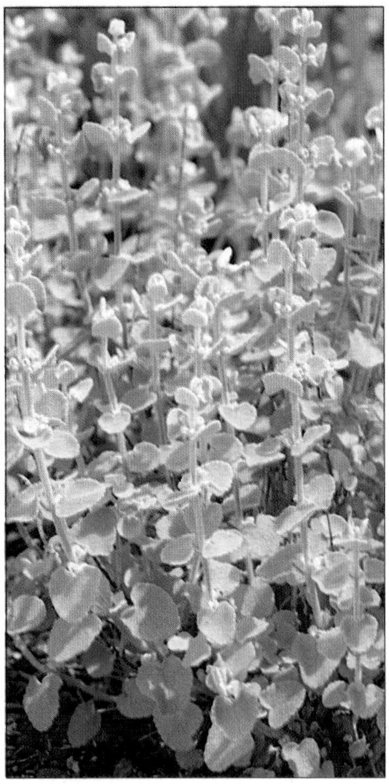

Ballota acetabulosa

B. acetabulosa ■ Compact, bushy subshrub with upright, white-woolly shoots and heart-shaped, round-toothed, grey-green leaves, to 5cm (2in) long. Small, 2-lipped, white-marked, purple-pink flowers, 1.5–2cm (½–¾in) long, with open funnel-shaped green calyces, to 2cm (¾in) across, are produced in mid- and late summer. ↕ 60cm (24in), ↔ 75cm (30in). S.E. Greece, Crete, W. Turkey. ❄❄

***B.* 'All Hallows Green'** ■ Bushy subshrub with heart-shaped, woolly, lime-green leaves, to 5cm (2in) long. Small, 2-lipped, pale green flowers with open funnel-shaped, green calyces, to 2cm (¾in) across, are produced in mid- and late summer. ↕ 60cm (24in), ↔ 75cm (30in). ❄❄❄ (borderline)

B. pseudodictamnus ■ 🏆 Mound-forming subshrub with ovate, yellowish grey-green leaves, to 3cm (1¼in) long, on sparsely branched, erect, woody-based, white-woolly stems. In late spring and early summer, bears 2-lipped, white or pinkish white flowers, 1.5cm (½in) long, with open funnel-shaped, pale green calyces, 2cm (¾in) wide. ↕ 45cm (18in), ↔ 60cm (24in). Greece, Crete, W. Turkey. ❄❄❄ (borderline)

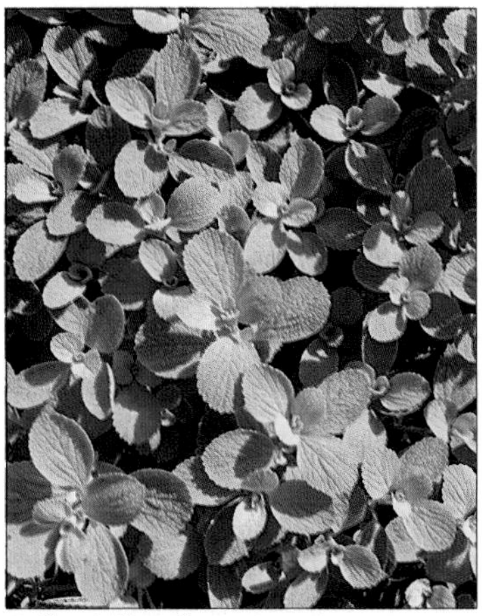

Ballota 'All Hallows Green'

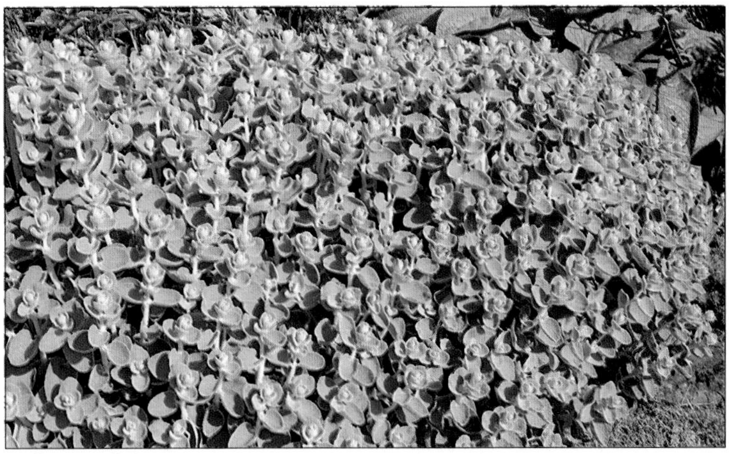

Ballota pseudodictamnus

▷**Balm** see *Melissa*
Bastard see *Melittis*
Bee see *Melissa officinalis, Monarda didyma*
Lemon see *Melissa officinalis*
▷**Balm of Gilead** see *Cedronella canariensis, Populus* x *candicans*
▷**Balsam** see *Impatiens*
▷**Balsam apple** see *Clusia major*
▷***Balsamita*** see *Tanacetum*
B. major see *T. balsamita*

BALSAMORHIZA

Balsam root

ASTERACEAE/COMPOSITAE

Genus of 10–14 species of perennials with fleshy, balsam-scented roots, from gravelly banks and cliffs in W. North America. Erect stems bear opposite, simple or pinnate leaves, mainly in basal rosettes, and solitary yellow flowerheads. Grow in a border or rock garden.
• **HARDINESS** Fully hardy, but liable to die back in wet winters.
• **CULTIVATION** Grow in well-drained, moderately fertile soil in full sun.
• **PROPAGATION** Sow seed in a cold frame in autumn. Divide in spring.
• **PESTS AND DISEASES** Trouble free.

B. sagittata. Clump-forming perennial with simple, heart- to arrow-shaped, entire, very white-hairy leaves, 15–50cm (6–20in) long, later almost hairless, with conspicuous midribs and long leaf-stalks. Flowerheads, 8–10cm (3–4in) across, with yellow disc- and ray-florets, and white-woolly involucres, are borne in late spring and early summer. ↕ 25–60cm (10–24in), ↔ 30cm (12in). Canada, N.W. USA. ❄❄❄

▷**Balsam root** see *Balsamorhiza*
▷**Bamboo** see *Bambusa*
Anceps see *Yushania, Y. anceps*
Black see *Phyllostachys nigra*
Buddha's belly see *Bambusa ventricosa*
Fishpole see *Phyllostachys aurea*
Fountain see *Fargesia nitida*
Giant timber see *Phyllostachys bambusoides*
Golden see *Phyllostachys aurea*
Heavenly see *Nandina domestica*
Hedge see *Bambusa multiplex*
Narihira see *Semiarundinaria fastuosa*
Noble see *Himalayacalamus falconeri*
Pygmy see *Pleioblastus pygmaeus*
Square-stemmed see *Chimonobambusa quadrangularis*

▷**Bamboo cont.**
Umbrella see *Fargesia murieliae*
Yellow-groove see *Phyllostachys aureosulcata*
Zigzag see *Phyllostachys flexuosa*
▷**Bamboos** see p.54

BAMBUSA

Bamboo

GRAMINEAE/POACEAE

Genus of 100–120 species of clump-forming, evergreen bamboos, occurring in forest and woodland in tropical and subtropical Africa, Asia, and Central and South America. Smooth, usually hollow canes produce slender branches at each node, bearing linear-lance-shaped leaves. They are cultivated for their foliage and, in some species, such as *B. ventricosa*, for their curious, swollen internodes. In frost-prone climates, grow in a temperate greenhouse or conservatory. In frost-free climates, *B. multiplex* is useful as a hedge or windbreak.
• **HARDINESS** Half hardy to frost tender.
• **CULTIVATION** Under glass, grow in loamless potting compost in bright indirect light. Maintain high humidity, and water moderately. To produce the swollen internodes, confine *B. ventricosa* and its allies to 13–18cm (5–7in) containers; water and fertilize sparingly. Outdoors, grow in moist, fertile, humus-rich soil, in a sheltered position in full sun or partial shade.
• **PROPAGATION** Divide established clumps in spring.
• **PESTS AND DISEASES** Emerging shoots are vulnerable to slugs.

B. glaucescens see *B. multiplex.*
B. multiplex, syn. *B. glaucescens* (Hedge bamboo). Variable bamboo with slender, arching canes, and up to 20 crowded, paired, linear-lance-shaped, mid-green leaves, to 15cm (6in) long, silvery beneath. ↕ 3–15m (10–50ft) (much smaller in containers), ↔ indefinite. China. ❄. **'Fernleaf'**, syn. 'Wang Tsai', has fern-like whorls of about 20 leaves, 2.5–4.5cm (1–1¾in) long. **'Wang Tsai'** see 'Fernleaf'.
B. ventricosa (Buddha's belly bamboo). Very vigorous bamboo with strong canes bearing whorls of 10–20 linear-lance-shaped, dark green leaves, to 12cm (5in) long. The internodes swell under poor growing conditions. ↕ 5–25m (15–80ft) outdoors, 2.5m (8ft) or more in containers, ↔ indefinite. S. China. ❀ (min. 7°C/45°F)

▷**Banana** see *Musa*
Abyssinian see *Ensete ventricosum*
Edible see *Musa acuminata* 'Dwarf Cavendish'
Ethiopian see *Ensete ventricosum*
Flowering see *Musa ornata*
Japanese see *Musa basjoo*
Scarlet see *Musa coccinea*
▷**Baneberry** see *Actaea*
Red see *A. rubra*
White see *A. alba*

BANKSIA

PROTEACEAE

Genus of about 70 species of evergreen trees and shrubs, occurring in temperate to tropical scrub and forest, mainly in Australia, with one in New Guinea. They are cultivated for their foliage and flowers. Alternate or whorled, linear to ovate or pinnate, leathery leaves are often boldly lobed or toothed. Cone-like flowerheads of crowded, slender florets are followed by woody fruit. In frost-prone areas, grow in a cool greenhouse. In frost-free areas, grow in a border or as specimen plants.
• **HARDINESS** Half hardy to frost tender. Many will survive short spells around 0°C (32°F).
• **CULTIVATION** Under glass, grow in equal parts loam-based potting compost (JI No.1), grit, and peat (or peat substitute), in full light and with good ventilation. In the growing season, water moderately and apply a half-strength, phosphate-free liquid fertilizer monthly; water sparingly in winter. Pot on or top-dress in spring. Outdoors, grow in well-drained, neutral to acid soil, low in phosphates and nitrates, in full sun. Pruning group 1 or 8.
• **PROPAGATION** Sow seed singly in small containers at 18°C (64°F) in spring. Take semi-ripe cuttings of smooth-leaved species in summer and root with bottom heat.
• **PESTS AND DISEASES** Outdoors, *Phytophthora* root rot may be fatal; plants may become chlorotic if soil contains too much phosphate or lime.

B. baxteri ■ Dense to loosely spreading shrub with alternate, fan-shaped leaves, 7–17cm (3–7in) long, with acutely triangular, brownish red lobes, maturing to deep green. From summer to autumn, produces spherical, greenish yellow flowerheads, 5–8cm (2–3in) across. ↕↔ 2–4m (6–12ft). Australia (Western Australia). ❄

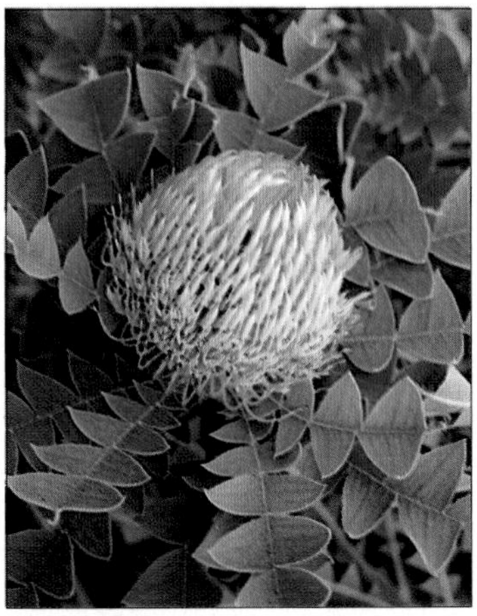

Banksia baxteri

B

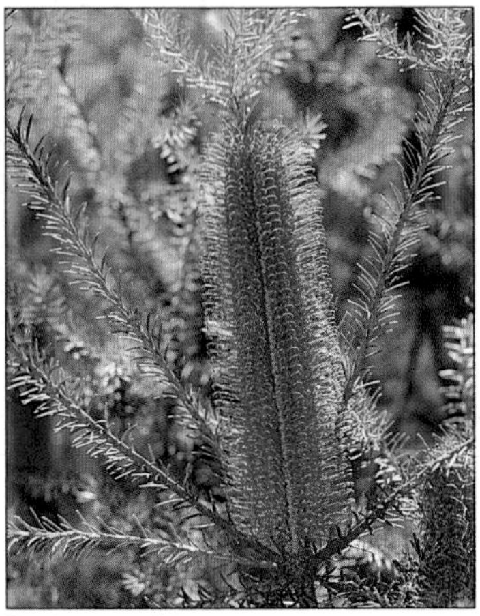

Banksia ericifolia

B. coccinea (Scarlet banksia). Erect, sparsely branched shrub with alternate, broadly heart-shaped, oblong to inversely heart-shaped, toothed leaves, to 10cm (4in) long, deep green above, white-downy beneath. Cylindrical scarlet flowerheads, to 8cm (3in) long, are produced from spring to summer. ↕4–8m (12–25ft), ↔ 1.5–4m (5–12ft). Australia (Western Australia). ❄

B. ericifolia ▣ (Heath banksia). Bushy shrub with crowded, alternate, linear, entire leaves, 2cm (¾in) long, glossy, mid- to deep green above, silvery beneath. Cylindrical, orange-yellow to orange-red or russet flowerheads, to 20cm (8in) long, are produced in autumn or winter. ↕3–6m (10–20ft), ↔ 2–4m (6–12ft). Australia (New South Wales). ❄

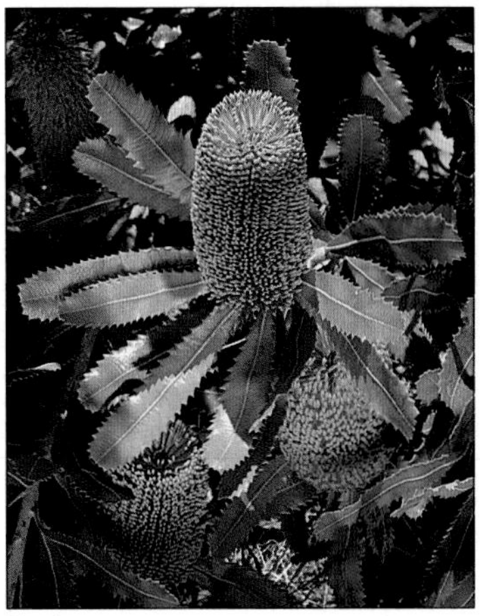

Banksia serrata

B. integrifolia ▣♀ (Coast banksia). Variable, vigorous, erect shrub or large tree, sparsely to moderately branched. Whorled, elliptic to obovate, entire, velvety, light brown leaves, to 10cm (4in) long, mature to mid-green above, white beneath. Cylindrical, pale yellow flowerheads, to 12cm (5in) long, are borne from late summer to autumn. ↕5–25m (15–80ft), ↔ 3–8m (10–25ft). Australia (Queensland to Victoria). ❄

B. menziesii ♀ (Firewood banksia, Menzies' banksia). Erect, then spreading, bushy shrub or tree with very downy young stems. Thick, alternate, narrowly oblong leaves, 15–30cm (6–12in) long, with shallow, irregular teeth and rust-red hairs, mature to semi-glossy or matt, deep or grey-green. From autumn to late spring, produces short, cylindrical to broadly ovoid flowerheads, 10–15cm (4–6in) long, varying from red ageing to yellow, to pink or bronze. ↕5–15m (15–50ft), ↔ 5–10m (15–30ft). Australia (Western Australia). ⊛ (min. 3–5°C/37–41°F)

B. serrata ▣♀ (Saw banksia). Erect then spreading shrub or tree with alternate, narrowly obovate to oblong, toothed leaves, 8–15cm (3–6in) long, downy and light red or reddish brown at first, then leathery, smooth, and semi-glossy, deep green. Cylindrical, greenish yellow to creamy grey flowerheads, 9–15cm (3½–6in) long, are produced from summer to late autumn. ↕3–20m (10–70ft), ↔ 2–8m (6–25ft). Australia (New South Wales, Victoria). ❄

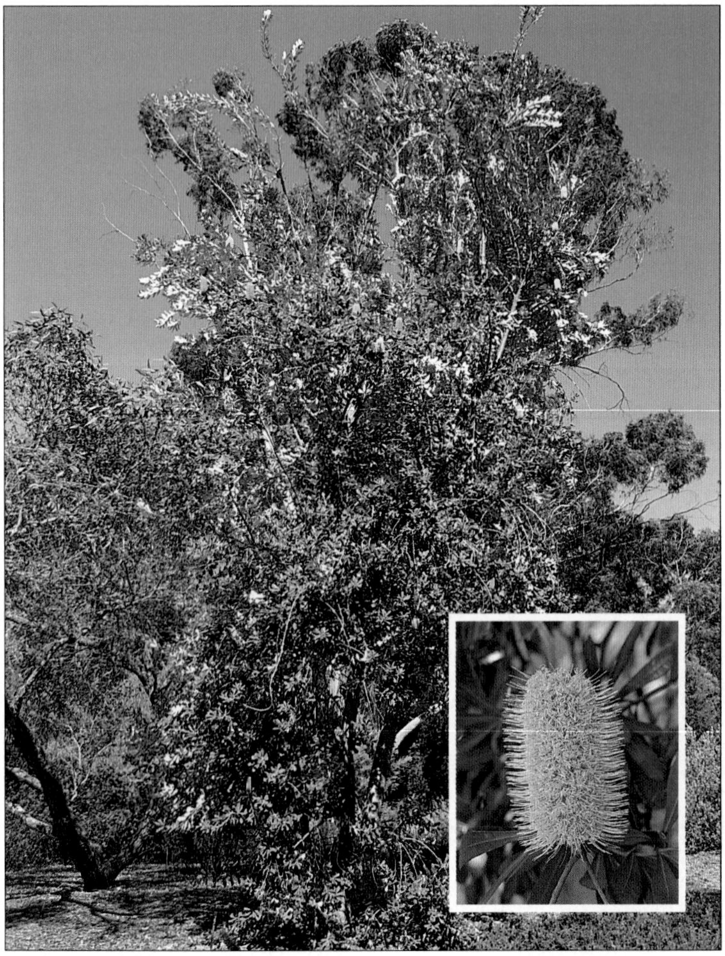

Banksia integrifolia (inset: flower detail)

▷**Banksia,**
Coast see *Banksia integrifolia*
Firewood see *Banksia menziesii*
Heath see *Banksia ericifolia*
Menzies' see *Banksia menziesii*
Saw see *Banksia serrata*
Scarlet see *Banksia coccinea*

▷**Banyan** see *Ficus benghalensis*
Australian see *F. macrophylla*
Malay see *F. microcarpa*

▷**Baobab tree** see *Adansonia digitata*

BAPTISIA

False indigo, Wild indigo

LEGUMINOSAE/PAPILIONACEAE

Genus of 20 or more species of erect or spreading perennials occurring in dry woodland and grassland in E. and S. USA, with a few in river valleys. They have alternate, fully divided, 3-palmate leaves and tall, branched stems bearing terminal or axillary racemes of pea-like flowers. The flowers are followed by large, often inflated pods. Grow in a border, wild garden, or dry, sunny bank.

- **HARDINESS** Fully hardy to frost hardy.
- **CULTIVATION** Grow in open, porous, preferably sandy soil in full sun.
- **PROPAGATION** Sow seed in containers in a cold frame as soon as ripe. Divide in early spring.
- **PESTS AND DISEASES** Trouble free.

B. alba. Erect, bushy perennial with palmate leaves, consisting of 3 obovate to narrowly elliptic-lance-shaped, glaucous leaflets, 2–5cm (2in) long. In early summer, bears racemes of up to 20 white flowers, to 2cm (¾in) long, sometimes with purple-marked standard petals. ↕60–120cm (2–4ft), ↔ 60cm (24in). S.E. USA. ❄❄❄

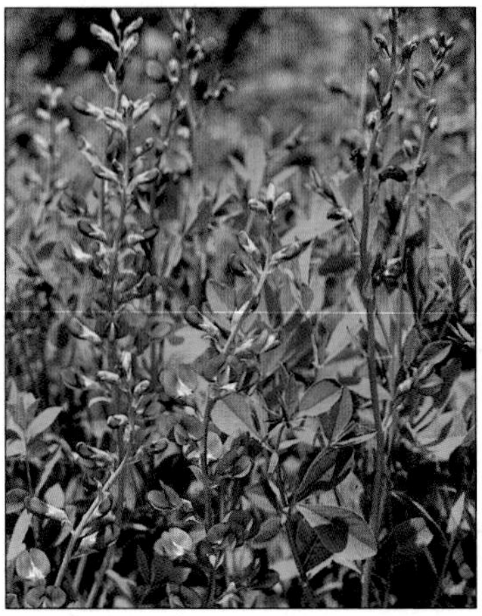

Baptisia australis

B. australis ▣♀ Gently spreading to erect perennial with glaucous stems and palmate, mid- to deep green leaves, each consisting of 3 ovate to inversely lance-shaped leaflets, to 4cm (1½in) long. In early summer, bears many-flowered racemes of dark blue flowers, to 3cm (1¼in) long, often flecked white or cream. ↕1.5m (5ft), ↔ 60cm (24in). E. USA. ❄❄❄

▷**Barbacenia elegans** see *Vellozia elegans*

▷**Barbados pride** see *Caesalpinia pulcherrima*

BARBAREA

St. Barbara's herb

BRASSICACEAE/CRUCIFERAE

Genus of about 12 species of biennials and perennials found in damp habitats in fertile, slightly acid to moderately alkaline soils, in temperate regions of the N. hemisphere. They have basal rosettes of entire or pinnatisect radical leaves and clasping stem leaves, and produce terminal racemes of cross-shaped, 4-petalled yellow flowers. A few are used as salad plants, and the double-flowered and variegated cultivars of *B. vulgaris* may be grown as ornamental plants at the front of a border.

- **HARDINESS** Fully hardy.
- **CULTIVATION** Grow in any moist but well-drained soil in full sun or partial shade.
- **PROPAGATION** Sow seed of biennials *in situ* as soon as ripe. Divide perennials in spring, or root softwood cuttings in early summer. *B. vulgaris* 'Variegata' breeds almost true from seed; discard green-leaved plants.
- **PESTS AND DISEASES** Flea beetles may damage the leaves.

B. vulgaris 'Variegata'. Rosette-forming biennial or short-lived perennial with 4- to 10-lobed basal leaves and simple stem leaves, both 5–12cm (2–5in) long, and mid- to deep green, variably splashed yellow. Cross-shaped yellow flowers are produced in racemes from early spring to early summer. Remove flowers unless seed is required. ↕25–45cm (10–18in), ↔ to 20cm (8in). ❄❄❄

▷**Barbed-wire plant** see *Tylecodon reticulatus*

▷**Barberry** see *Berberis*

BARKERIA

ORCHIDACEAE

Genus of about 10 species of deciduous, epiphytic orchids found at an altitude of 1,900–2,500m (6,200–8,000ft) in Central America. They produce stem-like, cylindrical or spindle-shaped pseudobulbs, with alternate, broadly linear to broadly ovate, slightly fleshy leaves and copious aerial roots. Flowers are borne in narrowly pyramidal or cylindrical, terminal racemes, rarely panicles, in early summer.

- **HARDINESS** Frost tender.
- **CULTIVATION** Cool-growing orchids. Grow in epiphytic orchid compost in a slatted basket. In summer, provide moist, shady conditions, water freely, applying fertilizer at every third watering, and mist once or twice a day.

Provide full light and keep dry in winter. See also p.46.
• **PROPAGATION** Divide when the plant fills the pot and "flows" over the sides.
• **PESTS AND DISEASES** Prone to red spider mites, aphids, and mealybugs.

B. lindleyana. Epiphytic orchid with cylindrical pseudobulbs and linear-lance-shaped to oblong-lance-shaped, grey-green leaves, 15cm (6in) long, with sharp-pointed tips. Bears white, lilac, or deep purple flowers, 6–7cm (2½–3in) across, in loose, terminal racemes in winter. ↕30cm (12in), ↔15cm (6in). Mexico to Costa Rica. ❅ (min. 11–13°C/52–55°F; max. 30°C/86°F)
B. skinneri. Epiphytic orchid with cylindrical pseudobulbs and elliptic to elliptic-lance-shaped, long, sharp-pointed, pale green leaves, 15cm (6in) long. Bears rich magenta to lilac flowers, 4cm (1½in) across, in terminal racemes or panicles, in winter. ↕30cm (12in), ↔15cm (6in). Guatemala. ❅ (min. 11–13°C/52–55°F; max. 30°C/86°F)

BARLERIA

ACANTHACEAE

Genus of about 250 species of evergreen perennials and shrubs occurring in scrub and forest in tropical and subtropical Africa and Asia, grown mainly for their spikes of tubular, 2-lipped flowers, which frequently have spiny bracts. The leaves are oblong, elliptic, or lance-shaped and are borne in opposite pairs. In frost-prone regions, grow in a temperate greenhouse. In frost-free areas, grow in a border or against a warm, sunny wall.
• **HARDINESS** Frost tender.
• **CULTIVATION** Under glass, grow in loam-based potting compost (JI No.3) with additional well-rotted compost, in full light, with shade from hot sun. When in growth, water freely and apply a balanced liquid fertilizer monthly; water sparingly in winter. Pot on or top-dress in spring. Outdoors, grow in fertile, moist but well-drained soil in a sunny site. Pruning group 2.
• **PROPAGATION** Sow seed at 16°C (61°F) in spring. Root softwood cuttings in late spring, or semi-ripe cuttings from non-flowering shoots in summer, with bottom heat.
• **PESTS AND DISEASES** Prey to red spider mites, whiteflies, and aphids under glass.

B. cristata ■ (Philippine violet). Erect to spreading, bushy, bristly-hairy shrub with oblong-elliptic, mid- to deep green leaves, to 10cm (4in) long. Bears small, stalkless, axillary spikes of light violet-blue, pink, or white flowers in summer. ↕90–120cm (3–4ft), ↔45–70cm (18–28in). India, Burma. ❅ (min. 10°C/50°F)
B. lupulina (Hop-headed barleria). Erect, bushy shrub with spiny stem nodes, and narrowly lance-shaped, bright green leaves, 10cm (4in) long, with pink to red main veins. In summer, bears terminal spikes, 4–8cm (1½–3in) long, with ovate bracts and yellow flowers. ↕60cm (24in), ↔40–60cm (16–24in). Mauritius. ❅ (min. 10°C/50°F)

▷**Barleria, Hop-headed** see *Barleria lupulina*

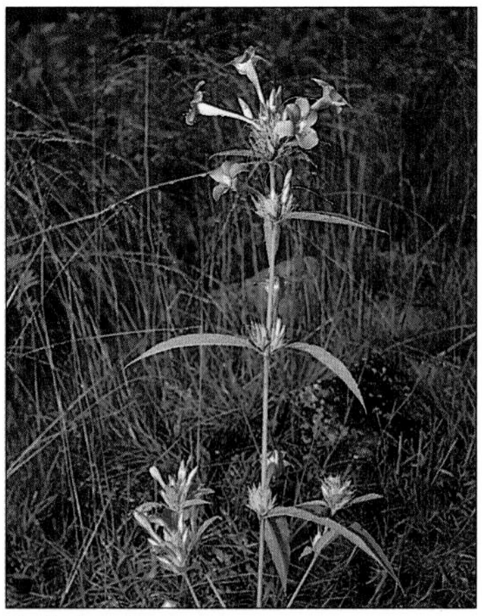
Barleria cristata

▷**Barley** see *Hordeum*
▷***Barosma pulchella*** see *Agathosma pulchella*
▷**Barrenwort** see *Epimedium*
▷***Bartlettina sordida*** see *Eupatorium sordidum*
▷***Bartonia aurea*** see *Mentzelia lindleyi*
▷**Basil** see *Ocimum basilicum*
Greek bush see *O. basilicum* var. *minimum*
Sweet see *O. basilicum*

BASSIA

CHENOPODIACEAE

Genus of about 26 species of annuals and perennials from disturbed land in S. Europe, Asia, and North America. They are cultivated for their habit, the feathery effect created by their alternate, very narrow, usually entire leaves, and their autumn tints. The flowers are inconspicuous. Plant in small groups in a bedding scheme, or to make a temporary low screen.
• **HARDINESS** Half hardy.
• **CULTIVATION** Grow in fertile, well-drained soil in a sheltered position in full sun. Trim untidy plants in summer.
• **PROPAGATION** Surface-sow seed at 16°C (61°F) in early or mid-spring, or sow *in situ* in late spring.
• **PESTS AND DISEASES** Trouble free.

B. scoparia* f. *trichophylla 🏆 syn. *Kochia trichophylla* (Burning bush, Summer cypress). Fast-growing, bushy, cone-shaped annual with close-set, narrowly lance-shaped to oblong, light green leaves, 5–8cm (2–3in) long, turning bright red or purple in late summer or autumn. ↕0.3–1.5m (1–5ft), ↔30–45cm (12–18in). Asia, North America. ✻

▷**Basswood** see *Tilia americana*
Carolina see *T. caroliniana*
▷**Bat flower** see *Tacca chantrierei, T. integrifolia*
▷**Bats-in-the-belfry** see *Campanula trachelium*

BAUERA

CUNONIACEAE

Genus of 3 species of evergreen shrubs occurring in light woodland in E. Australia. They are erect or prostrate, with slender, sometimes hairy branches bearing opposite, fully divided, 3-palmate, mid- or deep green leaves. Baueras are cultivated for their small, bowl-shaped, 4- to 10-petalled flowers, which are produced singly from the upper leaf axils. In frost-prone climates, grow in a cool greenhouse. In frost-free climates, they provide effective ground cover around shrubs and beneath trees.
• **HARDINESS** Frost tender.
• **CULTIVATION** Under glass, grow in a mix of equal parts loam, leaf mould, and sharp sand, in full light with shade from hot sun. During the growing season, water moderately and apply a balanced liquid fertilizer monthly; water sparingly in winter. Pot on or top-dress in late winter. Outdoors, grow in humus-rich, neutral to acid soil in partial shade. Pruning group 8.
• **PROPAGATION** Sow seed at 20–24°C (68–75°F) in spring. Root semi-ripe cuttings during late summer. Layer in spring.
• **PESTS AND DISEASES** Trouble free.

B. rubioides. Mat-forming to low, spreading, bushy, evergreen shrub bearing glossy, 3-palmate, deep green leaves, to 4cm (1½in) long, consisting of oblong to lance-shaped, often toothed leaflets. Solitary, bowl-shaped, pink or white flowers, to 2cm (¾in) across, are produced on long flower-stalks from the upper leaf axils, mainly from spring to summer. ↕0.15–3m (½–10ft), ↔0.6–3m (2–10ft). Australia (Queensland to Tasmania). ❅ (min. 3–5°C/37–41°F)

BAUHINIA

LEGUMINOSAE/PAPILIONACEAE

Genus of at least 250 species of evergreen or deciduous trees, shrubs, and perennial climbers from damp to dry forest and grassland in tropical and subtropical regions, grown mainly for their orchid-like flowers with 5 irregular petals. Leaves are alternate, simple, and often 2-lobed. In frost-prone areas, grow in a warm greenhouse; elsewhere, use as specimen plants or in a border.
• **HARDINESS** Frost tender.
• **CULTIVATION** Under glass, grow in loam-based potting compost (JI No.3) in full light. When in full growth, water freely and apply a balanced liquid fertilizer monthly; reduce water in winter. Pot on or top-dress in late winter. Outdoors, grow in fertile, moist but well-drained soil in full sun. Water freely during drought. Pruning group 12 for climbers; pruning group 1 (or 13 if wall-grown) for trees and shrubs.

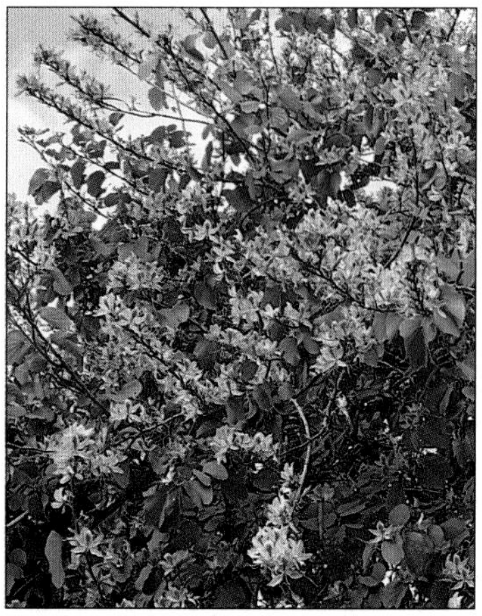
Bauhinia variegata

• **PROPAGATION** Sow seed at 16°C (61°F) in spring. Root semi-ripe cuttings in summer with bottom heat. Layer in spring.
• **PESTS AND DISEASES** Whiteflies, red spider mites, mealybugs, and aphids may be troublesome under glass.

B. corymbosa (Phanera). Evergreen, tendril climber with rust-red-hairy young shoots. Leaves, to 4cm (1½in) long, are rounded with heart-shaped bases and deeply 2-lobed tips, mid-green above, pale green beneath. In summer, produces dense, terminal racemes of fragrant, white or pink flowers, 3cm (1¼in) across. ↕4m (12ft) or more. S. China. ❅ (min. 7°C/45°F)
B. galpinii ■ syn. *B. punctata.* Spreading or semi-climbing, evergreen shrub with oval, notched or 2-lobed, light green leaves, 5cm (2in) long. Produces orange or red flowers, to 8cm (3in) across, in short, axillary racemes from spring to autumn. ↕2–3m (6–10ft), ↔1–3m (3–10ft). South Africa. ❅ (min. 7°C/45°F)
B. punctata see *B. galpinii.*
B. variegata ■ ♀ (Mountain ebony, Orchid tree). Spreading, deciduous tree bearing rounded, rich green leaves, 10–20cm (4–8in) long, with heart-shaped bases and deeply 2-lobed tips. From winter to summer, bears short, terminal racemes of light magenta to purple-blue flowers, 8–12cm (3–5in) across, sometimes white-variegated. ↕8–12m (25–40ft), ↔3–8m (10–25ft). E. Asia. ❅ (min. 7°C/45°F). **'Candida'** bears pure white flowers, occasionally suffused green.

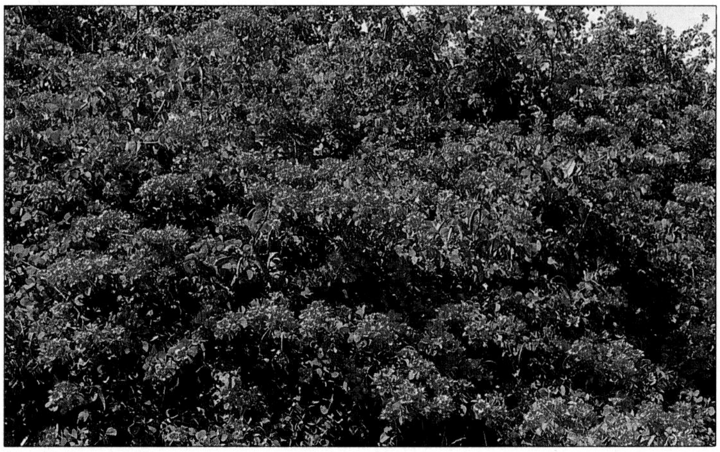
Bauhinia galpinii

▷ **Bay,**
Bull see *Magnolia grandiflora*
Loblolly see *Gordonia lasianthus*
Sweet see *Laurus nobilis, Magnolia virginiana*
▷ **Bay laurel** see *Laurus nobilis*
▷ **Bayonet, Spanish** see *Yucca aloifolia*
▷ **Bayonet plant** see *Aciphylla*
▷ **Bead plant** see *Nertera granadensis*
▷ **Bead-tree** see *Melia azedarach*
▷ **Bean,**
Egyptian see *Lablab purpureus*
Indian see *Lablab purpureus*
Snail see *Vigna caracalla*
▷ **Bean tree,**
Black see *Castanospermum australe*
Indian see *Catalpa bignonioides*
Lucky see *Erythrina caffra, E. lysistemon*
▷ **Bearberry** see *Arctostaphylos*
Alpine see *A. alpina*
Common see *A. uva-ursi*
▷ **Bear's breeches** see *Acanthus*
▷ **Bear's foot** see *Helleborus foetidus*

BEAUCARNEA

AGAVACEAE/DRACAENACEAE

Genus of about 24 species of evergreen shrubs and trees found in semi-desert and scrub from S. USA to Guatemala. Most have an expanded base and unbranched, palm-like stems with terminal tufts of strap-shaped, leathery leaves. They bear 6-tepalled flowers in terminal panicles. In frost-prone areas, grow in a temperate greenhouse. In frost-free, dry climates, grow as specimen plants.
• **HARDINESS** Frost tender.
• **CULTIVATION** Under glass, grow in loam-based potting compost (JI No.2) in full light. Water moderately in growth, sparingly in winter. Top-dress or pot on in spring. Outdoors, grow in fertile, sharply drained soil in full sun.
• **PROPAGATION** Sow seed at 18–21°C (64–70°F) or root offsets in spring.
• **PESTS AND DISEASES** Prey to scale insects and red spider mites under glass.

B. recurvata ▣ ♀ ◊ syn. *Nolina recurvata, N. tuberculata* (Bottle palm, Elephant foot tree, Ponytail). Evergreen tree with a flask-shaped base and an erect trunk that branches sparingly with age. Rosetted, mid- to deep green leaves, to 1.8m (6ft) long, are channelled and recurved. Tiny, mauve-tinted, creamy white flowers are produced in panicles 1m (3ft) long in summer. ↕ 4–8m (12–25ft), ↔ 2–4m (6–12ft). S.E. Mexico. ❄ (min. 7°C/45°F)

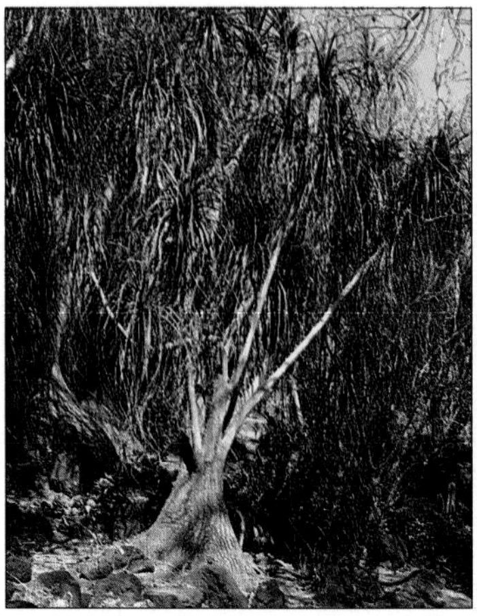

Beaucarnea recurvata

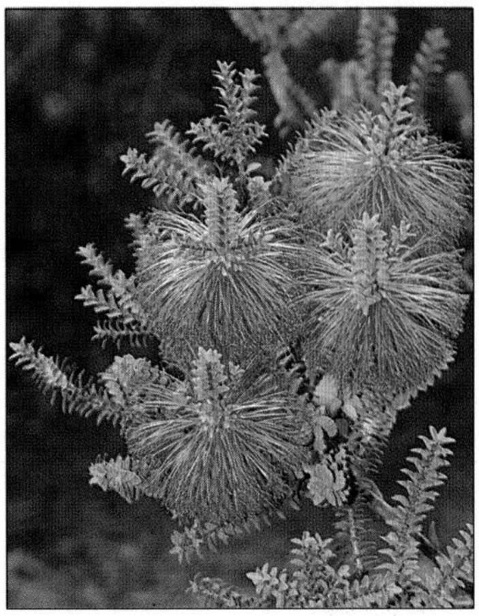

Beaufortia sparsa

BEAUFORTIA

MYRTACEAE

Genus of 18 species of evergreen shrubs occurring mainly on poor soils in scrub and forest in warm-temperate areas of Australia. They are cultivated for their terminal, brush-like heads of numerous small flowers, each consisting largely of a tuft of coloured stamens. Leaves are small, simple, and borne in opposite pairs, in most species tightly packed and overlapping to conceal the stems. In frost-prone regions, grow beaufortias in a cool greenhouse. In frost free climates, plant in a border or at the base of a warm, sunny wall; they may also be used as low windbreaks.
• **HARDINESS** Half hardy to frost tender.
• **CULTIVATION** Under glass, grow in a mix of equal parts loam, peat, and sand in full light, with good ventilation. Water freely during the growing season, sparingly in winter. Pot on or top-dress in early spring, or apply a half-strength, balanced liquid fertilizer monthly from spring to autumn. Outdoors, grow in poor, well-drained, neutral to acid soil in full sun. Pruning group 9.
• **PROPAGATION** Surface-sow seed at 13–16°C (55–61°F) in spring. Root semi-ripe cuttings in summer.
• **PESTS AND DISEASES** Prone to chlorosis and die-back in phosphate-rich soil.

B. sparsa ▣ (Swamp bottlebrush). Erect to spreading, evergreen shrub with upright to recurved, oval, mid- to deep green leaves, 1cm (½in) long. Bright orange-red flowerheads, 5–7cm (2–3in) long, are produced from summer to autumn. ↕ 2–3m (6–10ft), ↔ 1–2m (3–6ft). Australia (Western Australia). ❄ (min. 5°C/41°F)

BEAUMONTIA

APOCYNACEAE

Genus of 9 species of evergreen climbers occurring in temperate and tropical forest and scrub in China and from India to Vietnam. They are cultivated for their foliage and attractive, scented flowers. The leaves are opposite, entire, and usually oblong-ovate to ovate. The large, trumpet-shaped or bell-shaped flowers are produced in small, terminal and axillary corymbs, from late spring to summer. In frost-prone regions, grow beaumontias in a temperate or warm greenhouse. In frost-free regions, train them over a pergola or arbour, against a house wall, or through a tree.
• **HARDINESS** Frost tender, although *B. grandiflora* may survive short spells around 0°C (32°F).
• **CULTIVATION** Under glass, grow in loam-based potting compost (JI No.3) in full light. When in growth, water freely and apply a balanced liquid fertilizer monthly; water sparingly in winter. Top-dress in spring. Provide strong supports for the heavy, twining growth. Keep warm and humid in summer, but cool in winter, with night temperatures down to 7°C (45°F) to initiate flower-bud formation. Outdoors, grow in moist, fertile, humus-rich soil in full sun. Prune after flowering; pruning group 11 or 12.
• **PROPAGATION** Sow seed at 16°C (61°F) in spring. Root semi-ripe cuttings, preferably with a heel, in a propagating case with bottom heat in late summer. Layer in autumn or spring.
• **PESTS AND DISEASES** Red spider mites may be a problem under glass.

B. grandiflora ▣ (Herald's trumpet). Vigorous, evergreen, twining climber with broadly oblong-ovate, downy, reddish brown leaves, 10–25cm (4–10in) long, maturing to glossy, deep green. Trumpet-shaped, fragrant white flowers, 8–13cm (3–5in) long, with green bases, are borne in terminal and axillary corymbs from late spring to summer. ↕ 5–15m (15–50ft). India to Vietnam. ❄ (min. 5°C/41°F)

▷ **Beauty berry** see *Callicarpa*
▷ **Beauty bush** see *Kolkwitzia*
▷ **Bedstraw** see *Galium*
▷ **Beech** see *Fagus*
American see *Fagus grandifolia*
Antarctic see *Nothofagus antarctica*
Black see *Nothofagus solandri*
Common see *Fagus sylvatica*
Copper see *Fagus sylvatica* f. *purpurea*
Fern-leaved see *Fagus sylvatica* 'Aspleniifolia'
Japanese see *Fagus crenata*
Mountain see *Nothofagus solandri* var. *cliffortioides*
Myrtle see *Nothofagus cunninghamii*
Oriental see *Fagus orientalis*
Silver see *Nothofagus menziesii*
Southern see *Nothofagus*
Weeping see *Fagus sylvatica* f. *pendula*
▷ **Beefsteak plant** see *Iresine herbstii*
▷ **Beet** see *Beta*

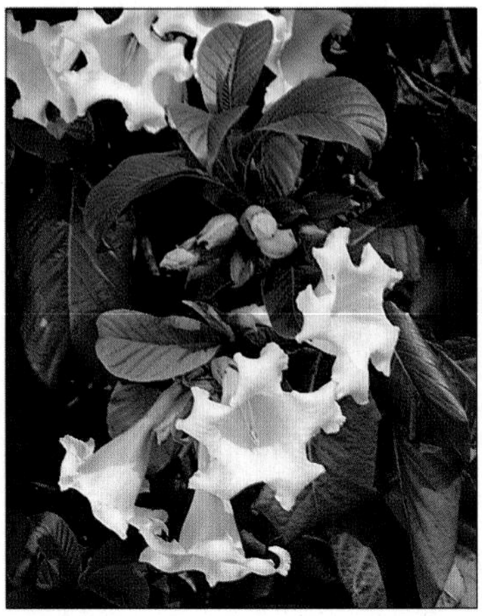

Beaumontia grandiflora

BEGONIA

BEGONIACEAE

Genus of about 900 species and many cultivars of more or less fleshy annuals, herbaceous perennials, evergreen shrubs, and climbers, including some succulents and epiphytes. They are widespread in tropical and subtropical regions, between approximately 15°N. and 15°S. of the equator. Begonias are variable in habit and may be fibrous-rooted, rhizomatous, or tuberous, the tubers becoming dormant in winter. Some are cultivated for their colourful flowers and others for their decorative, alternate, generally asymmetric, simple to compound leaves. The flowers are usually borne in axillary or terminal cymes or racemes. All begonias have flowers of both sexes on the same inflorescence: male flowers with 2–4 unequal petals, female flowers with 2–6 equal petals. In frost-prone areas, grow begonias as container plants in the home or conservatory; the Semperflorens and Tuberhybrida groups may be used for summer bedding. Most begonias are suitable for permanent outdoor cultivation only in relatively humid, tropical and subtropical regions, where they are grown in a bed or border.
For ease of reference, begonias may be divided into 7 informal groupings, based broadly on their growth habit and slightly differing cultivation needs.

Cane-stemmed begonias
Woody, fibrous-rooted, usually upright, evergreen perennials grown for their habit, foliage, and flowers. The species involved in their parentage are mostly from Brazil. The stems are slender and bamboo-like, with regularly spaced, swollen nodes. The often beautifully marked leaves are asymmetric, more or less ovate, and often deeply toothed to lobed. Showy flowers are borne mainly from early spring to summer. These begonias will not tolerate continuous, direct sunlight and tend to shed their lower leaves, especially if overwatered. To keep clothed to the base, cut back overlong canes to 2 or 3 buds in spring or early summer. Propagate by tip, leaf, or stem cuttings.
Rex-cultorum begonias
Mainly evergreen, usually rhizomatous perennials of variable habit, derived from crosses with *B. rex* and related species. Some involve crosses with tuberous begonias, and are not truly rhizomatous, showing a tendency to winter dormancy. They are grown for their foliage. The brilliantly coloured, obliquely ovate to ovate-lance-shaped leaves sometimes have spirally arranged basal lobes. Relatively inconspicuous single flowers, 1.5–2cm (½–¾in) across, are mainly borne in early spring. Grow in bright indirect light at an optimum of 21–24°C (70–75°F). Bright light deepens red leaf coloration, while lower light levels enhance the metallic sheen of many cultivars. To minimize the risk of rhizome rot, water by immersion of the containers. Propagate by seed, sections of rhizome, or leaf cuttings.
Rhizomatous begonias
Variable, mostly evergreen perennials with creeping, erect, or subsurface rhizomes, and small, single flowers

usually borne in winter or early spring. They are grown for their leaves, which are usually 7–30cm (3–12in) long, sometimes with spirally arranged basal lobes, and may be smooth, crested, or puckered, green or brown, often marked with silver. Hybrids derived from *B. bowerae*, the "eyelash begonia", have coloured leaves with fringed margins, and those derived from *B. imperialis* have unusual leaf surfaces and colours. Grow in bright filtered light with shade from hot sun, at an optimum of 19°C (66°F). To minimize the risk of rhizome rot, water by immersion of the containers. Some grow actively throughout the year; if so, continue watering moderately. Propagate by seed, leaf cuttings, or sections of rhizome.

Semperflorens begonias
Bushy, usually compact, fibrous-rooted, evergreen perennial hybrids, derived from *B. cucullata* var. *hookeri*, *B. schmidtiana*, and other species. They are grown for their leaves and flowers. Freely branching, soft, succulent stems bear generally rounded, bronze or green leaves, 3–10cm (1¼–4in) long. Single or double flowers, 1–2.5cm (½–1in) across, are borne throughout summer. In cold climates, plant when risk of frost has passed, in fertile, well-drained, humus-rich soil. These begonias flower well in partial shade, but tolerate all but direct overhead sunlight. Keep container plants just moist and well-ventilated in winter, at 10–15°C (50–59°F). In frost-free climates, treat as perennials and provide similar conditions outdoors, but lift and divide annually in spring. Propagate by seed or basal cuttings.

Shrub-like begonias
Mostly bushy, sometimes succulent, evergreen perennials with freely branching, erect or semi-erect stems. They are grown mainly for their leaves, which are hairless, hairy, or warty, with glossy or matt surfaces. The single, often small flowers are borne mainly from spring to summer. Under glass, maintain a winter minimum of 17°C (63°F) and provide moderate to bright winter light to enhance foliage colour; hairless and glaucous species and cultivars tolerate higher light levels than those with hairy leaves; all need shade from hot summer sun. To encourage compact growth, pinch out the growing tips twice during the growing season. Propagate by seed, or by tip, stem, or leaf cuttings.

Tuberous begonias (including the Tuberhybrida, Multiflora, and Pendula begonias)
Mostly upright, bushy, tuberous, winter-dormant perennials grown for their foliage and flowers. **Tuberhybrida** begonias (*B.* x *tuberhybrida*) are derived from Andean species, including *B. boliviensis*, *B. gracilis*, *B. pearcei*, and *B. veitchii*. They vary from pendent to upright, with sparsely branched, succulent stems, and pointed, glossy, bright to dark green leaves. Most are summer flowering and mainly double-flowered. The flowers are borne in small clusters consisting of 2 small female flowers and one showy, frequently double male flower. They produce flowers and top-growth annually from winter-dormant tubers. Several poorly defined subgroups are sometimes recognized, including the **Multiflora** begonias, with many small, single to double flowers, and the **Pendula** begonias, with trailing or pendulous stems. Under glass, provide bright, filtered light and good ventilation. Reduce humidity when flowering and pinch out small female flowers to prolong flowering. Treat bedding cultivars as for the Semperflorens begonias, but lift tubers in autumn before first frosts, and dry off. Dust with fungicide and store dormant tubers at 5–7°C (41–45°F). In spring, replant tubers, hollow side uppermost, in free-draining potting compost at 16–18°C (61–64°F). Propagate by seed, basal cuttings, or stem cuttings of side shoots. Some species may be increased by bulbils. Prone to vine weevil infestation.

BEGONIA GROUPS

Begonias are very varied in habit. The genus includes trailing, pendent, shrub-like, upright, and climbing species. Based partly on these habits, they may be divided into 7 broad groups.

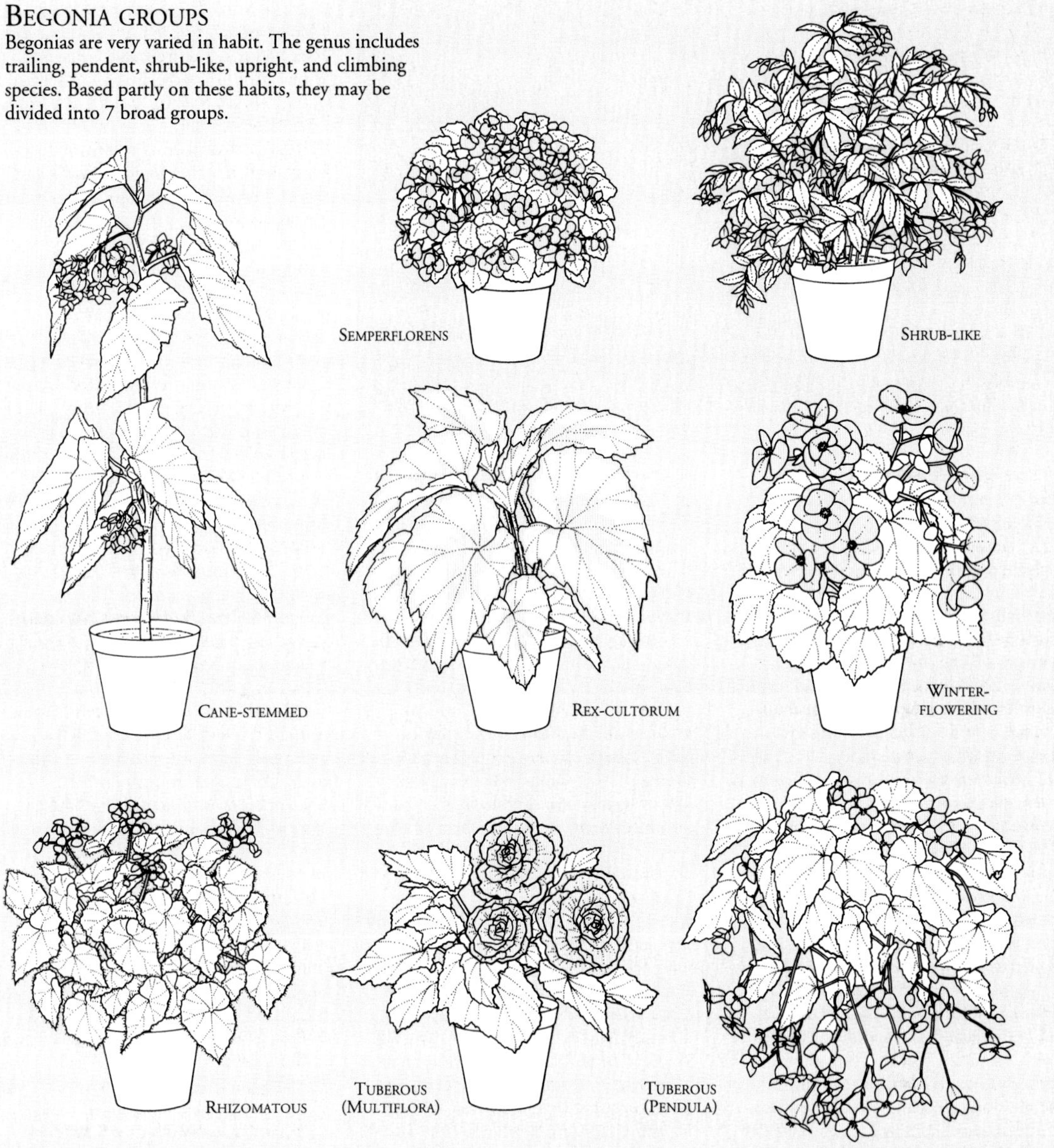

Winter-flowering begonias
Low-growing, compact, bushy, usually fibrous-rooted, evergreen perennials grown for their habit, foliage, and flowers. They have slender, succulent stems and asymmetric, green or bronze-flushed leaves, 5–8cm (2–3in) long, and bear a profusion of single, semi-double, or double flowers, generally from late autumn to early spring. Two broad groups are recognized: the Lorraine, Cheimantha, or Christmas begonias (*B.* x *cheimantha*), which are derived from *B. dregei* and *B. socotrana* and are usually single-flowered; and the Elatior and Rieger begonias which result from crosses between *B. socotrana* and various tuberous begonias. Grow in bright, filtered light, with the maximum available light in winter, at an optimum of 15–20°C (59–68°F), with relatively low humidity and good ventilation. Propagate by basal cuttings. Some winter-flowering begonias are very prone to mildew although the Rieger begonias show some resistance to this disease.

• **HARDINESS** Most are frost tender; a few are half hardy.
• **CULTIVATION** Under glass, grow all begonias in light, well-drained, neutral to slightly acid, loamless or loam-based potting compost (JI No.2) in bright light, with shade from direct sun. Water moderately when in growth, sparingly in winter; ensure the potting compost is never wet or waterlogged. Apply a balanced liquid fertilizer at alternate waterings when in full growth. Pot on annually in spring. For optimum growth, maintain at 19–23°C (66–73°F), with moderate humidity. Most will survive short periods at or just below 10°C (50°F), especially in dry compost, but all growth will cease and many will shed their leaves. Succulent begonias need a more porous medium, higher light levels, and drier conditions. The smallest begonias, including *B. imperialis* and *B. pustulata*, thrive in the high humidity and diffused light of a terrarium. Outdoors, grow begonias in fertile, well-drained, humus-rich, neutral to slightly acid soil in partial shade or good light, but out of direct sun. Further cultivation details are given under the individual groups.
• **PROPAGATION** Sow seed of species at 21°C (70°F) as soon as ripe, and seed of Tuberhybrida and Semperflorens hybrids in early spring. Root stem, tip, or leaf cuttings in spring or summer in a propagating case, in partial shade. Cut rhizomes into sections in summer. Root basal cuttings from tuberous begonias in spring, from winter-flowering begonias in early summer. Surface-sow bulbils on damp moss peat in spring. For further information, see the individual groups.
• **PESTS AND DISEASES** Vulnerable to caterpillars, mealybugs, mites, thrips, vine weevils, aphids, grey mould (*Botrytis*), powdery mildew, stem rot, and rhizome rot.

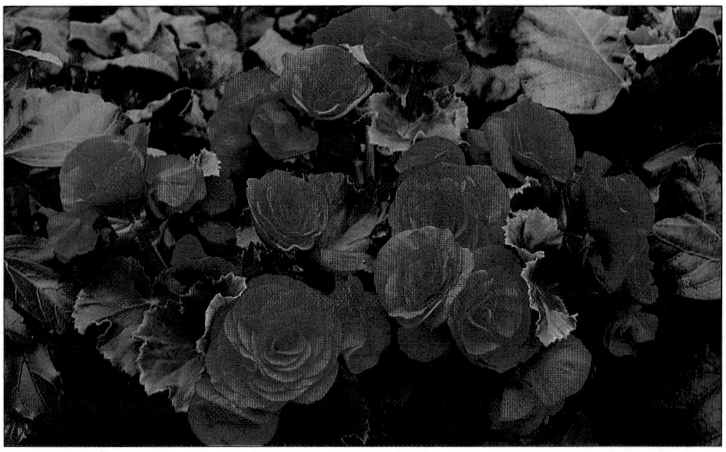

Begonia 'Azotus'

B. aconitifolia ■ syn. *B. sceptrum.* Cane-stemmed begonia bearing ovate, palmately 4- to 6-lobed leaves, 20cm (8in) long, which are dark green splashed with silver, with sunken red veins on the undersides. Panicles of pendent, pale pink or white flowers, to 5cm (2in) across, are produced in autumn. ↕ 1m (3ft), ↔ 30cm (12in). Brazil. ❄ (min. 10°C/50°F). **'Metallica'**, syn. 'Hildegard Schneider', produces bronze-tinted leaves with more pronounced silver markings.
B. albopicta ■ (Guinea-wing begonia). Semi-pendent to upright, freely branching cane-stemmed begonia. Ovate-lance-shaped, wavy-margined leaves, 8cm (3in) long, are glossy green and covered in silver spots above, pale green beneath. Produces panicles of pendent, green-white flowers, to 2cm (¾in) across, in summer. ↕ 60–100cm (24–39in), ↔ 30cm (12in). Brazil. ❄ (min. 10°C/50°F)
***B.* 'All Round'.** Semperflorens begonia with rounded, green or bronze leaves. In summer, produces weather-resistant, single flowers, 2cm (¾in) across, in pink, rose-pink, or white. ↕↔ to 40cm (16in). ❄ (min. 10–15°C/50–59°F)
***B.* 'Ambassador'.** Semperflorens begonia with rounded, mid-green leaves. Produces single, pink, scarlet, salmon-pink, rose-pink, or coral-pink flowers throughout summer. ↕↔ to 20cm (8in) ❄ (min. 10–15°C/50–59°F)
B. angularis see *B. stipulacea.*
***B.* 'Anniversary'** ■ Upright, strongly branched Tuberhybrida begonia with oval, mid-green leaves, to 20cm (8in) long. Golden flowers, 17cm (7in) across, with many broad, overlapping, slightly toothed petals, are produced in cymes in summer. ↕ 60cm (24in), ↔ 45cm (18in). ❄ (min. 10°C/50°F)
***B.* 'Apricot Cascade'** ■ Pendent Tuberhybrida begonia with oval, emerald-green leaves, to 20cm (8in) long. Double, pale apricot flowers, 7cm (3in) across, with toothed petals, are produced from early summer to mid-autumn. ↕↔ 60cm (24in). ❄ (min. 10°C/50°F)
***B.* 'Apricot Delight'** ■ Upright Tuberhybrida begonia bearing oval, mid-green leaves, to 20cm (8in) long. Pale apricot-orange flowers, 17cm (7in) across, with numerous, broad, delicately toothed, overlapping petals, are produced from early summer to mid-autumn. ↕ 60cm (24in), ↔ 45cm (18in). ❄ (min. 10°C/50°F)
B.* x *argenteoguttata ■ (*B. albopicta* x *B. olbia*) (Trout-leaved begonia). Shrub-like begonia with slender, strongly branched stems, and obovate, toothed, dark green leaves, to 15cm (6in) long, covered with silver spots above. Cream flowers, to 3–4cm (1¼–1½in) across, are freely produced in panicles, to 6cm (2½in) across, from spring to autumn. Garden origin. ↕ 75cm (30in), ↔ 60cm (24in). ❄ (min. 10°C/50°F)
***B.* 'Azotus'** ■ Winter-flowering begonia with ovate, dark green leaves. Double, cerise-pink flowers, to 4cm (1½in) across, are produced from late autumn to early spring. ↕ 20cm (8in), ↔ 15cm (6in). ❄ (min. 10°C/50°F)
***B.* 'Baby Perfection'.** Dwarf rhizomatous begonia with creeping rhizomes and ovate, deeply lobed, black-margined, pale green leaves, 4cm (1½in) long. Light pink flowers, 5mm (¼in) across, are profusely borne in spring. ↕ 10cm (4in), ↔ 18cm (7in). ❄ (min. 10°C/50°F)
***B.* 'Barcos'** ■ Winter-flowering begonia with ovate, very dark green leaves. Fully double, dark crimson flowers, to 4cm (1½in) across, are produced from late autumn to early spring. ↕ 23cm (9in), ↔ 20cm (8in). ❄ (min. 10°C/50°F)
***B.* 'Beatrice Hadrell'.** Vigorous rhizomatous begonia with star-shaped, almost black leaves, 13cm (5in) long, with green veins. Pink flowers, 4cm (1½in) across, are freely produced in winter. ↕ 20cm (8in), ↔ 22cm (9in). ❄ (min. 10°C/50°F)
***B.* 'Bethlehem Star'** ■ Rhizomatous begonia with ovate, entire, black-green leaves, 5cm (2in) long, each with a cream star at the centre. Light pink flowers, to 3cm (1¼in) across, are freely borne in winter. ↕ 25cm (10in), ↔ 30cm (12in). ❄ (min. 10°C/50°F)
***B.* 'Billie Langdon'** ■ Upright Tuberhybrida begonia with oval, mid-green leaves, to 20cm (8in) long. Pure white flowers, 18cm (7in) across, with broad, attractively veined petals, are freely borne in summer. ↕ 60cm (24in), ↔ 45cm (18in). ❄ (min. 10°C/50°F)
***B.* 'Bokit'.** Rhizomatous begonia with ovate, palmately lobed, dark green leaves, 7cm (3in) long, striped with dark brown and with spirally arranged basal lobes. Pinkish white flowers, to 4cm (1½in) across, are sparsely produced in winter. ↕ 26cm (10in), ↔ 35cm (14in). ❄ (min. 10°C/50°F)
B. bowerae ■ (Eyelash begonia). Rhizomatous begonia with ovate, entire, light green leaves, to 5cm (2in) long, marked with chocolate-brown and fringed with hairs. White flowers, 2cm (¾in) across, are produced in cymes from winter to early spring. ↕ 25cm (10in), ↔ 18cm (7in). Mexico. ❄ (min. 10°C/50°F)
***B.* 'Bridal Cascade'.** Pendent Tuberhybrida begonia with oval, mid-green leaves, to 20cm (8in) long. White flowers, to 8cm (3in) across, with narrow red margins, are produced in summer. ↕ 10cm (4in), ↔ 60cm (24in). ❄ (min. 10°C/50°F)
***B.* 'Burle Marx'** see *B. glazioui.*
***B.* 'Can-can'** ■ Upright Tuberhybrida begonia with oval, mid-green leaves, to 20cm (8in) long. Rich yellow flowers, 18cm (7in) across, composed of toothed petals with broad, red-picotee margins, are produced in summer. ↕ 90cm (36in), ↔ 45cm (18in). ❄ (min. 10°C/50°F)
***B.* 'Caravan'**, syn. *B.* 'Serlis'. Shrub-like begonia with upright stems and peltate, broadly ovate, soft, mid-green leaves, 20cm (8in) long, with a slightly felted appearance, and veins marked pale green. Small white flowers, 1cm (½in) across, are produced from early spring to late summer. ↕ 45cm (18in), ↔ 20cm (8in). ❄ (min. 10°C/50°F)
***B.* 'Carol Wilkins of Ballarat'.** Robust, upright Tuberhybrida begonia with oval, mid-green leaves, to 20cm (8in) long. Dark salmon-pink flowers, 13–15cm (5–6in) across, with broad, glaucous petals and rosebud centres, are freely borne in summer. ↕ 60cm (24in), ↔ 45cm (18in). ❄ (min. 10°C/50°F)
***B.* 'City of Ballarat'** ■ Strong-growing, upright Tuberhybrida begonia with oval, mid-green leaves, to 20cm (8in) long. In summer, produces bright orange flowers, 18cm (7in) across, with broad, slightly wavy, glaucous petals. ↕ 60cm (24in), ↔ 45cm (18in). ❄ (min. 10°C/50°F)
B. coccinea (Angelwing begonia). Cane-stemmed begonia, a parent of many hybrids. Ovate leaves, to 15cm (6in) long, are green with red margins above, dull red beneath. Coral-red flowers, to 3cm (1¼in) across, are profusely borne in red-stalked, pendent racemes in spring. Is an excellent houseplant if provided with sufficient light. ↕ 1.2m (4ft), ↔ 30cm (12in). Brazil. ❄ (min. 10°C/50°F)
***B.* Cocktail Series** ■ 🏆 Weather-resistant Semperflorens begonias with rounded bronze leaves. Single flowers, in a wide range of reds, pinks, and whites, including single colours and bicolours, are produced throughout summer. ↕ 20–30cm (8–12in), ↔ 30cm (12in). ❄ (min. 13°C/55°F)

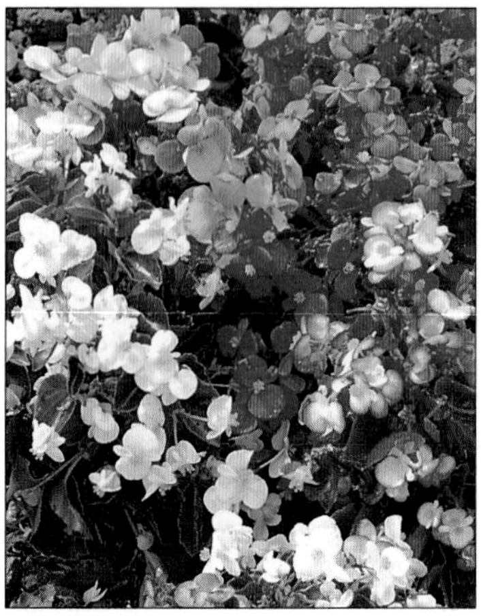

Begonia Cocktail Series

B. compta see *B. stipulacea.*
***B.* 'Corallina de Lucerna'** see *B.* 'Lucerna'.
***B.* 'Crestabruchii'** (Lettuce leaf begonia). Rhizomatous begonia with ovate, acute, mid-green leaves, 20cm (8in) long, with heavily crested margins. Small pink flowers, 5–8mm (¼–⅜in) across, are produced in late winter. ↕ 23cm (9in), ↔ 25cm (10in). ❄ (min. 10°C/50°F)
B. dichroa. Low-growing, somewhat pendent cane-stemmed begonia with ovate, bright green leaves, 12cm (5in) long. Orange flowers, 3cm (1¼in) across, are borne in panicles throughout the year. ↕ 35cm (14in), ↔ 25cm (10in). Brazil. ❄ (min. 10°C/50°F)
B. disticha see *B. stipulacea.*
B. dregei ■ (Maple-leaf begonia). Tuberous begonia with tall, flexible stems that have swollen nodes and break easily unless supported. Palmately lobed, maple-like leaves, to 7cm (3in) long, are green with purple veins above, red beneath, occasionally silver-speckled when young. Cymes of single white flowers, to 1.5cm (½in) across, cover the plant in late summer. ↕ 75cm (30in), ↔ 60cm (24in). South Africa. ❄ (min. 10°C/50°F), but may shed its leaves below 13°C (55°F).
***B.* 'Duartei'** ■ Rex-cultorum begonia with spirally arranged, obovate, red-hairy, dark green leaves, 17cm (7in) long, with darker green margins and a banding of silver streaks. Pink flowers are produced in spring. ↕↔ 60cm (24in). ❄ (min. 10°C/50°F)
***B.* 'Emerald Giant'.** Rex-cultorum begonia with creeping rhizomes and ovate, vibrant green leaves, 45cm (18in) long, banded with shades of brown. Pink flowers are produced in summer. ↕↔ 75cm (30in). ❄ (min. 10°C/50°F)
***B.* 'Enech'.** Rhizomatous begonia with ovate, entire, velvety, almost black leaves, 8cm (3in) long, with green veins, red bases, and maroon undersides. Small white flowers are produced in small sprays in spring. ↕ 15cm (6in), ↔ 18cm (7in). ❄ (min. 10°C/50°F)
***B.* 'Erythrophylla'**, syn. *B.* 'Feastii' (Beefsteak begonia). Rhizomatous begonia with thick, rounded, hairless leaves, 15cm (6in) long, glossy, mid- to dark green above and dark reddish brown beneath. Light pink flowers, to 2cm (¾in) across, are produced well above the foliage in late winter and early spring. Seldom attacked by pests. ↕ 20cm (8in), ↔ 30cm (12in). ❄ (min. 10°C/50°F)
***B.* 'Feastii'** see *B.* 'Erythrophylla'.
***B.* 'Flamboyant'** ■ Upright Tuberhybrida begonia with heart-shaped, mid-green leaves, to 15cm (6in) long. Single, dark scarlet flowers, 5cm (2in) across, are produced freely in summer. ↕ 17cm (7in), ↔ 15cm (6in). ❄ (min. 10°C/50°F)
B. foliosa ■ Shrub-like begonia with pendent stems, 45cm (18in) long, densely clothed with ovate, notched, mid-green leaves, 8mm (⅜in) long. White flowers, to 1.5cm (½in) across, are produced in panicles in autumn and spring. ↕ 45cm (18in), ↔ 30cm (12in). Colombia, Venezuela. ❄ (min.

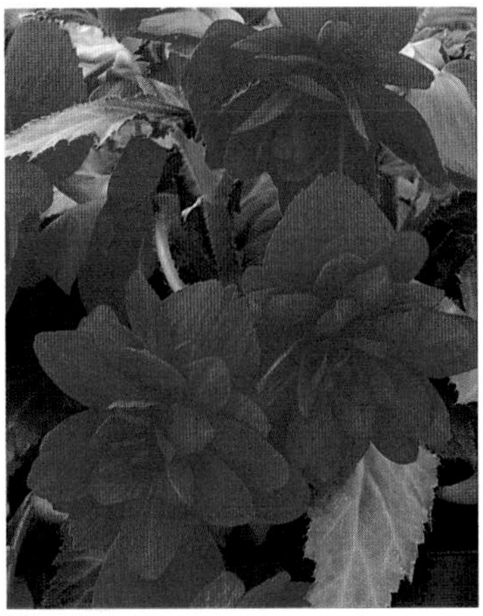

Begonia Illumination Series 'Illumination Orange'

10°C/50°F). **var. *miniata*** see *B. fuchsioides* var. *miniata*.
B. fuchsioides 🏆 (Fuchsia begonia). Shrub-like begonia with slender stems and oblong-ovate to sickle-shaped, toothed, shiny, mid-green leaves, 2.5cm (1in) long, flushed red when young. Fuchsia-like, pink to red flowers, to 3cm (1¼in) across, are produced in panicles in winter. ↕75cm (30in), ↔45cm (18in). Venezuela. ❀ (min. 10°C/50°F). **var. *miniata***, syn. *B. foliosa* var. *miniata*, is smaller, and produces bright red flowers; ↕45cm (18in), ↔30cm (12in).
***B.* 'Futta'** ▣ Winter-flowering begonia with ovate, mid-green leaves. Semi-double, mid-yellow flowers, to 4cm (1½in) across, with peach-pink margins, are produced from late autumn to early spring. ↕20cm (8in), ↔18cm (7in). ❀ (min. 10°C/50°F)
B. glazioui 🏆 syn. *B.* 'Burle Marx'. Rhizomatous begonia bearing obovate, mid-green leaves, 15cm (6in) long, with shiny, warty surfaces, which turn brown if grown in high light levels. White flowers, to 2cm (¾in) across, are produced in panicles, borne well above the foliage, in spring. ↕75cm (30in), ↔60cm (24in). Brazil. ❀ (min. 4°C/39°F)
***B.* 'Gloire de Lorraine'.** Winter-flowering begonia of the Lorraine group with inversely lance-shaped, shiny, bright green leaves. In winter, produces panicles, 15cm (6in) long, of mostly male, single, clear pink flowers, 2.5cm (1in) long. ↕45cm (18in), ↔60cm (24in). ❀ (min. 10°C/50°F)
B. goegoensis. Rhizomatous begonia with horizontal rhizomes and erect stems. Ovate-rounded, peltate, puckered, bronze-green leaves, 15cm (6in) or more long, have lighter green veins. From summer to autumn, produces small cymes of pink flowers, to 1cm (½in) across. ↕25cm (10in), ↔30cm (12in). Indonesia (Goego Island). ❀ (min. 10°C/50°F)
B. gracilis* var. *martiana, syn. *B. martiana* (Hollyhock begonia). Tuberous begonia with sparsely branched stems bearing obliquely heart-shaped, sharp-pointed, toothed, brownish green leaves, 4cm (1½in) long. Fragrant, rose-pink or white flowers, to 5cm (2in) across, are produced in racemes in summer. ↕75cm (30in), ↔35cm (14in). Mexico, Guatemala. ❀ (min. 10°C/50°F)
B. grandis* subsp. *evansiana. Tuberous begonia with bulb-like tubers, and branched stems bearing ovate, notched leaves, 10cm (4in) long, olive-green above, and pale green, occasionally red beneath. Bears pendent cymes of fragrant, pink or white flowers, to 3cm (1¼in) across, in summer. Axillary bulbils are produced in late summer. ↕50cm (20in), ↔30cm (12in). China to Malaysia, Japan. ✲. **var. *alba*** ▣ has erect cymes of pinkish white flowers.
B. haageana see *B. scharffii*.
***B.* 'Helene Harms'.** Upright Tuberhybrida begonia with ovate, mid-green leaves, to 20cm (8in) long. Produces a mass of semi-double, rich coppery yellow flowers, 5–7cm (2–3in) across, in summer. ↕13cm (5in), ↔15cm (6in). ❀ (min. 10°C/50°F)
***B.* 'Helen Lewis'** ▣ Upright Rex-cultorum begonia with ovate, silver-banded, dark wine-red leaves, to 15cm (6in) long. Creamy white flowers are produced in summer. ↕60cm (24in), ↔35cm (14in). ❀ (min. 10°C/50°F)
B. heracleifolia. Rhizomatous begonia with a short, thick rhizome, and rounded, palmately 7-lobed leaves, 15cm (6in) long, which are bronze-green above, red-green beneath. Fragrant, pinkish white flowers, 2.5–4cm (1–1½in) across, are profusely borne in panicles from spring to autumn. ↕45cm (18in), ↔35cm (14in). Mexico, Guatemala, El Salvador, Honduras. ❀ (min. 10°C/50°F). **var. *longipila*** has leaves which are dark reddish brown-green above, with pale green along the veins, and rust-red with pink veins beneath. **var. *nigricans*** has black-margined, mid-green leaves and red leaf-stalks. **var. *punctata*** has metallic-tinted leaves with dark brown marks above; Mexico. **'Sunderbruckii'** has bronze-streaked leaves with green along the veins, dark purple beneath, and pink flowers from winter to spring.
***B.* Hi Fi Series.** Very floriferous Semperflorens begonias with rounded, mid-green leaves. Single flowers, in pink, red, white, or brilliant rose-pink, are produced in summer. ↕↔20cm (8in). ❀ (min. 10°C/50°F)
***B.* Illumination Series.** Pendulous Tuberhybrida begonias with oval, mid- to dark green leaves, to 18cm (7in) long. Bears double, flattened, pale pink or orange flowers, to 8cm (3in) across, in arching cascades in summer. ↕60cm (24in), ↔30cm (12in). ❀ (min. 10°C/50°F). **'Illumination Orange'** ▣🏆 bears vivid orange flowers.
B. imperialis ▣ Rhizomatous begonia with ovate, toothed, light green leaves, 10cm (4in) long, with silvery green splashes along the main veins; the warty upper surfaces are covered with very fine hairs. White flowers, to 1.5cm (½in) across, are sparsely produced in panicles during winter. ↕13cm (5in), ↔23cm (9in). Mexico. ❀ (min. 10°C/50°F)
B. incana see *B. peltata*.
***B.* 'Ingramii'** ▣ Shrub-like begonia with erect, slender stems, pendent at the tips, and slender, ovate-lance-shaped, toothed, shiny, mid-green leaves, 7cm (3in) long. Produces dark pink flowers, to 3cm (1¼in) across, more or less continuously if grown in good light. Foliage burns if the light intensity is too high. ↕75cm (30in), ↔45cm (18in). ❀ (min. 10°C/50°F)

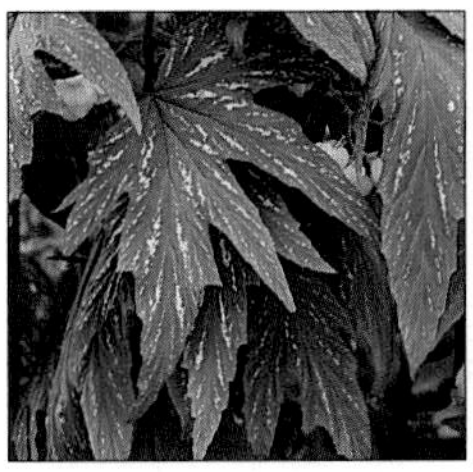

Begonia aconitifolia

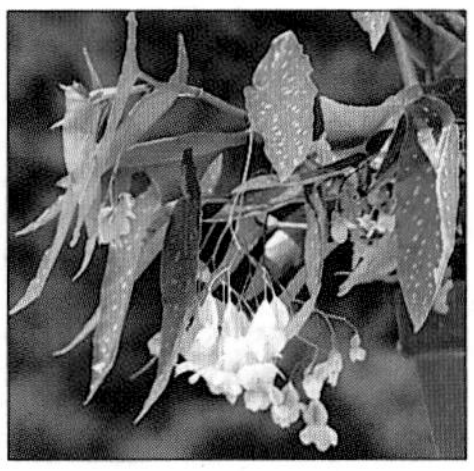

Begonia albopicta

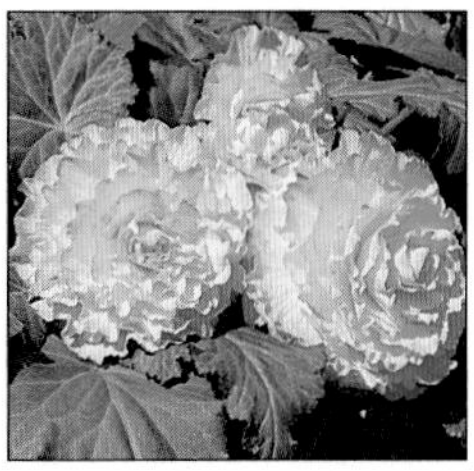

Begonia 'Anniversary'

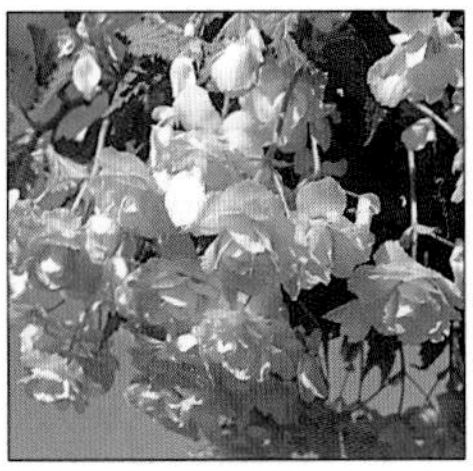

Begonia 'Apricot Cascade'

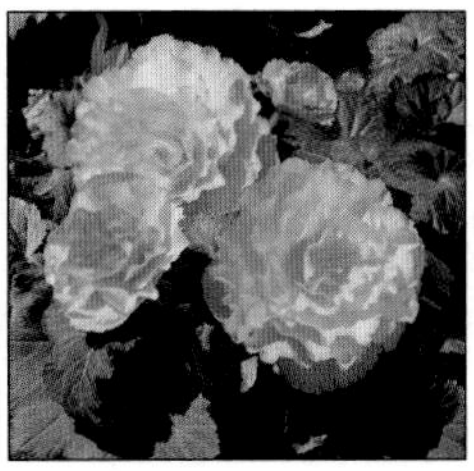

Begonia 'Apricot Delight'

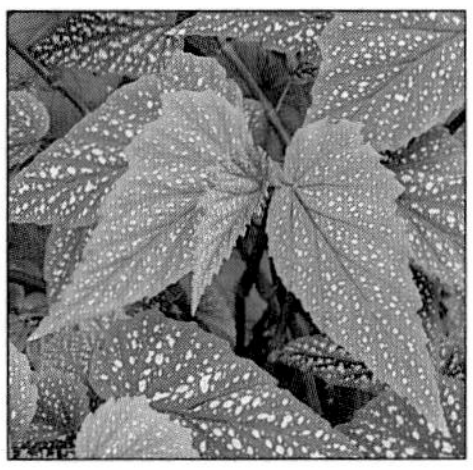

Begonia x *argenteoguttata*

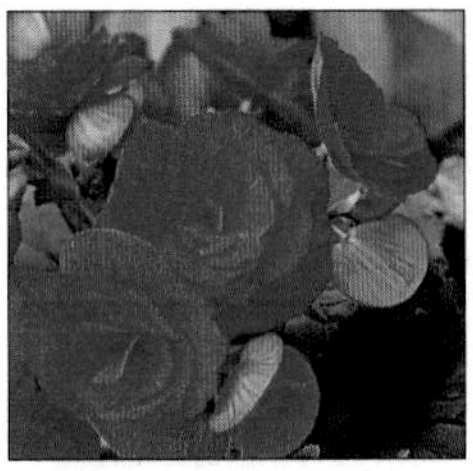

Begonia 'Barcos'

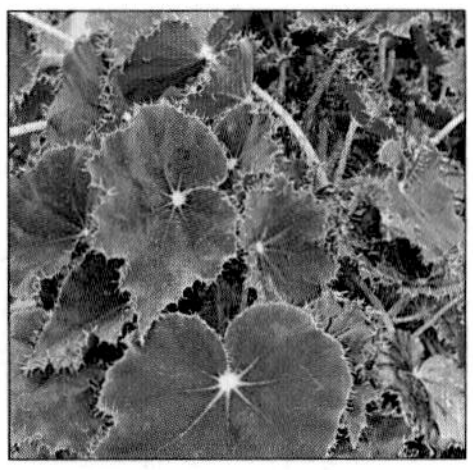

Begonia 'Bethlehem Star'

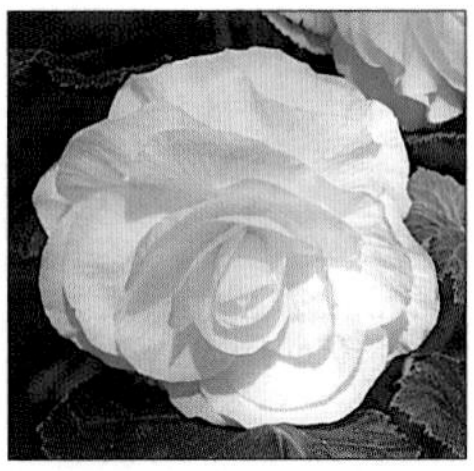

Begonia 'Billie Langdon'

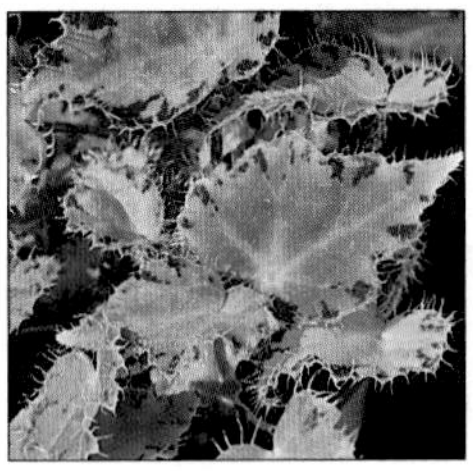

Begonia bowerae

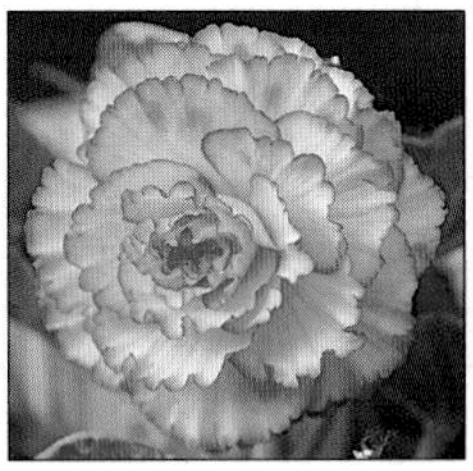

Begonia 'Can-can'

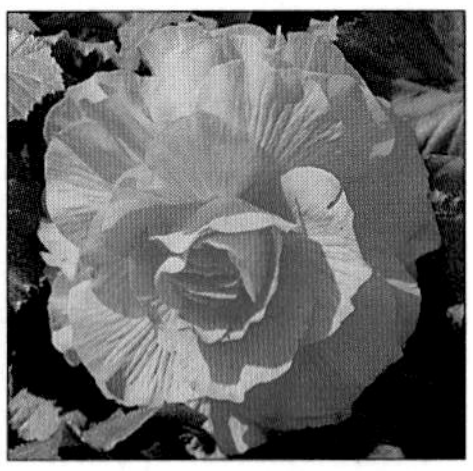

Begonia 'City of Ballarat'

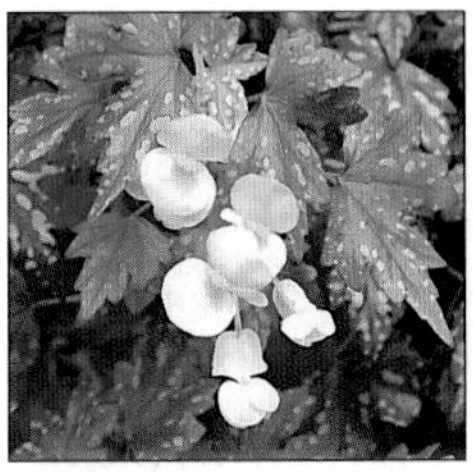

Begonia dregei

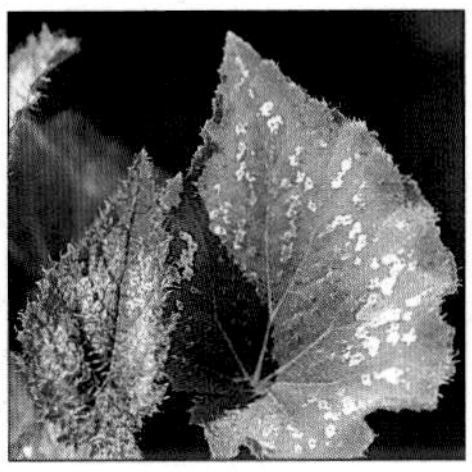

Begonia 'Duartei'

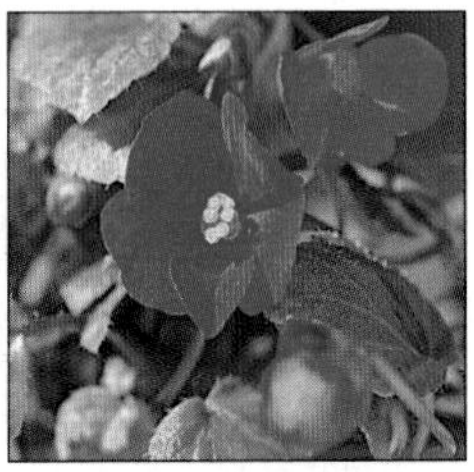

Begonia 'Flamboyant'

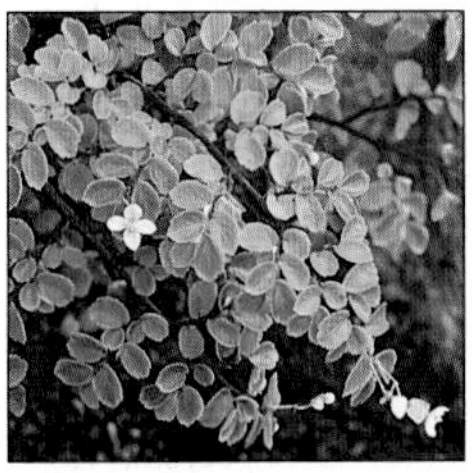

Begonia foliosa

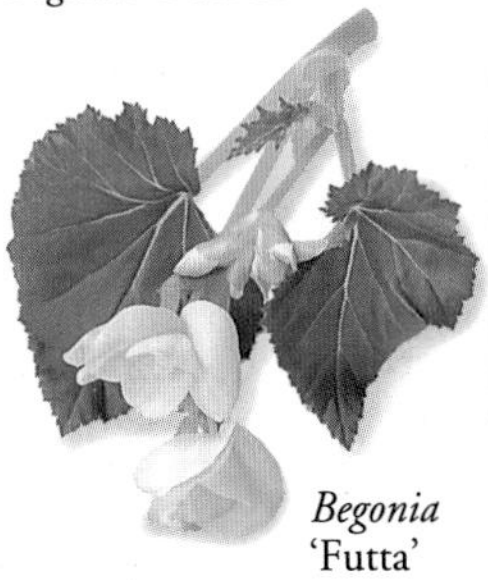

Begonia 'Futta'

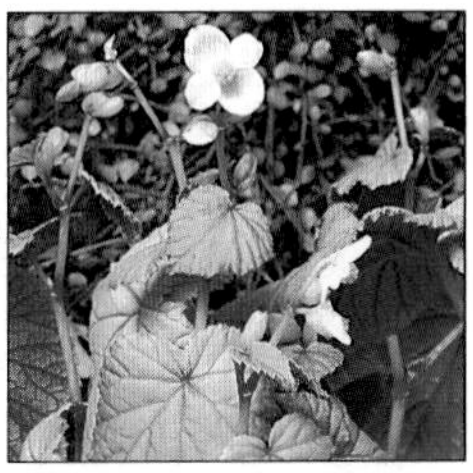

Begonia grandis subsp. *evansiana* var. *alba*

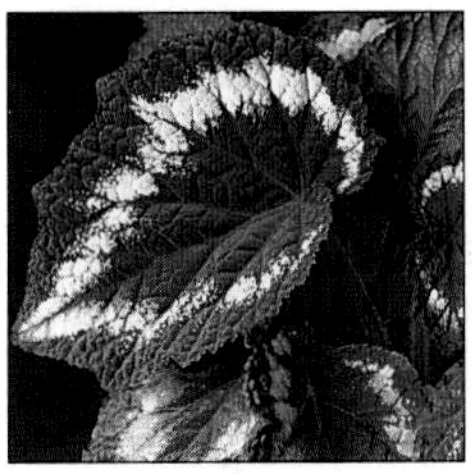

Begonia 'Helen Lewis'

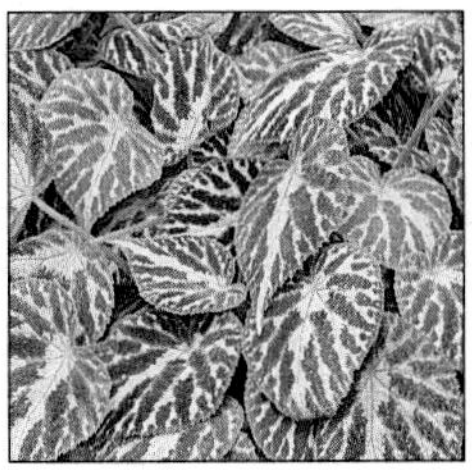

Begonia imperialis

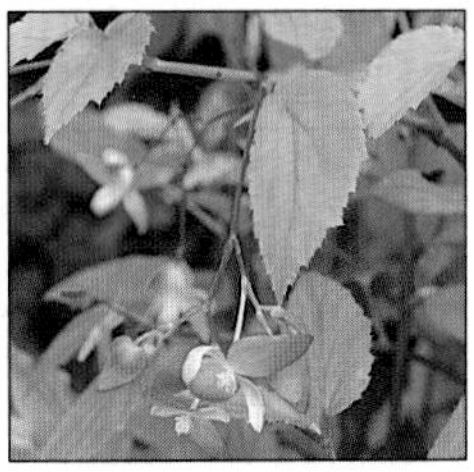

Begonia 'Ingramii'

***B.* 'Irene Nuss'** ■ ♀ Cane-stemmed begonia with ovate-oblique, wavy-margined, deeply lobed leaves, 20cm (8in) long, bronze above and red beneath. Dark coral-pink flowers, to 4cm (1½in) across, are freely produced in large, pendent panicles throughout summer. ↕75cm (30in), ↔60cm (24in). ❄ (min. 10°C/50°F)

***B.* 'Iron Cross'** see *B. masoniana.*

***B.* 'Jill Adair'.** Very compact shrub-like begonia with ovate-acute, slightly pleated, rich dark green leaves, 6cm (2½in) long, red-tinted beneath. White flowers, 2.5cm (1in) across, are freely produced well above the foliage throughout the year. ↕↔30cm (12in). ❄ (min. 10°C/50°F)

***B.* 'Kathleen Meyer'.** Miniature cane-stemmed begonia with lance-shaped-ovate, light green leaves, 5cm (2in) long, heavily splashed with white. Pink flowers, 5–8cm (2–3in) across, are freely produced from spring to summer. ↕35cm (14in), ↔23cm (9in). ❄ (min. 10°C/50°F)

***B.* 'Kleo'** ■ Winter-flowering begonia with ovate, dark green leaves. Semi-double, coral-pink flowers, to 4cm (1½in) across, with a hint of orange, are produced from late autumn to early spring. ↕20cm (8in), ↔18cm (7in). ❄ (min. 10°C/50°F)

***B.* 'Lime Swirl'.** Compact rhizomatous begonia with spirally arranged, deeply cut, bright green leaves, 13cm (5in) long, with wavy margins. Light pink flowers, 2.5–4cm (1–1½in) across, are freely produced in cymes, 15cm (6in) across, in very early spring. ↕35cm (14in), ↔30cm (12in). ❄ (min. 10°C/50°F)

***B.* 'Looking Glass'.** Cane-stemmed begonia with ovate, gently wavy-margined leaves, 15cm (6in) long, shallowly lobed, especially when young, glistening silvery bronze above, with olive-green veins, and burgundy-red beneath. Pink flowers, to 2cm (¾in) across, are sparsely produced in early summer. ↕90cm (36in), ↔45cm (18in). ❄ (min. 10°C/50°F)

***B.* 'Love Me'.** Winter-flowering begonia from the Lorraine Group with obovate, mid-green leaves. Single, coral-pink flowers, 2–4cm (¾–1½in) across, are profusely borne from late autumn to early spring. ↕45cm (18in), ↔25cm (10in). ❄ (min. 10°C/50°F)

***B.* 'Lucerna'**, syn. *B.* 'Corallina de Lucerna'. Vigorous cane-stemmed begonia with ovate, olive-green leaves, 20cm (8in) long, heavily marked with silvery white spots. Very large panicles, 25cm (10in) or more across, of single, rose-pink flowers, to 4cm (1½in) across, are borne mainly in summer. Remove the growing point to restrict height to about 1.5m (5ft), if required. ↕2–2.2m (6–7ft), ↔35cm (14in). ❄ (min. 10°C/50°F)

B. luxurians (Palm-leaf begonia). Shrub-like begonia with slightly hairy, mid-, dark, or bronze-green leaves, 25cm (10in) across, each with up to 16 lance-shaped leaflets. Leaves are borne, umbrella-like, at the top of erect, largely unbranched stems, to 15cm (6in) tall. From spring to summer, bears cymes, 10cm (4in) across, of many slightly fragrant, yellowish white flowers, 6mm (¼in) across. ↕75cm (30in), ↔60cm (24in). Brazil. ❄ (min. 10°C/50°F)

***B.* 'Mac's Gold'.** Creeping rhizomatous begonia with ovate, 5- to 7-palmate, light chocolate-brown and emerald-green leaves, 5cm (2in) across. Small, pale pink flowers are sparsely produced throughout the year. ↕20cm (8in), ↔25cm (10in). ❄ (min. 10°C/50°F)

***B.* 'Magic Lace'** ■ Rhizomatous begonia with spirally arranged, ovate, copper leaves, 10cm (4in) long, splashed silvery green. Light pink flowers, 3cm (1¼in) across, are produced in early spring. ↕25cm (10in), ↔30cm (12in). ❄ (min. 10°C/50°F)

***B.* 'Maid Marion'.** Upright Rex-cultorum begonia with spirally arranged, rounded, silvery pink leaves, 12cm (5in) long, which darken in colour when exposed to high light intensity. Sprays of small pink flowers are produced in early winter. ↕25cm (10in), ↔30cm (12in). ❄ (min. 10°C/50°F)

B. manicata ■ (Leopard begonia). Upright rhizomatous begonia characterized by a collar of red hairs around the stalks below the leaf-blades. Ovate to heart-shaped, toothed, glossy, light green leaves, 15cm (6in) long, are fringed with hairs. Panicles, to 5cm (2in) across, of pale pink flowers, to 1.5cm (½in) across, are produced well above the foliage in late winter. ↕60cm (24in), ↔35cm (14in). Mexico. ❄ (min. 10°C/50°F). **'Aureomaculata'** has glossy, light green leaves splashed with yellow. **'Crispa'**, syn. 'Cristata', has leaves with crested margins.

***B.* 'Margaritacea'.** Cane-stemmed begonia with ovate-acute, slightly wavy-margined, red-hairy, purple leaves, 12cm (5in) long, with a distinct silvery sheen. Pink flowers, to 2cm (¾in) across, are produced in late autumn. The very slender stems require staking. ↕60cm (24in), ↔45cm (18in). ❄ (min. 10°C/50°F)

B. martiana see *B. gracilis* var. *martiana.*

B. masoniana ■ ♀ syn. *B.* 'Iron Cross' (Iron-cross begonia). Rhizomatous begonia with ovate, sharp-pointed, warty, mid- to deep green leaves, 20cm (8in) long, which are red-hairy and overlaid with a black-brown mark resembling the German Iron Cross. Cymes of green-white flowers, to 2cm (¾in) across, are freely produced in summer. ↕50cm (20in), ↔45cm (18in). New Guinea. ❄ (min. 10°C/50°F)

B. mazae. Fibrous-rooted begonia with very slender, spreading, pendent stems. Ovate, sharp-pointed, bronze-green leaves, 7cm (3in) long, have pronounced red-brown markings along the veins. Fragrant pink flowers, to 1.5cm (½in) across, are profusely borne in cymes, to 10cm (4in) long, which cover the plant in early spring. ↕25cm (10in), ↔ indefinite. Mexico. ❄ (min. 10°C/50°F). **f. *viridis*** (Stitched-leaf begonia) has light green leaves with a pronounced, stitch-like, dark brown mark where each vein meets the margin.

***B.* 'Medora'.** Shrub-like begonia with strong, slender stems bearing lance-shaped, mid-green leaves, 6cm (2½in) long, marked with silver spots. Small panicles of pink flowers are freely produced in late summer. Prune regularly to restrict height to about 45cm (18in) and to encourage bushy growth. ↕90cm (36in), ↔30cm (12in). ❄ (min. 10°C/50°F)

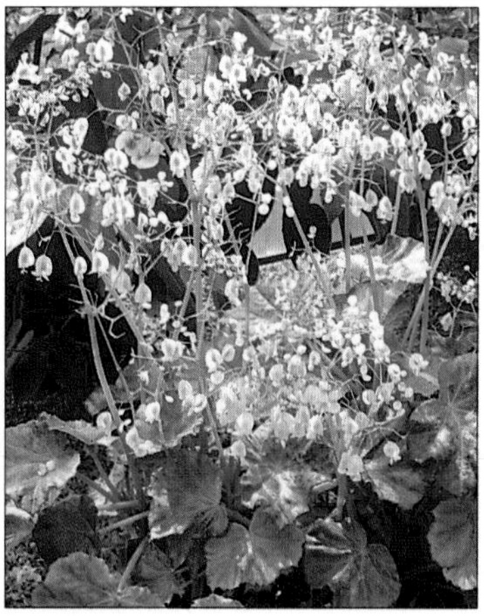

Begonia manicata

***B.* 'Merry Christmas'** ♀ ■ syn. *B.* 'Ruhrtal'. Rex-cultorum begonia with ovate, glossy, deep pink leaves, 20cm (8in) long, outlined in emerald-green, with darker red centres and margins. Pale rose-pink flowers are produced from autumn to early winter. ↕25cm (10in), ↔30cm (12in). ❄ (min. 10°C/50°F)

B. metallica ■ ♀ (Metallic-leaf begonia). Shrub-like begonia with ovate, red-hairy, dark green leaves, 18cm (7in) long, with a bright metallic sheen and sunken, dark reddish brown veins. Red-hairy, pink flowers, to 3.5cm (1½in) across, are produced in cymes in autumn. ↕90cm (36in), ↔60cm (24in). Brazil. ❄ (min. 10°C/50°F)

***B.* 'Midnight Sun'** ■ Compact shrub-like begonia with ovate leaves, 10cm (4in) long, pink when young and maturing to bright green. Sprays of white flowers, 4cm (1½in) across, are produced in summer. ↕30cm (12in), ↔45cm (18in). ❄ (min. 10°C/50°F)

***B.* 'Mini Merry'.** Miniature Rex-cultorum begonia with ovate, bright red leaves, to 7cm (3in) long, outlined in emerald-green, with darker red centres and margins. Pink flowers are produced in autumn. ↕12cm (5in), ↔15cm (6in). ❄ (min. 10°C/50°F)

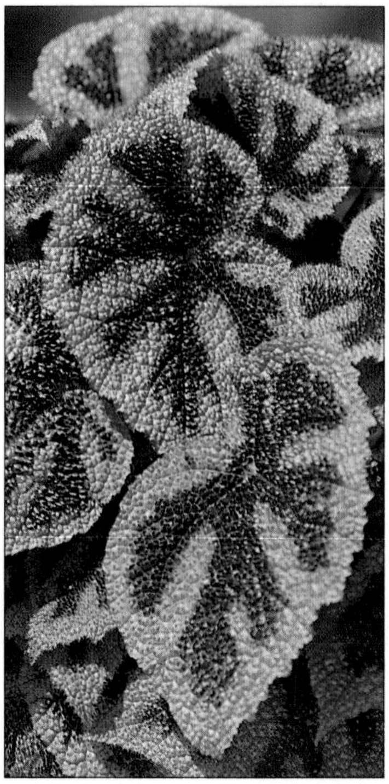

Begonia masoniana

***B.* 'Mme Richard Galle'.** Upright Tuberhybrida begonia with oval, mid-green leaves, to 18cm (7in) long. Numerous double, pink-orange flowers, 5–7cm (2–3in) across, are produced in summer. ↕25cm (10in), ↔20cm (8in). ❄ (min. 10°C/50°F)

***B.* 'Munchkin'** ■ ♀ Rhizomatous begonia with ovate leaves, 13cm (5in) long, bronze with dark green veins above, red beneath, and with crested margins covered in fine white hairs. Pink flowers, 1–2cm (½–¾in) across, are produced in cymes, to 10cm (4in) across, above the foliage in early spring. ↕↔20cm (8in). ❄ (min. 10°C/50°F)

B. nelumbiifolia ■ Rhizomatous begonia with rounded, peltate, mid-green leaves, to 30cm (12in) long, hairy beneath. Pinkish white flowers, to 1.5cm (½in) across, are sparsely produced in cymes in late winter. ↕45cm (18in), ↔60cm (24in). Mexico to Colombia. ❄ (min. 10°C/50°F). **'Red Veined'** has leaves with red veins.

***B.* Non Stop Series** ■ ♀ Upright, compact Tuberhybrida begonias with heart-shaped, mid-green leaves, 10–15cm (4–6in) long. Solitary, double flowers, to 8cm (3in) across, in apricot, bright red, orange, pink, white, or yellow, are borne in summer. ↕↔30cm (12in). ❄ (min. 10°C/50°F)

***B.* 'Norah Bedson'** ■ Rhizomatous begonia with red-speckled stems and ovate, sharp-pointed leaves, 5cm (2in) long, mottled chocolate and green, with red splashes beneath and tiny white hairs at the margins. Pink flowers, 3cm (1¼in) across, are produced in spring. ↕23cm (9in), ↔25cm (10in). ❄ (min. 10°C/50°F)

***B.* 'Oliver Twist'** ■ Rhizomatous begonia with ovate, crested, ruffled, mid-green leaves, 15cm (6in) long, with brown markings along the veins. Pink flowers, 4cm (1½in) across, are produced in winter. ↕45cm (18in), ↔25cm (10in). ❄ (min. 10°C/50°F)

B. olsoniae ■ Compact shrub-like begonia with ovate, blunt-based, bronze-tinted, lush green leaves, 12–20cm (5–8in) long, with prominent, creamy white veins and brownish red undersides. Pinkish white flowers, to 3cm (1¼in) across, are borne in cymes, 5cm (2in) across, well above the foliage at almost any time of year. ↕22cm (9in), ↔30cm (12in). Brazil. ❄ (min. 10°C/50°F)

***B.* 'Olympia White'** ■ Compact, weather-resistant Semperflorens begonia, a selection from the Olympia Series, with rounded, mid-green leaves. Neatly formed, single, pure white flowers, to 4cm (1½in) across, are borne in summer. ↕↔ to 20cm (8in). ❄ (min. 13°C/55°F)

***B.* 'Orange Cascade'.** Pendent Tuberhybrida begonia with freely branching stems and ovate, mid-green leaves, to 15cm (6in) long. Fully double, bright orange flowers, 7cm (3in) across, are profusely borne in summer. ↕↔60cm (24in). ❄ (min. 10°C/50°F)

***B.* 'Orange Rubra'** ■ Cane-stemmed begonia with lance-shaped, emerald-green leaves, 12cm (5in) long, sometimes faintly spotted with silver. Vivid orange flowers, 2–3cm (¾–1¼in) across, are produced at any time of year.

B

↕ 60cm (24in), ↔ 45cm (18in). ❀ (min. 10°C/50°F)
***B.* 'Organdy'** ■ Weather-resistant Semperflorens begonia with rounded, green or bronze leaves. In summer, bears single flowers, to 2cm (¾in) across, in a mix of white, pink, rose-pink, and scarlet. ↕↔ 15cm (6in). ❀ (min. 13°C/55°F)
***B.* 'Orpha C. Fox'** ■ Cane-stemmed begonia with ovate leaves, 15cm (6in) long, grey-green splashed with silver, and maroon beneath. Single, rose-pink flowers, to 3cm (1¼in) across, are produced throughout the year, but mainly in summer. ↕ 90cm (36in), ↔ 30cm (12in). ❀ (min. 10°C/50°F)
***B.* 'Pandora'.** Rex-cultorum begonia with ovate, dark green leaves, 13cm (5in) long, splashed with pink and silver. Produces pink flowers in autumn. ↕ 25cm (10in), ↔ 23cm (9in). ❀ (min. 10°C/50°F)
***B.* Party Fun Series.** Tall-growing, open Semperflorens begonias with rounded, mid-green leaves, to 12cm (5in) long. Single flowers, to 4cm (1½in) across, in scarlet, white, pink, and rose-pink, mixed and single, are produced in summer. ↕↔ to 30cm (12in). ❀ (min. 13°C/55°F)
B. paulensis. Rhizomatous begonia with rounded, peltate, glossy, mid-green leaves, 20cm (8in) long, with the surfaces between the radial veins covered with cross-veins. Creamy white flowers, 3.5–5cm (1½–2in) across, with red hairs, are produced in racemes to 10cm (4in) across in spring. ↕↔ to 30cm (12in). Brazil. ❀ (min. 13°C/55°F)
B. peltata, syn. *B. incana.* Fibrous-rooted, succulent, perennial begonia with slightly swollen, erect stems. Peltate, fleshy, ovate, mid-green leaves, 20cm (8in) long, have small, well-spaced, marginal teeth, and are densely white-hairy beneath. In spring, bears white or pink-flushed flowers, to 2.5cm (1in) across, in pendent panicles. ↕ 60cm (24in), ↔ 40cm (16in). Mexico, Guatemala. ❀ (min. 10°C/50°F)
***B.* 'Phyllomanica'** (Crazy-leaf begonia). Fibrous-rooted shrub-like begonia with thick, branched, shaggy-hairy stems and obliquely heart-shaped, toothed leaves, 15cm (6in) long, fringed with hairs, light green above, paler and with a few red hairs beneath. In winter or early spring, bears pale pink flowers, to 2cm (¾in) across, in panicles 8cm (3in) across. The adventitious plantlets on the stems, leaf-stalks, and leaves may be used for propagation. ↕ 1m (3ft), ↔ 45cm (18in). ❀ (min. 10°C/50°F)
***B.* 'Pickobeth'.** Compact cane-stemmed begonia with ovate, mid-green leaves, to 15cm (6in) long, heavily freckled with white spots, and bunched together along the stems. Rose-pink flowers, to 6cm (2½in) across, are borne in panicles in mid- and late spring. ↕ 75cm (30in), ↔ 35cm (14in). ❀ (min. 10°C/50°F)
***B.* 'Pink Avalanche'.** Loose, cascading Semperflorens begonia with rounded, mid-green leaves. Sterile, single pink flowers, to 4cm (1½in) across, are profusely and continuously produced throughout summer. ↕↔ to 30cm (12in). ❀ (min. 13°C/55°F)
***B.* 'Pin-up'** ■ 🏆 Erect, compact Tuberhybrida begonia with ovate, mid-green leaves, to 15cm (6in) long. Single white flowers, to 8cm (3in) across, with dark pink, picotee margins, are profusely borne in summer. ↕ 25cm (10in), ↔ 20cm (8in). ❀ (min. 13°C/55°F)
***B.* 'Potpourri'** ■ Trailing, pendent begonia with stems to 90cm (36in) long, and heart-shaped, vivid green leaves, 7cm (3in) long. Cascading panicles of fragrant white flowers, 3cm (1¼in) across, suffused salmon-pink towards the margins, are borne in winter. ↕↔ 30cm (12in). ❀ (min. 10°C/50°F)
***B.* 'Princess of Hanover'** ■ Rex-cultorum begonia with spirally arranged, ovate leaves, 20cm (8in) long, which are very dark green with a broad band of silvery white spots. Small, pale pink flowers are produced in autumn. ↕↔ 25–30cm (10–12in). ❀ (min. 10°C/50°F)
B. prismatocarpa. Rhizomatous begonia with obliquely ovate, lobed, bright green leaves, 3cm (1¼in) long. Produces cymes of small yellow flowers, to 2cm (¾in) across, throughout the year. ↕ 15–20cm (6–8in), ↔ 20–25cm (8–10in). Tropical West Africa. ❀ (min. 10°C/50°F)
B. procumbens see *B. radicans.*
B. pustulata. Rhizomatous begonia with broadly ovate, dark green, basal leaves, to 15cm (6in) long, which are warty and covered with tiny white hairs. Rose-pink flowers, to 1cm (½in) across, are borne in cymes in early summer. ↕ 15–20cm (6–8in), ↔ 20–25cm (8–10in). Mexico, Guatemala. ❀ (min. 10°C/50°F). **'Argentea'** ■ syn. *B.* 'Silver', has leaves with silvery white markings, and produces white flowers.
B. radicans 🏆 syn. *B. procumbens* (Shrimp begonia). Shortly rhizomatous begonia with slender, trailing stems, to 45cm (18in) long. Ovate to heart-shaped, acute, shiny leaves, 7cm (3in) across, are blue-green with white spots above, purple beneath, with slightly wavy margins. In midwinter, bears coral-red flowers, 2.5cm (1in) across, in panicles to 10cm (4in) across. Pinch out growing tips to encourage branching. ↕ 45cm (18in), ↔ 30cm (12in). Brazil. ❀ (min. 10°C/50°F)
***B.* rajah.** Rhizomatous begonia with ovate to heart-shaped, sharp-pointed, rich reddish brown leaves, to 10cm (4in) long, with deeply sunken green veins and puckered surfaces. Leaves become green in strong light. Pink flowers, 2cm (¾in) across, are produced in summer. Best maintained at 13–16°C (55–61°F). ↕ 15cm (6in), ↔ 18cm (7in). ❀ (min. 10°C/50°F)
B. rex (King begonia, Painted-leaf begonia). Rhizomatous begonia, the parent of the Rex-cultorum begonias. Ovate, warty leaves, 20cm (8in) long, are sparsely hairy and rich metallic-green, with a broad zone of silvery white above; the veins beneath and leaf-stalks are red and hairy. Bears panicles of pink flowers, to 2cm (¾in) across, in winter. N. India (Himalayas). ↕ 25cm (10in), ↔ 30cm (12in). ❀ (min. 10°C/50°F)
***B.* 'Roy Hartley'** ■ Upright Tuberhybrida begonia with ovate, mid-green leaves, to 15cm (6in) long. Double, soft pink flowers, 10cm (4in) across, tinged with salmon-pink, and with slightly toothed petals, are produced in summer. ↕ 60cm (24in), ↔ 45cm (18in). ❀ (min. 10°C/50°F)
***B.* 'Ruhrtal'** see *B.* 'Merry Christmas'.
B. sceptrum see *B. aconitifolia.*

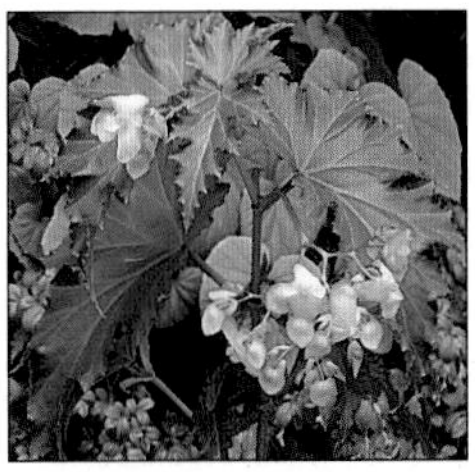
Begonia 'Irene Nuss'

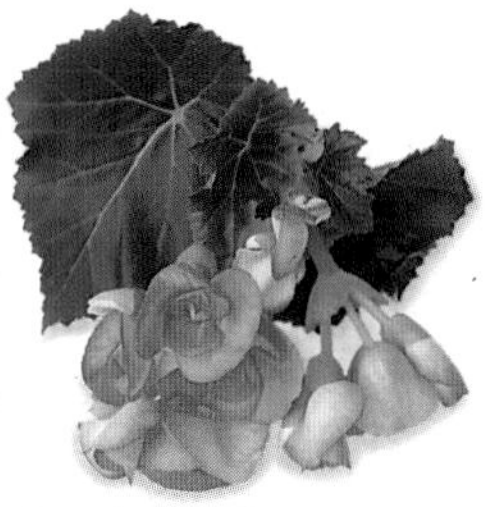
Begonia 'Kleo'

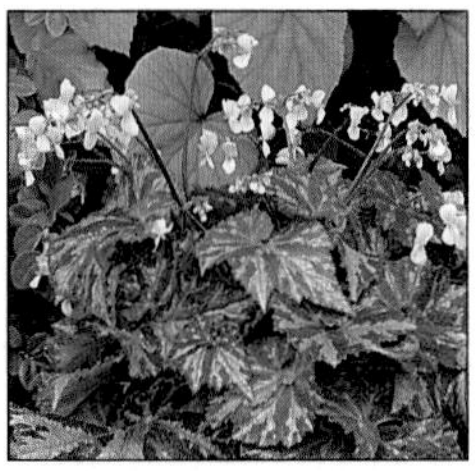

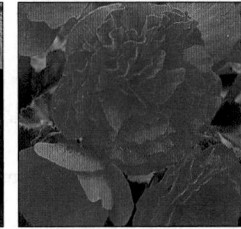
Begonia 'Magic Lace'

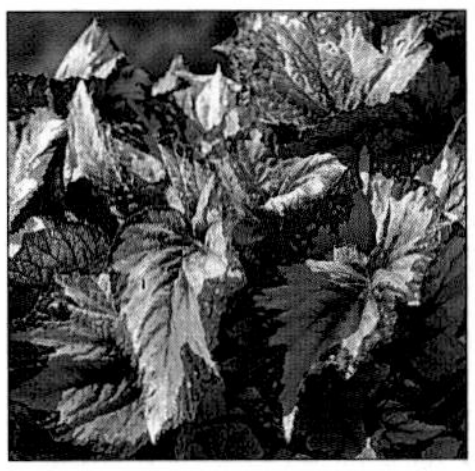
Begonia 'Merry Christmas'

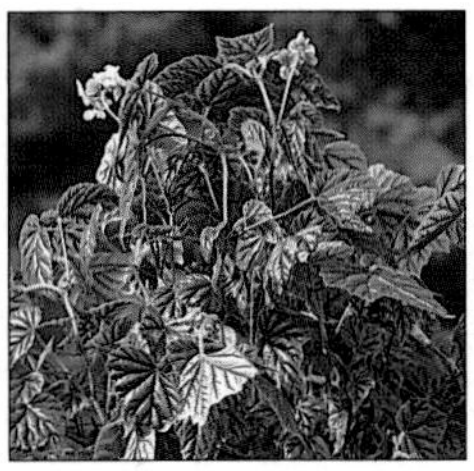
Begonia metallica

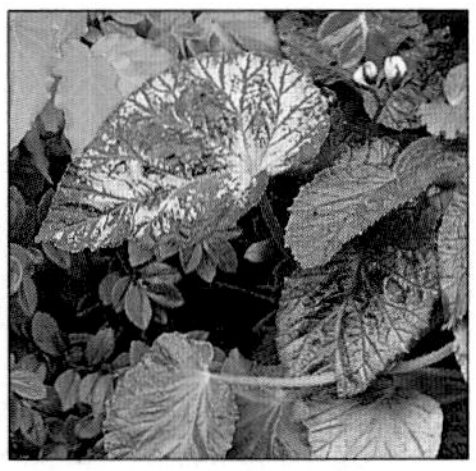
Begonia 'Midnight Sun'

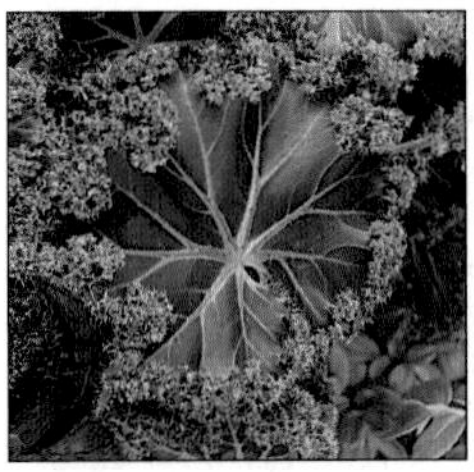
Begonia 'Munchkin'

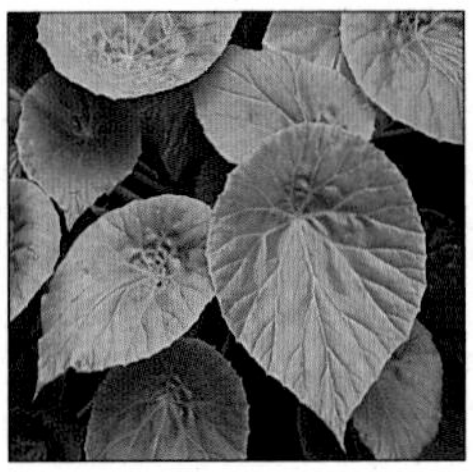
Begonia nelumbiifolia

Begonia Non Stop Series

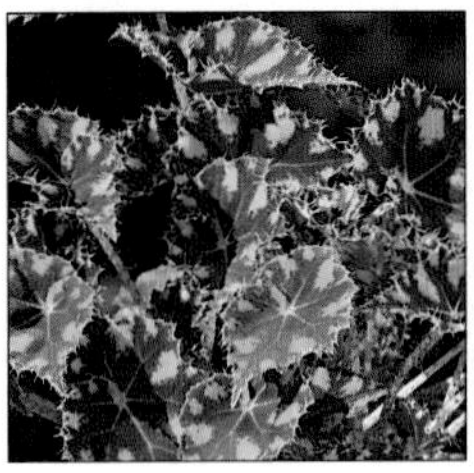
Begonia 'Norah Bedson'

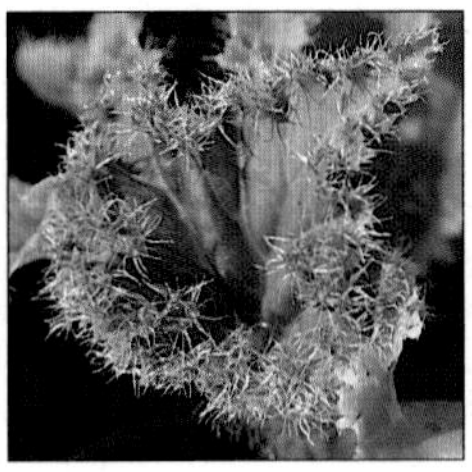
Begonia 'Oliver Twist'

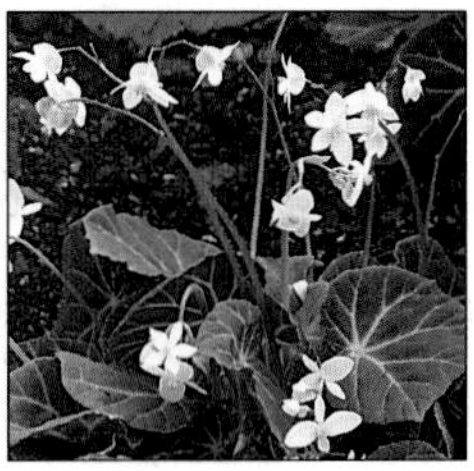
Begonia olsoniae

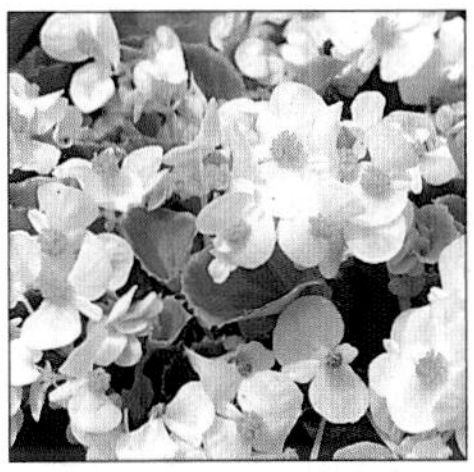
Begonia 'Olympia White'

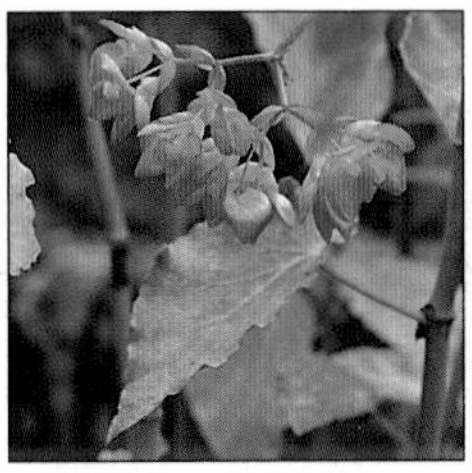
Begonia 'Orange Rubra'

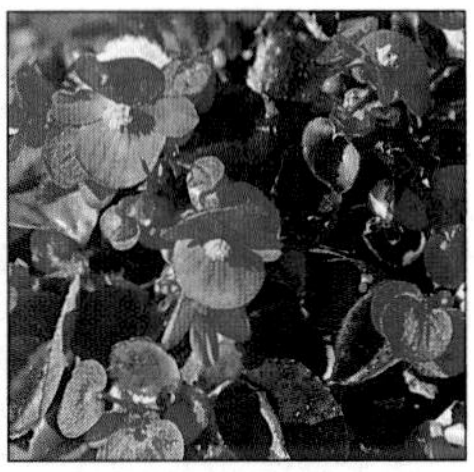
Begonia 'Organdy'

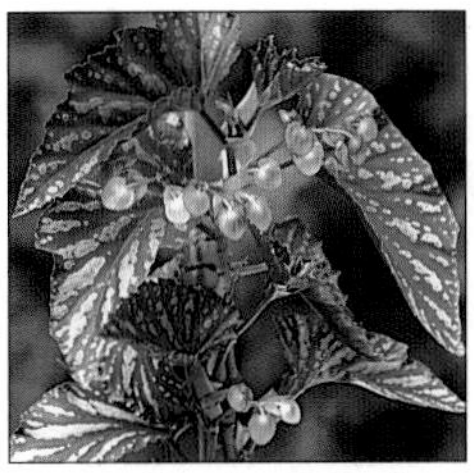
Begonia 'Orpha C. Fox'

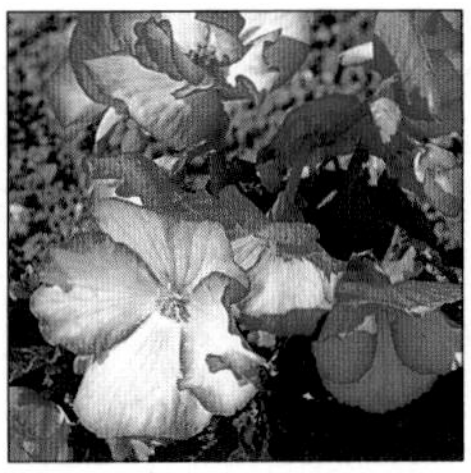
Begonia 'Pin-up'

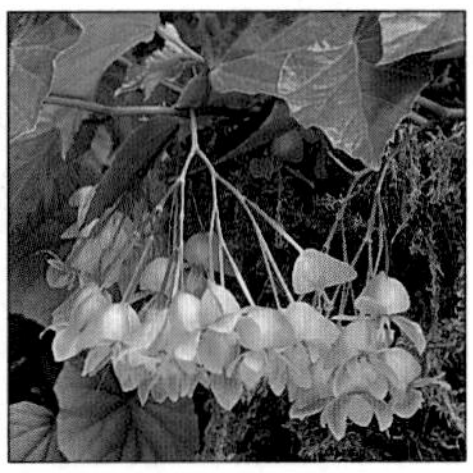
Begonia 'Potpourri'

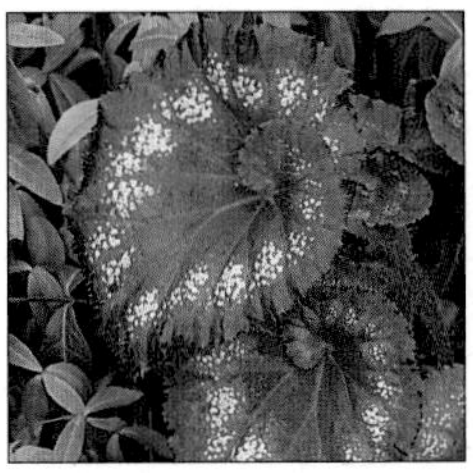
Begonia 'Princess of Hanover'

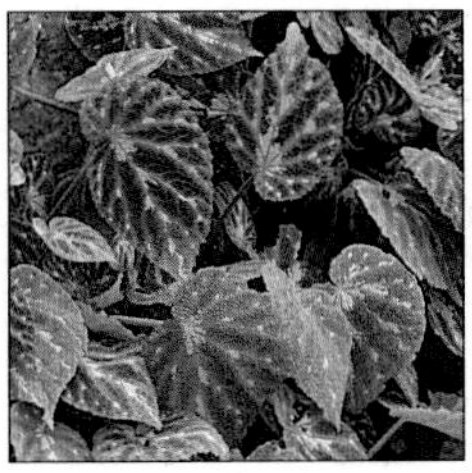
Begonia pustulata 'Argentea'

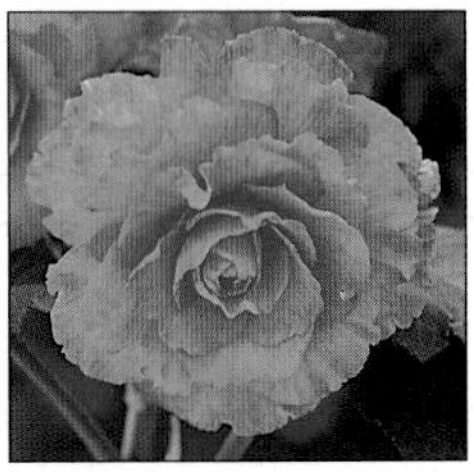
Begonia 'Roy Hartley'

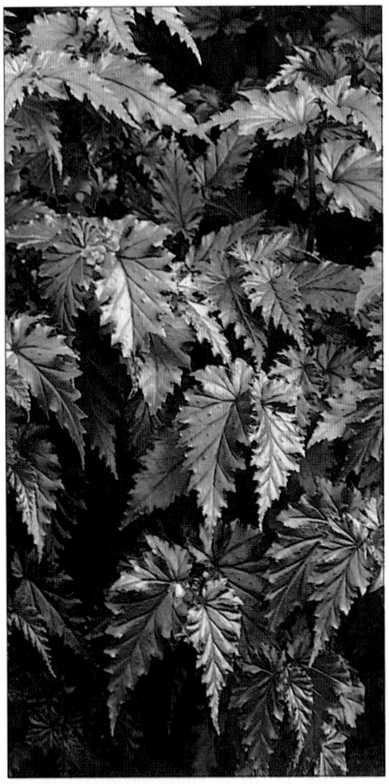

Begonia serratipetala

B. scharffii ▣ syn. *B. haageana*. Shrub-like begonia with obovate, tapered leaves, to 25cm (10in) long, bronze-green with red veins above, red beneath. Stems and leaves are covered with tiny white hairs. From winter to spring, bears panicles of pink-hairy, pink-white flowers, to 5cm (2in) across. ↕ 1.2m (4ft), ↔ 60cm (24in). Brazil. ❀ (min. 10°C/50°F)
***B.* 'Serlis'** see *B.* 'Caravan'.
B. serratipetala ▣ Shrub-like begonia bearing ovate, deeply toothed, reddish brown leaves, 8cm (3in) long, with wavy margins, slightly arched main veins, and raised pink spots. Single, rose-pink flowers, 2–3cm (¾–1¼in) across, are sparsely borne in panicles throughout the year. Water sparingly. ↕↔ 45cm (18in). New Guinea. ❀ (min. 13°C/55°F)
***B.* 'Silver'** see *B. pustulata* 'Argentea'.
***B.* 'Silver Queen'** ▣ 🏆 Rex-cultorum begonia with an erect rhizome bearing ovate, mainly silver leaves, 20cm (8in) long, with metallic purple centres. The leaves become dull purple in bright light. Pink flowers are produced in autumn. ↕ 30cm (12in), ↔ 45cm (18in). ❀ (min. 10°C/50°F)
***B.* 'Sophie Cecile'** 🏆 Cane-stemmed begonia with ovate-acute, slightly wavy-margined, deeply or palmately 7- to 9-lobed leaves, 20cm (8in) long, glossy green splashed with silver. Slightly fragrant pink flowers, 4cm (1½in) across, are freely produced in panicles from spring to summer. ↕ 1.3m (4½ft), ↔ 60cm (24in). ❀ (min. 10°C/50°F)
B. stipulacea, syn. *B. angularis*, *B. compta*, *B. disticha*, *B. zebrina*. Cane-stemmed begonia with slender, angular stems that require staking to remain erect. Ovate, sharp-pointed leaves, 10–15cm (4–6in) long, are fringed with hairs and slightly toothed, bright green above, but paler beneath. White flowers, to 1.5cm (½in) across, are freely produced in cymes throughout the year. ↕ 60cm (24in), ↔ 45cm (18in). Brazil. ❀ (min. 10°C/50°F)
B. sutherlandii ▣ 🏆 Tuberous begonia with long, slender, trailing stems and ovate-lance-shaped, slightly toothed, bright green leaves, to 15cm (6in) long, often with red veins. Orange flowers, to 2.5cm (1in) across, are freely produced in pendent panicles throughout summer. ↔ 45cm (18in). South Africa (KwaZulu/Natal), Tanzania. ✲ (borderline)
***B.* 'Thurstonii'** ▣ 🏆 Shrub-like begonia with ovate, sharp-pointed leaves, 15cm (6in) long, glossy green above, with sunken main veins, rich reddish brown beneath. The green colouring is lost in strong light. Panicles of small, single pink flowers, 4cm (1½in) across, are sparsely borne in summer. ↕ 2m (6ft), ↔ 45cm (18in). ❀ (min. 10°C/50°F)
***B.* 'Tingley Mallet'**. Cane-stemmed begonia with ovate, toothed, reddish brown leaves, to 13cm (5in) long, with slightly puckered surfaces, brown shading, fine hairs, and, frequently, silvery pink spots. Bears panicles, 6cm (2½in) across, of dark pink flowers, in early summer. ↕ 45cm (18in), ↔ 30cm (12in). ❀ (min. 10°C/50°F)
***B.* 'Tiny Bright'** ▣ Dwarf Rex-cultorum begonia with ovate-acute leaves, 8cm (3in) long, with red, green, and bronze bands. Pale pink flowers are sparsely produced from late summer to autumn. ↕ 10cm (4in), ↔ 12cm (5in). ❀ (min. 10°C/50°F)

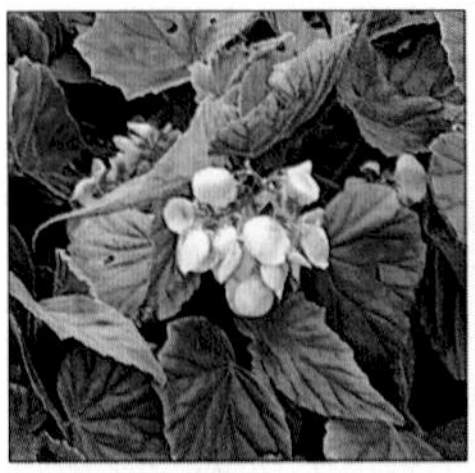

Begonia scharffii

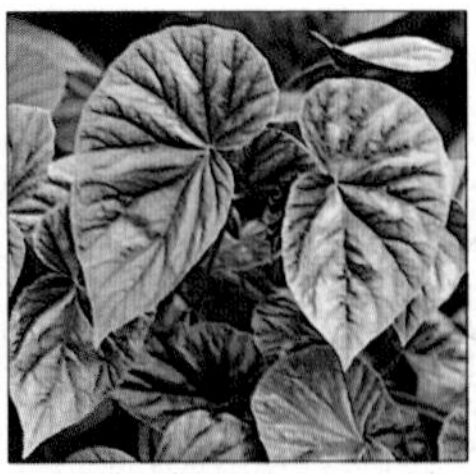

Begonia 'Thurstonii'

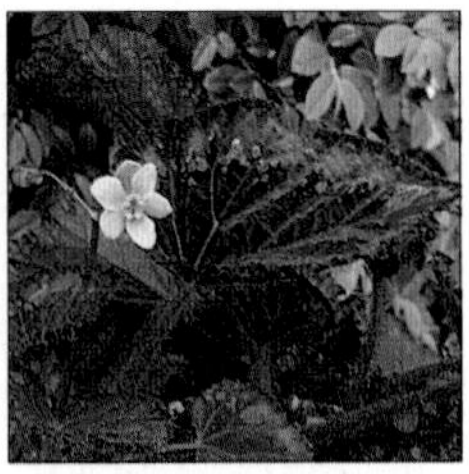

Begonia 'Tiny Bright'

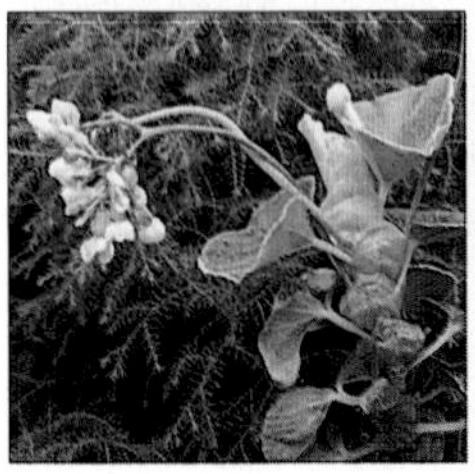

Begonia venosa

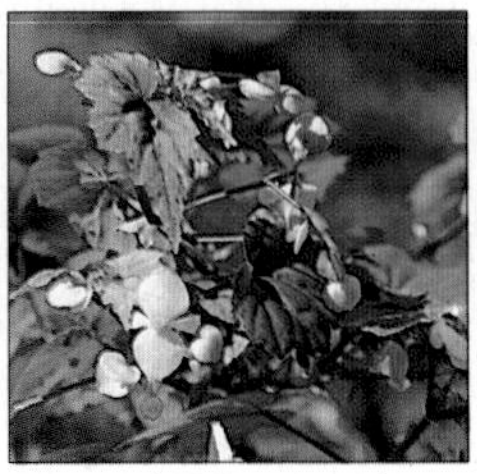

Begonia 'Weltoniensis'

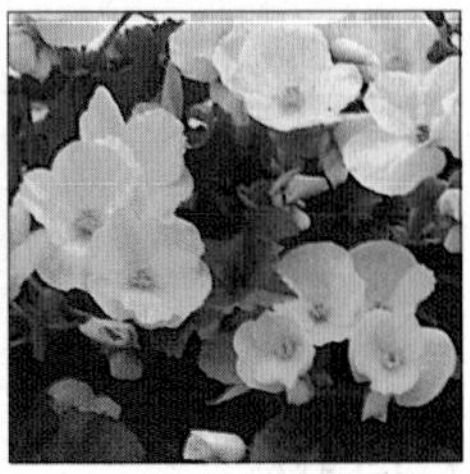

Begonia 'Yellow Melody'

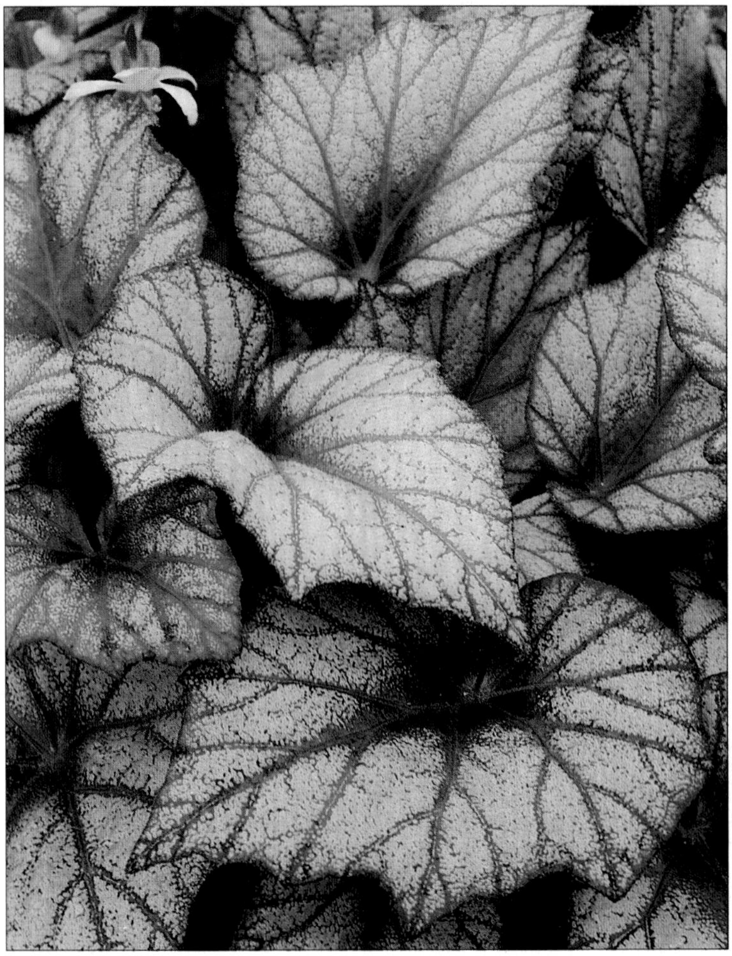

Begonia 'Silver Queen'

***B.* 'Tiny Gem'**. Shrub-like begonia with slender, semi-pendent stems bearing narrowly ovate, wavy-margined, mid-green leaves, 5cm (2in) long. Cascading umbels of small pink flowers, 2cm (¾in) across, are produced throughout the year. ↕ 17cm (7in), ↔ 22cm (9in). ❀ (min. 10°C/50°F)
***B.* 'Tweed'**. Rex-cultorum begonia bearing ovate leaves, 13cm (5in) long, with gently wavy and slightly lobed margins. A broad silver band separates the dark green centre of each leaf from a green-red marginal area, and the surface is covered with fine silvery hairs. Pink flowers are sparsely produced from late summer to autumn. ↕ 22cm (9in), ↔ 25cm (10in). ❀ (min. 10°C/50°F)
B. venosa ▣ Shrub-like begonia with stout, branched, succulent stems covered with persistent, veined stipules. Slightly convex, kidney-shaped, fleshy, white-hairy leaves, 6–7cm (2½–3in) long, have a frosted appearance. Long-stalked, fragrant white flowers, 1cm (½in) or more long, are produced in racemes, mainly from late summer to spring. ↕ 60–90cm (24–36in), ↔ 60cm (24in). Brazil. ❀ (min. 10°C/50°F)
B. versicolor. Rhizomatous begonia with ovate leaves, to 10cm (4in) long, with overlapping basal lobes; both surfaces are reddish brown, apple-green, and silver, with veins marked dark maroon, and very fine red hairs. Bears cymes of salmon-pink flowers, to 5cm (2in) across, sparsely and intermittently throughout the year. ↕ 15cm (6in), ↔ 30cm (12in). China. ❀ (18°C/64°F)
***B.* Victory Series**. Semperflorens begonias with rounded, mid-green leaves. Single flowers, to 4cm (1½in) across, are available in pink, rose-pink, scarlet, and white, or in a mix of these colours, and are borne in summer. ↕↔ to 25cm (10in). ❀ (min. 13°C/55°F)
***B.* 'Weltoniensis'** ▣ (Maple-leaf begonia). Upright, semi-tuberous begonia with lance-shaped, bright-green leaves, 7cm (3in) long, resembling maple leaves, with purple-red veining. Single pink flowers, to 3cm (1¼in) across, are profusely borne from early summer to mid-autumn. ↕ 45cm (18in), ↔ 30cm (12in). ❀ (min. 10°C/50°F)
***B.* 'Yellow Melody'** ▣ Winter-flowering begonia of the Elatior group bearing ovate, mid-green leaves, to 15cm (6in) long. Single, primrose-yellow flowers, 5cm (2in) across, with dark orange-yellow centres, are

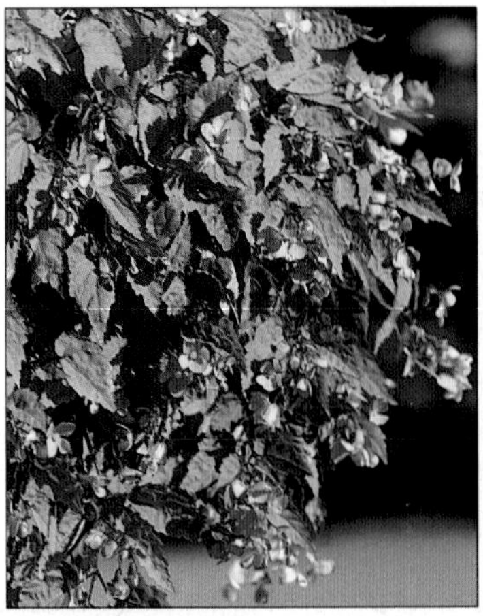

Begonia sutherlandii

BEGONIA

produced from late autumn to early spring. ↕ 20cm (8in), ↔ 18cm (7in). ❀ (min. 10°C/50°F)
B. zebrina see *B. stipulacea.*

▷ **Begonia,**
Angelwing see *Begonia coccinea*
Beefsteak see *Begonia* 'Erythrophylla'
Crazy-leaf see *Begonia* 'Phyllomanica'
Eyelash see *Begonia bowerae*
Fuchsia see *Begonia fuchsioides*
Guinea-wing see *Begonia albopicta*
Hollyhock see *Begonia gracilis* var. *martiana*
Iron-cross see *Begonia masoniana*
King see *Begonia rex*
Leopard see *Begonia manicata*
Lettuce leaf see *Begonia* 'Crestabruchii'
Maple-leaf see *Begonia dregei, B.* 'Weltoniensis'
Metallic-leaf see *Begonia metallica*
Painted-leaf see *Begonia rex*
Palm-leaf see *Begonia luxurians*
Shrimp see *Begonia radicans*
Stitched-leaf see *Begonia mazae* f. *viridis*
Trout-leaved see *Begonia* x *argenteoguttata*

BELAMCANDA

IRIDACEAE

Genus of 2 species of short-lived perennials with slender rhizomes, from sandy, coastal meadows and grassland in India, China, former USSR, and Japan. They have fans of sword-shaped leaves and branching stems that bear showy flowers with 6 tepals. Grow in a herbaceous border or large rock garden.
• **HARDINESS** Frost hardy; will tolerate short spells to -10°C (14°F) if given a deep, protective mulch in winter.
• **CULTIVATION** Grow in humus-rich, moist but well-drained soil that does not dry out in summer, in full sun or partial shade.
• **PROPAGATION** Sow seed in a cold frame in spring. Divide in spring.
• **PESTS AND DISEASES** Trouble free.

B. chinensis (Blackberry lily, Leopard lily). Clump-forming, rhizomatous perennial with sword-shaped, mid- to deep green leaves, 20cm (8in) long. In summer, bears a succession of up to 12 wide-opening flowers, 4cm (1½in) across, bright yellow to orange-red with maroon spots, followed by large black seeds. ↕ 45–90cm (18–36in), ↔ 20cm (8in). India, China, E. former USSR, Japan. ✻✻

▷ **Belle de nuit** see *Ipomoea alba*

BELLEVALIA

HYACINTHACEAE/LILIACEAE

Genus of 45 species of bulbous perennials from scrub and maquis in S. Europe and Asia, with strap-shaped, mid- to grey-green, basal leaves. They are valued for their racemes of bell-shaped flowers, similar to grape hyacinths (*Muscari*) but usually with constricted mouths, which are borne in spring and are mostly white, lilac, or violet-blue, often fading to brown. Grow in a rock garden or sunny border.
• **HARDINESS** Fully hardy to frost hardy.

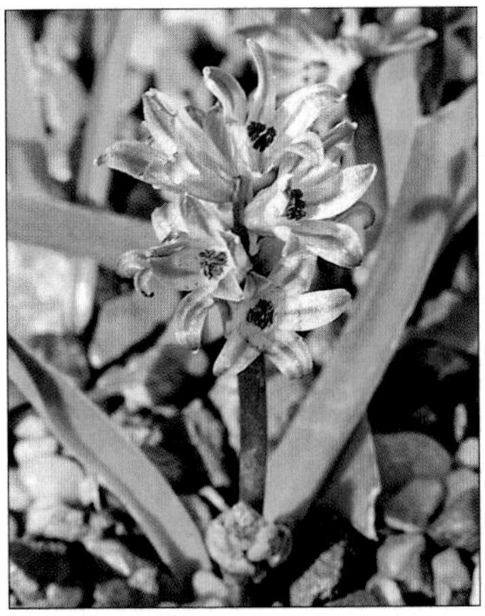
Bellevalia hyacinthoides

• **CULTIVATION** Plant 10cm (4in) deep in autumn in any well-drained soil in full sun. Divide congested clumps to maintain vigour. Most prefer to be kept dry in summer. *B. atroviolacea* and *B. hyacinthoides* are best in a bulb frame.
• **PROPAGATION** Sow seed in a cold frame in autumn. Remove offsets from mature bulbs while dormant in summer.
• **PESTS AND DISEASES** Trouble free.

B. atroviolacea. Bulbous perennial bearing strap-shaped, mid-green leaves, 10–30cm (4–12in) long. Dense racemes of deep violet-blue flowers, 1cm (½in) long, are produced in spring. ↕ 15–20cm (6–8in), ↔ 5cm (2in). Afghanistan. ✻✻✻
B. hyacinthoides ▣ syn. *Strangweja spicata.* Bulbous perennial with strap-shaped, fleshy, mid-green leaves, 15–45cm (6–18in) long, during autumn and winter. In spring, produces loose racemes of a few wide-opening flowers, 7–10mm (¼–½in) long, pale blue with deeper blue veins. ↕ 5–15cm (2–6in), ↔ 5cm (2in). Greece. ✻✻
B. pycnantha ▣ syn. *Muscari paradoxum* of gardens, *M. pycnantha.* Robust, bulbous perennial with strap-shaped, greyish green leaves, 15–45cm (6–18in) long. Navy-blue flowers, 7mm (¼in) long, with yellowish white rims, are produced in racemes in spring. ↕ 30cm (12in), ↔ 5cm (2in). Caucasus, E. Turkey, Iraq, Iran. ✻✻✻
B. romana, syn. *Hyacinthus romanus.* Bulbous perennial with strap-shaped, mid-green leaves, 15–30cm (6–12in) long. In spring, bears white flowers, to 8mm (⅜in) long, tinged green or

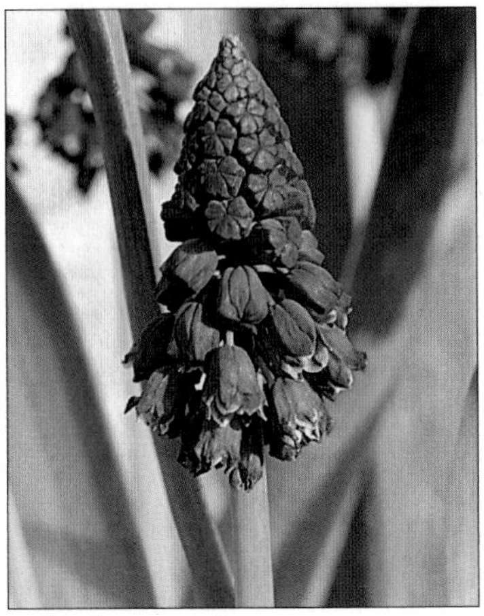
Bellevalia pycnantha

brown, in loose, conical racemes. ↕ 30cm (12in), ↔ 5cm (2in). Mediterranean (S. France to Greece). ✻✻✻

▷ **Bellflower** see *Campanula*
Adriatic see *Campanula garganica*
Bearded see *Campanula barbata*
Canary see *Canarina canariensis*
Chilean see *Lapageria rosea*
Chimney see *Campanula pyramidalis*
Clustered see *Campanula glomerata*
Dalmatian see *Campanula portenschlagiana*
Giant see *Ostrowskia*
Italian see *Campanula isophylla*
Milky see *Campanula lactiflora*
Nettle-leaved see *Campanula trachelium*
Peach-leaved see *Campanula persicifolia*
▷ **Bell heather** see *Erica cinerea*

BELLIS

Daisy

ASTERACEAE/COMPOSITAE

Genus of 15 species of rosette-forming, carpeting perennials from grassland in Europe and Turkey. They have oval to spoon-shaped leaves and solitary, long-stalked, white, pink, or deep reddish pink flowerheads. *B. perennis* has given rise to many cultivars, most commonly grown as biennials for spring bedding.
• **HARDINESS** Fully hardy.
• **CULTIVATION** Grow in well-drained, moderately fertile soil in full sun or partial shade. Dead-head to avoid self-seeding. For winter-flowering container plants, grow in loam-based potting compost (JI No.1), water moderately, and maintain at 4–7°C (39–45°F).
• **PROPAGATION** Sow seed in shallow drills outdoors in early summer, or at 10–13°C (50–55°F) in early spring. Divide in early spring or after flowering.
• **PESTS AND DISEASES** Trouble free.

B. perennis (Common daisy). Stoloniferous perennial with inversely lance-shaped to obovate or spoon-shaped, bright green leaves, 1–6cm (½–2½in) long. From late winter to late summer, produces flowerheads, 1–3cm (½–1¼in) across, with white ray-florets, often tinged maroon or pink, and yellow disc-florets. ↕↔ 5–20cm (2–8in). Europe, Turkey. ✻✻✻. **Habanera Series** cultivars bear pink, white, or red, long-petalled flowerheads, to 6cm (2½in) across, in early summer. **Pomponette Series** 🏆 cultivars bear double, pink, white, or red flowerheads, to 4cm (1½in) across, with quilled petals. **Roggli Series** cultivars flower early and prolifically, with semi-double, red, rose-pink, salmon-pink, or white flowerheads, to 3cm (1¼in) across. **Tasso Series** ▣ cultivars have double, pink, white, or red flowerheads, to 6cm (2½in) across, with quilled petals.

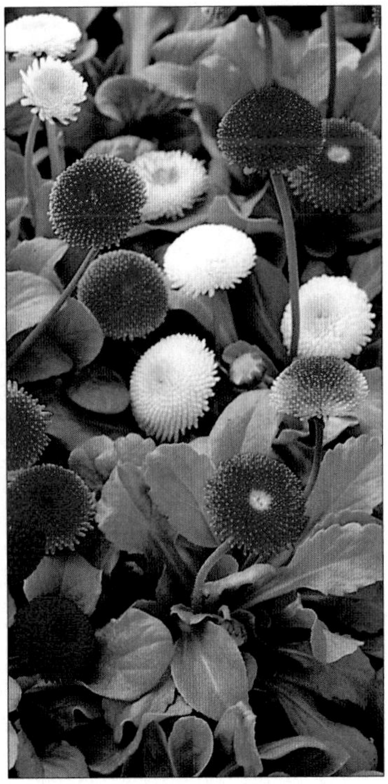
Bellis perennis Tasso Series

▷ **Bell pepper** see *Capsicum annuum* Grossum Group
▷ **Bells of Ireland** see *Moluccella laevis*
▷ ***Beloperone*** see *Justicia*
B. guttata see *J. brandegeeana*
▷ **Bent, Velvet** see *Agrostis canina*

BERBERIDOPSIS

FLACOURTIACEAE

Genus of one species of woody, evergreen, scandent climber from moist woodland in Chile, cultivated mainly for its clusters and racemes of spherical flowers. The leaves are ovate or heart-shaped, spiny, and alternate. Grow against a wall or train into a tree.
• **HARDINESS** Frost hardy.
• **CULTIVATION** Grow in humus-rich, neutral to acid, moist but well-drained soil, in a partially shaded, sheltered site. Protect the roots from frost with an autumn mulch. Pruning group 11, in spring, but only if essential.
• **PROPAGATION** Sow seed in containers in a cold frame in spring. Root semi-ripe cuttings in late summer. Layer in autumn.
• **PESTS AND DISEASES** Trouble free.

B. corallina ▣ (Coral plant). Weakly twining climber with ovate or heart-shaped, dark green leaves, to 10cm (4in) long, glaucous beneath, with small marginal spines. Spherical, dark red flowers, 1.5cm (½in) across, with stalks 5cm (2in) long, are produced both in pendent, terminal racemes and in 2- or 3-flowered clusters from the upper leaf axils from summer to early autumn. ↕ 5m (15ft). Chile. ✻✻

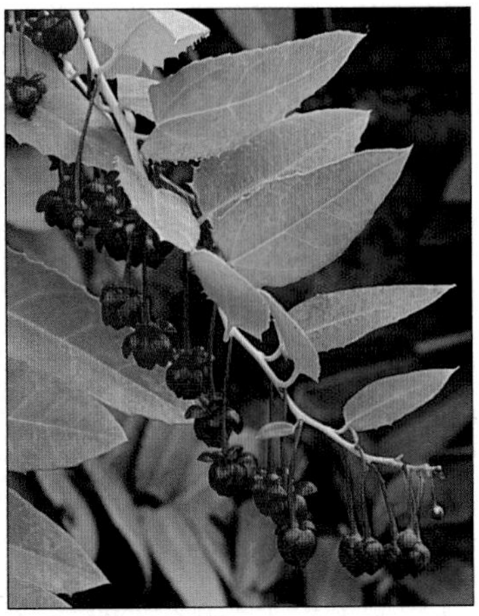
Berberidopsis corallina

BERBERIS

Barberry

BERBERIDACEAE

Genus of about 450 species of evergreen or deciduous shrubs from all parts of the N. hemisphere, N. and tropical Africa, and South America, that prefer rocky soils in mountain areas. Linear to very broadly ovate or obovate, entire or spine-toothed leaves are produced in the axils of stem spines, which are often borne in groups of 3, and persist on old, leafless stems. Barberries are cultivated for their foliage (ornamental or giving good autumn colour); racemes, panicles, or axillary clusters of yellow to dark orange flowers, cup-shaped with usually reflexed sepals; and colourful autumn fruits. They range from dwarf species and cultivars, suitable for a rock garden, to large shrubs that are effective in a border, as specimen shrubs, or as a hedge. All parts may cause mild stomach upset if ingested; contact with the spines may irritate skin.

• **HARDINESS** Fully hardy to frost hardy.

• **CULTIVATION** Grow in almost any well-drained soil in full sun or partial shade. Fruiting and autumn colour are better in sun. Evergreen species, pruning group 8; deciduous species, pruning group 2. Trim hedges after flowering.

• **PROPAGATION** Sow seed in a seedbed in early spring; many species cross freely in gardens, so seed-raised plants are often hybrids. Root softwood cuttings of deciduous barberries in summer; take semi-ripe cuttings of deciduous and evergreen ones in summer.

• **PESTS AND DISEASES** Powdery mildew and aphids may be troublesome.

B. aggregata. Compact, deciduous shrub with oblong-ovate, olive-green leaves, to 3cm (1¼in) long, sparsely toothed at the tips, blue-green beneath, and turning red in autumn. Pale yellow flowers, 7mm (¼in) across, are borne in dense axillary panicles, to 4cm (1½in) long, in late spring and early summer, followed by spherical to ovoid, grey-glaucous, red fruit, to 7mm (¼in) long. ↕ 1.5m (5ft), ↔ 2m (6ft). W. China (Gansu, Sichuan). ❄❄❄

B. x bristolensis ■ (*B. calliantha* x *B. verruculosa*). Dense, mound-forming, evergreen shrub with elliptic, spine-toothed leaves, to 4cm (1½in) long, glossy, dark green above, intensely glaucous beneath, some turning red in autumn or winter. Yellow flowers, 1cm (½in) or more across, are produced singly or in twos or threes from the leaf axils in late spring, followed by oblong-ovoid, blue-black fruit, 9mm (⅜in) long. ↕ 1.5m (5ft), ↔ 2m (6ft). Garden origin. ❄❄❄

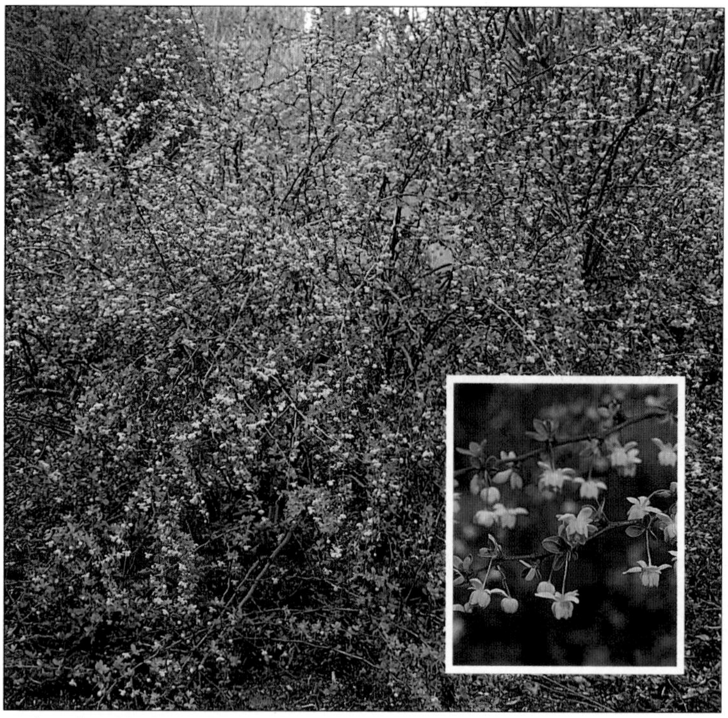

Berberis buxifolia (inset: flower detail)

B. buxifolia ■ Upright, evergreen or semi-evergreen shrub with arching branches and elliptic, spine-tipped, leathery, dark green leaves, to 2.5cm (1in) long. In mid- and late spring, dark orange-yellow flowers, to 1.5cm (½in) across, are produced singly or in pairs from the upper leaf axils, on stalks 2–2.5cm (¾–1in) long. They are followed by spherical, dark purple fruit, to 6–8mm (¼–⅜in) across. ↕ 2.5m (8ft), ↔ 3m (10ft). Chile, Argentina. ❄❄❄. **'Pygmaea'**, syn. var. *nana* of gardens, is compact, lacks spines, has leaves to 3cm (1¼in) long, and rarely produces flowers. ↕ 30cm (12in), ↔ 45cm (18in).

B. calliantha 🏆 Compact, evergreen shrub with holly-like, elliptic to oblong, spine-toothed leaves, to 6cm (2½in) long, glossy, dark green above, waxy-white beneath, and borne on red young shoots. Pale yellow flowers, to 2.5cm (1in) across, are produced singly, occasionally in twos or threes, from the upper leaf axils in late spring, followed by ovoid, blue-glaucous, black fruit, 1cm (½in) or more long. ↕ 75cm (30in), ↔ 90cm (36in). China (S.E. Tibet). ❄❄❄

B. candidula. Dense, mound-forming, evergreen shrub with elliptic to ovate, entire, spine-tipped leaves, to 3cm (1¼in) long, with inrolled margins, glossy, dark green above, waxy-white beneath. Produces solitary, bright yellow flowers, to 1.5cm (½in) across, from the upper leaf axils in late spring, followed by ovoid, white-glaucous, purple fruit, to 1cm (½in) long. ↕ 60cm (24in), ↔ 1.2m (4ft). W. China (Hubei). ❄❄❄

B. x carminea (*B. aggregata* x *B. wilsoniae*). Vigorous, semi-evergreen shrub with arching branches and narrowly obovate, slightly spiny, often greyish green leaves, to 3cm (1¼in) long. Bears spherical yellow flowers, to 7mm (¼in) across, in 10- to 16-flowered panicles, to 5cm (2in) long, in late spring and early summer, followed by dense clusters of ovoid-spherical, usually red or orange fruit, 1cm (½in) across. Garden origin. ↕ 1.5m (5ft), ↔ 2.5m (8ft). ❄❄❄. **'Barbarossa'** has bright red fruit. **'Buccaneer'** ■ bears spherical, glowing red fruit. **'Pirate King'** ■ has bright scarlet-red fruit.

B. 'Chenault' see *B.* 'Chenaultii'.

B. 'Chenaultii', syn. *B.* 'Chenault'. Spreading, dense, evergreen shrub with lance-shaped, wavy-margined, spine-toothed leaves, to 4cm (1½in) long, that are glossy, dark green above and glaucous beneath, often turning bronze in winter. Spherical yellow flowers, 1.5cm (½in) across, are produced in axillary clusters of 2–4 in late spring, followed by ovoid, blue-black fruit, 1cm (½in) long. ↕↔ 1.5m (5ft). ❄❄❄

B. 'Cherry Ripe'. Rounded, deciduous shrub with obovate, mainly entire leaves, to 2.5cm (1in) long, that are dull green above, grey-green beneath. Umbel-like clusters, to 10cm (4in) across, of 2–8 yellow flowers, to 1cm (½in) across, are produced freely in early summer. Broadly ovoid, creamy pink fruit, to 1cm (½in) long, turn bright cerise and last well into winter. ↕ 1.5m (5ft), ↔ 2m (6ft). ❄❄❄

B. coxii. Vigorous, dense, evergreen shrub with elliptic to ovate-elliptic, spine-toothed leaves, to 5cm (2in) long, that are glossy, dark green above and intensely glaucous beneath. Produces clusters of 3–6 pale yellow flowers, to 1cm (½in) across, in late spring, followed by oblong-ovoid, blue-glaucous, black fruit, 1cm (½in) long. ↕ 2m (6ft) or more, ↔ 3m (10ft). N.E. Burma. ❄❄❄

B. darwinii ■ 🏆 Vigorous, upright, evergreen shrub with obovate, spine-toothed, glossy, dark green leaves, 2–4cm (¾–1½in) long. Pendent racemes, to 5cm (2in) long, of 10–30 dark orange flowers, 5mm (¼in) across, are borne profusely in mid- and late spring, sometimes again in autumn, and are succeeded by spherical, blue-glaucous, black fruit, 7mm (¼in) across. ↕↔ 3m (10ft). Chile, Argentina. ❄❄❄. **'Flame'** has broad leaves, to 2cm (¾in) long, and produces rich orange-red flowers; ↕↔ 1.5m (5ft).

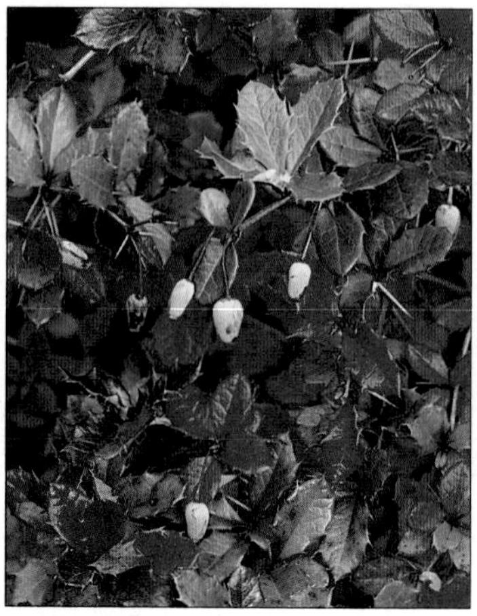

Berberis x *bristolensis*

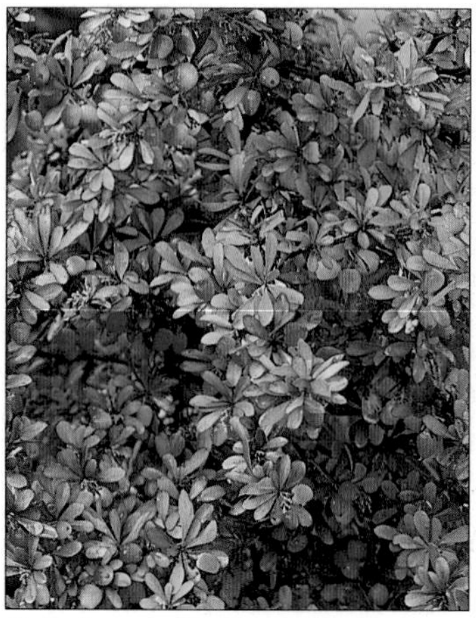

Berberis x *carminea* 'Buccaneer'

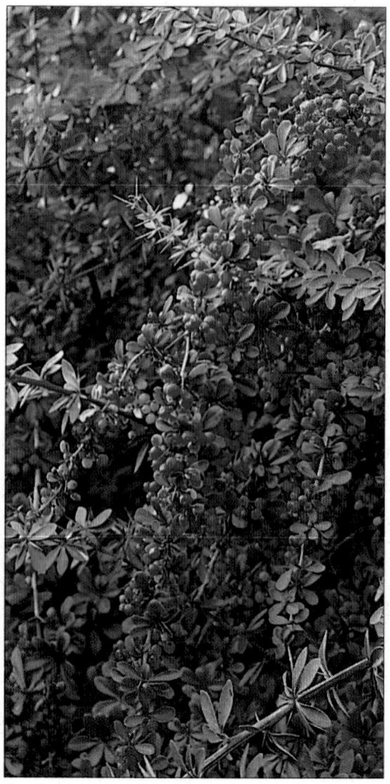

Berberis x *carminea* 'Pirate King'

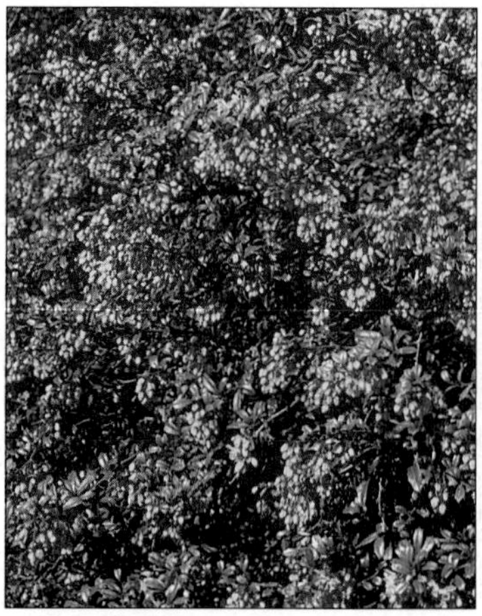

Berberis darwinii

B

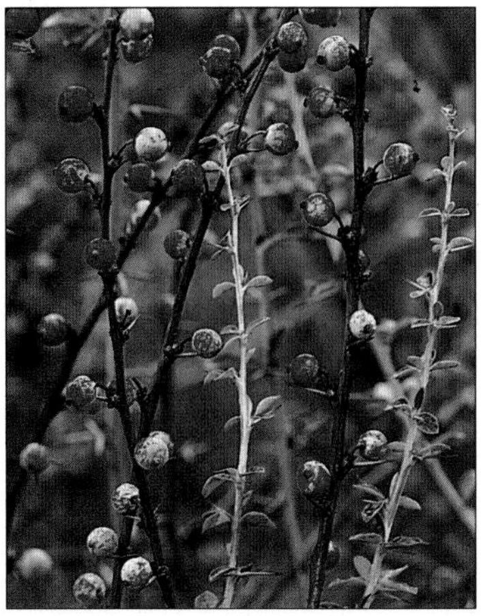

Berberis dictyophylla

B. *dictyophylla* ■ ♀ Vigorous, upright, deciduous shrub with reddish brown shoots covered in white bloom, and obovate to elliptic, entire or sometimes spine-toothed leaves, to 2cm (¾in) long, mid-green above, white beneath, and turning red in autumn. Bears pale yellow flowers, to 1.5cm (½in) across, singly or in twos from the upper leaf axils in late spring, followed by ellipsoid, white-glaucous, red fruit, to 1cm (½in) long. ↕ 2m (6ft), ↔ 1.5m (5ft). W. China (Yunnan, W. Sichuan). ❄❄❄
B. *empetrifolia* ■ Spreading, evergreen shrub with arching shoots and linear-elliptic, spine-tipped leaves, to 2.5cm (1in) long, dark green above, greyish beneath. Deep golden yellow flowers, 1cm (½in) across, are produced singly or in twos from the upper leaf axils in late spring, followed by spherical, blue-glaucous, black fruit, 7mm (¼in) across. ↕ 45cm (18in), ↔ 60cm (24in). Chile, Argentina. ❄❄❄
B. x *frikartii* 'Amstelveen' ♀ (*B. candidula* x *B. verruculosa*). Vigorous, compact, evergreen shrub with arching shoots and lance-shaped, glossy leaves, to 3cm (1¼in) long, dark green above, grey-white beneath. Yellow flowers, 1.5cm (½in) across, are produced in clusters of 2–4 from the upper leaf axils in late spring, followed by ovoid, blue-glaucous, black fruit, 1cm (½in) long. ↕ 1m (3ft), ↔ 1.5m (5ft). ❄❄❄. **'Telstar'** ♀ is flat-topped when mature; ↕ to 1.2m (4ft).
B. *gagnepainii* of gardens see *B. gagnepainii* var. *lanceifolia*.
B. *gagnepainii* var. *lanceifolia* ■ syn. *B. gagnepainii* of gardens. Dense,

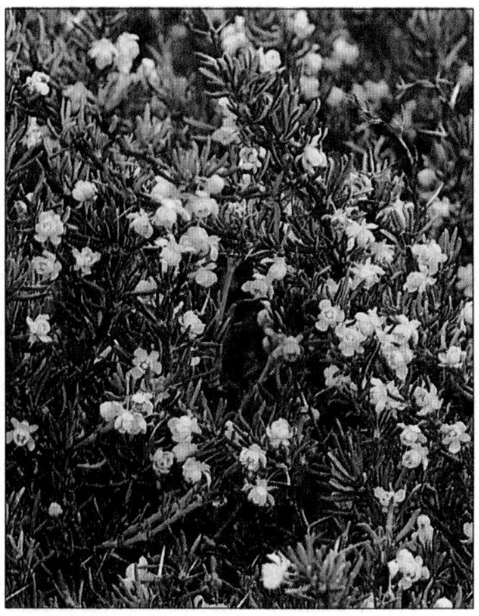

Berberis empetrifolia

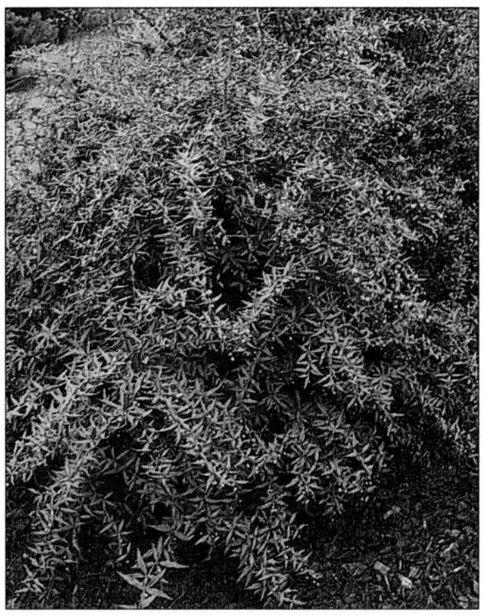

Berberis gagnepainii var. *lanceifolia*

evergreen shrub with spreading, semi-pendent branches and linear-lance-shaped, dark green leaves, to 10cm (4in) long, spine-toothed and wavy at the margins. Golden yellow flowers, 1cm (½in) across, are produced in clusters of 2–5 from the upper leaf axils in late spring and early summer, followed by oblong-ovoid, blue-black fruit, to 1cm (½in) long. Useful for hedging. ↕ 1.5m (5ft), ↔ 2m (6ft). W. China (Hubei, Sichuan). ❄❄❄
B. 'Goldilocks' ■ ♀ Very vigorous, upright then spreading, evergreen shrub with oblong-ovate, entire or slightly toothed leaves, to 5cm (2in) long, glossy, dark green above, paler beneath. Red-stalked, dark golden yellow flowers, 4mm (⅛in) across, are profusely borne in dense clusters, to 4cm (1½in) across, in mid- and late spring, followed by spherical, blue-black fruit, 8mm (⅜in) across. ↕ 4m (12ft), ↔ 3m (10ft). ❄❄❄
B. x *hybrido-gagnepainii* cultivars (*B. candidula* x *B. gagnepainii*). Evergreen shrubs with ovate to oblong-ovate or lance-shaped, bright green leaves, 2–5cm (¾–2in) long, sometimes tinted bluish or reddish green beneath. Clusters of yellow flowers, to 1cm (½in) across, are produced in late spring, followed by ovoid, grey-glaucous, black fruit, to 7mm (¼in) long. ↕ to 1.5m (5ft), ↔ to 2m (6ft) ❄❄❄. **'Minikin'** is compact, with slightly twisted, lance-shaped, bright green leaves, to 2cm (¾in) long, that are white beneath; ↕ 50cm (20in), ↔ 80cm (32in). **'Tottenham'** is more vigorous than 'Minikin', with arching shoots and oblong-ovate leaves, to 4cm (1½in)

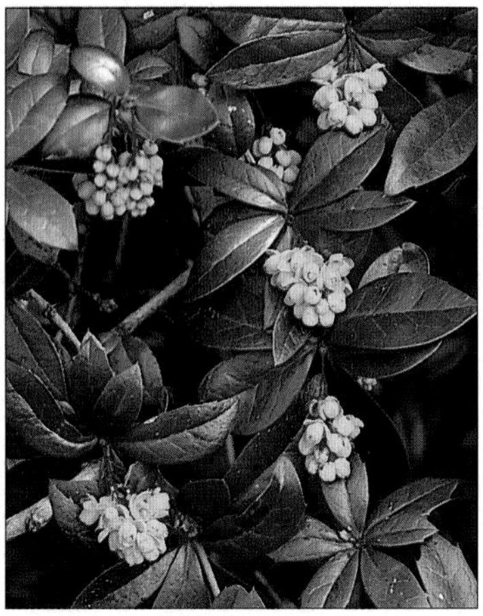

Berberis 'Goldilocks'

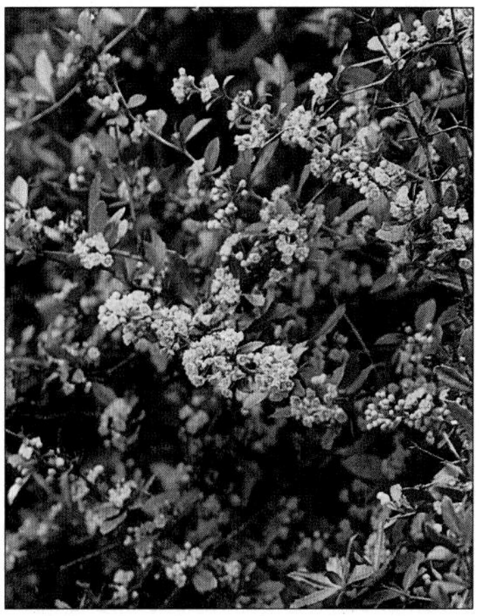

Berberis julianae

long, some turning red in autumn; ↔ 1.5m (5ft).
B. *hypokerina*. Evergreen shrub with arching, spineless, reddish green shoots, and rigid, elliptic, triangular-spined, grey-green leaves, to 15cm (6in) long, often white beneath. Produces lemon-yellow flowers, 1cm (½in) across, in dense clusters of 4–18 (rarely up to 25) in early summer, followed by ellipsoid, blue-glaucous, black fruit, to 1cm (½in) long. Grow in lime-free soil. ↕↔ 0.6–2.5m (2–8ft). W. China (Yunnan). ❄❄
B. x *interposita* 'Wallich's Purple'. Densely mound-forming, evergreen shrub with arching shoots and elliptic, sparsely spiny, glossy, mid-green leaves, to 2.5cm (1in) long, grey-green beneath, bronze-purple when young. Clusters of yellow flowers, 1.5cm (½in) across, are produced in late spring, followed by ellipsoid, slightly blue-glaucous, black fruit, 5cm (2in) long. ↕ 1.5m (5ft), ↔ 2m (6ft). ❄❄❄
B. *jamesiana*. Vigorous, upright, deciduous shrub with ovate, entire to finely toothed, olive-green leaves, to 10cm (4in) long, glaucous grey beneath, turning red in autumn. Pendent racemes, to 10cm (4in) long, of 20–40 yellow flowers, 5mm (¼in) across, are borne in early summer, followed by spherical, coral-red fruit, 1cm (½in) across. ↕ 2m (6ft), ↔ 1.5m (5ft). W. China (N.W. Yunnan). ❄❄❄
B. *julianae* ■ Dense, upright, evergreen shrub with rigid, obovate to elliptic leaves, to 4–8cm (1½–3in) long, that are glossy, deep green above, pale green beneath, with strongly spined margins. Up to 20 yellow or red-tinged flowers, 1cm (½in) across, are produced in clusters in late spring, and are succeeded by oblong, white-glaucous, black fruit, 8mm (⅜in) long. ↕↔ 3m (10ft). China. ❄❄❄. **'Lombart's Red'** has leaves tinged red beneath.
B. *linearifolia*. Upright, stiffly branched, evergreen shrub with obovate to inversely lance-shaped, glossy, dark green leaves, to 5cm (2in) long. Bears clusters of 2–4 rich orange to apricot flowers, 2cm (¾in) across, in late spring, followed by ellipsoid, blue-glaucous, black fruit, 1cm (½in) long. Chile, Argentina. ↕ 2m (6ft), ↔ 1.5m (5ft). ❄❄❄. **'Jewel'** ■ has clusters of 4–6 dark orange flowers that open from scarlet buds. **'Orange King'** ■ is vigorous, with arching shoots, leaves to 6cm (2½in) long, and less deeply

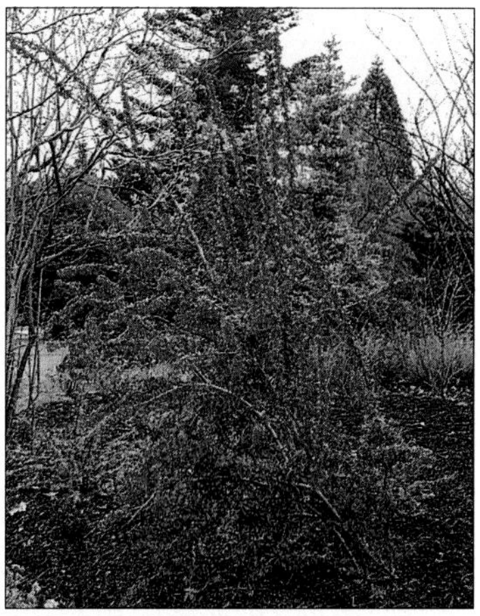

Berberis linearifolia 'Jewel'

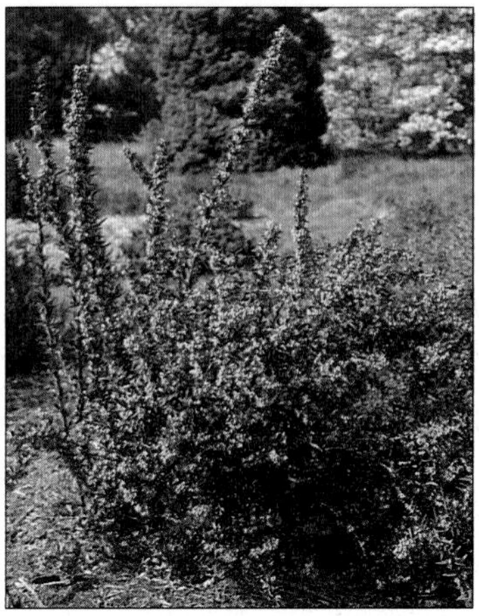

Berberis linearifolia 'Orange King'

coloured, slightly larger flowers than 'Jewel'; ↕↔ 2.5m (8ft).
B. x *lologensis* (*B. darwinii* x *B. linearifolia*). Strong-growing, spreading, evergreen shrub with arching shoots and spoon-shaped, spine-toothed, glossy, dark green leaves, to 5cm (2in) long. Clusters of 8–12 rich orange flowers, 3cm (1¼in) across, are produced in late spring, and often again from summer to autumn, followed by spherical, blue-black fruit, to 7mm (¼in) across. ↕↔ 4m (12ft). Argentina. ❄❄❄. **'Apricot Queen'** ♀ bears umbel-like racemes, to 5cm (2in) long, of 3–7 dark orange flowers in late spring and sporadically throughout summer; ↔ 3m (10ft). **'Mystery Fire'** bears abundant bright orange-yellow flowers. **'Stapehill'** ■ bears abundant rich orange flowers.

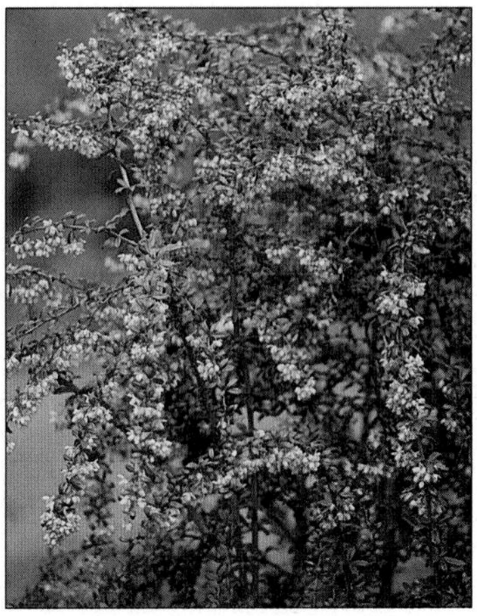

Berberis x *lologensis* 'Stapehill'

B

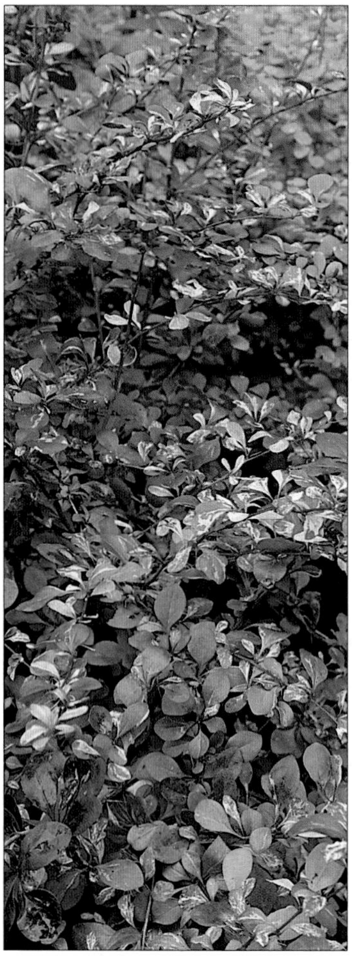

Berberis x *ottawensis* 'Silver Mile'

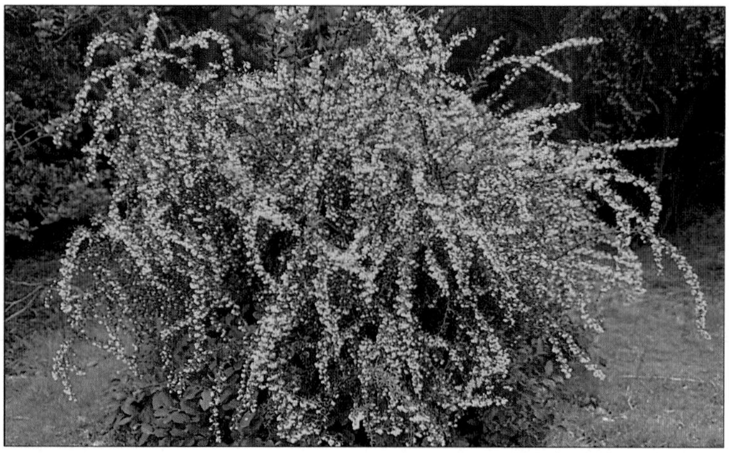

Berberis x *stenophylla*

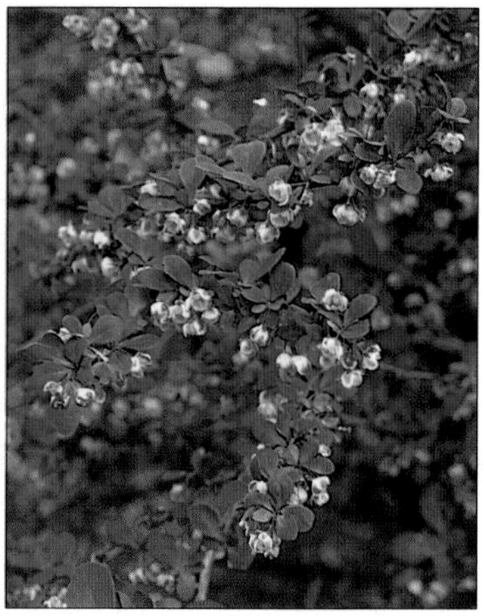

Berberis thunbergii f. *atropurpurea*

B.* x *ottawensis (*B. thunbergii* x *B. vulgaris*). Rounded, deciduous shrub with obovate, mainly entire, mid-green leaves, to 3cm (1¼in) long. Clusters of up to 10 red-tinged, pale yellow flowers, 8mm (⅜in) across, are borne in spring, followed by ovoid red berries, 8mm (⅜in) long. ↕↔ 2.5m (8ft). Garden origin. ❄❄❄. **'Purpurea'** see 'Superba'. **'Silver Mile'** ■ has dark red-purple leaves, flushed silvery grey, turning red in autumn. **'Superba'** ■🏆 syn. 'Purpurea', is vigorous, with red-purple leaves, turning crimson in autumn. Often used as a rootstock; grafted plants may produce purple-leaved basal shoots.

B. panlanensis see *B. sanguinea*.

***B.* 'Park Jewel'** see *B.* 'Parkjuweel'.

***B.* 'Parkjuweel'** 🏆 syn. *B.* 'Park Jewel'. Compact, semi-evergreen shrub with oblong-ovate, entire or slightly toothed, very glossy, mid- to dark green leaves, to 3cm (1¼in) long, some turning red in autumn. In late spring, bears yellow flowers, 8mm (⅜in) across, singly or in small clusters, to 2.5cm (1in) across. ↕2m (6ft), ↔ 2.5m (8ft). ❄❄❄

***B. polyantha* of gardens** see *B. prattii*.

B. prattii, syn. *B. polyantha* of gardens. Deciduous shrub with arching branches and densely clustered, obovate leaves, to 3cm (1¼in) long, that are glossy, mid-green above, grey beneath, with spine-tipped teeth. Bears lax, upright panicles, to 20cm (8in) long, of 8 yellow flowers in summer, followed by long-lasting, spherical, bright pink fruit, to 6mm (¼in) long. ↕↔ 3m (10ft). W. China (Sichuan). ❄❄❄

***B.* 'Red Jewel'** 🏆 Compact, semi-evergreen shrub (a sport of *B.* 'Parkjuweel') with oblong-ovate, entire or slightly toothed leaves, to 3cm (1¼in) long, dark bronze-red when young, mid- to dark green when mature. Yellow flowers, 8mm (⅜in) across, borne singly or in small clusters, to 2.5cm (1in) across, are produced in late spring. ↕2m (6ft), ↔ 2.5m (8ft). ❄❄❄

B.* x *rubrostilla see *B.* 'Rubrostilla'.

***B.* 'Rubrostilla'** 🏆 syn. *B.* x *rubrostilla*. Rounded, deciduous shrub with narrow, obovate, bright mid-green leaves, to 3cm (1¼in) long, with small, marginal spines. Umbel-like racemes of 2–4 yellow flowers, 7–9mm (¼–⅜in) across, on stalks 2.5cm (1in) long, are borne in profusion along the branches in summer, followed by oblong-ovoid, translucent, coral-red fruit, 1.5cm (½in) long. ↕1.5m (5ft), ↔ 2.5m (8ft). ❄❄❄

B. sanguinea, syn. *B. panlanensis*. Slow-growing, very dense, evergreen shrub with arching shoots and linear-lance-shaped, spine-toothed, grey-green leaves, to 6cm (2½in) long. Yellow flowers, to 1cm (½in) across, are borne in clusters of 2–7 in spring, followed by oblong black fruit, to 8mm (⅜in) long. ↕2.5m (8ft), ↔ 4m (12ft). W. China (Sichuan). ❄❄❄

B. sargentiana. Dense, upright, evergreen shrub with rigid, narrowly elliptic to oblong, strongly spined, glossy leaves, to 10cm (4in) long, dark green above and yellowish green beneath. Greenish yellow, sometimes red-tinged flowers, to 1cm (½in) across, are produced in clusters of 4–8 in late spring, and are succeeded by oblong-ellipsoid, blue-black fruit, to 6mm (¼in) long. ↕↔ 2m (6ft). W. China (Sichuan, Hubei). ❄❄❄

B.* x *stenophylla ■🏆 (*B. darwinii* x *B. empetrifolia*). Vigorous, evergreen shrub with long, arching branches and linear to narrowly elliptic, spine-tipped, dark green leaves, to 2.5cm (1in) long. Short, clustered racemes of 7–14 deep yellow flowers, to 1m (½in) across, are borne profusely along the branches in late spring, followed by spherical, blue-glaucous, black fruit, to 7mm (¼in) long. An excellent plant for hedging. ↕3m (10ft), ↔ 5m (15ft). Garden origin. ❄❄❄. **'Claret Cascade'** produces red young shoots and bronze-green young leaves; ↕↔ 1.2m (4ft). **'Coccinea'** is compact, with red flower buds and red-tinged flowers borne in clusters of 4–8; ↕1.2m (4ft), ↔ 1.5m (5ft). **'Corallina Compacta'** ■🏆 is compact, with leaves 6–8mm (¼–⅜in) long, and red-budded, light orange flowers; ↕↔ to 30cm (12in). **'Cornish Cream'** see 'Lemon Queen'. **'Cream Showers'** see 'Lemon Queen'. **'Irwinii'** is compact, with sharply toothed, glossy leaves and orange flowers; ↕↔ 1.5m (5ft). **'Lemon Queen'**, syn. 'Cornish Cream', 'Cream Showers', has dark green leaves, and produces creamy white flowers. **'Pink Pearl'** has leaves variegated white and pink, and pink flowers. Cut out reverted shoots as they occur; ↕↔ 1.5m (5ft).

B. temolaica. Very distinctive, deciduous shrub with arching stems, white-glaucous at first, later purple, and obovate to oblong, entire or few-spined, grey-green leaves, to 4.5cm (1¾in) long. Solitary, pale yellow flowers, 1.5cm (½in) across, are produced on stalks, 1.5cm (½in) long, in late spring, and are succeeded by ellipsoid, white-glaucous, red fruit, 1cm (½in) long. ↕2m (6ft), ↔ 3m (10ft). China (S.E. Tibet). ❄❄❄

B. thunbergii 🏆 Dense, rounded, deciduous shrub with obovate, entire leaves, to 3cm (1¼in) long, fresh green above and bluish green beneath, turning orange and red in autumn. Umbel-like racemes of 2–5, rarely solitary, red-tinged, pale yellow flowers, 1cm (½in) long, are produced along the branches in mid-spring, and are succeeded by ellipsoid, glossy red fruit, to 8mm (⅜in) long. Excellent for hedging. ↕1m (2ft) occasionally more, ↔ 2.5m (8ft). Japan. ❄❄❄. **f. *atropurpurea*** ■ produces dark red-purple or purplish bronze foliage, turning red in autumn. **'Atropurpurea Nana'** 🏆 syn. 'Crimson

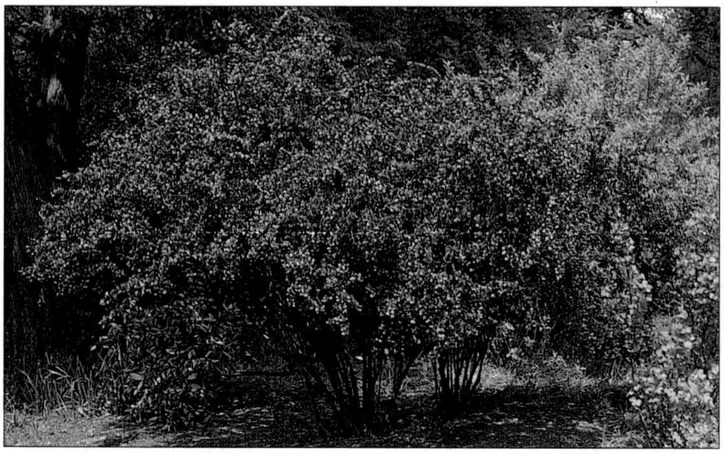

Berberis x *ottawensis* 'Superba'

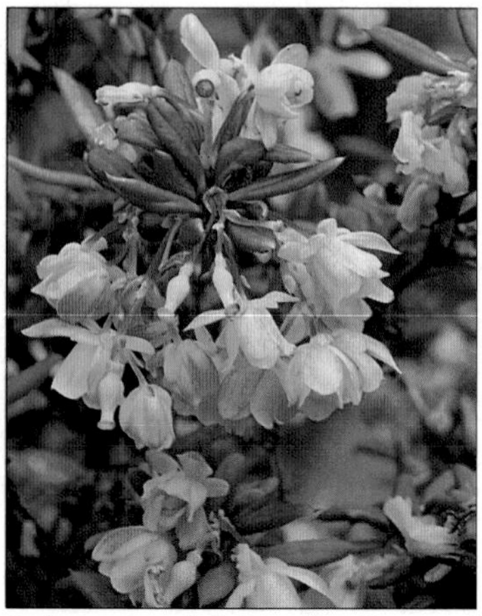

Berberis x *stenophylla* 'Corallina Compacta'

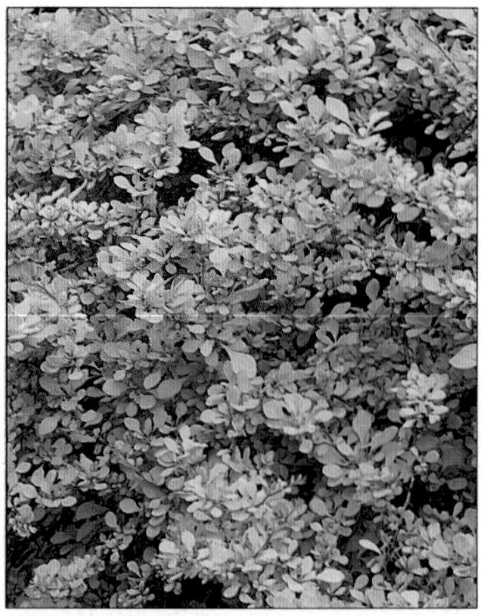

Berberis thunbergii 'Aurea'

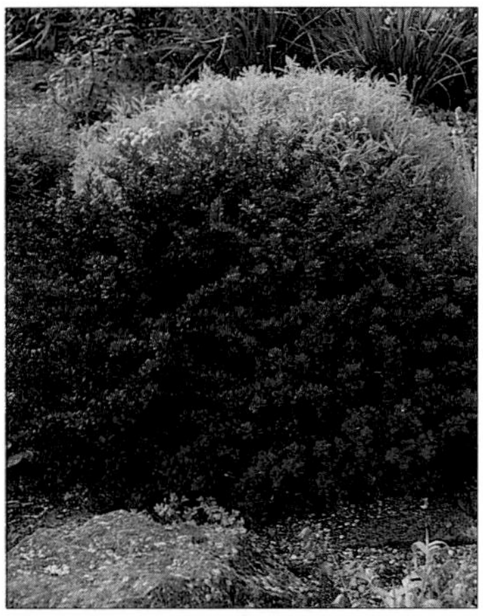

Berberis thunbergii 'Bagatelle'

Pygmy', 'Little Favourite', has red-purple foliage; ↕ 60cm (24in), ↔ 75cm (30in). **'Aurea'** ■ has bright yellow young foliage; ↕ 1.5m (5ft), ↔ 2m (6ft). **'Bagatelle'** ■ ♀ is very compact, with deep red-purple foliage; ↕ 30cm (12in), ↔ 40cm (16in). **'Crimson Pygmy'** see 'Atropurpurea Nana'. **'Dart's Red Lady'** ■ has very dark red-purple foliage, turning bright red in autumn. **'Erecta'** is upright when young, becoming open with age; ↕↔ 1.5m (5ft). **'Golden Ring'** ■ has purple leaves narrowly margined with golden yellow, turning red in autumn, and produces red fruit. **'Green Ornament'** is similar in habit to 'Erecta', with bronze young foliage and a profusion of red fruit. **'Helmond Pillar'** ■ is narrowly upright and has dark red-purple foliage; ↕ 1.5m

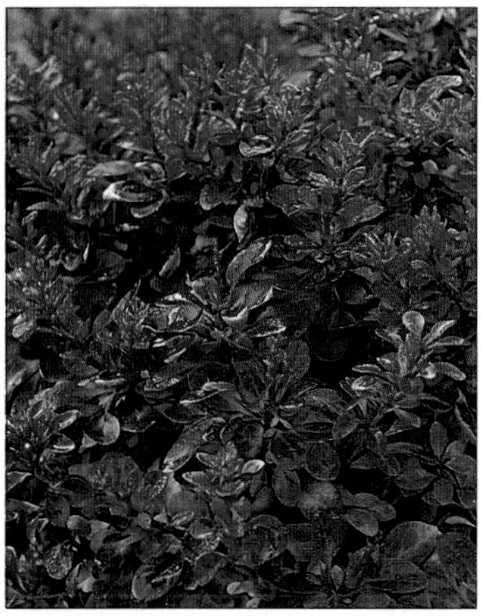

Berberis thunbergii 'Dart's Red Lady'

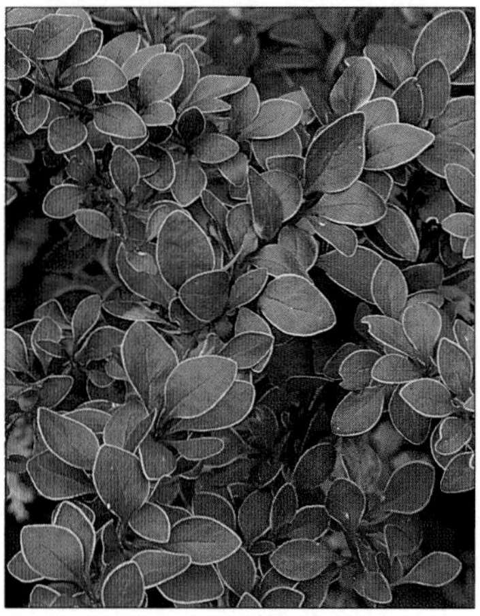

Berberis thunbergii 'Golden Ring'

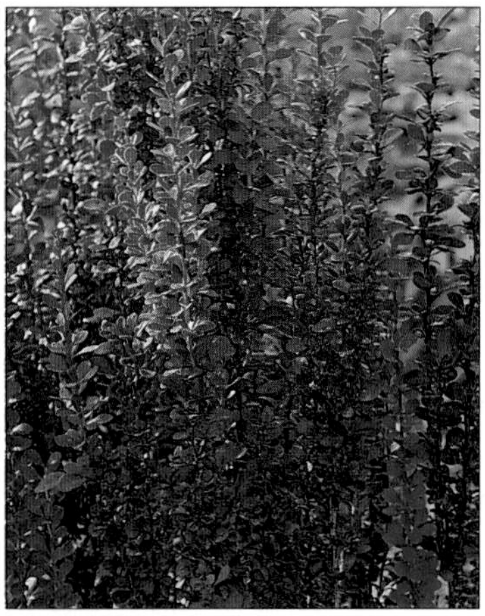

Berberis thunbergii 'Helmond Pillar'

(5ft), ↔ 60cm (24in). **'Kobold'** is very compact and fruits freely; ↕ 40cm (16in), ↔ 60cm (24in). **'Little Favourite'** see 'Atropurpurea Nana'. **'Pink Queen'** is similar to 'Rose Glow', but with more conspicuously variegated foliage. **'Red Pillar'** is similar in habit to 'Erecta', and has red-purple foliage. **'Rose Glow'** ■ ♀ has red-purple leaves flecked with white; but the first growth of the season shows no variegation. **'Silver Beauty'** is slow growing, with leaves mottled with creamy white; ↕ 60cm (24in), ↔ 90cm (36in). **'Sparkle'** is compact, with arching branches and good autumn colour, and fruits freely; ↕ 1.2m (4ft), ↔ 1.5m (5ft).
B. verruculosa ■ ♀ Compact, evergreen shrub with arching shoots and obovate to elliptic, spine-tipped leaves,

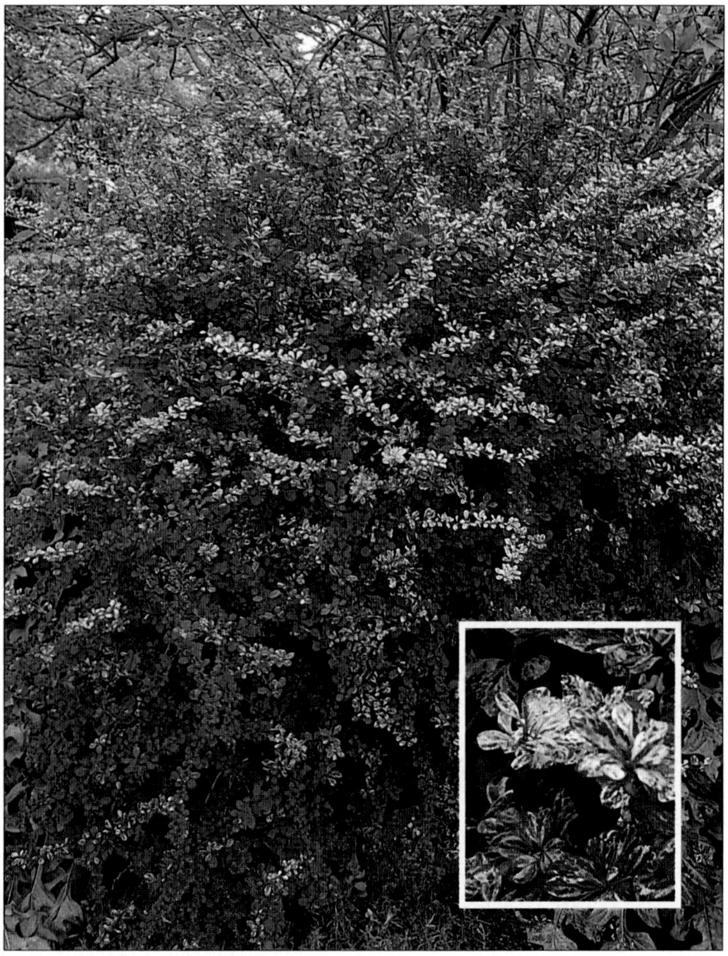

Berberis thunbergii 'Rose Glow' (inset: leaf detail)

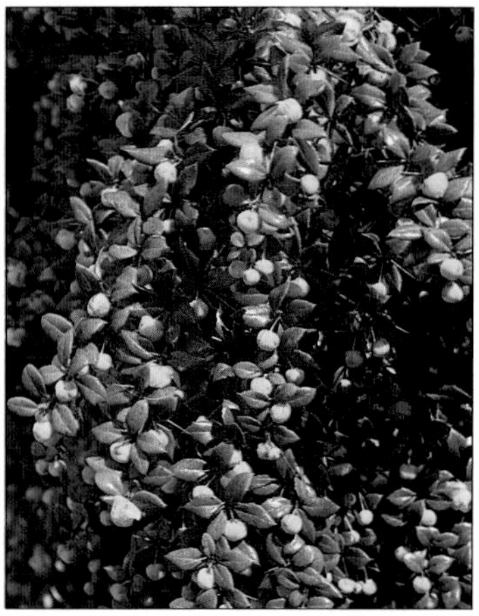

Berberis verruculosa

2–3cm (¾–1¼in) long, glossy, dark green above, grey-white beneath. Bears solitary, golden yellow flowers, 2cm (¾in) across, in late spring, followed by oblong-ovoid, white-glaucous, dark purple fruit, to 1cm (½in) long. ↕↔ 1.5m (5ft). W. China. ❄❄❄
B. wilsoniae ■ ♀ Dense, mound-forming, very spiny, semi-evergreen shrub with spreading, arching branches and obovate-spoon-shaped, usually entire, grey-green leaves, to 2.5cm (1in) long, that turn red and orange in autumn. Bears short panicles or clusters of 4–7 pale yellow flowers, 7–10mm (¼–½in) across, in summer, followed by spherical, translucent, coral-pink to pinkish red fruit, to 6mm (¼in) across. ↕ 1m (3ft), ↔ 2m (6ft). W. China. (W. Sichuan, Yunnan) ❄❄❄. **'Graciella'**,

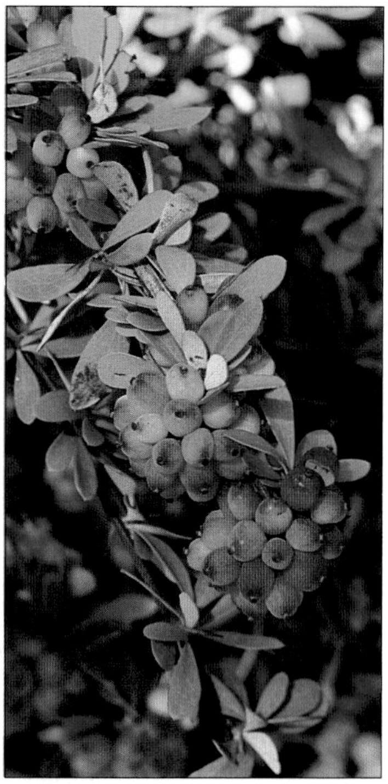

Berberis wilsoniae

syn. 'Marianne', has pale green leaves and red fruit; ↕ 50cm (20in), ↔ 90cm (36in). **'Marianne'** see 'Graciella'. **'Orangeade'** has carmine-red and orange-red fruit, 1cm (½in) across.

BERCHEMIA

RHAMNACEAE

Genus of about 12 species of deciduous climbers, rarely shrubs, from woodland in East Africa, E. Asia, and North and Central America. They have attractively veined, alternate, ovate to elliptic leaves, and terminal or axillary panicles of small flowers in summer. The fruits are fleshy. Train against a wall, fence, or pergola.

- **HARDINESS** Fully hardy to half hardy.
- **CULTIVATION** Grow in fertile soil in full sun or partial shade. Pruning group 11, in late winter or early spring.
- **PROPAGATION** Sow seed in containers in a cold frame in autumn or spring. Root semi-ripe cuttings in summer, or take root cuttings in winter. Layer in autumn or winter.
- **PESTS AND DISEASES** Trouble free.

B. racemosa. Twining, woody climber or spreading shrub, bearing ovate leaves, to 8cm (3in) long, dark green above, lighter or bluish green beneath, each with 7–9 pairs of prominent, parallel veins. Produces panicles, to 15cm (6in) long, of tiny green flowers in summer, followed by oblong red fruit, 10mm (½in) long, that ripen to black. ↕ 4m (12ft). Japan. ❄❄❄. **'Variegata'** has white-variegated leaves.
B. scandens (Rattan vine, Supple Jack). Vigorous, twining, woody climber bearing ovate, mid-green leaves, to 8cm (3in) long, each with 9–12 pairs of prominent, parallel veins. Bears panicles, 5cm (2in) long, of tiny green flowers in summer, followed by oblong, blue-black fruit, to 8mm (⅜in) long. ↕ 5m (15ft). S. USA to Central America. ❄❄❄

▷**Bergamot** see *Monarda, M. didyma*
Wild see *M. fistulosa*

B

BERGENIA *syn.* MEGASEA

Elephant-eared saxifrage, Elephant's ears

SAXIFRAGACEAE

Genus of 6–8 species of clump-forming, evergreen perennials from meadows, rocky moorland, and moist woodland in Central and E. Asia. They have tough, thick rhizomes and distinctive rosettes of alternate, simple, entire or toothed, obovate or oblong to broadly ovate, leathery, glossy leaves, many colouring well in winter. Panicle-like cymes of shallowly funnel-shaped to bell-shaped, 5-petalled flowers, usually 1.5–2.5cm (½–1in) across, on short, branched, often red or purple flower stems, are produced mainly in spring. Grow in a woodland garden or border.

• **HARDINESS** Fully hardy to frost hardy.

• **CULTIVATION** Grow in humus-rich, moist but well-drained soil in full sun or partial shade. Most dislike extremes of heat and drought, but will tolerate exposure and poor soil, which enhances their winter leaf colour. Mulch in autumn. Frost may damage early flowers, and the foliage of some species may die back in winter.

• **PROPAGATION** Seed-raised plants in gardens usually produce hybrids. Divide deteriorating clumps, or root rhizome sections from them, every 3–5 years in autumn or spring. Root sections of young rhizomes with one or more leaf rosettes after flowering or in autumn, in a sand frame or the open ground.

• **PESTS AND DISEASES** Susceptible to slugs, snails, and some caterpillars. Vine weevil and leaf spot may be a problem. Dry brown rot may affect the rhizomes.

***B.* 'Abendglut'**, syn. *B.* 'Evening Glow'. Clump-forming perennial with obovate, red-tinted, mid- to dark green leaves, 15cm (6in) long, ruby-red beneath, rich maroon in winter. Produces semi-double, magenta-crimson flowers on red flower stems in mid- and late spring. ↕20–30cm (8–12in), ↔45–60cm (18–24in). ❄❄❄

***B.* 'Baby Doll'.** Clump-forming perennial with obovate, bronze-tinted, mid-green leaves, 10cm (4in) long. In mid- and late spring, bears soft pink flowers, which darken with age. ↕30cm (12in), ↔45–60cm (18–24in). ❄❄❄

***B.* 'Ballawley'** ■ Clump-forming perennial with very broadly ovate, glossy, mid-green leaves, to 30cm (12in) long, turning bronze-purple in winter.

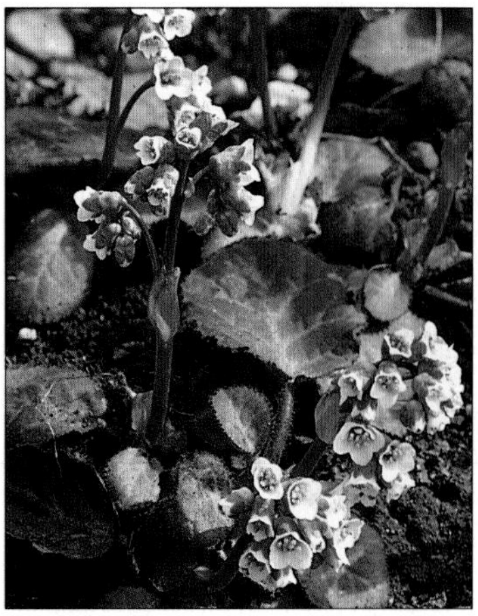

Bergenia ciliata

Red flower stems bear bright crimson flowers in mid- and late spring. Prefers a sheltered site. ↕60cm (24in), ↔45–60cm (18–24in). ❄❄❄

B. beesiana see *B. purpurascens.*

***B.* 'Beethoven'.** Free-flowering perennial with spoon-shaped, mid-green leaves, 25cm (10in) long. Produces white flowers, with red to greenish pink calyces, in mid- and late spring. ↕30–45cm (12–18in), ↔45–60cm (18–24in). ❄❄❄

***B.* 'Bell Tower'** see *B.* 'Glockenturm'.

***B.* 'Bressingham Bountiful'.** Compact perennial with broadly obovate to ovate, thin, dark green leaves, 18cm (7in) long, liable to frost damage but attractively margined with maroon, especially in winter. Bears nodding, rose-pink flowers in mid- and late spring, darkening as they age. ↕30–45cm (12–18in), ↔45–60cm (18–24in). ❄❄❄

***B.* 'Bressingham Salmon'.** Clump-forming perennial with obovate, bronze-tinted, deep green leaves, 15–18cm (6–7in) long, turning dark red in winter. Produces bright salmon-pink flowers in mid- and late spring. ↕30–45cm (12–18in), ↔45–60cm (18–24in). ❄❄❄

***B.* 'Bressingham White'** 🏆 Clump-forming perennial with robust, broadly obovate, deep green leaves, 15–18cm (6–7in) long. Pure white flowers are freely produced in mid- and late spring. ↕30–45cm (12–18in), ↔45–60cm (18–24in). ❄❄❄

B. ciliata ■ Clump-forming perennial with very broadly obovate, hairy, mid-green leaves, to 35cm (14in) long. In early spring, flower stems bear more or less erect flowers, that are pink, or white fading to pinkish white, with rose-pink calyces. In frost-prone areas, foliage dies back in winter. ↕30cm (12in), ↔45cm (18in). Himalayas, India (Assam). ❄❄❄ (borderline). **f. *ligulata*** has leaves with hairy margins and almost hairless surfaces, and produces very pale pink flowers with rose-red calyces.

B. cordifolia. Clump-forming perennial with rounded to heart-shaped, sometimes puckered, mid- to deep green leaves, 30cm (12in) long, tinted purple in winter. Bears pale rose-red to dark pink flowers on red flower stems in late winter and early spring. ↕60cm (24in), ↔75cm (30in). Russia (Siberia). ❄❄❄. **'Purpurea'** 🏆 has magenta-purple flowers and thicker, redder leaves.

B. crassifolia. Clump-forming perennial with oblong, obovate or broadly ovate, mid-green leaves, 9–18cm (3½–7in) long, with toothed margins, becoming red-tinged in exposed positions, especially in winter. Branched, reddish green flower stems bear nodding, pinkish purple flowers in late winter and early spring. ↕↔45cm (18in). Russia (Siberia). ❄❄❄. **var. *pacifica*** has slightly broader leaves and larger, red-purple flowers; ↕30cm (12in), ↔20cm (8in); Russia (Sikhote Alin mountains).

***B.* 'Eric Smith'.** Vigorous perennial with rounded-ovate, puckered, bronze-flushed, mid-green leaves, 20cm (8in) long, turning bronze-red in winter. Bears deep coral-pink flowers on strong, upright flower stems in mid- and late spring. ↕30–45cm (12–18in), ↔45–60cm (18–24in). ❄❄❄

***B.* 'Evening Glow'** see *B.* 'Abendglut'.

***B.* 'Glockenturm'**, syn. *B.* 'Bell Tower'. Free-flowering perennial with obovate-oblong, mid-green leaves, 15–18cm (6–7in) long. Deep reddish pink flowers are produced in mid- and late spring. ↕30–45cm (12–18in), ↔45–60cm (18–24in). ❄❄❄

B. milesii see *B. stracheyi.*

***B.* 'Morgenröte'** ■🏆 syn. *B.* 'Morning Red'. Clump-forming perennial with broadly obovate, deep green leaves, 13–15cm (5–6in) long. Bright reddish pink flowers are borne on strong red flower stems in mid- and late spring; repeat-flowers in cool summers. ↕30–45cm (12–18in), ↔45–60cm (18–24in). ❄❄❄

***B.* 'Morning Red'** see *B.* 'Morgenröte'.

***B.* 'Pugsley's Pink'.** Clump-forming perennial with obovate leaves, 15cm

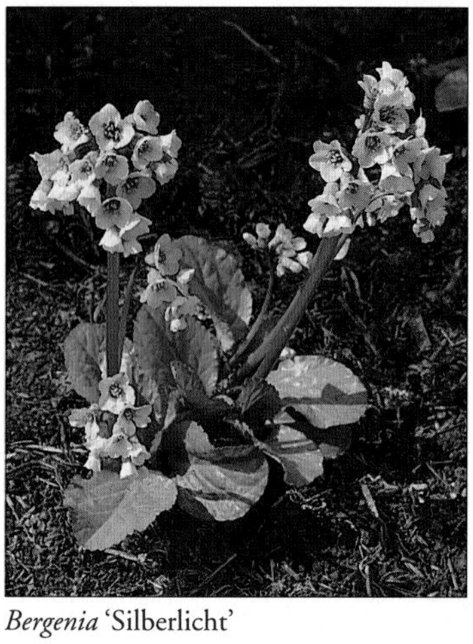

Bergenia 'Silberlicht'

(6in) long, mid-green above, reddish green beneath. Produces pink flowers, with brownish pink calyces, in mid- and late spring. ↕30–45cm (12–18in), ↔45–60cm (18–24in). ❄❄❄

B. purpurascens 🏆 syn. *B. beesiana.* Clump-forming perennial with elliptic or ovate-elliptic, deep green leaves, 7–25cm (3–10in) long, purple-red beneath, turning deep purple or beetroot-red in winter. Upright, reddish brown flower stems bear nodding to pendent, rich purple-red flowers in mid- and late spring. ↕45cm (18in), ↔30cm (12in). E. Himalayas, W. China, N. Burma. ❄❄❄

B.* x *schmidtii ■🏆 (*B. ciliata* x *B. crassifolia*). Vigorous perennial with broadly obovate to obovate-elliptic, rich green leaves, to 25cm (10in) long, narrowed at the base, with toothed margins, very sparsely fringed with hairs, and long leaf-stalks. Bright rose-pink flowers, nodding at first, then horizontal to erect, are borne in dense, short, panicle-like cymes in late winter and early spring. ↕30cm (12in), ↔60cm (24in). Garden origin. ❄❄❄

***B.* 'Schneekönigin'**, syn. *B.* 'Snow Queen'. Clump-forming perennial with rounded-obovate, mid-green leaves, 18–20cm (7–8in) long, with irregularly curled margins. Pale pink flowers are borne profusely in early and mid-spring, and darken as they age. ↕30–45cm (12–18in), ↔45–60cm (18–24in). ❄❄❄

***B.* 'Silberlicht'** ■🏆 syn. *B.* 'Silver Light'. Clump-forming perennial with broadly obovate, mid-green leaves, to 20cm (8in) long, with shallowly

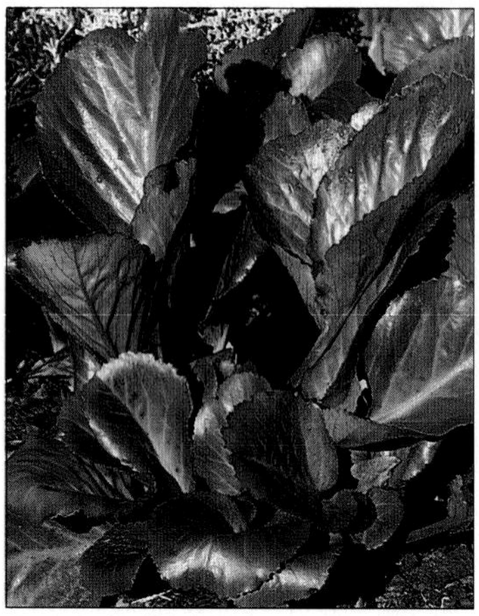

Bergenia 'Ballawley'

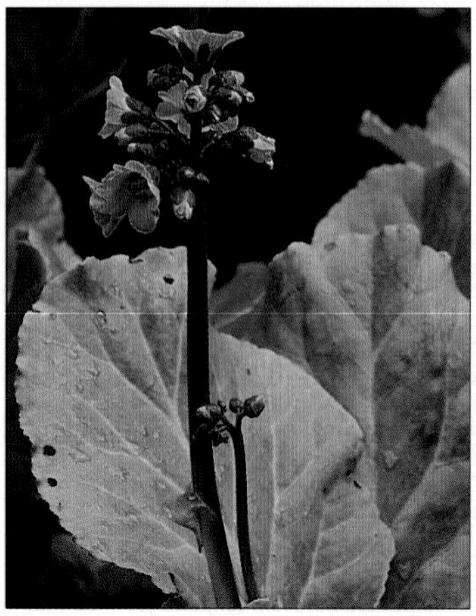

Bergenia 'Morgenröte'

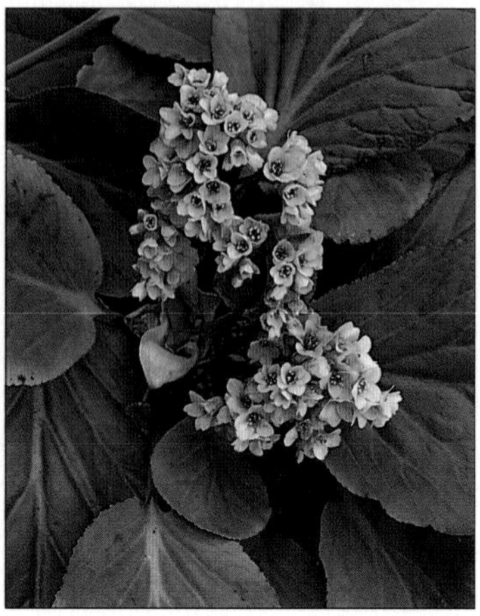

Bergenia x *schmidtii*

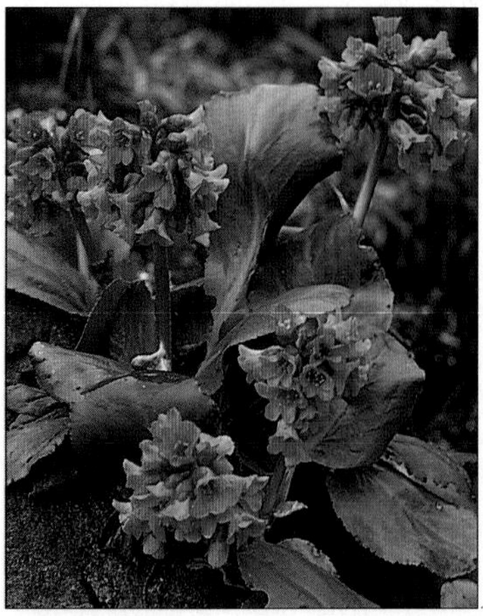

Bergenia stracheyi

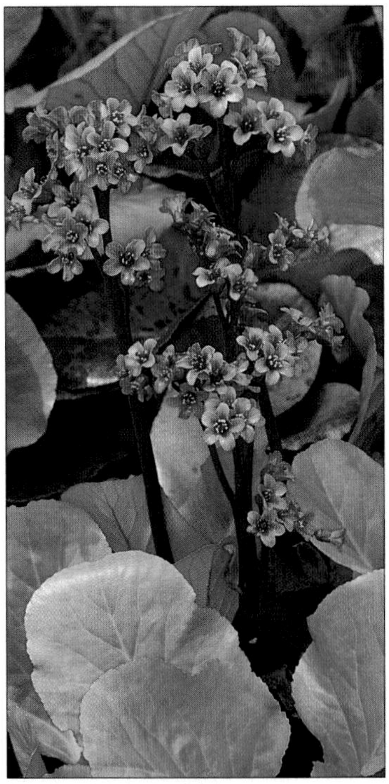

Bergenia 'Sunningdale'

scalloped margins. Bears white flowers, ageing to pink, with pink sepals, in early and mid-spring. ‡ 30–45cm (12–18in), ↔ 45–60cm (18–24in). ✻✻✻

***B.* 'Silver Light'** see *B.* 'Silberlicht'.

***B.* 'Snow Queen'** see *B.* 'Schneekönigin'.

B. stracheyi ▣ syn. *B. milesii.* Clump-forming perennial with erect, obovate, mid-green leaves, 6–20cm (2½–8in) long, wedge-shaped at the bases and hairy-margined. Nodding, fragrant pink flowers are produced on short flower stems in early spring. ‡ 15–30cm (6–12in), ↔ 30cm (12in). Tajikistan, Afghanistan, W. Himalayas. ✻✻✻. **f. *alba*,** syn. 'Alba', bears white flowers.

***B.* 'Sunningdale'** ▣ Clump-forming perennial with rounded-obovate, mid- to deep green leaves, 15–18cm (6–7in) long, red beneath, becoming copper-red in winter, especially in a sunny, exposed site. Rich lilac-magenta flowers are borne on red flower stems in early and mid-spring. ‡ 30–45cm (12–18in), ↔ 45–60cm (18–24in). ✻✻✻

***B.* 'Winter Fairy Tale'** see *B.* 'Wintermärchen'.

***B.* 'Wintermärchen',** syn. *B.* 'Winter Fairy Tale'. Clump-forming perennial with obovate to narrowly ovate, deep green leaves, 15cm (6in) long, red-purple beneath, with slightly twisted leaf-blades, red-tinged in winter. Bears dark rose-red flowers in early and mid-spring. ‡ 30–45cm (12–18in), ↔ 45–60cm (18–24in). ✻✻✻

BERGEROCACTUS

CACTACEAE

Genus of one species of perennial cactus from semi-desert areas of S. California, USA, and N.W. Mexico. It has funnel-shaped flowers produced laterally from the upper part of the stems in summer, and spherical, spiny fruit. In frost-prone areas, grow *B. emoryi* in a warm greenhouse for its golden-spined shoots. In warmer areas, grow in a desert garden.

• **HARDINESS** Frost tender.

• **CULTIVATION** Under glass, grow in standard cactus compost with additional sharp sand, in full light. During the growing season, water moderately and apply a nitrogen- and potash-based fertilizer monthly; keep completely dry in winter. Outdoors, grow in slightly enriched, sharply drained soil in full sun. See also pp.48–49.

• **PROPAGATION** Sow seed at 24°C (75°F) in early spring. Root 15cm- (6in-) long basal cuttings of new shoots in early or mid-spring, with bottom heat; keep barely moist.

• **PESTS AND DISEASES** Susceptible to mealybugs and root mealybugs.

B. emoryi, syn. *Cereus emoryi.* Perennial cactus branching freely from the base. Slender, erect or decumbent, pale green stems produce 14–20 or more, densely spiny, slightly warty ribs. Close-set areoles each produce 10–30 golden yellow spines, including 1–4 centrals. In summer, bears diurnal yellow flowers, 2–4cm (¾–1½in) across, with wool and spines in the axils of the ovaries and the short, scaly tubes. ‡ 60cm (24in), ↔ 45cm (18in). USA (S. California), N.W. Mexico. ⊛ (min. 16°C/61°F)

BERKHEYA

ASTERACEAE/COMPOSITAE

Genus of about 80 species of rosette-forming, often spiny-leaved biennials, perennials, evergreen subshrubs, and shrubs, found in open grassland and rocky areas in tropical Africa and South Africa. They are grown for their unusual foliage and long flowering period. Berkheyas are woody-based or tap-rooted, with pinnatisect, pinnatifid, or pinnate, prickly, thistle-like leaves, often white-hairy beneath, and spiny, involucral bracts. The daisy-like flowerheads are usually yellow. Grow in a sunny border or against a warm wall.

• **HARDINESS** Frost hardy.

• **CULTIVATION** Grow in fertile, well-drained soil, in a sheltered position in full sun. Protect from winter wet.

• **PROPAGATION** Sow seed in containers in a cold frame in autumn. Divide in spring; the divisions re-establish slowly.

• **PESTS AND DISEASES** Trouble free.

B. macrocephala ▣ Rosette-forming perennial with pinnatisect, narrowly oblong-ovate, very spiny, mid-green leaves, 30–45cm (12–18in) long, pale green beneath. In midsummer, erect,

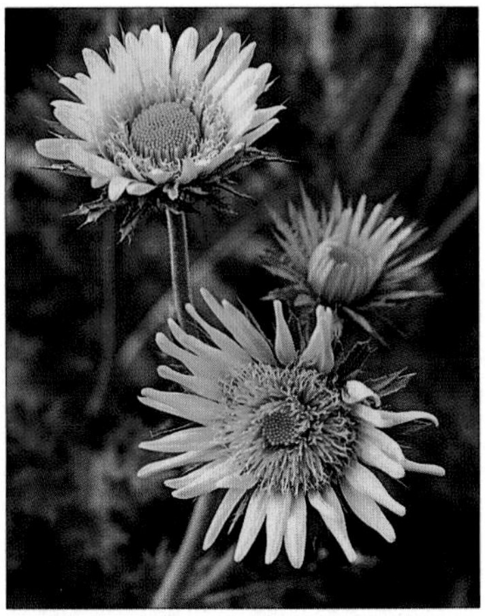

Berkheya macrocephala

branched stems bear a succession of bright yellow flowerheads, 10cm (4in) across, with paler yellow disc-florets and spiny bracts. ‡↔ 50–90cm (20–36in). South Africa (Kwazulu/Natal). ✻✻

B. purpurea. Rosette-forming perennial with oblong-lance-shaped, pinnatifid, spiny, mid-green basal leaves, to 45cm (18in) long, white-woolly beneath; upper stem leaves are pale green beneath and often slightly woolly. Corymbs of purple flowerheads, 7cm (3in) across, are produced in midsummer. ‡↔ 40–75cm (16–30in). South Africa (Orange Free State, Kwazulu/Natal, Eastern Cape), Lesotho. ✻✻

BERTOLONIA

MELASTOMATACEAE

Genus of about 14 species of low-growing, often creeping, evergreen perennials from forest in tropical South America, grown primarily for their variegated foliage. The leaves are simple, stalked, mostly ovate or ovate-oblong, prominently veined, velvety, and colourful, with scalloped margins. Shallowly cup- or saucer-shaped flowers, with 4 or 5 petals, are borne in corymb-like, terminal cymes. In frost-prone areas, grow in a bottle garden, terrarium, or warm greenhouse; elsewhere, use as low ground cover in a border.

• **HARDINESS** Frost tender.

• **CULTIVATION** Under glass, grow in loamless potting compost with added grit, in bright filtered light. In growth, water freely and maintain high humidity, but keep foliage dry. Keep just moist in winter. Outdoors, grow in humus-rich soil in partial shade.

• **PROPAGATION** Sow seed at 19–24°C (66–75°F) in spring. Root tip cuttings in spring, in a closed propagating case with bottom heat.

• **PESTS AND DISEASES** Trouble free.

B. marmorata. Decumbent or mound-forming perennial with ovate-oblong, hairy, bright green leaves, 5–8cm (2–3in) long, irregularly marked or banded with white, and deep purple beneath. Leaves may also be copper-green. Cymes, 10–13cm (4–5in) long, of saucer-shaped purple flowers, 2cm (¾in) across, are produced irregularly throughout the year. ‡ 10–15cm (4–6in), ↔ 25cm (10in) or more. Brazil. ⊛ (min. 16–19°C/61–66°F)

BESCHORNERIA

AGAVACEAE

Genus of about 7 species of clump-forming, rosetted, perennial succulents from semi-arid areas of Mexico. Leaves are linear to lance-shaped, arching, and often glaucous, with fleshy keels and very fine marginal teeth. Slightly arching, red-bracted racemes or panicles of pendent, tubular flowers are borne in late spring or summer. In frost-prone areas, grow in a temperate greenhouse; elsewhere, grow as specimen plants.

• **HARDINESS** Frost tender; may stand short periods down to 0°C (32°F).

• **CULTIVATION** Under glass, grow in standard cactus compost in full light. From late spring to autumn, water moderately and apply a balanced liquid fertilizer monthly; water sparingly in winter. Outdoors, grow in sharply

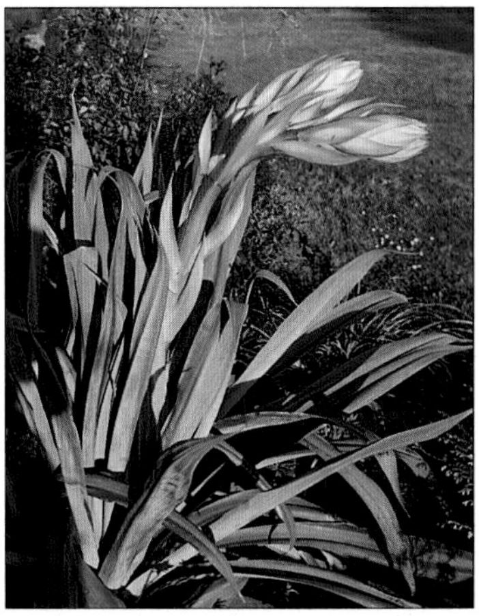

Beschorneria yuccoides

drained, humus-rich loam in full sun. See also pp.48–49.

• **PROPAGATION** Sow seed at 21°C (70°F) in early spring. Root offsets in early spring.

• **PESTS AND DISEASES** Scale insects may be a problem.

B. tubiflora. Perennial succulent with compact rosettes of slender, lance-shaped, fleshy, greyish green leaves, to 30cm (12in) long, roughened on both surfaces. Racemes, to 1m (3ft) long, with purplish red bracts and reddish green flowers, 4cm (1½in) long, are borne in late spring. ‡ 1m (3ft), ↔ 65cm (26in). Mexico. ⊛ (min. 7°C/45°F)

B. yuccoides ▣ ♀ Perennial succulent with compact rosettes of lance-shaped, fleshy, grey-green leaves, 50cm (20in) long, becoming glaucous with age. In summer, bears panicles, 1–1.5m (3–5ft) or more long, of vivid red bracts and yellow-tinted, bright green flowers, 7cm (3in) or more long, with spreading lobes. ‡ 1.5m (5ft), ↔ 1m (3ft) or more. Mexico. ✻ (borderline)

BESSERA

ALLIACEAE/LILIACEAE

Genus of 2 species of cormous perennials from rocky slopes, scrub, and grassland in Mexico. They are grown for their pendent, conical, brightly coloured flowers, produced in terminal umbels in summer or autumn. Leaves are basal and narrowly linear. In frost-prone areas, grow in a cool conservatory or at the base of a warm, sunny wall. In frost-free areas, grow in a sunny, open border.

• **HARDINESS** Half hardy.

• **CULTIVATION** Under glass, grow in loam-based potting compost (JI No.2) in full light. Water moderately in growth; keep dry once leaves die down. Outdoors, plant 6cm (2½in) deep in well-drained soil in full sun in spring. Keep dormant corms dry in winter.

• **PROPAGATION** Sow seed at 13–16°C (55–61°F) in spring, or remove offsets in autumn or winter.

• **PESTS AND DISEASES** Trouble free.

B. elegans (Coral drops). Cormous perennial with linear leaves, 60–80cm (24–32in) long. In late summer or autumn, bears umbels of up to 9 bright scarlet flowers, 3–4cm (1¼–1½in) across, creamy white within and with projecting stamens. ‡ 60cm (24in), ↔ 5cm (2in). S.W. and S.C. Mexico. ✻

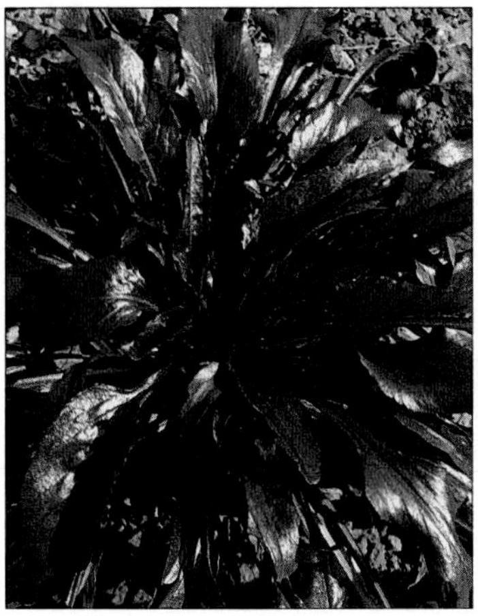

Beta vulgaris subsp. *cicla* 'MacGregor's Favourite'

BETA

Beet

CHENOPODIACEAE

Genus of 5 or 6 species of rosette-forming perennials and biennials from grassland and seashores in Europe and the Mediterranean. They have ovate to triangular-ovate, glossy, light or mid-green or reddish purple basal leaves, and lance-shaped stem leaves produced on stout leaf-stalks. Spike-like cymes of insignificant green flowers are produced in summer, with flowering accelerated by hot, dry conditions. The most commonly cultivated species of beet are grown as annual vegetables or fodder plants (mangold, beetroot, and chard), forming massively swollen roots. Some selections of *B. vulgaris* subsp. *cicla* produce attractive, ornamental foliage, and are useful for summer and winter colour contrast in a mixed border or annual bedding scheme.

• **HARDINESS** Fully hardy.

• **CULTIVATION** Grow in rich, light but moisture-retentive soil in full sun or partial shade. Water thoroughly during periods of drought in order to reduce the likelihood of flower and seed production (bolting).

• **PROPAGATION** Sow seed *in situ* in early spring or late summer.

• **PESTS AND DISEASES** Downy mildew and leaf spotting may be a problem in wet or humid conditions.

B. vulgaris* subsp. *cicla (Swiss chard). Ornamental biennial, grown as an annual for the decorative effect of its foliage. Produces clusters of upright, then arching, narrow, sometimes puckered, glossy, light or mid-green leaves, 23–30cm (9–12in) long, with bright red midribs and, in some selections, with the leaf-blades also red or purple-red. ↕23cm (9in), ↔ to 45cm (18in). ✲✲✲. **'Bull's Blood'** produces dark red foliage; ↕ to 45cm (18in). **'MacGregor's Favourite'** ▣ has brilliant blood-red foliage, and is less liable to bolt than most other cultivars. **'Vulcan'** has brilliant red foliage; ↕ to 45cm (18in).

▷ ***Betonica*** see *Stachys*
 B. officinalis see *S. officinalis*
▷ **Betony** see *Stachys*
 Water see *Scrophularia auriculata*
 Wood see *Stachys officinalis*

BETULA

Birch

BETULACEAE

Genus of about 60 species of deciduous trees and shrubs found in diverse habitats, including woodland, moors, mountains, and heathland, throughout the N. hemisphere. Leaves are alternate, toothed, usually ovate, and mid- to dark green. Male and female flowers are borne in separate catkins on the same plant in spring, the male catkins usually yellow-brown, pendent, and longer than the females, which are erect at first, becoming pendent. Birches are grown for their ornamental bark, colourful autumn foliage, attractive male catkins, and graceful, open habit. Many are suitable for a small garden, either as isolated specimens or in small groups.

• **HARDINESS** Fully hardy; most are tolerant of very exposed positions.

• **CULTIVATION** Grow in moderately fertile, moist but well-drained soil in full sun or light dappled shade. *B. alleghaniensis, B. grossa, B. lenta,* and *B. maximowicziana* prefer sheltered, woodland conditions. Pruning group 1.

• **PROPAGATION** Sow seed, of known wild origin only (most seed from cultivated plants will produce hybrids), in a seedbed in autumn. Root softwood cuttings in summer, or graft in winter.

• **PESTS AND DISEASES** Birch borers, birch leaf mining sawfly, birch rust, aphids, honey fungus, and mildew may cause problems. Leaves may become chlorotic on poor, shallow, chalky soil.

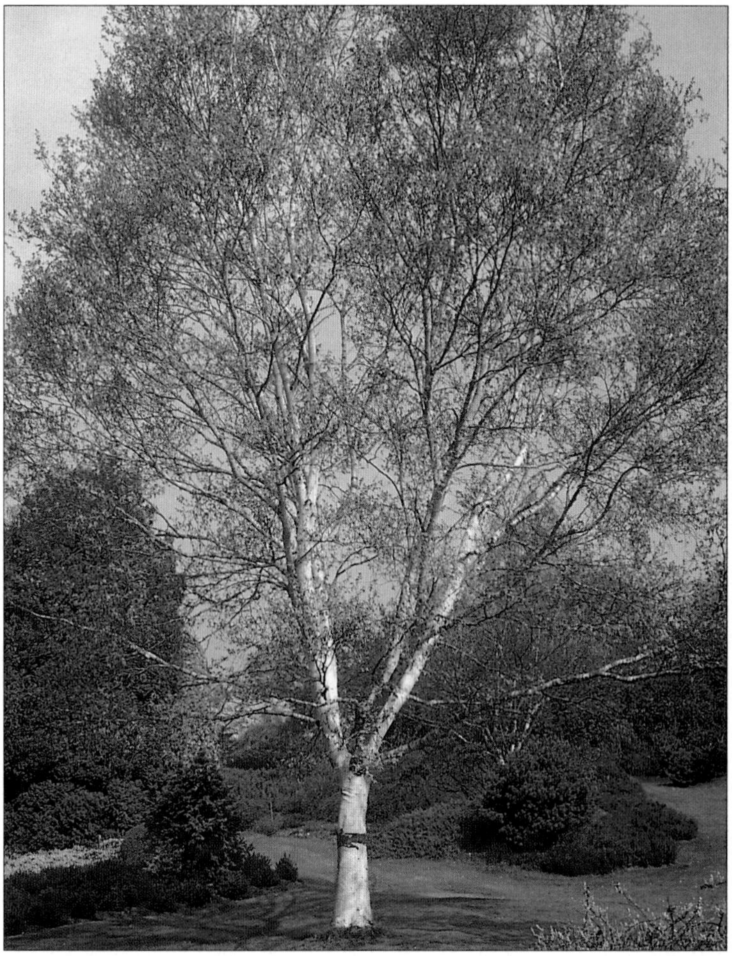

Betula ermanii

B. albosinensis ▣ 🏆 ♤ (Chinese red birch). Conical tree with peeling, orange-brown or brown bark, cream when newly exposed, often covered with a white-glaucous bloom when young. Ovate, tapered, glossy leaves, to 7cm (3in) long, are deep green above, lighter beneath, turning yellow in autumn. Yellow-brown male catkins, to 6cm (2½in) long, open with the young leaves. ↕25m (80ft), ↔ 10m (30ft). W. China. ✲✲✲. **var. *septentrionalis*** 🏆 has orange-brown bark and paler, dull leaves.

B. alleghaniensis ♤ syn. *B. lutea* (Yellow birch). Conical tree with peeling, yellow-brown bark. Ovate, matt, yellow-green leaves, to 14cm (5½in) long, become yellow in autumn and are borne on aromatic shoots. Yellow-brown male catkins, to 10cm (4in) long, are borne in early spring. ↕25m (80ft), ↔ 10m (30ft). E. North America. ✲✲✲

***B. costata* of gardens** see *B. ermanii* 'Grayswood Hill'.

B. ermanii ▣ ♤ (Erman's birch). Conical tree with rough, warty shoots and pinkish or creamy white bark with conspicuous lenticels. Ovate, tapered, dull, dark green leaves, 10cm (4in) long, are glandular beneath and turn yellow in autumn. Yellow-brown male catkins, to 10cm (4in) long, open as the young leaves emerge. ↕20m (70ft), ↔ 12m (40ft). Russia (Kamchatka), Japan, Korea. ✲✲✲. **'Grayswood Hill'** 🏆 syn. *B. costata* of gardens, is a vigorous clone, with pure white bark.

B. grossa ♤ (Japanese cherry birch). Conical tree with peeling, reddish grey bark, becoming dark grey on mature plants. Ovate, sharply toothed, matt, dark green leaves, to 10cm (4in) long, are borne on aromatic shoots and turn golden yellow in autumn. Produces yellow-brown male catkins, to 8cm (3in) long, in early spring. ↕25m (80ft), ↔ 10m (30ft). Japan. ✲✲✲

B. jacquemontii see *B. utilis* var. *jacquemontii.*

B. lenta ♤ (Cherry birch, Sweet birch). Conical tree with dark red bark that becomes grey and scaly on mature trunks. Aromatic shoots bear ovate, matt, yellow-green leaves, to 10cm (4in) long, which turn yellow in autumn. Produces yellow-brown male catkins, to 8cm (3in) long, in early spring. ↕15m (50ft), ↔ 12m (40ft). E. USA. ✲✲✲

B. lutea see *B. alleghaniensis.*

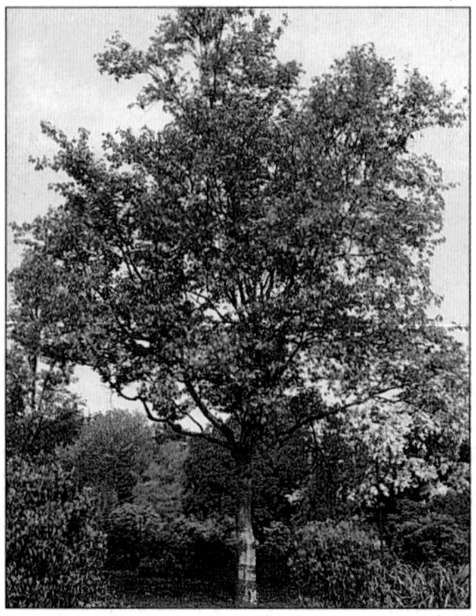

Betula albosinensis

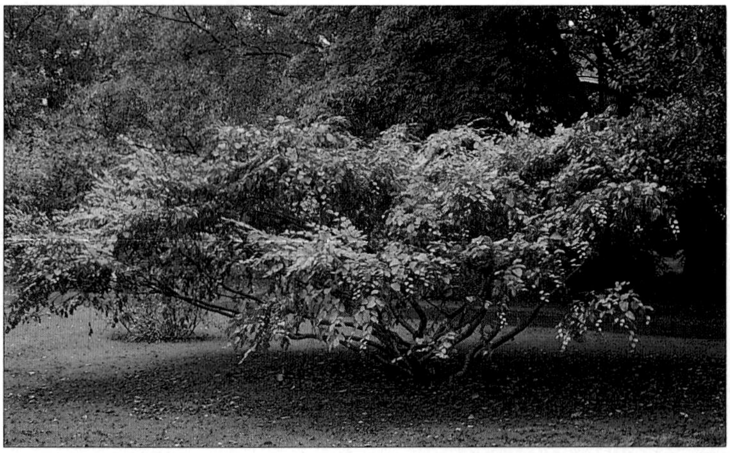

Betula medwedewii

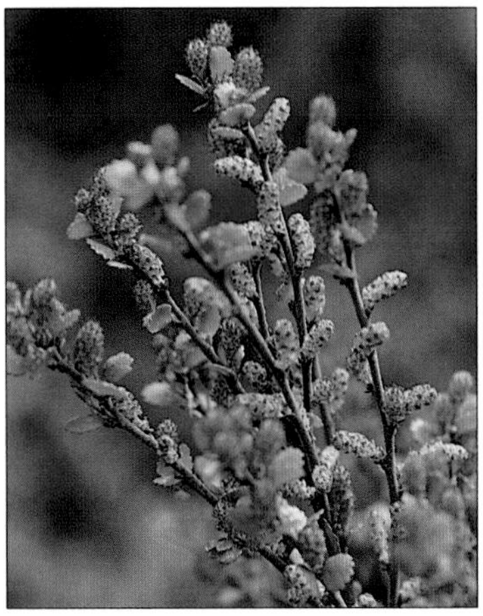

Betula nana

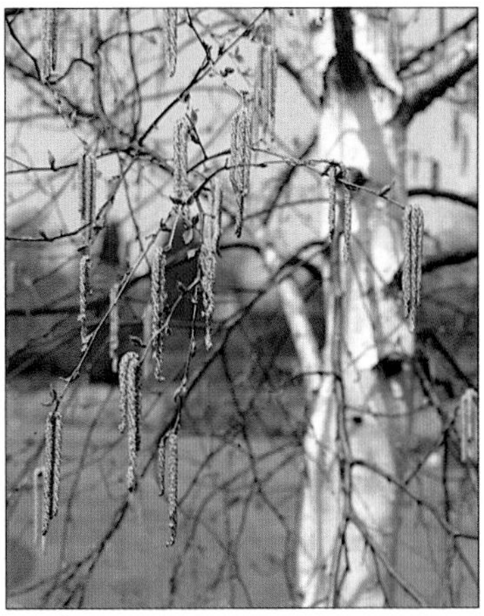

Betula papyrifera

B. maximowicziana ⌂ (Monarch birch). Broadly conical tree with pink-tinged, grey-white bark, peeling in horizontal strips, with conspicuous lenticels. Heart-shaped, deep green leaves, to 15cm (6in) long, turn yellow in autumn. Yellow-brown male catkins, to 12cm (5in) long, are produced in early spring. ↕25m (80ft), ↔12m (40ft). Japan, Kurile Islands. ✻✻✻
B. medwedewii ▣♀ (Transcaucasian birch). Compact shrub with upright branches spreading with age and bearing conspicuous, pointed, glossy winter buds. Ovate, glossy, dark green leaves, to 10cm (4in) long, turn yellow to yellow-brown in autumn. Produces yellow-brown male catkins, to 10cm (4in) long, in spring. ↕↔5m (15ft). Caucasus. ✻✻✻

B. nana ▣ (Arctic birch, Dwarf birch). Spreading shrub with rounded to kidney-shaped, finely toothed, glossy, mid-green leaves, to 2cm (¾in) long, turning yellow or red in autumn. Bears yellow-brown male catkins, to 1cm (½in) long, in spring. ↕60cm (24in), ↔1.2m (4ft). Subarctic N. America and Eurasia. ✻✻✻
B. nigra ▣♀⌂ (Black birch, River birch). Conical to spreading tree with shaggy, red-brown bark, peeling in layers when young, becoming blackish or grey-white and fissured on old trees. Diamond-shaped, glossy, mid- to dark green leaves, to 8cm (3in) long, glaucous beneath, turn yellow in autumn. Bears yellow-brown male catkins, to 8cm (3in) long, in early spring. ↕18m (60ft), ↔12m (40ft). E. USA. ✻✻✻

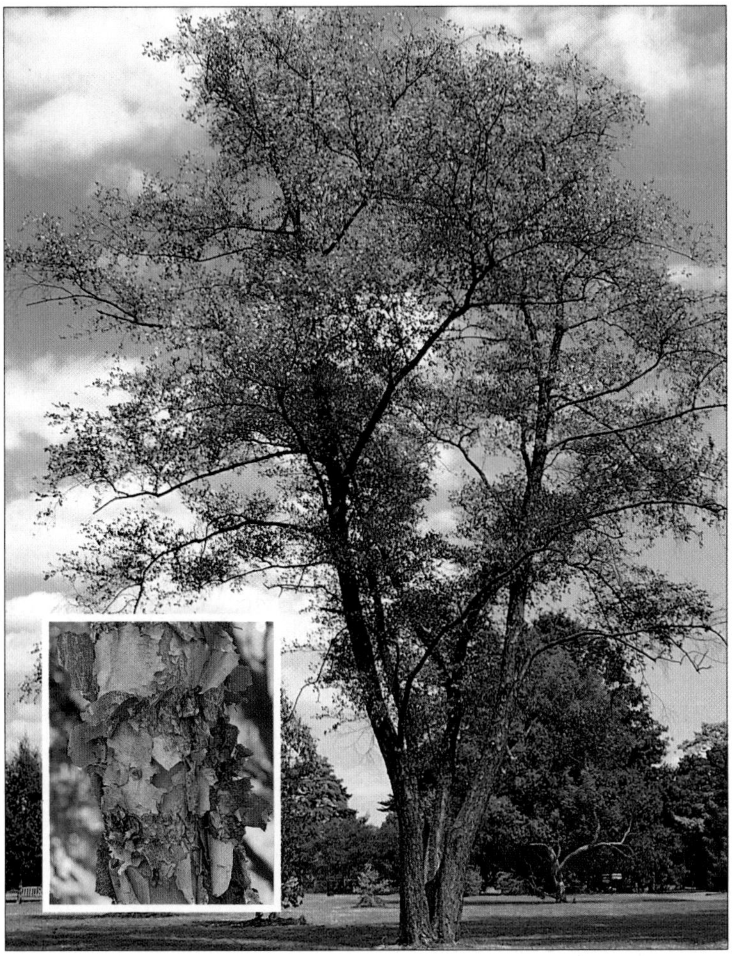

Betula nigra (inset: bark detail)

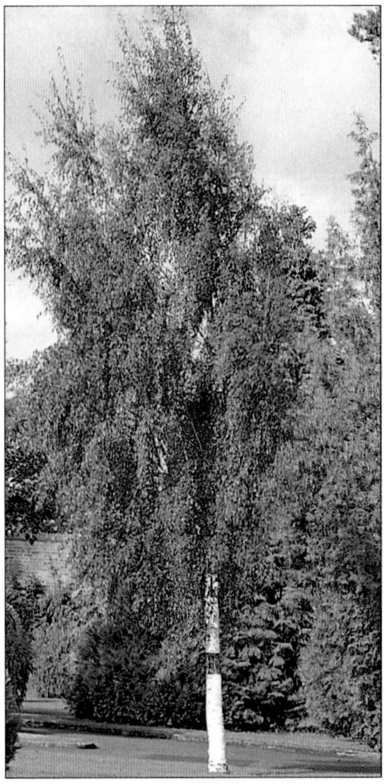

Betula pendula 'Laciniata'

B. papyrifera ▣⌂ (Canoe birch, Paper birch). Conical tree with white bark, peeling in thin layers and pale orange-brown when newly exposed. Ovate, dark green leaves, to 10cm (4in) long, turn yellow to orange in autumn. Produces yellow male catkins, to 10cm (4in) long, in early spring. ↕20m (70ft) or more, ↔10m (30ft). North America. ✻✻✻
B. pendula ♀◊ syn. *B. verrucosa* (Silver birch). Narrowly conical tree with pendent, warty branchlets and peeling white bark, which becomes marked with dark, rugged cracks at the base on older trees. Diamond-shaped, sharply toothed, mid-green leaves, to 6cm (2½in) long, turn yellow in autumn. Bears yellow-brown male catkins, to 6cm (2½in) long, in early spring. ↕25m (80ft), ↔10m (30ft). Europe, Russia (W. Siberia) ✻✻✻. **'Dalecarlica' of gardens** see 'Laciniata'. **'Fastigiata'** ◊ has upright branches; ↕20m (70ft), ↔6m (20ft). **'Golden Cloud'** has yellow foliage. Very hot sun may scorch the leaves; ↕6m (20ft), ↔5m (15ft). **'Laciniata'** ▣♀ syn. 'Dalecarlica' of gardens, has very pendulous branchlets and deeply cut leaves. **'Purpurea'** has purple-tinged bark and dark purple leaves; ↕10m (30ft), ↔3m (10ft). **'Tristis'** ▣♀ has slender branchlets and bark remaining white at the base. **'Youngii'** ▣♀⌓ (Young's weeping birch) is dome-shaped; ↕8m (25ft).
B. platyphylla* var. *japonica ◊ Narrowly conical tree with slightly pendent, warty branchlets, and bark creamy white to the base. Diamond-shaped, sharply toothed, yellowish green leaves, to 10cm (4in) long, are hairless beneath, and turn yellow in autumn. Bears yellow-brown male catkins, to 8cm (3in) long, in early spring. ↕20m (70ft), ↔12m (40ft). Japan. ✻✻✻. **var. *szechuanica*** see *B. szechuanica.* **'Whitespire'** is conical, with chalk-white bark, and is somewhat resistant to birch borer.
B. populifolia ◊ (Grey birch). Narrowly conical, sometimes multi-stemmed tree,

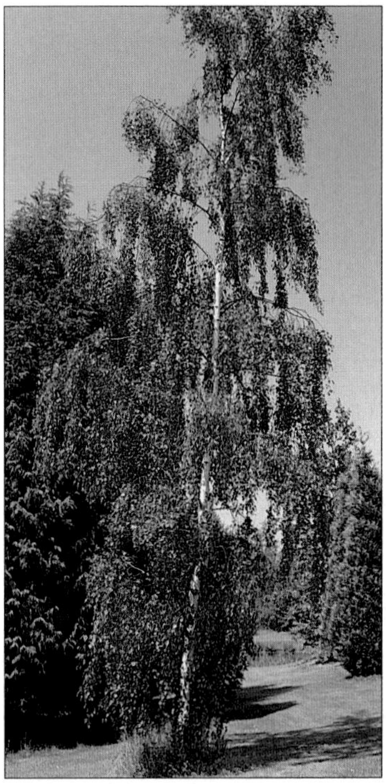

Betula pendula 'Tristis'

which is fast-growing, but usually short-lived. Branchlets are pendent and warty, and the grey-white bark, remaining white at the base, does not peel. Diamond-shaped, sharply toothed, glossy, yellowish green leaves, to 10cm (4in) long, end in long, slender points, and turn yellow in autumn. Bears yellow-brown male catkins, to 8cm (3in) long, in early spring. ↕10m (30ft), ↔3m (10ft). E. North America. ✻✻✻
B. pubescens ◊ (Downy birch). Narrowly conical tree with ascending branches, downy shoots, and peeling bark with conspicuous lenticels; bark remains white at the base. Diamond-shaped, sharply toothed, mid-green leaves, to 6cm (2½in) long, turn yellow in autumn. Produces pendent, yellow-brown male catkins, to 6cm (2½in) long, in early spring. Tolerates poor or wet, acid soils. ↕20m (70ft), ↔10m (30ft). Europe, N. Asia. ✻✻✻
B. szechuanica ⌂ syn. *B. platyphylla* var. *szechuanica* (Szechuan birch). Vigorous, conical tree with chalk-white bark when mature, and ovate, leathery, dark bluish green leaves, to 10cm (4in) long, turning golden yellow in autumn. Bears yellow-green male catkins, to 8cm

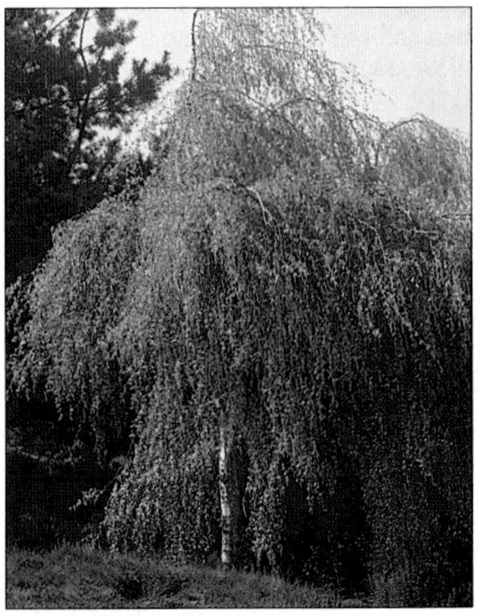

Betula pendula 'Youngii'

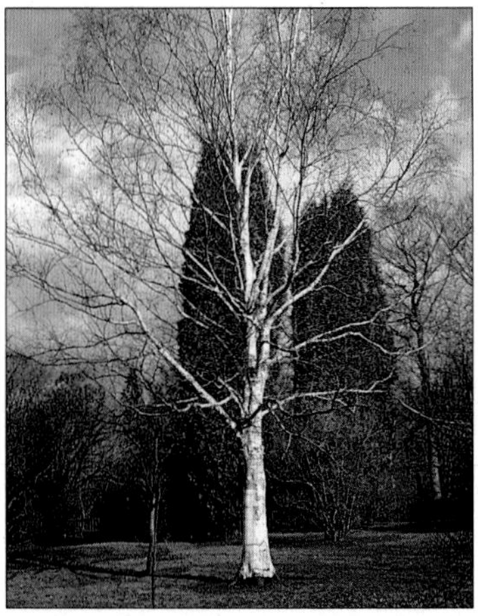

Betula utilis var. *jacquemontii* 'Jermyns'

(3in) long, in early spring. ↕ 20m (70ft), ↔ 10m (30ft). S.W. China. ❄❄❄
***B.* 'Trost's Dwarf'.** Slender-stemmed shrub with gracefully arching branches and ovate, mid-green leaves, to 5cm (2in) long, finely cut and divided into long, slender lobes. Not known to produce catkins. ↕↔ 1.5m (5ft). ❄❄❄
B. utilis △ (Himalayan birch). Variable tree with peeling, copper-brown or pinkish bark and ovate to oblong, tapered, dark green leaves, to 12cm (5in) long, that turn yellow in autumn. In early spring, produces yellow-brown male catkins, to 12cm (5in) long. ↕ 18m (60ft), ↔ 10m (30ft). China, Himalayas. ❄❄❄. Most often grown in one of the following forms. **var. *jacquemontii*** 🏆 syn. *B. jacquemontii*, has white bark; Himalayas. **var. *jacquemontii* 'Grayswood Ghost'** has brilliant white bark and very glossy leaves. **var. *jacquemontii* 'Jermyns'** ▣ is a vigorous clone, with pure white bark and larger catkins, 15cm (6in) or more long. **var. *jacquemontii* 'Silver Shadow'** ▣ 🏆 has bright white bark and pendent, dark green leaves, to 13cm (5in) long.
B. verrucosa see *B. pendula.*

BIARUM

ARACEAE

Genus of 15 species of small, tuberous perennials from open ground and maquis in the Mediterranean region and W. Asia. In autumn, they produce hooded, often malodorous spathes at ground level, followed by broadly ovate to spoon-shaped or lance-shaped leaves. They are best grown in a bulb frame or cold greenhouse, except *B. tenuifolium,* which may be grown outside at the base of a sunny wall, and increases rapidly.

• **HARDINESS** Fully hardy to frost hardy.

• **CULTIVATION** Plant dormant tubers 5cm (2in) deep in summer. Under glass, grow in equal parts loam, leaf mould, and sharp sand or grit, in full light. Keep warm and dry when dormant in summer; water regularly but sparingly when in leaf. Tubers may rot if overwatered. *B. tenuifolium* may be grown outside in light, open, sharply drained soil in full sun.

• **PROPAGATION** Sow seed at 13°C (55°F) in autumn or spring, and prick out seedlings as soon as possible. Separate tubers in summer.

• **PESTS AND DISEASES** Trouble free.

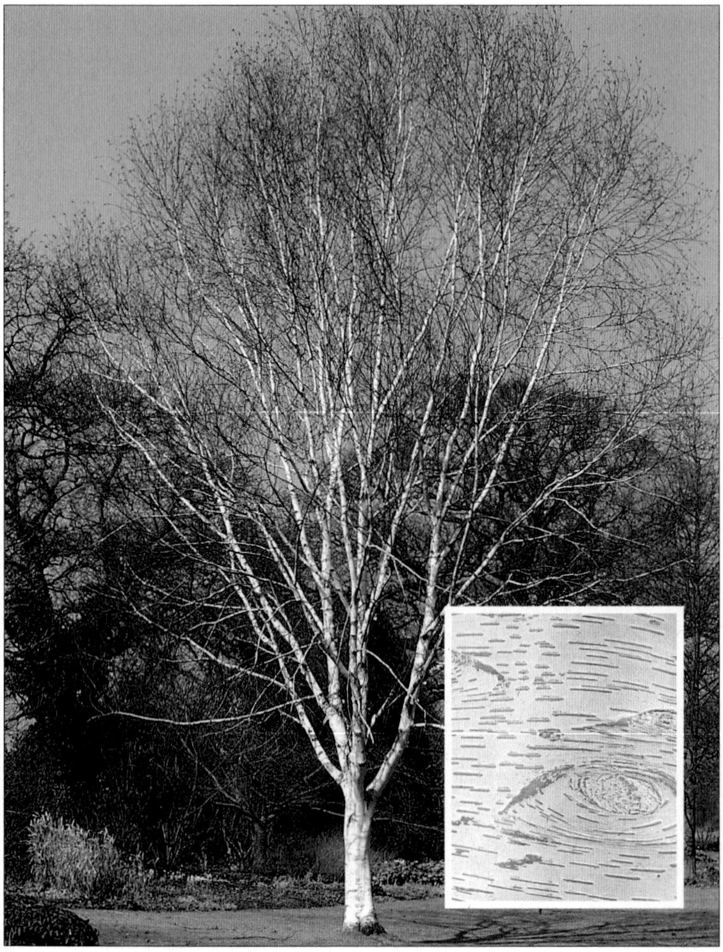

Betula utilis var. *jacquemontii* 'Silver Shadow' (inset: bark detail)

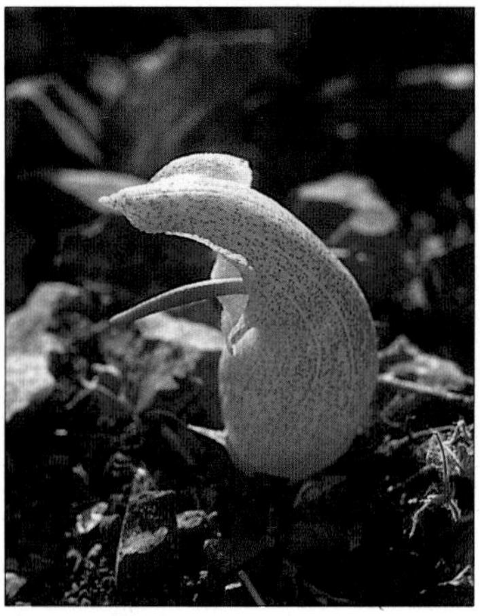

Biarum davisii

B. davisii ▣ Tuberous perennial producing open flask-shaped, sweet-scented, pink-spotted cream spathes, 5–6cm (2–2½in) long, enclosing slightly protruding, reddish brown spadices, in autumn. Spathes are followed by ovate, wavy-margined leaves, 7cm (3in) long. ↕ 7cm (3in), ↔ 5cm (2in). Crete, Turkey. ❄❄
B. eximium. Tuberous perennial bearing almost prostrate, recurved, deep purple spathes, 10–15cm (4–6in) long, revealing nearly black spadices, in autumn. Spathes are followed by narrowly ovate leaves, 17cm (7in) long. ↕ 8–10cm (3–4in), ↔ 5cm (2in). S. Turkey. ❄❄
B. tenuifolium. Tuberous perennial bearing narrow, often twisted, purple-flushed, pale green spathes, to 10cm (4in) long, and nearly black spadices, in autumn. Spathes are followed by lance-shaped to spoon-shaped leaves, 5–20cm (2–8in) long. ↕ 10–20cm (4–8in), ↔ 5cm (2in). Mediterranean. ❄❄❄

BIDENS

ASTERACEAE/COMPOSITAE

Genus of about 200 species of annuals, perennials, and deciduous shrubs occurring in grassland, wasteland, and among shrubs in Europe, tropical Africa, Asia, Australia, and temperate and tropical America. They have erect or spreading, opposite, simple or pinnate leaves, and flowerheads that are often terminal, or branched and cyme-like. Suitable for a container, hanging basket, gravel garden, or border. In frost-prone areas, grown as annuals.

• **HARDINESS** Fully hardy to frost tender.

• **CULTIVATION** Grow in reasonably fertile, moist but well-drained soil in full sun. Under glass, container plants will flower from mid-spring through to winter if grown in frost-free conditions.

• **PROPAGATION** Sow seed at 13–18°C (55–64°F) in spring. Root stem cuttings of perennials in spring or autumn, or divide when growth begins in spring.

• **PESTS AND DISEASES** Trouble free.

B. atrosanguinea see *Cosmos atrosanguineus.*
B. ferulifolia ▣ 🏆 Short-lived perennial, with 1- to 3-pinnate, fresh green leaves, to 8cm (3in) long, with lance-shaped leaflets. Slender, spreading stems produce daisy-like, golden yellow flowerheads, 3–4cm (1¼–1½in) across, from midsummer to autumn. ↕ to 30cm

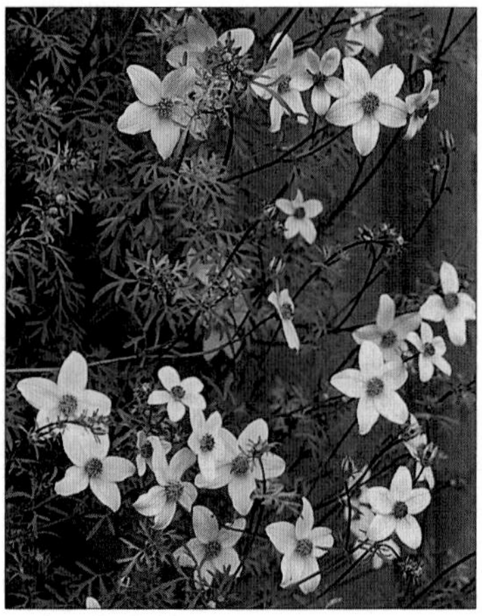

Bidens ferulifolia

(12in), ↔ indefinite. S. USA, Mexico. ❄❄. **'Golden Goddess'** has leaves with more slender segments and bears flowerheads 5cm (2in) across.

▷ **Bidi-bidi** see *Acaena*
▷ **Biennials** see pp.42–43

BIGNONIA *syn.* DOXANTHA

Cross vine

BIGNONIACEAE

Genus of one species of evergreen climber from moist forest in warm-temperate or tropical regions of North America. It is grown for its cymes of 2–5 trumpet-shaped flowers. Train against a wall or over a pergola or tree; in frost-prone areas, grow in a cool greenhouse.

• **HARDINESS** Half hardy; will survive light frost if against a sheltered wall.

• **CULTIVATION** Under glass, grow in loam-based potting compost (JI No.3) in full light with good ventilation. When in growth, water freely and apply a balanced liquid fertilizer monthly; water sparingly in winter. Pot on or top-dress in spring. Outdoors, grow in fertile, moist but well-drained soil in full sun. Pruning group 11, after flowering.

• **PROPAGATION** Sow seed at 18°C (64°F) in spring. Root leaf-bud cuttings in a propagating case with bottom heat in summer. Layer in autumn or spring.

• **PESTS AND DISEASES** Prey to mealy-bugs and red spider mites under glass.

B. capensis see *Tecoma capensis.*
B. capreolata, syn. *Doxantha capreolata.* Vigorous climber with opposite leaves, to 18cm (7in) long, usually consisting of 2 oblong-ovate to lance-shaped, wavy-margined leaflets and one tendril. Bears orange-red flowers, 4–5cm (1½–2in) long, in summer. ↕ 10m (30ft) or more. Canada (S. Ontario), E. USA. ❄
B. grandiflora see *Campsis grandiflora.*
B. jasminoides see *Pandorea jasminoides.*
B. pandorana see *Pandorea pandorana.*
B. radicans see *Campsis radicans.*
B. stans see *Tecoma stans.*
B. unguis-cati see *Macfadyena unguis-cati.*

▷ **Big tree** see *Sequoiadendron giganteum*
▷ **Bilberry** see *Vaccinium, V. myrtillus*
Dwarf see *V. caespitosum*
▷ ***Bilderdykia*** see *Fallopia*
B. aubertii see *F. aubertii*
B. baldschuanica see *F. baldschuanica*

BILLARDIERA

PITTOSPORACEAE

Genus of 8 species of evergreen, twining, perennial climbers occurring at forest margins and in moist to dry scrub in temperate to subtropical regions of Australia. They are cultivated for their usually bell-shaped, 5-petalled flowers, produced on the current year's growth, either singly or in small clusters in the upper leaf axils, and for their beautifully coloured berries. Leaves are alternate, small, entire, and often lance-shaped. In frost-prone areas, grow in a cool greenhouse or conservatory; elsewhere, grow over a pergola, against a house wall, or allow to scramble over vigorous shrubs.

• **HARDINESS** Frost hardy to half hardy; survive short spells at 0°C (32°F) in sheltered sites, but may lose some leaves.

• **CULTIVATION** Under glass, grow in lime-free (ericaceous) potting compost in bright filtered light. Water freely from spring to autumn, applying a balanced liquid fertilizer monthly; water sparingly in winter. Top-dress or pot on in late winter. Outdoors, grow in humus-rich, moist but well-drained, neutral to acid soil in a sunny or partially shaded, sheltered position. Pruning group 11; trim after flowering.

• **PROPAGATION** Sow seed at 13–15°C (55–59°F), ideally as soon as ripe in autumn, or in spring. Root softwood cuttings in early summer with bottom heat, or semi-ripe cuttings in late summer, both in a propagating case. Layer in autumn or spring.

• **PESTS AND DISEASES** Red spider mites may be troublesome under glass.

B. longiflora ▣ ♀ (Climbing blueberry, Purple apple berry). Slender, wiry-stemmed climber with linear-lance-shaped, deep green leaves, 1.5–4.5cm (½–1¾in) long. In summer, produces solitary, pendent, narrowly bell-shaped, pale green flowers, 2–3cm (¾–1¼in) long, followed by oblong-ovoid berries, 2cm (¾in) long, usually deep purple-blue, but sometimes purple, red, pink, or white. ↕ 2–3m (6–10ft). Australia (New South Wales to Tasmania). ❄❄

B. scandens (Common apple berry). Wiry-stemmed climber with ovate-lance-shaped, wavy-margined, deep green leaves, 1–5cm (½–2in) long. Solitary, bell-shaped, greenish yellow or violet to purple flowers, 1.5–2.5cm (½–1in) long, are produced mainly in late spring and early summer, followed by ellipsoid, olive-green berries, 2–3cm (¾–1¼in) long, which are occasionally flushed red. ↕ 2–5m (6–15ft). E. Australia. ❄

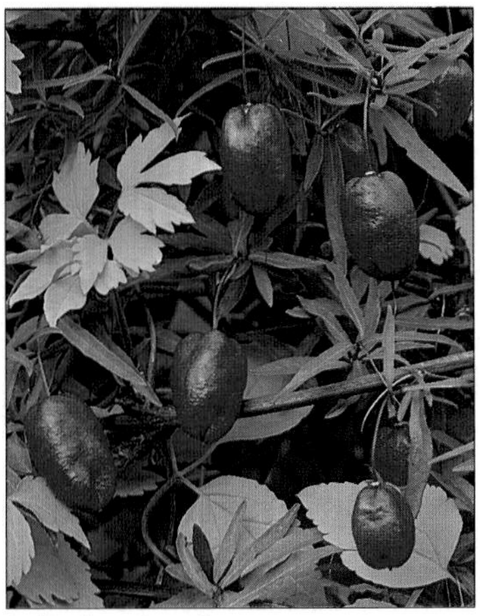

Billardiera longiflora

BILLBERGIA

BROMELIACEAE

Genus of about 60 species of rosette-forming, rhizomatous or suckering, evergreen, mainly epiphytic or rock-dwelling perennials (bromeliads) from scrub, woodland, and forest, up to an altitude of 1,700m (5,500ft), in S. Mexico, Central America, and N., E., and C. South America. They are cultivated for their erect or arching panicles or racemes of tubular, colourful but short-lived flowers. Many also have attractive leaves. In frost-prone areas, grow in a temperate greenhouse or as houseplants; in warm, humid areas, grow in a border.

• **HARDINESS** Frost hardy to frost tender.

• **CULTIVATION** Under glass, grow epiphytically or in containers of epiphytic bromeliad compost in bright indirect light. Keep the central funnel filled with fresh water. In growth, water freely and apply a well-balanced liquid fertilizer monthly; at other times, spray plants once a week with soft water. Outdoors, grow epiphytically or in humus-rich, sharply drained soil in partial shade. See also p.47.

• **PROPAGATION** Sow seed at 27°C (81°F) as soon as ripe. Root offsets in summer.

• **PESTS AND DISEASES** Scale insects may be troublesome.

B. amoena. Variable, rhizomatous bromeliad, generally epiphytic, with neat, tubular rosettes of 8–10 strap-shaped, mid-green, often white-spotted, sometimes red-flushed leaves, 30–60cm (12–24in) long. In summer, branched, arching, terminal inflorescences, 45cm (18in) long, with showy, deep red bracts, produce blue-tipped, green flowers, to 1.5cm (½in) long. ↕ to 60cm (24in), ↔ to 20cm (8in). E. Brazil. ❀ (min. 10°C/50°F)

B. distachia. Epiphytic bromeliad with short rhizomes and erect, cylindrical rosettes of 4 or 5 linear to lance-shaped, mid-green leaves, 25–90cm (10–36in) long, flushed purple, with short, widely spaced, marginal prickles. In summer, slightly arching panicles, 30cm (12in) long, bear short, lax branches of 7 or 8 green flowers, to 5cm (2in) long, with blue-tipped petals and sepals. ↕↔ 50cm (20in). E. Brazil. ❀ (min. 10°C/50°F)

***B.* Fantasia Group** ▣ ♀ (Marbled rainbow plant). Epiphytic bromeliads with urn-shaped rosettes of 6–8 narrowly lance-shaped, copper-green leaves, 30–45cm (12–18in) long, marbled creamy white and pink. Erect, white-felted, red-stalked inflorescences, to 40cm (16in) long, with red bracts, terminate in panicles, 12cm (5in) long, of violet-blue flowers, 6–8cm (2½–3in) long, in summer. ↕ 50cm (20in), ↔ 45cm (18in). ❀ (min. 10°C/50°F)

B. nutans ▣ (Friendship plant, Queen's tears). Variable, epiphytic bromeliad with short rhizomes and narrowly funnel-shaped rosettes of 12–15 linear or strap-shaped, pointed, sometimes red-flushed, grey-green leaves, to 70cm (28in) long, with smooth or finely toothed margins. In summer, slender, short-branched, red-bracted flower stems, to 15cm (6in) long, bear panicles, to 5cm (2in) long, of flowers with pale green petals margined blue and tipped darker green, and reflexed, rose-pink sepals with greenish blue margins. ↕ 50cm (20in), ↔ indefinite. S. Brazil, Paraguay, N. Argentina, Uruguay. ❄❄

B. porteana. Epiphytic bromeliad with short rhizomes and sturdy, tubular rosettes of 6–8 strap-shaped, grey-mottled, grey-green leaves, to 90cm (36in) long, with white cross-banding beneath and frequently spotted yellow. In summer, pendent, white-mealy racemes, to 40cm (16in) long, with papery red bracts, produce tubular, yellowish green flowers, 8cm (3in) long, with purple styles and stamens. ↕ 1m (3ft) or more, ↔ 50cm (20in). Brazil, Paraguay. ❀ (min. 10°C/50°F)

B. pyramidalis ▣ ♀ Epiphytic bromeliad with tubular rosettes of 5–13 strap-shaped, minutely toothed, fresh green leaves, to 50cm (20in) long. Dense panicles of erect, pale red flowers, 1.5–2cm (½–¾in) long, with reflexed blue tips, are borne terminally on white-mealy flower stems, to 12cm (5in) long, in summer. ↕ 50cm (20in), ↔ 25cm (10in). Brazil. ❀ (min. 10°C/50°F).

var. *concolor* has deeper red flowers without any blue coloration.

B. rhodocyanea see *Aechmea fasciata.*

B. vittata ♀ Epiphytic bromeliad with tubular rosettes of 8–10 lance- to strap-shaped, olive-green or grey-green leaves, 40–90cm (16–36in) or more long, with reflexed, spiny tips and grey cross-banding. In summer, narrowly pyramidal, pendent, red- or orange-bracted inflorescences, to 75cm (30in) long, bear 20 or more flowers, to 6cm (2½in) long, with orange sepals, white or pale green petals, and dark blue tips. ↕ to 1m (3ft), ↔ 40cm (16in). S.E. Brazil. ❀ (min. 10°C/50°F)

B.* x *windii ♀ (*B. decora* x *B. nutans*). Epiphytic bromeliad with broadly tubular rosettes of about 10 narrowly strap-shaped, toothed, white-mealy, mid-green leaves, to 70cm (28in) long, banded grey beneath. In summer, arching inflorescences, to 45cm (18in) long, produce numerous tuberous, red-margined, purple-tipped, green flowers, to 5cm (2in) long, among bright rose-pink bracts. ↕ 50cm (20in), ↔ 25cm (10in) or more. Garden origin. ❀ (min. 10°C/50°F)

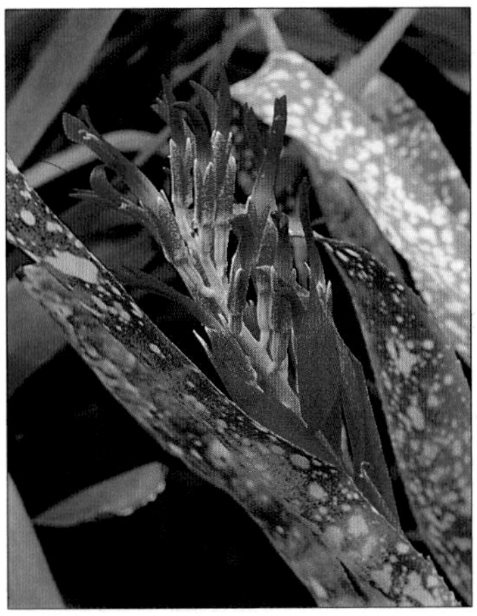

Billbergia Fantasia Group

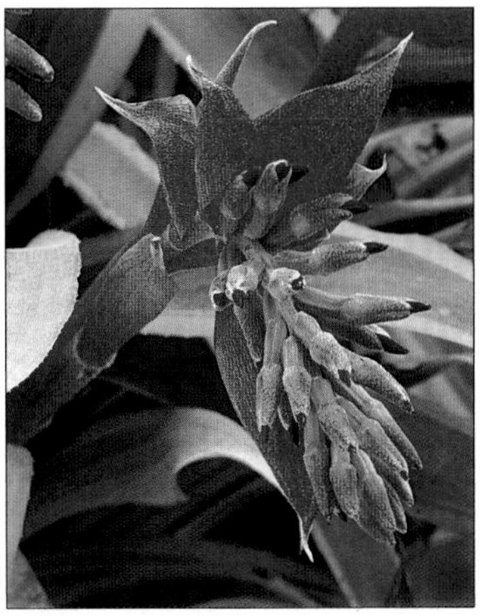

Billbergia pyramidalis

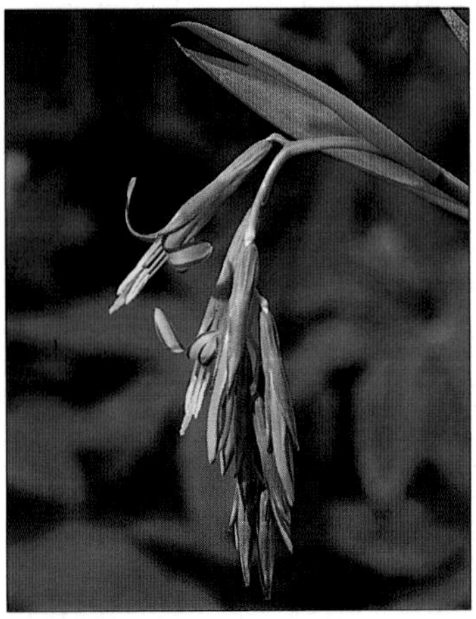

Billbergia nutans

▷ **Billy buttons** see *Craspedia*
▷ **Bindweed** see *Convolvulus*
▷ ***Biota orientalis*** see *Thuja orientalis*
▷ **Birch** see *Betula*
  Arctic see *B. nana*
  Black see *B. nigra*
  Canoe see *B. papyrifera*
  Cherry see *B. lenta*
  Chinese red see *B. albosinensis*
  Downy see *B. pubescens*
  Dwarf see *B. nana*
  Erman's see *B. ermanii*
  Grey see *B. populifolia*
  Himalayan see *B. utilis*
  Japanese cherry see *B. grossa*
  Monarch see *B. maximowicziana*
  Paper see *B. papyrifera*
  River see *B. nigra*
  Silver see *B. pendula*
  Sweet see *B. lenta*
  Szechuan see *B. szechuanica*
  Transcaucasian see *B. medwedewii*
  Yellow see *B. alleghaniensis*
  Young's weeping see *B. pendula* 'Youngii'
▷ **Bird catcher tree** see *Pisonia umbellifera*
▷ **Bird of paradise** see *Strelitzia*
▷ **Bird of paradise shrub** see *Caesalpinia gilliesii*
▷ **Bird's eye** see *Gilia tricolor*
▷ **Bird's eye bush** see *Ochna*
▷ **Bird's nest** see *Sansevieria trifasciata* 'Hahnii'
▷ **Birth root** see *Trillium erectum*
▷ **Birthwort** see *Aristolochia clematitis*
▷ **Bishop's cap** see *Astrophytum myriostigma, Mitella*
▷ **Bishop's mitre** see *Epimedium*
▷ **Bishop's wort** see *Stachys officinalis*

B

▷ **Bistort** see *Persicaria amplexicaulis, P. bistorta*
▷ ***Bistorta*** see *Persicaria*
B. amplexicaulis see *P. amplexicaulis*
▷ **Bittercress** see *Cardamine*
Trifoliate see *C. trifolia*
▷ **Bitternut** see *Carya cordiformis*
▷ **Bitterroot** see *Lewisia rediviva*
▷ **Bittersweet** see *Celastrus*
American see *C. scandens*
Climbing see *C. scandens*
Oriental see *C. orbiculatus*
▷ **Bitter vetch** see *Lathyrus linifolius* var. *montanus*
▷ **Bitterwort** see *Gentiana lutea*

BIXA

BIXACEAE

Genus of one species of evergreen tree from forest in tropical North and South America. It has alternate leaves and corymb-like panicles of dog-rose-like flowers, followed by bristly fruits. In frost-prone areas, grow *B. orellana* in a warm greenhouse or conservatory for its attractive fruit; in warmer climates, grow as a hedge or specimen tree, and for the seeds, which yield dye.

• **HARDINESS** Frost tender.
• **CULTIVATION** Under glass, grow in loam-based potting compost (JI No.3) in full light. Water freely in growth, sparingly in winter. Outdoors, grow in fertile, well-drained, humus-rich loam in full sun. Clip hedges in early spring before new growth begins. Pruning group 8 or 9 under glass; group 1 when grown outdoors as a tree.
• **PROPAGATION** Sow seed at 19–24°C (66–75°F) in spring, or root semi-ripe cuttings in summer.
• **PESTS AND DISEASES** Trouble free.

B. orellana ♀ (Achiote, Annatto, Lipstick tree). Intricately branched, evergreen tree with broad, ovate-heart-shaped, slender-pointed, smooth leaves, to 20cm (8in) long. From late summer to autumn, produces terminal panicles of 3–5 or more, open cup-shaped, 5-petalled, purple-tinted, white or pink flowers, to 5cm (2in) across, followed by ovoid, bristly, bright red or dark pink fruit, 5cm (2in) long, containing many dark red seeds. ↕ 7–10m (22–30ft), ↔ 3–5m (10–15ft), much less under glass. USA (Florida), West Indies, central and tropical South America. ❀ (min. 16–18°C/61–64°F)

▷ **Black-eyed Susan** see *Rudbeckia fulgida, R. hirta, Thunbergia alata*
▷ **Black pine,**
European see *Pinus nigra*
Japanese see *Pinus thunbergii*
▷ **Blackthorn** see *Prunus spinosa*
▷ **Blackwood** see *Acacia melanoxylon*
▷ **Bladdernut** see *Staphylea, S. pinnata*
▷ **Bladderpod** see *Physaria*
▷ **Bladderwort** see *Utricularia*

BLANDFORDIA

Christmas bells

BLANDFORDIACEAE/LILIACEAE

Genus of 4 species of rhizomatous perennials from swampy areas, acid heaths, and bogs on the Australian mainland and in Tasmania. They are cultivated for their racemes of showy, tubular flowers, produced in summer. The leaves are linear, sharp-pointed, and

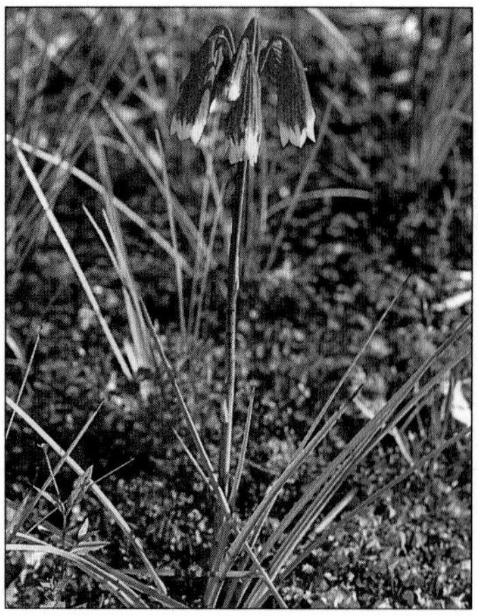

Blandfordia grandiflora

grey-green. In frost-prone areas, grow in a cool or temperate greenhouse. In frost-free areas, grow in a rock garden.

• **HARDINESS** Frost tender.
• **CULTIVATION** Under glass, plant rhizomes 5cm (2in) deep in autumn, in clay pots filled with lime-free (ericaceous) potting compost with additional sharp sand. Provide full light and good ventilation. When in growth, water moderately and apply a balanced liquid fertilizer monthly; keep dry during winter dormancy. Outdoors, grow in well-drained, humus-rich, acidic soil in full sun.
• **PROPAGATION** Sow seed at 13–16°C (55–61°F) in spring. Remove offsets after flowering.
• **PESTS AND DISEASES** Trouble free.

B. grandiflora ▣ Rhizomatous perennial with linear leaves, to 70cm (28in) long. In early summer, bears loose racemes of up to 10 red or red-and-yellow flowers, 4–6cm (1½–2½in) long. ↕ 60cm (24in), ↔ 15cm (6in). Australia. ❀ (min. 5°C/41°F)
B. punicea (Tasmanian Christmas bells). Rhizomatous perennial with linear leaves, to 35cm (14in) long. In summer, produces loose racemes of up to 25 flowers, 5cm (2in) long, pinkish red with yellow tips outside, yellow inside. ↕ 80–90cm (32–36in), ↔ 23cm (9in). Tasmania. ❀ (min. 5°C/41°F)

▷ **Blanket flower** see *Gaillardia, G. pulchella*
▷ **Blazing star** see *Liatris, Mentzelia lindleyi*

BLECHNUM

Hard fern

BLECHNACEAE

Genus of 150–200 species of usually evergreen, rhizomatous, terrestrial ferns found mostly in moist, sheltered, acid sites in temperate and tropical regions. The rhizomes are erect or creeping, often densely covered with black scales, and bear pinnate or pinnatifid, rarely simple, usually leathery fronds. Fertile fronds are generally erect, in the centres of the frond rosettes. Linear sori are arranged in 2 rows along the midrib of each frond lobe or segment. Some species form small "trunks". Grow in woodland, in a shady herbaceous border, or in a rock garden. In frost-prone areas, grow tender species in a warm greenhouse or conservatory.

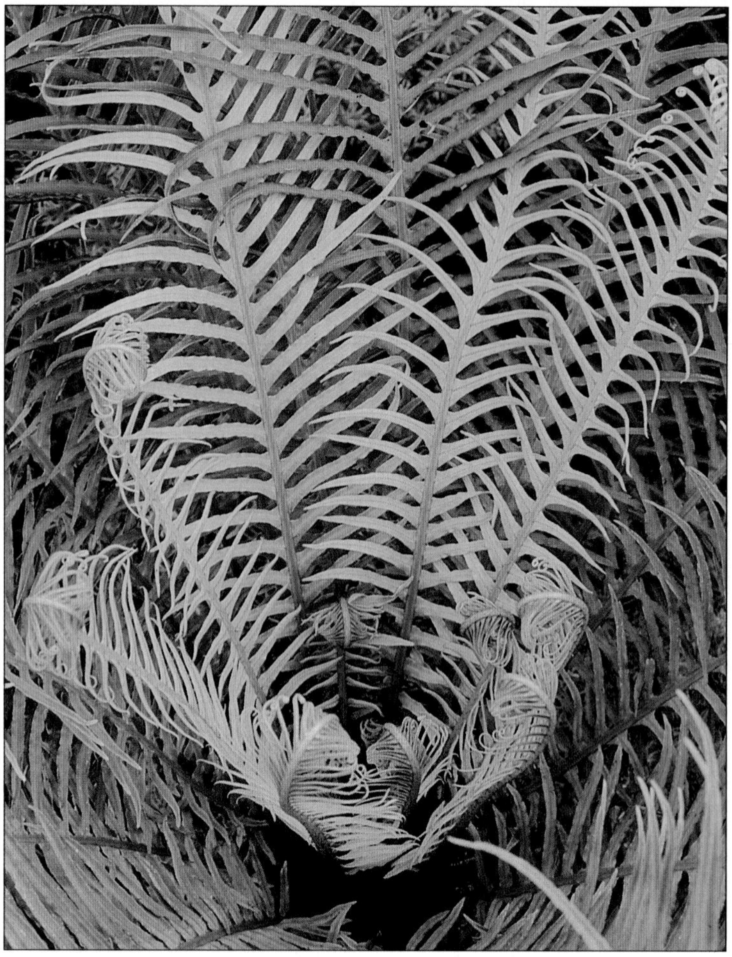

Blechnum gibbum

• **HARDINESS** Fully hardy to frost tender. *B. discolor* survives to -10°C (14°F) with some protection.
• **CULTIVATION** Under glass, grow in a mix of 1 part each lime-free loam, medium-grade bark, and charcoal, 2 parts sharp sand, and 3 parts coarse leaf mould. Provide bright filtered or indirect light, and moderate to high humidity with good ventilation. Fronds discolour if air circulation is poor and, in a dry atmosphere, they may scorch in full sun. Water freely when in growth, moderately in winter. Outdoors, grow in moist, humus-rich, acid soil in humid, partial or deep shade.
• **PROPAGATION** Sow spores in late summer. Divide *B. penna-marina* and *B. spicant* in spring; divisions of other species take some time to re-establish. See also p.51.
• **PESTS AND DISEASES** Trouble free.

B. alpinum see *B. penna-marina.*
B. brasiliense. Evergreen fern with upright, trunk-like rhizomes, to 30cm (12in) tall, and oblong-lance-shaped, pinnate, mid- to dark green fronds, 90cm (36in) tall, with finely toothed, linear pinnae. Fronds are reddish green when young. Similar to *B. gibbum,* but the fronds are narrower and the fertile fronds are similar to the sterile ones. ↕↔ 1–1.5m (3–5ft). Peru, Brazil. ❀ (min. 18°C/64°F)
B. chilense, syn. *B. cordatum, B. magellanicum.* Evergreen fern with a creeping rhizome, which may become erect and trunk-like. Ovate-lance-shaped, pinnate, dark green fronds, to 1m (3ft) long, have long, brown-scaly stalks. Sterile fronds have oblong, toothed pinnae; fertile ones have linear-lance-shaped pinnae. Often confused with *B. tabulare.* ↕ 0.9–1.8m (3–6ft), ↔ indefinite. Chile, Argentina. ✻✻✻
B. cordatum see *B. chilense.*
B. discolor (Crown fern). Evergreen fern with erect rhizomes, to 60cm (24in) tall, producing shuttlecocks of narrowly lance-shaped, lobed or pinnate to pinnatifid, glossy, dark green fronds, to 90cm (36in) long, in branching clusters. Sterile fronds have oblong pinnae and are whitish green beneath. Fertile fronds have ladder-like, narrow, linear pinnae, which are often wider and partially sterile towards the base of the fronds. Sometimes united with the closely related *B. nudum.* ↕↔ 0.3–1.2m (1–4ft). New Zealand. ✻✻

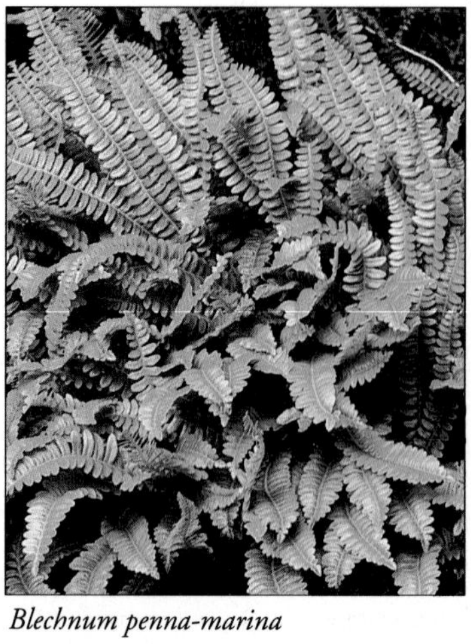

Blechnum penna-marina

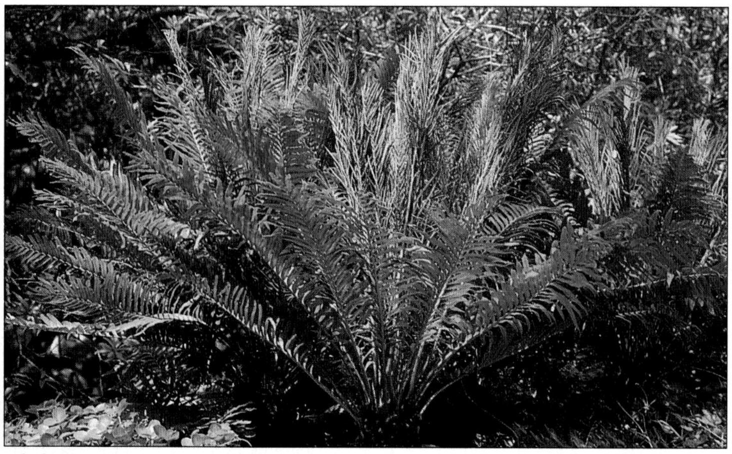

Blechnum tabulare

B. gibbum ■ syn. *Lomaria gibba.* Evergreen fern with upright, trunk-like rhizomes, to 90cm (36in) tall. Oblong-lance-shaped, pinnatisect, black-scaled, bright green fronds are usually 90cm (36in) long, but may reach 2m (6ft). Narrowly linear, entire lobes are erect, then spreading, each pair forming a V-shape along the frond. Sterile fronds have broader lobes than fertile ones. ↕↔ to 90cm (36in) or more. Fiji. ⊛ (min. 18°C/64°F)
B. magellanicum see *B. chilense.*
B. nudum. Evergreen fern with erect, occasionally trunk-like rhizomes, to 90cm (36in) tall, and lance-shaped-ovate, pinnate, mid- to dark green fronds. Sterile fronds are 40–100cm (16–39in) long, with narrowly linear pinnae. Fertile fronds are 20–70cm (8–28in) long, and are narrower, with more slender pinnae. Similar to *B. gibbum*, but pinnae are nearly perpendicular to the midribs. Sometimes united with the closely related *B. discolor.* ↕↔ to 1m (3ft). Australia. ✻✻
B. penna-marina ■ syn. *B. alpinum.* Evergreen fern with linear, pinnate or pinnatifid fronds arising in tufts from creeping rhizomes. Sterile fronds have oblong to triangular pinnae; fertile fronds have more widely spaced, narrowly linear to oblong pinnae. At least 2 variants are cultivated: one with glossy, dark green fronds, 20cm (8in) tall; the other smaller, 10–15cm (4–6in) tall, with matt, dark green fronds, which are reddish green when young. There is also a crested cultivar of the smaller form. ↕ 10–20cm (4–8in), ↔ indefinite. Australasia, S. South America. ✻✻✻
B. spicant ♀ (Hard fern). Evergreen fern with short, creeping rhizomes. Produces tufts of narrowly lance-shaped, pinnate, sometimes partly pinnatifid, dark green sterile fronds, 20–50cm (8–20in) long, with oblong pinnae. As they age, sterile fronds spread semi-horizontally to form a rosette around the taller fertile fronds; these are 30–60cm (12–24in) long, and have very narrowly linear, well separated pinnae. ↕ 20–50cm (8–20in), ↔ 60cm (24in) or more. Europe, N. Asia, North America. ✻✻✻
B. tabulare ■♀ Evergreen fern with erect rhizomes, to 60cm (24in) tall, and ovate, pinnate, dark green sterile fronds, 30–60cm (12–24in) long, with erect, then spreading, lance-shaped, paired pinnae, each pair forming a V-shape along the frond. Fertile fronds have linear, more closely set pinnae. ↕ to 1m (3ft), ↔ 60–120cm (2–4ft). South Africa, Madagascar, Australia, Falkland Islands, West Indies. ✻✻

▷**Bleeding heart** see *Dicentra spectabilis*
Wild see *D. formosa*

BLETILLA

ORCHIDACEAE

Genus of 9 or 10 species of deciduous, terrestrial orchids occurring in cool to temperate regions of China, Taiwan, and Japan. They have short rhizomes that develop corm-like pseudobulbs, partially underground, each pseudobulb producing 3 or 4 linear to obovate, folded leaves. Upright, terminal racemes of up to 12 narrowly bell-shaped flowers are borne from spring to early summer. Grow outdoors in a woodland garden, peat bed, or lath house, or, where temperatures fall below 0°C (32°F), in an alpine house or a cold greenhouse.
• **HARDINESS** Half hardy to frost tender.
• **CULTIVATION** Under glass, grow in loam-based potting compost (JI No.2) with added leaf mould, in bright filtered or bright indirect light. In summer, water freely, applying a quarter-strength balanced liquid fertilizer at every third watering. Keep dry in winter. Outdoors, grow in moist, well-drained, humus-rich soil in a sheltered site, with partial shade in summer. Mulch in winter, or lift and store dry and frost-free. See also p.46.
• **PROPAGATION** Divide in early spring.
• **PESTS AND DISEASES** Red spider mites, aphids, whiteflies, and mealybugs may be troublesome.

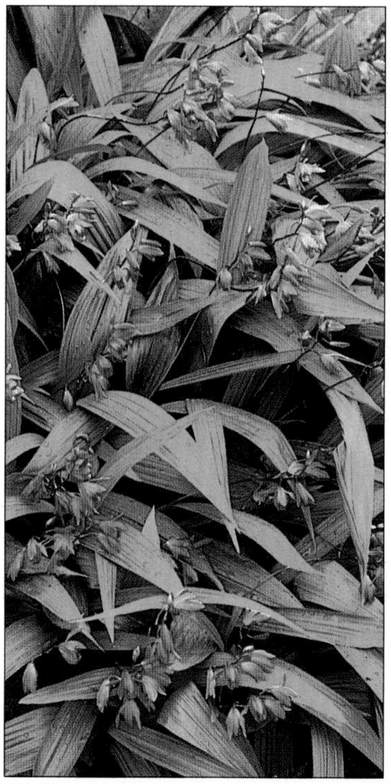

Bletilla striata

B. hyacinthina see *B. striata.*
B. striata ■ syn. *B. hyacinthina.* Terrestrial orchid with flattened pseudobulbs and oblong-lance-shaped leaves, 30–45cm (12–18in) long. Produces magenta flowers, 2.5cm (1in) across, from spring to early summer. ↕↔ 30–60cm (12–24in). China, Japan. ✻. **f. *alba*** has white flowers.

▷**Blood flower** see *Asclepias curassavica*
▷**Blood leaf** see *Iresine lindenii*
▷**Bloodroot** see *Sanguinaria*

BLOOMERIA

ALLIACEAE/LILIACEAE

Genus, related to *Allium* and *Brodiaea*, of 3 species of cormous perennials from scrub in North America. They have linear leaves with keeled tips and bear umbels of flattish, star-shaped flowers on leafless stems. Grow in a rock garden, on a raised bed, or in an alpine house.
• **HARDINESS** Frost hardy.
• **CULTIVATION** Plant corms 8cm (3in) deep in autumn in light, fertile, sandy soil in full sun or partial shade. Provide ample water while in growth; keep dry in summer after flowering. Excessive moisture encourages corms to rot. Under glass, grow in a mix of equal parts loam, leaf mould, and sharp sand.
• **PROPAGATION** Sow seed in containers in a cold frame as soon as ripe. Remove offsets in autumn.
• **PESTS AND DISEASES** Trouble free.

B. crocea. Cormous perennial with linear leaves, 10–15cm (4–6in) long, that die down at flowering time. In late spring and early summer, bears large, lax, spherical umbels of deep golden yellow flowers, 1.5–2cm (½–¾in) across, with a green or purple midrib on each tepal. ↕ 15–30cm (6–12in), ↔ 8cm (3in). USA (California). ✻✻

BLOSSFELDIA

CACTACEAE

Genus, closely related to *Parodia*, of one species of miniature, perennial cactus from rocky hills in semi-desert regions of the Bolivian and Argentinian Andes. It has tuberous rootstocks and flattened-spherical stems, which frequently offset to form cushions. Spineless areoles are scattered across the ribless stems and, in summer, those close to the crown produce funnel-shaped, diurnal flowers. These are followed by spherical fruits containing tiny, brownish red seeds. In frost-prone areas, grow *B. liliputana* in a temperate greenhouse. In frost-free areas, grow in a desert garden.
• **HARDINESS** Frost tender.
• **CULTIVATION** Under glass, grow in standard cactus compost in full light. When in growth, water moderately, applying half-strength, low-nitrogen fertilizer monthly; keep just moist from mid-autumn to early spring. Excess moisture may encourage root rot. Outdoors, grow in gritty, loamy soil in partial shade. See also pp.48–49.
• **PROPAGATION** Sow seed in early spring, or remove offsets in late spring or early summer; keep both at 21°C (70°F).
• **PESTS AND DISEASES** Susceptible to mealybugs.

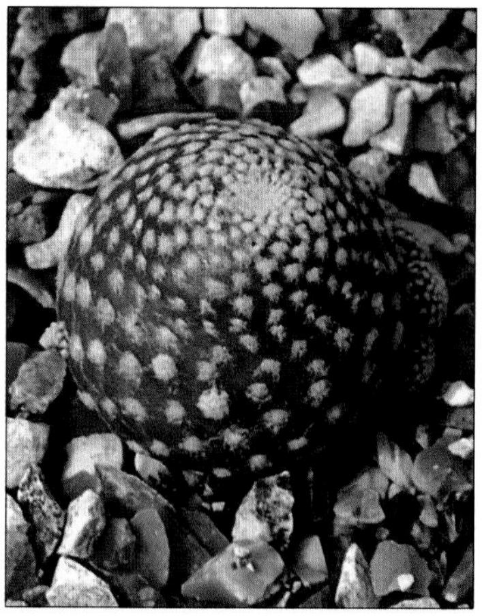

Blossfeldia liliputana

B. liliputana ■ syn. *Parodia liliputana.* Cushion-forming cactus with greyish or dark green stems, 2cm (¾in) high, and minute, woolly grey areoles. Produces open funnel-shaped, yellowish white flowers, 1cm (½in) across, in summer. ↕ 3–5cm (1¼–2in), ↔ to 6cm (2½in). Bolivia, Argentina. ⊛ (min. 17°C/63°F)

▷**Bluebell** see *Hyacinthoides*
Californian see *Phacelia campanularia*
English see *Hyacinthoides non-scripta*
New Zealand see *Wahlenbergia albomarginata*
Scottish see *Campanula rotundifolia*
Spanish see *Hyacinthoides hispanica*
Texan see *Eustoma grandiflorum*
▷**Bluebell creeper** see *Sollya heterophylla*
▷**Blue bells** see *Mertensia pulmonarioides*
▷**Blueberry** see *Vaccinium*
Box see *Vaccinium ovatum*
Climbing see *Billardiera longiflora*
Creeping see *Vaccinium crassifolium*
Highbush see *Vaccinium corymbosum*
Lowbush see *Vaccinium angustifolium* var. *laevifolium*
Swamp see *Vaccinium corymbosum*
▷**Blueblossom** see *Ceanothus thyrsiflorus*
Creeping see *C. thyrsiflorus* var. *repens*
▷**Bluebonnet, Texas** see *Lupinus texensis*
▷**Blue-bottle** see *Centaurea cyanus*
▷**Blue cohosh** see *Caulophyllum thalictroides*
▷**Blue-eyed Mary** see *Omphalodes verna*
▷**Blue-flowered torch** see *Tillandsia lindenii*
▷**Blue lace flower** see *Trachymene coerulea*
▷**Bluestem,**
Big see *Andropogon gerardii*
Little see *Schizachyrium scoparium*
▷**Bluets** see *Hedyotis*
Creeping *H. michauxii*
▷**Blushing bride** see *Serruria florida*
▷**Bobie-bobie** see *Phebalium squameum*
▷***Bocconia*** see *Macleaya*
B. cordata see *M. cordata*

B

B

BOENNINGHAUSENIA

RUTACEAE

Genus of one species of deciduous subshrub from woodland in the mountains of E. Asia. It is grown for its visually attractive, although unpleasantly scented leaves and its terminal panicles of small, delicate, 4-petalled flowers. Grow in a sheltered rock garden, in a shrub border, or against a warm wall.

- **HARDINESS** Frost hardy.
- **CULTIVATION** Grow in well-drained soil in full sun. In frost-prone areas, apply a deep winter mulch in autumn. Pruning group 6 in spring.
- **PROPAGATION** Sow seed in containers in a cold frame in autumn. Root softwood cuttings in summer.
- **PESTS AND DISEASES** Trouble free.

B. albiflora. Upright subshrub with alternate, 2- or 3-pinnate, dark green leaves, to 15cm (6in) long, consisting of 10–80 obovate leaflets. In late summer, produces cup-shaped, white or creamy white flowers, 1cm (½in) across, in panicles to 30cm (12in) long. ↕↔ 1m (3ft). Himalayas, China, Japan. ❄❄

▷**Boerboon, Weeping** see *Schotia brachypetala*
▷**Bogbean** see *Menyanthes trifoliata*
▷**Bog rosemary** see *Andromeda*
Common see *A. polifolia*
▷**Bog star** see *Parnassia*

BOLAX

APIACEAE/UMBELLIFERAE

Genus of 2 or 3 species of dense, cushion-forming, evergreen perennials, allied to *Azorella*, occurring in open, rocky areas of S. South America. They have tight rosettes of alternate, simple, very deeply 3-lobed leaves and umbels of insignificant, greenish white flowers. In the wild, they form large hummocks, to 60cm (24in) or more tall, by 1.2m (4ft) across, but seldom attain this size in cultivation. Grow as foliage plants in an alpine house, in a scree bed, or in tufa.

- **HARDINESS** Fully hardy.
- **CULTIVATION** Grow in any very sharply drained soil in full sun.
- **PROPAGATION** Sow seed (although seldom produced) in containers in a cold frame as soon as ripe. Remove and pot up offsets in spring.
- **PESTS AND DISEASES** Susceptible to red spider mites and aphids under glass.

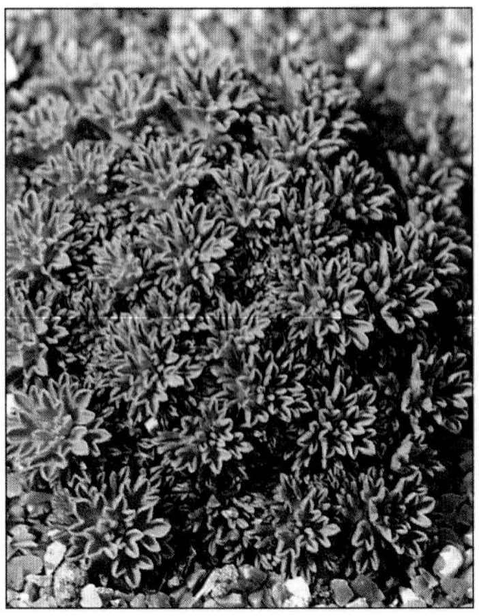

Bolax gummifera

B. glebaria see *B. gummifera.*
B. gummifera ■ syn. *Azorella glebaria, B. glebaria.* Slow-growing, compact perennial with rosettes of very deeply 3-lobed, leathery, dark blue-green leaves, to 6mm (¼in) long. The umbels, consisting of 3–20 tiny, greenish white flowers, borne in summer, are rarely produced. ↕ to 5cm (2in), sometimes to 15cm (6in), ↔ to 15cm (6in), sometimes to 25cm (10in). S. Chile, S. Argentina, Falkland Islands. ❄❄❄

BOLBITIS

LOMARIOPSIDACEAE

Genus of over 40 species of terrestrial, or almost scandent, epiphytic ferns usually found in flooded sites in tropical forest in Africa, Asia, and Central and South America. Creeping rhizomes produce entire and simple to pinnatifid or pinnate sterile fronds, often with plantlets near the tips. Fertile fronds are usually taller and narrower than sterile fronds, with black sporangia beneath. In frost-prone areas, they are best grown in the border of a warm greenhouse, to allow a free root run, but may also be grown in containers. In frost-free areas, grow in a bog garden or by a stream.

- **HARDINESS** Frost tender.
- **CULTIVATION** Under glass, grow in a mix of 1 part each of loam, medium-grade bark, and charcoal, 2 parts sharp sand, and 3 parts coarse leaf mould. Provide low light and high humidity. Water freely when in growth, sparingly in winter. Outdoors, grow in moist, humus-rich soil in partial or deep shade, in a sheltered, humid site.
- **PROPAGATION** Sow spores at 21°C (70°F) as soon as ripe. Root plantlets as soon as they appear. See also p.51.
- **PESTS AND DISEASES** Trouble free.

B. heteroclita ■ Variable, evergreen, rhizomatous, terrestrial or semi-epiphytic fern. Sterile, bright mid-green fronds, to 60cm (24in) or more long and usually elliptic, are simple, or pinnate with elliptic pinnae; most have a long, strongly developed, ovate-lance-shaped terminal segment, that produces a plantlet or roots down at the tip. Fertile fronds, 14–75cm (5½–30in) long, are usually pinnate, sometimes simple, with narrower pinnae than on sterile fronds; the lower surface is covered with felt-like sporangia. ↕ to 1m (3ft), ↔ 60cm (24in) or more. Tropical Asia. ⌂ (min. 16–21°C/61–70°F)

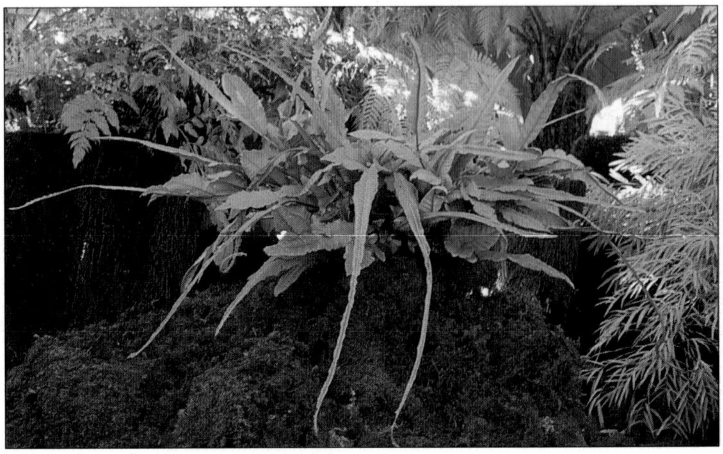

Bolbitis heteroclita

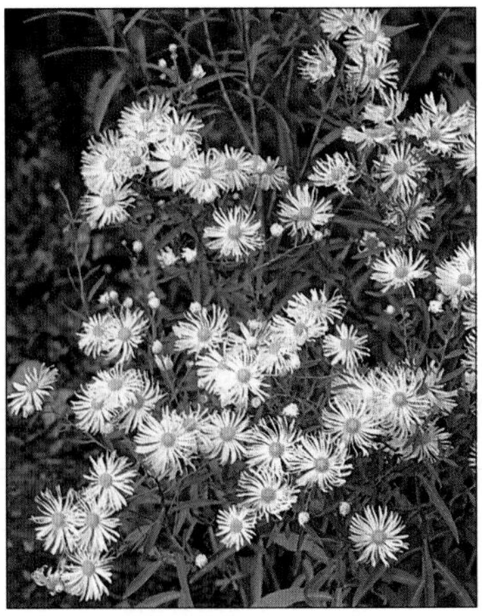

Boltonia asteroides

BOLTONIA

ASTERACEAE/COMPOSITAE

Genus of about 8 species of perennials from sunny, moist sites in North America. Erect, hairless stems branch towards the apex and bear alternate, inversely lance-shaped to lance-shaped, stalkless, sometimes finely toothed, blue-green or mid-green leaves. Small flowerheads of white, lilac, or pinkish purple ray-florets and yellow disc-florets are borne in panicles. Grow in a border or wild garden, or for cut flowers.

- **HARDINESS** Fully hardy.
- **CULTIVATION** Grow in fertile, moist but well-drained soil in full sun or partial shade. Divide every 2 or 3 years.
- **PROPAGATION** Sow seed in a cold frame in autumn. Divide in early spring.
- **PESTS AND DISEASES** Susceptible to mildew.

B. asteroides ■ Upright perennial with strong stems and inversely lance-shaped, finely toothed, slightly glaucous, blue-green leaves, 12cm (5in) long, becoming greener as they age. From late summer to mid-autumn, bears panicles, 10–15cm (4–6in) across, of flowerheads, 2cm (¾in) across, with white, lilac, or pinkish purple ray-florets. ↕ 2m (6ft), ↔ 1m (3ft). C. and E. USA. ❄❄❄. **var. *latisquama***, syn. *B. latisquama*, has flowerheads 2–3cm (¾–1¼in) across, with deep lilac-purple or white ray-florets. **'Snowbank'** has pure white ray-florets; ↕ to 1.5m (5ft).
B. latisquama see *B. asteroides* var. *latisquama.*

BOLUSANTHUS

South African wisteria

LEGUMINOSAE/PAPILIONACEAE

Genus of one species of deciduous tree from scrub and forest in Africa, grown mainly for its clustered racemes of brightly coloured, pea-like flowers. The alternate, pinnate leaves unfold after the flowers open. In frost-prone areas, grow *B. speciosus* in a cool greenhouse; it rarely flowers well in a container. In warmer regions, use as a specimen tree.

- **HARDINESS** Frost tender, but may survive short spells at 0°C (32°F).
- **CULTIVATION** Under glass, grow in loam-based potting compost (JI No.2) in full light. In growth, water moderately and apply balanced liquid fertilizer monthly; keep just moist in winter. Top-dress in late winter. Outdoors, grow in moderately fertile, well-drained soil in full sun. Pruning group 1.
- **PROPAGATION** Sow seed at 13–16°C (55–61°F) in spring.
- **PESTS AND DISEASES** Red spider mites may be troublesome under glass.

B. speciosus ♀ (Elephantwood). Spreading tree, briefly deciduous from late winter to spring, with silky-hairy, yellow-green leaves, to 15cm (6in) long, composed of 7–15 ovate-lance-shaped leaflets, maturing to glossy, pale green. Blue-violet flowers, 2cm (¾in) long, open in clustered racemes, to 25cm (10in) long, from late winter to spring. ↕ 4–6m (12–20ft), ↔ 2.5–4m (8–12ft). Angola, Zimbabwe, Mozambique, South Africa. ⌂ (min. 5°C/41°F)

BOMAREA

ALSTROEMERIACEAE/LILIACEAE

Genus of about 120 species of tuberous-rooted, usually deciduous, rarely semi-evergreen, twining and scandent climbers from scrub and forest margins in Mexico and South America. Leaves are alternate or spiralling, simple, and generally narrow. Tubular to bell-shaped, 6-tepalled flowers are borne in showy, terminal racemes or umbels. In frost-prone areas, grow in a cool greenhouse; elsewhere, use to clothe a pergola, arbour, or house wall. The naming of cultivated species is confused.

- **HARDINESS** Frost hardy to frost tender.
- **CULTIVATION** Under glass, grow in loam-based potting compost (JI No.3) with added sharp sand, in full light with shade from hot sun. Provide support. When in growth, water freely and apply a balanced liquid fertilizer monthly; keep just moist in winter. Pot on or top-dress in early spring. Outdoors, grow in fertile, moist but well-drained soil in full sun. Cut back dead growth and flowered stems to ground level in winter.
- **PROPAGATION** Sow seed at 13–16°C (55–61°F) in spring. Divide established plants in late winter or in early spring as growth begins.
- **PESTS AND DISEASES** Prey to red spider mites, whiteflies, and aphids under glass.

B. andimarcana, syn. *B. pubigera* of gardens. Scandent, erect, deciduous climber with lance-shaped, white-downy leaves, 5–12cm (2–5in) long, which appear almost grey. Umbels of up to 10

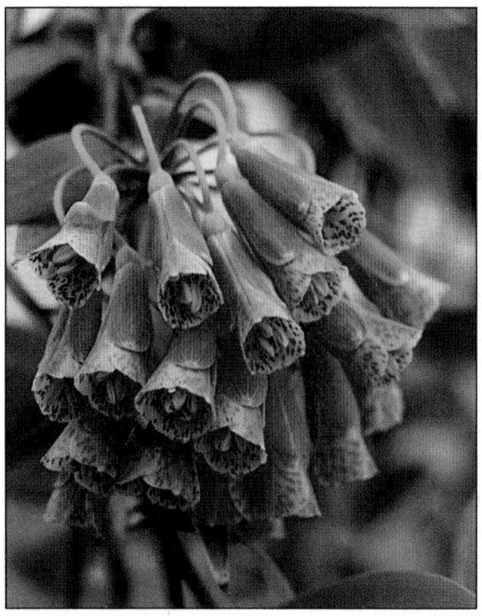
Bomarea caldasii

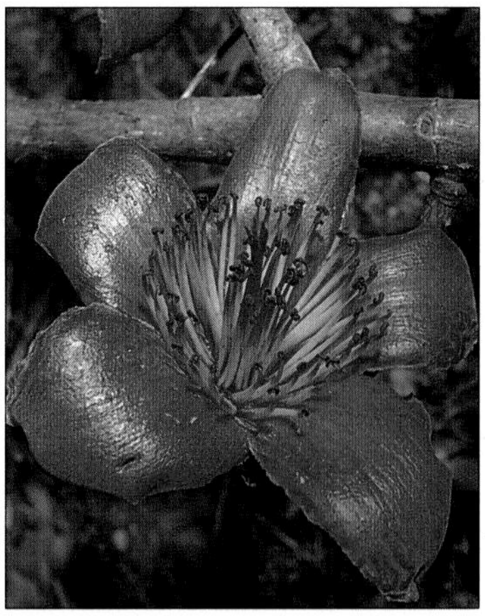
Bombax ceiba

pendent, tubular, pale yellow flowers, 4–5cm (1½–2in) long, suffused with light red and tipped with soft green, are produced intermittently from spring to autumn. ↕2–3m (6–10ft). Peru. ❄❄

B. caldasii ▣ 🍸 syn. *B. kalbreyeri* of gardens. Erect, deciduous, twining climber with narrowly oblong, light to mid-green leaves, 7–15cm (3–6in) long. From late spring to autumn, bears almost spherical umbels of 40 or more narrowly funnel-shaped flowers, 4–5cm (1½–2in) long, brick-red to orange on the outside, orange to yellow inside, spotted red, brown, or green. ↕3–4m (10–12ft). Colombia to Ecuador. ❄

B. edulis. Erect, deciduous, twining climber with lance-shaped, mid- to pale green leaves, 6–12cm (2½–5in) long, sometimes finely downy beneath. Loosely rounded umbels of 16–30 narrowly bell-shaped flowers, to 3.5cm (1½in) long, pink to light red on the outside, yellowish green flecked red inside, are produced from early summer to autumn. ↕2–3m (6–10ft). Mexico to Cuba, Peru. ❄❄ (borderline)

***B. kalbreyeri* of gardens** see *B. caldasii.*

***B. patacocensis* of gardens** see *B. racemosa.*

***B. pubigera* of gardens** see *B. andimarcana.*

B. racemosa, syn. *B. patacocensis* of gardens. Erect, red-stemmed, deciduous, twining climber with oblong-lance-shaped, mid-green leaves, to 13cm (5in) long, slightly hairy beneath. In summer, bears racemes of 40 or more narrowly bell-shaped, yellow-based, brown-spotted scarlet flowers, to 6cm (2½in) long. ↕3–5m (10–15ft). Colombia. ❄

BOMBAX

Silk cotton tree

BOMBACACEAE

Genus of 8 species of large, deciduous trees from moist tropical forest in Africa, Asia, and Australia. Alternate, fully divided, 3- to 7-palmate leaves, with stalked leaflets, unfold after the solitary, 5-petalled flowers open in spring. Oblong-ovoid fruit capsules, 15cm (6in) long, split to reveal silky seeds. In frost-prone areas, grow as foliage plants in a warm greenhouse (they seldom flower under glass). In warmer climates, grow as specimen trees and to provide shade.

- **HARDINESS** Frost tender.
- **CULTIVATION** Under glass, grow in loam-based potting compost (JI No.3) in full light. From spring to summer, water freely and apply a balanced liquid fertilizer monthly; keep almost dry while leafless. Outdoors, grow in humus-rich, fertile soil in full sun, with plenty of moisture in the growing season. Pruning group 1; will tolerate hard pruning to restrict size under glass.
- **PROPAGATION** Sow seed at 21–25°C (70–77°F) in spring. Root semi-ripe cuttings in summer with bottom heat.
- **PESTS AND DISEASES** Red spider mites may be a problem under glass.

B. ceiba ▣ ♀ syn. *B. malabaricum* (Red silk cotton tree). Erect to spreading tree with a spiny trunk when young and buttresses when mature. Rounded leaves, 30–50cm (12–20in) across, are divided into 3–7 obovate to lance-shaped leaflets. In spring, bears bright red flowers, 15cm (6in) across, with oblong-obovate, recurved, fleshy petals, each bloom with a dome-like brush of yellow-anthered stamens with pink filaments. ↕to 25m (80ft), ↔ 12–15m (40–50ft). India to S.E. Asia, N. Australia. ❀ (min. 13°C/55°F)

B. malabaricum see *B. ceiba.*

BONGARDIA

BERBERIDACEAE

Genus of one species of tuberous perennial found in dry uplands from Greece and Turkey to Pakistan. It is grown for its curious, spreading, pinnate leaves and its sprays of 5-petalled yellow flowers. *B. chrysogonum* may be grown in a warm site in a rock garden and is also suitable for cultivation in a bulb frame or alpine house.

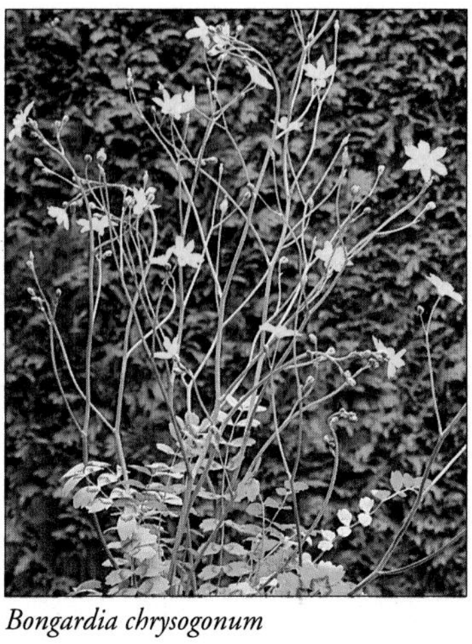
Bongardia chrysogonum

- **HARDINESS** Frost hardy.
- **CULTIVATION** Plant tubers 10–15cm (4–6in) deep in autumn in sharply drained, sandy soil in full sun. Water sparingly while in growth, and keep warm and dry when dormant. Tubers rot easily in wet conditions.
- **PROPAGATION** Sow seed in containers in a cold frame as soon as ripe.
- **PESTS AND DISEASES** Trouble free.

B. chrysogonum ▣ Tuberous perennial with pinnate, red-zoned, mid-green leaves, to 20cm (8in) long, with obovate or wedge-shaped leaflets. Bears open-branched inflorescences of star-shaped yellow flowers, 1.5cm (½in) across, in spring. ↕20–50cm (8–20in), ↔ 15cm (6in). Greece, Turkey, C. Asia, Afghanistan, Pakistan. ❄❄

▷ ***Bonifazia quezalteca*** see *Disocactus quezaltecus*

▷ **Boojum tree** see *Fouquieria columnaris*

▷ **Borage** see *Borago officinalis*

BORAGO

BORAGINACEAE

Genus of 3 species of annuals and perennials from rocky places in W., C., and E. Europe, and the Mediterranean. They have hairy stems and simple, alternate, roughly hairy leaves. Nodding blue flowers are produced in branching cymes. *B. officinalis* is a useful plant for dry places. *B. pygmaea* grows well in gravel or in a rock garden. Both species self-seed freely.

- **HARDINESS** Fully hardy to frost hardy.
- **CULTIVATION** Grow *B. officinalis* in any reasonably drained soil in full sun or partial shade. Grow *B. pygmaea* in moist soil in partial shade.
- **PROPAGATION** Sow seed *in situ* in spring. Divide *B. pygmaea* in spring, or root cuttings of young sideshoots in summer, overwintering in a cold frame.
- **PESTS AND DISEASES** Susceptible to powdery mildew.

B. laxiflora see *B. pygmaea.*

B. officinalis ▣ (Borage). Robust, freely branching annual with lance-shaped to ovate, bristly, dull basal leaves and stalkless, lance-shaped stem leaves, to 15cm (6in) long. Branched cymes of 5-petalled, star-shaped, bright blue flowers, to 2.5cm (1in) across, are borne over a long period in summer. ↕60cm (24in), ↔ 45cm (18in). Europe. ❄❄❄.

f. *alba* bears white flowers.

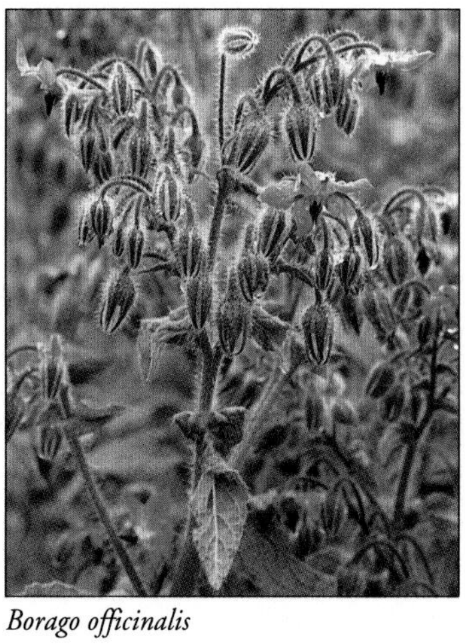
Borago officinalis

B. pygmaea, syn. *B. laxiflora.* Short-lived, rosette-forming perennial with ovate to lance-shaped, mainly basal leaves, 5–20cm (2–8in) long, and branched, decumbent stems. Loose cymes of bell-shaped, clear pale blue flowers, 9–15mm (⅜–½in) across, are produced from early summer to early autumn. ↕↔ to 60cm (24in). Corsica, Sardinia. ❄❄❄ (borderline)

B

BORASSUS

ARECACEAE / PALMAE

Genus of 7 species of robust, single-stemmed palms occurring in forest and near rivers in Africa, Madagascar, Saudi Arabia, Kuwait to S.E. Asia, the Malaysian islands, New Guinea, and Australia. Fan-like leaves are arranged in dense, terminal heads, and panicles of 3-petalled flowers develop among them. In frost-prone areas, grow young plants for their foliage in a warm greenhouse. In frost-free areas, use as specimen trees.

- **HARDINESS** Frost tender.
- **CULTIVATION** Under glass, grow in loamless potting compost in full light with shade from hot sun. In full growth, water freely and apply a balanced liquid fertilizer monthly; water sparingly in winter. Outdoors, grow in fertile, moist but well-drained soil in full sun, with some midday shade when young.
- **PROPAGATION** Sow seed at 24–29°C (75–84°F) in spring.
- **PESTS AND DISEASES** Red spider mites may be a problem under glass.

B. flabellifer ▣ 🌴 (Palmyra palm, Toddy palm, Wine palm). Tall palm

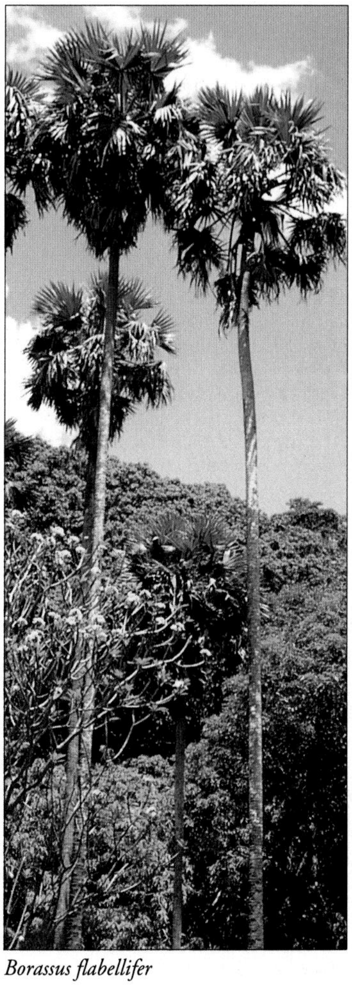
Borassus flabellifer

with a sturdy, mast-like stem, swollen at the base and often also about halfway up. Rounded to fan-shaped leaves, 2.5–3m (8–10ft) across, are composed of up to 80 slender, pointed, folded, rich green lobes. Bears cream flowers in panicles, to 1.5m (5ft) long, in spring or summer. ↕ to 20m (70ft), ↔ 5–6m (15–20ft). India, Sri Lanka, S.E. Asia, Malaysian islands, New Guinea. ❀ (min. 15–18°C/59–64°F)

BORONIA

RUTACEAE

Genus of about 95 species of evergreen shrubs from Australia, occurring on sandy heaths in scrub and light woodland. They are valued for their 4-petalled, cup- or bell-shaped, sometimes fragrant flowers, borne singly or in cymes or umbels. The opposite, lance-shaped to ovate, simple or compound leaves are often aromatic. In frost-prone areas, grow in a cool greenhouse and move outdoors during frost-free periods. In frost-free areas, grow in a border.

• **HARDINESS** Half hardy to frost tender; *B. megastigma* may survive short periods of light frost.

• **CULTIVATION** Under glass, grow in lime-free (ericaceous) potting compost in full light with shade from hot sun. Provide good ventilation. When in growth, water moderately, applying phosphate-free liquid fertilizer monthly; water sparingly in winter. Pot on or top-dress in early spring. Outdoors, grow in moist but well-drained, ideally sandy, neutral to acid soil in full sun or partial shade. *B. serrulata* prefers dappled shade; if grown in full sun, provide a cool root run. Pruning group 10, after flowering.

• **PROPAGATION** Sow seed at 16°C (61°F) in spring. Root semi-ripe cuttings in a propagating case with bottom heat in summer.

• **PESTS AND DISEASES** Red spider mites may be a problem under glass.

B. megastigma ▣ (Brown boronia, Scented boronia). Erect, dense shrub with aromatic leaves, 2cm (¾in) long, composed of 3, rarely 5, linear, soft-textured, mid- to deep green leaflets. Solitary, fragrant, pendent, bell-shaped flowers, 1cm (½in) wide, yellow-green to dark or reddish brown outside, yellow to yellow-green inside, are borne from the upper leaf axils in spring. ↕ 1–3m (3–10ft), ↔ 1–2m (3–6ft). Australia (Western Australia). ✲ (borderline).

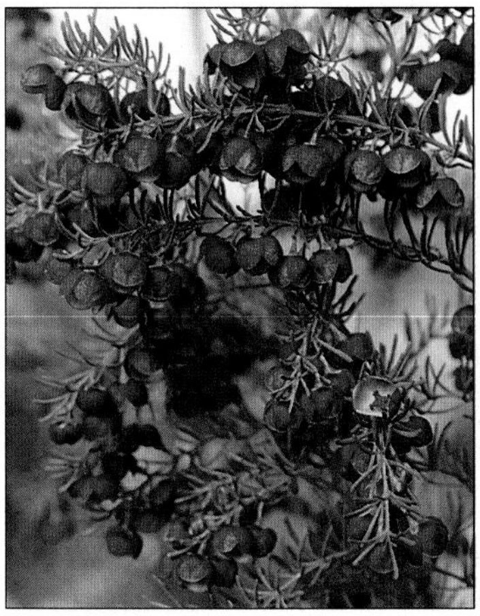

Boronia megastigma

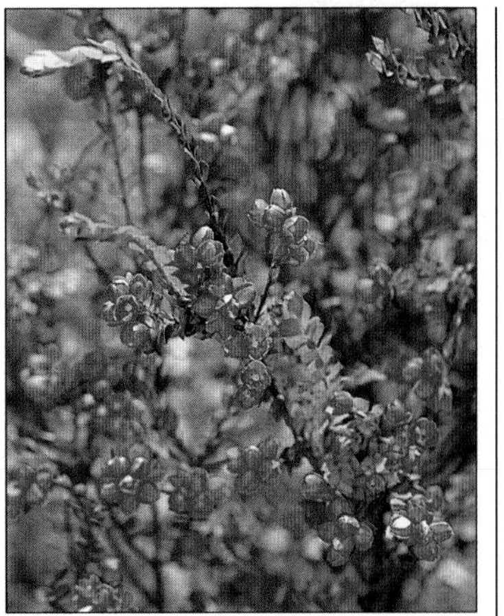

Boronia serrulata

'Heaven Scent' has strongly scented, chocolate-brown flowers. **'Lutea'** has strongly scented, clear greenish yellow flowers.

B. serrulata ▣ (Sydney rock rose). Bushy, erect then spreading shrub with broadly ovate, simple, finely toothed, aromatic, rich green leaves, 2cm (¾in) long. From late winter to summer, bears usually profuse, dense, terminal cymes of bell-shaped, fragrant, rich purplish pink or occasionally white flowers, to 1.5cm (½in) across. ↕ 45–90cm (18–36in), ↔ 1–1.5m (3–5ft). Australia (New South Wales). ❀ (min. 5°C/41°F)

▷ **Boronia,**
  Brown see *Boronia megastigma*
  Scented see *Boronia megastigma*
▷ ***Borzicactus*** see *Oreocereus*
  B. aurantiacus see *O. aurantiacus*
  B. celsianus see *O. celsianus*
  B. haynei see *O. haynei*
  B. leucotrichus see *O. hempelianus*
▷ ***Bothriochilus*** see *Coelia*
  B. bellus see *C. bella*

BOTHRIOCHLOA

GRAMINEAE/POACEAE

Genus of 30–40 species of spreading to erect, perennial grasses occurring in grassland in warm-temperate and tropical regions. The leaves are erect and lance-shaped, and the distinctive, finger-like, upright or ascending racemes vary from rich reddish purple to silver-grey. Suitable for a border. In frost-prone regions, grow as half-hardy annuals.

• **HARDINESS** Frost hardy to frost tender.

• **CULTIVATION** Grow in medium to light, well-drained soil in full sun.

• **PROPAGATION** Sow seed in containers in a cold frame in spring. Divide from mid-spring to early summer.

• **PESTS AND DISEASES** Trouble free.

B. saccharoides (Silver beard grass). Tufted grass with upright then arching, lance-shaped, silver- or blue-grey leaves, to 1.2m (4ft) long. Produces softly hairy, silver-grey inflorescences, 15cm (6in) long, in dense, finger-like racemes in late summer and early autumn. ↕ to 1.2m (4ft), ↔ 60cm (24in). North America to Brazil. ✲✲

▷ **Bo tree** see *Ficus religiosa*
▷ **Bottlebrush** see *Callistemon*
  Albany see *Callistemon speciosus*
  Alpine see *Callistemon pityoides, C. sieberi*

▷ **Bottlebrush cont.**
  Crimson see *Callistemon citrinus*
  Granite see *Melaleuca elliptica*
  Green see *Callistemon viridiflorus*
  Lemon see *Callistemon pallidus*
  Narrow-leaved see *Callistemon linearis*
  Natal see *Greyia sutherlandii*
  Pine see *Callistemon pinifolius*
  Scarlet see *Callistemon macropunctatus*
  Stiff see *Callistemon rigidus*
  Swamp see *Beaufortia sparsa*
  Tonghi see *Callistemon subulatus*
  Weeping see *Callistemon viminalis*
  White see *Callistemon salignus*
  Willow see *Callistemon salignus*
▷ **Bottletree** see *Brachychiton*

BOUGAINVILLEA

NYCTAGINACEAE

Genus of 14 species of evergreen shrubs and trees, and evergreen or partly deciduous, sometimes thorny climbers, from forest and thickets in tropical and subtropical South America. They are grown for their small, tubular flowers, each surrounded by 3 colourful, petal-like bracts, borne in large, axillary and terminal clusters. The alternate leaves are mainly ovate, slender-pointed, and entire. In frost-prone areas, grow in a temperate greenhouse; elsewhere, use on a pergola, arbour, arch, or a house wall.

• **HARDINESS** Half hardy to frost tender. *B.* x *buttiana*, *B. glabra*, and *B. spectabilis* may survive short spells down to 0°C (32°F) if kept fairly dry in winter; some leaves may be lost.

• **CULTIVATION** Under glass, grow in loam-based potting compost (JI No.3) in full light. From spring to autumn, water freely and apply a balanced liquid fertilizer monthly; keep just moist in winter. Pot on or top-dress in late winter. Outdoors, grow in fertile, well-drained soil in full sun. Pruning group 12: *B.* x *buttiana* and *B. glabra* in early spring; *B. spectabilis* after flowering.

• **PROPAGATION** Root softwood cuttings in early spring, or semi-ripe cuttings in summer, using a propagating case with bottom heat in frost-prone climates. In frost-free areas, root hardwood cuttings *in situ* in autumn. Layer in early autumn or spring.

• **PESTS AND DISEASES** Red spider mites, mealybugs, aphids, and whiteflies may be a problem under glass.

***B.* 'Ailsa Lambe'** see *B.* 'Mary Palmer'.
B.* x *buttiana (*B. glabra* x *B. peruviana*). Vigorous, evergreen climber with ovate, mid-green leaves, to 8cm (3in) long, lighter below. Large clusters of strongly waved floral bracts, 3–5cm (1¼–2in) long, in shades of golden yellow, purple, or red, are produced mainly from summer to autumn. ↕ 8–12m (25–40ft). Garden origin. ✲ (borderline). **'Apple Blossom'** see 'Audrey Grey'. **'Audrey Grey'**, syn. 'Apple Blossom', 'Jamaica White', has large, rounded, dark green leaves, to 13cm (5in) long, and white bracts with pink-flushed margins. **'Bridal Bouquet'** see 'Mahara Off-White'. **'California Gold'** see 'Golden Glow'. **'Crimson Lake'** see 'Mrs. Butt'. **'Golden Glow'**, syn. 'California Gold', 'Hawaiian Gold', has rich gold to pale yellow bracts. **'Hawaiian Gold'** see 'Golden Glow'. **'Jamaica White'** see

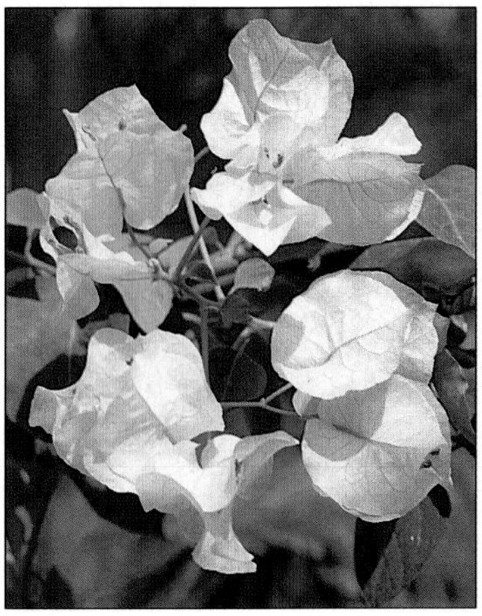

Bougainvillea glabra 'Snow White'

'Audrey Grey'. **'Limberlost Beauty'** see 'Mahara Off-White'. **'Mahara Off-White'**, syn. 'Bridal Bouquet', 'Limberlost Beauty', 'Tahitian Pink', has double, magenta-tipped white bracts. **'Mrs. Butt'** 🏆 syn. 'Crimson Lake', has crimson-shaded magenta bracts. **'Purple King'** see 'Texas Dawn'. **'Robyn's Glory'** see 'Texas Dawn'. **'Tahitian Pink'** see 'Mahara Off-White'. **'Texas Dawn'**, syn. 'Purple King', 'Robyn's Glory', is a sport of 'Mrs. Butt', with light purplish pink bracts and long, stout thorns.

B. glabra 🏆 Strong-growing, evergreen climber with elliptic, semi-glossy, mid- to deep green leaves, to 13cm (5in) long. Slightly wavy, white to magenta floral bracts, 4–6cm (1½–2½in) long, are borne mainly from summer to autumn. ↕ 5–8m (15–25ft). Brazil. ✲ (borderline). **'Sanderiana'** see 'Variegata'. **'Snow White'** ▣ has white bracts. **'Variegata'** ▣ syn. 'Sanderiana', has greyish green leaves margined with creamy white, and bright purple bracts.

***B.* 'Hawaiian Scarlet'** see *B.* 'Scarlett O'Hara'.

***B.* 'Helen Johnson'** see *B.* 'Temple Fire'.

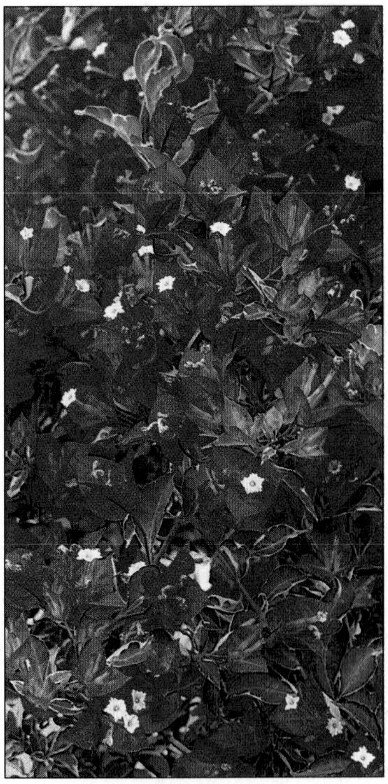

Bougainvillea glabra 'Variegata'

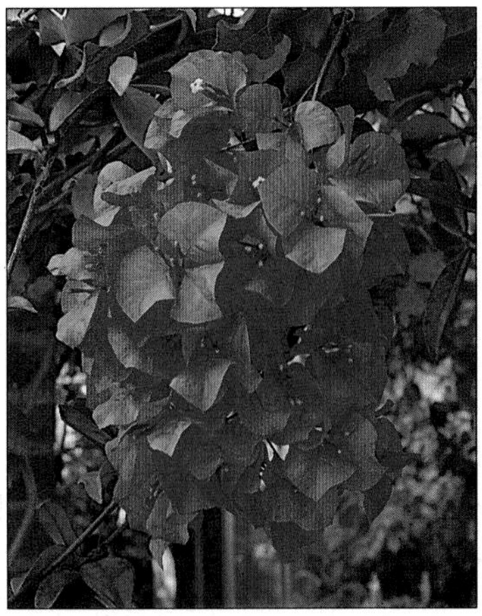

Bougainvillea 'Miss Manilla'

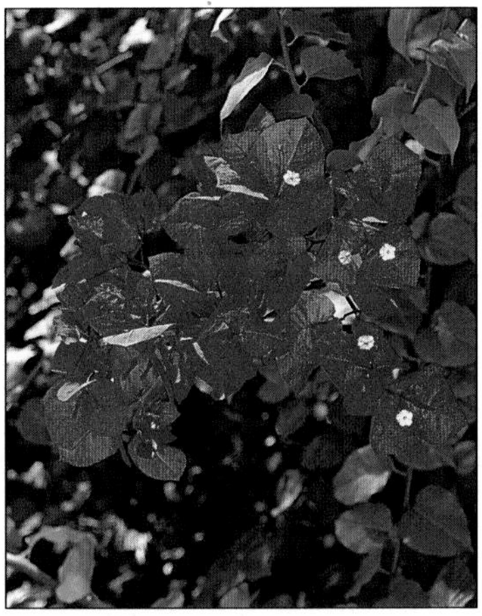

Bougainvillea 'Scarlett O'Hara'

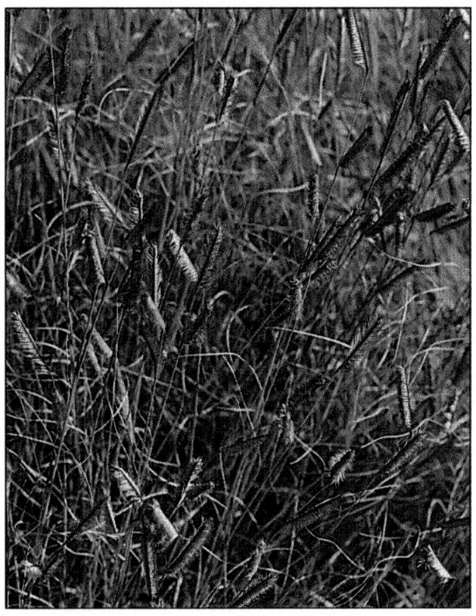

Bouteloua gracilis

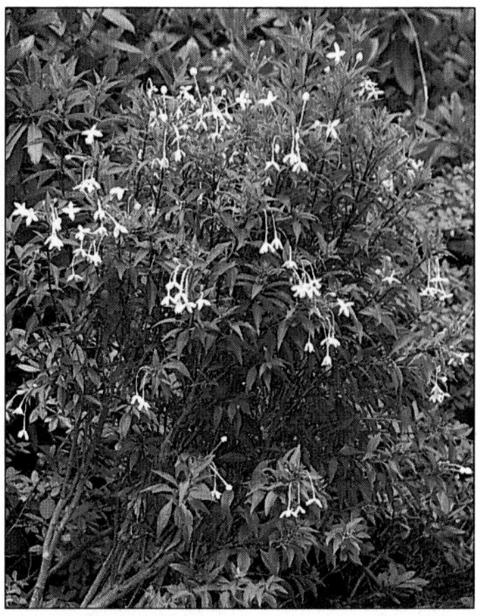

Bouvardia longiflora

***B.* 'Killie Campbell'** 🏆 Vigorous, evergreen climber with ovate, mid-green leaves, to 8cm (3in) long. Produces orange-bronze bracts, 3–5cm (1¼–2in) long, mainly from summer to autumn. ↕ 8–12m (25–40ft). ❄ (borderline)
***B.* 'La Jolla' of gardens.** Vigorous, evergreen climber with ovate, mid-green leaves, to 8cm (3in) long, and bright red bracts, 3–5cm (1¼–2in) long, produced mainly from summer to autumn. ↕ 8–12m (25–40ft). ❄ (borderline)
***B.* 'Mary Palmer'**, syn. *B.* 'Ailsa Lambe', *B.* 'Snow Cap', *B.* 'Surprise'. Vigorous, evergreen climber with ovate, mid-green leaves, to 8cm (3in) long; most leaves have a central yellow mark. Produces deep pink to white, or bicoloured bracts, 3–5cm (1¼–2in) long, mainly from summer to autumn. ↕ 8–12m (25–40ft). ❄ (borderline)
***B.* 'Miss Manilla'** ■ syn. *B.* 'Tango'. Vigorous, evergreen climber with ovate, mid-green leaves, to 8cm (3in) long. Produces pink bracts, 3–5cm (1¼–2in) long, mainly from summer to autumn. ↕ 8–12m (25–40ft). ❄ (borderline)
***B.* 'Raspberry Ice'** ■ syn. *B.* 'Tropical Rainbow'. Vigorous, compact, evergreen climber with ovate, cream-margined, deep green leaves, 8cm (3in) long. Bears bright cerise bracts, 3–5cm (1¼–2in) long, mainly from summer to autumn. ↕ 8–12m (25–40ft). ❄ (borderline)
***B.* 'San Diego Red'** see *B.* 'Scarlett O'Hara'.
***B.* 'Scarlett O'Hara'** ■ syn. *B.* 'Hawaiian Scarlet', *B.* 'San Diego Red'. Vigorous, evergreen climber with ovate, mid-green leaves, to 8cm (3in) long. Produces bright scarlet-cerise bracts, 3–5cm (1¼–2in) long, mainly from summer to autumn. ↕ 8–12m (25–40ft). ❄ (borderline)
***B.* 'Snow Cap'** see *B.* 'Mary Palmer'.
B. spectabilis. Vigorous, evergreen or almost deciduous climber with stems bearing down-curving thorns and ovate, downy, mid-green leaves, 10cm (4in) long. Purple or pink bracts, 5–6cm (2–2½in) long, are produced from spring to summer. ↕ 7–12m (22–40ft). Brazil. ❄ (borderline). **'Lateritia'** produces brick-red bracts, 3–3.5cm (1¼–1½in) long.
***B.* 'Surprise'** see *B.* 'Mary Palmer'.
***B.* 'Tango'** see *B.* 'Miss Manilla'.
***B.* 'Temple Fire'**, syn. *B.* 'Helen Johnson', *B.* 'Tom Thumb'. Shrubby, evergreen climber with ovate, mid-green leaves, to 8cm (3in) long. Produces mauve-purple bracts, 3–5cm (1¼–2in) long, mainly from summer to autumn. ↕ 8–12m (25–40ft). ❄ (borderline)
***B.* 'Tom Thumb'** see *B.* 'Temple Fire'.
***B.* 'Tropical Rainbow'** see *B.* 'Raspberry Ice'.

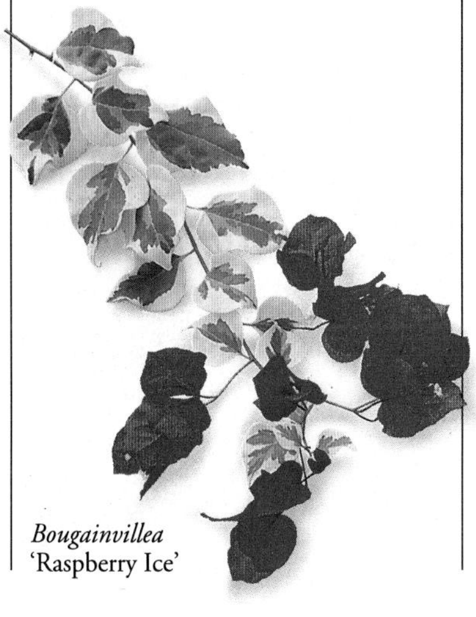

Bougainvillea 'Raspberry Ice'

▷ **Bouncing Bet** see *Saponaria officinalis*
▷ **Bourtree** see *Sambucus nigra*
▷ ***Boussingaultia*** see *Anredera*
***B. baselloides* of gardens** see *A. cordifolia*

BOUTELOUA

GRAMINEAE/POACEAE

Genus of 24–30 species of deciduous, rhizomatous or stoloniferous, annual and perennial grasses, largely found in open grassland and prairies in North, Central, and South America. They are cultivated for their unusual ornamental inflorescences: the flowers are borne in branched panicles with flattened, horizontally held spikes, which are said to resemble mosquitoes. The leaves are linear, and flat or folded. Grow as specimen plants, or in groups in a mixed or herbaceous border.

- **HARDINESS** Fully hardy.
- **CULTIVATION** Grow in medium to light, well-drained soil in full sun. Provide sharp drainage in areas where there is high winter rainfall; most species are intolerant of cold combined with winter wet. Cut back overwintered material in early spring, before new growth begins.
- **PROPAGATION** Sow seed in containers in a cold frame in spring. Divide clumps from mid-spring to early summer.
- **PESTS AND DISEASES** Trouble free.

B. gracilis ■ syn. *B. oligostachya*, *Chondrosum gracile* (Blue grama, Mosquito grass, Signal-arm grass). Clump-forming, perennial grass with short rhizomes and linear leaves, to 60cm (24in) long. In summer, produces panicles of 2–4 flower spikes, each with 40–90 tightly packed, brownish purple spikelets, to 5mm (¼in) long. ↕ to 60cm (24in), ↔ 30cm (12in). S. and W. USA, Mexico. ❄❄❄
B. oligostachya see *B. gracilis*.

BOUVARDIA

RUBIACEAE

Genus of about 30 species of evergreen shrubs and perennials occurring in scrub, thickets, woodland, and forest margins from tropical and subtropical S. USA to South America. They are valued for their salverform flowers, with 4 petal lobes, borne singly or in cymes or corymbs. Ovate or lance-shaped to oblong leaves are opposite or in whorls of 3 or more. In frost-prone areas, grow in a cool greenhouse; elsewhere, grow at the base of a house wall, or in a border.

- **HARDINESS** Frost tender.
- **CULTIVATION** Under glass, grow in loam-based potting compost (JI No.2) in bright filtered light. When in growth, water freely and apply a balanced liquid fertilizer monthly; keep just moist in winter. Pot on or top-dress in spring. Outdoors, grow in moist but well-drained, fertile soil in full sun with some midday shade. Pruning group 10, immediately after flowering.
- **PROPAGATION** Root softwood cuttings in spring or semi-ripe cuttings in summer, in a propagating case with bottom heat.
- **PESTS AND DISEASES** Whiteflies, mealybugs, and red spider mites may be troublesome under glass.

B. humboldtii see *B. longiflora*.
B. longiflora ■ syn. *B. humboldtii*. Erect to spreading, usually well-branched shrub with opposite, oblong to ovate leaves, to 4.5cm (1¾in) long. Long-tubed, fragrant white flowers, to 9cm (3½in) long, are borne singly or in axillary or terminal corymbs from late summer to early winter. ↕ 1m (3ft) or more, ↔ to 60cm (24in). Mexico. ⊛ (min. 5°C/41°F)
B. ternifolia ■ syn. *B. triphylla* (Scarlet trompetilla). Variable, erect, moderately branched shrub with opposite or whorled, ovate to lance-shaped leaves,

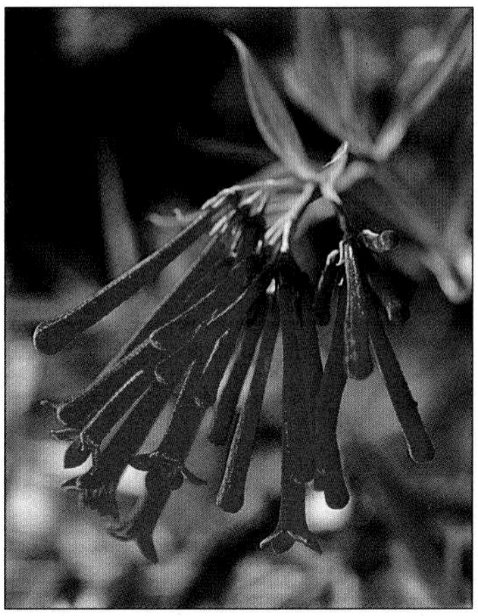

Bouvardia ternifolia

to 3cm (1¼in) long and softly hairy beneath. Bears dense, terminal corymbs of scarlet flowers, 3cm (1¼in) long, from late summer to winter. ↕ 60–90cm (24–36in), ↔ 30–60cm (12–24in). USA (Texas), Mexico. ⊛ (min. 5°C/41°F)
B. triphylla see *B. ternifolia*.

BOWENIA

BOWENIACEAE/ZAMIACEAE

Genus of 2 species of evergreen perennials (cycads) from forest in Australia. They are cultivated for their long-stalked, 2-pinnate, fern-like, dark green leaves. The insignificant, cone-like flower spikes are produced at ground level. In frost-prone climates, grow bowenias as houseplants or in a warm greenhouse. In frost-free climates, grow at the base of a wall, or in a courtyard garden, sheltered from heavy rainfall.

- **HARDINESS** Frost tender.
- **CULTIVATION** Under glass, grow in a mix of equal parts coarse bark, leaf mould, and sharp sand, in bright filtered light. When in growth, water freely and apply a balanced liquid fertilizer monthly; water sparingly in winter. Pot on or top-dress in spring. Outdoors, grow in well-drained, humus-rich soil in full sun or partial shade.
- **PROPAGATION** Sow seed at 24–26°C (75–79°F) in spring.
- **PESTS AND DISEASES** Red spider mites and scale insects may be a problem under glass.

B. spectabilis (Byfield fern). Fern-like cycad with 2 subterranean, bulbous trunks topped at ground level by sparse, erect leaf rosettes, each leaf to 2m (6ft) long and composed of many obliquely ovate, entire, leathery, glossy, dark green leaflets. Produces ovoid to spherical green flowerheads in summer. ↕↔ 1–2m (3–6ft). Australia (Queensland). ❀ (min. 15–18°C/59–64°F)

▷ **Bower plant** see *Pandorea jasminoides*

BOWIEA

HYACINTHACEAE/LILIACEAE

Genus of 2 or 3 species of perennial succulents occurring on low mountainsides in E. Africa and South Africa. Slender, succulent shoots arise from scaly bulbs, which enlarge with age to 20cm (8in) or more across, and often become exposed above soil level. Each bulb initially produces 1 or 2 very short-lived, linear, basal leaves. Thin, thread-like, freely branching, scrambling or climbing stems are produced after the short-lived leaves have died. Diurnal, 6-tepalled flowers are borne on short, fleshy stalks in terminal panicles, and are followed by ovoid, papery-coated fruits containing a few oblong, flattened, shiny black seeds. In frost-prone areas, grow bowieas in a warm greenhouse or as houseplants. In warmer climates, grow in a desert garden or in association with shrubs.

- **HARDINESS** Frost tender.
- **CULTIVATION** Under glass, plant the bulbs to one-quarter of their depth in standard cactus compost, in bright indirect light. When new growth is apparent, water sparingly; cease when the stems wither after flowering. Apply half-strength low-nitrogen fertilizer twice during the growing season. Outdoors, grow in sharply drained soil in full sun with some midday shade. See also pp.48–49.
- **PROPAGATION** Sow seed at 21°C (70°F) in early spring.
- **PESTS AND DISEASES** Mealybugs and aphids may be troublesome.

B. volubilis ■ Perennial succulent with a spherical brown bulb, which becomes pale green as it is exposed to light. Minute, linear leaves, 1mm (1/16in) long or less, soon disappear to be replaced by branching stems. Diurnal, star-shaped, greenish white flowers, 8mm (3/8in) across, are borne in twisting, terminal panicles in summer. ↕ 4m (12ft), ↔ indefinite. South Africa. ❀ (min. 13°C/55°F)

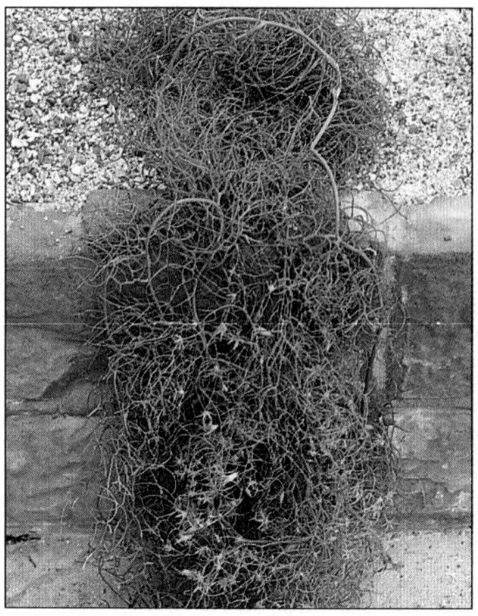

Bowiea volubilis

▷ **Bowman's root** see *Gillenia trifoliata*
▷ **Box** see *Buxus*
Balearic see *Buxus balearica*
Brush see *Lophostemon confertus*
Christmas see *Sarcococca*
Common see *Buxus sempervirens*
Creeping see *Mitchella repens*
Himalayan see *Buxus wallichiana*
Red see *Eucalyptus polyanthemos*
Small-leaved see *Buxus microphylla*
Sweet see *Sarcococca*
▷ **Box elder** see *Acer negundo*
▷ **Box thorn, Chinese** see *Lycium barbarum*
▷ **Boxwood** see *Buxus*
African see *Myrsine africana*

BOYKINIA

SAXIFRAGACEAE

Genus of approximately 10 species of perennials with short rhizomes, occurring in moist woodland and mountainous areas of Japan and North America. They have alternate, rounded to kidney-shaped, mid- to dark green basal leaves, sometimes bronze-tinted when young, with long leaf-stalks, and shorter-stalked or unstalked stem leaves. Crimson or white, 5-petalled flowers are produced in lax, corymb-like panicles. Grow in a shady woodland garden or wild garden.

- **HARDINESS** Fully hardy.
- **CULTIVATION** Grow in lime-free, cool, moist, humus-rich soil in partial shade. *B. jamesii* is best grown in an alpine house or in a crevice containing gritty but fertile, humus-rich, acid soil.
- **PROPAGATION** Sow seed in a cold frame as soon as ripe. Divide in spring.
- **PESTS AND DISEASES** Trouble free.

B. aconitifolia. Clump-forming perennial with 5- to 7-lobed, glandular-hairy, mid-green leaves, 5–15cm (2–6in) long, with broadly toothed margins. In early and midsummer, bears shallowly bell-shaped white flowers, to 1cm (1/2in) across, with yellowish white centres. ↕ 15–60cm (6–24in), ↔ 30cm (12in). E. USA. ✻✻✻
B. heucheriformis see *B. jamesii.*
B. jamesii ■ syn. *B. heucheriformis, Telesonix jamesii.* Mound-forming perennial with rosettes of slightly lobed, broadly toothed, glandular-hairy, mid-green leaves, 1–3cm (1/2–1 1/4in) long. Bears open bell-shaped, frilled, pinkish red flowers, to 2cm (3/4in) across, with green centres, in mid- and late spring. ↕↔ 15cm (6in). USA (Colorado). ✻✻✻

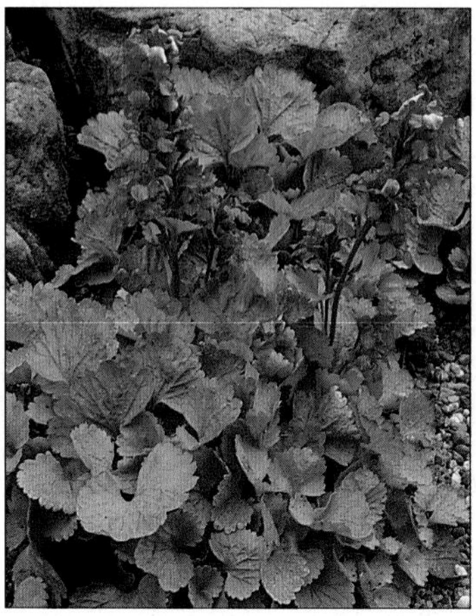

Boykinia jamesii

B. major. Clump-forming perennial with dark green leaves, 10–20cm (4–8in) long, with 5–7 coarsely cut lobes. Bears shallowly bell-shaped white flowers, 8–10mm (3/8–1/2in) across, in midsummer. ↕ 60–90cm (24–36in), ↔ 30cm (12in). W. USA. ✻✻✻
B. tellimoides see *Peltoboykinia tellimoides.*

▷ ***Brachychilum*** see *Hedychium*
B. horsfieldii see *H. horsfieldii*

BRACHYCHITON

Bottletree, Kurrajong

STERCULIACEAE

Genus of about 30 species of evergreen or deciduous trees, some with bottle-shaped trunks, from seasonally dry to moist tropical forest in Australia and Papua New Guinea. The leaves are alternate and entire to shallowly or palmately lobed. Unisexual, petalless flowers have 5 or 6 sometimes colourful tepals and are profusely borne in axillary or terminal, panicle-like cymes. In frost-prone areas, grow in a temperate or warm greenhouse. Elsewhere, grow as flowering specimen or shade trees.

- **HARDINESS** Frost tender.
- **CULTIVATION** Under glass, grow in loam-based potting compost (JI No.2) with additional sharp sand, in full light. When in growth, water moderately and apply a balanced liquid fertilizer monthly; water sparingly in winter. Pot on or top-dress in spring. Outdoors, grow in free-draining, fertile soil in full sun. Pruning group 1; need restrictive pruning under glass.
- **PROPAGATION** Sow seed at 16–18°C (61–64°F) as soon as ripe. Root semi-ripe cuttings in summer or hardwood cuttings in early autumn, both in a propagating case with bottom heat.
- **PESTS AND DISEASES** Red spider mites may be a problem under glass.

B. acerifolius ■ ◊ syn. *Sterculia acerifolia* (Flame kurrajong, Flame tree). Open-branched, evergreen or briefly deciduous tree with leathery, glossy, bright green leaves, 8–20cm (3–8in) long, which may be simple and ovate, or palmately 3- to 5-lobed, often on the same plant. Large, terminal, panicle-like cymes of bowl-shaped, bright coral-red flowers, 2cm (3/4in) across, are borne in summer, usually before the leaves. ↕ 15–35m (50–120ft), ↔ 8–12m (25–40ft). Australia (Queensland, New South Wales). ❀ (min. 10°C/50°F)
B. discolor ■ ♀ (Kurrajong, Queensland lacebark). Erect, semi-evergreen to fully deciduous tree with spreading branches and a thick trunk with light grey bark. Long-stalked, broadly ovate, 3- to 7-lobed, hairy, matt, mid-green leaves, 10–20cm (4–8in) long, are white-woolly on the undersides. Dense, axillary, panicle-like cymes of bell-shaped, pink or red flowers, 5cm (2in) wide, are borne from early summer to autumn. ↕ 10–30m (30–100ft), ↔ 5–15m (15–50ft). Australia (Queensland, New South Wales). ❀ (min. 10°C/50°F)
B. populneus ◊ syn. *Sterculia diversifolia* (Kurrajong). Broadly ovoid, densely branched, evergreen tree with ovate, lustrous, dark green leaves, 4–12cm

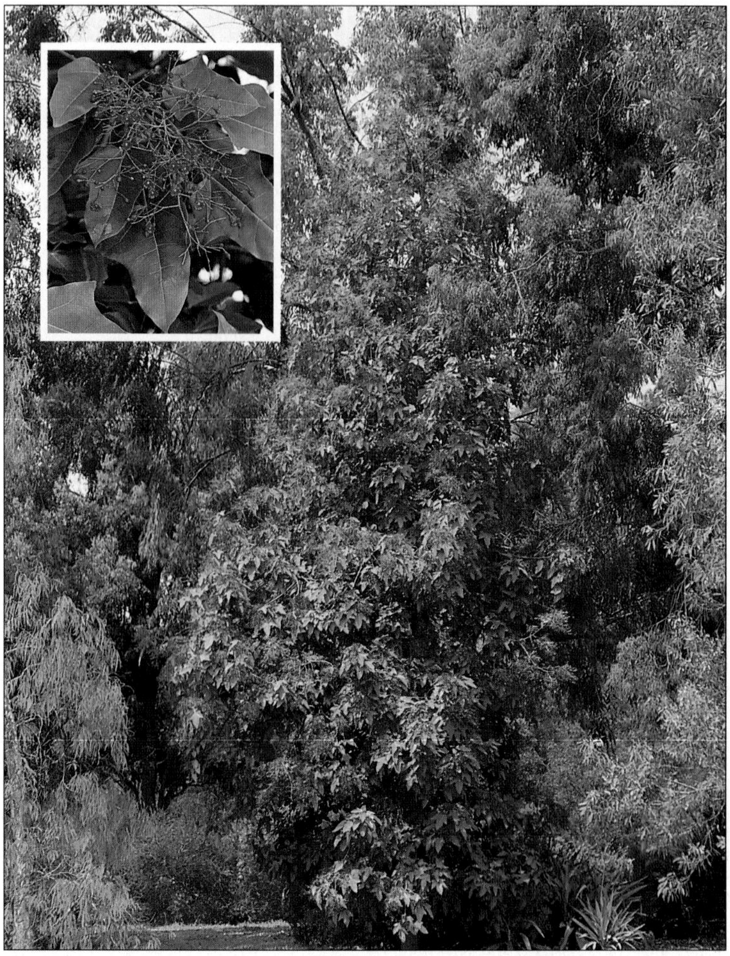

Brachychiton acerifolius (inset: leaf and flower detail)

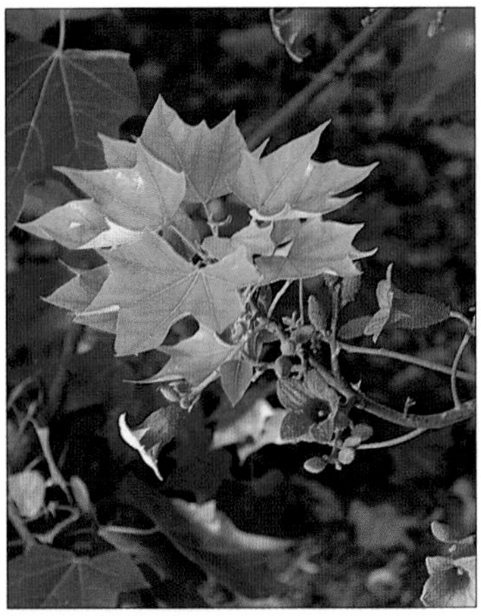

Brachychiton discolor

(1½–5in) long, varying from entire to 3- to 5-lobed on the same plant. In summer, produces terminal and axillary, panicle-like cymes of saucer-shaped, green, cream, or pink flowers, to 1.5cm (½in) across, spotted with brown or red and with spreading lobes. ↕ 6–20m (20–70ft), ↔ 3–6m (10–20ft). Australia (Northern Territory, Queensland to Victoria). ❀ (min. 10°C/50°F)

▷ ***Brachycome*** see *Brachyscome*

Brachyglottis

ASTERACEAE/COMPOSITAE

Genus of about 30 species of evergreen trees and shrubs, herbaceous perennials, and climbers, including several shrubby species once listed under *Senecio*, found in rocky places, scrub, grassland, and forest in New Zealand and Tasmania. They are cultivated for their attractive foliage and flowers: the alternate leaves are often dark green, frequently white- or buff-felted beneath; the daisy-like flowerheads, often with conspicuous ray-florets, are usually borne in racemes, corymbs, or panicles, rarely singly, in summer or autumn. Many are suitable for a shrub border, and the dwarfer species are ideal for a rock garden. Most thrive in coastal sites, where some are effective as hedges or as windbreaks.

- **Hardiness** Fully hardy to half hardy.
- **Cultivation** Grow in well-drained soil in full sun. Grow *B. hectoris* in fertile, moist soil in partial shade. Pruning group 8, if necessary.
- **Propagation** Root semi-ripe cuttings in summer.
- **Pests and diseases** Trouble free.

B. bidwillii, syn. *Senecio bidwillii*. Slow-growing, compact shrub with stout shoots and elliptic-oblong to obovate-oblong, leathery leaves, to 2.5cm (1in) long, glossy, dark green above and densely white-felted beneath. In summer, produces small, rayless white flowerheads in panicles to 5cm (2in) across. ↕ 1m (3ft), ↔ 1.2m (4ft). New Zealand (North Island). ❄❄
B. compacta, syn. *Senecio compactus*. Compact, mound-forming shrub with obovate to oblong, wavy-margined, white-hairy leaves, to 4cm (1½in) long, becoming hairless and dull, dark green above. In summer, bright yellow flowerheads, 3cm (1¼in) across, with conspicuous ray-florets, are borne in

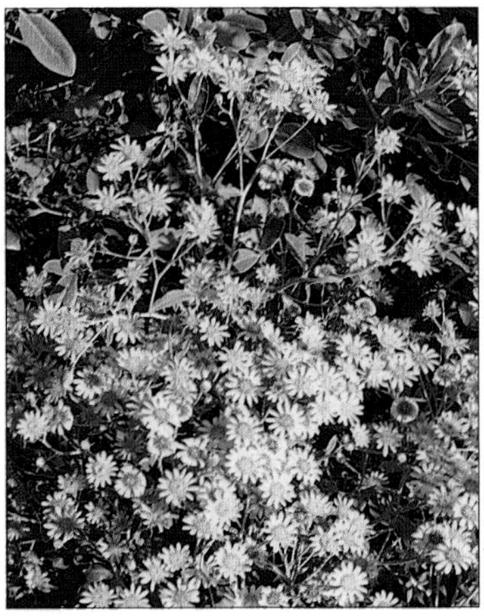

Brachyglottis Dunedin Hybrids 'Sunshine'

few-flowered racemes or singly. ↕ 1m (3ft), ↔ 2m (6ft). New Zealand (North Island). ❄❄
***B.* Dunedin Hybrids**, syn. *Senecio* Dunedin Hybrids, *S. laxifolius* of gardens, *S. greyi* of gardens. Spreading, bushy, mound-forming shrubs with obovate to elliptic, often wavy-margined, white-hairy, later hairless, mid- to dark green leaves, to 7cm (3in) long. Bears loose, terminal panicles of bright yellow flowerheads, to 3cm (1¼in) across, with conspicuous ray-florets, from summer to autumn. ↕ 1.5m (5ft), ↔ 2m (6ft) or more. ❄❄❄. **'Moira Read'**, syn. *Senecio* 'Moira Read', has elliptic, shallowly scalloped leaves, to 5cm (2in) long, initially white-hairy, then dark green, with irregular yellow variegation above; ❄❄. **'Sunshine'** ■🏆 syn. *Senecio* 'Sunshine', has elliptic, white-hairy leaves with shallowly scalloped margins, becoming dark green above.
B. elaeagnifolia ■ syn. *Senecio elaeagnifolius*. Vigorous, compact shrub with obovate to narrowly oblong, leathery, glossy, dark green leaves, to 9cm (3½in) long, distinctly veined and hairless above, white-felted below. Bears panicles, to 15cm (6in) across, of rayless yellow flowerheads, 1cm (½in) across, in summer. ↕ 3m (10ft), ↔ 5m (15ft). New Zealand (North Island). ❄❄
B. greyi, syn. *Senecio greyi*. Open, mound-forming shrub with ovate-oblong, shallowly scalloped leaves, to 8cm (3in) long, white-hairy at first, dark green above when mature. Bright yellow flowerheads, 3cm (1¼in) across, with

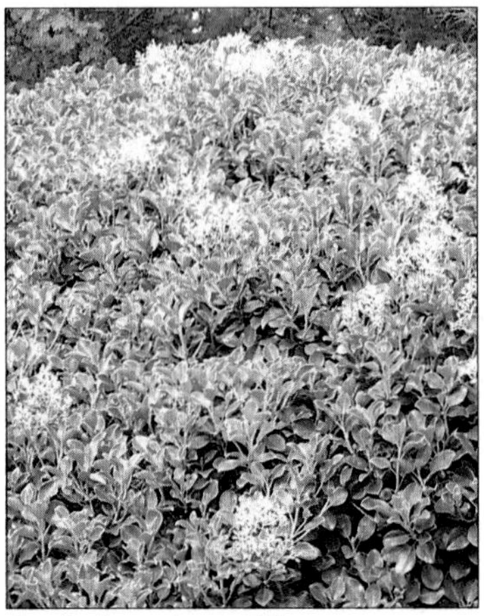

Brachyglottis elaeagnifolia

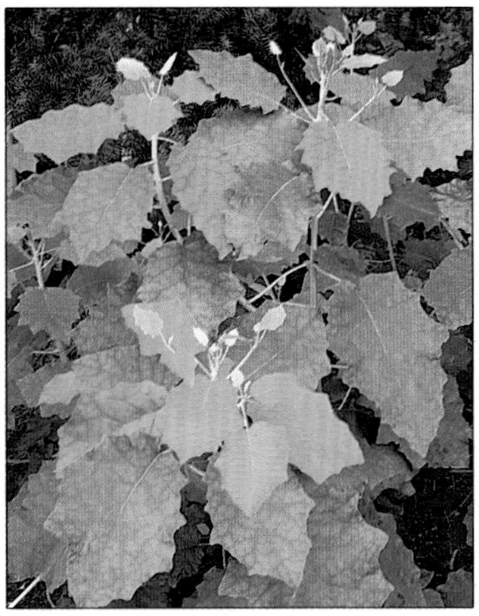

Brachyglottis repanda

conspicuous ray-florets, are produced in large, terminal corymbs from summer to early autumn. ↕ 2m (6ft), ↔ 3m (10ft). New Zealand (North Island). ❄❄
B. hectoris, syn. *Senecio hectoris*. Open, upright, semi-evergreen shrub with obovate, mid-green leaves, to 25cm (10in) long, lobed at the bases. Produces white flowerheads, 5cm (2in) across, with yellow disc-florets, in lax, terminal corymbs in midsummer. ↕ 4m (12ft), ↔ 3m (10ft). New Zealand (South Island). ❄❄
B. huntii 🗨 syn. *Senecio huntii*. Upright-branched shrub or sometimes small tree with densely clustered, elliptic-oblong, mid-green leaves, to 10cm (4in) long. Yellow flowerheads, 2cm (¾in) across, with conspicuous ray-florets, are borne in panicles, to 12cm (5in) across, in summer. ↕ 5m (15ft), ↔ 4m (12ft). New Zealand (Chatham Islands). ❄❄
B. laxifolia, syn. *Senecio laxifolius*. Laxly branched, mound-forming shrub with elliptic, entire or slightly scalloped leaves, to 6cm (2½in) long, white-hairy at first, becoming hairless and dark green above. Vivid yellow flowerheads, 2cm (¾in) across, with conspicuous ray-florets, are borne in loose panicles from summer to autumn. ↕ 1m (3ft), ↔ 2m (6ft). New Zealand (South Island). ❄❄
B. monroi, syn. *Senecio monroi*. Dense, many-branched shrub with obovate-oblong, leathery, olive-green leaves, to 4cm (1½in) long, tightly crisped at the margins, white beneath. In summer, produces yellow flowerheads, 2cm (¾in) across, with conspicuous ray-florets, in terminal corymbs. ↕ 1m (3ft), ↔ 2m (6ft). New Zealand (South Island). ❄❄❄
B. repanda ■ Spreading shrub with broadly oblong to ovate-oblong, wavy-margined, dark green leaves, to 25cm (10in) long, buff- or white-hairy beneath. Fragrant, creamy white flowerheads, 5mm (¼in) across, are produced in arching panicles, to 30cm (12in) long, in summer. ↕ 3m (10ft), ↔ 3m (10ft) or more. New Zealand. ❄
B. rotundifolia 🗨 syn. *Senecio reinholdii*, *S. rotundifolius*. Compact shrub or small tree with ovate, leathery, glossy, dark green leaves, to 10cm (4in) long, buff- or white-felted beneath. In early and midsummer, bears rayless yellow flowerheads, 1cm (½in) wide, in panicles to 20cm (8in) across. ↕↔ 1m (3ft). New Zealand (South Island). ❄❄

Brachyscome

syn. Brachycome
Swan river daisy

ASTERACEAE/COMPOSITAE

Genus of 60–70 species of annuals and deciduous and evergreen, often short-lived perennials, from damp grassland, bogs, and rocky habitats in alpine and subalpine areas of Australia, Tasmania, New Zealand, and New Guinea. They have very variable, often finely divided foliage, and produce masses of daisy-like flowerheads, with yellow disc-florets and usually purple, blue, or white ray-florets. Grow annuals in a border, in containers, for edging, or as bedding plants; use perennials in a rock garden. In frost-prone areas, grow half-hardy and frost-tender species in a cool greenhouse.

- **Hardiness** Frost hardy to frost tender.
- **Cultivation** Under glass, grow in loam-based potting compost (JI No.1) in full light. During the growing season, water freely and apply a balanced liquid fertilizer twice; keep moist in winter. Pinch out growing tips of young plants. Outdoors, grow in fertile, well-drained soil in a sheltered site in full sun.
- **Propagation** For annuals, sow seed at 18°C (64°F) in spring. For perennials, root basal cuttings in spring, or sow seed at 18°C (64°F) in spring or autumn, overwintering young plants under glass.
- **Pests and diseases** Slugs and snails may be a problem.

B. aculeata. Very variable, tufted, clump-forming, erect perennial with basal rosettes of spoon-shaped, mid-green leaves, 5–10cm (2–4in) long, and linear stem leaves, 2cm (¾in) long. Solitary, pale violet or white flowerheads, 2–2.5cm (¾–1in) across, are borne from midsummer to mid-autumn. ↕ 15–65cm (6–26in), ↔ to 60cm (24in). Australia. ❄❄
B. angustifolia. Prostrate to clump-forming, rhizomatous perennial with linear-elliptic to elliptic, entire or slightly lobed, mid-green, basal leaves, to 6cm (2½in) long. Bears solitary, blue, mauve, or pink flowerheads, to 2cm (¾in) across, from early spring to late summer. ↕ 35cm (14in), ↔ 60cm (24in). Australia. ❄❄. **var. *heterophylla*** has pinnatisect leaves.
B. iberidifolia ■ (Swan river daisy). Bushy or spreading, relatively drought-tolerant annual with pinnatisect, softly downy, grey-green leaves, to 14cm

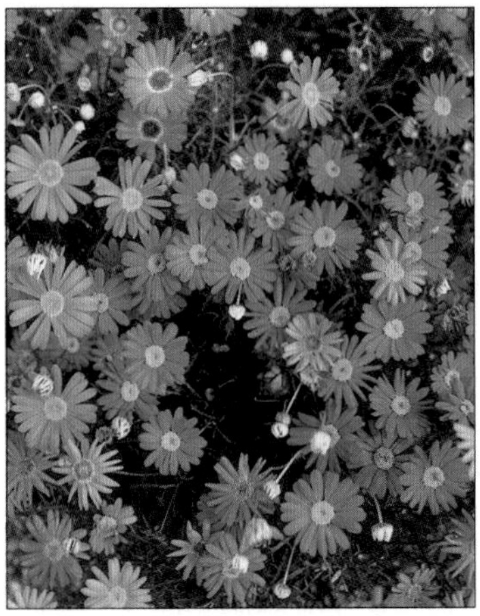

Brachyscome iberidifolia

B

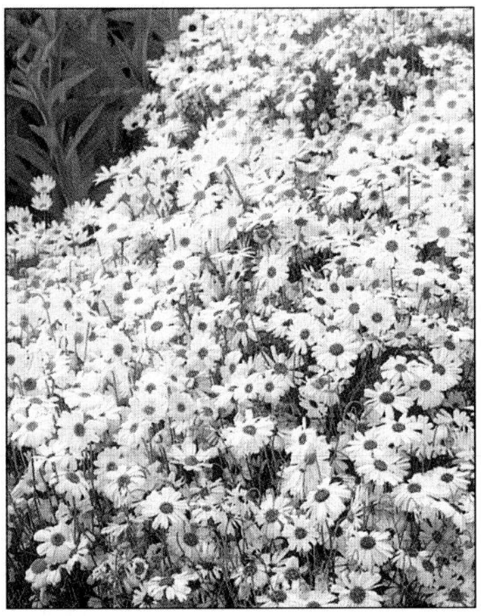

Brachyscome iberidifolia Splendour Series 'White Splendour'

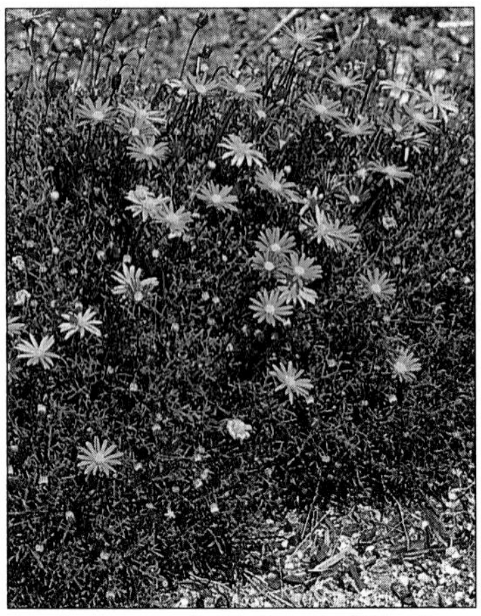

Brachyscome multifida 'Break O'Day'

(5½in) long. Bears fragrant, usually blue-purple, sometimes violet-pink or white flowerheads, to 4cm (1½in) across, in summer. ↕ to 45cm (18in), ↔ 35cm (14in). W. and S. Australia. ✲. Cultivars of **Splendour Series** have black-eyed, white, lilac-pink, or purple flowerheads; ↕ to 30cm (12in). **'White Splendour'** ■ has white flowerheads.
B. multifida (Rock daisy). Spreading, wiry annual with finely pinnatisect or 2-pinnatisect, bright green leaves, to 7cm (3in) long. From midsummer to mid-autumn, bears solitary, blue, pink, purple, mauve, or white flowerheads, 2cm (¾in) across. ↕↔ 45cm (18in). S.E. Australia. ✲. **'Break O'Day'** ■ has purple-pink flowerheads. **'Lemon Mist'** has soft pale yellow flowerheads.
B. nivalis. Variable, rosette-forming, loosely tufted, rhizomatous perennial bearing irregularly pinnatisect, mid-green leaves, 5–10cm (2–4in) long. Solitary white flowerheads, 3–4.5cm (1¼–1¾in) across, are produced in summer. ↕ to 20–30cm (8–12in), ↔ to 30cm (12in). Dry, rocky areas in Australia. ✲✲. **var. *alpina***, syn. *B. tadgellii*, has spoon-shaped leaves, and grows in marshy, boggy areas.
B. rigidula. Mound-forming, tufted, evergreen perennial with erect, branching stems and crowded, finely cut, mid-green leaves, 1–3cm (½–1¼in) long. Produces short-stemmed, pale to deep lavender-blue or purple-blue flowerheads, to 2.5cm (1in) across, from late spring to early autumn. ↕ 15cm (6in), ↔ to 20cm (8in). E. Australia, including Tasmania. ✲✲
B. tadgellii see *B. nivalis* var. *alpina*.

BRACHYSEMA

LEGUMINOSAE/PAPILIONACEAE

Genus of about 16 species of evergreen shrubs from sandy heaths, scrub, and light woodland in Australia. Alternate or opposite leaves are simple or reduced to scales or green stems. Inverted pea-like flowers are borne singly or in axillary clusters. In frost-prone areas, grow in a cool greenhouse. Elsewhere, grow in a shrub border or against a warm wall; use prostrate species for ground cover.
• **HARDINESS** Frost tender; may survive brief spells around 0°C (32°F).
• **CULTIVATION** Under glass, grow in loamless potting compost in full light. When in growth, water moderately and apply a low-phosphate liquid fertilizer monthly; water sparingly in winter. Outdoors, grow in poor to moderately fertile soil, low in phosphates, in full sun. Pruning group 8. Tip prune unflowered shoots in late winter, to encourage a bushy habit.
• **PROPAGATION** Sow seed at 13–15°C (55–59°F) in spring, after scarifying or soaking in hot water. Root semi-ripe cuttings in summer with bottom heat.
• **PESTS AND DISEASES** Prone to scale insects and red spider mites under glass.

B. acuminatum see *B. celsianum*.
B. celsianum, syn. *B. acuminatum*, *B. lanceolatum* (Swan river pea). Bushy, prostrate or semi-scandent, drought-tolerant shrub with usually opposite, lance-shaped leaves, to 10cm (4in) long, deep greyish green above, silver-hairy beneath. Produces red flowers, 2.5cm (1in) long, with silver-hairy calyces, either singly or in clusters of 2 or 3. Blooms over long periods, mainly from winter to spring. ↕ 0.3–1.5m (1–5ft), ↔ 1–2m (3–6ft). Australia (Western Australia). ⌂ (min. 5°C/41°F)
B. lanceolatum see *B. celsianum*.

BRACHYSTELMA

ASCLEPIADACEAE

Genus of about 50 species of perennial succulents from semi-arid areas of Africa and India. Most have fleshy, tuberous rootstocks and prostrate or erect, simple or branching stems with opposite, variably shaped leaves. In summer, star-shaped, 5-lobed flowers are borne singly, in pairs, or in few- to many-flowered, lateral or terminal umbels. In frost-prone areas, grow in a temperate

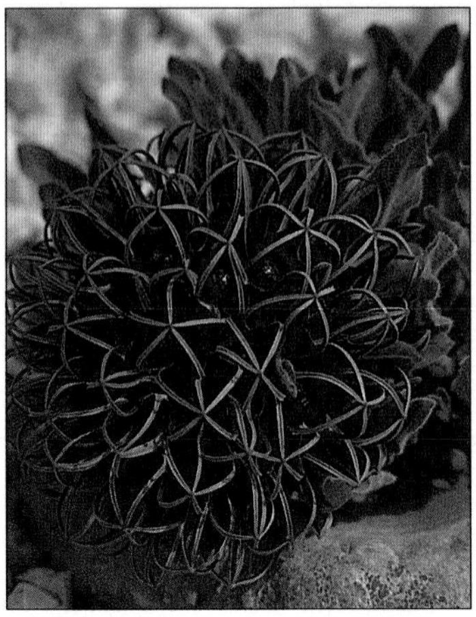

Brachystelma barberae

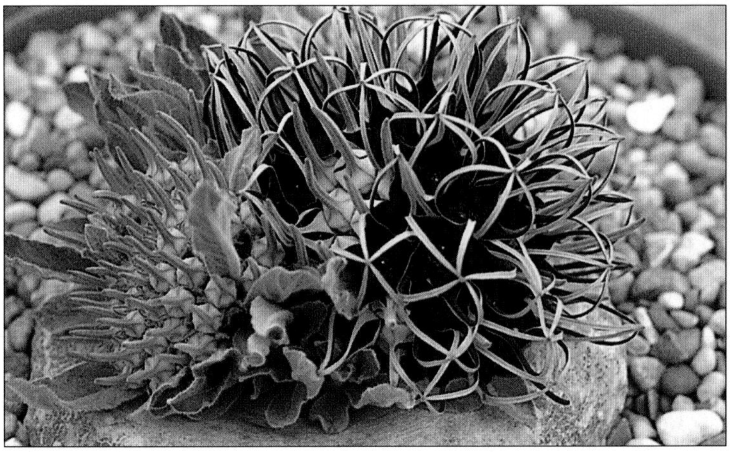

Brachystelma foetidum

greenhouse. In frost-free areas, grow in a desert garden or border.
• **HARDINESS** Frost tender.
• **CULTIVATION** Under glass, grow in equal parts loam, leaf mould, and sharp sand in bright filtered light. In growth, water moderately and apply half-strength, low-nitrogen fertilizer 2 or 3 times; keep dry at other times. Overwatering, particularly in winter, may encourage root rot. Outdoors, grow in gritty, humus-rich, sharply drained soil in partial shade. See also pp.48–49.
• **PROPAGATION** Sow seed at 21°C (70°F) in late spring, keeping the soil barely moist.
• **PESTS AND DISEASES** Mealybugs and root mealybugs may be a problem.

B. barberae ■ Very short-stemmed succulent with an ovoid-spherical rootstock, a flat, fleshy caudex, and linear, pointed, dark green leaves, 7–10cm (3–4in) or more long. In summer, bears spherical umbels, 10–12cm (4–5in) across, of 6 or more, yellow-centred, brownish purple flowers, 3cm (1¼in) across, with 3-angled lobes united at their tips. ↕ 10cm (4in), ↔ 14cm (5½in). South Africa (Eastern Cape). ⌂ (min. 10°C/50°F)
B. foetidum ■ Succulent with a flattened caudex bearing semi-erect, leafy stems with velvet-hairy branches clothed in ovate-spoon-shaped, pointed, wavy-margined, dark green leaves, 1–2.5cm (½–1in) long. Dark purplish brown flowers, 2.5–3cm (1–1¼in) across, are produced singly or in pairs in summer; the flower lobes are hairy on the outside, united to form a tube in the lower part, and narrowly triangular and spreading in the upper part. ↕ 15cm (6in), ↔ 12cm (5in). South Africa (Northern Transvaal, Eastern Transvaal). ⌂ (min. 10°C/50°F)

BRACTEANTHA

ASTERACEAE/COMPOSITAE

Genus of about 7 species of herbaceous perennials and annuals from open grassland and scrub in Australia. The stalkless, ovate to broadly lance-shaped, glandular-hairy leaves, 5–15cm (2–6in) long, are borne on erect, branching stems. Daisy-like flowerheads have papery, white, yellow, or pink involucral bracts and central yellow corollas. Grow in an annual border, or use to fill gaps in a mixed or herbaceous border. Low-growing cultivars may also be used for

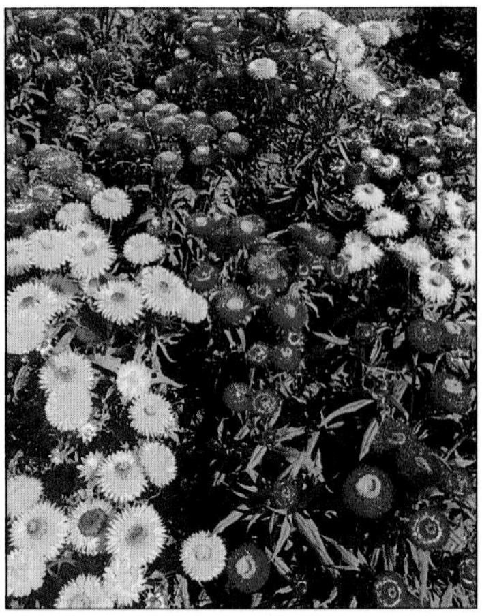

Bracteantha bracteata Bright Bikinis Series

edging, or in a window-box. *B. bracteata* is often grown for cutting and drying.
• **HARDINESS** Frost hardy to half hardy.
• **CULTIVATION** Grow in moderately fertile, moist but well-drained soil in full sun. Cultivars 90cm (36in) or more tall require staking.
• **PROPAGATION** Sow seed at 18°C (64°F) in spring.
• **PESTS AND DISEASES** Susceptible to downy mildew.

B. bracteata, syn. *Helichrysum bracteatum* (Golden everlasting, Strawflower). Erect annual or short-lived perennial with broadly lance-shaped, grey-green leaves, to 12cm (5in) long. From late spring to autumn, bears terminal, solitary, papery, bright white,

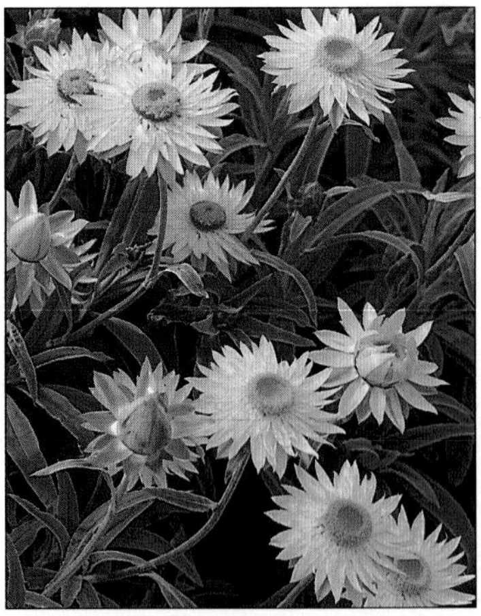

Bracteantha bracteata 'Dargan Hill Monarch'

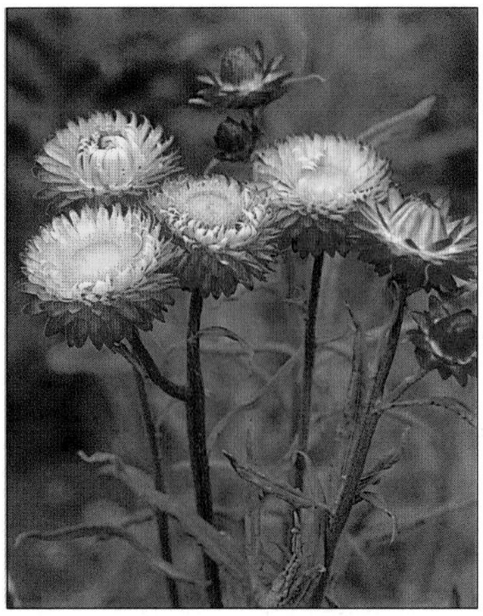

Bracteantha bracteata Monstrosum Series

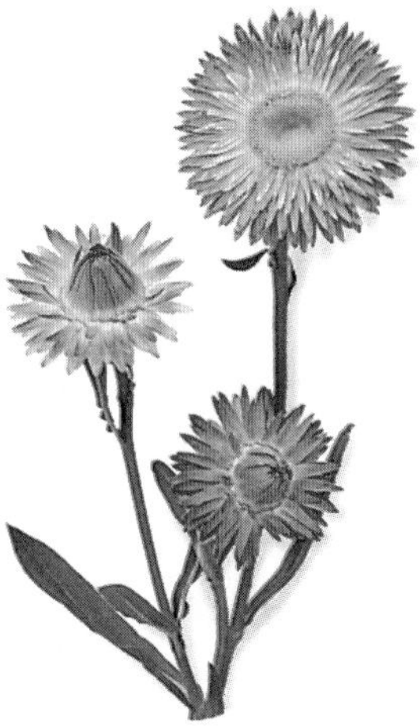

Bracteantha bracteata 'Silvery Rose'

yellow, pink, or red flowerheads, 2.5–8cm (1–3in) across. ↕ 1–1.5m (3–5ft), ↔ 30cm (12in). Australia. ❄. Cultivars of **Bright Bikinis Series** ▣ 🏆 have double, red, pink, orange, yellow, or white flowerheads, to 8cm (3in) across; ↕ to 30cm (12in). **'Dargan Hill Monarch'** ▣ has golden yellow flowerheads, 5–7cm (2–3in) across; ❄❄. **'Frosted Sulphur'** 🏆 has double, silvery, pale sulphur-yellow flowerheads; ↕ to 1m (3ft). **King Size Series** cultivars have fully double flowerheads, to 10cm (4in) across, in yellow, orange, red, pink, or silvery white (in single colours or a mix); ↕ 1m (3ft). **Monstrosum Series** ▣ cultivars have fully double flowerheads, to 8cm (3in) across, in pink, red, orange, yellow, or white; ↕ to 90cm (36in). **'Silvery Rose'** ▣ 🏆 has double, silvery rose-pink flowerheads; ↕ to 75cm (30in). **'Sky Net'** has pink-flushed, creamy white flowerheads, to 8cm (3in) across. **Tetraploid Double Series** cultivars are very vigorous, with pink, crimson-red, yellow, orange, or white flowerheads, to 8cm (3in) across; ↕ 1.5m (5ft)

BRAHEA

Hesper palm

ARECACEAE/PALMAE

Genus of 16 species of usually single-stemmed palms occurring on dry, open forest slopes in S. California, USA, and from Mexico to Guatemala. Long panicles of 3-petalled, bell-shaped flowers develop among dense, terminal heads of fan-like leaves. In frost-prone areas, grow young specimens for their foliage, as houseplants, or in a temperate greenhouse or conservatory. In warmer regions, use as specimen trees.

• **HARDINESS** Frost tender, but will withstand short periods at 0°C (32°F).

• **CULTIVATION** Under glass, grow in loam-based potting compost (JI No.2) in full light. When in growth, water moderately and apply a balanced liquid fertilizer monthly; water sparingly in winter. Pot on or top-dress in spring. Outdoors, grow in well-drained soil in full sun; will tolerate poor, dry soil.

• **PROPAGATION** Sow seed at 23–27°C (73–81°F) in spring.

• **PESTS AND DISEASES** Red spider mites and scale insects may be a problem.

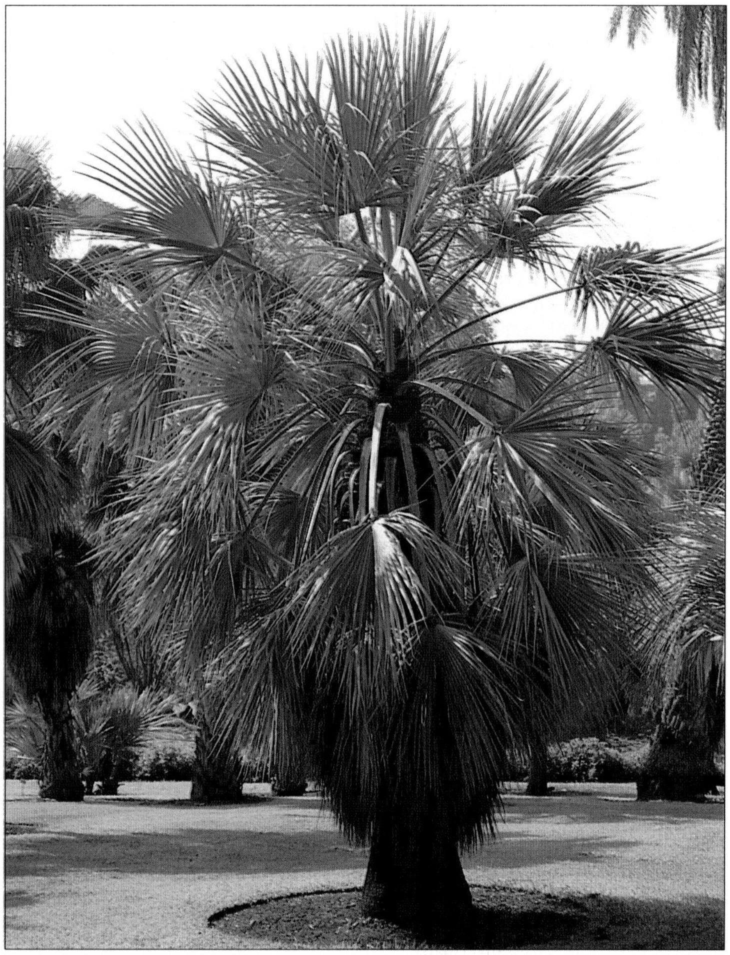

Brahea armata

B. armata ▣ 🌴 (Blue-fan palm, Blue hesper palm, Grey goddess palm). Erect palm with the trunk clothed in fibrous leaf bases. Fan-like, waxy-textured, blue-green leaves, 1–2m (3–6ft) across, with about 50 slender lobes, are borne on long, spiny stalks. In summer, bears arching panicles, 4m (12ft) long, of showy yellow flowers, 1.5cm (½in) across. ↕ to 15m (50ft), ↔ to 7m (22ft). USA (S. California), Mexico. ❁ (min. 5–15°C/41–59°F)

B. brandegeei 🌴 (San Jose hesper palm). Slender palm with a tapered trunk. Fan-like leaves, 1m (3ft) or more across, with about 50 narrow lobes, rich green above, tinted blue-grey beneath, are borne on long, spiny stalks. In summer, bears cream flowers, 7–10mm (¼–½in) across, in narrow panicles that are as long as the leaves. ↕ to 12m (40ft), ↔ to 5m (15ft). USA (S. California). ❁ (min. 5–15°C/41–59°F)

▷ **Brake** see *Pteris*
Jungle see *P. umbrosa*
Painted see *P. tricolor*
Shaking see *P. tremula*
Silver see *P. argyraea*
Spider see *P. multifida*
Sword see *P. ensiformis*
Tender see *P. tremula*

▷ ***Brassaia*** see *Schefflera*
B. actinophylla see *S. actinophylla*

BRASSAVOLA

ORCHIDACEAE

Genus of up to 20 species of evergreen, upright or horizontal to pendent, epiphytic or lithophytic orchids, found from sea level to 1,800m (6,000ft) in Central and South America. They have woody, creeping rhizomes that produce stem-like, narrowly cylindrical pseudobulbs, each with one cylindrical, apical leaf. Long-lasting, night-scented, white, ivory-white, or green flowers are borne singly or in short, often pendent racemes of up to 7 blooms from the base of the leaf, usually in summer.

• **HARDINESS** Frost tender.

• **CULTIVATION** Cool- to intermediate-growing orchids. Grow in epiphytic orchid compost in a slatted basket, or epiphytically on a bark slab. Provide moist, unshaded conditions all year. In summer, water freely, applying fertilizer at every third watering, and mist twice daily. Keep dry in winter. See also p.46.

• **PROPAGATION** Divide when plants fill their pots and "flow" over the sides.

• **PESTS AND DISEASES** Red spider mites, aphids, and mealybugs may be troublesome.

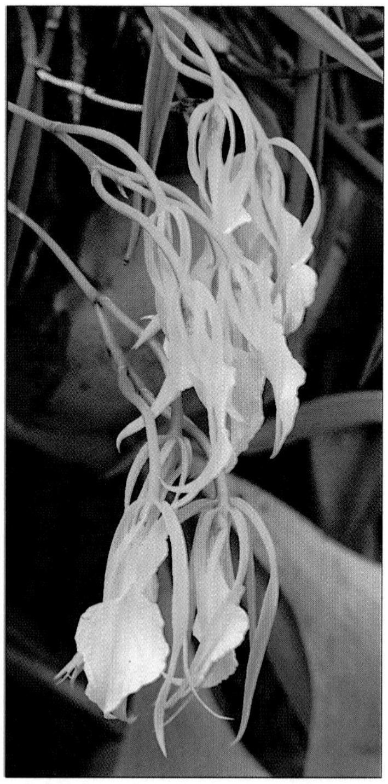

Brassavola nodosa

B. cucullata. Epiphytic orchid with small, stem-like pseudobulbs and pendent, cylindrical, glossy, dark green leaves, 25cm (10in) long. Solitary, occasionally 2 or 3, narrow-segmented, white or greenish yellow flowers, 8cm (3in) long, with green-tipped lips, are produced from autumn to winter. ↕ 40cm (16in), ↔ 30cm (12in). Mexico and West Indies, south to Ecuador. ❁ (min. 13°C/55°F; max. 30°C/86°F)

B. nodosa ▣ Epiphytic or lithophytic orchid with very small, stem-like pseudobulbs and stout, upright, cylindrical-linear, mid-green leaves, to 18cm (7in) long. In summer, bears racemes, to 15cm (6in) long, of 3–5 light green, ivory, or white flowers, 8cm (3in) across, with white lips and maroon-spotted throats. ↕↔ 18cm (7in). Mexico to Panama, Venezuela. ❁ (min. 13°C/55°F; max. 30°C/86°F)

▷ **Brass buttons** see *Cotula coronopifolia*

BRASSIA

ORCHIDACEAE

Genus of about 50 species of evergreen, epiphytic orchids, found at altitudes of 750–1,600m (2,500–5,200ft) in tropical regions of North, Central, and South America. They have horizontal to upright rhizomes and compressed, ovoid-spherical to cylindrical pseudobulbs, each with 1–3 strap-shaped to oblong-lance-shaped leaves. Racemes of up to 12 spider-like, fragrant, long-petalled, yellow to green flowers are borne laterally from the pseudobulb bases from spring to early summer.

• **HARDINESS** Frost tender.

• **CULTIVATION** Cool-growing orchids. Grow in epiphytic orchid compost in a pot or slatted basket, or epiphytically on a bark slab. In summer, provide moist, partially shaded, well-ventilated conditions; water freely, applying fertilizer at every third watering; and mist twice daily. Keep unshaded and almost dry in winter. See also p.46.

B

• **PROPAGATION** Divide when the plant fills the pot and "flows" over the sides, or pot up backbulbs separately.
• **PESTS AND DISEASES** Vulnerable to red spider mites, aphids, and mealybugs.

B. caudata. Epiphytic orchid with linear to elliptic-oblong pseudobulbs and 2 elliptic-oblong to inversely lance-shaped leaves, 30cm (12in) long. In autumn and spring, bears light green to orange-yellow flowers, often marked red-brown, in a suberect to arching raceme, 40–80cm (16–32in) long. ↕↔ 45cm (18in). USA (Florida), Mexico to Panama, West Indies to Bolivia and N. Brazil. ❅ (min. 11–13°C/52–55°F; max. 30°C/86°F)
B. lawrenceana (Spider orchid). Epiphytic orchid with oblong-ovate to oblong pseudobulbs and 2 narrowly oblong to elliptic-lance-shaped leaves, 40cm (16in) long. In spring, bears green or yellow flowers, with red-purple spots, in arching or pendent racemes, often 40cm (16in) or more long. ↕↔ 45cm (18in). Venezuela, Guyana, Surinam, N.E. Peru, N. Brazil. ❅ (min. 11–13°C/52–55°F; max. 30°C/86°F)
B. verrucosa 🏆 Epiphytic orchid with narrowly ovoid to oblong pseudobulbs and 2 elliptic-oblong to inversely lance-shaped, bright green leaves, 30cm (12in) long. In early summer, bears upright then arching racemes, to 75cm (30in) long, of yellow to green flowers, spotted red-brown, with white lips spotted dark green or red-brown. ↕↔ 75cm (30in). S. Mexico to Venezuela. ❅ (min. 11–13°C/52–55°F; max. 30°C/86°F)

BRASSICA

BRASSICACEAE/CRUCIFERAE

Genus of 30 species of annuals and evergreen biennials, perennials, or rarely subshrubs, occurring on rocky slopes, and waste and disturbed ground from the Mediterranean to temperate Asia. Most are erect, branching, tap-rooted plants, with oblong-ovate to rounded, entire or pinnately lobed, hairless, more or less glaucous leaves. They bear terminal racemes of cross-shaped, yellow or white flowers with 4 clawed petals, followed by long, narrow, beaked fruits. *Brassica* species have been developed to produce many edible vegetables, including cabbage, sprouts, cauliflower, and broccoli (all variants of *B. oleracea*), and turnip, Chinese cabbage, and oilseed rape. Most are grown in the vegetable garden, although some ornamental cabbages – with variegated pink, white, or green foliage – are used in a border or for a bedding display.
• **HARDINESS** Fully hardy, but flowerheads of edible vegetables may be damaged in severe winters.
• **CULTIVATION** Grow in fertile, well-drained, ideally lime-rich soil in full sun.
• **PROPAGATION** Sow seed *in situ* in spring, or under glass in early spring.
• **PESTS AND DISEASES** Susceptible to black leg, downy mildew, clubroot, aphids, whiteflies, root flies, flea beetles, caterpillars, leaf spots, powdery mildew, and white blister.

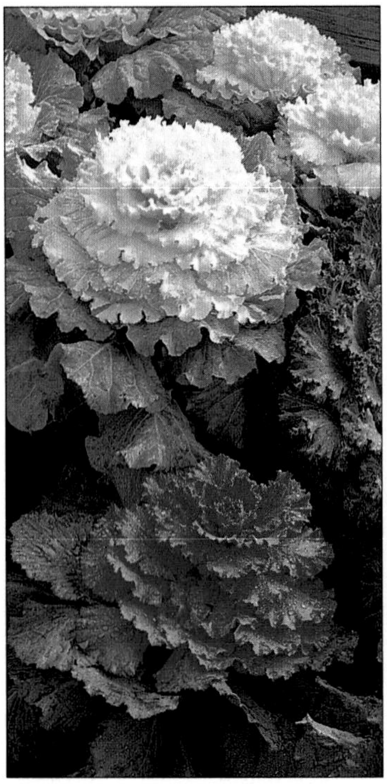

Brassica oleracea Osaka Series

***B. oleracea* cultivars.** Ornamental cabbage and kale cultivars grown as annuals for their rounded, loose rosettes of variously coloured foliage, suitable either for autumn or winter bedding or for containers. They are usually available as seed mixtures of rounded to ovate, plain or fringed, white, red, or pink leaves. Leaves produce the most vivid colours below 10°C (50°F). ↕↔ to 45cm (12–18in). ❄❄❄. **Osaka Series** ▣ cultivars are fast-growing, with wavy, bluish green outer leaves and compact, white, pink, or red centres; ↕ to 30cm (12in). **'Tokyo'** has neat, rounded, blue-green outer leaves and soft, pink, red, or white centres; ↕ to 25cm (10in).

x BRASSOCATTLEYA

ORCHIDACEAE

Bigeneric hybrid genus, a cross of *Brassavola* and *Cattleya*, consisting of several hundred evergreen, epiphytic orchids derived from Central American species. They have stout, club-shaped, sheathed pseudobulbs and 1 or 2 semi-rigid, oblong to oblong-lance-shaped, leathery leaves. Showy, fragrant flowers, with frilled lips, are borne in racemes arising from sheaths at the leaf bases in spring or autumn; each scape produces 1 or 2 flowers. These orchids are often loosely referred to as cattleyas.

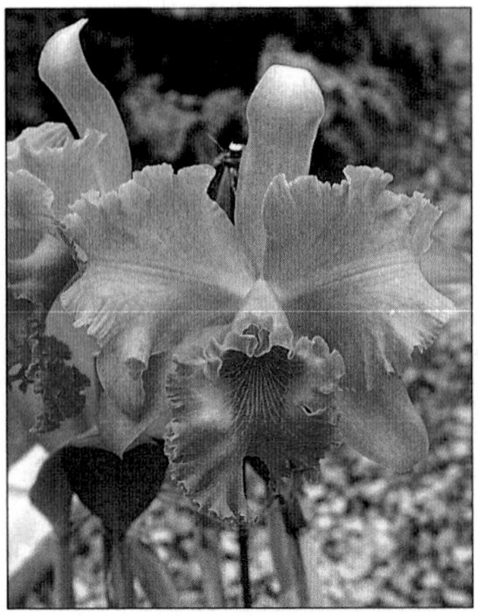

x *Brassocattleya* Mount Adams

• **HARDINESS** Frost tender.
• **CULTIVATION** Cool- to intermediate-growing orchids. Grow in epiphytic orchid compost in containers. In summer, provide moist, partially shaded conditions and water freely, applying fertilizer at every third watering. Keep unshaded and almost dry in winter. See also p.46.
• **PROPAGATION** Divide when the plant fills the pot and "flows" over the sides, or pot up backbulbs separately.
• **PESTS AND DISEASES** Scale insects, red spider mites, aphids, and mealybugs may be troublesome.

x *B.* Mount Adams ▣ (x *B.* Déesse x *Cattleya* Bob Betts). Epiphytic orchid with stout pseudobulbs and oblong-lance-shaped, mid-green leaves, 15cm (6in) long. Light rose-mauve flowers, 15cm (6in) across, with purple- and yellow-striped throats, are produced, usually in pairs, in spring or autumn. ↕ 30cm (12in), ↔ 45cm (18in). ❅ (min. 13°C/55°F; max. 28°C/82°F)

x BRASSOLAELIO-CATTLEYA

ORCHIDACEAE

Trigeneric hybrid genus, a cross of *Brassavola*, *Laelia*, and *Cattleya*, consisting of several hundred evergreen, epiphytic orchids derived from Central and South American species. They have stout, club-shaped, sheathed pseudobulbs and 1 or 2 semi-rigid, oblong to oblong-lance-shaped, leathery leaves. Colourful, fragrant flowers are produced in short inflorescences arising from sheaths at the leaf bases. Brassolaeliocattleyas resemble brassocattleyas, with which they are often associated.
• **HARDINESS** Frost tender.
• **CULTIVATION** As for *Brassocattleya*.
• **PROPAGATION** As for *Brassocattleya*.
• **PESTS AND DISEASES** As for *Brassocattleya*.

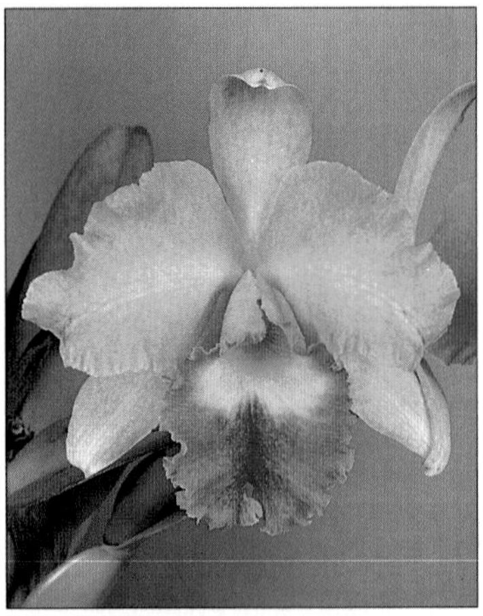

x *Brassolaeliocattleya* Hetherington Horace 'Coronation'

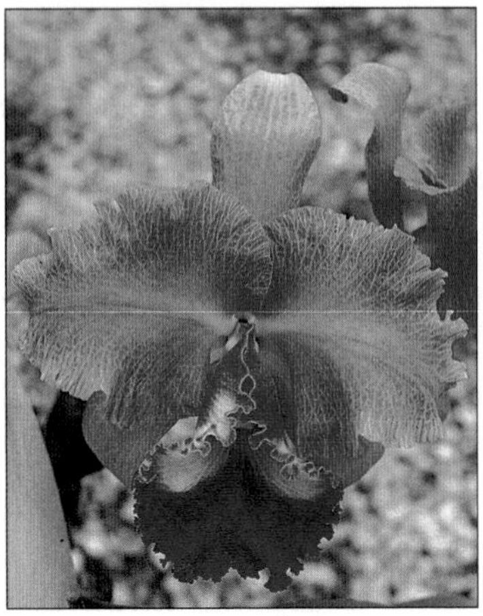

x *Brassolaeliocattleya* St. Helier

x *B.* Hetherington Horace 'Coronation' ▣ Epiphytic orchid with 1 or 2 oblong-lance-shaped, mid-green leaves, 15cm (6in) long. Soft lilac flowers, to 13cm (5in) across, with deep mauve lips and white-margined yellow throats, are produced in spring or autumn. ↕↔ 45cm (18in). ❅ (min. 13°C/55°F; max. 28°C/82°F)
x *B.* St. Helier ▣ (x *B.* Norman's Bay x x *B.* Sussex). Epiphytic orchid with 1 or 2 oblong-lance-shaped, mid-green leaves, 15cm (6in) long. Rich magenta flowers, 15–18cm (6–7in) across, 2 or 3 together, with mauve-purple and golden yellow lips, are produced in spring. ↕↔ 45cm (18in). ❅ (min. 13°C/55°F; max. 28°C/82°F)

▷ ***Bravoa geminiflora*** see *Polianthes geminiflora*
▷ **Breadfruit, Mexican** see *Monstera deliciosa*
▷ ***Brevoortia*** see *Dichelostemma*
▷ **Brewer spruce** see *Picea breweriana*

BREYNIA

EUPHORBIACEAE

Genus of about 25 species of evergreen shrubs and trees occurring in tropical forest and scrub in Asia, Australia, and the Pacific islands from New Caledonia to Hawaii. They are grown for their alternate, small, simple, colourful leaves, often in flattened, frond-like sprays. Insignificant, petalless flowers are succeeded by red berries. In frost-prone areas, grow as houseplants or in a warm greenhouse or conservatory; in warmer climates, plant in a border.
• **HARDINESS** Frost tender.
• **CULTIVATION** Under glass, grow in loam-based potting compost (JI No.2) in bright filtered light. When in full growth, water freely and apply a balanced liquid fertilizer monthly; water sparingly in winter. Pot on or top-dress in spring. Outdoors, grow in fertile, humus-rich soil, preferably in partial or light dappled shade. Pruning group 8; need restrictive pruning under glass. Pinch out stem tips when young.

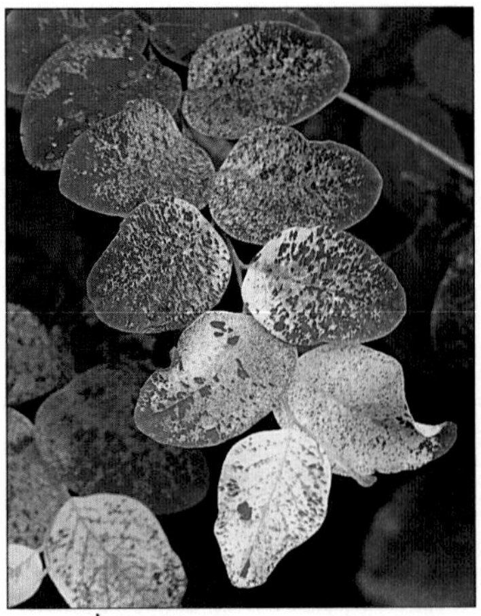

Breynia disticha

• **PROPAGATION** Root softwood cuttings in summer with bottom heat.
• **PESTS AND DISEASES** Red spider mites, whiteflies, and aphids may be a problem under glass.

B. disticha ■ syn. *B. nivosa, Phyllanthus nivosus* (Snow bush). Slender, evergreen shrub with zigzagged pink or red stems bearing ovate, dark green leaves, 2–5cm (¾–2in) long, with bold white variegation. ↕ 1m (3ft) or more, ↔ 60–100cm (24–39in). Pacific islands. ❀ (min. 15°C/59°F). **'Roseopicta'** has white- and pink-mottled leaves.
B. nivosa see *B. disticha.*

▷ **Briar,**
  Austrian see *Rosa foetida*
  Sweet see *Rosa eglanteria*
▷ **Bridal bouquet** see *Porana paniculata*
▷ **Bridal wreath** see *Francoa, Spiraea* 'Arguta', *Stephanotis floribunda*
▷ **Bride's bonnet** see *Clintonia uniflora*
▷ ***Bridgesia spicata*** see *Ercilla volubilis*

BRIGGSIA

GESNERIACEAE

Genus of at least 20 species of evergreen perennials from moist woodland in India, S. China, and S.E. Tibet. They produce basal rosettes of obovate or narrowly elliptic to lance-shaped, hairy leaves. Axillary, tubular flowers with 5 short petal lobes are borne singly or in cymes. In frost-prone regions, grow in an alpine house or cool greenhouse. In frost-free areas, grow in a rock garden.
• **HARDINESS** Frost tender.
• **CULTIVATION** Under glass, grow in loam-based potting compost (JI No.2) with additional leaf mould, in bright indirect light and with good ventilation. Water freely in summer, from below; keep moist in winter. Outdoors, grow in moist but well-drained, humus-rich soil in partial shade.
• **PROPAGATION** Surface-sow seed in containers of peaty seed compost in a cold frame in partial shade, in spring.
• **PESTS AND DISEASES** Susceptible to neck rot in winter, and aphids.

B. muscicola. Evergreen perennial with narrowly elliptic to lance-shaped, scalloped, pale green leaves, to 7cm (3in) long, clothed in silvery white hairs. In early summer, arching stems bear loose cymes of 2–6 tubular, soft yellow to orange-yellow flowers, to 2cm (¾in) long, marked purple within. ↕ 5–8cm (2–3in), ↔ to 15cm (6in). Bhutan, India (Assam), W. China. ❀ (min. 2°C/36°F)

BRIMEURA

HYACINTHACEAE/LILIACEAE

Genus of 2 species of bulbous perennials from meadows, maquis, and garigue in S.E. Europe. They are grown for their slender-stalked racemes of bell-shaped flowers, reminiscent of small bluebells, which are produced in spring. Leaves are basal and linear. Grow in a rock garden, beneath shrubs, or in an alpine house.
• **HARDINESS** Fully hardy.
• **CULTIVATION** Plant bulbs 5cm (2in) deep in autumn. Grow in humus-rich, well-drained soil in full sun or partial shade.

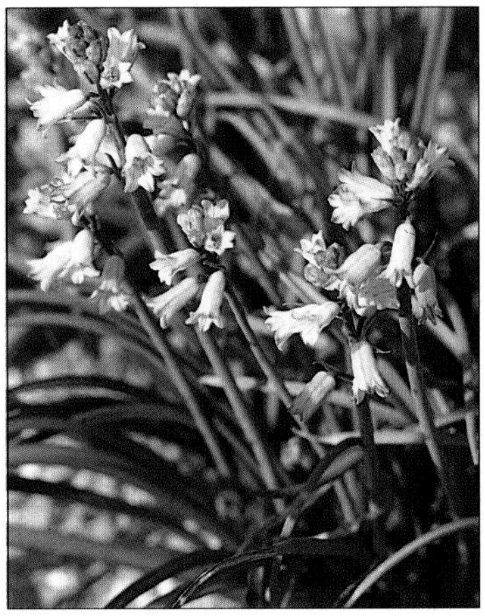
Brimeura amethystina

• **PROPAGATION** Sow seed in containers in a cold frame as soon as ripe. Divide clumps in summer.
• **PESTS AND DISEASES** Trouble free.

B. amethystina ■ syn. *Hyacinthus amethystinus.* Bulbous perennial with linear, channelled, bright green leaves, 10–30cm (4–12in) long. Bears loose, slender racemes of tubular-bell-shaped, pale to dark blue flowers, 1cm (½in) long, in spring. ↕ 10–20cm (4–8in), ↔ 5cm (2in). Pyrenees. ✻✻✻. **var. *alba*** bears white flowers.

▷ ***Brittonastrum*** see *Agastache*
  B. mexicanum see *A. mexicana*

BRIZA

Quaking grass

GRAMINEAE/POACEAE

Genus of 12–20 species of tufted, annual and perennial grasses occurring in open scrub and on a range of natural grassland in temperate regions of Europe and S.W. Asia. Attractive, long-lasting, loose or dense racemes or panicles of pendent, 4- to 20-flowered spikelets, animated by the slightest wind, are borne mostly in summer. The leaves are linear. Grow in a mixed or herbaceous border, or in a rock garden. The flowerheads are very popular for dried flower arrangements, used either in their natural colour or, very often, dyed.
• **HARDINESS** Fully hardy.
• **CULTIVATION** Grow annuals in any well-drained soil in full sun. Perennials tolerate a wide range of well-drained soil types in sun or partial shade.

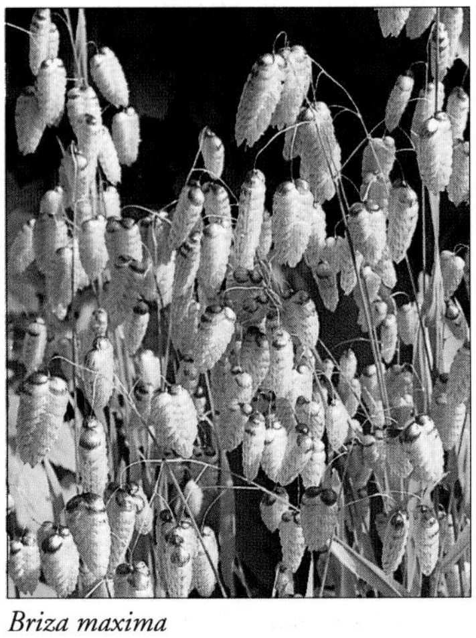
Briza maxima

• **PROPAGATION** Sow seed *in situ* in spring or autumn. Divide perennials from mid-spring to midsummer.
• **PESTS AND DISEASES** Trouble free.

B. maxima ■ (Greater quaking grass, Puffed wheat). Loosely tufted, erect, annual grass with linear, finely bristle-margined, pale green then straw-coloured leaves, to 20cm (8in) long. From late spring to late summer, produces loose, open panicles, to 10cm (4in) long, of 7- to 20-flowered, ovate to heart-shaped green spikelets, to 1cm (½in) long, which are tinged red-brown or purplish grey and become straw-coloured when ripe; they hang from hair-fine stalks. ↕ 45–60cm (18–24in), ↔ 25cm (10in). Mediterranean. ✻✻✻
B. media (Common quaking grass, Trembling grass). Perennial grass forming a dense tuft of linear, finely bristle-margined, blue-green leaves, to 15cm (6in) long. From late spring to midsummer, erect stems produce open, pyramidal panicles, to 18cm (7in) long, of 4- to 12-flowered, nodding, heart-shaped spikelets, to 1cm (½in) long; purple-tinted green at first, they later turn straw-coloured and are arranged like a rattlesnake's tail. ↕ 60–90cm (24–36in), ↔ 30cm (12in). Europe, W. Asia. ✻✻✻
B. minor (Lesser quaking grass). Erect, loosely tufted, annual grass with linear, finely bristle-margined, initially pale green, then straw-coloured leaves, to 15cm (6in) long. From early summer to early autumn, produces slender-stemmed panicles, to 20cm (8in) long, of 4- to 8-flowered, ovate spikelets, to 5mm (¼in) long; pale green initially and frequently purple-tinted, they later turn straw-coloured. ↕ to 45cm (18in), ↔ 25cm (10in). Europe, W. Asia. ✻✻✻

▷ **Broadleaf** see *Griselinia littoralis*

BRODIAEA

ALLIACEAE/LILIACEAE

Genus of 15 species of cormous perennials from grassland and dry woodland or scrub in W. USA and Mexico. They are grown for their funnel-shaped flowers, 2.5–4.5cm (1–1¾in) long, borne in umbels in spring or early summer. Long, basal leaves, 5–15cm (2–6in) long, are linear, blue-green or mid-green, and often die back before the flowers appear. Many similar cormous perennials, once listed as *Brodiaea*, are now classified under *Bloomeria, Dichelostemma*, and *Triteleia.* Suitable for a herbaceous border or rock garden, or an alpine house or bulb frame.
• **HARDINESS** Frost hardy.
• **CULTIVATION** Plant corms in groups 8cm (3in) deep in autumn. Grow in well-drained, light, fertile, sandy loam in full sun or partial shade. Water freely when in growth; keep warm and dry in summer when the corms have died down. In frost-prone areas, protect with a winter mulch.
• **PROPAGATION** Sow seed at 13–16°C (55–61°F) as soon as ripe. Remove offsets once they have become dormant.
• **PESTS AND DISEASES** Trouble free.

B. californica ■ Cormous perennial bearing large umbels of up to 12 widely funnel-shaped, violet, lilac, or pink

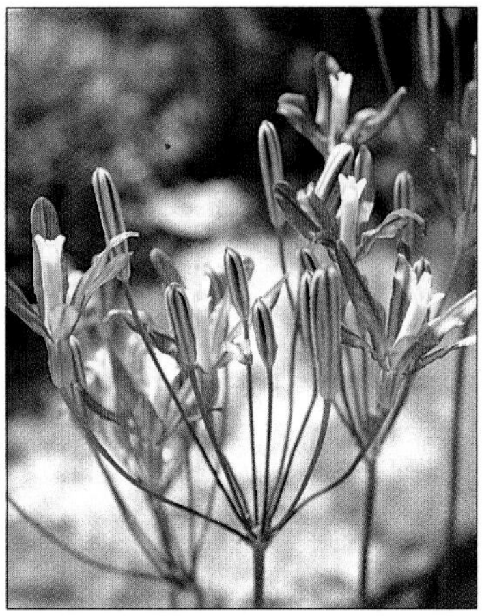
Brodiaea californica

flowers, on stalks 12cm (5in) long, in early summer. ↕ 50cm (20in), ↔ 8cm (3in). USA (N. California). ✻✻
B. capitata see *Dichelostemma pulchellum.*
B. congesta see *Dichelostemma congestum.*
B. coronaria, syn. *B. grandiflora.* Cormous perennial producing umbels of a few funnel-shaped, pale to deep purple flowers, with conspicuous cream stamens, on stalks to 5cm (2in) long, in early summer. ↕ 5–25cm (2–10in), ↔ 5cm (2in). W. USA. ✻✻
B. elegans. Cormous perennial producing umbels of up to 12 funnel-shaped, deep purple flowers, with strongly recurved tips, on stalks 5mm (¼in) long, in early summer. ↕ 10–50cm (4–20in), ↔ 5cm (2in). W. USA. ✻✻
B. grandiflora see *B. coronaria.*
B. hyacinthina see *Triteleia hyacinthina.*
B. ida-maia see *Dichelostemma ida-maia.*
B. ixioides see *Triteleia ixioides.*
B. lactea see *Triteleia hyacinthina.*
B. laxa see *Triteleia laxa.*
B. lutea see *Triteleia ixioides.*
B. peduncularis see *Triteleia peduncularis.*
B. pulchella see *Dichelostemma pulchellum.*
B. volubilis see *Dichelostemma volubile.*

▷ **Brodiaea, Twining** see *Dichelostemma volubile*

BROMELIA

BROMELIACEAE

Genus of at least 46 species of evergreen, rhizomatous or suckering, terrestrial, or rarely epiphytic perennials (bromeliads) occurring in woodland, scrub, or rocky areas, up to an altitude of 1,800m (6,000ft), in Central America, the West Indies, and South America. They form colonies of dense rosettes of linear to elliptic, rigid leaves with large, curved, marginal spines. Dense, cylindrical or conical inflorescences of white, red, or purple flowers are produced from the centres of the rosettes in summer, and are followed by ovoid yellow fruits containing large brown seeds. In frost-prone areas, grow in a warm greenhouse. In frost-free climates, they are suitable for a shady site or desert garden.
• **HARDINESS** Frost tender.
• **CULTIVATION** Under glass, grow in terrestrial bromeliad compost in full light. From spring to late autumn, water

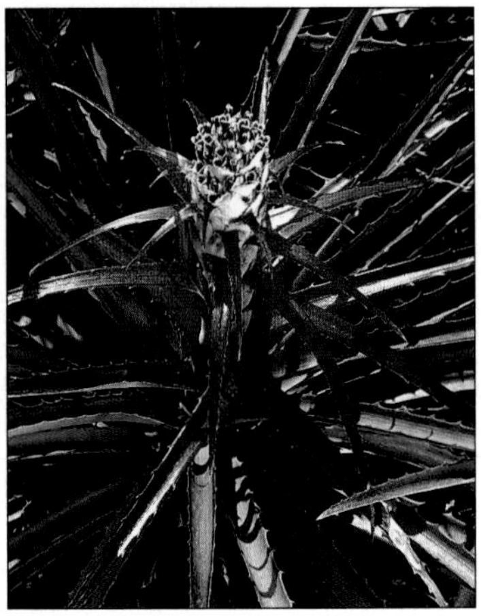

Bromelia balansae

freely and apply a low-nitrogen fertilizer 2 or 3 times; keep just moist at other times. Outdoors, grow in gritty, humus-rich, neutral to acid, well-drained soil in full sun, with some midday shade in summer. See also p.47.

• **PROPAGATION** Sow seed at 27°C (81°F) as soon as ripe. Divide in late spring or early summer.

• **PESTS AND DISEASES** Scale insects may be a problem, especially on young leaves.

B. balansae ■ (Heart of flame). Variable, terrestrial bromeliad with rosettes of 25–30 linear, wide-spreading, laxly spiny, often red-suffused, grey-green leaves, 1m (3ft) or more long, hairless above, with pale scales beneath. In summer, bears short-branched, cylindrical inflorescences, to 25cm (10in) long, of erect, tubular or cylindrical, white-margined violet flowers, 4.5cm (1¾in) long. ↕ to 1m (3ft), ↔ indefinite. Colombia, Brazil, Bolivia, Paraguay, N. Argentina. ❀ (min. 15°C/59°F)

B. laciniosa. Rhizomatous, terrestrial bromeliad with rosettes of up to 80 sword-shaped, recurved, laxly spiny, deep green leaves, 1m (3ft) long, brown-scaly above and white-scaly beneath. The shorter inner leaves turn bright red in sun. In summer, bears cylindrical panicles, to 70cm (28in) long, of erect, tubular or cylindrical purple flowers, to 5cm (2in) long. ↕ 1m (3ft), ↔ indefinite. N.E. Brazil. ❀ (min. 15°C/59°F)

▷**Bromeliad,**
Bird's-nest see *Nidularium*
Blushing see *Neoregelia carolinae, Nidularium fulgens*
▷**Bromeliads** see p.47
▷**Bromeliads, King of** see *Vriesea hieroglyphica*
▷**Brooklime** see *Veronica beccabunga*
▷**Broom** see *Cytisus, Genista, Ruscus, Spartium*
Butcher's see *Ruscus aculeatus*
Climbing butcher's see *Semele*
Common see *Cytisus scoparius*
Hedgehog see *Erinacea anthyllis*
Mount Etna see *Genista aetnensis*
Pineapple see *Cytisus battandieri*
Pink see *Notospartium carmichaeliae*
Portuguese see *Cytisus multiflorus*
Purple see *Chamaecytisus purpureus*
Spanish see *Spartium*
Warminster see *Cytisus* x *praecox* 'Warminster'
White Spanish see *Cytisus multiflorus*

BROUGHTONIA

ORCHIDACEAE

Genus of 5 species (possibly only one variable one) of evergreen, epiphytic orchids from Jamaica and Cuba, where they grow from sea level to 800m (2,600ft). They have 2 semi-rigid, narrowly oblong, dark green leaves, very short rhizomes, and tightly clustered and flattened-spherical to cylindrical pseudobulbs. In summer, racemes of brilliant crimson flowers are borne on long stems from the base of the leaves.

• **HARDINESS** Frost tender.

• **CULTIVATION** Cool- to intermediate-growing orchids. Grow in epiphytic orchid compost in a small container or epiphytically on a bark slab. In summer, provide moist conditions in bright filtered light, and water freely, applying fertilizer at every third watering. Keep almost dry in winter. See also p.46.

• **PROPAGATION** Divide when the plant fills the pot and "flows" over the sides.

• **PESTS AND DISEASES** Susceptible to red spider mites, aphids, and mealybugs.

B. sanguinea. Epiphytic orchid with flattened, subcylindrical pseudobulbs and 2 narrowly oblong, dark green leaves, 15–18cm (6–7in) long. In summer, stems to 50cm (20in) long produce up to 15 bright crimson, occasionally white or yellow flowers, 2.5cm (1in) across, with rose-purple lips. ↕ 50cm (20in), ↔ 15cm (6in). Jamaica. ❀ (min. 13°C/55°F; max. 30°C/86°F)

BROUSSONETIA

MORACEAE

Genus of about 7 species of deciduous trees and shrubs from woodland in E. Asia and Polynesia. They have alternate, entire or lobed, toothed leaves. Male and female flowers are borne on separate plants. *B. papyrifera*, the only widely cultivated species, is grown for its large leaves, pendent male catkins, and unusual fruit. It needs hot summers to ripen its wood and achieve tree stature, and then may be an attractive isolated specimen. Its tolerance of pollution, heat, and poor soil has made it a popular tree for urban locations. In areas with cool summers, it grows as a large shrub and is suitable for a shrub border.

• **HARDINESS** Fully hardy to frost tender.

• **CULTIVATION** Grow in almost any well-drained soil in full sun, sheltered from wind. Pruning group 1.

• **PROPAGATION** Sow seed in containers in a cold frame in autumn. Insert semi-ripe cuttings in late summer, and hardwood or root cuttings in winter. Transplant suckers in winter.

• **PESTS AND DISEASES** Susceptible to canker and leaf spot.

B. papyrifera ■ ♀ (Paper mulberry). Rounded, suckering tree or large shrub with ovate to deeply lobed, grey-green leaves, to 20cm (8in) long, which are roughly hairy above, softly hairy below. Male flowers with creamy anthers are borne in stout, pendent catkins, to 7cm (3in) long, in late spring and early summer. Female flowers, with slender purple stigmas, are produced in spherical heads, to 2cm (¾in) across,

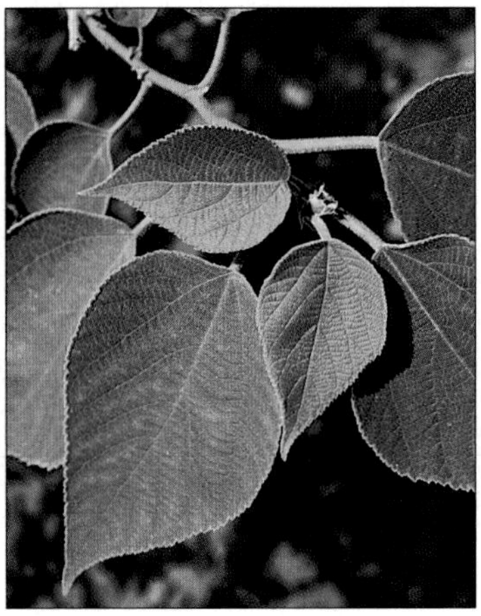

Broussonetia papyrifera

and develop into mulberry-like, sweet-tasting, edible, orange-red fruit in autumn. ↕↔ 8m (25ft). China, Korea, Japan. ❄❄❄ (borderline)

BROWALLIA

Amethyst violet, Bush violet

SOLANACEAE

Genus of 6 upright, bushy annuals and subshubby perennials from damp, shady areas and woodland in N. South America and the West Indies. They have slender, ovate to elliptic leaves and salverform, violet, purple, blue, or white flowers, with 5 broad, unequal lobes. In frost-prone areas, grow as short-lived container plants in a conservatory or in the home. In tropical climates, grow in a border or container.

• **HARDINESS** Frost tender.

• **CULTIVATION** Under glass, grow in loam-based potting compost (JI No.2) in full light, with shade from hot sun and good ventilation. When in full growth, water moderately and apply a balanced liquid fertilizer monthly; keep just moist in winter. Pinch out the growing tips to encourage bushy plants. Outdoors, grow in fertile, well-drained soil in full sun or partial shade.

• **PROPAGATION** Sow seed at 18°C (64°F) in early spring for summer-flowering plants and in late summer for winter- to spring-flowering plants.

• **PESTS AND DISEASES** Aphids and whiteflies may be a problem under glass.

B. americana, syn. *B. elata*. Variable, erect, bushy annual with usually ovate, pointed or blunt, slightly sticky, matt

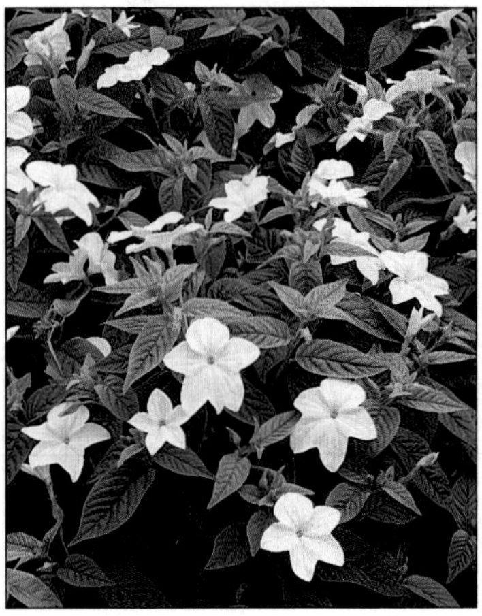

Browallia speciosa 'White Troll'

leaves, to 10cm (4in) long. In summer, bears single- or several-flowered, axillary inflorescences of violet to blue or white flowers, 5cm (2in) across. ↕↔ to 60cm (24in). Tropical South America. ❀ (min. 13–16°C/55–61°F)

B. elata see *B. americana.*

B. speciosa (Sapphire flower). Woody-based, bushy perennial, usually grown as an annual, with ovate or elliptic, rounded or pointed, slightly sticky, matt leaves, 10cm (4in) long. In summer, violet, blue, or white flowers, 5cm (2in) across, are borne singly or in small clusters from the leaf axils. ↕ 60cm (24in), ↔ 25cm (10in). Tropical South America. ❀ (min. 13–16°C/55–61°F). **'Blue Bells'** is compact, with violet-blue flowers; ↕ to 20cm (8in). **'Blue Troll'** is compact, with clear blue flowers; ↕ to 25cm (10in). **'Heavenly Bells'** bears pale sky-blue flowers, 6–7cm (2½–3in) across; ↕ 30cm (12in). **'Silver Bells'** is compact, with white flowers; ↔ 25–30cm (10–12in). **'Vanja'** ■ has deep blue flowers, to 7cm (3in) across, with white eyes. **'White Troll'** ■ has pure white flowers; ↕ to 25cm (10in).

BROWNEA

CAESALPINIACEAE/LEGUMINOSAE

Genus of at least 25 species of evergreen shrubs and trees found in tropical forest in South America, grown for their foliage and attractive flowerheads. Large, opposite, pinnate leaves emerge pink or red, speckled white, later turning deep green. Small, 4- or 5-petalled flowers are mixed with large coloured bracts in pompon-like, terminal inflorescences. In

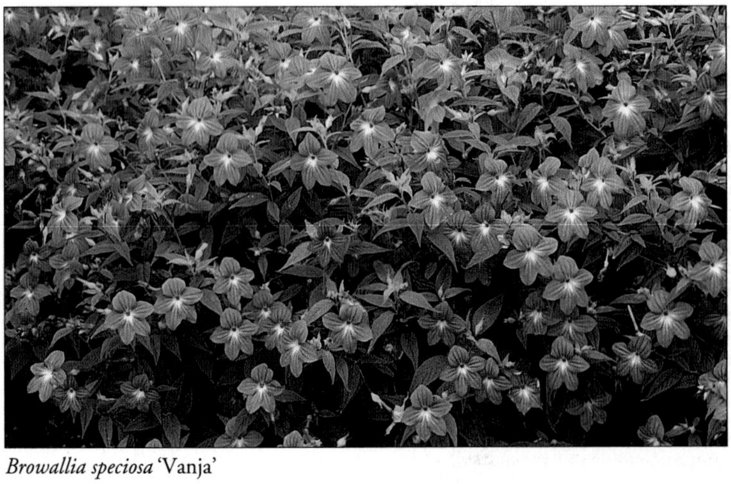

Browallia speciosa 'Vanja'

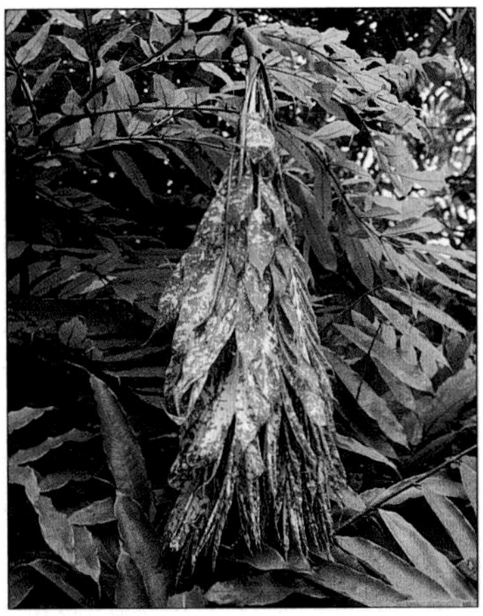

Brownea ariza

frost-prone areas, grow in a warm greenhouse; elsewhere grow as specimens.
• **HARDINESS** Frost tender.
• **CULTIVATION** Under glass, grow in loam-based potting compost (JI No.3) in full light. They need to be grown in a large container in order to flower. In growth, water freely and apply a balanced liquid fertilizer monthly; keep just moist in winter. Pot on or top-dress in early spring. Out-doors, grow in fertile, moist but well-drained soil in light dappled shade. Pruning group 1, but need restrictive pruning under glass.
• **PROPAGATION** Sow seed at 16°C (61°F) in spring. Root semi-ripe cuttings with bottom heat in summer. Layer in spring.
• **PESTS AND DISEASES** Red spider mites, mealybugs, and whiteflies may be a problem under glass.

B. ariza ▣ ♀ syn. *B. grandiceps*, *B. princeps*. Erect to spreading tree with pinnate leaves, 20–40cm (8–16in) long, consisting of 12 or more pairs of elliptic, bronze-red leaflets, pendent at first, then spreading. In summer, bears rounded, orange to red flowerheads, to 25cm (10in) across, with up to 50 flowers. ↕7–10m (22–30ft), ↔ 3–7m (10–22ft). Colombia. ✺ (min. 15°C/59°F)
B. grandiceps see *B. ariza*.
B. princeps see *B. ariza*.

BROWNINGIA
syn. AZUREOCEREUS
CACTACEAE

Genus of about 10 species of erect, tree-like, perennial cacti from hilly or low mountainous regions, principally in Peru and Chile. They branch freely towards the trunk base or from nearer the crown, like candelabra, with semi-pendent branches. The tubercled ribs produce prominently spiny areoles. Funnel-shaped, nocturnal flowers have short, rounded petals and densely scaly, often curved tubes. They are followed by spherical to ovoid, dry or juicy green fruits containing brown or black seeds. In frost-prone areas, grow in a conservatory or warm greenhouse; in warmer areas, use in a mixed cactus border or desert garden. They are large, architectural specimens when mature.
• **HARDINESS** Frost tender.
• **CULTIVATION** Under glass, grow in a mix of 4 parts standard cactus compost and 1 part lime chippings, in full light. From mid-spring to late summer, water freely and apply a low-nitrogen fertilizer every 3–4 weeks; keep completely dry at other times. Outdoors, grow in sharply drained, alkaline soil in full sun. See also pp.48–49.
• **PROPAGATION** Sow seed at 19–24°C (66–75°F) in early spring.
• **PESTS AND DISEASES** Aphids and mealybugs may be troublesome.

B. hertlingiana, syn. *Azureocereus hertlingianus*. Slow-growing cactus with a trunk, to 30cm (12in) thick, that generally branches, once it is 1m (3ft) tall, into thick, ascending, bluish green branches with 18 or more ribs. Tufted, grey-felted, yellowish brown areoles produce pale brown spines (4–7 radials, 1–3 centrals). Funnel-shaped purple flowers, 5cm (2in) across, white inside, are borne from the areoles near the stem tips in summer. ↕8m (25ft), ↔ to 1.5m (5ft). Peru, Chile. ✺ (min. 13°C/55°F)

BRUCKENTHALIA
ERICACEAE

Genus of one species of small, evergreen shrub occurring on lime-free soil in woodland and subalpine pastures in S.E. Europe. It has needle-like foliage, and bears terminal racemes of bell-shaped flowers from late spring to summer. Cultivated for its neat habit and attractive flowers, *B. spiculifolia* is suitable for a rock garden, and also associates well with heathers (*Calluna*, *Erica*), to which it is closely related.
• **HARDINESS** Fully hardy.
• **CULTIVATION** Grow in moist but well-drained, peaty, acid soil in full sun. Pruning group 10, after flowering.
• **PROPAGATION** Sow seed in containers in a cold frame in spring. Root semi-ripe cuttings in a closed propagating case with gentle bottom heat in summer.
• **PESTS AND DISEASES** Trouble free.

B. spiculifolia (Spike heath). Compact, evergreen shrub with whorls of linear, glossy, dark green leaves, to 5mm (¼in) long, which are borne on stiff, sparsely branched, upright stems. Dense, terminal racemes, to 3cm (1¼in) long, of bell-shaped, pale to deep pink, occasionally white flowers, 2–3cm (¾–1¼in) long, are produced from late spring to summer. Balkans. ↕15cm (6in), ↔ to 20cm (8in). ❄❄❄. **'Balkan Rose'** has deep pink flowers.

BRUGMANSIA
Angels' trumpets
SOLANACEAE

Genus of 5 species of evergreen shrubs and trees found in scrub and along streamsides from S. USA to South America. They are cultivated for their large, usually scented, solitary, pendent, tubular or trumpet-shaped flowers, with 5 usually reflexed, pointed lobes, borne from late spring to autumn. The leaves are alternate, simple, often toothed, and sometimes lobed. In frost-prone areas, grow in a temperate greenhouse or conservatory, and stand outside or plunge in a border for the summer. In milder areas, grow as specimen plants. All parts are highly toxic if ingested.
• **HARDINESS** Frost hardy to frost tender.
• **CULTIVATION** Under glass, grow in loam-based potting compost (JI No.3)

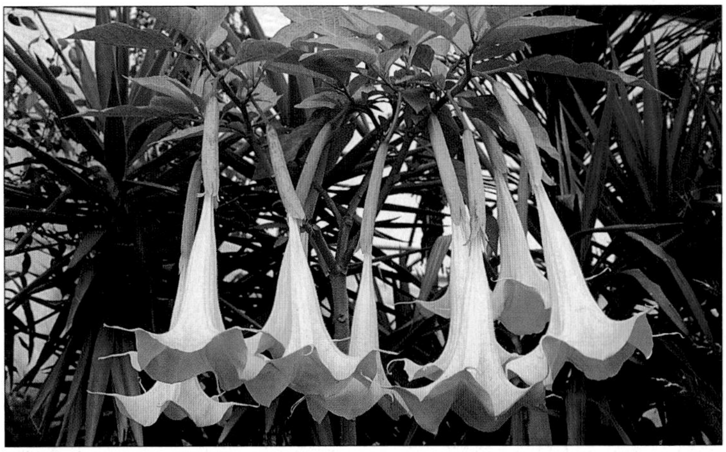

Brugmansia aurea

in full light. From spring to autumn, water freely and apply a balanced liquid fertilizer every 3–4 weeks; keep just moist in winter. Outdoors, grow in fertile, moist but well-drained soil in full sun. Pruning group 9, or 7 if required.
• **PROPAGATION** Sow seed at 16°C (61°F) in spring. Root semi-ripe cuttings with bottom heat in summer.
• **PESTS AND DISEASES** Red spider mites, whiteflies, and mealybugs may be a problem under glass.

B. arborea ♀ syn. *B. versicolor* of gardens, *Datura arborea* (Common angels' trumpets). Open shrub or tree with robust stems and elliptic-oblong to ovate, entire or coarsely toothed leaves, 15–30cm (6–12in) long. Trumpet-shaped, scented white flowers, to 15cm (6in) long, are borne from late spring to autumn. ↕2–4m (6–12ft) or more, ↔ 1.5–2.5m (5–8ft). Ecuador to N. Chile (Andes). ✺ (min. 7°C/45°F)
B. aurea ▣ ♀ syn. *Datura aurea*. Open shrub or tree with ovate leaves, 15–25cm (6–10in) long, coarsely toothed on young plants, entire on mature ones. Trumpet-shaped, night-scented, golden yellow to white flowers, to 24cm (10in) long, are borne mainly from summer to autumn. ↕5–10m (15–30ft), ↔ 2–4m (6–12ft). Colombia to Ecuador (Andes). ✺ (min. 7°C/45°F)
B. x candida ♀ (*B. aurea* x *B. versicolor*), syn. *Datura* x *candida*. Open shrub or tree with oblong-elliptic, entire to coarsely toothed, wavy-margined leaves, 30–60cm (12–24in) long. From summer to autumn, bears trumpet-shaped, night-scented flowers, to 30cm (12in) long, that may be white or soft yellow, ageing to white or, rarely, pink. ↕3–5m (10–15ft), ↔ 1.5–2.5m (5–8ft). Garden origin. ✺ (min. 7°C/45°F). **'Double White'** bears double white flowers. **'Grand Marnier'** ▣ 🏆 bears apricot flowers. **'Knightii'** 🏆 syn. 'Plena', bears hose-in-hose blooms. **'Plena'** see 'Knightii'.
***B. rosei* of gardens** see *B. sanguinea*.
B. sanguinea ▣ 🏆 ♀ syn. *B. rosei* of gardens, *Datura rosei* of gardens (Red angels' trumpets). Open shrub or tree with ovate-oblong, wavy-margined, coarsely toothed to entire leaves, to 18cm (7in) long. Tubular, unscented flowers, 15–25cm (6–10in) long, orange-red with yellow veins, are borne from late spring to autumn. ↕3–10m (10–30ft), ↔ 2–3m (6–10ft). Colombia to N. Chile. ✺ (min. 7°C/45°F)

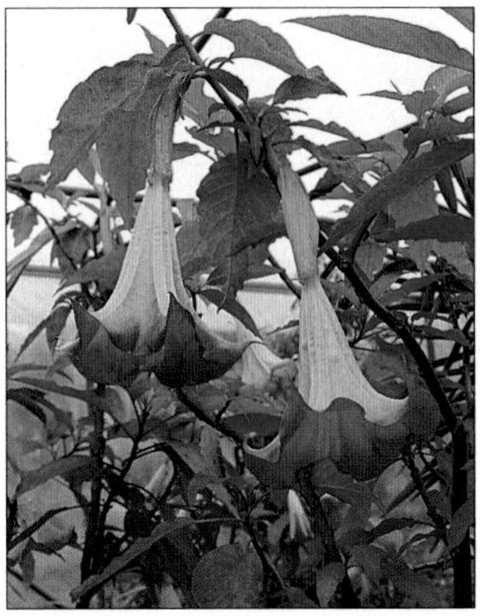

Brugmansia x *candida* 'Grand Marnier'

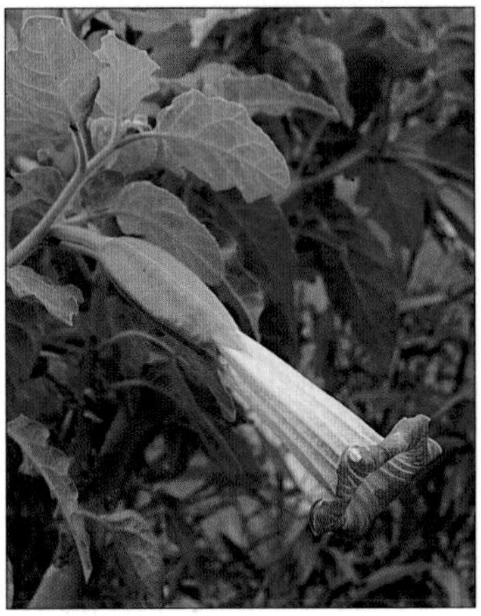

Brugmansia sanguinea

B. suaveolens 🏆 ♀ Vigorous shrub or tree with ovate-oblong to narrowly elliptic, hairless or hairy, entire leaves, to 20cm (8in) long. Tubular-bell-shaped, night-scented, white, sometimes yellow or pink flowers, 30cm (12in) long, are produced from early summer to autumn. ↕to 5m (15ft), ↔ 2.5–3m (8–10ft). S.E. Brazil. ✺ (min. 7°C/45°F)
B. versicolor ♀ Open shrub or tree with oblong-elliptic, hairless or slightly hairy, entire leaves, 20–50cm (8–20in) long. From late spring to autumn, produces trumpet-shaped flowers, 40cm (16in) or more long, that are usually white, but sometimes age to orange or peach-pink. ↕2–5m (6–15ft), ↔ 1.5–2.5m (5–8ft). Ecuador. ✺ (min. 7°C/45°F)
***B. versicolor* of gardens** see *B. arborea*.

B

BRUNFELSIA

SOLANACEAE

Genus of approximately 40 species of evergreen shrubs and small trees growing in light woodland and thickets in tropical North, Central, and South America. They are cultivated for their large, tubular, salverform flowers, each with 5 broad petal lobes. The alternate, simple leaves are elliptic to ovate, oblong, or spoon-shaped. In frost-prone climates, grow in a cool or temperate greenhouse. In frost-free climates, plant in a border.

- **HARDINESS** Frost tender.
- **CULTIVATION** Under glass, grow in loam-based potting compost (JI No.2) in bright indirect or filtered light. When in growth, water freely and apply a balanced liquid fertilizer every 3–4 weeks; water sparingly in winter. Pot on or top-dress in late winter. Outdoors, grow in fertile, humus-rich, moist but well-drained soil, in full sun with some midday shade. Pruning group 8; pinch out stem tips of young plants to promote branching.
- **PROPAGATION** Root softwood cuttings in spring or summer.
- **PESTS AND DISEASES** Susceptible to red spider mites and mealybugs under glass.

B. americana (Lady of the night). Erect to spreading shrub or small tree with elliptic to obovate, mid- to deep green leaves, 5–13cm (2–5in) long. Solitary, night-scented flowers, 8cm (3in) long, which age from white to creamy yellow, are produced during summer. ↕ 2–5m (6–15ft), ↔ 1–3m (3–10ft). West Indies. ❀ (min. 7°C/45°F)
B. calycina see *B. pauciflora.*
B. eximia see *B. pauciflora.*
B. pauciflora ♀ syn. *B. calycina, B. eximia* (Yesterday, today, and tomorrow). Bushy shrub with elliptic to oblong-lance-shaped, leathery, glossy, deep green leaves, 7–15cm (3–6in) long. Terminal or axillary cymes of up to 10 wavy-margined, pansy-like flowers, 3.5–5cm (1½–2in) across, opening purple and ageing almost to white, are borne from spring to summer. ↕ 1–3m (3–10ft), ↔ 0.5–1.5m (1½–5ft). Brazil. ❀ (min. 7°C/45°F). **'Floribunda'** is spreading, with freely borne flowers that open violet and age to purple; ↕ to 1.5m (5ft). **'Macrantha'** ■ has very large flowers, to 8cm (3in) across.

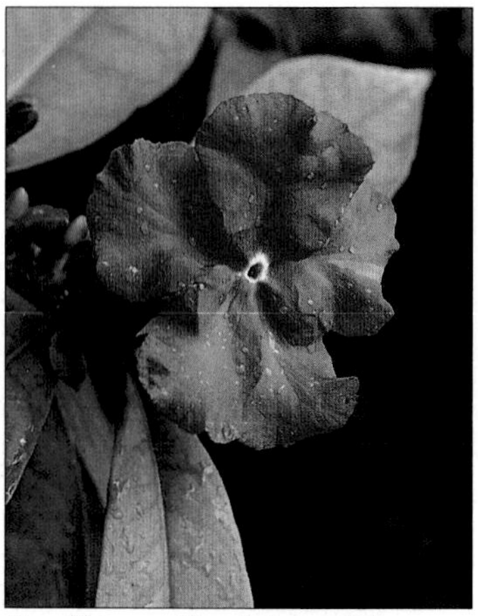

Brunfelsia pauciflora 'Macrantha'

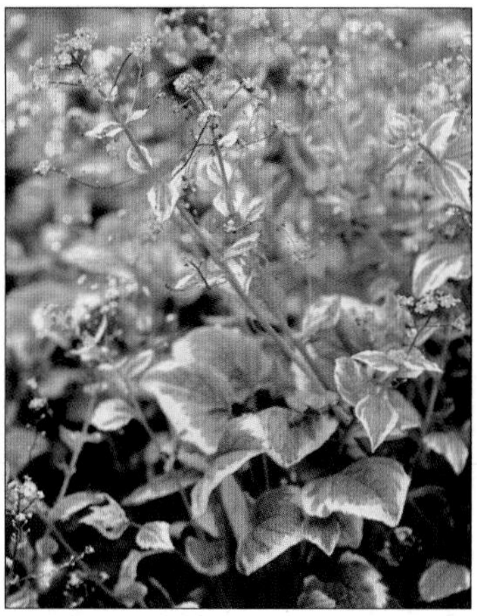

Brunnera macrophylla 'Dawson's White'

BRUNNERA

BORAGINACEAE

Genus of 3 species of rhizomatous perennials from woodland in E. Europe and N.W. Asia, valued for their flowers and ground-covering foliage. They have usually ovate, rough-hairy basal leaves and lance-shaped to ovate stem leaves. Terminal, cyme-like panicles of forget-me-not-like, purple-blue, rarely white flowers are borne in mid- and late spring. Grow in woodland or a border.

- **HARDINESS** Fully hardy.
- **CULTIVATION** Grow in moderately fertile, humus-rich, moist but well-drained soil, in a cool site.
- **PROPAGATION** In early spring, sow seed in containers in a cold frame, or divide. Take root cuttings of *B. macrophylla* in winter.
- **PESTS AND DISEASES** Trouble free.

B. macrophylla ♀ syn. *Anchusa myosotidiflora.* Rhizomatous perennial with softly hairy, mid- to deep green leaves. Basal leaves are ovate-heart-shaped, sharp-pointed, 5–20cm (2–8in) long, with long leaf-stalks; stem leaves are lance-shaped to elliptic-ovate. In mid- and late spring, produces bright blue flowers, to 7mm (¼in) across, in panicles 20cm (8in) or more long. ↕ 45cm (18in), ↔ 60cm (24in). Caucasus. ✻✻✻. **'Betty Bowring'** bears white flowers. **'Dawson's White'** ■ syn. 'Variegata', has wide, irregular, creamy white leaf margins. **'Hadspen Cream'** ♀ has irregular, creamy white leaf margins, narrower than those of 'Dawson's White'. **'Langtrees'** has leaves regularly spotted with silvery grey. **'Variegata'** see 'Dawson's White'.

▷ **x *Brunsdonna*** see x *Amarygia*
  x *B. parkeri* see x *A. parkeri*

BRUNSVIGIA

AMARYLLIDACEAE/LILIACEAE

Genus of about 20 species of bulbous perennials from grassland in South Africa, producing showy, terminal umbels of funnel-shaped flowers from late summer to autumn. Strap-shaped to oblong-ovate, basal leaves appear after or with the flowers. In frost-prone areas, grow in a cool greenhouse; in warmer areas, plant in a warm, sunny border or at the base of a warm, sunny wall.

- **HARDINESS** Half hardy to frost tender.
- **CULTIVATION** Under glass, plant in autumn in loam-based potting compost (JI No.2), with the neck of the bulb well above soil level. Provide full light, but shade lightly when in bloom. Water freely when in growth and sparingly as leaves wither; keep warm and dry when dormant. Repot or remove offsets only when congested. Outdoors, grow in sandy, sharply drained soil in full sun.
- **PROPAGATION** Sow seed at 18–21°C (64–70°F) as soon as ripe in sandy potting compost. Remove offsets in autumn before bulbs start into growth.
- **PESTS AND DISEASES** Vulnerable to leaf scorch, narcissus eelworm, mealybugs, aphids, whiteflies, and red spider mites.

B. josephinae. Perennial with very large bulbs. In autumn, bears umbels of up to 30 red flowers, 7cm (3in) long, with recurved tips. Strap-shaped, dark green leaves, 60–90cm (24–36in) long, appear after the flowers. ↕ 45–90cm (18–36in), ↔ 30cm (12in). South Africa. ✻

▷ ***Bryophyllum*** see *Kalanchoe*
  B. daigremontianum see *K. daigremontiana*
  B. tubiflorum see *K. delagoensis*
  B. uniflorum see *K. uniflora*
▷ **Buckeye** see *Aesculus*
  Bottlebrush see *A. parviflora*
  California see *A. californica*
  Ohio see *A. glabra*
  Red see *A. pavia*
  Yellow see *A. flava*
▷ **Buckler fern** see *Dryopteris*
  Broad see *D. dilatata*
  Narrow see *D. carthusiana*
▷ **Buckthorn,**
  Alder see *Rhamnus frangula*
  Common see *Rhamnus cathartica*
  Italian see *Rhamnus alaternus*
  Sea see *Hippophae rhamnoides*
▷ **Buckwheat,**
  Saffron see *Eriogonum crocatum*
  Wild see *Eriogonum*

BUDDLEJA syn. BUDDLEIA

BUDDLEJACEAE/LOGANIACEAE

Genus of about 100 species of evergreen, semi-evergreen, and deciduous shrubs, sometimes trees and climbers, and a few herbaceous perennials, from riversides, rocky areas, and scrub in Asia, Africa, and North and South America. They are cultivated for their panicles of small, tubular, usually fragrant flowers, and sometimes for their lance-shaped to broadly ovate, usually opposite leaves. All except the climbers are suitable for a mixed or shrub border; the frost-hardy species generally grow and flower best against a warm, sunny wall. In frost-prone areas, grow half-hardy and tender species in a cool greenhouse. *B. davidii* and several other species, such as *B. alternifolia* and *B. crispa* are attractive to insects.

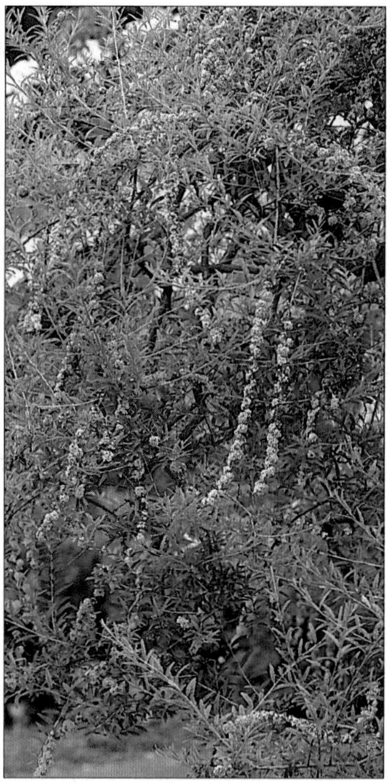

Buddleja alternifolia

- **HARDINESS** Fully hardy to frost tender.
- **CULTIVATION** Under glass, grow in loam-based potting compost (JI No.3) in full light with good ventilation. Water freely when in growth, sparingly in winter. Outdoors, grow in fertile, well-drained soil in full sun. Pruning group 6 for most; group 2 for *B. alternifolia, B. colvilei, B. farreri,* and *B. globosa* (although the last 3 need minimal pruning). Pruning group 13 for wall-trained plants: after flowering for those that bloom in spring or early summer, in spring for late-summer and autumn-flowering species.

BUDDLEJA INFLORESCENCES

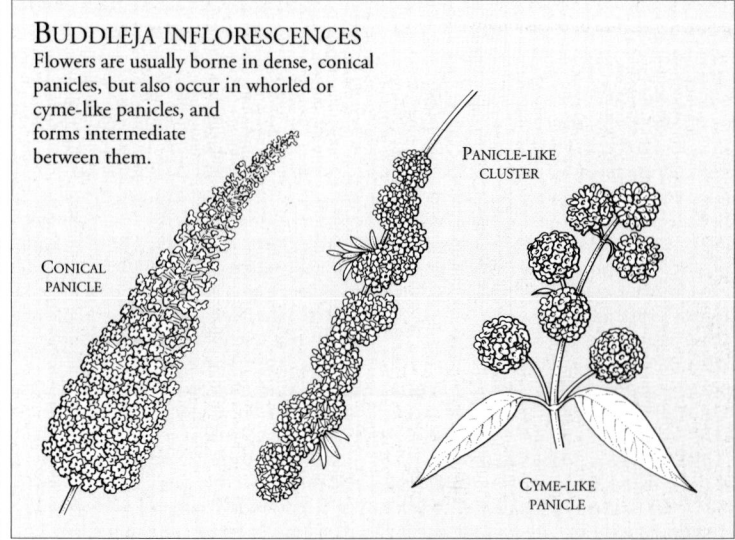

Flowers are usually borne in dense, conical panicles, but also occur in whorled or cyme-like panicles, and forms intermediate between them.

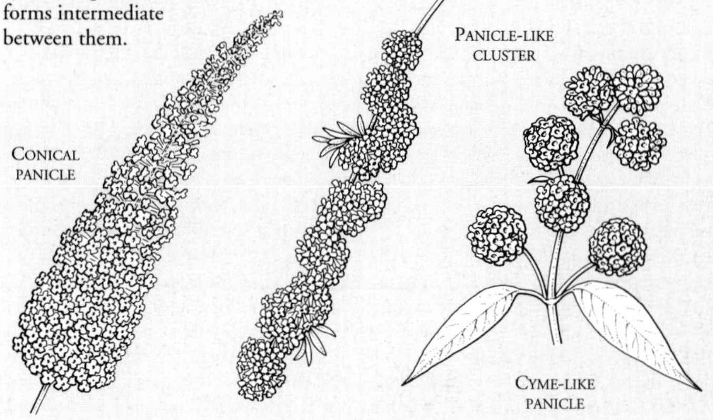

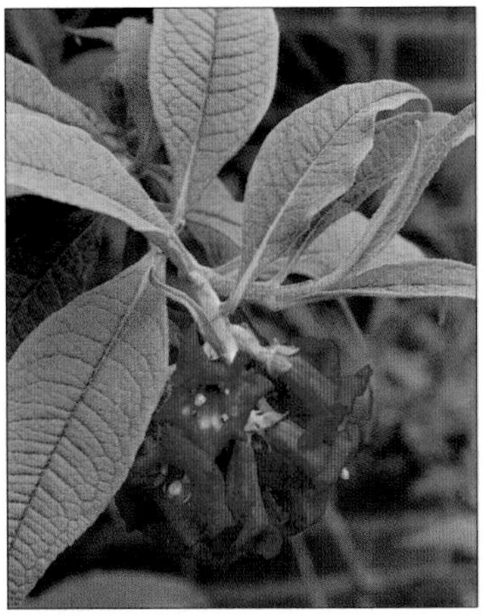

Buddleja colvilei 'Kewensis'

- **PROPAGATION** Root semi-ripe cuttings in summer. Root hardwood cuttings of *B. davidii* in autumn.
- **PESTS AND DISEASES** Prey to capsid bugs, caterpillars, figwort weevil, mullein moth, and red spider mites.

B. alternifolia ▣ ♀ Ϙ Deciduous shrub or small tree with slender, arching shoots and alternate, lance-shaped, dark green, occasionally silvery green leaves, to 7cm (3in) long. Dense, rounded clusters, 4cm (1½in) long, of intensely fragrant lilac flowers wreathe the branches of the previous year's growth in early summer. Trained as a standard, it is an excellent specimen plant. ↕↔ 4m (12ft). China. ❄❄❄
B. asiatica ♀ Evergreen shrub with arching white- or grey-woolly shoots and lance-shaped, dark green leaves, to 30cm (12in) long. Fragrant white flowers are produced in cyme-like panicles, to 25cm (10in) long, in late winter and early spring. ↕↔ 3m (10ft). Himalayas to S.E. Asia. ❄❄
B. auriculata. Upright, evergreen shrub with narrowly ovate-oblong, glossy, dark green leaves, to 12cm (5in) long, white beneath. Small, strongly fragrant, creamy white flowers, with orange or pink centres, are produced in axillary and terminal, cyme-like panicles, to 5cm (2in) long, from autumn to winter. ↕↔ 3m (10ft). South Africa. ❄❄
B. colvilei Ϙ Upright, stoutly branched, deciduous (sometimes semi-evergreen) shrub or small tree with elliptic-lance-shaped, dark green leaves, 12cm (5in) or more long. Bears tight, pendent, terminal, occasionally axillary

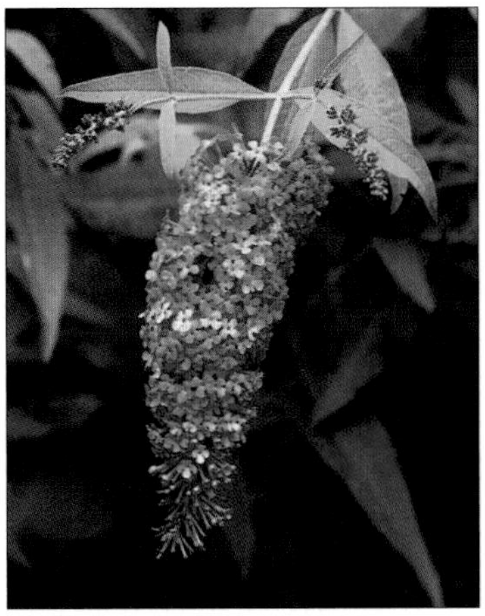

Buddleja davidii 'Empire Blue'

panicles, to 20cm (8in) long, of dark pink or red flowers in early summer. ↕↔ 6m (20ft). Himalayas. ❄❄❄.
'Kewensis' ▣ bears dark red flowers.
B. crispa ▣ Arching, deciduous shrub with white-woolly young shoots and broadly ovate-triangular, white-hairy leaves, to 12cm (5in) long. Fragrant, lilac-pink flowers are produced in dense, whorled, cyme-like, terminal and axillary panicles, to 10cm (4in) long, in mid- and late summer. ↕↔ 3m (10ft). Himalayas. ❄❄❄ (borderline)
B. davidii (Butterfly bush). Variable, fast-growing, deciduous shrub with long, arching shoots and lance-shaped, pointed, mid-green to grey-green leaves, to 25cm (10in) long. From summer to autumn, bears dense panicles, 30cm (12in) or more long, of fragrant, lilac to purple flowers. ↕ 3m (10ft), ↔ 5m (15ft). China, Japan. ❄❄❄. **'Black Knight'** ♀ bears dark purple-blue flowers. **'Charming'** bears lavender-pink flowers. **'Dartmoor'** ♀ has slender leaves with deeply cut margins and reddish purple flowers in open-branched panicles. **'Empire Blue'** ▣ ♀ has violet-blue flowers with orange eyes. **'Fascinating'** ▣ bears lilac-pink flowers in broad, tight panicles, 10cm (4in) or more across. **'Fortune'** bears soft lilac-blue flowers in slender panicles, to 40cm (16in) long. **'Glasnevin Blue'** see *B.* 'Glasnevin'. **'Harlequin'** ▣ has leaves that are yellow-margined when young, cream-margined when mature, and dark red-purple flowers. **'Nanho Blue'**, syn. 'Petite Indigo', has slender leaves and narrow panicles, to 15cm (6in) long, of pale lilac-blue flowers. **'Peace'** produces

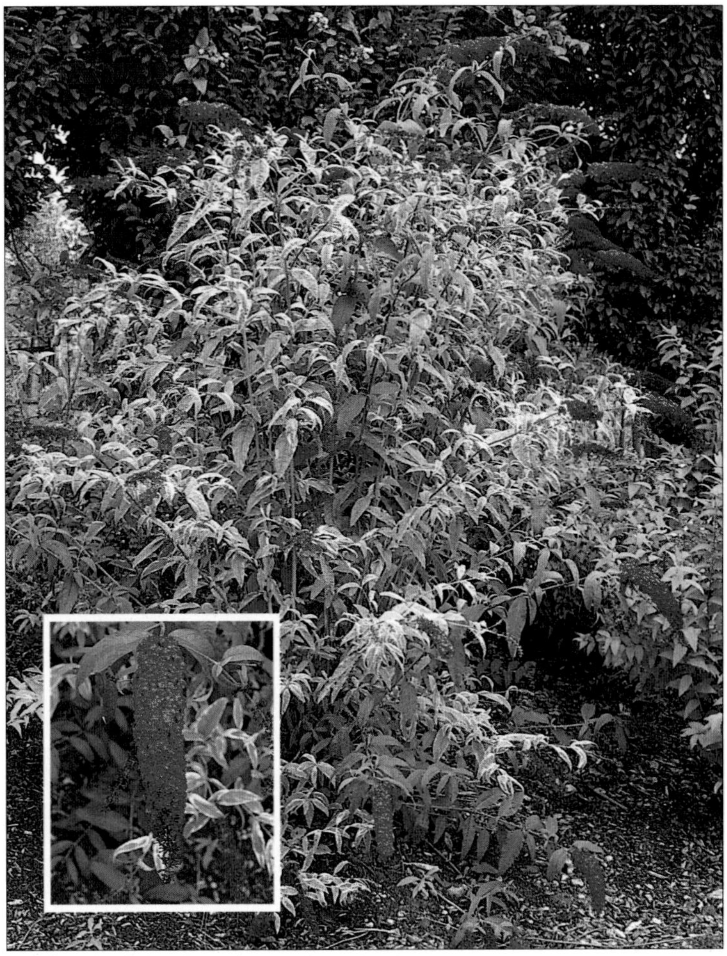

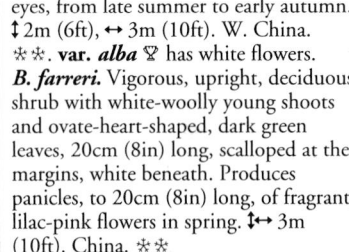

Buddleja davidii 'Harlequin' (inset: flower detail)

panicles, to 50cm (20in) long, of white flowers with orange eyes. **'Petite Indigo'** see 'Nanho Blue'. **'Pink Delight'** ♀ (a hybrid of *B. davidii*) has panicles, to 30cm (12in) long, of bright pink flowers with orange eyes. **'Pink Pearl'** has lilac-pink flowers with orange eyes. **'Royal Red'** ▣ ♀ has dark red-purple flowers in panicles to 50cm (20in) long. **'White Harlequin'** has leaves margined creamy white, and white flowers. **'White Profusion'** ▣ ♀ has yellow-eyed white flowers in panicles, to 40cm (16in) long.
B. fallowiana. Deciduous shrub with arching stems and lance-shaped, grey-white leaves, to 12cm (5in) long, mid-green beneath, and densely white-felted, particularly when young. Bears panicles, to 15cm (6in) long, of very fragrant, pale lavender-blue flowers, with orange eyes, from late summer to early autumn. ↕ 2m (6ft), ↔ 3m (10ft). W. China. ❄❄. **var. *alba*** ♀ has white flowers.
B. farreri. Vigorous, upright, deciduous shrub with white-woolly young shoots and ovate-heart-shaped, dark green leaves, 20cm (8in) long, scalloped at the margins, white beneath. Produces panicles, to 20cm (8in) long, of fragrant, lilac-pink flowers in spring. ↕↔ 3m (10ft). China. ❄❄
***B.* 'Glasnevin'**, syn. *B. davidii* 'Glasnevin Blue'. Spreading, semi-evergreen shrub with lance-shaped, dark green leaves, 20cm (8in) long, densely white-woolly beneath, grey-hairy when young. From late summer to autumn, bears fragrant, dark lilac-pink flowers in dense panicles, to 30cm (12in) long. ↕ 2.5m (8ft), ↔ 3m (10ft). ❄❄❄

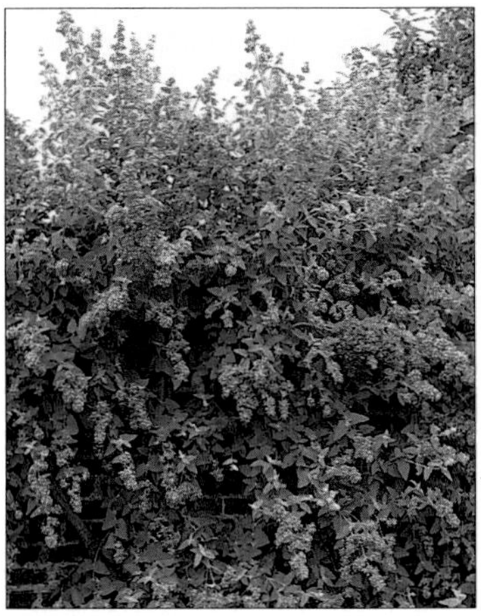

Buddleja crispa

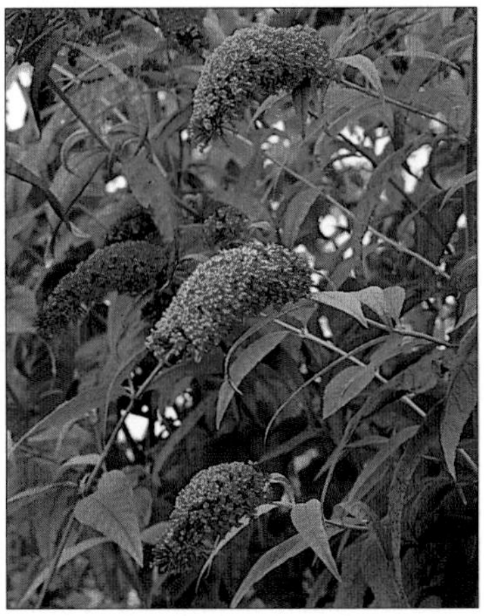

Buddleja davidii 'Fascinating'

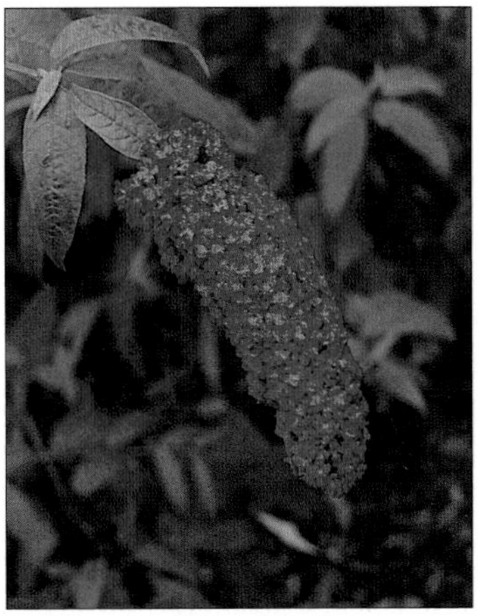

Buddleja davidii 'Royal Red'

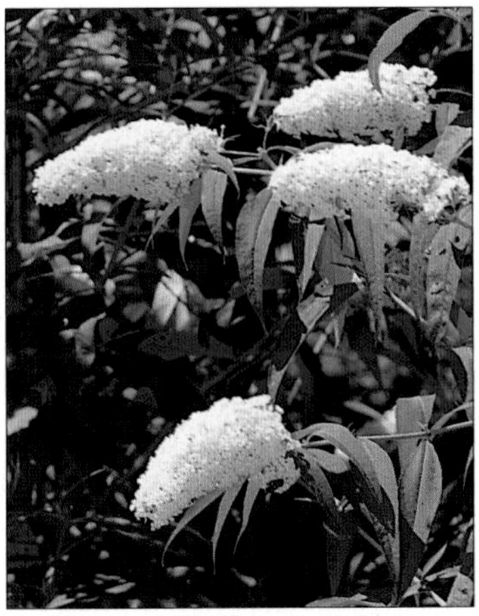

Buddleja davidii 'White Profusion'

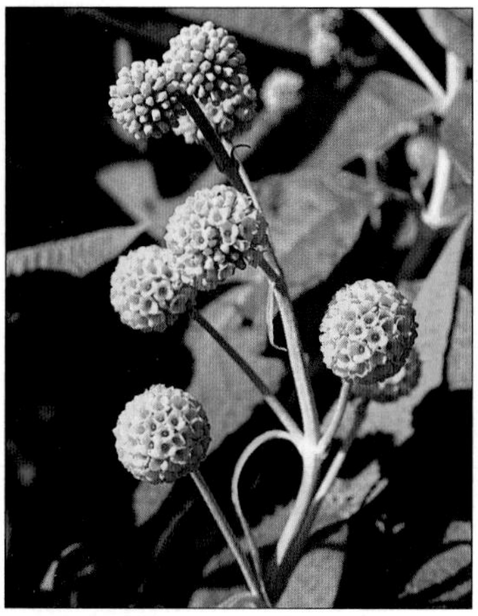

Buddleja globosa

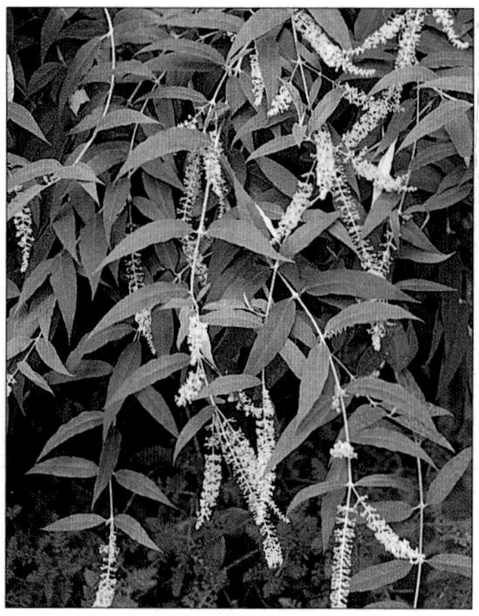

Buddleja madagascariensis

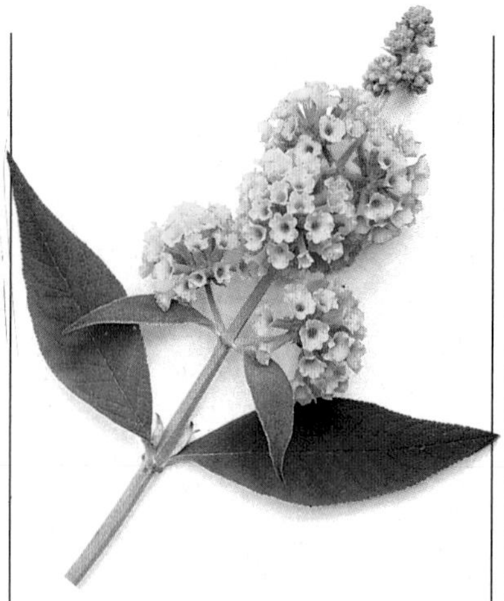

Buddleja x *weyeriana* 'Sungold'

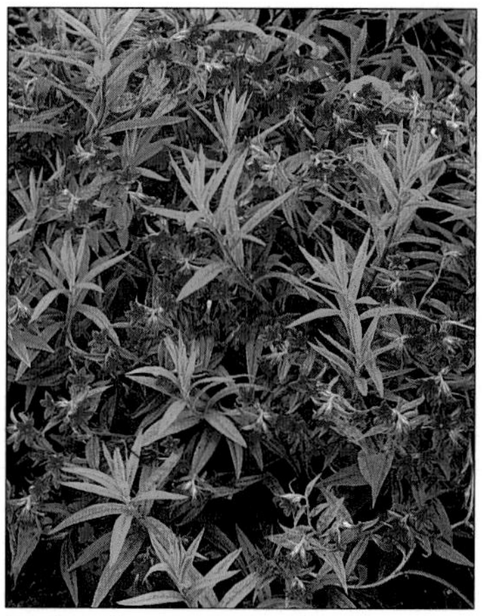

Buglossoides purpurocaerulea

B. globosa ■ ♀ (Orange ball tree). Rounded, stiffly branched, deciduous or semi-evergreen shrub with lance-shaped, deeply veined, dark green leaves, to 20cm (8in) long. Bears dense, rounded clusters, to 2cm (¾in) across, of fragrant, dark orange and yellow flowers in open panicles in early summer. ↕↔ 5m (15ft). Chile, Argentina. ❄❄
B. lindleyana ■ Upright, somewhat arching, slender-branched, deciduous shrub with ovate, dark green leaves, 10cm (4in) long, borne on square stems. Distinctly curved, dark violet flowers, 2cm (¾in) long, are borne in nodding panicles, to 20cm (8in) long, in late summer. ↕↔ 2m (6ft). China. ❄❄
***B.* 'Lochinch'** ♀ Spreading, vigorous, deciduous shrub with long, arching, grey-hairy shoots and lance-shaped, white-hairy, mid-green leaves, to 20cm (8in) long, that become greener with age. From late summer to autumn, bears fragrant, orange-eyed, violet-blue flowers in panicles to 20cm (8in) long. ↕ 2.5m (8ft), ↔ 3m (10ft). ❄❄❄
B. madagascariensis ■ syn. *B. nicodemia, Nicodemia madagascariensis.* Vigorous, strongly branched, evergreen shrub or lax climber with lance-shaped, deep green leaves, 5–14cm (2–5½in) long, white-felted beneath. From autumn to spring, bears bright orange-yellow flowers in slender, terminal panicles, 15–25cm (6–10in) long, sometimes followed by small, amethyst-purple berries. ↕↔ 2–4m (6–12ft). Madagascar. ❀ (min. 5–7°C/41–45°F)
B. nicodemia see *B. madagascariensis.*
B. nivea. Vigorous, upright, deciduous shrub with stout, densely white-woolly shoots and narrowly ovate leaves, to 20cm (8in) long, dark green above, white below. In late summer, bears slender panicles, to 15cm (6in) long, of pale lilac-blue or violet-blue flowers. ↕ 3m (10ft), ↔ 2.5m (8ft). China. ❄❄❄
B. officinalis. Upright, evergreen or semi-evergreen shrub with arching shoots and narrowly lance-shaped, dark green leaves, 15cm (6in) long, grey beneath. From winter to early spring, bears fragrant, yellow-eyed, lilac-pink flowers in arching panicles, to 30cm (12in) long. ↕↔ 2.5m (8ft). China. ❄❄
***B.* x *pikei* 'Hever'.** Spreading, branched, deciduous shrub with slender, arching shoots and opposite or alternate, ovate to oblong, grey-green leaves, to 15cm (6in) long, maturing to dark green. Fragrant, lilac-mauve flowers, with orange centres, are produced in arching panicles, to 30cm (12in) long, in late summer. ↕↔ 3m (10ft). ❄❄
B. salviifolia (South African sage wood). Arching, semi-evergreen shrub with sage-like, lance-shaped, grey-green leaves, to 10cm (4in) long, borne on very short stalks. Fragrant, pale lilac-blue flowers are produced in panicles, to 15cm (6in) long, in late autumn and early winter. ↕ 3m (10ft), ↔ 3m (10ft) or more. E. Africa, South Africa. ❄❄
***B.* 'West Hill'** ■ Vigorous, deciduous shrub with long, arching, grey-hairy shoots and lance-shaped, white-hairy, mid-green leaves, 20cm (8in) long. Fragrant, orange-eyed, pale lavender-blue flowers are produced in slender, arching panicles, to 20cm (8in) long, from late summer to autumn. ↕ 2.5m (8ft), ↔ 3m (10ft). ❄❄

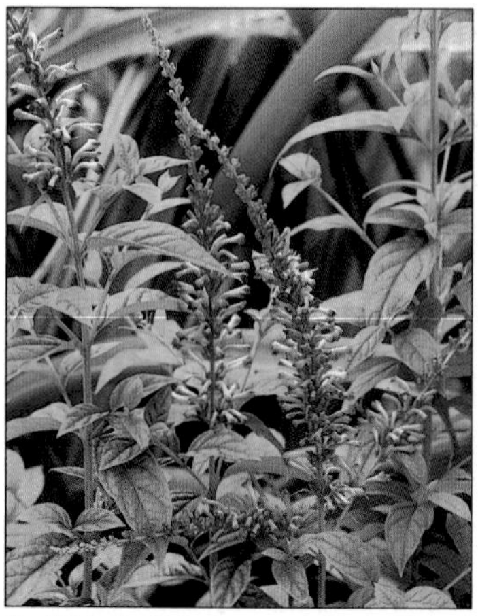

Buddleja lindleyana

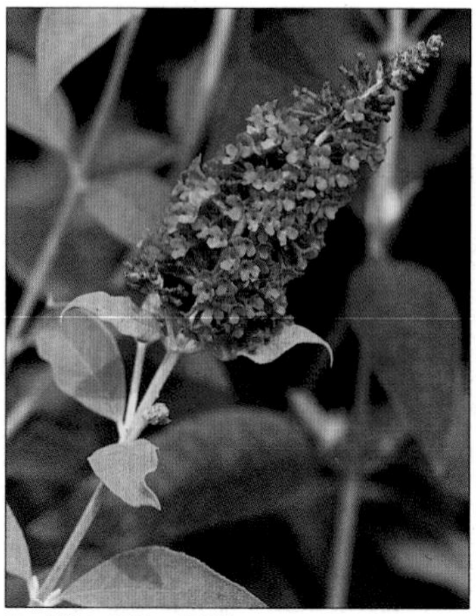

Buddleja 'West Hill'

B.* x *weyeriana (*B. davidii* x *B. globosa*). Spreading, deciduous shrub with long, arching shoots and lance-shaped, mid-green leaves, to 20cm (8in) long, both grey-hairy when young. Rounded clusters of fragrant yellow to violet flowers are produced in open, terminal panicles, to 30cm (12in) long, from summer to autumn. ↕ 4m (12ft), ↔ 3m (10ft). Garden origin. ❄❄❄. **'Golden Glow'** is vigorous, with loose clusters of mauve-flushed, orange-yellow flowers. **'Sungold'** ■ ♀ has dense heads of dark orange-yellow flowers.

▷**Buffalo berry** see *Shepherdia argentea*
▷**Buffalo-wood** see *Burchellia*
▷**Bugbane** see *Cimicifuga*
▷**Bugle** see *Ajuga*
  Blue see *A. genevensis*
  Pyramidal see *A. pyramidalis*
  Upright see *A. genevensis*

BUGLOSSOIDES

BORAGINACEAE

Genus, similar to *Lithospermum*, of about 15 species of hairy annuals, perennials, and evergreen or semi-evergreen subshrubs from sunny scrub and rocky slopes in W. and S. Europe, N. Africa, and parts of W. Asia. They have erect or decumbent stems, which sometimes root at the tips, and produce variable, simple, rough-hairy, mid- to dark green leaves and terminal cymes of small, salverform flowers. Grow in a border, rock garden, or wild garden.

• **HARDINESS** Fully hardy.
• **CULTIVATION** Grow in well-drained, fertile, neutral to alkaline soil in full sun with some midday shade.
• **PROPAGATION** Sow seed of annuals and perennials in containers in a cold frame in autumn or spring. Divide perennials in early spring. Root softwood cuttings of subshrubs in midsummer.
• **PESTS AND DISEASES** Trouble free.

B. gastonii. Rhizomatous perennial with erect stems and ovate-lance-shaped to lance-shaped, rough, mid-green leaves, to 6cm (2½in) long. In early summer, bears cymes of initially purple, later blue flowers, to 1.5cm (½in) long, with white throats. ↕ 30–45cm (12–18in), ↔ 30cm (12in). W. Pyrenees. ❄❄❄
B. purpurocaerulea ■ syn. *Lithospermum purpureocaeruleum.* Rhizomatous perennial with tip-rooting, decumbent, non-flowering stems and lance-shaped, dark green leaves, to 8cm (3in) long. In late spring and early summer, erect stems bear cymes of initially purple, later gentian-blue flowers, 1–2cm (½–¾in) long. ↕ to 60cm (24in), ↔ variable. W. Europe to N. Iran. ❄❄❄

BULBINE

ASPHODELACEAE/LILIACEAE

Genus of about 30 species of clump-forming, succulent and non-succulent, occasionally slightly woody-stemmed, sometimes bulbous or tuberous perennials, and one annual, occurring in desert grasslands in E. and South Africa, and Australia. They have linear to broadly lance-shaped, mid- to blue-green, basal leaves. Dense, terminal racemes of small, star-shaped to shallowly cup-shaped flowers, with conspicuously hairy stamens, are borne in spring or summer. In frost-prone areas, grow in a cool greenhouse. In frost-free areas, grow in a rock garden.

• **HARDINESS** Half hardy to frost tender; some withstand occasional light frost.
• **CULTIVATION** Under glass, grow in loam-based potting compost (JI No.2) with additional sharp sand, in full light with good ventilation. Water freely when in growth; keep dry in winter. Outdoors, grow in well-drained, sandy loam in full sun. Bulbines are tolerant of poor, dry soil.
• **PROPAGATION** Sow seed at 13–18°C (55–64°F) in early spring. Divide or root offsets in spring. Root stem cuttings of *B. frutescens* in summer.
• **PESTS AND DISEASES** Trouble free.

B. alooides. Clump-forming perennial with compact rosettes of lance-shaped, fleshy, mid-green leaves, 15–22cm (6–9in) long. Racemes, 20–30cm (8–12in) long, of star-shaped yellow flowers, to 4mm (⅛in) across, are produced in late spring. ↕ 30cm (12in), ↔ 15cm (6in). South Africa. ❀ (min. 5°C/41°F)
B. caulescens see *B. frutescens.*
B. frutescens, syn. *B. caulescens.* Succulent, branching, slightly woody-stemmed perennial with lance-shaped, blue-green, basal leaves, 4–22cm (1½–9in) long. Racemes, 15–30cm (6–12in) long, of star-shaped yellow flowers, 7–10mm (¼–½in) across, are borne in summer. ↕↔ 40cm (16in). South Africa. ❀ (min. 5°C/41°F)

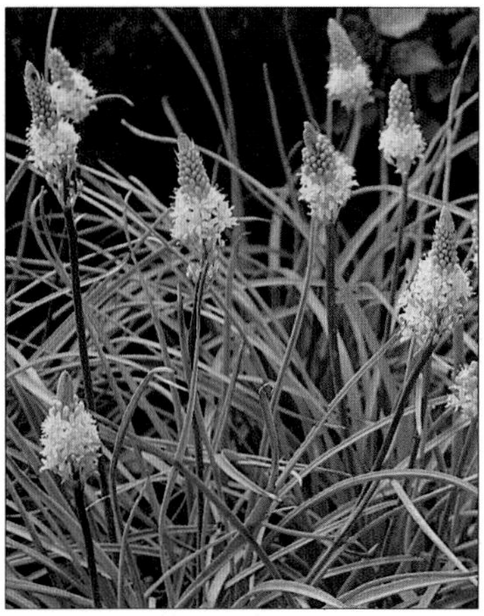

Bulbinella hookeri

BULBINELLA

ASPHODELACEAE/LILIACEAE

Genus of 20 species of robust perennials from grassland in South Africa and New Zealand. They have fleshy roots, and basal rosettes of succulent, grass-like leaves, 15–45cm (6–18in) long. In late winter, spring, or summer, they bear dense, terminal racemes of star-shaped or shallowly cup-shaped, occasionally monoecious flowers, usually to 1.5cm (½in) across. Grow in a rock garden or peat garden. In frost-prone areas, grow *B. cauda-felis* in an alpine house.
• **HARDINESS** Frost hardy to half hardy.
• **CULTIVATION** Grow in moist but well-drained, neutral to acid soil in full sun or partial shade. Mulch with leaf mould in winter. In an alpine house, grow in a mix of equal parts loam, leaf mould, and sharp sand.
• **PROPAGATION** Sow seed in a cold frame as soon as ripe. Divide in autumn.
• **PESTS AND DISEASES** Prey to whiteflies, red spider mites, and aphids under glass.

B. cauda-felis, syn. *B. setosa*. Robust perennial with leaves to 20cm (8in) long and racemes of bisexual yellow flowers, ageing to reddish brown, borne in late winter and early spring. ↕ 30cm (12in), ↔ 15cm (6in). South Africa. ❄
B. hookeri ■ Robust perennial with leaves 30cm (12in) long and racemes of bisexual yellow flowers borne from spring to summer. ↕ 60cm (24in), ↔ 30cm (12in). New Zealand. ❄❄
B. rossii. Robust perennial with leaves to 30cm (12in) long and racemes of unisexual yellow flowers produced in spring. ↕ 1.2m (4ft), ↔ 45cm (18in). New Zealand. ❄❄
B. setosa see *B. cauda-felis*.

BULBOCODIUM

COLCHICACEAE/LILIACEAE

Genus, related to *Colchicum*, of 2 species of cormous perennials from alpine meadows and dry grassland in S. and E. Europe. The funnel-shaped flowers, each with a single style, divided at the tip, and 6 free, clawed tepals, are borne in spring, just before or with the linear to lance-shaped, dark green leaves. Grow in a rock garden, or naturalize in turf.
• **HARDINESS** Fully hardy.
• **CULTIVATION** Plant corms 8cm (3in) deep in autumn, in humus-rich, well-drained soil in full sun.

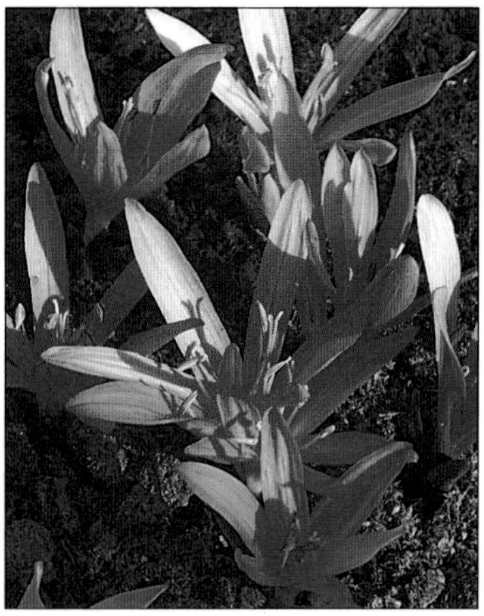

Bulbocodium vernum

• **PROPAGATION** Sow seed in containers in a cold frame in autumn or spring. Remove offsets in summer.
• **PESTS AND DISEASES** Trouble free.

B. vernum ■ Cormous perennial with 2 narrowly linear, glossy, dark green leaves, to 15cm (6in) long. Pinkish purple flowers, 4–8cm (1½–3in) long, are produced in spring. ↕ 4–8cm (1½–3in), ↔ 5cm (2in). Pyrenees, S.W. and W. central Alps. ❄❄❄

BULBOPHYLLUM

ORCHIDACEAE

Genus of 1,000–1,200 species of very variable, evergreen, epiphytic orchids from a range of habitats throughout tropical and subtropical regions. They have creeping or pendent rhizomes with angular pseudobulbs bearing 1 or 2 apical, ovate, oval, oblong-oval, or lance-shaped leaves. Flowers are borne at various times of the year, in basal racemes or umbels, occasionally singly. Many are pungent or sweet-smelling.
• **HARDINESS** Frost tender.
• **CULTIVATION** Cool- to intermediate-growing orchids. Grow in epiphytic orchid compost in a half-pot or slatted basket, or epiphytically on bark. In summer, provide high humidity and partial shade; water freely, applying fertilizer at every third watering, and mist twice daily. In winter, admit full light and keep dry. See also p.46.
• **PROPAGATION** Divide when the plant fills the pot and "flows" over the sides.
• **PESTS AND DISEASES** Susceptible to red spider mites, aphids, and mealybugs.

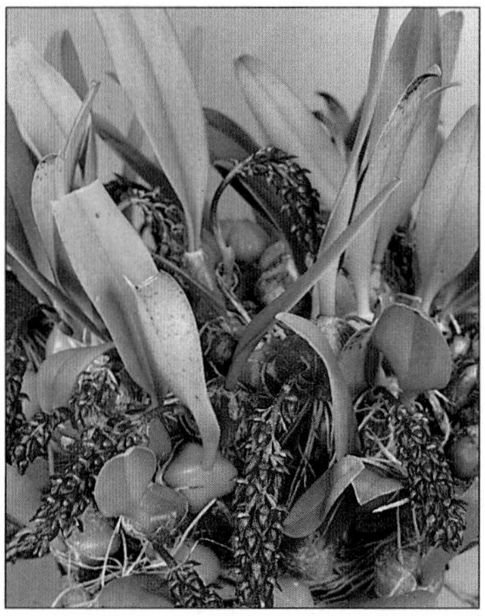

Bulbophyllum careyanum

B. careyanum ■ Epiphytic orchid with spherical to oblong pseudobulbs, each with one oblong or linear-oblong leaf, to 25cm (10in). In summer, bears dense, cylindrical, arching to pendent racemes, to 20cm (8in) long, of small, fragrant, orange-yellow or green flowers, suffused red-brown or purple, with violet lips. ↕ 25cm (10in), ↔ 30cm (12in). E. Himalayas, Burma, Thailand. ❀ (min. 13°C/55°F; max. 30°C/86°F)
B. guttulatum, syn. *Cirrhopetalum guttulatum*. Epiphytic orchid with ovoid pseudobulbs, each with one narrowly ovate leaf, 10cm (4in) long. Upright, umbel-like panicles, 15–25cm (6–10in) tall, of several small, purple-spotted, straw-yellow or green flowers, with pale purple lips, are produced in summer. ↕↔ 25cm (10in). India. ❀ (min. 13°C/55°F; max. 30°C/86°F)
B. lobbii. Epiphytic orchid with ovoid pseudobulbs, each with one narrowly oval leaf, 10cm (4in) long. In early summer, bears solitary, red-speckled, ochre-yellow flowers, 7–10cm (3–4in) across. ↕ 15cm (6in), ↔ 23cm (9in). N.E. India, S.E. Asia to the Philippines. ❀ (min. 13°C/55°F; max. 30°C/86°F)
B. medusae, syn. *Cirrhopetalum medusae*. Epiphytic orchid with ovoid pseudobulbs, each with one narrowly lance-shaped leaf, 15cm (6in) long. In summer, produces erect or arching flower stems bearing terminal umbels, to 15cm (6in) long, of small, white or cream flowers, spotted red or yellow. ↕ 20cm (8in), ↔ 23cm (9in). Thailand, Malaysia to Borneo and the Philippines. ❀ (min. 13°C/55°F; max. 30°C/86°F)

▷ **Bulbous plants** see pp.44–45
▷ **Bulrush** see *Typha*, *T. latifolia*
Lesser see *Typha angustifolia*
▷ **Bunny ears** see *Opuntia microdasys* var. *pallida*
▷ **Bunya-bunya** see *Araucaria bidwillii*

BUPHTHALMUM

ASTERACEAE/COMPOSITAE

Genus of 2 species of perennials found on rocky slopes, open woodland, and meadows in Europe and W. Asia. They have alternate, lance-shaped to obovate, entire or toothed leaves, and produce daisy-like yellow flowerheads from early summer to early autumn. Suitable for a border, a wild garden, or a grassy bank.
• **HARDINESS** Fully hardy.
• **CULTIVATION** Grow in poor, dry soil in full sun.

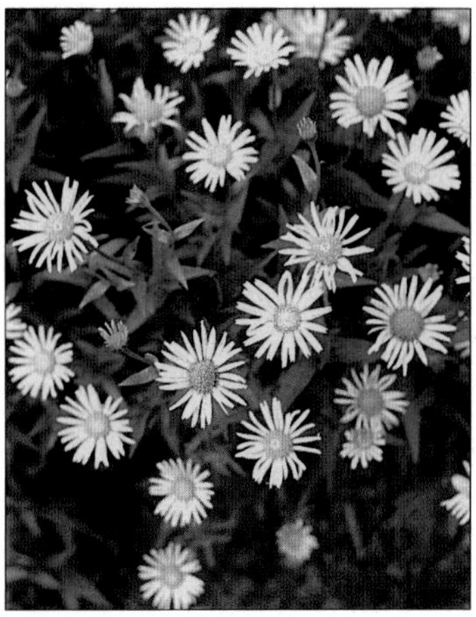

Buphthalmum salicifolium

• **PROPAGATION** Sow seed in containers in a cold frame in spring, or divide in early spring.
• **PESTS AND DISEASES** Trouble free.

B. salicifolium ■ Clump-forming perennial with narrowly obovate to lance-shaped, willow-like, dark green leaves, to 10cm (4in) long. From early summer to early autumn, erect, slender stems produce deep yellow flowerheads, 5–7cm (2–3in) across; these last well when cut. ↕ 60cm (24in), ↔ 45cm (18in). C. Europe. ❄❄❄
B. speciosum see *Telekia speciosa*.

BUPLEURUM

Thorow-wax

APIACEAE/UMBELLIFERAE

Genus of about 100 species of annuals, perennials, and evergreen or semi-evergreen shrubs. They are widely distributed in the N. hemisphere, with some species in southern Africa, and occur on dry, upland scrub, in moist areas, and among rocks. The variably shaped leaves are alternate, simple, and entire, often with conspicuous parallel veins. Umbels of star-shaped, yellow or green flowers are usually surrounded by involucres of leafy bracts. Grow in a flower border or shrub border. Plant the smaller species in a rock garden.
• **HARDINESS** Fully hardy to frost hardy.
• **CULTIVATION** Grow in any well-drained soil in full sun. Dead-head to avoid self-seeding. Grow *B. fruticosum* in a warm, sheltered site. Pruning group 9, if required; tolerates hard pruning.
• **PROPAGATION** Sow seed in containers in a cold frame in spring. Divide perennials in spring. Root semi-ripe cuttings of shrubs in summer.
• **PESTS AND DISEASES** Trouble free.

B. angulosum. Clump-forming, semi-evergreen perennial with linear-lance-shaped, blue-green basal leaves, 10–35cm (4–14in) long, and broader, heart-shaped, blue-green stem leaves, to 5cm (2in) long, clasping the upright, branching stems with their bases. In mid- and late summer, bears terminal umbels, 1cm (½in) across, comprising rings of 4–6 ovate, jade-green bracts surrounding clusters of tiny, star-shaped, yellowish or creamy green flowers. ↕↔ to 30cm (12in). Pyrenees, N.E. Spain. ❄❄❄.
B. fruticosum ■ (Shrubby hare's ear). Open, spreading but dense, evergreen

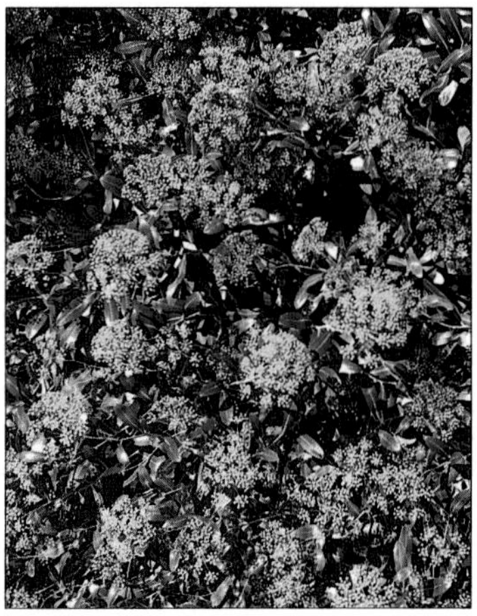

Bupleurum fruticosum

B

shrub with long, slender, mainly unbranched, erect shoots and narrowly obovate, blue-green leaves, to 8cm (3in) long. Small, star-shaped yellow flowers are borne in domed, terminal umbels, to 4cm (1½in) across, from midsummer to early autumn. Suitable for a coastal garden. ↕ 2m (6ft), ↔ 2.5m (8ft). Mediterranean. ❄❄❄ (borderline)

B. rotundifolium. Bushy, yellow-stemmed annual or short-lived perennial with stem-clasping, ovate to elliptic, or rounded, glaucous, mid-green leaves, 2–5cm (¾–2in) long, slightly pink-flushed when young. In summer, bears umbels, to 3cm (1¼in) across, of 4–8 greenish yellow bracts surrounding tiny, star-shaped, yellow-green flowers. ↕ 45–60cm (18–24in), ↔ 30cm (12in). C. and S. Europe, C. Asia. ❄❄. **'Green Gold'**, syn. 'Leprechaun Green Gold', has light green leaves and yellow flowers; ↕ to 45cm (18in).

BURCHARDIA

Milkmaids

COLCHICACEAE/LILIACEAE

Genus of 5 species of perennials from dry woodland and swamps in temperate Australia, grown for their umbels of 5–20, sometimes fragrant, star-shaped flowers. They have small corms, thick tuberous roots, and 1–5 linear, basal leaves, with a few leaves on the scapes in some species. In frost-prone areas, grow in a warm greenhouse or conservatory, or grow outdoors in a sunny border and lift and pot for winter storage. In warmer climates, grow in a border.

- **HARDINESS** Frost tender.
- **CULTIVATION** Under glass, grow in equal parts loam, leaf mould, and sharp sand in full light. Water freely when in growth, then sparingly as leaves wither, to store dry in winter. Pot on in spring. Outdoors, grow in humus-rich, moist but well-drained soil in full sun.
- **PROPAGATION** In spring, sow seed at 15–18°C (59–64°F) or pot up offsets.
- **PESTS AND DISEASES** Trouble free.

B. umbellata. Fleshy-rooted perennial with 1 or 2 linear, basal leaves, 4.5–6cm (1¾–2½in) long. In late spring and early summer, bears umbels of 2–9 fragrant, greenish white to white flowers, often tinged red outside, with purple anthers. ↕ 10–65cm (4–26in), ↔ 10–15cm (4–6in). Australia (except Northern Territory). ❀ (min. 10–13°C/50–55°F)

BURCHELLIA

Buffalo-wood

RUBIACEAE

Genus of one species of evergreen shrub from warm-temperate forests of South Africa, grown for its small, terminal heads of flowers. The leaves are opposite and ovate. In frost-prone climates, grow *B. bubalina* in a cool greenhouse; in warmer areas, grow in a border.

- **HARDINESS** Frost tender, but will tolerate short spells around 0°C (32°F).
- **CULTIVATION** Under glass, grow in loam-based potting compost (JI No.3) with full light and good ventilation. Water moderately throughout the year, applying a balanced liquid fertilizer monthly from spring to autumn. Pot on or top-dress in late winter. Outdoors,

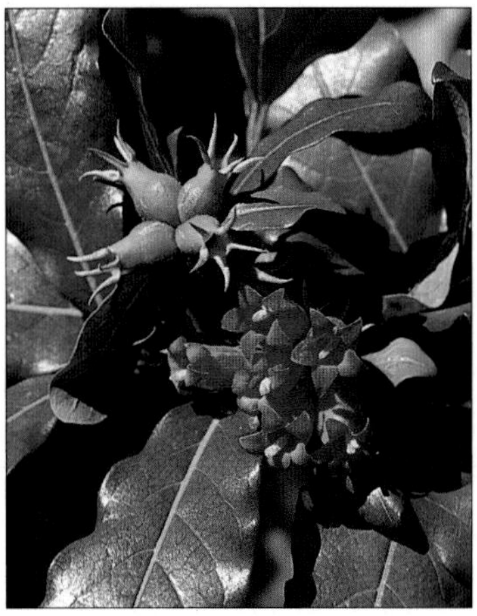

Burchellia bubalina

grow in moist but well-drained, fertile soil in full sun. Pruning group 8.

- **PROPAGATION** Root semi-ripe cuttings in a propagating case in summer, with gentle bottom heat.
- **PESTS AND DISEASES** Red spider mites, whiteflies, aphids, and mealybugs may be a problem under glass.

B. bubalina ▣ syn. *B. capensis* (Wild pomegranate). Erect to spreading shrub with ovate, glossy, dark green leaves, to 12cm (5in) long. From spring to summer, bears terminal clusters of 3–12 narrowly bell-shaped or tubular flowers, 2.5cm (1in) long, with 5 orange or scarlet petal lobes, ageing to red. These are followed by spherical, red to brown berries, 1.5cm (½in) across. ↕ 2–5m (6–15ft), ↔ 1–3m (3–10ft). South Africa. ❀ (min. 5°C/41°F)

B. capensis see *B. bubalina.*

▷ **Burnet** see *Sanguisorba*
 Canadian see *S. canadensis*
 Greater see *S. officinalis*

▷ **Burning bush** see *Bassia scoparia* f. *trichophylla, Dictamnus albus*

▷ **Burr, New Zealand** see *Acaena*

▷ **Burrawong** see *Macrozamia communis*

BURSERA

BURSERACEAE/PITTOSPORACEAE

Genus of about 40 species of variable, semi-evergreen, shrub- and tree-like perennials found in low, often hilly terrain from the Colorado Desert, USA, south to tropical Central America. They usually have stout trunks or stems; the succulent species are relatively fleshy. Pinnate, alternate leaves are clustered near the stem tips. Insignificant, usually white flowers are borne singly or in few-flowered cymes at the stem tips in summer, followed by single-seeded, capsular or fleshy fruits. Burseras may be treated as bonsai plants. In frost-prone areas, grow in a temperate greenhouse; in warmer areas, use in a desert garden.

- **HARDINESS** Frost tender.
- **CULTIVATION** Under glass, grow in a mix of 4 parts standard cactus compost and 1 part lime chippings in full light. When in growth, water freely and apply half-strength balanced liquid fertilizer monthly; keep completely dry in winter. Outdoors, grow in sharply drained, ideally alkaline soil in full sun. See also pp.48–49.
- **PROPAGATION** Sow seed at 21°C (70°F) in early spring. Root stem cuttings in late spring or early summer with bottom heat.
- **PESTS AND DISEASES** Aphids and, rarely, mealybugs may be troublesome.

B. microphylla (Elephant tree). Tree-like, perennial succulent with a stout, fleshy trunk and papery white bark, which readily peels off and exudes a milky white sap. Fern-like, pinnate leaves, 7–10cm (3–4in) long, have 30 or more oblong-linear leaflets, in opposite pairs. Cymes of star-shaped, yellow or white flowers, 1cm (½in) across, are produced in summer. ↕ to 5m (15ft), ↔ to 1.5m (5ft). USA (Colorado Desert). ❀ (min. 7–10°C/45–50°F)

▷ **Busy Lizzie** see *Impatiens, I. walleriana*

BUTEA

LEGUMINOSAE/PAPILIONACEAE

Genus of 4 species of deciduous trees, shrubs, and climbers from tropical forest in India, Sri Lanka, Burma, and Malaysia. They have large, long-stalked, alternate, fully divided, 3-palmate leaves and colourful, pea-like flowers in showy, terminal racemes or panicles. Only the trees are usually grown. In frost-prone areas, grow in a warm greenhouse; in warmer climates, use as specimen plants.

- **HARDINESS** Frost tender.
- **CULTIVATION** Under glass, grow in loam-based potting compost (JI No.3) in full light with high humidity. When in growth, water moderately and apply a balanced liquid fertilizer monthly; keep just moist in winter. Top-dress or pot on in spring. Outdoors, grow in moderately fertile soil in full sun. Pruning group 1, but need restrictive pruning under glass.
- **PROPAGATION** Sow seed at 18–24°C (64–75°F) in spring. Root semi-ripe cuttings in a propagating case with bottom heat in summer.
- **PESTS AND DISEASES** Red spider mites may be a problem under glass.

B. frondosa see *B. monosperma.*

B. monosperma ♀ syn. *B. frondosa* (Dhak, Flame of the forest, Palas). Strongly branched tree, twisting with age. Leathery, silky-backed leaves consist of 3 diamond-shaped to rounded leaflets, 10–20cm (4–8in) long, borne on stalks almost as long. Racemes, to 15cm (6in) long, of silver-hairy, rich vermilion flowers, 3–4cm (1¼–1½in) long, are borne along the bare branches from winter to spring. ↕ to 15m (50ft), ↔ 3–5m (10–15ft). India, Sri Lanka, Burma. ❀ (min. 16°C/61°F)

BUTIA

ARECACEAE/PALMAE

Genus of 8–12 species of monoecious, single-stemmed palms from cool, dry areas of S. Brazil, Paraguay, Uruguay, and Argentina. They bear panicles of 3-petalled, male and female flowers among dense, terminal heads of pinnate leaves. In frost-prone areas, grow young butias as houseplants or in a cool greenhouse or conservatory. In frost-free areas, grow as specimen trees.

- **HARDINESS** Half hardy to frost tender; withstand short periods near 0°C (32°F) in very dry, sunny climates.

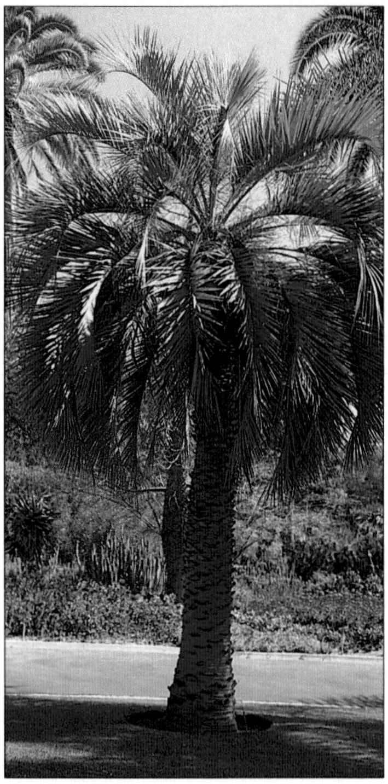

Butia capitata

- **CULTIVATION** Under glass, grow in loam-based potting compost (JI No.3) in bright filtered light. When in growth, water moderately and apply a balanced liquid fertilizer monthly. Keep just moist in winter. Pot on or top-dress in spring. Outdoors, grow in well-drained soil in full sun or partial shade.
- **PROPAGATION** Sow seed at 24–29°C (75–84°F) in spring.
- **PESTS AND DISEASES** Prey to red spider mites and scale insects under glass.

B. capitata ▣ 🌴 syn. *Cocos capitata* (Jelly palm). Slow-growing palm with a sturdy trunk often clothed with leaf bases. Strongly arching, narrowly elliptic to elliptic, blue-green-tinted, grey-green leaves, 2m (6ft) or more long, are comprised of many slender, leathery leaflets. Yellow flowers are borne in panicles, to 1.5m (5ft) long, in summer, followed by spherical to ovoid, yellow to purple fruit. ↕ 4–6m (12–20ft), ↔ 3–5m (10–15ft). S. Brazil, Uruguay, Argentina. ❀ (min. 5–10°C/41–50°F). **var. *nehrlingiana*** bears red-purple, female flowers and red fruit. **var. *pulposa*** has pulpy, edible yellow fruit.

BUTOMUS

Flowering rush, Water gladiolus

BUTOMACEAE

Genus of one species of rhizomatous, aquatic perennial widely distributed in Europe and W. Asia, often found at the margins of ponds or in shallow water with reedmaces (*Typha*). It produces long, twisted leaves and fragrant flowers. *B. umbellatus* is ideal for a large, decorative pond or wildlife pool.

- **HARDINESS** Fully hardy.
- **CULTIVATION** Grow in rich mud at the margins of ponds, or in water to 25cm (10in) deep, in full sun. If grown in a container, divide regularly to maintain free flowering. See also pp.52–53.
- **PROPAGATION** Sow seed in moist soil in a container half submerged in shallow water, in summer; after germination,

submerge the seedlings to a depth of 1cm (½in). Divide rhizomes in early spring when dormant. Remove root bulbils of divided plants in early spring and grow on in small containers of soil half submerged in water.
• **PESTS AND DISEASES** Water lily aphid may be troublesome.

B. umbellatus 🏆 Rush-like, marginal, aquatic perennial with long, twisted, radical, mid-green leaves, 1cm (½in) wide, turning bronze-purple then dark green as they extend, with sheathed, triangular bases. Spreading umbels, to 10cm (4in) across, of many cup-shaped, fragrant, rose-pink flowers, 1–2.5cm (½–1in) across, are borne well above the water in late summer. ↕ to 1.5m (5ft), ↔ 45cm (18in). Eurasia. ❄❄❄

▷**Butterbur** see *Petasites*
▷**Buttercup** see *Ranunculus*
  Bulbous see *R. bulbosus*
  Double creeping see *R. repens* 'Pleniflorus'
  Giant see *R. lyallii*
  Meadow see *R. acris*
  Persian see *R. asiaticus*
▷**Butterfly bush** see *Buddleja davidii*
▷**Butterfly flower** see *Schizanthus*
▷**Butterfly weed** see *Asclepias tuberosa*
▷**Butternut** see *Juglans cinerea*
▷**Butter tree** see *Tylecodon paniculatus*
▷**Butterwort** see *Pinguicula*
▷**Buttonbush** see *Cephalanthus occidentalis*
▷**Buttons, Blue** see *Succisa pratensis*
▷**Button-willow** see *Cephalanthus occidentalis*
▷**Buttonwood** see *Platanus occidentalis*

BUXUS

Box, Boxwood

BUXACEAE

Genus of about 70 species of evergreen shrubs and trees found in habitats ranging from rocky hills to woodland in Europe, Asia, Africa, and Central America. The leaves are opposite, linear-lance-shaped to almost rounded, entire, and leathery. In spring, small, axillary, star-shaped, yellow-green flowers of both sexes are borne on the same plant; several male flowers, with conspicuous yellow anthers, surround one female. Boxes are grown mainly for their foliage, which may be variegated, and for their ability to withstand clipping, which makes them ideal for hedging and topiary. Use dwarf boxes for edging,

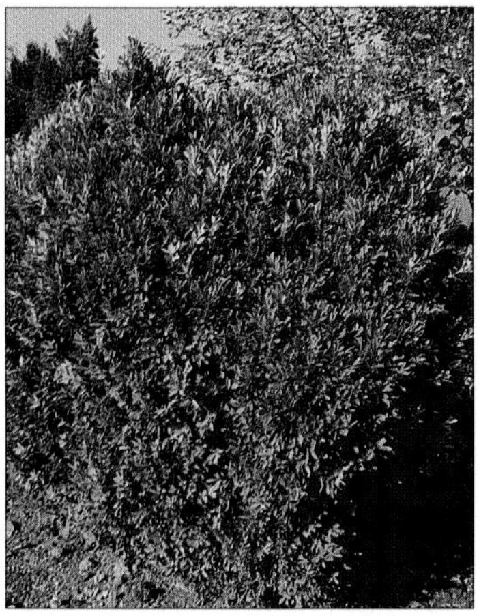
Buxus harlandii of gardens

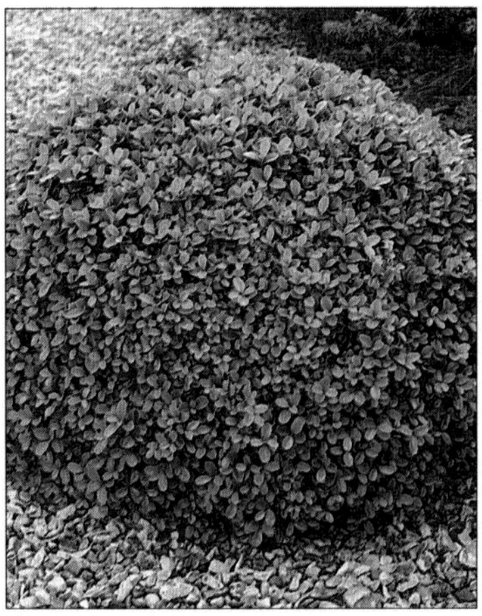

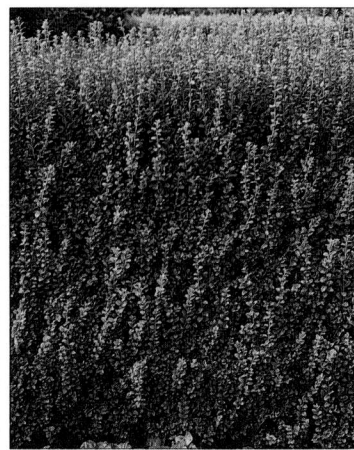
Buxus microphylla 'Green Pillow'

for ground cover, or in a rock garden. Contact with box sap may irritate skin.
• **HARDINESS** Fully hardy to frost hardy.
• **CULTIVATION** Grow in any fertile, well-drained soil, preferably in partial shade. They are tolerant of sun, but the combination of full sun and dry soil may encourage poor, dull foliage colour or scorching. Pruning group 8; trim hedges and edging plants in summer. Tolerant of hard, rejuvenative pruning in late spring, if followed by an application of fertilizer and a mulch.
• **PROPAGATION** Sow seed of *B. wallichiana* in containers in a cold frame in autumn. Root semi-ripe cuttings in summer. Graft in winter.
• **PESTS AND DISEASES** Box sucker and red spider mites may be troublesome.

B. balearica Q (Balearic box). Vigorous, broadly upright shrub or small tree with ovate to ovate-oblong, glossy, bright green leaves, to 4cm (1½in) long. ↕ 3m (10ft), ↔ 2.5m (8ft). Spain, Sardinia. ❄❄
***B.* 'Green Mountain'.** Dense, conical shrub with narrow, inversely lance-shaped, glossy, dark green leaves, 1.5cm (½in) long, somewhat blue-tinged at first. Excellent as a low hedge. ↕ 1.5m (5ft), ↔ 1m (3ft). ❄❄❄
***B. harlandii* of gardens** ▣ syn. *B. microphylla* var. *japonica*. Slow-growing, very dense, upright shrub with narrowly lance-shaped, mid- to deep green leaves, to 3cm (1¼in) long. The plant grown under this name is not the true *B. harlandii*, which is tender and native to S. China and Hong Kong. ↕ 1.5m (5ft), ↔ 1.2m (4ft). ❄❄❄

Buxus sempervirens 'Handsworthensis'

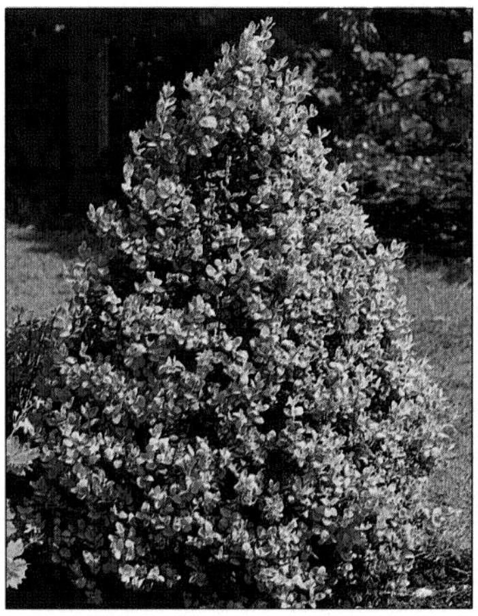
Buxus sempervirens 'Latifolia Maculata'

B. microphylla (Small-leaved box). Slow-growing, dense, rounded shrub with elliptic-oblong to inversely lance-shaped, dark green leaves, to 2cm (¾in) long, turning bronze in winter. ↕ 75cm (30in), ↔ 1.5m (5ft). Probably of garden origin. ❄❄❄. **'Compacta'** is very compact, dense, and slow-growing, with obovate, slightly recurved leaves, to 5mm (¼in) long; ↕↔ to 30cm (12in). **'Curly Locks'** has an open habit, and pale green leaves on twisted shoots; ↕ 1m (3ft), ↔ 1.2m (4ft). **'Green Jade'** has broadly ovate to rounded, pale green leaves, which are deeply notched at the tips; ↕ 60cm (24in), ↔ 1m (3ft). **'Green Pillow'** ▣ is very compact, dense, and slow-growing, with obovate, slightly recurved leaves; ↕ 45cm (18in), ↔ 1m (3ft). **var. *japonica*** see *B. harlandii* of gardens. **var. *koreana***, syn. *B. sinica* var. *insularis*, is very hardy; ↕ 60cm (24in), ↔ 75cm (30in); Korea, China. **'Morris Dwarf'** is slow-growing, forming a low, compact mound; ↕ 30cm (12in), ↔ 45cm (18in). **'Wintergreen'** is very hardy, and retains the dark green colour of its foliage in winter.
B. sempervirens 🏆Q (Common box). Bushy, rounded shrub or small tree with

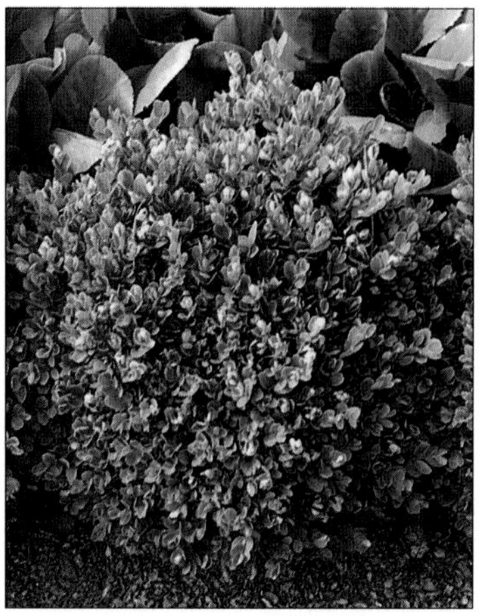
Buxus sempervirens 'Suffruticosa'

ovate to oblong, glossy, dark green leaves, to 3cm (1¼in) long, which are notched at the tips. ↕ 5m (15ft), ↔ 5m (15ft) or more. Europe, N. Africa, Turkey. ❄❄❄. **'Aureomarginata'** see 'Marginata'. **'Elegantissima'** 🏆 is very dense, with narrow, white-margined leaves, to 2cm (¾in) long; ↕↔ 1.5m (5ft). **'Handsworthensis'** ▣ is dense and upright, with leaves to 4cm (1½in) long. Very good as a hedge. **'Latifolia Maculata'** ▣🏆 is compact, with bright yellow young foliage, maturing to dark green marked yellow; ↕ 2.5m (8ft), ↔ 2m (6ft). **'Marginata'** ▣ syn. 'Aureomarginata', has yellow-margined, dark green leaves; ↕ 2.5m (8ft), ↔ 3m (10ft). **'Suffruticosa'** ▣🏆 is compact and very slow-growing. Excellent as a hedge; ↕ 1m (3ft), ↔ 1.5m (5ft). **'Vardar Valley'** forms a flat-topped mound, and has very dark green leaves; ↕ 1.5m (5ft).
B. sinica* var. *insularis see *B. microphylla* var. *koreana*.
B. wallichiana (Himalayan box). Open shrub with narrowly ovate-lance-shaped, glossy, bright green leaves, to 6cm (2½in) long, notched at the tips and borne on 4-angled shoots. ↕↔ 2.5m (8ft). N.W. Himalayas. ❄❄

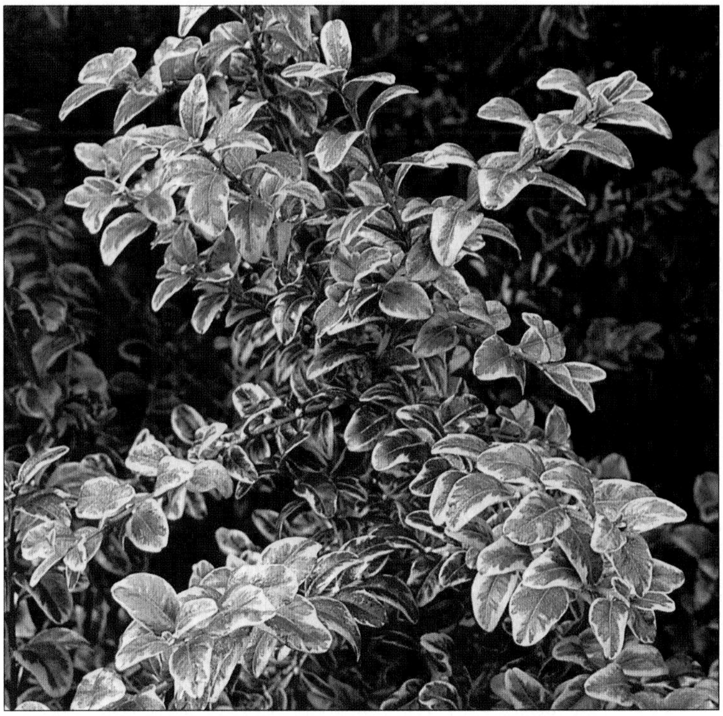
Buxus sempervirens 'Marginata'

C

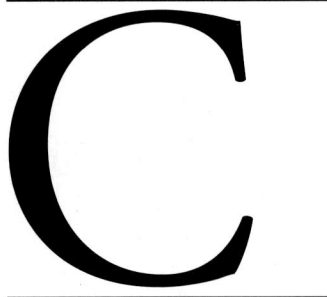

▷ **Cabbage palm** see *Cordyline, Livistona australis*
New Zealand see *Cordyline australis*
Saw see *Acoelorraphe wrightii*
▷ **Cabbage tree** see *Cordyline*

CABOMBA

CABOMBACEAE

Genus of 7 species of submerged aquatic perennials found in still water in tropical and subtropical areas of North and South America. Long, thin, branching stems produce opposite or whorled submerged leaves, divided into linear lobes, and alternate, peltate floating leaves with broadly ovate to narrowly elliptic leaf-blades. The solitary flowers, 1–4cm (½–1½in) across, are borne above the water on long stems. They are attractive aquarium oxygenators, valued for their feathery foliage.

• **HARDINESS** Frost tender.

• **CULTIVATION** In an aquarium, grow in full light in pots of coarse sand or grit in lime-free water without air-diffusers, as they dislike water movement. Most require a minimum temperature of 22°C (72°F), and water no deeper than 40cm (16in). *C. caroliniana* will over-winter at 18°C (64°F). See also pp.52–53.

• **PROPAGATION** Take stem tip cuttings, to 30cm (12in) long, in spring or early summer. Insert bunches of 5 or 6 cuttings into the aquarium soil.

• **PESTS AND DISEASES** Trouble free.

C. caroliniana ■ (Carolina water shield). Aquatic perennial with fan-shaped, sharp-pointed, dark green submerged leaves, to 7cm (3in) long, divided into 5 leaflets. The ovate, inversely lance-shaped to linear-oblong, sharp-pointed, mid-green floating leaves are 2cm (¾in) long. In summer, saucer-shaped, white or purple-pink flowers, 3–4cm (1¼–1½in) across, with 2 yellow spots at the base of each petal, are produced singly from the leaf axils, just above the water. ↔ indefinite. C. and S.E. USA. ❀ (min. 18°C/64°F)

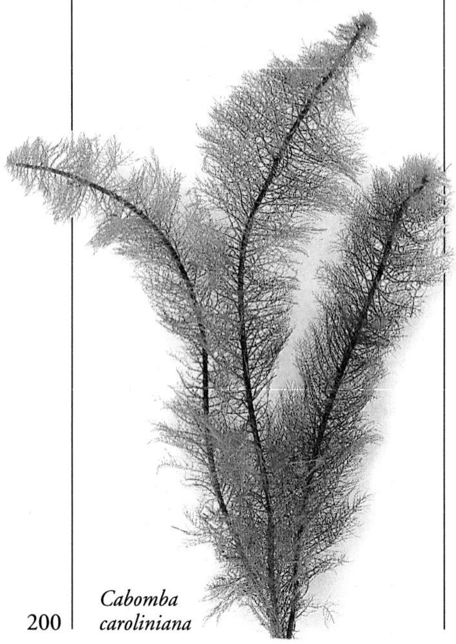

Cabomba caroliniana

▷ ***Cacalia*** see *Emilia*
C. coccinea see *E. coccinea*
C. sagittata see *E. coccinea*
C. sonchifolia see *E. sonchifolia*
▷ **Cacti** see pp.48–49
▷ **Cactus,**
Christmas see *Schlumbergera, S.* x *buckleyi*
Cotton-pole see *Opuntia vestita*
Crab see *Schlumbergera truncata*
Dumpling see *Lophophora williamsii*
Easter see *Hatiora rosea*
Goat's horn see *Astrophytum capricorne*
Golden barrel see *Echinocactus grusonii*
Gold lace see *Mammillaria elongata*
Grizzly bear see *Opuntia erinacea* var. *ursina*
Mistletoe see *Rhipsalis baccifera*
Old lady see *Mammillaria hahniana*
Old man see *Cephalocereus senilis*
Orchid see *Epiphyllum*
Peanut see *Echinopsis chamaecereus*
Rat's tail see *Aporocactus*
Saguaro see *Carnegiea gigantea*
Sand dollar see *Astrophytum asterias*
Scarlet ball see *Parodia haselbergii*
Sea-urchin see *Astrophytum asterias*
Silver ball see *Parodia scopa*
Snowball see *Mammillaria bocasana*
Snowball cushion see *Mammillaria candida*
Starfish see *Orbea variegata*
Toad see *Orbea variegata*
Turk's cap see *Melocactus*

CAESALPINIA

CAESALPINIACEAE/LEGUMINOSAE

Genus of 70 or more evergreen species of trees, scandent to climbing shrubs, and perennials found in scrub, lowland rainforest, and on rocky mountain slopes in tropical and subtropical areas. They are grown for their terminal racemes or panicles of 30–40 flowers, each 5-petalled and with protruding stamens, 5–7cm (2–3in) long, and for their alternate, 2-pinnate, fern-like leaves. In frost-prone areas, grow in a cool or temperate greenhouse. In frost-free regions, grow in a shrub border or as specimen plants.

• **HARDINESS** Half hardy to frost tender; *C. gilliesii* and *C. pulcherrima* may survive short spells around 0°C (32°F).

• **CULTIVATION** Under glass, grow in loam-based potting compost (JI No.3) with additional leaf mould, in full light. In the growing season, water moderately and apply a balanced liquid fertilizer monthly; water sparingly in winter. Pot on or top-dress in early spring. Outdoors, grow in moist but well-drained, fertile soil in full sun. Pruning group 8, or group 13 if wall-trained; plants under glass may need restrictive pruning after the first flush of flowers.

• **PROPAGATION** Sow seed at 13–18°C (55–64°F) in spring, after soaking in warm water for 24 hours. Root soft-wood cuttings in spring, or greenwood cuttings in summer.

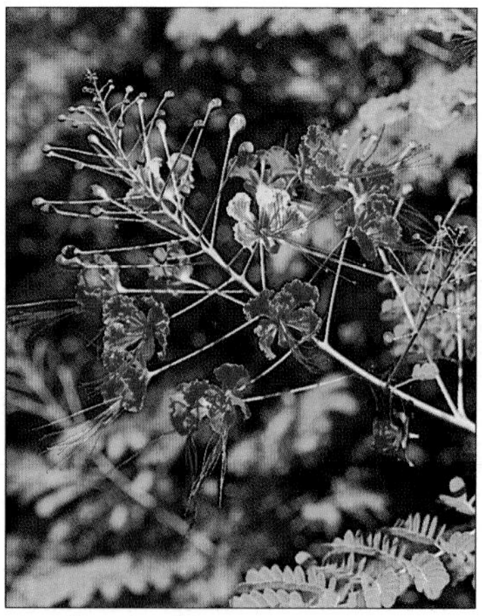

Caesalpinia pulcherrima

• **PESTS AND DISEASES** Prone to red spider mites, whiteflies, and mealybugs.

C. gilliesii ♀ syn. *Poinciana gilliesii* (Bird of paradise shrub). Erect to spreading shrub or small tree with 2-pinnate, mid- to dark green leaves, 20cm (8in) long, consisting of numerous oblong leaflets, 8mm (⅜in) long. Erect racemes, 15–30cm (6–12in) long, of up to 40 yellow flowers, to 3.5cm (1½in) across, with scarlet stamens, are borne in summer. ↕ 2–3m (6–10ft) or more, ↔ 1–2.5m (3–8ft). Argentina, Uruguay. ✲ (borderline)

C. pulcherrima ■ ♤ syn. *Poinciana pulcherrima* (Barbados pride). Erect shrub or small tree with long-stalked, 2-pinnate, light green leaves, 30cm (12in) or more long, composed of numerous elliptic to obovate leaflets, 8mm (⅜in) long. From spring to autumn, bears erect racemes, to 20cm (8in) long, of up to 40 irregularly bowl-shaped flowers, 3–4cm (1¼–1½in) across, with orange-yellow or yellow petals, orange-red sepals, and red stamens. ↕ 3–6m (10–20ft), ↔ 2–4m (6–12ft). Probably West Indies. ✲ (borderline)

CALADIUM

ARACEAE

Genus of 7 species of tuberous-rooted perennials from woodland margins in tropical South America. They are grown for their long-stalked, peltate, ovate to elliptic, broadly arrow- or lance-shaped leaves, which are variegated white, pink, or red. The greenish white spathes and spadices with green flowers are followed by white berries. In frost-prone areas, grow in a warm greenhouse; elsewhere, use as specimens in containers. Contact with all parts may irritate skin, and may cause mild stomach upset if ingested.

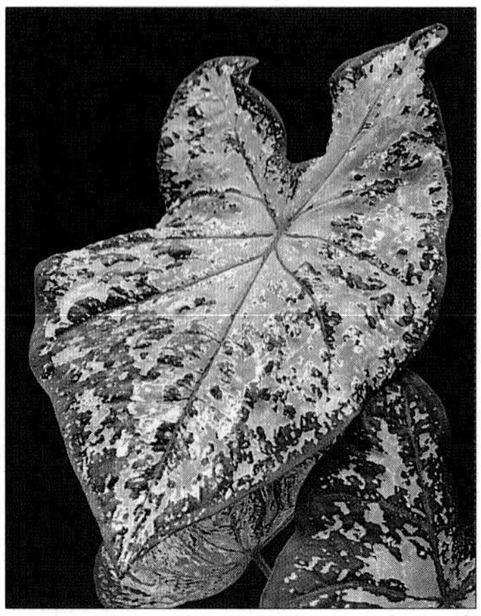

Caladium bicolor 'Pink Beauty'

• **HARDINESS** Frost tender.

• **CULTIVATION** Under glass, grow in loamless potting compost in bright filtered light. Pot up tubers in spring and provide high humidity at 21°C (70°F), not less than 13°C (55°F) when leaves develop. During the growing season, maintain high humidity, water freely, and apply a balanced liquid fertilizer monthly; reduce water in autumn. Keep dormant tubers almost dry at 13–16°C (55–61°F). Outdoors, grow in moist but well-drained, humus-rich, slightly acid soil in partial shade.

• **PROPAGATION** Divide tubers in spring; dust cut portions with fungicide.

• **PESTS AND DISEASES** Trouble free.

C. bicolor, syn. *C.* x *hortulanum* (Angel wings, Elephant's ears, Heart of Jesus). Tuberous-rooted perennial, the spherical tubers producing slender stems, 15cm (6in) long, with peltate, arrow- or lance-shaped, dark green leaves, 15–30cm (6–12in) long, streaked or spotted white, pink, or red. In spring, bears greenish white spathes to 23cm (9in) long. ↕ 15–30cm (6–12in), ↔ 13–20cm (5–8in). Garden origin. ❀ (min. 13°C/55°F). **'Candidum'** has white foliage with dark green veins. **'John Peed'** has leaves with dark red centres fading to broad, dark green margins. **'June Bride'** has silvery white leaves with green veins. **'Pink Beauty'** ■ has red-veined leaves, pink in the centres, with bright green, pink-speckled margins. **'Red Flash'** has white-marked green leaves with red veins and wide green margins.

C.* x *hortulanum see *C. bicolor.*

CALAMAGROSTIS

Reed grass, Smallweed

GRAMINEAE/POACEAE

Genus of about 250 species of sturdy, tufted, rhizomatous, perennial grasses widely distributed in temperate zones of the N. hemisphere, where they occur in marshland and damp woodland. They have linear, flat or channelled leaves and dense inflorescences borne in branching panicles. Ornamental cultivars are useful in a herbaceous or mixed border for their long-lasting, elegant inflorescences and architectural form. Some species may be invasive.

• **HARDINESS** Fully hardy.

• **CULTIVATION** Grow in moist, humus-rich soil in sun or partial shade, although they will tolerate all but the poorest soils. In early spring, before new growth begins, cut down to the ground all stems that were left for winter effect.

• **PROPAGATION** Divide in mid-spring.

• **PESTS AND DISEASES** Trouble free.

C.* x *acutiflora (*C. arundinacea* x *C. epigejos*) (Feather reed grass). Slow-spreading, clump-forming, perennial grass with arching, linear, flat, slightly glossy, mid-green leaves, 45–90cm (18–36in) long. Stiff, erect, unbranched stems bear soft, silvery bronze to pale purple-brown inflorescences in narrow panicles, 15–30cm (6–12in) long, in

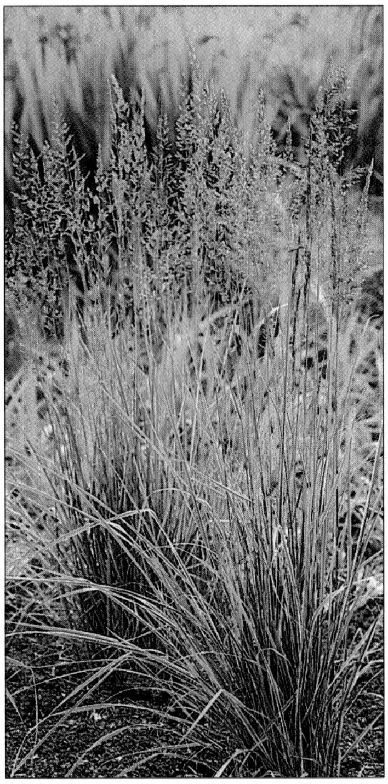

Calamagrostis x *acutiflora* 'Overdam'

mid- and late summer; these persist throughout winter. ❄❄❄. ↕0.6–1.8m (2–6ft), ↔ 0.6–1.2m (2–4ft). Europe, Russia. **'Karl Foerster'** has pink-bronze inflorescences that fade to buff or pale brown; ↕ to 1.8m (6ft), ↔ 60cm (24in). **'Overdam'** ▣ has leaves with pale yellow margins and stripes, which fade to pink-flushed white with age. Bears purplish inflorescences that become greyish pink. Forms looser clumps than 'Karl Foerster'; ↕ to 1.2m (4ft).

▷**Calamint** see *Acinos*, *Calamintha*
Alpine see *Acinos alpinus*
Lesser see *Calamintha nepeta*

CALAMINTHA

Calamint

LABIATAE/LAMIACEAE

Genus of 8 or more species of aromatic, sometimes rhizomatous perennials, some woody-based, found in grassland, scrub, and woodland in N. temperate regions. They have ovate to oblong, usually toothed leaves and bear axillary cymes of tubular, 2-lipped flowers, mainly in shades of blue, but pink or white in some species. Grow calamint in a rock garden, border, or an open woodland garden. The flowers attract bees.

• **HARDINESS** Fully hardy.
• **CULTIVATION** Grow in moist but well-drained, humus-rich soil in sun or partial shade.
• **PROPAGATION** Sow seed in containers in a cold frame in spring, or divide in early spring.
• **PESTS AND DISEASES** Powdery mildew may be a problem.

C. alpina see *Acinos alpinus.*
C. corsica see *Acinos corsicus.*
C. grandiflora, syn. *Clinopodium grandiflorum.* Rhizomatous, many-branched, bushy perennial with ovate, toothed leaves, 5cm (2in) long, dark green above and pale green beneath. Lax cymes of up to 5 pink flowers, 2.5–4cm (1–1½in) long, are borne in summer. Thrives in dappled shade. ↕↔ 45cm (18in). S. and S.E. Europe to Caucasus, Ukraine (Crimea), Turkey, Iran. ❄❄❄
C. nepeta (Lesser calamint). Aromatic, low-growing, erect perennial with ovate, often shallowly toothed, hairy, dark green leaves, to 4cm (1½in) long. Bears mauve, occasionally pink flowers, to 1.5cm (½in) long, in 5- to 15-flowered, branched cymes in summer. ↕ to 45cm (18in), ↔ 50–75cm (20–30in). S. and C. Europe, N.W. Africa, N. Turkey, Caucasus, Ukraine (Crimea). ❄❄❄

▷**Calamondin** see x *Citrofortunella microcarpa*

CALAMUS

ARECACEAE/PALMAE

Genus of about 370 species of spiny, evergreen, usually climbing, occasionally shrub-like, dioecious palms found in tropical forest in Africa and Asia, New Guinea, and from N.E. Australia to Fiji. The leaves are pinnate, sometimes ending in barbed whips, and have lance-shaped leaflets. The inflorescences, borne among the leaf sheaths, have tubular, spiny, persistent bracts. Male flowers are solitary and symmetrical; female flowers are paired with sterile males, and are often larger and followed by spherical yellow fruits, 1–3cm (½–1¼in) across. Many species are used in the construction of cane furniture. In frost-prone areas, grow young plants as houseplants, in a conservatory, or in a temperate greenhouse. In warmer areas, grow through shrubs or trees.

• **HARDINESS** Frost tender.
• **CULTIVATION** Under glass, grow in loam-based potting compost (JI No.3) in bright filtered light and high humidity. Throughout the summer, water freely and apply a balanced liquid fertilizer monthly; water more sparingly in winter. Outdoors, grow in moist but well-drained soil in partial shade.
• **PROPAGATION** Sow seed at 19–24°C (66–75°F) in spring.
• **PESTS AND DISEASES** Trouble free.

C. rotang 🌴–❄ (Rattan cane). Erect or climbing palm with solitary or clustered stems and alternate or nearly opposite, pinnate, light to mid-green leaves, 80cm (32in) long, composed of lance-shaped leaflets. Star-shaped, 3-pointed cream flowers, 1.5cm (½in) long, may be produced at any time during the year. ↕10m (30ft), ↔ 6–10m (20–30ft). S. India, Sri Lanka. ❀ (min. 10°C/50°F)

CALANDRINIA

PORTULACACEAE

Genus of about 150 species of annuals and short-lived, tufted to clump-forming, evergreen perennials, a few of which are succulent. They occur in hot, dry, open, rocky areas, and sometimes grassy or bare alpine steppe or scree, in W. North America, Central America to N.W. and W. South America, and also S. Australia. Although they often appear rosetted, the narrow, entire, usually fleshy leaves are alternate. The 5- to 7-petalled flowers, with 2 large sepals, are usually red, reddish purple, or white, and may be solitary or borne in semi-erect or pendent racemes or panicles on long stalks. In frost-prone areas, treat

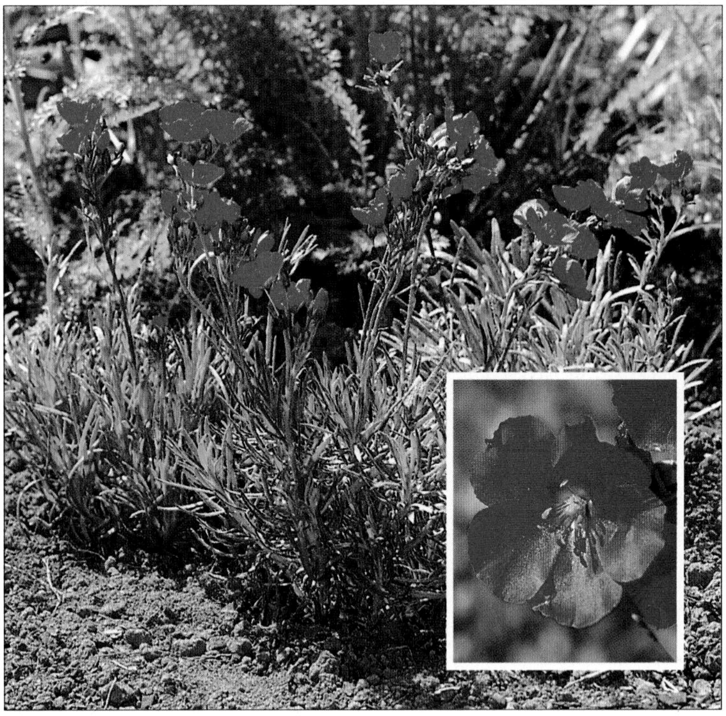

Calandrinia umbellata (inset: flower detail)

calandrinias as half-hardy annuals, or grow in a cool greenhouse. Elsewhere, grow on a sunny bank, or in a border, rock garden, scree bed, or alpine house.

• **HARDINESS** Frost hardy (but intolerant of winter wet) to frost tender.
• **CULTIVATION** Under glass, grow in a mix of equal parts loam, peat, leaf mould, and sand in full light. Water moderately when in growth (the high alpine species in particular are very sensitive to excess water) and apply a dilute, balanced liquid fertilizer monthly in summer; keep just moist in winter. Outdoors, grow in slightly acid, humus-rich, sharply drained soil in full sun. See also pp.48–49.
• **PROPAGATION** Sow seed at 16–18°C (61–64°F) in early spring or autumn, or take stem cuttings in spring. Propagate regularly.
• **PESTS AND DISEASES** Prone to aphids and red spider mites under glass. Young plants are vulnerable to slugs and snails.

C. caespitosa. Cushion-forming, variable, evergreen perennial with fleshy, linear to inversely lance-shaped, mid-green leaves, 0.5–3cm (¼–1¼in) long. The best variants have compact cushions of small-leaved rosettes, and bear cup-shaped, glossy magenta flowers, 1.5cm (½in) across, with greenish gold disc-florets, singly on short stems in summer. Less compact variants with golden orange or pale pink flowers also occur. ↕ to 7cm (3in), ↔ to 10cm (4in). Chile, Argentina, and Tierra del Fuego. ❄❄
C. ciliata. Semi-prostrate to semi-erect annual with fleshy, linear to spoon-shaped, grey-green leaves, 4cm (1½in) long, purple beneath, on spreading, erect stems. In late summer, bears solitary, purple, red, pink, or white flowers, to 2cm (¾in) across. Needs light soil in a sheltered site in full sun. ↕↔ to 30cm (12in). Ecuador, Peru. ❄
C. grandiflora. Clump-forming perennial succulent, often grown as an annual, with thick, elliptic, pointed, flat, smooth-margined, bright green leaves, to 20cm (8in) long. Racemes of numerous cup-shaped, pale reddish purple to magenta flowers, to 3cm (1¼in) across, are borne in summer. ↕ to 1m (3ft), ↔ 45cm (18in). Chile. ❀ (min. 6°C/43°F)
C. megarhiza* var. *nivalis see *Claytonia megarhiza* var. *nivalis.*
C. spectabilis. Shrubby, tufted perennial producing succulent branches, stems, and foliage. Pointed, softly hairy, smooth-margined, light to mid-green leaves, 3–4cm (1¼–1½in) long, are diamond- or spoon- to lance-shaped. In summer, bears solitary or paired, cup-shaped, vivid purple-red flowers, 5cm (2in) across. ↕60cm (24in), ↔ 45cm (18in). Chile. ❀ (min. 6°C/43°F)
C. umbellata ▣ (Rock purslane). Variable, loose, mound-forming, evergreen perennial, often treated as an annual, with semi-upright, branching stems and linear to linear-lance-shaped, very hairy, blue- or grey-green leaves, 2–4cm (¾–1½in) long. Produces loose panicles of 6–30 upturned, cup-shaped, crimson-magenta flowers, to 2cm (¾in) across, in summer. ↕↔ 15–20cm (6–8in). Chile, Argentina. ❄❄

CALANTHE

ORCHIDACEAE

Genus of 120–150 species of evergreen, semi-evergreen, or deciduous, rhizomatous, terrestrial, occasionally epiphytic orchids from sites in tropical and temperate Asia, Polynesia, and Madagascar, ranging from sea level and lowland forest to altitudes over 3,000m (10,000ft). The deciduous species are usually found in woodland or among shaded rocks. They have corm-like, sometimes angular, oblong-ellipsoid pseudobulbs, often partially exposed above the soil surface, and basal clusters of 2–5 mid- to dark green, folded leaves. Erect, loose to dense-flowered racemes of spurred flowers, each with a 3-lobed lip, are borne in spring, summer, or winter. *C. discolor* and *C. discolor* var.

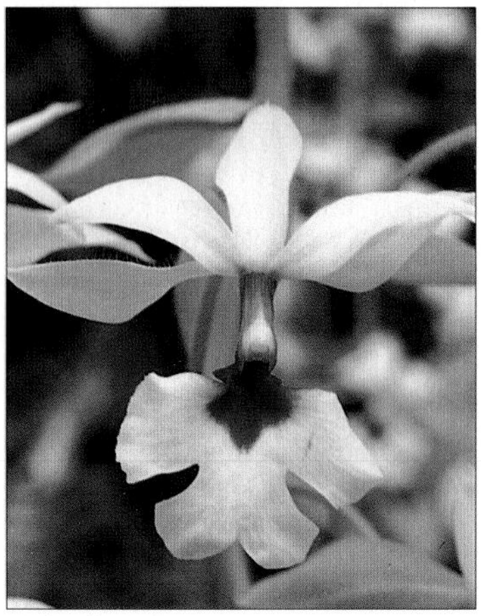

Calanthe vestita

bicolor are suitable for a rock garden or woodland garden; grow tender species in a warm greenhouse.

- **HARDINESS** Most are frost tender; *C. discolor* and its variants are frost hardy.
- **CULTIVATION** Cool- and warm-growing orchids. Under glass, grow in terrestrial orchid compost in bright filtered light and high humidity. In summer, water freely and apply a half-strength liquid fertilizer at every second or third watering. Avoid spraying the foliage, as it may become spotted. Water evergreen species sparingly in winter. Keep deciduous species completely dry when dormant, with a minimum of 10°C (50°F). Pot on annually. Outdoors, grow in coarse, well-drained, humus-rich soil in a sheltered site in partial or dappled shade. See also p.46.
- **PROPAGATION** For spring-flowering plants, divide pseudobulbs after flowering; otherwise, divide in early spring as new growth appears.
- **PESTS AND DISEASES** Prone to red spider mites, aphids, and mealybugs under glass; protect from slugs outdoors.

C. discolor. Evergreen or semi-evergreen, terrestrial orchid producing narrowly obovate to oblong leaves, 20–30cm (8–12in) long. In spring, bears up to 10 purple-brown to green flowers, 2.5–4cm (1–1½in) across, with pale rose-pink or white lips, in erect racemes, 40cm (16in) long. ↕ 15–30cm (6–12in), ↔ 30cm (12in). Korea, Japan, Taiwan. ✼✼. **var. *bicolor***, syn. *C. striata*, *C. striata* var. *bicolor*, produces flowers 3–4cm (1¼–1½in) across, the tepals sometimes suffused yellow.
f. *sieboldii*, syn. *C. sieboldii*, *C. sieboldii* var. *flava*, *C. striata* f. *sieboldii*, has clear yellow flowers.
C. sieboldii see *C. discolor* f. *sieboldii*.
C. sieboldii* var. *flava see *C. discolor* f. *sieboldii*.
C. striata see *C. discolor* var. *bicolor*.
C. striata* var. *bicolor see *C. discolor* var. *bicolor*.
C. striata* f. *sieboldii see *C. discolor* f. *sieboldii*.
C. tricarinata. Evergreen or semi-evergreen, terrestrial orchid producing broadly inversely lance-shaped to elliptic, strongly ribbed leaves, 18–30cm (7–12in) long. Racemes, 30–40cm (12–16in) long, of up to 15 nodding or pendent flowers, 2–4cm (¾–1½in) across, with greenish yellow to brown-green tepals, the lips purplish brown or red-brown, are borne from the leaf axils in spring. ↕↔ 50cm (20in). Himalayas, China, Japan, Taiwan. ❀ (min. 9°C/48°F; max. 27°C/81°F)
***C.* Veitchii** (*C. rosea* x *C. vestita*). Deciduous, terrestrial orchid with large, narrowly ovate leaves, to 90cm (36in) long. Many rose-pink flowers, 5cm (2in) across, with bright red lips, are borne in arching racemes, to 90cm (36in) tall, in winter, before the leaves emerge. ↕ 1.1m (3½ft), ↔ 1m (3ft). Garden origin. ❀ (min. 18°C/64°F; max. 30°C/86°F)
C. vestita ▣ Deciduous, terrestrial orchid with large, narrowly ovate to broadly lance-shaped leaves, to 90cm (36in) long. Arching racemes, to 90cm (36in) long, of up to 12 white or pale rose-pink flowers, 5cm (2in) across, with red to rose-pink or magenta lips, are borne in winter, before the leaves emerge. ↕ 1.1m (3½ft), ↔ 1m (3ft). Burma, Thailand, Cambodia, Laos, Vietnam, Indonesia (Sulawesi). ❀ (min. 18°C/64°F; max. 30°C/86°F)

CALATHEA

MARANTACEAE

Genus of about 300 species of evergreen, rhizomatous perennials found in humid forest and at forest margins in tropical Central and South America, and the West Indies. Most are clump-forming, with ovate to elliptic, shiny, long-stalked, pale to dark green leaves, often attractively patterned and red on the reverse; young plants may differ from mature plants in the size and colour of their foliage. Flowers, rarely produced in cultivation, are tubular with extended upper and lower lips, and are borne in racemes in summer. They have dense spikes of sheathed bracts with pairs of small flowers developing from openings in the sheaths. In frost-prone areas, grow in a warm or temperate greenhouse, or as houseplants; they will tolerate fairly low light levels. In warmer areas, grow in a border or among shrubs.

- **HARDINESS** Frost tender.
- **CULTIVATION** Under glass, grow in loamless or loam-based potting compost (JI No.2) in bright indirect or filtered light, with high humidity, draught-free conditions, and a constant temperature. When in growth, water freely and apply a balanced liquid fertilizer monthly; water moderately in winter. Pot on annually in late spring. Outdoors, grow in moist but well-drained, humus-rich soil in partial shade.
- **PROPAGATION** Divide clumps in late spring; keep plants in warm, humid conditions until re-established.
- **PESTS AND DISEASES** Aphids and red spider mites may be a problem. Bright light causes leaf scorch; dry air turns leaves brittle and brown at the margins.

***C. burle-marxii* 'Ice Blue'.** Clump-forming perennial with slightly arching or spreading, ovate leaf-blades, to 75cm (30in) long, on leaf-stalks to 30cm (12in) long. The leaves are bright green above with yellow-green midribs, and grey-green beneath with yellow midribs. Well-established plants bear ovoid flower spikes, 12–18cm (5–7in) long, with blue bracts and purple flowers. ↕ 80–150cm (32–60in), ↔ 1.2m (4ft). ❀ (min. 16–21°C/61–70°F)
C. discolor see *C. lutea*.
C. insignis see *C. lancifolia*.

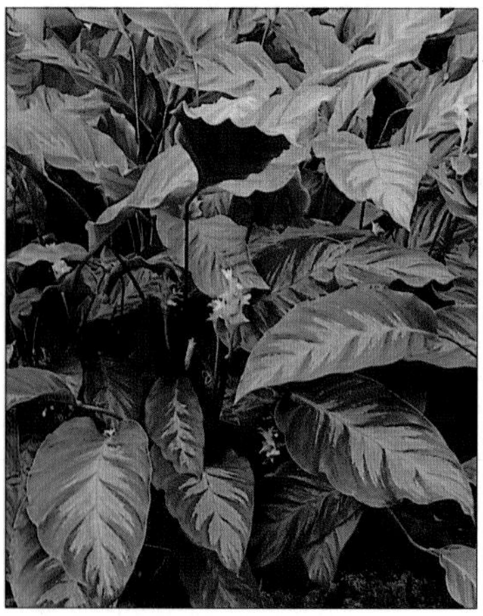

Calathea louisae

C. lancifolia ♀ syn. *C. insignis* (Rattlesnake plant). Clump-forming perennial with erect, linear to lance-shaped, wavy-margined leaf-blades, to 45cm (18in) long, on leaf-stalks to 30cm (12in) long. Leaves are pale green above, with darker green patches on either side of the midribs, and deep red-purple beneath. Yellow flowers are borne in conical spikes, 5–10cm (2–4in) long, in summer. ↕ 45–75cm (18–30in), ↔ 60cm (24in). Brazil. ❀ (min. 16–21°C/61–70°F)
C. lindeniana. Clump-forming perennial producing elliptic leaf-blades, 30–40cm (12–16in) long, on leaf-stalks to 30cm (12in) long. Leaves are dark green above with olive-green patches on each side of the midribs, green and red beneath. Pale yellow flowers are borne in ellipsoid spikes, to 10cm (4in) long. ↕ to 1m (3ft), ↔ 60cm (24in). Peru, N.W. Brazil. ❀ (min. 16–21°C/61–70°F)
C. louisae ▣ Clump-forming perennial producing elliptic-ovate, dark green leaf-blades, red beneath, and 15cm (6in) long, with silver-green feathering around the midribs, on leaf-stalks to 20cm (8in) long. White flowers are borne in conical spikes, 3–6cm (1¼–2½in) long. ↕ to 1m (3ft), ↔ 45cm (18in). Tropical Central and South America. ❀ (min. 16–21°C/61–70°F)
C. lutea, syn. *C. discolor*. Clump-forming perennial producing ovate to obovate leaf-blades, 1.7m (5½ft) long, bright green above, grey beneath, with raised lateral veins, on leaf-stalks to 15cm (6in) long. Yellow flowers are borne in ovoid spikes, 8–12cm (3–5in) long. ↕ to 2m (6ft), ↔ 1.2m (4ft). Tropical Central and South America. ❀ (min. 16–21°C/61–70°F)
***C. majestica* 'Roseolineata'**, syn. *C. ornata* 'Roseolineata'. Robust, clump-forming perennial, producing elliptic, unequal-sided leaf-blades, 30–40cm (12–16in) long, erect at first, then spreading, on leaf-stalks 20cm (8in) or more long. Leaves are deep olive-green above, with pairs of thin, rose-red, lateral stripes on opposite sides of the midribs, becoming white with age; the undersides are purple. Bears ovoid spikes, 5–8cm (2–3in) long, of white flowers with violet petal lobes. ↕ 2m (6ft), ↔ to 1m (3ft). ❀ (min. 16–21°C/61–70°F)
***C. majestica* 'Sanderiana'** see *C. sanderiana*.

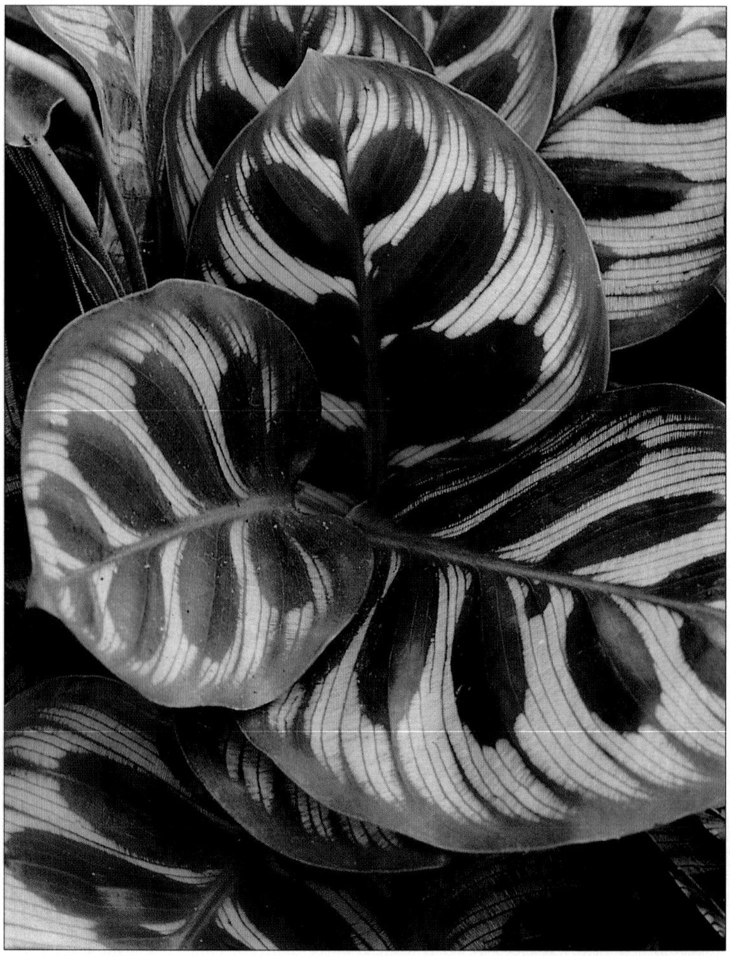

Calathea makoyana

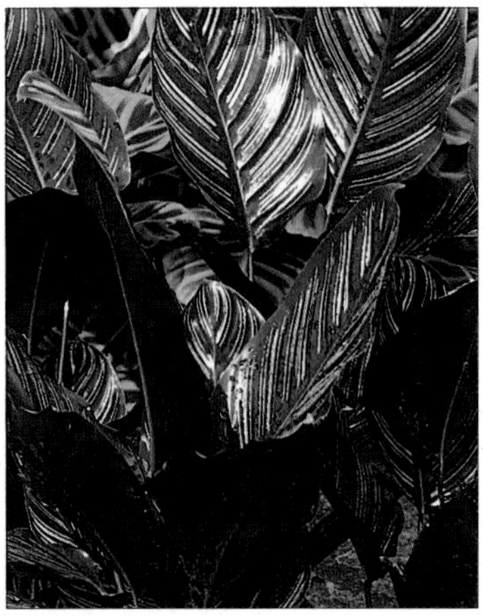

Calathea sanderiana

C. makoyana ■ 🏆 syn. *Maranta makoyana* (Cathedral windows, Peacock plant). Clump-forming, stemless perennial with erect, ovate leaf-blades, 20–30cm (8–12in) long, on leaf-stalks 15cm (6in) or more long. Leaves are pale green above, with oblong patches and fine lines of dark green along the lateral veins; the undersides are purple-tinged, with similar purple markings. Bears ovoid spikes, to 6cm (2½in) long, of white and purple flowers. ↕ 45cm (18in), ↔ 22cm (9in). E. Brazil. ❁ (min. 16–21°C/61–70°F)
C. oppenheimiana see *Ctenanthe oppenheimiana.*
***C. ornata* 'Roseolineata'** see *C. majestica* 'Roseolineata'.
C. ornata* var. *sanderiana see *C. sanderiana.*
C. picturata. Clump-forming perennial with elliptic leaf-blades, 20–25cm (8–10in) long, on leaf-stalks 20cm (8in) long. Leaves are deep olive-green above, marked with a wide silver line along each side of the midribs, and with a narrower, jagged silver line near the margins; the undersides are purple. White flowers are borne in cylindrical spikes, 10cm (4in) long. ↕↔ 35–40cm (14–16in). N.W. Brazil. ❁ (min. 16–21°C/61–70°F). **'Argentea'** produces leaves silvery white above, bright rich purple beneath; they have dark green margins.
C. roseopicta. Clump-forming perennial with rounded leaf-blades, to 20cm (8in) long, on leaf-stalks 3–10cm (1¼–4in) long. Leaves are dark green with pink midribs and feathered, pink or cream stripes between the midribs and margins; the undersides are red. Bears cylindrical spikes, 9cm (3½in) long, of white and violet flowers. ↕ 24cm (10in), ↔ 15cm (6in). N.W. Brazil. ❁ (min. 16–21°C/61–70°F)
C. sanderiana ■ syn. *C. majestica* 'Sanderiana', *C. ornata* var. *sanderiana, C.* 'Sanderiana'. Robust, clump-forming perennial with broadly elliptic, unequal-sided leaf-blades, 60cm (24in) long, on leaf-stalks 20cm (8in) or more long. Deep olive-green leaves have pairs of thin, rose-red, lateral stripes on either side of the midribs, becoming white on older leaves; the undersides are purple. White and violet flowers are borne in conical spikes, 5–8cm (2–3in) long, in summer. ↕ 3m (6ft), ↔ 1m (3ft). Peru. ❁ (min. 16–21°C/61–70°F)
***C.* 'Sanderiana'** see *C. sanderiana.*
C. veitchiana. Clump-forming perennial with ovate-elliptic, unequal-sided leaf-blades, 30cm (12in) long, on leaf-stalks 10–20cm (4–8in) or more long. Dark green leaves have feathery markings in 4 or more shades of green, and red undersides. Violet-flecked white flowers are borne in conical spikes, 7cm (3in) long. ↕ 1m (3ft), ↔ 60cm (24in). S.E. Brazil. ❁ (min. 16–21°C/ 61–70°F)
C. zebrina ■ 🏆 (Zebra plant). Clump-forming perennial with oblong-ovate to elliptic leaf-blades, 45cm (18in) or more long, on leaf-stalks 30cm (12in) long. Leaves are dark green and velvety above, purple-red beneath; they have yellow-green midribs, margins, and veins. Bears white to violet flowers in almost spherical spikes, 7–10cm (3–4in) long. ↕ 1m (3ft), ↔ 60cm (24in). S.E. Brazil. ❁ (min. 16–21°C/61–70°F). **'Humilior'** is compact, producing leaves with areas around the lateral veins that are olive-green above, grey-green beneath.

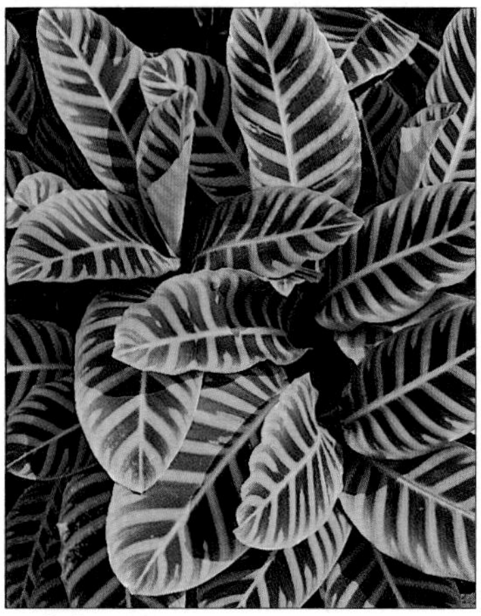

Calathea zebrina

CALCEOLARIA

Pouch flower, Slipper flower, Slipperwort

SCROPHULARIACEAE

Genus of some 300 species of annuals, biennials, perennials, and shrubs, some of them scandent, from diverse habitats ranging from dry scrub to alpine regions. They occur in temperate and tropical areas of Mexico, Central and South America (many in Peru and Chile), with some from the Falkland Islands. Leaves are opposite and whorled, or in rosettes. The slipper-like flowers are solitary or borne in few- to many-flowered panicles, racemes, corymbs, or cymes. They are usually yellow or purple, often heavily spotted in one or more contrasting colours, and 2-lipped, the upper lip small but often inflated, the lower lip large and pouched. In frost-prone areas, grow annuals, biennials, and shrubs in a temperate greenhouse or as summer bedding. The hardier, low-growing perennials (alpine species) are ideal for a rock garden, peat bed, or alpine house.

• **HARDINESS** Most are frost hardy to frost tender; some are fully hardy.

• **CULTIVATION** Under glass, grow in loam-based potting compost (JI No.2) in bright filtered light with good ventilation. In the growing season, water freely and apply a balanced liquid fertilizer every 3–4 weeks; water sparingly in winter. Outdoors, grow in light, moderately fertile, acid soil in sun or partial shade. They require cool, moist conditions to flower freely. Grow alpine species outdoors in moist but well-drained, very gritty soil in partial shade; protect from winter wet. In an alpine house, grow in loam-based potting compost (JI No.1), or in a mix of equal parts loam, leaf mould, and sharp sand; top-dress with grit. Pot on every second year in late spring.

• **PROPAGATION** Sow seed of hardy species in containers in a cold frame in autumn or early spring, or divide in spring. Root individual rosettes in early summer. Sow seed of *C. integrifolia* in spring or autumn, and seed of *C. mexicana* in late winter or early spring. Surface-sow seed of *C.* Herbeohybrida Group cultivars at 18°C (64°F) in late summer or spring. Root softwood cuttings of shrubby species in late spring or summer; increase good colour variants of *C. integrifolia* by rooting semi-ripe cuttings in late summer.

• **PESTS AND DISEASES** Under glass, especially in poorly ventilated conditions, prone to aphids, whiteflies, red spider mites, and fungal diseases, such as grey mould (*Botrytis*). Slugs and snails may be a problem outdoors.

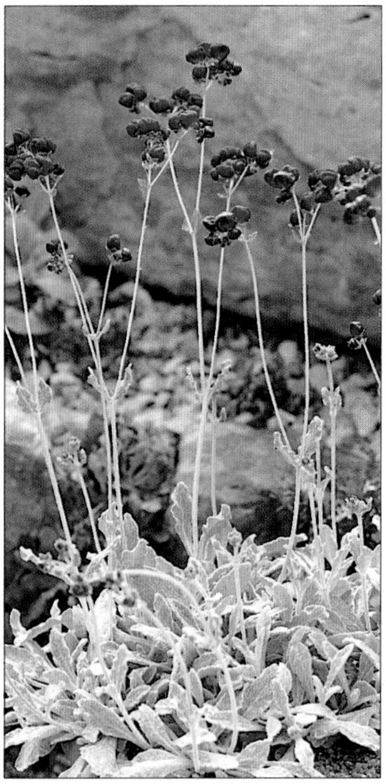

Calceolaria arachnoidea

C. acutifolia see *C. polyrrhiza.*
C. arachnoidea ■ Evergreen, rhizomatous, cushion- or mat-forming perennial with rosettes of lance-shaped to oblong-spoon-shaped, white-hairy leaves, 4–10cm (1½–4in) long, with winged leaf-stalks. Bears compact cymes of 2–5 deep purple flowers, to 1.5cm (½in) long, on slender, branching stems, from summer to autumn. Best in an alpine house. ↕ 20–25cm (8–10in), ↔ to 15cm (6in). Chile. ✻✻ (borderline)
C. biflora, syn. *C. plantaginea.* Evergreen, mat-forming, rhizomatous perennial with rosettes of ovate-lance-shaped to oblong, obovate, or diamond-shaped, toothed, dark green leaves, 2.5–10cm (1–4in) long. Bears loose racemes of 2–8 short-stemmed, bright yellow flowers, each to 2cm (¾in) long, over several months in summer. Suitable for a peat bed or shaded rock garden. ↕ 15–25cm (6–10in), ↔ to 20cm (8in). Chile, Argentina. ✻✻✻
C. darwinii, syn. *C. uniflora* var. *darwinii.* Rhizomatous, evergreen, rosetted perennial with oblong-spoon-shaped to diamond-shaped, wrinkled, glossy, dark green leaves, 3–4cm (1¼–1½in) long. In early summer, bears solitary yellow flowers, 2.5–3.5cm (1–1½in) long, each with a deep yellow lower lip, heavily freckled red-brown, and with a wide, horizontal white band at the junction of the throat and pouch. Best in an alpine house. ↕ 7–10cm (3–4in), ↔ to 12cm (5in). Argentina (S. Patagonia), Tierra del Fuego. ✻✻✻
***C.* Fruticohybrida Group** see *C. integrifolia* Fruticohybrida Group.
***C.* Herbeohybrida Group.** Bushy, compact biennials, normally grown as spring- or summer-flowering container plants, with opposite, ovate, softly hairy, mid-green leaves, 8–12cm (3–5in) or more long. ↕ 20–45cm (8–18in), ↔ 15–30cm (6–12in). ✻. There are 2 main subgroups: Grandiflora group cultivars have compact cymes of 5–15 flowers, to 8cm (3in) long, in red, yellow, orange, and bicolours, often marked with purple, red, or other colours; Multiflora group cultivars have cymes of 3–12 smaller, more numerous flowers, to 5cm (2in) long, in a range of colours. **Anytime Series** (Multiflora group) are compact, and flower in less than 16 weeks from sowing, at any time of year, given suitable conditions; ↕ to 20cm (8in). **'Bright Bikinis'** ■ (Multiflora group) bears dense cymes of yellow, orange, or red flowers in

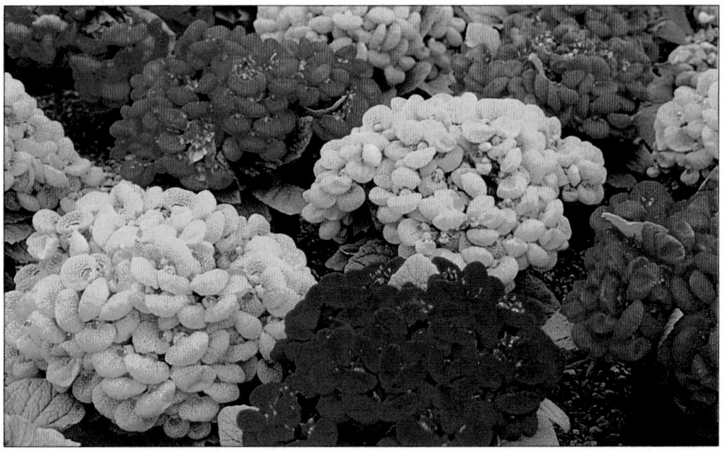

Calceolaria Herbeohybrida Group 'Bright Bikinis'

C

C

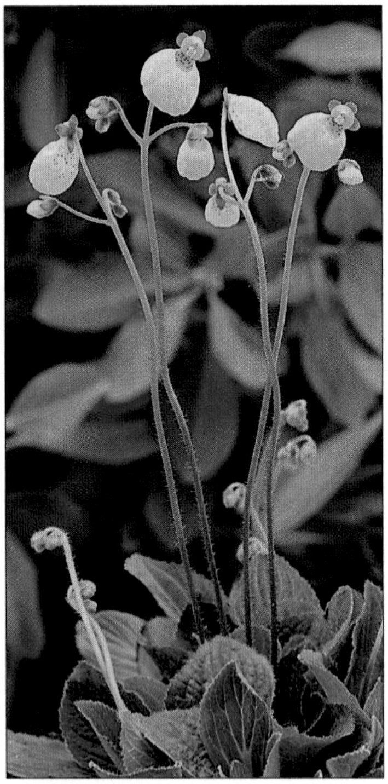

Calceolaria polyrrhiza

summer; ↕20cm (8in), ↔ 20cm (8in); ✻✻. **'Monarch'** (Grandiflora group) has light green leaves and red or yellow flowers, often marked orange-red or maroon; ↕30cm (12in), ↔ 25cm (10in).
C. integrifolia 🏆 syn. *C. rugosa.* Evergreen, subshrubby perennial, usually grown as an annual, with softly hairy young shoots. The opposite, linear-lance-shaped to ovate-lance-shaped leaves are finely toothed, grey-green, and 5cm (2in) or more long, frequently with reddish hairs beneath. Panicle-like cymes of 10–35 yellow flowers, to 2.5cm (1in) long, are borne over several months in summer. ↕ to 1.2m (4ft), ↔ 23–30cm (9–12in). Mexico. ✻. This species is the main parent of the **Fruticohybrida Group** of cultivars described below. **'Goldcut'** is tall-growing, and good for cut flowers; ↕30–40cm (12–16in). **'Golden Bunch'** is compact, with pale golden yellow flowers in early summer; excellent for containers or as bedding; ↕ to 25cm (10in). **'Midas'** is upright, bearing deep yellow, weather-resistant flowers in early summer; good for hanging baskets; ↕ to 25cm (10in). **'Sunshine'** 🏆 is similar to 'Midas', but flowers in midsummer.

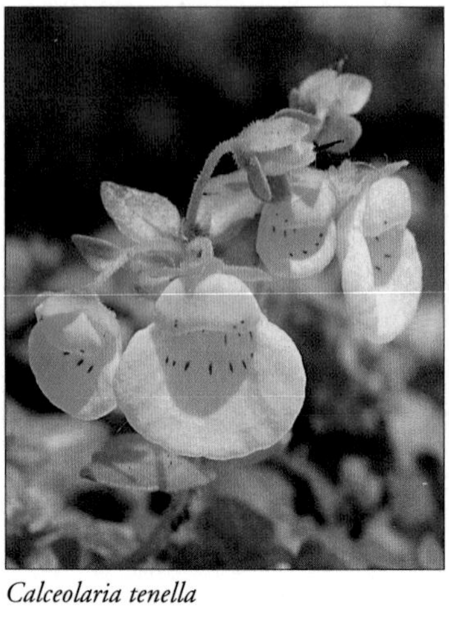

Calceolaria tenella

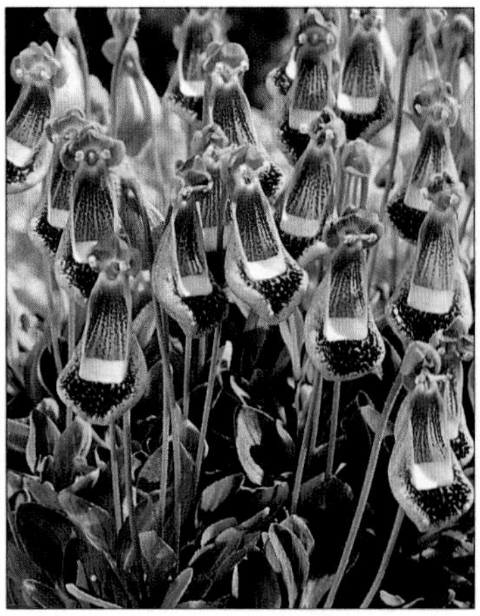

Calceolaria 'Walter Shrimpton'

Useful for bedding, hanging baskets, or containers; ↕ to 30cm (12in).
C. mexicana. Bushy, erect to spreading, softly hairy annual, with opposite, ovate to lance-shaped, pinnatifid, mid-green leaves, 2–7cm (¾–3in) long, often tinged purple beneath. Cymes of 3–5 pale to bright yellow, unspotted flowers, to 1.5cm (½in) long, are produced in summer. ↕20–50cm (8–20in), ↔ to 30cm (12in). Mexico to Bolivia. ✻
C. pavonii. Scandent, woody-based, evergreen, perennial climber with woolly stems. Winged leaf-stalks bear opposite, triangular-ovate, irregularly toothed, softly hairy, mid- to dark green leaves, 8–20cm (3–8in) long, heart-shaped at the bases. Cymes of 4–20 sulphur-yellow flowers, 2cm (¾in) long, with purple-marked throats, are borne in summer. ↕1.5–3m (5–10ft). Ecuador, Peru. ✻
C. plantaginea see *C. biflora.*
C. polyrrhiza ■ syn. *C. acutifolia.* Rhizomatous, mat-forming, evergreen perennial with opposite, oblong-ovate or lance-shaped, shallowly toothed, mid-green leaves, to 4.5cm (1¾in) long, crowded on the stems. In summer, bears cymes of 4–6 red-spotted yellow flowers, to 2.5cm (1in) long. ↕5cm (2in), ↔ to 20cm (8in). Chile, Argentina. ✻✻✻
C. rugosa see *C. integrifolia.*
C. scabiosifolia see *C. tripartita.*
***C.* Sunset Series.** Compact, rounded, evergreen, many-branched, sturdy-stemmed perennials producing opposite, ovate-lance-shaped, dark grey-green leaves, 10cm (4in) long. They bear red, yellow, orange, or bicoloured flowers, 2cm (¾in) long, from mid-spring to midsummer. ↕ to 30cm (12in), ↔ 23–30cm (9–12in). ✻✻
C. tenella ■ Mat-forming, creeping, evergreen perennial with slender stems clothed in broadly ovate, finely toothed, pale yellowish green leaves, to 1cm (½in) long. In summer, bears solitary or branched cymes of 3 broadly pouched, red-spotted yellow flowers, 7–9mm (¼–⅜in) long. ↕5cm (2in), ↔ to 30cm (12in) or more. Chile. ✻✻✻
C. tripartita, syn. *C. scabiosifolia.* Erect, evergreen perennial, usually grown as an annual, with softly hairy stems and leaves. The opposite, ovate, pinnatifid, toothed, mid-green leaves are 2–9cm (¾–3½in) long. In summer, bears cymes of 5–12 pale to bright to deep yellow, unspotted flowers, 5mm (¼in) long. ↕60cm (24in), ↔ 30cm (12in). Mexico to Peru. ✻

C. uniflora* var. *darwinii see *C. darwinii.*
***C.* 'Walter Shrimpton'** ■ Evergreen perennial, similar to *C. darwinii,* with rosettes of spoon- to diamond-shaped, glossy dark green leaves, 3–5cm (1¼–2in) long. In summer, bears cymes of 2–5 bronze-yellow flowers, to 2.5cm (1in) long, spotted rich brown, each with a horizontal white band at the junction of the throat and pouch, broader and bolder than in *C. darwinii.* ↕10cm (4in), ↔ 23cm (9in). ✻✻✻

CALENDULA

English marigold, Marigold, Pot marigold

ASTERACEAE/COMPOSITAE

Genus of 20–30 species of bushy, fast-growing annuals and woody-based, evergreen perennials, occurring in arable land, wasteland, and rocky habitats from S. Europe to North Africa. Leaves are alternate, simple, and aromatic. Daisy-like flowerheads, with orange or yellow ray-florets and yellow, orange, violet, purple, or brown disc-florets, are borne in a long succession over the summer and throughout autumn into mild winters. Many of the cultivars are excellent annuals for an informal border; the flowers last well when cut. They are also suitable for growing in containers in a cool conservatory.
• **HARDINESS** Fully hardy to half hardy.
• **CULTIVATION** Under glass, grow in loam-based potting compost (JI No.2) in full light; water moderately. Outdoors, grow in a well-drained, even poor soil in sun or partial shade. Dead-head to prolong flowering. If growing for cut flowers, pinch out terminal buds to encourage laterals.
• **PROPAGATION** Sow seed *in situ* in spring or autumn. Provide cloche protection for autumn-sown seedlings in frost-prone areas.
• **PESTS AND DISEASES** Aphids, powdery mildew, and cucumber mosaic virus may be a problem.

***C. officinalis* cultivars.** Fast-growing, erect, sometimes spreading annuals with inversely lance-shaped to spoon-shaped, softly hairy, aromatic leaves, to 15cm (6in) long. Daisy-like, single or double, orange, yellow, gold, cream, or apricot flowerheads, to 10cm (4in) across, many with dark disc-florets, are borne profusely from summer to autumn. ↕30–70cm (12–28in), ↔ 30–45cm (12–18in). ✻✻✻. **'Fiesta Gitana'** ■🏆

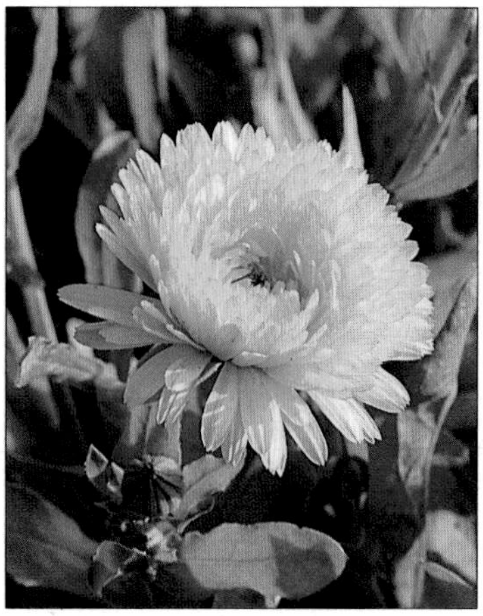

Calendula officinalis Pacific Beauty Series 'Lemon Queen'

is dwarf, with usually double flowerheads in pastel orange and yellow, including bicolours; ↕ to 30cm (12in). **Kablouna Series** cultivars are tall, with double orange, gold, or yellow flowerheads, each with a "crested" disc-floret of quilled petals; ↕ to 60cm (24in). **'Orange King'** has double, deep orange flowerheads; ↕ to 45cm (18in). **Pacific Beauty Series** cultivars have double flowerheads in an unusual colour range, including apricot-orange, primrose-yellow, cream, and bicolours, with red-brown disc-florets; ↕ to 60cm (24in); **'Lemon Queen'** ■ has double, lemon-yellow flowerheads; ↕ to 45cm (18in). **Prince Series** cultivars have double, golden yellow or orange flowerheads; **'Indian Prince'** has dark orange flowerheads, tinted reddish brown on the petals; good for cutting; ↕75cm (30in).

CALIBANUS

AGAVACEAE

Genus of one species of very slow-growing, perennial succulent from rocky grassland in C. and E. Mexico. It has a large, fibrous-rooted, spherical, corky-barked caudex, which, in the wild, sometimes grows partially above ground. The caudex develops tufts of grass-like, arching foliage, among which pinkish purple panicles of tiny flowers are borne. In frost-prone areas, grow *C. hookeri* in a temperate greenhouse; in warmer areas, grow outdoors in a desert garden.
• **HARDINESS** Frost tender.
• **CULTIVATION** Under glass, grow in standard cactus compost, with an

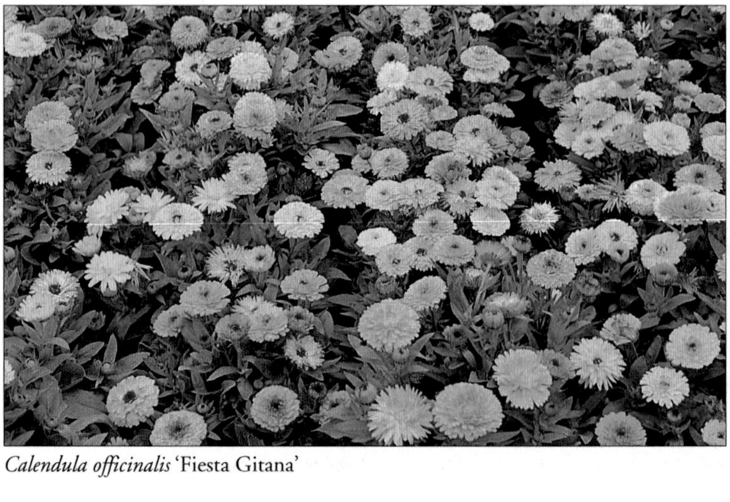

Calendula officinalis 'Fiesta Gitana'

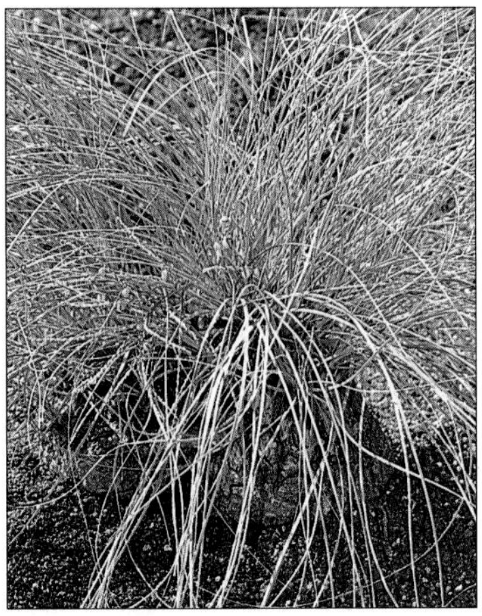
Calibanus hookeri

additional 25 per cent sharp sand, in full light. In the growing season, water freely and apply a low-nitrogen fertilizer monthly; keep just moist in winter. Outdoors, grow in very well-drained, gritty, alkaline, humus-rich soil in full sun. See also pp.48–49.
• **PROPAGATION** Sow seed at 19–24°C (66–75°F) in spring; keep moist.
• **PESTS AND DISEASES** Susceptible to scale insects in summer.

C. hookeri ▣ syn. *Dasylirion hartwegianum.* Perennial succulent with a spherical caudex, 30cm (12in) or more across, covered in thick, corky bark, and producing rosettes of 10–15 upright, then recurved, linear leaves, to 30cm (12in) long. Panicles, 50–60cm (20–24in) long, of cup-shaped, pinkish purple flowers, 5–8mm (¼–⅜in) across, are borne in summer. ↕ to 90cm (36in), ↔ 30cm (12in) or more. C. and E. Mexico. ❀ (min. 10°C/50°F)

▷**Calico bush** see *Kalmia latifolia*
▷**Calico flower** see *Aristolochia littoralis*
▷**Calico plant** see *Alternanthera bettzichiana*

CALLA

ARACEAE

Genus of one species of deciduous or semi-evergreen, marginal aquatic perennial from swamps, and lake and stream edges, in temperate regions of the N. hemisphere. *C. palustris* has glossy, dark green leaves and bears showy spathes, followed by dull red berries. It seldom exceeds 20–24cm (8–10in) in height and is excellent for softening the margins of a small to medium-sized pool. At depths of 5–7cm (2–3in), it spreads through shallow water or mud by creeping rhizomes, which may extend to 15–50cm (6–20in) and thicken to 3cm (1¼in) in diameter. Contact with the foliage may aggravate skin allergies.
• **HARDINESS** Fully hardy.
• **CULTIVATION** Grow in aquatic planting baskets in humus-rich, lime-free soil, or in mud in shallow, still or slow-moving water no deeper than 25cm (10in). Position in full sun to encourage flowering and fruiting. See also pp.52–53.
• **PROPAGATION** Sow seed in late summer in containers submerged to the rims in water. Divide rhizomes in spring.
• **PESTS AND DISEASES** Trouble free.

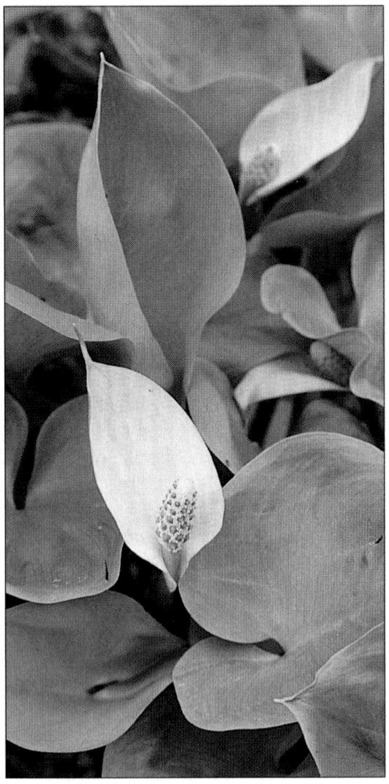
Calla palustris

C. palustris ▣ (Bog arum). Aquatic, rhizomatous perennial with upright, alternate, glossy, dark green leaves, to 20cm (8in) long, broadly ovate with heart-shaped bases. The basal leaves are arranged in 2 ranks on slender leaf-stalks growing from the rhizomes. In mid-summer, bears white-spathed inflorescences, 25cm (10in) tall; the spathes surround insignificant flower clusters. They are followed by clusters of dull red berries in autumn. ↕ 25cm (10in), ↔ 60cm (24in). N. and C. Europe, Asia, North America. ❄❄❄

CALLIANDRA

Powder-puff tree

LEGUMINOSAE/MIMOSACEAE

Genus of about 200 species of evergreen perennials, shrubs, and small trees from W. Africa, Madagascar, India, and tropical and subtropical North and South America, mainly found in dry sites at forest margins. Only the shrubs and trees are usually cultivated: they are valued for their attractive, alternate, pinnate or 2-pinnate leaves, and their spherical heads of few to many small, bell- or funnel-shaped flowers which have 10–100 colourful stamens, 1–4cm (½–1½in) long. In frost-prone areas, grow in a warm greenhouse; in warmer regions, grow in a shrub border.
• **HARDINESS** Frost tender.
• **CULTIVATION** Under glass, grow in loam-based potting compost (JI No.2) in full light with shade from hot sun. From early summer to autumn, water freely and apply a balanced liquid fertilizer monthly; water sparingly in winter. Outdoors, grow in well-drained, fertile soil in full sun. Pruning group 1, after flowering; plants under glass may need restrictive pruning.
• **PROPAGATION** Sow seed at 16–18°C (61–64°F) in spring. Root semi-ripe cuttings with bottom heat in summer. Layer in spring.
• **PESTS AND DISEASES** Prone to red spider mites and mealybugs under glass.

C. eriophylla ♀ Low-growing shrub or small tree producing 2-pinnate leaves, 7–12cm (3–5in) long, each pinna subdivided into 1 or 2 pairs of elliptic to ovate, dark green leaflets, often softly hairy beneath. In summer, bears axillary, spherical heads, to 3cm (1¼in) across, of pale to deep pink flowers, 1.5cm (½in) long, with reddish purple, sometimes white stamens. ↕ 1m (3ft), ↔ 80cm (32in). N. South America. ❀ (min. 13°C/55°F)
C. haematocephala ▣ ♀ syn. *C. inaequilatera.* Large, many-branched, spreading shrub or small tree with pinnate or 2-pinnate leaves, 30–45cm (12–18in) long; each leaf is composed of 5–10 pairs of sickle-shaped to elliptic, glossy, dark green leaflets. Axillary, spherical heads, to 7cm (3in) across, of usually red, sometimes pink or white flowers, 7–9mm (¼–⅜in) long, with prominent, bright red, pink, or white stamens, are borne in summer. ↕ 3–6m (10–20ft), ↔ 2–4m (6–12ft). Bolivia. ❀ (min. 13°C/55°F)
C. inaequilatera see *C. haematocephala.*
C. surinamensis ♀ Large, spreading shrub or small tree with 2-pinnate, pale green leaves, 10cm (4in) or more long, each pinna subdivided into 7–12 pairs of oblong-lance-shaped leaflets. Axillary heads, 5–8cm (2–3in) across, of yellow-green flowers, to 5mm (¼in) long, with conspicuous, white-based, deep red stamens, are produced from the leaf axils in summer. ↕ 3–8m (10–25ft), ↔ 2–5m (6–15ft). N. South America. ❀ (min. 13°C/55°F)
C. tweedii ♀ (Mexican flame bush). Large shrub or small tree producing 2-pinnate, mid-green leaves, 10–15cm (4–6in) long, each pinna divided into 15–20 pairs of narrowly oblong, often curved leaflets. Green or white flowers, to 5mm (¼in) long, with red stamens, are borne in axillary, spherical heads, 5–7cm (2–3in) across, from winter to spring. ↕ 2–5m (6–15ft), ↔ 1.5–2m (5–6ft), sometimes more. Brazil to Uruguay. ❀ (min. 13°C/55°F)

CALLIANTHEMUM

RANUNCULACEAE

Genus of about 10 species of perennials from alpine grassland, stony slopes, or coniferous forest in the mountains of C. Asia and C. and S. Europe. They have short rhizomes and produce rosettes of finely divided, pinnate leaves. In late spring, they bear white, pink, or mauve, buttercup-like flowers with 5–20 petals, usually solitary, but sometimes in 2- or 3-flowered racemes. Grow in a rock garden, scree bed, or alpine house.
• **HARDINESS** Fully hardy.
• **CULTIVATION** Under glass, grow in loam-based potting compost (JI No.1) with additional grit. Outdoors, grow in moist, humus-rich, gritty soil in full sun.
• **PROPAGATION** Sow seed as soon as ripe in containers in a cold frame; keep cool and shaded until germination. Divide as growth begins in spring.
• **PESTS AND DISEASES** Prone to aphids and red spider mites under glass.

C. coriandrifolium, syn. *C. rutifolium.* Prostrate perennial with erect rhizomes and rosettes of long-stalked, ovate-elliptic, pinnate leaves, 5–13cm (2–5in) long, with 5–7 linear-oblong, blue-green leaflets. In late spring, erect stems bear solitary (occasionally 2 or 3), 9- to 13-petalled white flowers, 2–3cm (¾–1¼in) wide, sometimes flushed pink outside, with greenish yellow centres. ↕↔ 10–20cm (4–8in). Mountains from N.W. Spain to S. Carpathians. ❄❄❄
C. rutifolium see *C. coriandrifolium.*

CALLICARPA

Beauty berry

VERBENACEAE

Genus of about 140 species of evergreen and deciduous shrubs and trees from woodland in mainly tropical and subtropical regions. They have opposite, simple leaves and bear dense, axillary cymes or panicles of numerous tiny,

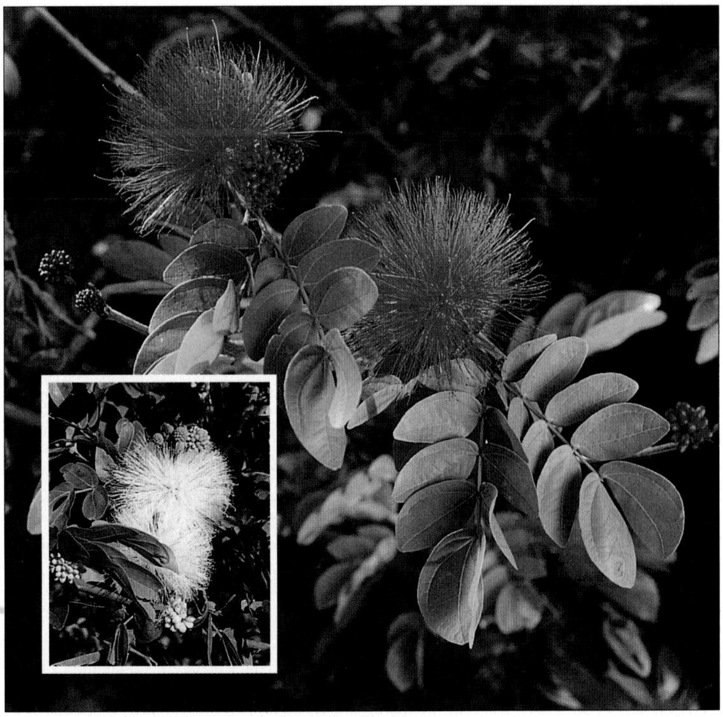
Calliandra haematocephala (inset: variant with white stamens)

C

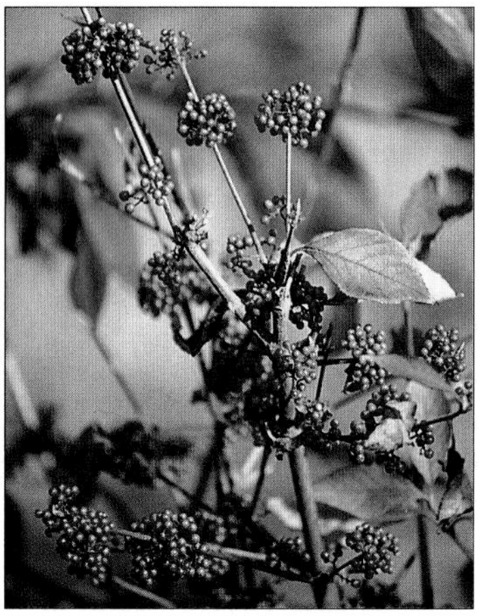

Callicarpa bodinieri var. *giraldii*

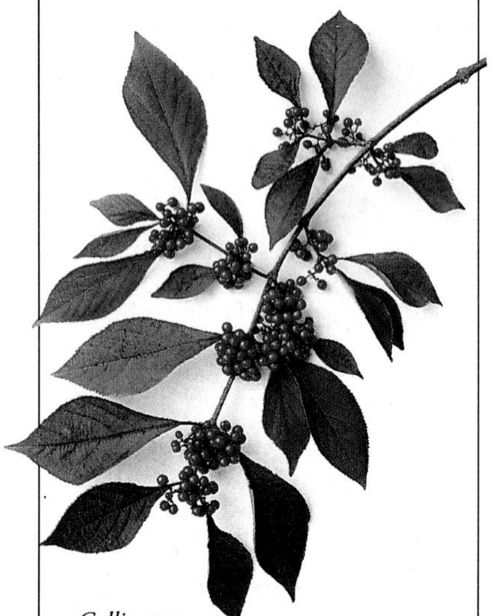

Callicarpa bodinieri var. *giraldii* 'Profusion'

white, pink, red, or purple flowers in summer. Grown mainly for their clusters of small but often highly coloured, spherical, bead-like fruits, 2–4mm (1⁄16–1⁄8in) across, they are ideal for a shrub border; they fruit most prolifically in long, hot summers and if planted in groups. In frost-prone areas, grow tender and half-hardy species in a cool greenhouse and move outdoors in summer.

• **HARDINESS** Fully hardy to frost tender.

• **CULTIVATION** Under glass, grow in loam-based potting compost (JI No.2) in full or bright filtered light. In the growing season, water freely and apply a balanced liquid fertilizer monthly; water sparingly in winter. Outdoors, grow in fertile, well-drained soil in sun or dappled shade. *C. dichotoma* thrives in areas with prolonged periods above 24°C (75°F). *C. japonica* 'Leucocarpa' may be cut back by severe weather but is seldom killed; it requires summer heat to ripen new wood. Pruning group 6.

• **PROPAGATION** Sow seed in containers in a cold frame in autumn or spring. Root softwood cuttings in spring, or semi-ripe cuttings with bottom heat in summer.

• **PESTS AND DISEASES** Trouble free.

C. bodinieri* var. *giraldii ■ Bushy, upright, deciduous shrub with elliptic to obovate, tapered, dark green leaves, to 18cm (7in) long. In midsummer, produces small pink flowers in cymes, to 3.5cm (1½in) across, from the leaf axils, followed by violet fruit in autumn. ↕3m (10ft), ↔2.5m (8ft). W. and C. China. ✻✻✻. **'Profusion'** ♀■ has bronze young leaves and pale pink flowers; it freely produces dark violet fruit.

C. dichotoma. Dense, upright, deciduous shrub with ovate to elliptic, tapered, bright green leaves, to 10cm (4in) long. Pale pink flowers are borne in axillary cymes, 1–2cm (½–¾in) across, in summer, followed by dark lilac fruit. ↕↔1.2m (4ft). China, Korea, Japan. ✻✻✻

***C. japonica* 'Leucocarpa'.** Bushy, deciduous shrub with narrowly oval to lance-shaped, tapered, pale green leaves, to 12cm (5in) long. White flowers are borne in axillary cymes, to 3cm (1¼in) across, in late summer, followed by white fruit. ↕↔1.5m (5ft). ✻✻✻

C. rubella. Evergreen or semi-evergreen, erect, open shrub with obovate to lance-shaped, yellow-green leaves, 10–15cm (4–6in) long, and downy beneath. Bears axillary cymes, to 5cm (2in) across, of small, purplish pink flowers in summer, followed by bright pinkish purple fruit. ↕1–3m (3–10ft), ↔1–2m (3–6ft). India to China, Malaysia. ✻

▷ ***Calliopsis tinctoria*** see *Coreopsis tinctoria*

CALLIRHOE

Poppy mallow

MALVACEAE

Genus of 8 species of annuals and tap-rooted perennials from prairies and grassland in the USA and Mexico. Their leaves are alternate and deeply palmately lobed. The 5-petalled, cup-shaped, mallow-like, brightly coloured flowers are produced from the upper leaf axils either singly or in short racemes. Poppy mallows will thrive in a hot, dry site in a border or rock garden.

• **HARDINESS** Fully hardy.

• **CULTIVATION** Grow in well-drained, sandy, loam soil in full sun. Protect from winter wet. Avoid damage to the tap root when planting.

• **PROPAGATION** Sow seed of annuals *in situ* in spring. Sow seed of perennials *in situ* in early spring, or root softwood cuttings in early summer.

• **PESTS AND DISEASES** Trouble free.

C. involucrata ■ (Prairie poppy mallow). Low-growing perennial with a carrot-like tap root, giving rise to procumbent, hairy stems, 15cm (6in) or more long, with rounded, 3- to 7-lobed leaves, 2.5–5cm (1–2in) long. From late spring to midsummer, long flower-stalks bear numerous erect, axillary, usually solitary flowers, 4.5–6cm (1¾–2½in) across, the petals cerise to purplish red with white bases. ↕↔30cm (12in). USA (Missouri to Texas). ✻✻✻

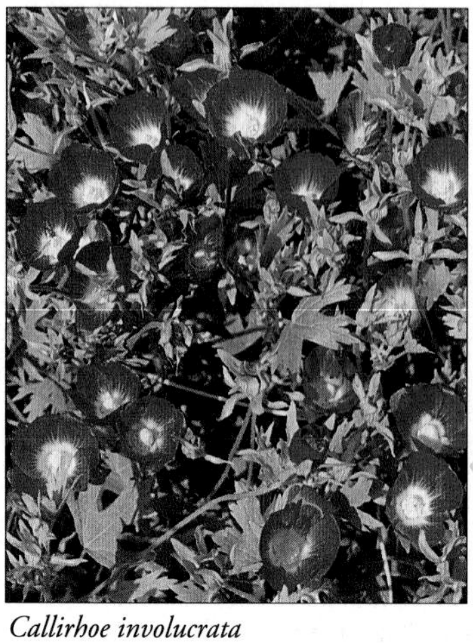

Callirhoe involucrata

CALLISIA *syn.* PHYODINA

COMMELINACEAE

Genus, related to *Tradescantia*, of about 20 species of creeping, spreading, or suberect, evergreen perennials, and (rarely) annuals, from forest margins in S.E. USA, Mexico, and tropical North and South America. They are valued for their attractive, alternate, succulent leaves. The flowers, borne in pairs in curled cymes or terminal panicles, are white or pink, with 3 sepals and 3 petals. In frost-prone regions, grow in hanging baskets in a temperate greenhouse or as houseplants; elsewhere, use as ground cover in a border.

• **HARDINESS** Frost tender.

• **CULTIVATION** Under glass, grow in 2 parts loam-based potting compost (JI No.2) to 1 part coarse grit in bright filtered or indirect light. In the growing season, water moderately and apply a balanced liquid fertilizer monthly; water sparingly in winter. Pot on only when very root-bound. Outdoors, grow in gritty, well-drained soil in partial shade.

• **PROPAGATION** Root tip cuttings, 6–7cm (2½–3in) long, in spring. Pot up several cuttings in an 8cm (3in) container to produce dense foliage cover quickly.

• **PESTS AND DISEASES** Trouble free.

C. elegans ♀ syn. *Setcreasea striata* (Striped inch plant). Decumbent, succulent perennial with 2-ranked, oval, pointed, olive-green leaves, 5–10cm (2–4in) long, purple beneath, and with longitudinal white stripes. From autumn to winter, bears paired, stemless white flowers, 1cm (½in) across, in terminal panicles or curled cymes, to 15cm (6in) long. ↕15cm (6in), ↔ to 1m (3ft). Guatemala, Honduras. ❀ (min. 10°C/50°F)

C. fragrans, syn. *Spironema fragrans* (Chain plant). Stoloniferous, succulent perennial with 2-ranked, elliptic to lance-shaped, shiny, light green leaves, purple beneath, and to 24cm (10in) long. Fragrant white flowers, 1cm (½in) across, are borne in terminal panicles, 8cm (3in) long, from winter to spring. ↕1.5m (5ft), ↔ to 1.5m (5ft). Mexico. ❀ (min. 10°C/50°F)

C. navicularis, syn. *Tradescantia navicularis* (Chain plant). Slow-growing, succulent perennial with tufts of dense foliage and long, trailing shoots rooting at the internodes. Broadly ovate to lance-shaped leaves, 2.5cm (1in) long, are dull copper-green above and purple-striped beneath. From summer to autumn, bears bright magenta flowers, 1.5–2cm (½–¾in) across, in curled cymes, 5cm (2in) long. ↕10cm (4in), ↔ to 30cm (12in). N.E. and E. Mexico. ❀ (min. 10°C/50°F)

C. repens ■ Variable, trailing perennial with stems rooting at the nodes to form mats of broadly ovate, bright green leaves, 1–4cm (½–1½in) long. White flowers, to 1cm (½in) across, are borne in spike-like, curled cymes, 3cm (1¼in) long, in autumn. ↕10cm (4in), ↔ to 1m (3ft). USA (Texas) to Argentina. ❀ (min. 10°C/50°F)

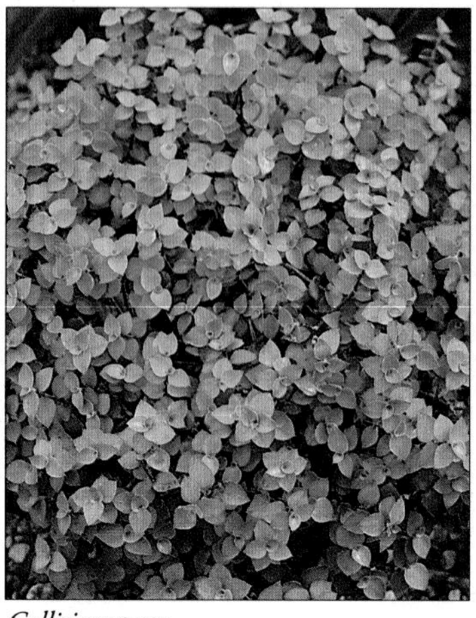

Callisia repens

CALLISTEMON

Bottlebrush

MYRTACEAE

Genus of 25 species or more of evergreen trees and shrubs from Australia, most occurring in moist soil in open or woodland sites. The simple, alternate, leathery leaves are cylindrical to broadly lance-shaped. Callistemons are grown for their colourful, terminal or axillary, bottlebrush-like spikes of numerous tiny, 5-petalled, long-stamened flowers, which may be red, purple, pink, white, green, or yellow. Grow at the base of a house wall or in a shrub border. In frost-prone climates, grow half-hardy and tender species in a cool greenhouse.

• **HARDINESS** Fully hardy to frost tender.

• **CULTIVATION** Under glass, grow in loam-based potting compost (JI No.2) in full light with good ventilation. In the growing season, water freely and apply a balanced liquid fertilizer monthly; water more sparingly in winter. Pot on or top-dress in early spring. Outdoors, grow in moist but well-drained, neutral to acid, moderately fertile soil in full sun. Pruning group 8; tolerates hard pruning.

• **PROPAGATION** Surface-sow seed on to moist compost at 16–18°C (61–64°F) in spring. Root semi-ripe cuttings in late summer.

• **PESTS AND DISEASES** Red spider mites, mealybugs, and scale insects may be a problem, especially under glass.

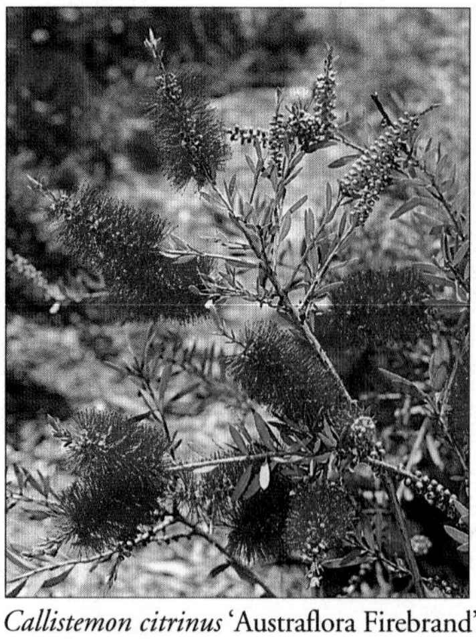

Callistemon citrinus 'Austraflora Firebrand'

***C.* 'Captain Cook'** ♀ syn. *C. viminalis* 'Captain Cook'. Dense, rounded shrub with lance-shaped, mid-green leaves, 2.5–4.5cm (1–1¾in) long. Bright red flowers are borne in spikes, 10–15cm (4–6in) long, from early summer to autumn. ↕↔ 2m (6ft). ❄❄
C. citrinus (Crimson bottlebrush). Variable shrub, often with arching branches, producing lance-shaped, dark green leaves, to 10cm (4in) long, with prominent oil glands. Brilliant crimson-red flowers in spikes, 5–15cm (2–6in) long, are borne freely in spring and summer. ↕↔ 1.5–8m (5–25ft). Australia (New South Wales, Victoria). ❄. **f. *albus*** see 'White Anzac'. **'Austraflora Firebrand'** ▣ is low and spreading, producing silvery pink young shoots and bright crimson flowers; ↕ 1.5–2m (5–6ft), ↔ 4m (10–12ft). **'Splendens'** ▣ ♀ has silky, pinkish red young shoots, broad leaves, and crimson flowers; ↕ 2–8m (6–25ft), ↔ 1.5–6m (5–20ft). **'White Anzac'**, syn. f. *albus*, bears white flowers, often tinged pink when mature; ↕↔ 1–3m (3–10ft).
***C.* 'King's Park Special'.** Spreading, bushy shrub with lance-shaped, smooth, deep green leaves, 5–8cm (2–3in) long. Bright red flowers are produced in profuse spikes, to 10cm (4in) long, in summer. ↕↔ 2–4m (6–12ft). ❄
C. linearis ♀ (Narrow-leaved bottlebrush). Spreading, dense to open shrub with linear, rigid, sharp-pointed, thick, dark green leaves, to 12cm (5in) long. Bears rich, matt red flowers in spikes, to 12cm (5in) long, from late spring to autumn. ↕ 2–4m (6–12ft), ↔ 3–5m (10–15ft). Australia (New South Wales). ❄
C. macropunctatus (Scarlet bottlebrush). Spreading, dense to open shrub with linear to narrowly oblong, pointed, glandular, mid-green leaves, 3–8cm (1¼–3in) long. Red flowers are borne in spikes, 10cm (4in) long, from early summer to autumn. ↕↔ 2–4m (6–12ft). Australia (South Australia, New South Wales, Victoria). ❄

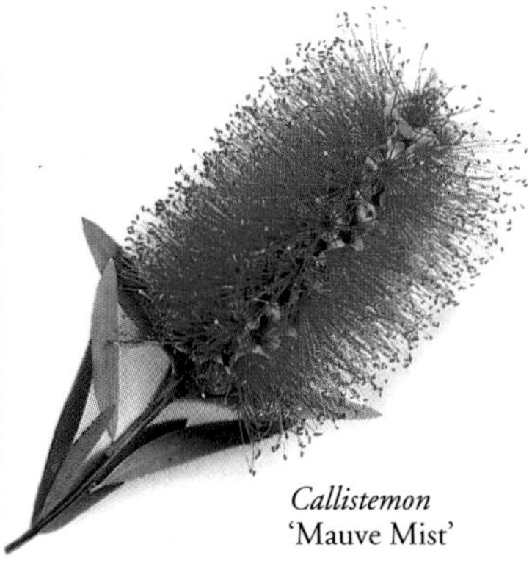

Callistemon 'Mauve Mist'

***C.* 'Mauve Mist'** ▣ Spreading shrub with narrowly oblong, mid-green leaves, 3–6cm (1½–2½in) long, tapered at each end. Mauve-pink flowers, fading with age, are borne in spikes, 10cm (4in) long, in summer. ↕↔ 2–4m (6–12ft). ❄
C. pallidus ▣ (Lemon bottlebrush). Erect to spreading shrub producing downy shoots and lance-shaped to broadly lance-shaped, densely glandular, dark green or grey-green leaves, to 10cm (4in) long. Cream to greenish yellow flowers are borne in spikes, 10cm (4in) long, from late spring to midsummer. ↕↔ 2–4m (6–12ft). Australia (Queensland to Tasmania). ❄. **'Candle Glow'**, syn. 'Austraflora Candleglow', produces spikes of lemon-yellow flowers.
C. paludosus see *C. sieberi.*
C. pinifolius (Pine bottlebrush). Spreading shrub with rigid, linear, sharply pointed, dark green leaves, to 10cm (4in) long. Yellow flowers are produced in spikes, 5–8cm (2–3in) long, during summer. ↕ 1.5m (5ft), ↔ 2.5m (8ft). Australia (New South Wales). ❄❄
C. pityoides (Alpine bottlebrush). Compact, usually upright shrub with densely arranged, linear, sharply pointed, dark green leaves, 2.5–4cm (1–1½in) long. Yellow flowers are produced in short spikes, 2–4cm (¾–1½in) long, in mid- and late summer. ↕ 1.5m (5ft), ↔ 1m (3ft). S.E. Australia. ❄❄❄

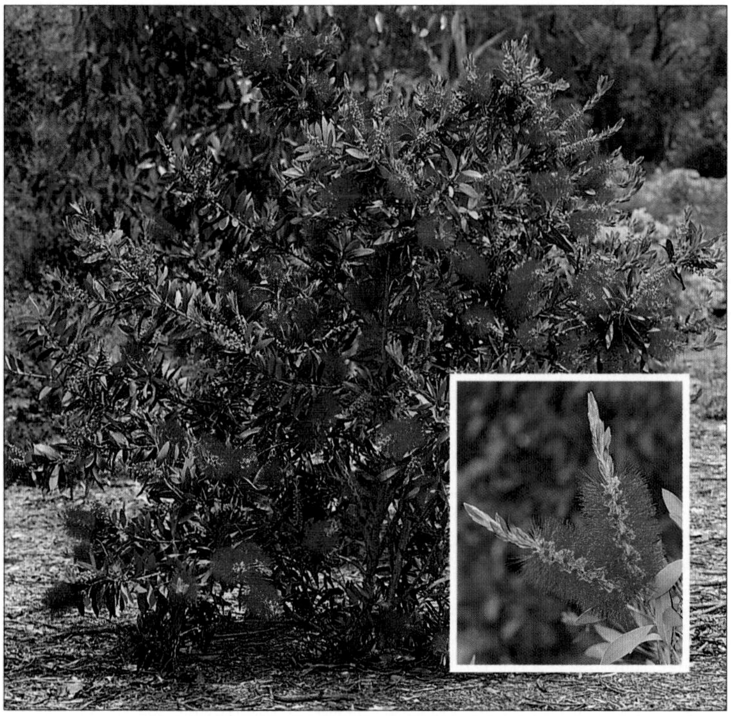

Callistemon citrinus 'Splendens' (inset: flower detail)

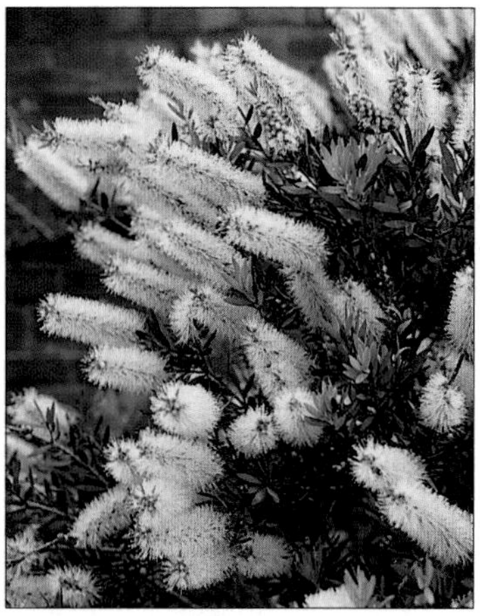

Callistemon pallidus

C. rigidus (Stiff bottlebrush). Bushy, stiff-stemmed shrub with linear to lance-shaped, matt, dark green leaves, to 15cm (6in) long. In summer, bears deep red flowers in numerous spikes, to 5cm (2in) long. ↕ 1–2.5m (3–8ft), ↔ 2–3m (6–10ft). Australia (Queensland, New South Wales). ❄
C. salignus ♀ ○ (White bottlebrush, Willow bottlebrush). Erect to spreading shrub or small tree with papery white bark and willow-like, narrowly lance-shaped, pale green leaves, to 10cm (4in) long. Bears green or white, sometimes red, pink, or mauve flowers in spikes, 3–5cm (1¼–2in) long, from late spring to midsummer. ↕ 5–15m (15–50ft), ↔ 3–5m (10–15ft). Australia (South Australia, New South Wales). ❄
C. sieberi ♀ syn. *C. paludosus* (Alpine bottlebrush). Small, spreading to semi-erect shrub with crowded, linear, rigid, dark green leaves, 4cm (1½in) long, with hard points. Bears creamy yellow flowers in spikes, 4–15cm (1½–6in) long, from late spring to summer. ↕↔ 1–2m (3–6ft). Australia (Queensland to Victoria). ❄❄. **'Summer Pink'** bears pink flowers.
C. speciosus (Albany bottlebrush). Erect, open shrub with lance-shaped to broadly lance-shaped, mid- to dark green leaves, to 15cm (6in) long. Deep red flowers are borne in dense spikes, to 15cm (6in) long, from late spring to autumn. ↕ 2–4m (6–12ft), ↔ 1–2m (3–6ft). Australia (Western Australia). ❄
C. subulatus (Tonghi bottlebrush). Evergreen shrub with arching shoots and linear, pointed, bright green leaves, to 4cm (1½in) long. Bright red flowers are borne in spikes, to 5cm (2in) long, in mid- and late summer. ↕ 1.5m (5ft), ↔ 2m (6ft). S.E. Australia. ❄❄❄
C. viminalis ○ (Weeping bottlebrush). Bushy shrub or small tree with arching or weeping stems and lance-shaped, glandular, mid- to dark green leaves, 2–6cm (¾–2½in) long. Bears bright red flowers in spikes, 10–20cm (4–8in) long, from late spring to midsummer. ↕ 2–10m (6–30ft), ↔ 1.5–4m (5–12ft). Australia (Queensland, New South Wales). ❄. **'Captain Cook'** see *C.* 'Captain Cook'. **'Rose Opal'** ▣ is compact, producing narrow leaves and spikes of deep red flowers that fade to rose-pink; ↕ 1.5–2m (5–6ft).
C. viridiflorus (Green bottlebrush). Compact shrub, usually of arching habit, with linear, sharply pointed, mid- to dark green leaves, 2–3cm (¾–1¼in)

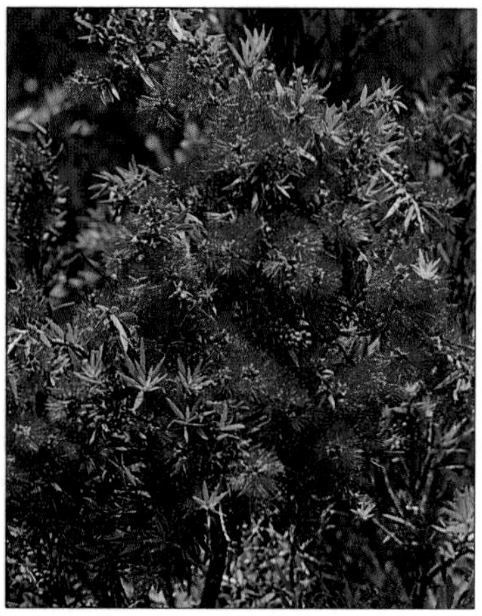

Callistemon viminalis 'Rose Opal'

long, densely arranged around the stems. Yellow-green flowers are borne in dense spikes, to 8cm (3in) long, in mid- and late summer. ↕ 1.5m (5ft), ↔ 2m (6ft). Australia (Tasmania). ❄❄

CALLISTEPHUS

China aster

ASTERACEAE/COMPOSITAE

Genus of one species of erect, bushy, fast-growing annual from stony slopes, wasteland, and cultivated fields in China. It has alternate, ovate-triangular or ovate, coarsely toothed leaves and solitary, daisy-like, single, semi-double, or double flowerheads, borne from late summer to autumn. Modern cultivars produce chrysanthemum-like, single to double flowers over a long season, in colours from indigo-blue, purple, and crimson to white. Use for bedding, in annual or informal borders, or in containers. In a frost-free site, they will bloom until midwinter. The cultivars provide long-lasting cut flowers.

- **HARDINESS** Half hardy.
- **CULTIVATION** Grow in a sheltered site in fertile, neutral to alkaline, moist but well-drained soil in full sun. Water in dry periods. Dead-head to prolong flowering. Tall cultivars require staking. Grow medium and dwarf cultivars for autumn flowering in 13–18cm (5–7in) containers of loam-based potting compost (JI No.2) in cool, well-ventilated conditions, with ample water.
- **PROPAGATION** Sow seed at 16°C (61°F) in early spring, or *in situ* in mid-spring. Sow seed for autumn-flowering container plants in early summer.
- **PESTS AND DISEASES** Prone to aster wilt, cucumber wilt, tomato spotted wilt, aphids, and cutworms.

***C. chinensis* cultivars.** Selections from *C. chinensis* are fast-growing, bushy annuals with ovate-triangular or ovate, coarsely toothed, mid-green leaves, to 8cm (3in) long. From late summer to autumn, they bear branching stems of single to fully double, chrysanthemum-like flowerheads, 7–12cm (3–5in) across, sometimes with quilled ray-florets, mainly in shades of purple- and violet-blue, but also in crimson, rose-pink, white, or occasionally yellow. ↕ 20–60cm (8–24in), ↔ 25–45cm (10–18in). ❄. **Comet Series** cultivars are dwarf and early flowering, with large, spreading, quill-petalled, double flowerheads in a range of colours,

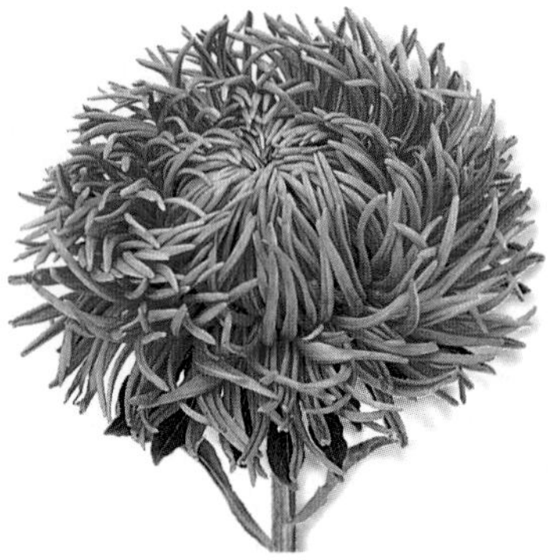

Callistephus chinensis Compliment Series 'Compliment Light Blue'

including white, pink, blue, purple, scarlet, and yellow; good for containers; ↕ to 24cm (10in), ↔ 20cm (8in). **Compliment Series** cultivars have large, spreading, quill-petalled, long-stemmed, double flowerheads in salmon-pink, light blue, and white; good for cut flowers; ↕ 70cm (28in), ↔ 20cm (8in); **'Compliment Light Blue'** ■ has double, pale violet-blue flowerheads with yellow disc-florets. **Duchesse Series** cultivars have incurved flowerheads in colours ranging from yellow to red and purple; good for cut flowers; ↕ 70cm (28in), ↔ 30cm (12in). **'Kyoto Pompon'** has small, weather-resistant, button-like, double flowerheads, in a range of colours, including yellow; ↕ to 60cm (24in), ↔ 45cm (18in). **'Matsumoto'** is tall and erect, bearing semi-double flowerheads with yellow disc-florets; it is good for cutting, weather-resistant, and partially wilt-resistant; ↕ to 75cm (30in). **Milady Series** ■ ♀ cultivars are sturdy-branched, bearing rounded, double flowerheads in rose-pink, rose-red, scarlet, blue, white, and mixed colours; they are ideal for bedding and partially wilt-resistant; ↕ to 30cm (12in), ↔ 25cm (10in). **Ostrich Plume Series** ■ cultivars have long stems and bear spreading, feathery, reflexed, double flowerheads, mainly in pinks and crimsons, from late summer to late autumn; good for cut flowers and partially wilt-resistant; ↕ to 60cm (24in), ↔ 30cm (12in). **Pinocchio Series** cultivars bear incurved, rounded, dense, double flowerheads in a wide colour range; good for bedding and edging; ↕ to 20cm (8in), ↔ 20cm (8in). **Pommax Series** cultivars are vigorous, tall, and compact, with spreading, narrow-petalled, double flowerheads in a wide

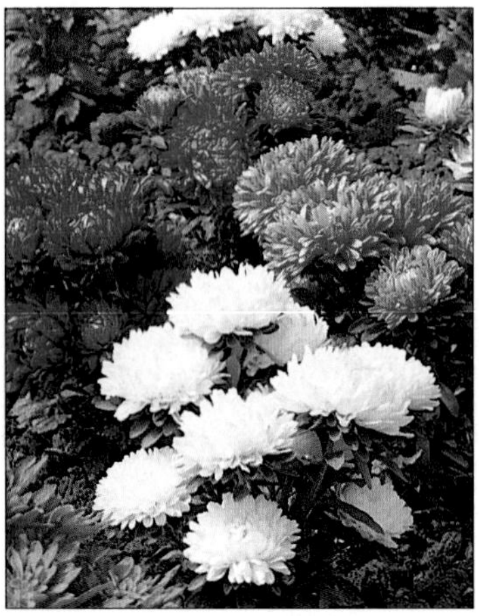

Callistephus chinensis Milady Series

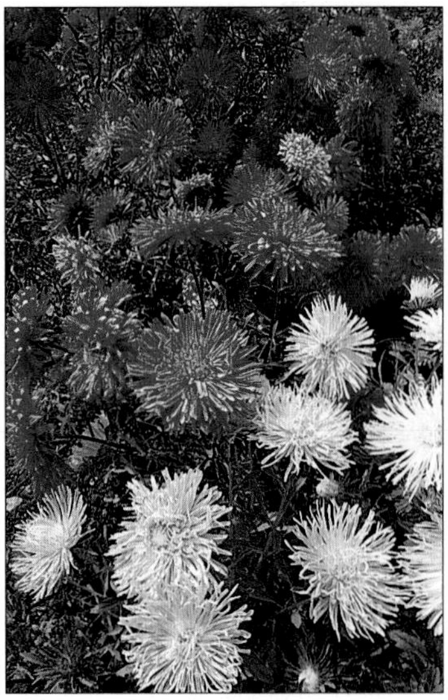

Callistephus chinensis Ostrich Plume Series

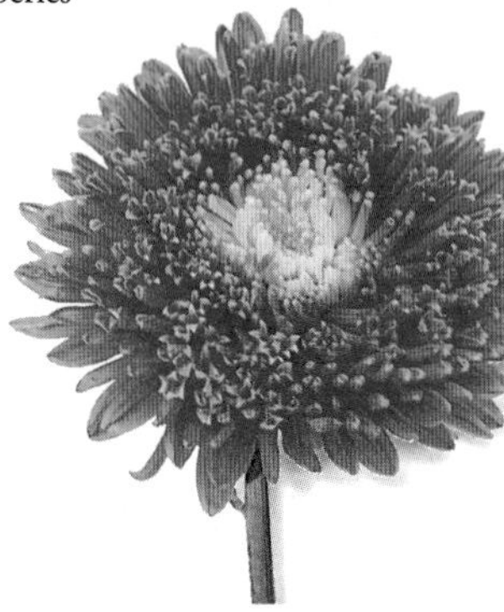

Callistephus chinensis Princess Series 'Giant Princess'

colour range, including blue, yellow, scarlet, white, and yellow; ↕ 60–70cm (24–28in), ↔ 30cm (12in). **Princess Series** cultivars have incurved, semi-double, quill-petalled flowerheads in a wide colour range; good for cutting and partially wilt-resistant; ↕ to 60cm (24in), ↔ 30cm (12in); **'Giant Princess'** is tall with semi-double, long-stemmed, red-purple flowerheads, their disc-florets tipped with yellow; ↕ 75cm (30in).

CALLITRICHE
Water starwort

CALLITRICHACEAE

Genus of 25 species of aquatic, sometimes terrestrial, herbaceous perennials from bogs and marshes in Europe, Asia, and North America. They grow in tight, submerged clumps or form a turf-like surface on wet soil. The floating leaves are opposite, and linear or spoon-shaped to rounded. The tangled submerged leaves are linear, and almost translucent in deeper water. The name "starwort" arises from the rosette-like arrangement of the leaves of some species. Minute, solitary flowers are produced in summer from the axils of both the floating and submerged leaves. Grow as oxygenating plants in ponds and cold-water aquaria.
• **HARDINESS** Fully hardy.
• **CULTIVATION** To control spread, grow in baskets of loamy soil or loam-based potting compost (JI No.1), topped with a layer of gravel, submerged 45–60cm (18–24in) deep, in sun or partial shade. In cold-water aquaria, grow in an inert medium in full light. See also pp.52–53.

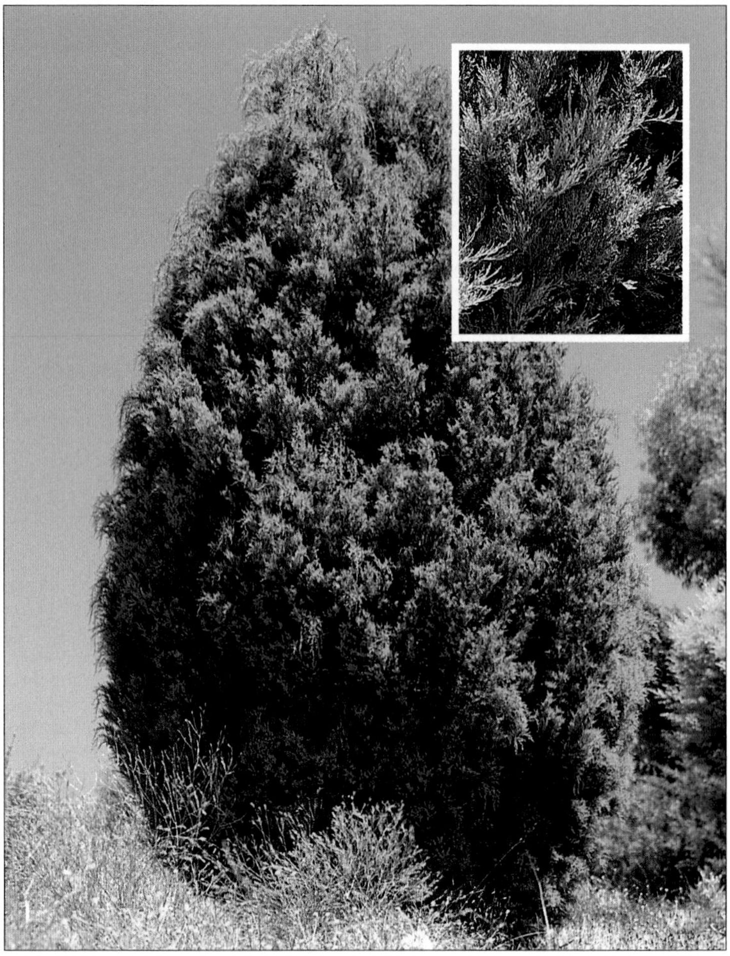

Callitris rhomboidea (inset: foliage detail)

• **PROPAGATION** In summer, take softwood cuttings of terminal shoots, 15–20cm (6–8in) long; bunch and weight them near the bases, and insert them into an aquatic planting basket or at the muddy bottom of a pond.
• **PESTS AND DISEASES** Waterfowl may feed on young growth in spring.

C. autumnalis see *C. hermaphroditica.*
C. hermaphroditica, syn. *C. autumnalis* (Autumn starwort). Submerged aquatic perennial producing linear, light green leaves, 3cm (1¼in) long, on thin, branching stems, to 50cm (20in) long. It does not develop floating "rosettes" and grows mainly towards the bottom of a pool. ↔ indefinite. Europe, North America. ❄❄❄

CALLITRIS
Cypress pine

CUPRESSACEAE

Genus of 14–17 species of evergreen, monoecious, coniferous large shrubs or trees from forest in Australia and New Caledonia. The scale-like adult leaves, 2–4mm (1/16–1/8in) long, have free tips but lie flat along the shoots in whorls of 3; the decurrent parts of the leaves form ridges and furrows on the shoots. Young leaves, 0.8–1.5cm (3/8–1/2in) long, are needle-like and arranged in whorls. The small, ovoid-conical to spherical female cones of most species each have a single whorl of 6 scales, hinged at the bases; male cones are cylindrical or oblong and are borne singly or in groups of 2 or 3. In frost-prone areas, grow tender species in a cool greenhouse or conservatory. In frost-free areas, grow cypress pines as windbreaks or specimen trees. They will tolerate drought, coastal conditions, and saline soils, and thrive in dry, temperate or warm Mediterranean climates.
• **HARDINESS** Frost hardy to frost tender.
• **CULTIVATION** Under glass, grow in loam-based potting compost (JI No.2) in full light, shaded from hot sun. When in growth, water freely and apply a balanced liquid fertilizer monthly; water sparingly in winter. Outdoors, grow in well-drained, sandy soil in full sun.
• **PROPAGATION** Sow seed at 13–18°C (55–64°F) in spring, or take root cuttings in late summer.
• **PESTS AND DISEASES** Trouble free.

C. cupressiformis see *C. rhomboidea.*
C. gunnii see *C. oblonga.*
C. oblonga ◊ syn. *C. gunnii* (Tasmanian cypress pine). Symmetrical shrub or small tree with erect branches, a dense crown, and blue-green or mid-green, keeled leaves. Ovoid-conical, shiny black female cones, 1.5–2cm (1/2–3/4in) long, with thick scales, are solitary or borne in groups. ↕ to 8m (25ft), ↔ 2–3m (6–10ft). Australia (Tasmania). ❄❄
C. rhomboidea ■ ◊ syn. *C. cupressiformis, C. tasmanica* (Oyster Bay cypress pine). Narrow, dense-crowned, large shrub or tree with bright green or blue-green leaves. Flattened-spherical, grey-brown female cones, 0.8–1.5cm (3/8–1/2in) across, with stout scales, are borne singly or in groups. ↕ 9–15m (28–50ft), ↔ 2–3m (6–10ft). Australia (Queensland to Tasmania, South Australia). ❄❄
C. tasmanica see *C. rhomboidea*

CALLUNA

Heather, Ling

ERICACEAE

Genus of one species of evergreen shrub found on acid moorland and lowland heaths from N. and W. Europe to Siberia, Turkey, Morocco, and the Azores. It bears dense racemes of bell-shaped flowers, in shades of red, purple, pink, or white. The calyces are normally 4-lobed, and longer than the corollas, but usually the same colour – features that help to distinguish heathers (*Calluna*) from heaths (*Erica*). Racemes on young plants may be short, 1–5cm (½–2in) long; medium, 5–10cm (2–4in); or long, over 10cm (4in). As plants age, the racemes become shorter. The leaves, borne in opposite and overlapping pairs, lying flat along the stems, are linear, slightly fleshy, and usually dark green, becoming purple-tinged in winter. There are more than 500 cultivars, all of which are good ground-cover plants. Heathers are very attractive to bees.

- **HARDINESS** Fully hardy.
- **CULTIVATION** Grow in an open site in well-drained, humus-rich, acid soil in full sun. Pruning group 10, in spring.
- **PROPAGATION** Root semi-ripe cuttings, 5cm (2in) long, in midsummer, or layer in spring.
- **PESTS AND DISEASES** Prone to fungal diseases, chiefly grey mould (*Botrytis*), *Phytophthora* root rot, and rhizoctonia, in warm wet conditions.

C. vulgaris, syn. *Erica vulgaris* (Ling, Scots heather). Variable, prostrate to erect shrub with green to grey, hairless or hairy leaves, 1–3mm (1/16–⅛in) long. Bell-shaped or tubular flowers, to 4mm (⅛in) long, are borne in short to long racemes from midsummer to late autumn. ↕ 10–60cm (4–24in), ↔ to 75cm (30in). N. and W. Europe to Russia (Siberia), Turkey, Morocco, the Azores. ❄❄❄. Unless stated otherwise, the following cultivars are erect with dark green leaves and single flowers. **'Alison Yates'** is compact but vigorous, with silvery grey foliage and long racemes of white flowers; ↕ 45cm (18in), ↔ 60cm (24in). **'Allegro'** ♀ is compact and vigorous, with medium racemes of ruby-red flowers; ↕ 50cm (20in), ↔ 60cm (24in). **'Annemarie'** ♀ bears long racemes of double, rose-pink flowers, good for cutting; ↕ 50cm (20in), ↔ 60cm (24in). **'Anthony Davis'** ▣ ♀ has green-grey leaves and long racemes of white flowers, good for cutting; ↕ 45cm (18in). **'Aureifolia'** see 'Hammondii Aureifolia'. **'Barbara Fleur'** produces medium racemes of pale crimson flowers; ↕ 45cm (18in), ↔ 55cm (22in). **'Beoley Gold'** ▣ ♀ has yellow foliage and medium racemes of white flowers; ↕ 35cm (14in). **'Beoley Silver'** has softly hairy silver foliage and medium racemes of white flowers; ↕ 40cm (16in), ↔ 60cm (24in). **'Blazeaway'** has gold foliage, turning bright red in winter, and medium racemes of lilac-mauve flowers; ↕ 35cm (14in), ↔ 60cm (24in). **'Boskoop'** ▣ has gold leaves, red-tinted orange in winter, and medium racemes of lilac-pink flowers. **'Clare Carpet'** is prostrate, with light green foliage and short racemes of pale pink flowers; ↕ 5cm (2in), ↔ 45cm (18in). **'County Wicklow'** ▣ ♀ is compact and semi-prostrate, with mid-green leaves and large, double, pale pink flowers in long racemes; ↕ 25cm (10in), ↔ 35cm (14in). **'Darkness'** ▣ ♀ has short racemes of crimson flowers; ↕ 25cm (10in), ↔ 35cm (14in). **'Dark Star'** ♀ is compact, with short racemes of semi-double, crimson flowers; ↕ 20cm (8in), ↔ 35cm (14in). **'Drum-ra'** has light green foliage and short racemes of white flowers; ↕ 20cm (8in). **'Elongata'** see 'Mair's Variety'. **'Elsie Purnell'** ▣ ♀ has grey-green leaves and long racemes of double, pale pink flowers, good for cutting; ↕ 40cm (16in), ↔ 75cm (30in). **'Firefly'** ▣ ♀ has terracotta foliage in summer, brick-red in winter, with short racemes of deep mauve flowers; ↕ 45cm (18in). **'Foxii Nana'** ▣ forms tight mounds of bright green foliage with short racemes of mauve flowers; ↕ 15cm (6in), ↔ 30cm (12in). **'Glenfiddich'** has copper-red leaves, turning bronze-red in winter, and medium racemes of mauve flowers; ↔ 40cm (16in). **'Golden Feather'** ▣ syn. 'Gold Feather', has gold foliage, turning reddish orange in winter, and bears short racemes of mauve flowers; ↕ 25cm (10in), ↔ 70cm (28in). **'Gold Haze'** ▣ ♀ syn. 'Golden Haze', has pale

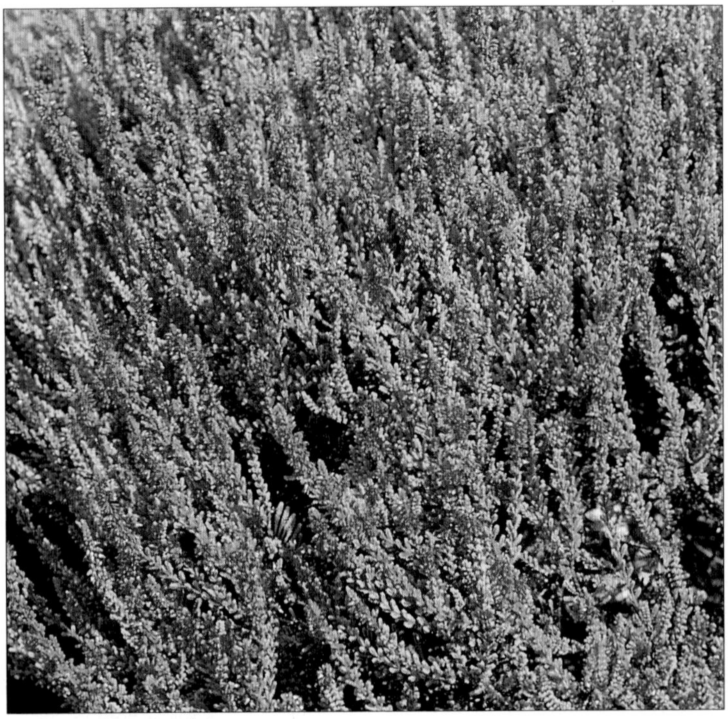

Calluna vulgaris 'Firefly'

yellow foliage and medium racemes of white flowers; ↔ 45cm (18in). **'Hamlet Green'** has yellowish grey-green leaves, becoming orange-yellow and green in winter, and short racemes of mauve flowers. **'Hammondii Aureifolia'**, syn. 'Aureifolia', 'Hammondii Aurea', has light green foliage tipped with yellow from spring to early summer, and short racemes of white flowers; ↔ 40cm (16in). **'H.E. Beale'**, syn. 'Pink Beale', has long racemes of double, pale pink flowers, good for cutting. **'Hirta'** is prostrate, with golden yellow foliage, yellow-green in winter, and bears short racemes of pink flowers; ↕ 10cm (4in), ↔ 30cm (12in). **'Inshriach Bronze'** has lemon-yellow leaves in spring, gold in summer, and bronze in winter, and bears medium racemes of lilac-pink flowers; ↕ 25cm (10in), ↔ 35cm (14in). **'J.H. Hamilton'** ▣ ♀ is dwarf, with medium racemes of double, deep pink flowers; ↕ 10cm (4in), ↔ 25cm (10in). **'John F. Letts'**, syn. 'J.F. Letts', is prostrate, with gold foliage, turning bronze then red and orange, and short racemes of pale lilac flowers; ↕ 10cm (4in), ↔ 25cm (10in). **'Johnson's Variety'** has mid-green leaves and medium racemes of purple-pink flowers from mid-autumn to midwinter; ↔ 60cm (24in). **'Joy Vanstone'** ♀ has straw-coloured foliage, turning orange in winter, and medium racemes of pink flowers. **'Kerstin'** has downy, deep lilac-grey leaves in winter, tipped pale yellow and red in spring, and short racemes of mauve flowers; ↔ 45cm (18in). **'Kinlochruel'** ▣ ♀ has bright green foliage, turning bronze in winter, and long racemes of double white flowers; ↕ 25cm (10in), ↔ 40cm (16in). **'Mair's Variety'** ♀ syn. 'Elongata', has mid-green leaves and long racemes of white flowers, good for cutting; ↕ 40cm (16in). **'Marinka'** see 'Red Carpet'. **'Marleen'** has medium racemes of purple-tipped white buds that do not open but persist late into autumn. **'Mullion'** ♀ has short racemes of lilac-pink flowers; ↕ 20cm (8in). **'Multicolor'** ▣ is compact with

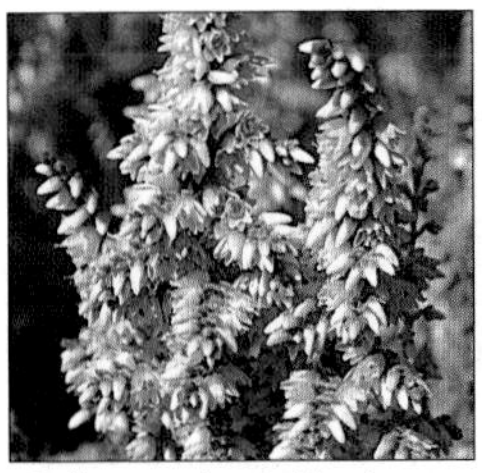

Calluna vulgaris 'Anthony Davis'

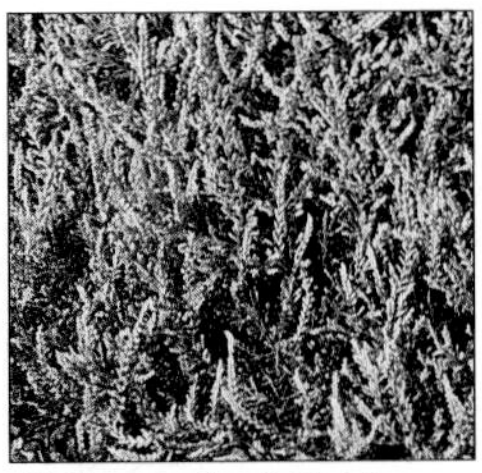

Calluna vulgaris 'Beoley Gold'

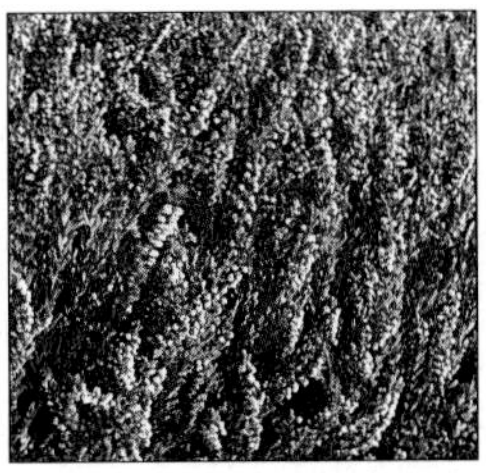

Calluna vulgaris 'Boskoop'

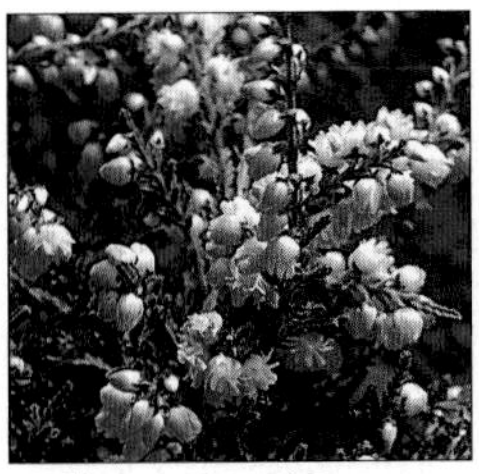

Calluna vulgaris 'County Wicklow'

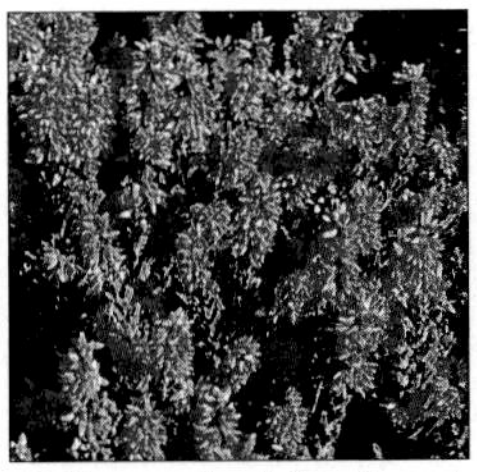

Calluna vulgaris 'Darkness'

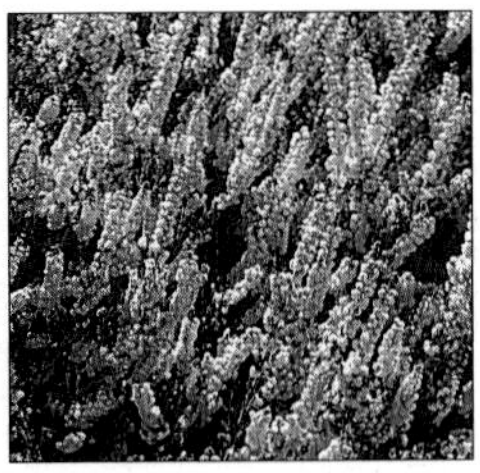

Calluna vulgaris 'Elsie Purnell'

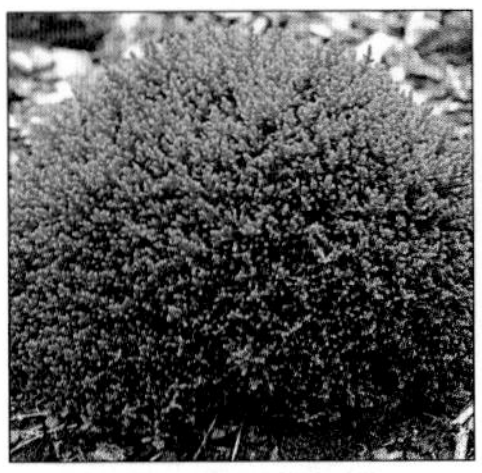

Calluna vulgaris 'Foxii Nana'

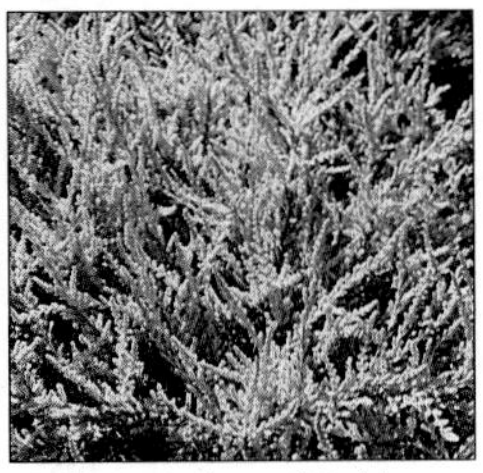

Calluna vulgaris 'Golden Feather'

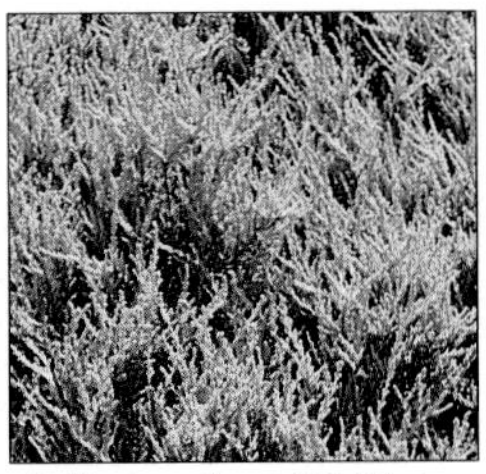

Calluna vulgaris 'Gold Haze'

Calluna vulgaris 'J.H. Hamilton'

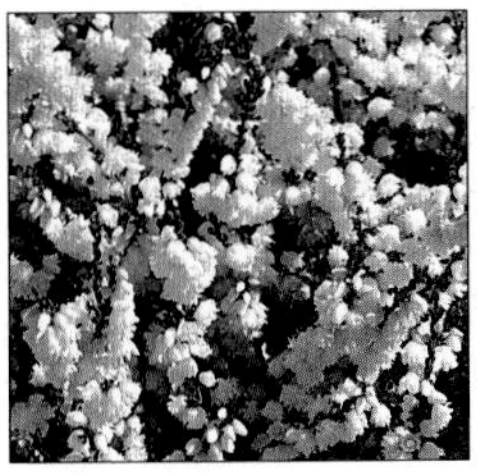

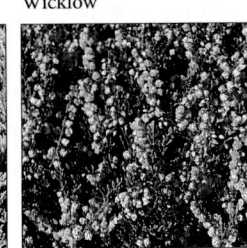

Calluna vulgaris 'Kinlochruel'

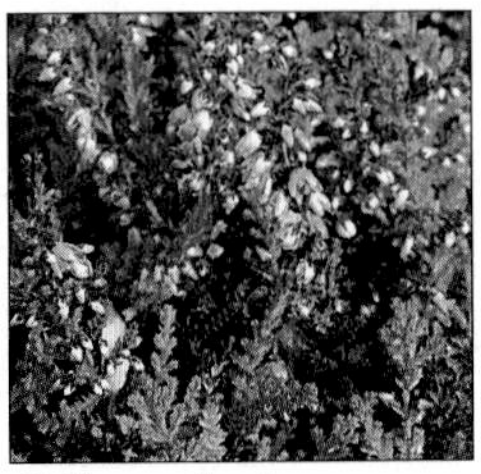

Calluna vulgaris 'Multicolor'

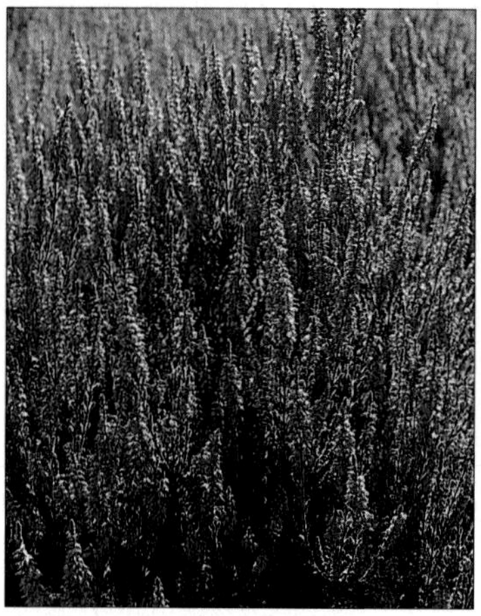

Calluna vulgaris 'Silver Knight'

copper foliage, usually flecked orange and red, and short racemes of mauve flowers; ↕ 10cm (4in), ↔ 25cm (10in). **'My Dream'** ▣ syn. 'Snowball', bears long racemes of double white flowers, good for cutting; ↕ 45cm (18in). **'Orange Queen'** 🏆 has bronze foliage in autumn, orange in winter, turning gold in summer, and bears short racemes of pink flowers. **'Peter Sparkes'** ▣ bears long racemes of double, rose-pink flowers, good for cutting, into late autumn; ↔ 55cm (22in). **'Pink Beale'** see 'H.E. Beale'. **'Red Carpet'**, syn. 'Marinka', is semi-prostrate, and chiefly grown for its foliage, which is orange-red in winter, gold in summer; it produces short racemes of mauve-pink flowers; ↕ 20cm (8in), ↔ 45cm (18in). **'Red Fred'** has brilliant red foliage in spring, persisting well into summer, and bears medium racemes of lilac-pink flowers; ↕ 35cm (14in), ↔ 45cm (18in). **'Red Star'** 🏆 has medium racemes of double, deep lilac-pink flowers in autumn; ↕ 40cm (16in), ↔ 60cm (24in). **'Robert Chapman'** ▣🏆 has gold foliage in summer, turning red in winter and spring, and produces medium racemes of purple flowers; ↕ 25cm (10in), ↔ 65cm (26in). **'Roland Haagen'** 🏆 syn. 'Rowland Heagan', is grown for its golden yellow foliage, turning bright orange in winter; it produces medium racemes of lilac-pink flowers; ↕ 15cm (6in), ↔ 35cm (14in). **'Rosalind, Underwood's Variety'** has yellow-green foliage, with yellow tips in autumn, winter, and spring, and bears medium racemes of pink flowers; ↔ 55cm (22in). **'Serlei Aurea'** 🏆 has dense, yellow-green foliage, tipped yellow in summer and autumn, and produces short racemes of white flowers; ↔ 40cm (16in). **'Silver Knight'** ▣ has downy grey foliage, deepening to purple-grey in winter, and medium racemes of mauve pink flowers; ↕ 40cm (16in). **'Silver Queen'** ▣🏆 is spreading with downy, silvery grey leaves, and short racemes of pale mauve flowers; ↕ 40cm (16in), ↔ 55cm (22in). **'Silver Rose'** 🏆 has silvery grey foliage, and bears medium racemes of lilac-pink flowers; ↕ 40cm (16in). **'Sir John Charrington'** 🏆 has golden yellow foliage in summer, turning orange and red in winter, and produces short racemes of mauve-pink flowers; ↕ 40cm (16in). **'Sirsson'** has gold leaves, turning bright orange-red in winter in cold, open sites, and bears medium racemes of pink flowers. **'Sister Anne'** 🏆 is compact and spreading, with grey-green foliage, becoming dull bronze in winter; it bears short racemes of mauve flowers; ↕ 10cm (4in), ↔ 25cm (10in). **'Snowball'** see 'My Dream'. **'Spring Charm'** see 'Spring Torch'. **'Spring Cream'** ▣🏆 is compact, with mid-green leaves, cream-tipped in spring, and short racemes of white flowers; ↕ 35cm (14in), ↔ 45cm (18in). **'Spring Torch'**, syn. 'Spring Charm', produces mid-green leaves with cream, orange, and red tips in spring, and short racemes of mauve flowers; ↕ 40cm (16in), ↔ 60cm (24in). **'Sunset'** 🏆 has golden yellow leaves in spring, turning orange in summer and red in winter, and bears short racemes of mauve-pink flowers; ↕ 25cm (10in). **'Tib'** ▣🏆 is fairly open in habit, bearing long racemes of double flowers in midsummer; ↔ 40cm (16in). **'Velvet Fascination'** has silvery grey foliage, and produces medium racemes of pure white flowers; ↕ 50cm (20in), ↔ 70cm (28in). **'White Lawn'** 🏆 is prostrate and trailing, producing bright green foliage and medium racemes of white flowers; ↕ 5cm (2in), ↔ 40cm (16in). **'Wickwar Flame'** 🏆 has gold leaves, turning red in winter, and bears medium racemes of mauve-pink flowers; ↕ 50cm (20in), ↔ 65cm (26in).

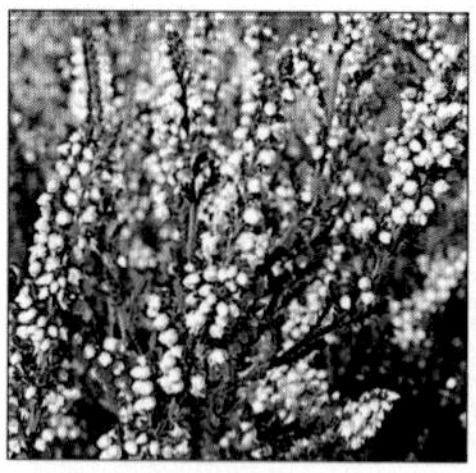

Calluna vulgaris 'My Dream'

Calluna vulgaris 'Peter Sparkes'

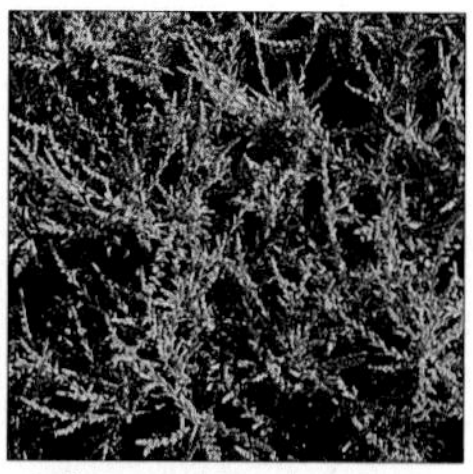

Calluna vulgaris 'Robert Chapman'

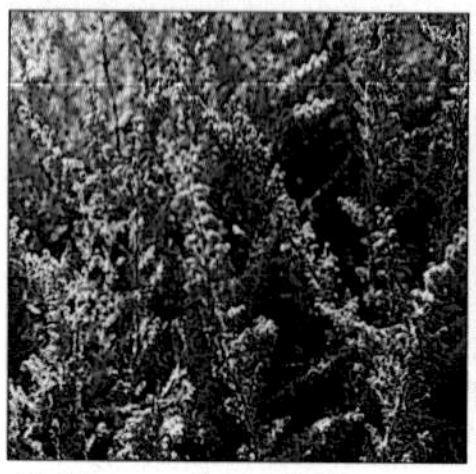

Calluna vulgaris 'Silver Queen'

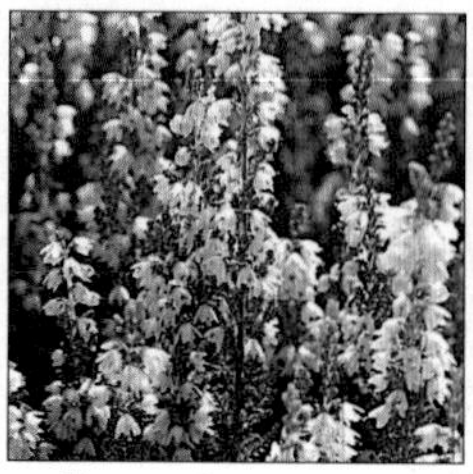

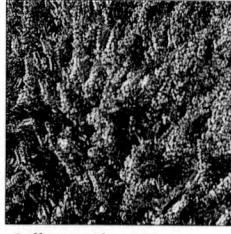

Calluna vulgaris 'Spring Cream'

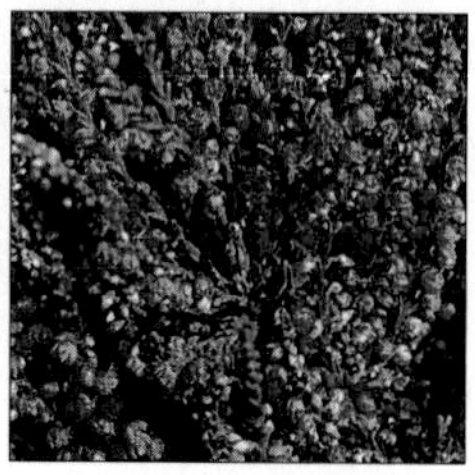

Calluna vulgaris 'Tib'

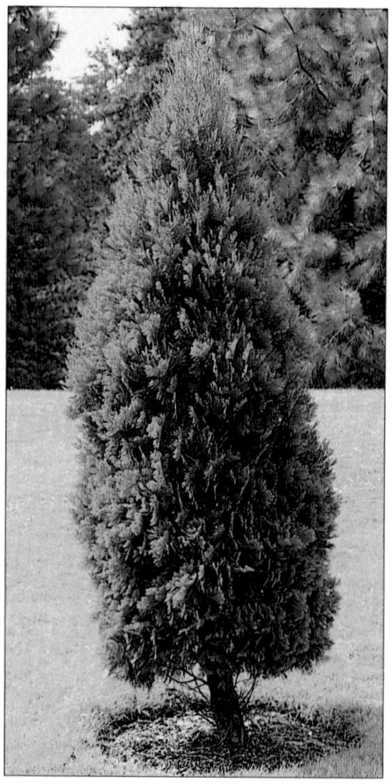

Calocedrus decurrens

CALOCEDRUS

Incense cedar

CUPRESSACEAE

Genus of 3 species of evergreen, monoecious conifers from dry, warm-temperate forest in S. China, Taiwan, Vietnam, and W. North America. The branchlets are arranged in 2 flattened rows; the decurrent, scale-like leaves appear 4-ranked, but are arranged in 2 pairs. The female cones have 6 scales, hinged at the bases, of which only the central pair is fertile, each scale bearing 2 seeds. Grow as specimen trees. In frost-prone areas, grow less hardy species in a cool greenhouse.

• **HARDINESS** Fully hardy to frost hardy.
• **CULTIVATION** Grow in any well-drained soil in sun or partial shade.
• **PROPAGATION** Sow seed in containers in a cold frame in spring, or root semi-ripe cuttings in late summer.
• **PESTS AND DISEASES** Trouble free.

C. decurrens ▣🏆◊ syn. *Heyderia decurrens, Libocedrus decurrens* (Incense cedar). Narrow-crowned, columnar tree in cultivation, but often with a wide crown and horizontal branches in the wild. Produces flat sprays of linear, glossy, dark green leaves, to 1cm (½in) long, with free tips. Pendent shoots bear erect, ovoid, yellow-brown female cones, 2–2.5cm (¾–1in) long, ripening red-brown. ↕ 20–40m (70–130ft), ↔ 2–9m (6–28ft). W. North America (Oregon to Baja California). ❄❄❄

C. macrolepis ◊ Narrow, conical tree with slightly larger and flatter, linear leaves than those of *C. decurrens*; they are 1.5cm (½in) long, bright green above, and glaucous beneath. Erect, ellipsoid, purple-tinted orange female cones, to 1.5cm (½in) long, are borne on pendent shoots. ↕ 30m (100ft), ↔ 8m (25ft). China (Yunnan, Hainan). ❄❄

▷ ***Calocephalus*** see *Leucophyta*
C. brownii see *L. brownii*

CALOCHONE

RUBIACEAE

Genus of 2 evergreen species, one a perennial climber, the other a shrub (not usually cultivated), found in forest in W. Africa. They have simple leaves, in opposite pairs, and are valued for their showy, tubular-based, 5-petalled flowers, which are borne in spherical heads at the ends of the shoots. Grow *C. redingii* in a warm greenhouse; in subtropical and tropical areas, it is suitable for training over large shrubs, through trees, or on house walls.

• **HARDINESS** Frost tender.
• **CULTIVATION** Under glass, grow in loam-based potting compost (JI No.3) in full light with shade from hot sun. In the growing season, water freely and apply a balanced liquid fertilizer monthly; water sparingly in winter. Pot on or top-dress in spring. Outdoors, grow in moist but well-drained, humus-rich, fertile soil in full sun. Pruning group 11, after flowering.
• **PROPAGATION** Root semi-ripe cuttings in summer.
• **PESTS AND DISEASES** Red spider mites may be a problem under glass.

C. redingii. Vigorous, twining climber producing ovate, bristly-hairy leaves, 15–20cm (6–8in) long, heart-shaped at the bases, and with wavy margins. Bears a profusion of flowers, 2cm (¾in) across, with greenish yellow tubes and bright-pink petals, from winter to spring. ↕ 10m (30ft) or more. Zaire. ❁ (min. 15°C/59°F)

CALOCHORTUS

Cat's ears, Fairy lantern, Mariposa tulip

LILIACEAE

Genus of about 60 species of bulbous perennials from grassland and open woodland in W. North America and Mexico. They are cultivated for their showy, tulip-like flowers, borne mainly in spring or early summer. The flowers have a distinctive nectary near the base of each inner petal, often with striking basal marks and conspicuous hairs inside. *C. luteus, C. superbus, C. venustus*, and *C. vestae* appear very similar, but differ in the shape of their nectaries. The leaves are mid- to grey-green; lower stem leaves are 20–70cm (8–28in) long, narrow, and linear to lance-shaped; upper stem leaves are

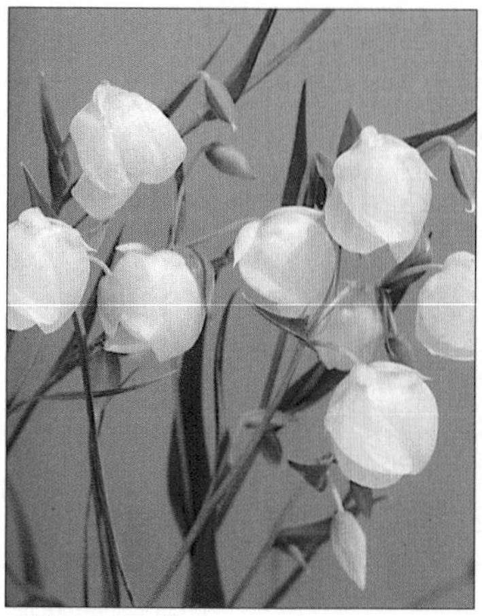

Calochortus albus

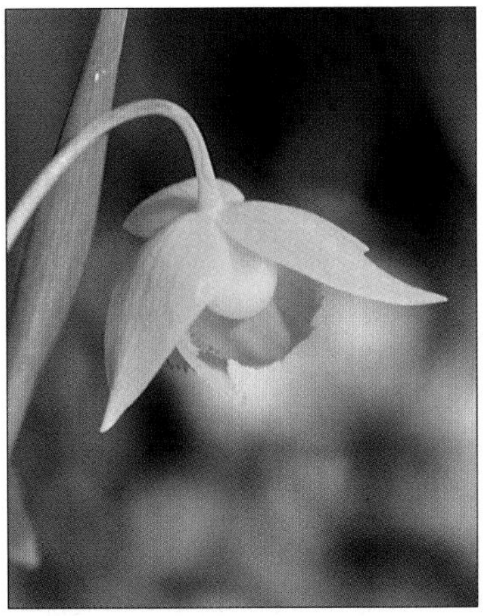
Calochortus amabilis

shorter, 10–30cm (4–12in) long. Best grown in a cold greenhouse or bulb frame as they are intolerant of wet when dormant in winter. In dry climates, grow in a mixed or herbaceous border.
• **HARDINESS** Frost hardy; *C. barbatus* is hardy to -10°C (14°F).
• **CULTIVATION** Plant bulbs 10–15cm (4–6in) deep in autumn. Under glass, grow in loam-based potting compost (JI No.1) with added grit, in full light. Water freely when in growth; water sparingly as the leaves die back; provide warm, dry conditions when dormant in late summer and early autumn. Pot on just before growth begins in autumn. Outdoors, grow in an open site in well-drained, sandy, loam soil in full sun. Protect from rain when dormant and in winter.
• **PROPAGATION** Sow seed in containers in a cold frame as soon as ripe, or remove offsets in late summer. Some species produce bulbils in the leaf axils; plant these in late spring or early summer.
• **PESTS AND DISEASES** Trouble free.

C. albus ■ Bulbous perennial with leaves 30–70cm (12–28in) long. From spring to early summer, branched stems bear 2 or more nodding, spherical to bell-shaped, sparsely hairy white flowers, 2–3cm (¾–1¼in) long, with crescent-shaped nectaries. ↕ 10–50cm (4–20in), ↔ 5cm (2in). USA (California). ❄❄
C. amabilis ■ Bulbous perennial producing leaves 20–50cm (8–20in) long. Branched stems bear 2 or more nodding, spherical to bell-shaped, deep yellow flowers, 1.5–2cm (½–¾in) long, from spring to early summer; the

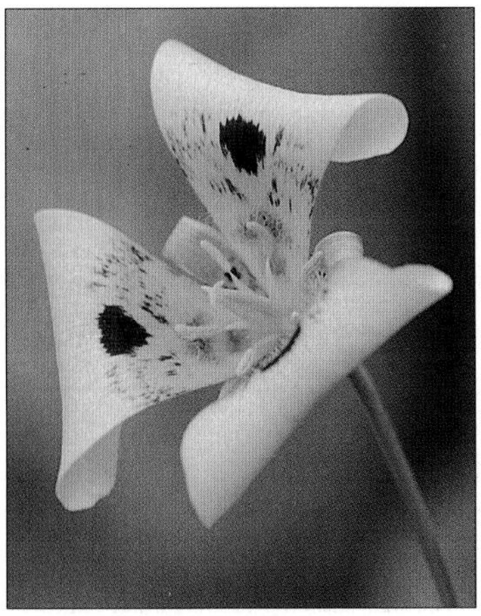
Calochortus luteus

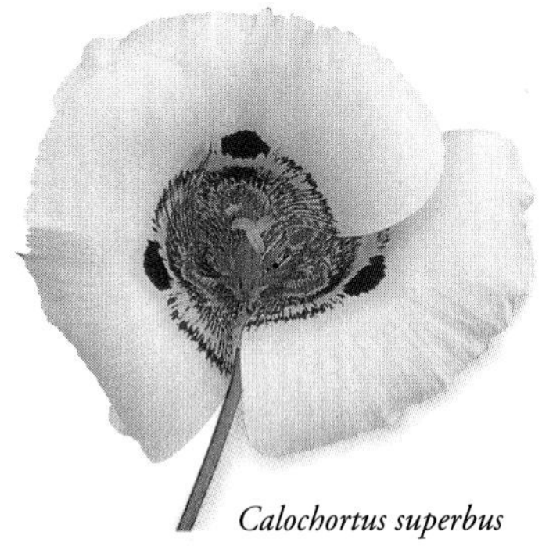
Calochortus superbus

conspicuous tepals, occasionally tinged green, have deeply crescent-shaped nectaries. ↕ 10–50cm (4–20in), ↔ 5cm (2in). USA (California). ❄❄
C. barbatus, syn. *Cyclobothra lutea.* Bulbous perennial with leaves 10–45cm (4–18in) long. In summer, branched, spreading stems bear 1 or 2 open cup-shaped flowers, 2–3cm (¾–1¼in) wide, usually mustard-yellow with purple hairs, but varying from yellow to purplish yellow. The nectaries are semi-circular. Sometimes produces bulbils. ↕ 15–30cm (6–12in), ↔ 5cm (2in). Mexico. ❄❄
C. luteus ■ (Yellow mariposa). Bulbous perennial with leaves 10–45cm (4–18in) long. In spring, branched stems bear 1–7 open bell-shaped flowers, 4–6cm (1½–2½in) across. Flowers are deep yellow; the insides have sparse, slender hairs and red-brown lines and marks. The nectaries are crescent-shaped. ↕ 20–50cm (8–20in), ↔ 8cm (3in). USA (California). ❄❄
C. macrocarpus. Bulbous perennial with leaves 20–50cm (8–20in) long. In summer, unbranched stems bear up to 3 erect, open cup-shaped purple flowers, 6–9cm (2½–3½in) across, usually with a deep purple ring inside, towards the bases of the petals. Narrow sepals extend beyond the petals. The nectaries are triangular. ↕ 20–50cm (8–20in), ↔ 5cm (2in). W. USA. ❄❄
C. superbus ■ Bulbous perennial producing leaves 10–40cm (4–16in) long. In late spring, branching stems bear 1–3 erect, cup-shaped, sparsely hairy, white, cream, lavender-blue, or yellow flowers, 5–8cm (2–3in) across, with a brown mark above the yellow base of each petal. The nectaries are V-shaped. ↕ 40–60cm (16–24in), ↔ 8cm (3in). USA (California). ❄❄
C. uniflorus. Bulbous perennial with very narrow leaves, 10–40cm (4–16in)

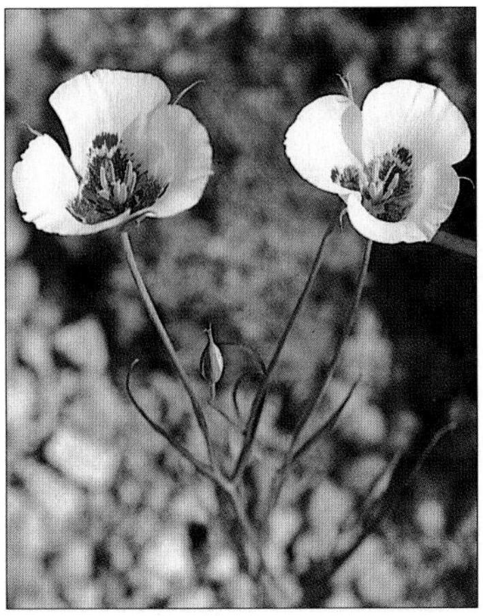
Calochortus venustus

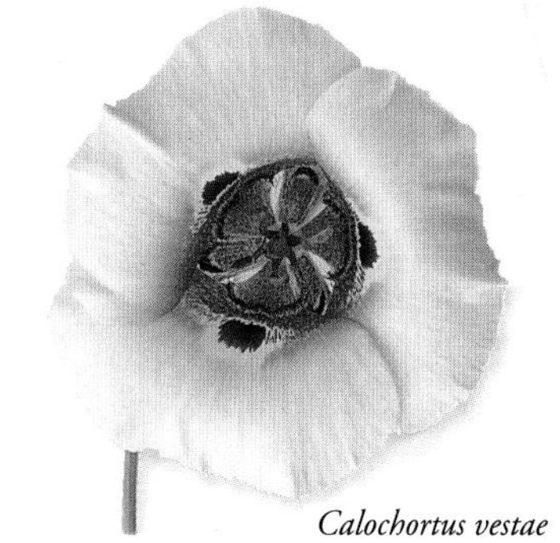
Calochortus vestae

long. Up to 5 erect, saucer-shaped, pale lilac flowers, 3.5–4.5cm (1½–1¾in) across, sparsely hairy and often with darker lilac marks inside, are borne on long, unbranched stems in summer. Has oblong nectaries. ↕ 10–15cm (4–6in), ↔ 5cm (2in). W. USA. ❄❄
C. venustus ■ Bulbous perennial with leaves 10–40cm (4–16in) long. From late spring to summer, branched stems bear 1–3 erect, cup-shaped flowers, 5–8cm (2–3in) across, varying from white to yellow, purple, or dark red, each with a yellow-ringed, dark red mark inside. The nectaries are rounded or diamond-shaped. ↕ 20–60cm (8–24in), ↔ 8cm (3in). USA (California). ❄❄
C. vestae ■ Bulbous perennial with leaves 15–45cm (6–18in) long. From late spring to summer, branched stems bear 1–6 erect, cup-shaped white flowers, 5–8cm (2–3in) across, sometimes tinged purple, with a yellow-ringed maroon mark at the base of each petal. The nectaries are double crescent-shaped. ↕ 30–50cm (12–20in), ↔ 8cm (3in). USA (California). ❄❄

CALOMERIA syn. HUMEA
Incense plant

ASTERACEAE/COMPOSITAE

Genus of about 14 species of strongly aromatic annuals and perennials found in varying habitats, from coastal mudflats to mountain forest, in Africa, Madagascar, and S. Australia. They have simple, alternate leaves and, in summer, bear large, branched, pyramidal panicles of tiny, tubular flowerheads. In frost-prone climates, grow incense plants as biennials in a conservatory or cool greenhouse, or use for summer bedding. In warmer regions, grow in a border or in specimen groups.
• **HARDINESS** Frost tender.

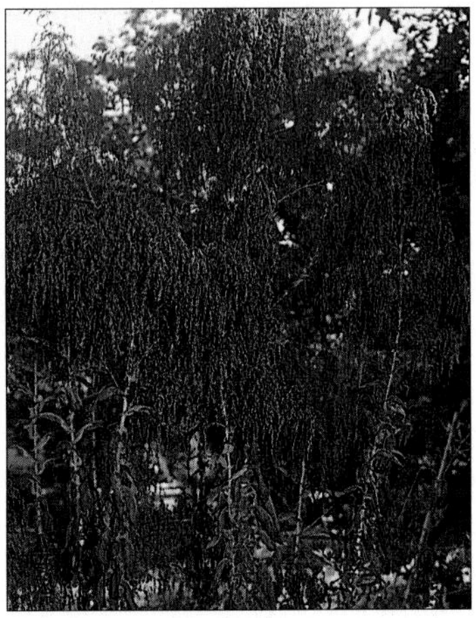
Calomeria amaranthoides

• **CULTIVATION** Under glass, grow in borders or containers of loam-based potting compost (JI No.3) in full light with good ventilation. When in growth, water moderately and apply a balanced liquid fertilizer every 3–4 weeks. Mist over to release fragrance. Keep just moist in winter. Outdoors, grow in fertile, well-drained soil in full sun.
• **PROPAGATION** Sow seed at 13–18°C (55–64°F) as soon as ripe.
• **PESTS AND DISEASES** Trouble free.

C. amaranthoides ■ syn. *Humea elegans* (Incense plant, Plume plant). Erect, branching, smooth to slightly hairy, aromatic perennial, usually grown as a biennial, with almost stem-clasping, ovate to lance-shaped leaves, to 25cm (10in) long. In summer, bears feathery panicles, to 1.2m (4ft) tall, of tiny, brownish pink to red flowerheads. Contact with the leaves may aggravate skin allergies. ↕ 1.2–2m (4–6ft), ↔ to 1m (3ft). Australia (New South Wales, Victoria). ❀ (min. 4°C/39°F)

▷ ***Calonyction aculeatum*** see *Ipomoea alba*

CALOSCORDUM
ALLIACEAE/LILIACEAE

Genus, related to *Allium*, of one species of bulbous perennial from mountainous regions of Asia. It has narrow leaves and bears umbels of tiny flowers in late summer, but does not have a pungent odour. *C. neriniflorum* is best grown in a sunny rock garden, or in an alpine house. In mild or frost-free areas, grow in thin grass on a sunny bank.
• **HARDINESS** Fully hardy.
• **CULTIVATION** Plant bulbs 7cm (3in) deep in spring. Grow in well-drained soil in full sun. Protect from excess winter wet.
• **PROPAGATION** Sow seed in containers in a cold frame in spring. Remove offsets after flowering.
• **PESTS AND DISEASES** Trouble free.

C. neriniflorum, syn. *Allium neriniflorum, Nothoscordum neriniflorum.* Bulbous perennial with 2–6 linear, channelled, pale green leaves, 8–15cm (3–6in) long, which die back as flowers are produced in late summer. Up to 20 star-shaped flowers, 4–7mm (⅛–¼in) across, the petals bright pink with dark midribs, are borne in erect, loose umbels, 5–7cm (2–3in) across. ↕ 25cm (10in), ↔ 5cm (2in). C. Asia, N. and W. China, Russia (Siberia). ❄❄❄

CALOTHAMNUS
Net bush

MYRTACEAE

Genus of about 25 species of evergreen shrubs found in Western Australia, usually in dry scrub and open forest. They are cultivated for their nodding flowers, 1–4cm (½–1½in) long, which have tiny petals and prominent, flattened bundles of long red stamens; they are produced in one-sided spikes or clusters, 2–25cm (¾–10in) long. The leaves are needle-like and leathery, and crowded on the stems, either irregularly or in whorls. In frost-prone regions, grow in a cool or temperate greenhouse; in warmer areas, grow in a shrub border.

C

C

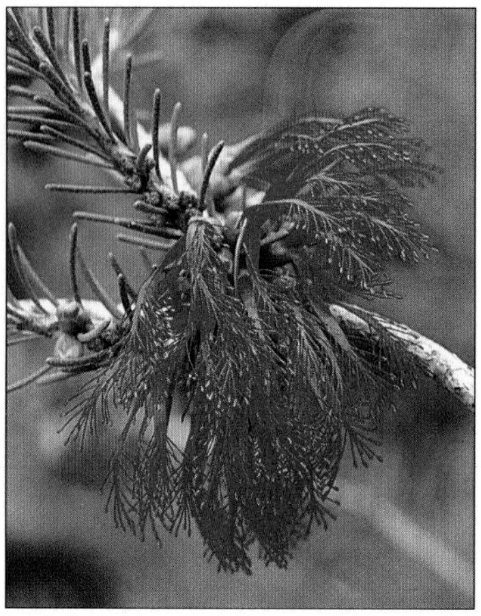

Calothamnus quadrifidus

• **HARDINESS** Frost tender.
• **CULTIVATION** Under glass, grow in loam-based potting compost (JI No.2) in full light with good ventilation. In the growing season, water moderately and apply a phosphate-free fertilizer every 4–6 weeks; water sparingly in winter. Pot on or top-dress in early spring. Outdoors, grow in well-drained, moderately fertile soil (very fertile soil diminishes flower production) in full sun. Pruning group 8, although pruning is seldom needed.
• **PROPAGATION** Surface-sow seed at 16–18°C (61–64°F) in spring. Root semi-ripe cuttings with bottom heat in late summer.
• **PESTS AND DISEASES** Scale insects may be a problem.

C. quadrifidus ■ (Common net bush). Erect to spreading shrub with linear, greyish to dark green or grey leaves, 3cm (1¼in) long. Bears irregular, axillary, one-sided spikes of rich red flowers, 2.5cm (1in) long, from late spring to autumn, often forming clusters, 20cm (8in) or more across, around the stems. ↕2–4m (6–12ft), ↔ 2–5m (6–15ft). Australia (Western Australia). ❀ (min. 5°C/41°F)

CALPURNIA

LEGUMINOSAE/PAPILIONACEAE

Genus of 10 or more species of evergreen shrubs and small trees from mountain forest in Africa and India. They are cultivated for their pendent racemes of yellow, pea-like flowers, which are produced from the leaf axils or at the ends of the shoots. The leaves are alternate and pinnate, with 3 to many pairs of leaflets. In frost-prone areas, grow in a temperate greenhouse. Elsewhere, use as specimen plants or as a colourful addition to a shrub border.
• **HARDINESS** Frost tender.
• **CULTIVATION** Under glass, grow in loam-based potting compost (JI No.3) in full light. During growth, water freely and apply a balanced liquid fertilizer monthly; water sparingly in winter. Pot on or top-dress in spring. Outdoors, grow in well-drained, fertile soil in full sun. Pruning group 8; plants under glass may need restrictive pruning.
• **PROPAGATION** Sow seed at 13–18°C (55–64°F) in spring; prick out seedlings as soon as possible.
• **PESTS AND DISEASES** Red spider mites may be a problem under glass.

C. aurea ♀ (East African laburnum, Natal laburnum). Erect shrub or small tree, usually spreading in habit, with pinnate leaves, 10–24cm (4–10in) long, composed of 3–12 pairs of ovate, fine-tipped leaflets, dark green above, paler beneath. Racemes, 8–18cm (3–7in) long, of up to 30 bright yellow flowers are borne from winter to spring. ↕2–10m (6–30ft), ↔ 1–4m (3–12ft). South Africa (mainly Eastern Cape), S. India. ❀ (min. 7°C/45°F)

CALTHA

Kingcup, Marsh marigold

RANUNCULACEAE

Genus of about 10 species of rhizomatous, marshland or marginal aquatic perennials and herbaceous, moisture-loving perennials, widespread in temperate and cold regions of the N. hemisphere. The leaves are generally heart- or kidney-shaped. Those grown as marginal water plants provide a display of cup-shaped, yellow or white flowers in spring. They are borne in terminal or axillary corymbs before the dense clumps of foliage are produced; a second flush of flowers is often produced in late summer. Although calthas are best grown at the water's edge, several will thrive in a mixed or herbaceous border, if the soil is kept moist. *C. introloba* is suitable for a peat bed, trough, or alpine house. There is considerable nomenclatural confusion over the limits of the species that are commercially available.
• **HARDINESS** Fully hardy to frost hardy.
• **CULTIVATION** Grow in an open site in rich, boggy soil in full sun at the water's edge; marsh marigolds will tolerate root restriction in aquatic planting baskets. *C. introloba* needs moist but well-drained, humus-rich soil in a cool site in partial shade. See also pp.52–53.
• **PROPAGATION** Sow seed as soon as ripe on permanently damp compost in a partially shaded cold frame. Divide in late summer or very early spring.
• **PESTS AND DISEASES** Prone to powdery mildew in summer.

C. introloba. Dwarf, tufted, marshland perennial with arrow-shaped, glossy, mid-green leaves, 2–2.5cm (¾–1in) long. In late winter, produces large, almost stemless white flowers, to 2.5cm (1in) across, flushed purple on the outside. ↕2.5cm (1in), ↔ to 7cm (3in). Mountains of Australia. ***
C. laeta see *C. palustris* var. *palustris.*

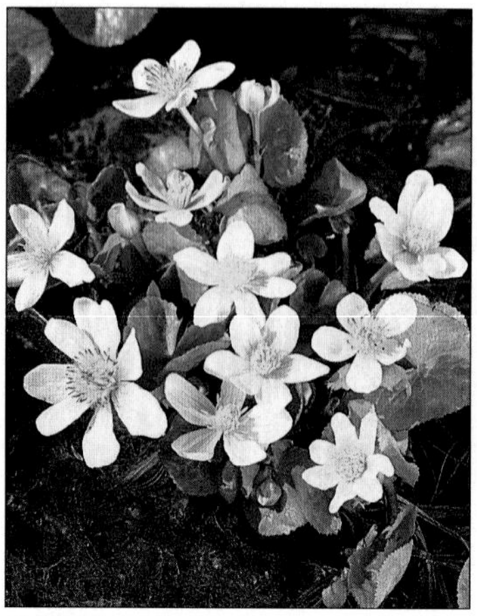

Caltha leptosepala

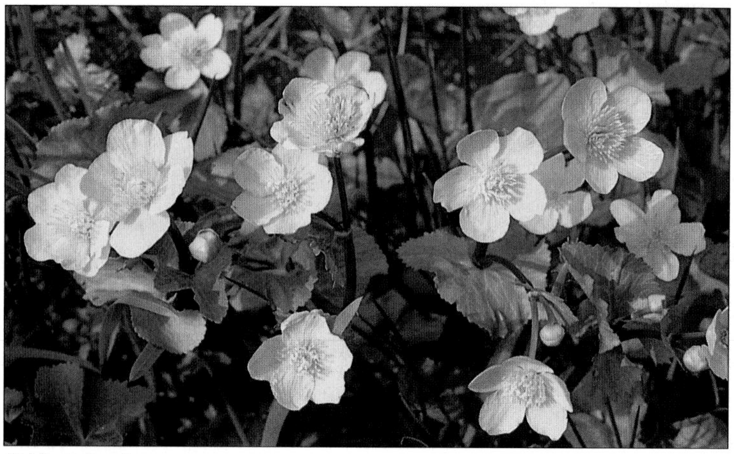

Caltha palustris

C. leptosepala ■ Marginal aquatic perennial with heart-shaped, radical, dark green leaves, to 6cm (2½in) long. Silvery white flowers, 2–3cm (¾–1¼in) across, open on leafless stems, 15–20cm (6–8in) tall, in spring. ↕↔ 30cm (12in). North America (Alaska to Alberta, south to Oregon, Utah, New Mexico). ***. **subsp. *howellii*** is compact, with broad leaves, to 8cm (3in) long, and white flowers, often in pairs; ↕20cm (8in); North America (Alaska to California).
C. palustris ■ ♀ (Kingcup, Marsh marigold). Variable, marginal aquatic perennial with decumbent rhizomes that produce kidney-shaped, toothed, dark green leaves, 4–10cm (1½–4in) long. In spring, stems 30–45cm (12–18in) tall, bear waxy yellow flowers, 4cm (1½in) across. May grow in water to 23cm (9in) deep for short periods, but prefers very shallow water or bog conditions. ↕10–40cm (4–16in), ↔ 45cm (18in). N. temperate regions. ***. **var. *alba*,** syn. 'Alba', is compact, bearing solitary white flowers with yellow stamens in early spring, often before the glossy foliage develops; ↕22cm (9in), ↔ 30cm (12in). **'Flore Pleno'** ■ ♀ has double yellow flowers; ↕↔ 25cm (10in). **var. *palustris*,** syn. *C. laeta*, *C. polypetala* of gardens (Giant marsh marigold), has creeping or decumbent rhizomes, rounded leaves, heart-shaped at the bases, and flowers to 8cm (3in) across; ↕60cm (24in), ↔ 70–75cm (28–30in). North America (Alaska to Oregon).
***C. polypetala* of gardens** see *C. palustris* var. *palustris*

▷**Caltrops, Water** see *Trapa natans*

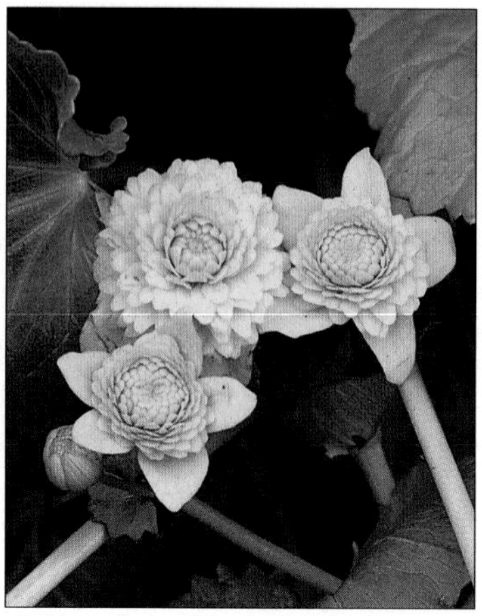

Caltha palustris 'Flore Pleno'

CALYCANTHUS

Allspice, Spicebush

CALYCANTHACEAE

Genus of 2 or 3 species of deciduous shrubs from woodland and streambanks in the USA. They are cultivated for their unusual, fragrant flowers, which have narrowly lance-shaped to elliptic petals and sepals, and resemble tiny water lilies; they are solitary, and are produced terminally or from the axils of the current year's shoots. The opposite, dark green leaves, 5–20cm (2–8in) long, are aromatic when crushed. Grow allspice in a shrub border or as specimen plants.
• **HARDINESS** Fully hardy.
• **CULTIVATION** Grow in fertile, moist, humus-rich soil in sun or, in warm climates, in partial shade. Some species may suffer frost damage in very cold winters. Pruning group 6.
• **PROPAGATION** Sow seed as soon as ripe or in autumn in an open frame. Root softwood cuttings in summer, layer in autumn, or remove suckers in spring.
• **PESTS AND DISEASES** Trouble free.

C. chinensis see *Sinocalycanthus chinensis.*
C. floridus (Carolina allspice, Common sweetshrub, Strawberry bush). Bushy, spreading shrub with oval or oblong, dark green leaves, to 12cm (5in) long, rough above, and sometimes turning yellow in autumn. Flowers, 4–5cm (1½–2in) across, with numerous strap-shaped, dark red petals, fading to brown at the tips, are borne in summer. ↕2.5m (8ft), ↔ 3m (10ft). S.E. USA. ***

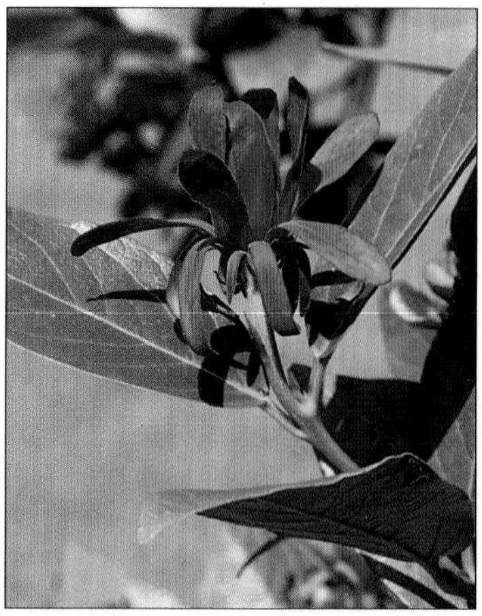

Calycanthus occidentalis

C. occidentalis ▣ (Californian allspice). Vigorous, spreading shrub with ovate to oblong-lance-shaped, dark green leaves, to 20cm (8in) long, rough above, and sometimes turning yellow in autumn. Dark red flowers, 5cm (2in) across, with linear, brown-tipped petals, are borne in summer. ↕3m (10ft), ↔4m (12ft). USA (California). ❄❄❄

CALYMMANTHIUM

CACTACEAE

Genus of 2 species of columnar, perennial cacti from hilly lowlands in Peru. The pale green stems, occasionally many-branched, have 3- to 5-angled, warty or scalloped ribs and small, spiny areoles. Tubular-bell-shaped, nocturnal, white to red flowers develop from a small, stem-like, fleshy receptacle tube bearing spiny areoles. This tube encloses the inner parts of the flower, and is split by the emerging perianth. Elongated, 4- or 5-angled, pale green fruits contain ovoid seeds. In frost-prone areas, grow in a warm greenhouse; elsewhere, use in a semi-desert garden.

• **HARDINESS** Frost tender.
• **CULTIVATION** Under glass, grow in standard cactus compost in full light with shade from hot sun. In growth, water moderately and apply a low-nitrogen liquid fertilizer monthly; keep dry at other times. Outdoors, grow in sharply drained, humus-rich soil in full sun. See also pp.48–49.
• **PROPAGATION** Sow seed at 19–24°C (66–75°F) in late spring, or root stem cuttings in summer.
• **PESTS AND DISEASES** Vulnerable to scale insects, mealybugs, and aphids.

C. substerile. Shrub-like cactus with ribbed stems bearing white areoles, each with 3–8 white or pale yellow radials, to 1cm (½in) long, and 1–6 white centrals, 1–5cm (½–2in) long. Nocturnal white flowers, to 11cm (4½in) long, with reddish brown outer petals, are borne in summer. ↕8m (25ft), ↔75cm (30in). N. Peru. ♛ (min. 13°C/55°F)

CALYPSO

ORCHIDACEAE

Genus of one species of deciduous, terrestrial orchid from Europe, Asia, and North America, found in damp woodland, bogs, and marshes. The ovoid corm produces a single, pleated leaf. Solitary, terminal, slipper-shaped flowers are borne in summer. In frost-prone climates, grow in a cold greenhouse or alpine house; in warmer regions, use in a rock, bog, or woodland garden.

• **HARDINESS** Frost hardy.
• **CULTIVATION** Cool-growing orchid. Under glass, grow in terrestrial orchid compost with added leaf mould and charcoal, in filtered light. Top-dress annually. Water freely in the growing season, more sparingly in winter. Outdoors, grow in moist, neutral to acid soil, enriched with leaf mould or bark chips, in partial shade. See also p.46.
• **PROPAGATION** Separate corms with great care in early spring.
• **PESTS AND DISEASES** Trouble free.

C. bulbosa ▣ Small, terrestrial orchid with one elliptic to oblong leaf, 12cm (5in) long. In summer, a slender stem,

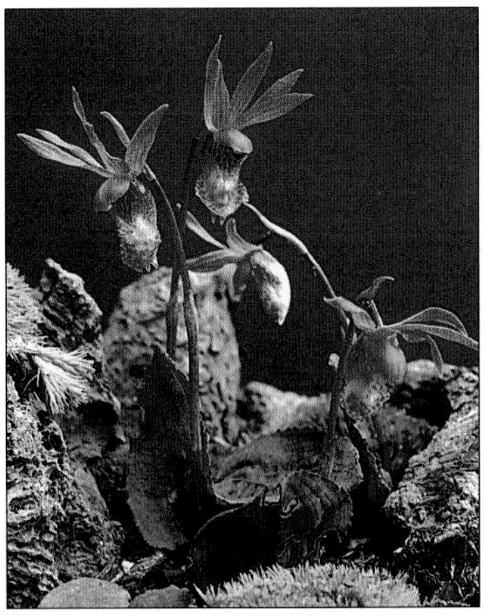

Calypso bulbosa

10–20cm (4–8in) tall, bears a solitary, nodding, fragrant flower, 2.5cm (1in) across; the reflexed sepals and petals are usually reddish purple, occasionally white; the lips are white. ↕20cm (8in), ↔15cm (6in). Scandinavia, Russia, Asia, North America. ❄❄

CALYTRIX

Starflower

MYRTACEAE

Genus of about 70 species of prostrate to erect, evergreen shrubs, usually found in open scrub or light, eucalyptus forest in Australia. The crowded, tiny leaves are alternate, opposite, or whorled. The star-shaped, 5-petalled, white to pink, purple, or yellow flowers, are borne singly from the leaf axils, and are often clustered at the branch ends. In frost-prone areas, grow in a cool greenhouse; elsewhere, use in a shrub border or as ground cover.

• **HARDINESS** Half hardy to frost tender.
• **CULTIVATION** Under glass, grow in loam-based potting compost (JI No.2) in full light with good ventilation. In the growing season, water freely, applying a phosphate-free liquid fertilizer monthly; water sparingly in winter. Pot on or top-dress in early spring. Outdoors, grow in well-drained, neutral to acid soil in full sun. Pruning group 10, after flowering.
• **PROPAGATION** Root semi-ripe cuttings with bottom heat in summer.
• **PESTS AND DISEASES** Trouble free.

C. alpestris (Snow myrtle). Many-branched, arching shrub with linear, spreading or sometimes reflexed, hairy, dark green leaves, 1–5mm (1/16–¼in) long. Bears profuse, often pink-budded white flowers, 5–10mm (¼–½in) across, from late spring to summer. ↕2–3m (6–10ft), ↔2–4m (6–12ft). Australia (South Australia, Victoria). ❄

▷**Camas, Death** see *Zigadenus venenosus*

CAMASSIA

Quamash

HYACYNTHACAEA/LILIACEAE

Genus of 5 or 6 species of bulbous perennials from damp, fertile meadowland in North America. Large, ovoid to spherical bulbs give rise to erect, narrow, linear, keeled, channelled, bright green, basal leaves. Loose or dense, terminal racemes of large, showy, star- or cup-shaped, blue, purple, or white flowers, each with 6 tepals, are borne on leafless stems among the leaves from late spring to summer; the dead tepals sometimes persist after capsules develop. Grow in a border or a wildflower meadow. Good for cut flowers. The bulbs of *C. quamash* were once an important food source for native Americans.

• **HARDINESS** Fully hardy to frost hardy.
• **CULTIVATION** Plant bulbs 10cm (4in) deep in autumn, in moist but well-drained, fertile, humus-rich soil in sun or partial shade. Do not allow soil to become waterlogged. Mulch in winter in areas with prolonged frosts.
• **PROPAGATION** Sow seed in containers in a cold frame as soon as ripe. Remove offsets when dormant in summer.
• **PESTS AND DISEASES** Trouble free.

C. cusickii. Bulbous perennial bearing large racemes, 20–40cm (8–16in) long, of shallowly cup-shaped, pale to deep steel-blue flowers, 5cm (2in) across, in late spring. The wavy-margined, linear leaves are 40–80cm (16–32in) long. ↕60–80cm (24–32in), ↔10cm (4in). USA (N.E. Oregon). ❄❄. **'Zwanenburg'** ▣ has deep blue flowers.
C. esculenta see *C. quamash.*
C. fraseri see *C. scilloides.*
C. leichtlinii ▣ ♀ Bulbous perennial with linear leaves, 20–60cm (8–24in) long. In late spring, bears racemes, 10–30cm (4–12in) long, of star-shaped, creamy white flowers, 5–7cm (2–3in) wide; the flower segments twist together as they fade. ↕60–130cm (24–54in), ↔10cm (4in). W. USA (Oregon). ❄❄. **'Semiplena'** ▣ is sterile, and bears semi-double, creamy white flowers in dense racemes, 20–50cm (8–20in) long. **subsp. *suksdorfii*** bears blue to violet flowers; W. North America (British Columbia to California). **subsp. *suksdorfii* 'Blau Donau'**, syn. subsp. *suksdorfii* 'Blue Danube', has violet flowers.
C. quamash, syn. *C. esculenta* (Quamash). Bulbous perennial with linear leaves, 20–50cm (8–20in) long.

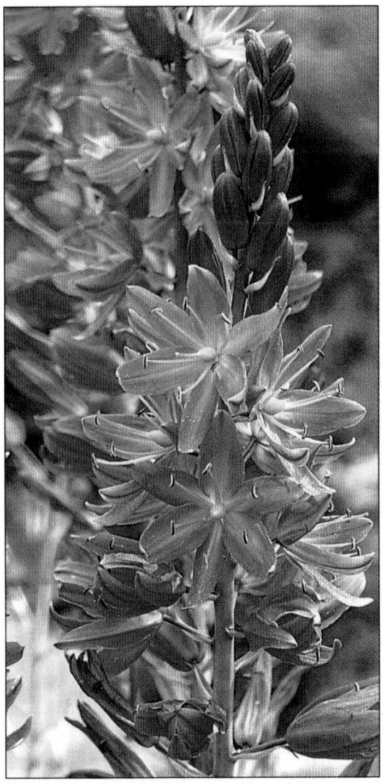

Camassia cusickii 'Zwanenburg'

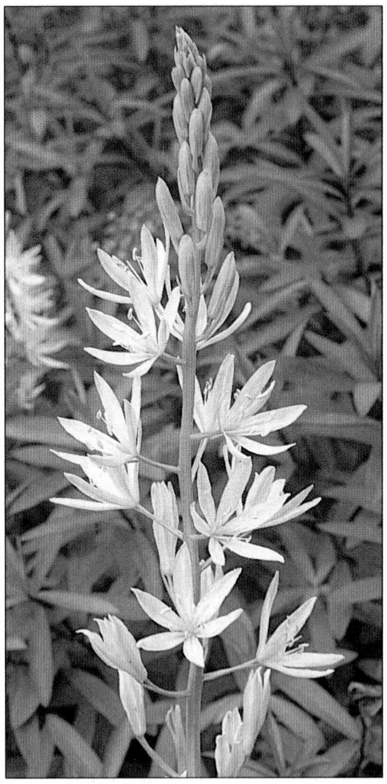

Camassia leichtlinii

Racemes, to 30cm (12in) long, of shallowly cup-shaped, bright blue flowers, 3–5cm (1¼–2in) across, are produced in late spring. Rapidly forms large clumps and is easily naturalized in grass, provided the soil is moist. ↕20–80cm (8–32in), ↔5cm (2in). Canada, USA. ❄❄. **'Orion'** produces larger racemes, 10–40cm (4–16in) long, of dark blue flowers; ↕60–80cm (24–32in).
C. scilloides, syn. *C. fraseri* (Wild hyacinth). Bulbous perennial producing linear leaves, 20–60cm (8–24in) long. Racemes, 8–15cm (3–6in) long, of star-shaped, violet, blue, or white flowers, 2–3cm (¾–1¼in) across, are borne in late summer. ↕20–80cm (8–32in), ↔10cm (4in). C. and E. USA. ❄❄

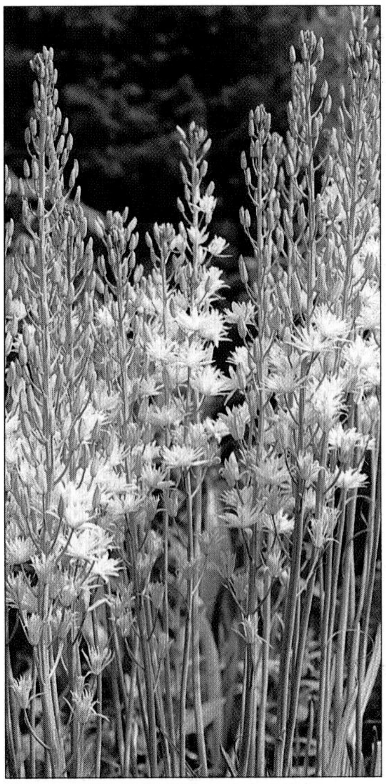

Camassia leichtlinii 'Semiplena'

C

CAMELLIA

THEACEAE

Genus of over 250 species of long-lived, evergreen shrubs and small trees, 1–20m (3–70ft) tall. They are found in acid soil in woodland areas from N. India and the Himalayas to China and Japan, and south to N. Indonesia, Java, and Sumatra. The usually glossy, mid- to dark green leaves are simple, alternate, and lance-shaped to elliptic, with toothed margins. Popular for their bold foliage and abundance of showy, white, pink, red, or yellow flowers, camellias have been extensively hybridized to produce a range of flower types (see panel, right). The flowers may be solitary, paired, or clustered, and are sometimes fragrant. In the following descriptions, flower sizes of cultivars have been defined as follows: miniature, to 6cm (2½in); small, 6–8cm (2½–3in); medium, 8–10cm (3–4in); large, 10–13cm (4–5in); very large, 13cm (5in) or more across.

Camellias are elegant shrubs for a border or a woodland garden; they also make excellent specimen plants, both outdoors in open ground or in containers. In frost-prone areas, grow half-hardy and tender species in a cool greenhouse. The flowers are suitable for cutting and exhibition.

• **HARDINESS** Fully hardy to frost tender.

• **CULTIVATION** Under glass, grow in lime-free (ericaceous) potting compost in bright filtered light. When in growth, water freely with soft water; water more sparingly in winter. Apply a balanced liquid fertilizer in mid-spring and again in early summer. Top-dress annually with shredded bark. Container-grown plants may be moved outdoors in summer to a partially shaded, sheltered site. Outdoors, grow in moist but well-drained, humus-rich, acid (pH5.5–6.5) soil; maintain a mulch, 5–7cm (2–3in) deep, of leaf mould or shredded bark.

Do not plant too deep; the top of the root ball should be level with the firmed soil. Position in partial or dappled shade, in a site sheltered from cold, dry winds and early morning sun; buds and flowers may be damaged by cold winds and late frosts. *C. sasanqua* cultivars will thrive in full sun once established, provided that the roots are kept cool. Water established plants in dry weather to prevent bud drop. Apply a balanced liquid fertilizer in mid-spring and again, if necessary, in early summer; do not overfeed. Protect from prolonged winter frosts with a thatch of straw or bracken litter. Pruning group 8; camellias tolerate hard pruning.

• **PROPAGATION** Root leaf bud or semi-ripe cuttings of the current year's growth from late summer to late winter, or graft in late winter.

• **PESTS AND DISEASES** Susceptible to aphids, scale insects, and vine weevils. A harmless sooty mould may grow on the honeydew produced by aphids and scale insects on the leaves. Virus diseases and leafy gall may blemish flowers and leaves. Leaf spot and honey fungus may also be a problem.

C. 'Black Lace' ■ Slow-growing, dense, upright shrub with ovate, dark green leaves, 8cm (3in) long, and large, formal double, black-red flowers, borne from early to late spring. ↕ 1.5–2.5m (5–8ft), ↔ 1–2.5m (3–8ft). ❄❄❄

C. 'Bonanza'. Strong-growing, upright shrub with ovate, dark green leaves, 6cm (2½in) long, and medium, loose peony-form red flowers, produced from mid-autumn to late winter. ↕ 1.8–3m (6–10ft), ↔ 1–2m (3–6ft). ❄❄❄

C. 'Chansonette'. Strong-growing shrub with elliptic, dark green leaves, 7cm (3in) long. Bears miniature, formal double, bright pink flowers from late autumn to late winter. ↕ 3–4m (10–12ft), ↔ 2–4m (6–12ft). ❄❄❄

C. chrysantha see *C. nitidissima.*

C. 'Cornish Snow' ■ 🏆 Fast-growing shrub with slender, arching branches and lance-shaped leaves, 5cm (2in) long, bronze when young, maturing to dark green. Bears a profusion of miniature, single white flowers, pink-tinged on opening, from midwinter to late spring. ↕ 3m (10ft), ↔ 1.5m (5ft). ❄❄❄

C. cuspidata. Erect, slender shrub with dark green, copper-tinted, lance-shaped to elliptic leaves, 5–9cm (2–3½in) long. From late winter to mid-spring, bears single white flowers, to 4cm (1½in) across. ↕↔ 3.5m (11ft). China. ❄❄❄

C. 'Dazzler' ■ Spreading shrub with fan-shaped branches and elliptic, dark green leaves, 5–7cm (2–3in) long. Medium, semi-double to loose peony-form, rose-red flowers are borne from late autumn to late winter. ↕ 2–3m (6–10ft), ↔ 1–2m (3–6ft). ❄❄❄

C. 'Dr. Clifford Parks' ■ 🏆 Upright shrub with oval, dark green leaves, 14cm (5½in) long, and very large, peony- or anemone-form, dark rose-red flowers, produced in mid-spring. ↕ 4m (12ft), ↔ 2.5m (8ft). ❄❄

C. 'Dream Girl'. Spreading shrub producing elliptic, dark green leaves, 16cm (6in) long. Large to very large, strongly scented, semi-double, salmon-pink flowers are borne from midwinter to early spring. Best grown in full sun. ↕ 2–4m (6–12ft), ↔ 1.2–2.5m (4–8ft). ❄❄❄

C. 'El Dorado'. Spreading shrub with elliptic, dark green leaves, 6–12cm (2½–5in) long, and large, loose peony-form, pale pink flowers, borne in early and mid-spring. ↕ 2–4m (6–12ft), ↔ 1.5–3m (5–10ft). ❄❄❄

C. 'Flower Girl'. Upright shrub with elliptic, dark green leaves, 12–18cm (5–7in) long, and large, scented, semi-double pink flowers, produced from midwinter to early spring. ↕ 2–4m (6–12ft), ↔ 1.2–2.5m (4–8ft). ❄❄❄

C. 'Francie L.' ■ Vigorous shrub with long, fan-shaped branches, ideal for training against a wall. Produces lance-shaped, dark green leaves, 6–10cm (2½–4in) long, and large, semi-double, salmon-red to deep rose-red flowers, from late winter to late spring. ↕ 5m (15ft), ↔ 6m (20ft). ❄❄❄

C. fraterna. Dense shrub producing small, elliptic, dark green leaves, 4–8cm (1½–3in) long, and fragrant, single, lilac-tinted white flowers, 2–3cm (¾–1¼in) across, in late winter and early spring. ↕ 5m (15ft), ↔ 1–3m (3–10ft). China. ❄

C. 'Freedom Bell' ■ Small, dense, rounded shrub with oval, glossy, dark green leaves, 9cm (3½in) long. Bears

CAMELLIA FLOWER FORMS

Camellia flowers may be **single**, with one row of up to 8 petals and prominent stamens, forming usually saucer-shaped, occasionally cup- or trumpet-shaped flowers; **semi-double**, with 2 or more rows of large outer petals, the centre regular, irregular, or composed of loose petals and stamens; **anemone-form**, with one or more rows of outer petals, and intermingling petaloids and stamens in the centre; **peony-form**, with a convex mass of irregular petaloids, petals, and stamens, or with irregular petals and petaloids and hidden stamens; **rose-form double**, with overlapping petals showing stamens in a concave centre when fully open; or **formal double**, with rows of overlapping petals and no stamens visible.

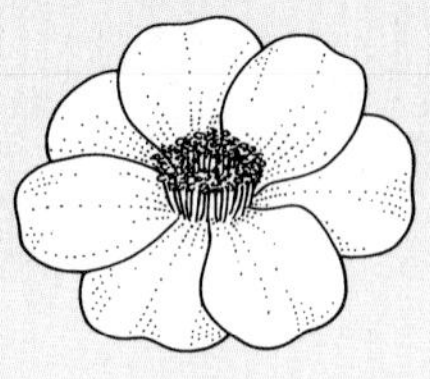
SINGLE

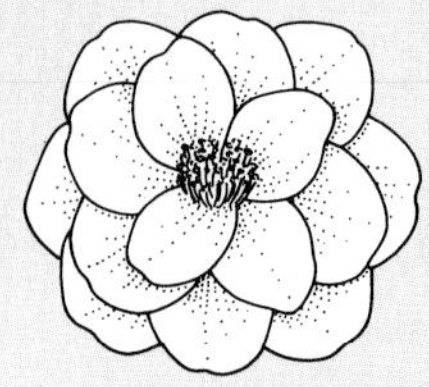
SEMI-DOUBLE

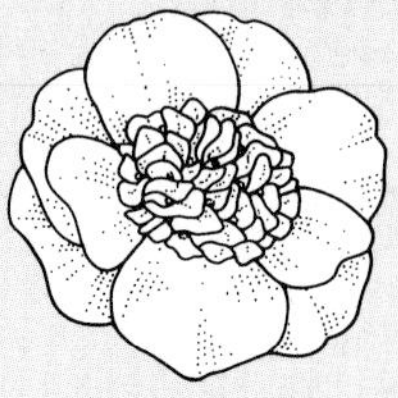
ANEMONE-FORM

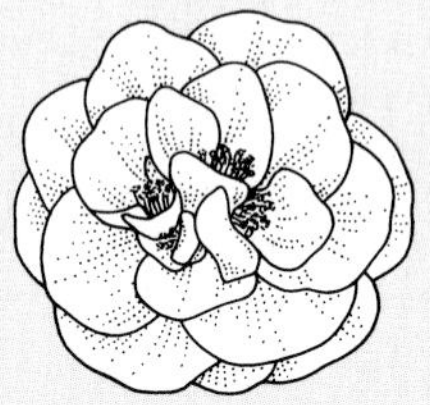
PEONY-FORM

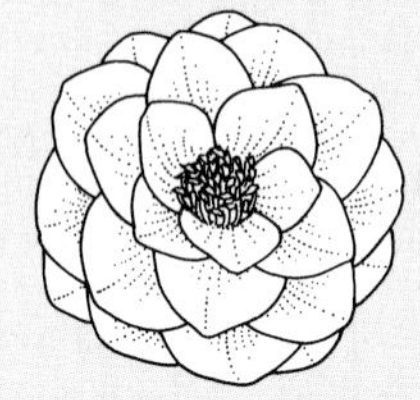
ROSE-FORM DOUBLE

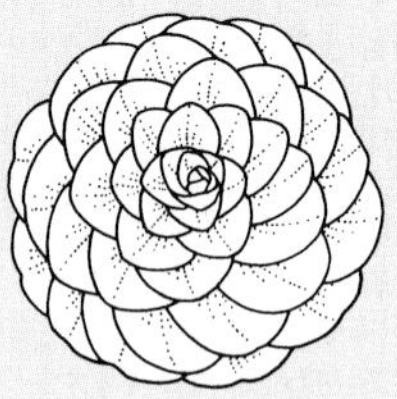
FORMAL DOUBLE

Camellia 'Black Lace'

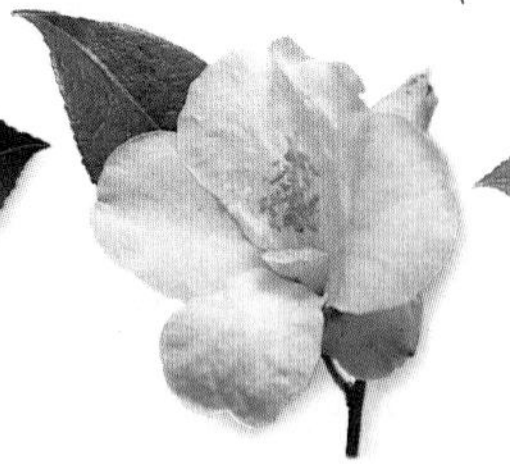
Camellia 'Cornish Snow'

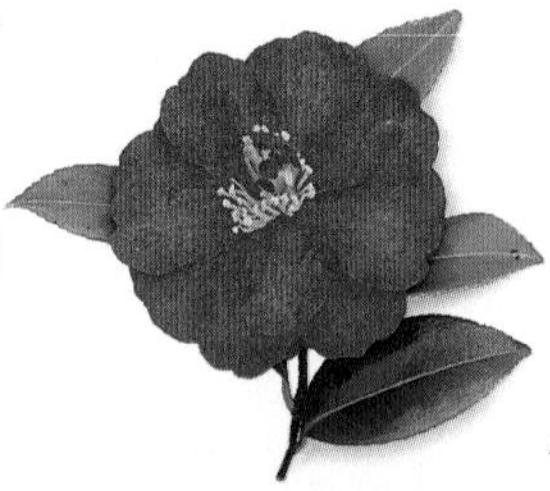
Camellia 'Dazzler'

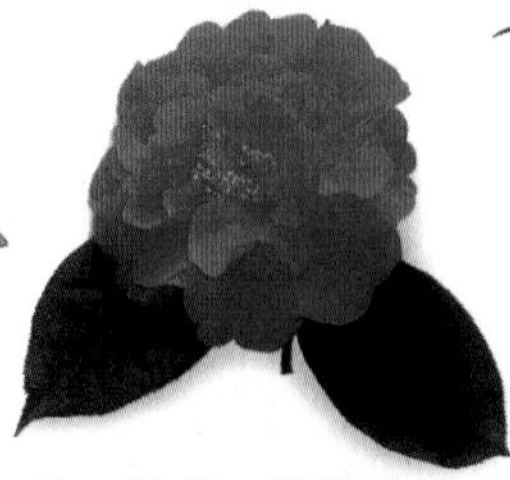
Camellia 'Dr. Clifford Parks'

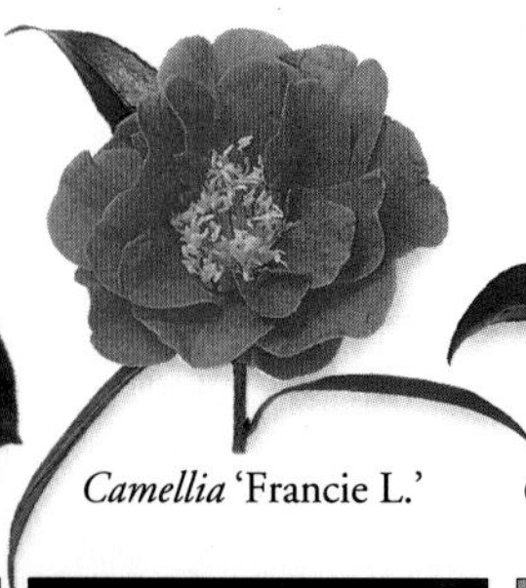
Camellia 'Francie L.'

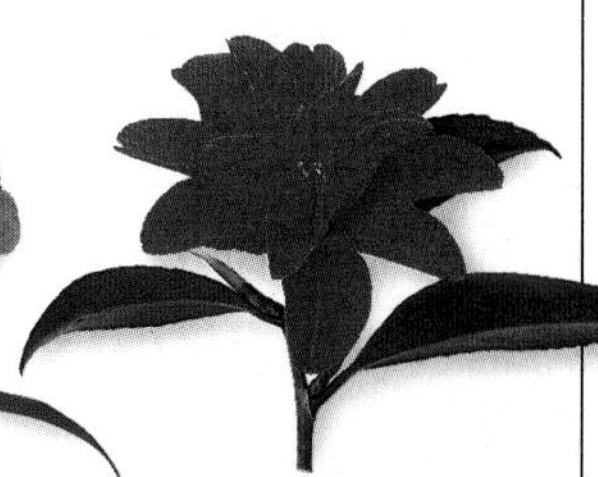
Camellia 'Freedom Bell'

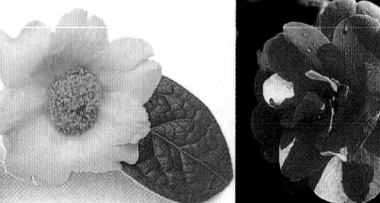

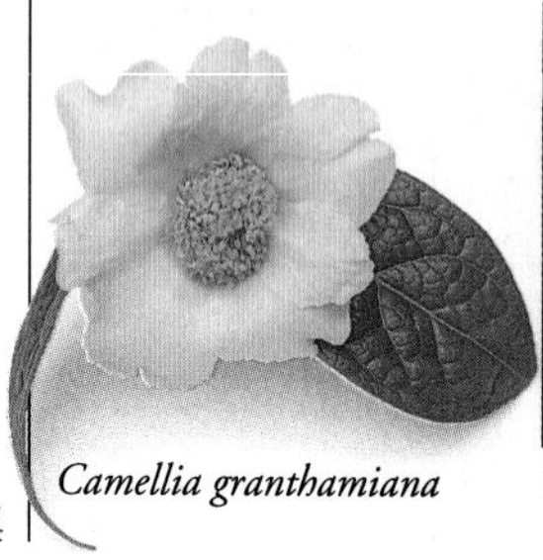
Camellia granthamiana

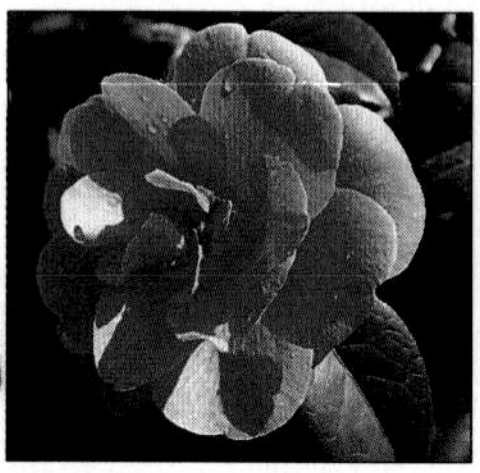
Camellia 'Inspiration'

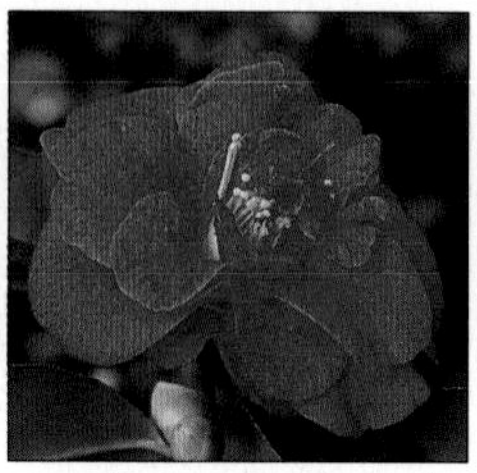
Camellia japonica 'Adolphe Audusson'

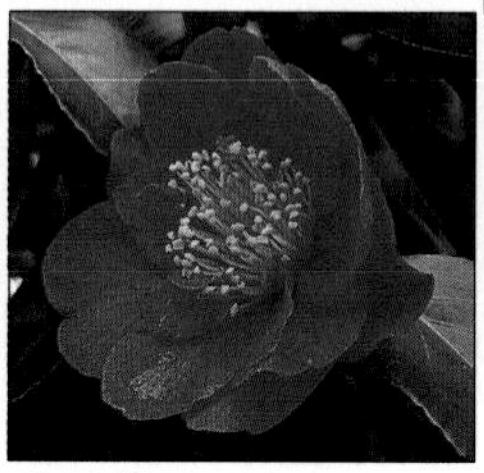
Camellia japonica 'Alexander Hunter'

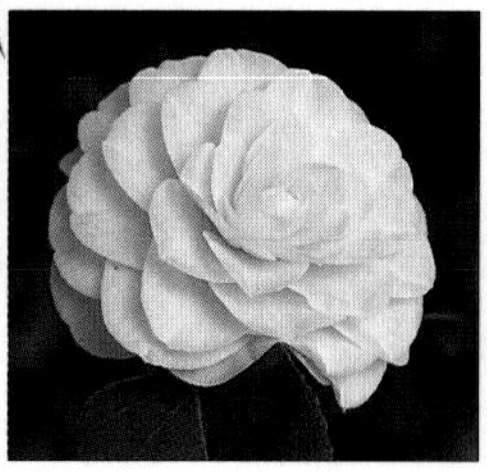
Camellia japonica 'Ave Maria'

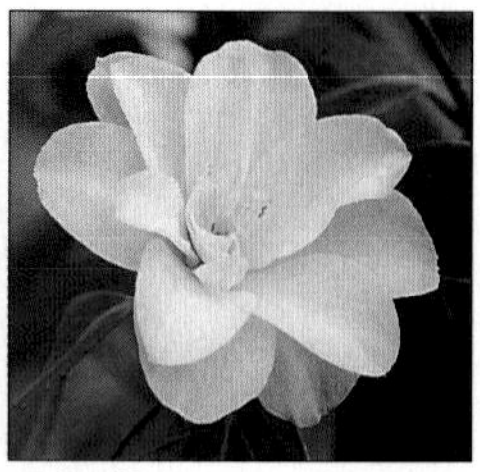
Camellia japonica 'Berenice Boddy'

medium, deeply cup-shaped, semi-double, bright red flowers from late winter to late spring. Excellent for a small garden. ↕↔ 2.2m (7ft). ✻✻✻
C. granthamiana ■ ♀ Large shrub or small tree producing distinctive, elliptic, dark green leaves, to 10cm (4in) long, with deeply impressed veins. Single white flowers, 12–14cm (5–5½in) across, open from brown buds in early and midwinter. ↕ 3m (10ft), ↔ 2m (6ft). Hong Kong. ✻
C. grijsii. Bushy shrub with elliptic to oval, dark green leaves, to 8cm (3in) long. Bears single white flowers, 2–3cm (¾–1¼in) across, sometimes scented, with 2-lobed petals, in late winter. ↕ 1–3m (3–10ft), ↔ 0.75–2m (2½–6ft). China. ✻
***C.* 'Harold L. Paige'.** Upright shrub with large, oval, dark green leaves, 12cm (5in) long, and bearing very large, rose-form double, bright red flowers, in mid-spring. ↕ 2–4m (6–12ft), ↔ 1.5–3m (5–10ft). ✻
***C.* 'Inspiration'** ■ ♀ ♀ Upright shrub or small tree producing oval, dark green leaves, 8cm (3in) long, and medium, semi-double, deep pink flowers, from midwinter to late spring. ↕ 4m (12ft), ↔ 2m (6ft). ✻✻✻
C. japonica ♀–♀ (Common camellia). Upright to spreading shrub or small tree with broadly elliptic, glossy, dark green leaves, 5–8cm (2–3in) long, and single red flowers, 3–4.5cm (1¼–1¾in) across. The species flowers in early spring, its cultivars over a much longer period, in mid- and late spring unless stated otherwise. ↕ 9m (28ft), ↔ 8m (25ft). China, Korea, Japan. ✻✻✻. **'Adolphe Audusson'** ■ ♀ is compact, bearing large, semi-double red flowers in early and mid-spring. **'Akashigata'** ♀ syn. 'Lady Clare', is a dense, strong-growing, rounded shrub with very large, semi-double, deep pink flowers with yellow stamens, borne from early to late spring. **'Alba Plena'** is erect, with light green foliage and medium, formal double white flowers. **'Alba Simplex'** is bushy, bearing medium, flat, single white flowers with a few pink flecks. **'Alexander Hunter'** ■ ♀ is upright, with upward-sweeping branches, bearing medium, single or semi-double crimson flowers with yellow stamens in early and mid-spring. **'Apollo'** see 'Paul's Apollo'. **'Augusto Leal de Gouveia Pinto'** is upright, bearing large, formal double, lavender-tinted red flowers, with white-edged petals, in early and mid-spring. In cooler climates, its flowers are more blue in colour. **'Ave Maria'** ■ is upright, with downward-sweeping branches, and bears miniature, formal double, soft pink flowers from early to late spring. **'Berenice Boddy'** ■ ♀ is a strong, bushy, very hardy shrub, of arching habit. The large, semi-double, clear pink flowers are darker on the outer petals and are borne from late winter to late spring. **'Betty Sheffield Supreme'** ■ is erect, with lance-shaped, slightly glossy leaves, 8–10cm (3–4in) long, and large, irregular, double white flowers, each petal margined in shades of rose-pink, borne in early and mid-spring; ↕ 2–4m (6–12ft), ↔ 1.5–3m (5–10ft). **'Bob Hope'** ♀ is a large, upright shrub with vigorous, dense growth and large, semi-double or loose peony-form, dark red flowers; ↕ 3m (10ft), ↔ 2m (6ft). **'Bob's Tinsie'** ■ ♀ has a dense, upright habit, and produces miniature, anemone-form, brilliant red flowers from early to late spring; ↕ 2m (6ft), ↔ 1m (3ft). **'Bokuhan'**, syn. 'Tinsie', is dwarf with spreading branches, and miniature, anemone-form flowers with red petals around a centre of white petaloids, borne from early winter to late spring; ↕ 1m (3ft), ↔ 60cm (24in). **'Chander's Elegans'** see 'Elegans'. **'Charlie Bettes'** is a large, dense, fast-growing shrub, bearing large, semi-double white flowers, with bright yellow stamens, from late winter to mid-spring. **'Charlotte de Rothschild'** ■ is slow-growing and spreading, producing medium, single white flowers, with prominent pale gold stamens, from early to late spring. **'C.M. Hovey'** ♀ is a large, arching shrub, with very large, flat, formal double, bright crimson or scarlet flowers. **'Commander Mulroy'** is upright and dense, with rounded to elliptic leaves and small, formal double, pure white flowers, pink in bud. It is an excellent container or patio plant. **'Contessa Lavinia Maggi'** see 'Lavinia Maggi'. **'Coquettii'** ■ ♀ syn. 'Glen 40', is an upright, slow-growing shrub with downward-sweeping branches. In early and mid-spring, bears profuse, medium to large, deep red flowers, sometimes

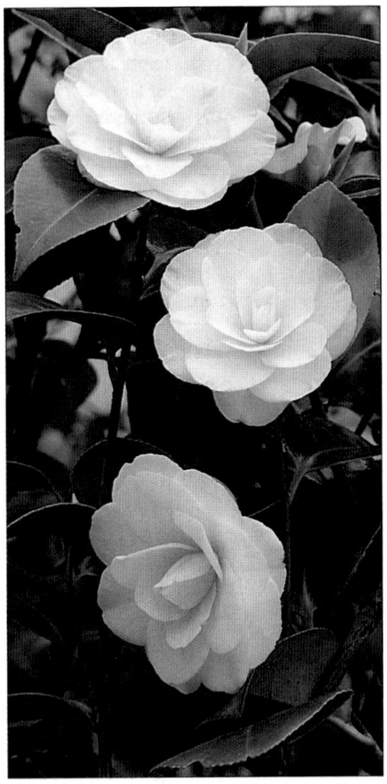
Camellia japonica 'Janet Waterhouse'

formal double, sometimes peony- or anemone-form. **'Dixie Knight'** is strong and bushy, with large, loose peony-form, dark red flowers. **'Dona Herzilia de Frietas Magalhaes'**, syn. 'Magellan', is a large, rounded shrub with medium, semi-double to anemone-form red flowers, variably suffused violet, borne in early and mid-spring. **'Donckelaeri'** see 'Masayoshi'. **'Dr. Burnside'** is moderately vigorous, with medium to large, semi-double or loose peony-form, dark red flowers, freely borne from early to late spring. **'Dr. Tinsley'** ♀ is compact and upright, bearing medium white flowers, suffused light pink, more strongly towards the petal margins. The flowers vary from semi-double to loose peony-form or formal double, and open from pink buds in early and mid-spring. **'Elegans'** ■ ♀ syn. 'Chander's Elegans', has spreading branches with wavy leaves, and bears large, anemone-form, rose-pink flowers. Leading branches should not be cut back. **'Elegans Supreme'** ■ is similar to 'Elegans', with wavy leaves and very large, anemone-form, deep salmon-pink flowers. **'Fimbriata'** is similar to 'Alba Plena', with medium, formal double white flowers with fringe-margined petals, borne in early and mid-spring. **'Glen 40'** see 'Coquettii'. **'Gloire de Nantes'** ■ ♀ is compact and upright, with medium, semi-double to incomplete double, rose-red flowers, borne from late autumn to late spring. **'Governor Mouton'** is vigorous, with medium, semi-double or loose peony-form red flowers, often marked white, in early and mid-spring. **'Grand Prix'** ♀ is vigorous, with very large, semi-double, brilliant red flowers with yellow stamens. **'Grand Slam'** ♀ is strong and upright, with large, mostly anemone-form, sometimes semi-double, dark red flowers. **'Guilio Nuccio'** ■ ♀ is a strong-growing, many-branched shrub with leaves 12–18cm (5–7in) long, and very large, semi-double, salmon-red flowers, with mustard-yellow stamens, borne from late winter to midsummer. **'Hagoromo'** ♀ syn. 'Magnoliiflora', is erect, bearing medium, semi-double, pale pink flowers in mid-spring. Good as a patio plant. **'Janet Waterhouse'** ■ is sturdy and upright, with medium white flowers, semi-double in hot climates or formal double in cooler conditions. **'Julia Drayton'** ■ syn. 'Mathotiana Purple King', 'Mathotiana Rubra', is upright and bears large, rose-form double or formal double crimson, purple-tinted flowers. **'Julia France'** is upright, with bold leaves, 8–12cm (3–5in) long, and large, semi-double, light pink flowers. **'Jupiter'** see 'Paul's Jupiter'. **'Kramer's Supreme'** ■ is compact and upright, bearing large to very large, flat, fragrant, full peony-form, rose-red flowers in late autumn and again in early and mid-spring. Grow in a cool greenhouse in winter and in cold areas; ✻✻✻ (borderline). **'Kumasaka'** is an upright shrub with formal double, occasionally peony-form, deep rose-pink flowers. **'Lady Clare'** see 'Akashigata'. **'Lady Loch'** ■ is a leafy, rounded shrub, bearing medium, peony-form pink flowers, with white picotee-margined petals, in spring. **'Lady Vansittart'** ■ is upright, with leaves 8–12cm (3–5in) long and medium, semi-double white flowers with rose-pink stripes; many specimens have

C

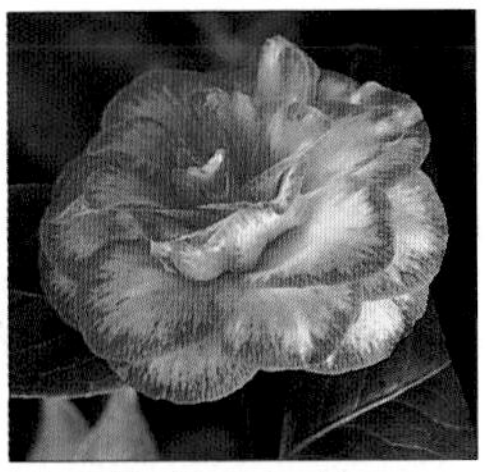
Camellia japonica 'Betty Sheffield Supreme'

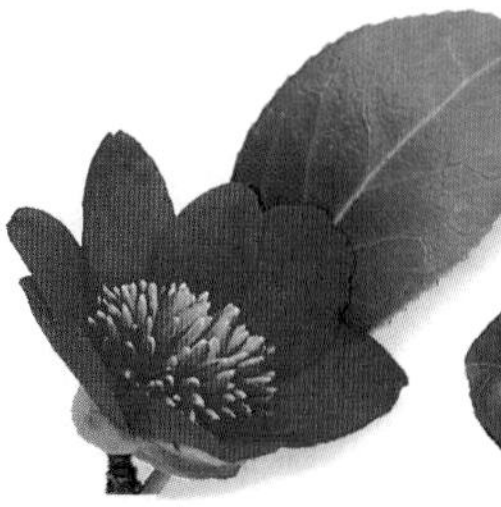
Camellia japonica 'Bob's Tinsie'

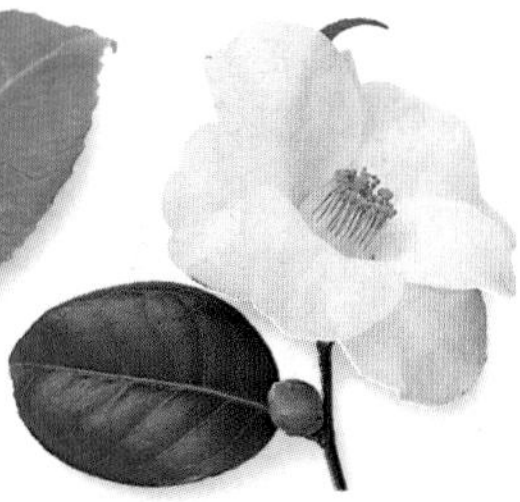
Camellia japonica 'Charlotte de Rothschild'

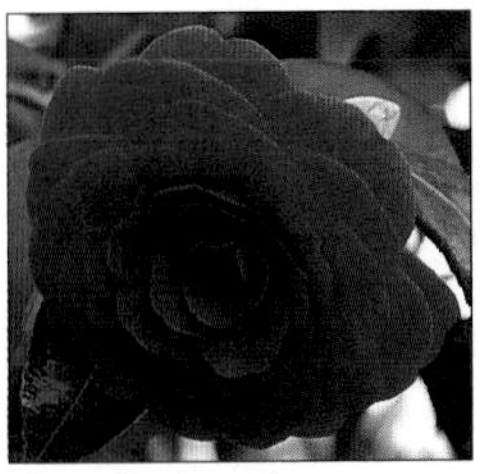
Camellia japonica 'Coquettii'

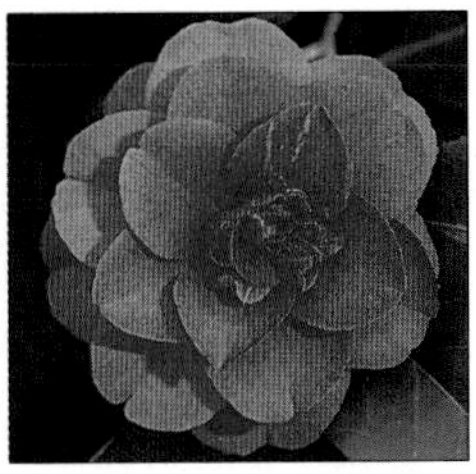
Camellia japonica 'Elegans'

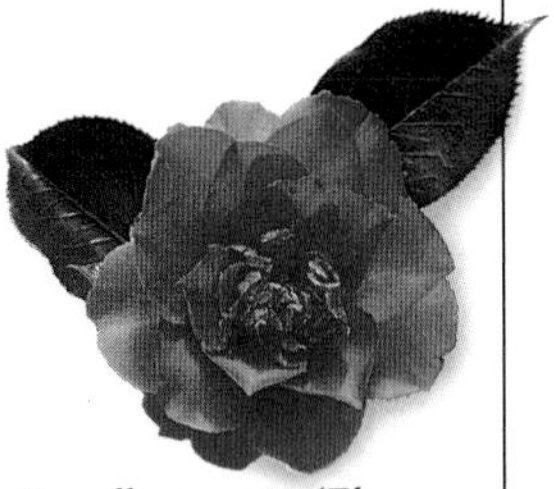
Camellia japonica 'Elegans Supreme'

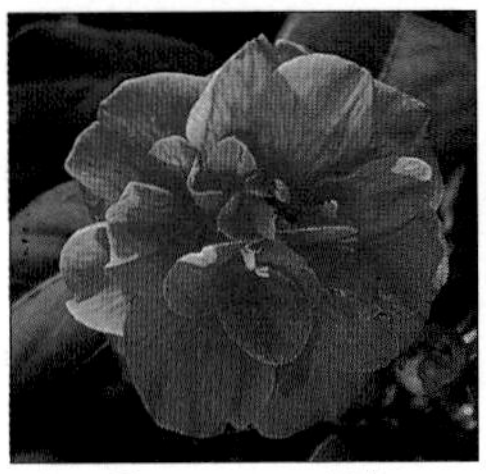
Camellia japonica 'Gloire de Nantes'

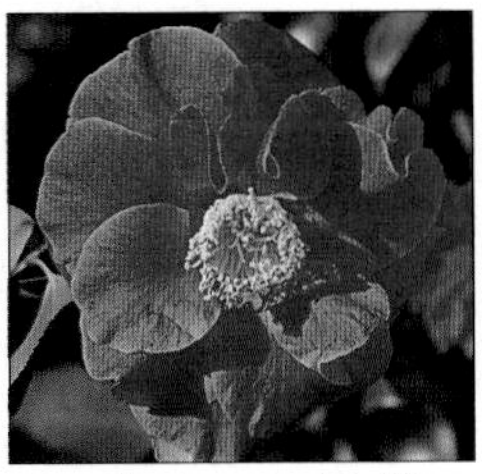
Camellia japonica 'Guilio Nuccio'

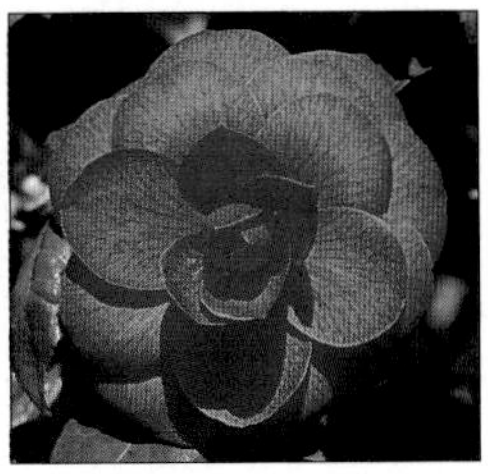
Camellia japonica 'Julia Drayton'

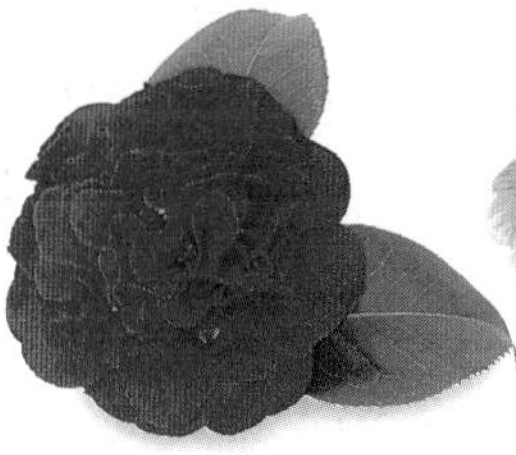
Camellia japonica 'Kramer's Supreme'

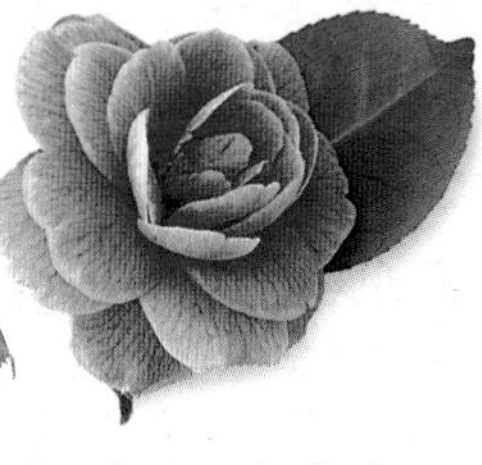
Camellia japonica 'Lady Loch'

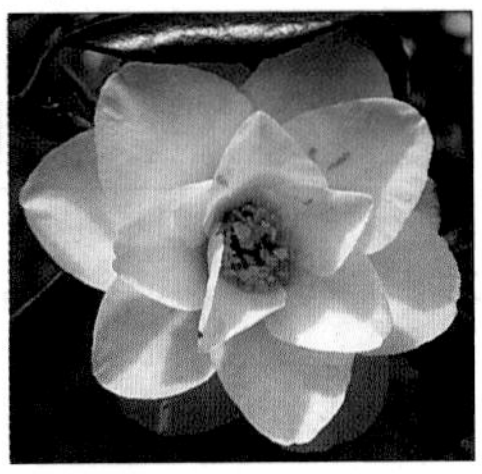
Camellia japonica 'Lady Vansittart'

CAMELLIA

stripes in 5 different colours, varying from white to red, on one shrub. The flowers are borne in early and mid-spring. **'Lavinia Maggi'** ■♀ syn. 'Contessa Lavinia Maggi', is a vigorous, spreading shrub, bearing medium, formal double white flowers, with red and pink stripes, in early and mid-spring. **'Lovelight'** ■ is vigorous and upright, with large leaves and large, semi-double white flowers, composed of broad petals around a small tuft of white and yellow stamens, from midwinter to mid-spring. **'Magellan'** see 'Dona Herzilia de Frietas Magalhaes'. **'Magnoliiflora'** see 'Hagoromo'. **'Man Size'** is spreading, bearing miniature, anemone-form white flowers in early and mid-spring. **'Margaret Davis Picotee'** ■ is upright, producing peony-form or formal double white flowers, with a narrow red margin to each petal. **'Mary Costa'** is upright, bearing large anemone-form white flowers, with elongated centres of yellow petaloids among incurved petals, from late winter to late spring. **'Masayoshi'** ♀ syn. 'Donckelaeri', is a vigorous shrub with oval-lance-shaped, dark green leaves and large, irregularly double white flowers, strongly marbled red, with some petals red or white-marbled red. **'Mathotiana Purple King'** see 'Julia Drayton'. **'Mathotiana Rubra'** see 'Julia Drayton'. **'Miss Charleston'** ♀ is upright, bearing very large, rich red flowers, peony-form in cool climates or semi-double in warmer areas, from early to late spring. **'Miss Universe'** ■ has a dense, spreading to upright habit, and from mid-spring to early summer bears large white flowers, which are formal double with notched petals in cool climates, and peony-form elsewhere. **'Mrs. D.W. Davis'** ■♀ is a broad, strong, upright shrub with very large, nodding, semi-double, soft pink flowers, borne from late winter to mid-spring. Best grown in a cool greenhouse. **'Nuccio's Gem'** is upright and dense in habit, bearing large, formal double white flowers, with spirally arranged petals, from late winter to mid-spring. Best grown in a cool greenhouse in frost-prone regions; outdoors, in temperate climates, the flowers are often irregular peony-form or semi-double; ✻✻✻ (borderline). **'Paul's Apollo'** ■ syn. 'Apollo', is spreading, bearing an abundance of showy, miniature, semi-double, rose-red flowers with yellow stamens, from early to late spring. **'Paul's Jupiter'** ■ syn. 'Jupiter', is a vigorous, upright shrub, bearing medium, single, carmine-rose flowers in early and mid-spring; the flowers have prominent yellow stamens with white filaments. **'Pink Perfection'** see *C. rusticana* 'Otome'. **'Primavera'** is a strong, upright shrub with medium to large, formal double white flowers. **'R.L. Wheeler'** ■♀ is a vigorous, rounded, open shrub with large, widely spaced leaves and very large, anemone-form or semi-double to incomplete double, brilliant red flowers, borne from early to late spring. **'Rubescens Major'** ■♀ is dense and upright, with distinctive, broad, rounded leaves and large, formal double or rose-form double crimson flowers, produced in mid-spring. **'Rudolph'** is upright, with medium, peony-form, brilliant red flowers, borne in early and mid-spring. **subsp. *rusticana* cultivars** see *C. rusticana* cultivars. **'Shiro Chan'** is similar to 'Elegans', and best grown in a cool greenhouse to protect its large, flat, anemone-form white flowers, initially pink at the petal bases, borne from early to late spring; ✻✻✻ (borderline). **'Sieboldii'** see 'Tricolor'. **'Something Beautiful'** is a strong, dense, erect shrub with miniature, formal double, pale pink flowers, the petals margined with burgundy-red, borne in early spring. **'Souvenir de Bahuaud-Litou'** ♀ is vigorous and upright, with medium, formal double, pale pink flowers in early spring. Best grown in a cool greenhouse; ✻✻✻ (borderline). **'Sylva'** is strong and upright, profusely bearing large, funnel-shaped, single, crimson-red flowers, with prominent, golden yellow stamens, in early spring. **'Tarô'an'** has a low, pendent habit, and medium, single, pale pink flowers, borne from late winter to mid-spring. Ideal for cascading over a bank, low wall, or stump. **'Tiffany'** is often vigorous and erect, but sometimes trailing, with large, peony-form, clear pink flowers. **'Tinsie'** see 'Bokuhan'. **'Tricolor'** ■♀ syn. 'Sieboldii', has bright green, crinkled, holly-like leaves, and produces medium, single or semi-double red flowers, striped pink and white, in early spring. Breeds almost true from seed. **'Ville de Nantes'**, similar to 'Masayoshi', is slow-growing and bushy, producing medium to large, semi-double red flowers with deeply fringed, white-marked petals, from early to late spring. **'White Nun'** ■ is a strong-growing shrub with slightly corrugated leaves and very large, flat, semi-double, pure white flowers, borne in mid-spring. **'Yours Truly'**, similar to 'Lady Vansittart', is upright, bearing small, trumpet-shaped flowers, crimson-streaked pink, with white-margined petals, in early and mid-spring.

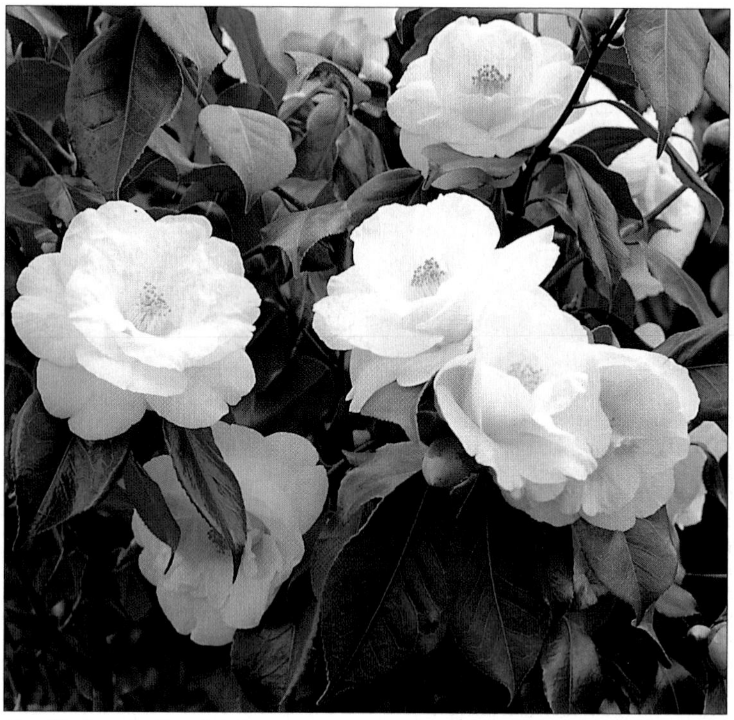
Camellia japonica 'Lovelight'

***C.* 'Jean Pursel'.** Strong-growing, upright shrub producing elliptic, dark green leaves, 15cm (6in) long. Very large, loose peony-form, purple-pink flowers are borne in mid-spring. ↕2–5m (6–15ft), ↔ 1.2–2.5m (4–8ft). ✻

***C.* 'Lasca Beauty'** ■♀ Open, stiffly branched, upright shrub with elliptic, dark green leaves, 13cm (5in) long, and very large, semi-double, pale pink flowers, borne in mid-spring. ↕2–5m (6–15ft), ↔ 1.5–3m (5–10ft). ✻

***C.* 'Leonard Messel'** ■♀ Very hardy, large, rounded, spreading shrub with oval, matt, dark green leaves, 8–15cm (3–6in) long. Large, loose, semi-double to peony-form, clear pink flowers are borne from early to late spring. Flowers tend to be semi-double under glass. ↕4m (12ft), ↔ 3m (10ft). ✻✻✻

***C.* 'Lila Naff'** ■ Strong, spreading shrub with smooth, elliptic to oval, dark green leaves, 10cm (4in) long. In mid-spring, bears very large, semi-double, clear silvery pink flowers. ↕2–7m (6–22ft), ↔ 1.2–2.5m (4–8ft). ✻

C. lutchuensis ♀ Spreading shrub or small tree with small, elliptic to oblong, bright green leaves, 4cm (1½in) long, covered with brown hairs. Bears scented, single white flowers, 1.5cm (½in) across, in late winter. ↕2–3m (6–10ft), ↔ 2–4m (6–12ft). Japan, Taiwan. ✻

***C.* x *maliflora*,** syn. *C. maliiflora*. Leafy shrub with elliptic, dark green leaves, 3.5–5cm (1½–2in) long. Bears peony-form flowers, 1.5–2cm (½–¾in) across, in 2 shades of pink, in early spring.

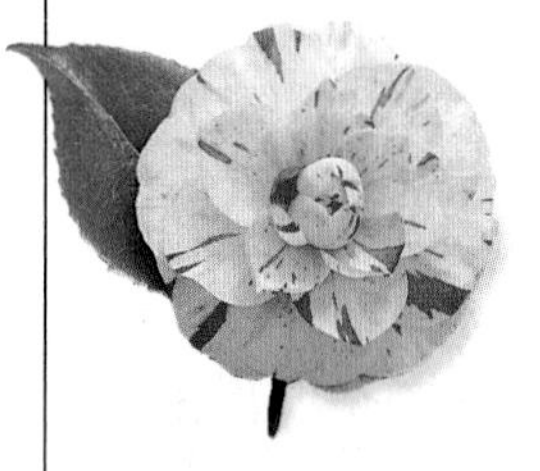
Camellia japonica 'Lavinia Maggi'

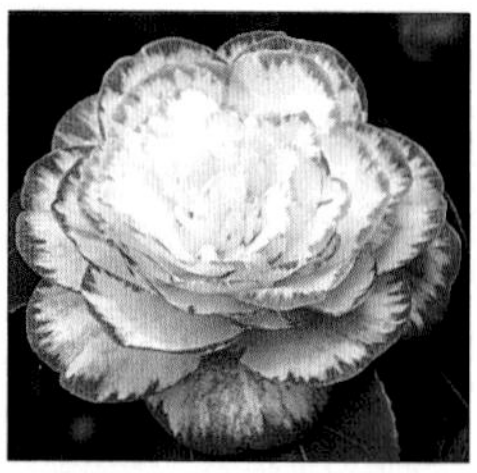
Camellia japonica 'Margaret Davis Picotee'

Camellia japonica 'Miss Universe'

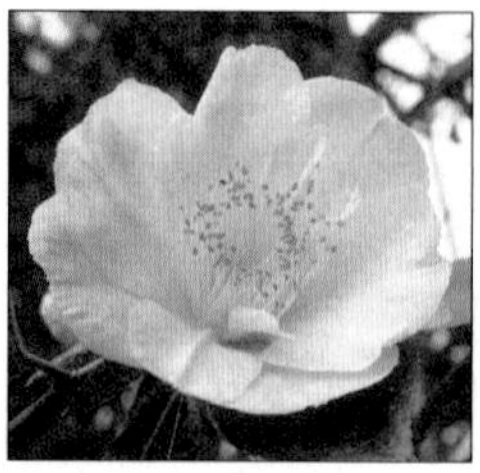
Camellia japonica 'Mrs. D.W. Davis'

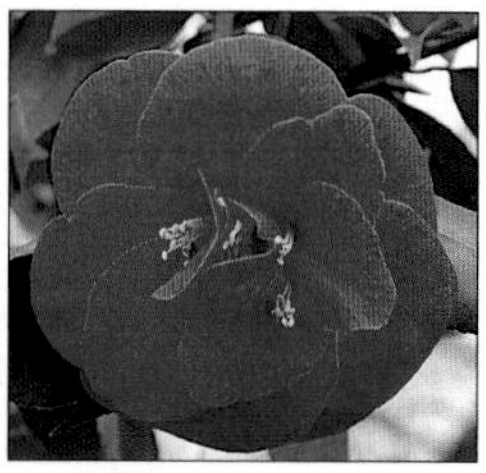
Camellia japonica 'Paul's Apollo'

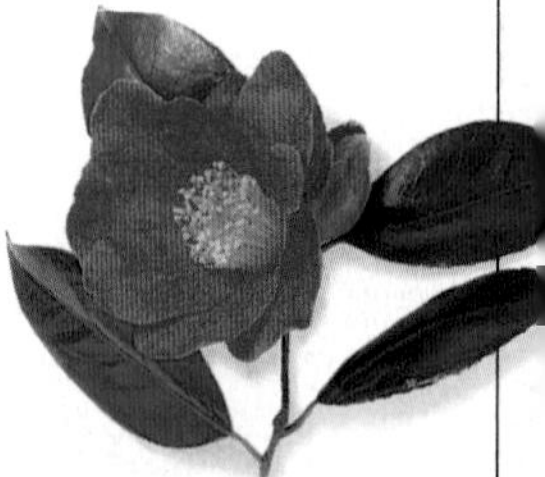
Camellia japonica 'Paul's Jupiter'

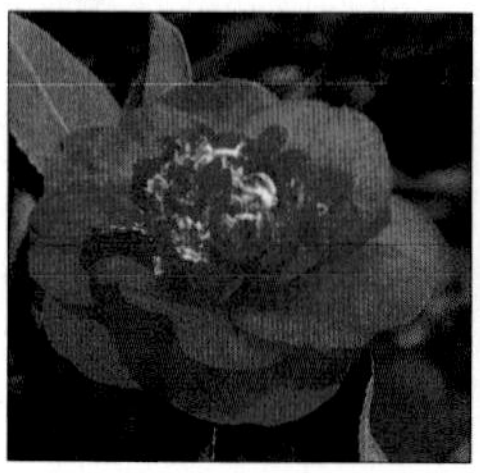
Camellia japonica 'R.L. Wheeler'

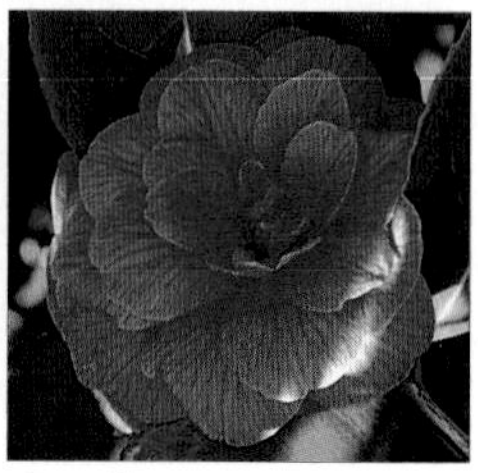
Camellia japonica 'Rubescens Major'

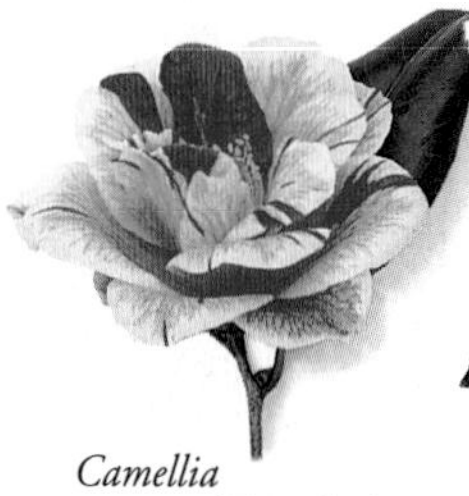
Camellia japonica 'Tricolor'

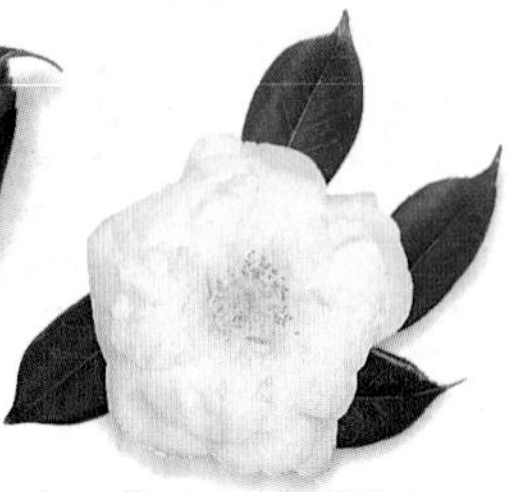
Camellia japonica 'White Nun'

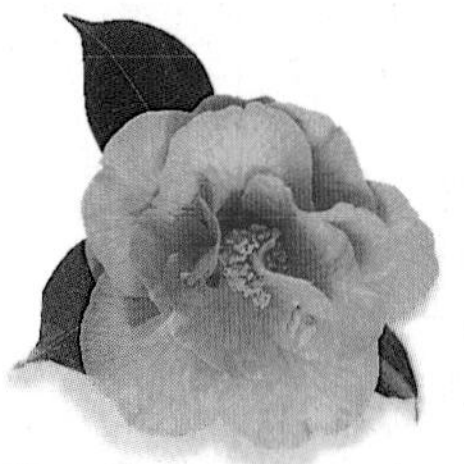
Camellia 'Lasca Beauty'

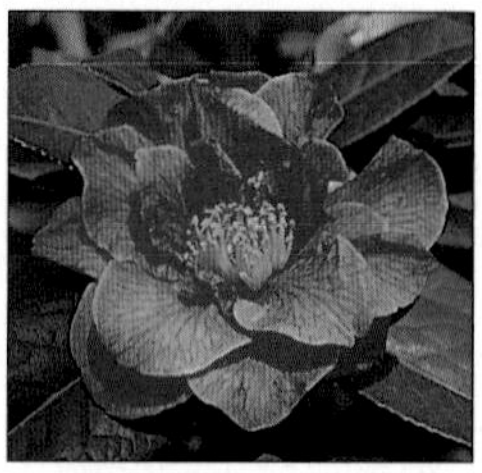
Camellia 'Leonard Messel'

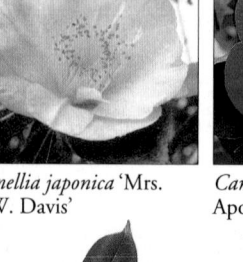

Good for training against a wall. ↕ 2.5m (8ft), ↔ 2m (6ft). Garden origin. ✻✻✻
C. maliiflora see *C.* x *maliflora.*
***C.* 'Nicky Crisp'.** Compact, slow-growing, rounded shrub with elliptic, dark green leaves, 8cm (3in) long, and large, semi-double, lavender-pink flowers borne from late winter to mid-spring. ↕↔ 1–2m (3–6ft). ✻✻✻
***C.* 'Night Rider'.** Upright shrub with narrowly elliptic, dark green leaves, 7cm (3in) long. Bears small, semi-double, dark red flowers from late winter to late spring; the yellow stamens remain when the petals drop. Unusual in appearance, the plant appearing to be suffused red, although the leaves are green. ↕ 2–4m (6–12ft), ↔ 1.2–2.5m (4–8ft). ✻✻✻
C. nitidissima ■ syn. *C. chrysantha.* Large shrub producing oval, dark green leaves, 8–11cm (3–4½in) long, with deeply indented veins. Fragrant, single yellow flowers, 2.5–5cm (1–2in) across, are borne from the leaf axils from early to late winter. Requires a warm, humid site in partial shade. ↕ 2–3m (6–10ft), ↔ 3m (10ft). S. China, Vietnam. ❀ (min. 7°C (45°F)
C. oleifera 🌳 Small, erect tree with slender branches and elliptic, oblong-elliptic, or obovate leaves, 3.5–9cm (1½–3½in) long, dark green above, light green beneath. In mid- and late autumn, bears scented, single white flowers, 5–6cm (2–2½in) across, occasionally 8–9cm (3–3½in) across. ↕ 7m (22ft), ↔ 3–4m (10–12ft). China. ✻✻✻
C. reticulata 🌳 Open-branched small tree or large shrub with broadly elliptic to oblong-elliptic, leathery leaves, 8–11cm (3–4½in) long, dark green above, paler beneath. In spring, bears single, rose-red flowers, to 11cm (4½in) across. ↕ to 15m (50ft), ↔ 5m (15ft). China. ✻. Flowers of cultivars vary from single to semi-double to peony-form, and are pink, red, or white; they are borne in mid-spring unless stated otherwise. **'Arch of Triumph'** ■🏆 is shrubby, with strong, erect growth, large leaves, and very large, loose peony-form, orange-tinted, crimson-pink flowers, to 17cm (7in) across; ↕ to 3m (10ft). **'Captain Rawes'** ■🏆 is a large, spreading shrub or small tree with very large, semi-double to loose peony-form, carmine-rose flowers, 14–17cm (5½–7in) across, borne in mid- and late

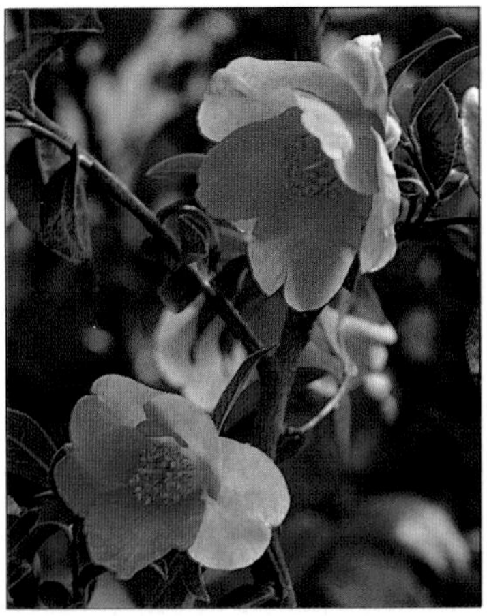
Camellia saluenensis

spring; ↕ to 10m (30ft). **'Curtain Call'** is a strong, spreading shrub with large, semi-double, deep coral-pink flowers, 15–17cm (6–7in) across. **'Elizabeth Johnstone'** 🌳 forms a small, erect tree with large, single, rose-pink flowers, to 11cm (4½in) wide, borne in early and mid-spring. **'Flore Pleno'** see 'Songzilin'. **'Mandalay Queen'** ■🏆 is a large, widely branching, erect shrub with broad leaves, and large, semi-double, deep rose-pink flowers, to 14cm (5½in) wide. **'Miss Tulare'** ■ is a large, strong-growing, many-branched shrub, bearing large, peony-form or rose-form double flowers, to 13cm (5in) across, with waxy, brilliant rose-red petals. **'Pagoda'** see 'Songzilin'. **'Robert Fortune'** see 'Songzilin'. **'Songzilin'**, syn. 'Flore Pleno', 'Pagoda', 'Robert Fortune', is an upright shrub bearing large, formal double or rose-form double, light red flowers, to 13cm (5in) across, in early and mid-spring. **'William Hertrich'** is a tall, open-growing shrub with very large, semi-double to loose peony-form, dark cherry-red flowers, to 17cm (7in) across.
C. rosiflora. Shrub of open, lax habit, producing elliptic to broadly elliptic leaves, 4.5–8cm (1¾–3in) long, dark green above, paler beneath. Single pink flowers, to 3.5cm (1½in) across, are borne in mid-spring. ↕ 2.5m (8ft), ↔ 1–2m (3–6ft). China. ✻✻✻
***C.* 'Royalty'** ■ Open, lax shrub with elliptic, glossy, dark green leaves, 11cm (4½in) long. In mid- and late spring, bears very large, semi-double, light red flowers. Train against a shady wall. ↕ 1m (3ft), ↔ 60cm (24in) ✻
***C. rusticana* cultivars**, syn. *C. japonica* subsp. *rusticana* cultivars (Snow camellia). Selections from the Japanese species *C. rusticana* have an erect to spreading habit and elliptic, dark green leaves, 5–12cm (2–5in) long. They bear single or double flowers, 3–4cm (1¼–1½in) across. ↕ 2–4m (6–12ft), ↔ 1–3m (3–10ft). ✻✻✻. **'Otome'**, syn. *C. japonica* 'Pink Perfection', *C. rusticana* 'Frau Minna Seidel', 'Pink Pearl', 'Usuôtome', bears many-petalled, formal double, pale pink flowers from late winter to mid-spring. **'Reigyoku'** has variegated leaves with distinctive gold "feathers", and bears small, single red flowers in early and mid-spring.
C. saluenensis ■ Freely branched shrub with narrowly ovate, glossy, dark green leaves, to 8cm (3in) long. In early and mid-spring, bears single, white, pink, pink-and-white, or pinkish red flowers, 3.5–5cm (1½–2in) across. ↕↔ 1–5m (3–15ft). China (Yunnan). ✻✻✻
C. sasanqua 🌳–🌳 Upright to spreading shrub or small tree with elliptic, oblong-elliptic, or broadly elliptic leaves, to 8cm (3in) long, dark green above, paler beneath. Bears fragrant, single, cup-shaped white flowers, 5–7cm (2–3in) across, in mid- and late autumn. Will tolerate sun; in cold areas may be grown in containers and taken indoors to flower. ↕ to 6m (20ft), ↔ to 3m (10ft). Japan. ✻✻✻. **'Cleopatra'** is low and compact, bearing medium, semi-double, rose-pink flowers. **'Mine-no-yuki'** is vigorous, with a willowy, spreading habit, and dark green leaves, 4cm (1½in) long. Bears small, double white flowers from mid-autumn to early winter. **'Narumigata'** ■🏆 is erect, with small, fragrant, single white, pink-tinged flowers. **'Navajo'** is upright, with large, semi-double white, red-margined flowers. **'Nodami-ushiro'** is erect and bushy, bearing large, single and semi-double, deep pink flowers. **'Shishigashira'** ■ has small, semi-double to rose-form double, pinkish red flowers. **'Yae-arare'** is spreading, and produces large, single flowers with reflexed, long pink-tipped white petals.
***C.* 'Satan's Robe'** ■🏆 Vigorous, erect shrub with broadly elliptic, glossy, dark

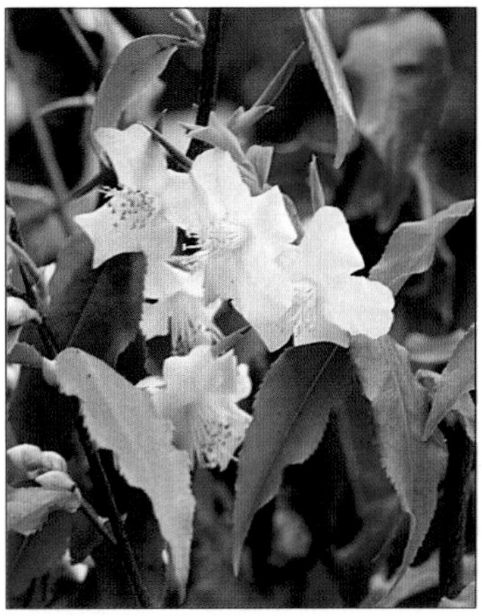
Camellia tsaii

green leaves, 12–16cm (5–6in) long. Large, semi-double, bright carmine-red flowers, with yellow stamens, are borne from early to late spring. ↕ 3–5m (10–15ft), ↔ 2–3m (6–10ft). ✻✻
***C.* 'Shiro-wabisuke'** ■ Rounded shrub with elliptic to oblong-elliptic, dark green leaves, 8–12cm (3–5in) long. From midwinter to early spring, bears small, fragrant, single white flowers. ↕↔ 1.4m (4½ft). ✻✻✻
***C.* 'Sparkling Burgundy'.** Spreading shrub with narrowly ovate, dark green leaves, 8–12cm (3–5in) long. Bears medium, peony-form, ruby-red flowers in early and midwinter. ↕ 1.5–3m (5–10ft), ↔ 1–2m (3–6ft). ✻✻✻
***C.* 'Spring Festival'** ■🏆 Narrow, upright shrub with elliptic, dark green leaves, 8–12cm (3–5in) long. In mid- and late spring, bears small, formal double pink flowers. ↕ 2–4m (6–12ft), ↔ 0.6–2m (2–6ft). ✻✻✻
C. taliensis 🌳 Spreading shrub or small tree with elliptic to broadly elliptic, bright green leaves, 9–15cm (3½–6in) long. From midwinter to late spring, produces single white flowers, 5–6cm (2–2½in) across. ↕ 2–7m (6–22ft), ↔ 2–4m (6–12ft). China (Yunnan). ✻
C. tsaii ■🏆🌳 Large, pendent shrub or small tree with oblong-elliptic, glossy, dark green leaves with wavy margins, to 9cm (3½in) long. Miniature, cup-shaped, single white flowers, 2cm (¾in) across, are produced from the leaf axils in mid- and late winter. ↕ to 10m (30ft),

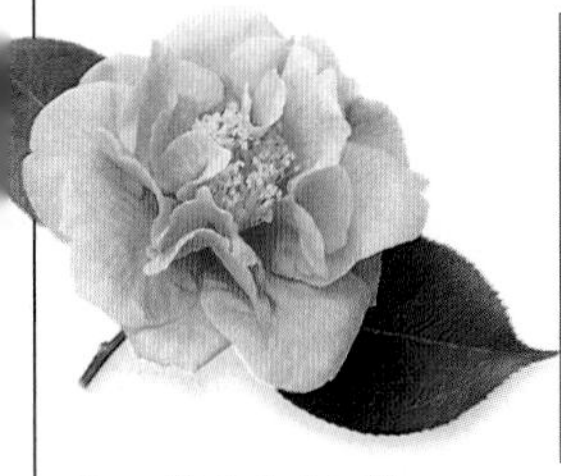
Camellia 'Lila Naff'

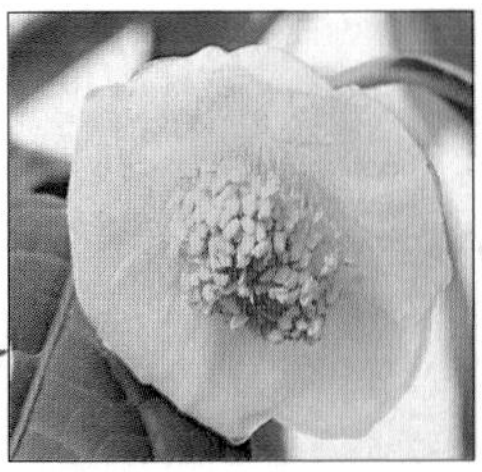
Camellia nitidissima

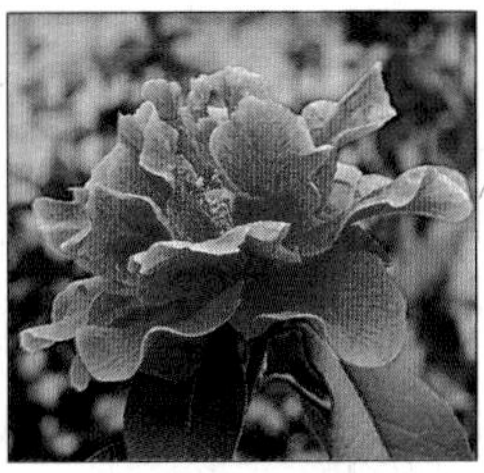
Camellia reticulata 'Arch of Triumph'

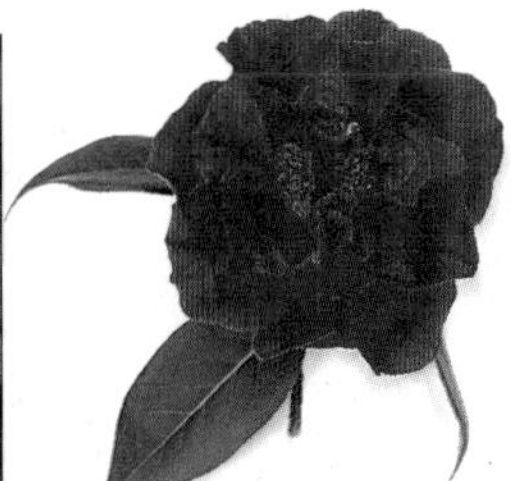
Camellia reticulata 'Captain Rawes'

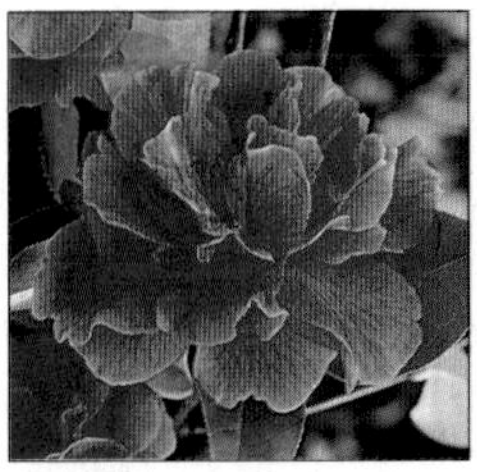
Camellia reticulata 'Mandalay Queen'

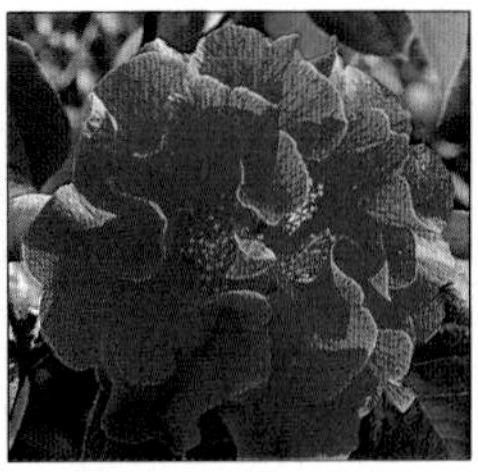
Camellia reticulata 'Miss Tulare'

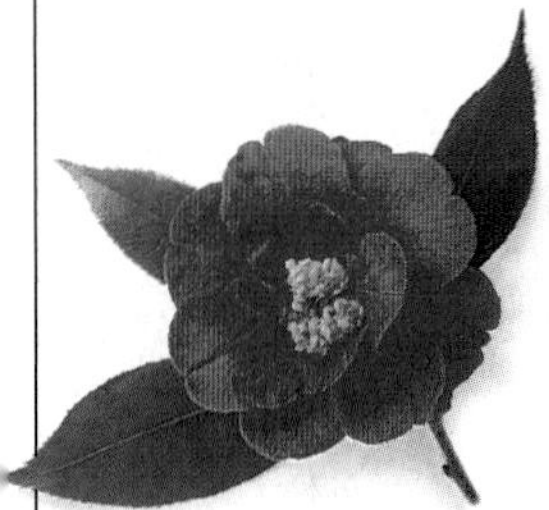
Camellia 'Royalty'

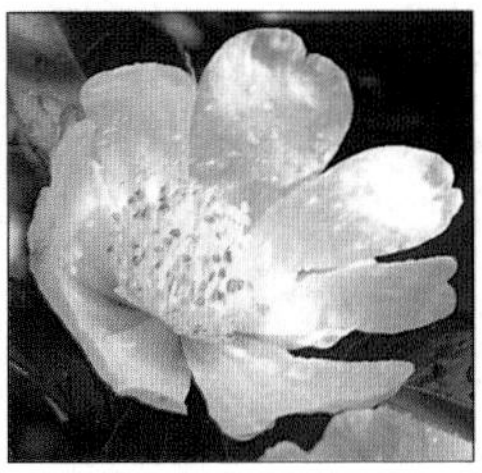
Camellia sasanqua 'Narumigata'

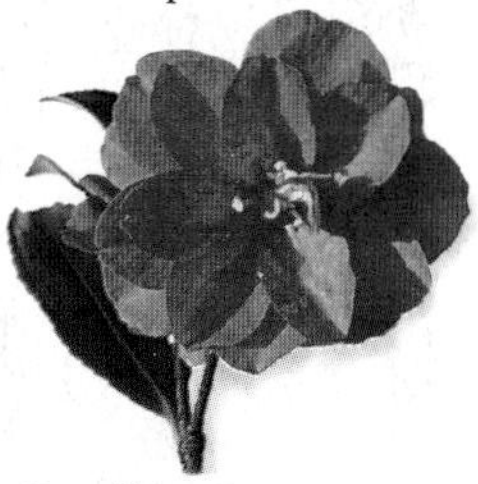
Camellia sasanqua 'Shishigashira'

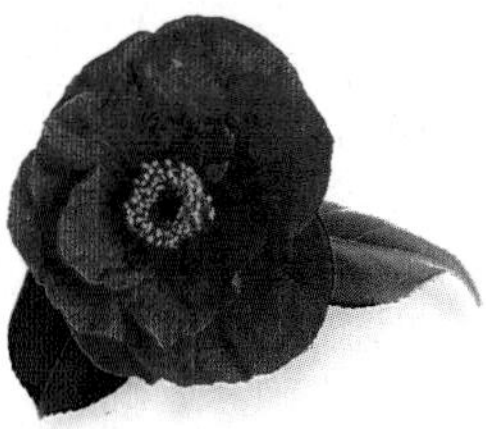
Camellia 'Satan's Robe'

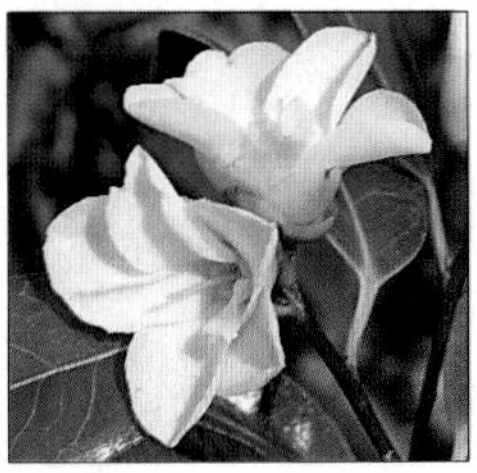
Camellia 'Shiro-wabisuke'

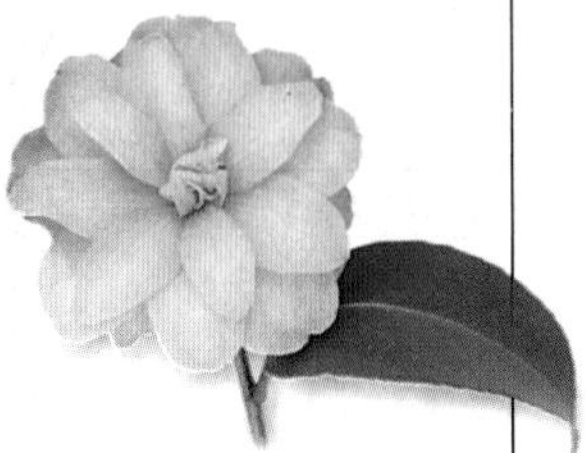
Camellia 'Spring Festival'

↔ to 5m (15ft). W. China, Burma, N. Vietnam. ❄

***C.* x *vernalis* cultivars.** Selections from *C.* x *vernalis* are erect to spreading shrubs with elliptic, dark green leaves, 5–14cm (2–5½in) long. They bear semi-double to double flowers, 6–8cm (2½–3in) across, in late winter and early spring (sometimes late autumn and early winter). ↕ 2–5m (6–15ft), ↔ 1–4m (3–12ft). ❄❄❄. **'Dawn'** see 'Ginryû'. **'Egao'** bears semi-double, deep pink flowers with bold yellow stamens. **'Ginryû'**, syn. 'Dawn', has semi-double or formal double, pink-tinged white flowers, in late winter and early spring. **'Star above Star'** ▣ bears semi-double flowers, with layers of reflexed, white or lavender-pink petals, in late winter and early spring. **'Yuletide'** has dense foliage and bears a profusion of single red flowers, with bright yellow stamens, in late autumn and early winter.

***C.* x *williamsii* cultivars.** Selections from *C.* x *williamsii* (*C. japonica* x *C. saluenensis*) are strong-growing shrubs with elliptic to broadly elliptic, glossy, bright green leaves, 6–10cm (2½–4in) long. They bear white to deep pink flowers in mid- and late spring, unless stated otherwise. They usually resemble *C. japonica* in their foliage and *C. saluenensis* in their flowers. ↕ 2–5m (6–15ft), ↔ 1–3m (3–10ft). ❄❄❄. **'Anticipation'** ▣🏆 is a narrow, upright shrub bearing very large, peony-form crimson flowers in late winter and early spring; ↕ 4m (12ft), ↔ 2m (6ft). **'Bow Bells'** ▣ is a dense shrub with small leaves, and profuse, medium, trumpet-shaped, single pink flowers borne from midwinter to mid-spring. Best grown against a shady wall; ↕ 4m (12ft). **'Bowen Bryant'** 🏆 is a wide, upright shrub with dark green foliage, and large, bell-shaped, semi-double, rose-pink

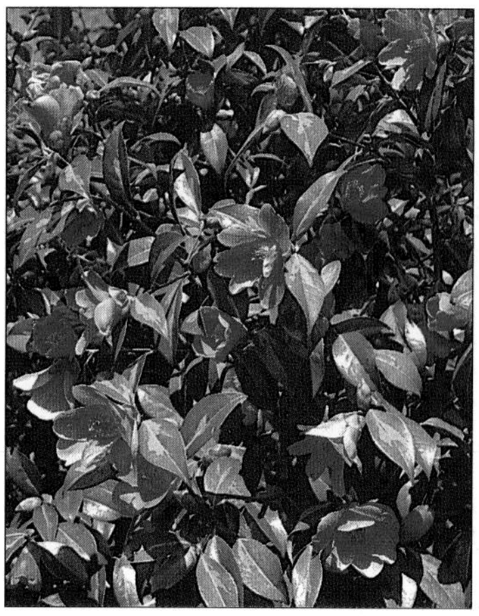

Camellia x *williamsii* 'Golden Spangles'

flowers borne from early to late spring. **'Brigadoon'** ▣🏆 is an open, rounded shrub with very large, semi-double, rose-pink, silver-tinged flowers with broad, downward-curving petals. **'Buttons 'n' Bows'** is compact, bearing small, formal double flowers in 2 shades of pink, from late winter to mid-spring. **'Caerhays'** ▣ is arching, with large leaves and large, anemone-form to loose peony-form, crimson-pink flowers, maturing purple; ↕ 2–4m (6–12ft), ↔ 1–3m (3–10ft). **'Debbie's Carnation'** is compact and erect, with medium, full peony-form, cerise-pink flowers borne from early to late spring; they drop whole when still coloured; ↕ 1.5–3m (5–10ft), ↔ 1–2m (3–6ft). **'Donation'** ▣🏆 is compact and erect, bearing large, semi-double pink flowers from late winter to late spring. In partial shade, its flowers are deeper in colour and last longer; ↕ 5m (15ft), ↔ 2.5m (8ft). **'Dream Boat'** ▣ has a spreading habit, and bears medium, formal double, pale purplish pink flowers, with incurved petals, in mid-spring. **'E.G. Waterhouse'** ▣ is a narrow, upright shrub with pale green foliage, and medium, formal double, pale pink flowers borne in mid-spring. **'Elsie Jury'** 🏆 is tall and upright, with well-spaced, spreading branches, and large, full peony-form pink flowers borne from early to late spring. **'E.T.R. Carlyon'** 🏆 has long, arching branches and bears medium, semi-double to rose-form, double white flowers. **'Francis Hanger'** ▣ is upright, bearing medium, single white flowers, with gold stamens, in early and mid-spring; ↕ 1.5m (5ft), occasionally more. **'Galaxie'** 🏆 is a rounded shrub bearing medium, formal double, light pink flowers, with thin red stripes and streaks, in mid-spring. **'Garden Glory'** is rounded and upright, with formal double or rose-form double, rich pink flowers produced in early and mid-spring. **'Gay Time'** is upright, with large, semi-double to loose peony-form, bright pink flowers, darker on the petal margins, borne in early and mid-spring. **'George Blandford'** ▣🏆 is vigorous, bearing medium, semi-double to peony-form, crimson-rose flowers; ↕ 4m (12ft), ↔ 4m (12ft). **'Golden Spangles'** ▣ a sport from 'Mary Christian', is upright, with a golden or yellow-green central zone on each leaf, and single, bright pinkish red flowers, 5–7cm (2–3in) across. **'J.C. Williams'** ▣🏆 has wide-sweeping branches and medium, single, pale pink flowers, with darker shading, in early and mid-spring. Good for training on a partially shaded wall. **'Joan Trehane'** ▣🏆 has strong, upright growth and large, rose-form double, rose-pink flowers. **'Julia Hamiter'** 🏆 is an open, spreading shrub, similar to 'Donation', bearing flat, medium, rose-form double flowers. The flowers have pink-flushed white petals, greenish white at the bases, surrounding cream petaloids. **'Jury's Yellow'** ▣ is narrow and erect, bearing medium, anemone-form white flowers, with centres of yellow petaloids. **'Lady's Maid'** is a vigorous shrub with medium, pendent, semi-double, bright pink flowers; ↕ 4m (12ft). **'Mary Christian'** ▣🏆 is upright, with dull, dark green foliage and trumpet-shaped, single, carmine-pink flowers, 5–7cm (2–3in) across, borne in late winter and early spring. **'Mary Larcom'** ▣ is a large, rounded, open shrub with broadly elliptic, blunt-tipped, dark green leaves and medium, single pink flowers; ↕ 4m (12ft). **'Mary Phoebe Taylor'** is strong-growing, with downward- and outward-sweeping branches and large, peony-form or semi-double, clear pink flowers. **'Mona Jury'** is an open shrub with medium, loose peony-form, apricot-pink flowers. **'St. Ewe'** ▣🏆 is a rounded shrub bearing large, trumpet-shaped, single, rose-pink flowers, in early and mid-spring. **'Tiptoe'** is an upright shrub producing medium, semi-double, pale pink flowers. **'Water Lily'** ▣🏆 is an upright shrub with large, formal double, deep rose-pink flowers. **'Wilber Foss'** ▣ is rounded, with dark green foliage and large, broad, peony-form, brilliant pink-red flowers; ↕ to 2m (6ft).

C. yuhsienensis 🗨 Rounded shrub or small tree with elliptic to oval, dark green leaves, to 9cm (3½in) long. Small, very fragrant, single white flowers, 5–7cm (2–3in) across, are produced in early and mid-spring. ↕ to 3m (10ft), ↔ 0.75–2m (2½–6ft). China (Hunan). ❄❄❄

▷**Camellia,**
Common see *Camellia japonica*
Snow see *Camellia rusticana* cultivars
▷**Camellia rose** see *Rosa laevigata*

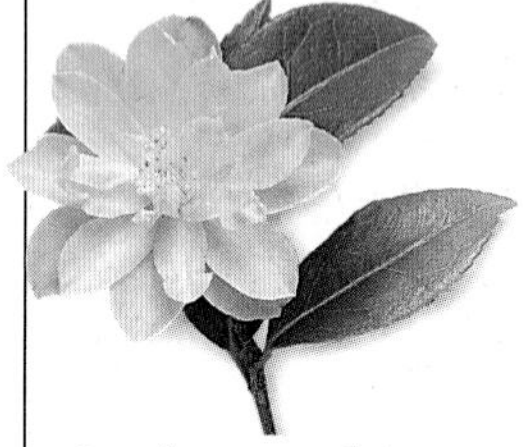

Camellia x *vernalis* 'Star above Star'

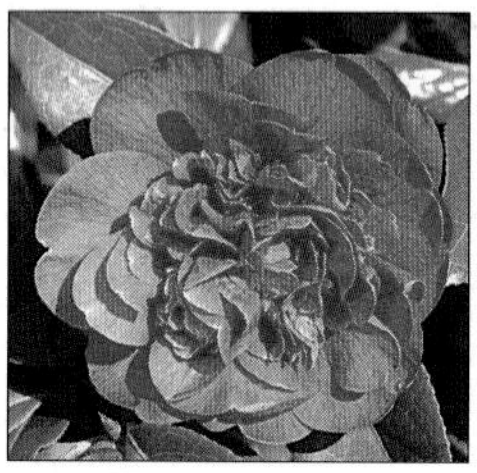

Camellia x *williamsii* 'Anticipation'

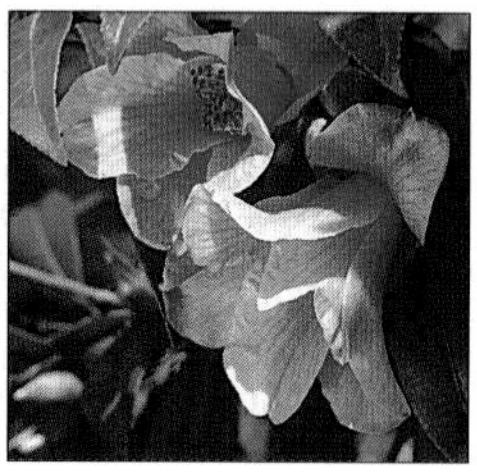

Camellia x *williamsii* 'Bow Bells'

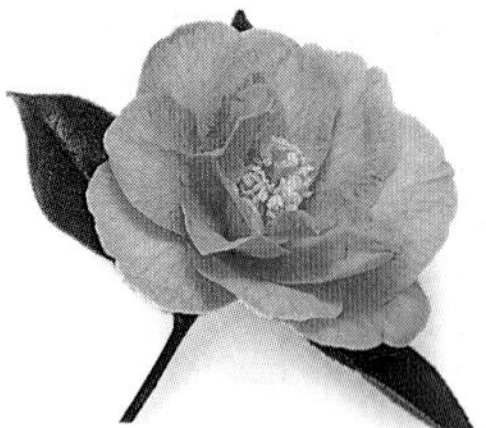

Camellia x *williamsii* 'Brigadoon'

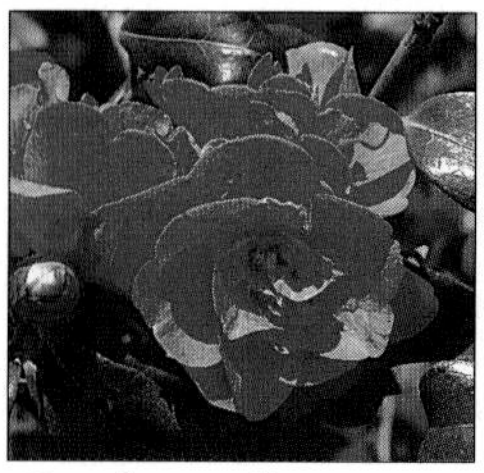

Camellia x *williamsii* 'Caerhays'

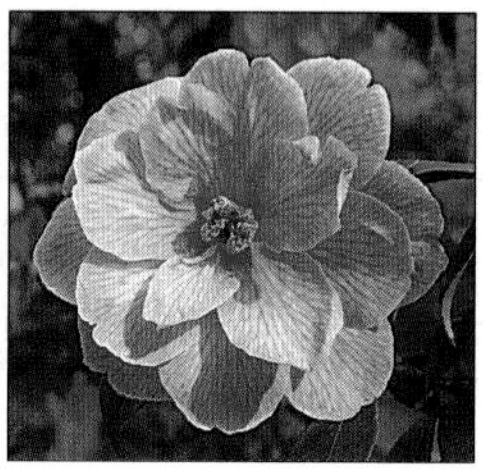

Camellia x *williamsii* 'Donation'

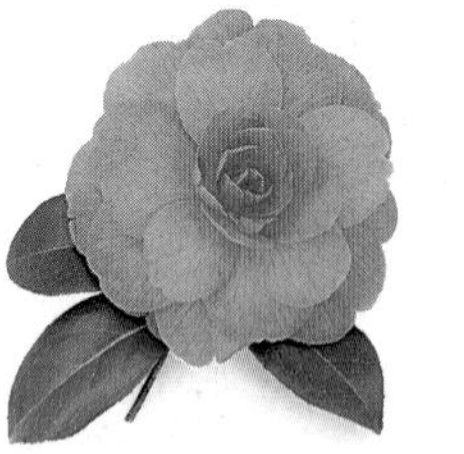

Camellia x *williamsii* 'Dream Boat'

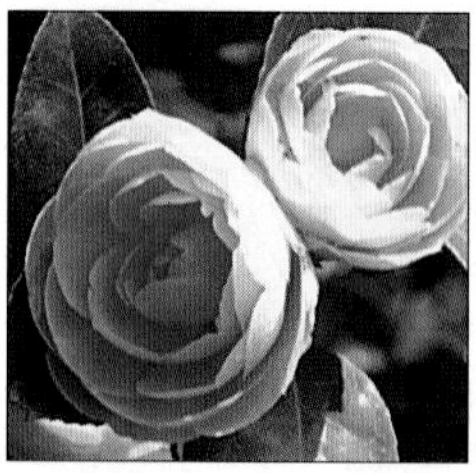

Camellia x *williamsii* 'E.G. Waterhouse'

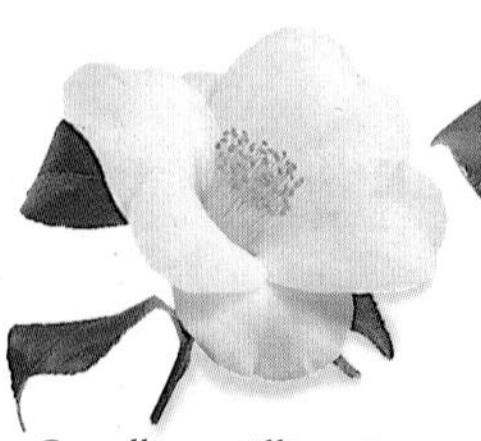

Camellia x *williamsii* 'Francis Hanger'

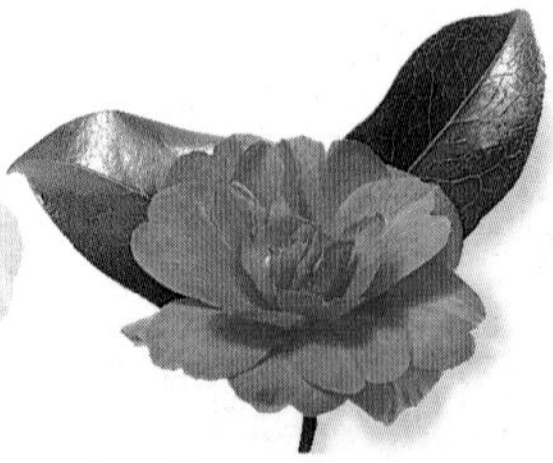

Camellia x *williamsii* 'George Blandford'

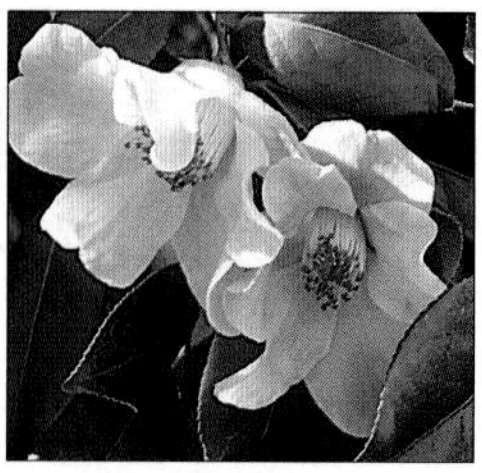

Camellia x *williamsii* 'J.C. Williams'

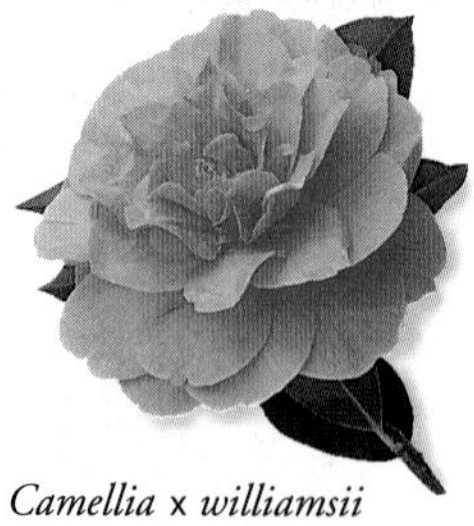

Camellia x *williamsii* 'Joan Trehane'

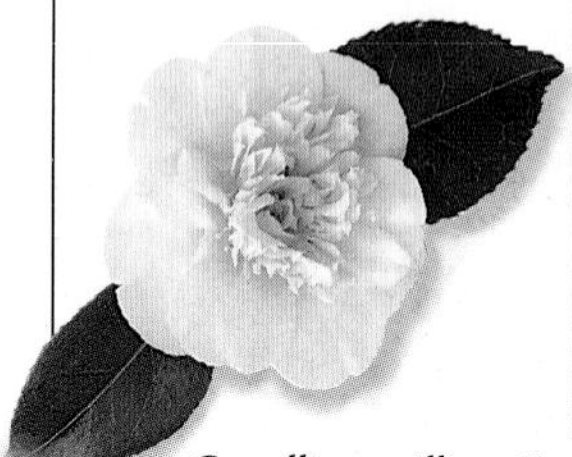

Camellia x *williamsii* 'Jury's Yellow'

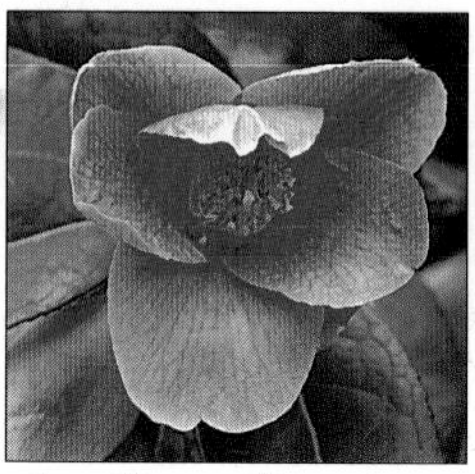

Camellia x *williamsii* 'Mary Christian'

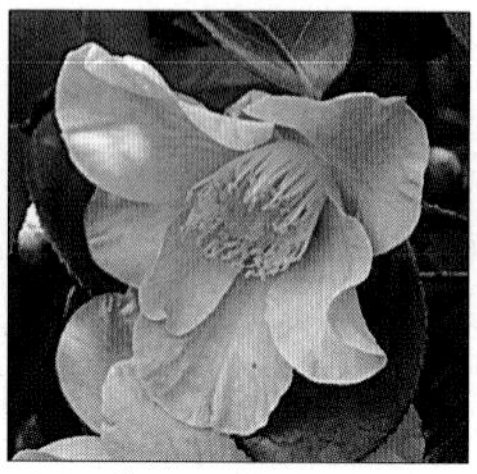

Camellia x *williamsii* 'Mary Larcom'

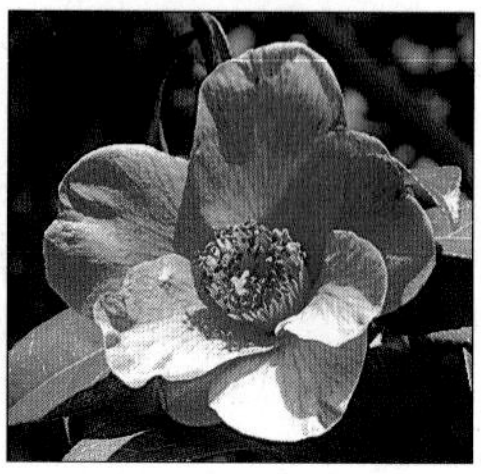

Camellia x *williamsii* 'St. Ewe'

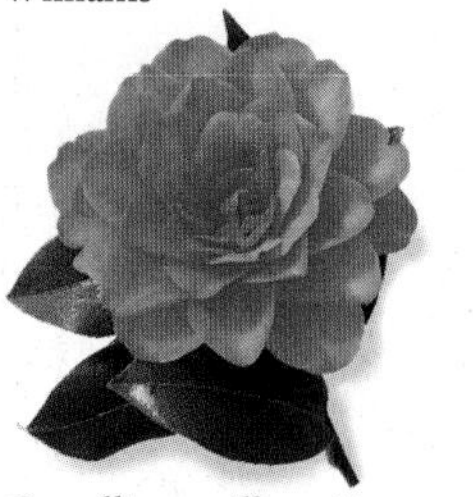

Camellia x *williamsii* 'Water Lily'

Camellia x *williamsii* 'Wilber Foss'

CAMPANULA

Bellflower

CAMPANULACEAE

Genus of about 300 species of annuals, biennials, and perennials, some of which are evergreen. They are distributed widely throughout temperate zones of the N. hemisphere, particularly in S. Europe and Turkey, and grow in diverse habitats, from high alpine rock crevices and scree to moorland, meadows, and woodland. Most species are easily cultivated and provide a long flowering display, blooming from late spring to late summer. The flowers are usually borne in panicles, racemes, or clustered heads, but are sometimes solitary. They vary from tubular to bell- or star-shaped, and may also be cup- or saucer-shaped. The entire or toothed leaves are alternate. Campanulas vary in habit from mat-forming, dwarf perennials to herbaceous species, 2m (6ft) tall.

Dwarf campanulas are ideal for a rock garden or alpine house, and many grow well on a wall or sunny bank. The taller perennials are excellent for a mixed or herbaceous border, or for naturalizing in a wildflower or woodland garden. In frost-prone regions, grow less hardy species, such as *C. isophylla*, in a conservatory or cool greenhouse.

• **HARDINESS** Fully hardy to frost tender.

• **CULTIVATION** For ease of reference, campanulas have been divided into the following cultivation groups:

1. Campanulas that need fertile, neutral to alkaline, moist but well-drained soil, in sun or partial shade; the delicate flower colours are best preserved in shade. *C. pyramidalis*, *C. sarmatica*, and *C. trachelium* thrive in dry soils, the first 2 in full sun, the last in partial shade. Taller species require staking. Cut back after flowering to prevent self-seeding and to encourage a second, less profuse flush of flowers.

2. Robust, rock-garden species, requiring moist but well-drained soil in sun or partial shade. Some thrive on a sunny wall or bank.

3. Species that enjoy the winter protection of deep, dry snow cover in their natural habitat and, in cultivation, will not tolerate winter wet. Grow in a scree bed, in tufa, in gritty, moist but sharply drained soil in a trough, or in an alpine house in loam-based potting compost (JI No.1) with up to one-third by volume of grit.

4. Tender perennials. In frost-prone areas, grow under glass in loam-based potting compost (JI No.2) in bright filtered light with good ventilation. In growth, water moderately and apply a balanced liquid fertilizer monthly; keep moist in winter. In frost-free areas, grow outdoors in an open site in well-drained, fertile soil in sun or partial shade. Cut dead stems to the base before winter.

• **PROPAGATION** Sow seed in containers in a cold frame in spring, except for alpines, which should be sown in an open frame in autumn. Divide in spring or autumn. Take basal cuttings of perennials in spring. To increase smaller species, take cuttings of new growth in early summer, or root rosettes of rosette-forming species in spring. Take tip cuttings of *C. isophylla* in early spring, and root with bottom heat.

• **PESTS AND DISEASES** Vulnerable to slugs and snails outdoors, and to aphids and red spider mites under glass. Some species, particularly *C. persicifolia* and its cultivars, are susceptible to rust. Vine weevil may affect *C. isophylla* and other tender species under glass. Powdery mildew may also be a problem.

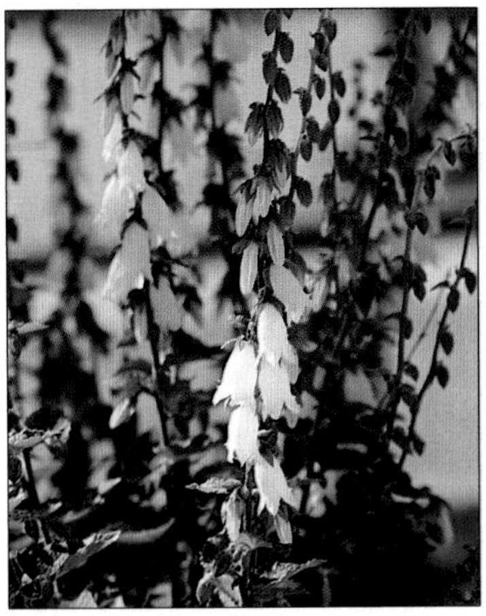

Campanula alliariifolia

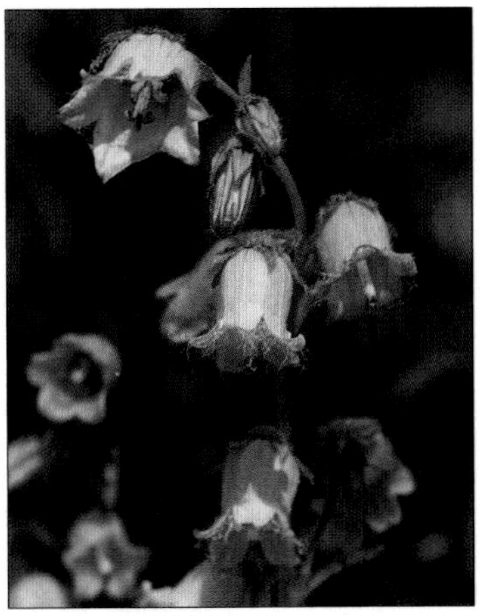

Campanula barbata

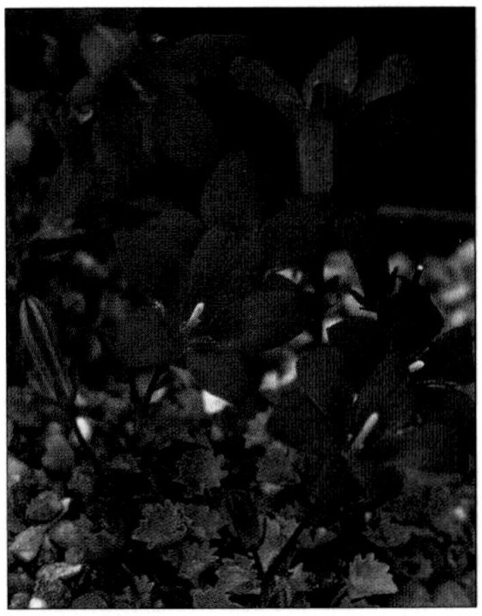

Campanula 'Birch Hybrid'

C. acutangula see *C. arvatica.*

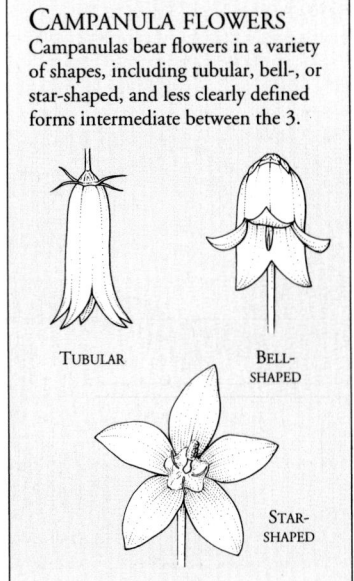

C. alliariifolia ▣ (Ivory bells). Vigorous, clump-forming perennial with heart-shaped, toothed, grey-hairy basal leaves, 8cm (3in) long. Leafy stems bear one-sided racemes of pendent, tubular-bell-shaped white flowers, 2cm (¾in) long, with sharply pointed petals, from midsummer to early autumn. Cultivation group 1. ↕ 30–60cm (12–24in), ↔ 45cm (18in). Caucasus, Turkey. ❄❄❄

***C. amabilis* 'Planiflora'** see *C. persicifolia* var. *planiflora.*

C. arvatica 🏆 syn. *C. acutangula.* Carpet-forming perennial with underground runners, and tufts of broadly ovate-heart-shaped, toothed, mid-green leaves, 5–8mm (¼–⅜in) long. Solitary, upturned, shallowly funnel-shaped, violet, pale blue, or white flowers, 2–4cm (¾–1½in) long, are borne on short stems in summer. Cultivation group 2. ↕ 8–10cm (3–4in), ↔ to 20cm (8in). N. Spain. ❄❄❄

C. aucheri. Densely tufted perennial with clustered rosettes of spoon-shaped to oblong, toothed, hairy, mid-green leaves, to 8cm (3in) long. In summer, upturned, open bell-shaped, deep violet-blue flowers, 2–5cm (¾–2in) across, are borne singly on spreading stems. Cultivation group 2 or 3. ↕ to 10cm (4in), ↔ 20cm (8in). E. Caucasus, Turkey, N. Iran. ❄❄❄

C. barbata ▣ (Bearded bellflower). Short-lived perennial or biennial with rosettes of narrowly lance-shaped to oblong, slightly toothed, hairy, pale to mid-green leaves, 6–8cm (2½–3in) long. In early summer, erect stems bear one-sided racemes of pendent, bell-shaped, lavender-blue, sometimes white flowers, 2–3cm (¾–1¼in) long, the petals fringed with white hairs. Cultivation group 2. ↕ to 30cm (12in), ↔ 20cm (8in). Mountains of Norway, Alps. ❄❄❄

C. bellardii see *C. cochleariifolia.*

C. betulaefolia see *C. betulifolia.*

C. betulifolia 🏆 syn. *C. betulaefolia, C. denticulata.* Tufted to clump-forming perennial with ovate to broadly ovate, toothed, dark green, purple-tinged leaves, 5–6cm (2–2½in) long. In early summer, corymbs of bell-shaped, pink-flushed white flowers, 2.5–3.5cm (1–1½in) long, with reflexed petal tips, open from pink or red buds. Cultivation group 2 or 3. ↕ to 8cm (3in), ↔ to 20cm (8in). Turkey (Anatolia). ❄❄❄

***C.* 'Birch Hybrid'** ▣🏆 Vigorous, prostrate, evergreen perennial with underground runners, and small, ovate-heart-shaped, toothed, bright green leaves, 1cm (½in) long. Bears abundant short racemes of open bell-shaped, mauve-blue flowers, 2cm (¾in) across, in summer. Cultivation group 2. ↕ 10cm (4in), ↔ to 50cm (20in) or more. ❄❄❄

CAMPANULA HABITS

Campanulas vary greatly in size and habit. They may be low, with a tufted, clump- or mat-forming, trailing, or spreading habit; or they may be tall and erect.

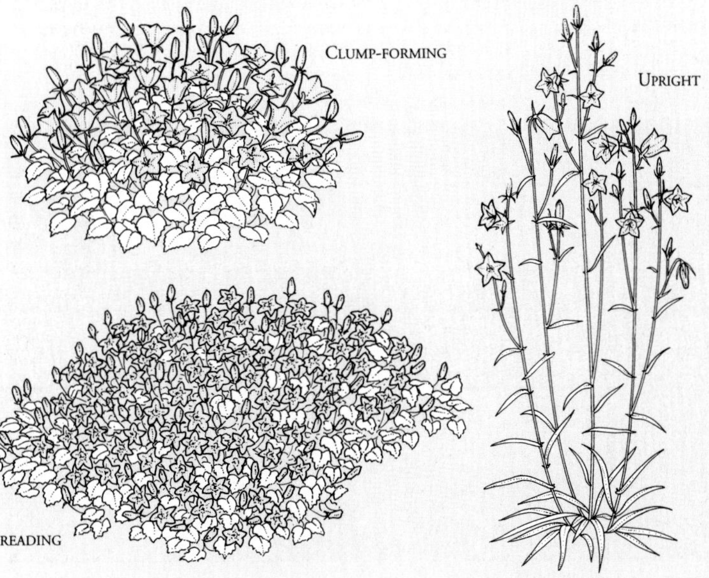

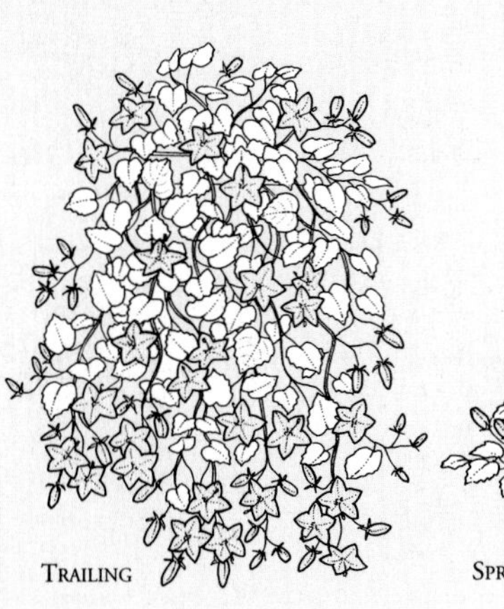

CAMPANULA FLOWERS

Campanulas bear flowers in a variety of shapes, including tubular, bell-, or star-shaped, and less clearly defined forms intermediate between the 3.

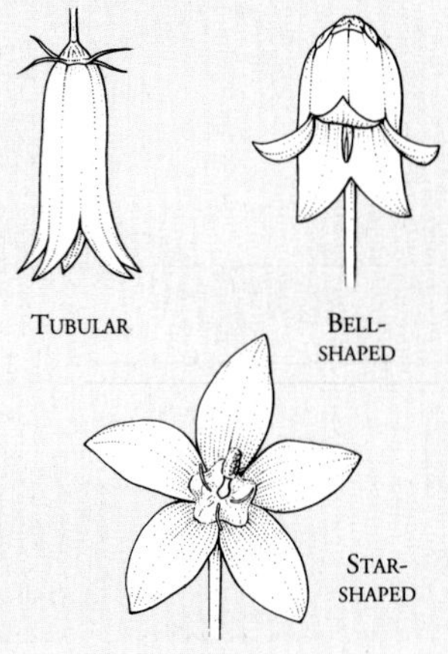

C

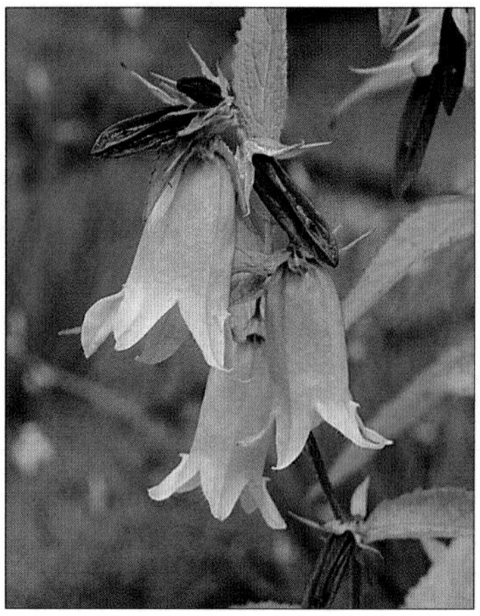
Campanula 'Burghaltii'

***C.* 'Burghaltii'** ■ 🏆 (*C. latifolia* x *C. punctata*). Mound-forming perennial with stalked, heart-shaped, toothed, mid-green basal leaves, to 9cm (3½in) long, and stalkless, much narrower stem leaves. In midsummer, bears racemes of pendent, tubular-bell-shaped flowers, to 10cm (4in) long, in an unusual greyish lavender-blue. Cultivation group 1. ↕60cm (24in), ↔ 30cm (12in). ❄❄❄
C. carpatica 🏆 Clump-forming, variable perennial with rounded to ovate or heart-shaped, toothed, mid-green, basal leaves, 2.5–5cm (1–2in) long. Many long, branched stems bear usually solitary, large, upturned, open bell-shaped, blue, violet-purple, or white flowers, 3cm (1¼in) or more across, over several months in summer. Cultivation group 2. ↕ to 30cm (12in), ↔ 30–60cm (12–24in) or more. C. Europe (Carpathians). ❄❄❄. **'Bressingham White'** ■ has large, pure white flowers, suffused blue-green at the bases; ↕ 15cm (6in). **'Jewel'** ■ is low-growing and compact, with bright purple-blue flowers; ↕ 10–15cm (4–6in). **'Turbinata'**, syn. var. *turbinata*, *C. turbinata*, is dwarf, with pale lavender-blue flowers borne singly on unbranched stems; ↕ 10–15cm (4–6in). **'Weisse Clips'**, syn. 'White Clips', produces abundant white flowers, and comes almost true from seed; ↕ 20cm (8in).
C. cashmeriana. Delicate, tufted, woody-based perennial with obovate to oblong, toothed, very hairy, grey-green leaves, to 1cm (½in) long, on slender, semi-erect, zigzagged, freely branching stems. Nodding, narrowly bell-shaped, pale lilac to grey-blue flowers, 1–2.5cm

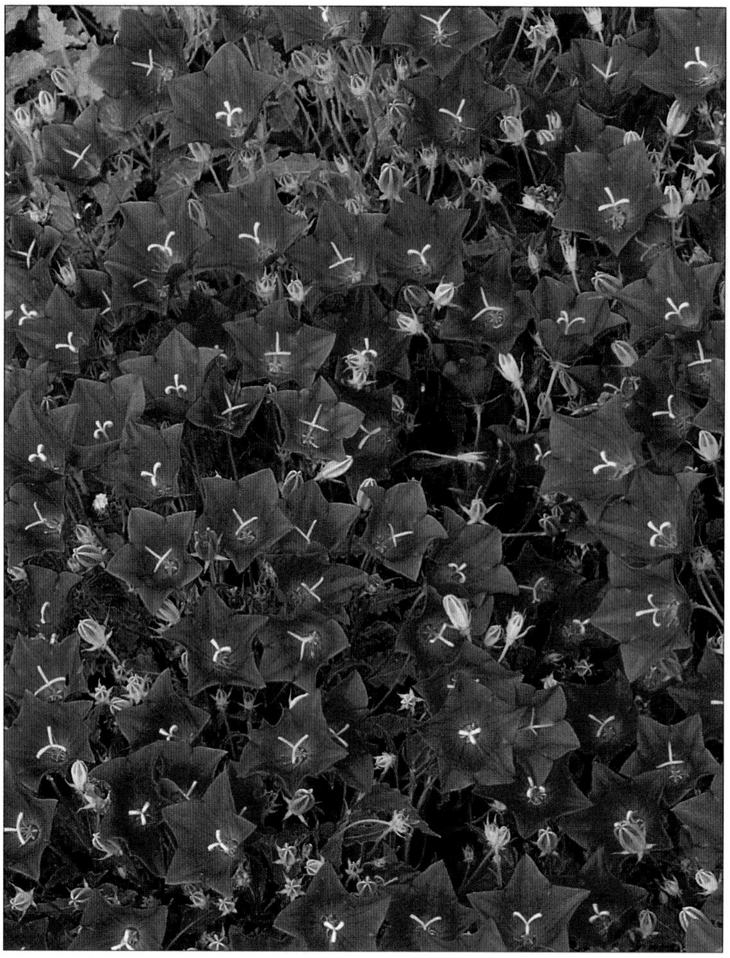
Campanula carpatica 'Jewel'

(½–1in) long, are produced singly from the leaf axils in summer. Best grown in an alpine house. Cultivation group 2 or 3. ↕ 10–15cm (4–6in), ↔ 15cm (6in). Afghanistan, India (Kashmir, Uttar Pradesh). ❄❄❄
C. chamissonis, syn. *C. dasyantha*, *C. pilosa*, *C. pilosa* var. *dasyantha*. Variable, rhizomatous perennial with rosettes of spoon-shaped to inversely lance-shaped, finely toothed, pale green leaves, to 4cm (1½in) long. In early summer, erect stems bear bell-shaped to tubular, blue, white-streaked flowers, 2–4cm (¾–1½in) long, usually singly but occasionally in few-flowered clusters. Cultivation group 2 or 3. ↕ 5–15cm (2–6in), ↔ to 20cm (8in). Japan to Alaska. ❄❄❄. **'Superba'** ■ 🏆 syn. 'Major', is very compact, with pale purple-blue flowers, to 4cm (1½in) long; ↕ 5cm (2in), ↔ 20cm (8in).
C. cochleariifolia ■ 🏆 syn. *C. bellardii*, *C. pusilla* (Fairies' thimbles). Creeping, tufted, rosette-forming perennial with slender rhizomes and oval to rounded-heart-shaped, toothed, bright green leaves, to 2cm (¾in) long. In summer, bears solitary, pendent, bell-shaped, white to lavender- or slate-blue flowers, 1.5cm (½in) long. Cultivation group 2. ↕ to 8cm (3in), ↔ to 30cm (12in) or more. European mountains. ❄❄❄. **'Elizabeth Oliver'** ■ produces double, pale lavender-blue flowers. **'Miranda'** bears single, grey-blue flowers. **'Miss Willmott'** has single, pale blue flowers, margined with silver.

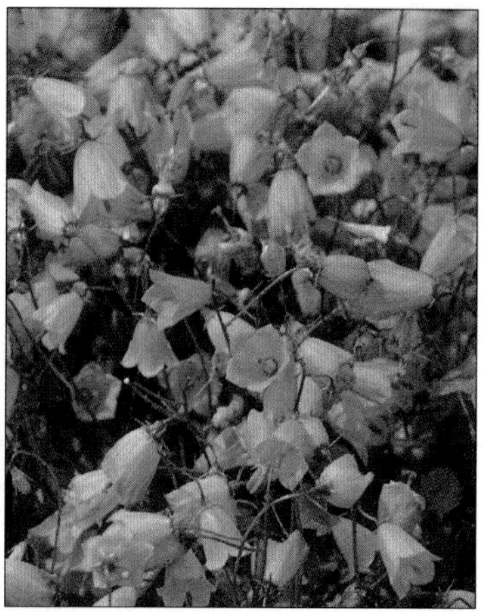
Campanula cochleariifolia

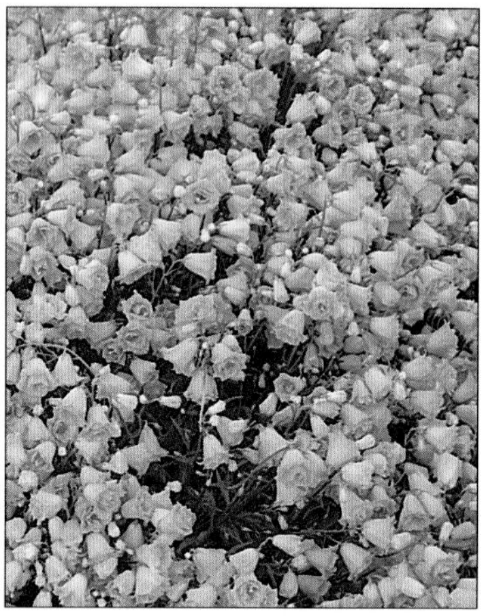
Campanula cochleariifolia 'Elizabeth Oliver'

C. dasyantha see *C. chamissonis*.
C. denticulata see *C. betulifolia*.
C. elatines* var. *garganica see *C. garganica*.
***C.* 'Elizabeth'** ■ syn. *C. takesimana* 'Elizabeth'. Rhizomatous perennial with rosettes of heart-shaped, toothed, mid-green leaves, 8cm (3in) long. In mid- and late summer, bears racemes of pendent, bell-shaped cream flowers, 5cm (2in) or more long, flushed reddish purple outside and spotted red inside. Cultivation group 1. ↕ 35–40cm (14–16in), ↔ 40cm (16in). ❄❄❄
C. excisa. Creeping, loose mat-forming perennial with upright, wiry stems bearing linear-lance-shaped, slender-pointed, entire, light green leaves, 2cm (¾in) long. In midsummer, produces

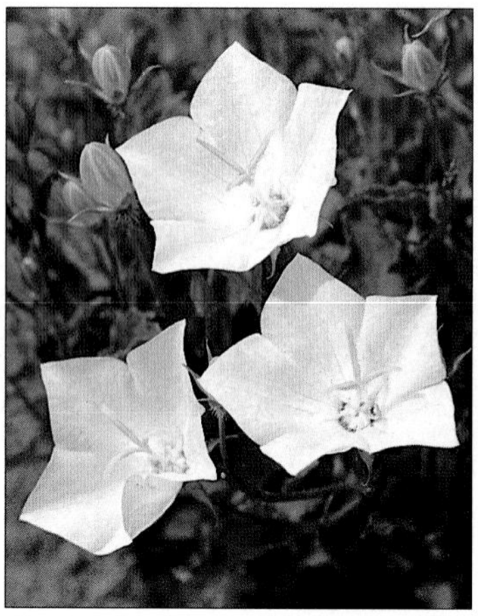
Campanula carpatica 'Bressingham White'

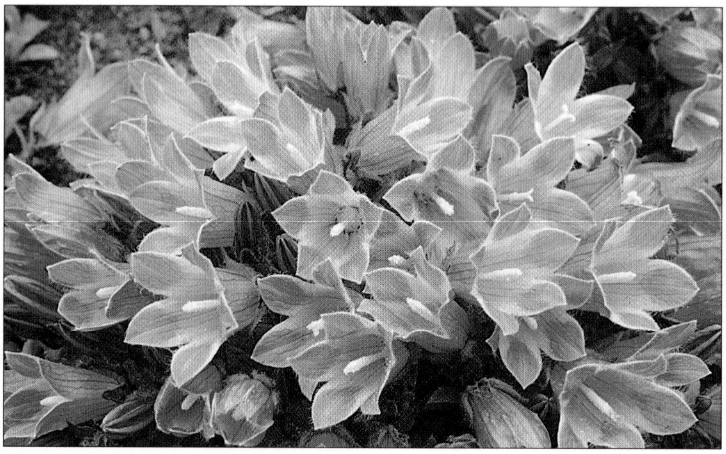
Campanula chamissonis 'Superba'

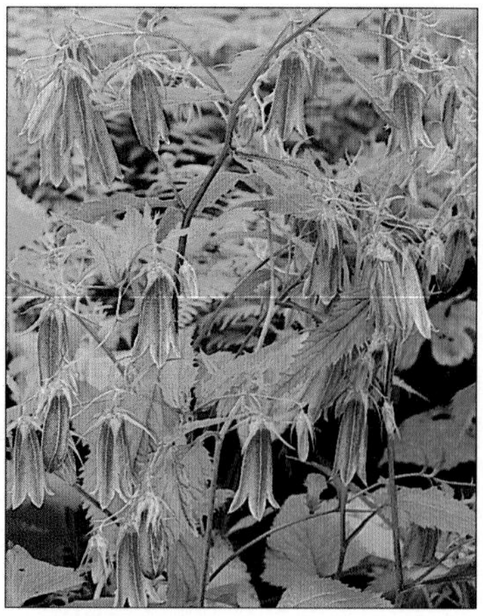
Campanula 'Elizabeth'

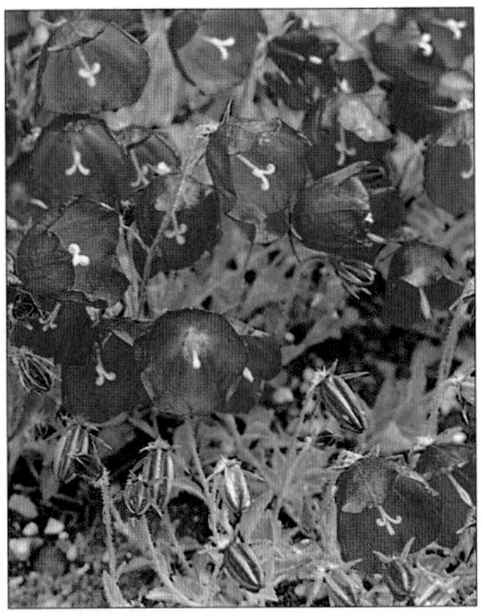

Campanula 'G.F. Wilson'

solitary (sometimes 2 or 3), pendent, bell-shaped, violet to lilac flowers, to 2.5cm (1in) long, with a round hole at the base of each lobe. Cultivation group 2 or 3. ↕ to 10cm (4in), ↔ to 20cm (8in). S.W. and S. Central Alps. ✻✻✻
C. garganica ♀ syn. *C. elatines* var. *garganica* (Adriatic bellflower). Spreading perennial with small, kidney-shaped or ovate-heart-shaped, toothed, mid-green basal leaves, 2.5–3.5cm (1–1½in) long, and heart-shaped, toothed stem leaves. Profuse racemes of star-shaped, bright blue to lilac flowers, 1–2cm (½–¾in) across, are produced in summer. Cultivation group 2. ↕ 5cm (2in), occasionally more, ↔ 30cm (12in) or more. S. Europe. ✻✻✻. **'Aurea'** see 'Dickson's Gold'. **'Dickson's Gold'**, syn. 'Aurea', has yellow leaves and blue flowers. **'W.H. Paine'** ♀ bears deep lavender-blue flowers with white centres.
***C.* 'G.F. Wilson'** ■ ♀ Compact, mound-forming perennial with slender runners and oval, toothed, pale yellow-green leaves, 2.5–5cm (1–2in) long. Bears solitary, semi-erect or nodding, cup-shaped, deep violet flowers, to 2.5cm (1in) across, in mid- and late summer. Cultivation group 2. ↕ to 10cm (4in), ↔ to 20cm (8in). ✻✻✻
C. glomerata (Clustered bellflower). Vigorous, variable, rhizomatous, hairy perennial, spreading to form clumps of erect, stiff stems and bearing numerous ovate to lance-shaped, round-toothed, dark green leaves, 5–10cm (2–4in) long. Dense, terminal racemes of tubular-bell-shaped flowers, 1.5–3.5cm (½–1½in) long, varying from violet to lavender-blue or white, are borne throughout

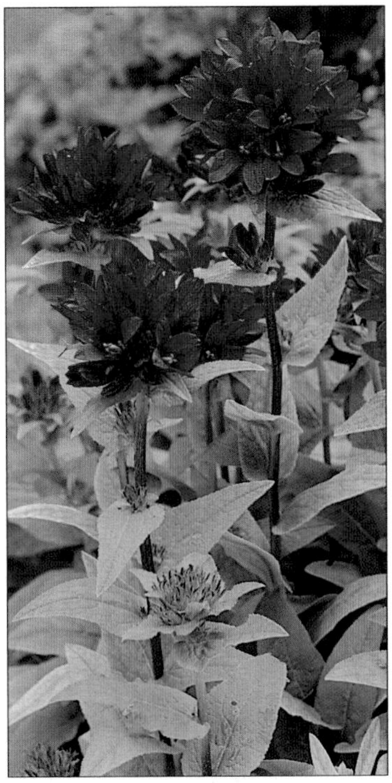

Campanula glomerata 'Superba'

summer. Cut back after flowering, to encourage a second flush. Cultivation group 1. ↕ 10–45cm (4–18in) or more, ↔ indefinite. Europe (excluding extreme N.), Turkey, W., C., and S. Asia. ✻✻✻. **'Crown of Snow'** see 'Schneekrone'. **var. *dahurica*** ■ has wide, deep purple flowers; ↕ to 75cm (30in). **'Joan Elliott'** has large violet flowers in early summer; ↕ 40cm (16in). **'Schneekrone'**, syn. 'Crown of Snow', bears dense clusters of white flowers, and breeds virtually true from seed; ↕ 50cm (20in). **'Superba'** ■ ♀ is vigorous, with purple-violet flowers; ↕ 60cm (24in).
C.* x *haylodgensis see *C.* x *haylodgensis* 'Plena'.
***C.* x *haylodgensis* 'Plena'**, syn. *C.* x *haylodgensis.* Spreading perennial with rounded to ovate or heart-shaped, toothed, mid-green leaves, 1–2cm (½–¾in) long. In mid- and late summer, bears clusters of rounded-bell-shaped, double, deep lavender-blue flowers, to 2.5cm (1in) across. Cultivation group 2. ↕ to 8cm (3in), ↔ 15cm (6in). Garden origin. ✻✻✻. **'Warley White'**, syn. *C. warleyensis,* has open, semi-double or double white flowers, to 4cm (1½in) across.

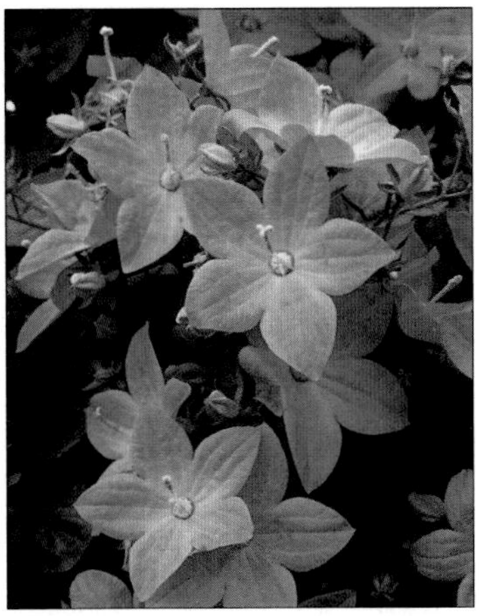

Campanula isophylla Kristal Hybrids 'Stella Blue'

C. isophylla ♀ (Falling stars, Italian bellflower, Star-of-Bethlehem). Trailing perennial with soft stems, becoming slightly woody at the bases, and small, heart-shaped, toothed, light green leaves, 6cm (2½in) long. Loose corymbs of numerous, upright, saucer-shaped, pale blue or pure white flowers, 3.5cm (1½in) across, are produced in mid-summer; flowers for 2–3 months. Excellent for containers and hanging baskets. Cultivation group 4. ↕ 15–20cm (6–8in), ↔ to 30cm (12in). N. Italy. ✻. **'Alba'** ■ ♀ produces pure white flowers. **Kristal Hybrids** are compact, long-blooming, and very free-flowering, producing strong stems and large flowers; they flower in early summer from late winter sowings. **'Stella Blue'** ■ is a compact Kristal Hybrid, producing star-shaped, bright violet-blue flowers; it is often cultivated as an annual for hanging baskets. **'Stella White'** is a Kristal Hybrid bearing star-shaped white flowers.
***C.* 'Joe Elliott'** ♀ Small, mound-forming perennial producing rounded-heart-shaped, slightly toothed, hairy, greyish green leaves, to 1.5cm (½in) long. Upright, bell- to funnel-shaped, lavender-blue flowers, 2–3cm (¾–1¼in) long, are borne singly or in small clusters of 2 or 3, just above the foliage in summer. Cultivation group 3. ↕ 8cm (3in), ↔ 20cm (8in). ✻✻✻
C. lactiflora ■ (Milky bellflower). Upright perennial producing thin, ovate to ovate-oblong, toothed, mid-green leaves, 5–12cm (2–5in) or more long. Conical panicles of open bell-shaped

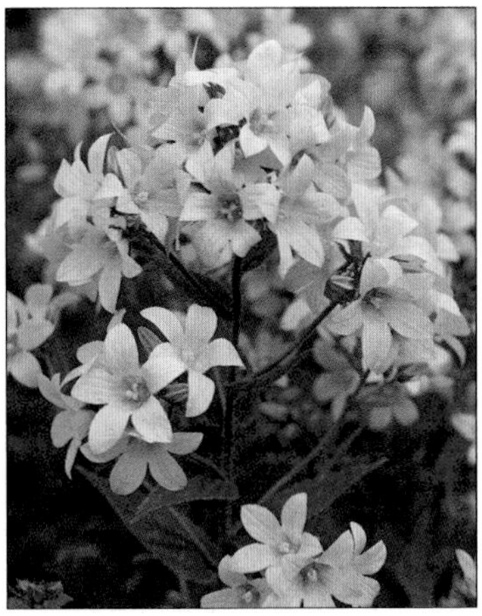

Campanula lactiflora 'Loddon Anna'

flowers, 1.5–2.5cm (½–1in) across, are borne on strongly branched, leafy stems from early summer to early autumn. The flowers are usually white to pale blue, sometimes lavender-blue, deep lilac-blue, or violet. Self-seeds freely, producing seedlings with some colour variation. May need staking in exposed sites. Cultivation group 1. ↕ 1.2–1.5m (4–5ft), ↔ 60cm (24in). Caucasus, Turkey. ✻✻✻. **'Alba'** produces pure white flowers. **'Loddon Anna'** ■ ♀ bears soft lilac-pink flowers. **'Pouffe'** is dwarf, forming a tight mound of foliage covered with profuse, pale lavender-blue flowers; ↕ 25cm (10in), ↔ 45cm (18in). **'Prichard's Variety'** ■ ♀ produces dark violet-blue flowers; ↕ to 75cm (30in). **'White Pouffe'** is similar to 'Pouffe', but with white flowers.
C. latifolia. Vigorous, upright perennial with stout, unbranched stems arising from basal clumps of ovate-oblong, long-stalked, rough-textured, toothed, mid-green leaves, 7–12cm (3–5in) long. Stem leaves are similar but stalkless and sharply pointed, decreasing in size towards the tops of the stems. In summer, flowers are produced singly or in twos or threes, from the axils of the upper leaves, forming narrow, leafy, spike-like racemes. The flowers are broadly tubular-bell-shaped, 4–6cm (1½–2½in) long, pale to deep violet or white, and have wide-spreading corolla lobes. Cultivation group 1. ↕ to 1.2m (4ft), ↔ 60cm (24in). Europe (except for the extreme N. and Mediterranean region), Caucasus, Turkey, Iran, W. Asia to India (Kashmir). ✻✻✻.

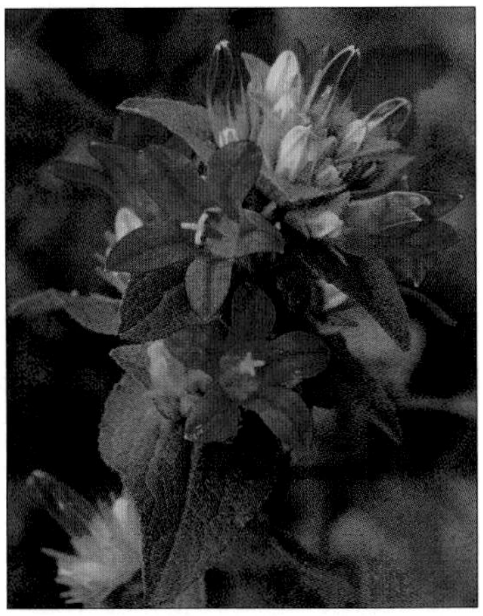

Campanula glomerata var. *dahurica*

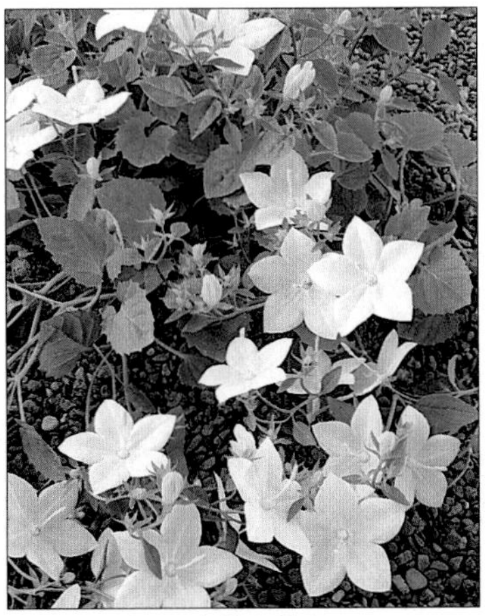

Campanula isophylla 'Alba'

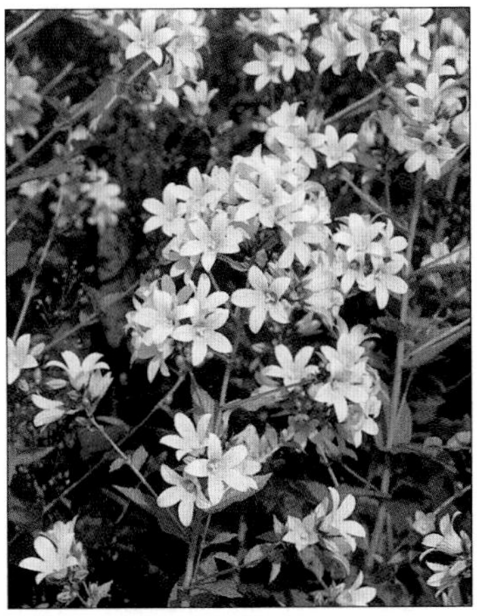

Campanula lactiflora

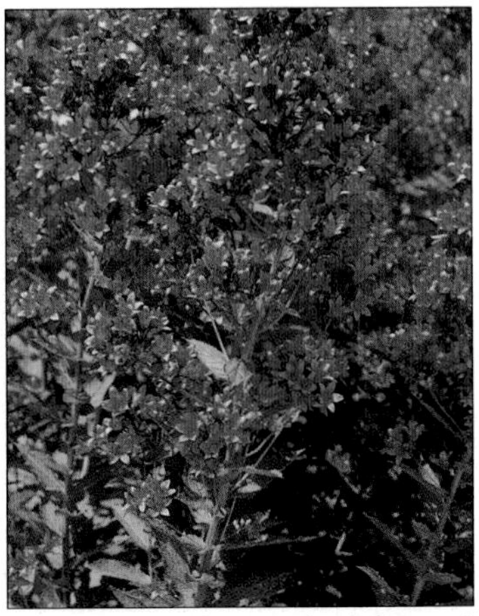

Campanula lactiflora 'Prichard's Variety'

C

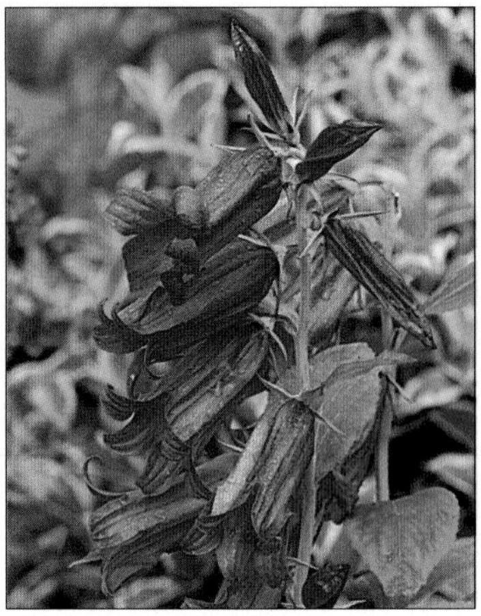
Campanula latifolia 'Brantwood'

'Brantwood' ■ bears deep violet flowers, and breeds almost true from seed; ↕75cm (30in). **'Gloaming'** produces pale smoke-blue flowers; ↕60cm (24in). **var. *macrantha*** has sparse foliage and dark blue flowers; ↕1m (3ft); Caucasus.
C. latiloba, syn. *C. persicifolia* subsp. *sessiliflora.* Clump-forming perennial with basal rosettes of broadly lance-shaped, toothed, mid-green leaves, 7–12cm (3–5in) long, and thick, erect stems. Short racemes of stalkless, shallowly cup-shaped, rich lavender-blue flowers, 3–5cm (1¼–2in) across, are borne in mid- and late summer. Cultivation group 1. ↕90cm (36in), ↔45cm (18in). N. Turkey. ✽✽✽. **'Hidcote Amethyst'** ■♀ has pale amethyst flowers with deeper purple shading. **'Percy Piper'** ♀ produces rich lavender-blue flowers; ↕75cm (30in).
C. medium (Canterbury bells). Slow-growing, clump-forming, downy biennial producing lance-shaped to elliptic, toothed, mid-green basal leaves, 12–15cm (5–6in) long, and smaller stem leaves. Lax racemes of single or double, bell-shaped, white, pink, or blue flowers, 2.5–4cm (1–1½in) long, open from spring to summer. Cultivation group 1. ↕60–90cm (24–36in), ↔30cm (12in). S. Europe. ✽✽✽. **'Bells of Holland'** ■ is dwarf, bearing single flowers in a variety of colours. May be grown as an annual; ↕40–45cm (16–18in). **'Calycanthema'**, syn. var. *calycanthema* (Canterbury bells, Cup and saucer) has single or double flowers, each surrounded by a large calyx the same colour as the petals. An additional,

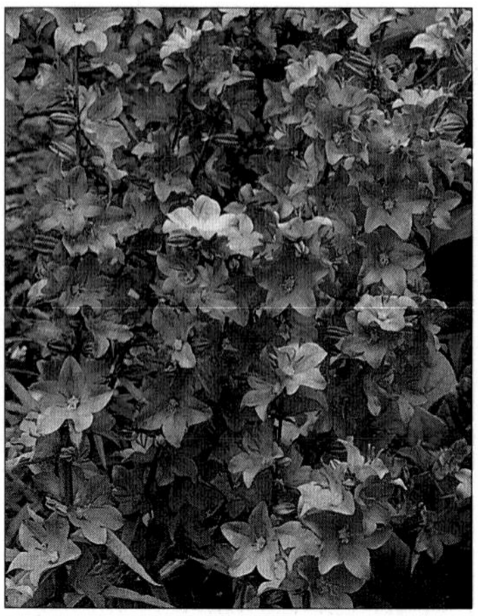
Campanula latiloba 'Hidcote Amethyst'

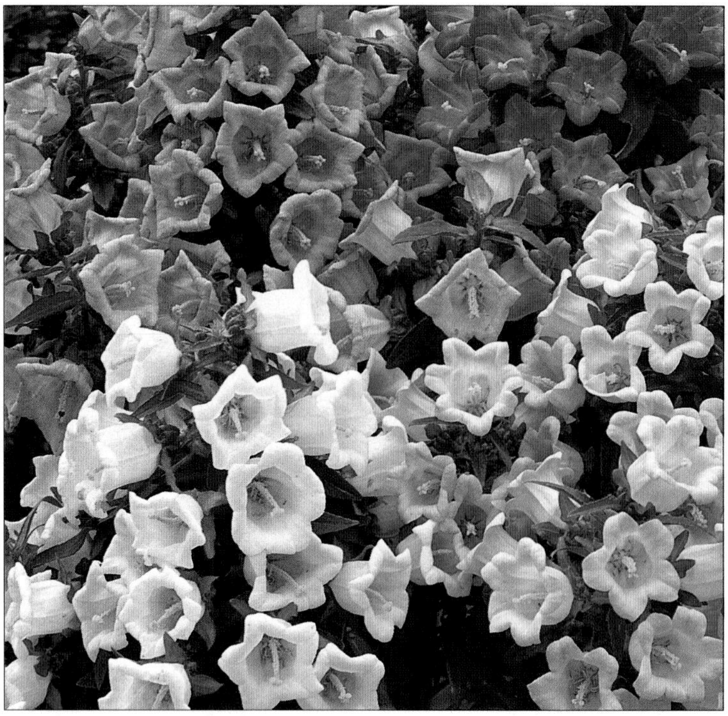
Campanula medium 'Bells of Holland'

flattened, lobed corolla forms a saucer-like rim at the base of the cup-like flowers; ↕to 75cm (30in).
C. morettiana. Small, tufted perennial with finely hairy, broadly ovate, coarsely toothed, mid-green leaves, to 2cm (¾in) long. Arching stems bear usually solitary, erect, tubular-bell-shaped, violet-blue flowers, 2–3cm (¾–1¼in) long, in late spring and early summer. Prefers alkaline soil. Cultivation group 3. ↕5cm (2in), ↔ to 10cm (4in). Rock crevices, mountains of N. Italy, W. Austria (Tyrol). ✽✽✽
C. muralis see *C. portenschlagiana.*
C. nitida see *C. persicifolia* var. *planiflora.*
***C. nitida* 'Planiflora'** see *C. persicifolia* var. *planiflora.*
C. ossetica see *Symphyandra pendula.*
C. persicifolia (Peach-leaved bellflower). Rosette-forming perennial with slender white rhizomes and ever-green, narrow, lance-shaped to oblong-obovate, toothed, bright green, basal leaves, 10–15cm (4–6in) long. Short, terminal racemes of 2 or 3, occasionally solitary, slightly pendent, cup-shaped flowers, to 5cm (2in) across, varying from white to lilac-blue, are produced on slender stems, or from the leaf axils, in early and midsummer. Cultivation group 1. ↕90cm (36in), ↔30cm (12in). S. Europe, to C. and S. Russia, W. and N. Asia. ✽✽✽. **'Alba Coronata'**, syn. 'Alba Plena', bears semi-double flowers with 2 or 3 rows of petals and enlarged, petaloid stamens; ↕45cm (18in). **'Boule de Neige'** bears double white flowers; ↕60cm (24in). **'Fleur de Neige'** ♀ produces large, shallowly cup-shaped white flowers with 3 rows of petals and petaloid stamens; ↕70cm (28in). **var. *planiflora***, syn. *C. amabilis* 'Planiflora', *C. nitida*, *C. nitida* 'Planiflora', *C. planiflora* (Willow-bell), is dwarf, with dense rosettes of inversely lance-shaped, wavy-margined, glossy, very dark green leaves, to 3cm (1¼in) long. In summer, bears erect racemes of widely bell-shaped blue flowers, 2–4cm (¾–1½in) across.
Cultivation group 2; ↕↔15cm (6in). **'Planiflora Alba'** has white flowers. Cultivation group 2; ↕↔15cm (6in). **'Pride of Exmouth'** bears semi-double, "cup-in-cup", purple-blue flowers, and is remontant; ↕60cm (24in). **subsp. *sessiliflora*** see *C. latiloba.* **'Telham Beauty'** ■ has light blue flowers, ↕7cm (3in) across; ↔90cm (36in).
C. pilosa see *C. chamissonis.*
C. pilosa* var. *dasyantha see *C. chamissonis.*
C. piperi. Slow-growing, tufted, rhizomatous perennial with rosettes of spoon- to lance-shaped, toothed, glossy mid-green leaves, to 2.5cm (1in) long. Solitary, shallowly bowl-shaped, bright blue flowers, 2cm (¾in) across, with red anthers, are borne in summer. Best

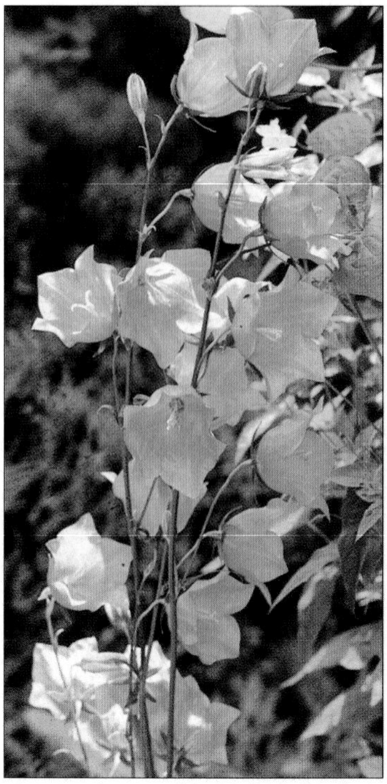
Campanula persicifolia 'Telham Beauty'

grown in an alpine house. Cultivation group 3. ↕to 5cm (2in), ↔ to 15cm (6in). N.W. USA (Olympic Mountains, in rock crevices). ✽✽✽
C. planiflora see *C. persicifolia* var. *planiflora.*
C. portenschlagiana ■♀ syn. *C. muralis* (Dalmatian bellflower). Robust, mound-forming, evergreen perennial with broadly kidney-shaped to ovate-heart-shaped, irregularly toothed, mid-green leaves, 2–4cm (¾–1½in) long. Erect or spreading, loosely branched panicles of tubular to funnel-shaped, deep purple flowers, to 2cm (¾in) long, are borne in mid- and late summer. Cultivation group 2. ↕to 15cm (6in), ↔ 50cm (20in) or more. Mountains of Croatia. ✽✽✽
C. poscharskyana ■ Vigorous perennial, spreading by underground runners, with toothed, rounded to ovate, mid-green leaves, to 2.5cm (1in) long, heart-shaped at the bases. Panicles of star-shaped, pale lavender flowers, 2–2.5cm (¾–1in) across, with white centres, are borne from summer to autumn. Cultivation group 2. ↕to 15cm (6in), ↔ to 60cm (24in). Mountains of Croatia, Bosnia & Herzegovina. ✽✽✽. **'Stella'** has bright violet flowers.
C. x pseudoraineri (*C. carpatica* 'Turbinata' x *C. raineri*). Variable, dense, clump-forming perennial, resembling *C. carpatica*, with ovate to rounded, or heart-shaped, toothed, hairy, grey-green, basal leaves, 1–2.5cm (½–1in) long. Solitary, large, upturned, open bell-shaped blue flowers, 3cm (1¼in) across, are borne on erect stems throughout the summer. Cultivation group 2. ↕to 12cm (5in), ↔ to 15cm (6in). Garden origin. ✽✽✽
C. pulla. Spreading perennial with underground runners and small rosettes of shallowly toothed, rounded-spoon-shaped, shiny, mid-green, basal leaves. Solitary, pendent, tubular-bell-shaped, deep violet or purple-blue flowers, to 2cm (¾in) long, are borne in late spring and early summer. Cultivation group 2 or 3. ↕to 5cm (2in), ↔ to 30cm (12in). N.E. Alps, Austria. ✽✽✽
C. punctata ■ Clump-forming perennial with creeping rhizomes and rosettes of ovate, toothed, slightly hairy, dark green leaves, 10–12cm (4–5in) long, heart-shaped at the bases. In early summer, erect stems bear short racemes of pendent, tubular-bell-shaped, creamy white to dusky pink flowers, 5cm (2in) long, red-spotted and hairy inside. Will

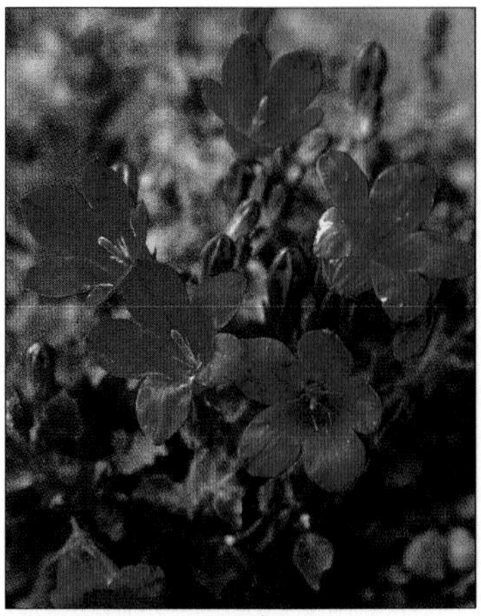
Campanula portenschlagiana

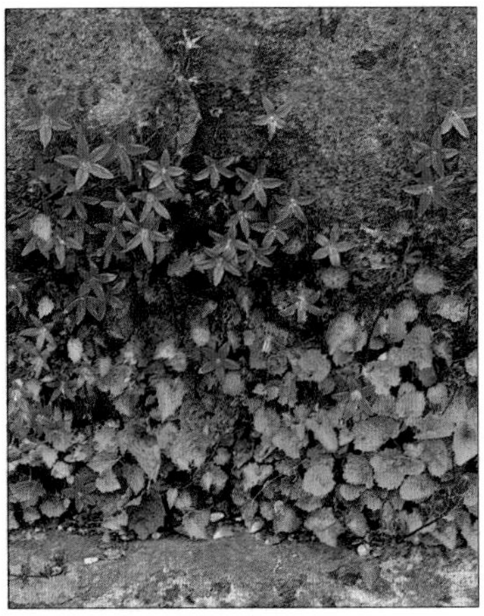
Campanula poscharskyana

thrive in fertile, sandy loam. Cultivation group 1. ↕30cm (12in), ↔ 40cm (16in). Russia (Siberia), Japan. ❄❄❄
C. pusilla see *C. cochleariifolia.*
C. pyramidalis (Chimney bellflower). Short-lived, erect perennial, best grown as a biennial. Loose rosettes of ovate-lance-shaped, toothed, light to mid-green leaves, 7–15cm (3–6in) long, give rise to tall stems with stalkless, lance-shaped leaves. Pyramidal racemes of cup-shaped, fragrant, light blue or white flowers, 4cm (1½in) across, are borne from late spring to summer. Prefers rich soil. Cultivation group 1. ↕ to 3m (10ft), ↔ 60cm (24in). N. Italy, N.W. Balkans. ❄❄. **'Alba'** has white flowers.
C. raineri ■ 🏆 Slow-spreading perennial with underground runners and obovate, toothed, hairy, grey-green leaves, 1–2.5cm (½–1in) long. In summer, bears solitary, upturned, open bell-shaped, pale lavender flowers, 3–4cm (1¼–1½in) across. Cultivation group 3. ↕ 5–8cm (2–3in), ↔ to 20cm (8in). Mountains of Switzerland, Italy. ❄❄❄
C. rotundifolia (Harebell, Scottish bluebell). Variable perennial with underground runners, and long-stalked, rounded to heart-shaped, finely toothed, light green basal leaves, 1cm (½in) long, and linear stem leaves. In summer, erect, slender stems bear lax, branched panicles of nodding, bell-shaped, dark blue to white flowers, to 2cm (¾in) long. May be naturalized in short turf. Cultivation group 2. ↕↔ 12–30cm (5–12in). Temperate N. hemisphere. ❄❄❄
C. sarmatica. Clump-forming perennial, similar to *C. alliariifolia* but less vigorous, with elongated, triangular-

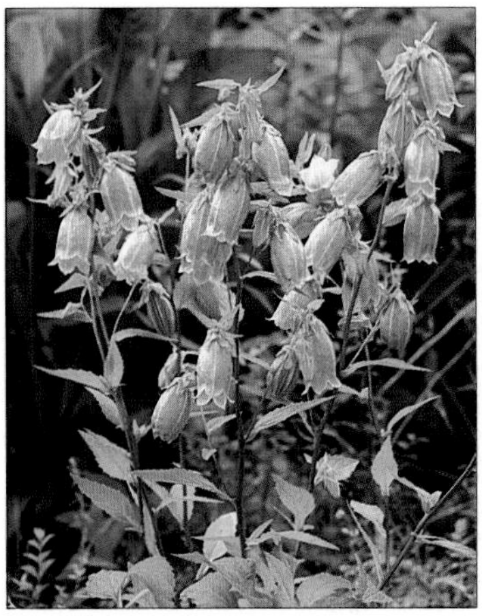
Campanula punctata

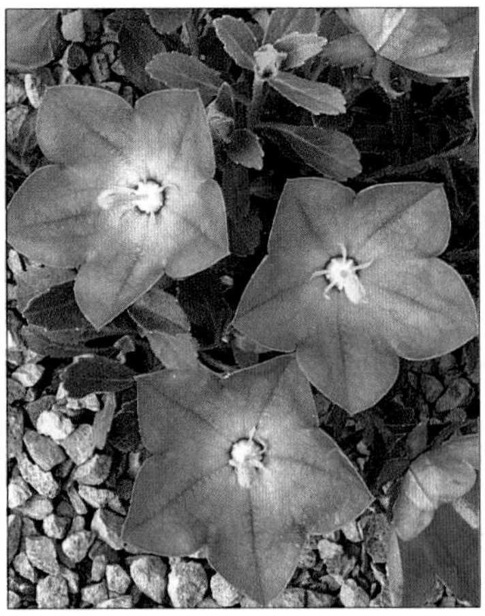
Campanula raineri

ovate, heart-shaped, toothed, wrinkled, grey-woolly, basal leaves, to 8cm (3in) long, with long leaf-stalks. Erect, unbranched, greyish green stems bear lax racemes of bell-shaped, hairy, light grey-blue flowers, 3–5cm (1¼–2in) long, from late spring to midsummer. Cultivation group 1. ↕ 50cm (20in), ↔ 40cm (16in). Caucasus. ❄❄❄
C. saxatilis 🏆 Tufted perennial with erect or spreading stems arising from a thick rootstock, and rosettes of spoon-shaped to inversely lance-shaped, entire or round-toothed, mid-green leaves, to 5cm (2in) long. In summer, long stems bear loose spikes or clusters of tubular, pale blue flowers, to 2cm (¾in) long, with darker veins. Cultivation group 3. ↕ 8cm (3in) or more, ↔ to 20cm (8in). Crete (in rock crevices). ❄❄❄
C. takesimana. Rapidly spreading, rhizomatous perennial with heart-shaped, toothed, glossy, mid-green leaves, to 8cm (3in) long, with winged leaf-stalks. In summer, bears arching, branched sprays of pendent, bell-shaped white flowers, 4–7cm (1½–3in) long, pink-flushed, and spotted maroon inside. Cultivation group 1. ↕ to 50cm (20in), ↔ to 1m (3ft). Korea. ❄❄❄
***C. takesimana* 'Elizabeth'** see *C.* 'Elizabeth'.
C. thyrsoides. Rosette-forming, bristly, monocarpic perennial or biennial with lance-shaped, wavy-margined, entire, mid-green leaves, 7–12cm (3–5in) long, the upper ones much narrower and stem-clasping. Dense, blunt-tipped, cylindrical spikes of cup-shaped, fragrant, lemon-yellow or creamy yellow flowers, 1.5–2.5cm (½–1in) long, are

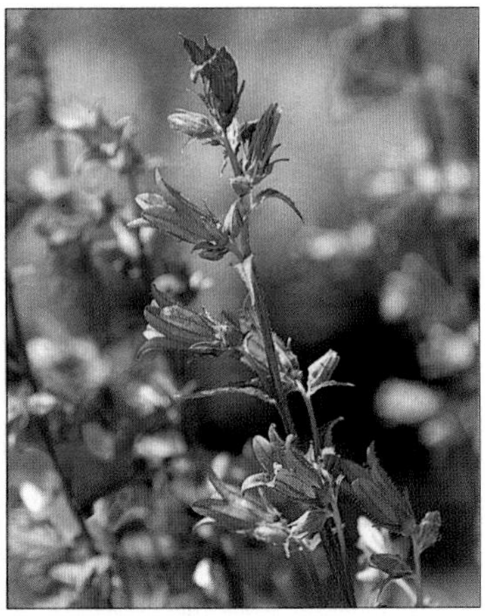
Campanula trachelium

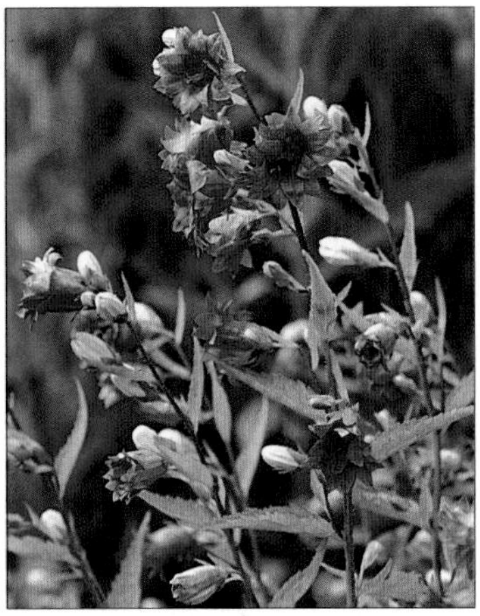
Campanula trachelium 'Bernice'

borne in mid- and late summer. Prefers light, alkaline soil. Cultivation group 1. ↕ 30–50cm (12–20in) or more, ↔ 23–30cm (9–12in). S. Europe. ❄❄❄
C. trachelium ■ (Bats-in-the-belfry, Nettle-leaved bellflower, Throatwort). Upright, woody-based perennial with ovate, sharply toothed, nettle-like, bristly, mid-green leaves, 5–12cm (2–5in) long. Stout, sometimes red-tinged stems bear short racemes of tubular, short-stalked, mid-blue to lilac, or white flowers, 2–3cm (¾–1¼in) long, from the leaf axils, in mid- and late summer. Cultivation group 1. ↕ 45–90cm (18–36in), ↔ 30cm (12in). Europe to Turkey and W. Asia, also N. Africa. ❄❄❄. **'Alba Flore Pleno'** has semi-double white flowers. **'Bernice'** ■ bears double, lilac-blue flowers.
C. turbinata see *C. carpatica* 'Turbinata'.
***C.* 'Van-Houttei'.** Clump-forming perennial with deeply notched, ovate to lance-shaped, scalloped, mid-green leaves, 9–10cm (3½–4in) long, with conspicuous veins. Pendent, tubular-bell-shaped mauve flowers, to 6cm (2½in) long, are produced on erect stems in early and midsummer. Cultivation group 1. ↕ 60cm (24in), ↔ 30cm (12in). ❄❄❄
C. vidalii see *Azorina vidalii.*
C. waldsteiniana. Tufted, clump-forming perennial with small, ovate-elliptic, toothed, bright green leaves, 1.5cm (½in) long. In late summer and early autumn, bears loose racemes of 3–5 upturned, star-shaped, mid-blue flowers, 2cm (¾in) across, on wiry stems. Cultivation group 3. ↕ to 10cm (4in), ↔ to 20cm (8in). Rock crevices and mountains in S. Croatia. ❄❄❄
C. wanneri see *Symphyandra wanneri.*
C. warleyensis see *C.* x *haylodgensis* 'Warley White'.
C. zoysii ■ Cushion-forming, tufted perennial producing small, obovate to ovate, toothed, glossy, mid-green leaves, 5–10mm (¼–½in) long. Erect stems each bear several pendent, tubular, clear blue to pale lavender-blue flowers, 1.5–2cm (½–¾in) long, contracted at the mouths, in midsummer. Needs very gritty, alkaline soil. Cultivation group 3. ↕ to 5cm (2in), ↔ to 10cm (4in). S.E. Alps. ❄❄❄

▷ ***Campelia zanonia*** see *Tradescantia zanonia*
▷ **Camphor tree** see *Cinnamomum camphora*

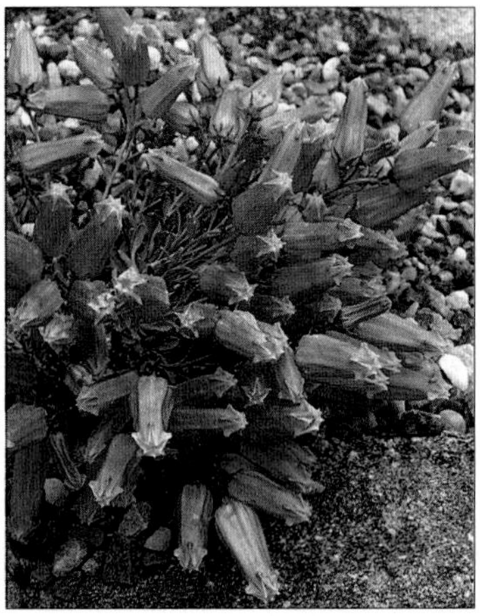
Campanula zoysii

▷ **Campion** see *Lychnis, Silene*
Alpine see *Lychnis alpina*
Double sea see *Silene uniflora* 'Flore Pleno'
Moss see *Silene acaulis*
Rose see *Lychnis coronaria*

CAMPSIS

Trumpet creeper, Trumpet vine

BIGNONIACEAE

Genus of 2 species of vigorous, woody, deciduous climbers, usually climbing by aerial roots, found in woodland in China and North America. They have opposite, pinnate leaves, with ovate leaflets, and showy, trumpet-shaped or funnel-shaped flowers, 6–8cm (2½–3in) long, borne in terminal panicles or cymes from late summer to autumn. Train against a wall, fence, or pillar, or on a tree.

- **HARDINESS** Fully hardy to frost hardy.
- **CULTIVATION** Grow in any moderately fertile, moist but well-drained soil. In frost-prone gardens, trumpet creepers are best grown against a warm wall in full sun. In warmer climates, they will tolerate a more exposed and shady site. Pruning group 12, in late winter or early spring. It may take 2 or 3 seasons to establish the main framework; train and tie in the shoots until the aerial roots have taken hold.
- **PROPAGATION** Sow seed in containers in a cold frame in autumn. Root leaf-bud cuttings in spring or semi-ripe cuttings in summer. Graft or insert root cuttings in winter.
- **PESTS AND DISEASES** Powdery mildew, leaf spot, scale insects, mealybugs, and whiteflies may be a problem.

C. chinensis see *C. grandiflora.*
C. grandiflora, syn. *Bignonia grandiflora, C. chinensis, Tecoma grandiflora* (Chinese trumpet creeper, Chinese trumpet vine). Vigorous climber with pinnate, mid- to dark green leaves, to 30cm (12in) long, composed of 7–9 ovate, coarsely toothed leaflets. Pendent, terminal panicles of 6–12 open funnel-shaped, dark orange to red flowers, with spreading lobes, are borne from late summer to autumn. It produces relatively few aerial roots and may need to be tied permanently to its support. ↕ 10m (30ft). China. ❄❄
C. radicans, syn. *Bignonia radicans, Tecoma radicans* (Common trumpet creeper). Vigorous climber with ovate, pinnate, dark green leaves, 2.5–10cm

C

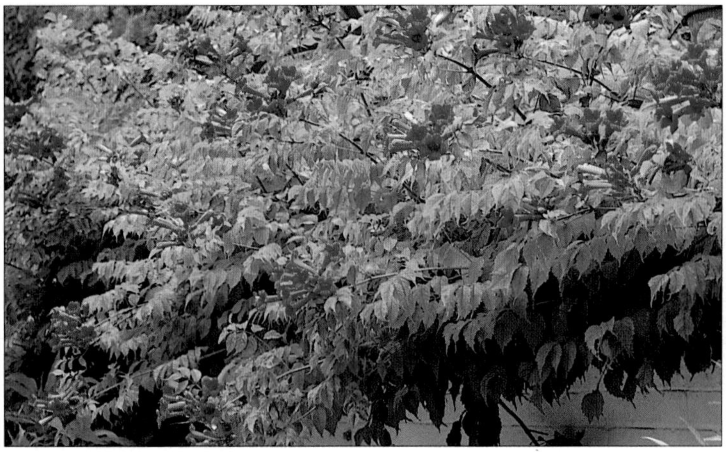

Campsis x *tagliabuana* 'Mme Galen'

(1–4in) long, composed of 7–11 toothed, ovate leaflets. Bears terminal cymes of 4–12 slender, tubular-trumpet-shaped, orange to red flowers from late summer to autumn. ↕ 10m (30ft) or more. S.E. USA. ❄❄. **f. *flava*** 🏆 syn. 'Yellow Trumpet', has yellow flowers.

***C.* x *tagliabuana* 'Mme Galen'** ▣ 🏆 Vigorous climber with pinnate, dark green leaves, to 30cm (12in) long, composed of 7–11 ovate leaflets. From late summer to autumn, bears terminal panicles of 6–12 trumpet-shaped, orange-red flowers. ↕ 10m (30ft) or more. ❄❄

▷ ***Camptosorus rhizophyllus*** see *Asplenium rhizophyllum*

CANANGA

ANNONACEAE

Genus of 2 species of evergreen trees occurring in tropical and subtropical forest from India to Australasia and the Pacific islands. They have alternate, simple leaves and are valued for their 6-petalled, scented flowers, produced in pendent clusters from the leaf axils. In frost-prone areas, grow in a warm greenhouse. In tropical climates, they are attractive street and specimen trees, and are cultivated commercially for their perfumed oil, which is distilled from the flowers.

• **HARDINESS** Frost tender.

• **CULTIVATION** Under glass, grow in loam-based potting compost (JI No.3) in bright filtered light with high humidity. Water freely in the growing season, applying a balanced liquid fertilizer monthly from summer to autumn; water sparingly but regularly in winter. Pot on or top-dress in spring. Outdoors, grow in moist, moderately fertile, humus-rich soil in partial shade. Pruning group 1; plants under glass may need restrictive pruning.

• **PROPAGATION** Sow seed at 21°C (70°F) in spring.

• **PESTS AND DISEASES** Red spider mites may be a problem under glass.

C. odorata ▣ 🌳 (Ilang-ilang, Macassar oil tree, Ylang-ylang). Spreading tree with arching to pendent branches and oblong-ovate, tapered, mid- to dark green leaves, 10–20cm (4–8in) long. Axillary, pendent clusters of strong-scented yellow flowers, 3–5cm (1¼–2in) across, with narrow, pointed petals, are borne in autumn. ↕ 10–20m (30–70ft), ↔ 4–8m (12–25ft). India to Australia (Queensland), Philippines. ❀ (min. 16°C/61°F)

CANARINA

CAMPANULACEAE

Genus of 3 species of herbaceous climbers, with thick, tuberous roots, found in forest and at forest margins in the Canary Islands and E. Africa. The leaves are opposite and simple or lobed. Canarinas are valued for their pendent, bell-shaped flowers, with 6 petal lobes, produced singly or in clusters from the upper leaf axils. In frost-prone regions, grow in a container or border in a cool greenhouse or conservatory; elsewhere, grow against a house wall or allow to scramble through low shrubs.

• **HARDINESS** Frost tender.

• **CULTIVATION** Under glass, grow in loam-based potting compost (JI No.3) in bright filtered light with good ventilation. Keep completely dry when foliage yellows in late spring; pot on in late summer while dormant and keep just moist until new growth begins; when in growth, water freely and apply a balanced liquid fertilizer every 2–3 weeks. Provide support. Outdoors, grow in fertile, well-drained soil in partial shade. Protect from summer rain when growth yellows, and keep the crowns dry until autumn.

• **PROPAGATION** Sow seed at 15–18°C (59–64°F) in autumn or spring. Take basal cuttings flush with the tubers in late winter or early spring as shoots are produced; root in a propagating case.

• **PESTS AND DISEASES** May be infested with whiteflies at high temperatures.

C. campanula see *C. canariensis.*

C. canariensis ▣ 🏆 syn. *C. campanula* (Canary bellflower). Scrambling, deciduous climber producing branching, scandent, robust stems and lance-shaped or 3-angled, shallowly lobed, mid-green leaves, 4–8cm (1½–3in) long. The bell-shaped, orange-red to orange-yellow flowers, 3–6cm (1¼–2½in) long, are attractively veined, and borne singly from the upper leaf axils from late winter to late spring. ↕ 1–1.5m (3–5ft), ↔ 60–90cm (24–36in). Canary Islands. ❀ (min. 5°C/41°F)

▷ **Canary bird bush** see *Crotalaria agatiflora*
▷ **Canary creeper** see *Tropaeolum peregrinum*
▷ **Candle plant** see *Plectranthus oertendahlii, Senecio articulatus*
Empress see *Senna alata*
▷ **Candlewood** see *Rothmannia capensis*
▷ ***Candollea*** see *Hibbertia*
C. cuneiformis see *H. cuneiformis*
▷ **Candytuft** see *Iberis*
Common see *I. umbellata*
▷ **Cane, Rattan** see *Calamus rotang*
▷ **Canebrake** see *Arundinaria gigantea*

CANISTRUM

BROMELIACEAE

Genus of 7 species of epiphytic or terrestrial, evergreen perennials (bromeliads) from forest in Brazil. The funnel-shaped leaf rosettes comprise strap-shaped, spiny-margined leaves, which are fine-scaly on the undersides. Dense, compound cymes, each consisting of a rounded flowerhead of green, yellowish green to white, yellow, or occasionally blue flowers in a "basket" of large, colourful bracts, are borne in summer. They are followed by spherical, greenish white fruits containing spindle-shaped seeds. In frost-prone climates, grow in a warm conservatory or greenhouse; in warmer areas, grow outdoors in a moist, shady site.

• **HARDINESS** Frost tender.

• **CULTIVATION** Under glass, grow epiphytically, or in epiphytic bromeliad compost, in bright filtered light with moderate humidity. In the growing season, water freely, applying a low-nitrogen fertilizer 3 or 4 times; keep just moist at other times. Outdoors, grow epiphytically in a tree or in humus-rich, sandy soil in partial shade. See also p.47.

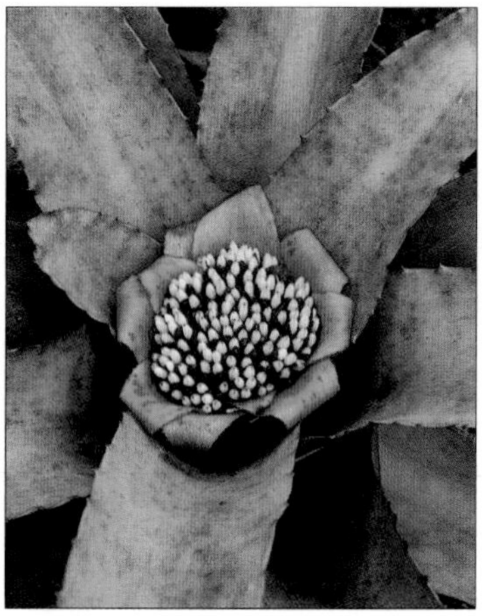

Canistrum lindenii var. *roseum*

• **PROPAGATION** Sow seed at 27°C (81°F) as soon as ripe. Remove offsets in early summer.

• **PESTS AND DISEASES** Scale insects may be a problem.

C. lindenii. Variable, epiphytic bromeliad with funnel-shaped rosettes, to 1m (3ft) across, of mid-green leaves, to 80cm (32in) long, often marked darker green. In summer, produces dense cymes of about 100 narrowly funnel-shaped, white-tipped green flowers surrounded by yellowish white or green bracts. ↕ to 1m (3ft) or more, ↔ 60–120cm (24–47in). Brazil. ❀ (min. 16°C/61°F). **var. *roseum*** ▣ has rose-pink to light red bracts.

CANNA

Indian shot plant

CANNACEAE

Genus of about 50 species of rhizomatous herbaceous perennials, mainly from forest margins and moist, open areas in forest in Asia and tropical North and South America. Cannas are cultivated for their large, alternate, paddle-shaped leaves, 30–60cm (12–24in) long in most species and cultivars; they are pinnately veined and sheathed at the bases. The racemes or panicles of brightly coloured flowers are also attractive, each asymmetric flower having 3 petals joined into a tube at the bases, 3 sepals, and showy stamens. The flowers are usually produced in pairs from the axil of each bract. Hundreds of hybrids have resulted from complex crosses between various species; they

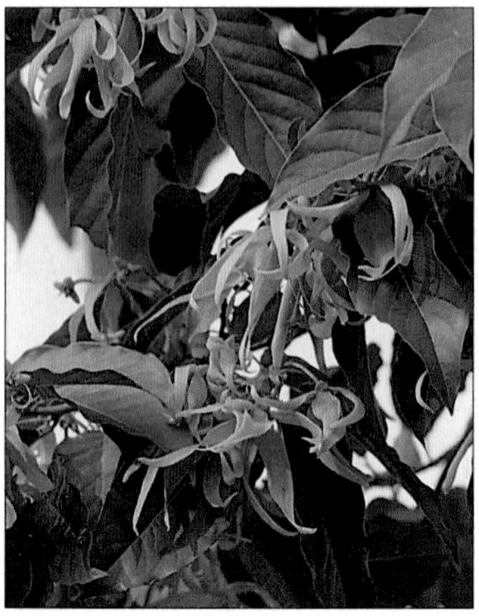

Cananga odorata

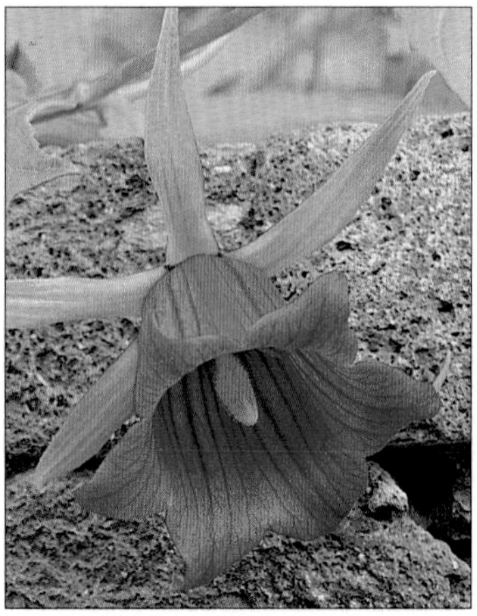

Canarina canariensis

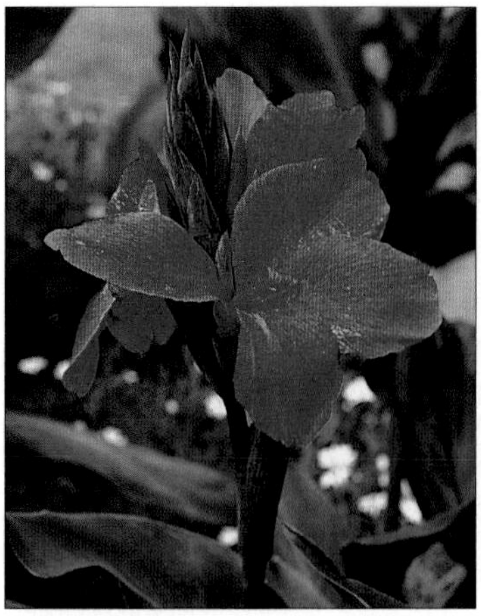

Canna 'Assaut'

are often grouped under the names *C. x generalis* and *C. x orchioides*. As the distinctions between these hybrid groups have been blurred by further inter-breeding these names have not been used in the descriptions below.

In frost-prone areas, use cannas in summer bedding and lift for winter, or grow in containers on a patio or in a cool conservatory or greenhouse. In warmer areas, grow in a border.

• **HARDINESS** Half hardy to frost tender.

• **CULTIVATION** Under glass, grow in loamless potting compost in full light with shade from hot sun. During the growing season, water freely and apply a phosphate-rich liquid fertilizer monthly. Outdoors, grow in a sheltered site in fertile soil in full sun; water freely in dry spells. Dead-head to promote continued flowering. In frost-prone regions, plant in early summer; when autumn frost blackens the foliage, remove the stems and leaves and lift the rhizomes for winter storage; store in barely moist peat or leaf mould in frost-free conditions. In areas that are frost-free or almost so, leave *in situ* and protect with a deep dry mulch.

• **PROPAGATION** Sow seed at 21°C (70°F) in spring or autumn. Chip seed or soak in warm water for 24 hours before sowing. Divide rhizomes into short sections, each with a prominent "eye", in early spring. Pot on and start into growth at 16°C (61°F); water sparingly at first.

• **PESTS AND DISEASES** Susceptible to red spider mites under glass. Slugs and caterpillars may be a problem outdoors.

***C.* 'Assault'** see *C.* 'Assault'.
***C.* 'Assault'** ■ syn. *C.* 'Assault'. Upright, rhizomatous perennial bearing purple-brown leaves, and racemes of gladiolus-like, orange-scarlet flowers, 7cm (3in) across, from midsummer to autumn. ↕ 1.8m (6ft), ↔ 50cm (20in). ✲
***C.* 'Black Knight'.** Erect, rhizomatous perennial producing bronze foliage. From midsummer to early autumn,

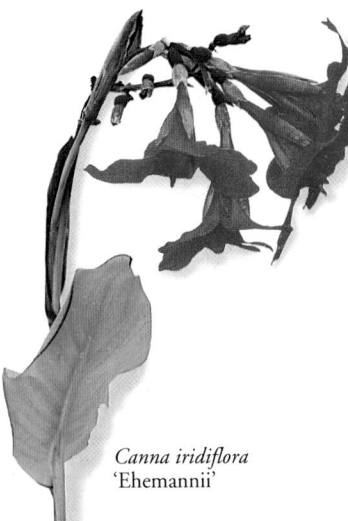

Canna iridiflora 'Ehemannii'

bears large racemes of gladiolus-like, very dark red flowers, 7cm (3in) across, with wavy petals. ↕ 1.8m (6ft), ↔ 50cm (20in). ✲
C. edulis see *C. indica.*
***C.* 'Endeavour'** ■ Erect, rhizomatous perennial producing blue-green leaves. Racemes of iris-like, bright soft red flowers, 5cm (2in) across, are borne from midsummer to early autumn. ↕ 1.5–2.2m (5–7ft), ↔ 50cm (20in). ✲
***C.* 'Erebus'.** Erect, rhizomatous perennial with dark green leaves. From midsummer to early autumn, bears racemes of gladiolus-like, dark red flowers, 8cm (3in) across. ↕ 1.8m (6ft), ↔ 50cm (20in). ✲
C. glauca. Slender, rhizomatous perennial with brittle rhizomes and narrowly ovate to elliptic, glaucous, blue-green leaves, 30–50cm (12–20in) long. Racemes of iris-like, pale lemon-yellow to dark yellow flowers, 7–9cm (3–3½in) across, are borne from mid-summer to early autumn. ↕ 1.5–2.2m (5–7ft), ↔ 50cm (20in). West Indies to Bolivia and Argentina. ✲
C. indica, syn. *C. edulis.* Rhizomatous perennial with ovate-lance-shaped to oblong, dark green, often bronze-tinted leaves, to 50cm (20in) long. Racemes or panicles of iris-like, bright red or soft orange flowers, 5–7cm (2–3in) across, are borne from midsummer to mid-autumn. ↕ 1.5–2.2m (5–7ft), ↔ 50cm (20in). Tropical and subtropical South America. ✲. **'Purpurea'** produces dark purple leaves.
C. iridiflora. Upright, rhizomatous perennial with broadly elliptic, dark bluish green leaves, to 1m (3ft) long. Pendent panicles of trumpet-shaped, bright cerise-pink flowers, 11cm (4½in) across, open from midsummer to early autumn. ↕ 3m (10ft), ↔ 50cm (20in). Peru. ✲. **'Ehemannii'** ■ has dark blue-green leaves with red margins, and bears panicles of waxy, bright pinkish red flowers, to 15cm (6in) across; ↕ 2m (6ft), ↔ 60cm (24in).
***C.* 'King Humbert'**, syn. *C.* 'Roi Humbert'. Erect, rhizomatous perennial with vivid purple leaves, and racemes of orchid-like, bright red flowers, 7cm (3in) across, borne from midsummer to early autumn. ↕ 1.8m (6ft), ↔ 50cm (20in). ✲
***C.* 'King Midas'** ■ Erect, rhizomatous perennial with dark green leaves. Sturdy racemes of gladiolus-like, golden yellow, orange-marked flowers, 7cm (3in) across, are borne from midsummer to early autumn. ↕ 1.5m (5ft), ↔ 50cm (20in). ✲
***C.* 'Louis Cayeux'.** Very free-flowering, rhizomatous perennial producing bright green leaves. Racemes of orchid-like, soft salmon-pink flowers, 10cm (4in) across, are borne from midsummer to early autumn. ↕ 1.5m (5ft), ↔ 50cm (20in). ✲
***C.* 'Lucifer'.** Dwarf, very free-flowering, rhizomatous perennial with mid-green leaves. From midsummer to early autumn, bears profuse racemes of iris-like flowers, 5cm (2in) across; tepals are red with yellow margins. ↕ 60cm (24in), ↔ 50cm (20in). ✲
***C. malawiensis* 'Variegata'** see *C.* 'Striata'.

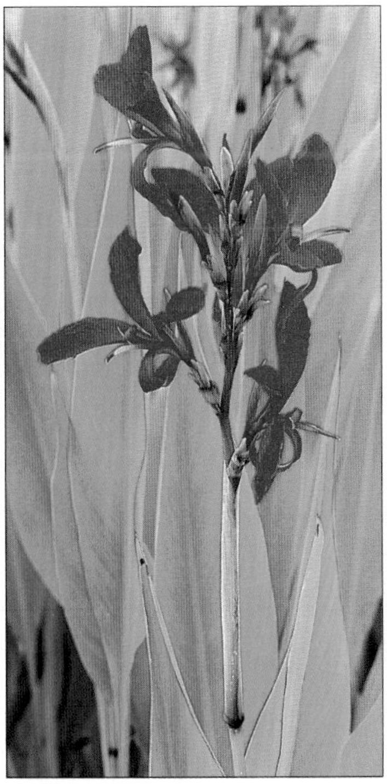

Canna 'Endeavour'

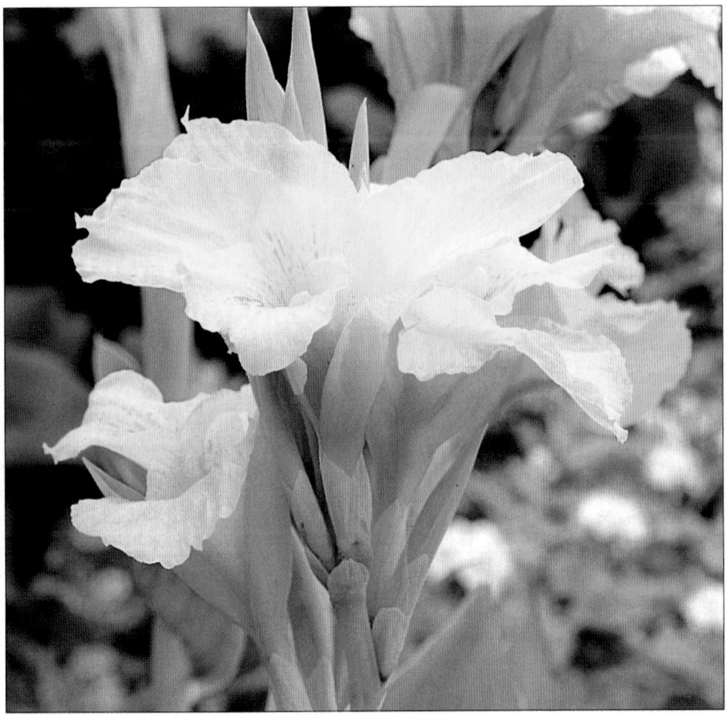

Canna 'King Midas'

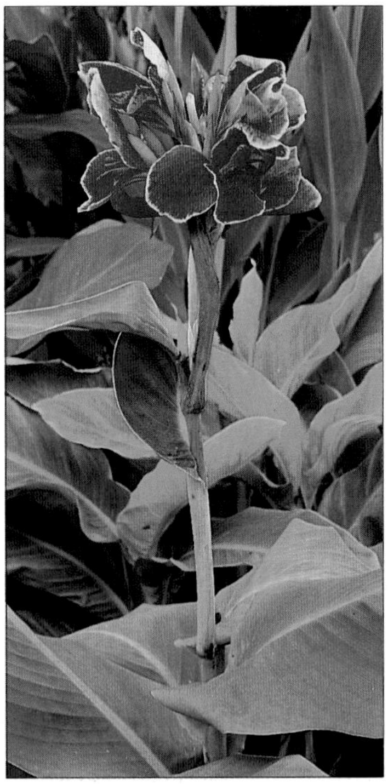

Canna 'Rosemond Coles'

***C.* 'Pfitzer's Chinese Coral'.** Upright, rhizomatous perennial with grey-green leaves. Abundant racemes of gladiolus-like, coral-pink flowers, 7cm (3in) wide, open from midsummer to early autumn. ↕ 80cm (32in), ↔ 50cm (20in). ✲
***C.* 'Picasso'.** Compact, rhizomatous perennial bearing blue-green leaves and racemes of gladiolus-like, yellow, red-spotted flowers, 7cm (3in) across, from midsummer to early autumn. Leaves and flowers are bleached by bright sun, so best grown in partial shade. ↕ 1.2m (4ft), ↔ 50cm (20in). ✲
***C.* 'President'.** Erect, rhizomatous perennial with glossy, blue-green leaves and racemes of gladiolus-like, rich scarlet flowers, 7cm (3in) across, borne from midsummer to early autumn. ↕ 1.2m (4ft), ↔ 50cm (20in). ✲
***C.* 'Roi Humbert'** see *C.* 'King Humbert'.
***C.* 'Rosemond Coles'** ■ Upright, rhizomatous perennial with large, mid-green leaves. From midsummer to early autumn, bears racemes of gladiolus-like red flowers, 7cm (3in) across, with yellow margins and yellow-spotted throats; the undersides of the petals are golden. ↕ 1.5m (5ft), ↔ 50cm (20in). ✲
***C.* 'Striata'**, syn. *C. malawiensis* 'Variegata'. Erect, rhizomatous perennial with dark red-purple stems and light green to yellow-green leaves, 25–50cm (10–20in) long, with bright yellow veins. Racemes of gladiolus-like orange flowers, 8cm (3in) across, are produced from midsummer to early autumn. ↕ 1.5m (5ft), ↔ 50cm (20in). ✲
***C.* 'Wyoming'.** Upright, rhizomatous perennial producing brown-purple leaves with darker purple veins. From midsummer to early autumn, bears racemes of gladiolus-like, frilled orange flowers, 10cm (4in) across, with apricot feathering and darker orange margins. ↕ 1.8m (6ft), ↔ 50cm (20in). ✲

▷ **Canterbury bells** see *Campanula medium, C. medium* 'Calycanthema'

CANTUA

POLEMONIACEAE

Genus of 6 species of evergreen, small trees and shrubs of arching, sometimes scandent habit, usually found in mountainous areas of South America. The alternate leaves are simple, and the showy, tubular, 5-lobed flowers, borne in terminal corymbs, are red, purple, violet, or white. In frost-prone areas, grow cantuas in a cool greenhouse. In frost-free climates, they are suitable for growing against a wall or pillar, or in a shrub border.

• **HARDINESS** Half hardy to frost tender. *C. buxifolia* can withstand short periods of frost if grown in a warm, sheltered position.

• **CULTIVATION** Under glass, grow in loam-based potting compost (JI No.3) in full light. Water freely during the growing season, applying a balanced liquid fertilizer monthly; water more sparingly in winter. Stand containers outdoors in summer. Top-dress or pot on in spring. The long, flexible stems require support. Outdoors, grow in fertile, moist but well-drained soil in a warm, sheltered site in full sun. Pruning group 11, after flowering.

• **PROPAGATION** Sow seed at 15–18°C (59–64°F) in spring. Root semi-ripe cuttings in summer.

• **PESTS AND DISEASES** Red spider mites and whiteflies may be a problem, particularly under glass.

C. buxifolia ■ syn. *C. dependens* (Sacred flower of the Incas). Upright, often semi-scandent shrub with elliptic to lance-shaped, lobed, softly hairy, mid-green leaves, 2.5–5cm (1–2in) long. In spring, bears terminal corymbs of long-tubed, pendent flowers, 6–7cm (2½–3in) long, the tubes pink to purple, the petal lobes red. ↕ 2–5m (6–15ft), ↔ 1.5–2.5m (5–8ft). Peru, Bolivia, N. Chile. ❄

C. dependens see *C. buxifolia.*

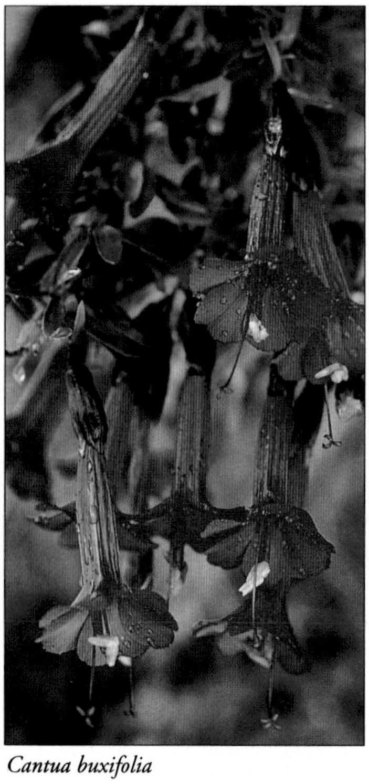

Cantua buxifolia

CAPSICUM

Chilli pepper, Pepper

SOLANACEAE

Genus of up to 10 species of erect or spreading, many-branched annuals and perennials from wasteland and lowland forest margins in tropical North and South America. They have entire leaves, which are alternate or borne in groups of 2 or 3 at the nodes. Tubular or bell-shaped, yellow, white, green-white, or purple-tinged flowers are produced singly or in clusters of 2 or 3 from the leaf axils. Capsicums are mostly cultivated as crop plants for their shiny, chambered, many-seeded, variably shaped fruits, which are green at first, often ripening to yellow, orange, or red. The genus includes bell peppers (pimentos) as well as hot chilli peppers. In frost-prone areas, capsicums with brightly coloured fruit are also used ornamentally as houseplants, for window-boxes and patio containers, or for a warm greenhouse or conservatory.

• **HARDINESS** Frost tender.

• **CULTIVATION** Under glass, grow in loam-based potting compost (JI No.2) in bright filtered light. When in growth, water freely and apply a balanced liquid fertilizer every 10 days until fruit begins to colour. Provide tall cultivars with support. In summer, maintain high humidity and temperatures of 21–25°C (70–77°F). Mist flowers daily with water to encourage fruiting. Outdoors, grow in fertile, well-drained soil enriched with garden compost or manure in full sun. Pinch out the growing tips of young plants to promote branching.

• **PROPAGATION** Sow seed at 21°C (70°F) in late winter.

• **PESTS AND DISEASES** Susceptible to viruses, fungal wilt, anthracnose, and powdery mildew. Red spider mites and aphids may be a problem under glass.

C. annuum* var. *acuminatum see *C. annuum.*

C. annuum, syn. *C. annuum* var. *acuminatum* (Chilli pepper, Paprika). Annual or short-lived perennial with alternate, lance-shaped to ovate, mid-green leaves, to 12cm (5in) long. Solitary, bell-shaped, white or yellow flowers, to 1.5cm (½in) across, are produced from the leaf axils in summer, or all year round, depending on the climate. The pendent, narrowly conical, twisted fruit, to 15cm (6in) long, are used fresh or dried. ↕ 1.5m (5ft), ↔ 50cm (20in). Tropical North and South America. ❀ (min. 4°C/39°F). Many cultivars are available. They are divided into 5 main groups, varying in shape, colour, and flavour. **Cerasiforme Group** (Cherry pepper) cultivars produce small, hot-flavoured, spherical fruit, 3–6cm (1¼–2½in) long, in shades of yellow, red, or purple. **Conioides Group** (Cone pepper) cultivars bear ornamental, hot-tasting, conical, erect fruit, to 5cm (2in) long, which are white or green at first, turning scarlet, crimson, or purple. **Fasciculatum Group** (Red cone pepper) cultivars bear hot-flavoured, clustered, upright, conical, bright red fruit, to 7cm (3in) long. **Grossum Group** (Bell pepper) cultivars include the salad peppers; they bear sweet, irregularly ovoid-bell-shaped green fruit, 10–12cm (4–5in) long, which ripen to yellow, crimson, or deep purple. **Longum Group** (Cayenne pepper, Chilli pepper) cultivars bear very hot-tasting, pendent, tapered fruit, 15–30cm (6–12in) long, in shades from red to black-purple; some also produce attractively variegated leaves.

CARAGANA

LEGUMINOSAE/PAPILIONACEAE

Genus of about 80 species of deciduous, often spiny shrubs or small trees found on dry soils in exposed sites from E. Europe to China. They are cultivated for their attractive leaves, which are alternate, pinnate, and often clustered, and their solitary or clustered, pea-like flowers, which are usually yellow, but sometimes white or pink. Flowers are followed in autumn by slender brown pods, 2–6cm (¾–2½in) long. Grow in a dry shrub border or use as windbreaks.

• **HARDINESS** Fully hardy.

• **CULTIVATION** Grow in well-drained, moderately fertile soil in full sun. Will thrive even in poor, dry soils in cold and exposed positions. Pruning group 1.

• **PROPAGATION** Sow seed in containers in an open frame as soon as ripe; pre-soak spring-sown seed in warm water. Root greenwood cuttings in late spring. Graft in late winter; *C. arborescens* 'Pendula' is usually top-grafted.

• **PESTS AND DISEASES** Trouble free.

C. arborescens (Pea tree). Erect, thorny shrub with pinnate, light green leaves, to 8cm (3in) long, composed of up to 12 elliptic leaflets. Pale yellow flowers, to 2cm (¾in) long, are borne singly or in small clusters in late spring. ↕ 6m (20ft), ↔ 4m (12ft). Russia (Siberia), N. China. ❄❄❄. **'Lorbergii'** 𝕍 has elegant leaves, with 10–14 long, linear-lance-shaped leaflets, and small flowers, to 1cm (½in) long. **'Nana'** ■ has a dwarf, congested habit and twisted shoots; ↕ 1.5m (5ft), ↔ 1m (3ft). **'Pendula'** has stiff, pendent shoots; ↕ 1.5m (5ft), ↔ 1.2m (4ft).

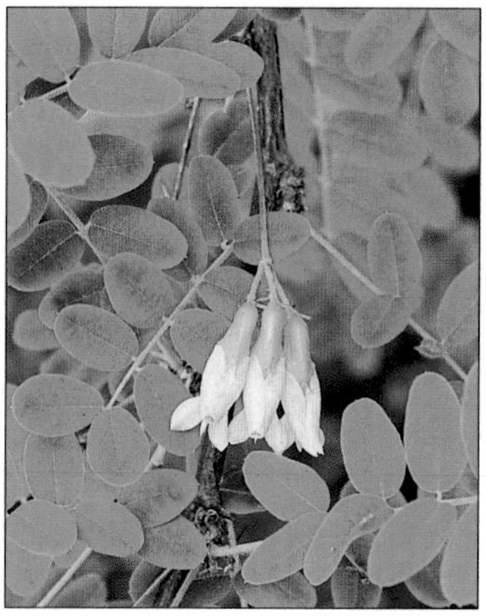

Caragana brevispina

C. brevispina ■ Spiny shrub with long, arching shoots, pink-tinged when young. Pinnate, softly hairy, mid-green leaves, to 10cm (4in) long, have up to 10 oblong to lance-shaped leaflets. In spring, produces clusters of 3 or 4 yellowish green flowers, to 2cm (¾in) long, becoming reddish yellow with age. ↕ 2–3m (6–10ft), ↔ 4m (12ft). N.W. Himalayas. ❄❄❄

C. frutex (Russian pea shrub). Shrub with upright, slender shoots and pinnate, dark green leaves, to 2.5cm (1in) long, each comprising 2 pairs of stalkless, ovate leaflets. Bright yellow flowers, to 2.5cm (1in) long, are produced singly from the leaf axils in late spring and early summer. ↕ 3m (10ft), ↔ 2.5m (8ft). S. former USSR, C. Asia. ❄❄❄

C. pygmaea. Low-growing, spiny shrub with arching or prostrate shoots and pinnate, mid-green leaves, 2–3cm (¾–1¼in) long, comprising 2 pairs of inversely lance-shaped leaflets. From late spring to summer, bears pendent yellow flowers, to 2.5cm (1in) long, singly along the shoots. ↕ 1m (3ft), ↔ 1.5m (5ft). Caucasus to E. Russia (Siberia) and China (Tibet). ❄❄❄

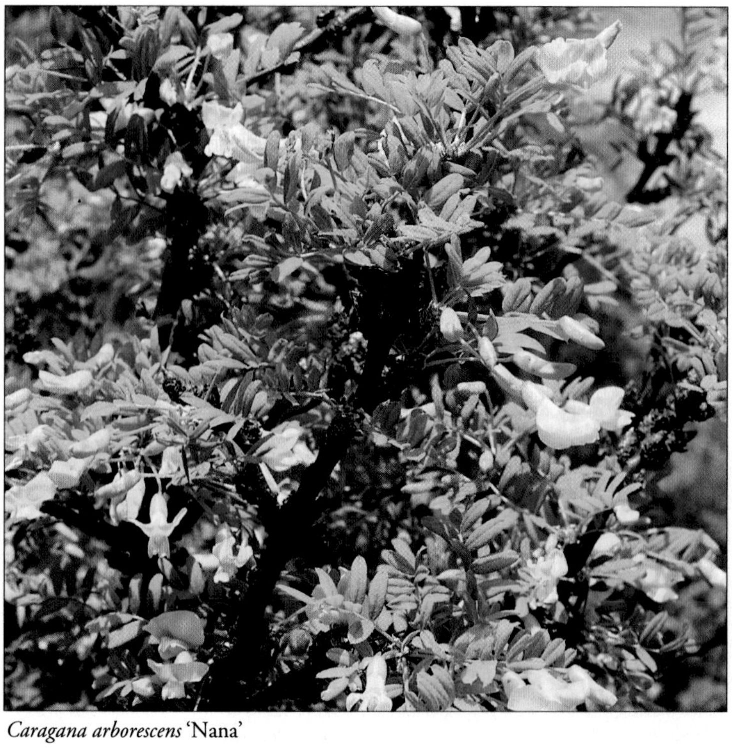

Caragana arborescens 'Nana'

CARALLUMA syn. FREREA

ASCLEPIADACEAE

Genus of 80–100 species of tufted or clump-forming, often stoloniferous, perennial succulents from dry areas of the Mediterranean, Africa, Socotra, the Arabian Peninsula, India, and Burma. They have succulent stems, producing leaves that are reduced to scales in most species. The open bell-shaped, 5-lobed, axillary or terminal flowers, solitary or in umbels, usually exude a pungent odour. The fruits are cylindrical, greyish green follicles containing tufted seeds. In frost-prone areas, grow in a warm greenhouse; in warm, dry climates, use outdoors in a semi-desert garden.

- **HARDINESS** Frost tender.
- **CULTIVATION** Under glass, grow in standard cactus compost in bright filtered light in summer and full light in winter. When in growth, water moderately and apply a low-nitrogen fertilizer monthly; water very sparingly in winter to avoid desiccation. Outdoors, grow in sharply drained, humus-rich, sandy soil in partial shade. See also pp.48–49.
- **PROPAGATION** Sow seed at 18–21°C (64–70°F) in late spring or early summer. Take stem cuttings in spring, allow calluses to form, then root in partial shade.
- **PESTS AND DISEASES** Prone to scale insects, mealybugs, root mealybugs, and black rot.

C. albocastanea see *Orbeopsis albocastanea.*
C. burchardii. Cushion-forming, leafless succulent with 4-angled, grey-green to bluish green stems with deep marginal teeth. Terminal umbels of up to 6 olive-green or reddish brown flowers, each to 1.5cm (½in) across, with white-hairy corolla lobes, are borne in summer. Canary Islands, Morocco. ↕ to 20cm (8in), ↔ to 18cm (7in). ❄ (min. 10°C/50°F)
C. dummeri see *Pachycymbium dummeri.*
C. europaea, syn. *Stapelia europaea.* Variable, leafless succulent with 4-angled, blunt-margined, grey-green stems, often spotted pale red. In summer, bears terminal umbels of 10 or more greenish yellow or reddish brown flowers, to 1.5cm (½in) across, the pointed yellow corolla lobes with reddish brown tips and purple stripes. ↕ 13cm (5in), ↔ to 20cm (8in). S. Italy, Spain, N. Africa. ❄ (min. 10°C/50°F)
C. frerei, syn. *Frerea indica.* Succulent with rounded, few-branched, prostrate or pendent, fleshy, pale green stems. The persistent, opposite, fleshy leaves, 2–3cm (¾–1¼in) long, are oblong or ovoid. In summer, bears solitary or paired, terminal, red-brown or maroon flowers, 2cm (¾in) across, with yellow- or white-marked lobes. ↕↔ to 12cm (5in). E. India. ❄ (min. 10°C/50°F)
C. joannis ■ Leafless succulent with erect or pendent, square to rounded, minutely toothed, purple-green stems. In summer, bears umbels of 2–10 flowers, each to 2.5cm (1in) across, with red-spotted, olive-yellow tubes and velvety purple lobes tipped with fine hairs. ↕ 10cm (4in) or more, ↔ 13cm (5in). Morocco. ❄ (min. 10°C/50°F)
C. lutea see *Orbeopsis lutea.*
C. pillansii see *Quaqua pillansii.*

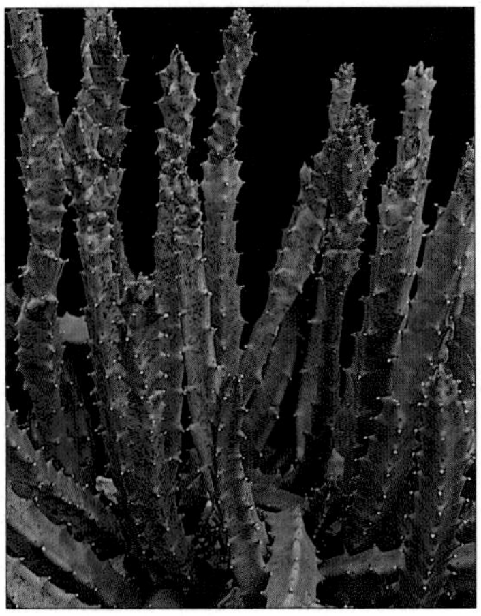
Caralluma joannis

▷**Caraway** see *Carum, C. carvi*

CARDAMINE syn. DENTARIA

Bittercress

BRASSICACEAE/CRUCIFERAE

Genus of about 150 species of annuals and perennials from cool, shady, damp habitats almost worldwide, but chiefly in the N. hemisphere. Some of the annuals are invasive garden weeds. The rootstock is fibrous or has scaly rhizomes. Cardamines have simple, pinnate or palmate leaves and unbranched stems bearing panicles or racemes (some short and congested) of 4-petalled, white, yellow, pink, lilac, or reddish violet flowers. Grow in a border, a rock garden, or in woodland.

- **HARDINESS** Fully hardy.
- **CULTIVATION** Grow in humus-rich, moist soil in full or partial shade.
- **PROPAGATION** Sow seed in containers in a cold frame in autumn or spring. Divide in spring or after flowering. Root leaf-tip cuttings of *C. pratensis* and its cultivars in midsummer; they may also form bulbils or plantlets in the axils of the leaflets.
- **PESTS AND DISEASES** Flea beetles and aphids may damage the leaves.

C. asarifolia. Stoloniferous, clump-forming perennial producing prostrate, rooting stems and simple, kidney-shaped, mid-green leaves, 10–15cm (4–6in) long. Compact racemes of white flowers, each 7–10mm (¼–½in) across, with violet anthers, are borne in late spring and early summer. ↕ 30–45cm (12–18in), ↔ to 60cm (24in). S. France, N. Italy. ✻✻✻
C. enneaphyllos ■ syn. *Dentaria enneaphyllos.* Spreading, rhizomatous perennial producing whorls of 2- to 4-ternate or 3- to 5-palmate, toothed, mid-green leaves, 10–12cm (4–5in) long, composed of ovate to lance-shaped leaflets. In late spring, bears lax panicles of pendent, white or yellowish white flowers, 2cm (¾in) or more across. ↕ 20–40cm (8–16in), ↔ 45–60cm (18–24in). W. Carpathians and E. Alps to S. Italy, N.W. Balkans. ✻✻✻
C. latifolia see *C. raphanifolia.*
C. pentaphyllos ■ syn. *Dentaria digitata, D. pentaphyllos.* Clump-forming, rhizomatous perennial with toothed, 5-palmate, mid-green leaves, 10–12cm (4–5in) long, composed of lance-shaped leaflets. Loose racemes of white, pale purple, or lilac flowers, to 2.5cm (1in) across, are borne in late spring and early summer. ↕ 30–50cm (12–20in), ↔ 30cm (12in). Pyrenees to S. Germany and N.W. Balkans. ✻✻✻
C. pratensis (Cuckoo flower, Lady's smock). Variable perennial with short rhizomes and rosettes of pinnate, grey-green to glossy, dark green leaves, to 15cm (6in) long, composed of 2–8 pairs of ovate to rounded or kidney-shaped leaflets, often producing plantlets. In late spring, bears panicles of purple, lilac, or white flowers, 1–3cm (½–1¼in) across. ↕ 30–45cm (12–18in), ↔ 30cm (12in). Europe, N. Asia, North America. ✻✻✻. **'Edith'** has pink buds, opening to double flowers that fade to white; ↕ 20cm (8in). **'Flore Pleno'** ■♀ forms compact clumps and freely produces plantlets in the basal leaf clusters; it has double, lilac-pink flowers; ↕ 20cm (8in).
C. raphanifolia, syn. *C. latifolia.* Rhizomatous, spreading perennial with pinnate, dark green leaves, 10–15cm (4–6in) long, composed of 1–6 pairs of ovate to rounded, toothed leaflets. Panicles of lilac, reddish violet, or white flowers, 1–2cm (½–¾in) across, are borne in early summer. ↕ 45–80cm (18–32in), ↔ 60cm (24in). Mountains of S. Europe. ✻✻✻
C. trifolia ■ (Trifoliate bittercress). Creeping perennial with short rhizomes and 3-palmate, dark green leaves, 2–3cm (¾–1¼in) long, with 3 rounded to diamond-shaped leaflets, red-tinted beneath. In late spring, produces short, congested racemes of open cup-shaped, yellow-anthered, white, occasionally pink flowers, 1–2cm (½–¾in) across. ↕ to 15cm (6in), ↔ to 30cm (12in). Mountainous, wooded areas in C. and S. Europe. ✻✻✻

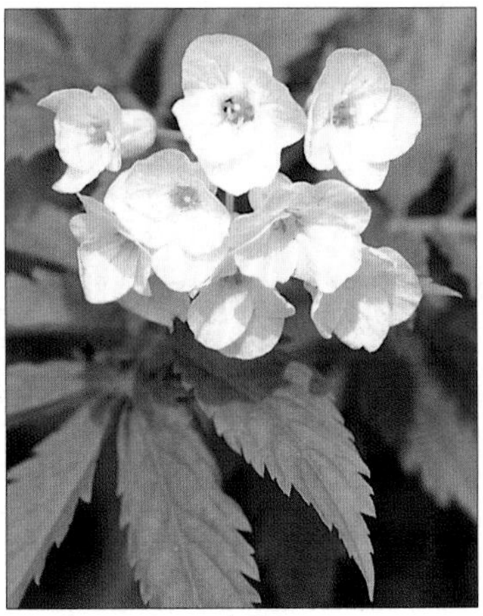
Cardamine enneaphyllos

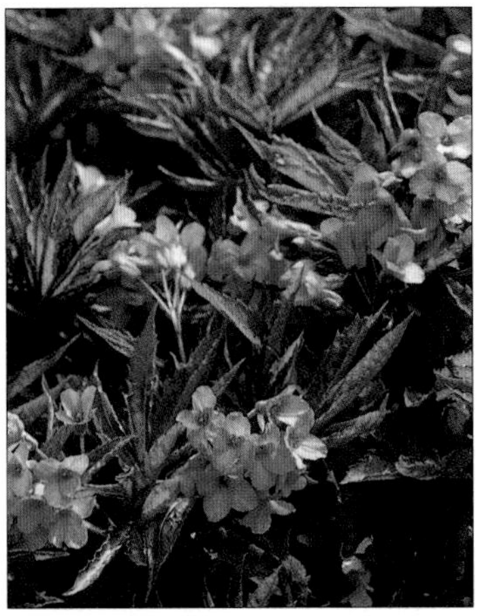
Cardamine pentaphyllos

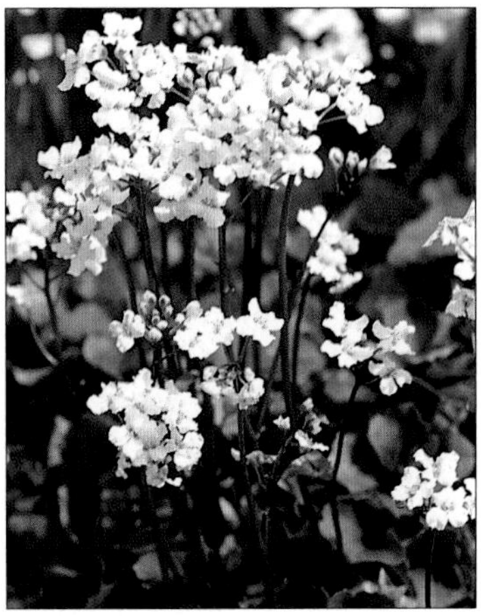
Cardamine trifolia

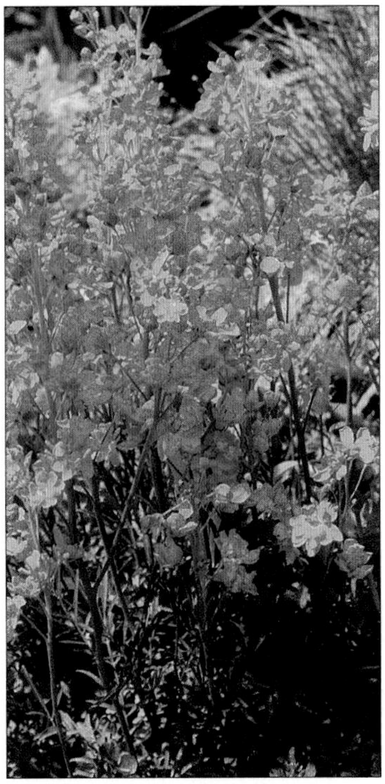
Cardamine pratensis 'Flore Pleno'

▷**Cardamom** see *Elettaria cardamomum*
▷**Cardinal climber** see *Ipomoea* x *multifida*
▷**Cardinal flower** see *Lobelia cardinalis, Sinningia cardinalis*
Blue see *Lobelia siphilitica*
▷**Cardinal's guard** see *Pachystachys coccinea*

CARDIOCRINUM

Giant lily

LILIACEAE

Genus of 3 species of large, bulbous, monocarpic perennials found in scrub and forest in the Himalayas, Japan, and China. They are cultivated for their spectacular, lily-like, trumpet-shaped flowers, borne in summer, and their attractive, heart-shaped, veined leaves. The flowers are followed by large, decorative, upright, oblong-ovoid, pale brown seed capsules, 5–6cm (2–2½in) long. The bulbs take several years to

C

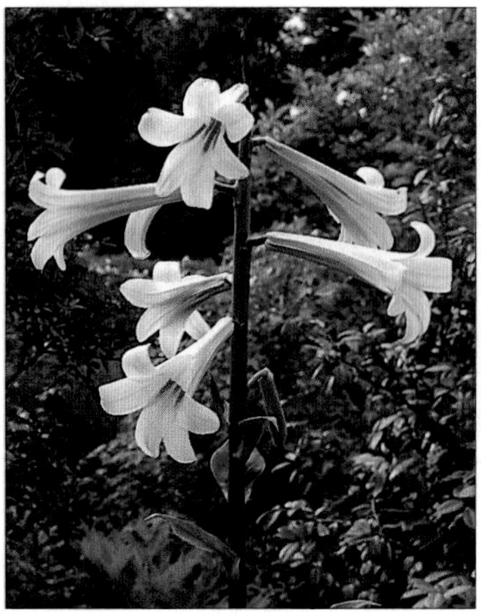

Cardiocrinum giganteum

reach maturity and die after flowering, leaving numerous offsets. Grow in woodland, or in a shaded, sheltered border.

- **HARDINESS** Fully to frost hardy; new growth that develops in early spring may need protection in frost-prone areas.
- **CULTIVATION** Plant bulbs just below the soil surface in autumn, in a cool, partially shaded, sheltered site in deep, fertile, humus-rich, moist but well-drained soil. Water freely in dry periods, but do not allow to become water-logged; giant lilies are intolerant of hot or dry conditions. Apply a balanced liquid fertilizer 2 or 3 times when in growth, to encourage the development of offsets. Top-dress annually with leaf mould. Provide a deep winter mulch.
- **PROPAGATION** Sow seed in deep trays in a cool, shaded bulb frame as soon as ripe. Remove offsets after flowering. Offsets may take 4–5 years to flower; seed-raised plants take 7 years or more.
- **PESTS AND DISEASES** Prone to lily viruses and slug damage.

C. cordatum, syn. *Lilium cordatum.* Bulbous perennial with broad, heart-shaped, dark green leaves, to 30cm (12in) long, stained maroon when young, borne on the lower part of the stems. In summer, stout, hollow stems bear congested, terminal racemes of 4–10, occasionally up to 20, trumpet-shaped, scented, creamy white flowers, to 15cm (6in) long, with purple marks on the lower tepals. ↕ 1.2–2m (4–6ft), ↔ 30cm (12in). Japan, Russia (Sakhalin). ❄❄❄

C. giganteum ■ ♀ syn. *Lilium giganteum.* Bulbous perennial with basal rosettes of large, broadly ovate, glossy, dark green leaves, to 45cm (18in) long. Smaller leaves are produced on the tall, stout flower stems, which in summer bear racemes of up to 20 large, nodding, trumpet-shaped, strongly scented white flowers, 15–20cm (6–8in) long, with maroon stripes inside. ↕ 1.5–4m (5–12ft), ↔ 45cm (18in). Himalayas, N.W. Burma, S.W. China. ❄❄❄.

var. *yunnanense* ■ has bronze-purple stems, leaves, and young shoots; the flowers are often tinted green; W. and C. China.

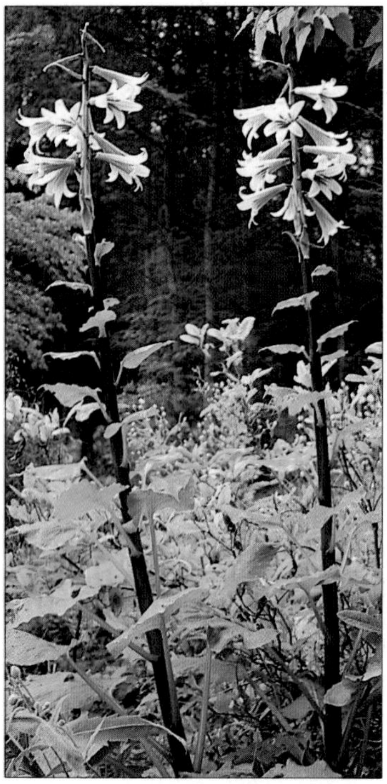

Cardiocrinum giganteum var. *yunnanense*

CARDIOSPERMUM

Heart seed

SAPINDACEAE

Genus of 14 species of evergreen, perennial, woody-stemmed tendril climbers from forest margins in tropical Africa, India, and North and South America. They are cultivated for their attractive, fern-like foliage and decorative, swollen seed pods. The alternate, 2-ternate leaves have deeply toothed or pinnatifid leaflets. Small flowers, with 4 unequal petals, are borne in stalked, axillary corymbs, each with a pair of opposite tendrils. In frost-prone areas, grow outdoors as half-hardy annuals, or in a temperate greenhouse. In warmer regions, train over a tall tree stump, archway, pergola, or arbour.

- **HARDINESS** Frost tender.
- **CULTIVATION** Under glass, grow in loam-based potting compost (JI No.3) in bright filtered light. In the growing season, water freely and apply a liquid fertilizer monthly; keep just moist in winter. Pot on or top-dress in spring. Outdoors, grow in fertile, moist but well-drained soil in full sun. Provide support. In early spring, thin out congested growth of plants grown as perennials.
- **PROPAGATION** Sow seed at 18–21°C (64–70°F) in spring. Root softwood cuttings in summer.
- **PESTS AND DISEASES** Aphids and whiteflies may be a problem under glass.

C. halicacabum (Balloon vine, Heart pea, Love-in-a-puff, Winter cherry). Slender, woody-based, evergreen tendril climber, normally grown as an annual or biennial. Leaves 15–20cm (6–8in) long are divided into 7–9 oblong-ovate, deeply toothed to pinnatifid, bright green leaflets. Tiny, greenish white flowers, 5mm (¼in) across, are borne from summer to autumn. They are followed by ovoid, membranous, 3-angled, balloon-like capsules, 2–3cm (¾–1¼in) long, which mature from light green to fawn. ↕ 3–4m (10–12ft). Tropical Africa, India, North and South America. ❀ (min. 7–10°C/45–50°F)

▷**Cardoon** see *Cynara cardunculus*

CAREX

Sedge

CYPERACEAE

Vast genus of 1,500 or more species of deciduous and evergreen, rhizomatous or tufted perennials from temperate and arctic zones, as well as high altitudes in tropical regions. Most species occur in bog, moorland, or damp woodland, or by water. Sedges are mainly cultivated for their variegated or colourful foliage, although some species have attractive inflorescences. The generally grass-like leaves are usually linear, 3-ranked, and with leaf bases sheathing the triangular stems, which are solid and without nodes. Sedges are mainly monoecious, occasionally dioecious, and bear panicles of small, grass-like flowers in short spikes. There are sedges for nearly every site in the garden.

- **HARDINESS** Most sedges originating from New Zealand and tropical areas, as well as *C. conica*, *C. morrowii*, and their cultivars, and *C.* 'Frosted Curls', are not reliably hardy where temperatures fall below -7°C (19°F) for long periods. All others described here are fully hardy.
- **CULTIVATION** Sedges have varying cultivation requirements. These are grouped as follows:

1. Most soils in sun or partial shade. Avoid extremes of wet or dry.
2. Fertile, moist but well-drained soil in sun or partial shade.
3. Fertile, moist or wet soil in sun or partial shade.
4. Moist but well-drained, alkaline soil in sun or partial shade.
5. Neutral to acid, lime-free soil in sun or partial shade.
In summer, cut out any dead leaves on evergreen species.

- **PROPAGATION** Sow seed of New Zealand species at 10–13°C (50–55°F) in early spring; expose those from Europe and North America to winter cold in a cold frame. Divide between mid-spring and early summer.

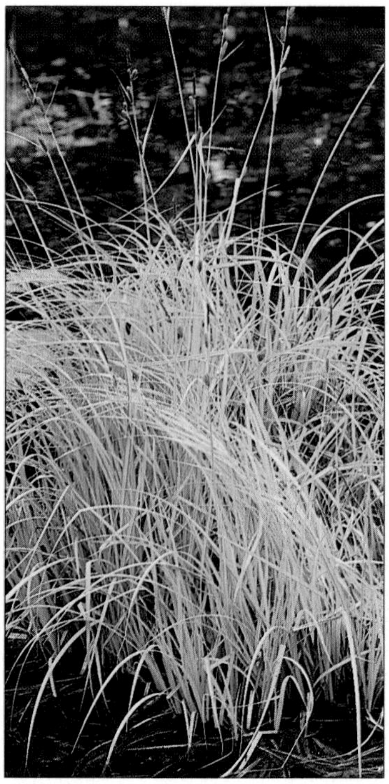

Carex elata 'Aurea'

- **PESTS AND DISEASES** Aphids sometimes infest the stem bases.

C. berggrenii. Miniature, evergreen perennial with short rhizomes, spreading slowly and forming loose tufts of short, blunt, blue-green, metallic-grey, or reddish brown leaves, to 5cm (2in) long. Small brown flower spikes, to 6mm (¼in) long, are borne on stems to 10cm (4in) long in midsummer. Cultivation group 2. ↕ 10cm (4in), ↔ 15cm (6in). New Zealand. ❄❄

C. buchananii (Leatherleaf sedge). Densely tufted, evergreen perennial of symmetrical, arching habit, with short rhizomes and orange-brown leaves, to 45cm (18in) long, curled at the tips. In mid- and late summer, produces brown flower spikes, 0.5–3cm (¼–1¼in) long, on lax stems, to 50cm (20in) long. Cultivation group 1. ↕ 50–75cm (20–30in), ↔ 90cm (36in). New Zealand. ❄❄

C. comans. Densely tufted, evergreen perennial forming tussocks of hair-like, pale yellow-green, pale grey, or reddish brown leaves, 25cm (10in) or more long. Inconspicuous brown flower spikes, 0.5–2.5cm (¼–1in) long, are produced on stems to 25cm (10in) long in mid- and late summer. Variants with warm brown foliage are commonly available. Cultivation group 1. ↕ 25–35cm (10–14in), ↔ 75cm (30in). New Zealand. ❄❄❄ (borderline)

***C. conica* 'Hime-kan-suge'** see *C. conica* 'Snowline'.

***C. conica* 'Snowline'**, syn. *C. conica* 'Hime-kan-suge'. Small, tufted, evergreen perennial with dark green, white-margined leaves, to 15cm (6in) long, forming dense, low, arching tufts. Small, dark brown-purple flower spikes, 1–2.5cm (½–1in) long, are produced on stems to 15cm (6in) long, in early summer. Cultivation group 2. ↕ 15cm (6in), ↔ 25cm (10in). ❄❄

***C. elata* 'Aurea'** ■ ♀ syn. *C. stricta* 'Aurea' (Bowles' golden sedge). Deciduous perennial with short rhizomes, forming a dense clump of gently arching, rich yellow leaves, 40–60cm (16–24in) long, narrowly margined in green. In late spring and early summer, stems 50cm (20in) or more long bear brown male flower spikes, to 2.5cm (1in) long, above 2 or 3 stalkless green female spikes, 1.5–4cm (½–1½in) long. Cultivation group 3. ↕ to 70cm (28in), ↔ 45cm (18in). ❄❄❄

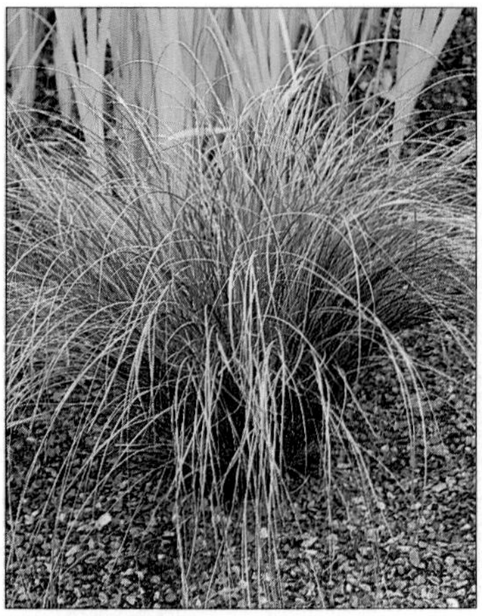

Carex flagellifera

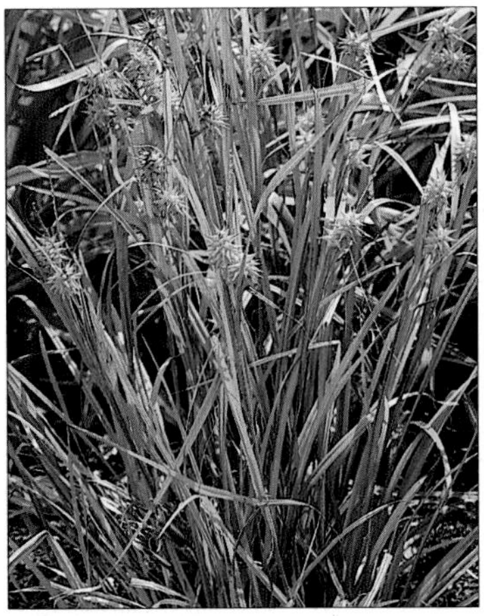

Carex grayi

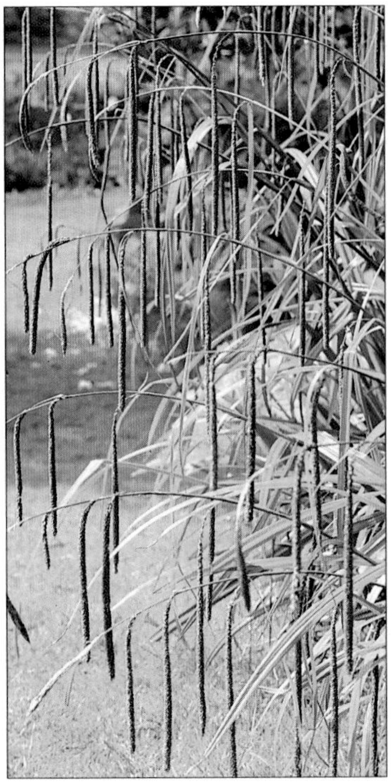

Carex pendula

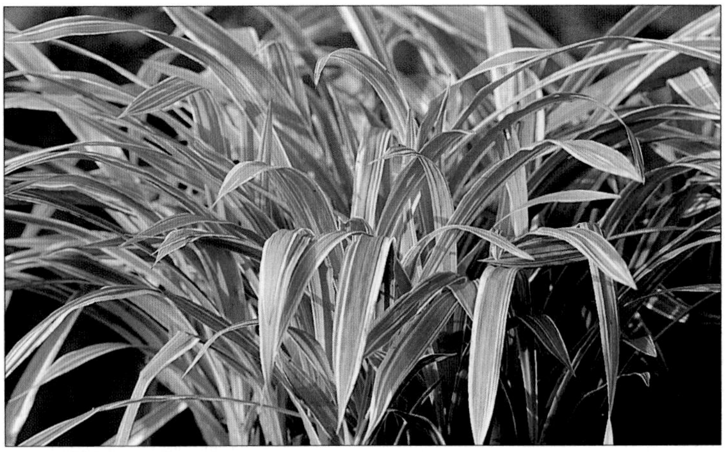

Carex siderosticha 'Variegata'

***C. firma* 'Variegata'.** Small, densely tufted, evergreen perennial with short rhizomes and short, stiff, pointed, shiny, blue-green leaves, to 10cm (4in) long, with bold, creamy yellow margins. In early summer, bears tiny, dark brown flower spikes, 5–10mm (¼–½in) long, on stems 7–10cm (3–4in) long. Cultivation group 4. ↕↔ 10cm (4in). ✼✼✼

C. flagellifera ▣ Densely tufted, evergreen perennial with short rhizomes. It is similar to *C. comans*, but taller and with broader green or reddish brown leaves, 40–70cm (16–28in) long. Stems bearing light brown flower spikes, 0.5–2.5cm (¼–1in) long, elongate to over 1m (3ft) as the red-brown fruit mature. Variants in cultivation often have red-brown foliage. Cultivation group 1. ↕ 1.1m (3½ft), ↔ 90cm (36in). New Zealand. ✼✼✼ (borderline)

***C.* 'Frosted Curls'.** Densely tufted, evergreen perennial with short rhizomes and arching, narrow, shiny, pale silvery green leaves, to 60cm (24in) long, curling at the tips. From early to late summer, bears small, inconspicuous, cylindrical green flower spikes, 5–10mm (¼–½in) long, on stems 45–60cm (18–24in) long. Cultivation group 1. ↕ 60cm (24in), ↔ 45cm (18in). ✼✼

C. grayi ▣ (Mace sedge). Deciduous, densely tufted perennial, with short rhizomes, forming strong, erect clumps of broad, rich green leaves, to 60cm (24in) long. Stems 60cm (24in) long bear mid-green flower spikes, 1.5–2cm (½–¾in) long, from early to late summer, followed by star-like, pale green seed heads; these resemble spiked clubs and are good for flower arranging. Cultivation group 3. ↕ to 75cm (30in), ↔ 60cm (24in). North America. ✼✼✼

***C. hachijoensis* 'Evergold'** ▣ 🏆 syn. *C. oshimensis* 'Evergold'. Tufted, evergreen perennial, with short rhizomes, forming a low mound of dark green leaves, to 25cm (10in) long, each with a broad; creamy yellow central stripe. In mid- and late spring, bears brown flower spikes, 1–3cm (½–1¼in) long, on stems to 15cm (6in) long. Often confused with *C. morrowii*. Cultivation group 2. ↕ 30cm (12in), ↔ 35cm (14in). ✼✼✼

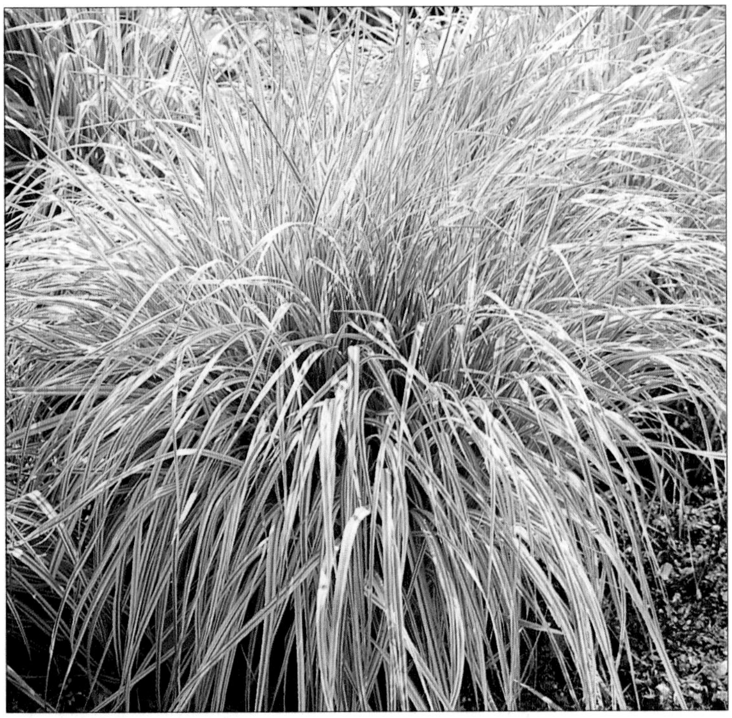

Carex hachijoensis 'Evergold'

***C. morrowii* 'Fisher'**, syn. *C. morrowii* 'Fisher's Form'. Clump-forming, evergreen perennial with broad, stiff, shiny, conspicuously cream-striped and cream-margined, mid-green leaves, 40cm (16in) long. Panicles of green and brown flower spikes, 2–5cm (¾–2in) long, are borne on stems 45cm (18in) long, in late spring. Cultivation group 2. ↕ 45–50cm (18–20in), ↔ 30cm (12in). ✼✼

***C. morrowii* 'Fisher's Form'** see *C. morrowii* 'Fisher'.

C. muskingumensis (Palm branch sedge). Loosely tufted, deciduous, gently spreading perennial with erect stems that bear horizontally held, bright green leaves, to 75cm (30in) long. In early and midsummer, produces golden brown flower spikes, 1.5–2.5cm (½–1in) long, on stems 60–75cm (24–30in) long. Cultivation group 3. ↕ 75cm (28in), ↔ 45cm (18in). North America. ✼✼✼

***C. oshimensis* 'Evergold'** see *C. hachijoensis* 'Evergold'.

C. pendula ▣ (Drooping sedge, Pendulous sedge, Weeping sedge). Tufted, evergreen perennial forming dense clumps of relatively wide, keeled, shiny, mid-green leaves, to 90cm (36in) long, and blue-green beneath. In late spring and early summer, arching stems, to 1.4m (4½ft) long, bear cylindrical, catkin-like, dark brown flower spikes, to 15cm (6in) long; erect at first, they become pendent with age. Cultivation group 3. ↕ to 1.4m (4½ft), ↔ to 1.5m (5ft). Europe, N. Africa. ✼✼✼

C. petriei. Densely tufted, evergreen perennial with short rhizomes and erect or arching, pale pinkish brown leaves, to 30cm (12in) long, with curled tips. In early and midsummer, bears stubby, red-brown flower spikes, 1–3cm (½–1¼in) long, on stems to 25cm (10in) long. Cultivation group 1. ↕ 25cm (10in), ↔ 15cm (6in). New Zealand. ✼✼

***C. pilulifera* 'Tinney's Princess'.** Deciduous perennial, similar to but more delicate than *C. hachijoensis* 'Evergold'. The leaves, to 10cm (4in) long, have broad, creamy yellow central stripes and narrow, dark green margins. In mid-spring, stems to 15cm (6in) long each bear a single, terminal, cylindrical brown male spike, 2–4cm (¾–1½in) long, and several red-brown female spikes, 2–4cm (¾–1½in) long, clustered just below the male. Cultivation group 5. ↕↔ 15cm (6in). ✼✼✼

***C. saxatilis* 'Ski Run'** (Variegated russet sedge). Loosely tufted, deciduous, strongly rhizomatous perennial, slowly forming a low carpet of curved, glossy, mid-green leaves, to 10cm (4in) long, each with a central white stripe. In late spring, flowering stems, to 10cm (4in) long, each bear a single, terminal, dark brown male spike, 0.5–1.5cm (¼–½in) long, above purple-brown female spikes, 0.5–2cm (¼–¾in) long. Cultivation group 3. ↕ to 15cm (6in), ↔ 30cm (12in) or more. ✼✼✼

***C. siderosticha* 'Variegata'** ▣ Slowly spreading, deciduous, rhizomatous perennial, forming clumps of relatively broad, linear-lance-shaped, pale green leaves, to 25cm (10in) long, margined and narrowly striped white, and pink-flushed at the bases. Slender, pale brown flower spikes, 3–5mm (⅛–¼in) long, open on stems to 30cm (12in) long, in late spring. Cultivation group 3. ↕ 30cm (12in), ↔ 40cm (16in) or more. ✼✼✼

***C. stricta* 'Aurea'** see *C. elata* 'Aurea'.

C. testacea. Densely tufted, evergreen perennial with arching leaves, to 60cm (24in) long, generally pale olive-green, but orange-brown on the surfaces that receive full light. Bears cylindrical, pale to dark brown flower spikes, to 2.5cm (1in) long, on stems 50–60cm (20–24in) long, in midsummer; stems later elongate in fruit to 1.5m (5ft). Cultivation group 1. ↕ to 1.5m (5ft), ↔ 60cm (24in). New Zealand. ✼✼

▷ **Caricature plant** see *Graptophyllum pictum*

CARISSA

APOCYNACEAE

Genus of about 20 species of evergreen, often spiny shrubs and small trees from dry, open woodland in tropical and subtropical Africa and Asia. The leaves are opposite, entire, and leathery. The tubular flowers, with 5 spreading petal lobes, are borne singly or in terminal or axillary cymes, and are followed by red or black, fleshy fruits. Although the flesh of these is edible and used for jam-making, the seeds are poisonous. In frost-prone regions, grow in a cool greenhouse or conservatory. In frost-free areas, grow outdoors in a shrub border, or as hedging.

C

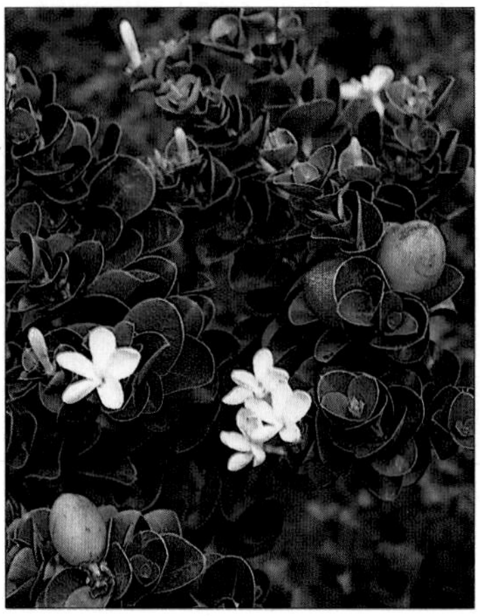

Carissa macrocarpa

• **HARDINESS** Mostly frost tender; *C. macrocarpa* and its cultivars may survive short spells around 0°C (32°F).
• **CULTIVATION** Under glass, grow in loam-based potting compost (JI No.3) in bright filtered light. When in growth, water moderately and apply a balanced liquid fertilizer monthly; water sparingly in winter. Top-dress or pot on in spring. Outdoors, grow in moderately fertile, well-drained soil in full sun; partial shade is tolerated. Pruning group 8; plants under glass may need restrictive pruning. Trim hedges after flowering.
• **PROPAGATION** Sow seed at 15–18°C (59–64°F) as soon as ripe or in spring. Root semi-ripe cuttings in summer.
• **PESTS AND DISEASES** Trouble free.

C. grandiflora see *C. macrocarpa.*
C. macrocarpa ▣ syn. *C. grandiflora* (Natal plum). Many-branched, spiny shrub with ovate, rich green leaves, to 7cm (3in) long. Fragrant, waxy, white, jasmine-like flowers, 5cm (2in) wide, are borne in terminal or axillary cymes, to 10cm (4in) long, in late spring; they are followed by plum-like, ovoid-ellipsoid, red to purple-black fruit, 5cm (2in) long. ↕ 2–3m (6–10ft) or more, ↔ 3m (10ft) or more. South Africa (KwaZulu/Natal). ❀ (min. 5°C/41°F). Various cultivars have been selected, including **'Fancy'**, which is erect and very free-flowering, with glossy, dark green leaves and orange-red fruit, and **'Tuttlei'** ▣ which is dwarf, semi-prostrate, and dense, and useful as ground cover or for containers; ↕ 1m (3ft), ↔ to 2m (6ft).
C. spectabilis see *Acokanthera oblongifolia.*

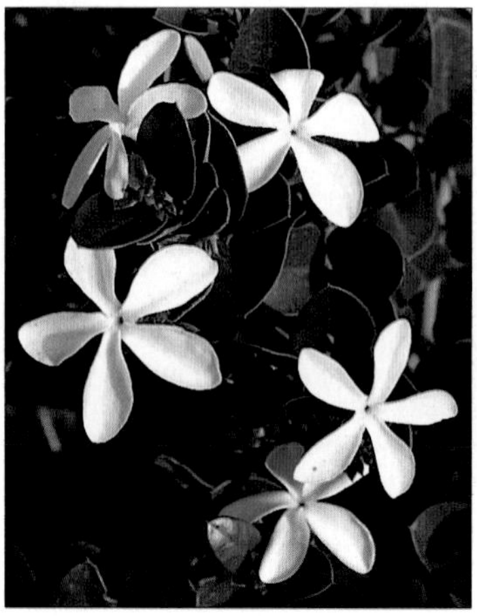

Carissa macrocarpa 'Tuttlei'

CARLINA

Carline thistle

ASTERACEAE/COMPOSITAE

Genus of about 28 species of annuals and perennials occurring in poor soils in Europe and Asia. The leaves form basal rosettes and are spiny and entire to pinnatisect. Large, solitary or cyme-like, occasionally stemless flowerheads are borne in summer; these have shiny, papery bracts and, in most species, are good for drying. The smaller species are suitable for a rock garden.
• **HARDINESS** Fully hardy.
• **CULTIVATION** Grow in poor, well-drained soil in full sun; soil must not become waterlogged or the stems will rot. The compact, stemless habit of *C. acaulis* is lost in fertile soils.
• **PROPAGATION** Sow seed in autumn *in situ*, or in containers in a cold frame.
• **PESTS AND DISEASES** Trouble free.

C. acaulis (Stemless Carline thistle). Clump-forming, short-lived perennial or monocarpic biennial with rosetted, pinnatifid to pinnatisect, elliptic-oblong, spiny-margined leaves, to 30cm (12in) long. Stemless flowerheads, to 10cm (4in) across, with silvery, off-white (sometimes pink-flushed) bracts surrounding a pale brown central disc, are borne in the centre of the rosettes in mid- and late summer. ↕ to 10cm (4in), ↔ to 25cm (10in). Alpine pastures of S. and E. Europe. ✻✻✻

CARLUDOVICA

CYCLANTHACEAE

Genus of 3 species of short-stemmed or stemless, palm-like perennials from woodland in tropical North and South America. The very long-stalked, rounded leaves are divided into several fan-like segments, each one deeply and narrowly lobed. Insignificant, fleshy, unisexual flowers are borne in cone-like spadices produced from the leaf axils in summer; they develop into showy red berries. In frost-prone climates, grow in a temperate or warm greenhouse, or plant outdoors in summer to lend a tropical effect to summer bedding. In tropical and subtropical regions, use in shady sites, especially beneath trees, where the handsome foliage may be displayed to best advantage. The large leaves are used to make panama hats.
• **HARDINESS** Frost tender.
• **CULTIVATION** Under glass, grow in loamless potting compost in full light with shade from hot sun. When in growth, water freely and apply a balanced liquid fertilizer monthly; water sparingly in winter. Pot on or top-dress in spring. Outdoors, grow in well-drained soil, ideally with some midday shade or in partial shade.
• **PROPAGATION** Sow seed at 18–21°C (64–70°F) in spring. Divide in spring.
• **PESTS AND DISEASES** Red spider mites may be a problem under glass.

C. palmata ▣ ✾ (Panama hat palm). Stemless, palm-like perennial with erect or suberect leaf-stalks, 1.5–3m (5–10ft) tall, and rounded leaf-blades, 40–80cm (16–32in) long. The leaf-blades have 3–5 segments, each with several rich green lobes, which are pendent at the

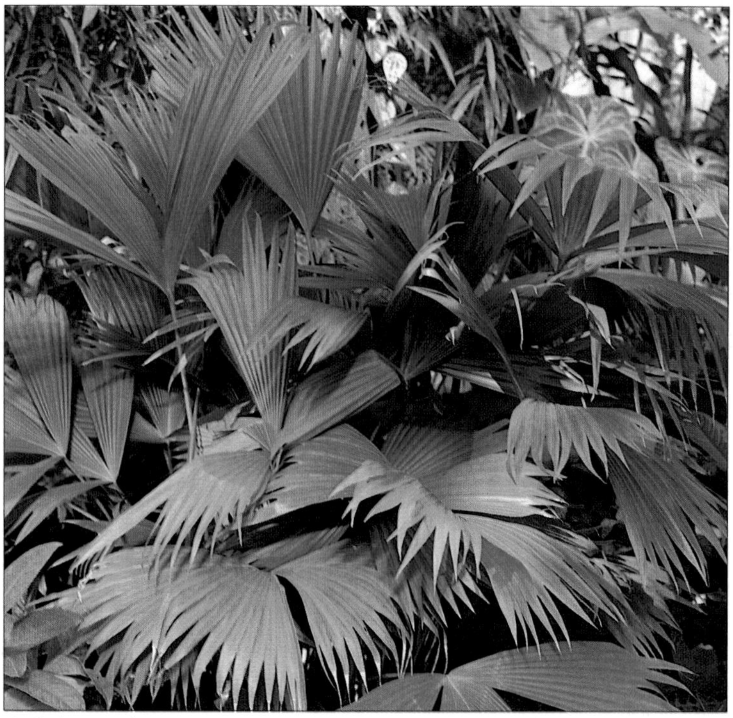

Carludovica palmata

tips. In summer, bears cylindrical to ellipsoid spathes enclosing yellowish to brownish green spadices that comprise groups of fleshy male flowers around individual female flowers. The spathes mature in autumn to about 15cm (6in) long, before they separate to disclose the bright red fruit. ↕ 2–3m (6–10ft), ↔ 1.5–3m (5–10ft). Central America to Bolivia. ❀ (min. 13–15°C/55–59°F)

CARMICHAELIA

LEGUMINOSAE/PAPILIONACEAE

Genus of about 40 species of deciduous shrubs, occasionally small trees, from New Zealand and Lord Howe Island. They are found in diverse habitats from coastal to mountain areas, including sand dunes, swamps, grassland, rocky places, woodland margins, streambanks, and lakesides. The seedlings have pinnate leaves, but mature plants are leafless or lose their leaves quickly. They are grown for their small, but usually profuse, often fragrant, pea-like flowers, borne in summer, sometimes singly, but mostly in dense, short racemes of 5–15, on cylindrical or flattened green shoots. They are attractive and unusual shrubs for a border or, in cooler areas, against a warm wall. Dwarf species, such as *C. enysii*, are suitable for a rock garden. In frost-prone areas, grow tender species in a cool greenhouse.
• **HARDINESS** Frost hardy to frost tender.
• **CULTIVATION** Grow in humus-rich, well-drained but not too dry soil, in sun or partial shade; *C. glabrata* requires acid soil. Shelter from cold winds, either against a wall or among other shrubs. Pruning group 1.
• **PROPAGATION** Sow seed in a cold frame in autumn; or sow seed, scarified or pre-soaked in hot water, in spring. Root semi-ripe cuttings in summer.
• **PESTS AND DISEASES** Trouble free.

C. enysii ▣ Dwarf, many-branched shrub, leafless when mature, with flattened, finely and longitudinally grooved shoots, to 2mm (1/16in) wide, which form a compact mound. Fragrant purple flowers, to 5mm (1/4in) long, with dark purple veins, are borne singly or in 2- to 5-flowered racemes, to 6cm (2½in) long, in midsummer. Often confused with the taller *C. orbiculata*, which grows to 10cm (4in) tall, and has wider stems. ↕ 5cm (2in), ↔ 5–30cm (2–12in). New Zealand (South Island). ✻✻
C. glabrata. Bushy, spreading shrub, leafy only when young, with flattened, pendent shoots, to 4mm (1/8in) across. Small, fragrant, purple-and-white flowers, to 5mm (1/4in) long, are borne in dense racemes, to 25cm (10in) long, in summer. ↕ 2m (6ft), ↔ 2.5m (8ft). New Zealand (South Island). ✻✻
C. odorata. Graceful shrub, leafless or nearly so when mature, with slender, flattened, pendent shoots, to 3mm (1/8in) across. Fragrant, lilac-pink flowers, to 2cm (3/4in) long, are borne in dense, erect racemes, 3–5cm (1¼–2in) long, in summer. ↕↔ 3m (10ft). New Zealand (North Island). ✻✻
C. williamsii ♀ Upright shrub or small tree, leafless or nearly so when mature, with broad, flattened shoots, to 1.5cm (½in) across. Relatively large, fragrant

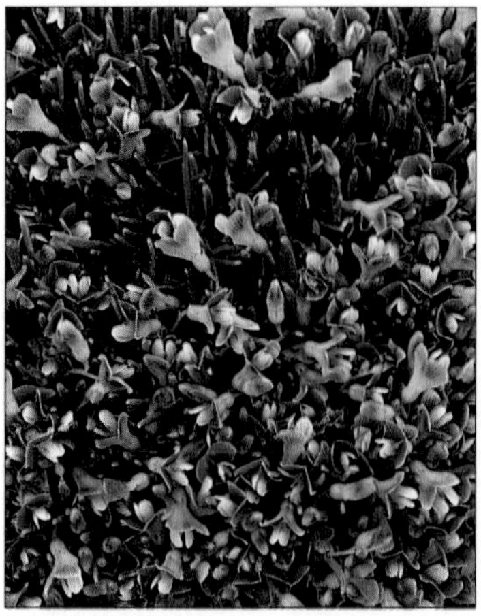

Carmichaelia enysii

flowers, 2.5cm (1in) long, creamy yellow, flushed with green and purple, are borne in racemes, 3–5cm (1¼–2in) long, in early and mid-spring. ↕ 3m (10ft) occasionally more, ↔ 2.5m (8ft). New Zealand (North Island). ❄❄

▷**Carnation** see *Dianthus*
Wild see *D. caryophyllus*

CARNEGIEA

CACTACEAE

Genus of one species of slow-growing, giant, perennial cactus from desert areas in the USA and N.W. Mexico. It sometimes attains only 1m (3ft) in height after 30 years; branching and flowering may not occur until plants reach 3–4m (10–12ft) tall. The large, funnel- to bell-shaped flowers, borne in early summer, open only in the morning. They are followed in autumn by ovoid-oblong, scaly, often spiny fruit containing glossy black seeds. In frost-prone areas, grow in a warm greenhouse; in warm, dry climates, grow in a desert garden.

• **HARDINESS** Frost tender.
• **CULTIVATION** Under glass, grow in a mix of 3 parts standard cactus compost and 1 part limestone chippings in full light, shaded from hot sun. When in growth, water freely and apply a low-nitrogen liquid fertilizer monthly; keep dry from mid-autumn to early spring. Outdoors, grow in sharply drained, humus-rich, gritty, slightly alkaline soil in full sun. See also pp.48–49.
• **PROPAGATION** Sow seed at 21°C (70°F) in early spring.
• **PESTS AND DISEASES** Trouble free.

C. gigantea ▣ (Saguaro cactus). Columnar, erect, slow-growing cactus with a tree-like trunk that eventually produces about 12 ascending branches with 12–24 (occasionally up to 30) ribs. The areoles bear grey or brown spines (12–16 radials and 3–6 centrals). In early summer, solitary, funnel- to bell-shaped, many-petalled white flowers, to 12cm (5in) long and across, are borne from felted, spineless areoles at the tips of the stems. ↕ to 16m (52ft), ↔ to 3m (10ft). USA (S. California, Arizona), N.W. Mexico. ❀ (min. 10°C/50°F)

CARPENTARIA

ARECACEAE/PALMAE

Genus of one species of single-stemmed palm from Queensland, Australia, found along riverbanks in rainforest. The prominent crownshaft bears dense, terminal clusters of pinnate leaves, and spreading or semi-pendent, many-branched panicles of 3-petalled flowers. In frost-prone areas, grow *C. acuminata* in a warm greenhouse, or use young specimens as houseplants. In frost-free climates, grow as a handsome specimen tree; it is frequently used as a street tree in N.E. Australia and Florida, USA.

• **HARDINESS** Frost tender.
• **CULTIVATION** Under glass, grow young plants in loam-based potting compost (JI No.3) in bright filtered light with high humidity. Water freely in growth, applying a balanced liquid fertilizer monthly; water sparingly in winter. Pot on or top-dress in spring. Outdoors, grow in fertile, humus-rich, moist but well-drained soil in full sun, but screen from hot sun when young.
• **PROPAGATION** Sow seed at 27°C (81°F) in spring.
• **PESTS AND DISEASES** Prone to scale insects and red spider mites under glass.

C. acuminata ▣ ♈ syn. *Kentia acuminata.* Medium-sized palm with a slender, smooth trunk ringed by old leaf scars. Arching, pinnate, dark green leaves, 2–4m (6–12ft) long, comprise many narrow, linear, abrupt- or ragged-ended leaflets. From spring to summer, bears cup-shaped cream flowers in panicles to 1.5m (5ft) long, followed by crimson fruit in persistent yellow calyces. ↕ 10–15m (30–50ft), ↔ 3–7m (10–22ft). Australia (Queensland). ❀ (min. 13–15°C/55–59°F)

CARPENTERIA

HYDRANGEACEAE/PHILADELPHACEAE

Genus of one species of evergreen shrub found in scrub on dry slopes and ridges, and in pine forest, in California, USA. It is valued mainly for its handsome leaves, which are opposite, leathery, and entire, and for its shallowly cup-shaped white flowers. *C. californica* is ideal for a shrub border or for growing against a wall.

• **HARDINESS** Frost hardy.
• **CULTIVATION** Grow in well-drained, not too dry soil in full sun; shelter from cold, dry, and strong winds. Pruning group 8; remove the oldest flowered shoots occasionally from the base.
• **PROPAGATION** Sow seed at 13–18°C (55–64°F) in autumn or spring. Root greenwood or semi-ripe cuttings in summer.
• **PESTS AND DISEASES** Fungal leaf spot may be a problem.

C. californica ▣ ♈ Upright, open shrub with peeling, pale brown bark and lance-shaped to narrowly ovate-oblong, glossy, dark green leaves, 10–12cm (4–5in) long. Cup-shaped, fragrant white flowers, 4–8cm (1½–3in) across, with central bosses of yellow stamens, are produced singly or in short terminal cymes from the upper leaf axils in early and midsummer. ↕ 2m (6ft), or more if trained against a wall, ↔ 2m (6ft). USA (California). ❄❄. **'Elizabeth'** is compact, bearing flowers to 2.5cm (1in) across. **'Ladham's Variety'** produces large flowers, to 8cm (3in) across.

▷**Carpet plant** see *Episcia*

CARPINUS

Hornbeam

BETULACEAE

Genus of 35–40 species of deciduous trees from woodland in Europe, Asia, and North America. They have alternate, prominently veined, entire or toothed leaves and, in spring, produce unisexual flowers in catkins; both male and female catkins are borne on the same plant. Hornbeams are cultivated for their elegant habit, ornamental foliage, autumn colour, and pendent, leafy-bracted racemes of fruit. They are attractive specimen trees for a park or woodland, and are excellent for hedging.

• **HARDINESS** Fully hardy.
• **CULTIVATION** Grow in moderately fertile, well-drained soil in sun or partial shade. Pruning group 1. Trim hedges of *C. betulus* in late summer. Hornbeams can withstand very hard pruning.
• **PROPAGATION** Sow seed in a seedbed in autumn. Root greenwood cuttings in early summer or bud in late summer. Graft in winter; top-graft *C. betulus* 'Pendula' to display its weeping habit.
• **PESTS AND DISEASES** Prone to coral spot, caterpillars, and aphids.

C. betulus ♈ ⌂–♀ (Common hornbeam). Pyramidal, later irregularly rounded tree with smooth, fluted grey bark and ovate, unequally toothed, mid-green leaves, 7–12cm (3–5in) long, turning yellow to orange in autumn. In spring, bears yellow male catkins, to 3cm (1¼in) long, and greenish female catkins, to 12cm (5in) long. Female catkins are followed by racemes, 3–6cm (1¼–2½in) long, of green fruit with prominent, 3-lobed bracts, maturing to yellow-brown. ↕ 25m (80ft), ↔ 20m (70ft). Europe, Turkey, Ukraine. ❄❄❄. **'Aspleniifolia'** ♀ has toothed leaves with deeply cut lobes. **'Columnaris'** ▯ is a slow-growing, densely branched, compact tree, spire-like when young; it becomes ovoid with age, but retains its

C

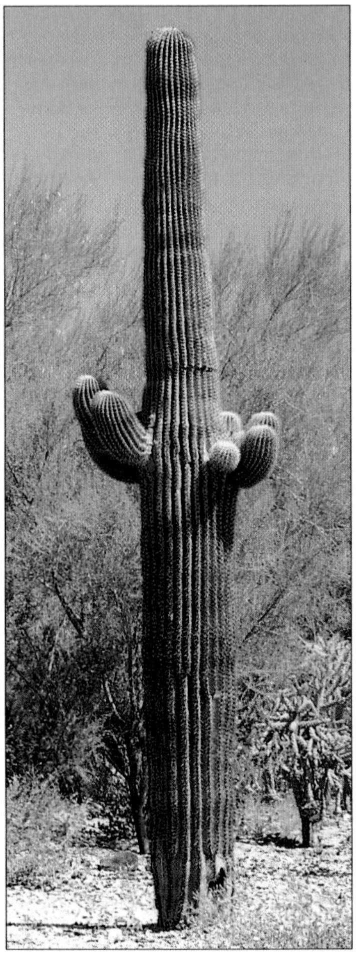

Carnegiea gigantea

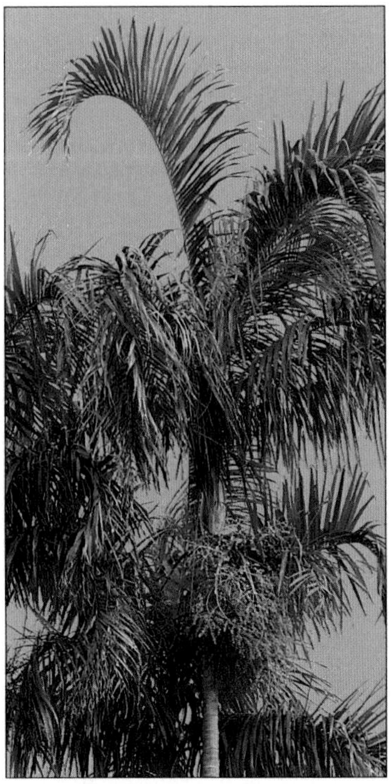

Carpentaria acuminata

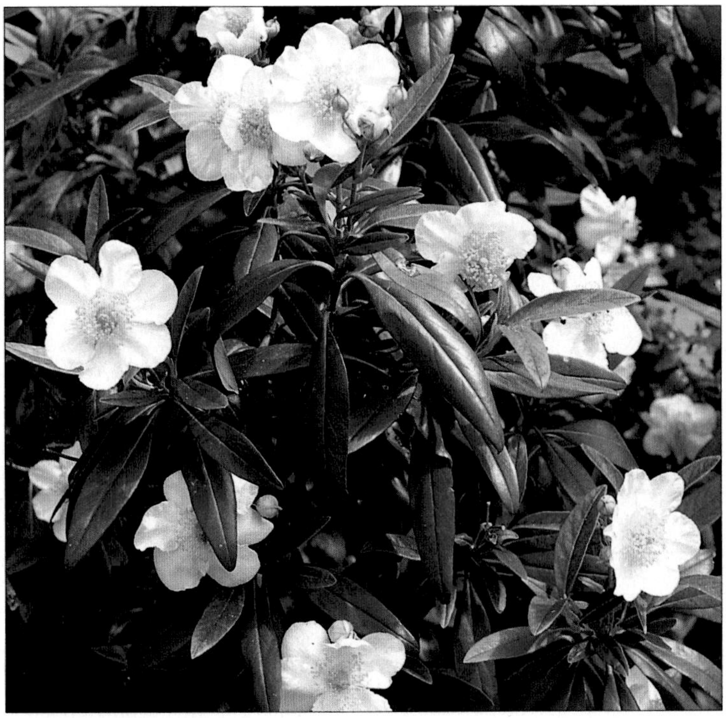

Carpenteria californica

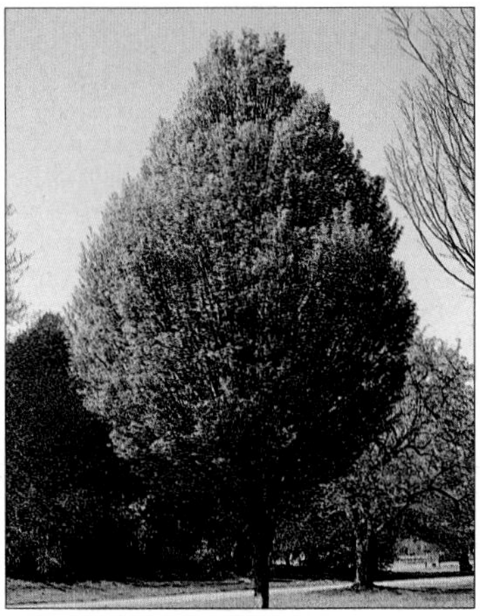

Carpinus betulus 'Fastigiata'

central leader; ↕ 10m (30ft), ↔ 6m (20ft). **'Fastigiata'** ■ ♀ ◊ syn. 'Pyramidalis', is narrow and upright, becoming broadly conical and more open with age; ↕ 15m (50ft), ↔ 12m (40ft). **'Frans Fontaine'** ◊ is similar to 'Fastigiata', but narrower when mature; ↕ 15m (50ft), ↔ 6m (20ft). **'Pendula'** ♀ is mound-forming, with pendent branches, and is best grown as a top-grafted standard; ↕ 2.5m (8ft), ↔ 4m (12ft). **'Pyramidalis'** see 'Fastigiata'.

C. caroliniana ♀ (American hornbeam). Spreading, occasionally shrubby tree with fluted, smooth grey bark. Ovate, sharply (sometimes doubly) toothed, slightly glaucous, blue-green leaves, 12cm (5in) long, are rounded or heart-shaped at the bases, turning yellow to orange-red in autumn. Male catkins are yellow and to 3.5cm (1½in) long. Mid-green female catkins, to 10cm (4in) long, are followed by racemes, 5–10cm (2–4in) long, of green fruit, maturing yellow-brown, with irregularly 3-lobed bracts; the central lobe is to 2.5cm (1in) wide. ↕ 12m (40ft), ↔ 15m (50ft). E. North America, Mexico. ❄❄❄

C. tschonoskii ♀ Spreading tree with pendent branch-tips and ovate, sharp-pointed, double-toothed, glossy leaves, to 7cm (3in) long, dark green above, mid-green beneath, and yellow in autumn. Male catkins are green and 1–2cm (½–¾in) long; female catkins are yellow-green, to 5cm (2in) long, and followed by pendent, green, later yellow-brown racemes of fruit, 5–7cm (2–3in) long, with ovate, toothed bracts. ↕↔ 12m (40ft). China, Korea, Japan. ❄❄❄

C. turczaninowii ■ ♀ Small, elegant tree, upright when young and later rounded, with slender shoots and ovate to broadly ovate, double-toothed, glossy, dark green leaves, to 5cm (2in) long, turning orange in autumn. Male catkins are green and 1–2.5cm (½–1in) long. Female catkins are yellow-green and to 5cm (2in) long; they are followed by racemes, 2.5–5cm (1–2in) long, of pendent, green, later yellow-brown fruit with ovate, unequal bracts, toothed on one side. ↕ 6–12m (20–40ft), ↔ 10m (30ft). China, Korea, Japan. ❄❄❄

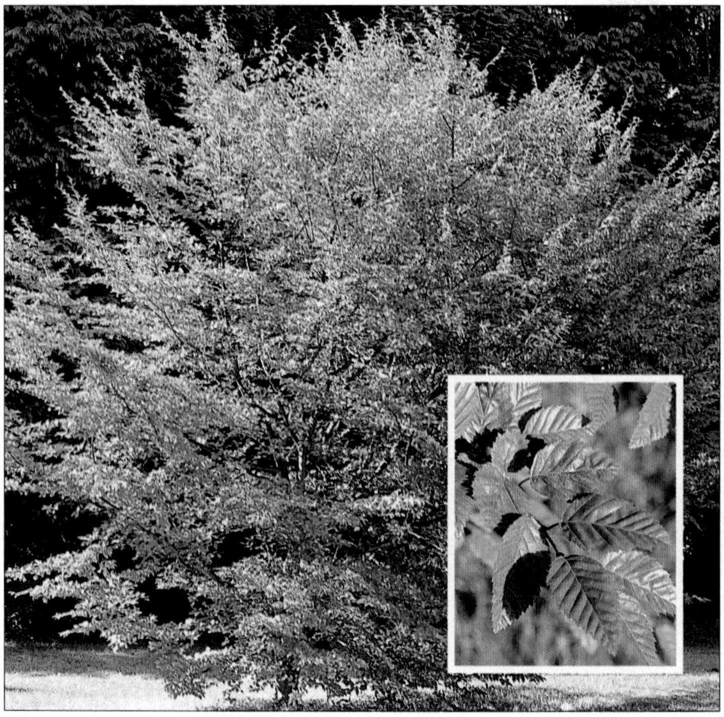

Carpinus turczaninowii (inset: leaf detail)

CARPOBROTUS

AIZOACEAE

Genus of 20–25 species of creeping, perennial succulents, mainly occurring in dry regions of South Africa, Australia (including Tasmania), Chile, and Mexico. They have prostrate, fleshy stems and pairs of finger-like, 3-angled, opposite, fleshy, smooth, sometimes spotted leaves, which are joined at the bases and usually keeled. Colourful, solitary, daisy-like, many-petalled, diurnal flowers are borne from late spring to early autumn and are followed by pear-shaped, fleshy fruits – those of *C. edulis* are used in preserves. In frost-prone areas, grow in a cool or temperate greenhouse, or treat as frost-tender annuals. In warmer areas, use as ground cover on a sandy, sunny bank or grow in a semi-desert garden. They are useful for binding and stabilizing sandy soils.

• **HARDINESS** Half hardy to frost tender.

• **CULTIVATION** Under glass, grow in a mix of 2 parts each loam and sharp sand and 1 part leaf mould in full light. In the growing season, water freely, and apply a balanced liquid fertilizer once annually, in early summer. Water very sparingly in winter. Outdoors, grow in poor, sharply drained, sandy, humus-rich soil in full sun. See also pp.48–49.

• **PROPAGATION** Sow seed at 15°C (59°F) in early spring or root stem cuttings in spring or summer.

• **PESTS AND DISEASES** Susceptible to mealybugs.

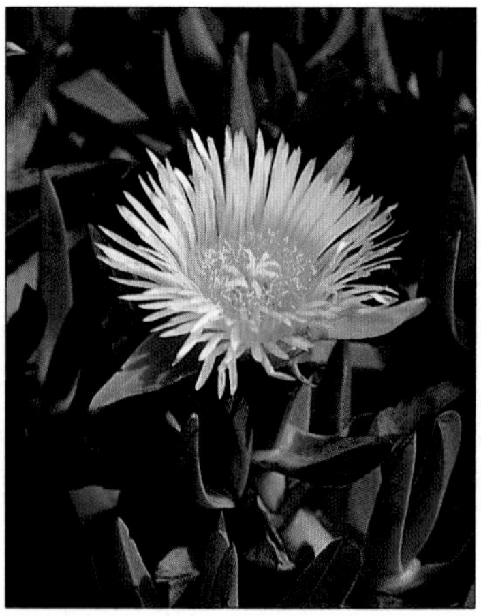

Carpobrotus edulis

C. acinaciformis. Succulent producing trailing stems, to 1.5m (5ft) or more long, with short, lateral branches. Sickle-shaped, strongly keeled, greyish green leaves, 9cm (3½in) long, have "blisters" at the bases of the upper sides. Daisy-like, bright reddish purple flowers, 12cm (5in) across, open after midday and are borne freely from late spring to early autumn. ↕ 15cm (6in), ↔ indefinite. South Africa (Eastern Cape, Western Cape, KwaZulu/Natal). ❄

C. edulis ■ (Hottentot fig, Kaffir fig). Widely spreading succulent with prostrate stems, 2m (6ft) or more long, rooting at intervals along their length, and sickle-shaped, slightly curved, dull, grey-green leaves, to 8cm (3in) long. Numerous, daisy-like yellow flowers, 8–12cm (3–5in) across, opening after noon and turning pinkish later in the day, are borne from late spring to early autumn. Produces edible, fig-like brown fruit. ↕ 15cm (6in), ↔ indefinite. South Africa (Eastern Cape, Western Cape, KwaZulu/Natal). ❀ (min. 7°C/45°F)

▷**Carrion flower** see *Stapelia*

CARTHAMUS

Safflower

ASTERACEAE/COMPOSITAE

Genus of 14 species of upright, hairy annuals and herbaceous perennials found in dry, open, sunny habitats in the Mediterranean and W. Asia. They have alternate, pinnatifid to pinnatisect, occasionally simple and shallowly lobed, spiny-margined leaves, and thistle-like, yellow, pink, purple, or violet flower-heads. *C. tinctorius* is the only widely cultivated species, and has been used for centuries as a source of red and yellow dye. It is a good "everlasting" flower for use in dried flower arrangements and is also excellent for growing in a border or herb garden.

• **HARDINESS** Fully hardy to half hardy.

• **CULTIVATION** Grow in any light, well-drained soil in full sun.

• **PROPAGATION** Sow seed at 10–15°C (50–59°F) from early to late spring.

• **PESTS AND DISEASES** Trouble free.

C. tinctorius (False saffron, Safflower). Erect annual producing simple, ovate to linear, wavy-margined or pinnatifid, often spiny-toothed, light greyish green basal leaves, 3–9cm (1¼–3½in) long; stem leaves are narrowly linear-lance-shaped and stem-clasping. In summer, bears loose corymbs of thistle-like flowerheads, to 4cm (1½in) across, with large basal "cups" of stiff green bracts, from which tasselled tufts of red, orange, or yellow ray-florets emerge. ↕ 30–60cm (12–24in), ↔ 30cm (12in). Probably W. Asia. ❄❄❄. **'Lasting White'** has creamy white flowers. **'Orange Ball'** produces orange flowers. **'Summer Sun'** has yellow flowers.

▷**Carthusian pink** see *Dianthus carthusianorum*

CARUM

Caraway

APIACEAE/UMBELLIFERAE

Genus of about 30 species of tap-rooted, upright biennials and perennials with 2- to 4-pinnate leaves and compound umbels of small white flowers. *C. carvi*, the only species cultivated, occurs in meadows, grassland and wasteland from Europe and North Africa to Siberia, Russia. It is grown in herb gardens for its scented, fern-like foliage and liquorice-flavoured seeds.

• **HARDINESS** Fully hardy.

• **CULTIVATION** Grow in deep, fertile, well-drained soil in full sun; caraway will tolerate heavier soils. Seed is borne in the second summer; harvest before it begins to darken, to avoid self-seeding. *C. carvi* self-seeds very freely.

• **PROPAGATION** Sow seed in rows *in situ* in late spring or late summer. Seedlings may be transplanted, but will bolt unless moved when very small.

• **PESTS AND DISEASES** Trouble free.

C. carvi (Caraway). Aromatic biennial with slender, ribbed stems and feathery, 2- or 3-pinnate, bright green leaves, 8–15cm (3–6in) long, comprising linear to linear-lance-shaped leaflets. Small white flowers are borne in compound umbels, to 4cm (1½in) across, in midsummer, followed by 5-ribbed fruit, 3–6mm (⅛–¼in) long, containing the liquorice-flavoured seeds. ↕ 60cm (24in), ↔ 30cm (12in). Europe to W. Asia. ❄❄❄

CARYA

Hickory

JUGLANDACEAE

Genus of about 25 species of deciduous trees, mostly found in woodland in E. Asia and North America. Hickories are valued for their foliage, which is pinnate and alternate, and often colours well in autumn, and for their sometimes ornamental bark. Flowers of both sexes are borne separately on the same plant in late spring and early summer: the males are produced in branched, pendent, yellow-green catkins, the females in small, terminal green spikes.

The autumn fruits are hard-shelled nuts, which in some species contain edible kernels, cultivated commercially as pecan nuts. Use hickories as specimen trees for a lawn or a woodland garden.

- **HARDINESS** Fully hardy except for *C. illinoinensis*, which tolerates only short periods below -12°C (10°F).
- **CULTIVATION** Grow in deep, fertile, moist but well-drained, humus-rich soil in sun or partial shade. Seedlings quickly develop a deep tap root and resent transplanting. Pruning group 1.
- **PROPAGATION** Sow seed *in situ* as soon as ripe; if sowing in a seedbed transplant seedlings as soon as possible. Graft cultivars of *C. illinoinensis* in winter.
- **PESTS AND DISEASES** Prone to crown gall, powdery mildew, and leaf spot.

C. cordiformis ■ 🏆 ♀ (Bitternut, Bitternut hickory, Swamp hickory). Broadly columnar tree with ornamental, ridged grey bark. Pinnate, mid-green leaves, 15–25cm (6–10in) or more long, with 5–9 ovate-lance-shaped leaflets, turn yellow in autumn. Produces unpalatable, thick-shelled, spherical nuts, to 4cm (1½in) long. ↕25m (80ft), ↔ 15m (50ft). E. North America. ❄❄❄

C. glabra ♀ (Hognut, Pignut, Pignut hickory). Spreading tree with furrowed grey, ornamental bark. Pinnate, mid-green leaves, 20–30cm (8–12in) long, with usually 5–7 ovate-lance-shaped to obovate leaflets, turn yellow in autumn. Produces obovoid, bitter-tasting, thin-shelled nuts, to 5cm (2in) long. ↕25m (80ft), ↔ 20m (70ft). E. USA. ❄❄❄

C. illinoinensis ♀ (Pecan). Rounded, tree with ornamental, furrowed grey

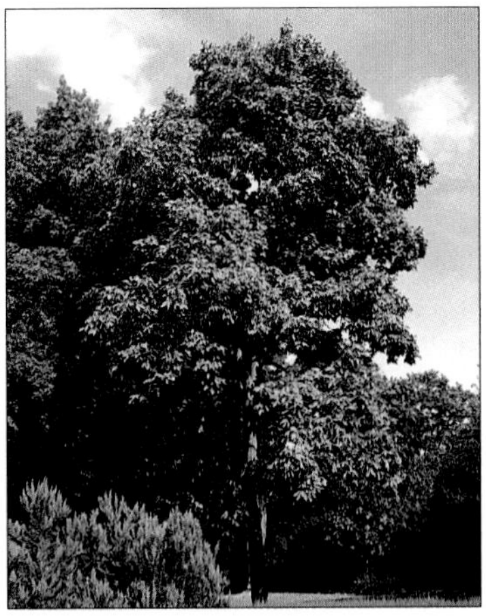

Carya ovata

bark. Pinnate, mid-green leaves, 30–50cm (12–20in) long, with usually 11–17 curved, oblong-lance-shaped leaflets, turn yellow in autumn. Oblong, thick-shelled nuts, to 6cm (2½in) long, are edible when ripe. In areas with warm summers, many cultivars are grown for their edible nuts. ↕30m (100ft), ↔ 20m (70ft). S. USA. ❄❄❄ (borderline)

C. ovata ■ 🏆 ♀ (Shagbark hickory). Broadly conical tree with ornamental, peeling, grey to brown bark. The pinnate, mid-green leaves, 20–35cm (8–14in) long, have usually 5 leaflets, the upper 3 obovate and the lower 2 ovate-lance-shaped to ovate; the leaves turn golden yellow in autumn. Thick-shelled nuts, to 6cm (2½in) long, are edible when ripe. ↕25m (80ft), ↔ 15m (50ft). E. North America. ❄❄❄

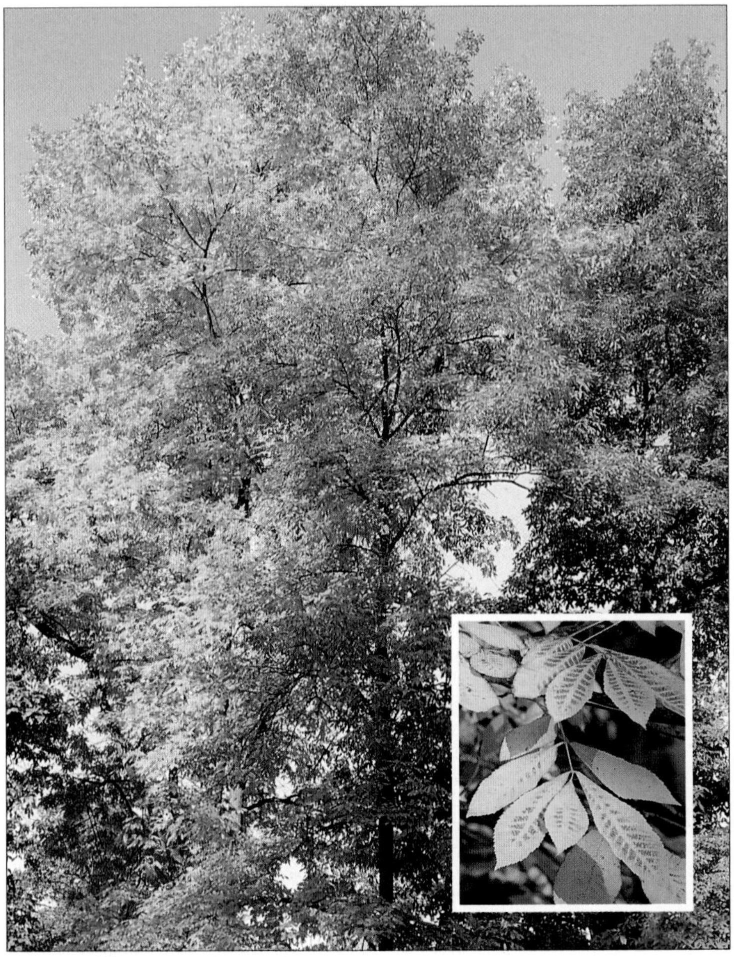

Carya cordiformis (inset: leaf detail)

CARYOPTERIS

VERBENACEAE

Genus of 6 species of aromatic, deciduous shrubs and perennials from a variety of habitats, including dry, hot slopes and woodland, in the Himalayas and mountains of E. Asia. They have opposite, simple, entire to toothed leaves and small, usually blue flowers borne in terminal or axillary panicles or cymes. Cultivated for their attractive, aromatic foliage and flowers, which are borne from late summer to autumn on the current year's shoots, they are ideal for a mixed or shrub border.

- **HARDINESS** Fully hardy to frost hardy.
- **CULTIVATION** Grow in moderately fertile, light, well-drained soil in full sun. Where temperatures fall to -15°C (5°F), plant against a warm, sunny wall, particularly if summers are cool. Pruning group 6.
- **PROPAGATION** Sow seed in autumn in containers in a cold frame. Root softwood cuttings in late spring or greenwood cuttings in early summer.
- **PESTS AND DISEASES** Capsid bugs may cause leaf distortion.

***C. x clandonensis* cultivars.** Selections derived from the dense, mound-forming shrub *C.* x *clandonensis* have ovate-lance-shaped, slightly toothed, grey-green leaves, to 5cm (2in) long, silver-hairy beneath. They bear axillary or terminal cymes of blue or purple-blue flowers, to 1cm (½in) across, in late summer and early autumn. ↕1m (3ft), ↔ 1.5m (5ft). ❄❄❄. **'Arthur Simmonds'** has dull, dark green leaves, silvery grey beneath, and bears bright purplish blue flowers. **'Dark Knight'** has silvery grey leaves and very dark blue flowers. **'Heavenly Blue'** 🏆 is erect, with intensely dark blue flowers. **'Kew Blue'** ■ has grey-green leaves, dull, dark green above, silvery grey beneath, and bears dark blue flowers. **'Worcester Gold'** ■ has warm yellow foliage and lavender-blue flowers.

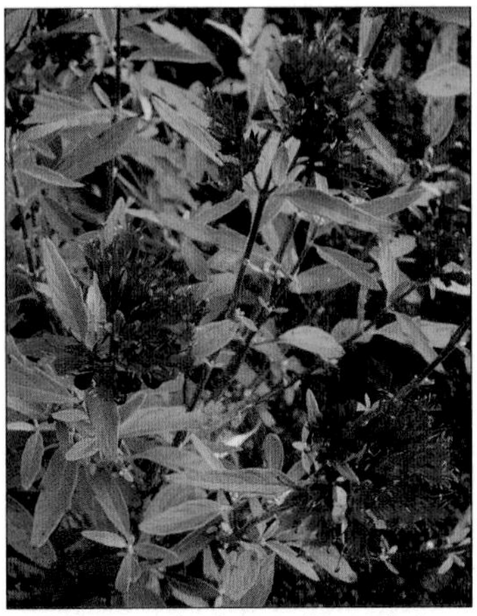

Caryopteris x *clandonensis* 'Kew Blue'

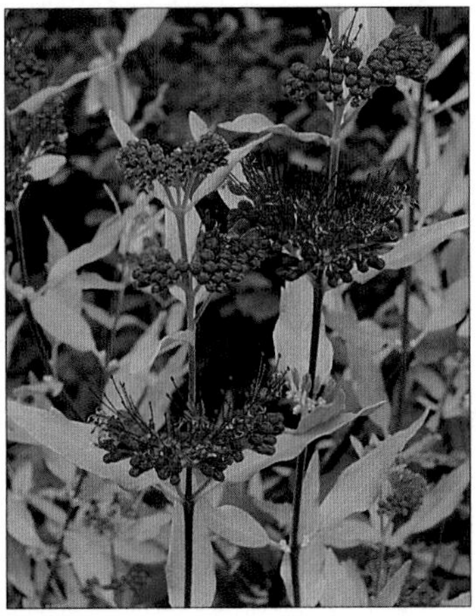

Caryopteris x *clandonensis* 'Worcester Gold'

C. incana, syn. *C. mastacanthus*. Dense, mound-forming shrub with aromatic, ovate, grey-green leaves, to 7cm (3in) long, sharply toothed at the margins. Bright violet-blue, occasionally white flowers, 7–8mm (¼–⅜in) across, are produced in rounded cymes from the upper leaf axils in autumn. ↕1.2m (4ft), ↔ 1.5m (5ft). China, Japan. ❄❄❄

C. mastacanthus see *C. incana*.

CARYOTA

Fish-tail palm

ARECACEAE/PALMAE

Genus of 12 species of single- and cluster-stemmed, monoecious, sometimes monocarpic palms from India and Sri Lanka to S.E. Asia, N. Australia, and the Solomon Islands. They occur in forest from sea level to 2,000m (7,000ft) in humid or monsoon climates. Huge, 2-pinnate leaves, each with a prominent sheathing base, are arranged in spirals on the upper part of each stem. The 3-petalled, cup-shaped flowers are borne in large, pendent panicles just below the lowest leaf. In frost-prone areas, grow in a temperate or warm greenhouse, or use young specimens as houseplants. In tropical regions, fish-tail palms are used as ornamental specimen trees; where they occur naturally, they provide sago, palm wine, and building materials.

- **HARDINESS** Frost tender.
- **CULTIVATION** Under glass, grow in loam-based potting compost (JI No.3) in bright filtered light and high humidity. Water freely when in growth, applying a balanced liquid fertilizer monthly; water sparingly in winter. Pot on or top-dress in spring. Outdoors, grow in fertile, humus-rich, moist but well-drained soil with midday shade.
- **PROPAGATION** Sow seed at 27°C (81°F) in spring.
- **PESTS AND DISEASES** Prone to scale insects and red spider mites under glass.

C. mitis ■ ❋ (Burmese fish-tail palm, Clustered fish-tail palm). Small to medium-sized palm with clustered

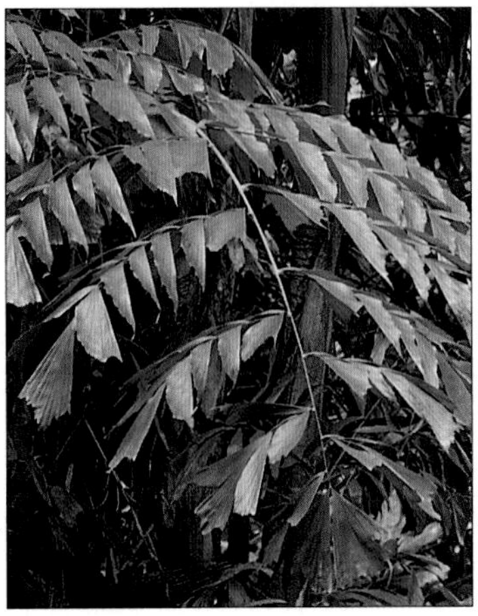

Caryota mitis

C

stems, at first clothed with fibrous leaf bases, later bare. The broadly linear, 2-pinnate, rich green leaves are 2–4m (6–12ft) long, with 6–60, fish-tail-like, asymmetrically 3-angled leaflets. Pendent panicles, 30cm (12in) or more long, of cream flowers, to 2cm (¾in) across, are borne in summer. ↕ 3–12m (10–40ft), ↔ 3–7m (10–22ft). Burma to Malaysian peninsula, Indonesia (Java), Philippines. ❀ (min. 15°C/59°F)
C. urens ☠ (Jaggery palm, Sago palm, Toddy palm, Wine palm). Medium-sized to large, fast-growing, monocarpic palm with a single, sturdy stem clothed with fibrous leaf bases. Arching, broadly linear, 2-pinnate, dark green leaves, to 6m (20ft) long, have 6–50 obliquely wedge-shaped leaflets, to 30cm (12in) long. Panicles, 2–4m (6–12ft) long, of cream flowers, 1–3cm (½–1¼in) across, are produced at the end of the tree's life, first at the top of the tree, then from each leaf axil downwards. The sugary sap is boiled down to make crude sugar (jaggery), or is distilled into toddy. ↕ 12–25m (40–80ft), ↔ to 10m (30ft). India, Sri Lanka, Malaysian peninsula. ❀ (min. 15°C/59°F)

▷ **Caspian locust** see *Gleditsia caspica*
▷ ***Cassandra*** see *Chamaedaphne*

CASSIA

CAESALPINIACEAE/LEGUMINOSAE

Genus of over 500 species of annuals and perennials, and deciduous, semi-evergreen, and evergreen shrubs and trees from moist woodland, riverbanks and scrub in tropical areas worldwide. They have pinnate leaves and 5-petalled, bowl-shaped flowers, borne in panicles or racemes, or occasionally singly. In frost-prone areas, grow in a temperate or warm greenhouse, or in a conservatory. In warmer climates, grow in a shrub border; use the trees as specimen plants.
• **HARDINESS** Fully hardy to frost tender.
• **CULTIVATION** Under glass, grow in loam-based potting compost (JI No.3) in full light. In the growing season, water freely and apply a balanced liquid fertilizer monthly. Top-dress or pot on in early spring. Outdoors, grow in deep, well-drained, moderately fertile soil in full sun. Pruning group 1; plants under glass need restrictive pruning after flowering.
• **PROPAGATION** Sow pre-soaked seed at 18–21°C (64–70°F) in spring. Root semi-ripe cuttings in summer.
• **PESTS AND DISEASES** Red spider mites and whiteflies may be troublesome under glass.

C. alata see *Senna alata.*
C. artemisioides see *Senna artemisioides.*
C. corymbosa see *Senna corymbosa.*
C. corymbosa* var. *plurijuga see *Senna* x *floribunda.*
C. didymobotrya see *Senna didymobotrya.*
C. fistula ▣ ♀ (Golden shower tree, Indian laburnum, Pudding pipe-tree, Purging cassia). Spreading, semi-evergreen to deciduous tree producing bright green leaves, to 60cm (24in) long, each with 6–16 ovate leaflets; the older leaves are shed in winter or during periods of drought. Fragrant, bright yellow flowers, to 4cm (1½in) across, are borne freely in pendent racemes,

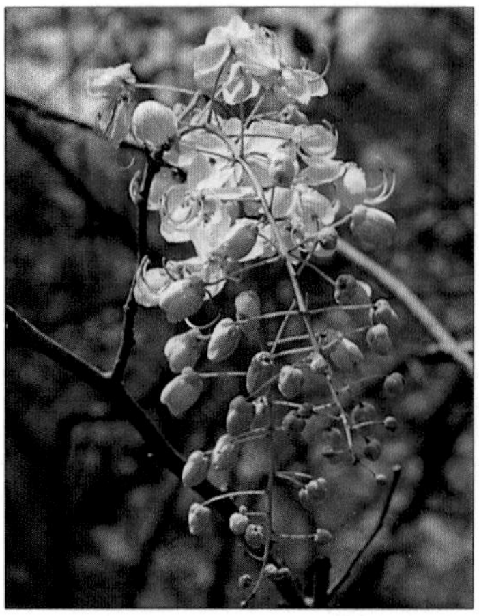
Cassia fistula

20–40cm (8–16in) long, from spring to summer. ↕ 8–12m (25–40ft), ↔ 3–5m (10–15ft). S.E. Asia, Pacific islands, Central and South America. ❀ (min. 15°C/59°F)
C.* x *floribunda see *Senna* x *floribunda.*
C. javanica ♀ (Pink shower). Many-branched, spreading, usually deciduous tree with densely downy young growth. The leaves, 40cm (16in) long, each have 16–34 elliptic to oblong-elliptic leaflets. Profuse pale pink, crimson, or buff-pink flowers, to 4cm (1½in) across, are borne in rigid racemes, 10cm (4in) or more long, from spring to summer. ↕ to 25m (80ft) or more, ↔ 3–6m (10–20ft). S.E. Asia. ❀ (min. 16°C/ 61°F)
C. siamea see *Senna siamea.*

▷ **Cassia,**
Purging see *Cassia fistula*
Silver see *Senna artemisioides*

CASSINIA

ASTERACEAE/COMPOSITAE

Genus of about 20 species of heather-like, evergreen shrubs, occasionally soft-stemmed, from Australia, New Zealand, and South Africa. In the wild, they are found from coastal areas to scrub and grassland in the mountains. Cassinias are cultivated for their neat leaves, which are alternate, narrow, and entire, and their small heads of often fragrant flowers, borne in terminal corymbs. They are suitable for a shrub border or heather garden.
• **HARDINESS** Fully hardy to frost hardy.
• **CULTIVATION** Grow in moderately fertile, well-drained, humus-rich soil in

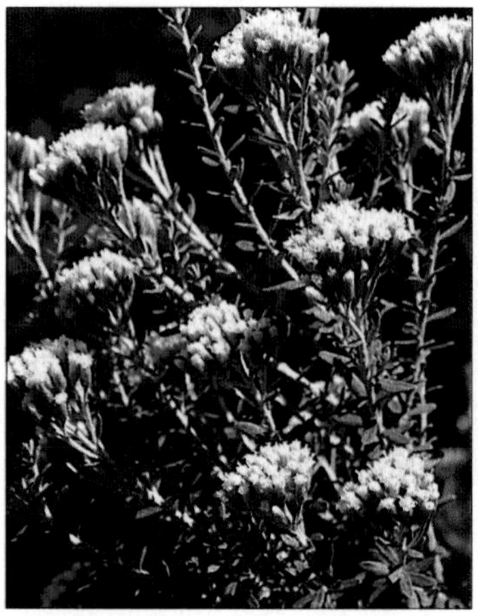
Cassinia leptophylla subsp. *vauvilliersii*

full sun. Pruning group 10, in spring.
• **PROPAGATION** Root semi-ripe cuttings in summer.
• **PESTS AND DISEASES** Trouble free.

C. fulvida see *C. leptophylla* subsp. *fulvida.*
C. leptophylla. Bushy, rounded, evergreen shrub with tiny, linear to spoon-shaped, dark green leaves, 2–10mm (⅛–⅜in) long, white- or yellowish white-hairy beneath, on sticky, white- or yellowish white-hairy shoots. In midsummer, bears small heads of tiny, funnel-shaped white flowers in terminal corymbs, to 8cm (3in) across. ↕ 2m (6ft), ↔ 2.5m (8ft). New Zealand. ❄❄❄. **subsp. *fulvida*,** syn. *C. fulvida* (Golden heather) has dark green leaves, yellow beneath, on sticky yellow shoots, giving the plant an overall golden appearance. **subsp. *vauvilliersii*** ▣ syn. *C. vauvilliersii*, has narrowly spoon-shaped to oblong-ovate leaves, and pure white flowers, to 8cm (3in) across; ↕↔ to 3m (10ft). **subsp. *vauvilliersii* var. *albida*** (Silver heather) has densely silver-white-hairy shoots and dark green leaves, densely silver-white-hairy beneath; white flowerheads are borne in dense corymbs, to 5cm (2in) across, in mid- and late summer; ↔ 1.5m (5ft); ❄❄.
C. vauvilliersii see *C. leptophylla* subsp. *vauvilliersii.*

CASSIOPE

ERICACEAE

Genus of 12 species of dwarf, evergreen shrubs from diverse habitats in arctic and alpine regions of N. Europe, N. Asia, and North America. They have 4 rows of tiny, overlapping, scale-like leaves, pressed flat to the whipcord-like stems, and bear solitary, axillary, bell- or urn-shaped flowers in late spring and early summer. Grow in a rock garden, on a peat bank, or in open areas in woodland.
• **HARDINESS** Fully hardy, although late frosts may destroy the flowers.
• **CULTIVATION** Grow in a sheltered site in moist, acid, humus-rich soil in partial shade or in an open, sunny site. *C. tetragona* tolerates some lime.
• **PROPAGATION** Sow seed in autumn in containers in an open frame. Root greenwood or semi-ripe cuttings in summer, preferably under mist. Prostrate species may be layered in autumn or early spring.
• **PESTS AND DISEASES** Trouble free.

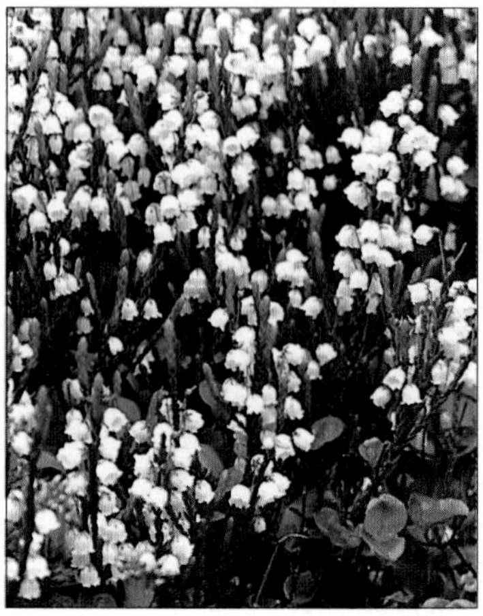
Cassiope 'Edinburgh'

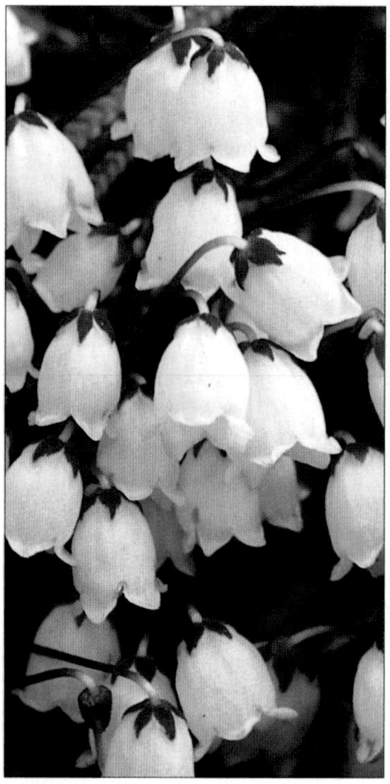
Cassiope lycopodioides

***C.* 'Edinburgh'** ▣ 🏆 Upright shrub with few-branched stems clothed in closely overlapping, lance-shaped, hairy-margined, dark green leaves, 2–4mm (1/16–⅛in) long, and slightly furrowed beneath. Nodding, bell-shaped white flowers, to 8mm (⅜in) across, with reflexed lobes and greenish brown calyces, are produced at the stem tips in late spring. ↕↔ to 25cm (10in). ❄❄❄
C. fastigiata. Lax, erect shrub bearing furrowed, lance-shaped, dark green leaves, to 4mm (⅛in) long, with fringed, silvery margins. In late spring, produces bell-shaped white flowers, 8mm (⅜in) across, with slightly reflexed lobes and green or red calyces. ↕ to 25cm (10in), ↔ to 20cm (8in). Himalayas. ❄❄❄
C. lycopodioides ▣ 🏆 Mat-forming shrub with slender, tangled stems and tiny, ovate, dark green leaves, to 2mm (1/16in) long. In late spring, bears axillary, short-stemmed, tubular-bell-shaped white flowers, 6mm (¼in) across, with red calyces and red leaf-stalks. ↕ to 8cm (3in), ↔ to 25cm (10in). Japan to USA (Alaska). ❄❄❄
C. mertensiana ▣ Dense, upright shrub with ovate-lance-shaped, dark green leaves, to 5mm (¼in) long. The bell-shaped, creamy white flowers, 7–8mm (¼–⅜in) across, have red or green calyces, and are produced from the leaf axils in spring. ↕ to 15cm (6in), ↔ to 25cm (10in). USA (California to Alaska). ❄❄❄. **var. *gracilis*** is mound-forming, slender, and free-flowering.
C. selaginoides. Many-branched shrub with stems densely clothed in minute, narrowly oblong, deeply furrowed, dark green leaves, to 2mm (1/16in) long. In late spring, pendent, bell-shaped white flowers, to 1cm (½in) across, with red calyces, are borne on long green flower-stalks, mainly at the stem tips. ↕↔ to 15cm (6in). W. China. ❄❄❄
C. tetragona. Upright shrub with 4-angled shoots clothed in oblong-lance-shaped, scale-like, leathery, dark green leaves, 3–5mm (⅛–¼in) long. Bears pendent, bell-shaped white flowers, to

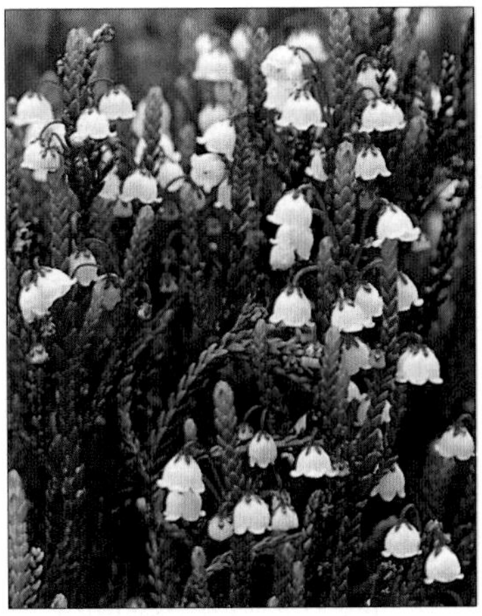

Cassiope mertensiana

6mm (¼in) across, with red calyces, in late spring. ↕ to 25cm (10in), ↔ to 20cm (8in). Arctic, subarctic Europe and North America. ❄❄❄
C. wardii. Lax, semi-upright shrub with 4-angled, few-branched stems and lance-shaped, hairy-margined, dark green leaves, to 5mm (¼in) long. Pendent, urn-shaped white flowers, 1cm (½in) across, flushed red inside at the bases, are borne close to the stem tips in late spring. Best grown in partial shade. ↕↔ to 15cm (6in). China (Tibet). ❄❄❄

CASTANEA

Chestnut, Sweet chestnut

FAGACEAE

Genus of about 12 species of deciduous trees and shrubs from woodland in S. Europe, Asia, North America, and N. Africa. They have alternate, oblong to oblong-elliptic or oval, veined, toothed leaves, and, in summer, bear small, heavily scented cream flowers in showy catkins from the leaf axils of young shoots. Chestnuts are valued for their bold foliage and spiny-husked, sometimes edible nuts, 2–6cm (¾–2½in) across. Grow as specimen trees or in woodland.
• **HARDINESS** Fully hardy.
• **CULTIVATION** Grow in deep, well-drained, slightly acid, loam soil in sun or partial shade. Most species tolerate dry, sandy soils; with the exception of *C. sativa*, they grow best in climates with long, hot summers. Pruning group 1.
• **PROPAGATION** Sow seed in a seedbed as soon as ripe. Graft in late winter, or bud in summer.
• **PESTS AND DISEASES** Susceptible to honey fungus and *Phytophthora* root rot. *C. dentata* is prone to chestnut blight.

C. dentata ♀ (American chestnut). Vigorous, rounded tree with spirally furrowed bark when old, and tapering, oblong-lance-shaped, toothed, matt mid-green leaves, to 25cm (10in) long. Edible fruit ripen in autumn. ↕ 30m (100ft), ↔ 15m (50ft). E. USA. ❄❄❄
C. mollissima ♀ (Chinese chestnut). Vigorous, spreading tree with spiral furrows in the bark when mature, and oblong to oval, toothed, glossy, mid-green leaves, to 20cm (8in) long, often softly downy beneath. Grown in North America for its edible fruit, borne in autumn. ↕↔ 20m (70ft). China. ❄❄❄
C. sativa ♀♀ (Spanish chestnut, Sweet chestnut). Vigorous, broadly columnar tree with spirally furrowed bark when old, and oblong, toothed, glossy, dark green leaves, to 20cm (8in) long. Bears edible fruit in autumn. ↕ 30m (100ft), ↔ 15m (50ft). S. Europe, N. Africa, S.W. Asia. ❄❄❄. **'Albomarginata'** ■ syn. 'Argenteomarginata', has leaves margined creamy white. **'Aspleniifolia'** has leaves deeply cut into slender lobes. Some cultivars, such as **'Marron de Lyon'**, are grown for their fruit.

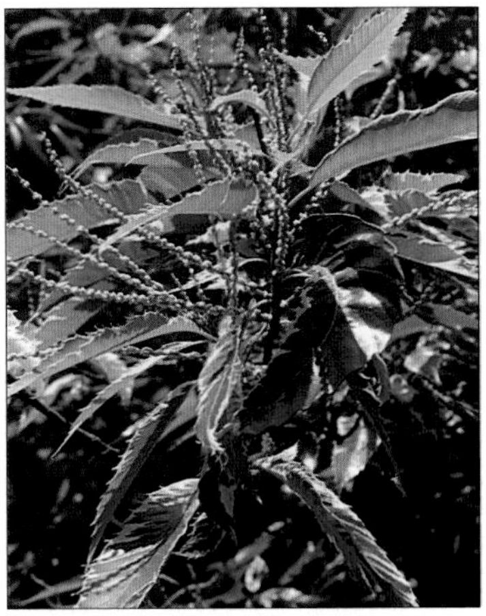

Castanea sativa 'Albomarginata'

CASTANOPSIS

FAGACEAE

Genus of about 110 species of evergreen trees and shrubs related to chestnuts (*Castanea*) and oaks (*Quercus*), from forest in warm regions of S.E. Asia. The leathery leaves are alternate and entire or toothed. The flowers are borne in erect, unisexual catkins, and are followed by nuts that develop inside prickly cases. They are useful specimen trees but may remain shrubby and achieve tree stature only in continental climates.
• **HARDINESS** Frost hardy to frost tender.
• **CULTIVATION** Grow in fertile, moist but well-drained, slightly acid soil in sun; shelter from cold, dry winds. Partial shade in climates with long, hot summers is tolerated. Pruning group 1.
• **PROPAGATION** Sow seed in containers in a cold frame as soon as ripe.
• **PESTS AND DISEASES** Trouble free.

C. chrysophylla see *Chrysolepis chrysophylla*.
C. cuspidata ♀ Spreading tree, often shrubby in cultivation, with attractive, pendent branches and ovate to oblong, tapered, usually entire leaves, to 10cm (4in) long, glossy, dark green above, bronze beneath. Small white flowers are borne in erect catkins, 5–7cm (2–3in) long, in summer. Acorn-like nuts enclosed in downy husks ripen in 2 years. ↕ 8m (25ft), ↔ 8m (25ft) or more. China, Japan. ❄❄

CASTANOSPERMUM

LEGUMINOSAE/PAPILIONACEAE

Genus of one species of evergreen tree from rainforest in Australia. It produces alternate, oval to lance-shaped, pinnate leaves and bears short, dense racemes of pea-like flowers. In frost-prone regions, grow in a temperate greenhouse; in warmer areas, it is a majestic specimen or shade tree, especially beside a lake or other water feature.
• **HARDINESS** Frost tender, but tolerates short periods at temperatures around 0°C (32°F).
• **CULTIVATION** Under glass, grow in loam-based potting compost (JI No.3) in full light, shaded from hot sun. Maintain moderate humidity. In the growing season, water freely and apply a balanced liquid fertilizer monthly; water more sparingly in winter. Pot on or top-dress in early spring. Outdoors, grow in deep, fertile, moist but well-drained soil in sun or partial shade. Pruning group 1; plants under glass may need restrictive pruning.
• **PROPAGATION** Sow seed at 13–18°C (55–64°F) as soon as ripe or in early spring.
• **PESTS AND DISEASES** Trouble free.

C. australe ♀ (Black bean tree, Moreton Bay chestnut). Open, spreading tree producing lustrous, dark green leaves, 30–45cm (12–18in) long, composed of 9–17 elliptic-oblong, slightly curved leaflets. Racemes of yellow, orange, or red flowers, 3–4cm (1¼–1½in) long, are borne from late spring to late summer. They are followed by thick pods, 10–25cm (4–10in) long, containing chestnut-like black seeds. ↕ 10–30m (30–100ft), ↔ 5–12m (15–40ft). N.E. Australia. ❄ (min. 7°C/45°F)

▷**Cast-iron plant** see *Aspidistra elatior*
▷**Castor oil plant** see *Ricinus communis*

CASUARINA

Australian pine, She oak

CASUARINACEAE

Genus of 40–70 species of evergreen, conifer-like trees and shrubs from Australia and the Pacific islands, where they thrive in a range of habitats from semi-desert to swamp forest. They are cultivated for their foliage, which is modified into minute scales or teeth arranged in a collar-like ring at each node. The tiny, petalless flowers are borne in single-sexed, cone-like spikes. Some species have nitrogen-fixing bacterial nodules on their roots. In frost-prone areas, grow young plants in a cool or temperate conservatory or greenhouse, or as houseplants. In frost-free climates, use Australian pines as specimen trees, windbreaks, or screens. They are tolerant of strong winds, coastal conditions, and wet or dry soils.
• **HARDINESS** Mostly frost tender, but *C. equisetifolia* and *C. torulosa* will tolerate short spells near to 0°C (32°F).
• **CULTIVATION** Under glass, grow in loam-based potting compost (JI No.2), with added sharp sand, in full light. When in growth, water freely and apply a balanced liquid fertilizer monthly; water more sparingly in winter. Pot on or top-dress in late winter. Outdoors, grow in fertile, moist but well-drained soil in full sun. Pruning group 1.
• **PROPAGATION** Sow seed at 13–18°C (55–64°F) in spring. Root semi-ripe cuttings in mid- or late summer.
• **PESTS AND DISEASES** Trouble free.

C. equisetifolia ♀ (Horsetail tree). Erect to spreading, open tree with pendent branch tips, grey-green shoots, and scale-like leaves, 1mm (1/16in) long, arranged in whorls of 6–8. The cylindrical to ovoid flower cones are 5mm (¼in) long. ↕ 5–15m (15–50ft), sometimes to 25m (80ft), ↔ 3–8m (10–25ft). E. Australia, Pacific islands. ❄ (min. 3–5°C/37–41°F)
C. torulosa ■♀–♀ (Forest oak). Slender, erect to spreading tree, sometimes with pendent shoots, and with corky bark. Scale-like leaves, 3–8mm (⅛–⅜in) long, arranged in whorls of 4, are pinkish when young, maturing to mid- or dark green. Some variants have light bronze to black-bronze foliage. Semi-spherical to cylindrical, bronze-green flower cones are 5–10mm (¼–½in) long. ↕ 8–25m (25–80ft), ↔ 5–10m (15–30ft). Australia (Queensland, New South Wales). ❄ (min. 3–5°C/37–41°F)

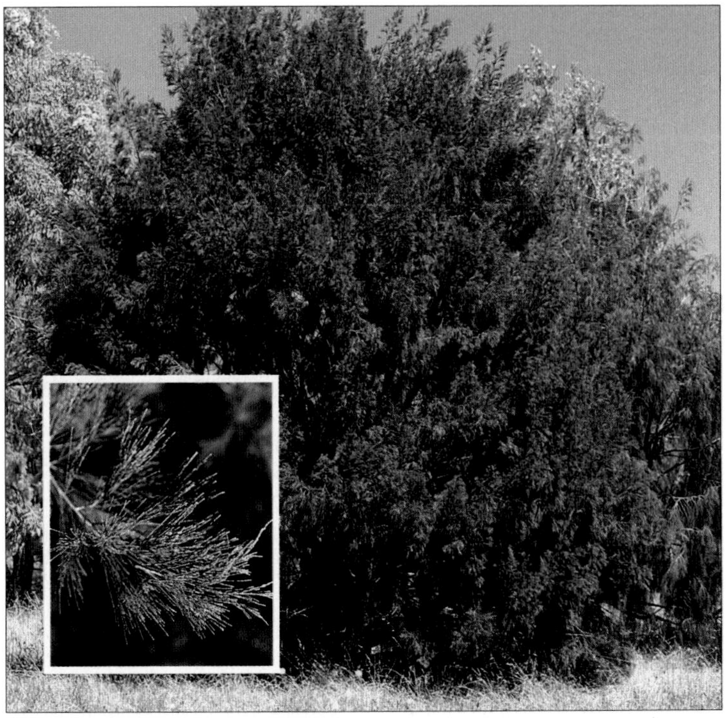

Casuarina torulosa (inset: leaf detail)

CATALPA

BIGNONIACEAE

Genus of 11 species of deciduous trees from E. Asia and North America, usually found on riverbanks and in woodland. Their large leaves are opposite or in whorls of 3. Catalpas are grown for their handsome foliage, for their large, bell-shaped, 2-lipped flowers, borne in upright, terminal panicles or racemes in mid- and late summer, and for their pendent, bean-like, narrowly cylindrical seed pods, which develop in autumn. Their wide-spreading habit and conspicuous flower panicles are seen to best advantage when they are grown as specimen trees. Those with coloured foliage are also effective in a shrub border; if pollarded or stooled annually, they produce large, ornamental leaves.

• **HARDINESS** Fully hardy.

• **CULTIVATION** Grow in fertile, moist but well-drained soil in full sun, sheltered from strong winds. Protect young plants from frost during very cold weather. Unripened wood is prone to frost damage. Pruning group 1, or group 7 if grown as a pollard.

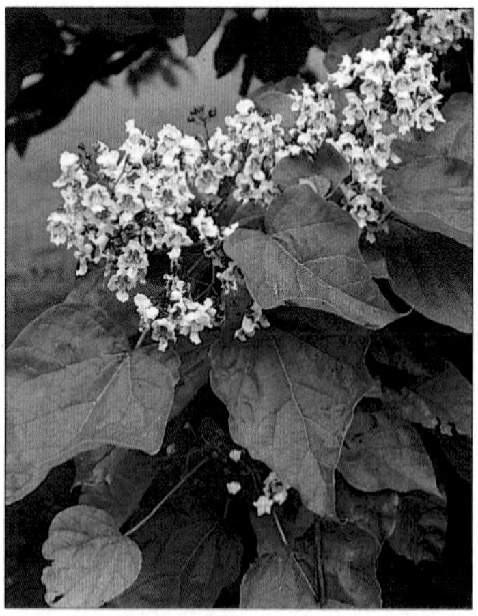

Catalpa bignonioides

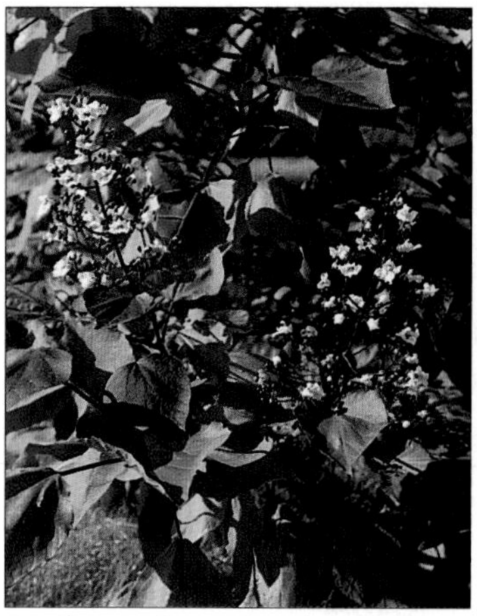

Catalpa x *erubescens* 'Purpurea'

• **PROPAGATION** Sow seed in a seedbed or in containers in an open frame in autumn. Root softwood cuttings in late spring or summer. Graft or insert root cuttings in winter. Bud in late summer.

• **PESTS AND DISEASES** Trouble free.

C. bignonioides ▣ ♀ ◌ (Indian bean tree, Southern catalpa). Spreading tree with broadly ovate, entire, mid-green leaves, heart-shaped at the bases, and to 25cm (10in) long. White flowers, to 5cm (2in) across, marked with yellow and purple-brown, are borne in upright panicles, 20–30cm (8–12in) tall. They are followed by slender pods, to 40cm (16in) long. ↕↔ 15m (50ft). S.E. USA. ✲✲✲. **'Aurea'** ▣ ♀ has bright yellow foliage, bronze when young; ↕↔ 10m (30ft). **'Nana'** is shrubby and rarely flowers; ↕ 1.8m (6ft), ↔ 1.5m (5ft). **'Purpurea'** see *C.* x *erubescens* 'Purpurea'.

***C.* x *erubescens* 'Purpurea'** ▣ ♀ ◌ syn. *C. bignonioides* 'Purpurea'. Spreading tree with broadly ovate leaves, 25–40cm (10–16in) long, with 3 shallow, tapered lobes, dark blackish purple when young, maturing to dark green. Bears white flowers, marked yellow and purple,

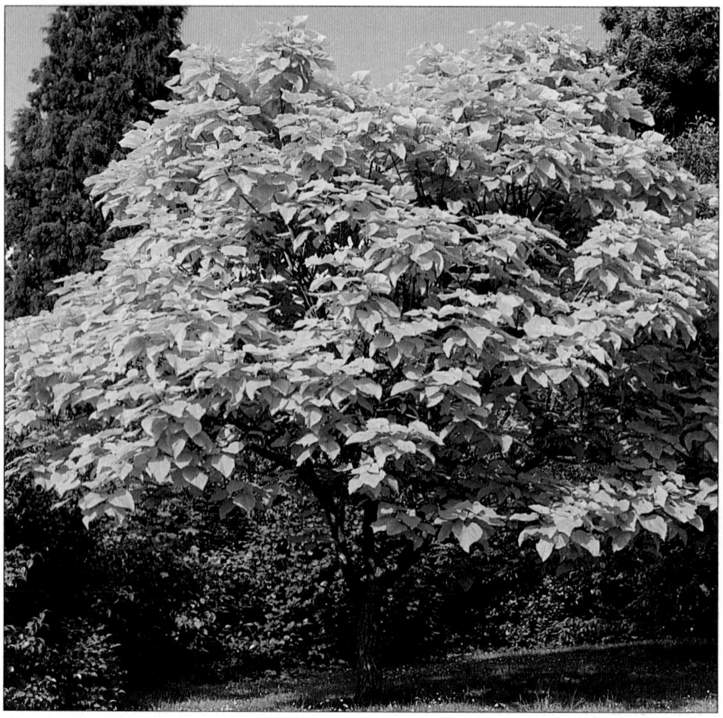

Catalpa bignonioides 'Aurea'

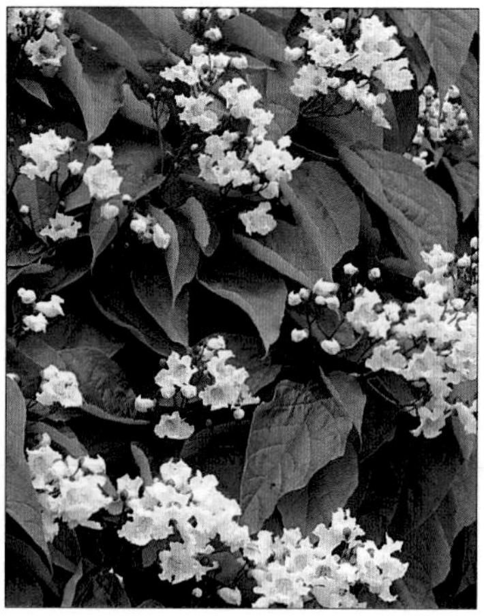

Catalpa speciosa

to 5cm (2in) across, in large, upright panicles, to 30cm (12in) tall. They are followed by slender pods, to 40cm (16in) long. ↕↔ 15m (50ft). ✲✲✲

C. ovata ◌ Spreading tree with broadly ovate, often 3-lobed, pale green leaves, to 25cm (10in) long. Upright panicles, to 25cm 10in) tall, of orange- and purple-marked, yellowish white flowers, to 3cm (1¼in) across, are followed by slender pods, to 30cm (12in) long. ↕↔ 10m (30ft). China. ✲✲✲

C. speciosa ▣ ◌ (Northern catalpa, Western catalpa). Spreading tree with broadly ovate, glossy, dark green leaves, to 30cm (12in) long, usually with 3 finely tapered lobes, densely hairy beneath. Large white flowers, to 6cm (2½in) across, marked with yellow and purple, are sparsely borne in upright panicles, 15–20cm (6–8in) tall. They are followed by slender pods, to 50cm (20in) or more long. ↕↔ 15m (50ft). USA. ✲✲✲

▷**Catalpa,**
Northern see *Catalpa speciosa*
Southern see *Catalpa bignonioides*
Western see *Catalpa speciosa*

CATANANCHE

Blue cupidone, Cupid's dart

ASTERACEAE/COMPOSITAE

Genus of 5 species of cornflower-like annuals and perennials occurring in dry meadows of the Mediterranean. They have linear to inversely lance-shaped, greyish green leaves, mainly in basal tufts, and are grown for their solitary flowerheads with strap-shaped, blue,

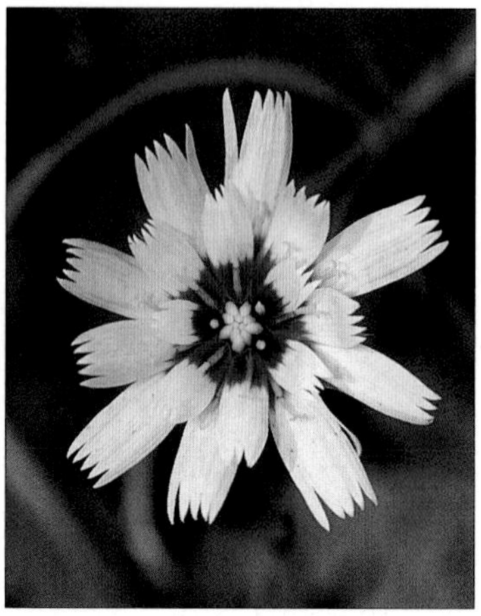

Catananche caerulea 'Bicolor'

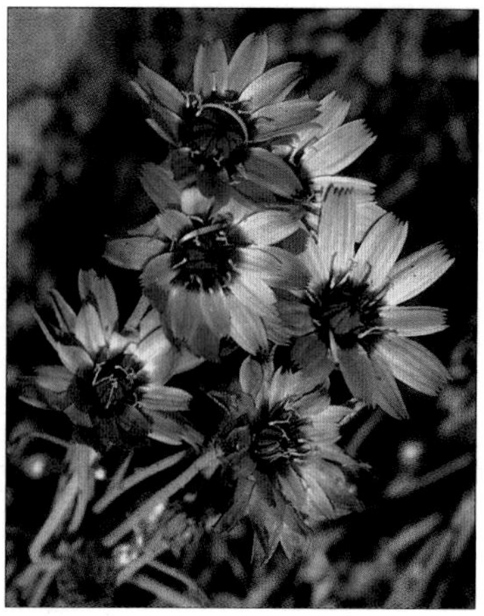

Catananche caerulea 'Major'

yellow, or white ray-florets and paper-like, silvery white bracts. Ideal for a sunny border; the flowers are also good for cutting and drying. *C. caespitosa* is best grown in an alpine house.

• **HARDINESS** Fully hardy.

• **CULTIVATION** Grow in any well-drained soil in full sun; *C. caerulea* is often short-lived in heavy soil. In an alpine house, grow *C. caespitosa* in loam-based potting compost (JI No.1), with additional grit, in full light.

• **PROPAGATION** Sow seed in containers in a cold frame in early spring or *in situ* in mid-spring. *C. caerulea* is best treated as an annual or a biennial; it usually flowers most freely in its second year. Divide in spring, or insert root cuttings in winter.

• **PESTS AND DISEASES** Powdery mildew may be a problem.

C. caerulea. Short-lived perennial with clumps of linear, grass-like, hairy leaves, to 30cm (12in) long. From midsummer to autumn, bears solitary, dark-centred, blue to lilac-blue flowerheads, 3–5cm (1¼–2in) across. ↕ 50–90cm (20–36in), ↔ 30cm (12in). S.W. Europe, Italy. ✲✲✲. **'Bicolor'** ▣ has white flowerheads with purple centres. **'Major'** ▣ ♀ has dark-centred, lilac-blue flowerheads, 5cm (2in) across; ↕ 45–50cm (18–20in). **'Perry's White'** has white flowerheads with cream centres.

C. caespitosa. Dwarf, mound-forming perennial with rosettes of hairy, linear leaves, to 7cm (3in) long. Produces solitary flowerheads, to 3cm (1¼in) across, with many pale to deep yellow ray-florets, on short stems in spring. ↕ 5–10cm (2–4in), ↔ 15–20cm (6–8in). Atlas Mountains. ✲✲✲

CATASETUM

ORCHIDACEAE

Genus of 50–70 species of deciduous, mainly epiphytic orchids from Central and South America, found from sea level to altitudes of 1,800m (6,000ft). They have stout, fleshy, ovoid to spindle-shaped pseudobulbs producing several alternately ranked, soft-textured, elliptic-lance-shaped to inversely lance-shaped leaves. Lateral, erect or pendent racemes of male and female flowers are borne on separate inflorescences from summer to autumn; occasionally flowers of both sexes are found on the same inflorescence.

• **HARDINESS** Frost tender.

• **CULTIVATION** Intermediate-growing orchids. Grow in epiphytic orchid compost in containers or slatted baskets. During summer, provide bright filtered light and high humidity with good ventilation. Water freely and apply a balanced liquid fertilizer at every third watering. In winter, remove shading and keep dry. Do not spray foliage as this may cause spotting. See also p.46.
• **PROPAGATION** Divide when the plant overflows its container.
• **PESTS AND DISEASES** Prone to red spider mites, aphids, and mealybugs.

C. pileatum. Deciduous, epiphytic orchid with ovoid to spindle-shaped pseudobulbs and lance-shaped leaves, 30cm (12in) long. Fragrant, pale yellow or creamy white flowers, 10cm (4in) across, sometimes flecked purple or red, are produced in racemes, to 40cm (16in) long, in summer. ↕30cm (12in), ↔45cm (18in). Ecuador, Colombia, Venezuela, Trinidad, Brazil. ❀ (min. 18°C/64°F; max. 30°C/86°F)

▷**Catchfly** see *Silene, Lychnis*
Alpine see *Lychnis alpina*
German see *Lychnis viscaria*
Nodding see *Silene pendula*

CATHARANTHUS

Madagascar periwinkle

APOCYNACEAE

Genus of 8 species of annuals and perennials from Madagascar, occurring in open scrub and at forest margins. The opposite leaves are simple and entire, and the 5-petalled, periwinkle-like flowers are solitary or borne in terminal cymes. Only *C. roseus* is widely cultivated. In frost-prone areas, grow as annual bedding, in a cool greenhouse or conservatory, or as a houseplant. In frost-free regions, grow in a bed or border.
• **HARDINESS** Frost tender.
• **CULTIVATION** Under glass, grow in loam-based potting compost (JI No.2) in full light with good ventilation. During the growing season, water moderately and apply a balanced liquid fertilizer monthly; water more sparingly in winter. Pot on or top-dress in late winter. Outdoors, grow in moderately fertile, well-drained soil in full sun. Plants under glass are best replaced every 2 years.
• **PROPAGATION** Sow seed at 13–18°C (55–64°F) in early spring. Root softwood cuttings in late spring or semi-ripe cuttings in summer.
• **PESTS AND DISEASES** Red spider mites and whiteflies may be a problem under glass.

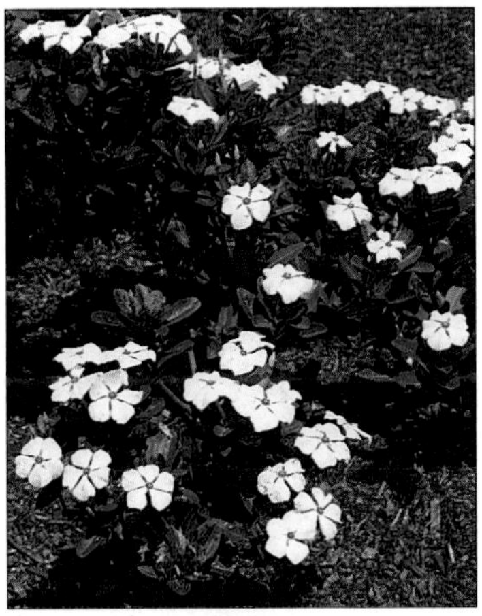

Catharanthus roseus

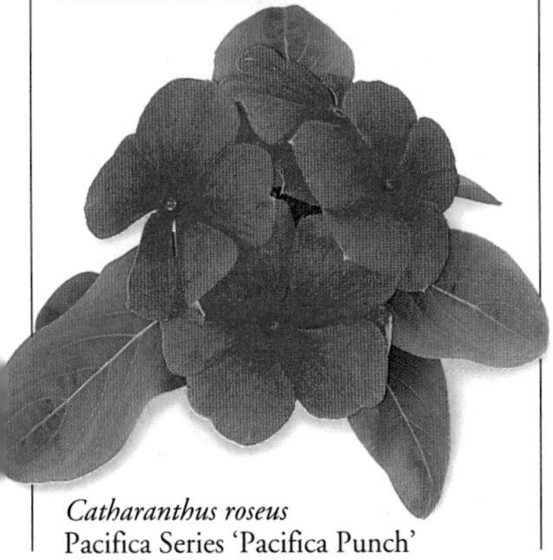

Catharanthus roseus
Pacifica Series 'Pacifica Punch'

C. roseus ■ ♀ syn. *Vinca rosea* (Madagascar periwinkle, Old maid). Woody-based, fleshy, evergreen perennial, erect at first, then spreading. It has stiff but slightly untidy stems and opposite, oblong-ovate, glossy, mid- to dark green leaves, to 5cm (2in) long, with paler midribs. Salverform, pink, rose-pink, red, or white flowers, to 4cm (1½in) across, are produced singly from the upper leaf axils, mainly from spring to summer. All parts may cause severe discomfort if ingested. ↕↔30–60cm (12–24in). Madagascar. ❀ (min. 5–7°C/41–45°F). **Cooler Series** cultivars are compact and branching, producing pastel to deep rose-pink and white flowers with broad, overlapping petals. **var. *ocellatus*** produces flowers with bright red eyes. **Pacifica Series** cultivars branch from the base, and bear large, lilac, pale pink, or white flowers in spring; some have white flowers with red eyes; ↕30–35cm (12–14in); **'Pacifica Punch'** ■ produces red, white, or rose-red flowers with deeper red centres.

▷***Cathcartia villosa*** see *Meconopsis villosa*
▷**Cathedral bell** see *Cobaea scandens*
▷**Cathedral windows** see *Calathea makoyana*
▷**Catherine's pincushion** see *Leucospermum catherinae*
▷**Catmint** see *Nepeta*

CATOPSIS

BROMELIACEAE

Genus, closely related to *Tillandsia*, of over 20 species of evergreen, epiphytic perennials (bromeliads) from lowland woodland, and rainforest. They occur up to altitudes of 2,000m (6,500ft) in S. North America, Central America, W., N., and E. South America, and the West Indies. The prominently sheathed leaves form funnel-shaped rosettes and are lance-shaped, smooth-margined, and often white-mealy. In summer, produces erect, arching, or pendent panicles of small, white or pale yellow flowers. Both male and female plants are needed to obtain fruit. In frost-prone areas, grow in a warm greenhouse or as houseplants. In warmer regions, grow in a moist, humid, outdoor site.
• **HARDINESS** Frost tender.
• **CULTIVATION** Under glass, grow epiphytically on bark or wood slabs, or in epiphytic bromeliad compost in bright filtered light. In summer, water moderately, mist frequently, apply a quarter-strength foliar fertilizer monthly and provide high humidity. Water sparingly at other times. Outdoors, grow epiphytically in humid conditions in partial shade. See also p.47.
• **PROPAGATION** Sow seed at 27°C (81°F) as soon as ripe. Root offsets in late spring with bottom heat in partial shade.
• **PESTS AND DISEASES** Susceptible to mealybugs and scale insects.

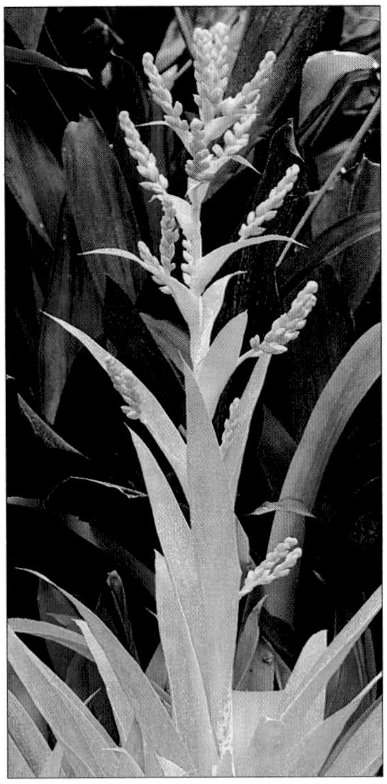

Catopsis hahnii

C. hahnii ■ Epiphytic bromeliad with dense rosettes of 12 or more white-mealy leaves, to 35cm (14in) long, tapering to fine tips. In summer, bears erect or arching panicles, 10–25cm (4–10in) long, with yellow bracts and white flowers, 7–9mm (¼–⅜in) long. ↕50cm (20in) or more, ↔20cm (8in). Mexico, Guatemala, El Salvador, Honduras, Nicaragua. ❀ (min. 16°C/61°F)

▷**Cat's claw vine** see *Macfadyena*
Common see *M. unguis-cati*
▷**Cat's ears** see *Antennaria, Calochortus*
▷**Cat's paw** see *Anigozanthos*
Common see *A. humilis*
▷**Cat's tail** see *Typha, T. latifolia*
Red-hot see *Acalypha hispida*
▷**Cat's whiskers** see *Tacca chantrierei*

CATTLEYA

ORCHIDACEAE

Genus of about 40 species of evergreen, epiphytic orchids from dry coastal areas to altitudes of 2,000m (7,000ft), often found along mountain streams, in Central and South America. They produce erect, stout to slender pseudobulbs on short rhizomes and 1 or 2 semi-rigid, leathery, oblong to broadly obovate, occasionally glaucous, mid- to dark green leaves. Large, showy flowers, with 3-lobed or entire lips usually surrounded by thick, bract-like sheaths, are borne in terminal racemes, or sometimes singly. Many hundreds of hybrids are available.
• **HARDINESS** Frost tender.
• **CULTIVATION** Cool to intermediate-growing orchids. Grow in epiphytic orchid compost in containers or orchid baskets. Provide high humidity, good ventilation, and bright filtered light or full light with shade from hot sun. In summer, water freely and apply a balanced liquid fertilizer at every third watering. In winter, remove shading and water more sparingly. See also p.46.
• **PROPAGATION** Divide when the plant overflows its container, or remove backbulbs and pot up separately.
• **PESTS AND DISEASES** Scale insects, red spider mites, aphids, and mealybugs may be a problem.

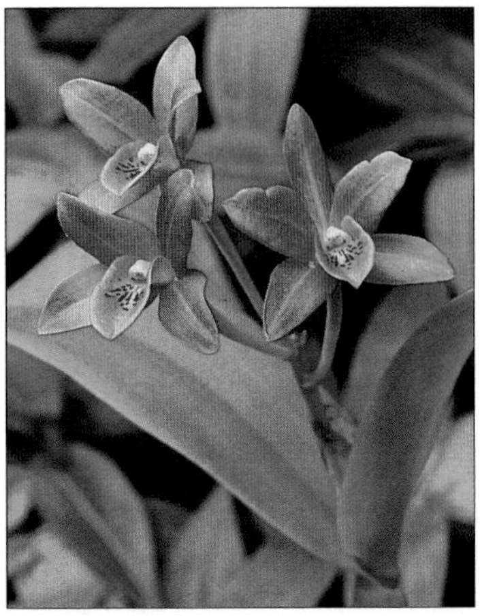

Cattleya aurantiaca

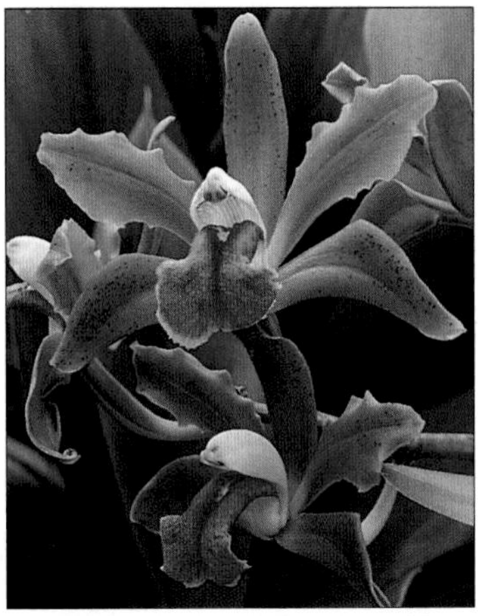

Cattleya bicolor

C. aurantiaca ■ Variable, epiphytic orchid with slender, narrowly cylindrical or spindle-shaped pseudobulbs and 2 ovate to elliptic leaves, 10–20cm (4–8in) long. Numerous bright orange, sometimes red or pale gold flowers, 4cm (1½in) across, often with dark red spots or streaks on the lips, are produced in racemes in summer. ↕↔30cm (12in). Central America. ❀ (min. 5°C/41°F; max. 30°C/86°F)
C. bicolor ■ Epiphytic orchid with cylindrical pseudobulbs producing 2 oblong leaves, 12–20cm (5–8in) long. Racemes of fragrant, yellow-green or brown flowers, 10cm (4in) across, with crimson lips, are borne from summer to autumn. ↕1.2m (4ft), ↔45cm (18in). Brazil. ❀ (min. 5°C/41°F; max. 30°C/86°F)

C

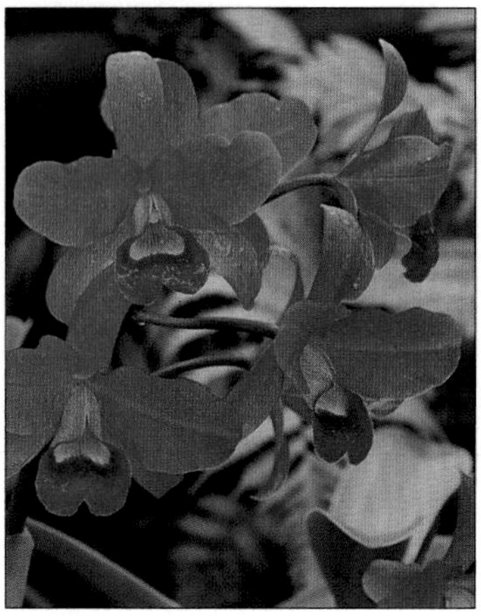

Cattleya bowringiana

C. bowringiana ▣ Epiphytic or terrestrial orchid producing cylindrical pseudobulbs and 2 narrowly oblong or elliptic-oblong, dark green leaves, 12–20cm (5–8in) long, glaucous at first. Long racemes of glossy, rose to magenta, white-throated flowers, 8cm (3in) across, with pale rose-purple and dark purple lips, open from autumn to winter. ↕ 1m (3ft), ↔ 45cm (18in). Guatemala, Belize. ❄ (min. 5°C/41°F; max. 30°C/86°F)
***C.* Chocolate Drop.** Epiphytic orchid with slender, oblong pseudobulbs and 2 oval leaves, 10–15cm (4–6in) long. In autumn, bears variable, chocolate-brown to reddish orange flowers, 5cm (2in) across, some with darker lips. ↕ 45cm (18in), ↔ 30cm (12in). ❄ (min. 5°C/41°F; max. 30°C/86°F)
C. dowiana. Epiphytic orchid with stout, oblong pseudobulbs producing one oblong leaf, to 30cm (12in) long. Racemes of fragrant yellow flowers, 12cm (5in) across, with crimson, gold-veined lips, are borne in autumn. ↕↔ 30cm (12in). Costa Rica, Colombia. ❄ (min. 5°C/41°F; max. 30°C/86°F)
C. forbesii. Epiphytic orchid with slender, oblong to cylindrical pseudobulbs and 2 oblong or narrowly elliptic leaves, to 15cm (6in) long. From spring to summer, bears racemes of fragrant, tawny pink to light green flowers, 7cm (3in) across, with yellow throats and a yellow stripe on the lips. ↕↔ 30cm (12in). Brazil. ❄ (min. 5°C/41°F; max. 30°C/86°F)
C. guttata. Epiphytic orchid producing cylindrical pseudobulbs and 2 lance-shaped or elliptic-oblong leaves, to 25cm (10in) long. In winter, produces

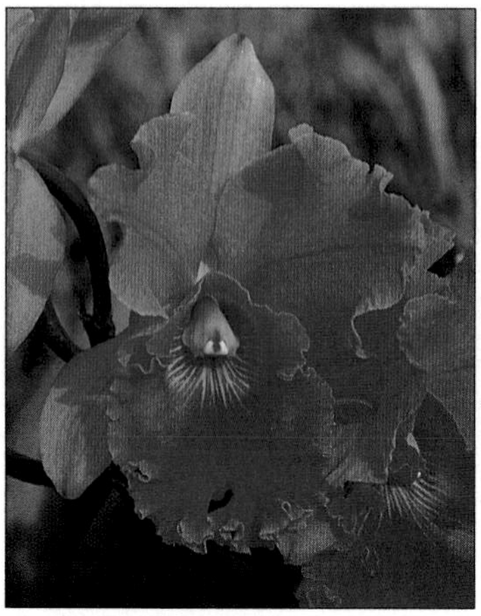

Cattleya J.A. Carbone

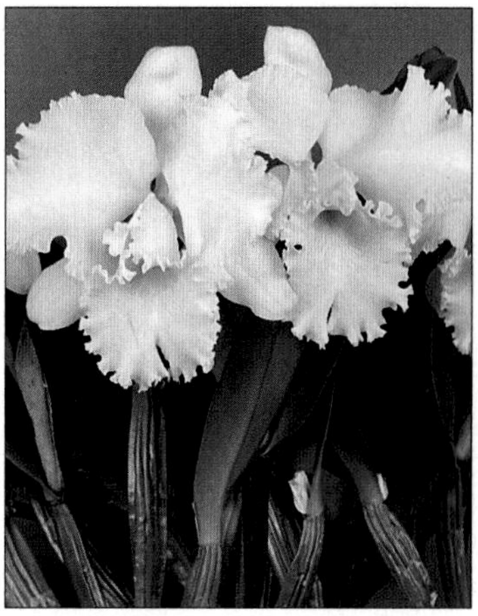

Cattleya José Marti

racemes of yellow- to lime-green flowers, to 7cm (3in) across, spotted red-brown, or banded purple; the 3-lobed lips are rose-purple to magenta. ↕ 1.2m (4ft), ↔ 60cm (24in). Brazil. ❄ (min. 5°C/41°F; max. 30°C/86°F)
***C.* J.A. Carbone** ▣ Epiphytic orchid with club-shaped pseudobulbs and one oblong leaf, 15cm (6in) long. In early summer, bears fragrant mauve flowers, 12cm (5in) across, with darker mauve lips. ↕ 20cm (8in), ↔ 45cm (18in). ❄ (min. 5°C/41°F; max. 30°C/86°F)
***C.* José Marti** ▣ syn. *C.* Mother's Favourite 'José Marti'. Epiphytic orchid with club-shaped pseudobulbs and one oblong leaf, 15cm (6in) long. Fragrant white flowers, 12cm (5in) across, with yellow throats, are borne in spring. ↕ 20cm (8in), ↔ 45cm (18in). ❄ (min. 5°C/41°F; max. 30°C/86°F)
C. labiata. Epiphytic orchid with club-shaped pseudobulbs and one oblong leaf, to 30cm (12in) long. Racemes of ruffled, pale rose-pink to lilac-magenta flowers, 15cm (6in) across, with purple, yellow-veined lips, are produced in autumn. ↕↔ 30cm (12in). Brazil. ❄ (min. 5°C/41°F; max. 30°C/86°F)
C. mossiae. Epiphytic orchid with club-shaped pseudobulbs and one oblong to ovate-oblong leaf, to 30cm (12in) long. In early summer, bears fragrant, light mauve, pink, or magenta flowers, 15cm (6in) across, with yellow-centred, white to lilac lips. ↕↔ 30cm (12in). Venezuela. ❄ (min. 5°C/41°F; max. 30°C/86°F)
***C.* Mother's Favourite 'José Marti'** see *C.* José Marti.
***C.* Nigritian 'King of Kings'.** Epiphytic orchid producing club-shaped pseudobulbs and one oblong leaf, 15cm (6in) long. Bears rich mauve flowers, 12cm (5in) across, with darker mauve lips, in autumn or spring. ↕ 20cm (8in), ↔ 45cm (18in). ❄ (min. 5°C/40°F; max. 30°C/86°F)
***C.* Portia 'Coerulea'.** Epiphytic orchid with club-shaped pseudobulbs and 1 or 2 oblong leaves, 15cm (6in) long. Bears blue-lilac flowers, 10cm (4in) across, in early summer. ↕↔ 30cm (12in). ❄ (min. 5°C/41°F; max. 30°C/86°F)
C. skinneri. Epiphytic orchid with cylindrical pseudobulbs and 2 oblong or elliptic-oblong leaves, to 30cm (12in) long. From winter to spring, bears many small, rose-purple to bright purple flowers, to 10cm (4in) across, the lips often white or cream. ↕↔ 30cm (12in). Mexico to Costa Rica, Guatemala. ❄ (min. 5°C/41°F; max. 30°C/86°F)
C. trianae. Epiphytic orchid with club-shaped pseudobulbs and one oblong leaf, 30cm (12in) long. Racemes of pure white or rose-white flowers, 20cm (8in) across, often purple-suffused, with pink and magenta lips, are borne from winter to spring. ↕↔ 30cm (12in). Colombia. ❄ (min. 5°C/41°F; max. 30°C/86°F)
C. walkeriana. Epiphytic orchid with stout, spindle-shaped pseudobulbs and one oblong leaf, 5–10cm (2–4in) long. Solitary (occasionally 2 or 3), rich amethyst or white flowers, 10cm (4in) across, with rose-pink or light magenta lips, are produced in spring. ↕ 12cm (5in), ↔ 15cm (6in). Brazil. ❄ (min. 5°C/41°F; max. 30°C/86°F)

CAULOPHYLLUM

BERBERIDACEAE

Genus of 2 (possibly only one) species of rhizomatous perennials found in mountain woodland, one in E. North America, the other in Japan. They bear racemes or panicles of small flowers, with sepals much larger than the petals. The fruits split open early to reveal berry-like seeds that turn from green to blue. The leaves develop with the flowers or just after they open, and immediately below them. Each leaf has 3 leaflets, which are ovate to obovate, 3-lobed, and conspicuously veined; they are occasionally 2-ternate. Grow in a woodland garden for their berries.
• **HARDINESS** Fully hardy.
• **CULTIVATION** Grow in moist, humus-rich, acid soil in partial or deep shade.
• **PROPAGATION** Sow seed in containers in an open frame as soon as ripe; germination may be slow and erratic. Divide in spring, before growth begins, or after flowering. Very slow to increase.
• **PESTS AND DISEASES** Trouble free.

C. thalictroides (Blue cohosh). Rhizomatous perennial with 3-palmate, mid-green leaves, produced singly or in pairs. In mid- and late spring, bears green- or yellow-brown flowers, 1cm (½in) across, with 6 long sepals and 6 short petals, the latter reduced to nectaries. Spherical seeds, to 1cm (½in) across, are deep, bright blue, sometimes glaucous. ↕ to 75cm (30in), ↔ 18cm (7in). North America (New Brunswick to Tennessee, and S. Carolina). ❄❄❄

CAUTLEYA

ZINGIBERACEAE

Genus of 5 or 6 species of rhizomatous perennials from shaded ravines among low, grassy vegetation and shrubs in the Himalayas. They have 2-ranked, lance-shaped to oblong leaves, and bear lax, terminal, spike-like racemes of complex, 2-lipped yellow flowers, with bold red bracts and sepals. Grow in a shaded mixed or herbaceous border, or in a woodland garden.
• **HARDINESS** Fully hardy to frost hardy.
• **CULTIVATION** Plant rhizomes 15cm (6in) deep in spring. Grow in moist, humus-rich soil in partial shade. Water freely in dry periods, and apply a thick mulch in autumn.
• **PROPAGATION** Sow seed at 13–18°C (55–64°F) in early spring, or divide in late spring after growth has just begun.
• **PESTS AND DISEASES** Slugs may damage the leaves.

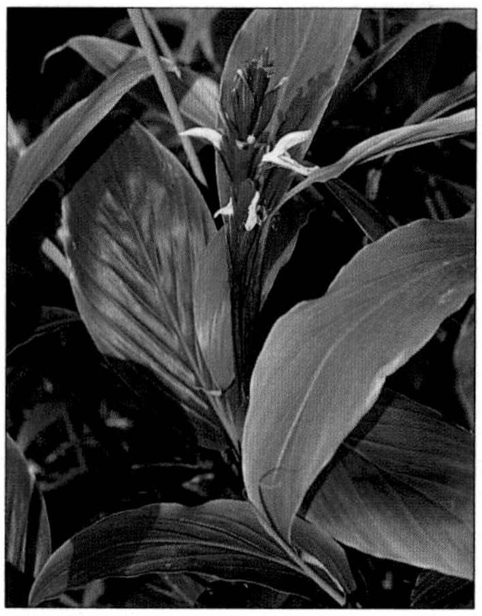

Cautleya spicata

C. spicata ▣ Rhizomatous perennial with broadly lance-shaped, hairless, mid-green leaves, to 35cm (14in) long. In late summer, produces stiff spikes of 2-lipped yellow flowers, 2.5cm (1in) long, with reddish green to maroon bracts. ↕ 60–90cm (24–36in), ↔ 45cm (18in). Himalayas. ❄❄❄ (borderline)

CAVENDISHIA

ERICACEAE

Genus of about 100 species of evergreen, small trees or shrubs from cloud forest in tropical South America. The leathery leaves are alternate, simple, and entire. They are cultivated mainly for their bell-shaped or tubular flowers, borne in axillary or terminal, simple or branched racemes. In frost-prone areas, grow in a cool or temperate greenhouse. In frost-free regions, grow in a shrub border or at the base of a house wall.
• **HARDINESS** Frost tender.
• **CULTIVATION** Under glass, grow in lime-free (ericaceous) potting compost in bright filtered light. In the growing season, water moderately and apply a balanced liquid fertilizer monthly; water more sparingly in winter. Top-dress or pot on in early spring. Outdoors, grow in moist but well-drained, humus-rich, neutral to acid soil in partial shade, or screened from full sun. Pruning group 8 or 9, but regular pruning is not necessary.
• **PROPAGATION** Sow seed at 15–18°C (59–64°F) in spring. Root semi-ripe cuttings in summer. Layer in spring or autumn.
• **PESTS AND DISEASES** Red spider mites and scale insects may be a problem under glass.

C. acuminata. Spreading shrub with arching to pendent branches, and ovate to oblong or lance-shaped leaves, 5–8cm (2–3in) long, pink when young but maturing to glossy, dark green. From autumn to early winter, produces clustered racemes, 3–6cm (1¼–2½in) long, of narrowly bell-shaped or tubular, crimson to scarlet flowers with green lobes, which are shielded in bud by large scarlet bracts. ↕ 1–2m (3–6ft), ↔ 1m (3ft). Colombia, Ecuador. ❄ (min. 5°C/41°F)

▷ **Cayenne pepper** see *Capsicum annuum* Longum Group
▷ ***Cayratia thomsonii*** see *Parthenocissus thomsonii*

CEANOTHUS

California lilac

RHAMNACEAE

Genus of about 55 species of deciduous and evergreen shrubs, more rarely small trees, mostly from W. North America, in particular California, but also from E. USA and Mexico, occurring from the coast to the mountains, usually in scrub and woodland on dry slopes. They have opposite or alternate, usually toothed leaves, and are cultivated for their small but profuse, blue, white, or pink flowers, to 3mm (1/8in) across, borne in terminal, lateral, or axillary cymes, racemes, or panicles. They are suitable for growing in a shrub border or against a sunny wall. Low-growing or prostrate species and cultivars are excellent as ground cover or in a large rock garden.

• **HARDINESS** Fully hardy to frost hardy.

• **CULTIVATION** Grow in fertile, well-drained soil in full sun, sheltered from strong, cold winds. California lilacs are lime tolerant, but may become chlorotic on shallow chalk soils. Most may be trained against a wall, where they can reach twice the height they would in an open site. Pruning group 8 after flowering for evergreens; group 6 in early spring for deciduous plants; group 13 if wall-trained. Mulch and apply a balanced liquid fertilizer after pruning.

• **PROPAGATION** Sow seed in a seedbed, or in containers in an open frame, in autumn; most species hybridize readily. Root greenwood cuttings of deciduous plants, and semi-ripe cuttings of evergreens, in mid- to late summer.

• **PESTS AND DISEASES** Susceptible to honey fungus.

***C. arboreus* 'Trewithen Blue'** ▣ 🏆 Vigorous, wide-spreading, evergreen shrub with alternate, broadly oval to rounded, shallowly toothed, dark green leaves, to 10cm (4in) long. In spring and early summer, bears fragrant, mid-blue flowers in large, pyramidal, terminal and lateral panicles, to 12cm (5in) long. ↕6m (20ft), ↔8m (25ft). ❄❄

***C.* 'A.T. Johnson'.** Vigorous, bushy, spreading, evergreen shrub with alternate, ovate, shallowly toothed, light green leaves, to 3cm (1¼in) long. Rich blue flowers are produced in lateral and terminal panicles, 5–6cm (2–2½in) long, over a long period in late spring and again from late summer to autumn. ↕↔2.5m (8ft). ❄❄

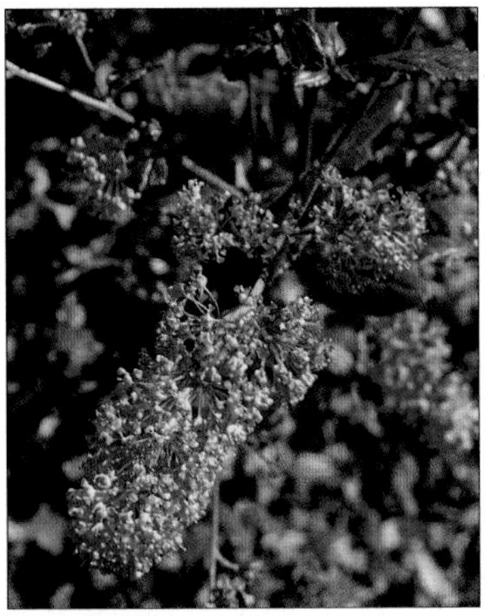

Ceanothus 'Autumnal Blue'

***C.* 'Autumnal Blue'** ▣ 🏆 Upright, evergreen shrub with alternate, elliptic, finely toothed, glossy, bright green leaves, to 5cm (2in) long. Rich sky-blue flowers are borne in large, lateral panicles, 8cm (3in) long, from late summer to autumn. ↕↔3m (10ft). ❄❄❄

***C.* 'Blue Jeans'.** Spreading, evergreen shrub with opposite, oblong, toothed, leathery, dark green leaves, 2–4cm (¾–1½in) long. Mid-blue flowers are freely borne in lateral and terminal, rounded cymes, to 2cm (¾in) across, in late spring. ↕↔2.5m (8ft). ❄❄

***C.* 'Blue Mound'** ▣ 🏆 Mound-forming, evergreen shrub with alternate, oblong, very finely toothed, glossy, dark green leaves, to 3cm (1¼in) long. In late spring, produces dark blue flowers in large, lateral cymes, 6–8cm (2½–3in) long. ↕1.5m (5ft), ↔2m (6ft). ❄❄

***C.* 'Burkwoodii'** 🏆 Bushy, compact, evergreen shrub with opposite, oval, toothed, glossy, dark green leaves, to 3cm (1¼in) long, and greyish beneath. Bright blue flowers are produced in dense lateral and terminal panicles, to 6cm (2½in) long, from late summer to autumn. ↕1.5m (5ft), ↔2m (6ft). ❄❄

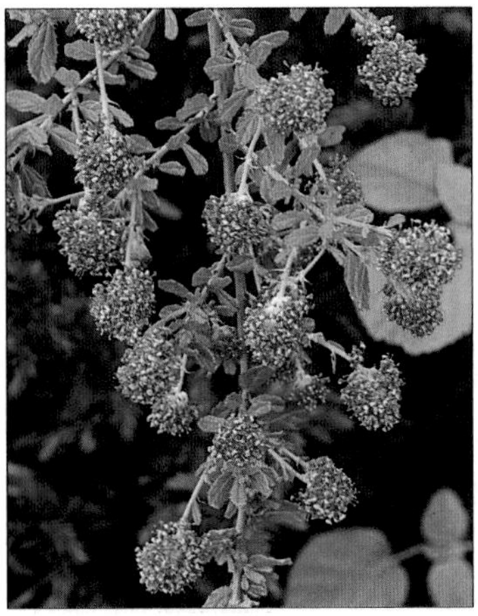

Ceanothus 'Cascade'

***C.* 'Burtonensis'.** Spreading, evergreen shrub with alternate, rounded, crinkled, dark green leaves, to 2cm (¾in) long. In late spring and early summer, bears dark blue flowers in dense, rounded, terminal and lateral cymes, to 3cm (1¼in) across. ↕2m (6ft), ↔4m (12ft). ❄❄

***C.* 'Cascade'** ▣ 🏆 Vigorous, evergreen, open shrub with arching branches and alternate, oblong, finely toothed, glossy, dark green leaves, to 5cm (2in) long. Bears a mass of powder-blue flowers in large, terminal and lateral panicles, to 6cm (2½in) long, from spring to early summer. ↕↔4m (12ft). ❄❄

***C.* 'Concha'** ▣ Dense, evergreen shrub with arching branches and alternate, oblong-elliptic, finely toothed, dark green leaves, to 5cm (2in) long. In late spring, reddish purple buds open to dark blue flowers in numerous rounded, terminal and lateral cymes, to 3cm (1¼in) across. ↕↔3m (10ft). ❄❄

***C.* 'Cynthia Postan'** ▣ syn. *C.* x *regius* 'Cynthia Postan'. Dense, rounded, evergreen shrub with alternate, oblong, finely toothed, glossy, dark green leaves, to 4cm (1½in) long, grey-green beneath. Rich blue flowers are profusely borne in dense, lateral cymes, 4–5cm (1½–2in)

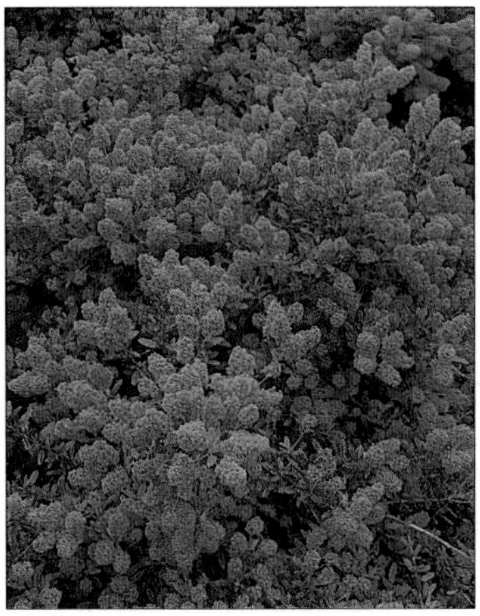

Ceanothus 'Concha'

long, in late spring and early summer. ↕↔2.5m (8ft). ❄❄

***C.* 'Dark Star'.** Arching, evergreen shrub with alternate, ovate, toothed, dark green leaves, to 1cm (½in) long, with deeply impressed veins. Honey-scented, dark purplish blue flowers are borne in rounded, terminal and lateral cymes, to 3cm (1¼in) across, in late spring. ↕2m (6ft), ↔3m (10ft). ❄❄

***C.* 'Delight'** 🏆 Vigorous, bushy, evergreen shrub with alternate, oblong, glossy, dark green leaves, to 2.5cm (1in) long. Dark blue flowers are produced in terminal and lateral panicles, to 6cm (2½in) long, in mid- and late spring. ↕3m (10ft), ↔5m (15ft). ❄❄

***C.* x *delileanus* 'Gloire de Versailles'** see *C.* 'Gloire de Versailles'.

C. dentatus*.** Densely branched, spreading, evergreen shrub with rigid shoots and alternate, tightly clustered, small, oblong-elliptic, toothed, dark green leaves, to 1cm (½in) long. In late spring, bears dark blue flowers in small, rounded, terminal or lateral cymes, to 2cm (¾in) across. ↕1.5m (5ft), ↔2m (6ft). USA (California). ❄❄. **var. *floribundus has broader leaves and more densely clustered flowers.

***C. divergens*.** Spreading, evergreen shrub with rigid, slender shoots and opposite, flat, holly-like, dark green leaves, to 2.5cm (1in) long, with smooth margins. In spring, purple-blue flowers open from red-purple buds in dense, rounded, lateral, umbel-like cymes, to 2cm (¾in) across. ↕1m (3ft), ↔1.5m (5ft). USA (California). ❄❄

***C.* 'Edinburgh'** 🏆 Vigorous, dense, upright, evergreen shrub with alternate,

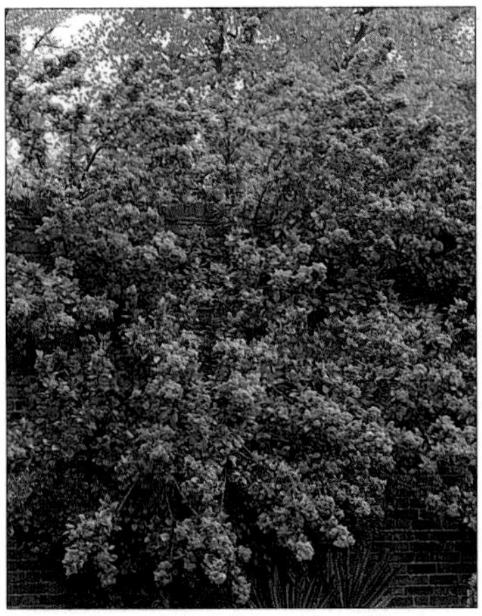

Ceanothus arboreus 'Trewithen Blue'

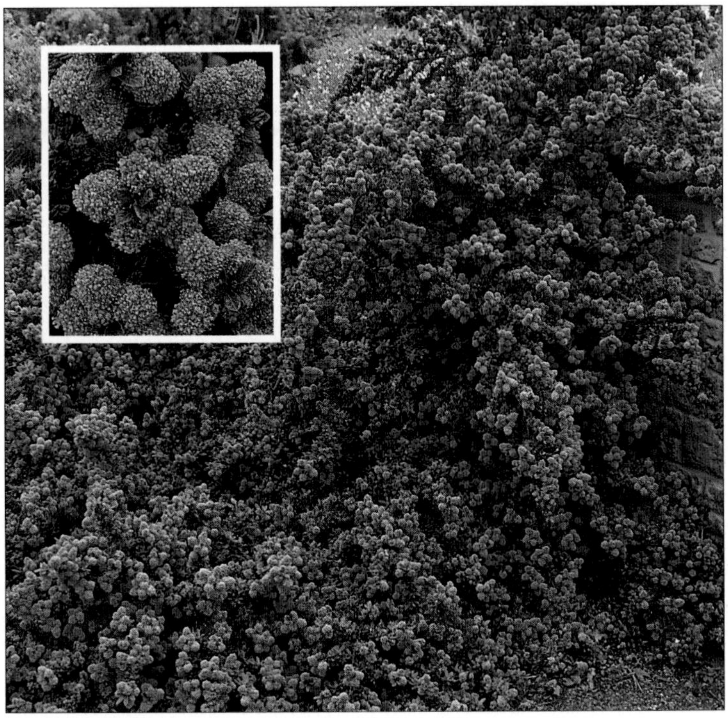

Ceanothus 'Blue Mound' (inset: flower detail)

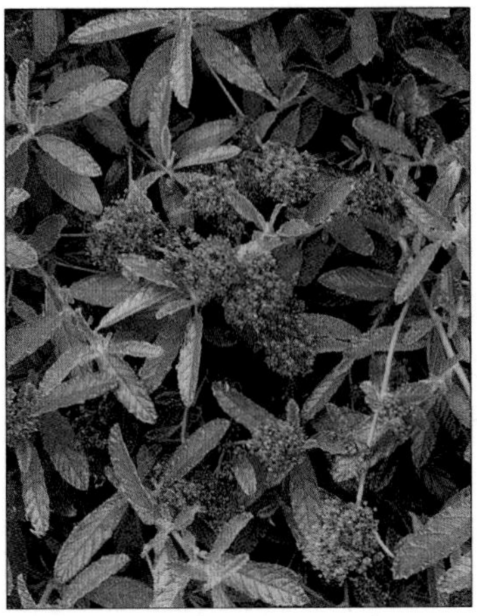

Ceanothus 'Cynthia Postan'

CEANOTHUS

C

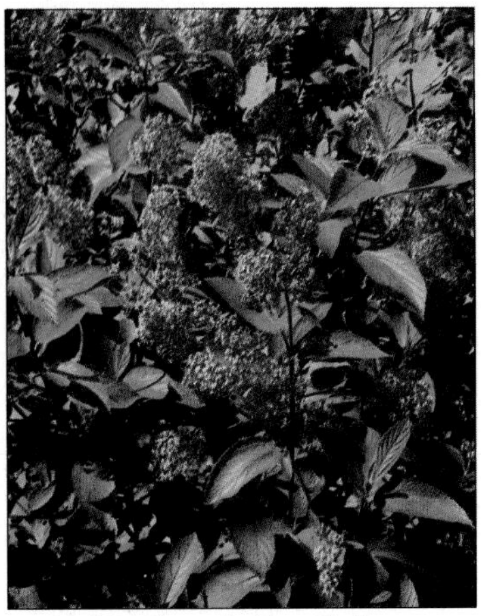

Ceanothus 'Gloire de Versailles'

oblong-ovate, toothed, olive-green leaves, to 7cm (3in) long. Produces rich blue flowers in lateral cymes, to 5cm (2in) long, from spring to early summer. ↕3m (10ft), ↔2.5m (8ft). ❄❄

***C.* 'Gentian Plume'.** Open, spreading, evergreen shrub with alternate, ovate-oblong, strongly veined, shallowly toothed, mid-green leaves, 8cm (3in) or more long. Deep sky-blue flowers are borne in large, open, terminal and axillary panicles, 12cm (5in) or more long, in late spring and often again in autumn. ↕↔4m (12ft). ❄❄

***C.* 'Gloire de Versailles'** ▣🏆 syn. *C.* x *delileanus* 'Gloire de Versailles'. Bushy, deciduous shrub with alternate, oval, finely toothed, dark green leaves, to 7cm (3in) long. From midsummer to autumn, bears pale blue flowers in large, terminal and axillary panicles, to 10cm (4in) or more long. ↕↔1.5m (5ft). ❄❄❄

C. gloriosus. Prostrate or decumbent, evergreen shrub with opposite, oblong-elliptic, holly-like, leathery leaves, to 4cm (1½in) long, dark green and hairless above, grey-hairy beneath, with strongly toothed margins. In late spring and early summer, bears deep blue to purple flowers in rounded, terminal, umbel-like cymes, to 5cm (2in) across. ↕30cm (12in), ↔3–4m (10–12ft). USA (California). ❄❄. **'Anchor Bay'** has dense growth and dark blue flowers; ↕50cm (20in), ↔2m (6ft). **'Emily Brown'** has small, very strongly toothed leaves, to 2.5cm (1in) long, and dark indigo flowers; ↕1m (3ft), ↔4m (12ft).

C. griseus (Carmel ceanothus). Vigorous, evergreen shrub producing alternate, ovate, glossy, dark green leaves, to 5cm (2in) long, grey-hairy beneath. Pale to dark blue flowers are borne in large, rounded, terminal and lateral panicles, to 7cm (3in) across, in late spring and early summer. ↕↔3m (10ft). USA (California). ❄❄. **var. *horizontalis* 'Yankee Point'** bears profuse bright blue flowers; ↕60–90cm (24–36in), ↔3m (10ft). **'Santa Ana'** is low-growing, with very dark blue flowers; ↕1.5m (5ft), ↔5m (15ft).

C. hearstiorum. Prostrate, evergreen shrub with alternate, deeply veined, oblong, toothed, dark green leaves, to 3cm (1¼in) long, white-hairy beneath. Bears rich, dark blue flowers in rounded, terminal and lateral cymes, 2.5cm (1in) across, in late spring and early summer. ↕30cm (12in), ↔2m (6ft). USA (California). ❄❄

***C.* 'Henri Désfosse'.** Bushy, deciduous shrub with alternate, oval, toothed, mid-green leaves, to 7cm (3in) long. From midsummer to autumn, bears dark blue flowers in large, terminal and lateral panicles, 8–12cm (3–5in) across. ↕↔1.5m (5ft). ❄❄❄

C. impressus (Santa Barbara ceanothus). Spreading, evergreen shrub with small, alternate, rounded to elliptic, deeply veined, dark green leaves, to 1cm (½in) long. Dark blue flowers are produced in rounded, terminal cymes, to 2.5cm (1in) across, in mid- and late spring. ↕1.5m (5ft), ↔2.5m (8ft). USA (California). ❄❄. **'Puget Blue'** is vigorous, with larger, elliptic-oblong leaves, to 2cm (¾in) long, and profuse dark blue flowers, borne in cymes to 3cm (1¼in) long; ↕↔3m (10ft).

C. incanus ▣ (Coast whitethorn). Spreading, stoutly branched, evergreen shrub with spiny, grey-glaucous shoots and alternate, ovate or broadly elliptic, entire or slightly toothed, grey-green leaves, to 6cm (2½in) long. In mid- and late spring, slightly fragrant, creamy white flowers are borne in lateral panicles, to 8cm (3in) long. ↕3m (10ft), ↔4m (12ft). USA (California). ❄❄

***C.* 'Italian Skies'** 🏆 Spreading, evergreen shrub with alternate, ovate, finely toothed, glossy, mid-green leaves, to 2cm (¾in) long. Bright blue flowers are borne in dense, conical, terminal and lateral cymes, to 7cm (3in) long, in late spring. ↕1.5m (5ft), ↔3m (10ft). ❄❄

***C.* 'Julia Phelps'.** Rounded, evergreen shrub producing small, alternate, oblong-elliptic, finely toothed, dark green leaves, to 2.5cm (1in) long. Violet flowers, opening from red-purple buds, are borne in dense, rounded, terminal and lateral cymes, to 3cm (1¼in) across, in late spring and early summer. ↕2m (6ft), ↔2.5m (8ft). ❄❄

***C.* 'Marie Simon'.** Upright, bushy, deciduous shrub with alternate, oval, toothed leaves, to 5cm (2in) long, borne on red stems. Pale pink flowers open in terminal panicles, to 7cm (3in) or more long, from midsummer to autumn. ↕↔1.5m (5ft). ❄❄❄

***C. papillosus* var. *roweanus*.** Bushy, spreading, evergreen shrub with slender, alternate, oblong to linear, dark green leaves, to 5cm (2in) long, covered on the margins of the upper surfaces with sticky glands. Dark blue to purple-blue flowers are produced in terminal and axillary racemes, 3–4cm (1¼–1½in) long, in mid- and late spring. ↕1.5m (5ft), ↔3m (10ft). USA (California). ❄❄

***C.* 'Perle Rose'** ▣ Bushy, deciduous shrub with alternate, oval, toothed, pale green leaves, to 5cm (2in) long. From midsummer to autumn, bears carmine-pink flowers in many terminal and lateral panicles, to 6cm (2½in) or more long. ↕↔1.5m (5ft). ❄❄❄

***C.* 'Pin Cushion'** ▣ Rounded, evergreen shrub with oblong-elliptic, dark green leaves, to 4cm (1½in) long. Mid- to light blue flowers are borne freely in terminal and axillary panicles, 5cm (2in) long, in late spring. ↕↔to 2m (6ft). ❄❄

C. purpureus (Hollyleaf ceanothus). Spreading, evergreen shrub with rigid shoots and opposite, holly-like, broadly elliptic to rounded, wavy-margined, spine-toothed, glossy, dark green leaves, to 2cm (¾in) long. In spring, red-purple

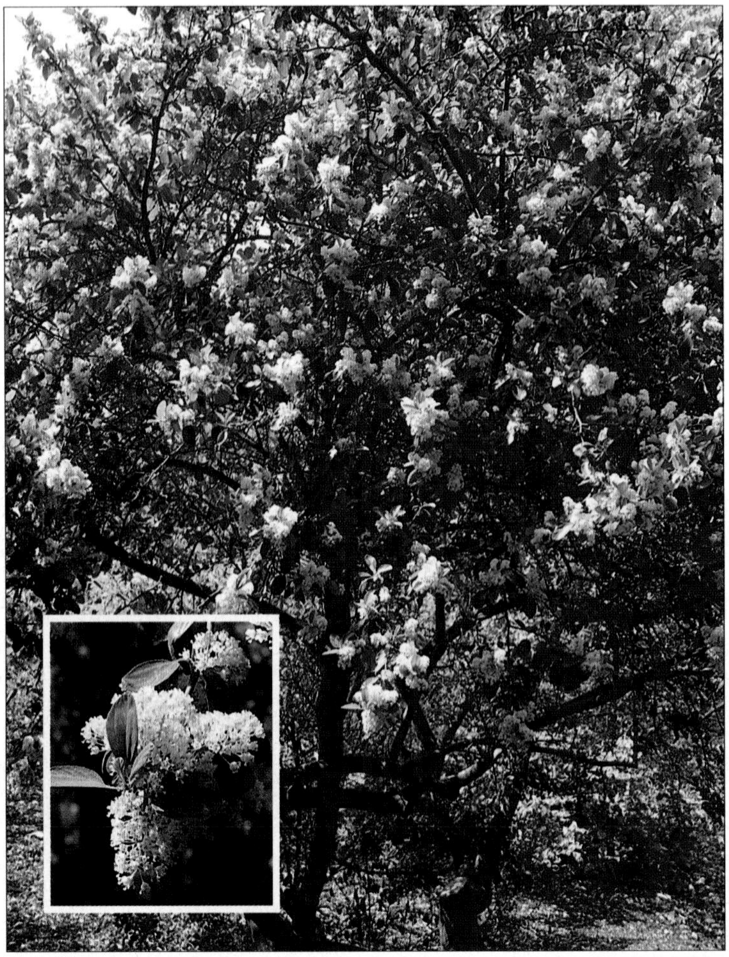

Ceanothus incanus (inset: flower detail)

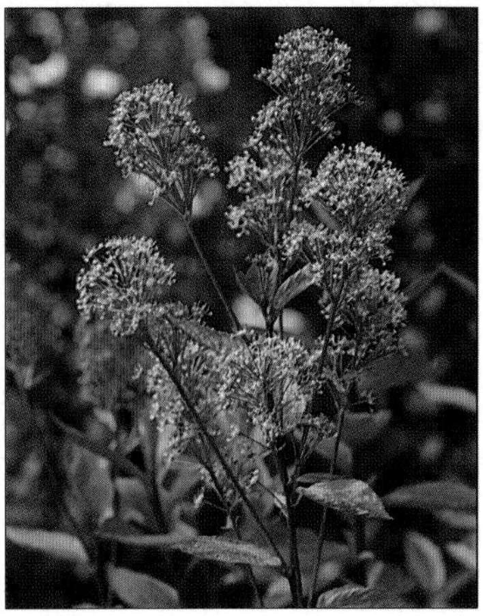

Ceanothus 'Perle Rose'

buds open to purple-blue flowers in dense, lateral, umbel-like cymes, to 4cm (1½in) across. ↕1.2m (4ft), ↔1.8m (6ft). USA (California). ❄❄

***C.* x *regius* 'Cynthia Postan'** see *C.* 'Cynthia Postan'.

C. repens see *C. thyrsiflorus* var. *repens.*

C. rigidus (Monterey ceanothus). Intricately branched, evergreen shrub producing small, opposite, wedge-shaped to rounded, obovate, toothed leaves, to 1cm (½in) long, glossy, mid-green above and softly downy beneath, clustered on rigid shoots. Bright blue to purple-blue flowers are borne in dense, lateral, umbel-like cymes, to 2cm (¾in) across, during late spring and early summer. ↕1.2m (4ft), ↔2m (6ft). USA (California). ❄❄. **'Snowball'** has white flowers.

***C.* 'Skylark'** ▣ Bushy, evergreen shrub with alternate, oblong-elliptic, finely toothed, glossy, mid-green leaves, to 5cm (2in) long. Dark blue flowers are borne in profuse, open, terminal and lateral panicles, 6–8cm (2½–3in) long, in late spring and early summer. ↕2m (6ft), ↔1.5m (5ft). ❄❄

***C.* 'Snow Flurries'.** Vigorous, upright, evergreen shrub with opposite, obovate, toothed, dark green leaves, 0.6–1.5cm (¼–½in) long, paler green beneath. Fragrant white flowers are borne in axillary panicles, 5cm (2in) long, from mid-spring to early summer. ↕↔1.2m (4ft). ❄❄

***C.* 'Southmead'** 🏆 Compact, bushy, evergreen shrub with alternate, oblong, finely toothed, dark green leaves, to 3cm (1¼in) long. In late spring and early summer, bears dark, rich blue flowers

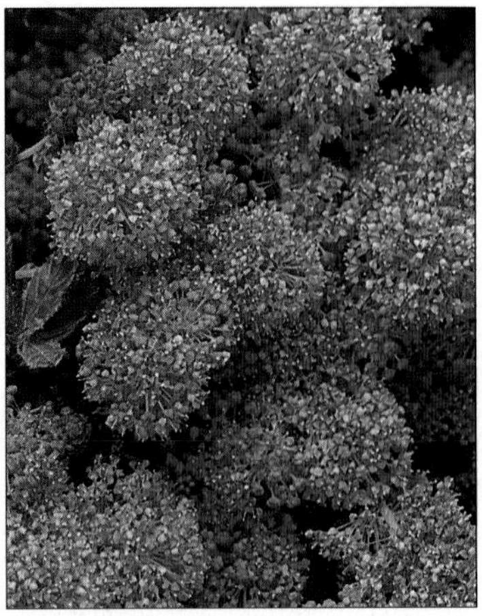

Ceanothus 'Pin Cushion'

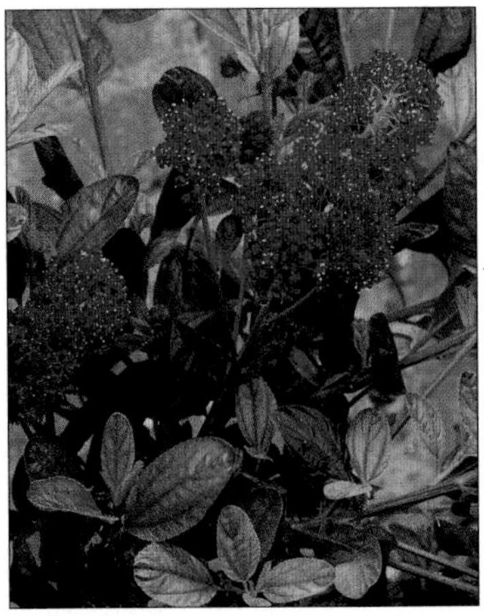

Ceanothus 'Skylark'

in oblong, lateral cymes, to 3cm (1¼in) long. ‡↔ 1.5m (5ft). ❄❄

C. thyrsiflorus (Blueblossom). Vigorous, upright, evergreen shrub with arching branches and alternate, ovate, toothed, glossy, mid-green leaves, to 4cm (1½in) long. In spring, bears pale to dark blue flowers in large, terminal and lateral panicles, 3–8cm (1¼–3in) long. ‡↔ 6m (20ft). USA (California, Oregon). ❄❄❄. **'Millerton Point'** has spreading branches and honey-scented, creamy white flowers in panicles to 9cm (3½in) long. **var. *repens*** 🏆 syn. *C. repens* (Creeping blueblossom), is low and spreading; ‡ 1m (3ft), ↔ 2.5m (8ft). USA (coastal N. California). **var. *repens* 'Ken Taylor'** is more prostrate; ‡ to 30cm (12in).

***C.* 'Topaze'.** Bushy, deciduous shrub producing alternate, oval, dark green leaves, to 7cm (3in) long. From mid-summer to autumn, bears dark indigo-blue flowers in large, terminal and axillary panicles, to 8cm (3in) long. ‡↔ 1.5m (5ft). ❄❄❄

C.* x *veitchianus (*C. griseus* x *C. rigidus*). Spreading, rigidly branched, evergreen shrub with small, alternate or opposite, wedge-shaped, toothed leaves, to 2cm (¾in) long, glossy, dark green above and grey-green-hairy beneath. Bears dark blue flowers in dense, rounded, lateral cymes, to 3cm (1¼in) long, in mid- and late spring. ‡↔ 3m (10ft). USA (California). ❄❄❄ (borderline)

▷**Ceanothus,**
 Carmel see *Ceanothus griseus*
 Hollyleaf see *Ceanothus purpureus*
 Monterey see *Ceanothus rigidus*
 Santa Barbara see *Ceanothus impressus*
▷**Cedar** see *Cedrus*
 Atlas see *Cedrus atlantica*
 Blue Atlas see *Cedrus atlantica* f. *glauca*
 Chilean incense see *Austrocedrus chilensis*
 Cyprus see *Cedrus brevifolia*
 Deodar see *Cedrus deodara*
 Incense see *Calocedrus, C. decurrens*
 Japanese see *Cryptomeria, C. japonica*
 Pencil see *Juniperus virginiana*
 Tasmanian see *Athrotaxis, A.* x *laxifolia*
 Western red see *Thuja plicata*
 White see *Thuja occidentalis*
▷**Cedar of Goa** see *Cupressus lusitanica*
▷**Cedar of Lebanon** see *Cedrus libani*
▷***Cedrela sinensis*** see *Toona sinensis*

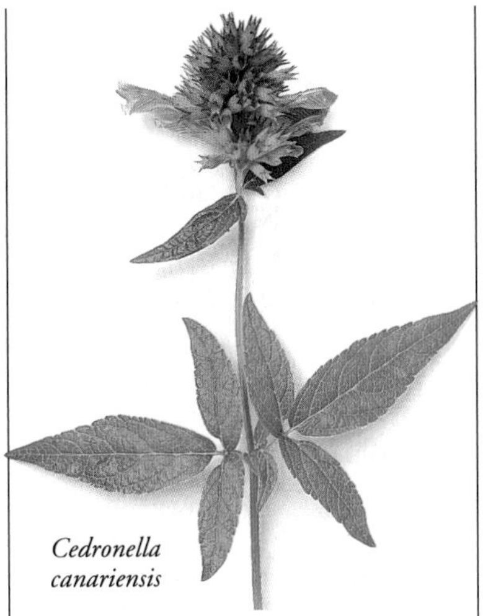

Cedronella canariensis

CEDRONELLA

LABIATAE/LAMIACEAE

Genus of one species of short-lived, woody-based perennial found on sunny, rocky slopes in the Canary Islands. It has alternate, 3-palmate leaves and 2-lipped flowers borne in long, terminal, whorled racemes. It is cultivated for its aromatic foliage, which is sometimes used in pot-pourri and herb teas. In frost-prone regions, *C. canariensis* is effective in a cool conservatory or greenhouse, or can be grown outdoors as an annual. In warmer areas, grow in a scented or herb garden.

- **HARDINESS** Frost tender.
- **CULTIVATION** Under glass, grow in loam-based potting compost (JI No.2) in full light. From spring to autumn, water moderately and apply a balanced liquid fertilizer monthly; water more sparingly in winter. Outdoors, grow in well-drained, fertile soil in full sun.
- **PROPAGATION** Sow seed at 15–18°C (59–64°F) in early spring. Root softwood cuttings in late spring.
- **PESTS AND DISEASES** Whiteflies may be a problem under glass.

C. canariensis ■ syn. *C. triphylla* (Balm of Gilead). Erect, woody-based, slender-stemmed perennial with aromatic, 3-palmate, mid-green leaves, 8–12cm (3–5in) long, emitting a cedar-like scent when touched. In midsummer, bears whorls of 2-lipped, white, pink, or lilac flowers, to 2cm (¾in) long. ‡ to 1.2m (4ft), ↔ 60cm (24in). Canary Islands. ❀ (min. 5°C/41°F)

C. mexicana see *Agastache mexicana*.

C. triphylla see *C. canariensis*.

CEDRUS

Cedar

PINACEAE

Genus of 4 species of monoecious, evergreen, coniferous trees found in forest in the W. Himalayas and the Mediterranean. Some authorities give *C. atlantica* and *C. brevifolia* subspecific rank under *C. libani*, but they are maintained here as species. The needle-like foliage is arranged in clusters on short shoots, which develop new whorls each year. Cones are produced terminally on short shoots. The male cones, borne in autumn, are erect, cylindrical, light brown, and to 7cm (3in) long. The female cones are erect, ovoid to oblong, cylindrical or barrel-shaped, green then brown, and to 12cm (5in) long; they ripen slowly over 2 years, then break up to release the seeds. With their large, spreading branches, cedars are majestic specimen trees, but need ample space if they are to achieve their full potential.

- **HARDINESS** Fully hardy.
- **CULTIVATION** Grow in a sunny, open site, in any well-drained soil, including chalk. If double leaders are produced, the weaker shoot should be cut out in autumn.
- **PROPAGATION** Sow seed in spring, after 21 days' moist pre-chill at 0–1°C (32–34°F). Graft selected cultivars in late summer or winter.
- **PESTS AND DISEASES** Very susceptible to honey fungus.

C. atlantica △ syn. *C. libani* subsp. *atlantica* (Atlas cedar). Conical, coniferous tree, later becoming more open, with fissured, silvery grey bark. Produces sharply pointed, roughly 4-sided, dark green to glaucous blue leaves, to 2.5cm (1in) long, in whorls of 30–45. Female cones, 6–10cm (2½–4in) long, are barrel-shaped and green, becoming pale brown. ‡ to 40m (130ft), ↔ to 10m (30ft). Atlas Mountains. ❄❄❄. **'Aurea'** is a slow-growing, conical tree with golden yellow foliage when young, maturing green. **f. *fastigiata*** ◊ is an upright, narrow-crowned tree with bluish green leaves. **f. *glauca*** ■ 🏆 △–◊ (Blue Atlas cedar) has vivid, glaucous blue foliage, silvery white at first. **'Glauca Pendula'** ⌓ has pendent, glaucous, blue-green foliage.

C. brevifolia 🏆 △ syn. *C. libani* subsp. *brevifolia* (Cyprus cedar). Open-crowned, coniferous tree with a narrow habit when young, becoming broader with age, and with fissured, silvery grey bark. Sharply pointed leaves, to 1.5cm (½in) long, are grey-green to mid-green, sometimes bluish green, and borne in whorls of 20–30. Cylindrical, green then pale brown female cones are 7–10cm (3–4in) long. ‡ 15–25m (50–80ft), ↔ to 12m (40ft). Cyprus. ❄❄❄

C. deodara 🏆 △ (Deodar cedar). Conical, coniferous tree with spreading branches, pendent shoot tips, and dark brown or black bark. The needle-like leaves, 4–5cm (1½–2in) long, are bright to glaucous, mid-green, and produced in whorls of 20–30. Glaucous, barrel-shaped female cones, 8–12cm (3–5in) long, are green at first, ripening to brown. ‡ to 40m (130ft), ↔ to 10m (30ft). W. Himalayas from W. Nepal to Afghanistan. ❄❄❄. **'Aurea'** ■ 🏆 is slow-growing with golden yellow foliage, becoming greener as it matures; ‡ 5m (15ft). **'Golden Horizon'** is vigorous and flat-growing, with yellow or yellowish green foliage if grown in sun, but blue-green leaves in shade.

C. libani ■ ⌓ (Cedar of Lebanon). Coniferous tree with wide-spreading branches, conical when young, flat-topped when old. The bark is black or brown with scaly fissures and ridges. Slightly flattened, 4-sided, sharply pointed, dark green to grey-green leaves, to 2.5cm (1in) long, are borne in whorls of 10–20. Barrel-shaped, dull green to brown female cones, broadest below the

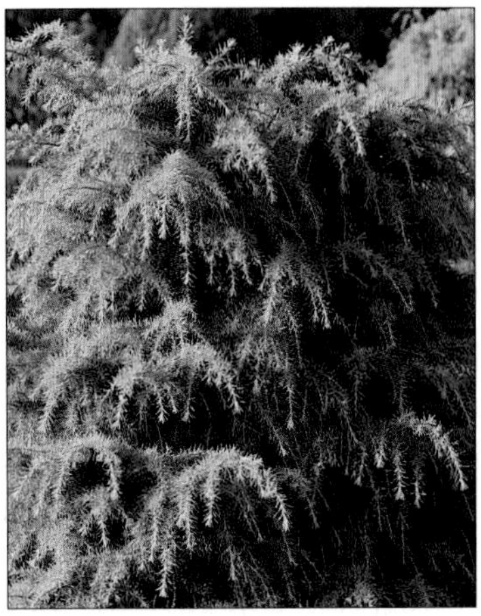

Cedrus deodara 'Aurea'

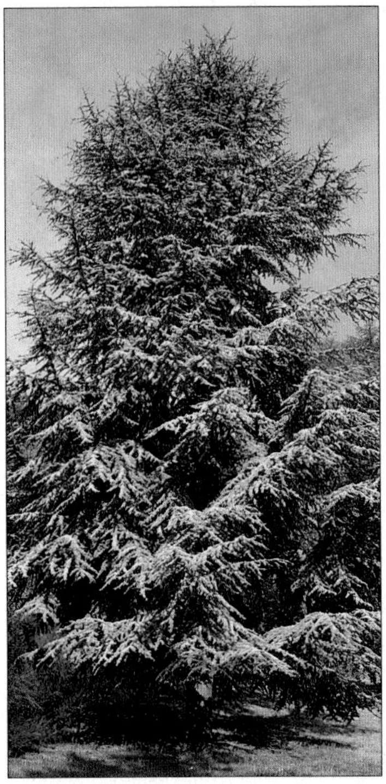

Cedrus atlantica f. *glauca*

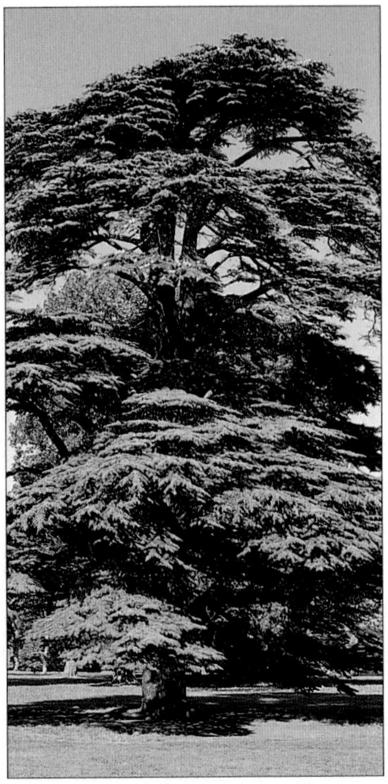

Cedrus libani

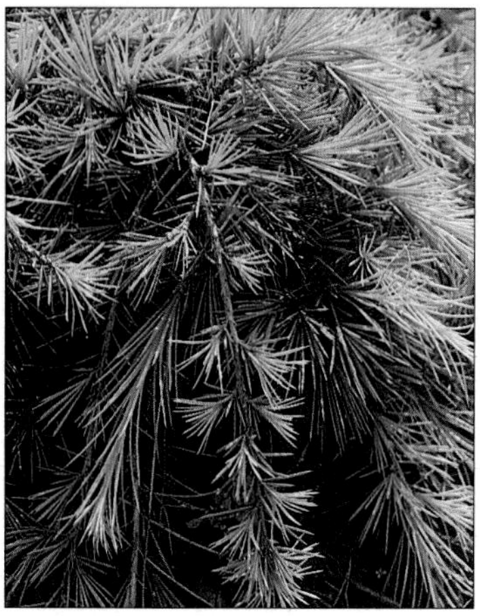

Cedrus libani 'Sargentii'

middle, are 8–12cm (3–5in) long. ↕↔ to 30m (100ft). Lebanon to Turkey. ❄❄❄. **subsp. *atlantica*** see *C. atlantica*. **subsp. *brevifolia*** see *C. brevifolia*. **'Sargentii'** ■♀ is slow-growing, with a pendent habit, and may be trained to make a rounded bush.

CEIBA

Silk cotton tree

BOMBACACEAE

Genus of 4 species of large, spiny-trunked, deciduous trees from tropical North and South America, Africa, and Asia, favouring moist sites in forest and rainforest. The handsome leaves are alternate and palmate, with entire or finely toothed leaflets. Conspicuous, 5-petalled flowers are borne singly or in axillary clusters on bare stems, and are followed by large seed pods containing seeds padded with white floss (kapok). In cool climates, grow young specimens as foliage plants in a warm greenhouse. In tropical regions, silk cotton trees are splendid specimen and shade trees.

- **HARDINESS** Frost tender.
- **CULTIVATION** Under glass, grow in large containers of loam-based potting compost (JI No.3) in full light shaded from hot sun. In the growing season, provide high humidity, water freely, and apply a balanced liquid fertilizer monthly; water sparingly when leafless. Outdoors, grow in fertile, humus-rich, moist but well-drained soil in full sun. Pruning group 1; plants under glass may need restrictive pruning.
- **PROPAGATION** Sow seed at 21–24°C (70–75°F) in spring. Root semi-ripe cuttings in summer.
- **PESTS AND DISEASES** Red spider mites often infest plants under glass.

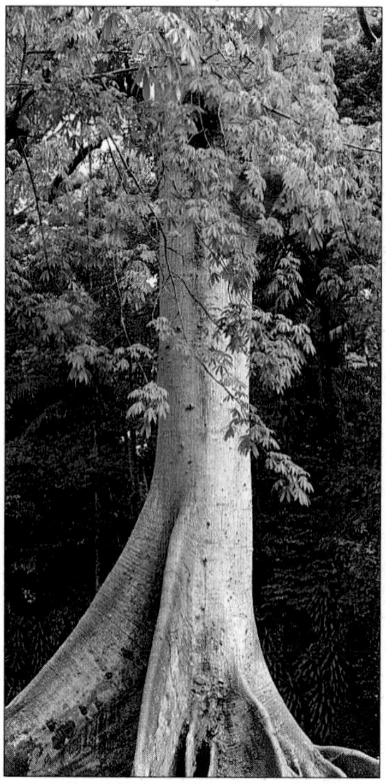

Ceiba pentandra

C. pentandra ■♀ (Kapok, White silk cotton tree). Tall tree, erect at first, then spreading, with a spiny trunk that eventually forms buttresses. Palmate, mid-green leaves, 8–15cm (3–6in) long, are comprised of 5–8 oblong-lance-shaped, entire leaflets. Clusters of cup-shaped, yellow, white, or pink flowers, 6cm (2½in) across, are produced from late winter to early spring, before the leaves expand. ↕ 25–70m (80–230ft), ↔ 5–25m (15–80ft). W. Africa (possibly introduced from South America). ❀ (min. 16°C/61°F)

▷**Celandine,**
Greater see *Chelidonium majus*
Lesser see *Ranunculus ficaria*

▷**Celandine poppy** see *Stylophorum diphyllum*

CELASTRUS

Bittersweet, Staff vine

CELASTRACEAE

Genus of about 30 species of deciduous, rarely evergreen shrubs and twining, woody climbers, with alternate, simple, usually toothed leaves. They are found worldwide but occur mainly in thickets and woodland in warm-temperate or subtropical regions. Their attraction as garden plants lies in their ornamental autumn fruits, which split when ripe to reveal coloured seeds. Male and female flowers, in terminal or axillary racemes, panicles, or cymes, are often borne on separate plants. Train against a wall, fence, or pergola, or through a tree.

- **HARDINESS** Fully hardy to frost tender.
- **CULTIVATION** Grow in well-drained soil in full sun; will tolerate partial shade. Plant one male with at least one female to ensure fruit production. The vigorous species need strong support; if grown up trees, these should be at least 10m (30ft) tall. Pruning group 11, in winter or early spring.
- **PROPAGATION** Sow seed in containers in an open frame as soon as ripe, or in spring. Insert root cuttings in winter, or semi-ripe cuttings in summer.
- **PESTS AND DISEASES** Trouble free.

C. articulatus see *C. orbiculatus*.
C. orbiculatus ■ syn. *C. articulatus* (Oriental bittersweet, Staff vine). Vigorous, woody, deciduous climber with broadly elliptic to rounded, scalloped to toothed, mid-green leaves, to 10cm (4in) long, turning yellow in autumn. Axillary cymes of small green flowers open in summer, followed by clusters of bead-like yellow fruit that open to expose pink to red seeds. ↕ 14m (46ft). E. Asia. ❄❄❄
C. scandens (American bittersweet, Climbing bittersweet, Staff tree, Staff

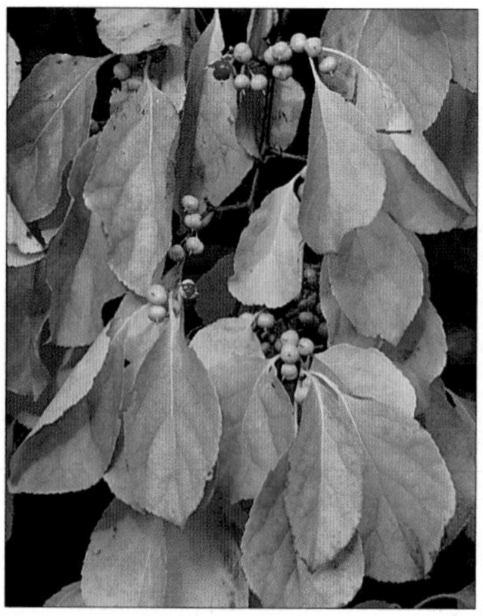

Celastrus orbiculatus

vine). Woody, deciduous climber bearing oval to ovate, toothed, mid-green leaves, 10cm (4in) long. In summer, produces small, yellow-green flowers in terminal panicles or racemes, followed by clusters of orange-yellow fruit with red seeds. ↕ 10m (30ft). E. North America. ❄❄❄

▷**Celery pine** see *Phyllocladus*

CELMISIA

New Zealand daisy

ASTERACEAE/COMPOSITAE

Genus of about 60 species of evergreen, mat- or rosette-forming perennials and subshrubs, mostly from grassland, moors, or scree at high altitudes in New Zealand and S.E. Australia. They often have silky, silvery foliage, and bear daisy-like, solitary flowerheads, usually with white ray-florets (occasionally flushed lilac or pale yellow) and yellow disc-florets, in late spring and summer. They are excellent free-flowering foliage plants for a rock garden or for growing among small shrubs; grow smaller species as specimens in pans in an alpine house. Celmisias thrive in cool, moist climates.

- **HARDINESS** Fully hardy.
- **CULTIVATION** Grow in moist but well-drained, slightly acid, humus-rich soil in sun or partial shade. Some species, especially *C. argentea* and *C. sessiliflora*, need protection from winter wet. In dry areas, shade from hot sun, and spray regularly during dry periods. In an alpine house, grow in a mix of equal parts lime-free loam, leaf mould, and sharp sand. Move pan-grown plants to a cool outdoor site in summer.
- **PROPAGATION** Sow seed in containers in an open frame as soon as ripe. Celmisias hybridize freely but often produce only a few viable seeds. Divide in spring, or root individual rosettes as cuttings in spring.
- **PESTS AND DISEASES** Prone to aphids and red spider mites under glass.

C. argentea. Cushion-forming perennial with densely packed, silver-woolly rosettes of linear leaves, to 1cm (½in) long. In late spring and early summer, bears almost stemless flower-heads, to 2.5cm (1in) across, with narrow, widely spaced white ray-florets, and yellow disc-florets. ↕ 2.5cm (1in), ↔ to 10cm (4in). New Zealand (South Island). ❄❄❄

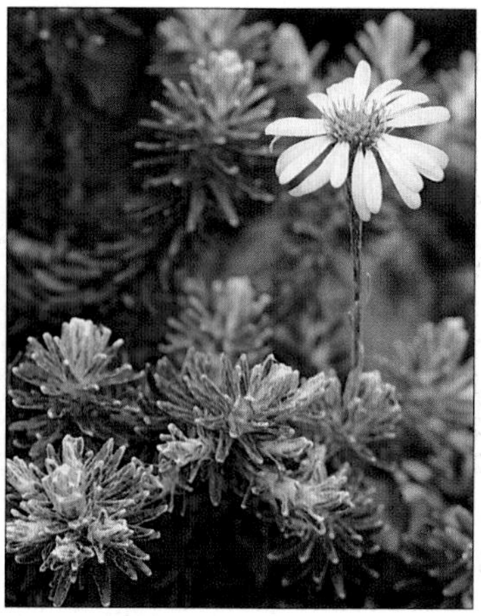

Celmisia ramulosa

C. asteliifolia. Clump-forming perennial with spreading to erect, linear silver leaves, to 8cm (3in) long. In spring, bears flowerheads to 2.5cm (1in) across, with white ray-florets and yellow disc-florets, on semi-erect, whitish green stems, to 20cm (8in) long. ↕ 15–20cm (6–8in), ↔ 30cm (12in). S.E. Australia, including Tasmania. ❄❄❄
C. bellidioides. Mat-forming perennial with rooting stems and small rosettes of obovate-oblong or spoon-shaped, dark green, leathery leaves, to 1.5cm (½in) long. In early summer, bears white-rayed flowerheads, to 2.5cm (1in) wide, with yellow disc-florets, on green stems to 3.5cm (1½in) long. ↕ to 5cm (2in), ↔ to 30cm (12in). New Zealand (South Island). ❄❄❄
***C. coriacea* of gardens** see *C. semicordata*.
C. gracilenta. Tufted perennial with erect to semi-prostrate, very narrow, linear leaves, to 10cm (4in) long, with recurved margins; they are dark green, mottled brown above, and silky white beneath. Flowerheads, to 2cm (¾in) across, with white ray-florets and yellow disc-florets, are borne on densely grey-woolly stems, to 20cm (8in) tall, in early summer. ↕↔ 20cm (8in). New Zealand. ❄❄❄
C. incana. Clump-forming subshrub with rosettes of obovate-oblong, brilliant white, silky-hairy leaves, 3–5cm (1¼–2in) long. Flowerheads, to 3.5cm (1½in) across, with numerous white ray-florets and yellow disc-florets, are borne on white-woolly stems, to 10cm (4in) long, in early summer. ↕ to 15cm (6in), ↔ to 20cm (8in). New Zealand. ❄❄❄

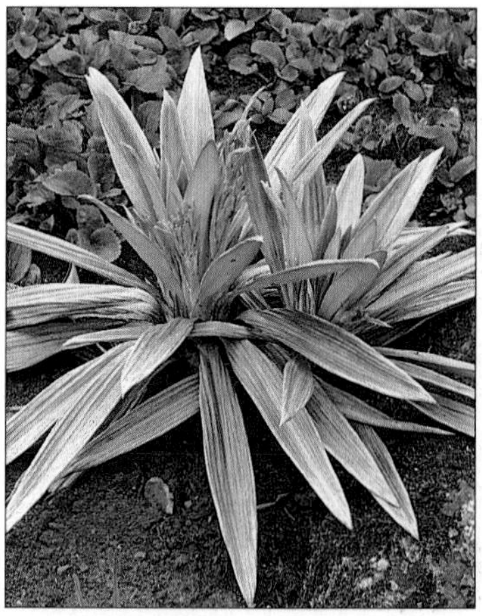

Celmisia semicordata

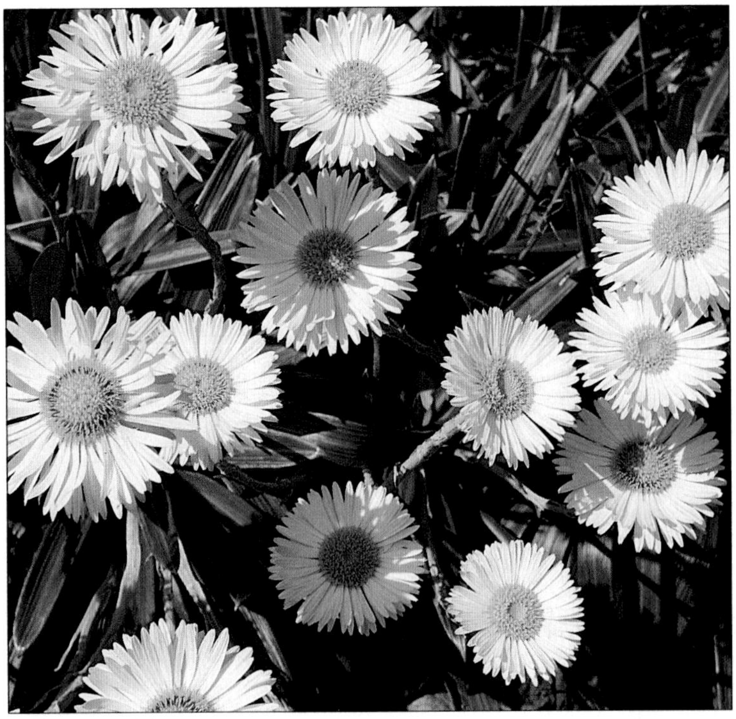
Celmisia spectabilis

C. ramulosa ■ Subshrub with branching stems and erect, overlapping, linear-oblong leaves, 8–10mm (⅜–½in) long, dark green above, densely white-woolly beneath. In late spring and early summer, bears flowerheads, 2.5cm (1in) across, with many white ray-florets and pale yellow disc-florets, on slender, sticky, whitish stems, 4–5cm (1½–2in) high. ↕↔ to 25cm (10in). New Zealand (South Island). ✻✻✻
C. semicordata ■ syn. *C. coriacea* of gardens. Clump-forming perennial with short rhizomes and erect, then recurved, sword- to lance-shaped, leathery, silky-hairy leaves, grey-green above, white beneath, to 30cm (12in) long. White-rayed flowerheads, to 8cm (3in) across, with yellow disc-florets, are borne on erect, whitish green stems, 30–40cm (12–16in) tall, in early and midsummer. ↕ to 50cm (20in), ↔ to 30cm (12in). New Zealand (South Island). ✻✻✻
C. sessiliflora. Cushion-forming perennial with rosettes of densely silver-woolly, sometimes olive-green, stiff, linear leaves, to 1.5cm (½in) long. Flowerheads, to 3cm (1¼in) across, with white ray-florets and yellow disc-florets, are produced on whitish green stems, 2.5–5cm (1–2in) long, in early summer. ↕ to 5cm (2in), ↔ to 20cm (8in). New Zealand (South Island). ✻✻✻
C. spectabilis ■ Tufted, clump-forming perennial with short rhizomes and narrowly oblong-lance-shaped, wide-spreading, leathery leaves, to 25cm (10in) long, glossy, dark green to silvery green above, and densely white- to buff-woolly beneath. Flowerheads, to 5cm (2in) across, with long white ray-florets and yellow disc-florets, are borne on densely whitish-woolly stems, 10–25cm (4–10in) long, in early summer. ↕↔ to 30cm (12in). New Zealand. ✻✻✻
C. walkeri ■ syn. *C. webbiana.* Subshrub with spreading, semi-decumbent, woody stems and terminal rosettes of linear-oblong, leathery, grey-green leaves, to 5cm (2in) long, densely white-woolly beneath. In early summer, white-rayed flowerheads, to 4cm (1½in) wide, with yellowish white disc-florets, are borne on slender, sticky green stems, to 20cm (8in) tall. ↕↔ to 30cm (12in). New Zealand (South Island). ✻✻✻
C. webbiana see *C. walkeri.*

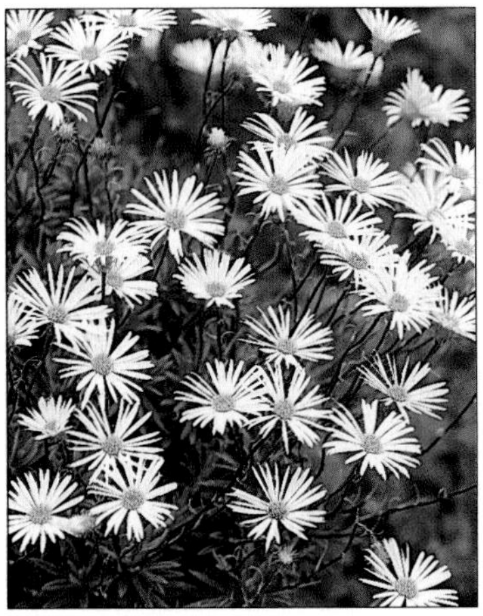
Celmisia walkeri

CELOSIA
Cockscomb
AMARANTHACEAE

Genus of 50–60 species of erect annuals, perennials, and shrubs from dry slopes, stony soils, and scrub in subtropical and tropical Asia, Africa, and North, Central and South America. Celosias have alternate, lobed or simple, oval to lance-shaped leaves and brightly coloured, terminal or axillary cymes of tiny flowers. The cultivars often have plume-like (Plumosa group) or crested (Cristata or Cockscomb group) inflorescences: the upright plumes of Plumosa group cultivars are frequently used for summer bedding schemes, while Cristata group cultivars, with their tightly clustered flowerheads, are used as summer-flowering container plants. Cristata

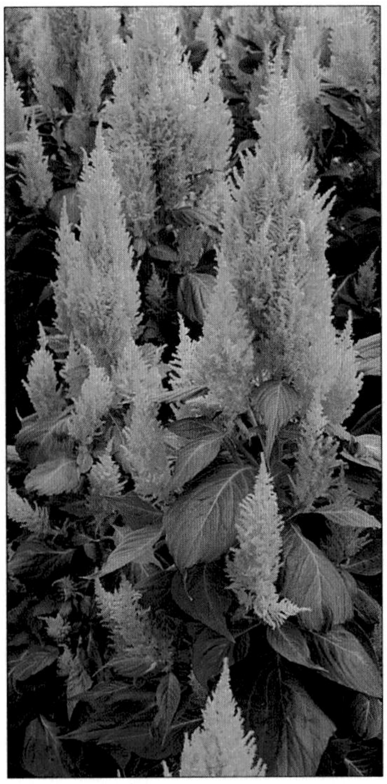
Celosia argentea Century Series 'Century Yellow'

group cultivars flower best in a warm greenhouse. Both groups are treated as annuals and discarded after flowering; they provide good cut flowers, either fresh or dried.
• **HARDINESS** Half hardy to frost tender.
• **CULTIVATION** Under glass, grow in loam-based potting compost (JI No.1) in full light with good ventilation; when in bloom, admit only bright filtered light to prolong flowering. Once the roots fill the container, water moderately but regularly, mist lightly, and apply a balanced liquid fertilizer every 2 weeks. Outdoors, after any danger of frost has passed, plant in moist but well-drained, fertile soil in a sheltered position in full sun; water freely in dry weather.
• **PROPAGATION** Sow seed at 18°C (64°F) from early to late spring.
• **PESTS AND DISEASES** Prone to foot and root rot, and fungal leaf spot diseases. Red spider mites, whiteflies, and aphids may be a problem under glass.

C. argentea. Upright, branching perennial, usually grown as an annual, with oval to lance-shaped, pale green leaves, to 15cm (6in) long. Flowers are

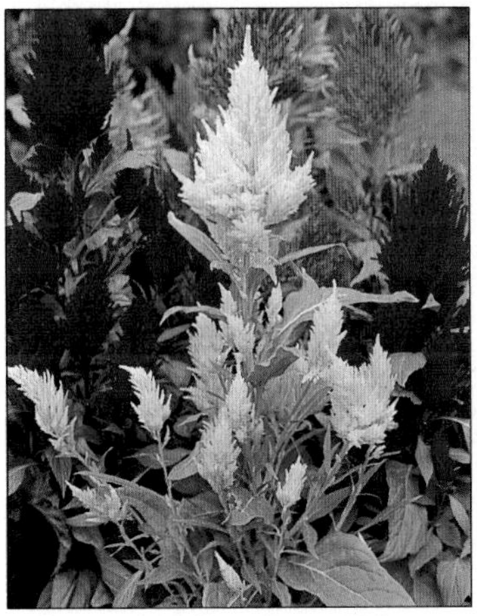
Celosia argentea 'Fairy Fountains'

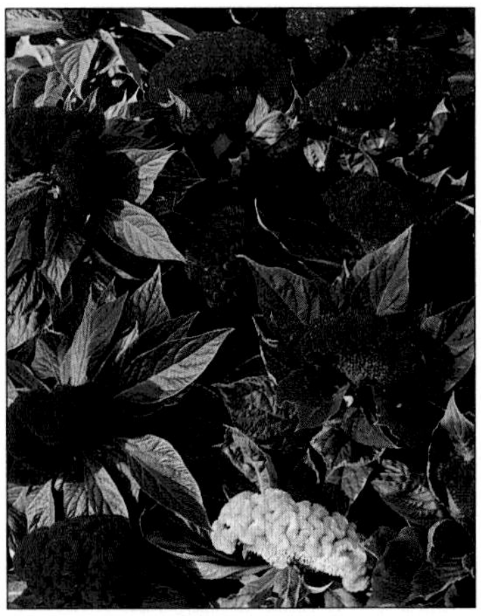
Celosia argentea Olympia Series

silvery white, and produced in dense, terminal spikes, 5–10cm (2–4in) long, in summer. ↕ to 60cm (24in), ↔ to 45cm (18in). Equatorial tropics in Asia, Africa, and North, Central, and South America. ✻. Cultivars also flower in summer and are available in red, orange, yellow, and cream. Plumosa group cultivars have open, feathery, pyramidal flowerheads, 10–25cm (4–10in) long; those in the Cristata or Cockscomb group are compact plants with crested, coral-like heads of tightly clustered flowers, 8–12cm (3–5in) across. **'Apricot Brandy'** (Plumosa group) is a many-branched cultivar producing deep orange flowerheads; ↕ to 50cm (20in). Cultivars of **Century Series** (Plumosa group) are among the most vigorous and widely cultivated, bearing vivid red, rose-pink, or yellow flowerheads; **'Century Yellow'** ■ is a vigorous cultivar with golden yellow flowerheads suitable for drying; ↕ to 45cm (18in). **'Fairy Fountains'** ■ (Plumosa group) has flowerheads in a range of pastel colours including pink, salmon-pink, and creamy yellow; ↕ to 40cm (16in). **Kimono Series** (Plumosa group) cultivars are dwarf, producing large flowerheads in bright colours including salmon-pink, rose-red, yellow, or creamy white; ↕ to 20cm (8in). Cultivars of **Kurume Series** (Cristata group) are available in a wide colour range, including gold, yellow, rose-pink, orange, scarlet, orange-red, and red-and-gold bicolours; the flowerheads, good for cutting, are to 20cm (8in) across; ↕ 1.2m (4ft). **'New Look'** (Plumosa group) has dark purple-green foliage and bears deep red flowerheads; ↕ to 45cm (18in). **Olympia Series** ■ (Cristata group) cultivars are dwarf, and bear flowerheads in colours including golden yellow, scarlet, light red, deep cerise and purple; ↕ to 20cm (8in).
C. spicata **Flamingo Series.** Cultivars from this series (derived from *C. spicata*) are upright and branching, with lance-shaped, mid-green leaves, 6–12cm (2½–5in) long. In summer, they bear compact, erect and cylindrical, barley-like spikes of flowers, 10–12cm (4–5in) long, pink towards the tips and silvery white at the bases. The flowers are excellent for both cutting and drying. ↕ to 18cm (7in), ↔ to 15cm (6in). ✻

▷ ***Celsia*** see *Verbascum*
C. acaulis see *V. acaule*
C. arcturus see *V. arcturus*

CELTIS

Hackberry, Nettle tree

ULMACEAE

Genus of about 70 species of deciduous and evergreen trees and shrubs from temperate and tropical regions in both hemispheres, usually found in woodland, on rocky slopes, or on riverbanks. Hackberries are grown for their form, habit, and foliage, which often colours well in autumn. They have alternate and usually toothed leaves. The small green, unisexual flowers are borne in spring; male flowers are produced in clusters at the base of twigs, while the females are produced singly or in twos or threes from the leaf axils, and are followed in autumn by spherical, fleshy berries. Use hackberries as lawn specimens or in a woodland garden. They grow best in continental climates with hot summers; in cool, maritime climates they often form small, multi-stemmed trees.

- **HARDINESS** Fully hardy.
- **CULTIVATION** In warm climates, grow in deep, fertile, well-drained soil in sun or partial shade. In cooler areas, hackberries thrive on dry soils and need a warm site in full sun. Pruning group 1.
- **PROPAGATION** Sow seed in a seedbed or open frame in autumn.
- **PESTS AND DISEASES** Trouble free.

C. australis ■ ○ (Southern nettle tree). Spreading, deciduous tree producing ovate to lance-shaped, rough, coarsely toothed leaves, to 15cm (6in) long; they are dark green above, downy and light green beneath, turning yellow in autumn. Bears edible red fruit, to 1cm (½in) across, ripening blackish brown. ↕↔ 20m (70ft). Mediterranean, S.W. Asia. ❄❄❄

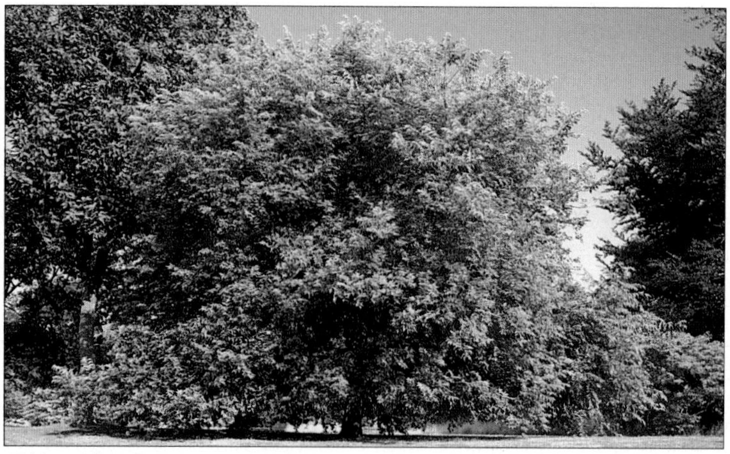

Celtis occidentalis

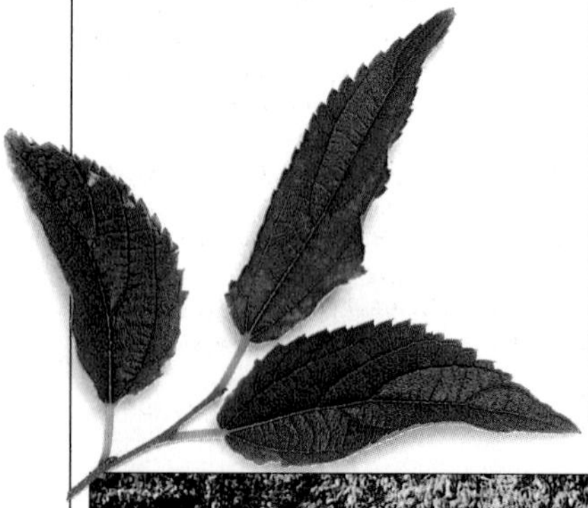

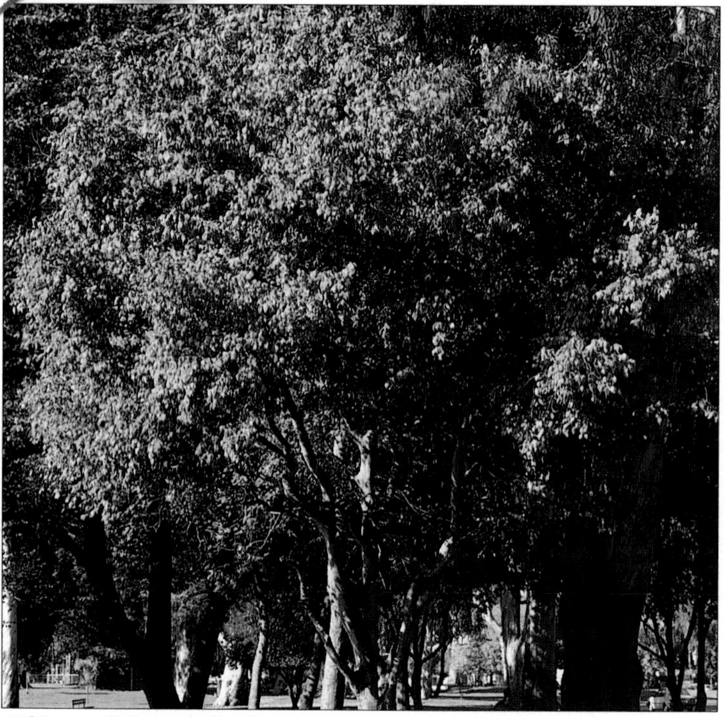

Celtis australis (inset: leaf detail)

C. laevigata ○ (Common hackberry, Mississippi hackberry, Sugar hackberry). Spreading, deciduous tree with ovate to lance-shaped, entire or sparsely toothed leaves, to 10cm (4in) long, dark green and hairless above, paler and softly hairy on the veins beneath. Sweet, edible, orange-red fruit, to 7mm (¼in) across, ripen to purple-black. ↕↔ 12m (40ft). S. USA. ❄❄❄

C. occidentalis ■ ○ (Hackberry, Sugarberry). Spreading, deciduous tree with broadly ovate to ovate-lance-shaped, sharply toothed leaves, to 12cm (5in) long, rounded to heart-shaped at the bases; they are glossy, mid-green above, paler green and sparsely softly hairy on the veins beneath. Sweet, edible fruit, to 1cm (½in) across, ripen from yellow or red to purple. ↕ 20m (70ft), ↔ 15m (50ft). E. North America. ❄❄❄

C. reticulata ○ (Western hackberry, Sugarberry). Spreading, deciduous tree or shrub producing thick, oblong to ovate, usually entire but sometimes toothed, dark green leaves, to 10cm (4in) long, bright green above, darker with downy veins beneath. Sweet, edible, orange-red fruit, to 1cm (½in) across, ripen to deep purple. ↕↔ 8m (25ft). S.W. USA. ❄❄❄

C. sinensis ○ Spreading, deciduous tree producing oblong to ovate leaves, to 8cm (3in) long, shallowly blunt-toothed except at the bases, glossy, dark green above, duller beneath, and hairless on both sides. Sweet, edible fruit, to 1cm (½in) across, are dark orange, ripening to red-brown. ↕↔ 12m (40ft). E. China, Korea, Japan. ❄❄❄

CENTAUREA

Hardheads, Knapweed

ASTERACEAE/COMPOSITAE

Genus of about 450 species of annuals, biennials, perennials, and subshrubs found in dry sites, including woodland, rocky mountain slopes, subalpine meadows, and sand dunes. They occur mainly in Europe and the Mediterranean, with a few in Asia, Australia, and North America. The simple leaves are pinnatisect or pinnatifid, and sometimes silver-hairy. They bear spherical or hemispherical flowerheads with tubular, usually deeply lobed florets, the outer ones often longer and more spreading than the rest. Each flowerhead has a conspicuous involucre, the bracts overlapping, fringed, and often with toothed or spiny, silvery white or black tips. Grow in a border or rock garden; some are ideal for naturalizing in grass or in a wildflower garden. Some frost-hardy perennials are grown as summer bedding annuals. For winter flowering, grow *C. cyanus* in containers. All are attractive to bees and butterflies.

- **HARDINESS** Fully hardy to frost hardy.
- **CULTIVATION** Grow in well-drained soil in full sun. *C. macrocephala* and *C. montana* and its cultivars require moist but well-drained soil in sun or partial shade; other perennials will tolerate some drought.
- **PROPAGATION** Sow seed of annuals *in situ* in spring, or in biodegradable containers to avoid root disturbance; seed of *C. cyanus* may be sown in early autumn to flower early the next year. Sow seed of perennials in containers in a cold frame in spring, and divide in spring or autumn. Sow seed of *C. montana* in late summer, or insert root cuttings in winter.
- **PESTS AND DISEASES** Powdery mildew may be a problem.

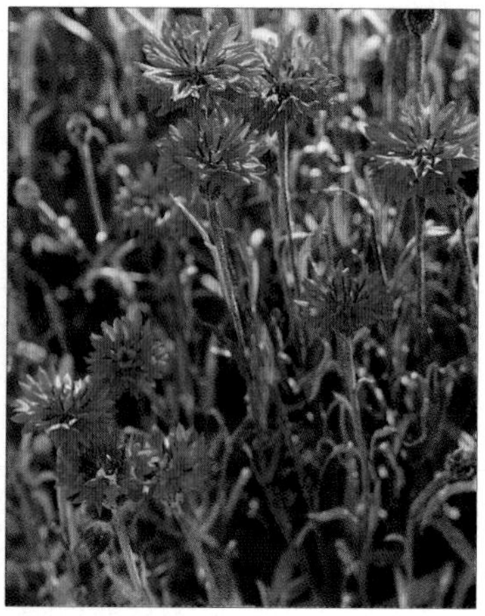

Centaurea cyanus

C. bella. Clump-forming perennial with densely white-woolly stems and obovate to fiddle-shaped, pinnatifid, feathery, light green leaves, to 12cm (5in) long, with elliptic to obovate lobes, the terminal lobes larger than the rest. Leaf undersides and flower stems are covered in fine white hairs. Pale pink to purple-pink flowerheads, to 4.5cm (1¾in) across, are borne in midsummer. ↕ 20–30cm (8–12in), ↔ 45cm (18in). Caucasus. ❄❄❄

C. benoistii. Clump-forming, woody-based perennial producing oblong-spoon-shaped, pinnatisect, mid-green leaves, to 6cm (2½in) long, with linear, sometimes toothed lobes. Pale pink or purple flowerheads, 3cm (1¼in) across, are borne in summer. ↕ 50–100cm (20–39in), ↔ 30–60cm (12–24in). Morocco. ❄❄❄

***C. candidissima* of gardens** see *C. cineraria.*

C. cineraria 🏆 syn. *C. candidissima* of gardens. Very variable, erect, or sometimes prostrate, evergreen perennial with sparsely branched stems. Lance-shaped to ovate, pinnatifid to 2-pinnatisect, grey-white leaves, 8–15cm (3–6in) long, with elliptic to lance-shaped lobes, are woolly on both sides. In summer, bears purple flowerheads, 1–2.5cm (½–1in) across. ↕ to 80cm (32in), ↔ 45cm (18in). W. and S. Italy, including Sicily. ❄❄❄

C. cyanus ■ (Blue-bottle, Cornflower). Erect annual with lance-shaped, entire

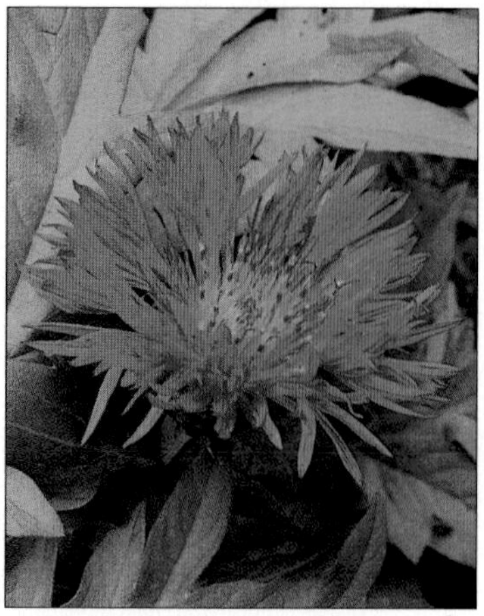

Centaurea dealbata 'Steenbergii'

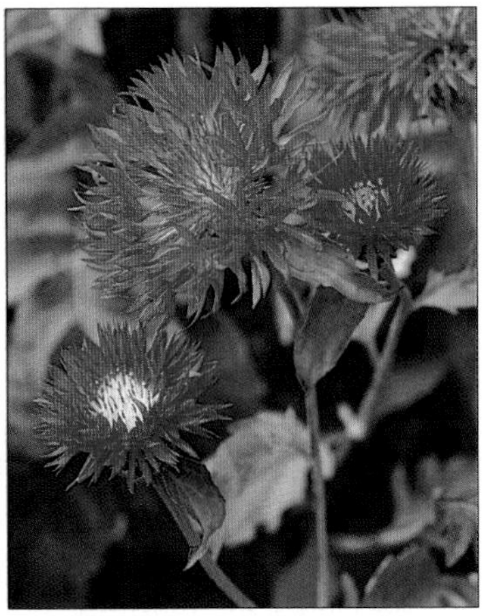

Centaurea hypoleuca 'John Coutts'

leaves, 10–20cm (4–8in) long, the lower leaves with a few pinnatifid lobes, and woolly-hairy beneath. Dark blue flowerheads, 2.5–4cm (1–1½in) across, with violet-blue inner florets, are borne from late spring to midsummer. ↕ 20–80cm (8–32in), ↔ 15cm (6in). N. temperate regions. ***. **Baby Series** cultivars are excellent in containers, and usually available with blue, white, or pink flowerheads; ↕ to 30cm (12in), ↔ 20cm (8in). **Florence Series** cultivars are compact, uniform, and many-branched, with flowerheads in cherry-red, pink, or white; ↕ to 35cm (14in), ↔ to 25cm (10in). **Standard Tall Group** cultivars produce flowerheads in a range of colours, including blue, white, pink, and shades of mauve and maroon; they are good for cut flowers; ↕ 1–1.2m (3–4ft), ↔ 25cm (10in).

C. dealbata. Clump-forming perennial with obovate, pinnatisect leaves, to 20cm (8in) long, light green above and grey-green beneath. White-centred pink flowerheads, to 4cm (1½in) across, are produced in midsummer. Requires staking, but easy to grow. Flowerheads are good for cutting. ↕ 90cm (36in), ↔ 60cm (24in). Caucasus. ***.

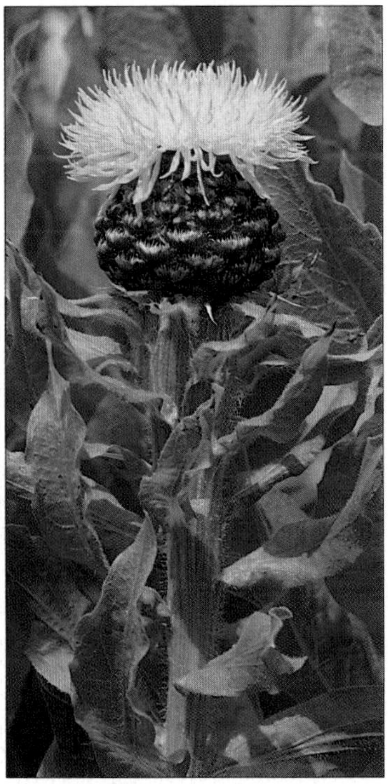

Centaurea macrocephala

'Steenbergii' ■ has dark carmine-pink flowerheads with white-tinged disc-florets; ↕ 60cm (24in).

C. hypoleuca. Clump-forming perennial with gently spreading roots and elliptic-lance-shaped, pinnatifid, wavy-margined leaves, 15–20cm (6–8in) long, light green above and grey-white beneath. Bears long-lasting, fragrant, pale to deep pink flowerheads, 6cm (2½in) across, in summer. ↕ 60cm (24in), ↔ 45cm (18in). Caucasus, Turkey, Iran. ***. **'John Coutts'** ■ has deep rose-pink flowerheads.

C. macrocephala ■ Clump-forming, robust perennial with broadly lance-shaped, pinnatifid, mid-green leaves, 15–20cm (6–8in) long, and stiff, leafy stems. In mid- and late summer, buds with fringed, glossy brown involucral bracts, open to deep, rich yellow flowerheads, 4.5–5cm (1¾–2in) across. ↕ to 1.5m (5ft), ↔ 60cm (24in). Caucasus, Turkey. ***

C. montana ■ Rhizomatous, mat-forming perennial with ovate to broadly lance-shaped, entire to pinnatifid, sometimes slightly toothed, mid-green leaves, 6cm (2½in) long, woolly beneath, with densely woolly stems. Blue flowerheads, 5cm (2in) across, with reddish violet florets, open from late spring to midsummer. Needs staking. ↕ 45cm (18in), ↔ 60cm (24in). Europe to Poland and N.W. Balkans. ***. **f. *alba*** has white flowerheads. **'Carnea'**, syn. 'Rosea', produces pink flowerheads. **'Parham'** has large, dark lavender-blue flowerheads. **'Rosea'** see 'Carnea'. **'Violetta'** bears dark violet flowerheads.

C. moschata see *Amberboa moschata.*

C. pulcherrima ■ Clump-forming perennial with lance-shaped to broadly lance-shaped, pinnatifid, silvery green leaves, to 25cm (10in) long. In midsummer, stiff, slender stems each bear a solitary flowerhead, to 5cm (2in) across, with silvery yellow involucral bracts and rose-pink or purple-pink florets. ↕ 30–40cm (12–16in), ↔ 60cm (24in). Caucasus, Turkey. ***

***C.* 'Pulchra Major'**, syn. *Leuzea centauroides.* Clump-forming perennial with numerous pinnatisect, narrowly ovate leaves, 15–45cm (6–18in) long, dark green above and grey-green beneath. In midsummer, tall stems bear striking buds, with bristly, glossy, silvery green bracts, which open to flowerheads, 8cm (3in) across, with bright purplish red florets. ↕ 1.2m (4ft), ↔ 60cm (24in). *** (borderline)

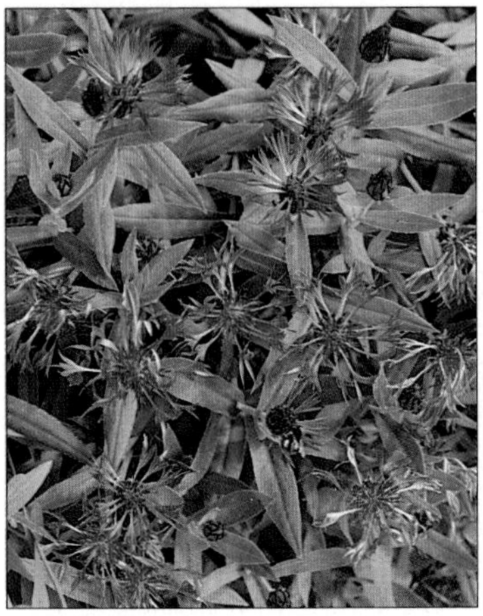

Centaurea montana

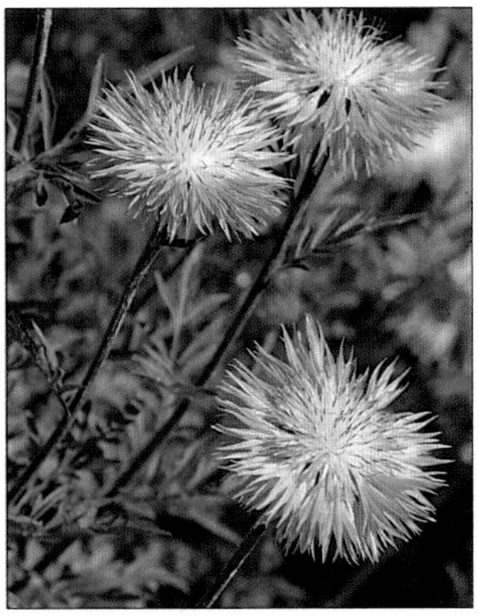

Centaurea pulcherrima

C. simplicicaulis. Rhizomatous perennial forming a dense mat of 2-pinnate, hairy, mid-green leaves, 5cm (2in) long, with 1–4 pairs of elliptic to rounded leaflets. In late spring and early summer, elongated buds, with white-tipped involucral bracts, open to silvery rose-pink flowerheads, 5cm (2in) across, on stiff, slender stems. ↕ to 25cm (10in), ↔ 60cm (24in). S. Caucasus, N. Turkey. ***

C. triumfettii* subsp. *stricta. Perennial with short rhizomes and narrowly lance-shaped, entire or slightly toothed, densely grey-woolly leaves, 10cm (4in) long. Solitary, terminal flowerheads, to 2.5cm (1in) across, with clear blue outer florets and reddish violet central florets, and brown, white-tipped bracts, are borne on axillary branches in early summer. ↕ 30cm (12in), ↔ 60cm (24in). C. and E. Europe, N. Balkans. ***

CENTAURIUM

syn. ERYTHRAEA

Centaury

GENTIANACEAE

Widely distributed genus of about 30 species of rosette-forming or tufted annuals, biennials, and perennials, from Europe, N. Africa, Australia, Chile, the USA, and W. Asia, often found in seaside habitats. Their leaves are mostly obovate to elliptic, grey-green to pale green, and 1–5cm (½–2in) long. Flat-topped cymes of upright, shallowly bell-shaped or salverform flowers are borne from early to late summer. Grow in a rock garden, trough, or alpine house.

- **HARDINESS** Fully hardy.
- **CULTIVATION** Grow in moist but well-drained soil in full sun. Centauries are often short-lived, so propagate regularly.
- **PROPAGATION** Sow seed in containers in a cold frame, as soon as ripe or in autumn. Divide in spring.
- **PESTS AND DISEASES** Prone to red spider mites and aphids under glass. Susceptible to slugs and snails outdoors.

C. erythraea (Common centaury). Variable, rosetted biennial or short-lived perennial with solitary or branching stems, and mostly basal, obovate to elliptic, grey-green leaves, 1–5cm (½–2in) long, with 3–7 prominent, parallel veins. In summer, stems 3–8cm (1¼–3in) long bear branched, flat-topped cymes of pink or pink-purple, salverform flowers, each to 1.5cm (½in) across. Thrives in sun or partial shade. ↕ to 8cm (3in), ↔ 2.5cm (1in). Dry grassland in Europe and W. Asia. ***

C. portense see *C. scilloides.*

C. scilloides, syn. *C. portense* (Perennial centaury). Evergreen, tufted perennial with short rhizomes and decumbent to upright stems bearing ovate-elliptic to oblong, glossy, pale green leaves, to 2cm (¾in) long. In early summer, produces cymes of open bell-shaped or salverform, bright pink flowers, 1–2cm (½–¾in) across, on stems 5–8cm (2–3in) long. Often self-seeds. ↕ to 8cm (3in), ↔ to 15cm (6in). W. Europe. ***

▷**Centaury** see *Centaurium*
Common see *C. erythraea*
Perennial see *C. scilloides*

CENTRADENIA

MELASTOMATACEAE

Genus of 4 or 5 species of evergreen perennials and small shrubs found at forest margins and in moist scrub in Mexico and Central America. They are grown mainly for their small, 4-petalled pink flowers, borne abundantly in terminal or axillary racemes or panicles, and for their attractive foliage. The leaves are entire, often strongly 3-veined, and arranged in opposite pairs; one leaf of each pair is usually smaller than the other. In frost-prone climates, grow in a warm greenhouse. In warmer areas, use in a shrub border.

- **HARDINESS** Frost tender.
- **CULTIVATION** Under glass, grow in loam-based potting compost (JI No.2) in bright filtered light. In growth, water freely, apply a balanced liquid fertilizer monthly, and provide high humidity; water moderately in winter. Top-dress or pot on in spring. Outdoors, grow in fertile, humus-rich, moist but well-drained soil in partial shade. Pruning group 9, after flowering.
- **PROPAGATION** Sow seed at 18–21°C (64–70°F) in spring. Root softwood cuttings in spring.
- **PESTS AND DISEASES** Red spider mites may be a problem under glass.

C. floribunda. Small, softly hairy shrub of open habit with lance-shaped leaves, 2.5–5cm (1–2in) long, mid- to dark green above and glaucous beneath, with reddish green veins. From winter to spring, bears small, lilac-pink flowers, white within, and 8mm (⅜in) across, in terminal panicles, to 10cm (4in) across. ↕↔ 30–90cm (12–36in). Mexico to Guatemala. ❀ (min. 13°C/55°F)

CENTRANTHUS

Valerian

VALERIANACEAE

Genus of 8–12 species of annuals and perennials, a few subshrubby, from dry, sunny slopes, often on chalky soils, in S. Europe, the Mediterranean, N.W. Africa, and S.W. Asia. They have erect, branched stems, simple or pinnate, opposite leaves, and funnel-shaped, red or white flowers, borne in terminal and axillary cymes. *C. ruber*, the only species in common cultivation, is valued for being free- and long-flowering. It is suitable for a border, but grows best on old walls and dry, stony banks. It is attractive to bees and other insects.

- **HARDINESS** Fully hardy to half hardy.

C

C

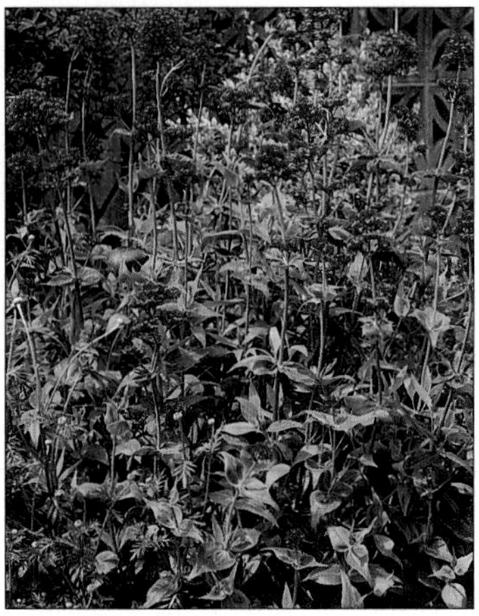

Centranthus ruber

• **CULTIVATION** Grow in well-drained, poor to moderately fertile, preferably chalk or lime soil in full sun. Dead-head regularly and replace every 3 or 4 years.
• **PROPAGATION** Sow seed in containers in a cold frame in spring. Divide perennials with care in early spring.
• **PESTS AND DISEASES** Trouble free.

C. ruber ■ (Red valerian). Clump-forming, woody-based, many-branched perennial producing simple, lance-shaped to ovate, slightly toothed or entire, fairly fleshy, glaucous, deep to mid-green leaves, to 8cm (3in) long. Dense cymes of small, funnel-shaped, fragrant, white, pale rose-pink, or dark crimson flowers, 1.5cm (½in) long, are borne from late spring to late summer. Self-seeds freely. ↕↔ to 1m (3ft). Mediterranean (S. Europe and N. Africa to Turkey). ❄❄❄

CEPHALANTHUS

RUBIACEAE

Widely distributed genus of about 10 species of deciduous and evergreen trees and shrubs found mainly by rivers in temperate and tropical regions of Africa, Asia, and North and Central America. They are grown for their ball-like, terminal or axillary heads of small, fragrant flowers. The leaves are opposite or whorled. Suitable for a shrub border; grow frost-tender species in a temperate greenhouse. The foliage may cause severe discomfort if ingested.
• **HARDINESS** Fully hardy to frost tender.
• **CULTIVATION** Grow in fertile, humus-rich, moist but well-drained, neutral to acid soil in full sun. Pruning group 6.
• **PROPAGATION** Sow seed of hardy species in containers in a cold frame in autumn. Take semi-ripe cuttings in summer, or hardwood cuttings in winter.
• **PESTS AND DISEASES** Trouble free.

C. occidentalis ♀ (Buttonbush, Button-willow, Honey-balls). Open-branched, deciduous shrub or small tree with oval to elliptic-lance-shaped leaves, to 18cm (7in) long. The glossy, mid-green leaves, with red veins and red midribs beneath, are opposite or arranged in whorls of 3, and emerge in late spring. Dense, rounded heads, to 2.5cm (1in) across, of small, very fragrant, tubular-funnel-shaped, white or cream flowers, are produced in late summer and early autumn. ↕2m (6ft), ↔2.5m (8ft), occasionally to 5m (15ft). North America, Mexico, Cuba. ❄❄❄. **var. *pubescens*** has oblong to ovate-lance-shaped leaves, and produces flowerheads to 5cm (2in) across. USA (Indiana to Texas).

CEPHALARIA

DIPSACACEAE

Genus of about 65 species of annuals and perennials, occurring in habitats ranging from meadows to mountain pastures, from Europe and Africa to C. Asia. They have opposite, pinnatifid or pinnatisect, toothed leaves and scabious-like, terminal flowerheads, usually pale yellow or white, with several rows of stiff involucral bracts. Grow at the back of a herbaceous border or in a wildflower garden.
• **HARDINESS** Fully hardy to half hardy.
• **CULTIVATION** Grow in fertile, moist but well-drained soil in sun or partial shade.
• **PROPAGATION** Sow seed in containers in a cold frame in early spring. Divide in early or mid-spring.
• **PESTS AND DISEASES** Trouble free.

C. alpina, syn. *Scabiosa alpina*. Clump-forming perennial with elliptic, pinnate or pinnatisect, basal leaves, 15–40cm (6–16in) long, consisting of 3–8 pairs of oblong-lance-shaped, toothed leaflets or lobes. Bears long-stalked, pale yellow flowerheads, 3cm (1¼in) or more wide, the outer florets larger than the rest, in early and midsummer. ↕to 2m (6ft), ↔60cm (24in). Jura mountains, S.W. and C. Alps, N. Apennines. ❄❄❄

C. gigantea ■ syn. *C. tatarica*, *Scabiosa gigantea*, *S. tatarica*. (Giant scabious, Yellow scabious). Clump-forming perennial producing pinnatisect, basal leaves, to 40cm (16in) long, with oblong to broadly lance-shaped, coarsely toothed lobes. In summer, stout, few-branched stems bear primrose-yellow flowerheads, 4–6cm (1½–2½in) across, the outer florets larger than the rest. ↕to 2.5m (8ft), ↔60cm (24in). Caucasus, N. Turkey. ❄❄❄

C. tatarica see *C. gigantea*.

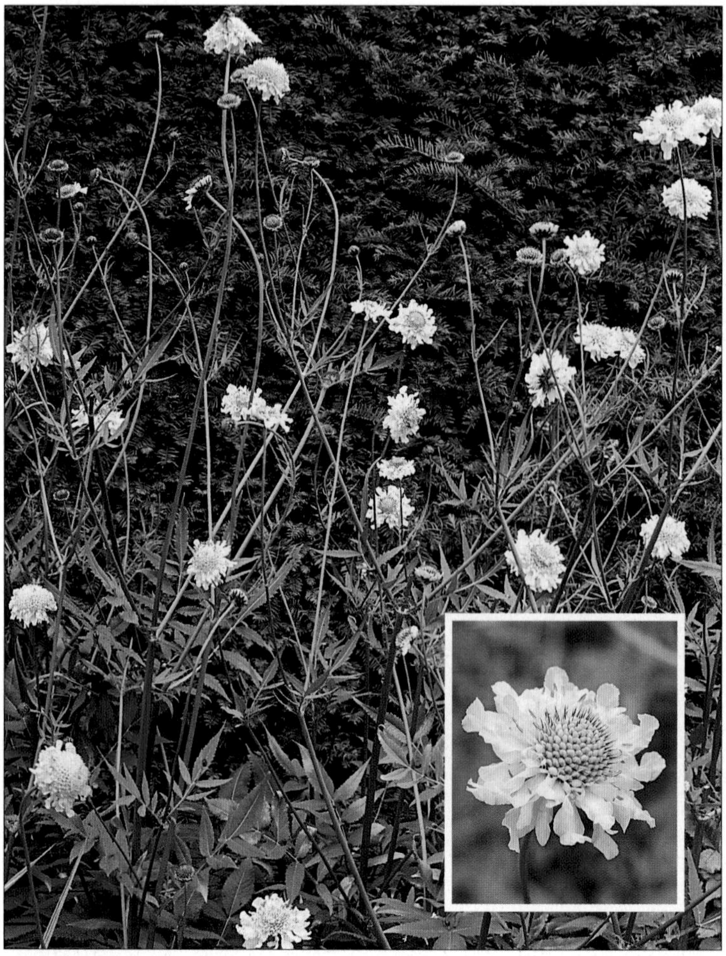

Cephalaria gigantea (inset: flowerhead detail)

CEPHALOCEREUS

CACTACEAE

Genus of 3 species of columnar, erect, occasionally branching, hairy, perennial cacti from rocky areas of C. Mexico. They have ribbed stems with closely set areoles and numerous spines. Mature plants develop woody growths that bear funnel-shaped flowers in summer, followed by ovoid, dry, hairy red fruits. In frost-prone regions, grow in a warm greenhouse or conservatory, or use as houseplants. In warm, dry climates, grow outdoors in a desert garden. Many species once included in *Cephalocereus* have been transferred to *Pilosocereus* and other genera.
• **HARDINESS** Frost tender.
• **CULTIVATION** Under glass, grow in a mix of 3 parts standard cactus compost and 1 part limestone chippings in full light. During the growing season, water moderately and apply a low-nitrogen liquid fertilizer monthly; keep plants completely dry in winter. Outdoors, grow in sharply drained, poor to moderately fertile, slightly alkaline soil in full sun. See also pp.48–49.
• **PROPAGATION** Sow seed at 19–24°C (66–75°F) in spring.
• **PESTS AND DISEASES** Susceptible to root mealybugs.

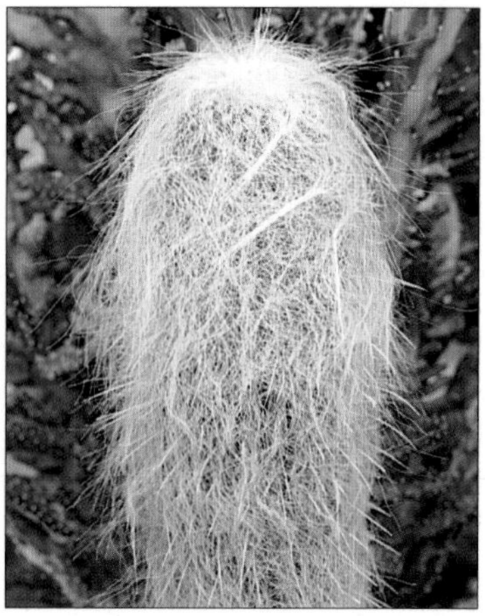

Cephalocereus senilis

C. euphorbioides see *Neobuxbaumia euphorbioides*.

C. senilis ■ (Old man cactus). Columnar cactus producing 20–30 ribs. The areoles bear long, twisting, bristly white hairs, that lengthen as the plant ages and almost cover the grey spines (3–5 centrals and 20–30 radials). Nocturnal pink flowers, 5cm (2in) long, are produced in summer. ↕12m (40ft), ↔ to 2m (6ft). C. Mexico. ❀ (min. 10°C/50°F)

CEPHALOPHYLLUM

AIZOACEAE

Genus of about 60 species of creeping, clump-forming or spreading, perennial succulents from sandy coastal regions of S.W. Africa and South Africa. They have fleshy, cylindrical to 3-angled leaves. Branched cymes of up to 3 many-petalled, large, daisy-like flowers, with yellow, red, purple, or white petals, and often with colourful stamens, open at about midday in summer. In frost-prone areas, grow in a cool or temperate greenhouse. In warm, dry regions, use as ground cover.
• **HARDINESS** Frost tender.
• **CULTIVATION** Under glass, grow in a mix of 2 parts each loam and sharp sand and 1 part leaf mould in full light; provide shade from hot sun and good ventilation. When in growth, water moderately and apply a low-nitrogen liquid fertilizer monthly. Keep plants almost dry at other times. Outdoors, grow in poor to moderately fertile, sharply drained, humus-rich soil in full sun. See also pp.48–49.
• **PROPAGATION** Sow seed at 13–18°C (55–64°F), or root cuttings, both in late spring.
• **PESTS AND DISEASES** Susceptible to aphids while flowering.

C. alstonii ■ Prostrate succulent with grey-green branches, 50cm (20in) or more long, and cylindrical, recurved, semi-erect, spotted, greyish green leaves, to 7cm (3in) long, the upper surfaces flattened. In summer, produces long-stemmed, ruby-red flowers, to 8cm (3in) across, with violet stamens. ↕10cm

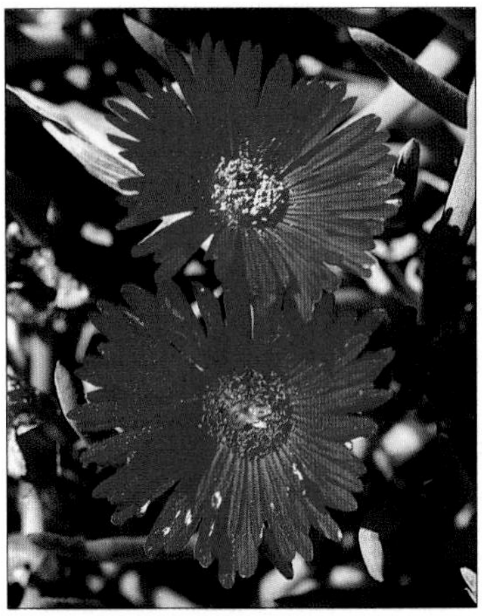

Cephalophyllum alstonii

(4in), ↔ indefinite. South Africa (Western Cape). ❀ (min. 7°C/45°F)
C. pillansii. Variable, prostrate, perennial succulent with greenish red, later grey branches, 30–40cm (12–16in) long, and cylindrical, recurved, spotted, dark green leaves, 2.5–20cm (1–8in) long. Short-stemmed, yellow, red-centred flowers, to 6cm (2½in) across, are borne in profusion in summer. ↕ 8cm (3in) or more, ↔ 60cm (24in). Namibia, South Africa (Western Cape, Northern Cape). ❀ (min. 7°C/45°F)

CEPHALOTAXUS

Plum yew

CEPHALOTAXACEAE

Genus of up to 9 species of evergreen, normally dioecious, occasionally monoecious, coniferous, small trees or shrubs from forest understorey in N.E. India, Burma, Vietnam, China, Korea, Japan, and Taiwan. The dark or mid-green foliage is yew-like, spreading, and 2-ranked on either side of the green shoots; the undersurfaces of the leaves have glaucous or silver bands. Male flowers are produced in spherical clusters from the axils on the undersides of the weaker shoots. Female plants produce fruits that consist of a single hard seed surrounded by a fleshy green covering. Plum yews grow well in shaded sites and are useful as hedges. They prefer cool, moist climates.

• **HARDINESS** Fully hardy.
• **CULTIVATION** Grow in fertile, moist but well-drained soil in partial shade, or in sun in cool, moist climates; will tolerate a range of soil types. Shelter from cold, dry winds. Trim hedges in early summer. Tolerant of hard clipping.
• **PROPAGATION** Sow seed in containers in a cold frame in autumn or in spring after stratification. Seed may take 2 years to germinate. Root greenwood or semi-ripe cuttings of terminal or epicormic shoots in summer or autumn; cuttings from sideshoots seldom develop satisfactorily.
• **PESTS AND DISEASES** Trouble free.

C. fortunei ⚠ (Fortune plum yew). Shrub or narrow-crowned, small, coniferous tree with whorled branches and shredding or scaly, red-brown bark. Linear or slightly curved, mid-green leaves, 4–9cm (1½–3½in) long, with 2 white bands beneath, are borne in flat or slightly V-shaped sprays. Ovoid to elliptic, olive-green fruit, to 2.5cm (1in) long, ripening to purple-brown, are borne on short stalks on female plants. ↕ to 10m (30ft), ↔ to 5m (15ft). C. and E. China. ❄❄❄
C. harringtoniana (Cowtail pine, Plum yew). Coniferous shrub, occasionally a small tree, with sharp-pointed, slightly curved or linear, dark green leaves, 4–6cm (1½–2½in) long, rising either side of the shoots in a wide V-shape. Female plants produce ovoid to obovoid, olive-green fruit, 3cm (1¼in) long, in autumn. ↕ 3–10m (10–30ft), ↔ 3–6m (10–20ft). Korea, Japan. ❄❄❄. **var. *drupacea*** ▣ 🏆 is a small tree with a wide, rounded crown and narrowly furrowed, partially peeling, dark grey bark. The leaves, 2.5–3.5cm (1–1½in) long, are arranged on each shoot in 2-ranks in a V-shape; ↔ 1–5m (3–15ft); Japan, C. and W. China. **'Fastigiata'** is a shrub, with erect branches and radially arranged leaves, to 8cm (3in) long; ↕↔ 5m (15ft).

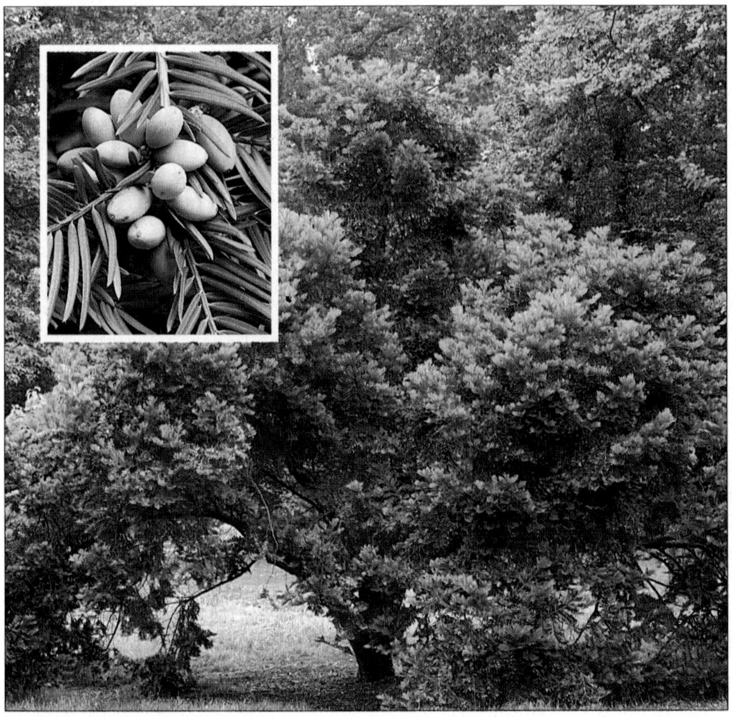

Cephalotaxus harringtoniana var. *drupacea* (inset: fruit detail)

CERARIA

PORTULACACEAE

Genus of 5 or 6 species of succulent, sometimes deciduous shrubs from hilly areas of Namibia and South Africa, with short, swollen trunks and often with waxy bark. They are grown for their thick, fleshy leaves, which are usually opposite, occasionally alternate, and for their small, funnel-shaped, white or pink flowers, borne singly or in clusters of 2–6 in summer. Both male and female plants are needed to obtain fruit. In frost-prone areas, grow in a temperate conservatory or greenhouse, or as house-plants. In warm, dry areas, grow in a border or desert garden.

• **HARDINESS** Frost tender.
• **CULTIVATION** Under glass, grow in a mix of 3 parts standard cactus compost and 1 part leaf mould in full light with shade from hot sun. When in growth, water moderately and apply a low-nitrogen fertilizer monthly. Keep almost dry at other times. Outdoors, grow in well-drained, poor to moderately fertile, humus-rich soil in a sheltered, sunny site. See also pp.48–49.
• **PROPAGATION** Sow seed at 19–24°C (66–75°F) as soon as ripe, or root stem cuttings in spring.
• **PESTS AND DISEASES** Susceptible to aphids early in the growing season.

C. pygmaea. Dwarf, succulent shrub with a short caudex bearing spreading, stiff, fleshy, often down-curving stems covered with thick, ovoid, fleshy, bluish green or yellow-green leaves, to 1.5cm (½in) long. Clusters of 2–5 pale pink flowers, 3–6mm (⅛–¼in) across, are produced in summer. ↕ 20cm (8in), ↔ 30cm (12in). Namibia, South Africa (Western Cape, Northern Cape). ❀ (min. 16°C/61°F)

CERASTIUM

CARYOPHYLLACEAE

Genus of up to 100 annuals and mainly carpet-forming or tufted perennials from temperate and arctic zones of Europe and North America. They are generally hairy, with tiny, star-shaped white flowers with 5 petals, deeply indented or cleft in 2, borne singly or in cymes. The leaves are usually simple, opposite, and entire. *Cerastium* species include many weeds; the species in cultivation are mainly vigorous and mat- or carpet-forming. Grow at the front of a border, on a wall, or in a large rock garden.

• **HARDINESS** Fully hardy.
• **CULTIVATION** Grow in any well-drained soil in full sun. *C. tomentosum* is useful for poor soil on dry, sunny banks.
• **PROPAGATION** Sow seed in containers in an open frame in autumn. Divide in spring; root stem tip cuttings in early summer.
• **PESTS AND DISEASES** Trouble free.

C. tomentosum ▣ (Snow-in-summer). Rampant, carpet- or mat-forming perennial producing linear or linear-lance-shaped, white- or silver-woolly leaves, 1–3cm (½–1¼in) long. Profuse cymes of star-shaped white flowers, to 2.5cm (1in) across, are borne in late spring and summer. ↕ 5–8cm (2–3in), ↔ indefinite. Italy, including Sicily, and widely naturalized elsewhere in Europe. ❄❄❄

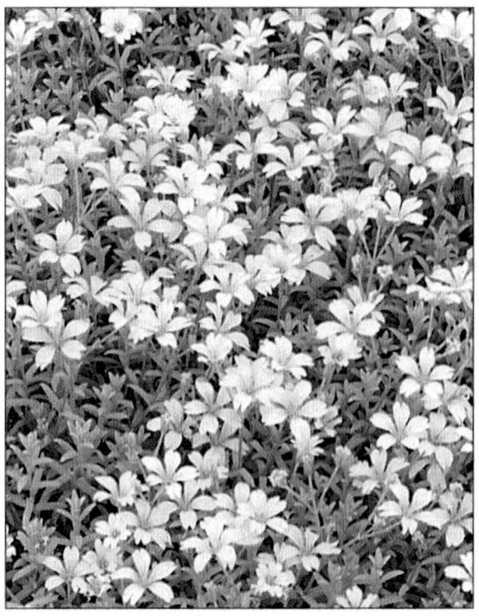

Cerastium tomentosum

CERATOPETALUM

CUNONIACEAE

Genus of 5 species of evergreen shrubs and trees from open woodland and rainforest in Australia and New Guinea. They are valued for their terminal and axillary panicles of 4- or 5-petalled flowers. After flowering, the calyces enlarge and become brightly coloured, producing a second, showier floral display. Leaves are simple or 3-palmate, and borne in opposite pairs. In frost-prone areas, grow in a cool greenhouse or conservatory. In frost-free climates, use as unusual specimen plants for a small garden.

• **HARDINESS** Frost tender.
• **CULTIVATION** Under glass, grow in loam-based potting compost (JI No.3) with additional leaf mould and sharp sand, in full light, with shade from hot sun. In the growing season, water moderately and apply a balanced liquid fertilizer monthly; reduce water in winter. Top-dress or pot on in spring. Outdoors, grow in moderately fertile, moist but well-drained soil in sun or partial shade. Pruning group 1; plants under glass may need restrictive pruning, after flowering.
• **PROPAGATION** Sow seed at 13–18°C (55–64°F) in spring. Root semi-ripe cuttings in summer (rooting may be slow).
• **PESTS AND DISEASES** Trouble free.

C. gummiferum 🏆 (New South Wales Christmas tree). Large shrub or small, bushy tree, erect at first then spreading, with 3-palmate leaves composed of narrowly oblong, shallowly toothed leaflets, to 7cm (3in) long, dark green above, paler beneath. Panicles, to 10cm (4in) or more long, of white flowers, 6mm (¼in) across, with enlarged, bright red calyces, to 1cm (½in) across, are produced in spring. ↕ 3–10m (10–30ft), ↔ 2–6m (6–20ft). Australia (New South Wales). ❀ (min. 5°C/41°F). **'Christmas Snow'** bears flowers with white calyces. **'White Christmas'** is similar to 'Christmas Snow', but has white-variegated leaves.

C

C

CERATOPHYLLUM
Hornwort
CERATOPHYLLACEAE

Genus of about 30 species of almost rootless, submerged aquatic perennials from Eurasia, N. and tropical Africa, and S. and E. USA, producing whorls of delicate, stalkless, linear, dark green leaves, 1–4cm (½–1½in) long, often crowded near the growing points. The minute, unisexual flowers are enclosed in axillary bracts, with both male and female flowers borne on the same plant. Hornworts are grown in cold-water aquaria for their delicate foliage, and are good oxygenators for a garden pool. They tolerate a wide range of water conditions.
• **HARDINESS** Fully hardy to frost tender.
• **CULTIVATION** Grow in water 60–90cm (24–36in) deep in full sun; hornworts will, however, tolerate shade. Grow in a pool, tub, or cold-water aquarium in full light. The almost rootless stems spread freely; some shoots may root in mud at the bottom of the water. *C. demersum* overwinters by modified terminal buds (turions), which sink to the bottom until spring, when they develop into young plants. See also pp.52–53.
• **PROPAGATION** Detach small pieces of stem, or turions, and float in water.
• **PESTS AND DISEASES** Algae may swamp the fragile lower leaves.

C. demersum (Hornwort). Submerged aquatic perennial producing slender, often rootless stems, 30–60cm (12–24in) long, with whorls of forked, brittle, dark green leaves, often borne more densely near the growing points. Tiny, cup-shaped flowers, the males white and 3mm (⅛in) across, the females green and 1mm (¹⁄₁₆in) across, are borne from the leaf axils in summer. ↔ indefinite. E. central Europe, Mediterranean, tropical Africa. ❄❄❄

CERATOSTIGMA
PLUMBAGINACEAE

Genus of about 8 species of deciduous and evergreen subshrubs and herbaceous perennials found in dry, open situations in N.E. tropical Africa, the Himalayas, China, and S.E. Asia. They are grown for their 5-lobed, salverform blue flowers, borne in terminal and axillary, spike-like clusters from late summer to autumn, and for their simple, alternate leaves, which turn red or bronze in autumn. Grow in a sunny, sheltered, mixed or shrub border, or against a warm, sunny wall. *C. plumbaginoides* is also suitable for ground cover and for a rock garden. The frost-tender species are best grown in a cold or cool greenhouse in frost-prone areas.
• **HARDINESS** Fully hardy to frost tender. Shrubby species are slightly less hardy than herbaceous species, but will usually regrow from the bases, if top growth is damaged in winter.
• **CULTIVATION** Grow in moderately fertile, light, moist but well-drained soil in full sun. Pruning group 10, for shrubby species, in early to mid-spring.
• **PROPAGATION** Root softwood cuttings in spring or semi-ripe cuttings in summer. Remove suckers in autumn or

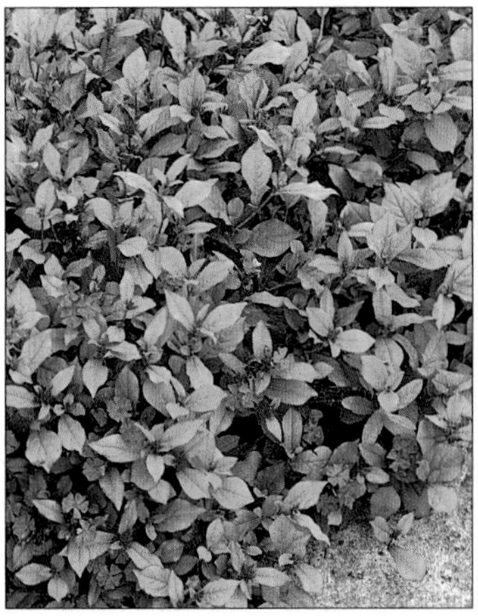
Ceratostigma plumbaginoides

spring. Layer in autumn. Overwinter young plants in frost-free conditions.
• **PESTS AND DISEASES** Powdery mildew may be a problem.

C. griffithii. Rounded, evergreen or semi-evergreen shrub with bristly red stems and obovate, densely bristly, purple-margined, mid-green leaves, to 3cm (1¼in) long, which turn red in autumn and winter. Bright blue flowers, to 3cm (1¼in) across, are borne in terminal, spike-like clusters from late summer to autumn. ↕ 1m (3ft), ↔ 1.5m (5ft). Himalayas. ❄❄
C. minus. Open-branched, deciduous shrub with slender, bristly, mid-green stems. Obovate to spoon-shaped, mid-green leaves, to 5cm (2in) long, are rounded at the tips and almost hairless above, but have bristly margins; they turn red in autumn. From late summer to autumn, bears dense, terminal or axillary, spike-like clusters of bright blue or purple-blue flowers, to 2cm (¾in) across and red-purple at the bases. ↕ 1m (3ft), ↔ 1.5m (5ft). W. China. ❄❄❄
C. plumbaginoides ■ ♀ syn. *Plumbago larpentiae.* Rhizomatous, spreading, woody-based perennial with upright, slender red stems and obovate, bright green leaves, to 9cm (3½in) long, with bristly, wavy margins, richly red-tinted in autumn. In late summer, bears terminal, spike-like clusters of brilliant blue flowers, to 2cm (¾in) across. ↕ to 45cm (18in), ↔ to 30cm (12in) or more. W. China. ❄❄❄
C. willmottianum ■ Open-branched, spreading, deciduous shrub with slender, bristly, mid-green stems. Lance-shaped to obovate, pointed, bristly, mid- to dark green, purple-margined leaves, to 5cm (2in) long, turn red in autumn. From late summer to autumn, bears pale to mid-blue flowers, 2.5cm (1in) across, with red-purple tubes, in terminal or axillary, spike-like clusters. ↕ 1m (3ft), ↔ 1.5m (5ft). W. China. ❄❄❄

CERATOZAMIA
ZAMIACEAE

Genus of 9 species of dioecious, evergreen cycads found in cloud forest, on dry upland, and among dense, tangled brushwood, from Mexico to Belize. They are palm-like in habit, with short, swollen trunks and rigid, pinnate, leathery leaves in lax, terminal rosettes or whorls. Cone-like male and female inflorescences ("cones") are borne on mature plants in summer: female cones are solitary, cylindrical, and dull green; male cones are slightly narrower and grey-green. In frost-prone areas, grow as houseplants or in a temperate or warm greenhouse. In warmer areas, use as specimen plants on a lawn or patio.
• **HARDINESS** Frost tender.
• **CULTIVATION** Under glass, grow in deep containers in a mix of equal parts loam, coarse sand, garden compost, and granulated bark in bright filtered or indirect light. In the growing season, water freely and apply a balanced liquid fertilizer monthly; water sparingly in winter. Pot on or top-dress in spring. Outdoors, grow in fertile, humus-rich, moist but well-drained, neutral to acid soil in partial or dappled shade.

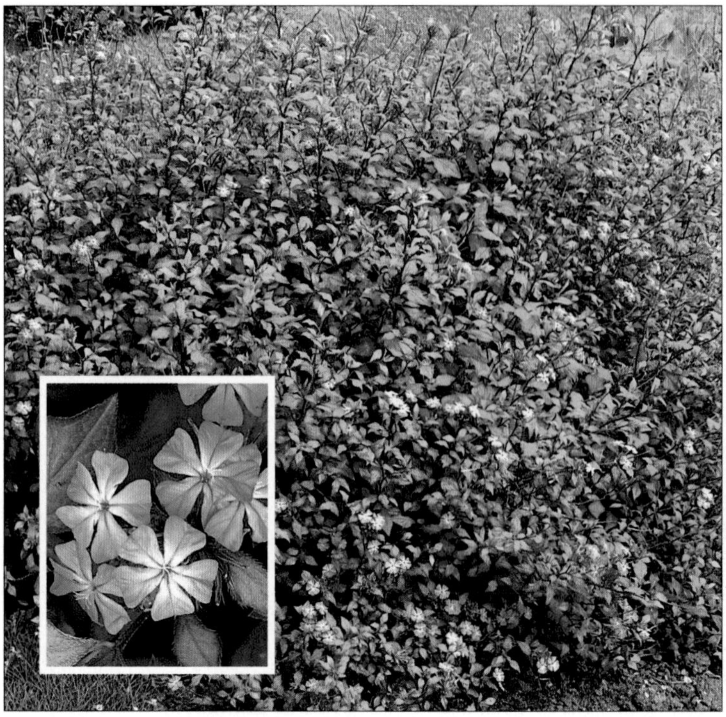
Ceratostigma willmottianum (inset: flower detail)

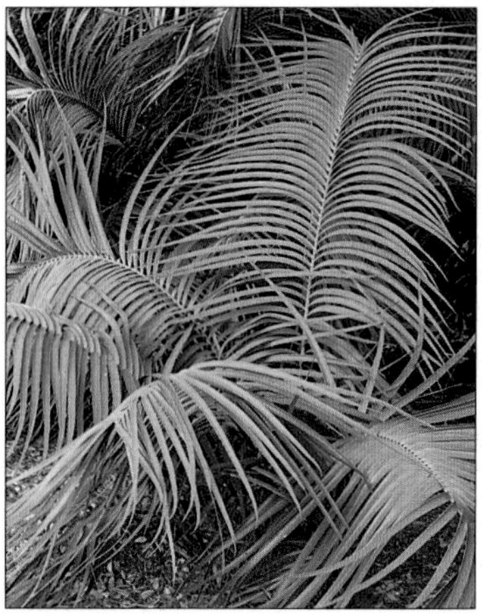
Ceratozamia mexicana

• **PROPAGATION** Sow seed at 21–30°C (70–86°F) in spring. If offsets develop, detach and pot them up in spring.
• **PESTS AND DISEASES** Prone to scale insects and mealybugs under glass.

C. mexicana ■ ❀ (Mexican horncone). Large cycad with almost columnar, usually single caudices. The arching, pinnate leaves are erect to spreading, 1–3m (3–10ft) long, and have up to 150 narrowly to broadly lance-shaped, light green leaflets. Flowering cones are borne in summer: green female cones, to 30cm (12in) long, have prominently horned scales; grey-green male cones, to 50cm (20in) long, have only rudimentary horns. ↕ to 2m (6ft), ↔ to 4m (12ft). Mexico. ⌂ (min. 16°C/61°F)

CERCIDIPHYLLUM
CERCIDIPHYLLACEAE

Genus of one species of deciduous tree from woodland in China and Japan. Tiny red flowers are borne in early spring, before the leaves; male and female flowers are produced on separate plants. *C. japonicum* is cultivated for its foliage, which provides particularly good autumn colour; it is best grown as a specimen tree in a woodland setting.
• **HARDINESS** Fully hardy. Young leaves may be damaged by late frost.
• **CULTIVATION** Grow in deep, fertile, humus-rich, moist but well-drained soil, preferably neutral to acid, in sun or dappled shade, sheltered from cold, dry winds. Plants often develop several main stems, but may be trained as central-leader standards. Pruning group 1.

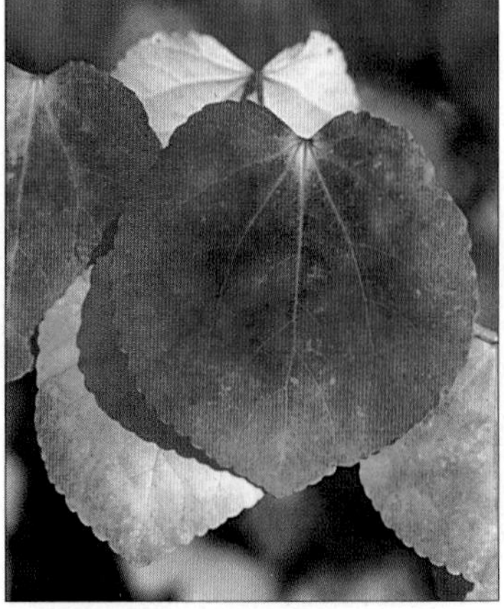
Cercidiphyllum japonicum

• **PROPAGATION** Sow seed in containers in an open frame as soon as ripe. Take basal cuttings in late spring and semi-ripe cuttings in midsummer.
• **PESTS AND DISEASES** Trouble free.

C. japonicum ▣ 𝕐 ♀ (Katsura tree). Pyramidal, later rounded, deciduous tree with vigorous shoots and opposite, sometimes alternate, ovate to rounded, mid-green leaves, to 10cm (4in) long. Bronze when young, the mid-green leaves turn yellow, orange, and red in autumn and colour best on acid soils. Fallen leaves smell of burnt sugar when crushed. ↕20m (70ft), ↔15m (50ft). China, Japan. ✻✻✻. **var. *magnificum*** 𝕐 syn. *C. magnificum*, is smaller, but with larger leaves, to 12cm (5in) long; ↕10m (30ft), ↔8m (25ft). Japan. **f. *pendulum*** ♀ syn. 'Pendulum', has a weeping habit, with slender, pendent branches; ↕6m (20ft), ↔8m (25ft).
C. magnificum see *C. japonicum* var. *magnificum*.

CERCIS

LEGUMINOSAE/PAPILIONACEAE

Genus of about 6 species of deciduous trees and shrubs found in woodland, at woodland margins, and on rocky hillsides in the Mediterranean, C. and E. Asia, and North America. They have alternate, heart-shaped, entire leaves and bear brightly coloured, pea-like flowers in stalkless clusters or short racemes in spring, followed by flattened pods. The flowers are normally produced on the previous year's wood either before or as the leaves unfold, but they may also be borne on wood that is several years old. Larger species are excellent specimen plants; grow smaller ones in a shrub border, or train against a wall.
• **HARDINESS** Fully hardy, but may be tender when young. Unripened wood is liable to frost damage.
• **CULTIVATION** Grow in fertile, deep, moist but well-drained, preferably loam soil in full sun or dappled shade. Plant in the final location when young; older plants resent transplanting. Pruning group 1; also group 7 for *C. canadensis* 'Forest Pansy'. For large foliage, pollard well-established plants in early spring.
• **PROPAGATION** Sow seed in containers in a cold frame in autumn. Root semi-ripe cuttings, or bud selected clones, in summer.
• **PESTS AND DISEASES** Canker, coral spot, *Verticillium* wilt, leafhoppers, and scale insects may be a problem.

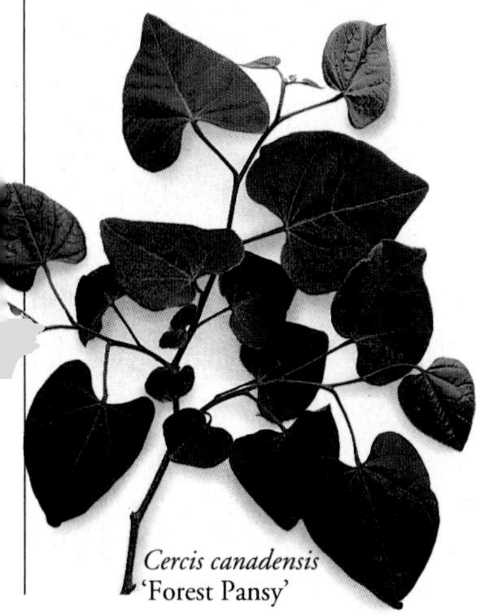
Cercis canadensis 'Forest Pansy'

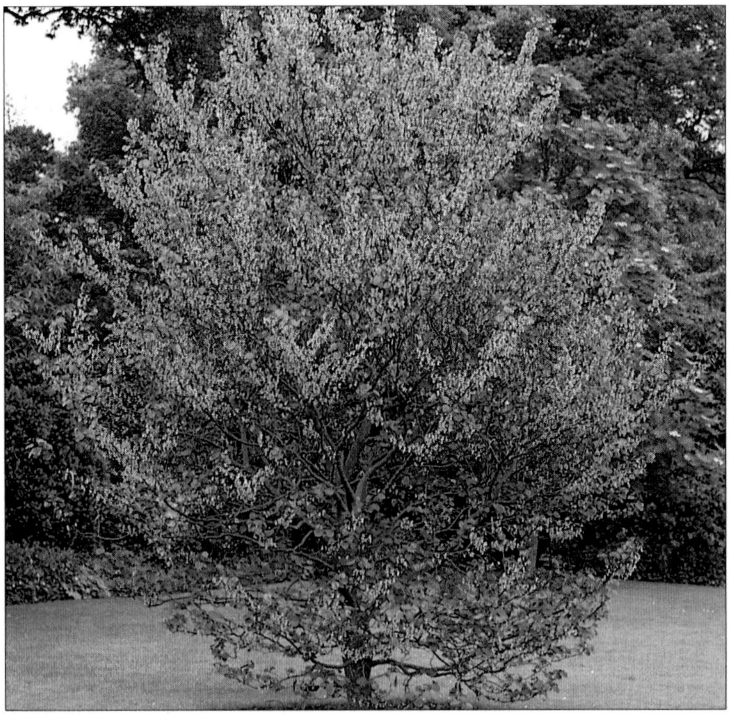
Cercis siliquastrum

C. canadensis ♀ (Eastern redbud). Spreading, often multi-stemmed tree with heart-shaped leaves, pointed at the tips, to 10cm (4in) long, bronze when young, turning yellow in autumn. Deep crimson, purple to pink, or occasionally white flowers, to 1cm (½in) long, are borne in clusters of 2–8 on bare stems, before the leaves. ↕↔10m (30ft). North America. ✻✻✻. **'Forest Pansy'** ▣ 𝕐 has dark red-purple leaves. **'Royal White'** bears a profusion of pure white flowers. **var. *texensis* 'Oklahoma'** syn. *C. reniformis* 'Oklahoma', has waxy, glossy, rich green leaves with rounded tips, and dark wine-red flowers; ↕↔5m (15ft).
C. chinensis ♀ (Chinese redbud). Densely branched shrub or small tree with erect shoots and rounded, glossy, leathery, rich green leaves, to 12cm (5in) long, with pointed tips, turning yellow in autumn. Bears clusters of 3–8 deep to lavender-pink flowers, to 1.5cm (½in) across, before the leaves. ↕6m (20ft), ↔5m (15ft). C. China. ✻✻✻. **'Avondale'** is compact with abundant dark purple-pink flowers; ↕to 3m (10ft).
C. occidentalis ♀ (California redbud, Western redbud). Spreading shrub or small tree, often multi-stemmed, with kidney-shaped, bluish green leaves, to 10cm (4in) long, that have rounded or notched tips, bronze at first, turning yellow in autumn. Dark purple-pink flowers, to 1.5cm (½in) across, are borne in clusters of 5 or 6, usually on year-old wood, before the leaves. ↕5m (15ft), ↔4m (12ft). S.W. USA. ✻✻✻
***C. reniformis* 'Oklahoma'** see *C. canadensis* var. *texensis* 'Oklahoma'.
C. siliquastrum ▣ 𝕐 ♀ (Judas tree). Spreading, sometimes multi-stemmed tree with inversely heart-shaped to kidney-shaped, glaucous, blue-green leaves, to 10cm (4in) long, with notched tips, bronze when young, turning yellow in autumn. Bears clusters of 3–6 magenta to pink, occasionally white flowers, 1.5–2cm (½–¾in) long, before and with the leaves, often on the main branches. ↕↔10m (30ft). S.E. Europe, S.W. Asia. ✻✻✻. **f. *albida***, syn. 'Alba', has white flowers. **'Bodnant'** ▣ has dark purple-pink flowers.

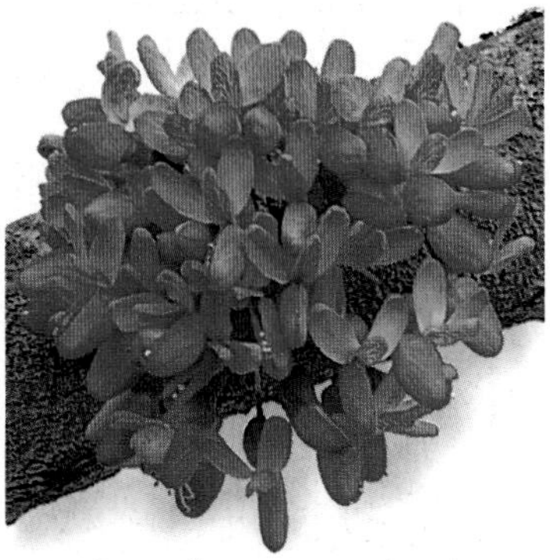
Cercis siliquastrum 'Bodnant'

CEREUS

CACTACEAE

Genus of about 25 species of tree-like or columnar, perennial cacti, mainly from rocky terrain in South America and the West Indies. They usually have 3–14 thick ribs and often woolly areoles bearing stout spines. Nocturnal, widely cup- or funnel-shaped flowers are borne from summer to early autumn, and are followed by ovoid, fleshy, red or yellow fruits containing glossy black seeds. In frost-prone areas, grow in a temperate greenhouse or conservatory. In warm, dry climates, use in a desert garden.
• **HARDINESS** Frost tender.
• **CULTIVATION** Under glass, grow in standard cactus compost in full light. In the growing season, water freely and apply a low-nitrogen liquid fertilizer monthly; keep almost dry in winter. Outdoors, grow in sharply drained, poor to moderately fertile, humus-rich, slightly acid soil in full sun. See also pp.48–49.
• **PROPAGATION** Sow seed at 19–24°C (66–75°F) in early spring, or root cuttings of young branches in late spring or early summer.

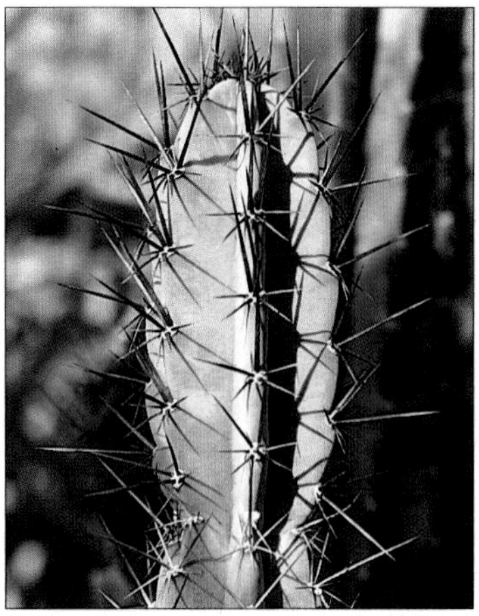
Cereus validus

• **PESTS AND DISEASES** Susceptible to mealybugs and scale insects.

C. chalybaeus. Columnar cactus with 5- or 6-ribbed, few-branched, often purple-tinged, glaucous, dark green stems. Brown-woolly areoles bear red then black spines (7–9 radials and 3 or 4 longer, thicker centrals). In summer, bears funnel-shaped flowers, to 20cm (8in) long; the inner petals are white, the perianth tubes and backs of the outer petals are purple or red. ↕3m (10ft), ↔70cm (28in). N. Argentina, Uruguay. ❁ (min. 7–10°C/45–50°F)
C. emoryi see *Bergerocactus emoryi.*
C. flagelliformis see *Aporocactus flagelliformis.*
C. forbesii see *C. validus.*
***C. peruvianus* of gardens** see *C. uruguayanus.*
C. silvestrii see *Echinopsis chamaecereus.*
C. spachianus see *Echinopsis spachiana.*
C. uruguayanus, syn. *C. peruvianus* of gardens. Tree-like, columnar cactus with 5- to 9-ribbed, few-branched, glaucous, dark green stems. Rounded, furrowed ribs bear brown areoles with reddish brown to black, occasionally yellowish spines (4–7 radials and 1 or 2 longer, thicker centrals). In summer, bears funnel-shaped flowers, 16cm (6in) long, with white inner petals and green-, brown-, or red-tipped white outer petals. ↕to 5m (15ft), ↔70cm (28in). S.E. Brazil to N. Argentina. ❁ (min. 7–10°C/45–50°F)
C. validus ▣ syn. *C. forbesii.* Tree-like, columnar cactus producing dull bluish green, then grey-green stems, with 4–7 often notched ribs. White-woolly areoles bear dark brown spines (5–7 radials and 1 or 2 longer, thicker centrals). Cup-shaped flowers, 25cm (10in) long, with white inner and red-pink outer petals, are borne in early autumn. ↕4m (12ft), ↔60cm (24in). Argentina. ❁ (min. 7–10°C/45–50°F)

▷**Ceriman** see *Monstera deliciosa*

CEROPEGIA

ASCLEPIADACEAE

Genus of up to 200 or more species of evergreen or semi-evergreen, erect, pendent, or climbing perennials from deserts to rainforests in tropical and subtropical areas of the Canary Islands, Africa, Madagascar, Asia, and Australia. Many are succulent, with fleshy, tuber-like caudices. The leaves are opposite

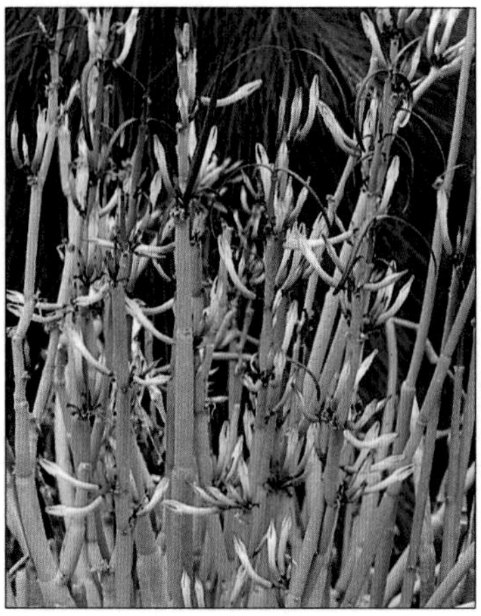

Ceropegia dichotoma

and in whorls of 3, varying from ovate-heart-shaped to lance-shaped or linear. The flowers are borne singly or in cymes in summer, and are often widely flared at the tips in the form of parachutes or lanterns. The fruits are cylindrical to lance-shaped, and the flat, silk-tufted seeds are contained in hairless follicles. In frost-prone areas, grow in a warm greenhouse or as houseplants, using pendent species in hanging baskets. In warm, dry climates, grow outdoors in a desert garden; train climbing species on trellis, a pergola, or other support.
• **HARDINESS** Frost tender.
• **CULTIVATION** Under glass, grow in a mix of 2 parts sharp sand and 1 part each loam, peat, and leaf mould in bright filtered light. When in growth, water moderately and apply a low-nitrogen liquid fertilizer 2 or 3 times. Keep plants dry at other times; over-watering and low temperatures will lead to basal rot of the caudices. Outdoors, grow in sharply drained, poor, humus-rich, loam soil, providing shelter from full sun. See also pp. 48–49.
• **PROPAGATION** Sow seed at 19–24°C (66–75°F) in early spring. Increase *C. linearis* subsp. *woodii* from stem bulbils. Take stem cuttings, 10–15cm (4–6in) long, in early summer; root in a sand and peat mix at 22–25°C (72–77°F), and keep moist.
• **PESTS AND DISEASES** Prone to aphids, scale insects, and sometimes mealybugs.

***C. devecchii* var. *adelaidae*.** Succulent climber with fleshy, grey-green, red-mottled stems, 1.2m (4ft) long, and ovate to 3-angled, scale-like, black-green leaves, to 4mm (⅛in) long. Solitary, tubular, red-spotted cream flowers, 3cm (1¼in) long, with broadly triangular, minutely hairy, green or pale red lobes, are borne in summer. ↕ 1.2m (4ft), ↔ 60cm (24in). Kenya, Tanzania. ❀ (min. 10°C/50°F)
C. dichotoma ■ Erect, semi-evergreen succulent producing grey-green stems, 30–100cm (12–39in) long, with linear, slightly fleshy, grey-green leaves, 2.5–8cm (1–3in) long. Bright yellow flowers with slightly curved, paler yellow tubes, 3cm (1¼in) long, and fully united lobes, to 1.5cm (½in) long, are borne singly or in cymes in summer. ↕ 1m (3ft), ↔ 60cm (24in). Canary Islands (Tenerife). ❀ (min. 10°C/50°F)
C. distincta* subsp. *haygarthii see *C. haygarthii*.
C. haygarthii, syn. *C. distincta* subsp. *haygarthii*. Climbing, semi-evergreen succulent with twining, pencil-like, fleshy stems, 40–130cm (16–51in) long, and ovate to elliptic, fleshy, mid-green leaves, 1.5cm (½in) or more long, heart-shaped at the bases. In summer, bears solitary, funnel-shaped, red-spotted, pale pink flowers, 2cm (¾in) or more long, slightly curved at the tubular bases, and with lobes that broaden upwards and unite to form stalks, surmounted by red, white-haired anthers. ↕ 1.2m (4ft), ↔ 60cm (24in). South Africa (Northern Cape, Eastern Cape, Western Cape). ❀ (min. 10°C/50°F)
C. linearis* subsp. *woodii ■🏆 syn. *C. woodii* (Hearts on a string, Rosary vine, Sweetheart vine). Pendent, evergreen, tuberous-rooted succulent with slender twining stems, to 1m (3ft) long. The heart-shaped, fleshy, mid-green leaves, to 1.5cm (½in) long, are purple beneath, and often have grey-green or purple markings above. Frequently produces bulbils from the leaf axils. Lantern-like, purplish brown flowers, 1–2cm (½–¾in) long, with pinkish green tubes margined with fine purple hairs, are borne singly in summer. ↕ 10cm (4in), ↔ indefinite. Zimbabwe to South Africa (Eastern Cape). ❀ (min. 10°C/50°F)
***C. nilotica*.** Twining, semi-evergreen succulent with rounded or 4-angled, fleshy, greyish green stems, 30–80cm (12–32in) long, and ovate, finely toothed, greyish green leaves, 2–4cm (½–1½in) long. In summer, bears cymes of flowers, 3–4cm (1¼–1½in) long, with yellowish white or pale green tubes, and triangular, purple-brown lobes, yellow-blotched at the bases. ↕ 75cm (30in), ↔ 60cm (24in). Sudan, Ethiopia, Kenya. ❀ (min. 10°C/50°F)
C. sandersoniae see *C. sandersonii*.
C. sandersonii, syn. *C. sandersoniae* (Fountain flower, Parachute plant). Twining, evergreen succulent with ovate-heart-shaped, fresh green leaves, 4–5cm (1½–2in) long, on light green stems, 40–140cm (16–55in) long. In summer, bears solitary, parachute-like, short-stalked green flowers, with broadly funnel-shaped tubes, to 5cm (2in) long, mottled darker green; the narrow lobes widen to unite at their upturned, white-haired margins, forming canopies to 2.5cm (1in) across. ↕ 1.2m (4ft), ↔ 60cm (24in). Mozambique, South Africa (KwaZulu/Natal). ❀ (min. 10°C/50°F)
C. woodii see *C. linearis* subsp. *woodii*.

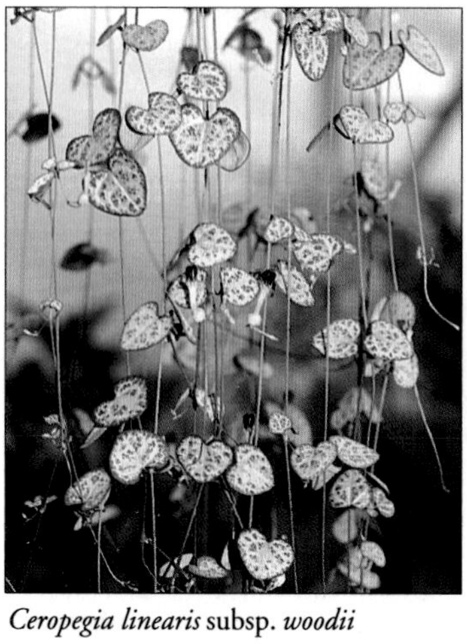

Ceropegia linearis subsp. *woodii*

CESTRUM

SOLANACEAE

Genus of about 175 species of evergreen and deciduous shrubs with alternate, simple, usually unpleasantly scented leaves, from woodland in Mexico and Central and South America. They are grown for their tubular to funnel-shaped, often fragrant flowers, borne in terminal or axillary cymes, followed by purple-red or red berries. Grow in a sheltered border or against a sunny wall. In frost-prone areas, grow tender species in a temperate or warm greenhouse or conservatory; container-grown plants may be moved outdoors in summer.
• **HARDINESS** Frost hardy to frost tender.
• **CULTIVATION** Under glass, grow in loam-based potting compost (JI No.3) in full light, with shade from hot sun and good ventilation. In the growing season, water moderately and apply a balanced liquid fertilizer monthly; water sparingly in winter. Outdoors, grow in fertile, well-drained soil in sun or partial shade. Provide support for scrambling species. Pruning group 8 for early-flowering evergreens; group 9 for late-flowering evergreens; and group 6 for deciduous plants. Plants under glass may need restrictive pruning; prune *C. aurantiacum* and *C. parqui* close to their bases annually in early spring.
• **PROPAGATION** Sow seed of frost-hardy species in containers in a cold frame in autumn; sow seed of tender species at 13–18°C (55–64°F) in spring. Root softwood cuttings of frost-hardy species, and semi-ripe cuttings of tender species, in summer.
• **PESTS AND DISEASES** Trouble free.

C. aurantiacum ■ Evergreen shrub, becoming scandent if not regularly pruned, with ovate to lance-shaped, smooth, light green leaves, to 11cm (4½in) long. Axillary and terminal, panicle-like cymes, to 10cm (4in) across, of tubular, bright orange flowers, to 3cm (1¼in) long, are borne from spring to early summer; they are followed by spherical, fleshy white berries. ↕ 2–3m (6–10ft), ↔ 1.5–2m (5–6ft). Venezuela to Guatemala. ❀ (min. 5°C/41°F)
C. elegans ■🏆 syn. *C. purpureum*. Vigorous, evergreen shrub with arching branches and ovate-oblong to lance-shaped, matt, mid-green leaves, to 10cm (4in) long. From summer to autumn, bears tubular, crimson to purple-red or

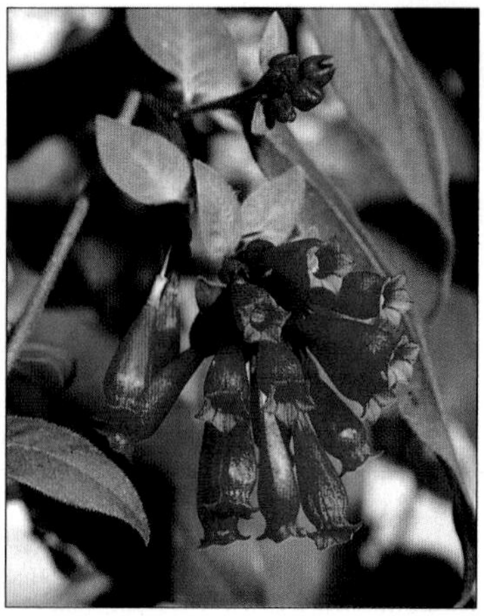

Cestrum elegans

pink flowers, to 2cm (¾in) long, in pendent, terminal, compound, panicle-like cymes, 10cm (4in) across; they are followed by purple-red berries. ↕↔ 3m (10ft). Mexico. ❀ (min. 5°C/41°F)
***C. fasciculatum*.** Strong-growing, evergreen shrub with arching branches and ovate to lance-shaped, wavy-margined, dark green leaves, to 7cm (3in) long. Tubular, bright red flowers, to 2cm (¾in) long, are borne in terminal, pendent cymes, to 8cm (3in) across, from spring to early summer; they are followed by purple-red berries. ↕↔ 2m (6ft). Mexico. ❄❄
C. 'Newellii' 🏆 Vigorous, evergreen shrub with arching branches and narrowly ovate, dark green leaves, to 10cm (4in) long. From summer to autumn, bears tubular crimson flowers, to 2cm (¾in) long, in dense, terminal, compound panicles, 8–12cm (3–5in) across, sometimes followed by purple-red berries. ↕↔ 3m (10ft). ❄❄
C. parqui ■🏆 (Willow-leaved jessamine). Upright, deciduous shrub, sometimes herbaceous in cold areas, with linear-lance-shaped to elliptic, mid-green leaves, to 12cm (5in) long. From summer to autumn, produces night-scented, tubular, bright yellow-green flowers, to 2.5cm (1in) long, with star-shaped mouths, in large, terminal and axillary cymes, to 13cm (5in) across; they are followed by violet-brown berries. ↕↔ 2m (6ft). Chile. ❄❄
***C. psittacinum*.** Scandent, evergreen shrub with alternate, elliptic to oblong, softly hairy, mid-green leaves, 5–12cm (2–5in) long, heart-shaped or rounded at the bases. Bears axillary and terminal

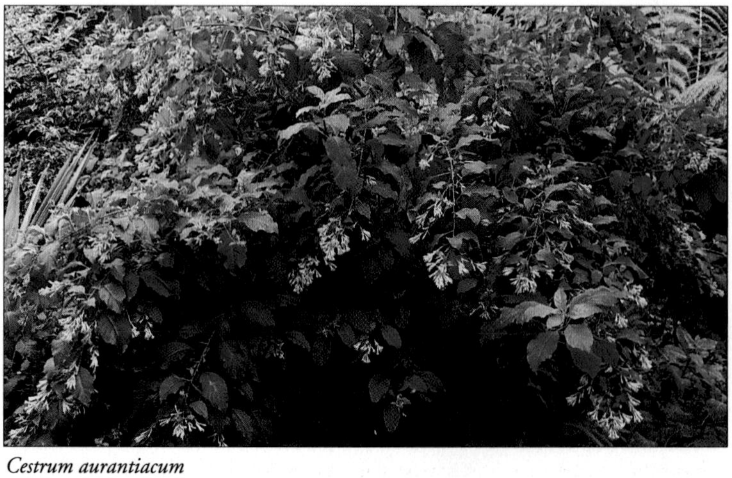

Cestrum aurantiacum

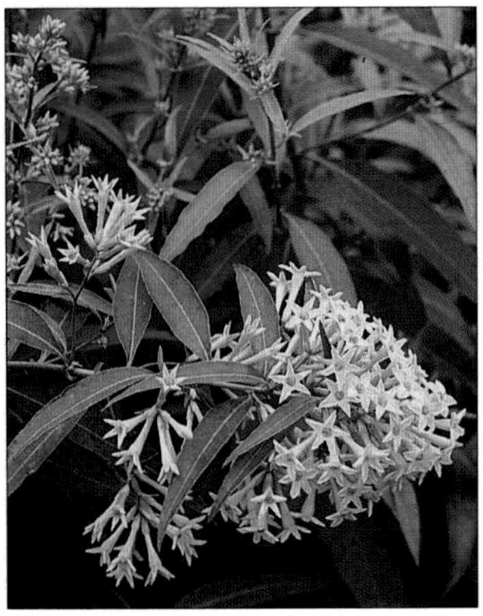

Cestrum parqui

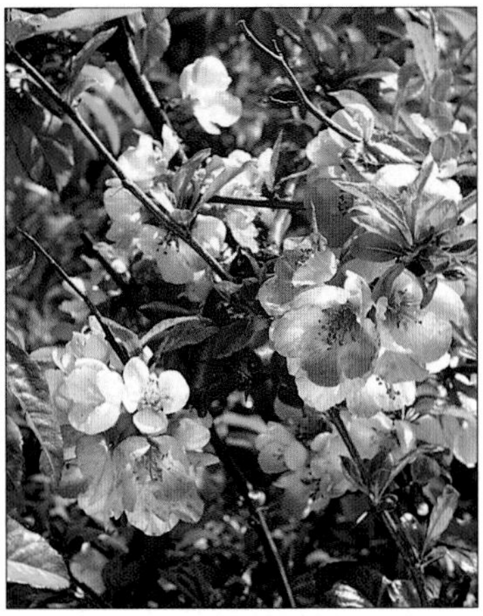

Chaenomeles speciosa 'Moerloosei'

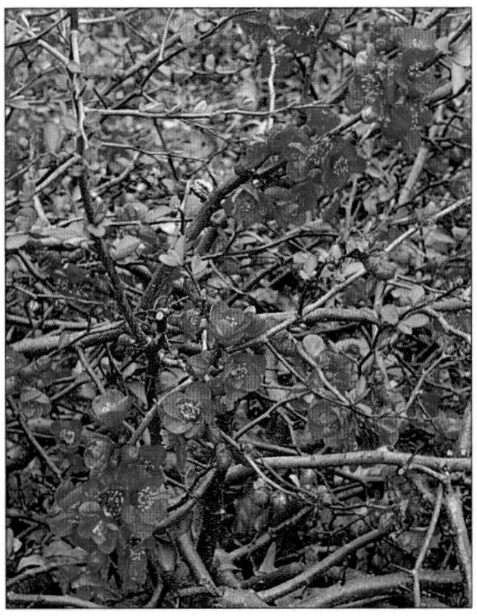

Chaenomeles x *superba* 'Crimson and Gold'

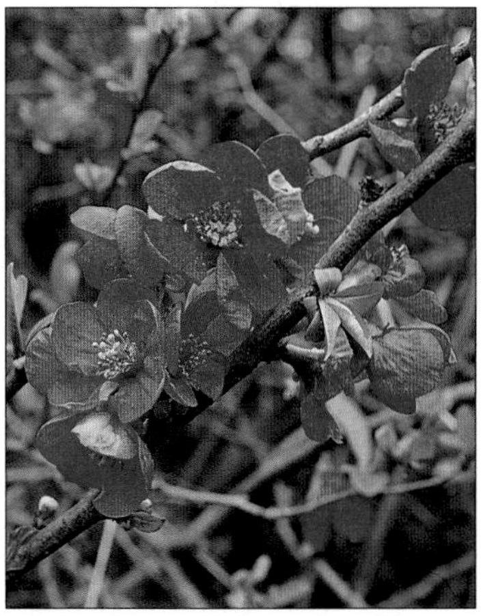

Chaenomeles x *superba* 'Pink Lady'

cymes of tubular to funnel-shaped, vivid orange flowers, 1.5cm (½in) long, in autumn, followed by ovoid black berries. ↕ 3m (10ft), ↔ 45cm (18in). Central America. ❄ (min. 10°C/50°F)
C. purpureum see *C. elegans*.
C. roseum. Erect, evergreen shrub with oblong to ovate, wavy-margined, softly hairy, mid-green leaves, to 10cm (4in) long. In summer, bears terminal cymes of tubular-funnel-shaped, rose-pink flowers, to 3cm (1¼in) long, with spreading lobes, followed by red berries. ↕↔ 2m (6ft). Mexico. ❄❄

▷ ***Ceterach*** see *Asplenium*
C. officinarum see *A. ceterach*

CHAENOMELES

Flowering quince, Japanese quince, Japonica

ROSACEAE

Genus of 3 species of deciduous, often spiny shrubs, one sometimes a small tree, from mountain woodland in China and Japan. They are cultivated for their early flowers, which are 5-petalled, cup-shaped, single to double, borne singly or in dense clusters, and for their apple-like, edible, aromatic, yellow to green, or purplish green fruits, produced in autumn, and palatable when cooked. The flowers are borne both before and with the alternately arranged, simple, toothed leaves. Grow in a shrub border, or on a bank, or train against a wall. Some flowering quinces, such as *C. japonica*, are useful as ground cover or low hedging.

- **HARDINESS** Fully hardy.
- **CULTIVATION** Grow in moderately fertile, well-drained soil in sun or partial shade. Suitable for a shaded wall, but bloom and fruit best in sun. Tolerant of lime, but may become chlorotic on very alkaline soils. Pruning group 2, or 13 if wall-trained.
- **PROPAGATION** Sow seed in containers in an open frame, or in a seedbed, in autumn. Root semi-ripe cuttings in summer. Layer in autumn.
- **PESTS AND DISEASES** Prone to canker, scale insects, and aphids.

***C.* x *californica* 'Enchantress'** ▣
Compact, spiny, upright shrub with lance-shaped, mid-green leaves, to 8cm (3in) long, light brown-woolly beneath when young. Dark rose-pink flowers, 5cm (2in) across, are produced in profuse clusters in spring, followed by large yellow fruit, to 6cm (2½in) long. ↕ 2.5m (8ft), ↔ 2m (6ft). ❄❄❄
C. cathayensis ♀ Vigorous, upright shrub or small tree with spiny shoots and lance-shaped, pointed, mid-green leaves, to 12cm (5in) long, often red-downy beneath when young. White, pink-flushed flowers, to 4cm (1½in) across, are borne in clusters of 2 or 3 blooms in early and mid-spring; they are followed by very large, yellow-green fruit, to 15cm (6in) long. ↕↔ 3m (10ft). China. ❄❄❄
C. japonica, syn. *C. maulei* (Japonica, Japanese quince, Maule's quince). Spreading, thorny shrub with obovate to rounded, glossy, mid-green leaves, to 5cm (2in) long. Abundant clusters of orange to red flowers, 4cm (1½in) across, are borne in spring, followed by yellow or yellow-flushed red fruit, 2.5–4cm (1–1½in) long. ↕ 1m (3ft), ↔ 2m (6ft). Japan. ❄❄❄
C. lagenaria see *C. speciosa*.
C. maulei see *C. japonica*.
C. speciosa, syn. *C. lagenaria, Cydonia speciosa, Pyrus japonica*. Vigorous, wide-spreading shrub with tangled, spiny branches and oval, glossy, dark green leaves, 4–9cm (1½–3½in) long. In spring, bears clusters of 2–4 scarlet to crimson flowers, 4.5cm (1¾in) across, followed by aromatic, green-yellow fruit, to 6cm (2½in) long. ↕ 2.5m (8ft), ↔ 5m (15ft). China. ❄❄❄. **'Apple Blossom'** see 'Moerloosei'. **'Falconnet Charlet'** has double, salmon-pink flowers. **'Moerloosei'** ▣🏆 syn. 'Apple Blossom', bears large white flowers, flushed dark pink. **'Nivalis'** has pure white flowers. **'Phylis Moore'** has large clusters of semi-double, light pink flowers. **'Port Eliot'** produces large red flowers. **'Simonii'** has large, double, dark blood-red flowers; ↕ 1m (3ft), ↔ 2m (6ft). **'Snow'** bears large white flowers. **'Umbilicata'** bears dark pink flowers.
C.* x *superba (*C. japonica* x *C. speciosa*). Rounded shrub with spiny, spreading branches and narrowly to broadly ovate or ovate-oblong, glossy, mid-green leaves, to 6cm (2½in) long. From spring to summer, bears clusters of cup-shaped, white, pink, orange-scarlet, or crimson to orange flowers, 3–4.5cm (1¼–1¾in) across; they are followed by green fruit, 5–7cm (2–3in) long, ripening to yellow. ↕ 1.5m (5ft), ↔ 2m (6ft). Garden origin. ❄❄❄. **'Cameo'** has double, peach-pink flowers. **'Crimson and Gold'** ▣🏆 is compact and spreading, and has dark red flowers with golden yellow anthers; ↕ 1m (3ft). **'Elly Mossel'** has large scarlet flowers. **'Etna'** is spreading, with dark scarlet flowers; ↔ 3m (10ft). **'Fire Dance'** is spreading, with large, bright red flowers. **'Knap Hill Scarlet'** 🏆 has large, bright red flowers. **'Nicoline'** ▣🏆 bears abundant large, sometimes semi-double scarlet flowers. **'Pink Lady'** ▣🏆 has very early, dark pink flowers. **'Rowallane'** 🏆 is low and spreading, with scarlet flowers; ↕ 1m (3ft).

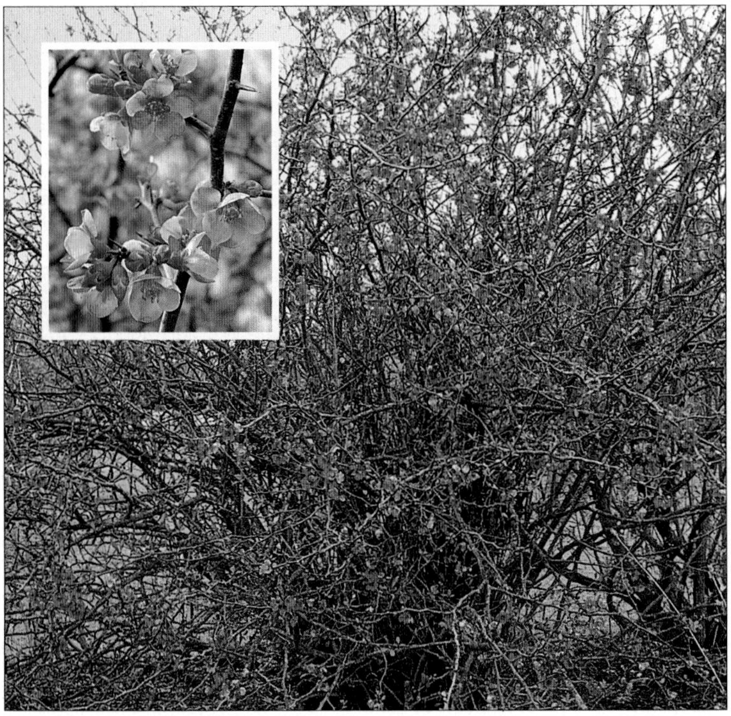

Chaenomeles x *californica* 'Enchantress' (inset: flower detail)

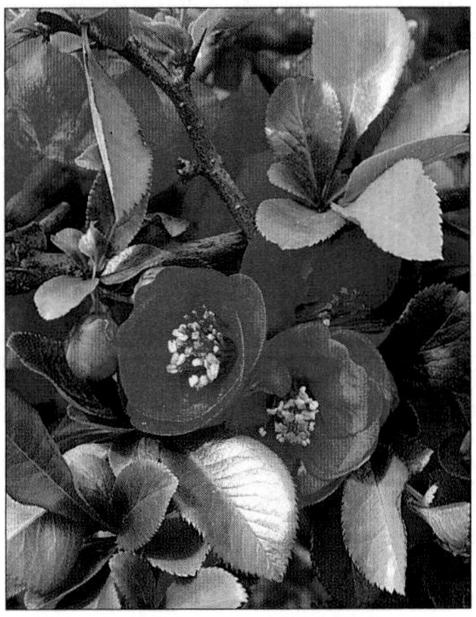

Chaenomeles x *superba* 'Nicoline'

CHAENORHINUM

Dwarf snapdragon

SCROPHULARIACEAE

Genus of about 20 species of annuals and perennials from dry, often stony soils in the Mediterranean region and in Turkey. They have branching, erect or spreading stems; 2-lipped, snapdragon-like flowers, produced either singly from the leaf axils or in terminal racemes; and opposite, simple, entire leaves. They are suitable for a rock garden, scree bed, or alpine house.

- **HARDINESS** Hardy to -10°C (14°F).
- **CULTIVATION** Grow in well-drained soil in full sun. Protect from winter wet.
- **PROPAGATION** Sow seed in containers in a cold frame in autumn. Separate rooted runners in spring.
- **PESTS AND DISEASES** Young growth is prone to damage from slugs and snails.

C. glareosum, syn. *Linaria glareosum*. Prostrate to upright, mat-forming perennial, spreading by runners, with scale-like, ovate to rounded, hairy, bluish green leaves, to 1.5cm (½in) long. Racemes of pale pinkish violet flowers, 1.5–2.5cm (½–1in) long, with yellow spurs and throats, are produced from early to late summer. ↕ 5cm (2in) if prostrate, ↕ 15–20cm (6–8in) when upright, ↔ to 20cm (8in). S. Spain. ✽✽

C

CHAEROPHYLLUM

APIACEAE/UMBELLIFERAE

Genus of about 35 species of tap-rooted or tuberous annuals, biennials, and perennials from meadows, hedgerows, and open woodland in N. temperate regions. They have fern-like, pinnate to 3-pinnate leaves and compound umbels of small, white, pink, or yellow flowers. Use in a border or a woodland garden; the leaves or roots of some (chervil) have culinary uses.

- **HARDINESS** Fully hardy.
- **CULTIVATION** Grow in moist, fertile soil in sun or partial shade.
- **PROPAGATION** Sow seed in containers in a cold frame as soon as ripe or in early spring.
- **PESTS AND DISEASES** Susceptible to damage from aphids, slugs, and snails. Powdery mildew may be a problem in dry spells.

C. aureum (Golden chervil). Clump-forming perennial with erect stems and mildly aniseed-flavoured, 3-pinnate, yellow-green leaves, 1–4cm (½–1½in) long, comprising lance-shaped, toothed or lobed leaflets. Umbels of white flowers, 5–10cm (2–4in) across, are borne in early summer. ↕ to 1.2m (4ft), ↔ 45cm (18in). C. and S. Europe, S.W. Asia. ✽✽✽

C. hirsutum. Upright, hairy perennial producing 2- or 3-pinnate, apple-scented, mid-green, sometimes purple-flushed leaves, 12–30cm (5–12in) long, with ovate to heart-shaped, toothed leaflets. Umbels of white flowers, 6cm (2½in) across, are borne from late spring to midsummer. ↕ 60cm (24in), ↔ 30cm (12in). Spain and France to S.W. Russia. ✽✽✽. **'Roseum'** ▣ syn. 'Rubrifolium', bears umbels of pink flowers.

▷**Chain fern** see *Woodwardia*
Asian see *W. unigemmata*
European see *W. radicans*
▷**Chain plant** see *Callisia fragrans*, *C. navicularis*
▷***Chamaecereus silvestrii*** see *Echinopsis chamaecereus*

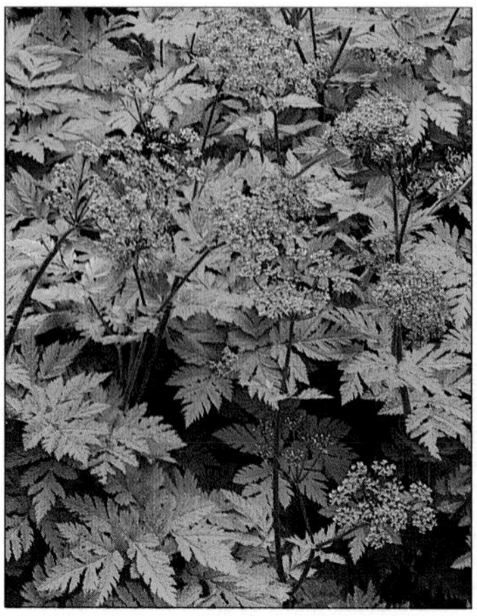

Chaerophyllum hirsutum 'Roseum'

CHAMAECYPARIS

Cypress

CUPRESSACEAE

Genus of 7 species of monoecious, evergreen, coniferous trees from forest in Taiwan, Japan, and North America. They have flattened sprays of scale-like, overlapping adult leaves, 1–5mm (1/16–¼in) long, and larger, ovate to linear juvenile leaves, 2–8mm (1/16–3/8in) long. The spherical or angular female cones have 2, occasionally 3–5 seeds on each shield-like scale, and most ripen in the first autumn. The spherical or ovoid male cones, usually 1–5mm (1/16–¼in) long, are borne in spring. Cypresses are used as specimen trees and for hedging; they have given rise to a vast number of cultivars, many dwarf or slow-growing and suitable for rock gardens or bonsai. Contact with the foliage may aggravate skin allergies.

- **HARDINESS** Fully hardy.
- **CULTIVATION** Tolerant of chalky soils but best grown in moist but well-drained, preferably neutral to slightly acid soil in full sun. Trim hedging from late spring to early autumn, but do not cut into older wood.
- **PROPAGATION** Sow seed in a seedbed outdoors in spring, or root semi-ripe cuttings in late summer. Some dwarf cultivars, especially those of *C. obtusa*, should be grafted in late winter or spring.
- **PESTS AND DISEASES** Susceptible to *Phytophthora* root rot, honey fungus, and *Coryneum* canker. Aphids may also be a problem.

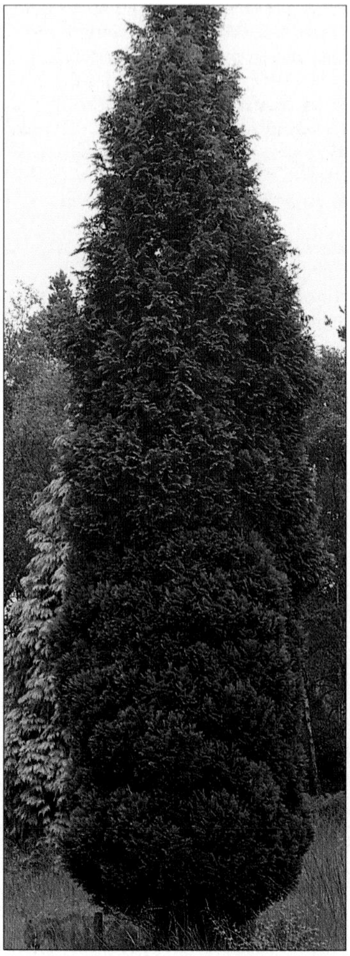

Chamaecyparis lawsoniana 'Columnaris'

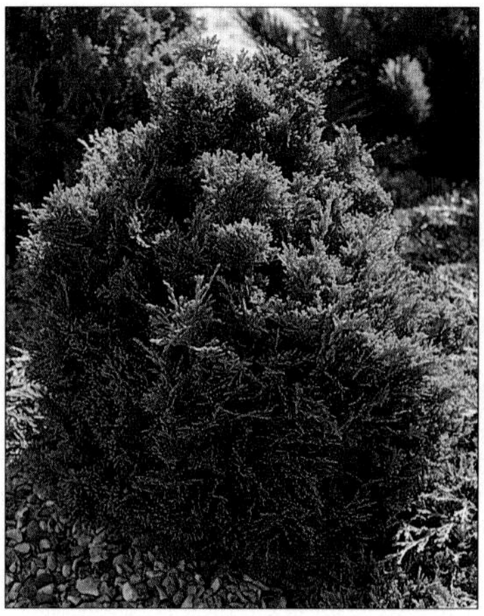

Chamaecyparis lawsoniana 'Gnome'

C. lawsoniana ▯ syn. *Cupressus lawsoniana* (Lawson cypress). Narrowly columnar, coniferous tree with a dense crown, a pendent leading shoot, and reddish brown bark forming rounded, scaly plates. Bright green mature leaves are arranged in opposite pairs; they are sharply pointed, with incurved tips and translucent central glands. Oblong male cones, 6–8mm (¼–3/8in) long, are bluish black in bud, opening brick-red. The wrinkled, reddish brown, sometimes glaucous female cones, to 1cm (½in) across, each have 8 scales. ↕ 15–40m (50–130ft), ↔ 2–5m (6–15ft). W. North America. ✽✽✽. **'Alumii'** ◊ has a narrow, conical habit, with erect sprays of blue-grey leaves, forming a billowing skirt of foliage at the base; ↕ 6–15m (20–50ft). **'Chilworth Silver'** ♀◊ is slow-growing and conical, with dense, blue-green juvenile foliage; ↕ to 1.5m (5ft). **'Columnaris'** ▣ has a columnar crown of pale blue-grey leaves; ↕ to 10m (30ft), ↔ 1m (3ft). **'Ellwoodii'** ♀ is a dense, conical shrub with erect branches and ovate, blue-grey young leaves; ↕ 3m (10ft). **'Fletcheri'** ♀ is similar to 'Ellwoodii' but larger, with greyer foliage; ↕ to 12m (40ft). **'Gnome'** ▣◯ is rounded and spreading, with bluish green foliage; ↕ 1m (3ft). **'Green Pillar'**, syn. 'Green Spire', has an upright habit with bright green foliage, good for low-maintenance hedges. **'Intertexta'** ▣♀ has hard, grey-green foliage in lax, pendent sprays. It eventually forms a tall tree and develops a crown with erratic, spreading branches. **'Kilmacurragh'** ♀ is a narrow-crowned tree with bright

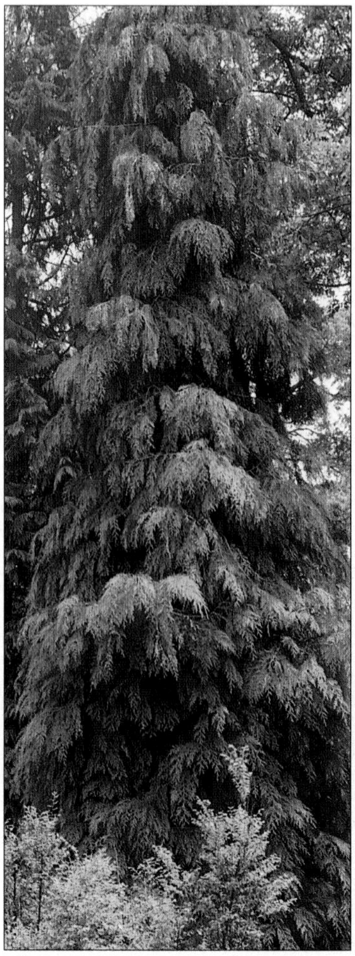

Chamaecyparis lawsoniana 'Intertexta'

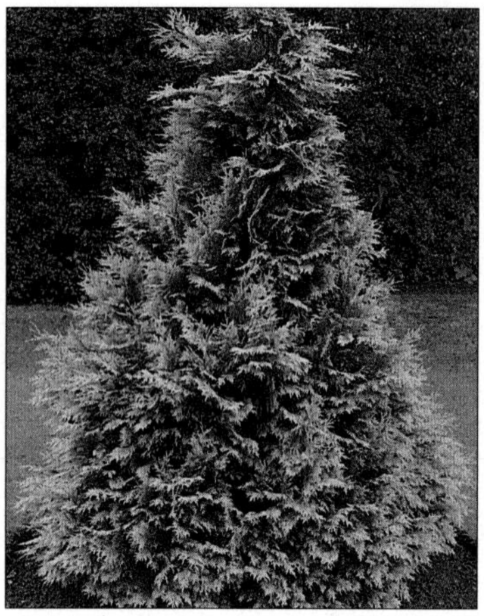

Chamaecyparis lawsoniana 'Lane'

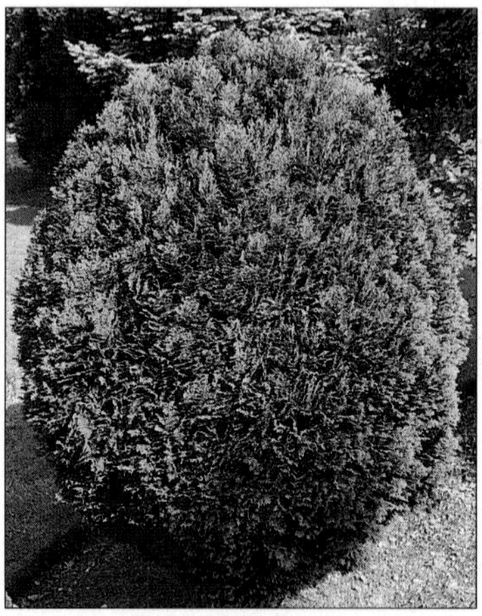

Chamaecyparis lawsoniana 'Minima'

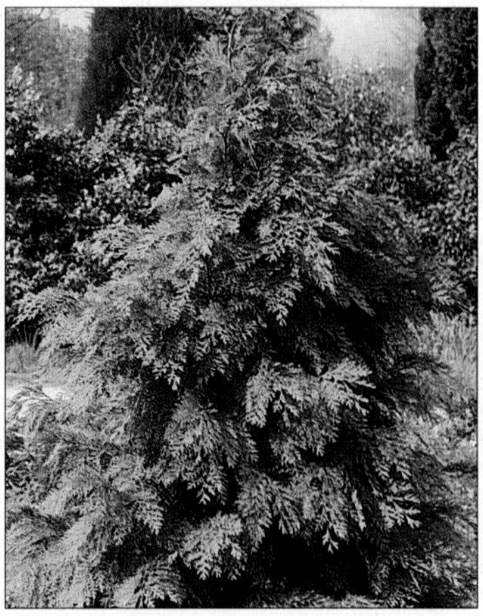

Chamaecyparis lawsoniana 'Pembury Blue'

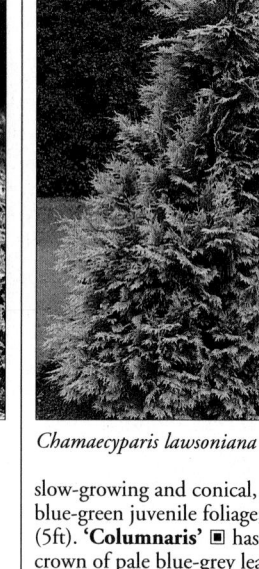

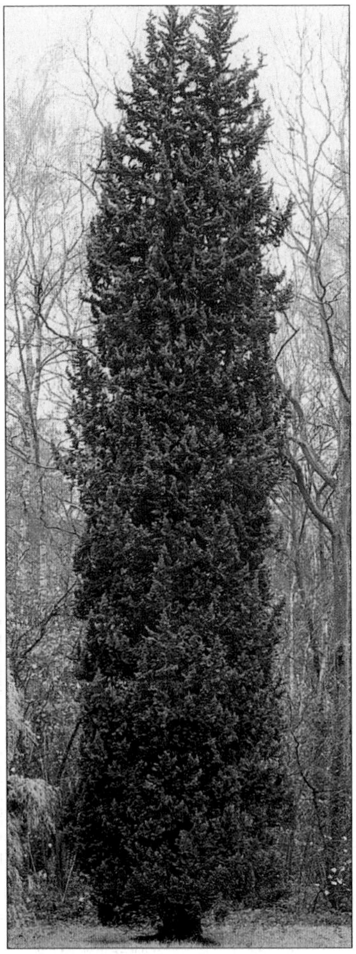

Chamaecyparis lawsoniana 'Wisselii'

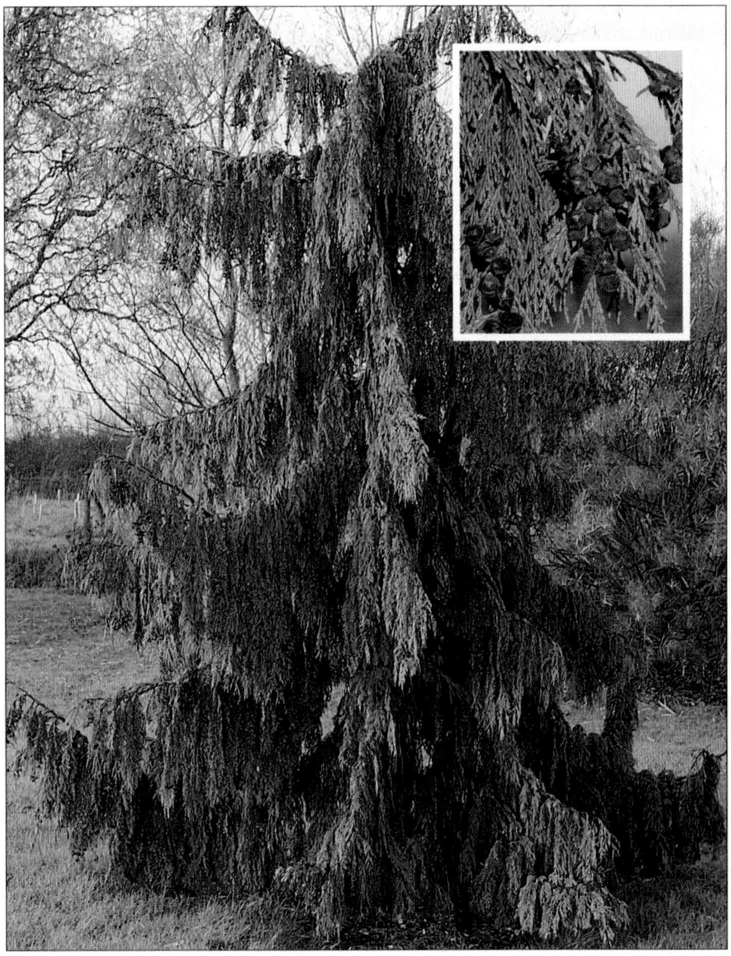

Chamaecyparis nootkatensis 'Pendula' (inset: cone detail)

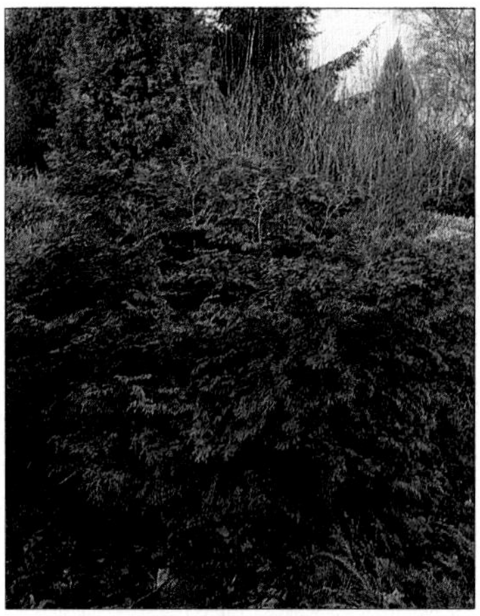

Chamaecyparis obtusa 'Pygmaea'

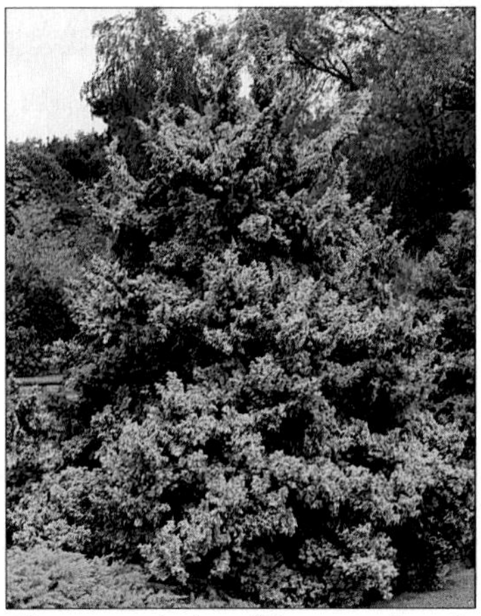

Chamaecyparis obtusa 'Tetragona Aurea'

green foliage; ↕10–15m (30–50ft). **'Lane'** ■ 𝕐 ◊ syn. 'Lanei', is narrowly conical, with leaves golden yellow above and green-yellow beneath. **'Lutea'** 𝕐 ◊ is narrowly columnar or conical, slow-growing at first, with pendent sprays of golden yellow foliage; ↕15–20m (50–70ft). **'Minima'** ■ ○–△ has a very dwarf, rounded to conical habit, with upswept branches and rounded sprays of bluish green foliage; ↕to 1.5m (5ft). **'Nana'** ◊ is similar to 'Minima' but forms a central trunk with yellow leaves; ↕to 2m (6ft). **'Pembury Blue'** ■ 𝕐 ◊ is a conical tree producing pendent sprays of bright blue-grey foliage; ↕to 15m (50ft). **'Pottenii'** ◊ has a spindle-shaped crown with a conical tip, and feathery, yellow- to grey-green foliage. **'Stardust'** 𝕐 ◊–△ is a slow-growing, narrowly to broadly conical tree with fern-like yellow foliage. **'Winston Churchill'** ◊ is a narrowly conical tree with golden foliage. **'Wisselii'** ■ 𝕐 ◊ is a narrowly conical tree with 3-dimensional sprays of blue-grey or blue-green foliage; it bears a mass of male cones in spring; ↕20–25m (70–80ft).

C. nootkatensis ◊ syn. *Cupressus nootkatensis* (Nootka cypress). Conical, occasionally columnar, coniferous tree with brown-grey bark, peeling in large plates, and sharply pointed, free-tipped, scale-like, dark green mature leaves arranged in long, pendent sprays. Green female cones, 1cm (½in) long, with a recurved central hook on each of the 4–6 scales, ripen in spring. Male cones are ovoid, brownish green, and 3mm (⅛in) long. ↕to 30m (100ft), ↔ to 8m (25ft). W. North America (Alaska to Oregon). ✱✱✱. **'Aurea'** ◊ has yellow foliage when young, maturing to yellow-green. **'Pendula'** ■ 𝕐 ⌓ has a pendent habit, with vertical sprays of hanging foliage and a gaunt, open crown when mature.

C. obtusa △ syn. *Cupressus obtusa* (Hinoki cypress). Broad, conical, coniferous tree with soft, stringy bark. Glandless, blunt, dark green mature leaves, with bright white bands beneath, are borne in 2 unequal pairs. The green, then brown, female cones are 1–2cm (½–¾in) across, and have 8–12 scales. Male cones are spherical, orange-brown, and 8–10mm (⅜–½in) across. A good specimen tree. ↕to 20m (70ft), ↔ to 6m (20ft). S. Japan. ✱✱✱. **'Crippsii'** ■ 𝕐 syn. 'Crippsii Aurea', is slow-growing with rich golden foliage. A fine specimen tree, best planted in full sun; ↕15m (50ft), ↔ 8m (25ft). **'Fernspray Gold'** is slow-growing, the branches clothed with short, rich golden yellow, fern-like leaves. **'Nana Aurea'** ■ 𝕐 is a flat-topped, dwarf shrub with golden yellow foliage, greener when grown in shade; ↕2m (6ft). **'Nana Gracilis'** 𝕐 has a dense, pyramidal habit with rich green foliage; ↕3m (10ft). **'Pygmaea'** ■ is a rounded, dwarf shrub with red-brown shoots and fan-shaped, bright green foliage, becoming brown over winter; ↕1.5m (5ft). **'Tempelhof'** is an ovoid or conical, dwarf shrub with yellow-green foliage, turning bronze in winter; ↕2.5m (8ft) **'Tetragona Aurea'** ■ 𝕐 has 4-ranked, golden yellow to bronze-yellow leaves, which are greener when grown in shade; ↕to 10m (30ft).

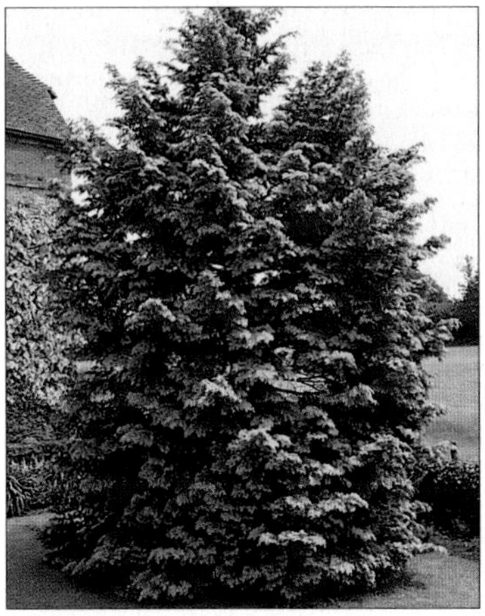

Chamaecyparis obtusa 'Crippsii'

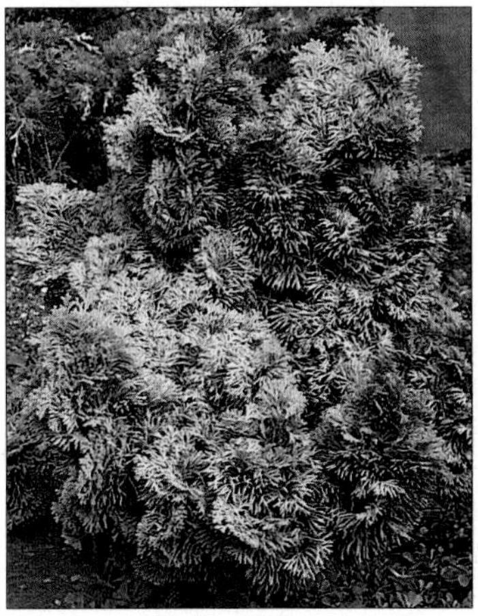

Chamaecyparis obtusa 'Nana Aurea'

C. pisifera △ syn. *Cupressus pisifera* (Sawara cypress). Initially broad, conical, coniferous tree with an open crown and hard, fissured, finely peeling, red-brown bark. Pairs of sharp-pointed, bright green mature leaves, marked white beneath, with small glands and free-spreading tips, are produced in flattened sprays. Angular female cones, to 7mm (¼in) long, are green, maturing to deep brown, with 6–8 scales. Black male cones are spherical, to 7mm (¼in) across. ↕to 20m (70ft), ↔ to 5m (15ft). S. Japan. ✱✱✱. **'Boulevard'** 𝕐 has soft, blue-green foliage. Needs a moist site; ↕10m (30ft). **'Filifera'** has slender, whip-like shoots, which are mostly unbranched, and dark green leaves. **'Filifera Aurea'** ■ 𝕐 is similar to 'Filifera' but has golden yellow leaves

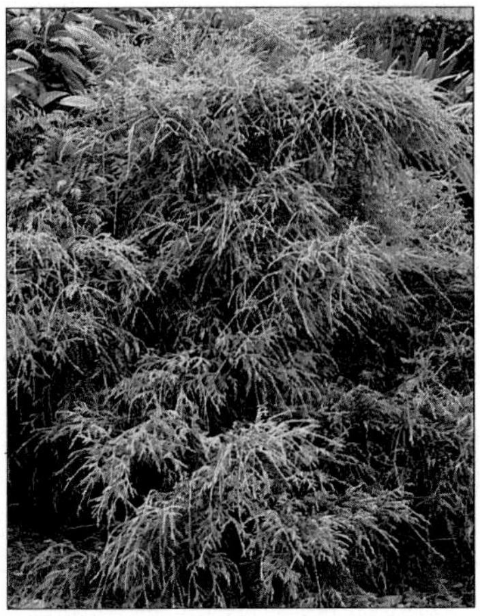

Chamaecyparis pisifera 'Filifera Aurea'

C

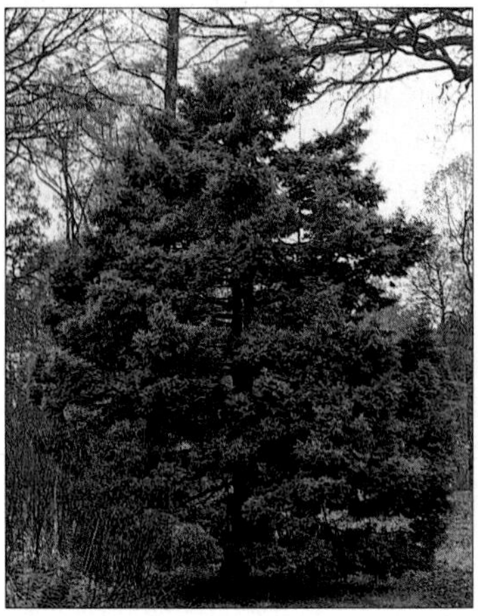

Chamaecyparis pisifera 'Squarrosa'

and is slower-growing; ↕ 12m (40ft). **'Plumosa'** is erect and broadly conical, with billowing foliage. The yellowish grey-green, semi-juvenile leaves, 2–4mm (1/16–1/8in) long, have free tips; ↔ 8m (25ft). **'Squarrosa'** ■ syn. 'Squarrosa Veitchii', has soft young leaves, 5–8mm (1/4–3/8in) long, with free tips. It is similar in habit to 'Plumosa' but tends to open up, losing the inner foliage.
C. thyoides ■ ◊ syn. *Cupressus thyoides* (White cypress). Narrowly conical, coniferous tree with dull red-brown or grey-brown bark. Sharply pointed, dark grey-green, sometimes glaucous mature leaves, with incurved tips and central glands, are produced on erratic sprays of fine shoots. The angular female cones, to 6mm (1/4in) across, are purple-black to red-brown, initially glaucous, and have 6–10 scales. Spherical male cones are brown, and to 7mm (1/4in) across. ↕ to 15m (50ft), ↔ to 4m (12ft). E. USA. ❄❄❄. **'Andelyensis'** is a neat, conical shrub with linear, bluish green leaves; ↕ to 3m (10ft).

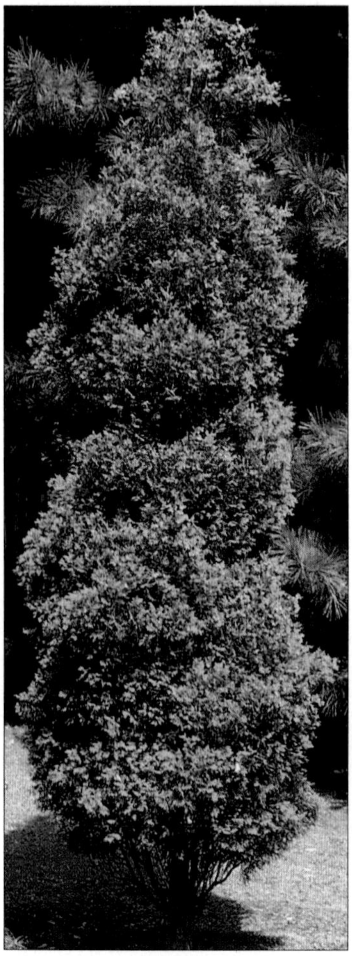

Chamaecyparis thyoides

CHAMAECYTISUS

LEGUMINOSAE/PAPILIONACEAE

Genus of about 30 species of evergreen and deciduous, occasionally spiny, small trees, shrubs, and subshrubs found mainly on hillsides and in open woodland, from sea level to 2,000m (7,000ft), in Europe and the Canary Islands. Some species were previously included in the genus *Cytisus.* They have alternate, 3-palmate leaves, sometimes with softly hairy leaflets, and are grown for their pea-like, usually yellow, sometimes purple-pink or white flowers, borne on short, axillary shoots or in terminal racemes or clusters. Grow on a sunny bank or in a shrub border, rock garden, trough, or raised bed. *C. purpureus* is sometimes top-grafted on to *Laburnum* understock to produce a small standard tree. In frost-prone areas, grow half-hardy species in a cool greenhouse or conservatory.

- **HARDINESS** Fully hardy to half hardy.
- **CULTIVATION** Tolerant of a range of soil types, including poor, dry soils, but not shallow soils over chalk. Best in moderately fertile, well-drained soil in full sun. Root disturbance is resented, so plant out directly from containers into the final location as soon as possible. Pruning group 3 or 10, after flowering, or in spring for *C. supinus. C. demissus* needs little pruning. Do not cut back hard as plants seldom recover fully.
- **PROPAGATION** Sow seed in containers in a cold frame in autumn or spring. Root semi-ripe cuttings in summer.
- **PESTS AND DISEASES** Red spider mites may be a problem under glass.

C. demissus 🏆 syn. *C. hirsutus* var. *demissus.* Slow-growing, prostrate, hairy shrublet with deciduous, 3-palmate, mid-green leaves, 0.6–1.5cm (1/4–1/2in) long, silky-hairy beneath, composed of oblong-obovate to inversely lance-shaped leaflets. Axillary clusters of 2–4 yellow flowers, to 3cm (1¼in) across, with brown keels and an involucre of brown bracts, are borne in late spring and early summer. Suitable for a rock garden or trough. ↕ 8cm (3in), ↔ 20cm (8in) or more. Greece. ❄❄❄

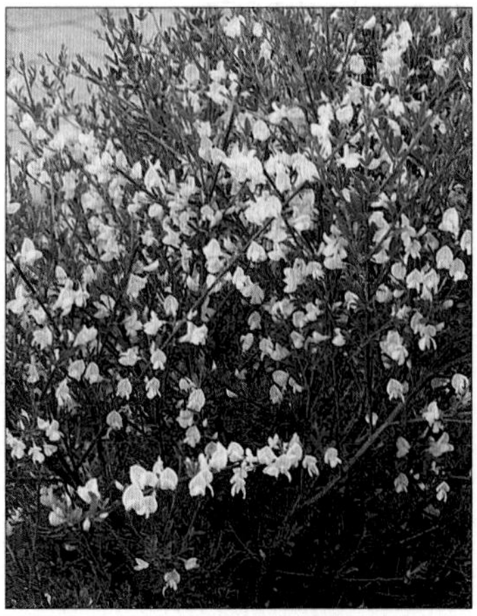

Chamaecytisus purpureus f. *albus*

C. hirsutus* var. *demissus see *C. demissus.*
C. purpureus, syn. *Cytisus purpureus* (Purple broom). Deciduous, dense, semi-erect shrub with smooth, branching stems and 3-palmate, dark green leaves, to 2.5cm (1in) long, with obovate leaflets. In early summer, bears axillary clusters of 2 or 3 pale pink to deep lilac flowers, to 2.5cm (1in) across, with darker throats. ↕ 45cm (18in), ↔ 60cm (24in). S.E. Europe. ❄❄❄. **f. *albus*** ■ has white flowers.
C. supinus, syn. *Cytisus supinus.* Bushy, rounded, deciduous shrub producing shoots covered with long, spreading hairs, and 3-palmate, mid-green leaves, to 4cm (1½in) long, with oblong-elliptic leaflets. Clusters of 2–8 bright yellow flowers, to 2.5cm (1in) across, are borne at the ends of the shoots from mid-summer to autumn. ↕↔ 1m (3ft). C. and S. Europe. ❄❄❄

CHAMAEDAPHNE

syn. CASSANDRA

ERICACEAE

Genus of one species of evergreen shrub found in moist, peaty soil, in bogs and at pond margins in N. temperate regions of Europe, Asia, and North America. It has alternate, glossy, dark green leaves and urn-shaped white flowers. Suitable for a peat or woodland garden.

- **HARDINESS** Fully hardy.
- **CULTIVATION** Grow in moist, peaty, acid soil in sun or dappled shade. Pruning group 8.
- **PROPAGATION** Root semi-ripe cuttings in summer.
- **PESTS AND DISEASES** Trouble free.

C. calyculata (Leatherleaf). Evergreen shrub with slender, arching shoots and obovate to oblong, leathery, glossy, dark green leaves, to 5cm (2in) long, scaly beneath. In spring, bears small, urn-shaped white flowers in arching, one-sided, leafy racemes, 4–12cm (1½–5in) long, at the ends of the shoots. ↕ 75cm (30in), ↔ 90cm (36in). N. Europe, N. Asia, North America. ❄❄❄. **'Nana'** is compact and free-flowering; ↕ 45cm (18in), ↔ 75cm (30in).

CHAMAEDOREA

ARECACEAE/PALMAE

Genus of about 100 species of mainly small palms from rainforest in Mexico and Central and South America. They are valued for their leaves, which are pinnate or resemble a fish's tail, often arching, either tufted or alternate, and borne on erect and flexible, sometimes scandent stems. Insignificant, 3-petalled flowers are borne in spikes or panicles, followed by small fruits, 0.6–1.5cm (1/4–1/2in) across. In frost-prone areas, grow as houseplants, or in containers or borders in a warm conservatory or greenhouse. In warmer areas, grow in a shaded border or courtyard.

- **HARDINESS** Frost tender.
- **CULTIVATION** Under glass, grow in loamless potting compost in bright filtered or indirect light, shaded from hot sun. In the growing season, water freely and apply a balanced liquid fertilizer monthly; water sparingly in winter. Pot on or top-dress in spring. Outdoors, grow in humus-rich, moist but well-drained, neutral to acid soil, in full or partial shade.
- **PROPAGATION** Sow seed in spring at not less than 25°C (77°F).
- **PESTS AND DISEASES** Prone to red spider mites, scale insects, and thrips under glass.

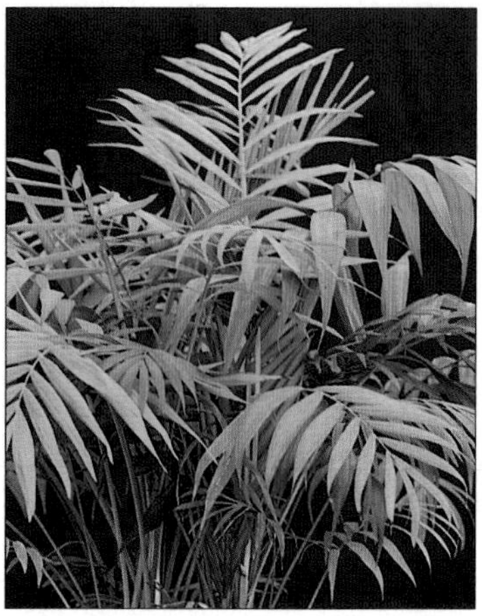

Chamaedorea elegans

C. elegans ■ 🏆 ✲ syn. *Neanthe bella* (Parlour palm). Slender-stemmed palm with a terminal tuft of pinnate, rich green leaves, to 60cm (24in) long, comprising 21–40 linear to lance-shaped leaflets. Tiny yellow flowers are borne in erect, simple or branched panicles, 15–30cm (8–12in) long, from spring to autumn, followed by small, spherical black fruit. ↕ 2–3m (6–10ft), ↔ 1–2m (3–6ft). Mexico, Guatemala. ⊛ (min. 16°C/61°F). **'Bella'** has a more compact tuft of leaves, and flowers freely.
C. metallica 🏆 ✲ (Miniature fish-tail palm). Very small palm with a single, cane-like stem and a terminal tuft of foliage. The semi-lustrous, deep bluish green leaves, 30–50cm (12–20in) long, are slightly puckered and shaped like a fish's tail. In summer, produces orange to red flowers in panicles 20–35cm (8–14in) long, just below the leaves,

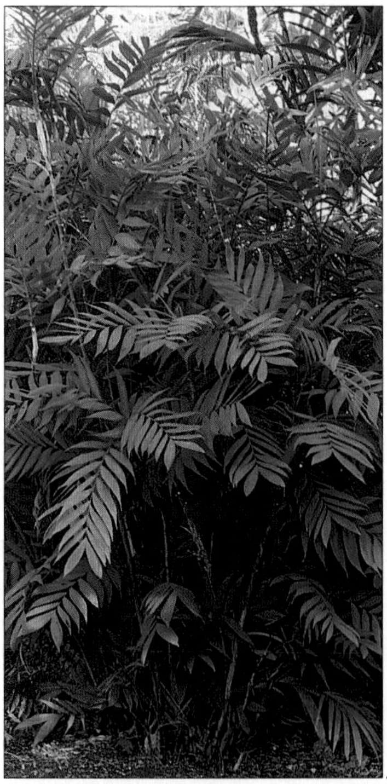

Chamaedorea microspadix

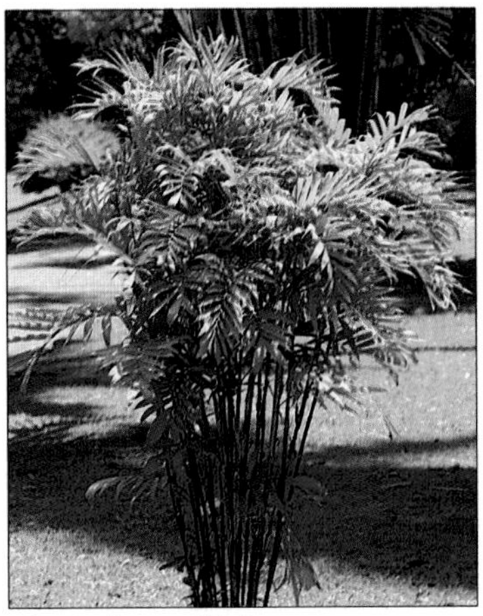

Chamaedorea seifrizii

followed by small, ovoid black fruit. ↕ to 1m (3ft), ↔ to 50cm (20in). Mexico. ❀ (min. 16°C/61°F)

C. microspadix ■ ✻ Small palm with groups of cane-like stems. Alternate, pinnate, blue-green leaves, 20–40cm (8–16in) long, have tubular, basal sheaths and 14–18 lance-shaped leaflets. In summer, cream to white flowers are borne in arching to pendent panicles, 15–23cm (6–9in) long, followed by small, spherical, orange-red fruit. ↕ to 3m (10ft), ↔ to 1.5m (5ft). E. Mexico. ❀ (min. 16°C/61°F)

C. seifrizii ■ ♀ ✻ (Reed palm). Small, clump-forming palm with flexible, cane-like stems that may be semi-scandent in mature or large specimens. Alternate or loosely clustered, pinnate, rich green leaves, to 60cm (24in) long, have 24–28 narrowly lance-shaped leaflets. Yellow flowers are borne in erect panicles, 15–25cm (6–10in) long, either on stalks or just above the foliage. The small, spherical fruit are black. ↕ 1–2m (3–6ft), ↔ 1–1.5m (3–5ft). Mexico (Yucatan). ❀ (min. 16°C/61°F)

CHAMAEMELUM

Chamomile

ASTERACEAE/COMPOSITAE

Genus of 4 species of aromatic annuals and perennials from grassy pastures and wasteland in Europe. The leaves are feathery, alternate, and pinnate then pinnatisect. The flowerheads are daisy-like, with yellow disc-florets and white ray-florets. *C. nobile* is grown for its medicinal flowers and for its foliage, which releases an apple-like fragrance when crushed. Close planting produces a dense sward, ideal for lawns and seats; the non-flowering cultivar *C. nobile* 'Treneague' is best for this purpose.

- **HARDINESS** Fully hardy.
- **CULTIVATION** Grow in an open site in well-drained, preferably light, sandy soil in full sun. To produce a lawn or seat, plant 12–15cm (5–6in) apart, and water freely until established. Cut the plants back regularly to encourage dense, compact growth; occasional rolling and treading of lawns will help to maintain an even surface.
- **PROPAGATION** Sow seed *in situ* or divide in spring. Increase *C. nobile* 'Treneague' by division.
- **PESTS AND DISEASES** Trouble free.

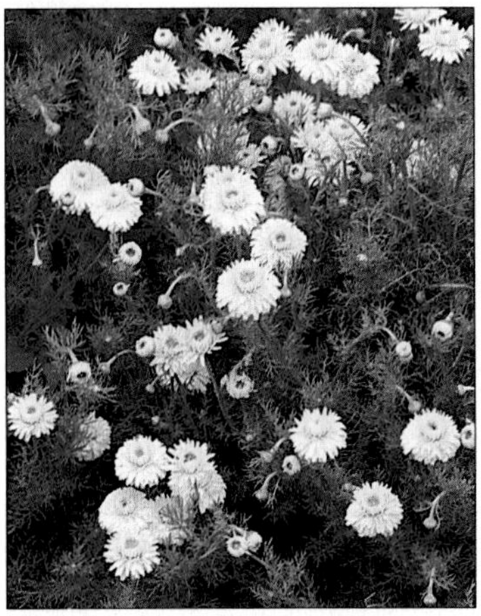

Chamaemelum nobile 'Flore Pleno'

C. nobile, syn. *Anthemis nobilis* (Lawn chamomile, Roman chamomile). Mat-forming, hairy, aromatic perennial with stalkless, oblong, fresh green leaves, to 5cm (2in) long, divided into thread-like segments. In summer, bears daisy-like flowerheads, 0.7–1.5cm (¼–½in) across, singly on long stalks. May be invasive. Contact with foliage may aggravate skin allergies. ↕ 30cm (12in), ↔ 45cm (18in). W. Europe. ✲✲✲. **'Flore Pleno'** ■ has double, button-like flowerheads, and is ideal for edging a herb border; ↕ 15cm (6in), ↔ 45cm (18in). **'Treneague'** is a low, tufted, non-flowering cultivar that roots where the decumbent stems touch the soil. It has strongly scented foliage, and is less vigorous than the species; ↕ 10cm (4in), ↔ 45cm (18in).

▷ ***Chamaenerion*** see *Epilobium*
C. angustifolium* f. *album see *E. angustifolium* f. *album*
▷ ***Chamaepericlymenum*** see *Cornus*
C. canadense see *C. canadensis*

CHAMAEROPS

Dwarf fan palm

ARECACEAE/PALMAE

Genus of one species of shrubby palm from dry scrub and rocky or sandy slopes in the W. Mediterranean region. Its pinnate leaves are densely borne in tufts or rosettes, and the tiny, 3-petalled flowers are produced in panicles from the lower leaf axils. In frost-prone areas, *C. humilis* is best grown in a cool greenhouse or as a houseplant. In warmer areas, use as a specimen plant for a small garden.

- **HARDINESS** Half hardy; may survive short spells just below 0°C (32°F).
- **CULTIVATION** Under glass, grow in loam-based potting compost (JI No.3) in full to bright indirect light. When in growth, water moderately and apply a balanced liquid fertilizer monthly; water sparingly in winter. Pot on or top-dress in spring. Outdoors, grow in well-drained, preferably moderately fertile soil in full sun; poor soil and partial shade is tolerated.
- **PROPAGATION** Sow seed at not less than 22°C (72°F) in spring, or separate suckers from established plants in late spring.
- **PESTS AND DISEASES** Red spider mites may be a problem under glass.

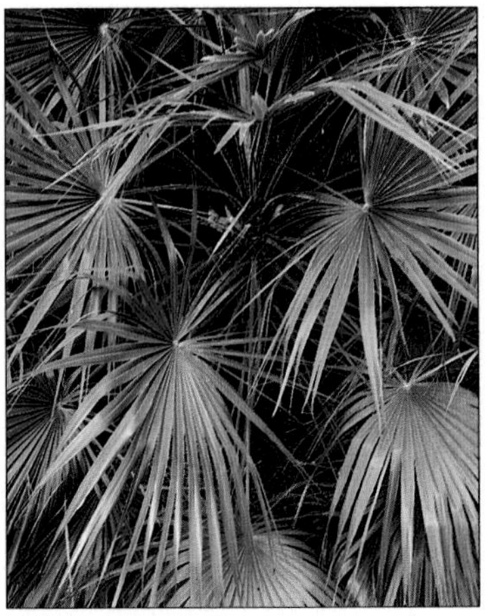

Chamaerops humilis

C. humilis ■ ♀ ✻ Bushy palm, producing suckers when mature, with broad, pinnate, bluish or greyish green leaves, 60–100cm (24–39in) long, composed of 12–15 linear leaflets. Yellow flowers are borne in dense, almost hidden panicles, to 35cm (14in) long, from spring to summer. ↕ 2–3m (6–10ft), ↔ 1–2m (3–6ft). Mediterranean. ✲

▷ ***Chamaespartium*** see *Genista*
C. sagittale see *G. sagittalis*
C. sagittale* subsp. *delphinense see *G. delphinensis*

CHAMELAUCIUM

MYRTACEAE

Genus of 21 species of evergreen shrubs from Western Australia, found on sandy heaths and in seasonally dry scrub. The narrow leaves are usually borne in opposite pairs, and the small, clustered flowers, for which these plants are valued, each have 5 rounded, spreading petals and a cup-shaped centre. In frost-prone areas, grow in a cool greenhouse or conservatory. In warmer climates, use to add colour and character to a shrub border or grow against a house wall; also useful for hedging.

- **HARDINESS** Most species are frost tender, but *C. uncinatum* will withstand short spells around 0°C (32°F).
- **CULTIVATION** Under glass, grow in lime-free (ericaceous) potting compost in full light with shade from hot sun. When in growth, water moderately, and apply a balanced liquid fertilizer monthly to well-established plants; water sparingly in winter. Pot on or top-dress in late winter. Outdoors, grow in sharply drained, neutral to acid, poor to moderately fertile, sandy soil in full sun.

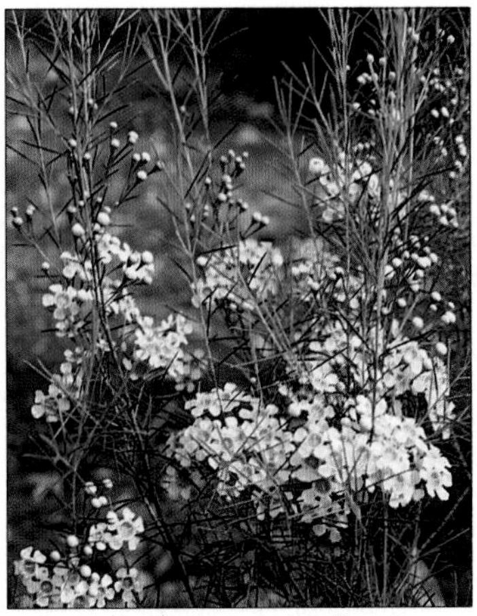

Chamelaucium uncinatum 'Album'

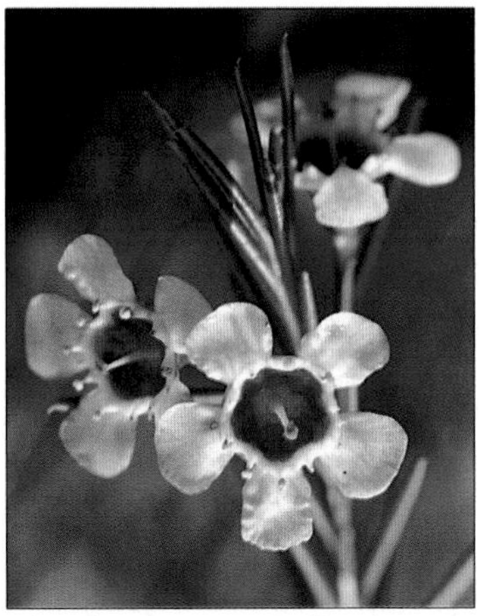

Chamelaucium uncinatum 'Bundara Excelsior'

Pruning group 8; plants under glass may need restrictive pruning.

- **PROPAGATION** Surface-sow seed at 13–18°C (55–64°F) in spring. Root greenwood cuttings in early summer or semi-ripe cuttings in late summer.
- **PESTS AND DISEASES** Root-rotting fungi may be a problem outdoors.

C. uncinatum (Geraldton wax). Large, erect to spreading, open shrub producing linear, 3-angled, dark green leaves, 2–4cm (¾–1½in) long, with hooked tips. Purple, mauve, red, pink, or white flowers, to 2.5cm (1in) across, are borne in abundant clusters, 5–10cm (2–4in) across, from spring to summer. Excellent for cut flowers; drought tolerant. ↕ 2–5m (6–15ft), ↔ 2–4m (6–12ft). Australia (Western Australia). ✲ (borderline). **'Album'** ■ bears pure white flowers. **'Bundara Excelsior'** ■ bears large pink blooms. **'Purple Pride'** has red-purple flowers.

▷ **Chamomile** see *Chamaemelum*
Lawn see *Chamaemelum nobile*
Ox-eye see *Anthemis tinctoria*
Roman see *Chamaemelum nobile*

CHASMANTHE

IRIDACEAE

Genus of 3 species of cormous perennials, related to *Crocosmia*, from semi-shaded sites in South Africa. They are valued for their attractive, spike-like racemes of hooded, tubular, orange or red flowers, borne from spring to summer. Their narrow, linear, lance- or sword-shaped, mid-green leaves form a flat, basal fan. Excellent for a mixed or herbaceous border.

- **HARDINESS** Fully hardy.
- **CULTIVATION** Grow in fertile, moist but well-drained soil in sun or partial shade. Cut down in late winter, before new growth begins.
- **PROPAGATION** Sow seed at 13–16°C (55–61°F) in spring, or divide in spring.
- **PESTS AND DISEASES** Trouble free.

C. aethiopica. Clump-forming, cormous perennial with lance-shaped or linear leaves, 40–60cm (16–24in) long. From spring to early summer, bears spike-like, one-sided racemes, 15–18cm (6–7in) long, of red or orange flowers, 8cm (3in) long, with maroon throats and yellow-striped tubes. ↕ to 70cm (28in), ↔ 5cm (2in). South Africa. ✲

C. floribunda. Clump-forming, cormous perennial producing lance-shaped leaves, 30–50cm (12–20in) long. Numerous bright orange or yellow flowers, to 8cm (3in) long, arranged in 2 ranks, are borne on branched spikes, 30cm (12in) long, in summer. ↕0.5–1.5m (20–60in), ↔ 15cm (6in). South Africa. ❄

CHASMANTHIUM

GRAMINEAE/POACEAE

Genus of about 6 species of perennial grasses, mostly from woodland in E. and C. USA, Mexico, and Central America. *C. latifolium*, the species most often cultivated, is bamboo-like with unusual flowerheads, which may be dried if cut before they are fully mature. Grow in a mixed or herbaceous border, or in a woodland garden.

- **HARDINESS** Fully hardy.
- **CULTIVATION** Grow in fertile, moist but well-drained soil in sun or partial shade. Cut down in late winter.
- **PROPAGATION** Sow seed in containers in a cold frame in spring, or divide between mid-spring and early summer.
- **PESTS AND DISEASES** Trouble free.

C. latifolium, syn. *Uniola latifolia* (Sea Oats, Spangle grass). Loosely tufted, spreading, perennial grass with broadly lance-shaped, arching, mid-green leaves, 10–25cm (4–10in) long, that turn yellow in winter. In late summer and early autumn, bears open panicles of flat, oblong-lance-shaped to broadly ovate green spikelets, 1cm (½in) long, ageing to brown, and breaking up at maturity. ↕1m (3ft), ↔ 60cm (24in). E. USA, N. Mexico. ❄❄❄

▷ **Chaste tree** see *Vitex agnus-castus*
▷ **Checkerberry** see *Gaultheria procumbens*
▷ **Checkerbloom** see *Sidalcea malviflora*
▷ **Cheesewood** see *Pittosporum undulatum*

CHEILANTHES

Lip fern

ADIANTACEAE

Genus of 150 or more species of mainly evergreen ferns, distributed worldwide. They are very drought-resistant, often growing between rocks, in near-deserts or deserts; the fronds shrivel in drought and recover after rain. They have erect or creeping rhizomes, producing dense clumps of small, pinnate to 3-pinnate, usually dull green fronds on shiny black stalks. The undersides of the leaf-blades may be white-mealy and covered with minute hairs or scales. Spores are formed at the margins of the frond segments, which curl under to protect them. In dry climates, grow in a scree bed, rock garden, or in a stone wall. Elsewhere, grow in containers in a cool or temperate greenhouse.

- **HARDINESS** Fully hardy to frost tender, but intolerant of excessive moisture.
- **CULTIVATION** Under glass, grow in a mix of equal parts loam-based potting compost (JI No.2), charcoal, and dolomitic limestone chippings, in full light. Provide low humidity and good ventilation. In the growing season, water sparingly (avoid wetting the foliage), and apply a half-strength, balanced

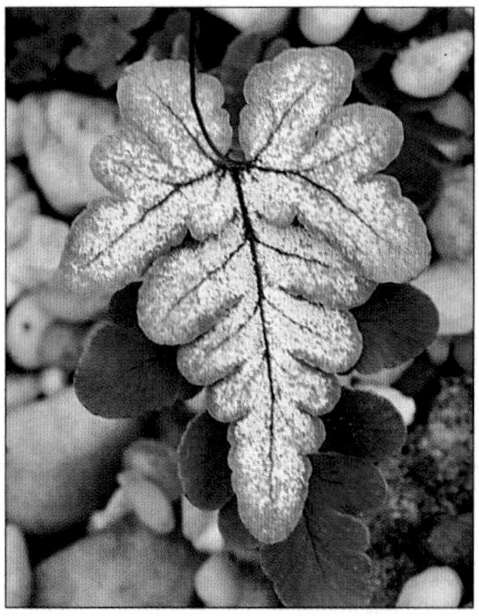

Cheilanthes argentea

liquid fertilizer monthly; keep almost dry in winter. Pot on every 2 or 3 years in spring. Outdoors, grow in sharply drained, gritty, humus-rich soil in full sun. Protect *C. fragrans* and *C. tomentosa* from winter rain.

- **PROPAGATION** Sow spores at 16°C (61°F) as soon as ripe. Divide in spring; this is less likely to be successful than sowing spores, because the rhizomes resent disturbance. See also p.51.
- **PESTS AND DISEASES** Fungal root rot may be a problem under glass.

C. argentea ■ Evergreen fern with erect or creeping rhizomes and long-stalked, 3-angled, 2- or 3-pinnate, dull green fronds, 15–25cm (6–10in) long, with linear segments; the undersides are white- or yellowish white-mealy. ↕20cm (8in), ↔ 30cm (12in). E. Asia. ❄❄❄
C. fragrans ■ Evergreen fern with erect rhizomes producing tufts of lance-shaped, 3-pinnate, mid-green fronds, 6–12cm (2½–5in) long; the fronds have rounded segments, hairless beneath. ↕15cm (6in), ↔ 20cm (8in). S. Europe, Canary Islands, N. Africa, W. Asia (on acid rocks). ❄❄❄ (borderline)
***C. lanosa* of gardens** see *C. tomentosa.*
C. tomentosa, syn. *C. lanosa* of gardens (Hairy lip fern). Evergreen fern with erect rhizomes. Lance-shaped, pinnatifid to 2-pinnate fronds, 15–30cm (6–12in) long, have rounded, dark grey-green segments, covered with silvery scales beneath. Stalks are purplish black with hair-like scales. ↕30cm (12in), ↔ 40cm (16in). USA (Pennsylvania to New Mexico, found on neutral or acid rocks). ❄❄❄ (borderline)

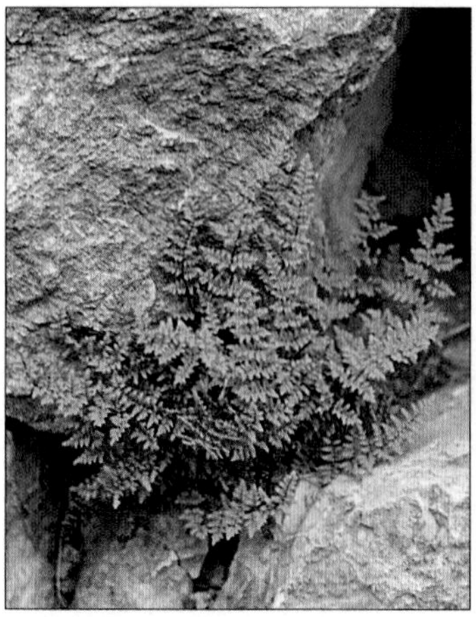

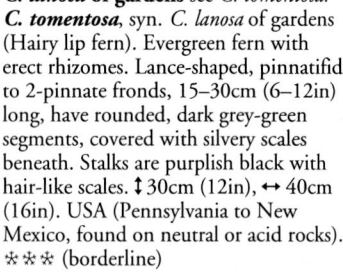

Cheilanthes fragrans

▷ ***Cheiranthus*** see *Erysimum*
C. x allionii see *E. x allionii*
C. cheiri see *E. cheiri*
***C. cheiri* 'Harpur Crewe'** see *E. x kewense* 'Harpur Crewe'

CHEIRIDOPSIS

AIZOACEAE

Genus of about 100 species of dwarf, clump-forming, perennial succulents occurring in periodically semi-arid regions of Namibia and South Africa. Smooth, velvety, fleshy leaves are produced in pairs, either entirely free or partially joined along most of their length. The daisy-like, solitary, mainly stalked flowers, borne in summer, are followed by ovoid green fruits, which contain pale brown seeds. In frost-prone areas, grow in a temperate greenhouse. In warm, dry climates, use in a border or raised bed.

- **HARDINESS** Frost tender.
- **CULTIVATION** Under glass, grow in a mix of 2 parts each loam and sharp sand and 1 part leaf mould, in full light. Provide low humidity. Water sparingly from summer to mid-autumn, applying a dilute, low-nitrogen liquid fertilizer at the beginning and end of this period; keep completely dry at other times. Outdoors, grow in gritty, humus-rich, sharply drained soil in full sun; protect from rain except when in full growth. See also pp.48–49.
- **PROPAGATION** Sow seed at 19–24°C (66–75°F), or root stem cuttings, in late spring or early summer.
- **PESTS AND DISEASES** Mealybugs may be a problem, particularly in dry weather.

C. candidissima see *C. denticulata.*
C. denticulata ■ syn. *C. candidissima.* Clump-forming succulent with paired, cylindrical, suberect, thick, greyish white leaves, to 10cm (4in) long, partially joined at the bases. Bears stalked yellow flowers, to 8cm (3in) across. ↕10cm (4in), ↔ indefinite. South Africa. ⌂ (min. 7°C/45°F)
C. purpurata see *C. purpurea.*
C. purpurea, syn. *C. purpurata.* Clump-forming succulent with pairs of angular, bluish or pinkish green leaves, to 6cm (2½in) long, flat on the upper surfaces and rounded and keeled beneath. Bears short-stalked, purplish pink or yellow flowers, 3.5cm (1½in) across. ↕10cm (4in), ↔ indefinite. South Africa, possibly Namibia. ⌂ (min. 7°C/45°F)

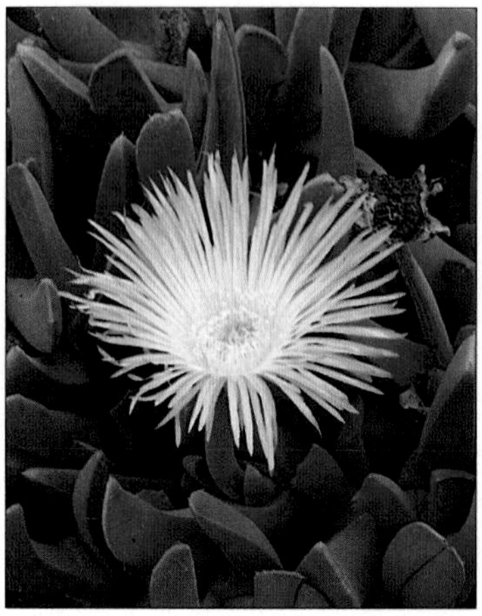

Cheiridopsis denticulata

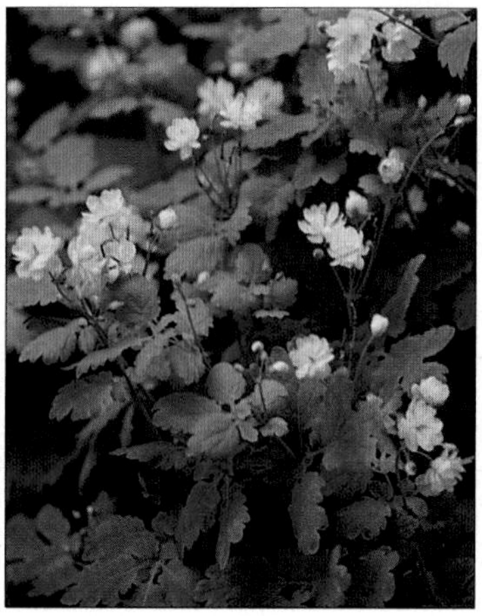

Chelidonium majus 'Flore Pleno'

CHELIDONIUM

PAPAVERACEAE

Genus of one species of variable biennial or short-lived perennial from woodland, scrub, wasteland, and rocky slopes in Europe and W. Asia. It has deeply pinnatifid or pinnatisect, hairless leaves, and bears umbels of poppy-like, bowl-shaped yellow flowers in summer. It is suitable for naturalizing in a wildflower garden or in light woodland. Contact with the orange-yellow sap may cause skin blisters.

- **HARDINESS** Fully hardy.
- **CULTIVATION** Easy to grow in any soil and in almost any situation, but prefers woodland conditions.
- **PROPAGATION** Sow seed *in situ* in early spring.
- **PEST AND DISEASES** Trouble free.

C. majus (Greater celandine). Clump-forming perennial with lobed to deeply pinnatifid or pinnatisect, scalloped, pale or slightly bluish green leaves, 10–25cm (4–10in) long. Loose, terminal umbels of 4-petalled yellow flowers, 2–2.5cm (¾–1in) across, are produced on upright, brittle stems in summer. Self-seeds profusely. ↕ to 60cm (24in), ↔ 20cm (8in). Europe, W. Asia. ❄❄❄.
'Flore Pleno' ■ has double yellow flowers.

CHELONE

Turtlehead

SCROPHULARIACEAE

Genus of about 6 species of perennials from moist woodland, prairies, and mountains of North America, valued for their strong growth and weather-resistant flowers. Turtleheads have a stiff, erect habit, and produce opposite pairs of simple, toothed, hairless leaves. The white, pink, or purple flowers, borne in short, dense, terminal racemes, from late summer to mid-autumn, are tubular and 2-lipped, with a beard on the inside of each lower lip. They are showy plants for a late summer border.

- **HARDINESS** Fully hardy.
- **CULTIVATION** Grow in deep, fertile, moist soil in an open site in partial shade or sun. Turtleheads will also grow in a bog garden, and tolerate heavy clay soil. Mulch in mid-spring with well-rotted manure or garden compost.
- **PROPAGATION** Sow seed in containers in a cold frame in early spring. Divide in

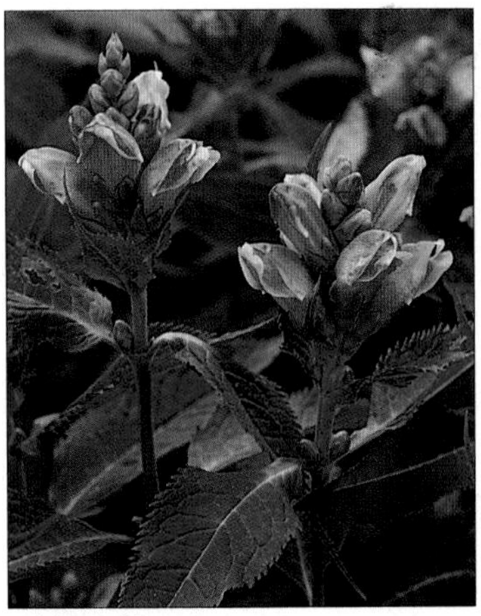

Chelone obliqua

spring. Root soft tip cuttings in late spring or early summer.

• **PESTS AND DISEASES** Susceptible to damage from slugs and snails.

C. barbata see *Penstemon barbatus.*
C. glabra, syn. *C. obliqua* var. *alba* (Turtlehead). Erect perennial with square stems and short-stalked, ovate to lance-shaped, mid-green leaves, 5–20cm (2–8in) long. Bears white or pink-tinged white flowers, 2.5cm (1in) long, with white beards. ↕60–100cm (24–39in), ↔ 45cm (18in). E. and S. North America. ❄❄❄
C. lyonii. Erect perennial with square stems and long-stalked, ovate to elliptic, toothed, mid-green leaves, 5–15cm (2–6in) long. Produces purple-pink flowers, 2.5cm (1in) long, with yellow beards. ↕ to 1.2m (4ft), ↔ 60cm (24in). Mountains of S.E. USA. ❄❄❄
C. obliqua ▣ Erect perennial with more rounded stems than other species, and short-stalked, broadly lance-shaped to lance-shaped-elliptic, toothed or incised, boldly veined, dark green leaves, 5–20cm (2–8in) long. Bears dark pink or purple flowers, to 2cm (¾in) long, with sparse yellow beards. ↕40–60cm (16–24in), ↔ 30cm (12in). C. and S.E. USA. ❄❄❄. **var. *alba*** see *C. glabra.*

▷**Cherry,**
Barbados see *Malpighia glabra*
Bell-flowered see *Prunus campanulata*
Bird see *Prunus padus*
Black see *Prunus serotina*
Brush see *Syzygium paniculatum*
Choke see *Prunus virginiana*
Christmas see *Solanum pseudocapsicum*
Cornelian see *Cornus mas*
False Jerusalem see *Solanum capsicastrum*
Fuji see *Prunus incisa*
Great white see *Prunus* 'Taihaku'
Ground see *Physalis*
Higan see *Prunus* x *subhirtella*
Hill see *Prunus jamasakura*
Holly-leaved see *Prunus ilicifolia*
Jerusalem see *Solanum pseudocapsicum*
Manchurian see *Prunus maackii*
Ornamental see *Prunus*
Pin see *Prunus pensylvanica*
Rosebud see *Prunus* x *subhirtella*
Saint Lucie see *Prunus mahaleb*
Sargent see *Prunus sargentii*
Taiwan see *Prunus campanulata*
Virginian bird see *Prunus virginiana*

▷**Cherry cont.**
Wild see *Prunus avium*
Wild rum see *Prunus serotina*
Winter see *Cardiospermum halicacabum, Solanum capsicastrum, S. pseudocapsicum*
Yoshino see *Prunus* x *yedoensis*
▷**Cherry laurel** see *Prunus laurocerasus*
▷**Cherry pie** see *Heliotropium arborescens*
▷**Chervil,**
Common see *Anthriscus cerefolium*
Golden *see Chaerophyllum aureum*
▷**Chestnut** see *Castanea*
American see *Castanea dentata*
Chinese see *Castanea mollissima*
Horse see *Aesculus, A. hippocastanum*
Moreton Bay see *Castanospermum australe*
Spanish see *Castanea sativa*
Sweet see *Castanea, C. sativa*
Water see *Trapa, T. natans*
▷***Chiapasia nelsonii*** see *Disocactus nelsonii*

CHIASTOPHYLLUM

CRASSULACEAE

Genus of one species of mat-forming, rhizomatous, succulent, evergreen perennial from shady, mountain habitats in the Caucasus. It is grown for its attractive, fleshy foliage and tiny yellow flowers in pendent racemes. Grow in a rock garden, border, or shaded rock and wall crevices.

• **HARDINESS** Fully hardy.
• **CULTIVATION** Grow in moist but well-drained, poor to moderately fertile soil in partial shade.
• **PROPAGATION** Sow seed in containers in a cold frame in autumn, or root sideshoot cuttings in early summer.
• **PESTS AND DISEASES** Susceptible to damage by slugs and snails.

C. oppositifolium ▣🏆 syn. *C. simplicifolium, Cotyledon simplicifolia.* Spreading, rhizomatous, evergreen perennial forming dense mats of ovate to rounded, scalloped or wavy-margined, fleshy, pale green leaves, 4–12cm (1½–5in) long. In late spring and early summer, long stems bear bell-shaped, deep yellow flowers, to 5mm (¼in) long, in dense, arching, branched racemes. ↕15–20cm (6–8in), ↔ 15cm (6in). Caucasus. ❄❄❄
C. simplicifolium see *C. oppositifolium.*

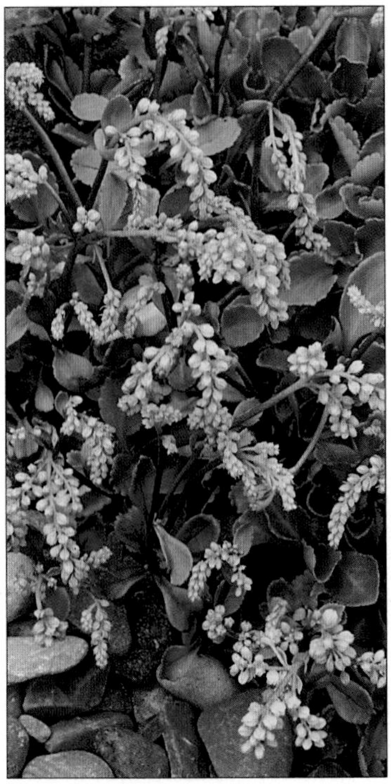

Chiastophyllum oppositifolium

▷**Chicory** see *Cichorium, C. intybus*
▷**Chile nut** see *Gevuina avellana*

CHILIOTRICHUM

ASTERACEAE/COMPOSITAE

Genus of 2 species of evergreen shrubs from temperate regions of South America, where they are found from sea level to the mountains. *C. diffusum* is grown for its rosemary-like leaves and daisy-like flowerheads, and is best suited to a sheltered, sunny shrub border. It thrives in coastal gardens.

• **HARDINESS** Frost hardy.
• **CULTIVATION** Grow in fertile, well-drained soil in full sun, with shelter from cold, dry winds. Pruning group 8.
• **PROPAGATION** Root semi-ripe cuttings in summer.
• **PESTS AND DISEASES** Trouble free.

C. amelloides see *C. diffusum.*
C. diffusum, syn. *C. amelloides.* Evergreen shrub with erect shoots and usually linear, oblong-lance-shaped to elliptic, glossy, dark green leaves, to 4cm (1½in) long, densely and alternately arranged around the stems. White flowerheads, to 5cm (2in) across, with yellow centres, are borne on flower-stalks to 10cm (4in) long, in late spring and early summer. ↕1m (3ft), ↔ 1.5m (5ft). S. Chile, S.W. Argentina, Falkland Islands. ❄❄

▷**Chilli pepper** see *Capsicum, C. annuum, C. annuum* Longum Group

CHIMAPHILA

Prince's pine

PYROLACEAE

Genus of about 6 species of evergreen, creeping perennials, related to *Pyrola*, found in cool-temperate woodland in Europe, Asia, and North America. They have slender, upright stems, and produce whorls of leathery leaves and nodding, white to pink flowers in terminal corymbs or umbels. They grow best in cool climates, and are ideal for a woodland garden, for shaded areas in a rock garden, or for growing on a peat terrace or bank.

• **HARDINESS** Fully hardy.
• **CULTIVATION** Grow in moist but well-drained, humus-rich, acid soil, enriched with leaf mould, in a cool site in partial or dappled shade. Not easy to establish.
• **PROPAGATION** Sow seed as soon as ripe on to lime-free (ericaceous) seed compost topped with damp sphagnum moss; keep in a cool, shaded frame until germination.
• **PESTS AND DISEASES** Prone to damage by slugs and snails.

C. maculata. Evergreen perennial, with a creeping, woody rootstock producing ovate to lance-shaped, leathery, white-veined, dark green leaves, to 7cm (3in) long, usually arranged in whorls of 3. Umbels of 3–5 open cup-shaped, white or pale pink flowers, to 1cm (½in) across, are borne on pendent flower-stalks in early summer. ↕ to 25cm (10in), ↔ to 20cm (8in). E. North America. ❄❄❄

C

CHIMONANTHUS

Wintersweet

CALYCANTHACEAE

Genus of 6 species of deciduous and evergreen shrubs occurring in woodland in China. They are cultivated for their unusual, many-petalled, open bowl-shaped, waxy, and very fragrant flowers, which are borne in winter before the young leaves emerge. Grow wintersweets as specimen plants or in a shrub border. They may also be trained against a sunny wall.

• **HARDINESS** Fully hardy, although unripened wood may be damaged by frost.
• **CULTIVATION** Grow in any fertile, well-drained soil in full sun. Pruning group 1, or group 13 if wall-trained; prune plants immediately after flowering.
• **PROPAGATION** Sow seed in containers in a cold frame as soon as ripe. Root softwood cuttings in summer.
• **PESTS AND DISEASES** Trouble free.

C. praecox (Wintersweet). Vigorous, broadly upright, deciduous shrub with entire, lance-shaped, glossy, mid-green leaves, to 20cm (8in) long, rough above, smooth beneath, arranged in opposite pairs. Pendent, fragrant, sulphur-yellow flowers, 2.5cm (1in) across, stained brown or purple inside, are produced on the bare shoots in winter. ↕4m (12ft), ↔ 3m (10ft). China. ❄❄❄. **'Concolor'** see 'Luteus'. **'Grandiflorus'** ▣🏆 has larger, deep yellow flowers, to 4.5cm (1¾in) long, conspicuously striped maroon inside. **'Luteus'** 🏆 syn. 'Concolor', bears clear yellow flowers which open widely. **'Parviflorus'** has pale yellow flowers to 1cm (½in) across.

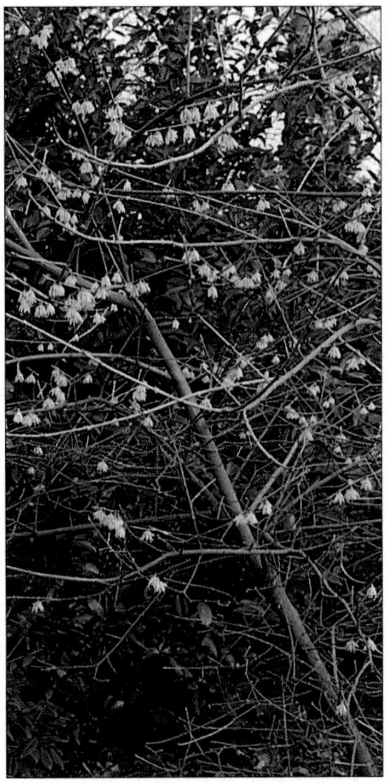

Chimonanthus praecox 'Grandiflorus'

C

CHIMONOBAMBUSA

GRAMINEAE/POACEAE

Genus of 6–20 species of small to medium-sized bamboos from deciduous woodland in S. and E. Asia, with running rhizomes, bright green leaves, and flowers borne in spike-like racemes. They are useful for planting as a screen or hedge, and grow well in a woodland garden. *C. quadrangularis* is cultivated for its unusual square canes, and elegant shape and foliage. Where temperatures fall below -10°C (14°F), grow less hardy species in a cool or temperate greenhouse or conservatory.

• **HARDINESS** Frost hardy to frost tender.
• **CULTIVATION** Grow in fertile, humus-rich, moist but well-drained soil in partial shade, with shelter from cold, dry winds.
• **PROPAGATION** Divide clumps, or take cuttings of sections of young rhizomes, in spring.
• **PESTS AND DISEASES** Emerging shoots are vulnerable to slug damage.

C. quadrangularis, syn. *Arundinaria quadrangularis* (Square-stemmed bamboo). Vigorous, spreading, rhizomatous bamboo, forming loose clumps of erect canes, often with sparse, small spines. Attractive, pendent, lance-shaped, dark green leaves, 20cm (8in) long, are produced from the prominent cane nodes. Older canes become square in cross-section, especially at the bases. ↕ to 9m (28ft), ↔ 1–2m (3–6ft). S.E. China, Taiwan. ✻✻

▷**China aster** see *Callistephus*
▷**Chincherinchee** see *Ornithogalum thyrsoides*
▷**Chinese-hat plant** see *Holmskioldia sanguinea*
▷**Chinese houses** see *Collinsia bicolor*
▷**Chinese lantern** see *Physalis alkekengi*
▷**Chinkapin, Golden** see *Chrysolepis chrysophylla*
▷**Chinquapin, Water** see *Nelumbo lutea*

CHIONANTHUS

Fringe tree

OLEACEAE

Genus of 100 or more species of evergreen and deciduous trees and shrubs found in a variety of habitats, including woodland and scrub, and on stream-banks and rocky outcrops. They occur mainly in tropical regions, including E. Asia, Korea, Japan, and E. USA. Cultivated for their terminal panicles of flowers, which have 4 slender white petals, and for their blue-purple or blue-black fruits, *Chionanthus* species are attractive specimen plants. They are also suitable for a shrub border. Some plants have only male or only female flowers, and therefore may not produce fruit.

• **HARDINESS** Fully hardy to frost tender.
• **CULTIVATION** Grow in any fertile, well-drained soil in full sun. Flowering and fruiting is best in areas with long, hot summers. Pruning group 1; remove the lower branches of *C. virginicus* to encourage a tree-like habit.
• **PROPAGATION** Sow seed in containers in a cold frame in autumn; germination may take up to 18 months.
• **PESTS AND DISEASES** Trouble free.

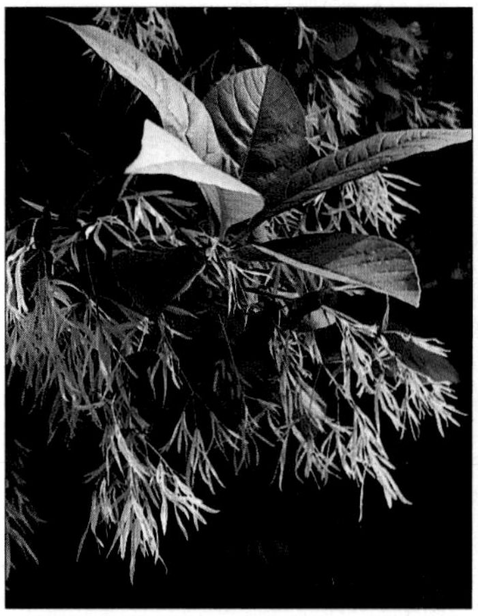

Chionanthus virginicus

C. retusus ⚲ (Chinese fringe tree). Spreading, deciduous shrub or small tree with peeling or deeply furrowed bark and opposite, usually elliptic, glossy leaves, 4–10cm (1½–4in) long, bright green above, softly white-hairy beneath. Fragrant white flowers are borne in erect panicles, 10–18cm (4–7in) long, in summer, followed by blue-black fruit, 1cm (½in) long. Lime-tolerant. ↕↔ 3m (10ft). China, Taiwan. ✻✻✻

C. virginicus ■ ⚲ (Fringe tree). Spreading, deciduous shrub, or sometimes small tree, with opposite, usually elliptic, glossy, dark green leaves, to 20cm (8in) long. Fragrant white flowers are borne in pendent panicles, to 20cm (8in) long, in summer; they are followed by small, blue-black fruit, 1.5cm (½in) long. Needs acid soil. ↕ 3m (10ft), ↔ 3m (10ft) or more. E. USA. ✻✻✻

CHIONOCHLOA

GRAMINEAE/POACEAE

Genus of about 20 species of evergreen, coarse, erect, tufted perennial grasses, mostly from New Zealand, found in alpine and subalpine grassland. The narrowly linear, deeply ridged leaves have persistent sheaths, similar to those of pampas grass (*Cortaderia*), to which this genus is related. The inflorescences bear several-flowered spikelets in loose, graceful panicles. *Chionochloa* species are cultivated for their strong, elegant shape, colourful foliage, and attractive flower-heads, which are excellent for dried flower arrangements if cut before fully mature. Grow as feature plants in a border or use as specimen plants.

• **HARDINESS** Most are frost hardy; *C. conspicua* will withstand falls in temperature to -10°C (14°F).
• **CULTIVATION** Grow in a sheltered site in light, fertile, moist but well-drained soil. Protect crowns from excessive winter wet. Cut out old, flowered stems at the bases in early winter.
• **PROPAGATION** Sow seed in containers in a cold frame in spring. Divide in spring.
• **PESTS AND DISEASES** Trouble free.

C. conspicua ■ syn. *Arundo conspicua, Cortaderia conspicua* (Plumed tussock grass). Robust, densely tufted, perennial grass, forming tussocks of stiff, arching, linear, red-brown-tinted, mid-green leaves, to 1.2m (4ft) long, often fringed with fine hairs at the bases. Strong, arching or erect stems bear large, open,

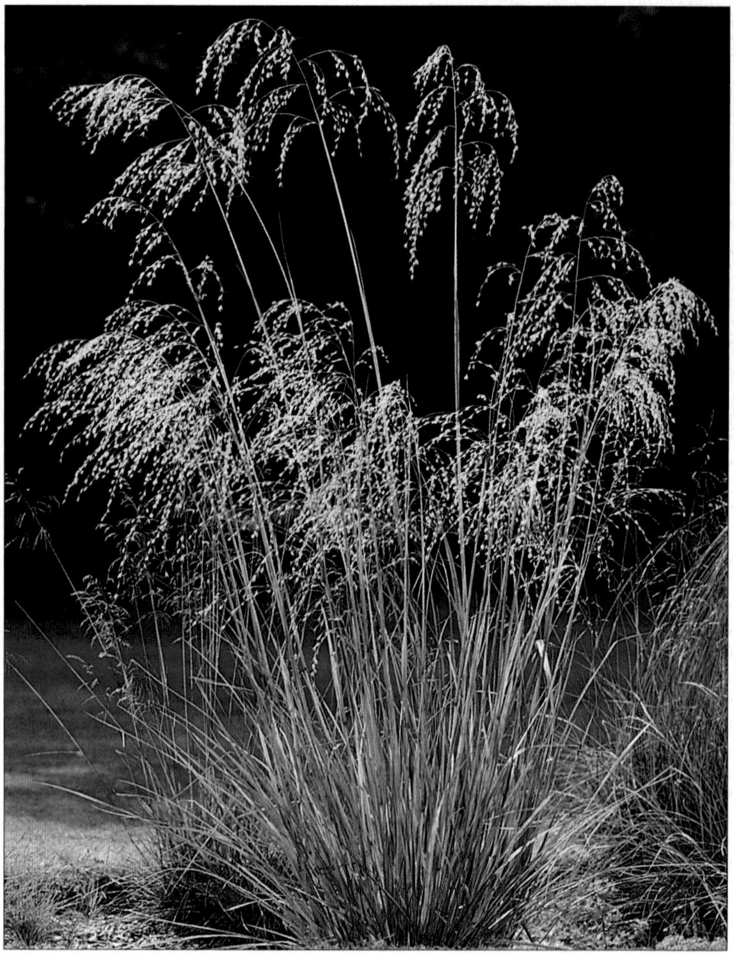

Chionochloa conspicua

pendent panicles, to 45cm (18in) long, of 3- to 7-flowered spikelets of creamy white flowers, each to 1.5cm (½in) long, in mid- and late summer. ↕ to 2m (6ft), ↔ 1m (3ft). New Zealand. ✻✻

CHIONODOXA

Glory of the snow

HYACINTHACEAE/LILIACEAE

Genus, related to *Scilla*, of 6 species of small, bulbous perennials from open mountainsides and forest in Crete, W. Turkey, and Cyprus. They bear racemes of star-shaped flowers in early spring, above linear, sometimes channelled, mid-green, basal leaves, to 28cm (11in) long. Grow in a rock garden, raised bed, or trough; most may also be grown under shrubs or trees, where they can spread. They self-seed freely. Their nomenclature is confused in commerce.

• **HARDINESS** Fully hardy to frost hardy.
• **CULTIVATION** Plant bulbs 8cm (3in) deep in autumn, in any well-drained soil in full sun. *C. nana* dislikes winter wet and is best grown in an alpine house.
• **PROPAGATION** Sow seed in containers in a cold frame as soon as ripe. Remove offsets in summer.
• **PESTS AND DISEASES** Trouble free.

C. cretica see *C. nana*.

C. forbesii ■ syn. *C. luciliae* of gardens, *C. siehei, C. tmolusi*. Bulbous perennial producing erect to spreading leaves, 7–28cm (3–11in) long. In early spring, bears racemes of 4–12 star-shaped blue flowers, 1–2cm (½–¾in) across, with white centres. ↕ 10–20cm (4–8in),

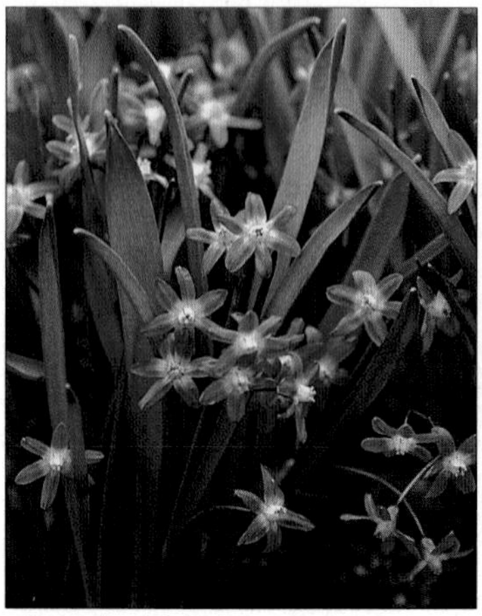

Chionodoxa forbesii

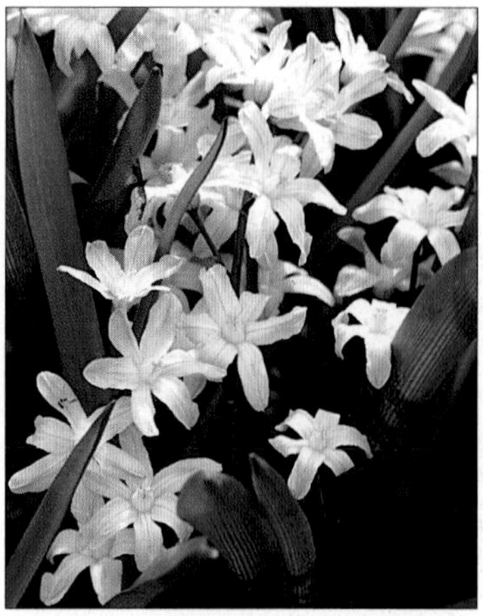

Chionodoxa forbesii 'Pink Giant'

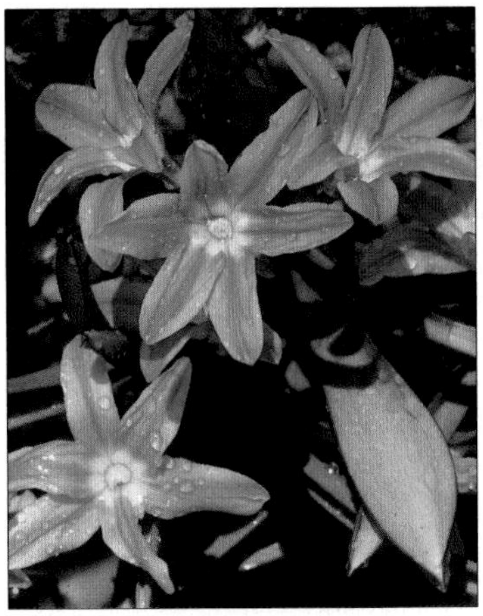

Chionodoxa luciliae

↔ 3cm (1¼in). W. Turkey. ❄❄❄. **'Pink Giant'** ▣ has pink flowers, 1.5cm (½in) across, with white centres.
C. gigantea see *C. luciliae.*
C. luciliae ▣🏆 syn. *C. gigantea.* Bulbous perennial with often recurved leaves, 7–20cm (3–8in) long. In early spring, bears racemes of up to 3 star-shaped blue flowers, 1–2cm (½–¾in) across, with white centres. Similar to *C. forbesii* but has fewer flowers, with slightly wider tepals. ↕ 15cm (6in), ↔ 3cm (1¼in). W. Turkey. ❄❄❄
***C. luciliae* of gardens** see *C. forbesii.*
C. nana, syn. *C. cretica.* Delicate, bulbous perennial with spreading leaves, 8–18cm (3–7in) long. In early spring, produces racemes of up to 3 star-shaped blue flowers, 6–10mm (¼–½in) across, with white centres. ↕ 15cm (6in), ↔ 3cm (1¼in). Greece (Crete). ❄❄
C. sardensis 🏆 Bulbous perennial with erect or spreading leaves, 7–20cm (3–8in) long. In early spring, bears racemes of up to 12 slightly pendent, star-shaped, deep clear blue flowers, 8–10mm (⅜–½in) across, with blue centres. ↕ 10–20cm (4–8in), ↔ 3cm (1¼in). W. Turkey. ❄❄❄
C. siehei see *C. forbesii.*
C. tmolusi see *C. forbesii.*

x CHIONOSCILLA

HYACINTHACEAE/LILIACEAE

Genus of one hybrid bulbous perennial, a cross between *Chionodoxa forbesii* and *Scilla bifolia*, with semi-erect, narrow, inversely lance-shaped, dark green, basal leaves. Grown for its short racemes of brilliant blue flowers in spring, it is suitable for a rock garden, trough, or raised bed, and for planting beneath trees or shrubs.

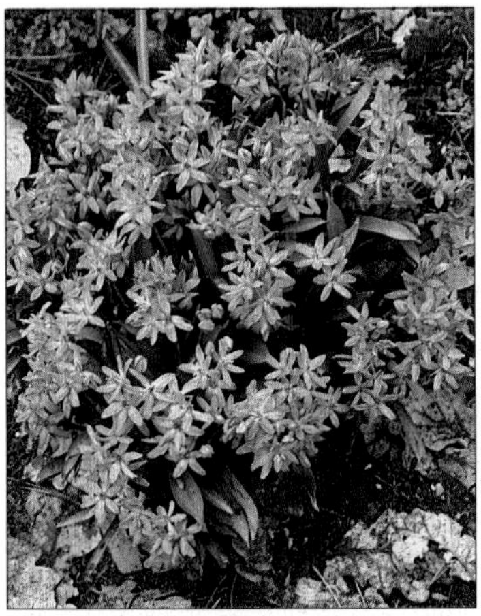

x *Chionoscilla allenii*

- **HARDINESS** Fully hardy.
- **CULTIVATION** Plant bulbs 7cm (3in) deep in autumn, in any well-drained soil in sun or partial shade.
- **PROPAGATION** Remove offsets in summer.
- **PESTS AND DISEASES** Trouble free.

x *C. allenii* ▣ Bulbous perennial with basal leaves, 7–15cm (3–6in) long, and short racemes, 6–12cm (2½–5in) long, of variable, star-shaped, mid- to deep blue flowers, 1–1.5cm (½in) across, borne in spring. Natural hybrid. ↕ 10–20cm (4–8in), ↔ 3cm (1¼in). Turkey. ❄❄❄. **'Fra Angelico'** has deep bright blue flowers.

CHIRITA

GESNERIACEAE

Genus of about 100 species of upright or mat-forming annuals and evergreen perennials from damp, semi-shaded sites in tropical Asia. They have fleshy stems and downy or bristly leaves in opposite pairs or whorls. The tubular or funnel-shaped flowers are either solitary or borne in many-flowered clusters from the leaf axils in summer and autumn. In frost-prone areas, grow in a warm greenhouse or conservatory; in tropical climates, grow in a damp, shady border.

- **HARDINESS** Frost tender.
- **CULTIVATION** Under glass, grow in loamless potting compost in bright filtered light, with high humidity and good air circulation. In the growing season, water moderately and apply a half-strength, balanced liquid fertilizer monthly. Water perennials more sparingly in winter. Outdoors, grow in well-drained, humus-rich, gritty soil in partial shade.
- **PROPAGATION** Sow seed at 19–24°C (66–75°F) in early spring; seed of *C. lavandulacea* may be sown in succession from late winter. *C. sinensis* may be increased by leaf cuttings, inserted in moist, sandy compost in a propagating case.
- **PESTS AND DISEASES** Prone to stem rot in damp conditions; water on the leaves causes discoloration and fungal rot.

C. lavandulacea ▣ Fast-growing, erect, usually unbranched annual with pairs of oblong-elliptic, softly hairy, light green leaves, 20cm (8in) long. In summer and autumn, bears a profusion of tubular, pale lavender-blue flowers, 2.5–4cm (1–1½in) across; each flower lasts only 2–3 days. At the coolest temperatures indicated, growth is more compact and the flowers last longer. ↕ 90cm (36in), ↔ 30cm (12in). Asia. ❀ (min. 13–21°C/55–70°F)

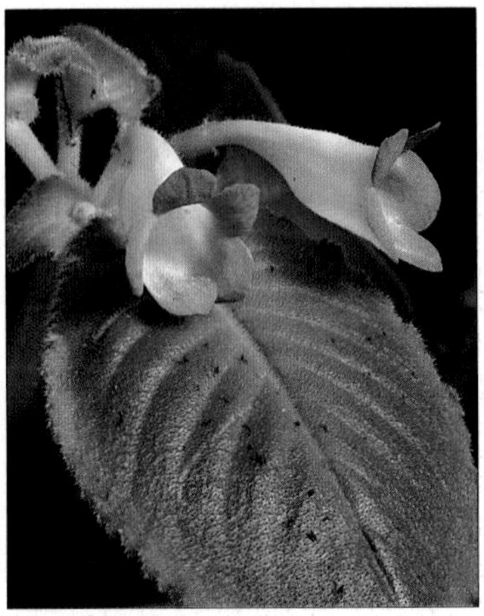

Chirita lavandulacea

C. sinensis 🏆 Evergreen perennial forming flat rosettes of thick, ovate-lance-shaped or elliptic, bristly-hairy, dark green leaves, sometimes heavily veined silver, 15–20cm (6–8in) long; they appear quilted, particularly at the margins. Occasionally produces tubular white flowers, 3cm (1¼in) long, marked yellow and suffused purple-pink. ↕ 5cm (2in), ↔ 35cm (14in). Himalayas, China, Hong Kong. ❀ (min. 13–21°C/55–70°F)

▷**Chittamwood** see *Cotinus obovatus*
▷**Chives** see *Allium schoenoprasum*
Chinese see *A. tuberosum*

CHLIDANTHUS

AMARYLLIDACEAE

Genus of one species of bulbous perennial found in the Andes in Peru. It is grown for its strongly scented flowers, borne in summer. In frost-prone areas, it is best grown in a cool or temperate greenhouse or conservatory. In areas that are virtually frost free, grow in a sheltered site outdoors, such as at the base of a sunny wall.

- **HARDINESS** Frost tender.
- **CULTIVATION** Plant with the nose of the bulb just above the soil surface in spring. Under glass, grow in loam-based potting compost (JI No.2) in full light. Water freely when in growth, reducing water as leaves wither; keep cool and dry in winter. Container-grown plants may be plunged outdoors in summer. Outdoors, grow in humus-rich, sandy, well-drained soil in a sheltered position; apply a dry mulch in winter.
- **PROPAGATION** Sow seed at 13–18°C (55–64°F) in spring. Remove offsets in spring.
- **PESTS AND DISEASES** Trouble free.

C. fragrans ▣ Bulbous perennial with semi-erect, narrow, linear, grey-green, basal leaves, 15–40cm (6–16in) long. In summer, leafless stems bear umbels of 3–5 trumpet-shaped, strongly scented, golden yellow flowers, 5cm (2in) wide. ↕ 30cm (12in), ↔ 8cm (3in). Peru (Andes). ❀ (min. 5–10°C/41–50°F)

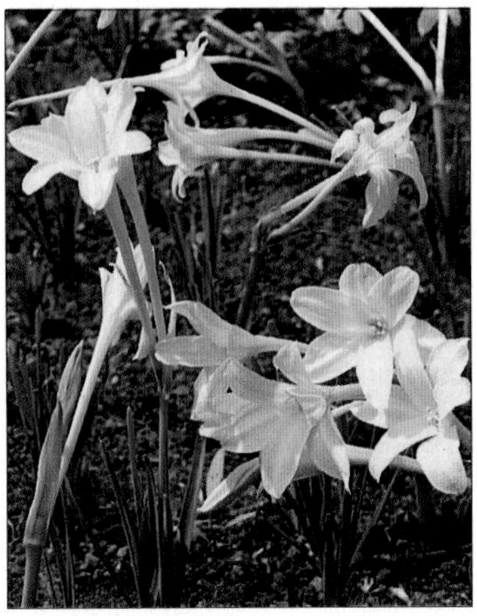

Chlidanthus fragrans

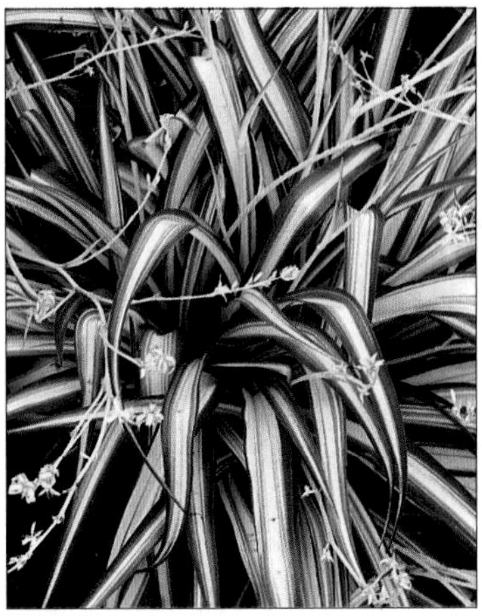

Chlorophytum comosum 'Vittatum'

CHLOROPHYTUM

ANTHERICACEAE/LILIACEAE

Genus of about 250 species of evergreen, rhizomatous perennials with fibrous or fleshy roots. Those in cultivation are from a variety of habitats in South Africa and W. Africa, and are clump-forming, with linear, lance-shaped, ovate, or strap-shaped, basal leaves. In summer, they bear arching racemes or panicles of tiny, 6-petalled flowers, and sometimes produce plantlets. In frost-prone areas, grow in containers and hanging baskets in a cool or temperate conservatory; they are also popular foliage houseplants, tolerant of a wide range of conditions. In warmer areas, use in a border or as ground cover.

- **HARDINESS** Frost tender.
- **CULTIVATION** Under glass, grow in loam-based potting compost (JI No.2) in bright indirect to full light, shaded from hot sun. Water freely in growth, moderately at other times. Outdoors, grow in any soil in sun or partial shade.
- **PROPAGATION** Sow seed at 18–20°C (64–68°F) in spring. Root plantlets, or divide, at any time except winter.
- **PESTS AND DISEASES** Trouble free.

C. capense. Clump-forming perennial with lance- or strap-shaped, bright green leaves, 25–60cm (10–24in) long. Bears tiny white flowers in racemes to 60cm (24in) long. Does not produce plantlets. ↕ 30cm (12in), ↔ 60cm (24in). South Africa. ❀ (min. 7°C/45°F)
***C. capense* of gardens** see *C. comosum.*
C. comosum, syn. *C. capense* of gardens (Ribbon plant, Spider plant). Clump-forming perennial with linear to linear-lance-shaped, fresh green leaves, 30cm (12in) long. Bears tiny white flowers in racemes, to 60cm (24in) long. Also produces plantlets. ↕ 15–20cm (6–8in), ↔ 15–30cm (6–12in). South Africa. ❀ (min. 7°C/45°F). **'Variegatum'** 🏆 produces leaves with white margins. **'Vittatum'** ▣🏆 has leaves with white or cream central stripes.
C. orchidastrum. Clump-forming perennial with oblong to inversely lance-shaped, often wavy-margined, glossy, mid-green leaves, 21–28cm (8–11in) long. Tiny, white, green-tinged flowers are borne in lax racemes, 25–40cm (10–16in) long. Does not produce plantlets. ↕ 15–20cm (6–8in), ↔ 15–30cm (6–12in). Sierra Leone. ❀ (min. 7°C/45°F)

C

CHOISYA

Mexican orange blossom

RUTACEAE

Genus of about 8 species of evergreen shrubs from canyons and rocky slopes in S.W. USA and Mexico. Choisyas are valued for their attractive, opposite, palmate, aromatic leaves, and for their fragrant, star-shaped white flowers, which are occasionally solitary, more often borne in terminal or axillary cymes or corymbs. They are best grown in a shrub border or against a wall.

• **HARDINESS** Fully hardy to frost hardy.
• **CULTIVATION** Grow in fertile, well-drained soil, preferably in full sun; less hardy species, such as *C. arizonica*, benefit from the shelter of a wall. Pruning group 8.
• **PROPAGATION** Root semi-ripe cuttings in summer.
• **PESTS AND DISEASES** Prone to snails.

C. arizonica. Erect shrub with slender branches, warty shoots, and mid- to dark green leaves comprising 5–10 linear, gland-margined leaflets, to 5cm (2in) long. In late spring, bears axillary corymbs of many pink-tinged white flowers, 2–3cm (¾–1¼in) across. ↕↔ 1m (3ft). USA (S. Arizona). ✻✻
***C.* 'Aztec Pearl'** ■ 🏆 Compact shrub with dark green leaves composed of 3–5 linear leaflets, to 8cm (3in) long. Pink-tinged white flowers, 2–3cm (¾–1¼in) across, are borne in axillary cymes of 3–6 blooms in late spring, and again in late summer and autumn. ↕↔ 2.5m (8ft). ✻✻✻

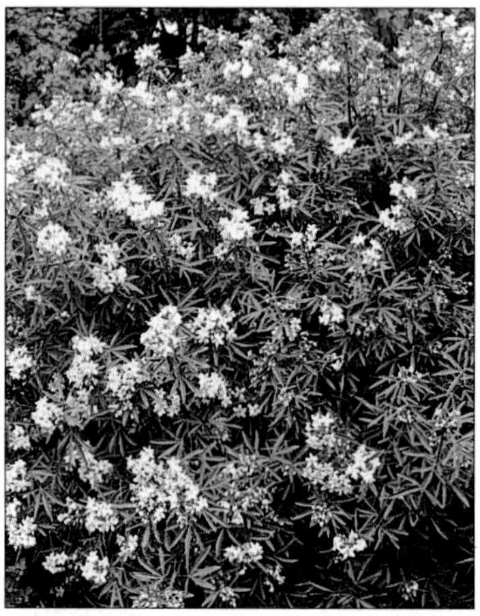
Choisya 'Aztec Pearl'

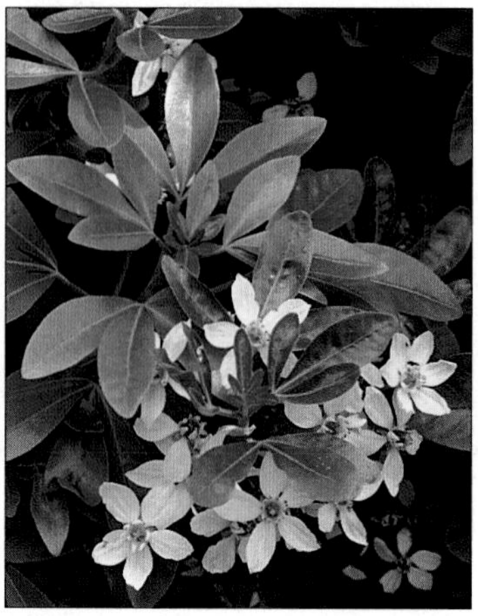
Choisya ternata

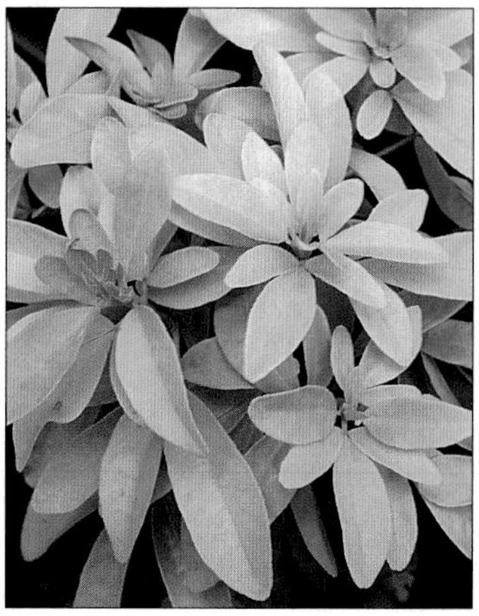
Choisya ternata 'Sundance'

C. ternata ■ 🏆 (Mexican orange blossom). Compact shrub with dark green leaves comprising 3 stalkless, obovate leaflets, 4–8cm (1½–3in) long. Axillary corymbs of 3–6 fragrant white flowers, 2.5–3cm (1–1¼in) across, are borne in late spring, and again in late summer and autumn. ↕↔ 2.5m (8ft). Mexico. ✻✻✻. **'Sundance'** ■ 🏆 has bright yellow young foliage, yellow-green when grown in partial shade; it rarely flowers.

▷ **Chokeberry** see *Aronia*
Black see *A. melanocarpa*
Purple see *A.* x *prunifolia*
Red see *A. arbutifolia*
▷ ***Chondrosum gracile*** see *Bouteloua gracilis*

CHORISIA

BOMBACACEAE

Genus of 2 species of semi-evergreen or deciduous, succulent trees from low-lying areas in the Windward Islands, Brazil, and Argentina. They have spiny, extremely fleshy trunks, alternate, 5- to 7-palmate leaves, and open funnel-shaped flowers borne in autumn. In frost-prone areas, grow in a warm greenhouse; elsewhere, use as specimen trees.

• **HARDINESS** Frost tender.
• **CULTIVATION** Under glass, grow in loam-based potting compost (JI No.3) in full light, shaded from hot sun, with good ventilation. Water moderately in growth, applying a balanced liquid fertilizer 2 or 3 times; keep dry at other times. Outdoors, grow in well-drained, neutral to acid, humus-rich soil in sun. Pruning group 1; plants under glass may need restrictive pruning in early spring.
• **PROPAGATION** Sow seed at 19–24°F (66–75°F) from spring to early summer.
• **PESTS AND DISEASES** Young plants are particularly vulnerable to scale insects.

C. speciosa ♤ (Floss silk tree). Broadly conical, slow-growing, semi-evergreen tree with long-stalked, pinnate leaves, to 12cm (5in) long, composed of 5–7 lance-shaped, often toothed leaflets. Open funnel-shaped, cream or white flowers, 10cm (4in) or more across, the upper parts of the petals reddish violet or yellowish white, are produced singly from the leaf axils in autumn. The pear-shaped, green then brown fruit contain seeds encased in silky floss. ↕ to 15m (50ft), ↔ to 1.5m (5ft). Brazil, Argentina. ❀ (min. 16°C/61°F)

CHORIZEMA

LEGUMINOSAE/PAPILIONACEAE

Genus of 18 species of evergreen, small shrubs and twining and scandent climbers found in semi-arid scrub and open woodland in Australia. They are cultivated for their brightly coloured, small, pea-like flowers, borne mostly in terminal racemes. The leathery leaves are usually alternate, and may be entire or prickle-toothed. In frost-prone areas, grow in a cool conservatory or greenhouse. In warmer areas, grow in a shrub border or as ground cover. Train climbing species over arches, arbours, or larger shrubs.

• **HARDINESS** Most are frost tender; *C. cordatum* and *C. ilicifolium* may survive brief spells close to 0°C (32°F).
• **CULTIVATION** Under glass, grow in loamless or loam-based potting compost (JI No.3), with additional sharp sand. Provide full light, with shade from hot sun, and good ventilation. When in growth, water moderately and apply a balanced liquid fertilizer monthly; water more sparingly in winter. Pot on in early spring. Outdoors, grow in humus-rich, neutral to slightly acid, moist but well-drained soil in full sun. Pruning group 8, or group 11 for climbing species; prune after flowering.
• **PROPAGATION** Sow seed at 13–18°C (55–64°F) in spring, after soaking in hot water. Root semi-ripe cuttings in summer.
• **PESTS AND DISEASES** Red spider mites may be a problem under glass.

C. cordatum 🏆 (Heart-leaved flame pea). Dense, low shrub or semi-scandent climber with ovate, leathery, mid- to dark green leaves, 2–5cm (¾–2in) long, heart-shaped at the bases, and with spine-like teeth. From late winter to late summer, freely bears orange-red and yellow flowers, 1.5cm (½in) across, with purplish pink keels, in terminal racemes, 8–15cm (3–6in) long. ↕↔ to 1.2m (4ft) or more. Australia (Western Australia). ❀ (min. 5–10°C/41–50°F)
C. ilicifolium ■ (Holly flame pea). Spreading, open shrub with slender branches and narrowly to broadly ovate, dark green leaves, 5–8cm (2–3in) long, with wavy, prickle-toothed margins. Orange-red and yellow flowers, 1cm (½in) across, with purplish pink keels, are produced in terminal and axillary racemes, 8–15cm (3–6in) long, from late winter to late summer. ↕↔ 1–3m (3–10ft). Australia (Western Australia). ❀ (min. 5–10°C/41–50°F)

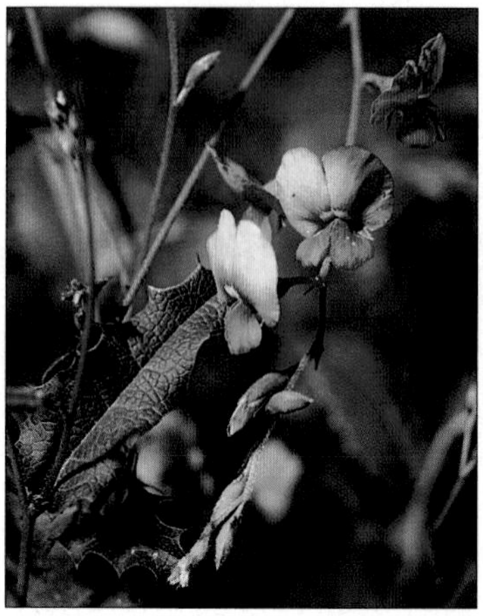
Chorizema ilicifolium

▷ **Chotito** see *Polyscias filicifolia*
▷ **Christmas bells** see *Blandfordia*
Tasmanian see *B. punicea*
▷ **Christmas berry tree** see *Schinus terebinthifolius*
▷ **Christmas pride** see *Ruellia macrantha*
▷ **Christmas rose** see *Helleborus niger*
▷ **Christmas tree** see *Metrosideros excelsus, Picea abies*
New South Wales see *Ceratopetalum gummiferum*
▷ **Christ's tears** see *Coix lacryma-jobi*
▷ **Christ's thorn** see *Euphorbia milii* var. *splendens, Paliurus spina-christi*

CHRYSALIDOCARPUS

Yellow palm

ARECACEAE/PALMAE

Genus of about 20 species of single- and cluster-stemmed palms from forest in areas with high rainfall in Madagascar and adjacent islands. The pinnate, arching leaves are arranged in terminal clusters; panicles of small, 3-petalled flowers are borne among them. In frost-prone areas, grow in a temperate or warm greenhouse, or as houseplants. In tropical or subtropical regions, grow as elegant specimen trees.

• **HARDINESS** Frost tender.
• **CULTIVATION** Under glass, grow in loam-based potting compost (JI No.3) in bright filtered or full light with shade from hot sun. Water freely when in growth, applying a balanced liquid fertilizer monthly; water sparingly in winter. Pot on or top-dress in spring. Outdoors, grow in fertile, moist but well-drained soil in sun or partial shade.
• **PROPAGATION** Sow seed at not less than 26°C (79°F) in spring.
• **PESTS AND DISEASES** Prone to scale insects and red spider mites under glass.

C. lutescens ■ 🏆 ✻ syn. *Areca lutescens, Dypsis lutescens* (Areca palm, Butterfly palm, Golden feather palm). Small palm with clustered stems, at first covered with yellow leaf bases. The leaves, 1–2m (3–6ft) long, have numerous slender, lance-shaped, usually yellow-green leaflets. In summer, bears yellow flowers in panicles to 60cm (24in) long. ↕ to 9m (28ft), ↔ to 6m (20ft). Madagascar. ❀ (min. 10–15°C/50–59°F)

▷ ***Chrysanthemopsis*** see *Rhodanthemum*

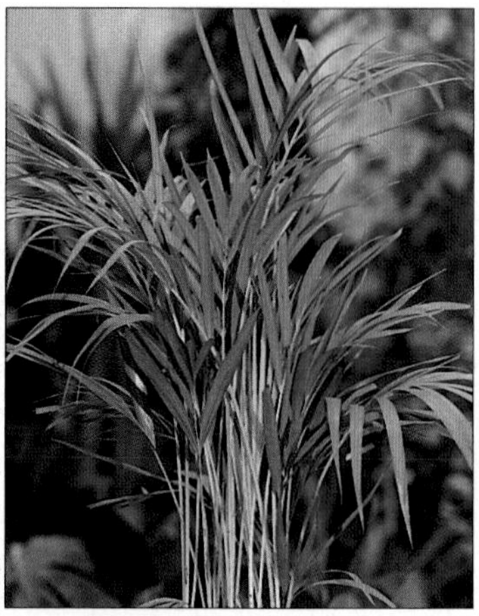
Chrysalidocarpus lutescens

CHRYSANTHEMUM

ASTERACEAE/COMPOSITAE

Genus of about 20 species of upright, bushy annuals and herbaceous perennials (some with woody bases), now almost all attributed by botanists to the genus *Dendranthema*, but here maintained under *Chrysanthemum* for the benefit of gardeners. The annual species come from the Mediterranean region, where they grow in dry fields and wasteland; the herbaceous perennials are from the Arctic, parts of N. and C. Russia, China, and Japan. The aromatic, alternate, ovate to lance-shaped, dark green leaves, 5–17cm (2–7in) long, are shallowly to deeply lobed or pinnatisect, occasionally entire, and often feathery.

Chrysanthemums are grown primarily for their showy flowerheads, 2.5–30cm (1–12in) across, which consist of ray-florets in a variety of colours, including yellow, white, pink, purple, and red, with yellow disc-florets; they are cultivated in a multiplicity of forms.

For ease of reference, chrysanthemums have been divided into the following groups:

Florists' chrysanthemums

These perennial cultivars are available in a wide range of forms and colours, and are grown for exhibition, the garden, and cutting. They are often categorized according to their flowerhead form (see panel below right), their flowering season – early (late summer and early autumn), mid-season (mid-autumn), or late (mid-autumn to midwinter) – and whether they are disbudded or non-disbudded (see below and panel below left). Disbudded chrysanthemums are classified by exhibitors into size groups. Non-disbudded chrysanthemums are categorized by both size and habit.

The early flowering spray chrysanthemums, reflexed cultivars, and pompon chrysanthemums are the best groups for outdoor use. Some mid-season reflexed cultivars are suitable for garden use, but most require protection from rain. Late-flowering cultivars are flowered in a temperate or warm greenhouse.

Disbudded – Disbudded chrysanthemums have all the flower buds on each shoot removed except for the terminal bud, in order to increase the size of the remaining bloom. For exhibition, those with incurved, intermediate, or reflexed flowers are restricted to 2 blooms per plant; in gardens, 4 or 5 blooms are allowed to develop. Single and anemone-centred flowers are reduced to 4–8 blooms for exhibition, and 10 or more for garden use and for cutting.

Non-disbudded – In non-disbudded chrysanthemums, the buds are usually allowed to develop freely. Non-disbudded chrysanthemums are grouped according to the following habits. **Spray chrysanthemums** produce several blooms per stem in a variety of flower forms: single, intermediate, reflexed, anemone-centred, pompon, spoon-shaped, or quill-shaped. They are grown mainly for garden decoration and for cutting. For exhibition, each plant is allowed to develop 4 or 5 stems, each bearing 5 or more flowerheads. Late-flowering sprays are restricted to 3 stems; for exhibition, each stem should bear 6 or 7 blooms or, if grown with controlled day length, 12 blooms per stem; for exhibition, the central bud of the spray is usually removed to give a more rounded outline. **Charm chrysanthemums** have a dwarf, bushy, domed to almost spherical habit, and bear hundreds of single flowerheads, to 2.5cm (1in) across. They do not need stopping or training, and are grown for indoor decoration, for exhibition, and as bonsai plants. **Cascade chrysanthemums** have similar flowerheads to charms but are trained as fans, pillars, pyramids, or cascades. They are grown for indoor decoration, for exhibition, and as bonsai plants. **Pompon chrysanthemums** are dwarf and bushy, producing 50 or more dense, spherical, or occasionally hemi-spherical flowerheads per plant. They are suitable for a border outdoors.

Rubellum Group chrysanthemums

These clump-forming, bushy perennials, with woody stem bases, are all named hybrids of *C. rubellum*, syn. *Dendranthema zawadskii*. They have pinnatisect leaves, often with a silvery cast, and bear single, semi-double, or double, yellow-centred flowerheads in a range of colours. Flowering in late summer and early autumn, they are excellent for a herbaceous border and for cutting.

Annual chrysanthemums

These chrysanthemums have a bushy, branched habit and bear clusters of mainly single, yellow or white flower-heads, some with contrasting zones of orange or red. They flower over a long period during spring and summer, or from summer to early autumn, and are suitable for an annual border, or for infilling in a herbaceous border. *C. segetum* is also suitable for a wildflower garden.

• **HARDINESS** Fully hardy to frost tender.

• **CULTIVATION** Grow early-flowering and mid-season florists' chrysanth-emums outdoors in a sheltered site in full sun in fertile, moist but well-drained, neutral to slightly acid soil, enriched with well-rotted manure. Apply a top-dressing of balanced fertilizer before planting, and plant out when any danger of frost has passed. Provide support and tie stems in with soft twine as growth proceeds. Stop plants at 15–20cm (6–8in) tall, by pinching out the growing tips to encourage the early production of flowering laterals. A second stop will produce greater numbers of smaller blooms. For exhibition purposes, select the required number of strong laterals and remove the remainder. Disbud gradually, removing unwanted flower buds as laterals reach about 2cm (¾in) long. The timing of stopping and disbudding varies with climate and growing conditions; specialist catalogues and National Chrysanthemum Society publications provide approximate dates.

Water freely in dry weather, and apply a balanced liquid fertilizer every 7–10 days from midsummer until buds begin to show colour. In mid- to late autumn, cut back flowered stems to 15–23cm (6–9in). Lift crowns and store over winter in loamless potting compost in frost-free conditions. In areas experiencing only light frosts, leave *in situ*, apply a deep, dry winter mulch, and cut back in early spring. Protect early and mid-season exhibition cultivars from rain and frost. White- and yellow-flowered cultivars may be adequately protected by greaseproof paper bags, put in place as buds begin to show colour.

DISBUDDED AND NON-DISBUDDED FORMS

Florists' chrysanthemums may be disbudded, leaving only one bud per stem. Non-disbudded plants produce flowerheads freely in sprays.

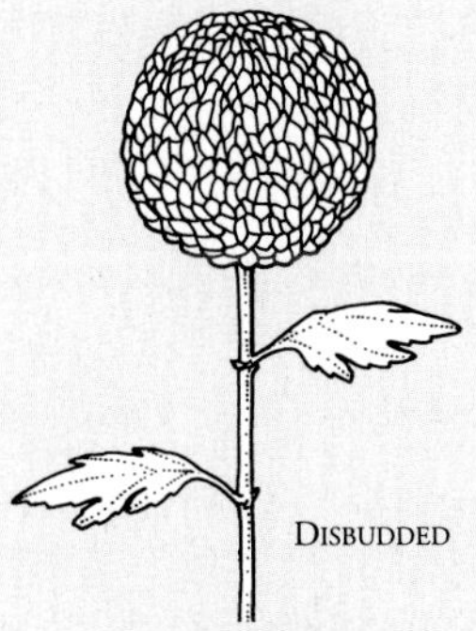

DISBUDDED

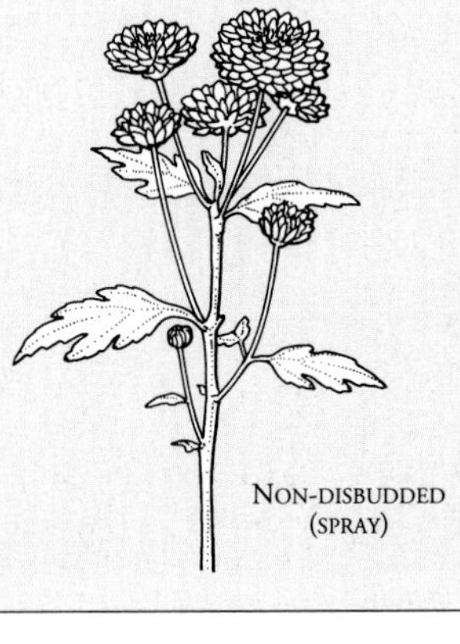

NON-DISBUDDED (SPRAY)

CHRYSANTHEMUM FLOWERHEAD FORMS

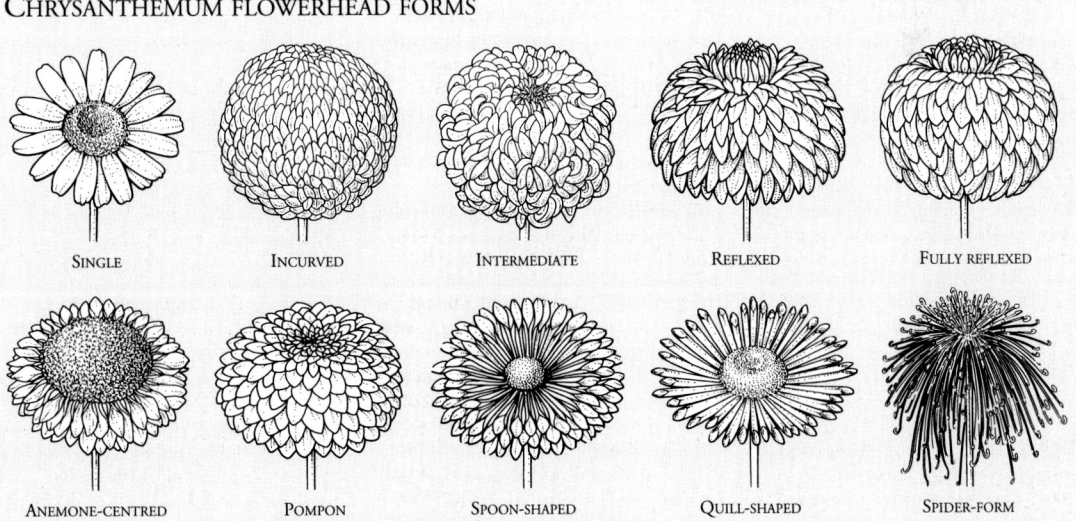

Single – Single flowerheads, which have up to 5 rows of flat ray-florets surrounding the central yellow, often green-centred discs.

Incurved – Fully double, spherical flowerheads with ray-florets opening from the bases and curving upwards.

Intermediate – Fully double, loose, spherical flowerheads with ray-florets mainly incurving but some lower ones reflexing.

Reflexed – Fully double flowerheads, similar to fully reflexed, but less compact, forming umbrella shapes.

Fully reflexed – Fully double, spherical flowerheads with ray-florets opening from the crown of each flower and curving downwards and inwards to touch the stem.

Anemone-centred – Single flowerheads with enlarged disc-florets that form dome-shaped centres, up to half the width or more of the flowerheads.

Pompon – Fully double, spherical flowerheads with tubular florets regularly and tightly packed, growing outwards from the crown.

Spoon-shaped – Double flowerheads with tubular ray-florets that open out at their tips to form spoon shapes.

Quill-shaped – Double flowerheads with tubular ray-florets that have a slanting opening at their tips, like that of a quill.

Spider-form – Double flowerheads with long, thin ray-florets; the outer ray-florets are more or less pendent, the inner ones curling upwards.

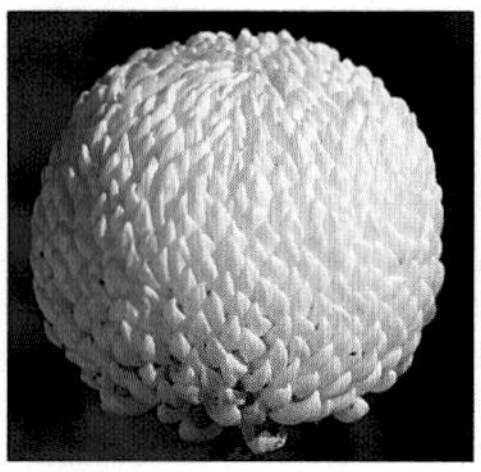
Chrysanthemum 'Alison Kirk'

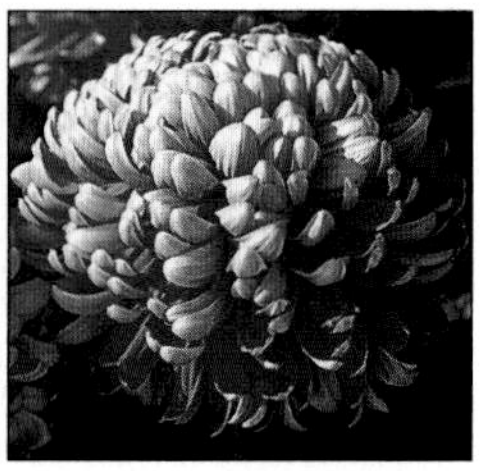
Chrysanthemum 'Autumn Days'

Chrysanthemum 'Beacon'

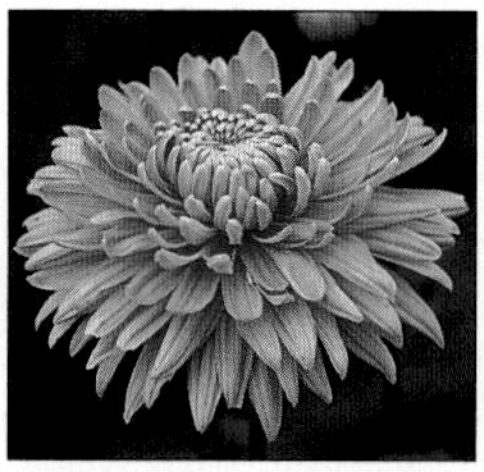
Chrysanthemum 'Brietner'

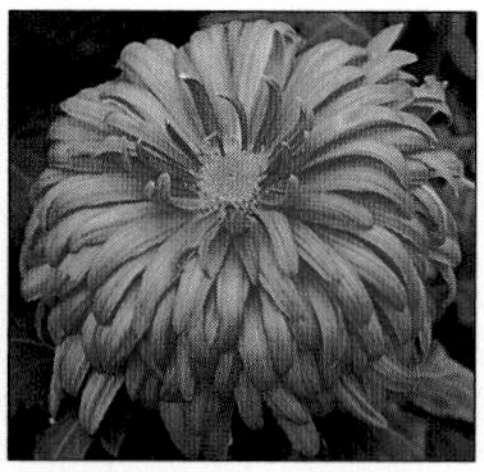
Chrysanthemum 'Bronze Hedgerow'

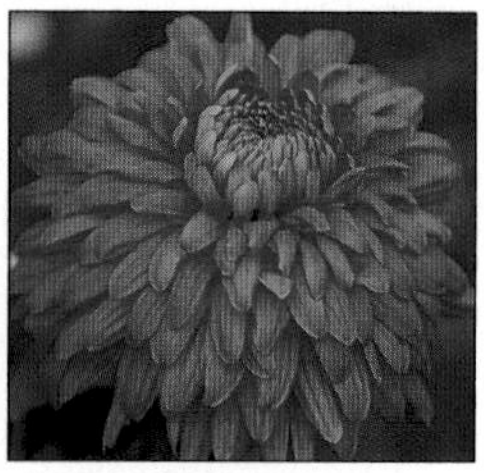
Chrysanthemum 'Bronze Yvonne Arnaud'

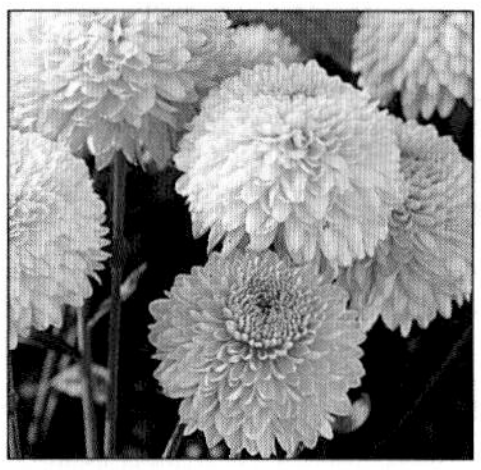
Chrysanthemum 'Buff Margaret'

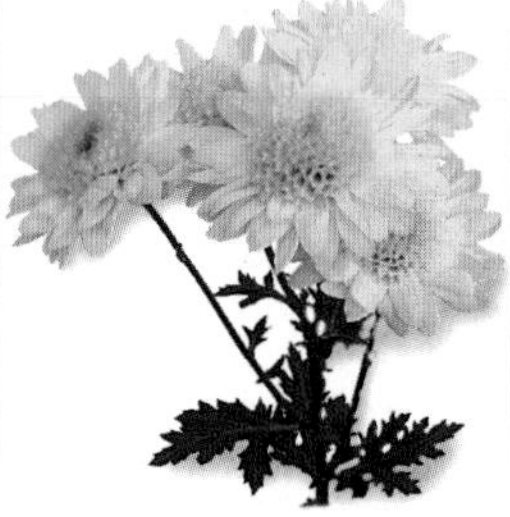
Chrysanthemum 'Cappa'

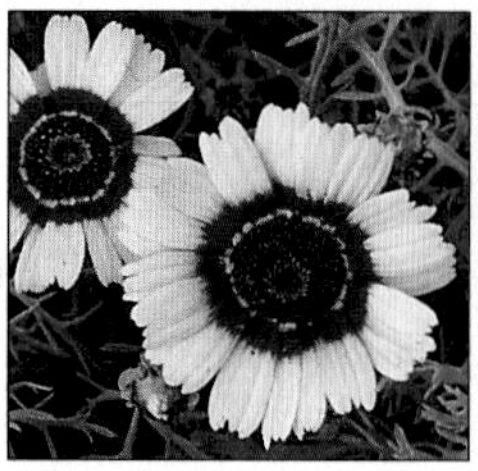
Chrysanthemum carinatum 'Court Jesters'

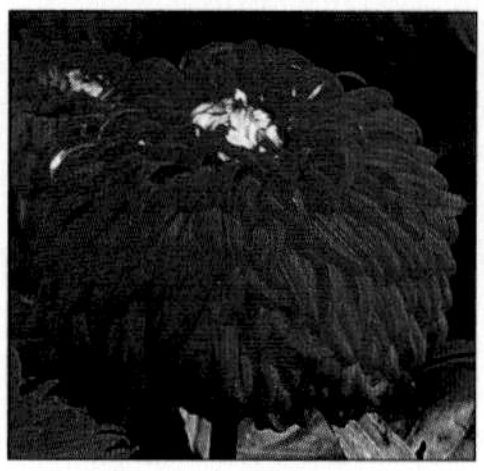
Chrysanthemum 'Cherry Chintz'

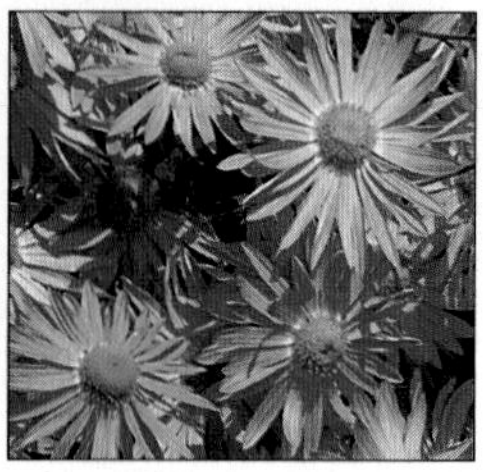
Chrysanthemum 'Clara Curtis'

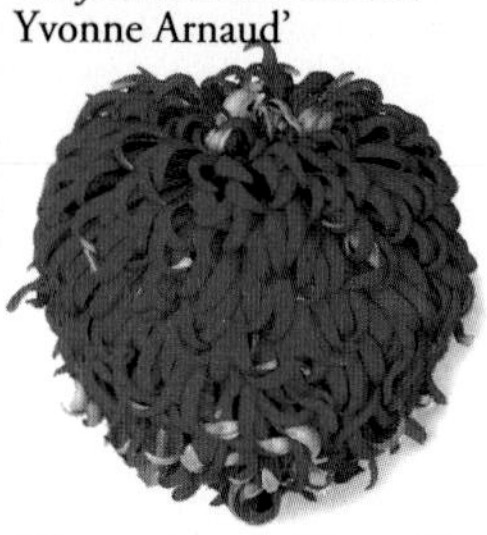
Chrysanthemum 'Cossack'

Cultivars of other colours, and all large-flowered cultivars of whatever colour, are best grown in an open-sided, polythene-covered lath house or in a cold greenhouse.

Grow late-flowering florists' chrysanthemums, including charms, cascades, and late-flowering sprays, in loam-based potting compost; use JI No.2 in 7.5cm (3in) containers, and pot on successionally to flower in 23–30cm (9–12in) containers of JI No.3, with the support of canes. Allow about 10 days between repotting and disbudding. Grow in a cold frame, bring into a warm greenhouse in early autumn, and provide bright filtered light with good ventilation and a winter minimum of 10°C (50°F). From midsummer onwards, water moderately and apply a balanced liquid fertilizer weekly.

Grow Rubellum Group and annual chrysanthemums in well-drained, moderately fertile soil in full sun.

• **PROPAGATION** Sow seed of charms and cascades at 13–16°C (55–61°F) in late winter or spring. Sow seed of Rubellum Group at 13–16°C (55–61°F) in spring, or divide in autumn or in early spring. Sow seed of annuals in containers in a cold frame in early spring, or *in situ* from spring to early summer; in frost-free areas, sow *in situ* in autumn for early flowering. Take basal cuttings of florists' chrysanthemums from over-wintered stools: for late-flowering cultivars, take cuttings in early or mid-winter; for other groups take in early spring. Root cuttings in loamless potting compost with dry sand on the surface, at around 16°C (61°F). Place in a cold frame after first potting; protect from frost and ventilate as weather allows. Harden off in mid-spring.

• **PESTS AND DISEASES** Vulnerable to aphids, earwigs, eelworms, capsid bugs, leaf miners, red spider mites, and white-flies. Prone to fungal rot, grey mould (*Botrytis*), powdery mildew, and white rust. Viruses may cause stunting, yellow markings, and puckering of leaves.

***C.* 'Alexis'.** Intermediate florists' chrysanthemum with light pink flower-heads, 18–20cm (7–8in) across when disbudded, borne in late autumn. Good for exhibition. ↕ 1.5m (5ft), ↔ 45–60cm (18–24in). ❄ (min. 10°C/50°F)

***C.* 'Alison Kirk'** ◼ Incurved florists' chrysanthemum with white flower-heads, 14cm (5½in) across when disbudded, borne in early autumn. Good for exhibition. ↕ 1.2m (4ft), ↔ 40cm (16in). ✲

C. alpinum see *Leucanthemopsis alpina.*

***C.* 'Amanda Whitmore'.** Anemone-centred florists' chrysanthemum bearing white flowerheads, to 15cm (6in) across when disbudded, in late autumn. Good for exhibition. ↕ 1.5m (5ft), ↔ 1m (3ft). ❄ (min. 10°C/50°F)

***C.* 'Amber Gigantic'.** Tightly incurved or loosely reflexed florists' chrysanth-emum, its form depending on the amount of warmth provided. Large amber flowerheads, 25–30cm (10–12in) across when disbudded, are borne in late autumn. ↕ 1.3m (4½ft), ↔ 30cm (12in). ❄ (min. 10°C/50°F)

***C.* 'Amethyst'.** Reflexed florists' chrysanthemum with purple blooms, 21cm (8in) across when disbudded, borne in late autumn. Good for exhibition. ↕ 1.2m (4ft), ↔ 30cm (12in). ❄ (min. 10°C/50°F)

C. atlanticum see *Rhodanthemum atlanticum.*

C. atratum see *Leucanthemum atratum.*

***C.* 'Autumn Days'** ◼ Intermediate or loosely incurved florists' chrysanth-emum with bronze flowerheads, 12cm (5in) across when disbudded, produced in early autumn. ↕ 1–1.2m (3–4ft), ↔ to 75cm (30in). ✲

C. balsamita see *Tanacetum balsamita.*

***C.* 'Beacon'** ◼ Intermediate florists' chrysanthemum bearing red, sometimes bronze flowerheads, to 18cm (7in) across when disbudded, in late autumn. Good for exhibition. ↕ 1.2m (4ft), ↔ 60cm (24in). ❄ (min. 10°C/50°F)

***C.* 'Bert Gibson'.** Reflexed florists' chrysanthemum producing light pink flowerheads, 18cm (7in) across when disbudded, in late autumn. Good for exhibition. ↕ 1.3m (4½ft), ↔ 45cm (18in). ❄ (min. 10°C/50°F)

***C.* 'Bill Wade'.** Intermediate to loosely incurved florists' chrysanthemum with pure white flowerheads, 18–20cm (7–8in) across when disbudded, borne in early autumn. Good for exhibition. ↕ 1.3m (4½ft), ↔ 60cm (24in). ✲

***C.* 'Brietner'** ◼ Reflexed florists' chrysanthemum producing pink flower-heads, to 12cm (5in) across when disbudded, in early autumn. Best used for garden decoration. ↕ to 1.2m (4ft), ↔ 75cm (30in). ✲

***C.* 'Bronze Fairie'** ◼ Pompon florists' chrysanthemum bearing many bronze flowerheads, 2.5cm (1in) across, in early autumn. ↕ 30–60cm (12–24in), ↔ 60cm (24in). ✲✲✲

***C.* 'Bronze Hedgerow'** ◼ Single florists' chrysanthemum with bronze flowerheads, 12cm (5in) across when disbudded, produced in late autumn. ↕ 1.5m (5ft), ↔ 75–100cm (30–39in). ❄ (min. 10°C/50°F)

***C.* 'Bronze Yvonne Arnaud'** ◼ Reflexed florists' chrysanthemum with bronze flowerheads, to 12cm (5in) across when disbudded, borne in early autumn. ↕ 1.2m (4ft), ↔ 60–75cm (24–30in). ✲

***C.* 'Buff Margaret'** ◼ Spray florists' chrysanthemum with reflexed, pale bronze flowerheads, 8–9cm (3–3½in) across, borne in early autumn. ↕ 1.2m (4ft), ↔ 60–75cm (24–30in). ✲✲✲

***C.* 'Cappa'** ◼ Spray florists' chrysanthemum with anemone-centred yellow flowerheads, 5–8cm (2–3in) across, borne in late autumn. ↕ 1.2m (4ft), ↔ 60–75cm (24–30in). ✲✲✲

C. carinatum, syn. *C. tricolor* (Painted daisy). Erect, fast-growing, branched annual chrysanthemum with almost succulent, pinnatisect, bright green leaves, to 10cm (4in) long. Long, stiff stems bear solitary, daisy-like, single, purple-eyed flowerheads, to 10cm (4in) across, from summer to early autumn. The flowerheads typically have yellow or white ray-florets, tinged red, with white zoning; a number of cultivars are available with flowerheads in shades of red, yellow, white, or purple, often with bold zoning on the ray-florets. ↕ 60cm (24in), ↔ 30cm (12in). Morocco. ✲. **'Court Jesters'** ◼ ♀ bears flowerheads to 8cm (3in) across, in brilliant colours from white and yellow to orange, scarlet, and maroon, zoned in orange or red. **'Polar Star'** has pale yellow flowerheads, zoned in orange.

C. catananche see *Rhodanthemum catananche.*

***C.* 'Cherry Chintz'** ◼ Fully reflexed florists' chrysanthemum with cherry-red flowerheads, to 13cm (5in) across when disbudded, produced in early autumn. ↕ to 1.3m (4½ft), ↔ 75cm (30in). ✲

***C.* 'Cherry Venice'.** Fully reflexed florists' chrysanthemum with deep salmon-pink flowerheads, 15cm (6in) across when disbudded, borne in early autumn. Use for exhibition. ↕ 1.2–1.3m (4–4½ft), ↔ 60–75cm (24–30in). ✲

***C.* 'Chessington'.** Intermediate to tightly incurved florists' chrysanthemum bearing white flowerheads, 18–20cm (7–8in) across when disbudded, in early autumn. Good for exhibition. ↕ 2–2.2m (6–7ft), ↔ 75cm (30in). ✲

***C.* 'Christina'.** Intermediate to loosely incurved florists' chrysanthemum bearing white flowerheads, to 14cm (5½in) across when disbudded, in early autumn. Use for exhibition. ↕ 1.3–1.5m (4½–5ft), ↔ 60–75cm (24–30in). ✲

***C.* 'Clara Curtis'** ◼ Rubellum Group chrysanthemum freely bearing long-lasting, single, clear pink flowerheads, to 7cm (3in) across, from late summer to mid-autumn. The flowers are pleasantly scented, with centres that turn from green to yellow as the disc-florets open. ↕ 75cm (30in), ↔ 60cm (24in). ✲✲✲

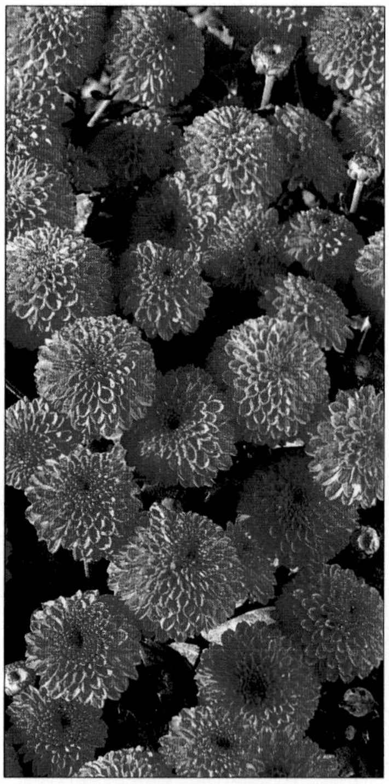
Chrysanthemum 'Bronze Fairie'

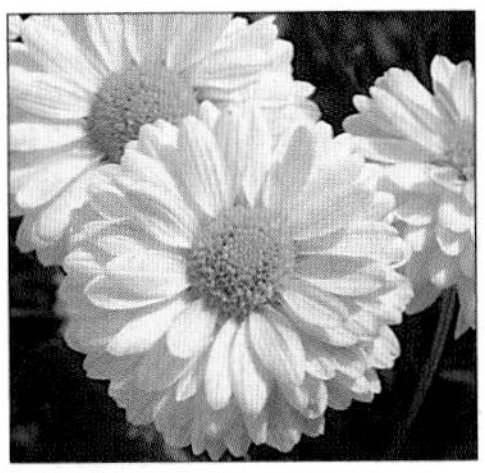
Chrysanthemum 'Dawn Mist'

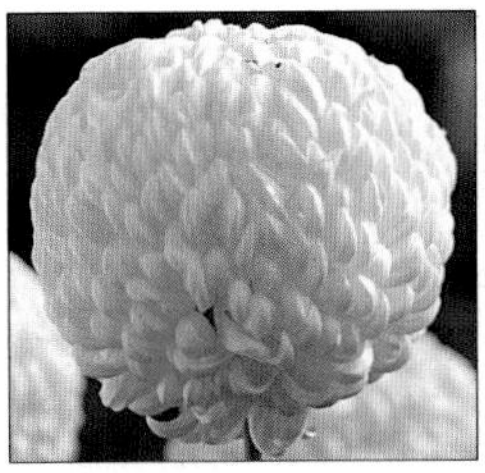
Chrysanthemum 'Discovery'

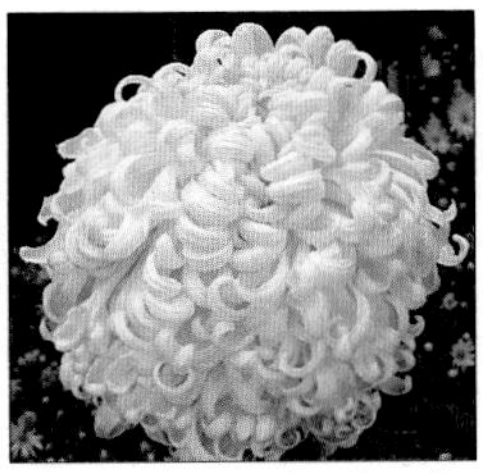
Chrysanthemum 'Duke of Kent'

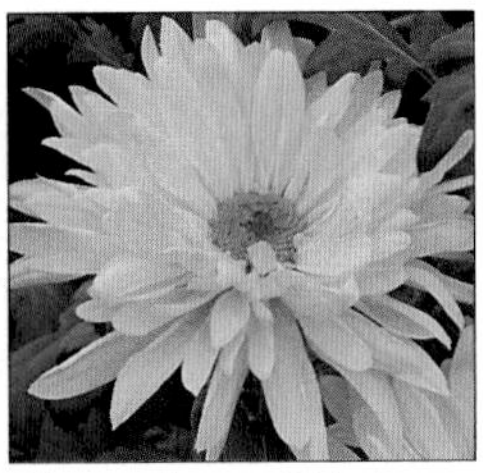
Chrysanthemum 'Edwin Painter'

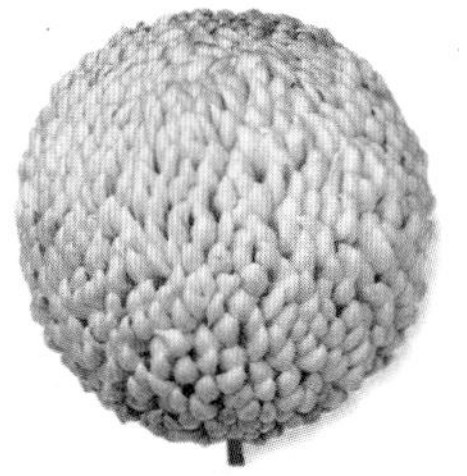
Chrysanthemum 'Fairweather'

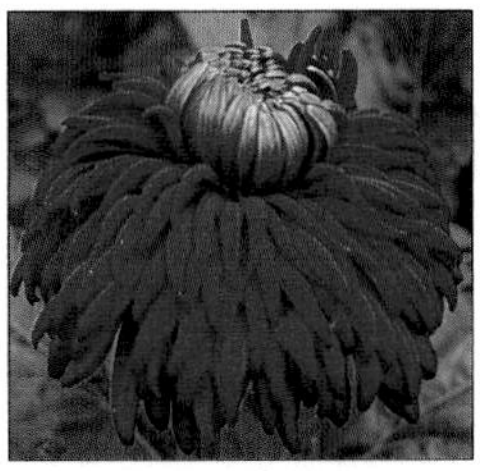
Chrysanthemum 'George Griffiths'

C

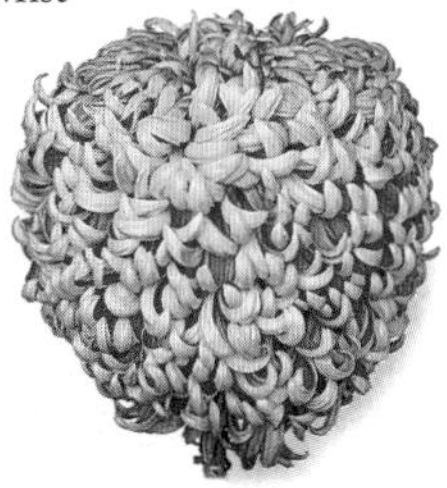
Chrysanthemum 'Golden Gigantic'

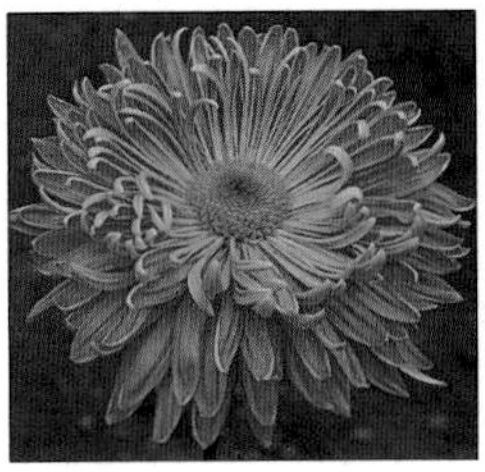
Chrysanthemum 'Golden Woolman's Glory'

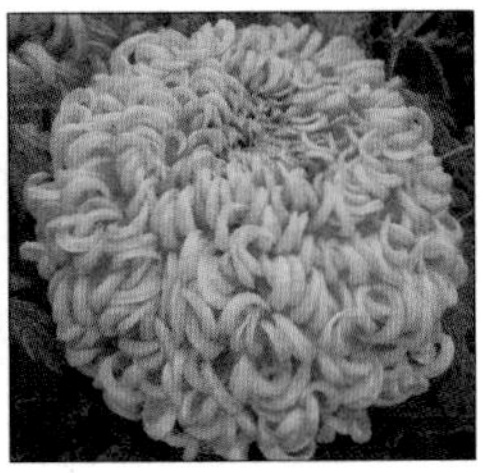
Chrysanthemum 'Green Satin'

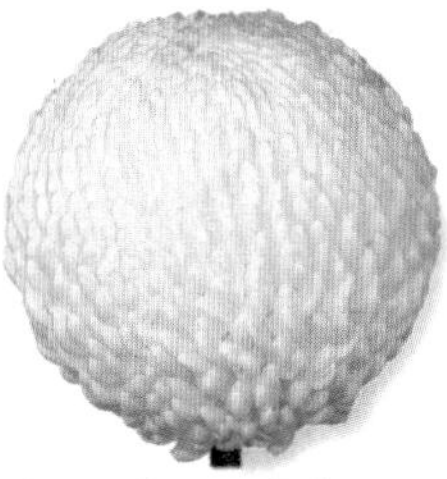
Chrysanthemum 'John Hughes'

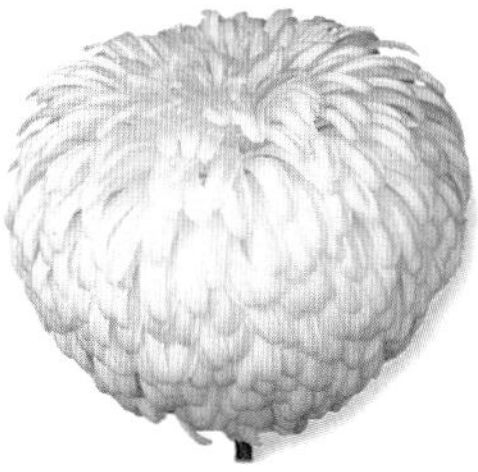
Chrysanthemum 'John Wingfield'

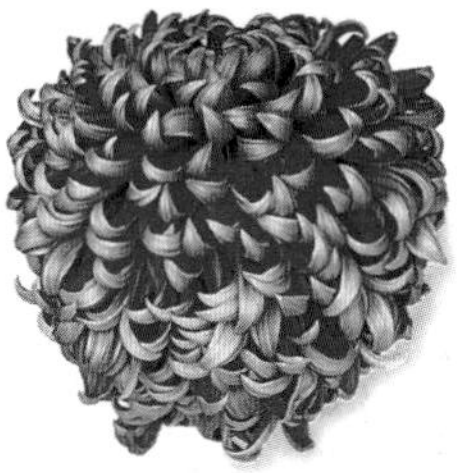
Chrysanthemum 'Keith Luxford'

C. coccineum see *Tanacetum coccineum.*
C. coronarium. Erect, vigorous, many-branched annual chrysanthemum with pinnatisect, fern-like, light green leaves, 5–7cm (2–3in) long. From spring to summer, bears daisy-like, single yellow flowerheads, to 5cm (2in) across. ↕ to 80cm (32in), ↔ to 40cm (16in). Mediterranean. ✻✻✻. **'Primrose Gem'** has primrose-yellow, golden-eyed flowerheads. ↕ to 30–45cm (12–18in).
***C.* 'Cossack'** ▣ Fully reflexed florists' chrysanthemum producing deep red flowerheads, 20cm (8in) across when disbudded, in late autumn. ↕ 1.2–1.3m (4–4½ft), ↔ 30cm (12in). ❀ (min. 10°C/50°F)
***C.* 'Cream Duke'.** Fully reflexed florists' chrysanthemum, a sport of 'Duke of Kent', bearing creamy white flowerheads, 25cm (10in) across when disbudded, in late autumn. Good for exhibition. ↕ 1.5m (5ft), ↔ 30cm (12in). ❀ (min. 10°C/50°F)
***C.* 'Cream John Hughes'.** Perfectly incurved florists' chrysanthemum with creamy white flowerheads, 12–14cm (5–5½in) across when disbudded, produced in late autumn. Good for exhibition. ↕ 1.2m (4ft), ↔ 60–75cm (24–30in). ❀ (min. 10°C/50°F)
***C.* 'Dawn Mist'** ▣ Spray florists' chrysanthemum with single, pale pink flowerheads, to 8cm (3in) across, produced in early autumn. ↕ 1.2m (4ft), ↔ 75–100cm (30–39in). ✻✻✻
C. densum see *Tanacetum densum* subsp. *amani.*
***C.* 'Discovery'** ▣ Intermediate to loosely incurved florists' chrysanthemum with light yellow flowerheads, 10–12cm (4–5in) across when disbudded, borne in early autumn. ↕ 1.2m (4ft), ↔ 75cm (30in). ✻
***C.* 'Dorridge Sun'.** Incurved florists' chrysanthemum with light yellow flowerheads, to 15cm (6in) across when disbudded, in late autumn. ↕ 1.3m (4½ft), ↔ 60cm (24in). ❀ (min. 10°C/50°F)
***C.* 'Duke of Kent'** ▣ Fully reflexed florists' chrysanthemum with white flowerheads, 25cm (10in) across when disbudded, produced in late autumn. Good for exhibition. ↕ 1.5m (5ft), ↔ 30cm (12in). ❀ (min. 10°C/50°F)
***C.* 'Edwin Painter'** ▣ Single florists' chrysanthemum producing yellow flowerheads, to 14cm (5½in) across when disbudded, in late autumn. ↕ 1.3–1.5m (4½–5ft), ↔ 75–100cm (30–39in). ❀ (min. 10°C/50°F)
***C.* 'Elsie Prosser'.** Fully reflexed florists' chrysanthemum with pink flowerheads, 25cm (10in) across when disbudded, produced in late autumn. Good for exhibition. ↕ 1.3–1.5m (4½–5ft), ↔ 30cm (12in). ❀ (min. 10°C/50°F)
***C.* 'Emperor of China'.** Rubellum Group chrysanthemum bearing double, silvery pink flowerheads, 5cm (2in) across, with quilled petals. While flowering, in late summer and early autumn, the leaves become red tinged. ↕ 1.2m (4ft), ↔ 60cm (24in). ✻✻✻
***C.* 'Enbee Wedding'** ♀ Spray florists' chrysanthemum with single, light pink flowerheads, to 8cm (3in) across, borne in early autumn. Good for exhibition. ↕ 1.2m (4ft), ↔ 75cm (30in). ✻✻✻
***C.* 'Fairie'.** Pompon florists' chrysanthemum with pink flowerheads, 4cm (1½in) across, borne in early autumn. ↕ 30–60cm (12–24in), ↔ 60cm (24in). ✻✻✻
***C.* 'Fairweather'** ▣ Incurved florists' chrysanthemum with pale purplish pink flowerheads, 14cm (5½in) across when disbudded, produced in late autumn. Good for exhibition. ↕ 1.1m (3½ft), ↔ to 75cm (30in). ❀ (min. 10°C/50°F)
C. gayanum see *Rhodanthemum gayanum.*
***C.* 'George Griffiths'** ▣ Fully reflexed florists' chrysanthemum bearing deep red flowerheads, to 14cm (5½in) across when disbudded, in early autumn. Good for exhibition. ↕ 1.3–1.5m (4½–5ft), ↔ 75cm (30in). ✻
***C.* 'Gigantic'.** Tightly incurved or loosely reflexed florists' chrysanthemum, its form depending on the amount of warmth provided; bears salmon-pink flowerheads, 25–27cm (10–11in) across when disbudded, in late autumn. Good for exhibition. ↕ 1.3m (4½ft), ↔ 30cm (12in). ❀ (min. 10°C/50°F)
***C.* 'Gillette'.** Incurved florists' chrysanthemum with cream flowerheads, 14cm (5½in) across when disbudded, borne in early autumn. ↕ 1.3m (4½ft), ↔ 45cm (18in). ✻
***C.* 'Ginger Nut'.** Intermediate florists' chrysanthemum producing light bronze flowerheads, to 14cm (5½in) across when disbudded, in early autumn; the flowerheads may close over at the top to become incurved. Good for exhibition. ↕ 1.2m (4ft), ↔ 60cm (24in). ✻
***C.* 'Golden Chalice'** ▣ Charm florists' chrysanthemum with single yellow flowerheads, 2.5cm (1in) across, borne in late autumn. Good for exhibition. ↕↔ 1m (3ft). ❀ (min. 10°C/50°F)
***C.* 'Golden Gigantic'** ▣ Tightly incurved or loosely reflexed florists' chrysanthemum, bearing large gold flowerheads, 25–27cm (10–11in) across when disbudded, in late autumn. Good for exhibition. ↕ 1.3m (4½ft), ↔ 30cm (12in). ❀ (min. 10°C/50°F)
***C.* 'Golden Woolman's Glory'** ▣ Single florists' chrysanthemum with gold flowerheads, 18cm (7in) across when disbudded, borne in late autumn. Good for exhibition. ↕ 1.3m (4½ft), ↔ 1m (3ft). ❀ (min. 10°C/50°F)
***C.* 'Green Satin'** ▣ Intermediate or loosely incurved florists' chrysanthemum with green flowerheads, 12cm (5in) across when disbudded, produced in late autumn. ↕ 1.2m (4ft), ↔ 60cm (24in). ❀ (min. 10°C/50°F)
C. haradjanii see *Tanacetum haradjanii.*
***C.* 'Hedgerow'.** Single florists' chrysanthemum with pink flowerheads, 12cm (5in) across when disbudded, produced in late autumn. ↕ 1.5m (5ft), ↔ 75–100cm (30–39in). ❀ (min. 10°C/50°F)

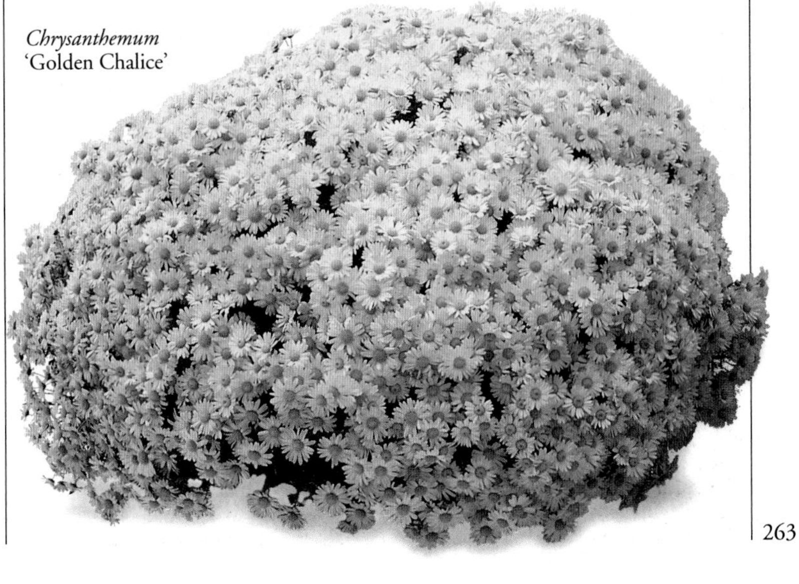
Chrysanthemum 'Golden Chalice'

***C.* 'Hilfred'.** Charm florists' chrysanthemum with a profusion of single white flowerheads, 2.5cm (1in) across, borne in late autumn. Good for exhibition. ↕↔ 1m (3ft). ❀ (min. 10°C/50°F)
C. hosmariense see *Rhodanthemum hosmariense.*
***C.* 'Idris'.** Incurved florists' chrysanthemum producing salmon-pink flowerheads, 21–25cm (8–10in) across when disbudded, in late autumn. ↕ 1.3m (4½ft), ↔ 45cm (18in). ❀ (min. 10°C/50°F)
***C.* 'Jessie Habgood'.** Reflexed florists' chrysanthemum producing large white flowerheads, 25cm (10in) or more across when disbudded, in late autumn. Good for exhibition. ↕ 2m (6ft), ↔ 45cm (18in). ❀ (min. 10°C/50°F)
***C.* 'John Hughes'** ▣ Incurved florists' chrysanthemum bearing white flowerheads, 12–14cm (5–5½in) across when disbudded, in late autumn. Good for exhibition. ↕ 1.2m (4ft), ↔ 60–75cm (24–30in). ❀ (min. 10°C/50°F)
***C.* 'John Wingfield'** ▣ Reflexed florists' chrysanthemum producing white, often pink-flushed flowerheads, 12cm (5in) across when disbudded, in late autumn. Good for exhibition. ↕ 1.5m (5ft), ↔ 45–60cm (18–24in). ❀ (min. 10°C/50°F)
***C.* 'Keith Luxford'** ▣ Incurved florists' chrysanthemum bearing pink flowerheads, 21–25cm (8–10in) across when

 CHRYSANTHEMUM

C

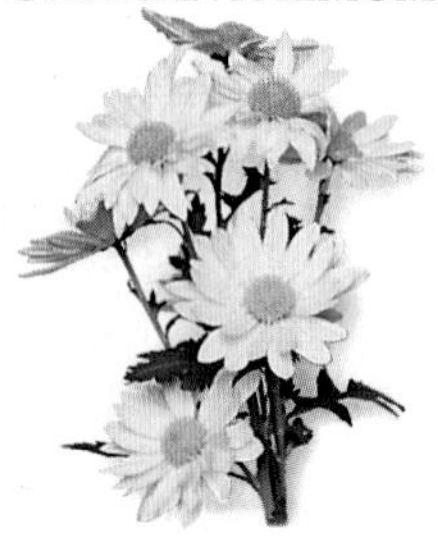
Chrysanthemum 'Lemon Rynoon'

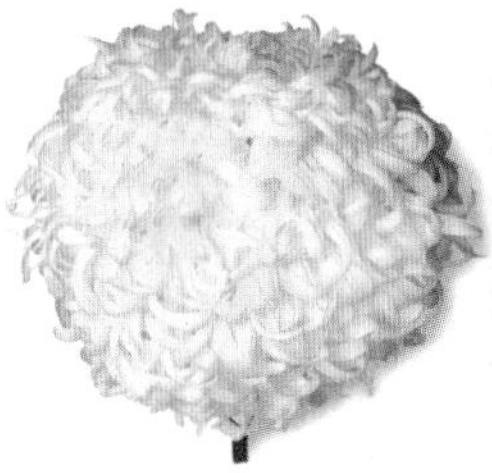
Chrysanthemum 'Lundy'

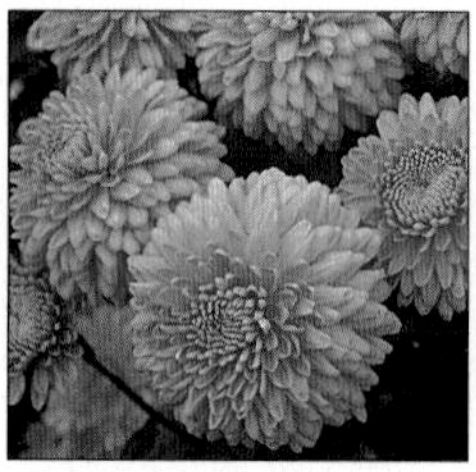
Chrysanthemum 'Madeleine'

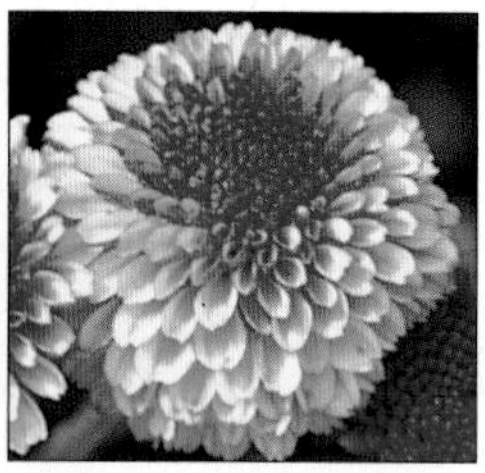
Chrysanthemum 'Maria'

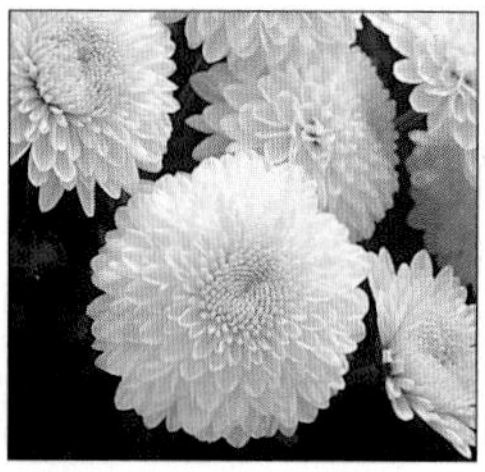
Chrysanthemum 'Marion'

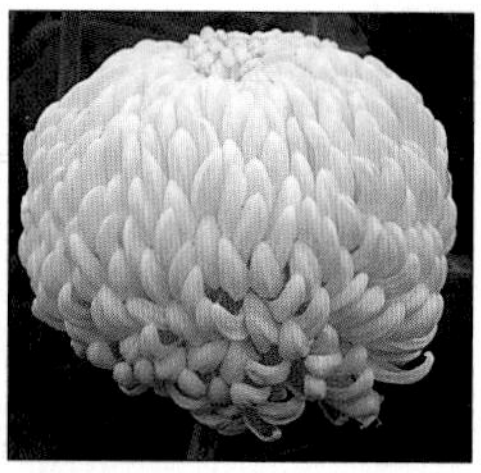
Chrysanthemum 'Marlene Jones'

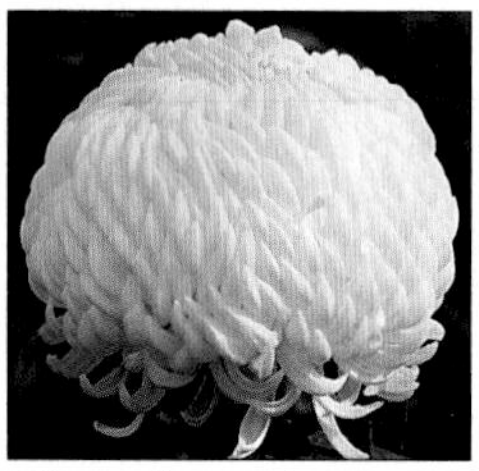
Chrysanthemum 'Michael Fish'

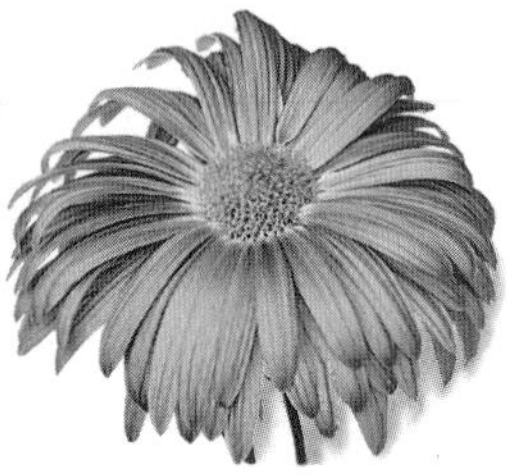
Chrysanthemum 'My Love'

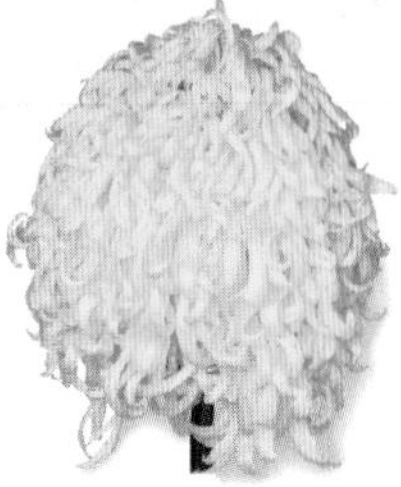
Chrysanthemum 'Nancye Furneaux'

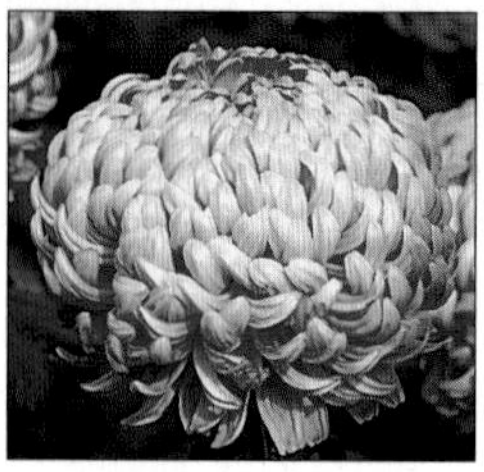
Chrysanthemum 'Oracle'

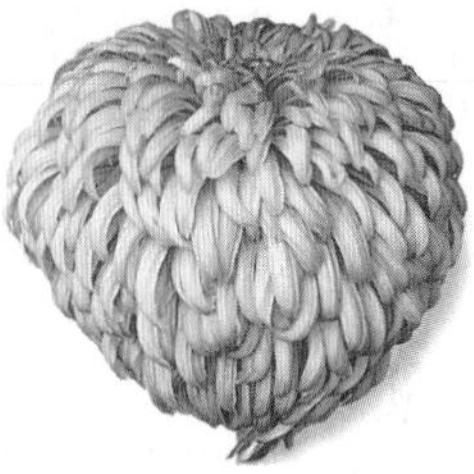
Chrysanthemum 'Patricia Millar'

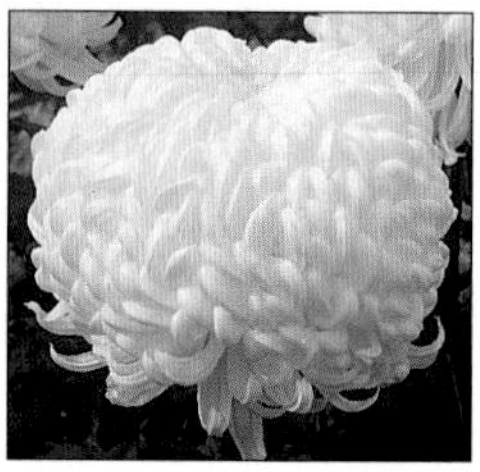
Chrysanthemum 'Pavilion'

disbudded, in late autumn. ↕1.5m (5ft), ↔45cm (18in). ❀ (min. 10°C/50°F)
***C.* 'Lemon Rynoon'** ■ Spray florists' chrysanthemum with single, pale lemon-yellow flowerheads, 8cm (3in) across, becoming white with age, borne in late autumn. ↕1.5m (5ft), ↔75–100cm (30–39in). ❀ (min. 10°C/50°F)
C. leucanthemum see *Leucanthemum vulgare.*
***C.* 'Lilac Prince'.** Reflexed florists' chrysanthemum bearing large pink flowerheads, 25cm (10in) or more across when disbudded, in late autumn. Good for exhibition. ↕1.5m (5ft), ↔45cm (18in). ❀ (min. 10°C/50°F)
***C.* 'Lundy'** ■ Fully reflexed florists' chrysanthemum with white flowerheads, 21–25cm (8–10in) across when disbudded, and often broader than they are deep, borne in late autumn. Good for exhibition. ↕1.5m (5ft), ↔45cm (18in). ❀ (min. 10°C/50°F)
***C.* 'Madeleine'** ■♀ Spray florists' chrysanthemum producing reflexed pink flowerheads, to 8cm (3in) across, in early autumn. Good for exhibition. ↕1.2m (4ft), ↔75cm (30in). ***
***C.* 'Majestic'.** Fully reflexed florists' chrysanthemum bearing light bronze flowerheads, 21–25cm (8–10in) across when disbudded, in late autumn. Good for exhibition. ↕1.3m (4½ft), ↔45cm (18in). ❀ (min. 10°C/50°F)
***C.* 'Malcolm Perkins'.** Intermediate florists' chrysanthemum with large yellow flowerheads, to 21cm (8in) across when disbudded, produced in early autumn. Good for exhibition. ↕1.6m (5½ft), ↔75cm (30in). *
C. maresii see *Rhodanthemum maresii.*
***C.* 'Margaret'** ♀ Spray florists' chrysanthemum bearing reflexed pink flowerheads, 8–9cm (3–3½in) across, in early autumn. Good for exhibition. ↕1.2m (4ft), ↔60–75cm (24–30in). ***
***C.* 'Maria'** ■ Pompon florists' chrysanthemum producing a profusion of pink flowerheads, to 4cm (1½in) across, in late summer and early autumn. ↕45cm (18in), ↔30–60cm (12–24in). ***
***C.* 'Marion'** ■ Spray florists' chrysanthemum bearing reflexed, pale yellow flowerheads, 9cm (3½in) across, in late summer. ↕1.2m (4ft), ↔75cm (30in). ***
***C.* 'Marlene Jones'** ■ Intermediate or loosely incurved florists' chrysanthemum with pale yellow flowerheads, to 15cm (6in) across when disbudded, borne in early autumn. Good for exhibition. ↕1m (3ft), ↔60cm (24in). ***
***C.* 'Mary Stoker'** ■ Rubellum Group chrysanthemum with single, rose-tinted, apricot-yellow flowerheads, 5cm (2in) across, produced in late summer and early autumn. The centres turn from green to yellow as the disc-florets open. ↕75cm (30in), ↔60cm (24in). ***
***C.* 'Mason's Bronze'.** Single florists' chrysanthemum producing bronze flowerheads, 12cm (5in) across when disbudded, in late autumn. Good for exhibition. ↕1.3–1.5m (4½–5ft), ↔1m (3ft). ❀ (min. 10°C/50°F)
***C. maximum* of gardens** see *Leucanthemum* x *superbum.*
***C.* 'Max Riley'** ♀ Fully incurved florists' chrysanthemum with yellow flowerheads, 12cm (5in) across when disbudded, produced in early autumn. Good for exhibition. ↕1.3m (4½ft), ↔75cm (30in). *

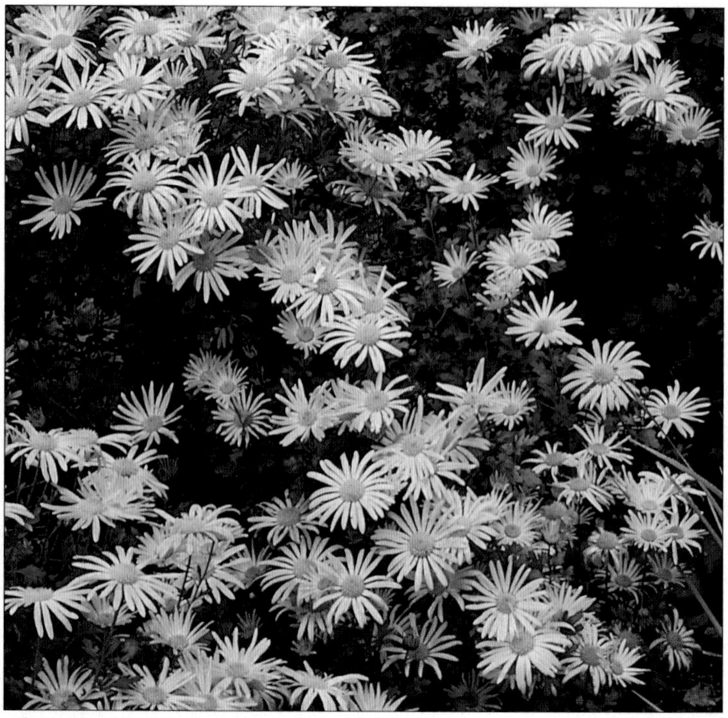
Chrysanthemum 'Mary Stoker'

***C.* 'Michael Fish'** ■ Intermediate or tightly incurved florists' chrysanthemum with white flowerheads, 15cm (6in) across when disbudded, borne in early autumn. Good for exhibition. ↕1.2m (4ft), ↔60–75cm (24–30in). *
***C.* 'Milady'.** Spray florists' chrysanthemum with anemone-centred white flowerheads, 9cm (3½in) across, produced in late autumn. Good for exhibition. ↕1.2m (4ft), ↔75cm (30in). ❀ (min. 10°C/50°F)
***C.* 'Mrs. Jessie Cooper'.** Rubellum Group chrysanthemum with semi-double red flowerheads, 9–10cm (3½–4in) across, produced in late summer and early autumn. ↕75cm (30in), ↔60cm (24in). ***
***C.* 'My Love'** ■ Single florists' chrysanthemum bearing salmon-pink flowerheads, 16cm (6in) across when disbudded, in late autumn. ↕1.5m (5ft), ↔75–100cm (30–39in). ❀ (min. 10°C/50°F)
***C.* 'Nancye Furneaux'** ■ Reflexed florists' chrysanthemum with yellow flowerheads, 21–25cm (8–10in) across when disbudded, borne in late autumn. Good for exhibition. ↕1.5m (5ft), ↔45cm (18in). ❀ (min. 10°C/50°F)
***C.* 'Nancy Perry'.** Rubellum Group chrysanthemum with semi-double, dark pink flowerheads, to 7cm (3in) across, produced in late summer and early autumn. ↕75cm (30in), ↔60cm (24in). ***
***C.* 'Nancy Sherwood'.** Single florists' chrysanthemum with yellow flowerheads, 14cm (5½in) across when disbudded, produced in late autumn. Good for exhibition. ↕1.3m (4½ft), ↔1m (3ft). ❀ (min. 10°C/50°F)
***C.* 'Oracle'** ■ Intermediate or loosely incurved florists' chrysanthemum producing pale bronze flowerheads, 12cm (5in) across when disbudded, in early autumn. Good for exhibition. ↕1.2m (4ft), ↔60–75cm (24–30in). *
C. pacificum see *Ajania pacifica.*
C. paludosum see *Leucanthemum paludosum.*
C. parthenium see *Tanacetum parthenium.*
***C.* 'Patricia Millar'** ■ Fully reflexed florists' chrysanthemum with light pink flowerheads, 13–14cm (5–5½in) across when disbudded, borne from early to late autumn. Use for exhibition. ↕1.3m (4½ft), ↔60–75cm (24–30in). *
***C.* 'Pavilion'** ■ Intermediate or loosely incurved florists' chrysanthemum with white flowerheads, 18cm (7in) across when disbudded, borne in early autumn. Good for exhibition. ↕1.3m (4½ft), ↔60–75cm (24–30in). *
***C.* 'Peach Brietner'** ■ Reflexed florists' chrysanthemum bearing peach-pink flowerheads, to 12cm (5in) across when disbudded, in early autumn. ↕to 1.2m (4ft), ↔75cm (30in). *
***C.* 'Peach Margaret'** ■♀ syn. *C.* 'Salmon Margaret'. Spray florists' chrysanthemum bearing reflexed, light salmon flowerheads, 8–9cm (3–3½in) across, in early autumn. ↕1.2m (4ft), ↔60–75cm (24–30in). ***
***C.* 'Pearl Celebration'.** Reflexed florists' chrysanthemum with large, light pink flowerheads, 18–21cm (7–8in) across when disbudded, borne in early autumn. Good for exhibition. ↕1.5m (5ft), ↔60–75cm (24–30in). *

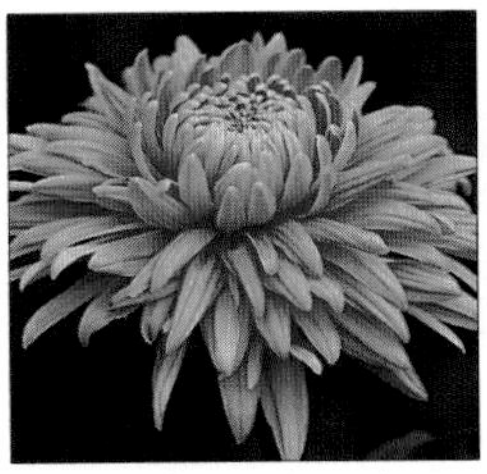
Chrysanthemum 'Peach Brietner'

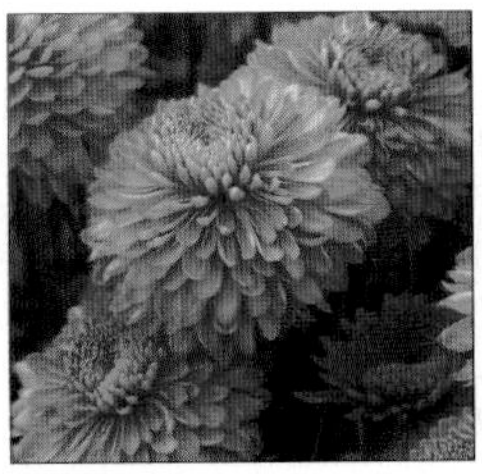
Chrysanthemum 'Peach Margaret'

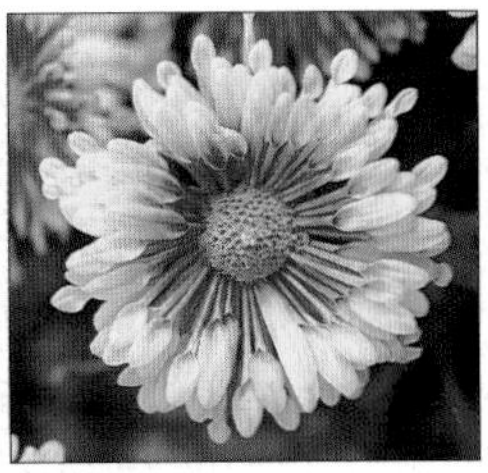
Chrysanthemum 'Pennine Alfie'

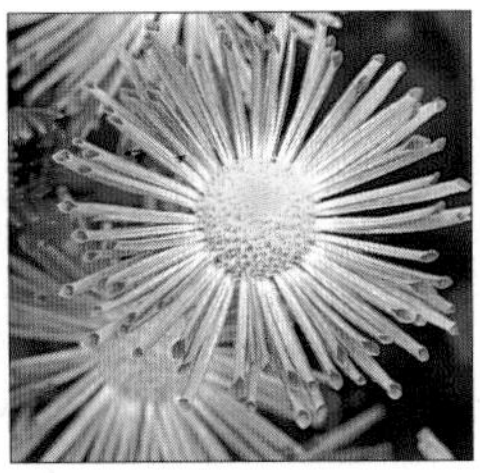
Chrysanthemum 'Pennine Flute'

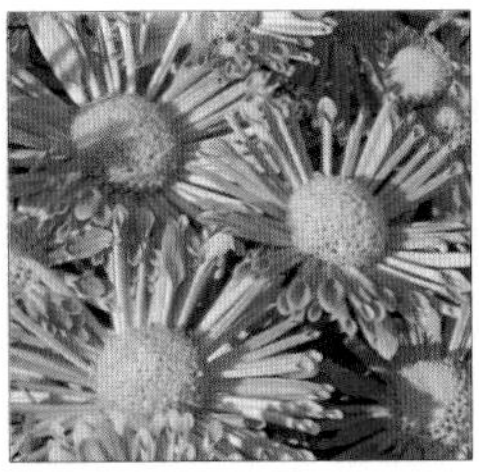
Chrysanthemum 'Pennine Jewel'

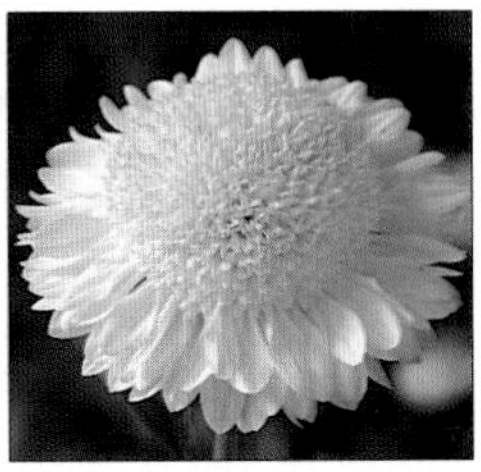
Chrysanthemum 'Pennine Oriel'

C

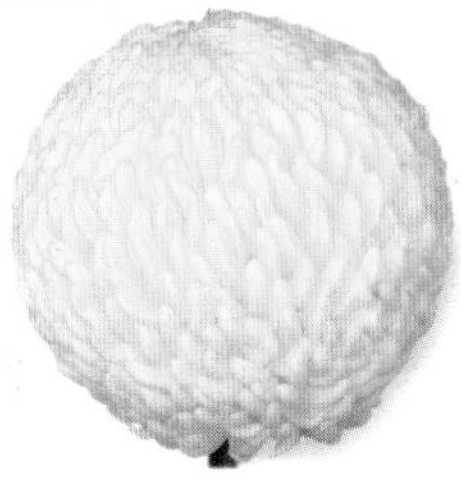
Chrysanthemum 'Primrose John Hughes'

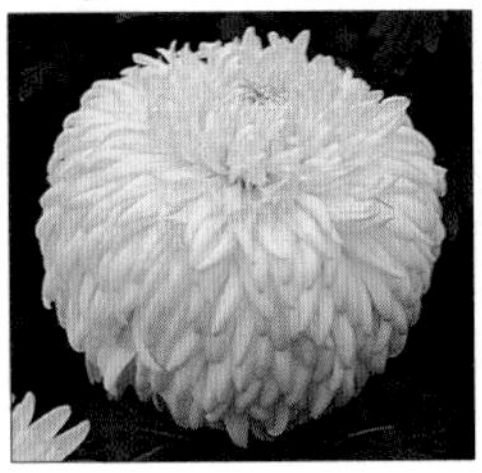
Chrysanthemum 'Primrose West Bromwich'

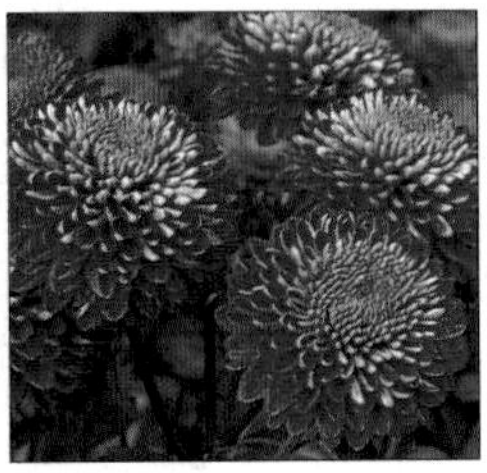
Chrysanthemum 'Purple Pennine Wine'

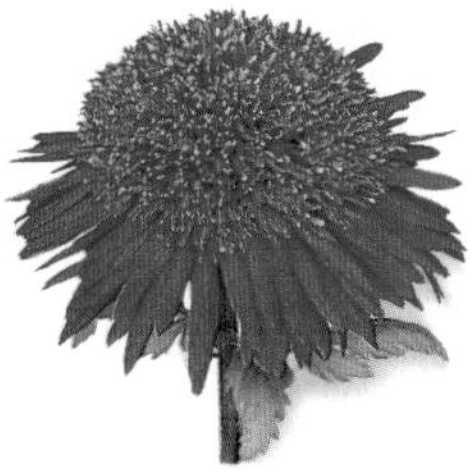
Chrysanthemum 'Raymond Mounsey'

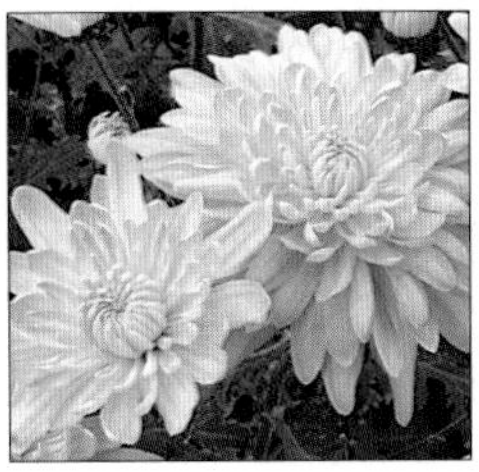
Chrysanthemum 'Roblush'

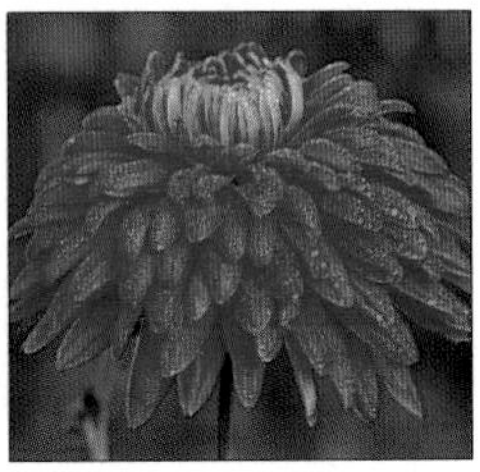
Chrysanthemum 'Rose Yvonne Arnaud'

C. pectinata see *Leucanthemopsis pectinata.*
C. 'Pennine Alfie' ■ Spray florists' chrysanthemum with spoon-shaped, light bronze flowerheads, 8cm (3in) across, produced in early autumn. ↕1.2m (4ft), ↔ 75cm (30in). ❄❄❄
C. 'Pennine Flute' ■♀ Spray florists' chrysanthemum with 4 or 5 stems of quill-shaped, purple-pink flowerheads, to 8cm (3in) across, produced in late summer and early autumn. ↕1.2m (4ft), ↔ 75cm (30in). ❄❄❄
C. 'Pennine Jade' ♀ Spray florists' chrysanthemum bearing numerous single, light bronze flowerheads, 8cm (3in) across, in early autumn. ↕1.2m (4ft), ↔ 1m (3ft). ❄
C. 'Pennine Jewel' ■ Spray florists' chrysanthemum with spoon-shaped, light bronze flowerheads, 8cm (3in) across, produced in early autumn. Good for exhibition. ↕1.2m (4ft), ↔ 60–75cm (24–30in). ❄❄❄
C. 'Pennine Oriel' ■ Spray florists' chrysanthemum bearing anemone-centred cream flowerheads, 9cm (3½in) across, with yellow centres in early autumn. Good for exhibition. ↕1.2m (4ft), ↔ 60–75cm (24–30in). ❄❄❄
C. 'Pennine Signal' ♀ Spray florists' chrysanthemum producing single red flowerheads, 9cm (3½in) across, in early autumn. ↕1.2m (4ft), ↔ 60–75cm (24–30in). ❄❄❄
C. 'Peter Rowe'. Incurved florists' chrysanthemum with yellow flowerheads, 12cm (5in) across when disbudded, produced in early autumn. Good for exhibition. ↕1.3m (4½ft), ↔ 60–75cm (24–30in). ❄
C. 'Pink Gin'. Spray florists' chrysanthemum producing reflexed, light purple flowerheads, 9cm (3½in) across, in late autumn. Good for exhibition. ↕1.2m (4ft), ↔ 75–100cm (30–39in). ❀ (min. 10°C/50°F)
C. 'Poppet' ♀ Pompon florists' chrysanthemum bearing a profusion of small yellow flowerheads, 4cm (1½in) across, in early autumn. ↕60cm (24in), ↔ to 75cm (30in). ❄❄❄
C. 'Primrose Alison Kirk'. Incurved florists' chrysanthemum with primrose-yellow flowerheads, 14cm (5½in) across when disbudded, borne in early autumn. Good for exhibition. ↕1.2m (4ft), ↔ 40cm (16in). ❄
C. 'Primrose Chessington'. Intermediate to tightly incurved florists' chrysanthemum with primrose-yellow flowerheads, 18–20cm (7–8in) across when disbudded, produced in early autumn. Good for exhibition. ↕2–2.2m (6–7ft), ↔ 75cm (30in). ❄
C. 'Primrose Jessie Habgood'. Reflexed florists' chrysanthemum with primrose-yellow flowerheads, 25cm (10in) or more across when disbudded, borne in late autumn. ↕2m (6ft), ↔ 45cm (18in). ❀ (min. 10°C/50°F)
C. 'Primrose John Hughes' ■ Perfectly incurved florists' chrysanthemum with primrose-yellow flowerheads, 12–14cm (5–5½in) across when disbudded, borne in late autumn. Good for exhibition. ↕1.2m (4ft), ↔ 60–75cm (24–30in). ❀ (min. 10°C/50°F)
C. 'Primrose Pennine Oriel'. Spray florists' chrysanthemum with anemone-centred, primrose-yellow flowerheads, 9cm (3½in) across, borne in early autumn. ↕1.2m (4ft), ↔ 60–75cm (24–30in). ❄❄❄
C. 'Primrose West Bromwich' ■ Fully reflexed florists' chrysanthemum bearing pale yellow flowerheads, 18cm (7in) across when disbudded, in mid-autumn. Good for exhibition. ↕1.5m (5ft), ↔ 75cm (30in). ❄
C. 'Primrose World of Sport'. Intermediate florists' chrysanthemum bearing primrose-yellow flowerheads, to 19cm (7in) across when disbudded, in early autumn. Good for exhibition. ↕1.5m (5ft), ↕75cm (30in). ❄
C. 'Purple Pennine Wine' ■♀ Spray florists' chrysanthemum with reflexed purple flowerheads, 8cm (3in) across, borne in early and mid-autumn. Good for exhibition. ↕1.2m (4ft), ↔ 75cm (30in). ❄❄❄
C. 'Raymond Mounsey' ■ Anemone-centred florists' chrysanthemum with red flowerheads, to 13cm (5in) across when disbudded, with domed, reddish bronze centres, produced in late autumn. Good for exhibition. ↕1.5m (5ft), ↔ 1m (3ft). ❀ (min. 10°C/50°F)
C. 'Rebecca Walker'. Intermediate florists' chrysanthemum producing large yellow flowerheads, 23cm (9in) across when disbudded, in early autumn. ↕2m (6ft), ↔ 75cm (30in). ❄
C. 'Red Amethyst'. Reflexed florists' chrysanthemum with vibrant, brilliant red flowerheads, 21cm (8in) across when disbudded, produced in late autumn. Good for exhibition. ↕1.2m (4ft), ↔ 30cm (12in). ❀ (min. 10°C/50°F)
C. 'Red Glory' see *C.* 'Red Woolman's Glory'.
C. 'Red Wendy' ♀ Spray florists' chrysanthemum producing reflexed red flowerheads, 8cm (3in) across, in early autumn. Bears 5 or 6 blooms per stem in perfect umbrella-form when grown with 4 stems per plant. Good for exhibition. ↕1.2m (4ft), ↔ 60–75cm (24–30in). ❄❄❄
C. 'Red Woolman's Glory', syn. *C.* 'Red Glory'. Single florists' chrysanthemum bearing red flowerheads, 21cm (8in) across when disbudded, in late autumn. ↕1.3m (4½ft), ↔ 1m (3ft). ❀ (min. 10°C/50°F)
C. 'Ringdove' ■ Charm florists' chrysanthemum producing abundant single pink flowerheads, 2.5cm (1in) across, in late autumn. ↕↔ 1m (3ft). ❀ (min. 10°C/50°F)
C. 'Robeam'. Spray florists' chrysanthemum with reflexed yellow flowerheads, to 8cm (3in) across, produced in late autumn. Good for exhibition. ↕1.5m (5ft), ↔ 75–100cm (30–39in). ❀ (min. 10°C/50°F)
C. 'Roblush' ■ Spray florists' chrysanthemum with reflexed, light pink flowerheads, to 8cm (3in) across, produced in late autumn. Good for exhibition. ↕1.5m (5ft), ↔ 75–100cm (30–39in). ❀ (min. 10°C/50°F)
C. 'Romark'. Spray florists' chrysanthemum producing reflexed white flowerheads, to 8cm (3in) across, in late autumn. Good for exhibition. ↕1.5m (5ft), ↔ 75–100cm (30–39in). ❀ (min. 10°C/50°F)
C. 'Rose My Love'. Single florists' chrysanthemum with deep salmon-pink flowerheads, 16cm (6in) across when disbudded, in late autumn. Good for exhibition. ↕1.5m (5ft), ↔ 75–100cm (30–39in). ❀ (min. 10°C/50°F)
C. 'Rose Yvonne Arnaud' ■ Reflexed florists' chrysanthemum with deep rose-

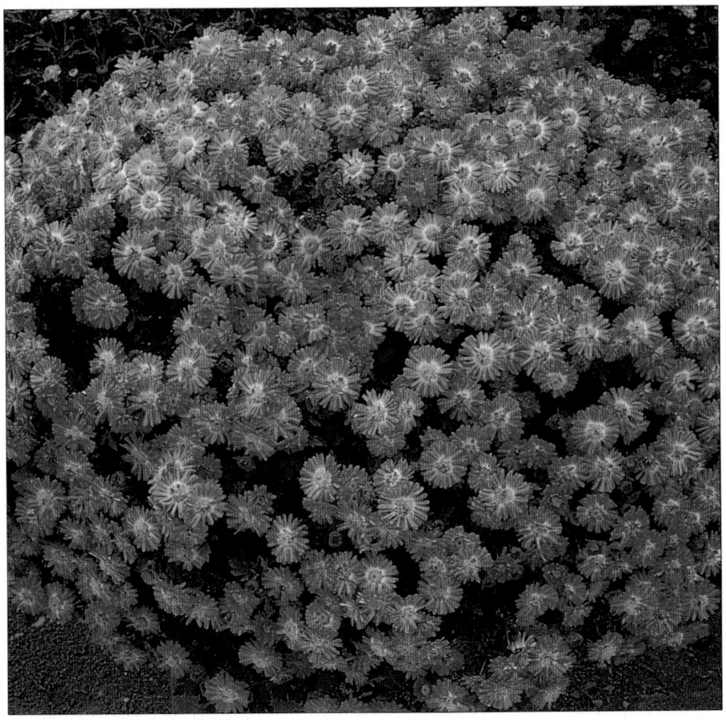
Chrysanthemum 'Ringdove'

CHRYSANTHEMUM

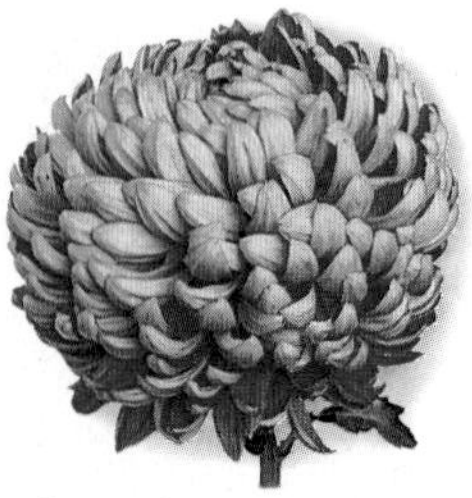

Chrysanthemum 'Roy Coopland'

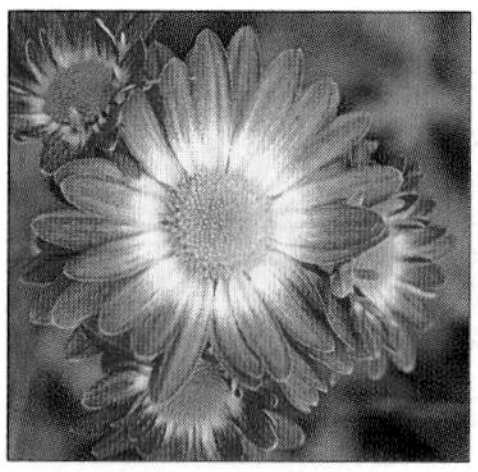

Chrysanthemum 'Rytorch'

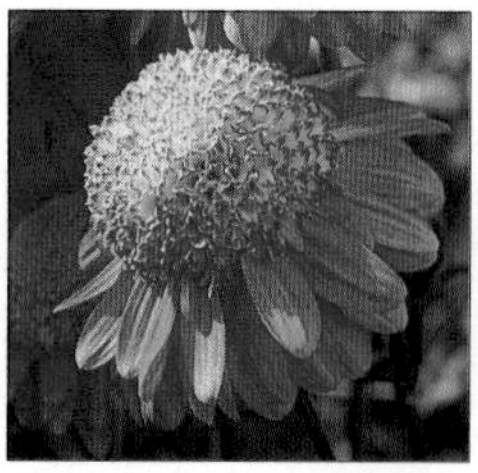

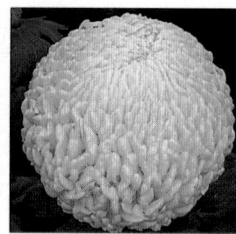

Chrysanthemum 'Sally Ball'

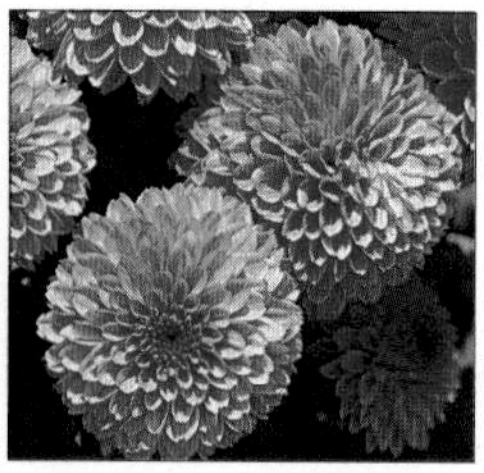

Chrysanthemum 'Salmon Fairie'

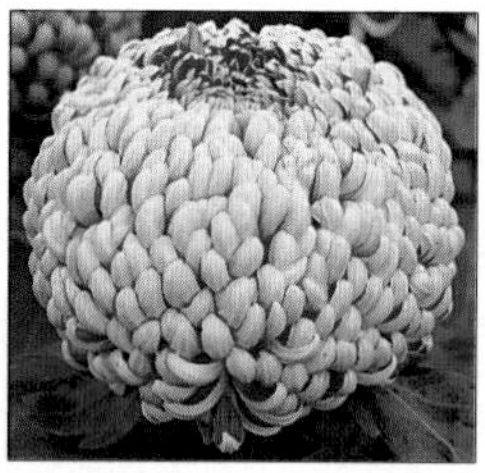

Chrysanthemum 'Salmon Fairweather'

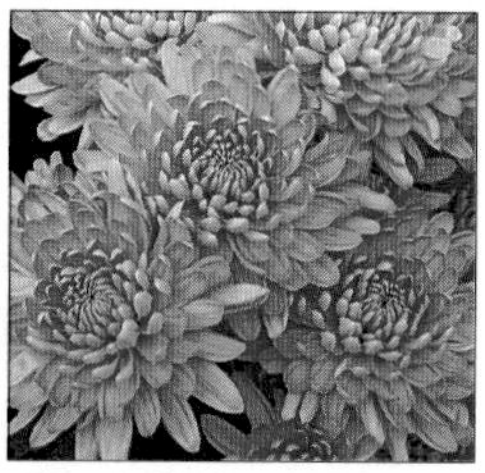

Chrysanthemum 'Satin Pink Gin'

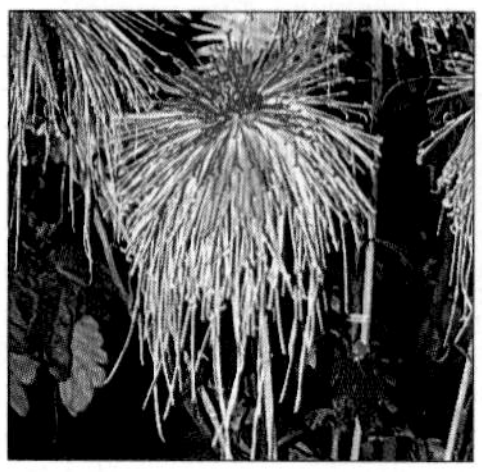

Chrysanthemum 'Senkyo Emiaki'

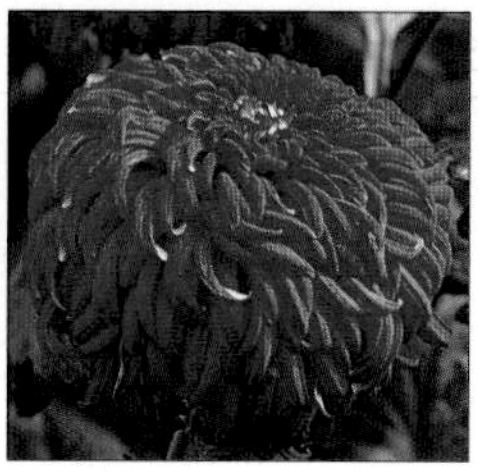

Chrysanthemum 'Sentry'

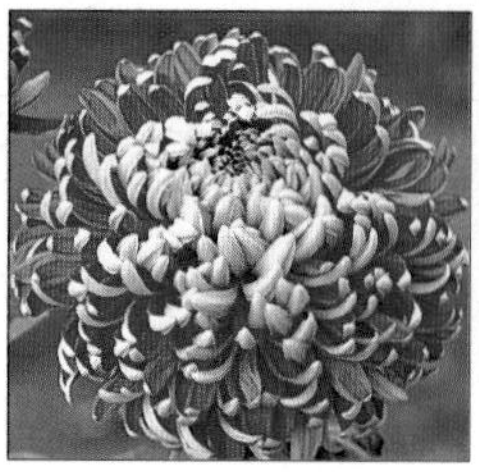

Chrysanthemum 'Skater's Waltz'

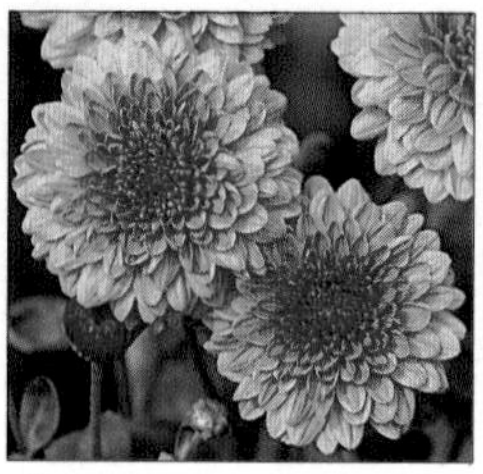

Chrysanthemum 'Wendy'

Chrysanthemum 'Yellow John Hughes'

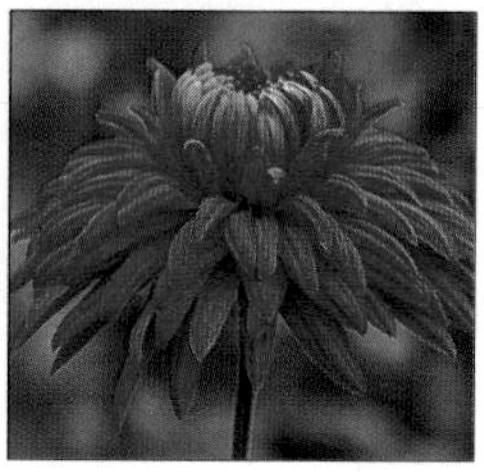

Chrysanthemum 'Yvonne Arnaud'

pink flowerheads, 12cm (5in) across when disbudded, produced in early autumn. ↕1.2m (4ft), ↔60–75cm (24–30in). ❄

***C.* 'Roy Coopland'** ▣ Intermediate to loosely incurved florists' chrysanthemum with bronze flowerheads, to 15cm (6in) across when disbudded, borne in late autumn. Good for exhibition. ↕1.4m (4½ft), ↔60cm (24in). ❀ (min. 10°C/50°F)

***C.* 'Ryflash'.** Spray florists' chrysanthemum producing single, deep red flowerheads, to 8cm (3in) across, in late autumn. Good for exhibition. ↕1.5m (5ft), ↔75–100cm (30–39in). ❀ (min. 10°C/50°F)

***C.* 'Rynoon'.** Spray florists' chrysanthemum bearing single, light pink flowerheads, to 8cm (3in) across, in late autumn. ↕1.5m (5ft), ↔75–100cm (30–39in). ❀ (min. 10°C/50°F)

***C.* 'Rytorch'** ▣ Spray florists' chrysanthemum with single, light bronze flowerheads, to 8cm (3in) across, with yellow centres, borne in late autumn. ↕1.5m (5ft), ↔75–100cm (30–39in). ❀ (min. 10°C/50°F)

***C.* 'Sally Ball'** ▣ Spray florists' chrysanthemum bearing a profusion of anemone-centred bronze flowerheads, 12cm (5in) across, in early autumn. ↕1.2m (4ft), ↔75cm (30in). ❄❄❄

***C.* 'Salmon Fairie'** ▣ Pompon florists' chrysanthemum bearing salmon-pink flowerheads, 4cm (1½in) across when disbudded, in late autumn. Good for exhibition. ↕30–60cm (12–24in), ↔ to 60cm (24in). ❄❄❄

***C.* 'Salmon Fairweather'** ▣ Incurved florists' chrysanthemum with salmon-pink flowerheads, 14cm (5½in) across when disbudded, borne in late autumn. Good for exhibition. ↕1.1m (3½ft), ↔ to 75cm (30in). ❀ (min. 10°C/50°F)

***C.* 'Salmon Margaret'** see *C.* 'Peach Margaret'.

***C.* 'Salmon Seychelle'.** Reflexed florists' chrysanthemum with salmon-pink flowerheads, 21cm (8in) across when disbudded, produced in late autumn. Good for exhibition. ↕1.5m (5ft), ↔45cm (18in) with one flowerhead grown; ↕ to 75cm (30in), with 2 flowerheads grown. ❀ (min. 10°C/50°F)

***C.* 'Salmon Venice'.** Reflexed florists' chrysanthemum with salmon-pink flowerheads, 15cm (6in) across when disbudded, borne in early autumn. Good for exhibition. ↕1.2–1.3m (4–4½ft), ↔60–75cm (24–30in) when grown with 2 or more flowerheads; ↕ to 1m (3ft) when grown with 3 or more flowerheads. ❄

***C.* 'Sam Oldham'.** Fully reflexed florists' chrysanthemum with large red flowerheads, to 18cm (7in) across when disbudded, produced in early autumn. Good for exhibition. ↕1.3m (4½ft), ↔60cm (24in). ❄

***C.* 'Satin Pink Gin'** ▣ Spray florists' chrysanthemum with reflexed, light pink flowerheads, 8cm (3in) across, produced in late autumn. Good for exhibition. ↕1.2m (4ft), ↔75–100cm (30–39in). ❀ (min. 10°C/50°F)

C. segetum ▣ (Corn marigold). Fast-growing, erect, fleshy annual chrysanthemum with oblong to obovate, grey-green leaves, 3–5cm (1¼–2in) long, entire towards the stem tips, pinnatisect lower down the stems. Solitary, single, daisy-like yellow flowerheads, to 5cm (2in) across, are produced in summer. Often included in wildflower seed mixtures. ↕ to 80cm (32in), ↔30cm (12in). Mediterranean. ❄❄❄. **'Eastern Star'** bears primrose-yellow flowerheads with brown central discs. **'Prado'** produces large, golden yellow flowerheads, to 8cm (3in) across, with dark brown central discs.

***C.* 'Senkyo Emiaki'** ▣ Spider-form florists' chrysanthemum bearing light pink flowerheads, 15cm (6in) across when disbudded, in early autumn. Good for exhibition. ↕30–60cm (12–24in), ↔ to 60cm (24in). ❀ (min. 10°C/50°F)

***C.* 'Sentry'** ▣ Reflexed florists' chrysanthemum bearing deep red flowerheads, 12cm (5in) across when disbudded, in early autumn. Good for exhibition. ↕1.2–1.3m (4–4½ft), ↔60–70cm (24–28in). ❄

C. serotinum see *Leucanthemella serotina.*

***C.* 'Seychelle'.** Reflexed florists' chrysanthemum with pink flowerheads, 21cm (8in) across when disbudded, borne in late autumn. Good for exhibition. ↕1.5m (5ft), ↔45–75cm (18–30in). ❀ (min. 10°C/50°F)

***C.* 'Silver Gigantic'.** Tightly incurved or loosely reflexed florists' chrysanthemum, its form depending on the amount of warmth provided. Bears silver flowerheads, 25–27cm (10–11in) across when disbudded, in late autumn. Good for exhibition. ↕1.3m (4½ft), ↔30cm (12in). ❀ (min. 10°C/50°F)

***C.* 'Skater's Waltz'** ▣ Loosely incurved florists' chrysanthemum with pink flowerheads, 15cm (6in) across when disbudded, borne in late autumn. Good for exhibition. ↕1.5m (5ft), ↔60–75cm (24–30in). ❀ (min. 10°C/50°F)

C.* x *superbum see *Leucanthemum* x *superbum.*

***C.* 'Susan Freestone'.** Fully reflexed florists' chrysanthemum producing yellow flowerheads, 15cm (6in) across when disbudded, in early autumn. Good for exhibition. ↕1.2m (4ft), ↔60cm (24in). ❄

***C.* 'Talbot Jo'** ▣ Spray florists' chrysanthemum bearing single pink

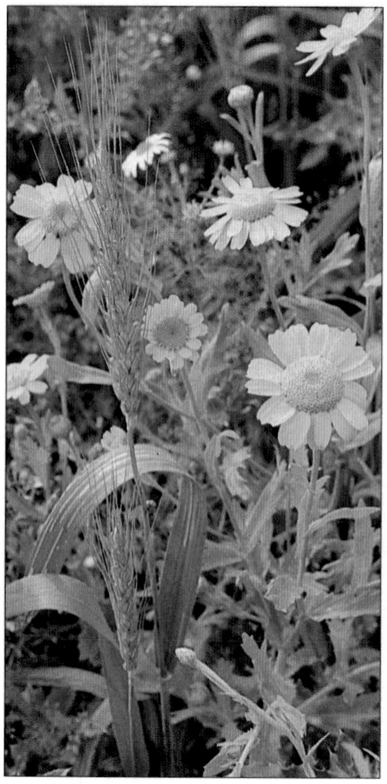

Chrysanthemum segetum

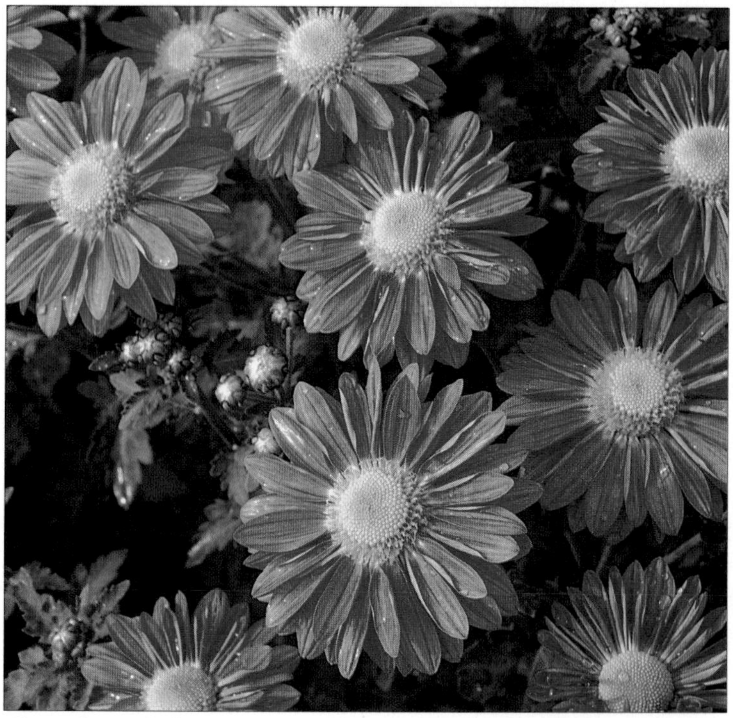

Chrysanthemum 'Talbot Jo'

flowerheads, 8cm (3in) across, in early autumn. Good for exhibition. ↕ 1.3m (4½ft), ↔ 75cm (30in). ❄❄❄
C. 'Tennis'. Intermediate florists' chrysanthemum with white flowerheads, to 12cm (5in) across when disbudded, borne in early autumn. Good for exhibition. ↕ 1.3m (4½ft), ↔ 60cm (24in). ❄
C. tricolor see *C. carinatum.*
C. uliginosum see *Leucanthemella serotina.*
C. 'Venice'. Reflexed florists' chrysanthemum bearing pink flowerheads, 15cm (6in) across when disbudded, in early autumn. Use for exhibition. ↕ 1.2–1.3m (4–4½ft), ↔ 60–100cm (24–39in). ❄
C. vulgare see *Tanacetum vulgare.*
C. 'Wendy' ▣ 🏆 Spray florists' chrysanthemum bearing reflexed, light bronze flowerheads, 8cm (3in) across, in early autumn. Good for exhibition. ↕ 1.2m (4ft), ↔ 60–75cm (24–30in) when grown with 4 stems. ❄❄❄
C. 'West Bromwich'. Reflexed florists' chrysanthemum with white flowerheads, 18cm (7in) across when disbudded, produced in mid-autumn. Good for exhibition. ↕ 1.5m (5ft), ↔ 75cm (30in) when disbudded. ❄
C. weyrichii see *Dendranthema weyrichii.*
C. 'White Fairweather'. Incurved florists' chrysanthemum with white flowerheads, 14cm (5½in) across when disbudded, borne in late autumn. Good for exhibition. ↕ 1.1m (3½ft), ↔ to 75cm (30in). ❀ (min. 10°C/50°F)
C. 'Wisley Bronze' ▣ Cascade florists' chrysanthemum bearing single bronze flowerheads, 6cm (2½in) across, in late autumn. Good for exhibition. ↕ 1.5m (5ft), ↔ 1m (3ft). ❀ (min. 10°C/50°F)

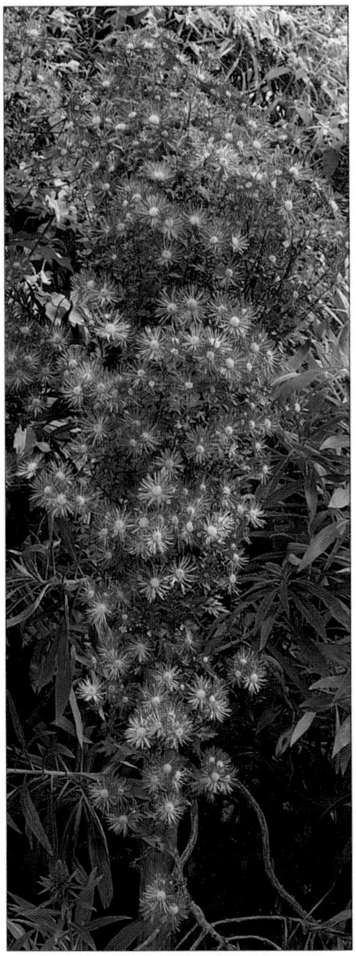
Chrysanthemum 'Wisley Bronze'

C. 'Woking Rose'. Intermediate florists' chrysanthemum producing rose-pink flowerheads, to 21cm (8in) across when disbudded, in late autumn. Good for exhibition. ↕ 1.5m (5ft), ↔ 45cm (18in). ❀ (min. 10°C/50°F)
C. 'Woolman's Glory'. Single florists' chrysanthemum with large bronze flowerheads, 21cm (8in) across when disbudded, borne in late autumn. Good for exhibition. ↕ 1.3m (4½ft), ↔ 1m (3ft) when disbudded to 4–6 flowerheads. ❀ (min. 10°C/50°F)
C. 'Woolman's Prince'. Incurved florists' chrysanthemum with large, light yellow flowerheads, to 15cm (6in) across when disbudded, borne in late autumn. Good for exhibition. ↕ 1.5m (5ft), ↔ 60cm (24in). ❀ (min. 10°C/50°F)
C. 'World of Sport'. Intermediate florists' chrysanthemum with large white flowerheads, 19cm (7in) across when disbudded, produced in early autumn. Good for exhibition. ↕ 1.5m (5ft), ↔ 75cm (30in). ❄
C. 'Yellow Ginger Nut'. Intermediate florists' chrysanthemum bearing yellow flowerheads, to 14cm (5½in) across when disbudded, sometimes closing over the top to become fully incurved, in early autumn. Good for exhibition. ↕ 1.2m (4ft), ↔ 60cm (24in). ❄
C. 'Yellow John Hughes' ▣ Incurved florists' chrysanthemum bearing yellow flowerheads, 12–14cm (5–5½in) across when disbudded, in late autumn. Good for exhibition. ↕ 1.2m (4ft), ↔ 60–75cm (24–30in). ❀ (min. 10°C/50°F)
C. 'Yellow John Wingfield'. Reflexed florists' chrysanthemum with yellow flowerheads, 12cm (5in) across when disbudded, borne in late autumn. Good for exhibition. ↕ 1.5m (5ft), ↔ 45–60cm (18–24in). ❀ (min. 10°C/50°F)
C. 'Yellow Pennine Oriel'. Spray florists' chrysanthemum with anemone-centred yellow flowerheads, 9cm (3½in) across, borne in early autumn. Good for exhibition. ↕ 1.2m (4ft), ↔ 60–75cm (24–30in). ❄❄❄
C. 'Yellow West Bromwich'. Fully reflexed florists' chrysanthemum with yellow flowerheads, 18cm (7in) across when disbudded, borne in mid-autumn. Good for exhibition. ↕ 1.5m (5ft), ↔ 75cm (30in). ❄
C. 'Yvonne Arnaud' ▣ Reflexed florists' chrysanthemum bearing reddish purple flowers, 14cm (5½in) across when disbudded, in early autumn. ↕ 1.2m (4ft), ↔ 60–75cm (24–30in). ❄

CHRYSOGONUM

ASTERACEAE/COMPOSITAE

Genus of one species of rhizomatous perennial, with leafy runners, occurring in rich woodland soils in E. USA. The flowerheads resemble those of small, single zinnias, and are produced over a very long period from early spring to late summer. *C. virginianum* is cultivated as attractive ground cover.
• **HARDINESS** Fully hardy.
• **CULTIVATION** Grow in moist but well-drained, humus-rich soil in sun or partial shade.
• **PROPAGATION** Sow seed in containers in a cold frame as soon as ripe. Divide or separate runners in spring or autumn.
• **PESTS AND DISEASES** Trouble free.

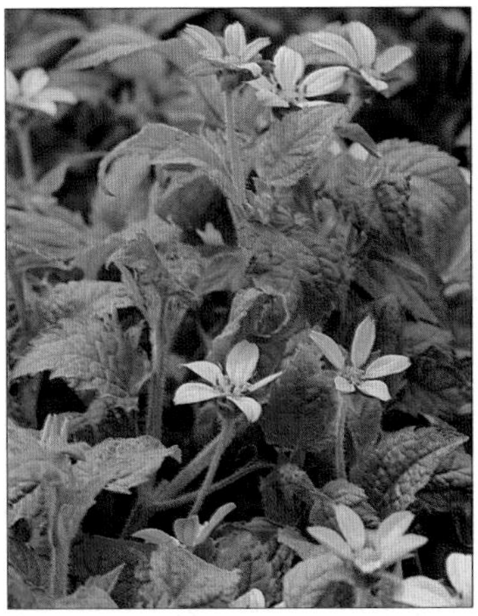
Chrysogonum virginianum

C. virginianum ▣ Creeping perennial with long, reddish green stalks and opposite, heart-shaped to ovate-oblong, hairy, mid-green leaves, 2.5–10cm (1–4in) long, with scalloped to toothed margins. From early spring to late summer, branched stems bear solitary, star-shaped yellow flowerheads, 4cm (1½in) across, from the upper leaf axils; they each have 5 large, triangular ray-florets around the central disc-florets. Evergreen in mild winters. ↕ 25cm (10in), ↔ 60cm (24in). E. USA. ❄❄❄

CHRYSOLEPIS

FAGACEAE

Genus of 2 species of evergreen trees and shrubs from hill and mountain slopes from California to Washington State, USA. They are grown mainly for their handsome foliage and attractive catkins and fruits. They grow best in maritime climates, and are excellent specimen plants for a large lawn.
• **HARDINESS** Fully hardy.
• **CULTIVATION** Grow in fertile, moist but well-drained, neutral or acid soil in sun or partial shade. Shelter from strong winds. Pruning group 8, or 1 for trees.
• **PROPAGATION** Sow seed as soon as ripe in a seedbed outdoors or in containers in an open frame.
• **PESTS AND DISEASES** Trouble free.

C. chrysophylla △ syn. *Castanopsis chrysophylla* (Golden chinkapin). Conical tree producing narrowly oval, tapered, dark green leaves, to 15cm (6in) long, densely golden hairy beneath. Fragrant, creamy white catkins are borne in summer, and are followed by spiny, chestnut-like fruit produced in the following summer. ↕ 12m (40ft), ↔ 12–30m (40–100ft). W. USA (Oregon, California). ❄❄❄

▷ ***Chrysopsis*** see *Heterotheca*
C. mariana see *H. mariana*
C. villosa see *H. villosa*

CHRYSOSPLENIUM

Golden saxifrage

SAXIFRAGACEAE

Genus of about 55 species of creeping annuals and perennials from Europe, Asia, and North America, often found in moist woodland and close to streams. They have rounded or kidney-shaped, toothed, light to dark green leaves, and flat, terminal cymes of shallowly cup-shaped flowers above leafy bracts. They are useful as ground cover in a shady border, bog garden, or woodland garden.

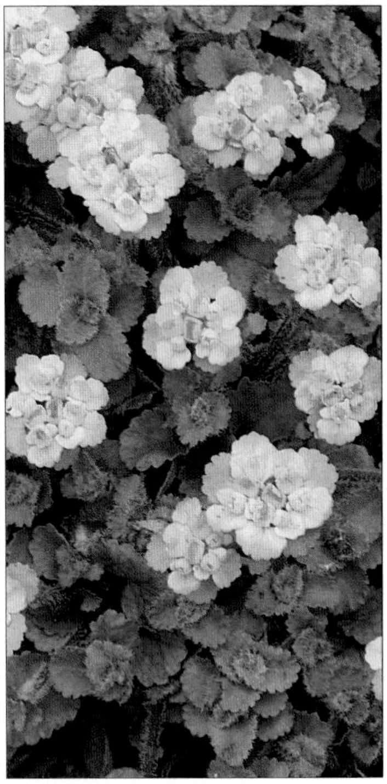
Chrysosplenium davidianum

• **HARDINESS** Fully hardy.
• **CULTIVATION** Grow in moist, poor to moderately fertile, humus-rich soil in a shady site.
• **PROPAGATION** Divide, or take soft tip cuttings, in spring.
• **PESTS AND DISEASES** Susceptible to damage by slugs and snails.

C. davidianum ▣ Rhizomatous, mat-forming perennial with erect, red-hairy stems. Broadly ovate-oblong leaves, 2–3cm (¾–1¼in) long, with scalloped margins, are mid- to dark green, densely white-hairy beneath, less so above. In late spring and early summer, bears greenish yellow flowers in cymes 3–5cm (1¼–2in) across, above pale green, leaf-like bracts. ↕ to 8cm (3in), ↔ 25cm (10in) or more. W. China. ❄❄❄

▷ **Chulta** see *Dillenia indica*

CHUSQUEA

GRAMINEAE/POACEAE

Genus of 90–100 species of evergreen, clump-forming bamboos occurring in upland woodland from Mexico to Chile. Chusqueas have cylindrical, smooth, glossy, pith-filled canes with 3 primary branches, borne alternately at the nodes, each branching densely and bearing linear to ovate or oval, pointed, mid- to dark green leaves. Use as specimen plants for a lawn or woodland garden.
• **HARDINESS** Fully hardy to frost tender.
• **CULTIVATION** Grow in humus-rich, leafy, moist but well-drained soil in sun or partial shade, sheltered from cold, dry winds.
• **PROPAGATION** Sow seed at 13–18°C (55–64°F) in spring. Divide clumps, or remove sections of rhizome with a stem and root, in spring.
• **PESTS AND DISEASES** Emerging shoots are prone to slug damage.

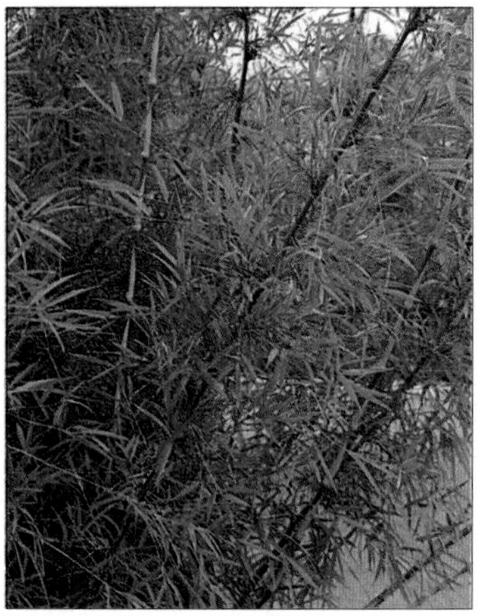

Chusquea culeou

C. culeou ■ 🏆 Graceful, erect bamboo, forming dense clumps of glossy, cylindrical, yellow-green to olive-green canes, to 3cm (1¼in) across, with long, tapered, papery white leaf sheaths; these are persistent for the first year, giving a striped appearance to the young canes. Clustered branches, 10–80cm (4–32in) long, arise alternately and almost encircle the white-waxy nodes; they bear numerous linear, tessellated, mid-green leaves, to 7cm (3in) long. As old leaves fall, branches and leaf-stalks persist, giving a whiskered look to the lower canes. ↕ to 6m (20ft), ↔ 2.5m (8ft) or more. Chile. ❄❄❄

CIBOTIUM

DICKSONIACEAE

Genus of about 10 species of evergreen tree ferns from forest in tropical and subtropical to warm-temperate regions. They have very large, finely divided, ovate to triangular fronds, growing in tufts from an erect, trunk-like rhizome, covered with golden brown hairs. In frost-prone climates, grow in a large, temperate or warm greenhouse or conservatory. Elsewhere, grow outdoors as imposing specimen plants.

• **HARDINESS** Frost tender.

• **CULTIVATION** Under glass, grow in 1 part each of loam, medium-grade bark, and charcoal, 2 parts sharp sand, and 3 parts coarse leaf mould. Provide bright filtered light and moderate humidity. In growth, water freely and apply a high-nitrogen liquid fertilizer monthly; in winter, water sparingly and admit maximum light. Top-dress or pot on in spring. If plants outgrow their site, they may be reduced in height by rooting the upper part of the stem in well-drained potting compost. Outdoors, grow in a humus-rich, moist but well-drained soil in partial shade.

• **PROPAGATION** Sow spores at 21°C (70°F) when ripe.

• **PESTS AND DISEASES** Trouble free.

C. glaucum ■ 🌴 (Hawaiian tree fern). Tree fern with an erect stem bearing ovate, 2-pinnate, mid-green fronds, 2–3m (6–10ft) long, glaucous beneath, with lance-shaped segments. The stem tips and bases of the frond-stalks are covered with hairs. ↕ 2–6m (6–20ft), ↔ 3–4m (10–12ft). USA (Hawaii). ❀ (min. 10°C/50°F)

C. regale 🌴 Tree fern with an erect stem crowned with ovate, 2-pinnate,

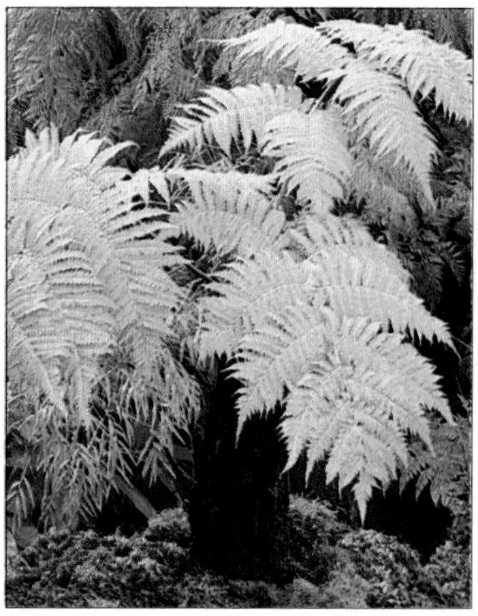

Cibotium glaucum

mid-green fronds, 3–4m (10–12ft) long, and glaucous beneath, divided into lance-shaped segments. The stem tips and bases of the frond-stalks are hairy. ↕ to 4m (12ft), ↔ 3–8m (10–25ft). Central America. ❀ (min. 10°C/50°F)

CICERBITA

ASTERACEAE/COMPOSITAE

Genus of about 20 species of erect perennials found in N. temperate zones in wooded ravines and subalpine and moist, grassy meadows. They have pinnatifid to pinnatisect, mid-green leaves, each with a large, 3-angled terminal lobe, and smaller, sharply pointed lateral lobes. The basal leaves are stalked, the smaller stem leaves are stalkless and stem-clasping; their sap is milky. Cicerbitas are grown for their corymb-like panicles of numerous dandelion-like flowers; these have strap-shaped florets in blue, violet, lilac, or occasionally yellow, and are borne on branched stems from midsummer to early autumn. They are suitable for a large mixed or herbaceous border, or for naturalizing in a wild garden.

• **HARDINESS** Fully hardy.

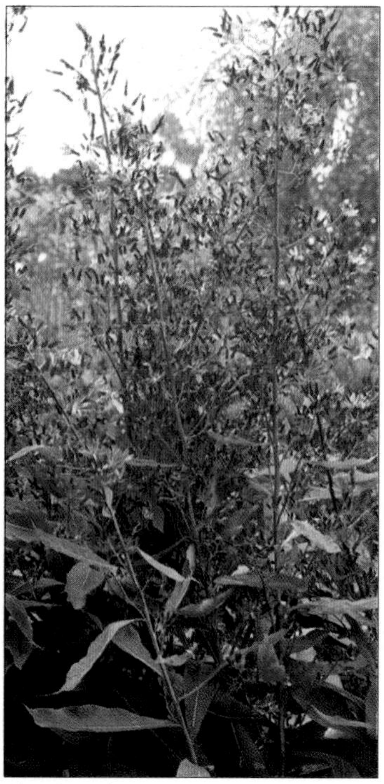

Cicerbita alpina

• **CULTIVATION** Grow in moist, fertile, humus-rich, neutral to acid soil in sun or partial shade. Dead-head to prevent self-seeding.

• **PROPAGATION** Sow seed in containers in early spring, or divide in early spring.

• **PESTS AND DISEASES** Mildew may be a problem.

C. alpina ■ syn. *Lactuca alpina, Mulgedium alpinum* (Mountain sow thistle). Clump-forming perennial producing mid-green, basal leaves, 8–25cm (3–10in) long, blue-green beneath. Erect, branching, softly hairy, reddish green stems bear elongated panicles of violet-blue flowerheads, 2cm (¾in) across, from midsummer to early autumn. ↕ to 2.5m (8ft), ↔ 60cm (24in). Norway, Scotland, Pyrenees, Alps, Apennines, mountains of Bulgaria, Carpathians. ❄❄❄

C. plumieri, syn. *Lactuca plumieri, Mulgedium plumieri.* Clump-forming, hairless perennial with mid-green, basal leaves, 5–60cm (2–24in) long, blue-green beneath. Erect, branching stems bear panicles of blue flowerheads, 3cm (1¼in) across, from midsummer to early autumn. ↕ to 1.3m (4½ft), ↔ 45cm (18in). Pyrenees, mountains of France, W. central Europe, S.W. Bulgaria. ❄❄❄

CICHORIUM

Chicory, Endive

ASTERACEAE/COMPOSITAE

Genus of about 8 species of annuals and perennials from dry, sunny sites in Europe, the Mediterranean, temperate Asia, and Ethiopia. They have large, variably toothed or pinnatifid, mid-green leaves, milky sap, and stems that branch at flowering to bear numerous thistle- or dandelion-like, usually blue, occasionally pink or white flowerheads, which close by midday. Several species are grown as salad plants. Contact with all parts of the plants may irritate skin or aggravate skin allergies.

• **HARDINESS** Fully hardy to frost hardy; *C. spinosum* may survive temperatures down to -10°C (14°F).

• **CULTIVATION** Grow in fertile, well-drained soil in full sun. *C. spinosum* needs sharply drained soil and protection from excessive winter wet.

• **PROPAGATION** Sow seed in containers in a cold frame in autumn or spring.

• **PESTS AND DISEASES** Prone to mildew, lettuce ringspot, rust, and slugs.

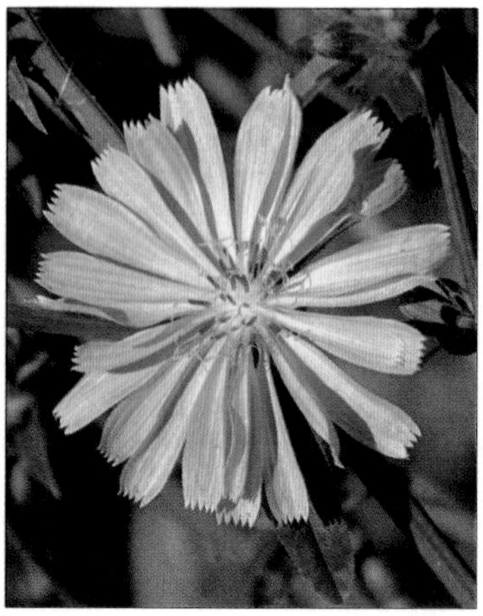

Cichorium intybus

C. intybus ■ 🏆 (Chicory). Clump-forming perennial with a large tap root and inversely lance-shaped, toothed, basal leaves, 7–30cm (3–12in) long. In summer, branched stems bear dandelion-like, terminal and axillary, clear blue, occasionally white or pink flowerheads, to 3.5cm (1½in) across. ↕ 1.2m (4ft), ↔ 60cm (24in). Mediterranean. ❄❄❄

C. spinosum. Dwarf perennial with a woody rootstock. Branching stems terminating in long green spines bear inversely lance-shaped, pinnatifid, glossy leaves, to 5cm (2in) long. In summer, produces thistle-like blue flowerheads, to 2cm (¾in) across, singly from the leaf axils, or in few-flowered terminal clusters. Best in an alpine house. ↕↔ to 20cm (8in). Mediterranean. ❄❄

▷**Cigar flower** see *Cuphea ignea*

CIMICIFUGA

Bugbane, Cohosh

RANUNCULACEAE

Genus of 18 species of erect, clump-forming perennials from N. temperate regions, usually found in moist, shady grassland, woodland, or scrub. They have alternate, ternate to 3-ternate leaves. The numerous, white or cream flowers, occasionally pink-tinged, and usually 1–2cm (½–¾in) long, have 2–5 small petals and prominent tufts of stamens. They are crowded together in slender, bottlebrush-like racemes or panicles, which are followed by greenish white, then brown, star-shaped follicles. Some are unpleasantly scented. They are suitable for a moist border or woodland.

• **HARDINESS** Fully hardy.

• **CULTIVATION** Grow in moist, fertile, preferably humus-rich soil in partial shade. Provide support.

• **PROPAGATION** Sow seed in containers in a cold frame as soon as ripe, to germinate the following spring. Divide in spring.

• **PESTS AND DISEASES** Trouble free.

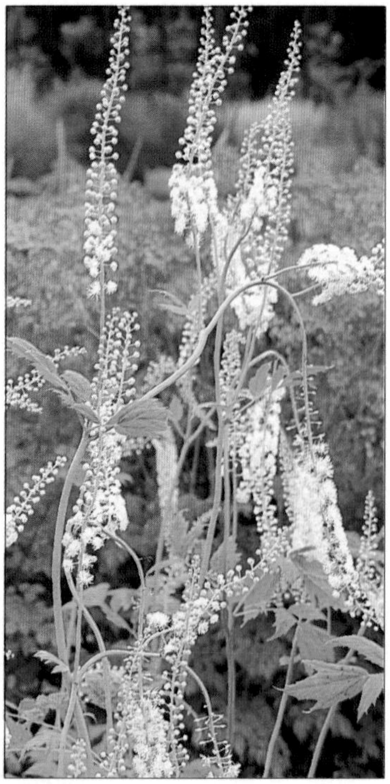

Cimicifuga simplex

C. acerina see *C. japonica*.
C. americana. Clump-forming perennial producing 2- or 3-ternate, toothed, basal leaves, to 50cm (20in) long, with 3-lobed, ovate to oblong leaflets, dark green above, mid-green beneath. Red-tinted white flowers, 5–12mm (¼–½in) long, are borne in lax, branched racemes, to 50cm (20in) long, from late summer to mid-autumn. ↕0.6–2.5m (2–8ft), ↔50–100cm (20–39in). E. USA. ❄❄❄
C. foetida. Clump-forming perennial with 2- or 3-ternate, toothed, mid-green, basal leaves, to 1m (3ft) long, usually with 3-lobed, oval or broadly ovate to elliptic leaflets. Pure white flowers, 5–12mm (¼–½in) long, are borne in branched racemes, to 60cm (24in) long, from late summer to mid-autumn. ↕0.6–2m (2–6ft), ↔50–80cm (20–32in). Russia (Siberia) to N. Mongolia. ❄❄❄
C. japonica, syn. *C. acerina*. Clump-forming perennial producing long-stalked, ternate or 2-ternate, toothed, hairy, dark green, basal leaves, 30–75cm (12–30in) long, with 3- to 5-lobed, ovate to broadly ovate leaflets. Pure white flowers, 0.5–1cm (¼–½in) long, are borne in erect racemes, to 35cm (14in) long, from late summer to mid-autumn. ↕60–90cm (24–36in), ↔60cm (24in). Japan. ❄❄❄
C. racemosa ♀ (Black snake root). Clump-forming perennial producing 2- or 3-ternate, occasionally ternate, dark green, basal leaves, to 40cm (16in) long, with oblong, often lobed or sharply toothed leaflets. In midsummer, slender, branched stems bear racemes, 60cm (24in) long, sometimes curved, of unpleasantly scented white flowers, 0.5–1.5cm (¼–½in) long. ↕1.2–2.2m (4–7ft), ↔60cm (24in). E. North America. ❄❄❄. **var. *cordifolia*** see *C. rubifolia*.
C. rubifolia, syn. *C. racemosa* var. *cordifolia*. Clump-forming perennial with ternate or 2-ternate, dark green, basal leaves, to 60cm (24in) long, composed of 3–17 broadly obovate leaflets, heart-shaped at the bases. In late summer, bears branched, sometimes curved racemes, to 60cm (24in) long, of creamy white flowers, to 1cm (½in) long. ↕30–140cm (12–55in), ↔60cm (24in). E. North America. ❄❄❄
C. simplex ▣ Clump-forming perennial with 3-ternate, light green to purplish green, basal leaves, 30–75cm (12–30in) long, composed of 27–81 ovate to rounded, irregularly lobed leaflets. In early and mid-autumn, unbranched, or occasionally branched, often arching stems bear white flowers, 2cm (¾in) long, in racemes 6–30cm (2½–12in) long. ↕1–1.2m (3–4ft), ↔60cm (24in). Russia (Kamchatka, Sakhalin, Siberia), China (W. China, Manchuria), Mongolia, Korea, Japan. ❄❄❄. **'Braunlaub'** has very dark green leaves; ↕60–90cm (24–36in). **'Brunette'** ▣ has very dark, brownish purple foliage, purple stems, and compact racemes, to 20cm (8in) long, of purple-tinted, off-white flowers. **'Elstead'** ♀ has purple-tinted buds that open to white flowers later than in other cultivars; ↕60–90cm (24–36in). **'White Pearl'** has arching stems bearing narrow racemes of green buds opening to white flowers over pale green leaves; ↕60–90cm (24–36in).

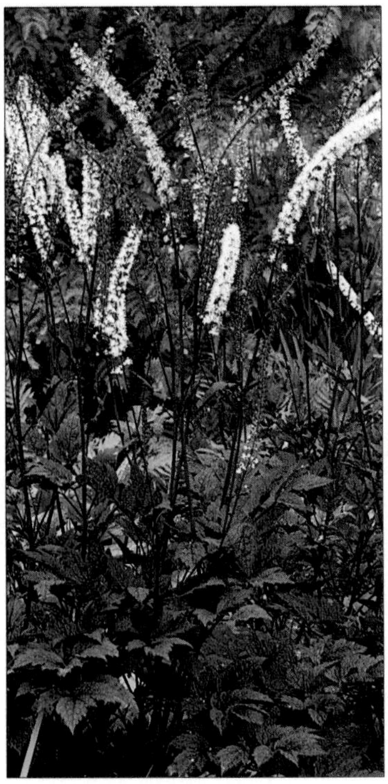
Cimicifuga simplex 'Brunette'

▷ ***Cineraria cruentus* of gardens** see *Pericallis* x *hybrida*
▷ **Cineraria, Florists'** see *Pericallis* x *hybrida*
▷ ***Cineraria* x *hybrida*** see *Pericallis* x *hybrida*
▷ ***Cineraria maritima*** see *Senecio cineraria*
▷ **Cinderella slippers** see *Sinningia regina*

CINNAMOMUM

LAURACEAE

Genus of about 250 species of evergreen trees and shrubs found in forest in E. and S.E. Asia and Australia. The opposite or almost opposite leaves are simple, leathery, and aromatic; the small, insignificant, 6-lobed flowers are borne in axillary or terminal panicles. In frost-prone areas, grow for their foliage in a temperate greenhouse. In frost-free areas, grow outdoors as shade or specimen trees.
• **HARDINESS** Frost tender; *C. camphora* will withstand occasional falls in temperature to 0°C (32°F).
• **CULTIVATION** Under glass, grow in loam-based potting compost (JI No.3) in full light with shade from hot sun. During the growing season, water freely and apply a balanced liquid fertilizer monthly; water more sparingly in winter. Pot on or top-dress in early spring. Outdoors, grow in fertile, moist but well-drained soil in sun or partial shade. Pruning group 1; plants under glass may need restrictive pruning after flowering or in spring.
• **PROPAGATION** Sow seed at 13–18°C (55–64°F) as soon as ripe, or in spring. Root semi-ripe cuttings in summer.
• **PESTS AND DISEASES** Scale insects may be a problem under glass.

C. camphora ♀ (Camphor tree). Erect to spreading tree with narrowly ovate, boldly veined, glossy leaves, to 10cm (4in) long, greenish red when young, then rich green. Small, bowl-shaped, greenish yellow flowers are borne in clusters 5–7cm (2–3in) across, from spring to summer, followed by black berries, 6–10mm (¼–½in) across. ↕20m (70ft) or more, ↔5–10m (15–30ft). Tropical S.E. and E. Asia, including Japan and Malaysia. ⌂ (min. 10°C/50°F)

▷ **Cinquefoil** see *Potentilla*
Himalayan see *P. atrosanguinea*
Marsh see *P. palustris*

CIONURA syn. MARSDENIA

ASCLEPIADACEAE

Genus of one species of semi-climbing, deciduous shrub occurring in rocky areas, river-gravels, and maritime sands in the E. Mediterranean. It is grown for its fragrant flowers. In frost-prone climates, grow in a cool conservatory or greenhouse; elsewhere, use outdoors against a sunny wall. Contact with the latex exuded by cut leaves and stems may irritate skin, and may cause severe discomfort if ingested.
• **HARDINESS** Frost hardy only in dry, sunny sites.
• **CULTIVATION** Under glass, grow in loam-based potting compost (JI No.3) in full light. Water freely in growth, applying a balanced liquid fertilizer monthly; keep just moist in winter. Outdoors, grow in moderately fertile, well-drained soil in a sunny, sheltered site. Pruning group 11, after flowering.
• **PROPAGATION** Sow seed at 13–18°C (55–64°F) in spring. Root semi-ripe cuttings in late summer.
• **PESTS AND DISEASES** Trouble free.

C. erecta, syn. *Marsdenia erecta*. Twining shrub with opposite, ovate-heart-shaped, grey-green leaves, to 6cm (2½in) long. Produces cymes of bowl-shaped white flowers, 1cm (½in) across, from the leaf axils in summer, followed by pointed fruit that open to release silky seeds. Balkans, Crete, Turkey, S.W. Asia. ↕3m (10ft) or more. ❄❄

▷ ***Cirrhopetalum guttulatum*** see *Bulbophyllum guttulatum*
▷ ***Cirrhopetalum medusae*** see *Bulbophyllum medusae*

CIRSIUM

ASTERACEAE/COMPOSITAE

Genus of about 200 species of biennials and perennials from a variety of habitats in N. temperate regions, including grassy mountain slopes, streamsides or moorland meadows, and dry or moist alpine and subalpine meadows. They have spiny leaves and bear heads of tubular, purple, red, yellow, or sometimes white flowers. Many are invasive, spreading by means of rhizomes, or self-seeding. Those listed here are useful border plants, or suitable for damp meadows in a wild garden.
• **HARDINESS** Fully hardy.
• **CULTIVATION** Grow in moist but well-drained soil in full sun. Dead-head to prevent self-seeding.
• **PROPAGATION** Sow seed in containers in a cold frame in spring. Divide perennials from autumn to spring.
• **PESTS AND DISEASES** Mildew may be a problem.

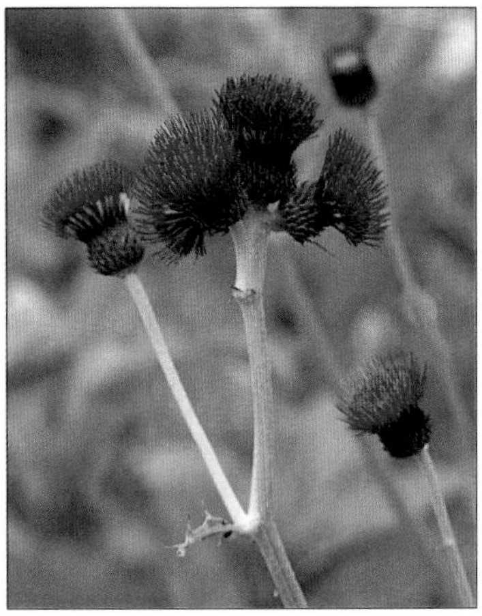
Cirsium rivulare 'Atropurpureum'

C. japonicum. Clump-forming biennial or perennial producing oblong-obovate, pointed, deeply lobed to pinnate, spiny, toothed, mid- to dark green leaves, to 30cm (12in) long. In late summer and early autumn, bears thistle-like, rose-pink to lilac flowerheads, 5cm (2in) across. ↕1–2m (3–6ft), ↔60cm (24in). Japan. ❄❄❄. **'Rose Beauty'** has deep carmine-red flowerheads.
C. rivulare. Clump-forming, spreading perennial with narrowly elliptic to oblong-lance-shaped, entire to pinnatifid, prickly, dark green leaves, to 45cm (18in) long, softly hairy beneath. Erect stems bear spherical, pincushion-like, deep crimson-purple to purple flowerheads, 3cm (1¼in) across, in early and midsummer. ↕1.2m (4ft), ↔60cm (24in). C. Europe into Russia, S.W. Europe. ❄❄❄. **'Atropurpureum'** ▣ has deep crimson flowerheads.

CISSUS

VITACEAE

Genus of about 350 species of evergreen perennials, shrubs, and climbers, some with succulent stems or roots, occurring in tropical and subtropical regions, at forest margins and in thickets. The leaves are alternate and may be simple, shallowly to deeply lobed, or 3- to 7-palmate. Insignificant, 4-petalled flowers are produced in compound, umbel-like cymes opposite the leaves or at the ends of the shoots. Dry, usually unpalatable berries, 0.3–3cm (⅛–1¼in) across, ripen to shades of blue, red, purple, or black. In frost-prone regions, grow as foliage houseplants, or in a cool or warm conservatory; most are suitable for hanging baskets. In warmer climates, use climbing species to clothe pergolas, arbours, walls, or tall tree stumps.
• **HARDINESS** Half hardy to frost tender.
• **CULTIVATION** Under glass, grow non-succulents in loam-based potting compost (JI No.2) in bright filtered or indirect light. Water freely when in growth, applying a balanced liquid fertilizer monthly; water sparingly in winter. Pot on or top-dress in spring. Grow succulent species in JI No.2 with added grit (up to one-third by volume), in full light. Water succulents moderately when in growth and keep them dry in winter. Outdoors, grow non-succulents in fertile, moist but well-drained soil in sun or partial shade; succulents need sharply drained soil and full sun. Pruning group 11, in spring;

C

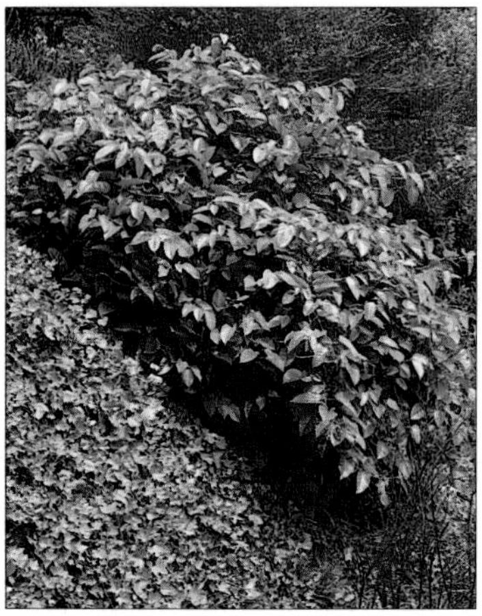

Cissus antarctica

pinch out young plants to encourage a bushy habit. See also pp.48–49.

• **PROPAGATION** For climbers and shrubs, root hardwood or greenwood cuttings in summer. For succulents, sow seed at 21°C (70°F) in spring, or take stem cuttings in early summer.

• **PESTS AND DISEASES** Red spider mites, whiteflies, and mealybugs may be a problem under glass.

C. antarctica ▣ 🏆 (Kangaroo vine). Climber with tendrils and broadly ovate, boldly toothed, leathery, glossy, rich green leaves, to 12cm (5in) long. Bears small green flowers in dense, axillary cymes, 3cm (1¼in) long, from spring to summer; they are followed by spherical black berries, 1cm (½in) across. ↕5–15m (15–50ft). N. Australia. ❁ (min. 5°C/41°F)
C. bainesii see *Cyphostemma bainesii.*
C. capensis see *Rhoicissus capensis.*
C. discolor ▣ Slender climber with red stems and tendrils. Ovate to lance-shaped leaves, 8–25cm (3–10in) long, with heart-shaped bases, are deep green with silver, grey, or pink zones between the veins above, maroon beneath. In summer, produces red-tinted green

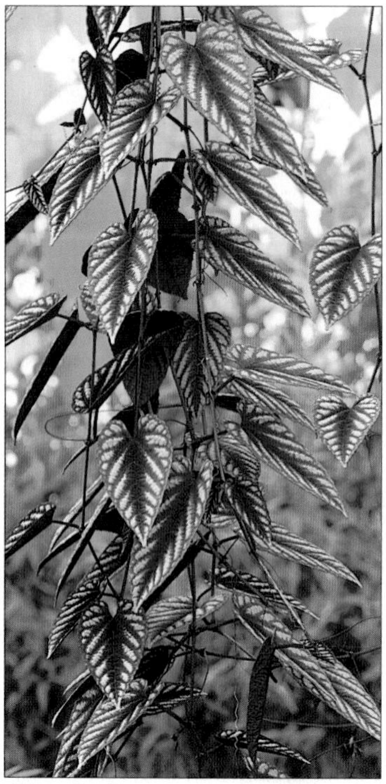

Cissus discolor

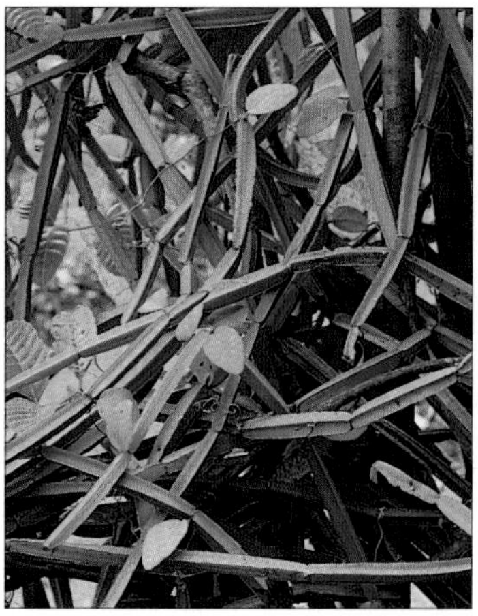

Cissus quadrangularis

flowers in small panicles, 5cm (2½in) long, followed by spherical, dark red fruit, 8mm (⅜in) across. ↕2–3m (6–10ft). S.E. Asia. ❁ (min. 5°C/41°F)
C. hypoglauca (Water vine). Vigorous, scandent climber with 5-palmate leaves, 5–8cm (2–3in) long, composed of ovate to lance-shaped leaflets, pale to deep green above, glaucous beneath. Small yellow flowers open in dense, axillary cymes, 4–6cm (1½–2½in) long, in summer, followed by blue-black berries, 1–2cm (½–¾in) across. ↕10–25m (30–80ft). Australia (New South Wales, Victoria). ❁ (min. 7°C/45°F)
C. juttae see *Cyphostemma juttae.*
C. quadrangularis ▣ Few-leaved, succulent climber with tendrils, thick, 4-angled stems, and thinner, wavy-margined, horny branches constricted at the nodes. Entire to 3-lobed, ovate to triangular, coarsely toothed, fleshy, mid-green leaves, 20cm (8in) or more long, develop from the nodes and opposite the tendrils. Small, green or yellow flowers open in cymes, 5cm (2in) long, in summer, followed by ovoid, reddish black fruit, 4–6mm (⅛–¼in) across. ↕3m (10ft). Tropical Africa, Arabian peninsula, E. India. ❁ (min. 15°C/59°F)
C. rhombifolia ▣ 🏆 syn. *Rhoicissus rhombifolia* (Grape ivy). Vigorous climber producing forked tendrils and 3-palmate, dark green leaves, to 15cm (6in) long, with ovate to diamond-shaped leaflets, boldly veined and coarsely toothed, with rust-red hairs beneath. In summer, bears hairy green flowers in cymes 3–7cm (1¼–3in) long, opposite the leaves, followed by blue-black berries, 0.5–1.5cm (¼–½in) across. ↕3m (10ft) or more. Tropical America. ❁ (min. 5°C/41°F). **'Ellen Danica'** 🏆 is compact and bushy but still vigorous, producing leaves with larger, deeply lobed leaflets; ↕1m (3ft).
C. striata, syn. *Ampelopsis sempervirens, Parthenocissus striata, Vitis striata* (Ivy of Uruguay). Slender, vigorous climber with tendrils and 3- to 5-palmate leaves, 4–7cm (1½–3in) long, composed of obovate, leathery, glossy, mid-green leaflets. In summer, bears green flowers in small cymes, 3cm (1¼in) long, opposite the leaves, followed by glossy black berries, 5–10mm (¼–½in) across. ↕10m (30ft). S. Brazil to Chile. ❄
C. voinieriana see *Tetrastigma voinierianum.*

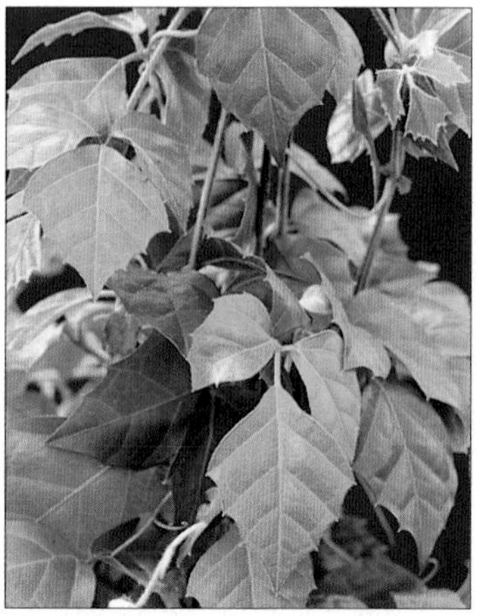

Cissus rhombifolia

CISTUS

Rock rose, Sun rose

CISTACEAE

Genus of about 20 species of evergreen shrubs occurring on dry, stony or rocky soils in the Canary Islands, N. Africa, Turkey, and S. Europe. They are grown for their showy, saucer-shaped, usually 5-petalled, white to dark pink flowers, borne singly or in terminal or axillary cymes from early to late summer; each bloom lasts only one day. They have opposite leaves. Rock roses are suitable for growing in a shrub border, on sunny banks, at the base of a wall, around paved areas, or in containers. They are often short-lived.

• **HARDINESS** Frost hardy.

• **CULTIVATION** Grow in poor to moderately fertile, well-drained soil in a sheltered site in full sun, planting after any danger of hard frosts has passed. Rock roses are generally lime-tolerant, but may become chlorotic with age on very chalky soils. Pinch back young plants after flowering to encourage a bushy habit. Pruning group 8 or 9; they do not respond well to hard pruning, and old, leggy plants are best replaced.

• **PROPAGATION** Sow seed in containers in a cold frame as soon as ripe or in spring. Root softwood or greenwood cuttings in summer.

• **PESTS AND DISEASES** Trouble free.

C. x aguilarii (*C. ladanifer* x *C. populifolius*). Rounded shrub with lance-shaped, 3-veined, wavy-margined, sticky, bright green leaves, to 10cm (4in) long. Solitary white flowers, to 8cm (3in) across, with golden yellow stamens, are borne in summer. ↕↔1.2m (4ft). S.W. Europe, N. Africa. ❄❄. **'Maculatus'** 🏆 has sticky leaves, and flowers with a dark red mark at the base of each petal.
C. albidus. Dense, bushy shrub with ovate to oblong, 3-veined, grey-white leaves, to 5cm (2in) long. Terminal cymes of 3–8 dark lilac-pink flowers, 5cm (2in) across, with yellow centres, are produced in summer. ↕↔1m (3ft). S.W. Europe, N. Africa. ❄❄
C. algarvensis see *Halimium ocymoides.*
***C.* 'Anne Palmer'.** Bushy shrub with erect, red-flushed shoots and lance-shaped, wavy-margined, deeply veined, dark green leaves, to 5cm (2in) long. Soft rose-pink flowers, to 7cm (3in) across, are borne singly or in small, terminal cymes of 2–4 blooms in summer. ↕↔1m (3ft). ❄❄
***C.* 'Blanche'.** Bushy shrub with lance-shaped leaves, 4–8cm (1½–3in) long, dark green above and grey-green beneath. Pure white flowers, to 10cm (4in) across, are produced singly from the leaf axils or in terminal cymes in summer. ↕↔1.5m (5ft). ❄❄
C. clusii, syn. *C. rosmarinifolius.* Mound-forming shrub with linear leaves, to 2.5cm (1in) long, dark green above and white beneath. Small white flowers, 2.5cm (1in) across, with yellow stamens, open in few-flowered, terminal cymes in summer. ↕30cm (12in), ↔60cm (24in). W. Mediterranean. ❄❄
C. x corbariensis ▣ 🏆 (*C. populifolius* x *C. salviifolius*) syn. *C.* x *hybridus.* Dense, bushy shrub with ovate, wavy-margined, dark green leaves, to 5cm (2in) long. From late spring to summer, red buds

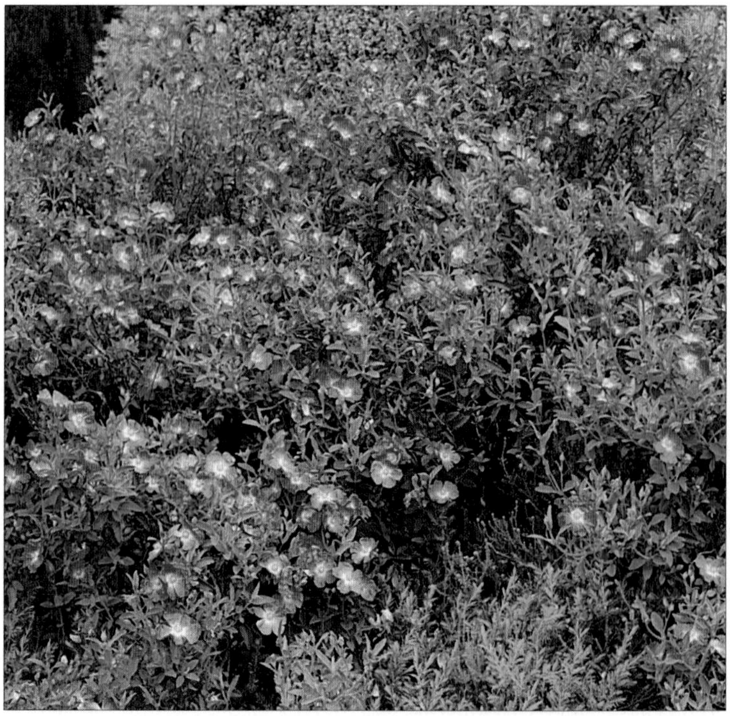

Cistus 'Peggy Sammons'

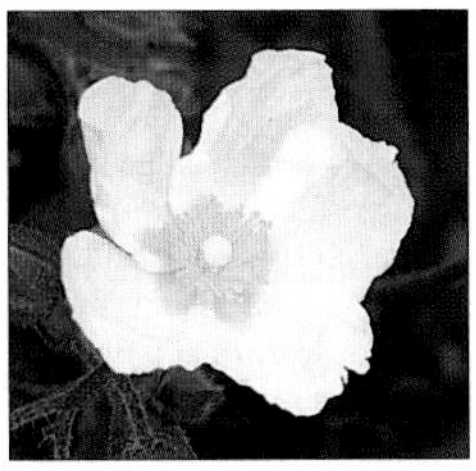
Cistus x *corbariensis*

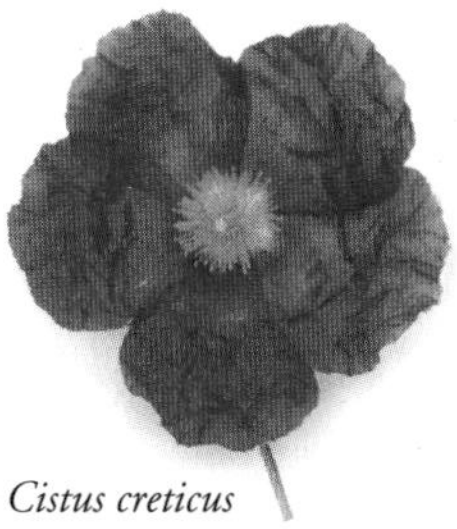
Cistus creticus

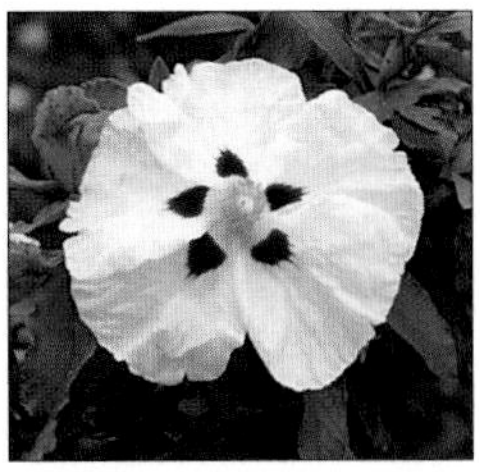
Cistus x *cyprius*

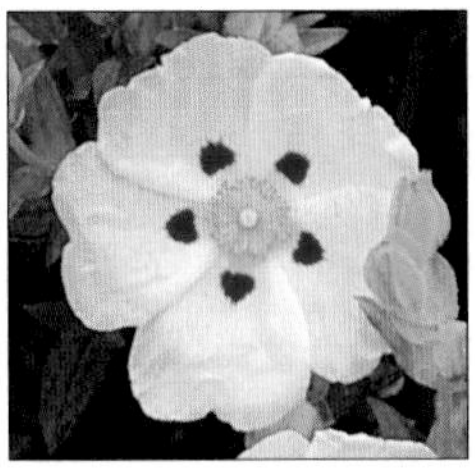
Cistus x *dansereaui* 'Decumbens'

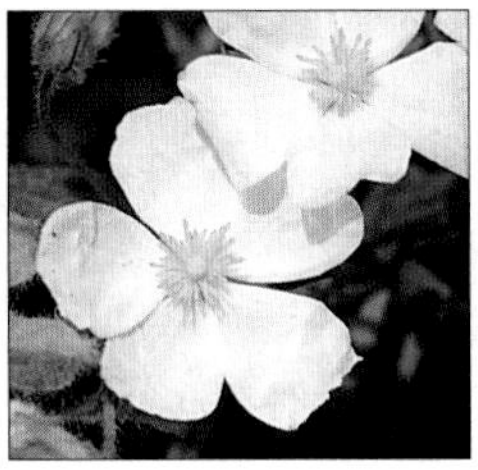
Cistus monspeliensis

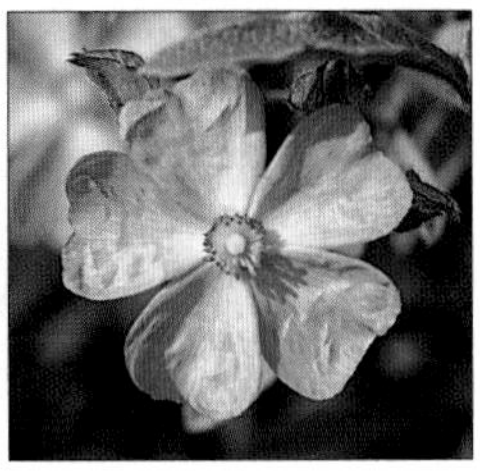
Cistus x *skanbergii*

open to white flowers, 4cm (1½in) across, with yellow centres and stamens, borne singly or in terminal cymes of 2 or 3 blooms. ↕ 1m (3ft), ↔ 1.5m (5ft). S. Europe. ✲✲
C. creticus ▣ syn. *C. incanus* subsp. *creticus.* Compact shrub with ovate to obovate, wavy-margined, deeply veined, mid-green leaves, to 7cm (3in) long. In summer, bears terminal cymes of 3–5 purple-pink flowers, to 6cm (2½in) across, with yellow stamens. ↕↔ 1m (3ft). E. Mediterranean. ✲✲
C. crispus. Rounded, bushy shrub with oblong to elliptic, grey-green leaves, to 4cm (1½in) long, deeply veined and wavy margined. In summer, produces terminal cymes of 2–5 purple-red flowers, to 6cm (2½in) across, with yellow stamens. ↕ 60cm (24in), ↔ 90cm (36in). W. Mediterranean. ✲✲.
'Sunset' see *C.* x *pulverulentus* 'Sunset'.
C.* x *cyprius ▣ ♀ (*C. ladanifer* x *C. laurifolius*). Bushy shrub with narrowly lance-shaped to oblong-lance-shaped, slightly wavy-margined, sticky, dark green leaves, to 10cm (4in) long. In summer, bears terminal cymes of 3–6 white flowers, to 7cm (3in) across, with yellow and crimson marks at the bases of the petals and yellow stamens. ↕↔ 1.5m (5ft). S.W. Europe. ✲✲
C.* x *dansereaui (*C. hirsutus* x *C. ladanifer*) syn. *C.* x *lusitanicus* of gardens. Upright shrub with sticky shoots and oblong-lance-shaped, dark green leaves, to 6cm (2½in) long. Terminal cymes of 3–6 white flowers, to 7cm (3in) across, with faint yellow and crimson marks at the base of each petal, are borne in summer. ↕↔ 1m (3ft). S.W. Europe. ✲✲. **'Decumbens'** ▣ ♀ is low and spreading; ↕ 60cm (24in).
***C.* 'Elma'** ♀ Vigorous, bushy shrub with lance-shaped, glossy, deep green leaves, to 10cm (4in) long. In summer, bears terminal cymes of 3–6 white flowers, to 10cm (4in) across, with yellow stamens. ↕↔ 2m (6ft). ✲✲
C.* x *florentinus (*C. monspeliensis* x *C. salviifolius*). Compact shrub with lance-shaped to elliptic-lance-shaped, wavy margined, grey-green leaves, to 4cm (1½in) long. White flowers, 4cm (1½in) across, with yellow centres, are produced in few-flowered, terminal cymes in summer. ↕ 1m (3ft), ↔ 1.5m (5ft). S. Europe, N. Africa. ✲✲

C. hirsutus. Mound-forming shrub with dense branches. Shoots and ovate to elliptic, dark green leaves, to 6cm (2½in) long, are covered with long white hairs. In summer, bears terminal cymes of 3–8 white flowers, 4cm (1½in) across, with yellow centres. ↕ 1m (3ft), ↔ 1.5m (5ft). S.W. Europe. ✲✲
C.* x *hybridus see *C.* x *corbariensis.*
C. incanus* subsp. *creticus see *C. creticus.*
C. ingwerseniana see x *Halimiocistus* 'Ingwersenii'.
C. ladanifer ♀ syn. *C. ladaniferus* (Common gum cistus, Laudanum). Upright shrub with linear-lance-shaped, sticky, aromatic, dark green leaves, to 10cm (4in) long. White flowers, to 10cm (4in) across, with yellow centres, sometimes with crimson marks at the base of each petal, are borne singly at the ends of short sideshoots in summer. ↕ 2m (6ft), ↔ 1.5m (5ft). S.W. Europe to N. Africa. ✲✲
C. ladaniferus see *C. ladanifer.*
C. laurifolius ♀ Upright shrub with ovate, sticky, aromatic, dark blue-green leaves, to 8cm (3in) long. In summer, bears erect, branched cymes of 3–8 white flowers, to 8cm (3in) across, with yellow centres. ↕↔ 2m (6ft). S.W. Europe. ✲✲
***C.* x *lusitanicus* of gardens** see *C.* x *dansereaui.*
C. monspeliensis ▣ (Montpellier rock rose). Bushy shrub with linear to lance-shaped, deeply veined, dark green leaves,

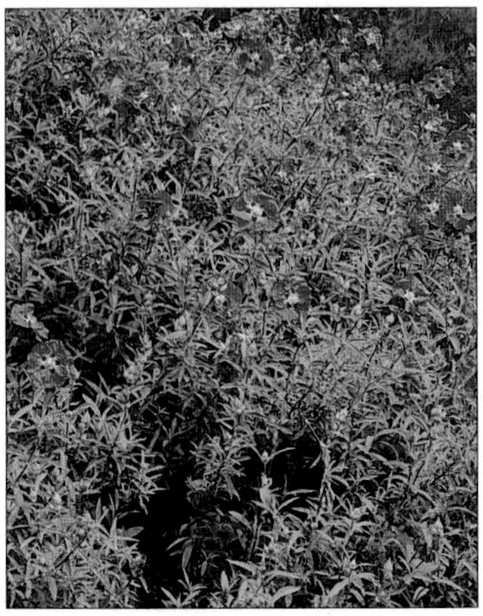
Cistus x *purpureus*

to 5cm (2in) long. Crowded, terminal and axillary cymes of 3–6 saucer-shaped white flowers, to 2.5cm (1in) across, with yellow stamens, are borne in summer. ↕ 1m (3ft), ↔ 1.5m (5ft). S.W. Europe, N. Africa. ✲✲
***C.* 'Paladin'.** Bushy shrub with lance-shaped leaves, to 10cm (4in) long, mid- to dark green above, grey-green beneath. Solitary white flowers, to 10cm (4in) across, marked dark red at the base of each petal, are produced in summer. ↕↔ 1.5m (5ft). ✲✲
C. parviflorus. Compact shrub with ovate, deeply veined, grey-green leaves, to 3cm (1¼in) long. Terminal and axillary cymes of 3–8 clear pink flowers, to 2.5cm (1in) across, are produced in summer. ↕ 1m (3ft), ↔ 1.5m (5ft). E. Mediterranean. ✲✲
***C.* 'Peggy Sammons'** ▣ ♀ Bushy, upright shrub with oval, grey-green leaves, to 6cm (2½in) long. In summer, bears profuse, terminal cymes of 3–8 pale purplish pink flowers, 6cm (2½in) across. ↕↔ 1m (3ft). ✲✲
C. populifolius. Rounded shrub with broadly ovate to heart-shaped, dark green leaves, to 9cm (3½in) long. In summer, produces cymes of 2–5 white flowers, to 5cm (2in) across, with yellow centres, from the upper leaf axils. ↕↔ 2m (6ft). S.W. Europe. ✲✲
***C.* x *pulverulentus* 'Sunset'**, syn. *C. crispus* 'Sunset'. Compact, spreading shrub with oblong, wavy-margined, greyish green leaves, to 5cm (2in) long. Profuse terminal cymes of 3–6 rose-pink flowers, 5cm (2in) across, with yellow centres, are borne in summer. ↕ 60cm (24in), ↔ 90cm (36in). ✲✲
C.* x *purpureus ▣ ♀ (*C. creticus* x *C. ladanifer*). Rounded shrub with upright, sticky, red-flushed shoots and narrowly oblong-lance-shaped to obovate, slightly wavy-margined, dark green leaves, to 5cm (2in) long. In summer, produces terminal cymes of 3 crinkled, dark pink flowers, to 7cm (3in) across, with maroon marks at the bases of the petals. ↕↔ 1m (3ft). S. Europe. ✲✲. **'Betty Taudevin'** has narrow, less wavy-margined leaves and brighter pink flowers, to 9cm (3½in) across.
***C. revolii* of gardens** see x *Halimiocistus sahucii.*
C. rosmarinifolius see *C. clusii.*
C. salviifolius. Bushy shrub with ovate, deeply veined, grey-green leaves, to 4cm (1½in) long. White flowers, to 5cm (2in) across, with yellow centres, are borne singly, or occasionally in few-flowered, axillary cymes, in summer. ↕ 75cm (30in), ↔ 90cm (36in). S. Europe. ✲✲. **'Prostratus'** is low and spreading, with smaller leaves, 2cm (¾in) long; ↕ 15–25cm (6–10in), ↔ 60–90cm (24–36in).
***C.* 'Silver Pink'.** Mound-forming shrub with lance-shaped, dark green leaves, to 7cm (3in) long, grey-green beneath. Silvery pink flowers, 8cm (3in) across, almost white in the centres, with prominent golden stamens, are borne in erect, terminal cymes of 3–5 blooms in summer. ↕ 75cm (30in), ↔ 90cm (36in). ✲✲
C.* x *skanbergii ▣ ♀ (*C. monspeliensis* x *C. parviflorus*). Compact shrub with narrowly oblong-lance-shaped, slightly wavy-margined, grey-green leaves, to 5cm (2in) long. In summer, profusely bears terminal cymes of 3–6 pale pink flowers, 2.5cm (1in) across. ↕ 75cm (30in), ↔ 90cm (36in). Greece. ✲✲
C. wintonensis see x *Halimiocistus wintonensis.*

▷**Cistus, Common gum** see *Cistus ladanifer*

C

x CITROFORTUNELLA

RUTACEAE

Hybrid genus of evergreen shrubs and trees, crosses of *Citrus* and *Fortunella.* The alternate, simple, leathery leaves may have narrow wings on the stalks. Saucer-shaped or shallowly cup-shaped, 5-petalled, waxy flowers are borne singly or in twos or threes from the leaf axils, and are followed by small, orange-like fruits. In frost-prone areas, grow in a cool or temperate greenhouse, or as houseplants; elsewhere, grow outdoors as specimen plants.

- **HARDINESS** Half hardy.
- **CULTIVATION** Under glass, grow in loam-based potting compost (JI No.2) in full light, with shade from hot sun, and good ventilation. When in growth, mist daily, water freely, and apply a balanced liquid fertilizer every 2–3 weeks; water sparingly in winter. Pot on or top-dress in winter. Outdoors, grow in neutral to acid, loamy, well-drained soil in full sun. Pruning group 1; plants under glass may need restrictive pruning in late winter or early spring.
- **PROPAGATION** Root semi-ripe cuttings in summer. Layer in early spring.
- **PESTS AND DISEASES** Red spider mites and scale insects may be a problem.

x *C. microcarpa* ▣ ♀ ◯ syn. x *C. mitis*, *Citrus mitis* (Calamondin, Panama orange). Large shrub or small, bushy tree, sometimes with a few short spines, and elliptic to broadly ovate, bright green leaves, 4–10cm (1½–4in) long. White flowers, 1.5cm (½in) across, are borne from spring to summer, followed by spherical, yellow then orange fruit, 2.5–4cm (1–1½in) across. ↕ 3–6m

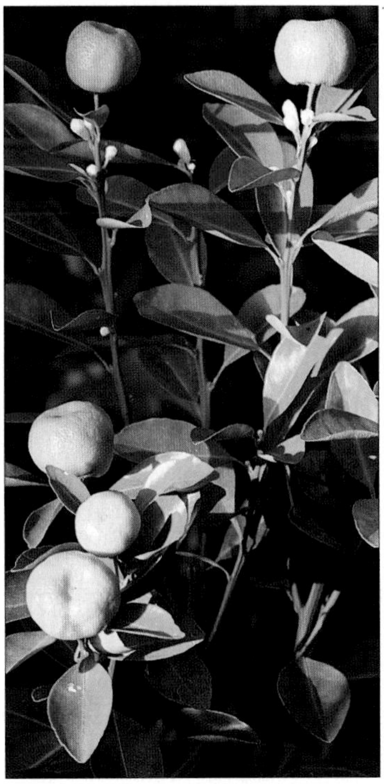
x *Citrofortunella microcarpa*

(10–20ft), ↔ 2–3m (6–10ft). Garden origin. ✻. **'Tiger'** produces leaves margined and streaked with white. **'Variegata'** has white-mottled leaves and green-variegated fruit.
x *C. mitis* see x *C. microcarpa.*

▷**Citron** see *Citrus medica.*

CITRUS

RUTACEAE

Genus of about 16 species of evergreen, often spiny trees and shrubs from open forest, thickets, and scrub in S.E. Asia and the larger islands in the E. Pacific. The leaves are alternate and simple, usually with winged stalks. Shallowly cup-shaped, 5-petalled, often scented white flowers, 2–5cm (1–2in) across, are borne in small, axillary racemes or corymbs. The familiar citrus fruits take about one year to mature. In frost-prone regions, grow in a cool or temperate greenhouse or conservatory. In warmer climates, grow as specimen plants, or in a fruit garden.

• **HARDINESS** Frost tender; but may survive short spells near to 0°C (32°F).
• **CULTIVATION** Under glass, grow in loam-based potting compost (JI No.2) in full light, shaded from hot sun. In growth, water freely, mist daily, and apply a balanced liquid fertilizer every 2–3 weeks; water sparingly in winter. Pot on or top-dress in late winter. Outdoors, grow in moist but well-drained, neutral to slightly acid soil in full sun. Pruning group 1; plants under glass may need restrictive pruning in winter or early spring.
• **PROPAGATION** Sow seed at 16°C (61°F) in spring; seedlings do not come true to type. Root semi-ripe cuttings in summer.
• **PESTS AND DISEASES** Prone to red spider mites, whiteflies, scale insects, and mealybugs under glass. Outdoors, *Phytophthora* root rot may be a problem.

C. aurantium ▣ ♀ (Seville orange). Spiny tree, with a rounded crown and ovate to ovate-oblong, mid-green leaves, 7–10cm (3–4in) long. From late spring to summer, bears fragrant white flowers, 2cm (¾in) across, singly or in pairs or clusters from the leaf axils; they are followed by slightly flattened-spherical, red-tinted orange fruit, 5–7cm (2–3in) long. ↕ 10m (30ft), ↔ 6m (20ft). S.E. Asia. ❅ (min. 3–5°C/37–41°F)
C. limon ▣ ♀ (Lemon). Large shrub or small, freely branching, spiny tree with narrowly ovate, finely toothed, light green leaves, 5–10cm (2–4in) long. From spring to summer, fragrant white flowers, 4–5cm (1½–2in) across, borne singly or in small cymes, open from red- or purple-tinted buds; they are followed by broadly ovoid yellow fruit, 7–15cm (3–6in) long. ↕ 2–7m (6–22ft), ↔ 1.5–3m (5–10ft). Asia. ❅ (min. 3–5°C/37–41°F). **'Meyer'**, syn. *C.* x *meyeri* (Meyer's lemon), is a compact hybrid of *C. limon*, with fragrant flowers and small, spherical fruit.
C. medica ♀ (Citron). Large shrub or small, spiny tree with elliptic-ovate, toothed, rich green leaves, 10–18cm (4–7in) long. Short racemes of white, purple-tinted flowers, 4cm (1½in) wide, open from spring to autumn, followed by ovoid to oblong, lemon-yellow fruit, to 30cm (12in) long. ↕ 3–5m (10–15ft),

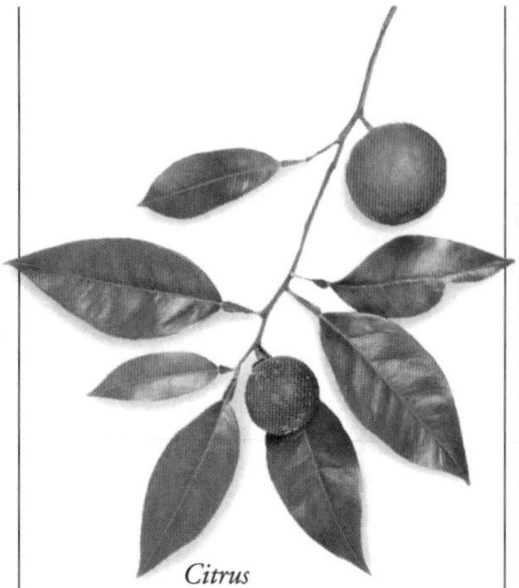

Citrus aurantium

↔ 2–3m (6–10ft). Probably S.W. Asia. ❅ (min. 3–5°C/37–41°F)
C.* x *meyeri see *C. limon* 'Meyer'.
C. mitis see x *Citrofortunella microcarpa.*
C. reticulata ♀ (Clementine, Mandarin, Tangerine). Rounded, sometimes spiny, large shrub or small tree with ovate to lance-shaped, deep green leaves, 3–4cm (1¼–1¾in) long. In spring, bears very fragrant white flowers, 2.5–4cm (1–1½in) across, in short racemes. Spherical orange fruit, 4–8cm (1½–3in) long, are borne from autumn to spring. ↕ 2–8m (6–25ft), ↔ 1.5–3m (5–10ft). S.E. Asia. ❅ (min. 3–5°C/37–41°F). **Satsuma Group** cultivars are more cold-resistant than other variants, and have thin-peeled, sweet orange fruit, to 5cm (2in) long.
***C. sinensis* 'Washington'** ♀ (Sweet orange). Large, rounded, bushy shrub or small tree with oval to elliptic, dark green leaves, 5–15cm (2–6in) long. In spring, bears fragrant white flowers, 4cm (1½in) across, singly or in racemes. Sweet orange fruit, 6–10cm (2½–4in) long, each with a secondary, embryonic fruit embedded at the apex, are borne in winter. ↕ 6–12m (20–40ft), ↔ 3–5m (10–15ft). ❅ (min. 3–5°C/37–41°F)

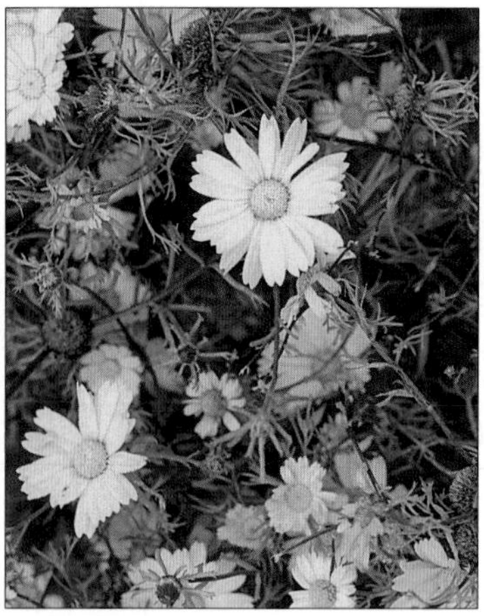

Cladanthus arabicus

CLADANTHUS

Palm Springs daisy

ASTERACEAE/COMPOSITAE

Genus of 4 species of hummock-forming, branched annuals occurring in dry pastures in Spain and N.W. Africa. They have much-divided, pinnatisect to 2-pinnatisect, alternate, aromatic, light green leaves. Daisy-like flowerheads are produced throughout the summer, and are useful as cut flowers. They are suitable for a window-box or flower border. In frost-prone climates, grow in a cool greenhouse for late winter flowering.

• **HARDINESS** Half hardy.
• **CULTIVATION** Under glass, grow in loam-based potting compost (JI No.2) in full light. Provide good ventilation and a minimum temperature of 7–10°C (45–50°F). In growth, water moderately and apply a balanced liquid fertilizer every 2–3 weeks. Outdoors, grow in light, moderately fertile, well-drained soil in full sun. Dead-head for continuous flowering.
• **PROPAGATION** Sow seed at 13–16°C (55–61°F), or *in situ*, in spring. For winter flowering, sow seed at 13–16°C (55–61°F) in autumn.
• **PESTS AND DISEASES** Trouble free.

C. arabicus ▣ Moderately fast-growing annual producing ovate, pinnatisect or 2-pinnatisect, light green leaves, to 3cm (1¼in) long, with linear lobes. Continuously branching laterals bear single, deep yellow flowerheads, to 5cm (2in) across, in summer. May self-seed. ↕ 40–60cm (16–24in), ↔ to 40cm (16in). S. Spain, N.W. Africa. ✻

CLADRASTIS

LEGUMINOSAE/PAPILIONACEAE

Genus of 5 species of deciduous trees found in woodland and on limestone cliffs in China, Japan, and the USA. They are grown for their terminal, erect or pendent panicles of pea-like flowers and colourful autumn foliage. The light to mid-green leaves are alternate and pinnate. They are excellent specimen trees for an open, but not exposed position. Flowering is best when wood is well ripened by long hot summers.

• **HARDINESS** Fully hardy.
• **CULTIVATION** Grow in fertile, well-drained soil in full sun; shelter from strong winds as the wood is very brittle. Pruning group 1, after flowering, or in late autumn or early winter.
• **PROPAGATION** Sow scarified seed outdoors in containers in an open frame, or in a seedbed, in autumn. Insert root cuttings in winter.
• **PESTS AND DISEASES** Trouble free.

C. kentukea see *C. lutea.*
C. lutea ▣ 𝕐 ♀ syn. *C. kentukea* (Yellow wood). Spreading tree with bright, light green leaves, to 30cm (12in) long, composed of 7–9 ovate or obovate leaflets, turning clear yellow in autumn. Pendent panicles of fragrant, white, yellow-marked flowers, to 3cm (1¼in) long, are produced in late spring and early summer. ↕ 12m (40ft), ↔ 10m (30ft). S.E. USA. ✻✻✻

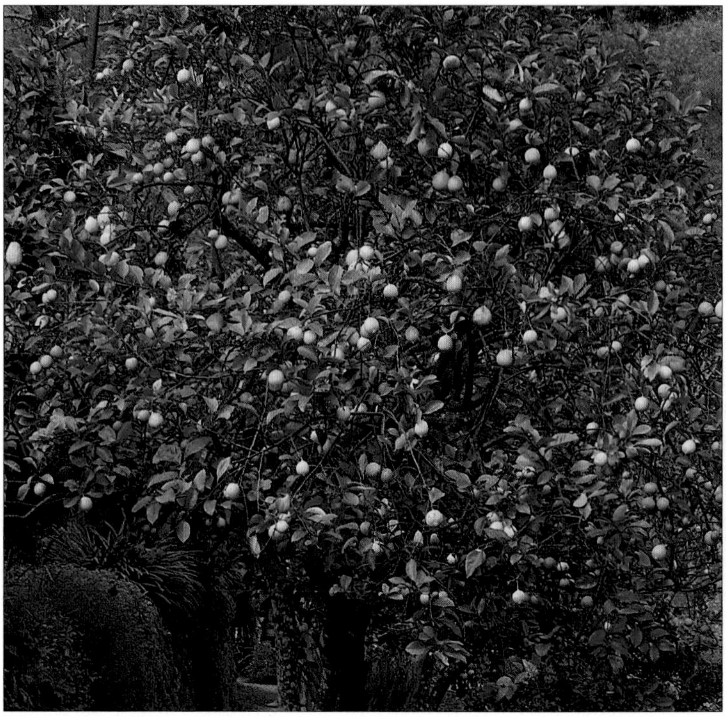

Citrus limon

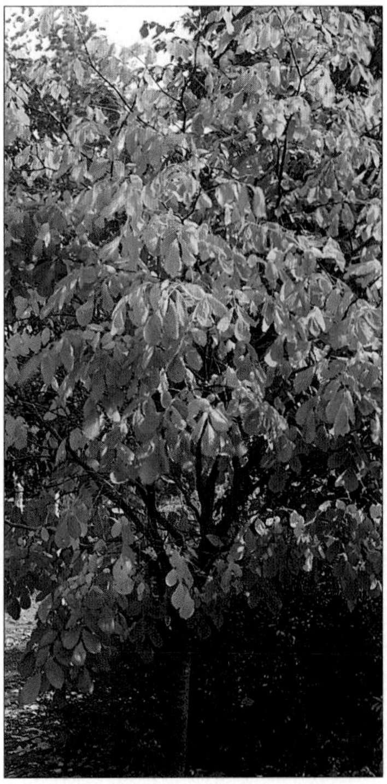

Cladrastis lutea

CLARKIA

syn. EUCHARIDIUM, GODETIA

ONAGRACEAE

Genus of about 36 species of vigorous, mostly slender-stemmed annuals found on dry, open slopes, from sea level to 2,400m (8,000ft), in W. North America and South America. They have oval or linear to elliptic, sometimes toothed leaves. Spreading, funnel-shaped, paper-thin, pastel-coloured flowers, with a satin-like texture, are borne in upright, leafy racemes in summer. Grow in an annual border. *Clarkia* species and cultivars are also good for cut flowers.

- **HARDINESS** Fully hardy.
- **CULTIVATION** Grow in moderately fertile, moist but well-drained, slightly acid soil in sun or partial shade. Very fertile soil encourages growth of foliage at the expense of flowers. They dislike hot, humid conditions.
- **PROPAGATION** Sow seed *in situ* in autumn or early spring. Protect autumn-sown seedlings with cloches over winter, and avoid transplanting.
- **PESTS AND DISEASES** Susceptible to foot, root, and stem rot.

C. amoena, syn. *Godetia amoena, G. grandiflora* (Satin flower). Erect annual with lance-shaped, sometimes toothed leaves, to 6cm (2½in) long. Fluted, single or double, lilac to reddish pink flowers, 5cm (2in) across, are borne in raceme-like clusters at the tips of long, leafy shoots in summer. ↕ to 75cm (30in), ↔ 30cm (12in). USA (California). ❄❄❄. Cultivars of **Grace Series** have single, lavender-pink, red, salmon-pink, or pink flowers with contrasting centres; ↕ to 50cm (20in). **Satin Series** cultivars are dwarf and bushy, with single flowers in various colours, many with white margins or contrasting centres; ↕ to 20cm (8in). **'Sybil Sherwood'** ■ has single, salmon-pink flowers, fading to white at the margins; ↕ to 45cm (18in).

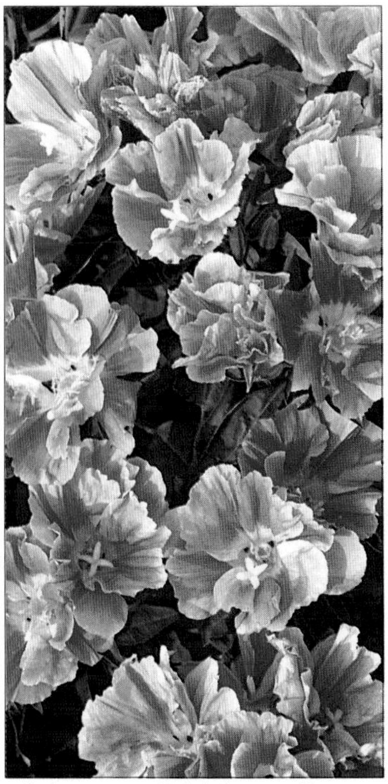

Clarkia amoena 'Sybil Sherwood'

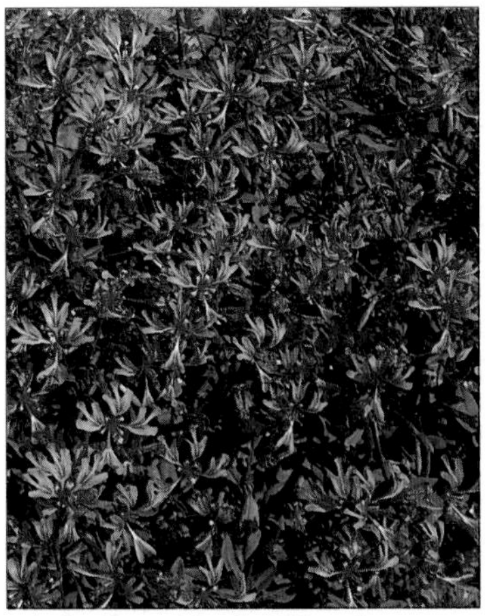

Clarkia breweri 'Pink Ribbons'

***C. breweri* 'Pink Ribbons'** ■ syn. *Eucharidium breweri* 'Pink Ribbons'. Erect to spreading annual bearing lance-shaped to linear, sometimes toothed leaves, to 5cm (2in) long. Scented, purplish pink flowers, to 5cm (2in) across, with 3-lobed, ribbon-like petals, are borne in raceme-like clusters at the tips of leafy shoots in summer. ↕ to 30cm (12in), ↔ to 23cm (9in). USA (California). ❄❄❄

C. elegans see *C. unguiculata.*

C. unguiculata, syn. *C. elegans.* Erect annual with lance-shaped, elliptic, or ovate leaves. In summer, bears solitary, lavender- to salmon-pink, purplish red, or dark red-purple, rarely white flowers, 1.5–4cm (½–1½in) across, from the upper leaf axils. ↕ 30–100cm (12–39in), ↔ 20cm (8in). USA (California). ❄❄❄. **Royal Bouquet Series** cultivars produce racemes, to 30cm (12in) long, resembling small hollyhocks, of evenly spaced, frilly, double, pink, red, or mauve flowers, to 5cm (2in) across, sometimes darker or paler at the bases; ↕ to 90cm (36in), ↔ to 30cm (12in).

▷ **Clary,**
Annual see *Salvia viridis*
Biennial see *Salvia sclarea*
Meadow see *Salvia pratensis*

CLAYTONIA

Purslane, Spring beauty

PORTULACACEAE

Genus of about 15 species of deciduous and evergreen, succulent perennials and some annuals or short-lived perennials. They occur mainly in mountainous areas, often in scree, in Australasia and W. North America. They have rosettes of fleshy, stalked basal leaves, and opposite, stalkless, often stem-clasping upper leaves. Small, 5-petalled, cup- or bowl-shaped, pink or white flowers are borne in terminal racemes in summer. Grow in an alpine house or a scree bed.

- **HARDINESS** Fully hardy.
- **CULTIVATION** Grow in gritty, humus-rich, sharply drained soil in full sun. Protect from excessive winter wet.
- **PROPAGATION** Sow seed in containers in an open frame in autumn.
- **PESTS AND DISEASES** Aphids may be a problem under glass.

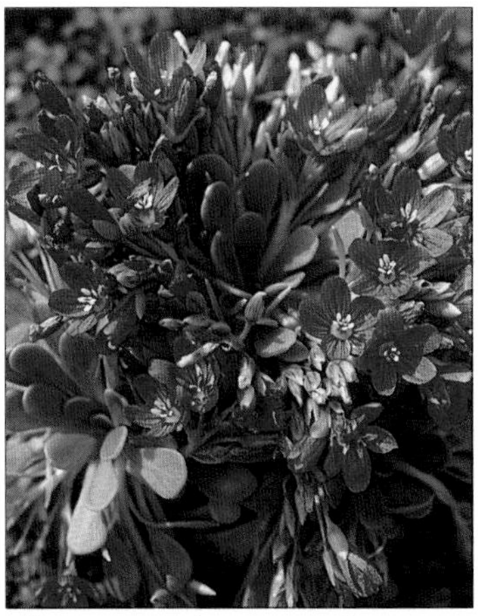

Claytonia megarhiza var. *nivalis*

C. megarhiza* var. *nivalis ■ syn. *Calandrinia megarhiza* var. *nivalis.* Short-lived, tap-rooted, evergreen perennial with spoon-shaped, fleshy, grey-green or deep green basal leaves, to 15cm (6in) long, and smaller, inversely lance-shaped to linear upper leaves. In early summer, shallowly cup-shaped, deep rose-pink flowers, 2–3cm (¾–1¼in) across, occasionally suffused yellow, are produced in dense racemes on short, branching stems. ↕ to 5cm (2in), ↔ to 15cm (6in). USA (Rocky Mountains). ❄❄❄

CLEISTOCACTUS

CACTACEAE

Genus of about 50 species of columnar, perennial cacti from mountainous areas, to 3,000m (10,000ft), in Peru, Bolivia, Paraguay, Argentina, and Uruguay, with cylindrical, fleshy stems bearing rounded ribs and dense spines. As they reach maturity (some in only 3–4 years), many species branch from the base and produce tubular, diurnal flowers. In frost-prone areas, grow in a warm greenhouse. In warmer climates, grow in a border with other cacti and succulents.

- **HARDINESS** Frost tender.
- **CULTIVATION** Under glass, grow in standard cactus compost in full light and with low humidity. In the growing season, water freely and apply a half-strength balanced liquid fertilizer every 5–6 weeks. Keep completely dry from mid-autumn to spring. Outdoors, grow in sharply drained, low fertility, humus-rich soil in full sun. See also pp.48–49.
- **PROPAGATION** Sow seed at 21°C (70°F) in early spring or summer. Root stem cuttings in early summer.
- **PESTS AND DISEASES** Mealybugs and root rot may be a problem.

C. brookei, syn. *C. wendlandiorum.* Semi-erect or spreading cactus with 22- to 25-ribbed, mid-green stems, 4–6cm (1½–2½in) thick, densely covered with bristle-like, slightly yellowish or greyish white spines. Red or orange flowers, 5cm (2in) long, are borne in summer. ↕ 65cm (26in), ↔ indefinite. Bolivia. ❀ (min. 10°C/50°F)

C. hyalacanthus ■ syn. *C. jujuyensis.* Erect cactus branching freely from the base. Greyish green stems, 4–6cm (1½–2½in) thick, have 17–25 ribs and are covered with bristle-like, hairy, brownish yellow or yellowish white spines. Bears pale red flowers, to 4cm (1½in) long, in summer. ↕ 1m (3ft) or more, ↔ 60cm (24in) or more. Bolivia, N.W. Argentina. ❀ (min. 10°C/50°F)

C. jujuyensis see *C. hyalacanthus.*

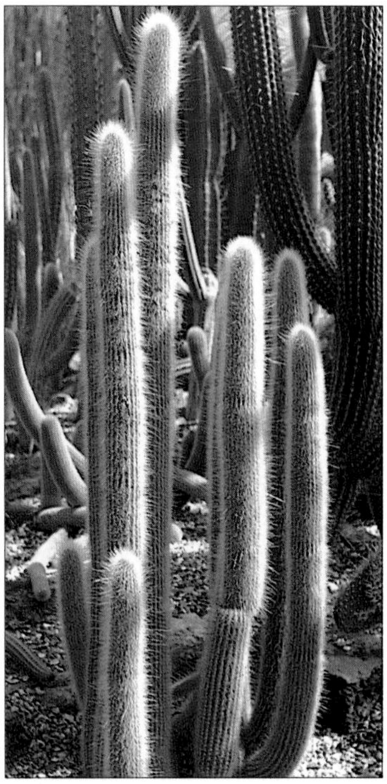

Cleistocactus hyalacanthus

C. smaragdiflorus. Erect, then decumbent cactus with 12- to 16-ribbed, mid-green stems, 4–6cm (1½–2½in) thick. Closely set areoles bear long, bristly, pale to dark brown spines. Green-tipped red flowers, to 5cm (2in) long, are produced in summer. ↕ 2m (6ft), ↔ indefinite. Bolivia, Paraguay, Argentina, Uruguay. ❀ (min. 10°C/50°F)

C. strausii ■ 🏆 (Silver torch). Erect cactus branching freely from the base. Light green stems, 4–8cm (1½–3in) thick, have about 25 ribs with densely arranged, bristle-like, snow-white spines. Bears carmine-red flowers, 8–9cm (3–3½in) long, in summer. ↕↔ 1m (3ft) or more. Bolivia. ❀ (min. 10°C/50°F)

C. wendlandiorum see *C. brookei.*

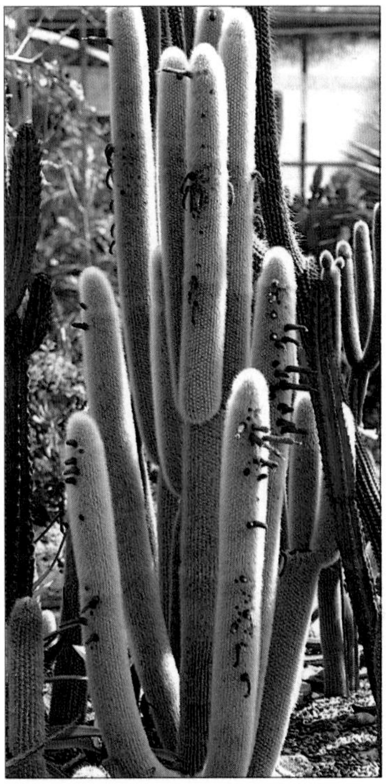

Cleistocactus strausii

C

CLEMATIS syn. ATRAGENE

Old man's beard, Traveller's joy, Virgin's bower

RANUNCULACEAE

Genus of more than 200 species of evergreen or deciduous, mainly semi-woody to woody, twining leaf-climbers and woody-based herbaceous perennials from the N. and S. hemispheres, including Europe, the Himalayas, China, Australasia, North America, and Central America. More than 400 mainly large-flowered cultivars are in cultivation. Due to the diversity of the species – which include short-growing herbaceous perennials, scandent or trailing shrubs, and climbers reaching 10–15m (30–50ft) in height – habit and leaf form vary greatly. The opposite, occasionally alternate, hairy to hairless leaves are simple, 3-palmate, or pinnate or 2-pinnate, with entire to irregularly cut margins. Climbing species attach to host plants or supporting structures by means of their leaf-stalks. More specific leaf information is given in the group descriptions below. The mostly bisexual, rarely unisexual flowers are borne singly or in cymes or panicles. They have 4–10 sepals (often referred to as petals) and vary greatly in shape and size (see panel below). Clematis are grown for their abundant flowers, often followed by decorative, filamentous, silvery grey seed heads. Some, such as *C. recta*, are scented. Use climbing species to clothe a wall, arbour, trellis, or pergola; they can also be grown over large shrubs or small trees. Grow herbaceous species in a mixed or herbaceous border.

For ease of reference, clematis may be divided into the following 3 groups, based on their cultivation requirements:

Group 1

Early-flowering species – bear flowers on the previous year's shoots in winter and early spring. They prefer a sheltered, sunny site with well-drained soil. Mid-green leaves are evergreen and glossy, or deciduous, usually divided into 3 leaflets, and either lance-shaped, to 12cm (5in) long, or simple, oblong, and fern-like, 5cm (2in) long. Flowers are single and either bell-shaped or open bell-shaped, 2–5cm (¾–2in) long, or saucer-shaped, 4–5cm (1½–2in) across. Fully hardy to frost hardy.

C. alpina, C. macropetala, ***and their cultivars*** – bear flowers on the previous year's shoots in spring and occasionally on new growth in summer. *C. alpina* and its variants are ideal for very cold, exposed sites. They are deciduous, having pale to mid-green leaves, 3–5cm (1¼–2in) long, with 3–5 lance-shaped to broadly oblong, toothed leaflets. Single, semi-double, or double, bell-shaped to open bell-shaped flowers, 3–7cm (1¼–3in) across, are followed by attractive seed heads from summer to autumn. Fully hardy to frost hardy.

C. montana ***and its cultivars*** – bear flowers on the previous year's ripened shoots in late spring. They are very vigorous, deciduous climbers, useful for clothing a large tree or building. Mid- to purplish green leaves, 5–8cm (2–3in) long, have 3 lance-shaped leaflets with pointed tips. Flowers are almost flat to saucer-shaped, and usually single, 5–7cm (2–3in) across. Fully hardy.

Group 2

Early- to mid-season, large-flowered cultivars – bear flowers in late spring and early summer on sideshoots arising from the previous year's growth, and in mid- and late summer at the tips of the current year's shoots. They are deciduous with pale to mid-green leaves, usually 10–15cm (4–6in) long and divided into 3 ovate or lance-shaped leaflets, or simple and ovate, to 10cm (4in) long. Flowers are upright, single, semi-double, or fully double, and mostly saucer-shaped, 10–20cm (4–8in) across. Fully hardy to frost hardy; severe winters may damage early top growth.

Group 3

Late, large-flowered cultivars – bear flowers on the current year's shoots in summer and early autumn. They are deciduous with pale to mid-green leaves, mostly 10–15cm (4–6in) long with 3 ovate or lance-shaped leaflets, or simple and ovate, to 10cm (4in) long. Flowers are single, outward-facing, and usually saucer-shaped, 7–15cm (3–6in) across. Fully hardy.

Late-flowering species and small-flowered cultivars – flower on the current year's shoots from summer to late autumn. They are generally deciduous with pale to dark green or grey-green leaves, 2–15cm (¾–6in) long, either pinnate or 2-pinnate, with lance-shaped leaflets, or simple and lance-shaped. Blooms are single or double, and saucer-shaped, star-shaped, bell-shaped, open bell-shaped, tulip-shaped, or tubular, 1–10cm (½–4in) across. Fully hardy to half hardy.

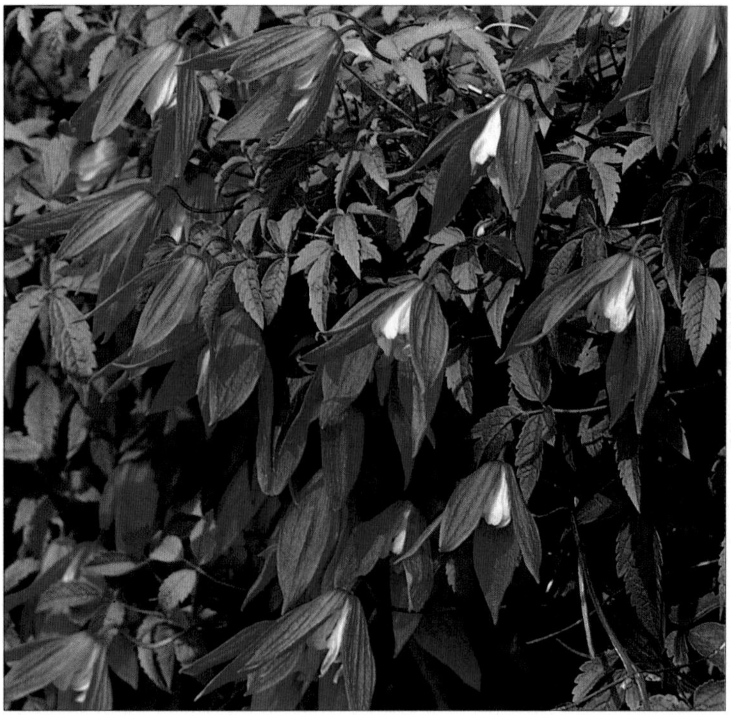

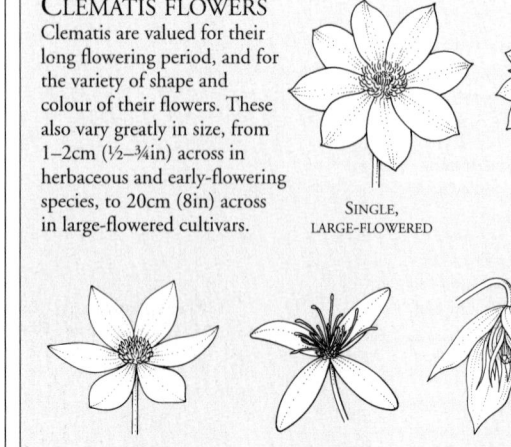

Clematis alpina

Herbaceous species and cultivars – bear flowers on the current year's shoots from midsummer to late autumn. They are suitable for a mixed border with perennials. The leaves are mid- to dark green or greyish green, either simple and lance-shaped to ovate or heart-shaped, 2.5–15cm (1–6in) long, some with toothed margins, or 2.5–8cm (1–3in) long with 3–5 lance-shaped to ovate leaflets. Single flowers are either saucer-shaped, 1–2cm (½–¾in) across, or bell-shaped or tubular, 1–4cm (½–1½in) long. Fully hardy to frost hardy.

• **HARDINESS** Fully hardy to half hardy. See also group descriptions above.

• **CULTIVATION** Grow in fertile, humus-rich, well-drained soil in sun or partial shade, with the roots and base of the plant in shade. Herbaceous species prefer full sun. Mulch all clematis in late winter with garden compost or well-rotted manure, avoiding the immediate crown. Plant climbing clematis with the top of the root ball about 8cm (3in) below the soil surface, to reduce risk of clematis wilt and encourage production of strong shoots from below soil level. After planting, cut back top growth of deciduous climbers to a strong pair of buds about 30cm (12in) above soil level. Provide strong support and tie in initially until plants begin to climb by themselves. Support herbaceous species and cultivars with twiggy brushwood.

Prune Group 1 clematis after flowering, removing dead or damaged stems and shortening others to their allotted space. This encourages production of new growth to flower in the following season. For Group 2 clematis, remove dead and damaged stems before growth begins in early spring, trimming all remaining stems back to where strong buds are visible. These buds provide a framework of second-year shoots which, in turn, produce sideshoots that flower in late spring and early summer. The flowers may then be removed. Young shoots bear more flowers later in the summer. For Group 3 clematis, cut back all the previous year's stems to a pair of strong buds, 15–20cm (6–8in) above soil level, before growth begins in early spring.

• **PROPAGATION** Sow seed of species as soon as ripe in containers in a cold frame. Divide or take basal cuttings of herbaceous species in spring. Root softwood cuttings in spring, or semi-ripe cuttings in early summer. Layer in late winter or early spring.

• **PESTS AND DISEASES** Clematis wilt may be a problem. Cutworms and voles may cut young stems. Aphids may attack young plants. Whiteflies may be a problem under glass.

***C.* 'Abundance'** ■ syn. *C. viticella* 'Abundance'. (Group 3) Late, small-flowered climber with light green leaves. From midsummer to late autumn, bears open bell-shaped, single, 4-sepalled, wine-red flowers, 6cm (2½in) across,

CLEMATIS FLOWERS

Clematis are valued for their long flowering period, and for the variety of shape and colour of their flowers. These also vary greatly in size, from 1–2cm (½–¾in) across in herbaceous and early-flowering species, to 20cm (8in) across in large-flowered cultivars.

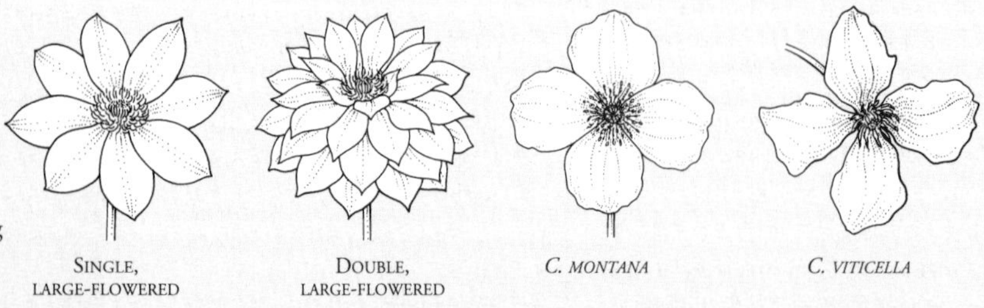

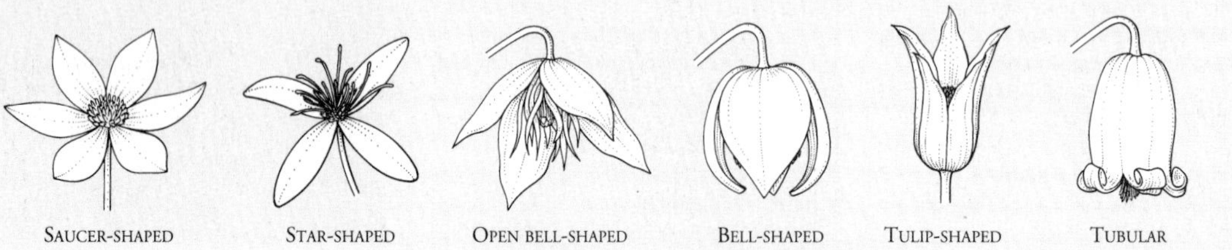

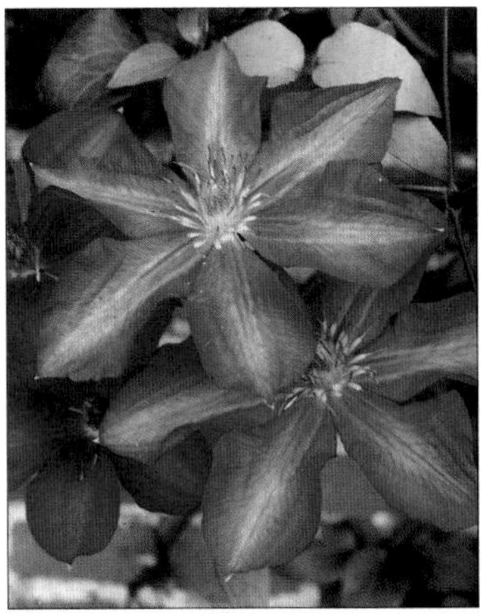
Clematis 'Ascotiensis'

with cream anthers. ↕ 3m (10ft), ↔ 1m (3ft). ❄❄❄
***C.* 'Alba Luxurians'** ■ ♀ syn. *C. viticella* 'Alba Luxurians'. (Group 3) Late, small-flowered climber with slightly grey-green foliage. From midsummer to late autumn, bears open bell-shaped, single flowers, 5–7cm (2–3in) across, with 4–6 green-tipped white sepals, sometimes faintly mauve-tinged when young, and small black anthers. ↕ 4m (12ft), ↔ 1.5m (5ft). ❄❄❄
C. alpina ■ ♀ (Alpine clematis). (Group 1) Early-flowering climber. Bears solitary, usually single, open bell-shaped blue flowers, 4–7cm (1½–3in) across, with white centres, from spring to early summer (occasionally also in mid- and late summer), followed by fluffy seed heads from late summer to autumn. ↕ 2–3m (6–10ft), ↔ 1.5m (5ft). Europe. ❄❄❄. **'Constance'** has semi-double, deep purplish pink flowers. **'Frances Rivis'** ♀ has slightly twisted, mid-blue flowers. **'Frankie'** has light to mid-blue flowers with cream petaloid stamens tipped pale blue. **'Helsingborg'** bears flowers with pointed, deep blue-purple sepals and light brown-purple petaloid stamens. **'Pamela Jackman'** has deep blue flowers with blue and cream anthers. **'Pink Flamingo'** is free-flowering, and has semi-double, pale pink flowers with veins darkening towards the bases, and cream anthers. **'Willy'** has pale pink flowers, the sepals darkening towards the bases, deeper pink undersides, and cream anthers.
C. armandii ■ (Group 1) Vigorous, evergreen, early-flowering climber bearing saucer-shaped, scented white flowers, 5cm (2in) across, with cream anthers, in axillary cymes in early spring. ↕ 3–5m (10–15ft), ↔ 2–3m (6–10ft). China. ❄❄. **'Apple Blossom'** has pink-tinged white flowers, with deeper pink undersides, fading to pinkish white, 4–6cm (1½–2in) across.
***C.* 'Asao'.** (Group 2) Compact, early, large-flowered climber producing single, creamy pink flowers, 10–13cm (4–5in) across, with deep pink sepal margins and yellow anthers, in late spring. Prefers partial shade. ↕ 2m (6ft), ↔ 1m (3ft). ❄❄❄
***C.* 'Ascotiensis'** ■ ♀ (Group 3) Vigorous, late, small- to large-flowered climber. Bears single, bright violet-blue flowers, 9–12cm (3½–5in) across, with pointed sepals and brownish green anthers, in summer. ↕ 3–4m (10–12ft), ↔ 1m (3ft). ❄❄❄
***C.* 'Barbara Dibley'.** (Group 2) Early, large-flowered climber bearing single, petunia-red flowers, 13–18cm (5–7in) across, with a darker central bar, pointed sepals, and red anthers, from early to late summer. The spring flowers are larger and darker in colour. ↕ 2.5m (8ft), ↔ 1m (3ft). ❄❄❄
***C.* 'Barbara Jackman'.** (Group 2) Early, large-flowered climber bearing single, mauve-blue flowers, 10cm (4in) across, with a magenta central band on each sepal and creamy yellow anthers, in summer. Fades in full sun. ↕ 2.5–3m (8–10ft), ↔ 1m (3ft). ❄❄❄
***C.* 'Beauty of Worcester'** ■ (Group 2) Early, large-flowered climber producing deep blue flowers, 12–16cm (5–6in) across, with creamy white anthers. Double flowers are produced in late spring; summer flowers are smaller and single. ↕ 2.5m (8ft), ↔ 1m (3ft). ❄❄
***C.* 'Bees' Jubilee'** ■ ♀ (Group 2) Compact, early, large-flowered climber flowering freely in late spring and early summer. Single flowers, 10–12cm (4–5in) across, are deep pink, fading with age, with a darker central band on each sepal and light brown anthers. Prefers partial shade. ↕ 2.5m (8ft), ↔ 1m (3ft). ❄❄❄
***C.* 'Belle of Woking'.** (Group 2) Early, large-flowered climber producing double, bluish white flowers, 8–12cm (3–5in) across, with cream anthers and sometimes green outer sepals, from late spring to late summer. Prefers full sun. ↕ 2.5m (8ft), ↔ 1m (3ft). ❄❄❄
***C.* 'Betty Corning'**, syn. *C. viticella* 'Betty Corning'. (Group 3) Late, small-flowered climber producing bell-shaped, slightly scented, single, pale lilac flowers, 5cm (2in) long, with recurved tips and cream anthers, from midsummer to late autumn. ↕ 2m (6ft), ↔ 1m (3ft). ❄❄❄
***C.* 'Bill MacKenzie'** ■ syn. *C. orientalis* 'Bill MacKenzie'. (Group 3) Vigorous, late, small-flowered climber (thought to be a hybrid between *C. orientalis* and *C. tangutica*). From midsummer to late autumn, bears abundant open bell-shaped, single yellow flowers, 8cm (3in) across, with red anthers, followed by large, fluffy seed heads. ↕ 7m (22ft), ↔ 2–3m (6–10ft). ❄❄❄
C. calycina see *C. cirrhosa*.
***C.* 'Cardinal Wyszynski'** see *C.* 'Kardynal Wyszynski'.
***C.* 'Carnaby'** ■ (Group 2) Compact, early, large-flowered climber. Single, mid- to dark pink flowers, 8–10cm (3–4in) across, with a darker central band on each sepal and red anthers, are borne in summer. From late summer to autumn, flowers have lighter bases and darker central bands. Fades in full sun. ↕ 2.5m (8ft), ↔ 1m (3ft). ❄❄❄
***C.* x *cartmanii* 'Joe'** (*C. marmoraria* x *C. ternifolia*). (Group 1) Bushy, trailing or low-climbing, evergreen shrub with purple-tinted branches bearing finely dissected, 2-ternate, leathery, deep green leaves, to 6cm (2½in) long. Cyme-like panicles of shallowly cup-shaped, pure white, male flowers, 3–4cm (1¼–1½in) across, with white anthers, are borne in early spring. Grow in a cold greenhouse or sheltered garden. ↕ to 1.5m (5ft) or more, if climbing. ↕ to 20cm (8in), ↔ to 50cm (20in), if allowed to spread. ❄❄
C. cirrhosa ■ syn. *C. calycina*. (Group 1) Evergreen, early-flowering climber with leaves slightly bronze beneath. Produces open cup-shaped cream flowers, to 6cm (2½in) long, sometimes red-flecked, either singly or in clusters, in late winter and early spring, followed by attractive seed heads. ↕ 2.5–3m (8–10ft), ↔ 1.5m (5ft). Europe. ❄❄. **var. *balearica*** has fragrant, pale cream flowers, speckled reddish brown; Balearic Islands. **'Freckles'** ♀ has creamy pink flowers, heavily speckled red inside.
***C.* 'Comtesse de Bouchaud'** ■ ♀ (Group 3) Strong-growing, late, large-flowered climber bearing single, bright mauve-pink flowers, 8–10cm (3–4in) across, with pale yellow anthers, in summer. ↕ 2–3m (6–10ft), ↔ 1m (3ft). ❄❄❄
***C.* 'Corona'.** (Group 2) Compact, early, large-flowered climber bearing single, light purplish pink flowers, 10–12cm (4–5in) across, with red anthers, in late spring and early summer. ↕ 2m (6ft), ↔ 1m (3ft). ❄❄❄
***C.* 'Countess of Lovelace'.** (Group 2) Early, large-flowered climber producing double, bluish lilac flowers, 10cm (4in) across, with cream anthers, in early summer. Single flowers, with pointed sepals, are borne on new shoots in late summer. ↕ 2m (6ft), ↔ 1m (3ft). ❄❄❄
***C. crispa*.** (Group 3) Deciduous, late-flowering climber. In summer, bears solitary, bell-shaped, single, lavender-blue flowers, 4–5cm (1½–2in) across, with white margins and recurved tips to the sepals, and cream anthers. ↕ 2.5m (8ft), ↔ 1m (3ft). S.E. USA. ❄❄❄
C. dioscoreifolia see *C. terniflora*.
***C.* 'Dr. Ruppel'** ■ ♀ (Group 2) Early, large-flowered climber. Single flowers, 10–15cm (4–6in) across, with deep rose-pink sepals with darker central bands and light chocolate anthers, are freely produced throughout summer. ↕ 2.5m (8ft), ↔ 1m (3ft). ❄❄❄
***C.* 'Duchess of Albany'** ■ ♀ syn. *C. texensis* 'Duchess of Albany'. (Group 3) Deciduous, late, small-flowered climber. From midsummer to autumn, bears tulip-shaped, deep pink flowers, 5cm (2in) long, with slightly darker central bands inside. ↕ 2.5m (8ft), ↔ 1.5m (5ft). ❄❄❄
C.* x *durandii ♀ (Group 3) Non-clinging, late-flowering, semi-climbing perennial. Solitary, saucer-shaped, single, deep indigo-blue flowers, 6–8cm (2½–3in) across, with distinctive, golden yellow anthers, are produced in summer. Requires staking. ↕ 1–2m (3–6ft), ↔ 1m (3ft). ❄❄
***C.* 'Edomurasaki'.** (Group 2) Vigorous, mid-season, large-flowered climber. In summer, bears single, dark violet-blue flowers, 12–15cm (5–6in) across, with deep red anthers. ↕ 3m (10ft), ↔ 1m (3ft). ❄❄
***C.* 'Elsa Späth'** ■ ♀ syn. *C.* 'Xerxes'. (Group 2) Early, large-flowered climber

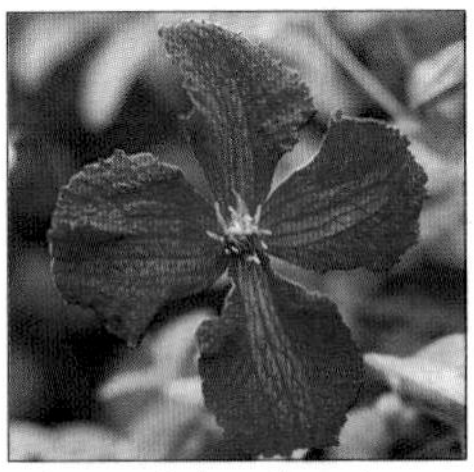
Clematis 'Abundance'

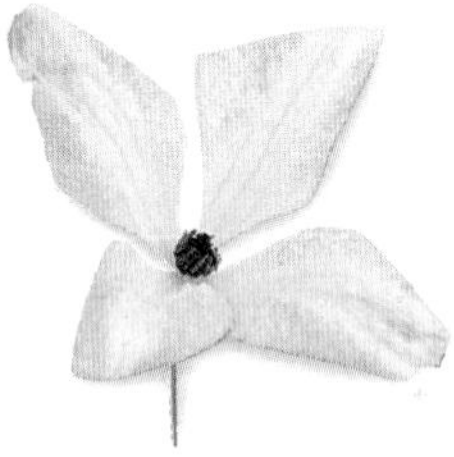
Clematis 'Alba Luxurians'

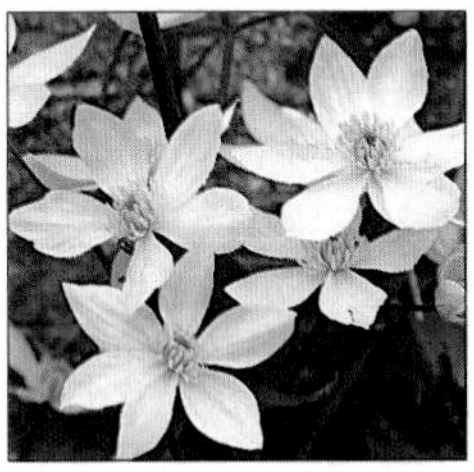
Clematis armandii

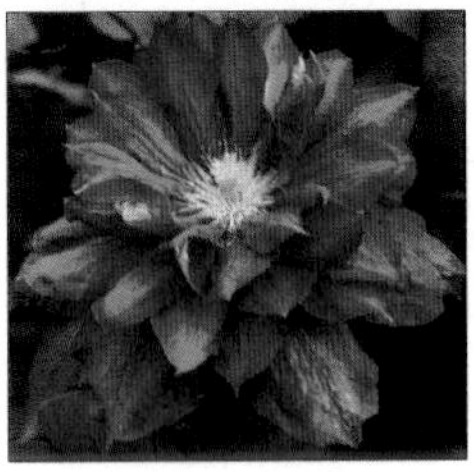
Clematis 'Beauty of Worcester'

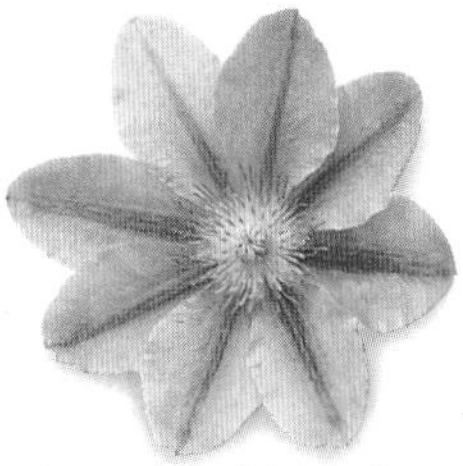
Clematis 'Bees' Jubilee'

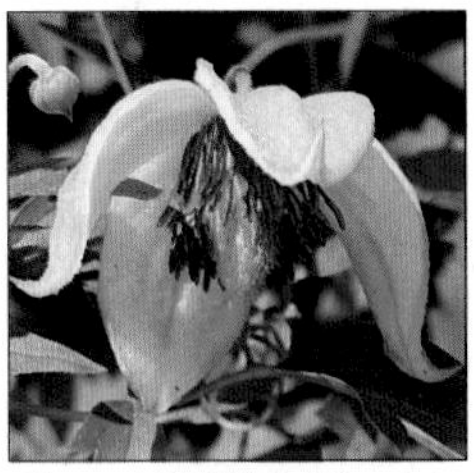
Clematis 'Bill MacKenzie'

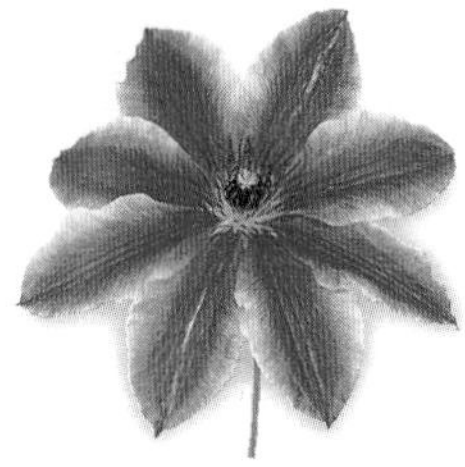
Clematis 'Carnaby'

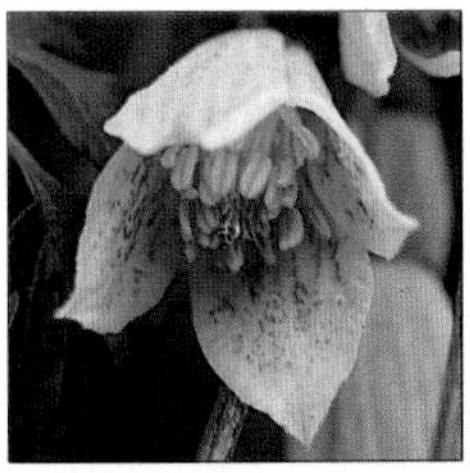
Clematis cirrhosa

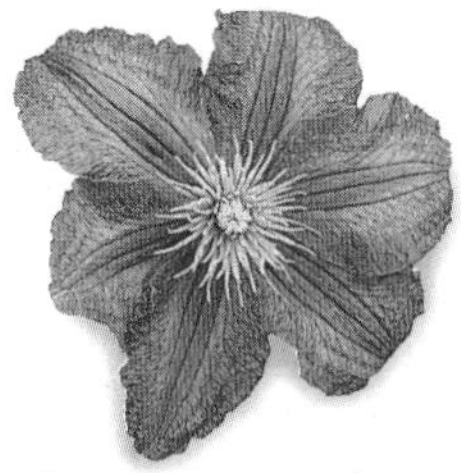
Clematis 'Comtesse de Bouchaud'

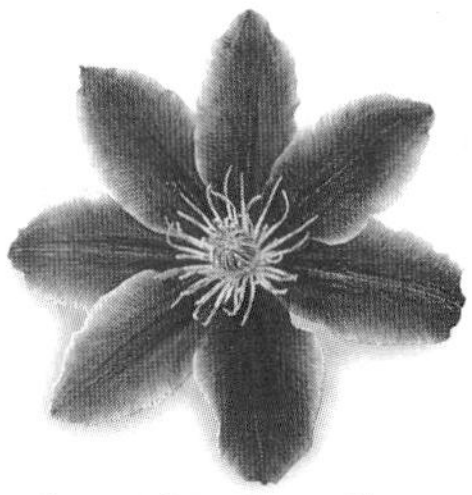
Clematis 'Dr. Ruppel'

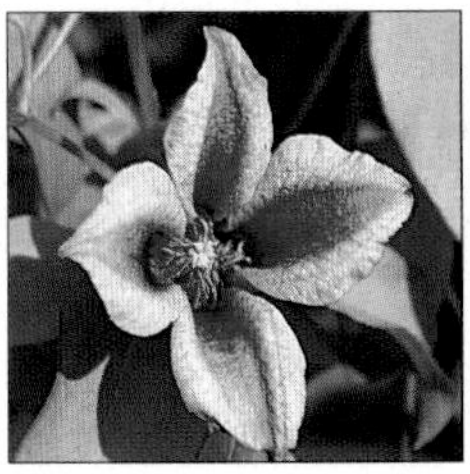
Clematis 'Duchess of Albany'

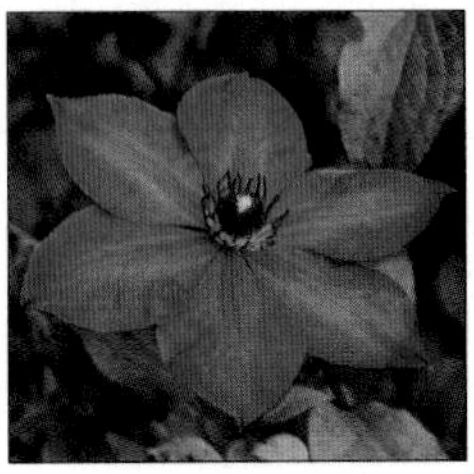
Clematis 'Elsa Späth'

C

C

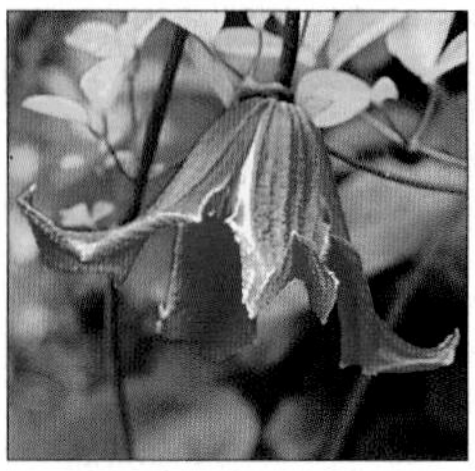
Clematis 'Etoile Rose'

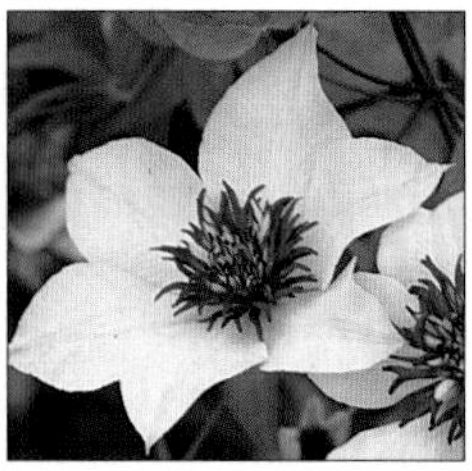
Clematis florida 'Sieboldii'

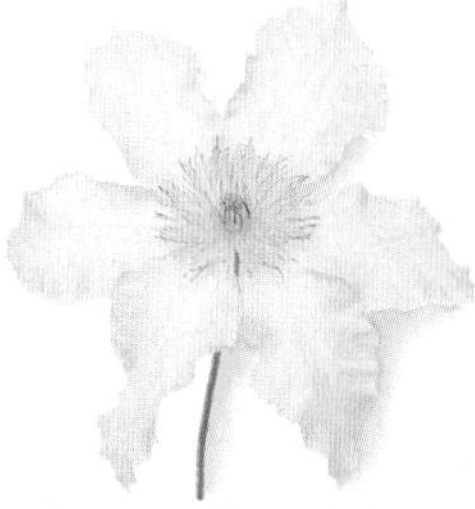
Clematis 'Gillian Blades'

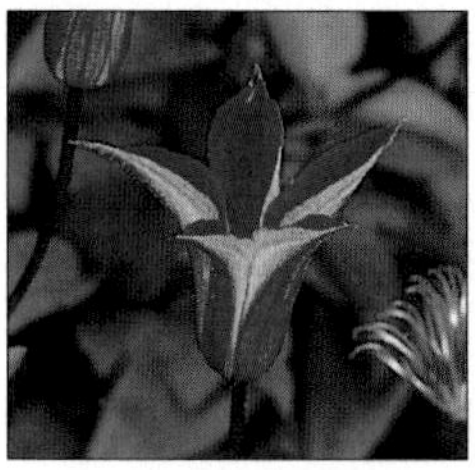
Clematis 'Gravetye Beauty'

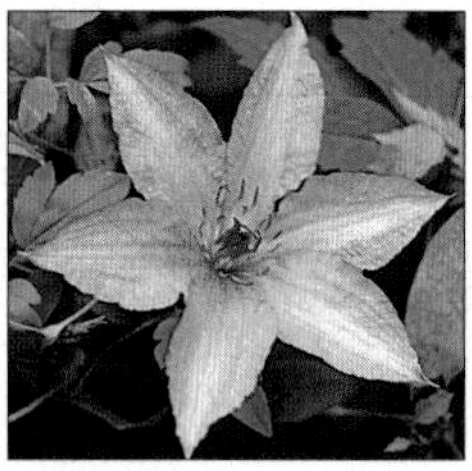
Clematis 'Hagley Hybrid'

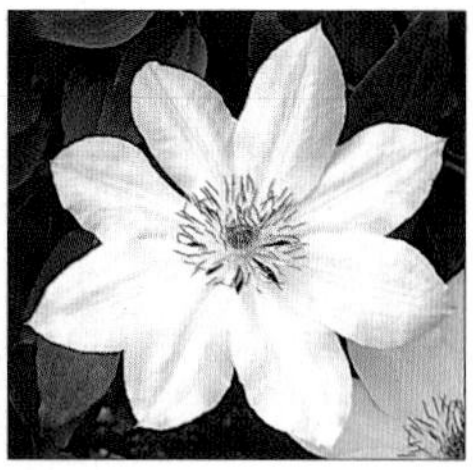
Clematis 'Henryi'

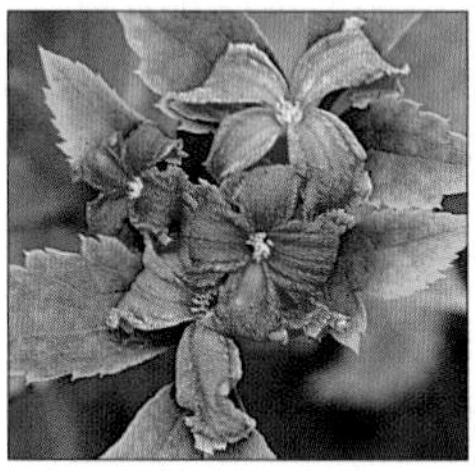
Clematis heracleifolia 'Wyevale'

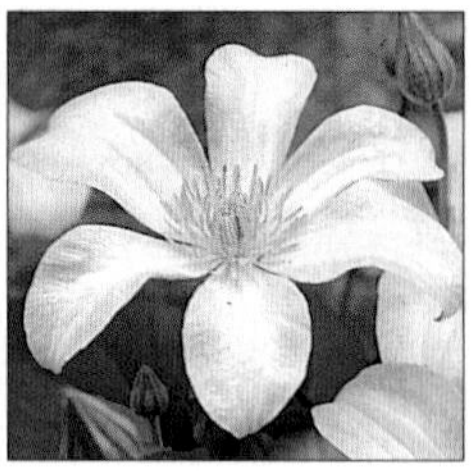
Clematis 'Huldine'

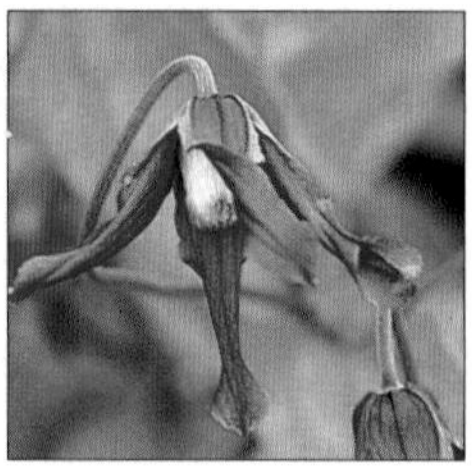
Clematis integrifolia

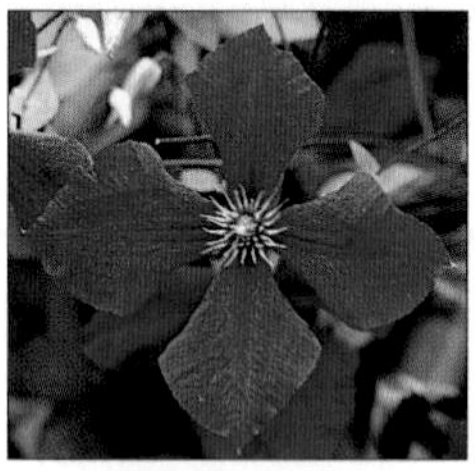
Clematis 'Jackmanii'

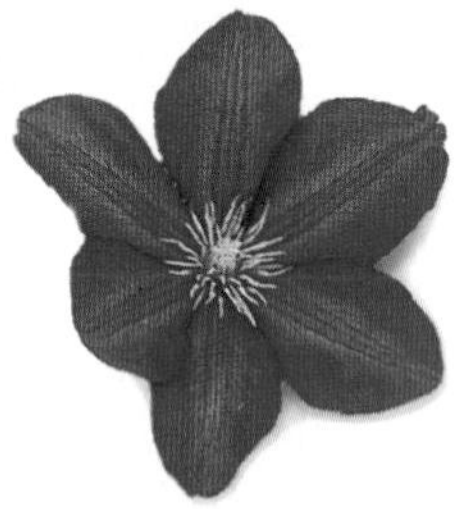
Clematis 'Jackmanii Rubra'

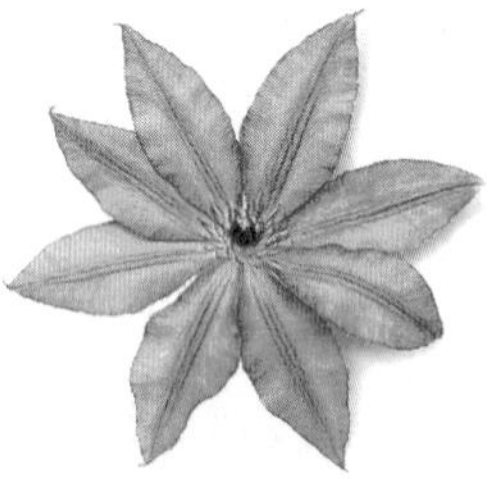
Clematis 'John Warren'

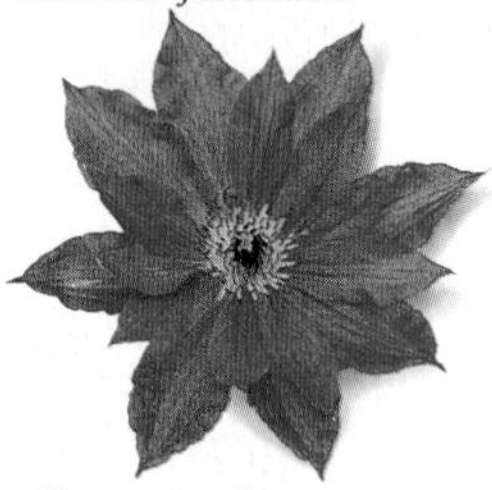
Clematis 'Kathleen Dunford'

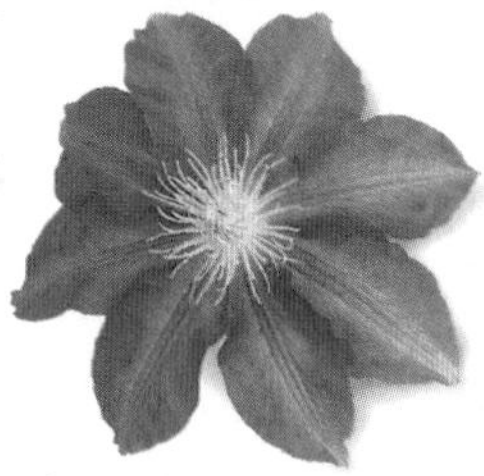
Clematis 'Lasurstern'

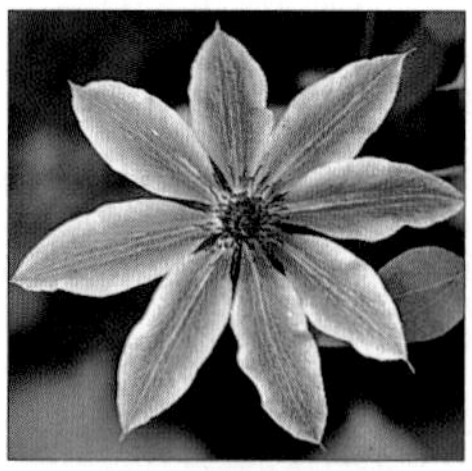
Clematis 'Lincoln Star'

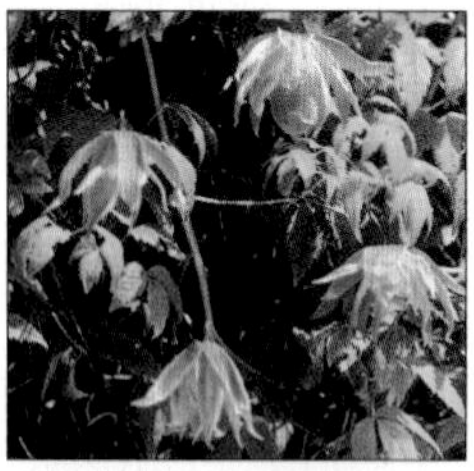
Clematis macropetala

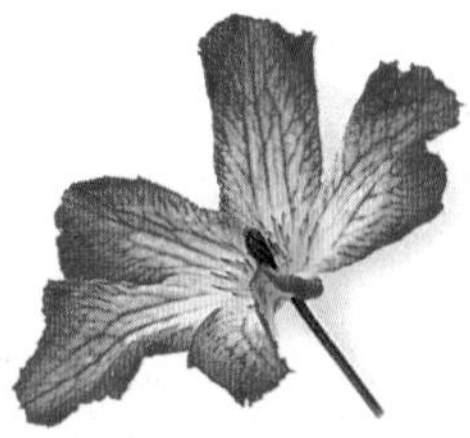
Clematis 'Minuet'

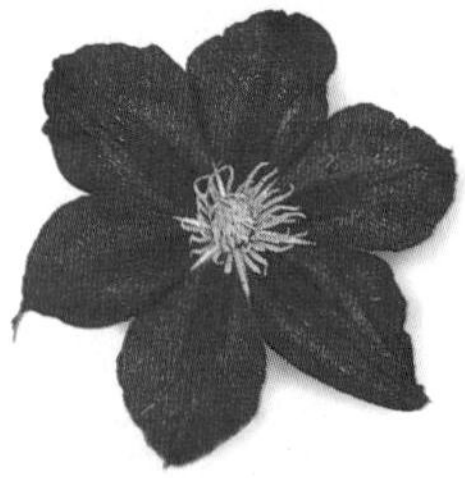
Clematis 'Mme Edouard André'

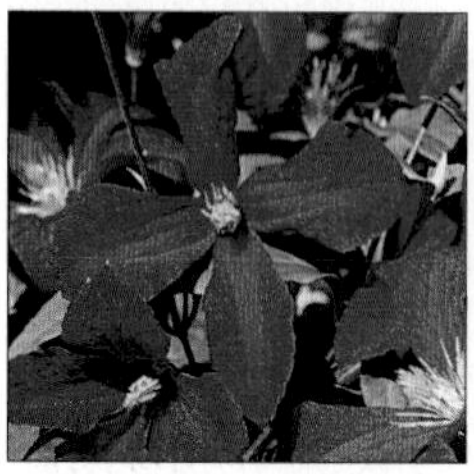
Clematis 'Mme Julia Correvon'

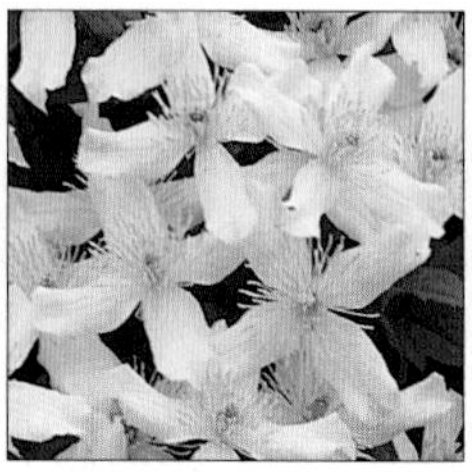
Clematis montana

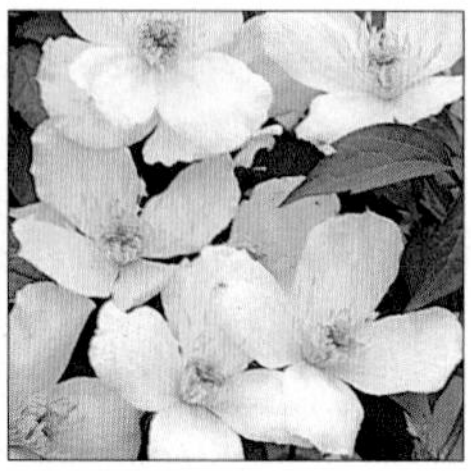
Clematis montana f. *grandiflora*

bearing single flowers, 12–16cm (5–6in) across, with overlapping, rich mauve-blue sepals and red anthers, from late spring to summer. ↕2–3m (6–10ft), ↔1m (3ft). ❄❄❄

C. x eriostemon. (Group 3) Late, small-flowered, woody-based, scandent climber. In summer and autumn, bears abundant solitary (sometimes 2 or 3), bell-shaped flowers, 8cm (3in) long, with very deep indigo-blue sepals, recurved at the tips, and creamy yellow anthers. ↕2.5m (9ft), ↔1m (3ft). Garden origin. ❄❄❄. **'Hendersonii'** has violet-blue sepals; ↕2–5m (6–15ft).

***C.* 'Ernest Markham'** ♀ (Group 3) Vigorous, late, small- to large-flowered climber. In summer, bears abundant, rich, vivid magenta flowers, 10cm (4in) across, with blunt-tipped sepals and light chocolate anthers. Prefers full sun. ↕3–4m (10–12ft), ↔1m (3ft). ❄❄❄

***C.* 'Etoile Rose'** ▣ syn. *C. texensis* 'Etoile Rose'. (Group 3) Late, small-flowered climber. From midsummer to autumn, bears numerous nodding, open bell-shaped, deep rose-pink flowers, 5cm (2in) across, with recurved tips, in clusters. ↕2.5m (8ft), ↔1m (3ft). ❄❄❄

***C.* 'Etoile Violette'** ▣♀ syn. *C. viticella* 'Etoile Violette'. (Group 3) Late, small-flowered climber freely producing single, nodding, saucer-shaped, violet-purple flowers, 7cm (3in) across, with contrasting yellow anthers, from midsummer to late autumn. ↕3–5m (10–15ft), ↔1.5m (5ft). ❄❄❄

***C. x fargesioides* 'Paul Farges'** ▣ syn. *C.* 'Summer Snow'. (Group 3) Very vigorous, late, small-flowered climber. Star-shaped flowers, 4cm (1½in) across, with white sepals and anthers, are borne from midsummer to autumn. ↕7–9m (21–28ft), ↔3m (10ft). ❄❄❄

C. flammula. (Group 3) Semi-evergreen or deciduous, late-flowering climber. Star-shaped, heavily scented white flowers, 3cm (1¼in) across, with cream anthers, are freely produced in panicle-like cymes from midsummer to autumn. Foliage is sometimes glaucous. Prefers a well-drained, sheltered, sunny site. ↕6m (20ft), ↔1m (3ft). S. Europe, N. Africa, W. Syria, Turkey. ❄❄

C. florida. (Group 2) Deciduous or semi-evergreen, mid-season to late-flowering, large-flowered climber. Bears single, white or creamy white flowers, to 14cm (5½in) across, singly or in cymes in late spring or summer. ↕to 4m (12ft), ↔1m (3ft). E. China, Japan. ❄❄. **var. *bicolor*** see 'Sieboldii'. **'Flore Pleno'** has fully double, greenish white flowers, to 12cm (5in) across. **'Sieboldii'** ▣ syn. var. *bicolor*, has single flowers, 7–10cm (3–4in) across, with creamy white sepals and large, domed bosses of rich purple stamens. Weak-growing; ↕2–2.5m (6–8ft).

***C.* 'General Sikorski'** ♀ (Group 2) Vigorous, mid-season, large-flowered climber. In early summer, bears single flowers, 10–15cm (4–6in) across, with overlapping blue sepals and creamy anthers. ↕3m (10ft), ↔1m (3ft). ❄❄❄

***C.* 'Gillian Blades'** ▣♀ (Group 2) Early, large-flowered climber. Single white flowers, 12–16cm (5–6in) across, with overlapping, wavy-margined sepals and cream anthers, appear in summer. ↕2.5m (8ft), ↔1m (3ft). ❄❄❄

***C.* 'Gipsy Queen'** ♀ (Group 3) Vigorous, late, large-flowered climber. Single flowers, 10–12cm (4–5in) across, with overlapping, velvety, violet-purple sepals and deep red anthers, are borne in summer. ↕3m (10ft), ↔1m (3ft). ❄❄❄

***C.* 'Gravetye Beauty'** ▣ syn. *C. texensis* 'Gravetye Beauty'. (Group 3) Late, small-flowered climber bearing tulip-shaped, rich crimson-red flowers, 5cm (2in) long, with paler bands outside, from midsummer to autumn. ↕2.5m (8ft), ↔1m (3ft). ❄❄❄

***C.* 'Guernsey Cream'.** (Group 2) Early, large-flowered climber bearing single flowers, 12cm (5in) across, with creamy yellow sepals and anthers, in early summer. Flowers are smaller and creamy white in late summer. Fades in full sun. ↕2.5m (8ft), ↔1m (3ft). ❄❄❄

***C.* 'Hagley Hybrid'** ▣ (Group 3) Vigorous, compact, late, large-flowered climber. Single flowers, 8–10cm (3–4in) across, with boat-shaped, pinkish mauve sepals and red anthers, are produced in summer. Fades in full sun. ↕2m (6ft), ↔1m (3ft). ❄❄❄

***C.* 'Henryi'** ▣♀ (Group 2) Vigorous, mid-season, large-flowered climber. Single flowers, 16–20cm (6–8in) across, with pointed, creamy white sepals and dark chocolate anthers, are produced in summer. ↕3m (10ft), ↔1m (3ft). ❄❄❄

***C. heracleifolia* 'Wyevale'** ▣ (Group 3) Woody-based perennial of open habit with toothed, deeply 3-lobed, light green leaves, 10–15cm (4–6in) long. Scented, tubular, light to mid-blue flowers, 4cm (1¼in) long, are produced in whorled racemes in summer. Needs support. ↕75cm (30in), ↔1m (3ft). ❄❄❄

***C.* 'H.F. Young'** ▣♀ (Group 2) Very free-flowering, compact, early, large-flowered climber. Bears single, warm blue flowers, 10cm (4in) across, with overlapping, violet-tinged sepals and cream anthers, in early summer. ↕2.5m (8ft), ↔1m (3ft). ❄❄❄

***C.* 'Horn of Plenty'** ♀ (Group 2) Compact, early, large-flowered climber. Rounded, single flowers, 12cm (5in) across, with lilac-mauve sepals fading to mauve-blue, and dark red anthers, are borne in early summer. ↕2.5m (8ft), ↔1m (3ft). ❄❄❄

***C.* 'Huldine'** ▣ (Group 3) Very vigorous, late, small-flowered climber bearing cup-shaped white flowers, 6cm (2½in) across, mauve beneath, with short creamy anthers, in summer. ↕3–5m (10–15ft), ↔2m (6ft). ❄❄❄

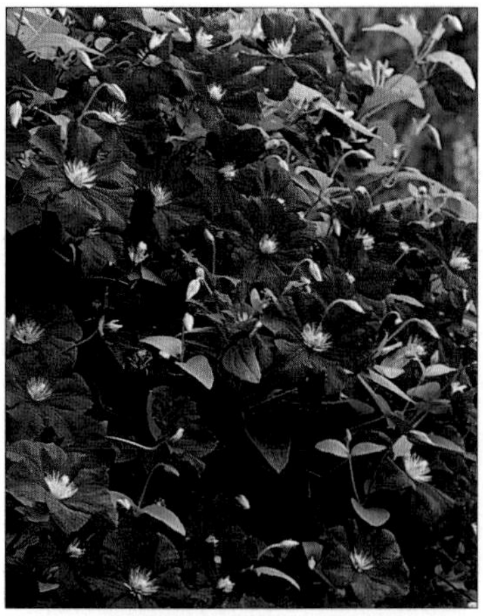
Clematis 'Etoile Violette'

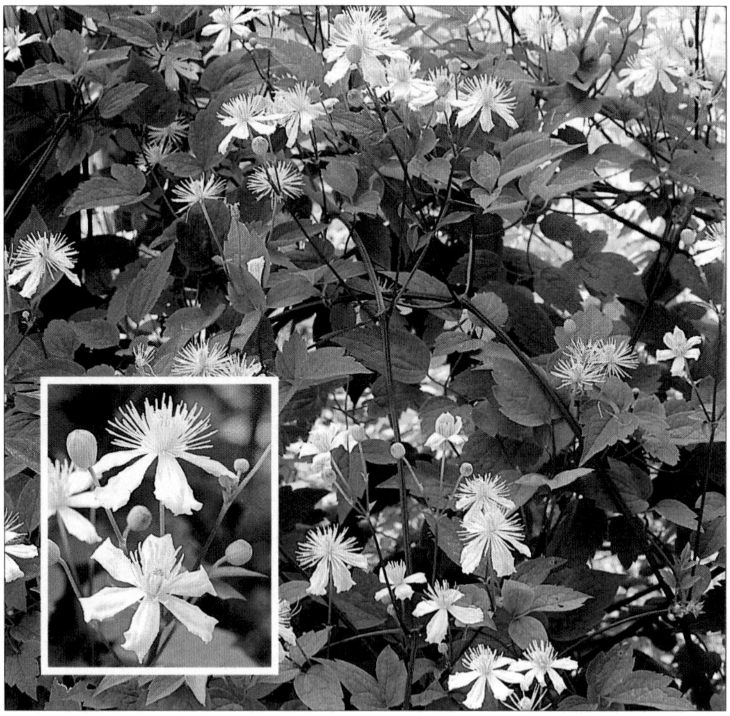

Clematis x *fargesioides* 'Paul Farges' (inset: flower detail)

C. integrifolia ▣ (Group 3) Herbaceous perennial with usually simple, inversely lance-shaped to elliptic leaves. Solitary, bell-shaped, mid-blue flowers, 5cm (2in) long, with 4 slightly twisted sepals and cream anthers, are borne in summer, followed by silvery brown seed heads. ↕↔ 60cm (24in). C. Europe. ✻✻✻
***C.* 'Jackmanii'** ▣ ♀ (Group 3) Late, large-flowered climber. In mid- and late summer, bears abundant single, velvety, dark purple flowers, 8–10cm (3–4in) across, with light greenish brown anthers. ↕ 3m (10ft), ↔ 1m (3ft). ✻✻✻
***C.* 'Jackmanii Alba'.** (Group 2) Vigorous, early, large-flowered climber. In early summer, bears semi-double flowers, 15cm (6in) across, with blue-tinged, milk-white, pointed sepals (and occasionally bluish grey-green outer sepals), and light chocolate anthers. Late-summer flowers are single and off-white. ↕ 3m (10ft), ↔ 1m (3ft). ✻✻✻
***C.* 'Jackmanii Rubra'** ▣ (Group 2) Early, large-flowered climber bearing semi-double flowers, 12cm (5in) across, with crimson-purple sepals and yellow anthers, in early summer, and single flowers in mid- and late summer. ↕ 2.5m (8ft), ↔ 1m (3ft). ✻✻✻
***C.* 'Jan Pawel II'**, syn. *C.* 'John Paul II'. (Group 3) Late, large-flowered climber. In summer, bears single, pink-tinged, off-white flowers, 8–10cm (3–4in) across, with red anthers. In late summer, each sepal has a central pink band. ↕ 3m (10ft), ↔ 1m (3ft). ✻✻✻
***C.* 'John Paul II'** see *C.* 'Jan Pawel II'.
***C.* 'John Warren'** ▣ (Group 2) Early, large-flowered climber. In early summer bears single flowers, 15–18cm (6–7in) across, with pointed, overlapping, pinkish grey sepals, with deep carmine-red veins and margins, and red anthers. ↕ 2.5–3m (8–10ft), ↔ 1m (3ft). ✻✻✻
***C.* 'Kakio'**, syn. C. 'Pink Champagne'. (Group 2) Compact, free-flowering, early, large-flowered climber. In early summer, bears rounded, single, purplish pink flowers, 10–15cm (4–6in) across, paler near the sepal centres, with yellow anthers. ↕ 2.5m (8ft), ↔ 1m (3ft). ✻✻
***C.* 'Kardynal Wyszynski'**, syn. *C.* 'Cardinal Wyszynski'. (Group 3) Free-flowering, late, large-flowered climber bearing single crimson flowers, 8–10cm (3–4in) across, with dark blackish red anthers, in summer. ↕ 2–3m (6–10ft), ↔ 1m (3ft). ✻✻✻
***C.* 'Kathleen Dunford'** ▣ (Group 2) Early, large-flowered climber bearing single or semi-double mauve flowers, 12cm (5in) across, with pointed sepals and red anthers, throughout summer. ↕ 2.5m (8ft), ↔ 1m (3ft). ✻✻✻
***C.* 'Lady Betty Balfour'.** (Group 3) Very vigorous, late, large-flowered climber producing single flowers, 12–15cm (5–6in) across, with rich purple sepals fading to purple-blue, and contrasting yellow anthers, in late summer and early autumn. Needs full sun. ↕ 3m (10ft), ↔ 1m (3ft). ✻✻✻
***C.* 'Lasurstern'** ▣ ♀ (Group 2) Early, large-flowered climber bearing single blue flowers, 12–15cm (5–6in) across, with wavy-margined, overlapping sepals and cream anthers, in early summer. ↕ 2.5m (8ft), ↔ 1m (3ft). ✻✻✻
***C.* 'Lincoln Star'** ▣ (Group 2) Early, large-flowered climber bearing single flowers, 10–12cm (4–5in) across, with raspberry-pink sepals and red anthers, in early summer. Later summer flowers are much paler, with central bands of pink and pale margins. Fades in full sun. ↕ 2–2.5m (6–8ft), ↔ 1m (3ft). ✻✻✻
***C.* 'Lord Nevill'** ♀ (Group 2) Early, large-flowered climber. In early summer, bears single flowers, 10–15cm (4–6in) across, with overlapping, deep blue sepals, minutely scalloped at the margins, and purple-red anthers. ↕ 2–3m (6–10ft), ↔ 1m (3ft). ✻✻✻
C. macropetala ▣ (Group 1) Early-flowering, deciduous climber bearing solitary, open bell-shaped, blue or violet-blue flowers, to 10cm (4in) across, from spring to early summer (occasionally from summer to early autumn), followed by silver seed heads. Flowers appear semi-double, having 4 long sepals with shorter petaloid stamens within: the outer stamens are blue and the inner ones cream. ↕ 2–3m (6–10ft), ↔ 1.5m (5ft). Russia (Siberia), Mongolia, China (Gansu). ✻✻✻. **'Blue Bird'** has open, semi-nodding, mauve-blue flowers, to 12cm (5in) across. **'Jan Lindmark'** has mauve flowers. **'Markham's Pink'** ▣ ♀ has sugar-pink flowers and pale to mid-green foliage. **'Rosy O'Grady'** has open, semi-nodding, pink-mauve flowers, 8cm (3in) across, with white petaloid stamens. **'White Swan'**, syn. *C.* 'White Swan', is compact with white flowers, to 8cm (3in) across, with cream petaloid stamens; ↔ 1m (3ft).
***C.* 'Marie Boisselot'** ♀ syn. *C.* 'Mme le Coultre'. (Group 2) Vigorous, mid-season, large-flowered climber. Single flowers, 15–18cm (6–7in) across, with overlapping white sepals and cream anthers, are produced from midsummer to late autumn. ↕ 3m (10ft), ↔ 1m (3ft). ✻✻✻
C. marmoraria. (Group 1) Early-flowering, tufted, sometimes suckering, dwarf, spreading shrub with stiff, 3-palmate, glossy, somewhat fern-like, dark green leaves, 1–4cm (½–1½in) long. In early and mid-spring, bears a profusion of long-stalked, erect, solitary or clustered, greenish white, unisexual, saucer-shaped flowers, 2.5cm (1in) across; the male flowers are larger and often whiter. Hybridizes freely with *C.* x *cartmanii.* Grow in an alpine house or rock garden. ↕ to 15cm (6in), ↔ to 25cm (10in). New Zealand (South Island). ✻✻
C. maximowicziana see *C. terniflora.*
***C.* 'Minuet'** ▣ ♀ syn. *C. viticella* 'Minuet'. (Group 3) Late, small-flowered climber bearing open bell-shaped, single white flowers, 5cm (2in) across, with pinkish purple veins and dark anthers, from midsummer to late autumn. ↕ 3m (10ft), ↔ 1m (3ft). ✻✻✻
***C.* 'Miss Bateman'** ♀ (Group 2) Compact, free-flowering, early, large-flowered climber. Rounded, single white flowers, 8–10cm (3–4in) across, with red anthers, are borne in early summer. ↕ 2.5m (8ft), ↔ 1m (3ft). ✻✻✻
***C.* 'Mme Baron Veillard'.** (Group 3) Very vigorous, late, large-flowered climber. Single, satin-like, lilac- to rose-pink flowers, 10cm (4in) across, with greenish, light brown anthers, are borne in late summer and early autumn. Needs full sun. ↕ 3–4m (10–12ft), ↔ 1m (3ft). ✻✻✻
***C.* 'Mme Edouard André'** ▣ ♀ (Group 3) Late, large-flowered climber freely producing single, deep red flowers, 8–10cm (3–4in) across, with silver undersides, pointed sepals, and yellow anthers, in midsummer. ↕ 2.5m (8ft), ↔ 1m (3ft). ✻✻✻
***C.* 'Mme Grangé'** ♀ (Group 3) Late, large-flowered climber. Single flowers, 10–13cm (4–5in) across, with boat-shaped, dusky purple sepals, with silver undersides and dark brown anthers, are produced in midsummer. Best against a light background. ↕ 3m (10ft), ↔ 1m (3ft). ✻✻✻
***C.* 'Mme Julia Correvon'** ▣ ♀ syn. *C. viticella* 'Mme Julia Correvon'. (Group 3) Late, large-flowered climber. From midsummer to late autumn, produces open bell-shaped, single, bright wine-red flowers, 7cm (3in) across, with slightly twisted sepals and yellow anthers. ↕ 3m (10ft), ↔ 1.5m (5ft). ✻✻✻
***C.* 'Mme le Coultre'** see *C.* 'Marie Boisselot'.
C. montana ▣ (Group 1) Early-flowering, very vigorous climber. Single white flowers, 5cm (2in) across, with creamy yellow anthers, either solitary or in short cymes, are produced very freely for about 4 weeks in late spring and early summer. ↕ 5–14m (15–46ft), ↔ 2–3m (6–10ft). W. and C. China, Himalayas. ✻✻✻. **'Alexander'** has large, light green leaves and white flowers, 8–10cm (3–4in) across. Prefers full sun; ↕ 7m (22ft), ↔ 3m (10ft). **'Elizabeth'** ♀ has large, purple-flushed, mid-green leaves and strongly scented, pale pink flowers, 7cm (3in) across, with yellow anthers; ↕ 7m (22ft), ↔ 3m (10ft). **f. *grandiflora*** ▣ ♀ syn. 'Grandiflora', is very vigorous, and has dark green leaves and white flowers, 8–10cm (3–4in) across, with cream anthers; ↕ 10m (30ft), ↔ 4m (12ft). **'Pink Perfection'** has purple-flushed, mid-green leaves and rounded, strongly scented pink flowers, 5–7cm (2–3in)

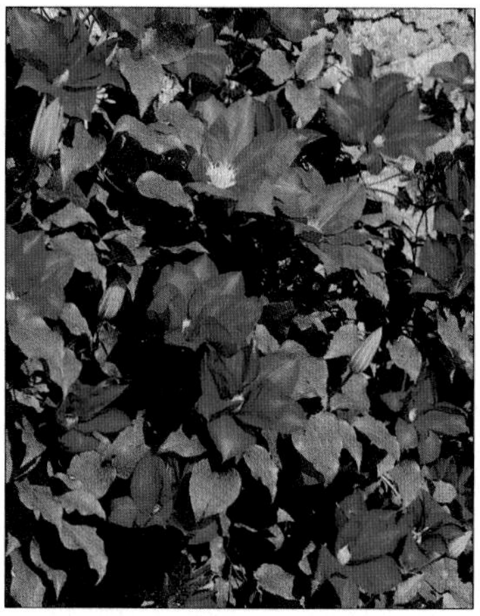

Clematis 'H.F. Young'

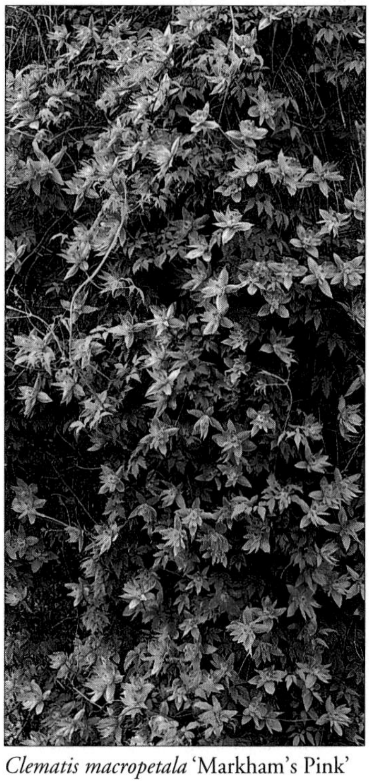

Clematis macropetala 'Markham's Pink'

across, with yellow anthers; ↕7m (22ft), ↔3m (10ft). **var. *rubens*** ■🏆 has purple-flushed, mid-green foliage and pink flowers, with cream anthers; ↕10m (30ft); China. **'Tetrarose'** ■🏆 has purplish green leaflets, with toothed margins, and produces satin-like pink flowers, 9cm (3½in) across, with large bosses of yellow anthers; ↕5m (15ft).
***C.* 'Mrs. Cholmondeley'** 🏆 (Group 2) Early, large-flowered climber bearing single, light lavender-blue flowers, 15–18cm (6–7in) across, with widely spaced sepals and light chocolate anthers, in early summer. ↕2–3m (6–10ft), ↔1m (3ft). ❄❄❄
***C.* 'Mrs. George Jackman'** 🏆 (Group 2) Compact, early, large-flowered climber producing semi-double, creamy white flowers, 10cm (4in) across, with light brown anthers, in early summer. ↕2.5m (8ft), ↔1m (3ft). ❄❄❄
***C.* 'Mrs. N. Thompson'.** (Group 2) Compact, early, large-flowered climber. Single, deep violet flowers, 10cm (4in) across, with vivid scarlet central bands and red anthers, are freely produced in early summer. ↕2.5m (8ft), ↔1m (3ft). ❄❄❄
***C.* 'Mrs. P.B. Truax'.** (Group 2) Compact, early, large-flowered climber. Produces single, periwinkle-blue flowers, 10–12cm (4–5in) across, with cream anthers, in early summer. ↕2.5m (8ft), ↔1m (3ft). ❄❄❄
***C.* 'Nelly Moser'** ■🏆 (Group 2) Compact, early, large-flowered climber. Single, pinkish mauve flowers, 12–16cm (5–6in) across, with darker central bands and red anthers, are borne in early summer. Flowers are paler in late summer. Fades in full sun. ↕2–3m (6–10ft), ↔1m (3ft). ❄❄❄
***C.* 'Niobe'** 🏆 (Group 2) Compact, early, large-flowered climber. Single, rich deep red flowers, 10–15cm (4–6in) across, with pointed sepals and yellow anthers, are freely borne throughout summer. ↕2–3m (6–10ft), ↔1m (3ft). ❄❄❄
***C. orientalis* 'Bill MacKenzie'** see *C.* 'Bill MacKenzie'.
***C. orientalis* 'Orange Peel'** see *C. tibetana* subsp. *vernayi* 'Orange Peel'.
C. paniculata see *C. terniflora.*
***C.* 'Perle d'Azur'** ■🏆 (Group 3) Vigorous, very free-flowering, late, small-flowered climber. Open bell-shaped flowers, 8cm (3in) across, with azure-blue sepals, recurved at the tips, and creamy green anthers, are borne from midsummer to autumn. ↕3m (10ft), ↔1m (3ft). ❄❄❄
***C.* 'Perrin's Pride'.** (Group 3) Late, large-flowered climber bearing rounded flowers, 8–10cm (3–4in) across, with rich mauve-purple sepals and greenish brown anthers, in summer. ↕2–3m (6–10ft), ↔1m (3ft). ❄❄❄

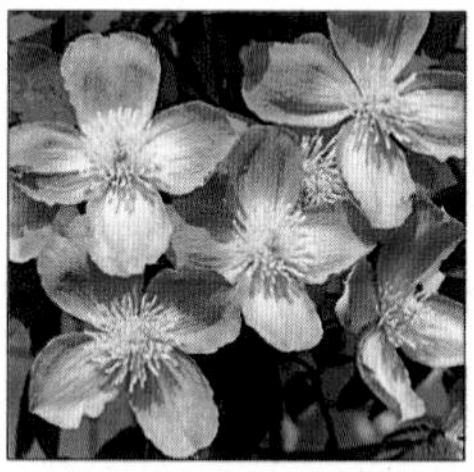
Clematis montana 'Tetrarose'

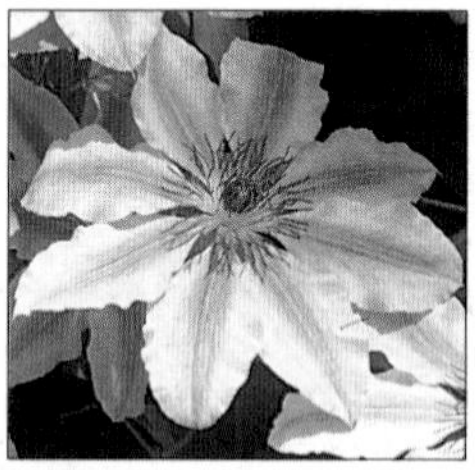
Clematis 'Nelly Moser'

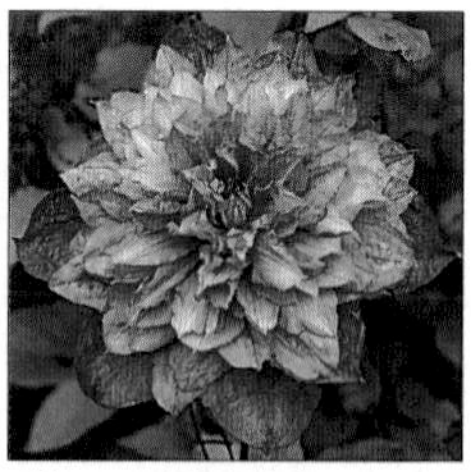
Clematis 'Proteus'

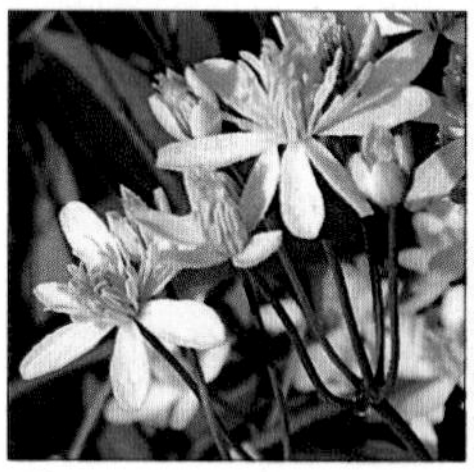
Clematis recta

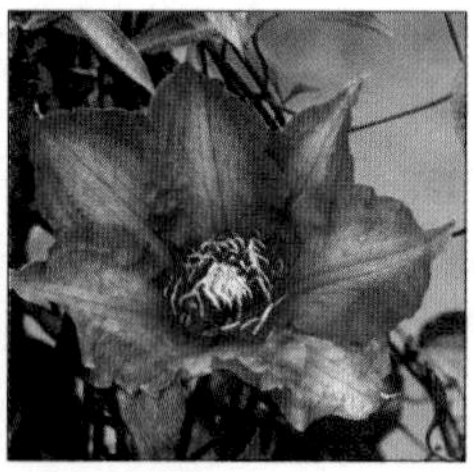
Clematis 'Richard Pennell'

Clematis 'Rouge Cardinal'

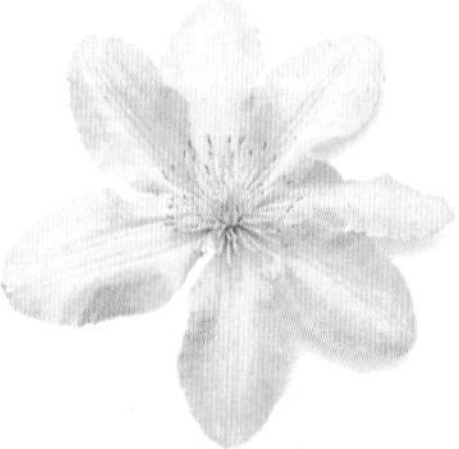
Clematis 'Silver Moon'

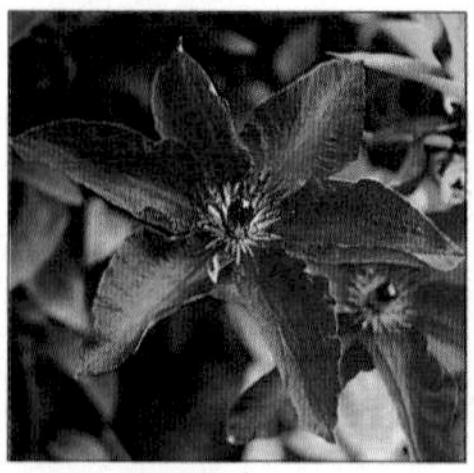
Clematis 'The President'

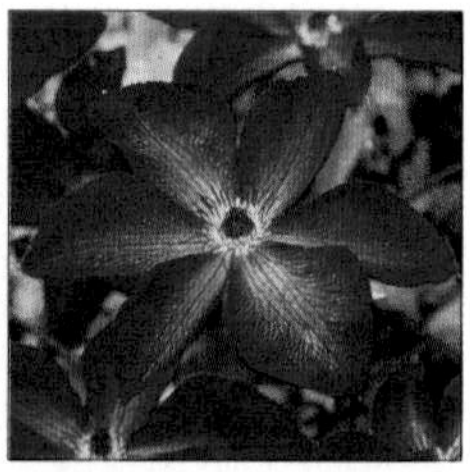
Clematis 'Venosa Violacea'

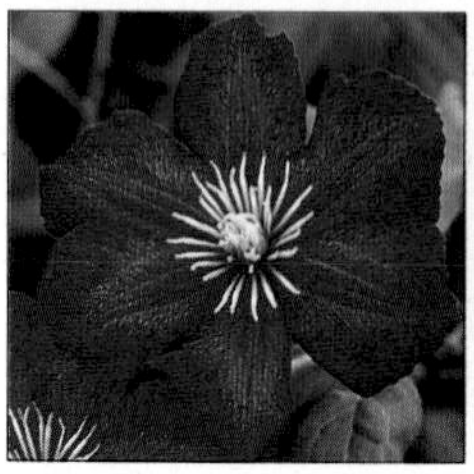
Clematis 'Ville de Lyon'

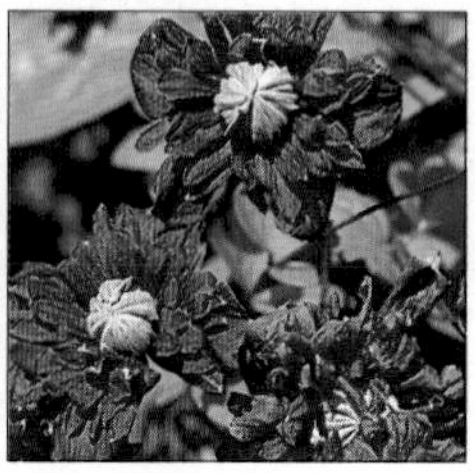
Clematis viticella 'Purpurea Plena Elegans'

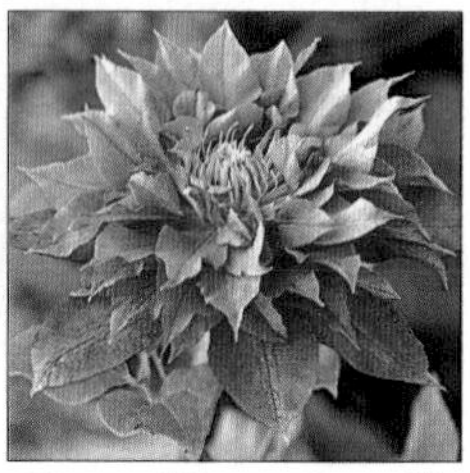
Clematis 'Vyvyan Pennell'

***C.* 'Pink Champagne'** see *C.* 'Kakio'.
***C.* 'Polish Spirit'** 🏆 syn. *C. viticella* 'Polish Spirit'. (Group 3) Late, small-flowered climber with dark green leaves. Saucer-shaped, single, rich purple-blue flowers, 5–8cm (2–3in) across, with red anthers, are freely produced from mid-summer to late autumn. ↕5m (15ft), ↔2m (6ft). ❄❄❄
***C. potaninii* var. *fargesii*.** (Group 3) Late-flowering climber. Saucer-shaped white flowers, 5cm (2in) across, with creamy yellow anthers, either solitary or borne in short cymes, are freely produced from midsummer to early autumn. ↕5m (15ft), ↔1.4m (4½ft). S.W. China. ❄❄❄
***C.* 'Proteus'** ■ (Group 2) Early, large-flowered climber. Double, mauve-pink flowers, 15cm (6in) across, paler towards the centres, with green outer sepals and cream anthers, are produced in early summer. From midsummer, flowers are single and pale mauve. ↕2.5–3m (8–10ft), ↔1m (3ft). ❄❄❄
***C.* 'Purpurea Plena Elegans'** see *C. viticella* 'Purpurea Plena Elegans'.
***C.* 'Ramona'.** (Group 2) Vigorous, early, large-flowered climber. Bears single, pale blue flowers, 10–15cm (4–6in) across, with dark red anthers, from midsummer to autumn. Prefers full sun. ↕3m (10ft), ↔1m (3ft). ❄❄❄
C. recta ■ (Group 3) Late-flowering, clump-forming, herbaceous perennial with grey-green foliage. Terminal panicles of small, star-shaped, heavily scented white flowers, 2cm (¾in) across, with cream anthers, are produced from midsummer to autumn, followed by attractive seed heads. Needs support. ↕1–2m (3–6ft), ↔75cm (30in). C. and S. Europe. ❄❄❄. **'Purpurea'** has purple young foliage.
C. rehderiana ■🏆 (Group 3) Vigorous, late-flowering climber producing panicles of tubular, cowslip-scented, single yellow flowers, 2cm (¾in) long, with creamy yellow anthers, from midsummer to late autumn. ↕6–7m (20–22ft), ↔2–3m (6–10ft). W. China. ❄❄❄
***C.* 'Richard Pennell'** ■🏆 (Group 2) Early, large-flowered climber bearing single, rich purple-blue flowers, 10–13cm (4–5in) across, with golden yellow anthers, in early summer. ↕2–3m (6–10ft), ↔1m (3ft). ❄❄❄
***C.* 'Rouge Cardinal'** ■ (Group 3) Late, large-flowered climber bearing single, glowing velvet-crimson flowers, 10cm (4in) across, with reddish brown anthers, in midsummer. Prefers full sun. ↕2–3m (6–10ft), ↔1m (3ft). ❄❄❄
***C.* 'Royalty'** 🏆 (Group 2) Compact, early, large-flowered climber. Bears semi-double, purple-mauve flowers, 10cm (4in) across, with yellow anthers, in early summer, followed by smaller, single flowers from midsummer to autumn. ↕2m (6ft), ↔1m (3ft). ❄❄❄
***C.* 'Royal Velvet'.** (Group 2) Compact, free-flowering, early, large-flowered climber. In early and midsummer, produces single flowers, 10–15cm (4–6in) across, with bluish, rich velvet-purple sepals, with darker central bands, and red anthers. ↕2–2.5m (6–8ft), ↔1m (3ft). ❄❄❄
***C.* 'Silver Moon'** ■🏆 (Group 2) Very compact, early, large-flowered climber. In early summer, produces single flowers, 10–15cm (4–6in) across, with overlapping, silver-mauve sepals and cream anthers. ↕2m (6ft), ↔1m (3ft). ❄❄❄
***C.* 'Snow Queen'.** (Group 2) Early, large-flowered climber. Single flowers, 15–18cm (6–7in) across, with pointed white sepals, tinged bluish pink, and red anthers, are borne in early summer. Late-summer flowers have hints of pink. ↕2.5m (8ft), ↔1m (3ft). ❄❄❄
***C. stans*.** (Group 3) Late-flowering, woody-based climber or herbaceous perennial. From late summer to mid-autumn, produces clusters of tubular, pale blue flowers, 3cm (1¼in) long, with cream anthers. ↕↔70cm (28in). Japan. ❄❄❄
***C.* 'Star of India'** 🏆 (Group 3) Vigorous, late, large-flowered climber. Deep purple-blue flowers, 8–10cm (3–4in) across, with deep carmine-red central bands and light brown anthers, are produced in midsummer. ↕3m (10ft), ↔1m (3ft). ❄❄❄
***C.* 'Summer Snow'** see *C.* x *fargesioides* 'Paul Farges'.
***C.* 'Sunset'.** (Group 3) Late, large-flowered climber bearing single, bright

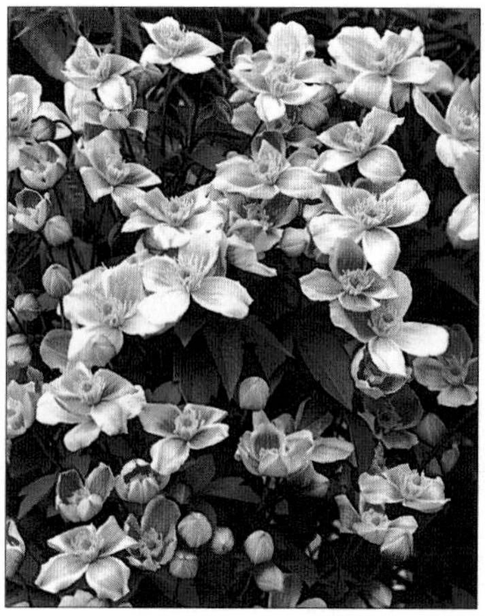
Clematis montana var. *rubens*

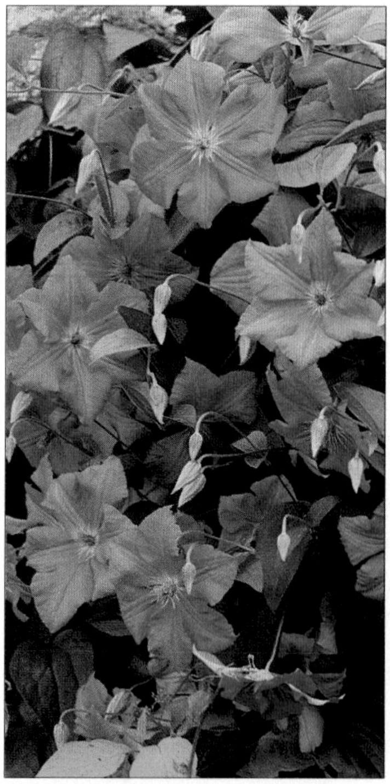
Clematis 'Perle d'Azur'

C

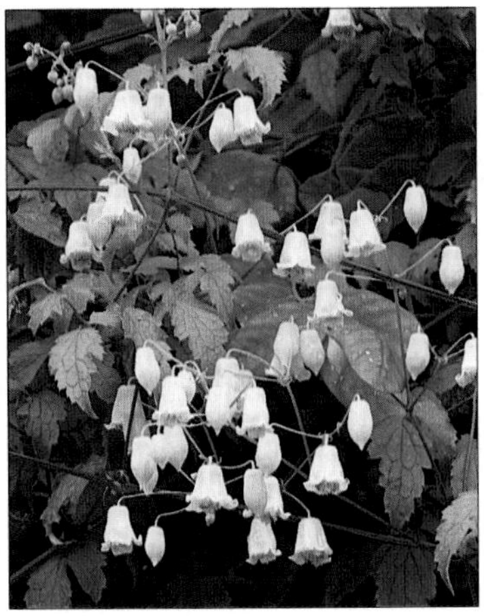

Clematis rehderiana

red flowers, 10–12cm (4–5in) across, with yellow anthers, in midsummer. ↕ 2.5m (8ft), ↔ 1m (3ft). ✻✻✻

***C.* 'Sylvia Denny'.** (Group 2) Early, large-flowered climber. Bears semi-double white flowers, 10cm (4in) across, with white anthers, in early summer. In late summer, flowers are single and 8cm (3in) across. ↕ 2.5m (8ft), ↔ 1m (3ft). ✻✻✻

C. tangutica ▣ (Group 3) Vigorous, late-flowering climber. Abundant, solitary, bell-shaped yellow flowers, 4cm (1½in) long, are produced from midsummer to late autumn, followed by fluffy seed heads. ↕ 5–6m (15–20ft), ↔ 2–3m (6–10ft). W. China. ✻✻✻

C. terniflora, syn. *C. dioscoreifolia*, *C. maximowicziana*, *C. paniculata*. (Group 3) Deciduous or semi-evergreen, late-flowering climber with deep green leaves, sometimes with silver central bands. Numerous star-shaped white flowers, 2–3cm (¾–1¼in) across, are borne in panicles from late summer to autumn, followed by attractive seed heads. Prefers full sun. ↕ 5–6m (15–20ft), ↔ 2–3m (6–10ft). Japan. ✻✻✻

C. texensis. (Group 3) Late-flowering climber. In summer, bears solitary, bell-shaped, reddish orange or scarlet flowers, 2–2.5cm (¾–1in) across, with thick sepals. ↕ 2m (6ft), ↔ 50cm (20in). USA. ✻✻✻. Many of the cultivars ascribed to *C. texensis* are of hybrid origin, and are listed here under their cultivar names. **'Duchess of Albany'** see *C.* 'Duchess of Albany'. **'Etoile Rose'** see *C.* 'Etoile Rose'. **'Gravetye Beauty'** see *C.* 'Gravetye Beauty'.

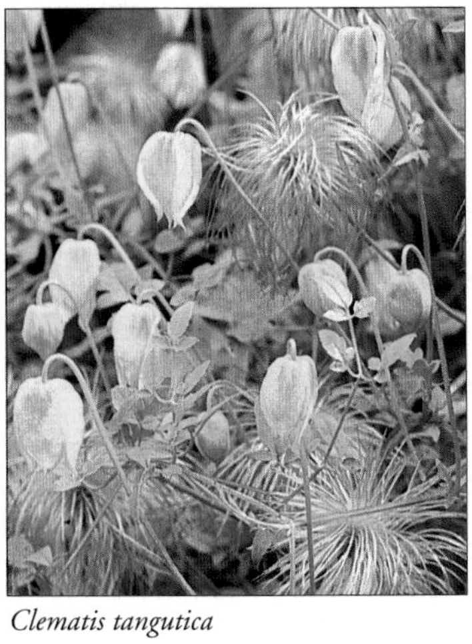

Clematis tangutica

***C.* 'The President'** ▣ ♀ (Group 2) Free-flowering, early, large-flowered climber bearing single, rich purple flowers, 10–15cm (4–6in) across, with silver undersides and red anthers, in early summer. ↕ 2–3m (6–10ft), ↔ 1m (3ft). ✻✻✻

***C. tibetana* subsp. *vernayi* 'Orange Peel'** ♀ syn. *C. orientalis* 'Orange Peel'. (Group 3) Vigorous, late, small-flowered climber. Bell-shaped, nodding flowers, 4cm (1½in) long, each with 4 thick yellow sepals and a dark centre, are produced from midsummer. Flowers are followed by attractive seed heads from late summer to winter. Often confused with other selections from the original collection in the wild. ↕ 6m (20ft), ↔ 2m (6ft). ✻✻✻

***C.* 'Venosa Violacea'** ▣ ♀ syn. *C. viticella* 'Venosa Violacea'. (Group 3) Late, small-flowered climber. Single, saucer-shaped, purple-veined white flowers, 8cm (3in) across, with boat-shaped sepals and bluish black anthers, are produced from midsummer to late autumn. ↕ 3m (10ft), ↔ 1m (3ft). ✻✻✻

***C.* 'Veronica's Choice'.** (Group 2) Early, large-flowered climber bearing semi-double, pale lavender-blue and mauve flowers, 10–15cm (4–6in) across, with cream anthers, in early summer. Later flowers are single. ↕ 2.5m (8ft), ↔ 1m (3ft). ✻✻✻

***C.* 'Victoria'.** (Group 3) Vigorous, late, large-flowered climber producing single, pinkish mauve flowers, 10cm (4in) across, with 4–6 sepals and light greenish brown anthers, in midsummer. ↕ 3m (10ft), ↔ 1m (3ft). ✻✻✻

***C.* 'Ville de Lyon'** ▣ (Group 3) Late, large-flowered climber. In midsummer, produces bright carmine-red flowers, 10–13cm (4–5in) across, with deeper-coloured sepal margins and yellow anthers. Best grown through an evergreen shrub, as lower foliage becomes scorched by late summer. ↕ 2–3m (6–10ft), ↔ 1m (3ft). ✻✻✻

***C.* 'Vino'.** (Group 2) Early, large-flowered climber. Single, purple-red flowers, 15cm (6in) across, with overlapping sepals and yellow anthers, are produced in early summer. ↕ 2–3m (6–10ft), ↔ 1m (3ft). ✻✻✻

C. viticella. (Group 3) Late, small-flowered, semi-woody climber. Solitary, open bell-shaped, blue, purple, or rose-red flowers, 4cm (1½in) across, with pale yellow anthers, are produced from midsummer to early autumn. ↕ 2–4m (6–12ft), ↔ 1.5m (5ft). Central S. Europe. ✻✻✻. Many of the cultivars ascribed to *C. viticella* are of hybrid origin, and are listed here under their cultivar names. **'Abundance'** see *C.* 'Abundance'. **'Alba Luxurians'** see *C.* 'Alba Luxurians'. **'Betty Corning'** see *C.* 'Betty Corning'. **'Etoile Violette'** see *C.* 'Etoile Violette'. **'Minuet'** see *C.* 'Minuet'. **'Mme Julia Correvon'** see *C.* 'Mme Julia Correvon'. **'Polish Spirit'** see *C.* 'Polish Spirit'. **'Purpurea Plena Elegans'** ▣ ♀ syn. *C.* 'Purpurea Plena Elegans', bears abundant double flowers, 5–8cm (2–3in) across, with many purplish mauve sepals, occasionally green outer sepals, and no anthers, from midsummer to late autumn; ↕ 3m (10ft), ↔ 1m (3ft). **'Venosa Violacea'** see *C.* 'Venosa Violacea'.

***C.* 'Vyvyan Pennell'** ▣ ♀ (Group 2) Early, large-flowered climber. In early summer, bears double lilac flowers, 10–13cm (4–5in) across, with central, lavender-blue rosettes, golden yellow anthers, and occasionally green outer sepals. Midsummer flowers are blue-mauve. ↕ 2–3m (6–10ft), ↔ 1m (3ft). ✻✻✻

***C.* 'Wada's Primrose'.** (Group 2) Early, large-flowered climber bearing single, creamy white flowers, 10–13cm (4–5in) across, with yellow anthers, in early summer. Fades in full sun. ↕ 2–2.5m (6–8ft), ↔ 1m (3ft). ✻✻✻

***C.* 'Warsaw Nike'** see *C.* 'Warszawska Nike'.

***C.* 'Warszawska Nike'**, syn. *C.* 'Warsaw Nike'. (Group 3) Late, large-flowered climber, freely producing rich velvet-purple flowers, 10cm (4in) across, with yellow anthers, in midsummer. ↕ 2–3m (6–10ft), ↔ 1m (3ft). ✻✻✻

***C.* 'W.E. Gladstone'.** (Group 2) Vigorous, early, large-flowered climber. Single, light blue flowers, 20cm (8in) across, with overlapping sepals and reddish brown anthers, are produced in mid- and late summer. ↕ 3m (10ft), ↔ 1m (3ft). ✻✻✻

***C.* 'White Swan'** see *C. macropetala* 'White Swan'.

***C.* 'Will Goodwin'** ♀ (Group 2) Early, large-flowered climber with a long flowering period. Bears single, pale blue flowers, 15cm (6in) across, with yellow anthers, from early to late summer. ↕ 3m (10ft), ↔ 1m (3ft). ✻✻✻

***C.* 'William Kennett'.** (Group 2) Early, large-flowered climber. Bears single, pale lavender-blue flowers, 10–12cm (4–5in) across, with dark red anthers, in early summer. Each sepal has a darker central band that fades as the flower matures. ↕ 2–3m (6–10ft), ↔ 1m (3ft). ✻✻✻

***C.* 'Xerxes'** see *C.* 'Elsa Späth'.

▷**Clematis, Alpine** see *Clematis alpina*
▷**Clementine** see *Citrus reticulata*

CLEOME

Spider flower

CAPPARIDACEAE

Genus of 150 species of bushy annuals and evergreen shrubs from sandy, free-draining soils on plains and in mountain valleys in tropical and subtropical zones worldwide. Only the annuals are commonly cultivated; they are valued for their terminal racemes of spider-like, 4-petalled flowers, with prominent stamens, which are borne above 3- to 7-palmate leaves. Grow in a summer flower border or as a seasonal filler for a mixed or herbaceous border. Flowers for cutting in summer may also be grown in a cool greenhouse.

- **HARDINESS** Half hardy to frost tender.
- **CULTIVATION** Under glass, grow in loam-based potting compost (JI No.2) in full light. In the growing season, water freely and apply a balanced liquid fertilizer every 3–4 weeks. Outdoors, grow in light, fertile, preferably sandy, free-draining soil in full sun. Dead-head to prolong flowering and water freely in dry weather.
- **PROPAGATION** Sow seed at 18°C (64°F) in spring. Harden off before planting when danger of frost has passed.
- **PESTS AND DISEASES** Aphids may infest young plants. Susceptible to whiteflies under glass.

C

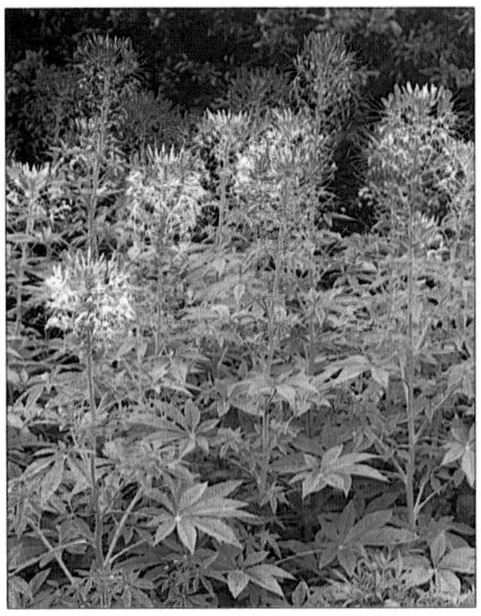

Cleome hassleriana 'Colour Fountain'

C. hassleriana, syn. *C. pungens* of gardens, *C. spinosa* of gardens (Spider plant). Erect annual with hairy stems and 5- to 7-palmate, minutely toothed, glandular-hairy leaves, to 12cm (5in) long, with ovate to lance-shaped leaflets and spines at the base of each leaf-stalk. Strongly scented, white to pink or purple flowers, to 3cm (1¼in) across, with oblong to rounded petals, are produced in dense, terminal racemes in summer. ↕ to 1.5m (5ft), ↔ to 45cm (18in). S. Brazil, Paraguay, Argentina, Uruguay. ❀ (min. 4°C/39°F). **'Colour Fountain'** ▣ has delicate, narrow-petalled, scented, pink, violet-pink, rose-red, or white flowers, to 10cm (4in) across; ↕ to 1.2m (4ft).

***C. pungens* of gardens** see *C. hassleriana*.

***C. spinosa* of gardens** see *C. hassleriana*.

CLERODENDRUM

VERBENACEAE

Genus of about 400 species of deciduous and evergreen trees, shrubs, and climbers, mainly found in woodland in tropical and subtropical regions, particularly in Africa and Asia. They are cultivated for their terminal or axillary cymes, panicles, or corymbs of showy, usually salverform, often fragrant flowers with cylindrical tubes and protruding stamens. The leaves are arranged in whorls or opposite pairs. The shrubs are suitable for a warm border. Train the climbers over a trellis, pergola, or other support. In frost-prone areas, grow half-hardy and frost-tender species in a warm greenhouse or conservatory.

- **HARDINESS** Fully hardy to frost tender.
- **CULTIVATION** Under glass, grow in a border or in large tubs of loam-based potting compost (JI No.3) in full light, with shade from hot sun and good ventilation in summer. In growth, water freely and apply a balanced liquid fertilizer monthly; water sparingly in winter. Outdoors, grow in fertile, humus-rich, moist but well-drained soil in full sun. Pruning group 11 for climbers (immediately after flowering); group 1 for deciduous shrubs or trees; group 9 for evergreen shrubs; group 6 for *C. bungei*. Shrubs under glass may need restrictive pruning.
- **PROPAGATION** Sow seed at 13–18°C (55–64°F) in spring. Remove suckers from shrubs or trees in autumn or

C

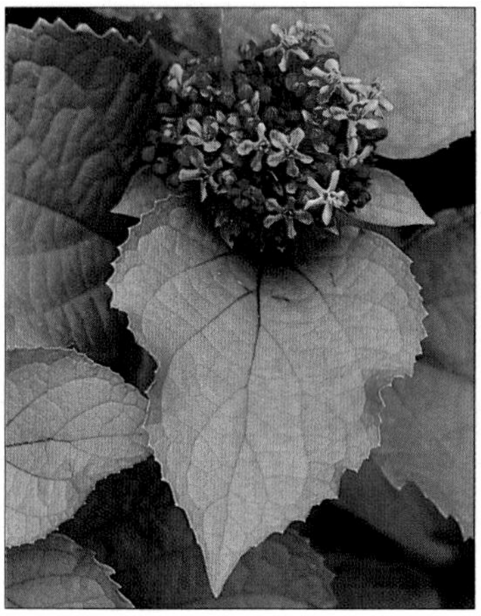
Clerodendrum bungei

spring. Root semi-ripe cuttings with bottom heat in summer. Insert root cuttings in winter.

• **PESTS AND DISEASES** Mealybugs, red spider mites, and whiteflies may be troublesome under glass.

C. bungei ■ 🏆 (Glory flower). Deciduous, suckering shrub producing upright shoots and opposite, ovate, toothed, dark green leaves, to 20cm (8in) long, tinged with purple when young. Salverform, very fragrant, dark pink flowers, each with 5 spreading lobes, are borne in rounded, terminal panicles, 12–15cm (5–6in) across, from late summer to autumn. ↕↔ 2m (6ft) or more. China. ❄❄

C. fallax see *C. speciosissimum.*

***C. fragrans* 'Pleniflorum'** see *C. philippinum.*

***C. myricoides* 'Ugandense'** see *C. ugandense.*

C. paniculatum (Pagoda flower). Erect, open, evergreen shrub bearing opposite, ovate, 5-lobed, deep green leaves, 10–15cm (4–6in) long, with heart-shaped bases; the upper leaves are toothed or entire. Salverform, long-tubed scarlet flowers are produced in terminal panicles, to 30cm (12in) long, from summer to autumn. ↕ 1–1.3m (3–4½ft), ↔ 60–90cm (24–36in). S.E. Asia. ❀ (min. 10–13°C/50–55°F)

C. philippinum, syn. *C. fragrans* 'Pleniflorum' (Glory bower). Erect, evergreen shrub with angular, downy stems and opposite, broadly ovate, toothed, mid- to deep green leaves, to 25cm (10in) long. Terminal corymbs, 7–10cm (3–4in) across, of many

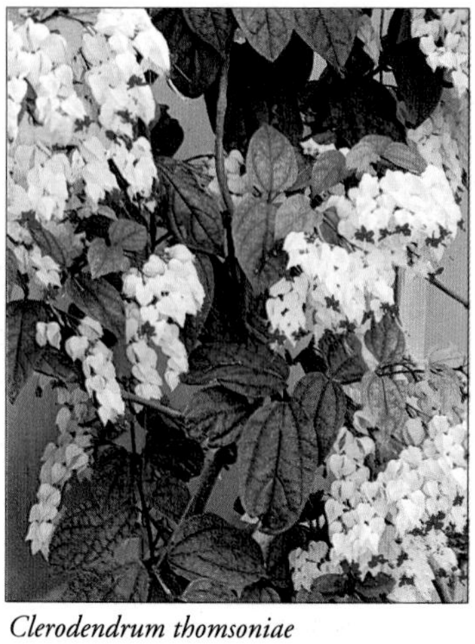
Clerodendrum thomsoniae

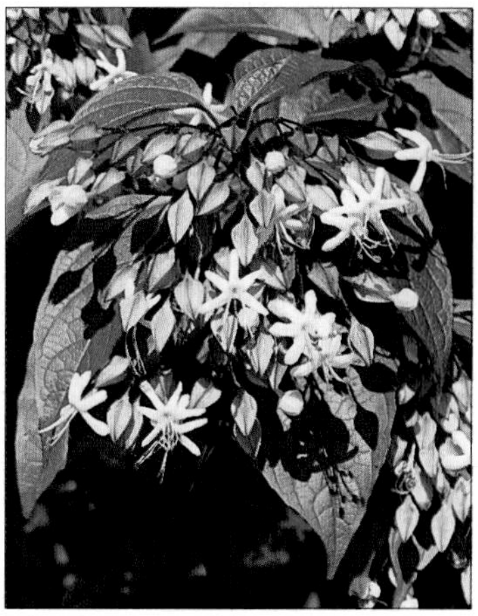
Clerodendrum trichotomum

fragrant, salverform, double, pink or white flowers, sometimes blue-tinted, are produced in summer. ↕ 2–3m (6–10ft), ↔ 1.5–2.5m (5–8ft). S. China. ❀ (min. 10–13°C/50–55°F)

C. speciosissimum, syn. *C. fallax* (Glory bower, Java glorybean). Erect, open, evergreen shrub with opposite, heart-shaped, corrugated, toothed, rich green leaves, to 30cm (12in) long. Bears tiered, terminal panicles, 20–30cm (8–12in) long, of salverform, bright scarlet flowers from summer to autumn. Bean-like fruit are dark blue. ↕ 1–4m (3–12ft), ↔ 1–2m (3–6ft). Indonesia (Java). ❀ (min. 10–13°C/50–55°F)

C. splendens 🏆 Twining, evergreen climber with opposite, ovate to elliptic, entire, more or less glossy, rich green leaves, to 18cm (7in) long. Salverform, bright scarlet flowers are produced in dense, terminal panicles, 10–13cm (4–5in) long, mainly in summer. ↕ 3m (10ft) or more. Tropical W. Africa. ❀ (min. 10–13°C/50–55°F)

C. thomsoniae ■ 🏆 (Glory bower). Twining, evergreen climber with opposite, ovate, entire, rich green leaves, to 17cm (7in) long. Terminal and axillary panicles, 10cm (4in) across, of flowers with bell-shaped, pure white calyces and rich crimson petals are produced freely in summer. ↕ to 4m (12ft). Tropical W. Africa. ❀ (min. 10–13°C/50–55°F)

C. trichotomum ■ ⚠ Upright, bushy, deciduous shrub or small tree with opposite, ovate, entire or sparsely toothed, dark green leaves, to 20cm (8in) long. From late summer to mid-autumn, bears salverform, fragrant white flowers with red sepals in erect, axillary cymes, to 20cm (8in) across; berries are bright blue. ↕↔ 5–6m (15–20ft). China, Japan. ❄❄❄. **var. *fargesii*** has bronze young leaves, and flowers with green sepals; China.

C. ugandense ■ syn. *C. myricoides* 'Ugandense' (Blue glory bower). Scandent, evergreen climber with opposite, elliptic to narrowly obovate, boldly toothed, bright green leaves, 7–10cm (3–4in) long. Bears terminal panicles, 10–15cm (4–6in) long, of 5-petalled, blue to violet, sometimes blue and white flowers, each with long lower lips, from summer to autumn. ↕ 3–4m (10–12ft). Tropical Africa. ❀ (min. 10°C/50°F)

CLETHRA

Summer-sweet, Sweet pepper bush, White alder

CLETHRACEAE

Genus of more than 60 species of deciduous and evergreen trees and shrubs, occurring in woodland, swamps, and rocky places in E. Asia and North America, with one species (*C. arborea*) from Madeira. The leaves are alternate, simple, obovate to oblong, rarely lance-shaped, finely to coarsely toothed, and mid- to dark green. Clethras are grown for their fragrant, bell- to cup-shaped, white or yellowish white flowers, borne in racemes or panicles, and are suitable for a woodland garden. In frost-prone areas, grow *C. arborea* in a cool greenhouse or conservatory; it may be moved outdoors during summer.

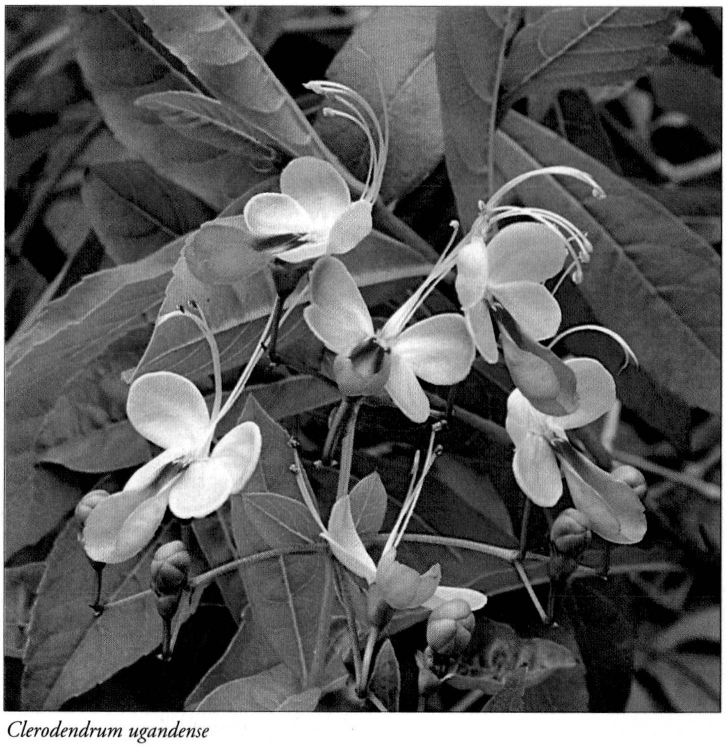
Clerodendrum ugandense

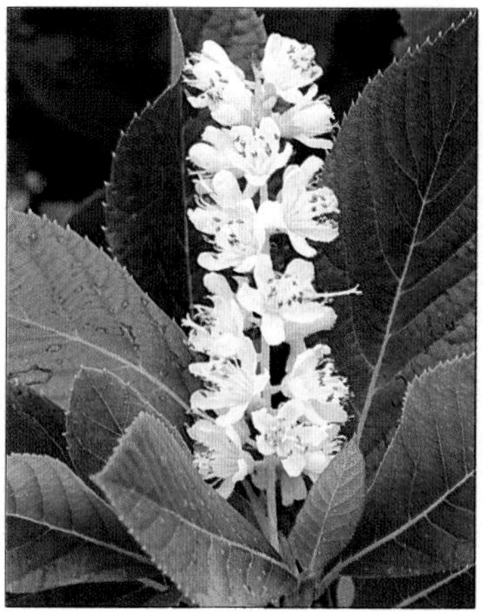
Clethra alnifolia

• **HARDINESS** Fully hardy to half hardy.

• **CULTIVATION** Under glass, grow in lime-free (ericaceous) potting compost in bright filtered light. In growth, water freely and apply a balanced liquid fertilizer monthly; water sparingly in winter. Outdoors, grow in acid, fertile, humus-rich, moist but well-drained soil in partial or dappled shade. Pruning group 1 for deciduous species. For *C. alnifolia* remove some of the old wood from the base in winter, leaving the strongest suckers as replacement growth. Pruning group 9 for *C. arborea*; needs restrictive pruning under glass.

• **PROPAGATION** Sow seed at 6–12°C (43–54°F) in spring or autumn, or sow seed of hardy species in containers outdoors in spring or autumn. Root greenwood cuttings of deciduous species in early summer and semi-ripe cuttings of evergreens in mid- or late summer.

• **PESTS AND DISEASES** Trouble free.

C. alnifolia ■ (Sweet pepper bush). Upright, suckering, deciduous shrub with oval, mid-green leaves, to 10cm (4in) long. In late summer and early autumn, bears bell-shaped, fragrant white flowers, to 1cm (½in) across, in dense, upright, terminal racemes, to 15cm (6in) long. ↕↔ 2.5m (8ft). E. USA. ❄❄❄. **'Paniculata'** 🏆 syn. *C. paniculata*, bears abundant white flowers in broad panicles, to 10cm (4in) across.

C. arborea ■ ⚠ (Lily of the valley tree). Broadly conical, evergreen shrub or tree with red young shoots and oval, dark green leaves, to 15cm (6in) long. Cup-shaped, very fragrant white flowers, to 8mm (⅜in) across, are produced in lax,

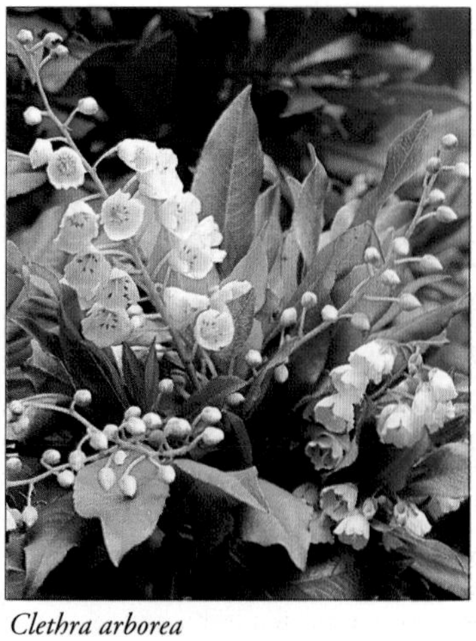
Clethra arborea

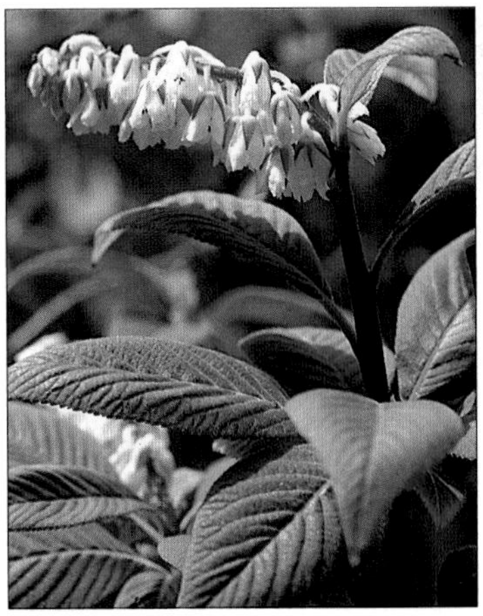

Clethra delavayi

terminal racemes, to 15cm (6in) long, from late summer to mid-autumn. ↕ 8m (25ft), ↔ 6m (20ft). Madeira. ✲
C. barbinervis 🏆 Upright, deciduous shrub with peeling bark when mature, and obovate-elliptic, dark green leaves, to 12cm (5in) long, turning red and yellow in autumn. Bell-shaped white flowers, to 8mm (3/8in) across, are produced in arching, terminal racemes, to 15cm (6in) long, from late summer to autumn. ↕↔ 3m (10ft). E. China to Japan. ✲✲✲
C. delavayi ▣ 🏆 Upright, deciduous shrub with arching shoots and lance-shaped, rich blue-green leaves, to 15cm (6in) long. Nodding, cup-shaped white flowers, 1.5cm (½in) across, produced in dense, terminal racemes, to 25cm (10in) long, open from pink buds in midsummer. ↕↔ 4m (12ft). W. China. ✲✲
C. fargesii. Upright, deciduous shrub with peeling bark on old stems, and slenderly tapered, ovate to lance-shaped, dark green leaves, to 12cm (5in) long, turning red and yellow in autumn. Produces cup-shaped white flowers, 6mm (¼in) across, in arching, terminal racemes, to 25cm (10in) long, from late summer to autumn. ↕↔ 3m (10ft). W. China. ✲✲✲
C. paniculata see *C. alnifolia* 'Paniculata'.

CLEYERA

THEACEAE

Genus of about 17 species of evergreen and deciduous trees and shrubs found in woodland from the Himalayas to Japan, and from Mexico to Central America. They have alternate, leathery, usually linear to ovate-oblong, mid- to dark green leaves. *Cleyera* species and cultivars are grown for their attractive foliage and bowl-shaped, pale yellow to creamy white flowers, which may be borne singly or in clusters from the leaf axils of the previous year's wood. Suitable for a warm, sheltered shrub border or for growing against a wall. In frost-prone areas, grow *C. japonica* 'Tricolor' in a cool greenhouse.

• **HARDINESS** Frost hardy to half hardy.
• **CULTIVATION** Under glass, grow in lime-free (ericaceous) potting compost in full light, with shade from hot sun. In growth, water freely and apply a balanced liquid fertilizer monthly; water sparingly in winter. Outdoors, grow in acid, moderately fertile, humus-rich, moist but well-drained soil in sun or partial shade, sheltered from cold, dry winds. Pruning group 8; may need restrictive pruning under glass.
• **PROPAGATION** Root semi-ripe cuttings in summer.
• **PESTS AND DISEASES** Susceptible to red spider mites and mealybugs under glass.

C. fortunei 'Variegata' see *C. japonica* 'Tricolor'.
C. japonica. Bushy, evergreen shrub with narrowly oblong to ovate-oblong, glossy, dark green leaves, to 10cm (4in) long. Bowl-shaped, fragrant, creamy white flowers, 1.5cm (½in) across, are produced singly or in threes from the leaf axils in summer, occasionally followed in autumn by small red fruit, 6–9mm (¼–3/8in) across, ripening to black. ↕↔ 3m (10ft). Burma, China, Korea, Japan. ✲✲. **'Tricolor'**, syn. *C. fortunei* 'Variegata', has young leaves tinged with pink, maturing to green with creamy white margins; ↕↔ 2m (6ft); ✲

CLIANTHUS

LEGUMINOSAE/PAPILIONACEAE

Genus of 2 species of evergreen, trailing or climbing shrubs or subshrubs found in semi-desert or warm-temperate scrub or woodland in Australia and New Zealand. They have alternate, pinnate, mid- to dark green leaves and showy flowers resembling lobsters' claws. In frost-prone climates, *C. formosus* is excellent for a hanging basket in a temperate greenhouse or conservatory; in warmer areas, grow in a raised bed or terrace planting. *C. puniceus* is suitable for training against a wall; in frost-prone areas, it needs the protection of a cool greenhouse or conservatory.

• **HARDINESS** Frost hardy to frost tender.
• **CULTIVATION** Under glass, grow in loam-based potting compost (JI No.3), with additional grit, in full light. In the growing season, provide moderate humidity, water freely (avoiding the foliage), and apply a balanced liquid fertilizer monthly; water sparingly and maintain low humidity in winter. Outdoors, grow in well-drained soil in full sun with shelter from cold, drying winds. If cut back by frost, *C. puniceus* often sprouts from the base in spring; provide a deep, dry winter mulch. Generally best with little pruning. *C. formosus* requires no regular pruning (except trimming). Pruning group 11

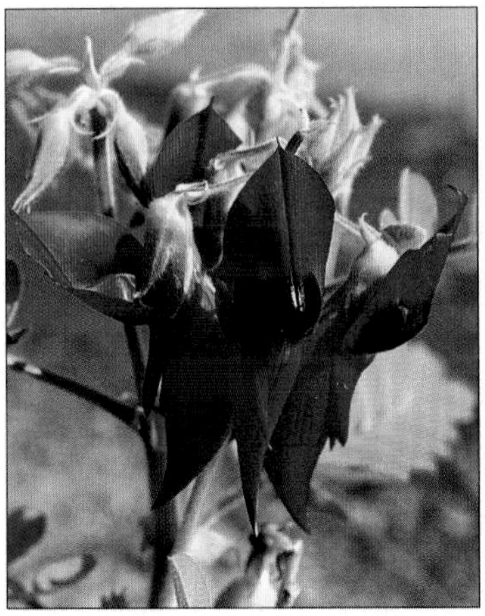

Clianthus formosus

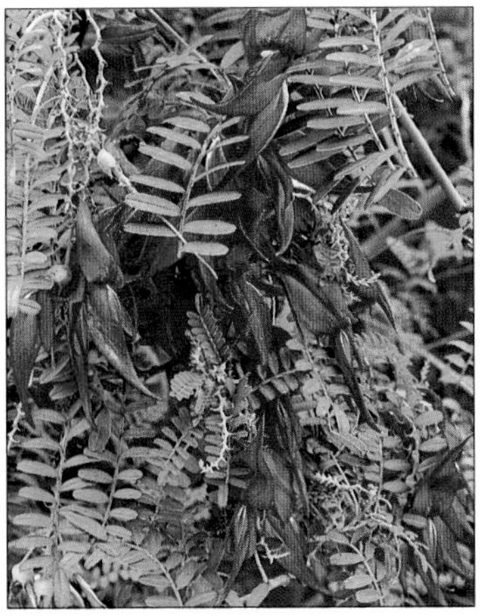

Clianthus puniceus

(or 13 if wall grown) for *C. puniceus* and cultivars, immediately after flowering; cut back flowered shoots by no more than one-third their length.
• **PROPAGATION** Sow seed at 13–18°C (55–64°F) in spring. Root semi-ripe cuttings of *C. puniceus* in summer. For hanging baskets, *C. formosus* is best grafted on to *Colutea arborescens* seedling rootstock in spring; on its own roots, it is very sensitive to overwatering.
• **PESTS AND DISEASES** Trouble free.

C. dampieri see *C. formosus*.
C. formosus ▣ syn. *C. dampieri* (Glory pea, Sturt's desert pea). Prostrate annual or short-lived perennial subshrub with densely silky-grey and downy leaves, 12–17cm (5–7in) long, with 9–21 oval leaflets. In summer, bears elongated, lobsterclaw-like, brilliant crimson and black flowers, 5–8cm (2–3in) long, in racemes 7–12cm (3–5in) long. ↕ to 20cm (8in), ↔ 1m (3ft) or more. N. Australia. ❀ (min. 7–10°C/45–50°F)
C. puniceus ▣ 🏆 (Glory pea, Lobster claw, Parrot's bill). Evergreen shrub with climbing shoots and dark green leaves, to 15cm (6in) long, with 13–25 narrowly oblong leaflets. From spring to early summer, bears lobsterclaw-like, brilliant red flowers, to 7cm (3in) long, in pendent racemes, to 15cm (6in) long. ↕ 4m (12ft), ↔ 3m (10ft). New Zealand (North Island). ✲✲. **f. albus** ▣ 🏆 has white flowers often flushed green. **f. albus 'White Heron'** bears abundant pure white flowers. **'Flamingo'** see 'Roseus'. **'Red Cardinal'** has brilliant scarlet flowers. **'Roseus'**, syn. 'Flamingo', has dark rose-pink flowers.

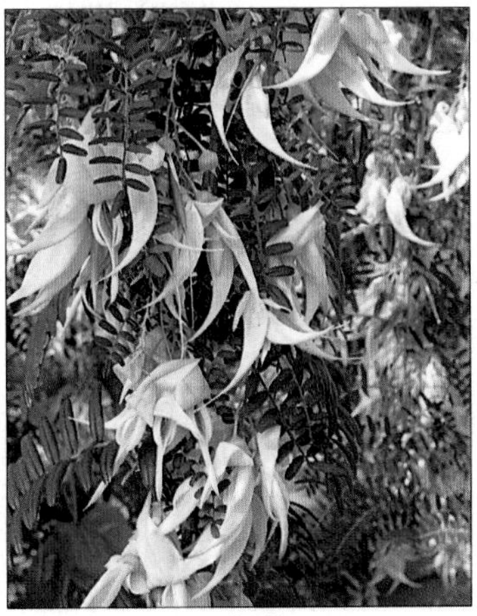

Clianthus puniceus f. *albus*

▷**Cliffbush** see *Jamesia americana*
▷**Climbers** see pp.36–37
▷***Clinopodium acinos*** see *Acinos arvensis*
▷***Clinopodium grandiflorum*** see *Calamintha grandiflora*

CLINTONIA

CONVALLARIACEAE/LILIACEAE

Genus of 5 species of rhizomatous herbaceous perennials from woodland in the Himalayas, E. Asia, and North America. They have basal clumps of elliptic to broadly ovate, entire, glossy, pale to mid-green leaves. Bell- to star-shaped flowers are borne on upright stems in racemes or umbels, or occasionally singly; they are followed by spherical, fleshy berries. Grow in a woodland garden.

• **HARDINESS** Fully hardy.
• **CULTIVATION** Grow in leafy, fertile, humus-rich, moist, neutral to acid soil in partial or full shade. Mulch with leaf mould or garden compost in spring.
• **PROPAGATION** Sow seed in containers of loamless seed compost in a cold frame in autumn. Divide in spring; plants may be slow to re-establish.
• **PESTS AND DISEASES** Slugs and snails may attack young growth.

C. alpina see *C. udensis*.
C. andrewsiana ▣ Clump-forming perennial with elliptic to broadly ovate, hairy-margined, glossy, rich green leaves, to 25cm (10in) long. In early summer, bears bell-shaped, pink-purple flowers, 2–2.5cm (¾–1in) long, in terminal umbels, sometimes with secondary umbels beneath, followed by deep blue berries. ↕ to 60cm (24in), ↔ to 25cm (10in). USA (California). ✲✲✲
C. borealis (Corn lily). Clump-forming perennial with inversely lance-shaped to obovate, glossy, pale green leaves, 10–30cm (4–12in) long, fringed with minute hairs. Bears loose, terminal umbels of nodding, bell-shaped, greenish yellow flowers, 1–2cm (½–¾in) long, in late spring and early summer, followed by blue or white berries. ↕ to 30cm (12in), ↔ to 20cm (8in). E. North America. ✲✲✲
C. udensis, syn. *C. alpina*. Clump-forming perennial with inversely lance-shaped to obovate or oblong, hairy-margined, glossy, mid-green leaves, 8–35cm (3–14in) long. In summer, bears bell-shaped, white, yellow-green,

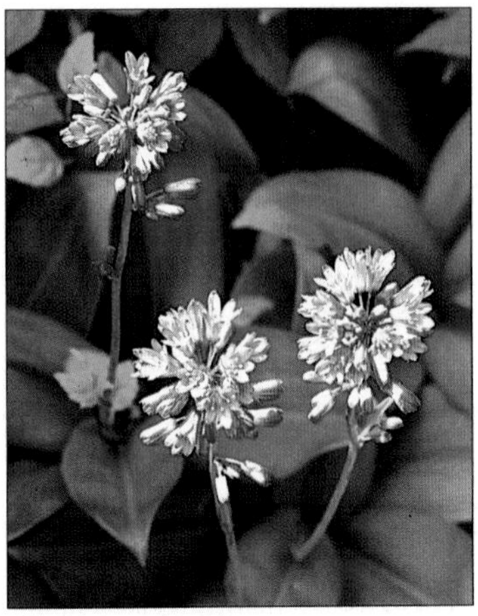

Clintonia andrewsiana

C

or pale lilac flowers, to 1cm (½in) long, in lax, terminal, umbel-like racemes, followed by deep blue-purple berries. ↕ to 30cm (12in), ↔ to 20cm (8in). Russia (Siberia), E. Himalayas, Japan. ❄❄❄

C. uniflora (Bride's bonnet, Queencup). Spreading perennial with inversely lance-shaped to obovate, glossy, mid-green leaves, 7–15cm (3–6in) long, hairy beneath. Erect, star-shaped, pure white flowers, to 2.5cm (1in) across, are produced singly in the upper leaf axils in late spring, followed by blue-black berries. ↕ 20cm (8in), ↔ 15cm (6in). W. North America. ❄❄❄

CLITORIA

LEGUMINOSAE / PAPILIONACEAE

Genus of 70 species of mainly evergreen perennials, shrubs, and climbers found in forest margins, thickets, and scrub in tropical regions. The leaves are alternate and pinnate or 3-palmate. Pea-like flowers, with incurved, keeled petals, are borne singly or in racemes from the leaf axils. Where temperatures fall below 16°C (61°F), grow in a warm greenhouse or conservatory; in warmer areas, grow on a trellis or through a vigorous tree or shrub.

- **HARDINESS** Frost tender.
- **CULTIVATION** Under glass, grow in loam-based potting compost (JI No.3) in full light. In the growing season, water moderately and apply a balanced liquid fertilizer monthly; water sparingly in winter. Pot on or top-dress in spring. Outdoors, grow in fertile, moist but well-drained, loamy soil in full sun. Provide support for climbers. Pruning group 11, in spring.
- **PROPAGATION** Sow seed at 19–24°C (66–75°F) in spring.
- **PESTS AND DISEASES** Susceptible to red spider mites and whiteflies under glass.

C. ternatea (Blue pea). Slender, trailing or scandent, evergreen climber, sometimes a short-lived perennial but often treated as an annual or biennial. Pinnate leaves, 6–12cm (2½–5in) long, each have 5–9 elliptic to ovate, rich green leaflets. Clear blue flowers, 3–5cm (1¼–2in) across, with yellow-tinted white centres, are produced singly or in pairs, from summer to autumn. ↕ to 3m (10ft), ↔ 2m (6ft) as a trailer. Tropical Asia. ❄ (min. 16°C/61°F)

CLIVIA

AMARYLLIDACEAE

Genus of 4 species of evergreen perennials from low-lying woodland, often by streams, in South Africa. They have swollen, bulb-like bases, and are grown for their erect, narrowly lance-shaped to strap-shaped, dark green, basal leaves and robust, tubular to trumpet-shaped, colourful flowers, borne in umbels on stout stems. In frost-prone areas, grow in a conservatory or warm greenhouse, or as houseplants. In hot climates, grow in a border or bed, or among shrubs. All parts of *C. miniata* may cause mild stomach upset if ingested, and the sap may irritate skin.

- **HARDINESS** Frost tender.
- **CULTIVATION** Under glass, grow in loam-based potting compost (JI No.2), with additional leaf mould and grit, in bright filtered or indirect light. In the growing season, water freely, applying a balanced liquid fertilizer weekly until the flower buds form; water very sparingly in winter. Outdoors, grow in fertile, humus-rich, well-drained soil in partial shade. Clivias resent root disturbance and need a restricted root run to encourage flowering.
- **PROPAGATION** Sow seed at 16–21°C (61–70°F) as soon as ripe. Divide in late winter or early spring.
- **PESTS AND DISEASES** Mealybugs may be troublesome.

C. caulescens. Evergreen perennial with strap-shaped leaves, to 1.8m (6ft) long. Umbels of 15–20 pendent, narrowly funnel-shaped, orange, red, or pinkish red flowers, 4–4.5cm (1½–1¾in) long, are produced from spring to summer. ↕ 50cm (20in), ↔ 30cm (12in). South Africa. ❄ (min. 10°C/50°F)

C. x cyrtanthiflora (*C. miniata* x *C. nobilis*). Evergreen perennial with strap-shaped leaves, 30–60cm (12–24in) long. From summer to autumn, bears umbels of 40–60 semi-pendent, trumpet-shaped, rich salmon-pink to yellowish green flowers, 4–7cm (1½–3in) long. ↕ 30–40cm (12–16in), ↔ 30cm (12in). South Africa. ❄ (min. 10°C/50°F)

C. gardenii. Evergreen perennial with narrowly lance-shaped leaves, 75cm (30in) long. Umbels of 10–20 pendent, narrowly funnel-shaped, often strongly curved, orange or red flowers, 4–6cm (1½–2½in) long, tipped with green, are produced from winter to spring. ↕ 45–75cm (18–30in), ↔ 30cm (12in). South Africa. ❄ (min. 10°C/50°F)

C. miniata ■ 🏆 Evergreen perennial with strap-shaped leaves, to 60cm (24in) long. Bears large umbels of up to 20 semi-pendent, open tubular to funnel-shaped, yellow, red, or orange flowers, 5–7cm (2–3in) long, from spring to summer. ↕ 45cm (18in), ↔ 30cm (12in). South Africa. ❄ (min. 10°C/50°F). **'Aurea'** 🏆 has yellow flowers.

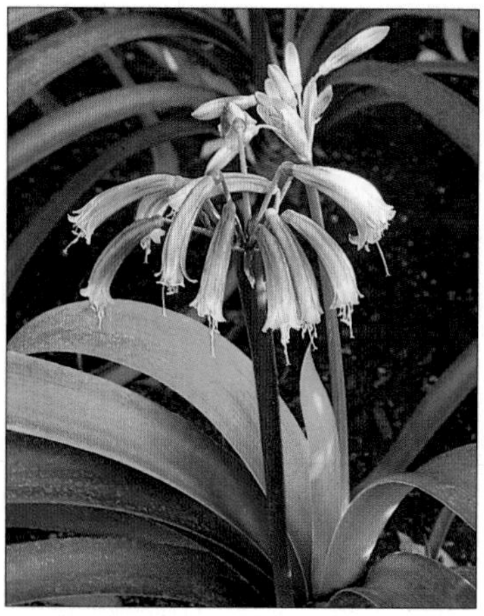

Clivia nobilis

C. nobilis ■ Evergreen perennial with strap-shaped leaves, 45cm (18in) long. Umbels of 40–60 semi-pendent, narrowly trumpet-shaped, red and yellow flowers, 2.5–4cm (1–1½in) long, tipped with green, are produced in spring and summer. ↕ 40cm (16in), ↔ 30cm (12in). South Africa. ❄ (min. 10°C/50°F)

▷ **Clock vine,**
Bengal see *Thunbergia grandiflora*
Bush see *Thunbergia erecta*
▷ **Clove** see *Syzygium aromaticum*
▷ **Clover** see *Trifolium*
Bush see *Lespedeza*
Crimson see *Trifolium incarnatum*
Dutch see *Trifolium repens*
Hairy canary see *Lotus hirsutus*
Italian see *Trifolium incarnatum*
Lucky see *Oxalis tetraphylla*
Water see *Marsilea, M. quadrifolia*
White see *Trifolium repens*
▷ **Club, Golden** see *Orontium*
▷ **Club moss** see *Lycopodium*
▷ **Club-rush** see *Schoenoplectus lacustris* subsp. *tabernaemontani* 'Zebrinus'
Round-headed see *Scirpoides holoschoenus*

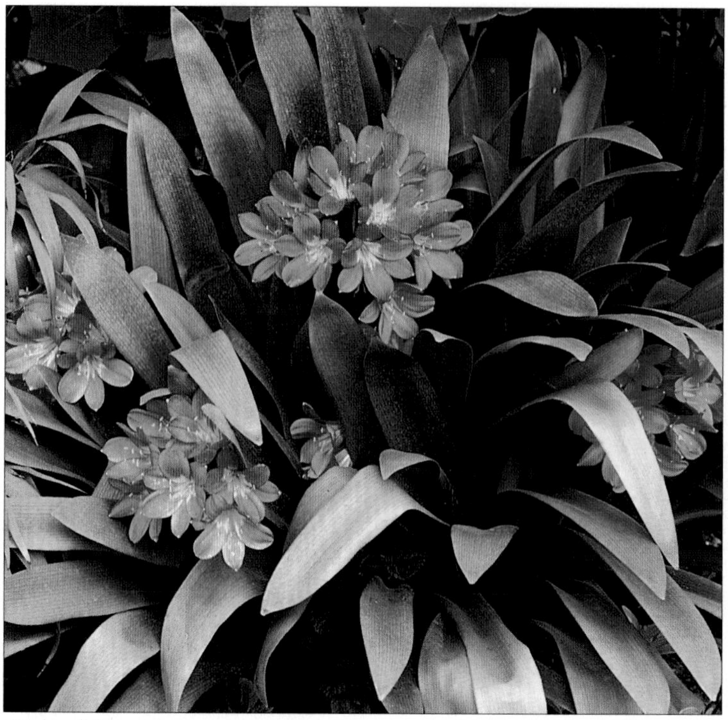

Clivia miniata

CLUSIA

GUTTIFERAE / HYPERICACEAE

Genus of about 145 species of evergreen trees and shrubs, some of which are epiphytic, found in forest from Florida, USA, to Mexico, the West Indies, and tropical South America. They are grown for their simple, leathery leaves, borne in opposite pairs, and for their 4- to 9-petalled, magnolia-like flowers, borne singly or in terminal clusters. In frost-prone areas, grow as foliage houseplants, or in a warm or temperate greenhouse. In humid tropical climates, they are suitable for a coastal garden, a shrub border, or for specimen planting.

- **HARDINESS** Frost tender.
- **CULTIVATION** Under glass, grow in loam-based potting compost (JI No.2), with additional sharp sand, in bright filtered light, with high humidity. From early summer to autumn, water freely and apply a balanced liquid fertilizer monthly; water moderately in winter. Top-dress or pot on in spring. Outdoors, grow in fertile, moist but well-drained soil in partial shade. Pruning group 1; tolerates restrictive pruning under glass.
- **PROPAGATION** Sow seed at 19–24°C (66–75°F) in spring. Root softwood cuttings with bottom heat in summer. Air layer in spring or summer.
- **PESTS AND DISEASES** Trouble free.

C. major ○ syn. *C. rosea* (Autograph tree, Balsam apple). Open, semi-epiphytic shrub or small tree with short-stalked, obovate, glossy, deep green leaves, 8–18cm (3–7in) long. Produces funnel-shaped, pink or creamy white flowers, 5–8cm (2–3in) across, in clusters of 1–3 in summer. ↕ 2–3m (6–10ft), ↔ 1–2m (3–6ft). Central to South America, W. Indies. ❄ (min. 16–18°C/61–64°F)

C. rosea see *C. major.*

CLYTOSTOMA

BIGNONIACEAE

Genus of 9 species of evergreen, perennial climbers found in forest in tropical North and South America. The mid- to dark green leaves, borne in opposite pairs, are composed of 2 (in rare cases, 3) leaflets and a tendril. They are cultivated for their foxglove-shaped flowers, produced in pairs or clusters from the leaf axils. In frost-prone areas, grow in a temperate or warm greenhouse. In warmer areas, grow as ground cover, or use to clothe a pergola, arbour, sunny wall, or tree.

- **HARDINESS** Frost tender.
- **CULTIVATION** Under glass, grow in a border or in large containers of loam-based potting compost (JI No.3), with added leaf mould and sharp sand; provide full light, with shade from hot sun, and moderate humidity. In growth, water freely and apply a balanced liquid fertilizer monthly; water moderately in winter. Top-dress or pot on in late winter or spring. Outdoors, grow in fertile, moist but well-drained soil in partial shade or full sun with some midday shade. Provide support for the climbing stems. Pruning group 11 after flowering; group 12 under glass, in early spring or after flowering.

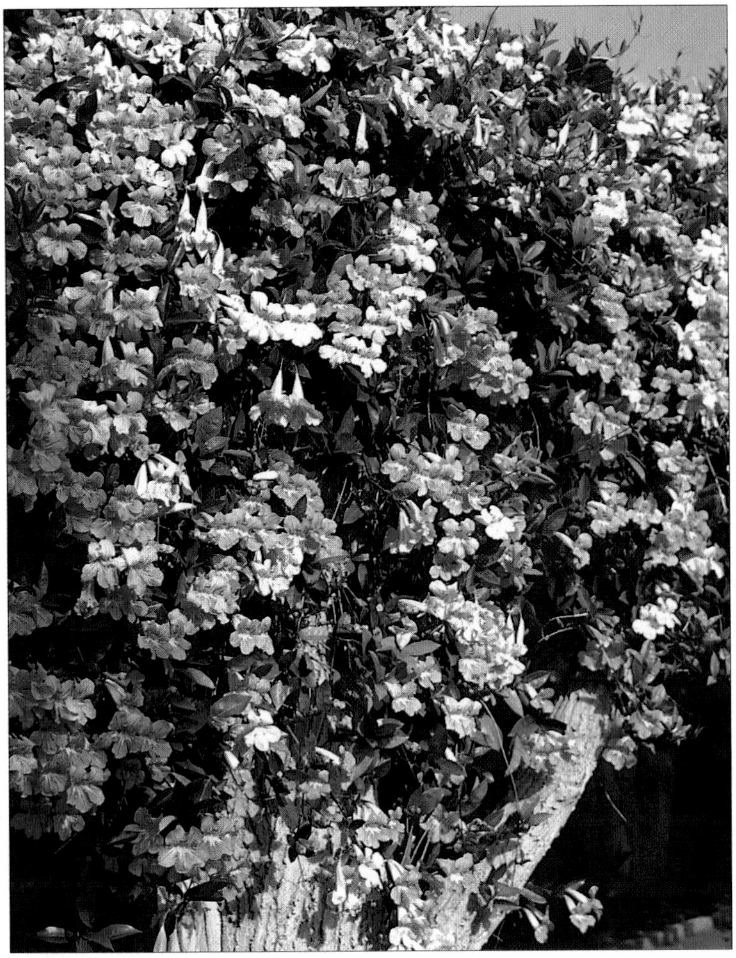

Clytostoma callistegioides

• **PROPAGATION** Sow seed at 13–18°C (55–64°F) in spring. Root short-jointed, lateral shoots in summer.
• **PESTS AND DISEASES** Red spider mites, whiteflies, and mealybugs may be a problem under glass.

C. callistegioides ▣ syn. *Pandorea lindleyana.* Vigorous, open climber, with oblong-elliptic, lustrous, deep green leaves, 8–10cm (3–4in) long, composed of 2 opposite leaflets and a tendril for climbing. Two-lipped purple flowers, 7cm (3in) long, with lilac-veined, often pale yellow tubes, are borne in summer. ↕ to 10m (30ft). S. Brazil to Argentina. ❀ (min. 7–10°C/45–50°F)

COBAEA

POLEMONIACEAE

Genus of about 20 species of woody, evergreen and herbaceous climbers found in forest and thickets from Mexico to tropical South America. They have alternate, pinnate leaves, each with a terminal, branched tendril. Large, 5-lobed, bell-shaped flowers are produced singly from the upper leaf axils. In frost-prone areas, grow in a cool greenhouse or conservatory, or outside as annuals. In warmer areas, use to clothe a pergola, arbour, sunny wall, or tree.
• **HARDINESS** Frost tender; *C. scandens* survives short periods near 0°C (32°F).
• **CULTIVATION** Under glass, grow in loam-based potting compost (JI No.2) in full light. In the growing season, water freely and apply a low-nitrogen liquid fertilizer monthly; water sparingly in winter. Top-dress or pot on in spring. Provide support. Outdoors, grow in moderately fertile, moist but well-drained soil in a sheltered site in full sun. Pruning group 11, after flowering or in late winter or early spring.
• **PROPAGATION** Sow seed at 18°C (64°F) in spring; plant out when danger of frost has passed. Root softwood cuttings with bottom heat in summer.
• **PESTS AND DISEASES** Susceptible to red spider mites under glass.

C. scandens ▣ (Cathedral bell, Cup and saucer plant). Vigorous, erect, dense, semi-woody, evergreen, perennial climber, grown as an annual. Each leaf, to 11cm (4½in) long, has 4 oblong-elliptic, rich green leaflets, 2 basal stipules, and a large, branched tendril with many tiny hooks. From summer to autumn, bears fragrant flowers, 5cm (2in) long, opening creamy green and ageing to purple. ↕ 10–20m (30–70ft). Mexico. ❀ (min. 5°C/41°F). **f. *alba*** has white flowers, ageing to creamy white.

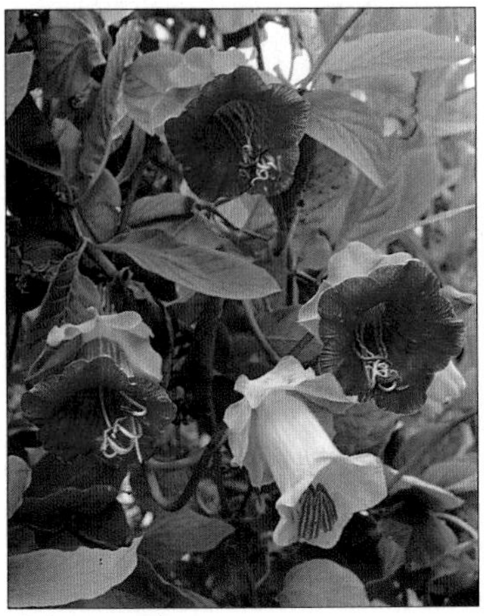

Cobaea scandens

COCCOTHRINAX

Thatch palm

ARECACEAE/PALMAE

Genus of 30–50 species of usually single-stemmed (rarely cluster-stemmed) palms occurring in dunes, scrub, and pine forest in Florida, USA, and the Caribbean. The 3-petalled flowers (with the petals and sepals fused into small, 6-pointed, star-like discs) are produced in panicles among terminal clusters of stalked, fan-shaped leaves, which have many slender, radiating lobes. In frost-prone climates, grow in a warm or temperate greenhouse, or as houseplants. Elsewhere, grow as specimen trees.
• **HARDINESS** Frost tender.
• **CULTIVATION** Under glass, grow in loam-based potting compost (JI No.3) in full light, with shade from hot sun. In the growing season, water freely, and apply a balanced liquid fertilizer monthly; water sparingly in winter. Pot on or top-dress in spring. Outdoors, grow in neutral to alkaline, fertile, moist but well-drained soil in full sun.
• **PROPAGATION** Sow seed at 24–27°C (75–81°F) in spring.
• **PESTS AND DISEASES** Red spider mites may be a problem under glass.

C. argentata ♈ (Florida silver palm). Single-stemmed palm with an erect grey trunk. Leaf-stalks, to 60cm (24in) long, bear lustrous, yellow-green leaf-blades, silvery white beneath, to 60cm (24in) across. Produces white flowers, 6–10mm (¼–½in) across, in panicles to 3m (10ft) long, in summer. ↕ to 8m (25ft), ↔ 2–3m (6–10ft). USA (Florida), Bahamas. ❀ (min. 13°C/55°F)
C. fragrans ♈ (Silver thatch). Single-stemmed palm with a slender trunk, at first bearing a fibrous webbing of old leaf bases, then smooth. The leaf-blades are light green above and silvery grey beneath, 40–60cm (16–24in) across, and borne on stalks of the same length. Produces fragrant yellow flowers, 6–8mm (¼–⅜in) across, in panicles to 2m (6ft) or more long, in summer. ↕ to 5m (15ft), ↔ 1.5–2.5m (5–8ft). Haiti, E. Cuba. ❀ (min. 13°C/55°F)

▷ ***Cochlearia armoracia*** see *Armoracia rusticana*

COCHLIODA

ORCHIDACEAE

Genus of about 6 species of evergreen, epiphytic orchids found at high altitudes in the Andes of Ecuador and Peru. One or two linear, dark green leaves, to 20cm (8in) long, are borne at the tip of each ovoid to conical pseudobulb. From late spring to summer, attractive, usually large, scarlet or bright pink flowers are borne in tall or short, arching racemes arising from the base of the pseudobulb.
• **HARDINESS** Frost tender.
• **CULTIVATION** Cool-growing orchids. Grow in epiphytic orchid compost in pots or slatted baskets. In summer, provide humid conditions with bright filtered light and good ventilation. Water freely, applying fertilizer at every third watering, and mist once or twice a day. In winter, admit full light and water sparingly. See also p.46.
• **PROPAGATION** Divide when the plant fills the container and "flows" over the sides.
• **PESTS AND DISEASES** Susceptible to red spider mites, aphids, and mealybugs.

C. noezliana. Epiphytic orchid with ovoid, compressed pseudobulbs. Racemes, 15–45cm (6–18in) long, of up to 12 rich scarlet flowers, 3.5cm (1½in) across, are produced in summer. ↕ 12cm (5in), ↔ 25cm (10in). Peru. ❀ (min. 10°C/50°F; max. 24°C/75°F)
C. rosea. Epiphytic orchid with ovoid, compressed pseudobulbs. Bears racemes, 13–40cm (5–16in) long, of up to 12 deep rose-pink flowers, 3.5cm (1½in) across, from spring to summer. ↕ 12cm (5in), ↔ 25cm (10in). Ecuador, Peru. ❀ (min. 10°C/50°F; max. 24°C/75°F)

COCHLOSPERMUM

BIXACEAE

Genus of 12–15 species of deciduous trees and shrubs from dry or seasonally dry forests of tropical Central and South America. They have alternate, palmately lobed or pinnatifid, long-stalked, mid- to dark green leaves, and are grown for their bowl- or cup-shaped, 5-petalled flowers, borne in terminal panicles before the new leaves unfold. In frost-prone areas, grow as foliage plants in a warm greenhouse. In warmer climates, grow as specimen plants.
• **HARDINESS** Frost tender.
• **CULTIVATION** Under glass, grow in loam-based potting compost (JI No.3), with added sharp sand, in full light and with low humidity. In growth, water moderately and apply a balanced liquid fertilizer monthly; keep just moist in winter. Pot on or top-dress in spring. Outdoors, grow in moderately fertile, well-drained soil in full sun. Pruning group 1, when leafless or immediately after flowering; needs restrictive pruning under glass.
• **PROPAGATION** Sow seed at 18–25°C (64–77°F) in spring. Root greenwood cuttings in early summer or semi-ripe cuttings in mid- to late summer, with bottom heat.
• **PESTS AND DISEASES** Red spider mites may be a problem under glass.

C. vitifolium ♀ (Wild cotton). Open, spreading tree with rounded, deeply 5-lobed, occasionally 3- to 7-lobed, rich green leaves, to 30cm (12in) across, with elliptic to narrowly obovate lobes. Cup-shaped, bright yellow flowers, 10–12cm (4–5in) across, with scarlet and orange stamens, are produced in panicles 15–30cm (6–12in) long, from winter to early summer. ↕ 12m (40ft), ↔ 10m (30ft). Mexico to Venezuela. ❀ (min. 15°C/59°F)

▷ **Cockies' tongues** see *Templetonia retusa*
▷ **Cockscomb** see *Celosia*
▷ **Cock's comb** see *Erythrina crista-galli*
▷ **Cockspur thorn** see *Crataegus crus-galli*
▷ **Coco-de-mer** see *Lodoicea*
▷ **Coconut** see *Cocos*
Double see *Lodoicea*

C

C

COCOS
Coconut

ARECACEAE/PALMAE

Genus of one species of single-stemmed palm from coastal tropical regions worldwide, possibly originating from the W. Pacific. Arching, pinnate leaves are borne in terminal heads. The 3-petalled flowers are produced in panicles from the leaf axils, followed by coconuts encased in thick, fibrous husks. In frost-prone areas, grow young specimens of *C. nucifera* as short-lived foliage plants in a warm greenhouse or conservatory, or as houseplants. In warmer areas, grow as a specimen or avenue tree.

• **HARDINESS** Frost tender.

• **CULTIVATION** Under glass, grow in loam-based potting compost (JI No.2) with additional sharp sand and fibrous organic matter, in full or bright filtered light with moderate humidity. In the growing season, water moderately and apply a balanced liquid fertilizer monthly; water sparingly in winter. Pot on or top-dress in spring. Outdoors, grow in fertile, humus-rich, moist but well-drained soil in full sun.

• **PROPAGATION** Sow seed at 27–30°C (81–86°F) in spring.

• **PESTS AND DISEASES** Susceptible to scale insects, mealybugs, and red spider mites under glass.

C. capitata see *Butia capitata*.
C. nucifera 🌴 Large palm with a swollen, tapered base, an often-leaning grey trunk, and pinnate, bright green leaves, 4–6m (12–20ft) long, with many linear leaflets. Small, bowl-shaped, fragrant, cream to yellow flowers are borne at intervals throughout the year, followed by ovoid fruit, each with a green to ochre-yellow or orange-red exterior covering a fibrous brown husk. ↕ 20–30m (70–100ft), ↔ to 12m (40ft). Coastal tropical regions. ❄ (min. 18°C/64°F). **'Nino'** is dwarf and compact, with very narrow, lustrous leaflets; ↕ to 3m (10ft), ↔ 1m (3ft).

▷ **Coco-yam** see *Colocasia esculenta*

CODIAEUM
Croton

EUPHORBIACEAE

Genus of 6 species of evergreen shrubs, trees, and perennials from Malaysia and the larger islands in the E. Pacific, found in open forest, thickets, and scrub. They produce attractive, alternate, linear to broadly ovate, simple or shallowly to deeply lobed, leathery, often variegated leaves. Tiny, star-shaped yellow flowers are produced in axillary racemes intermittently throughout summer. In frost-prone areas, grow in a warm or temperate greenhouse, or as houseplants. In tropical or subtropical climates, grow in a shrub border, a courtyard garden, or as an informal hedge or screen. Contact with the foliage may aggravate skin allergies.

• **HARDINESS** Frost tender.

• **CULTIVATION** Under glass, grow in loam-based potting compost (JI No.3) in full light, with shade from hot sun and high humidity. In growth, mist regularly, water freely, and apply a balanced liquid fertilizer every 2–3

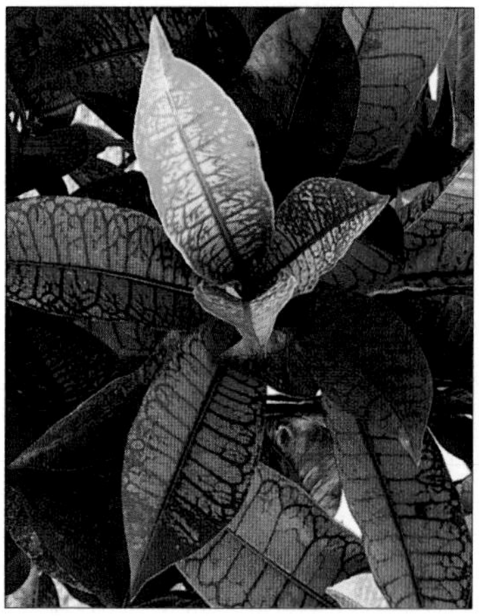

Codiaeum 'Baronne de Rothschild'

weeks; water sparingly with tepid water in winter. Draughts and fluctuating temperatures cause leaf drop. Top-dress or pot on in spring. Outdoors, grow in fertile, humus-rich, moist but well-drained soil in sun or partial shade. Pruning group 9; under glass, cut back leggy plants to within 8–12cm (3–5in) of soil level, and dust wounds with powdered charcoal.

• **PROPAGATION** Root softwood cuttings with bottom heat in summer, dipping the bases in charcoal to stop "bleeding". Air layer in spring.

• **PESTS AND DISEASES** Prone to scale insects and red spider mites under glass.

***C.* 'Baronne de Rothschild'** ▣ Upright, woody-based perennial with ovate or lance-shaped leaves, 20cm (8in) long, green and yellow when young, maturing to rich red. Produces white flowers, 5mm (¼in) across, in summer. Rarely flowers in cultivation. ↕↔ to 1.5m (5ft). ❄ (min. 8°C/46°F)
***C.* 'Flamingo'** ▣ Upright, evergreen shrub or woody-based perennial with ovate leaves, 15–25cm (6–10in) long. Young leaves are mid-green, with cream veins, turning yellow and maturing to red or purple. Produces yellow flowers, 5mm (¼in) across, in summer. Rarely flowers in cultivation. ↕ 1–2m (3–6ft), ↔ to 1m (3ft). ❄ (min. 8°C/46°F)
***C. variegatum* var. *pictum*.** Upright, woody-based perennial with thick, ovate to linear, leathery leaves, to 30cm (12in) long, often deeply lobed, in various colours, usually green and yellow when young, maturing to shades of red. White flowers, 5mm (¼in) across, are borne in summer. ↕ 1–2m (3–6ft), ↔ 0.6–1.5m (2–5ft). ❄ (min. 10–13°C/50–55°F). **'Andreanum'** is compact and bushy, with oval, pointed, copper-flushed leaves, 10–20cm (4–8in) long, with yellow veins and margins, maturing to reddish orange; ↕ to 1m (3ft) or more, ↔ to 60cm (24in). **'Commotion'** has oval, slightly lobed or fiddle-shaped, rich blue- and bright green leaves, 10–20cm (4–8in) long, variegated pink, yellow, and cream, and maturing to crimson; ↔ 60–120cm (24–48in). **'Evening Embers'** is dense and strong-growing, with oval, shallowly lobed, bluish black leaves, 15–25cm (6–10in) long, suffused and dashed red and green, with dark red veins; ↕ 1.5–2m (5–6ft), ↔ 75–150cm (30–60in). **'Imperiale'** is bushy, with elliptic leaves, 8–15cm (3–6in) long, which are almost entirely yellow at first,

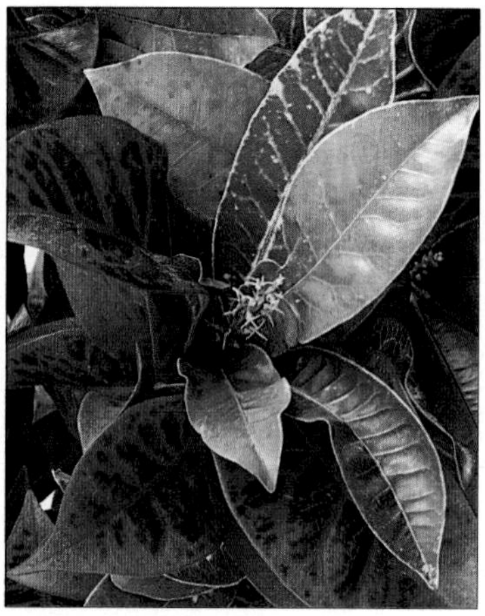

Codiaeum 'Flamingo'

turning orange to red with green midribs; ↕ to 1m (3ft), ↔ to 75cm (30in). **'Majesticum'** has arching to pendent branches and linear, deep to olive-green leaves, to 25cm (10in) long, with yellow midribs, maturing to crimson; ↕↔ 1m (3ft) or more. **'Mrs. Iceton'** has oval, blackish green leaves, 10–15cm (4–6in) long, with yellow markings between the veins, ageing to red and pink. **'Sunrise'** is strong-growing, with narrowly lance-shaped, rich green leaves, 10–20cm (4–8in) long, boldly veined and margined yellow, maturing to orange-red; ↔ 1–1.5m (3–5ft). **'Tortile'** has ribbon-like, spirally twisted, dark green leaves, 15–30cm (6–12in) long, which are variegated with orange-red; ↕↔ to 1m (3ft).

CODONANTHE

GESNERIACEAE

Genus of 13 species of epiphytic, creeping, evergreen shrubs and perennials found on forested hillsides from Mexico to S. Brazil. They have mainly elliptic to ovate or narrowly ovate, usually entire, fleshy leaves borne in opposite, equal- or very unequal-sized pairs. Flowers have curved corolla tubes, with wide yellow, sometimes red-speckled throats broadening to 5 petal lobes of white, pink, or pale or deep purple; they are solitary or borne in axillary cymes, and are followed by spherical, pink, red, or orange fruits. In frost-prone areas, grow in a warm greenhouse, or as houseplants in containers or hanging baskets. In tropical areas, grow epiphytically or beneath shrubs in a shady border.

• **HARDINESS** Frost tender.

• **CULTIVATION** Under glass, grow in loamless potting compost in bright filtered light, with moderate to high humidity. In growth, mist regularly, water freely with soft water, and apply a half-strength balanced liquid fertilizer monthly; water moderately in winter. Outdoors, grow in moist, open, moderately fertile, humus-rich soil in partial shade. Pruning group 11, after flowering. Prune only to restrict size.

• **PROPAGATION** Divide or root stem-tip cuttings at any time of year.

• **PESTS AND DISEASES** Mealybugs may be a problem.

***C. crassifolia*.** Epiphytic perennial with stems that are either prostrate and rooting at the nodes, or pendent. Elliptic to ovate, waxy, mid- to deep green leaves, 5cm (2in) or more long, have red glands beneath. Axillary cymes of 1–4 white flowers, 2–2.5cm (¾–1in) long, with yellow throats and sometimes pink-tinted petal lobes, are borne from spring to summer. ↕ 30cm (12in) or more, ↔ 60cm (24in) or more. Mexico to Brazil. ❄ (min. 15°C/59°F)
C. gracilis ▣ Epiphytic shrub with slender, prostrate or erect stems, bearing narrowly elliptic to ovate, stiffly and often sparsely hairy, mid- to deep green leaves, 2.5–4cm (1–1½in) long. In spring and summer, produces axillary cymes of 1 or 2 red- or maroon-spotted white flowers, 2cm (¾in) long, sometimes yellow at the bases. ↕↔ 30–90cm (12–36in). Brazil. ❄ (min. 15°C/59°F)

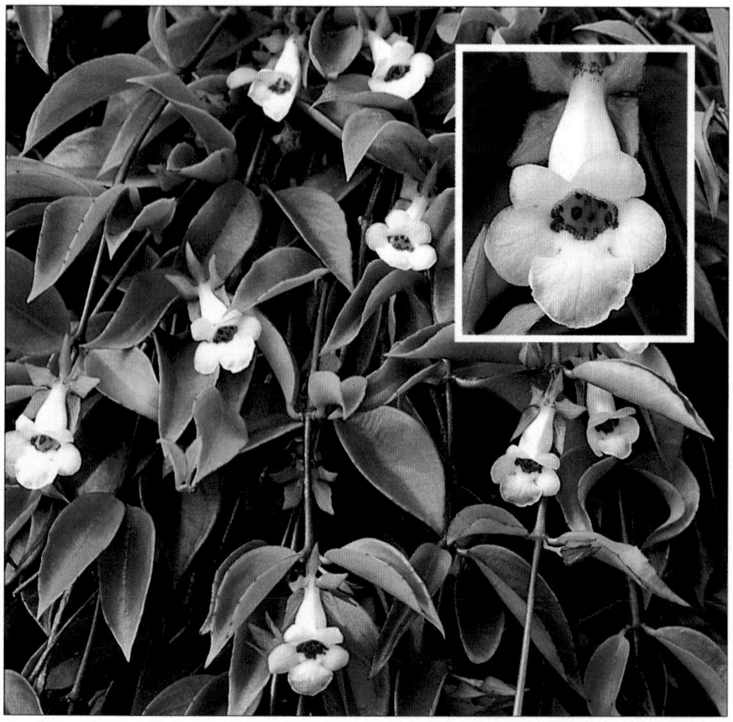

Codonanthe gracilis (inset: flower detail)

CODONOPSIS

CAMPANULACEAE

Genus of about 30 species of scandent or twining, mostly herbaceous perennials found on rocky mountain slopes or in alpine scrub from the Himalayas to Japan. Leaves are opposite or alternate, ovate or oblong to lance-shaped, and often malodorous when crushed. The flowers are usually solitary, terminal or axillary, nodding, and bell- or saucer-shaped, sometimes intricately marked inside. Grow smaller species in a rock garden, larger species in a herbaceous border or woodland garden, and scandent and twining species through small shrubs.

• **HARDINESS** Fully hardy to frost hardy.
• **CULTIVATION** Grow in light, fertile, humus-rich, moist but well-drained soil in sun or partial shade, with shelter from strong winds to protect the slender, brittle shoots. Those of *C. convolvulacea* are easily damaged; in very exposed areas grow in a cold greenhouse. Most species need light, twiggy support. In very cold areas, mulch in winter.
• **PROPAGATION** Sow seed in containers in a cold frame in autumn or spring.
• **PESTS AND DISEASES** Susceptible to attack by slugs and snails. Red spider mites may be a problem under glass.

C. clematidea ▣ Twining, herbaceous perennial climber with branching stems and alternate, narrowly ovate, slender-pointed, grey-green leaves, to 2.5cm (1in) long. Produces solitary, terminal, nodding, bell-shaped, pale greenish blue flowers, 2.5cm (1in) long, with yellow, blue, and black markings inside, in late summer. ↕ to 1.5m (5ft). C. Asia. ❄❄❄
C. convolvulacea ♀ Slender, twining, herbaceous perennial climber bearing opposite, ovate-lance-shaped to lance-shaped, mid-green leaves, 1–5cm (½–2in) long. Solitary, terminal, open bell- to saucer-shaped, violet-blue, occasionally white flowers, 3–5cm (1¼–2in) across, are produced in summer. ↕ to 2m (6ft). Himalayas, W. China. ❄❄❄
C. lanceolata ▣ syn. *C. ussuriensis.* Scandent herbaceous perennial with twining, purple-tinged stems and alternate, elliptic to oblong, mid-green leaves, to 5cm (2in) long. Solitary or paired, axillary, pendent, bell-shaped, mauve-flushed, greenish white flowers, spotted and striped violet inside, are

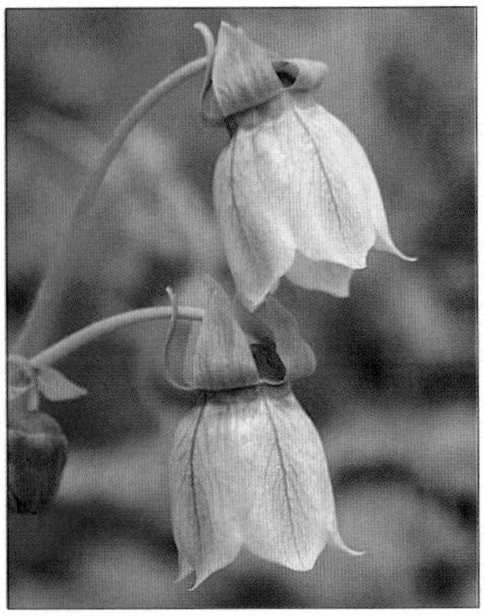

Codonopsis clematidea

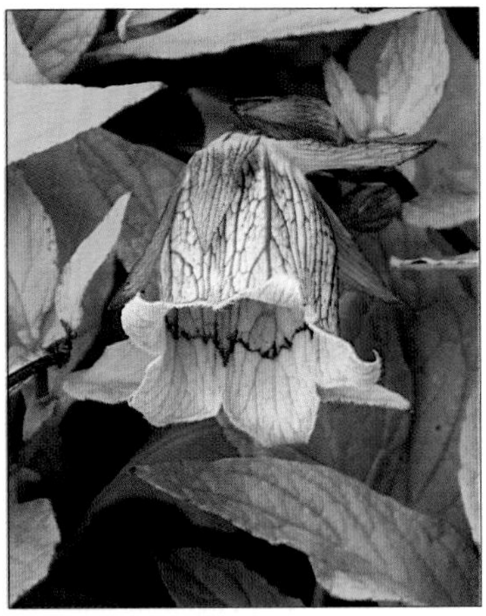

Codonopsis lanceolata

produced in autumn. ↕ 60–90cm (24–36in). China. ❄❄❄
C. meleagris. Upright, scandent herbaceous perennial with ovate, wavy, finely hairy, deep green leaves, 2–8cm (¾–3in) long, usually forming a basal rosette. In summer, branching stems bear solitary, axillary or terminal, nodding, bell-shaped, greenish blue flowers, heavily chequered purple and brown inside, 2.5–4cm (1–1½in) long. ↕↔ to 30cm (12in). China. ❄❄❄
C. ovata. Upright, non-twining herbaceous perennial with fleshy roots and mostly basal, opposite, ovate, very hairy, mid-green leaves, 1–3cm (½–1¼in) long. Solitary, terminal, tubular-bell-shaped, greenish blue flowers, 2.5–3cm (1–1¼in) long, chequered darker blue inside, are borne on slender stalks in mid- and late summer. Needs support. ↕↔ to 30cm (12in). W. Himalayas. ❄❄❄
C. tangshen. Herbaceous perennial climber with twining stems and alternate, broadly lance-shaped, fleshy, toothed, mid-green leaves, 2.5–6cm (1–2½in) long. Solitary, axillary or terminal, bell-shaped, yellow to olive-green flowers, with purple veins and spots inside, are produced in summer. ↕ 2m (6ft). W. China. ❄❄❄
C. ussuriensis see *C. lanceolata.*
C. vinciflora. Twining, herbaceous perennial climber with alternate or opposite, lance-shaped to ovate, thin-textured, mid-green leaves, 1.5–3.5cm (½–1½in) long, glaucous blue beneath. In early and midsummer, bears solitary, saucer-shaped, blue to bluish lilac flowers, 3–4.5cm (1¼–1¾in) across, terminally or on short lateral shoots. ↕ 1m (3ft). China. ❄❄❄

COELIA syn. BOTHRIOCHILUS

ORCHIDACEAE

Genus of 5 species of evergreen, epiphytic, terrestrial, or lithophytic orchids from Mexico to Panama, where they occur at altitudes up to 1,500m (5,000ft). They have short rhizomes and clusters of ovoid or ellipsoid, olive-green pseudobulbs; each produces up to 5 narrowly to broadly lance-shaped, folded, pale to mid-green leaves at the tip. The inflorescence is a short, basal raceme bearing 6 or more tubular-bell-shaped, fleshy, fragrant, cream, ivory-white, or buff flowers, with pink or violet marks.

• **HARDINESS** Frost tender.
• **CULTIVATION** Intermediate-growing orchids. Pot tightly in containers of epiphytic orchid compost. In summer, provide high humidity and bright filtered light, with generous ventilation; water moderately, applying fertilizer at every third watering. In winter, admit full light, and water more sparingly. See also p.46.
• **PROPAGATION** Divide when the plant fills the containers and "flows" over the sides.
• **PESTS AND DISEASES** Susceptible to red spider mites, aphids, and mealybugs.

C. bella, syn. *Bothriochilus bellus.* Epiphytic orchid with spherical to ovoid pseudobulbs, each producing 3 or 4 narrowly lance-shaped, pale green leaves, 45cm (18in) long. In early summer, up to 6 purple-tipped, ivory-white flowers, 2.5cm (1in) across, with lips marked golden orange, are borne in racemes 10–15cm (4–6in) long. ↕↔ 45cm (18in). Mexico, Guatemala, Honduras. ❀ (min. 13°C/55°F; max. 30°C/86°F)

COELOGYNE

ORCHIDACEAE

Genus of more than 100 species of evergreen, epiphytic orchids occurring from lowland forest to high altitudes in mountainous regions from India and S.E. Asia to the Pacific islands. They vary greatly in size, producing pseudobulbs with 2 linear to elliptic, leathery, pleated leaves. Flowers are borne in racemes, mainly from the centre of new growth, usually from spring to summer. Many species are fragrant. *C. cristata* may be grown as a houseplant.

• **HARDINESS** Frost tender.
• **CULTIVATION** Cool- to intermediate-growing orchids. Grow in epiphytic orchid compost in a container or slatted basket. In summer, provide moderate to high humidity, good ventilation, and bright filtered light; water freely, apply fertilizer at every third watering, and mist once or twice daily. In winter, admit full light and keep completely dry. Tropical species, such as *C. dayana* and *C. speciosa*, should be kept moist at a minimum temperature of 15°C (59°F) throughout the year. See also p.46.
• **PROPAGATION** Divide when the plant fills the containers and "flows" over the sides, or remove backbulbs in mid-spring and pot them up separately.
• **PESTS AND DISEASES** Susceptible to red spider mites, aphids, and mealybugs.

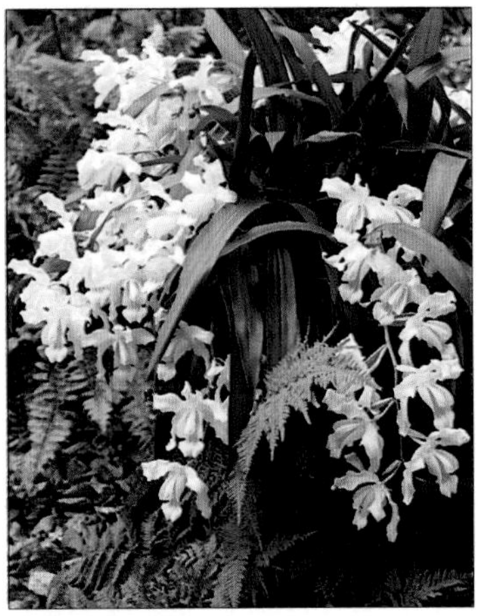

Coelogyne cristata

C. barbata. Epiphytic orchid with conical pseudobulbs and oblong-lance-shaped, semi-rigid leaves, to 45cm (18in) long. In summer, produces a succession of pure white flowers, 5cm (2in) across, with brown and white, fringed lips, in upright racemes. ↕↔ 45cm (18in). Bhutan, N.E. India. ❀ (min. 10°C/50°F; max. 30°C/86°F)
***C.* Burfordiense** (*C. asperata* x *C. pandurata*). Epiphytic orchid with flattened, ribbed pseudobulbs and elliptic-lance-shaped, semi-rigid, folded leaves, 60cm (24in) long. Many apple-green flowers, 10cm (4in) across, with black lacing on the lips, are borne in arching racemes in summer. ↕ 75cm (30in), ↔ 90cm (36in). ❀ (min. 10°C/50°F; max. 30°C/86°F)
C. cristata ▣ Epiphytic orchid with rounded pseudobulbs and lance-shaped leaves, to 30cm (12in) long. Pendent racemes of pure white, strongly fragrant flowers, 8cm (3in) across, with yellow-marked lips, are borne from winter to spring. ↕ 30cm (12in), ↔ 60cm (24in). E. Himalayas. ❀ (min. 10°C/50°F; max. 30°C/86°F)
C. dayana. Epiphytic orchid with conical pseudobulbs and lance-shaped, semi-rigid leaves, to 75cm (30in) long. From winter to spring, bears pendent racemes of many fragrant, pale yellow flowers, 5cm (2in) across, marked dark brown, with white-veined lips. ↕↔ 60cm (24in). Malaysia, Sumatra, Java, Borneo. ❀ (min. 15°C/59°F; max. 30°C/86°F)
C. flaccida ▣ Epiphytic orchid with conical pseudobulbs and lance-shaped, semi-rigid leaves, 20cm (8in) long. Bears racemes of strongly fragrant white flowers, 4cm (1½in) across, marked yellow on the central lobe of each lip and reddish brown on the lateral lobes, from winter to early summer. ↕ 25cm (10in), ↔ 30cm (12in). Himalayas. ❀ (min. 10°C/50°F; max. 30°C/86°F)
C. massangeana. Epiphytic orchid with conical pseudobulbs and elliptic-ovate, semi-rigid leaves, to 45cm (18in) long. From spring to early summer, fragrant,

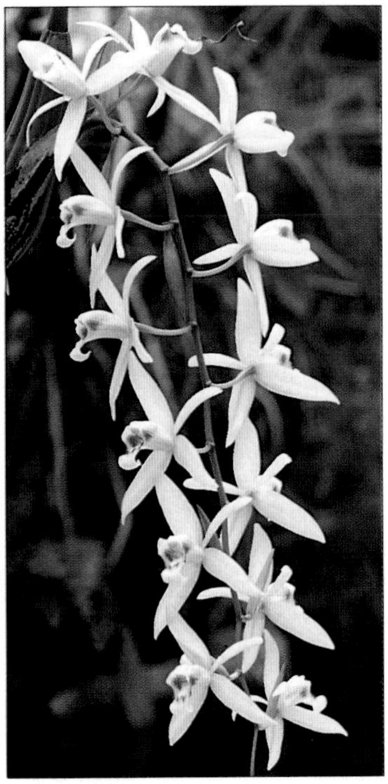

Coelogyne flaccida

C

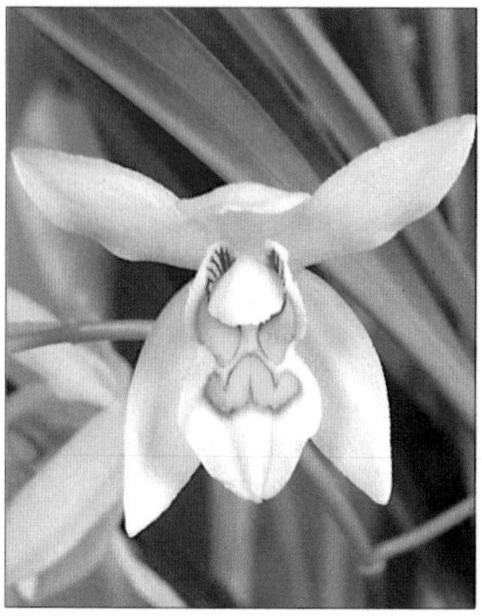

Coelogyne nitida

pale yellow flowers, 5cm (2in) across, with brown and yellow lips, are borne in pendent racemes. ‡↔ 60cm (24in). Malaysia, Sumatra, Java. ❀ (min. 15°C/59°F; max. 30°C/86°F)

C. nitida ▣ 🏆 syn. *C. ochracea.* Epiphytic orchid with oblong, shining pseudobulbs and elliptic-lance-shaped leaves, to 30cm (12in) long. From spring to early summer, bears racemes of strongly fragrant, pure white flowers, 2.5cm (1in) across, with orange and yellow lip markings. ‡ 25cm (10in), ↔ 30cm (12in). W. Himalayas, China, Burma, Thailand, Laos. ❀ (min. 10°C/50°F; max. 30°C/86°F)

C. ochracea see *C. nitida.*

C. pandurata. Epiphytic orchid with flattened, ribbed pseudobulbs and elliptic-lance-shaped, semi-rigid, folded leaves, to 60cm (24in) long. Bears pale green, fragrant flowers, 8cm (3in) or more across, with black lip markings, in long, arching racemes in summer. ‡ 75cm (30in), ↔ 90cm (36in). Malaysia, Borneo, Sumatra. ❀ (min. 15°C/59°F; max. 30°C/86°F)

C. speciosa ▣ Epiphytic orchid with conical pseudobulbs and elliptic or lance-shaped leaves, to 35cm (14in) long. Bears green-yellow to pale salmon-pink flowers, 7cm (3in) across, with reddish brown lips, in pendent racemes at any time of year. ‡ 30cm (12in), ↔ 60cm (24in). Sumatra, Java. ❀ (min. 15°C/59°F; max. 30°C/86°F)

▷ **Coffeeberry** see *Rhamnus californica*
▷ **Coffee tree** see *Polyscias guilfoylei*
Kentucky see *Gymnocladus dioica*
▷ **Cohosh** see *Cimicifuga*

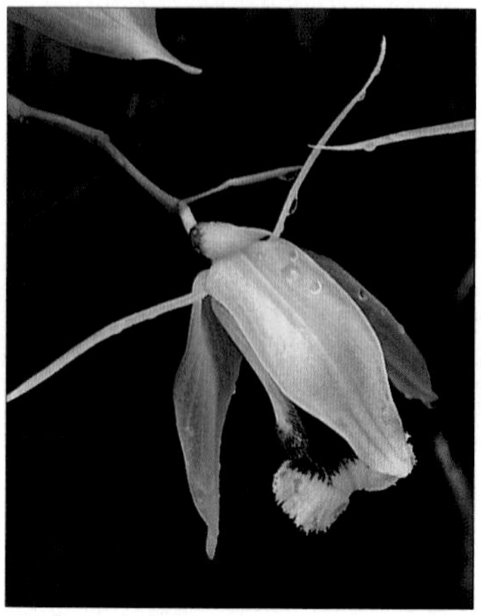

Coelogyne speciosa

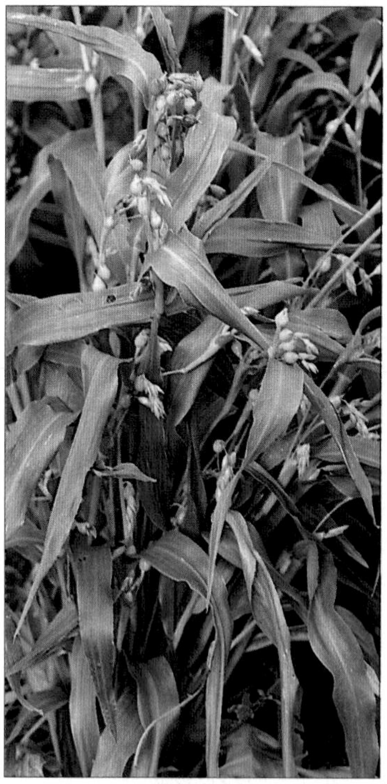

Coix lacryma-jobi

COIX

GRAMINEAE/POACEAE

Genus of about 5 species of monoecious, annual or perennial, often rhizomatous grasses, originating in E. Asia but widely naturalized in tropical regions throughout the world. The leaves are flat and narrowly lance-shaped. *Coix* species produce compound inflorescences, borne in the upper leaf axils, which consist of many racemes of separate male and female spikelets. Female flowers of *C. lacryma-jobi*, the only species commonly cultivated, produce hard, bead-like seeds, which are frequently used in the manufacture of rosaries. The teardrop-like shape of the seeds gives rise to the common names, Christ's or Job's tears. *C. lacryma-jobi* may be grown outdoors in both warm- and cool-temperate climates. It is suitable for an annual border or for infilling in a herbaceous border.

• **HARDINESS** Half hardy.

• **CULTIVATION** Grow in light to medium, fertile, moist but well-drained soil in a sheltered site in full sun. *C. lacryma-jobi* needs a long growing season to ripen fruit.

• **PROPAGATION** Sow seed at 13–16°C (55–61°F) in late winter or early spring, and plant out when danger of frost has passed. In warm areas, sow seed *in situ* in spring.

• **PESTS AND DISEASES** Trouble free.

C. lacryma-jobi ▣ (Christ's tears, Job's tears). Loosely tufted, annual grass with erect stems bearing bright green leaves, to 60cm (2ft) long. In early autumn, produces long-stalked, arching inflorescences with racemes of separate male and female spikelets, the latter giving rise to hard, shiny, ovoid-spherical seeds, to 1.5cm (½in) long, which are green at first, becoming pearly grey-purple when ripe. ‡ 45–90cm (18–36in), ↔ 30cm (12in) or more. S.E. Asia. ✻

COLCHICUM

Autumn crocus, Naked ladies

COLCHICACEAE/LILIACEAE

Genus of about 45 species of cormous perennials from alpine and subalpine meadows and stony hillsides in Europe, N. Africa, W. and C. Asia, N. India, and W. China. The basal, linear, strap-shaped, lance-shaped, or elliptic-ovate leaves, often ribbed or pleated, develop with or after the flowers. Conspicuous, usually goblet-shaped, sometimes fragrant flowers, with perianth tubes 1.5–7cm (½–3in) long, are borne in late summer, autumn, winter, or spring. Many large-flowered colchicums, with attractively tessellated flowers, bloom in autumn, mostly before the large leaves, which emerge from winter to early spring and persist until midsummer.

Grow large-leaved species among deciduous shrubs; *C. autumnale*, *C. speciosum*, and several other robust species may be naturalized in turf. The smaller species are suitable for a rock garden, scree bed, raised bed, or trough. Half-hardy species, and some of those with leaves present at flowering time, are best grown in a bulb frame or alpine house to protect them from excessive summer rainfall. All parts are highly toxic if ingested and, if in contact with skin, may cause irritation.

• **HARDINESS** Fully hardy to half hardy.

• **CULTIVATION** Plant 10cm (4in) deep in summer or early autumn. Colchicums have varying cultivation requirements, which, for ease of reference, may be grouped as follows:

1. Deep, fertile, well-drained soil that is not too dry, in an open site in full sun.

2. Gritty, sharply drained soil in a sunny raised bed or scree bed. In a bulb frame or alpine house, use a mix of equal parts loam, leaf mould, sharp sand, and grit in full light. Apply a low-nitrogen liquid fertilizer at the beginning of the growing season. Water moderately when in growth, avoiding the foliage and flowers; keep completely dry when dormant.

• **PROPAGATION** Sow seed in containers in an open frame as soon as ripe. Separate corms when dormant in summer.

• **PESTS AND DISEASES** Grey mould (*Botrytis*) and slugs may be a problem.

C. agrippinum ▣ 🏆 Cormous perennial, probably a hybrid between *C. autumnale* and *C. variegatum*, with semi-erect, linear-lance-shaped or strap-shaped, slightly wavy leaves, 9–15cm (3½–6in long). In early autumn, produces 1 or 2 narrowly funnel-shaped, heavily tessellated, deep purplish pink flowers with tepals 5cm (2in) long. Cultivation group 1. ‡ 8–10cm (3–4in), ↔ 8cm (3in). Unknown origin. ✻✻✻

C. alpinum. Cormous perennial with semi-erect, strap-shaped to linear-lance-shaped leaves, 8–15cm (3–6in) long. From late summer to autumn, produces 1 or 2 goblet-shaped, pale pink flowers with tepals 1.5–3cm (½–1¼in) long. Cultivation group 1 or 2. ‡ 6cm (2½in), ↔ 8cm (3in). France (including Corsica), Switzerland, Italy (including Sardinia). ✻✻✻

C. atropurpureum. Cormous perennial with erect, strap-shaped to narrowly lance-shaped leaves, 9–19cm (3½–7in) long. In autumn, bears 1–3 cup-shaped flowers, opening white, then turning dark magenta-red, with tepals 3–5cm (1¼–2in) long. Cultivation group 1 or 2. ‡↔ 5cm (2in). Unknown origin, probably Balkans. ✻✻✻

C. autumnale ▣ (Meadow saffron). Vigorous, cormous perennial bearing erect, linear-lance-shaped to broadly lance-shaped leaves, 14–35cm (5½–14in) long. In autumn, produces

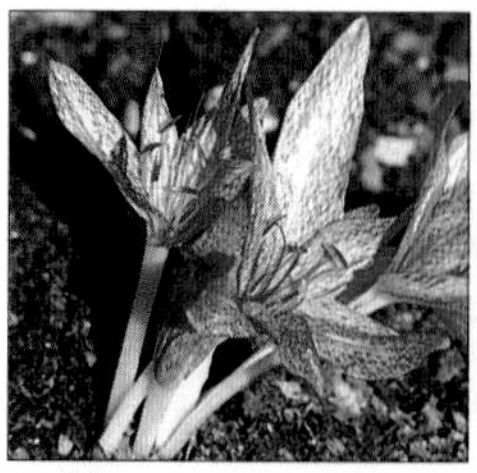

Colchicum agrippinum

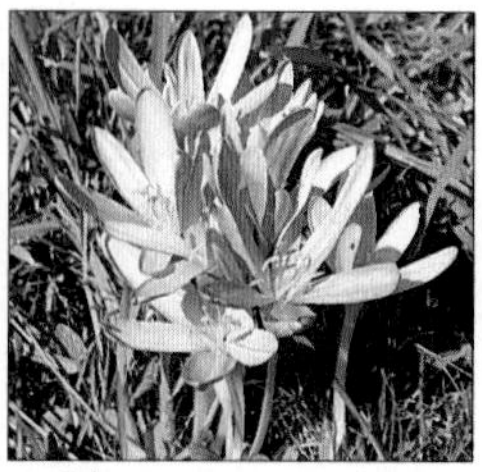

Colchicum autumnale

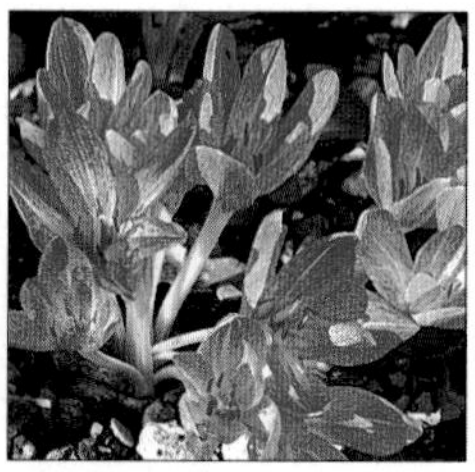

Colchicum bivonae

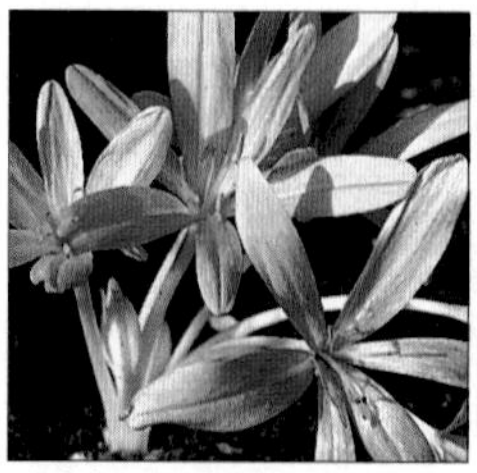

Colchicum byzantinum

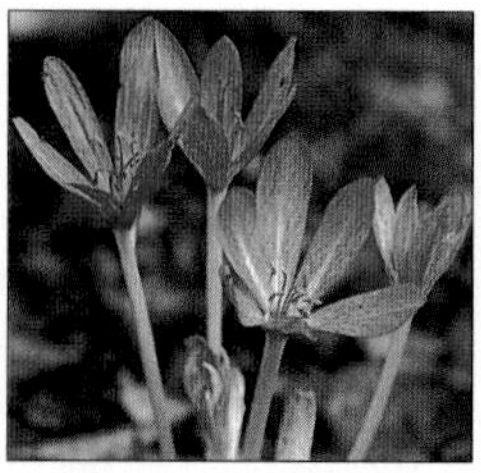

Colchicum cilicicum

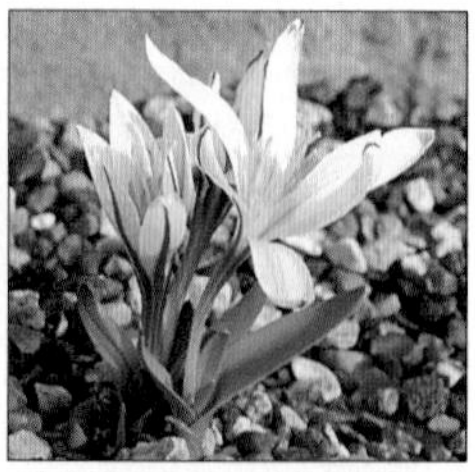

Colchicum kesselringii

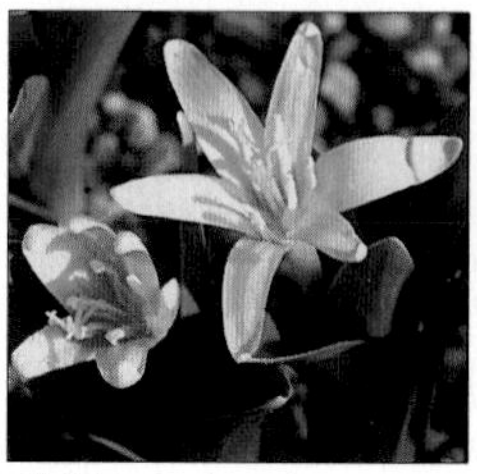

Colchicum luteum

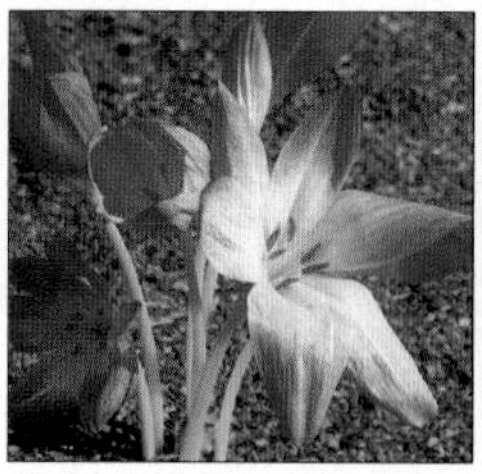

Colchicum 'The Giant'

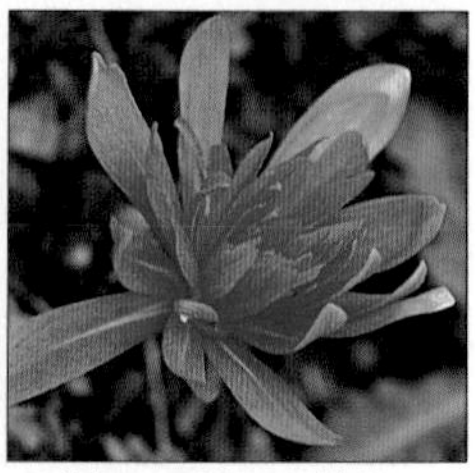

Colchicum 'Waterlily'

1–6 goblet-shaped, lavender-pink flowers, with tepals 4–6cm (1½–2½in) long. Cultivation group 1. ↕ 10–15cm (4–6in), ↔ 8cm (3in). Europe. ❄❄❄. **'Alboplenum'** has double white flowers with numerous narrow tepals. **f. *album*** has white flowers. **'Major'** see *C. byzantinum*. **'Pleniflorum'**, syn. 'Plenum', 'Roseum Plenum', has neat, rounded, double, pinkish lilac flowers, with tepals 5–7cm (2–3in) long. **'Plenum'** see 'Pleniflorum'. **'Roseum Plenum'** see 'Pleniflorum'.
***C.* 'Autumn Queen'** 🏆 Cormous perennial with semi-erect, broadly lance-shaped leaves, 18–25cm (7–10in) long. In early autumn, produces 1–4 goblet-shaped, fragrant flowers, with long perianth tubes, white throats, and rose-pink tepals, 4–8cm (1½–3in) long, strongly tessellated with deep purple. Cultivation group 1. ↕ 15cm (6in), ↔ 10cm (4in). ❄❄❄
C. baytopiorum. Cormous perennial with a horizontal corm and semi-erect, narrowly lance-shaped leaves, to 8cm (3in) long at flowering, 20–30cm (8–12in) long when mature. In autumn, produces 1–5 goblet-shaped, pinkish purple flowers, with tepals 2–4.5cm (¾–1½in) long. Cultivation group 1 or 2; best in an alpine house. ↕↔ 8cm (3in). W. Turkey. ❄❄❄ (borderline)
C. bivonae ▣ syn. *C. bowlesianum*, *C. sibthorpii*. Robust, cormous perennial with semi-erect, strap-shaped or linear-lance-shaped leaves, 12–30cm (5–12in) long. In autumn, produces 1–6 goblet-shaped, often fragrant, strongly tessellated, purplish pink flowers, with tepals 4–9cm (1½–3½in) long, often with white bases. Cultivation group 1. ↕ 15cm (6in), ↔ 10cm (4in). Italy to W. Turkey. ❄❄❄
C. boissieri, syn. *C. procurrens*. Cormous perennial with a horizontal corm and erect, narrowly linear leaves, 11–22cm (4½–9in) long. In autumn, produces 1 or 2 slender, goblet-shaped, pinkish lilac flowers, with tepals 2.5–5cm (1–2in) long. Cultivation group 2; best in a bulb frame. ↕ 3cm (1¼in), ↔ 5cm (2in). S. Greece, W. Turkey. ❄❄❄
C. bornmuelleri. Cormous perennial with semi-erect, narrowly elliptic leaves, 17–25cm (7–10in) long. In autumn, produces 1–6 funnel-shaped, pale to deep purplish pink flowers, with tepals 4.5–7cm (1¾–3in) long, and with purple-brown anthers. Often confused with *C. speciosum*, which has yellow anthers. Cultivation group 1. ↕ 15cm (6in), ↔ 10cm (4in). Turkey. ❄❄❄
***C. bornmuelleri* of gardens** see *C. speciosum*.
C. bowlesianum see *C. bivonae*.
C. byzantinum ▣🏆 syn. *C. autumnale* 'Major'. Vigorous, cormous perennial, probably a hybrid of *C. cilicicum*, with erect, strongly ribbed, elliptic or lance-shaped leaves, to 30cm (12in) long. In autumn, bears up to 20 open funnel-shaped, soft lilac flowers, with tepals 5cm (2in) long. Cultivation group 1. ↕ 12cm (5in), ↔ 10cm (4in). Origin unknown. ❄❄❄
C. cilicicum ▣ Cormous perennial bearing semi-erect, narrowly elliptic to elliptic-lance-shaped leaves, 30–40cm (12–16in) long. In autumn, produces 3–25 widely funnel-shaped, purplish pink flowers with blunt tepals, 4–7.5cm (1½–3in) long, sometimes deeper in colour towards the tips. Cultivation group 1. ↕ 10cm (4in), ↔ 8cm (3in). Turkey, Syria, Lebanon. ❄❄❄

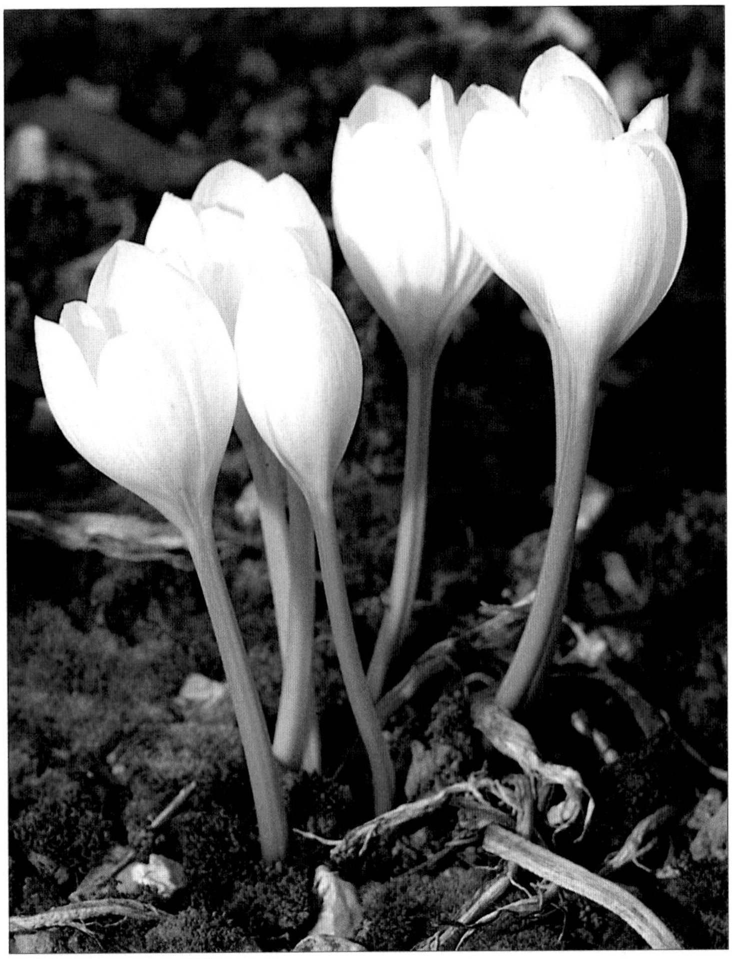
Colchicum speciosum 'Album'

***C.* 'Conquest'** see *C.* 'Glory of Heemstede'.
C. crociflorum see *C. kesselringii*.
C. cupanii. Cormous perennial with semi-erect, linear to linear-lance-shaped, very glossy leaves, 10cm (4in) long at flowering, to 15cm (6in) long when mature. Produces 1–12 widely goblet-shaped, pale to deep purplish pink flowers, with tepals 2–2.5cm (¾–1in) long, in autumn. Cultivation group 2; best in a bulb frame. ↕ 4cm (1½in), ↔ 5cm (2in). S. France, Italy, Greece (including Crete), N. Africa. ❄❄
C. doerfleri see *C. hungaricum*.
***C.* 'Glory of Heemstede'**, syn. *C.* 'Conquest'. Robust, cormous perennial with semi-erect, narrowly ovate leaves, 18–25cm (7–10in) long. Produces 1–6 goblet-shaped, strongly tessellated, fragrant, bright reddish purple flowers, with tepals 3–6cm (1¼– 2½in) long, in autumn. Cultivation group 1. ↕ 17cm (7in), ↔ 10cm (4in). ❄❄❄
C. hungaricum, syn. *C. doerfleri*. Cormous perennial with erect, narrowly linear-lance-shaped, hairy leaves, 3–10cm (1¼–4in) long at flowering, to 30cm (12in) long when mature. In late winter and early spring, produces up to 8 goblet-shaped, white or pinkish lilac flowers, with tepals 2–3cm (¾–1¼in) long. Cultivation group 2; best in an alpine house. ↕ 8cm (3in), ↔ 5cm (2in). Hungary, Balkans. ❄❄❄
C. kesselringii ▣ syn. *C. crociflorum*. Cormous perennial with semi-erect, linear-lance-shaped leaves, 1–2cm (½–¾in) long at flowering, 7–10cm (3–4in) long when mature. Produces up to 4 funnel-shaped white flowers, with tepals 1.5–3cm (½–1¼in) long, striped or suffused purple outside, in late winter and early spring. Cultivation group 2; best in an alpine house. ↕↔ 2.5cm (1in). C. Asia. ❄❄❄
***C.* 'Lilac Wonder'.** Robust, free-flowering cormous perennial with semi-erect, narrowly ovate leaves, 18–25cm (7–10in) long. Produces 4–10 goblet-shaped, deep lilac-pink flowers, with narrow tepals, 4–6cm (1½–2½in) long, in autumn. Cultivation group 1. ↕ 15cm (6in), ↔ 10cm (4in). ❄❄❄
C. luteum ▣ Cormous perennial with semi-erect, linear-lance-shaped leaves, 1–3cm (½–1¼in) long at flowering, 10–30cm (4–12in) long when mature. Produces up to 4 goblet-shaped golden flowers, with tepals 1.5–2.5cm (½–1in) long, in early spring. Cultivation group 2; best in a bulb frame. ↕↔ 8cm (3in). Afghanistan, N. India, Tibet. ❄❄
C. procurrens see *C. boissieri*.
***C.* 'Rosy Dawn'.** Robust, cormous perennial with semi-erect, ovate leaves, 18–25cm (7–10in) long. In autumn, produces 1–6 goblet-shaped then open trumpet-shaped, fragrant, pinkish violet flowers. Lightly tessellated tepals, 6–8cm (2½–3in) long, have prominent white centres. Cultivation group 1. ↕ 15cm (6in), ↔ 10cm (4in). ❄❄❄
C. sibthorpii see *C. bivonae*.
C. speciosum 🏆 syn *C. bornmuelleri* of gardens. Vigorous, cormous perennial producing semi-erect, narrowly elliptic to oblong-lance-shaped leaves, 18–25cm (7–10in) long. In autumn, produces 1–3 goblet-shaped flowers, with yellow anthers, often white throats, and pale to deep pinkish purple tepals, 4.5–8cm (1¾–3in) long. Cultivation group 1. ↕ 18cm (7in), ↔ 10cm (4in). Caucasus, N.E. Turkey, Iran. ❄❄❄. **'Album'** ▣🏆 has thick, weather-resistant, pure white flowers.
***C.* 'The Giant'** ▣ Robust, cormous perennial with semi-erect, narrowly ovate leaves, 18–25cm (7–10in) long. In autumn, produces a succession of up to 5 somewhat goblet-shaped, purplish violet flowers, with lightly tessellated tepals, to 8cm (3in) long, and white bases. Cultivation group 1. ↕ 20cm (8in), ↔ 10cm (4in). ❄❄❄
C. variegatum. Cormous perennial with horizontal, linear-lance-shaped or strap-shaped, wavy leaves, 9–15cm (3½–6in) long. In autumn, bears 1–3 widely funnel-shaped, short-tubed, strongly tessellated, violet-purple to pinkish purple flowers, with tepals 2–2.5cm (¾–1in) long. Cultivation group 2. ↕↔ 10cm (4in). Greece, S.W. Turkey. ❄❄
***C.* 'Violet Queen'.** Cormous perennial with semi-erect, broadly lance-shaped leaves, 18–25cm (7–10in) long. In early autumn, bears 1–5 funnel-shaped, strongly tessellated, fragrant, pinkish violet flowers with pointed tepals, 4–6cm (1½–2½in) long. Cultivation group 1. ↕ 15cm (6in), ↔ 10cm (4in). ❄❄❄
***C.* 'Waterlily'** ▣ Cormous perennial with semi-erect, narrowly ovate leaves, 18–25cm (7–10in) long. In autumn, produces up to 5 fully double, many-tepalled, pinkish lilac flowers, with tepals 4–7cm (1½–3in) long. Grows best where its blooms are supported by neighbouring plants. Cultivation group 1. ↕ 12cm (5in), ↔ 10cm (4in). ❄❄❄

COLEONEMA

RUTACEAE

Genus of 8 species of evergreen shrubs from open heathland and rocky slopes in South Africa. The alternate, usually short, linear to oblong or narrowly lance-shaped leaves are crowded on the stems, producing a feathery, heath-like effect. Small, star-shaped, 5-petalled flowers are produced singly, often profusely, at the ends of the shoots and from the leaf axils. In frost-prone areas, grow in a conservatory or cool greenhouse. In warmer climates, grow in a shrub border.

- **HARDINESS** Frost tender; *C. pulchrum* survives short periods near 0°C (32°F).
- **CULTIVATION** Under glass, grow in lime-free (ericaceous) potting compost in full light, with low humidity. Water moderately and apply a balanced liquid fertilizer monthly from spring to autumn; water sparingly in winter. Top-dress or pot on in spring. Outdoors, grow in moderately fertile, moist but well-drained, neutral to acid soil in full sun. Pruning group 10, after flowering.
- **PROPAGATION** Surface-sow seed at 13–16°C (55–61°F) in spring. Root semi-ripe cuttings with bottom heat in summer.

C. pulchrum. Freely branching shrub, erect at first then spreading, with linear, bright green leaves, 2–4cm (¾–1½in)

C

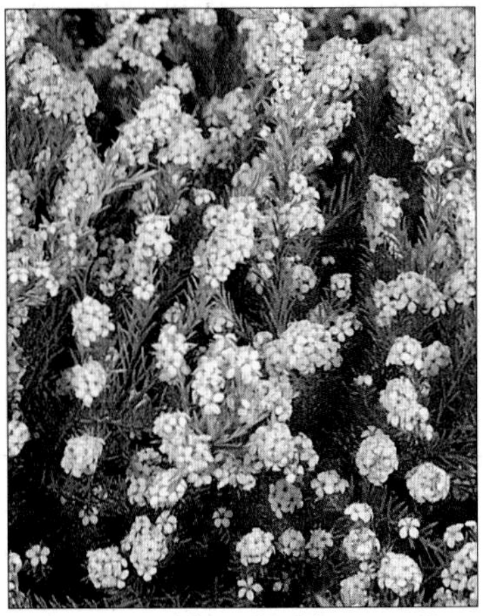

Coleonema pulchrum 'Golden Sunset'

long. Bears terminal and axillary, red or pink flowers, 9–13cm (3½–5in) across, with reflexed petals and darker eyes, from late spring to summer. ↕↔ 1–1.2m (3–4ft). South Africa. ❁ (min. 3–5°C/37–41°F). **'Golden Sunset'** ■ syn. 'Sunset Gold', has glowing, yellow-green leaves and white flowers.

▷ **Coleus** see *Solenostemon*
▷ ***Coleus blumei* var. *verschaffeltii*** see *Solenostemon scutellarioides*
▷ ***Coleus thyrsoideus*** see *Plectranthus thyrsoideus*

COLLETIA

RHAMNACEAE

Genus of 17 species of deciduous shrubs occurring in hillside scrub in temperate South America. The modified branches form succulent, cylindrical or flat, triangular, mid- to blue-green or grey-green spines, which point outwards from the shoots, with one terminal spine to each branch. The opposite leaves are sparse or wholly absent, particularly on mature plants; both the stems and leaves photosynthesize. Small, tubular or bell-shaped flowers, with tiny petals and conspicuous calyces, are produced singly or in many-flowered clusters, either on or below the spines. Grow in a sheltered shrub border or against a warm, sunny wall. In areas prone to severe frosts, grow in a cool greenhouse.

• **HARDINESS** Frost hardy.
• **CULTIVATION** Under glass, grow in loam-based potting compost (JI No.2) in full light, with good ventilation. In growth, water moderately and apply a balanced liquid fertilizer monthly; water sparingly in winter. Outdoors, grow in moderately fertile, well-drained soil in an open site in full sun, sheltered from cold, dry winds. Pruning group 1; tip-prune young plants to encourage bushiness. Tolerates moderately hard pruning.
• **PROPAGATION** Root semi-ripe cuttings of short sideshoots in late summer.
• **PESTS AND DISEASES** Trouble free.

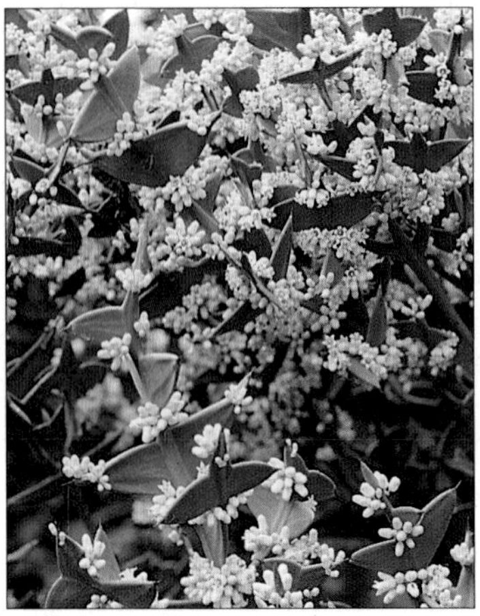

Colletia paradoxa

C. armata see *C. hystrix.*
C. cruciata see *C. paradoxa.*
C. hystrix, syn. *C. armata.* Stiffly branched, rounded, almost leafless shrub with cylindrical, sharp-pointed, grey-green spines, to 2.5cm (1in) long. Bears clusters of tubular, fragrant white flowers, 3mm (⅛in) long, on the spines, in late summer and early autumn. ↕↔ 3m (10ft). Chile. ❄❄. **'Rosea'** has white flowers opening from pink buds.
C. paradoxa ■ syn. *C. cruciata.* Spreading shrub with flattened, blue-grey spines, to 4cm (1½in) across, and few or no leaves. In autumn, clusters of tubular, fragrant white flowers, to 4mm (⅛in) long, are borne below the spines. ↕ 3m (10ft), ↔ 5m (15ft). Brazil, Uruguay. ❄❄

COLLINSIA

SCROPHULARIACEAE

Genus of 25 species of erect to spreading, slender-stemmed annuals from open woodland, fields, and low valleys in North America and Mexico. They produce opposite, ovate, oblong, or lance-shaped, sometimes softly hairy leaves. Whorled, asymmetrically 2-lipped, pink, white, blue, or bicoloured flowers are borne in racemes from spring to summer. Grow in an annual or mixed border, or in a wild garden; they provide long-lasting cut flowers.

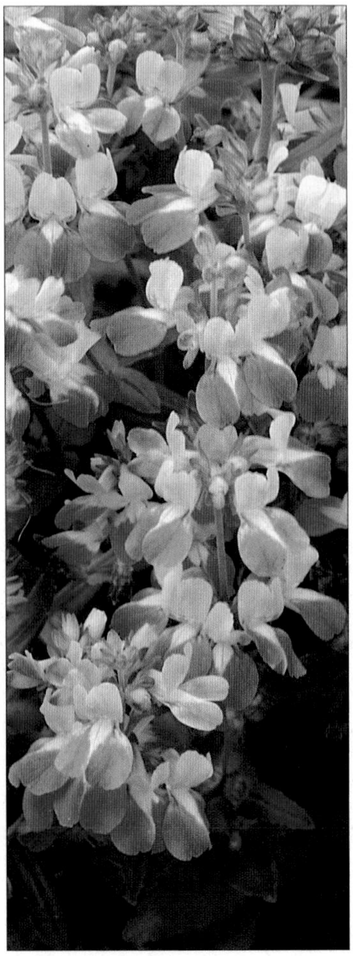

Collinsia bicolor

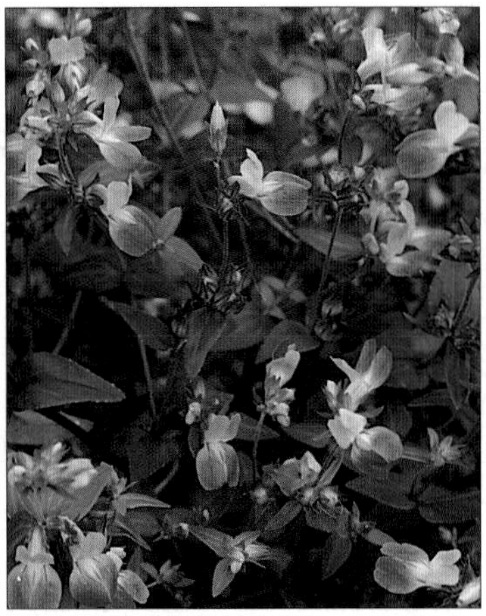

Collinsia grandiflora

• **HARDINESS** Fully hardy.
• **CULTIVATION** Grow in fertile, humus-rich, moist but well-drained soil in a sheltered, sunny to partially shaded site. Provide light twiggy support. Water in dry weather to prolong flowering.
• **PROPAGATION** Sow seed *in situ* in autumn or early spring, but delay thinning autumn sowings until the following spring.
• **PESTS AND DISEASES** Trouble free.

C. bicolor ■ syn. *C. heterophylla* (Chinese houses). Erect to spreading, weak-stemmed annual with ovate to lance-shaped, sometimes toothed, mid- to purplish green leaves, to 8cm (3in) long, heart-shaped at the bases. In summer, produces whorled racemes of flowers, to 3cm (1¼in) long, with upright, 2-lobed white upper lips, and lilac to pinkish purple lower lips, slanting outwards. ↕ to 60cm (24in), ↔ to 30cm (12in). USA (California). ❄❄❄. **'Candidissima'** has pure white flowers. **'Multicolor'** has flowers marked white, lilac, and purplish pink.
C. grandiflora ■ Erect, bushy, slender-stemmed annual with oval to lance-shaped or linear, toothed or entire, mid-green leaves, 4.5cm (1¾in) long. From spring to summer, bears whorled racemes of flowers, to 2.5cm (1in) long, with erect, 2-lobed, pale pinkish purple to pale purple upper lips, and deeper blue-purple, outward-slanting lower lips. ↕ 15–30cm (6–12in), ↔ 20–30cm (8–12in). W. North America (British Columbia to California). ❄❄❄
C. heterophylla see *C. bicolor.*

COLLOMIA

POLEMONIACEAE

Genus of 15 species of erect to spreading annuals and perennials found in habitats ranging from woodland to mountain screes, in North and South America. They are cultivated for their ovate to lance-shaped, entire to lobed leaves, and their small, funnel- to trumpet-shaped or tubular, 5-lobed, red, purple, blue, or pinkish yellow flowers, borne singly or in terminal cymes in summer. Grow *C. biflora* in an annual or mixed border. The flowers are attractive to bees.

• **HARDINESS** Fully hardy.
• **CULTIVATION** Grow in fertile, well-drained soil in full sun. During dry spells, water freely to prolong flowering.
• **PROPAGATION** Sow seed *in situ* in autumn or spring. Provide autumn-sown seedlings with cloche protection in frost-prone areas.
• **PESTS AND DISEASES** Trouble free.

C. biflora, syn. *C. cavanillesii.* Variable, softly hairy annual with lance-shaped leaves, to 6cm (2½in) long, toothed at the tips. Clusters of tubular scarlet flowers, to 1.5cm (½in) across, with 5 spreading lobes, are produced from the leaf axils at the stem tips in summer. ↕ to 60cm (24in), ↔ to 45cm (18in). Bolivia, Chile, Argentina. ❄❄❄
C. cavanillesii see *C. biflora.*

COLOCASIA

Taro

ARACEAE

Genus of 6 species of tuberous, deciduous or more or less evergreen perennials occurring in swampy or moist areas in tropical Asia, and widely grown there as a staple food. The upright, tuberous rootstocks produce rounded to arrow-shaped, mostly dark green leaves, sometimes with prominent veins. The inflorescences, which are rarely borne on cultivated plants, consist of small white spathes with spadices that develop fleshy, single-seeded, glossy green berries. In frost-prone areas, grow in a warm greenhouse, either in containers or at the margins of an indoor pool. In warmer areas, grow in moist conditions as foliage plants. All parts may cause mild stomach upset if ingested without cooking, and contact with the sap may irritate the skin.

• **HARDINESS** Frost tender.
• **CULTIVATION** Under glass, pot up tubers in spring in loamless potting compost, and bring into growth at 18°C (64°F). Provide bright filtered light and high humidity. In the growing season, water freely, applying a balanced liquid fertilizer monthly. Outdoors, grow in fertile, humus-rich, moist or wet, slightly acid soil in partial shade. Keep tubers dry and frost-free when dormant. See also pp.52–53.
• **PROPAGATION** Divide in winter or early spring.
• **PESTS AND DISEASES** Red spider mites, aphids, and whiteflies may be troublesome under glass.

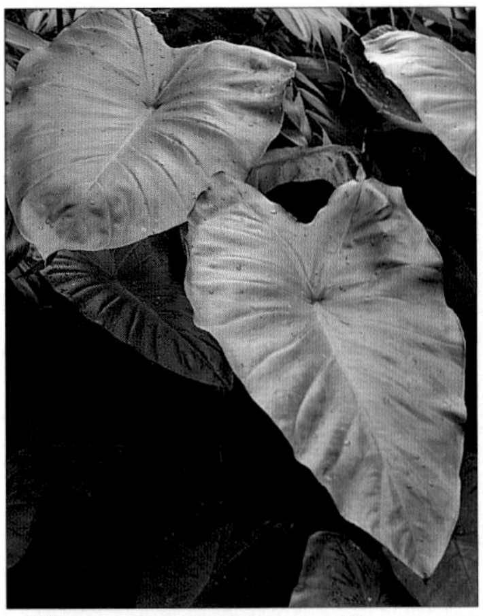

Colocasia esculenta 'Fontanesii'

C. antiquorum see *C. esculenta*.
C. esculenta ♀ syn. *C. antiquorum* (Coco-yam, Dasheen, Taro). Marginal aquatic perennial with ovate-heart-shaped to arrow-shaped, dark green leaf-blades, 60cm (24in) long, with leaf-stalks to 1m (3ft) long. ↕ 1.5m (5ft), ↔ 60cm (24in). Tropical E. Asia. ❀ (min. 1°C/34°F, or 21°C/70°F to remain evergreen). **'Fontanesii'** ■ has leaves with dark red to purple stalks, veins, and margins. **'Illustris'** (Imperial taro) has violet leaf-stalks and light green leaf-blades, marked blackish purple between the veins.

COLQUHOUNIA

LABIATAE/LAMIACEAE

Genus of 3 species of evergreen or semi-evergreen shrubs and subshrubs found in scrub and thickets in the Himalayas and China. The simple leaves, borne in opposite pairs, are finely toothed and light to dark green. Terminal spikes of showy, tubular, 2-lipped flowers are produced in axillary whorls. *C. coccinea* looks effective against a warm, sunny wall, or in a sheltered mixed border.

- **HARDINESS** Frost hardy.
- **CULTIVATION** Grow in poor to moderately fertile, well-drained soil in full sun, with shelter from cold, dry winds. May be cut back by hard frost, but will usually re-sprout from the base. Provide a deep, dry winter mulch. Pruning group 6.
- **PROPAGATION** Root softwood cuttings in summer.
- **PESTS AND DISEASES** Trouble free.

C. coccinea ■ ♀ Upright, evergreen or semi-evergreen subshrub bearing ovate-lance-shaped, finely toothed, aromatic, sage-green leaves, to 20cm (8in) long, woolly beneath. Whorls of tubular, 2-lipped, bright orange to scarlet (occasionally yellow) flowers, to 2.5cm (1in) long, are produced in terminal spikes in late summer. ↕↔ 2.5m (8ft). Himalayas, W. China. ❄❄

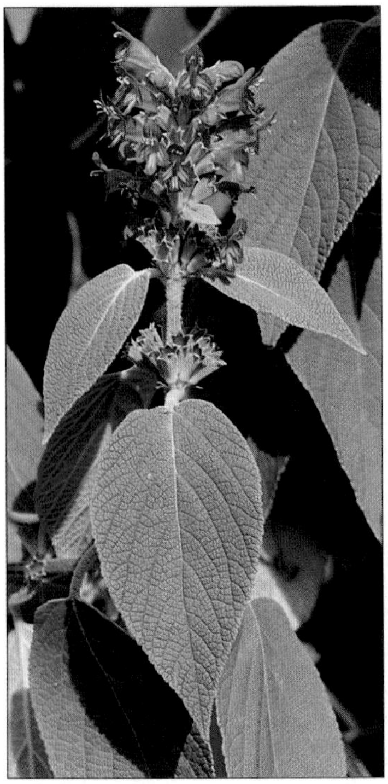

Colquhounia coccinea

▷ **Coltsfoot, Sweet** see *Petasites*
▷ **Columbine** see *Aquilegia*
Alpine see *A. alpina*
Rocky Mountain see *A. saximontana*

COLUMNEA

GESNERIACEAE

Genus of over 150 species of evergreen shrubs or subshrubs, with trailing or pendent shoots, and occasionally scandent climbers, found in moist woodland, rainforest, or cloud forest in the West Indies, Mexico, Central America, and tropical South America. In the wild, they are frequently epiphytic, and often branch where the stems are rooted into the humus; in cultivation, the stems tend to remain unbranched. They have pairs of usually ovate to elliptic, often hairy, dark green leaves. From spring to autumn, tubular flowers are borne singly or in small clusters from the leaf axils. They are 5-lobed, with the upper 2 petals joined to form a hood, and the stamens and style projecting beyond the hood. In frost-prone climates, grow as houseplants or in a warm greenhouse. In warm, humid areas, grow epiphytically or in a shaded position among trees and shrubs.

- **HARDINESS** Frost tender.
- **CULTIVATION** Under glass, grow in a moss-lined hanging basket or half-pot in loamless potting compost in bright filtered or indirect light. Mist regularly with tepid, soft water to maintain high humidity. When in full growth, water freely but carefully with soft water, applying quarter-strength, high-potash fertilizer at each watering. Overwatering may encourage root and stem rot. In winter, provide full light, water moderately, and avoid wetting the foliage. For maximum production of flowers, water sparingly in the 6 weeks preceding the normal flowering period; resume normal watering as flower buds appear. Outdoors, grow in coarse, open, moderately fertile, humus-rich soil in partial shade. To maintain vigorous growth, propagate every 2 or 3 years.
- **PROPAGATION** Root tip cuttings with bottom heat in spring.
- **PESTS AND DISEASES** Susceptible to mealybugs, aphids, and cyclamen mites.

C. x banksii ■ (*C. schiedeana* x *C. oerstediana*). Trailing subshrub with ovate to oblong-ovate, smooth, shiny, dark green leaves, 4cm (1½in) long,

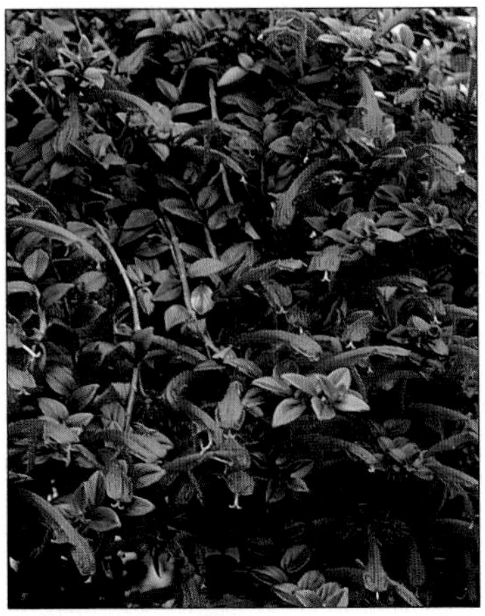

Columnea x *banksii*

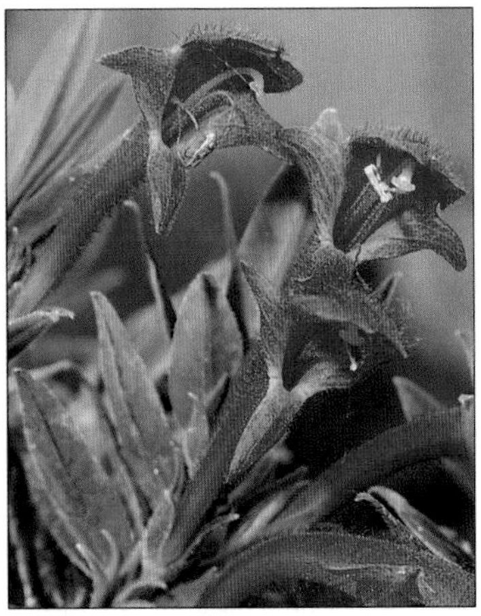

Columnea crassifolia

sparsely hairy beneath. Throughout the year, produces solitary, hairy, scarlet flowers, 6cm (2½in) long, with faint yellow lines in the throats. ↕ to 15cm (6in), ↔ trails to 1.2m (4ft). Garden origin. ❀ (min. 15°C/59°F)
C. crassifolia ■ Erect subshrub with narrowly elliptic, shiny leaves, dark green above, pale yellow-green and sparsely hairy beneath, to 10cm (4in) long. Bears solitary, hairy, bright scarlet flowers, to 10cm (4in) long, from spring to summer. ↕↔ 30cm (12in). Mexico, Guatemala. ❀ (min. 15°C/59°F)
C. gloriosa. Trailing subshrub with slender stems branching only at the base. Ovate or ovate-oblong, dark green leaves, 2.5cm (1in) long, are densely covered in fine purple hairs; the margins of the leaves are turned under, giving them a thickened appearance. From spring to summer, and intermittently throughout the rest of the year, bears solitary, hairy, fiery-red flowers, 8cm (3in) long, with yellow throats. ↕ 15cm (6in), ↔ trails to 1m (3ft). Central America. ❀ (min. 15°C/59°F)
C. microphylla. Trailing subshrub with thin stems bearing close-set, ovate to rounded, dark green leaves, to 1cm

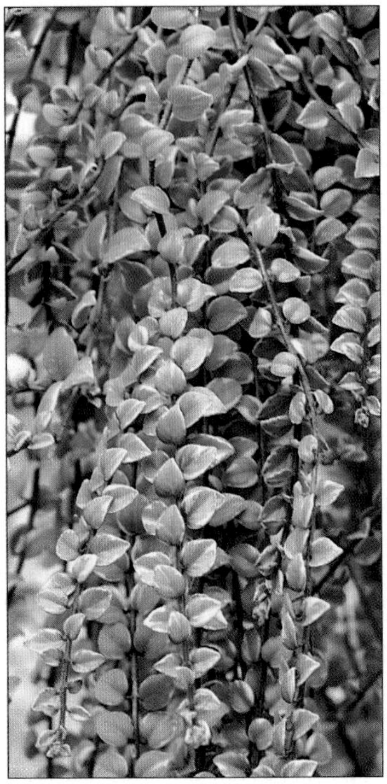

Columnea microphylla 'Variegata'

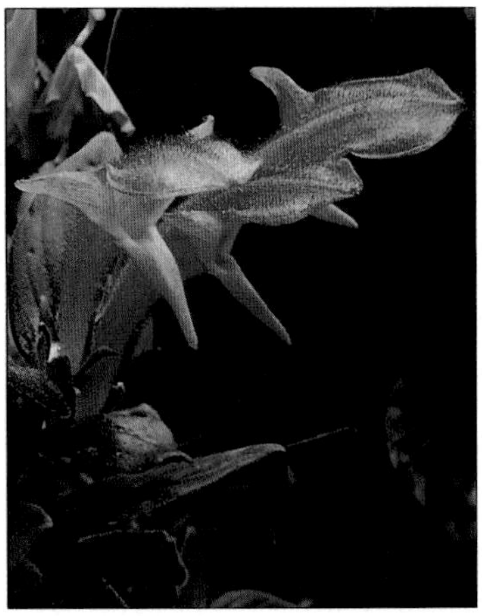

Columnea 'Robin'

(½in) long, covered in red-brown hairs. Bears solitary, hairy, scarlet flowers, 5–8cm (2–3in) long, with yellow throats, from spring to summer, and intermittently throughout the rest of the year. ↕ 15cm (6in), ↔ trails to 2m (6ft). Costa Rica. ❀ (min. 15°C/59°F). **'Variegata'** ■ has grey-green leaves with narrow cream margins.
C. 'Robin' ■ Vigorous, trailing subshrub with ovate, hairy, dark green leaves, 2–3cm (¾–1¼in) long. Numerous solitary, bright red flowers, 5–7cm (2–3in) long, are produced from early to late summer. ↕ 35cm (14in), ↔ 60cm (24in). ❀ (min. 15°C/59°F)
C. scandens. Trailing subshrub with slender stems bearing oblong to narrowly oblong or ovate-elliptic, dark green leaves, 5cm (2in) long, with red hairs at the margins. Bears sparsely hairy, red or yellow flowers, 6cm (2½in) long, either singly or in pairs, from spring to summer. ↕ to 15cm (6in), ↔ trails to 1m (3ft). Lesser Antilles. ❀ (min. 15°C/59°F). Several hybrids, including the following, have recently been named: **'Campus Sunset'** is vigorous and bushy, with ovate leaves, olive-green above, red beneath; bears yellow flowers, with red-margined lobes, in autumn. **'Early Bird'** is compact, with pointed leaves, 2.5cm (1in) long, and bears erect, yellow-throated orange flowers almost throughout the year; ↕ to 10cm (4in), ↔ trails to 35cm (14ft). **'Yellow Dancer'** is strong-growing, with yellow flowers.
C. 'Stavanger' ♀ (*C. microphylla* x *C.* x *vedrariensis*) (Norse fire plant). Very vigorous, freely branching, trailing subshrub bearing oval, lustrous, dark green leaves, 2cm (¾in) long. Solitary, hairy, bright scarlet flowers, 8–10cm (3–4in) long, are borne from spring to summer, and intermittently throughout the rest of the year. ↕ to 15cm (6in), ↔ to 60cm (24in). ❀ (min. 15°C/59°F)

COLUTEA

Bladder senna

LEGUMINOSAE/PAPILIONACEAE

Genus of about 25 species of deciduous shrubs, sometimes trees, found in dry soils in woodland and thickets, from S. Europe, E. Africa, Turkey, Iran, C. Asia, Afghanistan, Pakistan, and the Himalayas. They are grown for their pinnate leaves, with entire, usually elliptic to obovate leaflets, their pea-like, yellow to red-brown flowers, borne in

C

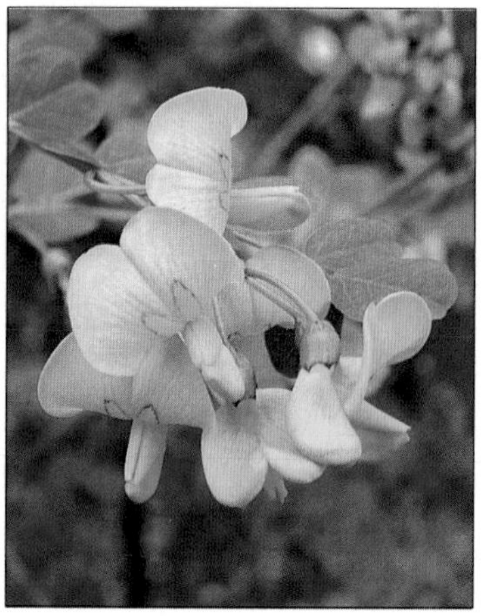

Colutea arborescens

few-flowered, axillary, long-stalked racemes, and their unusual, inflated, membranous, bladder-like fruits. Coluteas are suitable for a shrub border; those described are useful for an exposed site or dry, sunny bank. They tolerate poor, dry soils, coastal conditions, and urban pollution. Seeds may cause mild stomach upset if ingested.
• **HARDINESS** Fully hardy to frost hardy.
• **CULTIVATION** Grow in moderately fertile, well-drained soil in full sun. Pruning group 1 or 6; *C. arborescens* may be trained as a branched-head standard.
• **PROPAGATION** Sow seed in containers in a cold frame in autumn or spring. Root greenwood cuttings in early summer.
• **PESTS AND DISEASES** Trouble free.

C. arborescens ▣ (Bladder senna). Vigorous, shrub (rarely tree-like) with pinnate, pale green leaves, to 15cm (6in) long, with 5–6 pairs of broadly elliptic to ovate leaflets. Produces 3–8 yellow flowers, to 2cm (¾in) long, in racemes to 12cm (5in) long, over a long period in summer, followed by green, then translucent seed pods, to 8cm (3in) long. ↕↔ 3m (10ft). S. Europe. ❄❄❄
C. x media ▣ (*C. arborescens* x *C. orientalis*). Vigorous, bushy shrub with pinnate, blue-green leaves, to 15cm (6in) long, with 3–6 pairs of elliptic leaflets. From early to late summer, bears orange-brown flowers, to 1.5cm (¾in) long, sometimes flushed yellow in the centres, in racemes to 10cm (4in) long. Seed pods, to 8cm (3in) long, are greenish brown at first, then translucent. ↕↔ 3m (10ft). Garden origin. ❄❄❄
C. orientalis. Bushy, rounded shrub with pinnate, bluish green leaves, to 10cm (4in) long, with 3 or 4 pairs of obovate leaflets. In summer, produces 2–5 copper-red flowers, to 1.5cm (½in) long, with yellow markings, in racemes to 6cm (2½in) long, followed by pale brown then translucent seed pods, to 5cm (2in) long. ↕↔ 2m (6ft). Caucasus, N. Iran. ❄❄❄

COLUTEOCARPUS

BRASSICACEAE/CRUCIFERAE

Genus of one species of dwarf, tufted perennial, closely related to *Alyssum*, occurring in dry, rocky areas in the E. Mediterranean and Turkey. It has basal rosettes of oblong to lance-shaped leaves, terminal cymes of cross-shaped flowers, and inflated seed pods. *C. vesicarius* is suitable for an alpine house or scree bed. In cool, damp areas, seed pods are more reliably produced in an alpine house.
• **HARDINESS** Fully hardy to frost hardy.
• **CULTIVATION** Outdoors, grow in poor to moderately fertile, gritty, humus-rich, sharply drained soil in full sun. Protect from excessive wet. In an alpine house, grow in equal parts loam, leaf mould, and grit.
• **PROPAGATION** Sow seed in containers in a cold frame in autumn.
• **PESTS AND DISEASES** Susceptible to aphids and red spider mites under glass.

C. reticulatus see *C. vesicarius.*
C. vesicarius, syn. *Alyssum vesicaria, C. reticulatus.* Cushion-forming perennial with stiff, sharply toothed, glossy, mid-green leaves, to 8cm (3in) long. Loose, flat-topped, terminal cymes of golden yellow flowers, 1cm (½in) across, are produced on short stems in late spring, followed by papery, pale green seed pods, to 3cm (1¼in) long. ↕ to 8cm (3in), ↔ to 15cm (6in). E. Mediterranean. ❄❄❄ (borderline)

COLVILLEA

CAESALPINIACEAE/LEGUMINOSAE

Genus of one species of evergreen tree from forest in Madagascar. It has large, alternate, 2-pinnate leaves and produces showy, pea-like flowers in conspicuous, pendent racemes. In frost-prone areas, grow *C. racemosa* in a temperate greenhouse. In warmer climates, grow as a specimen tree.
• **HARDINESS** Half hardy.
• **CULTIVATION** Under glass, grow in loam-based potting compost (JI No.3) in full light, with shade from hot sun and moderate humidity. In growth, water freely and apply a balanced liquid fertilizer monthly; water sparingly in winter. Top-dress or pot on in spring. Outdoors, grow in fertile, moist but well-drained soil in full sun. Pruning group 1; needs restrictive pruning under glass, immediately after flowering.
• **PROPAGATION** Sow seed at 18°C (64°F) in spring.
• **PESTS AND DISEASES** Red spider mites may be a problem under glass.

C. racemosa ♀ Erect tree, often with a long trunk and spreading branches. Fern-like, 2-pinnate leaves, to 90cm (36in) long, have many small, elliptic to oblong leaflets. From late autumn to winter, produces scarlet flowers, 4.5cm (1¾in) across, in racemes to 30cm (12in) long. ↕ 8–15m (25–50ft), ↔ 3–5m (10–15ft). Madagascar. ❄

▷ ***Comarostaphylis*** see *Arctostaphylos*
C. diversifolia see *A. diversifolia*
▷ ***Comarum*** see *Potentilla*
C. palustre see *P. palustris*

COMBRETUM

COMBRETACEAE

Genus of about 250 species of evergreen or semi-evergreen, sometimes briefly deciduous trees and shrubs, some more or less scandent, occurring in forest and thickets in tropical regions worldwide (except Australia). Leaves, borne in opposite pairs or in whorls, are mainly ovate, or oblong to elliptic and entire. They are cultivated for their mostly small, tubular, 4- or 5-lobed flowers, borne in terminal and axillary racemes and panicles. In frost-prone areas, grow in a warm greenhouse or conservatory. In warmer climates, train on to a trellis or pergola.
• **HARDINESS** Frost tender.
• **CULTIVATION** Under glass, grow in a border or in large containers of loamless potting compost in bright filtered light, with full light in winter. Mist with tepid water as flower buds form. From spring to autumn, water freely and apply a balanced liquid fertilizer monthly; water moderately in winter. Top-dress or pot on in spring. Outdoors, grow in fertile, humus-rich, moist but well-drained soil, in partial shade. Pruning group 11 or 12, immediately after flowering.
• **PROPAGATION** Root semi-ripe cuttings with bottom heat in summer.
• **PESTS AND DISEASES** Red spider mites may be a problem under glass.

C. grandiflorum. Evergreen, more or less scandent shrub or semi-climber with ovate-elliptic, slender-pointed, smooth or downy leaves, 10–15cm (4–6in) long. Produces many short, dense, one-sided racemes of bright red flowers, 2cm (¾in) long, from autumn to winter. ↕ 4–6m (12–20ft), ↔ 2–4m (6–12ft). Gambia to Ghana. ❀ (min. 16°C/61°F)
C. paniculatum. Vigorous, usually open, semi-evergreen or briefly deciduous, scandent shrub or climber. The stems bear short spines and broadly elliptic to oblong, papery leaves, to 18cm (7in) long. Panicles of red flowers, 4cm (1½in) long, are produced in autumn. ↕ 10m (30ft) or more, ↔ 3–5m (10–15ft). Tropical Africa. ❀ (min. 16°C/61°F)

▷ **Comfrey** see *Symphytum*
Common see *S. officinale*
Tuberous see *S. tuberosum*

COMMELINA

Day flower, Widow's tears

COMMELINACEAE

Genus of 100 species of mat-forming or clump-forming annuals and fibrous- or tuberous-rooted perennials from forest floors in tropical and subtropical regions of southern Africa, Asia, and North, Central, and South America. The leaves are alternate and ovate, lance-shaped, or linear. Most species root at the leaf nodes as they spread. One-sided cymes of small, saucer-shaped, 3-petalled flowers are enclosed in folded, terminal, spathe-like bracts; flowers emerge one at a time, each lasting less than a day. Use *Commelina* species as permanent ground cover. In frost-prone areas, grow tender species in a cool greenhouse or outdoors in an annual border; frost-hardy species are suitable for a herbaceous border.
• **HARDINESS** Frost hardy to frost tender; crowns of some tender species may tolerate -3°C (27°F), perhaps lower, in well-drained soil.
• **CULTIVATION** Under glass, grow in loam-based potting compost (JI No.2) in bright filtered light. In growth, water moderately and apply a balanced liquid fertilizer monthly; water sparingly in winter. Outdoors, grow in fertile, well-drained soil in a warm, sheltered site in sun or partial shade. Provide a deep, dry,

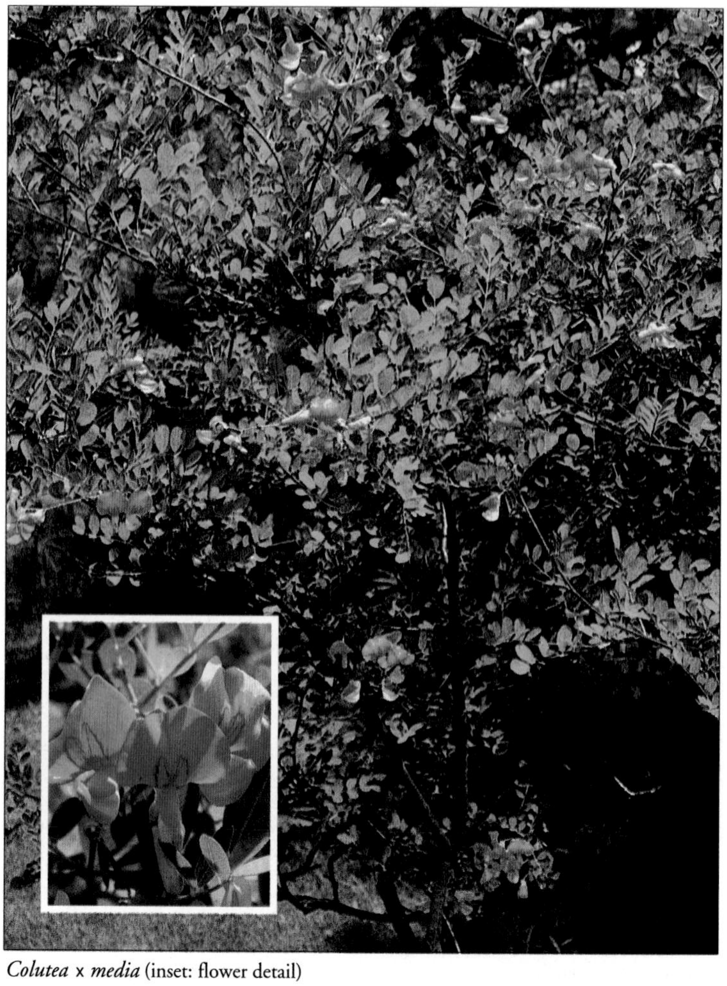

Colutea x *media* (inset: flower detail)

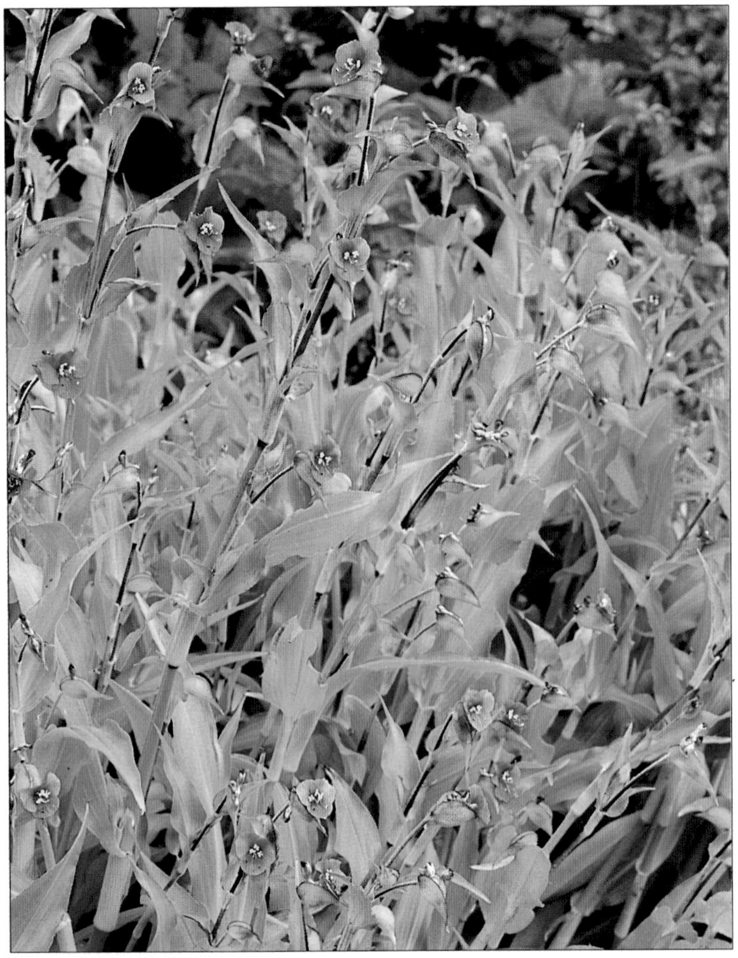

Commelina coelestis

winter mulch. In frost-prone climates, lift plants before the first frosts and overwinter in barely moist, frost-free conditions. Start into growth again in gentle heat in spring.
• **PROPAGATION** Sow seed at 13–18°C (55–64°F) in spring. Divide in spring.
• **PESTS AND DISEASES** Slugs and vine weevils may be a problem.

C. benghalensis. Creeping, fibrous-rooted perennial bearing ovate-lance-shaped to ovate leaves, to 7cm (3in) long. Cymes of blue or violet flowers, 1.5cm (½in) across, are borne in the upper leaf axils in summer. ↕ to 25cm (10in), ↔ indefinite. Tropical Asia, southern Africa. ❄ (borderline)
C. coelestis ◼ Vigorous, clump-forming, erect, tuberous perennial with hairy, fleshy stems bearing ovate-lance-shaped to oblong-lance-shaped, clasping leaves, 8–18cm (3–7in) long. From late summer to mid-autumn, freely produces cymes of vivid blue flowers, 2–3cm (¾–1¼in) across. Related to (and sometimes included in) *C. tuberosa.* ↕ to 90cm (36in), ↔ 45cm (18in). Central and South America. ❄❄. **var. *alba*** bears white flowers.
C. tuberosa. Mat-forming, procumbent, tuberous perennial bearing narrowly lance-shaped leaves, to 9cm (3½in) long. Cymes of green flowers, 3cm (1¼in) across, streaked with dark blue-purple, are produced in summer. ↕ to 20cm (8in), ↔ indefinite. Central and South America. ❄ (borderline)

▷**Compass plant** see *Silphium laciniatum*

CONANDRON

GESNERIACEAE

Genus of one species of rosette-forming, tuberous-rooted, evergreen perennial from Japan, found on wet, rocky cliffs in mountainous areas. Leaves are elliptic-ovate, coarsely toothed, wrinkled, and fleshy. Tubular flowers, with prominent stamens, are borne in nodding cymes on leafless stems in midsummer. In dry, cool-temperate climates, grow *C. ramondoides* in shaded, vertical crevices in a rock garden. In areas with cool, wet winters, grow in an alpine house.
• **HARDINESS** Frost hardy.
• **CULTIVATION** In an alpine house, grow in loam-based potting compost (JI No.2) with additional grit and leaf mould, in bright filtered light. In the growing season, water moderately with soft water, and apply a half-strength balanced liquid fertilizer monthly; water sparingly in winter. Outdoors, grow in moderately fertile, gritty, humus-rich, moist but well-drained, acid soil in partial shade. Protect from excessive winter wet.
• **PROPAGATION** Surface-sow seed in containers in a cold frame in spring; water seedlings from below by plunging pots to their rims in soft water. Root leaf cuttings in early summer.
• **PESTS AND DISEASES** Red spider mites and aphids may be troublesome under glass.

C. ramondoides. Hummock-forming perennial with glossy, mid-green leaves, to 30cm (12in) long. In midsummer, bears loose cymes of 10–40 tubular, deeply 5-lobed, white, lilac, or deep blue-purple flowers, to 1.5cm (½in) across, with orange centres, on stems to 20cm (8in) long. ↕ to 25cm (10in), ↔ to 20cm (8in). Japan (Honshu). ❄❄

▷**Cone bush** see *Isopogon*
▷**Coneflower** see *Echinacea, Rudbeckia*
Drooping see *Ratibida pinnata*
Grey-head see *Ratibida pinnata*
Prairie see *Ratibida*
Rose see *Isopogon dubius*
▷**Cone pepper** see *Capsicum annuum* Conioides Group
Red see *Capsicum annuum* Fasciculatum Group

CONGEA

VERBENACEAE

Genus of 7 species of evergreen, scandent shrubs and twining climbers found in forest and thickets in S.E. Asia. The leaves are opposite, entire, and ovate to elliptic or oblong. Congeas bear terminal panicles of tiny, tubular, 2-lipped flowers, borne in small clusters, ringed by several petal-like bracts. In frost-prone areas, grow in a warm greenhouse or conservatory. In warmer areas, grow on a trellis, pillar, or pergola.
• **HARDINESS** Frost tender.
• **CULTIVATION** Under glass, grow in loam-based potting compost (JI No.3) in full light, with shade from hot sun, and with good ventilation. In the growing season, water freely and apply a balanced liquid fertilizer monthly; water moderately in winter. Top-dress or pot on in spring. Provide support for the climbing stems. Outdoors, grow in fertile, humus-rich, moist but well-drained soil in full sun. Pruning group 11, immediately after flowering.
• **PROPAGATION** Sow seed at 16–20°C (61–68°F) in spring. Root semi-ripe cuttings in summer with bottom heat. Layer in spring.
• **PESTS AND DISEASES** Red spider mites may be a problem under glass.

C. tomentosa (Shower orchid). Evergreen climber with downy, purple and green, scandent or climbing stems. Leaves are ovate to elliptic or oblong and lightly hairy, to 20cm (8in) long. From winter to spring, bears panicles of white flowers in dense clusters, 5cm (2in) across, within groups of ovate to elliptic-oblong, violet or white bracts, densely covered with white hairs. ↕ 3–5m (10–15ft). Burma, Thailand. ❁ (min. 15°C/59°F)

CONICOSIA

AIZOACEAE

Genus of 10 species of semi-evergreen, spreading, perennial (in rare cases, biennial) succulents from arid regions of South Africa's Northern Cape, Eastern Cape, and Western Cape. The long, narrow, 3-angled to semi-cylindrical, fleshy, tufted, often dark-spotted leaves dry up after flowering, but persist after the solitary, long-stalked, daisy-like yellow flowers have faded. Green berries contain spherical, slightly keeled, smooth seeds. In frost-prone areas, grow in a temperate greenhouse. In warm, dry climates, they are suitable for growing outdoors in a desert garden.

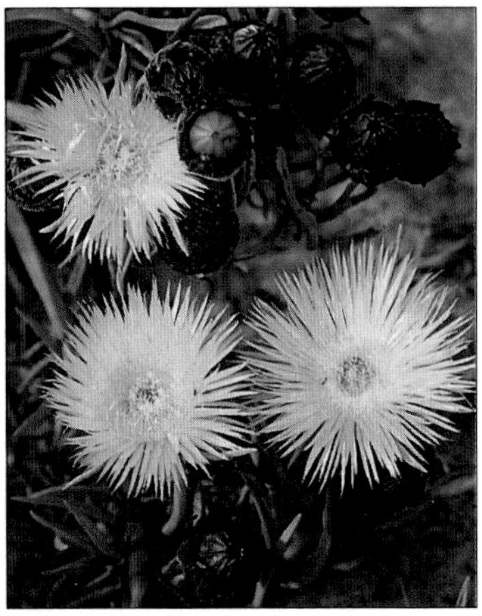

Conicosia pugioniformis

• **HARDINESS** Frost tender.
• **CULTIVATION** Under glass, grow in a mix of 2 parts each loam and sharp sand and 1 part leaf mould, in full light and with low humidity. At the beginning of the growing season, apply a balanced liquid fertilizer. Water moderately from early summer to autumn, and keep completely dry at other times of year. Outdoors, grow in humus-rich, not too fertile, well-drained soil in full sun. See also pp.48–49.
• **PROPAGATION** Sow seed at 21°C (70°F) in mid-spring.
• **PESTS AND DISEASES** Aphids may prove troublesome.

C. capensis. Perennial succulent with stems to 15cm (6in) or more long. These are crowned by 3-angled, grooved, spotted, bluish green leaves, to 40cm (16in) long, which are shorter on the prostrate, floral branches. Bears pale yellow flowers, 7cm (3in) across, in summer. ↕ 25cm (10in), ↔ 30cm (12in). South Africa (Northern Cape, Western Cape). ❁ (min. 7°C/45°F)
C. pugioniformis ◼ Perennial succulent with stems to 30cm (12in) long. These are crowned by 3-angled, greyish green leaves, to 20cm (8in) long, with grooved upper surfaces, reddish green at the bases. In late summer, bears glistening, bright yellow flowers, 7cm (3in) across. ↕ 40cm (16in), ↔ 30cm (12in). South Africa (Northern Cape, Western Cape). ❁ (min. 7°C/45°F)

CONIOGRAMME

ADIANTACEAE

Genus of 20 species of clump-forming, evergreen, semi-evergreen, or deciduous, terrestrial ferns from moist woodland in Asia. Creeping rhizomes produce pinnate to 3-pinnate, pale to dark green fronds with strap-shaped to ovate or oblong pinnae, pointed at the tips. Sporangia, not protected by indusia, are borne in rows on the undersides of the fronds. Suitable for growing in a shady border or woodland garden; in areas prone to hard frosts, grow half-hardy species in a cool greenhouse or conservatory.
• **HARDINESS** Fully hardy to half hardy.
• **CULTIVATION** Under glass, grow in 1 part each of loam, medium-grade bark, and charcoal, 2 parts sharp sand, and 3 parts coarse leaf mould. Provide bright filtered or indirect light and moderate humidity. In the growing season, water

freely, applying a half-strength balanced liquid fertilizer monthly; in winter, water moderately, keeping the foliage dry. Outdoors, grow in moist but well-drained, fertile, neutral to acid, leafy soil in partial shade. Provide shelter from strong winds.
• **PROPAGATION** Sow spores at 16°C (61°F) as soon as ripe. Divide rhizomes of well-established colonies in late spring. See also p.51.
• **PESTS AND DISEASES** Prone to slugs.

C. japonica (Bamboo fern). Deciduous, sometimes semi-evergreen fern with oblong to linear-lance-shaped fronds, 50–60cm (20–24in) long, which are pinnate at the tips and 2-pinnate at the bases. Narrowly ovate, pale green pinnae may have central yellow marks. ‡ 75cm (30in), ↔ 80cm (32in). E. Asia. ❄❄❄ (borderline)

CONOPHYTUM

AIZOACEAE

Genus of 290 species of dwarf, often slow-growing, clump-forming, perennial succulents, frequently with long roots, found in semi-desert areas with winter rainfall in Namibia and South Africa. Small, fleshy "bodies" comprise 2 united leaves with a central fissure, from which solitary, daisy-like flowers are produced, followed by small, ovoid, fleshy green fruits. After the flowers fade, the leaves gradually shrivel to papery sheaths; new leaves develop through the sheaths after the dormant period. In most climates they are grown in a warm greenhouse as they will not tolerate summer rainfall. In their native regions, grow in a raised bed or scree bed, or in a desert garden.
• **HARDINESS** Frost tender.
• **CULTIVATION** Under glass, grow in a mix of 2 parts loam to 1 part each sharp sand and leaf mould, in full light with low humidity. Water sparingly from late summer to early winter and again in spring; additional fertilizer is not needed. Keep completely dry from late spring to midsummer. Outdoors, grow in gritty, humus-rich, low-fertility soil in full sun. See also pp.48–49.
• **PROPAGATION** Surface-sow seed in late winter at 20–25°C (68–77°F) in moist, shady conditions; gradually increase light and reduce humidity after germination. Separate and root complete bodies in late summer.
• **PESTS AND DISEASES** Susceptible to aphids under glass.

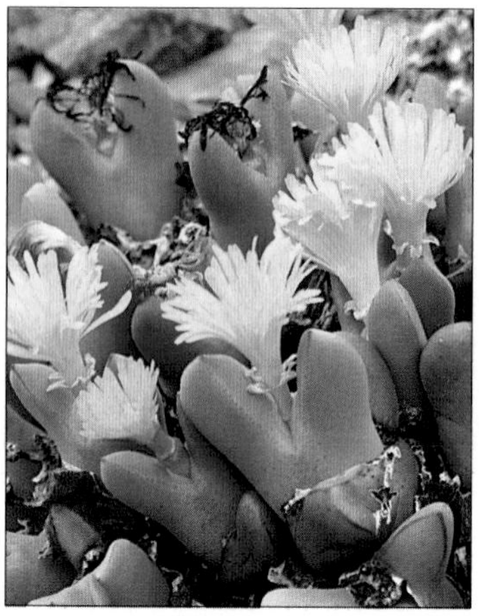
Conophytum bilobum

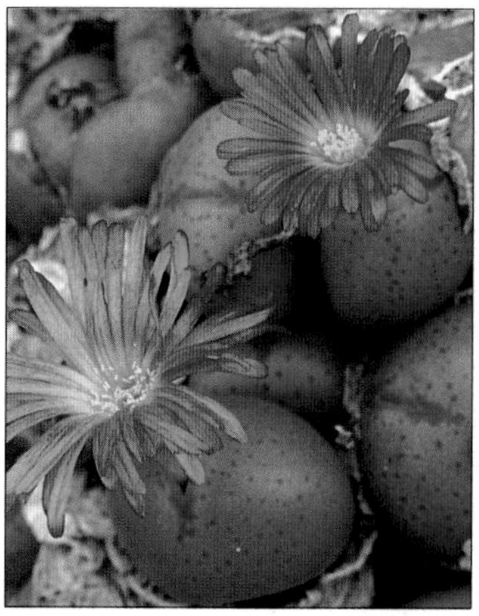
Conophytum notabile

C. bilobum ▣ Perennial succulent with flattened, heart-shaped, greyish green bodies, 2.5cm (1in) across, branching with age to form clusters. Bears yellow flowers, to 3cm (1¼in) across, in late summer. ‡ 5cm (2in), ↔ 15cm (6in). South Africa (Northern Cape, Western Cape). ❅ (min. 10°C/50°F)
C. longum see *Ophthalmophyllum longum.*
C. nanum. Perennial succulent with fleshy, minutely papillose, bright green leaves forming spherical bodies, to 7mm (¼in) across. Red-tipped white flowers, 1cm (½in) across, are produced in late summer. ‡ 2cm (¾in), ↔ 8cm (3in). South Africa (Northern Cape). ❅ (min. 10°C/50°F)
C. notabile ▣ Mat-forming, perennial succulent with generally ellipsoid, rounded, pale bluish green bodies, to 1cm (½in) across, each with a red dot on either side of the fissure. In late summer, bears brownish orange flowers, 2cm (¾in) across. ‡ 2.5cm (1in), ↔ 2cm (¾in). South Africa (Northern Cape, Western Cape). ❅ (min. 10°C/50°F)
C. obcordellum. Variable, mat-forming, perennial succulent with inversely conical, green-dotted, light green to grey bodies, to 2cm (¾in) across, with pinkish red sides. White flowers, to 1.5cm (½in) across, are produced in late summer. ‡ to 1.5cm (½in), ↔ to 7cm (3in). South Africa (Western Cape). ❅ (min. 10°C/50°F)
C. pillansii ▣ Perennial succulent with 1–3 joined, depressed obovoid, pale yellowish green bodies, 2cm (¾in) or more across, the tops marked with translucent green dots, the sides slightly

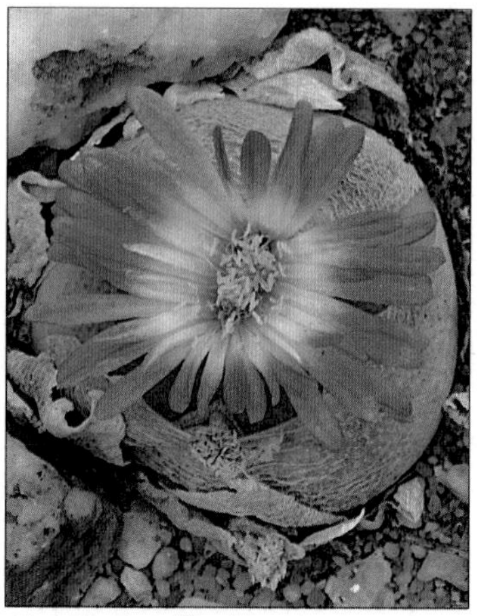
Conophytum pillansii

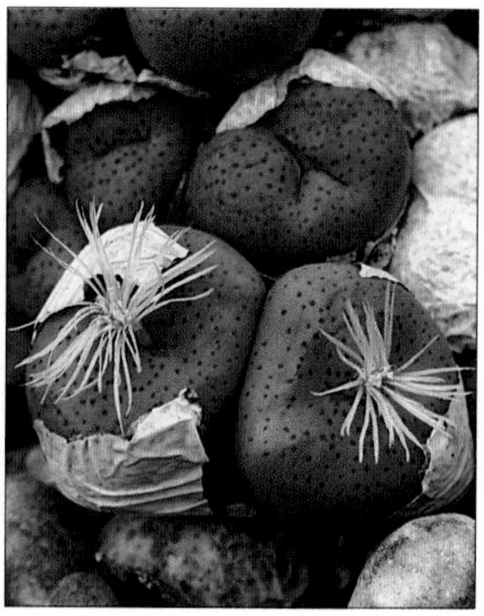
Conophytum truncatum

reddened. In late summer, bears pinkish purple flowers, 2.5cm (1in) across, sometimes with white bases. ‡ 2cm (¾in), ↔ to 7cm (3in). South Africa (Western Cape). ❅ (min. 10°C/50°F)
C. truncatum ▣ Variable, cushion-forming, perennial succulent with inversely conical, dark-spotted, greyish to bluish green bodies, 1.5cm (½in) across, with wide fissures. Yellowish or creamy white flowers, 1.5cm (½in) across, are produced in autumn. ‡ 1.5cm (½in), ↔ to 15cm (6in). South Africa (Eastern Cape, Western Cape). ❅ (min. 10°C/50°F)
C. velutinum. Mat-forming, perennial succulent with ovate, velvety, olive-green bodies, 8mm (⅜in) across, with convex tops and slightly depressed fissures. The bodies often arise from small, basal branches that are covered by the remains of papery leaf sheaths. Bears bright pinkish purple flowers, to 2cm (¾in) across, in late summer. ‡ 1.5cm (½in), ↔ 7cm (3in). South Africa (Northern Cape). ❅ (min. 10°C/50°F)
C. villetii. Clump-forming or solitary, perennial succulent with greyish green bodies, 1cm (½in) across, the upper lobes deeply divided. Pale pink flowers, 2cm (¾in) across, with deeper pink stripes, are produced from late summer to autumn. ‡ 2.5cm (1in), ↔ to 10cm (4in). Namibia, South Africa. ❅ (min. 10°C/50°F)

▷ ***Consolea falcata*** see *Opuntia falcata*

CONSOLIDA

Larkspur

RANUNCULACEAE

Genus of about 40 species of erect, slender-stemmed annuals, closely related to and sometimes included in the genus *Delphinium.* They occur in fallow fields and on stony slopes and steppes in S.E. Europe and from the W. Mediterranean region to C. Asia. The feathery, softly downy, mid- to dark green, usually rounded leaves are deeply pinnatisect, or palmate with numerous slender leaflets. Spurred, delphinium-like, pink, blue, or white flowers are produced in racemes or panicles in summer. The taller cultivars provide long-lasting cut flowers, which may also be dried. All are excellent for a cottage garden or annual border. Larkspur seeds are poisonous.
• **HARDINESS** Fully hardy.
• **CULTIVATION** Grow in light, fertile, well-drained soil in full sun. Water

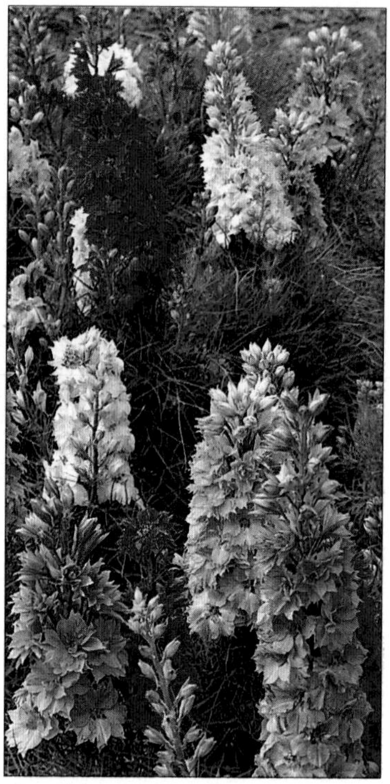
Consolida ajacis Dwarf Rocket Series

freely in dry weather. Provide twiggy support for tall cultivars. Dead-head to prolong flowering.
• **PROPAGATION** Sow seed *in situ* from early spring to early summer, or in autumn with cloche protection in frost-prone areas.
• **PESTS AND DISEASES** Slugs, snails, powdery mildew, and crown rot may cause problems.

C. ajacis, syn. *C. ambigua, Delphinium consolida* (Larkspur). Sparsely to well-branched annual with finely dissected, almost fern-like, palmate leaves, to 10cm (4in) long, with oblong to linear leaflets. In summer, bears upright, simple or branching, open to densely packed spikes, to 60cm (24in) tall, of spurred, single or rosette-like, double flowers, to 4cm (1½in) across, in rich tones or pastel shades of pink, white, or violet-blue. ‡ 30–120cm (12–48in), ↔ 23–30cm (9–12in). Mediterranean. ❄❄❄. **Dwarf Hyacinth Series** cultivars do not branch strongly at the bases, and bear double flowers in densely packed, blunt-tipped racemes. Grow in an exposed garden; ‡ 30–45cm (12–18in). **Dwarf Rocket Series** ▣ cultivars are compact, with double, blue, purple, white, or pink flowers; ‡ 30–50cm (12–20in), ↔ 15–25cm (6–10in). **Giant Imperial Series** cultivars branch strongly from the bases, and produce racemes of double flowers on long, straight stems. Good for cut flowers; ‡ 60–100cm (24–36in), ↔ 35cm (14in).
C. ambigua see *C. ajacis.*

CONVALLARIA

Lily-of-the-valley

CONVALLARIACEAE/LILIACEAE

Genus of 3 species, sometimes considered to be one variable species, of rhizomatous perennials found in light woodland, scrub, or alpine meadows in N. temperate regions. They have ovate-lance-shaped to elliptic, stalked, basal leaves. Pendent, bell-shaped, fragrant,

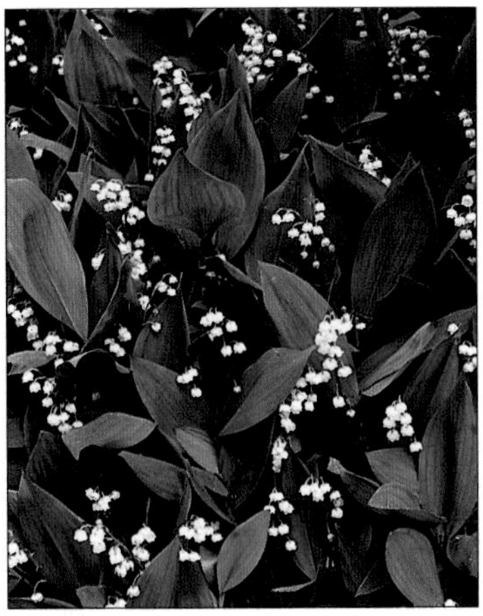

Convallaria majalis

mostly white flowers are produced in arching racemes. Grow in a wild or woodland garden, or use for ground cover in a damp, shady border. The seeds of *C. majalis* may cause mild stomach upset if ingested.
• **HARDINESS** Fully hardy.
• **CULTIVATION** Grow in leafy, fertile, humus-rich, moist soil in full or partial shade. Top-dress with leaf mould in autumn. For a fragrant indoor display, lift and pot up rhizomes in autumn, and force gently or allow them to grow at their own pace. Replant outdoors after flowering.
• **PROPAGATION** Sow seed in containers in a cold frame as soon as ripe, removing the flesh from the seeds before sowing. Separate rhizomes in autumn, keeping moist until established.
• **PESTS AND DISEASES** Susceptible to grey mould (*Botrytis*).

C. majalis ■ 🏆 Rhizomatous perennial producing tough, slender, creeping, branching rhizomes bearing pairs of ovate-lance-shaped to elliptic, stalked, hairless, basal leaves, 4–20cm (1½–8in) long. Arching racemes of pendent, spherical-bell-shaped, strongly scented, waxy white flowers, 0.5–1cm (¼–½in) across, are produced on leafless stems in late spring. ↕ 23cm (9in), ↔ 30cm (12in). N. temperate regions. ✲✲✲. **'Albostriata'** ■ has leaves longitudinally striped creamy white. **'Flore Pleno'** has double white flowers. **'Fortin's Giant'** is vigorous, with wide leaves, and flowers 8–15mm (⅜–½in) across; ↕ 30cm (12in). **'Hardwick Hall'** has broad leaves with very narrow, pale green

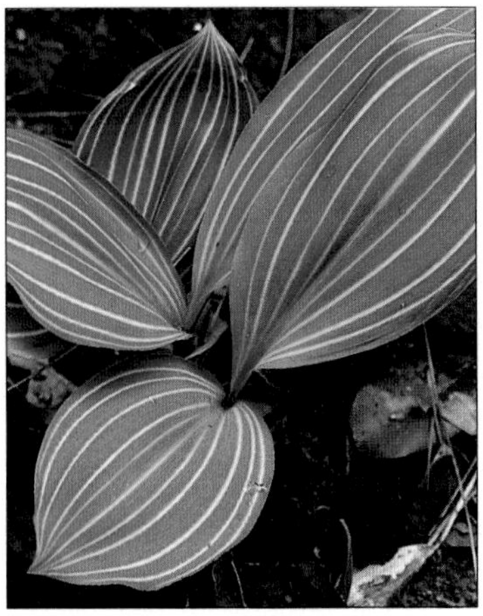

Convallaria majalis 'Albostriata'

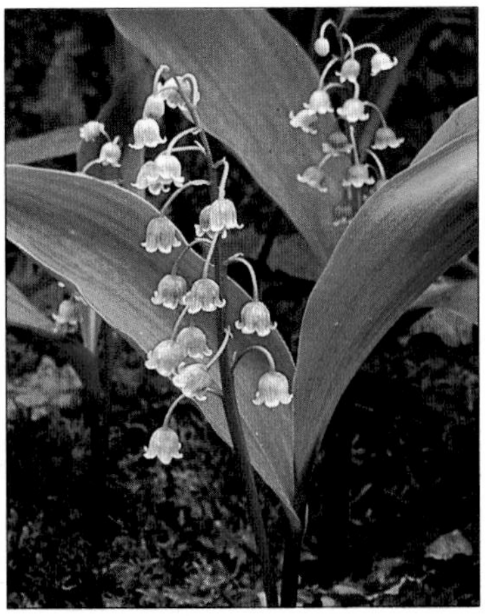

Convallaria majalis var. *rosea*

margins, and flowers 9–10mm (⅜–½in) across; ↕ 25cm (10in). **'Prolificans'** has panicle-like, branched inflorescences of sometimes slightly malformed flowers. **var. *rosea*** ■ has pale mauvish pink flowers; ↕ 20cm (8in).

CONVOLVULUS

Bindweed

CONVOLVULACEAE

Genus of about 250 species of upright, climbing, or scrambling annuals and perennials, and evergreen shrubs or subshrubs, occurring in diverse habitats in subtropical and temperate areas. They have mostly entire leaves and produce solitary or clustered, funnel- or trumpet-shaped flowers. Grow in a rock garden, on a sunny bank, or in a mixed or herbaceous border. In frost-prone areas, grow half-hardy and frost-tender species in a temperate greenhouse. In areas with cold, wet winters, grow *C. cneorum* and *C. sabatius* in containers, and move them into a cold greenhouse in winter. Species with running rootstocks can prove invasive.
• **HARDINESS** Fully hardy to frost tender.
• **CULTIVATION** Grow in poor to moderately fertile, gritty, well-drained soil in a sheltered site in full sun. Dead-head annuals to prolong flowering. Confine vigorous species by planting in a container plunged into the soil. In containers, use a loam-based potting compost (JI No.1), and water freely when in growth; keep just moist during winter. Pruning group 8 for *C. cneorum*.
• **PROPAGATION** Sow seed of annuals *in situ* in mid-spring, or in autumn with

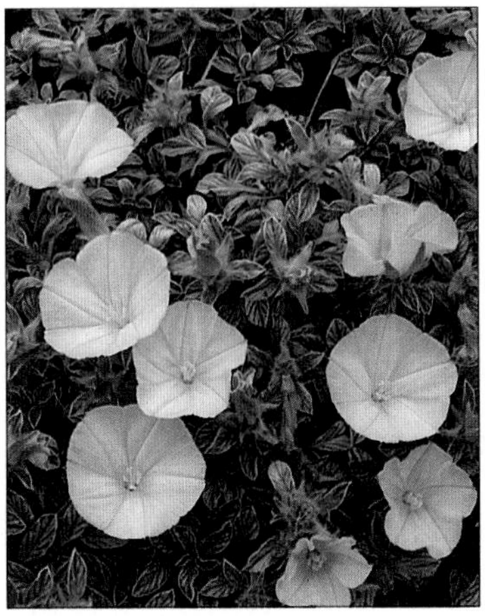

Convolvulus boissieri

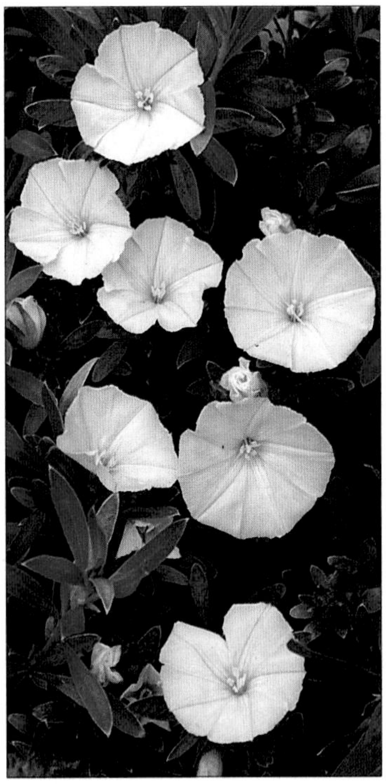

Convolvulus cneorum

cloche protection in frost-prone areas. For perennials, shrubs, and subshrubs, sow seed at 13–18°C (55–64°F) in spring; root softwood cuttings in late spring or greenwood cuttings in summer. Divide perennials in spring.
• **PESTS AND DISEASES** Susceptible to red spider mites and aphids under glass.

C. althaeoides. Vigorous, slender, climbing or trailing perennial with ovate to heart-shaped, shallowly to deeply lobed, hairy, silvery green leaves, to 3cm (1¼in) long. Axillary clusters of 1–3 widely funnel-shaped, clear pink flowers, to 4cm (1½in) across, are borne in mid- and late summer. Invasive, but suitable for a container. ↕ to 15cm (6in), ↔ indefinite. S. Europe. ✲✲✲. **subsp. *tenuissimus***, syn. *C. elegantissimus*, has more finely dissected leaves, with a covering of dense, soft, silvery hairs.
C. boissieri ■ syn. *C. nitidus*. Creeping, mat- or cushion-forming perennial with clustered, ovate, silky-hairy, silvery grey leaves, to 3cm (1¼in) long. Bears short-stemmed, axillary clusters of 1–4 funnel-shaped white, sometimes pink-flushed flowers, to 2cm (¾in) across, with small yellow centres, in early summer. Does not always flower freely. ↕ to 8cm (3in), ↔ 40cm (16in) or more. Spain. ✲✲✲
C. cneorum ■ 🏆 Compact, rounded, bushy shrub with inversely lance-shaped to linear, silky, silver-green leaves, 3–6cm (1¼–2½in) long. Funnel-shaped white flowers, to 4cm (1½in) across, with yellow centres, are borne from pink buds in axillary clusters from late spring to summer. ↕ 60cm (24in), ↔ 90cm (36in). C. and W. Mediterranean. ✲✲
C. elegantissimus see *C. althaeoides* subsp. *tenuissimus*.
C. mauritanicus see *C. sabatius*.
C. minor see *C. tricolor*.
C. nitidus see *C. boissieri*.
C. purpureus see *Ipomoea purpurea*.
C. sabatius ■ 🏆 syn. *C. mauritanicus*. Trailing, slender-stemmed, woody-based perennial with oblong to broadly ovate, mid-green leaves, to 3cm (1¼in) long. Produces a profusion of shallowly funnel-shaped, pale to deep lavender-blue flowers, 1.5–2.5cm (½–1in) across, in clusters of 1–3 from the leaf axils, from summer to early autumn. ↕ 15cm (6in), ↔ to 50cm (20in). Spain, Italy, North Africa. ✲✲
C. tricolor, syn. *C. minor*. Bushy, upright then spreading, red-stemmed annual or short-lived perennial with ovate to lance-shaped, dark green leaves, to 4cm (1½in) long. Solitary, open funnel-shaped, royal blue flowers, to 4cm (1½in) across, feathered white at the petal bases, with yellow eyes, are borne in long succession in summer; each bloom lasts only a day. ↕ 30–40cm (12–16in), ↔ 23–30cm (9–12in). Portugal to Greece, N. Africa. ✲✲✲.

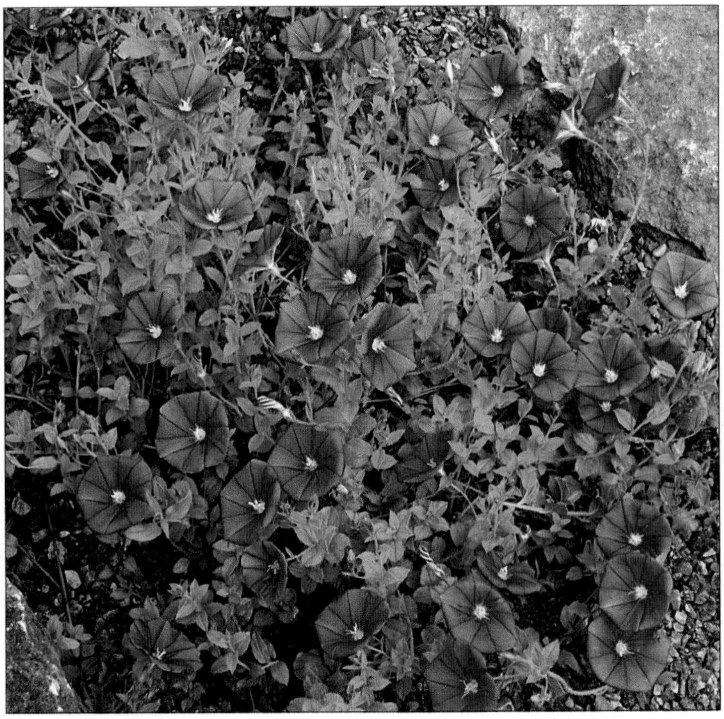

Convolvulus sabatius

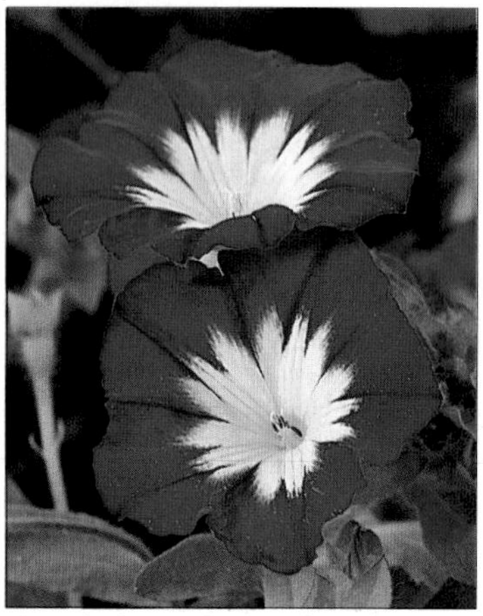

Convolvulus tricolor 'Royal Ensign'

'Royal Ensign' ■ produces deep blue flowers, to 5cm (2in) across; grow in a hanging basket; ↕ to 30cm (1ft).

▷ ***Cooperia*** see *Zephyranthes*

COPERNICIA

Wax palm

ARECACEAE/PALMAE

Genus of about 24 species of slow-growing, single-stemmed palms from savannah and forest, often in dry areas prone to periodic flooding, in Cuba, Hispaniola, and South America. Leaves, borne in dense, terminal clusters, are pinnate with the 10–60 leaflets arranged so that the leaves appear to be palmately lobed. On fading, the leaves remain in place, hanging down and forming a thatch-like skirt. The bowl-shaped, 3-petalled flowers are borne in panicles between the leaves. In frost-prone areas, grow as houseplants or in a warm greenhouse or conservatory. In warmer areas, use as specimen trees.
• **Hardiness** Frost tender.
• **Cultivation** Under glass, grow in loam-based potting compost (JI No.3) in full light, with shade from hot sun. In the growing season, water freely and applying a balanced liquid fertilizer monthly; water sparingly in winter. Pot on or top-dress in spring. Outdoors, grow in fertile, moist but well-drained soil in sun or partial shade.
• **Propagation** Sow seed at 23–27°C (73–81°F) in spring.
• **Pests and diseases** Red spider mites may be a problem under glass.

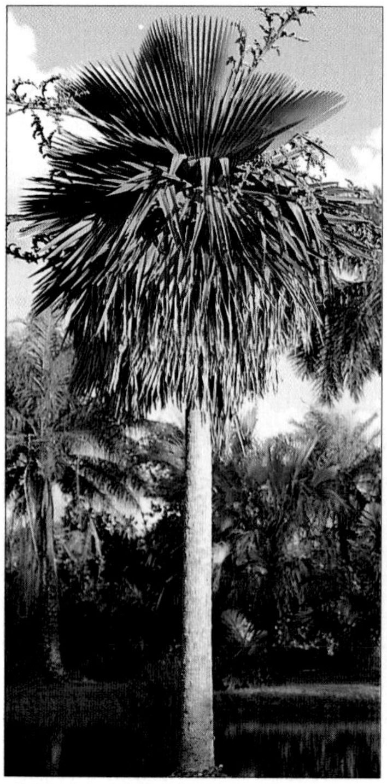

Copernicia macroglossa

C. macroglossa ■ 🌴 (Petticoat palm). Single-stemmed palm with a short, sturdy trunk covered in a skirt of dead leaves. Wedge-shaped leaflets, the outer ones with spiny margins, are stalkless or have very short stalks, and are usually deep green, to 1.4m (4½ft) long. Very small, greenish white flowers are borne in panicles that protrude beyond the leaf tips in summer. ↕ 5–7m (15–22ft), ↔ to 3m (10ft). Cuba. ⊛ (min. 13°C/55°F)

COPIAPOA

CACTACEAE

Genus of 10–20 species of slow-growing, solitary or clustered, perennial cacti from coastal deserts of N. Chile. The stems have warty ribs and spiny areoles. Funnel-shaped, diurnal flowers, mostly in shades of yellow, are borne from the densely woolly crowns in summer, followed by spherical green fruits with glossy black seeds. In frost-prone areas, grow as houseplants or in a warm greenhouse. In warmer areas, grow in a desert garden.
• **Hardiness** Frost tender.
• **Cultivation** Under glass, grow in a mix of 3 parts standard cactus compost and 1 part perlite in bright filtered light. From spring to early autumn, water moderately, applying a balanced liquid fertilizer monthly. Keep dry at other times. Outdoors, grow in gritty, poor soil in full sun, with some midday shade. See also pp.48–49.
• **Propagation** Sow seed at 19–24°C (66–75°F) in early spring. Remove offsets in summer.
• **Pests and diseases** Mealybugs may be a problem under glass.

C. barquitensis see *C. hypogaea.*
C. cinerea ■ Simple or clump-forming cactus producing spherical then cylindrical, 14- to 30-ribbed, greyish white stems, to 20cm (8in) across. Dark brown areoles bear 1 or 2 black or grey spines. Bright yellow flowers, 3.5cm (1½in) long, are produced in summer. ↕ to 70cm (3ft), rarely taller, ↔ to 40cm (16in). N. Chile. ⊛ (min. 10°C/50°F).
var. *gigantea*, syn. *C. haseltoniana*, bears completely grey stems with 20 or more very prominent ribs and dark brown spines; ↔ 20cm (8in).
C. haseltoniana see *C. cinerea* var. *gigantea.*
C. hypogaea, syn. *C. barquitensis.* Simple or clump-forming cactus with flattened-spherical, dark brownish green stems, 6–7cm (2½–3in) across, with 12 or more ribs. White-woolly areoles bear a few white radial spines. Yellow flowers, 2cm (¾in) long, are borne in summer. ↕ 4–7cm (1½–3in), ↔ 12cm (5in). N. Chile. ⊛ (min. 10°C/50°F)
C. krainziana ■ Clump-forming cactus with spherical, 13- to 24-ribbed, greyish green stems, to 12cm (5in) across. Grey areoles bear grey spines (10–12 radials and 14–20 centrals). Golden yellow flowers, 3.5cm (1½in) long, are produced in summer. ↕ 10cm (4in) or more, ↔ to 1m (3ft). N. Chile. ⊛ (min. 10°C/50°F)

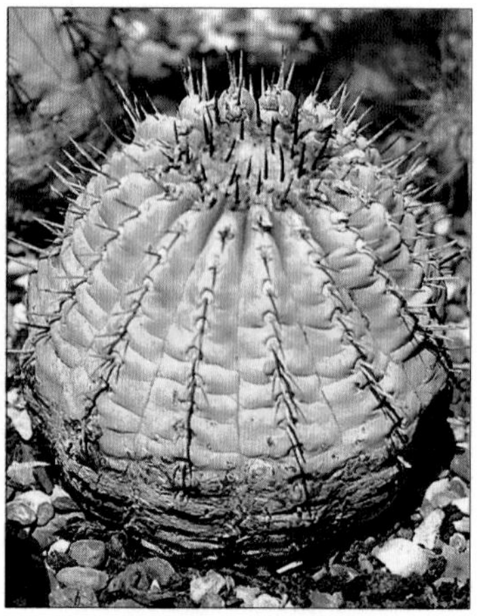

Copiapoa cinerea

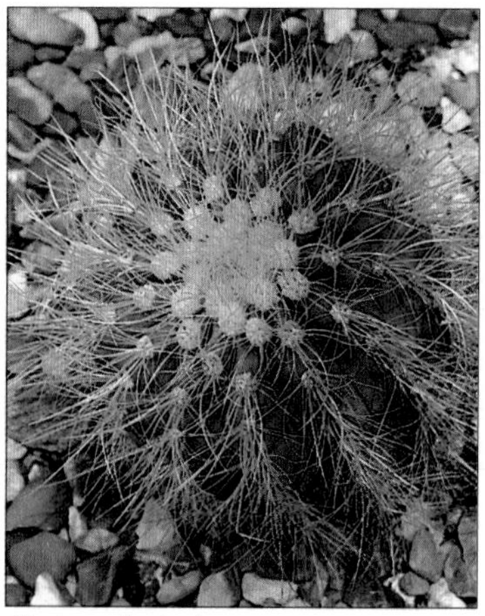

Copiapoa krainziana

▷ **Copper beech** see *Fagus sylvatica* f. *purpurea*
▷ **Copperleaf** see *Acalypha wilkesiana*

COPROSMA

RUBIACEAE

Genus of about 90 species of evergreen shrubs and small trees found in forest, swamp, grassland, and rocky areas, from sea level to mountainous regions, from Indonesia to Australia, New Zealand, and the Pacific islands. The opposite leaves are simple, linear to rounded, often leathery, and light to dark green, purple, or brown. The inconspicuous, usually dioecious, tubular or narrowly funnel-shaped flowers are borne singly or in cymes or clusters. Coprosmas are valued for their handsome foliage, and, where plants of both sexes are grown together, for their mainly spherical, brightly coloured, succulent berries, 4–10mm (⅛–½in) across, usually borne in autumn. Grow in a rock garden or shrub border. In frost-prone areas, grow half-hardy species and cultivars in a cool greenhouse or conservatory.
• **Hardiness** Frost hardy to half hardy.
• **Cultivation** Under glass, grow in loam-based potting compost (JI No.2) with additional grit in bright filtered light, with good ventilation. In growth, water freely and apply a balanced liquid fertilizer monthly; water moderately at other times. Outdoors, grow in neutral to slightly acid, moderately fertile, moist but well-drained soil in sun or partial shade. Pruning group 8.
• **Propagation** Sow seed in containers in a cold frame in spring. Root semi-ripe cuttings in late summer.
• **Pests and diseases** Trouble free.

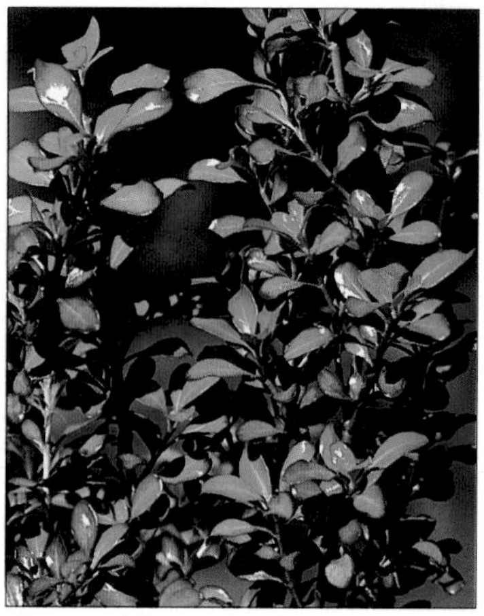

Coprosma 'Coppershine'

C. acerosa* f. *brunnea see *C. brunnea.*
C. baueri see *C. repens.*
C. baueriana see *C. repens.*
***C.* 'Beatson's Gold'.** Compact, rounded, female shrub with spreading branches and ovate, bright green leaves, to 1.5cm (½in) long, splashed yellow in the centres. Bright red berries are borne in autumn. ↕↔ 1.5m (5ft). ❄❄
***C.* 'Blue Pearls'.** Mat-forming female shrub with rigid, spreading branches and inversely lance-shaped, dark green leaves, to 1cm (½in) long. Translucent blue berries are produced in summer. ↕ 45cm (18in), ↔ 90cm (36in). ❄❄
***C.* 'Brunette'.** Bushy female shrub with ovate-oblong, glossy bronze leaves, 2.5cm (1in) long. Orange berries are borne in autumn. ↕↔ 1m (3ft). ❄❄
C. brunnea, syn. *C. acerosa* f. *brunnea.* Mat-forming, dioecious shrub with spreading, tangled, wiry shoots and slender, linear, brownish green leaves, to 1.5cm (½in) long. Translucent blue berries are produced on female plants in autumn. ↕ 45cm (18in), ↔ 2m (6ft). New Zealand. ❄❄
***C.* 'Chocolate Soldier'.** Erect, bushy, male shrub with oblong to oblong-ovate, very glossy, chocolate-brown to dark green leaves, 1–2cm (½–¾in) long. ↕ 1m (3ft), ↔ 45cm (18in). ❄

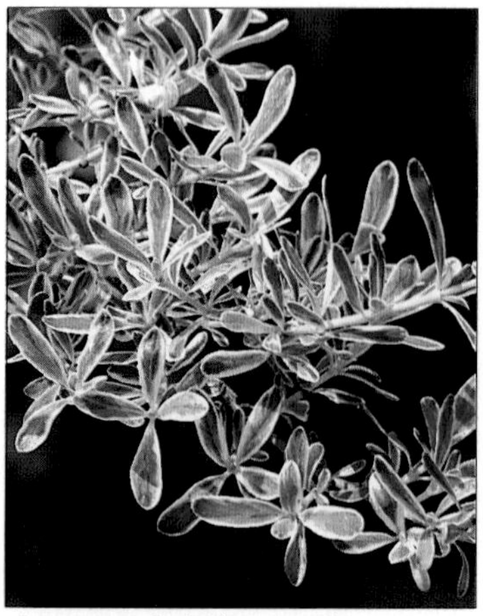

Coprosma x *kirkii* 'Variegata'

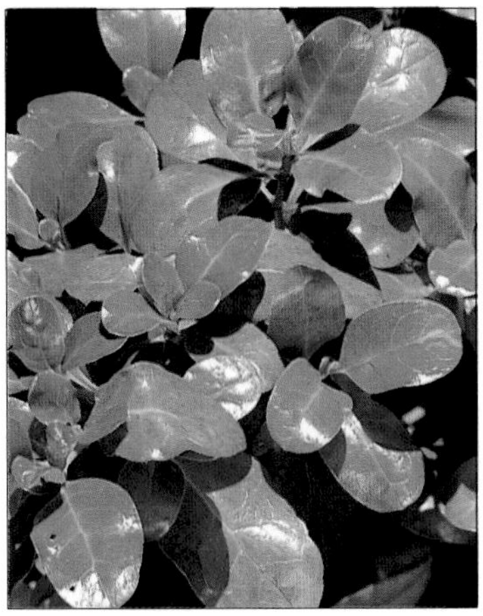
Coprosma repens

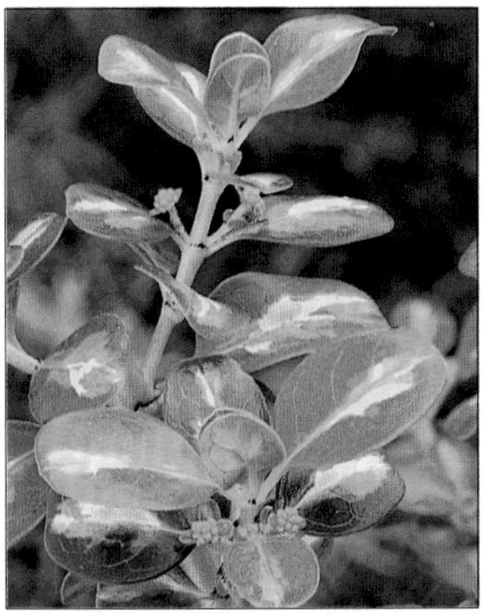
Coprosma repens 'Picturata'

***C.* 'Coppershine'** ▣ Bushy male shrub with narrowly ovate-oblong, glossy, dark green to purple leaves, suffused copper, 2.5cm (1in) long. ↕↔ 1m (3ft). ❄
C.* x *kirkii (*C. acerosa* x *C. repens*) Variants of this hybrid are of irregular, spreading habit. Arching branches bear linear-oblong, narrowly obovate, or lance-shaped, dark green leaves, to 4cm (1½in) long. In autumn, produces oblong-spherical, translucent or white berries, flushed or flecked red. ↕ 1.5m (5ft), ↔ 2m (6ft). New Zealand. ❄. **'Variegata'** ▣ is a spreading female shrub, with white-margined, grey-green leaves and white berries; ↕ 75cm (30in), ↔ 1.5m (5ft).
***C.* 'Kiwi-gold'.** Prostrate male shrub with elliptic to oblong, glossy, mid-green leaves, 3cm (1¼in) long, boldly splashed yellow. ↕ 25cm (10in), ↔ 1m (3ft). ❄❄
C. repens ▣♀ syn. *C. baueri*, *C. baueriana* (Looking glass plant). Large, dioecious shrub or small tree, sometimes prostrate, with broadly ovate-oblong, fleshy, glossy, deep green leaves, 2–8cm (¾–3in) long. Bears obovoid, orange-red berries, to 1cm (½in) long, from late summer to autumn. ↕ 0.6–8m (2–25ft), ↔ 1–3m (3–10ft). New Zealand. ❄. **'Exotica'** is a female version of 'Picturata'. **'Marble Queen'** ▣ is male, with leaves splashed creamy white. **'Picturata'** ▣ is male, and has leaves with deep cream to yellow centres and orange berries.
C. robusta. Vigorous, usually dioecious, erect then spreading shrub with elliptic, semi-glossy, dark green leaves, 7–12cm (3–5in) long. Ovoid, deep orange to yellow berries are produced in autumn. ↕ 4–6m (12–20ft), ↔ 2–4m (6–12ft). New Zealand. ❄. **'Variegata'** is male, with a central yellow blaze on each leaf. **'Williamsii Variegata'**, syn. 'Williamsii', is bisexual, with dark and light green marbled leaves, margined creamy yellow, and orange berries.

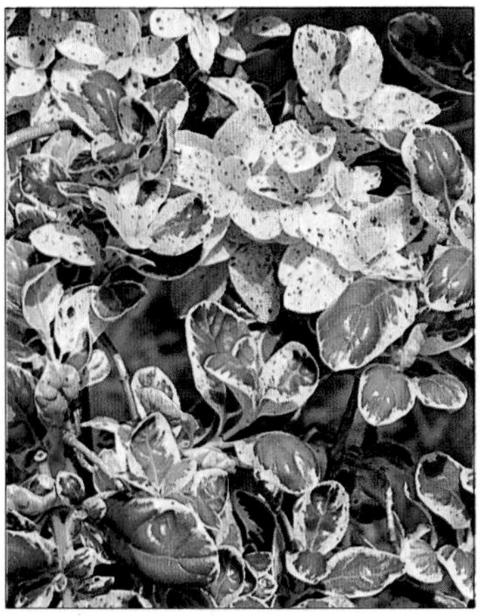
Coprosma repens 'Marble Queen'

COPTIS
Gold thread
RANUNCULACEAE

Genus of 10 species of low-growing, evergreen perennials from temperate, usually coniferous woodland and bogs in the N. hemisphere. They produce slender yellow rhizomes and basal, 3- to 5-palmate or finely palmately lobed leaves. Star-shaped flowers are borne on leafless stems above the foliage. Grow in a peat bed or woodland garden.
- **HARDINESS** Fully hardy.
- **CULTIVATION** Grow in moderately fertile, humus-rich, moist but well-drained, slightly acid soil in a sheltered site in full or partial shade.
- **PROPAGATION** Sow seed in a cold frame as soon as ripe, or divide in spring.
- **PESTS AND DISEASES** Trouble free.

C. quinquefolia. Rhizomatous, spreading, delicate perennial with long-stalked, 5-palmate leaves, to 2.5cm (1in) long, with obovate or diamond-shaped leaflets. Solitary, upturned white flowers are borne on stems 8–12cm (3–5in) long, in spring. ↕ to 12cm (5in), ↔ to 20cm (8in). Japan, Taiwan. ❄❄❄

▷**Coral bean** see *Erythrina herbacea*
▷**Coral bells** see *Heuchera sanguinea*
▷**Coralberry** see *Symphoricarpos orbiculatus*
▷**Coral bush** see *Templetonia retusa*
▷**Coral drops** see *Bessera elegans*
▷**Coral flower** see *Heuchera*
▷**Coral gem** see *Lotus berthelotii*
▷**Corallita** see *Antigonon*
White see *Porana paniculata*
▷**Coral pea** see *Hardenbergia, Kennedia*
Black see *Kennedia nigricans*
Dusky see *Kennedia rubicunda*
Purple see *Hardenbergia violacea*
▷**Coral plant** see *Berberidopsis corallina, Jatropha multifida, Russelia equisetiformis*
▷**Coral tree** see *Erythrina*
Common see *E. crista-galli*
▷**Coral vine** see *Antigonon*
Common see *Kennedia coccinea*

CORDYLINE
Cabbage palm, Cabbage tree
AGAVACEAE

Genus of 15 species of evergreen shrubs or tree-like, woody-stemmed perennials, the larger ones resembling palms, found on open hillsides and in scrub and open forest in S.E. Asia and the Pacific, including Australasia. The tufted or rosetted, leathery leaves are simple, entire, and lance-shaped to linear. Sweetly scented, shallowly cup-shaped, 6-tepalled flowers, 6–10mm (¼–½in) across, are produced in sometimes large, conspicuous, terminal panicles, followed by spherical, white, red, blue, or purple berries, 3–8mm (⅛–⅜in) across. In frost-prone areas, grow as houseplants or in a cool, temperate, or warm greenhouse or conservatory. In warmer areas, grow as specimen plants, in a mixed or shrub border, or in a courtyard garden.
- **HARDINESS** Half hardy to frost tender.
- **CULTIVATION** Under glass, grow in loamless or loam-based potting compost (JI No.2), with full light for green-leaved species, bright filtered or indirect light for variants with coloured foliage. In growth, water moderately and apply a balanced liquid fertilizer monthly; water sparingly in winter. Top-dress or pot on in spring. Outdoors, grow in fertile, well-drained soil in sun or partial shade.
- **PROPAGATION** Sow seed at 16°C (61°F) in spring. Remove well-rooted suckers in spring.
- **PESTS AND DISEASES** Scale insects and red spider mites may prove troublesome under glass.

C. australis ♀♆ syn. *Dracaena australis* (New Zealand cabbage palm). Erect, palm-like tree, branching sparingly with age. Arching, lance-shaped to linear leaves, 30–90cm (12–36in) long, are light green to almost yellow-green. In summer, mature trees bear tiny, creamy white flowers in broad panicles, 1m (3ft) or more long, followed by white or blue-tinted berries. ↕ 3–10m (10–30ft) or more, ↔ 1–4m (3–12ft). New Zealand. ❄. **'Albertii'** ▣♀ has matt-green leaves with red midribs, cream stripes, and pink margins. **'Atropurpurea'** has leaves flushed purple at the bases and on the main veins beneath. **'Doucettii'** has leaves with creamy white stripes and pink-flushed margins. **'Purple Tower'** has broad leaves, heavily flushed plum-purple. **'Purpurea'** is similar to 'Purple Tower' but has slightly paler leaves. **'Torbay Dazzler'** produces leaves with bold cream stripes and margins. **'Variegata'** ▣ has leaves longitudinally striped creamy white. **'Veitchii'** has leaves strongly flushed crimson at the bases and on the main veins beneath.
C. banksii ♆ Sparingly clump-forming or single-stemmed, erect shrub or, rarely, small tree with few branches and a crown of arching, strap-shaped, mid- to yellow-green leaves, 1m (3ft) or more long. White flowers are borne in broadly pyramidal panicles, 1–2m (3–6ft) long, in summer, followed by white or blue-tinted fruit. ↕ 3–4m (10–12ft), ↔ 2–3m (6–10ft). New Zealand. ❄
C. fruticosa, syn. *C. terminalis* (Good luck tree, Ti tree). Erect, suckering, clump-forming shrub with generally unbranched stems and strap-shaped, deep green leaves, 30–60cm (12–24in) long. In summer, produces white to purple flowers in loose panicles, 30–50cm (12–20in) long, followed by bright red berries. ↕ 2–5m (6–15ft), ↔ 1–2.5m (3–8ft). Tropical S.E. Asia, E. Australia, larger Pacific islands. ❁ (min. 13°C/55°F). **'Amabilis'** has broad, glossy, bronze and red leaves, with flecks of white and pink when mature. **'Baby Ti'** has leaf margins suffused copper-red; ↕↔ to 60cm (24in). **'Baptistii'** has broad, strongly recurved leaves streaked yellow and pink. **'Firebrand'**, syn. 'Red Dracaena', has compact heads of foliage, flushed deep red-purple. **'Guilfoylei'** has strongly tapered, recurved leaves streaked red, pink, and white, with white bases.

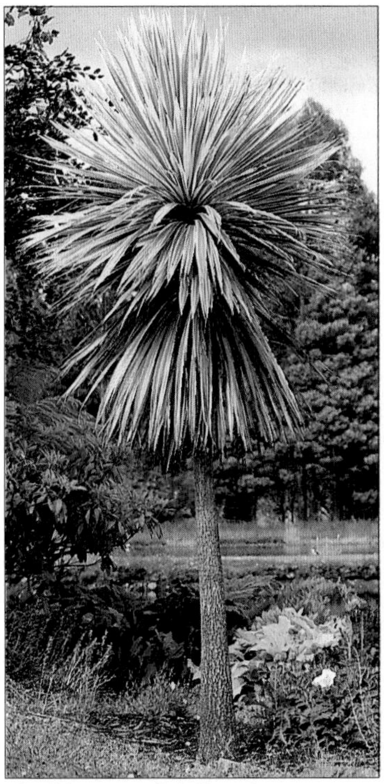
Cordyline australis 'Albertii'

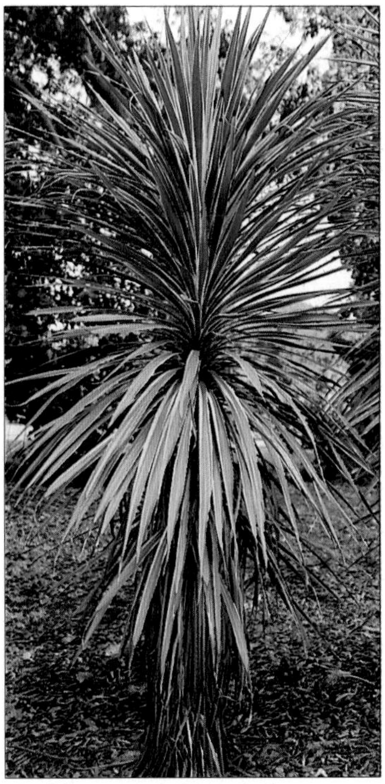
Cordyline australis 'Variegata'

C

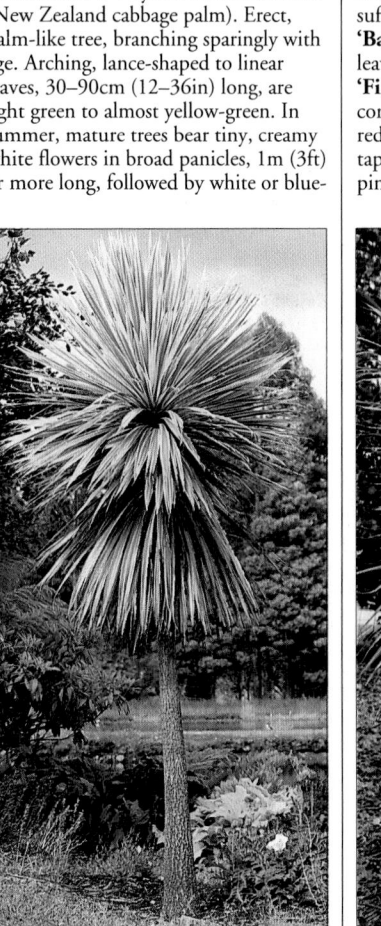

C

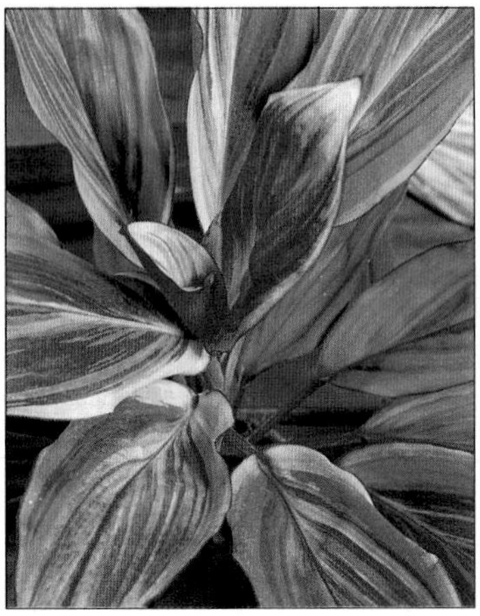

Cordyline fruticosa 'Tricolor'

'Hawaiian Bonsai' is compact, with dark crimson leaves; ↕ to 1m (3ft), ↔ to 60cm (24in). **'Margaret Storey'** is compact, with copper-flushed leaves splashed red and pink; ↕↔ 1m (3ft) or more. **'Mayi'** has red leaves when young, becoming deep green with red margins with age. **'Negri'** has deep copper-maroon foliage. **'Red Dracaena'** see 'Firebrand'. **'Tricolor'** ▣ has broad leaves boldly and very irregularly streaked and splashed in shades of red, pink, and cream.

C. indivisa ▣ 🌴 syn. *Dracaena indivisa.* Thick-stemmed tree with a few branches at the top when mature. Each branch bears a tuft of narrowly lance-shaped, mid- to light green leaves, 1–2m (3–6ft) long, with red-veins above and suffused blue-white beneath. Cream flowers are borne in dense panicles, to 1.6m (5½ft) long, in summer, followed by bluish purple berries. ↕ 6–10m (20–30ft), ↔ 2–4m (6–12ft). Mountain forests in New Zealand. ❄. **'Purpurea'** has leaves suffused bronze-purple.

C. stricta. Erect, suckering shrub with low-arching, linear, toothed, deep green leaves, 20–60cm (8–24in) long. In summer, produces lilac to violet flowers, with reflexed petals, in loose, pyramidal panicles, to 60cm (24in) long, followed by purple or almost black berries. ↕ 2–3m (6–10ft), ↔ 1–2m (3–6ft). Rainforest in Australia (Queensland to New South Wales). ⊛ (min. 13°C/55°F). **'Discolor'** has bronze-purple leaves. **'Grandis'** is generally larger and more robust; ↕ to 3.5m (11ft). **'Rubra'** has foliage suffused copper-red.

C. terminalis see *C. fruticosa.*

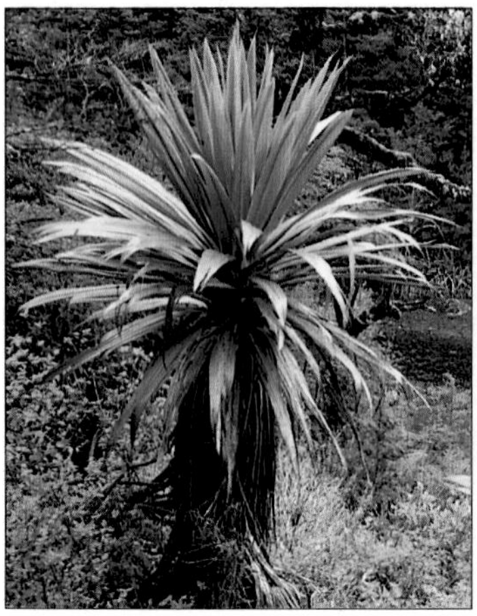

Cordyline indivisa

COREOPSIS

Tickseed

ASTERACEAE/COMPOSITAE

Genus of 80–100 species of hairless or softly hairy annuals and perennials, some becoming woody at the bases. They occur on prairies and in woodland in North and Central America, and Mexico. Most have upright stems and produce opposite leaves, which may be either simple and entire, pinnate, or palmate (either palmately lobed or fully divided, 3-palmate). Daisy-like, bright yellow flowerheads are borne on long stalks; they are good for cut flowers, and are attractive to bees. Grow in a sunny annual or herbaceous border. Some cultivars, although perennial, are grown as annuals; most flower freely in their first year from seed.

• **HARDINESS** Fully hardy to frost tender.

• **CULTIVATION** Outdoors, grow in fertile, well-drained soil in full sun or partial shade. Dead-head to prolong flowering. Support taller cultivars.

• **PROPAGATION** Sow seed of annuals *in situ*, in succession from early spring to early summer; sow perennials in a seedbed in mid-spring. Alternatively, sow seed at 13–16°C (55–61°F) in mid- or late winter; perennials will flower in the first year. Divide perennials in early spring. Root basal cuttings in spring.

• **PESTS AND DISEASES** Slugs and snails may prove troublesome.

C. auriculata. Rhizomatous perennial with erect, softly hairy stems bearing ovate to elliptic, entire or palmately lobed, mid-green leaves, to 12cm (5in) long. Solitary, bright yellow flowerheads, 5cm (2in) across, are borne from early to midsummer. ↕ to 80cm (32in), ↔ 60cm (24in). S.E. USA. ❄❄❄. **'Cutting Gold'** see 'Schnittgold'. **'Schnittgold'** ▣ syn. 'Cutting Gold', has vivid gold flowerheads. **'Superba'** produces bright orange-yellow flowerheads, 6cm (2½in) across, with maroon basal marks, from early to late summer; ↕ to 45cm (18in).

C. californica. Erect, branched, almost hairless annual with lance-shaped, entire to shallowly lobed, mostly basal, dark green leaves, to 15cm (6in) long. Produces solitary yellow flowerheads, to 3.5cm (1½in) across, in summer. ↕ to 45cm (18in), ↔ 23–30cm (9–12in). USA (California, S. Arizona), N.W. Mexico. ❄❄❄

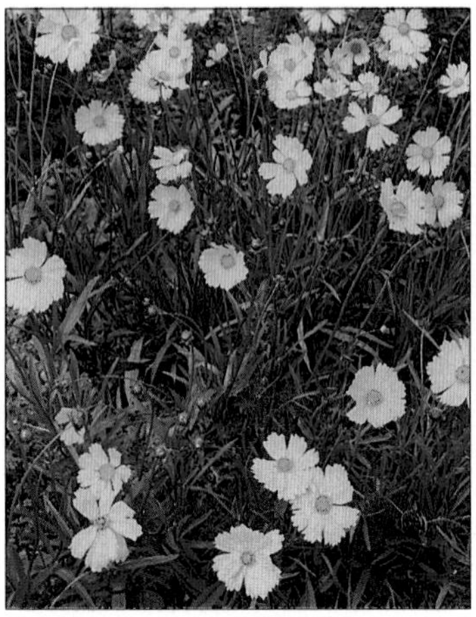

Coreopsis auriculata 'Schnittgold'

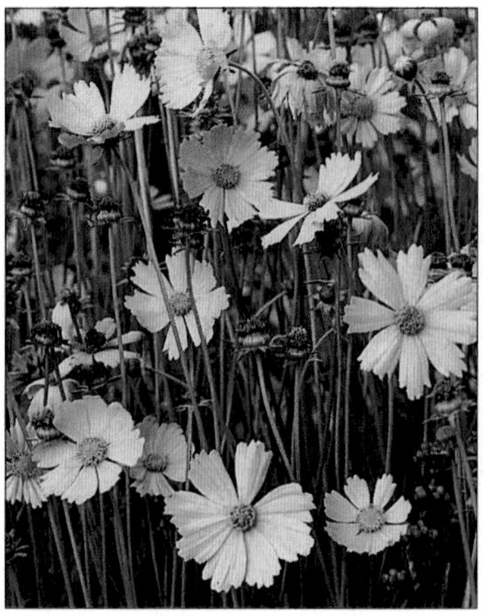

Coreopsis grandiflora 'Badengold'

C. grandiflora. Clump-forming, almost hairless perennial, often grown as an annual, with simple, lance-shaped or palmately lobed lower leaves, to 10cm (4in) long. Flowering stems produce 3- to 5-pinnate leaves with linear leaflets. From late spring to late summer, produces solitary flowerheads, to 6cm (2½in) across, consisting of golden yellow ray-florets, with unevenly cut outer margins, and darker yellow disc-florets. Excellent for cutting. Dislikes excessive heat. ↕ 45–90cm (18–36in), ↔ 45cm (18in). C. and S.E. USA. ❄❄❄. **'Badengold'** ▣ produces deep yellow flowerheads with orange centres; ↕ to 90cm (36in). **'Domino'** is a dwarf cultivar, producing yellow flowerheads; ↕ 40cm (16in). **'Early Sunrise'** ▣ is usually grown as an annual, and bears semi-double, deep yellow flowerheads, each flushed orange-yellow near the centre; ↕ to 45cm (18in). **'Gold Star'**, usually grown as an annual, bears golden yellow flowerheads and rolled or "quilled" petals; ↕ to 30cm (12in). **'Mayfield Giant'** has large, orange-yellow flowerheads, to 8cm (3in) across, and requires support; ↕ to 90cm (36in). **'Sunburst'** has double, rich yellow flowerheads. **'Sunray'** ▣, usually grown as an annual, has double, deep yellow flowerheads; ↕ 50–75cm (20–30in).

C. lanceolata ▣ Clump-forming, hairless perennial with usually entire, lance-shaped to inversely lance-shaped, mid-green leaves, to 15cm (6in) long. Flowering stems, with leaves only at the bases, produce solitary yellow flowerheads, 4–6cm (1½–2½in) across, from late spring to midsummer. ↕ to 60cm

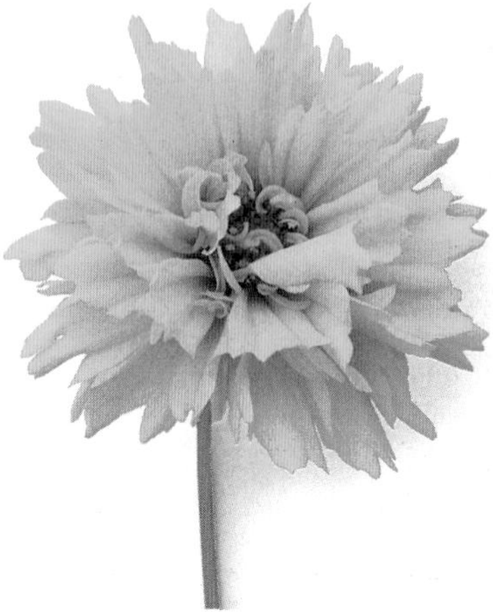

Coreopsis grandiflora 'Early Sunrise'

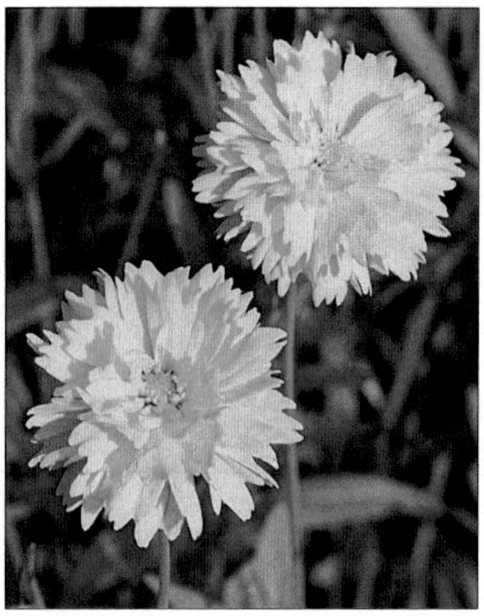

Coreopsis grandiflora 'Sunray'

(24in), ↔ 45cm (18in). C. and S. USA. ❄❄❄. **'Baby Sun'** see 'Sonnenkind'. **'Goldfink'** is a dwarf cultivar, bearing golden yellow flowerheads; ↕ to 25cm (10in). **'Sonnenkind'**, syn. 'Baby Sun', produces golden yellow flowerheads; ↕ 40cm (16in). **'Sterntaler'** produces yellow flowerheads with brown centres; ↕ to 40cm (16in).

C. tinctoria, syn. *Calliopsis tinctoria.* Erect, hairless, stiff-stemmed annual bearing mostly basal, mid- to dark green leaves, to 10cm (4in) long. Leaves are lance-shaped and either entire or pinnate or 2-pinnate with linear leaflets. In summer, produces solitary, bright yellow flowerheads, to 5cm (2in) across, shading to brown-red at the bases, with dark red disc-florets. Dark red, purple, and brown variants also occur; ↕ to 1.2m (4ft), ↔ 30–45cm (12–18in). North America. ❄❄❄. **'Mahogany Midget'** is a dwarf cultivar, with yellow-centred, rich mahogany-scarlet flowerheads; ↕ to 30cm (12in). **'Tiger Flower'** is a dwarf cultivar, producing flowerheads that vary from pure crimson to golden yellow, many of them speckled and striped with both colours; ↕ to 23cm (9in), ↔ to 20cm (8in).

C. verticillata ▣ Bushy, rhizomatous, slowly spreading, hairless perennial with numerous branched stems. Leaves are 3-pinnate, to 6cm (2½in) long, with linear, mid-green leaflets. Bears yellow flowerheads, to 5cm (2in) across, in loose corymbs in early summer. ↕ 60–80cm (24–32in), ↔ 45cm (18in). S.E. USA. ❄❄❄. **'Golden Shower'** see 'Grandiflora'. **'Grandiflora'** 🏆 syn. 'Golden Shower', has dark yellow

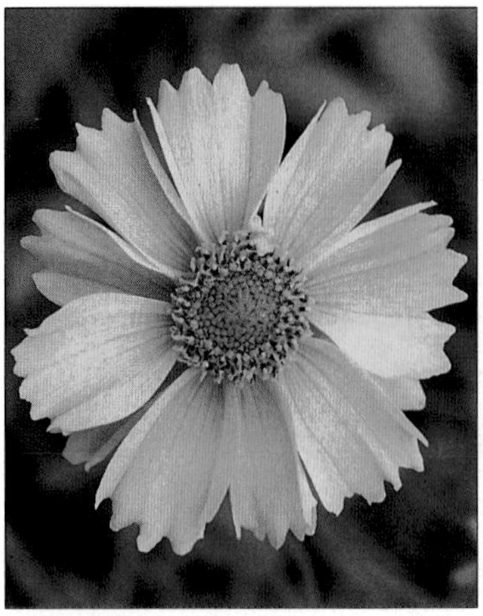

Coreopsis lanceolata

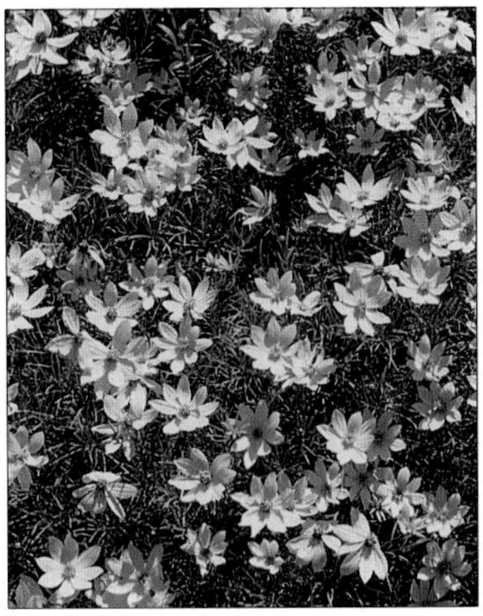

Coreopsis verticillata

flowerheads. **'Moonbeam'** has lemon-yellow flowerheads; ↕ to 50cm (20in). **'Zagreb'** has golden yellow flowerheads, and is drought-resistant; ↕ 25–30cm (10–12in), ↔ to 30cm (12in).

▷**Coriander** see *Coriandrum*

CORIANDRUM

Coriander

APIACEAE/UMBELLIFERAE

Genus of 2 species of annuals, with hairless, strongly aromatic foliage, occurring in scrub, wasteland, fallow fields, or steppes in the E. Mediterranean region. The basal leaves are ovate and either pinnate to 3-pinnate, with toothed, linear or oblong leaflets, or pinnatisect; the upper leaves are pinnate to 3-pinnate with linear leaflets. Terminal, compound umbels of small, cup-shaped, white or purple-flushed sterile flowers, surrounded by larger fertile flowers, are followed by spherical, ribbed fruits. Grow in a herb garden for the leaves and seeds, which are used in cooking.

- **HARDINESS** Fully hardy.
- **CULTIVATION** Grow in light, fertile, well-drained soil, in full sun for seed production or in partial shade for best leaf growth. Pick leaves throughout the growing season. Harvest seed when the fruits begin to change colour and become pleasantly aromatic.
- **PROPAGATION** Sow seed *in situ* in spring. May self-seed.
- **PESTS AND DISEASES** Susceptible to fungal wilt.

C. sativum. Aromatic annual with long-stalked, glossy, bright green leaves, 1cm (½in) long. From midsummer to autumn, 5-petalled, white or pale purple flowers are produced in umbels to 1.5cm (½in) across, followed by pale golden brown fruit. ↕ 50cm (20in), ↔ 20cm (8in). E. Mediterranean. ❄❄❄

CORIARIA

CORIARIACEAE

Genus of about 8 species of small trees or shrubs, usually deciduous, and rhizomatous, herbaceous or subshrubby perennials, which occur in warm-temperate climates in grassland, scrub, and woodland, often in mountainous regions. They are cultivated for their attractive habit, foliage, and fruits. Arching shoots bear opposite, simple, entire leaves. Small, insignificant green

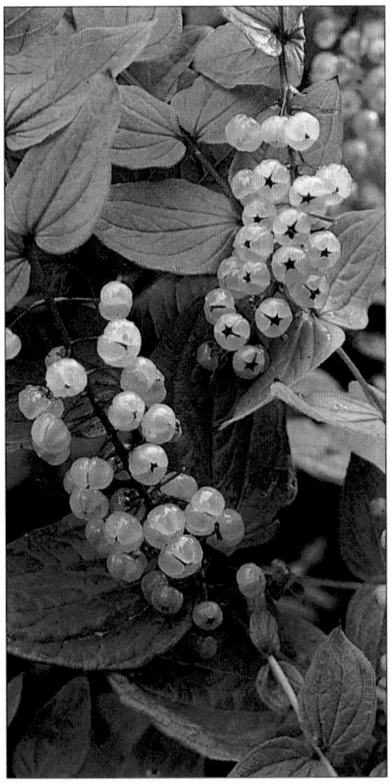

Coriaria terminalis var. *xanthocarpa*

flowers are produced in terminal or axillary racemes in spring, and followed by ornamental, fleshy, black, purplish black, red, or yellow fruits. In some species, male and female flowers are borne on different plants. *Coriaria* species are suitable for a shrub border or rock garden. In frost-prone climates, grow half-hardy and frost-tender species in a cool greenhouse. The leaves and fruits of some species may cause severe stomach upset if ingested; in other species, the fruits are edible, although the seeds are thought to be poisonous.

- **HARDINESS** Frost hardy to frost tender.
- **CULTIVATION** Grow in deep, moderately fertile, well-drained soil in a sheltered site in full sun. Provide a dry winter mulch in frost-prone areas. Pruning group 1 or 2.
- **PROPAGATION** Sow seed in containers in a cold frame as soon as ripe. Sow seed of tender species at 13–16°C (55–61°F) in spring. Divide rhizomatous species in spring. Root greenwood cuttings in summer.
- **PESTS AND DISEASES** Trouble free.

C. terminalis. Deciduous, rhizomatous subshrub with arching shoots bearing broadly lance-shaped, mid-green leaves, to 8cm (3in) long, turning red in autumn. Small green flowers are borne in terminal racemes, to 15cm (6in) long, in late spring, followed in late summer by spherical, fleshy, dark blackish red fruit, to 1cm (½in) across. ↕ 1m (3ft), ↔ 2m (6ft). W. China, Himalayas. ❄❄. **var. *xanthocarpa*** ■ has translucent yellow fruit.

▷**Corkscrew flower** see *Vigna caracalla*
▷**Cork tree, Amur** see *Phellodendron amurense*
▷**Corn cockle** see *Agrostemma*
▷**Cornel** see *Cornus*
Bentham's see *C. capitata*
Dwarf see *C. canadensis*
▷**Cornflower** see *Centaurea cyanus*
▷**Cornish heath** see *Erica vagans*
▷**Corn poppy** see *Papaver rhoeas*

CORNUS

syn. CHAMAEPERICLYMENUM, DENDROBENTHAMIA, THELYCRANIA

Cornel, Dogwood

CORNACEAE

Genus of about 45 species of mainly deciduous shrubs and small trees, and a few woody-based perennials, from grassland, thickets, woodland, rocky slopes, and swamps, mostly in N. temperate areas. The usually opposite, sometimes alternate leaves are lance-shaped-ovate to broadly ovate, and mid- to dark green. Small, star-shaped flowers are borne in terminal cymes, with or without bracts, in dense umbels with yellowish bracts that fall as the flowers open, or in dense clusters with conspicuous white or pink bracts. Those borne in cymes or umbels are followed by loose clusters of berries; those borne in clusters are followed by tight terminal clusters of berries or have the clusters united into compound, fleshy, strawberry-like fruits.

Dogwoods are grown for their showy bracts, elegant habit, fruits, and colourful autumn leaves; some are effective specimen trees or shrubs, especially in a woodland garden. Those with colourful winter shoots, grown as pollards, are useful for many situations, from a shrub border to a waterside garden. Use *C. canadensis* in woodland or for ground cover in a shrub border. The fruits of some species may cause mild stomach upset if ingested; contact with the leaf hairs may irritate skin.

- **HARDINESS** Fully hardy to frost hardy.
- **CULTIVATION** Grow "flowering dogwoods" (having large bracts), such as *C. capitata*, *C. florida*, *C. nuttallii*, and their hybrids, in fertile, humus-rich, well-drained, neutral to acid soil in sun or partial shade. *C. canadensis* prefers moist, acid soil. Others tolerate a range of soils and locations. Those grown for winter stems colour best in full sun. Pruning group 1; best with minimal pruning. Pruning group 7 for *C. alba*, *C. sanguinea*, and *C. stolonifera*.
- **PROPAGATION** Sow seed in a seedbed in autumn, or stratify and sow in spring. Divide *C. canadensis* in spring or autumn. Graft variegated cultivars of *C. alternifolia* and *C. controversa* in winter. Root greenwood cuttings in summer. Take hardwood cuttings of those grown for winter stems in autumn.
- **PESTS AND DISEASES** May be affected by anthracnose.

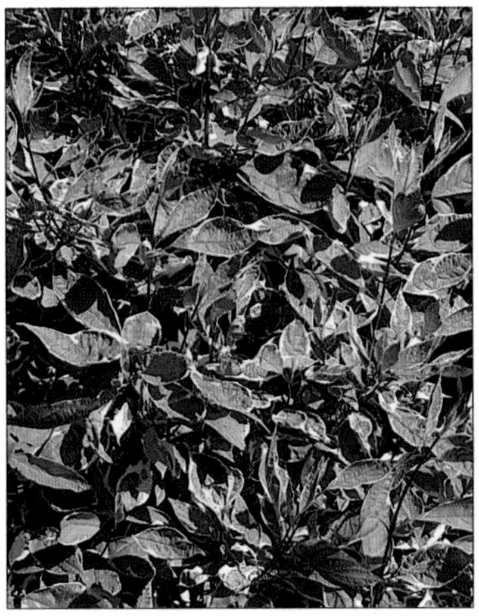

Cornus alba 'Elegantissima'

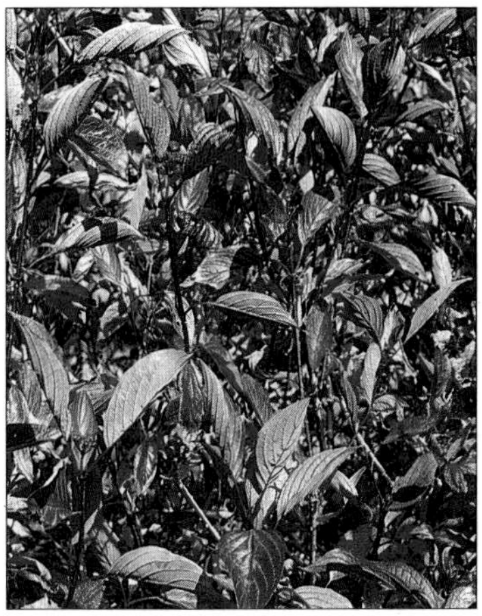

Cornus alba 'Kesselringii'

C. alba, syn. *Swida alba*, *Thelycrania alba* (Red-barked dogwood). Vigorous, upright, deciduous shrub with red winter shoots and ovate-elliptic, dark green leaves, to 10cm (4in) long, which turn red or orange in autumn. Bears white flowers in flat cymes, to 5cm (2in) across, in late spring and early summer. Ellipsoid fruit are white, often tinged blue. ↕↔ 3m (10ft). Siberia, N. China to Korea. ❄❄❄. **'Aurea'** has yellow leaves. **'Elegantissima'** ■ 🏆 has grey-green leaves, irregularly margined white. **'Gouchaultii'** has pink-flushed, yellow-margined leaves. **'Kesselringii'** ■ has blackish purple winter shoots and red and purple autumn leaves. **'Sibirica'** ■ 🏆 has bright red winter shoots and red autumn leaves. **'Spaethii'** ■ 🏆 has broadly yellow-margined leaves.

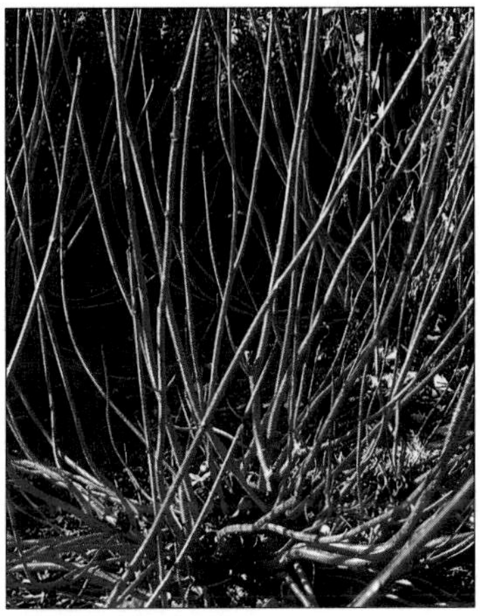

Cornus alba 'Sibirica'

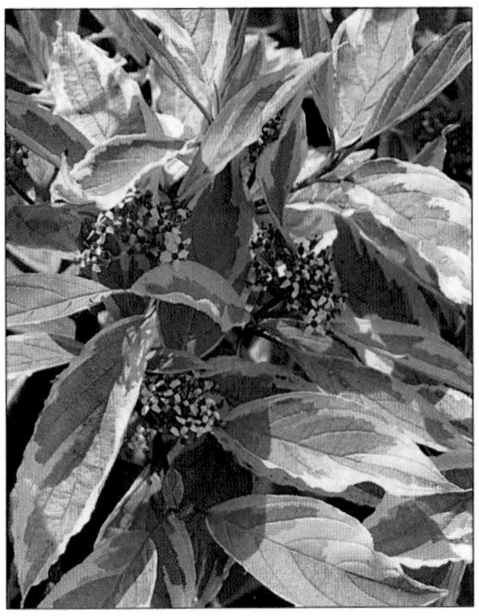

Cornus alba 'Spaethii'

CORNUS

C

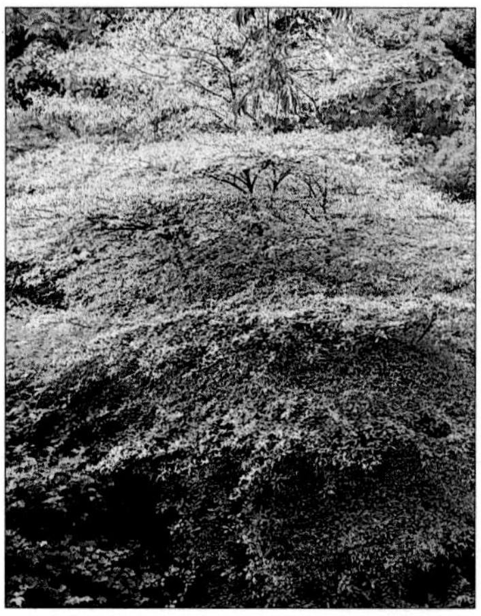

Cornus alternifolia 'Argentea'

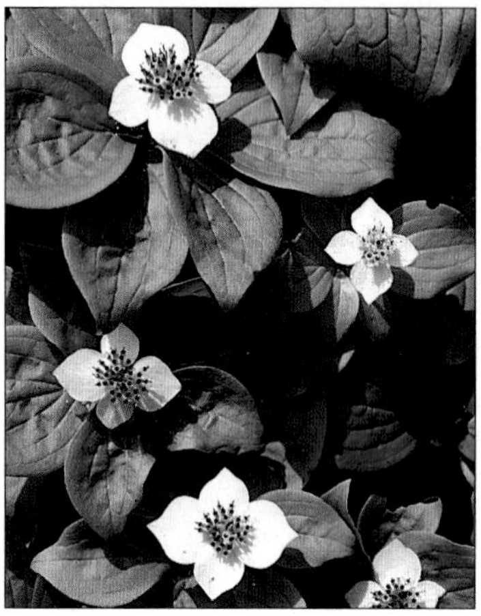

Cornus canadensis

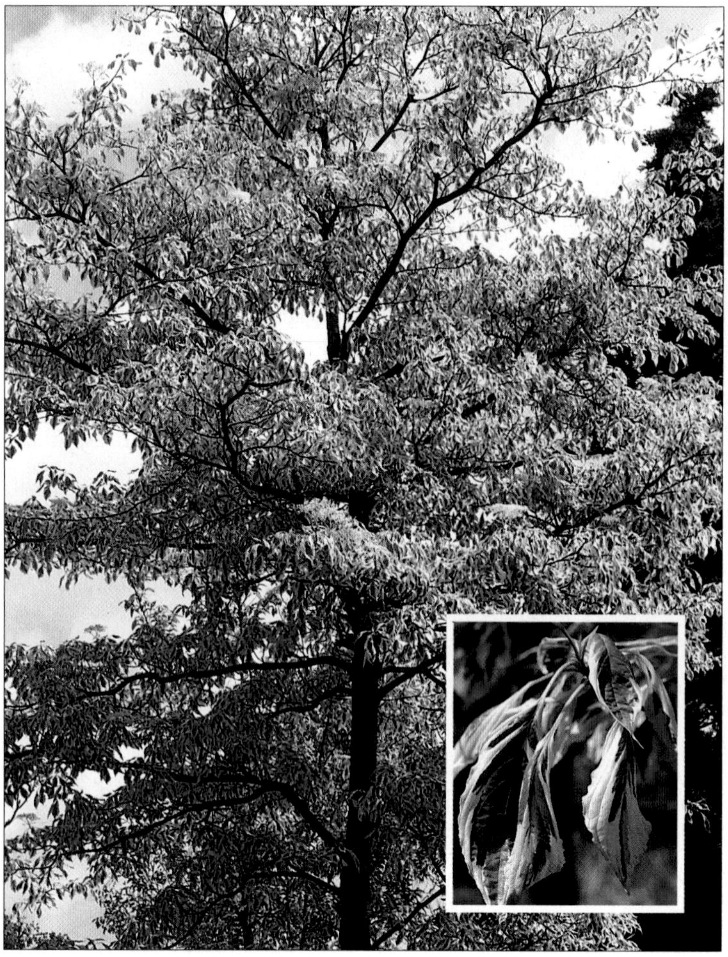

Cornus controversa 'Variegata' (inset: leaf detail)

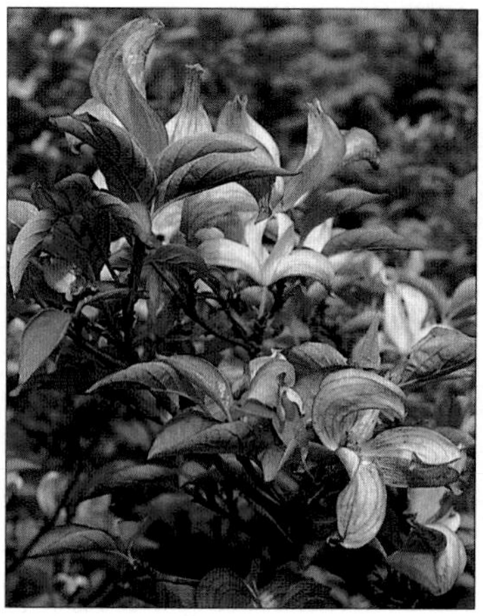

Cornus florida 'Spring Song'

C. alternifolia ♀ syn. *Swida alternifolia* (Green osier, Pagoda dogwood). Deciduous tree or multi-stemmed shrub with spreading, tiered branches. Alternate, ovate-elliptic, mid-green leaves, to 12cm (5in) long, turn red and purple in autumn. Small white flowers are borne in flat cymes, to 5cm (2in) across, in early summer, followed by spherical blue-black fruit. ↕↔ 6m (20ft). E. North America. ❄❄❄. **'Argentea'** ◘ 🏆 syn. 'Variegata', is a tiered shrub or small tree with white-margined leaves, to 8cm (3in) long; ↕ 3m (10ft), ↔ 2.5m (8ft).
C. amomum, syn. *Swida amomum.* Vigorous, spreading, deciduous shrub with dull red-purple winter shoots and ovate-elliptic, dark green leaves, to 12cm (5in) long, turning orange, red, or purple in autumn. White flowers are produced in arching cymes, to 6cm (2½in) across, in late spring and early summer, followed by spherical, metallic grey-blue fruit. ↕ 3m (10ft), ↔ 4m (12ft). E. North America. ❄❄❄
***C.* 'Ascona'**, syn. *C. nuttallii* 'Ascona'. Spreading, deciduous shrub producing purple winter shoots and ovate, mid-green leaves, to 12cm (5in) long, which turn orange, red, or purple in autumn. In late spring, green flowers are produced in flowerheads, 2cm (¾in) across, surrounded by 4 ovate, pointed white bracts, to 8cm (3in) long. ↕ 5m (15ft), ↔ 6m (20ft). ❄❄❄
C. canadensis ◘ 🏆 syn. *Chamaepericlymenum canadense* (Creeping dogwood, Dwarf cornel). Creeping, rhizomatous perennial with terminal whorls of oval or obovate to lance-shaped, mid-green leaves, 2–4cm (¾–1½in) long. In late spring and early summer, green flowers are borne in cymes, 1.5cm (½in) across, surrounded by 4–6 white, sometimes pink-flushed bracts, 1–2cm (½–¾in) long; flowers are followed by spherical, fleshy, bright red fruit. ↕ to 15cm (6in), ↔ indefinite. N. Asia, USA to Greenland. ❄❄❄
C. capitata ◘ ♀ syn. *Dendrobenthamia capitata* (Bentham's cornel). Spreading, bushy, evergreen tree or shrub with ovate to lance-shaped, grey-green leaves, to 12cm (5in) long. In summer, green flowers are produced in small, hemi-spherical heads, 1.5cm (½in) across, surrounded by 4–6 obovate, creamy white or yellowish white bracts, 4–5cm (1½–2in) long; flowers are followed by pendent, strawberry-like fruit. ↕↔ 12m (40ft). China, Himalayas. ❄❄
C. controversa ♀ syn. *Swida controversa.* Rounded, deciduous tree bearing spreading, tiered branches. Alternate, elliptic leaves, to 15cm (6in) long, glossy, dark green above and glaucous beneath, turn rich red and purple in autumn. White flowers are borne in large, flattish cymes, to 18cm (7in) across, in early summer, followed by spherical, blue-black fruit. ↕↔ 15m (50ft). China, Himalayas, Japan. ❄❄❄. **'Variegata'** ◘ 🏆 has leaves with bold, creamy white margins; ↕↔ 8m (25ft).
***C.* 'Eddie's White Wonder'** ◘ 🏆 △ Broadly conical, deciduous tree or multi-stemmed shrub with ovate, mid-green leaves, to 12cm (5in) long, turning orange, red, and purple in autumn. In late spring, purplish green flowers are produced in flowerheads, to 1cm (½in) across, surrounded by 4–6 ovate white bracts, to 8cm (3in) long. ↕ 6m (20ft), ↔ 5m (15ft). ❄❄❄
C. florida △ (Flowering dogwood). Conical, deciduous tree or shrub with broadly oval to ovate, often slightly twisted or curled, mid-green leaves, to 15cm (6in) long, which turn red and purple in autumn. In late spring, green flowers, tipped with yellow, are borne in flowerheads, to 1.5cm (½in) across, surrounded by 4 obovate, white to pink bracts, 4–5cm (1½–2in) long, joined at the tips as they open. ↕ 6m (20ft), ↔ 8m (25ft). E. North America. ❄❄❄. **'Cherokee Chief'** ◘ 🏆 has very dark ruby-pink bracts. **'Cherokee Princess'** produces abundant flowerheads with large white bracts, 6cm (2½in) long.

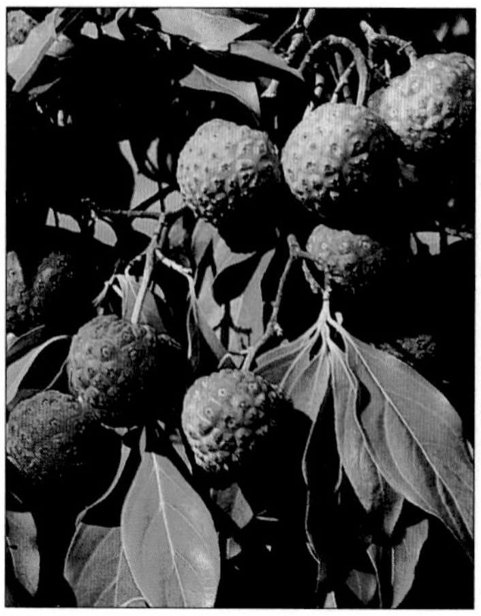

Cornus capitata

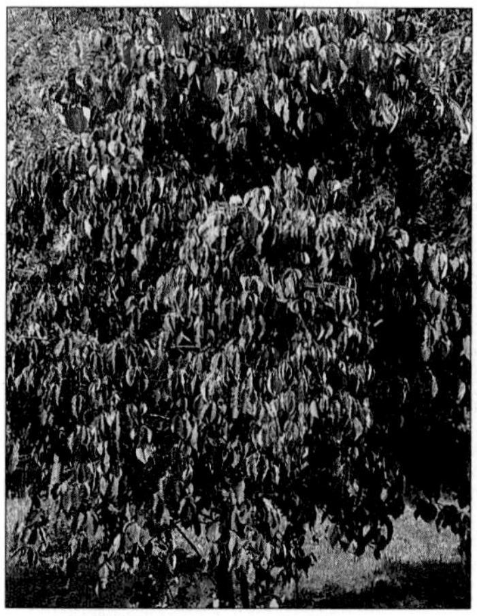

Cornus 'Eddie's White Wonder'

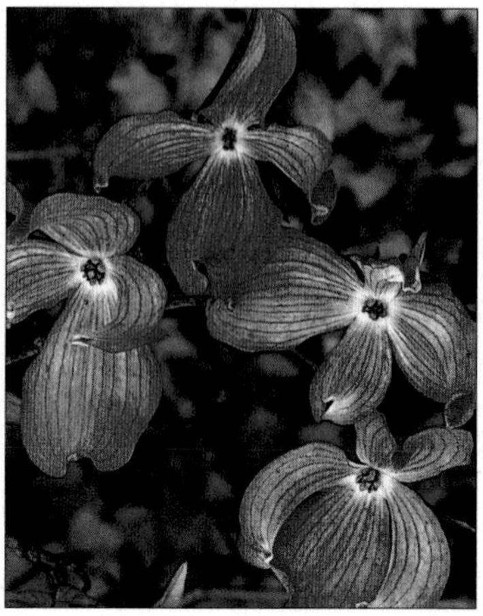

Cornus florida 'Cherokee Chief'

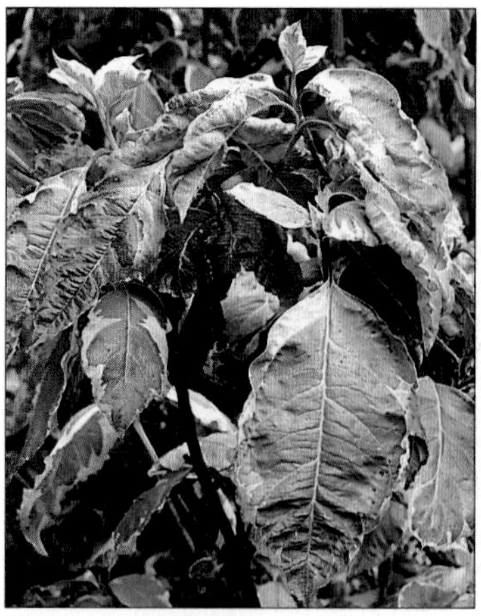

Cornus florida 'Welchii'

CORNUS

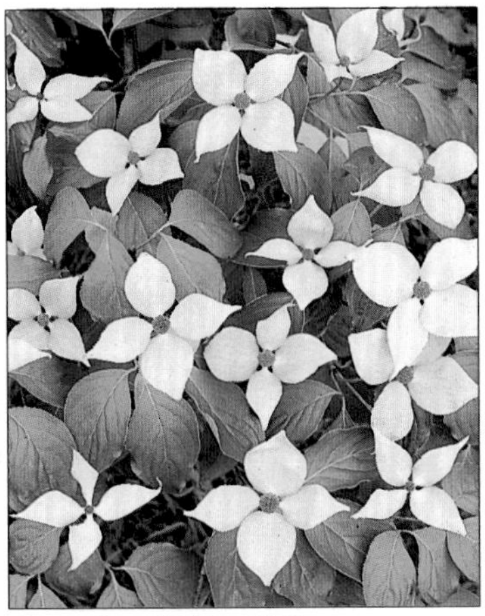

Cornus kousa 'China Girl'

'Cloud Nine' has large, overlapping white bracts, 6cm (2½in) long; it flowers freely, even when young. **'Hohman's Gold'** has leaves margined golden yellow, turning red-purple with scarlet margins in autumn, and produces white bracts; ↕3m (10ft), ↔4m (12ft). **'Rainbow'** is similar to 'Hohman's Gold', but compact and upright; ↕3m (10ft), ↔2.5m (8ft). **f. *rubra*** has pink bracts. **'Spring Song'** ▣ has deep rose-pink bracts. **'Tricolor'** see 'Welchii'. **'Welchii'** ▣ syn. 'Tricolor', is slow-growing, with white- and pink-margined, grey-green leaves, turning bronze-purple with rose-red margins in autumn, and white bracts. **'White Cloud'** is very free-flowering, and bears creamy white bracts.
C. kousa △ Broadly conical, deciduous tree with flaking bark and ovate, wavy-margined, dark green leaves, to 8cm (3in) long, turning deep crimson-purple in autumn. In early summer, green flowers are produced in flowerheads, to 1cm (½in) across, surrounded by 4 ovate-lance-shaped to ovate white bracts, 2.5–5cm (1–2in) long; flowers are followed by strawberry-like, fleshy red fruit. ↕7m (22ft), ↔5m (15ft). Korea, Japan. ✲✲✲. **'China Girl'** ▣ is very free-flowering, even when young. **var. *chinensis*** ▣♀ has smooth-margined leaves and large, tapered bracts, to 5cm (2in) long, which open creamy white and then turn white and eventually red-pink. **'Gold Star'** is shrubby, with leaves marked dark yellow in the centres, turning red with purple margins in autumn; bracts are white on opening, later becoming pink; ↕2.5m

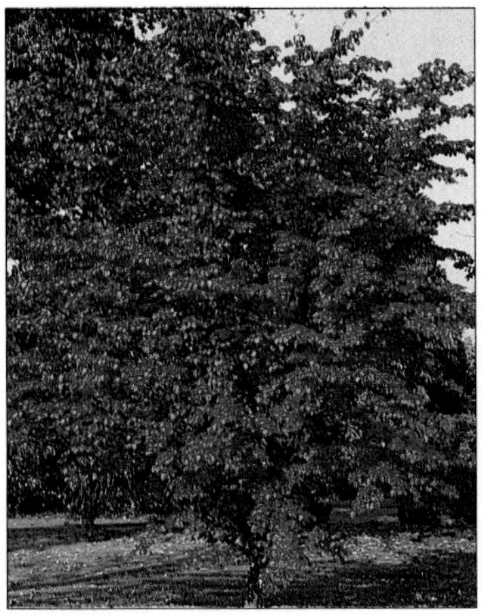

Cornus kousa var. *chinensis*

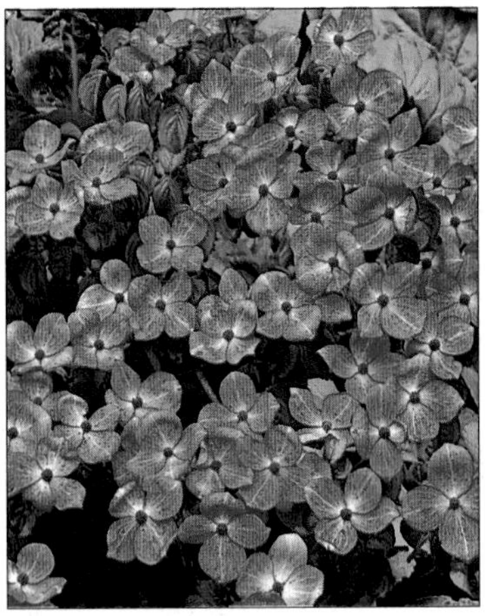

Cornus kousa 'Satomi'

(8ft), ↔2m (6ft). **'Milky Way'** flowers and fruits profusely. **'Satomi'** ▣♀ has dark red-purple autumn foliage and dark pink bracts. **'Snowboy'** has grey-green leaves with broad white margins, the leaves turning pink and red in autumn; ↕2.5m (8ft), ↔2m (6ft).
C. macrophylla ▣△ Broadly conical, deciduous tree with ovate, glossy, mid-green leaves, to 18cm (7in) long. Creamy white flowers are produced in broad, flattened heads, to 18cm (7in) across, in late summer; flowers are followed by spherical, blue-black fruit. ↕12m (40ft), ↔8m (25ft). China, Himalayas, Japan. ✲✲✲
C. mas ▣♀⚲ (Cornelian cherry). Vigorous, spreading, deciduous shrub or small tree with ovate, dark green leaves, to 10cm (4in) long, turning red-purple

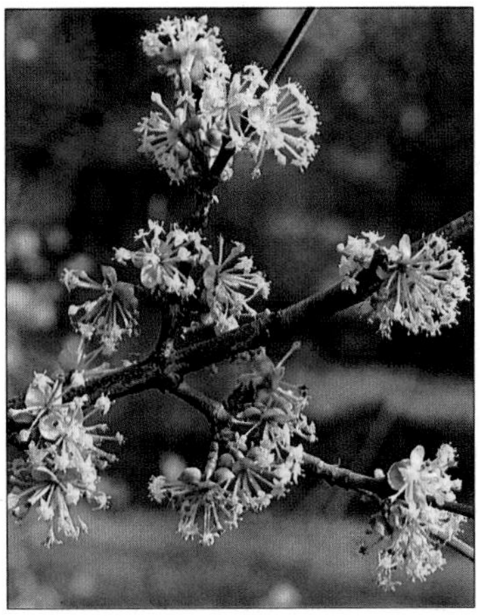

Cornus mas

in autumn. Yellow flowers are produced in small umbels, to 2cm (¾in) across, in late winter, before the leaves. Oblong-ellipsoid, fleshy, bright red fruit are produced in late summer, and are edible when ripe. ↕↔5m (15ft). Europe, W. Asia. ✲✲✲. **'Aurea'** has yellow juvenile leaves, maturing to mid-green. **'Aureoelegantissima'**, syn. 'Elegantissima', has leaves broadly margined yellow and pink; ↕2m (6ft), ↔3m (10ft). **'Elegantissima'** see 'Aureoelegantissima'. **'Variegata'** ♀ is compact, with white leaf margins and abundant fruit; ↕2.5m (8ft), ↔2m (6ft).
***C.* 'Norman Hadden'** ▣♀⚲ Spreading, semi-evergreen tree with arching branches and elliptic-ovate, mid-green leaves, to 8cm (3in) long, some turning yellow or pink in autumn.

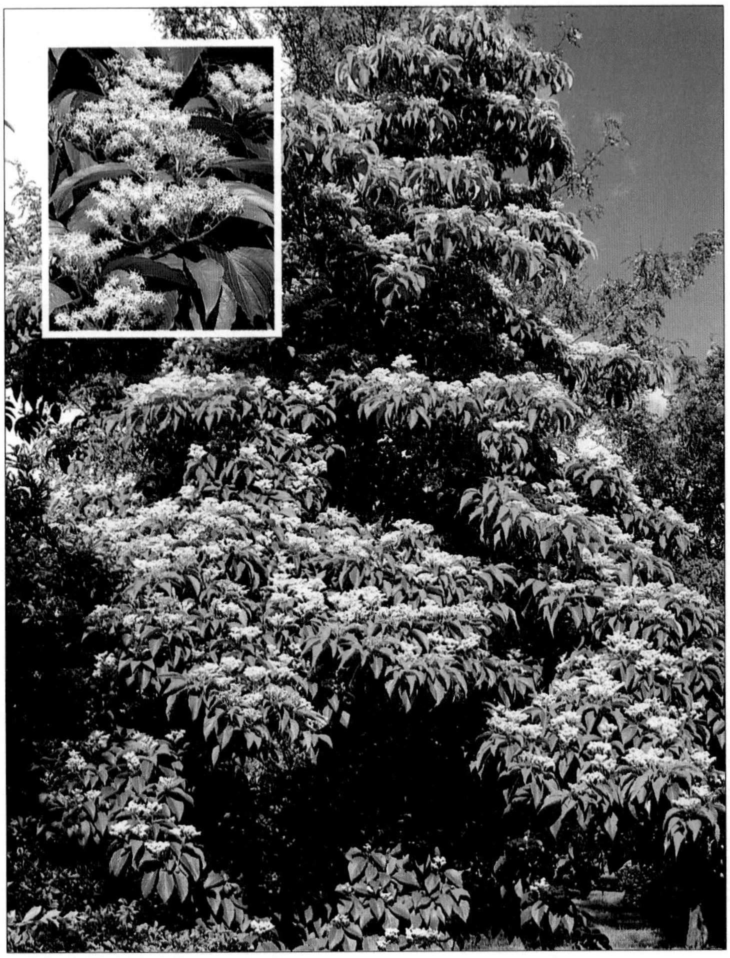

Cornus macrophylla (inset: flower detail)

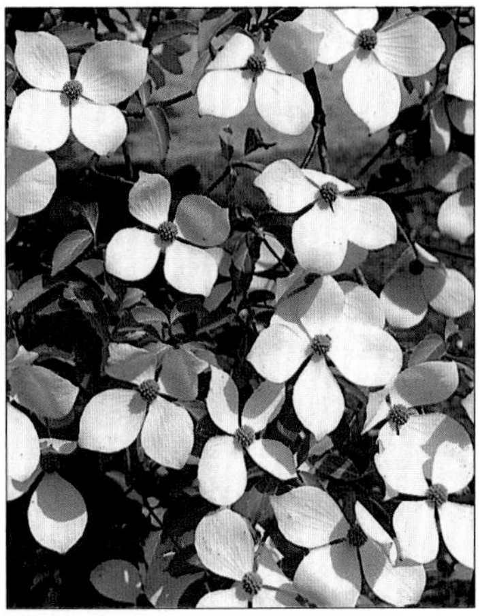

Cornus 'Norman Hadden'

In early summer, green flowers are produced in abundant flowerheads, 1cm (½in) across, surrounded by broadly elliptic cream bracts, 4cm (1½in) long, turning dark pink; they are followed by large, pendent, strawberry-like red fruit. ↕↔8m (25ft). ✲✲✲
C. nuttallii △ (Pacific dogwood). Conical, deciduous tree with oval to obovate, mid-green leaves, to 12cm (5in) long, sometimes turning red in autumn. In late spring, purple and green flowers are produced in flowerheads, to 1.5cm (½in) across, surrounded by 4–6, occasionally up to 8, broadly ovate to obovate, white or pink-tinged bracts, 4–8cm (1½–3in) long; flowers are followed by spherical, orange-red fruit. ↕12m (40ft), ↔8m (25ft). W. North America. ✲✲✲. **'Ascona'** see *C.* 'Ascona'. **'Colrigo Giant'** ▣ is very vigorous, with stout shoots, leaves to 15cm (6in) long, and spherical flowerheads with 6–8 bracts. **'Gold Spot'** has yellow-marked leaves.
C. officinalis. Vigorous, spreading, deciduous shrub with rough, flaking brown bark and ovate to elliptic, dark green leaves, to 10cm (4in) long, turning red-purple in autumn. Yellow flowers are produced in loose umbels, 2cm (¾in) or more across, in late winter, before the leaves open; they are followed by oblong-ellipsoid, edible, bright red fruit. ↕↔5m (15ft). China, Korea, Japan. ✲✲✲
***C.* 'Ormonde'** ⚲ Spreading, deciduous shrub or tree with oval, mid-green leaves, to 12cm (5in) long, turning orange, red, or purple in autumn. In late spring, purple and green flowers are

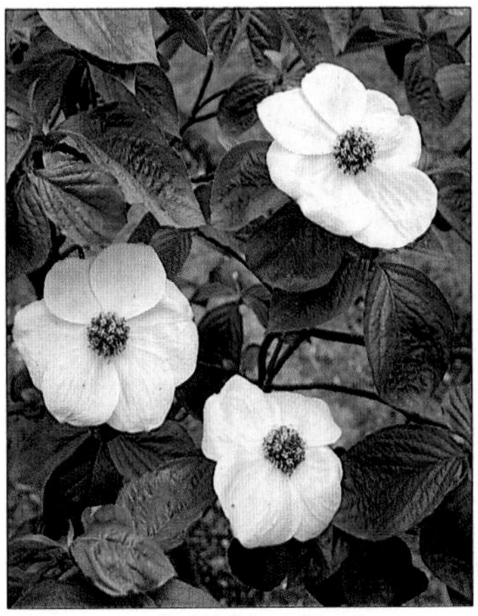

Cornus nuttallii 'Colrigo Giant'

C

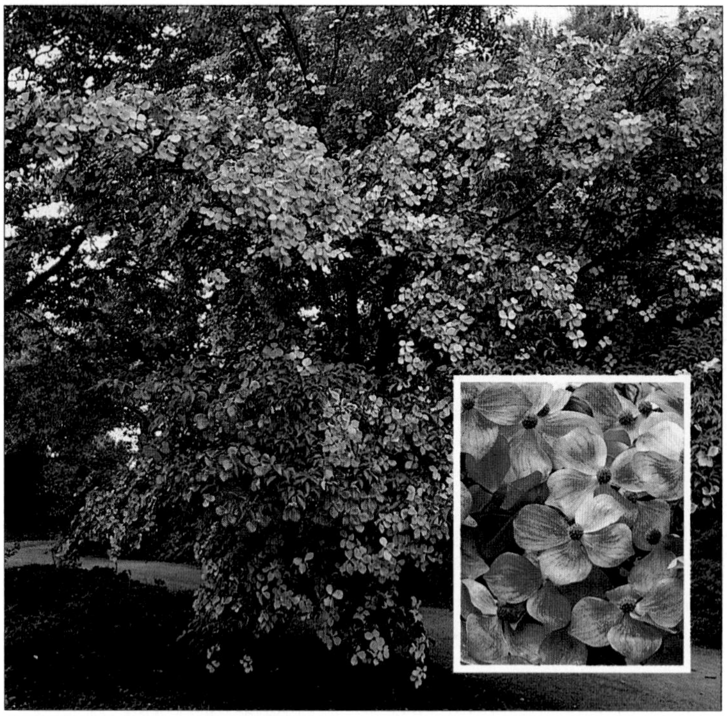

Cornus 'Porlock' (inset: flower detail)

produced in flowerheads, 1.5cm (½in) across, surrounded by usually 4, broadly elliptic, pink-tipped white bracts, 6cm (2½in) long. ↕4m (12ft), ↔6m (20ft). ❄❄❄

***C.* 'Porlock'** ▣ ♀ Spreading, semi-evergreen tree with elliptic to obovate, mid-green leaves, 5–7cm (2–3in) long. In late spring, purple and green flowers are produced in flowerheads, 1.5cm (½in) across, surrounded by ovate, white, then pink-red bracts, 7cm (3in) long. Very similar to *C.* 'Norman Hadden', but with narrower bracts, more tapered at their bases. ↕10m (30ft), ↔5m (15ft). ❄❄❄

C. sanguinea (Common dogwood). Upright, deciduous shrub with reddish green, sometimes entirely green, winter shoots and ovate, mid-green leaves, to 10cm (4in) long, turning red in autumn. White flowers are borne in dense, flat cymes, to 5cm (2in) across, in summer, followed by spherical, dull blue-black fruit. ↕3m (10ft), ↔2.5m (8ft). Europe. ❄❄❄. **'Viridissima'** has green winter shoots. **'Winter Beauty'** ▣ syn. 'Winter Flame', has bright orange-yellow and red winter shoots. **'Winter Flame'** see 'Winter Beauty'.

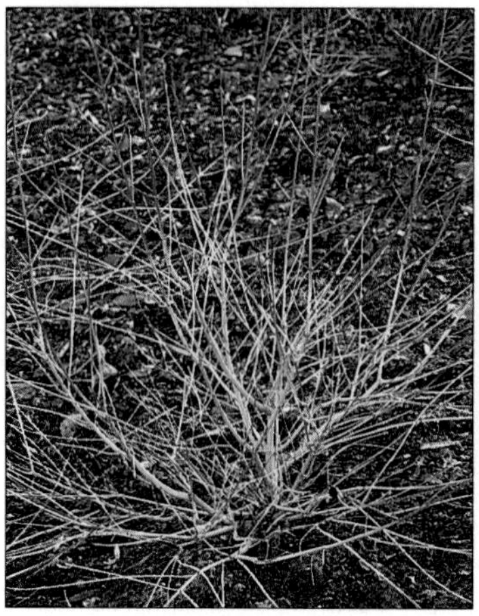

Cornus sanguinea 'Winter Beauty'

C. sericea see *C. stolonifera.*

C. stolonifera, syn. *C. sericea* (Red osier dogwood). Vigorous, suckering, deciduous shrub with dark red winter shoots. Ovate to lance-shaped, dark green leaves, to 12cm (5in) long, turn red or orange in autumn. In late spring and early summer, white flowers are borne in flat cymes, to 5cm (2in) across, followed by white fruit, often tinged blue. Tolerates wet soils. ↕2m (6ft), ↔4m (12ft). E. North America. ❄❄❄. **'Flaviramea'** ▣🏆 has bright yellow-green winter shoots. **'Kelseyi'**, syn. 'Kelsey's Dwarf', 'Nana', is compact, with red-tipped, yellow-green winter shoots; ↕75cm (30in), ↔1.5m (5ft). **'Kelsey's Dwarf'** see 'Kelseyi'. **'Nana'** see 'Kelseyi'.

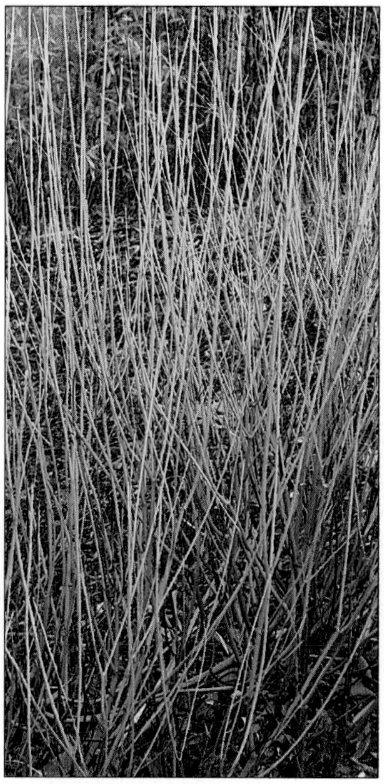

Cornus stolonifera 'Flaviramea'

COROKIA

CORNACEAE

Genus of 3 species of evergreen shrubs occurring in forests and rocky areas in New Zealand. They have alternate, linear to obovate leaves. Star-shaped, 5-petalled yellow flowers, 0.9–1.5cm (⅜–½in) across, are produced singly from the leaf axils or in short, terminal racemes, panicles, or clusters, followed by colourful autumn fruits. In frost-prone areas, grow *Corokia* species and cultivars as specimen plants in a sheltered shrub border or against a wall. In warmer coastal regions, they will tolerate an open site or partial shade, and may be used for hedging.

- **HARDINESS** Frost hardy.
- **CULTIVATION** Grow in fertile, well-drained soil, preferably in full sun, sheltered from cold, dry winds. Pruning group 8; will tolerate hard pruning to restrict growth, if required.
- **PROPAGATION** Root greenwood cuttings in early summer, or semi-ripe cuttings in mid- or late summer.
- **PESTS AND DISEASES** Trouble free.

C. buddlejoides (Korokio). Upright shrub with elliptic to linear-lance-shaped, glossy, dark green leaves, to 15cm (6in) long. Bears small, fragrant yellow flowers in terminal panicles, 2–5cm (¾–2in) long, in spring, followed by spherical, bright red-black fruit. ↕3m (10ft), ↔2m (6ft). New Zealand (North Island). ❄❄

C. cotoneaster ▣ (Wire-netting bush). Rounded, intricately branched shrub bearing interlacing shoots and broadly ovate to obovate, dark green leaves, to 1.5cm (½in) long. In late spring, small, fragrant yellow flowers are produced singly or in clusters of up to 4, from the leaf axils, followed by oblong-ellipsoid, red or yellow fruit. ↕↔2.5m (8ft). New Zealand. ❄❄

C. macrocarpa. Upright shrub with lance-shaped, leathery leaves, grey-green above and silvery beneath, to 8cm (3in) long. In early summer, small yellow flowers are borne in short racemes, to 4cm (1½in) long, from the leaf axils, followed by oblong-ellipsoid red fruit. ↕↔2m (6ft) or more. New Zealand (Chatham Island). ❄❄

C.* x *virgata ▣ (*C. cotoneaster* x *C. buddlejoides*). Upright shrub with spoon-shaped to inversely lance-shaped leaves, glossy, dark green above and

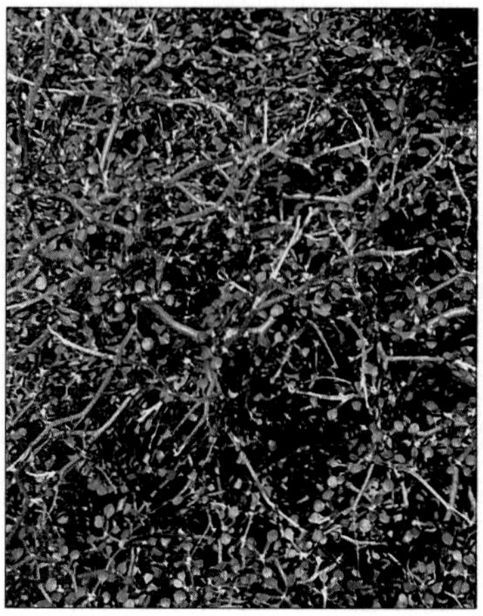

Corokia cotoneaster

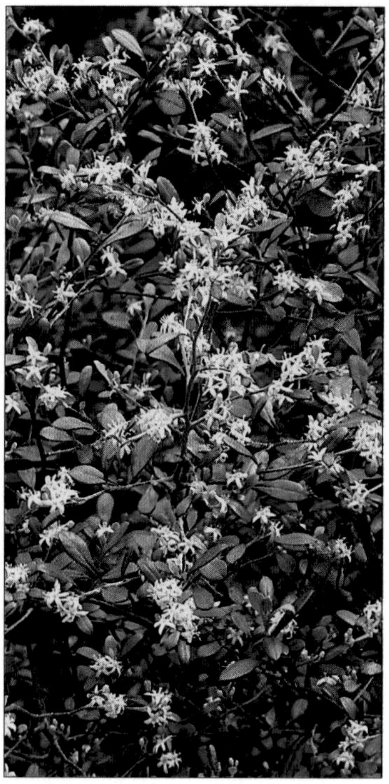

Corokia x *virgata*

white beneath, to 5cm (2in) long. In late spring, small, fragrant yellow flowers are produced in clusters of 3 from the leaf axils, followed by ovoid, yellow or orange fruit. ↕↔3m (10ft). New Zealand (North Island). ❄❄. **'Bronze King'** has bronze-tinged foliage. **'Bronze Lady'** has dark bronze leaves, to 4cm (1½in) long, and bright red fruit. **'Yellow Wonder'** is vigorous and bears golden yellow fruit.

CORONILLA

LEGUMINOSAE/PAPILIONACEAE

Genus of about 20 species of annuals, herbaceous perennials, and evergreen and deciduous shrubs from Europe and N. Africa, where they occur in habitats ranging from meadows to scrub, woodland and woodland margins, and cliffs. They are cultivated for their alternate, usually pinnate leaves and their often fragrant, pea-like flowers, borne in axillary umbels. Grow in a shrub border or at the base of a warm, sunny wall.

- **HARDINESS** Fully hardy to frost hardy.
- **CULTIVATION** Grow in light, moderately fertile, well-drained soil in full sun, sheltered from cold, dry winds.

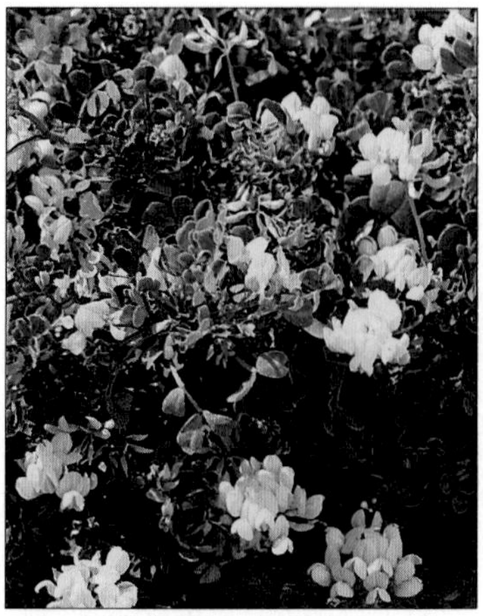

Coronilla valentina subsp. *glauca*

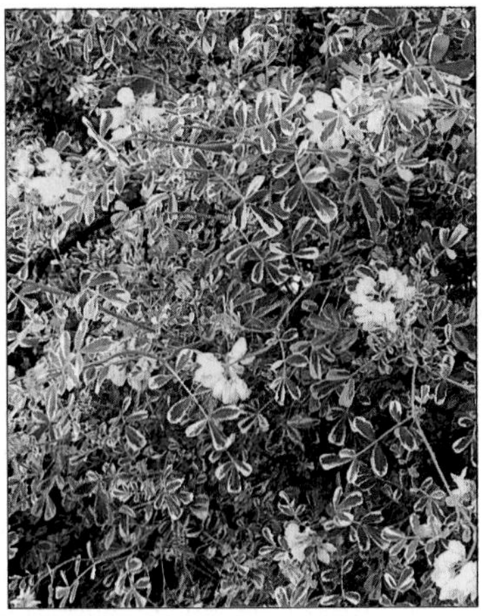

Coronilla valentina subsp. *glauca* 'Variegata'

Pruning group 1; cut back leggy plants almost to the bases to rejuvenate them in spring.

• **PROPAGATION** Sow seed in containers in a cold frame as soon as ripe, or stratify and sow at 10–13°C (50–55°F) in spring. Root greenwood cuttings in early summer or semi-ripe cuttings in late summer.

• **PESTS AND DISEASES** Trouble free.

C. emerus, syn. *Hippocrepis emerus* (Scorpion senna). Bushy, rounded, deciduous shrub with mid-green shoots and pinnate leaves, to 6cm (2½in) long, with up to 9 obovate leaflets. Slender-stalked, axillary umbels of 2 or 3 pale yellow flowers, 2cm (¾in) long, are produced from late spring to autumn, followed by slender, segmented pods, to 10cm (4in) long. ↕↔ 2m (6ft). C. and S. Europe. ❄❄❄

C. glauca see *C. valentina* subsp. *glauca*.

C. valentina. Dense, rounded, bushy, evergreen shrub with pinnate, bright green leaves, to 5cm (2in) long, with up to 13 obovate leaflets. Axillary umbels of 4–14 fragrant, bright yellow flowers, 1cm (½in) long, are produced in late winter and early spring, and again in late summer, followed by slender pods, to 5cm (2in) long. ↕↔ 1.5m (5ft). S. Portugal, Spain to Croatia (Dalmatia). ❄❄. **subsp. *glauca*** ■🏆 syn. *C. glauca*, is often more compact, and bears blue-green leaves with 5–7 leaflets; ↕↔ 80cm (32in); ❄❄❄ (borderline). **subsp. *glauca* 'Citrina'** 🏆 has pale yellow flowers. **subsp. *glauca* 'Variegata'** ■🏆 has leaves margined creamy white; ❄❄

CORREA

Australian fuchsia

RUTACEAE

Genus of about 20 species of evergreen shrubs and small trees found in scrub and open woodland in Australia. The opposite, simple leaves have star-shaped hairs and are aromatic when bruised. The mainly pendent, tubular to bell-shaped flowers, with 4 spreading or reflexed lobes, are produced singly or in few-flowered clusters. In frost-prone climates, grow in a cool greenhouse or conservatory. In warmer areas, grow in a shrub border or courtyard garden, or at the base of a house wall.

• **HARDINESS** Half hardy to frost tender.

• **CULTIVATION** Under glass, grow in lime-free (ericaceous) potting compost

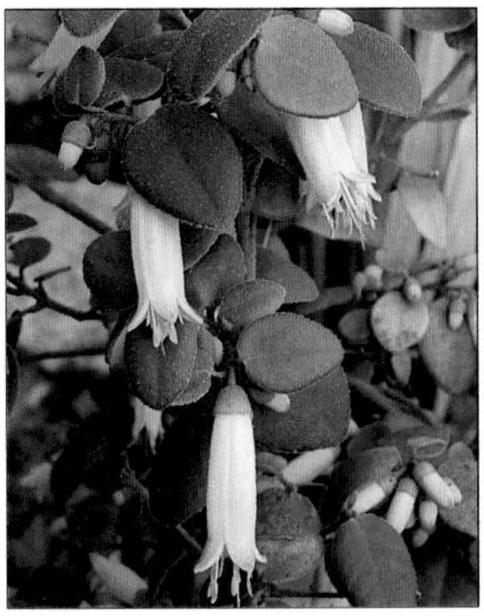

Correa backhouseana

in full light, with shade from hot sun, and with good ventilation. In the growing season, water moderately and apply a balanced liquid fertilizer monthly; water sparingly in winter. Top-dress or pot on in spring. Outdoors, grow in fertile, moist but well-drained, neutral to acid soil in full sun. *C. pulchella* and *C. reflexa* tolerate mildly alkaline soil. Pruning group 8.

• **PROPAGATION** Sow seed at 13–18°C (55–64°F) in spring. Root semi-ripe cuttings with bottom heat in summer.

• **PESTS AND DISEASES** Scale insects may be a problem under glass.

C. alba. Freely branching shrub with ovate, rich green leaves, 2–4cm (¾–1½in) long, smooth above, finely hairy beneath. From early summer to late autumn, bears short, bell-shaped, sometimes pink-tinted, waxy white flowers, to 1.5cm (½in) long, in few-flowered clusters. ↕ 2m (6ft), ↔ 1–2m (3–6ft). Australia (South Australia, New South Wales, Victoria, Tasmania). ❄. **'Pinkie'** is bushy and spreading, with hairy, rust-red stems and glossy, deep green leaves, grey-hairy beneath. From autumn to spring, produces clusters of dusky pink flowers, shortly tubular at first, then splitting into 4 reflexed petals. ↕ 1m (3ft), ↔ 1–1.5m (3–5ft).

C. backhouseana ■🏆 Dense, spreading shrub with hairy, rust-red twigs and oval, dark green leaves, 2–3cm (¾–1¼in) long, smooth above and hairy beneath. Produces small clusters of tubular, pale or reddish green or cream flowers, to 2.5cm (1in) long, from late

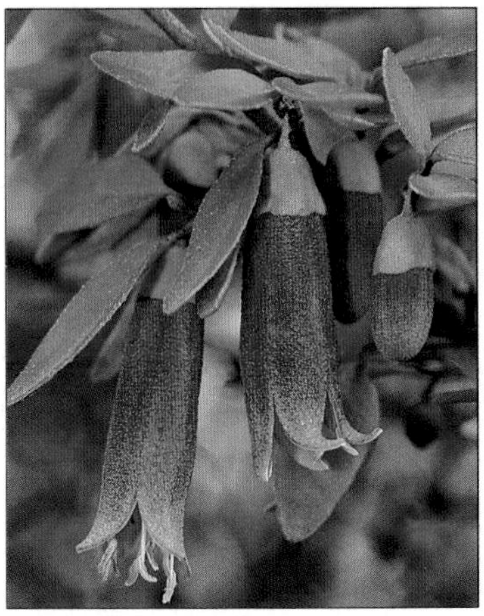

Correa 'Dusky Bells'

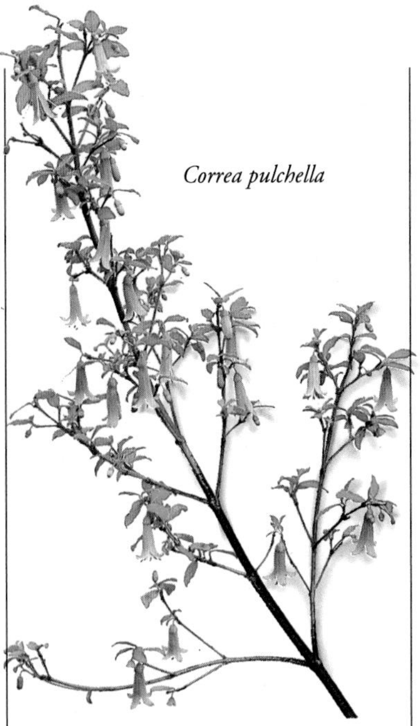

Correa pulchella

autumn to late spring. ↕ 1–2m (3–6ft), ↔ 1.5–2.5m (5–8ft). Australia (Victoria, Tasmania). ❄

***C.* 'Carmine Bells'** see *C.* 'Dusky Bells'.

***C.* 'Dusky Bells'** ■ syn. *C.* 'Carmine Bells', *C.* 'Pink Bells', *C.* 'Rubra'. Wide-spreading shrub with reddish brown stems and oval, mid- to deep green leaves, to 3.5cm (1½in) long. Tubular, dusky carmine-red flowers, to 2.5cm (1in) long, are borne in small clusters from autumn to spring. ↕ 30–90cm (12–36in), ↔ 1.5–3m (5–10ft). ❄

***C.* 'Harrisii'** see *C.* 'Mannii'.

***C.* 'Ivory Bells'.** Bushy, vigorous shrub with spreading, densely hairy stems and elliptic to ovate, matt, deep green leaves, 2–3cm (¾–1¼in) long. Clusters of tubular, ivory-white flowers, to 2cm (¾in) long, with recurved lobes, ageing to tan, are mainly produced from winter to summer. ↕ 1–2m (3–6ft), ↔ 2–3m (6–10ft). ❄

***C.* 'Mannii'** 🏆 syn. *C.* 'Harrisii'. Spreading shrub with broadly ovate leaves, 2–3cm (¾–1¼in) long, heart-shaped at the bases and dark green above, paler beneath. Tubular red flowers, to 2.5cm (1in) long, with reflexed petal tips, are borne in small clusters from autumn to spring. ↕ 1–2.5m (3–8ft), ↔ 2–3m (6–10ft). ❄

***C.* 'Pink Bells'** see *C.* 'Dusky Bells'.

C. pulchella ■ Freely branching, prostrate to almost erect shrub with oval to elliptic, smooth, bright green leaves, 1–2cm (½–¾in) long. Bears tubular, vermilion, orange, or pink to white flowers, to 2.5cm (1in) long, in small clusters from autumn to spring. ↕ 30–150cm (1–5ft), ↔ 0.9–2.5m (3–8ft). Australia (South Australia). ❄

C. reflexa 🏆 syn. *C. speciosa*. Erect to prostrate, loosely to compactly branched shrub bearing obovate-oblong to lance-shaped, rich green leaves, to 5cm (2in) long, white-felted beneath. Tubular to narrowly bell-shaped flowers are green, white, pink, or red, 2–2.5cm (¾–1in) long, sometimes with green or cream reflexed petal tips; they are produced in small clusters, mainly from autumn to spring. ↕ 0.3–3m (1–10ft), ↔ 1–3m (3–10ft). Australia (except Northern Territory). ❄

***C.* 'Rubra'** see *C.* 'Dusky Bells'.

C. speciosa see *C. reflexa*.

CORRYOCACTUS

syn. ERDISIA

CACTACEAE

Genus of about 20 species of trailing or erect, shrub-like, perennial cacti from semi-arid areas of S. and C. Peru, Bolivia, and N. Chile. Many branch from the bases to form large clumps, with cylindrical, ribbed stems bearing evenly spaced, spiny areoles. Solitary, funnel-shaped, diurnal, orange, red, or vivid yellow flowers are produced in summer, followed by spherical, spiny green fruits with small black or brown seeds. In frost-prone areas, grow in a temperate greenhouse, with a minimum temperature of 10°C (50°F). In warmer areas, grow in a desert garden.

• **HARDINESS** Frost tender.

• **CULTIVATION** Under glass, grow in standard cactus compost in full light, with shade from hot sun. From spring to summer, water moderately and apply a dilute, low-nitrogen liquid fertilizer monthly; keep completely dry at other times. Outdoors, grow in low-fertility, sharply drained, gritty, humus-rich soil in full sun. See also pp.48–49.

• **PROPAGATION** Sow seed at 21°C (70°F) in spring. Root stem cuttings in late spring or early summer.

• **PESTS AND DISEASES** Mealybugs, and occasionally aphids, may be a problem.

C. brachypetalus. Erect, clump-forming cactus with 7- or 8-ribbed, dull green stems branching from the base. White areoles bear 15–20 brownish black spines. Deep orange flowers, 4–6cm (1½–2½in) across, are produced in summer. ↕ 2–4m (6–12ft), ↔ 1m (3ft). S. Peru. ⌂ (min. 10°C/50°F)

C. erectus ■ syn. *Erdisia erecta*. Usually erect, clump-forming cactus with 5- or 6-ribbed, mid-green stems branching from the base, and pale brown or white areoles bearing yellowish white spines (10 or more radials and 1 or 2 centrals). Produces carmine-red or scarlet flowers,

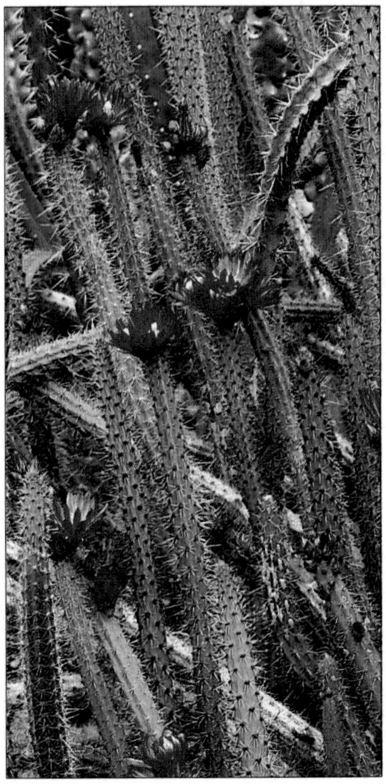

Corryocactus erectus

C

4–5cm (1½–2in) across, in summer. ↕ 1m (3ft) or more, ↔ 60cm (24in). S. Peru. ❄ (min. 10°C/50°F)

C. squarrosus, syn. *Erdisia squarrosa.* Erect, clump-forming cactus with 5- to 8-ribbed, deep green stems and brown areoles, each with about 11 yellow spines (1 radial and 10 centrals). Bright red, sometimes yellowish red flowers, 4cm (1½in) across, are produced in summer. ↕ 50cm (20in), ↔ 1m (3ft) or more. C. Peru. ❄ (min. 10°C/50°F)

▷**Corsican heath** see *Erica terminalis*

CORTADERIA

Pampas grass, Tussock grass

GRAMINEAE/POACEAE

Genus of about 23 species of evergreen or semi-evergreen, perennial grasses from grassland, often near water, in New Zealand, New Guinea, and South America. They form dense tussocks of stiff, flat, narrowly linear, often glaucous leaves with rough or sharp margins, and bear stout-stemmed, plume-like, silver, gold, or pale rose-pink flower panicles (usually with male and female spikelets on separate plants, but occasionally hermaphroditic). Female spikelets have long, silky hairs at the bases. The plumes may be used in fresh or dried flower arrangements. Grow at the back of a border or as free-standing specimens.

- **HARDINESS** Fully hardy to frost hardy.
- **CULTIVATION** Grow in fertile, well-drained soil in full sun, with ample space to develop. Protect crowns of young plants in their first winter. Cut and comb out the previous year's stems and dead foliage annually, in late winter or early spring, taking care to avoid the sharp leaf margins.
- **PROPAGATION** Sow seed at 13–18°C (55–64°F) in spring. Divide in spring.
- **PESTS AND DISEASES** Trouble free.

C. argentea see *C. selloana.*
C. conspicua see *Chionochloa conspicua.*
C. richardii (Toe toe). Densely tufted, clump-forming, evergreen, perennial grass with recurved, leathery, pale olive-green leaves, to 1.2m (4ft) long. In early and midsummer, arching stems, to 2.5m (9ft) tall, bear shaggy, pyramidal, creamy white or silvery white panicles, 60cm (24in) long, which persist into winter. ↕ to 2.5m (9ft), ↔ 1.8m (6ft). New Zealand. ❄❄
C. selloana, syn. *C. argentea* (Pampas grass). Densely tufted, clump-forming, evergreen, perennial grass with arching, glaucous, mid-green leaves, to 2.5m (8ft) or more long. In late summer, silky, silver, often pink- or purple-flushed spikelets are borne in pyramidal to oblong panicles, 45–90cm (18–36in) long, on erect stems. ↕ 2.5–3m (8–10ft), ↔ 1.5m (5ft) or more. Temperate South America. ❄❄❄. **'Albolineata'**, syn. 'Silver Stripe', is slow-growing and compact, with white-margined leaves and silvery white plumes; ↕ to 2m (6ft). **'Aureolineata'** ▣ ♀ syn. 'Gold Band', has rich yellow-margined leaves, ageing to dark golden yellow; ↕ to 2.2m (7ft). **'Gold Band'** see 'Aureolineata'. **'Pumila'** ♀ bears mid-green leaves and masses of erect, silvery yellow plumes; ↕ to 1.5m (5ft), ↔ 1.2m (4ft). **'Rendatleri'** has purplish pink panicles; ↕↔ to 2.5m (8ft). **'Silver Stripe'** see 'Albolineata'. **'Sunningdale Silver'** ▣ ♀ has strong, erect stems and dense, weather-resistant, silvery white plumes; ↕ 3m (10ft) or more, ↔ to 2.5m (8ft).

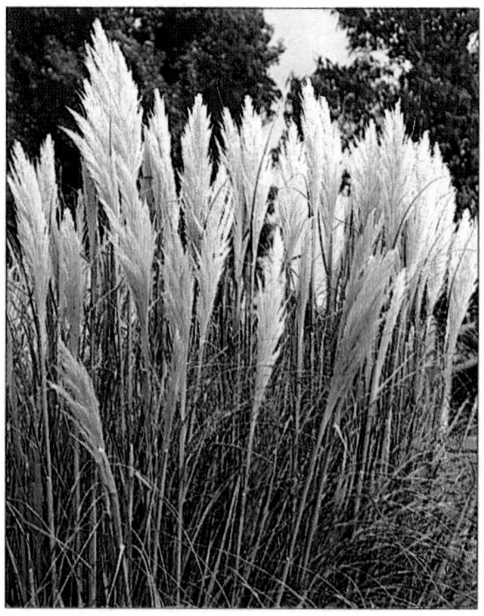
Cortaderia selloana 'Sunningdale Silver'

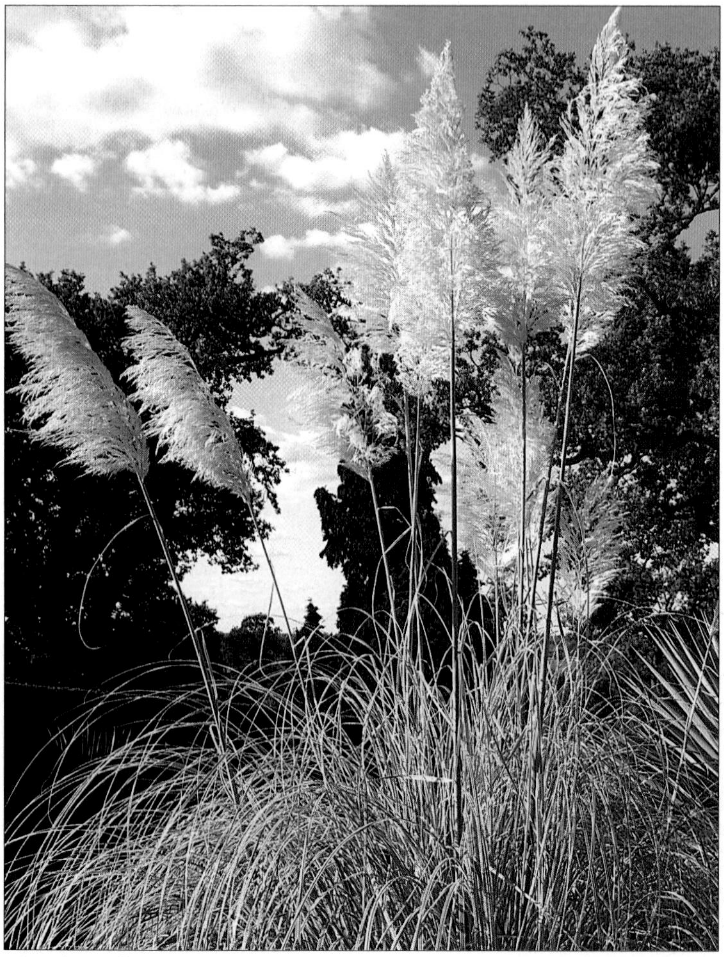
Cortaderia selloana 'Aureolineata'

CORTUSA

PRIMULACEAE

Genus of 8 species of herbaceous perennials occurring in mountain woodland from W. and C. Europe to N. Asia. They produce long-stalked, rounded to heart-shaped, basal leaves. One-sided umbels of funnel- to bell-shaped flowers are produced on slender stems above the foliage. *Cortusa* species are suitable for a woodland or rock garden; they will not thrive in hot, dry climates.

- **HARDINESS** Fully hardy.
- **CULTIVATION** Grow in moderately fertile, humus-rich, reliably moist but well-drained, slightly acid or alkaline soil in a cool position in partial shade.
- **PROPAGATION** Sow seed in containers in an open frame as soon as ripe. Divide in spring.
- **PESTS AND DISEASES** Slugs and snails may be a problem.

C. matthioli ▣ Clump-forming perennial with kidney-shaped to rounded, crinkled, rusty-hairy, deep green leaves, 12cm (5in) or more across, with coarsely toothed lobes. Pendent, broadly bell-shaped, magenta or purple-violet, occasionally white flowers, 1cm (½in) long, are borne in one-sided umbels on hairy stems, in late spring and early summer. ↕ 20–30cm (8–12in), ↔ to 15cm (6in). W. Europe. ❄❄❄

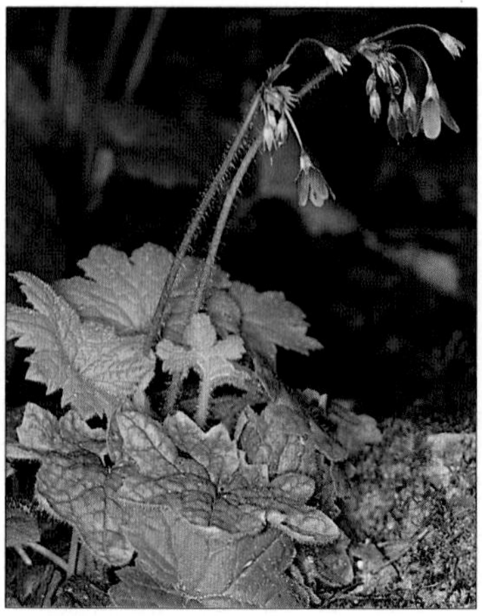
Cortusa matthioli

CORYDALIS

syn. PSEUDOFUMARIA

PAPAVERACEAE

Genus of about 300 species of fibrous- or fleshy-rooted annuals and biennials, and tuberous or rhizomatous perennials. Most are herbaceous; a few are evergreen. They occur in a range of habitats, with many from woodland or rocky, mountain sites, mostly in N. temperate regions. They have opposite or alternate stem leaves, which are compound, usually ternate to 3-ternate, sometimes pinnate to 3-pinnate, and sometimes triangular in outline. The leaflets are often finely divided, producing a fern-like appearance. Tubular flowers, borne in mostly terminal, sometimes axillary racemes, usually above the foliage, each have 4 petals: the outer pair with a spur and reflexed tips, the inner pair incurved to cover the stamens and style.

The sun-loving species are suitable for a rock garden or alpine house; grow shade-loving species in a peat bank, in a rock or woodland garden, or as underplanting in a shrub border. Some species need a period of dry dormancy in summer and protection from excessive winter wet; these are best grown in a bulb frame or alpine house.

- **HARDINESS** Fully hardy to frost hardy.
- **CULTIVATION** *Corydalis* species have varying cultivation requirements, which, for ease of reference, are grouped as follows:

1. Full sun or partial shade and fertile, well-drained soil. Often self-seed freely.
2. Full sun and sharply drained, moderately fertile soil in a rock garden. May tolerate partial shade.
3. Partial shade and moderately fertile humus-rich, moist but well-drained soil.
4. Grow in a bulb frame or alpine house, in equal parts loam, leaf mould, and grit. Resent excessive wet.

- **PROPAGATION** Sow seed in containers in an open frame as soon as ripe; germination may be erratic. Divide spring-flowering species in autumn, and summer-flowering species in spring.
- **PESTS AND DISEASES** Slugs and snails may be a problem. Aphids and red spider mites may prove troublesome under glass.

C. aitchisonii. Prostrate, tuberous perennial with clusters of ternate, blue-grey leaves, to 10cm (4in) long, with ovate leaflets. In spring, bears loose,

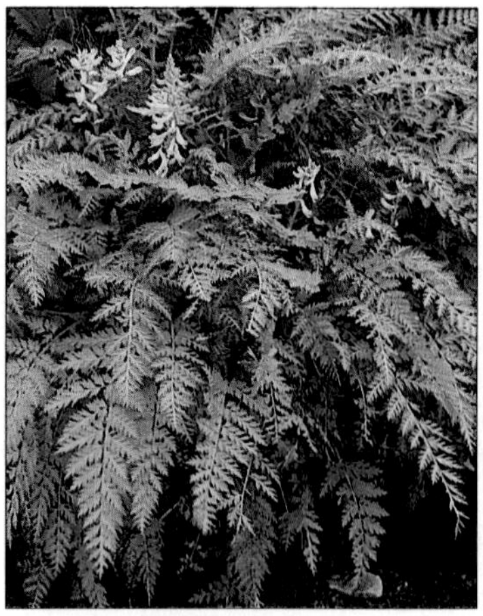
Corydalis cheilanthifolia

CORYDALIS

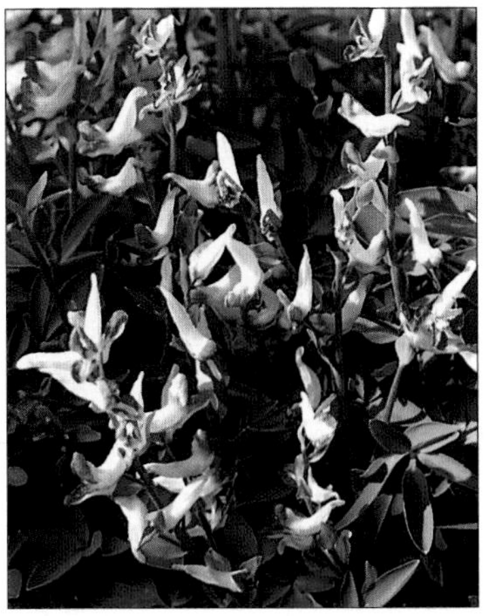
Corydalis diphylla

spike-like racemes of slender-tubed, golden yellow flowers, to 4cm (1½in) long, with curved spurs, on short stems. Cultivation group 4. ↕ 10cm (4in), ↔ 15cm (6in). Uzbekistan, Afghanistan. ❄❄❄

***C. ambigua* of gardens** see *C. fumariifolia.*

C. bracteata. Tuberous perennial with ternate, pale green leaves, to 10cm (4in) long, with broadly obovate leaflets deeply divided into linear lobes. In spring, produces racemes of pale yellow flowers, to 2.5cm (1in) long, with broad lower lips, usually with paler spurs to 1.5cm (½in) long, and with large, dissected bracts. Cultivation group 3. ↕ to 25cm (10in), ↔ 10cm (4in). C. Asia, Russia (Siberia). ❄❄❄

***C. bulbosa* of gardens** see *C. cava.*

C. cashmeriana. Tufted perennial with clusters of ovoid tubers. Bears ternate, bright green leaves, to 8cm (3in) long, with ovate leaflets finely divided into oblong or elliptic lobes. Dense racemes of 3–8 brilliant blue flowers, 1cm (½in) long, with curved spurs, are produced in summer. Prefers cool, moist climates. Cultivation group 3. ↕ 10–25cm (4–10in), ↔ 8–15cm (3–6in). Himalayas. ❄❄❄

***C. caucasica* var. *alba* of gardens** see *C. malkensis.*

C. cava ♀ syn. *C. bulbosa* of gardens. Hollow-tubered perennial with 2-ternate, pale green leaves, to 10cm (4in) long, with wedge-shaped, lobed leaflets. In early spring, bears dense racemes of purple or white flowers, to 2.5cm (1in) long, with downward-curving spurs, to 1cm (½in) long, and entire, scale-like bracts. Cultivation group 3. ↕ 10–20cm (4–8in), ↔ 10cm (4in). Europe. ❄❄❄

C. cheilanthifolia ■ Evergreen, fibrous-rooted, rosette-forming perennial with fern-like, 2- or 3-pinnate, bronze-tinted, light to mid-green leaves, 15–45cm (6–18in) long, with linear or linear-lance-shaped leaflets. Dense, spike-like racemes of straight-spurred, deep yellow flowers, to 1.5cm (½in) long, are borne from spring to summer. Self-seeds freely. Cultivation group 1. ↕ to 30cm (12in), ↔ to 25cm (10in). W. and C. China. ❄❄❄

C. diphylla ■ Tuberous perennial with semi-erect, long-stalked, 2- or 3-ternate, glaucous, mid-green leaves, to 8cm (3in) long, with linear-lance-shaped leaflets. In spring, bears loose, terminal racemes of 6–10 pale violet flowers, 2–3cm (¾–1¼in) long, with deeper violet or red-violet lips and upward-pointing white spurs, to 1cm (½in) long. Cultivation group 2. ↕ to 15cm (6in), ↔ to 10cm (4in). W. Himalayas. ❄❄❄

C. flexuosa ■ Erect, summer-dormant perennial with slender, fibrous rootstocks with small bulbils, and 2-ternate leaves, to 15cm (6in) long, with ovate, glaucous, light green leaflets, sometimes flushed purple. From late spring to summer, produces dense, terminal and axillary racemes of slender-tubed, brilliant blue flowers, to 2.5cm (1in) long, with white throats. Cultivation group 3. ↕ to 30cm (12in), ↔ 20cm (8in) or more. China (W. Sichuan). ❄❄❄

C. fumariifolia, syn. *C. ambigua* of gardens. Tuberous perennial with 2-ternate, slightly glaucous, mid-green leaves, to 7cm (3in) long, with entire, oval to obovate leaflets. From spring to early summer, bears loose, spike-like racemes of azure-blue, occasionally purple flowers, 2–3cm (¾–1¼in) long, with flattened, triangular spurs. Cultivation group 3. ↕ to 15cm (6in), ↔ to 10cm (4in). Russia (Kamchatka), China, Japan. ❄❄❄

C. halleri see *C. solida.*

C. ledebouriana. Tuberous perennial with ternate to 3-ternate, blue-green leaves, to 8cm (3in) long, with entire, elliptic to rounded leaflets. In spring, bears loose racemes of very pale purple flowers, to 7cm (3in) long, with dark purple lips and long, upward-curving spurs. Cultivation group 4. ↕ 10–15cm (4–6in), ↔ to 20cm (8in). Mainly Uzbekistan, also E. Afghanistan, N. Pakistan. ❄❄❄

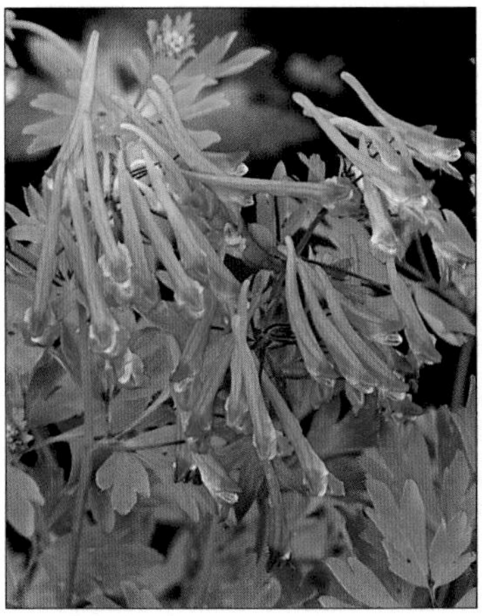
Corydalis flexuosa

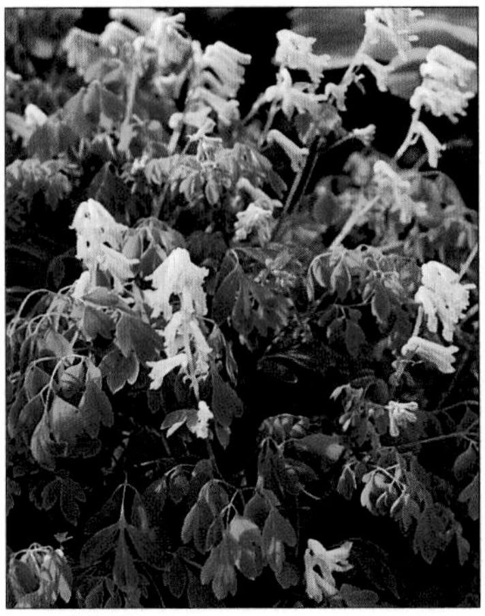
Corydalis lutea

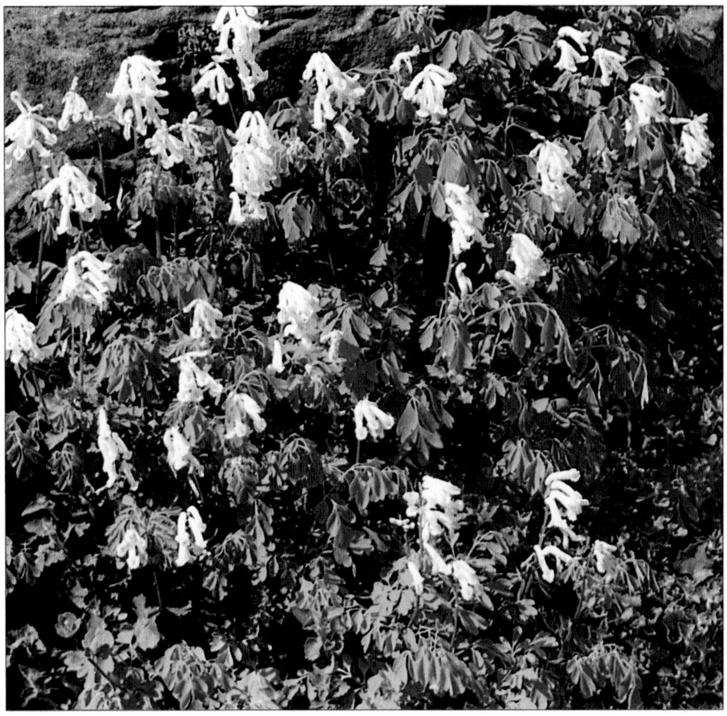
Corydalis ochroleuca

C. lutea ■ syn. *Pseudofumaria lutea.* Rhizomatous, mound-forming, evergreen perennial with fern-like, 2-ternate or 2- or 3-pinnate, arching leaves, 10–15cm (4–6in) long, with obovate, 3-lobed leaflets, pale green above, glaucous beneath. Bluntly spurred, golden yellow flowers, 1–2cm (½–¾in) long, are borne in terminal and axillary racemes of 6–16 flowers, in a long succession from late spring to early autumn. Self-seeds freely. Cultivation group 1, 2, or 3. ↕ 40cm (16in), ↔ 30cm (12in). Widespread in Europe. ❄❄❄

C. malkensis, syn. *C. caucasica* var. *alba* of gardens. Tuberous perennial producing ternate, pale green leaves, to 8cm (3in) long, with linear leaflets. Creamy white, occasionally blue flowers, to 2.5cm (1in) long, with broad lower lips and entire bracts, are produced in loose racemes in spring. Cultivation group 2 or 3. ↕ 8–15cm (3–6in), ↔ to 10cm (4in). Caucasus, Russia, N.E. Iran. ❄❄❄

C. nobilis. Rhizomatous, robust, deep-rooting perennial with much-divided, more or less stalkless, bluish green leaves, to 30cm (12in) long; the leaves are 2-pinnate at the bases, with wedge-shaped leaflets. In late spring, the upright stems bear dense, terminal racemes of up to 30 light yellow flowers, 2–2.5cm (¾–1in) long, each with a brown spot and a short, downward-pointing spur, and deeper yellow at the tips. Cultivation group 1. ↕ 60cm (24in), ↔ 45cm (18in). Russia (Siberia), E. Kazakhstan, N.W. China, Mongolia. ❄❄❄

C. ochotensis. Mound-forming, tap-rooted biennial bearing few long-stalked, 2- or 3-pinnate, light green leaves, 15cm (6in) long, with obovate to wedge-shaped, usually 2- or 3-lobed leaflets. Simple or branched racemes of up to 10 yellow flowers, 1.5–2cm (½–¾in) long, maroon at the tips, with tapering, downward-curving spurs, are produced from midsummer to late autumn. Cultivation group 1 or 3. ↕ 60cm (24in), ↔ 30cm (12in). N. China, Korea, Japan. ❄❄❄

C. ochroleuca ■ Evergreen, fibrous-rooted, clump-forming perennial with 2- or 3-pinnate, light green leaves, to 12cm (5in) long, with obovate leaflets. Compact, axillary racemes of creamy white flowers, to 1.5cm (½in) long, with yellow throats and downward-curving spurs, are produced from late spring to summer. Self-seeds freely. Cultivation group 1. ↕↔ to 30cm (12in). S.E. Europe. ❄❄❄

C. popovii ■ Tuberous perennial with 2- or 3-ternate, blue-green leaves, to 15cm (6in) long, with 3–9 ovate leaflets. In late spring, produces loose, upright racemes of outward-facing, pale violet to white flowers, to 4.5cm (1¾in) long, with deep red-purple lips and downward-curving spurs, to 2.5cm (1in) long. Cultivation group 4. ↕ to 15cm (6in), ↔ to 12cm (5in). C. Asia. ❄❄❄

C. rutifolia. Variable, tuberous perennial with tufted, 2-ternate, grey-green leaves, to 10cm (4in) long, with entire or finely cleft leaflets. In spring, bears violet flowers, to 2.5cm (1in) long, with dark purple lips and ascending, inflated spurs, in loose racemes just

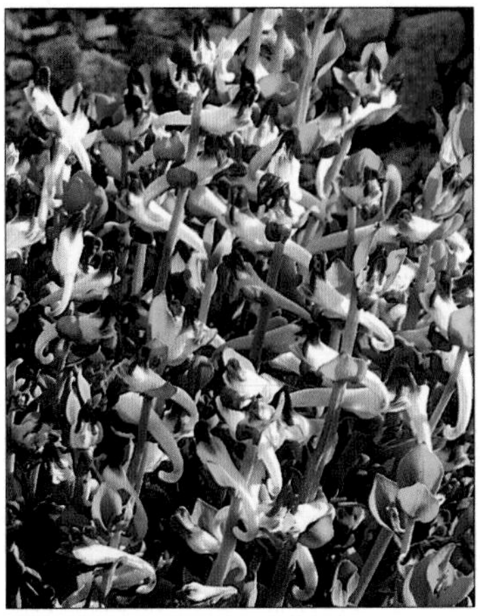
Corydalis popovii

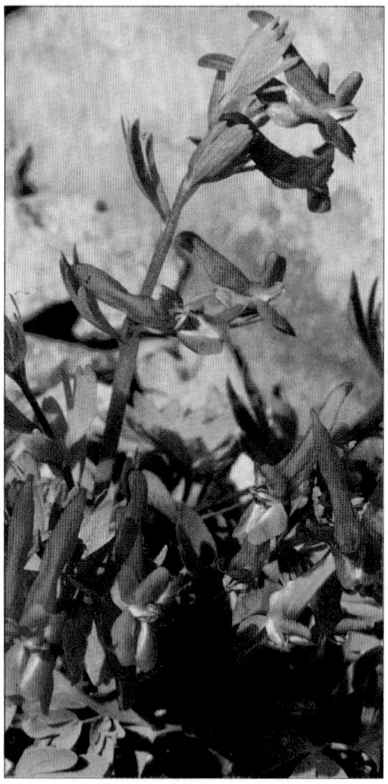

Corydalis solida 'George Baker'

above or among the leaves. Cultivation group 4. ↕ 8cm (3in), ↔ to 12cm (5in). Greece (Crete), Cyprus, E. Turkey. Lebanon, Iraq. ❄❄❄

C. saxicola, syn. *C. thalictrifolia.* Rhizomatous perennial with 2- or 3-pinnate, shiny, mid-green leaves, 35cm (14in) long, with obovate or ovate leaflets. Spreading racemes of short-spurred yellow flowers, to 2.5cm (1in) long, are produced from late spring to summer. Cultivation group 2 or 4. ↕ to 30cm (12in), ↔ to 20cm (8in). C. China. ❄❄

C. scouleri. Rhizomatous, spreading, deep-rooting perennial with upright stems bearing pinnatisect or 2- or 3-pinnate, greyish green leaves, to 35cm (14in) long, with ovate, entire or deeply cut lobes or leaflets. In late spring and early summer, produces racemes of 15–35 purplish pink or white flowers, 2.5cm (1in) long, with slender spurs. Cultivation group 3. ↕ to 90cm (36in), ↔ 45cm (18in). N.W. North America. ❄❄❄

C. solida 🏆 syn. *C. halleri*, *C. transsylvanica* of gardens (Fumewort). Variable, tuberous perennial with 2- or 3-ternate, grey-green leaves, to 8cm (3in) long, with deeply and unevenly dissected, narrowly to broadly ovate leaflets. In spring, produces dense, upright, spike-like racemes of numerous pale mauve-pink to red-purple or white flowers, to 2cm (¾in) long, with tapered, downward-curving spurs and lobed bracts. Cultivation group 2 (tolerates partial shade). ↕ to 25cm (10in), ↔ to 20cm (8in). N. Europe, Asia. ❄❄❄. **'George Baker'** ■ 🏆 syn. 'G.P. Baker', produces deep reddish salmon-pink flowers. Many similar seedlings from pink- or red-flowered variants of *C. solida* have recently been raised and named.

C. thalictrifolia see *C. saxicola.*

***C. transsylvanica* of gardens** see *C. solida.*

C. wilsonii ■ Evergreen perennial with a fleshy, tap-rooted rootstock and rosettes of pinnate, smooth, blue-green leaves, to 8cm (3in) long, with broadly oblong-elliptic leaflets. Loose racemes of short-spurred, green-tipped, canary-yellow flowers, to 2cm (¾in) long, are produced in spring. Suitable for an alpine house or shady wall. Cultivation group 4. ↕↔ 10–20cm (4–8in). C. China. ❄❄❄

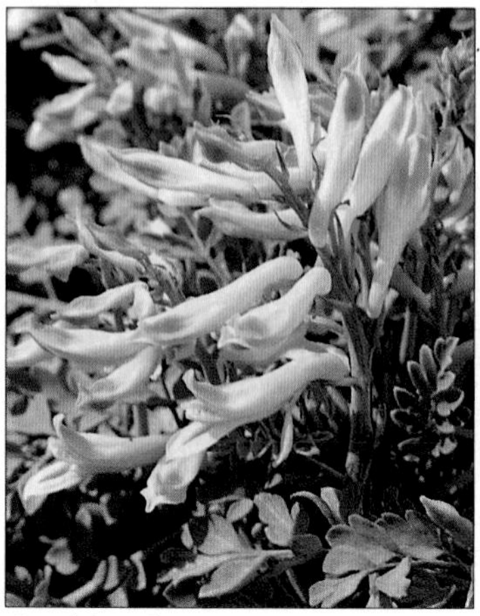

Corydalis wilsonii

CORYLOPSIS

HAMAMELIDACEAE

Genus of 7–10 species of deciduous shrubs and small trees found in woodland and scrub in the E. Himalayas, China, Taiwan, and Japan. They have alternate, simple, ovate to broadly ovate, toothed, pale to dark green leaves. Pendent racemes of 6–20 bell-shaped, fragrant yellow flowers are produced in spring, before the young leaves emerge. Grow in a woodland garden or shrub border.

• **HARDINESS** Fully hardy, although late frosts may damage the flowers.

• **CULTIVATION** Grow in fertile, moist but well-drained, acid soil in partial shade. Pruning group 1; prune immediately after flowering if required.

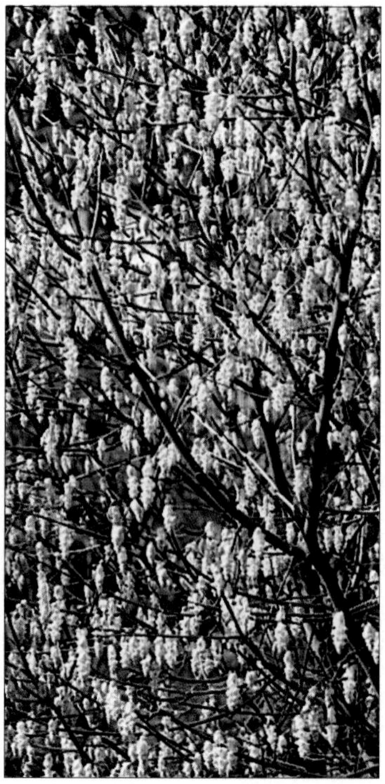

Corylopsis glabrescens

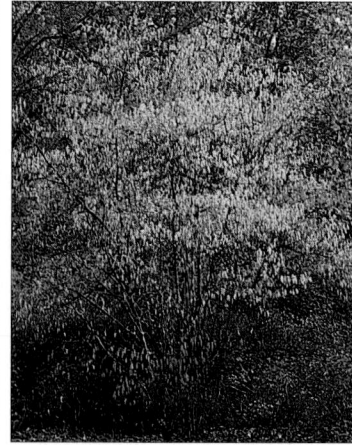

Corylopsis sinensis

• **PROPAGATION** Sow seed in containers in an open frame in autumn. Insert greenwood cuttings in summer. Layer in autumn.

• **PESTS AND DISEASES** Trouble free.

C. glabrescens ■ Open, spreading shrub with broadly ovate leaves, dark green above and blue-green beneath, to 10cm (4in) long. Pale yellow flowers are borne in pendent racemes, to 2.5cm (1in) long, in mid-spring. ↕↔ 5m (15ft). Korea, Japan. ❄❄❄

C. pauciflora 🏆 Bushy, spreading shrub with ovate, bright green leaves, to 7cm (3in) long, bronze when young. Bears abundant pale yellow flowers in pendent racemes, to 3cm (1¼in) long, in early and mid-spring. ↕ 1.5m (5ft), ↔ 2.5m (8ft). Japan, Taiwan. ❄❄❄

C. sinensis ■ syn. *C. willmottiae.* Vigorous, open, upright to spreading shrub with obovate to oblong leaves, to 10cm (4in) long, dark green above and blue-green beneath. Lemon-yellow flowers are produced in pendent racemes, to 8cm (3in) long, in mid-spring. ↕↔ 4m (12ft). China. ❄❄❄. **var. *calvescens* f. *veitchiana*** 🏆 syn. *C. veitchiana*, is upright, and produces pendent racemes, 9cm (3½in) long, of mid-yellow flowers with brick-red anthers; ↔ 2.5m (8ft). **'Spring Purple'** has dark plum-purple young foliage.

C. spicata. Open, spreading shrub with ovate to obovate leaves, dark green above and glaucous beneath, to 10cm (4in) long. Bears bright yellow flowers, with red to purple anthers, in slender, pendent racemes, to 15cm (6in) long, in spring. ↕ 2m (6ft), ↔ 3m (10ft). Japan. ❄❄❄

C. veitchiana see *C. sinensis* var. *calvescens* f. *veitchiana.*

C. willmottiae see *C. sinensis.*

CORYLUS

Hazel

BETULACEAE

Genus of 10–15 species of deciduous trees and shrubs from N. temperate regions, usually found in woodland. They have alternate, rounded or oval to ovate leaves, sometimes with heart-shaped bases. Hazels are grown for their foliage and yellow male catkins. Cultivars of *C. avellana* and *C. maxima* also produce edible nuts. Smaller hazels are best grown in a shrub border; the larger species and cultivars are excellent specimen trees.

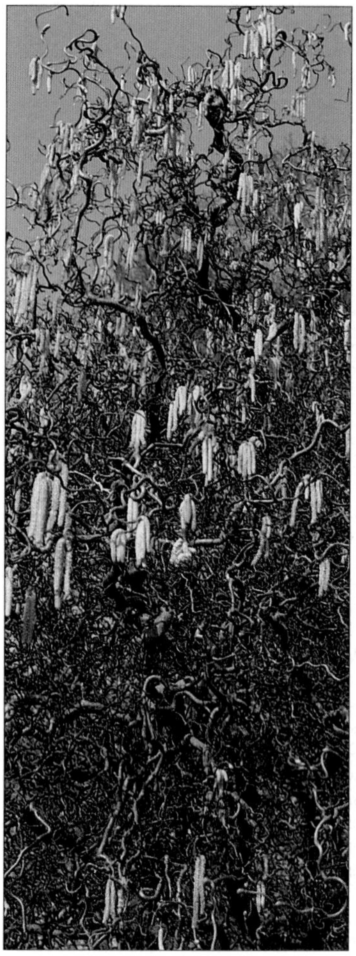

Corylus avellana 'Contorta'

• **HARDINESS** Fully hardy.

• **CULTIVATION** Grow in fertile, well-drained soil in sun or partial shade; they are ideal for chalky soils. Grow variants with coloured leaves in full sun. Remove suckers, which are produced particularly on grafted plants. Pruning group 1; also group 7 for *C. avellana* and *C. maxima.*

• **PROPAGATION** Sow seed in a seedbed as soon as ripe. Layer cultivars in autumn; graft in winter.

• **PESTS AND DISEASES** Caterpillars, mites, sawflies, and aphids may be troublesome. Honey fungus, silver leaf, and powdery mildew may be a problem.

***C. avellana* cultivars.** Upright or tree-like shrubs with broadly heart-shaped, round-tipped, toothed, mid-green leaves, to 10cm (4in) long. Pendent

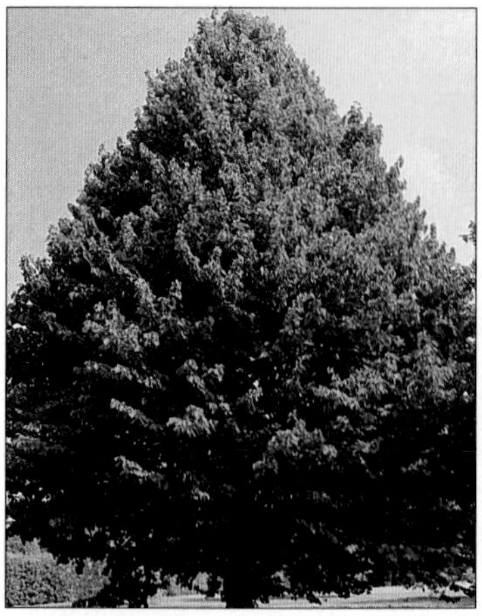

Corylus colurna

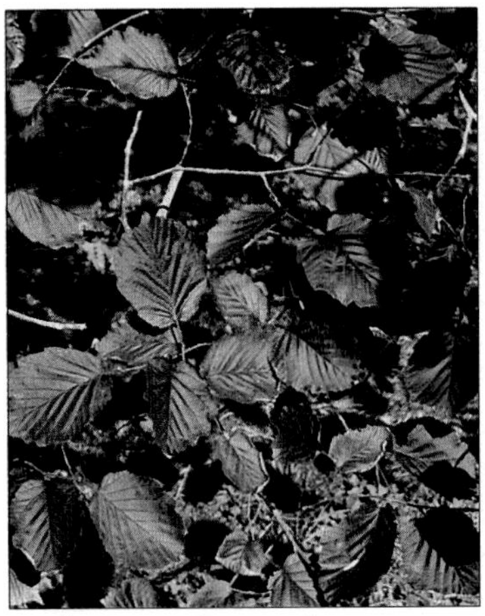
Corylus maxima 'Purpurea'

yellow catkins, 4–6cm (1½–2½in) long, are borne in late winter and early spring. ↕↔ 5m (15ft). Europe, Turkey. ❄❄❄.
'Aurea' has bright yellow young foliage, becoming yellow-green when mature.
'Contorta' ■ ♀ (Corkscrew hazel, Harry Lauder's walking stick) has strongly twisted shoots, which are particularly effective in winter, and is useful for flower arrangements.
C. colurna ■ ♀ ◊ (Turkish hazel). Conical tree with broadly oval, shallowly lobed, dark green leaves, to 12cm (5in) long, turning yellow in autumn. Pendent yellow catkins, 5–8cm (2–3in) long, are borne in late winter. Produces edible nuts, enclosed in deeply fringed husks, in autumn. ↕ 20m (70ft), ↔ 7m (22ft). S.E. Europe, W. Asia. ❄❄❄
C. maxima ◘ (Filbert). Upright shrub or tree with heart-shaped, mid-green leaves, to 14cm (5½in) long. Pendent yellow catkins, 5–8cm (2–3in) long, are borne in late winter. Produces edible nuts, enclosed in tubular husks, which ripen in autumn. ↕ 6m (20ft), ↔ 5m (15ft). S.E. Europe to Caucasus. ❄❄❄.
'Purpurea' ■ ♀ has dark purple foliage, and purple-tinged catkins and fruit husks; grow in full sun.

CORYNOCARPUS

CORYNOCARPACEAE

Genus of 48 species of evergreen trees from Australasia, New Guinea, Vanuatu, and New Caledonia, occurring in open woodland and thickets. Simple, entire, leathery leaves are arranged alternately or in spirals along the stems. Small, tubular, 5-petalled flowers are borne in terminal panicles or racemes, followed by plum-like fruits. In frost-prone areas, grow *Corynocarpus* species and cultivars in a temperate or warm greenhouse; in warmer climates, use as specimen trees, screens, or windbreaks, especially in a coastal garden.
• **HARDINESS** Frost tender.
• **CULTIVATION** Under glass, grow in loam-based potting compost (JI No.2) in full or bright filtered light, with good ventilation. In the growing season, water moderately and apply a balanced liquid fertilizer monthly; water sparingly in winter. Top-dress or pot on in spring. Outdoors, grow in fertile, moist but well-drained soil in sun or partial shade. Pruning group 1; plants under glass may need restrictive pruning.
• **PROPAGATION** Sow seed at not less than 15°C (59°F) in spring. Root semi-ripe cuttings with bottom heat in summer.
• **PESTS AND DISEASES** Prone to scale insects and red spider mites under glass.

C. laevigatus ■ ◊ (Karaka). Erect and bushy, then spreading tree with obovate to elliptic-oblong, lustrous, deep green leaves, 10–20cm (4–8in) long. When mature, produces tiny, greenish yellow flowers in stiff panicles, 10–20cm (4–8in) long, from spring to summer. Narrowly ovoid orange fruit, 4cm (1½in) long, ripen in autumn. ↕ 10–15m (30–50ft), ↔ 2–5m (6–15ft). Vanuatu, New Zealand. ⊛ (min. 10°C/50°F). **'Albovariegatus'** has leaves with white margins. **'Variegatus'** has yellow-margined leaves.

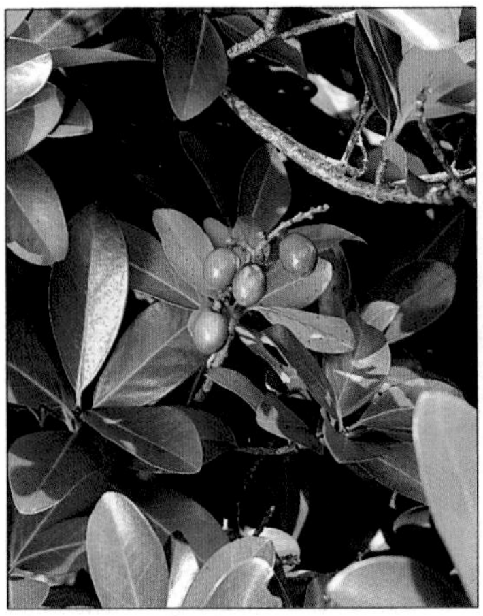
Corynocarpus laevigatus

CORYPHA

ARECACEAE/PALMAE

Genus of 8 species of monocarpic, single-stemmed palms from tropical Asia to N. Australia and the Malaysian islands. Pinnate leaves, which appear to be palmate, are borne in dense clusters. Bowl-shaped, 3-petalled flowers are produced in spectacular, terminal panicles. In frost-prone areas, grow as foliage houseplants or in a warm greenhouse; in warmer areas, grow as free-standing specimens on a lawn.
• **HARDINESS** Frost tender.
• **CULTIVATION** Under glass, grow in loam-based potting compost (JI No.3) in bright filtered light with moderate humidity. In the growing season, water moderately and apply a balanced liquid fertilizer monthly; water sparingly in winter. Pot on or top-dress in spring. Outdoors, grow in fertile, moist but well-drained soil in full sun.
• **PROPAGATION** Sow seed at 24–29°C (75–84°F) in spring.
• **PESTS AND DISEASES** Red spider mites and scale insects may be a problem under glass.

C. umbraculifera ■ ♀ (Talipot palm). Medium-sized to large palm with a sturdy trunk clad in old leaf bases. Leaf-stalks are 2–3m (6–10ft) long, with short, spiny teeth; the lustrous, rich green blades, 2.5–5m (8–15ft) across, have 70–120 segments. Creamy white flowers are borne in panicles, 6–8m (20–25ft) tall – the largest of all palm inflorescences; they first appear in spring at the end of the tree's life (usually between 20 and 30 years old). ↕ 15–25m (50–80ft), ↔ 7–14m (22–46ft). S. India, Sri Lanka. ⊛ (min. 15°C/59°F)

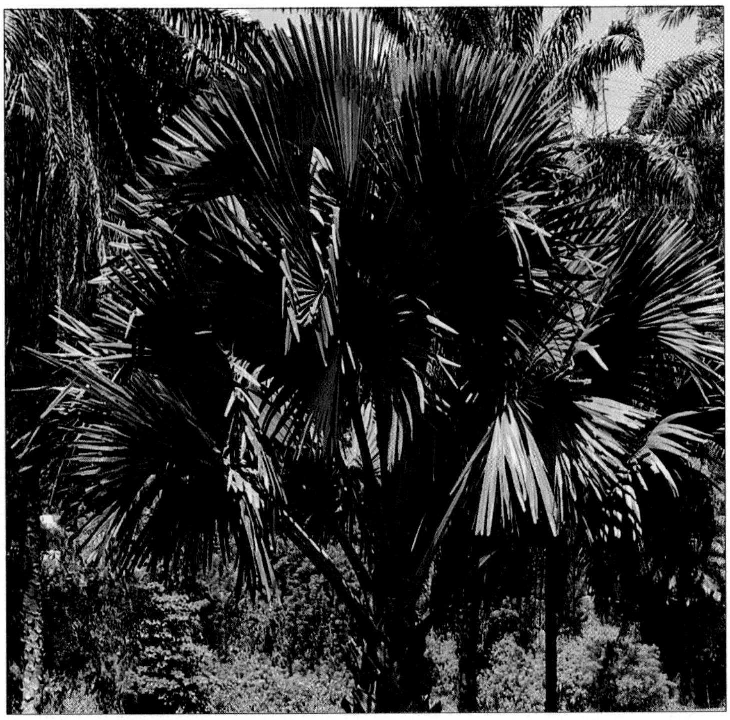
Corypha umbraculifera

CORYPHANTHA

CACTACEAE

Genus of 45 species of mostly spherical, occasionally cylindrical, warty, spiny, perennial cacti, occurring in semi-arid areas of S.W. USA and Mexico. In summer, solitary, funnel-shaped, diurnal flowers are produced from the bases of the furrows in the tubercle axils; these are followed by cylindrical green seed pods, which contain ovoid to kidney-shaped brown seeds. In frost-prone areas, grow as houseplants or in a warm greenhouse; in warmer climates, grow in a desert garden.

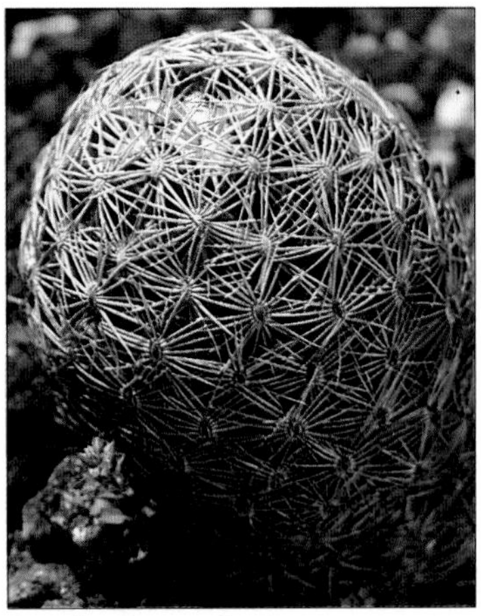
Coryphantha cornifera

• **HARDINESS** Frost tender.
• **CULTIVATION** Under glass, grow in standard cactus compost in full light. From spring to early autumn, water freely and apply a low-nitrogen liquid fertilizer monthly; keep completely dry at other times. Outdoors, grow in low-fertility, humus-rich, gritty, sharply drained soil in full sun. See also pp.48–49.
• **PROPAGATION** Sow seed at 19–24°C (66–75°F) in spring or early summer.
• **PESTS AND DISEASES** Mealybugs may be a problem under glass.

C. calochlora see *C. nickelsiae.*
C. conoidea see *Neolloydia conoidea.*
C. cornifera ■ Perennial cactus with spherical then columnar, dark to grey-green stems, covered with angular tubercles, each with an areole bearing curved, yellowish brown spines (7–12 radials and 1 central). Yellow flowers, 6cm (2½in) across, are produced in summer. ↕ to 12cm (5in), ↔ 8cm (3in). C. Mexico. ⊛ (min. 10°C/50°F)
C. elephantidens ■ Perennial cactus with flattened-spherical, glossy, mid-green stems, covered with long, very thick, furrowed and felted tubercles, and with white wool in the tubercle axils and at the crown. Each areole produces 6–8 curved, yellowish brown radial spines (no centrals). Deep pink flowers, 8–10cm (3–4in) across, with redder bases and mid-stripes, are produced in summer. ↕ 15cm (6in), ↔ to 20cm (8in). S.W. Mexico. ⊛ (min. 10°C/50°F)
C. macromeris. Variable, clump-forming cactus with spherical, greyish green stems with cylindrical tubercles.

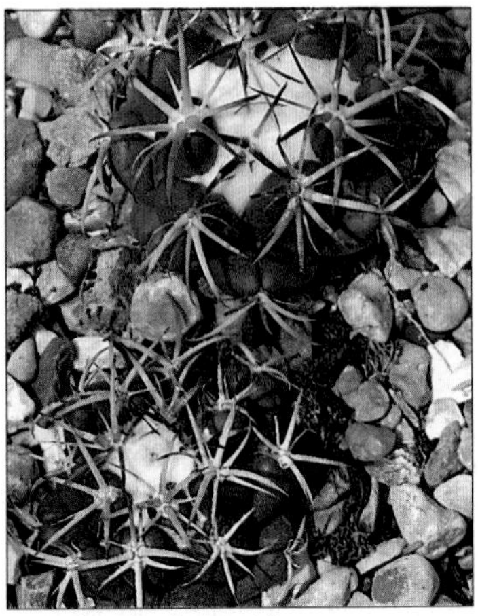
Coryphantha elephantidens

C

The areoles have straight or curved spines (15 red radials and 1–4 dark brown centrals). Deep pink to purple-red flowers, 8cm (3in) across, are produced in summer. ↕15cm (6in), ↔30cm (12in). S.W. USA, Mexico. ⊛ (min. 10°C/50°F)

C. nickelsiae, syn. *C. calochlora.* Clump-forming cactus producing ovoid, glaucous, pale green, later dark green stems with rounded tubercles. The areoles bear numerous straight or curved, yellowish white spines (12–15 radials and 3–5 centrals). Bears yellow flowers, 3–7cm (1¼–3in) across, with brownish purple outer segments, in summer. ↕↔8cm (3in). USA (Texas), Mexico. ⊛ (min. 10°C/50°F)

C. vivipara see *Escobaria vivipara.*

COSMOS

ASTERACEAE/COMPOSITAE

Genus of about 25 species of erect to spreading, freely branched annuals and perennials, found in scrub and meadows in S. USA and Central America. The leaves, borne in opposite pairs, may be simple, lobed, or pinnatisect to 3-pinnatisect or pinnate. *Cosmos* species and cultivars are grown for their large, showy, crimson-red, pink, or white flowerheads, which may be saucer-, bowl-, or open cup-shaped, and are borne on long stems, mainly in summer. Grow annual species and cultivars in an annual border or as fillers in a herbaceous border. Perennial species are excellent container or border plants.

- **HARDINESS** Frost hardy to frost tender.
- **CULTIVATION** Grow in moderately fertile, moist but well-drained soil in full sun. Dead-head to prolong flowering, leaving a few flowerheads on annual species, which often self-seed. Mulch *C. atrosanguineus* in autumn; in very cold areas, lift tubers before first frosts and keep frost-free during winter, packed in barely moist peat.
- **PROPAGATION** Sow seed at 16°C (61°F) in mid-spring, or *in situ* in late spring. Root basal cuttings of *C. atrosanguineus* with bottom heat in early spring.
- **PESTS AND DISEASES** Aphids, slugs, and grey mould (*Botrytis*) may prove troublesome.

C. atrosanguineus ▣ syn. *Bidens atrosanguinea.* Erect then spreading, tuberous perennial with reddish brown stems and spoon-shaped, pinnate to 2-pinnate, dark green leaves, 7–15cm (3–6in) long, with ovate-diamond-shaped, entire or toothed leaflets. Solitary, shallowly cup-shaped, chocolate-scented, velvet-textured, chocolate-maroon flowerheads, 4.5cm (1¾in) across, with slightly darker brown disc-florets, are produced from midsummer to autumn. ↕75cm (30in), ↔45cm (18in). Mexico. ❄❄

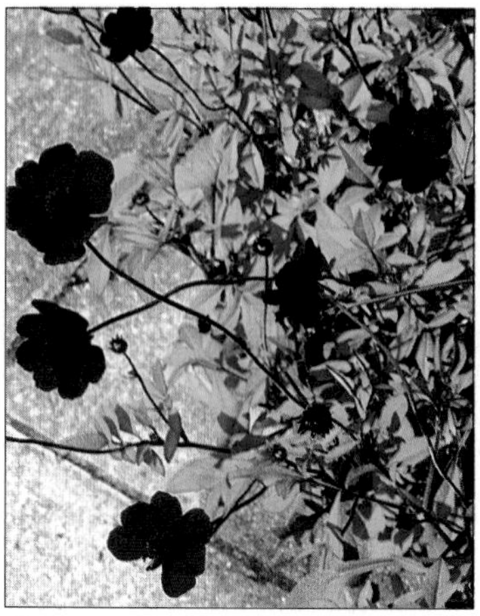

Cosmos atrosanguineus

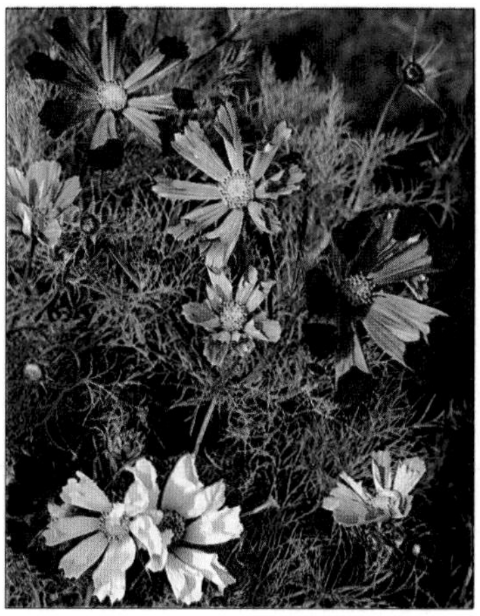

Cosmos bipinnatus 'Sea Shells'

C. bipinnatus. Erect, freely branching annual with pinnatisect, mid-green leaves, to 30cm (12in) long, with linear segments. Produces solitary, bowl- or saucer-shaped, white, pink, or crimson flowerheads, 8cm (3in) across, with yellow centres, throughout summer. ↕to 1.5m (5ft), ↔45cm (18in). Mexico. ❄. **'Candy Stripe'** has white flowerheads with a variable, dark crimson picotee margin to each floret, some flecked also in crimson, and with the occasional pure crimson bloom; ↕to 90cm (36in). **'Sea Shells'** ▣ has carmine-red, pink, or white flowerheads, with florets curiously "quilled" or rolled into tubes; ↕to 90cm (36in). **Sensation Series** cultivars bear pink or white flowerheads, sometimes more than 9cm (3½in) across, in late spring; ↕to 90cm (36in). Cultivars of **Sonata Series** 🏆 are dwarf, with flowerheads in carmine-red, pink, or white, and are especially suitable for an exposed garden; ↕↔30cm (12in). The series includes **'Sonata White'** ▣, which has pure white flowers; ↕to 45cm (18in), ↔30cm (12in).

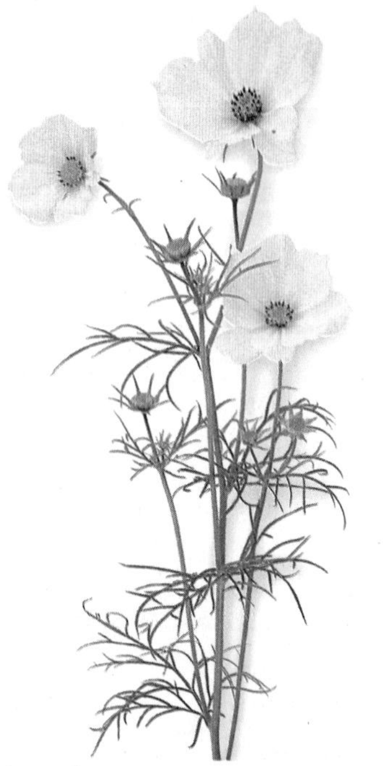

Cosmos bipinnatus 'Sonata White'

C. sulphureus. Erect, bushy, hairy-stemmed annual with 2- or 3-pinnatisect, mid-green leaves, to 18cm (7in) long, with linear lobes. Open bowl-shaped, orange or yellowish red flowerheads, with black centres, are borne in clusters, 3.5–6cm (1½–2½in) across, throughout summer. ↕1.4m (4½ft), ↔45cm (18in). Mexico. ⊛ (min. 5°C/41°F). **'Butterkist'**, syn. 'Lemon Cream', 'Lemon Peel', 'Yellow Garden', bears semi-double yellow flowerheads, to 6cm (2½in) across, in late summer or early autumn; ↕to 75cm (30in). **Ladybird Series** cultivars have less feathery foliage and semi-double flowerheads, 4–8cm (1½–3in) across, in yellow, orange, or scarlet; ↕30–40cm (12–16in), ↔20cm (8in). **'Lemon Cream'** see 'Butterkist'. **'Lemon Peel'** see 'Butterkist'. **'Yellow Garden'** see 'Butterkist'.

▷**Costmary** see *Tanacetum balsamita*

COSTUS

ZINGIBERACEAE

Genus of over 90 species of mostly clump-forming, rhizomatous perennials with an open, lax habit found on forest floors in tropical Africa, Asia, Australia, and North, Central, and South America. The spirally arranged, somewhat fleshy leaves are inversely lance-shaped, lance-shaped, or elliptic. *Costus* species are cultivated for their showy, solitary or paired, white, yellow, orange, pink, or red flowers with basal bracts, usually produced in dense, terminal heads on leafy shoots or sometimes on leafless shoots. The flowers are tubular, each with 3 petals, usually of equal size. Where temperatures fall below 18°C (64°F), grow in a warm greenhouse. In humid tropical climates, grow in a shady border.

- **HARDINESS** Frost tender.
- **CULTIVATION** Under glass, grow in lime-free (ericaceous) potting compost, ideally planted directly into a border, in bright indirect light with high humidity. From spring to summer, water freely and apply a balanced liquid fertilizer monthly; reduce water in autumn, and water sparingly in winter. Pot on or replant in spring. Outdoors, grow in moist but well-drained, fertile, acid soil in full or partial shade.
- **PROPAGATION** Sow seed at 20°C (68°F) as soon as ripe. Divide in spring.
- **PESTS AND DISEASES** Red spider mites may be troublesome under glass.

C. cuspidatus see *C. igneus.*

C. igneus, syn. *C. cuspidatus* (Fiery costus). Erect then spreading perennial producing elliptic, long-pointed leaves, 10–20cm (4–8in) long, dark green above and reddish green beneath. Bears terminal, deep yellow or orange flowers, 5cm (2in) across, at any time of year. ↕40cm (16in), ↔45cm (18in). Brazil. ⊛ (min. 18°C/64°F)

C. malortieanus ▣ (Spiral ginger). Erect perennial with broadly elliptic or obovate, mid-green leaves, to 20cm (8in) long, with darker bands or stripes above and shiny pale green beneath. Deep yellow flowers, 5cm (2in) across, with brown- or red-banded lips, are produced in dense, terminal heads at any time of year. ↕↔1m (3ft). Central America. ⊛ (min. 18°C/64°F)

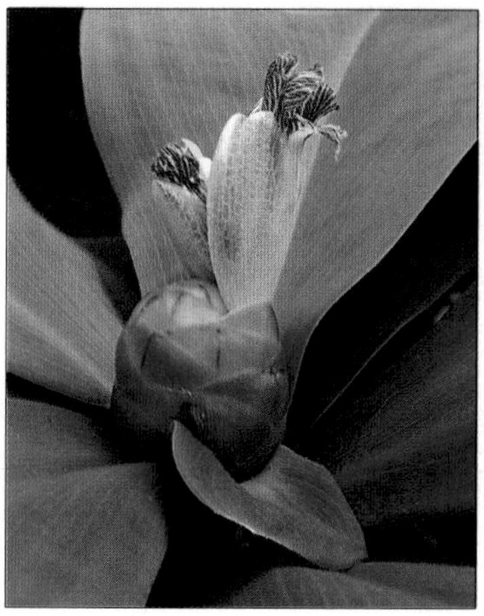

Costus malortieanus

C. speciosus (Crepe ginger). Erect perennial with narrowly elliptic, mid-green leaves, 12–25cm (5–10in) long. Orange- or yellow-centred, white or pink flowers, 5cm (2in) across, are produced in terminal heads, 12cm (5in) long, with red bracts, at any time of year. ↕2.5m (8ft), ↔1m (3ft). S.E. Asia to New Guinea. ⊛ (min. 18°C/64°F)

C. spicatus. Erect perennial with cane-like stems and narrowly elliptic, mid-green leaves, 30cm (12in) long. Yellow and pink flowers, 5cm (2in) across, with red to yellow lips, are produced in terminal heads at any time of year. ↕2.5m (8ft), ↔1m (3ft). West Indies (Hispaniola). ⊛ (min. 18°C/64°F)

▷**Costus, Fiery** see *Costus igneus*

COTINUS

Smoke bush

ANACARDIACEAE

Genus of 2 species of deciduous trees and shrubs occurring in rocky habitats from the Mediterranean region to China and in S. USA. They are cultivated for their alternate, broadly elliptic to rounded, green or purple leaves, which colour well in autumn, and for their plume-like panicles of small, ovoid fruits, which appear in late summer. Inconspicuous flowers are borne in filamentous panicles in summer, producing a smoke-like appearance. Grow in a shrub border or as specimen plants, or plant in groups, which look particularly effective in autumn.

- **HARDINESS** Fully hardy.
- **CULTIVATION** Grow in moderately fertile, moist but well-drained soil in full sun or partial shade. Purple-leaved forms colour best in full sun. Pruning group 1; or group 7 to produce large foliage.
- **PROPAGATION** Sow seed in containers in a cold frame in autumn. Layer in spring. Root softwood cuttings in summer.
- **PESTS AND DISEASES** Susceptible to *Verticillium* wilt. Powdery mildew may affect purple-leaved forms.

C. americanus see *C. obovatus.*

C. coggygria 🏆 ♀ syn. *Rhus cotinus* (Smoke bush, Venetian sumach). Bushy

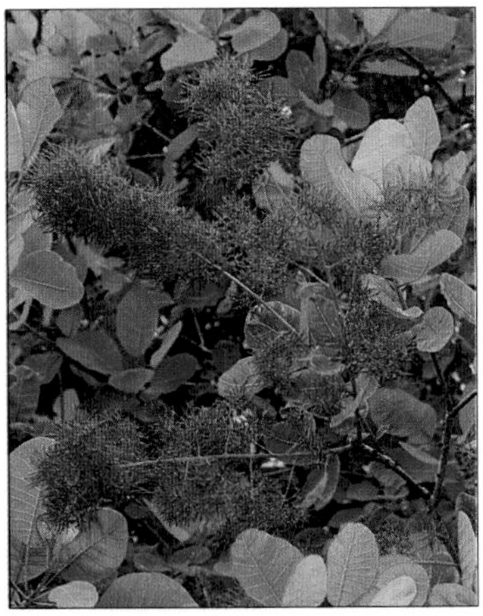

Cotinus coggygria f. *purpureus*

tree or shrub with oval, mid-green leaves, to 7cm (3in) long, turning yellow to orange and red in autumn. Fruiting panicles, to 15cm (6in) long, are green at first, becoming fawn then grey as they mature. ↕↔ 5m (15ft). S. Europe to C. China. ❄❄❄. **'Flame'** see *C.* 'Flame'. **'Notcutt's Variety'** has wine-red foliage and purple-pink fruiting panicles. **f. *purpureus*** ▣ produces light to mid-green leaves, turning orange to red in autumn, and purplish pink inflorescences. **'Royal Purple'** ♀ bears dark red-purple foliage, turning scarlet in autumn.

***C.* 'Flame'** ▣ ♀ ♤ syn. *C. coggygria* 'Flame'. Vigorous, bushy, small tree or shrub producing oval, light green leaves, to 10cm (4in) long, which turn brilliant orange-red in autumn. Fruiting panicles

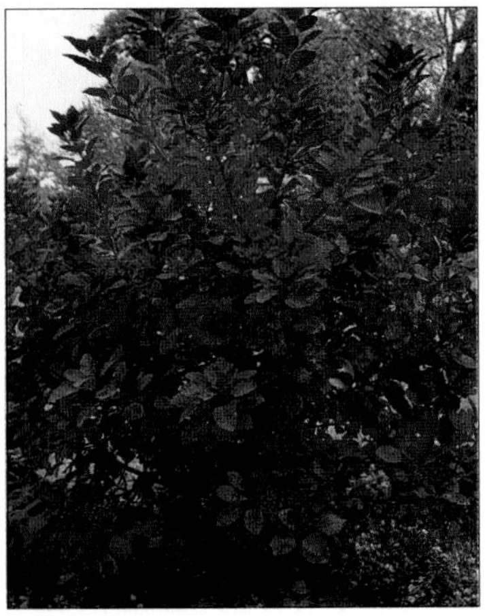

Cotinus 'Grace'

are purple-pink. ↕ 6m (20ft), ↔ 5m (15ft). ❄❄❄

***C.* 'Grace'** ▣ ♀ ♤ Bushy, vigorous shrub or small tree with oval purple leaves, to 10cm (4in) long, turning brilliant, translucent red in late autumn. Fruiting panicles are purple-pink. ↕ 6m (20ft), ↔ 5m (15ft). ❄❄❄

C. obovatus ♀ ♤ syn. *C. americanus*, *Rhus cotinoides* (American smoke tree, Chittamwood). Broadly conical shrub or small tree with obovate to oval leaves, to 12cm (5in) or more long, pinkish bronze when young, turning brilliant orange, red, and purple in autumn. Large, plume-like, pinkish grey fruiting panicles, to 30cm (12in) long, are borne in summer and persist into autumn. ↕ 10m (30ft), ↔ 8m (25ft). S.E. USA. ❄❄❄

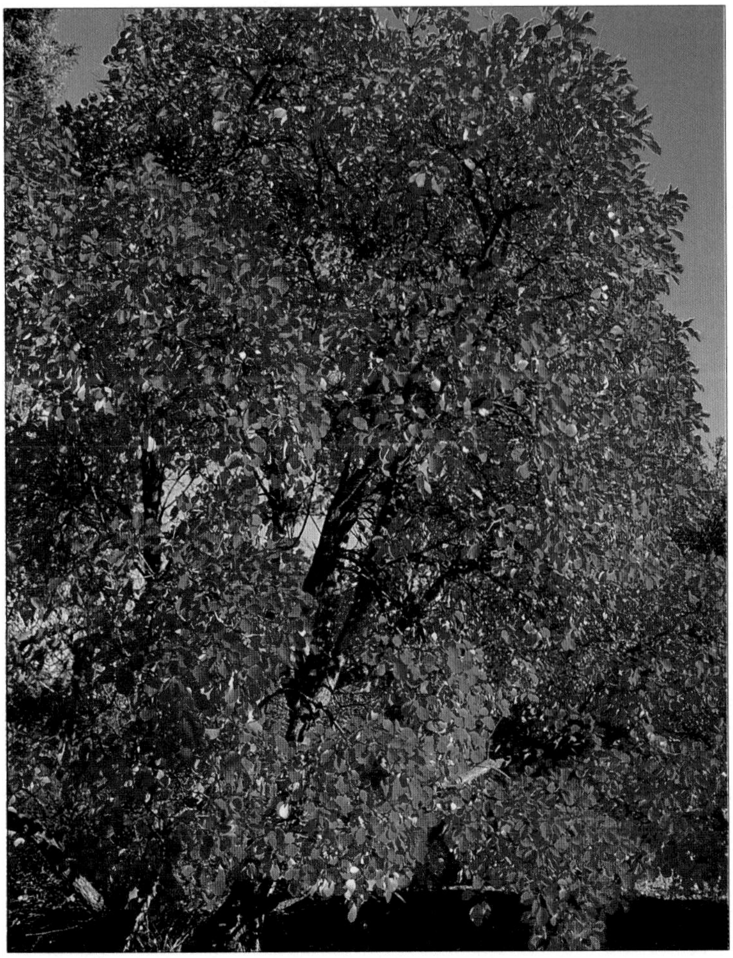

Cotinus 'Flame'

COTONEASTER

ROSACEAE

Genus of more than 200 species of deciduous, semi-evergreen, or evergreen shrubs and trees from woodland and rocky areas in N. temperate regions of Europe, Asia, and N. Africa. They have alternate, lance-shaped to narrowly elliptic, broadly ovate, or rounded leaves. Saucer- to shallowly cup-shaped, white to deep pink flowers, borne singly or in cymes from spring to summer, are followed in autumn by ornamental, spherical to ovoid or obovoid fruits. Grow in a shrub border or as a hedge or screen; some are ideal for wall training. Dwarf species are suitable for a rock garden. Many prostrate species provide good ground cover; some may be trained as weeping standards. Seeds may cause mild stomach upset if ingested.

• **HARDINESS** Fully hardy.

• **CULTIVATION** Grow in moderately fertile, well-drained soil; most will tolerate dry positions. Deciduous species prefer full sun. Large and medium-sized evergreens thrive in sun or partial shade, but need protection from cold, dry winds in areas with prolonged periods below -10°C (14°F). Dwarf evergreens fruit more prolifically in full sun. Most need little regular pruning but will tolerate hard renovation pruning. Pruning group 1 for deciduous species; group 8 for evergreens; group 13 for wall-trained shrubs. Prune formal hedges and wall-trained plants back to the fading flowers or nearest berry cluster in mid- or late summer. Trim again lightly in early autumn if fresh growth obscures fruit display.

• **PROPAGATION** Sow seed in containers in a cold frame as soon as ripe, in autumn; some species are apomictic and come true from seed. Root semi-ripe cuttings of evergreen and semi-evergreen species in late summer; root greenwood cuttings of deciduous species in early summer.

• **PESTS AND DISEASES** Susceptible to fireblight and honey fungus. May be infested by aphids, woolly aphids, scale insects, and webber moth caterpillars.

C. acutifolius. Upright, deciduous shrub with arching shoots and ovate, dark green leaves, to 5cm (2in) long. Short cymes of pink-tinged white flowers are borne in summer, followed by obovoid red fruit, 8–10mm (3/8–1/2in) long. ↕↔ 3m (10ft). China. ❄❄❄

C. adpressus ♀ Prostrate, deciduous shrub with broadly ovate to obovate, wavy-margined, dull green leaves, 1cm (1/2in) long, turning red in autumn. In summer, bears red-tinged white flowers singly or in pairs, followed by spherical, bright red fruit, to 7mm (1/4in) long. ↕ 30cm (12in), ↔ 2m (6ft). W. China. ❄❄❄. **var. *praecox*** see *C. nanshan.*

C. affinis ♤ Vigorous, rounded to broadly columnar, deciduous shrub or small tree with peeling bark and elliptic, dark green leaves, 4–10cm (1 1/2–4in) long. White flowers, borne in large cymes in early summer, are followed by cylindrical, dark purple-black fruit, 0.9–1.5cm (3/8–1/2in) long. ↕ 5m (15ft), ↔ 4m (12ft). Himalayas. ❄❄❄

C. apiculatus. Vigorous, more or less prostrate, deciduous shrub bearing

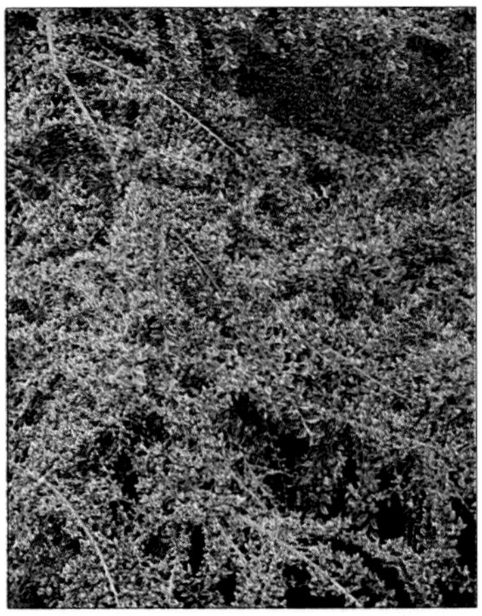

Cotoneaster atropurpureus 'Variegatus'

rounded, wavy-margined, glossy, mid-green leaves, 1–2cm (1/2–3/4in) long, turning red to purple-red in autumn. Solitary, red-tinged white flowers are borne in summer, followed by spherical red fruit, 1cm (1/2in) long. ↕ 1m (3ft), ↔ 2.5m (8ft). China (Sichuan). ❄❄❄

C. atropurpureus. Compact, prostrate or ascending, deciduous shrub with arching branches, and broadly ovate, slightly wavy-margined, glossy, mid-green leaves, to 1cm (1/2in) long, turning dark red-purple in autumn. Solitary, black-based red flowers are borne in summer, followed by almost spherical, bright orange-red fruit, 4–5mm (1/8–1/4in) long. ↕ 50–100cm (20–39in), ↔ 2.5m (8ft). China (Hubei). ❄❄❄. **'Variegatus'** ▣ ♀ syn. *C. horizontalis* 'Variegatus', is less vigorous, with white-margined leaves, turning pink and red in autumn; ↕ 45cm (18in), ↔ 90cm (36in).

***C.* 'Autumn Fire'** see *C.* 'Herbstfeuer'.

C. bullatus* var. *macrophyllus see *C. rehderi.*

C. cashmiriensis ▣ ♀ syn. *C. cochleatus* of gardens, *C. melanotrichus*, *C. microphyllus* var. *cochleatus* of gardens. Compact, prostrate, evergreen shrub with elliptic, glossy, dark green leaves, to 1cm (1/2in) long. Bears usually solitary white flowers, pink in bud, in summer, followed by almost spherical, dark red fruit, 6–8mm (1/4–3/8in) long. Ideal as ground cover. ↕ 30cm (12in), ↔ 2m (6ft). Himalayas (Kashmir). ❄❄❄

***C. cochleatus* of gardens** see *C. cashmiriensis.*

C. congestus, syn. *C. pyrenaicus*. Dense, mound-forming or prostrate, evergreen shrub with obovate, dull pale green

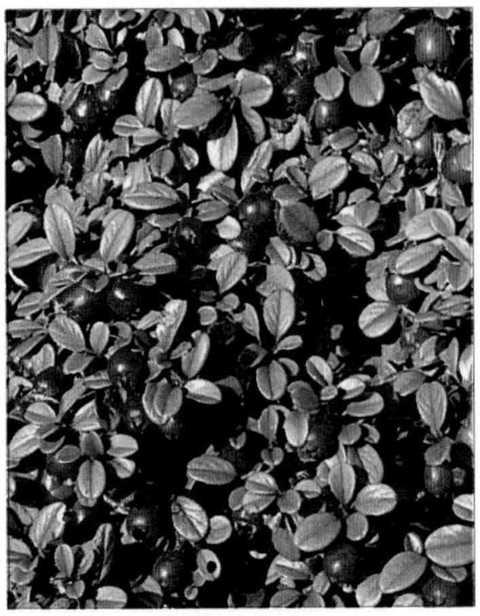

Cotoneaster cashmiriensis

C

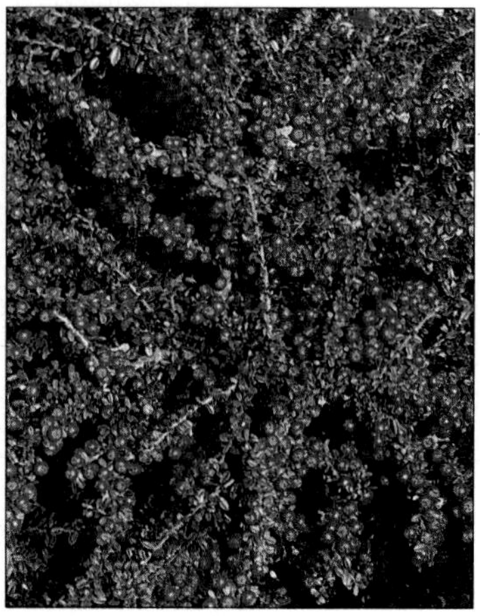
Cotoneaster conspicuus

leaves, 5–15mm (¼–½in) long. Solitary white flowers are borne in summer, followed by spherical, bright red fruit, 6–10mm (¼–½in) long. Excellent in a rock garden. ↕70cm (28in), ↔ 90cm (36in). Himalayas. ✻✻✻
C. conspicuus ▣ ♀ syn. *C. conspicuus* var. *decorus*. Dense, mound-forming, evergreen shrub with narrowly elliptic, slightly shiny, dark green leaves, 0.5–2cm (¼–¾in) long. White flowers are produced singly or occasionally in cymes of up to 5 in summer; they are followed by spherical, shiny red fruit, 7–9mm (¼–⅜in) long, which often last well into winter. ↕1.5m (5ft), ↔ 2–2.5m (6–8ft). S.E. Tibet. ✻✻✻. **'Red Glory'** is erect and vigorous, producing dark red fruit; ↕2m (6ft).
C. conspicuus* var. *decorus see *C. conspicuus*.
***C.* 'Coral Beauty'.** Dense, mound-forming, evergreen shrub with arching branches and obovate to oblong, glossy, dark green leaves, to 1cm (½in) long. Cymes of white flowers are borne in summer, followed by profuse, spherical, bright orange fruit, to 9mm (⅜in) long. Ideal as ground cover. ↕1m (3ft), ↔ 2m (6ft). ✻✻✻

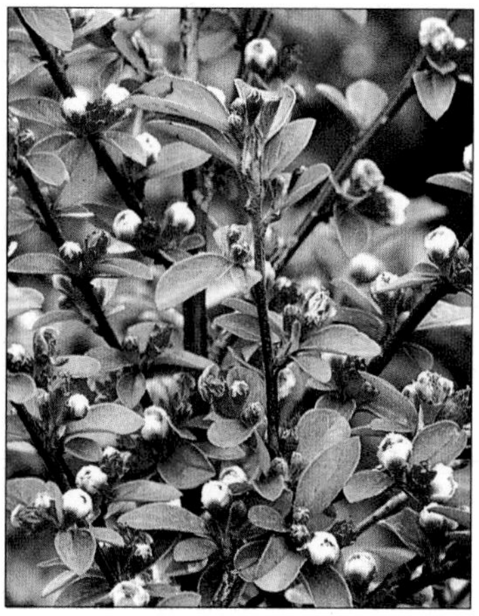
Cotoneaster divaricatus

***C.* 'Cornubia'** ▣ ♀ ○ Vigorous, arching, semi-evergreen shrub or tree bearing narrowly elliptic, dark green leaves, to 12cm (5in) long, some of which turn bronze in winter. Cymes of white flowers are produced in summer, followed by abundant, almost spherical, bright red fruit, to 7mm (¼in) long. ↕↔ 6m (20ft). ✻✻✻
C. dammeri ♀ Vigorous, prostrate, evergreen shrub with long, spreading shoots and broadly obovate to elliptic, mid- to dark green leaves, 1.5–3cm (½–1¼in) long. White flowers are solitary or borne in 2- to 4-flowered cymes in early summer, followed in autumn by almost spherical red fruit, to 7mm (¼in) long. ↕20cm (8in), ↔ 2m (6ft). China (Hubei). ✻✻✻. **'Major'** has rounded, dark green leaves, to 3.5cm (1½in) long. **'Streibs Findling'** see *C. procumbens*.
***C. dielsianus*.** Erect, deciduous, occasionally semi-evergreen shrub with slender, arching shoots bearing ovate to obovate leaves, to 4cm (1½in) long, dark green above and yellowish grey-hairy beneath, turning red in autumn. In summer, bears cymes of 3–7 pink-tinged white flowers, followed by almost

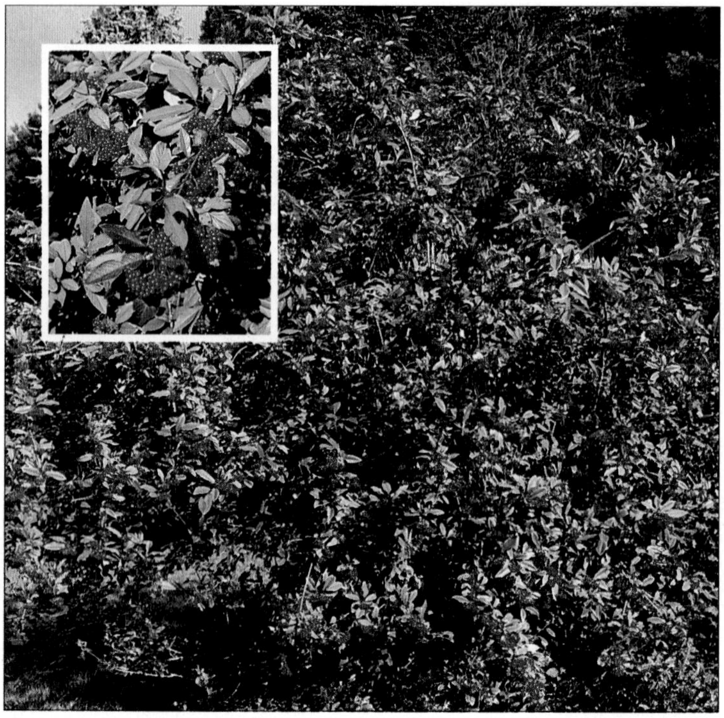
Cotoneaster 'Cornubia' (inset: fruit detail)

spherical, glossy red fruit, 6mm (¼in) long. ↕↔ 2.5m (8ft). China. ✻✻✻
C. distichus see *C. nitidus*.
C. divaricatus ▣ Densely branched, erect, rounded, deciduous shrub with ovate to elliptic, glossy, dark green leaves, 0.8–2.5cm (⅜–1in) long, turning red in autumn. Pink-tinged white flowers are solitary or produced in 2- to 4-flowered cymes in summer, followed by ellipsoid to cylindrical, dark red fruit, 7–9mm (¼–⅜in) long. ↕2.5m (8ft), ↔ 3m (10ft). China (Hubei). ✻✻✻
***C.* 'Exburiensis'.** Vigorous, arching, evergreen shrub with narrowly pointed, elliptic-lance-shaped, deeply veined, mid-green leaves, to 12cm (5in) long. Large cymes of white flowers, borne in early summer, are followed by almost spherical, pale yellow fruit, 5mm (¼in) long, becoming pink-tinged in winter. ↕↔ 5m (15ft). ✻✻✻
***C. floccosus* of gardens** see *C. salicifolius*.
C. franchetii*.** Spreading to erect, evergreen or semi-evergreen shrub with arching branches, and elliptic to ovate leaves, to 3.5cm (1½in) long, grey-green above and white beneath. White flowers, suffused red, with erect petals, are produced in 5- to 15-flowered cymes in summer, followed by obovoid, bright orange-red fruit, 6–9mm (¼–⅜in) long. ↕↔ 3m (10ft). China (Yunnan). ✻✻✻. **var. *sternianus see *C. sternianus*.
C. frigidus ▣ ♀–○ Deciduous tree or large shrub, upright when young, later spreading, with peeling bark and narrowly elliptic to obovate, wavy-margined, dull green leaves, to 15cm (6in) long. Large cymes of 20–60 white flowers are borne in summer, followed by almost spherical, bright red fruit, 6mm (¼in) long. ↕↔ 10m (30ft). Himalayas. ✻✻✻. **'Fructu Luteo'** ▣ has creamy yellow fruit.
***C. glaucophyllus*.** Spreading, evergreen or semi-evergreen shrub with ovate or elliptic, mid-green leaves, 3–8cm (1¼–3in) long, glaucous beneath. Cymes of 15–40 white flowers are produced in midsummer, followed in late autumn by obovoid, orange-red fruit, to 7mm (¼in) long. ↕↔ 3m (10ft). China (Yunnan). ✻✻✻
***C.* 'Gnom'** ▣ syn. *C.* 'Gnome', *C. salicifolius* 'Gnom'. Prostrate, dense, evergreen shrub bearing narrowly lance-shaped, dark green leaves, to 3cm (1¼in) long. Cymes of white flowers are produced in early summer, followed by spherical red fruit, to 5mm (¼in) long. Excellent as ground cover. ↕30cm (12in), ↔ 2m (6ft). ✻✻✻
***C.* 'Gnome'** see *C.* 'Gnom'.
***C.* 'Herbstfeuer'**, syn. *C.* 'Autumn Fire'. Evergreen shrub, prostrate at first, later mound-forming, with lance-shaped, dark green leaves, to 6cm (2½in) long, some turning bright red in autumn. Cymes of 5–12 white flowers are borne in early summer, followed by spherical, bright red fruit, to 5mm (¼in) long. ↕1m (3ft), ↔ 3m (10ft). ✻✻✻
C. horizontalis ▣ ♀ Spreading, deciduous shrub with branches forming a herringbone pattern. Rounded to broadly elliptic, glossy, dark green leaves, to 1cm (½in) long, turn red in autumn. In late spring, bears pink-tinged white flowers singly or in pairs. Spherical fruit, to 6mm (¼in) long, are bright red. ↕1m (3ft), ↔ 1.5m (5ft).

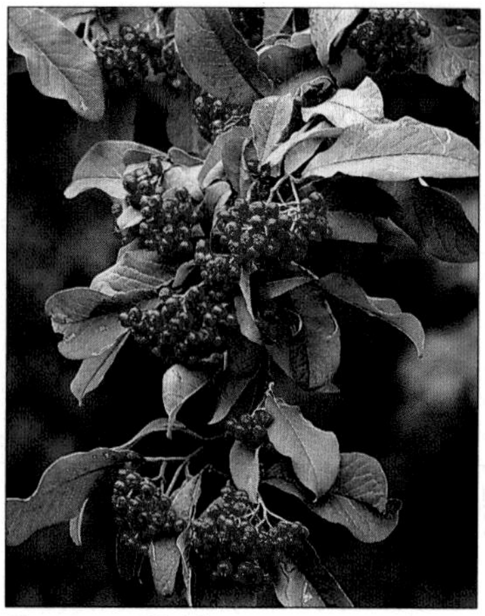
Cotoneaster frigidus

W. China. ✻✻✻. **var. *perpusillus*** see *C. perpusillus*. **'Variegatus'** see *C. atropurpureus* 'Variegatus'.
***C. hupehensis*.** Deciduous shrub with slender, arching branches and elliptic to ovate, dark green leaves, to 3.5cm (1½in) long. Cymes of 5–10 white flowers are borne from late spring to summer, followed by spherical, bright red fruit, to 1cm (½in) or more long. ↕2.5m (8ft), ↔ 4m (12ft). W. China (Hubei). ✻✻✻
***C.* 'Hybridus Pendulus'.** Prostrate, evergreen or semi-evergreen shrub with elliptic-lance-shaped, dark green leaves, to 8cm (3in) long. Small cymes of white flowers are borne in early summer, followed by almost spherical, bright red fruit, 5mm (¼in) long. Forms a small tree with weeping branches when grown as a standard. ↕↔ 2m (6ft). ✻✻✻
C. hylmoei, syn. *C. salicifolius* var. *rugosus* of gardens. Rounded, evergreen shrub with arching shoots and elliptic-lance-shaped, deeply veined, tapered, dark green leaves, to 7cm (3in) long. Cymes of small white flowers, opening from pink buds, are borne in summer, followed by long-lasting, spherical, bright red fruit, 6–8mm (¼–⅜in) long. ↕2.5m (8ft), ↔ 4m (12ft). W. China. ✻✻✻
C. integrifolius, syn. *C. microphyllus* of gardens, *C. thymifolius*. Stiffly branched, compact, evergreen shrub with obovate to oblong, glossy, dark green leaves, to 1cm (½in) long. Solitary white flowers are borne in early summer, followed by spherical, dark reddish pink fruit, 8–10mm (⅜–½in) long. ↕1m (3ft), ↔ 1.5m (5ft). Himalayas. ✻✻✻

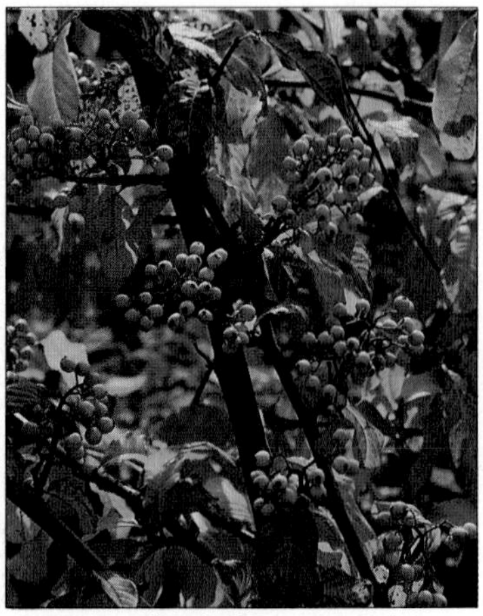
Cotoneaster frigidus 'Fructu Luteo'

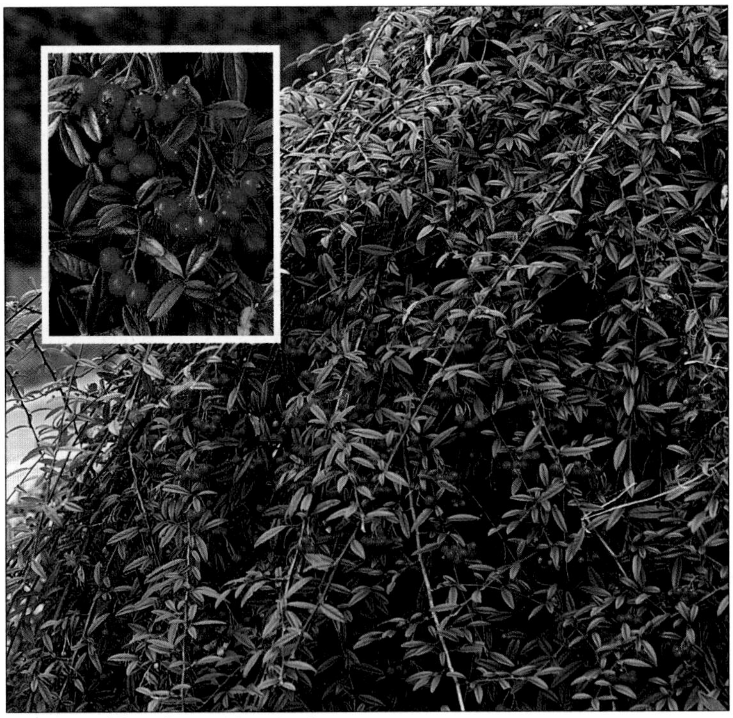

Cotoneaster 'Gnom' (inset: fruit detail)

C. lacteus ▣ 🏆 Dense, evergreen shrub with arching branches bearing obovate or broadly elliptic, deeply veined leaves, 3.5–9cm (1½–3½in) long, dark green above and yellow-white felted beneath. Bears cymes of up to 100 milky white flowers in summer, followed by obovoid red fruit, 6mm (¼in) long, which persist over winter. May be grown as a hedge. ↕↔ 4m (12ft). China (Yunnan). ❄❄❄
C. linearifolius, syn. *C. microphyllus* var. *thymifolius* of gardens. Compact, rounded, evergreen shrub with rigid branches. Oblong to inversely lance-shaped, glossy, dark green leaves, 4–7mm (⅛–¼in) long, are glaucous beneath and notched at the tips. Solitary white flowers, pink in bud, are borne in early summer, followed by spherical, dark red fruit, 4–5mm (⅛–¼in) long. ↕↔ 60–90cm (24–36in). Nepal. ❄❄❄
C. melanotrichus see *C. cashmiriensis.*
***C. microphyllus* var. *cochleatus* of gardens** see *C. cashmiriensis.*
***C. microphyllus* of gardens** see *C. integrifolius.*
***C. microphyllus* var. *thymifolius* of gardens** see *C. linearifolius.*
C. multiflorus. Vigorous, deciduous shrub with long, arching branches and ovate to rounded leaves, to 5cm (2in) long, dull yellowish green above and sparsely hairy, mid-green beneath. Cymes of 10–20 white flowers are borne in late spring, followed by abundant spherical red fruit, to 1cm (½in) long, from late summer to autumn. ↕↔ 5m (15ft). Kazakhstan. ❄❄❄
***C. multiflorus* of gardens** see *C. purpurascens.*
C. nanshan, syn. *C. adpressus* var. *praecox.* Prostrate, spreading, deciduous shrub with rounded, very wavy-margined, mid-green leaves, 1–2.5cm (½–1in) long, turning red in autumn. Paired or single, pinkish white or red-flushed white flowers are produced in late spring, followed by large, almost spherical, bright red fruit, to 1cm (½in) long. ↕ 1m (3ft), ↔ 2m (6ft). W. China (Sichuan, Yunnan). ❄❄❄
C. nitidus, syn. *C. distichus.* Wide-spreading or erect, deciduous or semi-evergreen shrub with stiff branches bearing rounded, glossy, dark green leaves, to 1cm (½in) long. Solitary, pink-tinged white flowers are produced in summer; flowers are followed by long-lasting, obovoid to almost spherical, bright red fruit, to 6mm (¼in) long. ↕ 2.5m (8ft), ↔ 4m (12ft). China (Yunnan), Himalayas. ❄❄❄
C. perpusillus, syn. *C. horizontalis* var. *perpusillus.* Prostrate, deciduous shrub with branches forming a herringbone pattern. Rounded, glossy, dark green leaves, to 8mm (⅜in) long, turn red in autumn, but remain longer than those of *C. horizontalis.* In summer, bears solitary, pink-tinged white flowers. Almost spherical fruit, 4–5mm (⅛–¼in) long, are bright red. ↕ 30cm (12in), ↔ 2m (6ft). China (Hubei). ❄❄❄
***C.* 'Pink Champagne'.** Vigorous, arching, evergreen shrub with narrowly elliptic-lance-shaped, pointed, deeply veined, mid-green leaves, to 12cm (5in) long. Large cymes of white flowers are borne in early summer, followed by spherical, pale yellow fruit, 5mm (¼in) long, which turn pink in late autumn. ↕↔ 5m (15ft). ❄❄❄
C. procumbens ▣ syn. *C. dammeri* 'Streibs Findling'. Prostrate, evergreen shrub, occasionally forming a low mound. Broadly obovate, dull dark green leaves, to 1cm (½in) long, are purplish when young. Solitary white flowers are borne in summer, followed by almost spherical red fruit, to 6mm (¼in) long. ↕ 10cm (4in), ↔ 2m (6ft). China. ❄❄❄
***C. prostratus* of gardens** see *C. rotundifolius.*
C. purpurascens ▣ ♀ syn. *C. multiflorus* of gardens. Erect shrub or small tree with arching branches and ovate to rounded, mid-green leaves, 2–6cm (¾–2½in) long, paler beneath, and hairy when young. In mid- and late spring, bears cymes of white flowers, followed by long-lasting, pear-shaped or spherical red fruit, 6mm (¼in) long. ↕↔ 3–4m (10–12ft). Russia (Siberia), China. ❄❄❄
C. pyrenaicus see *C. congestus.*
C. rehderi, syn. *C. bullatus* var. *macrophyllus.* Vigorous, deciduous shrub with long, arching shoots and ovate to oblong-elliptic, pointed, deeply veined, dark green leaves, to 15cm (6in) long, turning red in autumn. Cymes of up to 30 pink-tinged white flowers are borne in early summer, followed by obovoid to almost spherical, bright red fruit, 8–10mm (⅜–½in) long. ↕ 5m (15ft), ↔ 3m (10ft). China (Sichuan). ❄❄❄
***C.* 'Rothschildianus'** ▣ 🏆 Vigorous, arching, evergreen shrub with narrowly elliptic-lance-shaped, tapered, deeply veined, pale green leaves, to 10cm (4in) long. Bears large cymes of white flowers in early summer, followed by spherical, golden yellow fruit, 5mm (¼in) long, produced over a long period in autumn. ↕↔ 5m (15ft). ❄❄❄
C. rotundifolius, syn. *C. prostratus* of gardens. Spreading, evergreen shrub with arching branches and broadly elliptic to obovate-elliptic, glossy, dark green leaves, to 2cm (¾in) long. Solitary flowers are borne in late spring, followed by spherical, dark pinkish red fruit, 7–10mm (¼–½in) long. ↕ 1.5m (5ft), ↔ 3m (10ft). Himalayas. ❄❄❄
***C.* 'Sabrina'** see *C. splendens.*
C. salicifolius, syn. *C. floccosus* of gardens. Vigorous, evergreen shrub with arching branches and elliptic-lance-shaped, dark green leaves, to 10cm (4in) long. Bears cymes of 30–100 white flowers in summer, followed by almost spherical, shiny, bright red fruit, 5mm (¼in) long. ↕↔ 5m (15ft). China. ❄❄❄. **'Gnom'** see *C.* 'Gnom'. **var. *rugosus* of gardens** see *C. hylmoei.*
C. serotinus ♀ Arching, open, evergreen shrub or small tree with elliptic or obovate-elliptic leaves, 2.5–7cm (1–3in) long, dark green above and pale green (softly downy at first) beneath. Cymes of up to 40 white flowers are borne in mid- and late summer, followed in autumn by obovoid to almost spherical, bright red fruit, 6mm (¼in) long. ↕ 10m (30ft), ↔ 3–4m (10–12ft). W. China (Yunnan). ❄❄❄

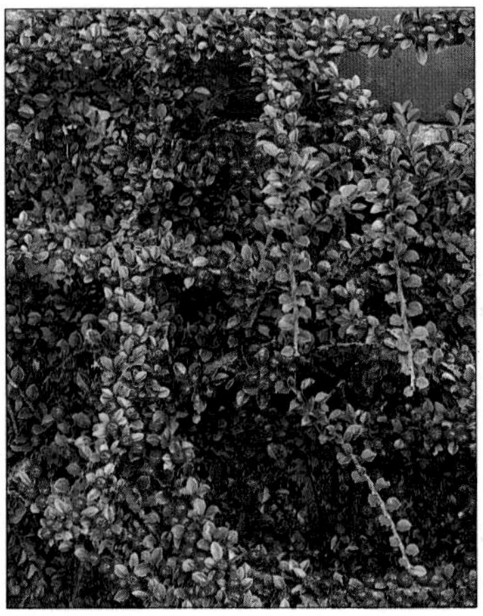

Cotoneaster horizontalis

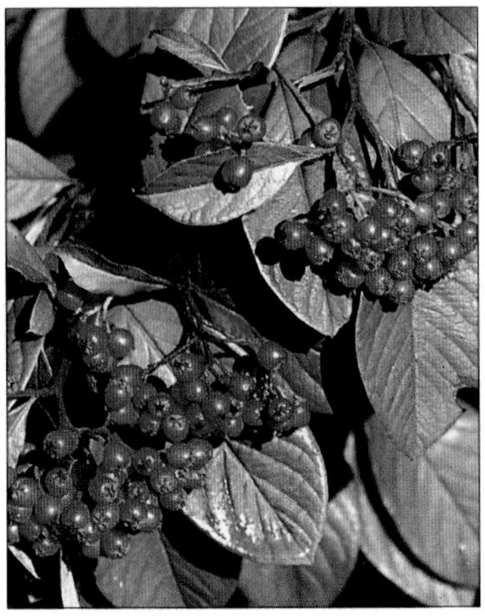

Cotoneaster lacteus

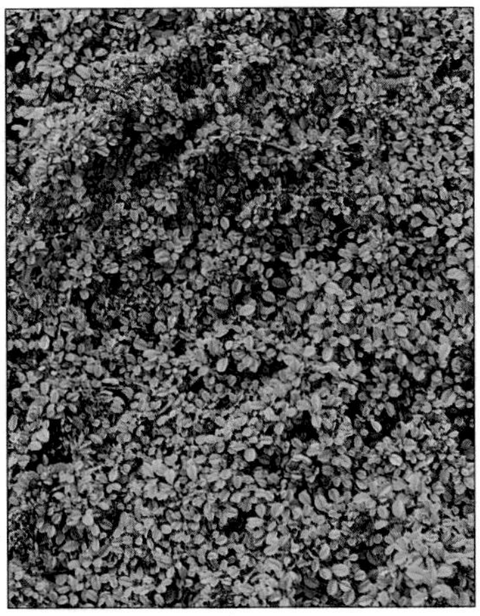

Cotoneaster procumbens

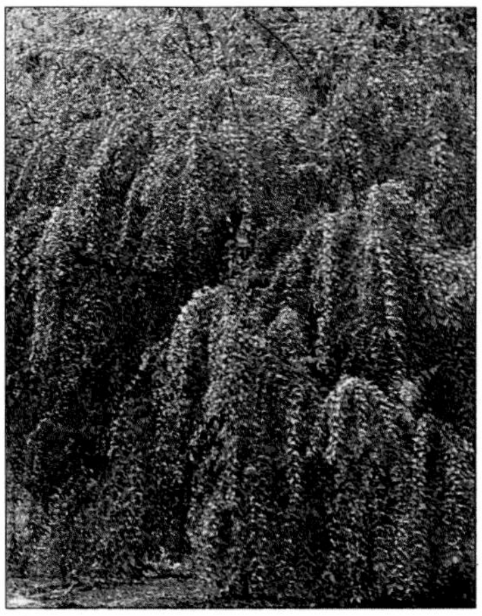

Cotoneaster purpurascens

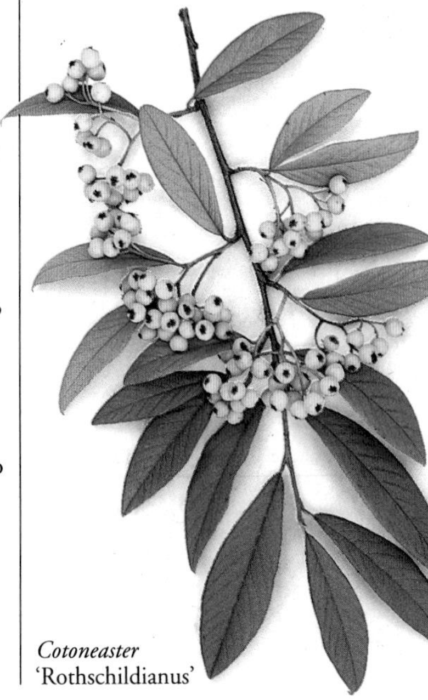

Cotoneaster 'Rothschildianus'

C

C

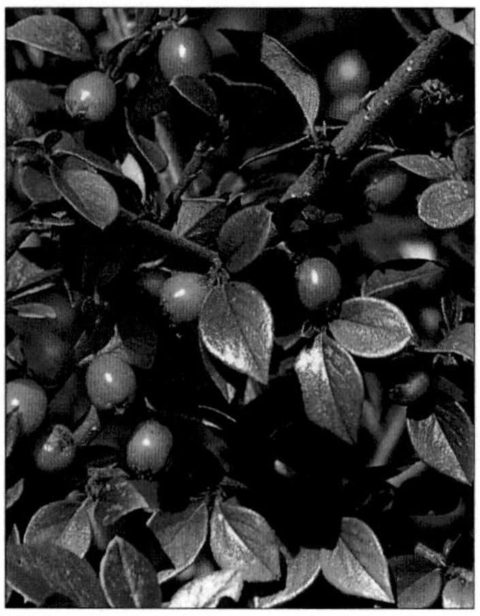

Cotoneaster simonsii

C. simonsii ▣ ♀ Upright, deciduous or semi-evergreen shrub. Broadly ovate, glossy, dark green leaves, to 3cm (1¼in) long, turn red in autumn. Bears pink-tinged white flowers singly or in few-flowered cymes in summer. Obovoid fruit, 8–10mm (⅜–½in) long, are bright orange-red. ↕2.5m (8ft), ↔ 2m (6ft). India (Sikkim), Bhutan. ❄❄❄
***C.* 'Skogholm'**, syn. *C.* 'Skogsholmen'. More or less prostrate, evergreen shrub with ovate to oblong, glossy, dark green leaves, to 2cm (¾in) long. White flowers are borne singly or in few-flowered cymes in late spring, followed by sparse, spherical, bright red fruit, 6–8mm (¼–⅜in) long. Good as ground cover. ↕60cm (24in), ↔ 3m (10ft). ❄❄❄
***C.* 'Skogsholmen'** see *C.* 'Skogholm'.
C. splendens ♀ syn. *C.* 'Sabrina'. Rounded, deciduous shrub with arching branches bearing broadly elliptic to rounded, glossy, mid-green leaves, to 2cm (¾in) long, turning red in autumn. Bears cymes of 3 (occasionally up to 7) pink-suffused white flowers, margined rose-pink, in early summer, followed by almost spherical, bright orange fruit, 9–10mm (⅜–½in) long. ↕2m (6ft), ↔ 2.5m (8ft). China (Sichuan). ❄❄❄
C. sternianus ▣ ♀ syn. *C. franchetii* var. *sternianus*. Vigorous, upright, evergreen or semi-evergreen shrub with arching branches and elliptic, glossy, dark green leaves, 2.5–6cm (1–2½in) long, white-woolly beneath. Erect cymes of up to 15 pink-tinged white flowers are produced in summer, followed by spherical, bright, deep orange-red fruit, 8–10mm (⅜–½in) long. Grow as a hedge. ↕↔ 3m (10ft). China (Yunnan). ❄❄❄

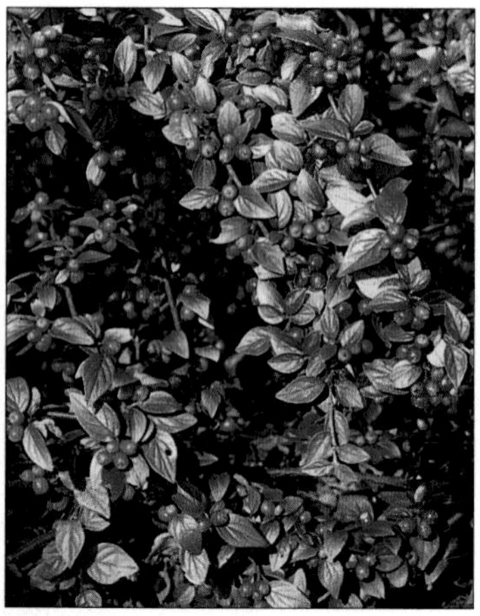

Cotoneaster sternianus

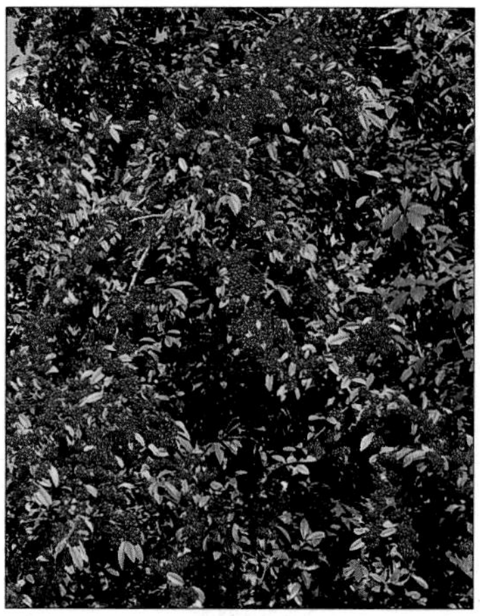

Cotoneaster x *watereri* 'John Waterer'

C. thymifolius see *C. integrifolius*.
***C.* 'Valkenburg'.** Dense, spreading, semi-evergreen shrub with ovate, glossy, mid-green leaves, to 2cm (¾in) long, turning orange, red, and yellow in autumn. In late spring, pink-suffused white flowers are produced singly or in few-flowered cymes, followed by ellipsoid to cylindrical red fruit, 7–9mm (¼–⅜in) long. ↕2m (6ft), ↔ 4m (12ft). ❄❄❄
***C.* x *watereri* 'John Waterer'** ▣ ♀ Vigorous, evergreen or semi-evergreen shrub or small tree with arching branches and lance-shaped, dark green leaves, to 10cm (4in) long. Large cymes of 30–50 white flowers are borne in summer, followed by almost spherical red fruit, 9mm (⅜in) long. ↕↔ 5m (15ft). ❄❄❄

▷**Cotton, Wild** see *Cochlospermum vitifolium*
▷**Cotton grass** see *Eriophorum*
Broad-leaved see *E. latifolium*
Common see *E. angustifolium*
▷**Cotton lavender** see *Santolina chamaecyparissus*
▷**Cottonwood** see *Populus*
Black *P. trichocarpa*
Eastern see *P. deltoides*

COTULA

ASTERACEAE/COMPOSITAE

Genus of about 55 species of prostrate, tufted, or creeping, rhizomatous annuals and perennials, mostly found in moist areas in N. and E. Africa, South Africa, Australia, Mexico, and South America. They are grown mainly for their aster-like flowerheads. In some species, the male and female florets are borne in separate heads. *Cotula* species are also grown for their mainly alternate, sometimes opposite or rosette-forming leaves, which are usually pinnate or lobed, occasionally entire, and mostly silver or fresh green. *C. coronopifolia* is suitable for a pond margin, a bog garden, or a damp border; in areas prone to hard frosts, grow as an annual. Alpine species are suitable for a rock garden.
• **HARDINESS** Frost hardy to half hardy.
• **CULTIVATION** Grow in moist, humus-rich, moderately fertile soil in full sun. Dead-head to prolong flowering.
• **PROPAGATION** Surface-sow seed at 13–18°C (55–64°F) in spring. Lift and divide plants in autumn; in frost-prone areas, overwinter in a cold frame.
• **PESTS AND DISEASES** Trouble free.

C. atrata see *Leptinella atrata*.
C. coronopifolia (Brass buttons). Moisture-loving annual or short-lived perennial with numerous creeping, semi-prostrate, hairless, succulent stems and linear, lobed or coarsely toothed, strongly scented, fresh green leaves, 5–12cm (2–5in) long. Bears button-like, bright yellow flowerheads, 1cm (½in) across, on slender stalks in summer. May be grown in water to 15cm (6in) deep. ↕15cm (6in), ↔ 30cm (12in). South Africa. ❄❄

COTYLEDON

CRASSULACEAE

Genus of 9 species of compact, often clump-forming, perennial succulents and evergreen subshrubs from desert or shaded areas in E. Africa, the Arabian Peninsula, and southern Africa. They are grown for their foliage and flowers. The stalked, fleshy leaves are borne in opposite pairs. Tubular to bell-shaped, generally pendent, red, yellow, or orange flowers are borne in crowded, terminal panicles, mostly in late summer and autumn. In frost-prone areas, grow in a temperate greenhouse or as houseplants. Elsewhere, grow in a desert garden.
• **HARDINESS** Frost tender.
• **CULTIVATION** Under glass, grow in standard cactus compost in full light, with shade from hot sun. In the growing season, water moderately, avoiding the foliage, and apply a dilute, low-nitrogen liquid fertilizer monthly; keep completely dry in winter. Outdoors, grow in gritty, low-fertility, humus-rich, sharply drained soil in full sun with some midday shade. See also pp.48–49.
• **PROPAGATION** Sow seed at 19–24°C (66–75°F), or root stem cuttings, in spring or summer.
• **PESTS AND DISEASES** Prone to aphids.

C. alternans see *Adromischus maculatus*.
C. cooperi see *Adromischus cooperi*.
C. ladismithensis ▣ syn. *C. tomentosa* var. *ladismithensis*. Bushy, often semi-prostrate succulent with many branches, fleshy and hairy above, woody beneath. Thick, oblong, round-tipped, softly hairy, mid-green leaves, 5cm (2in) long, have 2–4 soft teeth. In autumn, bears tubular, brownish red flowers, to 1.5cm (½in) long, in a fleshy inflorescence, 9cm (3½in) long. Often considered a variety of *C. tomentosa*. ↕30cm (12in), ↔ to 20cm (8in). South Africa (Western Cape). ❀ (min. 7°C/45°F)

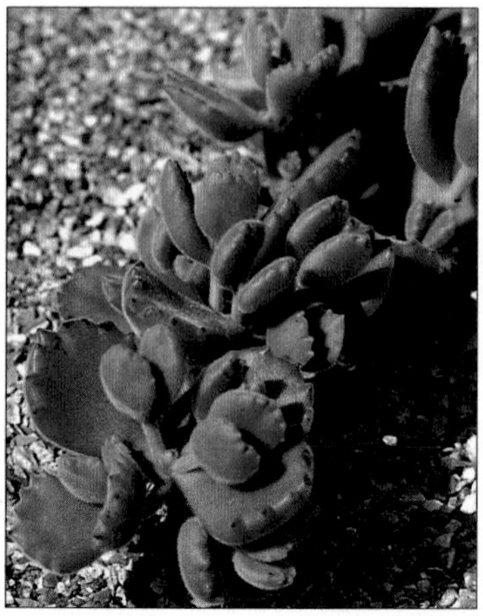

Cotyledon ladismithensis

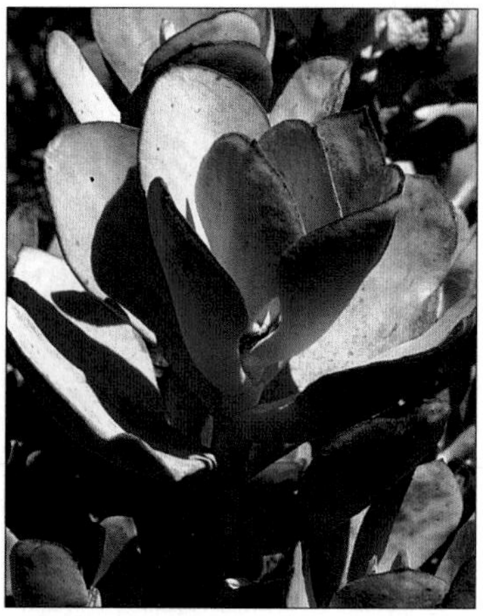

Cotyledon orbiculata

C. maculata see *Adromischus maculatus*.
C. oblonga see *C. orbiculata* var. *oblonga*.
C. orbiculata ▣ Shrubby, erect, freely branching succulent with thick, fleshy stems and ovoid, white-frosted-waxy, white or grey leaves, to 14cm (5½in) long. Bears tubular, red or yellowish red flowers, 1.5–2cm (½–¾in) long, in fleshy inflorescences, to 70cm (28in) long, from late summer to autumn. ↕to 1m (3ft), ↔ 50cm (20in). Angola, Namibia, South Africa (Northern Cape, Western Cape). ❀ (min. 7°C/45°F).
var. *oblonga* ▣ syn. *C. oblonga*, *C. undulata*, is decumbent to suberect, with densely packed, obovate to inversely lance-shaped, thick, fleshy, wavy-margined, white-frosted leaves and yellowish red or orange flowers.
C. paniculata see *Tylecodon paniculatus*.
C. reticulata see *Tylecodon reticulatus*.
C. simplicifolia see *Chiastophyllum oppositifolium*.
***C. tomentosa*.** Compact, woody-based, perennial succulent with slender, loose stems and thick, obovoid, grey-green leaves, to 5cm (2in) long, covered with a dense felt of dark hairs at the tips. From late summer to autumn, bears pendent, tubular red flowers, to 1.5cm (½in) long, with long, recurved lobes, in panicles to 20cm (8in) long. ↕to 30cm (12in), ↔ 12cm (5in). South Africa (Western Cape). ❀ (min. 7°C/45°F).
var. *ladismithensis* see *C. ladismithensis*.
C. undulata see *C. orbiculata* var. *oblonga*.
C. wallichii see *Tylecodon papillaris* subsp. *wallichii*.
C. zeyheri see *Adromischus cristatus* var. *zeyheri*.

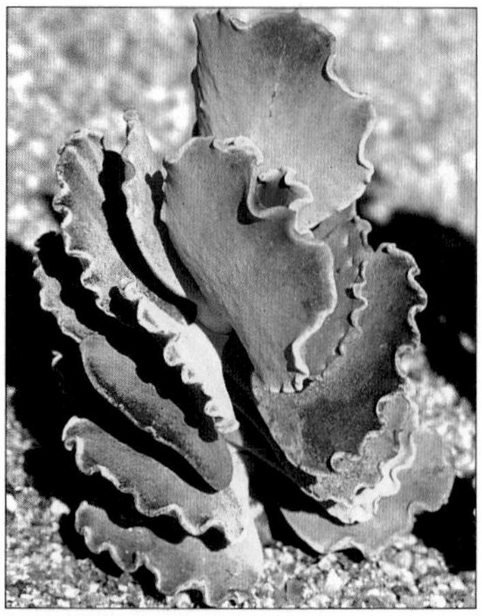

Cotyledon orbiculata var. *oblonga*

▷ **Couch,**
  Hairy see *Elymus hispidus*
  Onion see *Arrhenatherum elatius* subsp. *bulbosum* 'Variegatum'
▷ **Cowberry** see *Vaccinium vitis-idaea*
▷ **Cow itch tree** see *Lagunaria patersonii*
▷ **Cow parsley** see *Anthriscus sylvestris*
▷ **Cowslip** see *Primula veris*
  American see *Dodecatheon*
  Blue see *Pulmonaria angustifolia*
  Cape see *Lachenalia*
  Giant see *Primula florindae*
  Himalayan see *Primula sikkimensis*
  Jerusalem see *Pulmonaria officinalis*
  Virginia see *Mertensia pulmonarioides*
▷ **Crab apple** see *Malus*
  Common see *M. sylvestris*
  Japanese see *M. floribunda*
  Manchurian see *M. baccata* var. *mandschurica*
  Siberian see *M. baccata*
  Wild see *M. sylvestris*
  Wild sweet see *M. coronaria*

CRAMBE

BRASSICACEAE/CRUCIFERAE

Genus of about 20 species of imposing, often woody-based annuals and perennials from rocky mountain slopes and coastal sand dunes, and in open grassland, in Europe, Turkey, C. Asia, and tropical Africa. They have large, simple to pinnatisect basal leaves and erect, often thick stems, which are usually leafless or bear smaller leaves. Numerous tiny, scented, cross-shaped, white or pale yellow flowers are borne in large racemes or panicles. *Crambe* species are cultivated for their handsome foliage and elegant inflorescences, which are attractive to bees. They are suitable for a herbaceous border or a wild or woodland garden, and thrive in coastal sites. The leafy stems of *C. maritima* are often eaten as a vegetable; developing stems may be blanched from late winter to spring.
• **HARDINESS** Fully hardy.
• **CULTIVATION** Grow in deep, fertile, well-drained soil in full sun, although they will tolerate poor soils and partial shade. Provide shelter from strong winds.
• **PROPAGATION** Sow seed in containers in a cold frame in spring or autumn. Divide in early spring, or insert root cuttings in winter.
• **PESTS AND DISEASES** Susceptible to clubroot and soil-borne black rot (especially *C. maritima*).

C. cordifolia ■ ♀ Clump-forming perennial forming a mound of long-stalked, kidney-shaped to ovate, puckered, toothed, bristly, dark green leaves, to 35cm (14in) or more across, which die down in mid- or late summer. Strong stems bear white flowers in many-branched panicles, to 1.5m (5ft) across, in late spring and midsummer. ↕ to 2.5m (8ft), ↔ 1.5m (5ft). Caucasus. ✻✻✻
C. maritima (Sea kale). Spreading, mound-forming perennial with ovate, irregularly pinnatifid, twisted, glaucous, blue-green leaves, to 30cm (12in) long. Thick stems bear white flowers in dense racemes, to 60cm (24in) across, in early summer. ↕ 75cm (30in), ↔ 60cm (24in). Coastal areas of N. and W. Europe, Black Sea. ✻✻✻

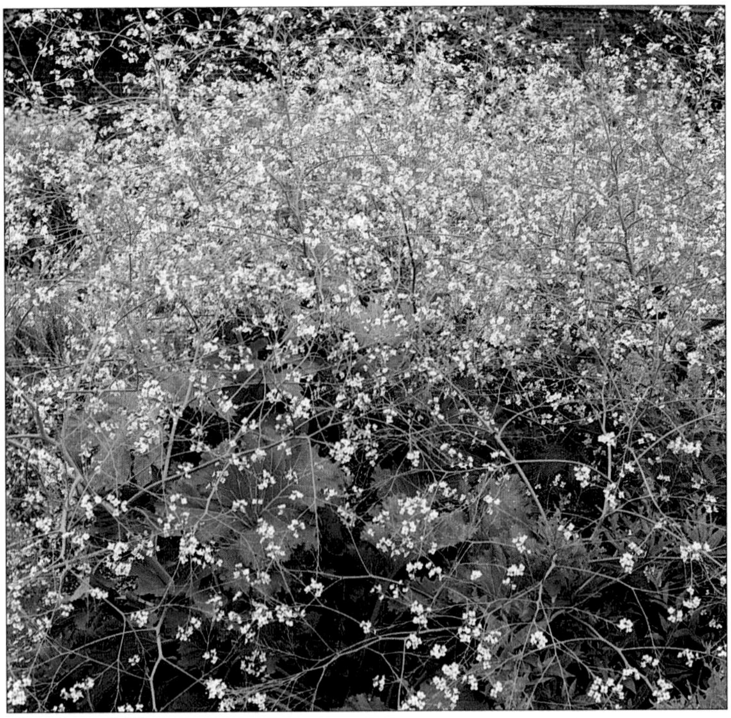

Crambe cordifolia

▷ **Cranberry** see *Vaccinium*, *V. macrocarpon*
▷ **Crane flower** see *Strelitzia reginae*
▷ **Cranesbill** see *Geranium*
  Armenian see *G. psilostemon*
  Bloody see *G. sanguineum*
  Dusky see *G. phaeum*
  Meadow see *G. pratense*
  Wood see *G. sylvaticum*

CRASPEDIA

Bachelor's buttons, Billy buttons

ASTERACEAE/COMPOSITAE

Genus of 8 species of annuals and perennials from mountainous regions of Australia, Tasmania, and New Zealand. They are grown mainly for their dense, hemispherical flowerheads of tiny, cup-shaped flowers, surrounded by leafy bracts and borne on stiff, unbranched stems. They are also cultivated for their basal rosettes of elliptic, obovate, spoon-shaped, or linear, hairy, mid-green to silvery white leaves. Grow perennial species in a rock garden or scree bed. In damp, frost-prone areas, most are best in an alpine house; grow *C. globosa* in an annual border. The flowerheads are useful for dried flower arrangements.
• **HARDINESS** Fully hardy to half hardy.
• **CULTIVATION** Grow annuals in any well-drained soil in full sun. Grow perennials in sharply drained, low-fertility, humus-rich, gritty soil in full sun; protect from excessive winter wet. Under glass, grow in a mix of equal parts loam, leaf mould, and sharp sand, with a top-dressing of grit. Water freely when in growth (avoiding the foliage) and keep just moist in winter.
• **PROPAGATION** Sow seed of annuals and perennials at 13–18°C (55–64°F) in spring. Divide perennials in spring.
• **PESTS AND DISEASES** Slugs and snails may attack young growth. Red spider mites may be troublesome under glass.

C. glauca, syn. *C. richea*. Tufted, rosette-forming perennial with inversely lance-shaped to linear, usually white-hairy, grey-green leaves, to 15cm (6in) long. Solitary flowerheads, to 3cm (1¼in) across, of yellow or cream florets, are borne on stiff stems in summer. ↕ 40cm (16in) or more, ↔ 20cm (8in). S. Australia. ✻✻✻ (borderline)
C. globosa (Bachelor's buttons, Drumsticks). Rosette-forming, white-woolly perennial, usually grown as an annual, with narrowly strap-shaped, light green leaves, to 30cm (12in) long, covered in white hairs. Mustard-yellow flowerheads, to 3cm (1¼in) across, are produced in summer at the tips of long, rigid, hairy stems. ↕ 60–90cm (24–36in), ↔ to 12cm (5in). Australia (W. Victoria, New South Wales). ✻✻✻
C. incana. Densely white-woolly perennial bearing basal rosettes of obovate to spoon-shaped, mid-green leaves, to 10cm (4in) long. Dense, bright yellow flowerheads, to 3cm (1¼in) across, are produced in summer. ↕ 20–30cm (8–12in), ↔ 15cm (6in). New Zealand. ✻✻
C. richea see *C. glauca*.
C. uniflora ■ (Bachelor's buttons). Rosette-forming annual or perennial with long-stalked, woolly, obovate or lance-shaped, mid-green basal leaves, to 12cm (5in) long, and white-woolly, lance-shaped, clasping stem leaves, 6cm (2½in) long. Clear yellow flowerheads, to 4cm (1½in) across, are produced in summer. ↕ to 45cm (18in), ↔ 35cm (14in). S. Australia, Tasmania, New Zealand. ✻

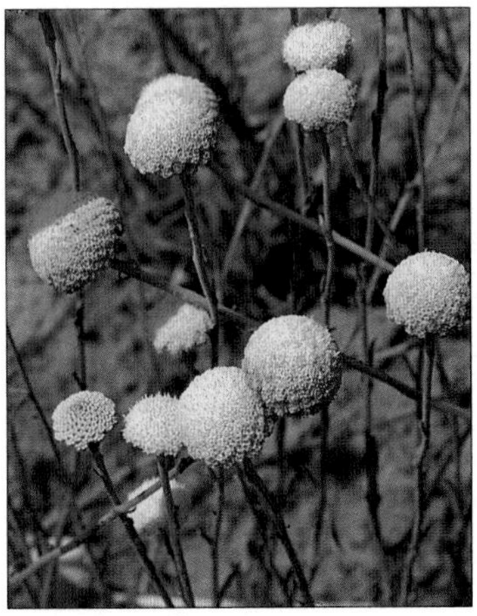

Craspedia uniflora

CRASSULA

CRASSULACEAE

Genus of about 150 species of annual and perennial succulents and evergreen, succulent shrubs and subshrubs, ranging from dwarf to tall, tree-like plants, and found in dry to moist, high to low areas in Africa, Madagascar, and Asia, but mostly in South Africa. They are grown mainly for their fleshy, usually opposite leaves, which vary greatly in shape, size, and texture, and are also cultivated for their tubular or star- or funnel-shaped flowers, borne in dense, terminal, cyme-like inflorescences. In frost-prone areas, grow as houseplants, or in a cool or temperate greenhouse. In warm, dry climates, grow in a border with other succulents or in a desert garden.
• **HARDINESS** Half hardy to frost tender.
• **CULTIVATION** Under glass, grow in standard cactus compost in full light; a few need bright filtered or indirect light. From spring to autumn, apply balanced liquid fertilizer monthly and water moderately; water sparingly in winter. Outdoors, grow in moderately fertile to poor, humus-rich, sharply drained soil in full sun; *C. capitella* subsp. *thyrsiflora*, *C. hemisphaerica*, and *C. schmidtii* prefer partial shade. See also pp.48–49.
• **PROPAGATION** Sow seed at 15–18°C (59–64°F) in early spring. Root stem or leaf cuttings in spring or summer.
• **PESTS AND DISEASES** Mealybugs, vine weevils, and aphids may be a problem.

C. arborescens ■ (Silver jade plant). Shrub-like succulent with a stout, branched stem and broadly elliptic to obovate, greyish green leaves, 3.5–7cm (1½–3in) long, often with red margins, or red-spotted above. From autumn to winter, bears star-shaped pink flowers, to 1cm (½in) across. ↕ 4m (12ft), ↔ to 2m (6ft). South Africa (Western Cape, Eastern Cape, KwaZulu/Natal). ❀ (min. 5–7°C/41–45°F)
***C. arborescens* of gardens** see *C. ovata*.
***C. argentea* of gardens** see *C. ovata*.
C. capitella* subsp. *thyrsiflora, syn. *C. corymbosula*, *C. thyrsiflora*. Variable, erect, sparingly branched, perennial

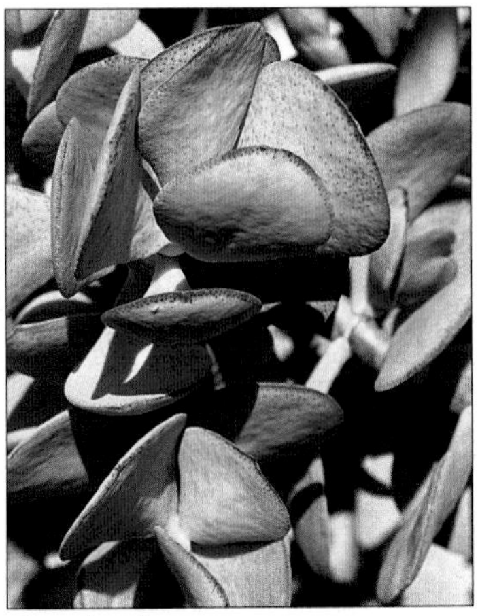

Crassula arborescens

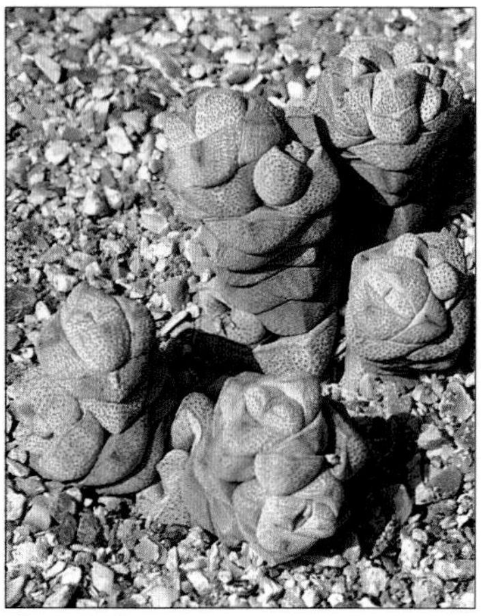
Crassula deceptor

succulent. Ovate to linear-lance-shaped, hairy-margined, grey-green leaves, 3–7cm (1¼–3in) long, are spotted dark green or red. Star-shaped white flowers, 6–8mm (¼–⅜in) across, are produced in autumn. ↕ to 30cm (12in), ↔ 15cm (6in). Namibia, South Africa (Eastern Transvaal, Orange Free State, KwaZulu/Natal, Northern Cape, Eastern Cape). ❀ (min. 5–7°C/41–45°F)

C. coccinea, syn. *Rochea coccinea.* Erect, succulent subshrub with elliptic to ovate, pointed, dull green, often red-tinged leaves, to 2.5cm (1in) long, densely arranged in 4 rows on red stems. Tubular, bright red, occasionally white flowers, to 4.5cm (1¾in) long, are borne from summer to autumn. ↕ 60cm (24in), ↔ to 40cm (16in). South Africa (Northern Cape, Western Cape, Eastern Cape). ❀ (min. 5–7°C/41–45°F)

C. corymbosula see *C. capitella* subsp. *thyrsiflora.*

C. deceptor ■ syn. *C. deceptrix.* Perennial succulent, sometimes branching from the base, with 4-ranked, thick, ovate, greenish grey leaves, 1.5cm (½in) long, with minute, raised dots and lines. Bears funnel-shaped, cream to pale yellow or pink flowers, to 5mm (¼in) across, in spring. ↕↔ 10cm (4in). South Africa (Northern Cape, Western Cape). ❀ (min. 5–7°C/ 41–45°F)

C. deceptrix see *C. deceptor.*

C. falcata see *C. perfoliata* var. *minor.*

C. hemisphaerica. Tufted, perennial succulent with a short stem, crowned by a dense, hemispherical rosette of 4-ranked, obovate, recurved, grey-green leaves, 1–5cm (½–2in) long, with fine white hairs. Bears tubular white flowers,

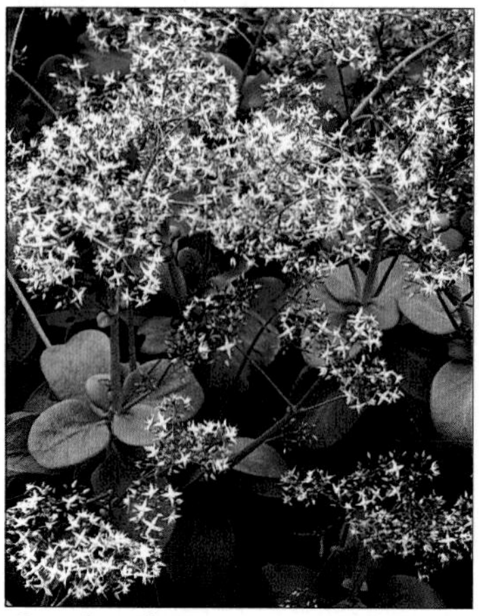
Crassula multicava

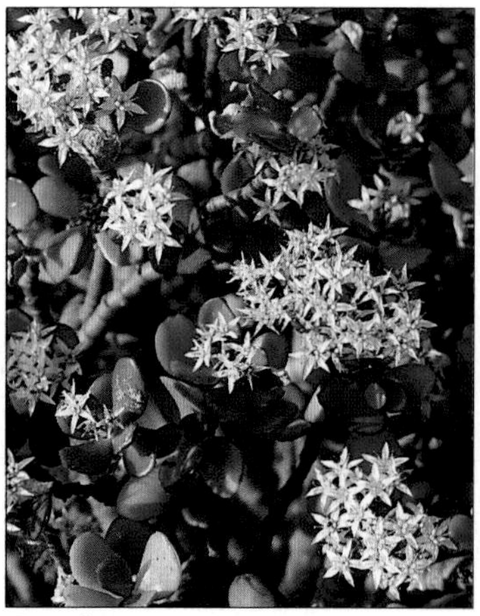
Crassula ovata

3mm (⅛in across), in spring. ↕ 5–15cm (2–6in), ↔ to 18cm (7in). South Africa (Northern Cape, Western Cape). ❀ (min. 5–7°C/41–45°F)

C. lactea. Semi-erect or prostrate, succulent subshrub. Short branches bear inversely lance-shaped, pointed, glossy, dark green leaves, 3–7cm (1¼–3in) long, margined with white dots. Small, star-shaped, scented, yellow-white, pink-flushed flowers, to 5mm (¼in) across, are produced in winter. ↕ 20–30cm (8–12in), ↔ 1m (3ft) or more. South Africa (Eastern Cape, KwaZulu/Natal). ❀ (min. 5–7°C/41–45°F)

C. lycopodioides see *C. muscosa.*

***C. maculata* of gardens** see *Adromischus maculatus.*

C. multicava ■ Freely branching, bushy or prostrate, perennial succulent with oblong-ovate to elliptic, minutely spotted and pitted, grey-green or glossy, mid-green leaves, 2–7cm (¾–3in) long. Star-shaped, pinkish white flowers, to 6mm (¼in) or more across, open in spring. ↕ 30–40cm (12–16in), ↔ to 1m (3ft). South Africa (Northern Transvaal, Eastern Transvaal, KwaZulu/Natal). ❀ (min. 5–7°C/41–45°F)

C. muscosa, syn. *C. lycopodioides* (Lizard tail). Spreading, perennial succulent, forming a dense bush, with triangular to ovate, scale-like, densely 4-ranked, mid-green leaves, tinged yellow, grey, or brown, 2–8mm (1/16–⅜in) long. Bears minute, tubular, greenish yellow flowers, to 3mm (⅛in) across, singly or in few-flowered, axillary clusters, in spring. ↕ 10–30cm (4–12in), ↔ 20cm (8in). South Africa (Northern Cape, Western Cape). ❀ (min. 5–7°C/41–45°F)

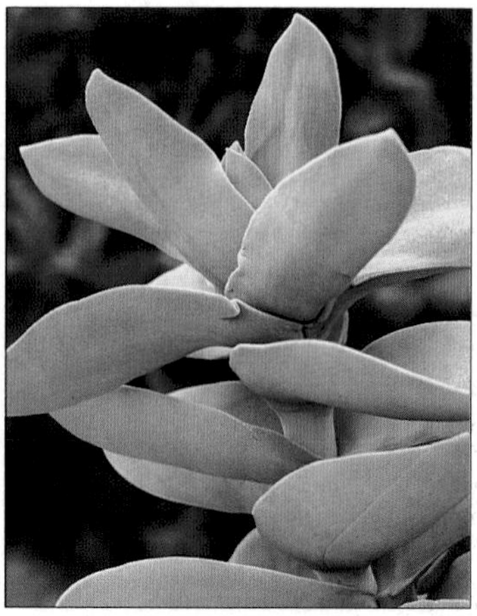
Crassula perfoliata var. *minor*

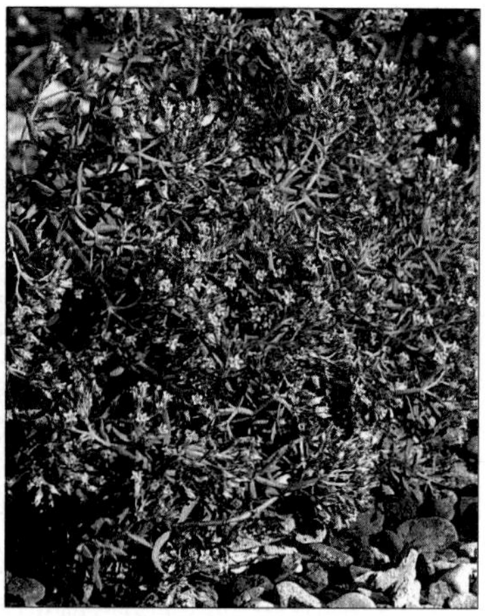
Crassula sarcocaulis

C. orbicularis, syn. *C. rosularis.* Tufted, perennial succulent with flat rosettes of elliptic to inversely lance-shaped, hairy-margined, glossy, mid-green leaves, 1.5–5cm (½–2in) long. Star-shaped white flowers, 4–8mm (⅛–⅜in) across, are produced from summer to autumn. ↕ 15–25cm (6–10in), ↔ to 30cm (12in). South Africa (KwaZulu/Natal). ❀ (min. 5–7°C/41–45°F)

C. ovata ■♀ syn. *C. arborescens* of gardens, *C. argentea* of gardens, *C. portulacea* (Jade plant, Jade tree). Erect, many-branched, succulent shrub with a thick, fleshy stem and elliptic, glossy, mid-green leaves, sometimes red-margined, 2–4cm (¾–1½in) long. Bears star-shaped, white to pale pink flowers, to 8mm (⅜in) across, in autumn. ↕ 2m (6ft) or more, ↔ 1m (3ft) or more. South Africa (Northern Cape, Western Cape, Eastern Cape, KwaZulu/Natal, Northern Transvaal, Eastern Transvaal). ❀ (min. 5–7°C/41–45°F)

C. perfoliata* var. *falcata see *C. perfoliata* var. *minor.*

C. perfoliata* var. *minor ■♀ syn. *C. falcata, C. perfoliata* var. *falcata, Rochea falcata* (Propeller plant). Erect, perennial succulent with fleshy stems and thick, triangular-lance-shaped, curving grey leaves, 10cm (4in) long. Star-shaped, scented, scarlet, pink, or white flowers, to 1cm (½in) across, are borne in late summer. ↕ 1m (3ft), ↔ 75cm (30in). South Africa (Eastern Cape). ❀ (min. 5–7°C/41–45°F)

C. portulacea see *C. ovata.*

C. pyramidalis ♀ Semi-erect, perennial succulent with stems forming leafy columns and 4 neat ranks of ovate, flat,

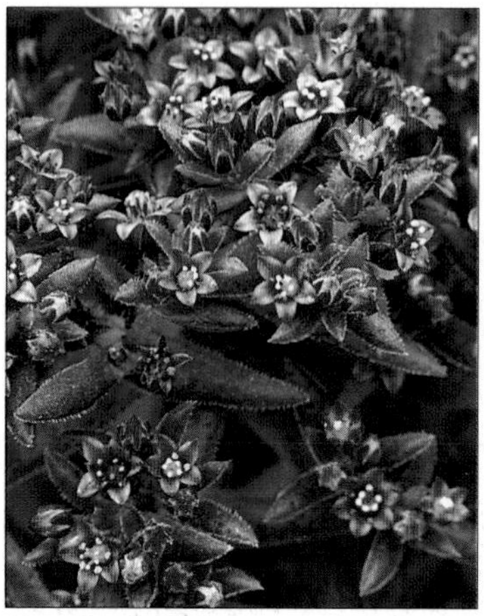
Crassula schmidtii

mid-green leaves, 4–12cm (1½–5in) long. In autumn, each stem is crowned by creamy white flowers, to 1cm (½in) across. ↕ 3–8cm (1¼–3in) or more, ↔ 10cm (4in). South Africa (Northern Cape). ❀ (min. 5–7°C/41–45°F)

C. rosularis see *C. orbicularis.*

C. rupestris ♀ Erect, spreading, or semi-prostrate, perennial succulent with thick, ovate-lance-shaped, brownish red leaves, 3–15mm (⅛–½in) long, often with red margins. In summer, bears star-shaped, white or pink flowers, to 6mm (¼in) across, in axillary cymes. ↕ 50cm (20in), ↔ 40cm (16in). South Africa (Northern Cape, Western Cape, Eastern Cape). ❀ (min. 5–7°C/41–45°F)

C. sarcocaulis ■ syn. *Sedum sarcocaule.* Bushy, perennial succulent with fleshy stems and branches, bearing elliptic-lance-shaped, sharply tapering, red-tinted, mid-green leaves, 1–3cm (½–1¼in) long. Produces star-shaped, malodorous, white or pink flowers, to 4–5mm (⅛–¼in) across, in summer. ↕ 30cm (12in) or more, ↔ 30cm (12in). South Africa (Eastern Cape, KwaZulu/Natal), Lesotho. ✲✲

C. schmidtii ■ Mat-forming, perennial succulent with erect, hairy, green or red stems bearing loose rosettes of narrowly lance-shaped, flat, pitted and spotted, dark green leaves, 3–4cm (1¼–1½in) long, margined with white hairs. Star-shaped, bright purplish pink flowers, to 4mm (⅛in) across, are produced in winter. ↕ 10cm (4in), ↔ 30cm (12in). South Africa (Western Cape, Eastern Cape, Kwazulu/Natal). ❀ (min. 5–7°C/41–45°F)

C. socialis ■ Tufted, perennial succulent bearing short, dense rosettes of 4-ranked, obovate to ovate, horny-margined, light green leaves, 6mm (¼in) long, with rounded undersides. Bears star-shaped white flowers, to 6mm (¼in) across, in spring. ↕ 6cm (2½in), ↔ indefinite. South Africa (Eastern Cape). ❀ (min. 5–7°C/41–45°F)

C. thyrsiflora see *C. capitella* subsp. *thrysiflora.*

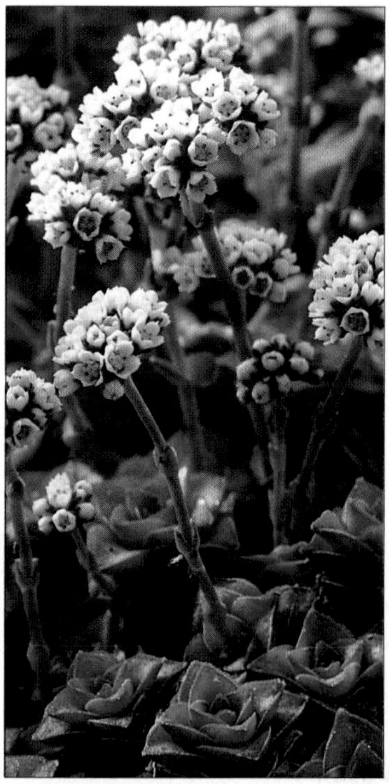
Crassula socialis

CRATAEGUS

Hawthorn

ROSACEAE

Genus of 200 or more species of usually spiny, deciduous, sometimes semi-evergreen trees and shrubs occurring in woodland and scrub in N. temperate regions. The leaves are alternate, simple or lobed, mostly ovate or obovate, and mid- to dark green; some species produce good autumn colour. The white to deep pink flowers are usually shallowly cup-shaped and mostly borne in flat or rounded corymbs at the ends of short, leafy shoots, although, rarely, they may be solitary. Fruits, produced in autumn, consist of fleshy exteriors with bony nutlets; they are mostly red but may also be black, yellow, or bluish green. Hawthorns are valued for their long season of interest and their extreme hardiness. They are particularly useful specimen trees for a town, coastal, or exposed garden. *C. laevigata* and *C. monogyna* are also used for hedging. The seeds may cause mild stomach upset if ingested.

- **HARDINESS** Fully hardy.
- **CULTIVATION** Grow in any (except waterlogged) soil in full sun or partial shade. Pruning group 1. Trim hedges after flowering or in autumn.
- **PROPAGATION** Remove seed from flesh as soon as ripe and sow in a seedbed or in containers in an open frame. Stratify and sow seed in a seedbed in spring (germination may take 18 months). Bud cultivars in midsummer, or graft in winter.
- **PESTS AND DISEASES** Caterpillars, aphids, gall midges, fireblight, honey fungus, rust, and powdery mildew may be troublesome.

C. cordata see *C. phaenopyrum.*

C. crus-galli ♀ (Cockspur thorn). Spreading, deciduous tree with curved thorns, 3–8cm (1¼–3in) long. Obovate, leathery, glossy, dark green leaves, to 10cm (4in) long, turn bright crimson in autumn. Bears many-flowered corymbs of white flowers, to 1.5cm (½in) across, with pink anthers, in early summer, followed by long-lasting, spherical, dark red fruit, to 1cm (½in) across. ↕8m (25ft), ↔ 10m (30ft). E. USA. ❄❄❄

C. ellwangeriana ♀ Spreading, spiny, deciduous tree with ovate, sharply toothed and lobed, mid-green leaves, to 8cm (3in) long, turning orange and red in autumn. Corymbs of 9–10 white flowers, to 2cm (¾in) across, with red anthers, are produced in late spring, followed by oblong-ellipsoid, glossy crimson fruit, to 1.5cm (½in) long. ↕↔ 6m (20ft). E. USA. ❄❄❄

C. flava ♀ (Yellow haw). Spreading, spiny, deciduous shrub or small tree with ovate to obovate, often 3-lobed, dark green leaves, to 5cm (2in) long. Corymbs of 3–7 white flowers, 1cm (½in) across, are borne in late spring and early summer, followed by spherical or pear-shaped, yellow-green fruit, to 1cm (½in) across. ↕6m (20ft), ↔ 8m (25ft). E. USA. ❄❄❄

C. laciniata ▣ ♀ syn. *C. orientalis.* Compact, spreading, sparsely thorny, deciduous tree with triangular to diamond-shaped, 5- to 9-lobed, dark green leaves, to 5cm (2in) long. In late spring and early summer, bears corymbs of up to 12 white flowers, to 1.5cm (½in) across, with red anthers, followed by spherical, downy, orange-red to red fruit, to 1.5cm (½in) across. ↕↔ 6m (20ft). S.E. Europe, W. Asia. ❄❄❄

C. laevigata ♀ syn. *C. oxyacantha* of gardens (May, Midland hawthorn). Rounded, thorny, deciduous tree with ovate, shallowly 3- to 5-lobed, glossy, mid- green leaves, to 5cm (2in) long. Corymbs of up to 10 white to pink flowers, 1cm (½in) across, are produced in late spring, followed by spherical to ovoid red fruit, 0.6–1.5cm (¼–½in) long. ↕↔ to 8m (25ft). Europe to India, N. Africa. ❄❄❄. **'Coccinea Plena'** see 'Paul's Scarlet'. **'Crimson Cloud'** has large, bright red flowers, 2cm (¾in) across, with white centres. **'Paul's Scarlet'** ▣ 🏆 syn. 'Coccinea Plena', bears profuse, double, dark pink flowers. **'Plena'** has double white flowers, ageing to pink. **'Rosea Flore Pleno'** 🏆 bears double pink flowers.

***C. x lavallei* 'Carrierei'** 🏆 ♀ Strong-growing, spreading, thorny, semi-evergreen tree with obovate, toothed, glossy, dark green leaves, to 10cm (4in), long, turning red in late autumn and winter. In early and midsummer, bears erect, many-flowered corymbs of white flowers, to 2cm (¾in) across. Long-lasting, ellipsoid or spherical, orange-red fruit, 2cm (¾in) long, ripen in late autumn. ↕7m (22ft), ↔ 10m (30ft). ❄❄❄

C. macrosperma* var. *acutiloba ▣ ♀ Spreading, thorny, deciduous tree with ovate to elliptic, sharply toothed, dark green leaves, to 8cm (3in) long, with 5 broadly triangular, toothed lobes. Corymbs of 5–12 white flowers, to 1.5cm (½in) across, with red anthers, are produced in late spring; they are followed by obovoid, bright red fruit, 1.5cm (½in) long. ↕6m (20ft), ↔ 8m (25ft). E. North America. ❄❄❄

C. monogyna ♀ (Common hawthorn, May, Quick, Quickthorn). Rounded, deciduous tree with numerous thorns and broadly ovate to diamond-shaped, deeply 3- to 7-lobed, glossy leaves, to 5cm (2in) long, dark green above and paler beneath. Flat corymbs of 6–12 fragrant white flowers, to 1.5cm (½in) across, with pink anthers, are borne in late spring, followed by spherical, ovoid, or ellipsoid, glossy, dark red fruit, 6mm (¼in) long. Suitable as a hedge. ↕10m (30ft), ↔ 8m (25ft). Europe. ❄❄❄. **'Biflora'** (Glastonbury thorn) produces both foliage and flowers in mild winter weather, as well as in spring. **'Stricta'** ♀ is narrow and columnar, with erect branches; ↔ 4m (12ft).

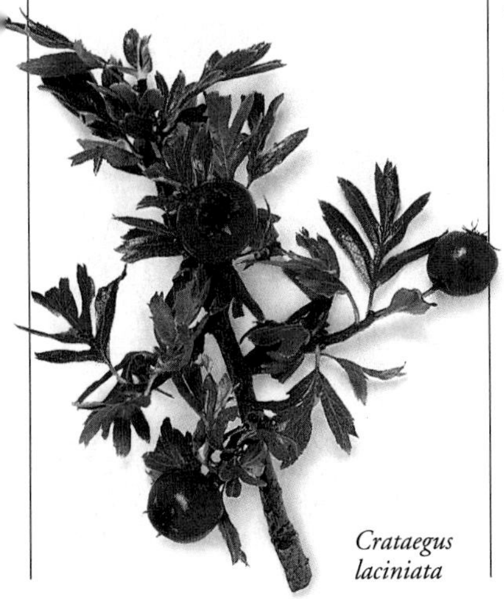

Crataegus laciniata

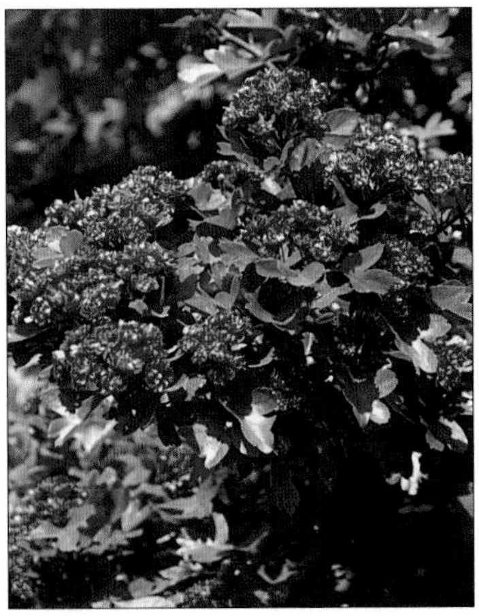

Crataegus laevigata 'Paul's Scarlet'

***C. x mordenensis* cultivars** ♀ Compact, rounded, thornless, deciduous trees with obovate, deeply 2- to 4-lobed, mid-green leaves, to 7cm (3in) long. In late spring, bear many-flowered corymbs of white or pink flowers, 1.5cm (½in) across, in late spring. Spherical, red-pink fruit, to 1cm (½in) long, are rarely produced. ↕↔ 6m (20ft). ❄❄❄. **'Snowbird'** has fragrant, double white flowers. **'Toba'** has pink-tinged white flowers, ageing to pink.

C. orientalis see *C. laciniata.*

***C. oxyacantha* of gardens** see *C. laevigata.*

C. pedicellata ▣ ♀ Spreading, thorny, deciduous tree. Broadly ovate, dark green leaves, to 10cm (4in) long, with 4–5 pairs of shallow, sharply toothed lobes, turn orange and red in autumn. Loose, many-flowered corymbs of white flowers, to 2cm (¾in) across, with red anthers, are produced in late spring, followed by pear-shaped, bright red fruit, 2cm (¾in) long. ↕↔ 6m (20ft). E. North America. ❄❄❄

***C. persimilis* 'Prunifolia'** 🏆 ♀ syn. *C. x prunifolia.* Rounded, deciduous tree producing stout thorns and obovate, glossy, deep green leaves, to 8cm (3in) long, which turn orange and red in autumn. In early summer, produces dense, rounded, many-flowered corymbs of white flowers, to 2cm (¾in) across, with pink anthers, followed by spherical, bright red fruit, 1.5cm (½in) long. ↕8m (25ft), ↔ 10m (30ft). ❄❄❄

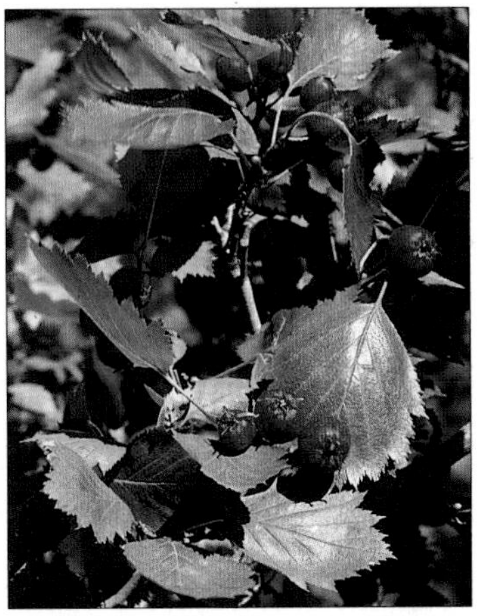

Crataegus macrosperma var. *acutiloba*

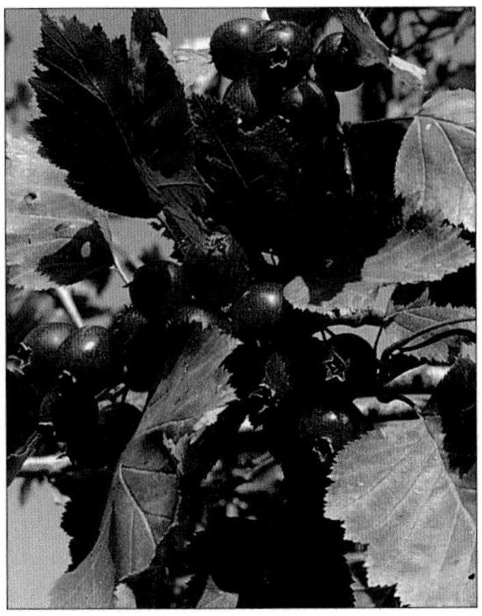

Crataegus pedicellata

C. phaenopyrum ♀ syn. *C. cordata* (Washington thorn). Rounded, slender, thorny, deciduous tree. The maple-like, deeply 3-lobed leaves, to 7cm (3in) long, are triangular with heart-shaped bases, and glossy, mid-green, turning orange to red in autumn. In early and midsummer, bears many-flowered corymbs of white flowers, 1cm (½in) across, with pink anthers, followed by long-lasting, spherical, glossy, bright red fruit, 6mm (¼in) long. ↕↔ 10m (30ft). S.E. USA. ❄❄❄

C. x prunifolia see *C. persimilis* 'Prunifolia'.

***C. punctata* 'Ohio Pioneer'** ♀ Spreading, almost thornless, deciduous tree with obovate, dark green leaves, to 10cm (4in) long. Many-flowered corymbs of white flowers, 2cm (¾in) across, with pink anthers, are borne in spring, followed by slightly pear-shaped to spherical, dark red fruit, 2–2.5cm (¾–1in) long. ↕8m (25ft), ↔ 10m (30ft). ❄❄❄

C. tanacetifolia ♀ (Tansy-leaved thorn). Rounded to broadly upright, usually thornless, deciduous tree with stout shoots and obovate to diamond-shaped, grey-green leaves, to 2.5cm (1in) long, with 5–7 narrowly oblong, finely divided lobes. Rounded corymbs of 6–8 fragrant white flowers, to 2.5cm (1in) across, with red anthers, are borne in midsummer, followed by spherical, aromatic, orange-yellow fruit, 2–2.5cm (¾–1in) across. ↕10m (30ft), ↔ 8m (25ft). W. Asia. ❄❄❄

***C. viridis* 'Winter King'** ♀ Round-headed, deciduous tree with a few slender thorns, to 4cm (1½in) long. The ovate or oblong, toothed or shallowly lobed, glossy, mid-green leaves, to 6cm (2½in) long, turn red in autumn. In late spring, bears many-flowered corymbs of white flowers, to 2cm (¾in) across, with pale yellow anthers, followed by spherical red fruit, 6–9mm (¼–⅜in) long, which last through winter. ↕12m (40ft), ↔ 6m (20ft). ❄❄❄

▷ ***Crawfurdia speciosa*** see *Gentiana speciosa*
▷ **Creamcups** see *Platystemon, P. californicus*
▷ **Creeping buttons** see *Peperomia rotundifolia*
▷ **Creeping Charlie** see *Pilea nummulariifolia*
▷ **Creeping devil** see *Stenocereus eruca*
▷ **Creeping Jenny, Golden** see *Lysimachia nummularia* 'Aurea'

C

C

CREMANTHODIUM

ASTERACEAE/COMPOSITAE

Genus of about 50 species of perennials, mostly found in cool, moist conditions, in scrub and on open slopes at high altitudes in India, Tibet, and China. They have often kidney-shaped, usually rosetted basal leaves and upright stems with bract-like leaves. They are grown for their usually pendent, daisy-like flowerheads, borne singly or in simple, few-flowered racemes or corymbs. Grow in woodland, a rock garden, or an alpine house. They grow best in cool climates with snow cover in winter.

- **HARDINESS** Fully hardy.
- **CULTIVATION** Grow in moderately fertile, humus-rich, moist but well-drained soil in partial shade. In areas without snow cover, protect with a deep, winter mulch. In an alpine house, grow in a mix of equal parts loam, leaf mould, and grit.
- **PROPAGATION** Sow seed in containers in an open frame as soon as ripe.
- **PESTS AND DISEASES** Slugs and snails may damage outdoor plants. Prone to aphids and red spider mites under glass.

C. reniforme, syn. *Senecio reniformis.* Rosette-forming perennial with kidney-shaped, toothed, glossy, mid-green leaves, 15–20cm (6–8in) long. In summer, solitary, pendent, cone-shaped flowerheads, to 7cm (3in) across, with narrow, tapering, pale yellow ray-florets and brown disc-florets, are produced on stout stems, to 20cm (8in) long. ↕20cm (8in), ↔15cm (6in). India (Sikkim) to Bhutan and Nepal. ❄❄❄

▷**Crepe flower** see *Lagerstroemia indica*
▷**Crepe myrtle** see *Lagerstroemia indica*
Giant see *L. speciosa*
Queen's see *L. speciosa*

CREPIS

Hawk's beard

ASTERACEAE/COMPOSITAE

Genus of about 200 species of annuals and perennials found in dry grassland, on stony slopes, and among mountain screes and rocks throughout the N. hemisphere. Although some species are persistent weeds, others are cultivated for their dandelion-like flowerheads, borne singly or in simple or compound, many-flowered racemes, corymbs, or panicles. They have one or several, mainly branched stems, and usually produce flattened, basal rosettes of entire to pinnatifid leaves. Those species grown as ornamental plants are suitable for a rock garden.

- **HARDINESS** Fully hardy.
- **CULTIVATION** Grow in any well-drained soil in full sun.
- **PROPAGATION** Sow seed in an open frame as soon as ripe. Insert root cuttings from lateral roots (not tap roots) in winter. Most species self-seed freely.
- **PESTS AND DISEASES** Trouble free.

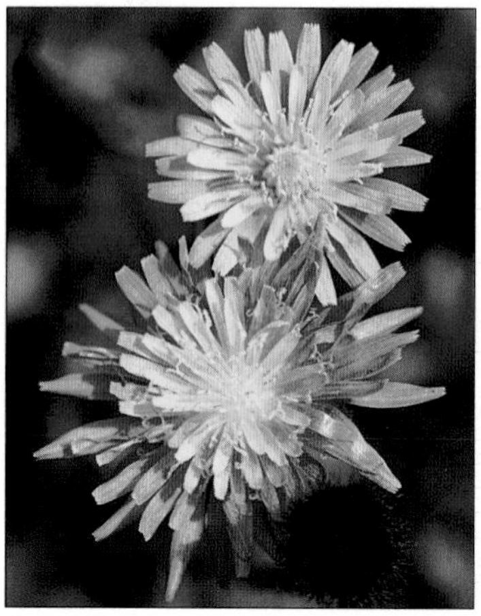

Crepis aurea

C. aurea ▣ Rosette-forming, tap-rooted perennial with obovate to inversely lance-shaped, toothed or cleft, light green leaves, to 10cm (4in) long. Usually solitary, golden orange flowerheads, 3cm (1¼in) across, are borne on stems clothed in black and white hairs, from summer to autumn. ↕10–30cm (4–12in), ↔ to 30cm (12in). Alps, mountainous areas of Italy, S. and W. Balkans. ❄❄❄

C. incana 🏆 (Pink dandelion). Rosette-forming perennial with inversely lance-shaped, pinnatisect, usually densely grey-hairy leaves, 3–13cm (1¼–5in) long. In late summer, bears bright, clear pink to magenta-pink flowerheads, 3cm (1¼in) across, in many-flowered corymbs. Needs full sun. ↕↔ to 30cm (12in). S. and S.E. Greece. ❄❄❄

C. rubra. Rosette-forming annual or short-lived perennial with mostly basal, inversely lance-shaped, toothed, slightly puckered and hairy, pale green leaves, to 15cm (6in) long. Pinkish red flowerheads, to 2.5cm (1in) across, are borne singly or in pairs on stiff, slightly arching stems from spring to summer. ↕30–40cm (12–16in), ↔15cm (6in). Balkans, S. Italy, Greece (Crete). ❄❄❄. **var. *alba*** has white flowers.

▷**Cress,**
Indian see *Tropaeolum majus*
Rock see *Arabis*
Stone see *Aethionema*
▷***Crinitaria*** see *Aster*

CRINODENDRON

ELAEOCARPACEAE

Genus of 2 species of evergreen shrubs and trees from forests in Chile. They are cultivated for their foliage and flowers. The alternate, dark green leaves are narrowly elliptic to narrowly oblong or ovate. Pendent, bell-, lantern-, or urn-shaped, red or white flowers are borne singly or in pairs. Grow in a sheltered woodland garden or against a sheltered wall; they will tolerate an exposed site in mild areas. They may also be grown in a cool greenhouse or conservatory, where they will flower earlier.

- **HARDINESS** Hardy to -7°C (19°F).
- **CULTIVATION** Grow in fertile, moist but well-drained, humus-rich, acid soil in partial shade, or in full sun with the roots kept cool and shaded. *C. patagua* tolerates drier conditions and prefers full sun. Shelter from cold, drying winds. Restrict pruning to removal of dead wood in late spring. Pruning group 9 for *C. patagua*; group 8 for *C. hookerianum.*
- **PROPAGATION** Root greenwood cuttings in early summer, or semi-ripe cuttings in late summer.
- **PESTS AND DISEASES** Trouble free.

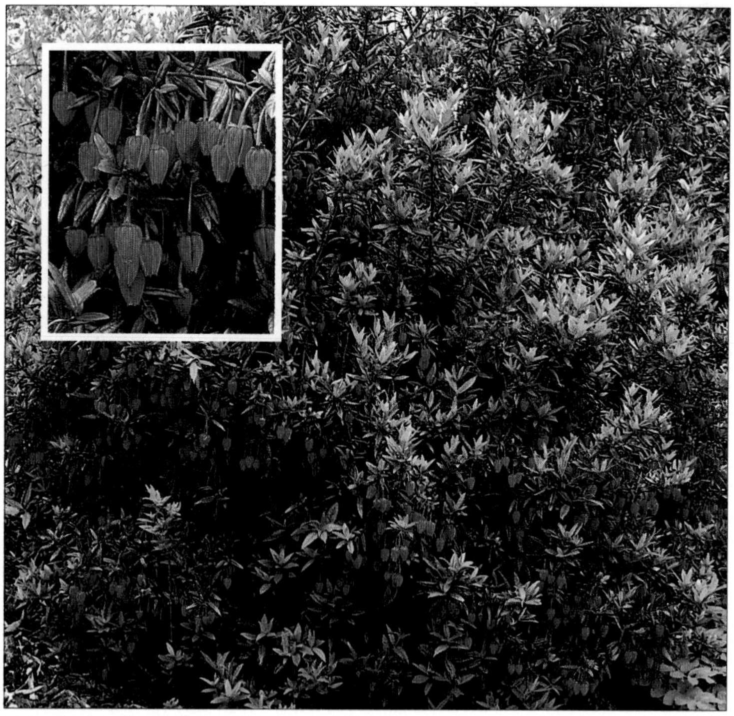

Crinodendron hookerianum (inset: flower detail)

C. hookerianum ▣🏆◐ syn. *Tricuspidaria lanceolata* (Lantern tree). Stiffly branched shrub, rarely a small tree, with upright shoots bearing narrowly elliptic to narrowly oblong, pointed, toothed, dark green leaves, to 10cm (4in) long. Lantern- or urn-shaped, fleshy-petalled, scarlet to deep carmine-pink flowers, 2–2.5cm (¾–1in) long, are produced from late spring to late summer. The young growth and flower buds may be damaged by hard frosts. ↕6m (20ft), ↔5m (15ft). Chile. ❄❄

C. patagua ◐–● Vigorous, upright shrub, rarely a small tree, bearing ovate, glossy, dark green leaves, to 7cm (3in) long. Bell-shaped, scented flowers, 2.5cm (1in) long, with fringed white petals, are produced in late summer. ↕8m (25ft), ↔5m (15ft). Chile. ❄❄

▷**x *Crinodonna*** see x *Amarcrinum*
x *C. corsii* see x *A. memoria-corsii*

CRINUM

AMARYLLIDACEAE

Genus of approximately 130 species of deciduous or evergreen, bulbous perennials found at streamsides and lake margins throughout tropical regions and South Africa. They are grown for their umbels of large, showy, funnel-shaped, long-tubed, often scented flowers, borne on leafless stems from spring to autumn. Leaves are basal, usually long, strap-shaped, and light to mid-green. Grow in a warm, sheltered border. In frost-prone areas, grow tender species in a temperate or warm greenhouse. All parts may cause severe discomfort if ingested; contact with the sap may irritate skin.

- **HARDINESS** Fully hardy to frost tender.
- **CULTIVATION** Plant in spring, with the neck of the bulb just above soil level. Under glass, grow in loam-based potting compost (JI No.2) with additional sharp sand and well-rotted manure, in full or bright filtered light. Water freely when in growth; keep moist after flowering. Pot on only when absolutely necessary, in early spring. Outdoors, grow in deep, fertile, humus-rich, moist but well-drained soil in full sun.
- **PROPAGATION** Sow seed at 21°C (70°F) as soon as ripe. Remove offsets in spring.
- **PESTS AND DISEASES** Trouble free.

C. americanum (Florida swamp lily). Deciduous, clump-forming perennial, spreading by stolons, with curved, sparingly toothed, mid-green leaves, to 75cm (30in) long. Umbels of up to 6 white flowers, 10–13cm (4–5in) long, with purple or brown backs, are borne from spring to autumn. ↕50cm (20in), ↔15cm (6in). S. USA. ❁ (min. 10°C/50°F). **'Miss Elsie'** has leaves to 1.2m (4ft) long; flowers, with brown-flushed backs, are borne from spring to summer.

C. asiaticum ▣ (Poison bulb). Deciduous, clump-forming perennial with semi-erect, mid-green leaves, to 1.2m (4ft) long, grouped at the top of a false stem. Bears umbels of 20 or more narrow-tepalled, fragrant white flowers, 10cm (4in) long, from spring to summer. ↕60cm (24in), ↔15cm (6in). Tropical S.E. Asia. ❁ (min. 10°C/50°F)

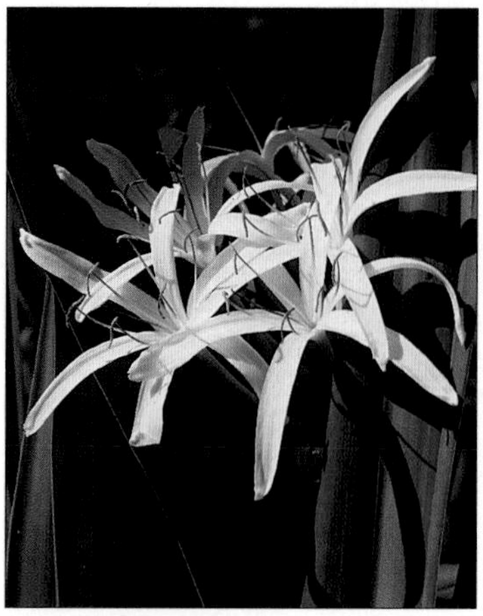

Crinum asiaticum

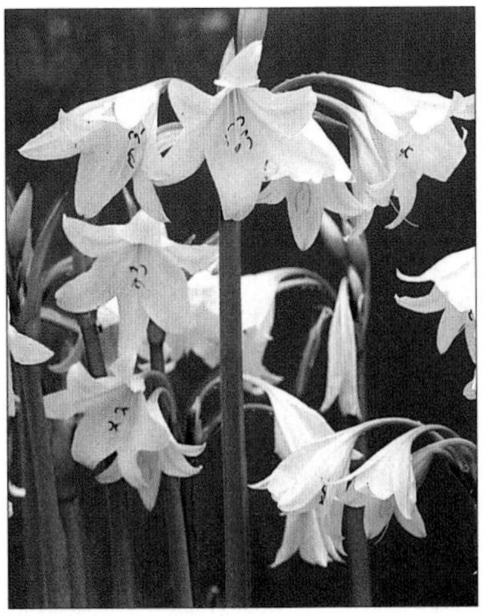

Crinum x *powellii* 'Album'

C. bulbispermum, syn. *C. longifolium.* Deciduous perennial bearing curved, light to mid-green leaves, 60–90cm (24–36in) long. In summer, produces umbels of 6–12 fragrant, white or pink flowers, 7–15cm (3–6in) long, flared at the tips, with a dark red central stripe on each tepal. Easily grown in a sheltered border. ↕ 60cm (24in), ↔ 15cm (6in). South Africa. ❄❄

C. longifolium see *C. bulbispermum.*

C. macowanii (Pyjama lily). Deciduous perennial with curved, mid-green leaves, 90cm (36in) long, with wavy margins. In autumn, bears umbels of 10–15 fragrant, white or pink flowers, to 10cm (4in) long, flared at the tips, with a dark red central stripe on each tepal. ↕ 60cm (24in), ↔ 15cm (6in). C. and E. Africa, South Africa. ❄

C. moorei. Deciduous perennial bearing light to mid-green leaves, 90cm (36in) long, grouped at the top of a long, false stem. Umbels of 6–12 fragrant flowers, 8cm (3in) long, either white or in shades of pink, are produced in autumn. ↕ 90cm (36in), ↔ 30cm (12in). South Africa. ❄

C.* x *powellii 🏆 (*C. bulbispermum* x *C. moorei*). Deciduous perennial with a long bulb neck bearing arching, light to mid-green leaves, to 1.5m (5ft) long. Umbels of up to 10 widely flared, fragrant, pale to mid-pink flowers, to 10cm (4in) long, are produced from late summer to autumn. ↕ 1.5m (5ft), ↔ 30cm (12in). Garden origin. ❄❄❄ (borderline). **'Album'** ■ has pure white flowers.

CROCOSMIA

syn. ANTHOLYZA, CURTONUS

Montbretia

IRIDACEAE

Genus of 7 species of clump-forming, cormous perennials from grassland in South Africa. Erect, linear-lance-shaped leaves are mostly ribbed or sometimes pleated, mainly mid-green, sometimes pale green or brownish green, usually 60–100cm (24–36in) long. They are grown for their funnel-shaped, brightly coloured flowers, borne from mid- to late summer in often branched spikes on wiry stems. Grow at the edge of a shrub border or in clumps in a herbaceous border. The flowers are excellent for cutting.

- **HARDINESS** Fully hardy to frost hardy.
- **CULTIVATION** Plant 8–10cm (3–4in) deep in spring, in moderately fertile, humus-rich, moist but well-drained soil in sun or partial shade. In frost-prone areas, plant near a wall; mulch in the first winter and in periods of prolonged frost. Lift and divide congested clumps in spring to maintain vigour.
- **PROPAGATION** Sow seed in containers in a cold frame as soon as ripe. Divide in spring, just before growth starts.
- **PESTS AND DISEASES** Red spider mites may be troublesome.

C. aurea. Cormous perennial with pale green leaves, 50–70cm (20–28in) long. Erect or occasionally branched spikes of pale to dark orange flowers, 5cm (2in) long, arranged in 2 rows, are produced in early summer. ↕ 80–90cm (32–36in), ↔ 8cm (3in). South Africa. ❄❄

***C.* 'Bressingham Blaze'.** Cormous perennial with large clumps of pleated, mid-green leaves. In late summer, bears brilliant orange-red flowers, 5–6cm (2–2½in) long, with yellow throats, in spikes 60–80cm (24–32in) long. ↕ 75–90cm (30–36in), ↔ 8cm (3in). ❄❄

***C.* 'Citronella' of gardens** see *C.* 'Golden Fleece'.

C.* x *crocosmiiflora (*C. aurea* x *C. pottsii*) (Montbretia). Robust, sometimes invasive, variable cormous perennial with pale green leaves, 60–80cm (24–32in) long. Thin, slightly arching, sometimes branched spikes of orange or yellow flowers, 3–5cm (1¼–2in) long, are produced in summer. ↕ 60cm (24in), ↔ 8cm (3in). South Africa. ❄❄❄

***C.* 'Emberglow'.** Cormous perennial with mid-green leaves. Dark red flowers, 5–8cm (2–3in) long, arranged in 2 rows in arching, freely branching spikes, are produced in summer. ↕ 60–75cm (24–30in), ↔ 8cm (3in). ❄❄

***C.* 'Emily McKenzie'**, syn. *C.* 'Lady McKenzie'. Cormous perennial with mid-green leaves. In late summer, bears branched spikes of usually downward-facing, broad-petalled, bright orange flowers, 4–5cm (1½–2in) long, with mahogany throat markings. ↕ 60cm (24in), ↔ 8cm (3in). ❄❄

***C.* 'Firebird'.** Robust, cormous perennial with mid-green leaves. In summer, bears upward-facing, bright orange-red flowers, 5–8cm (2–3in) long, in spreading, mostly unbranched spikes. ↕ 80cm (32in), ↔ 8cm (3in). ❄❄

***C.* 'Fire King' of gardens** see *C.* 'Jackanapes'.

***C.* 'George Davison' of gardens** see *C.* 'Golden Fleece'.

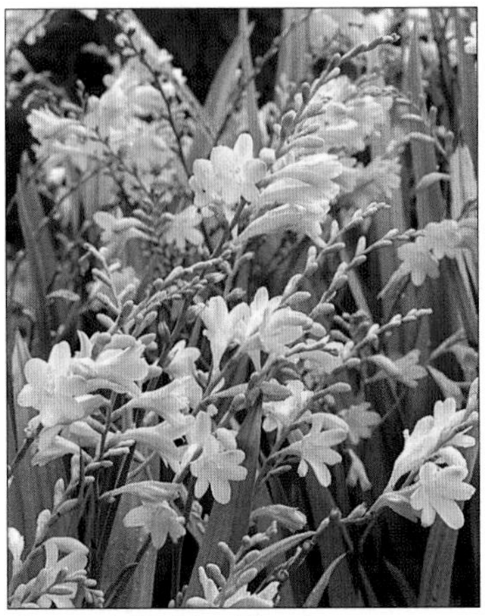

Crocosmia 'Golden Fleece'

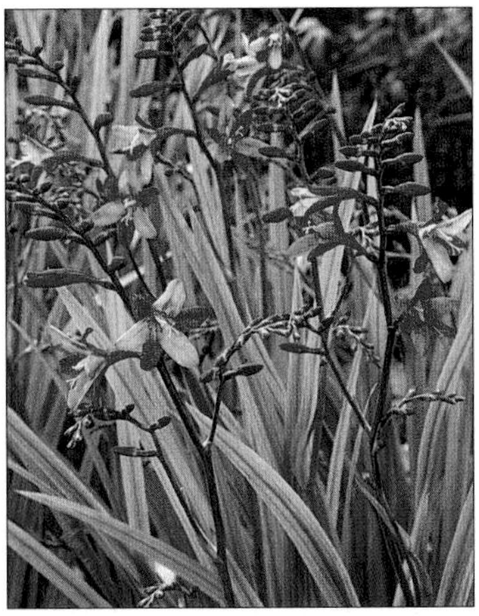

Crocosmia 'Jackanapes'

***C.* 'Golden Fleece'** ■ syn. *C.* 'Citronella' of gardens, *C.* 'George Davison' of gardens. Cormous perennial with mid-green leaves. In late summer, bears slightly arching, freely branched spikes of lemon-yellow flowers, to 5cm (2in) long. ↕ 60–75cm (24–30in), ↔ 8cm (3in). ❄❄

***C.* 'Jackanapes'** ■ syn. *C.* 'Fire King' of gardens. Cormous perennial with mid-green leaves. Arching, many-branched stems of bicoloured, orange-red and yellow flowers, 2–3cm (¾–1¼in) long, are produced in late summer. ↕ 40–60cm (16–24in), ↔ 8cm (3in). ❄❄

***C.* 'Lady Hamilton'.** Cormous perennial with mid-green leaves. In late summer, golden yellow flowers, 3–4cm (1¼–1½in) long, with apricot-yellow

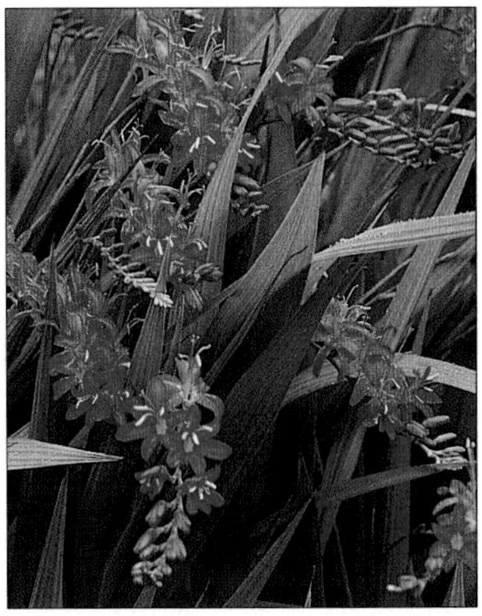

Crocosmia masoniorum

centres, are produced in erect, branched spikes. ↕ 60–75cm (24–30in), ↔ 8cm (3in). ❄❄

***C.* 'Lady McKenzie'** see *C.* 'Emily McKenzie'.

***C.* 'Lucifer'** ■🏆 Robust, cormous perennial bearing pleated, mid-green leaves. Upward-facing, bright tomato-red flowers, to 5cm (2in) long, are produced in bold, slightly arching, sparsely branched spikes in midsummer. ↕ 1–1.2m (3–4ft), ↔ 8cm (3in). ❄❄

C. masoniorum ■🏆 Robust, cormous perennial bearing pleated, mid-green leaves, 60–100cm (24–39in) long. In midsummer, bears upward-facing, orange-red flowers, 5cm (2in) long, in arching, usually unbranched spikes. ↕ 1.2m (4ft), ↔ 8cm (3in). South Africa. ❄❄❄ (borderline)

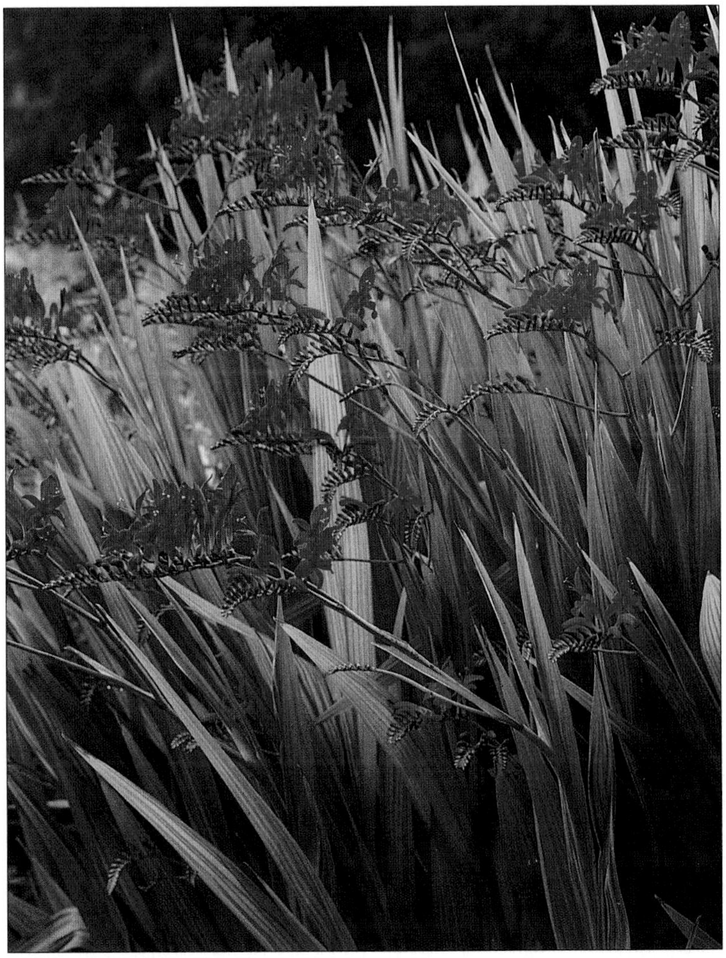

Crocosmia 'Lucifer'

C

C

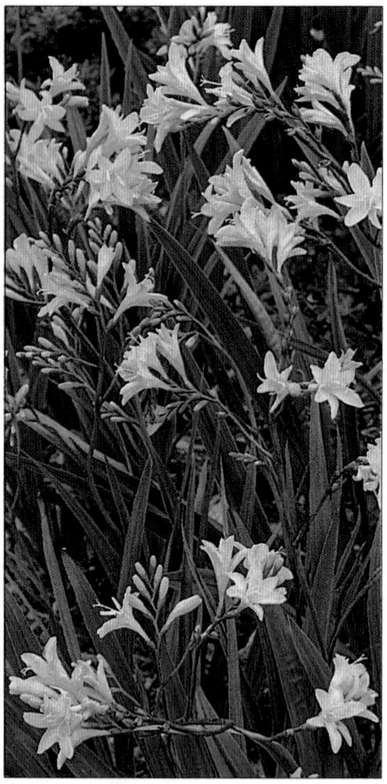

Crocosmia 'Solfatare'

C. paniculata, syn. *Antholyza paniculata, Curtonus paniculatus.* Cormous perennial producing strongly pleated, olive green leaves, to 1m (3ft) long. In late summer, downward-curved orange flowers, to 6cm (2½in) long, are borne alternately on branched, zigzagged stems. ↕1.5m (5ft), ↔10cm (4in). South Africa. ❄❄
C. rosea see *Tritonia disticha.*
***C.* 'Solfatare'** ▣ ♀ syn. *C.* 'Solfaterre'. Cormous perennial with bronze leaves. Apricot-yellow flowers, 3cm (1¼in) long, are borne on arching, branched stems in midsummer. ↕60–70cm (24–28in), ↔8cm (3in). ❄❄
***C.* 'Solfaterre'** see *C.* 'Solfatare'.
***C.* 'Spitfire'.** Cormous perennial with mid-green leaves. Upward-facing, bright orange-red flowers, 3.5cm (1½in) long, are borne on arching, branched stems in late summer. ↕70–90cm (28–36in), ↔8cm (3in). ❄❄
***C.* 'Star of the East'** ▣ Cormous perennial with mid-green leaves. From late summer to early autumn, produces horizontal-facing, clear orange flowers, 3.5cm (1½in) long, each with a paler orange centre, on branched stems. ↕70cm (28in), ↔8cm (3in). ❄❄

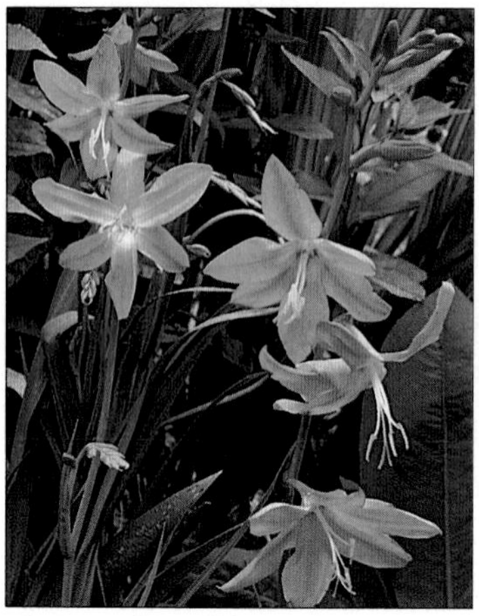

Crocosmia 'Star of the East'

CROCUS

IRIDACEAE

Genus of about 80 species of dwarf, cormous perennials found in a wide range of habitats, including woodland, scrub, and meadows, from coastal to subalpine areas in C. and S. Europe, N. Africa, the Middle East, C. Asia, and W. China. The small, mainly goblet-shaped flowers (4 or more per corm) open in autumn or early spring to reveal inner tepals in often contrasting colours. The 6 tepals forming the bowl of the flower are usually each 2–5cm (¾–2in) long, while the perianth tube may be up to 15cm (6in) long. The styles are either 3-branched (with expanded or frilled ends), 6-branched, or multi-branched (with more than 6 branches). Semi-erect, linear to linear-lance-shaped leaves, mostly mid-green with pale silvery green central stripes, usually appear at the same time as or soon after the flowers and elongate markedly as the flowers fade. In some autumn-flowering species, flowers appear before the leaves.

Chrysanthus Hybrids are selections of *C. biflorus* or *C. chrysanthus*, or hybrids between these two species. They have grey- to mid-green leaves, to 15cm (6in) long, borne with or after the flowers. Up to 4 flowers, each 5–10cm (2–4in) long, are produced in spring.

Grow crocuses in drifts at the front of a mixed or herbaceous border, or in a rock garden, raised bed, or trough; the most vigorous are useful for naturalizing in short turf. Some need a dry summer dormancy, and these are best grown in a bulb frame or alpine house.

• **HARDINESS** Fully hardy to frost hardy.
• **CULTIVATION** Plant crocuses 8–10cm (3–4in) deep: spring-flowering ones in autumn, and autumn-flowering ones in late summer. Crocuses have varying cultivation requirements, which, for ease of reference, are grouped as follows:
1. Full sun and gritty, poor to moderately fertile, well-drained soil.
2. Full light in a bulb frame or alpine house, in a mix of equal parts loam, leaf mould, and grit or sharp sand. In the growing season, water freely and apply a low-nitrogen fertilizer monthly; keep completely dry in summer dormancy.
3. Sun or partial shade and moderately fertile, humus-rich, moderately moist but well-drained soil.
• **PROPAGATION** Collect seed as soon as ripe, just before the seed capsule splits, and sow immediately in containers in a cold frame. Leave seedlings in containers for 2 years before planting out. Many crocuses self-seed freely. Remove cormlets during dormancy.
• **PESTS AND DISEASES** Mice, voles, and squirrels may feed on the corms. Birds sometimes pick off flowers. Corms in storage are prone to rots and moulds.

***C.* 'Advance'.** Early spring-flowering Chrysanthus Hybrid producing several pale yellow flowers, suffused violet-bronze outside and golden yellow inside. Cultivation group 1. ↕7cm (3in), ↔5cm (2in). ❄❄❄
***C. aerius* of gardens** see *C. biflorus* subsp. *pulchricolor.*
C. ancyrensis ▣ Late winter- and early spring-flowering crocus, producing 5 or more, rounded, bright yellow or orange flowers, 1.5–3cm (½–1¼in) long, which have long perianth tubes. Cultivation group 1. ↕↔5cm (2in). C. and N. Turkey, W. China (Tien Shan). ❄❄❄

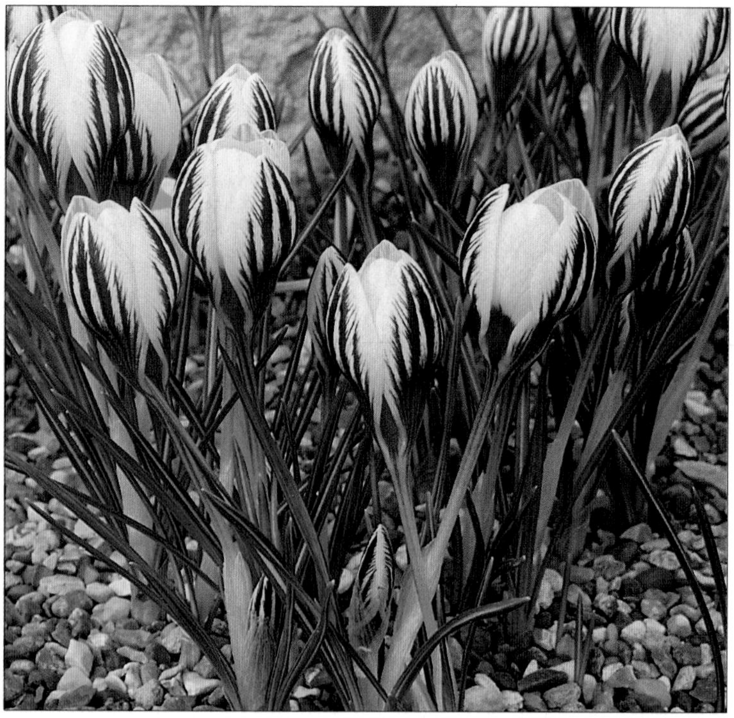

Crocus 'Gipsy Girl'

C. angustifolius ♀ syn. *C. susianus* (Cloth of gold crocus). Spring-flowering crocus producing grey-green leaves and 1 or 2 narrow, orange-yellow flowers, 1.5–3.5cm (½–1½in) long. Outer tepals are suffused or almost wholly marked deep bronze, and recurve strongly when flowers are fully open. Cultivation group 1 or 2. ↕↔5cm (2in). S. Ukraine (including Crimea), Armenia. ❄❄❄
C. asturicus see *C. serotinus* subsp. *salzmannii.*
C. aureus see *C. flavus.*
C. banaticus ▣ ♀ syn. *C. iridiflorus.* Early autumn-flowering crocus with very distinctive, solitary flowers. Large, lilac to purple outer tepals, to 5cm (2in) long, open wide; smaller inner tepals, to 3cm (1¼in) long, remain erect and are usually paler. The style is divided into a mass of lilac or white branches. Dark green leaves, without central stripes, are borne after the flowers. Slow to increase, and best propagated by seed. Cultivation group 3. ↕10cm (4in), ↔5cm (2in). N.E. former Yugoslavia, Romania, S.W. Ukraine. ❄❄❄
C. baytopiorum. Spring-flowering crocus with 1or 2 rounded, clear blue-turquoise flowers, 2–3cm (¾–1¼in) long. Cultivation group 2. ↕5cm (2in), ↔2.5cm (1in). S.W. Turkey. ❄❄❄
C. biflorus ▣ Very variable, early spring-flowering crocus producing 1–4 yellow-throated flowers, to 3cm (1¼in) long, in shades of lilac-blue or white, the outer tepals sometimes striped purple or brownish purple. Cultivation group 1. ↕6cm (2½in), ↔5cm (2in). Italy, S. former Yugoslavia, Greece, Bulgaria, Turkey, Iran, S. Ukraine (Crimea), Armenia, Caucasus. ❄❄❄. **subsp. *alexandri*** has white flowers, the outer tepals heavily marked deep purple; S.W. Bulgaria, former Yugoslavia. **subsp. *pulchricolor***, syn. *C. aerius* of gardens, has rich blue-purple flowers, stained dark violet near the bases, with deep yellow throats; N.W. Turkey. **subsp. *weldenii* 'Fairy'** has white flowers, the outer tepals dusted violet.
***C.* 'Blue Bird'.** Spring-flowering Chrysanthus Hybrid with pale blue flowers, heavily marked violet outside, with golden yellow throats. Cultivation group 1. ↕7cm (3in), ↔5cm (2in). ❄❄❄
***C.* 'Blue Pearl'** ♀ Spring-flowering Chrysanthus Hybrid producing yellow-throated white flowers with soft lilac-blue outer tepals. Cultivation group 1. ↕7cm (3in), ↔5cm (2in). ❄❄❄
C. boryi ♀ Autumn-flowering crocus producing up to 4 well-rounded, creamy white flowers, to 5cm (2in) long, sometimes veined or flushed mauve outside, with the leaves. Cultivation group 2. ↕8cm (3in), ↔5cm (2in). Greece (including Crete). ❄❄
C. cancellatus. Very variable, autumn-flowering crocus with 1–3 slender, pale blue flowers, to 6cm (2½in) long, striped violet outside. Grey-green leaves are usually absent but may just be visible at flowering. Cultivation group 2. This description applies to subsp. *cancellatus*, the most commonly cultivated variant, found in S. Turkey, Lebanon, and S. Israel; other subspecies occur in Greece, S. former Yugoslavia, Lebanon, Jordan, Iraq, and Iran. ↕↔5cm (2in). ❄❄❄
C. cartwrightianus ▣ ♀ Autumn- and early winter-flowering crocus with 1–5 open goblet-shaped, fragrant, pale to deep lilac or white flowers, 1.5–3cm (½–1¼in) long, veined dark purple. Leaves appear with or shortly after the flowers. Cultivation group 2, but may be grown outside in a sunny, very well-drained situation. ↕↔5cm (2in). Greece (including Crete). ❄❄❄. **f. *albus*** ♀ has white flowers, and is often cultivated.
C. chrysanthus ♀ Late winter- and early spring-flowering crocus with dull green leaves and up to 4 rounded, scented flowers, 1.5–4cm (½–1½in) long, which vary from cream to deep golden yellow, often suffused or veined

bronze-maroon outside. Cultivation group 1. ↕5cm (2in), ↔4cm (1½in). Former Yugoslavia, Greece, Albania, Macedonia, Bulgaria, W., C., and S. Turkey. ❄❄❄

C. clusii see *C. serotinus* subsp. *clusii.*

C. corsicus ■ 🏆 Spring-flowering crocus with 1 or 2 slender, scented flowers, 2–3.5cm (¾–1½in) long, bright lilac inside and paler lilac, striped violet or purple outside, with bright orange styles. Leaves are deep green. Cultivation group 1 or 2. ↕8–10cm (3–4in), ↔4cm (1½in). France (Corsica). ❄❄❄

***C.* 'Cream Beauty'** 🏆 Compact, spring-flowering Chrysanthus Hybrid producing rich cream flowers with pale greenish brown bases and deep golden yellow throats. Cultivation group 1. ↕7cm (3in), ↔5cm (2in). ❄❄❄

C. cvijicii ■ Spring-flowering crocus producing solitary flowers, 2–4cm (¾–1½in) long, usually golden yellow but sometimes white or cream. Leaves are only just visible at flowering. Cultivation group 2. ↕10cm (4in), ↔4cm (1½in). S. former Yugoslavia, N. Greece, E. Albania. ❄❄❄

C. dalmaticus ■ Late winter- and early spring-flowering crocus with solitary, rounded, pale lilac flowers, 1.5–3.5cm (½–1½in) long. Outer tepals have a silver or biscuit-brown overlay, lightly veined with purple. Cultivation group 1. ↕8cm (3in), ↔4cm (1½in). Former Yugoslavia, N. Albania. ❄❄❄

***C.* 'Dutch Yellow'** 🏆 syn. *C.* 'Golden Yellow', *C.* x *luteus* 'Dutch Yellow'. Vigorous, spring-flowering crocus with 2–5 orange-yellow flowers, 3–5cm (1¼–2in) long. Suitable for naturalizing in grass. Cultivation group 1. ↕8–10cm (3–4in), ↔5cm (2in). ❄❄❄

***C.* 'E.A. Bowles'** ■ 🏆 Spring-flowering Chrysanthus Hybrid with compact, rich lemon-yellow flowers, the outer tepals with bronze-green bases and purple feathering. Cultivation group 1. ↕7cm (3in), ↔5cm (2in). ❄❄❄

***C.* 'Elegance'.** Tall, spring-flowering Chrysanthus Hybrid with large, bright golden yellow flowers with large brown marks outside. Cultivation group 1. ↕8–10cm (3–4in), ↔5cm (2in). ❄❄❄

***C. etruscus* 'Zwanenburg'** ■ Late winter- and spring-flowering crocus with 1 or 2 lilac-blue flowers, 3–4cm (1¼–1½in) long, the outsides washed silver or biscuit-brown with faint purple veining. Cultivation group 1. ↕8cm (3in), ↔4cm (1½in). ❄❄❄

***C.* 'Eyecatcher'.** Spring-flowering Chrysanthus Hybrid with grey-white flowers, heavily marked deep purple outside. Cultivation group 1. ↕7cm (3in), ↔5cm (2in). ❄❄❄

C. flavus, syn. *C. aureus.* Spring-flowering crocus producing 1–4 scented, orange-yellow flowers, 2–3.5cm (¾–1½in) long. Cultivation group 1. ↕8cm (3in), ↔5cm (2in). S. former Yugoslavia, C. and N. Greece, N.W. and W. Turkey, Romania. ❄❄❄

C. gargaricus. Spring-flowering crocus with tiny corms, 5mm (¼in) across, and solitary, slender, bright orange-yellow flowers, 1.5–4.5cm (½–1¾in) long. Non-stoloniferous and may be difficult to grow. Cultivation group 3. ↕4cm (1½in), ↔2.5cm (1in). N.W. Turkey. ❄❄❄. **subsp. *herbertii*** ■ increases by stolons and may form large clumps. Easier to grow; cultivation group 2 or 3.

***C.* 'Gipsy Girl'** ■ Spring-flowering Chrysanthus Hybrid producing large yellow flowers with purple stripes and feathering outside. Cultivation group 1. ↕7cm (3in), ↔5cm (2in). ❄❄❄

***C.* 'Golden Yellow'** see *C.* 'Dutch Yellow'.

C. goulimyi ■ 🏆 Autumn-flowering crocus producing 1–3 rounded, scented, lilac flowers, 1.5–4cm (½–1½in) long, with long, slender perianth tubes. Leaves are borne with the flowers. Cultivation group 1 or 2. ↕10cm (4in), ↔5cm (2in). S. Greece. ❄❄❄

C. hadriaticus 🏆 syn. *C. hadriaticus* var. *chrysobelonicus.* Autumn-flowering crocus producing 1–3 white flowers, 2–4.5cm (¾–1¾in) long, with the leaves. Flowers have conspicuous yellow throats and may be lightly feathered with lilac at the bases; the style is divided into 3 bright red branches. Cultivation group 1 or 2. ↕8cm (3in), ↔4cm (1½in). Greece. ❄❄❄

C. hadriaticus* var. *chrysobelonicus see *C. hadriaticus.*

***C. imperati* 'De Jager'** ■ Late winter- and early spring-flowering crocus with 1 or 2 flowers, 3–4.5cm (1¼–1¾in) long, with long perianth tubes. Flowers are rich violet-purple inside and biscuit-brown outside, with pronounced violet stripes. Leaves are shiny and dark green. Cultivation group 1. ↕10cm (4in), ↔4cm (1½in). ❄❄❄

C. iridiflorus see *C. banaticus.*

C. korolkowii (Celandine crocus). Late winter- and early spring-flowering crocus with 3–5 slender, scented, shiny, golden yellow flowers, 2–3.5cm (¾–1½in) long. Cultivation group 2, although may be grown outside. Needs a dry summer dormancy. ↕10cm (4in), ↔5cm (2in). Uzbekistan, Tajikistan, N. and E. Afghanistan, N. Pakistan. ❄❄❄

C. kotschyanus ■ 🏆 syn. *C. zonatus.* Vigorous, autumn-flowering crocus with large, irregular, flattened corms. Solitary, long-tubed, pale lilac flowers, 3–4.5cm (1¼–1¾in) long, are borne before the leaves. Each short-stemmed flower has a ring of yellow dots around the throat and creamy white stamens. Cultivation group 1 or 2. Needs a dry summer dormancy. ↕6–8cm (2½–3in), ↔5cm (2in). Turkey, N.W. Syria, Lebanon. ❄❄❄. **var. *leucopharynx*** has flowers with white throats.

***C.* 'Ladykiller'** ■ 🏆 Spring-flowering Chrysanthus Hybrid producing white flowers heavily marked deep purple outside. Cultivation group 1. ↕7cm (3in), ↔5cm (2in). ❄❄❄

C. laevigatus 🏆 Late autumn- and early winter-flowering crocus with 1–3 often fragrant, white to lilac flowers, 1.5–3cm (½–1¼in) long, sometimes yellow or biscuit-coloured outside, often heavily feathered with deep violet-purple. Deep green leaves are borne with the flowers. Suitable for naturalizing in grass. Cultivation group 1 or 2. ↕4–8cm (1½–3in), ↔4cm (1½in). Greece (including Crete). ❄❄❄

C. longiflorus ■ 🏆 Autumn-flowering crocus with 1 or 2 pale to deep lilac, strongly fragrant flowers, 2–4.5cm (¾–1¾in) long, often lightly feathered outside, with bright orange-red styles. Leaves, with white central stripes, appear with the flowers. Cultivation group 2. ↕8–10cm (3–4in), ↔3cm (1¼in). S.W. Italy (including Sicily), Malta. ❄❄❄

***C.* x *luteus* 'Dutch Yellow'** see *C.* 'Dutch Yellow'.

C. malyi ■ 🏆 Spring-flowering crocus with slightly grey-green leaves and 1 or 2 white flowers with long perianth tubes, pointed tepals, 2–4cm (¾–1½in) long, sometimes faintly suffused purple at the bases, and yellow throats. Cultivation group 2. ↕8cm (3in), ↔4cm (1½in). W. former Yugoslavia. ❄❄❄

C. medius ■ 🏆 Late autumn-flowering crocus producing solitary, vivid purple, or sometimes paler flowers, 2.5–5cm (1–2in) long, with long perianth tubes and bright orange-red styles; flowers appear just before the leaves. Cultivation group 1. ↕8cm (3in), ↔2.5cm (1in). S.E. France, N.W. Italy. ❄❄❄

C. minimus ■ Late spring-flowering crocus with 1 or 2 mid- to deep lilac-purple flowers, 2–3cm (¾–1¼in) long, with long perianth tubes. Outer tepals

C

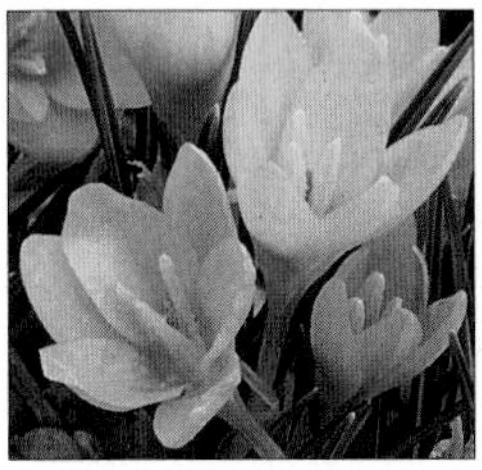
Crocus ancyrensis

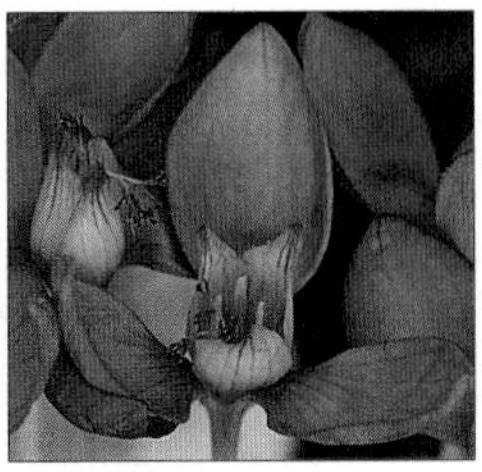
Crocus banaticus

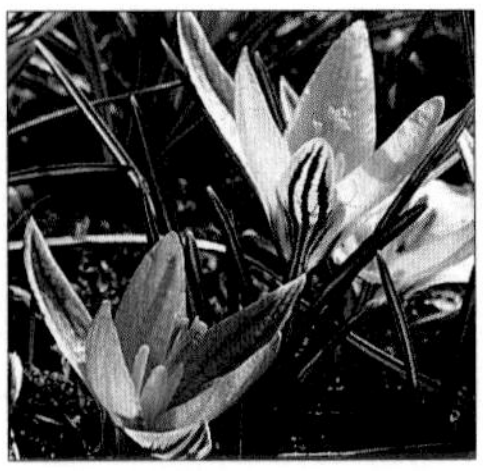
Crocus biflorus

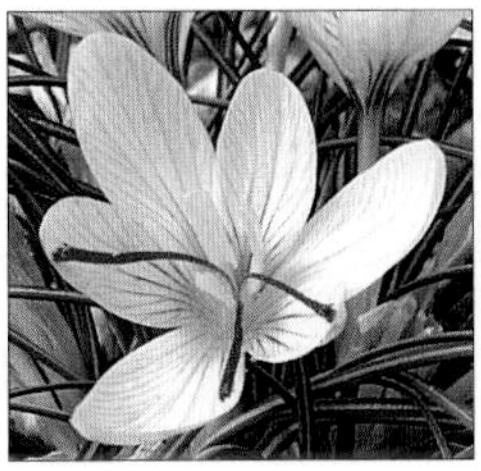
Crocus cartwrightianus

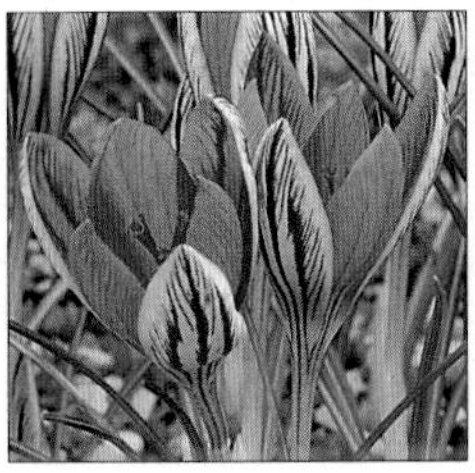
Crocus corsicus

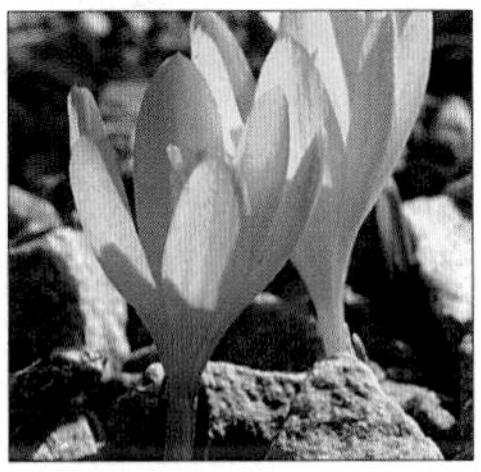
Crocus cvijicii

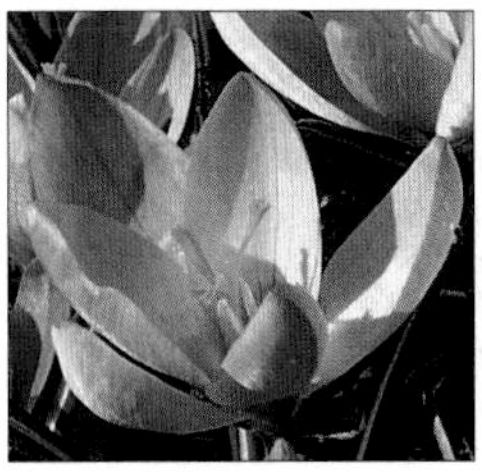
Crocus dalmaticus

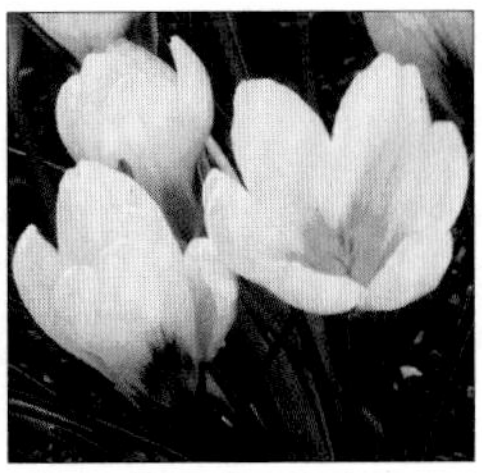
Crocus 'E.A. Bowles'

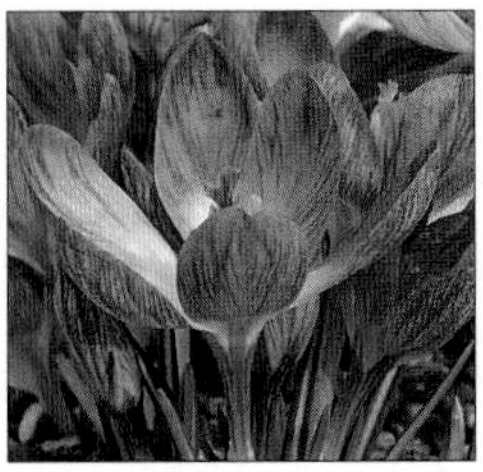
Crocus etruscus 'Zwanenburg'

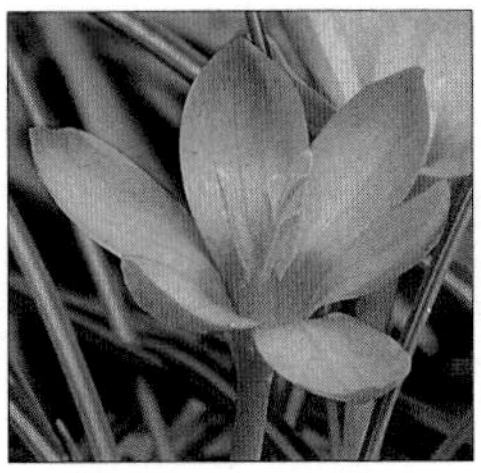
Crocus gargaricus subsp. *herbertii*

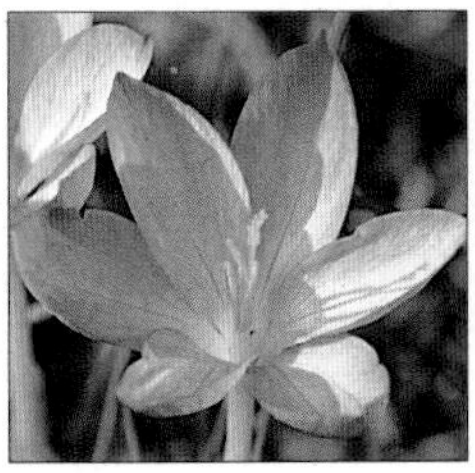
Crocus goulimyi

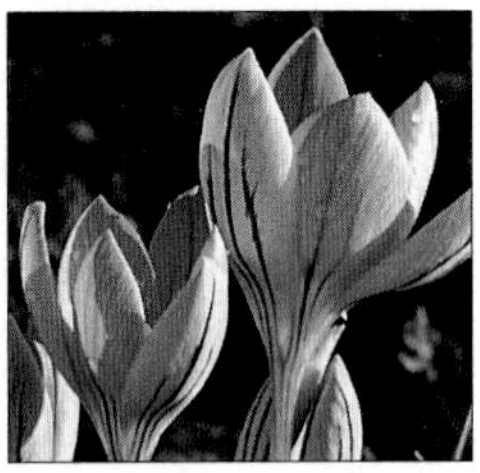
Crocus imperati 'De Jager'

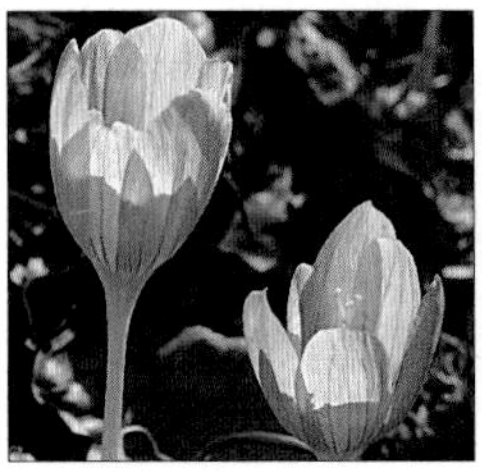
Crocus kotschyanus

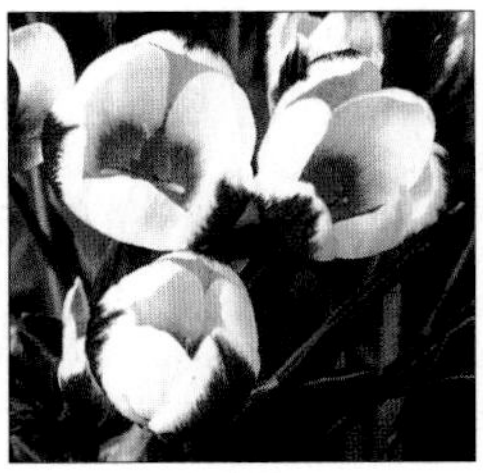
Crocus 'Ladykiller'

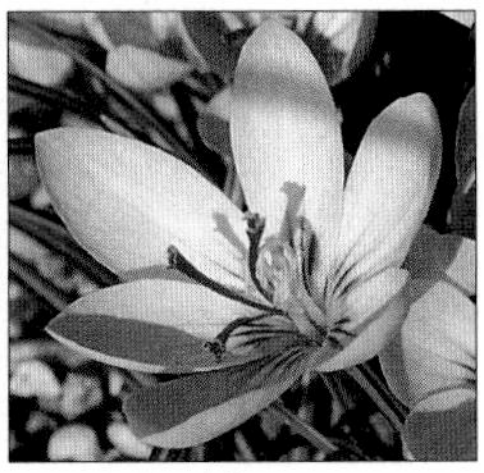
Crocus longiflorus

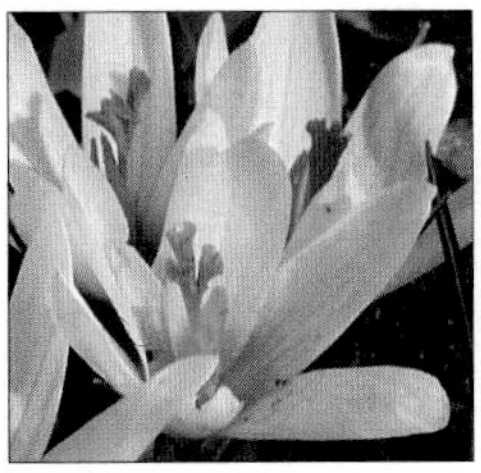
Crocus malyi

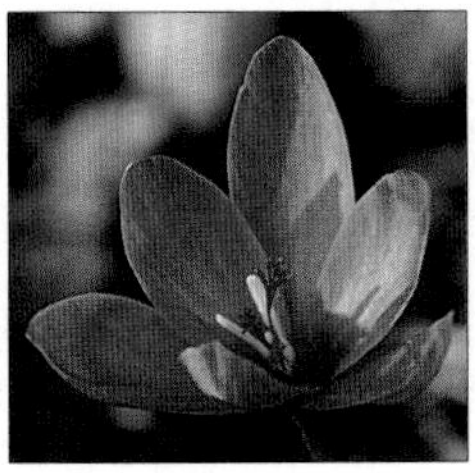
Crocus medius

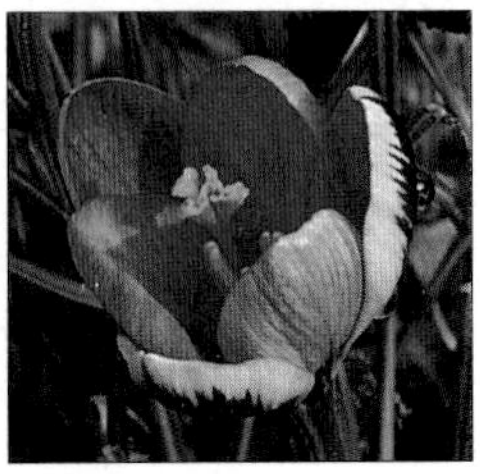
Crocus minimus

C

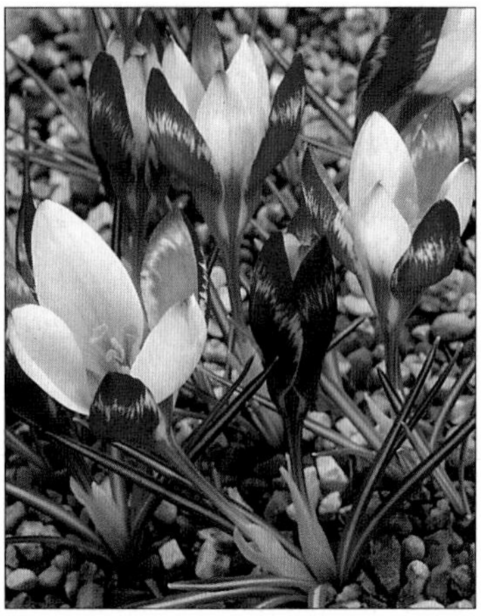
Crocus sieberi 'Hubert Edelsten'

are veined, stained, or feathered with dark violet, often on a buff or yellow base. Cultivation group 1. ↕ 8cm (3in), ↔ 2.5cm (1in). France (S. Corsica), Italy (Sardinia). ❄❄❄
C. niveus. Autumn-flowering crocus producing 1 or 2 flowers when the leaves are just present. The flowers, 3–6cm (1¼–2½in) long, vary from white to lilac with yellow throats and long, white, yellow, or purple-brown perianth tubes. The orange styles are much-divided and very conspicuous. Cultivation group 2, but may be grown outside. Needs a dry summer dormancy. ↕ 10–15cm (4–6in), ↔ 4cm (1½in). S. Greece. ❄❄❄
C. nudiflorus. Autumn-flowering crocus producing solitary, long-tubed, rich purple flowers, 3–6cm (1¼–2½in) long, before the leaves. Spreads by stolons and is suitable for naturalizing in grass. Cultivation group 3. ↕ 15–26cm (6–10in), ↔ 5cm (2in). S.W. France, N. and E. Spain. ❄❄❄
C. ochroleucus ■ ♀ Late autumn-flowering crocus producing 1–3 creamy white flowers, 2–3.5cm (¾–1½in) long, with conspicuous yellow throats and long perianth tubes. Leaves appear with, or shortly after the flowers. Increases freely by offsets and is suitable for naturalizing in grass. Cultivation group 1 or 2. ↕ 5cm (2in), ↔ 2.5cm (1in). S.W. Syria, Lebanon, N. Israel. ❄❄❄
C. olivieri. Spring-flowering crocus with spreading leaves, producing 1–4 long-tubed, pale lemon-yellow to deep orange flowers, 1.5–3.5cm (½–1½in) long, with undivided styles. Cultivation group 1. ↕ 5cm (2in), ↔ 4cm (1½in). S.E. Romania, S. Albania, Macedonia, S. Bulgaria, Greece, Turkey (except E. Turkey). ❄❄❄. **subsp. *balansae*** has much-divided styles, and outer tepals striped or heavily suffused bronze; Greece (Samos, Chios), W. Turkey.
C. oreocreticus. Autumn-flowering crocus producing 1–5 rich lilac flowers, 1.5–3cm (½–1¼in) long, each with dark purple veins and a silvery wash on the outside. Leaves are only just present at flowering. Increases easily from seed. Cultivation group 2. ↕↔ 5cm (2in). Greece (Crete). ❄❄❄
***C.* 'Princess Beatrix'** see *C.* 'Prinses Beatrix'.
***C.* 'Prinses Beatrix'**, syn. *C.* 'Princess Beatrix'. Spring-flowering Chrysanthus Hybrid producing compact, clear blue flowers with yellow bases. Cultivation group 1. ↕ 7cm (3in), ↔ 5cm (2in). ❄❄❄
C. pulchellus ■ ♀ Autumn- to early winter-flowering crocus producing 1, occasionally 2, long-tubed, goblet-shaped flowers, 3–6cm (1¼–2½in) long, before the leaves. Flowers are pale lilac-blue, lightly veined violet, with deep yellow throats and white anthers. Very similar to *C. speciosus*, with which

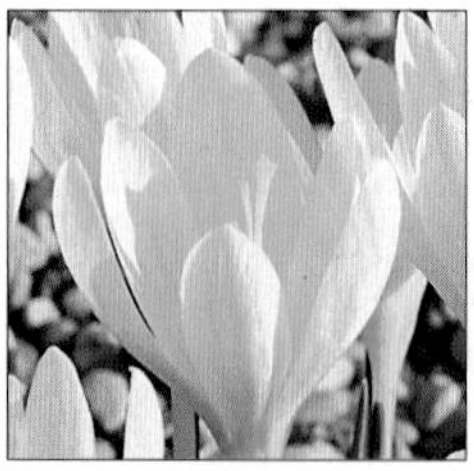
Crocus ochroleucus

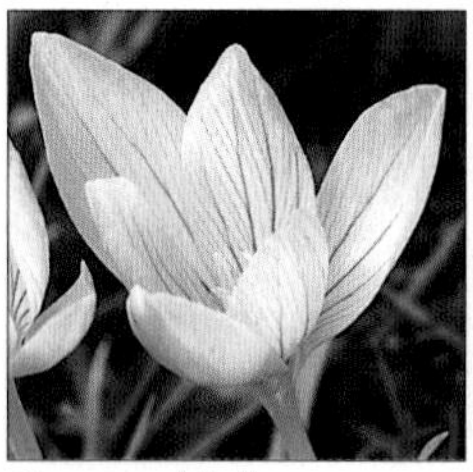
Crocus pulchellus

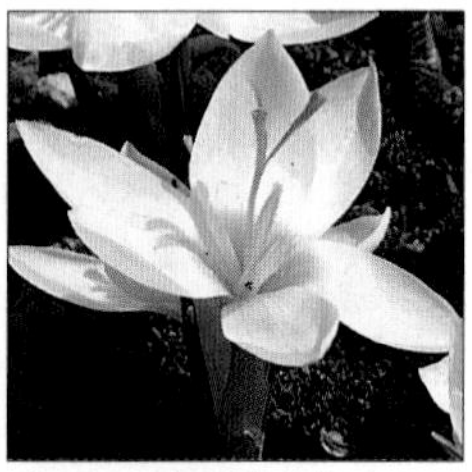
Crocus sieberi 'Bowles' White'

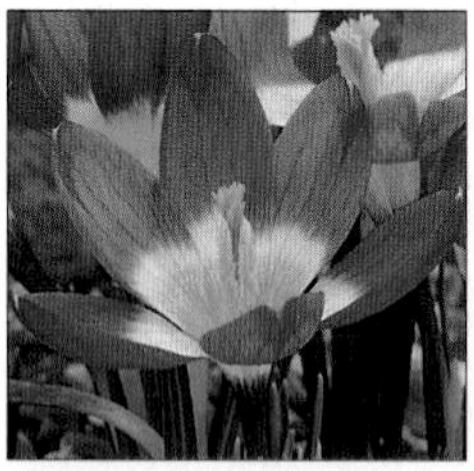
Crocus sieberi subsp. *sublimis* f. *tricolor*

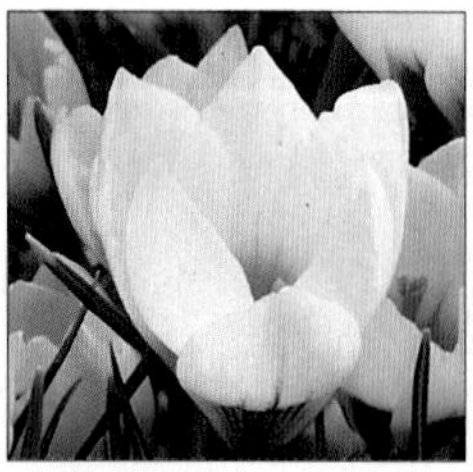
Crocus 'Snow Bunting'

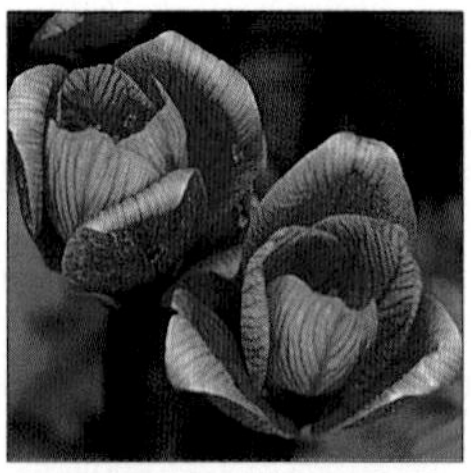
Crocus speciosus 'Oxonian'

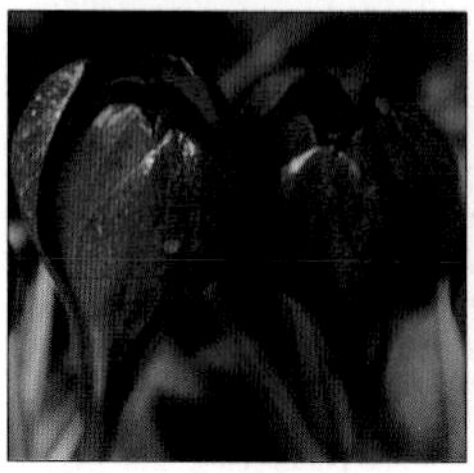
Crocus tommasinianus 'Ruby Giant'

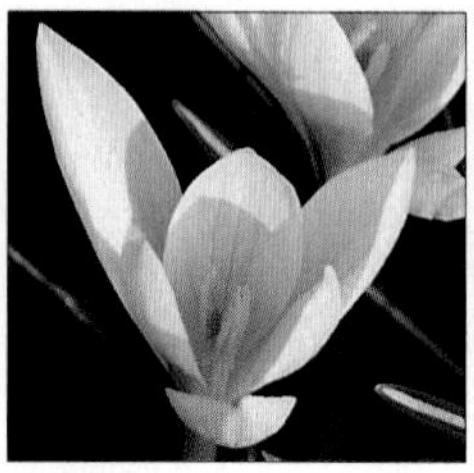
Crocus vernus subsp. *albiflorus*

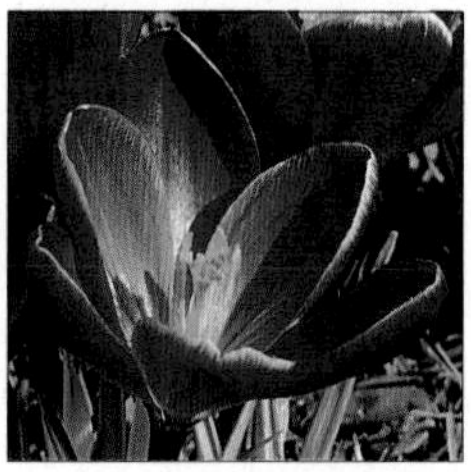
Crocus vernus 'Purpureus Grandiflorus'

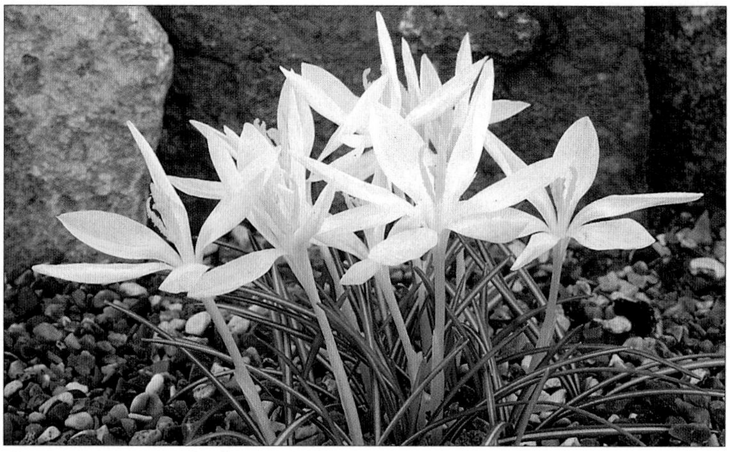
Crocus tommasinianus f. *albus*

it hybridizes. Suitable for naturalizing in grass. Cultivation group 1. ↕ 10–12cm (4–5in), ↔ 4cm (1½in). S. former Yugoslavia, N. Greece, S. Bulgaria, Turkey. ❄❄❄. **'Zephyr'** see *C.* 'Zephyr'.
C. reticulatus. Late winter- and early spring-flowering crocus producing 1 or 2 cup-shaped, fragrant, white or lilac flowers, 1.5–3.5cm (½–1½in) long, with light yellow throats inside. Outer tepals have 3–5 longitudinal, deep violet bands. Grey-green leaves have white central stripes. Cultivation group 2. ↕ to 10cm (4in), ↔ 8cm (3in). N.E. Italy to S. Turkey and N. Caucasus. ❄❄❄
C. salzmannii see *C. serotinus* subsp. *salzmannii.*
C. sativus, syn. *C. sativus* var. *cashmirianus* (Saffron crocus). Autumn-flowering crocus producing 1–5 widely open, rich lilac flowers, to 5cm (2in) long, with dark purple veins. Dull green leaves are borne with or shortly after the flowers. Saffron is obtained from the long, conspicuous, 3-branched, deep red style. Sterile, increasing only by division. Cultivation group 1 or 2. ↕↔ 5cm (2in). Origin uncertain; it is probably an ancient selection of *C. cartwrightianus.* ❄❄❄. **var. *cashmirianus*** see *C. sativus.*
C. serotinus. Autumn-flowering crocus with solitary, pale to deep lilac flowers, 2.5–4cm (1–1½in) long, sometimes veined darker lilac, with long perianth tubes and white or very pale yellow throats. Dark green leaves are sometimes present at flowering. Cultivation group 2. ↕ 5–8cm (2–3in), ↔ 4cm (1½in). S. Portugal. ❄❄❄. **subsp. *clusii*** ♀ syn. *C. clusii*, produces leaves as the flowers fade; cultivation group 1, with added humus; ↕ 5–8cm (2–3in), ↔ 4cm (1½in); Portugal, N.W. and S.W. Spain. **subsp. *salzmannii***, syn. *C. asturicus, C. salzmannii*, flowers earlier, producing larger, pale lilac flowers when leaves are only just present; N., C., and S. Spain, Gibraltar, N. Africa.
C. sieberi ♀ Vigorous, late winter- and early spring-flowering crocus with 1–3 scented, rich pinkish lilac-blue, yellow-throated flowers, 2–3cm (¾–1¼in) long. Cultivation group 1. ↕ 5–8cm (2–3in), ↔ 2.5cm (1in). Greece. ❄❄❄. **'Albus'** see 'Bowles' White'. **'Bowles' White'** ■ ♀ syn. 'Albus', produces white flowers, 3–4.5cm (1¼–1¾in) long, with deep golden yellow throats, in early spring. **'Firefly'** has abundant, lilac flowers. **'Hubert Edelsten'** ■ ♀ has pale lilac flowers, 3–4.5cm (1¼–1¾in) long, with rich purple outer tepals, each with a bold white line. **subsp. *sieberi*** produces white flowers, marked purple outside, from spring to early summer; cultivation group 2; ↕ 4cm (1½in); Greece (Crete). **subsp. *sublimis* f. *tricolor*** ■ ♀ has narrow flowers, each with 3 distinct bands of lilac, white, and golden yellow. **'Violet Queen'** has deep violet flowers with pointed tips.
***C.* 'Skyline'.** Spring-flowering Chrysanthus Hybrid producing clear blue flowers, lightly veined darker blue outside. Cultivation group 1. ↕ 7cm (3in), ↔ 5cm (2in). ❄❄❄
***C.* 'Snow Bunting'** ■ ♀ Spring-flowering Chrysanthus Hybrid with white flowers, lightly feathered grey-blue outside. Cultivation group 1. ↕ 7cm (3in), ↔ 5cm (2in). ❄❄❄
C. speciosus ♀ Autumn-flowering crocus producing solitary flowers before the leaves. Long-tubed flowers, 3–6cm (1¼–2½in) long, in shades of violet-blue with deeper blue veins, have much-divided, bright orange styles. Increases rapidly by seed and offsets; suitable for naturalizing in grass. Cultivation group 1. ↕ 10–15cm (4–6in), ↔ 5cm (2in). N. and C. Turkey, N. Iran, S. Ukraine (Crimea), Caucasus, C. Asia. ❄❄❄. **f. *albus*** ♀ syn. 'Albus', has pure white flowers. **'Conqueror'** has deep blue flowers, 4–7cm (1½–3in) long. **'Oxonian'** ■ has violet-mauve flowers with dark violet bases and tubes.
***C.* 'Spring Pearl'.** Spring-flowering Chrysanthus Hybrid with bronze-yellow flowers, feathered purple-brown outside. Cultivation group 1. ↕ 7cm (3in), ↔ 5cm (2in). ❄❄❄
C. susianus see *C. angustifolius.*
C. tommasinianus ♀ Late winter- to spring-flowering crocus producing 1 or 2 slender flowers, 2–4.5cm (¾–1¾in) long, with long white perianth tubes. Flowers vary from pale silvery lilac to shades of reddish purple; outer tepals are often overlaid silver. Increases freely by seed and offsets; suitable for naturalizing in grass. Cultivation group 1. ↕ 8–10cm (3–4in), ↔ 2.5cm (1in). S. Hungary, S. former Yugoslavia, N.W. Bulgaria. ❄❄❄. **f. *albus*** ■ has white flowers. **'Barr's Purple'** has purple flowers, silvery outside. **'Ruby Giant'** ■ is clump-forming, with sterile, rich reddish purple flowers. **'Whitewell Purple'** increases rapidly and has reddish purple flowers, silver mauve inside.
C. tournefortii ♀ Late autumn- to winter-flowering crocus. Solitary, long-

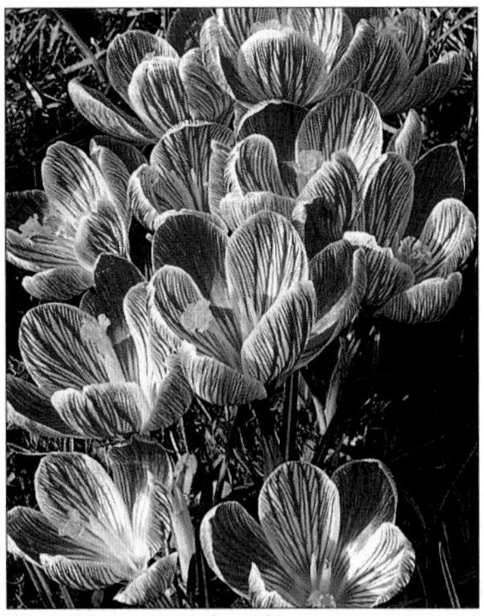
Crocus vernus 'Pickwick'

tubed, widely open, pale lilac flowers, 1.5–3.5cm (½–1½in) long, have much-divided orange styles and white anthers. Flowers, borne with the leaves, remain open at night. Cultivation group 1 or 2. ↕ 5–8cm (2–3in), ↔ 4cm (1½in). S. Greece (including Crete, Cyclades). ❄❄❄
C. vernus (Dutch crocus). Spring- to early summer-flowering crocus producing solitary flowers, 3–6cm (1¼–2½in) long, in white or shades of lilac or purple. Suitable for naturalizing in grass. Cultivation group 1. ↕ 10–12cm (4–5in), ↔ 5cm (2in). W. Russia, Poland, Czech Republic, Slovakia, Austria, former Yugoslavia, Hungary, Romania, Italy. ❄❄❄. **subsp. *albiflorus*** ■ has pointed, white or occasionally purple flowers, and is more difficult to cultivate; France, Spain (Pyrenees), Switzerland, Italy (including Sicily), Germany, Austria, Czech Republic, Slovakia, former Yugoslavia, Albania. **'Flower Record'** has pale violet flowers. **'Haarlem Gem'** has lilac flowers, silvery grey outside. **'Jeanne d'Arc'**, syn. 'Joan of Arc', has white flowers with deep purple bases and faint purple feathering. **'Joan of Arc'** see 'Jeanne d'Arc'. **'Pickwick'** ■ has white flowers, striped pale and dark lilac, with dark purple bases. **'Purpureus Grandiflorus'** ■ has abundant violet flowers with purple bases. **'Queen of the Blues'** has lilac-blue flowers. **'Remembrance'** has shiny violet flowers. **'Vanguard'** produces pale lilac flowers, grey outside, in late winter.
***C.* 'Zephyr'** 🏆 syn. *C. pulchellus* 'Zephyr'. Autumn-flowering crocus producing solitary, long-tubed, pale lilac flowers, 2–4cm (¾–1½in) long, before the leaves. Cultivation group 1. ↕ 10–12cm (4–5in), ↔ 5cm (2in). ❄❄❄
C. zonatus see *C. kotschyanus.*
***C.* 'Zwanenburg Bronze'** 🏆 Spring-flowering Chrysanthus Hybrid producing yellow flowers, almost completely suffused dark reddish brown outside. Cultivation group 1. ↕ 7cm (3in), ↔ 5cm (2in). ❄❄❄

▷ **Crocus,**
Autumn see *Colchicum*
Celandine see *Crocus korolkowii*
Chilean blue see *Tecophilaea cyanocrocus*
Cloth of gold see *Crocus angustifolius*
Dutch see *Crocus vernus*
Saffron see *Crocus sativus*

CROSSANDRA

ACANTHACEAE

Genus of about 50 species of evergreen shrubs and subshrubs from forest margins of the Arabian Peninsula, tropical Africa, Madagascar, India, and Sri Lanka. They have whorls of hairless or softly hairy, usually entire, obovate, ovate, elliptic, or lance-shaped leaves. Salverform flowers, each with a long corolla tube and 5 usually orange or red lobes, are borne in terminal or axillary, 4-sided spikes with prominent bracts. In frost-prone areas, grow in a temperate or warm greenhouse; a few may be used as houseplants. In tropical areas, grow in a shrub border.
• **HARDINESS** Frost tender.
• **CULTIVATION** Under glass, grow in loamless or loam-based potting compost (JI No.3) in full light from autumn to spring, and in bright filtered light in summer. Provide moderate to high humidity. In growth, water freely with soft water and apply a balanced liquid fertilizer monthly; water sparingly in winter. Pinch out growing points when young to encourage bushy growth. Outdoors, grow in fertile, humus-rich, well-drained soil in full sun. Pruning group 8; plants under glass need restrictive pruning in late winter.
• **PROPAGATION** Sow seed at 16°C (61°F) in early spring. Root semi-ripe cuttings with bottom heat in early spring.
• **PESTS AND DISEASES** Trouble free.

C. infundibuliformis ■ syn. *C. undulifolia* (Firecracker flower). Erect subshrub with slender stems and ovate to lance-shaped, wavy-margined, glossy, mid-green leaves, 5–12cm (2–5in) long. Fan-shaped, orange-yellow to salmon-pink flowers, to 3cm (1¼in) across, are borne in usually axillary, cone-shaped spikes, 10cm (4in) long, with downy bracts, at any time of year. ↕ 1m (3ft), ↔ 60cm (24in). S. India, Sri Lanka. ❀ (min. 15°C/59°F). **'Mona Walhead'** is much more compact, with lustrous green leaves and deep salmon-pink flowers; ↕ 50cm (20in), ↔ 30cm (12in).
C. nilotica ■ Erect subshrub with elliptic, softly hairy, mid-green leaves, the few basal leaves 6cm (2½in) long, and the stem leaves 10cm (4in) long. Fan-shaped, vivid red to orange flowers, 2.5cm (1in) across, are produced in dense, axillary or terminal spikes, to 7cm

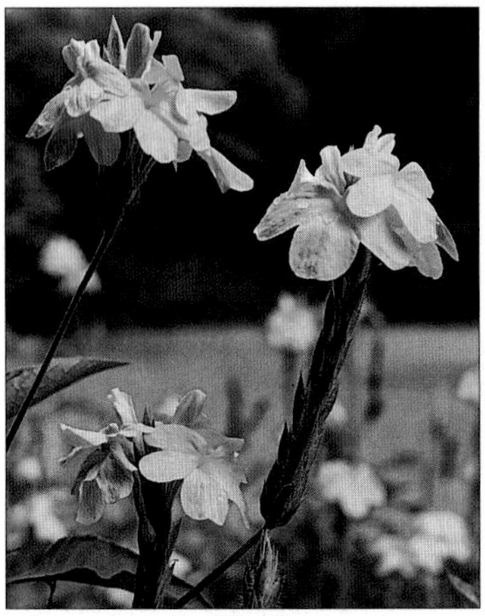
Crossandra infundibuliformis

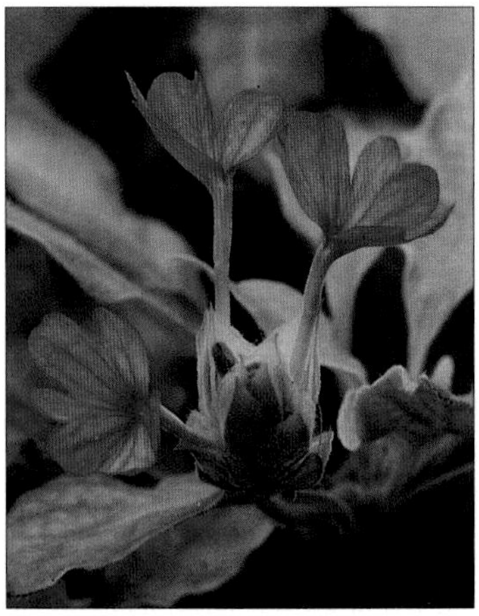
Crossandra nilotica

(3in) long, with hairy bracts, at any time of year. ↕ 30–60cm (12–24in), ↔ to 35cm (14in). Tropical Africa. ❀ (min. 15°C/59°F)
C. pungens. Dense subshrub with oblong, white-veined, dull green leaves, 5–14cm (2–5½in) long. Produces fan-shaped orange flowers, to 4cm (1½in) across, in congested, axillary or terminal spikes, 10cm (4in) long, with bristly, sometimes spiny bracts, at any time of year. ↕ 60cm (24in), ↔ 50cm (20in). Tropical Africa. ❀ (min. 15°C/59°F)
C. undulifolia see *C. infundibuliformis.*

▷ **Cross-leaved heath** see *Erica tetralix*

CROTALARIA

Rattlebox

LEGUMINOSAE/PAPILIONACEAE

Genus of about 600 species of annuals, perennials, and evergreen shrubs from scrub, grassland, and open forest in tropical and subtropical zones worldwide, particularly in E. and S. tropical Africa. The alternate leaves are simple or 3- to 7-palmate. Pea-like flowers are borne in terminal or axillary racemes, followed by inflated seed pods. In frost-prone areas, grow the perennials and shrubs in a temperate greenhouse. In warm, dry climates, grow against a warm, sunny wall or in a border. Annuals are easy to cultivate in a border.
• **HARDINESS** Frost tender.
• **CULTIVATION** Under glass, grow in loam-based potting compost (JI No.2) in full light with shade from hot sun, and with good ventilation. In the growing season, water freely, and apply a balanced liquid fertilizer monthly; water sparingly in winter. Top-dress or pot on in spring. Outdoors, grow in fertile, moist but well-drained soil in full sun. Pruning group 8; plants under glass need restrictive pruning after flowering.
• **PROPAGATION** Sow seed at 15–18°C (59–64°F) in spring. Root semi-ripe cuttings with bottom heat in summer.
• **PESTS AND DISEASES** Red spider mites and whiteflies may prove troublesome under glass.

C. agatiflora ■ (Canary bird bush). Erect to spreading shrub with 3-palmate leaves, 5–8cm (2–3in) long, with ovate to elliptic-lance-shaped, mid- to deep green leaflets. Yellow- to olive-green flowers, 3.5–5cm (1½–2in) long, are borne in terminal racemes, 25–40cm (10–16in) long, mainly in summer,

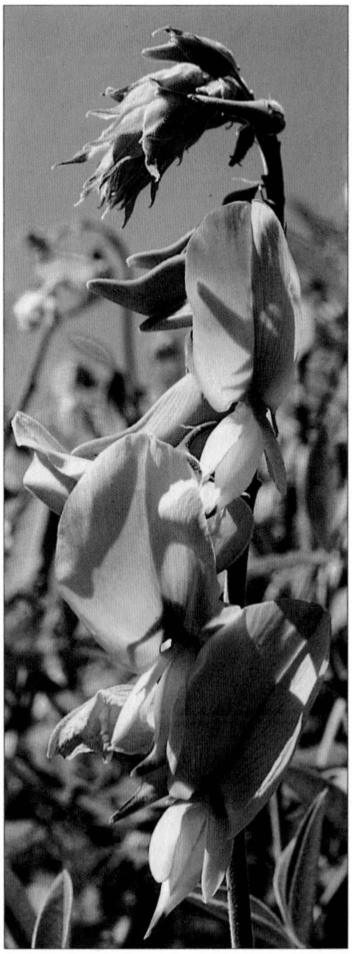
Crotalaria agatiflora

followed by large, rattle-like seed pods. ↕ 2–3m (6–10ft), ↔ 1–2m (3–6ft). Uganda to Zimbabwe, highlands of Kenya. ❀ (min. 7–10°C/ 45–50°F)

▷ **Croton** see *Codiaeum*

CROWEA

RUTACEAE

Genus of 3 species of evergreen shrubs and woody-based perennials found in scrub and open woodland in Australia. The alternate, linear to elliptic leaves are simple and glandular. The usually solitary, sometimes paired, axillary or terminal, star-shaped flowers have 5 wide, spreading petals. In frost-prone areas, grow in a cool greenhouse or conservatory; in warmer climates, use in a shrub border or courtyard garden.
• **HARDINESS** Frost tender; *C. exalata* survives short periods near 0°C (32°F).
• **CULTIVATION** Under glass, grow in loam-based potting compost (JI No.2) in full light with shade from hot sun, and with good ventilation. In growth, water moderately, applying a balanced liquid fertilizer monthly from spring to autumn; water sparingly in winter. Top-dress or pot on in spring. Outdoors, grow in fertile, moist but well-drained soil in full sun, with some midday shade, or in partial shade. Pruning group 10, after flowering.
• **PROPAGATION** Sow seed at 16–18°C (61–64°F) in early spring. Root semi-ripe cuttings with bottom heat in summer.
• **PESTS AND DISEASES** Scale insects may be a problem under glass.

C

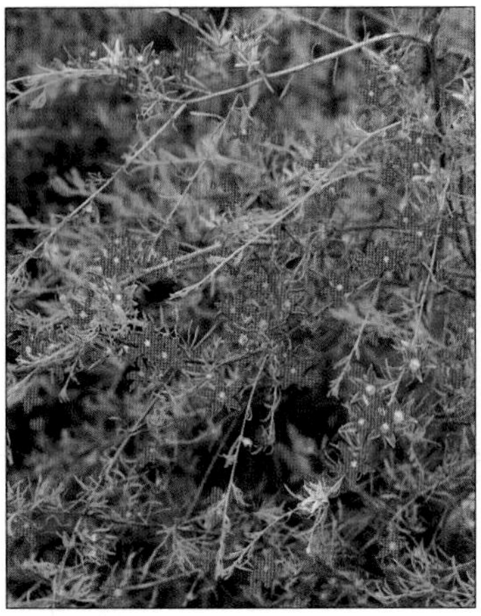
Crowea exalata

C. exalata ■ Open-branched shrub producing linear to narrowly obovate, mid-green leaves, 2–5cm (¾–2in) long, which smell of aniseed when bruised. Abundant pink or, rarely, white flowers, 2cm (¾in) across, are produced singly from the leaf axils, from late spring to autumn. ↕ 30–90cm (12–36in), ↔ 0.5–1.5m (20–60in). Australia (New South Wales, Victoria). ❀ (min. 5°C/41°F)
C. saligna. Open-branched shrub with slender stems bearing narrowly elliptic, deep green leaves, 4–8cm (1½–3in) long, with recurved margins. From summer to late autumn, produces solitary, waxy pink flowers, 3.5cm (1½in) across, from the leaf axils. ↕↔ 1–1.5m (3–5ft). Australia (New South Wales). ❀ (min. 5°C/41°F)

▷ **Crowfoot** see *Ranunculus*
Water see *R. aquatilis*
▷ **Crown imperial** see *Fritillaria imperialis*
▷ **Crown of thorns** see *Euphorbia milii*
▷ ***Crucianella*** see *Phuopsis*
C. stylosa see *P. stylosa*
▷ **Cruel plant** see *Araujia sericifera*
▷ ***Cryptanthopsis navioides*** see *Orthophytum navioides*

CRYPTANTHUS
Earth star, Starfish plant
BROMELIACEAE

Genus of about 20 species of mostly stemless, evergreen, mainly dwarf, terrestrial perennials (bromeliads) found in soil or on rocks in dry, forest regions, at altitudes up to 1,600m (5,000ft), in E. Brazil. The strap- to spoon-shaped, wavy-margined, sometimes attractively zoned leaves are borne in flat, star-like rosettes. In some species, offsets form in the leaf axils; others produce them from stolons. In summer, inconspicuous, star-shaped, often scented, white or greenish white, occasionally pale yellow flowers are produced in sunken, corymb-like inflorescences at the centre of each rosette. Where temperatures fall below 15–20°C (59–68°F), grow in a warm greenhouse, as houseplants, or in a bottle garden; in humid, tropical areas, grow in a bed or border.
• **HARDINESS** Frost tender.
• **CULTIVATION** Under glass, grow in terrestrial bromeliad compost, in full or bright filtered light with moderate to high humidity. In the growing season, water moderately but carefully, mist regularly with tepid soft water, and apply a dilute fertilizer monthly; reduce water slightly in winter. Outdoors, grow in moist but well-drained, moderately fertile, acid soil, enriched with fibrous organic matter, in partial or dappled shade. See also p.47.
• **PROPAGATION** Sow seed at 27°C (81°F) as soon as ripe. Remove offsets in early summer.
• **PESTS AND DISEASES** Susceptible to root rot.

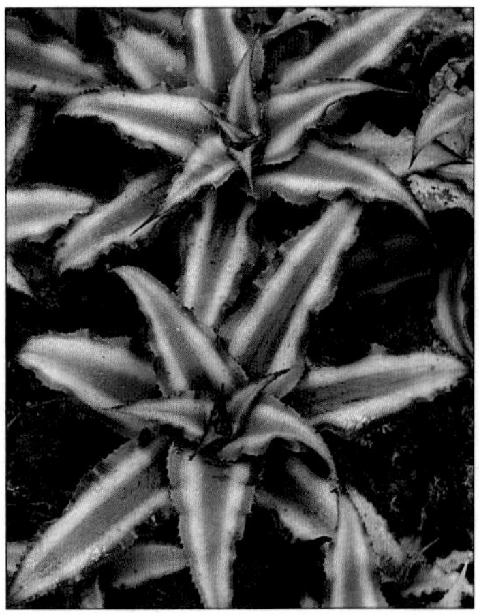
Cryptanthus bivittatus

C. acaulis (Green earth star). Stemless or short-stemmed, clump-forming bromeliad with rosettes of 10–15 narrowly lance-shaped, wavy-margined, minutely toothed leaves, 13cm (5in) long; leaves are mid-green and scaly above, densely white-scaly beneath. Corymbs of 5 or 6 or more, scented white flowers, 4cm (1½in) long, are produced in summer. ↕ to 10cm (4in), ↔ indefinite. E. Brazil. ❀ (min. 20°C/68°F). **'Ruber'**, syn. var. *ruber*, has leaves tinged brownish red.
C. beuckeri. Stemless or very short-stemmed, clump-forming bromeliad with loose, often irregular rosettes of 10–20 broadly lance-shaped to narrowly ovate, tapering, wavy-margined, toothed, pink-flushed, dull green leaves, to 15cm (6in) long, white mottled above and grey scaly beneath. Corymbs of 3–6 white or greenish white flowers, 3cm (1¼in) long, are produced in summer. ↕↔ to 15cm (6in). E. Brazil. ❀ (min. 20°C/68°F)
C. bivittatus ■ 🏆 Stemless bromeliad with low, spreading rosettes of about 20 strap-shaped, wavy-margined, toothed, dark green leaves, to 18cm (7in) long, striped white or pink. Few-flowered corymbs of white flowers, 2.5cm (1in) long, are produced in summer. ↕ to 10cm (4in), ↔ to 25cm (10in). E. Brazil. ❀ (min. 20°C/68°F)

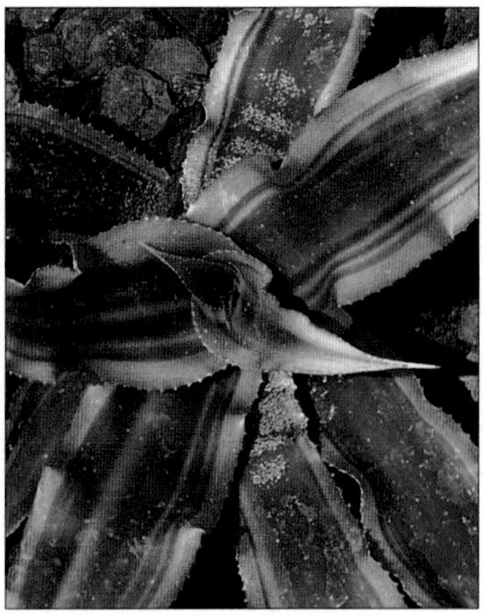
Cryptanthus 'Pink Starlight'

C. bromelioides (Rainbow star). Short-stemmed, stoloniferous bromeliad with rosettes of 10–20 strap-shaped, minutely toothed, stiff, olive-green to bronze leaves, to 35cm (14in) long, often wavy-margined, and stems to 60cm (24in) long. Dense corymbs of white flowers, 4cm (1½in) long, are produced in summer. ↕ 30–40cm (12–16in), ↔ indefinite. E. Brazil. ❀ (min. 20°C/68°F). **'Tricolor'** ■ 🏆 syn. var. *tricolor*, has olive-green leaves with white and red longitudinal stripes.
C. fosterianus 🏆 Stemless or short-stemmed bromeliad with almost flat, widely spreading rosettes of up to 12 strap-shaped, long-pointed, wavy-margined, toothed, brownish green or reddish brown leaves, to 30cm (12in) long, cross-banded purplish brown or greyish brown above and grey scaly beneath. In summer, white flowers, 1cm (½in) long, are produced in corymbs, each consisting of a 3- or 4-flowered outer cluster and a 2-flowered inner cluster. ↕ to 12cm (5in), ↔ to 60cm (24in). E. Brazil. ❀ (min. 20°C/68°F)
***C.* 'Pink Starlight'** ■ Stemless, spreading bromeliad with rosettes of about 15 strap-shaped, wavy-margined leaves, to 8cm (3in) long, striped olive-green and white, and strongly suffused deep pink. In summer, inconspicuous, slightly scented white flowers, 3cm (1¼in) long, are borne in few-flowered corymbs. ↕ 20cm (8in), ↔ 35cm (14in) or more. ❀ (min. 20°C/68°F)
C. zonatus 🏆 (Zebra plant). Stemless bromeliad with rosettes of 8–15 strap-shaped, mid-green leaves, to 20cm (8in) long, with grey-brown cross-banding above and densely white-scaly beneath. White flowers, 3cm (1¼in) long, are produced in few-flowered corymbs in summer. ↕ to 12cm (5in), ↔ to 40cm (16in). E. Brazil. ❀ (min. 20°C/68°F). **'Zebrinus'** ■ has dark grey-green leaves with pronounced white cross-banding.

x CRYPTBERGIA
BROMELIACEAE

Hybrid genus, between *Cryptanthus* and *Billbergia*, of rosette-forming, evergreen, terrestrial perennials (bromeliads). The narrowly triangular, arching, olive-green to bronze outer leaves (shading to wine-red in the centre in some variants) are much longer than the inner ones, which tend to form a cup. In summer, cryptbergias usually bear small corymbs of tubular white flowers, with spreading lobes, from the centres of the rosettes. Most offset freely. In frost-prone areas, grow in a warm greenhouse or as foliage houseplants; in warmer climates, grow in a bed or at the front of a border.
• **HARDINESS** Frost tender.
• **CULTIVATION** Under glass, grow in terrestrial bromeliad compost in bright filtered light, with moderate humidity. In the growing season, water freely, applying a dilute fertilizer monthly; water sparingly at other times. Outdoors, grow in moist but well-drained, moderately fertile, acid soil, enriched with fibrous organic matter, in partial shade. See also p.47.
• **PROPAGATION** Remove offsets in spring.
• **PESTS AND DISEASES** Whiteflies and scale insects may prove troublesome under glass.

x *C.* 'Rubra' ■ Clump-forming bromeliad producing basal rosettes of dark green leaves, to 50cm (20in) long, turning copper-red in the lower halves, and with minutely scaly undersurfaces. In full light, the foliage intensifies to bronze-red. Small clusters of short-lived white flowers, to 1cm (½in) across, are occasionally produced in summer. ↕↔ 30cm (12in). ❀ (min. 13°C/55°F)

▷ ***Cryptocereus anthonyanus*** see *Selenicereus anthonyanus*

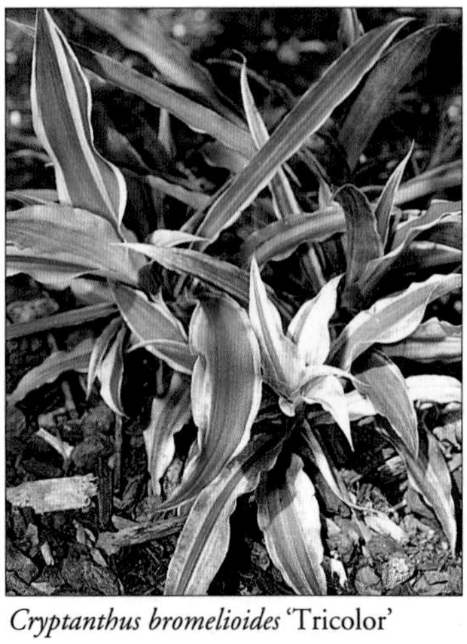
Cryptanthus bromelioides 'Tricolor'

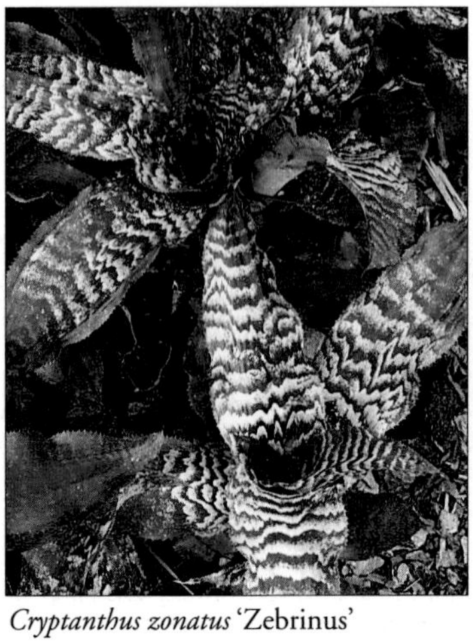
Cryptanthus zonatus 'Zebrinus'

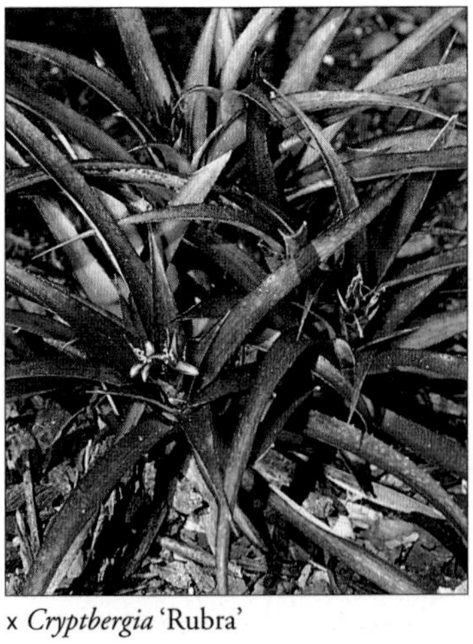
x *Cryptbergia* 'Rubra'

CRYPTOCORYNE

Water trumpet

ARACEAE

Genus of 50 species of slow-growing, rhizomatous, evergreen, marginal aquatic perennials from tropical S. and S.E. Asia. They are grown for their stiff, broadly ovate to lance-shaped, leathery leaves, which are mostly submerged. Minute, orange, red, or purple to almost black flowers are produced in a tubular spathe that projects above the surface of the water in mature plants. The flowers contain olfactory glands that give off a dung-like scent; this attracts insects, which crawl down the inside of the spathe, where they become trapped and pollinate the female flowers. In frost-prone areas, grow in a tropical aquarium or in the margins of an indoor pool in a warm greenhouse. In warmer areas, grow in the margins of an outdoor pool.

• **HARDINESS** Frost tender.

• **CULTIVATION** In an indoor pool, grow in aquatic planting baskets of inert medium, in full light, in water 15–30cm (6–12in) deep, and feed with sachets of proprietary aquatic plant fertilizer. In an outdoor pool, grow in baskets of humus-rich, sandy soil, or plant directly into the mud at the pond margin, in full sun or partial shade. In an aquarium, grow in containers of sharp sand and leave undisturbed. Provide full light until established; thereafter, they will tolerate bright filtered light. Maintain the water temperature at 20–30°C (68–86°F). See also pp.52–53.

• **PROPAGATION** Remove offsets in spring, or divide rhizomes in spring or early summer, and plant 1–2cm (½–¾in) deep.

• **PESTS AND DISEASES** Slight changes in external conditions, such as light and temperature, or in water chemistry, may cause the leaves to become soft and translucent.

C. beckettii. Submerged aquatic perennial with narrowly ovate to ovate, olive-green to dark brown leaves, 15cm (6in) long, with violet leaf-stalks. The twisted flower spathes, to 12cm (5in) tall, dull yellow on the outside and purplish brown inside, with blackish purple collars, are produced intermittently, only when growth is above the water surface, but most often in winter. ↕↔ 15cm (6in). S. and S.E. Asia. ❀ (min. 15°C/59°F)

C. spiralis. Submerged aquatic perennial, variable in habit, with linear-lance-shaped, dark green leaves, 10–15cm (4–6in) long. The purple spathes, to 24cm (10in) tall, are twisted at first, later becoming straight, and are produced intermittently throughout the year. ↕ 25cm (10in), ↔ 15cm (6in). India. ❀ (min. 15°C/59°F)

CRYPTOMERIA

Japanese cedar

TAXODIACEAE

Genus of 1 (possibly 2) species of evergreen, monoecious, coniferous tree from forests of China and Japan. It is cultivated for its conical or columnar habit, its thick, fibrous, red-brown bark, and its narrowly wedge-shaped, light to dark green leaves, which point forwards

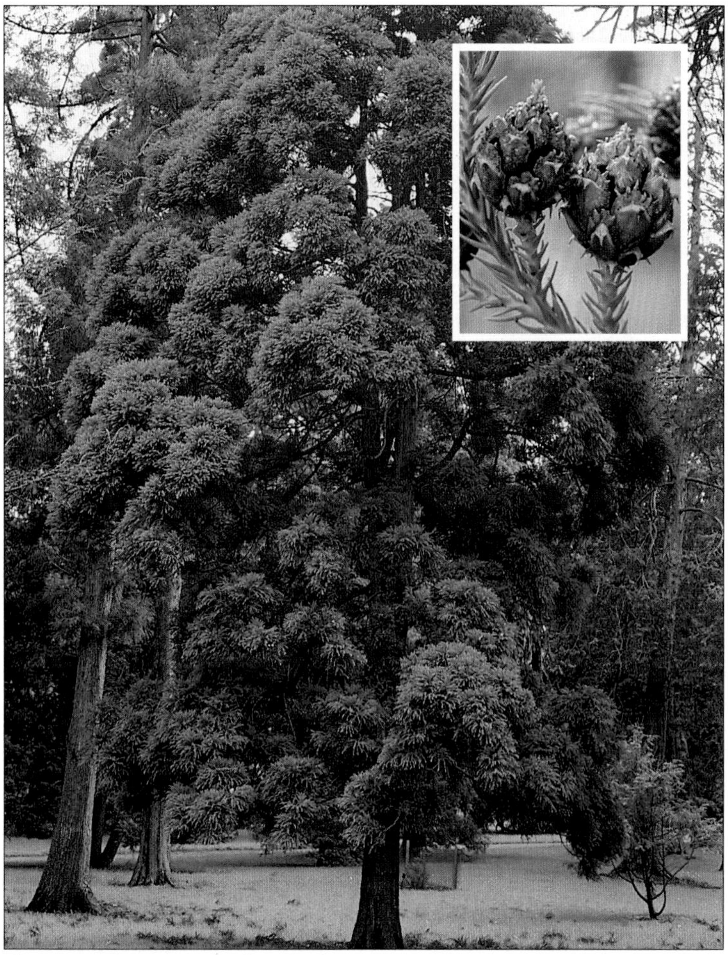

Cryptomeria japonica (inset: fruit detail)

in 5-ranked spirals around the shoots. Solitary, spherical female cones, 1–3cm (½–1¼in) long, have shield-like scales, each with a central point and triangular teeth. The ovoid male cones, 1cm (½in) long, are clustered at the shoot tips. Grow both species and cultivars as specimen trees; the dwarf cultivars are effective accent plants for a conifer collection, with heaths or heathers. *Cryptomeria* is one of the few conifer genera that will coppice successfully.

• **HARDINESS** Fully hardy.

• **CULTIVATION** Tolerates most well-drained soils, including chalky ones, although it grows best in deep, fertile, moist but well-drained, humus-rich soil in a sheltered site in full sun or partial shade. Needs no formal pruning. To coppice or restore untidy specimens,

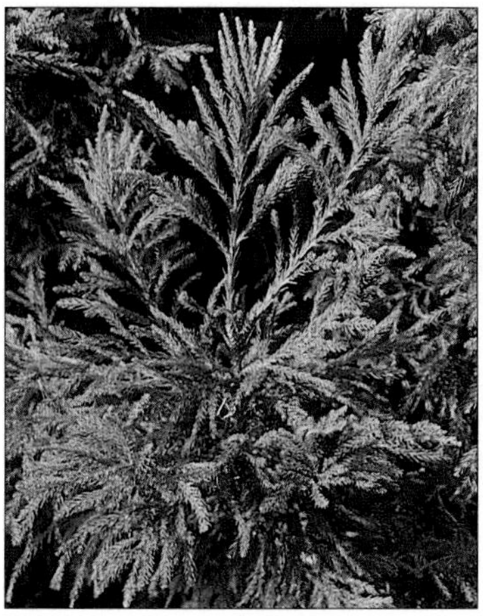

Cryptomeria japonica 'Cristata'

cut back to within 60–90cm (24–36in) of ground level in spring.

• **PROPAGATION** Sow seed in containers in a cold frame or in a seedbed in spring. Root ripewood cuttings in late summer or early autumn.

• **PESTS AND DISEASES** Trouble free.

C. fortunei see *C. japonica* var. *sinensis*.

C. japonica ▣ ♀ ◊ (Japanese cedar). Conical or columnar, coniferous tree with mid-to deep green leaves, 0.5–1.5cm (¼–½in) long, and brown female cones, each scale with 3–5 seeds. ↕ to 25m (80ft), ↔ to 6m (20ft). Japan. ✼✼✼. **'Bandai-sugi'** ♀ is a rounded, irregular shrub, with dense foliage that turns bronze in winter; ↕ 2m (6ft). **'Cristata'** ▣ syn. 'Sekka-sugi', is narrow and conical, with several shoots fused

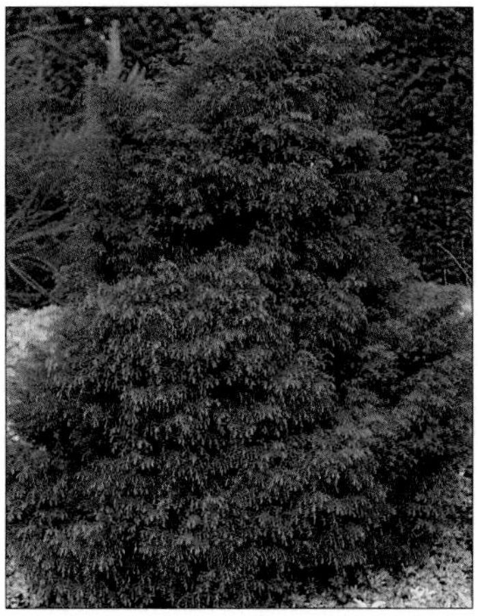

Cryptomeria japonica 'Elegans Compacta'

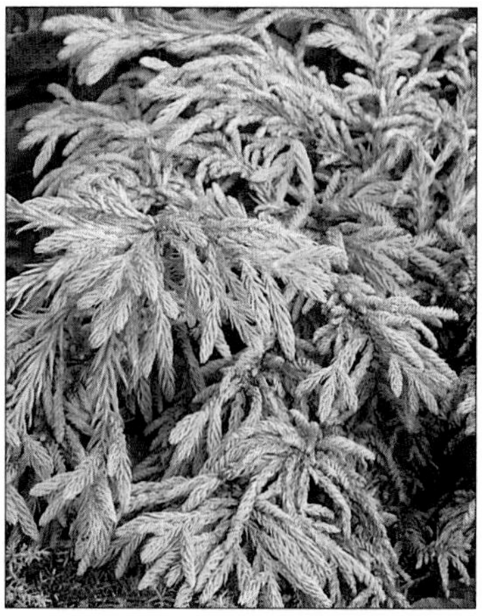

Cryptomeria japonica 'Spiralis'

and flattened into "cockscombs"; ↕ 8m (25ft), ↔ 5m (15ft). **'Elegans'** ◊ has soft, bluish green juvenile foliage, to 2.5cm (1in) long, turning red-brown in winter; leaves are well spaced on the shoots but dense in overall effect; ↕ 6–10m (20–30ft). **'Elegans Compacta'** ▣ ♀ is a conical shrub with soft, glossy, dark green juvenile leaves, turning bronze in winter; ↕ 2–4m (6–12ft). **'Pyramidata'** ◊ is narrowly columnar; ↕ to 4m (12ft), ↔ 40cm (16in). **'Sekkan-sugi'** is moderately slow-growing with creamy yellow leaves, turning almost white in winter. **'Sekka-sugi'** see 'Cristata'. **var. *sinensis***, syn. *C. fortunei*, is conical, becoming rounded when mature, with an open crown and billowing branches (more pendent than those of *C. japonica*), and yellow-green leaves; female cones have only 2 seeds per fertile scale; S. China. **'Spiralis'** ▣ syn. 'Yore-sugi', is a dense shrub or small tree, producing spirally curved and twisted, inward-pointing leaves; ↕ to 6m (20ft). **'Yore-sugi'** see 'Spiralis'.

▷ ***Cryptostemma calendulaceum*** see *Arctotheca calendula*

CTENANTHE

MARANTACEAE

Genus of about 15 species of rosette-forming, evergreen, rhizomatous perennials from damp forest floors and thickets in Costa Rica and Brazil. They are grown for their ovate to obovate, lance-shaped, or inversely lance-shaped, yellowish to dark green leaves, marked dark or light green, silver, or yellow. The basal leaves have longer stalks than the stem leaves. Irregularly shaped, tubular, white or yellow flowers are borne in short, terminal racemes or spikes. In frost-prone areas, grow in a warm greenhouse or as houseplants. In tropical and subtropical areas, they are suitable for growing in a shaded bed or border.

• **HARDINESS** Frost tender.

• **CULTIVATION** Under glass, grow in loamless or loam-based potting compost (JI No.2) in bright filtered or bright indirect light, with high humidity. Maintain constant temperatures and draught-free conditions. In growth, mist with soft water, water freely, and apply a balanced liquid fertilizer every 3 or 4 weeks. Water moderately in winter. Repot annually in late spring or early

C

C

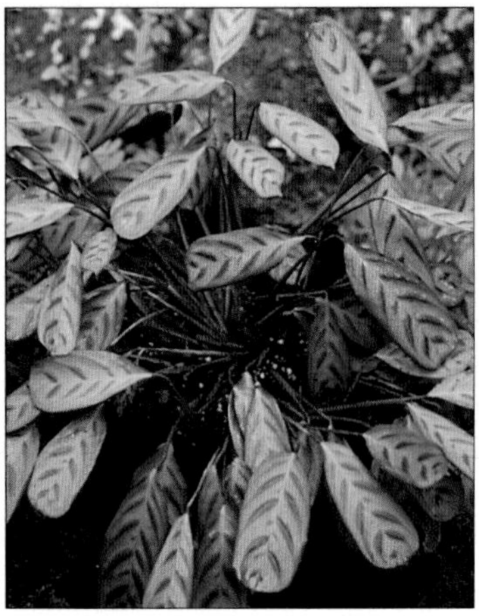

Ctenanthe burle-marxii

summer. Outdoors, grow in moist, fertile, humus-rich soil in partial shade.
• **PROPAGATION** Sow seed at 19–24°C (66–75°F) as soon as ripe or in spring. Divide in spring.
• **PESTS AND DISEASES** Mealybugs may be a problem under glass.

C. burle-marxii ■ Evergreen perennial with softly hairy, purple-tinged green stems. Ovate to obovate-oblong, hairless leaves, pale green above and deep purple beneath, have sickle-shaped, dark green markings, prominent main veins, and leaf bases of unequal size. The stem leaves, 14cm (5½in) long, are much larger than the basal leaves. White flowers are borne in inconspicuous spikes intermittently throughout the year. ↕ to 60cm (24in), ↔ 35cm (14in). Brazil. ❀ (min. 13°C/55°F)
C. compressa. Evergreen perennial with wiry stems and slender-pointed, linear-oblong to oblong-ovate, waxy leaves, 35cm (14in) long, mid-green above and greyish green beneath. Spikes of yellowish green flowers are produced irregularly throughout the year. ↕ 60cm (24in), ↔ 35cm (14in). S.E. Brazil. ❀ (min. 13°C/55°F)
C. lubbersiana ♀ Evergreen perennial with widely branched stems and linear to linear-oblong leaves, 30cm (12in) long, deep green with irregular yellow streaks above, pale green beneath. Spikes of white flowers are borne intermittently throughout the year. ↕ 2m (6ft), ↔ 1m (3ft). Brazil. ❀ (min. 13°C/55°F)
C. oppenheimiana, syn. *Calathea oppenheimiana.* Vigorous, bushy, evergreen perennial with lance-shaped, leathery leaves, 40cm (16in) long, dark green with V-shaped silver patterns above and wine-red beneath. Spikes of white flowers appear irregularly throughout the year. ↕ 1m (3ft), ↔ 60cm (24in). E. Brazil. ❀ (min. 13°C/55°F).
'Tricolor' ■ ♀ (Never-never plant) has foliage with irregular, creamy white and pale and dark green markings.
C. setosa. Vigorous, evergreen perennial with inversely lance-shaped, mid-green leaves, 12–18cm (5–7in) long, with the tips bent over, sometimes margined or sparsely striped white. Inconspicuous, pale yellow flowers are borne in spikes at any time of year. ↕ 1.5m (5ft), ↔ 1m (3ft). S.E. Brazil. ❀ (min. 13°C/55°F)

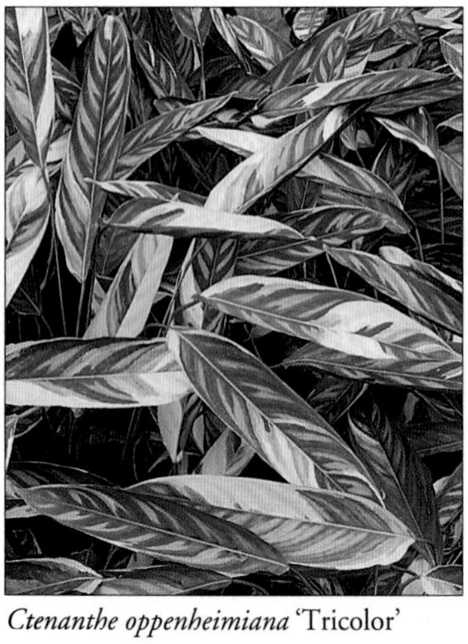

Ctenanthe oppenheimiana 'Tricolor'

▷ **Cuckoo flower** see *Cardamine pratensis*
▷ **Cucumber,**
Serpent see *Trichosanthes cucumerina* var. *anguina*
Squirting see *Ecballium*
▷ **Cucumber tree** see *Magnolia acuminata*
▷ ***Cudrania*** see *Maclura*
C. tricuspidata see *M. tricuspidata*
▷ **Culver's root** see *Veronicastrum virginicum*
▷ **Cumin** see *Cuminum, C. cyminum*

CUMINUM

Cumin

APIACEAE/UMBELLIFERAE

Genus of 2 species of slender annuals found in open maquis and garigue, and on cultivated ground, from the eastern Mediterranean to C. Asia. The 2-ternate leaves consist of thread-like segments. Compound umbels, with few rays bearing small, irregularly shaped, white to pale pink flowers, are followed by oblong-ovoid, ridged, finely hairy fruits. *C. cyminum* is grown for its aromatic fruit, which are used in cooking. Grow in a herb or vegetable garden.
• **HARDINESS** Half hardy.
• **CULTIVATION** Grow in fertile, well-drained soil in full sun. Need 3–4 warm months in summer for good seed production; harvest seed in late summer.
• **PROPAGATION** In frost-free areas, sow seed *in situ* in early spring. In cool-temperate areas, sow seed at 13–18°C (55–64°F) in late winter or early spring, and plant out in late spring.
• **PESTS AND DISEASES** Trouble free.

C. cyminum (Cumin). Slender, spreading annual with ovate, 2-ternate, blue-green leaves, to 10cm (4in) long, with narrowly linear segments. In mid-summer, produces white to pale pink flowers in umbels to 2.5cm (1in) across, followed by ovoid-oblong, ribbed, grey-green fruit, 5mm (¼in) long, containing pale brown seeds. ↕↔ 30cm (12in). E. Mediterranean. ✲

CUNNINGHAMIA

China fir

TAXODIACEAE

Genus of 2 or 3 species of evergreen, monoecious, coniferous trees from forests of China and Taiwan. They have thick, fibrous, red-brown bark and stiff, sharply pointed, narrowly lance-shaped, mid- to dark green leaves, densely arranged in 2 ranks in the same plane. Solitary female cones are brown and spherical to ovoid-conical; spherical, yellow-brown male cones are borne in clusters. They are closely related to the redwoods (*Sequoia*), although the foliage is similar to that of the monkey puzzle tree (*Araucaria araucana*). Grow as a specimen tree.
• **HARDINESS** Fully hardy.
• **CULTIVATION** Grow in any moist but well-drained soil, including deep soils over chalk, in full sun or dappled shade. Shelter from cool, drying winds. Best in a moist climate, otherwise old foliage may turn brown and persist. Tolerates coppicing. Young plants may be slow to form a leader; if so, grow as a multi-stemmed specimen, or cut back in spring and train in the strongest resulting shoot as the new leader.
• **PROPAGATION** Sow seed in containers in a cold frame in spring. Root ripe-wood cuttings in summer.
• **PESTS AND DISEASES** Trouble free.

C. lanceolata ■ ◊–◊ syn. *C. lanceolata* var. *sinensis* (China fir). Narrowly to broadly upright or conical, coniferous tree, developing a rounded, domed top. Lance-shaped, glossy, bright green leaves, to 7cm (3in) long, each with a raised midrib and 2 white bands beneath, are decurrent on the green shoots. Ovoid-conical, green-brown female cones are 3–4cm (1¼–1½in) long. ↕ to 20m (70ft) or more, ↔ to 6m (20ft). China. ✲✲✲. **var. *sinensis*** see *C. lanceolata.*

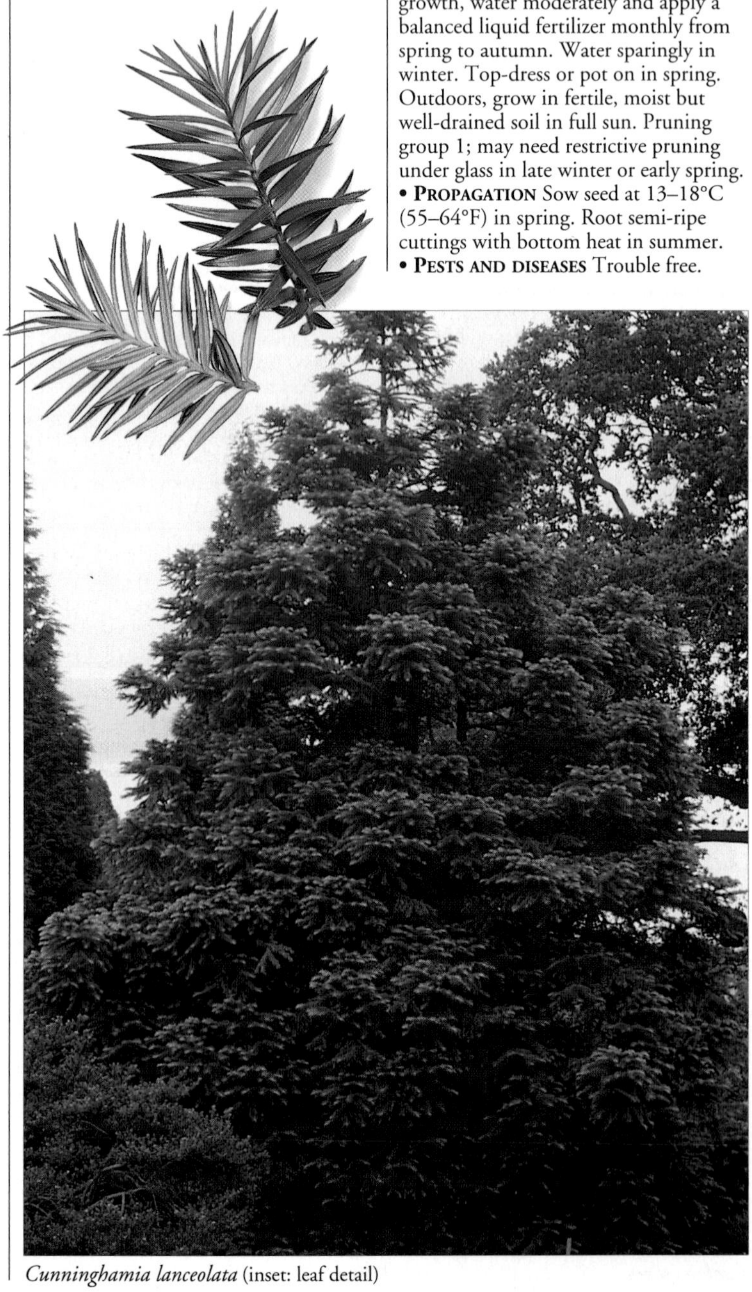

Cunninghamia lanceolata (inset: leaf detail)

CUNONIA

CUNONIACEAE

Genus of 15 species of evergreen trees occurring in damp sites in South Africa and New Caledonia. The pinnate or 3-palmate, thick, leathery, mid- to dark green leaves are borne in opposite pairs. Star-shaped, 5-petalled flowers are produced in dense, axillary racemes. In frost-prone climates, grow *C. capensis* as a foliage plant in a temperate greenhouse or conservatory; in warmer areas, it is an effective specimen or shade tree.
• **HARDINESS** Half hardy to frost tender; *C. capensis* may survive short periods near 0°C (32°F).
• **CULTIVATION** Under glass, grow in loam-based potting compost (JI No.2) in full light, with shade from hot sun. In growth, water moderately and apply a balanced liquid fertilizer monthly from spring to autumn. Water sparingly in winter. Top-dress or pot on in spring. Outdoors, grow in fertile, moist but well-drained soil in full sun. Pruning group 1; may need restrictive pruning under glass in late winter or early spring.
• **PROPAGATION** Sow seed at 13–18°C (55–64°F) in spring. Root semi-ripe cuttings with bottom heat in summer.
• **PESTS AND DISEASES** Trouble free.

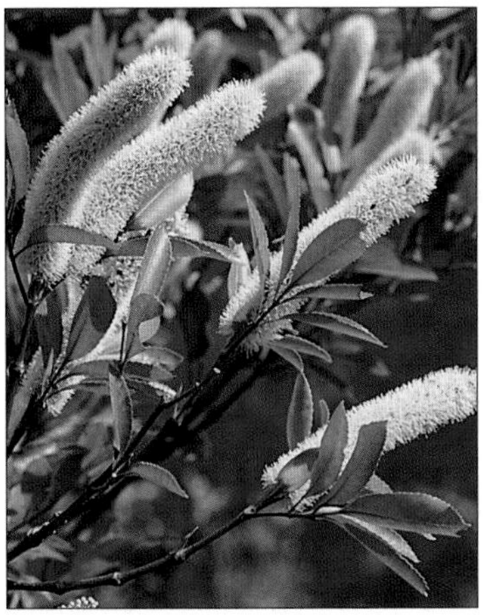

Cunonia capensis

C. capensis ▣ ♀ (African red alder). Freely branched tree with pinnate, rich green leaves, 20–40cm (8–16in) long, with 5–9 lance-shaped to oblong, toothed leaflets, to 10cm (4in) long. Bears fragrant, cream to white flowers in opposite, paired racemes, to 15cm (6in) long, in late summer. ↕ 10–18m (30–60ft), ↔ 3–6m (10–20ft). South Africa. ❀ (min. 7°C/45°F)

▷ **Cup and saucer** see *Campanula medium* 'Calycanthema'
▷ **Cup and saucer plant** see *Cobaea scandens*
▷ **Cup flower** see *Nierembergia*

CUPHEA

LYTHRACEAE

Genus of more than 250 species of annuals, short-lived, sometimes subshrubby, evergreen perennials, and evergreen shrubs, from woodland clearings and pasture in S.E. USA, Mexico, and subtropical and tropical Central and South America. Many species have sticky, glandular hairs. Mainly opposite, ovate to lance-shaped, entire or slightly toothed leaves are mid- to dark green. Irregularly shaped, tubular flowers are borne singly or in often leafy racemes or panicles. In frost-prone areas, grow as houseplants or in a temperate greenhouse or conservatory, or use as annuals and grow in a summer bedding or annual border. In warmer climates, grow in a shrub border or bed.

• **HARDINESS** Half hardy to frost tender.

• **CULTIVATION** Under glass, grow in loam-based potting compost (JI No.2) in full light with shade from hot sun and in moderate humidity. In the growing season, water freely and apply a balanced liquid fertilizer every 3 or 4 weeks; water sparingly in winter. Outdoors, grow in moderately fertile, well-drained soil in full sun or partial shade. Pruning group 10, in spring.

• **PROPAGATION** Sow seed at 13–16°C (55–61°F) in early spring, or *in situ* in late spring. Divide, or root softwood cuttings of perennials with bottom heat, in late spring.

• **PESTS AND DISEASES** Susceptible to aphids and whiteflies.

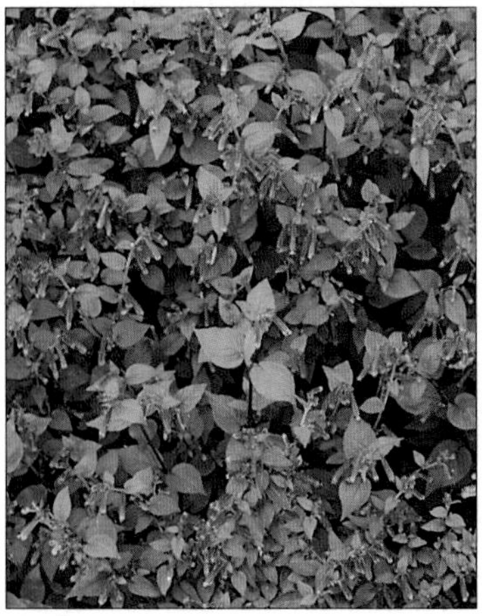

Cuphea cyanea

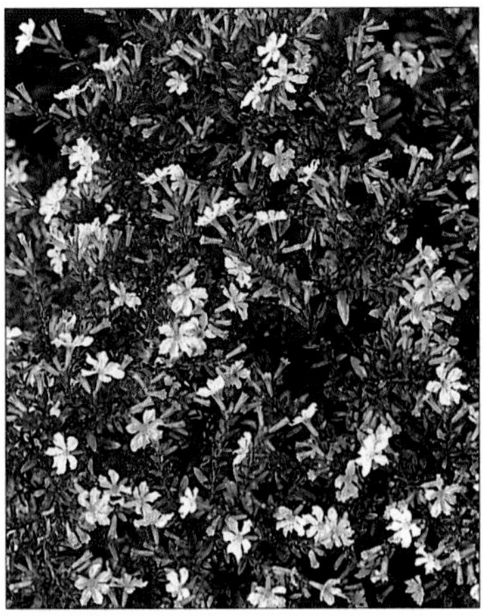

Cuphea hyssopifolia

C. cyanea ▣ Freely branching, soft-stemmed shrub or subshrub with sticky, glandular-hairy shoots and long-stalked, ovate, mid- to deep green leaves, 5–8cm (2–3in) long. From late spring to autumn, produces terminal racemes of green-tipped, orange-red flowers, 2–3cm (¾–1¼in) long, each with 2 small, deep violet-blue petals. ↕↔ to 1m (3ft) or more. Mexico. ❀ (min. 7°C/45°F)

C. hyssopifolia ▣ ♀ (False heather). Bushy, rounded shrub with slender, downy stems and densely borne, narrowly lance-shaped, dark green leaves, 0.6–2.5cm (¼–1in) long. Produces short racemes of 1–3 light pink-purple, pink, or white flowers, to 1cm (½in) long, with 6 spreading petals, from the upper leaf axils, mainly from summer to autumn. ↕ 30–60cm (12–24in), ↔ 20–80cm (8–32in). Mexico, Guatemala. ❀ (min. 7°C/45°F)

C. ignea ▣ ♀ syn. *C. platycentra* (Cigar flower). Spreading, freely branching, soft-stemmed shrub or subshrub, often grown as an annual, with lance-shaped to narrowly oblong, glossy, bright green leaves, 3–8cm (1¼–3in) long. From late spring to autumn, slender, deep red flowers, 2–3cm (¾–1¼in) long, each with a dark red band, a white rim, and 2 tiny black-purple petals, are borne singly from the upper leaf axils. ↕ 30–75cm (12–30in), ↔ 30–90cm (12–36in). Mexico to Jamaica. ❀ (min. 7°C/45°F). **'Variegata'** has mid-green leaves flecked cream and lime-green.

C. lanceolata. Bushy, purple-stemmed subshrub with glandular-hairy, sticky stems and foliage. Lance-shaped to oval, pointed leaves are mid-green and white-hairy, to 8cm (3in) long. Solitary, 6-petalled, deep violet flowers, to 4cm (1½in) long, constricted at the necks, then flaring into unequally sized upper and lower lips, are borne from the upper leaf axils from summer to autumn. ↕ to 65cm (26in), ↔ to 45cm (18in) (in containers). C. Mexico. ✻

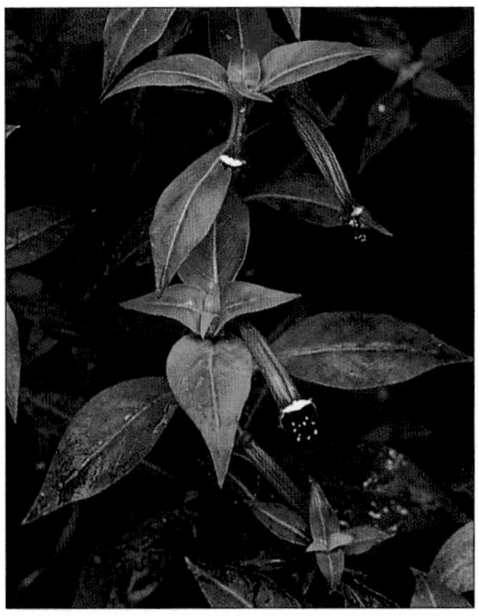

Cuphea ignea

C. llavea* var. *miniata. Bushy subshrub with bristly stems and ovate to lance-shaped, mid-green leaves, to 8cm (3in) long. In early summer, bears terminal racemes of 2-petalled, vermilion flowers, 3.5cm (1½in) long, flared at the mouths and with greenish purple calyces. ↕ 45cm (18in), ↔ 15cm (6in). Mexico. ✻

***C. llavea* var. *miniata* of gardens** see *C.* x *purpurea.*

***C. llavea* of gardens** see *C.* x *purpurea.*

***C. miniata* of gardens** see *C.* x *purpurea.*

C. platycentra see *C. ignea.*

C.* x *purpurea (*C. llavea* x *C. procumbens*), syn. *C. llavea* var. *miniata* of gardens, *C. llavea* of gardens, *C. miniata* of gardens. Bushy subshrub, often grown as an annual, with sticky, glandular-hairy stems and foliage. Red stems bear ovate to lance-shaped, pointed, dark green leaves, to 8cm (3in) long. From spring to autumn, produces terminal racemes of 2-petalled, pink to red flowers, to 3cm (1¼in) long, which flare at the mouths. ↕ 30–60cm (12–24in), ↔ 23–45cm (9–18in). Garden origin. ✻. **'Avalon'** has purple flowers. **'Firefly'** has cherry-red flowers.

▷ **Cupidone, Blue** see *Catananche*
▷ **Cupid's bower** see *Achimenes*
▷ **Cupid's dart** see *Catananche*
▷ **Cup of gold** see *Solandra maxima*
▷ **Cup plant** see *Silphium perfoliatum*

x CUPRESSOCYPARIS

CUPRESSACEAE

Hybrid genus, between *Chamaecyparis* and *Cupressus*, of fast-growing, columnar, evergreen, coniferous trees. They produce flattened sprays of scale-like, dark green leaves, to 3mm (⅛in) long. Female cones are spherical; male cones are ovoid, yellow, and 2–3mm (1/16–⅛in) long. Grow as specimen trees or use for hedging. Contact with the foliage may aggravate skin allergies.

• **HARDINESS** Fully hardy.

• **CULTIVATION** Grow in any deep, well-drained soil in full sun or partial shade. Needs no formal pruning. Trim hedging 2 or 3 times in the growing season (without cutting back into the old wood), with the last cut in late summer or early autumn.

• **PROPAGATION** Root semi-ripe cuttings in late summer.

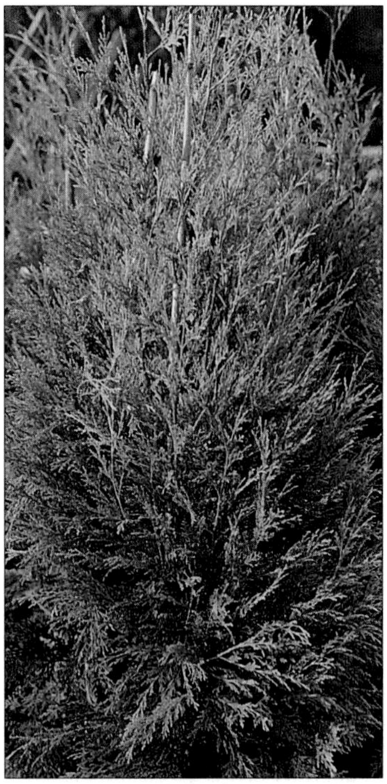

x *Cupressocyparis leylandii* 'Castlewellan'

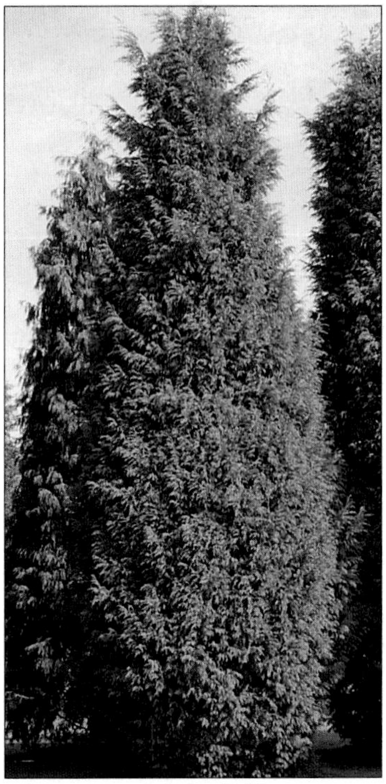

x *Cupressocyparis leylandii* 'Haggerston Grey'

• **PESTS AND DISEASES** May be affected by honey fungus. *Coryneum* canker may cause the death of twigs and ultimately entire trees. Aphids may cause dieback.

x *C. leylandii* ◊ syn. *Cupressus leylandii* (Leyland cypress). Tapering, coniferous tree with smooth bark, becoming stringy with age, and flat sprays of pointed, dark green, grey-tinged leaves. Dark brown female cones, 1.5–2cm (½–¾in) across, each have 8 scales. ↕ to 35m (120ft), ↔ to 5m (15ft). Garden origin. ✻✻✻. **'Castlewellan'** ▣ syn. 'Galway Gold', produces plume-like sprays of yellow foliage; ↕ 25m (80ft). **'Galway Gold'** see 'Castlewellan'. **'Haggerston Grey'** ▣ ♀ is the most popular cultivar, and has

C

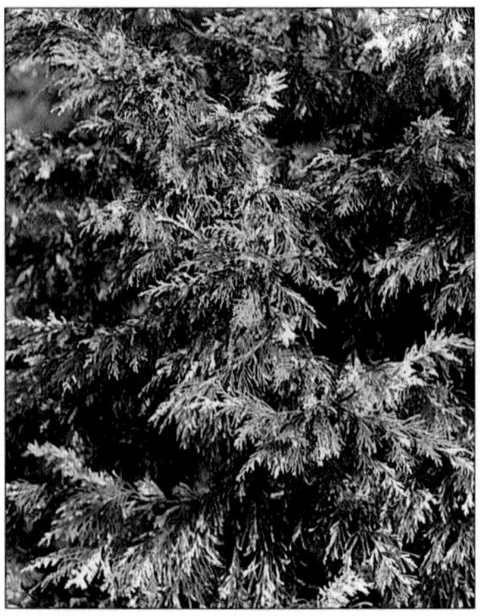

x *Cupressocyparis leylandii* 'Harlequin'

grey-green foliage. **'Harlequin'** ■ syn. 'Variegata', a sport of 'Haggerston Grey', has patches of ivory-white foliage. **'Leighton Green'** is narrow, with fresh green foliage. **'Naylor's Blue'** has blue-grey foliage, which is especially attractive after rain. **'Robinson's Gold'** ♀ has bronze-yellow foliage in spring, maturing to golden yellow and lime-green. **'Variegata'** see 'Harlequin'.
x *C. notabilis* ♀ ◊ Narrowly conical, coniferous tree with upswept branches, red-brown bark, and acute, blue-grey leaves, borne in sparse sprays. Purple female cones, 1.5cm (½in) across, each have 4–8 scales. ↕ to 15m (50ft), ↔ to 6m (20ft). Garden origin. ❄❄❄

CUPRESSUS

Cypress

CUPRESSACEAE

Genus of about 24 species of evergreen, monoecious, coniferous trees from the N. hemisphere, found in dry, open hillside forest. The paired, overlapping, forward-pointing, scale-like leaves vary from rounded to pointed at the tips. The mature bark often breaks off into curling or rounded scales. Small, spherical to ovoid female cones, to 4cm (1½in) long, ripen in the second year but usually persist on the tree, and have 5–20 seeds per scale. Ovoid green male cones, 2–3mm (1/16–1/8in) long, are borne at the shoot tips. Cypresses tolerate dry conditions and are excellent specimen trees. *C. macrocarpa* may be used as a hedge or screen. In frost-prone areas, grow *C. torulosa* 'Cashmeriana' in a cool greenhouse or conservatory.

- **HARDINESS** Fully hardy to half hardy.
- **CULTIVATION** Under glass, grow in loam-based potting compost (JI No.3) in full light, with good ventilation. Outdoors, grow in any well-drained soil (including alkaline and acid soils) in full sun. Shelter from cold, drying winds. Trim hedges in late spring, without cutting back into the old wood.
- **PROPAGATION** Sow seed in a seedbed, or in containers in a cold frame, in spring. Root semi-ripe cuttings in late summer.
- **PESTS AND DISEASES** May be affected by honey fungus. *Coryneum* canker may cause the death of twigs and ultimately entire trees. Aphids may cause dieback.

C. abramsiana ◊ Vigorous, conical, coniferous tree with deeply furrowed, dark grey bark and sparse sprays of

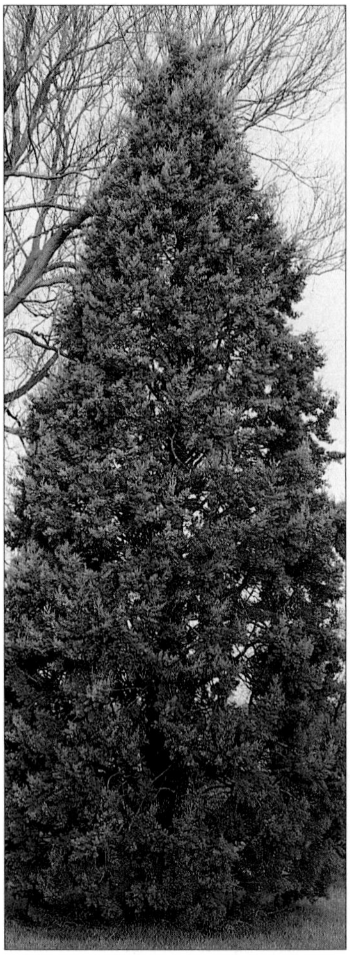

Cupressus arizonica var. *glabra*

pointed, bright green, glandless leaves, 2mm (1/16in) long. Spherical, shiny brown to grey-buff female cones, to 3.5cm (1½in) across, each have 6 scales. ↕ to 20m (70ft), ↔ to 6m (20ft). USA (California). ❄❄❄
C. arizonica* var. *glabra ■ ◊ syn. *C. glabra* (Smooth cypress). Conical, coniferous tree with smooth, reddish purple bark. Pointed, glaucous, blue-grey leaves, 2mm (1/16in) long, are arranged in dense sprays. Dorsal resin glands form white flecks on the foliage. Spherical, prickly brown female cones, 2.5cm (1in) across, each have 6 or 8 scales. ↕ 10–15m (30–50ft), ↔ 4–5m (12–15ft). S.W. USA. ❄❄❄
C. bakeri ◊ (Baker cypress). Conical, coniferous tree with reddish grey or grey bark, splitting into thin scales. Pointed, aromatic, grey-green leaves, 2mm (1/16in) long, with prominent, dorsal resin glands, are borne in sparse sprays. Spherical, greyish brown female cones, 1.5cm (½in) across, each have 6–8 scales and prominent curved prickles. ↕ to 15m (50ft), ↔ to 5m (15ft). USA (Oregon, N. California). ❄❄❄
C. cashmeriana see *C. torulosa* 'Cashmeriana'.
C. glabra see *C. arizonica* var. *glabra*.
C. goveniana* var. *pygmaea ◊–◊ Shrubby, narrowly conical to columnar, coniferous tree with exfoliating, rough, grey or brown bark. Pointed, dark green, glandless leaves, 2mm (1/16in) long, which are lemon-scented when crushed, are borne in plume-like sprays. Spherical, prickly brown female cones, less than 2cm (¾in) across, usually have 6 scales each. ↕ to 10m (30ft), ↔ to 4m (12ft). USA (Mendocino County, California). ❄❄❄
C. guadalupensis ◊–◊ (Guadalupe cypress). Narrowly conical then ovoid, coniferous tree with red-brown bark that cracks into small flakes. Slender, blunt or pointed, blue-green leaves, 3mm (1/8in) long, borne in slender sprays, have resin glands that are fragrant when crushed. Spherical brown female cones, 3–4cm (1¼–1½in) across, each have 8–10 scales and a prominent dorsal prickle. ↕ to 15m (50ft), ↔ to 3–4m (10–12ft). USA (S. California). ❄❄. **'Glauca'** has glaucous, grey-green leaves.
C. lawsoniana see *Chamaecyparis lawsoniana*.
C. leylandii see x *Cupressocyparis leylandii*.
C. lindleyi see *C. lusitanica*.
C. lusitanica ◊–◊ syn. *C. lindleyi* (Cedar of Goa, Mexican cypress). Conical to columnar, coniferous tree with brown bark, shallowly fissured into fibrous spirals. Bears scarcely scented, glandless, grey-green or blue-green leaves, 2–3mm (1/16–1/8in) long, with free, pointed tips, in spreading sprays. Spherical, glaucous blue then shiny brown female cones, 1.5cm (½in) across, each have 6–8 scales and conical prickles. ↕ to 20m (70ft), ↔ to 6m (20ft). Mexico to Guatemala. ❄❄❄. **'Glauca Pendula'** has pendent sprays of bright blue-green foliage.
C. macrocarpa ◊–◊ (Monterey cypress). Coniferous tree, narrowly conical to columnar and spiky-topped when young, becoming very wide-spreading with age, with shallowly ridged bark. Pointed, dark to bright green, glandless, lemon-scented leaves, 2mm (1/16in) long, are borne in erect or spreading, plume-like sprays. Spherical brown female cones, 2.5–3cm (1–1¼in) across, each have 8–10 scales that lack a prominent prickle. ↕ to 30m (100ft), ↔ 4–12m (12–40ft). USA (Monterey County, California). ❄❄❄. **'Goldcrest'** ■ ♀ ◊–◊ is narrowly conical, with dense, rich golden yellow foliage; ↕ to 5m (16ft), ↔ 2.5m (8ft).

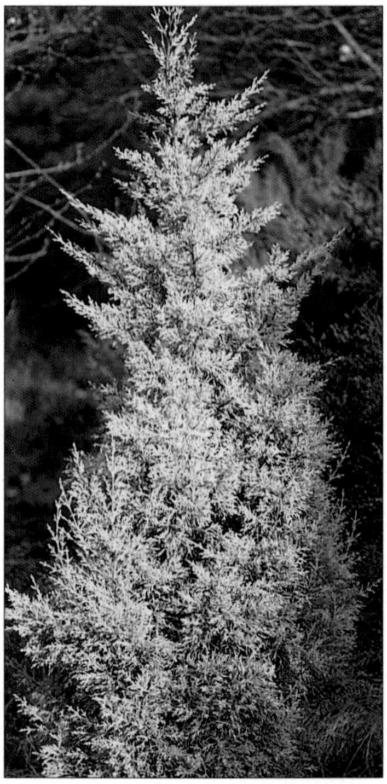

Cupressus macrocarpa 'Goldcrest'

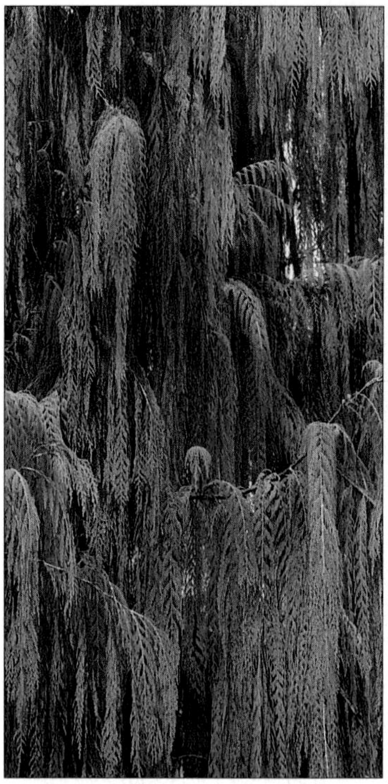

Cupressus torulosa 'Cashmeriana'

C. nootkatensis see *Chamaecyparis nootkatensis*.
C. obtusa see *Chamaecyparis obtusa*.
C. pisifera see *Chamaecyparis pisifera*.
C. sempervirens ◊–◊ (Italian cypress, Mediterranean cypress). Narrowly conical or columnar to broadly spreading, coniferous tree. Horizontal branches bear dense sprays of grey-green or dark green, glandless leaves, to 1mm (1/16in) long, usually with rounded, abruptly pointed tips (but with free, pointed tips on strong shoots). Spherical to ovoid, prickly brown female cones, 2.5–3.5cm (1–1½in) long, each have 8–14 scales. ↕ to 20m (70ft), ↔ 1–6m (3–20ft). E. Mediterranean to Iran. ❄❄❄. **'Stricta'** ♀ ◊ is narrowly upright, sometimes forming a very narrow, almost pencil-like tree, with fused and flattened branches; ↔ to 3m (10ft). **'Swane's Gold'** ♀ ◊ is narrowly upright, with pale yellow or greenish yellow leaves; ↕ to 6m (20ft), ↔ 1m (3ft).
C. thyoides see *Chamaecyparis thyoides*.
***C. torulosa* 'Cashmeriana'** ■ ♀ ◊–◊ syn. *C. cashmeriana* (Kashmir cypress). Coniferous tree, conical when young, becoming broad and columnar when mature, with fibrous, red-brown bark. Bright, glaucous blue, glandless leaves, 2–3mm (1/16–1/8in) long, with free, pointed tips, to 2mm (1/16in) long, are borne in long, flat, pendent sprays. Spherical, prickly, green-brown female cones, 1.5cm (½in) across, each have 8–10 scales. ↕ to 30m (100ft), ↔ to 10m (30ft). Probably Himalayas. ❄

CURCUMA

ZINGIBERACEAE

Genus of 40 species of reed-like, rhizomatous perennials, which often have fleshy roots and thick, aromatic rhizomes. They are found in seasonally drought-prone areas of tropical Asia and Australia. The leaves are narrowly ovate to oblong. Cone-like, terminal inflorescences are formed from often colourful bracts. Very small, 3-petalled,

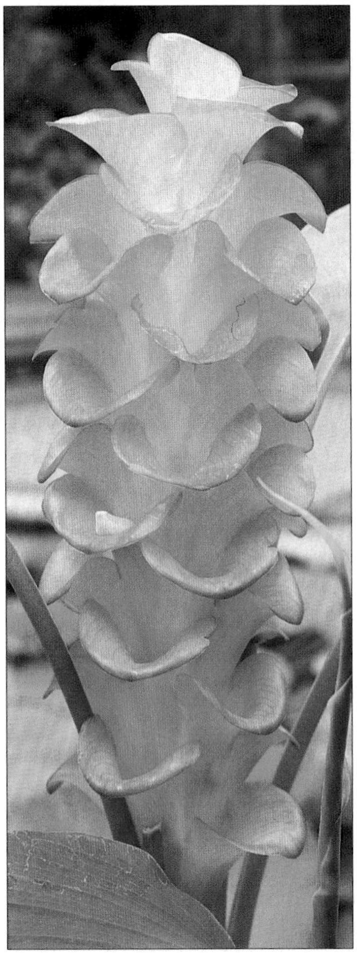

Curcuma roscoeana

tubular flowers are often obscured by the bracts. Where temperatures fall below 18°C (64°F), grow in a warm greenhouse; in tropical areas, use as ground cover. The rhizomes of some species are used as spices and in cooking.
• **HARDINESS** Frost tender.
• **CULTIVATION** Under glass, grow in loam-based potting compost (JI No.2) in bright filtered light, with moderate humidity. In growth, water freely and apply a balanced liquid fertilizer monthly. In winter dormancy, keep almost dry at 12°C (54°F). Pot on in spring. Outdoors, grow in fertile, moist but well-drained soil in partial shade.
• **PROPAGATION** Sow seed at 20°C (68°F) as soon as ripe. Divide in spring.
• **PESTS AND DISEASES** Trouble free.

C. petiolata (Queen lily). Upright perennial with a brown or brownish yellow rhizome, pale yellow inside, and up to 6 oblong leaves, 25cm (10in) long, with leaf-stalks of almost equal length. Yellow and white flowers, 1cm (½in) long, are borne at any time of year in terminal spikes, 15cm (6in) long, with deep violet upper bracts and green, occasionally violet lower bracts. ↕60cm (24in), ↔45cm (18in). Malaysia. ❀ (min. 18°C/64°F)
C. roscoeana ▣ Erect perennial with a brown rhizome, white inside, and ovate, shiny, mid-green leaves, 15–30cm (6–12in) long, with deep green veins. In summer, bears bright yellow flowers, 1cm (½in) long, with orange bracts, in terminal spikes, 20cm (8in) long. ↕to 90cm (36in), ↔45cm (18in). Malaysia. ❀ (min. 18°C/64°F)

▷**Currant,**
Buffalo see *Ribes odoratum*
Flowering see *Ribes, R. sanguineum*
Fuchsia-flowered see *Ribes speciosum*
Indian see *Symphoricarpos orbiculatus*
▷**Curry plant** see *Helichrysum italicum* subsp. *serotinum*
▷***Curtonus*** see *Crocosmia*
C. paniculatus see *C. paniculata*
▷**Cushion bush** see *Leucophyta*

CYANANTHUS

CAMPANULACEAE

Genus of about 25 species of tufted, perennials occurring in cool, moist, mountainous areas in the Himalayas and W. China. They have prostrate stems radiating from a cluster of stout, almost woody roots, and alternate, linear to broadly rounded leaves, which are toothed, lobed, or entire, and often hairy. Terminal, usually solitary, broadly funnel-shaped, blue, violet, or yellow, occasionally white flowers each have 5 spreading lobes and short tubes. Grow in a rock garden, scree bed, peat bed, or trough, or in an alpine house.
• **HARDINESS** Fully hardy.
• **CULTIVATION** Grow in poor to moderately fertile, humus-rich, moist but well-drained, preferably neutral to slightly acid soil in partial shade. In an alpine house, grow in loam-based potting compost (JI No.1) with added grit and leaf mould; keep plants cool and shaded in summer.
• **PROPAGATION** Sow seed in containers in an open frame as soon as ripe or in early spring. Root softwood cuttings in late spring or early summer.
• **PESTS AND DISEASES** Susceptible to red spider mites and aphids under glass.

***C. integer* of gardens** see *C. microphyllus.*
C. lobatus ▣ ♀ Spreading perennial with obovate, deeply lobed, fleshy, dull green leaves, 1cm (½in) long, with wedge-shaped bases. In late summer, produces solitary, bright blue-purple flowers, 2–4cm (¾–1½in) across, with spreading lobes and dark brown, shaggy-hairy calyces. ↕5cm (2in), ↔ to 30cm (12in). Himalayas to China (Yunnan). ❄❄❄
C. microphyllus ♀ syn. *C. integer* of gardens. Mat-forming perennial with slender red stems, clothed in ovate to oblong-elliptic, dark green leaves, 2–8mm (1/16–3/8in) long, with the margins rolled under. In late summer, bears solitary, violet-blue flowers, 2.5cm (1in) across, with tufts of white hair at the throats. ↕to 2.5cm (1in), ↔ to 25cm (10in). Nepal to S.W. Tibet. ❄❄❄

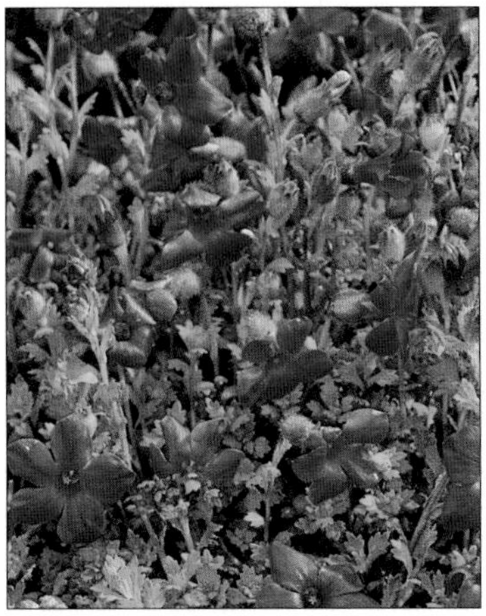

Cyananthus lobatus

CYANOTIS

COMMELINACEAE

Genus of about 30 species of low-growing, evergreen perennials, related to *Tradescantia*, but more succulent and with greater tolerance of dry conditions. They occur in upland forest and rocky areas in Africa and Asia. The trailing stems, to 30cm (12in) long, are almost hidden by hairy, densely 2-ranked, lance-shaped to broadly ovate or oblong leaves. One-sided cymes of short-lived, shallowly cup-shaped, 3-petalled, purple, violet, or blue flowers are borne in summer. In frost-prone areas, grow in a temperate greenhouse or conservatory, in hanging baskets, or as houseplants. In warmer climates, grow in a herbaceous bed or border.
• **HARDINESS** Frost tender.
• **CULTIVATION** Under glass, grow in loam-based potting compost (JI No.2) in full light, with shade from hot sun, and with low humidity. Water moderately at all times. During active growth, apply a balanced liquid fertilizer monthly; excessive feeding causes soft, untypical growth. Outdoors, grow in sharply drained, moderately fertile soil in full sun, with some midday shade.
• **PROPAGATION** Root stem-tip cuttings with bottom heat in spring.
• **PESTS AND DISEASES** Trouble free.

C. kewensis ♀ (Teddy bear plant). Spreading perennial with lance-shaped, fleshy leaves, to 5cm (2in) long, dark green above and red beneath, densely covered with short, felted, ginger-brown hairs. Cymes of up to 8 pink-purple flowers, 8mm (3/8in) across, are borne in summer. ↕12cm (5in), ↔30cm (12in). S. India. ❀ (min. 10°C/50°F)
C. somaliensis ▣ ♀ (Pussy ears). Spreading perennial with oblong-linear, pointed, arching, leathery, deep olive-green leaves, 4cm (1½in) long, slightly purple-flushed and with whisker-like white hairs. Bears cymes of mauve-blue flowers, 5mm (¼in) across, with prominent golden stamens, in summer; these are only occasionally produced in cultivation. ↕15cm (6in), ↔40cm (16in). Somalia. ❀ (min. 10°C/50°F)

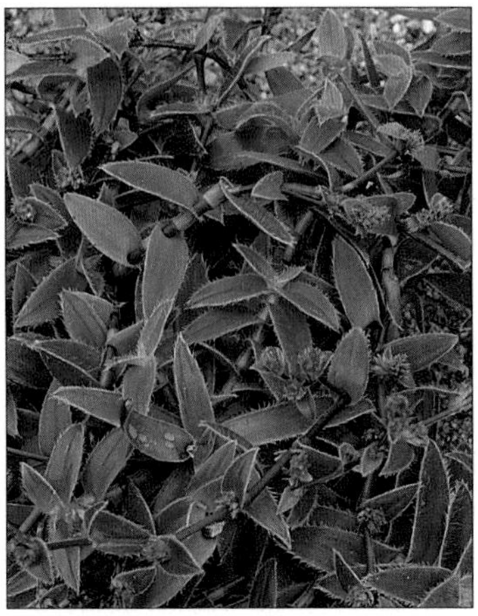

Cyanotis somaliensis

CYATHEA *syn.* ALSOPHILA

Tree fern

CYATHEACEAE

Genus of 600 or more species of evergreen tree ferns, mainly from forested mountain ranges in tropical and subtropical regions of the S. hemisphere. Cyatheas may reach over 20m (70ft) tall, some relatively quickly. They have a pole-like, fibrous trunk, consisting of an erect rhizome clad in roots, topped by large, pinnate, 2-pinnate, or pinnatifid fronds, which develop in flushes; the crowns of uncurling fronds are densely covered by white, brown, or black scales. The stems bear characteristic scars of old fronds. Grow as specimen plants in a shady site. In frost-prone areas, grow in a cool, temperate, or warm greenhouse.
• **HARDINESS** Half hardy to frost tender.
• **CULTIVATION** Under glass, grow in large containers in a mix of 1 part each of loam, sharp sand, and charcoal, and 3 parts coarse leaf mould or peat. Provide bright filtered light and moderate to high humidity. In growth, water freely, applying a balanced liquid fertilizer monthly; water sparingly in winter. Outdoors, grow in fertile, moist but well-drained soil in dappled or partial shade, or full sun in moist soil. Outdoors and under glass, damp down trunk and leaves regularly on hot days.
• **PROPAGATION** Sow spores at 15–18°C (59–64°F) as soon as ripe.
• **PESTS AND DISEASES** *Rhizoctonia* on young plants may be a problem.

C. australis ♈ syn. *Alsophila australis.* Tree fern producing a stem covered with frond scars and, towards the base, dense wiry roots. Ovate, 2-pinnate, dark green fronds, to 4m (12ft) long, have lance-shaped or linear segments and shiny brown scales. ↕1–3m (3–10ft), ↔3–5m (10–15ft). E. Australia. ❄
***C. australis* of gardens** see *C. cooperi.*
C. cooperi ▣ ♈ syn. *Alsophila australis* of gardens, *C. australis* of gardens. Fast-

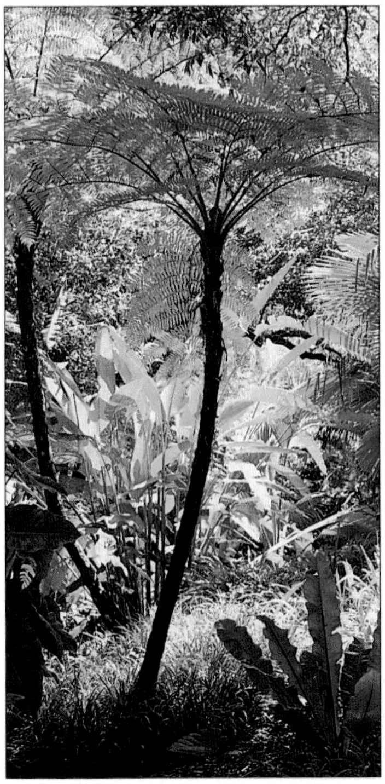

Cyathea cooperi

C

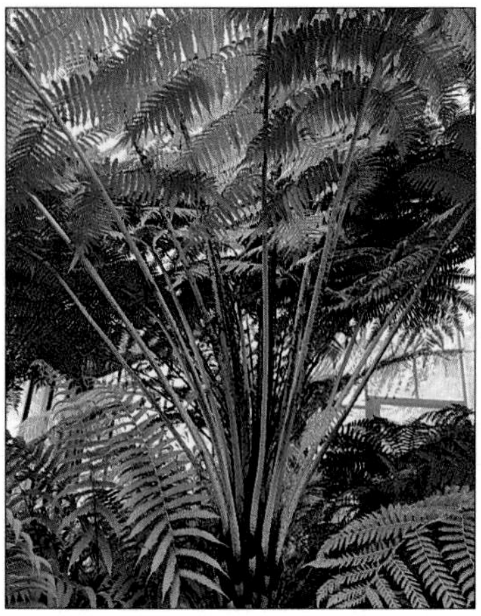
Cyathea dealbata

growing tree fern with a slender stem. Narrowly ovate, 2-pinnate, mid-green fronds, to 4m (12ft) long, have lance-shaped or linear segments. Scales on the frond stalks are white. ↕ 2–5m (6–15ft), ↔ 3–4m (10–12ft). Australia. ❀ (min. 10°C/50°F)

C. dealbata ▣ 🌴 Tree fern with an attractive glaucous bloom, both on the frond bases covering the stem and on the undersides of the fronds. Narrowly ovate, 2-pinnate, mid- to deep green fronds, to 3m (10ft) long, have oblong-lance-shaped segments. Scales are shining, dark brown. ↕ to 10m (30ft), ↔ 1–3m (3–10ft). New Zealand. ✻

C. howeana 🌴 Tree fern with a slender trunk and narrowly ovate, 2-pinnate, scaly-hairy, light green fronds, to 3m (10ft) long, with deeply toothed or pinnatifid segments. ↕ to 2m (6ft), ↔ 3–4m (10–12ft). Australia (Lord Howe Island). ❀ (min. 10°C/50°F)

C. medullaris ▣ 🌴 (Black tree fern, Sago fern). Wide-spreading tree fern with a black stem and a rosette of 2- or 3-pinnate fronds, 3–6m (10–20ft) long, deep green above and paler beneath, with narrowly oblong, finely tapering segments. Black stalks are scaly-hairy. ↕ 10–15m (30–50ft), ↔ 3–6m (10–20ft). Australia (Victoria to Tasmania), New Zealand. ✻

C. smithii 🌴 Upright tree fern with a stout, tapering stem and a rosette of oblong-lance-shaped, 2- or 3-pinnate fronds, 1–2m (3–6ft) long, with yellow-green stalks and toothed, narrowly oblong segments, bright mid-green above and pale green beneath. ↕ to 8m (25ft), ↔ to 4m (12ft). New Zealand. ✻

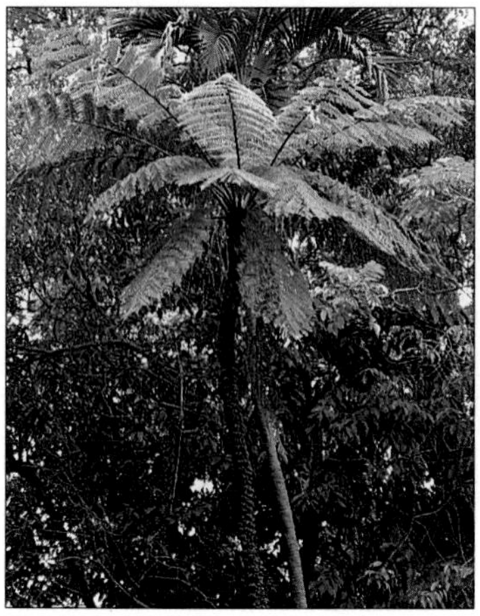
Cyathea medullaris

CYATHODES

EPACRIDACEAE

Genus of about 175 species of heath-like evergreen shrubs and small trees found in alpine and subalpine regions of Australia, Tasmania, and New Zealand, and in various habitats in Malaysia, New Guinea, and Polynesia. They have usually small, overlapping, linear, linear-oblong to lance-shaped, elliptic, or inversely lance-shaped leaves, the new growth often flushed pink or bronze. Small, tubular, unisexual or bisexual flowers are either solitary or borne in terminal racemes; they are followed by fleshy, colourful fruits, 8–10mm (3/8–1/2in) across, although fruiting is not always reliable in cultivation. Some species, including *C. colensoi*, are suitable for a rock garden, a peat terrace, or a shrub border. In frost-prone areas, grow half-hardy or frost-tender species in a cool or temperate greenhouse.

• **HARDINESS** Frost hardy to frost tender.

• **CULTIVATION** Grow in moist but well-drained, fertile, humus-rich, acid soil in partial shade, although they will tolerate full sun in cooler climates, where soil remains reliably moist in the growing season. Provide shelter from cold, drying winds. Pruning group 8.

• **PROPAGATION** Sow seed in containers in a cold frame in autumn; germination may take up to 3 years. Root greenwood cuttings in early summer, or semi-ripe cuttings in late summer.

• **PESTS AND DISEASES** Trouble free.

C. colensoi, syn. *Leucopogon colensoi*, *Styphelia colensoi*. Prostrate or decumbent shrub with stiff, upright shoots clothed in narrowly oblong, smooth, grey-green leaves, to 9mm (3/8in) long, fringed with fine hairs. White flowers, 6mm (1/4in) long, are borne in erect racemes at the tips of young growth in spring, occasionally followed by spherical, white to deep crimson fruit, 4–5mm (1/8–1/4in) across. ↕↔ 30cm (12in). New Zealand. ✻✻

C. fraseri see *Leucopogon fraseri*.

CYBISTAX

BIGNONIACEAE

Genus of 3 species of deciduous or semi-evergreen trees and shrubs occurring in forest from Mexico to Paraguay. The palmate leaves, with 5–7 short-stalked leaflets, are borne in opposite pairs. Funnel-shaped, 5-lobed flowers are borne in showy, terminal panicles. In frost-prone areas, grow in a temperate or warm greenhouse. In warmer climates, grow as specimen or shade trees.

• **HARDINESS** Frost tender.

• **CULTIVATION** Under glass, plant directly into a greenhouse border in loam-based potting compost (JI. No.3) in full light, and with moderate to high humidity. In the growing season, water freely and apply a balanced liquid fertilizer monthly; water sparingly in winter. Top-dress or pot on in spring. Outdoors, grow in fertile, moist but well-drained soil in full sun. Pruning group 1; plants under glass need restrictive pruning, when leafless or immediately after flowering.

• **PROPAGATION** Sow seed at 15–18°C (59–64°F) in spring. Root semi-ripe cuttings with bottom heat in summer. Air layer in early spring.

• **PESTS AND DISEASES** Susceptible to red spider mites and whiteflies under glass.

C. donnell-smithii ♀ syn. *Tabebuia donnell-smithii* (Primavera). Spreading to round-headed, deciduous tree, with 5- to 7-palmate, mid- to light green leaves, to 35cm (14in) long. Lax panicles, 15–30cm (6–12in) long, of foxglove-like yellow flowers, 3–4cm (1¼–1½in) long, are borne on the bare branches in spring. ↕ 18–25m (60–80ft), ↔ 5–10m (15–30ft). Mexico, Guatemala. ❀ (min. 10–15°C/50–59°F)

▷ **Cycad,**
Ferocious blue see *Encephalartos horridus*
Lebombo see *Encephalartos lebomboensis*
Modjadji see *Encephalartos transvenosus*
Natal see *Encephalartos natalensis*
Prickly see *Encephalartos altensteinii*
Suurberg see *Encephalartos longifolius*
▷ **Cycads** see p.50

CYCAS

Fern palm, Sago palm

CYCADACEAE

Genus of about 15 species of cycads found mainly on dry, stony slopes and in semi-desert and dry, open woodland (and, rarely, at rainforest margins) from Madagascar to S. and S.E. Asia, Australia, and the Pacific islands. They have whorls of pinnate, stiff, leathery leaves, with linear-lance-shaped to sickle-shaped leaflets. Dioecious inflorescences arise from the centres of the leaf rosettes. The large male inflorescences are cone-like, up to 80cm (32in) tall, and usually covered in woolly hairs; the female inflorescences consist of loosely arranged, modified leaves, to 30cm (12in) long, bearing ovules on the margins. *Cycas* species are generally cultivated for their palm-like appearance. In frost-prone climates, grow in a temperate or warm greenhouse, or as foliage houseplants. In warmer climates, they make excellent specimen plants.

• **HARDINESS** Frost tender; *C. revoluta* will survive short periods near to 0°C (32°F) if given some protection.

• **CULTIVATION** Under glass, grow in a mix of equal parts loam, garden compost, and coarse bark with additional grit and charcoal, and a slow-release fertilizer. Provide full light, with shade from hot sun, and moderate humidity. In the growing season, water moderately; reduce humidity and water in winter. Pot on or top-dress in spring. Outdoors, grow in fertile, moist but well-drained soil in full sun.

• **PROPAGATION** Sow seed at 15–29°C (59–84°F) in spring. Remove and pot up suckers in spring.

• **PESTS AND DISEASES** Susceptible to red spider mites, mealybugs, and scale insects under glass. *Cycas* species may be damaged by chemical pesticides; use soft soap or biological controls.

C. circinalis ▣ 🌴 (False sago, Fern palm, Sago palm). Erect cycad with a robust stem, thickened towards the base

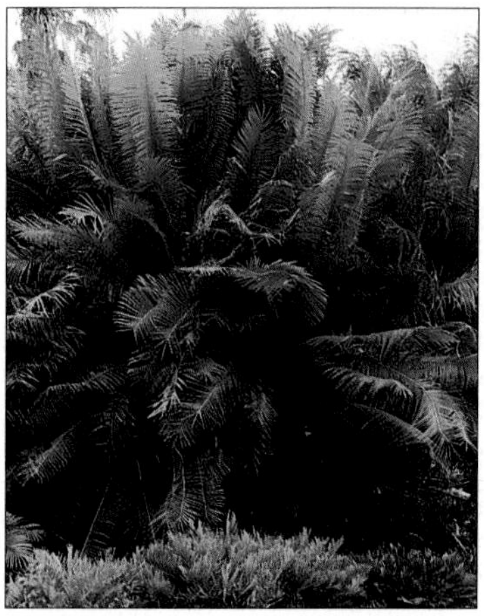
Cycas circinalis

and bearing pale bands of old leaf scars. Leaves are pinnate, 1.5–3m (5–10ft) long, with up to 100 narrowly lance-shaped, glossy, rich green leaflets. Cone-like inflorescences are brown; the males to 45cm (18in) long, females to 30cm (12in) long. Female inflorescences produce ovoid red fruit, to 6cm (2½in) long. ↕ to 6m (20ft), ↔ 3–6m (10–20ft). S.E. India. ❀ (min. 13°C/55°F)

C. media 🌴 (Zamia palm). Erect cycad with a robust stem, rarely branched, bearing rings of pale leaf scars. Spreading leaves, ascending at first, are pinnate, to 1.5m (5ft) long, consisting of linear, bright green leaflets. Cone-like inflorescences are brown; the males to 50cm (20in) long, the females to 40cm (16in) long. Female inflorescences produce broadly ellipsoid, orange-red fruit, 2–4cm (¾–1½in) long. ↕ to 5m (15ft), ↔ to 3m (10ft). Australia (Queensland). ❀ (min. 13°C/55°F)

C. revoluta ▣ ♀ ❋ (Japanese sago palm). Robust-stemmed cycad, erect at first but gradually reclining with age, and suckering and branching when mature. Arching leaves, 0.75–1.5m (30–60in) long, are pinnate, with up to 125 sickle-shaped, glossy, dark green leaflets. Ovoid, woolly, golden brown inflorescences are produced on mature plants but seldom on those grown in containers. The male inflorescences, to 40cm (16in) long, are pineapple-scented; females, 20cm (8in) long, produce ovoid yellow fruit, 3–4cm (1¼–1½in) long. ↕ 1–2m (3–6ft) or more, ↔ 1–2m (3–6ft) or more. Japan (including Ryukyu Islands). ❀ (min. 7–10°C/45–50°F)

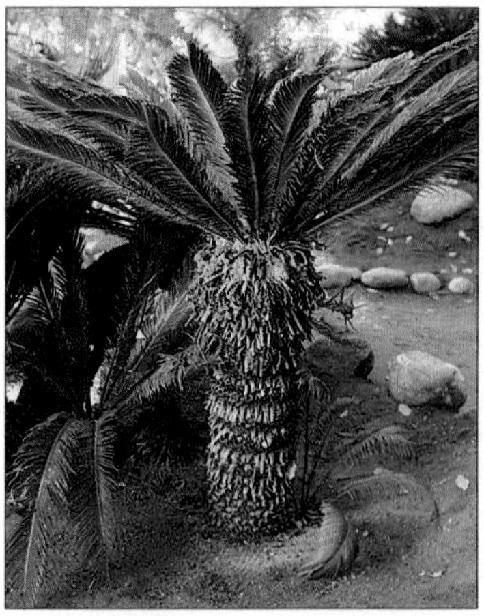
Cycas revoluta

CYCLAMEN

Sowbread

PRIMULACEAE

Genus of about 19 species of tuberous perennials found in habitats ranging from alpine woodland and damp woods to dry sands and maquis, from the Mediterranean east to Iran and south to Somalia. Leaves are rounded to heart-shaped, sometimes toothed or lobed, often with silver zones or light and dark patterns above, and purplish red below. Leaves of autumn-flowering species last through winter to spring. The nodding, sometimes fragrant flowers, 1–3cm (½–1¼in) long, each have 5 reflexed, twisted petals, varying from white to pink and carmine-red, often with darker "mouths" (perianth tube rims). Flowers may be borne at almost any time of year, depending on the species. In most species, the flower-stalk coils on to the soil surface after flowering to release the ripe seeds. *C. persicum* has been selected extensively to produce a wide colour and size range, the flowers often much larger than those of the wild species.

Grow fully hardy species and cultivars in a rock garden, border, or raised bed. Frost-hardy to frost-tender cyclamens (with the exception of *C. parviflorum*), need a warm, dry summer dormancy; outside Mediterranean climates, they are best grown in a cool greenhouse, alpine house, or bulb frame. Cultivars of *C. persicum* are excellent in a conservatory or as houseplants. All parts may cause severe discomfort if ingested.

• **HARDINESS** Fully hardy to frost tender.

• **CULTIVATION** For ease of reference, cultivation requirements may be divided into 3 groups, as follows:

1. Plant 3–5cm (1¼–2in) deep. Grow in moderately fertile, humus-rich, well-drained soil in partial shade, under trees or shrubs, to avoid excessive summer moisture. Mulch annually with leaf mould as leaves wither; in areas with prolonged frost, provide a deep, loose mulch. Do not allow *C. parviflorum* and *C. purpurascens* to dry out.

2. Plant 2–2.5cm (¾–1in) deep, or with the tops of the tubers just at the soil surface. Grow in a mix of equal parts loam, leaf mould, peat, and sharp sand in an alpine house or bulb frame; grow half-hardy species in a cool greenhouse, in bright filtered light with moderate humidity. In growth, water moderately. Reduce water and humidity as leaves fade; keep completely dry in dormancy. Apply a low-nitrogen liquid fertilizer every 6–8 weeks when in full leaf.

3. (*C. persicum* and its cultivars). Plant with the tops of the tubers just above the soil surface. Grow in loam-based potting compost (JI No.2) in bright filtered light (full light in winter), with moderate humidity and an even winter temperature of 13–16°C (55–61°F). Avoid draughts and hot, dry air. When in full leaf, water moderately (avoiding the crown), and apply a low-nitrogen liquid fertilizer every 2 weeks. Reduce water as leaves wither after flowering; keep dry when dormant (about 2–3 months). Resume watering and feeding as new growth appears. When tubers fill the pot, repot when dormant.

• **PROPAGATION** Sow seed as soon as ripe, in darkness, at 6–12°C (43–54°F). Sow seed of *C. persicum* at 12–15°C (54–59°F): sow seed of open-pollinated cultivars in late summer to flower in about 14 months; sow seed of other cultivars from late winter to mid-spring to flower in autumn of the same year. Before sowing, soak all seed in water for at least 10 hours and rinse thoroughly.

• **PESTS AND DISEASES** Mice or squirrels may be a problem. Prone to red spider mites, vine weevil, cyclamen mite, and grey mould (*Botrytis*) under glass.

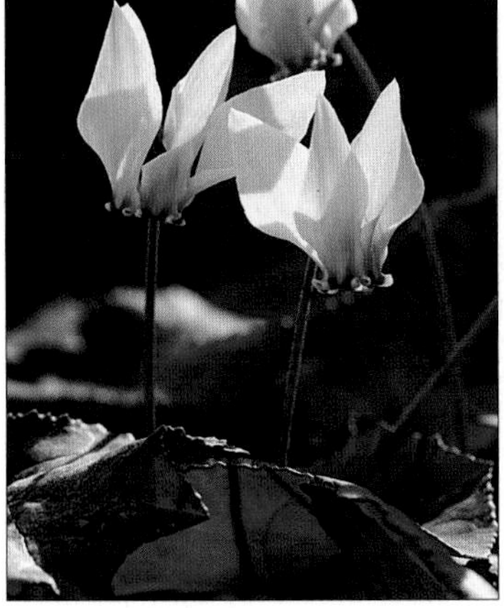

Cyclamen africanum

C. abchasicum see *C. coum* subsp. *caucasicum*.

C. africanum ▣ Tuberous perennial with heart-shaped, bright green leaves, to 10cm (4in) long, with paler green markings. Produces flowers, 2–3.5cm (¾–1½in) long, in shades of pink with deep maroon mouths, just before the leaves in autumn. Cultivation group 2; cool greenhouse. ↕ 12–15cm (5–6in), ↔ 23cm (9in). Algeria. ✻

C. alpinum see *C. trochopteranthum*.

C. balearicum. Tuberous perennial with scallop-margined, heart-shaped, mid-green or grey-green leaves, heavily silvered above, maroon beneath, to 9cm (3½in) long, usually smaller. Delicate, strongly fragrant, white or pale pink flowers, to 1.5cm (½in) long, with fine pink veins, are borne with the leaves in spring. Cultivation group 2. ↕ 5cm (2in), ↔ 5–8cm (2–3in). Balearic Islands. ✻✻

C. caucasicum see *C. coum* subsp. *caucasicum*.

C. cilicium ▣ ♀ Tuberous perennial with rounded or heart-shaped, strongly patterned, mid-green leaves, 1.5–5cm (½–2in) long, often purplish beneath.

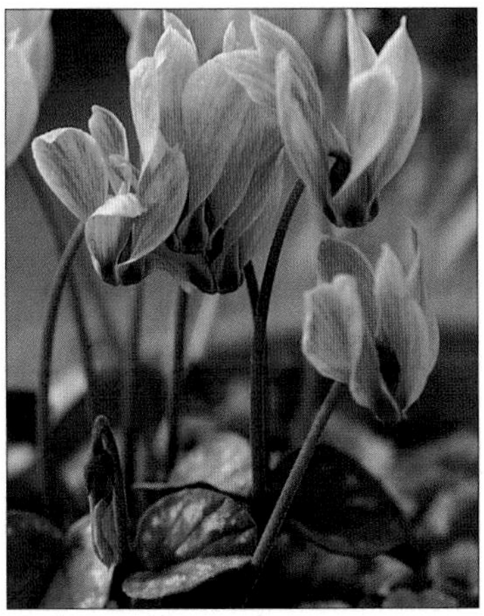

Cyclamen cilicium

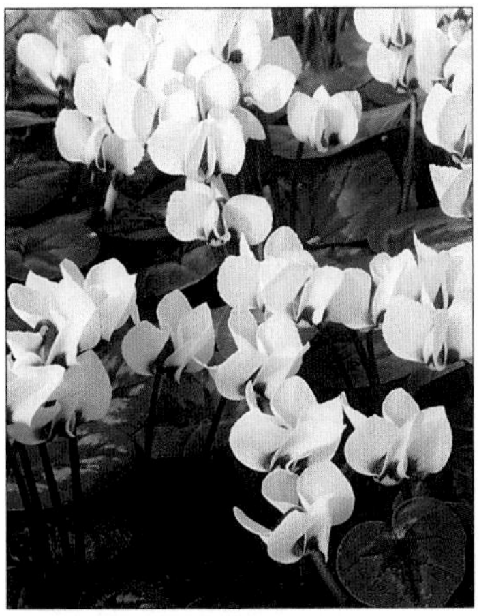

Cyclamen coum f. *albissimum*

Slender, white or pink flowers, 1–2cm (½–¾in) long, stained dark carmine-red at the mouths, are borne with the leaves in autumn. Cultivation group 1 or 2. ↕ 5cm (2in), ↔ 8cm (3in). S. Turkey. ✻✻. **f. album** has white flowers.

C. coum ♀ Tuberous perennial with rounded leaves, 2.5–6cm (1–2½in) long, either shiny, unmarked, and deep green, or deep green with silver patterns. Compact flowers, 0.8–1.5cm (⅜–½in) long, varying from white to shades of pink and carmine-red, with dark carmine-red stains above white-rimmed mouths, are produced with the leaves in winter or early spring. Cultivation group 1. ↕ 5–8cm (2–3in), ↔ 10cm (4in). Bulgaria, Caucasus, Turkey, Lebanon. ✻✻✻. **f. albissimum** ▣ syn. 'Album', bears white flowers with dark carmine-red marks at the mouths. **subsp. caucasicum**, syn. *C. abchasicum*, *C. caucasicum*, has pinkish lilac flowers, to 1.5cm (½in) long, and heart-shaped, silver-marked leaves, with scalloped margins. **Pewter Group** ▣ ♀ is a variable, vigorous selection, with leaves almost entirely silvered above.

C. creticum. Tuberous perennial with heart-shaped, greyish green leaves, to 4cm (1½in) long, with silver markings. Slender, fragrant, white or very pale pink flowers, 1.5–2.5cm (½–1in) long, are borne with the leaves in spring. Cultivation group 2. ↕ 5–8cm (2–3in), ↔ 8–10cm (3–4in). Greece (Crete). ✻✻

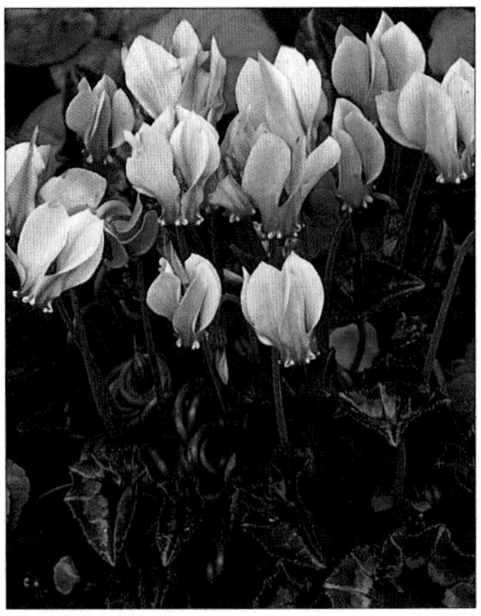

Cyclamen hederifolium

C. cyprium. Tuberous perennial with heart-shaped, toothed leaves, to 5cm (2in) or more long, patterned light grey-green. Bears very fragrant white flowers, to 2.5cm (1in) long, marked carmine-red at the mouths, with the leaves in autumn. Cultivation group 2. ↕ 5–8cm (2–3in), ↔ 15cm (6in). Cyprus. ✻✻

C. europaeum see *C. purpurascens*.

C. fatrense see *C. purpurascens*.

C. graecum. Tuberous perennial with long, fleshy roots and heart-shaped, deep green leaves, 5–14cm (2–5½in) long, marked silver and light green. Pink to carmine-red flowers, 1.5–2.5cm (½–1in) long, with darker markings at the mouths, are borne just before the leaves in autumn. Cultivation group 2; best in a large container. ↕ 8–10cm (3–4in), ↔ 15cm (6in). Greece, Aegean Islands, Turkey, Cyprus. ✻✻. **f. album** has pure white flowers.

C. hederifolium ▣ ♀ syn. *C. neapolitanum*. Tuberous perennial with

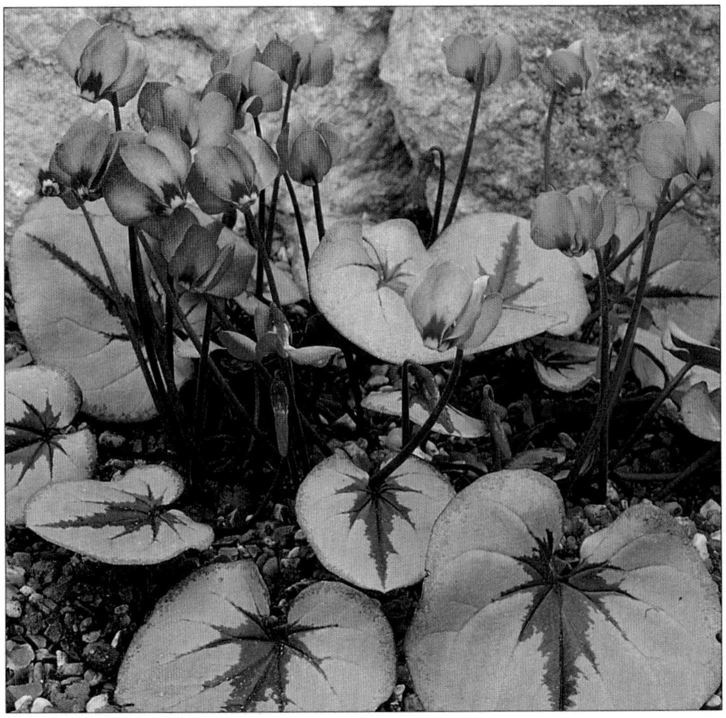

Cyclamen coum Pewter Group

C

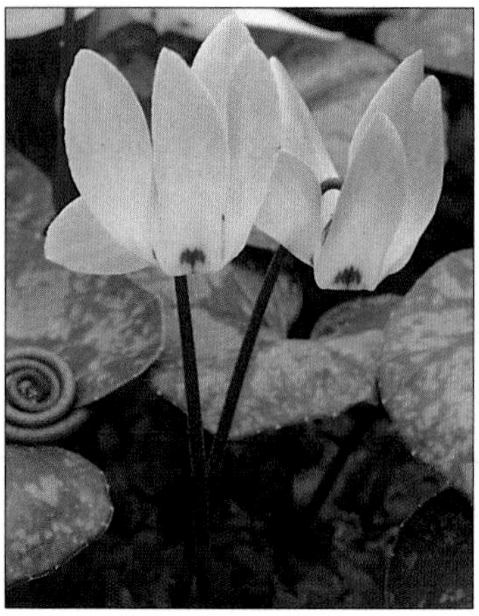

Cyclamen libanoticum

large, flattened tubers and clumps of very variable, triangular to heart-shaped, pointed, patterned, mid- to dark green leaves, 5–15cm (2–6in) long, often purplish green beneath. Sometimes scented flowers, to 2.5cm (1in) long, in shades of pink, with deep maroon marks at the apexes of the mouths, are produced in mid- and late autumn before the leaves. Self-seeds freely. Cultivation group 1. ↕ 10–13cm (4–5in), ↔ 15cm (6in). Mediterranean (Italy to Turkey). ✻✻✻. **f. *albiflorum*** has pure white flowers without basal marks.
C. libanoticum ■ ♀ Tuberous perennial bearing rounded-heart-shaped, shallowly lobed, dull green leaves, 8cm (3in) long, patterned with lighter green,

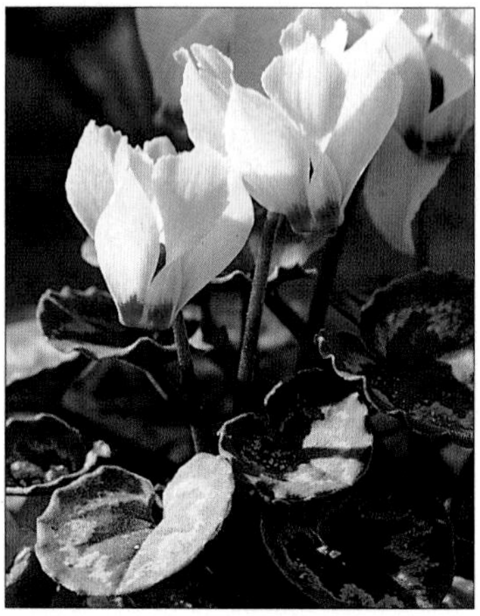

Cyclamen mirabile

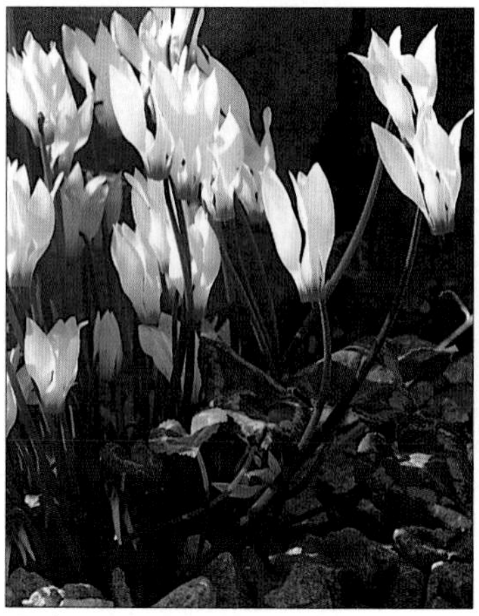

Cyclamen persicum

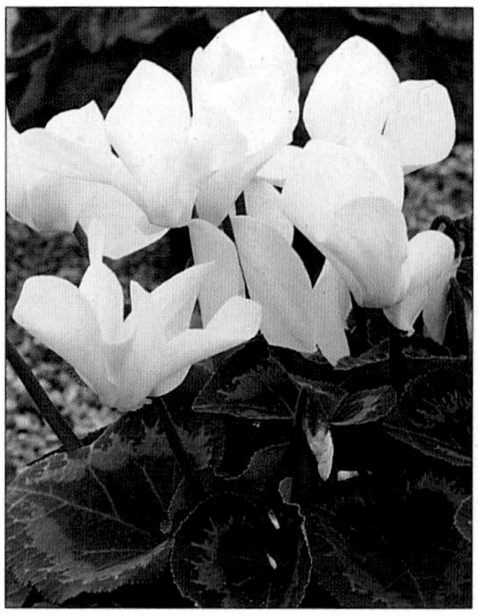

Cyclamen persicum Sierra Series 'Sierra White'

in winter. Pale to mid-pink flowers, to 3cm (1¼in) long, white at the bases, with bold carmine-red marks at the mouths, are produced with the leaves from winter to early spring. Cultivation group 2; cool greenhouse. ↕ 10cm (4in), ↔ 15cm (6in). Lebanon. ✻
C. mirabile ■ ♀ Tuberous perennial with heart-shaped leaves, to 3.5cm (1½in) long, with scalloped margins, mid-green above and purplish red beneath; they often have pink marks on the upper surfaces when they first expand. Slender, pale pink flowers, to 2cm (¾in) long, with fringed petals and maroon marks at the mouths, are produced with the leaves in autumn. Cultivation group 2. ↕ 8cm (3in), ↔ 8–10cm (3–4in). S.W. Turkey. ✻✻
C. neapolitanum see *C. hederifolium.*
C. parviflorum. Tuberous perennial with rounded, dull, deep green leaves, to 3.5cm (1½in) long, often smaller. Pink flowers, to 1cm (½in) long, stained dark pink at the mouths, are borne with the leaves in early spring. Cultivation group 1 or 2. ↕ 2.5–4cm (1–1½in), ↔ 5–8cm (2–3in). N.E. Turkey. ✻✻
C. persicum ■ Tuberous perennial with heart-shaped leaves, 2.5–14cm (1–5½in) long, deep green, often silver-marbled above and pale or purplish green beneath. Sweet-scented, pink, red, or white flowers, 1–2cm (½–¾in) or more long, are produced on tall, slender stems, with the leaves, from early winter to early spring. Cultivation group 2 if grown outdoors; cultivation group 3 under glass and for all cultivars. ↕ to 20cm (8in), ↔ 15cm (6in). S.E.

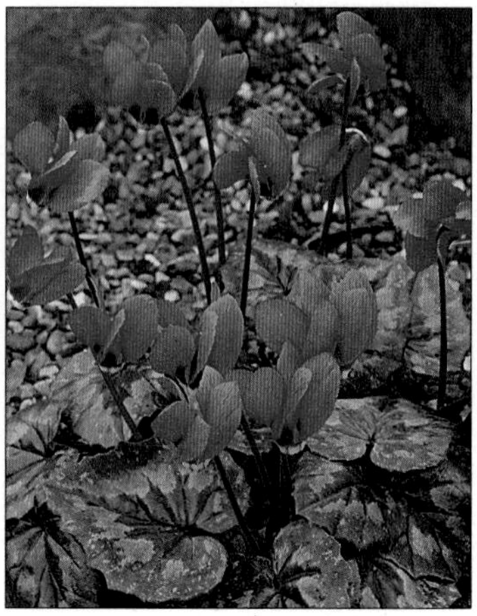

Cyclamen pseudibericum

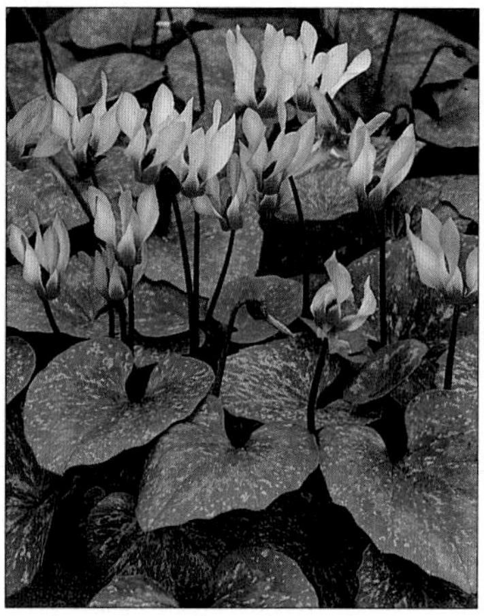

Cyclamen repandum subsp. *peloponnesiacum*

Mediterranean, N. Africa. ❀ (min 10°C/50°F). **Halios Series** cultivars have blunt-toothed, dark green leaves, 10–14cm (4–5½in) across, with silver marbling. A succession of flowers, 5–7cm (2–3in) long, in white, pink, scarlet, lilac, or purple, is borne from late summer to autumn; ↕ 30cm (12in), ↔ 18cm (7in). **Mirabelle Series** cultivars have small flowers, to 4cm (1½in) across, in deep or light salmon-pink, lilac, purple, scarlet, or white; ↕ 15cm (6in). **Miracle Series** cultivars have pink, salmon-pink, scarlet, or white flowers, 5–8cm (2–3in) long; ↕ to 15cm (6in). **'Scentsation'** is open-pollinated and produces strongly scented flowers, 5–8cm (2–3in) long, in pink, carmine-red, or crimson; ↕ 15cm (6in), ↔ 23cm (9in). **Sierra Series** cultivars have marbled foliage and flower in late winter, bearing flowers 5–8cm (2–3in) long in colours including white, pink, salmon-pink, scarlet, lilac, or purple; ↕ 23cm (9in), ↔ 20cm (8in); the series includes **'Sierra White'** ■ with clear white flowers. **'Victoria'** is open-pollinated, and has ruffled white flowers, 5–8cm (2–3in) long, with bright cherry-red margins and mouths; ↕↔ to 30cm (12in)
C. pseudibericum ■ ♀ Tuberous perennial with heart-shaped, silvery, dark green leaves, to 7cm (3in) long, lightly to conspicuously marked with silvery grey or grey-green. Fragrant, bright magenta flowers, to 2.5cm (1in) long, with darker, white-rimmed mouths, are borne with the leaves from winter to spring. Cultivation group 2. ↕ 10–15cm (4–6in), ↔ 8–10cm (3–4in). Turkey. ✻✻
C. purpurascens ♀ syn. *C. europaeum, C. fatrense.* Evergreen, sometimes deciduous, tuberous perennial with rounded to heart-shaped, shiny, dark green leaves, to 8cm (3in) long, sometimes faintly mottled silvery green above, and purplish red below. Broad-mouthed, very strongly scented, rich to pale carmine-red flowers, to 2cm (¾in) long, are produced with the leaves in mid- and late summer. Prefers alkaline conditions. Cultivation group 1 or 2. ↕ 10cm (4in), ↔ 8–10cm (3–4in). C. and E. Europe. ✻✻✻
C. repandum. Tuberous perennial bearing heart-shaped to triangular leaves, to 13cm (5in) long, dark green with grey-green patterning or speckles. Slender, fragrant, rich carmine-red flowers, to 2cm (¾in) long, are borne with the leaves in mid- and late spring. Cultivation group 1 or 2. ↕ 10–15cm (4–6in), ↔ 10–13cm (4–5in). S. France (including Corsica), Italy, former Yugoslavia, Greece. ✻✻✻ (borderline). **subsp. *peloponnesiacum*** ■ ♀ has scallop-margined leaves with heavy silver speckling and paler pink flowers with darker pink zones around the mouths.
C. rohlfsianum. Tuberous perennial with heart-shaped, strongly scalloped, shiny, bright green leaves, to 11cm (4½in) long, patterned silvery green. Often scented pink flowers, to 2.5cm (1in) long, with deep maroon mouths and projecting anthers, are produced with the leaves in autumn. Cultivation group 2; cool greenhouse. ↕ 10–13cm (4–5in), ↔ 15cm (6in). Libya. ✻
C. trochopteranthum, syn. *C. alpinum.* Tuberous perennial with rounded to heart-shaped, dark green, silver-marked leaves, 2.5–5cm (1–2in) long. Fragrant, white, pink, or carmine-red flowers, to 1.5cm (½in) long, with propeller-like, twisted petals, are produced with the leaves in late winter and early spring. Cultivation group 2. ↕ 5–8cm (2–3in), ↔ 8–10cm (3–4in). S.W. Turkey. ✻✻

▷ ***Cyclobothra lutea*** see *Calochortus barbatus*

CYCNOCHES

Swan orchid

ORCHIDACEAE

Genus of about 12 species of deciduous, epiphytic orchids from Central and South America, occurring at altitudes to 1,000m (3,250ft). They have elongated, spindle-shaped to cylindrical, fleshy pseudobulbs, and produce soft, folded, strap-shaped to ovate leaves in summer. Swan-like flowers, which may be male or female, are borne in arching or pendent racemes from nodes on the upper portion of the pseudobulbs, in early summer. The sex of the flowers is determined by the light level: in poor light, inflorescences of male flowers are usually produced. Female inflorescences develop in brighter conditions.

- **HARDINESS** Frost tender.
- **CULTIVATION** Warm-growing orchids. Grow in epiphytic orchid compost in deep containers or baskets. In summer, provide bright filtered light and moderate humidity; water moderately, applying fertilizer at every third watering, and keep foliage dry. Provide full light in winter; keep completely dry when dormant. See also p.46.
- **PROPAGATION** Divide pseudobulbs when growth recommences in spring.
- **PESTS AND DISEASES** Red spider mites, whiteflies, and mealybugs may be troublesome under glass.

C. egertonianum. Epiphytic orchid with cylindrical to spindle-shaped pseudobulbs and strap-shaped leaves, 7–21cm (3–8in) long. From summer to autumn, bears racemes of brown- or purple-spotted, green or greenish brown, sometimes yellow or white, rarely pink female flowers, 5cm (2in) across. Dark purple male flowers are smaller. ↕ 40cm (16in), ↔ 45cm (18in). Belize, Costa Rica, Guatemala, Nicaragua. ❀ (min. 18–20°C/64–68°F; max. 30°C/86°F)

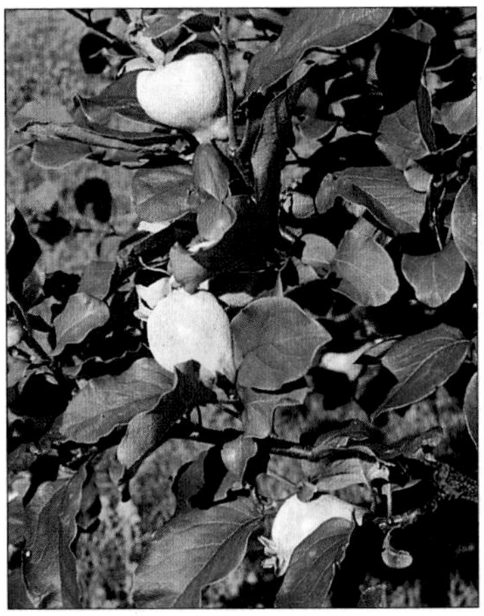

Cydonia oblonga 'Vranja'

CYDONIA

Quince

ROSACEAE

Genus of one species of deciduous tree or shrub occurring at woodland margins and on rocky slopes in S.W. Asia. The elliptic to ovate leaves are arranged alternately. Attractive, shallowly bowl-shaped flowers are followed by pear-like, ornamental fruit, which are edible when cooked. *C. oblonga* should not be confused with the flowering quinces (*Chaenomeles*). In regions with cold summers or winter temperatures that fall below -15°C (5°F), fan train *C. oblonga* against a wall. In warmer climates, it is excellent as a free-standing specimen; it fruits best in areas with long, hot summers.

• **HARDINESS** Fully hardy.

• **CULTIVATION** Grow in fertile, moist but well-drained soil in full sun. Pruning group 1; group 13 in winter, if fan-trained. In the first 3 or 4 winters, establish a framework of fruiting spurs; thereafter, prune only to remove badly placed shoots or to relieve overcrowding.

• **PROPAGATION** Sow seed of the species in a seedbed in autumn. Insert greenwood cuttings in early summer, or semi-ripe cuttings in mid- or late summer. May also be propagated from hardwood cuttings in autumn or early winter. Bud cultivars in summer, or bottom graft on to seedling quince stocks in late winter.

• **PESTS AND DISEASES** Susceptible to quince leaf blight, brown rot, fireblight, and mildew.

C. oblonga ♀ (Common quince). Rounded tree or shrub with crowded branches bearing broadly ovate, dark green leaves, grey-downy beneath, to 10cm (4in) long. Solitary, pale pink to white flowers, 5cm (2in) across, are produced from the leaf axils in late spring. Aromatic, edible, light golden yellow fruit, 8cm (3in) long, which ripen in autumn, are used for flavouring and in preserves. ↕↔ 5m (15ft). S.W. Asia. ❄❄❄. **'Lusitanica'**, syn. 'Portugal', is vigorous, producing dark yellow fruit, 10cm (4in) long, covered in grey down. **'Maliformis'** produces almost spherical fruit. **'Portugal'** see 'Lusitanica'. **'Vranja'** ■🏆 has very fragrant, pale green fruit, which ripen to golden yellow.

C. sinensis see *Pseudocydonia sinensis.*

C. speciosa see *Chaenomeles speciosa.*

CYMBIDIUM

ORCHIDACEAE

Genus of about 50 species of evergreen, epiphytic, lithophytic, or terrestrial orchids from temperate and tropical areas in India, China, Japan, S.E. Asia, and Australia. They have spherical to ovoid pseudobulbs and 8–10 long, narrowly oval to linear leaves. Flowers are borne in long or short racemes from the bases, mainly in spring. Hundreds of winter- or spring-flowering hybrids have been produced. Grow as houseplants or in a cool or temperate greenhouse; in Mediterranean climates, they may also be grown in a lath house. Contact with the foliage may aggravate skin allergies.

• **HARDINESS** Frost hardy to frost tender.

• **CULTIVATION** Cool-growing orchids. Pot firmly into epiphytic or terrestrial orchid compost with added charcoal and bone meal. In summer, provide bright filtered light and good ventilation. Water moderately, applying fertilizer at every third watering, and mist once or twice a day. In winter, place in full light and water sparingly. See also p.46.

• **PROPAGATION** Divide in early and mid-spring when pot-bound, or remove backbulbs and pot up after flowering.

• **PESTS AND DISEASES** Red spider mites, aphids, whiteflies, and mealybugs may prove troublesome.

C. aloifolium, syn. *C. pendulum.* Epiphytic orchid with small, ovoid pseudobulbs and fleshy, semi-rigid, linear leaves, 30–60cm (12–24in) long. Bears numerous, pale yellow to cream flowers, 4.5cm (1¾in) across, with dark red stripes on the tepals and lips, in pendent racemes from late winter to spring. ↕ 30cm (12in), ↔ 45cm (18in). E. Himalayas to S. China and Malaysia. ❄ (min. 10°C/50°F; max. 24°C/75°F)

C. bicolor. Epiphytic orchid with small, ovoid pseudobulbs and fleshy, semi-rigid, linear leaves, 30cm (12in) long. Numerous creamy white flowers, 4.5cm (1¾in) across, with purple-spotted lips, are produced in pendent racemes in autumn. ↕ 30cm (12in), ↔ 45cm (18in). E. Himalayas to S. China and Indonesia. ❄ (min. 10°C/50°F; max. 24°C/75°F)

***C.* Christmas Angel 'Cooksbridge Sunburst'** (*C.* Angelica x *C.* Lucy Moore). Terrestrial orchid with ovoid pseudobulbs and linear leaves, 75cm (30in) long. Bright yellow flowers, 10cm (4in) across, with spotted lips, are borne

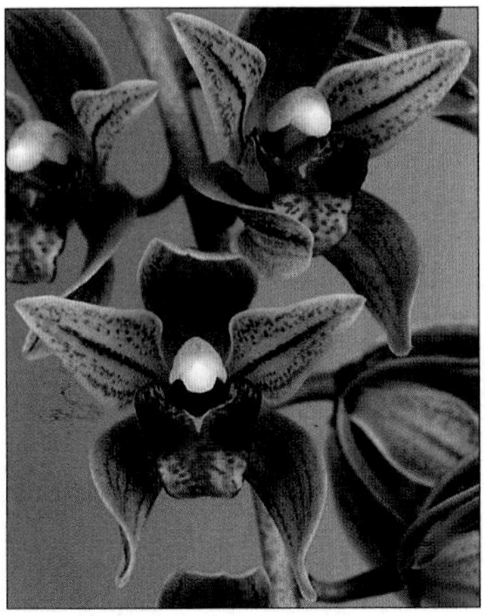

Cymbidium devonianum

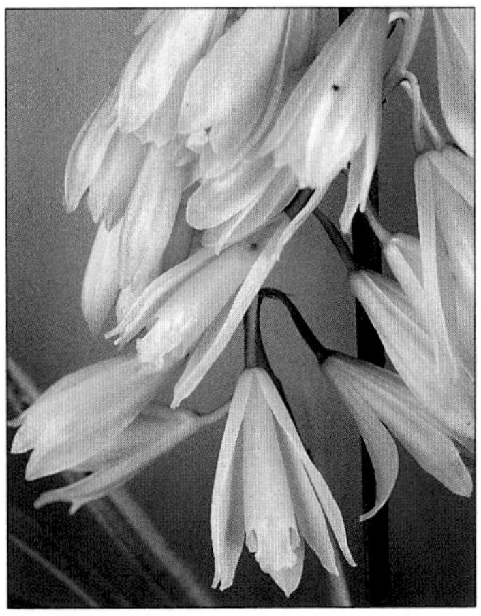

Cymbidium elegans

in pendent racemes in winter. ↕ 75cm (30in), ↔ 90cm (36in). ❄ (min. 10°C/50°F; max. 24°C/75°F)

C. devonianum ■ Epiphytic orchid with small, ovoid pseudobulbs and oval leaves, 30–60cm (12–24in) long. From spring to summer, bears olive-brown to yellow-green flowers, 4cm (1½in) across, with dull purple lips, in pendent racemes. ↕↔ 30cm (12in). N.E. India, N. Thailand. ❄ (min. 10°C/50°F; max. 24°C/75°F)

C. eburneum. Epiphytic orchid with very small pseudobulbs and linear leaves, 40–60cm (16–24in) long. In winter, bears upright racemes of white flowers, 8cm (3in) across, with yellow-stained lips. ↕ 50cm (20in), ↔ 60cm (24in). Himalayas, N. Burma, S.W. China. ❄ (min. 10°C/50°F; max. 24°C/75°F)

C. elegans ■ syn. *Cyperorchis elegans.* Epiphytic orchid with slender, ovoid pseudobulbs and narrowly oval leaves, 50cm (20in) long. Corn-yellow flowers, 5cm (2in) long, are produced in dense, pendent racemes from autumn to winter. ↕ 50cm (20in), ↔ 60cm (24in). Himalayas, S.W. China. ❄ (min. 10°C/50°F; max. 24°C/75°F)

C. ensifolium. Lithophytic or terrestrial orchid with ovoid pseudobulbs and linear leaves, 30cm (12in) long. In summer, produces upright racemes of greenish yellow flowers, 2.5cm (1in) across, with white lips irregularly spotted red-brown. ↕↔ 30cm (12in). India, China, Japan, S.E. Asia. ❄ (min. 10°C/50°F; max. 24°C/75°F)

C. grandiflorum see *C. hookerianum.*

C. hookerianum ■ syn. *C. grandiflorum.* Epiphytic or lithophytic

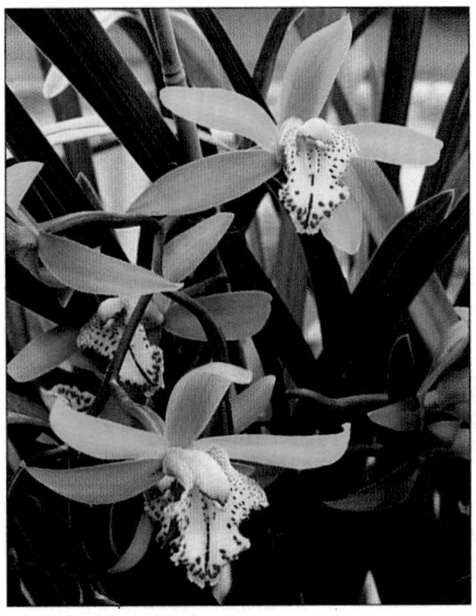

Cymbidium hookerianum

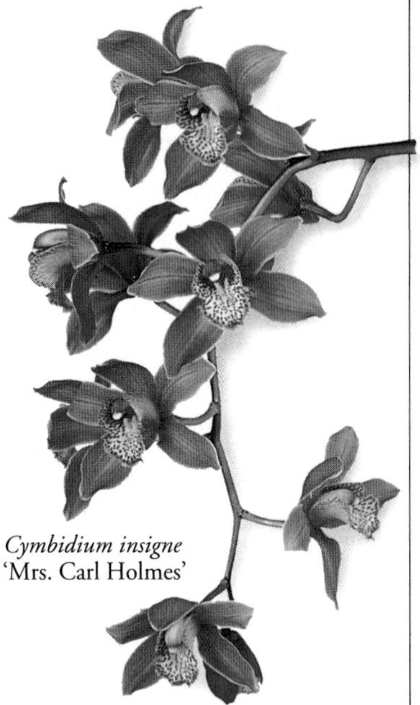

Cymbidium insigne 'Mrs. Carl Holmes'

orchid with ovoid pseudobulbs and linear leaves, 60cm (24in) long. In early winter, bears fragrant, deep apple-green flowers, 9–13cm (3½–5in) across, with purple- or yellow-spotted white lips, in arching racemes. ↕ 60cm (24in), ↔ 90cm (36in). Himalayas, S.W. China. ❄ (min. 10°C/50°F; max. 24°C/75°F)

C. insigne. Lithophytic or terrestrial orchid with ovoid pseudobulbs and linear leaves, 50–100cm (20–39in) long. Bears upright racemes of white or white-flushed pink flowers, 8cm (3in) across, with white-flushed, pink-spotted lips, in spring. ↕ 90cm (36in), ↔ 60cm (24in). Vietnam, N. Thailand, S. China. ❄ (min. 10°C/50°F; max. 24°C/75°F). **'Mrs. Carl Holmes'** ■ has rose-pink flowers with red-spotted white lips.

***C.* Kings Loch** (*C.* King Arthur x *C.* Loch Lomond). Terrestrial orchid with ovoid pseudobulbs and linear leaves, 75cm (30in) long. Numerous green flowers, 8cm (3in) across, are borne in upright racemes in winter. ↕ 60cm (24in), ↔ 90cm (36in). ❄ (min. 10°C/50°F; max. 24°C/75°F). **'Miniature Yellow'** ■ has yellow flowers marked dark red on the lips.

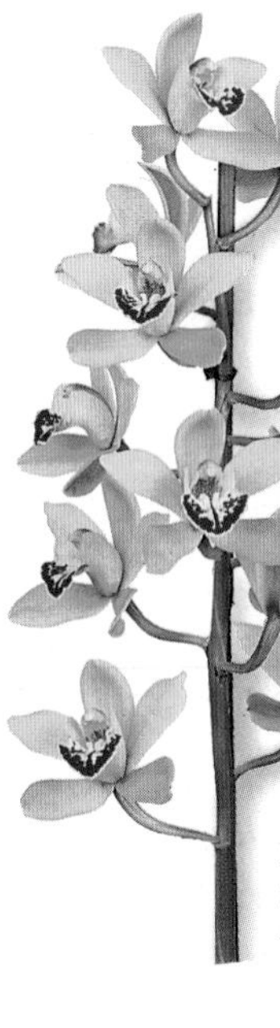

Cymbidium King's Loch 'Miniature Yellow'

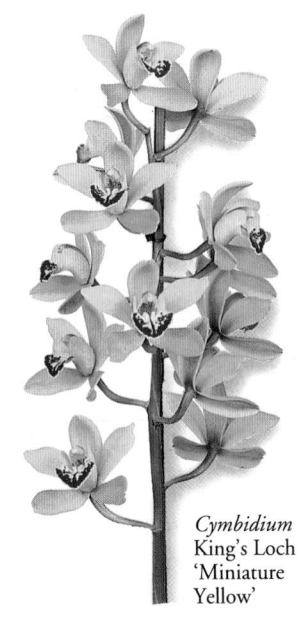

C

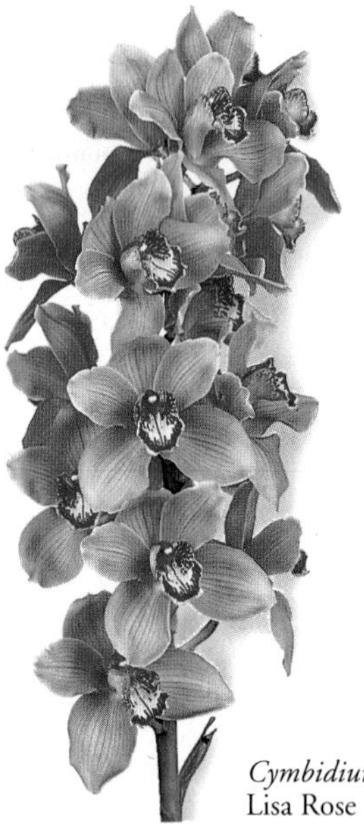

Cymbidium Lisa Rose

C. Lisa Rose ■ (*C.* Keera x *C.* Sylvania). Terrestrial orchid with ovoid pseudobulbs and linear leaves, 75cm (30in) long. Up to 12 rose-pink flowers, 10cm (4in) across, with yellowish white and deep red lips, are borne in upright racemes in winter. ↕60cm (24in), ↔90cm (36in). ❄ (min. 10°C/50°F; max. 24°C/75°F)
C. lowianum. Epiphytic orchid with ovoid pseudobulbs and linear leaves, 60–75cm (24–30in) long. Greenish yellow flowers, 9–12cm (3½–5in) across, with red-banded lips, are borne in arching racemes in spring. ↕↔90cm (36in). Burma, Thailand, S.W. China. ❄ (min. 10°C/50°F; max. 24°C/75°F)
C. New Dimension (*C.* Mavourneen x *C.* Sussex Moor). Terrestrial orchid with ovoid pseudobulbs and narrowly oval leaves, 75cm (30in) long. Pale green flowers, 10cm (4in) across, are produced in upright racemes in winter. ↕60cm (24in), ↔90cm (36in). ❄ (min. 10°C/50°F; max. 24°C/75°F). **'Standard White'** ■ has white flowers with pink-flushed petals, and yellow and white lips with red markings.
C. pendulum see *C. aloifolium.*
C. Pontac 'Mont Millais' ■ (*C.* Hamsey x *C.* Memoria Doctor Borg).

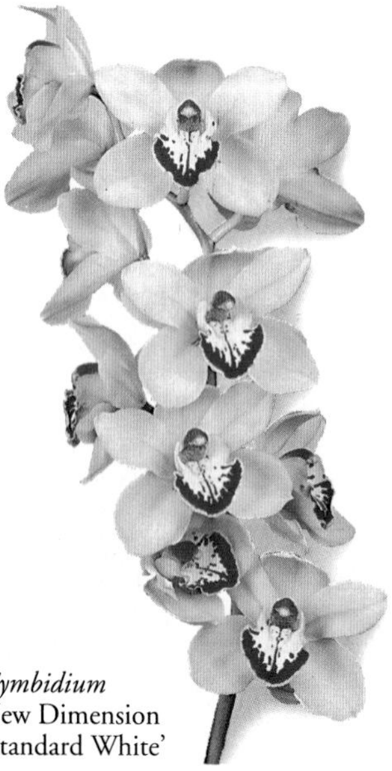

Cymbidium New Dimension 'Standard White'

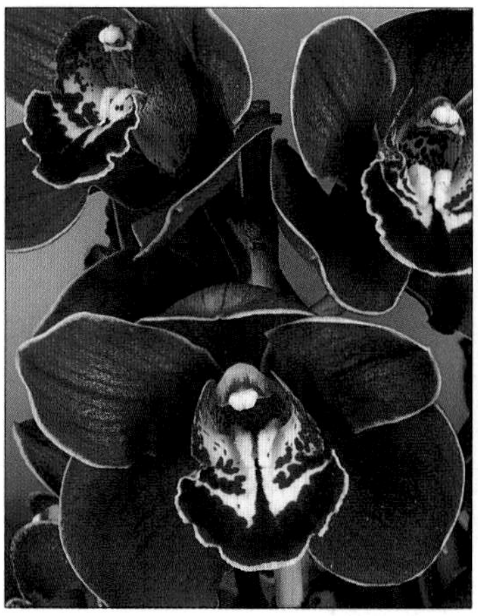

Cymbidium Pontac 'Mont Millais'

Terrestrial orchid with ovoid pseudobulbs and linear leaves, 75cm (30in) long. Bears dark red flowers, 10cm (4in) across, with red-banded white lips, in long, upright racemes in winter. ↕↔90cm (36in). ❄ (min. 10°C/50°F; max. 24°C/75°F)
C. Portelet Bay ■ (*C.* Caithness x *C.* Snowsprite). Terrestrial orchid with ovoid pseudobulbs and linear leaves, 75cm (30in) long. White flowers, 8cm (3in) across, with white-based, deep red lips, are borne in upright racemes in winter. ↕60cm (24in), ↔90cm (36in). ❄ (min. 10°C/50°F; max. 24°C/75°F)
C. Rosehill (*C.* Hamsey x *C.* Vieux Rose). Terrestrial orchid with ovoid pseudobulbs and linear leaves, 75cm (30in) long. Deep pink flowers, 10cm (4in) across, are borne in upright racemes in winter. ↕60cm (24in), ↔90cm (36in). ❄ (min. 10°C/50°F; max. 24°C/75°F)
C. St. Helier 'Trinity' (*C.* Mavourneen x *C.* New Dimension). Terrestrial orchid with ovoid pseudobulbs and narrowly oval leaves, 75cm (30in) long. Yellow-green flowers, 10cm (4in) across, with clear white lips, are produced in upright racemes from winter to spring. ↕↔90cm (36in). ❄ (min. 10°C/50°F; max. 24°C/75°F)
C. Showgirl ■🏆 (*C.* Alexanderi x *C.* Sweetheart). Terrestrial orchid with spherical pseudobulbs and linear leaves, to 45cm (18in) long. Pink-flushed white flowers, 6cm (2½in) across, with red flecks and stripes on the lips, are borne in upright racemes from winter to spring. ↕↔45cm (18in). ❄ (min. 10°C/50°F; max. 24°C/75°F)

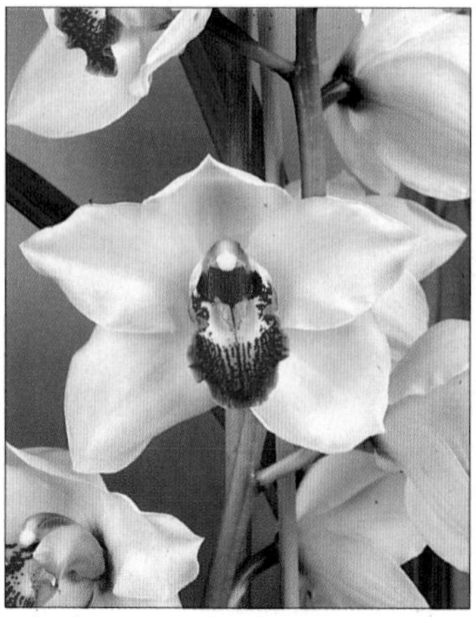

Cymbidium Portelet Bay

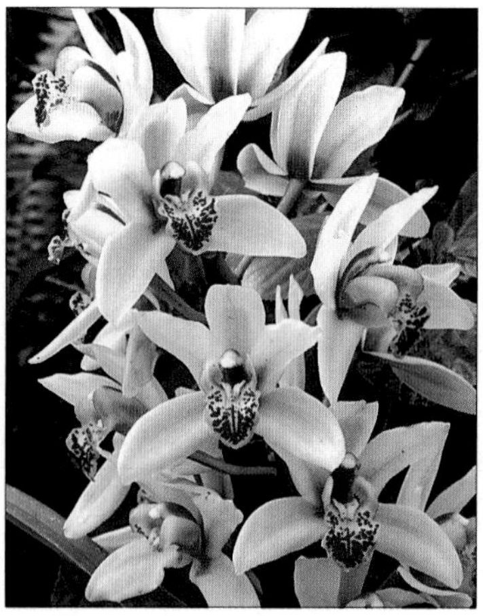

Cymbidium Showgirl

C. Strathbraan ■ (*C.* New Dimension x *C.* Putana). Terrestrial orchid with spherical pseudobulbs and linear leaves, to 45cm (18in) long. Very pale pink to rose-pink flowers, 6cm (2½in) across, with red flecks and margins on the lips, are borne in upright racemes in winter. ↕↔45cm (18in). ❄ (min. 10°C/50°F; max. 24°C/75°F)
C. Strathdon 'Cooksbridge Noel' ■🏆 (*C.* Kurun x *C.* Nip). Terrestrial orchid with spherical pseudobulbs and linear leaves, to 45cm (18in) long. Dusky red-pink flowers, 6cm (2½in) across, with yellow lips marked deep red and pale pink, are borne in upright racemes in winter. ↕↔45cm (18in). ❄ (min. 10°C/50°F; max. 24°C/75°F)
C. Strathkanaid (*C.* Hamsey x *C.* Nip). Terrestrial orchid with rounded pseudobulbs and linear leaves, to 45cm (18in) long. Upright racemes of dark pinkish red flowers, 6cm (2½in) across, are produced in winter. ↕↔45cm (18in). ❄ (min. 10°C/50°F; max. 24°C/75°F)
C. Thurso ■ (*C.* Miretta x *C.* York Meredith). Terrestrial orchid with ovoid pseudobulbs and linear leaves, 75cm (30in) long. Bears upright racemes of mid-green flowers, 10cm (4in) across, with red stripes and flecks on the lips, in winter. ↕60cm (24in), ↔90cm (36in). ❄ (min. 10°C/50°F; max. 24°C/75°F)
C. Tiger Tail (*C.* Alexanderi x *C. tigrinum*). Terrestrial orchid with ovoid pseudobulbs and linear leaves, 30cm (12in) long. Brown-shaded, lemon-yellow flowers, 6cm (2½in) across, are borne in upright racemes in early winter. ↕↔30cm (12in). ❄ (min. 10°C/50°F; max. 24°C/75°F)

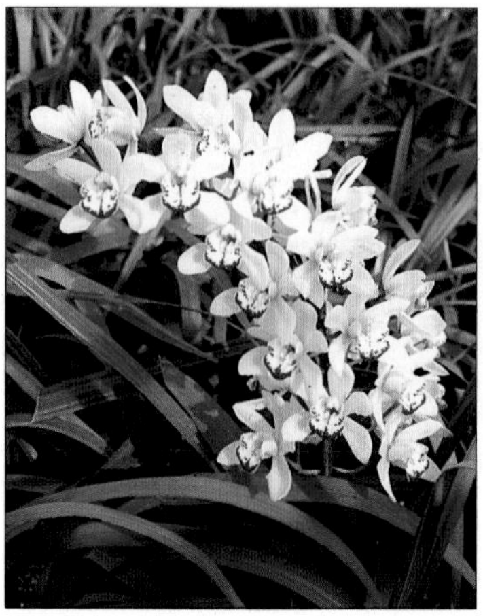

Cymbidium Strathbraan

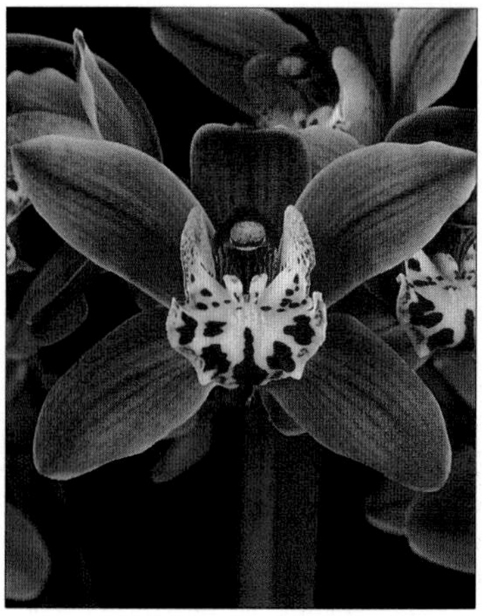

Cymbidium Strathdon 'Cooksbridge Noel'

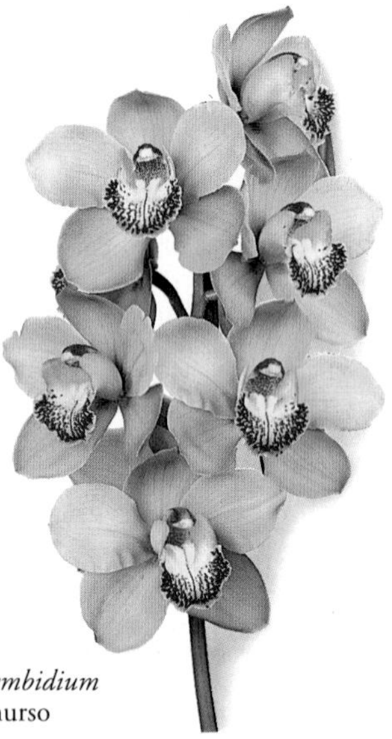

Cymbidium Thurso

C. tigrinum. Lithophytic orchid with almost spherical pseudobulbs and narrowly oval leaves, 23cm (9in) long. Olive-green to yellow flowers, to 5cm (2in) across, with purple lines, spots, and margins on the lips, are produced in upright racemes in autumn. ↕25cm (10in), ↔15cm (6in). Burma, N.E. India. ❄ (min. 10°C/50°F; max. 24°C/75°F)
C. tracyanum ■ Epiphytic orchid with ovoid pseudobulbs and linear leaves, 60–75cm (24–30in) long. Strongly fragrant, yellow-green flowers, 9cm (3½in) across, boldly striped brown, with cream or yellow lips flecked purple-brown, are borne in arching racemes in

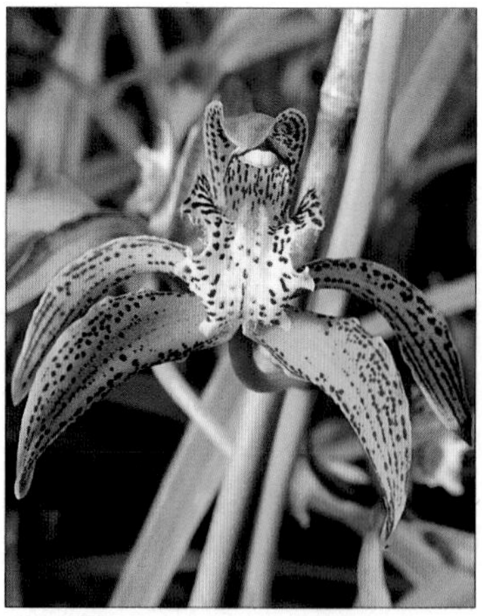

Cymbidium tracyanum

autumn. ↕↔ 90cm (36in). N. Burma, N. Thailand, China (S. Yunnan). ❀ (min. 10°C/50°F; max. 24°C/75°F)
C. Vieux Rose 'Del Park' (*C.* Babylon x *C.* Rio Rita). Terrestrial orchid with ovoid pseudobulbs and linear leaves, 75cm (30in) long. Light pink flowers, 10cm (4in) across, with heavily red-spotted lips, are borne in upright racemes in spring. ↕↔ 90cm (36in). ❀ (min. 10°C/50°F; max. 24°C/75°F)

CYMBOPOGON

GRAMINEAE/POACEAE

Genus of about 56 species of sturdy, aromatic, tufted, evergreen, perennial grasses, occurring in warm-temperate, subtropical, and tropical Africa and Asia, often in savannah grassland. They are grown for their linear to lance-shaped, mid- to bluish green leaves, and their loose or compact, many-branched flowering panicles, borne at the ends of the branches. The panicles consist of spikelets borne in short, paired, spike-like racemes, which are enclosed in spathe-like bracts. In frost-prone areas, grow in a conservatory or warm greenhouse and move outdoors in summer; in warmer climates, use in a mixed or grass border. *Cymbopogon* species contain essential oils that have medicinal, culinary, and cosmetic uses.
• **HARDINESS** Frost tender.
• **CULTIVATION** Under glass, grow in loam-based potting compost (JI No.2) in full light, with moderate humidity. In the growing season, water freely; water sparingly in winter. Repot in early spring. Outdoors, grow in fertile, moist but well-drained soil in full sun.
• **PROPAGATION** Sow seed at 13–18°C (55–64°F) in early spring. Divide in late spring.
• **PESTS AND DISEASES** Trouble free.

C. citratus (Lemon grass). Densely tufted, clump-forming, perennial grass with hollow, cane-like stems and erect to arching, linear, rough-margined, strongly lemon-scented, pale blue-green leaves, to 90cm (36in) long. In late summer and early autumn, bears loose, branching flowering panicles, to 5cm (2in) long. Does not flower freely under glass. ↕ to 1.5m (5ft), ↔ 90cm (36in). S. India, Sri Lanka. ❀ (min. 10°C/50°F)

CYNARA

ASTERACEAE/COMPOSITAE

Genus of about 10 species of clump-forming, thistle-like perennials found on well-drained, sunny slopes and grassland in the Mediterranean region, N.W. Africa, and the Canary Islands. Many are imposing plants, with pinnatifid or 2-pinnatifid, silvery or greyish green leaves and tall, spherical flowerheads, borne singly or in corymbs. *Cynara* species are statuesque plants, suitable for a herbaceous border. The flowerhead bracts, leaf-stalks, and midribs of some species are edible. The thistle-like flowerheads are also useful for dried flower arrangements, and attract bees.
• **HARDINESS** Fully hardy to frost hardy.
• **CULTIVATION** Grow in fertile, well-drained soil in full sun, sheltered from strong winds. For best foliage effects, remove the flowering stems as they emerge in summer. Where temperatures

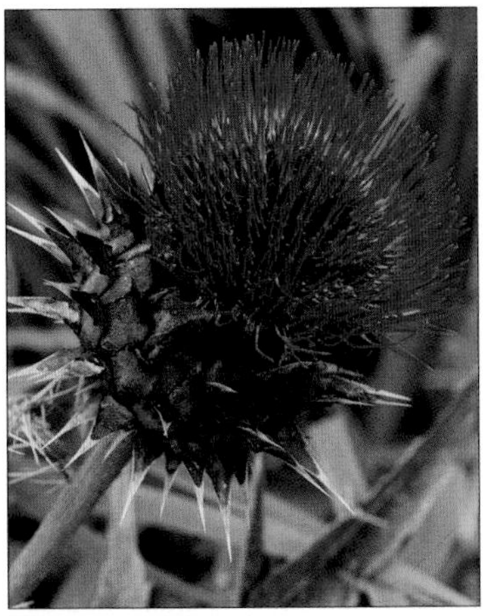

Cynara cardunculus

fall below -15°C (5°F), protect the rootstock with a dry winter mulch.
• **PROPAGATION** Sow seed in containers in a cold frame, or divide in spring. Insert root cuttings in winter.
• **PESTS AND DISEASES** Susceptible to grey mould (*Botrytis*), slugs, and aphids.

C. cardunculus ▣ 🏆 (Cardoon). Clump-forming perennial with pinnatifid or 2-pinnatifid, usually spiny, silvery grey leaves, to 50cm (20in) long, with ovate to linear-lance-shaped segments and deep basal lobes. From early summer to early autumn, purple flowerheads, 4–8cm (1½–3in) across, are produced on grey-woolly stems. Blanched leaf-stalks and midribs are edible. ↕ 1.5m (5ft), ↔ 1.2m (4ft). S.W. Mediterranean, Morocco. ❄❄❄
C. scolymus (Globe artichoke). Clump-forming perennial with deeply lobed or pinnatifid, grey-green leaves, to 80cm (32in) long, with pointed segments, grey-hairy above, densely white-woolly beneath. In early autumn, bears purple flowerheads, 8–15cm (3–6in) across, with large involucral bracts. The flowerheads (in bud) are eaten as a vegetable. Probably a variant of *C. cardunculus* but horticulturally distinct. ↕ to 2m (6ft), ↔ 1.2m (4ft). Origin unknown. ❄❄❄

CYNOGLOSSUM

Hound's tongue

BORAGINACEAE

Genus of about 55 species of annuals, biennials, and short-lived perennials from grassy places and rocky slopes in temperate regions and tropical uplands. They have alternate, narrowly lance-shaped to oblong or ovate, rough leaves, often clasping the stems, the lower ones stalked. They are cultivated for their usually blue, sometimes purple, rose-pink, or white flowers, similar to forget-me-nots (*Myosotis*), each with a short, tubular corolla and 5 widely spreading lobes, produced in one-sided, terminal cymes over a long period from spring to autumn. Grow in a mixed, herbaceous, or annual border.
• **HARDINESS** Fully hardy to half hardy.
• **CULTIVATION** Grow in moderately fertile, moist but well-drained soil in sun or partial shade. Plants become coarse and leafy and may not flower well in soil that is too fertile; they do not thrive in heavy clay soils.
• **PROPAGATION** Sow seed of perennials in containers in a cold frame in autumn

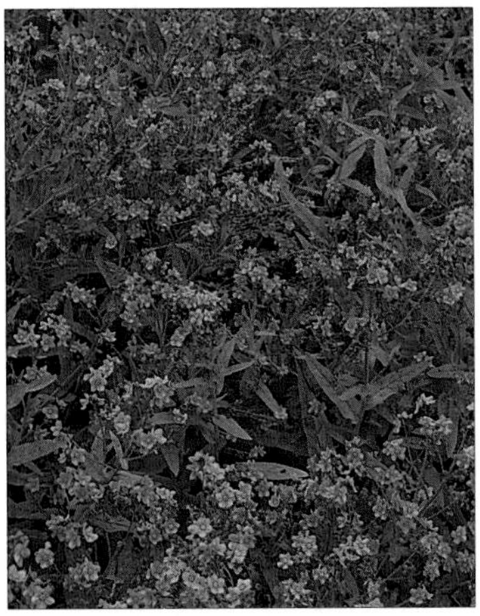

Cynoglossum amabile 'Firmament'

or spring. Sow seed of annuals and biennials *in situ* in mid-spring. Divide perennials in spring.
• **PESTS AND DISEASES** Prone to mildew.

C. amabile 🏆 (Chinese forget-me-not). Slow-growing, upright, bushy annual or biennial with obovate to lance-shaped, hairy, grey-green leaves, to 20cm (8in) long. Terminal cymes of pendent, sky-blue, sometimes white or pale pink flowers, 5–10mm (¼–½in) across, are produced in late summer. ↕ 45–60cm (18–24in), ↔ to 30cm (12in). E. Asia. ❄❄❄. **'Firmament'** ▣ is compact, with deep blue flowers and grey-hairy leaves; ↕ to 40cm (16in).
C. longiflorum see *Lindelofia longiflora*.
C. nervosum ▣ (Hound's tongue). Clump-forming, erect, bushy perennial with bristly stems and narrowly oblong-lance-shaped, softly hairy or bristly, bright green leaves: the basal leaves to 4cm (1½in) long, the lower stem leaves to 12cm (5in). Many-flowered cymes of azure-blue flowers, 1cm (½in) across, are produced from mid-spring to mid-summer. ↕↔ 60cm (24in). W. Pakistan, N.W. India (including Kashmir). ❄❄❄
C. officinale (Hound's tongue). Softly hairy biennial that in its first year forms a basal rosette of elliptic-oblong, grey-green leaves, 12cm (5in) long. In the second summer, ascending, leafy stems bear loose cymes of dull dark purple flowers, 6mm (¼in) across. ↕ 50–70cm (20–28in), ↔ 30–50cm (12–20in). Europe, W. Asia. ❄❄❄
C. wallichii. Upright, bushy, densely white-hairy annual or biennial with obovate to lance-shaped, prominently veined, mid-green leaves, to 18cm (7in) long. Dense, terminal cymes of pendent, pale to dark blue flowers, to 4mm (⅛in) across, are produced from spring to summer. ↕ 60–90cm (24–36in), ↔ to 45cm (18in). C. and S. Asia. ❄❄
C. zeylanicum. Upright, bushy annual or biennial with elliptic to oblong, densely brown- or yellow-hairy, mid-green leaves, to 20cm (8in) long. Bears terminal cymes of pendent, blue to white flowers, to 5mm (¼in) across, in summer. ↕ to 85cm (34in), ↔ to 45cm (18in). Afghanistan to Sri Lanka and Japan. ❄

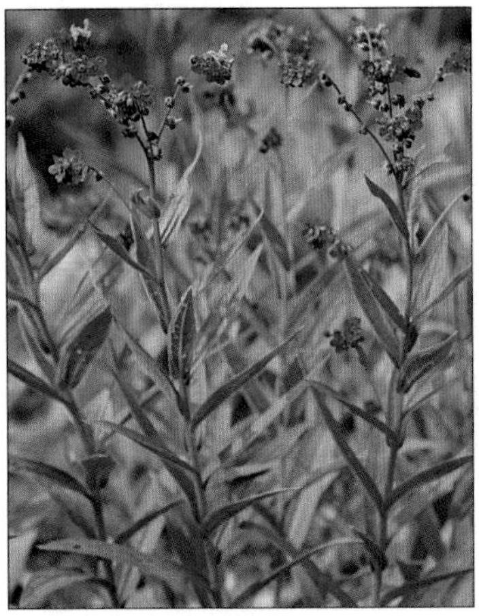

Cynoglossum nervosum

CYPELLA

IRIDACEAE

Genus of 15 species of bulbous perennials occurring in grassland and woodland, often near streams, in Central and South America. They are cultivated for their curious, iris-like flowers, each with 3 spreading outer tepals and 3 much smaller, incurved inner ones, borne singly or in terminal corymbs. Individual flowers are short-lived but are produced in succession over long periods in winter or summer. Leaves are linear-lance-shaped and pleated. In frost-prone areas, grow in a cool greenhouse or conservatory; in warmer climates, grow at the base of a warm wall or in a rock garden.
• **HARDINESS** Half hardy to frost tender.
• **CULTIVATION** Plant 8cm (3in) deep. Under glass, grow in 2 parts loam-based potting compost (JI No.2) to 1 part grit, in bright filtered light with good ventilation. In the growing season, water freely and apply a low-nitrogen liquid fertilizer monthly until flowers begin to form; keep dry and frost-free when dormant. Outdoors, grow in humus-rich, sandy soil, in a warm, sunny site. Either plant in autumn and protect with a mulch in winter, or plant in spring. Alternatively, in cold areas, lift bulbs after flowering and store in a frost-free place over winter.
• **PROPAGATION** Sow seed as soon as ripe at 7–13°C (45–55°F). Remove offsets when dormant, in late winter or spring if outdoors, or in summer or autumn, just before growth begins, if under glass.
• **PESTS AND DISEASES** Trouble free.

C. herbertii ▣ Bulbous perennial with linear-lance-shaped, pleated leaves, 15–30cm (6–12in) long, borne on the lower part of the stem. A succession of

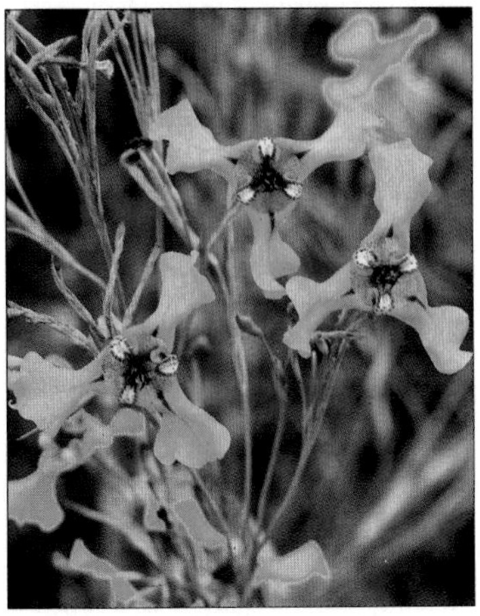

Cypella herbertii

C

flowers, 4–6cm (1½–2½in) across, with broad, mustard-yellow outer tepals and purple-spotted or lined inner ones, is produced in summer. ↕30–50cm (12–20in), ↔ 5cm (2in). Argentina, Uruguay. ❄

C

▷ ***Cyperorchis elegans*** see *Cymbidium elegans*

CYPERUS

CYPERACEAE

Genus of about 500–600 species of sedge- or grass-like annuals and evergreen, rhizomatous perennials, found almost exclusively in wet habitats throughout tropical and subtropical areas, with a small number in cool-temperate regions. They are grown for their foliage and unusual inflorescences. The cylindrical, 3-angled, or winged, often leafy stems, bear grass-like, linear leaves. Terminal, usually linear spikelets of hermaphroditic flowers have leaf-like bracts beneath, which in most species give the inflorescence a typically umbrella-like form. Grow at the margins of a pool or in a bog garden. In frost-prone areas, grow tender species as houseplants, in a temperate greenhouse or conservatory, or as marginal plants in an indoor pool.

- **HARDINESS** Fully hardy to frost tender.
- **CULTIVATION** Under glass, grow in loam-based potting compost (JI No.2 or 3) in bright filtered light. Stand containers in shallow trays of water to ensure ample moisture and high humidity at all times. In summer, apply a balanced liquid fertilizer monthly. To grow as a marginal in an indoor pool, grow in a watertight tub or bowl of loamy soil, top-dressed with a 2.5cm (1in) layer of gravel. Set at the pond edge with the gravel surface about 2.5–5cm (1–2in) below water level. Outdoors, *C. eragrostis* thrives in most soils, not necessarily damp ones, in sun or partial shade. It will usually self-seed, even if the parent plant is killed in extreme cold. Grow *C. longus* as a marginal plant, in water 15–30cm (6–12in) deep, or in moist soil in a sunny or partially shaded border. Cut back dead material in late autumn. In subtropical and tropical areas, grow all species outdoors as for *C. longus*.
- **PROPAGATION** Sow seed in permanently moist seed compost in spring; hardy species in containers in a cold frame, tender species at 18–21°C (64–70°F). Divide both tender and hardy species in spring. Plantlets will develop on the leafy inflorescences of some tender species if they are placed upside down in water.
- **PESTS AND DISEASES** Trouble free.

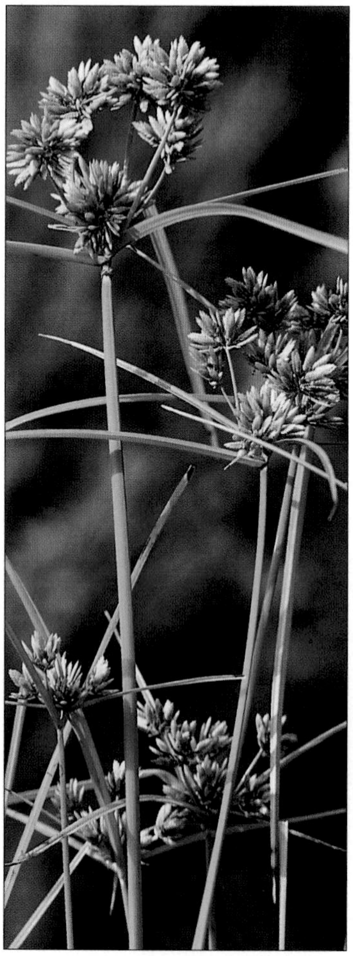

Cyperus eragrostis

C. albostriatus, syn. *C. diffusus* of gardens, *C. elegans* of gardens. Densely tufted perennial with slender, woody rhizomes and firm, thin, winged stems. Mid-green leaves, to 60cm (24in) long, have pale, prominent veins. From midsummer to early autumn, bears pale greenish yellow to pale brown spikelets in loose, compound umbels, 5–20cm (2–8in) across, above 6–9 leafy bracts, 0.8–1.5cm (⅜–½in) long. ↕60cm (24in), ↔ 30cm (1ft). Southern Africa. ❀ (min. 10°C/50°F). **'Variegatus'** has stems, leaves, and bracts conspicuously variegated with white stripes of varying widths; ↕60–90cm (24–36in).
C. alternifolius (Umbrella plant). Densely tufted perennial with woody rhizomes and no basal leaves. Numerous winged, dark green stems each bear a terminal whorl of 11–25 deep green, arching, leaf-like bracts, 10–15cm (4–6in) long. From summer to autumn, the stems are topped by small spikelets of pale yellow-brown flowers in compound umbels, to 12cm (5in) across. ↕45–90cm (18–36in), ↔ 40cm (16in). Madagascar. ❀ (min. 5°C/41°F)
***C. alternifolius* of gardens** see *C. involucratus*.
***C. diffusus* of gardens** see *C. albostriatus*.
***C. elegans* of gardens** see *C. albostriatus*.

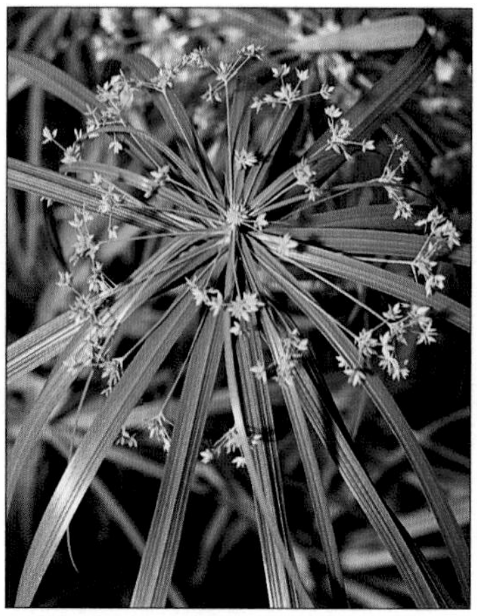

Cyperus involucratus

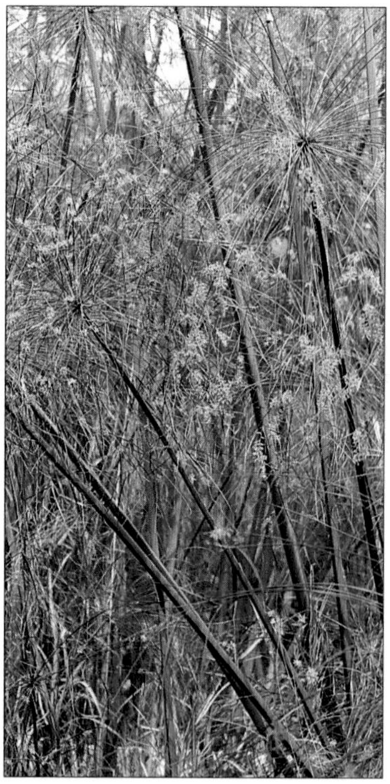

Cyperus papyrus

C. eragrostis ■ syn. *C. vegetus* (American galingale). Loosely tufted, shortly rhizomatous perennial with stout, winged stems bearing net-veined, rough-margined, bright green leaves, to 90cm (36in) long, which are V-shaped in section. From midsummer to early autumn, produces spherical clusters of pale green spikelets in spreading, compound umbels, 2.5cm (1in) across, above 5–8 linear bracts, 8–10cm (3–4in) long. Good for drying. ↕60–90cm (24–36in), ↔ 45cm (18in). W. USA, warm-temperate South America. ❄❄
C. flabelliformis see *C. involucratus*.
C. involucratus ■ 🏆 syn. *C. alternifolius* of gardens, *C. flabelliformis* (Umbrella grass). Clump-forming, tufted perennial with 12–28 leafy bracts in an umbrella-spoke arrangement, on 3-angled stems. Short, basal leaves are reduced to sheaths, 5cm (2in) long. In summer, produces 14–32 rays bearing tiny clusters of yellow flowers, which turn brown after producing pollen. ↕↔ 60–75cm (24–30in). Widely cultivated and naturalized throughout Africa. ❀ (min. 5–10°C/41–50°F)
C. longus (Galingale). Loosely tufted perennial with long, knotted rhizomes and stiff, erect, 3-angled stems. Each stem produces 2 or 3 arching, rough-margined, glossy, bright green leaves, 0.6–1.5m (2–5ft) long, grooved above, paler and sharply keeled beneath. In late summer and early autumn, bears red-brown spikelets in loose umbels, to 7cm (3in) across, above 2–6 leaf-like bracts that are often longer than the inflorescence. ↕0.6–1.5m (2–5ft), ↔ 1m (3ft) or more. Europe, N. Africa, S.W. and C. Asia. ❄❄❄
C. papyrus ■ (Egyptian paper rush, Papyrus). Clump-forming perennial with tall, 3-angled, pithy, leafless stems. Globe-like compound umbels of 100–200 thread-like rays, 12–30cm (5–12in) long, each ending in a tiny brown flower, become pendent with age. Ancient Egyptians flattened and dried the stems to make a form of paper. Needs high humidity. ↕2m (6ft), ↔ 0.6–1.2m (2–4ft). Egypt to tropical Africa. ❀ (min. 5–10°C/41–50°F).
C. vegetus see *C. eragrostis*.

CYPHOMANDRA

Tree tomato

SOLANACEAE

Genus of about 30 species of perennials and evergreen shrubs, trees, and climbers from the margins of dry forests in tropical America. Leaves are simple, occasionally 3-lobed, or compound, and arranged alternately. Star-, bowl-, or saucer-shaped flowers, each with 5 petal lobes, may be produced singly or in racemes or panicles from the upper leaf axils. Tomato-like, spherical to oblong-ellipsoid fruits, produced from summer to winter, are palatable only when fully ripe. In frost-prone climates, grow in a cool or temperate greenhouse; in warmer areas, use in a shrub border, courtyard garden, or fruit garden.

- **HARDINESS** Frost tender.
- **CULTIVATION** Under glass, grow in loam-based potting compost (JI No.3) in full or bright filtered light, with moderate humidity. In the growing season, water freely, applying a balanced liquid fertilizer monthly; water sparingly in winter. Top-dress or pot on in spring. Outdoors, grow in fertile, moist but well-drained soil in sun or partial shade. Pruning group 8; tip-prune when young. Plants under glass need restrictive pruning in late winter.
- **PROPAGATION** Sow seed at 13–18°C (55–64°F) in spring. Root greenwood cuttings with bottom heat in early summer.
- **PESTS AND DISEASES** Susceptible to whiteflies and red spider mites under glass.

C. betacea ■ ♀ syn. *C. crassicaulis*. Sparingly, robustly branched, small tree or large shrub with ovate to heart-shaped, softly downy, almost fleshy, mid- to deep green leaves, to 30cm (12in) long. From spring to summer, star- or bowl-shaped, white to pale buff-pink flowers, 2.5cm (1in) across, are produced in axillary racemes, 10–15cm (4–6in) long, followed by ellipsoid, brick- to orange-red, edible fruit, 5–6cm (2–2½in) long. ↕2–3m (6–10ft), ↔ 1–2m (3–6ft). Peru. ❀ (min. 5–7°C/41–45°F)
C. crassicaulis see *C. betacea*.

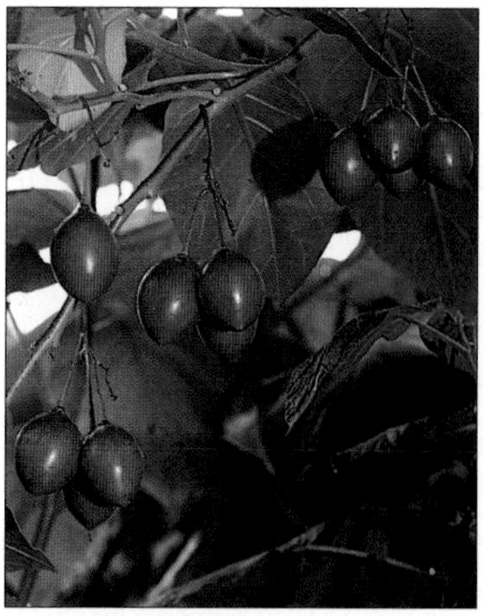

Cyphomandra betacea

CYPHOSTEMMA

VITACEAE

Genus of about 150 species of prostrate or climbing, often deciduous, perennial succulents from semi-desert areas of Africa and Madagascar. They sometimes have trunk-like caudices, often with peeling "bark", and produce fleshy branches, with the leaves clustered at their tips. The leaves may be pinnate or 3- to 7-palmate, occasionally simple. In some species, resin exudes from the leaf undersides. Corymbs of pendent, cup-shaped to cylindrical flowers are borne in summer, followed by ovoid fruits, which usually contain only one seed each. In frost-prone areas, grow in a warm greenhouse; in warmer climates, grow in a desert garden.

- **HARDINESS** Frost tender.
- **CULTIVATION** Under glass, grow in standard cactus compost in full light with low humidity. In growth, water sparingly, and apply a low-nitrogen fertilizer 2 or 3 times; keep completely dry once the leaves have fallen. Outdoors, grow in poor to moderately fertile, humus-rich, sharply drained soil, in full sun. See also pp.48–49.
- **PROPAGATION** Sow seed at 18–21°C (64–70°F) in spring. Root basal cuttings in spring.
- **PESTS AND DISEASES** Mealybugs may be a problem under glass.

C. bainesii, syn. *Cissus bainesii*. Deciduous, perennial succulent with a spherical or bottle-shaped caudex, which is often divided into 2 thick branches with peeling, pale yellow or green bark. Resinous, usually 3-pinnate leaves, to 12cm (5in) long, with lance-shaped, toothed, fleshy, silvery green leaflets, are silver-hairy when young. Flat-topped cymes of cup-shaped, yellowish green flowers, 1cm (½in) across, are produced in summer, followed by red fruit. ↕↔ 60cm (24in). S.W. Africa. ❁ (min. 10°C/50°F)

C. juttae ▣ syn. *Cissus juttae*. Deciduous, perennial succulent with very swollen stems and branches, which have peeling, yellowish green bark. Oval, 3-palmate, coarsely toothed, resinous, glossy, mid-green leaves, to 15cm (6in) long, are often red-tinted. Cymes of cylindrical, yellowish green flowers, 1cm (½in) across, are produced in summer, followed by red fruit. ↕↔ 2m (6ft). S. Namibia. ❁ (min. 10°C/50°F)

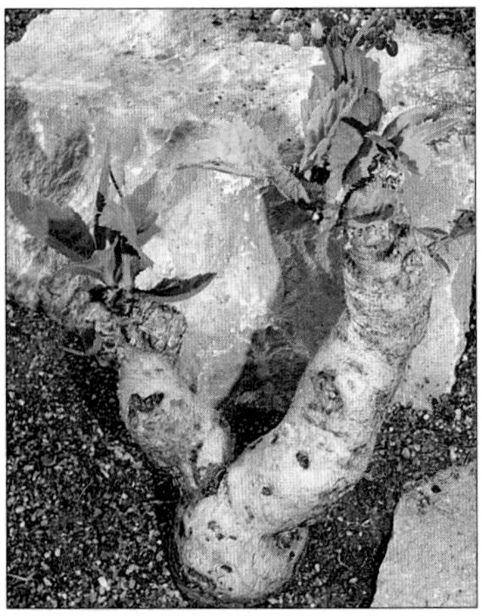

Cyphostemma juttae

▷**Cypress** see *Chamaecyparis, Cupressus*
Baker see *Cupressus bakeri*
Guadalupe see *Cupressus guadalupensis*
Hinoki see *Chamaecyparis obtusa*
Italian see *Cupressus sempervirens*
Kashmir see *Cupressus torulosa* 'Cashmeriana'
Lawson see *Chamaecyparis lawsoniana*
Leyland see x *Cupressocyparis leylandii*
Mediterranean see *Cupressus sempervirens*
Mexican see *Cupressus lusitanica*
Monterey see *Cupressus macrocarpa*
Nootka see *Chamaecyparis nootkatensis*
Pond see *Taxodium distichum* var. *imbricarium*
Sawara see *Chamaecyparis pisifera*
Smooth see *Cupressus arizonica* var. *glabra*
Summer see *Bassia scoparia* f. *trichophylla*
Swamp see *Taxodium, T. distichum*
White see *Chamaecyparis thyoides*
▷**Cypress pine** see *Callitris*
Oyster Bay see *C. rhomboidea*
Tasmanian see *C. oblonga*
▷**Cypress spurge** see *Euphorbia cyparissias*

CYPRIPEDIUM

Lady's slipper orchid

ORCHIDACEAE

Genus of about 35 species of deciduous, terrestrial orchids found in dry woodland or marshy places in temperate areas of the N. hemisphere, and in S. Asia and Mexico. They have slender rhizomes and several soft, folded, ovate to fan-shaped leaves, which are either spirally arranged or borne in opposite pairs. The flowers, produced singly or in terminal racemes of up to 12 flowers in summer, each have 3 spreading, white, pink, red, or purple tepals, and a slipper-shaped, yellow, white, pink, or dark purple pouch (an adaptation of the lip), hence the common name. *Cypripedium* species are suitable for a shady rock garden, peat bed, or woodland garden.

- **HARDINESS** Fully hardy to half hardy.
- **CULTIVATION** Grow in moist, fertile, leafy, humus-rich, neutral to acid soil, in a sheltered site, in light dappled or partial shade. *C. calceolus* prefers slightly alkaline soil; *C. reginae* prefers acid soil. Provide an annual winter mulch of leaf mould. See also p.46.

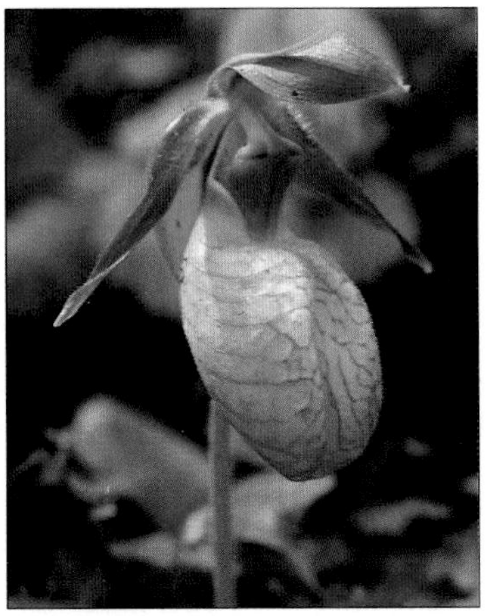

Cypripedium acaule

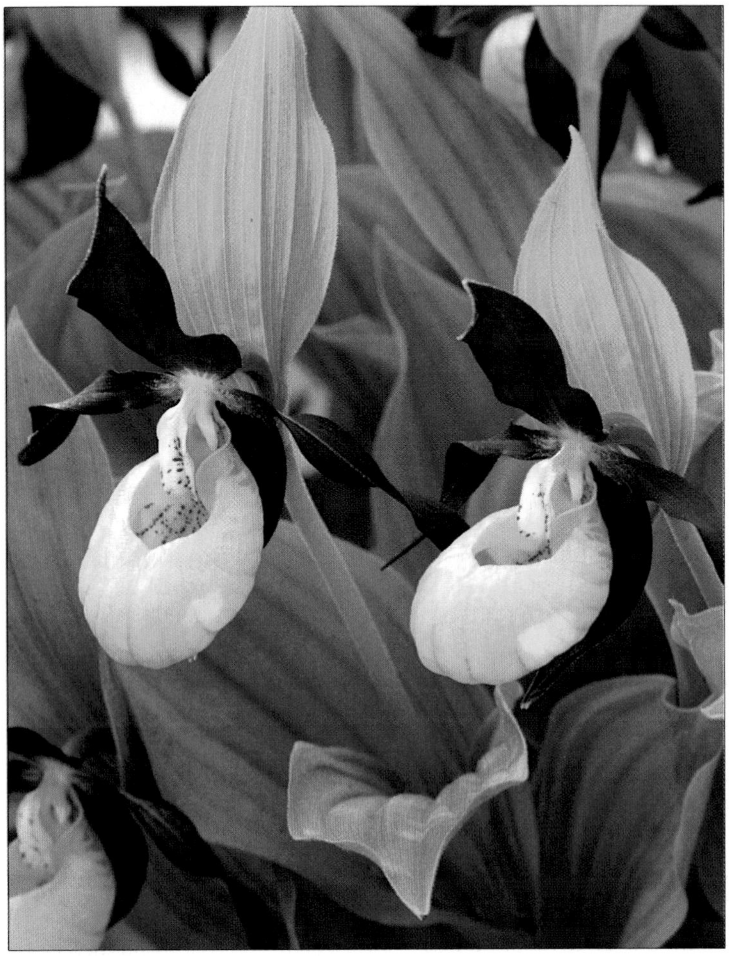

Cypripedium calceolus

- **PROPAGATION** Divide carefully in early or mid-spring, and replant immediately. Some of the soil from the root ball, which contains beneficial fungi, should be planted with each division.
- **PESTS AND DISEASES** Susceptible to grey mould (*Botrytis*) and slugs.

C. acaule ▣ Terrestrial orchid with 2 elliptic leaves, 10–23cm (4–9in) long. Solitary, nodding, light greenish brown flowers, 5cm (2in) long, with pink lips, are borne on upright stems in summer. ↕↔ 23cm (9in). Canada, E. USA. ❄❄❄

C. calceolus ▣ (Lady's slipper orchid). Terrestrial orchid with 3–5 ovate to elliptic leaves, 5–20cm (2–8in) long. In summer, bears purple-brown flowers, 9cm (3½in) long, with twisted petals and large, deep yellow lips, singly or in pairs on upright stems. ↕↔ 40cm (16in). Europe, Asia, North America. ❄❄❄

C. macranthon ▣ Terrestrial orchid with 3 or 4 ovate to elliptic leaves, 8–15cm (3–6in) long. Usually solitary, violet to purple-red or greenish brown flowers, 8cm (3in) across, with arching and downward-pointing tepals, are produced on upright stems in summer. ↕ 45cm (18in), ↔ 30cm (12in). N. Mongolia, N. and W. China, Korea, Japan. ❄❄❄

C. reginae ▣ (Showy lady's slipper orchid). Terrestrial orchid with 3–7 ovate to lance-shaped leaves, 10–23cm (4–9in) long. White flowers, almost 10cm (4in) long, with rose-pink lips, are borne singly or in pairs on upright stems in summer. ↕ 75cm (30in), ↔ 30cm (12in). E. North America. ❄❄❄

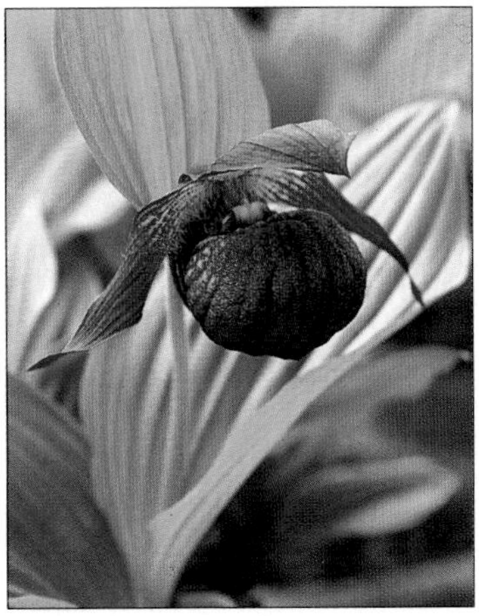

Cypripedium macranthon

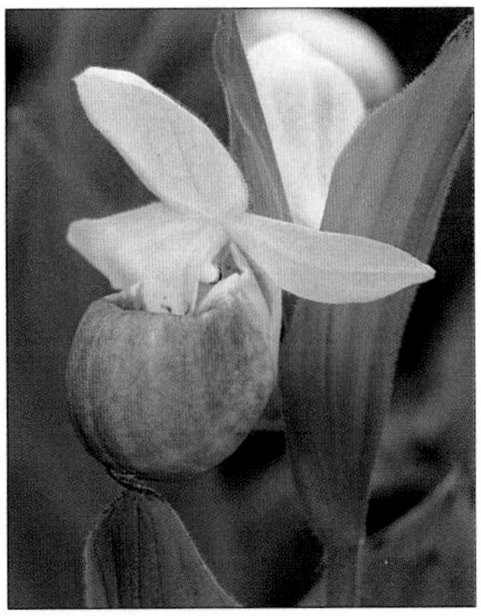

Cypripedium reginae

CYRILLA

CYRILLACEAE

Genus of one species of spreading, deciduous, semi-evergreen, or evergreen shrub or tree, found in moist woodland from S.E. USA to N. South America and Brazil. It is grown for its colourful autumn foliage, arranged alternately or occasionally in whorls, and for its long racemes of small, cup-shaped flowers, 5mm (¼in) long. *C. racemiflora* varies in hardiness according to its origin. In frost-prone climates, it is important to select stock from the northerly parts of the range to ensure that plants are hardy. Grow in a sheltered shrub border. In milder areas (particularly with hot summers), it grows vigorously and is evergreen.

- **HARDINESS** Fully hardy to half hardy.
- **CULTIVATION** Grow in fertile, humus-rich, moist but well-drained, acid soil in sun or partial shade, sheltered from cold, drying winds. Pruning group 9.
- **PROPAGATION** Sow seed in containers in a cold frame as soon as ripe in autumn. Root semi-ripe cuttings in summer. Insert root cuttings in winter.
- **PESTS AND DISEASES** Trouble free.

C. racemiflora Q (Leatherwood). Rounded shrub or, rarely, small tree with inversely lance-shaped to obovate, glossy, dark green leaves, to 10cm (4in) long, turning orange and red in autumn. From late summer to autumn, produces small, fragrant white flowers in slender, axillary racemes, to 15cm (6in) long. ↕↔ 1.2m (4ft). S.E. USA to Brazil (including West Indies). ❄❄❄ for plants from S.E. USA; ❄ for plants from Brazil.

CYRTANTHUS

Fire lily

AMARYLLIDACEAE

Genus of about 50 species of clump-forming, bulbous perennials from grassland to forest and cliffs in Africa. Most cultivated species are from South Africa. Usually deciduous, sometimes semi-evergreen, lance- to strap-shaped, mostly mid-green, basal leaves may be present or absent at flowering. Umbels of showy, tubular or tubular-bell-shaped to funnel-shaped flowers are produced on leafless stems mainly from spring to autumn. In frost-prone areas, grow in a cool or temperate greenhouse, or as a houseplant. Elsewhere, grow in a border or at the base of a warm, sunny wall.

- **HARDINESS** Frost hardy to frost tender.
- **CULTIVATION** Under glass, plant bulbs with the neck at soil level in loam-based potting compost (JI No.2), with added leaf mould and sharp sand, in bright filtered or full light with shade from hot sun. Water freely when in active growth, sparingly in winter; when dormant, keep deciduous species barely moist at not less than 5–10°C (41–50°F). In summer, apply a dilute, balanced liquid fertilizer every 2–3 weeks. Outdoors, plant at twice the bulb's depth in moderately fertile, humus-rich, well-drained soil in full sun.
- **PROPAGATION** Sow seed at 13–18°C (55–64°F) when ripe. Remove offsets in spring.
- **PESTS AND DISEASES** Trouble free.

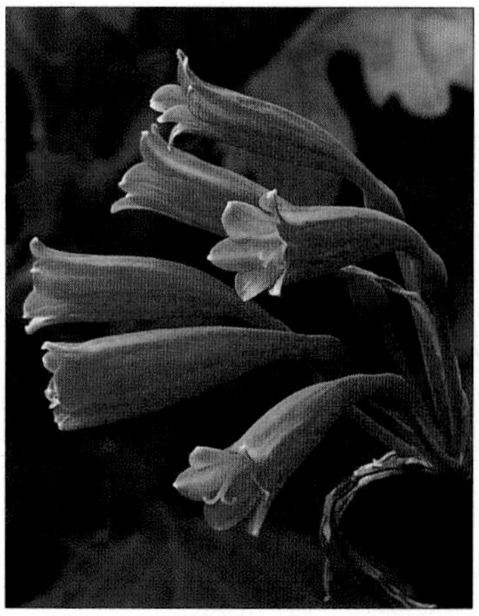

Cyrtanthus brachyscyphus

C. brachyscyphus ▣ syn. *C. parviflorus.* Deciduous perennial with semi-erect, lance-shaped, bright green leaves, 30cm (12in) long. From spring to summer, produces 6–12 narrowly tubular, slightly curved red flowers, 2.5–3cm (1–1¼in) long. ↕ 20–30cm (8–12in), ↔ 10cm (4in). S.E. South Africa. ❄

C. breviflorus, syn. *Anoiganthus breviflorus, A. luteus.* Deciduous perennial with erect, lance-shaped leaves, 20cm (8in) long. Up to 20 bell-shaped yellow flowers, to 3cm (1¼in) long, are produced at any time of year. ↕ 20cm (8in), ↔ 10cm (4in). South Africa (widespread). ❄❄ (borderline)

C. elatus ▣♀ syn. *C. purpureus, Vallota speciosa* (Scarborough lily). Deciduous perennial with erect, strap-shaped leaves, 20–45cm (8–18in) long. Produces up to 9 open funnel-shaped, bright scarlet flowers, 7–10cm (3–4in) long, in late summer. Easily grown on a window-sill. ↕ 30–60cm (12–24in), ↔ 10cm (4in). South Africa (Western Cape). ❄. **'Delicata'** has soft salmon-pink flowers.

C. falcatus. Deciduous perennial with broadly strap-shaped, curved leaves, to 25cm (10in) long. Up to 10 pendent, funnel-shaped red flowers, 6cm (2½in) long, are produced in spring. ↕ 30cm (12in), ↔ 10cm (4in). South Africa. ❄

C. mackenii* var. *cooperi ▣ Deciduous perennial with semi-erect, linear leaves, to 30cm (12in) long. From spring to summer, bears 4–10 narrowly tubular, scented, yellow or cream flowers, 5cm (2in) long. ↕ 20–30cm (8–12in), ↔ 10cm (4in). South Africa (Eastern Cape). ❄

C. obliquus. Deciduous perennial with strap-shaped, curved leaves, 20–60cm (8–24in) long. From winter to early summer, bears umbels of 6–12 funnel-shaped, bicoloured yellow and red, slightly green-tinged flowers, 7cm (3in) long. ↕ 30–60cm (12–24in), ↔ 8cm (3in). South Africa (S. KwaZulu/Natal, Eastern Cape). ❄

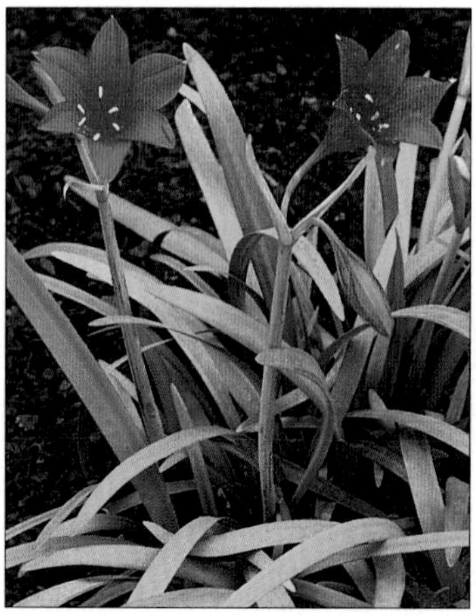

Cyrtanthus elatus

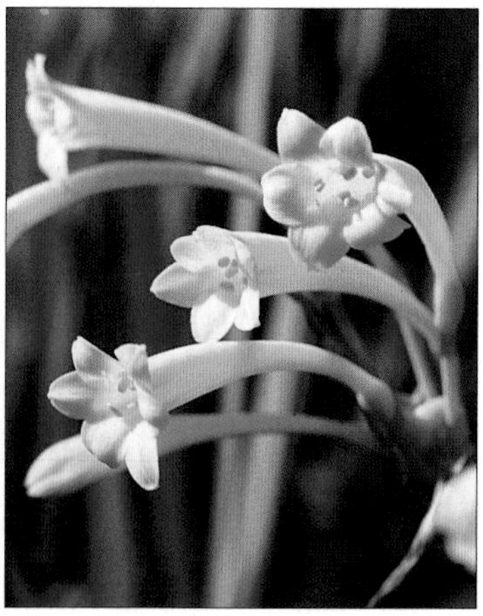

Cyrtanthus mackenii var. *cooperi*

C. parviflorus see *C. brachyscyphus.*

C. purpureus see *C. elatus.*

C. sanguineus. Deciduous perennial with semi-erect, strap-shaped leaves, to 40cm (16in) long. In summer, produces 1 or 2, rarely 3, open funnel-shaped, bright scarlet flowers, 8–10cm (3–4in) long. ↕ 30–50cm (12–20in), ↔ 10cm (4in). South Africa. ❄

▷ ***Cyrtochilum macranthum*** see *Oncidium macranthum*

CYRTOMIUM

syn. PHANEROPHLEBIA

DRYOPTERIDACEAE

Genus of 12 species of evergreen or deciduous ferns from often moist, rocky areas or woodland in C. and E. Asia. They have erect rhizomes and pinnate, leathery fronds with sickle-shaped, sharp-pointed pinnae. Sori, each with a peltate indusium, are scattered over the undersides of the pinnae. Most species have distinctive fronds, which provide strong contrast to more lacy ferns. Grow in a shady border or a rock garden. *C. falcatum* is also a handsome houseplant.

- **HARDINESS** Fully hardy to frost hardy.
- **CULTIVATION** Grow in moderately fertile, humus-rich, moist but well-drained soil in partial to full shade. In frost-prone areas, plant *C. falcatum* in the shelter of a rock and cover the crown with straw in winter. Under glass, grow in 1 part each loam, medium-grade bark, and charcoal, 2 parts sharp sand, and 3 parts coarse leaf mould, in bright indirect light. In growth, water freely and apply a dilute liquid fertilizer every 2 weeks; water moderately in winter.
- **PROPAGATION** Sow spores at 16°C (61°F) in late summer. See also p.51.
- **PESTS AND DISEASES** Trouble free.

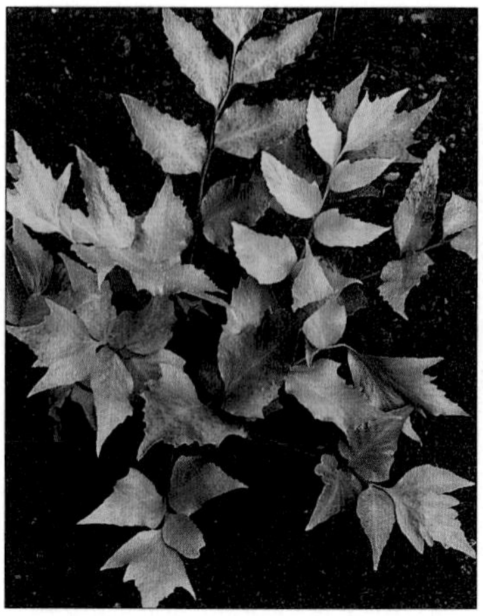

Cyrtomium falcatum

C. falcatum ▣♀ syn. *Phanerophlebia falcata* (Japanese holly fern). Evergreen fern, often deciduous in harsh climates. Spreading, glossy, dark green fronds, 20–60cm (8–24in) long, have holly-like pinnae, 4–6cm (1½–2½in) long. ↕ 60cm (24in), ↔ 1.1m (3½ft). Japan. ❄❄. **'Cristatum'**, syn. 'Mayi', has heavily crested frond tips and twisted pinnae tips; it is reluctant to spore. **'Mayi'** see 'Cristatum'. **'Rochfordianum'** has deeply cut pinnae margins.

C. fortunei, syn. *Phanerophlebia fortunei.* Evergreen fern with erect, dull, pale green fronds, 30–60cm (12–24in) long, with broadly sickle-shaped pinnae, 2.5–5cm (1–2in) long. ↕ 60cm (24in), ↔ 40cm (16in). E. Asia. ❄❄❄

C. macrophyllum (Large-leaved holly fern). Evergreen fern with spreading, broad fronds, 20–50cm (8–20in) long, with ovate to ovate-oblong pinnae, 10–20cm (4–8in) long. ↕ 45cm (18in), ↔ 60cm (24in). E. Asia. ❄❄❄

CYRTOSTACHYS

ARECACEAE/PALMAE

Genus of 8 or 9 species of single- or cluster-stemmed palms occurring in swampy ground and tropical forest from Malaysia, Indonesia (Sumatra), and Borneo to New Guinea and the Solomon Islands. Terminal clusters of ascending, pinnate leaves are borne above distinct crownshafts. Small, bowl-shaped, 3-petalled flowers are produced in panicles between the leaf clusters. In frost-prone climates, grow *C. lakka* as a

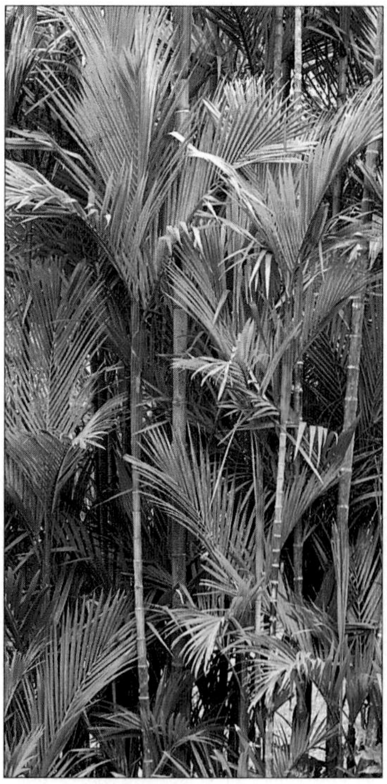

Cyrtostachys lakka

houseplant or in a warm greenhouse; in humid tropical areas, use as a specimen tree or in a courtyard garden.
• **HARDINESS** Frost tender.
• **CULTIVATION** Under glass, grow in loamless or loam-based potting compost (JI No.2) in bright filtered light, with moderate humidity. In growth, water freely, applying a balanced liquid fertilizer monthly; water moderately in winter. Pot on or top-dress in spring. Outdoors, grow in fertile, moist but well-drained soil in sun or partial shade.
• **PROPAGATION** Sow seed at 27°C (81°F) in spring. Remove and pot up suckers in spring.
• **PESTS AND DISEASES** Scale insects and red spider mites may be troublesome under glass.

C. lakka ■ ✻ (Lipstick palm, Sealing wax palm). Clump-forming, cluster-stemmed palm with erect, slender stems. Each stem is topped by a scarlet crown-shaft and a head of erect to ascending leaves, to 1.5m (5ft) long, with scarlet stalks and midribs, and many linear, mid-green leaflets, grey-tinted beneath. Panicles of bowl-shaped green flowers, 1cm (½in) long, are produced in summer. ↕ to 5m (15ft), ↔ to 3m (10ft). Malaysian Peninsula, Indonesia (Sumatra), Borneo. ⊛ (min. 16°C/61°F)

CYSTOPTERIS

Bladder fern

DRYOPTERIDACEAE/WOODSIACEAE

Genus of 10–20 species of deciduous, rhizomatous ferns found among calcareous rocks in temperate and sub-tropical areas. Very finely divided, lance-shaped or triangular fronds, usually pinnate or 2- to 4-pinnate to pinnatifid, arise from creeping or erect rhizomes; the sori are protected by bladder-shaped indusia, giving rise to the common name. Grow in a rock garden or shady fern border, or in an alpine house.
• **HARDINESS** Fully hardy.
• **CULTIVATION** Grow in fertile, moist but well-drained soil in partial shade. Shelter from cold, drying winds. Under glass, grow in 1 part each of loam, medium-grade bark, charcoal, and limestone chippings, 2 parts sharp sand, and 3 parts coarse leaf mould.
• **PROPAGATION** Sow spores at 16°C (61°F), or plant bulbils in late summer. Alternatively, divide rhizomes in spring. See also p.51.
• **PESTS AND DISEASES** Trouble free.

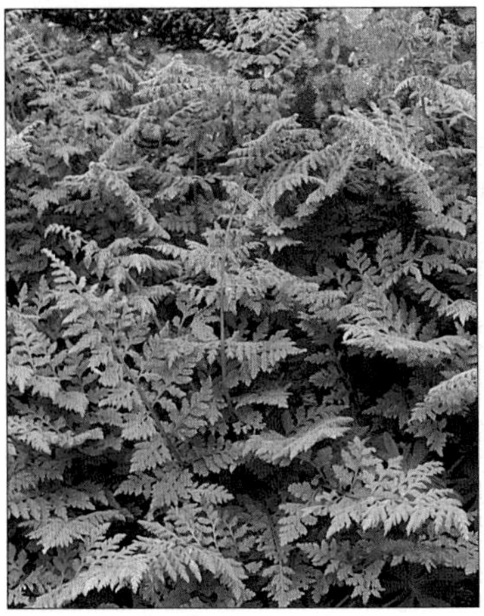
Cystopteris fragilis

C. bulbifera. Delicate, rosette-forming fern with erect rhizomes and tufts of erect, lance-shaped, 2-pinnate, pale green fronds, to 75cm (30in) long, with lance-shaped to linear-oblong segments. Bulbils develop beneath the often red-tinged midribs. Establishes quickly. ↕ 30cm (12in), ↔ 20cm (8in). North America. ❄❄❄
C. dickieana (Dickie's fern). Clump-forming fern with erect rhizomes and tufts of lance-shaped, 2- or 3-pinnate, grey-green fronds, 10–25cm (4–10in) or more long, with rounded lobes at the tips, and overlapping, ovate to oblong-lance-shaped segments. ↕ 15cm (6in), ↔ 20cm (8in). Europe. ❄❄❄
C. fragilis ■ (Brittle bladder fern). Clump-forming fern with erect rhizomes and tufts of lance-shaped, 2- or 3-pinnate, pale grey-green fronds, 15–45cm (6–18in) long, with oblong-lance-shaped segments, sharply pointed at the frond tips; frond segments do not overlap. ↕↔ 20cm (8in). Mainly N. temperate regions, Chile. ❄❄❄

▷ ***Cytisophyllum sessilifolium*** see *Cytisus sessilifolius*

CYTISUS syn. ARGYROCYTISUS

Broom

LEGUMINOSAE/PAPILIONACEAE

Genus of about 50 species, similar to *Genista*, of deciduous to evergreen shrubs, rarely small trees, from Europe, W. Asia, and N. Africa, found in well-drained soils, usually in open sites, from high mountains to scrub and heathland at lower altitudes. Brooms have alternate, usually 3-palmate, occasionally simple, mostly mid-green leaves, but are occasionally leafless when mature. They are cultivated for their abundant pea-like, sometimes very fragrant flowers, borne singly or in terminal or leafy, axillary racemes or clusters. Flowers are followed by linear or oblong, usually mid-green, often hairy or downy seed pods. The smaller species and cultivars are suitable for a rock garden or raised bed. Grow larger brooms in a shrub border; use prostrate variants as ground cover. In frost-prone regions, grow *C.* x *spachianus* as a houseplant, or in a conservatory or cool greenhouse. All parts, especially the seeds, may cause mild stomach upset if ingested.
• **HARDINESS** Fully hardy to frost tender.
• **CULTIVATION** Under glass, grow in loam-based potting compost (JI No.2) in full light. In the growing season, water freely and apply a balanced liquid fertilizer monthly; water sparingly in winter. Outdoors, grow in moderately fertile, well-drained soil in full sun. Provide less hardy species with shelter from cold, drying winds. Brooms thrive in poor, acid soils. Most are also lime-tolerant, but often become chlorotic on shallow chalk soils. Plant directly from containers when small; they resent transplanting. Pruning group 1 or 3; do not cut into the old wood. Prune *C. nigricans* in early spring. Prostrate and decumbent species generally need minimal pruning.
• **PROPAGATION** Sow seed in containers in a cold frame in autumn or spring. Root ripewood cuttings in midsummer, and semi-ripe cuttings in late summer.
• **PESTS AND DISEASES** Gall mites may be a problem.

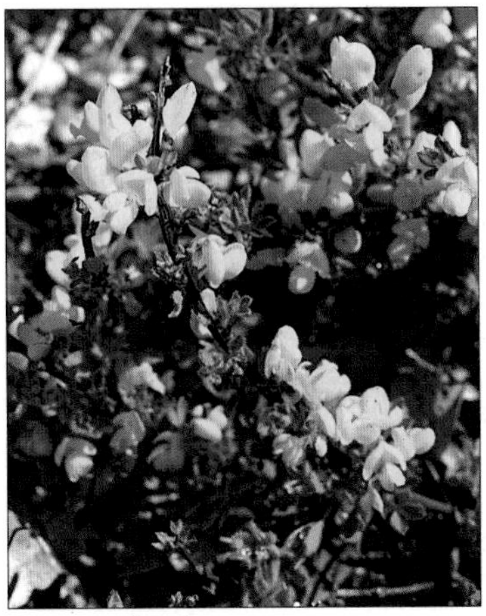
Cytisus ardoinoi

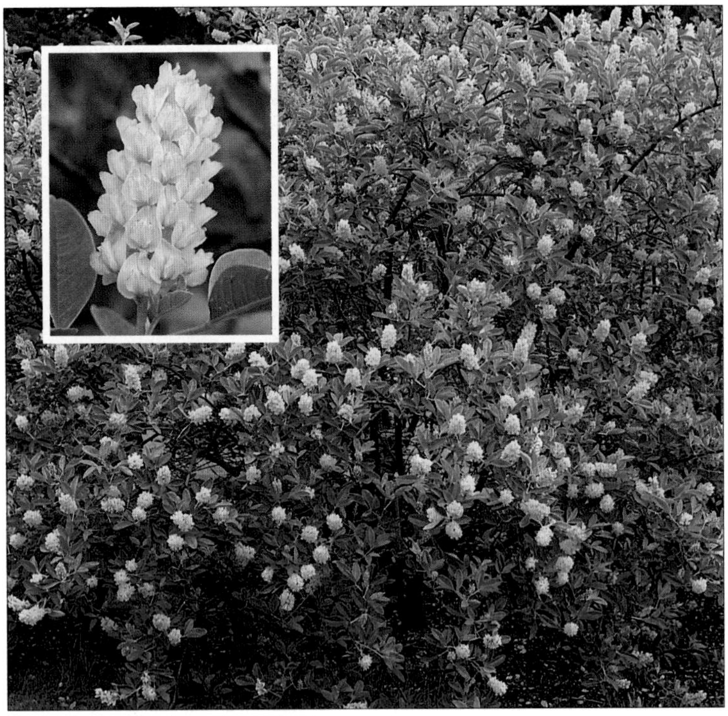
Cytisus battandieri (inset: flower detail)

***C. albus* of gardens** see *C. multiflorus*.
C. ardoinoi ■ ♀ Semi-prostrate, hummock-forming, deciduous shrub with arching, ridged stems and 3-palmate leaves, 8mm (⅜in) long. Axillary clusters of 1–3 bright yellow flowers, 1cm (½in) long, are borne from late spring to summer. ↕↔ 20–60cm (8–24in). Maritime Alps. ❄❄❄
C. battandieri ■ ♀ syn. *Argyrocytisus battandieri* (Pineapple broom). Vigorous, upright, tree-like deciduous shrub, spreading with age, with 3-palmate, silvery grey leaves, to 10cm (4in) long. Dense, upright, terminal racemes, to 15cm (6in) long, of pineapple-scented yellow flowers, 1.5–2cm (½–¾in) long, are produced in mid- and late summer. Tolerates an open but not exposed position. Pruning group 1. ↕↔ 5m (15ft). Morocco. ❄❄
C.* x *beanii ■ ♀ (*C. ardoinoi* x *C. purgans*). Semi-procumbent, deciduous shrub with arching, cylindrical stems and simple, linear, hairy leaves, to 1cm (½in) long. In spring, rich yellow flowers, 0.8–1.5cm (⅜–½in) long, are produced in axillary clusters of 1–3. ↕ to 60cm (24in), ↔ to 1m (3ft). Garden origin. ❄❄❄
***C.* 'Burkwoodii'** ♀ Rounded, bushy, deciduous shrub with slender shoots and 3-palmate leaves, 1–2cm (½–¾in) long. Dark pink flowers, 2cm (½in) long, with yellow-margined crimson wings, are produced in axillary clusters in late spring and early summer. ↕↔ 1.5m (5ft). ❄❄❄
***C. canariensis* of gardens** see *C.* x *spachianus*.
***C.* 'Cornish Cream'.** Bushy, spreading, deciduous shrub with slender, arching shoots and 3-palmate leaves, 1–2cm (½–¾in) long. In late spring and early summer, abundant flowers, 2.5cm (1in) long, in a mixture of creamy yellow and white, are produced in axillary clusters. ↕↔ 1.5m (5ft). ❄❄❄
C. decumbens, syn. *Genista decumbens*. Ascending or prostrate, deciduous shrub with wiry, branching stems and simple, oblong, finely hairy, stalkless leaves, 0.6–2cm (¼–¾in) long. Produces axillary clusters of 1–3 brilliant yellow flowers, 0.9–1.5cm (⅜–½in) long, in late spring and early summer. ↕ 10–30cm (4–12in), ↔ to 1m (3ft). S. Alps, Italy (Apennines). ❄❄❄

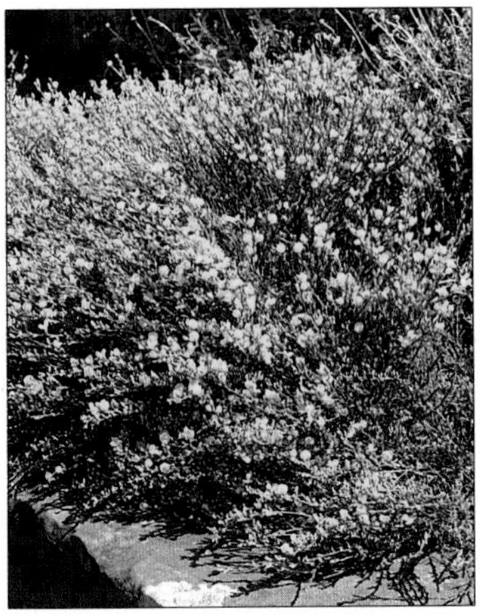
Cytisus x *beanii*

C

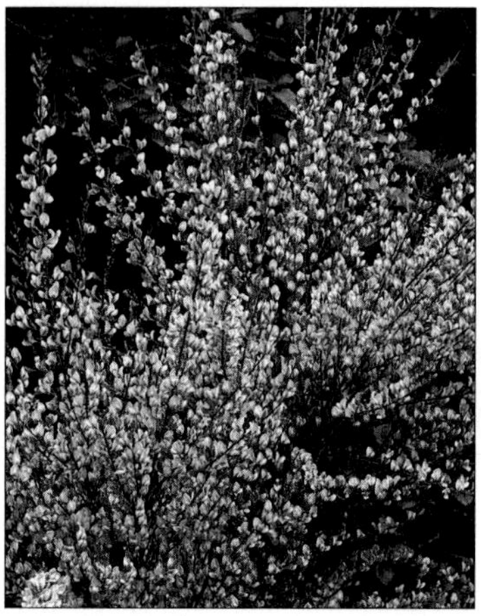

Cytisus 'Hollandia'

***C.* 'Dragonfly'.** Compact, deciduous shrub with slender, arching shoots and 3-palmate leaves, to 1cm (½in) long. Dark yellow flowers, 1.5cm (½in) long, with crimson wings, are produced in axillary clusters in late spring and early summer. ↕↔ 1.5m (5ft). ✲✲✲

***C.* 'Firefly'.** Rounded, bushy, deciduous shrub with slender, arching shoots and 3-palmate leaves, 1–2cm (½–¾in) long. In late spring and early summer, bears axillary racemes of abundant yellow flowers, 1.5cm (½in) long, with wings marked dark bronze-red. ↕↔ 1.5m (5ft). ✲✲✲

***C.* 'Golden Sunlight'.** Rounded, deciduous shrub producing slender, arching branches and 3-palmate leaves, 1–2cm (½–¾in) long. Abundant pale gold flowers, 1.5cm (½in) long, are borne in axillary racemes in late spring and early summer. ↕↔ 1.5m (5ft). ✲✲✲

***C.* 'Hollandia'** ▣ ♀ Rounded, deciduous shrub with slender, arching branches and 3-palmate leaves, 1–2cm (½–¾in) long. Abundant cream and dark pink flowers, 1.5cm (½in) long, are borne in axillary clusters in late spring and early summer. ↕↔ 1.5m (5ft). ✲✲✲

***C.* 'Johnson's Crimson'.** Rounded, deciduous shrub with long, arching shoots and 3-palmate leaves, 1–2cm (½–¾in) long. In late spring and early summer, produces axillary clusters of abundant carmine-red flowers, to 2cm (¾in) long, with pink wings. ↕↔ 1.5m (5ft). ✲✲✲

C.* x *kewensis ♀ (*C. ardoinoi* x *C. multiflorus*). Prostrate, deciduous shrub with arching stems, clothed in 3-palmate, softly hairy leaves, to 2cm

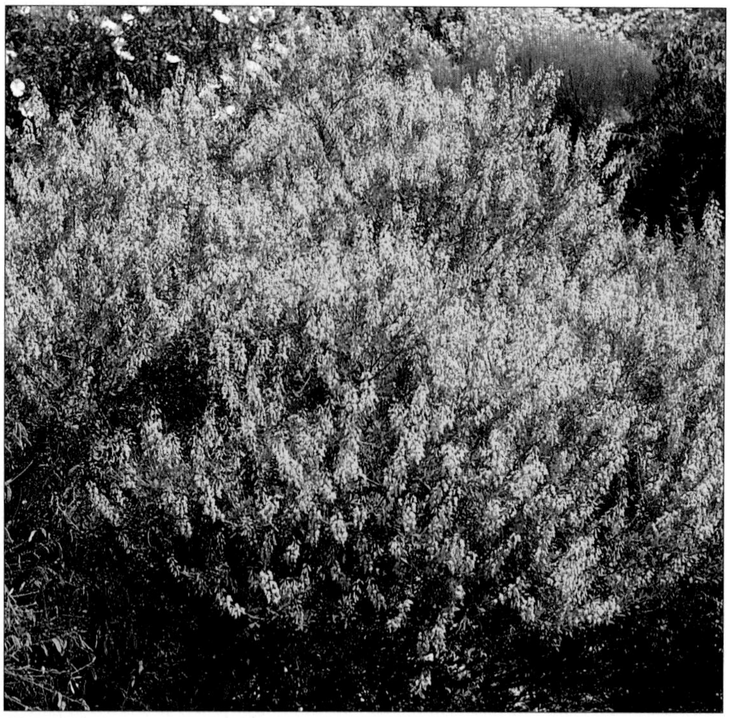

Cytisus nigricans

(¾in) long. Axillary racemes of 1–3 cream flowers, 1.5cm (½in) long, are produced along the lengths of downy branches in late spring. ↕ 30cm (12in), ↔ to 1.5m (5ft). Garden origin. ✲✲✲

***C.* 'Killiney Red'.** Compact, deciduous shrub with arching branches and 3-palmate leaves, 1–2cm (½–¾in) long. Abundant rich red flowers, 1.5cm (½in) long, with darker wings, are borne in axillary clusters in late spring and early summer. ↕ 1.2m (4ft), ↔ 1.5m (5ft). ✲✲✲

***C.* 'Lena'** ♀ Compact, spreading, deciduous shrub with 3-palmate leaves, 0.8–1.5cm (⅜–½in) long. In late spring and early summer, produces axillary clusters of dark yellow flowers, to 2cm (¾in) long, with the backs of the standards and wings bright red. ↕ 1.2m (4ft), ↔ 1.5m (5ft). ✲✲✲

C. leucanthus see *C. multiflorus*.

***C.* 'Maria Burkwood'.** Vigorous, spreading, deciduous shrub with slender, arching shoots and 3-palmate leaves, 1–2cm (½–¾in) long. Carmine-red flowers, 1.5cm (½in) long, with copper-bronze wings, are produced in axillary clusters in late spring and early summer. ↕↔ 1.5m (5ft). ✲✲✲

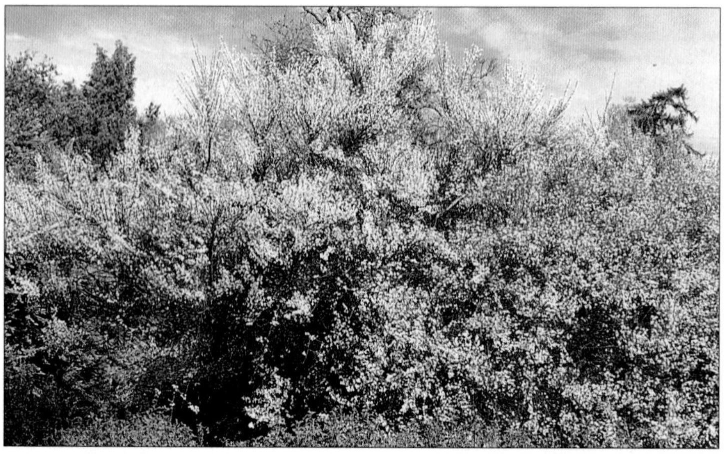

Cytisus multiflorus

C. multiflorus ▣ ♀ syn. *C. albus* of gardens, *C. leucanthus* (Portuguese broom, White Spanish broom). Upright then spreading, deciduous shrub with 3-palmate or simple, linear-oblong leaves, to 1cm (½in) long. Abundant white flowers, to 1.5cm (½in) long, are borne in axillary clusters in late spring and early summer. ↕ 3m (10ft), ↔ 2.5m (8ft). Portugal, Spain. ✲✲✲

C. nigrescens see *C. nigricans*.

C. nigricans ▣ syn. *C. nigrescens*, *Lembotropis nigricans*. Erect, deciduous shrub with upright shoots and 3-palmate leaves, to 2.5cm (1in) long. Yellow flowers, 1.5cm (½in) long, are produced in slender, terminal racemes in late summer. ↕ 1.5m (5ft), ↔ 1m (3ft). C. and S.E. Europe. ✲✲✲

***C.* 'Porlock'** ♀ Vigorous, arching, semi-evergreen shrub with upright shoots and 3-palmate leaves, 1–2cm (½–¾in) long. Terminal racemes of very fragrant, clear yellow flowers, 2cm (¾in) long, are produced in spring and, rarely, in mild weather in winter. ↕↔ 3m (10ft). ✲✲

C.* x *praecox (*C. multiflorus* x *C. purgans*). Compact, deciduous shrub with arching shoots and simple leaves, to 2cm (¾in) long. Produces axillary clusters of abundant pale yellow flowers, 1–2cm (½–¾in) long, in mid- and late spring. ↕ 1.2m (4ft), ↔ 1.5m (5ft). Garden origin. ✲✲✲. **'Allgold'** ▣ ♀ produces dark yellow flowers. **'Warminster'** ▣ ♀ (Warminster broom) has creamy yellow flowers.

C. purpureus see *Chamaecytisus purpureus*.

C. scoparius (Common broom). Upright, deciduous shrub with slender, arching shoots and usually 3-palmate leaves, 1–2cm (½–¾in) long. Abundant bright yellow flowers, 1.5–2.5cm (½–1in) long, are produced in axillary clusters in late spring. ↕↔ 1.5m (5ft). W. Europe. ✲✲✲. **f. *andreanus*** ♀ has yellow flowers, splashed red on the backs of the wings. **subsp. *maritimus***, syn. var. *prostratus*, is low-growing,

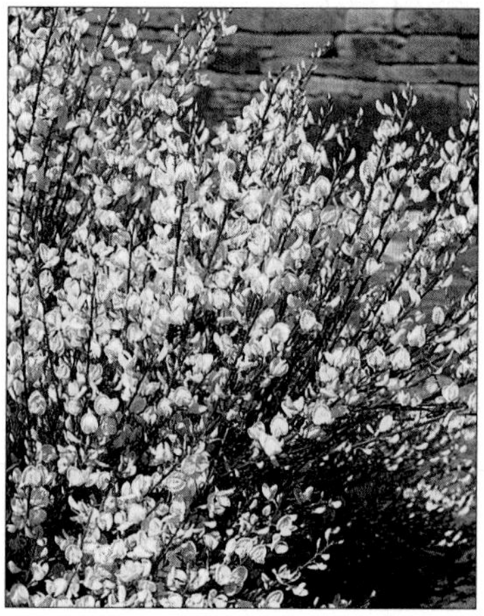

Cytisus x *praecox* 'Allgold'

forming a dense mound, with grey-green leaves; ↕ 20cm (8in), ↔ 1.5m (5ft). **'Moonlight'** is compact, with large, pale sulphur-yellow flowers, 1.5cm (½in) long; ↕↔ 75cm (30in). **var. *prostratus*** see subsp. *maritimus*.

C. sessilifolius, syn. *Cytisophyllum sessilifolium*. Bushy, deciduous shrub with angled shoots and more or less stalkless, 3-palmate leaves, 0.8–2cm (⅜–¾in) long. Yellow flowers, 1cm (½in) long, are produced in short, terminal racemes in early summer. ↕↔ 1.5m (5ft). S. France, E. Spain, Italy. ✲✲✲

C.* x *spachianus ♀ (*C. canariensis* x *C. stenopetalus*), syn. *C. canariensis* of gardens, *Genista fragrans* of gardens, *G.* x *spachiana*. Vigorous, evergreen shrub with upright, later arching branches and 3-palmate leaves, to 4cm (1½in) long. Bears slender, terminal racemes of very fragrant, golden yellow flowers, 1cm (½in) long, in late winter and early spring. ↕↔ 3m (10ft). Garden origin. ✲

C. supinus see *Chamaecytisus supinus*.

***C.* 'Windlesham Ruby'.** Rounded, bushy, deciduous shrub with slender, arching shoots and 3-palmate leaves, 1–2cm (½–¾in) long. Abundant rich red flowers, 1.5cm (½in) long, are borne in axillary racemes in late spring and early summer. ↕↔ 1.5m (5ft). ✲✲✲

***C.* 'Zeelandia'** ♀ Rounded, bushy, deciduous shrub with slender, arching shoots and 3-palmate leaves, 1–2cm (½–¾in) long. Abundant creamy white and lilac-pink flowers, to 2cm (¾in) long, are borne in axillary clusters in late spring and early summer. ↕↔ 1.5m (5ft). ✲✲✲

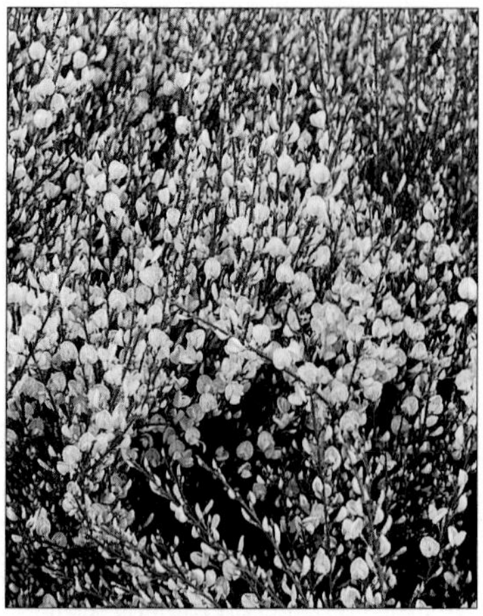

Cytisus x *praecox* 'Warminster'

D

DABOECIA

ERICACEAE

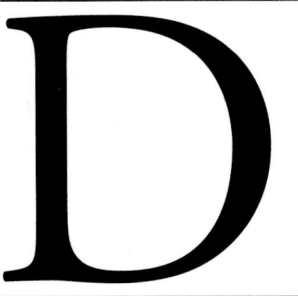

Genus of 2 species of evergreen shrubs from W. Ireland, W. France, N.W. Spain, N. Portugal, and the Azores; they occur from coastal cliffs to mountain heathland. Urn-shaped flowers are borne in racemes above alternate, lance-shaped to elliptic, usually dark green leaves. Use for ground cover in a heather garden or grow among other ericaceous shrubs. In frost-prone climates, grow half-hardy species in a cool greenhouse.

- **HARDINESS** Fully hardy to half hardy. *D. x scotica* is hardy to -10°C (14°F).
- **CULTIVATION** Under glass, grow in lime-free (ericaceous) potting compost in full light. In growth, water freely, applying a balanced liquid fertilizer monthly. Water sparingly in winter. Outdoors, grow in well-drained, acid soil in full sun; will tolerate neutral soil and partial shade. Pruning group 10, in early to mid-spring.
- **PROPAGATION** Root semi-ripe cuttings in midsummer.
- **PESTS AND DISEASES** Susceptible to *Phytophthora* root rot.

D. azorica, syn. *D. cantabrica* subsp. *azorica* (Azores heath). Compact shrub bearing narrowly elliptic leaves, 5–8mm (¼–⅜in) long, dark green above and silvery grey beneath, with recurved margins. Produces spherical-urn-shaped, ruby-crimson, sometimes paler flowers, 8mm (⅜in) long, in racemes 5cm (2in)

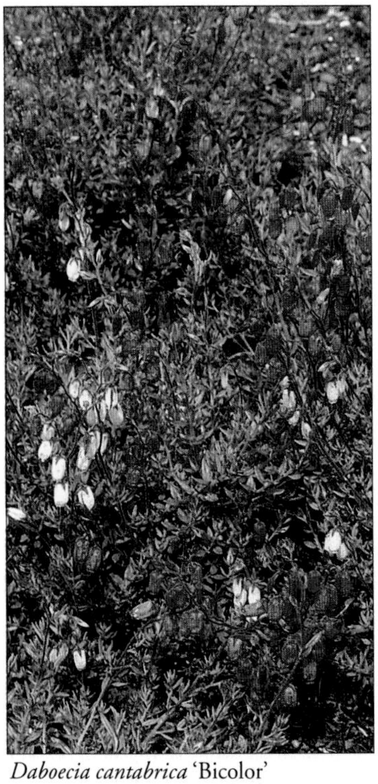

Daboecia cantabrica 'Bicolor'

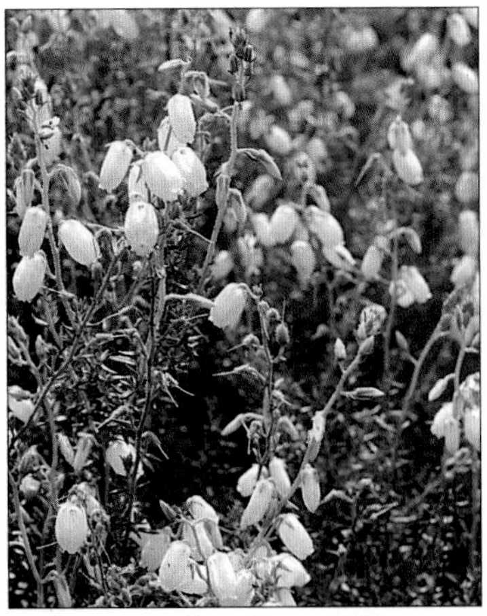

Daboecia cantabrica 'Snowdrift'

long, in early summer. ↕ 20cm (8in), ↔ 40cm (16in). Azores. ❄. **f. *albiflora*** has white flowers.

D. cantabrica, syn. *D. polifolia* (Cantabrian heath, St. Dabeoc's heath). Prostrate to erect shrub bearing lance-shaped to oval leaves, 7–10mm (¼–½in) long, usually dark green and lustrous above and densely silver-hairy beneath. Produces ovoid-urn-shaped, pinkish purple flowers, 1cm (½in) long, in racemes 10cm (4in) long, from early summer to mid-autumn. ↕ 25–40cm (10–16in), ↔ 65cm (26in). W. Europe. ❄❄❄. **subsp. *azorica*** see *D. azorica*. **'Bicolor'** ▣🏆 has mid-green foliage and white, pink, and beetroot-red flowers, some striped, often on the same raceme. **'Praegerae'** has mid-green leaves, which may be deciduous in hard winters, and glowing, deep cerise flowers; ↕ 40cm (16in), ↔ 70cm (28in); ❄ (borderline). **'Snowdrift'** ▣ has white flowers and bright green leaves. **'Waley's Red'** 🏆 syn. 'Whalley', has glowing, deep magenta flowers; ↔ 50cm (20in).

D. polifolia see *D. cantabrica*.

D. x scotica (*D. azorica* x *D. cantabrica*). Compact shrub with elliptic to elliptic-ovate, dark green leaves, 6–9mm (¼–⅜in) long. Racemes, 10cm (4in) long, of ovoid-urn-shaped, crimson to lilac-pink or white flowers, 9mm (⅜in) long, are borne from late spring to mid-autumn. ↕ 25cm (10in), ↔ 40cm (16in). Garden origin. ❄❄. **'Silverwells'** 🏆 produces mid-green foliage and white flowers; ↕ 15cm (6in), ↔ 35cm (14in). **'William Buchanan'** ▣🏆 produces purple-crimson flowers; ↕ 35cm (14in), ↔ 55cm (22in).

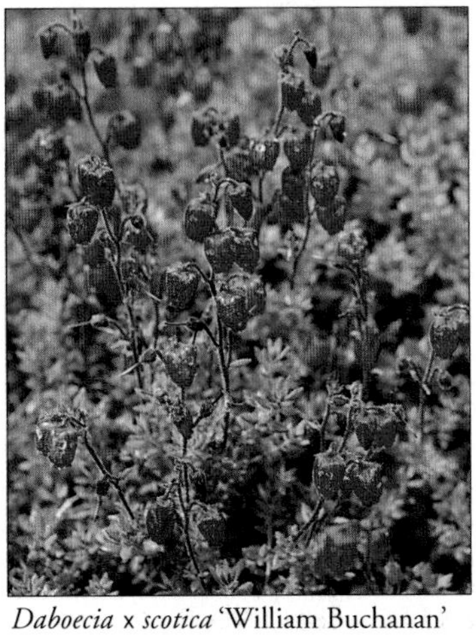

Daboecia x *scotica* 'William Buchanan'

DACRYDIUM

PODOCARPACEAE

Genus of 25–30 species of dioecious, evergreen, coniferous trees and shrubs found in habitats ranging from swamps to dry, mountainous areas in subtropical S.E. Asia, W. Pacific islands, and New Zealand. They have linear juvenile leaves and spirally arranged, scale-like adult leaves, which lie flat along the shoots. The male cones are cylindrical and borne in short, axillary spikes; female cones are erect and terminal. In areas with humid summers and mild, damp winters, grow as specimen plants or in a shrub border; in frost-prone areas, grow in a cool greenhouse or conservatory.

- **HARDINESS** Frost hardy to frost tender.
- **CULTIVATION** Under glass, grow in loam-based potting compost (JI No.3) in full or bright filtered light, with high humidity. In summer, water freely and apply a balanced liquid fertilizer monthly; water sparingly in winter. Outdoors, grow in moist but well-drained, humus-rich soil in sun or partial shade.
- **PROPAGATION** Sow seed in containers in a cold frame, or root semi-ripe cuttings from mid- to late summer.
- **PESTS AND DISEASES** Trouble free.

D. cupressinum ◊ (Rimu). Conical, later rounded, coniferous tree with dark green foliage. Pointed, linear juvenile leaves, to 7mm (¼in) long, are arching or pendent; scale-like adult leaves are up to 3mm (⅛in) long. Female cones each contain a single, blue-black seed with a red or orange aril. ↕ to 10m (30ft), ↔ 3–10m (10–30ft). New Zealand. ❄❄

DACTYLIS

GRAMINEAE/POACEAE

Genus of 2 species of evergreen, perennial grasses from open grassland in Europe, N. Africa, and Asia. They have linear leaves and one-sided panicles of compressed, pale green spikelets. *D. glomerata* 'Variegata' looks best at the front of a border or in a rock garden.

- **HARDINESS** Fully hardy.
- **CULTIVATION** Grow in fertile, well-drained soil in sun or partial shade.
- **PROPAGATION** Divide in early or mid-spring.
- **PESTS AND DISEASES** Trouble free.

***D. glomerata* 'Variegata'.** Densely tufted, clump-forming, perennial grass with linear, white-variegated leaves, to 15cm (6in) long. Pale green spikelets in one-sided panicles, 5cm (2in) long, are borne on stems 25cm (10in) long, throughout summer. ↕ to 45cm (18in) in flower, ↔ 25cm (10in). ❄❄❄

DACTYLORHIZA

Marsh orchid, Spotted orchid

ORCHIDACEAE

Genus of about 30 species of tuberous, deciduous, terrestrial orchids found in meadows, heathland, or marshy stream-sides in Europe, N. Africa, Asia, and North America. They have finger-like, flattened tubers and linear to lance-shaped, fleshy, usually mid-green, sometimes spotted leaves, 10–20cm (4–8in) long. Purple, lilac-purple, red, pink, or white flowers, with green, sometimes purplish bracts, are borne in dense, upright, terminal racemes, mostly 5–15cm (2–6in) long. Grow in a rock or woodland garden, or in meadowland.

- **HARDINESS** Fully hardy.
- **CULTIVATION** Grow in moist but well-drained, humus-rich, leafy soil in partial shade. See also p.46.
- **PROPAGATION** Divide in early spring.
- **PESTS AND DISEASES** Trouble free.

D

D. elata 🏆 syn. *Orchis elata* (Robust marsh orchid). Terrestrial orchid with 6–10 linear to ovate-lance-shaped, sometimes brown- or purple-spotted leaves. Deep purple flowers, with long, protruding bracts, are produced in racemes 10–25cm (4–10in) long, in late spring. ↕ to 60cm (24in), ↔ 15cm (6in). S.W. Europe. ❄❄❄

D. foliosa ▣🏆 syn. *D. maderensis*, *Orchis maderensis*. Robust, terrestrial orchid with 4–6 lance-shaped leaves, sometimes brown- or purple-spotted. Pink to bright purple flowers, with bracts protruding or just hidden, are produced in racemes 5–13cm (2–5in) long, in late spring and early summer. ↕ 60cm (24in), ↔ 15cm (6in). Madeira. ❄❄❄

D. fuchsii, syn. *D. maculata* subsp. *fuchsii*. Terrestrial orchid with 8–12 lance-shaped, purple-spotted leaves. Pale pink to white or mauve flowers, marked deep red or purple, are produced in late spring and early summer. ↕ 20–60cm (8–24in), ↔ 10cm (4in). Europe, W. Asia. ❄❄❄

D. maculata (Heath spotted orchid). Terrestrial orchid with 5–12 lance-shaped, plain or brown- or purple-spotted leaves. Bears white, rose-pink, red, or mauve flowers from mid-spring to late summer. ↕ 15–60cm (6–24in), ↔ 15cm (6in). Europe, N. Africa. ❄❄❄. **subsp. *fuchsii*** see *D. fuchsii*.

D. maderensis see *D. foliosa*.

▷ **Daffodil** see *Narcissus*
Autumn see *Sternbergia*
Hoop-petticoat see *Narcissus bulbocodium*
Peruvian see *Hymenocallis narcissiflora*
Queen Anne's double see *Narcissus* 'Eystettensis'
Sea see *Pancratium maritimum*
Tenby see *Narcissus obvallaris*
White hoop-petticoat see *Narcissus cantabricus*
Wild see *Narcissus pseudonarcissus*

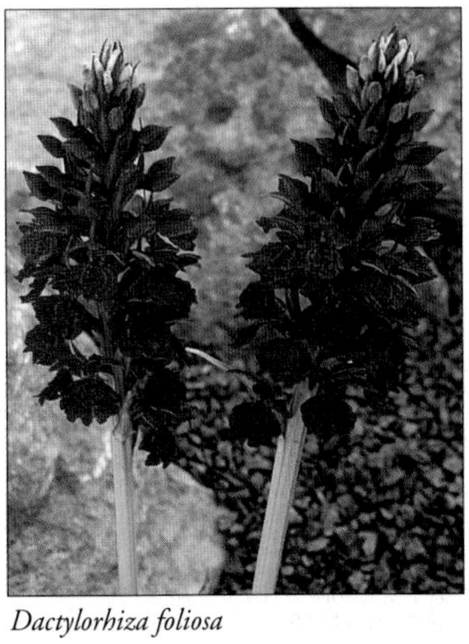

Dactylorhiza foliosa

DAHLIA

DAHLIA

ASTERACEAE/COMPOSITAE

Genus of about 30 species – and some 20,000 cultivars, predominantly derived from *D. pinnata* and *D. coccinea* – of bushy, usually tuberous-rooted perennials from mountainous areas of Mexico and Central America. The mid- to dark green leaves, 20–50cm (8–20in) long, are usually pinnate, the toothed, oval leaflets having rounded tips, or are sometimes pinnatifid to pinnatisect. Dahlias are grown for their flowerheads, cultivated in a variety of forms (see panel below), and in colours from white to red, orange to yellow, and pink to dark purple. They flower from mid-summer to autumn (until the first frosts in cool-temperate regions), when many other plants are past their best. Although often informally divided into 2 types – tall-growing "border" dahlias and low-growing "bedding" dahlias – all are good for garden display and cutting. Many, especially the giant-flowered dahlias, are also suitable for exhibition. Bedding dahlias, which may be raised from seed and treated as annuals, flower from early or midsummer to autumn, particularly if dead-headed, and are suitable for massed plantings, for edging a border, or for growing in a container. Those grown for exhibition or cutting look best in rows on their own, free from competition with other plants.

Most dahlias are classified according to the form of their flowerheads. In addition, the groups most commonly grown for exhibition are classified by the width of the flowerhead (see table below), although the precise dimensions may vary according to the specifications of the various national dahlia societies.

EXHIBITION FLOWERHEAD SIZES

GIANT	over 25cm (10in)
LARGE	20–25cm (8–10in)
MEDIUM	15–20cm (6–8in)
SMALL	10–15cm (4–6in)
MINIATURE	less than 10cm (4in)

Single-flowered dahlias
Flowerheads are open-centred, with 1 or 2 rows of ray-florets, which may overlap, surrounding a central cluster of tiny disc-florets. Flowerheads are usually less than 10cm (4in) across.

Waterlily dahlias
Flowerheads are double with relatively few, broad ray-florets, which are either flat, or slightly incurved or recurved along their margins, giving the blooms a flattened, shallow appearance. Blooms are classified by size, and range from miniature- to giant-flowered.

DAHLIA GROUPS

Most dahlias are divided into groups determined by the form of their flowerheads. Those groups commonly cultivated for exhibition purposes – waterlily, ball, semi-cactus, cactus, and decorative – are also classified by size (see table above).

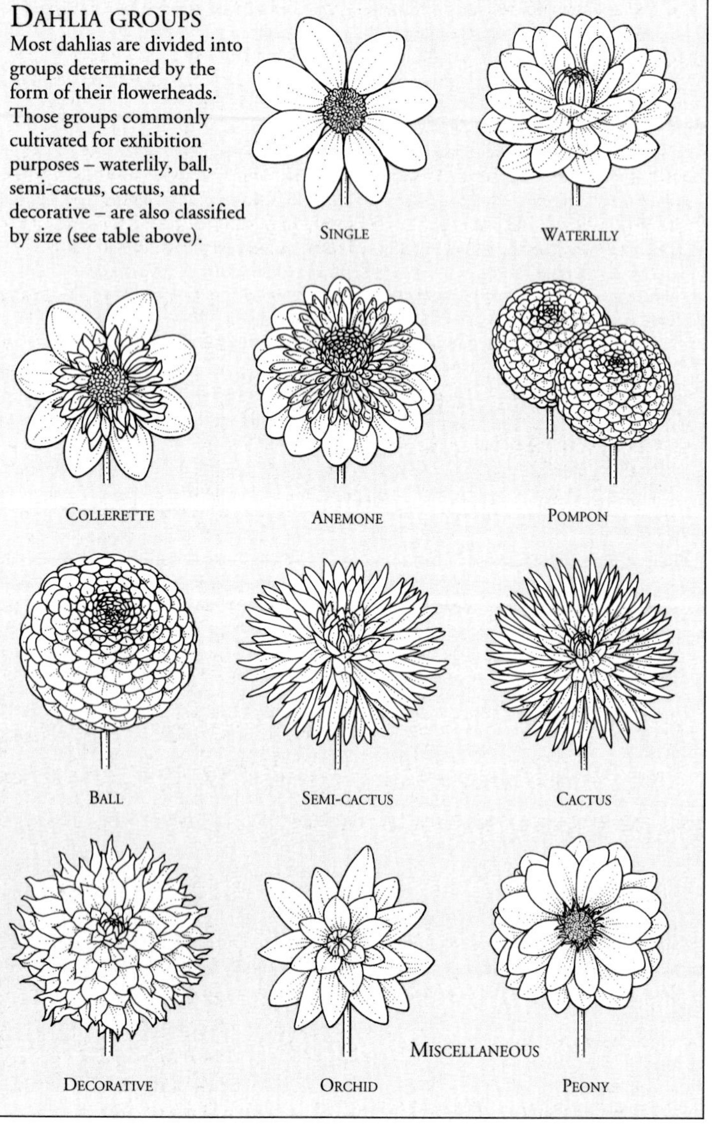

Collerette dahlias
Flowerheads have an outer, single row of usually flat ray-florets, which may overlap, surrounding an inner ring of shorter florets (the collar) around a central disc. Flowerheads are usually 10–15cm (4–6in) across.

Anemone-flowered dahlias
Flowerheads are double with one or more rings of usually flattened ray-florets surrounding a dense group of upward-pointing, tubular florets, which are longer than the disc-florets of single-flowered dahlias. Flowerheads are usually 10–15cm (4–6in) across.

Pompon dahlias
Pompons are similar to ball dahlias but more spherical, with florets incurved for the whole of their length. Flowerheads are no more than 5cm (2in) across.

Ball dahlias
Flowerheads are fully double, ball-shaped, or slightly flattened at the top. The ray-florets are spirally arrranged, incurved for more than half of their length, and blunt or rounded at the tips. Blooms are classified by size, and range from miniature- to small-flowered.

Semi-cactus dahlias
Blooms are fully double with slightly pointed ray-florets, broader at the base than those of cactus dahlias. They are recurved for up to half of their length towards the petal tips, and either straight or curling towards the centre. Blooms are classified by size, ranging from miniature- to giant-flowered.

Cactus dahlias
Flowerheads are fully double with long, narrow, pointed ray-florets, strongly recurved for more than half of their length, and either straight or curling towards the centre of the bloom. Blooms are classified by size, and range from miniature- to giant-flowered.

Decorative dahlias
Flowerheads are fully double, showing no central disc, with ray-florets that are broad, generally flat or slightly incurved at their margins, sometimes slightly twisted, and usually with blunt points. Blooms are classified by size, and range from miniature- to giant-flowered.

Miscellaneous dahlias
Dahlias that do not fall into any of the above groups may be classified into informal groups, including orchid-, chrysanthemum-, and peony-flowered, and star and lilliput dahlias.

• **HARDINESS** Frost hardy to frost tender.
• **CULTIVATION** Grow in fertile, humus-rich, well-drained soil in full sun. All dahlias benefit from a high-nitrogen liquid fertilizer every week in early summer, then a high-potash fertilizer every week from midsummer to early autumn. Bedding dahlias need no staking or disbudding: simply pinch out the growing point to encourage bushiness, and dead-head as the flowers fade. For taller dahlias, insert canes or stakes at planting time; when plants are about 40cm (16in) tall, pinch out the growing tips to encourage branching. For giant blooms, restrict plants to 3–5 flowering stems; for smaller blooms, allow 7–10 flowering stems. To produce high-quality blooms, remove the 2 pairs of buds developing in the leaf axils below the terminal bud; for giant blooms, remove 3 pairs. Dead-head as the flowers fade. In mid-autumn, preferably when the foliage has been blackened by the first frosts, cut back stems to 15cm (6in), and lift the tubers. Gently brush off the soil, and place upside down in frost-free conditions to dry naturally. Dust with fungicide, then pack in boxes of peat or dry sand and store over winter in a well-ventilated, frost-free place. Check periodically for fungal infection, cut out any damaged tissue, and re-treat with fungicide, then return to store. In frost-free areas, dahlias may be left in the ground over winter, but where occasional frosts are expected, apply a deep, dry mulch.
• **PROPAGATION** Sow seed of bedding dahlias in trays at 16°C (61°F) in early spring; harden off and plant out when all danger of frost has passed. Take basal shoot cuttings from tubers started into growth in late winter or early spring under glass, and root in a propagating case. Alternatively, start tubers into growth in early spring and, when shoots are 2cm (¾in) long, divide tubers into 2 or 3 pieces, each with a shoot; plant these out, 12cm (5in) deep, after all danger of frost has passed.
• **PESTS AND DISEASES** Aphids, capsid bugs, red spider mites, caterpillars, earwigs, and slugs may be troublesome. Also prone to powdery mildew, mosaic virus, tomato spotted wilt virus, and rotting of tubers in store.

***D.* 'Abingdon Ace'.** Small-flowered decorative dahlia with dark red blooms on strong stems. Good for exhibition. ↕ 1.2m (4ft), ↔ 60cm (24in). ✲

***D.* 'Abridge Natalie'** ▣ Small-flowered waterlily dahlia bearing blooms in blends of light and dark pink, with a touch of yellow at the base of each petal. ↕ 1.1m (3½ft), ↔ 60cm (24in). ✲

***D.* 'Abridge Patricia'.** Small-flowered waterlily dahlia producing blooms in blends of lilac and white on strong, slender stems. ↕ 1.2m (4ft), ↔ 60cm (24in). ✲

***D.* 'Alfred C'.** Giant-flowered semi-cactus dahlia with blooms in blends of orange and bronze. Good for exhibition. ↕ 1.3m (4½ft), ↔ 60cm (24in). ✲

***D.* 'Alloway Cottage'** ▣ Medium-flowered decorative dahlia producing very full, formal blooms in soft yellow, with a touch of lavender-blue on the tip of each petal. Good for exhibition. ↕ 1.2m (4ft), ↔ 60cm (24in). ✲

***D.* 'Alltami Alpine'.** Medium-flowered decorative dahlia bearing white blooms, each with a touch of lavender-blue in the centre. Good for exhibition. ↕ 1.5m (5ft), ↔ 75cm (30in). ✲

***D.* 'Alltami Apollo'.** Short-growing, giant-flowered semi-cactus dahlia producing waxy white blooms. Good for exhibition. ↕ 1.1m (3½ft), ↔ 60cm (24in). ✲

***D.* 'Alltami Cherry'.** Small-flowered ball dahlia with vivid, cherry-red blooms. Good for exhibition. ↕ 1.1m (3½ft), ↔ 60cm (24in). ✲

***D.* 'Alltami Classic'.** Medium-flowered decorative dahlia bearing clear yellow blooms on strong, compact stems. Good for exhibition. ↕ 1.2m (4ft), ↔ 60cm (24in). ✲

***D.* 'Alltami Corsair'** ▣ Very free-flowering, medium-flowered semi-cactus dahlia with blooms in very rich, unfading crimson. Good for exhibition. ↕ 1.3m (4½ft), ↔ 60cm (24in). ✲

D. 'Alltami Cosmic' ▣ Large-flowered decorative dahlia producing rich orange blooms, each with a pink tinge in the centre. Good for exhibition. ↕1.5m (5ft), ↔ 75cm (30in). ❄
D. 'Alva's Doris' ▣ ♀ Very free-flowering, small-flowered cactus dahlia bearing blood-red blooms on strong stems. Good for exhibition. ↕1.2m (4ft), ↔ 60cm (24in). ❄
D. 'Alva's Supreme' ▣ Giant-flowered decorative dahlia with blooms in soft yellow. Good for exhibition. ↕1.3m (4½ft), ↔ 60cm (24in). ❄
D. 'Apricot Honeymoon Dress' ▣ Small-flowered decorative dahlia with apricot blooms. Good for exhibition. ↕1.2m (4ft), ↔ 60cm (24in). ❄
D. 'Athalie'. Small-flowered cactus dahlia bearing dark pink blooms with bronze blends. Good for exhibition. ↕1.1m (3½ft), ↔ 60cm (24in). ❄
D. 'Barberry Carousel' ▣ Small-flowered ball dahlia bearing blooms in blends of lilac and purple with a white base to each petal. Good for exhibition. ↕1.2m (4ft), ↔ 60cm (24in). ❄
D. 'Bern'. Dwarf bedding dahlia bearing double, bright red blooms, to 10cm (4in) across. ↕60cm (24in), ↔ 45cm (18in). ❄
D. 'Berwick Wood'. Medium-flowered decorative dahlia bearing purple-pink blooms on strong stems. Good for exhibition. ↕1.3m (4½ft), ↔ 60cm (24in). ❄
D. 'Biddenham Strawberry'. Small-flowered decorative dahlia. Blooms are bright red with a touch of carmine-red and a splash of creamy yellow at the base of each petal. ↕1.2m (4ft), ↔ 60cm (24in). ❄
D. 'Biddenham Sunset'. Strong-stemmed, medium-flowered semi-cactus dahlia with blooms in blends of deep orange-red, with a yellow base to each petal. ↕1.3m (4½ft), ↔ 60cm (24in). ❄
D. 'Bishop of Llandaff' ▣ Peony-flowered (miscellaneous group) dahlia with semi-double, bright red blooms, 5–6cm (2–2½in) across, bright yellow anthers, and black-red foliage. ↕1.1m (3½ft), ↔ 45cm (18in). ❄
D. 'B.J. Beauty' ▣ Very free-flowering, medium-flowered decorative dahlia bearing pure white blooms. Good for exhibition. ↕1.2m (4ft), ↔ 60cm (24in). ❄
D. 'Black Monarch'. Giant-flowered decorative dahlia with oxblood-red blooms, shading to crimson. ↕1.2m (4ft), ↔ 60cm (24in). ❄
D. 'Bonaventure'. Giant-flowered decorative dahlia with blooms in blends of bronze and yellow. Good for exhibition. ↕1.3m (4½ft), ↔ 60cm (24in). ❄
D. 'Border Princess'. Strong-stemmed, very free-flowering, small-flowered cactus dahlia, often used for bedding, with golden bronze blooms. ↕to 60cm (24in), ↔ 45cm (18in). ❄
D. 'Boy Mick'. Medium-flowered decorative dahlia bearing yellow blooms on strong stems. Good for exhibition. ↕1.2m (4ft), ↔ 60cm (24in). ❄
D. 'Candy Cupid'. Miniature-flowered ball dahlia producing lavender-pink blooms. Good for exhibition. ↕1.1m (3½ft), ↔ 60cm (24in). ❄
D. 'Charlie Kenwood'. Miniature-flowered decorative dahlia bearing bright lavender-pink blooms with a white base to each petal. ↕1.1m (3½ft), ↔ 60cm (24in). ❄
D. 'Charlie Two' ▣ Medium-flowered decorative dahlia with yellow blooms. Good for exhibition. ↕1.3m (4½ft), ↔ 60cm (24in). ❄
D. 'Chimborazo' ▣ Very free-flowering collerette dahlia, each bloom with dark maroon outer petals surrounding a yellow collar and central disc. ↕1.2m (4ft), ↔ 60cm (24in). ❄
D. 'Christopher Nickerson'. Medium-flowered semi-cactus dahlia bearing gold-tipped, rich yellow blooms. Good for exhibition. ↕1.2m (4ft), ↔ 60cm (24in). ❄
D. 'Christopher Taylor' ▣ Strong-stemmed, small-flowered waterlily dahlia producing red blooms with silver undersides. ↕1.1m (3½ft), ↔ 60cm (24in). ❄
D. 'Clair de Lune' ▣ Collerette dahlia, each bloom with an outer ring of clear to pale yellow petals, a cream inner ring and centre, and deep yellow anthers. ↕1.1m (3½ft), ↔ 60cm (24in). ❄
D. 'Coltness Gem'. Bushy, dwarf bedding dahlia, grown as an annual, producing single, yellow-eyed flowerheads, 5–7cm (2–3in) across, in colours including white, yellow, apricot-yellow, scarlet-red, purple, and pink, many zoned with a second colour. ↕↔ 45cm (18in). ❄
D. 'Comet'. Anemone-flowered dahlia bearing dark velvet-red blooms. ↕1.1m (3½ft), ↔ 60cm (24in). ❄
D. 'Connie Bartlam'. Medium-flowered decorative dahlia producing salmon-pink blooms with a gold tip to each petal. Good for exhibition. ↕1.2m (4ft), ↔ 60cm (24in). ❄
D. 'Conway' ▣ ♀ Small-flowered semi-cactus dahlia bearing blooms in blends of dusky purple with a hint of buff. Begins flowering in early summer. ↕1.1m (3½ft), ↔ 60cm (24in). ❄
D. 'Corton Olympic' ▣ Giant-flowered decorative dahlia producing orange blooms on strong stems. Good for exhibition. ↕1.2m (4ft), ↔ 60cm (24in). ❄
D. 'Cream Alva's'. Giant-flowered decorative dahlia with cream blooms. Good for exhibition. ↕1.3m (4½ft), ↔ 60cm (24in). ❄
D. 'Cryfield Bryn'. Very free-flowering, small-flowered semi-cactus dahlia producing clear yellow blooms. ↕1.1m (3½ft), ↔ 60cm (24in). ❄

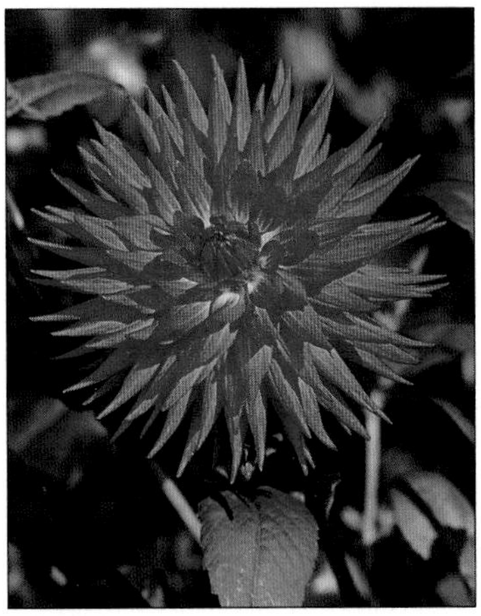
Dahlia 'Conway'

D. 'Cryfield Keene'. Large-flowered semi-cactus dahlia with light pink blooms. Good for exhibition. ↕1.2m (4ft), ↔ 60cm (24in). ❄
D. 'Daddy's Choice' ▣ Strong-growing, small-flowered semi-cactus dahlia bearing pale lemon-yellow blooms with a pale lilac tinge. ↕1.3m (4½ft), ↔ 60cm (24in). ❄
D. 'Daleko Jupiter'. Giant-flowered semi-cactus dahlia with blooms in blends of rose-red to pink-yellow, held well above the foliage. Good for exhibition. ↕1.3m (4½ft), ↔ 60cm (24in). ❄
D. 'Dana Iris' ▣ ♀ Outstanding, small-flowered cactus dahlia with red blooms. Good for exhibition. ↕1.3m (4½ft), ↔ 60cm (24in). ❄
D. 'Dandy' ▣ Bushy bedding dahlia grown as an annual. Flowerheads, to 7cm (3in) across, each with a collar-like ring of lighter, quilled petals around the central disc, are produced in many

Dahlia 'Abridge Natalie'

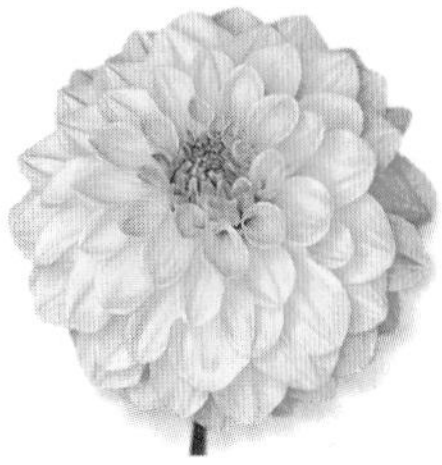
Dahlia 'Alloway Cottage'

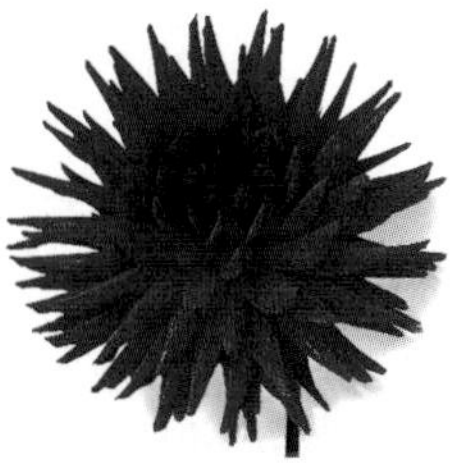
Dahlia 'Alltami Corsair'

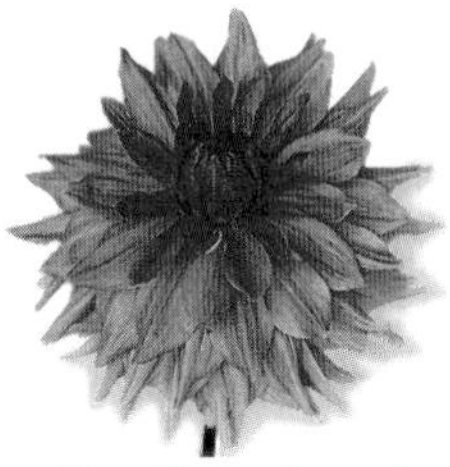
Dahlia 'Alltami Cosmic'

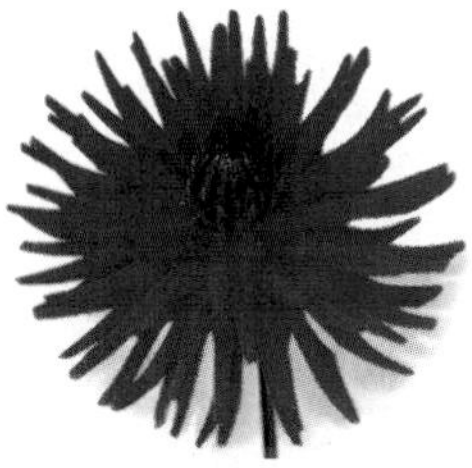
Dahlia 'Alva's Doris'

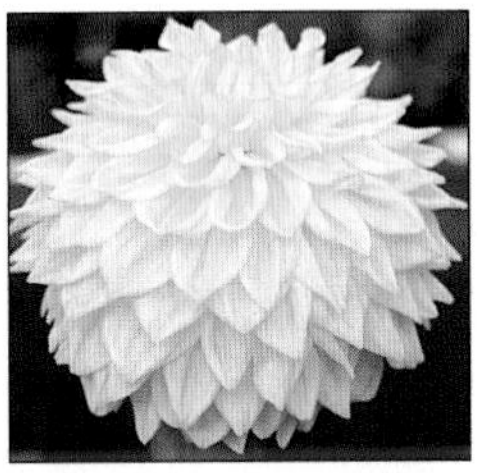
Dahlia 'Alva's Supreme'

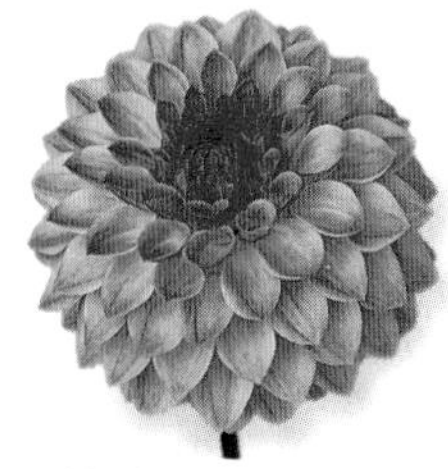
Dahlia 'Apricot Honeymoon Dress'

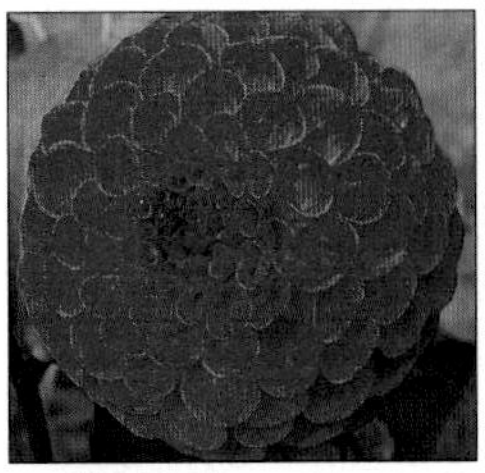
Dahlia 'Barberry Carousel'

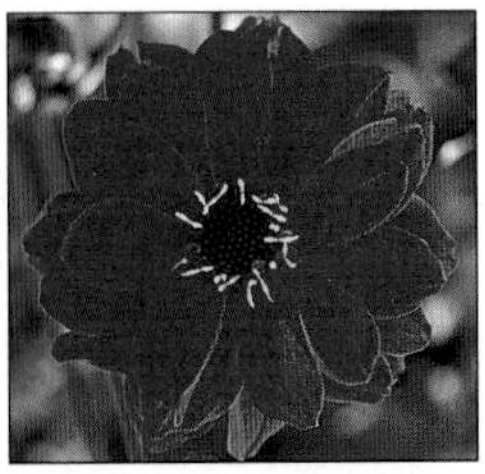
Dahlia 'Bishop of Llandaff'

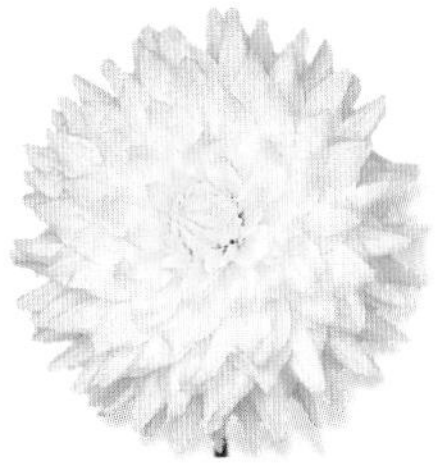
Dahlia 'B.J. Beauty'

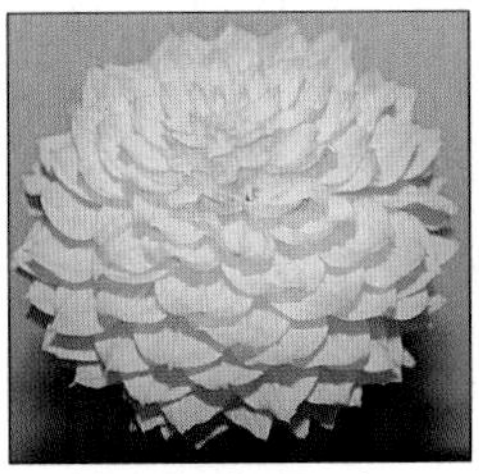
Dahlia 'Charlie Two'

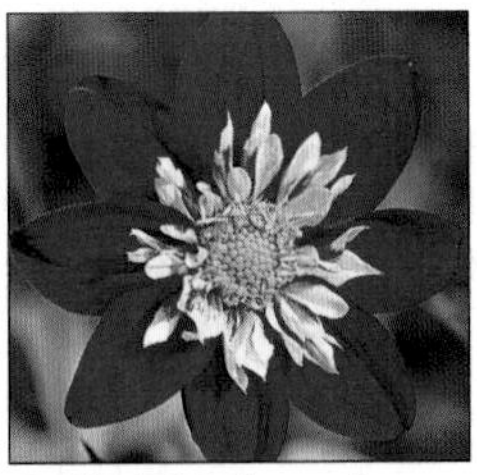
Dahlia 'Chimborazo'

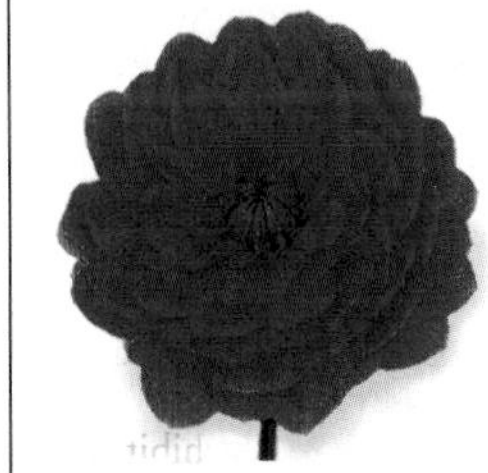
Dahlia 'Christopher Taylor'

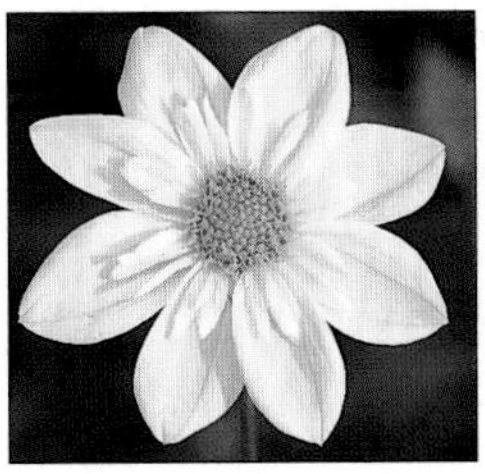
Dahlia 'Clair de Lune'

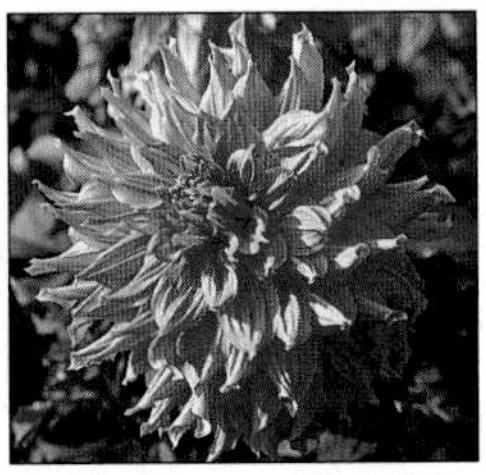
Dahlia 'Corton Olympic'

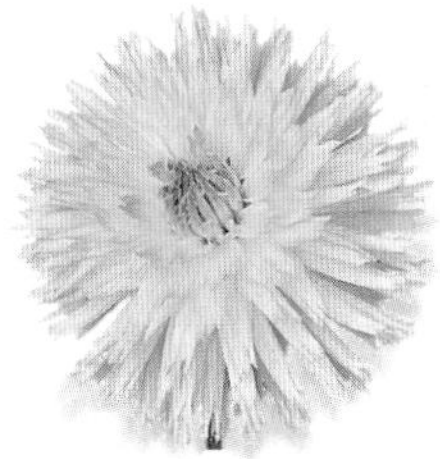
Dahlia 'Daddy's Choice'

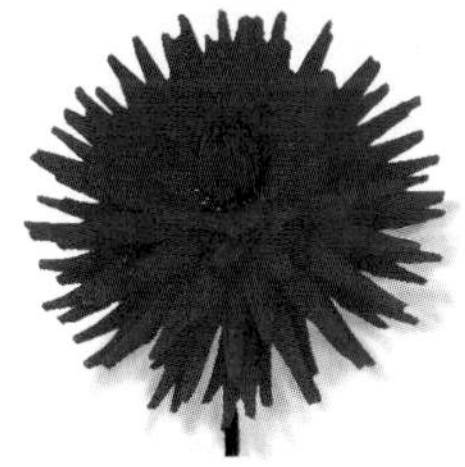
Dahlia 'Dana Iris'

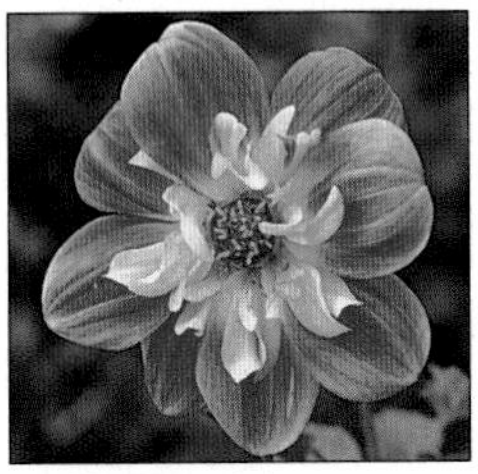
Dahlia 'Dandy'

D

colours, including white, yellow, pink, and red. ↕↔ to 60cm (24in). ✻
***D.* 'Davenport Honey'** ▣ Miniature-flowered decorative dahlia with amber blooms. Good for exhibition. ↕ 1.2m (4ft), ↔ 60cm (24in). ✻
***D.* 'Davenport Lesley'.** Miniature-flowered decorative dahlia with bright scarlet blooms. Good for exhibition. ↕ 1.3m (4½ft), ↔ 60cm (24in). ✻
***D.* 'Davenport Pride'.** Medium-flowered semi-cactus dahlia bearing apricot-orange blooms on strong stems. ↕ 1.1m (3½ft), ↔ 60cm (24in). ✻
***D.* 'Davenport Sunlight'** ▣ Medium-flowered semi-cactus dahlia with vivid yellow blooms held well above the foliage. Good for exhibition. ↕ 1.2m (4ft), ↔ 60cm (24in). ✻
***D.* 'Debra Ann Craven'.** Giant-flowered semi-cactus dahlia bearing deep red blooms, with a velvet texture, held well above the foliage on strong stems. Good for exhibition. ↕ 1.3m (4½ft), ↔ 60cm (24in). ✻
***D.* 'Diablo'** ♀ Bushy, fast-growing, free-flowering, dwarf bedding dahlia grown as an annual. Mainly double flowerheads, 5–7cm (2–3in) across, in colours ranging from white and yellow to pink, red, or orange, are borne above dark bronze leaves. ↕ 15–18cm (6–7in), ↔ 30–35cm (12–14in). ✻
***D.* 'Doc van Horn'.** Large-flowered semi-cactus dahlia. Dark pink blooms have a gold sheen. Good for exhibition. ↕ 1m (3ft), ↔ 60cm (24in). ✻
***D.* 'Dr. Caroline Rabbett'.** Small-flowered decorative dahlia bearing blooms in blends of yellow and orange on strong stems. ↕ 1.5m (5ft), ↔ 60cm (24in). ✻
***D.* 'Easter Sunday'** ▣ Collerette dahlia producing creamy white blooms, each with a central yellow disc. Blooms are held well above the foliage. ↕ 1.1m (3½ft), ↔ 60cm (24in). ✻
***D.* 'Eastwood Moonlight'.** Medium-flowered semi-cactus dahlia with pale yellow blooms on strong stems. Good for exhibition. ↕ 1.1m (3½ft), ↔ 60cm (24in). ✻
***D.* 'Edna C'.** Medium-flowered decorative dahlia that produces clear yellow blooms with reflexed petals. Good for exhibition. ↕ 1.2m (4ft), ↔ 60cm (24in). ✻
***D.* 'Emmerdale'.** Small-flowered cactus dahlia producing red-tipped yellow blooms. ↕ 1m (3ft), ↔ 45cm (18in). ✻
***D.* 'Ernest Pitt'.** Small-flowered decorative dahlia producing salmon-pink blooms with a yellow base to each petal. Good for exhibition. ↕ 1m (3ft), ↔ 45cm (18in). ✻
***D.* 'Evelyn Rumbold'.** Giant-flowered decorative dahlia producing purple blooms on very strong, long stems. ↕ 1.3m (4½ft), ↔ 60cm (24in). ✻
***D.* 'Fascination'** ▣♀ Peony-flowered (miscellaneous group) dwarf bedding dahlia with dark bronze foliage and light purplish pink flowerheads, to 10cm (4in) across. ↕ 60cm (24in), ↔ 45cm (18in). ✻
***D.* 'Figaro'.** Fast-growing, dwarf bedding dahlia, grown as an annual, producing double, sometimes semi-double flowerheads, 5–7cm (2–3in) across, in mixed colours, including white, yellow, red, and pink. ↕↔ to 40cm (16in). ✻
***D.* 'Frank Hornsey'** ▣ Strong-stemmed, small-flowered decorative dahlia that produces blooms in blends of yellow-bronze and apricot. Good for exhibition. ↕ 1.2m (4ft), ↔ 60cm (24in). ✻
***D.* 'Freestyle'.** Small-flowered cactus dahlia with vivid purple blooms held well above the foliage. ↕ 1.1m (3½ft), ↔ 60cm (24in). ✻
***D.* 'Garden Festival'.** Small-flowered waterlily dahlia bearing red blooms with yellow tips and margins. ↕ 1.3m (4½ft), ↔ 60cm (24in). ✻
***D.* 'Gateshead Festival'** ▣ Small-flowered decorative dahlia bearing peach to orange blooms with lemon-yellow petal bases. Good for exhibition. ↕ 1.2m (4ft), ↔ 60cm (24in). ✻
***D.* 'Gay Princess'** ▣ Small-flowered waterlily dahlia bearing shimmering, lilac-pink blooms on strong stems well above the foliage. ↕ 1.5m (5ft), ↔ 75cm (30in). ✻
***D.* 'Geerlings Indian Summer'** ♀ syn. *D.* 'Indian Summer'. Very free-flowering, small-flowered cactus dahlia producing red blooms. ↕ 1.2m (4ft), ↔ 60cm (24in). ✻
***D.* 'Gerrie Hoek'.** Very free-flowering, small-flowered waterlily dahlia with silvery pink blooms on strong stems. ↕ 1.2m (4ft), ↔ 60cm (24in). ✻
***D.* 'Gilt Edge'** ▣ Very free-flowering, compact, medium-flowered decorative dahlia bearing dark pink blooms, with yellow-tipped ray-florets, on strong stems. ↕ 1.1m (3½ft), ↔ 60cm (24in). ✻
***D.* 'Glorie van Heemstede'** ▣♀ Very free-flowering, small-flowered waterlily dahlia bearing yellow blooms on strong stems. ↕ 1.3m (4½ft), ↔ 60cm (24in). ✻
***D.* 'Golden Impact'.** Medium-flowered semi-cactus dahlia with deep yellow blooms. Good for exhibition. ↕ 1.3m (4½ft), ↔ 60cm (24in). ✻
***D.* 'Grenidor Pastelle'** ▣ Medium-flowered semi-cactus dahlia bearing salmon-pink blooms with cream petal bases. Good for exhibition. ↕ 1.3m (4½ft), ↔ 60cm (24in). ✻
***D.* 'Hallmark'.** Pompon dahlia bearing white flowerheads, with lilac petal margins, held well above the leaves. ↕ 1.1m (3½ft), ↔ 60cm (24in). ✻
***D.* 'Hamari Accord'** ▣♀ Large-flowered semi-cactus dahlia producing pale, clear yellow blooms held well above the foliage on strong stems. Good for exhibition. ↕ 1.2m (4ft), ↔ 60cm (24in). ✻
***D.* 'Hamari Bride'** ▣♀ Medium-flowered semi-cactus dahlia with pure white blooms. Good for exhibition. ↕ 1.2m (4ft), ↔ 60cm (24in). ✻
***D.* 'Hamari Gold'** ▣♀ Giant-flowered decorative dahlia bearing deep gold-bronze blooms. Good for exhibition. ↕ 1.2m (4ft), ↔ 60cm (24in). ✻
***D.* 'Hamari Katrina'** ▣ Large-flowered semi-cactus dahlia with very pale lemon-yellow blooms. Good for exhibition. ↕ 1.3m (4½ft), ↔ 60cm (24in). ✻
***D.* 'Hamilton Lillian'** ♀ Small-flowered decorative dahlia bearing bronze blooms with light pink blends. ↕ 1.2m (4ft), ↔ 60cm (24in). ✻
***D.* 'Hans Ricken'** ▣ Small-flowered waterlily dahlia bearing bright yellow blooms on strong stems. ↕ 1.1m (3½ft), ↔ 60cm (24in). ✻
***D.* 'Hayley Jane'** ▣ Small-flowered semi-cactus dahlia producing white blooms heavily tipped with purplish pink. ↕ 1.3m (4½ft), ↔ 60cm (24in). ✻
***D.* 'Highgate Lustre'** ▣ Medium-flowered semi-cactus dahlia with bright orange blooms. ↕ 1.3m (4½ft), ↔ 60cm (24in). ✻
***D.* 'Highgate Torch'** ▣ Strong-growing, medium-flowered semi-cactus dahlia with blooms in an unusual shade of orange verging on flame-red, held well above the foliage. ↕ 1.2m (4ft), ↔ 60cm (24in). ✻
***D.* 'Hillcrest Hillton'.** Large-flowered semi-cactus dahlia with weather-resistant, deep rich yellow blooms. Good for exhibition. ↕ 1.5m (5ft), ↔ 75cm (30in). ✻
***D.* 'Hillcrest Royal'** ▣♀ Medium-flowered cactus dahlia with rich purple blooms, with incurving petals, on strong stems. ↕ 1.1m (3½ft), ↔ 60cm (24in). ✻
***D.* 'Honeymoon Dress'.** Small-flowered decorative dahlia producing

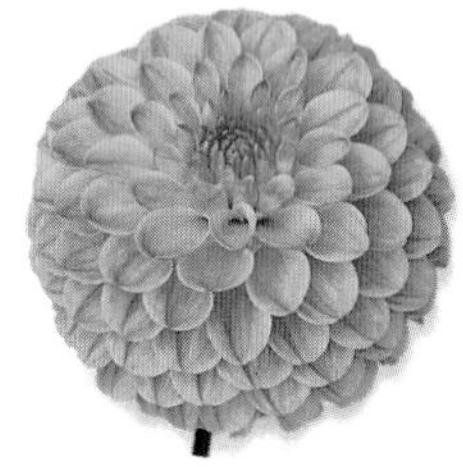
Dahlia 'Davenport Honey'

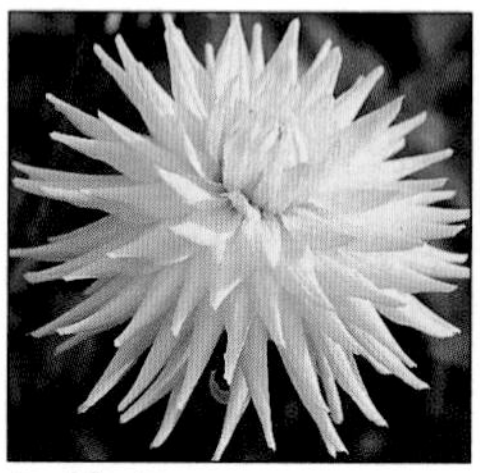
Dahlia 'Davenport Sunlight'

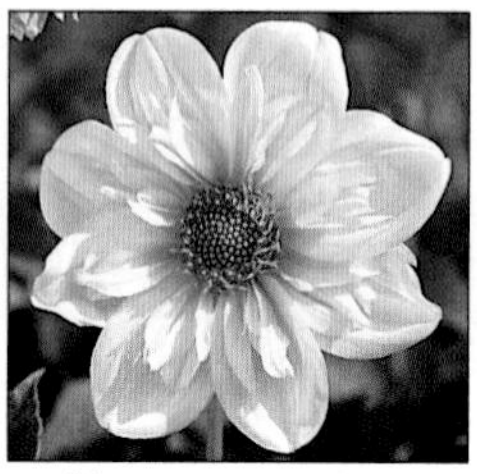
Dahlia 'Easter Sunday'

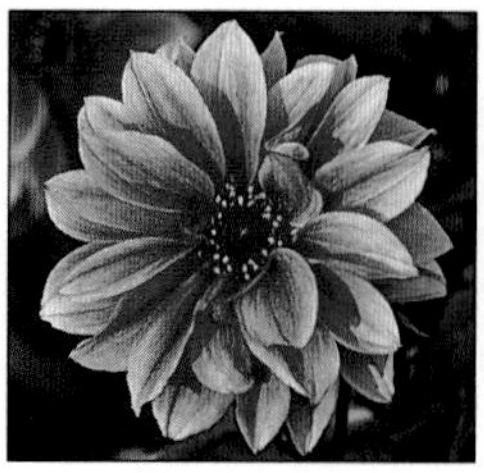
Dahlia 'Fascination'

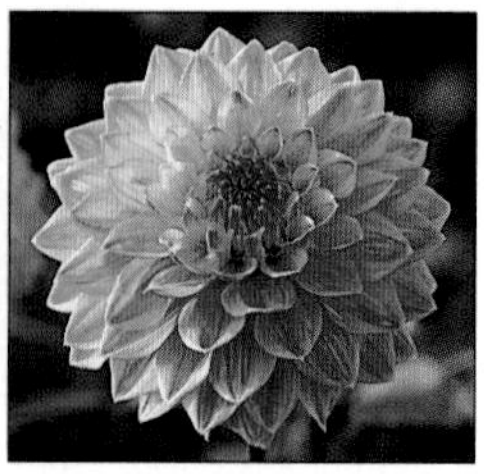
Dahlia 'Frank Hornsey'

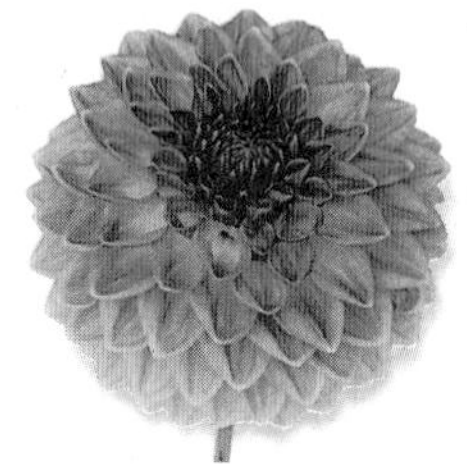
Dahlia 'Gateshead Festival'

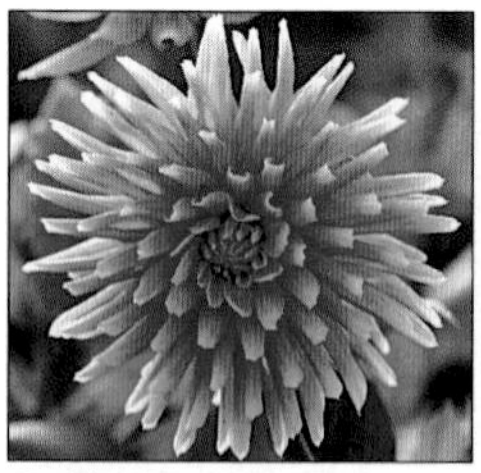
Dahlia 'Gay Princess'

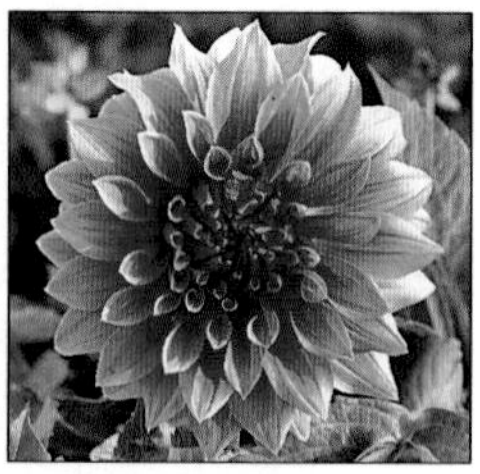
Dahlia 'Gilt Edge'

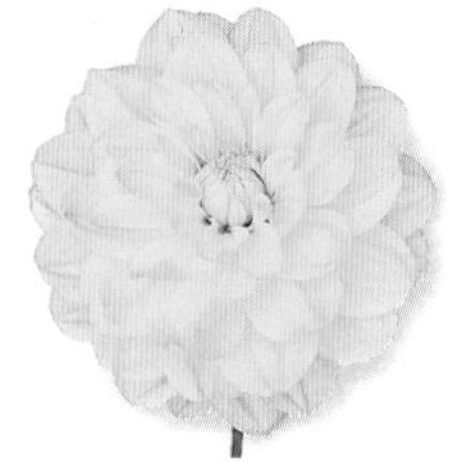
Dahlia 'Glorie van Heemstede'

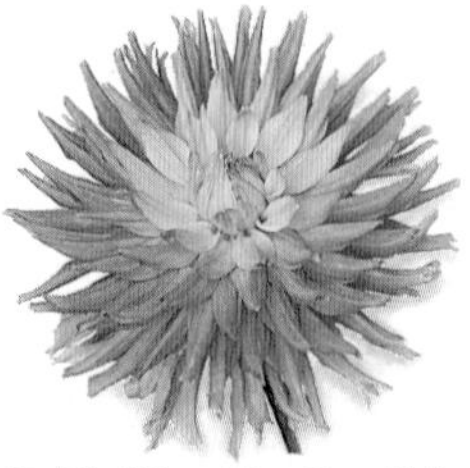
Dahlia 'Grenidor Pastelle'

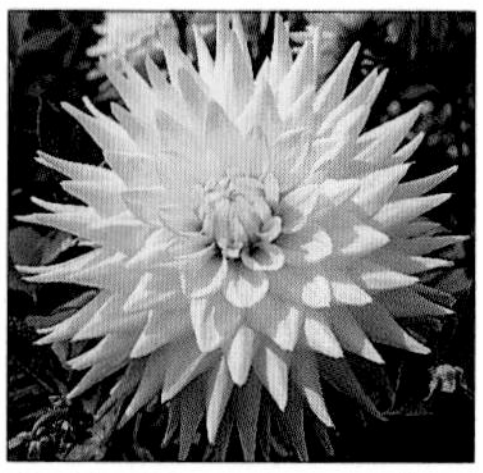
Dahlia 'Hamari Accord'

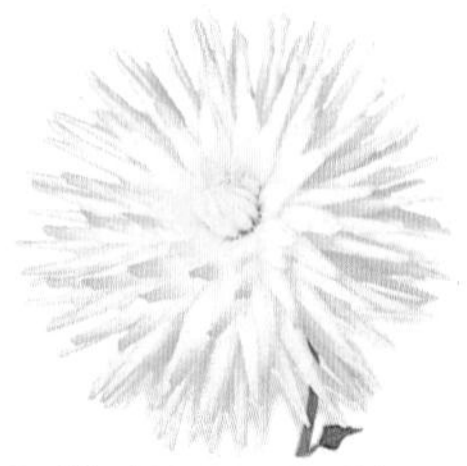
Dahlia 'Hamari Bride'

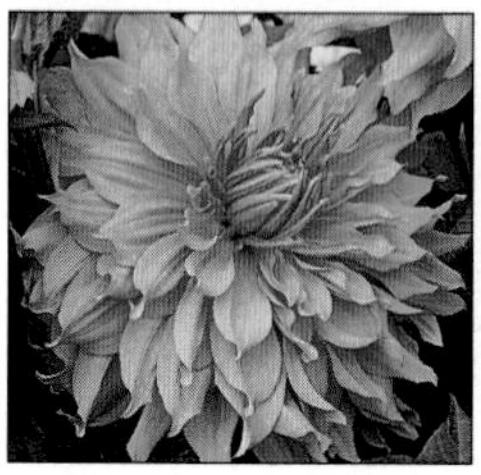
Dahlia 'Hamari Gold'

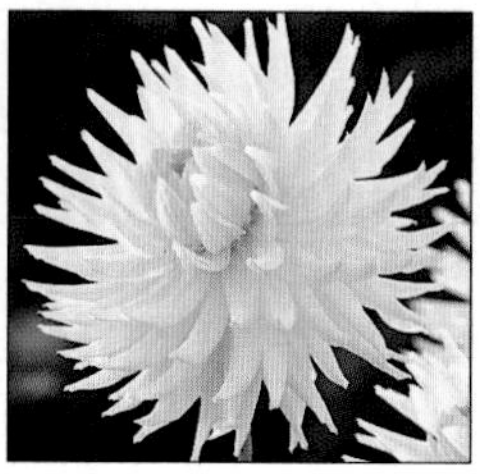
Dahlia 'Hamari Katrina'

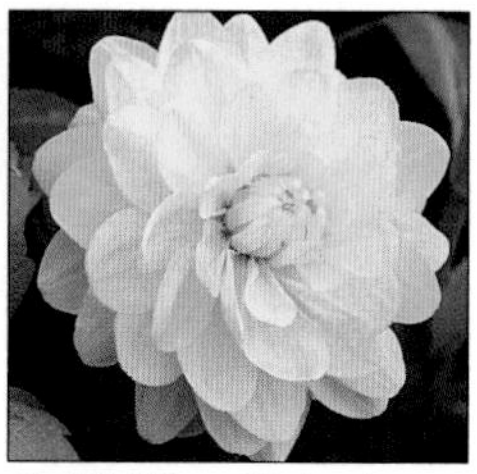
Dahlia 'Hans Ricken'

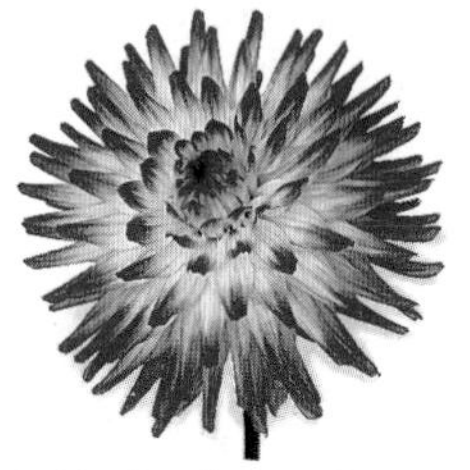
Dahlia 'Hayley Jane'

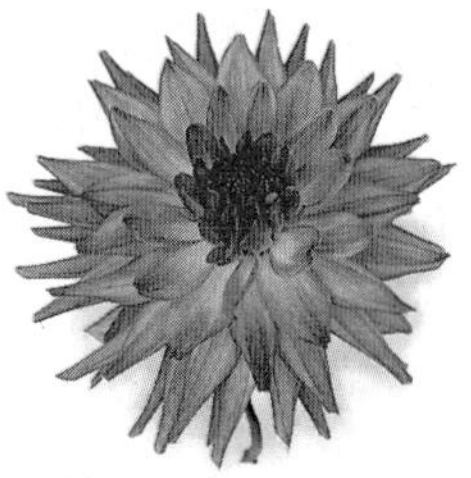
Dahlia 'Highgate Lustre'

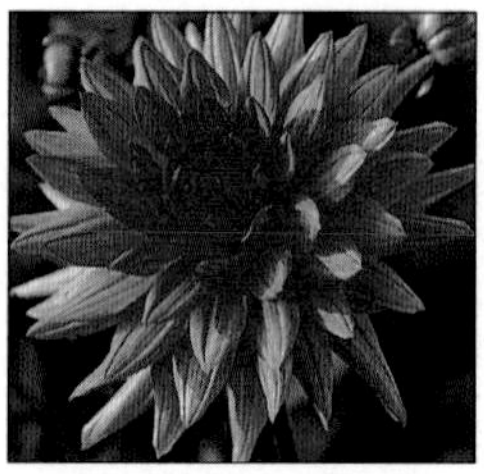
Dahlia 'Highgate Torch'

pure salmon-pink blooms with a gold base to each petal. Good for exhibition. ↕ 1.1m (3½ft), ↔ 60cm (24in). ✻

***D.* 'Hugh Mather'** ▣ Very free-flowering, miniature-flowered waterlily dahlia producing orange-amber blooms on strong, slender stems. Best not disbudded. ↕ 1.1m (3½ft), ↔ 60cm (24in). ✻

***D.* 'Inca Dambuster'.** Very strong-growing, giant-flowered semi-cactus dahlia with blooms in the palest yellow verging on white. Good for exhibition. ↕ 1.3m (4½ft), ↔ 60cm (24in). ✻

***D.* 'Indian Summer'** see *D.* 'Geerlings Indian Summer'.

***D.* 'Jeanette Carter'** ▣🏆 Miniature-flowered decorative dahlia with pale yellow blooms, sometimes flushed pink in the centres. ↕ 1.1m (3½ft), ↔ 60cm (24in). ✻

***D.* 'Jescot Julie'** ▣ Orchid-flowered (miscellaneous group) dahlia producing burnt-orange blooms, 6–8cm (2½–3in) across, plum beneath. ↕ 1m (3ft), ↔ 45cm (18in). ✻

***D.* 'Jill Doc'.** Medium-flowered decorative dahlia. The rich orange blooms are shaded with amber. Good for exhibition. ↕ 1.2m (4ft), ↔ 60cm (24in). ✻

***D.* 'Jim Branigan'** ▣ Large-flowered semi-cactus dahlia with bright red blooms held well above the foliage. Good for exhibition. ↕ 1.3m (4½ft), ↔ 60cm (24in). ✻

***D.* 'Jocondo'.** Giant-flowered decorative dahlia bearing blooms in bright reddish purple on strong stems. Good for exhibition. ↕ 1.2m (4ft), ↔ 60cm (24in). ✻

***D.* 'John Prior'** ▣ Small-flowered decorative dahlia with wine-red blooms on erect stems. Good for exhibition. ↕ 1.2m (4ft), ↔ 60cm (24in). ✻

***D.* 'John Street'** 🏆 Compact, small-flowered waterlily dahlia with bright scarlet blooms held well above the foliage on strong, thin stems. ↕ 1m (3ft), ↔ 45cm (18in). ✻

***D.* 'Karenglen'** 🏆 Miniature-flowered decorative dahlia bearing well-formed, vibrant orange-scarlet flowerheads. Good for exhibition. ↕ 1.1m (3½ft), ↔ 60cm (24in). ✻

***D.* 'Kathryn's Cupid'** ▣ Miniature-flowered ball dahlia with peach blooms. Good for exhibition. ↕ 1.2m (4ft), ↔ 60cm (24in). ✻

***D.* 'Kay Helen'** 🏆 Very free-flowering pompon dahlia with light pink blooms held well above the foliage. Good for exhibition. ↕ 1.1m (3½ft), ↔ 60cm (24in). ✻

***D.* 'Kenora Fireball'.** Miniature-flowered ball dahlia bearing cerise-red blooms, with a yellow base to each petal, on strong stems. Good for exhibition. ↕ 1m (3ft), ↔ 45cm (18in). ✻

***D.* 'Kidd's Climax'.** Giant-flowered decorative dahlia with gold-suffused pink blooms. Good for exhibition. ↕ 1.1m (3½ft), ↔ 60cm (24in). ✻

***D.* 'Kiwi Gloria'** ▣ Very free-flowering, small-flowered cactus dahlia with white blooms suffused lavender-pink. ↕ 1.2m (4ft), ↔ 60cm (24in). ✻

***D.* 'Klankstad Kerkrade'.** Small-flowered cactus dahlia with pale lemon-yellow blooms. Good for exhibition. ↕ 1.2m (4ft), ↔ 60cm (24in). ✻

***D.* 'Lady Kerkrade'** ▣ Small-flowered cactus dahlia bearing purple-lilac blooms, with creamy white petal bases, on strong stems. Good for exhibition. ↕ 1.2m (4ft), ↔ 60cm (24in). ✻

***D.* 'Lady Linda'.** Very vigorous, very free-flowering, small-flowered decorative dahlia bearing well-formed, primrose-yellow blooms, held well above the foliage. Good for exhibition. ↕ 1.2m (4ft), ↔ 60cm (24in). ✻

***D.* 'Lady Sunshine'** ▣ Compact, small-flowered cactus dahlia with very bright, clear yellow blooms on strong stems. ↕ 1.1m (3½ft), ↔ 60cm (24in). ✻

***D.* 'L'Ancresse'.** Miniature-flowered ball dahlia bearing neat white blooms with a hint of lavender-blue on each petal margin. Good for exhibition. ↕ 1.1m (3½ft), ↔ 60cm (24in). ✻

***D.* 'Lavender Athalie'** ▣ Small-flowered cactus dahlia with lavender-pink blooms held well above the foliage. Good for exhibition. ↕ 1.3m (4½ft), ↔ 60cm (24in). ✻

***D.* 'Liberator'.** Giant-flowered decorative dahlia with velvet-red blooms held well above the foliage on strong stems. ↕ 1.1m (3½ft), ↔ 60cm (24in). ✻

***D.* 'Lifesize'.** Large-flowered decorative dahlia with canary-yellow blooms. Good for exhibition. ↕ 1.1m (3½ft), ↔ 60cm (24in). ✻

***D.* 'Light Music'.** Large-flowered cactus dahlia that produces lilac blooms. Good for exhibition. ↕ 1.2m (4ft), ↔ 60cm (24in). ✻

***D.* 'Lilian Ingham'.** Small-flowered cactus dahlia with rose-red blooms. ↕ 1.1m (3½ft), ↔ 60cm (24in). ✻

***D.* 'Linda's Chester'.** Small-flowered cactus dahlia with yellow blooms overlaid with bronze at the petal tips. Good for exhibition. ↕ 1.2m (4ft), ↔ 60cm (24in). ✻

***D.* 'Love's Dream'.** Small-flowered waterlily dahlia with sparsely petalled, light raspberry-red blooms shading to salmon-pink, borne on long, strong stems. ↕ 1.5m (5ft), ↔ 60cm (24in). ✻

***D.* 'Majestic Kerkrade'** ▣ Small-flowered cactus dahlia bearing soft salmon-pink blooms with a yellow base to each petal. Good for exhibition. ↕ 1.2m (4ft), ↔ 60cm (24in). ✻

***D.* 'Mark Damp'.** Large-flowered semi-cactus dahlia with light orange blooms on strong stems well above the foliage. Flowers early. Good for exhibition. ↕ 1.1m (3½ft), ↔ 60cm (24in). ✻

***D.* 'Mark Hardwick'** ▣ Compact, giant-flowered decorative dahlia producing bright deep yellow blooms on strong stems. Good for exhibition. ↕ 1.1m (3½ft), ↔ 60cm (24in). ✻

***D.* 'Match'.** Small-flowered semi-cactus dahlia producing purple-splashed white blooms well above the foliage on strong stems. ↕ 1.2m (4ft), ↔ 60cm (24in). ✻

D. merckii. Tuberous-rooted perennial with many-branched stems and pinnate or 2-pinnate, mid-green leaves, to 40cm (16in) long. Saucer-shaped, single, purple to pink or white flowerheads, to 8cm (3in) across, with purple or yellow disc florets, and with often arching flower stalks, are produced from summer to autumn, either in cyme-like racemes or singly from the leaf axils. ↕ to 2m (6ft), ↔ 1m (3ft). Mexico. ✻✻✻ (borderline)

***D.* 'Mistill Beauty'.** Small-flowered cactus dahlia. Dark pink blooms, with a yellow base to each petal, are held well above the foliage. Good for exhibition. ↕ 1.2m (4ft), ↔ 60cm (24in). ✻

***D.* 'Mi Wong'** ▣ Pompon dahlia bearing white blooms suffused pink. Good for exhibition. ↕ 1.1m (3½ft), ↔ 60cm (24in). ✻

***D.* 'Moor Place'** ▣ Outstanding pompon dahlia with wine-red blooms. Good for exhibition. ↕ 1.1m (3½ft), ↔ 60cm (24in). ✻

***D.* 'Neal Gillson'** ▣ Medium-flowered decorative dahlia bearing rich corn-yellow blooms, suffused apricot, on strong stems. Good for exhibition. ↕ 1.3m (4½ft), ↔ 60cm (24in). ✻

***D.* 'Nina Chester'** ▣ Strong-stemmed, small-flowered decorative dahlia bearing white blooms with a hint of lilac at the tip of each petal. Good for exhibition. ↕ 1.1m (3½ft), ↔ 60cm (24in). ✻

***D.* 'Noreen'** ▣ Pompon dahlia with pure pink blooms. Good for exhibition. ↕ 1m (3ft), ↔ 45cm (18in). ✻

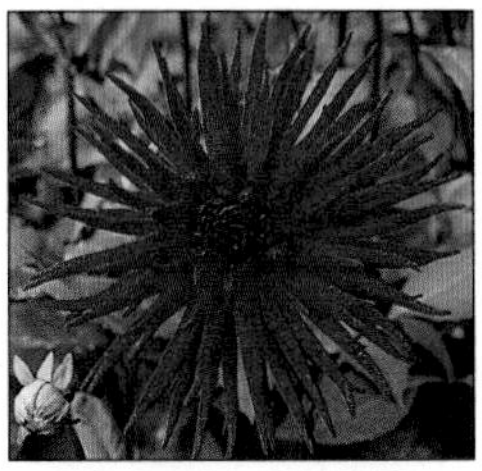
Dahlia 'Hillcrest Royal'

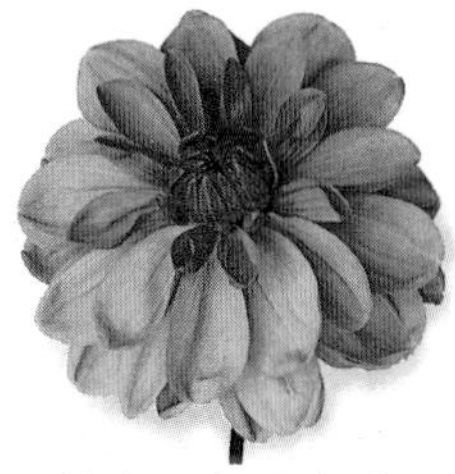
Dahlia 'Hugh Mather'

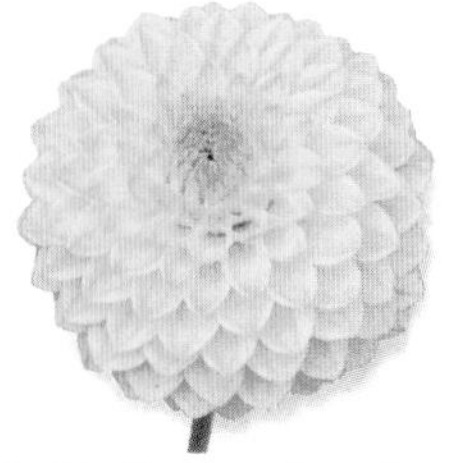
Dahlia 'Jeanette Carter'

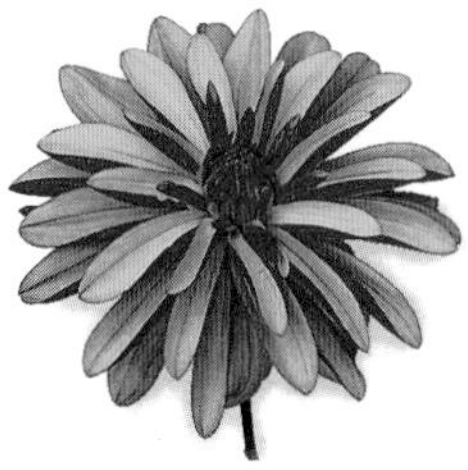
Dahlia 'Jescot Julie'

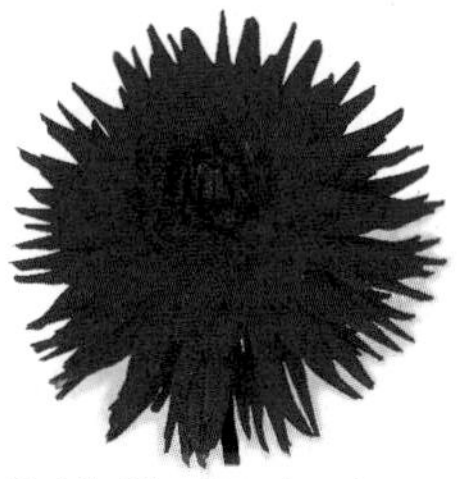
Dahlia 'Jim Branigan'

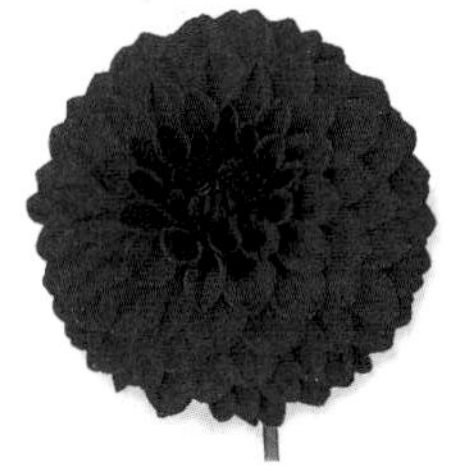
Dahlia 'John Prior'

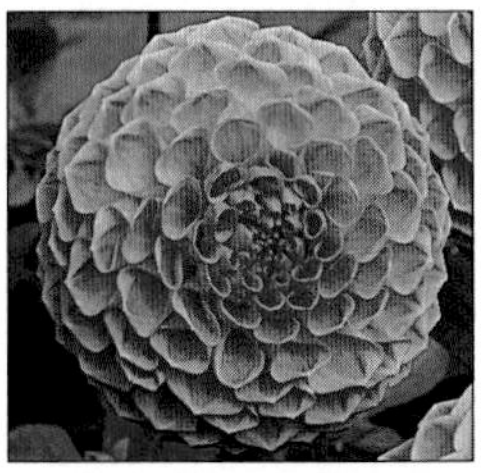
Dahlia 'Kathryn's Cupid'

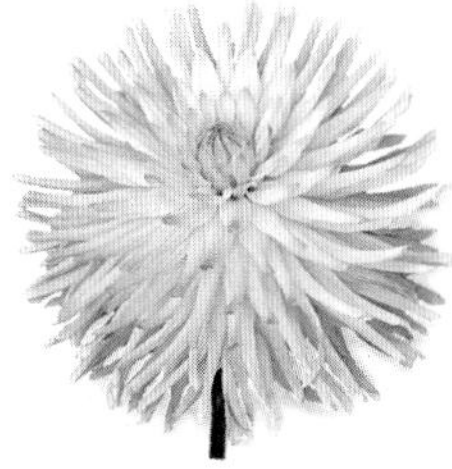
Dahlia 'Kiwi Gloria'

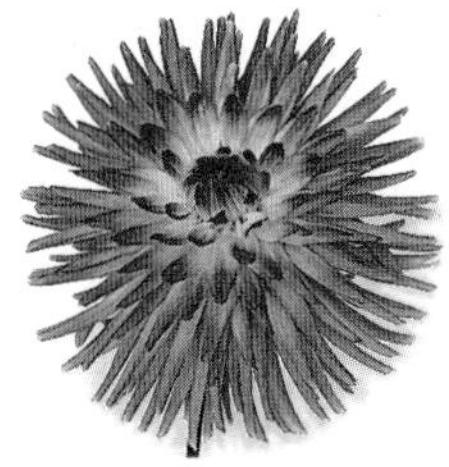
Dahlia 'Lady Kerkrade'

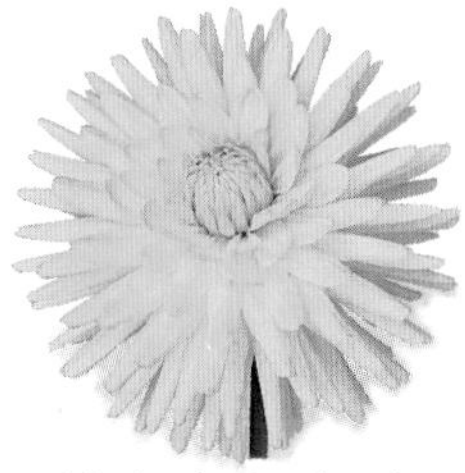
Dahlia 'Lady Sunshine'

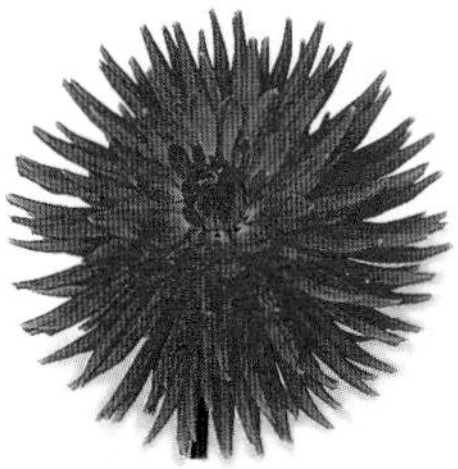
Dahlia 'Lavender Athalie'

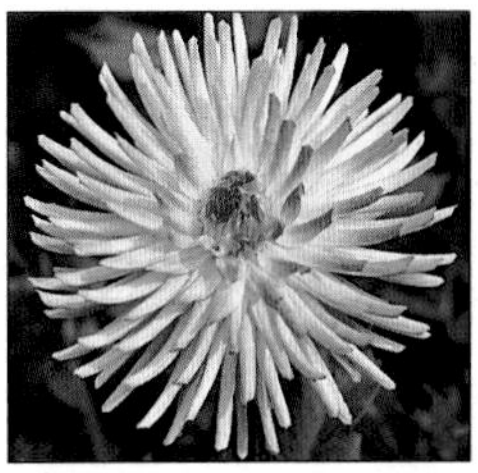
Dahlia 'Majestic Kerkrade'

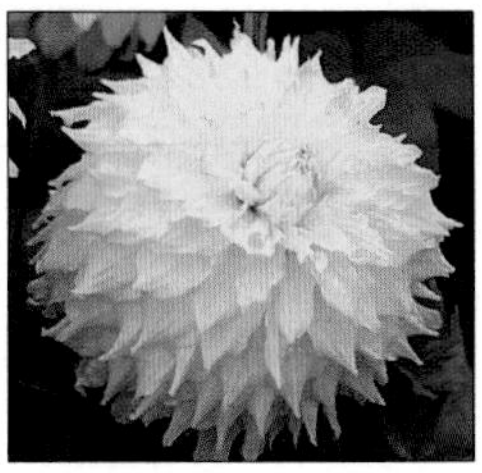
Dahlia 'Mark Hardwick'

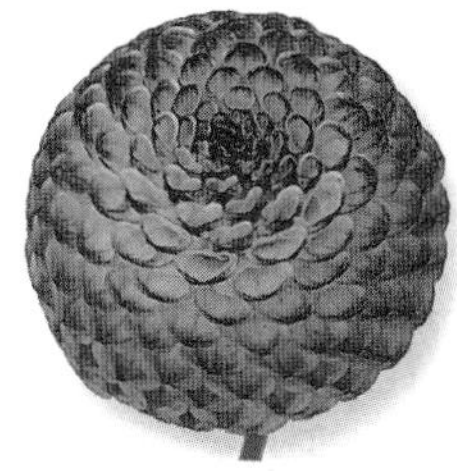
Dahlia 'Mi Wong'

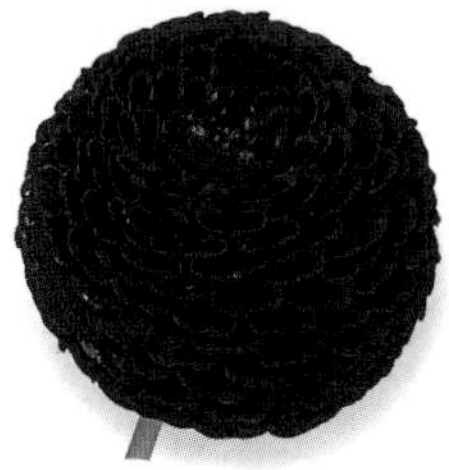
Dahlia 'Moor Place'

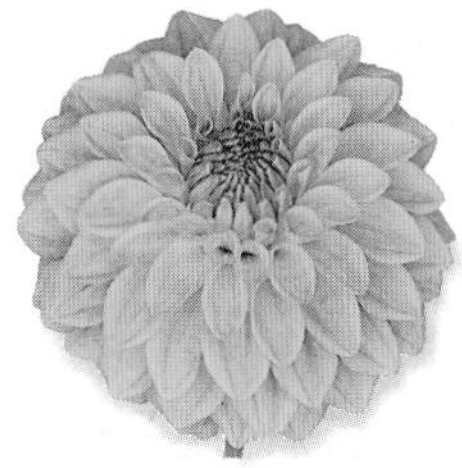
Dahlia 'Neal Gillson'

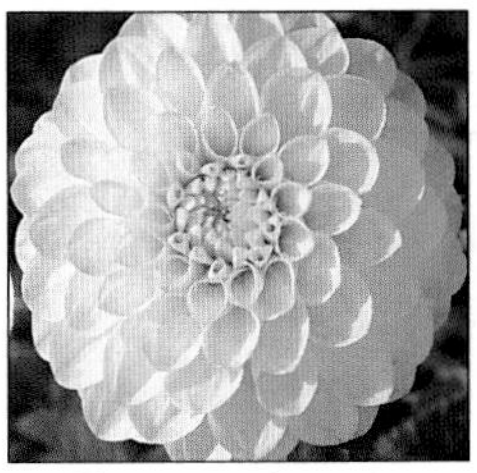
Dahlia 'Nina Chester'

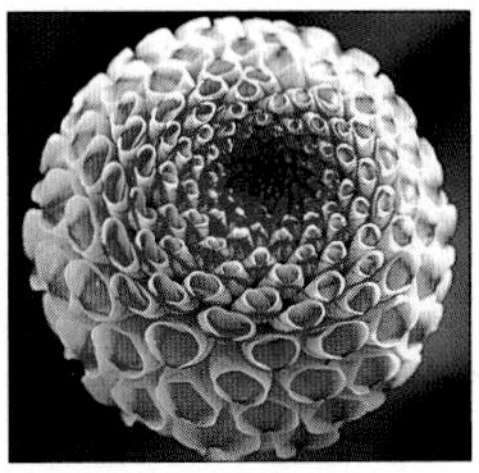
Dahlia 'Noreen'

D. 'Pamela'. Small-flowered waterlily dahlia producing golden amber blooms with few petals. ↕ 1m (3ft), ↔ 45cm (18in). ✻

D. 'Pearl of Heemstede' ■ ♀ Low-growing, very free-flowering, small-flowered waterlily dahlia bearing pale silvery pink blooms on long, thin stems. ↕ 1m (3ft), ↔ 45cm (18in). ✻

D. 'Periton'. Miniature-flowered ball dahlia bearing dark red blooms. ↕ 1.1m (3½ft), ↔ 60cm (24in). ✻

D. 'Piccolo'. Compact, fast-growing, single-flowered, dwarf bedding dahlia, grown as an annual. Flowerheads, 5–7 cm (2–3in) across, in a range of clear, bright, mixed colours, including shades of red, rose-pink, yellow, and white, are borne in summer and autumn. ↕↔ 30cm (12in). ✻

D. 'Pink Cloud'. Small-flowered semi-cactus dahlia producing blooms in blends of light and dark pink on long, strong stems. ↕ 1.2m (4ft), ↔ 60cm (24in). ✻

D. 'Pink Frank Hornsey'. Small-flowered decorative dahlia producing clear lilac-pink flowerheads with white blends. Good for exhibition. ↕ 1.2m (4ft), ↔ 60cm (24in). ✻

D. 'Pink Jupiter' ■ Giant-flowered semi-cactus dahlia producing deep pinkish mauve blooms. Good for exhibition. ↕ 1.3m (4½ft), ↔ 60cm (24in). ✻

D. 'Pink Kerkrade'. Small-flowered cactus dahlia producing deep lilac-pink blooms. Good for exhibition. ↕ 1.2m (4ft), ↔ 60cm (24in). ✻

D. 'Pink Pastelle' ♀ Medium-flowered semi-cactus dahlia producing dark pink blooms. Good for exhibition. ↕ 1.2m (4ft), ↔ 60cm (24in). ✻

D. 'Pink Shirley Alliance' ■ Small-flowered cactus dahlia producing soft lilac-pink blooms. ↕ 1.2m (4ft), ↔ 60cm (24in). ✻

D. 'Pink Symbol'. Medium-flowered semi-cactus dahlia bearing blooms in blends of lilac-pink, with a yellow base to each petal. ↕ 1.3m (4½ft), ↔ 60cm (24in). ✻

D. 'Polar Sight' ■ Giant-flowered cactus dahlia with pure white blooms. Good for exhibition. ↕ 1.3m (4½ft), ↔ 60cm (24in). ✻

D. 'Pontiac' ■ Very free-flowering, small-flowered cactus dahlia producing bright pink blooms overlaid with salmon-pink. ↕ 1.2m (4ft), ↔ 60cm (24in). ✻

D. 'Porcelain'. Small-flowered waterlily dahlia producing almost translucent, white blooms delicately shaded with violet-lilac. ↕ 1.3m (4½ft), ↔ 60cm (24in). ✻

D. 'Preston Park' ■ ♀ Single-flowered, dwarf bedding dahlia producing nearly black foliage and bright scarlet flowerheads, each with a purple centre and prominent yellow anthers, on short stems. ↕↔ 45cm (18in). ✻

D. 'Purple Joy'. Medium-flowered decorative dahlia with deep purple blooms held well above the foliage. Good for exhibition. ↕ 1.2m (4ft), ↔ 60cm (24in). ✻

D. 'Red Admiral'. Miniature-flowered ball dahlia that produces mid-red blooms held well above the foliage. Good for exhibition. ↕ 1.2m (4ft), ↔ 60cm (24in). ✻

D. 'Red Sensation'. Medium-flowered decorative dahlia bearing bright orange-red blooms, with slightly reflexed petals. Good for exhibition. ↕ 1.1m (3½ft), ↔ 60cm (24in). ✻

D. 'Redskin'. Dwarf bedding dahlia grown as an annual. Semi-double or double flowerheads, 5cm (2in) across, in a broad range of colours, including scarlet-red, lilac-pink, and orange, are held above bronze foliage. ↕↔ 45–60cm (18–24in). ✻

D. 'Reginald Keene'. Large-flowered semi-cactus dahlia producing orange flowerheads with flame-red blends. Good for exhibition. ↕ 1.2m (4ft), ↔ 60cm (24in). ✻

D. 'Rhonda' ■ Pompon dahlia producing white blooms with a touch of lilac on the margin of each petal. Good for exhibition. ↕ 1.1m (3½ft), ↔ 60cm (24in). ✻

D. 'Risca Miner'. Small-flowered ball dahlia with deep purple blooms. Good for exhibition. ↕ 1.1m (3½ft), ↔ 60cm (24in). ✻

D. 'Rokesley Mini' ■ Very free-flowering, miniature-flowered cactus dahlia bearing pure white blooms. ↕ 1m (3ft), ↔ 45cm (18in). ✻

D. 'Rose Jupiter'. Giant-flowered semi-cactus dahlia with rose-pink blooms. Good for exhibition. ↕ 1.3m (4½ft), ↔ 60cm (24in). ✻

D. 'Rothesay Superb' ■ Very free-flowering, miniature-flowered ball dahlia bearing bright scarlet blooms on strong stems. ↕ 1.1m (3½ft), ↔ 60cm (24in). ✻

D. 'Rotonde'. Small-flowered cactus dahlia producing deep salmon-pink blooms with incurving petals, resembling incurved chrysanthemums. ↕ 1.1m (3½ft), ↔ 60cm (24in). ✻

D. 'Ruby Wedding' ■ Miniature-flowered decorative dahlia producing ruby red blooms. ↕ 1m (3ft), ↔ 60cm (24in). ✻

D. 'Ruskin Belle'. Medium-flowered semi-cactus dahlia producing purplish pink blooms. Good for exhibition. ↕ 1m (3ft), ↔ 45cm (18in). ✻

D. 'Ruskin Diane' ■ Small-flowered decorative dahlia with well-formed, clear yellow blooms. Good for exhibition. ↕ 1.2m (4ft), ↔ 60cm (24in). ✻

D. 'Rustig'. Medium-flowered decorative dahlia producing pale yellow blooms on strong stems well above the foliage. Good for exhibition. ↕ 1.2m (4ft), ↔ 60cm (24in). ✻

D. 'Salmon Athalie'. Small-flowered cactus dahlia that produces blooms in pale salmon-pink with a touch of yellow at the base of each petal. Good for exhibition. ↕ 1.3m (4½ft), ↔ 60cm (24in). ✻

D. 'Salmon Keene'. Large-flowered semi-cactus dahlia with deep, salmon-pink blooms. Good for exhibition. ↕ 1.2m (4ft), ↔ 60cm (24in). ✻

D. 'Sara G'. Large-flowered semi-cactus dahlia producing light pink blooms, with yellow blends at the petal bases, on strong stems. Good for exhibition. ↕ 1.2m (4ft), ↔ 60cm (24in). ✻

D. 'Scarlet Beauty'. Small-flowered waterlily dahlia with scarlet blooms. ↕ 1.1m (3½ft), ↔ 60cm (24in). ✻

D. 'Scarlet Comet' ■ Anemone-flowered dahlia bearing scarlet blooms with upright, tubular disc-florets. ↕ 1.1m (3½ft), ↔ 60cm (24in). ✻

D. 'Scottish Relation' ♀ Small-flowered semi-cactus dahlia producing vivid purple blooms with cream petal bases. Good for exhibition. ↕ 1.1m (3½ft), ↔ 60cm (24in). ✻

D. 'Senzoe Ursula' ■ Small-flowered decorative dahlia that produces violet blooms with a white base to each petal. Good for exhibition. ↕ 1.2m (4ft), ↔ 60cm (24in). ✻

D. 'Shirley Alliance' ■ Small-flowered cactus dahlia bearing soft orange blooms with a gold base to each petal. Good for exhibition. ↕ 1.3m (4½ft), ↔ 60cm (24in). ✻

D. 'Silver City'. Large-flowered decorative dahlia with waxy white blooms. Good for exhibition. ↕ 1.1m (3½ft), ↔ 60cm (24in). ✻

D. 'Small World' ■ Pompon dahlia with pure white blooms. Good for exhibition. ↕ 1.1m (3½ft), ↔ 60cm (24in). ✻

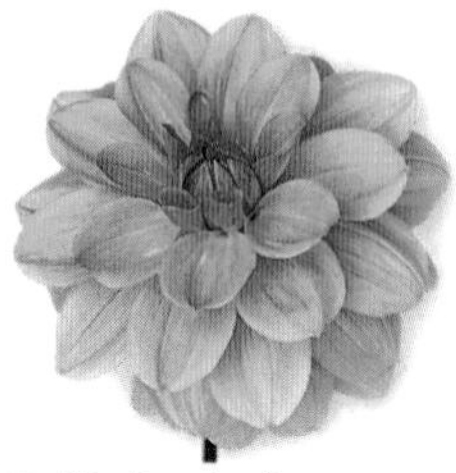
Dahlia 'Pearl of Heemstede'

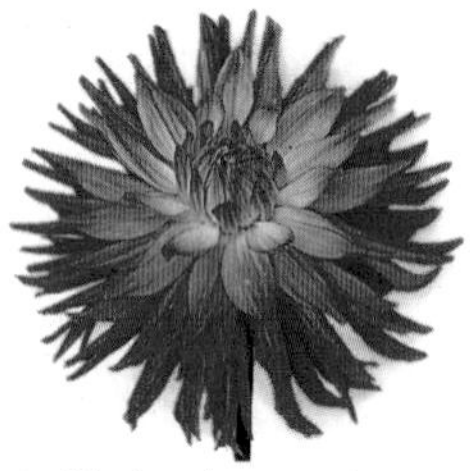
Dahlia 'Pink Jupiter'

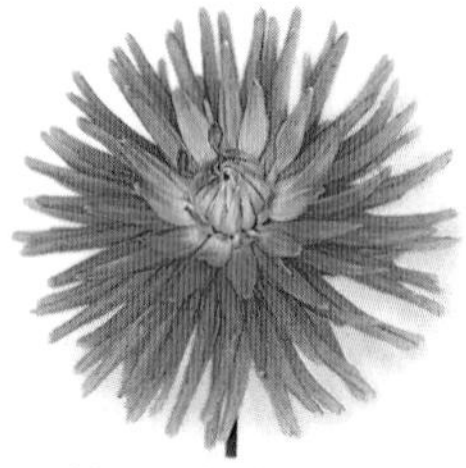
Dahlia 'Pink Shirley Alliance'

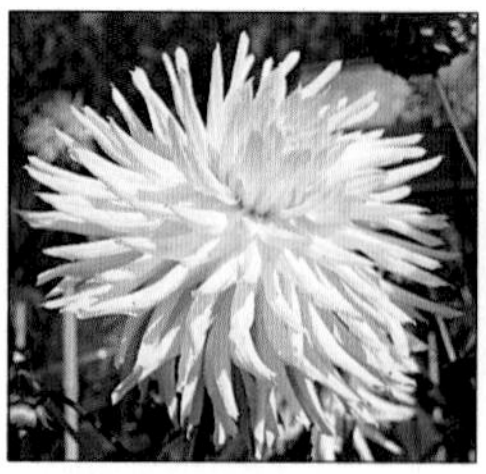
Dahlia 'Polar Sight'

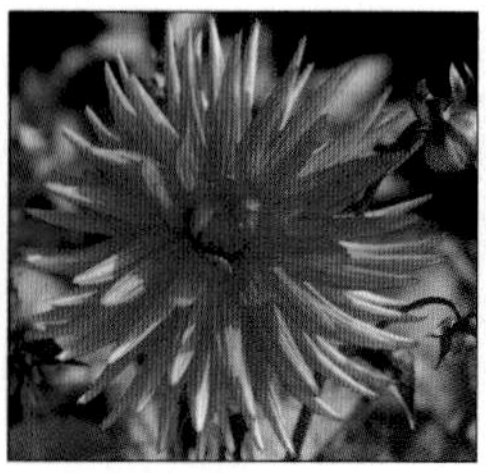
Dahlia 'Pontiac'

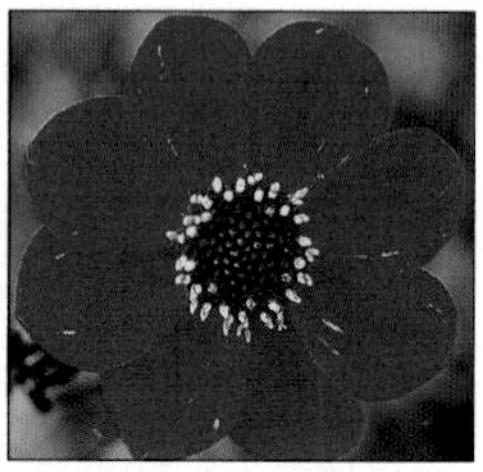
Dahlia 'Preston Park'

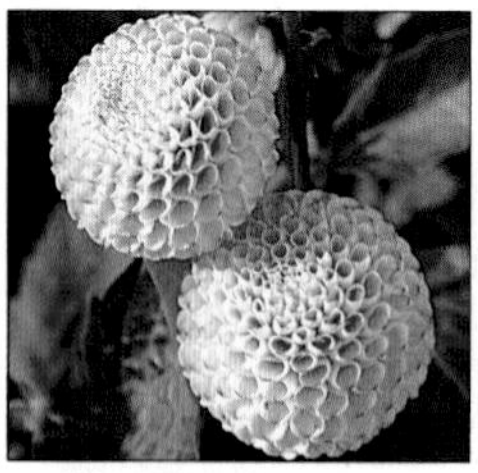
Dahlia 'Rhonda'

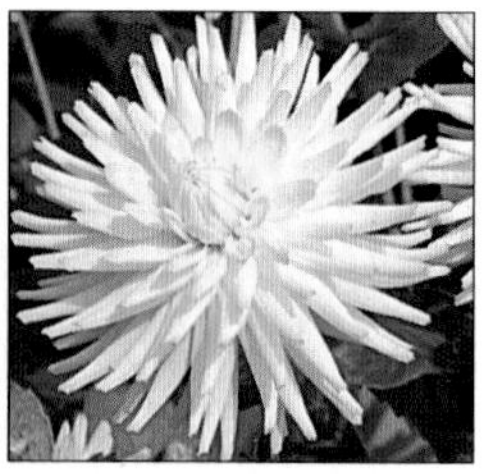
Dahlia 'Rokesley Mini'

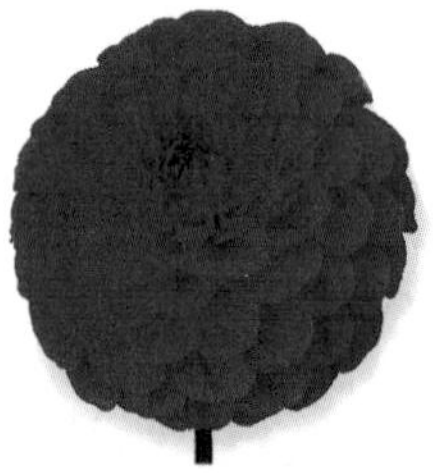
Dahlia 'Rothesay Superb'

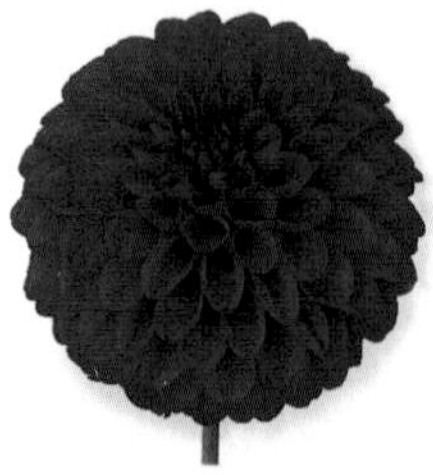
Dahlia 'Ruby Wedding'

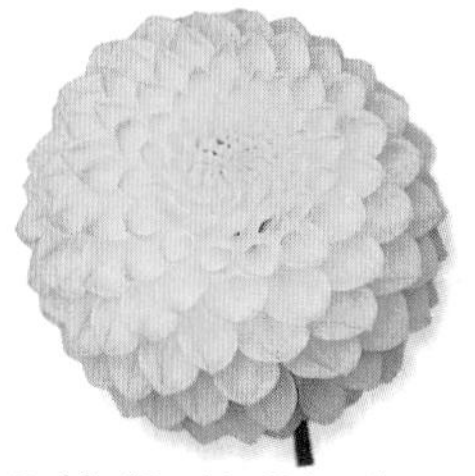
Dahlia 'Ruskin Diane'

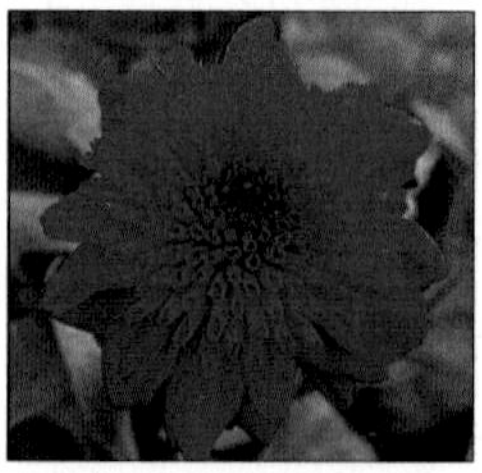
Dahlia 'Scarlet Comet'

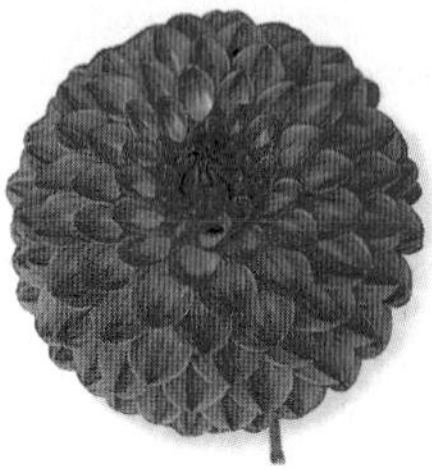
Dahlia 'Senzoe Ursula'

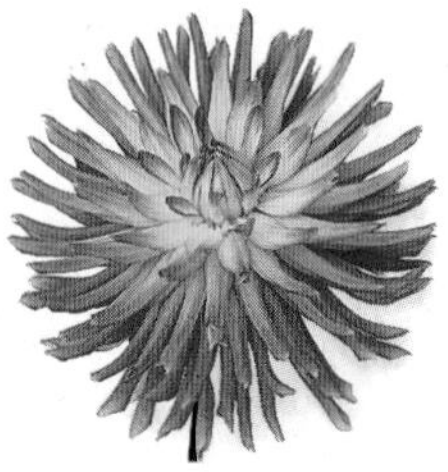
Dahlia 'Shirley Alliance'

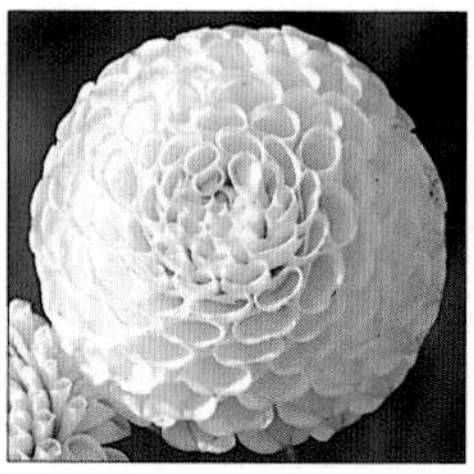
Dahlia 'Small World'

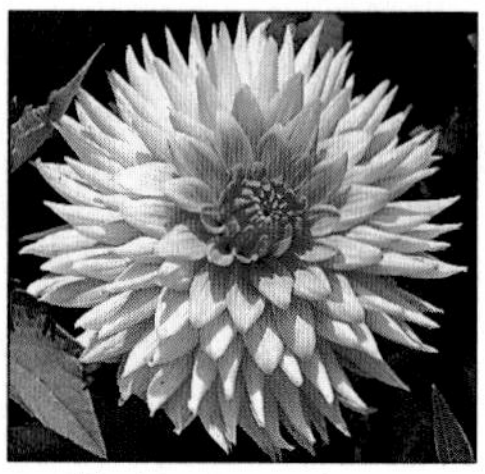
Dahlia 'So Dainty'

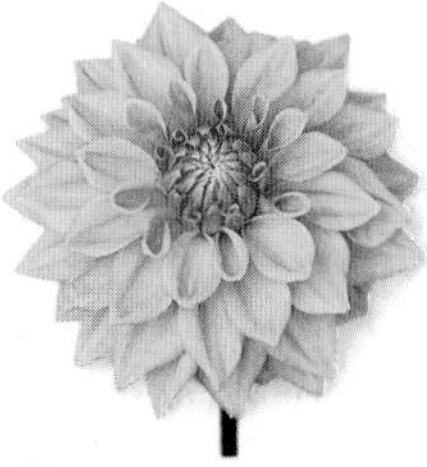
Dahlia 'Trengrove Tauranga'

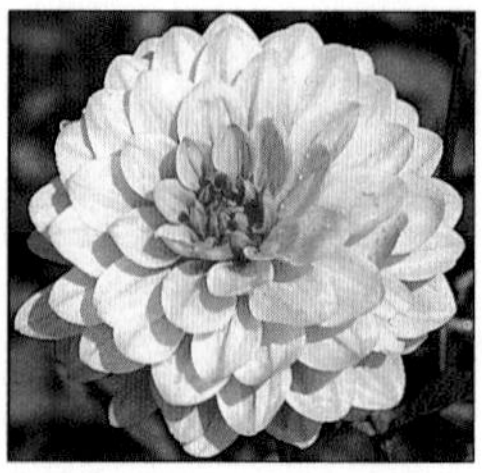
Dahlia 'Vicky Crutchfield'

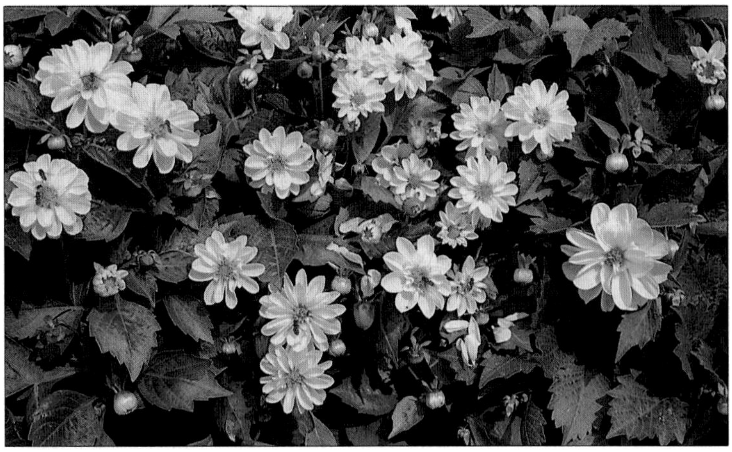
Dahlia 'Sunny Yellow'

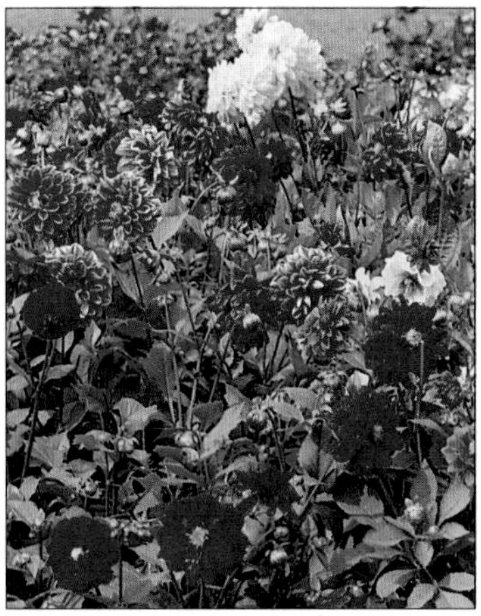
Dahlia Unwins Dwarf Group

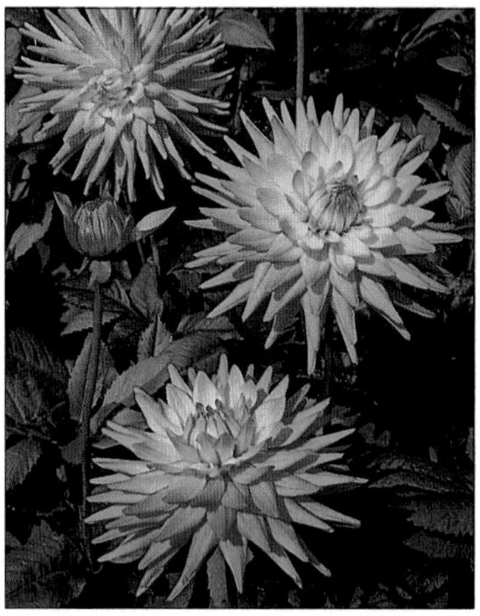
Dahlia 'Wootton Impact'

***D.* 'So Dainty'** ▣ ♀ Miniature-flowered semi-cactus dahlia producing golden bronze blooms, with an apricot tinge, on strong stems. Good for exhibition. ↕ 1.1m (3½ft), ↔ 60cm (24in). ❄
***D.* 'Sunny Yellow'** ▣ ♀ Bushy, fast-growing, dwarf bedding dahlia, grown as an annual, producing semi-double to double, bright yellow flowerheads, 5–7cm (2–3in) across. ↕↔ 45–50cm (18–20in). ❄
***D.* 'Sunray Glint'.** Medium-flowered semi-cactus dahlia producing bright pink blooms with pale lemon-yellow at the base of each petal. Good for exhibition. ↕ 1.2m (4ft), ↔ 60cm (24in). ❄
***D.* 'Susannah Yorke'.** Small-flowered waterlily dahlia producing soft rose-pink blooms with few petals. ↕ 1.1m (3½ft), ↔ 45cm (18in). ❄
***D.* 'Swanvale'.** Small-flowered decorative dahlia producing clear yellow blooms on long, firm stems. ↕ 1.3m (4½ft), ↔ 60cm (24in). ❄
***D.* 'Temptress'.** Small-flowered cactus dahlia bearing light lavender-blue blooms with white petal bases. Good for exhibition. ↕ 1.1m (3½ft), ↔ 60cm (24in). ❄
***D.* 'Trelawny'.** Giant-flowered decorative dahlia producing large-petalled, bronze-red flowerheads and distinctive, leathery, very dark green leaves with well-spaced, prominent veins. ↕ 1.2m (4ft), ↔ 60cm (24in). ❄
***D.* 'Trengrove Jill'.** Medium-flowered decorative dahlia with deep bronze blooms held well above the foliage on strong stems. ↕ 1.3m (4½ft), ↔ 60cm (24in). ❄
***D.* 'Trengrove Summer'.** Medium-flowered decorative dahlia with shining yellow blooms. Good for exhibition. ↕ 1.2m (4ft), ↔ 60cm (24in). ❄
***D.* 'Trengrove Tauranga'** ▣ Medium-flowered decorative dahlia with blooms in shades of bronze. ↕ 1.2m (4ft), ↔ 60cm (24in). ❄
***D.* Unwins Dwarf Group** ▣ Bushy, dwarf bedding dahlias, grown as annuals, producing semi-double to double flowerheads, to 10cm (4in) across, in a range of bright colours, including yellow, red, and white, some flushed with a second colour. ↕↔ to 60cm (24in). ❄
***D.* 'Vantage'.** Giant-flowered semi-cactus dahlia with large-petalled, deep yellow blooms borne well above the foliage on very strong stems. Good for exhibition. ↕ 1.3m (4½ft), ↔ 60cm (24in). ❄
***D.* 'Vicky Crutchfield'** ▣ Small-flowered waterlily dahlia producing shell-pink flowerheads with slightly curled petals. ↕ 1.1m (3½ft), ↔ 60cm (24in). ❄
***D.* 'Vigor'.** Very free-flowering, small-flowered waterlily dahlia producing pale yellow blooms on strong stems. ↕ 1.2m (4ft), ↔ 60cm (24in). ❄
***D.* 'Wanda's Capella'** ▣ Giant-flowered decorative dahlia with bright yellow blooms. Good for exhibition. ↕ 1.2m (4ft), ↔ 60cm (24in). ❄
***D.* 'Wanda's Moonlight'.** Giant-flowered decorative dahlia with yellow blooms. Good for exhibition. ↕ 1.2m (4ft), ↔ 60cm (24in). ❄
***D.* 'Wendy's Place'.** Pompon dahlia with bright purple blooms. Good for exhibition. ↕ 1.1m (3½ft), ↔ 60cm (24in). ❄
***D.* 'Whale's Rhonda'.** Pompon dahlia bearing bright purple blooms with light silver undersides. Good for exhibition. ↕ 1m (3ft), ↔ 45cm (18in). ❄
***D.* 'White Alva's'** ▣ Giant-flowered decorative dahlia with pure white blooms held well above the foliage on strong stems. Good for exhibition. ↕ 1.2m (4ft), ↔ 60cm (24in). ❄
***D.* 'White Klankstad'** ▣ Small-flowered cactus dahlia that produces white blooms. ↕ 1.2m (4ft), ↔ 60cm (24in). ❄
***D.* 'White Linda'.** Small-flowered decorative dahlia bearing white blooms with a touch of light lavender-blue. Good for exhibition. ↕ 1.2m (4ft), ↔ 60cm (24in). ❄
***D.* 'White Moonlight'.** Medium-flowered semi-cactus dahlia with white blooms. Good for exhibition. ↕ 1.2m (4ft), ↔ 60cm (24in). ❄
***D.* 'White Perfection'.** Very free-flowering, giant-flowered decorative dahlia producing pure white blooms with a neat petal formation. ↕ 1.2m (4ft), ↔ 60cm (24in). ❄
***D.* 'White Rustig'.** Medium-flowered decorative dahlia with white blooms. Good for exhibition. ↕ 1.2m (4ft), ↔ 60cm (24in). ❄
***D.* 'White Swallow'.** Small-flowered semi-cactus dahlia with white blooms borne on strong stems. Good for exhibition. ↕ 1.1m (3½ft), ↔ 60cm (24in). ❄
***D.* 'Willo's Surprise'.** Pompon dahlia with wine-red blooms. Good for exhibition. ↕ 1.1m (3½ft), ↔ 60cm (24in). ❄
***D.* 'Wootton Cupid'** ▣ ♀ Miniature-flowered ball dahlia with sugar-pink blooms held well above the foliage on strong stems. Good for exhibition. ↕ 1.1m (3½ft), ↔ 60cm (24in). ❄
***D.* 'Wootton Impact'** ▣ ♀ Medium-flowered semi-cactus dahlia producing blooms in shades of bronze held well above the foliage on strong stems. Good for exhibition. ↕ 1.2m (4ft), ↔ 60cm (24in). ❄
***D.* 'Yellow Frank Hornsey'.** Small-flowered decorative dahlia bearing bright yellow blooms with a touch of bronze on each petal. ↕ 1.2m (4ft), ↔ 60cm (24in). ❄
***D.* 'Yellow Hammer'** ▣ ♀ Single-flowered, dwarf bedding dahlia producing yellow flowerheads above bronze foliage. ↕ 60cm (24in), ↔ 45cm (18in). ❄
***D.* 'Yellow Spiky'** ▣ Medium-flowered semi-cactus dahlia bearing yellow blooms overlaid with bronze. Good for exhibition. ↕ 1.3m (4½ft), ↔ 60cm (24in). ❄
***D.* 'Yelno Enchantment'** ▣ Small-flowered waterlily dahlia producing blooms in shades of peach-pink with a touch of apricot. ↕ 1.2m (4ft), ↔ 60cm (24in). ❄
***D.* 'Yelno Firelight'** ▣ Small-flowered waterlily dahlia producing red and yellow blooms, with a neat petal formation, on strong stems. ↕ 1.2m (4ft), ↔ 60cm (24in). ❄
***D.* 'Yelno Royal'.** Small-flowered waterlily dahlia producing red-purple blooms, with a neat petal formation, on strong stems. ↕ 1.2m (4ft), ↔ 60cm (24in). ❄
***D.* 'Yelno Velvena'.** Small-flowered waterlily dahlia producing deep maroon blooms on strong stems. ↕ 1.2m (4ft), ↔ 60cm (24in). ❄
***D.* 'Zorro'** ▣ Giant-flowered decorative dahlia producing bright blood-red blooms. Good for exhibition. ↕ 1.2m (4ft), ↔ 60cm (24in). ❄

▷ **Daily dew** see *Drosera*

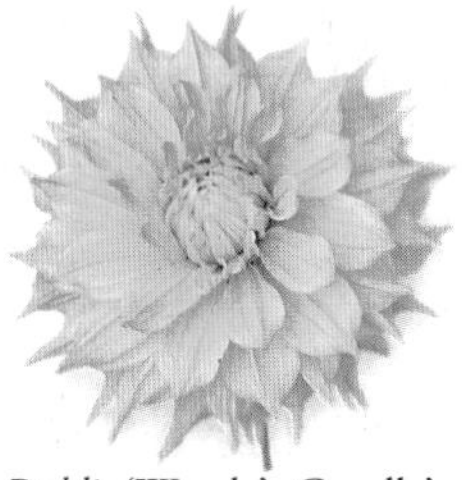
Dahlia 'Wanda's Capella'

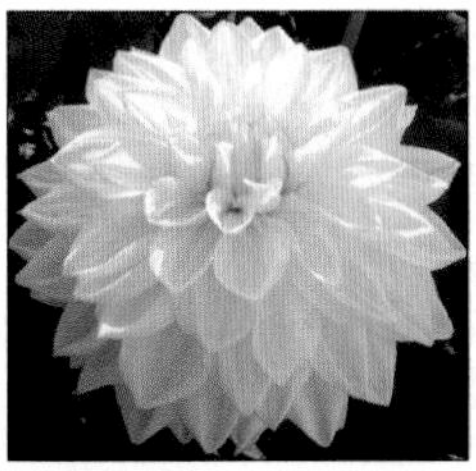
Dahlia 'White Alva's'

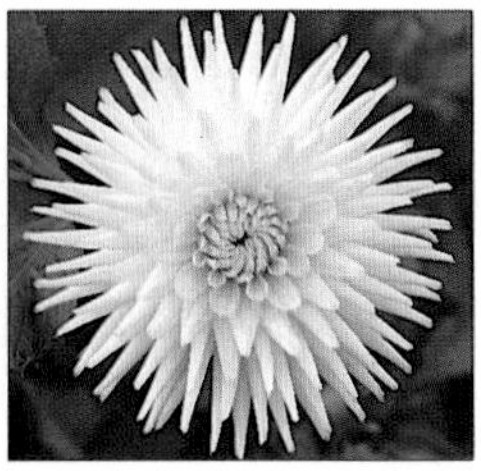
Dahlia 'White Klankstad'

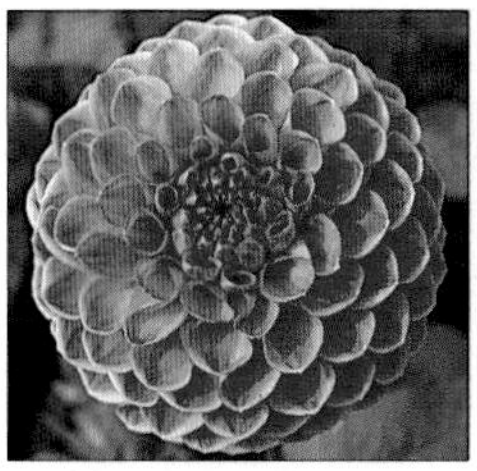
Dahlia 'Wootton Cupid''

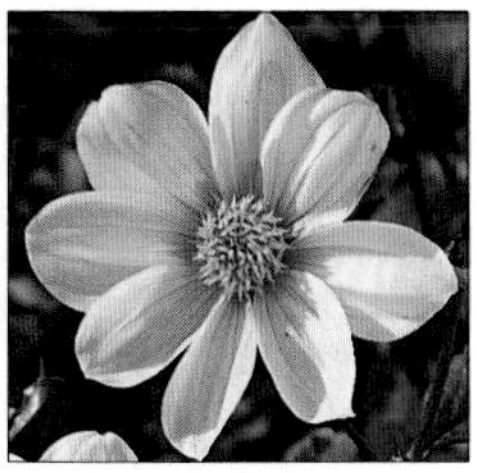
Dahlia 'Yellow Hammer'

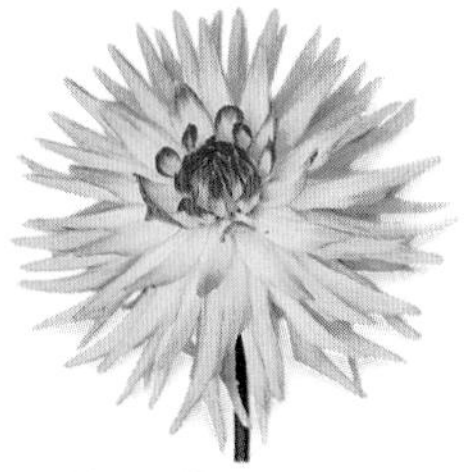
Dahlia 'Yellow Spiky'

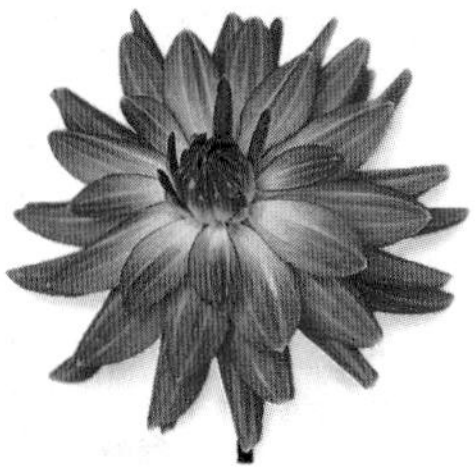
Dahlia 'Yelno Enchantment'

Dahlia 'Yelno Firelight'

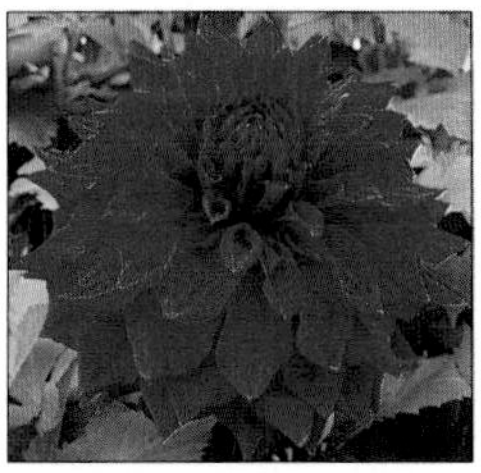
Dahlia 'Zorro'

D

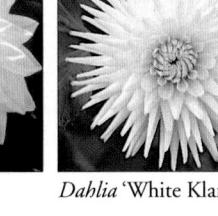

DAIS

THYMELAEACEAE

Genus of 2 species of deciduous or evergreen shrubs and trees from forest margins and damp, wooded slopes in Madagascar and South Africa. They have alternate or opposite, obovate to oblong-elliptic leaves, and are grown for their terminal umbels of tubular flowers, with 5 spreading lobes. Grow in a border or as specimen plants. In frost-prone areas, grow in a cool greenhouse.

• **HARDINESS** Half hardy to frost tender.

• **CULTIVATION** Under glass, grow in loam-based potting compost (JI No.2) in full light. In growth, water freely and apply balanced liquid fertilizer monthly; keep just moist in winter. Top-dress or pot on in spring. Outdoors, grow in fertile, moist but well-drained soil in full sun. Pruning group 1.

• **PROPAGATION** Sow seed at 16–18°C (61–64°F) in spring. Root semi-ripe cuttings with bottom heat in summer. Detach suckering shoots when dormant.

• **PESTS AND DISEASES** Red spider mites may infest greenhouse plants.

D. cotinifolia ▣ ◌ Bushy, rounded shrub or small tree, deciduous in cool climates but evergreen in warm areas, with obovate to ovate or oblong, glossy, bluish green leaves, 4–7cm (1½–3in) long. In summer, bears erect, rounded umbels, 3–5cm (1¼–2in) across, of up to 15 fragrant, lilac or lilac-pink flowers, 1.5cm (½in) long. ↕ 1.5–3m (5–10ft), ↔ 2–4m (6–12ft). Madagascar, South Africa. ❄ (borderline)

▷ ***Daiswa*** see *Paris*
D. polyphylla see *P. polyphylla*

▷ **Daisy** see *Bellis*
African see *Arctotis, Dimorphotheca*
Barberton see *Gerbera jamesonii*
Blue see *Felicia, F. amelloides*
Blue-eyed African see *Arctotis venusta*
Common see *Bellis perennis*

▷ **Daisy cont.**
Dahlberg see *Thymophylla tenuiloba*
Globe see *Globularia*
Kingfisher see *Felicia bergeriana*
Livingstone see *Dorotheanthus, D. bellidiformis*
Marlborough rock see *Pachystegia insignis*
Michaelmas see *Aster novi-belgii*
New Zealand see *Celmisia*
Ox-eye see *Leucanthemum vulgare*
Painted see *Chrysanthemum carinatum, Tanacetum coccineum*
Palm Springs see *Cladanthus*
Rain see *Dimorphotheca pluvialis*
Rock see *Brachyscome multifida*
Shasta see *Leucanthemum* x *superbum*
Star see *Lindheimera, L. texana*
Swan river see *Brachyscome, B. iberidifolia*
Transvaal see *Gerbera jamesonii*

▷ **Daisy bush** see *Olearia*

▷ **Damask rose** see *Rosa* x *damascena*

DAMASONIUM

Starfruit

ALISMATACEAE

Genus of 6 species of marginal aquatic, herbaceous perennials, closely related to water plantains (*Alisma*), found in the N. hemisphere and Australia. The long-stalked, linear-oblong, often floating leaves have prominent midribs. Whorls of shallowly cup-shaped, white or pink flowers are borne in umbels, racemes, or panicles. The clusters of ellipsoid fruits grow in radiating, star-like whorls, hence the common name. Grow in the shallow margins of a small pool.

• **HARDINESS** Frost hardy if rootstocks are submerged.

• **CULTIVATION** Grow in full sun, in water no deeper than 15cm (6in), or in wet mud at the side of still water.

• **PROPAGATION** Sow seed in seed trays or containers half-submerged in shallow trays of water, as soon as ripe or in the following spring if kept damp. Divide rhizomes when dormant.

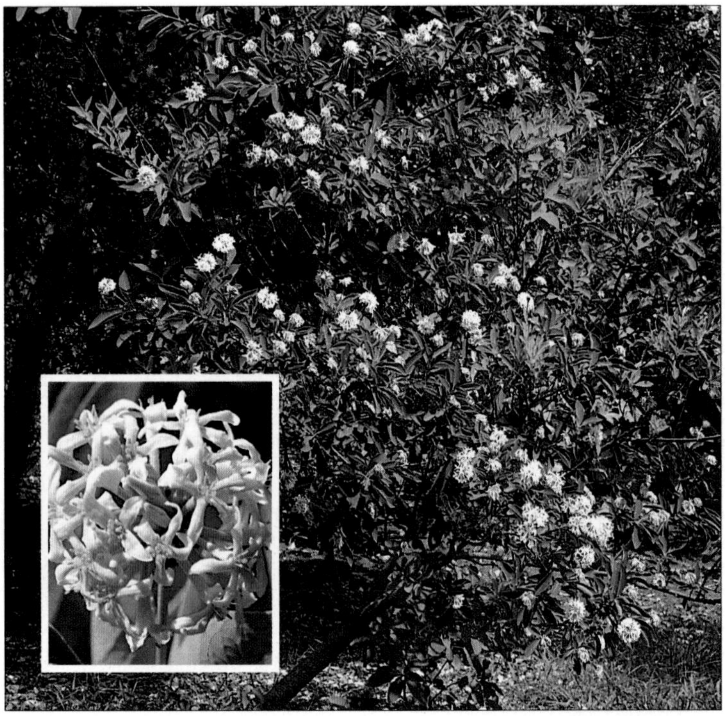

Dais cotinifolia (inset: flower detail)

• **PESTS AND DISEASES** Larvae of certain moths, particularly the brown china-mark moth, may feed on the leaves.

D. alisma. Variable, marginal aquatic perennial with oblong or ovate-oblong, floating leaves, 8cm (3in) long, which are produced from congested rhizomes. Numerous white flowers, 6–8mm (¼–⅜in) across, with a yellow spot at the base of each petal, are produced in whorled panicles, 3–7cm (1¼–3in) long, in late spring and early summer. The star-shaped fruit are 5–12mm (¼–½in) across. ↕↔ 15–20cm (6–8in). W., S., and S.E. Europe. ❄❄

D. californicum. Marginal aquatic, rhizomatous perennial with erect or floating, linear-oblong to ovate leaves, 10cm (4in) long. Numerous white or pink flowers, 4–6mm (⅛–¼in) across, are borne in whorled panicles, to 45cm (18in) long, in late spring and early summer. ↕ 45cm (18in), ↔ 40cm (16in). S. USA. ❄❄

▷ ***Dammara*** see *Agathis*

DAMPIERA

GOODENIACEAE

Genus of about 70 species of soft-stemmed herbaceous perennials or deciduous or evergreen subshrubs from heath to high mountains in Australia. The variable, alternate leaves are often densely woolly. Flowers are usually blue and have a split corolla tube, the 3 lower petals spreading, the upper 2 widely separated and erect; they are solitary or borne in cymes, panicles, or racemes. Suckering species are useful for ground cover. In frost-prone areas, grow tender species in a temperate greenhouse.

• **HARDINESS** Half hardy to frost tender.

• **CULTIVATION** Under glass, grow in loam-based potting compost (JI No.2) in full light with some midday shade. In growth, water freely and apply a balanced liquid fertilizer monthly; keep just moist in winter. Outdoors, grow in well-drained, neutral to acid soil in sun or partial shade. *D. hederacea* and *D. diversifolia* grow well in partial shade.

• **PROPAGATION** Divide rootstocks and separate suckers of perennials in spring; root semi-ripe cuttings in summer.

• **PESTS AND DISEASES** Trouble free.

D. diversifolia ▣ Densely branched, suckering, prostrate perennial. The lance-shaped to inversely lance-shaped, hairless, leathery leaves, to 3cm (1¼in) long, are entire or minutely toothed. Solitary, dark blue flowers, 1cm (½in) across, on short peduncles, are produced from the leaf axils in summer. ↕ 1m (3ft), ↔ 2m (6ft). Australia (Western Australia). ❀ (min. 7°C/45°F)

D. hederacea. Procumbent perennial with ovate, often lobed, hairless leaves, to 4cm (1½in) long, broadly ovate to heart-shaped at the bases and densely woolly beneath. The upper leaves are smaller. Bears 3–7 pale to rich blue or white flowers, to 1cm (½in) long, softly hairy on the outside, in slender cymes, to 5cm (2in) long, from midwinter to midsummer. ↕ 30cm (12in), ↔ 1m (3ft). Australia (Western Australia). ❄

D. linearis. Erect or spreading, suckering perennial with blunt-tipped, obovate to elliptic, entire or toothed,

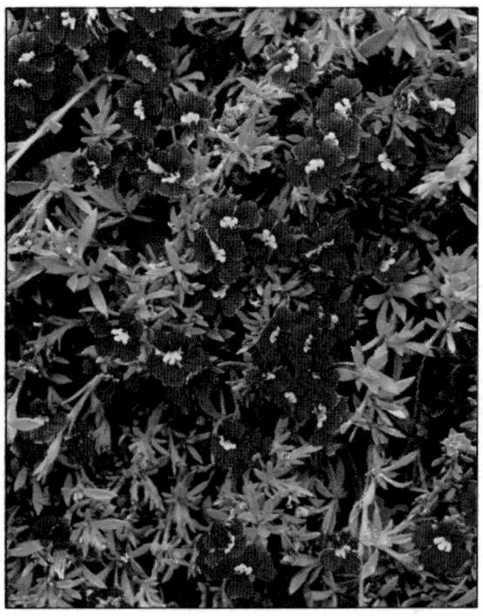

Dampiera diversifolia

stalkless, leathery leaves, 4cm (1½in) long. Produces 1–7 blue flowers, 1.5cm (½in) across, in cymes to 5cm (2in) long, in summer. ↕ 30cm (12in), ↔ 1m (3ft). Australia (Western Australia). ❀ (min. 10°C/50°F)

D. rosmarinifolia (Wild rosemary). Erect or procumbent, suckering, evergreen subshrub with densely woolly stems and blunt-tipped, linear-oblong or oblong, entire, silver leaves, 2.5cm (1in) long. Bears solitary, deep blue, rarely pink flowers, 1.5cm (½in) across, in summer. ↕ 50cm (20in), ↔ 1m (3ft). Australia (South Australia, Victoria). ❀ (min. 10°C/50°F)

D. trigona. Erect or spreading perennial or evergreen subshrub with narrowly elliptic to linear, entire to minutely toothed, hairless leaves, 5cm (2in) long. Usually solitary, blue, violet-blue, or white flowers, to 1.5cm (½in) across, are produced in summer. ↕ 20–75cm (8–30in), ↔ 40–120cm (16–48in). Australia (Western Australia). ❀ (min. 10°C/50°F)

DANAE

LILIACEAE/RUSCACEAE

Genus of one species of clump-forming, shrub-like, evergreen, rhizomatous perennial found in woodland in Turkey and Iran. Upright then arching, branched shoots bear flattened, leaf-like stems. Small, greenish yellow flowers are followed by red berries. Valued for its attractive foliage, stems, and fruit, *D. racemosa* is suitable for light woodland or a shrub border.

• **HARDINESS** Frost hardy.

• **CULTIVATION** Grow in fertile, moist but well-drained soil in sun or shade, sheltered from strong winds. Cut old shoots back to ground level in spring.

• **PROPAGATION** Sow seed in containers in a cold frame in autumn. Divide from autumn to early spring.

• **PESTS AND DISEASES** Trouble free.

D. racemosa ♈ (Alexandrian laurel). Shrub-like perennial with slender green shoots and alternate, lance-shaped to ovate-lance-shaped, tapering, glossy, leaf-like stems, to 10cm (4in) long. Terminal racemes, 5cm (2in) long, of 5–8 small, greenish yellow flowers are borne in early summer. Berries are orange-red or red, 6mm (¼in) across. ↕↔ 1m (3ft). Turkey, Iran. ❄❄

▷ **Dandelion, Pink** see *Crepis incana*

DAPHNE

THYMELAEACEAE

Genus of about 50 species of deciduous, semi-evergreen, or evergreen shrubs from Europe, N. Africa, and temperate and subtropical Asia, found in habitats ranging from lowland woodland to mountains. They are grown mainly for their 4-lobed, tubular, usually fragrant, terminal or axillary flowers, borne singly or in short racemes or clustered heads, and varying from red-purple to pink, white, yellow, lavender-pink, and lilac. Daphnes are also sometimes grown for their foliage, fruit, or upright, rounded, or prostrate habit. The simple, linear to ovate, entire leaves are alternate, rarely opposite, and hairless to softly hairy. The spherical to ovoid fruits, 2–10mm (1/16–1/2in) across, may be fleshy or dry, and white, pink, orange, red, or purple-black. Grow in a rock garden, a shrub border, or in woodland. All parts, including the seed, are highly toxic if ingested, and contact with the sap may irritate skin.

- **HARDINESS** Fully hardy to frost hardy.
- **CULTIVATION** Grow in moderately fertile, humus-rich, well-drained but not dry soil. Mulch to keep roots cool. Most prefer slightly alkaline to slightly acid soil in sun or partial shade. *D. arbuscula* and *D. genkwa* need full sun, while *D. laureola* and *D. pontica* tolerate deep shade. All resent transplanting. Pruning group 1 or 8; keep to a minimum.
- **PROPAGATION** Sow seed in containers in a cold frame as soon as ripe. Insert softwood cuttings in early and mid-summer, and semi-ripe and evergreen cuttings in mid- or late summer. Graft in winter or layer in spring.
- **PESTS AND DISEASES** Aphids, leaf spot, grey mould (*Botrytis*), and viruses may be troublesome.

D. acutiloba. Erect, sometimes spreading, evergreen shrub with oblong-lance-shaped to inversely lance-shaped, leathery, glossy, bright green leaves, to 10cm (4in) long. Bears terminal clusters of 5–7 white, usually scented flowers, to 1.5cm (1/2in) across, in summer, followed by fleshy, spherical red fruit. ↕↔ 1.5m (5ft). W. and C. China. ❄❄❄

D. alpina ▣ Upright, compact, deciduous shrub with downy shoots and obovate to inversely lance-shaped, hairy, grey-green leaves, 1–4cm (1/2–11/2in) long. Bears terminal clusters of 4–10

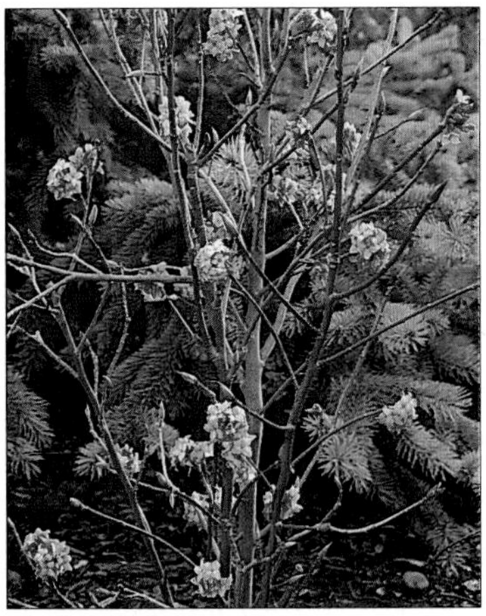

Daphne bholua 'Gurkha'

fragrant white flowers, to 1cm (1/2in) across, in late spring and early summer, followed by fleshy, spherical, orange-red fruit. ↕↔ to 60cm (24in). C. and S. Europe. ❄❄❄

D. arbuscula ♀ Dwarf, semi-prostrate, evergreen shrub with linear to linear-oblong, leathery, glossy, dark green leaves, to 2cm (3/4in) long. In late spring and early summer, produces dense terminal clusters of 3–30 very fragrant, deep pink flowers, to 1.5cm (1/2in) across, followed by dry, ovoid, greyish white fruit. ↕ to 15cm (6in), ↔ to 45cm (18in). Czech Republic and Slovakia (Carpathians). ❄❄❄

D. bholua. Upright, rarely spreading, deciduous or evergreen shrub with narrowly elliptic to inversely lance-shaped, leathery, dark green leaves, to 10cm (4in) long. Terminal clusters of 7–15 richly fragrant white flowers, to 1.5cm (1/2in) across, flushed purple-pink, are produced in late winter, followed by fleshy, spherical, blackish purple fruit. ↕ 2–4m (6–12ft), ↔ 1.5m (5ft). E. Himalayas. ❄❄. **'Gurkha'** ▣♀ is deciduous; ❄❄❄. **'Jacqueline Postill'** ▣♀ is evergreen, with intensely fragrant flowers, to 2cm (3/4in) across, deep purple-pink outside and white within; ❄❄❄ (borderline)

D. blagayana ▣ Prostrate, trailing, evergreen or semi-evergreen shrub with broadly ovate to obovate, leathery, dark green leaves, 3–5cm (11/4–2in) long. In spring, bears terminal clusters of 20–30 fragrant, creamy white flowers, to 1cm (1/2in) across, followed by fleshy, spherical, white or pink fruit. ↕ to 40cm (16in), ↔ 1m (3ft). Balkans. ❄❄❄

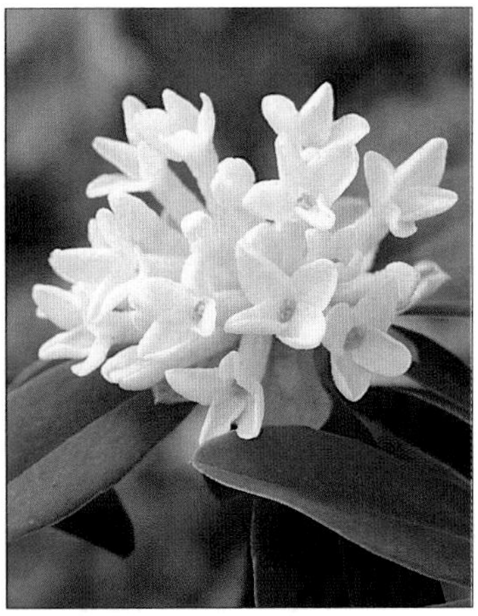

Daphne blagayana

***D. x burkwoodii* cultivars.** Upright, densely branched, semi-evergreen shrubs with linear to inversely lance-shaped, mid-green leaves, to 4cm (11/2in) long. Bears terminal clusters of up to 16 fragrant white flowers, 8mm (3/8in) across, flushed pink to pale purplish pink, in late spring, and sometimes again in autumn. ↕↔ 1–1.5m (3–5ft). ❄❄❄. **'Albert Burkwood'** is rounded, usually broader than tall, and has pink-flushed white flowers; ↕ 75cm (30in), ↔ 1m (3ft). **'Astrid'** ▣ has narrow, creamy white leaf margins. **'Carol Mackie'** has leaves margined golden yellow, later creamy white. **'G.K. Argles'** has leaves with golden yellow margins. **'Lavenirii'** is spreading, and has deep purple-pink flowers with light pink lobes and deep pink throats; ↕ 1m (3ft), ↔ 1.3m (41/2ft). **'Somerset'** ▣ is vase-shaped and has purple-pink flowers with light pink lobes; ↕ 1.5m (5ft), ↔ 1m (3ft). **'Somerset Variegated'** has broad cream leaf margins.

D. caucasica. Upright, deciduous shrub with inversely lance-shaped to linear-lance-shaped, hairless, pale green leaves, to 7cm (3in) long. Produces terminal and axillary clusters of up to 20 fragrant white flowers, to 1.5cm (1/2in) across, in late spring and early summer, followed by fleshy, spherical black fruit (red in one variant). ↕↔ 1.5m (5ft). Caucasus, Georgia, Armenia, Azerbaijan. ❄❄❄

D. cneorum ▣ (Garland flower). Low-growing, evergreen shrub with trailing, branching stems and smooth, inversely lance-shaped leaves, 1–2cm (1/2–3/4in) long, dark green above and grey-green beneath. Bears abundant dense, terminal

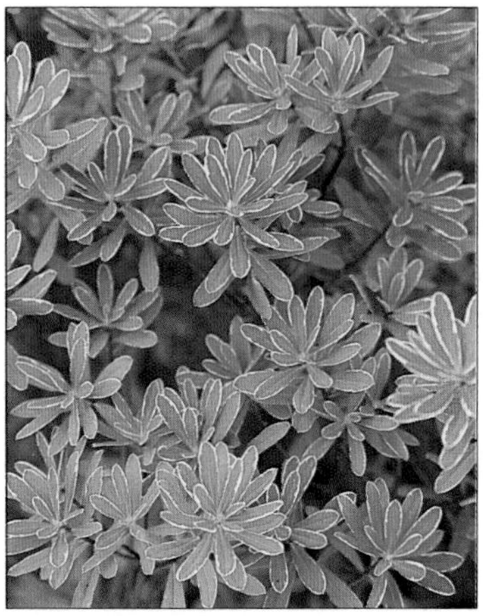

Daphne x *burkwoodii* 'Astrid'

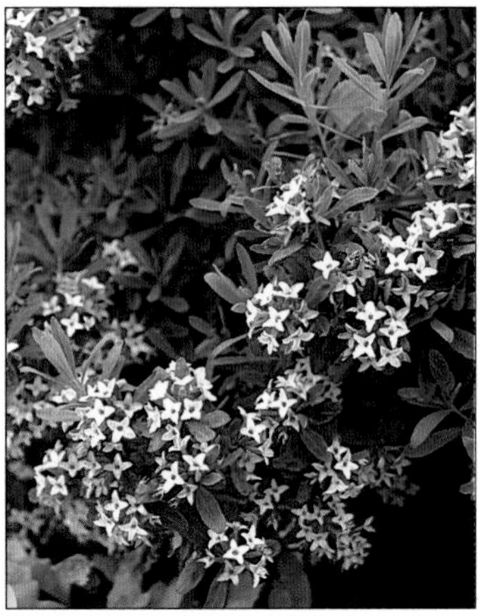

Daphne x *burkwoodii* 'Somerset'

clusters of 6–20 strongly scented, pale to deep rose-pink, occasionally white flowers, to 1cm (1/2in) long, in late spring. ↕ 15cm (6in) or more, ↔ to 2m (6ft). Mountains of C. and S. Europe. ❄❄❄. **'Eximia'** ♀ is vigorous, with crimson buds and deep rose-pink flowers, to 1cm (1/2in) long; ↕ to 20cm (8in). **var. *pygmaea*** is very compact, with leaves 6–8mm (1/4–3/8in) long; ↕ to 10cm (4in), ↔ to 30cm (12in); Alps (S.E. France, N. Italy).

D. collina, syn. *D. sericea* Collina Group. Domed, many-branched, dense, evergreen shrub with obovate, glossy, mid-green leaves, 2–4cm (3/4–11/2in) long, hairy beneath. In late spring and early summer, bears terminal clusters of up to 15 strongly fragrant, deep purplish pink flowers, to 8mm (3/8in)

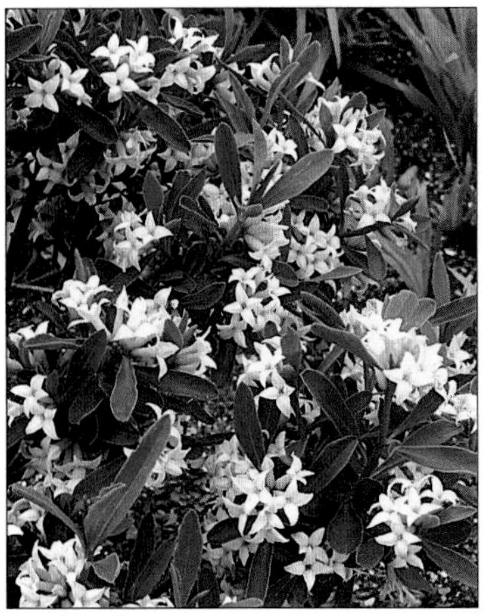

Daphne alpina

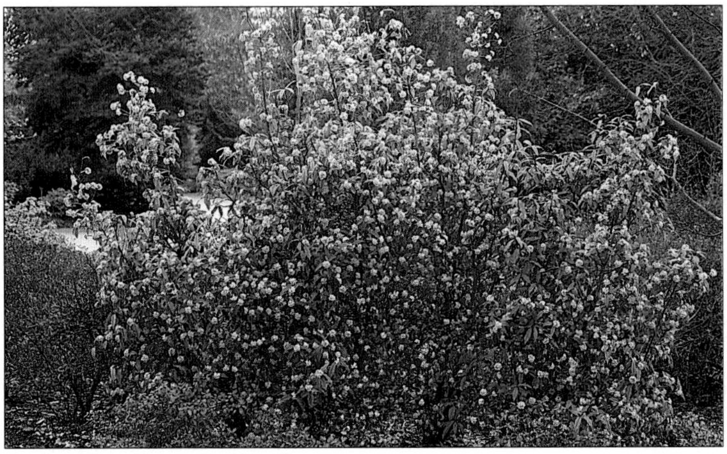

Daphne bholua 'Jacqueline Postill'

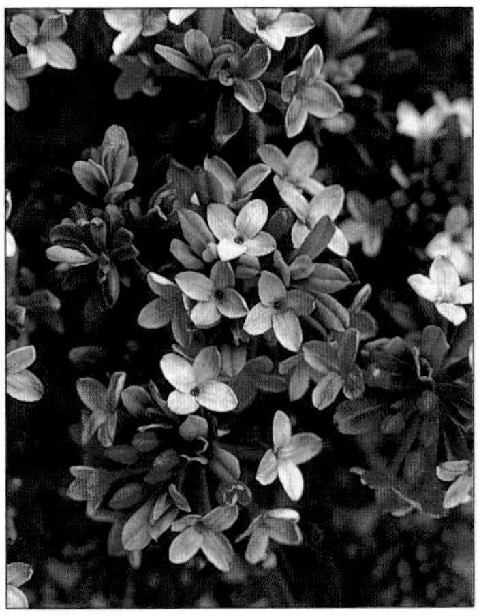

Daphne cneorum

D

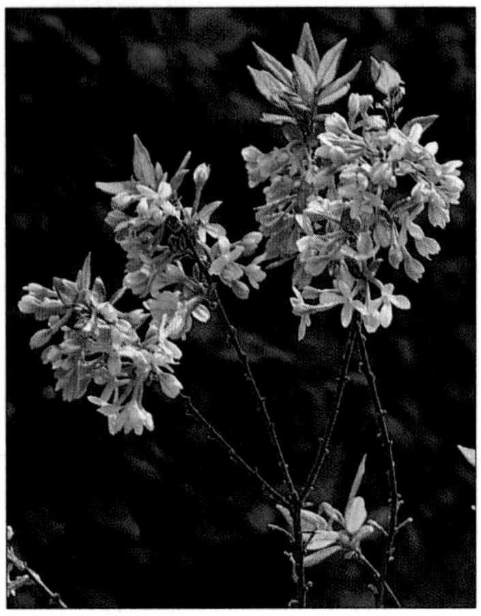

Daphne genkwa

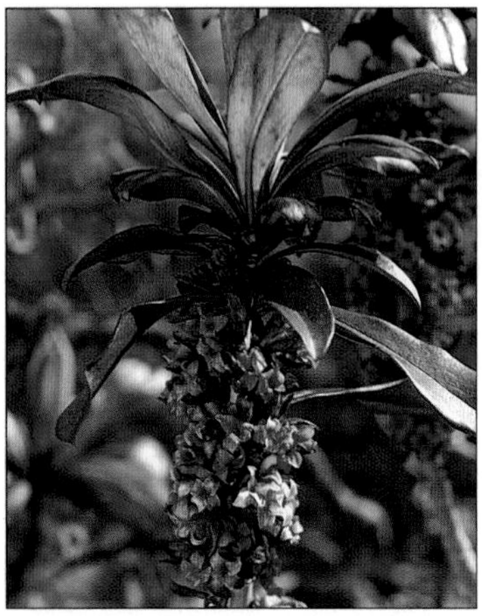

Daphne x *houtteana*

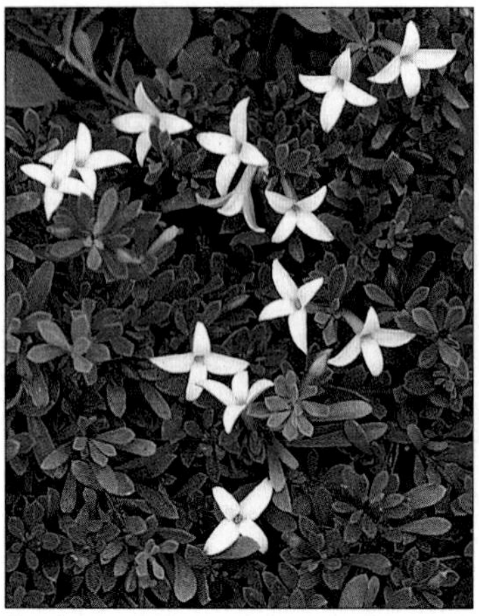

Daphne jasminea

across, with silky-haired tubes, and becoming paler with age. The fleshy, spherical fruit are orange-red. ↕↔ to 50cm (20in). S. Italy. ✻✻✻

D. genkwa ■ Upright, open, deciduous shrub with opposite, occasionally alternate, lance-shaped to ovate, mid-green, initially silky leaves, to 7cm (3in) long. Axillary clusters of 2–7 fragrant lilac flowers, 0.6–2cm (¼–¾in) across, are borne before the leaves, in mid- and late spring. The dry, ovoid fruit are greyish white. ↕↔ 1.5m (5ft). China (W. Hubei). ✻✻✻

D. giraldii. Upright, bushy, deciduous shrub bearing inversely lance-shaped, slightly glaucous, pale green leaves, to 6cm (2½in) long. Produces terminal clusters of 4–8 fragrant, golden yellow flowers, 8mm (⅜in) across, in early summer; flowers are followed by fleshy, spherical red fruit. ↕↔ 60cm (24in). China. ✻✻✻

D. glandulosa see *D. oleoides.*

D. gnidium. Upright, evergreen shrub with linear to obovate-oblong, pointed, leathery, grey-green leaves, to 5cm (2in) long. Bears terminal and axillary panicles of 10 or more fragrant, creamy white flowers, to 6mm (¼in) across, from late spring to autumn, followed by fleshy, spherical red fruit. ↕ 1.5m (5ft), ↔ 1.2m (4ft). Coastal areas of Spain to Greece, N. Africa, Canary Islands. ✻✻

D.* x *houtteana ■ (*D. laureola* x *D. mezereum*). Erect, semi-evergreen shrub with inversely lance-shaped, glossy, dark green leaves, suffused purple, to 9cm (3½in) long. Bears axillary clusters of 2–5 purple-pink flowers, 6mm (¼in) across, in early spring. ↕ 1.2m (4ft), ↔ 1.5m (5ft). Garden origin. ✻✻✻

D. jasminea ■ Semi-prostrate, occasionally upright, many-branched, evergreen shrub with scattered, oblong-obovate, hairless, grey-green or blue-green leaves, to 1cm (½in) long. Terminal pink buds, in pairs (rarely in groups of 3), open to fragrant, sometimes pink-flushed, white or cream flowers, to 8mm (⅜in) across, from late spring to summer. ↕ 10–30cm (4–12in), ↔ to 30cm (12in). S.E. Greece (including Crete), Libya. ✻✻✻

D. jezoensis ■ Slow-growing, rounded, upright, summer-deciduous shrub with inversely lance-shaped leaves, to 9cm (3½in) long, slightly shiny above, pale green at first, later mid-green. Bears up to 10 fragrant, golden yellow flowers, to 1.5cm (½in) across, in terminal clusters, from winter to early spring, followed by fleshy, spherical red fruit. ↕ 45cm (18in), ↔ 60cm (24in). N. Japan. ✻✻✻

***D.* 'Kilmeston'.** Semi-prostrate, evergreen shrub with narrowly ovate, leathery, dark green leaves, 1.5cm (½in) long. Terminal clusters of 6–12 fragrant, mid-pink flowers, 8–12mm (⅜–½in) across, are produced in early and mid-spring and sporadically in early and midsummer. ↕ 30cm (12in), ↔ 40cm (16in). ✻✻✻

D. laureola (Spurge laurel). Bushy, evergreen shrub with obovate to inversely lance-shaped, leathery, glossy, dark green leaves, to 8cm (3in) long. In late winter and early spring, bears axillary clusters of up to 10 slightly fragrant, pale green or yellow-green flowers, to 8mm (⅜in) across, followed by fleshy, ovoid black fruit. ↕ 1m (3ft),

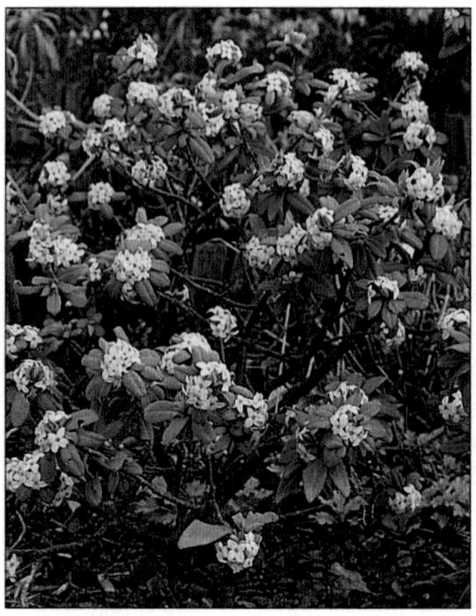

Daphne jezoensis

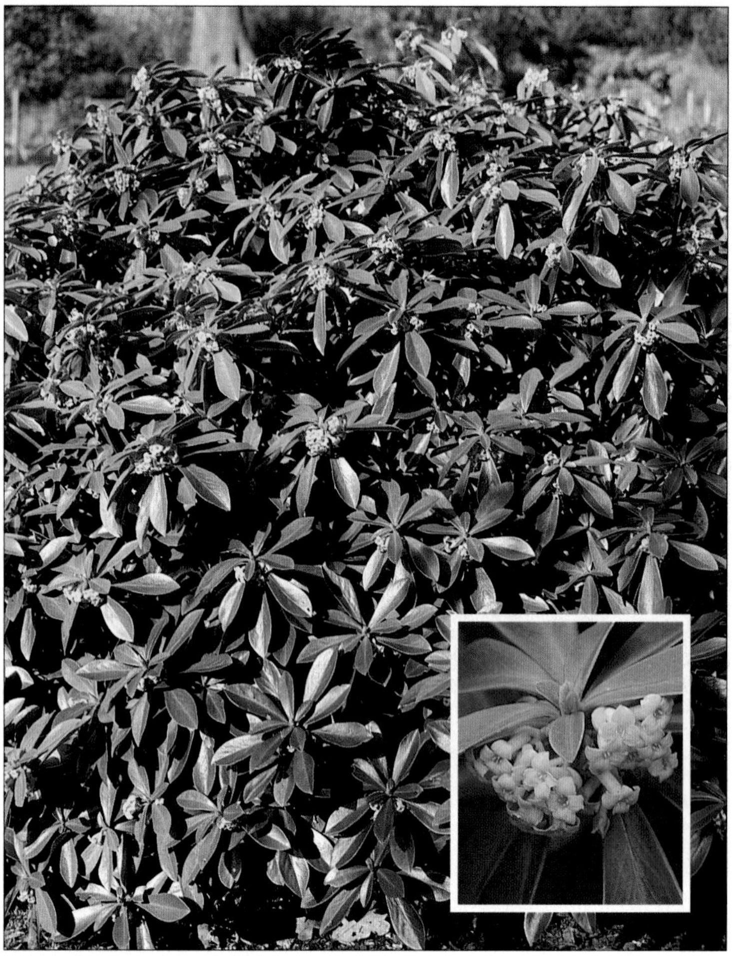

Daphne laureola subsp. *philippi* (inset: flower detail)

↔ 1.5m (5ft). W. to S.E. Europe, Sicily, Corsica, North Africa, Azores. ✻✻✻. **subsp. *philippi*** ■ is semi-prostrate, mildly suckering, and compact, with leaves to 6cm (2½in) long and flowers to 5mm (¼in) across; ↕ 45cm (18in), ↔ 60cm (24in). Pyrenees.

D. longilobata. Erect, sometimes spreading, evergreen shrub with oblong-lance-shaped to inversely lance-shaped, leathery, glossy, mid-green leaves, to 10cm (4in) long. Bears terminal clusters of 5–7 fragrant, softly hairy white flowers, 1.5cm (½in) across, above new growth in early summer, followed by abundant, fleshy, spherical, glossy red fruit. ↕↔ 1.5m (5ft). W. China, S.E. Tibet. ✻✻✻. **'Peter Moore'** has grey-green leaves with creamy white margins.

***D.* x *mantensiana* 'Manten'.** Dwarf, rounded, evergreen shrub with oblong to obovate, glossy, mid-green leaves, to 3.5cm (1½in) long. Terminal clusters of up to 12 fragrant, purple-pink flowers, to 1cm (½in) across, paler within, are borne in late spring and early summer, and often again from summer to autumn. ↕↔ 75cm (30in). ✻✻✻

D. mezereum ■ (Mezereon). Upright, deciduous shrub with inversely lance-shaped, pale green to soft grey-green leaves, to 12cm (5in) long. Lateral clusters of 2–4 fragrant, pink to purplish pink flowers, to 6mm (¼in) long, are borne in late winter and early spring, before the leaves, followed by fleshy, spherical red fruit. ↕ 1.2m (4ft), ↔ 1m (3ft). Europe, Caucasus, Turkey, Siberia. ✻✻✻. **f. *alba*** has creamy white flowers and yellow fruit. **'Bowles' Variety'** ■ syn. 'Bowles' White', is very vigorous and upright, with pure white flowers and yellow fruit; ↕ to 2m (6ft).

D.* x *napolitana 🏆 (*D. cneorum* x *D. sericea*), syn. *D. neapolitana.* Compact, densely branched, evergreen shrub with inversely lance-shaped to narrowly obovate, glossy, dark green leaves, to 3.5cm (1½in) long, greyish green beneath. Bears terminal clusters of 6–8 (occasionally up to 16) fragrant, rose-pink flowers, to 8mm (⅜in) across, in spring, with further flushes from summer to autumn. ↕↔ 75cm (30in). Garden origin. ✻✻

D. neapolitana see *D.* x *napolitana.*

D. odora. Rounded, evergreen shrub with inversely lance-shaped to narrowly oval, leathery, glossy, deep green leaves, to 8cm (3in) long. Bears fragrant, deep purple-pink and white flowers, to 1.5cm

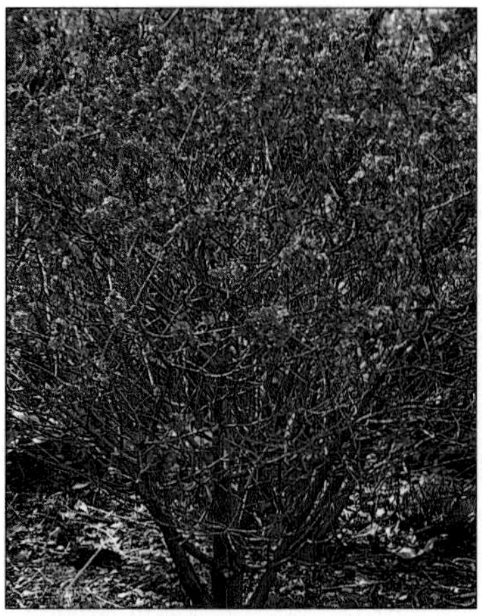

Daphne mezereum

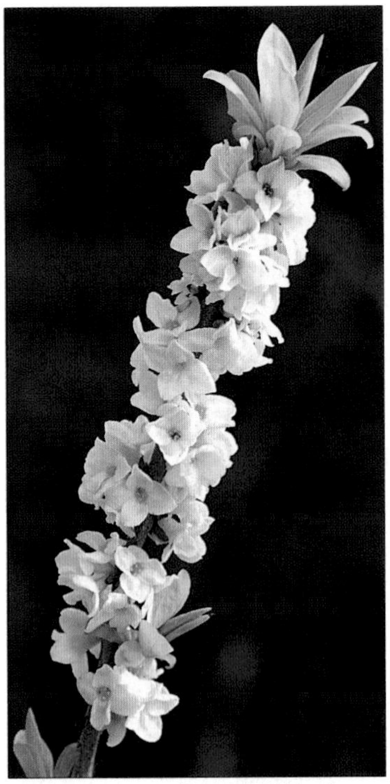

Daphne mezereum 'Bowles' Variety'

(½in) across, in terminal, sometimes axillary clusters of 10–15 or more, from midwinter to early spring, followed by fleshy, spherical red fruit. ↕↔ 1.5m (5ft). China, Japan. ❄❄. **f. *alba*,** syn. var. *leucantha*, bears white or creamy white flowers. **'Aureomarginata'** ▣ syn. 'Marginata', has leaves with narrow, irregular yellow margins, and red-purple flowers, paler and sometimes almost white within. **var. *leucantha*** see f. *alba*. **'Marginata'** see 'Aureomarginata'.

D. oleoides, syn. *D. glandulosa*. Slow-growing, variable, evergreen shrub with spreading branches and elliptic to obovate, leathery, grey-green leaves, 1–4.5cm (½–1¾in) long. Produces terminal clusters of up to 8 usually scented, sometimes pink-tinged, creamy white flowers, to 1.5cm (½in) across, in early summer, followed by downy, fleshy orange fruit. ↕ 20cm (8in), ↔ to 25cm (10in). S. Europe, N. Africa, Turkey, Caucasus. ❄❄❄

***D. petraea* 'Grandiflora'** ▣ 🏆 Slow-growing, very compact, many-branched, evergreen shrub with narrowly spoon-shaped, leathery, shiny, dark green leaves, to 1cm (½in) long. Bears dense, terminal clusters of 3–5 or more,

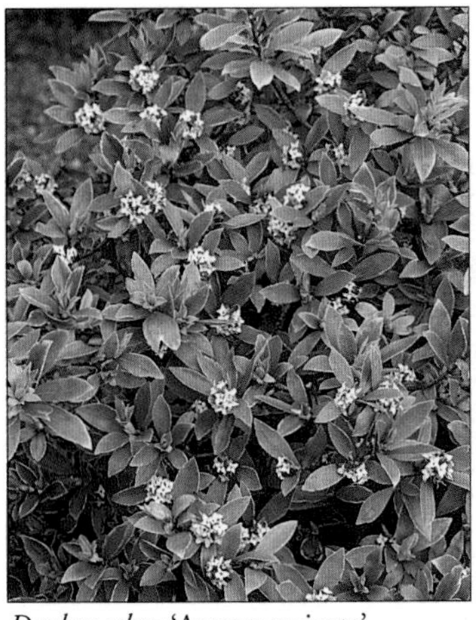

Daphne odora 'Aureomarginata'

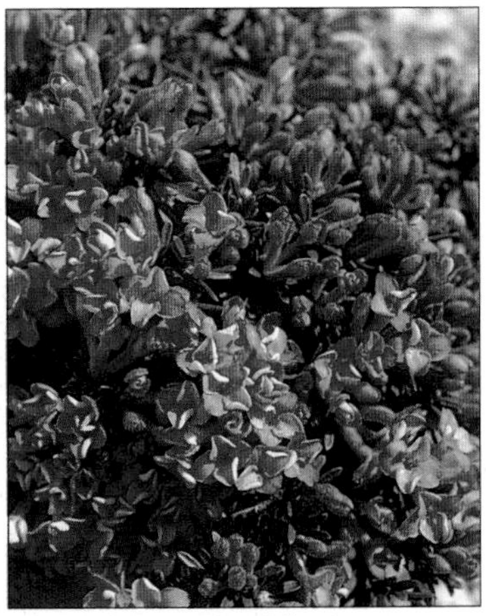

Daphne petraea 'Grandiflora'

scented, deep rose-pink flowers, to 1cm (½in) across, in late spring. ↕ 10cm (4in), ↔ to 25cm (10in). ❄❄❄

D. pontica 🏆 Spreading, evergreen shrub with obovate, pointed, glossy, dark green leaves, to 10cm (4in) long. Clusters of up to 10 pairs of fragrant, yellow-green flowers, to 2cm (¾in) across, with slender, pointed lobes, are borne at the base of overlapping shoots, in mid- and late spring, followed by fleshy, ovoid black fruit. ↕ 1m (3ft), ↔ 1.5m (5ft). S.E. Europe, N. Turkey, S.E. Bulgaria, Caucasus. ❄❄❄

D. retusa ▣ 🏆 syn. *D. tangutica* Retusa Group. Compact, dwarf, evergreen shrub with inversely lance-shaped to elliptic, leathery, glossy, dark green leaves, to 5cm (2in) long, notched at the tips. Bears terminal clusters of up to 10 or more fragrant flowers, to 1cm (½in) across, purple-red outside, white within, in late spring and early summer; flowers are followed by fleshy, spherical red fruit. ↕↔ 75cm (30in). W. China (W. Sichuan, Yunnan). ❄❄❄

D. sericea 🏆 Compact or open, rounded, evergreen shrub with inversely lance-shaped, obovate, or narrowly elliptic, dark green leaves, to 5cm (2in) long, glossy above, softly hairy beneath. Terminal and axillary clusters of up to 15 fragrant, purple-pink and white flowers, to 1cm (½in) across, fading to buff, are produced in late spring. ↕↔ 50cm (20in). Italy (including Sicily), Greece (Crete), S. and W. Turkey, Syria, Caucasus. ❄❄. **Collina Group** see *D. collina*.

D. tangutica 🏆 Upright, open to dense, evergreen shrub with inversely lance-shaped, oblong or elliptic, leathery, dull, dark green leaves, to 7cm (3in) long, with pointed or notched tips. Terminal clusters of 6–8 fragrant, purple- or pink-flushed white flowers, to 1cm (½in) across, are produced in late spring and early summer, followed by fleshy, spherical red fruit. ↕↔ 1m (3ft). Tibet, China (Gansu, Hubei, Sichuan), possibly Taiwan. ❄❄❄. **Retusa Group** see *D. retusa*.

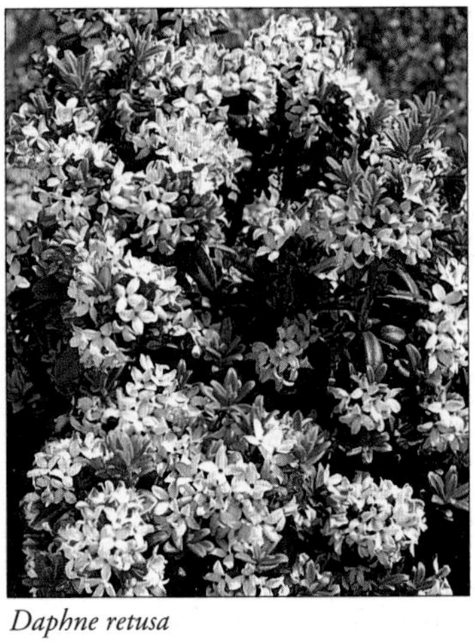

Daphne retusa

DAPHNIPHYLLUM

DAPHNIPHYLLACEAE

Genus of about 15 species of evergreen trees and shrubs found in woodland in E. Asia, grown for their handsome foliage. The alternate, rhododendron-like leaves often appear whorled at the ends of the shoots. Inconspicuous, petalless, pink, green, or yellow flowers are borne in short racemes, the male and female on separate plants. The rounded or ovoid, fleshy fruits have large, hard, blue-black seeds. Grow in a large shrub border or woodland garden. In frost-prone areas, grow frost-tender and half-hardy species in a temperate greenhouse.

- **HARDINESS** Frost hardy to frost tender.
- **CULTIVATION** Grow in moist but well-drained, humus-rich soil in sun or partial shade. Provide shelter from cold, drying winds. Pruning group 8; tolerates hard pruning.
- **PROPAGATION** Insert semi-ripe or evergreen cuttings in late summer.
- **PESTS AND DISEASES** Trouble free.

D. himalense* subsp. *macropodum see *D. macropodum*.

D. macropodum Q syn. *D. himalense* subsp. *macropodum*. Dense, rounded shrub or small tree with narrowly oval to oblong, leathery, dark green leaves, to 20cm (8in) long, glaucous beneath. Axillary racemes of small, petalless, deep purple-pink male or green female flowers are borne on separate plants in late spring and early summer. ↕↔ 6m (20ft). China, Korea, Japan. ❄❄

DARMERA syn. PELTIPHYLLUM

SAXIFRAGACEAE

Genus of one species of rhizomatous perennial from mountain streamsides in woodland in W. USA. With its large, bold, peltate leaves, which appear after the star-shaped, white to pink flowers, *D. peltata* forms an imposing, umbrella-like clump for a pond or streambank.

- **HARDINESS** Fully hardy, but flowers may be damaged by late frosts.
- **CULTIVATION** Grow in moist or boggy soil (although it will tolerate drier conditions), in sun or partial shade.
- **PROPAGATION** Sow seed in containers in a cold frame in spring or autumn, or divide in spring.
- **PESTS AND DISEASES** Trouble free.

D. peltata ▣ 🏆 syn. *Peltiphyllum peltatum*. Slowly spreading, rhizomatous perennial with leaf-stalks to 2m (6ft) long, and peltate, rounded, deeply lobed, coarsely toothed, conspicuously veined, dark green leaves, to 60cm (24in) across, that turn red in autumn. Rounded cymes of numerous 5-petalled, white to bright pink flowers, to 1.5cm (½in) across, are borne on flower stems to 2m (6ft) long in late spring. ↕ to 2m (6ft), ↔ 1m (3ft) or more. USA (S.W. Oregon to N.W. California). ❄❄❄

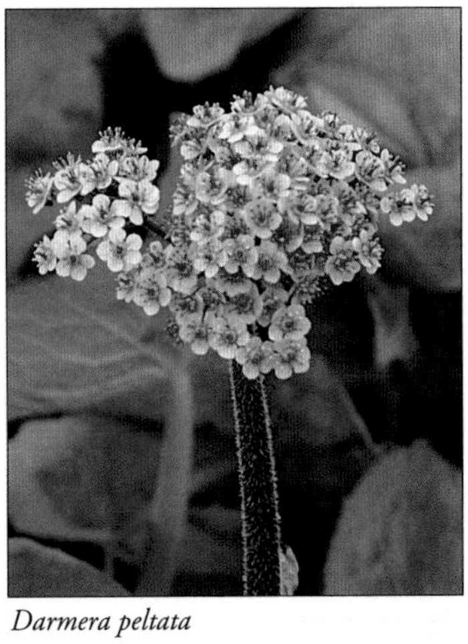

Darmera peltata

D

DARWINIA

MYRTACEAE

Genus of at least 60 species of evergreen, heather-like shrubs found on heaths, on sandy plains, and in scrub in Australia. They are grown for their dense, terminal heads of tiny, petalless flowers, enclosed by sometimes large, petal-like, colourful bracts. The crowded, opposite, linear to rounded leaves are small and sometimes aromatic. In frost-prone areas, grow in a cool greenhouse. In warmer areas, plant at the base of a wall or in a border.

- **HARDINESS** Frost tender.
- **CULTIVATION** Under glass, grow in loamless potting compost in full light, with shade from hot sun, and good ventilation. In the growing season, water moderately, applying a low-nitrogen liquid fertilizer monthly; keep just moist in winter. Top-dress or pot on in spring. Outdoors, grow in humus-rich, well-drained, sandy soil in full sun. Pruning group 10, after flowering.
- **PROPAGATION** Sow seed at not less than 16°C (61°F) in spring. Root semi-ripe cuttings in summer, with bottom heat. Layer in spring.
- **PESTS AND DISEASES** Scale insects may be a problem.

D. citriodora ▣ (Lemon-scented myrtle). Erect to spreading, bushy shrub with narrowly ovate to lance-shaped, lemon-scented, grey-green leaves, 1–2cm (½–¾in) long, sometimes heart-shaped at the bases, with slightly

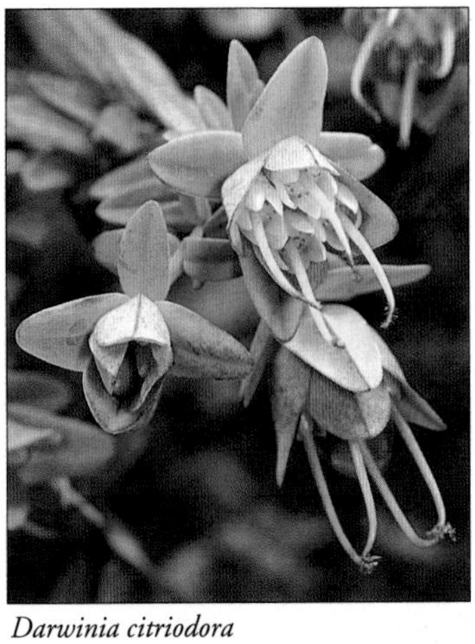

Darwinia citriodora

recurved margins. Produces pendent to erect flowerheads, 2.5–3cm (1–1¼in) across, with prominent, bell-shaped, orange-red and green outer bracts, usually in spring. ↕ 0.5–2m (20–72in), ↔ 1–2.5m (3–8ft). Western Australia. ❀ (min. 5°C/41°F)

▷ **Dasheen** see *Colocasia esculenta*

DASYLIRION

DRACAENACEAE/LILIACEAE

Genus of 18 species of yucca-like, evergreen shrubs, trees, and perennial succulents found in dry, mountainous areas and deserts in S. USA and Mexico. They have thick, woody stems and bear narrowly lance-shaped, mostly spiny-margined leaves, usually about 1m (3ft) long, in dense, terminal rosettes. Mature plants bear star- or bell-shaped flowers, to 2mm (1⁄16in) across, in long, narrow panicles intermittently throughout summer. Male and female flowers are borne on separate plants. In frost-prone areas, grow in a temperate or warm greenhouse or conservatory. Elsewhere, use at the base of a wall or as a focal feature on a lawn or in a desert garden.

• **HARDINESS** Frost tender, although mature plants may withstand several degrees of frost if kept dry.

• **CULTIVATION** Under glass, grow in a mix of 2 parts each loam and sand and 1 part each leaf mould and peat (or peat substitute). Provide full light with low humidity. From early spring to autumn, water freely, applying a balanced liquid fertilizer monthly; water sparingly in winter. In summer, move containerized specimens outside. Outdoors, grow in well-drained soil in a sheltered site in full sun. See also pp.48–49.

• **PROPAGATION** Sow seed at 21°C (70°F) in spring.

• **PESTS AND DISEASES** Susceptible to scale insects.

D. acrotrichum ■ syn. *D. gracile.* Evergreen shrub, eventually forming a trunk 0.9–1.5m (3–5ft) high. Upright then arching, fibrous-tipped, pale green leaves are margined with hooked yellow spines. Dense, narrow inflorescences, 2.5–4m (8–12ft) long, of star-shaped white flowers are produced in summer. ↕ 3.5–6m (11–20ft), ↔ to 2.2m (7ft). Mexico. ❀ (min. 10°C/50°F)

D. gracile see *D. acrotrichum.*

D. hartwegianum see *Calibanus hookeri.*

D. longissimum (Mexican grass plant). Tree-like succulent with erect then spreading, entire, 4-angled, stiff, slightly fleshy, olive-green leaves, 1.5m (5ft) or more long, on a trunk 1–2m (3–6ft) tall. Dense inflorescences, 1.5–5m (5–15ft) long, of bell-shaped white flowers, are produced in summer. ↕ to 4m (12ft) or more, ↔ 1.5m (5ft). E. Mexico. ❀ (min. 7°C/45°F)

D. texanum. Tall, evergreen shrub with semi-pendent, glossy, mid-green leaves margined with yellow spines, which fade to brown. Leaves persist when dead, usually concealing the trunk, 3m (10ft) tall. Dense inflorescences, to 1.5m (5ft) long, of bell-shaped white flowers are produced in early summer. ↕ to 5m (15ft), ↔ to 3m (10ft). USA (Texas), N. Mexico. ❀ (min. 7°C/45°F)

D. wheeleri ♈ Small, evergreen tree bearing flexible, ribbed, slightly fleshy,

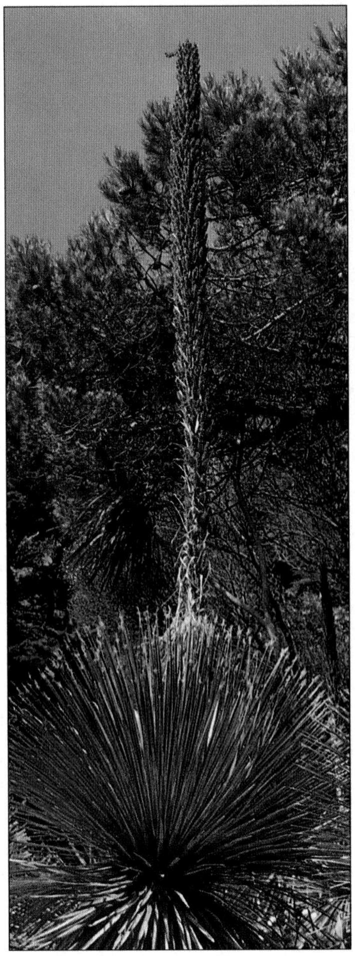

Dasylirion acrotrichum

glaucous silver leaves, with fine, hooked, yellow to rust-brown marginal spines, on a trunk 1–1.5m (3–5ft) tall. Bell-shaped white flowers are produced in inflorescences 2.5–4m (8–12ft) tall, in summer. ↕ 3.5–6m (11–20ft), ↔ 1m (3ft) or more. USA (Arizona, Texas). ❀ (min. 7°C/45°F)

▷ **Date palm** see *Phoenix dactylifera*
  Canary Island see *P. canariensis*
  Miniature see *P. roebelenii*
  Pigmy see *P. roebelenii*

▷ ***Datura arborea*** see *Brugmansia arborea*

▷ ***Datura aurea*** see *Brugmansia aurea*

▷ ***Datura* x *candida*** see *Brugmansia* x *candida*

▷ ***Datura rosei* of gardens** see *Brugmansia sanguinea*

▷ ***Daubentonia*** see *Sesbania*
  D. punicea see *S. punicea*

DAVALLIA

DAVALLIACEAE

Genus of 34 species of mostly epiphytic ferns found by streams or on rocks in the W. Mediterranean region, N. Africa, from China to Japan, and from tropical Asia to Australia and the Pacific islands. Creeping surface rhizomes, densely covered with scales, produce triangular, usually finely dissected, shiny fronds, which, in many species, are short-lived and deciduous. The sori are marginal or submarginal, with tubular to urn-shaped indusia. In frost-prone climates, *Davallia* species are suitable for a warm or cool greenhouse or bathroom; they look particularly effective when grown

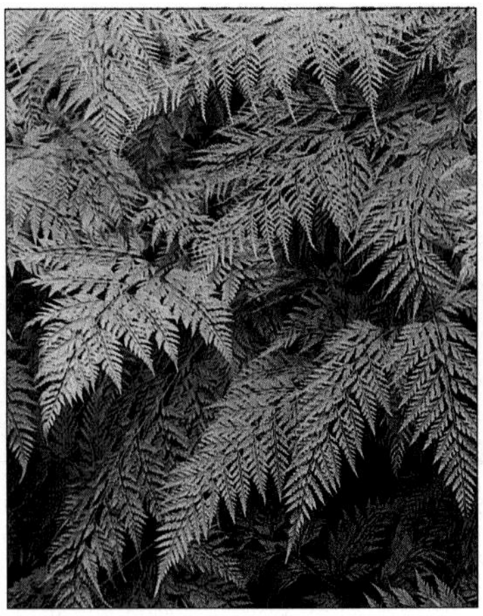

Davallia fejeensis

in hanging baskets, and their cut fronds may also be used in flower arranging. In warmer climates, grow in a moist, shaded site.

• **HARDINESS** Most are half hardy to frost tender; *D. mariesii* is hardy to -7°C (19°F) if protected in winter.

• **CULTIVATION** Under glass, grow in equal parts coarse leaf mould or peat substitute (or peat), moss, bark, sharp sand, charcoal, and pine needles, in bright indirect light with high humidity. In summer, water moderately and mist frequently; water sparingly in winter. Outdoors, grow epiphytically, or in moist, open, leafy soil in partial shade.

• **PROPAGATION** Sow spores of hardy species at 15°C (59°F), and tender species at 21°C (70°F), as soon as ripe. Divide rhizomes in spring, ensuring each division has roots. See also p.51.

• **PESTS AND DISEASES** Trouble free.

D. bullata. Deciduous fern with thin, long-trailing rhizomes covered with dark brown or black scales with toothed white margins. Bears 3- or 4-pinnate, pale green fronds, 15–20cm (6–8in) long, with narrowly triangular or linear segments. ↕ 20–35cm (8–14in), ↔ 50–80cm (20–32in) or more. India, China. ❀ (min. 10°C/50°F)

D. canariensis ♀ (Hare's foot fern). Deciduous or semi-evergreen fern with thick, succulent rhizomes covered with dark brown scales. Produces broad, 3- to 4-pinnate, mid-green fronds, 20–50cm (8–20in) long, with narrowly triangular or linear segments. ↕ 20–50cm (8–20in), ↔ 30–100cm (12–39in). S.W. Europe, N.W. Africa. ❀ (min. 5°C/41°F)

D. fejeensis ■ (Rabbit's foot fern). Evergreen fern with thick, tough rhizomes covered with mid- to dark brown scales pressed tightly to the surface, with long, curly hairs on the margins. Produces very broad, 3- to 4-pinnate, mid-green fronds, 20–100cm (8–39in) long, with linear segments. ↕ 20–100cm (8–39in), ↔ 40–150cm (16–60in). Fiji. ❀ (min. 10°C/50°F). **'Major'** has fronds 60–120cm (2–4ft) long; ↔ to 1.2m (4ft).

D. mariesii ■ ♀ (Squirrel's foot fern). Deciduous fern with thin, creeping rhizomes covered with brown scales. Broad, very finely cut, 3- or 4-pinnate, mid-green fronds, 20–30cm (8–12in) long, have narrowly triangular or linear segments. ↕ 15cm (6in), ↔ indefinite. E. Asia, Japan. ✲✲

DAVIDIA

Dove tree, Ghost tree, Handkerchief tree

CORNACEAE/DAVIDIACEAE

Genus of one species of deciduous tree found in woodland in China, with small ellipsoid flowerheads surrounded by showy white bracts, which give rise to the common name. Its bark is smooth and mid-grey, and the leaves are simple, alternate, and broadly ovate. Grow *D. involucrata* as a specimen tree.

• **HARDINESS** Fully hardy.

• **CULTIVATION** Grow in fertile, moist but well-drained soil in sun or partial shade, with shelter from strong winds. Pruning group 1; maintain a strong central leader in the formative years.

• **PROPAGATION** Sow the whole fruit in a seedbed, or in containers in an open frame, as soon as ripe. Germination normally occurs in spring after 2 winters outdoors. Seed-raised plants may not flower for up to 10 years. Insert leaf-bud cuttings in early autumn, or hardwood cuttings in winter.

• **PESTS AND DISEASES** Trouble free.

D. involucrata ■ ♀ ♤ Conical tree with broadly ovate, sharp-pointed, toothed, red-stalked leaves, to 16cm (6in) long, with heart-shaped bases, mid-green above and softly hairy beneath. In late spring, produces dense, pendent, ellipsoid heads, to 2cm (¾in) across, of small male flowers, each with red-purple anthers and a single, ovoid green ovary. Each flower is surrounded by a pair of leafy, spherical white bracts of unequal size. Pendent, ridged fruit are greenish brown, 4cm (1½in) across.

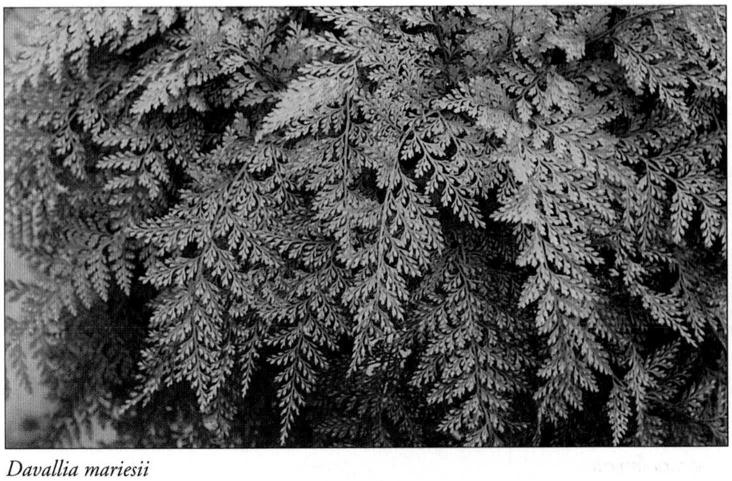

Davallia mariesii

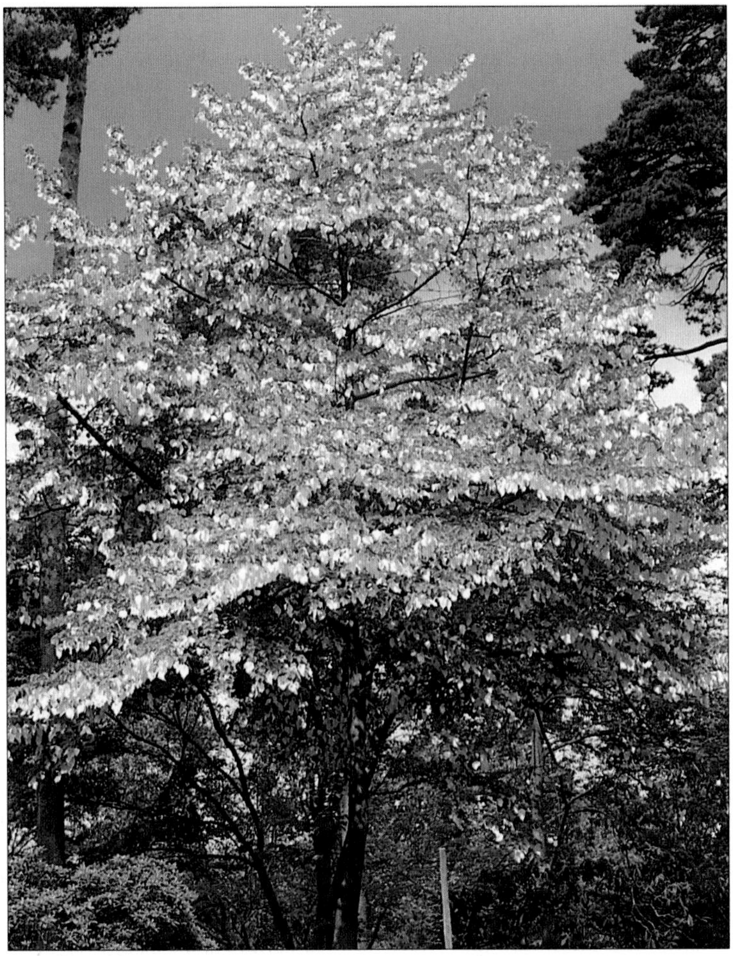
Davidia involucrata

↕15m (50ft), ↔ 10m (30ft). S.W. China. ❄❄❄. **var. *vilmoriniana*** 🏆 has almost hairless leaves, yellow-green or glaucous above, dark green beneath.

▷**Dawn flower, Blue** see *Ipomoea indica*
▷**Day flower** see *Commelina*
▷**Daylily** see *Hemerocallis*
▷**Dead nettle** see *Lamium*
Pyrenean see *Horminum pyrenaicum*

DECAISNEA

LARDIZABALACEAE

Genus of 2 species of deciduous shrubs from woodland in the Himalayas and W. China. They are cultivated for their bold, alternate, pinnate leaves, borne on stout shoots, and their unusual, bean-like, pendent fruits. The bell-shaped flowers are petalless. Grow *D. fargesii* in a shrub border or woodland garden.

- **HARDINESS** Fully hardy, although late frosts may damage young foliage.
- **CULTIVATION** Grow in fertile, moist but well-drained soil in sun or partial shade, with shelter from strong winds. Pruning group 1.
- **PROPAGATION** Sow seed in containers in an open frame in autumn.
- **PESTS AND DISEASES** Trouble free.

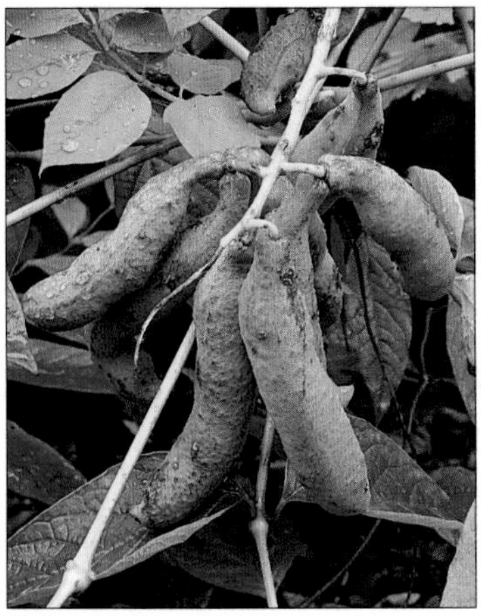
Decaisnea fargesii

D. fargesii ■ Upright, sparsely branched shrub with stout, hairless shoots bearing pinnate leaves, to 90cm (36in) long, dark green above, glaucous, mid-green beneath, with 13–25 ovate to elliptic leaflets. Bears pendent panicles, to 45cm (18in) long, of bell-shaped, petalless, green or yellow-green flowers in early summer, followed by pendent, cylindrical, dull, deep blue fruit, to 10cm (4in) long, in autumn. ↕↔ 6m (20ft). W. China. ❄❄❄ (borderline)

DECARYA

DIDIEREACEAE

Genus of one species of deciduous, succulent shrub or small tree occurring from sea level to 500m (1,600ft) or more in Madagascar. It has zigzag twigs, borne on spreading branches, which produce a small, inversely heart-shaped leaf and 2 spines from each node, and a single cyme of small, cup-shaped white flowers in summer. In frost-prone areas, grow *D. madagascariensis* in a warm greenhouse. In warmer areas, grow at the base of a wall or in a courtyard garden.

- **HARDINESS** Frost tender.
- **CULTIVATION** Under glass, grow in loam-based potting compost (JI No.2) with 10 per cent additional grit, in full light and low humidity. In the growing season, water moderately, applying a low-nitrogen liquid fertilizer monthly; keep just moist at other times. Outdoors, grow in sharply drained soil in full sun. See also pp.48–49.
- **PROPAGATION** Sow seed at 21°C (70°F), or take stem cuttings from spring to summer.
- **PESTS AND DISEASES** Susceptible to scale insects.

D. madagascariensis ♀ Succulent shrub or small tree with a straight, brownish green trunk branching from the sides and base, and inversely heart-shaped, fleshy, spiny, dull, mid-green leaves, to 5mm (¼in) long. A single cyme, 5–7cm (2–3in) long, of small white flowers is produced in summer. ↕6–8m (20–25ft), ↔ indefinite. S.W. Madagascar. ❁ (min. 13°C/55°F)

DECUMARIA

HYDRANGEACEAE

Genus of 2 species of woody, evergreen or deciduous climbers, occurring in China and S.E. USA, where they grow on forest trees. They climb by aerial roots, and produce opposite pairs of attractive, ovate to oblong, glossy, dark green leaves. Slightly fragrant, white or yellowish white flowers, each with 10 small petals and 20–30 stamens in a "brush", are produced in terminal corymbs or panicles. Grow *Decumaria* species at the base of a sheltered wall, or train into a tree. *D. barbara* is also useful for ground cover.

- **HARDINESS** Frost hardy.
- **CULTIVATION** Grow in reasonably fertile, preferably loamy, well-drained soil in sun or partial shade. Provide shelter in all but mild areas. Pruning group 13, if wall-grown; otherwise needs minimal pruning.
- **PROPAGATION** Root semi-ripe cuttings in late summer or early autumn.
- **PESTS AND DISEASES** Trouble free.

D. barbara. Deciduous climber with ovate to ovate-oblong, glossy, dark green leaves, to 10cm (4in) long. In summer, white flowers are produced in corymbs, to 8cm (3in) across. ↕10m (30ft). S.E. USA. ❄❄

D. sinensis. Evergreen climber with narrowly obovate to ovate, glossy, dark green leaves, to 7cm (3in) long. Yellow or creamy white flowers are produced in pyramidal panicles, to 8cm (3in) across, in late spring and early summer. ↕2m (6ft) or more. C. China. ❄❄

DEINANTHE

HYDRANGEACEAE

Genus of 2 species of rhizomatous perennials, related to hydrangeas, found in moist, shady woodland in China and Japan. They produce short rhizomes and upright stems. The opposite leaves are ovate or obovate to elliptic, toothed, crinkled, hairy, and slightly glossy, mid- to dark green. Terminal panicles of showy, pendent, cup-shaped, waxy, fertile flowers with 5 fleshy petals and numerous stamens, and a few sterile outer flowers without petals, are borne in mid- and late summer. Suitable for a woodland or peat garden.

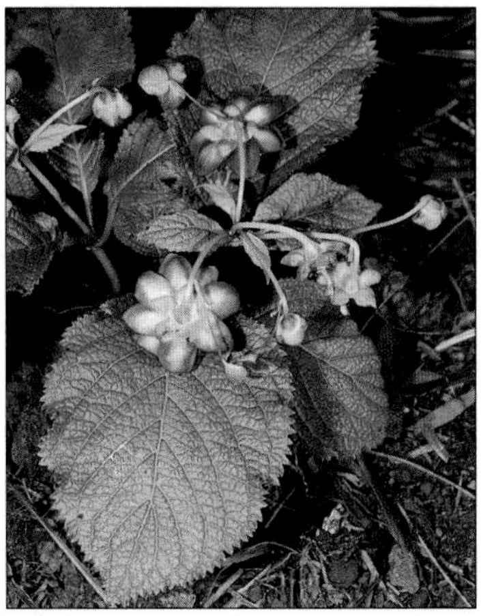
Deinanthe caerulea

- **HARDINESS** Fully hardy.
- **CULTIVATION** Grow in moist, humus-rich soil in partial shade, with shelter from cold, drying winds. Will not tolerate heat or drought.
- **PROPAGATION** Sow seed in containers in a cold frame as soon as ripe, although germination is uncertain and seedlings take several years to reach flowering size. Divide in early spring; divisions are slow to re-establish.
- **PESTS AND DISEASES** Slugs may damage young shoots.

D. bifida. Clump-forming perennial with obovate to elliptic, mid-green leaves, to 20cm (8in) long, distinctly notched at the tips. White flowers, 1–2cm (½–¾in) across, have yellow stamens. ↕40cm (16in), ↔45cm (18in). Japan. ❄❄❄

D. caerulea ■ Clump-forming perennial, usually with 2 pairs of ovate to elliptic, sharp-pointed, conspicuously veined, mid- to dark green leaves, to 15cm (6in) long. Mauve to violet-blue flowers, 2–4cm (¾–1½in) across, have grey-blue or blue stamens. ↕↔ 45cm (18in). C. China (Hubei). ❄❄❄

▷***Delairea odorata*** see *Senecio mikanioides*

DELONIX

CAESALPINIACEAE/LEGUMINOSAE

Genus of 10 species of deciduous, semi-evergreen, or evergreen trees from open, dry forest in Madagascar, tropical Africa, and India. They have elegant, alternate, 2-pinnate, fern-like leaves, and produce large, terminal, corymb-like racemes of irregularly shaped, 5-petalled flowers. In frost-prone areas, grow in a temperate greenhouse as foliage plants, since they rarely flower in a container. In warmer areas, they make effective specimen or shade trees.

- **HARDINESS** Frost tender.
- **CULTIVATION** Under glass, grow in loam-based potting compost (JI No.3) in full light. In the growing season, water freely, applying a balanced liquid fertilizer monthly; keep just moist in winter. Top-dress or pot on in spring. Outdoors, grow in fertile, moist but well-drained soil in full sun, with shelter from strong winds. Pruning group 1; tolerates hard pruning under glass.

D

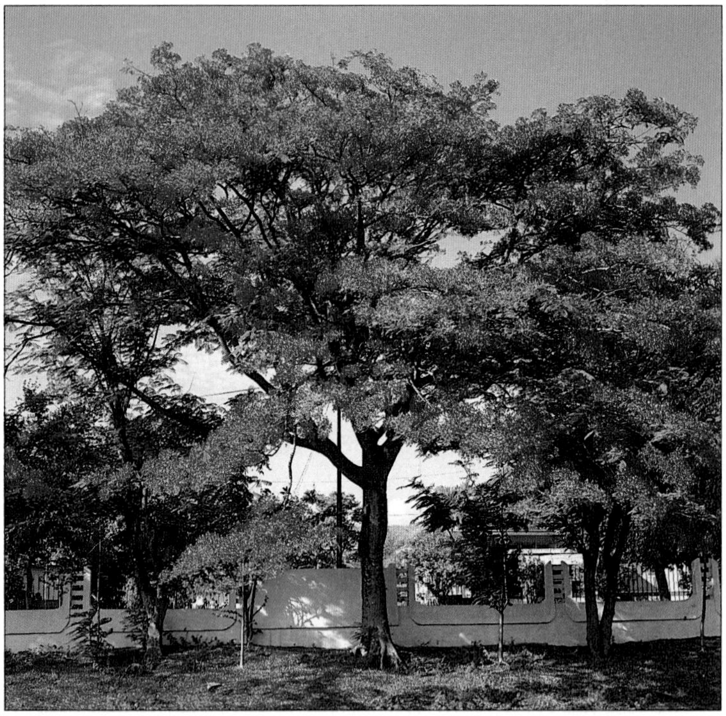

Delonix regia

• **PROPAGATION** Sow seed at 18–21°C (64–70°F) in spring. Root semi-ripe cuttings in summer, with bottom heat.
• **PESTS AND DISEASES** Susceptible to red spider mites and whiteflies under glass.

D. regia ■ ♀ syn. *Poinciana regia* (Flamboyant tree, Flame tree). Semi-evergreen tree (fully deciduous in areas with a long, dry season). It has a wide-spreading, dome-shaped crown and broadly ovate, 2-pinnate, bright-green leaves, 30–50cm (12–20in) long, each pinna divided into 10–25 pairs of elliptic to oblong leaflets. From spring to summer, bears many scarlet flowers, 10–13cm (4–5in) across, the standard petals pale yellow and striped with red. ↕ to 10m (30ft), ↔ 5–10m (15–30ft). Madagascar. ❀ (min. 7°C/45°F)

DELOSPERMA

AIZOACEAE

Genus of about 150 or more species of evergreen or semi-evergreen, succulent shrubs and mat-forming, succulent perennials (some with annual shoots from a tuberous caudex) found in hilly lowlands in C., E., and southern Africa.

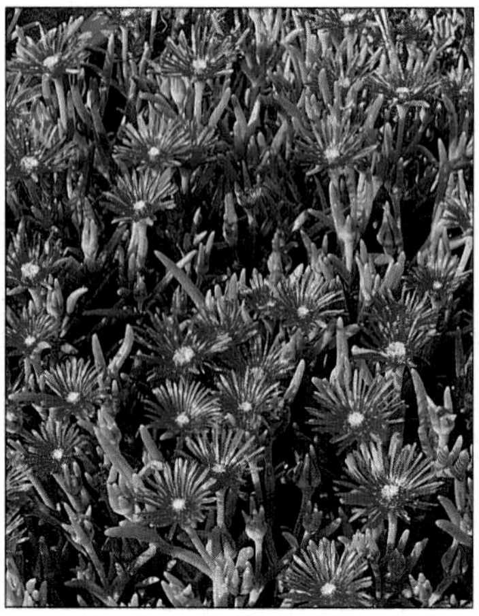

Delosperma aberdeenense

The triangular to cylindrical, fleshy leaves are borne in opposite pairs; the daisy-like flowers are produced singly or in open cymes in summer. In frost-prone areas, grow in a temperate greenhouse or as houseplants; elsewhere, grow in a desert garden or border.
• **HARDINESS** Frost hardy to frost tender; *D. cooperi* can survive to -8°C (18°F).
• **CULTIVATION** Under glass, grow in standard cactus compost in full light, with good but draught-free ventilation. In growth, water moderately, applying fertilizer every 3 weeks; keep dry at other times. Outdoors, grow in sharply drained soil in a sheltered site in full sun. See also pp.48–49.
• **PROPAGATION** Sow seed at 21°C (70°F), or take stem cuttings in spring or summer.
• **PESTS AND DISEASES** Susceptible to mealybugs and greenfly.

D. aberdeenense ■ Dense, evergreen, succulent shrub with minutely warty, often prostrate branches with thick, semi-cylindrical, pointed, mid-green leaves, 1–2cm (½–¾in) long. Solitary, purplish red flowers, 1.5cm (½in) across, are freely produced in summer. ↕ to 12cm (5in), ↔ indefinite. South Africa (Western Cape, Eastern Cape). ❀ (min. 5°C/41°F)
D. cooperi. Creeping, mat-forming, subshrubby, succulent perennial with cylindrical, warty, light green leaves, to 5cm (2in) long. Solitary, glossy magenta flowers, to 5cm (2in) across, with white anthers, are produced in mid- and late summer. ↕ 5cm (2in), ↔ 60cm (24in) or more. South Africa (Orange Free State). ❄❄
D. velutinum. Compact, bushy, semi-evergreen, succulent shrub with curved, warty-bristly branches and broadly cylindrical, tapering, pale green leaves, to 1.5cm (½in) long, keeled beneath. Solitary white flowers, 1.5cm (½in) across, are produced in summer. ↕ 5cm (2in), ↔ indefinite. South Africa (KwaZulu/Natal). ❀ (min. 5°C/41°F)

DELPHINIUM

RANUNCULACEAE

Genus of about 250 species of annuals, biennials, and perennials found mainly in mountainous areas worldwide, except Australia and the polar regions. They are grown for their spikes, racemes, or occasionally panicles of shallowly cup-shaped, sometimes hooded, spurred, single to fully double flowers, often known as "florets". Most have fibrous or fleshy roots, although some are tuberous. The basal leaves, mostly to 20cm (8in) long, are toothed and deeply or shallowly 3- to 5-lobed, occasionally 7-lobed. Grow tall delphiniums in a mixed border or island bed, and dwarf ones in a rock garden. All parts may cause severe discomfort if ingested, and contact with foliage may irritate skin.

For ease of reference, delphinium cultivars have been grouped as follows:

Belladonna Group
Upright, branching perennials with palmately lobed leaves. Wiry stems bear loose, branched spikes of elf cap-shaped, single flowers, 2cm (¾in) or more across, with spurs up to 3cm (1¼in) long, in early and late summer. ↕ 1–1.2m (3–4ft), ↔ to 45cm (18in).
Elatum Group
Clump-forming perennials with fleshy crowns producing flowering spikes in early and midsummer, and sometimes again in autumn if cut back. The spikes bear numerous single, semi-double, or double flowers, with 5 large outer sepals and an "eye" formed by 8 inner sepals. The flowers, at least 6cm (2½in) across, are usually larger at the base of the spike. Each stem also bears lateral shoots, flowering after the main spike, with slightly smaller flowers. Elatum Group cultivars are the most common garden delphiniums. They fall into 3 height categories: small, to 1.5m (5ft); medium, 1.7m (5½ft); and tall, 2m (6ft). Spreads are usually in the range 60–90cm (24–36in).
Pacific Hybrids
Similar to Elatum Group cultivars, but grown as annuals or biennials. At one time they were raised from hand-pollinated, line-bred seed to produce selections with clear, brightly coloured flowers; today, they are cross-pollinated and less uniform. The short-lived flowers are large, to 7cm (3in) across, and semi-double, and are produced on spikes in early and midsummer. ↕ 1.7m (5½ft), ↔ to 75cm (30in).

• **HARDINESS** Fully hardy.
• **CULTIVATION** Grow in fertile, well-drained soil in full sun, with shelter from strong winds. Except for the dwarf perennials, most delphiniums need staking: the low-growing cultivars with twiggy, brushwood support; the taller, large-flowered ones with stout canes. Insert supports no later than mid-spring, or when the plants reach 30cm (12in) high. To ensure good-quality flower spikes, thin shoots when 7cm (3in) high; leave a minimum of 2 or 3 shoots on young plants and 5–7 strong shoots on well-established ones. In growth, water all plants freely, applying a balanced liquid fertilizer every 2–3 weeks. Dead-head by cutting spent flower spikes back to small, flowering sideshoots. Cut all growth to ground level after it has withered in autumn.
• **PROPAGATION** Sow seed at 13°C (55°F) in early spring. For Elatum and Belladonna Group cultivars, take pencil-thick basal cuttings, 7–10cm (3–4in) long, with solid heels, from close to the crown in early spring.
• **PESTS AND DISEASES** Susceptible to slugs, snails, leaf miners, delphinium moth caterpillars, leaf blotch, powdery mildew, crown rot (on mature plants), and occasionally cucumber mosaic virus.

***D.* 'Alice Artindale'.** Small Elatum Group perennial bearing neat, button-like, fully double mauve flowers, to 3cm (1¼in) or more across, margined with blue, on narrow spikes. Good for cut flowers. ❄❄❄
***D.* 'Andenken an August Koenemann'** see *D.* 'Wendy'.
***D.* 'Astolat'.** Pacific Hybrid perennial with lilac and pink flowers. ❄❄❄
***D.* 'Bellamosum'** ■ Belladonna Group perennial with deep gentian-blue flowers. ❄❄❄
***D.* 'Berghimmel'.** Tall Elatum Group perennial producing short, slim, wind-resistant stems and single, clear sky-blue

DELPHINIUM INFLORESCENCES

Delphiniums are grown for their showy spikes of colourful summer flowers. The spikes are variable in height and shape: those produced by the Belladonna Group hybrids are loose and branched, while the tallest spikes (to 2m/6ft high) are produced by hybrids of the Elatum Group. Pacific Hybrids are similar to Elatum Group cultivars, although they are not as tall.

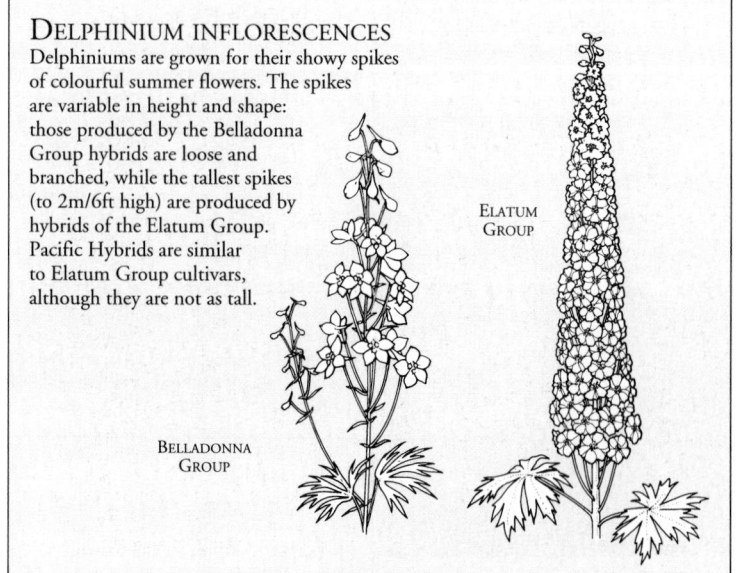

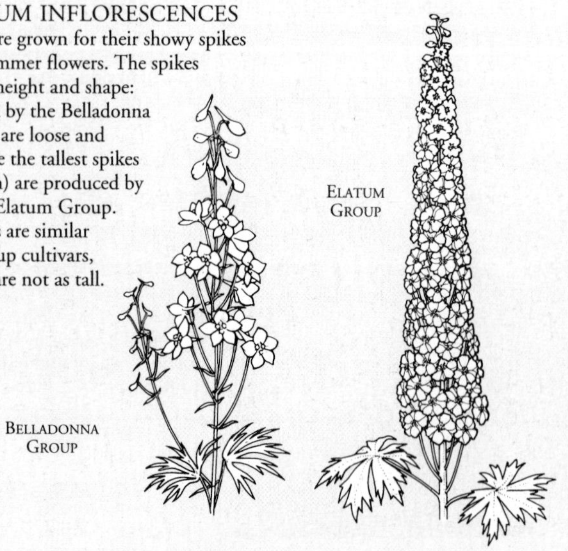

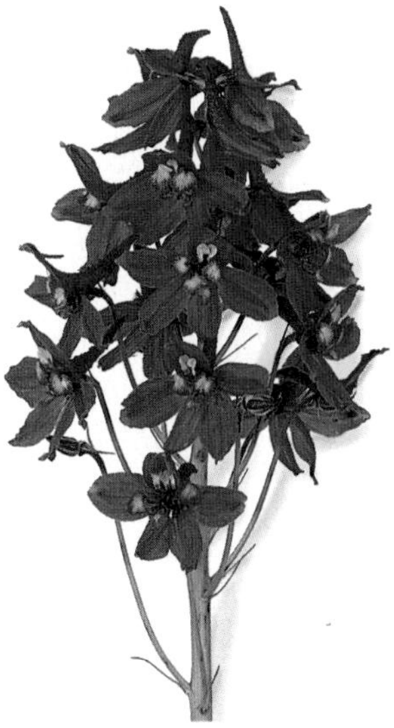

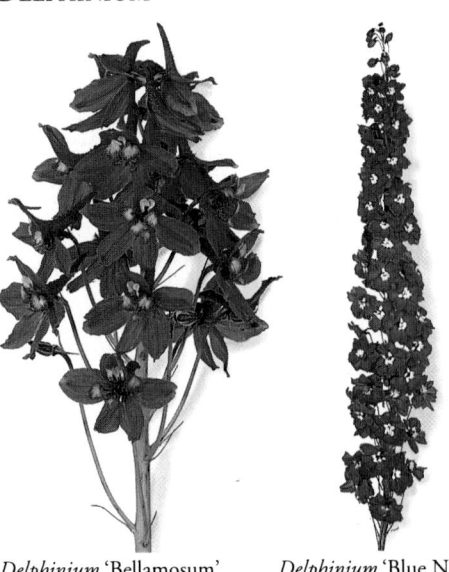

Delphinium 'Bellamosum'

Delphinium 'Blue Nile'

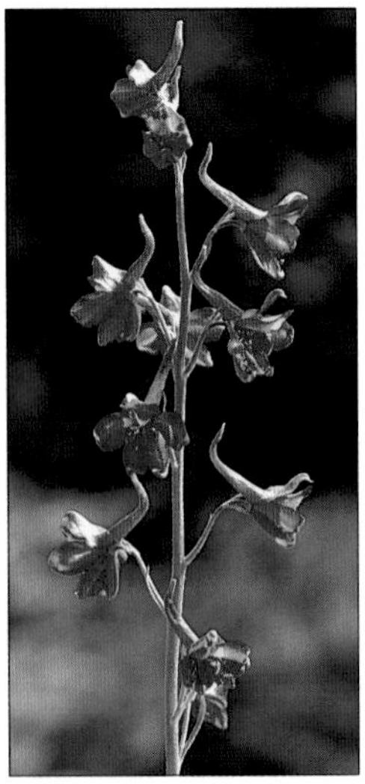

Delphinium cardinale

Delphinium 'Cliveden Beauty'

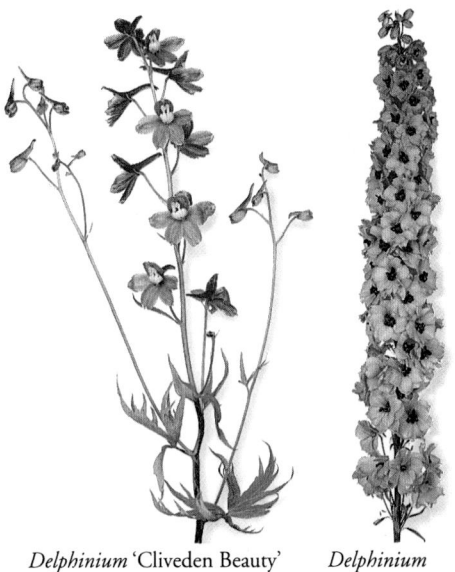

Delphinium 'Conspicuous'

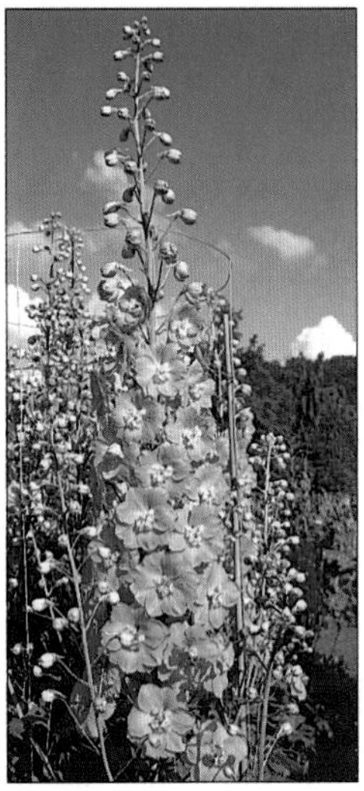

Delphinium 'Emily Hawkins'

D

flowers with white eyes; the lower florets are often still in good condition as the top ones open. ✻✻✻
D. 'Black Knight'. Pacific Hybrid perennial bearing deep purple flowers with black eyes. ✻✻✻
D. 'Blue Bees' ▣ Belladonna Group perennial producing clear blue flowers with white eyes. ✻✻✻
D. 'Blue Dawn' 🏆 Medium Elatum Group perennial bearing semi-double, pale blue flowers, with a touch of pink, and small, dark brown eyes. ✻✻✻
D. 'Blue Jay'. Pacific Hybrid perennial with deep blue flowers. ✻✻✻
D. 'Blue Nile' ▣🏆 Medium Elatum Group perennial. Semi-double, bright mid-blue flowers have white eyes. ✻✻✻
D. 'Bruce' ▣🏆 Tall Elatum Group perennial bearing semi-double, violet-purple flowers, paler towards the centres, with dark brown eyes. ✻✻✻
D. brunonianum. Upright perennial with hairy stems and deeply 3- to 5-lobed leaves. In early summer, bears racemes of hooded, single, short-spurred, hairy, blue to purple flowers, 3–5cm (1¼–2in) across, with black-purple eyes and heavy veining. ↕↔ 20cm (8in). Pakistan to S.W. Tibet. ✻✻✻
D. 'Butterball' ▣ Small Elatum Group perennial. Semi-double, rich light cream flowers have deep yellow eyes. ✻✻✻
D. 'Cameliard'. Pacific Hybrid perennial with deep purple flowers, shading to blue at the frilly sepal margins, and creamy white eyes. ✻✻✻
D. 'Can-can'. Small Elatum Group perennial bearing fully double flowers. The sepals are light mauve with darker veining and frilled margins; outer sepals have dark blue margins. ✻✻✻
D. cardinale ▣ Short-lived perennial with deeply 3- to 5-lobed leaves. Bears loose racemes of elf cap-shaped, stout-spurred, single scarlet flowers, 2cm (¾in) across, with yellow centres, in early summer. ↕ 2m (6ft), ↔ 45cm (18in). USA (California), Mexico (Baja California). ✻✻✻
D. 'Casablanca'. Belladonna Group perennial with white flowers. ✻✻✻
D. cashmerianum. Perennial with rounded, toothed, shallowly 5- to 7-lobed leaves. In early and late summer, bears single, dark purple-blue flowers, 3–4cm (1¼–1½in) across, in open panicles. ↕ 30–40cm (12–16in), ↔ 15cm (6in). N. India to China. ✻✻✻
D. 'Cassius'. Medium Elatum Group perennial with semi-double, deep blue flowers overlaid with purple and with brown-tinged eyes. ✻✻✻
D. 'Chelsea Star'. Medium Elatum Group perennial bearing semi-double, rich velvety violet flowers with white eyes. ✻✻✻
D. chinense see *D. grandiflorum.*
D. 'Cliveden Beauty' ▣ Belladonna Group perennial with sky-blue flowers. ✻✻✻
D. consolida see *Consolida ajacis.*
D. 'Conspicuous' ▣🏆 Small Elatum Group perennial bearing semi-double, lilac-mauve flowers with prominent brown eyes. ✻✻✻
D. 'Crown Jewel'. Small Elatum Group perennial bearing semi-double, pink-tinged, pale blue flowers with prominent brown eyes. ✻✻✻
D. 'Emily Hawkins' ▣🏆 Medium Elatum Group perennial producing neat, semi-double, light violet flowers with fawn eyes. ✻✻✻

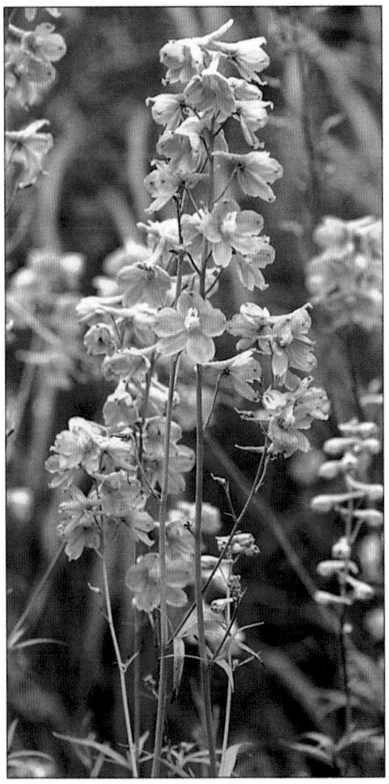

Delphinium 'Blue Bees'

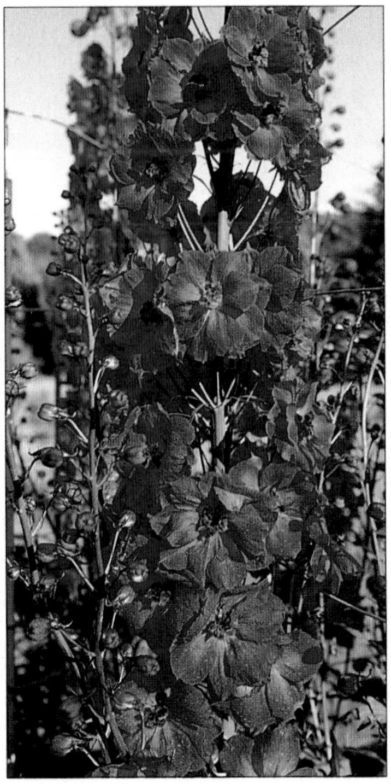

Delphinium 'Bruce'

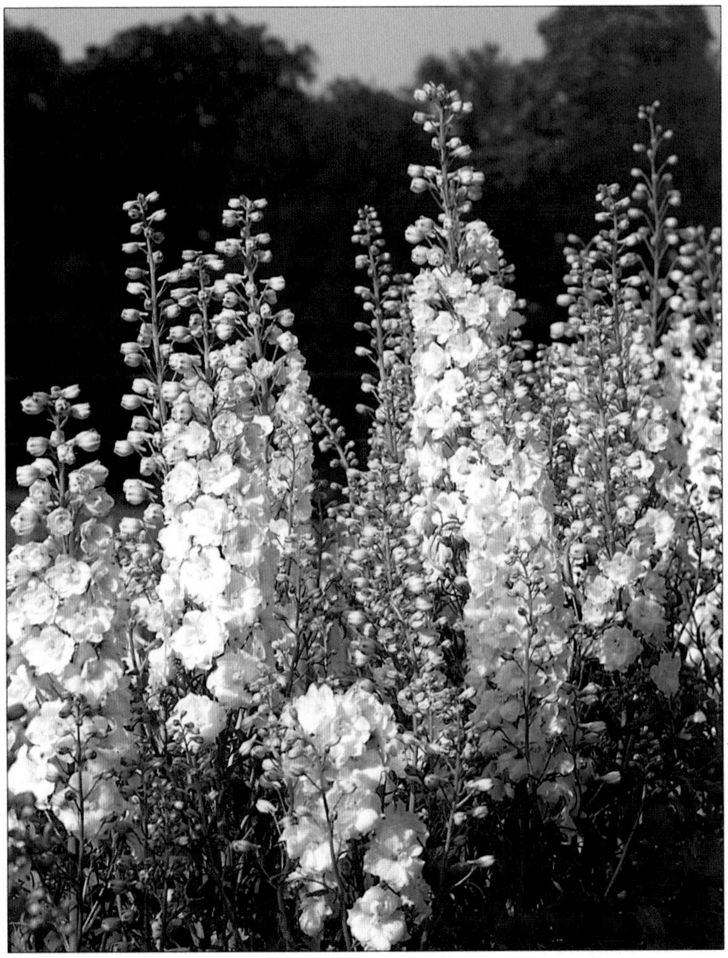

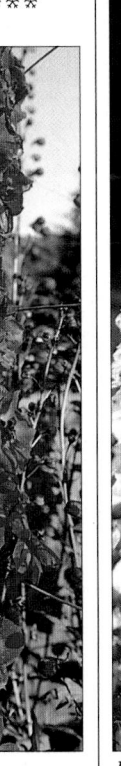

Delphinium 'Butterball'

D

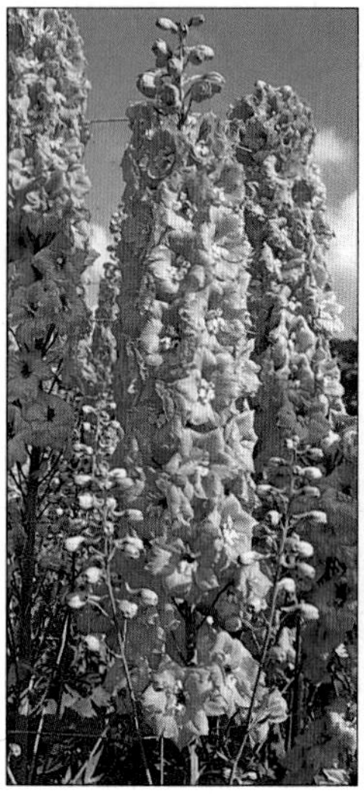
Delphinium 'Fanfare'

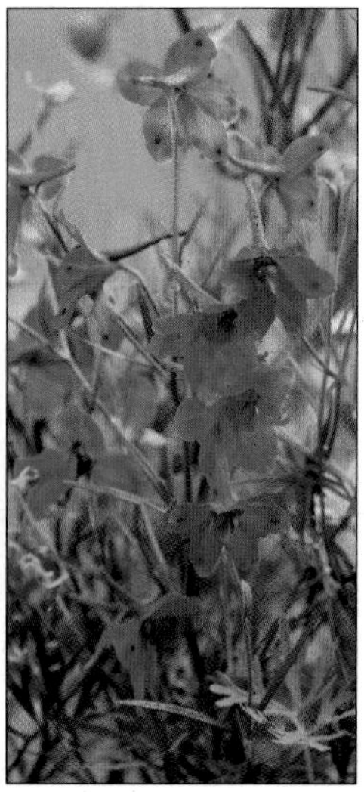
Delphinium grandiflorum 'Blue Butterfly'

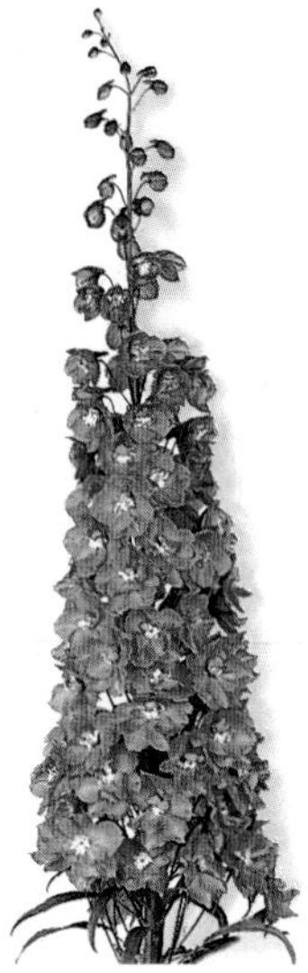
Delphinium 'Langdon's Royal Flush'

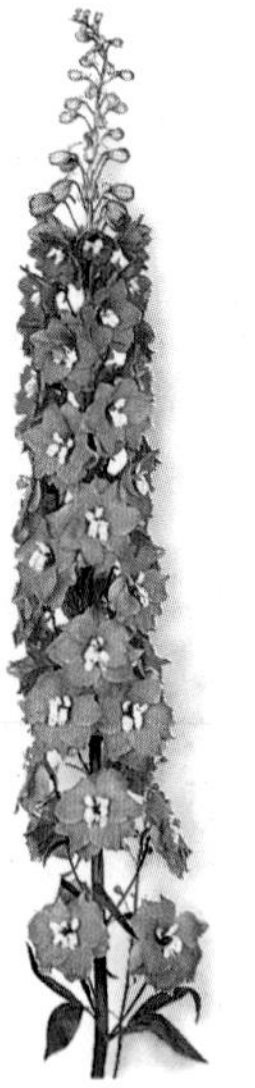
Delphinium 'Lord Butler'

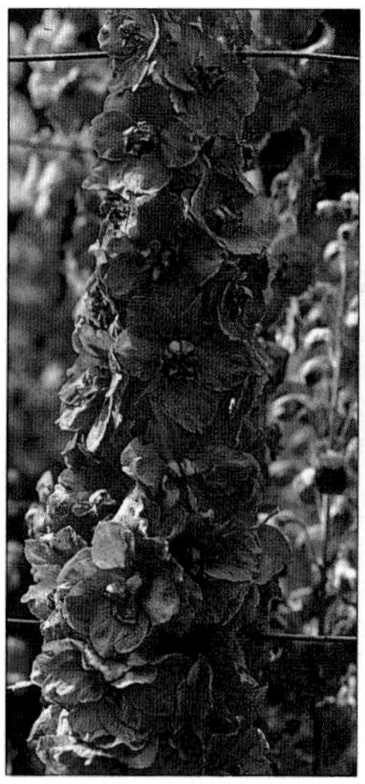
Delphinium 'Mighty Atom'

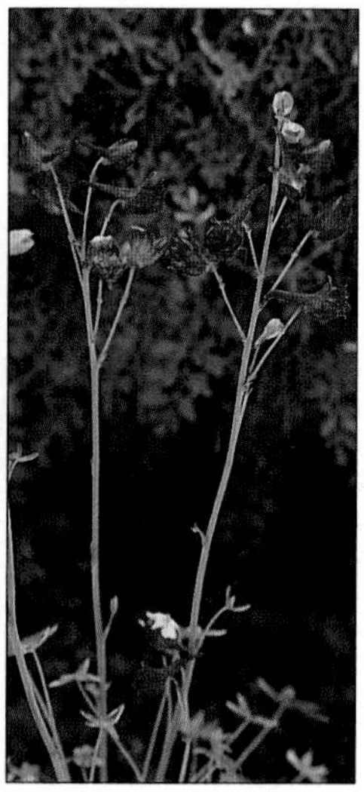
Delphinium nudicaule

***D.* 'Fanfare'** ▣ 🏆 Very tall Elatum Group perennial bearing semi-double, silvery mauve flowers with white eyes. ↕2.2m (7ft). ❄❄❄
***D.* 'Faust'** 🏆 Tall Elatum Group perennial with semi-double, deep cornflower-blue flowers, overlaid with purple, and with indigo eyes. ❄❄❄
***D.* 'Fenella'** 🏆 Small Elatum Group perennial bearing semi-double, gentian-blue flowers with black eyes. ❄❄❄
***D.* 'Finsteraarhorn'.** Medium Elatum Group perennial with short, slim, wind-resistant stems and single, dark gentian-blue flowers with black eyes. The lower florets are often still in good condition as the top ones open. ❄❄❄
***D.* 'Galahad'.** Pacific Hybrid perennial with pure white flowers. ❄❄❄
***D.* 'Gillian Dallas'** 🏆 Small Elatum Group perennial producing semi-double, slate-grey flowers with a hint of mauve and white eyes. ❄❄❄
***D.* 'Giotto'** 🏆 Medium Elatum Group perennial bearing semi-double flowers with clear violet inner sepals, gentian-blue outer sepals, and light yellowish brown eyes. ❄❄❄
***D.* 'Gletscher Wasser'.** Medium Elatum Group perennial with short, slim, wind-resistant stems and single, light ice-blue flowers. The lower florets are often still in good condition as the top ones open. ❄❄❄
***D.* 'Gordon Forsyth'.** Tall Elatum Group perennial producing semi-double, amethyst-purple flowers with grey-brown eyes. ❄❄❄
***D. grandiflorum*,** syn. *D. chinense.* Short-lived perennial usually grown as an annual. The elf cap-shaped, single, blue, violet, or white flowers, 3.5cm (1½in) across, are produced in open panicles in early summer. Leaves are 5-lobed, with each lobe further divided into narrow segments. ↕20–50cm (8–20in), ↔23–30cm (9–12in). Siberia, Mongolia, China, Japan. ❄❄❄. **'Album'** produces white flowers. **'Blauer Zwerg'** is upright and produces gentian-blue flowers; ↕to 20cm (8in). **'Blue Butterfly'** ▣ is stocky, and produces bright blue flowers. **'Sky Blue'** bears flowers with almost pure white sepals, turning very pale blue, with dark veins beneath.
***D.* 'Guinevere'.** Pacific Hybrid perennial producing pale purple flowers, tinged pink with white eyes. ❄❄❄
***D.* 'Jubelruf'.** Tall Elatum Group perennial producing short, slim, wind-resistant stems bearing semi-double, bright mid-blue flowers with white eyes. The lower florets are often still in good condition as the top ones open. ❄❄❄
***D.* 'King Arthur'.** Pacific Hybrid perennial bearing plum-purple flowers with white eyes. ❄❄❄
***D.* 'Lancelot'.** Pacific Hybrid perennial with purplish pink flowers. ❄❄❄
***D.* 'Langdon's Royal Flush'** ▣ Small Elatum Group perennial bearing semi-double, pale mauve-pink flowers with white or pale yellow eyes. ❄❄❄
***D.* 'Loch Leven'** 🏆 Medium Elatum Group perennial bearing semi-double, mid-blue flowers with white eyes. ❄❄❄
***D.* 'Lord Butler'** ▣ 🏆 Small Elatum Group perennial with semi-double, mid-blue flowers, flushed mauve at the centres, with white eyes. ❄❄❄
***D.* 'Mighty Atom'** ▣ 🏆 Small Elatum Group perennial bearing semi-double, mid-violet flowers with brown-streaked eyes. May develop fused and flattened stems, especially if overfertilized. ❄❄❄
***D.* 'Min'** 🏆 Medium Elatum Group perennial bearing semi-double, very pale purple flowers, suffused and veined with deeper purple; the brown eyes are striped with pale purple. ❄❄❄
***D.* 'Moerheimii'.** Belladonna Group perennial with white flowers. ❄❄❄
***D.* 'Mother of Pearl'** see *D.* 'Perlmutterbaum'.
D. muscosum. Perennial with rounded, 3- to 7-lobed, finely divided, softly hairy leaves, on long stalks. Bears single, dark blue to dark violet flowers, 3–4cm (1¼–1½in) across, in racemes in early and midsummer. ↕↔10–15cm (4–6in). Bhutan. ❄❄❄
***D.* 'Nachtwache'.** Tall Elatum Group perennial with short, slim, wind-resistant stems and semi-double, violet-blue flowers with white eyes. The lower florets are often still in good condition as the top ones open. ❄❄❄
D. nudicaule ▣ Short-lived perennial, often grown as an annual, with fleshy, 3- to 5-lobed leaves on long stalks. Half-closed, funnel-shaped, single, bright vermilion-red, orange-red, or yellow flowers, to 2cm (¾in) across, with red to yellow throats, are produced in open panicles on sturdy, unbranched stems in midsummer. ↕20–60cm (8–24in), ↔20cm (8in). USA (California). ❄❄❄
***D.* 'Percival'.** Pacific Hybrid perennial producing white flowers with black eyes. ❄❄❄
***D.* 'Pericles'.** Medium Elatum Group perennial producing semi-double, pale sky-blue flowers. The white eyes have a few cream hairs. ❄❄❄
***D.* 'Perlmutterbaum'**, syn. *D.* 'Mother of Pearl'. Tall Elatum Group perennial producing semi-double, light blue and soft pink, bicoloured flowers, with brown eyes, on short, slim, wind-resistant stems. The lower florets are often still in good condition as the top ones open. ❄❄❄
***D.* 'Piccolo'.** Belladonna Group perennial with bright gentian-blue flowers. ❄❄❄

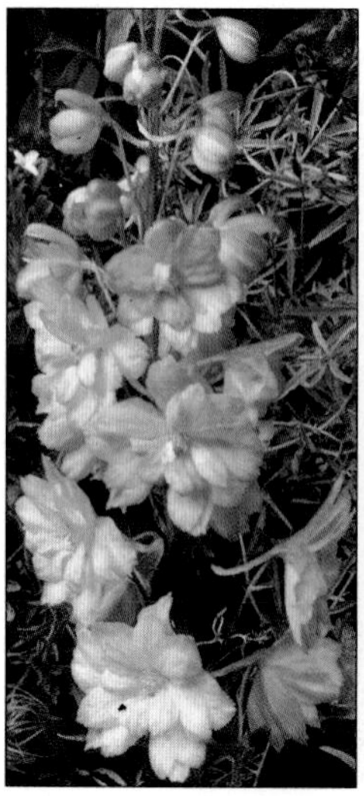
Delphinium 'Princess Caroline'

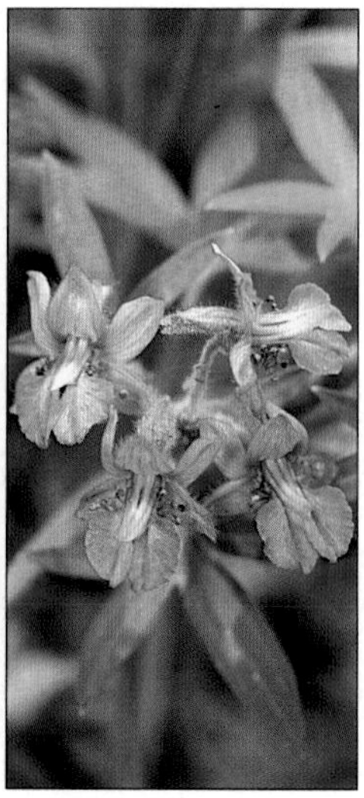
Delphinium requienii

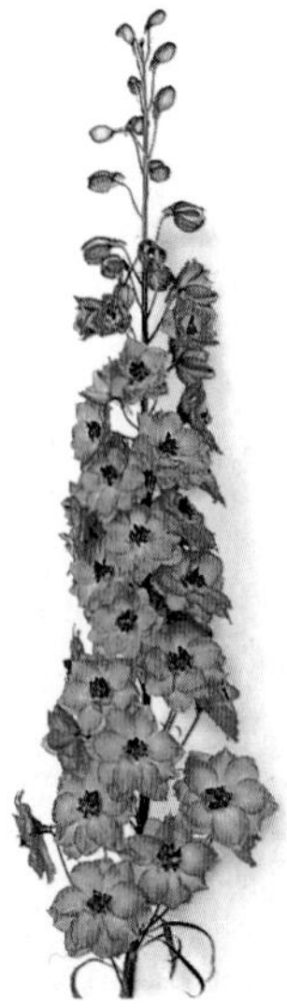
Delphinium 'Rosemary Brock'

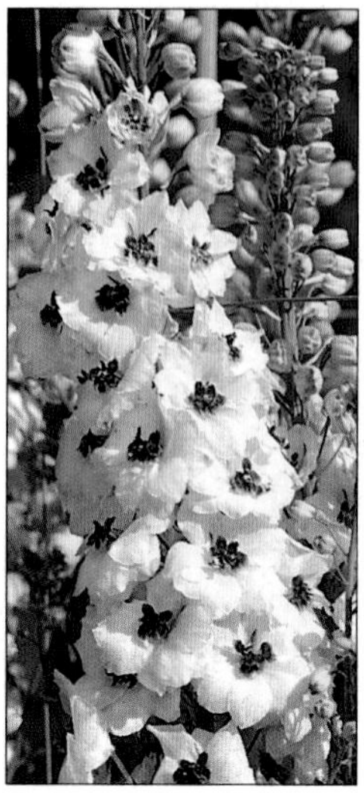
Delphinium 'Sandpiper'

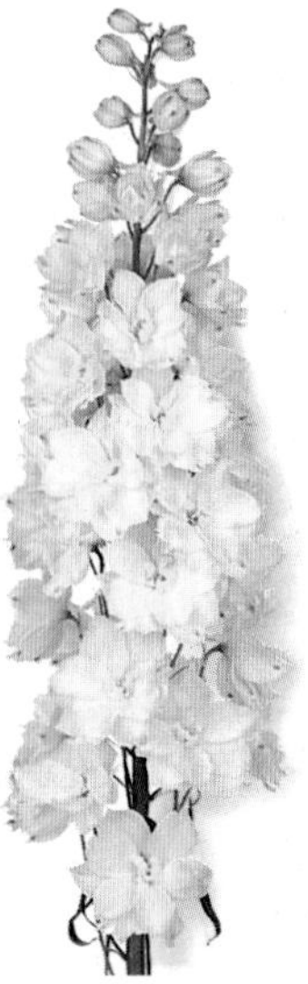
Delphinium 'Sungleam'

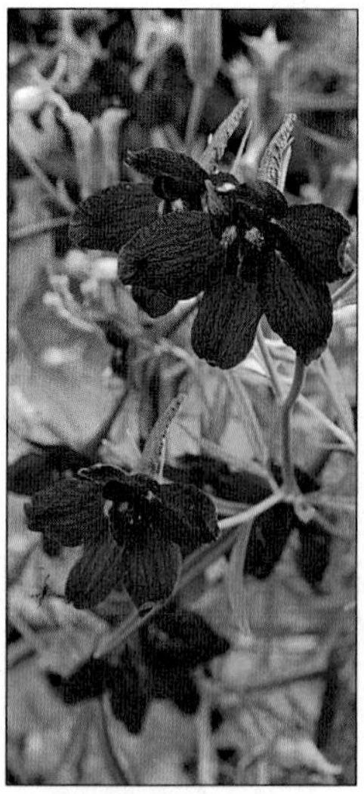
Delphinium tatsienense

D. 'Princess Caroline' ■ Perennial selected from hybrids of *D. cardinale*, *D. elatum*, and *D. nudicaule* cultivars. Bears semi-double, coral-pink flowers, 3–6cm (1¼–2½in) across, in short racemes in early summer. ↕ 1.1m (3½ft), ↔ 60cm (24in). ❄❄❄
D. requienii ■ Vigorous annual or biennial with 5- to 7-lobed, glossy leaves. In early summer, produces many branched spikes of elf cap-shaped, green and mauve-grey flowers, 1cm (½in) across, with prominent purple anthers. ↕ 30–100cm (12–39in), ↔ 45cm (18in). S. France (including Iles d'Hyères and Corsica), Italy (Sardinia). ❄❄❄
D. 'Rosemary Brock' ■ ♀ Small Elatum Group perennial bearing semi-double, deep dusky pink flowers with darker sepal tips and margins, and brown eyes with yellow hairs. ❄❄❄
D. x *ruysii* 'Pink Sensation'. Short-lived, upright perennial with small, glossy, finely divided, 3- to 5-lobed leaves. Nodding, yellowish pink buds, on short, straight, slim spikes, open to elf cap-shaped, dusty pink flowers, 2cm (¾in) across, from summer to autumn. ↕ 1m (3ft), ↔ 60cm (24in). ❄❄❄
D. 'Sandpiper' ■ ♀ Small Elatum Group perennial producing semi-double white flowers with dark brown eyes. ❄❄❄
D. semibarbatum, syn. *D. zalil.* Short-lived, tuberous perennial with 5-lobed leaves, further divided into narrow segments. In early and midsummer, bears unbranched spikes of elf cap-shaped, sulphur-yellow flowers, 1.5cm (½in) across, with orange tips to the central sepals. ↕ 1m (3ft), ↔ 23cm (9in). Afghanistan, Iran. ❄❄❄
D. 'Skyline'. Small Elatum Group perennial with semi-double, sky-blue flowers tinged pink near the centres, the large white eyes tinted blue. ❄❄❄
D. 'Spindrift' ♀ Medium Elatum Group perennial with semi-double, pale cobalt-blue flowers with creamy white eyes; sepals and eyes are suffused lilac. Variable in colour: the sepals often have turquoise and green tinges. ❄❄❄
D. 'Summer Skies'. Pacific Hybrid perennial producing light sky-blue flowers. ❄❄❄
D. 'Sungleam' ■ ♀ Small Elatum Group perennial. Semi-double cream flowers, deeper cream near the margins, have pale sulphur-yellow eyes. ❄❄❄
D. tatsienense ■ Perennial with deeply divided, 3- to 7-lobed leaves. In early and midsummer, branched stems bear panicles of elf cap-shaped, bright cornflower-blue flowers, 2.5–5cm (1–2in) across, with hooded eyes and azure tips to the sepals. ↕ 20–60cm (8–24in), ↔ 30cm (12in). W. China (including E. Tibet). ❄❄❄
D. 'Tiddles' ♀ Small Elatum Group perennial with fully double, slate-mauve flowers. ❄❄❄
D. 'Turkish Delight'. Medium Elatum Group perennial producing semi-double, pale pinkish mauve flowers with white eyes. ❄❄❄
D. 'Völkerfrieden'. Strong-growing Belladonna Group perennial with deep blue flowers. ❄❄❄
D. 'Wendy', syn. *D.* 'Andenken an August Koenemann'. Belladonna Group perennial with gentian-blue flowers. ❄❄❄
D. zalil see *D. semibarbatum.*

DENDRANTHEMA

ASTERACEAE/COMPOSITAE

Genus of 20 species of erect perennials from Europe and C. and E. Asia, found in very variable habitats, from seashores to mountain summits. They were previously included in and commonly grown as *Chrysanthemum*, but are now considered distinct. Alternate, mostly rounded, aromatic, fleshy, mid- to dark green leaves are palmately 5-lobed. Disc- or bowl-shaped, white, yellow, pink, or purple flowerheads, 1–8cm (½–3in) across, are produced singly or in loose corymbs. Grow in a herbaceous or mixed border, a rock garden, or a scree bed. All parts may cause mild stomach upset if ingested, and contact with the foliage may aggravate skin allergies.
• **HARDINESS** Fully hardy.
• **CULTIVATION** Grow in fertile, moist but well-drained soil in full sun. Tall plants may need staking in exposed situations.
• **PROPAGATION** Sow seed in containers in an open frame in autumn. Divide after flowering in autumn, or in spring.
• **PESTS AND DISEASES** Trouble free.

D. pacificum see *Ajania pacifica.*
D. weyrichii, syn. *Chrysanthemum weyrichii.* Mat-forming, rhizomatous perennial with rounded, 5-lobed, fleshy, mid- to dark green leaves, 5–10cm (2–4in) long. The smaller stem leaves are inversely lance-shaped and usually pinnatifid. Daisy-like flowerheads, to 5cm (2in) across, with pink or white ray-florets and yellow disc-florets, are produced in autumn. ↕ to 30cm (12in), ↔ 45cm (18in). Russia (Kamchatka, Sakhalin). ❄❄❄

▷ ***Dendrobenthamia*** see *Cornus*
D. capitata see *C. capitata*

DENDROBIUM

ORCHIDACEAE

Genus of about 900–1,400 species of deciduous, semi-evergreen, or evergreen, epiphytic and terrestrial orchids widely distributed from India and S.E. Asia to New Guinea, Australia, and the Pacific islands; they occur in low-altitude rain-forest or montane forest over 2,000m (7,000ft). Elongated, stem-like pseudobulbs, sometimes branched, bear linear or lance-shaped to ovate leaves, either at the ends of the stems or 2-ranked. Single- to many-flowered racemes or panicles of showy flowers are produced from nodes along the stems, mainly in spring.
• **HARDINESS** Frost tender.
• **CULTIVATION** Cool-growing orchids. Grow epiphytically on a bark slab, or in epiphytic orchid compost in a container or slatted basket. From late spring to summer, grow in humid, partial shade; water freely, adding fertilizer at every third watering, and mist twice daily. Admit full light from autumn to early spring; keep dry in winter. They resent disturbance and flower best in small containers. Provide support for the flowering stems. See also p.46.
• **PROPAGATION** Divide when plant fills and "overflows" the container. For deciduous species, take stem cuttings of the older stems, each with one or more dormant buds, and lay them on damp moss in humid conditions. Pot up individually when rooted, usually after a few months.
• **PESTS AND DISEASES** Susceptible to red spider mites, aphids, and mealybugs.

D. aggregatum see *D. lindleyi.*
D. amethystoglossum. Semi-evergreen, epiphytic orchid with upright pseudobulbs and oval-oblong leaves, 10cm (4in) long. White flowers, to 3cm (1¼in) across, with bright amethyst lips, are borne in crowded racemes, 12cm (5in) long, from winter to spring. ↕ 60–90cm (24–36in), ↔ 15cm (6in). Philippines. ❀ (min. 10°C/50°F; max. 30°C/86°F)
D. aphyllum ■ syn. *D. pierardii.* Deciduous, epiphytic orchid with pendent, slender pseudobulbs and lance-shaped to linear-lance-shaped, fleshy leaves, 12cm (5in) long. Pale mauve-pink flowers, 5cm (2in) across, with primrose yellow lips, are borne in pairs in spring. ↕ 1m (3ft), ↔ 15cm (6in). Himalayas, S.W. China to Malaysia. ❀ (min. 10°C/50°F; max. 30°C/86°F)
D. bigibbum. Semi-evergreen, epiphytic orchid with upright pseudobulbs and oblong-lance-shaped, leathery leaves, to 12cm (5in) long. In spring, produces white, lilac-purple, mauve, or pink flowers, to 6cm (2½in) across, in racemes 10–40cm (4–16in) long, from the upper nodes. ↕ 1m (3ft) or more, ↔ 15cm (6in). Australia (Queensland). ❀ (min. 13°C/55°F; max. 30°C/86°F). **var. *phalaenopsis***, syn. *D. phalaenopsis*, has white flowers, flushed light pinkish mauve at the tips and on the lips.
D. chrysanthum ■ Evergreen, epiphytic orchid producing pendent pseudobulbs, 1–2m (3–6ft) long, with lance-shaped leaves, 10–20cm (4–8in) long, along their lengths. Deep golden yellow flowers, 4cm (1½in) across, are borne in pendent racemes, 4–20cm (1½–8in) long, in spring. ↕ 1–2m (3–6ft), ↔ 45cm (18in). E. Himalayas to Burma, Thailand. ❀ (min. 10°C/50°F; max. 30°C/86°F)
D. densiflorum. Evergreen, epiphytic orchid with 4-angled pseudobulbs and narrowly elliptic or lance-shaped leaves, to 16cm (6in) long. In spring, golden yellow flowers, 5cm (2in) across, are produced in dense, pendent racemes, to 26cm (10in) long, from the upper nodes. ↕↔ 30cm (12in). Himalayas, Burma, Vietnam, Thailand. ❀ (min. 10°C/50°F; max. 30°C/86°F)

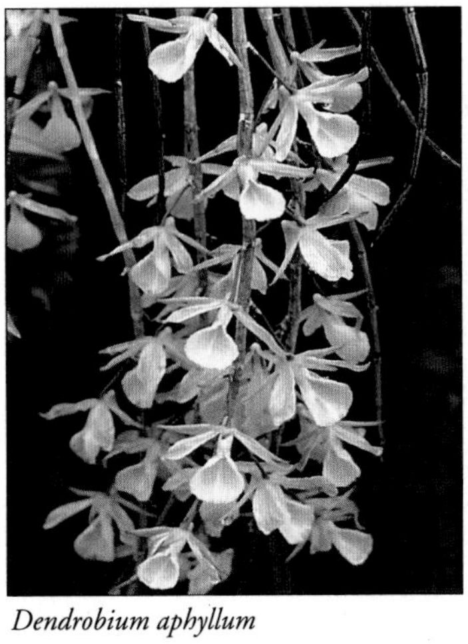
Dendrobium aphyllum

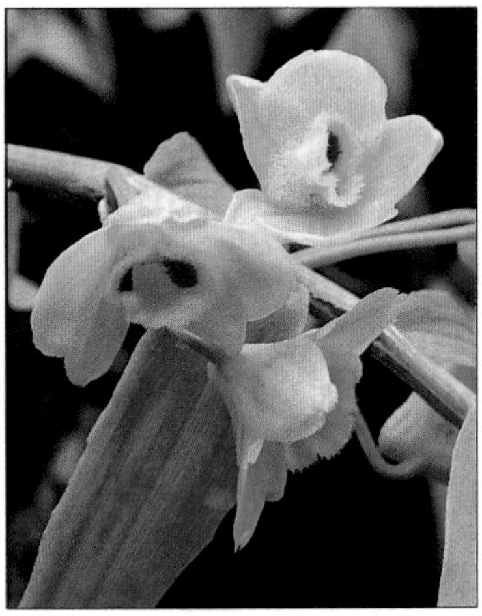
Dendrobium chrysanthum

D. fimbriatum. Evergreen, epiphytic orchid with slender, spindle-shaped pseudobulbs bearing oblong to lance-shaped leaves, 8–15cm (3–6in) long, with pointed tips. In spring, golden yellow or orange-yellow flowers, to 6cm (2½in) across, with fringed lips, are produced in pendent racemes, to 18cm (7in) long, from the upper nodes. ↕ 45cm (18in), ↔ 30cm (12in). Himalayas, Burma, Thailand, Malaysia, Vietnam, Laos, S. China. ❀ (min. 10°C/50°F; max. 30°C/86°F)
D. infundibulum ■ ♀ Semi-evergreen, epiphytic orchid with cylindrical, hairy pseudobulbs and ovate-oblong leaves, to 12cm (5in) long. From spring to summer, produces pure white flowers, 8cm (3in) across, with yellow throat markings, in racemes to 20cm (8in) long, from the upper halves of the pseudobulbs. ↕ 60cm (24in), ↔ 15cm (6in). Burma, Thailand. ❀ (min. 10°C/50°F; max. 30°C/86°F)
D. kingianum ♀ Evergreen, epiphytic orchid with narrowly ovate to narrowly obovate leaves, to 10cm (4in) long, produced from the upper portions of the narrowly conical pseudobulbs. In spring, fragrant, white, pink, mauve, purple, or red flowers, to 4cm (1½in) across, are produced in racemes 7–15cm (3–6in) long, from the pseudobulb tips. ↕↔ 15cm (6in). Australia (New South Wales, Queensland). ❀ (min. 13°C/55°F; max. 30°C/86°F)
D. lindleyi, syn. *D. aggregatum.* Evergreen, epiphytic orchid with spindle-shaped pseudobulbs, each bearing a single, oval leaf, 5–8cm (2–3in) long. Bright yellow or pale golden yellow

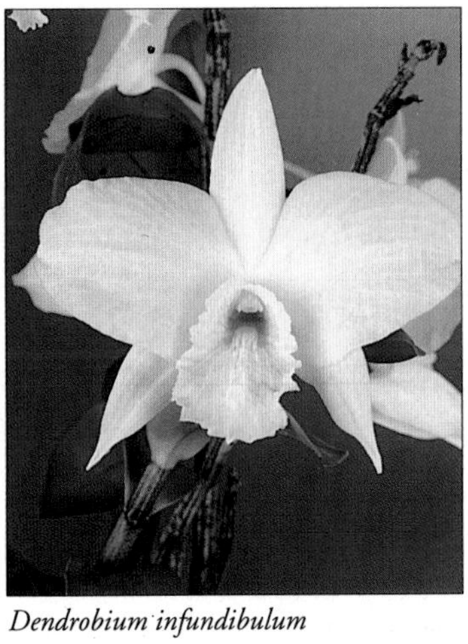
Dendrobium infundibulum

D

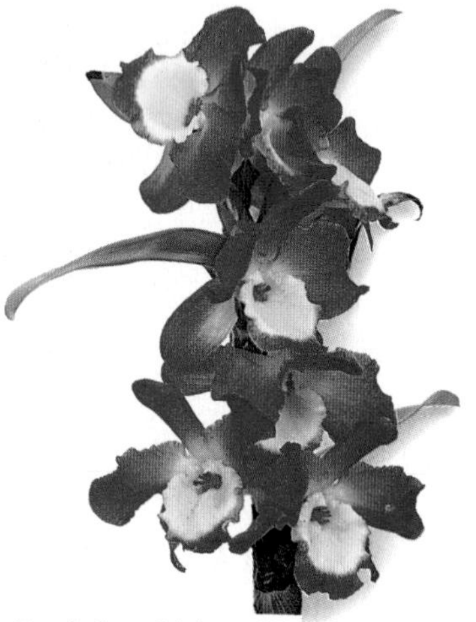

Dendrobium Malones 'Hope'

flowers, to 4cm (1½in) across, are produced in pendent racemes, 10–30cm (4–12in) long, in spring. ↕10cm (4in), ↔15cm (6in). Himalayas, Laos, Vietnam, Cambodia, S.W. China, Burma, Thailand. ❄ (min. 10°C/50°F; max. 30°C/86°F)

D. loddigesii. Deciduous, epiphytic orchid with cylindrical pseudobulbs, becoming pendent, and oblong, fleshy leaves, 7cm (3in) long. Pale rose-pink flowers, 5cm (2in) across, each with an orange disc on the fringed lip, are produced singly from the nodes in spring, usually after the leaves have fallen. ↕↔15cm (6in). S.W. China. ❄ (min. 10°C/50°F; max. 30°C/86°F)

D. longicornu. Semi-evergreen, epiphytic orchid with slender, black-hairy pseudobulbs bearing linear-lance-shaped leaves, 7cm (3in) long. Racemes of 1–3 fragrant white flowers, 5cm (2in) across, with red and yellow markings on the fringed lips, are produced from the upper halves of the leafy stems in spring. ↕30cm (12in), ↔15cm (6in). Himalayas, Burma, Thailand. ❄ (min. 10°C/50°F; max. 30°C/86°F)

***D.* Malones 'Hope'** ■ Evergreen orchid bearing oblong leaves, 10cm (4in) long. Dark pink flowers, 7cm (3in) across, with white-margined yellow lips, are produced in pairs in spring. ↕60cm (24in), ↔30cm (12in). ❄ (min. 10°C/50°F; max. 30°C/86°F)

***D.* Momozono 'Princess'** ■ Evergreen orchid bearing oblong leaves, 10cm (4in) long. Dark pink flowers, 7cm (3in) across, fading to white in the centres, and with white and pink marks on the lips, are produced in pairs in

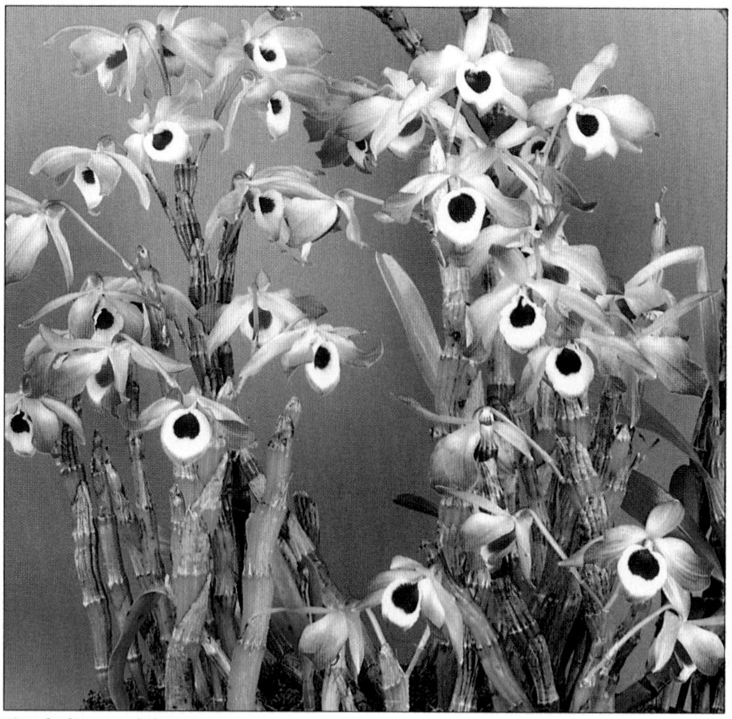

Dendrobium nobile

spring. ↕60cm (24in), ↔30cm (12in). ❄ (min. 10°C/50°F; max. 30°C/86°F)

D. moschatum. Evergreen, epiphytic orchid with cylindrical pseudobulbs and lance-shaped leaves, to 15cm (6in) long. Produces pale yellow flowers, 8cm (3in) across, with a pink flush and 2 maroon marks on each cupped lip, in racemes to 20cm (8in) long, from the upper nodes, in spring. ↕1.2m (4ft), ↔60cm (24in). Himalayas, Burma, Thailand, Laos. ❄ (min. 10°C/50°F; max. 30°C/86°F)

D. nobile ■ ♀ Semi-evergreen, epiphytic orchid with cylindrical to club-shaped pseudobulbs and lance-shaped to ovate-lance-shaped leaves, 7–12cm (3–5in) long. Pale rose-pink flowers, 6cm (2½in) across, tipped with amethyst and with a maroon mark on each lip, are produced in pairs in spring. ↕45cm (18in), ↔15cm (6in). Himalayas, S. China, Taiwan. ❄ (min. 10°C/50°F; max. 30°C/86°F)

D. ochreatum. Deciduous, epiphytic orchid with stout, cylindrical, decumbent pseudobulbs, 10–13cm (4–5in) long, and lance-shaped leaves, 10–17cm (4–7in) long. Rich golden yellow flowers, 7cm (3in) across, with a maroon mark on each lip, are produced in pairs in spring. ↕↔15cm (6in). E. Himalayas, Burma, Thailand, Laos. ❄ (min. 10°C/50°F; max. 30°C/86°F)

***D.* Oriental Paradise** ■ Evergreen orchid bearing oblong leaves, 10cm (4in) long. White flowers, 7cm (3in) across, with dark pink notches on the petals and red and yellow marks on the lips, are borne in pairs in spring. ↕60cm (24in), ↔30cm (12in). ❄ (min. 10°C/50°F; max. 30°C/86°F)

D. phalaenopsis see *D. bigibbum* var. *phalaenopsis.*

D. pierardii see *D. aphyllum.*

D. speciosum. Evergreen, semi-epiphytic orchid with stout, cylindrical or club-shaped pseudobulbs bearing ovate or oblong leaves, to 25cm (10in) long, at the apexes. In spring, produces fragrant, creamy white flowers, to 8cm (3in) across, that do not open widely, in dense racemes, to 60cm (24in) long, from the pseudobulb tips. ↕45cm (18in), ↔30cm (12in). Australia (New South Wales, Queensland, Victoria). ❄ (min. 13°C/55°F; max. 30°C/86°F)

***D.* Spiral Gem 'Universal Topaz'** ■ Evergreen orchid producing narrowly ovate leaves, 10–25cm (4–10in) long. Produces racemes 30cm (12in) long of 6–9 green-yellow flowers, 8–12mm (⅜–½in) across, with red lips, from winter to spring. ↕25–35cm (10–14in), ↔1m (3ft). ❄ (min. 10°C/50°F; max. 30°C/86°F)

D. wardianum. Deciduous, epiphytic orchid with jointed, cylindrical pseudobulbs, becoming pendent, and lance-shaped leaves, 8–12cm (3–5in) long. White flowers, to 10cm (4in) across, with purple-tipped segments and yellow and maroon marks on the lips, are produced in pairs from spring to autumn. ↕30cm (12in), ↔15cm (6in). E. Himalayas, S.W. China, Burma, Thailand. ❄ (min. 10°C/50°F; max. 30°C/86°F)

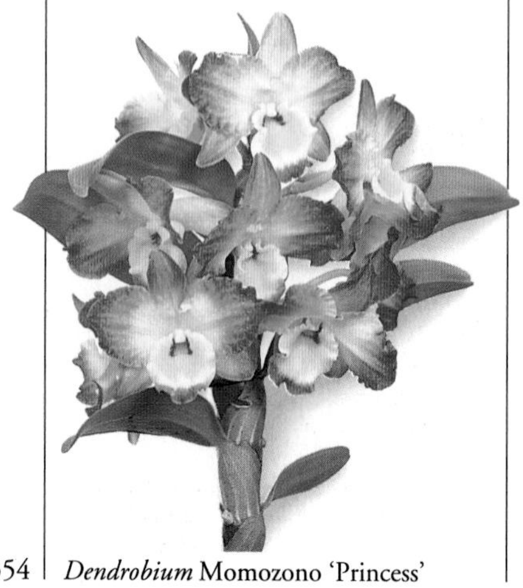

Dendrobium Momozono 'Princess'

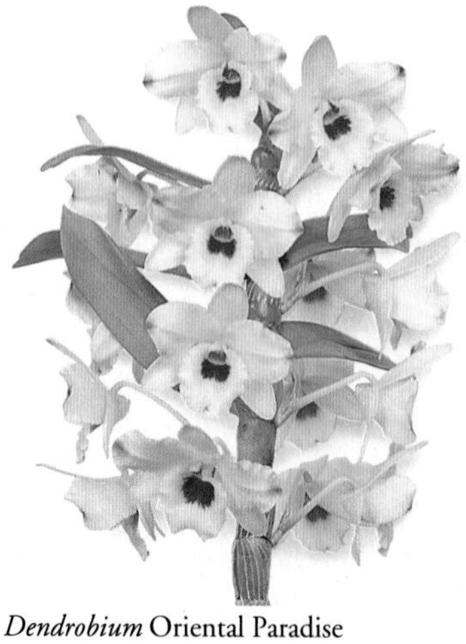

Dendrobium Oriental Paradise

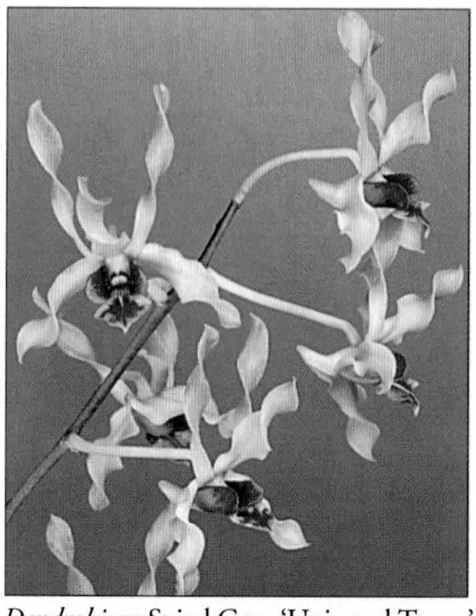

Dendrobium Spiral Gem 'Universal Topaz'

DENDROCALAMUS

GRAMINEAE/POACEAE

Genus of about 30 species of giant, clump-forming, evergreen, rhizomatous bamboos from tropical and subtropical S. and E. Asia. They have thick canes and lance-shaped, downy or bristly leaf-blades. In their native regions, these huge bamboos are used in the construction industry; the hollowed stems are used in irrigation systems and to make paper pulp. They are suitable for specimen plantings or may be used for making a bamboo grove. In frost-prone areas, they are sometimes grown in a warm greenhouse or in interior landscapes in a public space.

- **HARDINESS** Frost tender.
- **CULTIVATION** Under glass, grow in loam-based potting compost (JI No.3), enriched with leaf mould, in bright filtered light with high humidity. Water freely in summer, moderately in winter. Outdoors, grow in fertile, humus-rich, moist but well-drained soil in sun or partial shade.
- **PROPAGATION** Divide established clumps in spring. Cut sections of young culms in spring, then place horizontally in sphagnum moss in a closed, heated propagating case.
- **PESTS AND DISEASES** Trouble free.

D. giganteus, syn. *Sinocalamus giganteus* (Kyo-Chiku). Robust, clump-forming bamboo producing rapidly spreading rhizomes and erect, later gracefully arching, hairy-jointed canes that eventually reach 35cm (14in) wide. The lance-shaped, smooth, minutely toothed leaf-blades, to 55cm (22in) long, arise from the cane joints and clasp the canes at their bases. ↕25–30m (80–100ft), ↔3–4m (10–12ft). S.E. Asia. ❄ (min. 5°C/41°F)

DENDROCHILUM

Golden chain orchid

ORCHIDACEAE

Genus of about 120–150 species of evergreen, epiphytic orchids from S.E. Asia and New Guinea, often found on trees and rocks by rivers at altitudes of 700–2,000m (2,300–7,000ft). Ovoid to cylindrical pseudobulbs produce 1 or 2 lance-shaped-elliptic leaves. Golden chain orchids are valued for their chain-like racemes of fragrant, dainty, star-shaped flowers, borne in early summer.

- **HARDINESS** Frost tender.
- **CULTIVATION** Cool-growing orchids. Grow in epiphytic orchid compost in a container. In summer, provide humid,

shaded conditions; water freely and apply fertilizer at every third watering. In winter, admit full light and water very sparingly. See also p.46.
• **PROPAGATION** Divide when plant "overflows" the container, or remove backbulbs and pot up separately.
• **PESTS AND DISEASES** Susceptible to red spider mites, aphids, and mealybugs.

D. glumaceum. Epiphytic orchid with ovoid pseudobulbs, each bearing one narrowly elliptic leaf, to 30cm (12in) long. Star-shaped white flowers, to 2cm (¾in) across, do not open widely. They are produced densely from the axils of conspicuous white bracts, in 2 rows on pendent racemes, from the centre of the new growth. ↕ to 50cm (20in), ↔ 30cm (12in). Philippines. ⚘ (min. 13°C/55°F; max. 30°C/86°F)

DENDROMECON
Tree poppy

PAPAVERACEAE

Genus of 1 or 2 species of evergreen shrubs and small trees found in scrub on dry, rocky slopes in S.W. USA and Mexico. *D. rigida* is cultivated for its lance-shaped, simple, leathery, glaucous leaves, arranged alternately along the stems, and for its showy, poppy-like, fragrant flowers. It looks best grown against a wall, but may be grown in a cool greenhouse in cold regions.
• **HARDINESS** Frost hardy, but may survive short periods at temperatures below -5°C (23°F) if protected.
• **CULTIVATION** Grow in well-drained soil in full sun. Pruning group 13, if wall-trained.
• **PROPAGATION** Sow seed at 10–13°C (50–55°F) in autumn or spring. Root softwood cuttings in summer, or insert root cuttings in winter.
• **PESTS AND DISEASES** Trouble free.

D. rigida ■ Spreading shrub with rigid, upright shoots and lance-shaped, leathery, glaucous, grey-green leaves, to 10cm (4in) long. Solitary, poppy-like, fragrant yellow flowers, to 7cm (3in) across, are produced from spring to autumn. ↕↔ 3m (10ft). USA (California), Mexico. ❄❄

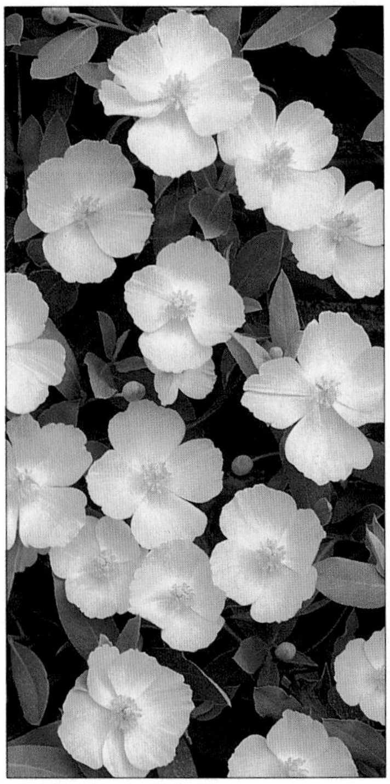

Dendromecon rigida

DENMOZA

CACTACEAE

Genus of 2 species of spherical to columnar, perennial cacti from hillsides in Argentina. They have very thick stems and densely spiny ribs. Tubular flowers are produced mainly near the top of the stems, the style and stamens protruding in a cluster from each almost closed throat. Spherical, scaly fruits have woolly tufts, which later fall, and large, helmet-shaped black seeds. In frost-prone areas, grow in a warm greenhouse. In warmer climates, grow in a border with other succulents.
• **HARDINESS** Frost tender.
• **CULTIVATION** Under glass, grow in standard cactus compost in full light and low humidity. In growth, water moderately and apply fertilizer monthly; keep completely dry at other times. Outdoors, grow in sharply drained, gritty soil in full sun. See also pp.48–49.
• **PROPAGATION** Sow seed at 21°C (70°F) in spring or early summer.
• **PESTS AND DISEASES** Mealybugs and root mealybugs may be troublesome, especially in containers.

D. rhodacantha. Spherical cactus with 15–30 deeply furrowed ribs. Areoles have brownish red spines (8–10 radials and usually 1 central). Diurnal, tubular red flowers, 7cm (3in) long, are borne in summer. ↕ 15–30cm (6–12in), ↔ 16cm (6in). N.W. and W. Argentina. ⚘ (min. 10°C/50°F)

DENNSTAEDTIA

DENNSTAEDTIACEAE

Genus of about 70 species of deciduous ferns found mainly in woodland in tropical regions. In spring, erect, lance-shaped or roughly triangular fronds, usually 2- or 3-pinnate, arise from a creeping rhizome, soon forming colonies that may become invasive. Sori develop along the margins of the frond segments, and are covered by cup-shaped indusia. Use *Dennstaedtia* species for ground cover in a shady border. In frost-prone areas, grow tender species in a cool or warm greenhouse.
• **HARDINESS** Fully hardy to frost tender.
• **CULTIVATION** Under glass, grow in 1 part each of loam, medium-grade bark, and charcoal, 2 parts sharp sand, and 3 parts coarse leaf mould. Provide bright filtered light. Water freely in growth, sparingly in winter. Pot on regularly. Outdoors, grow in moist, humus-rich, acid soil in deep to light dappled shade.
• **PROPAGATION** Sow spores at 15°C (59°F) for hardy species, and 21°C (70°F) for tender species, as soon as ripe. Divide in spring. See also p.51.
• **PESTS AND DISEASES** Trouble free.

D. davallioides. Spreading fern with long-creeping rhizomes. Broadly triangular, mid-green fronds, 40–70cm (16–28in) long, are 4- or 5-pinnate with linear segments. ↕ 75cm (30in), ↔ indefinite. Australia (Queensland, New South Wales, Victoria). ❄

D. punctiloba (North American hay-scented fern). Fern with long-creeping rhizomes. Erect to arching, yellow-green fronds, 15–45cm (6–18in) long, are lance-shaped and 2- or 3-pinnate, with linear segments. May be invasive. ↕ 45cm (18in), ↔ indefinite. North America. ❄❄❄

▷ ***Dentaria*** see *Cardamine*
D. digitata see *C. pentaphyllos*
D. enneaphyllos see *C. enneaphyllos*
D. pentaphyllos see *C. pentaphyllos*
▷ ***Derwentia*** see *Parahebe*

DESCHAMPSIA
Hair grass

GRAMINEAE/POACEAE

Genus of about 50 species of tufted or tussock-forming, herbaceous or evergreen, perennial grasses. They are widely distributed in arctic and temperate zones, found in damp meadows, moorland, and woodland clearings, and on high mountains in tropical regions. The leaves are thread-like, linear, or oblong. Grown for their habit and graceful, airy panicles, they are suitable for a mixed, herbaceous, or shrub border, or for a wildflower or rock garden. The flowerheads of the taller species are useful for fresh or dried flower arrangements.
• **HARDINESS** Fully hardy.
• **CULTIVATION** Grow in dry to damp, neutral to acid soil in sun or partial shade. Incorporate garden compost before planting in dry soils. Remove flowerheads before new growth begins in early spring.
• **PROPAGATION** Sow seed *in situ* in spring or autumn, or divide in mid-spring or early summer.
• **PESTS AND DISEASES** Trouble free.

D. cespitosa (Tufted hair grass, Tussock grass). Dense, tussock-forming, evergreen grass with rigid, linear, rough, mid-green leaves, to 60cm (24in) long. Produces airy, arching panicles, to 45cm (18in) long, of glistening, silver-tinted purple spikelets, from early to late summer. ↕ to 2m (6ft), ↔ 1.2–1.5m (4–5ft). Eurasia, tropical Africa. ❄❄❄. **'Fairy's Joke'** see var. *vivipara*. **'Golden Dew'** see 'Goldtau'. **'Golden Veil'** see 'Goldschleier'. **'Goldschleier'**, syn. 'Golden Veil', has dark green leaves and spikelets that age to bright silvery yellow; ↕↔ to 1.2m (4ft). **'Goldtau'** ■ syn. 'Golden Dew', is more compact, with silvery reddish brown spikelets that age to golden yellow; ↕↔ to 75cm (30in). **var. *vivipara***, syn. 'Fairy's Joke', produces young plantlets in place of seed, eventually weighing the slender culms to the ground; ↕↔ to 1.2m (4ft).

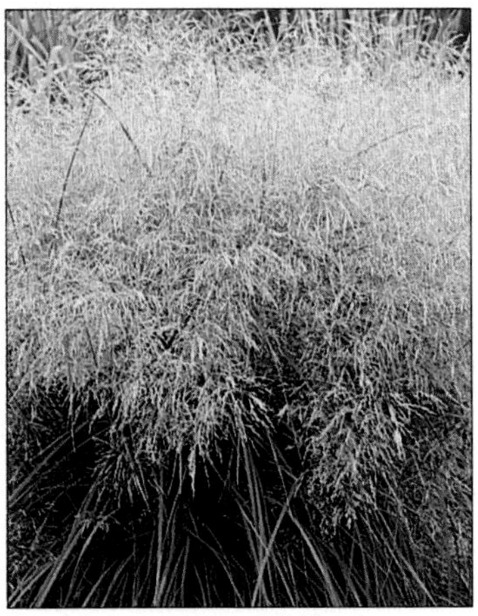

Deschampsia cespitosa 'Goldtau'

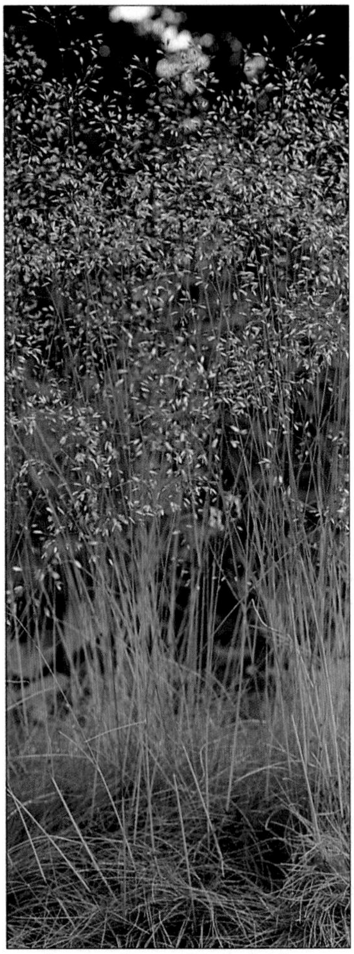

Deschampsia flexuosa 'Tatra Gold'

D. flexuosa, syn. *Aira flexuosa* (Wavy hair grass). Tufted, often rhizomatous, evergreen grass with thread-like, smooth, bluish green leaves, to 20cm (8in) long. Open panicles, to 12cm (5in) long, of glistening, silver-tinted, purple or brown spikelets are borne on wavy stalks in early and midsummer. Prefers acid soil. ↕ to 60cm (24in), ↔ 30cm (12in). Europe, Asia, N.E. USA, South America. ❄❄❄. **'Tatra Gold'** ■ syn. 'Aurea', has arching, bright yellow-green leaves and bronze-tinted inflorescences; ↕ 50cm (20in).

▷ **Desert candle** see *Eremurus*
▷ **Desert pea, Sturt's** see *Clianthus formosus*
▷ **Desert rose** see *Adenium*

DESFONTAINIA

DESFONTAINIACEAE/LOGANIACEAE

Genus of one species of evergreen shrub from rainforest and mountain slopes in the Andes, cultivated for its holly-like, opposite leaves and its showy, solitary, tubular flowers. In areas of high rainfall, *D. spinosa* will tolerate open situations, but in drier places a cool, sheltered shrub border or peat garden is essential.
• **HARDINESS** Frost hardy.
• **CULTIVATION** Grow in moist, peaty, lime-free soil in cool, dappled shade, with shelter from cold, drying winds. Pruning group 9.

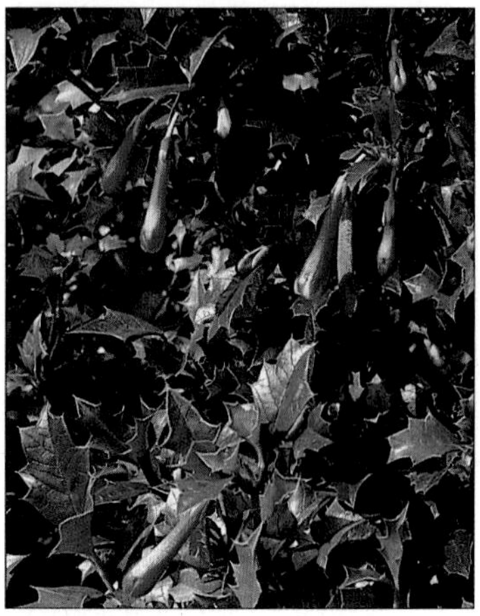

Desfontainia spinosa

• **PROPAGATION** Insert semi-ripe cuttings in summer.
• **PESTS AND DISEASES** Trouble free.

D. spinosa ■ 🏆 Dense, bushy shrub with oval or ovate, spiny, glossy, dark green leaves, to 6cm (2½in) long. Pendent, yellow-tipped red flowers, to 4cm (1½in) long, are produced from the upper leaf axils from midsummer to late autumn. ↕↔ 2m (6ft). Andes (from Colombia to Straits of Magellan). ❄❄

DESMODIUM

LEGUMINOSAE/PAPILIONACEAE

Genus of more than 450 species of deciduous shrubs, subshrubs, and herbaceous perennials from tropical and subtropical regions. They are grown for their loose, terminal or axillary panicles or racemes of small, pea-like, white to purple flowers. The alternate leaves are pinnate to 3-palmate. Grow against a wall. In frost-prone areas, grow half-hardy and frost-tender species in a temperate greenhouse.
• **HARDINESS** Fully hardy to frost tender.
• **CULTIVATION** Grow in well-drained soil in full sun. Pruning group 4 or 6.
• **PROPAGATION** Sow seed in containers in a cold frame in autumn. Insert softwood cuttings in late spring.
• **PESTS AND DISEASES** Trouble free.

D. elegans ■ syn. *D. tiliifolium.* Upright subshrub with leaves to 25cm (10in) long, composed of 3 obovate leaflets, dark green above and grey and hairy beneath. Terminal panicles, 20cm (8in) long, of pea-like, lilac to deep pink flowers are produced from late summer to autumn. ↕↔ 1.5m (5ft). Himalayas, China. ❄❄
D. praestans see *D. yunnanense.*
D. tiliifolium see *D. elegans.*
D. yunnanense, syn. *D. praestans.* Vigorous, spreading shrub with pale green leaves, 10–20cm (4–8in) long, downy, grey-green beneath, composed of 1 broadly ovate central leaflet and 2 much smaller lateral ones; they are occasionally reduced to a single, large, central leaflet. Pea-like purple flowers are produced in terminal panicles, to 40cm (16in) long, in late summer. ↕↔ 4m (12ft). S.W. China. ❄❄

DEUTZIA

HYDRANGEACEAE/SAXIFRAGACEAE

Genus of about 60 species of mainly deciduous shrubs, found in scrub and woodland from the Himalayas to E. Asia. Many have peeling bark, especially when mature. Leaves, usually to 7cm (3in) long, are opposite, ovate to lance-shaped, and mainly toothed. Numerous 5-petalled, cup- to star-shaped, often fragrant, white to pink flowers are borne in axillary or terminal racemes, panicles, cymes, or corymbs from mid-spring to midsummer. All are suitable for a shrub border; the larger ones are also good specimen plants. In colder regions, grow frost-hardy deutzias against a wall or among trees and other shrubs.
• **HARDINESS** Fully hardy to frost hardy.
• **CULTIVATION** Grow in reasonably fertile, not too dry soil, preferably in full sun; some will tolerate partial shade. Pruning group 2.
• **PROPAGATION** Sow seed in containers in a cold frame in autumn. Insert softwood cuttings in summer; root hardwood cuttings in autumn.
• **PESTS AND DISEASES** Trouble free.

***D.* 'Candelabra'.** Upright, arching shrub with broadly lance-shaped, bright green leaves. Bears star-shaped white flowers, to 2.5cm (1in) across, in dense, upright panicles, 6–8cm (2½–3in) long, in mid- and late spring. ↕ 1m (3ft), ↔ 1.5m (5ft). ❄❄❄
D. chunii see *D. ningpoensis.*
D. compacta. Spreading shrub with lance-shaped to inversely lance-shaped, tapered leaves, to 6cm (2½in) long, dark green above and grey-green beneath. In midsummer, produces compact, corymb-like panicles, 5cm (2in) across,

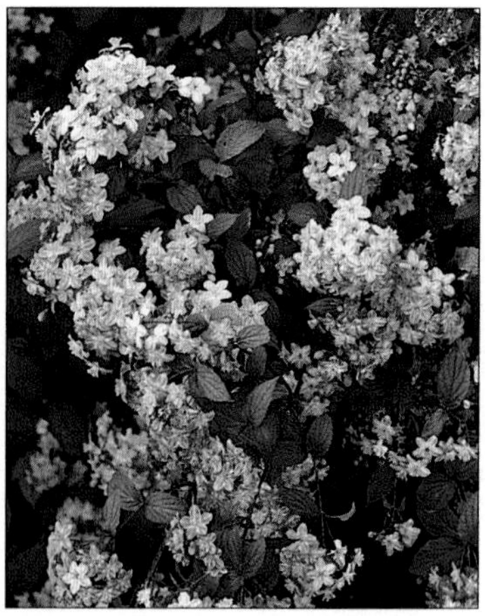

Deutzia x *elegantissima* 'Rosealind'

of cup-shaped, fragrant white flowers, 1cm (½in) across. ↕ 2m (6ft), ↔ 2.5m (8ft). China. ❄❄❄. **'Lavender Time'** produces lilac flowers, fading with age.
***D.* 'Contraste'.** Bushy shrub with arching branches and narrowly ovate, dark green leaves. Star-shaped, wavy-petalled, yellow-anthered, pink to purplish pink flowers, to 2.5cm (1in) across, with deep pink bands on the backs of the petals, are produced in corymb-like panicles, 5–7cm (2–3in) across, in early summer. ↕ 1.5m (5ft), ↔ 1.2m (4ft). ❄❄❄
***D. crenata* var. *nakaiana* 'Nikko'** ■ Compact shrub with lance-shaped, rich green leaves, 3–6cm (1¼–2½in) long, turning red-purple in autumn. Produces racemes or panicles, 10–15cm (4–6in) long, of star-shaped white flowers, 1.5cm (½in) across, in summer. Suitable for a rock garden. ↕ 60cm (24in), ↔ 1.2m (4ft). ❄❄❄
***D. discolor* 'Major'.** Spreading shrub with arching branches and narrowly ovate-oblong, mid-green leaves, to 10cm (4in) long. Produces star-shaped, pink-flushed white flowers, 1.5–2.5cm (½–1in) across, in corymbs, 8cm (3in) across, in late spring and early summer. ↕ 1.5m (5ft), ↔ 2m (6ft). ❄❄❄
***D.* x *elegantissima* 'Rosealind'** ■ 🏆 Compact, rounded, upright shrub with ovate to ovate-oblong, dull, mid-green leaves. Star-shaped, pink-flushed white flowers, 2cm (¾in) across, are produced in corymb-like cymes, 4–8cm (1½–3in) across, in late spring and early summer. ↕ 1.2m (4ft), ↔ 1.5m (5ft). ❄❄❄
D. gracilis ■ Bushy, erect shrub with lance-shaped to ovate, tapered, bright

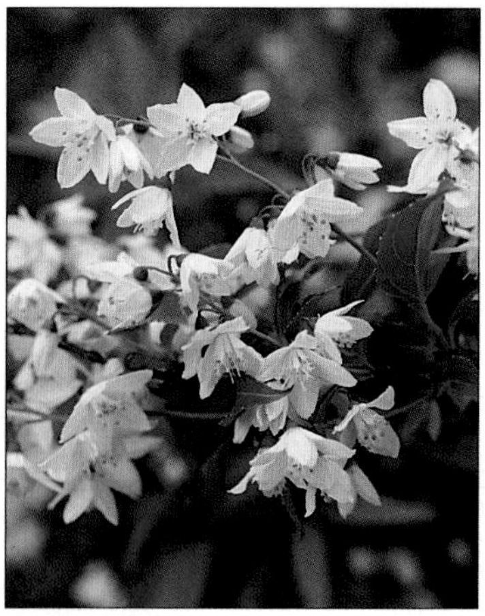

Deutzia gracilis

green leaves, to 6cm (2½in) long. Fragrant, star-shaped white flowers, to 2cm (¾in) across, are produced in upright racemes, 5–7cm (2–3in) long, from spring to early summer. ↕↔ 1m (3ft). Japan. ❄❄❄
***D.* 'Joconde'.** Bushy, upright shrub with narrowly ovate, long-pointed, mid-green leaves. Panicles, 5–7cm (2–3in) long, of cup-shaped, yellow-anthered white flowers (purple in bud), 2.5–3cm (1–1¼in) across, streaked purple on the backs of the wavy petals, are produced in summer. ↕↔ 1.5m (5ft). ❄❄❄
D.* x *kalmiiflora (*D. parviflora* x *D. purpurascens*). Open shrub with arching branches and narrowly oval, mid-green leaves, 4–7cm (1½–3in) long. Bears star-shaped, deep pink flowers, to 2cm (¾in) across, paler inside, in upright

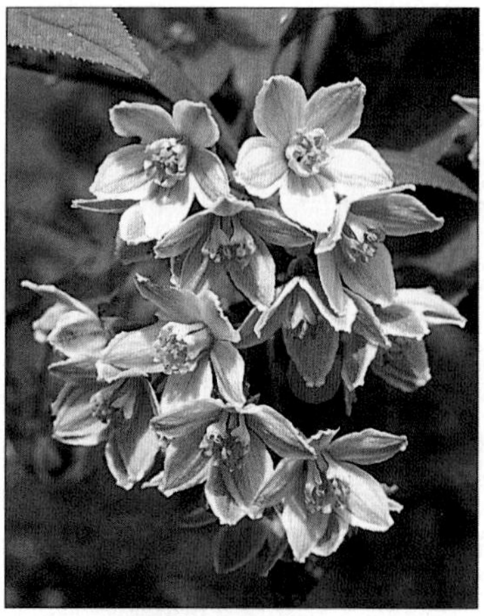

Deutzia longifolia 'Veitchii'

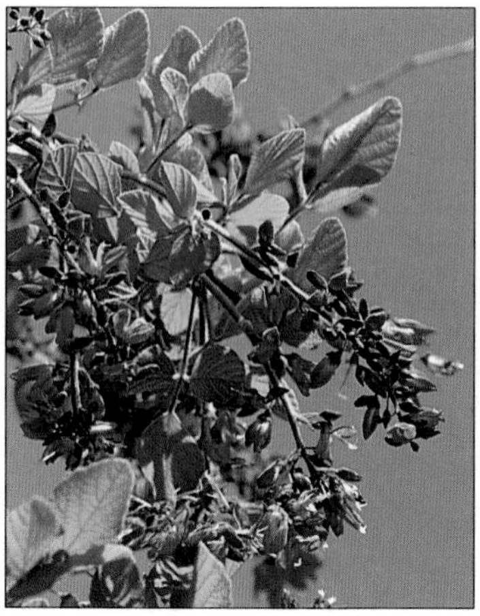

Desmodium elegans

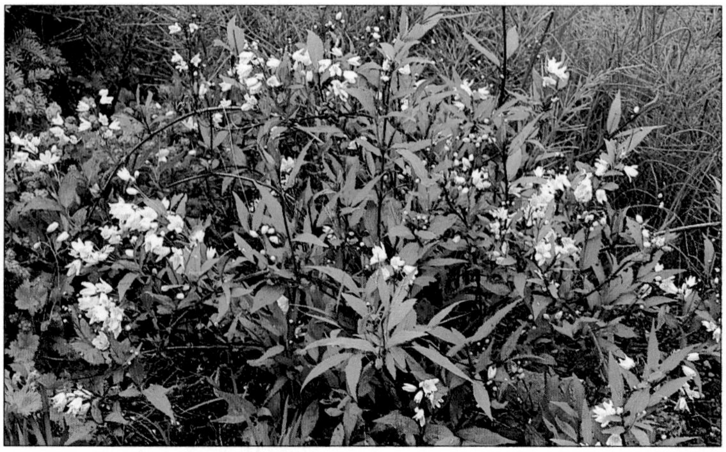

Deutzia crenata var. *nakaiana* 'Nikko'

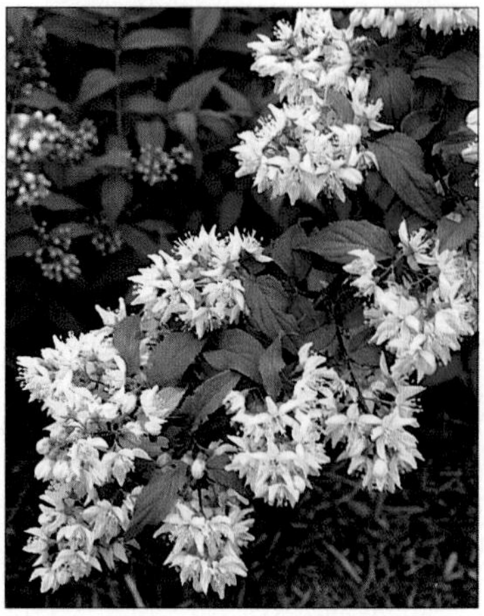

Deutzia x *magnifica* 'Staphyleoides'

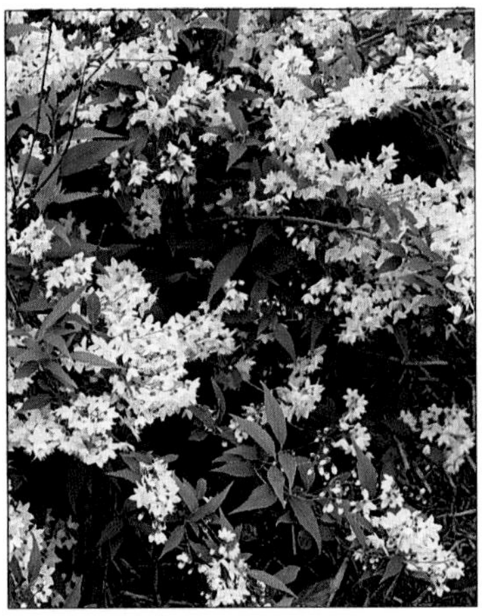

Deutzia monbeigii

panicles, 5–7cm (2–3in) long, in early summer. ↕↔ 1.5m (5ft). Garden origin. ✻✻✻

D. longifolia. Spreading shrub with arching branches and lance-shaped, grey-green leaves, to 12cm (5in) long. Panicle-like cymes, 5–7cm (2–3in) long, of star-shaped white flowers, to 2.5cm (1in) across, purple-pink on the backs of the petals, are borne in early and midsummer. ↕ 2m (6ft), ↔ 3m (10ft). W. China (Sichuan, Yunnan). ✻✻✻. **'Veitchii'** ▣ 🏆 has deep lilac-pink flowers, to 3cm (1¼in) across, with white margins.

***D.* 'Magicien'.** Bushy, upright shrub with narrowly ovate, mid-green leaves. In early summer, bears panicles, 5–7cm (2–3in) long, of cup-shaped flowers, 2.5cm (1in) across, pink inside, white

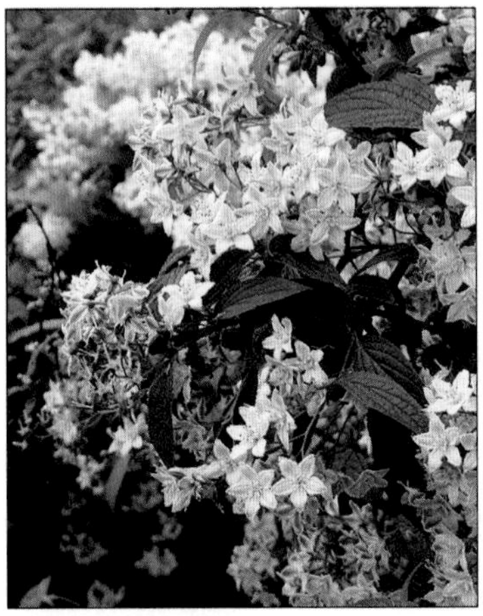

Deutzia 'Mont Rose'

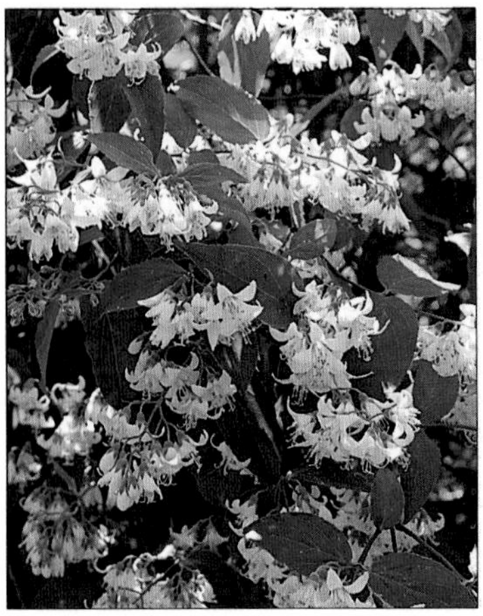

Deutzia ningpoensis

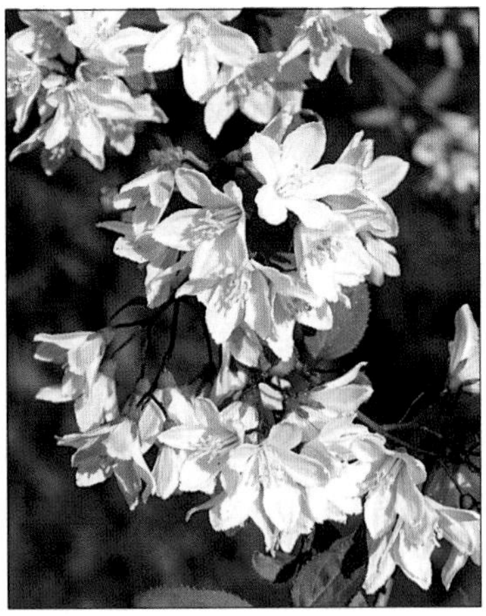

Deutzia x *rosea*

with deep pink stripes outside, and with yellow anthers. ↕↔ 1.5m (5ft). ✻✻✻

***D.* x *magnifica* 'Staphyleoides'** ▣ Vigorous, upright shrub with arching branches and ovate-oblong, bright green leaves, to 10cm (4in) long, hairy below. In early summer, bears star-shaped white flowers, 2–2.5cm (¾–1in) across, with recurved petals, in panicles 10cm (4in) long. ↕ 3m (10ft), ↔ 2m (6ft). ✻✻✻

D. monbeigii ▣ Arching shrub with slender shoots and ovate-lance-shaped, dark green leaves, to 5cm (2in) long, white hairy beneath. Bears star-shaped white flowers, to 1.5cm (½in) across, in corymbs, 6cm (2½in) across, in early and midsummer. ↕ 1.2m (4ft), ↔ 1.5m (5ft). S.W. China (Yunnan). ✻✻✻

***D.* 'Mont Rose'** ▣ Bushy, upright shrub with narrowly ovate, dark green leaves. Star-shaped, purple-pink flowers, to 1.5cm (½in) across, with wavy petals and yellow anthers, are produced in panicles, 2–3cm (¾–1¼in) long, in early summer. ↕↔ 1.2m (4ft). ✻✻✻

D. ningpoensis ▣ syn. *D. chunii*. Open shrub with slender, lance-shaped to ovate, generally entire, mid-green leaves, densely hairy beneath. Panicles, to 10cm (4in) long, of star-shaped white or pink-tinged flowers, to 1cm (½in) across, are produced in summer. ↕↔ 2m (6ft). E. China (Zhejiang, Anhui). ✻✻✻

D. pulchra. Upright shrub with arching branches and peeling, orange-brown bark. Lance-shaped to narrowly ovate, entire or toothed, dark green leaves are densely hairy, to 10cm (4in) long. Bears star-shaped, pink-tinged white flowers, to 2cm (¾in) across, in slender, pendent panicles, to 12cm (5in) long, in late

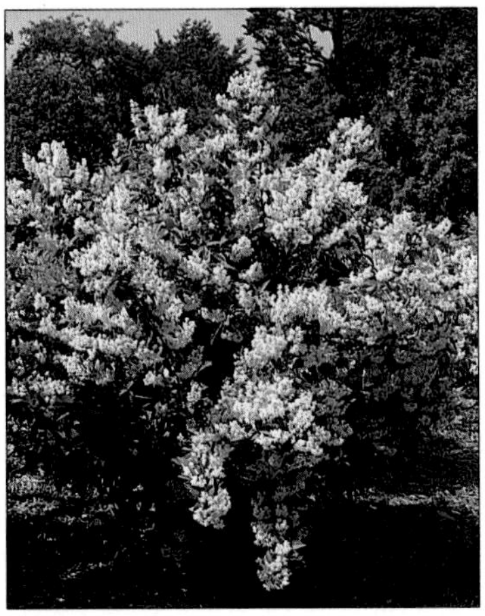

Deutzia scabra

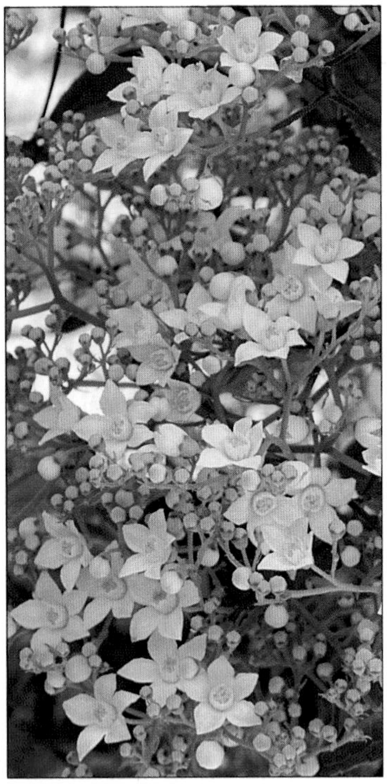

Deutzia setchuenensis var. *corymbiflora*

spring and early summer. ↕ 2.5m (8ft), ↔ 2m (6ft). Taiwan, Philippines. ✻✻

D.* x *rosea ▣ (*D. gracilis* x *D. purpurascens*). Compact, rounded, bushy shrub with ovate-lance-shaped to ovate-oblong, dark green leaves. In early summer, bears a profusion of star-shaped white flowers, to 1.5cm (½in) across, pink- to red-tinged outside, in broad, corymb-like panicles, 5–7cm (2–3in) long. ↕↔ 1.2m (4ft). Garden origin. ✻✻✻. **'Campanulata'** has bell-shaped white flowers, 2cm (¾in) across.

D. scabra ▣ Upright shrub with arching shoots, peeling, pale brown bark when mature, and broadly ovate, dark green leaves, to 8cm (3in) long. Produces dense, upright, cylindrical panicles, 8–16cm (3–6in) long, of star-shaped, single, honey-scented, white or pink-tinged flowers, to 1.5cm (½in) across, in early and midsummer. ↕ 3m (10ft), ↔ 2m (6ft). Japan. ✻✻✻. **'Candidissima'** produces double white flowers. **'Pride of Rochester'** has double white flowers tinged with pink.

D. setchuenensis* var. *corymbiflora ▣ 🏆 Upright shrub with peeling, pale brown bark when mature, and ovate to lance-shaped, long-pointed, grey-green leaves, to 11cm (4½in) long. In early and midsummer, produces cup-shaped white flowers, to 1.5cm (½in) across, in corymbs 7–10cm (3–4in) across. ↕ 2m (6ft), ↔ 1.5m (5ft). W. China. ✻✻

▷ **Devil flower** see *Tacca chantrierei*
▷ **Devil-in-a-bush** see *Nigella, N. damascena*
▷ **Devil's apples** see *Mandragora officinarum*
▷ **Devil's bit scabious** see *Succisa pratensis*
▷ **Devil's claw, Common** see *Proboscidea louisianica*
▷ **Devil's tongue** see *Amorphophallus, A. konjac*
▷ **Devil's walking stick** see *Aralia spinosa*
▷ **Dewdrop, Golden** see *Duranta erecta*
▷ **Dhak** see *Butea monosperma*

DIANELLA

LILIACEAE/PHORMIACEAE

Genus of 25–30 species of variable, evergreen, rhizomatous perennials, sometimes with fibrous roots, found in subtropical and temperate woodland, heath, or more open areas in E. Africa, Madagascar, E. Asia, W. Pacific, and Australasia. They are grown for their loose panicles of slightly pendent, star-shaped, usually blue flowers, followed by spherical or oblong-ovoid berries. Grass-like, linear to lance-shaped leaves are radical or borne in 2 ranks on the stems, which are usually 40–80cm (16–32in) tall, although they may reach 2m (6ft). Grow in a woodland garden or a warm, sheltered border. In frost-prone areas, grow tender species in a cool greenhouse, preferably in a border.

- **HARDINESS** Frost hardy to frost tender.
- **CULTIVATION** Under glass, grow in loam-based potting compost (JI No.2), in full light with shade from hot sun. In the growing season, water freely and apply a balanced liquid fertilizer weekly; keep just moist in winter. Outdoors, grow in moderately fertile, humus-rich, well-drained, neutral to acid soil in a sheltered site in sun or partial shade.
- **PROPAGATION** Sow seed at 13–16°C (55–61°F), or divide in spring.
- **PESTS AND DISEASES** Trouble free.

D. caerulea. Tufted or mat-forming perennial with broadly lance-shaped, keeled, stiff leaves, to 75cm (30in) long, with rough margins. Panicles, to 30cm (12in) long, of pendent, star-shaped, blue, blue-green, or white flowers, 1–2cm (½–¾in) long, with conspicuous yellow anthers, are produced in early summer, followed by spherical, shiny blue berries, 7–12mm (¼–½in) long. ↕ 60cm (24in), ↔ 30cm (12in). E. Australia, New Guinea. ✻✻

D. tasmanica ▣ Tufted perennial forming clumps of strap-shaped, stiff, rough-margined leaves, to 1.2m (4ft) long, sometimes also producing tall, cane-like stems with tufts of smaller leaves at the top. Branching panicles, to 60cm (24in) long, of star-shaped, lavender-blue to violet flowers, to 2cm (¾in) across, with pale yellow anthers, are borne in early summer, followed by persistent, oblong-ovoid, dark blue berries, to 2cm (¾in) long. ↕ to 1.2m (4ft), ↔ 45cm (18in). S.E. Australia (including Tasmania). ✻✻

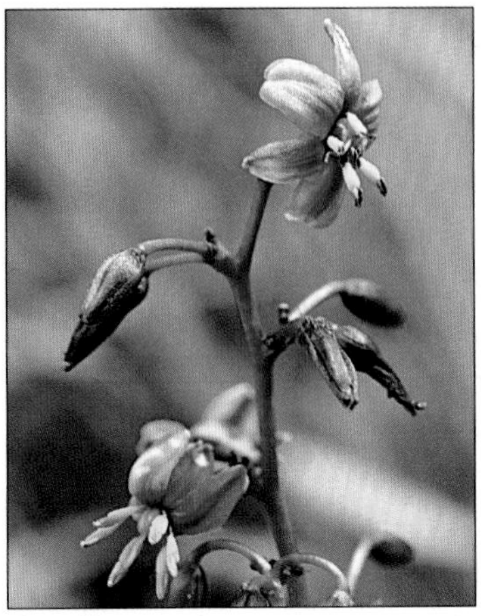

Dianella tasmanica

DIANTHUS

Carnation, Pink

CARYOPHYLLACEAE

Genus of over 300 species of low-growing, evergreen subshrubs and perennials, annuals, and biennials – including the popular bedding plant *D. barbatus* (Sweet William) – found in mountains and meadows in Europe, Asia, and southern Africa. The tens of thousands of cultivars, bred for garden use and exhibition, are usually divided into several subgroups, described below. The leaves of all *Dianthus* species and cultivars are linear to lance-shaped, mostly pointed, and often blue-grey or grey-green with a waxy bloom. Leaves of the alpine species are 1.5–5cm (½–2in) long; those of carnations and larger pinks may be up to 13cm (5in) long.

Carnations and pinks are similar in habit and flower, although pinks are smaller and frequently have fewer petals, often distinctively patterned. Both are grown mainly for their flowers, borne in profusion over a long period in summer, and exceptionally long-lasting when cut. The blooms are often fragrant (referred to as "clove-scented"), and are solitary or borne in few- to many-flowered, terminal, cyme-like umbels or cymes. Each flower has a short tubular base and usually 5 spreading tepals (fully double cultivars have up to 60); these are sometimes toothed or fringed, and bearded.

For exhibition purposes, carnations and pinks are grouped according to the colouring and marking of their flowers (see panel below). Carnations and pinks are also divided into the following broader subgroups:

Border carnations
Fully hardy, annual or evergreen, perennial border plants, also good for cutting. In midsummer, each stem bears 5 or more double flowers, to 8cm (3in) across, with no fewer than 25 petals. These are of the self, fancy, or picotee types, and may be clove-scented.
↕45–60cm (18–24in), ↔40cm (16in).

Perpetual-flowering carnations
Half-hardy, evergreen perennials; they are usually grown under glass for cut flowers, and for exhibition. Flowers, produced throughout the year, are double, to 10cm (4in) across, and are of the self, fancy, or picotee types. Modern cultivars are often scented, although few of the older ones are fragrant.
↕90–150cm (3–5ft), ↔30cm (12in).

Malmaison carnations
Half-hardy, evergreen perennials, derived from *D.* 'Souvenir de la Malmaison', grown for their intensely fragrant flowers. Under glass and in conservatories, they bloom sporadically throughout the year, producing large, double flowers, to 13cm (5in) across. Most Malmaisons are selfs, with thick stems and broad, curled leaves. They generally produce blooms with such a large number of petals that the calyces split, and are usually disbudded to leave only the crown bud on each stem.
↕50–70cm (20–28in), ↔40cm (16in).

Old-fashioned pinks
Fully hardy, evergreen perennials, grown for border decoration and cutting. Most form compact mounds, although some are more open in habit. They bloom for 2–3 weeks in early summer, bearing 4–6 usually clove-scented, single, semi-double, or double flowers per stem, each 3.5–6cm (1½–2½in) across; these may be selfs, bicolours, or laced. The sterile "Mule" pinks are crosses between *D. barbatus* and border carnations.
↕25–45cm (10–18in), ↔30cm (12in).

Modern pinks
Fully hardy, evergreen perennials, grown for border decoration and cutting, most forming compact mounds. Flowers, 3.5–6cm (1½–2½in) across, are single, semi-double, or double, usually with 4–6 but occasionally 1–3 flowers per stem, and with 2 or 3 flushes of bloom from early summer to autumn; they may be selfs, bicolours, fancies, or laced, and some are clove-scented.
↕25–45cm (10–18in), ↔40cm (16in).

Alpine pinks
Fully hardy, evergreen, alpine species, and cultivars derived from them, with a neat, mat- or cushion-forming habit. They grow easily at the edge of a border or in a rock garden, raised bed, trough, or alpine house. Single, semi-double, or double flowers, 1–4cm (½–1½in) across, borne in summer, are solitary or in few-flowered clusters and often clove-scented. Many have grey foliage.
↕8–10cm (3–4in), ↔20cm (8in).

CARNATIONS AND PINKS

For exhibition purposes, carnations and pinks are classified as: self-coloured (**selfs**), which are of any one colour; **fancies**, with stripes, flakes, or flecks that contrast with the ground colour; **picotee** carnations, usually white or yellow, each petal margined in a contrasting colour; **bicolour** pinks, which have a central zone or eye of contrasting colour; and **laced** pinks, which have a contrasting centre and each petal margined in the same colour.

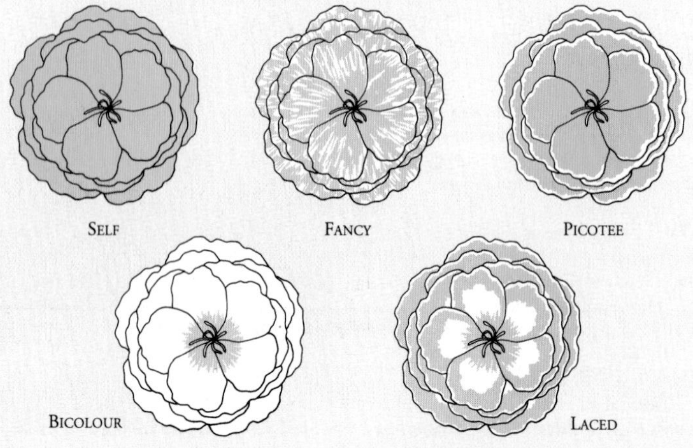

• **HARDINESS** Fully hardy, except for perpetual-flowering and Malmaison carnations, which are half hardy.
• **CULTIVATION** All fully hardy *Dianthus* species and cultivars prefer well-drained, neutral to alkaline soil, in full sun, although *D. glacialis*, *D. microlepis*, and *D. pavonius* prefer acid conditions.

Alpine species benefit from the sharp drainage of a raised bed, wall, or trough. Grow annual and biennial pinks in full sun in well-drained, neutral to acid soil, enriched with well-rotted manure and top-dressed with a balanced granular fertilizer. Discard after flowering. Grow biennials in well-drained, neutral to alkaline soil in full sun. Provide twiggy support in exposed areas. Remove flower stems after flowering to induce a second crop in the following year.

Plant young border carnations and pinks in soil enriched with well-rotted manure or garden compost, and apply a balanced fertilizer in spring. Do not bury the lowest leaves. Support border carnations in late spring, using thin canes or twigs, 75cm (30in) long, and wire rings. In the first year, remove only the small bud below each crown bud; second-year plants need moderate disbudding; disbud 3-year-old border carnations to leave 1 or 2 buds per stem.

Grow perpetual-flowering and Malmaison carnations under glass at 7–10°C (45–50°F) in loam-based potting compost (JI No.2). Stop cuttings to leave 6 pairs of leaves. Admit full light in winter, and bright filtered light in summer with good ventilation at all times. Provide low humidity in winter. To prevent formation of split calyces, prevalent in older cultivars, avoid fluctuating temperatures, erratic watering, and overfertilizing. In spring and summer, water moderately and apply a balanced liquid fertilizer every 10 days; water sparingly in autumn and winter. Support flowering stems with rings and 1.2m (4ft) canes. Disbud gradually over several days, to leave only the crown buds. Dead-head all *Dianthus* species and cultivars to maintain a compact habit or to prolong flowering.
• **PROPAGATION** Sow seed of alpine species in containers in a cold frame from autumn to early spring. Sow seed of annuals at 13–15°C (55–59°F) in early spring. Sow biennials *in situ* in autumn or at 13°C (55°F) in early spring to flower in the same year. Take cuttings from non-flowering shoots of perennial *Dianthus* species and pinks in summer, and of perpetual-flowering and Malmaison carnations in late winter. Layer border carnations after flowering.
• **PESTS AND DISEASES** Aphids and slugs may weaken garden plants. Aphids, thrips, tortrix moth caterpillars, and red spider mites may damage carnations under glass. Rust affects the leaves and stems of carnations and pinks, and of *D. barbatus*. Virus diseases and *Fusarium* wilt are easily transmitted by aphids.

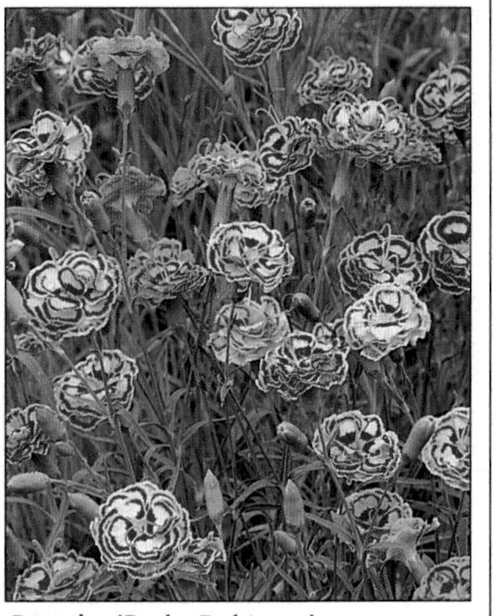

Dianthus 'Becky Robinson'

***D.* 'A.J. MacSelf'** see *D.* 'Dad's Favourite'.
***D.* 'Aldridge Yellow'.** Self border carnation producing double, pale yellow flowers on stiff stems. ❄❄❄
***D.* 'Alice'** ■ Bicolour modern pink. Clove-scented, semi-double, ivory-white flowers have dark crimson eyes. ❄❄❄
***D.* 'Alice Forbes Improved'.** Fancy border carnation producing double, pure white flowers with pinkish mauve stripes. ❄❄❄
***D.* 'Allen's Maria'** see *D.* 'Maria'.
D. alpinus ♀ (Alpine pink). Short-lived, cushion-forming perennial with glossy, dark green leaves, to 3cm (1¼in) long. Bears solitary, single, pale-spotted, deep pink to crimson flowers, 2.5–4cm (1–1½in) across, with bearded, toothed petals, in summer. Best in humus-rich soil. ↕8cm (3in), ↔ to 10cm (4in). S.E. European Alps. ❄❄❄. **'Joan's Blood'** ■♀ bears deep magenta-pink flowers with crimson centres.
D. amurensis. Short-lived, upright, mat-forming, loosely branched perennial with bright green leaves, to 5cm (2in) long. Terminal cymes of 1–3 single, deep purplish pink to mauve flowers, 1–2.5cm (½–1in) across, with darker centres and deeply toothed, bearded petals, are produced in summer. ↕ to 40cm (16in), ↔ to 30cm (12in). E. Asia. ❄❄❄
***D.* 'Annabelle'.** Alpine pink bearing masses of solitary, clove-scented, double, cerise-pink flowers. ❄❄❄
D. arenarius. Tufted, slender perennial with bright green leaves, to 4cm (1½in) long. Produces solitary, deeply fringed, bearded, single white flowers, to 2.5cm (1in) across, often purple at the bases, in summer. ↕↔ to 30cm (12in). N. and E. Europe. ❄❄❄
D. armeria ♀ (Deptford pink). Basal-rosetted, stiffly hairy annual or biennial with dark green leaves, 5cm (2in) long. In summer, bears dense, terminal cymes, 3–6cm (1¼–2½in) across, of numerous single, toothed, bearded, bright rose-pink flowers, to 1.5cm (½in) across, with prominent bracts, dotted pale pink at the bases. ↕ to 40cm (16in), ↔45cm (18in). Europe, W. Asia. ❄❄❄
D. barbatus (Sweet William). Bushy, short-lived perennial, grown as a biennial, with light to mid-green leaves, to 10cm (4in) long, sometimes deep bronze-green. In late spring and early summer, leafy bracts surround dense, flat, terminal clusters, 8–12cm (3–5in) across, of many small, single, sweet-

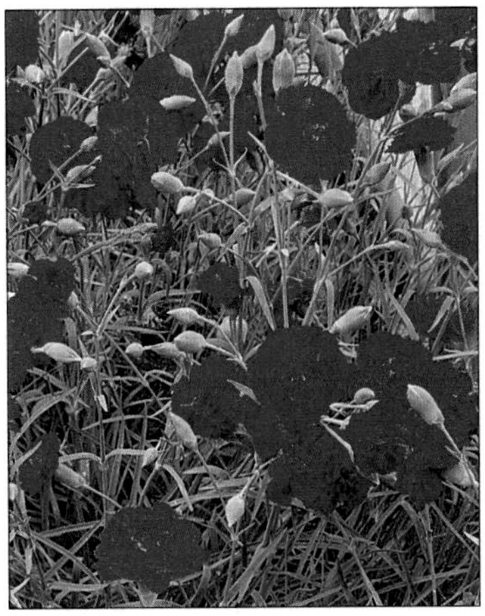
Dianthus 'Bovey Belle'

scented, purple-red, pink, salmon-pink, or white flowers, sometimes bicoloured, each petal bearded and dotted with a paler colour at the base. ↕ to 70cm (28in), ↔ to 30cm (12in). S. Europe. ❄❄❄. **'Dunnet's Dark Crimson'** has deep bronze-green foliage and blood-red flowers; ↕ to 60cm (24in). **'Giant Auricula-eyed'** has bicoloured crimson, red, purple, rose-pink, or salmon-pink flowers, with well-defined, pale centres; ↕ to 60cm (24in). **'Indian Carpet'** has crimson, purple, or pink flowers, with many bicolours; ↕ 15–22cm (6–9in). **Monarch Series** cultivars have flowers in pink, white, crimson-red, or purple, many flushed and patterned with contrasting colours or with well-defined centres; ↕ to 60cm (24in). **Roundabout Series** ◼ cultivars are bushy, with flowers in a range of single colours and bicolours, and may be grown as hardy annuals; ↕ 20cm (8in). **'Super Duplex Double'** has double and semi-double flowers in crimson, purple, red, or pink. Good for cutting; ↕ 45cm (18in). **'Wee Willie'** has crimson, rose-pink, or white flowers, and may be grown as a hardy annual; ↕ 10–15cm (4–6in).

***D.* 'Becky Robinson'** ◼🏆 Laced modern pink bearing clove-scented, double, warm pink flowers with ruby-red centres and margins. ❄❄❄

***D.* 'Bombardier'.** Alpine pink with solitary, double, scarlet flowers. ❄❄❄

***D.* 'Bookham Fancy'** ◼ Fancy border carnation. Bears double, bright yellow

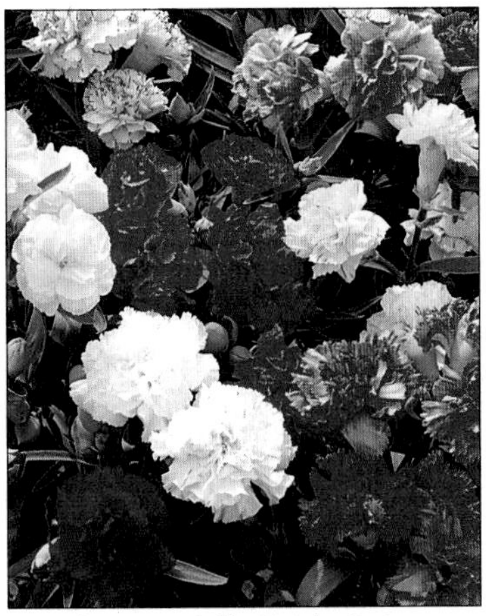
Dianthus caryophyllus Knight Series

flowers, with red-purple margins and flecks, on short, stiff stems. ❄❄❄

***D.* 'Bookham Perfume'.** Self border carnation with clove-scented, double, clear crimson flowers. ❄❄❄

***D.* 'Bourboule'** see *D.* 'La Bourboule'.

***D.* 'Bovey Belle'** ◼🏆 Vigorous, self modern pink producing long-stemmed, clove-scented, double, bright deep pink flowers. ❄❄❄

***D.* 'Brympton Red'.** Laced old-fashioned pink producing single, bright crimson flowers with deeper crimson stripes. ❄❄❄

D. caesius see *D. gratianopolitanus.*

***D.* 'Carolyn Hardy'.** Self perpetual-flowering carnation with clove-scented, pale lavender-pink flowers. ❄

D. carthusianorum (Carthusian pink). Tufted perennial with usually pale green leaves, 2cm (¾in) long. In summer, bears flattened, terminal clusters, 3–5cm (1¼–2in) across, of toothed, bearded, single, deep red-pink, occasionally white flowers, to 2cm (¾in) across, on slender stems. ↕ to 40cm (16in), ↔ to 20cm (8in). S. and C. Europe. ❄❄❄

D. caryophyllus (Wild carnation). Loosely tufted, woody perennial with flattened, soft mid-green leaves, to 15cm (6in) long, with conspicuous sheaths. Bears loose cymes, 5cm (2in) across, of 1–5 strongly fragrant, single, toothed, bright pink-purple flowers, to 1.5cm (½in) across, on stiff stems in summer. ↕ to 80cm (32in), ↔ 15–23cm (6–9in). Mediterranean. ❄❄❄. **Floristan Series** cultivars are biennials producing double flowers in single colours, including yellow, salmon-pink, scarlet, and white, with some picotees. Good for cut flowers; ↕ to 75cm (30in), ↔ to 30cm (12in). Cultivars of **Knight Series** ◼ are dwarf, very bushy, and grown as annuals, with double flowers; colours include crimson, yellow, white, and orange, with some picotees; ↕ to 30cm (12in), ↔ to 23cm (9in). **Lillipot Series** cultivars are dwarf, bushy, and grown as annuals or biennials, with double flowers in colours including lavender-pink, purple, yellow, scarlet, and orange, with some bicolours; ↕ 20–25cm (8–10in), ↔ 20cm (8in). **'Scarlet Luminette'** is grown as an annual or biennial, with double, bright scarlet flowers. Best in a cold greenhouse; ↕ to 45cm (18in), ↔ to 23cm (9in).

***D.* 'Catherine Glover'.** Fancy border carnation. Double, bright yellow flowers have scarlet margins and bars. ❄❄❄

***D.* 'Charles Musgrave'** see *D.* 'Musgrave's Pink'.

***D.* 'Cheryl'** see *D.* 'Houndspool Cheryl'.

D. chinensis (Chinese pink, Indian pink). Bushy, short-lived, hairy perennial or biennial, usually grown annually from seed. Leaves are pale to mid-green, up to 8cm (3in) long. In summer, bears loose, terminal cymes, to 8cm (3in) across, of up to 15 single pink, red, or white flowers, often with purple eyes, fringed to nearly half their lengths and often intricately patterned. ↕ to 70cm (28in), ↔ 16–23cm (6–9in). China. ❄❄❄. Cultivars of **Baby Doll Series** have large, single, patterned flowers, mainly crimson to white; ↕ 15–20cm (6–8in). Cultivars of **Carpet Series** have single, self-coloured flowers in crimson, rose-pink, or white; the series includes **'Fire Carpet'** ◼ which has scarlet flowers; ↕ to 20cm (8in). **Heddewigii Group 'Colour Magician'** is compact and free-flowering, with small, single flowers that age from clear white to rose-pink; ↕ to 25cm (10in). **'Parfait'** bears small, weather-resistant, single, lightly fringed flowers, with some bicolours, throughout summer; ↕ to 30cm (12in). **'Persian Carpet'** is compact and free-flowering, with flowers in carmine-red, pink, or rose-red, together with white; ↕ 10cm (4in).

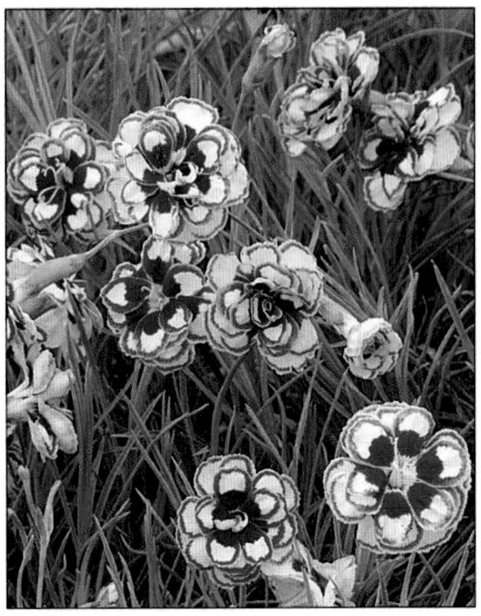
Dianthus 'Dad's Favourite'

***D.* 'Clara'** ◼ Fancy perpetual-flowering carnation bearing clear yellow flowers, striped salmon-pink. ❄

***D.* 'Clara's Lass'** ◼ Fancy perpetual-flowering carnation with pure white flowers, striped salmon-pink. ❄

***D.* 'Constance Finnis'** see *D.* 'Fair Folly'.

***D.* 'Coronation Ruby'** ◼🏆 Laced modern pink with clove-scented, double, warm pink flowers, with ruby-red margins and centres. ❄❄❄

***D.* 'Cream Sue'** ◼ Self perpetual-flowering carnation producing cream flowers. ❄

***D.* 'Crompton Princess'** ◼ Self perpetual-flowering carnation with perfectly formed, pure white flowers. ❄

***D.* 'Dad's Favourite'** ◼ syn. *D.* 'A.J. MacSelf'. Laced old-fashioned pink. Semi-double white flowers have ruby-red margins and purple centres. ❄❄❄

D. deltoides 🏆 (Maiden pink). Mat-forming perennial with narrow, dark green leaves, 1–1.5cm (½in) long. Usually solitary, single flowers, to 2cm (¾in) across, with toothed, bearded petals, are borne on upright, leafy stems in summer. Flowers are white, deep pink, or red, often with darker eyes. ↕ to 20cm (8in), ↔ 30cm (12in) or more. Europe, Asia. ❄❄❄. **'Leuchtfunk'**, syn. 'Flashing Light' ◼ produces numerous brilliant cerise flowers.

***D.* 'Doris'** ◼🏆 Bicolour modern pink producing scented, double, pale pink flowers with dark pink centres. ❄❄❄

D

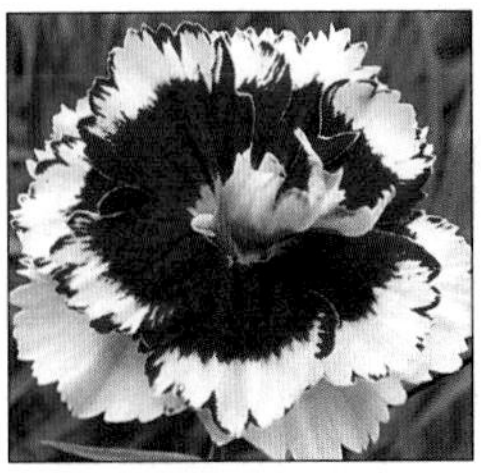
Dianthus 'Alice'

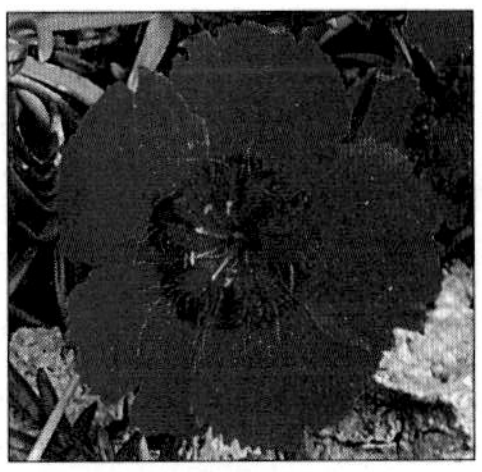
Dianthus alpinus 'Joan's Blood'

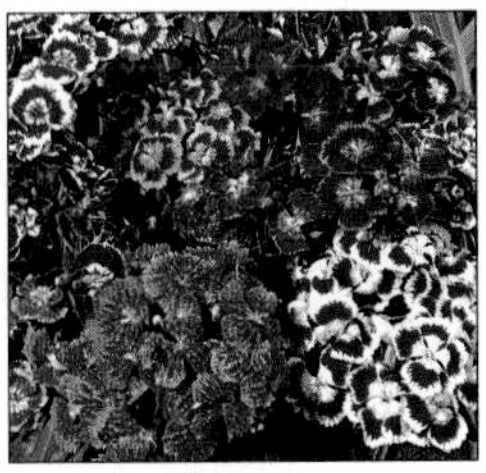
Dianthus barbatus Roundabout Series

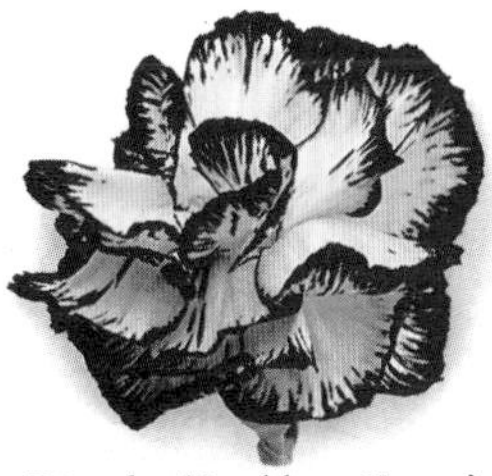
Dianthus 'Bookham Fancy'

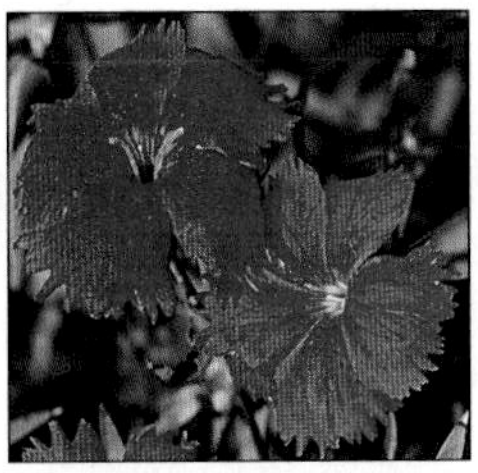
Dianthus chinensis Carpet Series 'Fire Carpet'

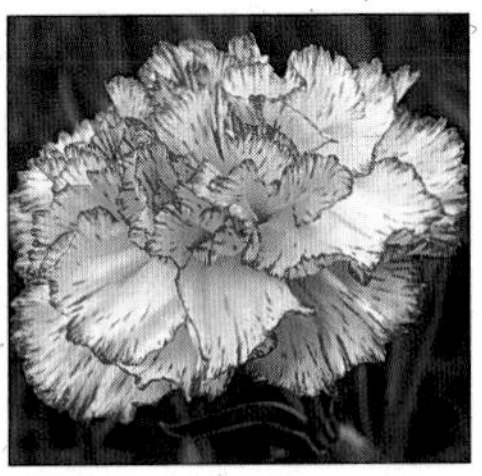
Dianthus 'Clara'

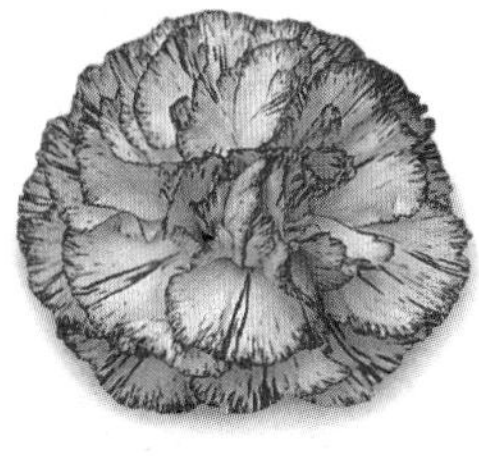
Dianthus 'Clara's Lass'

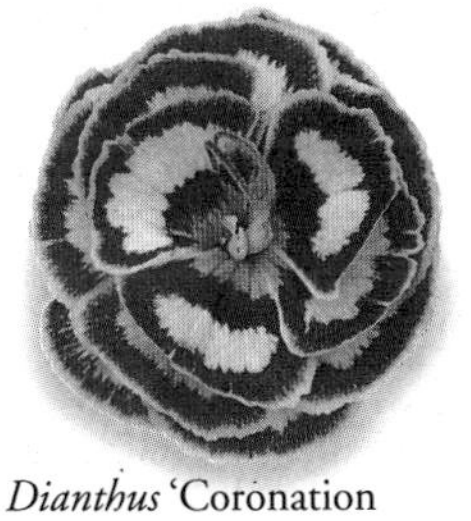
Dianthus 'Coronation Ruby'

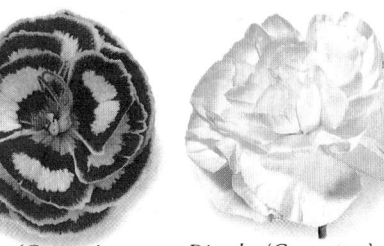

Dianthus 'Cream Sue'

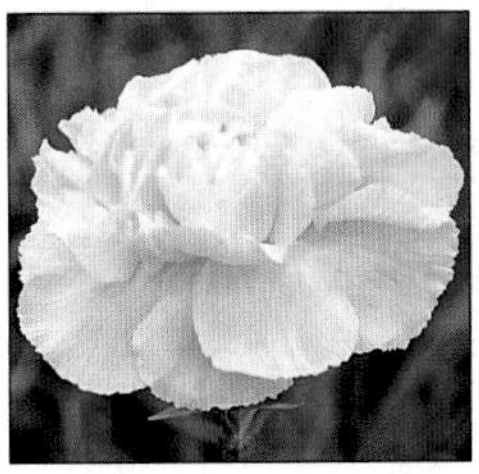
Dianthus 'Crompton Princess'

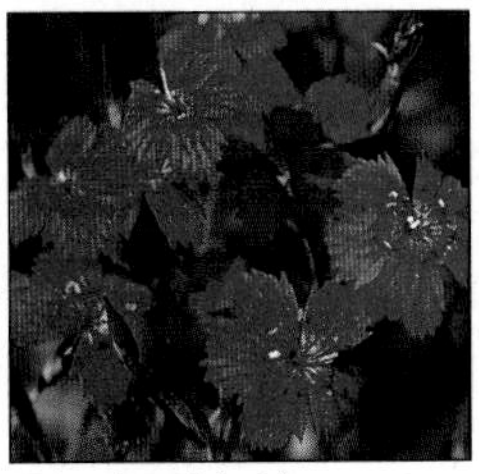
Dianthus deltoides 'Leuchtfunk'

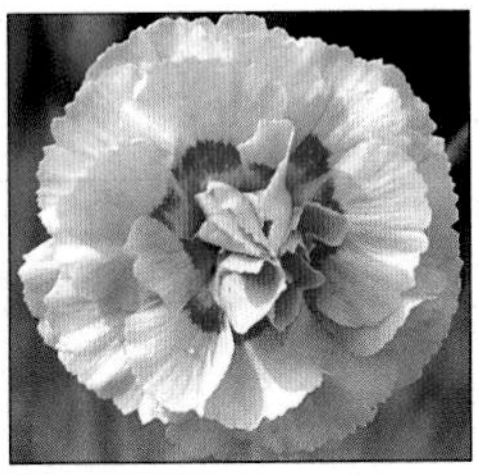
Dianthus 'Doris'

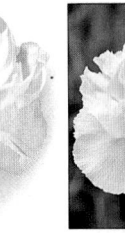

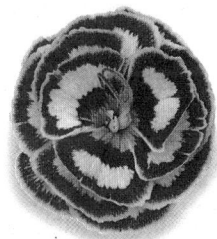

DIANTHUS

D

D. 'Duchess of Westminster' ■ Vigorous, self Malmaison carnation producing salmon-pink flowers with stronger calyces than most Malmaison carnations. ❄
D. 'Earl of Essex'. Bicolour old-fashioned pink producing double, rose-pink flowers with darker eyes. ❄❄❄
D. 'Emile Paré'. Self old-fashioned "Mule" pink with bright green foliage and clusters of double, salmon-pink flowers. ❄❄❄
D. erinaceus ■ Cushion-forming perennial with stiff, mid-green leaves, to 2cm (¾in) long. Solitary, occasionally paired pink flowers, 1.5cm (½in) across, with toothed, bearded petals, are produced on short stems in summer. (Flowers are generally sparsely produced in cool climates.) ↕ 5cm (2in), ↔ 50cm (20in) or more. Mountainous regions of Turkey. ❄❄❄
D. 'Eva Humphries'. Picotee border carnation producing double, white flowers with very narrow purple margins. ❄❄❄
D. 'Excelsior'. Self old-fashioned pink producing clove-scented, double, pink flowers with fringed petals. ❄❄❄
D. 'Fair Folly', syn. *D.* 'Constance Finnis'. Laced old-fashioned pink producing single white flowers with strawberry-pink centres and margins. ❄❄❄
D. Festival Series (*D. barbatus* x *D. chinensis*). Bushy, short-lived perennials, usually grown as annuals or biennials, with bright green leaves, 8–12cm (3–5in) long. They produce terminal clusters, 8–10cm (3–4in) across, of small, single pink, red, or white flowers, in summer. ↕ 20–35cm (8–14in), ↔ 23cm (9in). ❄❄❄
D. 'Fiery Cross'. Self border carnation producing perfectly formed, double, bright scarlet flowers. ❄❄❄

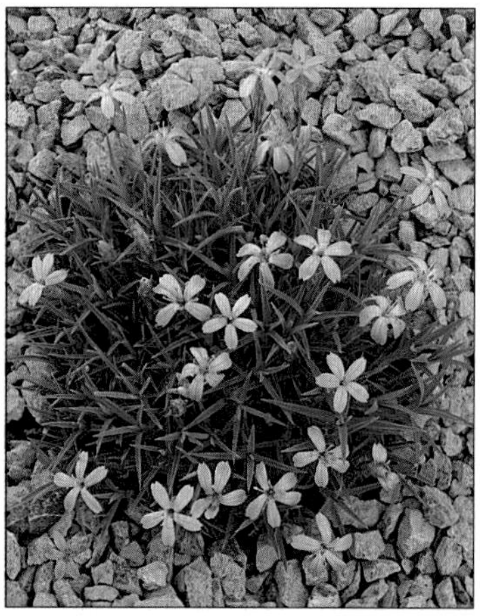

Dianthus erinaceus

D. 'Forest Treasure' ■ Fancy border carnation with double white flowers, flecked red-purple. ❄❄❄
D. 'Freckles'. Fancy modern pink of dwarf habit with clove-scented, well-formed, double, bright pink flowers, flecked and spotted scarlet. ❄❄❄
D. glacialis. Compact, densely tufted, cushion-forming perennial with soft, glossy, dark green leaves, to 1.5cm (½in) long. Usually solitary, short-stemmed, single, pale to deep pink flowers, to 2cm (¾in) across, with finely toothed, bearded petals, are produced in summer. ↕ 5cm (2in), ↔ 15cm (6in). E. Alps. ❄❄❄
D. 'Golden Cross' ■ Self border carnation with well-formed, double, bright yellow flowers borne on short, stiff stems. ❄❄❄
D. 'Gran's Favourite' ■🏆 Laced modern pink with short-stemmed, clove-scented, double white flowers with mauve centres and margins. ❄❄❄
D. gratianopolitanus 🏆 syn. *D. caesius* (Cheddar pink). Mat-forming perennial with grey-green leaves, to 5cm (2in) long. Solitary, very fragrant, single, deep pink flowers, to 3cm (1¼in) across, with slightly bearded, toothed petals, are produced in summer. ↕ to 15cm (6in), ↔ to 40cm (16in). N.W. and C. Europe. ❄❄❄
D. 'Green Eyes' see *D.* 'Musgrave's Pink'.
D. haematocalyx. Compact, cushion-forming perennial with grey-green leaves, 2.5–5cm (1–2in) long. Bears terminal clusters, 2–6cm (¾–2½in) across, of 1–4 single flowers, 1.5–2.5cm (½–1in) across, with toothed, bearded, deep pink petals, tinged with yellow on the reverse, in summer. ↕ to 12cm (5in), ↔ to 20cm (8in). Balkan Peninsula, mountains in N. Greece. ❄❄❄
D. 'Hannah Louise'. Picotee border carnation of neat but vigorous habit. Double, bright yellow flowers have broad scarlet margins. ❄❄❄
D. 'Happiness'. Fancy border carnation with double, primrose-yellow flowers, and scarlet stripes and margins. ❄❄❄
D. 'Harmony'. Fancy border carnation producing double grey flowers, striped cerise. ❄❄❄
D. 'Haytor' see *D.* 'Haytor White'.
D. 'Haytor White' ■🏆 syn. *D.* 'Haytor'. Self modern pink with perfectly formed, clove-scented, double, pure white flowers. ❄❄❄
D. 'Hidcote'. Alpine pink producing clusters of 1–3 double, deep red flowers. ❄❄❄
D. 'Houndspool Cheryl', syn. *D.* 'Cheryl'. Self modern pink with double, currant-red flowers. ❄❄❄
D. 'Houndspool Ruby' ■🏆 syn. *D.* 'Ruby', *D.* 'Ruby Doris'. Bicolour modern pink with double, rose-pink flowers with currant-red centres. ❄❄❄
D. Ideal Series (*D. barbatus* x *D. chinensis*). Bushy, short-lived perennials, usually grown as annuals or biennials and producing bright green leaves, 8–12cm (3–5in) long. In summer, bear terminal clusters, 10–12cm (4–5in) across, of small, single flowers in a range of vivid, single colours, including deep violet-blue, purple-pink, and crimson-red, some flushed with a different colour. ↕ 20–35cm (8–14in), ↔ 23cm (9in). ❄❄❄. **'Cherry Picotee'** ■ has flowers with white picotee margins and cherry-red eyes.
D. 'Inchmery'. Self old-fashioned pink with double, pale lavender-pink flowers. ❄❄❄
D. 'Inshriach Dazzler' 🏆 Alpine pink bearing solitary, short-stemmed, single, deep carmine-red flowers with fringed petals. ❄❄❄
D. 'Irene Della-Torré' 🏆 Fancy border carnation with clove-scented, double, pure white flowers, margined and lightly striped bright pink. ❄❄❄
D. 'Jacqueline Ann' 🏆 Fancy perpetual-flowering carnation producing clove-scented white flowers, flecked cerise. ❄
***D. japonicus* Ginza Series.** Bushy, erect, short-lived perennials, usually grown as annuals, with blunt-tipped, light to mid-green leaves, 4–5cm (1½–2in) long. Dense, flat terminal clusters, 7–12cm (3–5in) across, of small, toothed, single lilac to deep rose-pink flowers are produced in summer. ↕↔ 45cm (18in). ❄❄❄ (borderline)
D. 'Joanne'. Self perpetual-flowering carnation with deep cerise flowers. ❄
D. 'Joanne's Highlight'. Self perpetual-flowering carnation producing light pink flowers. ❄
D. 'Joe Vernon'. Self perpetual-flowering carnation with clove-scented, rich purple flowers. ❄
D. 'Joy'. Self modern pink with semi-double, carmine-red flowers on strong stems. ❄❄❄
D. 'La Bourbille' see *D.* 'La Bourboule'.

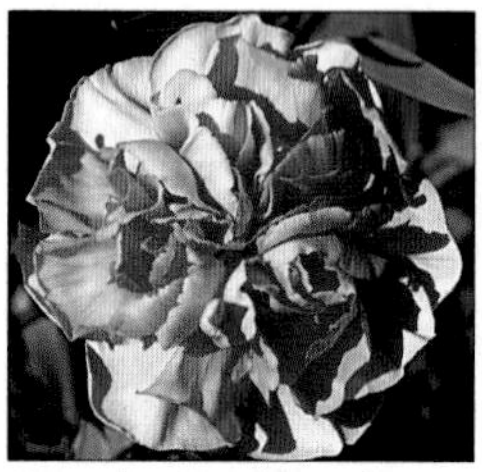

Dianthus 'Duchess of Westminster'

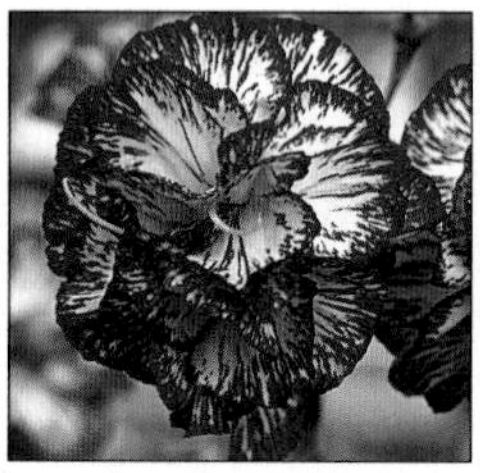

Dianthus 'Forest Treasure'

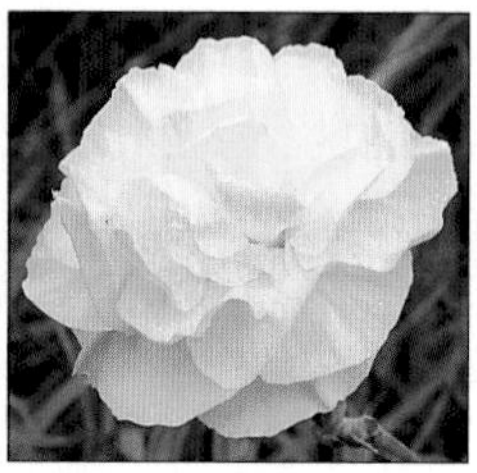

Dianthus 'Golden Cross'

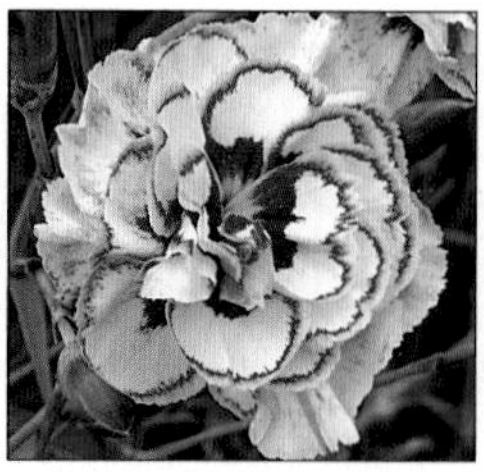

Dianthus 'Gran's Favourite'

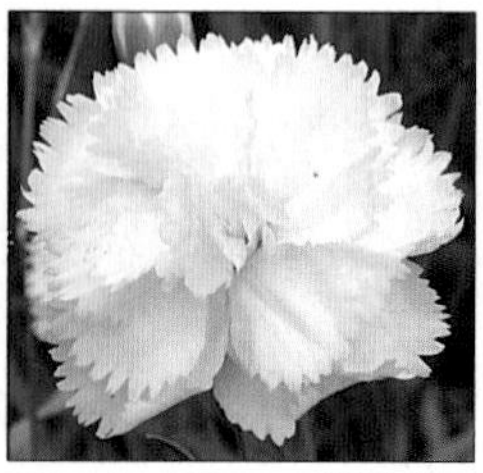

Dianthus 'Haytor White'

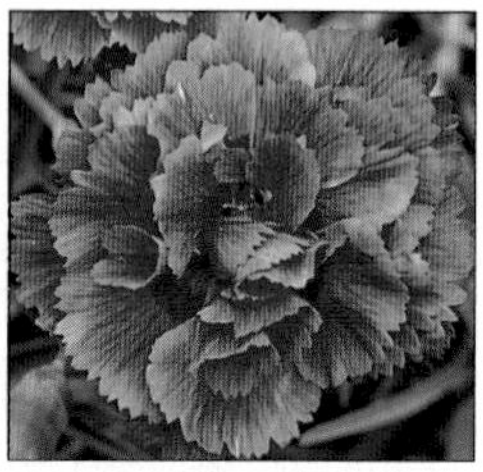

Dianthus 'Houndspool Ruby'

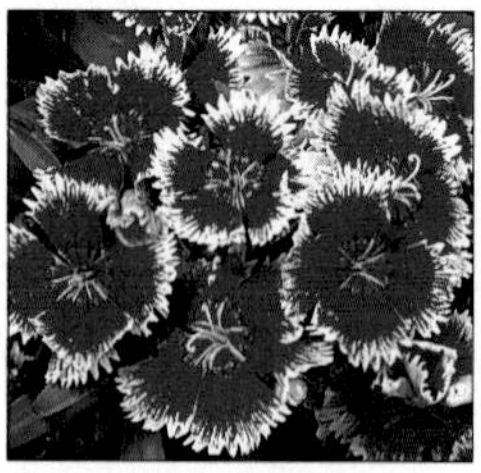

Dianthus Ideal Series 'Cherry Picotee'

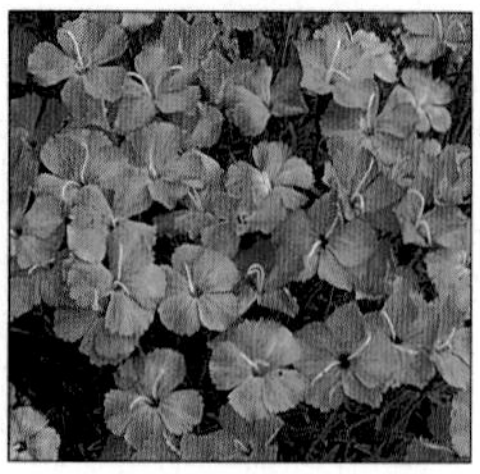

Dianthus 'La Bourboule'

Dianthus 'Laced Monarch'

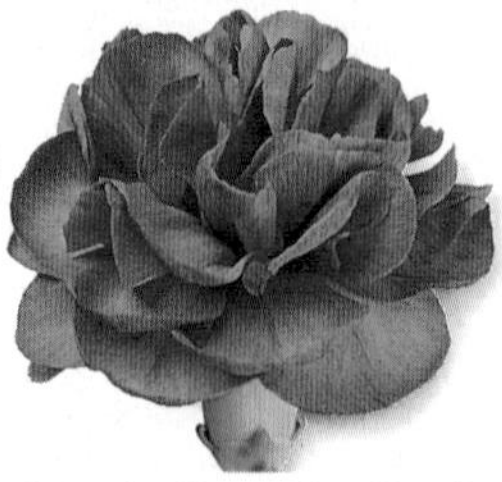

Dianthus 'Lavender Clove'

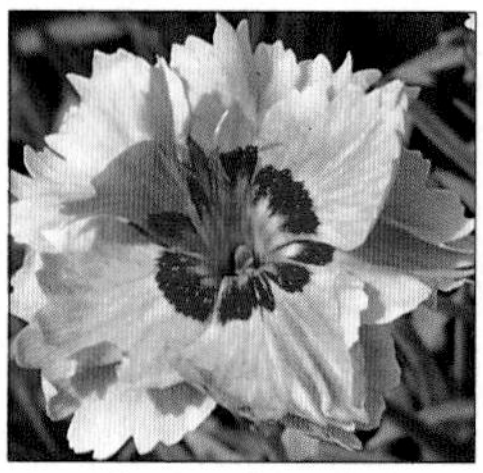

Dianthus 'Little Jock'

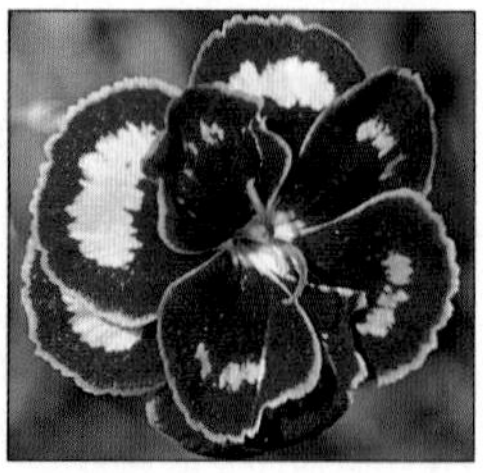

Dianthus 'London Brocade'

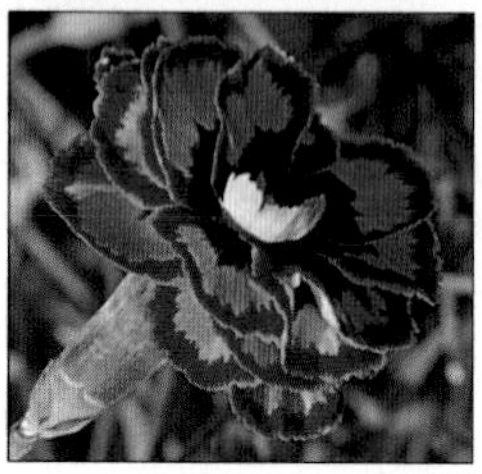

Dianthus 'London Delight'

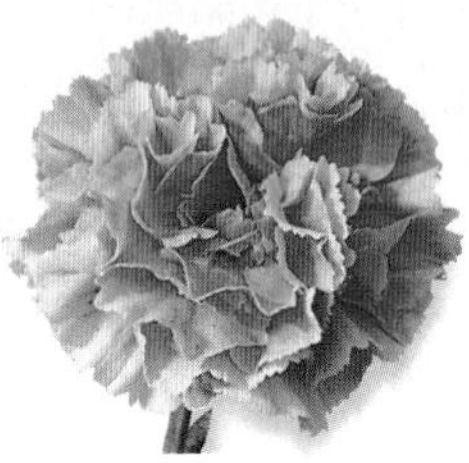

Dianthus 'Marmion'

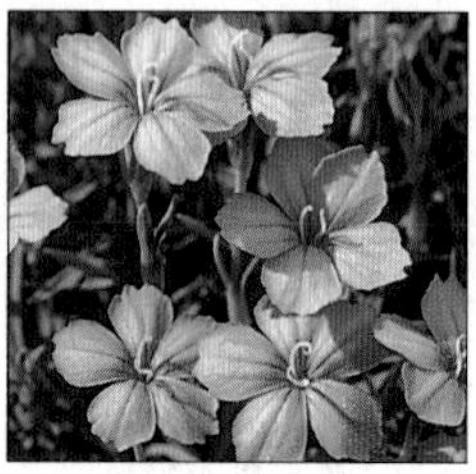

Dianthus microlepis

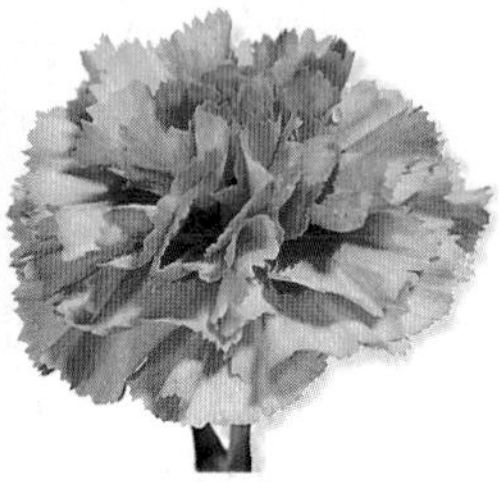

Dianthus 'Monica Wyatt'

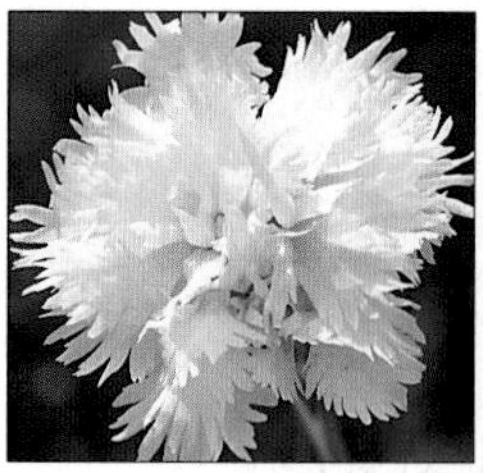

Dianthus 'Mrs. Sinkins'

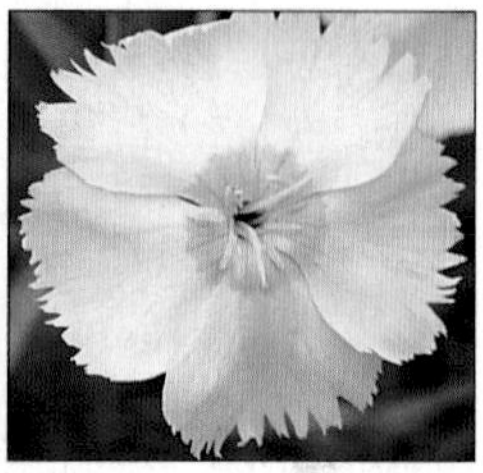

Dianthus 'Musgrave's Pink'

***D.* 'La Bourboule'** ■ ♀ syn. *D.* 'Bourboule', *D.* 'La Bourbille'. Alpine pink with clusters of clove-scented, single, clear pink flowers with fringed petals. ❄❄❄

***D.* 'Laced Monarch'** ■ Laced modern pink producing double pink flowers with deep red centres and margins. ❄❄❄

***D.* 'Laced Prudence'** see *D.* 'Prudence'.

***D.* 'Lavender Clove'** ■ Vigorous self border carnation producing large, clove-scented, double, greyish lavender-pink flowers. ❄❄❄

***D.* 'Leslie Rennison'.** Fancy border carnation with clove-scented, double flowers, a blend of purple and rose-pink, creating a "shot-silk" effect. ❄❄❄

***D.* 'Little Jock'** ■ Alpine pink with very short-stemmed, solitary, clove-scented, semi-double, maroon-eyed, pale pink flowers with deeply fringed petals. ❄❄❄

***D.* 'London Brocade'** ■ Laced modern pink bearing clove-scented, double pink flowers with crimson centres and margins. ❄❄❄

***D.* 'London Delight'** ■ Laced modern pink with clove-scented, semi-double, pale pink flowers with maroon centres and margins. ❄❄❄

***D.* 'Manon'.** Self perpetual-flowering carnation producing salmon-pink flowers. ❄

***D.* 'Maria',** syn. *D.* 'Allen's Maria'. Bicolour modern pink producing clove-scented, double, pale pink flowers with cochineal-pink centres. ❄❄❄

***D.* 'Marmion'** ■ Malmaison carnation bearing flowers in deep warm pink with broad, blush-pink margins and stronger calyces than most Malmaisons. ❄

D. microlepis ■ Neat, cushion-forming perennial with tufts of silvery grey to green leaves, to 2cm (¾in) long. Solitary, single pink or purple flowers, 1.5cm (½in) across, with slightly toothed petals, are borne just above the leaves in early summer. ↕ 5cm (2in), ↔ to 15cm (6in). Mountains in Bulgaria. ❄❄❄

***D.* 'Monica Wyatt'** ■ ♀ Bicolour modern pink with clove-scented, double, pale lavender-pink flowers, centred magenta. ❄❄❄

D. monspessulanus (Fringed pink). Loosely tufted perennial with soft, grey-green leaves, to 1.5cm (½in) long. Terminal cymes, 2–6cm (¾–2½in) across, of 2–7 fragrant white or pink flowers, with deeply fringed petals, are produced on slender stems in summer. ↕ to 50cm (20in), ↔ to 20cm (8in). Mountains in C. and S. Europe. ❄❄❄

***D.* 'Mrs. Sinkins'** ■ Self old-fashioned pink producing double, fringed white flowers. Grown for its powerful scent, although the flowers are shaggy with split calyces. ❄❄❄

***D.* 'Murcia'.** Self perpetual-flowering carnation producing orange-yellow flowers. ❄

***D.* 'Musgrave's Pink'** ■ syn. *D.* 'Charles Musgrave', *D.* 'Green Eyes'. Bicolour old-fashioned pink producing clove-scented, single white flowers with green eyes. ❄❄❄

D. myrtinervius ■ Dense, mat-forming perennial with bright green leaves, to 5mm (¼in) long. Numerous solitary, single, deep pink flowers, 1cm (½in) across, with pale eyes, are produced just above the leaves in summer. Best in scree. ↕ to 5cm (2in), ↔ to 20cm (8in). Balkans, Macedonia, N. Greece. ❄❄❄

D. neglectus see *D. pavonius.*

***D.* 'Nina'** ■ Self perpetual-flowering carnation with smooth-margined crimson flowers. ❄

***D. nitidus* of gardens** see *D. scardicus.*

***D.* 'Old Blush',** syn. *D.* 'Souvenir de la Malmaison'. Self Malmaison carnation producing large, blush-pink flowers. ❄

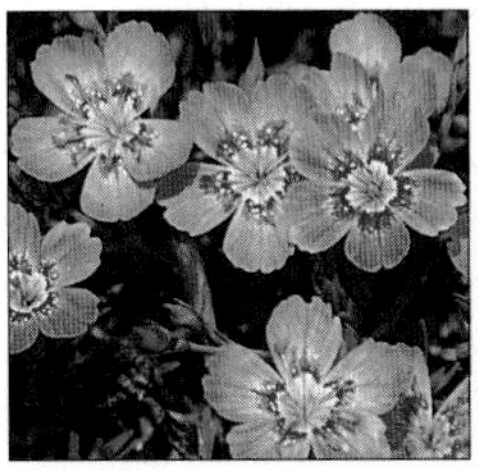
Dianthus myrtinervius

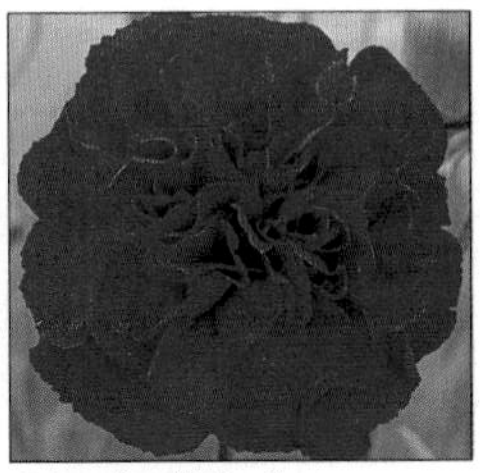
Dianthus 'Nina'

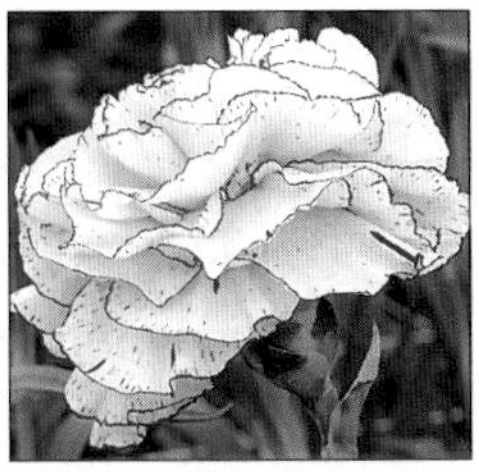
Dianthus 'Pierrot'

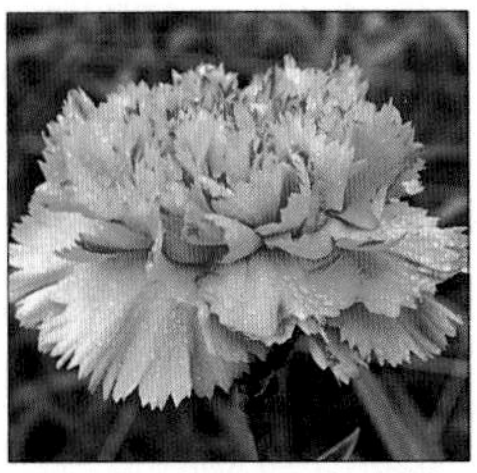
Dianthus 'Raggio di Sole'

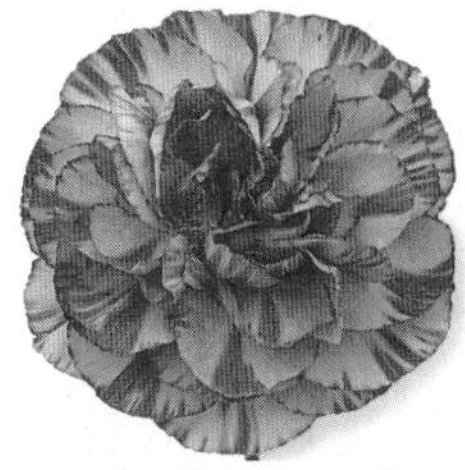
Dianthus 'Sandra Neal'

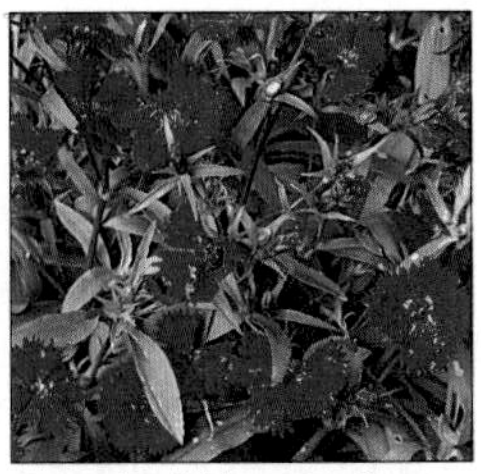
Dianthus Telstar Series 'Telstar Crimson'

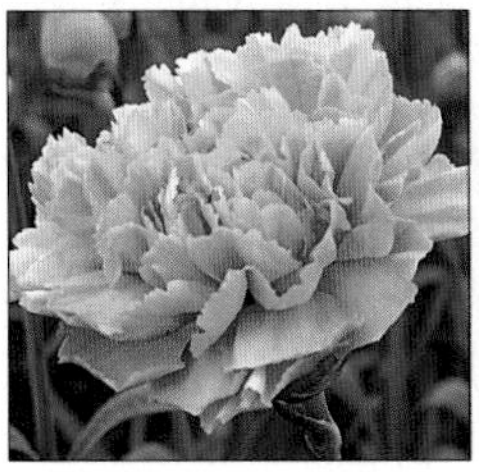
Dianthus 'Truly Yours'

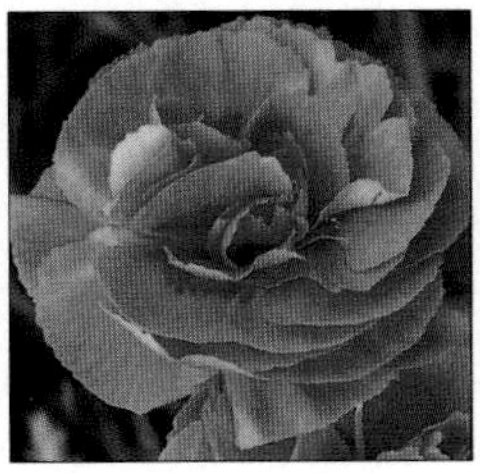
Dianthus 'Valda Wyatt'

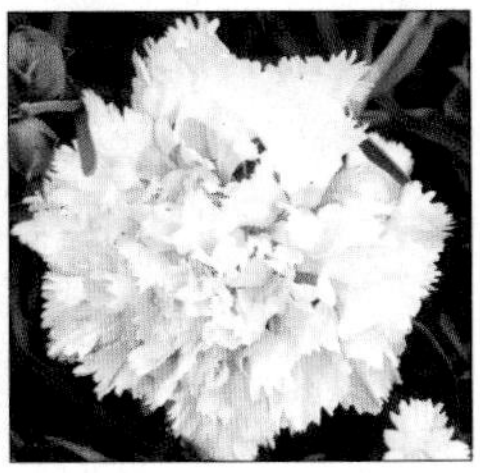
Dianthus 'White Ladies'

D. pavonius ♀ syn. *D. neglectus.* Mat-forming perennial with basal, grey-green leaves, to 4cm (1½in) long. Produces usually solitary, occasionally 2 or 3, toothed, bearded, single, pale to deep pink flowers, to 3cm (1¼in) across, buff-coloured on the reverses, in summer. ↕ 8cm (3in), ↔ to 20cm (8in). S.W. Alps. ❄❄❄

***D.* 'Peter Wood'** ♀ Fancy border carnation producing double, light pink flowers, striped and flaked with bright red. ❄❄❄

D. petraeus, syn. *D. suendermannii.* Variable, mat-forming perennial with stiff, basal, mid-green leaves, to 2.5cm (1in) long. Usually solitary, fragrant, single white flowers, 8–10mm (⅜–½in) across, with toothed or notched petals, are produced in summer. ↕ 15cm (6in), ↔ to 20cm (8in). S.E. Europe, Balkan peninsula, Romania. ❄❄❄

***D.* 'Pierrot'** ■ Picotee perpetual-flowering carnation producing pale lilac flowers with deep purple margins. ❄

***D.* 'Pike's Pink'** ♀ Alpine pink with solitary, double, clove-scented, pale pink flowers, darker zoned at the bases. ↕ 15cm (6in). ❄❄❄

***D.* 'Pink Calypso'** see *D.* 'Truly Yours'.

***D.* 'Princess of Wales'.** Self Malmaison carnation producing large, salmon-pink flowers. ❄

***D.* 'Prudence',** syn. *D.* 'Laced Prudence'. Laced modern pink of neat habit, producing double, pale pink flowers with crimson centres and margins. ❄❄❄

***D.* 'Raggio di Sole'** ■ Fancy perpetual-flowering carnation with bright orange flowers with red flecks. ❄

***D.* 'Ron's Joanne'.** Fancy perpetual-flowering carnation with light cerise flowers, marked very pale pink. ❄

***D.* 'Ruby'** see *D.* 'Houndspool Ruby'.

***D.* 'Ruby Doris'** see *D.* 'Houndspool Ruby'.

***D.* 'Sam Barlow'.** Bicolour old-fashioned pink producing clove-scented, double white flowers with deep purple centres. ❄❄❄

***D.* 'Sandra Neal'** ■ ♀ Fancy border carnation with double, golden apricot flowers, flaked deep rose-pink. ❄❄❄

***D.* 'Santa Claus'.** Picotee border carnation producing double, pale yellow flowers with light crimson margins. ❄❄❄

D. scardicus, syn. *D. nitidus* of gardens. Domed, cushion-forming perennial with dark green leaves, 2cm (¾in) long. Bears solitary, short-stemmed, single pink flowers, to 1.5cm (½in) across, in summer. ↕ 10cm (4in), ↔ to 15cm (6in). Mountains of Slovenia and E. Albania. ❄❄❄

***D.* 'Scarlet Joanne'.** Self perpetual-flowering carnation producing scarlet flowers. ❄

***D.* 'Souvenir de la Malmaison'** see *D.* 'Old Blush'.

D. subacaulis ■ Mat-forming or densely tufted perennial with basal, dark green leaves, to 1.5cm (½in) long. Bears solitary, single, deep pink flowers, to 1.5cm (½in), or occasionally 2cm (¾in) across, with entire or finely toothed, rounded petals, on very short stems in summer. ↕ 5cm (2in), ↔ to 10cm (4in). Mountains in S.W. Europe. ❄❄❄

D. suendermannii see *D. petraeus.*

D. superbus. Loosely tufted perennial with mid-green leaves, to 8cm (3in)

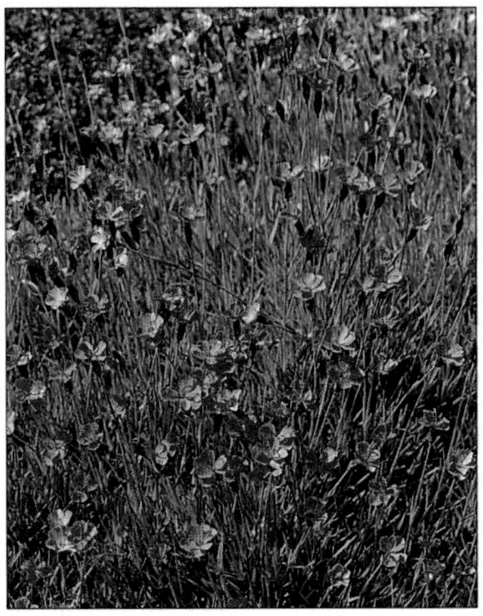
Dianthus subacaulis

long. Upright, slender, terminally branching stems bear fragrant, single, purplish pink flowers, 4–6cm (1½–2½in) across, with deeply fringed petals, either singly or in pairs at the ends of the shoots, in summer. ↕↔ to 20cm (8in). Mountains of Europe and Asia. ❄❄❄

***D.* 'Tayside Red'.** Self Malmaison carnation with very large, brick-red flowers. ❄

D. Telstar Series (*D. barbatus* x *D. chinensis*). Bushy, short-lived perennials, usually grown as annuals or biennials, with dark green leaves, 5–8cm (2–3in) long. In summer, they bear terminal clusters, 5–8cm (2–3in) across, of small, weather-resistant, single flowers, in separate, strong shades of pink, red, or white, including some bicolours and picotees. ↕ 20–25cm (8–10in), ↔ 23cm (9in). ❄❄❄. **'Telstar Crimson'** ■ has deep blood-red flowers. **'Telstar Picotee'** is a very free-flowering red picotee. **'Telstar White'** bears white flowers with a slight pink blush.

***D.* 'Thora'.** Self Malmaison carnation producing pale pink flowers, fading to white. ❄

***D.* 'Tony Langford'.** Fancy perpetual-flowering carnation with lavender-pink flowers, margined and flecked carmine-red. ❄

***D.* 'Truly Yours'** ■ syn. *D.* 'Pink Calypso'. Self perpetual-flowering carnation with salmon-pink flowers. ❄

***D.* 'Valda Wyatt'** ■ ♀ Bicolour modern pink bearing clove-scented, double, lavender-pink flowers, slightly deeper in colour at the centres. ❄❄❄

***D.* 'Valencia'.** Self perpetual-flowering carnation with bronze-yellow flowers. ❄

***D.* 'White Ladies'** ■ Bicolour old-fashioned pink producing clove-scented, double, fringed white flowers with light green centres. ❄❄❄

***D.* 'White Sim',** syn. *D.* 'White William Sim'. Self perpetual-flowering carnation producing white flowers. ❄

***D.* 'Whitesmith'** ♀ Self border carnation of neat habit, producing clove-scented, double, pure white flowers. ❄❄❄

***D.* 'White William Sim'** see *D.* 'White Sim'.

***D.* 'Widecombe Fair'.** Bicolour modern pink with strongly clove-scented, double, peach-apricot flowers, opening to blush-pink. ❄❄❄

***D.* 'William Sim'.** Tall, self perpetual-flowering carnation producing scarlet flowers. ❄

D

DIASCIA

SCROPHULARIACEAE

Genus of about 50 species of annuals and semi-evergreen, occasionally evergreen, sometimes suckering perennials found mainly in mountains in southern Africa. Erect, semi-erect or prostrate stems bear opposite, ovate or heart-shaped to elliptic or linear, toothed, mainly mid-green leaves. Diascias are valued for their long flowering season; they produce terminal racemes of tubular, 5-lobed flowers, the lower lobes broad, the paired upper lobes having 2 backward-pointing spurs and a translucent yellow "window" at each base. Grow at the front of a border, on a sunny bank, or in a rock garden.

- **HARDINESS** Most are hardy to -8°C (18°F).
- **CULTIVATION** Grow in fertile, moist but well-drained soil in full sun. Water in dry periods. Dead-head regularly.
- **PROPAGATION** Sow seed at 16°C (61°F) as soon as ripe or in early spring. Divide suckering species in spring. Take softwood cuttings in spring, or semi-ripe cuttings in summer. Overwinter young plants under glass.
- **PESTS AND DISEASES** May be damaged by slugs and snails.

D. anastrepta. Decumbent, mat-forming perennial with ovate leaves, to 2.5cm (1in) long. Bears loose racemes of nodding, deep pink flowers, to 2cm (¾in) across, with upward-curving spurs and purple-marked "windows", on slender stems in summer. ↕ 25–40cm (10–16in), ↔ to 50cm (20in). South Africa (Drakensberg Mountains). ❄❄

***D.* 'Blackthorn Apricot'** ▣ Mat-forming perennial with narrowly heart-shaped, tapering, leaves, 2–3cm (¾–1¼in) long. From summer to autumn, bears loose racemes of apricot flowers, 1.5–2cm (½–¾in) across, with small, narrow "windows" and almost straight, downward-pointing spurs.

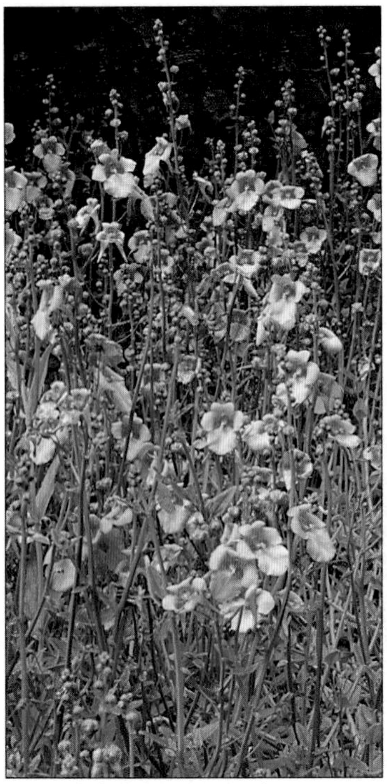

Diascia 'Blackthorn Apricot'

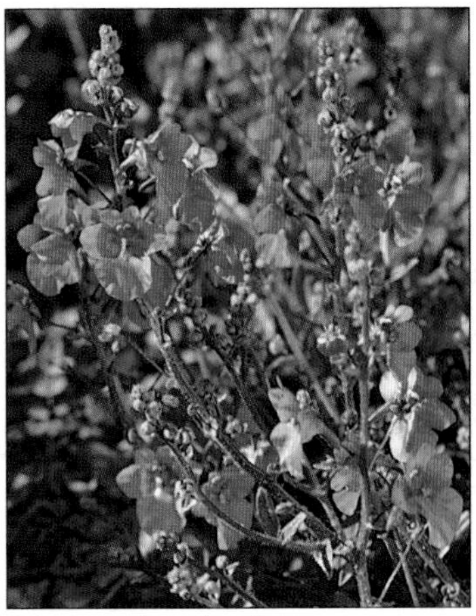

Diascia cordata of gardens

Probably a selection of *D. barberae.* ↕ 25cm (10in), ↔ to 50cm (20in). ❄❄

***D. cordata* of gardens** ▣ Mat-forming perennial with branching stems and heart-shaped, tapering, pale green leaves, 1.5–2cm (½–¾in) long. From early summer to early autumn, bears loose racemes of long-stalked, deep pink flowers, 2cm (¾in) across, with small, narrow "windows" and slightly curved, downward-pointing spurs. Probably a selection of *D. barberae.* ↕ 15cm (6in), ↔ to 50cm (20in). South Africa. ❄❄

D. elegans see *D. vigilis.*

D. felthamii see *D. fetcaniensis.*

D. fetcaniensis, syn. *D. felthamii.* Creeping perennial with ovate, hairy leaves, 2.5cm (1in) long, heart-shaped at the bases. Loose racemes of rose-pink flowers, 2cm (¾in) long, with concave "windows" and incurved, downward-pointing spurs, are produced from summer to early autumn. ↕ 25cm (10in), ↔ to 50cm (20in). South Africa, Lesotho (Drakensberg Mountains). ❄❄

***D.* 'Hector Harrison'** see *D.* 'Salmon Supreme'.

D. integerrima, syn. *D. integrifolia.* Creeping perennial with slender, wiry, upright stems bearing linear to oblong-lance-shaped, sparsely toothed leaves, 2–2.5cm (¾–1in) long. Loose racemes of purplish pink flowers, 2cm (¾in) long, with broad, horizontal lower lips, concave "windows", and downward-pointing, incurved spurs, are produced in summer. ↕ 30cm (12in) or more, ↔ to 50cm (20in). South Africa. ❄❄

D. integrifolia see *D. integerrima.*

D. rigescens ▣🏆 Trailing perennial with stiff, erect and semi-erect,

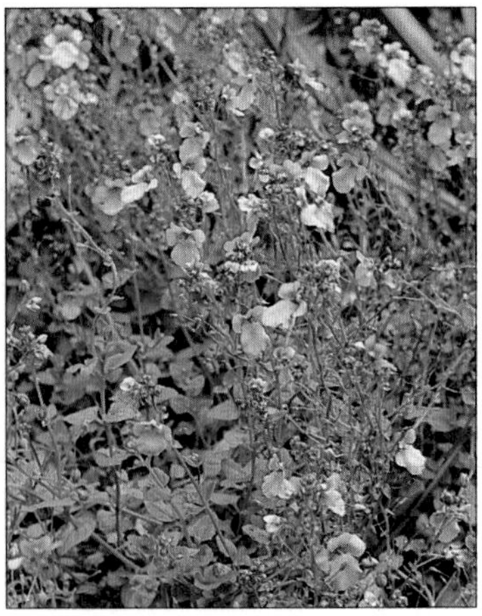

Diascia 'Salmon Supreme'

branching stems and heart-shaped, deeply toothed, mainly stalkless leaves, 4cm (1½in) long. Produces tall, dense racemes of mid- to deep pink flowers, 2cm (¾in) across, with small, round "windows" and short, incurved spurs, in summer. ↕ 30cm (12in), ↔ to 50cm (20in). South Africa. ❄❄

***D.* 'Ruby Field'** 🏆 Mat-forming perennial with short, wiry stems clothed in heart-shaped leaves, 2.5–4cm (1–1½in) long. Masses of rich salmon-pink flowers, 1cm (½in) long, with small, narrow "windows" and spurs curving inwards and downwards, are produced from summer to autumn. ↕ 25cm (10in), ↔ to 60cm (24in). ❄❄

***D.* 'Rupert Lambert'.** Mat-forming perennial with narrowly elliptic to ovate, pointed, shallowly toothed leaves, 2.5–4cm (1–1½in) long. Long racemes of deep pink flowers, 2.5cm (1in) long, with double "windows" and long, parallel spurs, are produced from summer to autumn. ↕ 25cm (10in), ↔ to 50cm (20in). ❄❄

***D.* 'Salmon Supreme'** ▣ syn. *D.* 'Hector Harrison'. Mat-forming perennial with heart-shaped, sparsely toothed leaves, 2.5–4cm (1–1½in) long. Dense racemes of pale apricot flowers, 1.5cm (½in) long, with very small, deeply concave "windows" and short, straight, downward-pointing spurs, are produced from summer to autumn. ↕ 15cm (6in), ↔ to 50cm (20in). ❄❄

D. vigilis 🏆 syn. *D. elegans.* Vigorous, creeping, prostrate perennial with ovate-lance-shaped, fleshy, deeply toothed leaves, 2.5–4cm (1–1½in) long. Loose racemes of clear pink flowers, 2–2.5cm (¾–1in) long, with deep-set yellow and maroon "windows" and short, incurved spurs, are produced from early summer to early autumn. One of the hardiest and most free-flowering species. ↕ 30cm (12in), ↔ to 60cm (24in). South Africa, Lesotho (Drakensberg Mountains). ❄❄

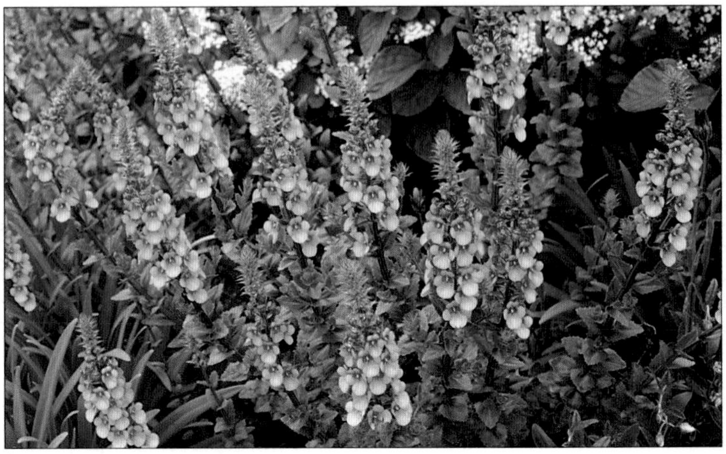

Diascia rigescens

DICENTRA

FUMARIACEAE/PAPAVERACEAE

Genus of 20 or more species of annuals and perennials from Asia and North America, often found in moist habitats, including woodland, especially in mountainous areas. The perennial species may be rhizomatous or tuberous, or have fleshy tap roots. The hairless, sometimes silvery grey leaves are fern-like and much divided. Pendent, heart-shaped flowers, in red, pink, white, purple, or yellow, are borne in panicles or racemes, often arching, or are occasionally solitary. Some species are excellent woodland plants or useful border plants; the smaller species are best in a rock garden or alpine house. All parts of the plant may cause mild stomach upset if ingested. Contact with the foliage may aggravate skin allergies.

- **HARDINESS** Fully hardy, although early growth may be damaged by frost.
- **CULTIVATION** Grow most species and cultivars in moist, fertile, humus-rich soil, preferably neutral or slightly alkaline, in partial shade. *D. chrysantha* needs a dry, sunny site; *D. spectabilis* tolerates sun in reliably moist soil. Grow *D. peregrina* in sharply drained, volcanic soil or very gritty potting compost in a scree bed or alpine house.
- **PROPAGATION** Sow seed in containers in a cold frame as soon as ripe or in spring. Divide carefully in early spring or after the leaves have died down. Insert root cuttings of *D. spectabilis* in winter. Hybrids self-seed to produce a wide range of seedlings that vary widely in foliage and flower characteristics.
- **PESTS AND DISEASES** Slugs may cause damage.

***D.* 'Adrian Bloom'.** Clump-forming, rhizomatous perennial with pinnate, grey-green leaves, 10–50cm (4–20in) long. Nodding racemes of narrow, dark carmine-red flowers, 3cm (1¼in) long, are produced in late spring and intermittently to early autumn. ↕ 35cm (14in), ↔ 45cm (18in). ❄❄❄

***D.* 'Bacchanal'** ▣ Rhizomatous perennial with finely lobed, grey-green

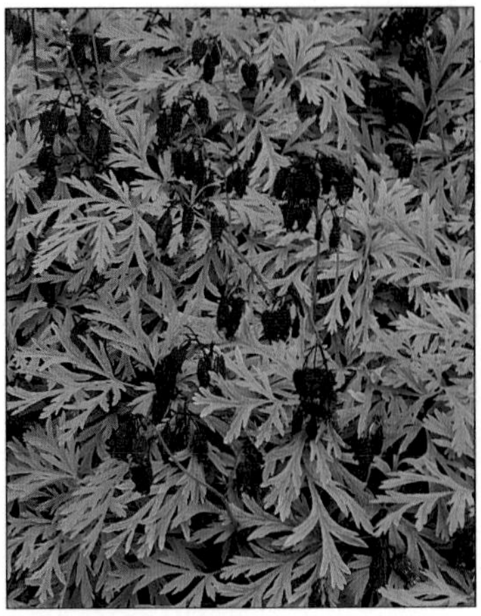

Dicentra 'Bacchanal'

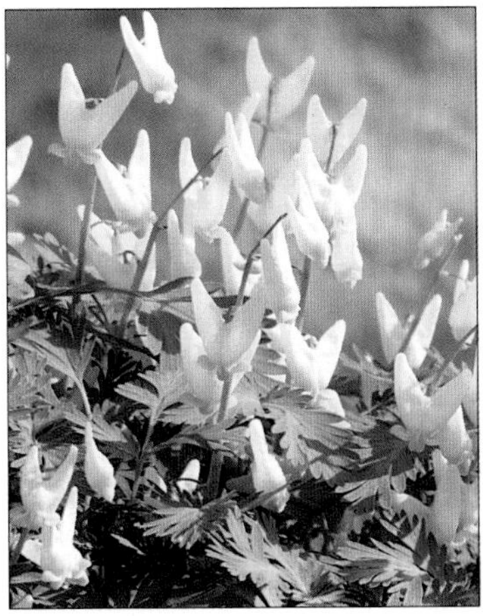

Dicentra cucullaria

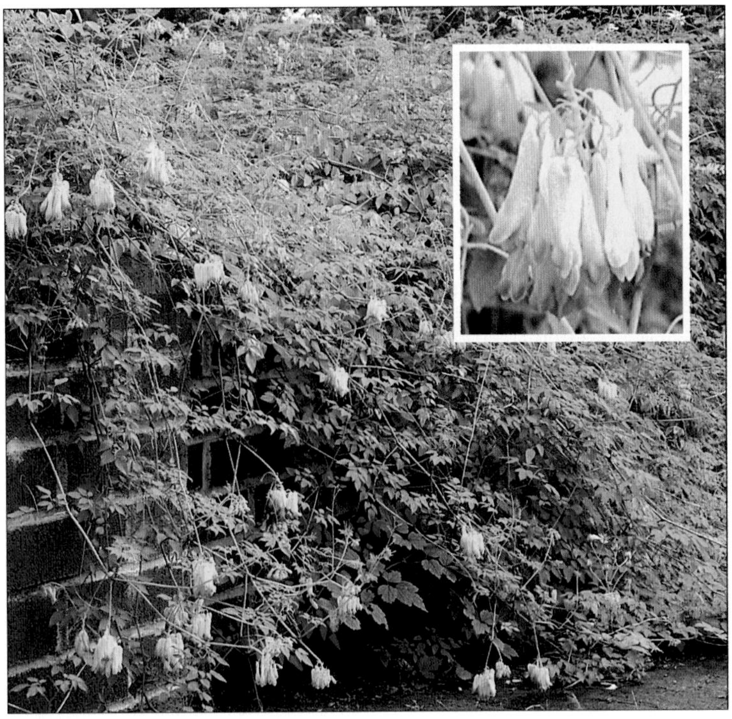

Dicentra scandens (inset: flower detail)

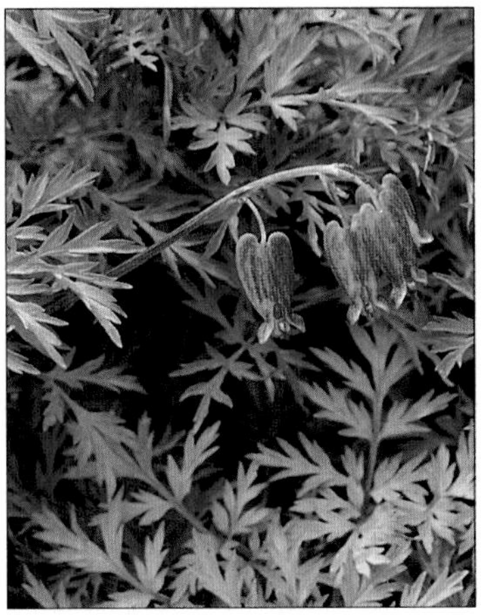

Dicentra 'Stuart Boothman'

leaves, 1–2cm (½–¾in) long. Racemes of dusky crimson flowers, 2.5cm (1in) long, are produced in mid- and late spring. ↕45cm (18in), ↔60cm (24in). ❄❄❄

***D.* 'Boothman's Variety'** see *D.* 'Stuart Boothman'.

***D.* 'Bountiful'.** Clump-forming, rhizomatous perennial with red-tinged stems bearing pinnate, mid-green leaves, 10–50cm (4–20in) long. In late spring and intermittently to early autumn, bears nodding racemes or panicles of purplish pink flowers, 1.5–2.5cm (½–1in) long. ↕30cm (12in), ↔45cm (18in). ❄❄❄

D. chrysantha (Golden eardrops). Upright perennial with 2-pinnate, glaucous, mid-green leaves, 10–45cm (4–18in) long, with linear, lobed leaflets. Numerous golden yellow flowers, 1–2cm (½–¾in) long, are produced in upright panicles, to 30cm (12in) long, from midsummer to early autumn. ↕1–1.5m (3–5ft), ↔45cm (18in). W. USA (S. Oregon to dry chaparral of S. California). ❄❄❄

D. cucullaria ▣ (Dutchman's breeches). Compact, clump-forming, tuberous perennial with 3-ternate, blue-green leaves, 10–25cm (4–10in) long, deeply lobed or divided into linear to elliptic leaflets. Racemes of white, rarely pink-flushed, yellow-tipped flowers, 1–2cm (½–¾in) long, on arching stems, are borne in early spring. Needs gritty, humus-rich soil in partial shade. Dies down quickly after flowering and should be kept almost dry in summer, when dormant. ↕to 20cm (8in), ↔to 25cm (10in). E. North America (Nova Scotia to Kansas and N. Carolina). ❄❄❄

***D. eximia*.** Clump-forming, rhizomatous perennial with red-tinged stems bearing pinnate, mid- to grey-green leaves, 15–50cm (6–20in) long, with lance-shaped to oblong or ovate lobes. In late spring and intermittently to early autumn, nodding racemes or panicles of deep rose-pink buds open to narrow pink, purple-pink, or white flowers, 1.5–3cm (½–1¼in) long, with reflexed outer petals. ↕60cm (24in), ↔45cm (18in). E. USA. ❄❄❄

***D. eximia* of gardens** see *D. formosa.*

D. formosa*,** syn. *D. eximia* of gardens (Wild bleeding heart). Wide-spreading, rhizomatous perennial with abundant, lobed, basal leaves, 15–50cm (6–20in) long, mid-green above, glaucous beneath. Deep rose-pink buds, borne high above the foliage in branching racemes, open to pink flowers, 1–2.5cm (½–1in) long, fading almost to white, in late spring and early summer. Self-seeds freely. ↕45cm (18in), ↔60–90cm (24–36in). W. North America. ❄❄❄. **var. *alba has white flowers. **subsp. *oregona*,** syn. *D. oregona*, has more glaucous leaves and soft bluish pink flowers. USA (Oregon, California).

***D.* 'Langtrees'** ♀ Vigorous, rhizomatous perennial with abundant, lobed, silvery grey leaves, to 30cm (12in) long. Bears pink-tinted white flowers, 1–2cm (½–¾in) long, in racemes from mid-spring to early or midsummer. ↕30cm (12in), ↔45cm (18in). ❄❄❄

***D.* 'Luxuriant'** ♀ Spreading perennial with lobed, mid- to deep green leaves, to 30cm (12in) long. Racemes of red flowers, 1.5–2.5cm (½–1in) long, are produced from mid-spring to early or midsummer. ↕30cm (12in), ↔45cm (18in). ❄❄❄

***D. macrantha*.** Spreading perennial with 2-ternate, coarsely toothed, pale to yellow-green leaves, 20–30cm (8–12in) long, divided into ovate leaflets, borne on yellowish green stalks. Bears narrow, creamy yellow flowers, 8cm (3in) long, solitary or in short racemes, in late spring. May be damaged by cold, drying winds and late frosts. ↕60cm (24in), ↔45cm (18in). E. China. ❄❄❄

D. oregona see *D. formosa* subsp. *oregona.*

***D.* 'Pearl Drops'.** Rhizomatous perennial with lobed, glaucous, blue-green leaves, to 30cm (12in) long. Racemes of pink-tinted white flowers, 1cm (½in) long, are produced from mid-spring to early or midsummer. ↕30cm (12in), ↔45cm (18in). ❄❄❄

***D. peregrina*.** Tuft-forming perennial with deeply cut and finely lobed, blue-green leaves, 4–16cm (1½–6in) long. Short-stemmed racemes of purple-tipped pink, white, or purple flowers, 1.5–2.5cm (½–1in) long, are produced in early summer. ↕to 7cm (3in), ↔to 10cm (4in). E. Siberia, China, Japan. ❄❄❄

D. scandens ▣ syn. *D. thalictrifolia.* Climbing perennial with slender stems and deeply lobed, mid-green leaves, 15–35cm (6–14in) long, divided into ovate to lance-shaped leaflets. White or yellow, sometimes purple- or pink-tipped flowers, 2–2.5cm (¾–1in) long, are borne in long racemes on leafy peduncles in summer. ↕↔1m (3ft). Himalayas. ❄❄❄ (borderline)

***D.* 'Silver Smith'.** Clump-forming, rhizomatous perennial with pinnate, blue-green leaves, 10–50cm (4–20in) long. In late spring and intermittently to early autumn, bears nodding racemes or panicles of pink-flushed, creamy white flowers, 1.5–2cm (½–¾in) long. ↕↔45cm (18in). ❄❄❄

D. spectabilis ▣♀ (Bleeding heart, Dutchman's breeches, Lyre flower). Clump-forming perennial with thick, fleshy roots and 2-ternate, pale green leaves, 15–40cm (6–16in) long, with ovate, sometimes cut or lobed leaflets. Arching, fleshy stems produce racemes of flowers, 2–3cm (¾–1¼in) long, with rose-pink outer petals and white inner ones, in late spring and early summer. ↕to 1.2m (4ft), ↔45cm (18in). Siberia, N. China, Korea. ❄❄❄. **f. *alba*** ▣♀ is more robust, and produces pure white flowers until midsummer.

***D.* 'Spring Morning'.** Clump-forming, rhizomatous perennial with finely cut, mid- to dark green leaves, 10–50cm (4–20in) long. Bears nodding racemes or panicles of light pink flowers, 2–3cm (¾–1¼in) long, in late summer and intermittently to early autumn. ↕30cm (12in), ↔45cm (18in). ❄❄❄

***D.* 'Stuart Boothman'** ▣♀ syn. *D.* 'Boothman's Variety'. Spreading, rhizomatous perennial with 3-palmate, blue-grey leaves, 10–20cm (4–8in) long, with narrow leaflets. From mid-spring to early or midsummer, bears deep pink flowers, 1.5–2.5cm (½–1in) long. ↕30cm (12in), ↔40cm (16in). ❄❄❄

D. thalictrifolia see *D. scandens.*

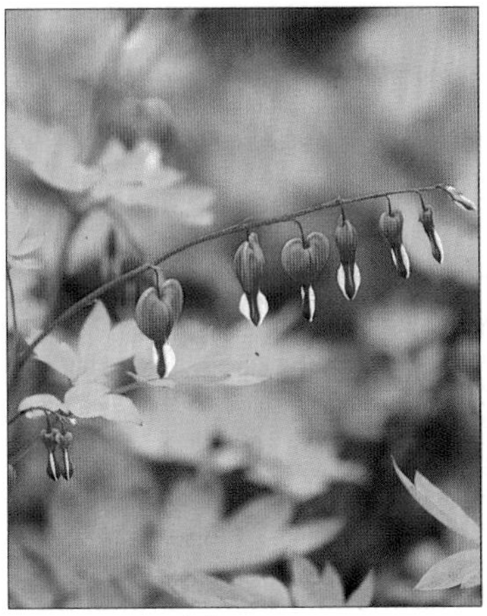

Dicentra spectabilis

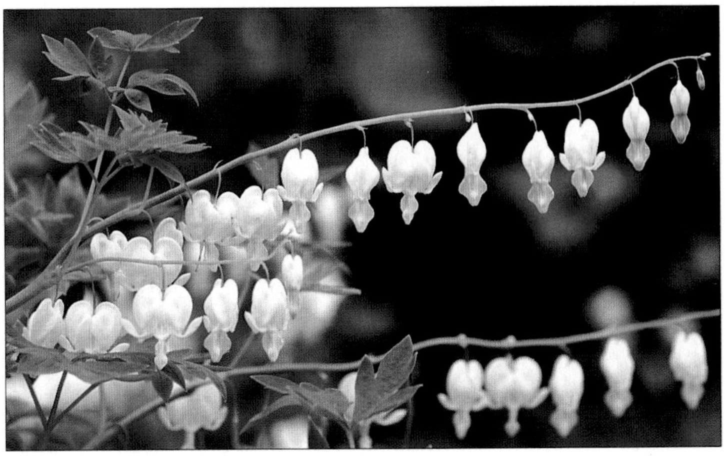

Dicentra spectabilis f. *alba*

D

DICHELOSTEMMA

syn. BREVOORTIA

ALLIACEAE/LILIACEAE

Genus of 7 species of cormous perennials found in chaparral and grassland in W. North America. They are grown for their umbels or racemes of tubular to bell-shaped flowers, clustered at the ends of long, thin stems. Narrow, grass-like leaves, 30cm (12in) long, produced in spring, die off as the flowers open. Grow in a warm, sheltered border or, in cool climates with damp summers, in a bulb frame or cold greenhouse to ensure a warm, dry dormancy.

• **HARDINESS** Frost hardy.
• **CULTIVATION** Plant 10cm (4in) deep in autumn, in well-drained soil in full sun. Keep warm and dry after flowering.
• **PROPAGATION** Sow seed at 13–16°C (55–61°F) as soon as ripe, or remove offsets in late summer.
• **PESTS AND DISEASES** Trouble free.

D. congestum, syn. *Brodiaea congesta.* Cormous perennial producing dense racemes, 5cm (2in) across, of numerous tubular, lilac-blue flowers, 2cm (¾in) long, in early summer. Similar to *D. pulchellum* but flower stalks are joined at the base. ↕40–90cm (16–36in), ↔5cm (2in). USA (Washington, Oregon, California). ❄❄
D. ida-maia ■ syn. *Brodiaea ida-maia* (Californian firecracker). Cormous perennial bearing umbels, 6cm (2½in) across, of up to 8 pendent, narrowly tubular, crimson flowers, 2–3cm (¾–1¼in) long, with short, reflexed sepals with greenish yellow tips, in summer. Excellent for cutting. Requires a dormant season to ripen the corm, so best grown in an alpine house or cold frame. ↕20–30cm (8–12in), ↔5cm (2in). USA (Oregon, California). ❄❄
D. pulchellum, syn. *Brodiaea capitata, B. pulchella.* Cormous perennial bearing dense umbels, 5cm (2in) across, of many tubular, lilac-blue flowers, 1.5cm (½in) long, in early summer. ↕30–60cm (12–24in), ↔5cm (2in). USA (Oregon, California). ❄❄
D. volubile, syn. *Brodiaea volubilis* (Twining brodiaea). Scrambling, cormous perennial producing umbels, 8cm (3in) across, of many tubular pink or pinkish mauve flowers, 2cm (¾in) long, in summer. Needs support. ↕to 1.5m (5ft), ↔5cm (2in). USA (California). ❄❄

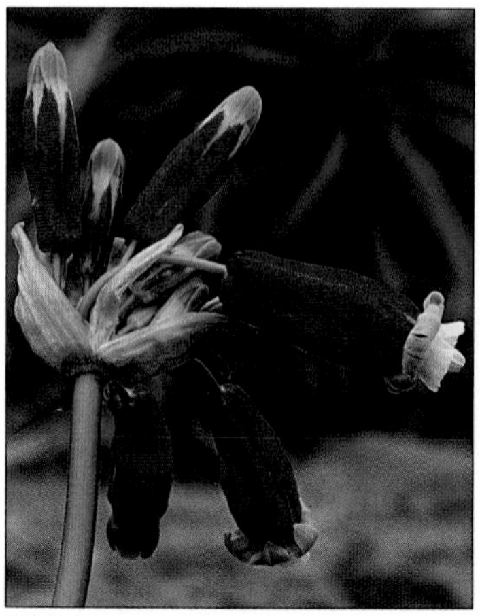

Dichelostemma ida-maia

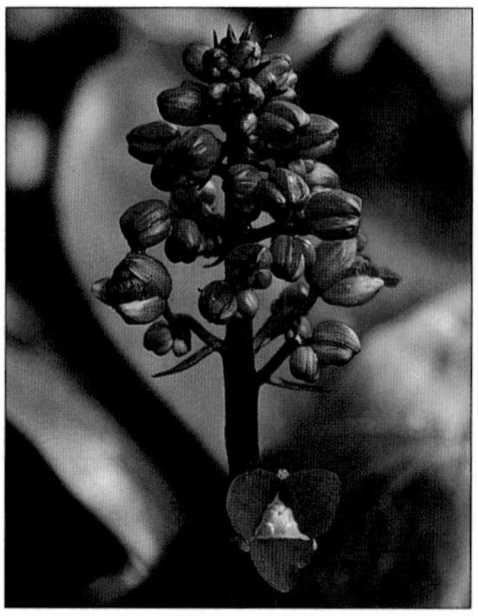

Dichorisandra reginae

DICHORISANDRA

COMMELINACEAE

Genus of about 25 species of robust, erect, soft-stemmed, evergreen perennials from woodland in tropical North, Central, and South America. The linear to elliptic leaves are spirally arranged or 2-ranked, and the angular, cup-shaped flowers, with 3 sepals and 3 intense blue or sometimes white petals of unequal size, are borne in terminal or axillary racemes, followed by fleshy, orange-red fruit. In frost-prone areas, grow in a warm greenhouse; in warmer climates, use in a border.

• **HARDINESS** Frost tender.
• **CULTIVATION** Under glass, grow in loam-based potting compost (JI No.3) in bright filtered light and high humidity. In the growing season, water freely and apply a balanced liquid fertilizer monthly; keep just moist in winter. Outdoors, grow in well-drained, fertile soil in partial shade.
• **PROPAGATION** Divide or root stem cuttings at any time.
• **PESTS AND DISEASES** Mealybugs may be troublesome.

D. reginae ■ Erect perennial with fleshy, rhizomatous roots and 2-ranked, elliptic, dark green leaves, 18cm (7in) long, suffused with reddish purple when young, often streaked with silver, and purple beneath. White flowers, to 2cm (¾in) across, violet-blue on the upper half of the petals, are borne in compact racemes, 15–20cm (6–8in) long, from summer to autumn. ↕↔30cm (12in). Peru. ❀ (min. 12°C/54°F)
D. thyrsiflora. Erect perennial with short, rhizomatous roots and spirally arranged, elliptic-lance-shaped, lustrous, dark green leaves, 20–30cm (8–12in) long. Deep violet flowers, 1–2cm (½–¾in) across, are produced in dense racemes, 13–20cm (5–8in) long, in autumn. ↕2.5m (8ft), ↔1m (3ft). Brazil. ❀ (min. 12°C/54°F)

DICKSONIA

CYATHEACEAE/DICKSONIACEAE

Genus of about 25 species of evergreen or semi-evergreen ferns, usually with upright, trunk-like rhizomes or caudices, but occasionally creeping in habit. They are found in sheltered, upland forest in temperate and tropical regions of S.E. Asia, Australasia, and South America.

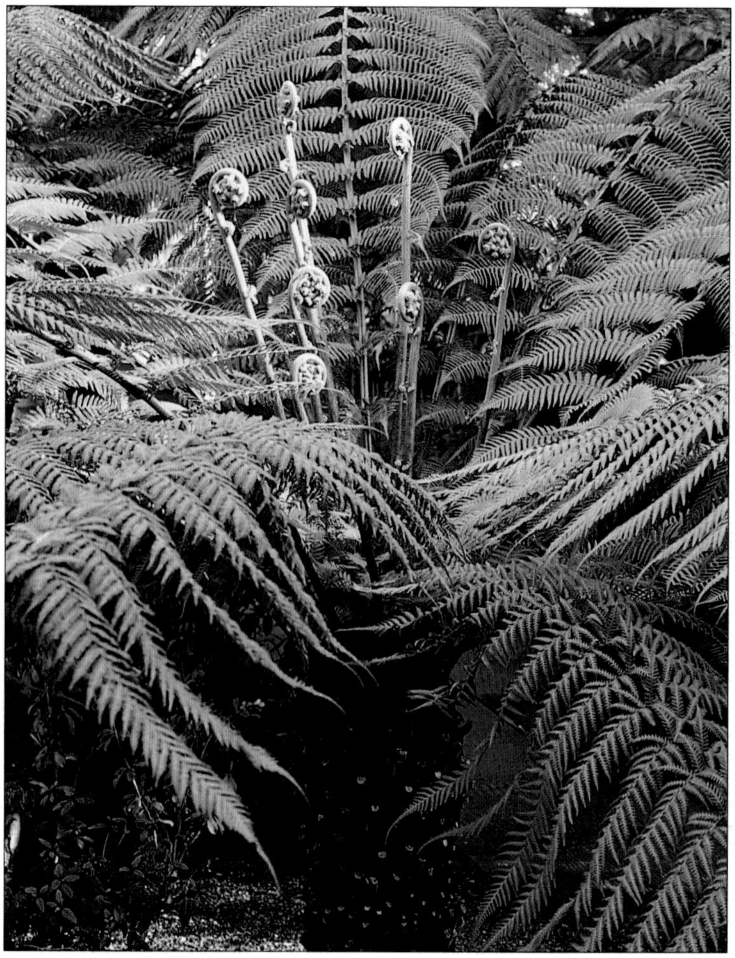

Dicksonia antarctica

The often massive rhizomes or caudices are usually clothed in old leaf bases and fibrous roots, and crowned with spreading, 2- to 4-pinnate or pinnatifid, leathery fronds. The sori are round and form along the margins of the segments, on the underside, each protected by an indusium. *Dicksonia* species are fine specimen plants, whether in a cool greenhouse or conservatory, or outdoors in frost-free areas.

• **HARDINESS** Frost hardy to frost tender.
• **CULTIVATION** Under glass, grow in a mix of 1 part each loam, medium-grade bark, and charcoal, 2 parts sharp sand, and 3 parts coarse leaf mould, in bright filtered light with moderate humidity; if possible, move plants outside during summer. In growth, water freely, applying a high-nitrogen liquid fertilizer monthly; keep just moist and admit full light in winter. Top-dress or pot on annually in spring. Outdoors, grow in humus-rich, acid soil in partial or full shade. In hot, dry weather, hose the rhizomes or caudices with water daily.
• **PROPAGATION** Sow spores at 15–16°C (59–61°C) as soon as ripe. See also p.51.
• **PESTS AND DISEASES** Trouble free.

D. antarctica ■ 🏆 ♣ (Man fern, Soft tree fern, Woolly tree fern). Tree-like fern, evergreen in mild climates, with an erect rhizome, covered with a thick mass of roots, forming a trunk up to 60cm (24in) across. The 2- or 3-pinnate fronds, to 3m (10ft) long, are pale green when young and darken with age. ↕to 6m (20ft) (usually considerably less), ↔4m (12ft). E. Australia (including Tasmania). ❄❄

DICLIPTERA

ACANTHACEAE

Genus of 150 species of annuals, soft-stemmed or woody, evergreen sub-shrubs, perennials, and climbers with angled stems, found in many tropical or warm-temperate regions. They are grown for their opposite, lance-shaped to rounded, velvety, grey-green leaves and their slender, tubular, 2-lipped, brightly coloured flowers, borne in terminal and axillary clusters with prominent, colourful bracts. Grow in a border; in frost-prone areas, grow as a houseplant or in a warm greenhouse.

• **HARDINESS** Frost tender.
• **CULTIVATION** Under glass, grow in loam-based potting compost (JI No.3)

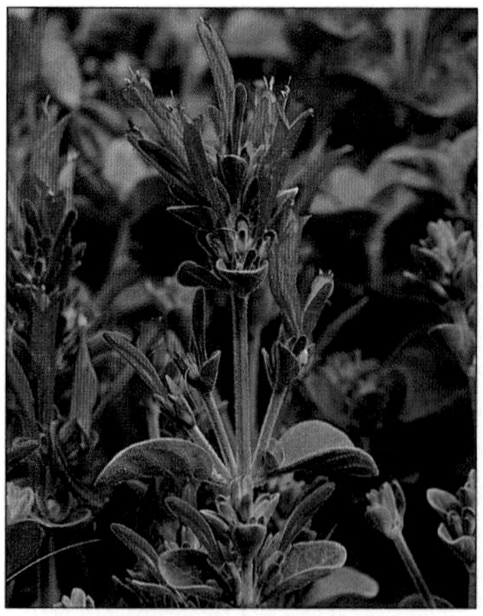

Dicliptera suberecta

in full light with shade from hot sun. In the growing season, water freely and apply a balanced liquid fertilizer every 3–4 weeks; keep just moist in winter. Outdoors, grow in moderately fertile, well-drained soil in sun or partial shade. Cut back leggy plants after flowering.
• **PROPAGATION** Root softwood cuttings in spring, or greenwood cuttings in summer.
• **PESTS AND DISEASES** Trouble free.

D. suberecta ■ syn. *Jacobinia suberecta, Justicia suberecta.* Erect or arching subshrub with slender stems and ovate, dull, mid-green leaves, 4–8cm (1½–3in) long, covered in grey down. Bears orange-red flowers, 3.5cm (1½in) long, in axillary and terminal clusters, in summer. ↕ 60cm (24in), ↔ 45cm (18in). Uruguay. ❀ (min. 13°C/55°F)

DICRANOSTIGMA

PAPAVERACEAE

Genus of 3 species of annuals and perennials found on mountain slopes, especially screes, in the Himalayas and W. and C. China. They produce basal rosettes of pinnatifid leaves, arising from a deep rootstock, and terminal, poppy-like flowers. Use in an informal border, or in a wildflower or rock garden.
• **HARDINESS** Fully hardy.
• **CULTIVATION** Grow in well-drained, humus-rich soil in partial shade. Will tolerate sun in cool climates, if the soil remains moist during growth.
• **PROPAGATION** Sow seed in containers in a cold frame as soon as ripe; self-seeds freely.
• **PESTS AND DISEASES** May be damaged by slugs and snails.

D. lactucoides. Rosette-forming perennial with elliptic to inversely lance-shaped, pinnatifid, 4- to 7-lobed, blue-green leaves, 12–25cm (5–10in) long. Deep yellow or orange flowers, 5cm (2in) across, are borne on sparsely leafy stems in summer. ↕ to 60cm (24in), ↔ 35cm (14in). Himalayas. ✻✻✻

DICTAMNUS

RUTACEAE

Genus of one species of woody-based perennial, with several geographical variants, native to open woodland, dry grassland, and rocky sites, in C. and S. Europe, and from S. and C. Asia to China and Korea. It has pinnate, ash-

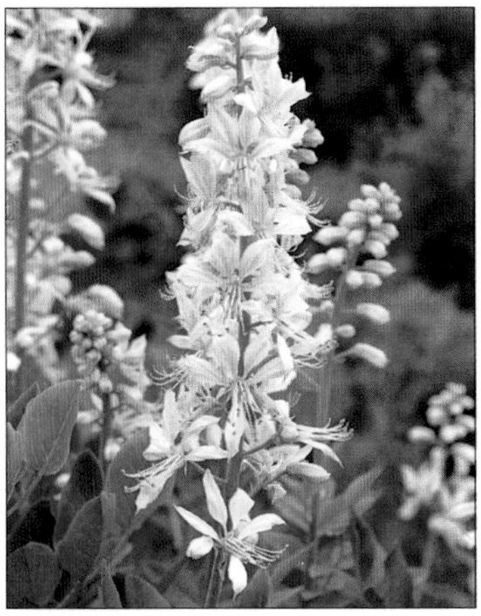

Dictamnus albus

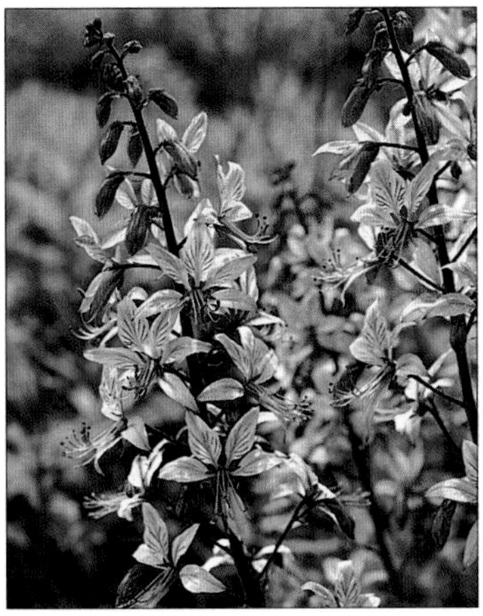

Dictamnus albus var. *purpureus*

like, alternate leaves, each with 3–6 pairs of leaflets and a single terminal leaflet. The 5-petalled, asymmetrical flowers, with long, projecting stamens, are borne in long, open racemes. They, and the unripe fruit, produce an aromatic, volatile oil, which may be ignited in hot weather. *D. albus* is suitable for a border. Its foliage, roots, and seeds may cause mild stomach upset if ingested, and contact with the foliage may cause photodermatitis.
• **HARDINESS** Fully hardy.
• **CULTIVATION** Grow in any dry, well-drained, moderately fertile soil in full sun or partial shade.
• **PROPAGATION** Sow seed in containers in a cold frame as soon as ripe. Divide in autumn or spring, although the woody rootstock does not re-establish easily.
• **PESTS AND DISEASES** Trouble free.

D. albus ■♀ syn. *D. fraxinella* (Burning bush, Dittany). Clump-forming perennial with pinnate, leathery, lemon-scented leaves, to 35cm (14in) long, with lance-shaped to ovate leaflets. White or pinkish white flowers, 2–2.5cm (¾–1in) across, with darker veins, are produced in early summer. ↕ 40–90cm (16–36in), ↔ 60cm (24in). C. and S. Europe to N. China, Korea. ✻✻✻. **var. *purpureus*** ■♀ has purple-mauve flowers with darker veins.
D. fraxinella see *D. albus.*

DICTYOSPERMA

Princess palm

ARECACEAE/PALMAE

Genus of one species of monoecious, single-stemmed palm from Mauritius and the Réunion Islands. Pinnate leaves are produced in a terminal head above a distinct crownshaft, and 3-petalled, cup-shaped flowers, arranged in groups of 3 (2 male and 1 female), develop in simple panicles between them. *D. album* is an effective specimen tree. In frost-prone areas, grow in a warm greenhouse.
• **HARDINESS** Frost tender.
• **CULTIVATION** Under glass, grow in loam-based potting compost (JI No.3) in bright filtered light. In the growing season, water freely, applying a balanced liquid fertilizer monthly; keep just moist in winter. Pot on or top-dress in spring. Outdoors, grow in fertile, moist but well-drained soil in sun or partial shade, with shelter from scorching winds.
• **PROPAGATION** Sow seed at 24–29°C (75–84°F) in spring.

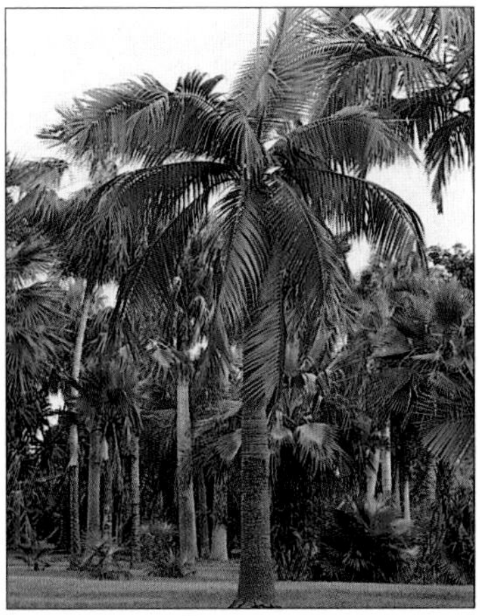

Dictyosperma album

• **PESTS AND DISEASES** Red spider mites may be troublesome under glass.

D. album ■🌴 Single-stemmed palm with a closely ringed, dark brown to grey trunk, sometimes wider at the base, with a woolly, red-brown to whitish grey crownshaft. Arching, pinnate leaves, to 3m (10ft) long, have up to 140 lance-shaped, often divided, mid- to dark green leaflets with yellow midribs and dark veins when young. Leaf-stalks are orange-yellow above, yellow-striped beneath. Bears yellow male flowers in panicles, to 1m (3ft) long, in summer, followed by ovoid, purplish black fruit, to 2cm (¾in) long. ↕ 20m (70ft), ↔ to 6m (20ft). Mauritius, Réunion Islands. ❀ (min. 16°C/61°F). **var. *conjugatum*** has maroon to red male flowers.

▷ ***Didiscus*** see *Trachymene*
D. coeruleus see *T. coerulea*

DIDYMOCHLAENA

DRYOPTERIDACEAE

Genus of one species of evergreen fern from tropical Africa, America, and Polynesia, occurring in woodland and by streams. It produces tufts of glossy, mid-green fronds, tinged with rose-pink or red when young. Grow *D. truncatula* in a shady border; in frost-prone areas, grow in a warm greenhouse or as houseplants.
• **HARDINESS** Frost tender.
• **CULTIVATION** Under glass, grow in 1 part each of loam, medium-grade bark, and charcoal, 2 parts sharp sand, and 3 parts coarse leaf mould, in bright filtered light with high humidity. In growth, water freely, applying a balanced liquid fertilizer monthly; keep just moist in winter. Outdoors, grow in moist, humus-rich soil in partial shade.
• **PROPAGATION** Sow spores at 21°C (70°F) as soon as ripe; divide established plants in spring. See also p.51.
• **PESTS AND DISEASES** Trouble free.

D. lunulata see *D. truncatula.*
D. truncatula ■ syn. *D. lunulata.* Evergreen fern with erect rhizomes and triangular, 2-pinnate fronds, 60–150cm (2–5ft) long, with simple, obliquely ovoid-diamond-shaped segments. ↕↔ to 1m (3ft). Tropical and southern Africa, Fiji, Argentina. ❀ (min. 10°C/50°F)

DIEFFENBACHIA

Dumb cane, Mother-in-law's tongue

ARACEAE

Genus of about 30 species of evergreen perennials found in tropical forest in North and South America and the West Indies. Most cultivars are derived from *D. seguine*, now thought to include *D. maculata*, a name still used commercially. They are grown for their handsome, large, mainly paddle-shaped, oblong, or ovate, fleshy leaves, often heavily marked yellow or white and borne on sheathed stalks. As the lower leaves are shed, scars are left on the erect, thick, cane-like stems, although some modern cultivars are virtually stemless. Inflorescences with creamy spathes are produced intermittently throughout the year, although seldom in cultivation. In frost-prone areas, grow in a warm greenhouse or conservatory, or as houseplants; elsewhere, grow in a border. All parts may cause severe discomfort if ingested, and contact with sap may irritate skin.
• **HARDINESS** Frost tender.
• **CULTIVATION** Under glass, grow in loam-based potting compost (JI No.3) in bright filtered light with high humidity. In the growing season, water moderately, applying a balanced liquid fertilizer monthly; mist daily in summer. Water sparingly and admit full light in winter. Pot on each spring. Outdoors, grow in fertile, moist but well-drained soil in partial shade.
• **PROPAGATION** Root tip cuttings in spring or summer, or take stem sections, each with a growth bud, and lay flat on the surface of the compost. Alternatively, increase by air layering.

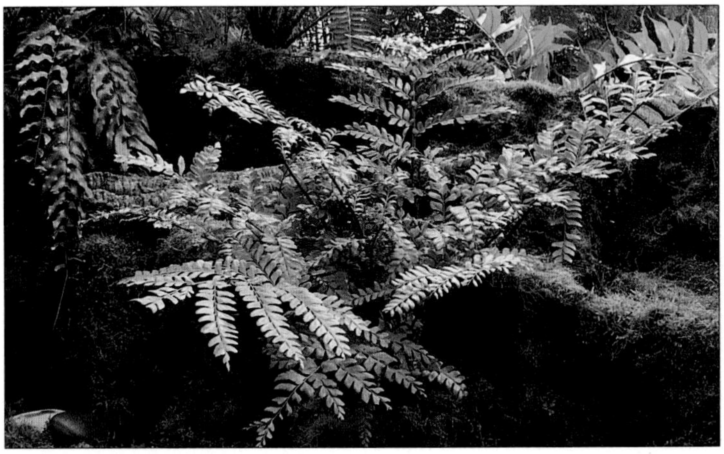

Didymochlaena truncatula

D

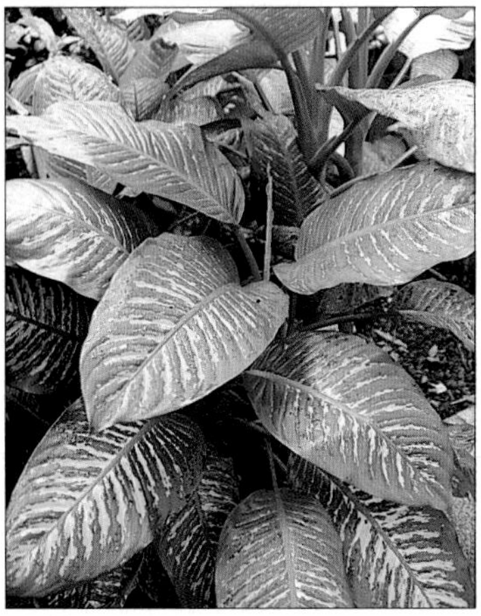
Dieffenbachia seguine 'Amoena'

• **PESTS AND DISEASES** Soft new growth is susceptible to infestation by aphids.

***D. amoena* of gardens** see *D. seguine* 'Amoena'.
***D.* 'Exotica'** see *D. seguine* 'Exotica'.
D. maculata see *D. seguine, D. seguine* 'Maculata'.
***D. maculata* 'Hi-colour'** see *D. seguine* 'Tropic Snow'.
***D. maculata* 'Snow Queen'** see *D. seguine* 'Tropic Snow'.
***D. maculata* 'Tropic Topaz'** see *D. seguine* 'Tropic Snow'.
***D.* 'Memoria'** see *D. seguine* 'Memoria Corsii'.
D.* x *memoria-corsii see *D. seguine* 'Memoria Corsii'.
***D.* 'Pia'** see *D. seguine* 'Pia'.
D. picta see *D. seguine.*

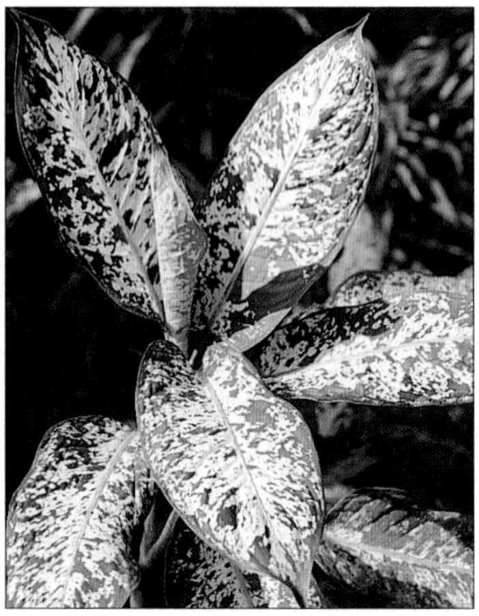
Dieffenbachia seguine 'Exotica'

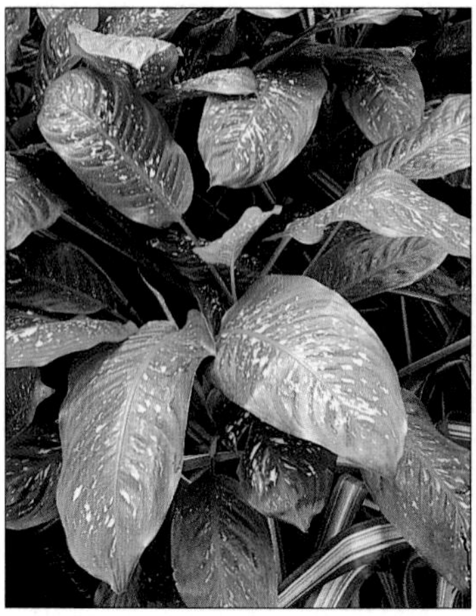
Dieffenbachia seguine 'Maculata'

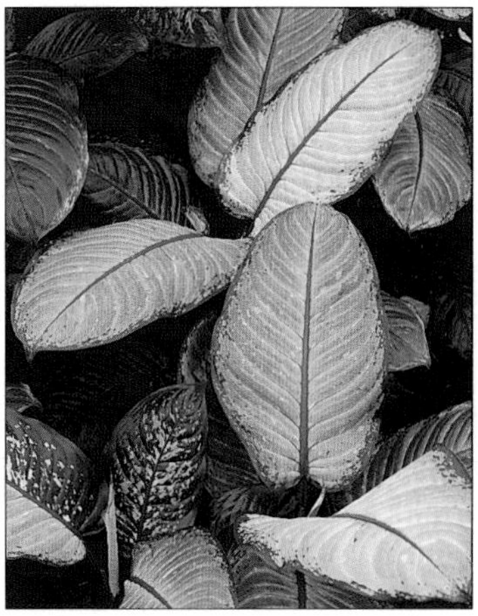
Dieffenbachia seguine 'Rudolph Roehrs'

D. seguine, syn. *D. maculata, D. picta.* Robust perennial with alternate, broadly ovate to oblong or lance-shaped leaves, 30–45cm (12–18in) long, evenly spread along the stem. They are glossy, dark green, sparsely spotted white, with white midribs. ↕ 1–3m (3–10ft), ↔ 60cm (24in). Brazil. ❀ (min. 15°C/59°F). **'Amoena'** ▣ syn. *D. amoena* of gardens, has oblong-ovate leaves, 15–35cm (6–14in) long, with creamy white bands and marbling between the veins; ↕ to 2m (6ft). **'Exotica'** ▣ syn. *D.* 'Exotica', *D. maculata* 'Exotica', is virtually stemless, with oblong-ovate leaves, heavily and irregularly white-variegated between the veins and on the midribs; ↕ 1m (3ft), ↔ 40cm (16in). **'Maculata'** ▣ syn. *D. maculata*, has bright green leaves, 25cm (10in) long, heavily veined and spotted creamy white, and mottled leaf-stalks; ↕ 1.2m (4ft) or more, ↔ 1m (3ft). **'Memoria'** see 'Memoria Corsii'. **'Memoria Corsii'**, syn. *D.* 'Memoria', *D.* x *memoria-corsii*, 'Memoria', has elliptic to oblong, grey-green leaves, that darken with age, with large, dark green patches, darker veining, and sparse white spots; ↕ 1m (3ft), ↔ 40cm (16in). **'Pia'**, syn. *D. maculata* 'Pia', *D.* 'Pia', is virtually stemless, with oblong-lance-shaped white leaves, tinged pale green and deep green margins; ↕ 40cm (16in), ↔ 30cm (12in). **'Roehrsii'** see 'Rudolph Roehrs'. **'Rudolph Roehrs'** ▣ syn. *D. maculata* 'Rudolph Roehrs', 'Roehrsii', has ovate to elliptic leaves, mostly creamy yellow or chartreuse-green, spotted white, with dark green midribs and margins; ↕ 1m (3ft) or more, ↔ 40cm (16in). **'Tropic Snow'**, syn. *D. maculata* 'Hi-colour', *D. maculata* 'Snow Queen', *D. maculata* 'Tropic Snow', *D. maculata* 'Tropic Topaz', *D.* 'Tropic Snow', is virtually stemless, with thick, ovate, mid-green leaves, with sage-green markings and cream feathering. ↕ 1.2m (4ft).
***D.* 'Tropic Snow'** see *D. seguine* 'Tropic Snow'.

DIERAMA

Angel's fishing rod, Wandflower

IRIDACEAE

Genus of 44 species of evergreen, cormous perennials usually found in moist, mountainous or submountainous grassland in Ethiopia, E. and S. tropical Africa, and South Africa. Gladiolus-like corms, produced annually, form chains of old corms on top of one another.

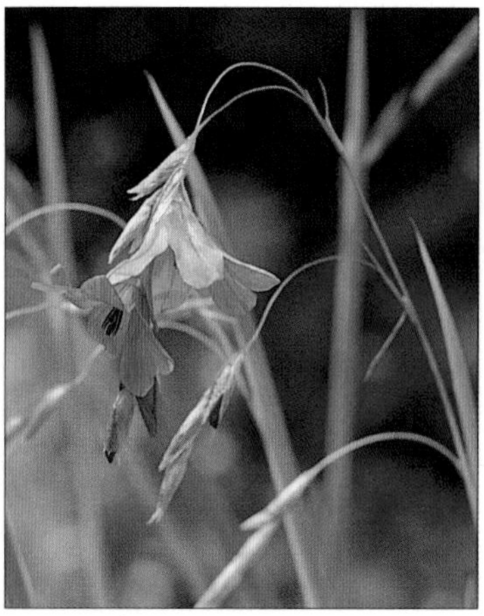
Dierama dracomontanum

Basal tufts of semi-erect to erect, thin, grass-like, mid- to grey-green leaves, to 90cm (36in) long, are overtopped in summer by a succession of pendent, funnel- or bell-shaped flowers, borne in spikes on long, slender, arching stems. Hybrids between *D. dracomontanum* and *D. pulcherrimum* are sometimes known as Slieve Donard Hybrids, a name wrongly applied to mixed seedlings. In frost-prone areas, grow half-hardy species in a cool greenhouse. Elsewhere, grow tall species at the back of a border or by a pool or stream, and dwarf species in a rock garden or at the front of a border.
• **HARDINESS** Frost hardy to half hardy; well-established clumps may tolerate temperatures to -10°C (14°F).
• **CULTIVATION** Plant corms 5–7cm (2–3in) deep in spring. Under glass, grow in loam-based potting compost (JI No.2) in full light. In growth, water freely. Outdoors, grow in humus-rich, well-drained soil in a sheltered site in full sun, watering freely during the growing season. Divisions and young plants are slow to establish, but once settled are trouble free.
• **PROPAGATION** Sow seed in a seedbed or in containers in a cold frame as soon as ripe, or divide in spring.
• **PESTS AND DISEASES** Trouble free.

D. dracomontanum ▣ syn. *D. pumilum* of gardens. Clump-forming, cormous perennial. Produces arching stems of bell-shaped, light to rose-pink or light coral-pink to red, occasionally purple-pink or mauve flowers, 2–3cm (¾–1¼in) long, in summer. ↕ 60cm

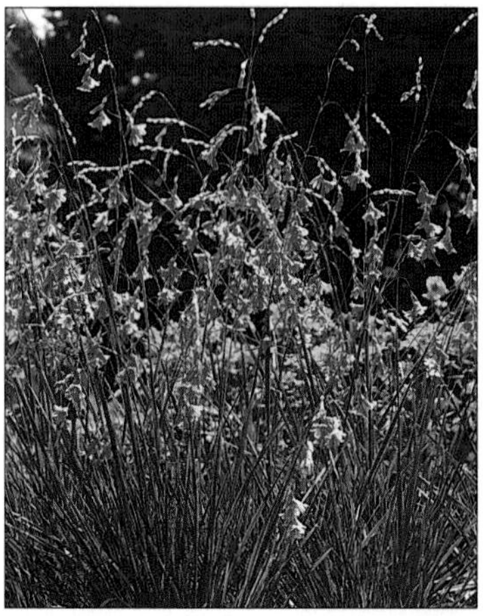
Dierama 'Miranda'

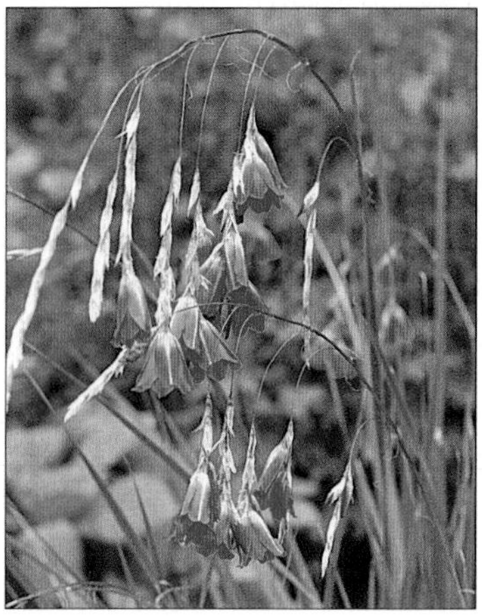
Dierama pulcherrimum

(24in), occasionally to 1m (3ft), ↔ 30cm (12in). South Africa. ❄❄
D. ensifolium see *D. pendulum.*
D. luteoalbidum. Cormous perennial producing narrowly bell-shaped, white or creamy yellow flowers, 3–5cm (1¼–2in) long, in summer. ↕ 60–90cm (24–36in), ↔ 30cm (12in). South Africa (KwaZulu/Natal). ❄
***D.* 'Miranda'** ▣ Clump-forming, cormous perennial. Bell-shaped, bright pink flowers, 3–4cm (1¼–1½in) long, are produced in summer. ↕ 75–90cm (30–36in), ↔ 30cm (12in). ❄❄
D. pendulum, syn. *D. ensifolium.* Tufted, clump-forming, cormous perennial. Bears clustered spikes of wide, open bell-shaped, purple-pink flowers, 3–5cm (1¼–2in) long, in summer. ↕ 1–2m (3–6ft), ↔ 60cm (24in). South Africa (Western and Eastern Cape). ❄❄
D. pulcherrimum ▣ Cormous perennial bearing dense, pendent spikes of tubular-bell-shaped, pale to deep magenta-pink, occasionally purple-red or white flowers, 3.5–6cm (1½–2½in) long, in summer. ↕ 1–1.5m (3–5ft), ↔ 60cm (24in). Zimbabwe, South Africa. ❄❄. **'Blackbird'** has deep wine-purple flowers, 4–5cm (1½–2in) long.
***D. pumilum* of gardens** see *D. dracomontanum.*
***D.* 'Titania'.** Clump-forming, cormous perennial producing bell-shaped, pale pinkish red flowers, 3–5cm (1¼in–2in) long, in summer. ↕ 60cm (24in), ↔ 30cm (12in). ❄❄

DIERVILLA

Bush honeysuckle

CAPRIFOLIACEAE

Genus of 3 species of suckering, deciduous shrubs from North America, found in light woodland. They are valued for their attractive habit and tubular, 2-lipped yellow flowers, borne in axillary or terminal cymes. Leaves are simple, oblong-lance-shaped to ovate, toothed, and opposite. Grow in a shrub border or light woodland garden.
• **HARDINESS** Fully hardy.
• **CULTIVATION** Grow in fertile, well-drained soil in sun or partial shade. Mulch well. Pruning group 6.
• **PROPAGATION** Separate suckers in late winter. Root softwood cuttings in summer.
• **PESTS AND DISEASES** Trouble free.

D. sessilifolia. Thicket-forming shrub, spreading by suckers. Ovate-lance-shaped, mid-green leaves, 6–18cm (2½–7in) long, are tapered at the tips and bronze tinged when young. Sulphur-yellow flowers, to 1.5cm (½in) long, are produced in terminal cymes, to 7cm (3in) across, in summer. ↕ 1–1.5m (3–5ft), ↔ 1.5m (5ft). S.E. USA. ✻✻✻

DIETES

IRIDACEAE

Genus of 6 species of evergreen, rhizomatous perennials from C., E., and S.E. tropical Africa, South Africa, and Lord Howe Island, Australia, occurring in open grassland, dry bushland, moist forest margins, and mountain cliffs. They have erect, linear to sword-shaped, leathery, basal leaves. Branching stems bear a succession of flat, individually short-lived, iris-like flowers, from spring to summer. In frost-prone areas, grow in a cool greenhouse or conservatory. In warmer climates, grow outdoors in a border.

- **HARDINESS** Half hardy.
- **CULTIVATION** Under glass, grow in loam-based potting compost (JI No.2) in full light and good ventilation. In growth, water freely, applying balanced liquid fertilizer monthly; reduce water after flowering to keep just moist when dormant. Outdoors, grow in moist but well-drained soil in full sun or partial shade. Tolerates poor, dry soils. The flowering stems of *D. iridioides* should not be cut back after flowering.
- **PROPAGATION** Sow seed at 13–15°C (55–59°F) in autumn or spring. Divide rhizomes after flowering, although they may be difficult to establish.
- **PESTS AND DISEASES** Trouble free.

D. bicolor ■ Rhizomatous perennial with narrowly sword-shaped, pale green, basal leaves, 60cm (24in) long. Pale to deep yellow flowers, 4cm (1½in) across, are produced from spring to summer. The 3 larger tepals each have a brown mark at the base. ↕ 60–90cm (24–36in), ↔ 30cm (12in). South Africa. ✻

D. iridioides, syn. *D. vegeta*. Rhizomatous perennial with a fan of sword-shaped, dark green, basal leaves, 60cm (24in) long. White flowers, 5–6cm (2–2½in) across, with a yellow mark at the centre of each of the 3 larger tepals, are produced from spring to summer. ↕ 30–60cm (12–24in), ↔ 30cm (12in). South Africa, E. Africa to Kenya. ✻

D. vegeta see *D. iridioides*.

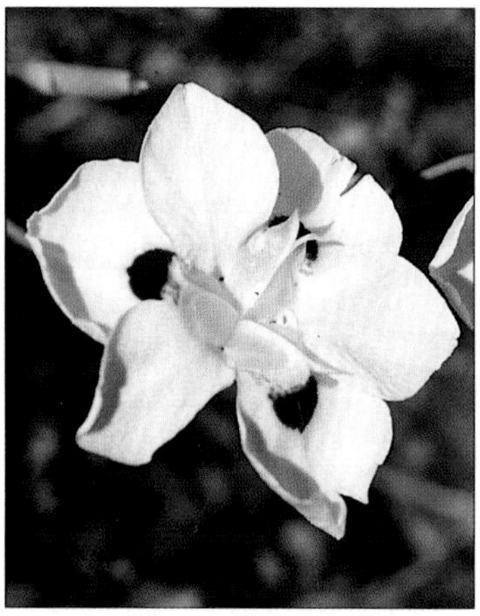

Dietes bicolor

DIGITALIS

Foxglove

SCROPHULARIACEAE

Genus of about 22 species of biennials and short-lived perennials from Europe, N.W. Africa, and C. Asia, found in open woodland, with a few occurring in subalpine meadows and on stony, grassy slopes. They produce simple, mainly oblong to lance-shaped to obovate, entire or toothed, mostly mid-green leaves. They have one or more basal leaf rosettes with smaller, alternate stem leaves. Inflated, tubular-bell-shaped, somewhat 2-lipped flowers, often spotted inside, are produced in tall, sometimes branched, often closely packed racemes, usually on one side of the stems. Most foxgloves are imposing plants, suitable for a border or for naturalizing in woodland. All parts may cause severe discomfort if ingested. Contact with foliage may irritate skin.

- **HARDINESS** Fully hardy to frost hardy.
- **CULTIVATION** Grow in almost any soil and situation, except very wet or very dry, although most prefer humus-rich soil in partial shade. Some species self-seed profusely, so, unless seedlings are required, dead-head after flowering.
- **PROPAGATION** Sow seed in containers in a cold frame in late spring. Seed of *D. purpurea* may also be sown *in situ* in late spring.
- **PESTS AND DISEASES** Leaves are susceptible to leaf spot and powdery mildew.

D. ambigua see *D. grandiflora*.

D. davisiana ■ Rhizomatous perennial with linear-lance-shaped, finely toothed, hairless, mid-green leaves, 7–12cm (3–5in) long. Pale yellow flowers, 3–4cm (1¼–1½in) long, with orange veins, are produced in loose-flowered racemes in early summer. ↕ to 70cm (28in), ↔ 45cm (18in). Turkey. ✻✻

D. dubia. Rosette-forming perennial with lance-shaped, wrinkled, entire or shallowly toothed, dark green leaves, 3–12cm (1¼–5in) long, hairless above and downy beneath. Bears few-flowered racemes of purplish pink or white flowers, 3.5–4cm (1½–1½in) long, heavily spotted inside, in early summer. ↕ 45cm (18in), ↔ 30cm (12in). Spain (Balearic Islands). ✻✻

D. eriostachya see *D. lutea*.

D. ferruginea (Rusty foxglove). Rosette-forming, robust biennial or perennial with oblong to oblong-lance-shaped, entire, dark green leaves, 5–20cm (2–8in) long, sometimes slightly hairy beneath. Bears racemes of golden brown flowers, 3.5cm (1½in) long, with red-brown veins inside and sepals with translucent margins, in midsummer. ↕ to 1.2m (4ft), ↔ 45cm (18in). S. and S.E. Europe, Hungary, Balkans, Turkey, Lebanon, Caucasus. ✻✻✻

D. grandiflora ■ ♀ syn. *D. ambigua*, *D. orientalis* (Yellow foxglove). Clump-forming biennial or perennial with ovate-oblong, finely toothed, conspicuously veined, usually hairless, often glossy, mid-green leaves, 7–25cm (3–10in) long. Racemes of well-spaced, pale yellow flowers, 4–5cm (1½–2in) long, with brown veins inside, are produced in early and midsummer.

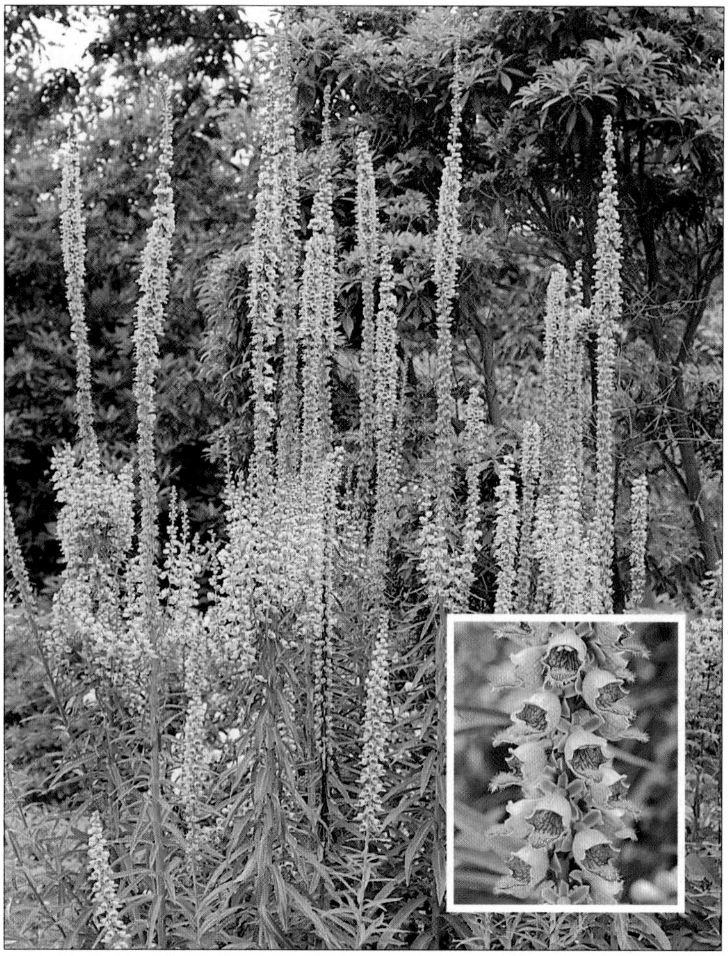

Digitalis davisiana (inset: flower detail)

↕ to 1m (3ft), ↔ 45cm (18in). C. and S. Europe to Siberia, Turkey. ✻✻✻

D. kishinskyi see *D. parviflora*.

D. laevigata. Clump-forming, hairless perennial with obovate, mid-green basal leaves and linear-lance-shaped stem leaves, 5–25cm (2–10in) long. Loose racemes of horizontally borne, brown-yellow flowers, to 3.5cm (1½in) long, each with a white lower lip, and reddish brown veins and speckles inside, open in midsummer. ↕ to 1m (3ft), ↔ 45cm (18in). W. and C. Balkans. ✻✻✻

D. lanata ♀ Clump-forming biennial or perennial with oblong-lance-shaped or inversely lance-shaped, mid-green leaves, to 12cm (5in) long, hairless beneath or with toothed margins. Dense, leafy racemes of pale cream or fawn flowers, 3cm (1¼in) long, each with brown or violet-brown veins and a lighter cream lower lip, are produced from mid- to late summer. ↕ 60cm (24in), ↔ 30cm (12in). Italy, Balkans, Hungary, Turkey. ✻✻✻

D. lutea, syn. *D. eriostachya*. Clump-forming perennial with oblong to inversely-lance-shaped, toothed to almost entire, hairless, glossy, dark green leaves, 5–20cm (2–8in) long. Slender racemes of narrow, pale yellow flowers, 1–2.5cm (½–1in) long, are produced in early and midsummer. Prefers alkaline soil. ↕ 60cm (24in), ↔ 30cm (12in). S.W. central Europe to Italy, N.W. Africa. ✻✻✻

D. x mertonensis ■ ♀ (*D. grandiflora* x *D. purpurea*). Robust, clump-forming perennial with ovate-lance-shaped to lance-shaped, toothed, conspicuously

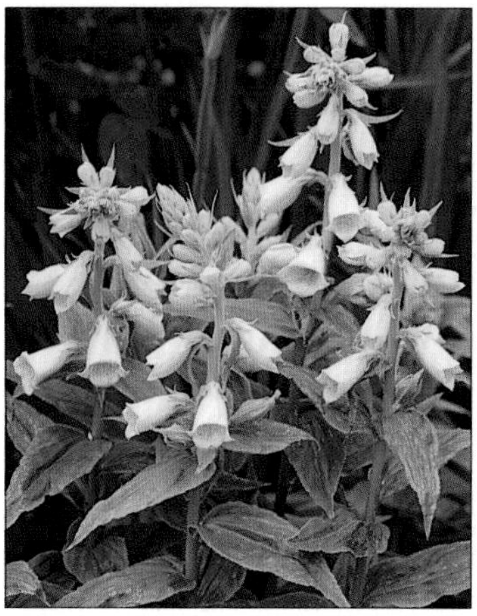

Digitalis grandiflora

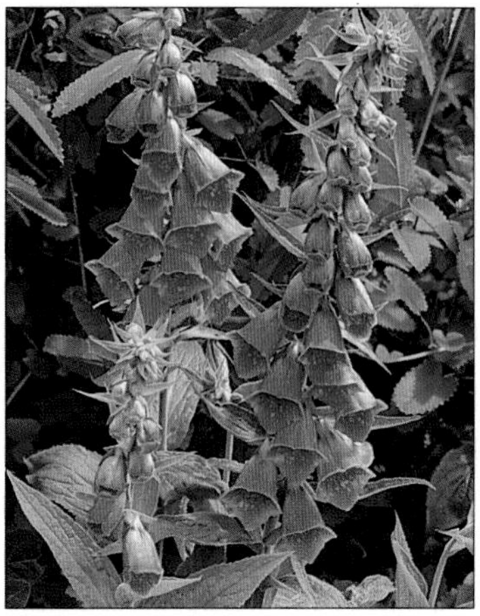

Digitalis x *mertonensis*

D

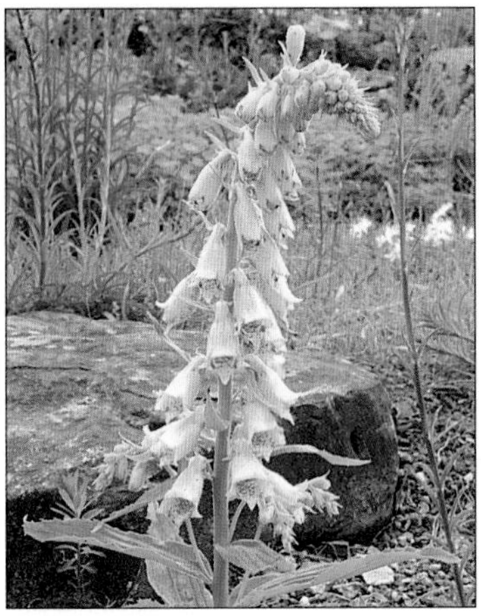
Digitalis obscura

veined, glossy, dark green leaves, 7–30cm (3–12in) long, slightly hairy beneath. Bears racemes of pinkish buff flowers, to 6cm (2½in) long, in late spring and early summer. Comes true from seed. ↕ to 90cm (36in), ↔ 30cm (12in). Garden origin. ❄❄❄
D. obscura ▣ Subshrubby perennial with lance-shaped to linear, entire, hairless, grey-green leaves, 8–15cm (3–6in) long. Racemes of rust-brown to yellow or orange-yellow flowers, 2–3cm (¾–1¼in) long, with red veins and spotting inside, are produced from late spring to midsummer. ↕ 30–120cm (12–48in), ↔ 45cm (18in). Spain. ❄❄
D. orientalis see *D. grandiflora*.
D. parviflora, syn. *D. kishinskyi*. Clump-forming perennial with oblong to inversely-lance-shaped to lance-shaped, entire or slightly toothed, leathery, softly hairy, dark green leaves, 8–20cm (3–8in) long. Dark orange-brown flowers, 1–2cm (½–¾in) long, each with a purple-brown lip, are produced in dense racemes in early summer. ↕ 60cm (24in), ↔ 30cm (12in). N. Spain. ❄❄❄
D. purpurea (Common foxglove). Rosette-forming, very variable, hairy biennial or short-lived perennial with ovate to lance-shaped, usually toothed, dark green, sometimes white-woolly leaves, 10–25cm (4–10in) long. Tall, one-sided spikes of purple, pink, or white flowers, to 6cm (2½in) long, spotted maroon to purple inside, are produced in early summer. Best grown annually from seed. ↕ 1–2m (3–6ft), ↔ to 60cm (24in). S.W. and W. central Europe. ❄❄❄. **f. *albiflora*** ▣ ♀ has white flowers. **'Dwarf Sensation'** is compact, with densely packed flowers, to 8cm (3in) long; ↕ 1.2m (4ft). **Excelsior Hybrids** ▣ ♀ bear flowers in pastel shades of creamy yellow, white, purple, or pink, held horizontally and arranged evenly around each spike. Good for cut flowers. **Foxy Hybrids** produce flowers in carmine-red, pink, creamy yellow, or white, heavily spotted maroon, and may be grown as annuals; ↕ to 90cm (36in). **'Gloxinioides'** has horizontally held, wide-open, frilly-margined flowers in salmon-pink, creamy yellow, purple, or pink, richly spotted and blotched inside; ↕ 2m (6ft) or more. **'Sutton's Apricot'** ♀ has apricot-pink flowers.

▷**Dill** see *Anethum, A. graveolens*

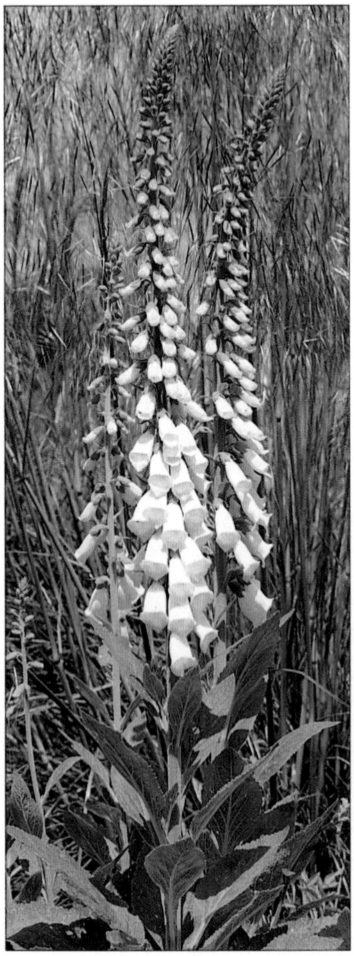
Digitalis purpurea f. *albiflora*

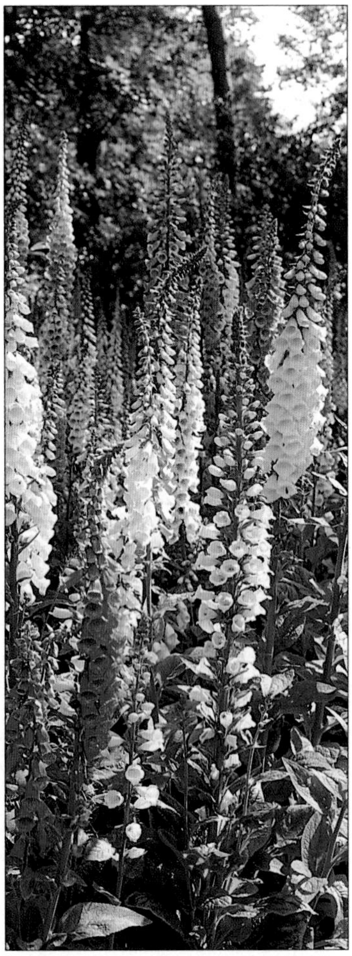
Digitalis purpurea Excelsior Hybrids

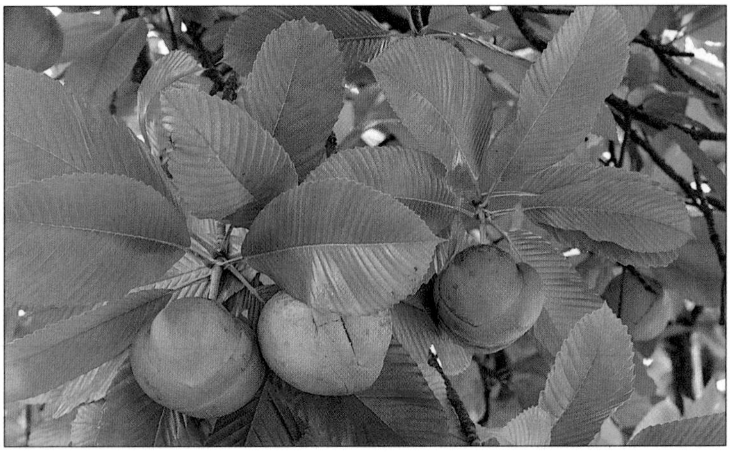
Dillenia indica

DILLENIA

DILLENIACEAE

Genus of about 60 species of magnolia-like, evergreen or briefly deciduous shrubs and trees usually found in forest from Asia to Australia. They are grown for their flowers and their large, alternate, usually ovate to rounded, conspicuously veined leaves. The 5-petalled, saucer- to cup-shaped flowers are solitary or borne in racemes or panicles; they are followed by edible, fleshy, star-shaped to spherical fruits in enlarged calyces. In frost-prone areas, grow *D. indica* in a temperate or warm greenhouse; in warmer regions, it is an effective specimen or shade tree.

- **HARDINESS** Frost tender.
- **CULTIVATION** Under glass, grow in loam-based potting compost (JI No.3), with additional sharp sand, in full light. In growth, water freely and apply a balanced liquid fertilizer monthly; water sparingly in winter. Top-dress or pot on in spring. Outdoors, grow in fertile, humus-rich, moist but well-drained, neutral to acid soil in full sun. Pruning group 1; under glass, may need light restrictive pruning after flowering.
- **PROPAGATION** Sow seed at 16–18°C (61–64°F) in spring. Root semi-ripe cuttings with bottom heat in summer.
- **PESTS AND DISEASES** Trouble free.

D. indica ▣ ♀ (Chulta). Bushy shrub or spreading tree with elliptic-oblong, toothed, lustrous, bright, dark green leaves, 30cm (12in) or more long, boldly patterned with sunken veins. Solitary, cup-shaped white flowers, 20cm (8in) or more across, are produced from the upper leaf axils in summer, followed by spherical, yellowish green fruit, to 10cm (4in) across. ↕ 15m (50ft), ↔ 10–15m (30–50ft). India to Java. ❀ (min. 15°C/59°F)

DILLWYNIA

LEGUMINOSAE/PAPILIONACEAE

Genus of 15 species of evergreen shrubs from dry scrub, heath, and sandy plains in Australia. They are grown for their pea-like flowers, with large wing petals, which are borne singly, or in terminal or axillary racemes or corymbs. The small, alternate, linear leaves are often crowded. Grow in a border or rock garden. In frost-prone areas, grow in a cool greenhouse.

- **HARDINESS** Generally frost tender, but *D. floribunda* and *D. sericea* may be half hardy in a sheltered site.
- **CULTIVATION** Under glass, grow in loam-based potting compost (JI No.3) with additional sharp sand, in full light and with good ventilation. In the growing season, water moderately and apply a balanced liquid fertilizer monthly; water sparingly in winter. Top-dress or pot on in spring. Outdoors, grow in moist but well-drained, poor to moderately fertile soil in sun or partial shade. Pruning group 10, after flowering.
- **PROPAGATION** Sow seed at 18–21°C (64–70°F) in spring after soaking in hot water. Root semi-ripe cuttings with bottom heat in summer.
- **PESTS AND DISEASES** Red spider mites may infest greenhouse plants.

D. floribunda. Freely branching, softly hairy shrub with crowded, linear, warty, mid- to deep green leaves, 5–15mm (¼–½in) long. Produces a profusion of yellow, or yellow and orange flowers, 7mm (¼in) across, in leafy, spike-like, terminal and axillary racemes, mainly from spring to summer. ↕↔ 1–1.5m (3–5ft). Australia (Queensland, New South Wales). ❄ (borderline)
D. sericea. Erect, freely branching shrub with silky-white-hairy shoots bearing linear, warty, usually mid- to deep green leaves, 7–12mm (¼–½in) long. Spike-like terminal racemes of single or paired flowers, 1.5cm (½in) across, in shades of yellow and red, apricot, orange, or pink, are produced from spring to summer. ↕ 60–120cm (2–4ft), ↔ 0.9–1.5m (3–5ft). Australia (Queensland to South Australia and Tasmania). ❄ (borderline)

DIMORPHOTHECA

African daisy

ASTERACEAE/COMPOSITAE

Genus of 7 species of low-branching, erect annuals or evergreen, subshrubby perennials occurring in open, semi-arid, sandy areas in tropical Africa and South Africa, closely related to *Osteospermum* and at one time considered to include species now placed in that genus. All produce alternate, obovate to inversely lance-shaped, entire to pinnatisect, wavy-margined, toothed leaves, and daisy-like flowerheads, on stiff stems, that close in dull weather. They are attractive container, bedding, or border plants, flowering from summer until

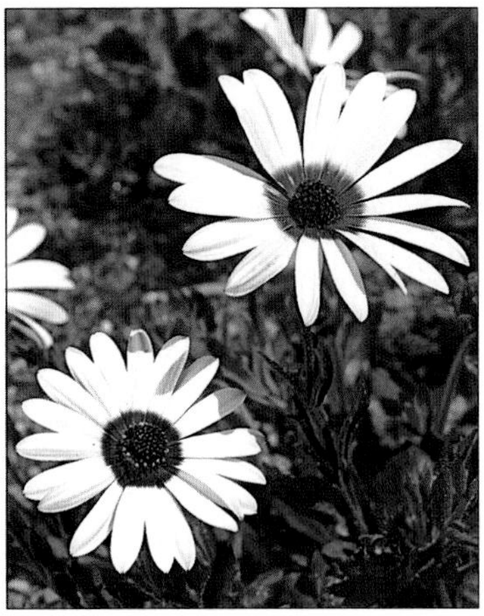
Dimorphotheca pluvialis

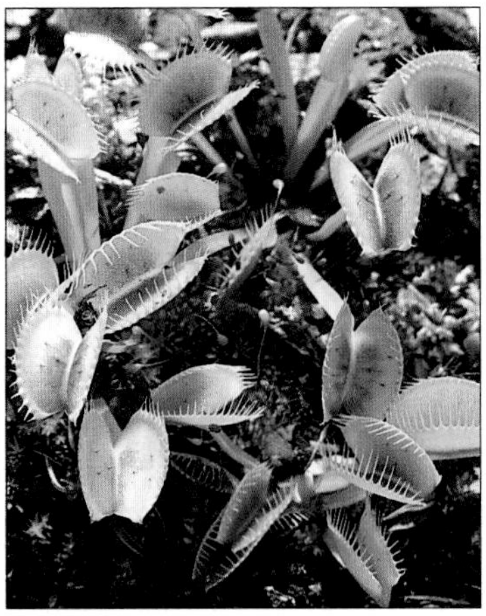
Dionaea muscipula

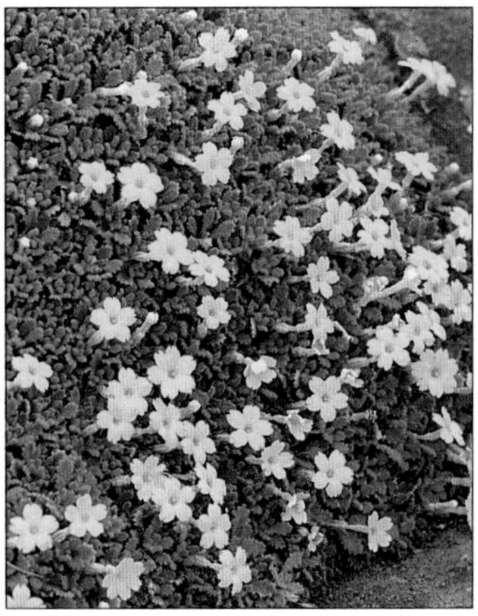
Dionysia aretioides

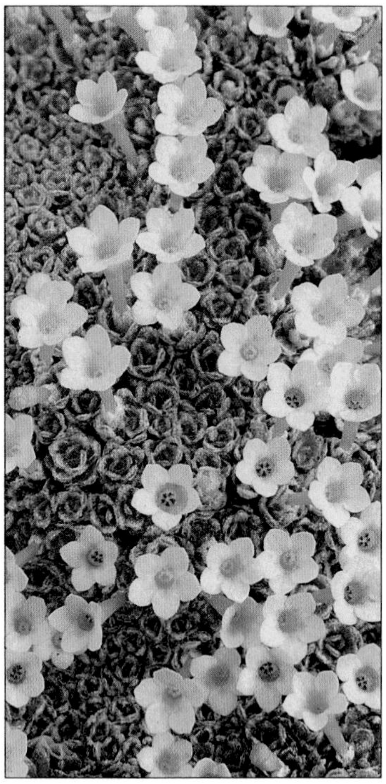
Dionysia tapetodes

first frosts. The perennial species may also be treated as annuals.
• **HARDINESS** Half hardy.
• **CULTIVATION** Grow in light, well-drained, fertile soil in full sun, in a sheltered position. Dead-head regularly to prolong flowering.
• **PROPAGATION** Sow seed at 18°C (64°F) in early spring and plant out seedlings when danger of frost has passed, or sow *in situ* in mid-spring.
• **PESTS AND DISEASES** Grey mould (*Botrytis*) may be a problem.

D. annua see *D. pluvialis.*
***D. aurantiaca* of gardens** see *D. sinuata.*
***D. barberae* of gardens** see *Osteospermum jucundum.*
D. ecklonis see *Osteospermum ecklonis.*
D. pluvialis ■ syn. *D. annua* (Rain daisy, Weather prophet). Erect, hairy annual with obovate to inversely lance-shaped, coarsely toothed or pinnatifid, aromatic, dark green leaves, to 10cm (4in) long. In summer, produces single white flowerheads, to 6cm (2½in) across, violet-blue beneath, with violet-purple zoning at the bases of the ray florets and violet-brown central discs. ↕ to 40cm (16in), ↔ 15–30cm (6–12in). Namibia, South Africa. ❄. **'Glistening White'** has white flowerheads, tinged with violet. **'Tetra Polar Star'** has white flowerheads, to 7cm (3in) across, with deep violet-blue central discs.
D. sinuata, syn. *D. aurantiaca* of gardens (Star of the veldt). Erect annual with oblong to lance-shaped, coarsely toothed, aromatic, mid-green leaves, to 10cm (4in) long. In summer, bears white, yellow, orange, or pink flower-heads, to 4 cm (1½in) across, often tinged violet-blue, with violet-brown central discs. ↕↔ to 30cm (12in). South Africa. ❄

DIONAEA

Venus fly trap

DROSERACEAE

Genus of one species of insectivorous perennial found in bogs in coastal areas of North and South Carolina, USA. It has hinged, rounded, 2-lobed leaves, with stiff marginal spines and 3 or 4 sensitive hairs in the centre of each lobe. When an insect, attracted by the plant's nectar, touches the hairs, the hinge mechanism is triggered, and the leaves close, trapping the insect. Cup-shaped flowers are borne in umbel-like cymes. In frost-prone areas, grow *D. muscipula* in a conservatory or as a houseplant; elsewhere, grow in a bog garden.
• **HARDINESS** Half hardy; needs 5°C (41°F) to start into growth.
• **CULTIVATION** Under glass, grow in an acidic mix of equal parts moss peat and lime-free sand in full or bright filtered light. Keep wet by standing in a saucer with 1cm (½in) of soft water. Growth ceases in autumn, leaving swollen leaf bases in a bulb-like structure below soil level; keep just moist when dormant. Pot on each spring as new growth appears. Outdoors, grow in moist, acid soil in full sun. To encourage "trap" production, pinch out emerging flower stems and remove dead "traps".
• **PROPAGATION** Sow seed at 10–13°C (50–55°F) in spring; place the container in a water tray to keep the potting compost moist. Germination is often very slow. Divide in spring, or take leaf cuttings in late spring or early summer.
• **PESTS AND DISEASES** Trouble free.

D. muscipula ■ (Venus fly trap). Very variable, rosette-forming perennial with rounded, yellow-green to red leaves with winged stalks. Each leaf has 2 hinged lobes with 15–20 stiff, marginal spines. Winter and early summer leaves are 8cm (3in) long, with "traps" 2.5cm (1in) long; many plants also produce summer leaves, to 15cm (6in) long, with "traps" 3cm (1¼in) long and flatter, narrower stalks. In early and midsummer, bears 3–10 white flowers, 1cm (½in) across, in umbel-like cymes on bare stems, 30cm (12in) or more tall. ↕ 15–45cm (6–18in), ↔ 15cm (6in). USA (North Carolina and South Carolina). ❄

DIONYSIA

PRIMULACEAE

Genus of 42 species of tufted or cushion-forming, subshrubby, evergreen perennials found on shady cliffs in arid mountainous areas of C. Asia. The leaves, usually oblong to spoon-shaped, often with a woolly coating (farina) beneath, are borne in rosettes at the ends of branching shoots. Long-tubed, 5-petalled, salverform flowers, with spreading lobes, are solitary or borne in umbels in spring or early summer. They may be pin- or thrum-eyed and, except for *D. involucrata,* both variants must be grown together to produce seed. Grow in an alpine house or outdoors in tufa, protected from excess rainfall.
• **HARDINESS** Fully hardy.
• **CULTIVATION** Under glass, grow in a mix of 3 parts grit and 1 part each loam and leaf mould, with a deep collar of grit around the neck of the plant; provide full light and good ventilation. When in growth, water freely from below, keeping the collar dry; water sparingly in winter. Outdoors, grow in tufa in full sun. Water the material into which the plants are plunged; the leaves and plant collar must be kept dry.
• **PROPAGATION** Sow seed in containers in a cold frame as soon as ripe. Take cuttings of single rosettes in summer, and root in a propagating case, watering only from below.
• **PESTS AND DISEASES** Very susceptible to grey mould (*Botrytis*), especially if overwatered or poorly ventilated. May be infested with aphids.

D. aretioides ■ 🏆 Cushion-forming perennial with dense rosettes of linear-oblong to narrowly spoon-shaped, softly hairy, grey-green leaves, to 7mm (¼in) long, with turned-back margins, yellow- or white-mealy beneath. Produces numerous solitary, stemless, scented, bright yellow flowers, to 1cm (½in) across, with notched petals, in early spring. Relatively easy to grow. ↕ 7cm (3in), ↔ to 30cm (12in). N. Iran. ❄❄❄
D. involucrata. Dense, cushion-forming perennial with obovate to broadly spoon-shaped, finely toothed, dark green leaves, 4–12mm (⅛–½in) long. In early summer, bears stalked umbels of violet or violet-purple flowers, 7–15mm (¼–½in) across, with white eyes that darken with age. Relatively easy to grow. ↕ 7cm (3in), ↔ to 10cm (4in). N.E. Afghanistan and Tajikistan (Pamir Mountains). ❄❄❄
D. michauxii ■ Dense, cushion-forming perennial with tight, rounded rosettes of oblong to oblong-spoon-shaped, silver-grey-hairy leaves, to 3mm (⅛in) long. In spring, the cushions are studded with stemless yellow flowers, to 6mm (¼in) across. ↕ 5cm (2in), ↔ to 15cm (6in). S.W. Iran. ❄❄❄
D. microphylla. Dense, cushion-forming perennial with hard, compact rosettes of entire, obovate to rounded, often sharp-pointed, grey-green leaves, to 2mm (1/16in) long, with a mealy yellow coating beneath. In early summer, bears short-stemmed umbels of white-eyed, pale to deep violet flowers, to 1cm (½in) across, with darker petal bases. ↕ 5cm (2in), ↔ to 15cm (6in). N.W. Afghanistan. ❄❄❄
D. tapetodes ■ Tight, cushion-forming perennial with rosettes of oblong, obovate, or spoon-shaped, glandular, mid-green leaves, to 4mm (⅛in) long, sometimes with a dense, woolly white or yellow farina beneath. Bears masses of solitary, stemless, long-tubed, sometimes scented yellow flowers, to 1cm (½in) across, in late spring and early summer. Relatively easy to grow. ↕ 5cm (2in), ↔ to 20cm (8in). Turkmenistan, N.E. Iran, C. Afghanistan. ❄❄❄

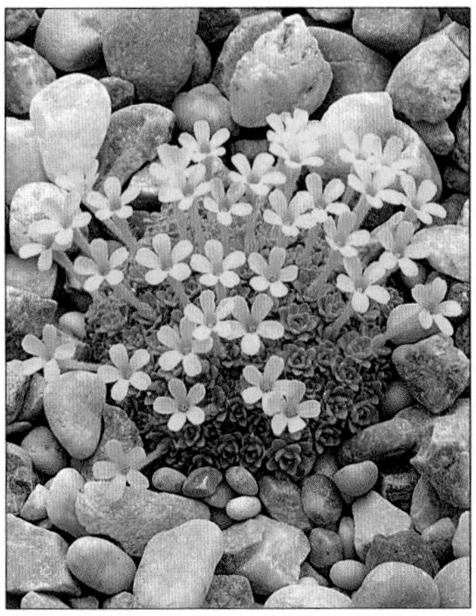
Dionysia michauxii

DIOON

ZAMIACEAE

Genus of 10 species of dioecious, ever-green, palm-like cycads, with strong, woody stems, found on steep, rocky slopes or in open woodland in Central America. The stiff, leathery leaves are pinnate with many slender leaflets. Large, elliptic-ovoid, woolly female cones are produced in the centre of the terminal leaf rosettes; the male cones are cylindrical and smaller. Grow as specimen plants. In frost-prone areas, *Dioon* species need the protection of a temperate or warm greenhouse.

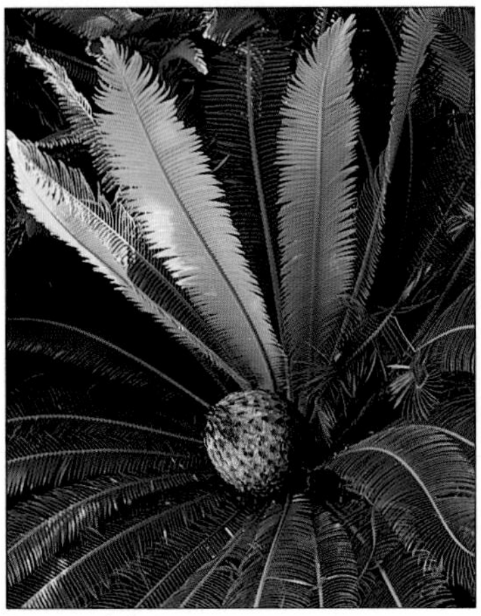

Dioon edule

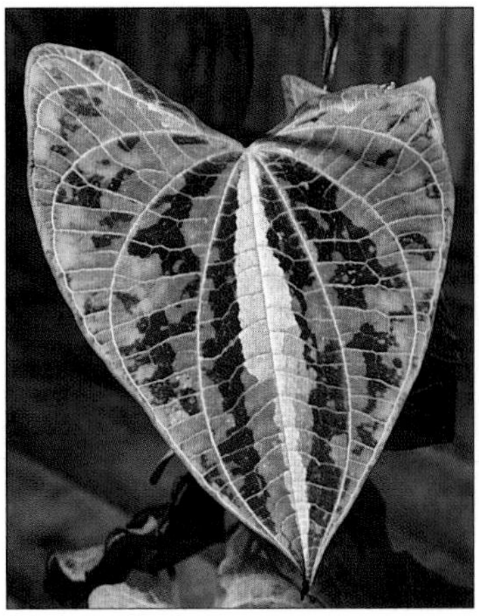

Dioscorea discolor

- **HARDINESS** Frost tender.
- **CULTIVATION** Under glass, grow in a mix of equal parts fibrous loam, coarse bark, and garden compost, in full light with shade from hot sun. In the growing season, water *D. edule* freely and *D. spinulosum* moderately, applying a balanced liquid fertilizer monthly. Water sparingly in winter. Top-dress or pot on in spring. Outdoors, grow most species in fertile, moist but well-drained, humus-rich, neutral to acid soil in full sun. *D. spinulosum* prefers partial shade, high humidity, and neutral to slightly alkaline soil.
- **PROPAGATION** Sow seed at 24–32°C (75–90°F) in spring in very sandy potting compost.
- **PESTS AND DISEASES** Scale insects may be a problem under glass.

D. edule ■ Ŧ (Mexican fern palm). Very slow-growing cycad with a robust, solitary stem, inclining with age. Semi-erect leaves, 0.9–1.5m (3–5ft) long, have up to 200 linear-lance-shaped, sharp-tipped, hairy, grey- to bluish green leaflets, the lower ones almost spine-like. Female cones, to 30cm (12in) long, are rarely produced in cultivation. ↕ to 1.8m (6ft), ↔ 1.5–2.5m (5–8ft). Mexico. ❅ (min. 13°C/55°F)
D. spinulosum Ŧ One of the tallest cycads, with a slender stem, inclining with age. Arching to ascending leaves, 1–2m (3–6ft) long, have up to 150 lance-shaped, spiny-toothed leaflets, downy and grey-blue initially, maturing to mid-green. Grey to brown female cones, 30cm (12in) or more long, are borne in summer. ↕ to 15m (50ft), ↔ to 4m (12ft). Mexico. ❅ (min. 13°C/55°F)

DIOSCOREA

DIOSCOREACEAE

Genus of 600 species of tuberous, deciduous or evergreen, monoecious or dioecious, climbing perennials, some of which are succulent, from tropical forest and relatively dry, often arid areas in tropical and subtropical regions, and from woodland and open scrub in temperate areas. In a few species, the tubers are at or above ground level and covered with bosses of corky bark, resembling a caudex. The stems are mostly woody based and often become vine-like, with alternate, occasionally opposite, simple or palmate leaves, and axillary racemes of small, bell-shaped, 6-tepalled flowers. Some species produce bulbils in the leaf axils. Use to clothe a pillar or pergola; *D. elephantipes* is also suitable for a desert garden. In frost-prone areas, grow tender species in a temperate or warm greenhouse or conservatory.

- **HARDINESS** Fully hardy to frost tender.
- **CULTIVATION** Under glass, grow in loam-based potting compost (JI No.3) in bright filtered light. Provide support. In the growing season, water freely, applying a balanced liquid fertilizer monthly; keep just moist at other times. Outdoors, grow in fertile, humus-rich soil in partial shade. Under glass, *D. elephantipes* needs full light and gritty, sharply drained potting compost, top-dressed with grit. In growth, water moderately; reduce water as the stems wither to keep completely dry when dormant. Outdoors, provide sharply drained soil in full sun. Pruning group 11, in spring, if necessary to restrict size.
- **PROPAGATION** Sow seed at 19–24°C (66–75°F), or plant bulbils in spring. Divide tubers when dormant. Root cuttings of young shoots as they arise from the tuber in spring.
- **PESTS AND DISEASES** Prone to aphids.

D. discolor ■ (Ornamental yam). Moderately vigorous, erect, evergreen, twining climber with slightly angled stems. Heart-shaped or ovate, pointed leaves, 10–15cm (4–6in) long, are velvety olive-green, marbled silver, paler green, and brown, and have silvery pink veins above, purple beneath. In summer, produces green flowers, 2mm (1/16in) across. ↕ 2–3m (6–10ft). Tropical South America. ❅ (min. 13–15°C/ 55–59°F)

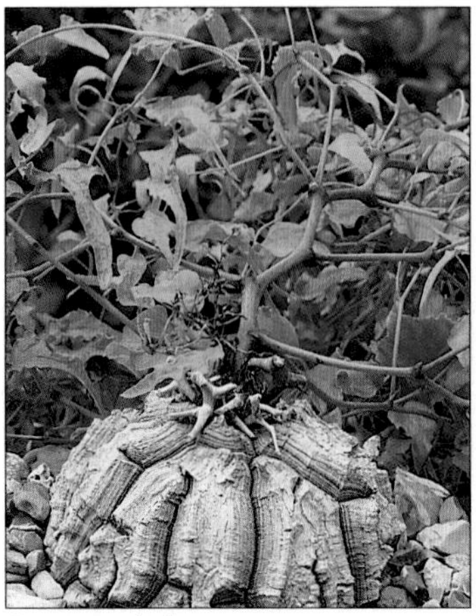

Dioscorea elephantipes

D. elephantipes ■ syn. *Testudinaria elephantipes* (Elephant's foot). Slow-growing, deciduous, climbing perennial with a partially buried, pyramidal or hemispherical, woody tuber, to 90cm (3ft) across, divided into angled, corrugated fissures. Blue-green leaves, to 6cm (2½in) long, are heart- or kidney-shaped. Dark-spotted, greenish yellow flowers, 4mm (⅛in) across, are borne in summer. ↕↔ 1m (3ft). South Africa. ❅ (min. 7–10°C/45–50°F)

▷ ***Diosphaera*** see *Trachelium*
D. asperuloides see *T. asperuloides*

DIOSPYROS

EBENACEAE

Genus of 475 species of deciduous or evergreen trees and shrubs found in forest in tropical, subtropical, and warm-temperate regions worldwide. They are grown for their attractive habit, their bold, alternate, lance-shaped to broadly ovate, simple, often glossy leaves (sometimes with heart-shaped bases), and their fleshy fruits. Bell- or urn-shaped, male and female flowers are usually borne on separate plants, on the previous year's wood. Although some female cultivars of *D. kaki* produce fruit without a male, pollination will generally result in larger crops. In cool-temperate climates, the species and cultivars described here make attractive specimen trees, but most need long, warm summers to fruit well. If growing for fruit, train *D. kaki* as an espalier on a warm, sunny wall, or in frost-prone climates, in a cool greenhouse.

- **HARDINESS** Fully hardy to frost tender.
- **CULTIVATION** Under glass, grow in loam-based potting compost (JI No.3) in full light. In the growing season, water freely, applying a balanced liquid fertilizer monthly; water sparingly in winter. Outdoors, grow in deep, fertile, well-drained, loamy soil in full sun, preferably sheltered from cold, drying winds and late frosts. Pruning group 1.
- **PROPAGATION** Sow seed in containers in an open frame as soon as ripe. Graft cultivars of *D. kaki* in winter.
- **PESTS AND DISEASES** Trouble free in cool climates; in warmer regions and under glass, mealybugs, leaf rollers, and scale insects may be troublesome.

D. kaki ○ (Chinese persimmon, Japanese persimmon, Kaki). Spreading, deciduous tree with oval, glossy, dark green leaves, to 20cm (8in) long, which turn yellow to orange-red and purple in autumn. Small, bell-shaped, pale yellow flowers, to 1.5cm (½in) across, are produced in summer. Female plants bear edible, conical to spherical yellow to orange fruit, to 8cm (3in) across. ↕ 10m (30ft), ↔ 7m (22ft). China. ❄❄.
'Hachiya' ■ is female, with conical, orange-red fruit, 8cm (3in) long.
D. lotus (Date plum) ○ Spreading, deciduous tree with lance-shaped, elliptic, or oval, glossy, dark green leaves, to 12cm (5in) long. Bears tiny, bell-shaped, red-tinged green flowers in mid- to late summer, followed (on female plants) by inedible, spherical to ovoid, yellow to purple fruit, to 2cm (¾in) across. ↕ 10m (30ft), ↔ 6m (20ft). S.W. Asia to China. ❄❄❄

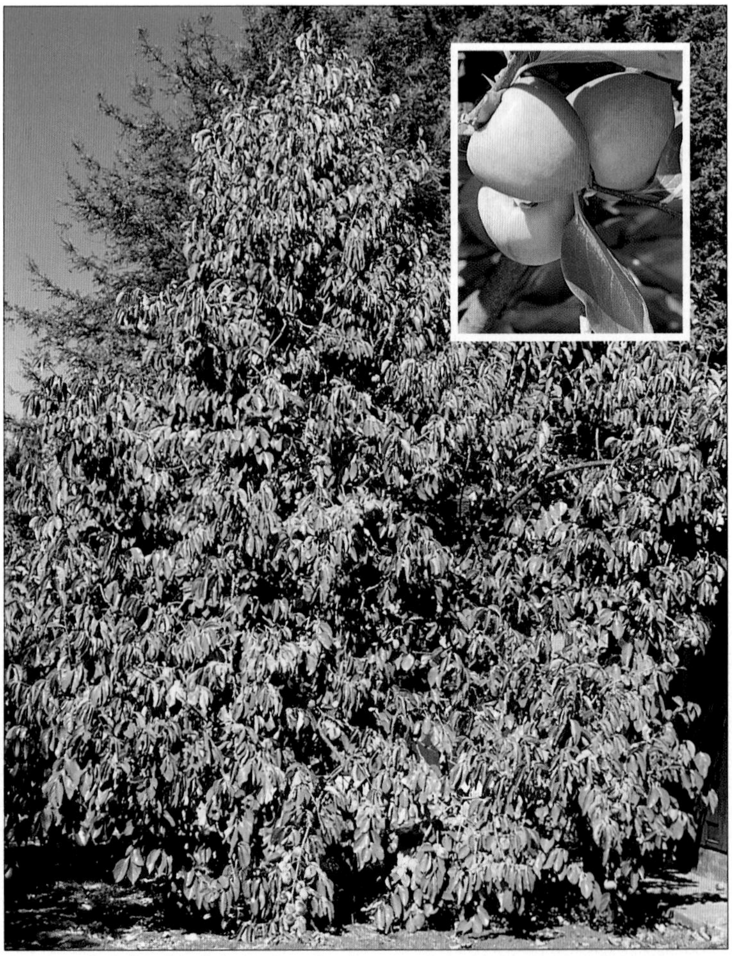

Diospyros kaki 'Hachiya' (inset: fruit detail)

DIPCADI

HYACINTHACEAE/LILIACEAE

Genus of 55 species of small, bulbous perennials found in dry, rocky areas in S. and W. Europe and N. and southern Africa. Leaves are linear to strap-shaped, and the narrowly bell-shaped or tubular flowers, reminiscent of bluebells, are borne in loose racemes. Grow in a rock garden; where winters are cold and wet, grow in an alpine house or bulb frame.

- **HARDINESS** Frost hardy.
- **CULTIVATION** Plant bulbs 5cm (2in) deep in winter or early spring. Under glass, grow in a mix of equal parts loam, leaf mould, and sharp sand in full light. In growth, water freely; reduce water as leaves wither, and keep dry during summer dormancy. Outdoors, grow in light, well-drained soil in full sun.
- **PROPAGATION** Sow seed in containers in a cold frame as soon as ripe. Remove offsets during summer dormancy.
- **PESTS AND DISEASES** Trouble free.

D. serotinum. Bulbous perennial with narrowly linear, grey- or light green, basal leaves, to 30cm (12in) long. In spring, bears racemes of tubular bronze, green, or dull orange-red flowers, 2.5cm (1in) long, with spreading or reflexing tips, on leafless stems, 45cm (18in) long. ↕ 10–45cm (4–18in), ↔ 5cm (2in). S.W. Europe, N. Africa. ❄❄

DIPELTA

CAPRIFOLIACEAE

Genus of 4 species of deciduous shrubs found in scrub and woodland in C. and W. China. They are valued for their peeling bark, their fragrant, tubular to bell-shaped flowers, borne singly or in short corymbs, and for the papery bracts that surround the fruits. The simple, ovate to oval-lance-shaped, pointed leaves are borne in opposite pairs. Grow as a specimen or in a large shrub border.

- **HARDINESS** Fully hardy.
- **CULTIVATION** Grow in fertile, well-drained, preferably alkaline soil in sun or partial shade. Pruning group 2.
- **PROPAGATION** Sow seed in a seedbed in autumn or spring. Root softwood cuttings in summer.
- **PESTS AND DISEASES** Trouble free.

D. floribunda ■ Upright, multi-stemmed shrub with pale brown bark and ovate to oval-lance-shaped, sharp-pointed, pale green leaves, to 10cm (4in) long. Produces terminal and axillary corymbs of 1–6 tubular, yellow-marked, pale pink flowers, to 3cm (1¼in) long, in late spring and early summer. ↕↔ 4m (12ft). C. and W. China. ❄❄❄

D. yunnanensis. Arching shrub with pale brown bark and ovate-lance-shaped, pointed, glossy, mid-green leaves, to 12cm (5in) long. Corymbs of 1–4 tubular, orange-marked white flowers, to 2.5cm (1in) long, are borne on short, leafy stems in late spring. ↕ 3m (10ft), ↔ 4m (12ft). W. China. ❄❄❄

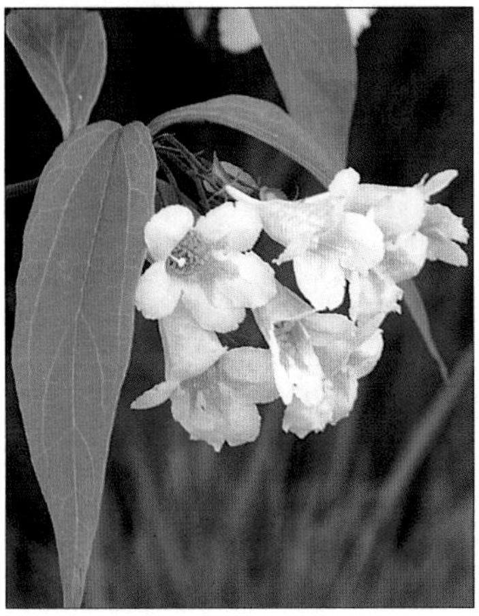

Dipelta floribunda

DIPHYLLEIA

BERBERIDACEAE

Genus of 2 or 3 species of rhizomatous perennials found in woodland and by mountain streams in Japan and North America. They produce large, peltate, dark green leaves and terminal cymes of 6-petalled, bowl-shaped white flowers that quickly lose their petals. Grow in a woodland or peat garden.

- **HARDINESS** Fully hardy.
- **CULTIVATION** Grow in moist, leafy, or humus-rich soil in full or partial shade, preferably sheltered from wind.
- **PROPAGATION** Sow seed in containers in a cold frame as soon as ripe. Divide rhizomes in spring.
- **PESTS AND DISEASES** Slugs and snails eat resting buds and young growth.

D. cymosa (Umbrella leaf). Rhizomatous perennial with cleft radical leaves, 30–60cm (12–24in) across, each segment with 5–7 shallow, pointed, toothed lobes. Upright flowering stems each bear 2 deeply 2-lobed leaves, to 40cm (16in) across. Bears flowers to 2cm (¾in) across in umbel-like cymes in late spring and early summer, followed by blue berries, 1cm (½in) across, on red stalks. ↕ to 1m (3ft), ↔ 30cm (12in). USA (S. Appalachians). ❄❄❄

▷ ***Diplacus*** see *Mimulus*
D. glutinosus see *M. aurantiacus*
▷ ***Dipladenia*** see *Mandevilla*
D. boliviensis see *M. boliviensis*
D. splendens see *M. splendens*

DIPLARRHENA

syn. DIPLARRENA

IRIDACEAE

Genus of 2 species of rhizomatous, evergreen perennials from moist, grassy mountain slopes in S.E. Australia and Tasmania. They form basal tufts of long, flat, linear to sword-shaped leaves, and the usually unbranched flowering stems produce clusters of fragrant, short-lived, iris-like flowers, enclosed by 2 bracts. Grow in a sheltered herbaceous border, at the base of a house wall, or in a cool greenhouse or conservatory.

- **HARDINESS** Frost hardy; may survive to -10°C (14°F) in well-drained soil.
- **CULTIVATION** Under glass, grow in loamless potting compost in bright filtered light. Water freely when in growth, sparingly in winter. Outdoors, grow in moist but well-drained, sandy, humus-rich, neutral to acid soil in full sun, or partial shade in a hot site.
- **PROPAGATION** Sow seed in containers in a cold frame in autumn or spring, or divide in spring.
- **PESTS AND DISEASES** Trouble free.

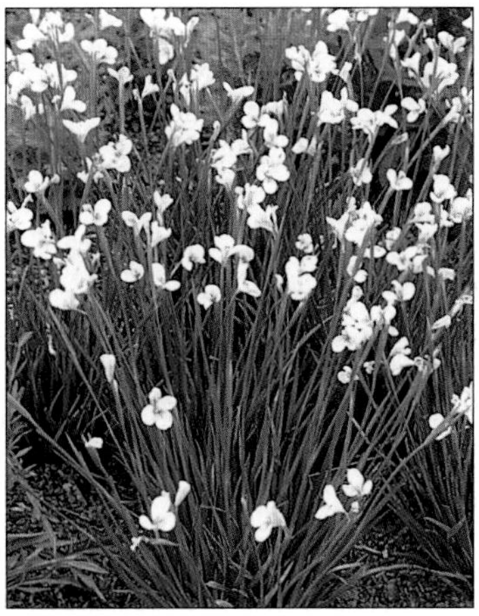

Diplarrhena moraea

D. moraea ■ Tufted perennial with short rhizomes and linear to sword-shaped, dark green, sometimes slightly glaucous, basal leaves, 45cm (18in) long. Bears a succession of 3–6 white flowers, 4–6cm (1½–2½in) across, the inner tepals marked with yellow and purple, in late spring and early summer. ↕ 60cm (24in), ↔ 23cm (9in). S.E. Australia, Tasmania. ❄❄

DIPLAZIUM

ATHYRIACEAE/DRYOPTERIDACEAE

Genus of about 350 terrestrial or epiphytic, evergreen ferns, often with trunk-like rhizomes, found worldwide, in tropical, and warm- or cool-temperate forest. The pinnate to 3-pinnate or simple fronds, arise from erect or sometimes creeping rhizomes. Spores, formed in single or often V-shaped, double lines along the veins on the lower surfaces of the fronds, are covered by indusia when young. In frost-prone areas, grow in a warm greenhouse; elsewhere, use in a moist, sheltered site.

- **HARDINESS** Frost tender.
- **CULTIVATION** Under glass, grow in a mix of 1 part each loam, medium-grade bark, and charcoal, 2 parts sharp sand, and 3 parts coarse leaf mould. Provide bright filtered light and high humidity. Water freely when in growth, sparingly in winter. Pot on annually in spring. Outdoors, grow in humus-rich, moist but well-drained soil in partial shade.
- **PROPAGATION** Sow spores at 21°C (70°F) as soon as ripe. Separate underground runners of species such as *D. esculentum* in spring.
- **PESTS AND DISEASES** Snails, slugs, and various insects often cause serious damage to tender young fronds.

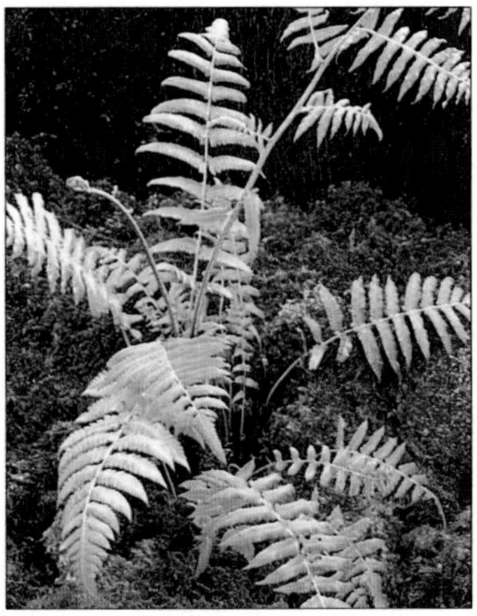

Diplazium esculentum

D. esculentum ■ Evergreen fern, which spreads by underground runners. Ovate-triangular, pinnate or 2-pinnate, leathery, dark green fronds, to 60cm (24in) long, with oblong-lance-shaped segments, are produced in tufts from an erect, stem-like rhizome. ↕↔ to 1m (3ft). S.E. Asia, Polynesia. ⌂ (min. 8–10°C/46–50°F)

▷ ***Diplocyathus ciliata*** see *Orbea ciliata*

D

DIPSACUS

Teasel

DIPSACACEAE

Genus of 15 species of hairy or prickly biennials or short-lived perennials from damp grassland and woodland in Europe, N. Africa, and Asia. The simple or pinnatifid, toothed or cut leaves are borne in opposite pairs, with the bases of the upper leaves usually forming a "cup" around each stem. In the second summer, teasels bear cone-shaped flowerheads on long, upright, branching stems. Grow in a wild garden or wild-flower border; the dried flowerheads are good in floral arrangements.

- **HARDINESS** Fully hardy.
- **CULTIVATION** Grow in any moderately fertile soil, including heavy clay, in sun or partial shade. Flowerheads should be harvested for air-drying from mid- to late summer.
- **PROPAGATION** Sow seed *in situ* in autumn or spring.
- **PESTS AND DISEASES** Prone to aphids.

D. fullonum ■ syn. *D. sylvestris.* Prickly biennial producing a basal rosette of simple, oblong-lance-shaped, toothed, dark green leaves, 30cm (12in) or more long, covered in spiny pustules; these leaves usually wither before flowers appear. Paired lance-shaped leaves are borne on upright stems in the second summer, each pair joined at the base to form a cup. Oblong-ovoid, thistle-like, pinkish purple or white flowerheads, 3–8cm (1¼–3in) long, with stiff, curved, prickly bracts, are borne in mid- and late summer. ↕ 1.5–2m (5–6ft), ↔ 30–80cm (12–32in). Europe, Asia. ❄❄❄

D. sylvestris see *D. fullonum.*

▷ ***Dipteracanthus*** see *Ruellia*

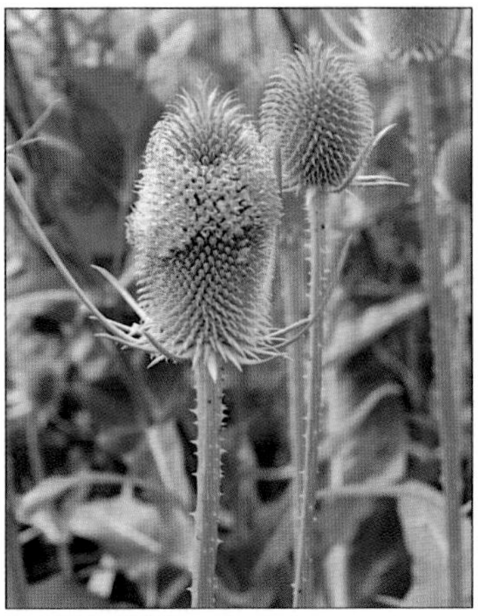

Dipsacus fullonum

D

DIPTERONIA

ACERACEAE

Genus of 2 species of deciduous trees and shrubs found in woodland in C. and S. China. *D. sinensis* is grown for its pinnate leaves, produced in opposite pairs, and for its large clusters of winged, red-brown fruit. Small, greenish white flowers are produced in erect terminal panicles in summer. Grow in a large shrub border or woodland garden.

• **HARDINESS** Fully hardy.
• **CULTIVATION** Grow in fertile, moist but well-drained, loamy soil in sun or partial shade. Pruning group 1.
• **PROPAGATION** Sow seed in a seedbed in autumn. Layer in late spring or early summer; shoots often layer naturally. Insert softwood cuttings in summer.
• **PESTS AND DISEASES** Trouble free.

D. sinensis ⚲ Spreading tree or shrub with pinnate leaves, to 30cm (12in) long, with 7–11 ovate or lance-shaped, toothed leaflets. Bears erect, pyramidal panicles, 15–30cm (6–12in) long, of small, greenish white flowers in summer, followed by large clusters of flat, winged, red-brown fruit, 2.5cm (1in) across, ripening to brown-red in autumn. ↕↔ 10m (30ft). C. China. ✻✻✻

DIRCA

THYMELEACEAE

Genus of 2 species of deciduous shrubs found in woodland in E. North America and on wet slopes in evergreen forest on rocky hills in California, USA. The oval to obovate or broadly elliptic leaves are simple, entire, and alternate. They are cultivated for their early, *Daphne*-like flowers, borne on bare branches in axillary clusters of 2 or 3 in early spring. Grow in a sheltered shrub border.

• **HARDINESS** Fully hardy.
• **CULTIVATION** Grow in moist but well-drained, humus-rich soil in partial shade. Provide shelter from frosts, which may spoil the early flowers. Pruning group 1.
• **PROPAGATION** Sow seed in a seedbed in autumn. Layer in autumn or spring.
• **PESTS AND DISEASES** Trouble free.

D. palustris (Leatherwood). Upright shrub with fibrous bark and very flexible shoots bearing oval to obovate leaves, to 7cm (3in) long, mid-green above, blue-green beneath. Narrowly funnel-shaped, pale yellow flowers, 1cm (½in) long, are borne in clusters of 3 in early spring. ↕↔ 1.5m (5ft). E. North America. ✻✻✻

DISA

ORCHIDACEAE

Genus of approximately 100 species of deciduous, occasionally evergreen, terrestrial orchids found at low to high altitudes, often by running water, in tropical C. and E. Africa, South Africa, and Madagascar. They have tuberous, sometimes also stoloniferous roots. The erect stems, with ovate to lance-shaped or linear leaves, bear one to many richly coloured flowers, with hooded upper and spreading lower perianth segments, in terminal racemes or corymbs.

• **HARDINESS** Frost tender.

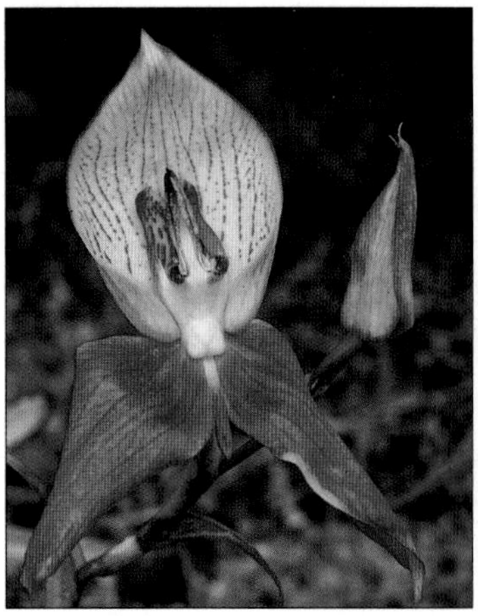

Disa uniflora

• **CULTIVATION** Cool-growing orchids. Grow in a mix of equal parts peat, perlite, and chopped sphagnum moss, and cover the compost surface with sphagnum moss. In summer, provide cool, humid, shady conditions. In the growing season, water freely with soft water, to keep the roots continually moist, but avoid wetting the leaves, which are prone to black rot; keep cool and dry in winter. Do not fertilize. Repot annually after new growth has started. See also p.46.
• **PROPAGATION** Divide plants when repotting.
• **PESTS AND DISEASES** Red spider mites may be troublesome.

D. grandiflora see *D. uniflora*.
***D.* Kirstenbosch Pride** (*D. cardinalis* x *D. uniflora*). Hybrid terrestrial orchid producing a basal rosette of lance-shaped leaves, 7–15cm (3–6in) long. Racemes of up to 8 scarlet and orange-red flowers, 7cm (3in) across, are produced on tall stems in late summer. ↕ 90cm (36in), ↔ 20cm (8in). ❀ (min. 5°C/41°F; max. 24°C/75°F)
D. uniflora ▣ syn. *D. grandiflora*. Terrestrial orchid with lance-shaped leaves, to 25cm (10in) long. Produces short racemes of up to 3, or very rarely 10, brilliant scarlet flowers, 8–12cm (3–5in) across, with red and gold veining, in midsummer. ↕ 60cm (24in), ↔ 20cm (8in). South Africa (Northern Cape, Western Cape, Eastern Cape). ❀ (min. 5°C/41°F; max. 24°C/75°F)

DISANTHUS

HAMAMELIDACEAE

Genus of one species of deciduous shrub found in woodland and mountains in China and Japan. It is grown for its striking autumn colour, graduating from yellow through red to purple, and displaying all these shades at once. The ovate to rounded leaves are alternate, and the slightly fragrant, spidery flowers are borne in pairs in mid-autumn as the leaves fall. Grow *D. cercidifolius* as a specimen in a woodland garden.

• **HARDINESS** Fully hardy, but late frosts may damage young growth.
• **CULTIVATION** Grow in humus-rich, moist but well-drained, lime-free soil in sun or partial shade, sheltered from strong winds. Pruning group 1.
• **PROPAGATION** Sow seed in a seedbed in autumn or spring. Layer in spring.
• **PESTS AND DISEASES** Trouble free.

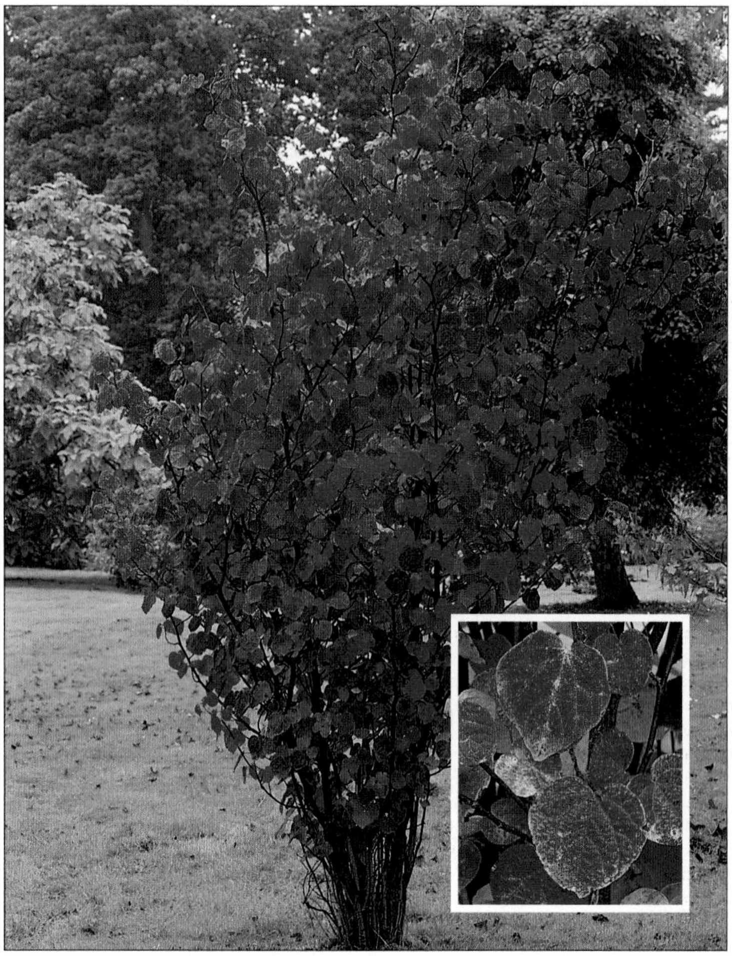

Disanthus cercidifolius (inset: leaf detail)

D. cercidifolius ▣ 🏆 Rounded shrub with ovate to rounded, glaucous, blue-green leaves, to 10cm (4in) long, with heart-shaped bases, turning yellow, orange, red, and purple in autumn. Slightly fragrant, axillary, spidery, bright rose-red flowers, 2cm (¾in) across, are produced in mid-autumn. ↕↔ 3m (10ft). C. China, Japan. ✻✻✻

DISCARIA

RHAMNACEAE

Genus of about 15 species of spiny, deciduous shrubs and small trees from Australia, New Zealand, and temperate South America, found in rocky places and scrub, and closely allied to *Colletia*. They produce opposite or clustered, mainly elliptic to obovate or oblong leaves, opposite pairs of spines on stiff or flexuous branches, and star- or bell-shaped flowers, often with petals absent. *Discaria* species are grown for their numerous thick spines and their abundant, densely clustered flowers. In warm climates, they are suitable for an open shrub border; in cooler conditions, they grow best at the base of a warm, sunny, sheltered wall.

• **HARDINESS** Fully hardy to frost hardy.
• **CULTIVATION** Grow in fertile, well-drained soil in full sun. In cold regions, shelter from hard frost and cold, drying winds. Pruning group 1, after flowering.
• **PROPAGATION** Sow seed in containers in a cold frame in autumn or spring. Insert greenwood cuttings in early summer or semi-ripe cuttings in late summer.
• **PESTS AND DISEASES** Trouble free.

D. toumatou ⚲ (Wild Irishman). Large shrub or small tree bearing cylindrical, flexuous, slender green stems; numerous slender, opposite green spines, to 5cm (2in) long, are borne at right-angles to the stems. Obovate to narrowly oblong, glossy leaves, to 2cm (¾in) long, borne below the spines on year-old shoots, fall early. Bears dense clusters of star-shaped, greenish white flowers, 3mm (⅛in) across, composed of 4 or 5 small sepals, in late spring. ↕ 2.5m (8ft), ↔ 3m (10ft). New Zealand. ✻✻

DISCOCACTUS

CACTACEAE

Genus of 5–7 species of ribbed, spherical, perennial cacti from hilly lowlands in Brazil, E. Bolivia, and N. Paraguay. Most have prominent areoles and strong, often horny spines. Mature plants develop a woolly and bristly-spiny cephalium, from which funnel-shaped or tubular, salverform, scented, white or pink flowers, 5–10cm (2–4in long), are produced at night in summer. The berries contain minute black seeds. Suitable for a desert garden. In frost-prone areas, grow in a warm greenhouse or as houseplants.

• **HARDINESS** Frost tender.
• **CULTIVATION** Under glass, grow in standard cactus compost in full light. In the growing season, water moderately, applying a nitrogen- and potassium-based fertilizer every 3 weeks. Keep completely dry from autumn to early spring. Outdoors, grow in sharply drained, mineral soil, low in organic matter, in full sun. See also pp.48–49.

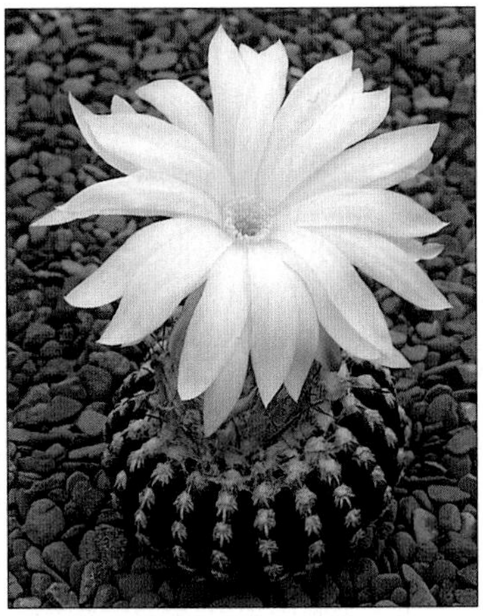

Discocactus horstii

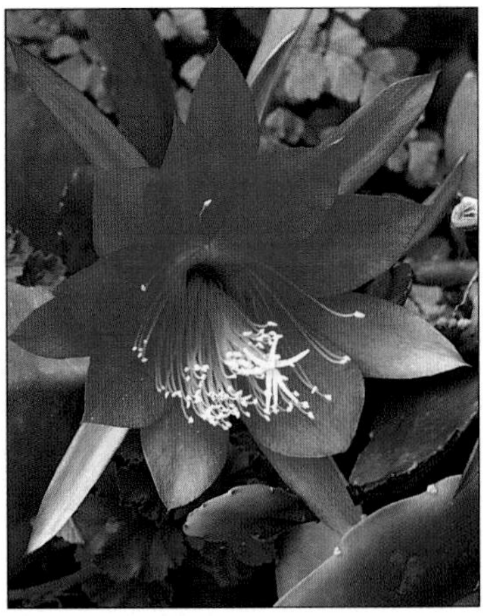

Disocactus nelsonii

• **PROPAGATION** Sow seed at 21–24°C (70–75°F) in spring or early summer.
• **PESTS AND DISEASES** Vulnerable to mealybugs.

D. hartmannii, syn. *Echinocactus hartmannii.* Flattened-spherical to spherical cactus with a white-woolly, tufted cephalium, 15–22 dark green ribs, and well-spaced areoles bearing blackish brown spines (6–12 radials and 1 central). Funnel-shaped, many-petalled white flowers, to 10cm (4in) across, are produced in summer. ↕10cm (4in), ↔ to 25cm (10in). Brazil, N. Paraguay. ❄ (min. 16°C/61°F)
D. horstii ■ Flattened-spherical cactus with a white-woolly cephalium, 15–22 prominent, brownish green to purple-brown ribs, and close-set areoles, each bearing 8–10 minute, greyish white to chalky white radial spines. Open funnel-shaped white flowers, to 8cm (3in) across, are produced in summer. ↕2–3cm (¾–1¼in), ↔ to 6cm (2½in). E. Brazil. ❄ (min. 16°C/61°F)
D. placentiformis, syn. *D. tricornis.* Flattened-spherical cactus, sometimes producing offsets, with a white-woolly cephalium, 10–16 light to dark green or blue-green ribs, and few areoles, bearing brownish white spines (3–8 curved radials and often a shorter, straight central). Funnel-shaped white flowers, to 9cm (3½in) across, are borne in summer. ↕5–10cm (2–4in), ↔ 10cm (4in). E. Brazil. ❄ (min. 16°C/61°F)
D. tricornis see *D. placentiformis.*

DISOCACTUS

CACTACEAE

Genus of 10 species of freely branching, epiphytic or rock-dwelling, perennial cacti, found in rainforest in subtropical and tropical Central and South America, and the West Indies. They have cylindrical primary stems, rounded in cross-section, and flattened lateral stems. Funnel-shaped or tubular, diurnal flowers, sometimes sweetly scented, are borne on marginal areoles, followed by spherical to ovoid, usually white or greenish white fruits with black seeds. In frost-prone areas, grow in a container or hanging basket in a warm greenhouse; in warmer regions, grow epiphytically.
• **HARDINESS** Frost tender.
• **CULTIVATION** Under glass, grow in acidic, epiphytic cactus compost in bright filtered light and low humidity. In the growing season, water freely, applying fertilizer in spring and again in late autumn; keep just moist in winter. Outdoors, grow epiphytically in partial shade. See also pp.48–49.
• **PROPAGATION** Sow seed at 27°C (81°F) as soon as ripe in loamless seed compost, in a closed case and filtered light; keep the compost moist. Root stem cuttings in late spring.
• **PESTS AND DISEASES** Vulnerable to mealybugs.

D. alatus, syn. *Pseudorhipsalis alata.* Freely branching cactus with pendent primary stems, to 5m (15ft) across, bearing broadly linear to lance-shaped or oblong, leaf-like, flat, scalloped-wavy lateral stems. Open funnel-shaped, yellowish cream or greenish white flowers, 1.5cm (½in) across, are borne in late spring. ↕30cm (12in), ↔ 15cm (6in). Jamaica. ❄ (min. 16°C/61°F)
D. amazonicus, syn. *Wittia amazonica, Wittiocactus amazonicus.* Freely branching cactus bearing oblong-lance-shaped, leaf-like, flattened stems, 15–30cm (6–12in) long, with coarsely toothed margins and prominent mid-ribs. Bears tubular magenta flowers, 2–3cm (¾–1¼in) across, in late spring. ↕45cm (18in), ↔ 20cm (8in). N.W. Peru, Colombia. ❄ (min. 16°C/61°F)
D. biformis, syn. *Phyllocactus biformis.* Freely branching cactus with cylindrical primary stems, to 20cm (8in) long, bearing linear or narrowly oblong lateral stems with toothed margins. Narrowly funnel-shaped, deep red to magenta flowers, 5–6cm (2–2½in) long, are produced in early spring. ↕↔ 20cm (8in). Guatemala, Honduras. ❄ (min. 16°C/61°F)
D. eichlamii, syn. *Phyllocactus eichlamii.* Freely branching cactus with slender primary stems, to 75cm (30in) long, bearing narrowly lance-shaped, toothed, flattened lateral stems. Funnel-shaped, carmine-red flowers, to 6cm (2½in) long, are borne in early spring. ↕30cm (12in), ↔ 45cm (18in). Guatemala. ❄ (min. 16°C/61°F)
D. macranthus, syn. *Pseudorhipsalis macrantha.* Bushy cactus producing a cylindrical base and pendent, strap-shaped, slightly toothed stems, to 90cm (36in) across. Bears numerous tubular-salverform, sweetly scented flowers, 6cm (2½in) across, pink-purple at the bases, with pale orange-brown outer tepals, lemon-yellow inside, in late winter and early spring. ↕60cm (24in), ↔ 30cm (12in). S. Mexico. ❄ (min. 16°C/61°F)
D. nelsonii ■ ♀ syn. *Chiapasia nelsonii.* Freely branching cactus with cylindrical primary stems, to 1.5m (5ft) long, and pendent, inversely lance-shaped, slightly toothed, flattened lateral stems. Funnel-shaped, scented, purplish pink flowers, 9–11cm (3½–4½in) across, are borne from spring to early summer. ↕50cm (20in) or more, ↔ 25cm (10in). Mexico to Honduras. ❄ (min. 16°C/61°F)
D. quezaltecus, syn. *Bonifazia quezalteca.* Freely branching cactus with primary stems, to 80cm (32in) long, flattened at the top, and toothed, leaf-like lateral stems. Tubular-salverform, pale purple to purple-red flowers, 9cm (3½in) across, are borne from spring to early summer. ↕60cm (24in), ↔ 30cm (12in). Guatemala. ❄ (min. 16°C/61°F)

DISPOROPSIS

CONVALLARIACEAE/LILIACEAE

Genus of 4 species, closely allied to *Polygonatum*, of rhizomatous, evergreen perennials, occurring in upland forest in S.E. China. Mottled, dark green stems bear lance-shaped-elliptic, waxy leaves, which gradually die back as new growth is fully formed. Pendent, narrowly bell-shaped flowers are solitary or produced in pairs from the leaf axils. Grow in a woodland garden or peat bed.
• **HARDINESS** Fully hardy.
• **CULTIVATION** Grow in moist but well-drained, humus-rich, leafy soil in partial shade.
• **PROPAGATION** Sow seed in containers in a cold frame in autumn or spring, or divide rhizomes in spring.
• **PESTS AND DISEASES** Trouble free.

D. pernyi ■ syn. *Polygonatum cyrtonema* of gardens. Rhizomatous perennial with lance-shaped to elliptic, glossy, dark green leaves, to 12cm (5in) long. Lemon-scented white flowers, 2cm (¾in) long, with pale green outer tips that are slightly reflexed, are produced singly or in pairs in early summer. ↕40cm (16in), ↔ 30–40cm (12–16in). S.E. China. ✱✱✱

DISPORUM *syn.* PROSARTES

Fairy bells

CONVALLARIACEAE/LILIACEAE

Genus of 10–20 species of rhizomatous perennials occurring in woodland in the Himalayas, E. and S.E. Asia, and temperate North America. The mid- to dark green leaves are ovate to lance-shaped, stalkless or with short stalks, usually hairless, and borne alternately on sparsely branched stems. Often pendent, narrowly bell-shaped, tubular, open trumpet-shaped, or cup-shaped, white to green-yellow, purple-red, or brown-red flowers, 1–3cm (½–1¼in) long, are usually borne in few-flowered umbels, occasionally singly. They are followed by orange, red, or black berries. Grow in a woodland garden or on a peat bank. In frost-prone areas, grow half-hardy and tender species in a cool greenhouse.
• **HARDINESS** Fully hardy to frost tender.
• **CULTIVATION** Grow in cool, moist, well-drained, humus-rich soil in partial shade. *D. smithii* tolerates deep shade.
• **PROPAGATION** Sow seed in containers in a cold frame in autumn; alternatively, divide rhizomes in spring, before or as growth begins.

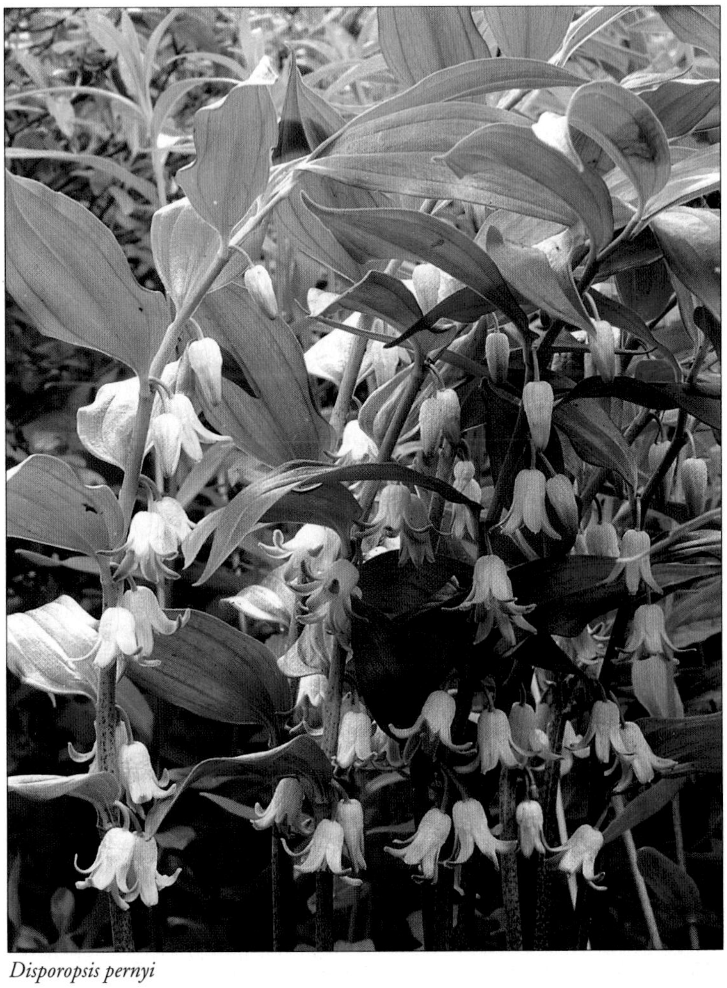

Disporopsis pernyi

D

D

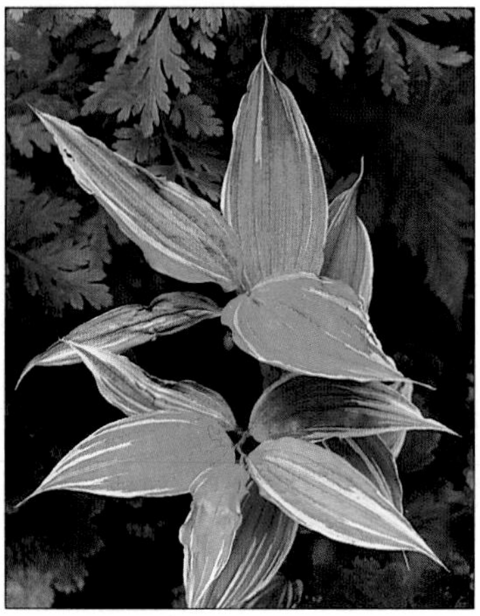

Disporum sessile 'Variegatum'

• **PESTS AND DISEASES** Slugs and vine weevils may be troublesome.

D. cantoniense. Clump-forming, rhizomatous perennial bearing lance-shaped leaves, 5–15cm (2–6in) long. Bears umbels of 3–6 pendent, tubular, purplish red, brownish red, or white flowers, on short stalks, in late spring and early summer, followed in early autumn by black-red berries. ↕ to 90cm (36in), ↔ 30cm (12in). Himalayas, China, S.E. Asia. ❄ (borderline)
D. flavens. Clump-forming, rhizomatous perennial bearing lance-shaped leaves, 5–15cm (2–6in) long. In early spring, 1–3 pendent, tubular, soft yellow flowers are produced on axillary stalks, followed in early autumn by black berries. ↕ to 75cm (30in), ↔ 30cm (12in). Korea. ❄❄❄
D. hookeri. Clump-forming, rhizomatous perennial producing ovate to lance-shaped leaves, 3–14cm (1¼–5½in) long, with heart-shaped bases, hairy on the margins and on the veins beneath. Umbels of up to 3 pendent, tubular-bell-shaped, greenish cream flowers, with slightly spreading tepals, are produced in late spring, followed in early autumn by orange-red berries. ↕ to 90cm (36in), ↔ 45cm (18in). N.W. USA. ❄❄❄
D. lanuginosum. Clump-forming, rhizomatous perennial with ovate-lance-shaped leaves, 3–12cm (1¼–5in) long, with narrow, pointed tips, downy beneath. Umbels of up to 3 open trumpet-shaped, pale yellowish white or greenish white flowers, with narrow tepals, are borne in late spring, followed in early autumn by black or red berries. ↕ 30–90cm (12–36in), ↔ 30cm (12in). Central E. USA. ❄❄❄
D. sessile. Spreading, rhizomatous perennial with almost stalkless, oblong or oblong-lance-shaped leaves, 5–15cm (2–6in) long. Each stem produces 2 or 3 flower stalks, each bearing up to 3 pendent, tubular, green-tipped white or very pale cream flowers in late spring and early summer, followed in early autumn by black berries. ↕ 60cm (24in), ↔ 60cm (24in) or more. Japan. ❄❄❄. **'Variegatum'** ▣ has leaves broadly and variously striped white; ↕ 45cm (18in), ↔ 90cm (36in) or more.
D. smilacinum. Sparsely branched, rhizomatous perennial with oblong to elliptic-ovate leaves, 4–7cm (1½–3in) long. Stems, 15–40cm (6–16in) long, produce 1 or 2 pendent or semi-pendent, cup-shaped white flowers in mid- and late spring. ↕ to 40cm (16in), ↔ 30cm (12in). Korea, Japan. ❄❄❄
D. smithii ▣ Clump-forming, rhizomatous perennial with red-tinged stems and ovate to ovate-lance-shaped leaves, 5–12cm (2–5in) long, rounded to heart-shaped at the bases. Umbels of 2–6 pendent, tubular-bell-shaped, greenish white flowers are borne from early to late spring; flowers are followed in late summer by orange berries. ↕ 30–60cm (12–24in), ↔ 30cm (12in). W. North America (British Columbia to California). ❄❄❄

DISTICTIS

BIGNONIACEAE

Genus of 9 species of climbing, evergreen perennials from Mexico and the West Indies, usually among thickets and at forest margins. They are valued for their colourful, tubular to trumpet-shaped or salverform flowers, produced in small, terminal racemes or panicles. The opposite leaves consist of 2 ovate-lance-shaped leaflets and a 3-branched tendril. In frost-prone climates, grow in a cool greenhouse; in warmer regions, train on a pergola or wall, or grow through trees.
• **HARDINESS** Frost tender, although *D. buccinatoria* may survive short periods near to or below 0°C (32°F).
• **CULTIVATION** Under glass, grow in loam-based potting compost (JI No.3) in full light. Support with wires or trellis and tie in as growth proceeds. In the growing season, water freely, applying fertilizer monthly; water sparingly in winter. Top-dress or pot on in spring. Outdoors, grow in fertile, moist but well-drained soil in full sun. Pruning group 11, in early spring.
• **PROPAGATION** Sow seed at 16–18°C (61–64°F) in spring. Root semi-ripe cuttings with bottom heat in summer. Layer in early spring.
• **PESTS AND DISEASES** Red spider mites and whiteflies may be troublesome under glass.

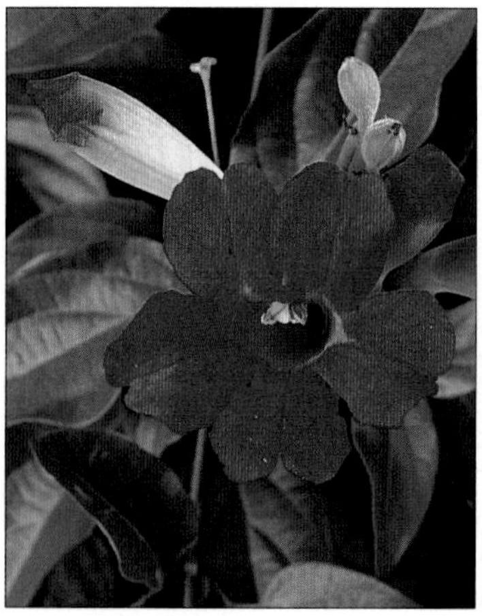

Distictis buccinatoria

D. buccinatoria ▣ syn. *Phaedranthus buccinatorius.* Vigorous climber bearing ovate-lance-shaped, mid- to deep green leaflets, to 10cm (4in) long. Tubular-salverform, purple-red flowers, to 8cm (3in) long, with yellow towards the bases, are borne in racemes, 15–25cm (6–10in) long, from summer to autumn. ↕ 10–25m (30–80ft). Mexico. ❄ (borderline)

DISTYLIUM

HAMAMELIDACEAE

Genus of about 6–8 species of evergreen shrubs and trees found in woodland in E. Asia. They have alternate, obovate or ovate to lance-shaped, leathery, usually dark green leaves, and petalless, male and bisexual flowers in axillary spikes or racemes. *D. racemosum* is valued for its simple, glossy foliage, borne on arching branches, and for its unusual flowers. Grow in a sheltered position among trees and other shrubs.
• **HARDINESS** Frost hardy to frost tender.
• **CULTIVATION** Grow in moist but well-drained, humus-rich soil in partial shade, sheltered from strong, cold, drying winds. Pruning group 1, but pruning is not usually necessary.
• **PROPAGATION** Sow seed in containers in a cold frame as soon as ripe. Insert semi-ripe cuttings in summer.
• **PESTS AND DISEASES** Trouble free.

D. racemosum ♀ Spreading shrub or tree with obovate to narrowly oblong, leathery, glossy, dark green leaves, 3–7cm (1¼–3in) long. Small flowers are produced in upright racemes, 2.5–5cm (1–2in) long, in late spring and early summer; they lack petals but have conspicuous, 5-parted red calyces and purple stamens. ↕ 2–3m (6–10ft) (tree to 25m/80ft in the wild), ↔ 3m (10ft). S. Japan. ❄❄

▷**Dittany** see *Dictamnus albus*
Cretan see *Origanum dictamnus*

▷***Dizygotheca elegantissima*** see *Schefflera elegantissima*
▷**Dock** see *Rumex*
Bloody see *Rumex sanguineus*
Prairie see *Silphium*
Red-veined see *Rumex sanguineus*
▷**Dockmackie** see *Viburnum acerifolium*

DOCYNIA

ROSACEAE

Genus of 2 species of evergreen, semi-evergreen, or deciduous trees and shrubs, occurring in woodland in the Himalayas and E. Asia. The oblong to ovate or lance-shaped leaves, borne alternately, are either entire or toothed. Bowl-shaped, white or pinkish white flowers are produced in umbels of 2–6. *D. delavayi* is an attractive flowering specimen tree or shrub, suitable for a sheltered site.
• **HARDINESS** Frost hardy.
• **CULTIVATION** Grow in fertile, well-drained soil in sun or partial shade. Provide protection from strong winds. Pruning group 1, but pruning is not usually necessary.
• **PROPAGATION** Sow seed in containers in a cold frame in autumn or spring.
• **PESTS AND DISEASES** Susceptible to fireblight. Caterpillars may also be troublesome.

D. delavayi ♀ Spreading, semi-evergreen to deciduous tree with tiered branches, spiny, blackish green shoots, and alternate, narrowly to broadly ovate-lance-shaped, usually entire, toothed, dark green leaves, to 7cm (3in) long. (On young seedlings, leaves are hawthorn-like and deeply lobed.) Produces umbels of 2–4 bowl-shaped white flowers, to 2.5cm (1in) across, from pink buds in spring, followed by small, apple-like yellow fruit, 4cm (1½in) across, in autumn. ↕↔ 8m (25ft). China (Sichuan, Yunnan). ❄❄

DODECATHEON

American cowslip, Shooting stars

PRIMULACEAE

Genus of 14 species of perennials mostly found in damp grassland or high alpine meadows, occasionally in woodland, in North America. They have basal rosettes of ovate to inversely lance-shaped, spoon-shaped, or oblong, usually hairless leaves. Umbels of pendent, cyclamen-like flowers are produced on arching stems, the petals acutely reflexed, displaying long, pointed styles. American cowslips become dormant in summer, after flowering. They are suitable for a woodland or rock garden.
• **HARDINESS** Most are fully hardy, although *D. clevelandii* may be damaged by early frosts.
• **CULTIVATION** Grow in moist but well-drained, humus-rich soil in sun or partial shade, with abundant moisture in the growing season; grow *D. dentatum* and *D. pulchellum* in moist shade. During summer dormancy, keep *D. clevelandii* and *D. hendersonii* in a bulb frame.
• **PROPAGATION** Sow seed in containers in an open frame as soon as ripe; the seed needs exposure to cold before it will germinate. Divide in spring.
• **PESTS AND DISEASES** Young leaves may be eaten by slugs and snails.

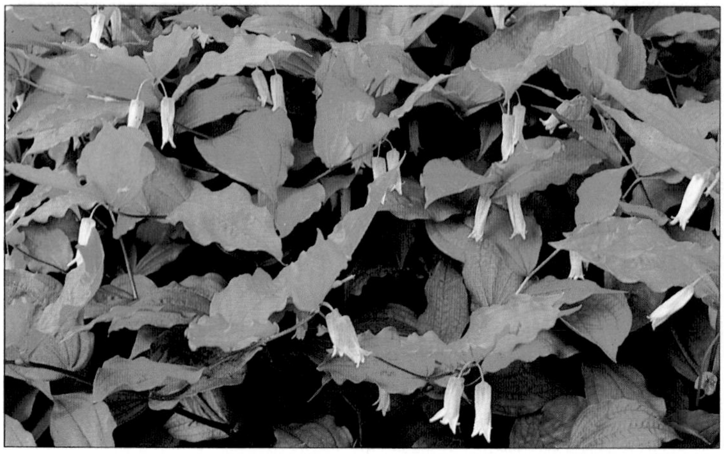

Disporum smithii

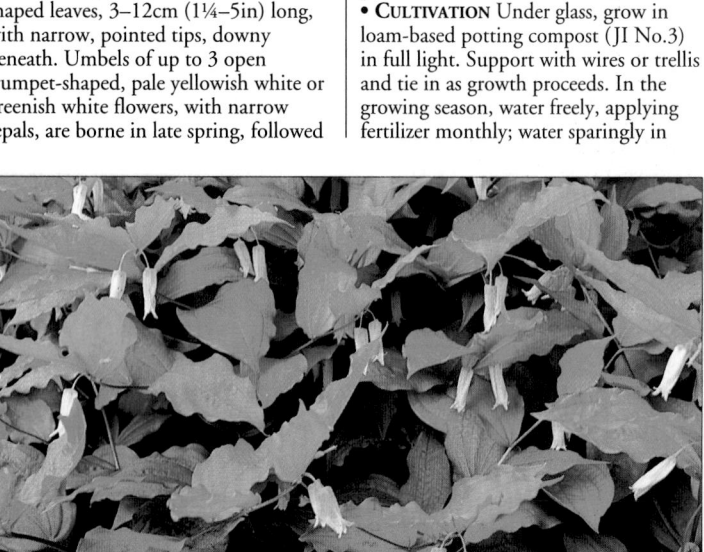

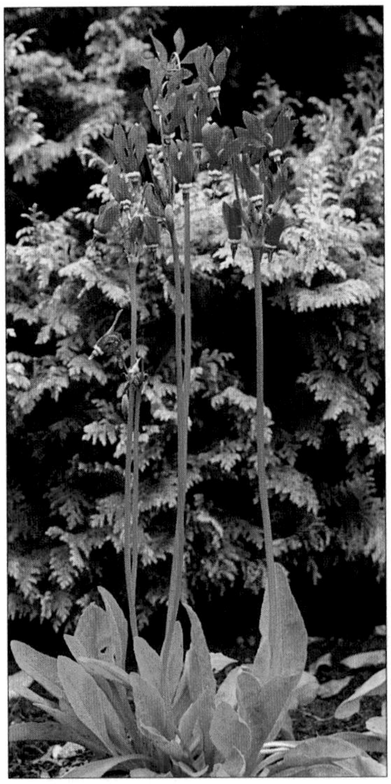

Dodecatheon clevelandii

D. amethystinum see *D. pulchellum.*
D. clevelandii ▣ Rosette-forming perennial with spoon-shaped to ovate, irregularly toothed, fleshy, pale green leaves, to 6cm (2½in) long. Produces umbels of up to 20 reddish purple flowers, to 2cm (¾in) long, with yellow tubes, spotted purple at the throats, in early spring. ↕ to 40cm (16in), ↔ to 15cm (6in). USA (California). ❄❄❄ (borderline). **subsp. *insulare*** flowers in late spring; ❄❄❄
D. dentatum ▣ 🏆 Clump-forming perennial with rosettes of long-stalked, oblong-lance-shaped, sometimes toothed, pale to mid-green leaves, to 8cm (3in) long. In late spring, bears umbels of 2–5 slender-stemmed white flowers, 1–2cm (½–¾in) long, sometimes purple-spotted at the petal bases, with prominent, dark purple anthers. ↕↔ to 20cm (8in). W. North America. ❄❄❄
D. hendersonii 🏆 syn. *D. latifolium* (Mosquito bills, Sailor caps). Rosette-forming perennial with oblong-ovate, fleshy, dark green leaves, to 6cm (2½in) long. Sturdy stems produce umbels of 1–5 dark-centred, purplish pink flowers, 1.5–2.5cm (½–1in) long, each with a

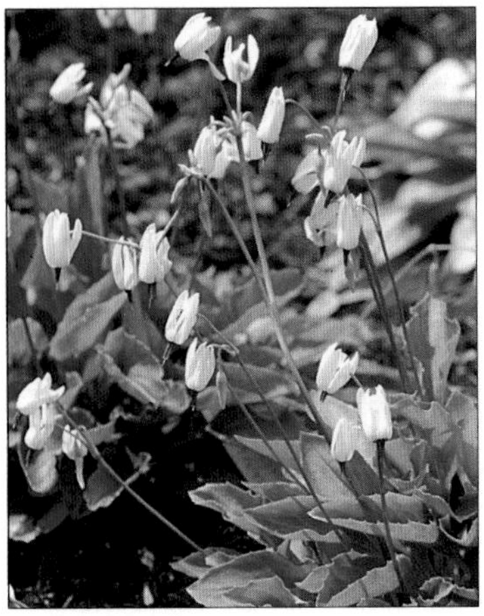

Dodecatheon dentatum

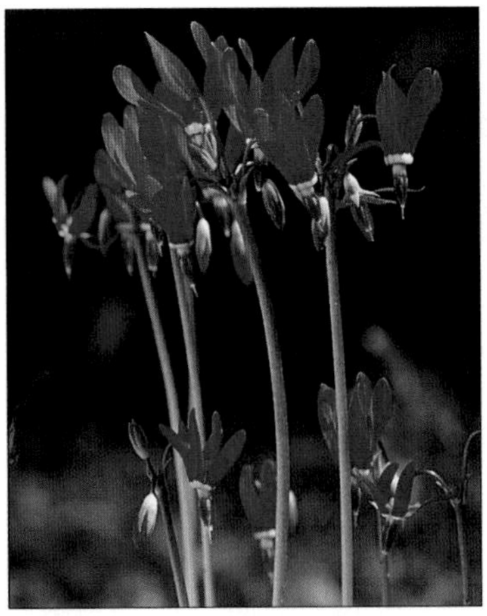

Dodecatheon pulchellum 'Red Wings'

white ring at the base, in early summer. ↕ 40cm (16in), ↔ 25cm (10in). USA (California). ❄❄❄
D. latifolium see *D. hendersonii.*
D. meadia 🏆 syn. *D. pauciflorum* (Shooting star). Variable, clump-forming perennial with ovate, toothed, pale to mid-green leaves, to 25cm (10in) long. Umbels of up to 15 magenta-pink flowers, 1.5–2cm (½–¾in) long, are borne on strong stems in mid- and late spring. ↕ 40cm (16in), ↔ 25cm (10in). N.W. USA. ❄❄❄. **f. *album*** 🏆 has creamy white flowers, with dark centres, and yellow styles and anthers.
D. pauciflorum see *D. meadia.*
***D. pauciflorum* of gardens** see *D. pulchellum.*
D. pulchellum 🏆 syn. *D. amethystinum, D. pauciflorum* of gardens, *D. radicatum.* Clump-forming perennial with ovate-spoon-shaped, mid-green leaves, to 20cm (8in) long. Umbels of up to 20 dark-centred, deep cerise-pink flowers, 1–2cm (½–¾in) long, are produced in mid- and late spring. ↕ to 35cm (14in), ↔ to 15cm (6in). High altitudes in W. North America. ❄❄❄. **'Red Wings'** ▣ has oblong-ovate, soft, pale green leaves, and produces deep magenta-pink flowers, 1–2cm (½–¾in) long, on strong stems in late spring and early summer; ↔ 20cm (8in).
D. radicatum see *D. pulchellum.*

DODONAEA

SAPINDACEAE

Genus of 50–60 species of evergreen shrubs and small trees found in tropical and subtropical regions, but primarily in Australia, where they grow in dry, open forest, thickets, and scrub. They are grown mainly for their needle-like or oblong to broadly ovate or obovate, simple or pinnate, leathery leaves, dotted with glands and spiralling or scattered along the stems. The insignificant, petal-less flowers, with 3- to 5-lobed calyces, are borne in terminal and axillary cymes, male and female on separate plants. The fruits are membranous, 3-angled or 3-winged (sometimes up to 6-winged), often colourful capsules. In frost-prone areas, grow in a cool greenhouse. Elsewhere, use as a hedge or in a border. *D. viscosa* tolerates drought and exposure to wind, salt, and atmospheric pollution.
• **HARDINESS** Frost tender; *D. viscosa* survives short spells near to 0°C (32°F).
• **CULTIVATION** Under glass, grow in loam-based potting compost (JI No.2)

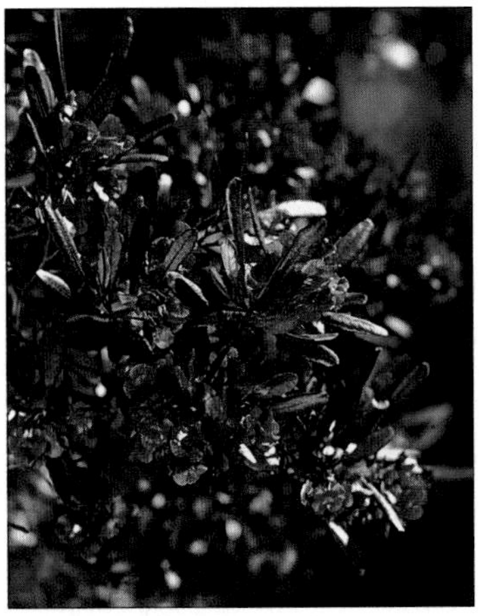

Dodonaea viscosa 'Purpurea'

in full light. In growth, water freely and apply a balanced liquid fertilizer monthly; water sparingly in winter. Top-dress or pot on in spring. Outdoors, grow in moderately fertile, moist but well-drained soil in full sun. Pinch out tips of young shoots to encourage bushy growth. Pruning group 1: clip hedges lightly in spring.
• **PROPAGATION** Sow seed at no less than 18°C (64°F) in spring. Root semi-ripe cuttings with bottom heat in summer.
• **PESTS AND DISEASES** Red spider mites may infest greenhouse plants.

D. viscosa ◊ (Hop bush). Vigorous, erect to spreading shrub or small tree with elliptic to almost obovate, simple, yellow to mid-green leaves, 7–13cm (3–5in) long, with irregular, wavy margins. Bears 2- or 3-winged, pink to reddish brown, light brown, purple, or yellow capsules, 2–2.5cm (¾–1in) across, from summer to autumn. ↕ 1–5m (3–15ft), ↔ 1–3m (3–10ft). Coastal regions in tropics and subtropics worldwide. ❄ (borderline). **'Purpurea'** ▣ has leaves strongly suffused purplish red.

▷ **Dog violet** see *Viola canina*
  Common see *V. riviniana*
  Western see *V. adunca*
▷ **Dog's-tooth violet** see *Erythronium*
  European see *E. dens-canis*
▷ **Dogwood** see *Cornus*
  Common see *C. sanguinea*
  Creeping see *C. canadensis*
  Flowering see *C. florida*
  Pacific see *C. nuttallii*
  Pagoda see *C. alternifolia*
  Red-barked see *C. alba*
  Red osier see *C. stolonifera*
▷ ***Dolichos*** see *Lablab*
  D. lablab see *L. purpureus*
  D. niger see *L. purpureus*
  D. purpureus see *L. purpureus*
▷ ***Dolichothele baumii*** see *Mammillaria baumii*
▷ ***Dolichothele camptotricha*** see *Mammillaria camptotricha*
▷ **Doll's eyes** see *Actaea alba*

DOMBEYA

STERCULIACEAE

Genus of 200–300 species of evergreen or deciduous shrubs and trees from Africa and Madagascar to the Mascarene Islands, found in habitats ranging from tropical woodland to upland scrub. Leaves are alternate, simple, and lobed or unlobed, often heart-shaped, with long stalks. Dombeyas are grown mainly for their 5-petalled, white, pink, yellow, or red flowers, resembling those of mallows (*Malva*); they are produced in dense, axillary, terminal, or umbel-like cymes on long, nodding or pendent stalks. In frost-prone areas, grow in a warm greenhouse; elsewhere, use outdoors as a specimen or in a border.
• **HARDINESS** Frost tender.
• **CULTIVATION** Under glass, grow in loam-based potting compost, in bright filtered light or in full light with shade from hot sun. In the growing season, water freely, applying a balanced liquid fertilizer monthly; water sparingly in winter. Top-dress or pot on in spring. Outdoors, grow in fertile, moist but well-drained soil in sun or partial shade. Pruning group 6 (deciduous), 8 (evergreen); plants under glass may need restrictive pruning.
• **PROPAGATION** Sow seed at 18–21°C (64–70°F) in spring. Root semi-ripe cuttings with bottom heat in summer.
• **PESTS AND DISEASES** Susceptible to red spider mites and whiteflies under glass.

D. burgessiae, syn. *D. mastersii.* Strong-growing, open, evergreen shrub with softly hairy young stems and broadly ovate to rounded (heart-shaped at the bases), 3- to 5-lobed or unlobed, downy, mid-green leaves, 11–22cm (4½–9in) long. Axillary corymbs or cymes, 10cm (4in) or more across, of fragrant, red- or pink-veined white flowers, 5–8cm (2–3in) across, are borne from late summer to autumn. ↕ 2–4m (6–12ft), ↔ 1.5–3m (5–10ft). Kenya to South Africa. ❀ (min. 10°C/50°F)
D. x cayeuxii ▣ ◊ (*D. burgessiae* x *D. wallichii*). Vigorous, evergreen shrub or small tree with bristly-hairy stems and ovate to heart-shaped, acute, toothed, hairy, mid- to dark green leaves, 20–30cm (8–12in) long. Produces pink flowers, 3–4cm (1¼–1½in) across, in many-flowered, spherical, umbel-like cymes, 10–13cm (4–5in) across, usually from autumn to spring. ↕ 3–5m (10–15ft), ↔ 2–3m (6–10ft). Garden origin. ❀ (min. 10°C/50°F)
D. mastersii see *D. burgessiae.*
D. wallichii ◊ Evergreen shrub or tree of variable habit but generally freely branching, with sturdy, downy stems. The broadly ovate to rounded, toothed, bright green leaves, 15–20cm (6–8in) long, softly hairy beneath, have pointed tips and heart-shaped bases. Deep pink or red flowers, 3–5cm (1¼–2in) across,

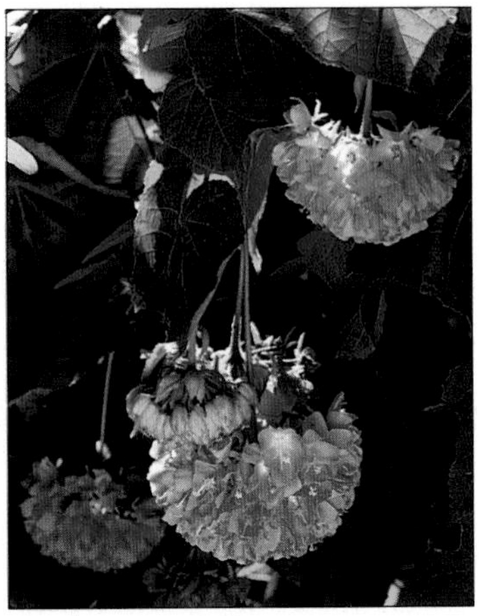

Dombeya x *cayeuxii*

are borne in dense, umbel-like cymes, 10–15cm (4–6in) across, mainly from winter to spring. ↕ 6–10m (20–30ft), ↔ 2.5–5m (8–15ft). E. Africa, Madagascar. ❀ (min. 10°C/50°F)

▷ ***Dondia*** see *Hacquetia*
D. epipactis *see H. epipactis*

D

DOODIA

BLECHNACEAE

Genus of about 11 species of usually evergreen, terrestrial ferns found mainly in damp, sunny or partially shaded sites, often rocky woodland margins, in Australasia. Fronds, produced in tufts from short, creeping rhizomes, are lance-shaped, pinnate or pinnatifid, and usually pink tinged when young. Fertile fronds are often more erect than sterile fronds, with slightly narrower divisions. The sori are covered by curved indusia. *Doodia* species are easy to grow, thriving in a rock garden or sheltered border; in frost-prone areas, grow tender and half-hardy species in a cool greenhouse.

• **HARDINESS** Frost hardy to frost tender.
• **CULTIVATION** Under glass, grow in a mix of 1 part each loam, medium-grade bark, and charcoal, 2 parts sharp sand, and 3 parts coarse leaf mould. Provide bright filtered light and moderate humidity. Water freely when in growth. In winter, admit full light and water sparingly. Outdoors, grow in moist, acid soil in sheltered partial shade. In frost-prone areas, cover crowns with a straw mulch in winter.
• **PROPAGATION** Sow spores at 15°C (59°F) as soon as ripe. Divide in late spring. See also p.51.
• **PESTS AND DISEASES** Trouble free.

D. media (Common rasp fern). Tufted, evergreen fern with suberect rhizomes, and lance-shaped to inversely lance-shaped, leathery, dark green fronds, 30–60cm (12–24in) long, pinnatifid at the tips and pinnate towards the bases, often with brown midribs. Ovate-heart-shaped pinnae have a firm, prickly texture and very finely toothed margins. ↕ 30–40cm (12–16in), ↔ 50–100cm (20–39in). Australia, New Zealand, Pacific Islands to Hawaii. ❄❄

DORONICUM

Leopard's bane

ASTERACEAE/COMPOSITAE

Genus of about 35 species of deciduous, rhizomatous or tuberous perennials from woodland, scrub, meadows, heathland, and rocky sites in Europe, S.W. Asia, and Siberia. They have alternate, elliptic to ovate basal leaves, with heart-shaped bases, and lance-shaped to ovate or oblong stem leaves. The daisy-like yellow flowerheads are borne singly or in cyme-like corymbs. Grow in a border or naturalize in a woodland garden. The flowers are also good for cutting.

• **HARDINESS** Fully hardy.
• **CULTIVATION** Grow in moist, humus-rich soil in partial or dappled shade. *D. orientale* and its cultivars are prone to root rot in wet areas, and need moist but well-drained, reasonably fertile, preferably sandy soil in partial shade.
• **PROPAGATION** Sow seed in containers in a cold frame in spring. Alternatively, divide in early autumn.

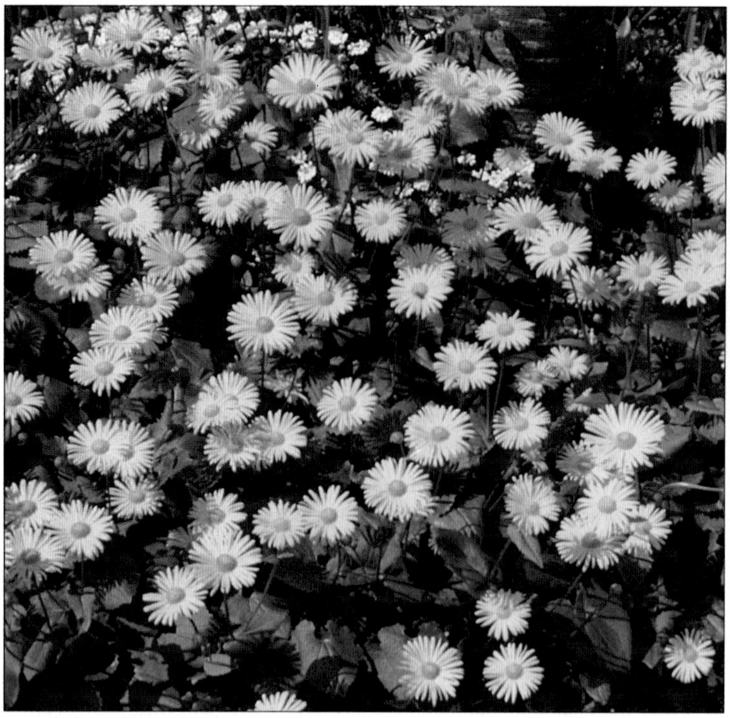

Doronicum columnae 'Miss Mason'

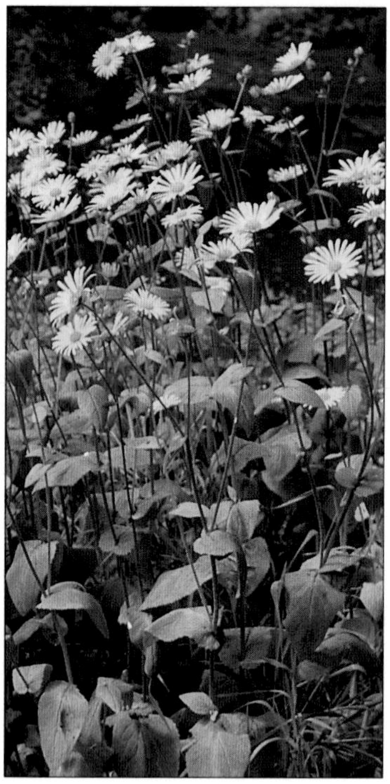

Doronicum pardalianches

• **PESTS AND DISEASES** Leaf spot and root rot may be troublesome, and some species are susceptible to powdery mildew.

D. austriacum. Clump-forming, rhizomatous perennial bearing ovate-oblong, toothed, hairy basal leaves, 13cm (5in) long, heart-shaped at the bases, usually at or just after flowering; the stem leaves are smaller, narrower, and either entire or minutely toothed. Produces corymbs of yellow flowerheads, 3.5–6cm (1½–2½in) across, on slender, branched stems, in late spring and early summer. ↕↔ to 1.2m (4ft). Mountain woodland in C. and S. Europe, Turkey. ❄❄❄
D. caucasicum see *D. orientale.*

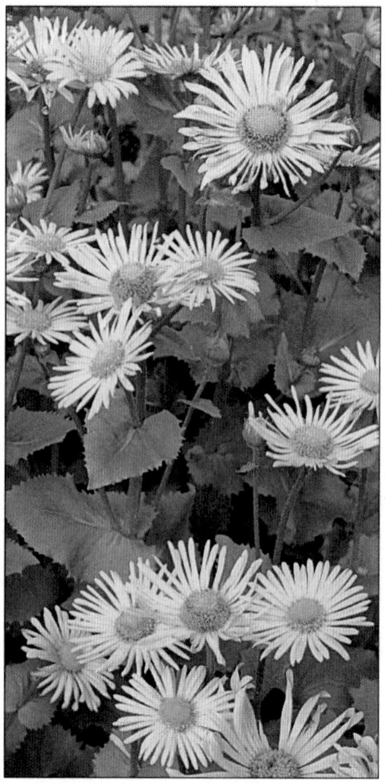

Doronicum x *excelsum* 'Harpur Crewe'

D. columnae, syn. *D. cordatum.* Clump-forming, rhizomatous perennial bearing clustered, ovate-rounded to heart-shaped, toothed, hairy or hairless, scalloped basal leaves, 3–8cm (1¼–3in) long, and elliptic to ovate-lance-shaped stem leaves. Slender stems bear solitary yellow flowerheads, 2–7cm (¾–3in) across, from mid-spring to early summer. ↕ 12–60cm (5–24in), ↔ 30cm (12in). Mountains of S. and E. Europe. ❄❄❄. **'Miss Mason'** ■ 🏆 has bright yellow flowerheads, 8cm (3in) across, held well above the foliage, in mid- and late spring; ↔ 60cm (24in).
D. cordatum see *D. columnae, D. pardalianches.*
***D.* x *excelsum* 'Harpur Crewe'** ■ syn. *D. plantagineum* 'Excelsum', *D. plantagineum* 'Harpur Crewe'. Rhizomatous perennial bearing ovate-elliptic, entire, softly hairy basal leaves, to 12cm (5in) long, heart-shaped at the bases; the stem leaves are ovate-lance-shaped and toothed. In spring, branched stems bear 3 or 4 golden yellow flowerheads, to 10cm (4in) across. ↕↔ to 60cm (24in). ❄❄❄
D. orientale, syn. *D. caucasicum.* Slowly spreading, rhizomatous perennial with

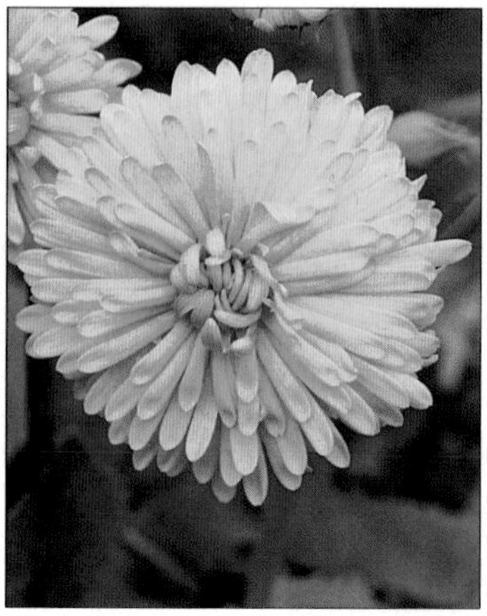

Doronicum orientale 'Frühlingspracht'

ovate-elliptic, gently scalloped, sparsely hairy basal leaves, 6–10cm (2½–4in) long, with heart-shaped bases, and a few elliptic to ovate-lance-shaped stem leaves. Produces solitary, golden yellow flowerheads, 2.5–5cm (1–2in) across, on slender stems in mid- and late spring. ↕ to 60cm (24in), ↔ 90cm (36in). S.E. Europe, Caucasus, Turkey, Lebanon. ❄❄❄. **'Finesse'** has slender ray-florets and long stems, comes true from seed, and is good for cutting; ↕ to 50cm (20in). **'Frühlingspracht'** ■ syn. 'Spring Beauty', has double flowerheads; ↕ to 40cm (16in). **'Gerhard'** produces double, lemon-yellow flowerheads with greenish yellow centres. **'Goldzwerg'** has golden yellow ray-florets; ↕ 25cm (10in). **'Magnificum'** has flowerheads 4–5cm (1½–2in) across, and comes true from seed; ↕ 50cm (20in). **'Spring Beauty'** see 'Frühlingspracht'.
D. pardalianches ■ syn. *D. cordatum.* Spreading, rhizomatous perennial with ovate to rounded, toothed, softly hairy basal leaves, 7–12cm (3–5in) long, with heart-shaped bases, and ovate to lance-shaped stem leaves. Corymbs of light yellow flowerheads, 3–5cm (1¼–2in) across, are borne on branching, softly hairy stems, from late spring to mid-summer. ↕ 90cm (36in), ↔ 60–90cm (24–36in) or more. W. and C. Europe to S. central Europe. ❄❄❄.
'Goldstrauss' flowers very freely.
D. plantagineum. Spreading, rhizomatous perennial with ovate-elliptic, entire or weakly toothed, hairy basal leaves, 5–11cm (2–4½in) long, and lance-shaped stem leaves. Branched stems bear golden yellow flowerheads, 3–5cm (1¼–2in) across, in late spring. Leaves die back soon after flowering. ↕ 80cm (32in), ↔ 45cm (18in). W. Europe to N. France. ❄❄❄.
'Excelsum' see *D.* x *excelsum* 'Harpur Crewe'. **'Harpur Crewe'** see *D.* x *excelsum* 'Harpur Crewe'.
'Strahlengold' flowers freely from spring to summer; the foliage persists in summer. Resists mildew and root rot.

DOROTHEANTHUS

Ice plant, Livingstone daisy

AIZOACEAE

Genus of 10 species of low-growing, basally branching, succulent annuals from open, sandy or rocky areas in South Africa. They have opposite or alternate, narrowly linear to spoon-shaped leaves, glistening with small, crystal-like structures. In summer, they produce numerous long-stalked, daisy-like, white, yellow, orange, pink, or red flowers that close in dull weather. Grow as border edging, to fill gaps in paving, or on a dry slope.

• **HARDINESS** Half hardy.

• **CULTIVATION** Grow in well-drained, preferably low-fertility, sandy soil in full sun. Dead-head to prolong flowering.

• **PROPAGATION** Sow seed at 16–19°C (61–66°F) in late winter or early spring. In frost-prone climates, harden off seedlings, and plant out when danger of hard frosts has passed.

• **PESTS AND DISEASES** Slugs, greenfly, snails, and foot rot may be troublesome.

D. bellidiformis, syn. *D. littlewoodii, Mesembryanthemum criniflorum* (Livingstone daisy). Low-growing annual bearing alternate, cylindrical, obovate to spoon-shaped, fleshy, light green leaves, to 7cm (3in) long. Solitary flowers, to 4cm (1½in) across, in white, crimson, rose-red, orange-gold, or buff-yellow, some zoned in a contrasting colour, are freely borne in summer. Plants with striped, light pink flowers, to 2.5cm (1in) across, and white throats, are sometimes listed as *D. littlewoodii.* ↕10–15cm (4–6in), ↔ 30cm (12in). South Africa (Western Cape). ✲. **'Lunette'**, syn. 'Yellow Ice', produces red-centred, soft yellow flowers. **'Magic Carpet'** ▣ produces pink, purple, cream, orange, or white flowers. **'Yellow Ice'** see 'Lunette'.

D. gramineus, syn. *Mesembryanthemum tricolor.* Erect, red-stemmed annual with opposite, linear, bright green leaves, to 5cm (2in) long, rounded on the lower surfaces. Bears solitary, crimson to deep rose-pink or white flowers, to 2.5cm (1in) across, with a dark central disc, in summer. ↕10cm (4in), ↔ to 30cm (12in). South Africa (Western Cape). ✲

D. littlewoodii see *D. bellidiformis.*

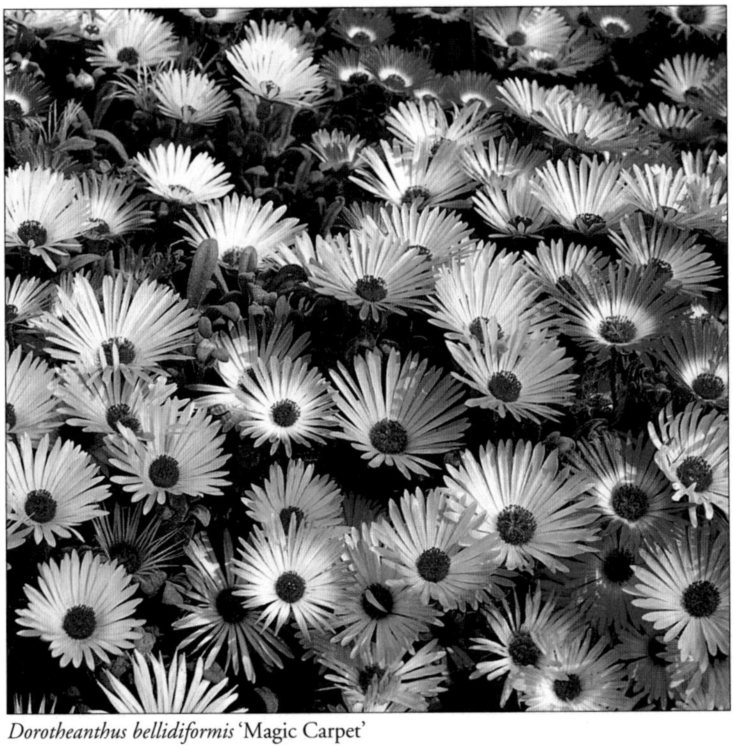

Dorotheanthus bellidiformis 'Magic Carpet'

DORSTENIA

MORACEAE

Genus of about 170 species of rhizomatous or shrubby perennials, a small number of which are succulent, from lowlands in the Arabian Peninsula, N.E. Africa, Madagascar, India, and tropical South and Central America. In many species, the rhizome is thick and tuber-like, and the caudex fleshy and thick, with leaves that are sometimes scale-like, especially on the upper nodes. The insignificant, petalless flowers and, later, ovoid green fruits are embedded in disc-shaped receptacles, produced from the upper leaf axils. In frost-prone areas, grow in a warm greenhouse for their bonsai-like growth, or use as ground cover beneath greenhouse staging. Elsewhere, grow in a desert garden. All parts are harmful if ingested.

• **HARDINESS** Frost tender.

• **CULTIVATION** Under glass, grow in a mix of equal parts loam, peat (or peat substitute), leaf mould, and gritty sand, in full light. In the growing season, water freely, applying fertilizer monthly; keep just moist in winter. Outdoors, grow in sharply drained, gritty, humus-rich soil in full sun. See also pp.48–49.

• **PROPAGATION** Sow seed at 21–24°C (70–75°F) in spring or summer.

• **PESTS AND DISEASES** Susceptible to scale insects.

D. foetida ▣ Erect or semi-prostrate, subshrubby succulent with a flattened caudex, thick, fleshy branches, and oblong-lance-shaped or obovate, spirally arranged leaves, 3–14cm (1¼–5½in) long. Circular, greenish white "flowers",

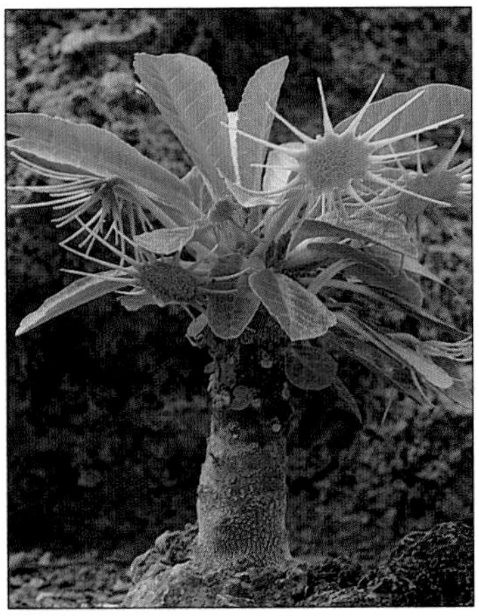

Dorstenia foetida

2cm (¾in) across, shaped like spinning-tops, with 6–10 bract-like "tentacles", are produced in summer. ↕15–30cm (6–12in), ↔ indefinite. Saudi Arabia. ❀ (min. 16°C/61°F)

DORYANTHES

Spear lily

DORYANTHACEAE/LILIACEAE

Genus of 2 species of perennial succulents mainly from coastal, open *Eucalyptus* forests of E. Australia. They are grown for their loosely rosetted, linear to lance-shaped leaves, with long, cylindrical points, and huge, terminal inflorescences of tubular flowers, with spreading tips, borne on mature plants. Grow as specimen plants. In frost-prone areas, grow on a patio (overwinter under glass) or in a cool greenhouse.

• **HARDINESS** Frost tender, although mature plants may withstand several degrees of frost if kept dry.

• **CULTIVATION** Under glass, grow in loam-based potting compost (JI No.2) in full light. In growth, water freely, applying a balanced liquid fertilizer monthly; keep just moist in winter. Outdoors, grow in humus-rich, well-drained soil in sun, with plenty of water in the growing season, although they will tolerate poor soils, some drought, and partial shade. See also pp.48–49.

• **PROPAGATION** Sow seed at 10–13°C (50–55°F) in spring. Sow bulbils, occasionally produced on flower stems, when mature. Separate suckers produced after flowering.

• **PESTS AND DISEASES** Trouble free.

D. excelsa. Succulent with erect clusters of 100 or more curving, linear or lance-shaped, dark green leaves, to 2.5m (8ft) long. Flowering stems, to 5m (15ft) long, bear many short, erect, linear-lance-shaped leaves and dense, spherical racemes, to 70cm (28in) across, of tubular red flowers, 10cm (4in) long, enclosed within leafy bracts, in late summer. ↕5–6m (15–20ft), ↔ to 2.5m (8ft). Australia (New South Wales). ❀ (min. 2°C/36°F)

D. palmeri ▣ Succulent with rosettes of upright then arching, linear or lance-shaped, lush, bright green leaves, 2.5–3m (8–10ft) long. Flowering stems, 3–4m (10–12ft) long, are also erect then arching. Along the upper halves, they bear smaller, linear-lance-shaped leaves and dense, oblong panicles, to 1m (3ft) long, of tubular, rich red or red-brown

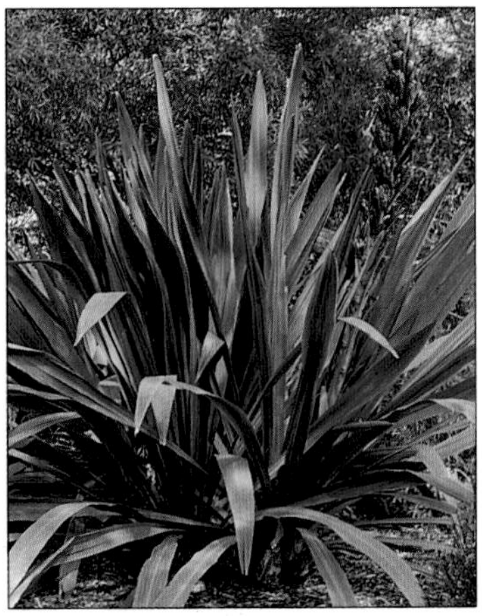

Doryanthes palmeri

flowers, 4–6cm (1½–2½in) long, pale red or white inside, enclosed in deep red bracts, in late spring. ↕2.5m (8ft), ↔ to 3m (10ft). Australia (Queensland, N. New South Wales). ❀ (min. 2°C/36°F)

▷ ***Dorycnium*** see *Lotus*
 D. hirsutum see *L. hirsutus*

DORYOPTERIS

ADIANTACEAE / PTERIDACEAE

Genus of about 25 species of evergreen ferns from dry, open areas or woodland in tropical regions. The tufted fronds, borne on erect or creeping rhizomes, have arrow-shaped, pedate, or palmate, sometimes pinnatifid blades on long, shining, black stalks. Grow in a warm, shady, sheltered border. In frost-prone areas, grow in a warm greenhouse.

• **HARDINESS** Frost tender.

• **CULTIVATION** Under glass, grow in a mix of 1 part loam, 2 parts sharp sand, and 3 parts leaf mould, in bright filtered light and moderate humidity. Water moderately when in full growth, sparingly in winter. Outdoors, grow in well-drained soil in partial shade.

• **PROPAGATION** Sow spores at 21°C (70°F) as soon as ripe, or divide mature plants in spring. Pot up "bulblets" from fronds of *D. palmata* when 3–4cm (1¼–1½in) across. See also p.51.

• **PESTS AND DISEASES** Trouble free.

D. elegans see *Hemionitis elegans.*

D. palmata, syn. *D. pedata* var. *palmata.* Evergreen fern bearing broadly ovate, dark green fronds, 20–60cm (8–24in) long, very deeply palmately lobed with 10–15 or more lobes. Proliferous buds ("bulblets") are borne at the frond bases. ↕ to 35cm (14in), ↔ 30–50cm (12–20in). West Indies, C. and W. tropical South America to Peru and Brazil. ❀ (min. 8–10°C/46–50°F)

D. pedata* var. *palmata see *D. palmata.*

▷ **Douglas fir** see *Pseudotsuga menziesii*
 Blue see *P. menziesii* var. *glauca*
▷ ***Douglasia*** see *Androsace, Vitaliana*
 D. laevigata see *Androsace laevigata*
 D. vitaliana see *Vitaliana primuliflora*
▷ **Dove tree** see *Davidia*
▷ ***Doxantha*** see *Bignonia, Macfadyena*
 D. capreolata see *Bignonia capreolata*
 D. unguis-cati see *Macfadyena unguis-cati*

DRABA

Whitlow grass

BRASSICACEAE/CRUCIFERAE

Genus of about 300 species of annuals and mat- or cushion-forming, evergreen or semi-evergreen perennials found in scree and other rocky, mountainous areas in arctic and northern temperate regions and temperate South America. They have rosettes of mainly linear to ovate, oblong, or spoon-shaped leaves, and small, cross-shaped flowers, borne in terminal racemes, in spring or early summer. Grow in a rock garden, scree bed, or alpine house, or in tufa.

- **HARDINESS** Fully hardy.
- **CULTIVATION** Grow in gritty, sharply drained soil in full sun. Protect from excessive winter rain. Grow the densest cushion plants in an alpine house, in a mix of equal parts loam, leaf mould, and grit, with a layer of grit or small stones around the neck of the plant. Avoid wetting the foliage at all times.
- **PROPAGATION** Sow seed in containers in an open frame in autumn; they need exposure to cold to germinate. Root rosettes of larger species in late spring.
- **PESTS AND DISEASES** Susceptible to aphids and red spider mites under glass.

D. aizoides (Yellow whitlow grass). Mat- or cushion-forming, semi-evergreen perennial bearing rosettes of linear-lance-shaped, bristle-margined, dark green leaves, to 1.5cm (½in) long. Dense racemes of 4–18 bright yellow flowers, 8–12mm (⅜–½in) across, are produced on stems 5–10cm (2–4in) long, in late spring. ↕ 10cm (4in), ↔ to 25cm (10in). UK, C. and S. Europe to Carpathians. ✽✽✽

D. bryoides see *D. rigida* var. *bryoides*.

D. dedeana ▣ Woody-based, cushion-forming, evergreen perennial with dense rosettes of linear-oblong, fringed and bristle-tipped, grey-green or bright green leaves, to 6mm (¼in) long. From spring to early summer, bears dense racemes of 3–10 white flowers, 8–10mm (⅜–½in) across, flushed pale violet at the bases, on stems to 8cm (3in) long. ↕ to 8cm (3in), ↔ to 15cm (6in). N. and E. Spain (mountains). ✽✽✽

D. longisiliqua 🏆 Cushion-forming, evergreen perennial with firm rosettes of obovate, grey-hairy leaves, 6–8mm (¼–⅜in) long. Short, dense racemes of 3–14 yellow flowers, to 1cm (½in) across, are borne on stems 5–8cm

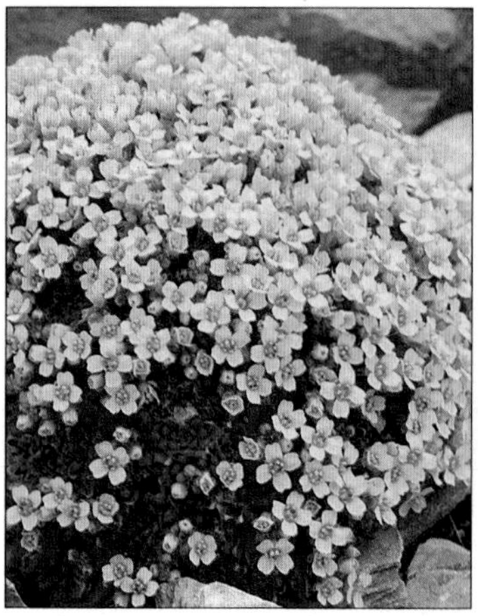

Draba mollissima

(2–3in) long, in spring. Grow in an alpine house or scree bed. ↕ 9cm (3½in), ↔ to 25cm (10in). Caucasus. ✽✽✽

D. mollissima ▣ Hummock-forming, evergreen perennial with rosettes of oblong, very hairy, grey-green leaves, to 6mm (¼in) long, forming a dense, domed cushion. In late spring, produces tight racemes of 6–8 bright yellow flowers, to 8mm (⅜in) across, on stems to 8cm (3in) long. Grow in an alpine house. ↕ 8cm (3in), ↔ to 20cm (8in). Caucasus. ✽✽✽

D. rigida. Hummock-forming, evergreen perennial with rosettes of linear to obovate, spreading, dark green, hairy-margined leaves, 3–6mm (⅛–¼in) long. In late spring, bears corymb-like racemes of 5–20 bright yellow flowers, 4–5mm (⅛–¼in) across, on stems to 5cm (2in) long. Grow in an alpine house. ↕ to 5cm (2in), ↔ to 20cm (8in). Turkey (Anatolia). ✽✽✽. **var. *bryoides***, syn. *D. bryoides*, has smaller rosettes; leaves, to 2mm (¹⁄₁₆in) long, have inrolled margins; ↕ 3cm (1¼in), ↔ to 15cm (6in). Caucasus, Georgia, Armenia.

DRACAENA

AGAVACEAE/DRACAENACEAE

Genus of 40 species of sparsely branched, evergreen shrubs and trees from forest, scrub, and dry, open slopes. They occur in the Canary Islands and throughout tropical Africa, but mainly in W. Africa, with one species in South America. These striking architectural plants produce usually lance- to strap-shaped, leathery, glossy leaves, which are

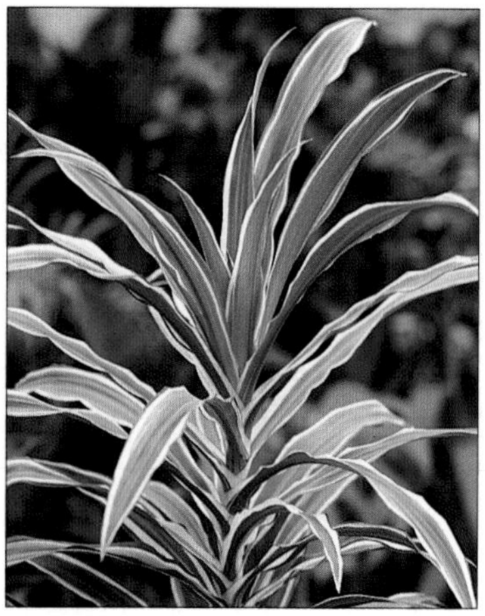

Dracaena fragrans Deremensis Group 'Warneckei'

spirally arranged and often crowded at the stem tips. Small flowers, with tubular bases and 6 spreading tepals, are borne in terminal panicles, followed by red or yellow berries. Grow as specimen plants or in a border. In frost-prone areas, grow in a warm or temperate greenhouse, or as houseplants.

- **HARDINESS** Frost tender.
- **CULTIVATION** Under glass, grow in loam-based potting compost (JI No.3) in full light, with shade from hot sun and moderate humidity. Green-leaved plants tolerate slightly lower light levels. From spring to autumn, water freely, applying a balanced liquid fertilizer monthly; water sparingly in winter. Top-dress or pot on in spring. Outdoors, grow in moderately fertile, moist but well-drained soil in full sun. Regular pruning is not necessary. If growth is weak, cut back to within 15cm (6in) of the base in spring.
- **PROPAGATION** Sow seed at 18–21°C (64–70°F) in spring, although variegated cultivars will not come true. Root semi-ripe cuttings and leafless stem sections with bottom heat in summer.
- **PESTS AND DISEASES** Red spider mites, thrips, and scale insects may be troublesome under glass.

D. australis see *Cordyline australis*.

D. deremensis see *D. fragrans* Deremensis Group.

***D. deremensis* 'Souvenir de Schrijver'** see *D. fragrans* Deremensis Group 'Warneckei'.

D. draco ▣ ♈ (Dragon tree). Robust, slow-growing, eventually widely branched tree, resembling an inside-out umbrella in outline when mature. Tufted or rosetted, glaucous, mid- to dark green leaves, 30–60cm (12–24in) long, are linear-lance-shaped and spine-tipped. Mature plants produce terminal panicles, to 30cm (12in) long, of white-tinged green flowers in summer, followed by large, spherical, orange-red fruit. ↕ 3–10m (10–30ft) or more, ↔ 2–8m (6–25ft) or more. Canary Islands. ❀ (min. 13°C/55°F)

D. fragrans ♀ Erect, evergreen shrub or small tree, very sparsely branched when young, with spreading to strongly arching, inversely lance-shaped, keeled, mid-green leaves, 20–120cm (8–48in) long, confined to upper parts of the stems. When mature, bears strongly scented white flowers in erect to

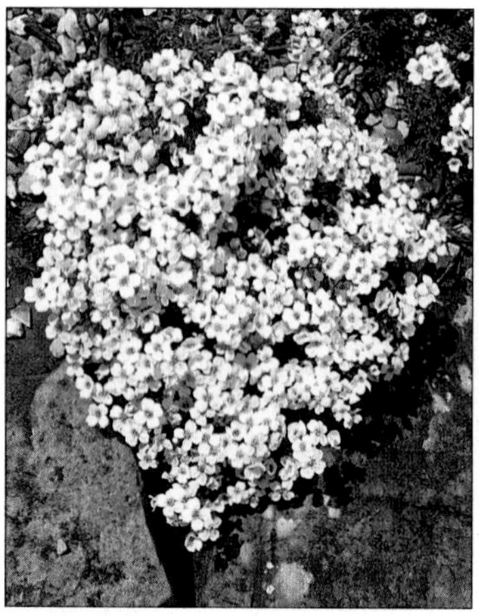

Draba dedeana

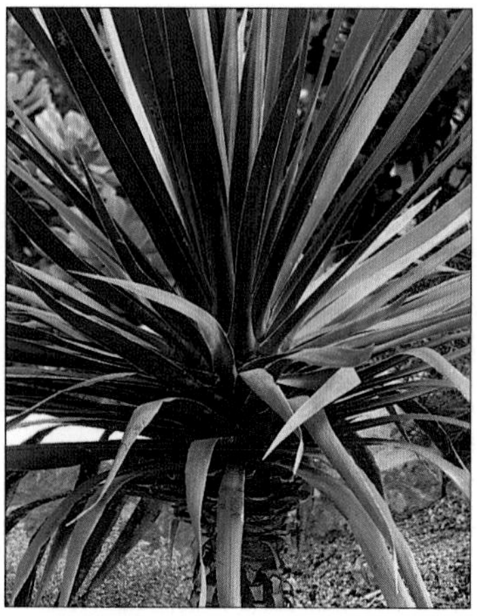

Dracaena draco

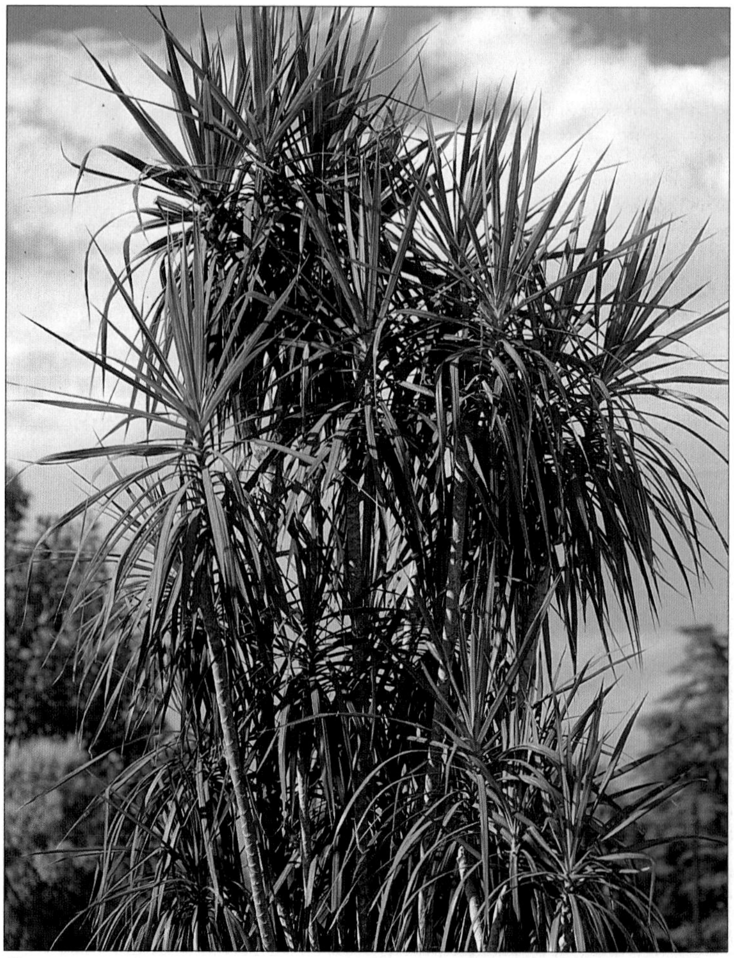

Dracaena marginata

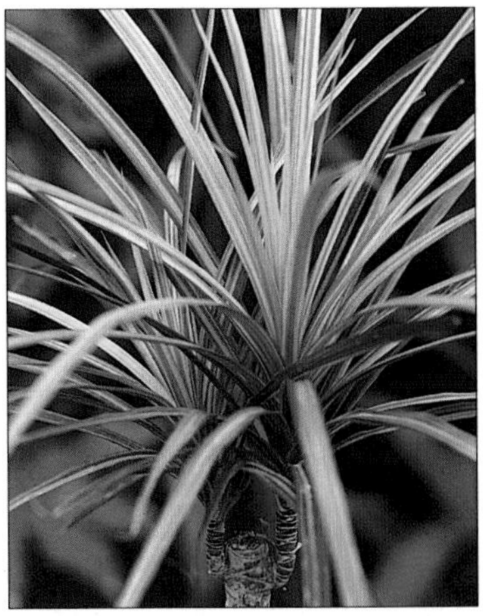

Dracaena marginata 'Tricolor'

arching, branched or unbranched, terminal panicles, to 50cm (20in) long, in summer, followed by spherical, orange-red fruit. ↕ 5–15m (15–50ft), ↔ 1–3m (3–10ft). W., C., and E. Africa. ❀ (min. 13°C/55°F).
Deremensis Group, syn. *D. deremensis*, includes cultivars with different patterns of longitudinal leaf striations of varying colours and widths. **Deremensis Group 'Warneckei'** ▣ ♀ syn. *D. deremensis* 'Souvenir de Schrijver', *D. deremensis* 'Warneckei', has dark grey-green leaves, 40–60cm (16–24in) long, with narrow lighter streaks, dark green margins, and near-central, longitudinal white stripes. **'Massangeana'** ♀ has recurved, dull green leaves, 20–60cm (8–24in) long, with greyish green streaks and a broad, longitudinal, yellow-green band, interspersed with narrow, grey-green stripes.
D. indivisa see *Cordyline indivisa.*
D. marginata ▣ ♀ ◊ Erect, slow-growing shrub or small tree, often unbranched at first, then branching and spreading. Spreading, linear-lance-shaped, recurved, red-margined, dark green leaves, 30–60cm (12–24in) long, are densely borne on upper parts of the stems. Mature plants produce terminal panicles, 40–50cm (16–20in) across, of white flowers in summer, followed by yellow berries. ↕ 2–5m (6–15ft), ↔ 1–3m (3–10ft). Réunion Islands. ❀ (min. 13°C/55°F). **'Tricolor'** ▣ has leaves with cream marginal stripes shaded red at the edges.
D. sanderiana ▣ ♀ (Ribbon plant). Slender, erect shrub with cane-like stems that branch sparingly to moderately from the base. Arching, slightly wavy, lance-shaped, glossy, rich green leaves, 15–25cm (6–10in) long, tapering to false stalks, have bold, longitudinal, silvery white stripes. Not known to flower in cultivation. ↕ to 1.5m (5ft), ↔ 40–80cm (16–32in). Cameroon. ❀ (min. 13°C/55°F)

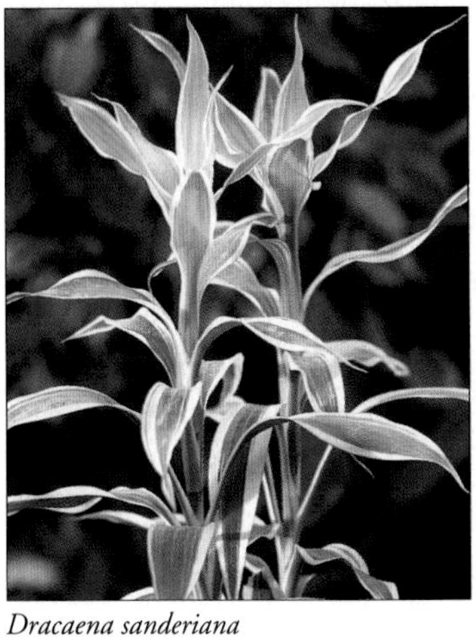

Dracaena sanderiana

DRACOCEPHALUM

Dragon's head

LABIATAE/LAMIACEAE

Genus of 50 species of annuals, perennials, and dwarf, evergreen shrubs found in a range of habitats, from dry, sunny steppes and rocky, grassy slopes to dry woodland, mostly in Eurasia, but also in N. Africa and N. USA. They are grown for their whorls of sage-like, tubular, 2-lipped flowers produced in upright, terminal or axillary racemes, 7–30cm (3–12in) or more long, in summer. They have square stems, and opposite, often aromatic, mainly linear to broadly ovate, entire or toothed, lobed or pinnatisect, mid-green leaves, usually 1.5–8cm (½–3in) long. Grow in a border or rock garden; some species are also suitable for naturalizing in partial shade. Annuals may be used to fill gaps in mixed plantings.

- **HARDINESS** Fully hardy.
- **CULTIVATION** Grow in well-drained, moderately fertile soil in full sun with some midday shade. *D. forrestii* requires sharply drained soil with some protection from excessive winter wet. *D. ruyschiana* tolerates dry soils.
- **PROPAGATION** Sow seed of annuals *in situ* in mid-spring, thinning as required. Divide or sow seed of perennials in containers in a cold frame in autumn or spring, or root basal cuttings of young growth in mid- or late spring.
- **PESTS AND DISEASES** Occasionally affected by rust and mildew.

D. argunense ▣ syn. *D. ruyschiana* var. *speciosum, D. speciosum.* Clump-forming perennial with oblong-lance-shaped to linear-lance-shaped, entire, minutely glandular, hairy leaves, 5–7cm (2–3in) long. Bluish purple flowers, to 4.5cm (1¾in) long, are borne in softly hairy, whorled, terminal racemes among ovate-lance-shaped stem leaves in midsummer. ↕ 45cm (18in), ↔ 30cm (12in). China, N.E. Asia. ❄❄❄
D. forrestii. Rhizomatous perennial with obovate, pinnatisect leaves, 1.5–2cm (½–¾in) long, with 2 or 3 pairs of tightly inrolled, linear segments. Slender, very leafy, white-hairy stems bear dense, whorled racemes of softly white-hairy, deep purple-blue flowers, 2–3cm (¾–1¼in) long, from late summer to mid-autumn. ↕ to 50cm (20in), ↔ 30cm (12in). China (Yunnan). ❄❄❄
D. govanianum see *Nepeta govaniana.*
D. grandiflorum. Upright, rhizomatous perennial with long-stalked, oblong-elliptic, toothed radical leaves, 2–5cm (¾–2in) long, and smaller, broadly ovate, scalloped, stalkless stem leaves. Bears short, spike-like racemes of hooded, intense deep blue flowers, to 4cm (1½in) long, with darker spots on the lower lips, in summer. ↕ 30cm (12in), ↔ 20cm (8in). Siberia. ❄❄❄
D. moldavica, syn. *D. moldavicum.* Erect, bushy, slightly hairy, aromatic annual with oblong-lance-shaped to ovate-triangular, toothed, grey-green leaves, 1.5–4cm (½–1½in) long. Slender, spike-like racemes of whorled, unevenly 2-lipped, hairy, violet-blue to purple flowers, to 2.5cm (1in) long, are produced in summer. ↕ 30–60cm (12–24in), ↔ 30cm (12in). E. and C. Europe, C. Asia, Siberia, China. ❄❄❄. **f. album** has white flowers.
D. moldavicum see *D. moldavica.*
D. ruyschiana, syn. *D. ruyschianum* (Siberian dragon's head). Clump-forming, bushy perennial with linear-lance-shaped, entire, hairless leaves, 3.5–6cm (1½–2½in) long, with inrolled margins, and erect, often downy stems. Short spikes of blue-purple flowers, to 2.5cm (1in) long, are borne in mid- and late summer. ↕ to 60cm (24in), ↔ 30cm (12in). C. Europe to Siberia. ❄❄❄. **var. *japonicum*** has white flowers shaded blue; Japan. **var. *speciosum*** see *D. argunense.*
D. ruyschianum see *D. ruyschiana.*
D. sibiricum see *Nepeta sibirica.*
D. speciosum see *D. argunense.*
D. tanguticum. Clump-forming, variable perennial bearing ovate, pinnatisect, aromatic leaves, 2.5–8cm (1–3in) long, with 5–7 narrowly linear divisions. Produces whorled, spike-like racemes of long-lasting, deep violet-blue flowers, 2–3cm (¾–1¼in) long, from midsummer to early autumn. ↕ 40cm (16in), ↔ 30cm (12in). S.W. China. ❄❄❄

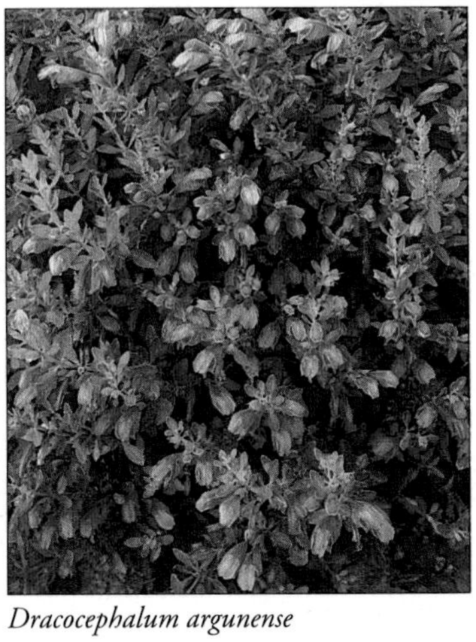

Dracocephalum argunense

DRACULA

ORCHIDACEAE

Genus of about 60 species of evergreen, epiphytic orchids from around 2,000m (7,000ft) in the Andean regions of South America and adjacent highlands of Central America. They produce short, slender stems along creeping rhizomes, each stem having a single, lance-shaped to obovate, dark green leaf. The flowers are borne singly or in erect, or more usually pendent, arching racemes. The sepals are fused into wide, star-shaped cups, with the free parts of the sepals like long "tails". The lip has a short claw and a cup (or pouched blade).

- **HARDINESS** Frost tender.
- **CULTIVATION** Cool-growing orchids. Grow in epiphytic orchid compost in a slatted basket. In summer, provide humid, shady conditions, and water moderately, applying fertilizer at every third watering. Water sparingly in winter to avoid root rot. See also p.46.
- **PROPAGATION** Divide when the plant fills the pot and "flows" over the sides.
- **PESTS AND DISEASES** Prey to red spider mites, aphids, whiteflies, and mealybugs.

D. bella. Epiphytic orchid with oblong to lance-shaped leaves, 12–20cm (5–8in) long. Flowers, 10–25cm (4–10in) long, densely spotted brown, with greenish yellow bases, long-tailed sepals, and small white lips, are borne singly, from winter to summer. ↕↔ 25cm (10in). Colombia. ❀ (min. 10°C/50°F; max. 24°C/75°F)
D. chimaera. Robust, epiphytic orchid with elliptic to obovate leaves, 15–25cm (6–10in) long. In winter, the erect or ascending stems each bear a succession of 3–8 densely spotted, dark maroon flowers, 12cm (5in) long, with yellow or greenish yellow bases, long-tailed sepals, and small cream lips. ↕ to 60cm (24in), ↔ 20cm (8in). Colombia. ❀ (min. 10°C/50°F; max. 24°C/75°F)
D. erythrochaete. Epiphytic orchid with elliptic to obovate leaves, 15–25cm (6–10in) long. Bears 1–3 cream flowers, 10cm (4in) across, with red-purple spotting and purple tails, on long, erect to pendent stems, from autumn to winter. ↕ 40–60cm (16–24in), ↔ 20cm (8in). Costa Rica to Colombia. ❀ (min. 10°C/50°F; max. 24°C/75°F)

DRACUNCULUS

ARACEAE

Genus of 3 species of tuberous perennials from the Mediterranean, Madeira, and the Canary Islands found on waste ground, rocky areas, and hill-sides, with pedate, sometimes white-mottled, dark green leaves. They are grown for their distinctive but foul-smelling, often very large, flat or curved spathes, borne in spring or summer. Although not reliably hardy, they grow well in open glades in sheltered wood-land or at the base of a sunny wall.

- **HARDINESS** Frost hardy.
- **CULTIVATION** Plant tubers 15cm (6in) deep in autumn or spring in humus-rich, well-drained soil that dries out in summer. Grows best in full sun but will tolerate partial shade. Protect with a winter mulch.
- **PROPAGATION** Separate offsets in autumn or spring.
- **PESTS AND DISEASES** Trouble free.

D. vulgaris ▣ syn. *Arum dracunculus* (Dragon arum). Tuberous perennial

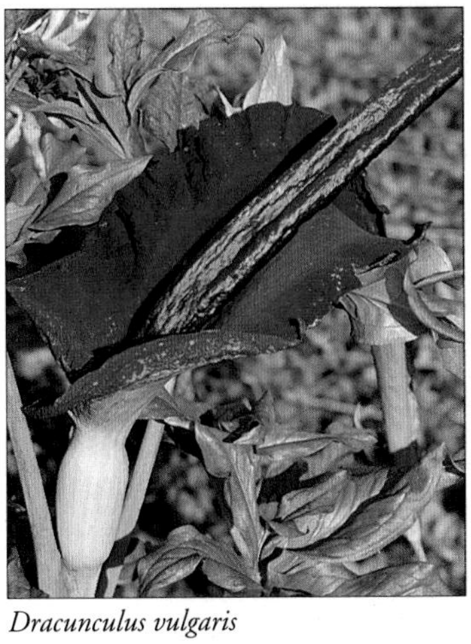

Dracunculus vulgaris

D

with pedate, dark green, basal leaves, 30cm (12in) or more long, marked purple-brown. In spring or summer, foul-smelling, maroon-purple spathes, 60–100cm (24–39in) long, with erect, almost black spadices, are borne above the leaves. ↕ to 1.5m (5ft), ↔ 60cm (24in). C. and E. Mediterranean. ❄❄

▷ **Dragonhead, False** see *Physostegia virginiana*
▷ **Dragon's head** see *Dracocephalum*
 Siberian see *D. ruyschiana*
▷ **Dragon's mouth** see *Horminum pyrenaicum*
▷ **Dragon tree** see *Dracaena draco*

DREGEA syn. WATTAKAKA

ASCLEPIADACEAE

Genus of 3 or more species of twining, woody, evergreen climbers found in tropical forest from South Africa to China, with opposite, heart-shaped to pointed ovate or lance-shaped leaves. They are cultivated for their small, bowl-shaped, fragrant, yellow or white flowers, produced in stalked umbels from the leaf axils. Grow *D. sinensis* against a sheltered wall.
• **HARDINESS** Frost hardy.
• **CULTIVATION** Grow in well-drained soil in sun or partial shade. Tie young shoots to their supports until they begin to twine. Pruning group 11, after flowering; remove dead wood in early spring.
• **PROPAGATION** Sow seed in containers in a cold frame in spring. Take stem cuttings in summer or autumn.
• **PESTS AND DISEASES** Trouble free.

D. sinensis, syn. *Wattakaka sinensis.* Twining climber with ovate-heart-shaped leaves, to 10cm (4in) long, mid-green above and grey-downy beneath. Produces fragrant, creamy white flowers, to 1.5cm (½in) across, pale pink and speckled red within, in umbels 6cm (2½in) across, in summer, followed by slender, paired seed pods, to 7cm (3in) long. ↕ 3m (10ft). China. ❄❄

▷ ***Drejerella*** see *Justicia*
 D. guttata see *J. brandegeeana*
▷ ***Drepanostachyum falconeri*** see *Himalayacalamus falconeri*

DRIMYS syn. TASMANNIA

WINTERACEAE

Genus of about 30 species of evergreen shrubs and trees from woodland and mountains in Malaysia, Australasia, and Central and South America. They are grown for their handsome, usually elliptic to inversely lance-shaped, aromatic leaves, arranged alternately on the branches, and terminal, umbel-like clusters of small, star-shaped, sometimes unisexual flowers. Grow in a woodland garden or in a sheltered position among other trees and shrubs.
• **HARDINESS** Frost hardy.
• **CULTIVATION** Grow in fertile, moist but well-drained soil in sun or partial shade. Shelter from cold, drying winds. Pruning group 8; cut out dead or damaged wood in spring.
• **PROPAGATION** Sow seed in containers in a cold frame in autumn. Insert semi-ripe cuttings in summer.
• **PESTS AND DISEASES** Trouble free.

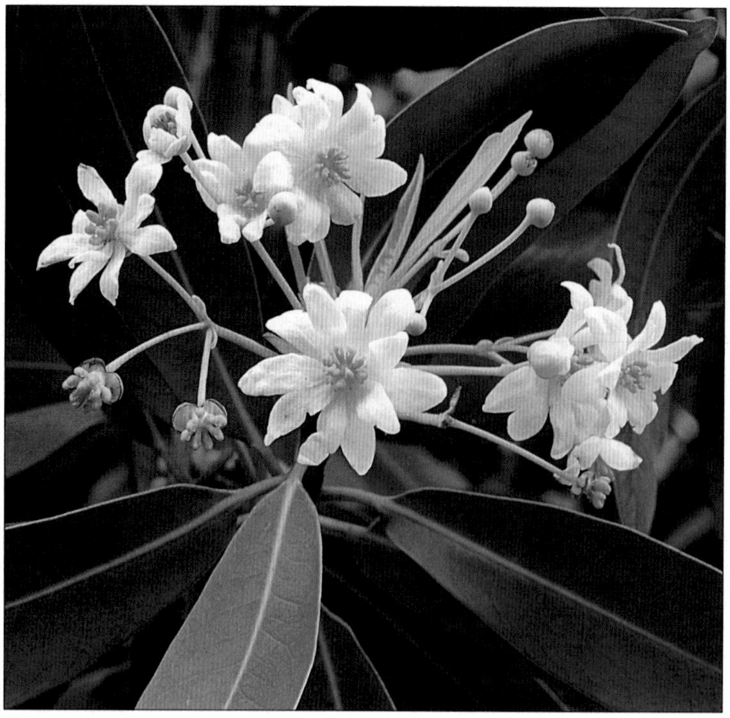

Drimys winteri

D. aromatica see *D. lanceolata.*
D. colorata see *Pseudowintera colorata.*
D. lanceolata ♀ syn. *D. aromatica, Tasmannia aromatica* (Mountain pepper). Dense, upright shrub or tree with deep red shoots and elliptic to inversely lance-shaped, leathery, glossy, dark green leaves, to 8cm (3in) long. Clusters of 7–18 white flowers, 1.5cm (½in) across, are produced in mid- and late spring. ↕ 4m (12ft), ↔ 2.5m (8ft). S.E. Australia, Tasmania. ❄❄
D. winteri ◼♀ syn. *Wintera aromatica* (Winter's bark). Vigorous, upright tree or shrub with aromatic bark and oblong-elliptic to narrowly inversely lance-shaped, leathery leaves, to 20cm (8in) long, dark green above, blue-white beneath. Produces large umbels of 5–20 fragrant, ivory-white flowers, 2.5cm (1in) across, from spring to early summer. ↕ 15m (50ft), ↔ 10m (30ft). Mexico, Chile, Argentina. ❄❄. **var. *andina*** is dwarf, and flowers when 30–40cm (12–16in) tall; ↕↔ 90–100cm (36–39in). Andes of Chile, Argentina.

▷ **Dropwort** see *Filipendula vulgaris*

DROSANTHEMUM

AIZOACEAE

Genus of about 90 species of erect or prostrate, succulent shrubs from semi-desert regions of Namibia and South Africa. They have slender, rough stems clad in minute, fine hairs, and leaves, triangular to cylindrical in cross-section, densely covered with papillae. Daisy-like, white or red flowers, produced singly or in threes, open after midday in summer. In frost-prone areas, grow in a cool greenhouse and transfer outdoors in summer; in warmer climates, grow outdoors in a desert garden or in a border with other succulents.
• **HARDINESS** Frost tender.
• **CULTIVATION** Under glass, grow in standard cactus compost in full light. From spring to summer, water freely, applying a balanced liquid fertilizer monthly; keep just moist at other times. Outdoors, grow in sharply drained soil in full sun. See also pp.48–49.
• **PROPAGATION** Sow seed at 16–19°C (61–66°F), or take stem cuttings from spring to summer.
• **PESTS AND DISEASES** Susceptible to aphids while flowering.

D. hispidum ◼ Bushy, succulent shrub with erect then spreading, roughly hairy branches, which frequently root where they touch the ground. Cylindrical, fleshy, glossy, pale green to reddish green leaves, to 2.5cm (1in) long, are covered with transparent papillae. In summer, bears solitary, glossy-petalled, deep purplish red flowers, to 3cm (1¼in) across. ↕ 15cm (6in), ↔ 1m (3ft). Namibia, South Africa (Western Cape). ❀ (min. 5°C/41°F)
D. speciosum. Bushy, succulent shrub with erect, spotted stems and curved, semi-cylindrical, fleshy leaves, 1.5cm (½in) long, covered with glistening papillae. Solitary, orange-red flowers, to 5cm (2in) across, with green centres, are produced in summer. South Africa (Western Cape). ↕ 30–40cm (12–16in), ↔ 30cm (12in). ❀ (min. 5°C/41°F)

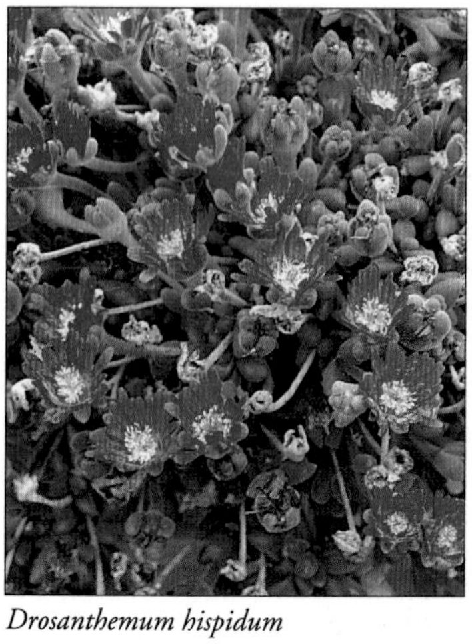

Drosanthemum hispidum

DROSERA

Daily dew, Sundew

DROSERACEAE

Genus of about 100 species of rosette-forming or scrambling, evergreen or herbaceous, insectivorous perennials, also including some annuals, found in poor, acid, boggy soil throughout the world, but mainly in Australia. Leaves are alternate or whorled, often long-stalked, and linear to rounded, the blades covered and fringed with gland-tipped, red or green hairs, which trap and digest insects. The small flowers are usually 5-petalled, most often white, pink, or purple, and are solitary or borne in racemes or panicles. In frost-prone areas, grow in a cool greenhouse; in warmer climates, use in a bog garden.
• **HARDINESS** Fully hardy to frost tender.
• **CULTIVATION** Under glass, grow in a mix of equal parts moss peat (or peat substitute) and sand in full light, with shade from hot sun. Keep continually moist by standing in a saucer of soft (lime-free) water. Outdoors, grow in wet, peaty, acid, nutritionally poor soil in full sun.
• **PROPAGATION** Sow seed at 10–13°C (50–55°F) as soon as ripe. Take cuttings from young, fully developed leaves, or take root cuttings when dormant.
• **PESTS AND DISEASES** Trouble free.

D. capensis (Cape sundew). Evergreen perennial with loose, basal rosettes of linear-oblong to spoon-shaped leaves, 3–6cm (1¼–2½in) long, covered in glandular red or green hairs. Racemes of 6–20 rounded, rose-pink flowers, 2cm (¾in) across, are borne from spring to autumn, and sometimes into winter. ↕ 20–30cm (8–12in), ↔ to 15cm (6in). Southern Africa. ❀ (min. 2°C/36°F)

▷ **Drumsticks** see *Craspedia globosa, Isopogon*
 Broad-leaf see *Isopogon anemonifolius*
▷ **Drunkard's dream** see *Hatiora salicornioides*

DRYANDRA

PROTEACEAE

Genus of about 60 species of evergreen shrubs and small trees found on sandy heath, on dry, rocky and sandy coasts, and in scrub in Australia. They are grown for their foliage and their very colourful flowerheads, both of which are suitable for dried flower arrangements. Leaves are alternate, sometimes whorled, linear to ovate, leathery, usually very boldly toothed, and often pinnatifid. Spherical to ovoid, often thistle-like flowerheads, borne at the ends of the shoots, consist of many slender, usually yellow florets enclosed by overlapping, sometimes coloured bracts. In frost-prone areas, grow in a cool greenhouse; elsewhere, grow in a border, against a warm wall, or in a sunny courtyard.
• **HARDINESS** Frost tender; *D. formosa* survives short periods near 0°C (32°F).
• **CULTIVATION** Under glass, use 1 part loam-based potting compost (JI No.1) and 3 parts of a 50/50 mix of grit and peat (or peat substitute), and grow in full light. In the growing season, water moderately and apply a half-strength,

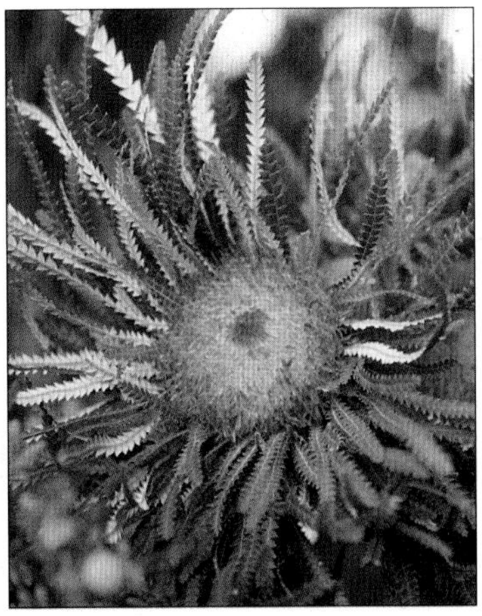

Dryandra formosa

phosphate-free fertilizer monthly; water sparingly in winter. Top-dress or pot on in spring. Outdoors, grow in sharply drained, neutral to acid soil of low fertility (or at least with low levels of phosphates), in full sun. Pruning group 1 or 8.

• **PROPAGATION** Sow seed at not less than 18°C (64°F) in spring, ideally singly, in small containers. Root softwood cuttings with bottom heat in summer; rooting may be slow.

• **PESTS AND DISEASES** In warm areas, *Phytophthora* root rot may be fatal. In soil containing too much phosphate, plants may become chlorotic.

D. formosa ■ ♀ (Showy dryandra). Erect, moderately bushy shrub or small tree. Crowded, linear, mid- to dark green leaves, to 20cm (8in) long, with triangular, teeth-like lobes, are sometimes downy beneath. Spherical, bright yellow-orange flowerheads, to 10cm (4in) across, are produced from spring to early summer. ↕ 2–3m (6–10ft), ↔ 2–5m (6–15ft). Australia (Stirling Range to Albany Mountains, Western Australia). ❄ (borderline)

▷ **Dryandra, Showy** see *Dryandra formosa*

DRYAS

Mountain avens

ROSACEAE

Genus of 3 species of prostrate, evergreen subshrubs found on cliffs and rock ledges in alpine and arctic regions of the N. hemisphere. They are grown for their oak-like, leathery, wrinkled, dark green leaves, 3–4cm (1¼–1½in) long, and white downy beneath. Solitary, cup- to bell-shaped, 8-petalled flowers are followed by fluffy seed heads. They are easily cultivated carpeting plants, useful for a rock garden, wall, or border edge.

• **HARDINESS** Fully hardy.

• **CULTIVATION** Grow in well-drained, humus-rich, preferably gritty soil in sun or partial shade.

• **PROPAGATION** Sow seed in containers in a cold frame as soon as ripe, or take softwood cuttings in early summer. Lift and transplant rooted stems in spring.

• **PESTS AND DISEASES** Trouble free.

D. drummondii. Mat-forming subshrub with elliptic to obovate, coarsely scalloped leaves, to 4cm (1½in) long, and nodding, bell-shaped, pale

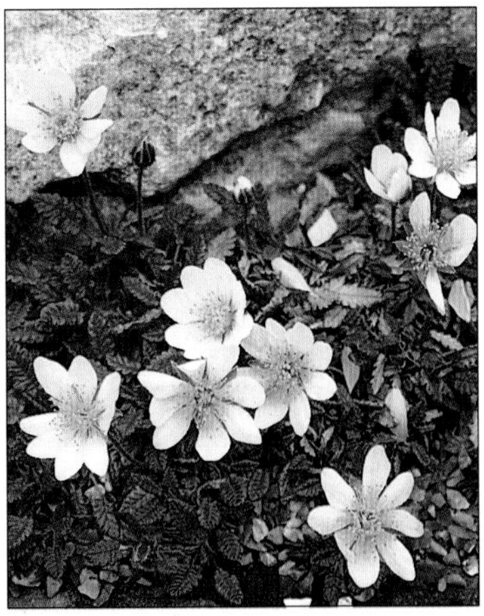

Dryas octopetala

yellow flowers, 1.5–2.5cm (½–1in) across, in early summer. ↕ 10cm (4in), ↔ 1m (36in) or more. North America. ❄❄❄. **'Grandiflora'** bears large flowers, to 2.5cm (1in) across.

D. octopetala ■ ♀ (Mountain avens). Mat-forming subshrub with oblong-elliptic to ovate, scalloped leaves, to 4cm (1½in) long. Upward-facing, cup-shaped, creamy white flowers, to 4cm (1½in) across, with yellow stamens, are produced in late spring and early summer. ↕ 10cm (4in), ↔ 1m (36in) or more. N. Europe. ❄❄❄

D.* x *suendermannii ♀ (*D. drummondii* x *D. octopetala*). Mat-forming subshrub with oblong-elliptic to ovate, scalloped leaves, to 4cm (1½in) long. Produces slightly nodding, cup-shaped flowers, to 3cm (1¼in) across, pale yellow in bud, becoming pale creamy yellow, from spring to early summer. ↕ 10cm (4in), ↔ 1m (36in) or more. Garden origin. ❄❄❄

DRYNARIA

POLYPODIACEAE

Genus of 20 epiphytic, evergreen ferns found in tropical forest and scrub in tropical Africa, S.E. Asia, and Australia, with thick, creeping rhizomes and 2 types of frond. Basal fronds are papery, oak-like in shape, stalkless, and sterile. They turn brown quickly and form a "nest" in which humus collects. The taller, stalked, more upright fertile fronds remain green. They are either deeply pinnate, with linear pinnae, or pinnatisect; small groups of spores form on the undersides. The pinnae are often

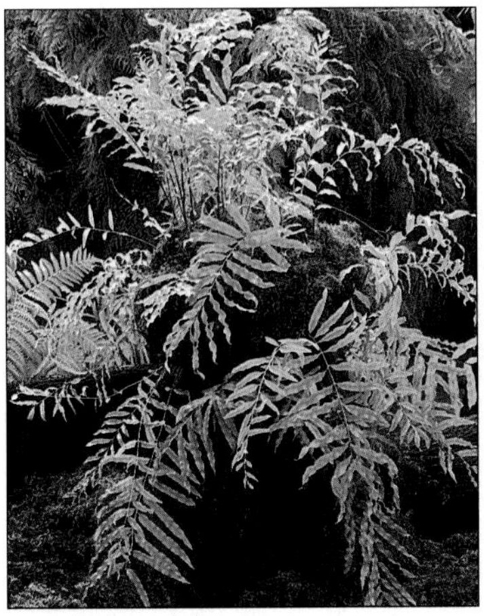

Drynaria rigidula

shed in dry periods, leaving long, bare midribs. All fronds, even when fresh, have a thin, leathery texture. In frost-prone areas, grow in a warm greenhouse; elsewhere, grow epiphytically.

• **HARDINESS** Frost tender.

• **CULTIVATION** Under glass, grow in a mix of equal parts medium-grade bark, perlite, and charcoal, in a hanging basket, or epiphytically on bark or a tree-fern slab, with a moss pad at the base. In summer, provide bright filtered light with high humidity and good ventilation, and water freely. Admit full light and water sparingly in winter. Repot in early spring. Outdoors, grow epiphytically on a tree trunk in humid, partial shade.

• **PROPAGATION** *D. rigidula* increases readily from spores, sown at 21°C (70°F) as soon as ripe; other species are less easy to propagate from spores. Divide the rhizomes of large specimens in spring, and make sure that each portion has at least one growing tip. See also p.51.

• **PESTS AND DISEASES** Scale insects may infest fronds.

D. quercifolia. Clump-forming, epiphytic fern with ovate, shallowly lobed basal fronds, and narrowly ovate, deeply pinnatisect, dark green fertile fronds, to 1m (36in) tall, which have linear-lance-shaped pinnae. Spores are formed in small sori in double rows running from midrib to margins. ↕ to 1m (3ft), ↔ 1m (3ft). S.E. Asia, Australia. ❀ (min. 10°C/50°F)

D. rigidula ■ Clump-forming, epiphytic fern producing elongated, deeply lobed basal fronds, and ovate, pinnate, dark green fertile fronds, to 1.5m (5ft) tall. Young fronds are covered in soft down that often persists until the fronds wither. Spores form in a single row of sori between midrib and margins. ↕ to 1m (3ft), ↔ to 1.5m (5ft). India, S. China, Polynesia, New Guinea, Australia. ❀ (min. 10°C/50°F)

DRYOPTERIS

Buckler fern

DRYOPTERIDACEAE

Genus of about 200 species of terrestrial ferns found mainly in temperate regions of the N. hemisphere, where they grow in woodland, by streams or lakes, and among mountain rocks. Most are deciduous, but in mild winters some stay green in sheltered sites. Pinnate to

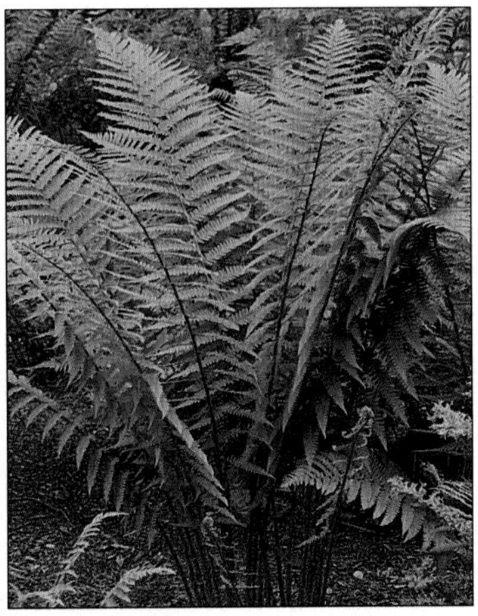

Dryopteris affinis

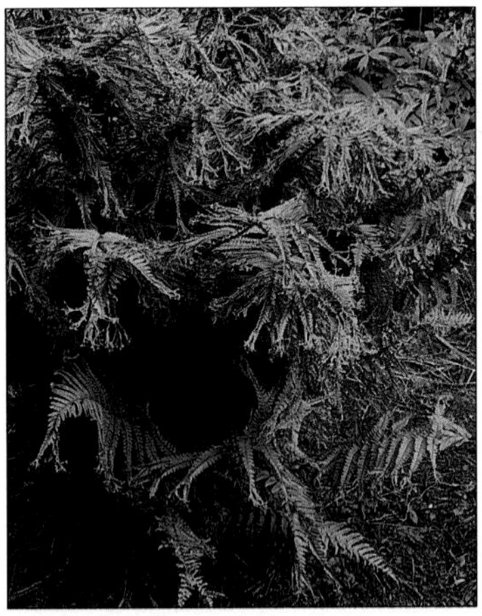

Dryopteris affinis Polydactyla Group 'Mapplebeck'

4-pinnate, sometimes pinnatisect fronds form "shuttlecocks" in most cultivated species. Spores are produced in kidney-shaped sori. The foliage looks effective with most herbaceous plants and shrubs; in frost-prone areas, grow tender species in a cool greenhouse.

• **HARDINESS** Mostly fully hardy; some species are frost hardy or frost tender.

• **CULTIVATION** Grow in moist, humus-rich soil in partial shade and a sheltered site. *D. affinis* and its cultivars will tolerate more sun and wind than other species.

• **PROPAGATION** Sow spores at 15°C (59°F) as soon as ripe. Except in *D. affinis*, sporelings of cultivars differ in appearance from the parent. Divide mature plants in spring or autumn. See also p.51.

• **PESTS AND DISEASES** Trouble free, but moth larvae may feed on spores.

D. affinis ■ ♀ syn. *D. borreri*, *D. pseudomas* (Golden male fern). Virtually evergreen fern producing a shuttlecock of lance-shaped, 2-pinnate or pinnatisect fronds, 20–80cm (8–32in) tall, from an erect rhizome. Fronds are pale green as they unfurl in spring, in striking contrast to the scaly, golden brown midribs; they mature to dark green and often remain green through winter. Distinguished from *D. filix-mas* by a dark spot where each pinna joins the midrib. ↕↔ 90cm (36in). Europe to Himalayas. ❄❄❄. **'Crispa Congesta'** see 'Crispa Gracilis'. **'Crispa Gracilis'**, syn. 'Crispa Congesta', is dwarf and evergreen, with congested fronds and pinnae twisted at the tips; ↕↔ 30cm (12in). **'Cristata'**, syn. 'Cristata The King', has arching fronds, 10–15cm (4–6in) across, with crested tips and pinnae, and is the most handsome of numerous selected cultivars. **'Cristata Angustata'** is similar to 'Cristata', but the fronds are 5cm (2in) wide. **'Cristata The King'** see 'Cristata'. **Polydactyla Group 'Mapplebeck'** ■ has semi-erect fronds, with large, fingered crests at the tips, broader than the fronds; pinnae are also finger-crested; ↕↔ 1.2m (4ft).

***D. atrata* of gardens** see *D. cycadina.*

D. austriaca see *D. dilatata.*

D. borreri see *D. affinis.*

D. carthusiana (Narrow buckler fern). Usually deciduous, delicate fern with a slowly creeping rhizome producing a tuft of narrowly lance-shaped, 2- or 3-pinnate, pale green fronds, to 60cm

D

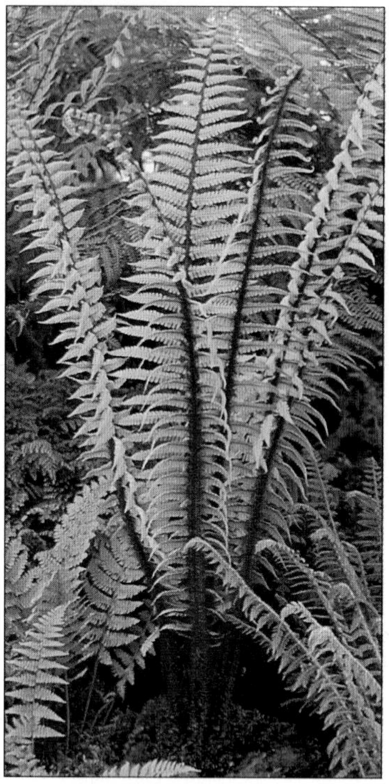

Dryopteris wallichiana

(24in) long, with uniformly pale scales on the midribs. ↕ to 60cm (24in), ↔ 30cm (12in). Europe (damp woods, marshy areas). ❄❄❄. **'Cristata'** has crested pinnae and frond tips.

D. x complexa (*D. affinis* x *D. filix-mas*). Semi-evergreen fern, similar to *D. affinis*, with fronds 1m (3ft) tall. ↕↔ 1m (3ft). Garden origin. ❄❄❄. **'Crispa Angustata'** has crisped fronds; ↕ 60cm (24in), ↔ 45cm (18in). **'Stablerae'** has narrow pinnae; ↕ 1.2m (4ft).

D. cycadina, syn. *D. atrata* of gardens, *D. hirtipes*. Deciduous fern with an erect rhizome producing a shuttlecock of lance-shaped, pinnate, bright green fronds, 45cm (18in) tall, with green midribs. ↕ 60cm (24in), ↔ 45cm (18in). N. India to China, Taiwan, Japan. ❄❄❄

D. dilatata, syn. *D. austriaca* (Broad buckler fern). Usually deciduous fern with a shuttlecock of broadly triangular-lance-shaped, 2- or 3-pinnate, dark green fronds, to 1.5m (5ft) tall and 40cm (16in) wide, arising from an erect rhizome. Frond midribs and stalks are covered in conspicuous, dark brown scales with darker centres. ↕ 90cm (3ft), ↔ 1.2m (4ft). N.W. and C. Europe. ❄❄❄. **'Crispa Whiteside'** has prettily crisped fronds. **'Lepidota Cristata'** is crested, with narrower fronds, 20cm (8in) wide, more finely divided pinnules, and paler brown scales; ↕ 60–90cm (24–36in), ↔ 45cm (18in).

D. erythrosora 𝕐 Usually deciduous fern with a slow-creeping rhizome producing a tuft of triangular, 2- or 3-pinnate fronds, 25–60cm (10–24in) long; these are copper-red when young, slowly turning slightly shiny, dark green. Midribs are green; young sori are often red. A striking border fern, suitable for a protected, moist site. ↕ 60cm (24in), ↔ 38cm (15in). China, Japan. ❄❄❄

D. filix-mas 𝕐 (Male fern). Deciduous fern forming a large clump of lance-shaped, 2-pinnate or pinnatifid, mid-green fronds, 1–1.2m (3–4ft) tall, with green midribs, arising from a crown of large rhizomes. ↕↔ 1m (3ft). Europe, North America. ❄❄❄. **'Barnesii'** has long, narrow fronds; ↕↔ 1.2m (4ft). **'Crispa Cristata'** has crested fronds, and pinnae that are both crested and crisped; ↕ 60cm (24in). **'Grandiceps Wills'** is a striking plant: the tip of each frond has a heavy crest as wide as the frond, and the pinnae are also finely crested; ↕↔ 90cm (36in). **Linearis Group** cultivars have narrower pinna divisions than the species, giving a delicate, airy look; the Group includes **'Linearis Cristata'**, which has crested pinnae and frond tips; ↕ 90cm (36in), ↔ 60cm (24in).

D. goldieana (Goldie's fern). Deciduous fern with a slow-creeping rhizome producing tufts of long-stalked, broadly oval, 2-pinnate, pale green fronds, 1.2m (4ft) tall, with green midribs. ↕ 1.2m (4ft), ↔ 60cm (24in). North America. ❄❄❄

D. hirtipes see *D. cycadina.*

D. pseudomas see *D. affinis.*

D. wallichiana ▣ 𝕐 (Wallich's wood fern). Deciduous fern producing an erect rhizome and a shuttlecock of lance-shaped, 2-pinnate or pinnatisect, dark green fronds, yellow-green when young, 90cm (36in) or more long. Midribs are covered with dark brown or black scales, providing wonderful colour contrasts in spring. ↕ 90cm (36in), sometimes to 1.8m (6ft), ↔ 75cm (30in). Himalayas. ❄❄❄

DUCHESNEA

ROSACEAE

Genus of 6 species of low-growing, more or less evergreen perennials from damp, shady woodland and streamsides in S. and E. Asia. The 5-petalled flowers are yellow and strawberry-like, as are the fruits that follow, although these are unpalatable. Rooting runners may be invasive in warm areas, but the fully divided, 3-palmate, conspicuously veined, toothed, strawberry-like leaves provide useful ground cover. *D. indica* also looks effective when grown as a houseplant, especially in a hanging basket.

• **HARDINESS** Fully hardy.

• **CULTIVATION** Grow in any soil and position, although they prefer humus-rich, woodland soil in full or partial shade.

• **PROPAGATION** Sow seed in containers in a cold frame in autumn or spring, or detach and replant rooted plantlets at almost any time of year.

• **PESTS AND DISEASES** Slugs and snails may eat fruits.

D. indica ▣ syn. *Fragaria indica* (Indian strawberry, Mock strawberry). Rosette-forming, more or less evergreen perennial producing numerous short runners that root at the nodes. The 3-palmate, hairy leaves, to 10cm (4in) long, have obovate leaflets. Bears solitary yellow flowers, to 2.5cm (1in) across, surrounded by large green calyces and epicalyces, in early and late summer, followed by unpalatable, bright red fruit, to 2cm (¾in) long. ↕ 10cm (4in), ↔ 1.2m (4ft) or more. India, China, Japan. ❄❄❄. **'Harlequin'** has red-tinged foliage speckled with white.

▷**Duck plant** see *Sutherlandia frutescens*
▷**Duck potato** see *Sagittaria latifolia*

DUDLEYA

CRASSULACEAE

Genus of 40 species of basal-rosetted, perennial succulents, closely related to *Echeveria,* mainly from hilly and low mountainous areas of S. and S.W. USA and N. and N.W. Mexico. Often low-growing, they produce dense rosettes of ovate to linear, succulent leaves. In spring or early summer, tubular, bell-, or star-shaped, yellow, white, or red flowers are borne in panicles from the leaf axils. In frost-prone areas, grow as houseplants or in a cool or temperate greenhouse; in warmer climates, use in a border with other succulents.

• **HARDINESS** Frost tender.

• **CULTIVATION** Under glass, grow in standard cactus compost in full or bright filtered light. During growth, water moderately, applying fertilizer monthly; water sparingly in summer when plants are semi-dormant. Outdoors, grow in sharply drained, humus-rich, moderately fertile soil in full sun. See also pp.48–49.

• **PROPAGATION** Sow seed at 16°C (61°F) in early spring, or take stem cuttings from spring to summer.

• **PESTS AND DISEASES** Vulnerable to mealybugs.

D. attenuata. Variable, perennial succulent with stems branching to form large rosettes of slender, linear-inversely-lance-shaped, fleshy, silvery grey leaves, 2–10cm (¾–4in) long; the stem leaves are linear-lance shaped. Produces tubular, yellowish red flowers, 2cm (¾in) across, in panicles, 5–20cm

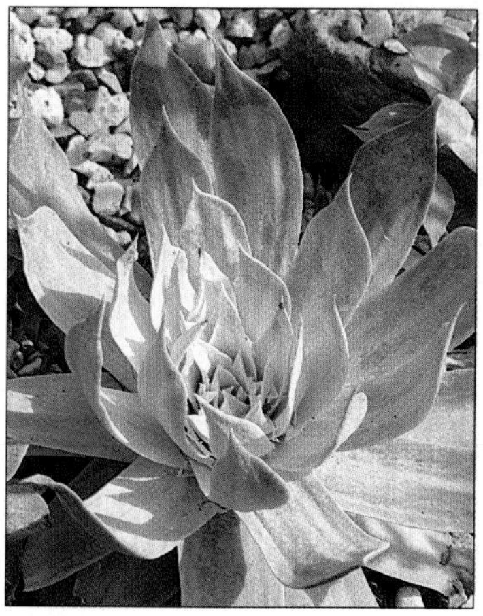

Dudleya pulverulenta

(2–8in) tall, in spring or early summer. ↕ 10–15cm (4–6in), ↔ to 40cm (16in). USA (California), Mexico. ❁ (min. 7°C/45°F). **subsp. *orcuttii*** has pink-flushed white flowers.

D. pulverulenta ▣ Variable, perennial succulent with an unbranched, silvery grey stem, often very thick and fleshy. Oblong to obovate-spoon-shaped, tapering, fleshy, silvery grey leaves are 7–30cm (3–12in) long. Star-shaped, red to yellow flowers, 2–3cm (¾–1¼in) across, are borne in panicles, 40–80cm (16–32in) tall, in spring or early summer. ↕ 30cm (12in) or more, ↔ to 55cm (22in). USA (California), N. Mexico. ❁ (min. 7°C/45°F)

D. traskiae. Perennial succulent with a short, branching stem and oblong, pointed, fleshy, silvery grey leaves, 4–15cm (1½–6in) long. Star-shaped yellow flowers, 2cm (¾in) across, are produced in panicles, to 30cm (12in) or more tall, in spring or early summer. ↕ 20cm (8in), ↔ 25cm (10in). USA (Santa Barbara Island, California). ❁ (min. 7°C/45°F)

▷**Dumb cane** see *Dieffenbachia*
▷**Dungwort** see *Helleborus foetidus*

DURANTA

VERBENACEAE

Genus of about 30 species of evergreen trees and shrubs found in tropical S. USA and Central and South America, in scrub, thickets, and open woodland. Simple, mainly ovate, often toothed leaves are opposite or sometimes in whorls. They are grown for their salver-

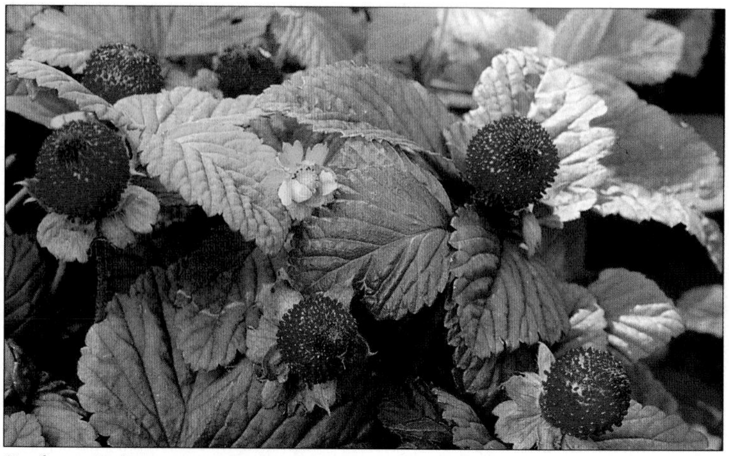

Duchesnea indica

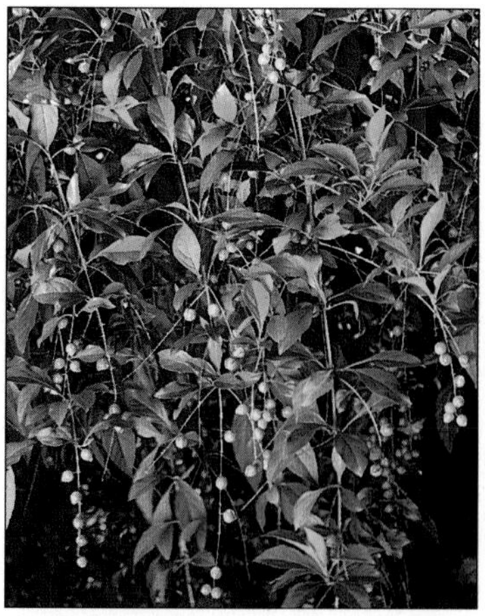

Duranta erecta

form flowers, borne in terminal or axillary racemes or panicles, followed by attractive, spherical berries. In frost-prone areas, grow in a temperate greenhouse; in warmer climates, use in a border, or as a hedge or windbreak.
• **HARDINESS** Frost tender.
• **CULTIVATION** Under glass, grow in loam-based potting compost (JI No.3) in full light, with shade from hot sun. During growth, water freely, applying a balanced liquid fertilizer every 2 weeks; water sparingly in winter. Top-dress or pot on in spring. Outdoors, grow in moist but well-drained, moderately fertile soil in full sun. Pruning group 1; plants under glass may need restrictive pruning in late winter.
• **PROPAGATION** Sow seed at 18–21°C (64–70°F) in spring. Root semi-ripe cuttings with bottom heat in summer. Layer in early spring.
• **PESTS AND DISEASES** Susceptible to red spider mites, mealybugs, and whiteflies under glass.

D. erecta ■ ♀ syn. *D. plumieri, D. repens* (Golden dewdrop, Pigeon berry, Sky flower). Erect to spreading, bushy shrub or small tree with ovate to obovate, sparsely to boldly toothed, usually rich green leaves, to 7cm (3in) long. Axillary, pendent panicles, 10–15cm (4–6in) long, of small, blue, lilac-blue, purple, or white flowers, are produced mainly in summer, followed by yellow fruit, to 1cm (½in) across. ↕3–6m (10–20ft), ↔ 2–3m (6–10ft). USA (Florida) to Brazil. ❄ (min. 10°C/50°F)
D. plumieri see *D. erecta.*
D. repens see *D. erecta.*

▷**Dusty miller** see *Lychnis coronaria*
▷**Dutchman's breeches** see *Dicentra cucullaria, D. spectabilis*
▷**Dutchman's pipe** see *Aristolochia, A. macrophylla*

DUVALIA

ASCLEPIADACEAE

Genus of about 19 species of prostrate or semi-erect, mainly leafless, clump-forming, perennial succulents from hilly lowlands of the Arabian Peninsula, E. Africa, and southern Africa. They have toothed stems, each with 4–6 blunt, warty ribs separated by transverse furrows. Star-shaped, stalked flowers have 5 fleshy lobes, recurved at the tips, and are solitary or produced in clusters

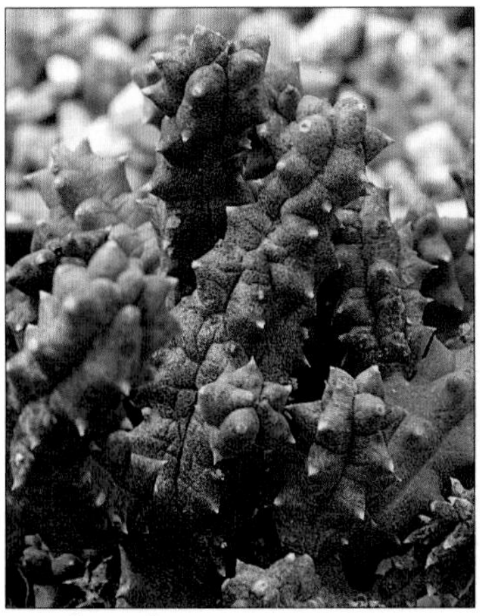

Duvalia corderoyi

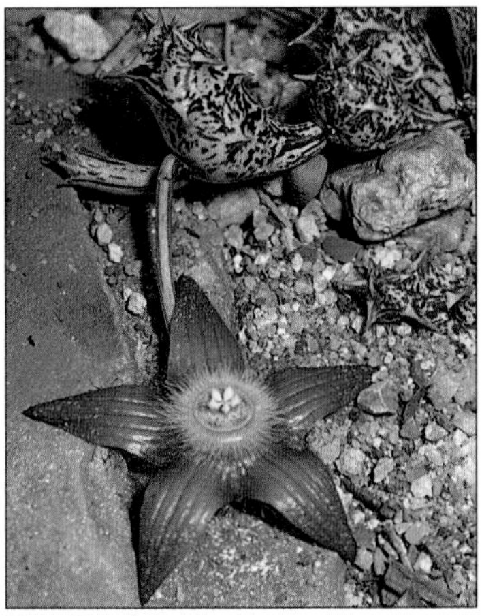

Duvalia sulcata

at the base of the stems, from late spring to summer. In frost-prone areas, grow in a warm greenhouse; in warmer climates, grow outdoors with other succulents.
• **HARDINESS** Frost tender.
• **CULTIVATION** Under glass, grow in standard cactus compost in bright filtered light. In the growing season, water moderately, and apply fertilizer monthly; keep almost completely dry when dormant. Overwatering may encourage black rot. Outdoors, grow in sharply drained, humus-rich, gritty soil in partial shade. See also pp.48–49.
• **PROPAGATION** Sow seed at 21–24°C (70–75°F), or take stem cuttings from spring to summer.
• **PESTS AND DISEASES** Susceptible to mealybugs and black rot.

D. corderoyi ■ Semi-erect succulent with short, somewhat rounded, 6-ribbed, leafless, green or purple stems. Produces 2–4 dull olive-green flowers, to 5cm (2in) across, covered with soft purple hairs, in summer. ↕ to 5cm (2in), ↔ indefinite. South Africa (Northern Cape). ❄ (min. 10°C/50°F)
D. maculata. Prostrate succulent with oblong, leafless, dark green stems, each with 4 or 5 ribs and prominent, pointed teeth. Bears 4–8 olive-green or dark reddish brown flowers, 2cm (¾in) across, with lobes spotted red-brown, and the white tubes spotted maroon, in summer. ↕ to 5cm (2in), ↔ indefinite. Namibia, South Africa (Western Cape). ❄ (min. 10°C/50°F)
D. sulcata ■ Prostrate succulent with 4-ribbed, leafless, whitish green stems with purple spots and prominent teeth. Clusters of 1–3 reddish brown flowers, 4.5cm (1¾in) across, with 5-furrowed, hairy-based lobes, covered with pale reddish hairs, are produced from late spring to summer. ↕ to 7cm (3in), ↔ indefinite. Arabian Peninsula. ❄ (min. 10°C/50°F)

▷***Duvernoia*** see *Justicia*
D. adhatodoides see *J. adhatoda*

DYCKIA

BROMELIACEAE

Genus of over 100 species of rosette-forming, stemless, evergreen, succulent, terrestrial perennials (bromeliads) from South America, found in rocky areas, especially near coasts, and in mountains at altitudes up to 2,000m (6,500ft). They have linear to lance-shaped or short, triangular, spiny-margined, stiff, often grey-scaly leaves, and tubular, sulphur-yellow to orange flowers, produced laterally from the rosettes in racemes or panicles, generally in spring. Many species develop a trunk-like stem, while some are mat-forming. In areas where temperatures drop below 10°C (50°F), grow as houseplants or in a temperate or warm greenhouse; in warmer regions, grow in a desert garden.
• **HARDINESS** Frost tender.
• **CULTIVATION** Under glass, grow in terrestrial bromeliad compost in full light. From late spring to autumn, water moderately, applying fertilizer monthly; keep completely dry in winter. Outdoors, grow in sharply drained, gritty, humus-rich soil in full sun. See also p.47.
• **PROPAGATION** Sow seed at 27°C (81°F) in early spring. Divide clumps in late spring or early summer.
• **PESTS AND DISEASES** Scale insects may be troublesome.

D. argentea see *Hechtia argentea.*
D. fosteriana ■ Bromeliad with dense, flat rosettes of lance-shaped, grey-scaly leaves, 9–17cm (3½–7in) long, with sharp, recurved marginal spines. Densely scaly racemes, 45cm (18in) long, of bright orange flowers, 2.5cm (1in) long, are produced in late spring. ↕ 20cm (8in), ↔ 12cm (5in). E. Brazil. ❄ (min. 10°C/50°F)
D. platyphylla. Bromeliad with spreading rosettes of thick, narrowly triangular, dark green leaves, to 23cm (9in) long, hairless above, with white scales pressed flat against the undersides.

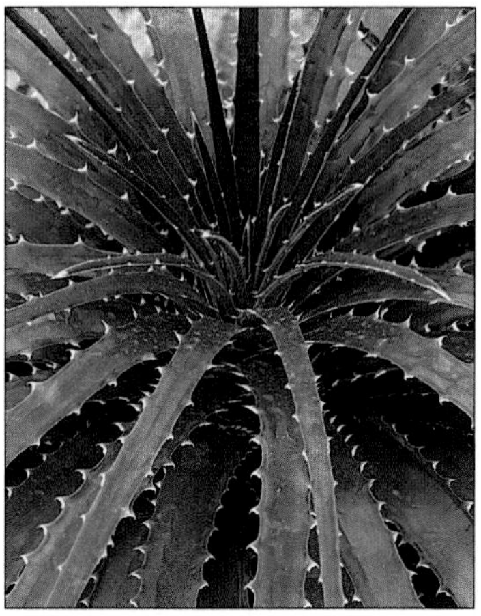

Dyckia remotiflora

Lax racemes, 80cm (32in) long, of bright yellow flowers, 2.5cm (1in) long, are produced in late spring. ↕ 30cm (12in), ↔ 40cm (16in). E. Brazil. ❄ (min. 10–13°C/50–55°F)
D. remotiflora ■ Bromeliad with dense rosettes of very narrowly triangular, arching, dark green leaves, 10–25cm (4–10in) long, covered with grey scales, especially on the undersides, and with hooked marginal spines. Loose, sparsely hairy panicles, to 1m (36in) long, with lateral spikes of dark orange flowers, 2cm (¾in) long, are borne in late spring. ↕ 30cm (12in), ↔ 30–50cm (12–20in). S. Brazil, Uruguay. ❄ (min. 10°C/50°F)

▷**Dyer's greenweed** see *Genista tinctoria*
▷***Dypsis lutescens*** see *Chrysalidocarpus lutescens*

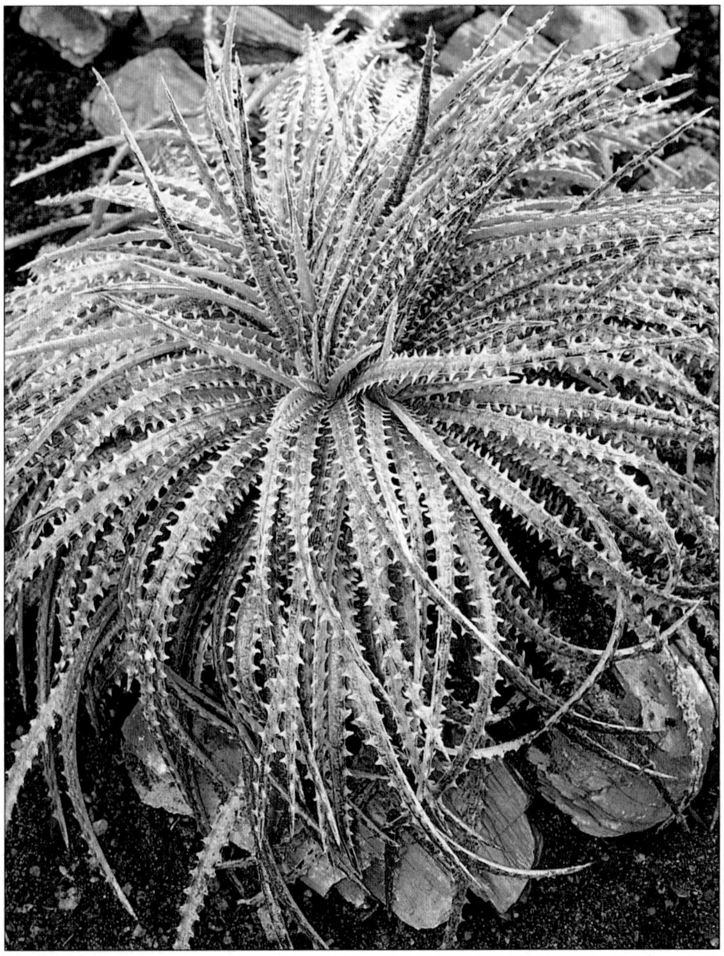

Dyckia fosteriana

D

E

E

▷ **Earth star** see *Cryptanthus*
Green see *C. acaulis*
▷ **Eaton's firecracker** see *Penstemon eatonii*
▷ **Ebony, Mountain** see *Bauhinia variegata*

EBRACTEOLA

AIZOACEAE

Genus of 5 species of very fleshy, mat- or clump-forming, perennial succulents from low-lying hills in Namibia. They have extremely thick rootstocks and 3-sided, sometimes spotted, bluish green leaves. Solitary, almost stalkless, daisy-like, terminal flowerheads are borne in summer. In frost-prone areas, grow as ground cover in a warm greenhouse; in warm, dry climates, grow in a desert garden or in a raised bed.

• **HARDINESS** Frost tender.
• **CULTIVATION** Under glass, grow in standard cactus compost in full light. When in growth, water moderately and apply a low-nitrogen liquid fertilizer monthly; keep dry at other times. Outdoors, grow in sharply drained soil in full sun. See also pp.48–49.
• **PROPAGATION** Sow seed at 19–24°C (66–75°F) in spring or summer, or take cuttings of stem sections in early summer.
• **PESTS AND DISEASES** Trouble free.

E. derenbergiana, syn. *Mesembryanthemum derenbergianum*, *Ruschia derenbergiana*. Mat- or cushion-forming succulent with a very thick tap root, 20cm (8in) long, producing fleshy stems, each with 2 or 3 pairs of 3-sided, densely spotted, light blue-green leaves, 3–4cm (1¼–1½in) long, bluntly margined, with the sides hatchet-shaped above. Daisy-like, pale pink flowers, 2–2.5cm (¾–1in) across, are borne in summer. ↕ to 7cm (3in), ↔ indefinite. Namibia. ❀ (min. 10°C/50°F)

ECBALLIUM

Squirting cucumber

CUCURBITACEAE

Genus of one species of trailing or bushy, bristly-hairy, monoecious perennial found in rough, dry ground from the Mediterranean to S. Russia. The female flowers give rise to touch-sensitive fruit that squirt out seeds over great distances when ripe. It is usually grown for the curiosity value of its fruit. Needs an open, sunny site. In frost-prone areas, treat as a half-hardy annual.

• **HARDINESS** Half hardy.
• **CULTIVATION** Grow in well-drained, poor to moderately fertile soil in full sun.
• **PROPAGATION** Sow seed at 18°C (64°F) in early spring, and plant out

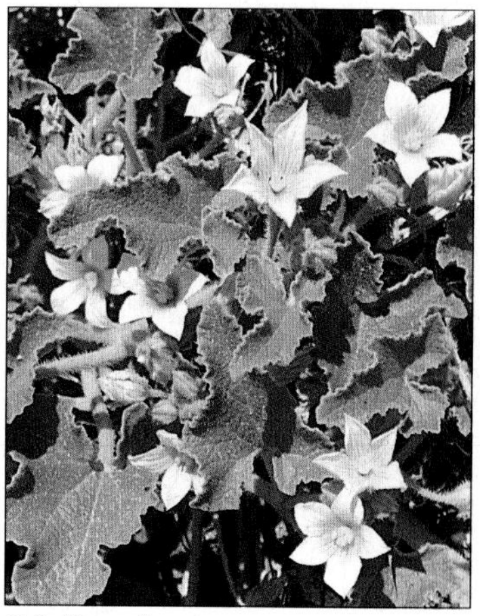

Ecballium elaterium

seedlings when risk of frost has passed.
• **PESTS AND DISEASES** Under glass, aphids and red spider mites may be a problem.

E. elaterium ■ Bushy or trailing perennial with long, bristly-hairy stems and ovate-triangular, palmately 5-lobed, dark greyish green leaves, 5–15cm (2–6in) long, with shallow, wavy-margined lobes, rough-textured above, downy on the undersides. In summer, produces widely funnel-shaped, pale yellow flowers, to 2.5cm (1in) across, sometimes with deeper yellow centres. Male flowers are produced in racemes; female flowers are solitary. Ovoid to cylindrical, hairy, blue-green fruit, to 5cm (2in) long, enclose many seeds in watery mucilage. ↕ to 50cm (20in), ↔ 1m (3ft) or more. Mediterranean. ✽

▷ ***Eccremocactus bradei*** see *Weberocereus bradei*

ECCREMOCARPUS

Chilean glory flower

BIGNONIACEAE

Genus of 5 species of evergreen or herbaceous, climbing perennials from scrub and forest margins in Chile and Peru. They are grown for their colourful, terminal racemes of lopsidedly tubular flowers. The leaves are opposite and 2-pinnate, each with a terminal, branched tendril. In frost-prone areas, grow in a cool greenhouse, or outside as annuals. In warmer areas, grow as short-lived perennials, to clothe an arch, pergola, or house wall, or to clamber through a large shrub or small tree.

• **HARDINESS** Frost hardy to frost tender.
• **CULTIVATION** Under glass, grow in well-drained, loam-based potting compost (JI No.2) in full light. When in growth, water freely and apply a balanced liquid fertilizer monthly; water sparingly in winter. Outdoors, grow in fertile, well-drained soil in full sun. Provide support. Pruning group 11, in early spring.
• **PROPAGATION** Sow seed at 13–16°C (55–61°F) in late winter or early spring. Root tip cuttings with bottom heat in spring or summer.
• **PESTS AND DISEASES** Prone to red spider mites and whiteflies under glass.

E. scaber ■ ♀ (Chilean glory flower). Slender, fast-growing, evergreen climber with sharply 4-angled stems, erect at

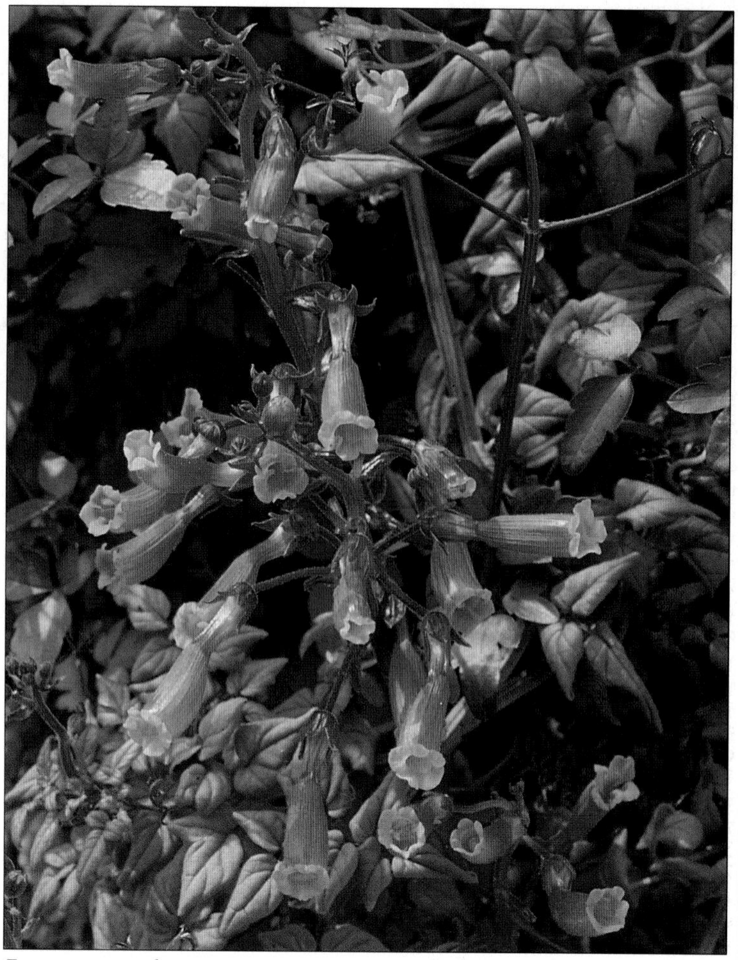

Eccremocarpus scaber

first, then branching and spreading. Pinnate leaves, 5–7cm (2–3in) long, have small, ovate, boldly veined, light green, sometimes grey-tinted leaflets. From late spring to autumn, bears tubular, orange-red flowers, to 2.5cm (1in) long, swollen near the mouths, in racemes 10–15cm (4–6in) long. ↕ 3–5m (10–15ft), sometimes more. Chile. ✽✽ (borderline). **Anglia Hybrids** is a mixed colour selection that produces red, pink, orange, or yellow flowers. **f. *aureus*** has golden yellow blooms. **f. *carmineus*,** syn. 'Ruber', has carmine-red flowers. **f. *roseus*** has bright pink to light red flowers. **'Ruber'** see f. *carmineus.*

ECHEVERIA

CRASSULACEAE

Genus of about 150 species of evergreen succulents and evergreen, occasionally deciduous subshrubs found in dry, often semi-desert areas in Texas, USA, Mexico, and from Central America to the Andes. The often spectacularly colourful leaves, usually in rosettes, are fleshy, alternate, and may be linear to cylindrical, spoon-shaped, or broadly triangular. The flowers have erect or spreading petal lobes, often slightly spreading at the tips or constricted at the mouths, and occasionally angled or keeled tubes. They are borne in racemes, cymes, or panicles, on long stalks from the leaf axils. In frost-prone areas, grow as houseplants or in a temperate greenhouse. Compact species may be used as annuals in carpet bedding. In warmer climates, plant outdoors in a border with other succulents.

• **HARDINESS** Frost tender.
• **CULTIVATION** Under glass, grow in standard cactus compost in full light. While in growth, water moderately and apply a half-strength balanced liquid fertilizer monthly; keep just moist in winter. Stand containerized plants outdoors during the frost-free months. Outdoors, grow in moderately fertile to poor, well-drained soil in full sun. See also pp.48–49.
• **PROPAGATION** Sow seed at 16–19°C (61–66°F) as soon as ripe. Root stem or leaf cuttings in late spring, or separate offsets in spring.
• **PESTS AND DISEASES** Prone to greenfly, vine weevil larvae, and mealybugs.

E. agavoides ■ ♀ Often clump-forming, very short-stemmed succulent with solitary or tufted rosettes of thick, ovate to ovate-triangular, sharply pointed, waxy, pale green leaves, 3–9cm (1¼–3½in) long, with transparent, often reddish brown margins. From spring to early summer, bears ovoid, yellow-tipped red flowers, to 1.5cm (½in) long, yellow inside, in one-sided cymes, to 50cm (20in) long. ↕ 15cm (6in), ↔ 30cm (12in) or more. Mexico. ❀ (min. 7°C/45°F)
E. ciliata. Short-stemmed, hairy succulent with dense rosettes of wedge-shaped to obovate, bristle-tipped, dark green leaves, to 5cm (2in) long, often margined red. In early summer, bears ovoid, green then red or yellow-red flowers, 1.5cm (½in) long, in one-sided cymes, 4–14cm (1½–5½in) long. ↕ to 17cm (7in), ↔ to 10cm (4in). Mexico. ❀ (min. 7°C/45°F)

E. cooperi see *Adromischus cooperi.*
E. crenulata. Short-stemmed succulent with loose rosettes of broadly obovate-diamond-shaped, pointed, pale green leaves, to 30cm (12in) long, with or without bristle tips, and with wavy or flat, red or red-brown margins. From early summer to winter, bears ovoid, yellowish red flowers, 1.5cm (½in) long, yellow inside, in panicle-like cymes, to 1m (3ft) long. ↕ 30cm (12in) or more, ↔ 50cm (20in). Mexico. ❄ (min. 7°C/45°F)
E. cuspidata. Stemless succulent with dense rosettes of oblong-obovate, flat, rather thin, somewhat glaucous, grey-green leaves, 7cm (3in) long, that are blunt with small points, and suffused and tipped red-bronze. From spring to early summer, bears one-sided cymes, to 40cm (16in) long, of purplish red to deep pink flowers, 1.5cm (½in) long, with conical tubes. ↕ 12–15cm (5–6in), ↔ 15cm (6in). Mexico. ❄ (min. 7°C/45°F)
E. derenbergii 🏆 Short-stemmed succulent with dense tufts or rosettes of wedge-shaped to obovate, thick, bristle-tipped, intensely white-frosted, light green leaves, to 4cm (1½in) long, tipped and margined red. From late winter to early summer, produces racemes, to 10cm (4in) long, of ovoid-bell-shaped yellow flowers, to 1.5cm (½in) long, with red petal lobes. ↕ 10cm (4in), ↔ to 30cm (12in). Mexico. ❄ (min. 7°C/45°F)
E. elegans ■ 🏆 Stemless or short-stemmed, clump-forming succulent with rounded rosettes of obovate to spoon-shaped, sometimes red-margined, silvery blue leaves, 3–6cm (1¼–2½in) long. From late winter to early summer, produces solitary, one-sided cymes, to 25cm (10in) long, of ovoid, yellow-tipped pink flowers, 1cm (½in) long, yellow-orange inside. ↕ 5cm (2in), ↔ 50cm (20in). Mexico. ❄ (min. 7°C/45°F)
E.* x *fruticosa see x *Pachyveria glauca.*
E. gibbiflora. Simple-stemmed or few-branched succulent that produces terminal rosettes of obovate-spoon-shaped, pointed, wavy-margined, grey-green leaves, to 35cm (14in) long, often tinged reddish brown. Panicle-like cymes, to 1m (3ft) long, of ovoid-bell-shaped, pale red flowers, to 2cm (¾in) long, yellow inside, are borne from late summer to winter. ↕ 30cm (12in), ↔ 15cm (6in). Mexico. ❄ (min. 7°C/45°F). **'Carunculata'** has wart-like protuberances on the upper leaf surfaces, causing the margins to curl and twist. **'Metallica'** bears white- or red-margined, purple-green leaves maturing to green-bronze.

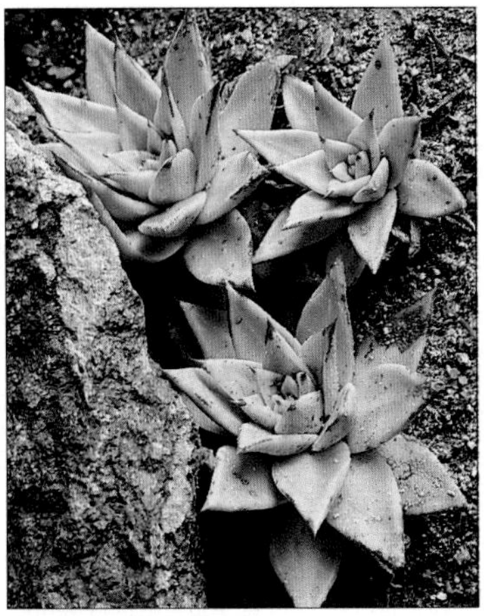
Echeveria agavoides

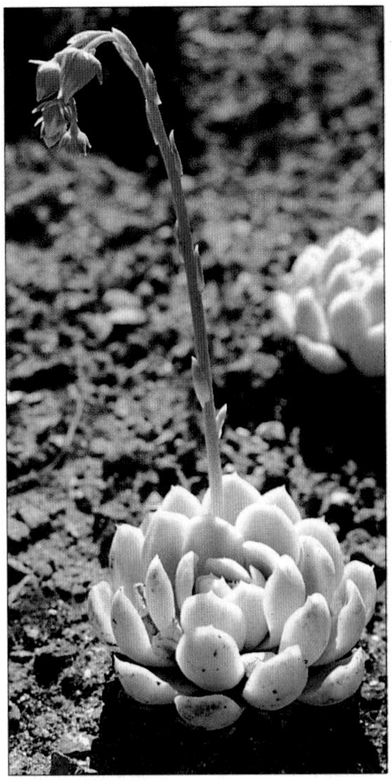
Echeveria elegans

E. goldieana. Stemless or very short-stemmed, clump-forming succulent with dense rosettes of broadly obovate, thick, glossy, mid-green leaves, to 4cm (1½in) long, blunt with small points. From spring to early summer, produces racemes, 40cm (16in) long, of pitcher-shaped, nodding pink flowers, to 1.5cm (½in) long, with greenish yellow tips. ↕ 6cm (2½in), ↔ to 12cm (5in). Mexico. ❄ (min. 7°C/45°F)
E. harmsii 🏆 syn. *Oliveranthus elegans.* Bushy succulent with softly hairy branches, each branch crowned with a rosette of narrow, inversely lance-shaped, pointed, slightly hairy, red-margined, light green leaves, 2–5cm (¾–2in) long. In spring, produces urn-shaped, orange-tipped red flowers, 3cm (1¼in) long, yellow inside, in racemes to 20cm (8in) long. ↕↔ 30cm (12in). Mexico. ❄ (min. 7°C/45°F)
E. nodulosa. Erect then prostrate succulent covered in minute, prickly-tipped white papillae. Thick, obovate-spoon-shaped leaves, 5cm (2in) long, light green with red margins and keels, are arranged in loose rosettes or scattered. From early summer to autumn, produces ovoid-angular, yellow-tipped red flowers, 1.5cm (½in) long, yellow inside, in racemes to 30cm (12in) long. ↕ 30cm (12in), ↔ to 40cm (16in). S. Mexico. ❄ (min. 7°C/45°F)

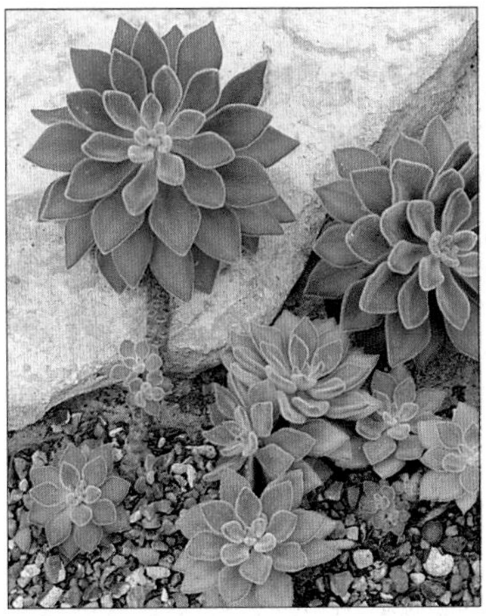
Echeveria pilosa

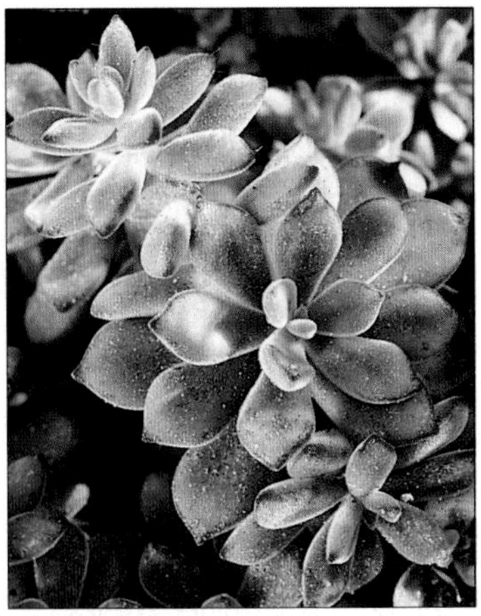
Echeveria pulvinata

E. peacockii. Stemless or short-stemmed succulent producing dense rosettes of obovate-oblong, slightly tapering, pointed or bristle-tipped, white-frosted leaves, to 7cm (3in) long, with red tips and margins. In early summer, bears ovoid, deep red or red-pink flowers, to 1.5cm (½in) long, in one-sided cymes, 30cm (12in) or more long. ↕ to 12cm (5in), ↔ 25cm (10in). Mexico. ❄ (min. 7°C/45°F)
E. pilosa ■ Short-stemmed, sparsely branched or unbranched succulent, densely covered with white hairs. Reddish brown stems bear loose rosettes of thick, spoon-shaped, mid-green leaves, 7cm (3in) long, with wedge-shaped ends. From spring to summer, produces ovoid flowers, to 1.5cm (½in) long, dull orange-red outside, yellow inside and on the tips, in raceme-like cymes, 30cm (12in) long. ↕ 10cm (4in), ↔ 40cm (16in). Mexico. ❄ (min. 7°C/45°F)
E. pulvinata ■ 🏆 (Plush plant). Bushy succulent with brown-felted stems, each producing a lax rosette of spoon-shaped-obovate, fine-pointed, thick, softly white-hairy, mid-green leaves, 2.5–6cm (1–2½in) long, the margins turning red in autumn. From winter to early summer, produces loose panicles, 20–30cm (8–12in) long, of ovoid to urn-shaped, red-keeled, yellow or yellow-red flowers, to 2cm (¾in) long. ↕ 30cm (12in), ↔ 50cm (20in). S. Mexico. ❄ (min. 7°C/45°F)

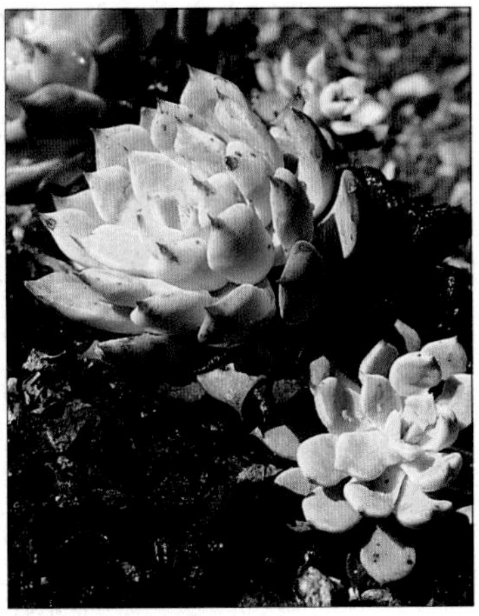
Echeveria secunda

E. secunda ■ Short-stemmed, clump-forming succulent with often decumbent, dense, basal rosettes of spoon- to wedge-shaped, blunt, bristle-tipped, glaucous, pale green to grey leaves, to 5cm (2in) long, with red tips and margins. In late spring and early summer, produces ovoid red flowers, to 1.5cm (½in) long, yellow inside, in one-sided cymes, to 30cm (12in) long. ↕ 4cm (1½in), ↔ 30cm (12in). Mexico. ❄ (min. 7°C/45°F)
E. setosa 🏆 (Mexican firecracker). Stemless succulent with dense, nearly spherical rosettes of inversely lance-shaped to spoon-shaped, pointed, bristle-tipped, mid-green leaves, 8cm (3in) long, densely covered with white hairs. From late spring to summer, urn-shaped, yellow-tipped red flowers, 1cm (½in) or more long, yellow inside, are produced in one-sided cymes, to 30cm (12in) long. ↕ 4cm (1½in), ↔ 30cm (12in). Mexico. ❄ (min. 7°C/45°F)

ECHIDNOPSIS

ASCLEPIADACEAE

Genus of about 20 species of very variable, perennial succulents from low hillsides in Saudi Arabia, Oman, Yemen, and tropical E. Africa and South Africa. They have branching, prostrate to erect, spherical to short-columnar stems, each with 6- to 20-angled, dark green ribs, usually divided into hexagonal tubercles. Tiny, grey-green leaves are short-lived, sometimes persisting as white spines on the tubercles. Saucer- to bell-shaped, 5-lobed, fleshy flowers, with whorled, cup-shaped corollas, are borne in clusters, mainly at the stem tips. In frost-prone areas, grow as houseplants or in a warm greenhouse; in warm, dry climates, grow outdoors in a border with other succulents.

- **HARDINESS** Frost tender.
- **CULTIVATION** Under glass, grow in a mix of equal parts loam-based potting compost (JI No.2) and grit, in full light and with good ventilation. In growth, water moderately and apply a balanced liquid fertilizer monthly; water very sparingly in winter. Outdoors, grow in moderately fertile, sharply drained soil in full sun. See also pp.48–49.
- **PROPAGATION** In spring or summer, sow seed at 21–24°C (70–75°F), or take stem cuttings ensuring the cut surface forms a complete callus before inserting.
- **PESTS AND DISEASES** Vulnerable to black rot if overwatered, especially if temperatures fall below 16°C (61°F).

E. chrysantha see *E. scutellata* subsp. *planiflora.*
E. dammanniana. Erect or curved succulent with 8-angled, ribbed stems, each rib divided into small, irregular tubercles. From late spring to summer, produces clusters of 2–5 flowers, to 1cm (½in) wide; the cup-shaped corollas and spreading lobes vary from yellow, densely spotted with purplish maroon, to purplish maroon; the coronas are yellowish purple. ↕ 20cm (8in), ↔ to 25cm (10in). N. Ethiopia. ❄ (min. 16°C/61°F)

E

E. scutellata. Erect or prostrate succulent with 8- to 9-angled, ribbed stems, each rib divided into hexagonal-conical tubercles. In late spring, bears solitary or paired flowers, to 1cm (½in) wide: the saucer- to bell-shaped corollas are yellow or yellowish green (often with purple mottling on the exterior), with triangular to ovoid-triangular, minutely warty lobes; the coronas are yellow, with red-spotted throats. ↕ to 30cm (12in), ↔ indefinite. Saudi Arabia, Yemen, Somalia. ❀ (min. 16°C/61°F). **subsp. *planiflora***, syn. *E. chrysantha*, has 8- to 15-angled, ribbed stems, and flowers varying in colour from brown, suffused yellow near the centres, to bright yellow with pale green outsides; coronas vary from yellow to red-brown; Ethiopia, Djibouti, Somalia.

ECHINACEA

Coneflower

ASTERACEAE/COMPOSITAE

Genus of about 9 species of bold, stiff perennials from dry prairies, gravelly hillsides, and open woodland in C. and E. North America, usually with thick, black rootstocks and short rhizomes. Erect, hairy stems bear linear-lance-shaped to ovate, entire, toothed, or deeply pinnatifid, bristly, dark green leaves. Solitary, daisy-like, purple, red, or pink flowerheads, with pointed, stiff scales on the undersides and prominent, ovoid or cone-shaped, brownish yellow to orange central discs, are produced terminally on stout, sometimes sparsely branched stems. Grow in a herbaceous border or in open woodland.

- **HARDINESS** Fully hardy.
- **CULTIVATION** Grow in deep, well-drained, humus-rich soil in full sun, although they will tolerate some shade. Cut back stems as the blooms fade to encourage further flower production.
- **PROPAGATION** Sow seed at 13°C (55°F) in spring. Divide in autumn or spring, although they resent a lot of disturbance. Insert root cuttings from late autumn to early winter.
- **PESTS AND DISEASES** Trouble free.

E. angustifolia. Erect perennial with lance-shaped to linear, hairy, entire leaves, to 15cm (6in) long, the stem leaves stalkless. In early summer, produces flowerheads, to 15cm (6in) across, with conical, orange-brown discs and narrow, arching, pink or purple-pink, occasionally white ray-florets,

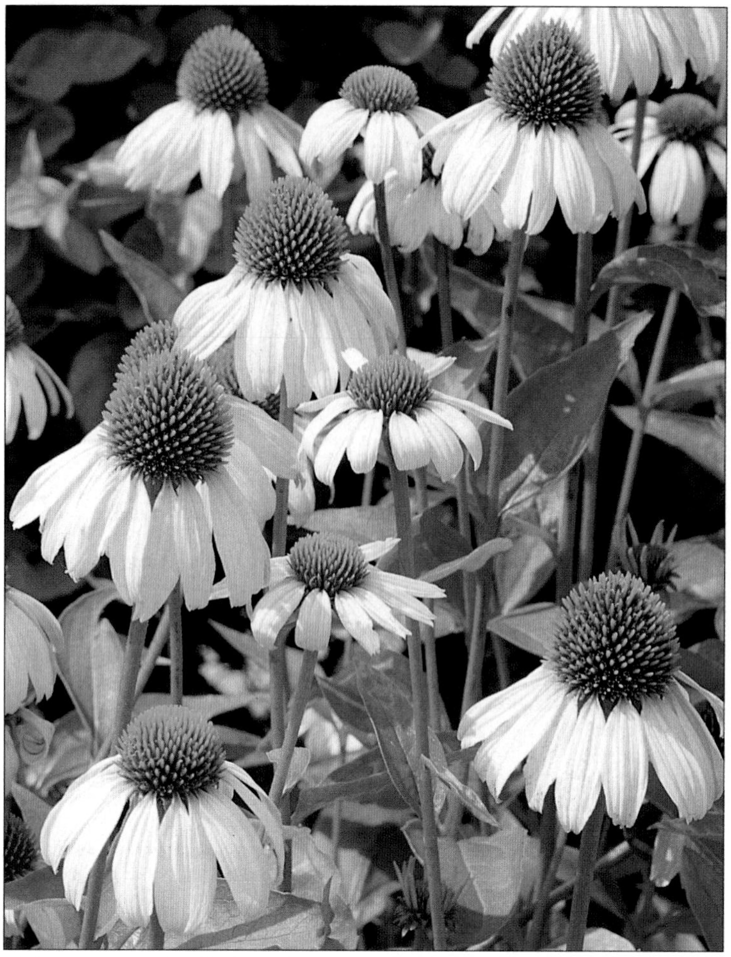

Echinacea purpurea 'White Lustre'

3–4.5cm (1¼–1¾in) long. ↕ to 1.2m (4ft), ↔ 45cm (18in). North America (S. Canada to Texas). ❄❄❄

E. purpurea, syn. *Rudbeckia purpurea.* Erect perennial with smooth, sometimes rough-hairy, red-tinted green stems, ovate, toothed, rough-hairy basal leaves, 15cm (6in) long, and ovate-lance-shaped, toothed stem leaves. From mid-summer to early autumn, bears flower-heads to 12cm (5in) across, with golden brown, cone-shaped discs and partly reflexed, purplish red ray-florets, 3–8cm (1¼–3in) long. ↕ to 1.5m (5ft), ↔ 45cm (18in). USA (Michigan S. to Virginia, Louisiana, and Georgia). ❄❄❄. **'Bright Star'** see 'Leuchtstern'. **'Leuchtstern'**, syn. 'Bright Star', has purple-red flowerheads; ↕ to 80cm (32in). **Lustre Hybrids** have clear purple, red-purple, or white flowerheads; ↕ 80–120cm (2½–4ft). **'Magnus'** has flowerheads to 18cm (7in) across, with dark orange discs, the ray-florets deep purple and more horizontal than in other cultivars. **'Robert Bloom'** ◼ has prominent, dark orange-brown discs and mauve-crimson ray-florets. **'The King'** has arching, pinkish crimson ray-florets and ovate, orange-brown discs. **'White Lustre'** ◼ has creamy white flowerheads with orange-brown discs; ↕ to 80cm (32in). **'White Swan'** has white flowerheads, to 11cm (4½in) across, with orange-brown discs; ↕ to 60cm (24in).

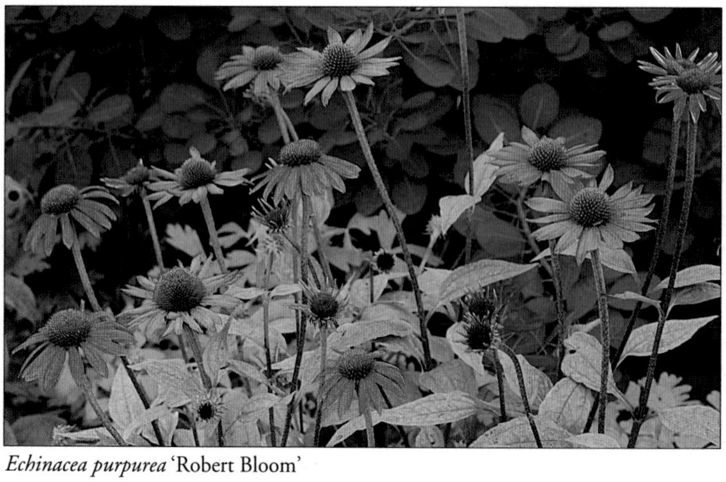

Echinacea purpurea 'Robert Bloom'

ECHINOCACTUS

CACTACEAE

Genus of about 15 species of slow-growing, spherical, barrel-shaped, or columnar, perennial cacti from low, open scrubland in S.W. USA and Mexico. They have prominent, heavily spined ribs and large areoles forming densely woolly crowns, from which rings of diurnal, bell-shaped, yellow, pink, red, or magenta flowers develop in summer on mature plants. Ovoid, white-woolly fruits contain large black or dark brown seeds. In frost-prone areas, grow in a warm greenhouse; elsewhere, plant in a desert garden.

- **HARDINESS** Frost tender.
- **CULTIVATION** Under glass, grow in standard cactus compost in full light. From mid-spring to early autumn, water freely and apply a half-strength balanced liquid fertilizer every 4 weeks; keep totally dry at other times of the year. Outdoors, grow in fertile, well-drained soil in full sun. See also pp.48–49.
- **PROPAGATION** Sow seed at 21°C (70°F) in spring.
- **PESTS AND DISEASES** Vulnerable to mealybugs, especially when young.

E. asterias see *Astrophytum asterias.*
E. capricornis see *Astrophytum capricorne.*
E. chilensis see *Neoporteria chilensis.*
E. grusonii ◼ (Golden barrel cactus, Mother-in-law's cushion). Spherical, eventually elongating cactus with a bright green stem bearing 20–40 sharply angled ribs. Yellow areoles produce golden yellow spines (8–10 radials and 3–5 centrals). Bears bright yellow flowers, 4–6cm (1½–2½in) long, in summer. ↕ to 60cm (24in), ↔ to 80cm (32in). C. Mexico. ❀ (min. 10°C/50°F)
E. hartmannii see *Discocactus hartmannii.*
E. horizonthalonius. Spherical to columnar cactus with a blue-green or grey-green stem bearing 7–13 often spirally arranged ribs. Brown areoles produce brown spines (6–9 radials and 1 central). Rose-red or pink flowers, 5–7cm (2–3in) long, darker near their bases, are produced in summer. ↕ to 25cm (10in), ↔ to 40cm (16in). USA (W. Texas, New Mexico), N. Mexico. ❀ (min. 10°C/50°F)
E. ingens see *E. platyacanthus.*
E. myriostigma see *Astrophytum myriostigma.*
E. ornatus see *Astrophytum ornatum.*
E. platyacanthus, syn. *E. ingens.* Spherical cactus with a fresh green stem bearing 20–60 very pronounced ribs. Grey areoles produce greyish brown or yellow-brown spines (about 4 radials and 3 or 4 centrals). In summer, bears golden yellow flowers, 3–6cm (1¼–2½in) long, with brown-tipped outer tepals. ↕↔ to 1m (3ft). C. and N. Mexico. ❀ (min. 10°C/50°F)
E. polycephalus ◼ Spherical, often elongating, clump-forming cactus with 13- to 21-ribbed, grey-green stems. Whitish grey areoles bear reddish brown spines (4–8 flattish radials and 4 centrals). In summer, produces yellow flowers, 5–6cm (2–2½in) long, the outer tepals with pink midribs. ↕ to 70cm (28in), ↔ 25cm (10in). USA (California, S. Utah, N. Arizona), N. Mexico. ❀ (min. 10°C/50°F)
E. ritteri see *Aztekium ritteri.*
E. scheeri see *Sclerocactus scheeri.*
E. texensis, syn. *Homalocephala texensis.* Flattened-spherical or barrel-shaped

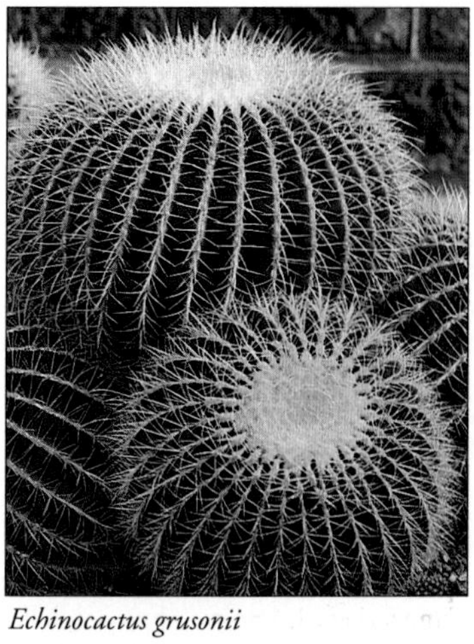

Echinocactus grusonii

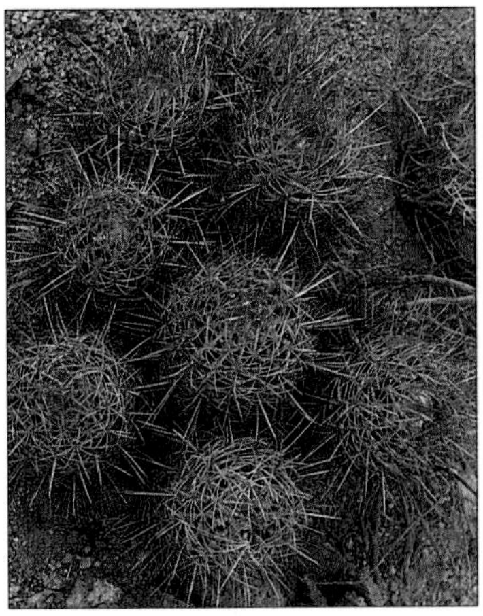

Echinocactus polycephalus

cactus with a 13- to 27-ribbed, greyish green stem. Well-spaced, white-woolly areoles bear red-brown spines (6 or 7 radials and 1 thicker central). Bears satiny, pale reddish pink flowers, 5–6cm (2–2½in) long, with pink to orange-red throats and paler, irregular margins, in summer. ↕ to 15cm (6in), ↔ to 30cm (12in). USA (Texas, S. New Mexico), N.E. Mexico. ❄ (min. 10°C/50°F)
E. uncinatus see *Sclerocactus uncinatus.*

ECHINOCEREUS

CACTACEAE

Genus of about 45 species of simple or clump-forming, perennial cacti found in lowland deserts to open, dry uplands in S. and S.W. USA and Mexico. They produce spherical to cylindrical, prominently ribbed stems and are noted for their very colourful, diurnal flowers, which are generally large and usually funnel- or bell-shaped. In frost-prone areas, grow on a sunny window-sill or in a cool or temperate greenhouse; in warmer areas, plant in a desert garden.

- **HARDINESS** Frost tender.
- **CULTIVATION** Under glass, grow in standard cactus compost in full light. From mid-spring to early autumn, water freely and apply a half-strength balanced liquid fertilizer monthly; keep totally dry at other times. Outdoors, grow in well-drained soil in full sun. See also pp.48–49.
- **PROPAGATION** Sow seed at 21°C (70°F) in early spring. Root stem cuttings in spring or summer.
- **PESTS AND DISEASES** Vulnerable to mealybugs and scale insects.

E. baileyi see *E. reichenbachii* var. *baileyi.*
E. brandegeei. Erect or decumbent, clump-forming cactus with cylindrical, 6- to 8-ribbed, warty, dull, pale green stems, 4–6cm (1½–2½in) thick. Yellowish green areoles bear yellowish red or yellowish white spines (12 radials and 4 centrals). Produces bell-shaped, purplish pink flowers, to 7cm (3in) long, with red throats, in early summer. ↕ 1m (3ft), ↔ to 50cm (20in). Mexico (Baja California). ❄ (min. 7°C/45°F)
E. cinerascens. Clump-forming cactus with spherical to cylindrical, 5- to 12-ribbed, sometimes warty, bright green stems, 4–7cm (1½–3in) thick. Bright green areoles bear yellowish white or red spines (8–10 radials and 1–4 centrals). Funnel-shaped, bright pink or purple

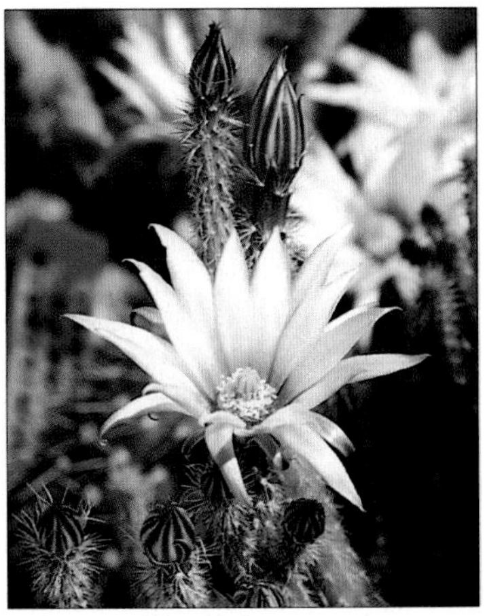

Echinocereus leucanthus

flowers, 6–10cm (2½–4in) across, with paler, greenish pink throats, are borne in early summer. ↕ 10–60cm (4–24in), ↔ to 1m (3ft). N., C., and E. Mexico. ❄ (min. 7°C/45°F)
E. engelmannii. Semi-erect, clump-forming cactus with cylindrical, 10- to 14-ribbed, densely spiny, mid-green stems, 4–8cm (1½–3in) thick. Large, mid-green areoles bear variously coloured spines (10–12 radials and 2–6 longer centrals). Produces broadly funnel-shaped, purple-red to magenta or lavender-pink flowers, 7cm (3in) across, in early summer. ↕ 5–60cm (2–24in), ↔ to 45cm (18in). S.W. USA, N.W. Mexico. ❄ (min. 7°C/45°F)
E. fendleri. Simple or clump-forming cactus with ovoid to cylindrical, variably warty, 9- to 18-ribbed, dull or brownish green stems, 4–8cm (1½–3in) thick. Green areoles bear brown spines (about 8 radials and 1 longer central). From spring to early summer, produces broadly bell-shaped, purplish violet or purple-magenta to white flowers, 9cm (3½in) long, which darken towards the sometimes green-tinged centres and have jagged petal margins. ↕ 8–50cm (3–20in), ↔ to 30cm (12in). USA (S. Utah, Arizona, New Mexico), N.W. Mexico. ❄ (min. 7°C/45°F)
E. knippelianus. Erect, simple or clustering cactus with spherical, almost ovoid, dark green stems, to 8cm (3in) thick, offsetting from the base, with 5–8 rounded ribs divided by broad furrows. Small green areoles bear 1–3 bristly, short-lived, yellow radial spines. Funnel-shaped, pink, lavender-pink, purple, or white flowers, to 4cm (1½in) long, are borne from spring to early summer. ↕ to 20cm (8in), usually smaller, ↔ 15cm (6in). N.E. Mexico. ❄ (min. 7°C/45°F)
E. leucanthus ■ syn. *Wilcoxia albiflora.* Clambering cactus, freely branching from the base, with cylindrical, 8- to 12-ribbed, dark green stems, to 6mm (¼in) thick. Brown areoles bear 10–12 yellow, sometimes almost black radial spines. Wide-spreading, funnel-shaped white flowers, 2–4cm (¾–1½in) long, with greenish brown throats, and sometimes pale pink midstripes, are borne in early summer. ↕ to 1m (3ft), ↔ 30cm (12in). N.W. Mexico. ❄ (min. 7°C/45°F)
E. maritimus. Variable, erect, clump-forming cactus with spherical or slightly cylindrical, 8- to 10-ribbed, greenish grey stems, 2.5cm (1in) thick. Bright green areoles bear greyish white or red, later greyish yellow to grey spines (9 or 10 radials and 1–4 longer centrals). Funnel-shaped, brown- or red-tinged yellow flowers, 4cm (1½in) long, are produced in early summer. ↕ 15cm (6in), ↔ indefinite. N.W. Mexico. ❄ (min. 7°C/45°F)
E. pectinatus. Erect, simple or eventually sparsely branched cactus with spherical or cylindrical, 12- to 23-ribbed, mid-green stems, 7–10cm (3–4in) thick. Mid-green areoles produce comb-like, pinkish white spines (up to 30 radials and 3 shorter centrals). In late spring and early summer, bears funnel-shaped, pale pinkish lavender, sometimes magenta or yellow flowers, 7–12cm (3–5in) long, green at the bases, with white or maroon throats. ↕ 8–35cm (3–14in), ↔ 20cm (8in). S.W. USA, N. Mexico. ❄ (min. 7°C/45°F)
E. pentalophus ■ syn. *E. procumbens.* Prostrate or erect, clump-forming cactus with cylindrical, 4- to 8-ribbed, pale to dark green stems, 2cm (¾in) thick. White areoles bear about 6 yellow or white radial spines. Bell-shaped, lilac to carmine-red or bright pink-magenta flowers, to 10cm (4in) long, with white or yellow throats, rarely entirely white, develop in early summer. ↕ 20cm (8in), ↔ 60cm (24in). USA (Texas), E. and N.E. Mexico. ❄ (min. 7°C/45°F)
E. procumbens see *E. pentalophus.*
E. pulchellus ■ Erect, simple or clustering cactus that branches at the base. Spherical or hemispherical, grey to bluish green stems, 4–5cm (1½–2in) thick, have 11–13 low, warty ribs. White areoles bear 3 or 4 yellow to grey radial spines. Widely spreading, funnel-shaped, bright rose-pink, pink, magenta,

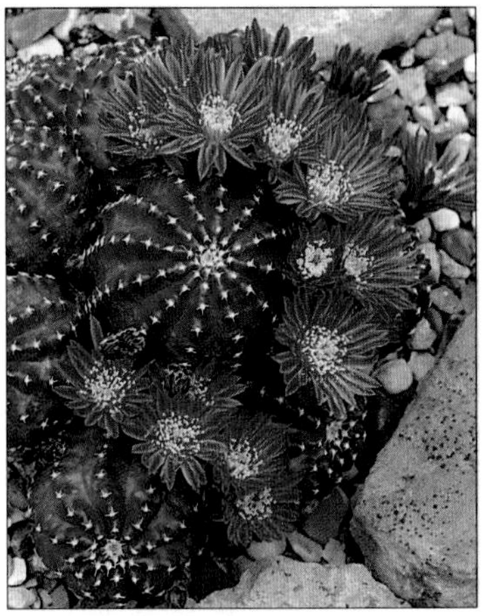

Echinocereus pulchellus

or white flowers, 4cm (1½in) long, with white margins, are produced in late spring and early summer. ↕ 5cm (2in), ↔ 15cm (6in). N. and S. central Mexico. ❄ (min. 7°C/45°F)
E. reichenbachii ♀ Variable, erect cactus with usually simple, spherical to cylindrical, light to dark green stems, to 10cm (4in) thick, with up to 19 ribs. Light to dark green areoles bear 12–40 white or brown radial spines. Bears broadly funnel-shaped, pink to purple or magenta flowers, 7cm (3in) across, with darker throats, from spring to early summer. ↕ to 35cm (14in), ↔ 20cm (8in). USA (Kansas, Oklahoma, Texas), N. Mexico. ❄ (min. 7°C/45°F). **var. *baileyi***, syn. *E. baileyi*, is sparsely branched, with 12–15 ribs. Areoles bear up to 14 radial spines and sometimes 1–3 centrals. Rich pink flowers have darker petal bases. ↕↔ to 20cm (8in). USA (Oklahoma, Texas).
E. schmollii ■ syn. *Wilcoxia schmollii.* Usually erect, simple or sparsely branched cactus with a tuberous rootstock and cylindrical, purplish green stems, 2cm (¾in) thick, with 8–10 warty ribs. Light to dark green areoles bear numerous hair-like white radial spines. Produces funnel-shaped, pinkish purple or bright pink flowers, 3.5cm (1½in) long, in early summer. ↕ 30cm (12in) or more, ↔ 25cm (10in). E. Mexico. ❄ (min. 7°C/45°F)
E. subinermis ♀ Erect, simple or sparsely clustered cactus with spherical then cylindrical, 5- to 8-ribbed, shallow-furrowed, bluish green or dark green stems, 7–9cm (3–3½in) thick at the bases. Dark green areoles bear yellow

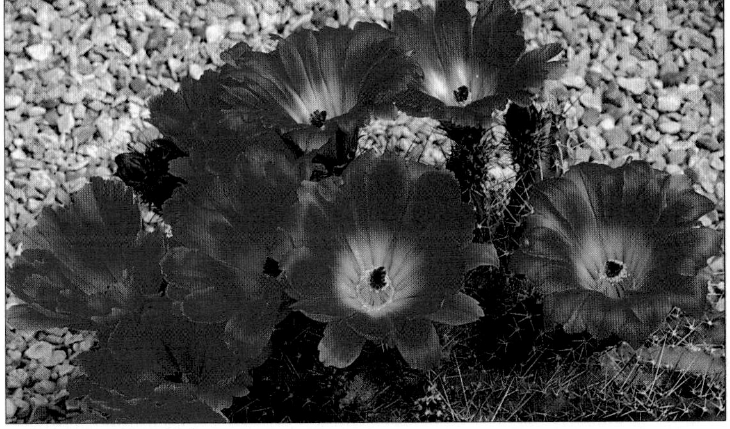

Echinocereus pentalophus

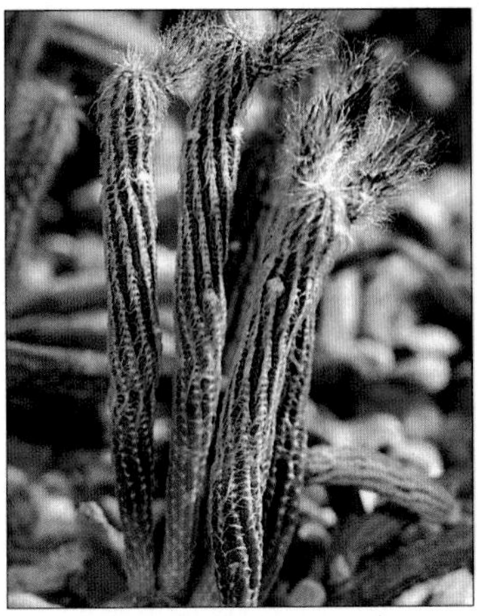

Echinocereus schmollii

E

E

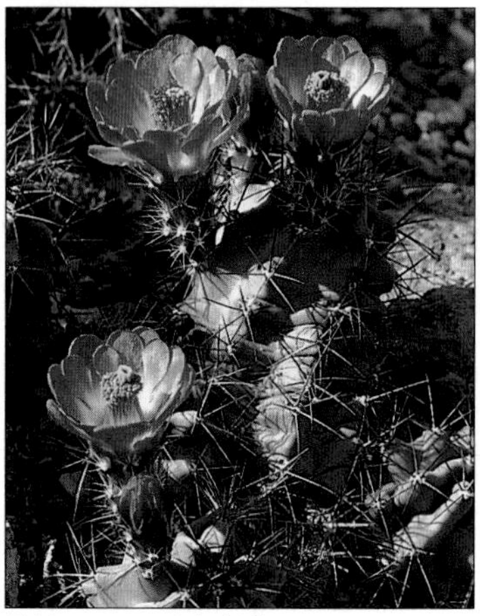

Echinocereus triglochidiatus var. *paucispinus*

spines (3–8 radials and often 1 central). Produces broadly funnel-shaped, bright yellow flowers, 8cm (3in) long, in early summer. ↕↔ to 30cm (12in). N., N.W., and C. Mexico. ❁ (min. 7°C/45°F)

E. triglochidiatus. Very variable, erect, simple or clustering cactus with ovoid to cylindrical, 6- to 12-ribbed, sometimes warty, dark green stems, 5–15cm (2–6in) thick. Dark green, woolly areoles bear pale brown spines (3–16 radials and often 1 central). Funnel-shaped, bright red flowers, to 8cm (3in) long, are produced from spring to early summer. ↕ 30cm (12in), ↔ 15cm (6in). S. USA, N. Mexico. ❁ (min. 7°C/45°F). **var. *paucispinus*** ■ has 6- or 7-ribbed stems, 10cm (4in) thick. Areoles bear 4–6 radial spines and no centrals. Orange-red flowers, 7cm (3in) long, are produced in spring. ↕ 20cm (8in), ↔ to 50cm (20in). USA (Texas).

▷ ***Echinofossulocactus*** see *Stenocactus*
E. coptonogonus see *S. coptonogonus*
E. lamellosus see *S. crispatus*
E. multicostatus see *S. multicostatus*
E. pentacanthus see *S. obvallatus*
E. violaciflorus see *S. obvallatus*
▷ ***Echinomastus macdowellii*** see *Thelocactus macdowellii*

ECHINOPS

Globe thistle

ASTERACEAE/COMPOSITAE

Genus of about 120 species of perennials, biennials, and annuals found in hot, gravelly slopes and dry grassland from C. and S. Europe to C. Asia, India, and the mountains of tropical Africa. Globe thistles have simple, entire or pinnatifid to pinnatisect, spiny foliage, usually greyish white and woolly. They bear spherical, white, grey, or blue, terminal flowerheads with bristly bracts. Undemanding plants, they are suitable for a large border or wild garden. They are also good for cutting and drying.

- **HARDINESS** Fully hardy to frost hardy.
- **CULTIVATION** Best grown in poor, well-drained soil in full sun, but will grow in almost any soil in full sun or partial shade. Dead-head to prevent self-seeding.
- **PROPAGATION** Sow seed in a seedbed in mid-spring. Divide perennials from autumn to spring, or insert root cuttings in winter.
- **PESTS AND DISEASES** Susceptible to infestation by aphids.

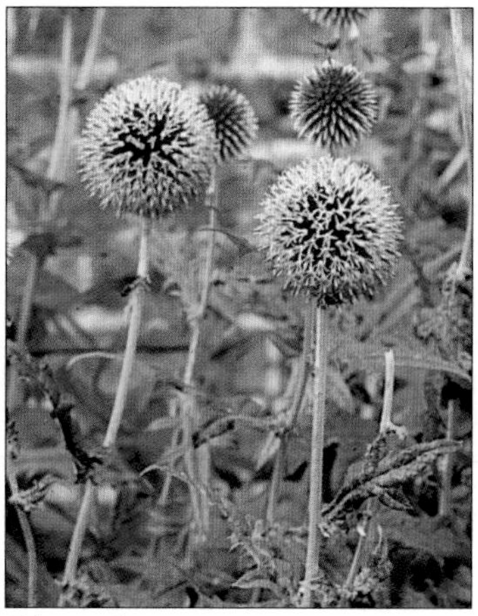

Echinops bannaticus

E. bannaticus ■ Clump-forming perennial with densely grey-woolly stems and ovate to elliptic, subentire to 2-pinnatisect, spiny, hairy, grey-green leaves, to 25cm (10in) long. Produces spherical, blue-grey to blue flowerheads, 2.5–5cm (1–2in) across, in mid- and late summer. ↕ 0.5–1.2m (1½–4ft), ↔ 60cm (24in). S.E. Europe. ❄❄❄. **'Blue Globe'** has dark blue flowerheads, 6cm (2½in) across, and blooms again if stems are cut back after flowering; ↕ to 1m (3ft). **'Taplow Blue'** 🏆 has bright blue flowerheads.

E. giganteus. Imposing perennial with erect, woolly stems and obovate to lance-shaped, pinnatifid, bristly leaves, 45cm (18in) long, which are white-hairy beneath. In midsummer, produces solitary, sometimes several, spherical, greyish blue flowerheads, 20cm (8in) across. ↕ to 5m (15ft), ↔ 75cm (30in). Ethiopia. ❄❄

E. niveus. Slender but sturdy, clump-forming perennial with lance-shaped to elliptic, deeply pinnatisect, spiny leaves, 7–20cm (3–8in) long, with linear segments, mid-green above, densely white-woolly beneath. In late summer, grey stems bear spherical, blue-grey or white flowerheads, 3.5–8cm (1½–3in) across. ↕ to 1.8m (6ft), ↔ 60cm (24in). W. Himalayas. ❄❄❄

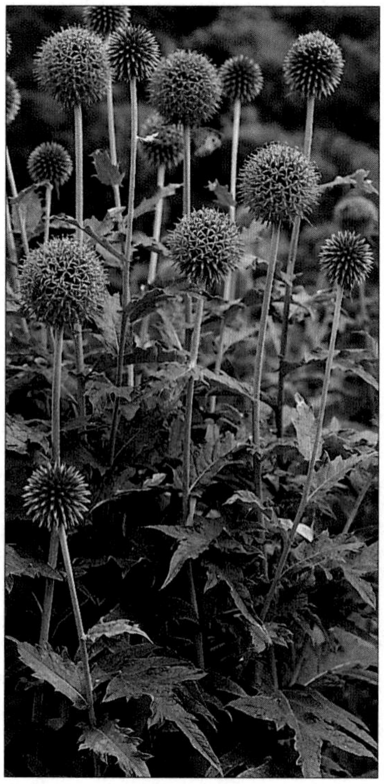

Echinops ritro 'Veitch's Blue'

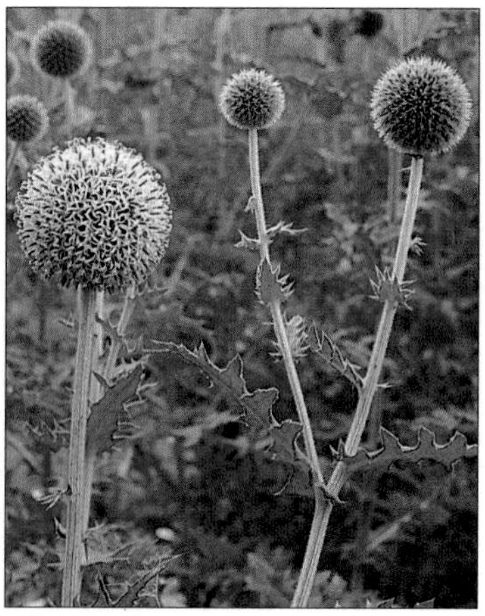

Echinops sphaerocephalus

E. ritro 🏆 Compact, clump-forming perennial with oblong-elliptic, pinnatifid to pinnatisect, stiff, spiny leaves, to 20cm (8in) long, dark green and cobwebby above, white-downy beneath. In late summer, bears spherical flowerheads, 2.5–4.5cm (1–1¾in) across, metallic-blue before the florets open, maturing to a brighter blue. ↕ to 60cm (24in), ↔ 45cm (18in). S. central and S.E. Europe to C. Asia. ❄❄❄. **'Veitch's Blue'** ■ is remontant, with slightly darker blue flowerheads, and is good for cutting; ↕ to 90cm (36in).

E. sphaerocephalus ■ Vigorous, clump-forming perennial with oblong-elliptic, pinnatifid or 2-pinnatifid to pinnatisect, spiny, grey-green leaves, to 35cm (14in) long, hairy beneath. Spherical, silvery grey flowerheads, 3–6cm (1¼–2½in) across, are borne on stout grey stems in mid- and late summer. ↕ to 2m (6ft), ↔ 90cm (36in). C. and S. Europe, Caucasus, Russia (Siberia). ❄❄❄

ECHINOPSIS

CACTACEAE

Genus of 50–120 species of sometimes shrubby or tree-like, perennial cacti occurring in South America, in habitats ranging from lowland deserts to upland dry scrub. They have mainly spherical stems with straight ribs and spiny areoles. Large, trumpet-shaped to almost bell-shaped flowers are produced laterally or near the ends of the stems from spring to summer. On species native to mountainous regions to 3,000m (10,000ft) high, the flowers are white, yellow, red, purple, or pink, and open during the day; on plants that grow naturally at much lower altitudes, the flowers are mainly white or pale pink, and open at night. In frost-prone areas, grow as houseplants or in a temperate or warm greenhouse. In warmer areas, grow in a desert garden.

- **HARDINESS** Frost tender.
- **CULTIVATION** Under glass, grow in standard cactus compost in full light. In growth, water freely and apply a nitrogen- and potassium-based fertilizer monthly; keep completely dry in winter. Outdoors, grow in well-drained soil in full sun. See also pp.48–49.
- **PROPAGATION** Sow seed at 21°C (70°F) in spring, or remove offsets in spring or summer.
- **PESTS AND DISEASES** Spherical species are particularly prone to mealybugs.

E. backebergii ■ syn. *Lobivia backebergii*. Simple or clump-forming cactus with spherical to obovoid, mid- to dark green stems, 4–5cm (1½–2in) thick, bearing about 15 spirally notched ribs. White-woolly areoles produce 3–7 red-brown, later grey radial spines, sometimes curved or hooked. In summer, bears diurnal, carmine-red or violet flowers, 5cm (2in) long, with paler throats. ↕↔ 5cm (2in). E. Bolivia, S. Peru. ❁ (min. 10°C/50°F)

E. candicans ■ syn. *Trichocereus candicans*. Erect or semi-prostrate, clump-forming cactus with cylindrical to hemispherical, bright, light green stems, 16cm (6in) thick, bearing 9–11 prominent ribs. Large white areoles produce yellowish brown spines (10–14 radials and 1 or more centrals). Nocturnal, fragrant white flowers, 18–25cm (7–10in) long, are produced in summer. ↕ to 60cm (24in), ↔ to 50cm (20in). W. Argentina. ❁ (min. 10°C/50°F)

E. chamaecereus, syn. *Cereus silvestrii*, *Chamaecereus silvestrii*, *Lobivia silvestrii* (Peanut cactus). Clump- or mat-forming cactus with spreading, branching, cylindrical, mid-green stems, 9–15mm (⅜–½in) thick, with 6–9 ribs. Areoles produce 10–15 bristly, white or brownish white radial spines. Bears diurnal, funnel-shaped, bright orange-scarlet flowers, to 7cm (3in) long, in summer. ↕ to 10cm (4in), ↔ 30–60cm (12–24in). Argentina. ❁ (min. 5°C/41°F)

E. cinnabarina, syn. *Lobivia cinnabarina*. Simple cactus with flattened-spherical to spherical, dark green stems, to 15cm (6in) thick, bearing about 20 notched, acutely warty ribs. White areoles produce light brownish grey spines (8–12 radials and

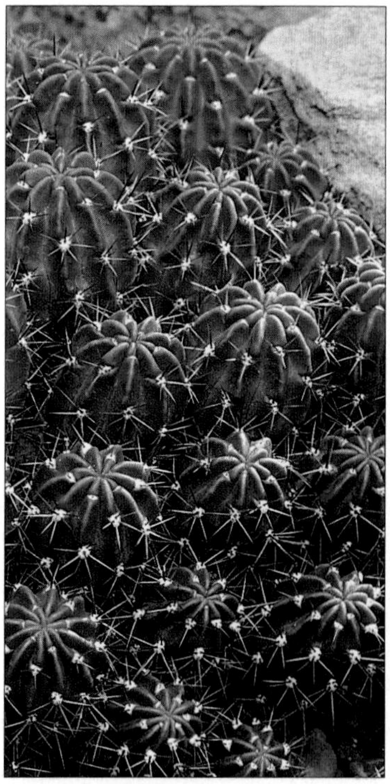

Echinopsis backebergii

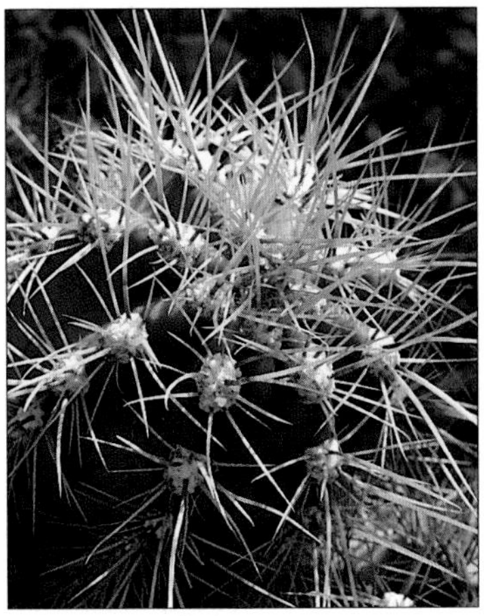

Echinopsis candicans

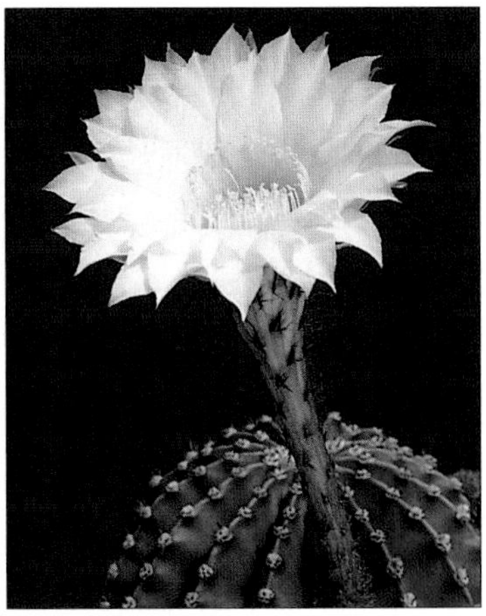

Echinopsis oxygona

2 or 3 stouter centrals). Diurnal, short-tubed, rich scarlet flowers, 4cm (1½in) long, are produced from spring to summer. ↕↔ to 15cm (6in). Bolivia. ❄ (min. 10°C/50°F)

E. eyriesii ♀ Spherical, later cylindrical cactus, occasionally offsetting and clustering, with mid-green stems, 10–15cm (4–6in) thick, bearing 11–18 ribs separated by sharp furrows. Grey areoles bear short, dark brown, almost black spines (up to 10 radials and 4–8 centrals). White flowers, 17–25cm (7–10in) long, open in late afternoon in summer. ↕ to 30cm (12in), ↔ to 15cm (6in). N. Argentina to Uruguay, S. Brazil. ❄ (min. 10°C/50°F)

E. ferox, syn. *Lobivia ferox*. Simple cactus with spherical, 15- to 30-ribbed, pale grey-green stems, to 30cm (12in) thick. Grey areoles produce initially brown, then grey spines (8–12 radials and about 3 centrals). Diurnal white, rarely pink flowers, 7–11cm (3–4½in) long, are borne in summer. ↕↔ 30cm (12in) or more. Bolivia to N. Argentina. ❄ (min. 10°C/50°F)

E. huascha, syn. *Trichocereus huascha, T. grandiflorus*. Offsetting, erect to semi-prostrate cactus with many-branched, 12- to 18-ribbed, dark green stems, 5–8cm (2–3in) thick. Whitish brown areoles bear dark yellow to brown spines (9–11 radials and 1 or 2 centrals). Diurnal, golden yellow or red flowers, 7–10cm (3–4in) long, are produced in summer. ↕↔ to 1m (3ft). Argentina. ❄ (min. 10°C/50°F)

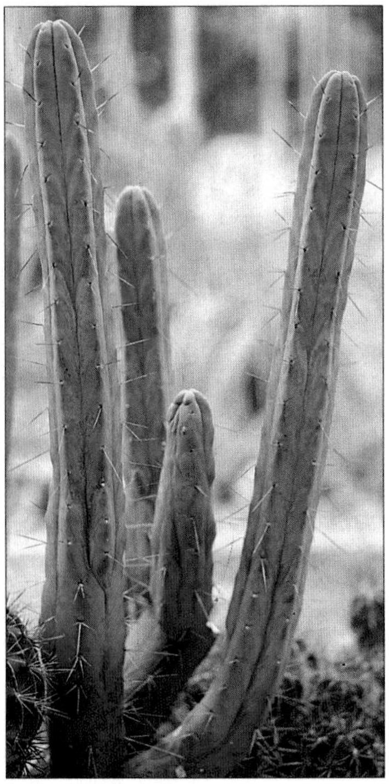

Echinopsis lageniformis

E. lageniformis ■ syn. *Trichocereus bridgesii*. Tree-like cactus with columnar, somewhat glaucous, pale to dark green stems, to 15cm (6in) thick, bearing 4–8 rounded ribs. Grey areoles produce 2–6 yellow radial spines. Bears nocturnal white flowers, 18cm (7in) long, in summer. ↕ 2m (6ft) or more, ↔ 20cm (8in) or more. Bolivia. ❄ (min. 10°C/50°F)

E. maximiliana, syn. *Lobivia caespitosa*. Clump-forming cactus with depressed-spherical to obovoid or cylindrical, pale green stems, 6–8cm (2½–3in) thick, each with 12–17 ribs divided by cross-furrows into hatchet-shaped tubercles. White areoles bear brown spines (7–12 radials and 1 longer, up-curving central). Diurnal, red or scarlet flowers, 5–8cm (2–3in) long, with orange-yellow throats, and sometimes darker-tipped inner tepals, are produced in summer. ↕↔ 7cm (3in). S. Peru, N. Bolivia. ❄ (min. 10°C/50°F)

E. multiplex see *E. oxygona*.

E. oxygona ■ syn. *E. multiplex*. Clustering cactus with spherical or cylindrical, 12- to 15-ribbed, mid-green stems, to 20cm (8in) thick, offsetting from the base and sides. Large, white-woolly areoles bear yellowish brown spines (10–15 radials and 2–7 longer centrals). In summer, produces diurnal flowers, to 20cm (8in) long, with dark reddish brown tubes and pink-flushed white outer petals. ↕ 25–30cm (10–12in), ↔ to 30cm (12in). N. Argentina, Uruguay, S. Brazil. ❄ (min. 10°C/50°F)

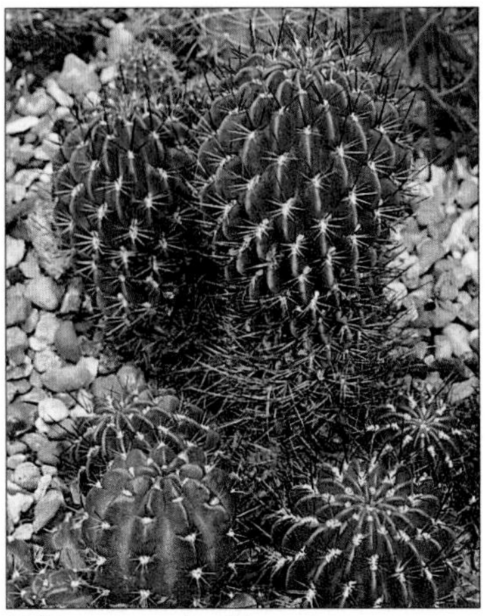

Echinopsis pentlandii

E. pentlandii ■ syn. *Lobivia pentlandii*. Clump-forming cactus with spherical to obovoid, mid-green stems, to 15cm (6in) thick, bearing 15 or more warty ribs. Grey areoles produce brown spines (5–15 radials and sometimes 1 central). Diurnal, yellow, orange, pink, red, or purple flowers, 5–7cm (2–3in) long, with white throats, are produced from spring to summer. ↕ to 15cm (6in), ↔ 30cm (12in). S. Peru, N. Bolivia. ❄ (min. 10°C/50°F)

E. rhodotricha. Simple or clump-forming cactus with spherical, then cylindrical, 8- to 13-ribbed, mid-green stems, 9cm (3½in) thick. White-felted areoles bear brown-tipped, pale yellow spines (4–7 radials and sometimes 1 longer central). Diurnal white flowers, 15cm (6in) long, are produced from spring to summer. ↕ 30cm (12in), ↔ 20cm (8in). Paraguay, N.E. Argentina. ❄ (min. 10°C/50°F)

E. schickendantzii, syn. *Trichocereus shaferi*. Shrub-like cactus with oblong to cylindrical, bright green stems, 6cm (2½in) thick, bearing about 14–18 prominent ribs. White areoles produce about 10 yellow radial spines. White flowers, to 20cm (8in) long, are produced by day or night in summer. ↕ to 30cm (12in), ↔ 12cm (5in). W. Argentina. ❄ (min. 10°C/50°F)

E. spachiana ■ syn. *Cereus spachianus, Trichocereus spachianus*. Shrub-like cactus with cylindrical, 10- to 15-ribbed, dark green stems, to 6cm (2½in) thick, branching freely from the base. Areoles are initially yellow, later becoming grey, and bear yellowish brown spines (8–10 radials and often 2 or 3 centrals). Nocturnal flowers, to 20cm (8in) long, produced in midsummer, have white inner segments and green outer ones. ↕ 1–2m (3–6ft), ↔ 75cm (30in) or more. Argentina. ❄ (min. 10°C/50°F)

E. spiniflora, syn. *Acanthocalycium violaceum*. Simple cactus with a spherical to short-cylindrical and decumbent, dull green stem, 15cm (6in) thick, bearing about 15–20 ribs. Grey areoles produce slender, yellowish brown spines (12 or more radials and 3 or 4 longer centrals). Diurnal, erect, pale violet, pink, or white flowers, 4–5cm (1½–2in) long, with green tubes, are produced in summer. ↕ to 60cm (24in), ↔ 13cm (5in). W. Argentina. ❄ (min. 10°C/50°F)

E. thionantha, syn. *Acanthocalycium aurantiacum*. Simple cactus with spherical to cylindrical, 9- to 16-ribbed, dark greyish green stems, 10–15cm (4–6in) thick. White areoles produce dark, almost blackish brown spines (5–10 radials and occasionally 1 longer central). Diurnal, bright yellow, red, or white flowers, 5cm (2in) long, with yellowish orange inner throats, are borne in summer. ↕↔ 5–12cm (2–5in). N.W. Argentina. ❄ (min. 10°C/50°F)

▷ ***Echinospartum*** see *Genista*
▷ ***Echioides longiflorum*** see *Arnebia pulchra*

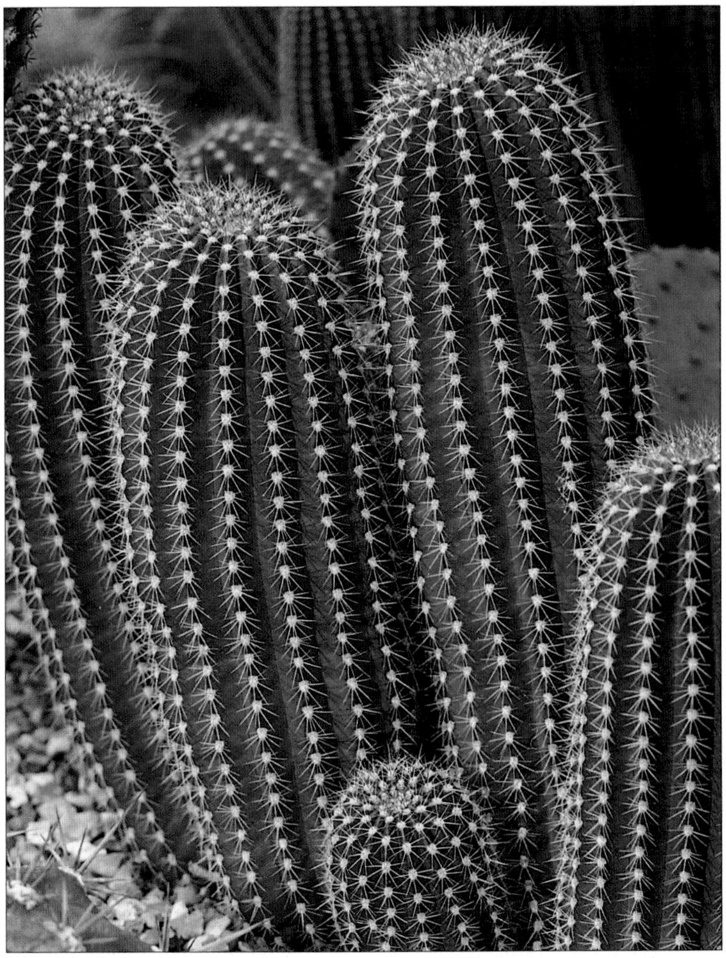

Echinopsis spachiana

E

ECHIUM

BORAGINACEAE

Genus of 40 species of rosette-forming, stiffly hairy annuals and evergreen biennials, perennials (some monocarpic), and shrubs, from stony hillsides, cliffs, open woodland, and grassy steppes in Europe, the Canary Islands, the Mediterranean, Africa, and W. Asia. They are grown for their often one-sided, cyme-like panicles or spikes of roughly funnel-shaped, sometimes bell-shaped, blue, purple, yellow, white, or red flowers, usually 1–2cm (½–¾in) long, borne mainly in summer. The bristly-hairy, usually stalkless leaves are borne in basal rosettes and on the flower stems. Grow echiums in an annual, mixed, or herbaceous border. In frost-prone climates, grow tender species in a cool greenhouse. All parts may cause mild stomach upset if ingested; contact with the foliage may irritate skin.

• **HARDINESS** Fully hardy to frost tender.

• **CULTIVATION** Under glass, grow in loam-based potting compost (JI No.3) in full light. Water freely when in growth, sparingly in winter. Outdoors, grow in moderately fertile, well-drained soil in full sun. In frost-prone areas, protect perennial species *in situ* with horticultural fleece in winter.

• **PROPAGATION** Sow seed of perennial and biennial species at 13–16°C (55–61°F) in summer, overwintering seedlings at 5–7°C (41–45°F). Sow seed of annuals in spring, either *in situ* or under glass. Root semi-ripe cuttings of shrubby perennials in midsummer.

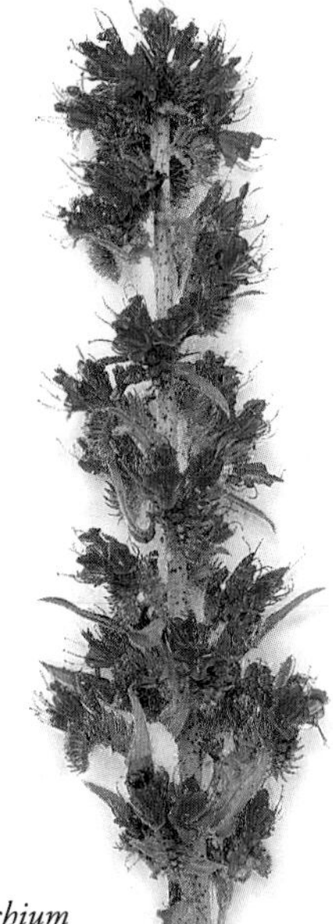

Echium vulgare

• **PESTS AND DISEASES** Outdoors, slugs may attack young growth. Under glass, whiteflies and red spider mites may be a problem.

E. bourgaeanum see *E. wildpretii.*
E. candicans ■ syn. *E. fastuosum* (Pride of Madeira). Open, usually rounded, woody-based biennial with rosetted, lance-shaped, softly white-hairy, prominently veined leaves, 15–25cm (6–10in) long. Bears dense, cylindrical, panicle-like cymes, to 30cm (12in) long, of many narrowly funnel-shaped, white, bluish white, or deep purple-blue flowers, mainly from spring to summer. ↕1.5–2.5m (5–8ft), ↔ 1.5–2m (5–6ft). Madeira. ❀ (min. 5–7°C/41–45°F)
E. fastuosum see *E. candicans.*
E. pininana, syn. *E. pinnifolium.* Rosette-forming biennial or short-lived perennial with elliptic-lance-shaped, densely and roughly silver-hairy leaves, to 7cm (3in) long. In mid- and late summer, each rosette produces a panicle-like cyme, 1.5–4m (5–12ft) long, of funnel-shaped blue flowers with large bracts. ↕ to 4m (12ft), ↔ 90cm (36in). Canary Islands. ❄❄
E. pinnifolium see *E. pininana.*
E. vulgare ■ (Viper's bugloss). Bushy, upright, bristly biennial with narrowly lance-shaped to linear, toothed, white bristly-hairy leaves, to 15cm (6in) long. In early summer, produces short, dense spikes or cymes, 30cm (12in) long, of broadly bell-shaped flowers, purple in bud, violet-blue (occasionally pink or white) in flower, each bloom with a prominent, hairy green calyx. Suitable for an annual border or wildflower garden. ↕60–90cm (24–36in), ↔ to 30cm (12in). Europe. ❄❄❄. **'Blue Bedder'** ■ has light blue flowers, ageing to bluish pink; ↕ to 45cm (18in). **Dwarf Hybrids** bear flowers in pink, purple, lilac-blue, or white, often with darker streaks; ↕ to 45cm (18in).
E. wildpretii, syn. *E. bourgaeanum.* Woody-stemmed, unbranched biennial or short-lived perennial with a dense rosette of narrowly lance-shaped, silver-hairy, light green leaves, to 20cm (8in) long. From late spring to summer, produces a dense, column-like cyme, 90cm (36in) or more long, of funnel-shaped red flowers. ↕ to 2m (6ft), ↔ 60cm (24in). Canary Islands. ❄

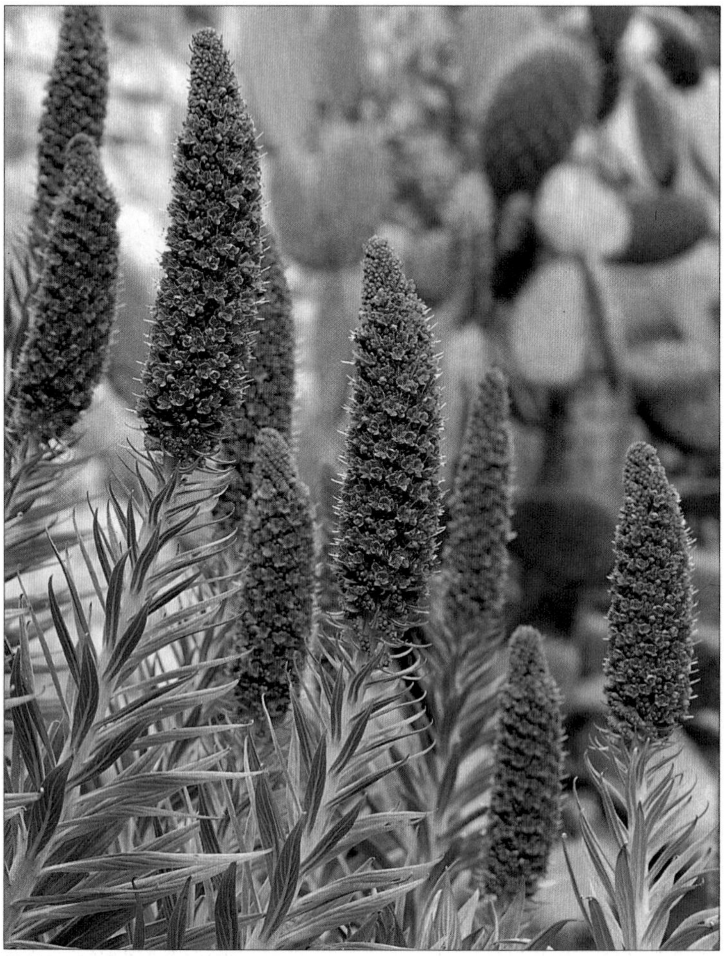

Echium candicans

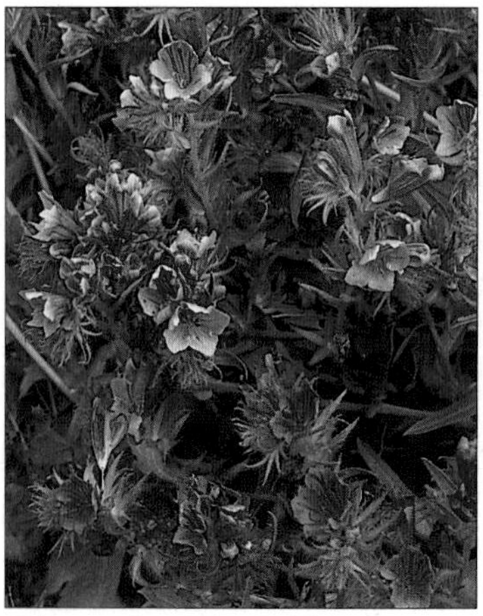

Echium vulgare 'Blue Bedder'

▷**Edelweiss** see *Leontopodium, L. alpinum*
Brazilian see *Sinningia canescens*
New Zealand see *Leucogenes*

EDGEWORTHIA

Paper bush

THYMELAEACEAE

Genus of 3 species of deciduous or evergreen shrubs with papery bark, found in woodland in the Himalayas and China. The alternate, simple, narrowly oblong or lance-shaped to ovate or oblong, entire, tough, usually hairy leaves are clustered at the branch tips. The only widely cultivated species, *E. chrysantha*, is valued for its tubular flowers, each with 4 spreading lobes. In frost-prone areas, grow against a warm wall or in a cool greenhouse; elsewhere, grow in a shrub border or woodland garden.

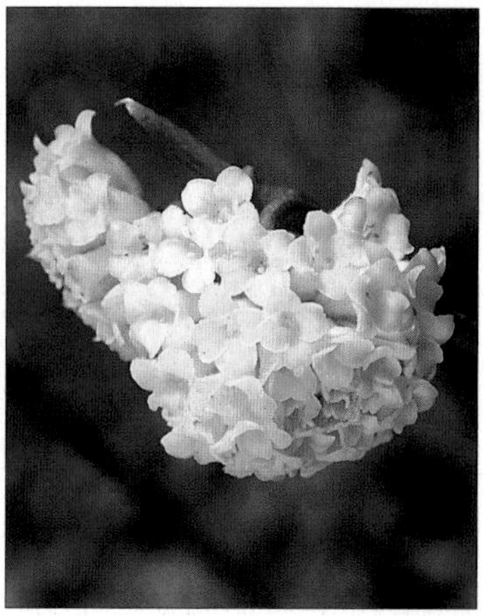

Edgeworthia chrysantha

• **HARDINESS** Frost hardy to frost tender. Severe frost may damage the flowers.

• **CULTIVATION** Under glass, grow in loam-based potting compost (JI No.3) in bright filtered light. When in growth, water freely, applying a balanced liquid fertilizer monthly; water sparingly in winter. Outdoors, grow in moist but well-drained, humus-rich, loamy soil in full sun or light dappled shade. Pruning group 1.

• **PROPAGATION** Sow seed in containers in a cold frame in autumn. Insert semi-ripe cuttings in summer.

• **PESTS AND DISEASES** Trouble free.

E. chrysantha ■ syn. *E. papyrifera.* Open, rounded, deciduous shrub with supple shoots and lance-shaped to ovate, dark green leaves, to 15cm (6in) long. Small, fragrant yellow flowers, densely covered with silky white hairs, are borne in spherical heads, 3.5–5cm (1½–2in) across, in late winter and early spring. ↕↔ 1.5m (5ft). China. ❄❄
E. papyrifera see *E. chrysantha.*

EDITHCOLEA

ASCLEPIADACEAE

Genus of 1 or 2 species of perennial succulents, closely related to *Caralluma,* from low-lying hills in Yemen, Ethiopia, Somalia, Kenya, and Tanzania. The long, 5-angled stems are very fleshy and may be erect or decumbent. Solitary, colourful, star-shaped flowers, with short-tubed, 5-lobed corollas and fleshy, erect coronas, open during the day from summer to early autumn. Leaves are scale-like and short-lived. In frost-prone areas, grow in a warm greenhouse. In warm, dry areas, grow outdoors in a desert garden.

• **HARDINESS** Frost tender.

• **CULTIVATION** Under glass, grow in equal parts loam-based potting compost (JI No.2) and grit in full light. From late spring to mid-autumn, water moderately and apply a balanced liquid fertilizer monthly; keep barely moist when dormant. Prone to stem rot if overwatered. Outdoors, grow in sharply drained, moderately fertile soil in full sun. See also pp.48–49.

• **PROPAGATION** Sow seed at 21–24°C (70–75°F) in spring. Root stem cuttings in spring or summer.

• **PESTS AND DISEASES** Trouble free.

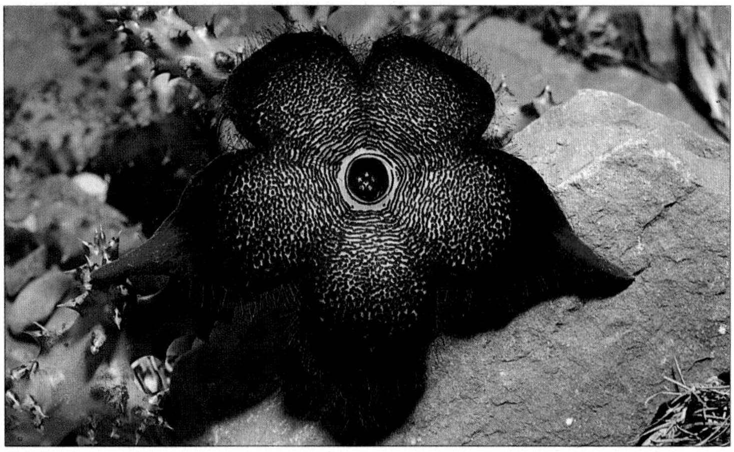

Edithcolea grandis

E. grandis ■ Variable, decumbent to semi-erect succulent with greyish green stems, 2.5cm (1in) thick, bearing very sharp, thorn-like brown teeth. Stalked, hairy-margined, reddish brown flowers, 10–13cm (4–5in) across, with pale creamy yellow spots and stripes and purple centres, are borne near the stem tips from summer to early autumn. ↕30cm (12in), ↔ 13cm (5in). Yemen, Ethiopia, Somalia, Kenya, Tanzania. ❀ (min. 16°C/61°F)

EDRAIANTHUS

Grassy bells

CAMPANULACEAE

Genus of about 24 species of generally short-lived, herbaceous and evergreen perennials, closely allied to, and sometimes included in *Wahlenbergia*. They occur in well-drained, sunny habitats, sometimes in mountainous areas, from the Mediterranean region to the Caucasus. Delicate, bell-shaped flowers, surrounded by leafy bracts, are produced singly or in terminal heads in summer. The tufted, grass-like leaves usually arise from a central rootstock and, in winter, plants are often reduced to a small, resting bud, which is just visible on each rootstock. Suitable for a rock garden, scree bed, trough, alpine house, or dry wall.

• **HARDINESS** Fully hardy.

• **CULTIVATION** Grow in light, sharply drained, humus-rich, preferably alkaline soil in full sun. Resting buds are susceptible to winter wet.

• **PROPAGATION** Sow seed in containers in an open frame in autumn, or take softwood cuttings from sideshoots in early summer.

• **PESTS AND DISEASES** Susceptible to aphids and red spider mites under glass, and to slugs and snails outdoors.

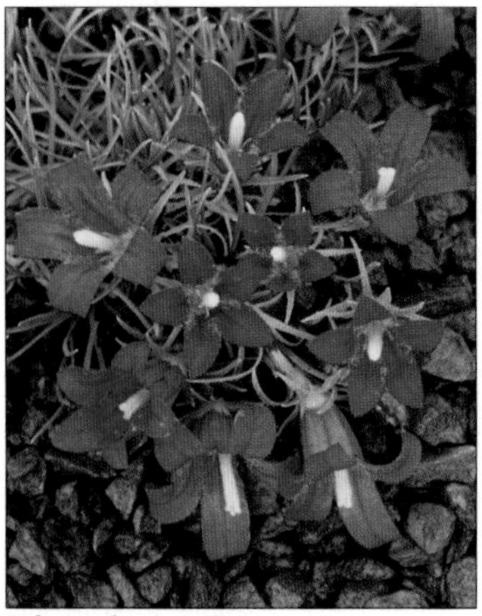

Edraianthus pumilio

E. graminifolius ♀ Tufted, herbaceous or semi-evergreen perennial with rosettes of linear to narrowly spoon-shaped, mid-green leaves, to 3.5cm (1½in) long, downy and sometimes bristly above. In early and midsummer, erect stems, to 7cm (3in) long, bear spherical heads of upturned, bell-shaped, deep purple flowers, 2.5cm (1in) long, each with a whorl of conspicuous, ovate, long-pointed bracts. ↕↔ to 15cm (6in). Balkans, C. and S. Italy, Sicily. ✻✻✻

E. pumilio ■♀ syn. *Wahlenbergia pumilio.* Cushion-forming, herbaceous perennial with compact tufts of narrowly linear, finely hairy, silvery green leaves, to 1cm (½in) long. In early summer, produces solitary, almost stemless, upturned, bell-shaped, pale to deep violet flowers, 1cm (½in) long. ↕2.5cm (1in), ↔ to 15cm (6in). S. Croatia (Dalmatia). ✻✻✻

E. serpyllifolius, syn. *Wahlenbergia serpyllifolia.* Tight mat-forming, evergreen perennial with tufts of linear-spoon-shaped, dark green leaves, to 2cm (¾in) long, with finely hairy margins. In early summer, spreading leafy stems, 2.5–12cm (1–5in) long, bear solitary, upturned, bell-shaped, deep violet flowers, to 2cm (¾in) long. ↕ to 5cm (2in), ↔ to 15cm (6in). Croatia (Dalmatia), Bosnia & Herzegovina, Albania. ✻✻✻. **'Major'** has flowers to 2.5cm (1in) long.

▷ ***Edwardsia microphylla*** see *Sophora microphylla*

EGERIA

HYDROCHARITACEAE

Genus of 2 species of semi-evergreen and evergreen, marginal to deep-water aquatic perennials found in still or slow-moving water in South America. Multi-branched stems bear linear to narrowly oblong leaves in whorls or opposite pairs. Cymes of 2–5 white, 3-parted male flowers, and much smaller females, are borne within tubular, translucent spathes in summer. Use as oxygenators in a cold-water or tropical aquarium; *E. densa* will overwinter in ponds outdoors in all but the coldest winters.

• **HARDINESS** Hardy to 1°C (34°F).

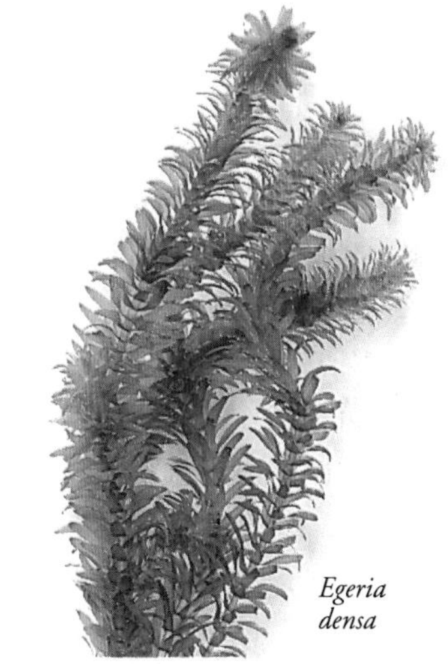

Egeria densa

• **CULTIVATION** In an aquarium, grow in an inert, sandy medium in full light maintaining a temperature of 5–18°C (41–64°F). Outdoors, grow in full sun in water 30–90cm (12–36in) deep, rooted into the muddy bottom, or in an aquatic basket of loam-based potting compost (JI No.2) topped off with shingle. Trim regularly to encourage fresh young growth. See also pp.52–53.

• **PROPAGATION** Insert stem cuttings into the pond or aquarium sediment. Allow stems to float just under the water surface; when roots develop, plant in the bottom of a pond or aquarium.

• **PESTS AND DISEASES** Young shoots may be nibbled by snails or fish.

E. densa ■ syn. *Anacharis densa, Elodea densa.* Submerged, sometimes floating, aquatic perennial with many-branched stems, to 90cm (36in) long, bearing numerous whorls of stalkless, linear leaves, to 2.5cm (1in) long, with long, sharp-pointed tips. Tubular spathes, 2cm (¾in) long, of small but showy white male flowers are borne above the water surface in summer. ↔ indefinite. South America. ✻ (borderline)

▷ **Eggs and bacon** see *Pultenaea procumbens*

EHRETIA

BORAGINACEAE/EHRETIACEAE

Genus of about 50 species of deciduous and evergreen trees and shrubs from Africa, Asia, and North and South America, mainly in woodland. They are grown for their spreading habit, ridged or furrowed bark, simple, entire or toothed, alternate leaves, and terminal panicles of small, 5-lobed, tubular to bell-shaped or star-shaped, scented flowers. Ideal for a woodland garden. In frost-prone areas, grow tender species in a cool or temperate greenhouse.

• **HARDINESS** Frost hardy to frost tender.

• **CULTIVATION** Grow in moderately fertile, well-drained soil in full sun or partial shade, sheltered from cold, drying winds. Pruning group 1.

• **PROPAGATION** Sow seed in containers in a cold frame as soon as ripe. Insert softwood cuttings in summer.

• **PESTS AND DISEASES** Trouble free.

E. dicksonii ■⚲ Spreading, deciduous tree with deeply ridged, grey-brown bark and elliptic to oblong-elliptic, glossy, dark green leaves, to 20cm (8in) long, rough-hairy above, velvety-hairy beneath. In late spring and early summer, bears tubular-bell-shaped white flowers in flattish panicles, 5–10cm (2–4in) across. ↕↔ 10m (30ft). China, Taiwan, Japan (Ryukyu Islands). ✻✻

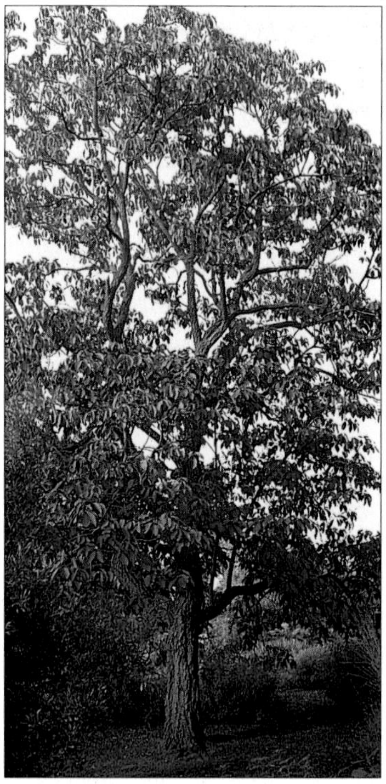

Ehretia dicksonii

EICHHORNIA

Water hyacinth

PONTEDERIACEAE

Genus of 7 species of rhizomatous, marginal to deep-water aquatic perennials, rarely annuals, from lakes, canals, rivers, and streams in subtropical and tropical South America. Submerged leaves are linear to strap-shaped and arranged in 2 ranks; floating and aerial leaves are stalked, mainly obovate, rounded, or heart-shaped, and borne in rosettes. Showy, funnel-shaped flowers are borne in terminal spikes, each within a leafy sheath. Grow in a greenhouse pool, in a tropical aquarium, or outdoors in a decorative pool. In frost-prone areas, overwinter under glass.

• **HARDINESS** Hardy to 1°C (34°F).

• **CULTIVATION** Under glass, provide full light with an air temperature of 13–16°C (55–61°F). Aquarium plants need 30–40cm (12–16in) of head space to grow well. Outdoors, grow on open water in full sun. In frost-prone areas, introduce plants on to the water surface when danger of frost has passed. Overwinter on trays of moist, loamless compost, at a minimum of 15°C (59°F) in full light. See also pp.52–53.

• **PROPAGATION** Detach offshoots at any time of year.

• **PESTS AND DISEASES** Trouble free.

E. azurea. Floating or submerged aquatic perennial with a thick stem that floats or roots in mud. Bears linear to strap-shaped submerged leaves, 10cm (4in) long, arranged in 2 ranks, and rounded-heart-shaped to diamond-shaped floating leaves, 10cm (4in) long, in rosettes to 20cm (8in) or more across. Pale blue flowers, 5–7cm (2–3in) long,

E

with yellow-spotted, dark purple throats, are borne in spikes 5–15cm (2–6in) long, throughout summer. ↕ 10–12cm (4–5in), ↔ 45cm (18in). Subtropical and tropical South America. ✻ (borderline)

E. crassipes, syn. *E. speciosa* (Water hyacinth). Floating aquatic perennial with a thick, floating or anchored stem bearing rosettes of rounded to ovate leaves, to 15cm (6in) across, with inflated, shiny, pale green stalks. Long, purplish green roots hang down 30cm (12in) in the water. Pale blue to violet flowers, 3cm (1¼in) across, have yellow markings on the upper petals and are borne in spikes 15cm (6in) tall, in summer. ↕↔ 45cm (18in). Tropical South America. ✻ (borderline)

E. speciosa see *E. crassipes*.

ELAEAGNUS

ELAEAGNACEAE

Genus of about 45 species of deciduous or evergreen shrubs or trees mainly from Asia, but a few from S. Europe and North America, growing wild in thickets and dry places. They are cultivated for their often silvery leaves, which are alternate and lance-shaped to ovate or oblong, and for the small, tubular or bell-shaped, sometimes intensely fragrant flowers, produced in clusters from the leaf axils. The flowers are followed by edible, sometimes colourful berries, 1–2.5cm (½–1in) long. Grow in a shrub border or as specimen shrubs; evergreens are also suitable as a hedge.

- **HARDINESS** Fully hardy.
- **CULTIVATION** Grow in fertile, well-drained soil, ideally in full sun, although evergreens will grow well in partial shade. All tolerate dry soil and coastal winds, but may become chlorotic on shallow, chalky soil. Pruning group 1 or 2 (deciduous), or 9 (evergreens). Remove reverted shoots on variegated cultivars.
- **PROPAGATION** Sow seed in a cold frame in autumn. Insert greenwood cuttings in late spring or early summer, or semi-ripe cuttings of deciduous species in midsummer. Insert semi-ripe cuttings of evergreens in summer, or graft in late winter. Remove rooted suckers of deciduous species in autumn.
- **PESTS AND DISEASES** Susceptible to coral spot.

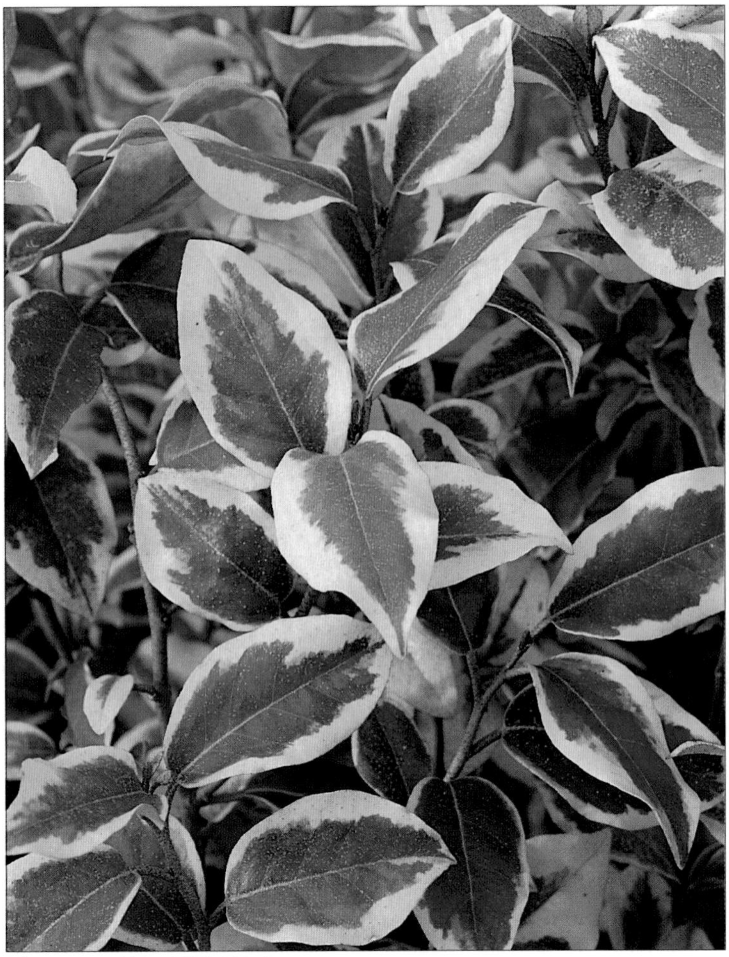

Elaeagnus x *ebbingei* 'Gilt Edge'

E. angustifolia ♀ ⚲ (Oleaster). Deciduous shrub or tree with spreading, red-tinted, sometimes spiny branches, covered with silvery scales, and willow-like, lance-shaped leaves, to 10cm (4in) long, dark green above, silver-scaly beneath. In summer, produces yellowish white flowers, to 1cm (½in) long, followed in autumn by silver-scaly yellow fruit. ↕↔ 6m (20ft). S. Europe to C. Asia, Himalayas, China. ✻✻✻. **'Quicksilver'** ▣ ♀ syn. *E.* 'Quicksilver', is a fast-growing, open, pyramidal, suckering shrub with silvery shoots, elliptic to lance-shaped, tapered, very silver-scaly leaves, to 5cm (2in) long, and yellow flowers produced from silvery buds; ↕↔ 4m (12ft).

E. commutata (Silver berry). Thicket-forming, deciduous shrub, spreading by suckers, with upright, red-brown shoots and broadly elliptic leaves, to 7cm (3in) long, completely covered with silvery scales. Pendent, silver-scaly, yellowish white flowers, 1cm (½in) long, are produced in late spring, followed in autumn by silver-mealy red fruit. ↕ to 4m (12ft), ↔ 2m (6ft). North America. ✻✻✻

***E.* x *ebbingei* cultivars.** Dense, rounded to spreading, evergreen shrubs with elliptic, leathery leaves, to 10cm (4in) long, glossy, dark or metallic sea-green on the upper surfaces, silver-scaly beneath. Silver-scaly, creamy white flowers, 1cm (½in) long, are produced in autumn. ↕↔ 4m (12ft). Garden origin. ✻✻✻. **'Gilt Edge'** ▣ ♀ has leaves with dark green centres and conspicuous, golden yellow margins. **'Limelight'** ▣ has silvery young leaves, which become marked with yellow and pale green in the centres; ↕↔ 3m (10ft).

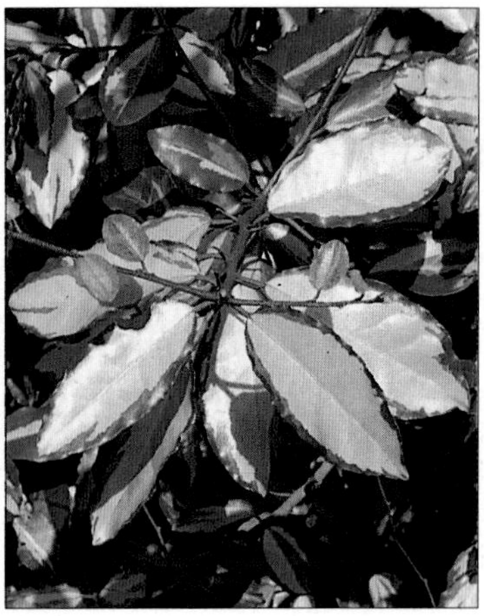

Elaeagnus pungens 'Maculata'

'The Hague' produces silvery young leaves maturing to dark green above; ↕↔ 5m (15ft).

E. macrophylla. Vigorous, spreading, evergreen shrub with silvery white-scaly branches when young. Broadly ovate to elliptic leaves, to 10cm (4in) long, are very silver-scaly when young, becoming glossy, dark green above. Silver-scaly cream flowers, to 1cm (½in) long, are produced in autumn and followed by scaly red fruit. ↕ 3m (10ft), ↔ 5m (15ft). Korea, Japan. ✻✻✻

E. pungens. Dense, slightly spiny, evergreen shrub with young branches covered in brown scales. Oblong-elliptic to oblong, lustrous, dark green leaves, to 10cm (4in) long, are often wavy-margined; the undersides are tinged white and brown-scaly. Bears pendent, silvery white flowers, 1cm (½in) long, in autumn, followed by brown fruit that ripen to red. ↕ 4m (12ft), ↔ 5m (15ft). Japan. ✻✻✻. **'Argenteovariegata'** see 'Variegata'. **'Aureovariegata'** see 'Maculata'. **'Dicksonii'** has leaves with broad, golden yellow margins; ↕↔ 3m (10ft). **'Frederici'** ▣ is slow-growing, and has small, narrow, creamy yellow leaves, 3–4cm (1¼–1½in) long, with narrow, glossy, dark green margins; ↕↔ 2m (6ft). **'Goldrim'**, syn. 'Golden Rim', has glossy, dark green leaves with narrow, bright yellow margins. **'Maculata'** ▣ ♀ syn. 'Aureovariegata', has leaves boldly marked dark yellow in the centres. **'Variegata'**, syn. 'Argenteovariegata', has leaves with narrow, creamy yellow margins.

***E.* 'Quicksilver'** see *E. angustifolia* 'Quicksilver'.

E.* x *reflexa (*E. glabra* x *E. pungens*). Vigorous, semi-scandent, sparsely thorny, evergreen shrub with long shoots and ovate to ovate-lance-shaped, glossy, deep green leaves, to 6cm (2½in) long, intensely brown-scaly beneath. Silvery white flowers, 1cm (½in) long, are borne in autumn. Will climb if supported. ↕ 4m (12ft), ↔ 6m (20ft). Garden origin. ✻✻✻

E. umbellata ▣ ⚲ Vigorous, frequently wide-spreading, deciduous shrub or small tree with brown-scaly, often spiny shoots. Elliptic to ovate-oblong, wavy-margined leaves, to 10cm (4in) long, are silvery at first, maturing to bright green above. Silvery yellow-white flowers, 1cm (½in) long, are borne in late spring and early summer, followed by silvery fruit that turn red in autumn. ↕↔ 5m (15ft). Himalayas, China, Japan. ✻✻✻.

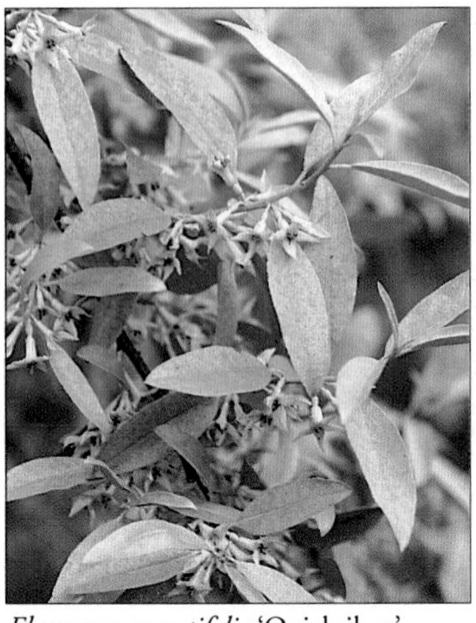

Elaeagnus angustifolia 'Quicksilver'

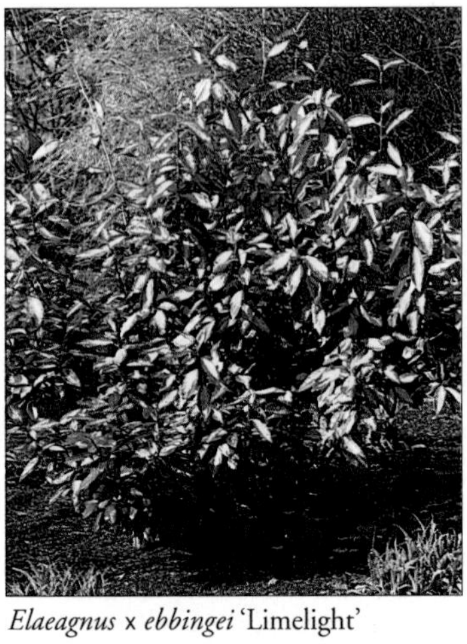

Elaeagnus x *ebbingei* 'Limelight'

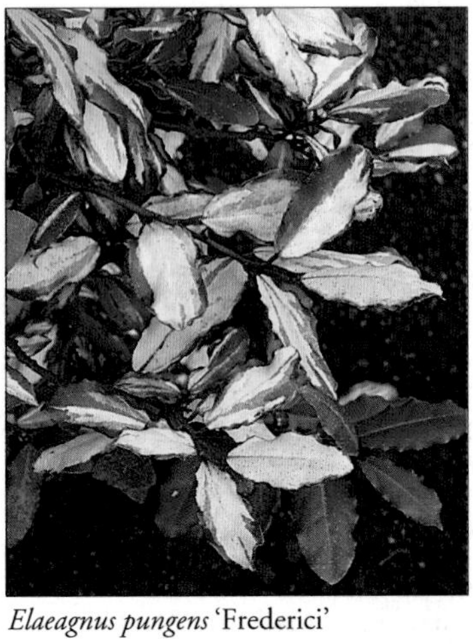

Elaeagnus pungens 'Frederici'

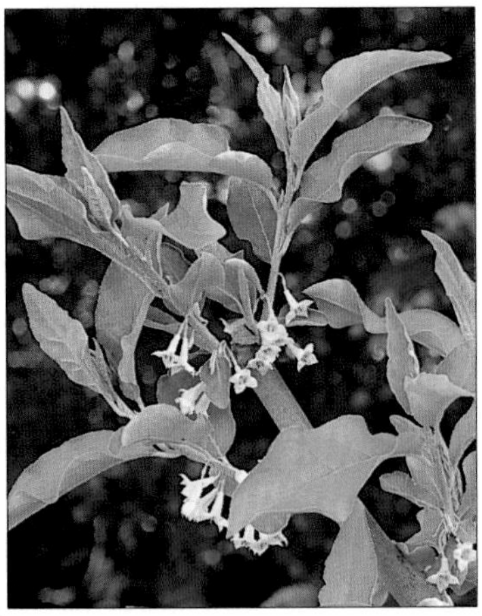

Elaeagnus umbellata

'Titan' is a dense, upright, branched cultivar, with silver-tinged, olive-green leaves and bright yellow flowers; ↕4m (12ft), ↔ 2m (6ft).

ELAEIS

Oil palm

ARECACEAE/PALMAE

Genus of 2 species of single-stemmed, monoecious palms occurring on moist, sandy soils in open forest in tropical regions of America and Africa. Large, pinnate leaves are borne in terminal clusters, the dead ones hanging down like a skirt before falling. The 3-petalled flowers are produced in panicles from the leaf axils. In frost-prone areas, grow young oil palms in a warm greenhouse; elsewhere, use as lawn specimens.

• **HARDINESS** Frost tender.
• **CULTIVATION** Under glass, grow in loam-based potting compost (JI No.3) in full light. When in growth, water freely and apply a balanced liquid fertilizer monthly; water sparingly in winter. Pot on or top-dress in spring. Outdoors, grow in fertile, moist but well-drained soil in full sun.
• **PROPAGATION** Soak seed for 7 days and sow at 19–24°C (66–75°F) in spring. Germination is slow.
• **PESTS AND DISEASES** Red spider mites may be troublesome under glass.

E. guineensis ♆ (African oil palm, Macaw fat palm). Erect palm with much of its stem covered with old, fibrous leaf bases. Bears a dense crown of arching leaves, 2.5–5m (8–15ft) long, composed of numerous, more or less pendent, crowded, slender, linear, rich green leaflets, held in differing planes along the midribs. Yellow flowers are borne intermittently throughout the year in separate male and female panicles, 30–45cm (12–18in) long. Females develop large, rounded bunches of ovoid fruit, rich in commercially valuable oil. ↕ to 18m (60ft), ↔ 5–9m (15–28ft). Tropical Africa. ❄ (min. 18°C/64°F)

ELAEOCARPUS

ELAEOCARPACEAE

Genus of 60 species of evergreen shrubs and trees occurring in forest and thickets from E. Asia to Indonesia and Malaysia, and from Australasia and the Pacific. They are grown for their axillary racemes of small, 3- to 5-petalled, bell-shaped, fringed, usually fragrant flowers,

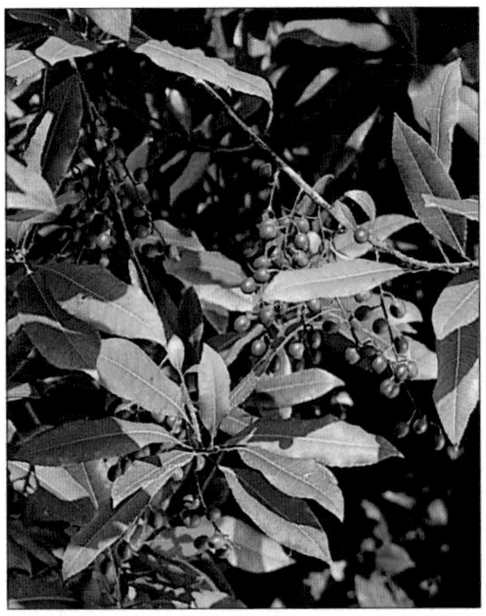

Elaeocarpus cyaneus

and for their colourful berries. The mainly alternate leaves are lance-shaped to broad-ovate or oblong, leathery, and entire or toothed. In frost-prone areas, grow in a cool greenhouse; in warmer areas, grow as specimen plants or in a shrub border.

• **HARDINESS** Frost tender; *E. cyaneus* may survive short spells near 0°C (32°F).
• **CULTIVATION** Under glass, grow in well-drained, loam-based potting compost (JI No.3) in full light. From spring to autumn, water freely and apply a balanced liquid fertilizer monthly; water sparingly in winter. Top-dress or pot on in spring. Outdoors, grow in fertile, humus-rich, moist but well-drained, neutral to acid soil in full sun. Pruning group 1.
• **PROPAGATION** Root semi-ripe cuttings with bottom heat in summer (rooting may be slow).
• **PESTS AND DISEASES** Prone to whiteflies and red spider mites under glass.

E. cyaneus ▣ ◐–○ syn. *E. reticulatus.* Erect to spreading tree or shrub bearing oblong-elliptic to oblong-lance-shaped, conspicuously veined and shallowly toothed, shiny, dark green leaves, 10–15cm (4–6in) long. Small, fragrant, white or pink flowers are produced in racemes, to 10cm (4in) long, from spring to summer. Long-lasting, lustrous, deep blue berries, 8–15mm (⅜–½in) long, ripen from autumn to winter. ↕6–15m (20–50ft), ↔ 2–5m (6–15ft). Australia (Queensland to Victoria). ❄ (min. 5°C/41°F)
E. reticulatus see *E. cyaneus.*

ELATOSTEMA *syn.* PELLIONIA

URTICACEAE

Genus of about 50 species of evergreen perennials and subshrubs, some with succulent or partly woody stems, widely distributed in tropical and subtropical Asia, where they grow in forest clearings. Cultivated for their decorative leaves, which are alternate, 2-ranked, linear to rounded, entire or toothed, and heavily marked with silver and bronze. The inflorescences are relatively insignificant. Trailing species are ideal for a hanging basket or as ground cover. In frost-prone areas, grow as houseplants or in a warm greenhouse; elsewhere, grow in a border or under trees and shrubs.

• **HARDINESS** Frost tender.
• **CULTIVATION** Under glass, grow in loamless potting compost in bright

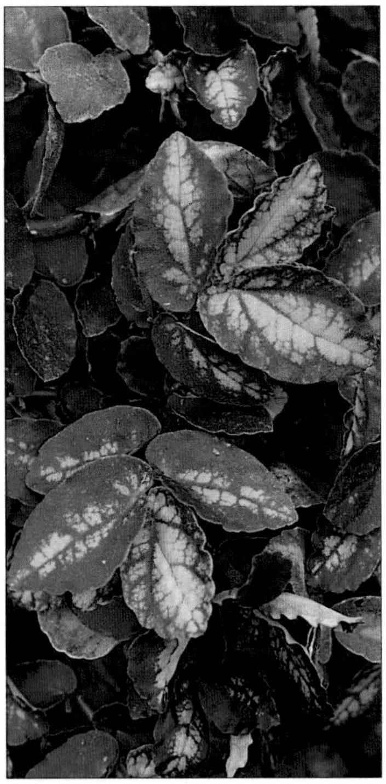

Elatostema repens

indirect light. When in growth, water freely and apply a balanced liquid fertilizer monthly; water moderately in winter. Outdoors, grow in humus-rich, fertile soil in deep shade. Shorten shoots in spring or summer to maintain shape.
• **PROPAGATION** Root cuttings at any time of year.
• **PESTS AND DISEASES** Trouble free.

E. pulchra, syn. *Pellionia pulchra.* Creeping and trailing, evergreen perennial with fleshy, purple-tinged stems, and oblong to broadly elliptic, dark green leaves, 2–5cm (¾–2in) long, tinged purple beneath, with very dark green midribs and veins above. ↕8cm (3in), ↔ 45cm (18in). Vietnam. ❄ (min. 13°C/55°F)
E. repens ▣ ♀ syn. *Pellionia daveauana, P. repens.* Creeping, evergreen perennial with fleshy, greenish pink stems. Wavy-margined leaves, to 6cm (2½in) long, are oblong, elliptic, or sometimes rounded. They are dark blackish green above, marked grey and paler green, and often bronze-flushed; beneath, they are often tinged pink, with purple margins. ↕10cm (4in), ↔ to 60cm (24in). S.E. Asia. ❄ (min. 13°C/55°F)

▷**Elder** see *Sambucus*
 American see *Sambucus canadensis*
 Black see *Sambucus nigra*
 Box see *Acer negundo*
 Common see *Sambucus nigra*
 European see *Sambucus nigra*
 Ground see *Aegopodium*
 Red-berried see *Sambucus racemosa*
 Variegated ground see *Aegopodium podagraria* 'Variegatum'
 Yellow see *Tecoma stans*
▷**Elderberry** see *Sambucus nigra*
▷**Elecampane** see *Inula helenium*
▷**Elephant foot tree** see *Beaucarnea recurvata*
▷**Elephant's ear** see *Philodendron domesticum*
▷**Elephant's ear plant** see *Alocasia*
▷**Elephant's ears** see *Bergenia, Caladium bicolor*
▷**Elephant's foot** see *Dioscorea elephantipes*
▷**Elephant's tusk** see *Proboscidea*
▷**Elephant tree** see *Bursera microphylla, Pachycormus discolor*
▷**Elephantwood** see *Bolusanthus speciosus*

ELETTARIA

ZINGIBERACEAE

Genus of 4 species of evergreen, rhizomatous perennials from tropical rainforest in India, Sri Lanka, Malaysia, and Sumatra. The rhizomes produce erect, reed-like shoots with 2 ranks of linear to lance-shaped leaves. Separate, horizontal flowering shoots, bearing large-bracted spikes of lipped, 3-petalled flowers, are followed by spherical or ellipsoid seed capsules. The only widely cultivated species, *E. cardamomum,* produces aromatic fruit used as a spice. It needs tropical conditions to fruit well, but in temperate regions is still an attractive foliage plant for a warm greenhouse. In frost-free areas, grow in a shady bed or border.

• **HARDINESS** Frost tender.
• **CULTIVATION** Under glass, grow in fertile, loam-based potting compost (JI No.2) with additional leaf mould or granulated bark, in bright filtered light with high humidity. When in growth, water freely and apply a balanced liquid fertilizer monthly; water sparingly in winter. Pot on in spring and remove flowered stems. Outdoors, grow in fertile, open, humus-rich soil, in full sun with some midday shade.
• **PROPAGATION** Sow seed at 19–24°C (66–75°F) as soon as ripe. Divide in spring.
• **PESTS AND DISEASES** Susceptible to mosaic virus and thrips in tropical areas.

E. cardamomum (Cardamom). Evergreen perennial with thick rhizomes bearing upright shoots with linear-lance-shaped, pointed, dark green leaves, 60cm (24in) long, paler and softly hairy beneath. During summer, almost prostrate shoots bear loose panicles, to 60cm (24in) long, of violet-veined white flowers, 2cm (¾in) long, with yellow-margined, or pink-, lilac-, or violet-striped lips, followed by aromatic, pale green capsules, each containing 15–20 seeds. ↕↔ to 3m (10ft) (much smaller in containers). India. ❄ (min. 10°C/50°F)

ELEUTHEROCOCCUS

syn. ACANTHOPANAX

ARALIACEAE

Genus of about 30 species of mainly deciduous trees and shrubs, sometimes climbers, from scrub and woodland in E., S., and S.E. Asia. They have alternate, 3- to 7-palmate leaves, and bear terminal, simple or compound umbels of small, 5-petalled, greenish white flowers from spring to summer, followed by ivy-like, spherical to ellipsoid, black or purple-black fruits. Grown for their foliage and autumn fruits, they are useful as specimens or in a shrub border.

• **HARDINESS** Fully hardy.
• **CULTIVATION** Grow in well-drained soil, ideally in full sun; *E. sieboldianus* thrives in poor, dry soil and will tolerate shade. Pruning group 1.

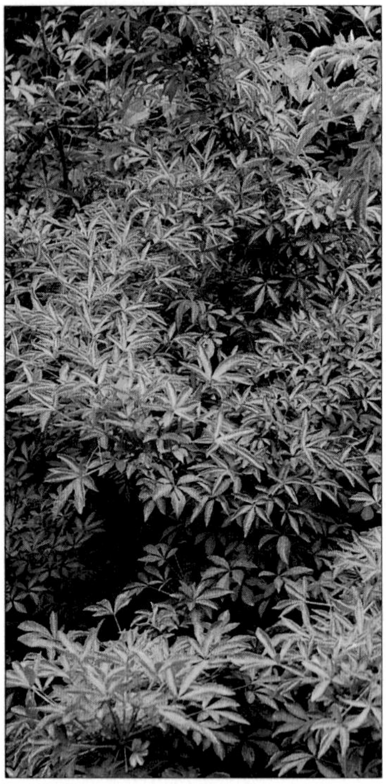

Eleutherococcus sieboldianus

• **PROPAGATION** Sow seed in a seedbed in autumn or spring. Insert greenwood cuttings in early summer, or take root cuttings in winter. Separate suckers in winter.
• **PESTS AND DISEASES** Trouble free.

E. pictus see *Kalopanax septemlobus.*
E. sieboldianus ◼ syn. *Acanthopanax sieboldianus.* Spiny, sometimes scandent shrub bearing slender, arching, cane-like branches. Bright green, 5- to 7-palmate leaves have ovate or obovate, toothed leaflets, to 9cm (3½in) long. Solitary umbels of star-shaped, greenish white flowers are borne in late spring and early summer, followed by spherical black fruit, to 8mm (⅜in) across. ↕↔ 2.5m (8ft). E. China. ❄❄❄. **'Variegatus'** has leaflets margined with creamy white.

▷ **Elkwood** see *Magnolia tripetala*
▷ ***Elliottia*** see *Tripetaleia*
E. paniculata see *T. paniculata*
▷ **Elm** see *Ulmus*
American white see *Ulmus americana*
Camperdown see *Ulmus glabra* 'Camperdownii'
Caucasian see *Zelkova carpinifolia*
Chinese see *Ulmus parvifolia*
Cornish see *Ulmus minor* 'Cornubiensis'
Cornish golden see *Ulmus minor* 'Dicksonii'
Dickson's golden see *Ulmus minor* 'Dicksonii'
Dutch see *Ulmus* x *hollandica*
English see *Ulmus procera*
European field see *Ulmus minor*
Exeter see *Ulmus glabra* 'Exoniensis'
Goodyer's see *Ulmus minor* subsp. *angustifolia*
Huntingdon see *Ulmus* x *hollandica* 'Vegeta'
Jersey see *Ulmus minor* 'Sarniensis'
Siberian see *Ulmus pumila*
Smooth-leaved see *Ulmus minor*
Wheatley see *Ulmus minor* 'Sarniensis'
Wych see *Ulmus glabra*

ELODEA

Pondweed

HYDROCHARITACEAE

Genus of 12 species of submerged aquatic perennials occurring in fresh water from North America to subtropical South America. The erect, spreading stems and lance-shaped to linear or ovate, bright green leaves, borne in whorls of 3, provide excellent cover for fish fry; they are also good oxygenators. Tiny, solitary flowers are produced within axillary spathes. Grow in a garden pond; the less vigorous species are suitable for an aquarium.
• **HARDINESS** Fully hardy to frost tender.
• **CULTIVATION** Outdoors, grow in loamy soil, in an aquatic planting basket in a pond in full sun. Trim back periodically throughout summer and prune hard in autumn to within 30cm (12in) of the container. Grow *E. callitrichoides* in an aquarium in an inert medium, with full light and a water temperature of 5–22°C (41–72°F); it dies back rapidly at higher temperatures. See also pp.52–53.
• **PROPAGATION** Take stem cuttings, 15–30cm (6–12in) long, in summer.
• **PESTS AND DISEASES** Trouble free.

E. callitrichoides. Submerged aquatic perennial with slender, spreading stems, 3–4m (10–12ft) long. Forms dense masses of linear to narrowly lance-shaped or ovate, finely toothed, bright, pale green leaves, 8–15mm (⅜–½in) long. Floating, petalless white flowers, 2mm (1/16in) across, are produced in summer. ↔ indefinite. Temperate South America. ❄
E. canadensis (Canadian pondweed). Submerged aquatic perennial with brittle, branching stems, 3–4m (10–12ft) long, bearing lance-shaped to ovate, finely toothed, flat, translucent, bright, dark green leaves, 0.5–1cm (¼–½in) long, which curl slightly downwards. Floating, petalless, purple-tinged green flowers, 8mm (⅜in) across, borne among the leaves in summer, have long, thread-like stalks. Too vigorous for an aquarium. ↔ indefinite. North America. ❄❄❄
***E. crispa* of gardens** see *Lagarosiphon major.*
E. densa see *Egeria densa.*

ELSHOLTZIA

LABIATAE/LAMIACEAE

Genus of about 35 species of annuals, perennials, and semi-evergreen or deciduous shrubs and subshrubs occurring on dry, open hillsides and roadsides in C. and E. Asia. They are valued for their aromatic foliage and their slender panicles or racemes of 2-lipped, tubular flowers. The leaves are opposite and lance-shaped to ovate-elliptic. Grow in a herbaceous or shrub border. In frost-prone areas, grow tender species in a cool greenhouse.
• **HARDINESS** Frost hardy to frost tender.
• **CULTIVATION** Grow in any well-drained, fertile soil in full sun. Pruning group 6.
• **PROPAGATION** Sow seed at 13°C (55°F) as soon as ripe. Insert softwood cuttings in summer.
• **PESTS AND DISEASES** Trouble free.

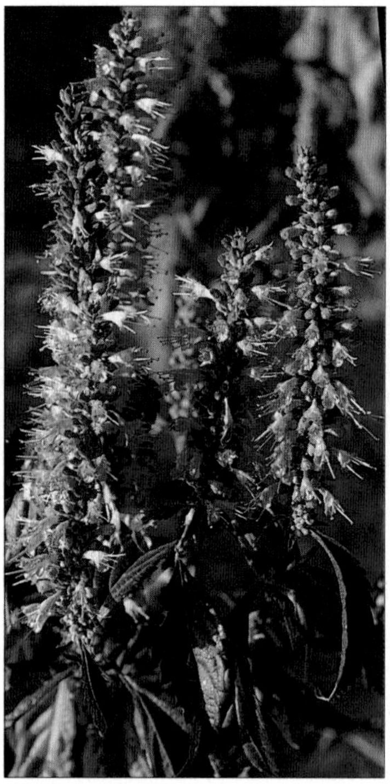

Elsholtzia stauntonii

E. stauntonii ◼ Open, rounded, deciduous subshrub with lance-shaped to ovate-elliptic, toothed, mint-scented, mid-green leaves, to 15cm (6in) long, turning red in autumn. From late summer to autumn, produces terminal racemes or panicles, 10–20cm (4–8in) long, of very small, purple-pink flowers. ↕↔ 1.5m (5ft). China. ❄❄

ELYMUS

Wild rye

GRAMINEAE/POACEAE

Genus of about 150 species of tufted or rhizomatous, mainly perennial grasses, widely distributed throughout N. and S. temperate regions, and often occurring on sandy soils. They have linear, flat or occasionally rolled leaves, and stout or slender, bristled flower spikes consisting of flattened, stalkless spikelets, arranged alternately along the flower stalks. The genus includes the invasive *E. repens* (couch grass or twitch), but those species described here are not invasive. Most are useful in a rock garden, or in a mixed or herbaceous border.
• **HARDINESS** Fully hardy.
• **CULTIVATION** Grow in any moderately fertile, moist but well-drained soil in full sun. *E. canadensis* tolerates damp conditions. Cut back to ground level in late autumn, or leave those species with good winter leaf colour until late winter.
• **PROPAGATION** Sow seed *in situ* in autumn or spring. Divide from mid-spring to early summer.
• **PESTS AND DISEASES** May be attacked by rust.

E. arenarius see *Leymus arenarius.*
E. canadensis (Canadian wild rye). Loosely tufted, perennial grass with erect stems bearing linear, flat or rolled, rough-textured or slightly bristly, green to blue-green leaves, 20–35cm (8–14in) long. In late summer and early autumn, produces dense green flower spikes, 20–25cm (8–10in) long, nodding at the tips; 2- to 5-flowered spikelets, with reddish brown bristles, are arranged alternately in groups of 4 along each spike. ↕ 1.2–1.8m (4–6ft), ↔ 60cm (24in). Temperate North America. ❄❄❄
***E. glaucus* of gardens** see *E. hispidus.*
E. hispidus, syn. *E. glaucus* of gardens (Hairy couch, Intermediate wheatgrass). Loosely tufted, perennial grass with erect or arching, linear, inrolled, bristly, pale silvery blue leaves, 10–20cm (4–8in) long. In early and midsummer, upright stems bear slender, insignificant flower spikes of blunt, 3- to 8-flowered spikelets. ↕ to 75cm (30in), ↔ 40cm (16in). Temperate Eurasia. ❄❄❄
E. magellanicus. Densely tufted, mound-forming, perennial grass with linear, flat or folded, intense blue leaves, to 5cm (2in) long. Lax, almost prostrate flower spikes, 19cm (7in) long, comprising 2- to 7-flowered spikelets, are borne throughout summer. ↕ 15cm (6in), ↔ 30cm (12in). Temperate S. Chile and S. Argentina. ❄❄❄
E. racemosus see *Leymus racemosus.*

EMBOTHRIUM

Chilean fire bush

PROTEACEAE

Genus of 8 species of evergreen trees and shrubs occurring in forest in the C. and S. Andes of South America. They are cultivated for their showy, tubular, waxy flowers, which split into 4 recurved and coiling, narrow, twisted lobes, and are borne in terminal and axillary racemes. The alternate, simple leaves are lance-shaped to elliptic or oblong, entire, and leathery. Grow in a woodland garden or in a sheltered site. In areas where frosts are light and infrequent, they will tolerate more open sites and are good specimen trees.
• **HARDINESS** Fully hardy to frost hardy.
• **CULTIVATION** Grow in fertile, humus-rich, moist but well-drained, neutral to acid soil in full sun or partial shade. Shelter from cold, drying winds. Pruning group 1.

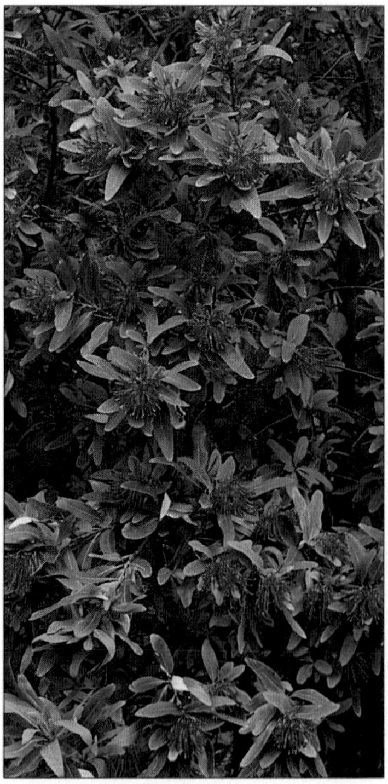

Embothrium coccineum

• **PROPAGATION** Sow seed at 13–16°C (55–61°F) in spring. Root greenwood cuttings in early summer, or semi-ripe cuttings in mid- or late summer, with bottom heat. Insert root cuttings or remove suckers in late winter.
• **PESTS AND DISEASES** Red spider mites may infest plants under glass.

E. coccineum ■ ♀ (Chilean fire bush, Flame flower). Upright, freely branching, suckering tree or shrub with oblong to narrowly lance-shaped, mid- to deep green leaves, to 12cm (5in) long. Scarlet, rarely yellow flowers, 3–4.5cm (1¼–1¾in) long, are produced in dense racemes, to 10cm (4in) long, in late spring and early summer. ↕ 10m (30ft) or more, ↔ 5m (15ft) or more. S. Chile. ❄❄. **var. *lanceolatum* 'Norquinco'** ♕ syn. var. *lanceolatum* 'Norquinco Form', var. *lanceolatum* 'Norquinco Valley', has narrowly lance-shaped leaves; ❄❄❄ (borderline)

▷**Emerald creeper** see *Strongylodon macrobotrys*
▷**Emerald feather** see *Asparagus densiflorus* 'Sprengeri'

EMILIA syn. CACALIA
Tassel flower

ASTERACEAE/COMPOSITAE

Genus of about 24 species of rosette-forming annuals from disturbed ground or stony slopes, to 3,500m (11,500ft) high, in tropical Africa, India, and Polynesia. The lower leaves are lance-shaped-oblong or pinnatifid, stalkless or with winged stalks; the upper leaves are oblong to ovate, and clasp the stems. In summer, stiff, slender, leafy stems bear upright, tassel-like, red, yellow, purple-red, or orange flowerheads, singly or in corymbs. Grow in an annual border in hot and dry, or coastal areas. The flowers are good for cutting and drying.
• **HARDINESS** Half hardy.
• **CULTIVATION** Grow in well-drained soil in full sun. Dead-head to prolong flowering.
• **PROPAGATION** Sow seed at 13–18°C (55–64°F) in mid-spring, or *in situ* in late spring.
• **PESTS AND DISEASES** Trouble free.

E. coccinea, syn. *Cacalia coccinea, C. sagittata, E. flammea, E. javanica* (Flora's paintbrush). Smooth to slightly hairy, rosette-forming annual with mid-green leaves, to 14cm (5½in) long; the lower leaves are stalkless and entire to toothed. In summer, fluffy, orange-red or scarlet flowerheads, to 1.5cm (½in) across, are produced singly or in loosely clustered corymbs. ↕ 45–60cm (18–24in), ↔ 30–60cm (12–24in). Tropical Africa. ❄
E. flammea see *E. coccinea*.
E. javanica see *E. coccinea*.
E. sonchifolia, syn. *Cacalia sonchifolia*. Smooth to slightly hairy, rosette-forming annual with toothed, mid- to grey-green leaves, to 10cm (4in) long; the lower leaves have winged stalks, the upper leaves are smaller and almost arrow-shaped. In summer, bears loosely clustered corymbs of fluffy, purple-red flowerheads, to 1.5cm (½in) across. Tropical Africa and Asia. ↕ 45–60cm (18–24in), ↔ 30–60cm (12–24in). ❄. **'Lutea'** has yellow flowerheads.

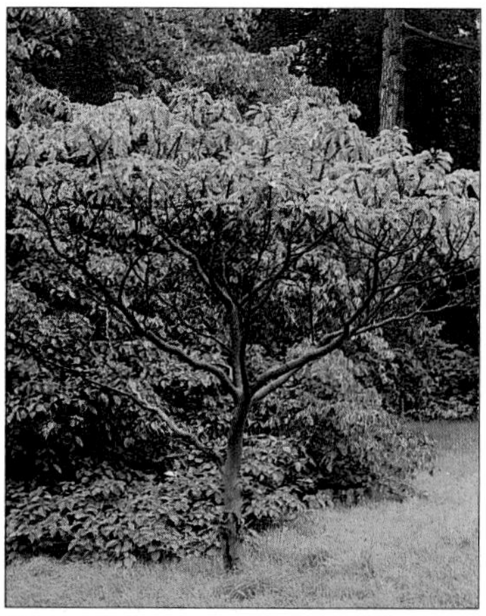

Emmenopterys henryi

EMMENOPTERYS

RUBIACEAE

Genus of 2 species of deciduous trees from forest in E. Asia. They are valued for their spreading habit and opposite, large, ovate to broadly elliptic, leathery leaves. Terminal panicles of funnel- or bell-shaped white flowers, also a notable feature, are produced on mature trees during prolonged periods of over 24°C (75°F). Grow in woodland or as specimen plants.
• **HARDINESS** Fully hardy when mature.
• **CULTIVATION** Grow in fertile, humus-rich, moist but well-drained soil in full sun. Shelter from cold, drying winds. Pruning group 1.
• **PROPAGATION** Insert greenwood cuttings in early or midsummer.
• **PESTS AND DISEASES** Trouble free.

E. henryi ■ ♀ Spreading tree with elliptic-oblong to elliptic-ovate leaves, to 20cm (8in) long, dark green above, paler and softly hairy beneath, bronze-purple when young. In summer, bears funnel-shaped white flowers, 2.5cm (1in) across, with 5 spreading lobes, some bearing a large white bract, in panicles to 18cm (7in) long by 25cm (10in) wide. ↕↔ 12m (40ft). W. and C. China, S.E Asia. ❄❄❄

▷**Empress tree** see *Paulownia tomentosa*
▷**Emu bush** see *Eremophila*
Common see *E. glabra*
Spotted see *E. maculata*

ENCEPHALARTOS

ZAMIACEAE

Genus of about 25 species of slow-growing, dioecious cycads, some palm-like, others with a short or buried stem, from open, dry forest and scrub and open, rocky slopes in C. and southern Africa. The pinnate leaves, whorled in terminal crowns, have spiny stalks and hard, leathery, often spiny-toothed leaflets. Cone-like male and female inflorescences ("cones") are borne within the leaf rosettes: male cones are more or less cylindrical; female cones are usually oblong to ovoid. In frost-prone areas, grow in a temperate or warm greenhouse; in warmer areas, they are striking plants for a garden or courtyard.
• **HARDINESS** Frost tender.
• **CULTIVATION** Under glass, grow in deep containers in equal parts loam, coarse sand, and granulated bark, with added slow-release fertilizer, in bright filtered light. During the growing season, water freely and apply a balanced liquid fertilizer monthly; water moderately in winter. Pot on or top-dress in spring. Grow *E. horridus* in full light and water sparingly in winter. Outdoors, grow in fertile, humus-rich, well-drained, neutral to slightly acid soil in partial or light dappled shade. *E. horridus* needs full sun.
• **PROPAGATION** Sow seed at 24–30°C (75–86°F) in spring, in a very sandy mix. Remove offsets in spring.
• **PESTS AND DISEASES** Cycad weevils may be a problem. Scale insects may infest greenhouse plants.

E. altensteinii ■ ⚲ (Prickly cycad). Palm-like cycad with an erect stem and straight to arching leaves, 2–3.5m (6–11ft) long, composed of numerous, narrowly oblong, bright green leaflets, sparsely toothed at the margins. Produces yellow-green flowering cones, usually in summer. ↕↔ 4–7m (12–22ft). South Africa (Eastern Cape). ⌂ (min. 16°C/61°F)
E. caffer ✱ (Kaffir bread). Cycad with a buried stem, to 40cm (16in) long, only the growing point at or above soil level. Upright then arching leaves, to 1m (3ft) long, are composed of linear-lance-shaped, sometimes sparsely toothed, bright green leaflets. Bears greenish yellow flowering cones, mainly in summer. ↕ to 1m (3ft), ↔ to 2m (6ft). South Africa. ⌂ (min. 16°C/61°F)
E. ferox ✱ Palm-like cycad with a short trunk and spreading leaves, 1–1.8m (3–6ft) long, composed of narrowly oblong to oblong-ovate, lustrous, deep green leaflets, with spiny teeth. Mature specimens bear flowering cones in summer: male cones are red; females range from pink to bright red. ↕ to 1m (3ft), ↔ 1.8–3m (6–10ft). South Africa. ⌂ (min. 13°C/55°F)
E. horridus ■ ✱ (Ferocious blue cycad). Cycad with a stem that is buried at first, then gradually elongates to about 60cm (24in) tall. Erect, ascending then arching leaves, to 1m (3ft) long, with recurved tips, are composed of numerous lance-shaped, spine-tipped and lobed, rich blue-green leaflets. Produces red-brown flowering cones, usually in summer. ↕ 1–1.4m (3–4½ft), ↔ to 2m (6ft). South Africa. ⌂ (min. 16°C/61°F)

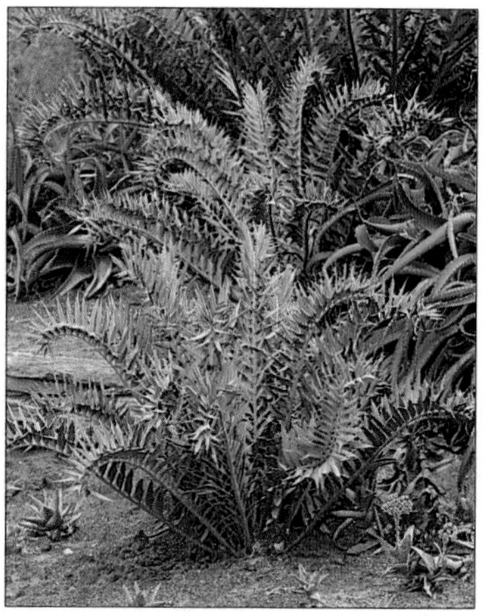

Encephalartos horridus

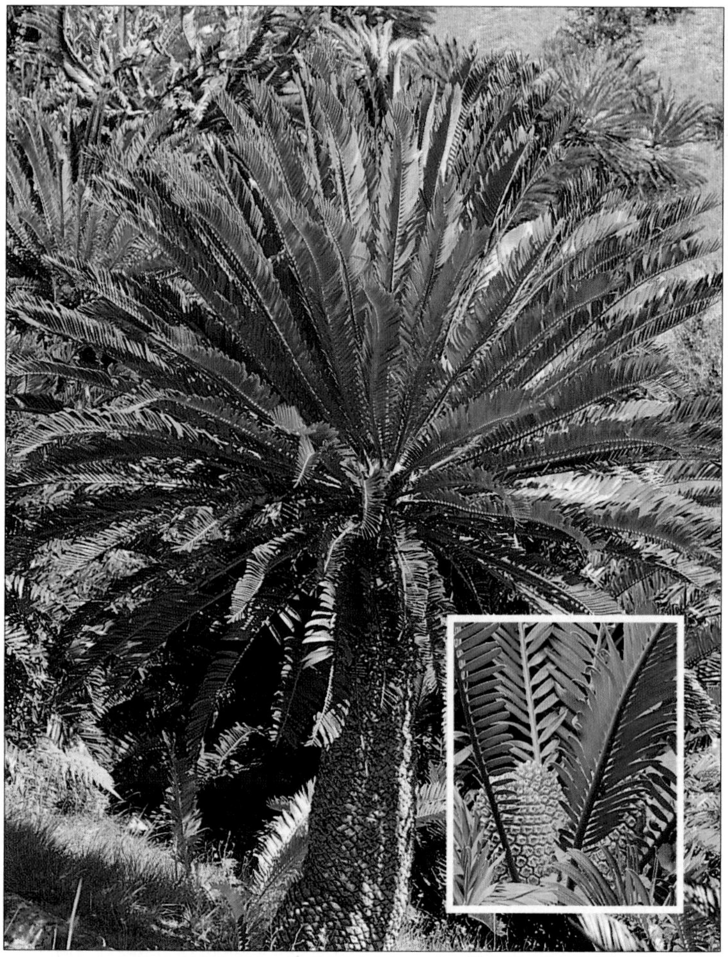

Encephalartos altensteinii (inset: cone detail)

E

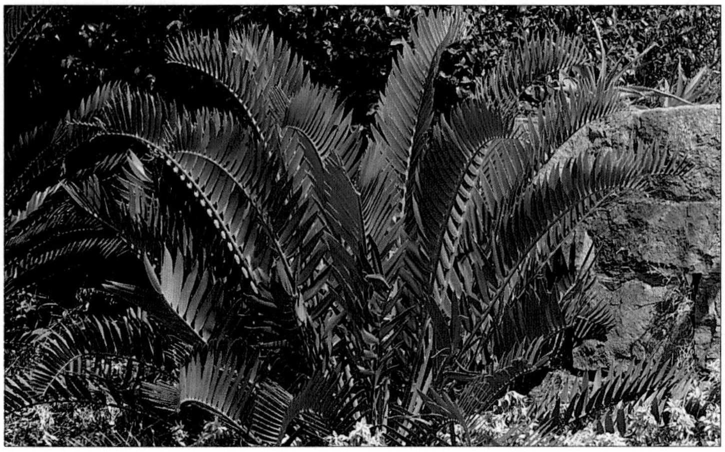

Encephalartos longifolius

E. humilis. Cycad with a buried stem, usually with only the growing tip above ground, or occasionally elongating to 30cm (12in) tall. Strongly arching, twisted leaves, 30–50cm (12–20in) long, with recurved tips, are divided into numerous linear to lance-shaped leaflets, softly hairy at first, then smooth, deep green. Brownish grey flowering cones are produced mainly in summer. ↕ 10–40cm (4–16in), ↔ 60–100cm (24–39in). South Africa (Eastern Transvaal). ❀ (min. 16°C/61°F)

E. lebomboensis ✾ (Lebombo cycad). Palm-like cycad with an erect stem and bright green leaves, 1–3m (3–10ft) long, composed of many overlapping, lance-shaped leaflets, each with a few well-spaced teeth. Produces pink to apricot-yellow flowering cones, usually in summer. ↕ 3–6m (10–20ft), ↔ 2–6m (6–20ft). South Africa (Northern Transvaal, Eastern Transvaal, KwaZulu/Natal), Swaziland, Mozambique. ❀ (min. 16°C/61°F)

E. longifolius ■ ✾ (Suurberg cycad). Palm-like cycad with a robust, erect trunk and arching, glossy, deep green, occasionally bluish green leaves, 1–2m (3–6ft) long, composed of overlapping, lance-shaped, sometimes sparsely toothed leaflets. Mature specimens bear red-hairy, greenish brown flowering cones in summer. ↕ 2–4m (6–12ft), ↔ 3.5m (11ft). South Africa (Eastern Cape). ❀ (min. 13°C/55°F)

E. natalensis ✾ (Natal cycad). Palm-like cycad with a usually erect stem and deep green leaves, 2.5–3.5m (8–11ft) long, with broadly lance-shaped, entire or sparsely spiny-toothed leaflets. Brown flowering cones, woolly at first, mature to deep yellow, and are borne in summer. ↕ to 4m (12ft), occasionally 6m (20ft), ↔ 2–3m (6–10ft). South Africa (Eastern Transvaal, KwaZulu/ Natal). ❀ (min. 16°C/61°F)

E. transvenosus ✾ (Modjadji cycad). Palm-like cycad with an erect stem and arching, lustrous, deep green leaves, 1.5–2.5m (5–8ft) long, composed of broadly lance-shaped leaflets, each with a few small teeth. Produces golden brown flowering cones, woolly when young, usually in summer. ↕ 5–8m (15–25ft), ↔ 3–5m (10–15ft). South Africa (Northern Transvaal, Eastern Transvaal). ❀ (min. 16°C/61°F)

E. villosus ■ Cycad with a buried stem, only the growing point at or above ground level. Arching, deep green leaves, to 3m (10ft) long, are composed of numerous, narrowly lance-shaped, entire or sparsely toothed leaflets, more or less hairy beneath, the lowest leaflets reduced to spines. Bears yellow flowering cones in summer. ↕ 1.5–3m (5–10ft), ↔ 3–6m (10–20ft). South Africa (Northern Transvaal, Eastern Transvaal, KwaZulu/Natal, Eastern Cape), Swaziland. ❀ (min. 16°C/61°F)

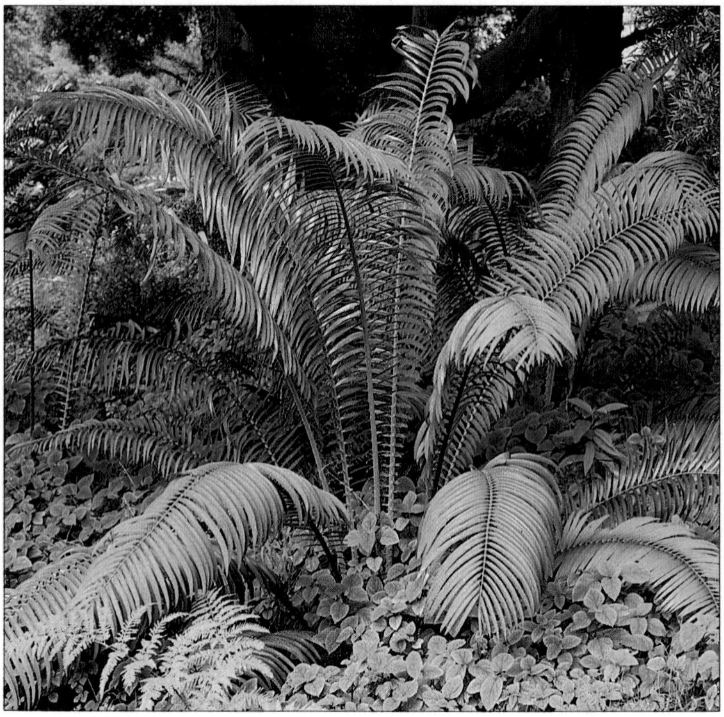

Encephalartos villosus

ENCYCLIA

ORCHIDACEAE

Genus of approximately 150 species of mainly evergreen, epiphytic orchids found in the USA and from Mexico and the West Indies south to tropical N. South America, occurring in forest from sea level to 3,000m (10,000ft). They have fleshy pseudobulbs, which may be rounded or elongated, and usually 2 narrowly oblong to strap-shaped or linear to elliptic, fleshy or leathery leaves. Attractive, variable, often fragrant flowers are produced from the apexes of the pseudobulbs, mainly in late spring or summer but often intermittently throughout the year.

- **HARDINESS** Frost tender.
- **CULTIVATION** Cool-growing orchids. Grow in epiphytic orchid compost in a slatted basket, in bright filtered light, or full light with shade from hot sun. In active growth, water freely and apply fertilizer at every third watering. Keep dry in winter. See also p.46.
- **PROPAGATION** Divide when plants overflow their containers, or remove backbulbs and pot up separately.
- **PESTS AND DISEASES** Susceptible to red spider mites, aphids, and mealybugs.

E. alata. Evergreen orchid with conical to ovoid pseudobulbs and strap-shaped to narrowly elliptic, mid-green leaves, 15cm (6in) long, often flushed red-purple. Fragrant, pale green or yellow-green flowers, 5cm (2in) across, marked purple or red-brown with the lips veined with dark red, are borne in racemes to 1.5m (5ft) long, mostly in summer. ↕ 1.5m (5ft), ↔ 45cm (18in). S. Mexico to Costa Rica. ❀ (min. 11–12°C/ 52–54°F; max. 30°C/86°F)

E. brassavolae. Evergreen orchid with elongated, ovoid to spindle-shaped or pear-shaped pseudobulbs and narrowly oblong leaves, 14–28cm (5½–11in) long. Yellow-green to brown flowers, 8cm (3in) across, with purple-tipped white lips, are produced in racemes 15–100cm (6–39in) long, from summer to autumn. ↕ 60cm (24in), ↔ 45cm (18in). S. Mexico to W. Panama. ❀ (min. 11–12°C/52–54°F; max. 30°C/86°F)

E. citrina. Semi-evergreen orchid with ovoid, conical, or spindle-shaped pseudobulbs and narrowly elliptic to elliptic, pendent, glaucous, grey-green leaves, 18–26cm (7–10in) long. Solitary, occasionally 2, pendent, fleshy, fragrant, bright lemon-yellow flowers, to 8cm (3in) across, are borne from spring to early summer. Requires drier conditions than other species. ↕ 30cm (12in), ↔ 23cm (9in). Mexico. ❀ (min. 11–12°C/52–54°F; max. 30°C/86°F)

E. cochleata ■ Evergreen orchid with flattened pear-shaped to ellipsoid pseudobulbs and elliptic to lance-shaped leaves, 20–35cm (8–14in) long. Ribbon-like flowers, 10cm (4in) long, with twisted, pale green sepals and petals, dark purple lips flushed yellowish green, and white bases with deep purple veins, are produced in racemes to 50cm (20in) long, intermittently throughout the year. ↕↔ 45cm (18in). USA (Florida) to Mexico, Colombia, Venezuela. ❀ (min. 11–12°C/52–54°F; max. 30°C/86°F)

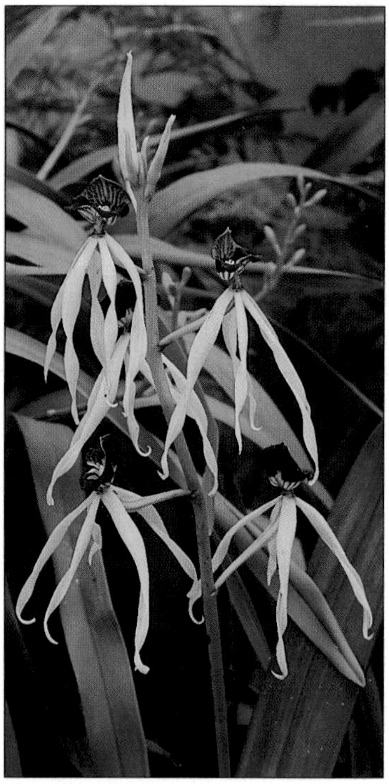

Encyclia cochleata

E. cordigera. Evergreen orchid with conical to ovoid pseudobulbs and semi-rigid, narrowly elliptic leaves, to 45cm (18in) long. Fragrant, brown, purple-brown, or purple-green flowers, to 5cm (2in) across, with cream lips streaked pink or magenta, are borne in racemes to 75cm (30in) long, from spring to summer. ↕ 45cm (18in), ↔ 30cm (12in). S. Mexico, Central America, Colombia, Venezuela. ❀ (min. 11–12°C/52–54°F; max. 30°C/86°F)

E. fragrans. Evergreen orchid with elongated, narrowly ovoid to ellipsoid pseudobulbs, each bearing a single oblong-strap-shaped to elliptic leaf, 35cm (14in) long. Fragrant, cream to greenish white flowers, to 3.5cm (1½in) across, with red-striped lips held uppermost, are borne in racemes to 20cm (8in) long, from spring to summer. ↕ 23cm (9in), ↔ 15cm (6in). S. Mexico, Central America to Brazil, Greater Antilles. ❀ (min. 11–12°C/52–54°F; max. 30°C/86°F)

E. mariae. Evergreen orchid with conical pseudobulbs and narrowly oblong leaves, 13cm (5in) long. In summer, bears racemes, 5–27cm (2–11in) long, of 2–4 pendent, yellow to olive-green flowers, to 6cm (2½in) long, with large, papery white lips, and green veins in the throats. ↕ 18cm (7in), ↔ 15cm (6in). E. Mexico. ❀ (min. 11–12°C/52–54°F; max. 30°C/86°F)

E. radiata. Evergreen orchid with ellipsoid to ovoid pseudobulbs and elliptic to lance-shaped leaves, to 35cm (14in) long. Fragrant, cream or greenish white flowers, 3.5cm (1½in) across, with violet-lined lips held uppermost, are produced in racemes to 20cm (8in) long, from autumn to winter. ↕ 25cm (10in), ↔ 30cm (12in). C. and S. Mexico, Guatemala, Honduras, Costa Rica. ❀ (min. 11–12°C/52–54°F; max. 30°C/86°F)

E. vitellina. Evergreen orchid with ovoid to conical pseudobulbs and lance-shaped to elliptic, grey-green leaves, to 22cm (9in) long. Brilliant orange or vermilion flowers, 4cm (1½in) across, with orange- to red-tipped yellow lips, develop in racemes 12–30cm (5–12in) long, from spring to summer. ↕ 23cm (9in), ↔ 15cm (6in). S. Mexico, Guatemala. ❀ (min. 11–12°C/52–54°F; max. 30°C/86°F)

▷ **Endive** see *Cichorium*
▷ ***Endymion*** see *Hyacinthoides*
E. non-scriptus see *H. non-scripta*
E. hispanicus see *H. hispanica*

ENKIANTHUS

ERICACEAE

Genus of about 10 species of mainly deciduous shrubs, occasionally trees, occurring in scrub and woodland from the Himalayas to Japan. They are grown for their terminal umbels or corymb-like racemes of bell- or urn-shaped flowers, usually 5–9mm (¼–⅜in) long, borne from mid-spring to early summer, and for their simple, lance-shaped to elliptic-obovate, usually toothed, alternate leaves, which turn various shades of red in autumn. Best grown in an open site in a woodland garden.

• **HARDINESS** Fully hardy.
• **CULTIVATION** Grow in humus-rich, moist but well-drained, acid to neutral soil in full sun or partial shade. Pruning group 1.
• **PROPAGATION** Sow seed at 18–21°C (64–70°F) in late winter or early spring. Insert semi-ripe cuttings in summer. Layer in autumn.
• **PESTS AND DISEASES** Trouble free.

E. campanulatus ■ ♀ Spreading, tree-like, deciduous shrub with whorled branches and obovate-elliptic, toothed, dull green leaves, to 6cm (2½in) long, clustered at the tips of the shoots and turning orange-yellow to red in autumn. Bears pendent, corymb-like racemes of 5–15 bell-shaped, creamy yellow flowers, veined pink to red, in late spring and early summer. ↕↔ 4–5m (12–15ft). Japan. ✻✻✻. **f. *albiflorus*** has white flowers. **'Hiraethlyn'** bears

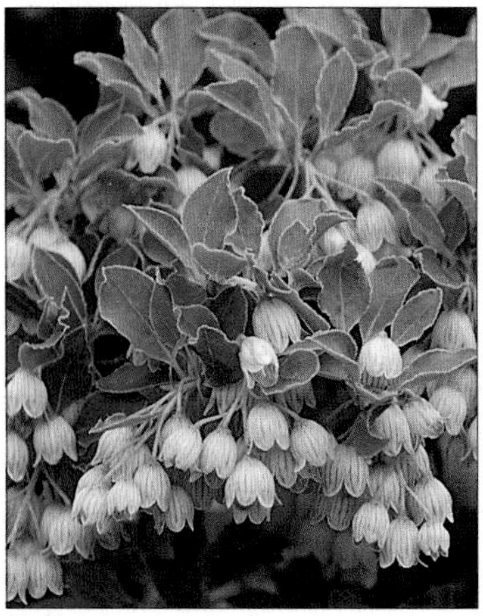

Enkianthus campanulatus

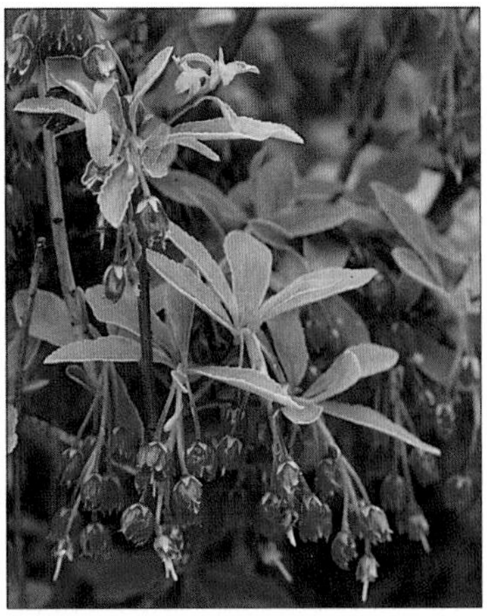

Enkianthus cernuus var. *rubens*

cream flowers with dark red veins. **var. *palibinii*** has dark red flowers.

E. cernuus* var. *rubens ■ ♀ Bushy, deciduous shrub with dense clusters of obovate, toothed, bright green leaves, to 5cm (2in) long, tinged purple in summer and turning dark red-purple in autumn. In late spring and early summer, produces slender, pendent racemes of 5–12 broadly bell-shaped, rich red flowers, with finely toothed mouths. ↕↔ 2.5m (8ft). Japan. ✻✻✻

E. chinensis. Upright, deciduous shrub with elliptic to elliptic-oblong, toothed, bright green leaves, to 7cm (3in) long, softly hairy along the midribs above, glaucous and hairless beneath, turning orange and red in autumn. Pendent, corymb-like racemes of 12–24 bell-shaped, creamy yellow flowers, with pink veins, are produced in late spring. ↕ to 3.5m (11ft), ↔ 2m (6ft). China, N. Burma. ✻✻✻

E. deflexus ■ ♀ Vigorous, upright, deciduous shrub or small tree with red shoots and oval to obovate, bright green leaves, to 7cm (3in) long, downy beneath, turning orange and red in autumn. Umbels of 8–20 relatively large, broadly bell-shaped, pink-veined cream flowers, 1.5cm (½in) across, are produced in late spring and early summer. ↕ 2.5–4m (8–12ft) (sometimes more), ↔ 3m (10ft). Himalayas, W. China. ✻✻✻

E. perulatus ■ ♀ Compact, deciduous shrub with red-tinted young branches. Elliptic to obovate, toothed, mid-green leaves, to 5cm (2in) long, clustered at the ends of the shoots, are downy on the midribs beneath and turn brilliant red in

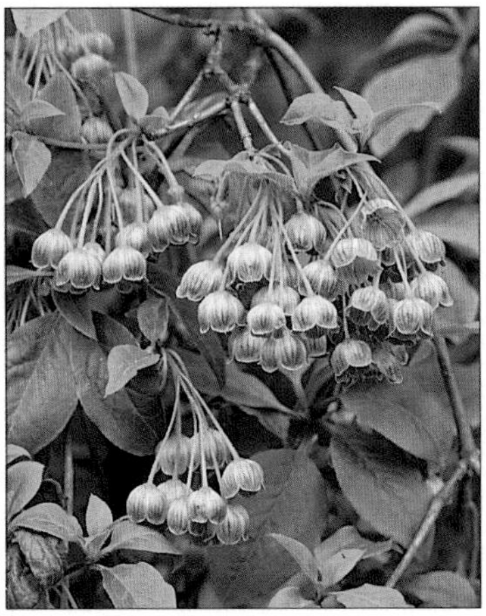

Enkianthus deflexus

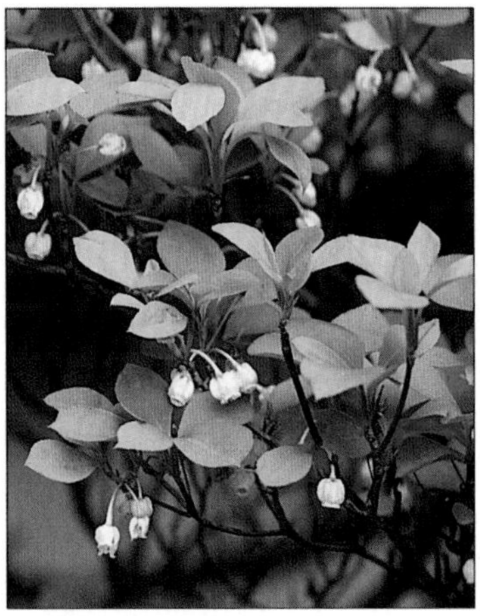

Enkianthus perulatus

autumn. Produces pendent umbels of up to 10 urn-shaped white flowers in mid-spring. ↕↔ to 2m (6ft). Japan. ✻✻✻

ENSETE

MUSACEAE

Genus of 7 species of banana-like, monocarpic, evergreen perennials from lower mountain slopes in tropical Africa and Asia. They have large, paddle-shaped leaves growing from trunk-like pseudostems, which are formed by the bases of the old leaf-stalks. Cup-shaped flowers are produced in pendent, terminal inflorescences among large bracts. Fruits are banana-like but dry and unpalatable. In frost-prone areas, grow in a temperate greenhouse, or plunge outdoors during summer to provide subtropical effects in summer bedding. In frost-free climates, grow as specimen plants or in a courtyard.

• **HARDINESS** Frost tender.
• **CULTIVATION** Under glass, grow in loam-based potting compost (JI No.3) in full light with shade from hot sun. Keep well-ventilated. When in growth, water freely and apply a balanced liquid fertilizer monthly. Outdoors, grow in humus-rich soil in full sun or partial shade. Lift plunged plants before first frosts, cut back long roots, and reduce top-growth to the newest 2 or 3 leaves. Cut the dead leaves no lower than the base of each leaf-blade.
• **PROPAGATION** Sow seed at 18–21°C (64–70°F) in spring, after soaking in tepid water for 24 hours. Germination is erratic.
• **PESTS AND DISEASES** Red spider mites and aphids may be a problem, especially under glass.

E. ventricosum ■ syn. *Musa arnoldiana, M. ensete* (Abyssinian banana, Ethiopian banana). Fast-growing, banana-like perennial with huge, paddle-shaped, bright olive-green leaves, to 6m (20ft) long, produced from the centre of the plant, with thick midribs that are bright red beneath. White flowers, concealed within arching cylinders of bronze-red bracts, are borne in inflorescences 1–1.2m (3–4ft) long, in summer. ↕ 6m (20ft) or more, ↔ to 5m (15ft). Ethiopia to Angola. ❀ (min. 7°C/45°F). **'Maurelii'** has leaves tinged red above, especially along the margins, and dark red leaf-stalks.

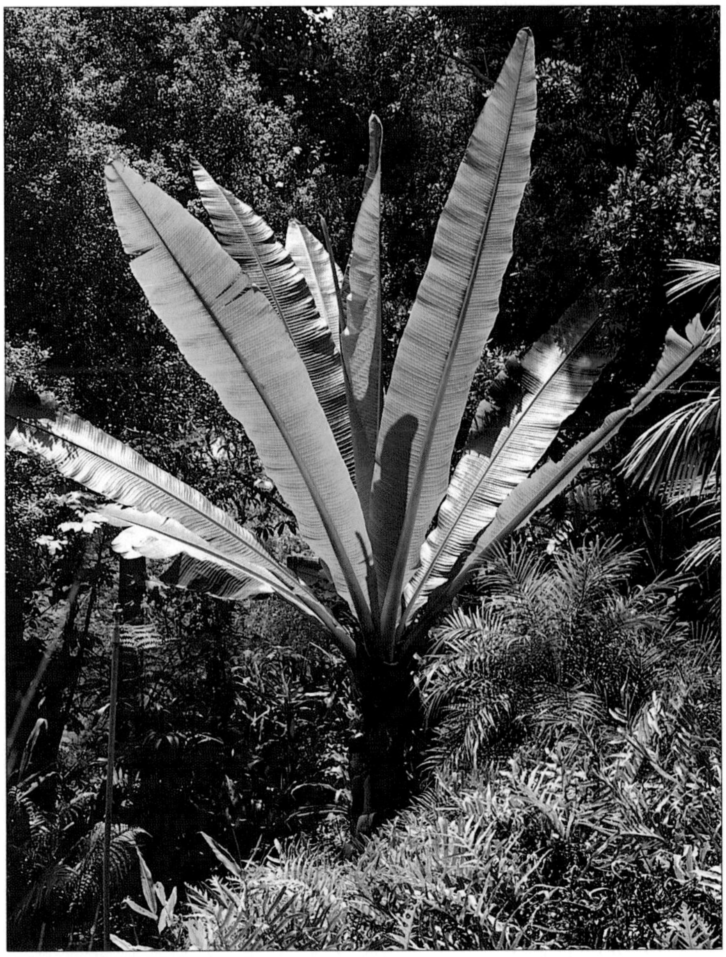

Ensete ventricosum

E

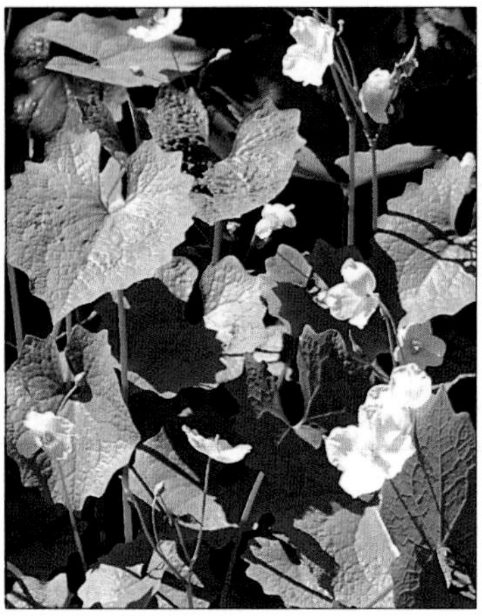

Eomecon chionantha

EOMECON

Snow poppy

PAPAVERACEAE

Genus of one species of rhizomatous perennial occurring on riverbanks in E. China. It has slightly fleshy leaves and nodding, poppy-like flowers. Grow as ground cover on a moist, shady bank, in a shrub border, or in a rock garden.
• **HARDINESS** Fully hardy.
• **CULTIVATION** Grow in humus-rich, moist but well-drained soil in light shade, or in full sun where the soil does not dry out in summer. May spread rapidly in fertile soil.
• **PROPAGATION** Sow seed in containers in a cold frame in spring. Divide, or separate rooted runners, both in spring.
• **PESTS AND DISEASES** Sometimes damaged by slugs and snails.

E. chionantha ■ Vigorous, spreading perennial with heart- to kidney- or arrow-shaped, leathery, dull grey-green leaves, to 10cm (4in) across. Upright, branching stems bear loose panicles of poppy-like, glistening white flowers, to 5cm (2in) across, from late spring to midsummer. ↕ to 40cm (16in), ↔ indefinite. E. China. ❄❄❄

EPACRIS

EPACRIDACEAE

Genus of 35 species of evergreen, heather-like shrubs occurring on heaths, open slopes, and scrub in Australia, New Zealand, and New Caledonia. They are cultivated for their often showy, tubular, cylindrical to bell-shaped, 5-lobed flowers, which are freely produced, usually in leafy, terminal racemes. The linear-lance-shaped to broadly ovate, mid- or dark green leaves are alternate or spiralling, and usually crowded on the stems. In frost-prone areas, grow in a cool greenhouse. In warmer areas, grow in a border or a large rock garden.
• **HARDINESS** Frost hardy to frost tender.
• **CULTIVATION** Under glass, grow in lime-free (ericaceous) potting compost in full light with shade from hot sun. From spring to autumn, water freely and apply a half-strength, balanced liquid fertilizer monthly. Water moderately in winter. Outdoors, grow in poor to moderately fertile, humus-rich, moist but well-drained, neutral to acid soil in full sun with some midday shade. Pruning group 10, after flowering.

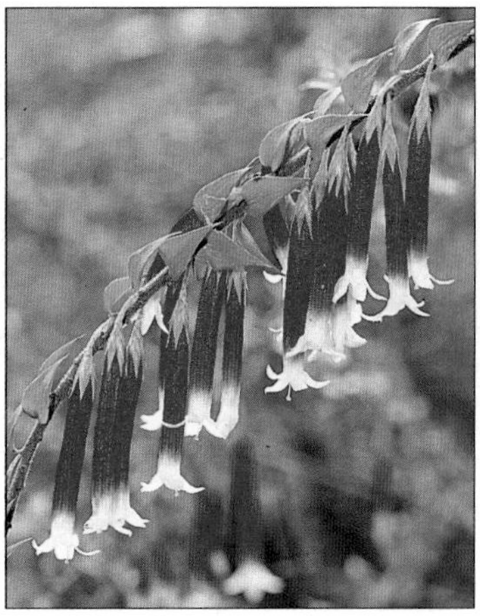

Epacris longiflora

• **PROPAGATION** Surface-sow seed at 13–16°C (55–61°F) in spring; germination is slow and usually erratic, taking between 3 and 6 months. Root semi-ripe cuttings with bottom heat in summer.
• **PESTS AND DISEASES** Scale insects may infest greenhouse plants.

E. impressa (Common Australian heath). Erect to spreading, often slender, evergreen shrub with narrowly ovate, deep green leaves, to 1.5cm (½in) long, tapering to prickle-like tips. Pendent, cylindrical, red, pink, or white flowers, 2cm (¾in) long, are borne in slender, erect, terminal racemes, 10cm (4in) or more long, from spring to summer. ↕ 30–120cm (12–48in), occasionally to 1.8m (6ft), ↔ 30–90cm (12–36in). Australia (New South Wales to Tasmania). ❄
E. longiflora ■ Erect or spreading, evergreen shrub, often irregular in habit, with broadly to narrowly ovate, broadly pointed, deep green leaves, to 1cm (½in) long. Pendent, cylindrical, white-tipped red flowers, 1–4cm (½–1½in) long, are produced singly from the leaf axils and in raceme-like, terminal spikes, to 4cm (1½in) long, mainly from spring to summer. ↕ 0.5–1.5m (20–60in), ↔ 1–2m (3–6ft). S.W. Australia. ❄. **'White Sport'** produces white flowers.

▷ **Epaulette tree** see *Pterostyrax hispida*

EPHEDRA

EPHEDRACEAE

Genus of about 40 species of usually dioecious, evergreen shrubs, occasionally climbers, occurring in dry, rocky sites from the Mediterranean to China, and in North and South America. They have green shoots and tiny, scale-like leaves, and are valued for their spherical fruits, which, on female plants, follow the tiny flowers. Grow as ground cover in a shrub border or rock garden. In frost-prone areas, grow tender species in a cold greenhouse or alpine house.
• **HARDINESS** Fully hardy to frost tender.
• **CULTIVATION** Grow in poor to moderately fertile, sharply drained soil in full sun.
• **PROPAGATION** Sow seed of hardy species in containers in an open frame in autumn; sow seed of tender species at 13–16°C (55–61°F) in spring. Divide in autumn or spring.
• **PESTS AND DISEASES** Trouble free.

E. gerardiana. Dense, thicket-forming shrub with upright, jointed, deep green shoots. Bears insignificant, yellowish green flowers in summer. Spherical red fruit, 1cm (½in) across, ripen in autumn. ↕ 60cm (24in), ↔ 3m (10ft) or more. Himalayas, China. ❄❄❄

EPIDENDRUM

ORCHIDACEAE

Genus of about 750 species of highly varied, evergreen orchids, including epiphytes, lithophytes, and terrestrials. They are widespread in tropical North, Central, and South America, some thriving in montane forests to an altitude of 1,000m (3,250ft). Most produce cylindrical, leafy stems that may be either tall and reed-like or short and fleshy; others have pseudobulbs. The leaves vary greatly. The flowers are produced in usually terminal, umbel-like racemes or panicles, which are a continuation of the leafy stems, or they are occasionally borne from the bases.
• **HARDINESS** Frost tender.
• **CULTIVATION** Cool- to intermediate-growing orchids. Grow in containers of epiphytic or terrestrial orchid compost; provide support for long, scrambling stems. In summer, provide bright filtered light and high humidity; water freely, applying fertilizer at every third watering, and mist once or twice daily. Provide full light and water sparingly in winter. Keep species with pseudobulbs dry in winter. See also p.46.
• **PROPAGATION** Divide when the plants overflow their containers. Root plantlets of *E. ibaguense* as soon as they have developed vigorous roots.
• **PESTS AND DISEASES** Susceptible to red spider mites, aphids, and mealybugs.

E. ciliare. Epiphytic orchid with leafy, pseudobulb-like stems, and 1 or 2 oblong-elliptic, leathery, mid-green leaves, to 15cm (6in) long. Fragrant, white-lipped, pale yellow-green or pale yellow flowers, 9cm (3½in) across, sometimes with fringed lobes, are produced in terminal racemes, to 30cm (12in) long, mostly in winter. ↕ 50cm (20in), ↔ 30cm (12in). Mexico to N. South America, West Indies. ⊛ (min. 13°C/55°F; max. 30°C/86°F)
E. conopseum. Epiphytic orchid with slender, leafy stems and 1–3 narrowly oblong to linear-lance-shaped, rigid, leathery, often purple-flushed, mid-green leaves, 9cm (3½in) long. In summer, bears fragrant, often purple-tinged, light grey-green flowers, 2cm (¾in) across, in terminal sub-umbels, to 16cm (6in) long. ↕ 20cm (8in), ↔ 15cm (6in). USA (Florida) to Mexico. ⊛ (min. 13°C/55°F; max. 30°C/86°F)
E. difforme ■ Epiphytic orchid with flattened, fleshy, leafy stems and oblong to elliptic-lance-shaped, fleshy to leathery, glossy, yellowish green leaves, to 11cm (4½in) long. Fragrant, pale green, green-yellow, or white, almost translucent flowers, to 3cm (1¼in) across, are produced in clustered racemes, to 15cm (6in) across, in summer. ↕ 35cm (14in), ↔ 30cm (12in). USA (Florida), West Indies, Mexico, Central America, Ecuador, Peru, Brazil. ⊛ (min. 13°C/55°F; max. 30°C/86°F)
E. ibaguense, syn. *E. radicans.* Terrestrial orchid with tall, rambling, leafy stems and ovate-oblong to oblong, leathery, yellowish green leaves, 15cm (6in) long. Bright red, occasionally orange or yellow flowers, 4cm (1½in) across, are produced year-round in dense, terminal racemes, to 70cm (28in) long. ↕ 2m (6ft), ↔ 1m (3ft). West Indies, Mexico, Central America, Colombia, Venezuela, Guyana, Peru. ⊛ (min. 13°C/55°F; max. 30°C/86°F)
E. nocturnum. Epiphytic orchid with leafy stems and 1 or 2 oblong-lance-shaped to elliptic, leathery, glossy, mid-green leaves, to 15cm (6in) long. Night-scented, white-lipped, pale yellow-green flowers, 6cm (2½in) across, sometimes with fringed lobes, are produced singly or in pairs in succession from summer to autumn. ↕ 60cm (24in), ↔ 30cm (12in). West Indies, USA (Florida), Central

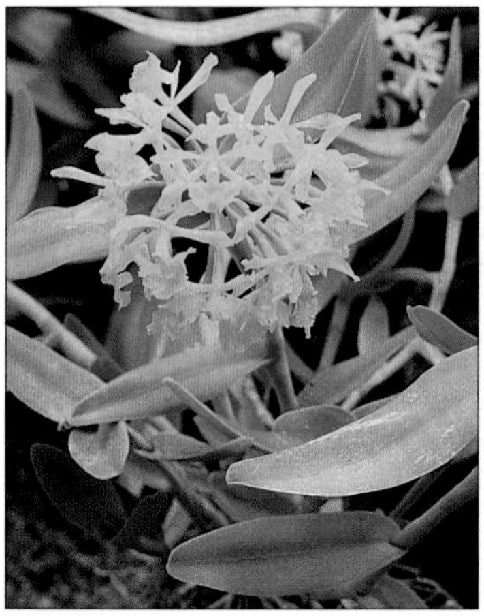

Epidendrum difforme

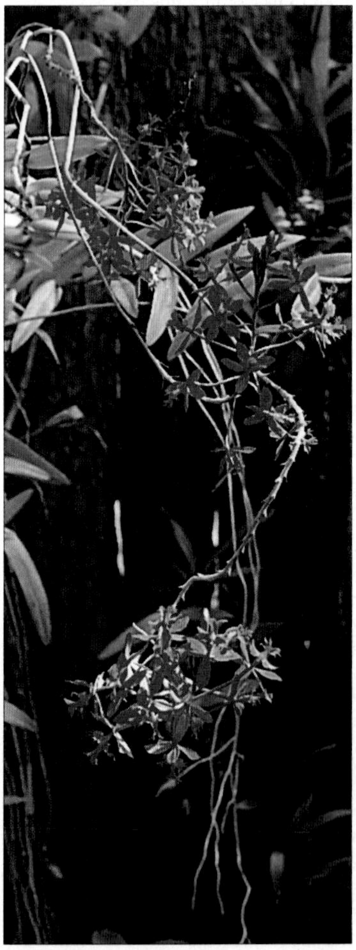

Epidendrum x *o'brienianum*

America, N. South America. ❀ (min. 13°C/55°F; max. 30°C/86°F)
E.* x *o'brienianum ▣ (*E. evectum* x *E. ibaguense*). Epiphytic orchid with tall, rambling, leafy stems and semi-rigid, ovate-oblong to oblong, leathery, yellowish green leaves, 15cm (6in) long. Terminal racemes, 80–90cm (32–36in) long, of long-lasting, bright orange-red or orange flowers, 4cm (1½in) across, are borne more or less continuously. ↕↔ 1m (3ft). Garden origin. ❀ (min. 13°C/55°F; max. 30°C/86°F)
E. pseudepidendrum. Epiphytic orchid with leafy stems and inversely lance-shaped, leathery, glossy, mid-green leaves, to 20cm (8in) long. Distinctive, fleshy green flowers, 5cm (2in) long, with protruding, bright orange lips with finely fringed lobes, are produced in few-flowered, pendent racemes, to 15cm (6in) long, from summer to autumn. ↕ 1m (3ft), ↔ 60cm (24in). Costa Rica, Panama. ❀ (min. 13°C/55°F; max. 30°C/86°F)
E. radicans see *E. ibaguense.*
E. secundum. Epiphytic orchid with leafy stems and ovate-lance-shaped, leathery, mid-green leaves, to 14cm (5½in) long. Rose-pink flowers, 2.5cm (1in) across, with deeply 3-lobed lips marked white and yellowish white, are produced in racemes to 75cm (30in) long throughout summer and autumn. ↕ 60cm (24in), ↔ 30cm (12in). West Indies, tropical South America. ❀ (min. 13°C/55°F; max. 30°C/86°F)
E. stamfordianum. Epiphytic orchid with spindle-shaped, leafy stems and 4–6 linear- to elliptic-oblong, leathery, mid-green leaves, to 18cm (7in) long. In summer, fragrant, white-lipped, yellow-green to pale bronze flowers, 5cm (2in) across, mottled red-brown or purple, are produced in racemes or panicles, to 60cm (24in) long, from the bases of the leafy stems. ↕ 30cm (12in), ↔ 60cm (24in). Guatemala. ❀ (min. 13°C/55°F; max. 30°C/86°F)

EPIGAEA syn. ORPHANIDESIA

ERICACEAE

Genus of 3 species of prostrate, evergreen shrubs and subshrubs from woodland in Turkey, Japan, and North America. They are grown for their short, axillary or terminal clusters or racemes of small, urn-shaped, funnel-shaped, or tubular-bell-shaped flowers, borne in spring, and for their ovate to oblong, entire, tough, prominently veined, dark green leaves, produced from rusty-hairy branches. Grow in a shaded niche in a rock garden, peat bed, or woodland garden. In areas that are prone to early frosts, grow in an alpine house.
• **HARDINESS** Mainly fully hardy. *E. gaultherioides* is hardy to -10°C (14°F).
• **CULTIVATION** Grow in humus-rich, moist, acid soil in deep or partial shade. In an alpine house, *E. gaultherioides* requires lime-free (ericaceous) potting compost and indirect light.
• **PROPAGATION** Surface-sow seed at 10–13°C (50–55°F) as soon as ripe; keep warm and moist until germination. Water seedlings from below with soft water. Separate rooted layers or take greenwood cuttings in early summer.
• **PESTS AND DISEASES** May be infested with whiteflies and red spider mites under glass.

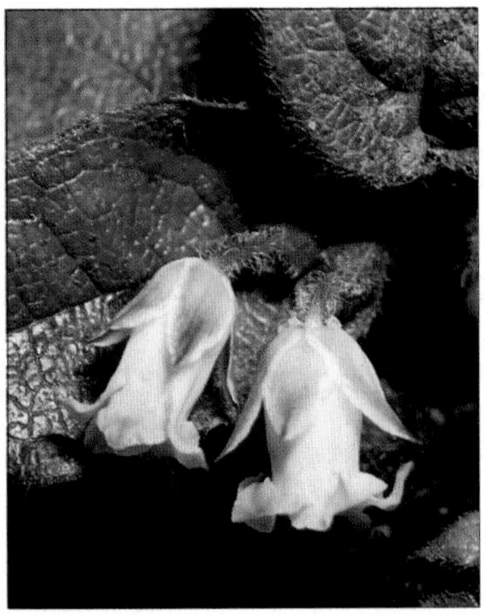
Epigaea asiatica

E. asiatica ▣ Creeping, stem-rooting shrub with oblong to elliptic, leathery, dark green leaves, 3.5–10cm (1½–4in) long, heart-shaped at the bases and with finely bristly margins. Stems and leaves are clothed in fine brown hairs. In late spring, bears short, pendent, axillary or terminal racemes of slightly fragrant, tubular-bell-shaped, light to mid-pink flowers, 1cm (½in) long, often with white tubes. ↕ to 10cm (4in), ↔ to 20cm (8in). Japan. ❄❄❄
E. gaultherioides, syn. *Orphanidesia gaultherioides.* Prostrate subshrub with ovate to oblong, leathery, dark green leaves, 8–12cm (3–5in) long, with bristly veins and margins. Bears widely funnel-shaped, shell-pink flowers, to 5cm (2in) across, in axillary clusters in spring. Needs shade. ↕ to 10cm (4in), ↔ to 30cm (12in). N.E. Turkey. ❄❄
E. repens (Mayflower, Trailing arbutus). Creeping subshrub with ovate-oblong, sparsely bristly-hairy, glossy, dark green leaves, to 8cm (3in) long, heart-shaped at the bases, borne on hairy, rooting stems. In spring, produces fragrant, urn-shaped white flowers, to 1.5cm (½in) long, occasionally pink-flushed, in dense, raceme-like, terminal clusters. ↕ to 8cm (3in), ↔ to 30cm (12in). North America. ❄❄❄

EPILOBIUM

syn. CHAMAENERION
Willow herb

ONAGRACEAE

Genus of about 200 species of annuals, biennials, herbaceous and semi-evergreen perennials (some of which are stoloniferous), and semi-evergreen subshrubs. They are widely distributed in temperate regions on waste and disturbed ground, stony slopes, river gravels, and subalpine screes and meadows. They are grown for their 4-petalled, pink or white flowers, produced singly or in leafy racemes from the leaf axils, usually over long periods from summer to autumn. The leaves are linear to broadly ovate. Wind-borne seeds and spreading rhizomes make many species invasive, but those described here are garden worthy. Grow in a rock garden or herbaceous border. *E. glabellum* is good as ground cover.
• **HARDINESS** Fully hardy.
• **CULTIVATION** Grow in humus-rich, moist but well-drained soil in full sun or partial shade. Alpine species may need some midday shade. Dead-head for repeat flowering and to prevent seeding.
• **PROPAGATION** Sow seed in containers in a cold frame as soon as ripe or in spring. Divide in autumn or spring. Take softwood cuttings from sideshoots in spring.
• **PESTS AND DISEASES** Vulnerable to slugs and snails, rust, and powdery mildew.

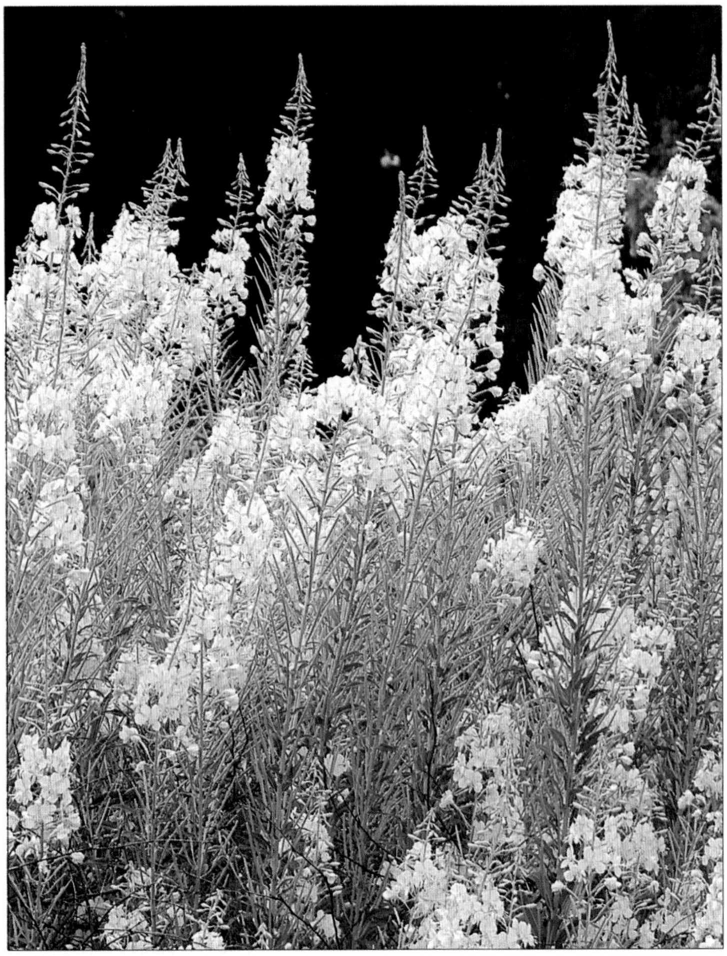
Epilobium angustifolium f. *album*

E. angustifolium* f. *album ▣ syn. *Chamaenerion angustifolium* f. *album, E. angustifolium* var. *leucanthum.* Strongly spreading, rhizomatous perennial with linear-lance-shaped, sometimes wavy, willow-like, pale to mid-green leaves, 2.5–20cm (1–8in) long. From midsummer to early autumn, bears racemes of open saucer-shaped white flowers, to 1.5cm (½in) across, with green sepals. Self-seeds freely. ↕ to 1.5m (5ft), ↔ 1m (3ft) or more. N. hemisphere. ❄❄❄
E. angustifolium* var. *leucanthum see *E. angustifolium* f. *album.*
E. californicum see *Zauschneria californica.*
E. canum see *Zauschneria californica* subsp. *cana.*
E. chlorifolium* var. *kaikourense. Clump-forming, woody-based perennial with ovate to broadly ovate, finely toothed, bronze-green leaves, 1–3cm (½–1¼in) long. In summer, upright, branching stems bear racemes of long-tubed, white or pale pink flowers, 1.5cm (½in) across, with spreading lobes. ↕ to 30cm (12in), ↔ to 15cm (6in). New Zealand. ❄❄❄
E. crassum. Prostrate, creeping perennial with narrowly obovate, finely toothed, slightly fleshy, glossy, mid-green leaves, 1–4cm (½–1½in) long, pink-flushed beneath. In summer, bears solitary, open cup-shaped, pink-veined white flowers, 1.5cm (½in) across. Grow in partial shade. ↕ to 10cm (4in), ↔ to 20cm (8in). New Zealand. ❄❄❄
E. dodonaei. Spreading perennial with a woody rootstock and upright stems bearing linear, toothed, bristly-hairy, mid-green leaves, to 2.5cm (1in) long. Throughout summer, bears cup-shaped, deep pinkish purple flowers, to 3.5cm (1½in) across, in loose, terminal racemes. ↕ 30–90cm (12–36in), ↔ to 20cm (8in). C. and S. Europe to W. Asia. ❄❄❄
***E. glabellum* of gardens** ▣ Mat- or clump-forming, semi-evergreen perennial with elliptic to ovate, finely

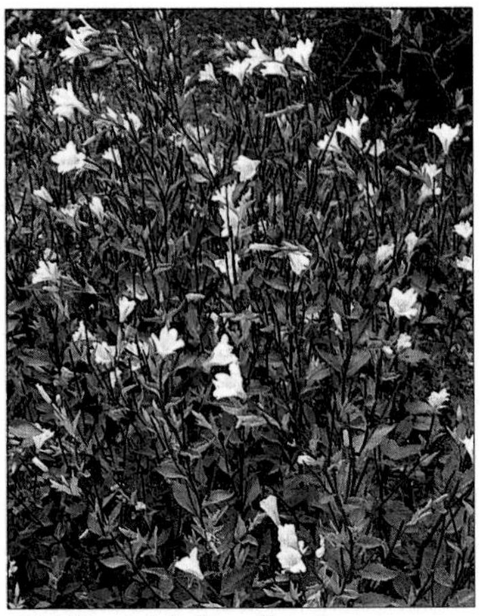
Epilobium glabellum of gardens

E

toothed, bronzed, deep green leaves, to 2cm (¾in) long, on bristly-hairy, often red-tinted stems, 5–40cm (2–16in) long. Outward-facing, cup-shaped, creamy white or pink flowers, 2.5cm (1in) across, are borne singly on slender, branching stems in summer. Prefers cool, damp shade. ↕↔ to 20cm (8in). New Zealand. ❄❄❄

E. latifolium. Spreading, rhizomatous perennial with ovate-elliptic, glaucous, mid-green leaves, 1–7cm (½–3in) long. Funnel-shaped, pink or white to pink-purple flowers, to 3cm (1¼in) across, with crimson sepals, are produced in short, leafy racemes from midsummer to early autumn. ↕↔ 45cm (18in). N. Eurasia, North America. ❄❄❄

E. septentrionale see *Zauschneria septentrionalis.*

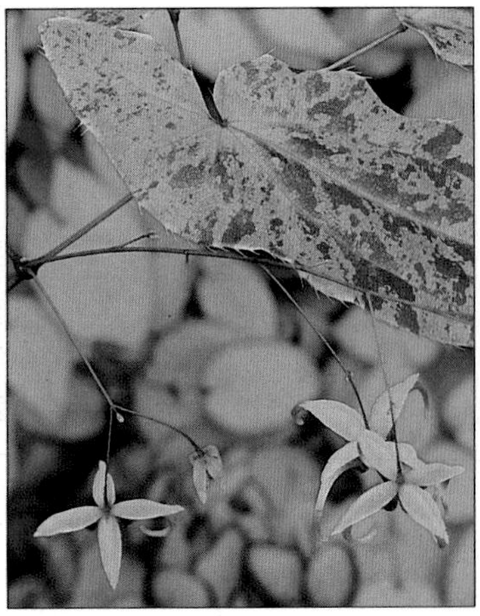
Epimedium acuminatum

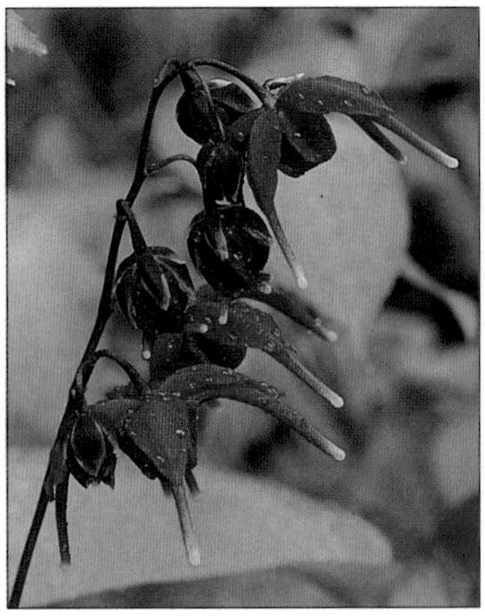
Epimedium grandiflorum 'Crimson Beauty'

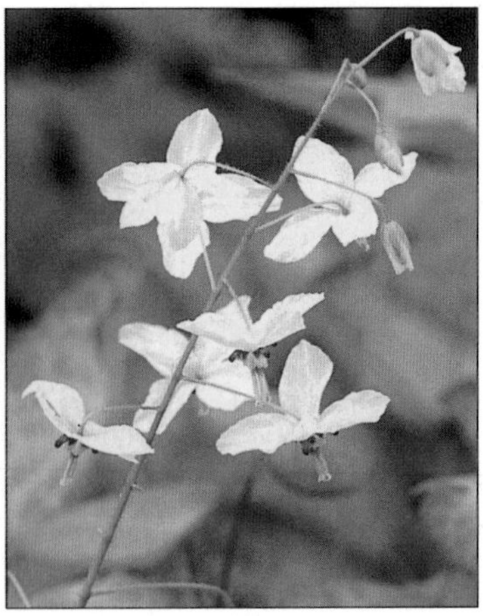
Epimedium x *perralchicum*

EPIMEDIUM

Barrenwort, Bishop's Mitre

BERBERIDACEAE

Genus of 30–40 species of evergreen and deciduous, rhizomatous perennials from the Mediterranean to temperate E. Asia, occurring in woodland, scrub, and shady, rocky places. They have mainly basal, 2- or 3-ternate, sometimes pinnate, leathery leaves, unequally heart-shaped at the bases and pointed at the tips, with more or less spiny margins. The leaves are sometimes bronze-tinted in spring, and often colour well in autumn. Some species are deciduous in autumn, others retain old leaves until the new leaves are produced. Small, mainly saucer- to cup-shaped, yellow, beige, white, pink, red, or purple flowers, often with spurs, are borne in lax racemes, or sometimes in panicles, from spring to early summer. Grow as ground cover under trees or shrubs, or in a border; the smaller species are suitable for a rock garden.

- **HARDINESS** Fully hardy, although frost may damage young flowers and foliage.
- **CULTIVATION** Grow in fertile, humus-rich, moist but well-drained soil in partial shade, with shelter from cold, dry winds. *E. perralderianum* tolerates part-day sun where soils remain moist; *E.* x *versicolor* tolerates full sun and slightly drier soils. Except for *E. perralderianum*, most provide the best display of foliage and flowers if the old leaves are clipped back in late winter or early spring, before flower spikes form. Provide a deep winter mulch where frosts are prolonged or severe.
- **PROPAGATION** Sow seed in containers in a cold frame as soon as ripe. Divide in autumn or after flowering. Root rhizome cuttings under glass in winter; plant out after all danger of frost has passed.
- **PESTS AND DISEASES** Vine weevil and mosaic virus may be a problem.

E. acuminatum ■ Clump-forming, evergreen, rhizomatous perennial with leaves divided into 3 obliquely lance-shaped to narrowly ovate leaflets, 3–18cm (1¼–7in) long, with spiny, marginal teeth, the lower 2 leaflets with very unequally lobed bases. Young leaves are mid-green, marked reddish brown and mauve, becoming glaucous beneath. Long-spurred, usually pale purple to purple-pink flowers, 3–4cm (1¼–1½in) across, are produced from mid-spring to early summer. ↕ 30cm (12in), ↔ 45cm (18in). W. and C. China. ❄❄❄

E. alpinum. Clump-forming, deciduous, rhizomatous perennial with leaves divided into 5–9 ovate, spiny-margined, bright green leaflets, 5–9cm (2–3½in) long, often colouring crimson in winter. Produces almost spurless flowers, 0.9–1.5cm (⅜–½in) across, with brownish red sepals and yellow petals, in mid- and late spring. ↕ 15–30cm (6–12in), ↔ 30cm (12in). S. Europe. ❄❄❄

E.* x *cantabrigiense (*E. alpinum* x *E. pubigerum*). Clump-forming, evergreen, rhizomatous perennial with long-stalked, mid-green leaves, each divided into 7–17 ovate, few-spined leaflets, 5–10cm (2–4in) long, persistently softly hairy beneath and variably coloured in autumn. Numerous spurless, pinkish beige and yellow flowers, to 1cm (½in) across, are produced well above the foliage in mid- and late spring. ↕ 30–60cm (12–24in), ↔ 60cm (24in). Garden origin. ❄❄❄

E. davidii ■ Clump-forming, evergreen, rhizomatous perennial with leaves divided into 3, occasionally 5, ovate to ovate-lance-shaped leaflets, 3–7cm (1¼–3in) long, copper when young, becoming fresh green later. Pale to deep yellow flowers, 2–3cm (¾–1¼in) across, with curved yellow spurs, are produced from mid-spring to early summer. ↕ 30cm (12in), ↔ 45cm (18in). W. China. ❄❄❄

E. diphyllum. Clump-forming, evergreen or semi-evergreen, rhizomatous perennial bearing leaves divided into 2

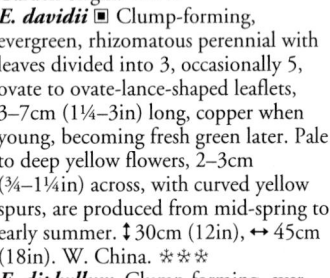

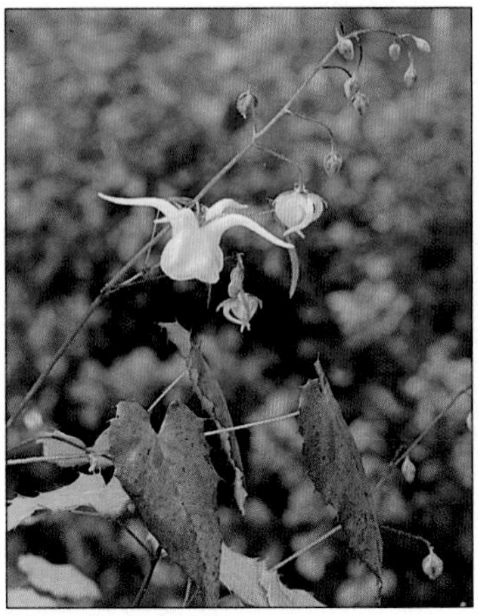
Epimedium davidii

broadly ovate to heart-shaped, light green leaflets, 2–5cm (¾–2in) long, with a few marginal spines. Bears spurless, pendent, bell-shaped, pure white flowers, 1cm (½in) across, in mid- and late spring. ↕ to 25cm (10in), ↔ 30cm (12in). Japan. ❄❄❄

E. grandiflorum 🏆 syn. *E. macranthum.* Clump-forming, deciduous, rhizomatous perennial bearing leaves 30cm (12in) long, with usually 9 ovate-heart-shaped, spiny-margined, light green leaflets, 3–6cm (1¼–2½in) long, flushed bronze when young. Pendent, white, yellow, pink, or purple flowers, 2.5–4.5cm (1–1¾in) across, with spurs 2.5cm (1in) long, are produced in mid- and late spring. ↕ 20–30cm (8–12in), ↔ 30cm (12in). China (S. Manchuria), N. Korea, Japan. ❄❄❄. **'Crimson Beauty'** ■ has copper markings on young leaves and copper-crimson flowers. **f. *flavescens*,** syn. *E. koreanum*, bears pale yellow flowers; Korea. **'Lilac Fairy'** see 'Lilafee'. **'Lilafee'** ■ syn. 'Lilac Fairy', has purple-tinted young leaves and violet-purple flowers; ↕ 20–25cm (8–10in). **'Nanum'** 🏆 has white flowers; ↕ 7cm (3in). **'Rose Queen'** 🏆 has dark bronze-purple young leaves and deep rose-pink flowers with long, white-tipped spurs. **f. *violaceum*,** syn. 'Violaceum', bears purple-and-white flowers. **'White Queen'** 🏆 produces large, pure white flowers, 4.5cm (1¾in) across.

E. koreanum see *E. grandiflorum* f. *flavescens.*

E. leptorrhizum. Slowly spreading, evergreen, rhizomatous perennial

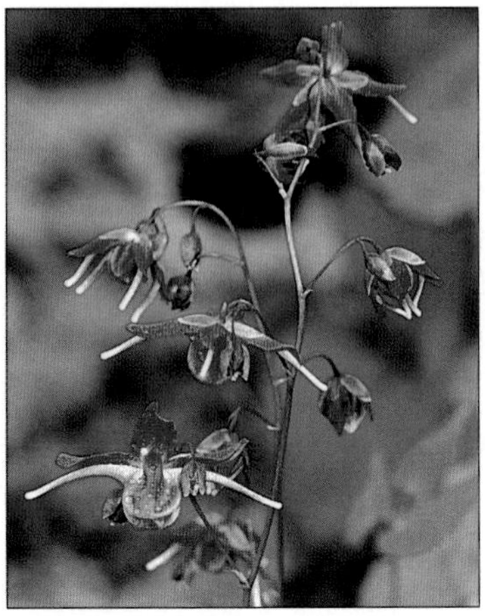
Epimedium grandiflorum 'Lilafee'

bearing 3-ternate, rarely simple, spiny-margined, red-stalked leaves with ovate-lance-shaped, conspicuously veined leaflets, 7–11cm (3–4½in) long, heart-shaped at the bases and with long, pointed tips. Young leaves are bronze-brown with red hairs beneath, especially along the veins, maturing to mid-green and remaining hairy only on the veins beneath. From mid-spring to early summer, produces white flowers, to 4cm (1½in) across, suffused lilac-pink, with spurs 2cm (¾in) long. ↕ 12–30cm (5–12in), ↔ 45cm (18in). China. ❄❄❄

E. macranthum see *E. grandiflorum.*

E.* x *perralchicum ■ 🏆 (*E. perralderianum* x *E. pinnatum* subsp. *colchicum*). Robust, clump-forming, evergreen, rhizomatous perennial with glossy, deep green leaves, bronze when young; each leaf is divided into 9, occasionally only 3, ovate, spiny-margined leaflets, 8cm (3in) long, often with overlapping lobes at the base. Pendent, bright yellow flowers, to 2cm (¾in) across, with very short brown spurs, are produced in mid- and late spring. ↕ 40cm (16in), ↔ 60cm (24in). Garden origin. ❄❄❄. **'Fröhnleiten'**

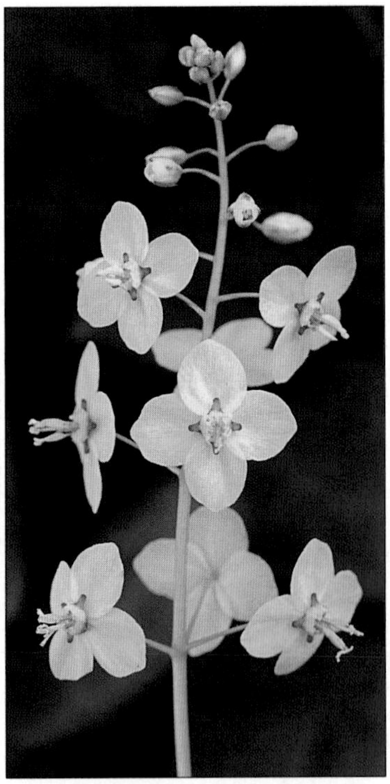
Epimedium pinnatum subsp. *colchicum*

produces elongated leaflets with more dense marginal spines, and flowers to 2.5cm (1in) across. **'Wisley'** has flowers to 2.5cm (1in) across; ↕60cm (24in).
E. perralderianum. Gently spreading, evergreen, rhizomatous perennial forming a bold, dense clump of leaves, each leaf divided into usually 3 ovate, conspicuously toothed leaflets, 5–8cm (2–3in) long, bronze when young, maturing to glossy, dark green. Bright yellow flowers, to 2cm (¾in) across, with short brown spurs, are produced in mid- and late spring. ↕30cm (12in), ↔60cm (24in). Algeria. ❄❄❄
E. pinnatum. Slowly spreading, evergreen, rhizomatous perennial bearing 2-ternate or sometimes pinnate leaves with ovate, spiny-margined, white- or red-hairy, later hairless, dark green leaflets, 5–10cm (2–4in) long. Produces bright yellow flowers, to 2cm (¾in) across, with brownish purple spurs, in late spring and early summer. ↕↔20–30cm (8–12in). N. Iran. ❄❄❄. **subsp. *colchicum*** ■ ♀ syn. subsp. *elegans*, is slow-growing, its shorter rhizomes making a denser clump. The leaves are divided into 5, more rounded, less spiny leaflets, 6–13cm (2½–5in) long. Flowers with brown or yellow spurs are borne in spring. ↕30–40cm (12–16in), ↔25cm (10in). Caucasus to N.E. Turkey.
E. pubigerum ■ Clump-forming, evergreen, rhizomatous perennial producing leaves with up to 9 ovate to rounded, spiny, glossy, mid-green leaflets, 4–8cm (1½–3in) long, heart-shaped at the bases, hairy beneath. Creamy white, sometimes yellowish white flowers, to 1cm (½in) across, are borne well above the foliage in mid- and late spring. ↕↔45cm (18in). Bulgaria, Turkey to W. Georgia. ❄❄❄
E. x rubrum ♀ (*E. alpinum* x *E. grandiflorum*). Slowly spreading, clump-forming, deciduous, rhizomatous perennial. Bears 2-ternate leaves with ovate, pointed, thin, spiny-toothed leaflets, 6–10cm (2½–4in) long, flushed red when young, turning red and reddish brown in autumn, and remaining through winter. Crimson and pale yellow flowers, to 2cm (¾in) across, with short spurs, are produced in mid- and late spring. ↕↔30cm (12in). Garden origin. ❄❄❄
***E. stellulatum* 'Wudang Star'.** Clump-forming, evergreen perennial with a short, creeping rhizome and 2-ternate leaves with ovate, spine-toothed, glossy, mid-green leaflets, 6–10cm (2½–4in) long. In spring, bears panicles of star-shaped white flowers, 1.5cm (½in) across, with prominent yellow stamens. ↕↔25–35cm (10–14in). ❄❄❄
E. sutchuenense. Clump-forming, evergreen, rhizomatous perennial with 3-ternate leaves comprised of narrowly ovate, mid-green leaflets, 5–8cm (2–3in) long, heart-shaped at the bases, pointed at the tips, and sparsely grey-hairy above. Long-spurred, rose-pink flowers, 2cm (¾in) across, sometimes purple-tinted, are borne in mid- and late spring. ↕↔30cm (12in). China. ❄❄❄
E. x versicolor (*E. grandiflorum* x *E. pinnatum* subsp. *colchicum*). Clump-forming, evergreen, rhizomatous perennial with leaves usually divided into 5–15 ovate-heart-shaped, spine-toothed leaflets, 5–9cm (2–3½in) long,

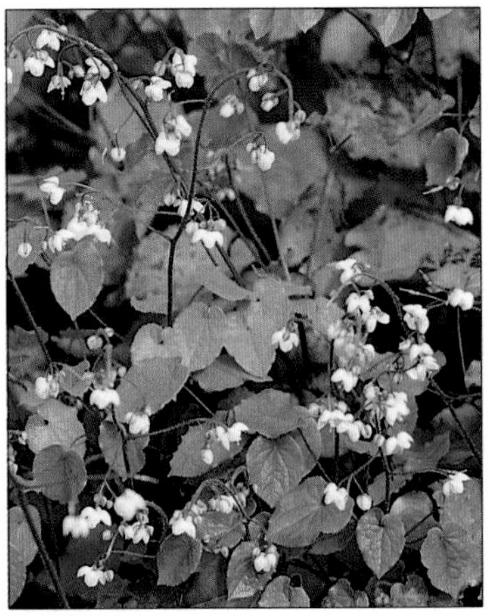
Epimedium pubigerum

copper-red and brown when young, turning mid-green. Bears pink and yellow flowers, 0.6–2cm (¼–¾in) across, with red-tinted spurs, in mid- and late spring. ↕↔30cm (12in). Garden origin. ❄❄❄. **'Cupreum'** has copper-red flowers. **'Neosulphureum'** has pale yellow flowers and 3–9 leaflets per leaf. **'Sulphureum'** ♀ has 5–11 leaflets per leaf, and bears slightly darker yellow flowers and longer spurs than 'Neosulphureum'; ↔1m (3ft).
var. *versicolor* ■ has small flowers, 6–10mm (¼–½in) across, with deep reddish pink sepals and yellow petals.
E. x warleyense ■ (*E. alpinum* x *E. pinnatum* subsp. *colchicum*). Spreading, clump-forming, evergreen, rhizomatous perennial with leaves divided into 5–9 ovate, sparsely spiny,

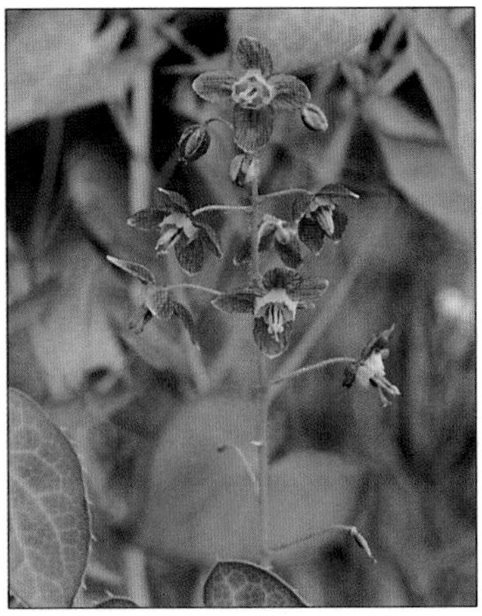
Epimedium x *warleyense*

mid-green leaflets, 7–12cm (3–5in) long, hairy beneath, and tinted red in spring and autumn. Produces yellow flowers, 1.5cm (½in) across, with reddish orange sepals, in mid- and late spring. ↕to 50cm (20in), ↔75cm (30in). Garden origin. ❄❄❄.
'Orangekönigin' makes a denser clump and has slightly paler orange sepals.
E. x youngianum (*E. diphyllum* x *E. grandiflorum*). Clump-forming, deciduous, rhizomatous perennial with leaves divided into 2–9 leaflets, 2–8cm (¾–3in) long, on red-tinted leaf-stalks; leaflets are narrowly ovate, mid-green, thin, wavy-margined, almost spineless, hairy, becoming hairless beneath, with one leaflet distinctly larger. In mid- and late spring, produces greenish white or pale rose-pink flowers, 1.5–2cm

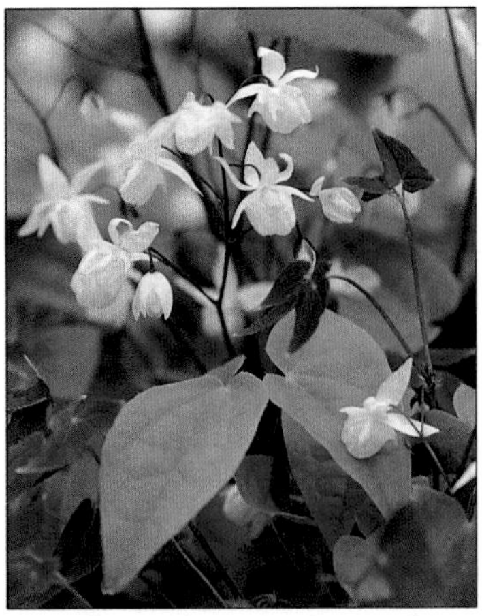
Epimedium x *youngianum* 'Niveum'

(½–¾in) long, sometimes with spurs. ↕20–30cm (8–12in), ↔30cm (12in). Garden origin. ❄❄❄. **'Lilacinum'** see 'Roseum'. **'Merlin'** has purple-flushed young leaves, and bears spurred, dusky mauve flowers, 2cm (¾in) across.
'Niveum' ■ ♀ bears pure white flowers, to 1cm (½in) across, sometimes spurred, and often produces very colourful young foliage. **'Roseum'**, syn. 'Lilacinum', has variable foliage and dusky pink to purple flowers.

EPIPACTIS

Helleborine

ORCHIDACEAE

Genus of 24 species of rhizomatous, terrestrial, herbaceous orchids, mainly found in temperate areas of the N. hemisphere, often occurring in marshes, alpine meadows, rich woodland, or on dunes; a few are tropical species from Africa, Thailand, and Mexico. They usually have ribbed, lance-shaped to ovate leaves, arranged spirally or in 2 ranks. The spurless flowers are borne in loose or dense spikes on twisted stalks. The upper segments of each flower spread or curve inwards to form a "helmet", and the 2-parted lower lip unites at the base to form a "cup", with a heart-shaped or triangular lobe beneath. Grow in a damp, shady border, or in a wild or woodland garden.

- **HARDINESS** Fully hardy.
- **CULTIVATION** Grow in fertile, humus-rich, moist but well-drained soil in partial or deep shade. May spread freely in ideal conditions. See also p.46.
- **PROPAGATION** Divide in early spring, ensuring that each piece of rhizome has at least one growing point.
- **PESTS AND DISEASES** Vulnerable to slugs and snails.

E. gigantea (Giant helleborine). Rhizomatous orchid with upright stems bearing lance-shaped to ovate leaves, to 20cm (8in) long. From spring to early summer, produces loose, terminal spikes of up to 15 nodding, bright greenish yellow flowers, to 2cm (¾in) across, each with a leafy bract beneath; the lips and upper lobes are veined maroon, the widely spreading, yellow lateral lobes are veined brownish purple. ↕30–40cm (12–16in), ↔to 1.5m (5ft). S.W. USA. ❄❄❄

▷ ***Epiphyllanthus obovatus*** see *Schlumbergera opuntioides*

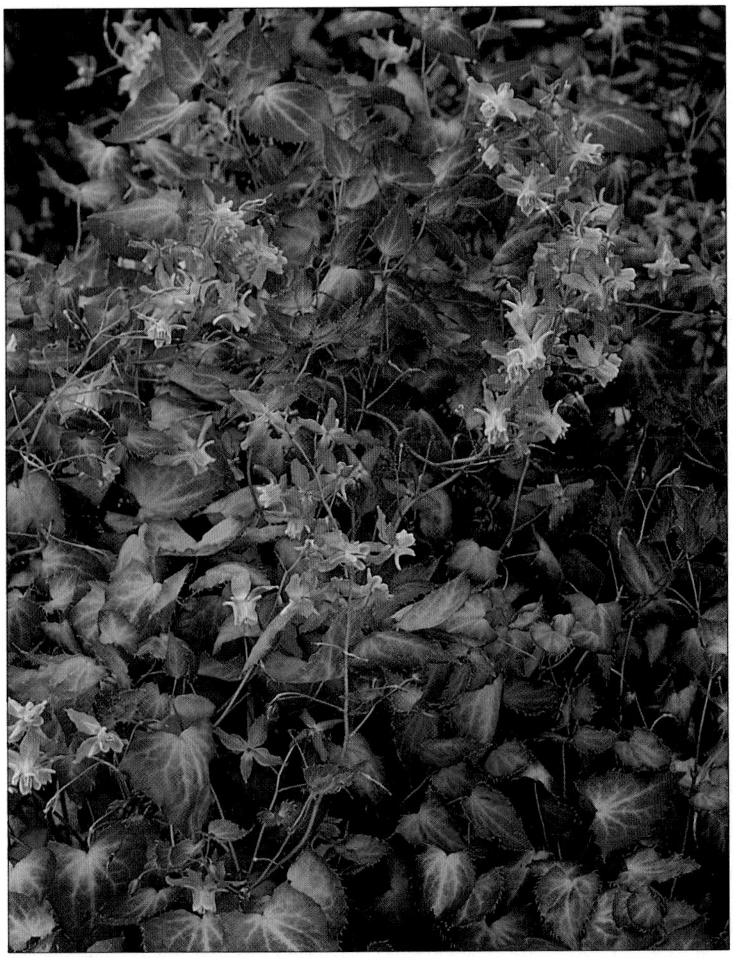
Epimedium x *versicolor* var. *versicolor*

E

E

EPIPHYLLUM

Orchid cactus

CACTACEAE

Genus of about 20 species of mostly epiphytic, perennial cacti occurring mainly in rainforest from S. Mexico to Argentina, and also in the West Indies. The strap-shaped, cylindrical, flattened, often deeply toothed, fleshy green stems and branches become 2-ribbed when mature, and bear small, usually spineless areoles. The mainly funnel-shaped flowers, 8–30cm (3–12in) long, are often sweetly scented and last for 2 or more days; many are nocturnal. In areas where temperatures drop below 10°C (50°F), grow as houseplants or in a warm greenhouse. In warmer climates, plant in a shaded courtyard.

- **HARDINESS** Frost tender. They require a minimum temperature of 10°C (50°F) for most of the year but, for successful cultivation, the temperature should be increased to 15°C (59°F) in early spring.
- **CULTIVATION** Under glass, grow in epiphytic cactus compost in bright filtered light, with moderate to high humidity. From mid-spring to late summer, water freely and apply a high-potash fertilizer every 2 weeks as flower buds form; keep just moist in winter. Outdoors, grow in fertile, sharply drained soil in light dappled or partial shade. See also pp.48–49.
- **PROPAGATION** Sow seed at 21°C (70°F) in spring or early summer. Take stem cuttings in early summer.
- **PESTS AND DISEASES** Vulnerable to mealybugs and aphids.

E. ackermannii see *Nopalxochia ackermannii.*

E. anguliger. Erect, bushy, many-branched, epiphytic cactus with partly cylindrical, partly flattened, deeply toothed, mid-green stems, 4–8cm (1½–3in) wide. From late spring to summer, produces diurnal, funnel-shaped, scented flowers, 15cm (6in) long, with narrow, wide-spreading, golden or lemon-yellow outer tepals and white inner tepals. ↕ to 75cm (30in). ↔ 45cm (18in). S. Mexico. ❄ (min. 10–15°C/50–59°F)

E. chrysocardium, syn. *Marniera chrysocardium, Selenicereus chrysocardium.* Erect then semi-pendent, or scandent, epiphytic cactus with very deeply toothed, flattened, mid-green stems, to 30cm (12in) wide, forming lobes 3–4cm (1¼–1½in) wide, the areoles sometimes with 2 or 3 bristles each. In late winter or spring, produces nocturnal, funnel-shaped flowers, 30cm (12in) or more long, that have dull purple outer tepals, white inner tepals, tubes that are pale green below, dull purple above, and golden yellow stamens. ↕ to 2m (6ft), ↔ 75cm (30in). S. Mexico. ❄ (min. 10–15°C/50–59°F)

E. crenatum ▣ Erect, bushy, semi-epiphytic cactus with a cylindrical main stem and leaf-like, greyish green branches, 12cm (5in) wide, the margins wavy and toothed. Diurnal, funnel-shaped, fragrant, creamy white flowers, 20cm (8in) long, with green, pink, or pale yellow outer segments, are produced in summer. ↕↔ to 3m (10ft). S. Mexico to Honduras. ❄ (min. 10–15°C/50–59°F)

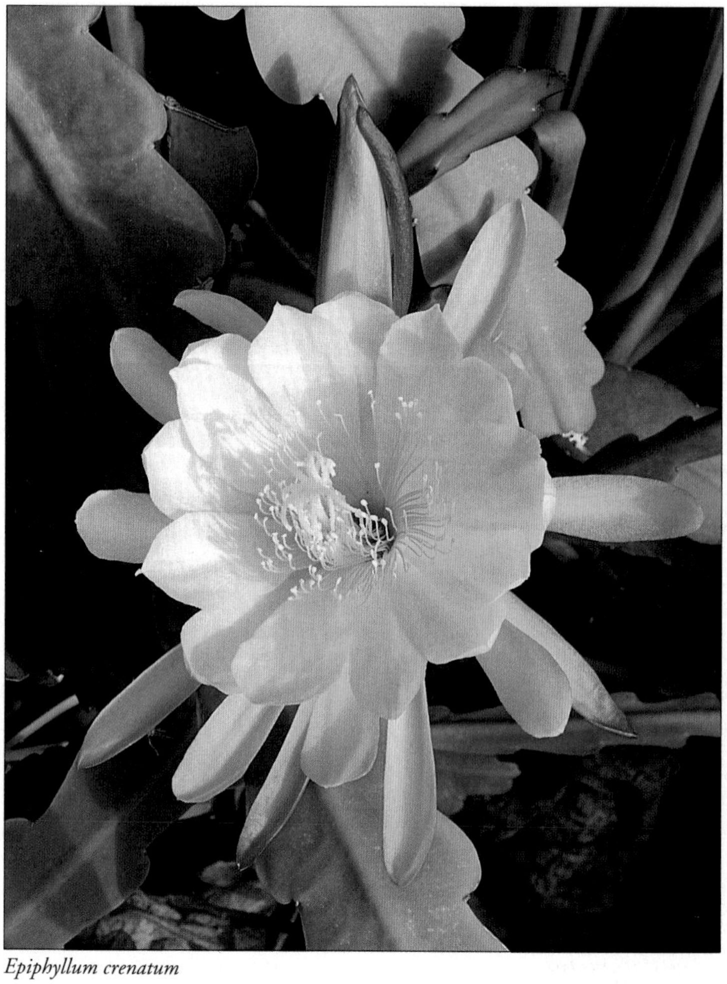

Epiphyllum crenatum

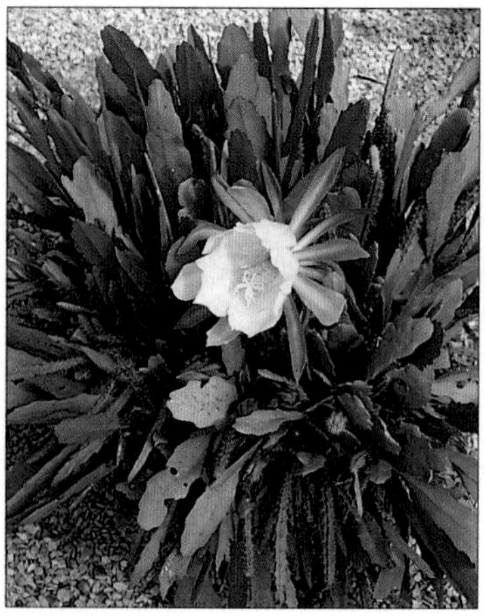

Epiphyllum laui

E. hookeri, syn. *E. strictum.* Erect, bushy, scandent, epiphytic cactus with flattened, coarsely toothed, bluish green stems, 8cm (3in) wide. Nocturnal, star-shaped, creamy or yellowish white flowers, to 25cm (10in) long, with red-tinged, pale green outer segments, are produced in midsummer. Resembles *E. phyllanthus* but has broader flowers. ↕ 2m (6ft), ↔ 50cm (20in). S. Mexico to Costa Rica, Trinidad. ❄ (min. 10–15°C/50–59°F)

E. laui ▣ Erect, bushy, epiphytic cactus with flattened, often red-tinged, glossy, mid-green stems, 10cm (4in) wide, sometimes 4-angled or cylindrical, with slightly toothed margins. Bears diurnal or nocturnal, funnel-shaped, scented white flowers, 18cm (7in) long, with brown outer segments, in early summer. ↕ 30cm (12in), ↔ to 50cm (20in). S. Mexico. ❄ (min. 10–15°C/50–59°F)

E. macdougallii see *Nopalxochia macdougallii.*

E. oxypetalum. Erect or semi-erect, many-branched, epiphytic cactus with cylindrical, mid-green stems and thin, leaf-like, elliptic, sharp-pointed, scalloped branches, 12cm (5in) wide. Nocturnal, funnel-shaped white flowers, 25–30cm (10–12in) long, with long, curved, arching tubes and very pale purplish white outer segments, are produced from late spring to summer. ↕ 3m (10ft), ↔ 1m (3ft). Mexico, Guatemala, Venezuela, Brazil. ❄ (min. 10–15°C/50–59°F)

E. phyllanthus. Semi-erect, bushy, semi-epiphytic cactus with cylindrical stems and leaf-like, linear, blunt or pointed, stiff, scalloped, mid-green branches, 7cm (3in) wide, with prominent midribs and purple-shaded margins. In summer, bears nocturnal, funnel-shaped, glistening white or pale yellowish white flowers, 25–30cm (10–12in) long, with green- or red-tinged outer tepals and slender green tubes. ↕ 2m (6ft), ↔ 60cm (24in). Panama, Colombia, Ecuador, Peru, Brazil. ❄ (min. 10–15°C/50–59°F)

E. pumilum. Semi-erect or pendent, epiphytic cactus with long, leaf-like, mid-green stems, 3–8cm (1¼–3in) wide, often tapering to a point. In summer, produces nocturnal, funnel-shaped, scented, creamy white flowers, 8–12cm (3–5in) long, with red outer tepals, white inner tepals, and green tubes. ↕↔ 50cm (20in) or more. Guatemala. ❄ (min. 10–15°C/50–59°F)

E. strictum see *E. hookeri.*

EPIPREMNUM

ARACEAE

Genus of 8 species of evergreen, root-clinging climbers, with juvenile and adult phases, found in forest from S.E. Asia to the W. Pacific. They are grown for their attractive, alternate leaves, which may be entire to pinnate, sometimes on the same plant. Spikes of tiny, petalless flowers are enclosed in spathes. In frost-prone areas, grow in a temperate or warm greenhouse, or as houseplants. In warmer areas, grow against a wall, over a pergola, or through trees. All parts may cause severe discomfort if ingested, and contact with the sap of *E. aureum* may irritate skin.

- **HARDINESS** Frost tender.
- **CULTIVATION** Under glass, grow in loam-based potting compost (JI No.3) in full or bright filtered light. During the growing season, water freely and apply a balanced liquid fertilizer every month; water moderately in winter. Provide the support of a moss pole. Outdoors, grow in fertile, moist but well-drained soil in full sun or partial shade. Pruning group 11, in early spring. Tip-prune in spring to promote branching.
- **PROPAGATION** Root leaf-bud or stem-tip cuttings with bottom heat in summer. Layer in spring or summer.
- **PESTS AND DISEASES** Scale insects and red spider mites may be troublesome under glass.

E. aureum, syn. *Scindapsus aureus* (Devil's ivy, Golden pothos). Strong-growing climber that, when young, has ovate, entire, glossy, bright green leaves, 10–30cm (4–12in) long, heart-shaped at the bases, and dashed or striped white, cream, or yellow. Mature plants have deeply lobed leaves, to 80cm (32in) long, and bear green flowering spathes, 15cm (6in) long, in summer. ↕ 8–12m (25–40ft). Solomon Islands. ❄ (min. 15°C/59°F). **'Exotica'** has lance-shaped, matt, dark green leaves, to 20cm (8in) long, slanted at the bases, and mottled with silver. **'Marble Queen'** ▣ has mainly white leaves, heavily flecked and splashed with yellow, cream, and green; ↕ 1–3m (3–10ft).

***E. pictum* 'Argyraeum'** ▣ syn. *Scindapsus pictus* 'Argyraeus'. Slow-growing climber cultivated in its juvenile phase, when it has ovate, entire leaves, 7–10cm (3–4in) long, heart-

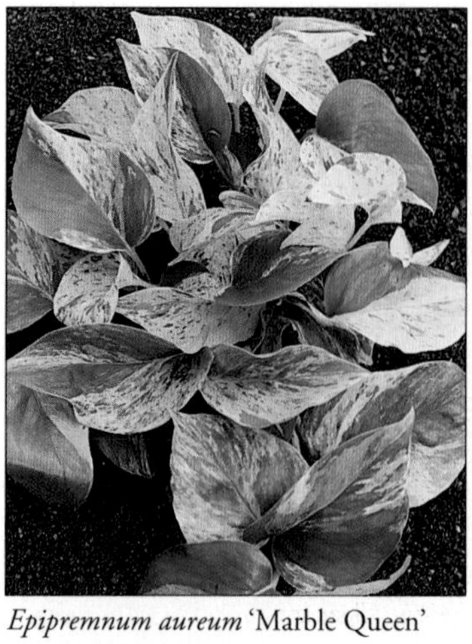

Epipremnum aureum 'Marble Queen'

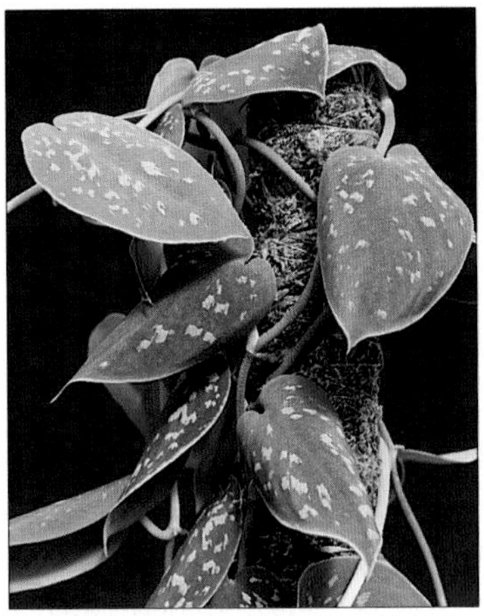

Epipremnum pictum 'Argyraeum'

shaped at the bases, satin-textured and deep green above, with irregular silver spots, paler and unspotted beneath. ↕45–90cm (18–36in) if trained on a support, 1–2m (3–6ft) or more if grown against a wall or through a tree. ❄ (min. 15°C/59°F)

EPISCIA syn. ALSOBIA

Carpet plant, Flame violet

GESNERIACEAE

Genus of 6 species of creeping, stoloniferous, mat-forming, epiphytic or terrestrial, evergreen perennials found in tropical forest and rocky habitats from Mexico to South America. They are grown for their soft, colourful foliage and salverform, 5-lobed flowers, which are borne singly or in small racemes from the leaf axils, from spring to autumn. Opposite, oblong to oblong-elliptic, hairy, often puckered leaves are produced in rosettes or whorls. In frost-prone areas, grow as houseplants, in a conservatory or terrarium, or in hanging baskets; elsewhere, use as ground cover.
- **HARDINESS** Frost tender.
- **CULTIVATION** Under glass, grow in loamless potting compost with added perlite or vermiculite, in bright filtered light, with high humidity. In growth, water moderately, applying a quarter-strength, balanced liquid fertilizer at each watering. Keep just moist in winter. Outdoors, grow in fertile, humus-rich, moist but sharply drained soil in partial shade.
- **PROPAGATION** Surface-sow seed at about 20–25°C (68–77°F) as soon as ripe or in early spring. Divide, separate plantlets, or root stem cuttings with bottom heat, in early or midsummer.
- **PESTS AND DISEASES** Aphids may infest young growing tips.

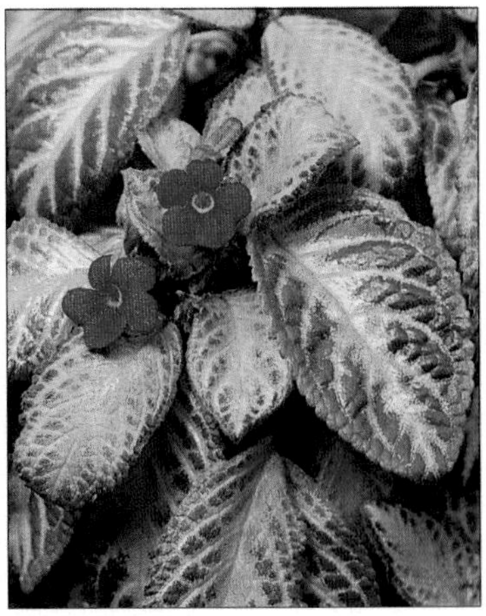

Episcia cupreata

***E.* 'Cleopatra'** ■ Mat-forming, terrestrial perennial with reddish green stolons and ovate, light green leaves, to 10cm (4in) long, suffused and marked creamy white, and with down-turned, broad pink margins. Axillary racemes of 3–5 orange-red flowers, to 5cm (2in) long, are produced from spring to autumn. ↕18cm (7in), ↔40cm (16in). ❄ (min. 15°C/59°F)

E. cupreata ■ Variable, mat-forming, terrestrial perennial with elliptic, toothed, deep copper-green leaves, to 9cm (3½in) long, purple beneath. Red and yellow flowers, to 6cm (2½in) long, sometimes spotted purple in the throats, are borne in axillary racemes of 3 or 4 from spring to autumn. ↕15cm (6in), ↔ indefinite. Colombia, Venezuela, Brazil. ❄ (min. 15°C/59°F). **'Acajou'** has dark tan leaves netted with silvery green, and freely produces orange-red flowers. **'Metallica'** has copper leaves, each with a central silver band and metallic-pink margins, and produces flame-red flowers. **'Tropical Topaz'** produces pale green leaves and bright yellow flowers.

***E.* 'Cygnet'**, syn. *Alsobia* 'Cygnet'. Vigorous, trailing, terrestrial perennial with elliptic to ovate, velvety, light green leaves, 10cm (4in) long. Purple-spotted white flowers, 2cm (¾in) across, are produced in twos in the leaf axils from spring to summer. ↕15cm (6in), ↔30cm (12in). ❄ (min. 13°C/55°F)

E. dianthiflora ■ syn. *Alsobia dianthiflora*. Creeping, terrestrial perennial bearing elliptic to ovate, toothed, dark green leaves, to 4cm (1½in) long, often veined purple-red. Solitary white flowers, to 3cm (1¼in) across, with purple spots at the bases and very deeply and finely fringed lobes, are produced from spring to summer. ↕15cm (6in), ↔30cm (12in). Mexico, Costa Rica. ❄ (min. 13°C/55°F)

E. lilacina. Variable, mat-forming, epiphytic or terrestrial perennial bearing ovate, scalloped, copper-green leaves, 5cm (2in) long, with fresh green midribs and veins, and purple undersides. White flowers, to 4.5cm (1¾in) long, with lavender-blue throats, are produced in axillary racemes of up to 4 from spring to autumn. ↕15cm (6in), ↔40cm (16in). Costa Rica. ❄ (min. 15°C/59°F). **'Cuprea'** has deep copper leaves, with narrow silver markings around the midribs, and white-centred, lavender-blue flowers.

***E.* 'Pink Panther'.** Mat-forming, terrestrial perennial with ovate, lime-green leaves, to 12cm (5in) long. Axillary racemes of 3–5 rose-pink flowers, to 6cm (2½in) long, are produced from spring to autumn. ↕18cm (7in), ↔45cm (18in). ❄ (min. 15°C/59°F)

***E.* 'Silver Skies'.** Mat-forming, terrestrial perennial bearing ovate leaves, to 3cm (1¼in) long, with silvery green centres and broad, mid-green margins. Axillary racemes of 3–5 red flowers, 5cm (2in) long, are produced from spring to autumn. ↕18cm (7in), ↔35cm (14in). ❄ (min. 15°C/59°F)

EPITHELANTHA

CACTACEAE

Genus of one very variable species of perennial cactus occurring in S. USA and Mexico, mainly on calcareous soils. The stems are thickly covered with rows of small tubercles, usually spirally arranged. Small, tufted areoles bear numerous white spines; the areoles at the apexes elongate slightly when producing the small, funnel-shaped, white or pale orange to pink flowers. In frost-prone areas, grow in a warm greenhouse; in warm, dry climates, grow in a desert garden or on a raised bed.
- **HARDINESS** Frost tender.
- **CULTIVATION** Under glass, grow in standard cactus compost, with added limestone chippings, in full light. From spring to autumn, water moderately and apply low-nitrogen fertilizer every 4–5 weeks; keep completely dry at other times. Outdoors, grow in poor to moderately fertile, sharply drained soil in full sun. See also pp.48–49.
- **PROPAGATION** Sow seed at 21°C (70°F) in early spring, or graft on to species of *Cereus*.
- **PESTS AND DISEASES** Vulnerable to root mealybugs under glass.

E. micromeris ■ Solitary or clump-forming, spherical to obovoid, greyish green cactus with diurnal, funnel-shaped, white or pale orange to pink flowers, 1cm (½in) across, borne in groups of 2 or 3 or more in summer. ↕4cm (1½in), ↔4–8cm (1½–3in). S. USA, Mexico. ❄ (min. 10°C/50°F)

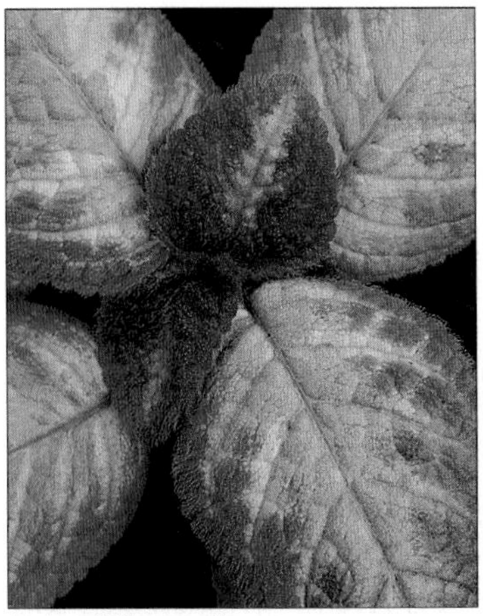

Episcia 'Cleopatra'

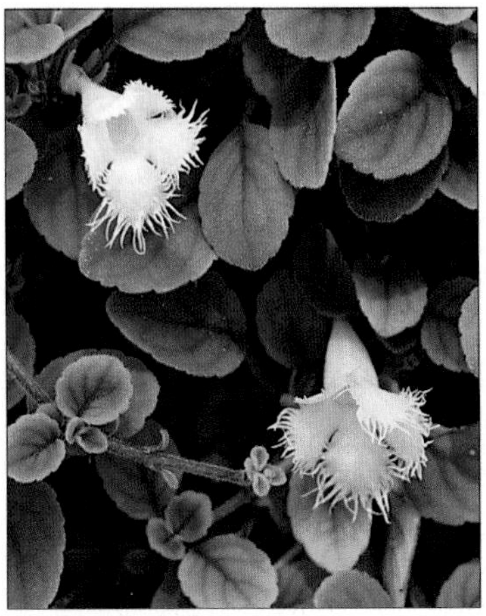

Episcia dianthiflora

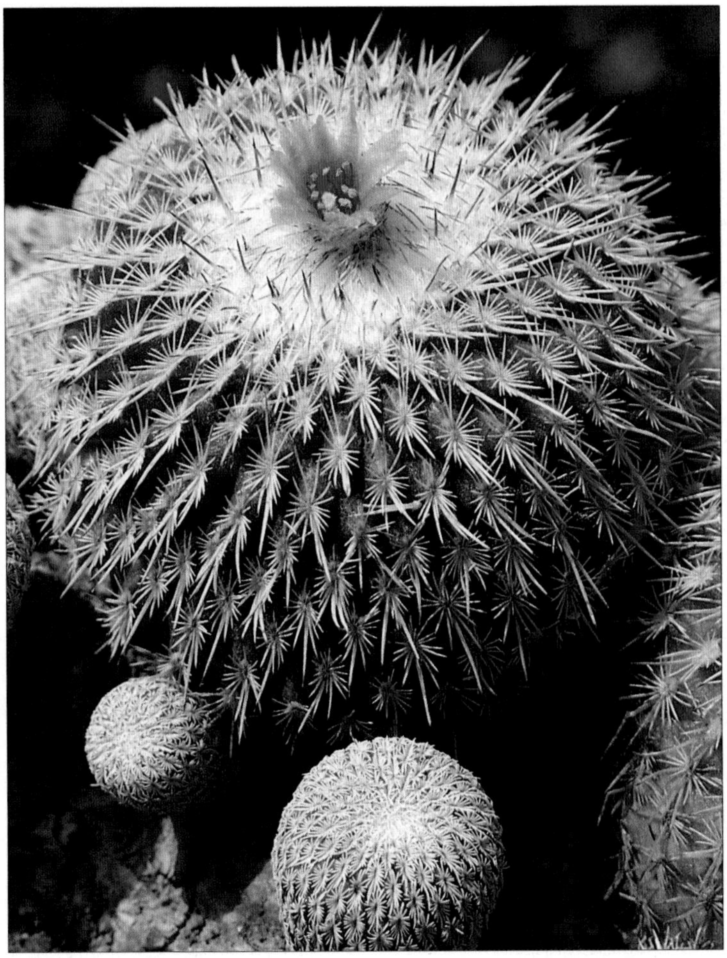

Epithelantha micromeris

E

Eragrostis

Love grass

GRAMINEAE/POACEAE

Genus of approximately 250 species of clump-forming, annual and perennial grasses widely distributed throughout tropical and temperate regions of the world. They occur on cultivated or disturbed ground, often on sandy soils. The narrowly linear leaves are flat or rolled. Dense or open, sparsely to many-branched panicles of small, flattened, closely overlapping spikelets are borne on slender, upright stems from summer to autumn. Grow as specimen plants, in a mixed or herbaceous border, or in a rock garden. In frost-prone climates, grow half-hardy species in a cool greenhouse. The inflorescences are useful for cut flower arrangements.

• **Hardiness** Fully hardy to half hardy. *E. curvula* is frost hardy but will tolerate brief spells down to -10°C (14°F).

• **Cultivation** Grow in medium to light, poor to moderately fertile, well-drained soil in a warm, sunny site. In late winter or early spring, before new growth begins, cut back any stems and foliage left for winter interest.

• **Propagation** Sow seed in containers in a cold frame in spring, or divide between mid-spring and early summer.

• **Pests and diseases** Trouble free.

E. curvula. Densely tufted, mound-forming, perennial grass with arching, narrowly linear, rolled or slightly open, rough-textured, dark green leaves, to 30cm (12in) long. In late summer and early autumn, bears erect or nodding, open panicles, to 30cm (12in) long, consisting of closely overlapping, 3- to 18-flowered, dark olive-grey spikelets, to 1.5cm (½in) long, which persist through winter. ↕↔ 1.2m (4ft). Southern Africa, India. ❄❄

Eranthemum

ACANTHACEAE

Genus of approximately 30 species of woody-based perennials and evergreen shrubs occurring in forest and scrub in tropical Asia. They are cultivated for their tubular, 5-lobed flowers, which are produced in terminal or axillary spikes or panicles in winter. The leaves are opposite, lance-shaped to broadly ovate, simple, entire or toothed, and often prominently veined. In frost-prone regions, grow in a warm greenhouse or conservatory, or as houseplants. In humid, subtropical climates, they may be grown outdoors and are particularly useful in a lightly shaded border.

• **Hardiness** Frost tender.

• **Cultivation** Under glass, grow in loam-based potting compost (JI No.3) in bright filtered light. From spring to autumn, water moderately and apply a balanced liquid fertilizer every month; water sparingly in winter. Top-dress or pot on in spring. Outdoors, grow in fertile, moist but well-drained soil in full sun. Pruning group 8; may need restrictive pruning under glass.

• **Propagation** Root softwood cuttings with bottom heat in late spring or early summer.

• **Pests and diseases** Whiteflies may be troublesome under glass.

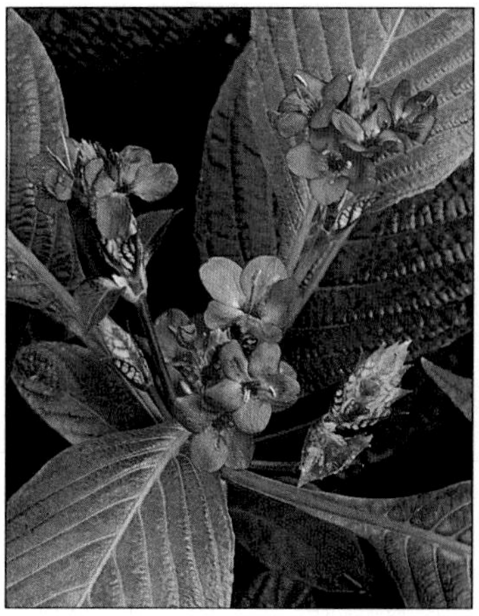

Eranthemum pulchellum

E. atropurpureum see *Pseuderanthemum atropurpureum.*

E. nervosum see *E. pulchellum.*

E. pulchellum ■ syn. *E. nervosum* (Blue sage). Open shrub with elliptic, slender-pointed, occasionally toothed, boldly veined, lustrous, deep green leaves, 10–20cm (4–8in) long. In winter, rich blue flowers, 3cm (1¼in) long, are produced in spikes to 8cm (3in) long, or sometimes clustered into panicles. ↕90–120cm (3–4ft), ↔ 60–90cm (24–36in). India. ❀ (min. 13°C/55°F)

Eranthis

Winter aconite

RANUNCULACEAE

Genus of about 7 species of small, clump-forming perennials with knobbly tubers, occurring in damp woodland and shady places in Eurasia. They are grown for their cup-shaped flowers, borne in late winter and early spring. Stem leaves 0.5–1.5cm (¼–½in) or more long, often finely dissected, form ruffs immediately below the flowers; basal leaves, 1.5–3cm (½–1¼in) or more long, are palmately lobed or pinnate. Most species are best grown around deciduous shrubs or trees where they will form carpets of flowers and may naturalize in grass; *E. pinnatifida* is best grown in an alpine house or sheltered peat bed. All parts may cause mild stomach upset if ingested, and contact with the sap may irritate skin.

• **Hardiness** Fully hardy to frost hardy.

• **Cultivation** Grow in fertile, humus-rich soil that does not dry out in summer, in full sun or light dappled shade. Plant tubers 5cm (2in) deep in autumn. Overdried tubers may be difficult to establish.

• **Propagation** Sow seed in containers in a cold frame in late spring. Separate tubers in spring after flowering.

• **Pests and diseases** Prone to smuts. Slugs may eat the foliage.

E. cilicica. Clump-forming, tuberous perennial with bright yellow flowers, 2–4cm (¾–1½in) across, produced above ruffs of finely dissected, glossy, bronze-tinged, mid-green leaves in early spring. Similar to *E. hyemalis* but with more numerous leaf lobes and slightly larger flowers. ↕5–8cm (2–3in), ↔ 5cm (2in). Turkey to Afghanistan. ❄❄❄

E. hyemalis ■ ♀ (Winter aconite). Clump-forming, tuberous perennial producing bright yellow flowers, 2–3cm

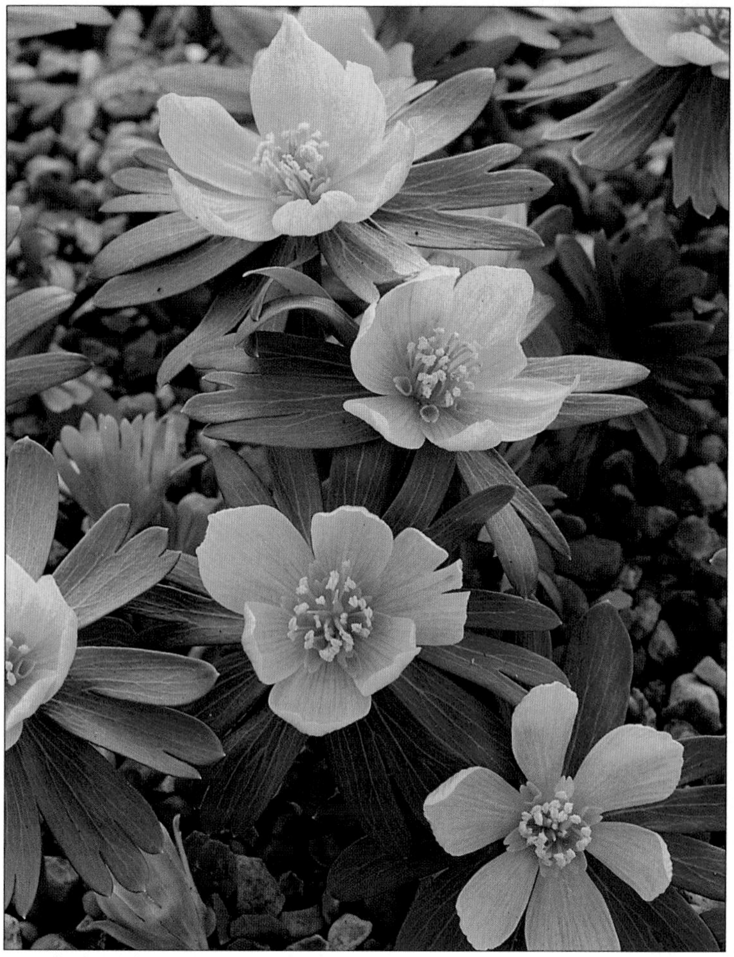

Eranthis hyemalis

(¾–1¼in) across, each above a ruff of dissected, bright green leaves, in late winter and early spring. Quickly forms large colonies, particularly in alkaline soils. ↕5–8cm (2–3in), ↔ 5cm (2in). S. France to Bulgaria. ❄❄❄

E. keiskei see *E. pinnatifida.*

E. pinnatifida, syn. *E. keiskei.* Clump-forming, tuberous perennial bearing white flowers, 2cm (¾in) across, above ruffs of pinnate leaves, in early spring. ↕↔ 5cm (2in). Japan. ❄❄❄

***E. x tubergenii* 'Guinea Gold'** ♀ (*E. cilicica* x *E. hyemalis*). Vigorous, clump-forming, sterile, tuberous perennial with golden flowers, 2–3cm (¾–1¼in) across, each above a ruff of dissected, bronze-green leaves, in late winter. ↕8–10cm (3–4in), ↔ 5cm (2in). ❄❄❄

Ercilla

PHYTOLACCACEAE

Genus of 2 species of root-clinging, climbing, evergreen perennials from temperate North and South America, growing wild in open woodland and forest margins. The alternate leaves are simple, ovate-heart-shaped to oblong, and leathery. Small, petalless flowers are produced in short, axillary spikes. *Ercilla* species provide excellent ground cover if allowed to spread; otherwise grow on a shady wall, or through trees.

• **Hardiness** Frost hardy; *E. volubilis* may tolerate temperatures to -10°C (14°F) if wood is well-ripened.

• **Cultivation** Grow in fertile, moist but well-drained soil in full sun or partial shade, with protection from cold, drying winds. Pruning group 11, after flowering. Tie in to a support until the adhesive roots become established and can support the mature plant.

• **Propagation** Root semi-ripe cuttings in summer, with bottom heat. Layer in early spring.

• **Pests and diseases** Scale insects may be troublesome under glass.

E. spicata see *E. volubilis.*

E. volubilis, syn. *Bridgesia spicata, E. spicata.* Vigorous, freely branching climber with ovate-heart-shaped to oblong, lustrous, deep green leaves, 4–5cm (1½–2in) long, with a pattern of pale veins. Mature plants produce an abundance of green or purple flower spikes, to 4.5cm (1¾in) long, mainly in spring, sometimes followed by deep purple berries. ↕6–10m (20–30ft). Peru, Chile. ❄❄

▷ ***Erdisia*** see *Corryocactus*
E. erecta see *C. erectus*
E. squarrosa see *C. squarrosus*

Eremophila

Emu bush

MYOPORACEAE

Genus of about 180 species of evergreen perennials, shrubs, and trees occurring on open slopes and in scrub and light woodland in Australia. They are grown for their tubular-based, 2-lipped flowers, produced singly from the uppermost leaf axils, giving the appearance of leafy racemes in some species. Leaves are simple, entire, and linear to rounded, and may be alternate or opposite, or occasionally whorled. In frost-prone areas, grow in a temperate or cool greenhouse. In warmer, drier areas, plant in a courtyard garden, in a border, or at the base of a warm, sunny wall.

• **HARDINESS** Half hardy to frost tender. *E. glabra* and *E. maculata* may survive short periods at about 0°C (32°F) if they are kept fairly dry.

• **CULTIVATION** Under glass, grow in loam-based potting compost (JI No.3) in full light. When in growth, water freely and apply a balanced liquid fertilizer monthly. At other times, water sparingly. Top-dress or pot on in spring. Outdoors, grow in moderately fertile, sharply drained soil in full sun. Pruning group 8; may need restrictive pruning under glass.

• **PROPAGATION** Sow seed at 13–16°C (55–61°F) in spring, first soaking for several days; germination may take 2 weeks to 2 years or more. Root semi-ripe cuttings in a shaded cold frame in summer.

• **PESTS AND DISEASES** Scale insects may be a problem under glass.

E. alternifolia. Rounded shrub with alternate, very narrow, cylindrical, recurved, mid-green leaves, to 3.5cm (1½in) long. Solitary pink flowers, 3–4cm (1¼–1½in) long, with darker spots, are produced on slender stalks from spring to summer. ↕↔ 3m (10ft). Australia (except Tasmania). ❄
E. glabra (Common emu bush, Fuchsia bush). Prostrate, or erect to spreading shrub with alternate, elliptic to narrowly lance-shaped, densely hairy or hairless, mid-green leaves, 2–5cm (¾–2in) long. Solitary, red, orange, yellow, or green flowers, 3cm (1¼in) long, are borne mainly from early spring to autumn. ↕ to 1.5m (5ft), ↔ 1–3m (3–10ft). Australia (except Tasmania). ❄ (borderline).
'Murchison River' has silvery foliage and bright red flowers.
E. maculata (Spotted emu bush). Dense shrub with alternate, linear-lance-shaped to ovate-lance-shaped, mid- to grey-green leaves, to 5cm (2in) long, which are hairless when mature. Solitary, red to purple, pink, or almost white flowers, 2–3.5cm (¾–1½in) long, often spotted with cream or yellow, are produced from winter to late spring or early summer. ↕ 0.5–2.5m (1¾–8ft), ↔ 1–2m (3–6ft). Australia (except Tasmania). ❄ (borderline). **'Aurea'** ■ has light to mid-green leaves, and produces yellow flowers.

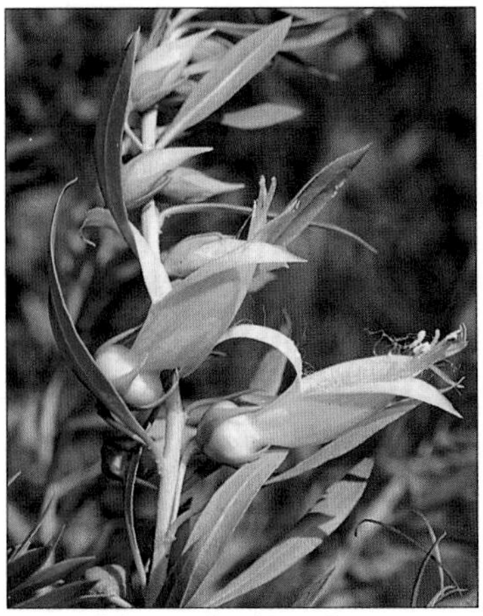
Eremophila maculata 'Aurea'

EREMURUS

Desert candle, Foxtail lily

ASPHODELACEAE/LILIACEAE

Genus of about 40–50 species of clump-forming, fleshy-rooted perennials found in dry grassland and semi-desert in W. and C. Asia. Leafless flowering stems, usually one per crown, each produce a dense raceme of star-shaped, usually pink, white, or yellow flowers, with conspicuous stamens. Tufted rosettes of folded, linear to lance-shaped, basal leaves die back to the conical crown after flowering. Grow in a border; need winter cold to induce flowering.

• **HARDINESS** Fully hardy, although young growth is frost tender.

• **CULTIVATION** Grow in fertile, sandy, well-drained loam in full sun, with shelter from wind. Mulch with garden compost in autumn, avoiding the crown. Protect young growth with a dry mulch. Provide support in exposed sites.

• **PROPAGATION** Sow seed in containers in a cold frame in autumn, or at 15°C (59°F) in late winter. Divide after flowering.

• **PESTS AND DISEASES** Susceptible to slug damage.

E. aitchisonii. Tufted perennial with narrowly lance-shaped, rough-margined, glossy, grass-green leaves, 30–60cm (12–24in) long. Pale pink flowers, to 3cm (1¼in) across, are borne in racemes 30cm (12in) long in early summer. ↕ 1–2m (3–6ft), ↔ 1m (3ft). Tajikistan, Afghanistan. ❄❄❄
E. aurantiacus see *E. stenophyllus* subsp. *aurantiacus.*
E. bungei see *E. stenophyllus* subsp. *stenophyllus.*
E. himalaicus ■ Tufted perennial with strap-shaped, bright green leaves, 30cm (12in) long. Bears white flowers, 2.5cm (1in) across, in racemes to 90cm (36in) long in late spring and early summer. ↕ 1.2–2m (4–6ft), ↔ 60cm (24in). Kashmir, N.W. Himalayas. ❄❄❄

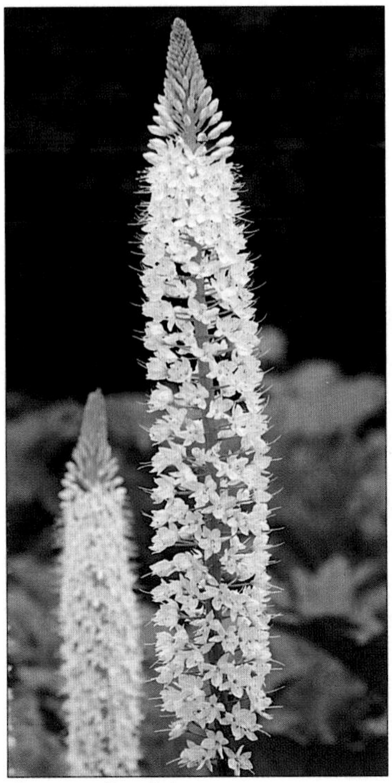
Eremurus himalaicus

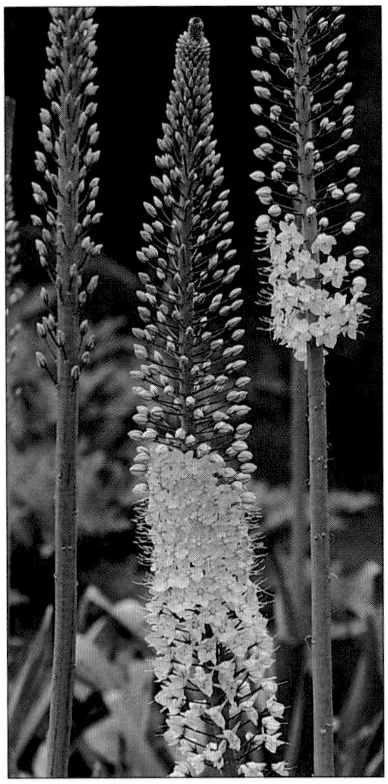
Eremurus robustus

E. 'Himrob'. Tufted perennial with lance-shaped, blue-green leaves, 60–100cm (24–39in) long. In early and midsummer, bears very pale pink flowers, 2–3cm (¾–1¼in) across, in racemes to 60cm (24in) long. ↕ to 1.2m (4ft), ↔ 90cm (36in). ❄❄❄
***E. x isabellinus* cultivars** (*E. olgae* x *E. stenophyllus*). Robust, tufted perennials with lance-shaped, mid-green leaves, 15–30cm (6–12in) long. In early summer, variously coloured flowers, 2–4cm (¾–1½in) across, are borne in racemes 20–50cm (8–20in) long. ↕ to 1.5m (5ft), ↔ 90cm (36in). ❄❄❄.
'Cleopatra' has orange flowers. **'Feuerfackel'**, syn. 'Fire Torch', has orange-red flowers. **'Fire Torch'** see 'Feuerfackel'. **'Isobel'** bears rose-pink flowers tinged with orange. **'Rosalind'** bears bright pink flowers. **'Sahara'** has sandy-copper flowers. **'Schneelanze'**, syn. 'Snow Lance', has greenish white flowers. **'Snow Lance'** see 'Schneelanze'.
E. robustus ■ Tufted perennial with strap-shaped, rough-margined, bluish green leaves, to 1.2m (4ft) long. In early and midsummer, pale pink flowers, to 4cm (1½in) across, with brown-marked bases and yellow stamens, are borne in racemes 75–120cm (2½–4ft) long. ↕ to 3m (10ft), ↔ 1.2m (4ft). C. Asia (Tien Shan and Pamir Mountains). ❄❄❄
E. spectabilis. Tufted perennial with strap-shaped, often rough-margined, greyish green leaves, 30–40cm (12–16in) long. In midsummer, bears racemes, to 1m (3ft) long, of sulphur-yellow flowers, 2cm (¾in) across, with orange-red stamens. ↕ 1.2–2m (4–6ft), ↔ 60cm (24in). Turkey, Lebanon, Iraq, Iran, W. Pakistan. ❄❄❄
E. stenophyllus ■ Tufted perennial with narrowly linear, rough-margined, sometimes softly hairy, greyish green leaves, 24cm (10in) long. In early and midsummer, bears racemes, 15–30cm (6–12in) long, of dark yellow flowers, to 2cm (¾in) across, fading to orange-brown. ↕ 1m (3ft), ↔ 60cm (24in). C. Asia, Iran, W. Pakistan. ❄❄❄.

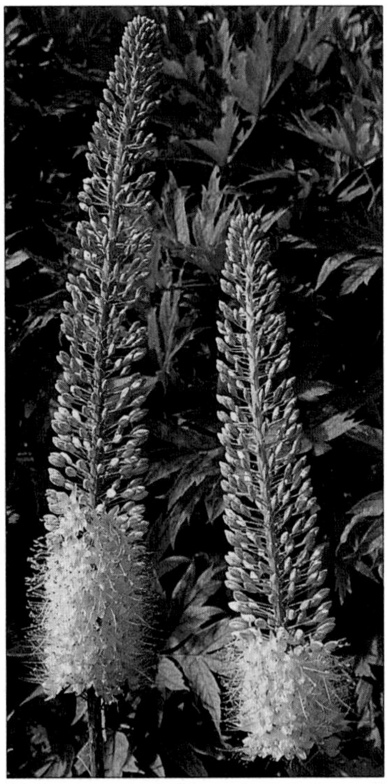
Eremurus stenophyllus

subsp. *aurantiacus*, syn. *E. aurantiacus*, has hairy flower stems; Tajikistan, Afghanistan, Pakistan. **subsp. *stenophyllus*,** syn. *E. bungei*, has leaves to 35cm (14in) long, and brighter yellow flowers; ↕ to 1.5m (5ft), ↔ 75cm (30in); C. Asia, Iran.

ERIA

ORCHIDACEAE

Genus of over 500 species of evergreen, epiphytic, sometimes terrestrial orchids from tropical Asia, Malaysia to Papua New Guinea, Australia, Polynesia, and adjacent islands. They occur in varied habitats, including montane forest. Most have ellipsoid to narrowly cylindrical, pseudobulb-like stems producing 2 or more linear to narrowly elliptic, mid- to dark green leaves. Small, *Dendrobium*-like flowers are borne in terminal or axillary racemes.

• **HARDINESS** Frost tender.

• **CULTIVATION** Cool-growing orchids. Under glass, grow in containers of epiphytic orchid compost. In summer, provide humid, well-ventilated, shady conditions and water freely, applying fertilizer at every third watering. At other times, provide full light and water sparingly. Do not mist at the start of the growing season. See also p.46.

• **PROPAGATION** Divide when plants overflow their containers.

• **PESTS AND DISEASES** Susceptible to red spider mites, aphids, and mealybugs.

E. coronaria, syn. *Trichosma suavis.* Terrestrial or epiphytic orchid with slender, pseudobulb-like stems and 2 broadly lance-shaped, thinly fleshy leaves, to 15cm (6in) long. Fragrant, waxy cream flowers, 2.5–4cm (1–1½in) wide, with yellow and red markings on the lips, are borne in terminal racemes, 20cm (8in) long, in summer. ↕↔ 23cm (9in). India. ❁ (min. 10°C/50°F; max. 30°C/86°F)

▷ ***Erianthus*** see *Saccharum*

ERICA

Heath

ERICACEAE

Genus of over 700 species of prostrate to tree-like, evergreen shrubs occurring in a variety of habitats from wet moorland to dry heathland in Europe, temperate Africa (mainly confined to S. of the Limpopo River in South Africa), and temperate W. and C. Asia. The whorled, rarely opposite, mainly linear leaves are tightly curled back, and usually 3–10mm (⅛–½in) long, although in some of the larger species they may be 2cm (¾in) long. The usually bell- to urn-shaped flowers, 0.2–4cm (1⁄16–1½in) long, develop in terminal racemes (sometimes leafy, and often spike-like), umbels, or panicle-like heads, or in 2- to 5-flowered, axillary clusters or whorls, on short lateral branches produced on the previous year's growth. The flowers may be distinguished from those of heathers (*Calluna*) by the prominent corollas and usually green calyces.

Hardy species are widely grown as ground cover, either on their own or with other ericaceous plants or dwarf conifers, and provide colour throughout the year. Tree-like species are excellent specimen plants. In frost-prone areas, grow the tender species in a cool greenhouse; in warmer climates, grow in a heather garden or among other shrubs.

• **HARDINESS** Fully hardy to frost tender.

• **CULTIVATION** Grow in well-drained, acid soil in an open site in full sun; most winter- and spring-flowering European species, and the summer-flowering *E. manipuliflora*, *E. terminalis*, *E. vagans*, and *E.* x *williamsii* will tolerate alkaline soil. Under glass, grow in lime-free (ericaceous) potting compost with added sharp sand, in full light and with good ventilation at all times. In the growing season, water freely and apply a half-strength balanced liquid fertilizer every 4 weeks; water moderately when not in flower. Pruning group 10, after flowering; group 8 for tree-like species.

• **PROPAGATION** Root semi-ripe cuttings in mid- or late summer. Mound-layer in spring.

• **PESTS AND DISEASES** Susceptible to fungal attack, chiefly from *Phytophthora* root rot, *Pythium*, and *Rhizoctonia*, in warm, wet conditions.

E. arborea (Tree heath). Upright shrub with needle-like, dark green leaves, grooved beneath. In spring, bears bell-shaped, honey-scented, greyish white flowers, 4mm (⅛in) long, in pyramidal, leafy racemes, 20–40cm (8–16in) long. ↕ to 6m (20ft), ↔ 3m (10ft). S.W. Europe, Mediterranean, N. Africa, mountains of central E. Africa. ❄❄❄ (borderline). **'Albert's Gold'** 🏆 syn. *E.* x *veitchii* 'Albert's Gold', has golden foliage but seldom bears flowers; ↕ 2m (6ft), ↔ 80cm (32in). **var. *alpina*** ■ 🏆 produces white flowers in dense, cylindrical racemes; ↕ 2m (6ft), ↔ 85cm (34in). ❄❄❄. **'Estrella Gold'** 🏆 bears white flowers above compact, lime-green foliage tipped bright yellow; ↕ 1.2m (4ft), ↔ 75cm (30in).

E. australis ■ 🏆 (Spanish heath). Erect, open shrub with linear, dark green leaves, channelled beneath. From mid-spring to early summer, bears tubular to

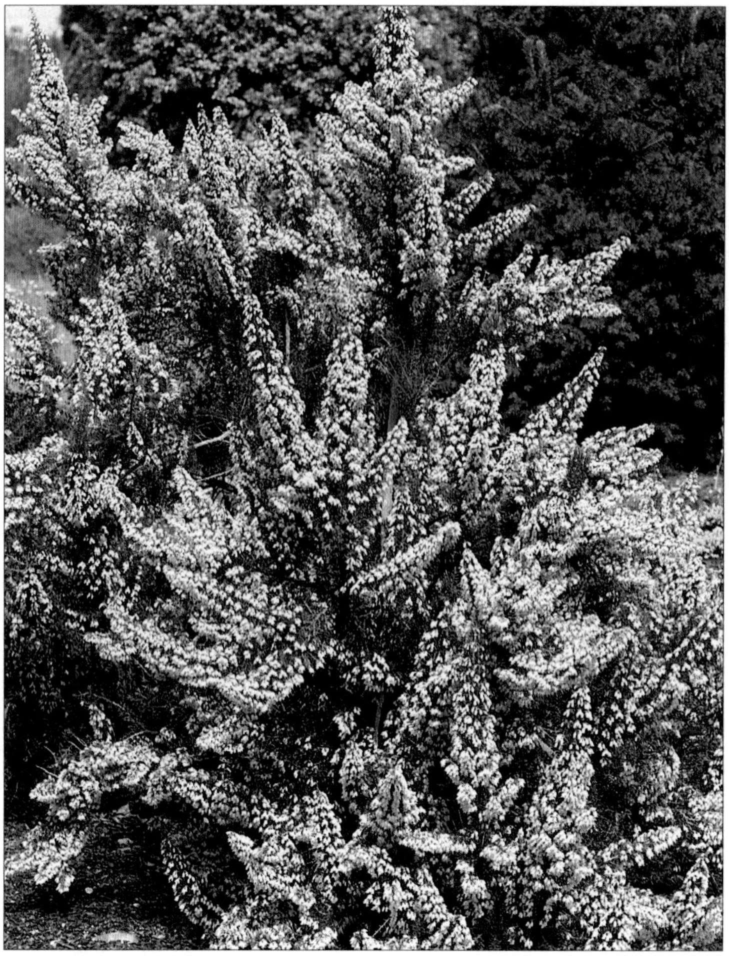

Erica arborea var. *alpina*

bell-shaped, purplish pink flowers, to 9mm (⅜in) long, in umbel-like racemes, 20cm (8in) long. Prone to damage by wind or snow. ↕ to 2m (6ft), ↔ to 1m (3ft). Portugal, W. Spain, Tangier. ❄❄. **'Mr. Robert'** 🏆 produces white flowers. **'Riverslea'** 🏆 bears lilac-pink flowers.

E. baccans. Robust, erect, many-branched shrub with linear, sea-green leaves. From winter to spring, bears axillary whorls, 2.5cm (1in) long, each with 4 almost spherical, deep pink flowers, 6mm (¼in) across, with constricted throats and keeled, dark pink sepals. ↕ to 2.5m (8ft), ↔ to 1m (3ft). South Africa (Western Cape). ❄

E. blenna. Stout, upright shrub with linear-lance-shaped, mid-green leaves, grooved beneath. Urn-shaped to ovoid-conical, sticky, bright orange flowers, 0.9–1.5cm (⅜–½in) long, constricted at the mouths, with green throats and lobes, are borne on axillary shoots, to 3cm (1¼in) long, mainly from winter to spring. ↕ to 1.2m (4ft), ↔ to 80cm (32in). South Africa (Western Cape). ❄

E. canaliculata ■ 🏆 (Channelled heath). Erect shrub with linear leaves, mid-green above, paler with fine hairs beneath. From winter to early spring, produces panicle-like whorls, to 30cm (12in) long, of cup-shaped, pale pink to near-white flowers, 4mm (⅛in) across, with white sepals and very dark brown anthers. ↕ to 2m (6ft), ↔ to 1.2m (4ft). South Africa (Western Cape, Eastern Cape). ❄

E. carnea, syn. *E. herbacea* (Alpine heath, Winter heath). Low, spreading shrub with linear, dark green leaves.

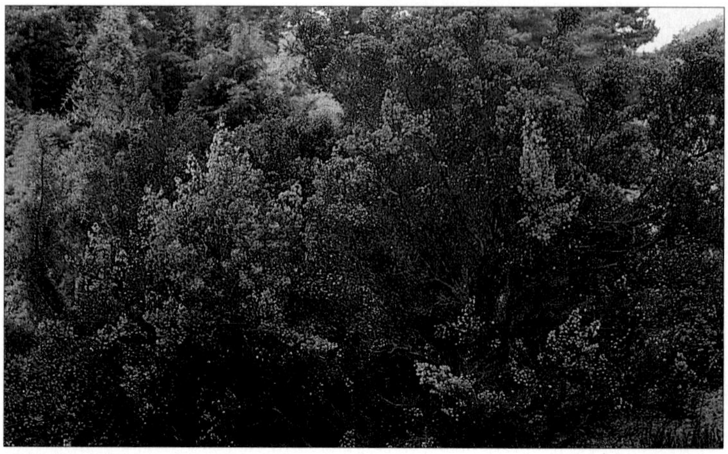

Erica australis

Bears one-sided racemes, 7cm (3in) long, of narrowly urn-shaped, purple-pink flowers, 6–9mm (¼–⅜in) long, in late winter and early spring. Tolerates mildly alkaline soil and some shade. ↕ 20–25cm (8–10in), ↔ to 55cm (22in). C. Alps, N.W. Italy, N.W. Balkans, E. Europe. ❄❄❄. Unless otherwise stated, the following cultivars have mid- to dark green foliage, and bear purplish pink flowers from winter to mid-spring; ↕ 15cm (6in), ↔ 45cm (18in). **'Adrienne Duncan'** 🏆 has bronze-hued foliage, and flowers from midwinter to mid-spring; ↔ 35cm (14in). **'Altadena'** has yellow foliage tipped pink and bronze, and bears lilac-pink flowers, deepening to purplish pink; ↔ 35cm (14in). **'Ann Sparkes'** ■ 🏆 has dark golden foliage with bright bronze tips in spring, and rose-pink flowers, darkening to purplish pink; ↔ 25cm (10in). **'Barry Sellers'** has yellow foliage, turning orange in cold weather, and produces deep pink flowers, ageing to magenta; ↔ 30cm (12in). **'Challenger'** 🏆 produces bold magenta flowers. **'December Red'** ■ bears flowers that open pink and deepen to purplish pink. **'Eileen Porter'** ■ bears magenta flowers with cream sepals; ↕↔ 20cm (8in). **'Foxhollow'** ■ 🏆 has bronze-tipped yellow foliage, deepening to orange-red in very cold weather; ↔ 40cm (16in). **'Golden Starlet'** 🏆 bears white flowers, and lime-green foliage that turns glowing yellow in summer; ↔ 40cm (16in). **'King George'** produces deep pink flowers, and is one of the first to bloom in early winter; ↔ 25cm (10in). **'Lesley Sparkes'** ■ has mid-green foliage tipped with salmon-pink and gold, particularly in spring; ↔ 25cm (10in). **'March Seedling'** flowers until late spring; ↔ 50cm (20in). **'Mr. Reeves'** see *E.* x *darleyensis* 'Darley Dale'. **'Myretoun Ruby'** 🏆 syn. 'Myreton Ruby', has pink flowers that deepen to crimson with age. **'R.B. Cooke'** 🏆 bears masses of pink flowers, ageing to mauve. **'Springwood Pink'** is trailing, and bears pink flowers that turn deeper pink with age; ↔ 40cm (16in). **'Springwood White'** ■ 🏆 is vigorous and trailing, with masses of white flowers above bright green foliage. **'Urville'** see 'Vivellii'. **'Vivellii'** ■ 🏆 syn. 'Urville', has bronze leaves and purplish pink flowers that darken to magenta; ↔ 35cm (14in). **'Westwood Yellow'** 🏆 is more upright than other yellow-foliaged cultivars, and bears shell-pink flowers; ↔ 30cm (12in). **'White Glow'** see *E.* x *darleyensis* 'White Glow'. **'White Perfection'** see *E.* x *darleyensis* 'White Perfection'.

E. cerinthoides ■ (Erica heath, Fire heath). Erect shrub with linear, grey-green leaves, which are variably softly hairy and usually glandular. Tubular, bright red, sometimes pale pink or white flowers, 2–3.5cm (¾–1½in) long, with slightly constricted throats and inflated bases, are borne in umbels 2–3.5cm (¾–1½in) across from winter to spring, and occasionally throughout the year. ↕ to 1.5m (5ft), ↔ to 1m (3ft). South Africa, Swaziland. ❄

E. ciliaris (Dorset heath). Spreading shrub with ovate to lance-shaped, usually glandular leaves, grey-green or dark green above, white beneath. From midsummer to mid-autumn, produces

ERICA

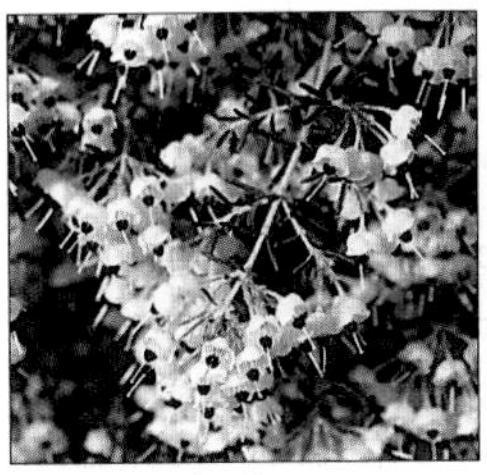
Erica canaliculata

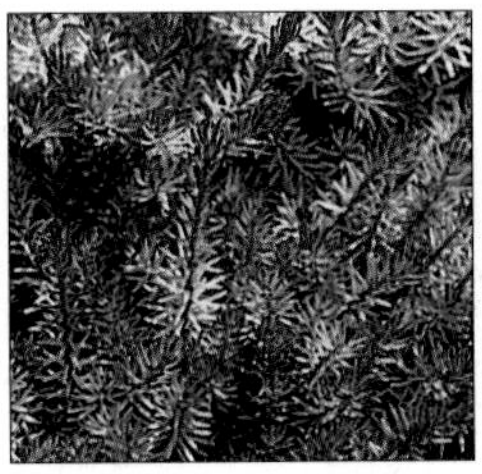
Erica carnea 'Ann Sparkes'

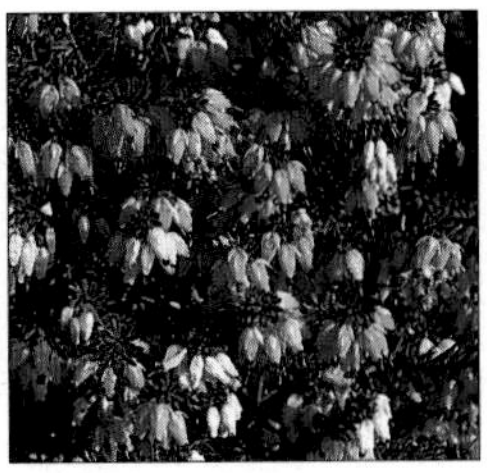
Erica carnea 'December Red'

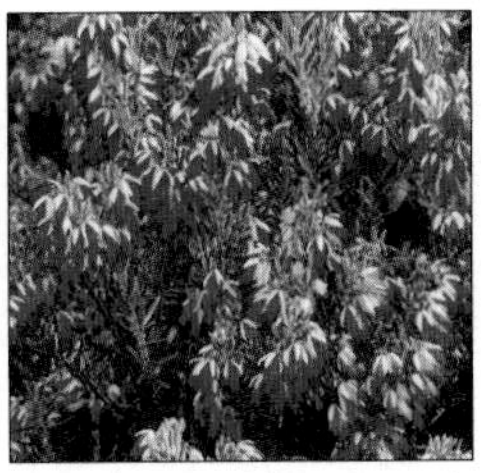
Erica carnea 'Eileen Porter'

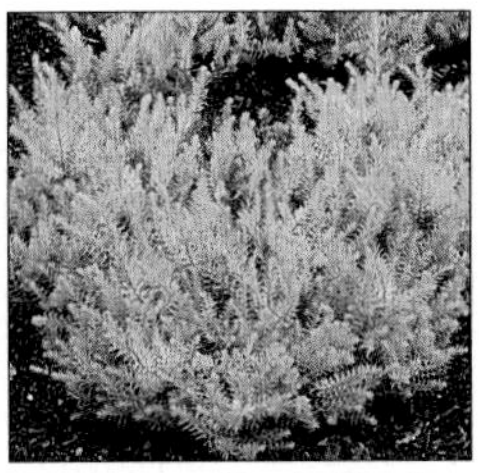
Erica carnea 'Foxhollow'

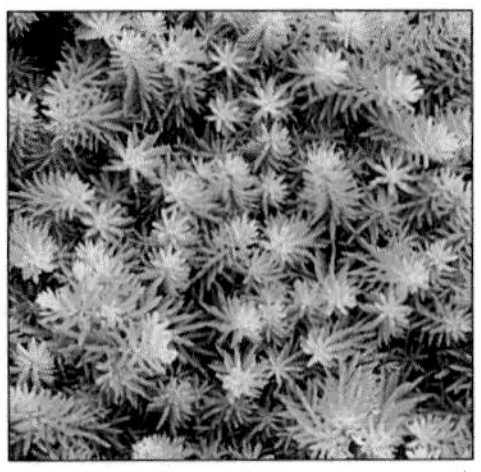
Erica carnea 'Lesley Sparkes'

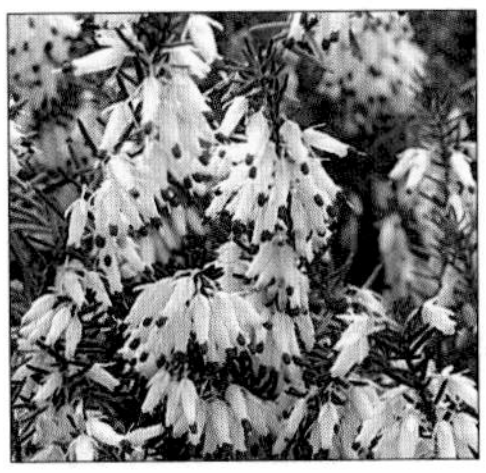
Erica carnea 'Springwood White'

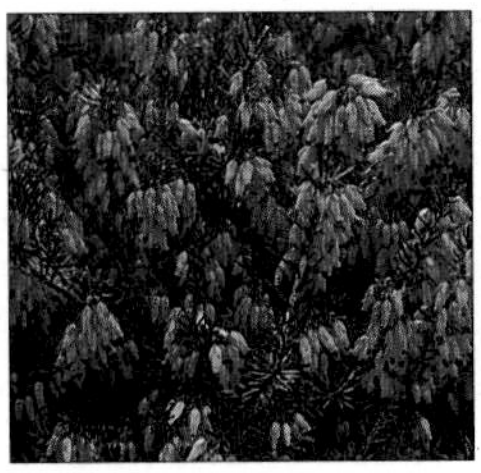
Erica carnea 'Vivellii'

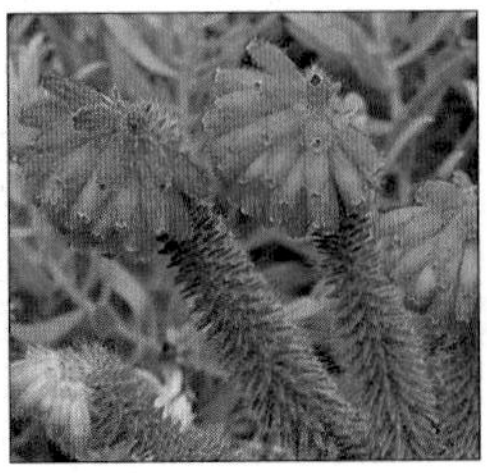
Erica cerinthoides

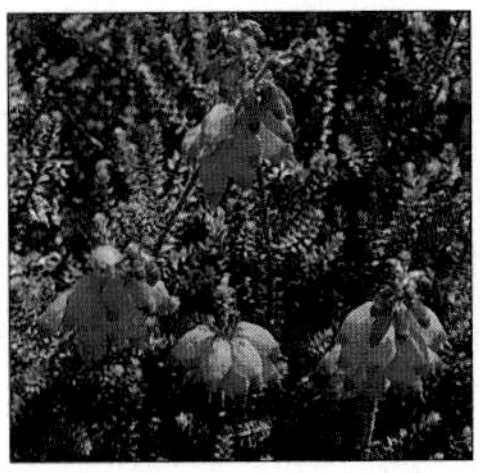
Erica ciliaris 'Corfe Castle'

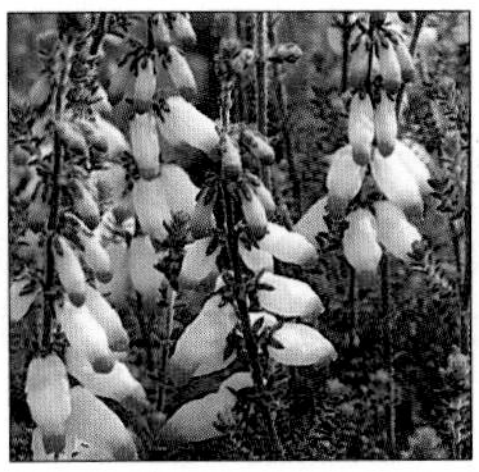
Erica ciliaris 'David McClintock'

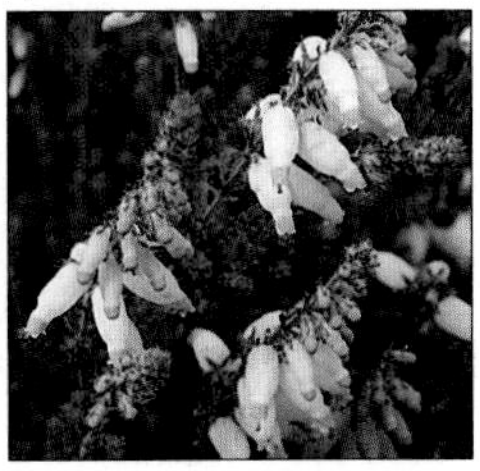
Erica ciliaris 'White Wings'

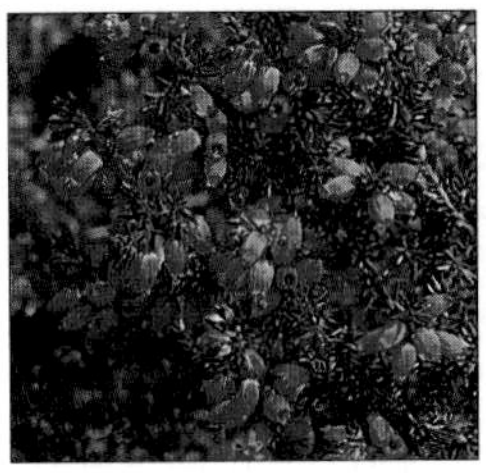
Erica cinerea 'C.D. Eason'

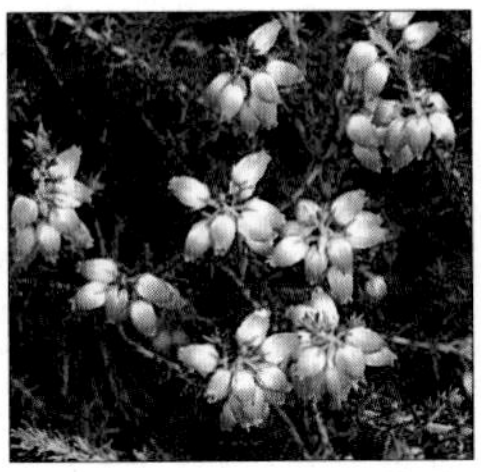
Erica cinerea 'Eden Valley'

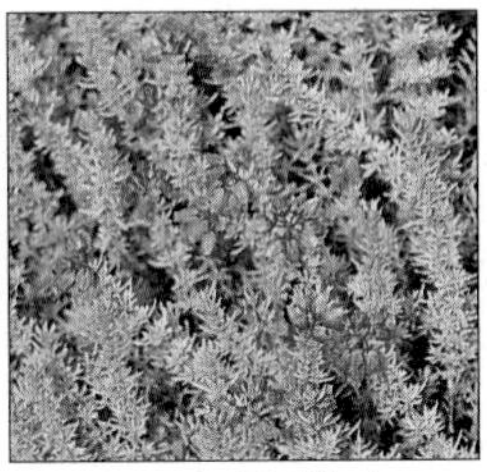
Erica cinerea 'Fiddler's Gold'

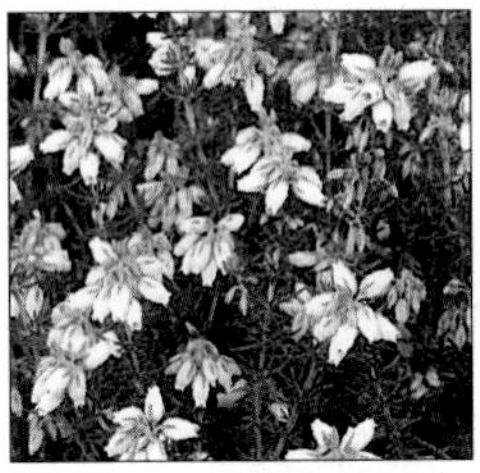
Erica cinerea 'Hookstone White'

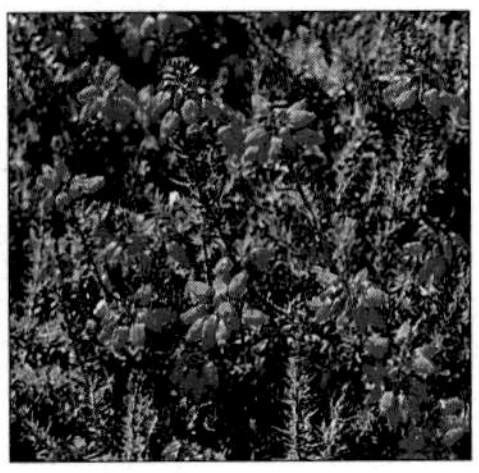
Erica cinerea 'Purple Beauty'

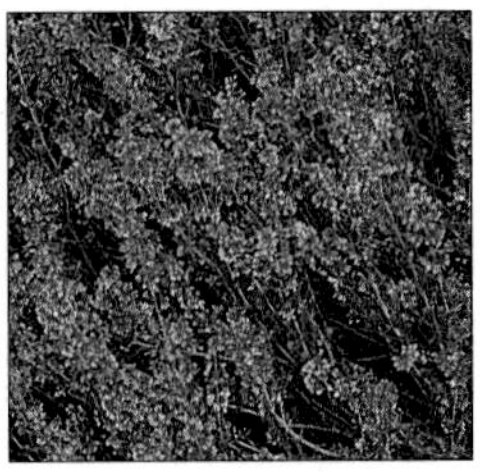
Erica cinerea 'Yvonne'

E

racemes, 7cm (3in) long, of urn-shaped, usually lilac-pink flowers, to 1cm (½in) long, sharply constricted at the mouths. May be damaged in very severe winters. ↕35–60cm (14–24in), ↔ to 50cm (20in). Europe. ❄❄❄. **'Aurea'** has straw-yellow foliage in summer, deepening in winter; ↕25cm (10in). **'Corfe Castle'** ▣🏆 bears distinctive, rose-pink flowers, and mid-green foliage that turns bronze-green in winter; ↕22cm (9in), ↔ 35cm (14in). **'David McClintock'** ▣🏆 bears flowers with white bases and purplish pink mouths; ↕ to 40cm (16in), ↔ 45cm (18in). **'White Wings'** ▣ bears white flowers; ↕15cm (6in), ↔ 45cm (18in).

E. cinerea (Bell heather). Compact shrub with usually linear, strongly rolled-back, dark bottle-green leaves. Urn-shaped, white, pink, or purple flowers, to 7mm (¼in) long, are borne in racemes 5cm (2in) long from early summer to early autumn. ↕60cm (24in), ↔ to 80cm (32in). Europe. ❄❄❄. **'Alba Major'** bears white flowers and mid-green foliage; ↕30cm (12in), ↔ 55cm (22in). **'C.D. Eason'** ▣🏆 has bright magenta flowers, and is good ground cover; ↕25cm (10in), ↔ 50cm (20in). **'Contrast'** bears beetroot-red flowers; ↕25cm (10in), ↔ 45cm (18in). **'Eden Valley'** ▣🏆 has lavender-pink flowers, shading to white at the bases, and mid-green foliage; ↕20cm (8in), ↔ 50cm (20in). **'Fiddler's Gold'** ▣🏆 has lilac-pink flowers, and golden yellow foliage that deepens to red; ↕25cm (10in), ↔ 45cm (18in). **'Foxhollow Mahogany'** bears ruby-red flowers, and is good for ground cover; ↕20cm (8in), ↔ 50cm (20in). **'Glencairn'** ▣ bears magenta flowers, and has dark green foliage with red tips, which are especially pronounced in spring; ↕30cm (12in), ↔ 50cm (20in). **'Golden Hue'** 🏆 produces amethyst flowers, and pale yellow foliage tipped orange in winter; ↕35cm (14in), ↔ 70cm (28in). **'Hookstone White'** ▣🏆 produces white flowers in racemes 7–12cm (3–5in) long, above mid-green foliage; ↕35cm (14in), ↔ 65cm (26in). **'Janet'** bears shell-pink flowers above compact, light green foliage; ↕20cm (8in), ↔ 30cm (12in). **'Lime Soda'** bears a profusion of soft lavender-pink flowers above lime-green foliage; ↕35cm (14in), ↔ 55cm (22in). **'Peñaz'** bears masses of bright ruby-red flowers; ↕25cm (10in), ↔ 40cm (16in). **'Pentreath'** 🏆 produces a neat carpet of beetroot-red flowers; ↕30cm (12in), ↔ 55cm (22in). **'Pink Ice'** 🏆 syn. 'Pink Lace', is dwarf and twiggy, with clear rose-pink flowers, and deep green foliage that is bronze when young and in winter; ↕20cm (8in), ↔ 35cm (14in). **'Pink Lace'** see 'Pink Ice'. **'Purple Beauty'** ▣ bears bright, deep pinkish purple flowers; ↕30cm (12in), ↔ 55cm (22in). **'Rock Pool'** has golden yellow foliage turning orange-red in winter, and produces a few short racemes, 3cm (1¼in) long, of mauve flowers; ↕15cm (6in), ↔ 30cm (12in). **'Romiley'** ▣ bears magenta flowers, and provides neat ground cover; ↕25cm (10in), ↔ 55cm (22in). **'Rosabella'** bears magenta flowers in racemes 7–10cm (3–4in) long, and is good ground cover; ↕30cm (12in), ↔ 60cm (24in). **'Windlebrooke'** ▣🏆 bears golden yellow foliage turning orange-red in winter; ↕15cm (6in), ↔ 45cm (18in). **'Yvonne'** ▣ produces salmon-pink flowers with deeply cut corollas; ↕35cm (14in), ↔ 45cm (18in).

E. codonodes see *E. lusitanica*.

E. corsica see *E. terminalis*.

E. crawfordii see *E. mackaiana*.

E. cruenta (Blood-red heath). Upright, loosely branched shrub with linear, dark green leaves. Terminal, whorled, leafy racemes, 10cm (4in) long, of tubular, blood-red flowers, 2–2.5cm (¾–1in) long, are produced from spring to early autumn. ↕1m (3ft), ↔ 70cm (28in). South Africa (Western Cape). ❄❄

E. curviflora (Water heath). Erect shrub with linear to linear-lance-shaped, mid-green leaves. Tubular, usually hairy, red, orange, yellow, or pink flowers, 2–4cm (¾–1½in) long, are flared at the mouths. They are usually borne singly, occasionally in terminal clusters of 3 or 4, at any time of year, but most often from winter to spring. Prefers wet soil. ↕ to 1.5m (5ft), ↔ to 1m (3ft). South Africa (Western Cape, Eastern Cape). ❄

E. x darleyensis (*E. carnea* x *E. erigena*) (Darley Dale heath). Bushy shrub with lance-shaped, mid-green leaves. In late winter and early spring, bears racemes, 10cm (4in) long, of urn-shaped to cylindrical, white to rose-pink flowers, 5mm (¼in) long. Suitable for any well-drained soil. Particularly good ground cover. ↕ to 60cm (24in), ↔ to 75cm (30in). Garden origin. ❄❄❄. The following cultivars are ↕30cm (12in), ↔ 60cm (24in), unless otherwise stated.

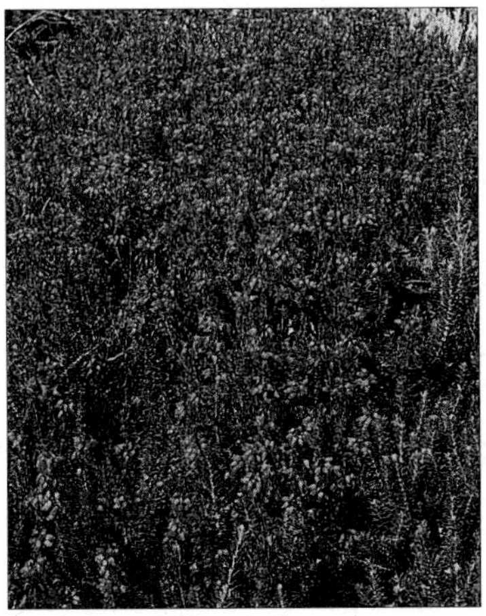
Erica cinerea 'Glencairn'

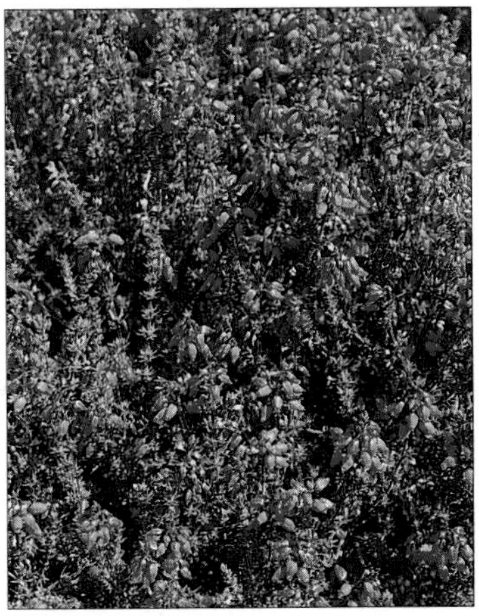
Erica cinerea 'Romiley'

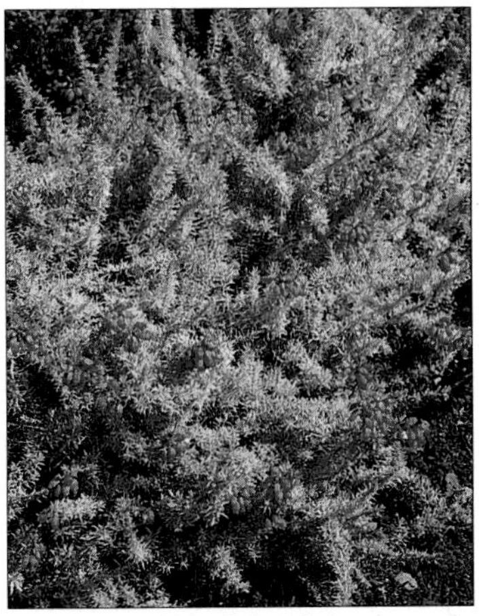
Erica cinerea 'Windlebrooke'

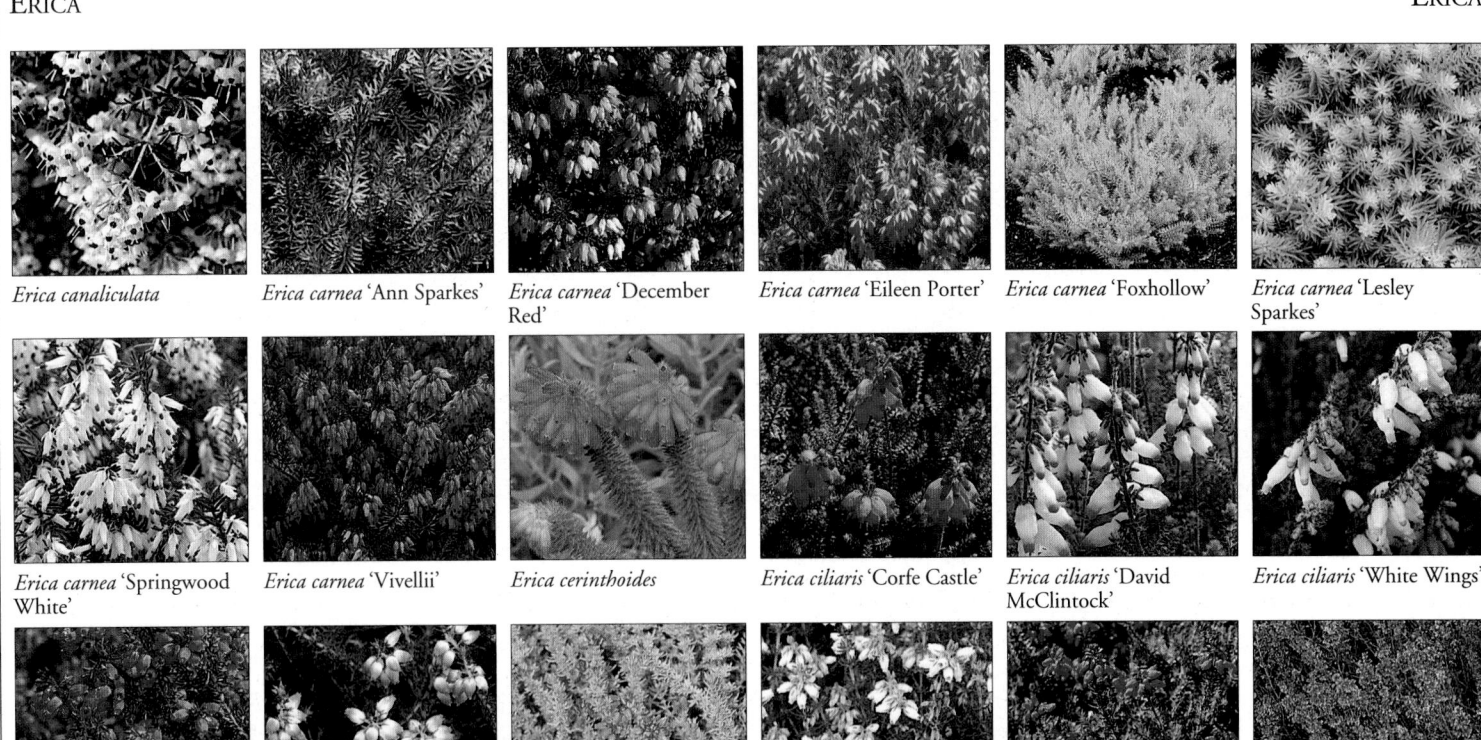

ERICA

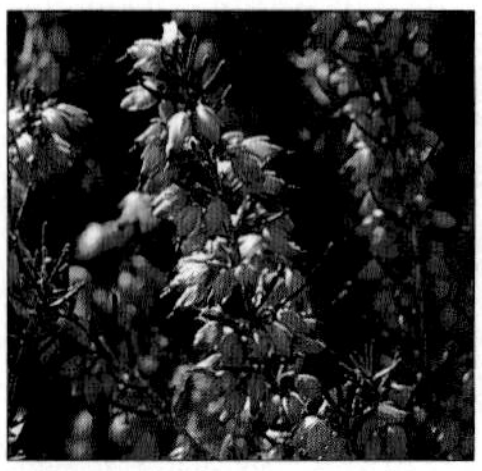
Erica x *darleyensis* 'Archie Graham'

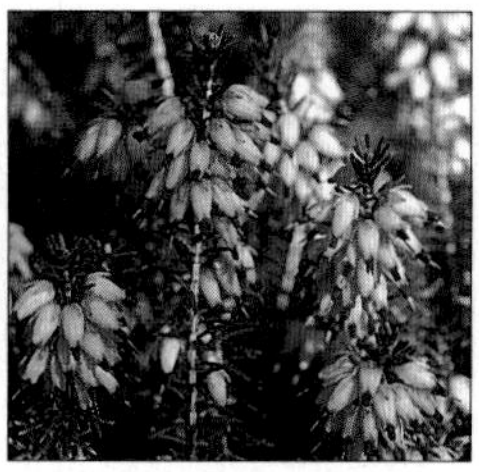
Erica x *darleyensis* 'Darley Dale'

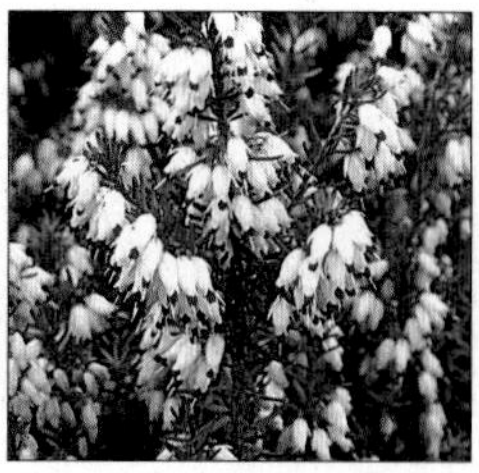
Erica x *darleyensis* 'Jenny Porter'

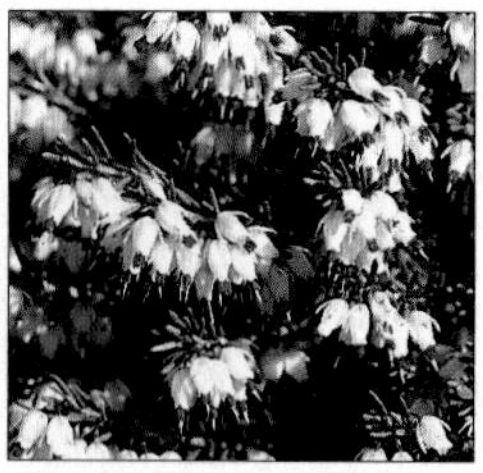
Erica x *darleyensis* 'White Glow'

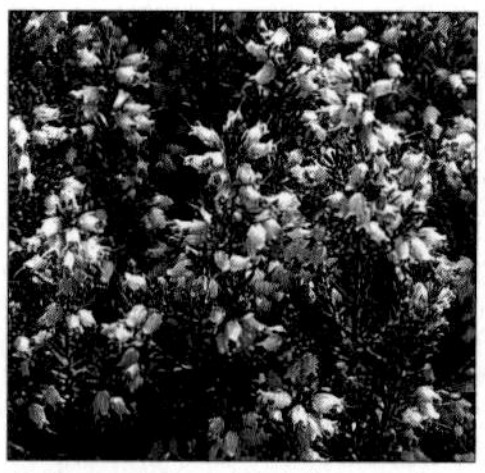
Erica erigena 'Brightness'

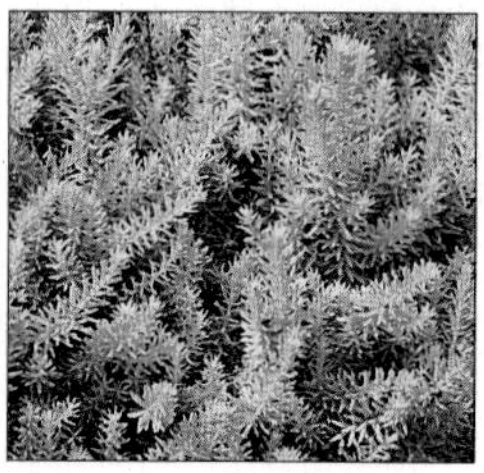
Erica erigena 'Golden Lady'

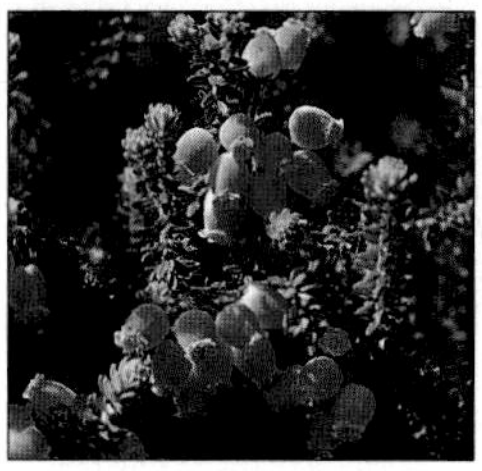
Erica mackaiana 'Plena'

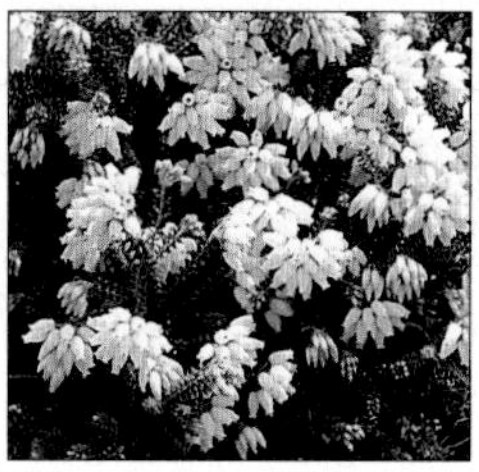
Erica mackaiana 'Shining Light'

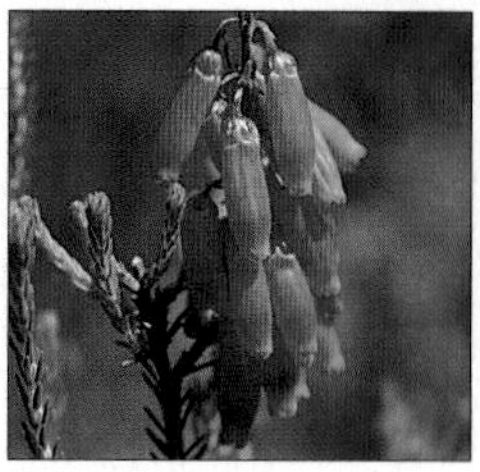
Erica mammosa

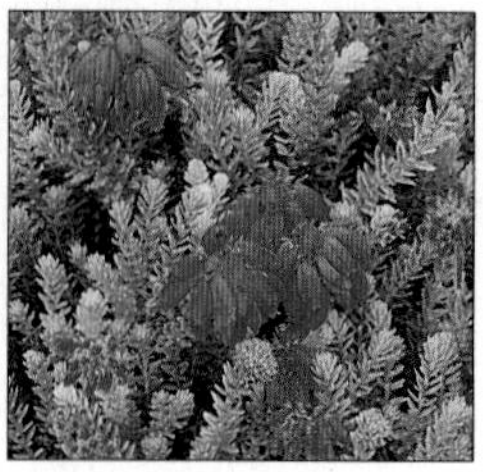
Erica x *stuartii* 'Irish Lemon'

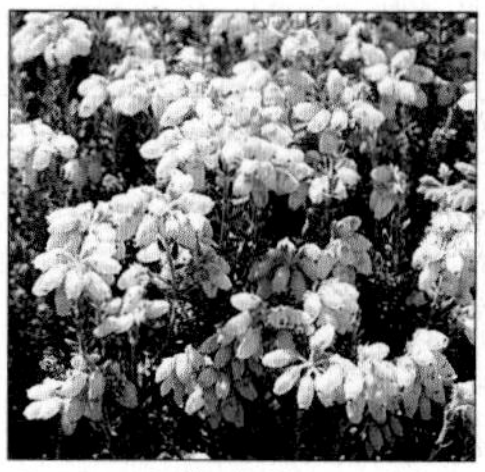
Erica tetralix 'Alba Mollis'

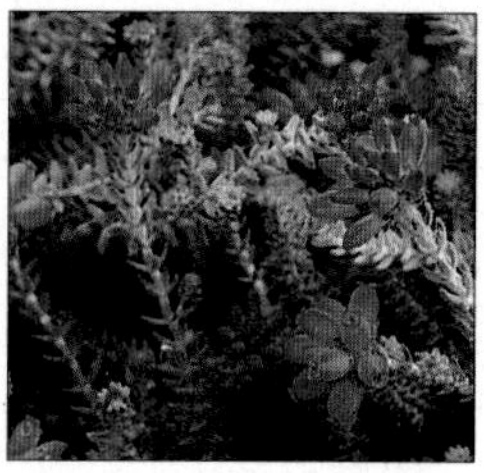
Erica tetralix 'Pink Star'

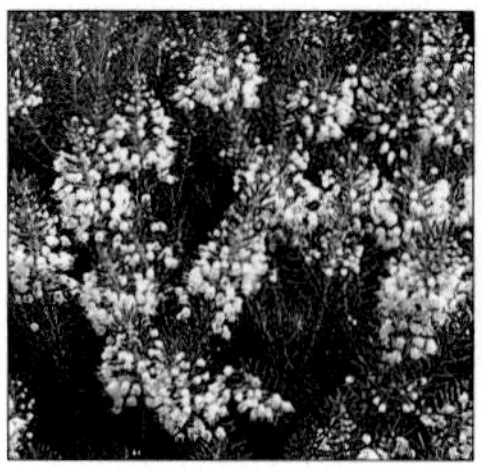
Erica vagans 'Lyonesse'

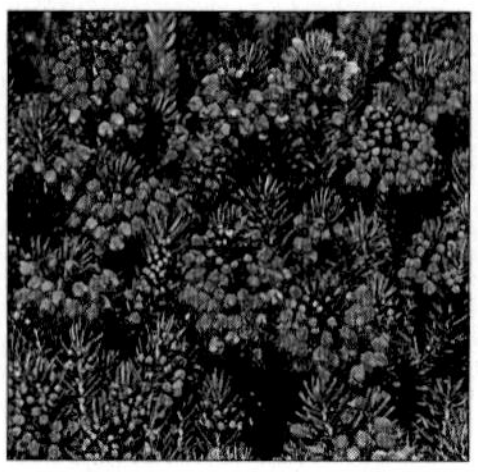
Erica vagans 'Mrs. D.F. Maxwell'

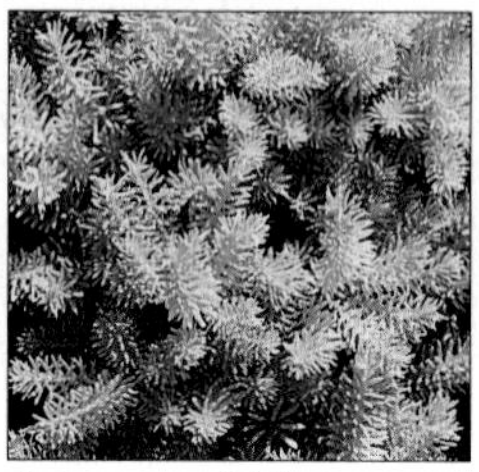
Erica vagans 'Valerie Proudley'

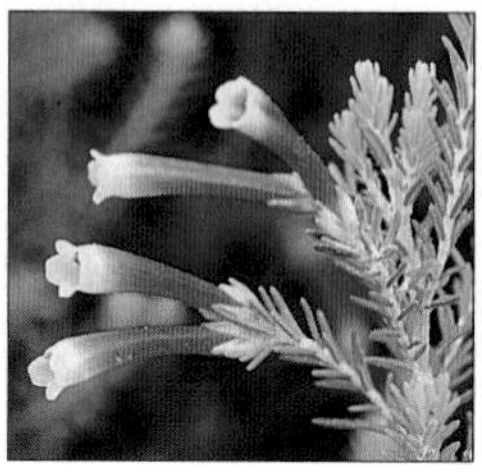
Erica versicolor

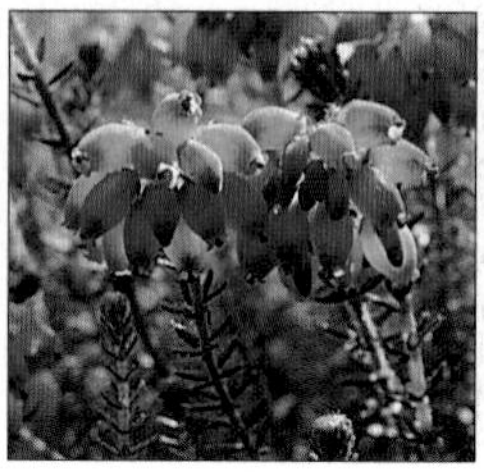
Erica x *watsonii* 'Dawn'

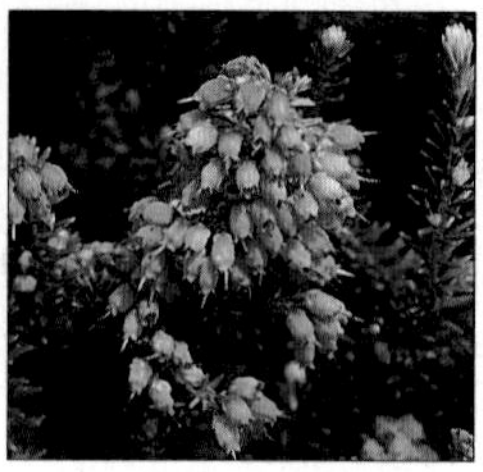
Erica x *williamsii* 'P.D. Williams'

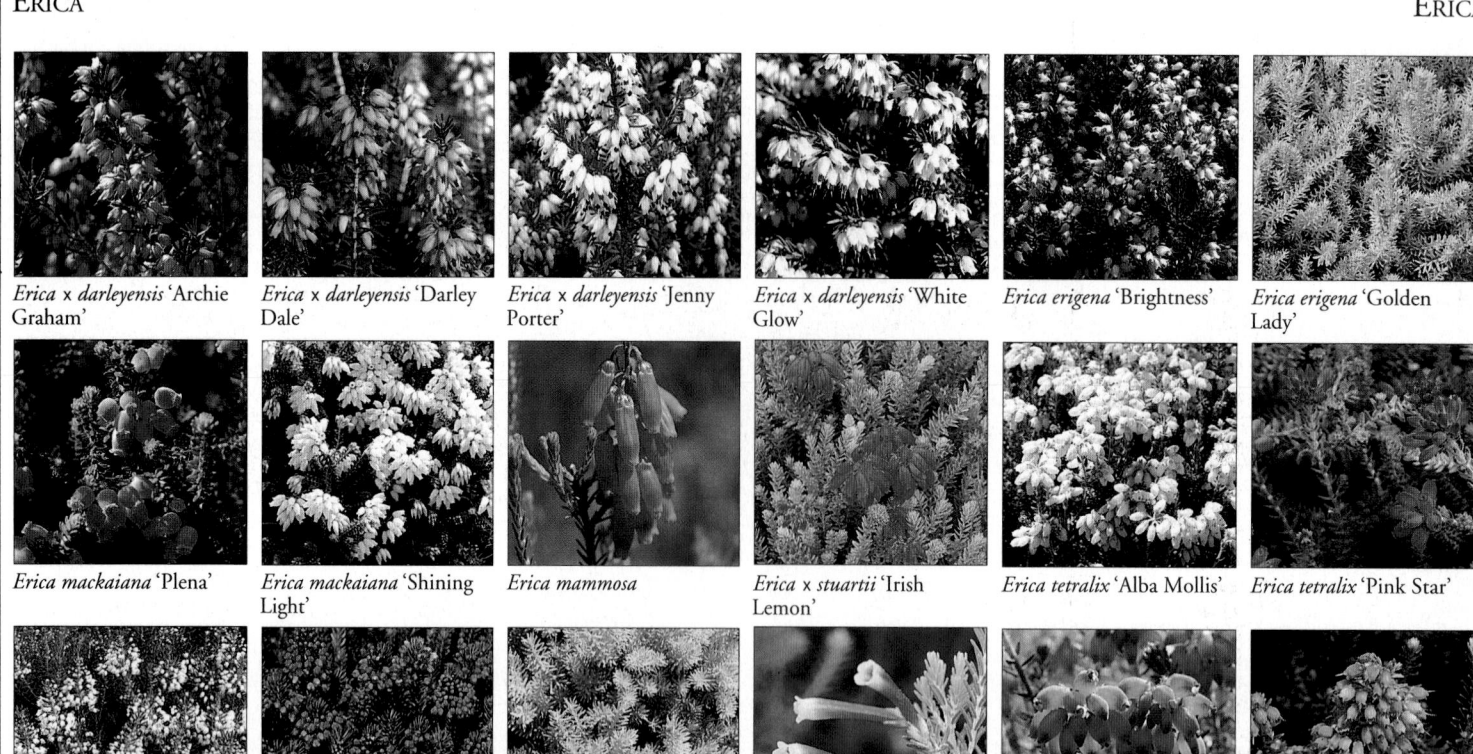

'Archie Graham' ■ has pink flowers, ageing to purplish pink; ↕ 50cm (20in). **'Darley Dale'** ■ syn. 'Darleyensis', 'Pink Perfection', *E. carnea* 'Mr. Reeves', has foliage tipped cream in spring, and shell-pink flowers that darken with age; ↔ 55cm (22in). **'Darleyensis'** see 'Darley Dale'. **'Ghost Hills'** 🏆 has light green foliage, tipped cream in spring; ↔ 80cm (32in). **'Jack H. Brummage'**, syn. 'J.H. Brummage', *E. erigena* 'Jack H. Brummage', produces yellow-orange leaves and purplish pink flowers. **'Jenny Porter'** ■🏆 has foliage with pale cream tips in spring, and pinkish white flowers. **'J.W. Porter'** 🏆 has dark green foliage, tipped red and cream in spring, and purplish pink flowers; ↕ 25cm (10in), ↔ 40cm (16in). **'Kramer's Rote'** 🏆 syn. 'Kramer's Red', has bronze-green foliage and magenta flowers. **'Molten Silver'** see 'Silberschmelze'. **'Pink Perfection'** see 'Darley Dale'. **'Silberschmelze'**, syn. 'Molten Silver', 'Silver Beads', has white flowers, and foliage that is faintly cream-tipped in spring, later deep green, and tinged red in winter; ↕ 35cm (14in), ↔ 80cm (32in). **'Silver Beads'** see 'Silberschmelze'. **'White Glow'** ■ syn. 'White Gown', *E. carnea* 'White Glow', is compact, and bears masses of white flowers; ↕ 25cm (10in), ↔ 50cm (20in). **'White Gown'** see 'White Glow'. **'White Perfection'** 🏆 syn. *E. carnea* 'White Perfection', produces pure white flowers and bright green foliage; ↕ 40cm (16in), ↔ 70cm (28in).

E. erigena, syn. *E. hibernica*, *E. mediterranea* (Irish heath, Mediterranean heath). Upright shrub with brittle stems and linear, dark green leaves. From winter to spring, produces urn-shaped to cylindrical, honey-scented, deep lilac-pink flowers, 5mm (¼in) long, in racemes 4cm (1½in) long. Good for low hedges in areas free from heavy snowfall. ↕ to 2.5m (8ft), ↔ to 1m (3ft). Ireland, S.W. France, Spain, Portugal, Tangier. ❄❄❄. **'Brightness'** ■ has purple-green foliage in winter, becoming glaucous green in summer, and bears lilac-pink flowers in spring; ↕↔ 50cm (20in); ❄❄. **'Golden Lady'** ■🏆 has bright golden yellow foliage, which may be burnt by cold wind; ↕ 30cm (12in), ↔ 40cm (16in). **'Irish Dusk'** 🏆 has dark grey-green leaves, and produces rose-pink flowers from late autumn to late spring; ↕ 60cm (24in), ↔ 45cm (18in). **'Irish Lemon'** see *E.* x *stuartii* 'Irish Lemon'. **'Jack H. Brummage'** see *E.* x *darleyensis* 'Jack H. Brummage'. **'Mediterranea Superba'** see 'Superba'. **'Superba'**, syn. 'Mediterranea Superba', bears strongly scented, shell-pink flowers, deepening with age, in mid- and late spring. Suitable as a hedge; ↕ 1.8m (6ft), ↔ 50cm (20in). **'W.T. Rackliff'** 🏆 is compact, with rich green foliage, and produces masses of white flowers in spring; ↕ 75cm (30in), ↔ 55cm (22in).

E. glandulosa. Untidy shrub with overlapping, linear, light green leaves. Gland-tipped hairs on leaves and stems make the plant sticky to touch. Axillary clusters, 1.5cm (½in) across, of 2–5 tubular flowers, 4–10mm (⅛–½in) long, in shades of pink, are borne mainly from autumn to spring. ↕ to 60cm (24in), ↔ to 90cm (36in). South Africa (Western Cape, Eastern Cape). ❄

E. gracilis. Compact shrub with linear, deep green leaves. From autumn to spring, bears whorls, 1cm (½in) long, of 4 urn-shaped, pale pink to cerise flowers, 4mm (⅛in) long. ↕↔ 50cm (20in). South Africa (Western Cape, Eastern Cape). ❄

E. herbacea see *E. carnea.*

E. hibernica see *E. erigena.*

E.* x *hiemalis. Usually upright shrub with linear, light green leaves. From late autumn to winter, bears tubular, pink-suffused white flowers, 1.5cm (½in) long, in dense racemes, 10cm (4in) long. ↕↔ 60cm (24in). Garden origin. ❄

***E. hybrida* 'Irish Lemon'** see *E.* x *stuartii* 'Irish Lemon'.

E. lusitanica 🏆 syn. *E. codonodes* (Portuguese heath). Erect shrub with feathery, linear, mid-green leaves. From winter to spring, tubular to bell-shaped white flowers, 5mm (¼in) long, opening from pink buds, are borne in branched racemes, 25cm (10in) long. Prefers acid soil. ↕ to 3m (10ft), ↔ to 1m (3ft). S.W. France, Portugal, W. Spain. ❄❄. **'George Hunt'** has bright yellow leaves; it requires a sheltered site.

E. mackaiana, syn. *E. crawfordii, E. mackaii, E. mackayana* (Mackay's heath). Decumbent to erect shrub with oblong-lance-shaped, hairy-tipped leaves, which are dark green and sometimes slightly hairy above, white beneath. From summer to early autumn, produces umbels, 1cm (½in) across, of urn-shaped, bright pink flowers, to 7mm (¼in) long, with constricted mouths. Needs damp soil. ↕ to 50cm (20in), ↔ to 75cm (30in). Ireland, Spain. ❄❄❄. **'Dr. Ronald Gray'**, syn. *E. tetralix* 'Dr. Ronald Gray', has hairless, bright green leaves and pure white flowers; ↕ 15cm (6in), ↔ 35cm (14in). **'Plena'** ■ syn. *E. tetralix* 'Plena', produces double magenta flowers. Good ground cover; ↕ 15cm (6in), ↔ 40cm (16in). **'Shining Light'** ■🏆 has grey-green foliage, and bears masses of white flowers, 8mm (⅜in) long; ↕ 25cm (10in), ↔ 55cm (22in).

E. mackaii see *E. mackaiana.*

E. mackayana see *E. mackaiana.*

E. mammosa ■ Erect shrub with linear to lance-shaped, dark green leaves. From spring to summer, bears tubular, dark red, orange-red, pink, green, or white flowers, 1.5–2.5cm (½–1in) long, in clustered, terminal racemes, 7cm (3in) long. ↕ to 1.5m (5ft), ↔ to 2m (6ft). South Africa (Western Cape). ❄

E. manipuliflora, syn. *E. verticillata* of gardens (Whorled heath). Erect to spreading shrub with linear, sharply pointed, mid-green leaves. From late summer to autumn, bears irregular racemes, 10cm (4in) long, of cylindrical to bell-shaped, rose-pink flowers, 4mm (⅛in) long. ↕ to 1m (3ft), ↔ to 1.1m (3½ft). E. Mediterranean. ❄❄. **subsp. *anthura* 'Heaven Scent'** 🏆 bears sprays of strongly scented, lilac-pink flowers; ↔ 60cm (24in); ❄❄❄

E. mediterranea see *E. erigena.*

E. nana. Dwarf, prostrate, sometimes erect shrub with linear, mid-green leaves. In autumn, bears whorls, to 2cm (¾in) long, of 3 tubular yellow flowers, to 2cm (¾in) long, with spreading, green-tipped lobes. Good in containers. ↕ usually 20–25cm (8–10in), sometimes to 50cm (20in), ↔ to 1m (3ft). South Africa (Western Cape). ❄

E. pageana. Erect shrub with linear, mid-green leaves. In late winter and early spring, short branches bear groups of 3 or 4 bell-shaped, rich yellow flowers, 8–10mm (⅜–½in) long, in dense, spike-like racemes, 10cm (4in) long. ↕ to 60cm (24in), ↔ to 30cm (12in). South Africa (Western Cape). ❄

E. patersonia (Mealie heath). Erect shrub with linear, mid-green leaves. In late winter and early spring, bears dense, spike-like racemes, 8cm (3in) long, of tubular yellow flowers, 1.5–2cm (½–¾in) long, in groups of 4. ↕ to 90cm (36in), ↔ to 60cm (24in). South Africa (Western Cape). ❄

E. perspicua ■ (Prince of Wales heath). Variable shrub with overlapping, linear, grey-green leaves. Translucent, tubular flowers, 1–2cm (½–¾in) long, in white, pink and white, red and white, purple and white, or red, are borne in loose, spike-like racemes, 8cm (3in) long, mainly from early autumn to winter. Needs damp soil. ↕ to 2m (6ft), ↔ to 1m (3ft). South Africa (Western Cape). ✻

E. peziza (Kapokkie heath). Upright, many-branched shrub with linear, mid-green leaves. In spring, bears racemes, 5cm (2in) long, of cup-shaped white flowers, 5mm (¼in) across, covered with woolly hairs. ↕↔ 60cm (24in). South Africa (Western Cape). ✻

E.* x *praegeri see *E.* x *stuartii.*

E. quadrangularis. Compact, well-rounded shrub with linear, mid-green leaves. From late winter to summer, bears whorls, 2cm (¾in) long, of 4 cup-shaped flowers, 2–3mm (1/16–⅛in) long, ranging from white through pink to red. ↕ 60cm (24in), ↔ 45cm (18in). South Africa (Western Cape). ✻

E. scoparia (Besom heath). Untidy, erect shrub with linear, dark green leaves. In summer, tiny, bell-shaped, greenish brown flowers, to 3mm (⅛in) long, are borne in spike-like racemes, 6cm (2½in) long. ↕ to 2m (6ft), ↔ to 1m (3ft). S.W. France, Spain, N. Africa, Canary Islands. ✻✻✻. **'Minima'** is compact, and bears a few brownish green flowers in late spring and early summer; ↕ 25cm (10in), ↔ 80cm (32in).

E. sessiliflora. Upright shrub with erect to spreading, linear, mid-green leaves. Bears congested, spike-like racemes, to 6cm (2½in) long, of tubular, greenish white flowers, 1.5–3cm (½–1¼in) long, from late winter to spring. Sepals eventually turn red, producing tight fruiting heads that remain on the plant for several years. ↕ to 2m (6ft), ↔ to 1m (3ft). South Africa (Western Cape, Eastern Cape). ✻

E. speciosa. Sturdy, erect, many-branched shrub with linear, mid-green leaves. Spike-like racemes, 9cm (3½in) long, of tubular, pink- or red-based flowers, 2–3cm (¾–1¼in) long, with white, green, or yellow lobes, are borne in whorls of 3, or occasionally singly, from early spring to early autumn. ↕ to 1.2m (4ft), ↔ to 1m (3ft). South Africa (Western Cape, Eastern Cape). ✻

E. stricta see *E. terminalis.*

E.* x *stuartii (*E. mackaiana* x *E. tetralix*), syn. *E.* x *praegeri.* Erect shrub with oblong, glandular, grey-green leaves. Throughout summer and autumn, produces umbels of urn-shaped pink flowers, 8mm (⅜in) long, which are contracted at the mouths. Needs moist soil. ↕ 25cm (10in), ↔ 50cm (20in). Ireland (Donegal, Connemara). ✻✻✻. **'Irish Lemon'** ■♀ syn. *E. erigena* 'Irish Lemon', *E. hybrida* 'Irish Lemon', has brilliant lemon-yellow spring growth, and bears mauve flowers from late spring to summer.

E. subdivaricata. Spreading shrub with linear, usually hairy, mid-green leaves. Whorls of 4 cup-shaped, honey-scented, occasionally pink-flushed, white flowers, 4mm (⅛in) long, are produced in the leaf axils from early summer to late autumn. Requires damp soil. ↕ 50–80cm (20–32in), ↔ to 1m (3ft). South Africa (Western Cape). ✻

E. terminalis ♀ syn. *E. corsica*, *E. stricta* (Corsican heath). Erect shrub with linear, glossy, dark green leaves. Bears umbels of urn-shaped, lilac-pink flowers, 7mm (¼in) long, from midsummer to early autumn. The faded flowers have a russet hue all winter. Good as a hedge, or as a specimen plant if pruned hard when young. ↕↔ to 1m (3ft). Europe, S.W. Mediterranean. ✻✻✻

E. tetralix (Cross-leaved heath). Dwarf, spreading shrub with lance-shaped to linear-oblong, often glandular, usually grey-green leaves, white beneath, arranged in whorls of 4 to form crosses. From midsummer to mid-autumn, bears umbels of urn-shaped, pale pink flowers, 9mm (⅜in) long, with constricted mouths. Prefers moist soil. ↕ to 30cm (12in), ↔ 50cm (20in). W. Europe. ✻✻✻. **'Alba Mollis'** ■♀ has silvery grey leaves and pure white flowers; ↕ 20cm (8in), ↔ 30cm (12in). **'Con Underwood'** ♀ bears magenta flowers; ↕ 25cm (10in). **'Dr. Ronald Gray'** see *E. mackaiana* 'Dr. Ronald Gray'. **'Pink Star'** ■♀ bears lilac-pink flowers in star-like patterns; ↕ 20cm (8in), ↔ 35cm (14in). **'Plena'** see *E. mackaiana* 'Plena'.

E. umbellata (Dwarf Spanish heath). Compact shrub with linear, grey-green leaves. In late spring and early summer, bears umbels of bell-shaped to ovoid mauve flowers, 6mm (¼in) long, with conspicuous, dark brown anthers. Grows in any soil. ↕ 35–80cm (18–32in), ↔ 55cm (22in). Portugal, W. Spain, Tangier. ✻✻

E. vagans (Cornish heath, Wandering heath). Vigorous, spreading shrub with decumbent to ascending stems and linear, dark green leaves. Cylindrical to bell-shaped, pink, mauve, or white flowers, to 4mm (⅛in) long, are borne in racemes 14cm (5½in) long, from mid-

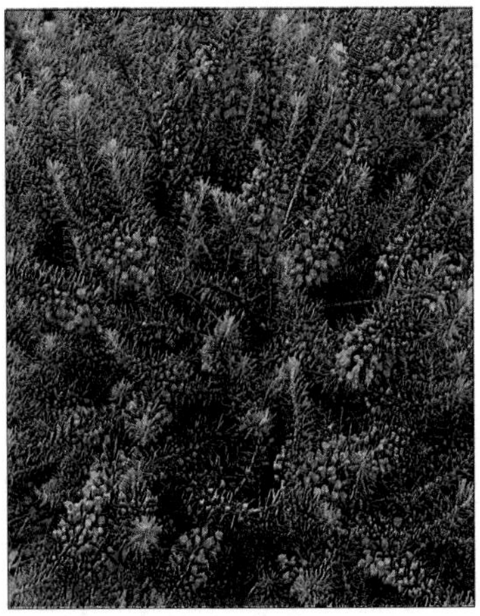

Erica vagans 'Birch Glow'

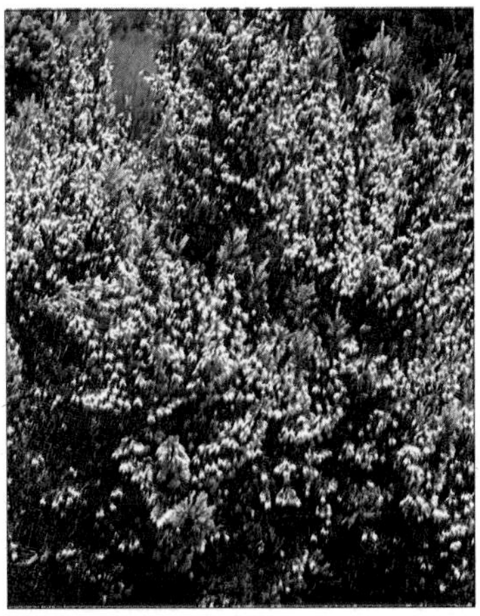

Erica x *veitchii* 'Exeter'

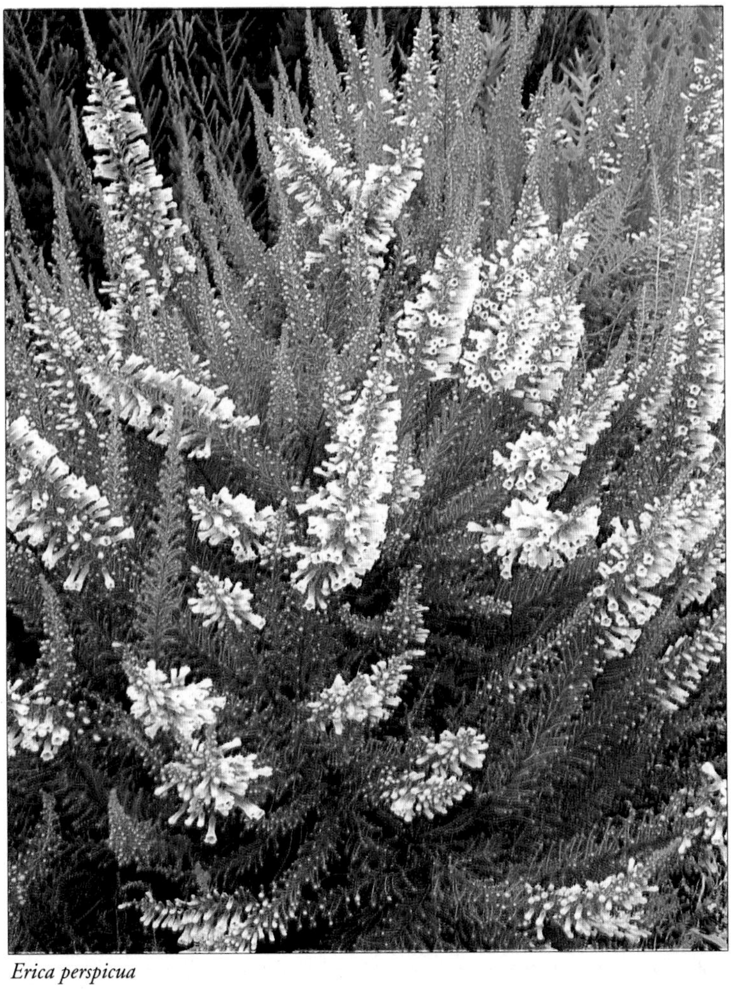

Erica perspicua

summer to mid-autumn. Grows in any well-drained soil. ↕ 40–80cm (16–32in), ↔ to 80cm (32in). Ireland, UK (Cornwall), W. France, Spain. ✻✻✻. **'Birch Glow'** ■♀ has deep rose-pink flowers; ↕ 30cm (12in), ↔ 50cm (20in). **'French White'** bears masses of off-white flowers; ↕ 40cm (16in), ↔ 60cm (24in). **'Lyonesse'** ■♀ has bright green leaves and pure white flowers; ↕ 25cm (10in), ↔ 50cm (20in). **'Mrs. D.F. Maxwell'** ■♀ bears deep rose-pink flowers; ↕ 30cm (12in), ↔ 45cm (18in). **'St. Keverne'** has clear pink flowers; ↕ 40cm (16in), ↔ 45cm (18in). **'Valerie Proudley'** ■♀ bears bright yellow foliage and white flowers; ↕ 15cm (6in), ↔ 30cm (12in).

***E.* 'Valerie Griffiths'.** Spreading shrub with linear, yellow leaves, deepening to golden yellow in winter. Bears racemes, 5–10cm (2–4in) long, of bell-shaped, pale pink flowers, to 4mm (⅛in) long, from summer to early autumn. Tolerates mildly alkaline soil. ↕ 40cm (16in), ↔ 55cm (22in). ✻✻✻

E.* x *veitchii (*E. arborea* x *E. lusitanica*) (Veitch's heath). Erect, open shrub with linear, mid-green leaves. From late winter to spring, bears leafy racemes, 30cm (12in) long, of cylindrical-spherical white flowers, to 4mm (⅛in) long. Tolerates mildly alkaline soil. ↕ to 2.2m (7ft), ↔ 65cm (26in). Garden origin. ✻✻. **'Albert's Gold'** see *E. arborea* 'Albert's Gold'. **'Exeter'** ■ bears masses of scented flowers in spring; ↕ 1.9m (6ft).

E. versicolor ■ Erect shrub with linear, mid-green leaves. Bears dense, spike-like racemes, 3cm (1¼in) long, of tubular flowers, 2–3cm (¼–1¼in) long, in whorls of 3, usually with red tubes and green to white tips; flowers mainly from autumn to early winter. ↕ to 3m (10ft), ↔ 1m (3ft). South Africa (Western Cape). ✻

***E. verticillata* of gardens** see *E. manipuliflora.*

E. vestita. Erect shrub with densely packed, linear, mid-green leaves. Bears spike-like racemes, 3cm (1¼in) long, of arching, tubular, red to dark pink, or white flowers, 1.5–2.5cm (½–1in) long, from spring to late summer. ↕↔ to 90cm (36in). South Africa (Western Cape). ✻

E. vulgaris see *Calluna vulgaris.*

E.* x *watsonii (*E. ciliaris* x *E. tetralix*) (Watson's heath). Compact, spreading shrub with linear, greyish green leaves. In summer, produces dense racemes, 1cm (½in) long, of urn-shaped pink flowers, to 1cm (½in) long, with constricted mouths. ↕ to 40cm (16in), ↔ to 85cm (34in). UK (Cornwall). ✻✻✻. **'Dawn'** ■♀ has red spring growth that turns golden, and bears deep pink flowers from midsummer to mid-autumn; ↕ 20cm (8in).

E.* x *williamsiana see *E.* x *williamsii.*

E.* x *williamsii (*E. tetralix* x *E. vagans*), syn. *E.* x *williamsiana* (Williams' heath). Decumbent to ascending shrub with linear, mid-green leaves, tipped bright yellow in spring. Bears dense racemes, 4cm (1½in) long, of bell-shaped, lilac-pink flowers, to 3mm (⅛in) long, from midsummer to late autumn. ↕ to 75cm (30in), ↔ 45cm (18in). UK (Cornwall). ✻✻✻. **'P.D. Williams'** ■♀ has yellow-tipped spring growth that lasts well into summer; ↕ to 30cm (12in).

E

ERIGERON

Fleabane

ASTERACEAE/COMPOSITAE

Genus of about 200 species of annuals, biennials, and perennials found in dry grassland and mountainous areas, with a very wide distribution, but occurring especially in North America. They range from low-growing alpine species to taller, bushy, clump-forming plants. All have simple, rarely lobed or dissected, usually oblong to lance-shaped or spoon-shaped, mainly basal leaves; the leaves on the stems are usually shorter and narrower. Leaf descriptions below are of basal leaves unless otherwise stated. Fleabanes are grown for their daisy-like, single to semi-double, mainly yellow-centred, white, pink, blue, or purple, sometimes yellow or orange flowerheads, which are borne singly or in corymbs over long periods, mainly in summer. Herbaceous hybrids have leaves 6–15cm (2½–6in) long, and flowerheads that are are mostly 4–6cm (1½–2½in) across. Grow in a mixed or herbaceous border, especially in a coastal or rock garden. The flowerheads last well as cut flowers if they are picked when fully open.

- **HARDINESS** Fully hardy.
- **CULTIVATION** Grow in fertile, well-drained soil that does not dry out in summer, in full sun with some midday shade. The smaller alpine species need sharp drainage and protection from excessive winter wet. Most taller species and hybrids need staking. Dead-head to encourage further flowering. Cut back to ground level in autumn to retain neat growth. Divide every 2 or 3 years (*E.* 'Dimity' every other year) in late spring, and discard the woody crowns.
- **PROPAGATION** Sow seed in containers in a cold frame in mid- or late spring. Divide, or root basal cuttings, in spring.
- **PESTS AND DISEASES** Powdery mildew affects some hybrids in dry conditions. *E. aurantiacus* is susceptible to slugs.

E. alpinus ■ Clump-forming perennial with narrowly elliptic to spoon-shaped, hairy leaves, to 8cm (3in) long. In summer, slender stems, to 20cm (8in) long, produce solitary, or groups of 2 or 3, lilac-blue to red-purple flowerheads, to 3.5cm (1½in) across, with yellow disc-florets. ↕ to 25cm (10in), ↔ to 20cm (8in). Mountains of C. and S. Europe. ❄❄❄

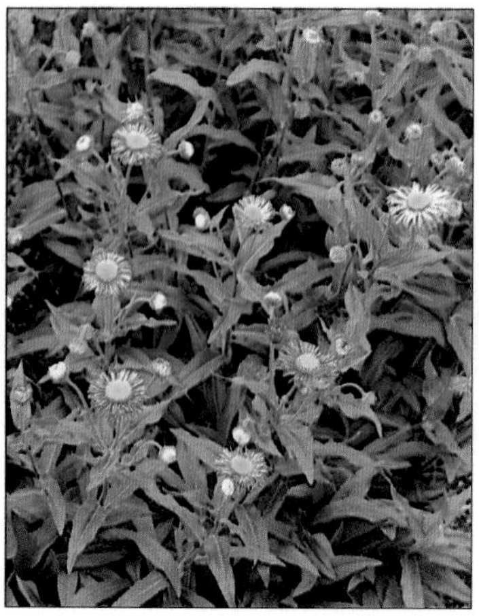

Erigeron alpinus

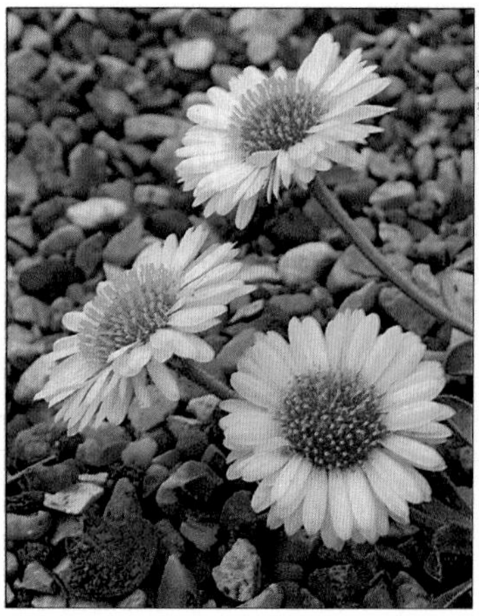

Erigeron aureus 'Canary Bird'

E. aurantiacus. Mat- to clump-forming perennial with elliptic to spoon-shaped, velvety leaves, to 10cm (4in) long. Over long periods in summer, stout, leafy stems produce solitary, brilliant orange flowerheads, to 5cm (2in) across, with yellow disc-florets. ↕↔ to 30cm (12in). Mountains of Turkestan. ❄❄❄

E. aureus. Short-lived, mound-forming perennial with tufts of broadly elliptic to spoon-shaped, hairy, grey-green leaves, to 8cm (3in) long. In summer, solitary, deep golden yellow flowerheads, 2cm (¾in) or more across, are produced on stems 5cm (2in) long. ↕ 5–10cm (2–4in), rarely to 20cm (8in), ↔ to 15cm (6in). Mountains of W. North America. ❄❄❄. **'Canary Bird'** ■ is a longer-lived perennial, and produces bright canary-yellow flowerheads; ↕ to 10cm (4in).

***E.* 'Azure Fairy'** see *E.* 'Azurfee'.

***E.* 'Azurfee'**, syn. 'Azure Fairy'. Clump-forming perennial with inversely lance-shaped leaves. Produces corymbs of semi-double, yellow-centred, lavender-blue flowerheads in early and mid-summer. ↕↔ 45cm (18in). ❄❄❄

***E.* 'Black Sea'** see *E.* 'Schwarzes Meer'.

***E.* 'Charity'** ■ Clump-forming perennial with lance-shaped leaves. In early and midsummer, semi-double, yellow-centred, light lilac-pink flower-heads are produced singly or in groups of 2 or 3. ↕ 60cm (24in), ↔ 45cm (18in). ❄❄❄

***E. chrysopsidis* 'Grand Ridge'** 🏆 Dense, mat- to hummock-forming perennial with linear, grey-green leaves, 2–8cm (¾–3in) long. Masses of short-stemmed, deep yellow flowerheads, 3–5cm (1¼–2in) across, are borne, usually singly, over very long periods in summer. ↕ to 5cm (2in), ↔ to 20cm (8in). ❄❄❄

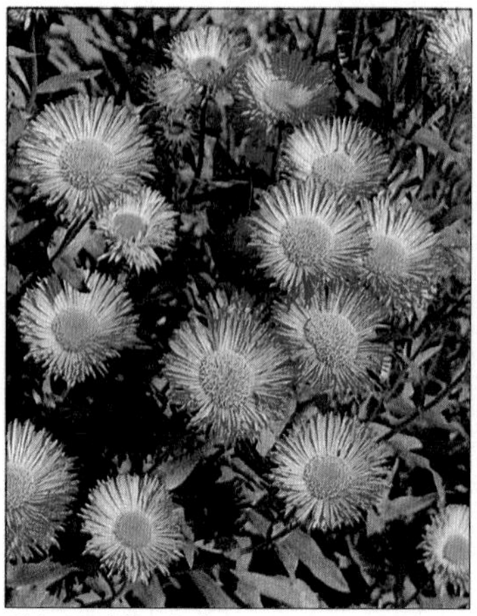

Erigeron 'Charity'

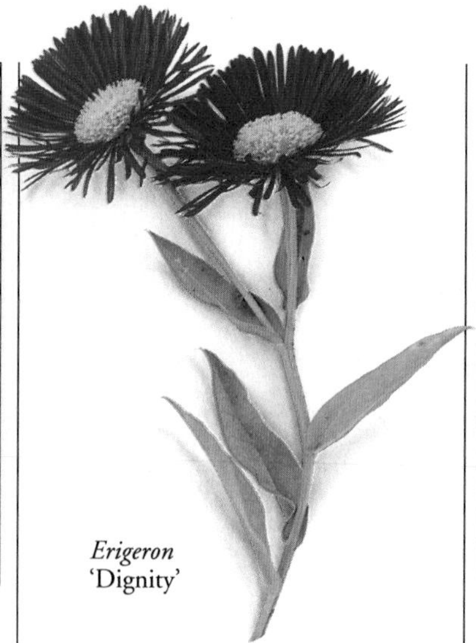

Erigeron 'Dignity'

E. compositus. Tufted, loose cushion-forming perennial with fan-shaped, 3- or 4-ternate, lobed or dissected, hairy, grey-green leaves, 2–6cm (¾–2½in) long. In summer, bears solitary, yellow-centred, white, pink, or very pale blue flowerheads, to 2cm (¾in) across. May self-seed excessively. ↕ to 15cm (6in), ↔ to 10cm (4in). Greenland, Canada, W. North America. ❄❄❄

***E.* 'Darkest of All'** see *E.* 'Dunkelste Aller'.

***E.* 'Dignity'** ■ Clump-forming perennial with lance-shaped to spoon-shaped leaves. Solitary, yellow-centred, violet-mauve flowerheads are produced in early and midsummer. ↕ 50cm (20in), ↔ 45cm (18in). ❄❄❄

***E.* 'Dimity'.** Clump-forming perennial making a low mound of lance-shaped leaves. In early and midsummer, bears solitary, semi-double, orange-centred, bright pink flowerheads, with fine ray-florets, tinted orange in bud. ↕ 25cm (10in), ↔ 30cm (12in). ❄❄❄

***E.* 'Dunkelste Aller'** ■ 🏆 syn. *E.* 'Darkest of All'. Clump-forming perennial with lance-shaped, greyish green leaves. In early and midsummer, produces corymbs of semi-double, yellow-centred, dark violet flowerheads, with long ray-florets. ↕ 60cm (24in), ↔ 45cm (18in). ❄❄❄

***E.* 'Felicity'.** Clump-forming perennial with lance-shaped leaves. Produces corymbs of large, single, yellow-centred pink flowerheads in early and mid-summer. ↕ 60cm (24in), ↔ 50cm (20in).. ❄❄❄

***E.* 'Foersters Liebling'** 🏆 Clump-forming perennial with lance-shaped, greyish green leaves. Corymbs of semi-double, yellow-centred, deep reddish pink flowerheads, with numerous closely packed ray-florets, are produced in early and midsummer. ↕ 60cm (24in), ↔ 45cm (18in). ❄❄❄

***E.* 'Gaiety'** ■ Clump-forming perennial with lance-shaped leaves. Corymbs of semi-double, yellow-centred, bright pink flowerheads are produced very freely in early and midsummer. ↕ 60cm (24in), ↔ 45cm (18in). ❄❄❄

E. glaucus (Beach aster). Tufted perennial with succulent-looking stems and inversely lance-shaped, obovate, or broadly spoon-shaped, more or less glaucous leaves, 12–15cm (5–6in) long, with blunt points. Semi-double flower-heads, 3.5–6cm (1½–2½in) across, with thin, pale mauve ray-florets and yellow, later brown disc-florets, are solitary or produced on sparsely branched stems, from late spring to midsummer. ↕ 30cm (12in), ↔ 45cm (18in). USA (Oregon, California). ❄❄❄. **'Elstead Pink'** ■ produces lilac-pink flowerheads.

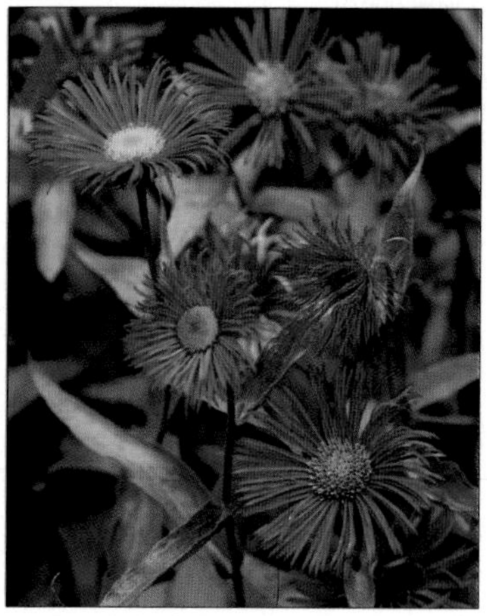

Erigeron 'Dunkelste Aller'

E. karvinskianus 🏆 syn. *E. mucronatus.* Carpeting, rhizomatous, woody-based, vigorously spreading perennial with lax, branching stems and elliptic-lance-shaped, hairy, grey-green leaves, to 4cm (1½in) long. In summer, produces abundant yellow-centred flowerheads, 2cm (¾in) across, either singly or in loose corymbs of 2–5, opening white and fading through pink to purple. Suitable for a wall or paving crevices. ↕ 15–30cm (6–12in), ↔ 1m (3ft) or more. Mexico to Panama. ❄❄❄. **'Profusion'** ■ is very floriferous, and bears flowerheads with pink or white ray-florets. Excellent for a hanging basket, window-box, or container. ↕ 20–30cm (8–12in), ↔ to 50cm (20in).

E. mucronatus see *E. karvinskianus.*

***E.* 'Pink Jewel'** see *E.* 'Rosa Juwel'.

E. pinnatisectus. Tufted perennial with linear, pinnatisect, hairy leaves, to 2cm (¾in) long. In summer, produces solitary, blue to purple flowerheads, 2.5cm (1in) or more across, with bright yellow to orange disc-florets. Suitable for a rock garden. ↕ to 20cm (8in), ↔ to 15cm (6in). C. USA. ❄❄❄

***E.* 'Prosperity'.** Erect, clump-forming perennial with lance-shaped leaves. Corymbs of almost double, yellow-centred, mauve-blue flowerheads are

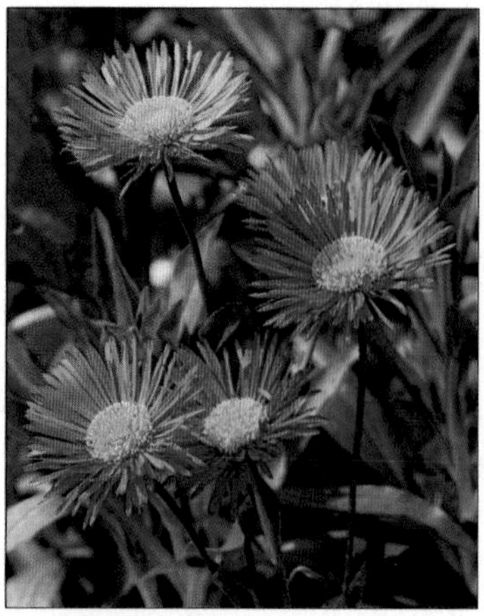

Erigeron 'Gaiety'

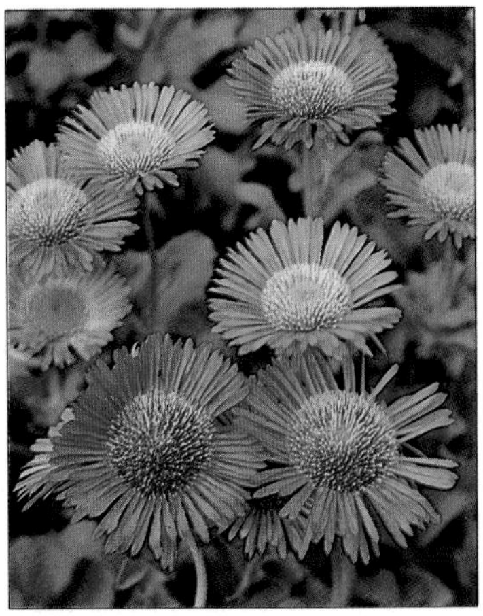

Erigeron glaucus 'Elstead Pink'

produced in early and midsummer. ↕↔ 45cm (18in). ✲✲✲
***E.* 'Quakeress'** ■ Strong-growing, clump-forming perennial with lance-shaped, greyish green leaves. Produces corymbs of single, yellow-centred, pink-flushed white flowerheads in early and midsummer. ↕ 60cm (24in), ↔ 45cm (18in). ✲✲✲
***E.* 'Red Sea'** see *E.* 'Rotes Meer'.
***E.* 'Rosa Juwel'**, syn. *E.* 'Pink Jewel'. Clump-forming perennial with lance-shaped leaves. Corymbs of semi-double, yellow-centred, pale but bright pink flowerheads are produced in early and midsummer. ↕ 60cm (24in), ↔ 45cm (18in). ✲✲✲
***E.* 'Rotes Meer'**, syn. *E.* 'Red Sea'. Upright, clump-forming perennial with spoon-shaped leaves. Corymbs of semi-double, deep dark red flowerheads are produced in midsummer. ↕↔ 60cm (24in). ✲✲✲
***E.* 'Schwarzes Meer'**, syn. *E.* 'Black Sea'. Clump-forming perennial with lance-shaped leaves. Bears corymbs of semi-double, yellow-centred, deep violet flowerheads in early and midsummer. ↕ 60cm (24in), ↔ 45cm (18in). ✲✲✲
***E.* 'Serenity'** ■ Somewhat lax, clump-forming perennial with lance-shaped leaves. Produces corymbs of semi-double, yellow-centred, violet-mauve flowerheads in early and midsummer. ↕ 75cm (30in), ↔ 45cm (18in). ✲✲✲
E. speciosus. Clump-forming perennial with mostly hairless leaves, to 15cm (6in) long, with fringed, hairy margins; the basal leaves are inversely lance-shaped to inversely spoon-shaped, the stem leaves are lance-shaped to ovate. In

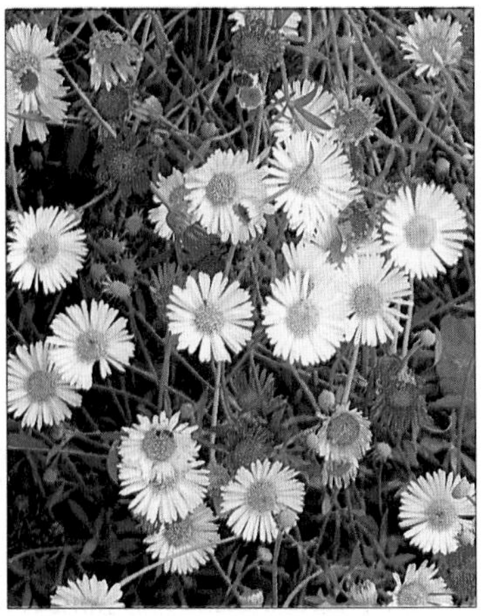

Erigeron karvinskianus 'Profusion'

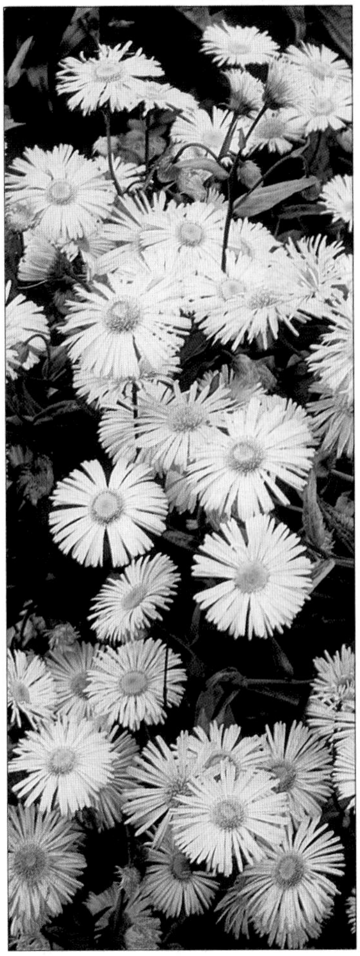

Erigeron 'Quakeress'

early and midsummer, produces yellow-centred, lavender-blue to lilac flowerheads, 4cm (1½in) across, in corymbs to 10cm (4in) across. ↕↔ 60cm (24in). Canada to N.W. USA. ✲✲✲
E. uniflorus. Clump-forming perennial with spoon-shaped, initially sparsely hairy leaves, to 5cm (2in) long. From summer to early autumn, produces solitary, white to pale lilac flowerheads, 1.5cm (½in) across. Suitable for a rock garden. ↕ to 15cm (6in), ↔ to 10cm (4in). Mountains of N. Europe, N. Asia, North America. ✲✲✲
***E.* 'Wuppertal'.** Clump-forming perennial with lance-shaped leaves. Produces corymbs of semi-double, yellow-centred, dark lilac flowerheads in early and midsummer. ↕ 60cm (24in), ↔ 45cm (18in). ✲✲✲

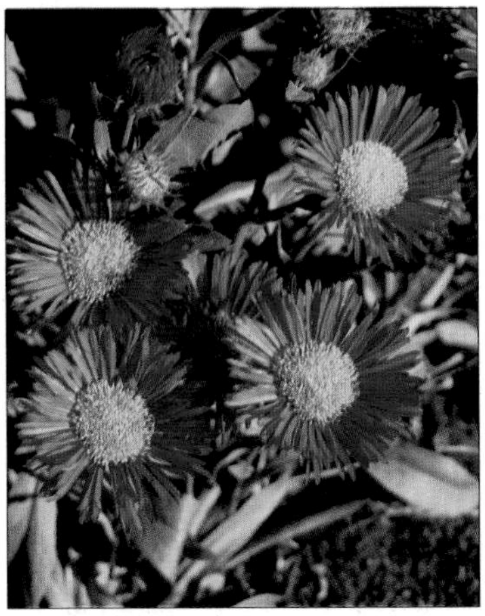

Erigeron 'Serenity'

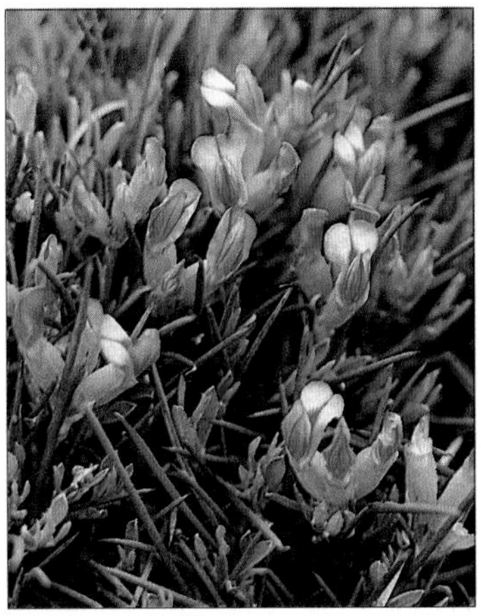

Erinacea anthyllis

ERINACEA

LEGUMINOSAE/PAPILIONACEAE

Genus of one species of dense, compact, evergreen subshrub from exposed, stony habitats in calcareous mountains in S.W. Europe and Morocco. It has stiff, sharp spines, simple or 3-palmate leaves, and axillary, pea-like, 2-lipped flowers. Long-lived and slow-growing, it flowers in profusion once established. Grow in a rock garden, scree bed, or raised bed.
• **HARDINESS** Fully hardy.
• **CULTIVATION** Grow in deep, gritty, sharply drained soil in full sun.
• **PROPAGATION** Sow seed in containers in an open frame in autumn. Root greenwood cuttings in late spring or early summer.
• **PESTS AND DISEASES** May be infested by red spider mites under glass.

E. anthyllis ■ 🏆 syn. *E. pungens* (Hedgehog broom). Mound-forming subshrub with spine-tipped, intricately branching stems and simple or 3-palmate, dark grey-green leaves, to 1cm (½in) long, with inversely lance-shaped leaflets. In late spring and early summer, bears clusters of 2–4 violet-blue flowers, to 2cm (¾in) long, with white-marked standard petals. ↕ to 30cm (12in), ↔ to 1m (3ft). E. Pyrenees to W. Mediterranean, Morocco. ✲✲✲
E. pungens see *E. anthyllis.*

ERINUS

Fairy foxglove

SCROPHULARIACEAE

Genus of 2 species of semi-evergreen perennials with rosettes of inversely lance-shaped to wedge-shaped, toothed leaves and terminal racemes of tubular flowers with 5 spreading lobes. Growing wild in rocky mountains in North Africa and C. and S. Europe, they are ideal for a rock garden, a wall, or paving crevices.
• **HARDINESS** Fully hardy.
• **CULTIVATION** Grow in light to moderately fertile, well-drained soil in full sun or partial shade.
• **PROPAGATION** Sow seed *in situ* or in containers in an open frame in autumn. Frequently self-seeds. Root rosettes as cuttings in spring.
• **PESTS AND DISEASES** Trouble free.

E. alpinus ■ 🏆 Short-lived, tufted perennial with inversely lance-shaped to wedge-shaped, sticky leaves, 0.5–2cm

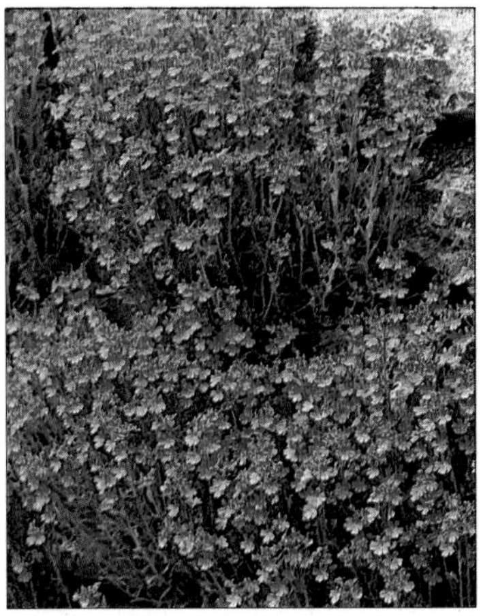

Erinus alpinus

(¼–¾in) long. Bears short racemes of 2-lipped, pink, purple, or white flowers, to 1cm (½in) across, from late spring to summer. ↕ 8cm (3in), ↔ 10cm (4in). C. and S. Europe. ✲✲✲. **'Dr. Hähnle'** has deep crimson flowers.

ERIOBOTRYA

ROSACEAE

Genus of about 30 species of evergreen shrubs and trees from woodland in the Himalayas and E. Asia. They have alternate, simple, lance-shaped to broadly elliptic, often toothed, leathery leaves and small, 5-petalled flowers in broad, pyramidal panicles. In frost-prone areas, grow in a cool greenhouse; frost-hardy species may also be grown against a sunny wall. In warmer areas, grow as specimens. *E. japonica* is also grown commercially for its fruit.
• **HARDINESS** Frost hardy to frost tender.
• **CULTIVATION** Under glass, grow in loam-based potting compost (JI No.3) in full light, with good ventilation. In growth, water moderately and apply a balanced liquid fertilizer monthly; water sparingly in winter. Outdoors, grow in fertile, well-drained soil in a sheltered site in full sun. Pruning group 1; may need restrictive pruning under glass.
• **PROPAGATION** Sow seed at 13–16°C (55–61°F) in spring. Insert semi-ripe cuttings in summer.
• **PESTS AND DISEASES** Susceptible to mealybugs and leaf blight under glass.

E. japonica ■ 🏆 ◯ (Loquat). Vigorous, spreading shrub or tree with stout shoots and bold, inversely lance-shaped to

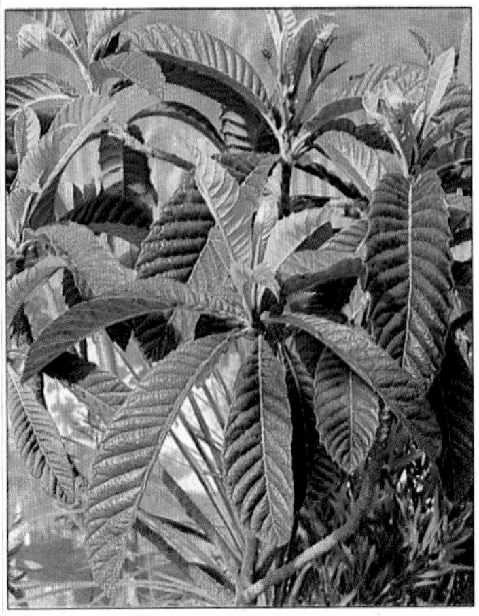

Eriobotrya japonica

narrowly obovate, sharp-pointed, strongly veined, dark green leaves, to 30cm (12in) long, glossy above. Bears large panicles of fragrant white flowers from autumn to winter, followed in spring by spherical to pear-shaped, edible, orange-yellow fruit, 4cm (1½in) across. ↕↔ 8m (25ft). China, Japan. ❄❄

▷ ***Eriocactus*** see *Parodia*
E. apricus see *P. concinna*
E. leninghausii see *P. leninghausii*
▷ ***Eriocereus jusbertii*** see *Harrisia jusbertii*
▷ ***Eriocereus martianus*** see *Aporocactus martianus*
▷ ***Eriocereus pomanensis*** see *Harrisia bonplandii*

E

ERIOGONUM

St. Catherine's lace, Wild buckwheat

POLYGONACEAE

Genus of approximately 150 species of annuals, perennials, and evergreen shrubs and subshrubs, occurring mostly in desert and mountains in W. USA. They are cultivated for their beautiful, often white-woolly foliage and their dense heads, umbels, or cymes of small, long-lasting flowers, cupped in involucres of toothed or lobed bracts. They range from compact, cushion-forming plants with linear to ovate or rounded leaves in basal rosettes, to large shrubs with opposite, alternate, or whorled leaves. Grow the smaller, rosette-forming species in a rock garden or alpine house, the larger ones in a shrub border. In frost-prone areas, grow tender species in a cool greenhouse or conservatory.

• **HARDINESS** Fully hardy to frost tender.

• **CULTIVATION** Under glass, grow in a mix of equal parts loam-based potting compost (JI No.1) and grit, in full light. In growth, water moderately and apply a balanced liquid fertilizer monthly; water sparingly at other times. Outdoors, grow in poor to gritty, moderately fertile, sharply drained soil in full sun; protect from winter wet. Dead-head unless seed is required. In an alpine house, grow in 1 part leaf mould and 2 parts each loam and grit or sharp sand. Pruning group 1.

• **PROPAGATION** Sow seed of hardy species in containers in an open frame in autumn. Sow seed of tender species in spring at 13–16°C (55–61°F). Root individual rosettes of cushion-forming species as cuttings in spring or early summer. Water only from below. Root semi-ripe cuttings of shrubs in summer.

• **PESTS AND DISEASES** Prone to aphids and red spider mites under glass.

E. arborescens ■ Domed, loose or open shrub with oblong or linear leaves, 2–3cm (¾–1¼in) long, borne in tufts at the ends of the branches; leaves are smooth and mid- to deep green above, densely white-woolly beneath, with margins rolled under. From early summer to autumn, produces dense, terminal cymes, 5–15cm (2–6in) across, of white to pale pink flowers. ↕↔ 0.6–1.5m (2–5ft). USA (California). ❀ (min. 5°C/41°F)

E. crocatum (Saffron buckwheat). Branching subshrub or woody-based perennial with broadly ovate to elliptic, white-felted, mid-green leaves, to 3.5cm (1½in) long. In late spring and early

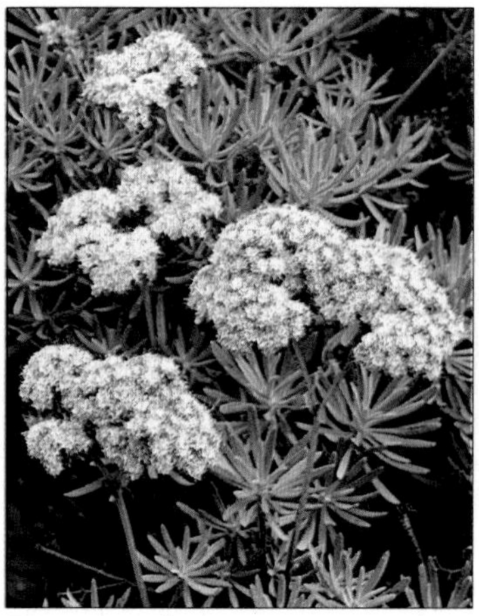

Eriogonum arborescens

summer, bears tiny, bright yellowish green flowers in dense cymes, to 8cm (3in) across. Best in an alpine house. ↕ 30–40cm (12–16in), ↔ to 40cm (16in). USA (California). ❄❄

E. fasciculatum. Rounded shrub with spreading branches that bear tufts of narrowly oblong to linear-lance-shaped leaves, 0.5–1.5cm (¼–½in) long, deep green above, white-woolly beneath, with inrolled margins. White, sometimes pink-tinted flowers are produced in loose, terminal heads, 3–10cm (1¼–4in) across, in summer. ↕ 30–60cm (12–24in), ↔ 90cm (36in). USA (California, Nevada, Utah). ❄❄

E. giganteum (St. Catherine's lace). Freely branching, rounded shrub with oblong to oblong-ovate, leathery leaves, 3–10cm (1¼–4in) long, densely white-downy beneath, smoother and grey above, mainly grouped towards the stem tips. In summer, produces heads of small white flowers in dense cymes, 20–30cm (8–12in) across. ↕↔ 1–2m (3–6ft). S.W. USA (Santa Catalina and adjacent islands). ❀ (min. 5°C/41°F)

E. gracilipes, syn. *E. kennedyi* subsp. *gracilipes* (Sulphur flower). Woody-based, mat-forming perennial with oval to oval-lance-shaped, white-woolly, greenish grey leaves, to 8mm (⅜in) long, with margins rolled under. In early and midsummer, umbels, to 1cm (½in) across, of pink-tinted white flowers that darken with age are borne on stems to 10cm (4in) long. Best in a scree bed or alpine house. ↕ to 8cm (3in), ↔ to 12cm (5in). USA (Sierra Nevada). ❄❄❄

E. kennedyi* subsp. *gracilipes see *E. gracilipes.*

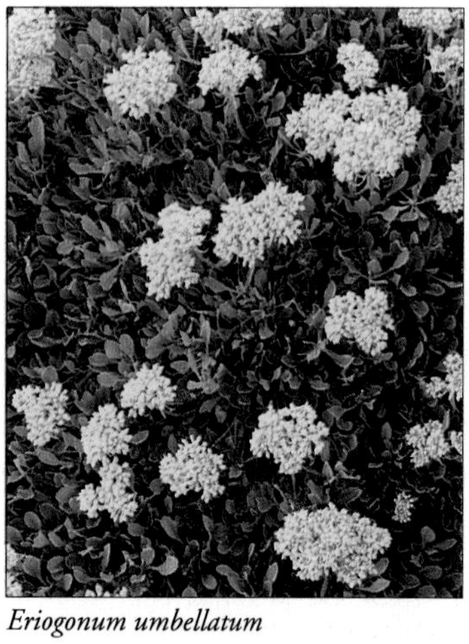

Eriogonum umbellatum

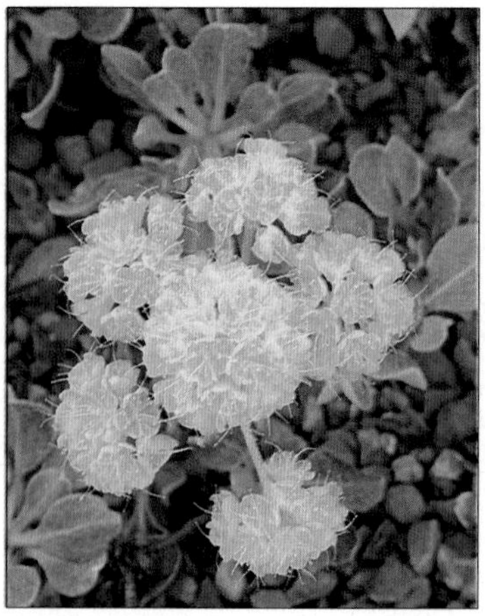

Eriogonum umbellatum var. *torreyanum*

E. ovalifolium. Cushion- or mat-forming, woody-based perennial with long-stalked, spoon-shaped, silver-hairy leaves, 0.5–1.5cm (¼–½in) long. In summer, stems, to 20cm (8in) long, bear dense, spherical heads, to 2cm (¾in) across, of cream or yellow flowers, sometimes maturing to pink-purple. Suitable for an alpine house. ↕ to 5cm (2in), ↔ to 20cm (8in). USA (Oregon to Nevada). ❄❄❄

E. torreyanum see *E. umbellatum* var. *torreyanum.*

E. umbellatum ■ (Sulphur flower). Spreading, mat-forming perennial or subshrub with rosettes of spoon-shaped or ovate leaves, to 2cm (¾in) long, mid-green above, white-woolly beneath. In mid- and late summer, produces umbels, 3–6cm (1¼–2½in) across, of cream to sulphur-yellow flowers that become tinted copper-red with age, on stems to 25cm (10in) long. Not always free-flowering. ↕ to 30cm (12in), ↔ to 1m (3ft). S.W. Canada to USA (E. Rocky Mountains). ❄❄❄. **var. *torreyanum*** ■ syn. *E. torreyanum,* is a long-lived, upright, domed shrub with hairless, dark green leaves. In mid-summer, produces abundant, noticeably bracted, bright yellow flowerheads on stems 5–10cm (2–4in) long. USA (S. Oregon to N. California).

ERIOPHORUM

Cotton grass

CYPERACEAE

Genus of 20 species of rapidly spreading, evergreen, rhizomatous, bog, marsh, or marginal aquatic perennials found in Europe, southern Africa, and North America. They have slender, needle-like, tough leaves, and produce tufted umbels of many-flowered spikelets in summer. Effective beside a wildlife pool or in a bog garden.

• **HARDINESS** Fully hardy.

• **CULTIVATION** Grow in acid soil alongside shallow water, or in an aquatic planting basket of peaty soil in a small pool, in full sun and with ample room. Capable of surviving in water to 5cm (2in) deep.

• **PROPAGATION** Divide established clumps in spring.

• **PESTS AND DISEASES** Trouble free.

E. angustifolium ■ (Common cotton grass). Marginal aquatic perennial with a long rootstock, short, distinctly angled stems, and linear, grooved, mainly basal

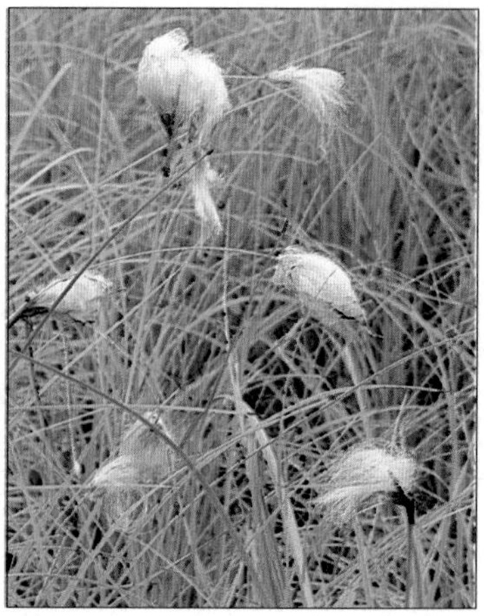

Eriophorum angustifolium

leaves, 15–30cm (6–12in) long, with long, sharp-pointed tips. In summer, produces umbels of 3–7 pendent, downy, tufted white spikelets, 3–5cm (1¼–2in) across. ↕ 30–45cm (12–18in), sometimes to 75cm (30in), ↔ indefinite. N. Europe (including Arctic), Russia (Siberia), North America. ❄❄❄

E. latifolium (Broad-leaved cotton grass). Marginal aquatic perennial with tufted rhizomes, 3-angled stems, and linear, flat, grooved, mainly basal leaves, 20–40cm (8–16in) long, with long, sharp-pointed tips. In summer, produces umbels of 3–7 pendent, tufted, downy white spikelets, 3–5cm (1¼–2in) across, with purplish green scales. Similar to *E. angustifolium,* but has broader leaves. ↕ 30–45cm (12–18in), ↔ indefinite. Europe, Turkey, Russia (Siberia), North America. ❄❄❄

ERIOPHYLLUM

Golden yarrow, Woolly sunflower

ASTERACEAE/COMPOSITAE

Genus of about 12 species of annuals, perennials, and subshrubs occurring mostly in open, sandy scrub, often in mountainous areas, in W. North America. They have alternate, deeply toothed or pinnatifid, white-hairy leaves, and bear cymes or corymbs of daisy-like flowerheads on upright stems, mainly in summer. Grow in a rock garden, at the front of a border, on a dry wall, or in paving crevices. *E. lanatum* may overwhelm smaller alpines and should be sited with care.

• **HARDINESS** Fully hardy to frost hardy.

• **CULTIVATION** Grow in light, poor to moderately fertile, sharply drained soil in full sun. Cut back after flowering to keep compact.

• **PROPAGATION** Sow seed in containers in an open frame in autumn, or divide in spring.

• **PESTS AND DISEASES** Susceptible to slugs and snails; birds use the foliage as nesting material.

E. lanatum ■ Variable, vigorous, clump-forming perennial with erect or decumbent stems and white-woolly, silvery grey leaves. The basal leaves, to 8cm (3in) long, are spoon-shaped to inversely lance-shaped, and entire or lobed; the smaller stem leaves are pinnatifid, or narrow and entire. Bears a succession of daisy-like, bright yellow flowerheads, 2–4cm (¾–1½in) across, singly or in loose corymbs, over long

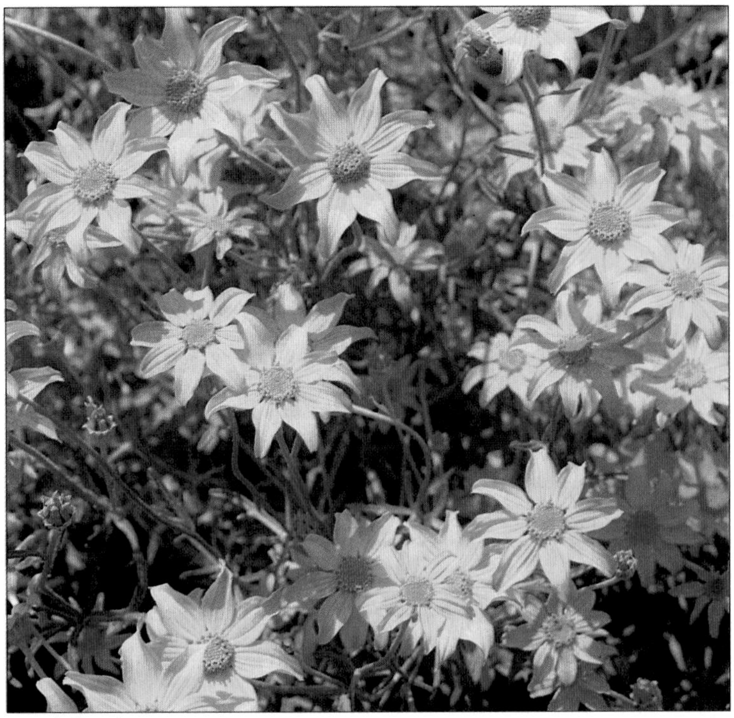

Eriophyllum lanatum

periods from late spring to summer. Drought-tolerant. ↕↔ 20–60cm (8–24in), rarely to 90cm (36in). North America (British Columbia to N. California and W. Montana). ✻✻✻.
var. *monoense*, syn. *E. lutescens,* is almost cushion-forming, with spoon-shaped, entire or 3-toothed leaves, to 2cm (¾in) long. Best variant for a rock garden; ↕ to 25cm (10in), ↔ to 1m (3ft). USA (California, Nevada, Wyoming).
E. lutescens see *E. lanatum* var. *monoense.*

ERIOSTEMON
Waxflower

RUTACEAE

Genus of 33 species of evergreen shrubs or small trees from open, rocky slopes, scrub, and open forest in Australia. They are grown mainly for their star-shaped, usually 5-petalled, waxy, white, pink to red, blue, or mauve flowers, which are solitary or borne in terminal or axillary racemes or cymes. The leaves are alternate, flat to cylindrical, linear to rounded, often warty, and strongly aromatic. In frost-prone areas, grow in a cool greenhouse; elsewhere, plant in a shrub border or against a house wall.
• **HARDINESS** Half hardy to frost tender; *E. australasius* and *E. myoporoides* may survive short periods of light frost, if growth is well ripened in summer.
• **CULTIVATION** Under glass, grow in lime-free (ericaceous) potting compost in full light. During the growing season, water freely and apply a low-phosphate liquid fertilizer monthly; water sparingly in winter. Top-dress or pot on in spring. Outdoors, grow in fertile, moist soil in full sun. Pruning group 1; may need restrictive pruning under glass.
• **PROPAGATION** Sow pre-soaked seed at 10–13°C (50–55°F) in spring. Root semi-ripe cuttings in summer with bottom heat. Germination is often erratic and rooting of cuttings slow.
• **PESTS AND DISEASES** Scale insects may be a problem.

E. australasius (Pink wax flower). Erect, freely branching shrub with angular, minutely hairy stems and narrowly elliptic or oblong to obovate, nearly hairless, glandular, leathery leaves, to 7cm (3in) long. From spring to autumn, bears solitary, pink to mauve-pink, sometimes white flowers, 4cm (1½in) wide, usually in profusion, at the shoot tips. ↕ 1–2m (3–6ft), ↔ 0.6–1.5m (2–5ft). Australia (Queensland to New South Wales). ✻ (borderline)
E. myoporoides (Long-leaf wax flower). Erect, bushy shrub with usually cylindrical, warty stems and elliptic or oblong to broadly obovate, warty leaves, 5–12cm (2–5in) long, deep green above, paler beneath. From autumn to spring or summer, pink buds open to white flowers, to 2.5cm (1in) across, borne in axillary cymes, to 10cm (4in) long. ↕ 1.5–5m (5–15ft), ↔ 1–2.5ft (3–8ft). Australia (Queensland to Victoria). ✻ (borderline). **'Clearview Pink'** has red flowerbuds and pink-tinted petals.
E. trachyphyllus ■ ◊ Bushy tree or shrub with cylindrical, hairless, warty stems. Elliptic to obovate-oblong leaves, to 5cm (2in) long, are thin, papery, hairless, and finely wrinkled. In winter or early spring, bears solitary white to pink flowers, 1.5cm (1½in) across, with fleshy, fringed sepals and long stamens, from the leaf axils. ↕ to 7m (22ft), ↔ 2.5m (8ft). Australia (New South Wales, Victoria). ❀ (min. 5°C/41°F)

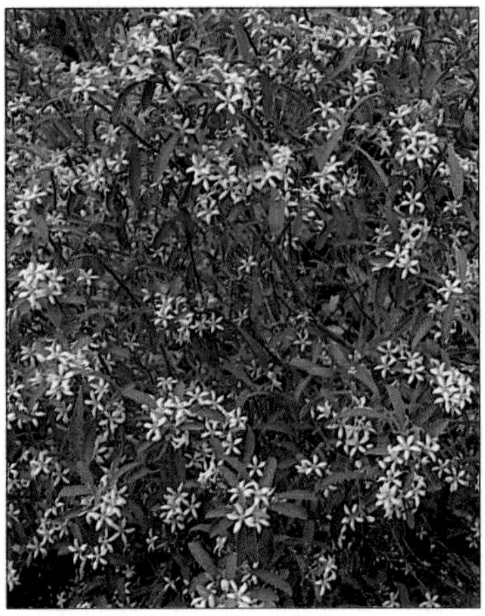

Eriostemon trachyphyllus

ERITRICHIUM
Alpine forget-me-not

BORAGINACEAE

Genus of approximately 30 species of low-growing, tufted or cushion-forming perennials found mostly in high-altitude scree and rock crevices in Europe, the Himalayas, and North America. They are grown mainly for their short, axillary or terminal, raceme-like cymes of blue, occasionally white flowers, similar to forget-me-nots (*Myosotis*), which are produced from spring to early summer. The leaves are alternate, usually elliptic to linear, softly hairy, and grey-green. *E. nanum* and the American cushion-forming species are very challenging container plants for an alpine house; other species may be grown in a scree bed or trough, or in tufa.
• **HARDINESS** Fully hardy.
• **CULTIVATION** In an alpine house, grow in a mix of 3 parts grit, 1 part loam, and 1 part leaf mould, with a deep collar of grit or pieces of rock wedged around the neck of the plants. Provide full light and good ventilation. Water freely during the growing season by immersing the containers to their rims in water; avoid wetting the foliage. Keep just moist in winter. Outdoors, grow in poor, sharply drained soil in full sun, with protection from winter wet.
• **PROPAGATION** Sow seed in containers in an open frame in autumn. Water seedlings very carefully from below. Root basal stem cuttings in summer.
• **PESTS AND DISEASES** Prone to aphids and red spider mites under glass.

E. canum, syn. *E. rupestre, E. sericeum, E. strictum.* Tufted perennial covered in silky hairs, with upright stems sparsely clothed in stalkless, lance-shaped to linear, grey-green leaves, 3–4cm (1¼–1½in) long. Broad, raceme-like cymes of short-tubed, salverform, pure soft blue flowers, to 7mm (¼in) across, are produced in summer. Self-seeds freely in scree. ↕ 15cm (6in), ↔ to 10cm (4in). W. Himalayas. ✻✻✻
E. nanum ■ Cushion-forming perennial with rosettes of elliptic or inversely lance-shaped to linear, densely silky-hairy, silvery grey-green leaves, to 1cm (½in) long. In late spring and early summer, short-tubed, salverform, yellow-eyed, azure-blue flowers, 5–8mm (¼–⅜in) across, are borne in raceme-like cymes. ↕ 5cm (2in), ↔ 7cm (3in). Alps, USA (Rocky Mountains). ✻✻✻
E. rupestre see *E. canum.*
E. sericeum see *E. canum.*
E. strictum see *E. canum.*

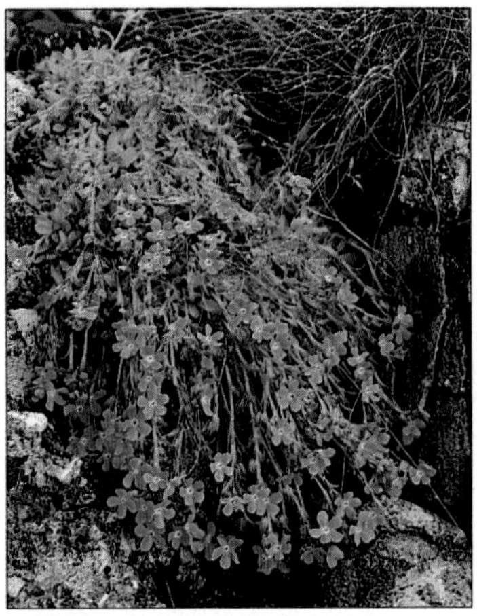

Eritrichium nanum

ERODIUM
Heron's bill, Stork's bill

GERANIACEAE

Genus of approximately 60 species of annuals, perennials, and evergreen and deciduous subshrubs occurring in rocky habitats, mainly in the calcareous mountains of Europe and C. Asia, but also in N. Africa, North and South America, and temperate Australia. They are valued for their attractive foliage and long flowering period. The leaves are opposite or alternate, and lobed, pinnate, or pinnatisect. In summer, the 5-petalled flowers are produced singly from the leaf axils or in terminal umbels; they range from pink to purple, occasionally yellow or white, and resemble *Geranium* flowers (except they have 5, not 10, stamens). Grow in a rock garden, trough, or alpine house; plant the taller and more robust species at the front of a herbaceous border.
• **HARDINESS** Fully hardy to frost hardy.
• **CULTIVATION** Grow in gritty, humus-rich, sharply drained, neutral to alkaline soil in full sun. Protect the smallest species from excessive winter wet. In an alpine house, grow in equal parts loam, leaf mould, and grit.
• **PROPAGATION** Sow seed in containers in an open frame as soon as ripe. Divide in spring. Root basal stem cuttings in late spring or early summer.
• **PESTS AND DISEASES** Trouble free.

E. chamaedryoides see *E. reichardii.*
***E. chamaedryoides* 'Roseum'** see *E.* x *variabile* 'Roseum'.
E. cheilanthifolium ■ syn. *E. petraeum* subsp. *crispum.* Compact, mound-forming perennial with ovate-oblong, 2-pinnatifid, crinkled, greyish green leaves, 2–5cm (¾–2in) long. In summer, bears umbels of up to 5 flat-faced, red-veined, pale pink or white flowers, to 2.5cm (1in) across, stained reddish purple at the bases of the 2 upper petals. ↕ to 20cm (8in), ↔ to 30cm (12in). S. Spain, North Africa. ✻✻✻

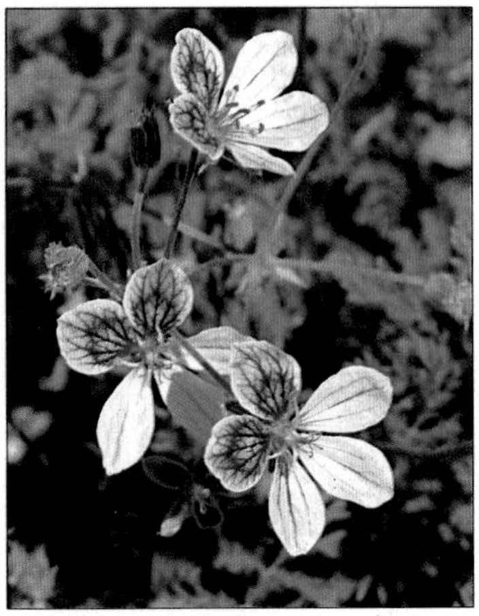

Erodium cheilanthifolium

E

E

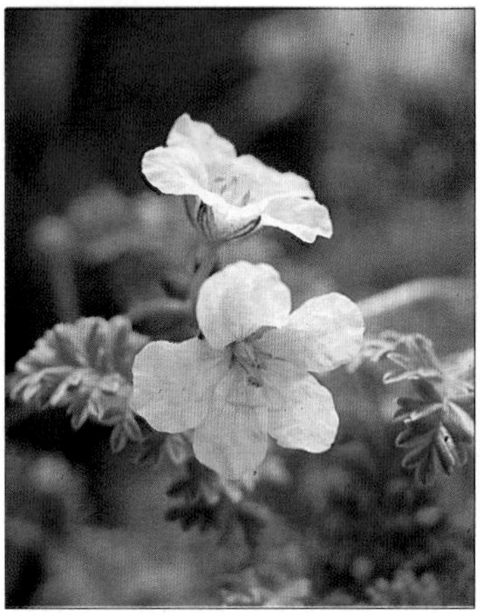
Erodium chrysanthum

E. chrysanthum ■ Dense, tufted, mound-forming perennial with ovate, 2-pinnate, finely dissected, silvery green leaves, to 3.5cm (1½in) long, each with oblong to lance-shaped leaflets. In summer, branching stems bear umbels of 2–7 saucer-shaped, sulphur-yellow, dioecious flowers, to 2cm (¾in) across. ↕ to 15cm (6in), ↔ to 40cm (16in). Greece. ✻✻✻
E. corsicum ■ Mat-forming perennial with ovate, crumpled, silver-downy, grey-green leaves, 1.5cm (½in) long, with scalloped margins. From late spring to summer, short, branched stems bear umbels of 1–3 saucer-shaped, rose-pink flowers, to 2cm (¾in) across, with darker veins. ↕ 8cm (3in), ↔ to 20cm (8in). Sea cliffs of Corsica and Sardinia. ✻✻✻ (borderline)

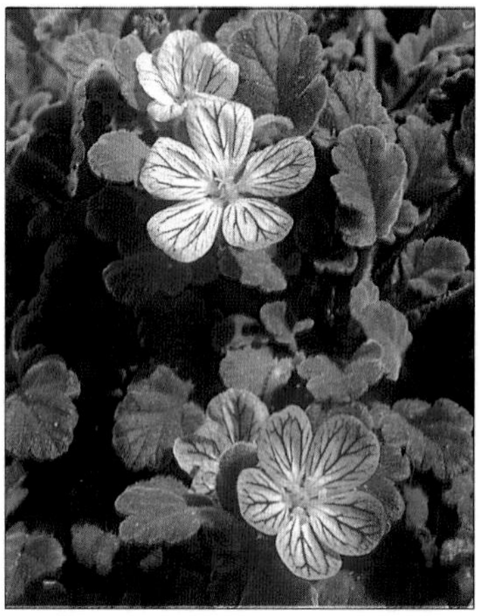
Erodium corsicum

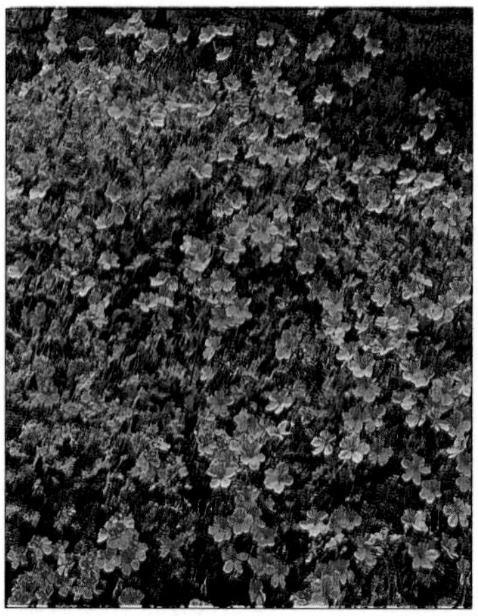
Erodium glandulosum

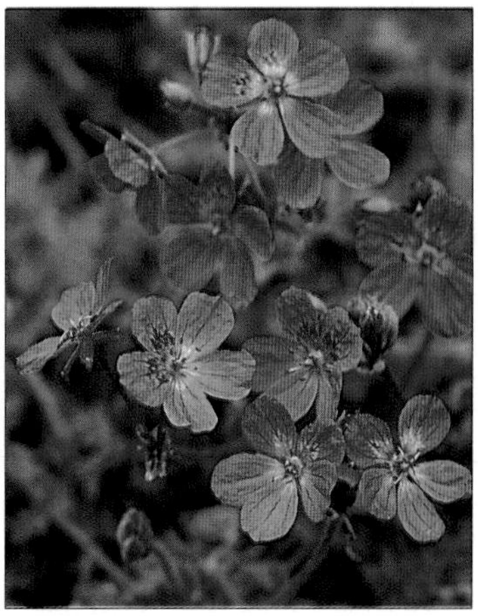
Erodium manescaui

E. glandulosum ■ ♀ syn. *E. macradenum*, *E. petraeum* subsp. *glandulosum*. Compact, tufted perennial bearing ovate-oblong, 2-pinnatifid, silvery, basal leaves, 4–10cm (1½–4in) long, with oblong to lance-shaped divisions. In summer, produces umbels of up to 5 saucer-shaped, lilac-pink flowers, to 2.5cm (1in) across, usually marked dark purple on the 2 upper petals. ↕ 10–20cm (4–8in), ↔ to 20cm (8in). Pyrenees, N. Spain. ✻✻✻
E. macradenum see *E. glandulosum*.
E. manescaui ■ syn. *E. manescavii*. Clump-forming perennial with pinnate, lance-shaped to ovate-lance-shaped, toothed, hairy, mid-green, basal leaves, to 30cm (12in) long, with ovate leaflets. Long-stalked umbels of 5–20 saucer-shaped, magenta-purple flowers, to 3cm (1¼in) across, with darker spots on the upper 2 petals, are profusely borne from early summer to early autumn. Self-seeds freely. ↕ 20–45cm (8–18in), ↔ 20cm (8in). Pyrenees. ✻✻✻
E. manescavii see *E. manescaui*.
E. petraeum* subsp. *crispum see *E. cheilanthifolium*.
E. petraeum* subsp. *glandulosum see *E. glandulosum*.
E. reichardii, syn. *E. chamaedryoides*. Mound-forming perennial with heart-shaped, scalloped, slightly downy, dark green leaves, to 1.5cm (½in) long. Bears solitary, saucer-shaped, red-veined white flowers, 8mm (⅜in) wide, on very short stems in summer. ↕ 5–7cm (2–3in), ↔ to 15cm (6in). Majorca, Corsica. ✻✻✻ (borderline)
E. x variabile (*E. corsicum* x *E. reichardii*). Spreading or cushion-forming perennial with ovate, scalloped or lobed, mid-green leaves, to 2cm (¾in) long, heart-shaped at the bases. In summer, bears solitary, single or double, deep red flowers, to 1cm (½in) across, veined maroon. ↕ to 12cm (5in), ↔ to 30cm (12in). Garden origin. ✻✻✻.
'Flore Pleno' has narrowly ovate, scalloped, dark to grey-green leaves, and rounded, double, deep pink flowers, with darker veining, from spring to autumn. **'Ken Aslet'** ■ has prostrate stems and single, deep pink flowers.
'Roseum' ♀ syn. *E. chamaedryoides* 'Roseum', has deep pink flowers with darker veining; ↕ to 8cm (3in).

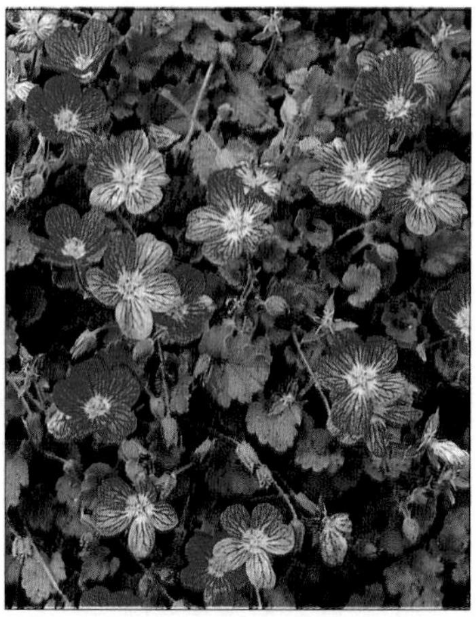
Erodium x *variabile* 'Ken Aslet'

▷ ***Erpetion*** see *Viola*
E. hederaceum see *V. hederacea*
E. reniforme see *V. hederacea*
▷ ***Ervatamia coronaria*** see *Tabernaemontana divaricata*

Eryngium

Eryngo, Sea holly

APIACEAE/UMBELLIFERAE

Genus of 230 species of hairless annuals, biennials, and deciduous and evergreen perennials. Those that are native to dry, rocky places and coastal areas in Europe, N. Africa, Turkey, C. Asia, China, and Korea usually have tap roots, ovate to heart-shaped, often divided leaves, and congested heads of blue or white flowers, with conspicuous bracts. Those that are from often wet and marshy grassland in Mexico, Brazil, Argentina, and warm-temperate regions of North, Central, and South America, usually have fibrous roots, sword-shaped, evergreen foliage, less showy, greenish white (occasionally purplish brown) flowers, and small bracts. Most eryngiums form basal rosettes, the leaves often spiny and with silvery white veins, and bear crowded, hemispherical to cylindrical, thistle-like umbels of stalkless flowers on branched stems.

Eryngiums are striking plants for naturalizing; some also provide long-lasting displays for a border. They may be dried for arrangements; cut the stems before the flowers are fully open.

• **Hardiness** Fully hardy to frost hardy; frost-hardy American species tolerate temperatures down to -10°C (14°F), although leaves may be damaged if temperatures drop below -7°C (19°F).
• **Cultivation** Eryngiums have varying cultivation requirements. For ease of reference, these have been grouped as follows:
1. Grow in dry, well-drained, poor to moderately fertile soil in full sun, with protection from winter wet.
2. Grow in moist, well-drained, fertile soil in full sun.
• **Propagation** Sow seed in containers in a cold frame as soon as ripe. Divide in spring, although they are slow to re-establish. Insert root cuttings of perennials in late winter.
• **Pests and diseases** Prone to root rot, slugs, snails, and powdery mildew.

E. agavifolium, syn. *E. bromeliifolium* of gardens. Rosette-forming, evergreen perennial with broadly sword-shaped, prominently and sharply toothed, glossy, deep green basal leaves, 40–75cm (16–30in) long. In late summer, lightly branched stems bear cylindrical umbels, 5cm (2in) long, of greenish white flowers, with entire to spiny-toothed bracts, 6mm (¼in) long. Cultivation group 2. ↕ 1–1.5m (3–5ft), ↔ 60cm (24in). Argentina. ✻✻
E. alpinum ■ ♀ Rosette-forming, tap-rooted herbaceous perennial with ovate to heart-shaped, spiny-toothed, mid-green basal leaves, 8–15cm (3–6in) long, and palmately 3-lobed stem leaves. From midsummer to early autumn, branched stems, steel-blue near the apex, bear cylindrical umbels, to 4cm (1½in) long, of steel-blue or white flowers, with pinnatifid, softly spiny bracts, to 6cm (2½in) long. Cultivation group 1, but soil not too dry. ↕ 70cm (28in), ↔ 45cm (18in). Europe (Jura, Alps, mountains of W. and C. Balkans). ✻✻✻.
'Amethyst' has smaller, violet-blue flowerheads, 2.5cm (1in) long.
E. amethystinum. Clump-forming, tap-rooted herbaceous perennial with obovate, pinnate, spiny, leathery, mid-green basal leaves, 10–15cm (4–6in) long, with oblong leaflets, and palmately 3-lobed upper leaves. In mid- and late summer, branching, silvery blue stems bear cylindrical umbels, 2–3cm (¾–1¼in) long, of steel-blue to amethyst flowers, with lance-shaped, spiny, silvery green bracts, to 5cm (2in) long. Cultivation group 1. ↕↔ 70cm (28in). Italy, Sicily, Balkans. ✻✻✻
E. bourgatii ■ Clump-forming, tap-rooted herbaceous perennial with rounded, pinnatifid or 2-pinnatifid, spiny, conspicuously silver-veined, dark green basal leaves, to 7cm (3in) long. In mid- and late summer, branching blue stems bear blue, or often grey-green

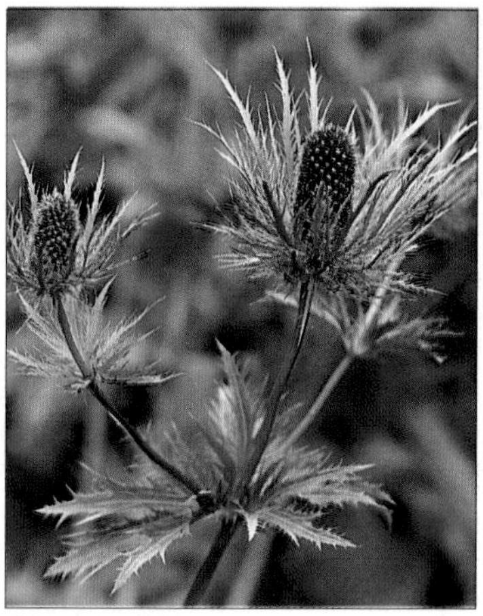
Eryngium alpinum

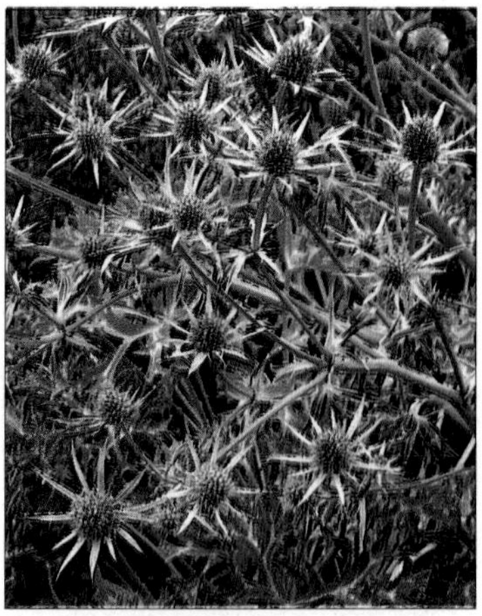
Eryngium bourgatii

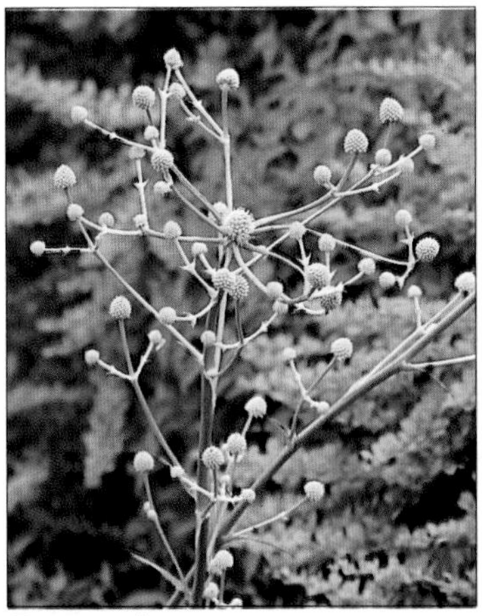
Eryngium eburneum

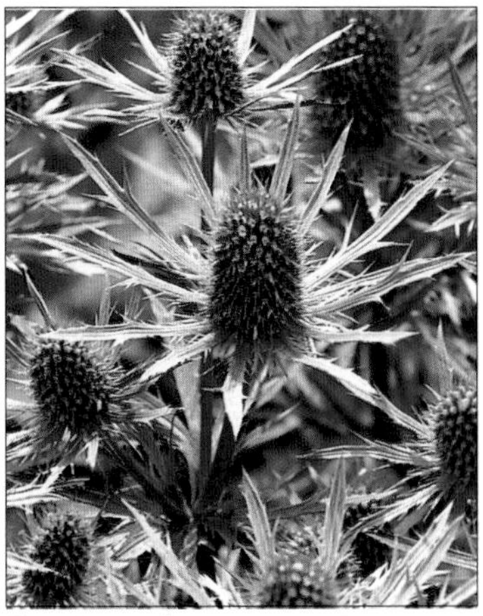
Eryngium x *oliverianum*

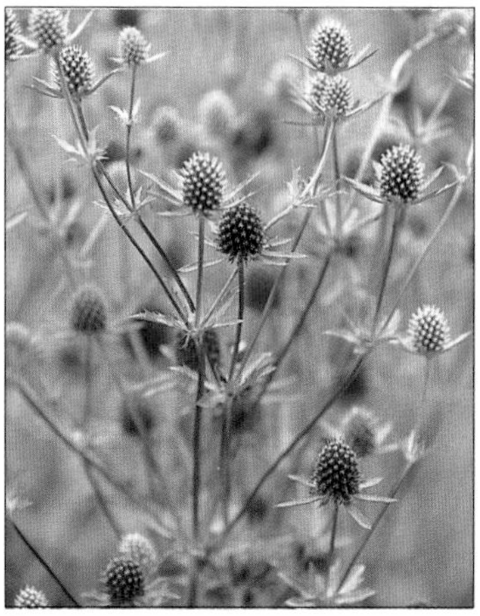
Eryngium x *tripartitum*

flowers in cylindrical umbels, 1–3cm (½–1¼in) long, with lance-shaped, blue-tinged, silver bracts, to 6cm (2½in) long. Cultivation group 1. ↕15–45cm (6–18in), ↔ 30cm (12in). Spain (Pyrenees). ❄❄❄. **'Oxford Blue'** ♀ has darker, silvery blue flowerheads.
***E. bromeliifolium* of gardens** see *E. agavifolium.*
E. decaisneanum see *E. pandanifolium.*
E. delaroux see *E. proteiflorum.*
E. eburneum ▣ syn. *E. paniculatum.* Clump-forming, evergreen perennial with narrowly linear, spiny-toothed, mid-green leaves, to 1m (3ft) long. In late summer, arching, branched, pale green stems bear groups of spherical-cylindrical umbels, 1–2cm (½–¾in) long, composed of whitish green flowers, with linear-lance-shaped, spine-tipped bracts, to 2cm (¾in) long. Cultivation group 2. ↕to 1.5m (5ft), ↔ 60cm (24in). Temperate South America. ❄❄
E. giganteum ▣ ♀ (Miss Willmott's ghost). Rosette-forming, tap-rooted, short-lived herbaceous perennial with heart-shaped, mid-green basal leaves, 7–16cm (3–6in) long, and ovate, sometimes lobed, scalloped to toothed, spiny stem leaves. In summer, branched inflorescences comprise cylindrical umbels, to 6cm (2½in) long, of initially pale green, then steel-blue flowers, with ovate, toothed, silvery grey bracts, to 6cm (2½in) long, both prickly. Cultivation group 1. ↕90cm (36in), ↔ 30cm (12in). Caucasus, Iran. ❄❄❄. **'Silver Ghost'** has narrower, very silvery white bracts; ↕to 60cm (24in).
E.* x *oliverianum ▣ ♀ (*E. alpinum* x *E. giganteum*). Clump-forming, tap-rooted herbaceous perennial with ovate, slightly 3-lobed, spiny-toothed, dark green basal leaves, 8–16cm (3–6in) long, with conspicuous veins and heart-shaped bases, and palmately 4- or 5-lobed stem leaves. From midsummer to early autumn, branched blue stems bear cylindrical umbels, 4cm (1½in) long, of flowers, with linear, spiny bracts, to 6cm (2½in) long, both bright silver-blue, sometimes tinted purple with age. Cultivation group 1. ↕90cm (36in), ↔ 45cm (18in). Garden origin. ❄❄❄
E. pandanifolium, syn. *E. decaisneanum.* Tufted, clump-forming, evergreen perennial with linear to sword-shaped, silvery green leaves, 1–2m (3–6ft) long, with slender marginal spines. Bears cylindrical umbels, 1cm (½in) long, of purplish brown flowers, with shorter, ovate bracts, 1.5cm (½in) long, from late summer to mid-autumn. Cultivation group 2. ↕to 4m (12ft), ↔ to 2m (6ft). Brazil to Argentina. ❄❄
E. paniculatum see *E. eburneum.*
E. planum. Clump-forming, tap-rooted, evergreen perennial with oblong to ovate-oblong, toothed, dark green basal leaves, 5–10cm (2–4in) long, with heart-shaped bases, spiny, palmately lobed, blue-tinted stem leaves; both are somewhat leathery. From midsummer to early autumn, strong, branching stems bear numerous spherical-cylindrical umbels, 1–2cm (½–¾in) long, of light blue flowers, with linear, spiky, blue-green bracts, 2.5cm (1in) long. Cultivation group 1. ↕90cm (36in), ↔ 45cm (18in). C. and S.E. Europe to C. Asia. ❄❄❄. **'Blauer Zwerg'**, syn. 'Blue Dwarf', has intense blue flowers; ↕to 50cm (20in).
E. proteiflorum ▣ syn. *E. delaroux.* Rosette-forming, tap-rooted, evergreen perennial with narrowly linear, spiny-margined, silvery green basal leaves, 10–30cm (4–12in) long, with white midribs. In early and mid-autumn, branching stems bear cylindrical umbels, 2.5–7cm (1–3in) long, of greyish blue flowers, with linear to lance-shaped, spiny-margined, silvery white bracts, to 10cm (4in) long. Cultivation group 1, or grow in a container. ↕90cm (36in), ↔ 60cm (24in). Mexico. ❄❄
E.* x *tripartitum ▣ ♀ Clump-forming, tap-rooted herbaceous perennial with narrowly ovate, 3-lobed, toothed, dark green leaves, 6–12cm (2½–5in) long, with a few marginal spines. From mid-summer to early autumn, many-branched stems bear spherical-cylindrical umbels, 1–2cm (½–¾in) long, of violet-blue flowers, with narrowly lance-shaped, grey-blue bracts, to 3.5cm (1½in) long. Cultivation group 1. ↕60–90cm (24–36in), ↔ 50cm (20in). Probably Mediterranean origin. ❄❄❄
E. variifolium ▣ Clump-forming, tap-rooted, evergreen perennial with rosettes of ovate, toothed, spiny, slightly fleshy, dark green leaves, 5cm (2in) long, heart-shaped at the bases and marbled with white veins that are broadest in the leaf centre. In mid- and late summer, stiff, branching stems bear cylindrical umbels, 3cm (1¼in) long, of grey-blue to pale blue flowers, with longer, sharply pointed, silvery white bracts, to 4cm (1½in) long. Suitable for a rock garden. Cultivation group 1, but soil not too dry. ↕30–40cm (12–16in), ↔ 25cm (10in). Morocco. ❄❄❄ (borderline)
E. yuccifolium. Rosetted, tap-rooted, evergreen perennial with sword-shaped, spiny-margined, blue-grey leaves, 20–100cm (8–39in) long. From mid-summer to early autumn, strong, lightly branched stems bear cylindrical umbels, 2–4cm (¾–1½in) long, of whitish green to pale blue flowers, with shorter, ovate, grey-green bracts, 9mm (⅜in) long. Cultivation group 1. ↕1.2m (4ft), ↔ 60cm (24in). S. and E. USA. ❄❄
E.* x *zabelii (*E. alpinum* x *E. bourgatii*). Clump-forming, tap-rooted, semi-evergreen perennial with heart-shaped, spiny-toothed, dark green basal leaves, 8–12cm (3–5in) long. Blue stems bear deeply 3-lobed leaves. In mid- and late summer, bears spherical-cylindrical umbels, 2–4cm (¾–1½in) across, of long-lasting, intense blue or violet flowers, with rigid, spiny-toothed, green-tipped blue bracts, 6cm (2½in) long. ↕60–75cm (24–30in), ↔ 45cm (18in). Garden origin. ❄❄❄. **'Violetta'** has umbels, to 5cm (2in) long, of violet-blue flowers and silvery blue bracts.

▷ **Eryngo** see *Eryngium*

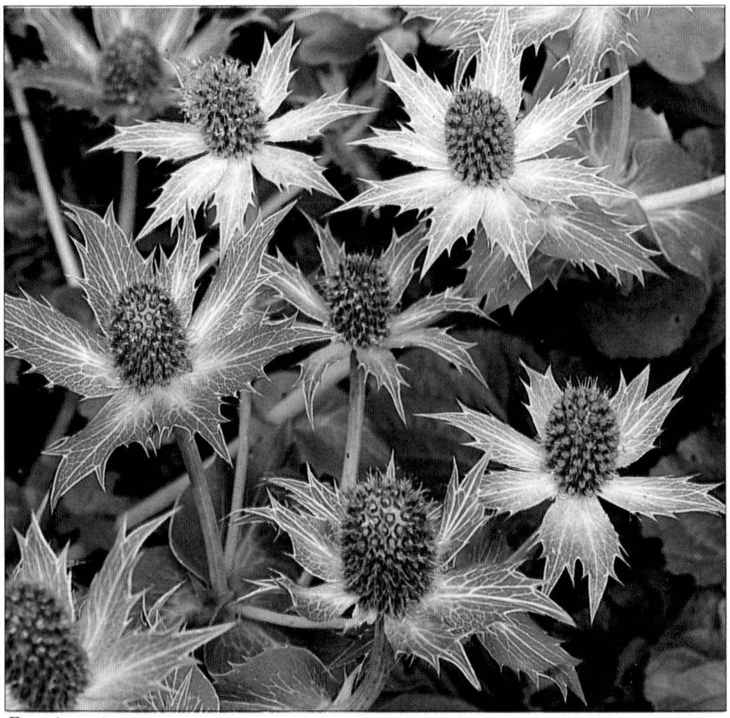
Eryngium giganteum

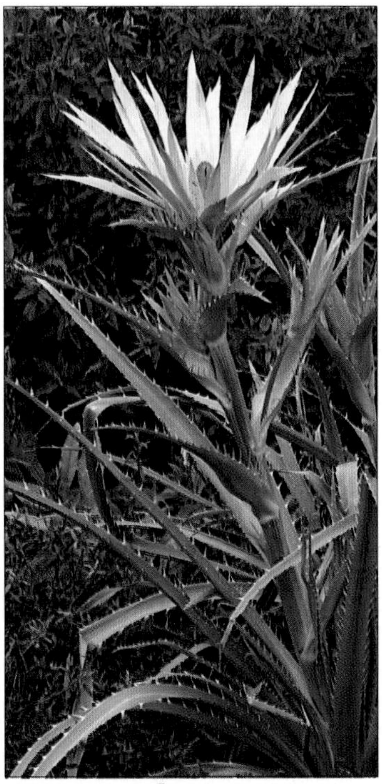
Eryngium proteiflorum

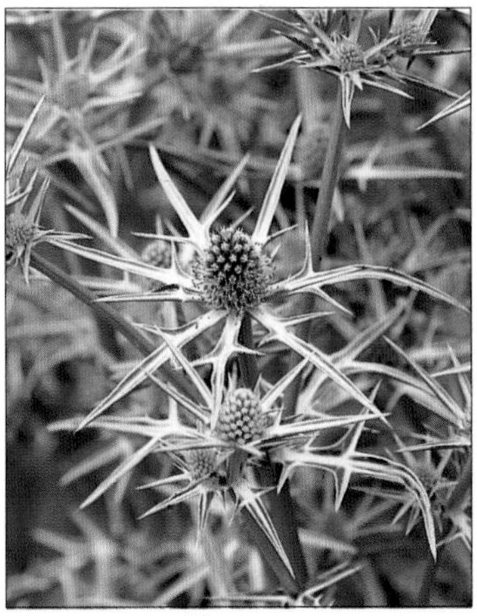
Eryngium variifolium

E

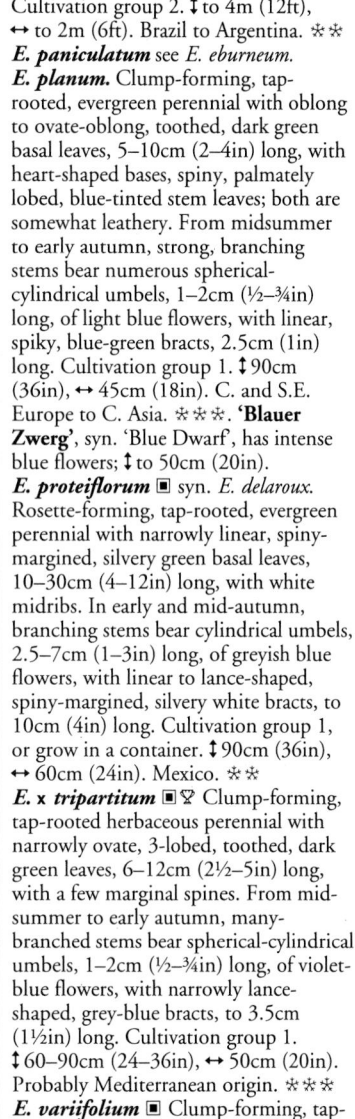

ERYSIMUM syn. CHEIRANTHUS

Wallflower

BRASSICACEAE/CRUCIFERAE

Genus, now including *Cheiranthus,* of about 80 species of annuals, biennials, and mainly evergreen perennials, often woody based, found mostly on well-drained, calcareous soil from Europe to N. Africa, W. and C. Asia, and N. America. They are cultivated for their often yellow flowers, to 2.5cm (1in) across, each with 4 petals arranged in a cross, borne in dense, usually elongating, corymb-like racemes. Most wallflowers produce inversely lance-shaped, toothed, softly hairy leaves, 3–12cm (1¼–5in) long. Many are ideal for a rock garden or wall, the front of a sunny border, or a raised bed. The biennials are popular as spring bedding plants or in a border.

- **HARDINESS** Fully hardy to frost hardy.
- **CULTIVATION** Grow in poor to moderately fertile, well-drained, neutral or, ideally, alkaline soil in full sun. Trim perennials lightly after flowering to prevent plants becoming leggy.
- **PROPAGATION** Sow seed of perennials in containers in a cold frame in spring. Take nodal or heeled softwood cuttings from shrubby perennials in spring or summer. Sow seed of biennials in a seedbed from late spring to early summer, grow on in a nursery bed, and transplant to flowering positions in mid-autumn. Provide cloche protection where frosts are severe or prolonged.
- **PESTS AND DISEASES** Susceptible to fungal and bacterial diseases including clubroot, mildew, leaf spot, root rot, and mosaic virus. May suffer damage from slugs, snails, and flea beetles.

E.* x *allionii ▣ 🏆 syn. *Cheiranthus* x *allionii* (Siberian wallflower). Tufted, short-lived, evergreen perennial, grown as a biennial, with lance-shaped, coarsely toothed leaves, to 8cm (3in) long. In spring, produces spice-scented, brilliant orange flowers, to 1cm (½in) across, in short racemes. ↕ 50–60cm (20–24in), ↔ to 30cm (12in). Garden origin. ❄❄❄

E. asperum (Western wallflower). Erect, rarely branched, short-lived, evergreen perennial or biennial with linear to lance-shaped, usually entire leaves, to 12cm (5in) long. From spring to early summer, bears short racemes of open, copper-yellow flowers, to 2.5cm (1in)

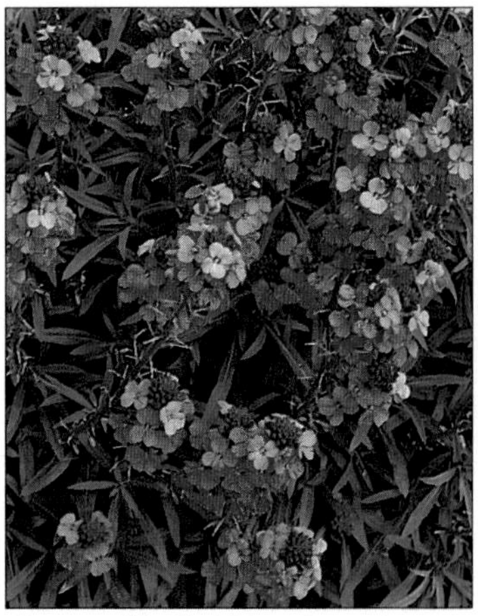

Erysimum 'Bowles' Mauve'

across. ↕ to 30cm (12in), ↔ to 25cm (10in). North America (British Columbia to Washington, Minnesota, Kansas). ❄❄❄

***E.* 'Bowles' Mauve'** ▣ 🏆 syn. *E.* 'E.A. Bowles'. Vigorous, subshrubby, evergreen perennial with narrowly lance-shaped, grey-green leaves. Bears mauve flowers, to 1.5cm (½in) across, in long racemes from late winter to summer. ↕ to 75cm (30in), ↔ 60cm (24in). ❄❄❄

***E.* 'Bredon'** ▣ 🏆 Sturdy, mound-forming, evergreen perennial with inversely lance-shaped, bluish green leaves. Reddish brown buds open to rich yellow flowers, to 2cm (¾in) across, in long racemes from mid-spring to early summer. ↕ 30cm (12in), ↔ 45cm (18in). ❄❄❄

***E.* 'Butterscotch'.** Mounded, subshrubby, evergreen perennial with inversely lance-shaped leaves. Produces orange-yellow flowers, to 1.5cm (½in) across, in long racemes from late spring to midsummer. ↕ 30cm (12in), ↔ 60cm (24in). ❄❄❄

E. cheiri, syn. *Cheiranthus cheiri* (Wallflower). Subshrubby, short-lived, evergreen perennial, grown as a biennial, forming mounds of lance-shaped to obovate-lance-shaped, dark green leaves, to 23cm (9in) long, the margins entire or with well-spaced teeth. Open, sweet-scented, bright yellow-orange flowers, to 2.5cm (1in) across, are produced in short racemes in spring. ↕ 25–80cm (10–32in), ↔ 30–40cm (12–16in). S. Europe. ❄❄❄. Cultivars of **Bedder Series** ▣ are dwarf and compact, with flowers in golden yellow, primrose-

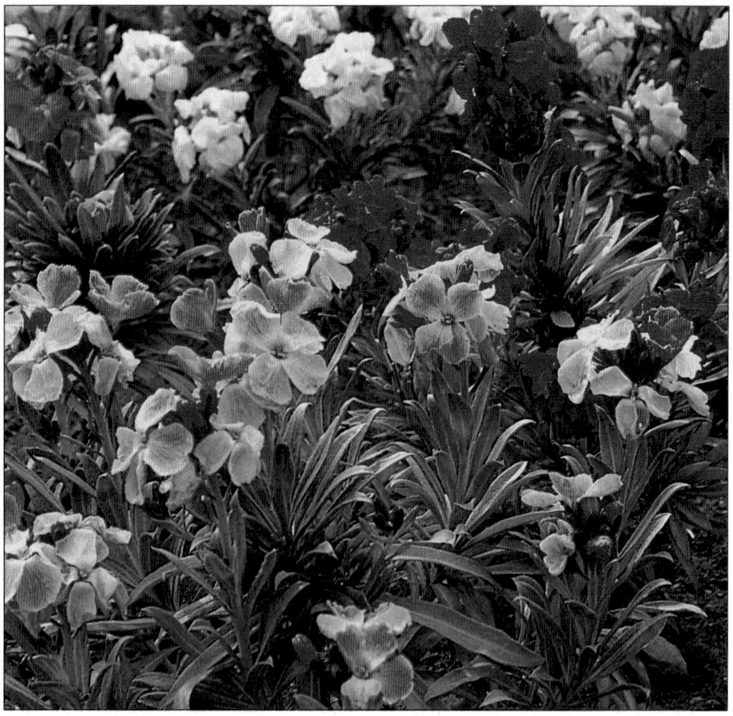

Erysimum cheiri Bedder Series

yellow, orange, or scarlet-red; ↕ to 30cm (12in). **Bedder Series 'Orange Bedder'** freely bears orange flowers; ↕ 23–30cm (9–12in), ↔ 25–30cm (10–12in). **'Blood Red'** ▣ bears deep red flowers. Cultivars of **Fair Lady Series** produce flowers in pale pink, yellow, and creamy white, with some reds. **'Fire King'** bears orange-red flowers. **'Harlequin'** is compact and uniform, and bears flowers in golden yellow, orange, cream, scarlet, crimson, intermediate pastel shades, and bicolours; ↕ to 25cm (10in). **'Harpur Crewe'** see *E.* x *kewense* 'Harpur Crewe'. **'Ivory White'** produces creamy white flowers.

***E.* 'Constant Cheer'** 🏆 Bushy, evergreen perennial with inversely lance-shaped, dark green leaves. Dusky orange-red flowers, to 1.5cm (½in) across, becoming purple, are produced in short racemes from mid-spring to early summer. ↕ to 30cm (12in), ↔ 60cm (24in). ❄❄❄

***E.* 'E.A. Bowles'** see *E.* 'Bowles' Mauve'.

***E.* 'Golden Jubilee'.** Robust, clump-forming, semi-evergreen perennial with narrowly lance-shaped, dark green leaves. From late spring into summer, bears short racemes of soft golden yellow flowers, to 1.5cm (½in) across. ↕ 25cm (10in), ↔ to 40cm (16in). ❄❄❄

***E.* 'Jacob's Jacket'.** Bushy, evergreen perennial with inversely lance-shaped, dark green leaves. From early to late spring, bears short racemes of flowers, to 1.5cm (½in) across, that open bronze-tinted, become more orange, and finally turn lilac, with blooms in all shades present at the same time. ↕ 30cm (12in), ↔ 45cm (18in). ❄❄❄

***E.* 'John Codrington'** ▣ Bushy, evergreen perennial with inversely lance-shaped leaves. Short racemes of pale yellow flowers, to 1.5cm (½in) across, shaded brown and purple, are produced in mid- and late spring. ↕ 25cm (10in), ↔ 30cm (12in). ❄❄❄

***E.* 'Jubilee Gold'.** Bushy, evergreen perennial with inversely lance-shaped leaves. Golden yellow flowers, to 1.5cm (½in) across, are produced in short racemes in mid- and late spring. ↕ to 40cm (16in), ↔ 45cm (18in). ❄❄❄

E.* x *kewense (*E. bicolor* x *E. cheiri*). Bushy, upright, woody-based, evergreen perennial with branched stems and narrowly lance-shaped or inversely lance-shaped, entire, grey-green leaves,

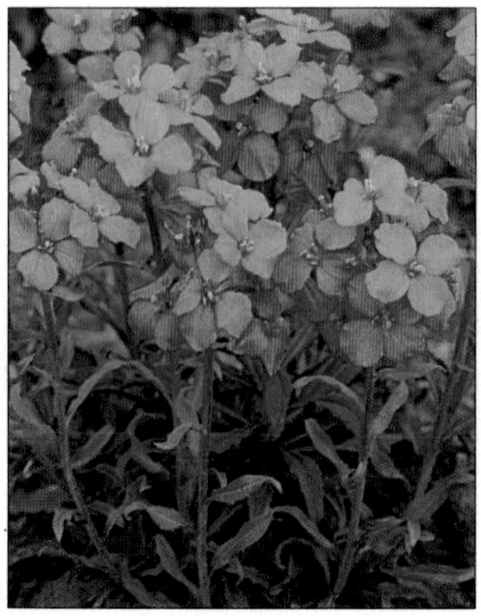

Erysimum x *allionii*

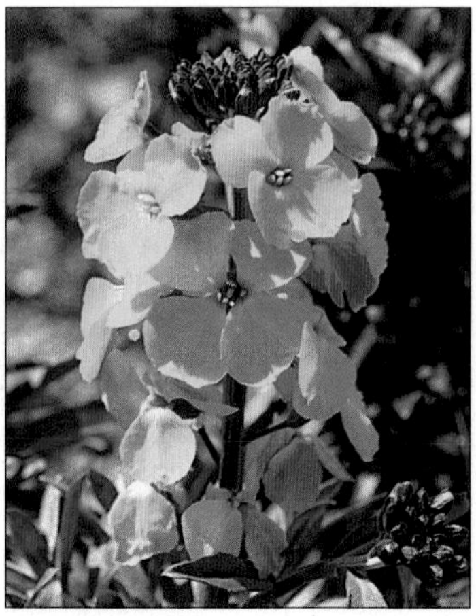

Erysimum 'Bredon'

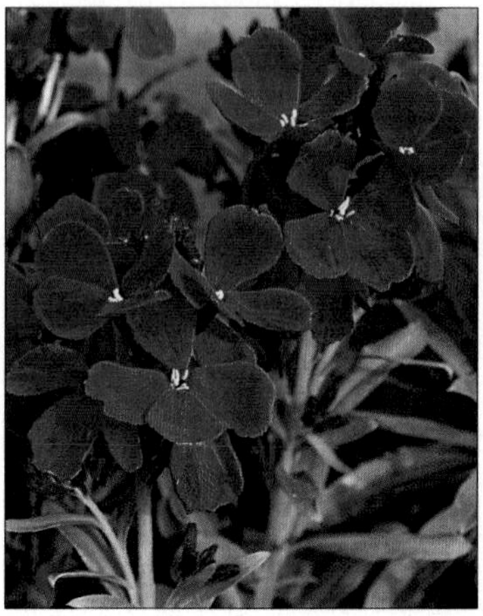

Erysimum cheiri 'Blood Red'

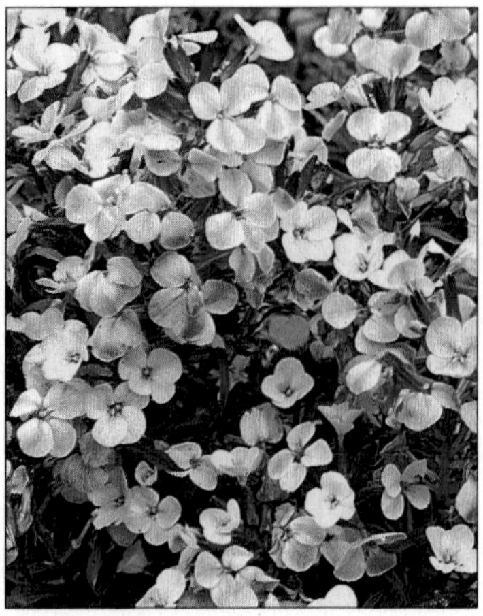

Erysimum 'John Codrington'

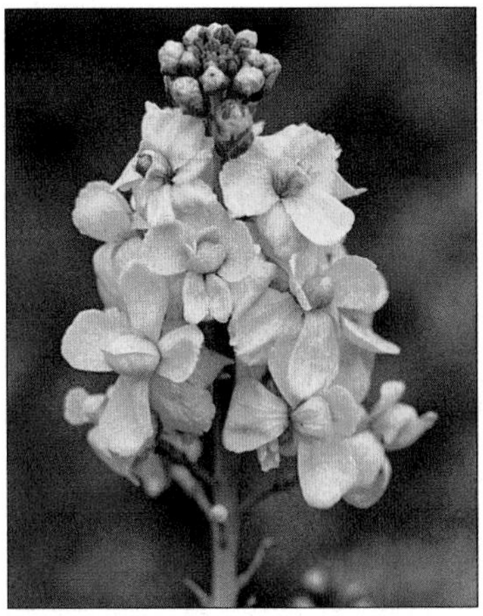

Erysimum x *kewense* 'Harpur Crewe'

5–8cm (2–3in) long. From late winter to early summer, bears short racemes of fragrant flowers, 2.5cm (1in) across, initially yellowish orange to bronze, turning light purple. ↕ to 40cm (16in), ↔ 30cm (12in). Garden origin. ❄❄❄.
'Harpur Crewe' ▣ 🏆 syn. *Cheiranthus cheiri* 'Harpur Crewe', *E. cheiri* 'Harpur Crewe', produces double yellow flowers; ↕ 30cm (12in), ↔ 60cm (24in).
'Variegatum' bears cream-variegated leaves.
E. kotschyanum. Densely tufted, evergreen perennial with crowded clusters of linear, usually toothed, pale green leaves, 1cm (½in) long. In summer, produces compact racemes of open, yellow to golden orange flowers, 1cm (½in) across. ↕ 10cm (4in), ↔ to 20cm (8in). Turkey. ❄❄❄
E. linifolium. Mat-forming, woody-based, evergreen perennial with narrowly linear-lance-shaped, entire, wavy, greyish green leaves, 2–9cm (¾–3½in) long. From mid-spring to early autumn, numerous slender, unbranched stems bear long racemes of open, lilac or lavender-blue flowers, 1–2cm (½–¾in) across. Prone to frost damage. ↕ 12–70cm (5–28in), ↔ 25cm (10in). N. Portugal, C. Spain. ❄❄❄.
'Bicolor' produces both pinkish violet and white flowers. **'Variegatum'** ▣ syn. *E.* 'Sissinghurst Variegated', is more tufted, with mauve flowers and white-variegated leaves; ↕↔ 45cm (18in).
***E.* 'Moonlight'** ▣ Mat-forming, evergreen perennial with inversely lance-shaped leaves. Short racemes of pale sulphur-yellow flowers, to 1.5cm (½in) across, are produced from early spring to

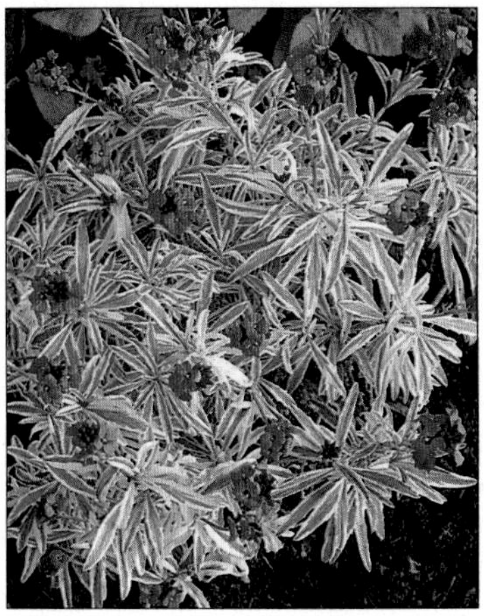

Erysimum linifolium 'Variegatum'

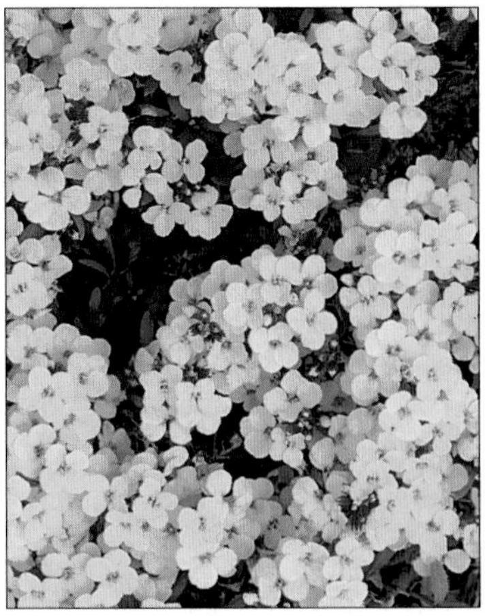

Erysimum 'Moonlight'

early summer. ↕ 25cm (10in), ↔ 45cm (18in). ❄❄❄
E. perofskianum. Rosette-forming biennial or short-lived, evergreen perennial, grown as an annual, with lance-shaped, sometimes finely toothed, greyish green leaves, 5–10cm (2–4in) long. Open, golden orange or red-orange flowers, to 2cm (¾in) across, are borne in long racemes in summer. ↕ 15–40cm (6–16in), ↔ to 25cm (10in). Afghanistan, Pakistan. ❄❄❄
***E.* 'Rufus'.** Bushy, not robust, evergreen perennial with inversely lance-shaped leaves. Rich orange-brown flowers, 1.5–2cm (½–¾in) across, are borne in long racemes from early to late spring. ↕ 15cm (6in), ↔ 30cm (12in). ❄❄❄
***E.* 'Sissinghurst Variegated'** see *E. linifolium* 'Variegatum'.
***E.* 'Sprite'.** Mat-forming, evergreen perennial with inversely lance-shaped leaves. Pale yellow flowers, to 1cm (½in) across, are borne in short racemes from early to late spring. ↕ 20cm (8in), ↔ 45cm (18in). ❄❄❄
***E.* 'Wenlock Beauty'** 🏆 Bushy, evergreen perennial with inversely lance-shaped leaves. From early to late spring, bears bronze-shaded, mauve and buff-yellow flowers, to 1.5cm (½in) across, in long racemes. ↕↔ 45cm (18in). ❄❄❄

▷ ***Erythraea*** see *Centaurium*

ERYTHRINA

Coral tree

LEGUMINOSAE / PAPILIONACEAE

Genus of over 100 species of deciduous, semi-evergreen, or evergreen, usually spiny, trees, shrubs, subshrubs, and woody-based perennials found in woodland and thickets, and on open slopes, in tropical regions worldwide. They are grown for their pea-like, 5-petalled flowers with long standard petals, borne singly or in clusters in the leaf axils, or in axillary or terminal racemes, on often leafless stems. Leaves are alternate and 3-pinnate, with the terminal leaflet larger than the others and sometimes differently shaped. Grow as specimen plants. In cool-temperate areas, grow half-hardy and frost-tender species in a cool or temperate greenhouse.
• **HARDINESS** Frost hardy to frost tender. *E. crista-galli* and *E. herbacea* may survive down to -10°C (14°F) if protected with a thick mulch.
• **CULTIVATION** Under glass, grow in loam-based potting compost (JI No.3) in full light. From spring to autumn, water freely and apply a balanced liquid fertilizer monthly. Outdoors, grow in fertile, moist but well-drained soil in full sun. Pruning group 1; may need restrictive pruning under glass.
• **PROPAGATION** Sow seed at 21–24°C (70–75°F) in spring. Root softwood cuttings in early summer, or semi-ripe cuttings in late summer, both with bottom heat.
• **PESTS AND DISEASES** Prone to red spider mites and mealybugs under glass.

E.* x *bidwillii ▣ (*E. crista-galli* x *E. herbacea*). Large, deciduous subshrub or shrub in warm regions, woody-based herbaceous perennial in cool ones. Robust, sparsely branched, spiny stems bear light to mid-green leaves, divided into 3 ovate-oblong leaflets, 20cm (8in) long. In summer, bears dark red flowers, to 5cm (2in) long, in small, axillary clusters of 3, or in terminal racemes, 30–60cm (12–24in) long. ↕ 2–4m (6–12ft), ↔ 1.5–3m (5–10ft). Garden origin. ❄
E. caffra 🌳 (Cape kaffirboom, Lucky bean tree). Wide-spreading, semi-evergreen tree with sometimes prickly branches, and prickly-stalked leaves divided into 3 broadly ovate leaflets, the longest to 9cm (3½in) long. In spring, bears dense, terminal racemes, to 15cm (6in) long, of orange-scarlet flowers, 5cm (2in) long, with broad, strongly arching standard petals. ↕ 12–18m (40–60ft), ↔ 10–15m (30–50ft). E. South Africa. ❀ (min. 5°C/41°F)
E. crista-galli ▣ 🏆 🌳 (Cock's comb, Common coral tree). Open, deciduous tree in warm regions, woody-based perennial in cool ones. Branches bear stout spines. Leathery leaves, including the prickly stalks, are 30cm (12in) or more long, with 3 triangular leaflets to 10cm (4in) long; the largest leaflet is ovate-oblong. Deep red flowers, 5–6cm (2–2½in) long, are borne in terminal racemes, 30–60cm (12–24in) or more long, from summer to autumn. ↕ 6–9m (20–28ft), ↔ 3–4m (10–12ft) as a tree; ↕ 1.5–2.5m (5–8ft), ↔ 1–1.5m (3–5ft) as a woody perennial. E. Bolivia to Argentina. ❄❄
E. herbacea (Coral bean). Semi-herbaceous, woody-based perennial with a thick, woody rootstock. Leaves are divided into 3 ovate to lance-shaped or arrow-shaped leaflets, 5–10cm (2–4in) long. From midsummer to early autumn, bears deep scarlet flowers, to

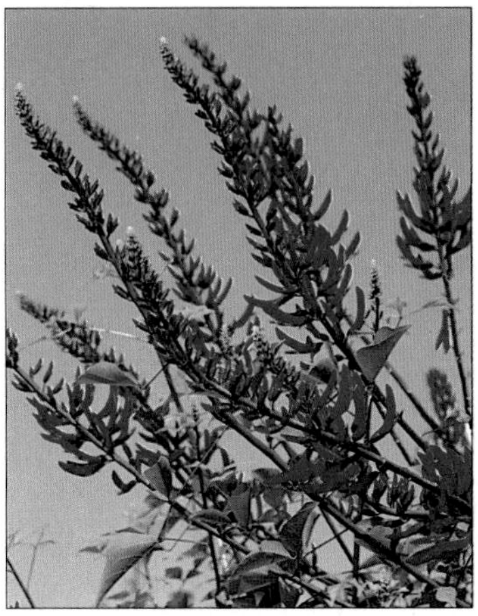

Erythrina x *bidwillii*

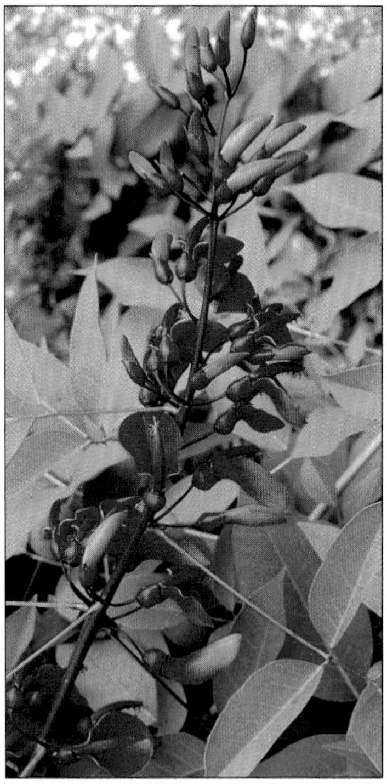

Erythrina crista-galli

5cm (2in) long, with narrow standard petals, in terminal racemes, to 60cm (24in) long. ↕ to 1m (3ft), ↔ 60cm (24in). S.E. USA, Mexico. ❄❄
E. lysistemon 🌳 (Lucky bean tree, Transvaal kaffirboom). Open, semi-evergreen tree. Leaves, including the long, sometimes prickly stalks, are to 22cm (9in) long, with 3 ovate, tapering leaflets to 7cm (3in) long. In summer, bears compact, terminal racemes, to 20cm (8in) long, of bright scarlet flowers, 6cm (2½in) long. ↕ 7–10m (22–30ft), ↔ 3–5m (10–15ft). South Africa. ❀ (min. 5°C/41°F)
E. variegata ▣ 🌳 Spreading, deciduous tree with many robust branches scattered with prickles. Leaves, including the long stalks, are 25–40cm (10–16in) long, with 3 ovate to broadly diamond-shaped leaflets, 15–20cm (6–8in) long, usually rich green, and often variegated light green and yellow along the main veins. Scarlet or crimson flowers, 5–6cm (2–2½in) long, are borne in dense, terminal racemes, to 20cm (8in) long, in summer. ↕ 18–25m (60–80ft), ↔ 8–15m (25–50ft). E. Africa to India, China, Taiwan, Malaysia, and parts of Polynesia. ❀ (min. 7°C/45°F)

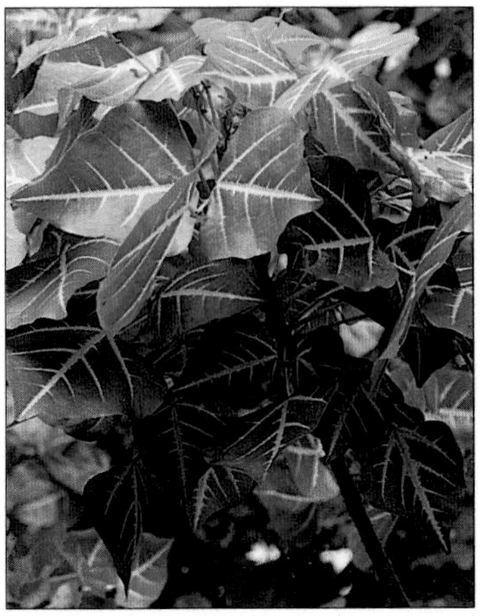

Erythrina variegata

ERYTHRONIUM

Dog's-tooth violet, Trout lily

LILIACEAE

Genus of about 22 species of clump-forming perennials, with long-pointed, tooth-like bulbs. They occur in habitats ranging from deciduous woodland to open mountain meadows in Europe, Asia, and North America. From spring to early summer, slender, upright stems produce 1–10 pendent flowers, usually 3–6cm (1¼–2½in) across, in shades of purple, violet, pink, yellow, or white, each with conspicuous stamens and 6 pointed, recurved tepals. Broadly elliptic to ovate-elliptic, paired, usually semi-erect, basal leaves, 3–35cm (1¼–14in) long, are glossy to glaucous, mid- to dark green, in some species heavily marbled bronze. Grow in clumps under deciduous trees and shrubs, or in a rock garden. *E. dens-canis* may be naturalized in thin grass.

- **HARDINESS** Fully hardy.
- **CULTIVATION** Plant bulbs at least 10cm (4in) deep in autumn, in fertile, humus-rich, well-drained soil that does not dry out, in light dappled or partial shade. Bulbs must be kept slightly damp during storage and before planting.
- **PROPAGATION** Divide established clumps after flowering.
- **PESTS AND DISEASES** May be damaged by slugs.

E. americanum ■ (Yellow adder's tongue). Stoloniferous, bulbous perennial bearing horizontal, narrowly elliptic, mid- to deep green leaves, to

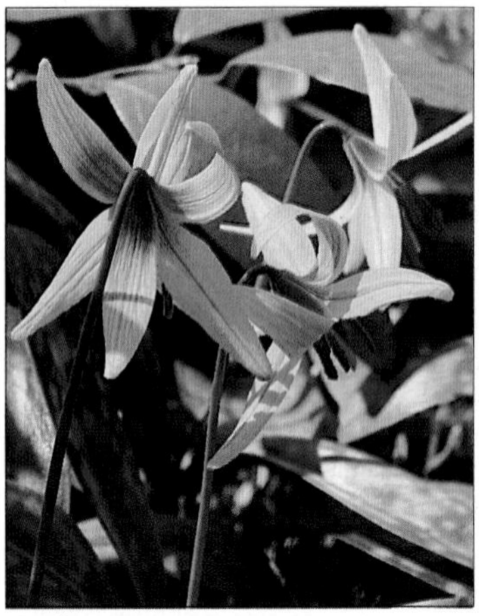

Erythronium americanum

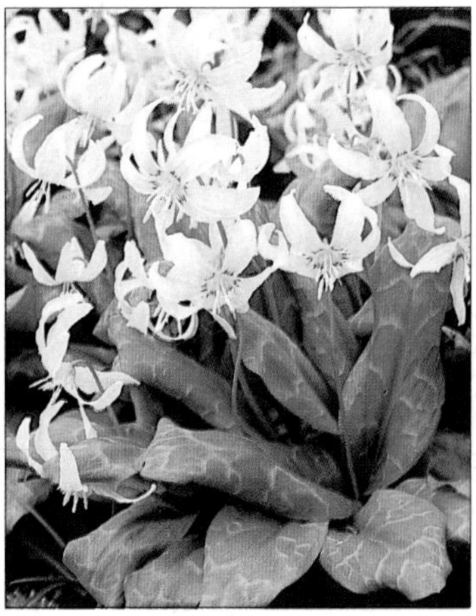

Erythronium californicum 'White Beauty'

15cm (6in) long, with purple-brown marbling. Solitary, sulphur-yellow flowers, 3–5cm (1¼–2in) across, with reddish yellow or purple outsides and purple, yellow, or brown anthers, are produced in spring. Often shy to flower. ↕8–15cm (3–6in), ↔ 10cm (4in). E. North America. ✽✽✽

E. californicum ■ ♀ Bulbous perennial with elliptic, dark green leaves, 3–7cm (1¼–3in) long, lightly mottled brownish green. In spring, each stem produces 1–3 creamy white flowers, 5–7cm (2–3in) across, with brownish orange central markings, white anthers, and stamens with rounded filaments. ↕15–35cm (6–14in), ↔ 10cm (4in). USA (California). ✽✽✽. **'White Beauty'** ■ ♀ syn. *E.* 'White Beauty', is vigorous, with a rusty red basal ring in each flower; it increases well by offsets.

***E.* 'Citronella'.** Vigorous, bulbous perennial with elliptic, bronze-mottled, slightly glossy, mid-green leaves. In spring, each stem bears up to 10 clear yellow flowers with dark yellow anthers. Similar to *E.* 'Pagoda', but flowers slightly later. ↕20–35cm (8–14in), ↔ 10cm (4in). ✽✽✽

E. dens-canis ■ ♀ (European dog's-tooth violet). Bulbous perennial with elliptic-oblong, mid-green leaves, 10–15cm (4–6in) long, marbled purplish brown. In spring, bears solitary, white, pink, or lilac flowers, to 3–4cm (1¼–1½in) across, with purple or blue-purple anthers. ↕10–15cm (4–6in), ↔ 10cm (4in). Europe, Asia. ✽✽✽. **'Lilac Wonder'** has rich purple flowers, with a brown basal spot on each petal forming a conspicuous central ring.

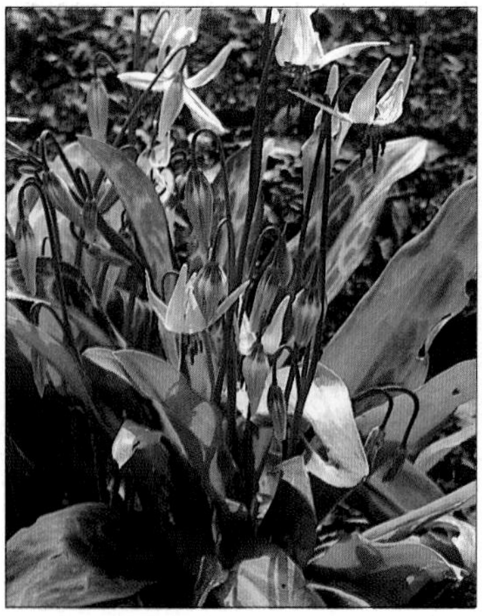

Erythronium hendersonii

'Pink Perfection' produces clear pink flowers, 3–5cm (1¼–2in) across, in early spring. **'Purple King'** bears rich plum-coloured flowers, striped white and brown in the centres. **'Snowflake'** bears pure white flowers. **'White Splendour'** produces white flowers with brown centres, in early spring.

E. grandiflorum. Bulbous perennial with elliptic, bright mid-green leaves, 10–20cm (4–8in) long. In spring, each stem bears 1–3 golden yellow flowers, 5cm (2in) across, with distinctive, 3-lobed stigmas and white, yellow, or red-black anthers. ↕15–30cm (6–12in), ↔ 10cm (4in). W. USA. ✽✽✽

E. hartwegii see *E. multiscapoideum.*

E. hendersonii ■ Bulbous perennial with elliptic, wavy-margined, lightly brown-banded, dark green leaves, 10–20cm (4–8in) long. In spring, each stem bears up to 10 pale lilac flowers, 5cm (2in) across, with purple anthers and deep purple, sometimes yellow centres. Best in partial shade in soil that dries out in summer. ↕15–35cm (6–14in), ↔ 8cm (3in). USA (S.W. Oregon, N.W. California). ✽✽✽

E. japonicum ■ Bulbous perennial with elliptic, mid- to deep green leaves, 10–15cm (4–6in) long, lightly marbled purplish brown. In spring, bears solitary, pale to rich violet flowers, 3–5cm (1¼–2in) across, with darker centres and purple anthers. ↕10–15cm (4–6in), ↔ 8cm (3in). Japan. ✽✽✽

***E.* 'Joanna'.** Bulbous perennial bearing elliptic, slightly glossy, mid-green leaves, with brown marbling. In spring, each stem produces up to 8 pink-flushed, creamy yellow flowers with pale yellow

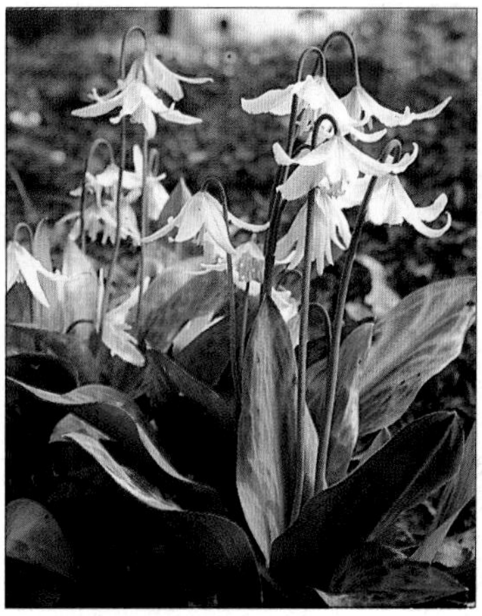

Erythronium oregonum

anthers. ↕25–30cm (10–12in), ↔ 8cm (3in). ✽✽✽

***E.* 'Kondo'.** Vigorous, bulbous perennial with elliptic, bronze-mottled, mid-green leaves; the mottling fades after flowering. In spring, each stem bears 2–5, sometimes up to 10, scented, green-suffused, lemon-yellow flowers, with red-brown centres and deep yellow anthers. ↕15–35cm (6–14in), ↔ 10cm (4in). ✽✽✽

E. multiscapoideum, syn. *E. hartwegii, E. purdyi.* Bulbous perennial with elliptic, lightly brown-mottled, dark green leaves, 3.5–10cm (1½–4in) long. In spring, each branched flower stem produces solitary, red-flushed buds that open into creamy white flowers, 4–6cm (1½–2½in) across, with white anthers and yellow or yellowish green centres. Similar to *E. californicum*, but the flower stem branches at or just below ground. ↕15–35 (6–14in), ↔ 10cm (4in). USA (Sierra Nevada). ✽✽✽

E. oregonum ■ Vigorous, bulbous perennial with elliptic, shiny, brown-mottled, mid- to deep green leaves, 12–15cm (5–6in) long. In spring, each stem bears up to 6 creamy white flowers, 4–7cm (1½–3in) across, with yellow centres sometimes surrounded by orange-brown marks, and bright yellow anthers. Similar to *E. californicum*, but stamens have wide, flattened, thread-like filaments. ↕15–35cm (6–14in), ↔ 10cm (4in). North America (British Columbia to Oregon). ✽✽✽

***E.* 'Pagoda'** ■ ♀ Very vigorous, bulbous perennial with elliptic, strongly bronze-mottled, glossy, deep green leaves. In spring, the stems each bear

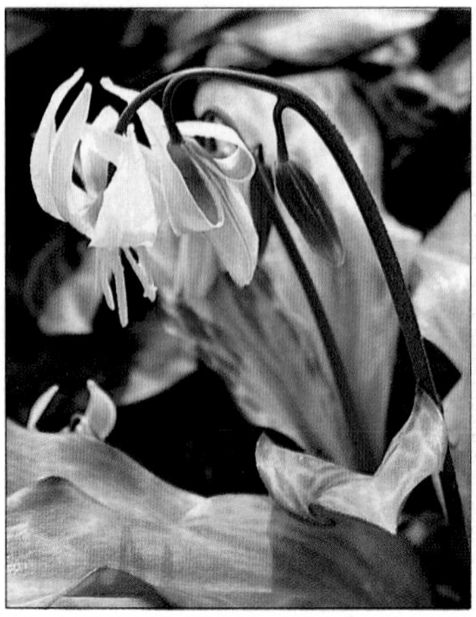

Erythronium californicum

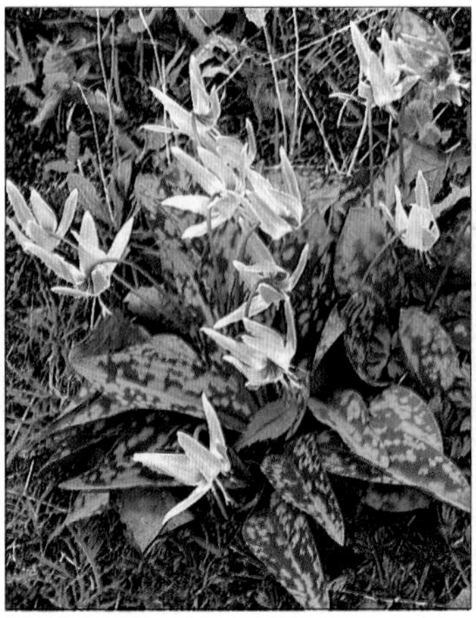

Erythronium dens-canis

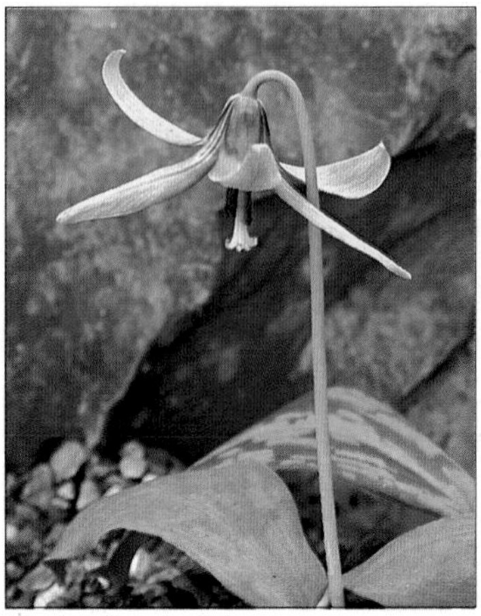

Erythronium japonicum

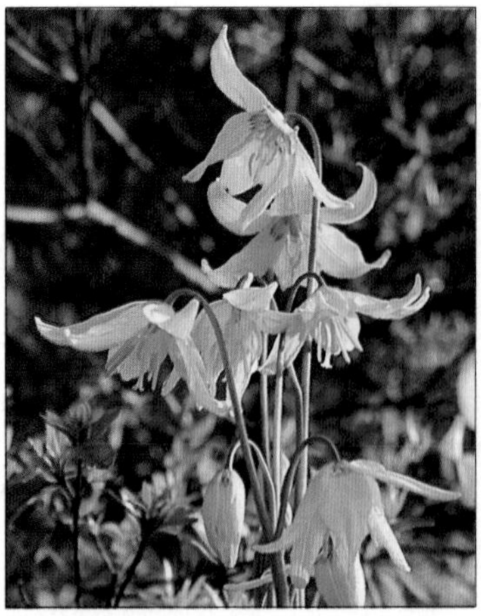

Erythronium 'Pagoda'

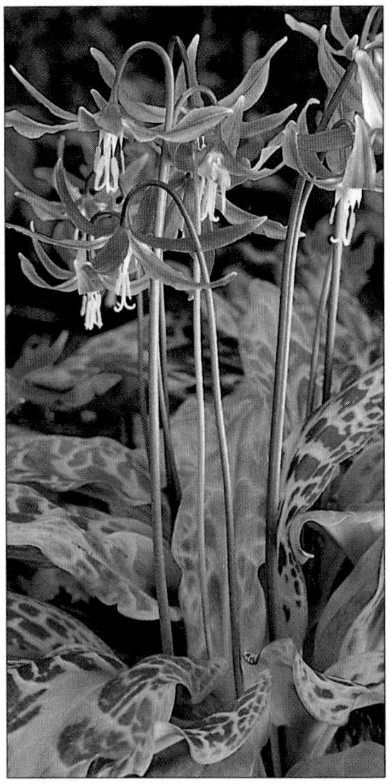

Erythronium revolutum

2–5, sometimes up to 10, sulphur-yellow flowers, with brown central rings and deep yellow anthers. ↕15–35cm (6–14in), ↔ 10cm (4in). ❄❄❄
E. purdyi see *E. multiscapoideum.*
E. revolutum ■ 🏆 (American trout lily). Bulbous perennial with elliptic, wavy-margined, deep green leaves, 15–20cm (6–8in) long, strongly mottled dark brown. In mid-spring, each stem bears up to 4 lilac-pink flowers, 4–7cm (1½–3in) across, with yellow central rings and yellow anthers. Sometimes slow to establish, but may self-seed freely once it has. ↕20–30cm (8–12in), ↔ 10cm (4in). USA (N. California, Vancouver Island). ❄❄❄. **'Pink Beauty'** has deep lavender-pink flowers.
E. tuolumnense ■ 🏆 Vigorous, bulbous perennial with elliptic, often slightly wavy-margined, pale to mid-green leaves, 20–30cm (8–12in) long. In spring, bears up to 4, occasionally up to 7, green-veined, bright yellow flowers, 3–5cm (1¼–2in) across, with yellow anthers, in a cluster towards the top of each stem. ↕20–35cm (8–14in), ↔ 8cm (3in). USA (C. California). ❄❄❄
***E.* 'White Beauty'** see *E. californicum* 'White Beauty'.

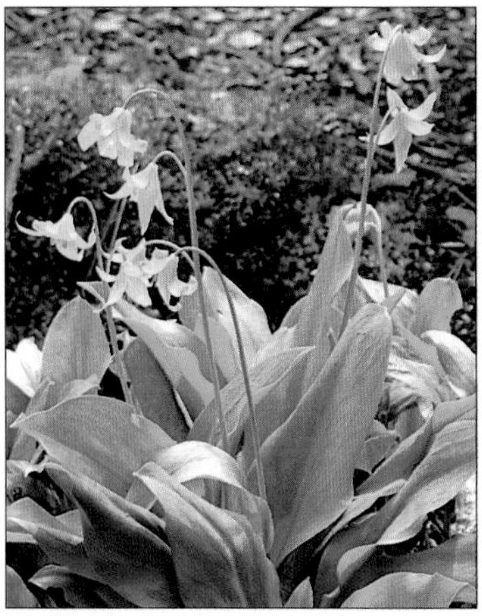

Erythronium tuolumnense

ESCALLONIA

ESCALLONIACEAE/GROSSULARIACEAE

Genus of about 50–60 species of mostly evergreen shrubs or, more rarely, small trees, found in woodland and scrub, and often on mountains, in South America. They are grown for their usually alternate, occasionally whorled, bold, often narrowly to broadly oval, glossy leaves, and for their mainly terminal racemes or panicles of tubular, salver-form, chalice-shaped, or saucer-shaped, 5-petalled, white to pink or red flowers, with spreading or erect lobes. They flower freely over a long period, mainly in summer. Grow in a shrub border, against a wall, or as a hedge, screen, or windbreak – particularly near coasts.

- **HARDINESS** Fully hardy to half hardy; many half-hardy and frost-hardy species and cultivars may survive temperatures below -5°C (23°F) if planted against a sunny wall.
- **CULTIVATION** Grow in fertile, well-drained soil in full sun, and shelter from cold, drying winds. Pruning group 9.
- **PROPAGATION** Take softwood cuttings in early summer, semi-ripe cuttings in late summer, and hardwood cuttings from late autumn to winter.
- **PESTS AND DISEASES** Trouble free.

***E.* 'Apple Blossom'** ■ 🏆 Compact, bushy, evergreen shrub with elliptic, glossy, dark green leaves, to 5cm (2in) long. In early and midsummer, bears short racemes of chalice-shaped, apple-blossom-pink flowers, 2–2.5cm (¾–1in) across, with white centres. ↕↔ 2.5m (8ft). ❄❄
E. bifida ■ syn. *E. montevidensis.* Vigorous, upright, evergreen shrub with narrowly oval to obovate or spoon-shaped, finely toothed, glossy, dark green leaves, to 7cm (3in) long. Bears pure white flowers, to 2cm (¾in) across, with tubular then spreading petals, in panicles to 15cm (6in) long from late summer to autumn. Grow against a wall in cold areas. Brazil, Uruguay. ↕3m (10ft), ↔ 2.5m (8ft). ❄❄
***E.* 'C.F. Ball'.** Vigorous, erect, open, evergreen shrub with broadly oval to obovate, deeply toothed, glossy, dark green leaves, to 6cm (2½in) long. Bears tubular, bright rich red flowers, to 2cm (¾in) long, in short racemes throughout summer. ↕↔ 2.5m (8ft). ❄❄❄
***E.* 'Donard Radiance'** 🏆 Vigorous, compact, evergreen shrub with obovate, coarsely toothed, glossy, dark green leaves, to 4cm (1½in) long. Chalice-shaped, rich pink flowers, to 2cm (¾in) across, are produced in short racemes in early and midsummer. ↕↔ 2.5m (8ft). ❄❄
***E.* 'Donard Seedling'** ■ Vigorous, evergreen shrub with arching shoots and obovate to narrowly oval, glossy, dark green leaves, to 2.5cm (1in) long. Produces masses of saucer-shaped, pink-tinted white flowers, 1cm (½in) across, opening from pink buds, in short racemes in early and midsummer. ↕↔ 2.5m (8ft). ❄❄❄
***E.* 'Edinensis'** 🏆 Evergreen shrub with arching shoots and oblong, glossy, dark green leaves, to 2cm (¾in) long. Short racemes of saucer-shaped, pinkish red flowers, to 1cm (½in) across, red in bud, are borne in early and midsummer. ↕2m (6ft), ↔ 3m (10ft). ❄❄❄
***E.* 'Iveyi'** 🏆 Upright, evergreen shrub with oval to elliptic, glossy, dark green leaves, to 7cm (3in) long, often bronze-tinted in cold weather. From mid- to late summer, bears chalice-shaped, fragrant, pure white flowers, to 1cm (½in) across, in conical panicles, 13–16cm (5–6in) long, and 10cm (4in) wide at the bases. ↕↔ 3m (10ft). ❄❄
***E.* 'Langleyensis'** ■ 🏆 Evergreen or semi-evergreen shrub with slender, arching shoots and obovate to narrowly oval, glossy, dark green leaves, to 2.5cm (1in) long. Bears a profusion of saucer-shaped, bright rose-red flowers, to 1cm (½in) across, in short racemes in early and midsummer. ↕2m (6ft), ↔ 3m (10ft). ❄❄❄

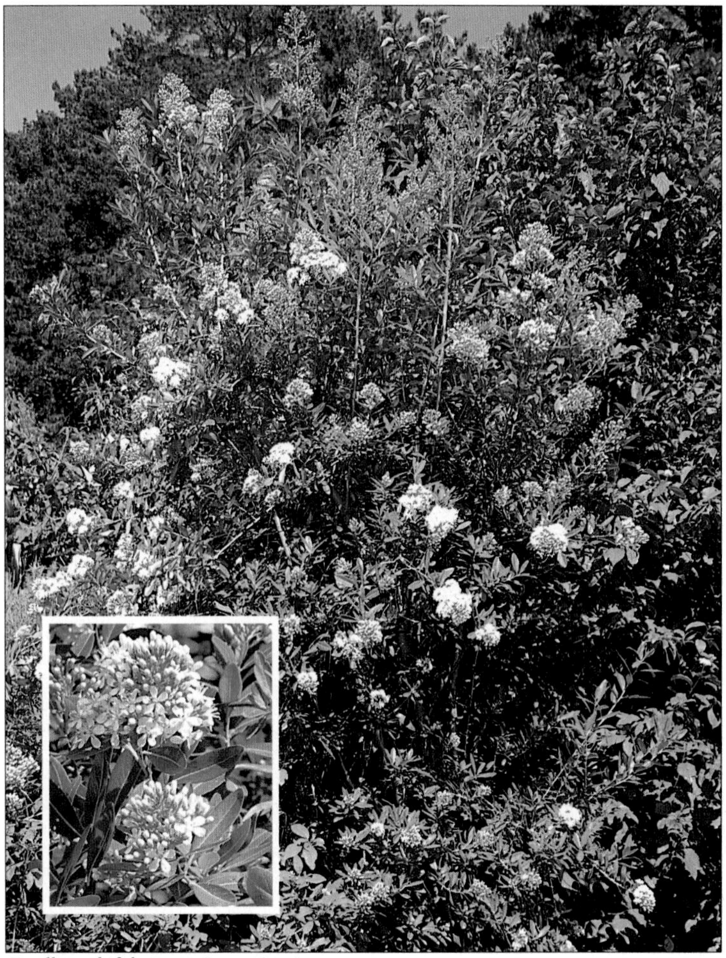

Escallonia bifida (inset: flower detail)

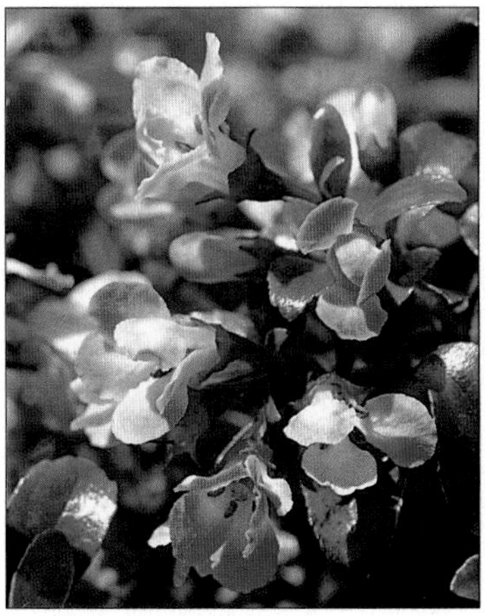

Escallonia 'Apple Blossom'

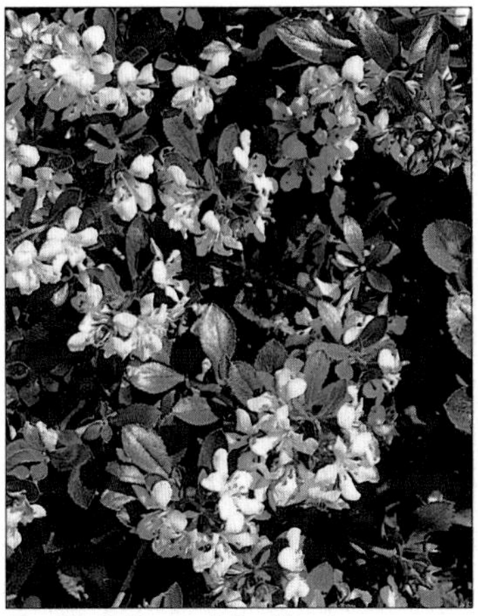

Escallonia 'Donard Seedling'

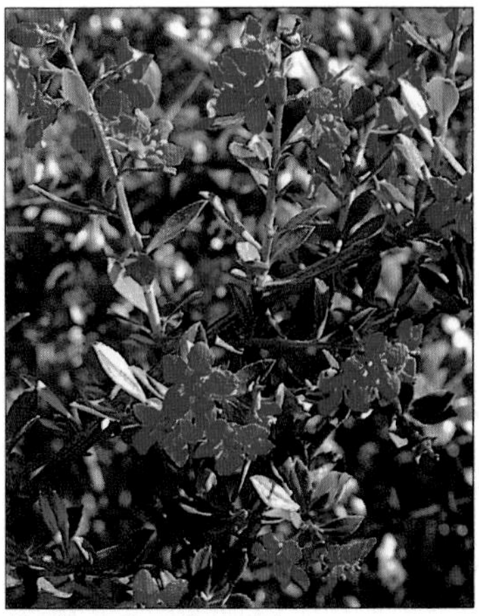

Escallonia 'Langleyensis'

E

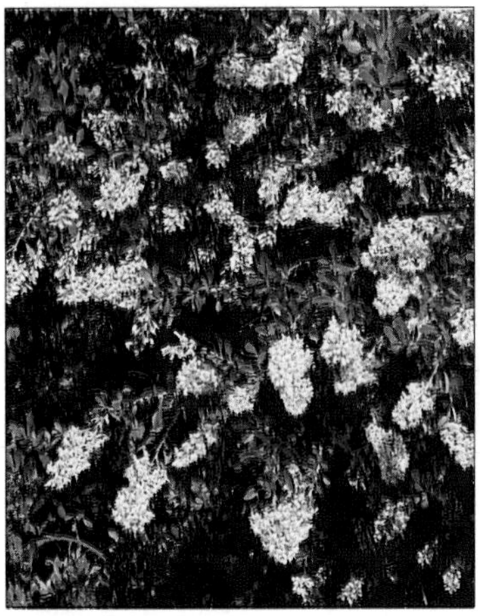

Escallonia leucantha

E. leucantha ■ Upright, tree-like, evergreen shrub with narrowly obovate to inversely lance-shaped, toothed, glossy, dark green leaves, to 2.5cm (1in) long. In midsummer, tubular, creamy white flowers, to 1cm (½in) long, are borne in panicle-like inflorescences, to 30cm (12in) long, and 8–18cm (3–7in) wide at the bases. ↕ 3m (10ft), ↔ 2.5m (8ft). Chile, Argentina. ❄❄
E. montevidensis see *E. bifida*.
***E.* 'Peach Blossom'** ♀ Vigorous, bushy, evergreen shrub with arching shoots and elliptic, glossy, dark green leaves, to 4cm (1½in) long. In early and midsummer, bears short racemes of chalice-shaped, white-centred, peach-pink flowers, to 2.5cm (1in) across. ↕↔ 2.5m (8ft). ❄❄
***E.* 'Pride of Donard'** ■ ♀ Erect, compact, evergreen shrub with ovate,

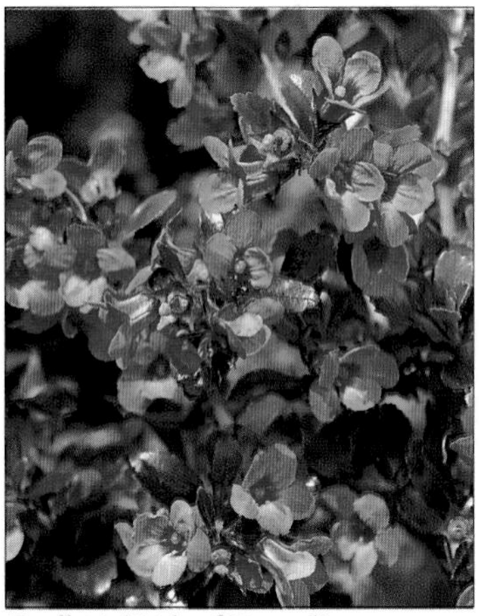

Escallonia 'Pride of Donard'

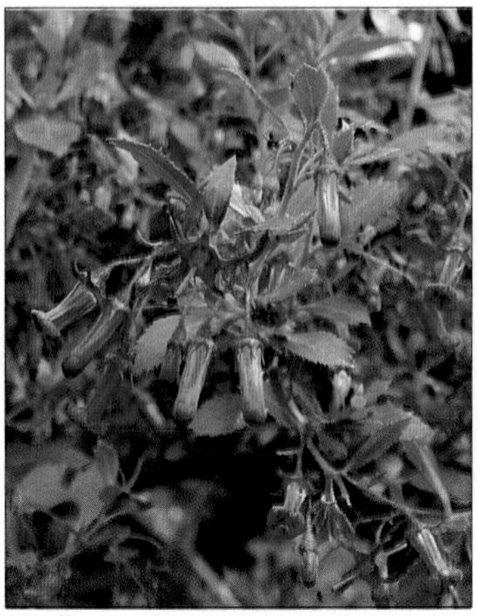

Escallonia rubra 'Woodside'

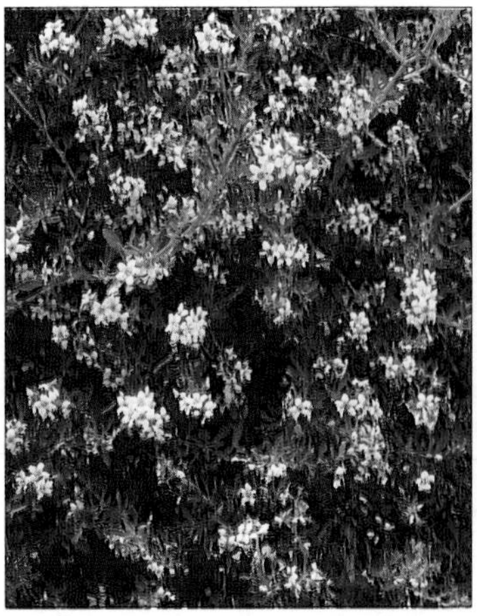

Escallonia virgata

glossy, dark green leaves, to 2.5cm (1in) long. Bears chalice-shaped, rich, light red flowers, to 2.5cm (1in) across, in short racemes in early and midsummer. ↕ 1.5m (5ft), ↔ 2.5m (8ft). ❄❄
***E.* 'Red Elf'.** Compact, evergreen shrub of spreading habit with broadly oval to obovate, glossy, dark green leaves, to 2.5cm (1in) long. Bears tubular, dark crimson flowers, to 1cm (½in) long, in short racemes in early and midsummer. ↕ 2.5m (8ft), ↔ 4m (12ft). ❄❄
E. rubra. Vigorous, variable, evergreen shrub with peeling brown bark and elliptic to broadly ovate or obovate, toothed, glossy, dark green leaves, to 6cm (2½in) long. Bears loose panicles, to 10cm (4in) long, of tubular, dark crimson to pink flowers, 1cm (½in) long, in abundance from summer to early autumn. ↕↔ to 5m (15ft). Chile, Argentina. ❄❄❄. **'Crimson Spire'** ♀ is erect, with deep crimson flowers, to 2cm (¾in) long; excellent for a coastal garden or as a hedge. **var. *macrantha*** is similar to 'Crimson Spire' but less erect, with broadly oval or obovate leaves, to 8cm (3in) long, and tubular, bright rose-red flowers, to 1.5cm (½in) long; ↕↔ 3m (10ft). **'Pygmaea'** see 'Woodside'. **'Woodside'** ■ syn. 'Pygmaea', is dwarf, compact, and rounded, with crimson flowers. Tends to revert to *E. rubra*, of which it is a sport. Cut out vigorous shoots when seen; ↕ 75cm (30in), ↔ 1.5m (5ft).
E. virgata ■ Deciduous shrub with arching branches and obovate, finely toothed, glossy, dark green leaves, to 2cm (¾in) long. Axillary racemes, to 5cm (2in) long, of salverform white flowers, to 1cm (½in) long, are borne close to the tips of the branches in early and midsummer. ↕ 2m (6ft), ↔ 2.5m (8ft). Chile, Argentina. ❄❄

ESCHSCHOLZIA

California poppy

PAPAVERACEAE

Genus of 8–10 species of slender, erect, basally branching annuals and perennials from grassy, open areas in W. North America. They have finely divided, fern-like, light to blue-green foliage. Solitary, shallowly cupped, paper-thin, 4-petalled (rarely 5- to 8-petalled), poppy-like flowers, in red, orange, or yellow, are borne in spring or summer; they close in dull weather. Grow in an annual border, or in a gravel or rock garden. Good for cut flowers.

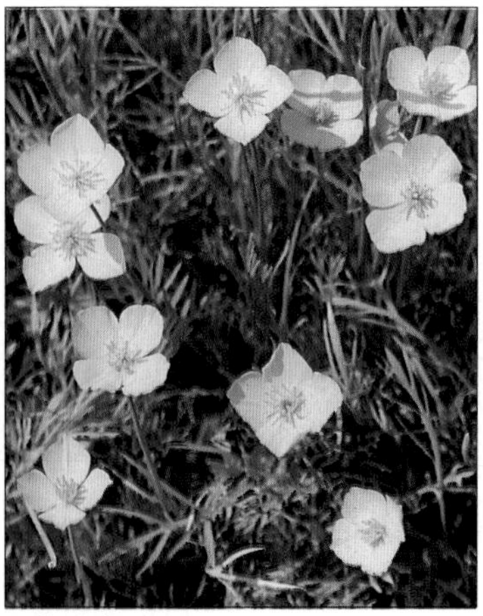

Eschscholzia caespitosa

- **HARDINESS** Fully hardy.
- **CULTIVATION** Grow in poor, well-drained soil in full sun.
- **PROPAGATION** Sow seed *in situ* in mid-spring or early autumn. Sow in succession for a continuous display.
- **PESTS AND DISEASES** Trouble free.

E. caespitosa ■ ♀ Tufted annual with finely divided, almost thread-like leaves, 10–12cm (4–5in) long. In summer, produces numerous, scented, single, bright yellow flowers, 3–5cm (1¼–2in) across. ↕↔ to 15cm (6in). USA (C. California). ❄❄❄. **'Sundew'** bears lemon-yellow flowers.
E. californica ■ ♀ (California poppy). Variable, mat-forming, frequently hairy annual with lance-shaped, finely cut leaves, 15–20cm (6–8in) long. In summer, bears numerous single, predominantly orange, sometimes also red, yellow, or white flowers, to 7cm (3in) across, followed by long, curved seed pods. ↕ to 30cm (12in), ↔ to 15cm (6in). USA (Oregon to coastal California). ❄❄❄. **'Ballerina'** bears fluted, semi-double or double, red, pink, yellow, or orange flowers. **'Dali'** ♀ is compact, with scarlet flowers; ↕ 25cm

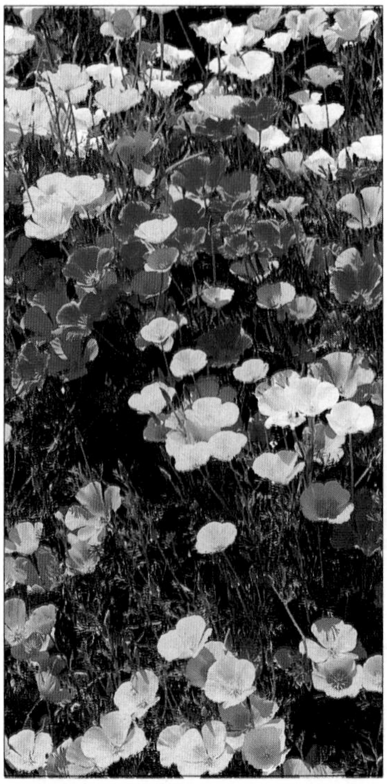

Eschscholzia californica

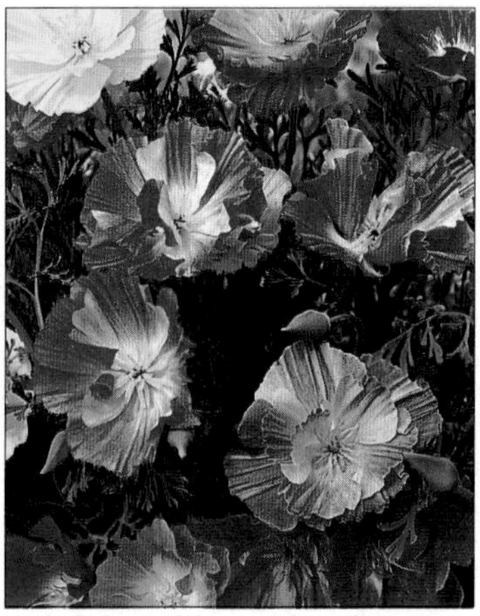

Eschscholzia californica Thai Silk Series

(10in). **'Monarch Art Shades'** bears semi-double or double, orange, yellow, apricot-yellow, creamy yellow, or red flowers, with frilled petals. Cultivars of **Thai Silk Series** ■ are compact, with single or semi-double, fluted, bronze-tinged flowers in red, pink, or orange; ↕ 20–25cm (8–10in).

ESCOBARIA

CACTACEAE

Genus of about 17 species of small, mainly spherical to cylindrical, solitary or clustering, perennial cacti from low-lying areas, semi-desert, and arid, uncultivated land in S. Canada, USA, N. Mexico, and Cuba. The stems are studded with tubercles (each with a furrow immediately above it) and very spiny, generally white areoles. In summer, diurnal, mostly bell-shaped flowers are produced from the areoles of young tubercles at or around the crowns. In frost-prone areas, grow in an indoor or bowl garden, or in a temperate greenhouse; in warm, dry areas, grow in a raised bed or desert garden.

- **HARDINESS** Frost tender.
- **CULTIVATION** Under glass, grow in standard cactus compost in full light. In the growing season, water moderately and apply a low-nitrogen fertilizer every 4–5 weeks; keep dry at other times. Outdoors, grow in poor to moderately fertile, sharply drained soil in full sun. See also pp.48–49.
- **PROPAGATION** Sow seed at 19–24°C (66–75°F) in spring, or divide offsets in summer.
- **PESTS AND DISEASES** Susceptible to mealybugs.

E. asperispina, syn. *Neobesseya asperispina*. Solitary cactus with a spherical, dull, bluish green stem, 6cm (2½in) thick, and conical tubercles. Areoles bear 9 or 10 greyish white radial spines. Bell-shaped flowers, 3cm (1¼in) long, with wide-spreading, whitish yellow petals, each with a pale brown or olive-green mid-stripe, are produced in summer. ↕↔ 6cm (2½in). N. Mexico. ❀ (min. 7°C/45°F)
E. sneedii. Clustering cactus with cylindrical stems, 2–8cm (¾–3in) thick, studded with minute, conical tubercles. Areoles bear 30–60 red radial spines, which turn white. In summer, produces pale pink, pinkish brown, or magenta flowers, to 2cm (¾in) long, with a pink mid-stripe on each petal. ↕ 6cm (2½in),

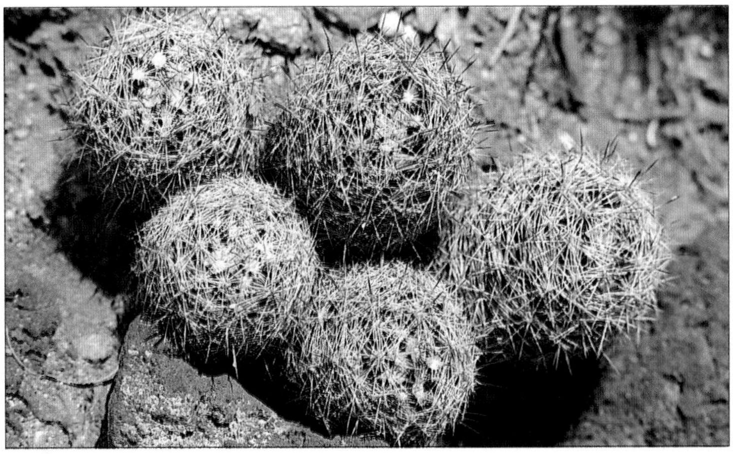

Escobaria vivipara

↔ indefinite. S.W. USA. ❄ (min. 7°C/45°F)
E. vivipara ■ syn. *Coryphantha vivipara.* Solitary or clustering cactus with depressed-spherical to short-cylindrical, white-woolly grey stems, 2.5–5cm (1–2in) thick, with cylindrical tubercles. Areoles bear brown spines (12–40 radials and 2–12 centrals). Wide-spreading, almost daisy-like, pink, magenta, purple, or occasionally white flowers, 3.5cm (1½in) long, are borne in summer. ↕ to 13cm (5in), ↔ indefinite. S. Canada to N. Mexico. ❄ (min. 7°C/45°F)

▷ ***Esmeralda sanderiana*** see *Euanthe sanderiana*

ESPOSTOA

CACTACEAE

Genus of 10 species of columnar, often tree-like, slow-growing, perennial cacti, some of which branch from near their bases to form clumps. They occur in hilly regions of S. Ecuador, Peru, and Bolivia. The straight-ribbed, dark to greyish green stems and branches are covered with areoles bearing numerous

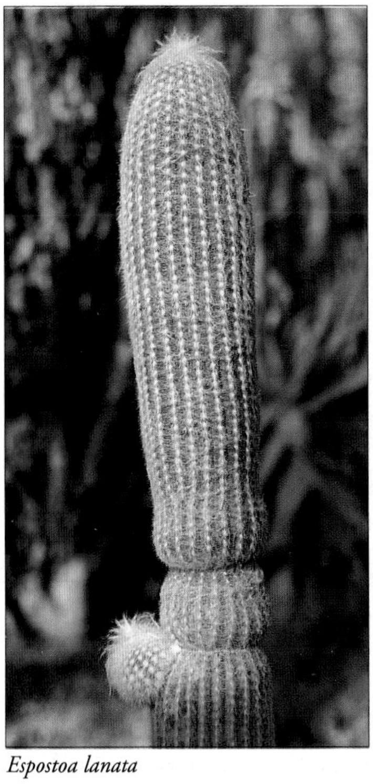

Espostoa lanata

spines. As they mature, most species produce a long pseudocephalium that bears cup-shaped to tubular, usually nocturnal flowers in summer. In frost-prone areas, grow as houseplants or in a temperate greenhouse. In warm, dry areas, plant outdoors in a desert garden.
• **HARDINESS** Frost tender.
• **CULTIVATION** Under glass, grow in standard cactus compost in full light. From spring to summer, water moderately and apply a low-nitrogen fertilizer every 4–5 weeks; keep dry at other times. Outdoors, grow in poor to moderately fertile, sharply drained soil in full sun. See also pp.48–49.
• **PROPAGATION** Sow seed at 21°C (70°F) in early spring.
• **PESTS AND DISEASES** Trouble free.

E. lanata ■ Tree-like or shrubby cactus with a columnar, 20- to 30-ribbed, mid-green stem, 10–15cm (4–6in) thick. The stem is densely covered with white areoles that bear short, usually yellowish white, occasionally red, yellow, brown, or purple spines and long, silky white hairs. Produces cup-shaped, white to purple flowers, 4–8cm (1½–3in) long, in summer. ↕ 1.5m (5ft), ↔ 60cm (24in). S. Ecuador, Peru. ❄ (min. 5–10°C/ 41–50°F)
E. melanostele. Shrubby, erect cactus with a columnar, 20- to 30-ribbed, greyish green stem, 10cm (4in) thick, with close-set brown areoles and initially yellow, later black spines. In summer, bears tubular white, sometimes yellow or brown flowers, 5cm (2in) long. ↕ 2m (6ft), ↔ 10cm (4in). C. Peru. ❄ (min. 5–10°C/41–50°F)
E. senilis. Shrubby or tree-like cactus with simple, or occasionally branched, 18- to 25-ribbed, dark green stems, 5–7cm (2–3in) thick. White areoles bear white spines. Solitary, tubular purple flowers, 3–4cm (1¼–1½in) long, are produced in summer. ↕ 2–3m (6–10ft), ↔ 60cm (24in). Peru. ❄ (min. 5–10°C/41–50°F)

ETLINGERA

ZINGIBERACEAE

Genus of 57 species of rhizomatous, evergreen or semi-evergreen perennials occurring in forest margins from Sri Lanka to New Guinea. They have cane-like stems, linear to inversely lance-shaped leaves, and produce torch-like inflorescences at the top of leafless stalks. The inflorescences are composed of overlapping, thick, waxy, usually colourful bracts, with relatively insignificant flowers often concealed in the lower bracts. *E. elatior* is the only widely cultivated species. In frost-prone areas, grow in a warm greenhouse; in warmer areas, grow in a bed or border.
• **HARDINESS** Frost tender.
• **CULTIVATION** Under glass, grow in loam-based potting compost (JI No.3) with added bark and leaf mould, preferably in a border, in bright filtered light. In the growing season, water freely and apply a balanced liquid fertilizer monthly. Outdoors, grow in fertile, humus-rich, well-drained soil in full sun or light dappled shade.
• **PROPAGATION** Sow seed at 20°C (68°F) as soon as ripe. Divide in spring or summer.
• **PESTS AND DISEASES** Trouble free.

E. elatior, syn. *Nicolaia elatior* (Philippine waxflower, Torch ginger). Upright, rhizomatous, evergreen perennial with linear-lance-shaped leaves, to 85cm (34in) long, dark green above, purplish green beneath. In summer, stems 1.5m (5ft) tall bear cone-shaped inflorescences, to 30cm (12in) long, composed of deep pink, sterile bracts, to 12cm (5in) long, and crimson, 3-petalled flowers with white or yellow margins, produced from the smaller, paler, lower bracts. ↕ 6m (20ft), ↔ 3m (10ft). Indonesia (Java, Sulawesi); widely naturalized in the tropics. ❄ (min. 16°C/61°F)

EUANTHE

ORCHIDACEAE

Genus of one species of monopodial, evergreen, epiphytic orchid, closely allied to the genus *Vanda*. It occurs mainly at sea level in the Philippines. Its upright stem is clothed in leaf bases and has 2 rows of strap-shaped leaves. Long aerial roots appear near the bases where the leaves have been shed, and racemes of flowers are produced from the leaf axils in autumn. *E. sanderiana* hybridizes readily with *Vanda* species.
• **HARDINESS** Frost tender.
• **CULTIVATION** Warm-growing orchid. Grow in epiphytic orchid compost, made with coarse bark, in a slatted basket. In summer, provide high humidity and bright filtered light, water freely, adding fertilizer at every third watering, and mist once or twice a day. In winter, admit full light and water more sparingly. See also p.46.
• **PROPAGATION** When they have their own roots, remove the growths that are occasionally produced from the bases and pot them up separately.
• **PESTS AND DISEASES** Red spider mites, aphids, and mealybugs may be troublesome.

E. sanderiana, syn. *Esmeralda sanderiana, Vanda sanderiana.* Epiphytic orchid with semi-rigid, strap-shaped, recurved, leathery leaves, 30cm (12in) long, with central grooves. Racemes, 25–35cm (10–14in) long, of 6–10 delicately coloured, white-flushed pink flowers, 10cm (4in) or more across, with red veining, are produced well above the leaves in autumn. ↕↔ 45cm (18in). Philippines. ❄ (min. 16°C/61°F; max. 32°C/90°F)

EUCALYPTUS

Gum, Ironbark

MYRTACEAE

Genus of over 500 species of evergreen trees and shrubs found in all but the driest habitats, mainly in Australia, but also in the Philippines, Malaysia, Indonesia, Papua New Guinea, and Melanesia. They are valued for their often aromatic foliage and their attractive bark. Young plants (and sucker shoots) generally have opposite leaves, developing alternate ones as they mature. The petalless flowers, composed of many showy, usually white or creamy yellow, sometimes red stamens, are usually borne in umbels. Most gum trees are best planted as specimens. In frost-prone areas, grow half-hardy and tender species in a cool greenhouse and stand them outside in summer.
• **HARDINESS** Fully hardy to frost tender.
• **CULTIVATION** Outdoors, grow in fertile, neutral to slightly acid soil that does not dry out, in full sun; shelter from cold, drying winds. Under glass, grow in loam-based potting compost (JI No.3), with added sharp sand, in full light with good ventilation. In growth, water freely and apply a balanced liquid fertilizer monthly; water sparingly in winter. Pruning group 1 or, for the best display of juvenile foliage, group 7; may need restrictive pruning under glass.
• **PROPAGATION** Sow seed at 13–18°C (55–64°F) in spring or summer.
• **PESTS AND DISEASES** Prone to silver leaf, oedema, and suckers (psyllids).

E. camaldulensis ♀ (Red river gum). Spreading, usually dense tree with a smooth, grey or whitish blue trunk, sometimes streaked or tinted reddish pink. Juvenile leaves are ovate to broadly lance-shaped, and grey-green; adult leaves, to 30cm (12in) long, are lance-shaped to narrowly lance-shaped, and usually mid-green, sometimes grey-green. Produces umbels of 7–11 white flowers, mainly in summer. ↕ 15–50m (50–160ft), ↔ 15–35m (50–120ft). Australia (except Tasmania). ✲
E. coccifera ■ ♀ (Mount Wellington peppermint, Tasmanian snow gum). Spreading tree with peeling, white or white-grey bark, which is sometimes yellow or pink when young. Rounded, mid-green juvenile leaves are followed by peppermint-scented, elliptic, grey-

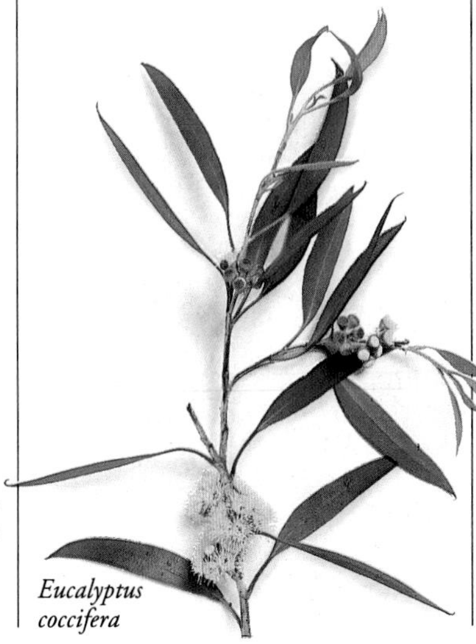

Eucalyptus coccifera

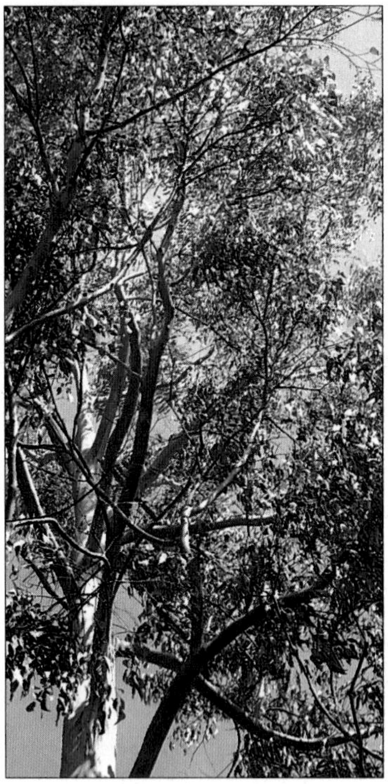

Eucalyptus dalrympleana

green adult leaves, to 10cm (4in) long. Bears umbels of 3, sometimes up to 9, white or creamy white flowers in summer. ↕ 18m (60ft), ↔ 7m (22ft). Australia (Tasmania). ❄❄❄

E. dalrympleana ▣ ♀ ◊ (Broad-leaved kindling bark, Mountain gum). Vigorous, broadly columnar tree with smooth, creamy white bark. Ovate, light green to blue-green juvenile leaves are followed by narrowly lance-shaped, bright green adult leaves, to 20cm (8in) long. Bears umbels of 3, sometimes up to 7, white flowers from late summer to autumn. Will tolerate chalk soil. ↕ 20m (70ft), ↔ 8m (25ft). S.E. Australia. ❄❄❄ (borderline)

E. delegatensis ◊ Broadly conical tree with peeling bark, rough and grey to brown on the lower half of the trunk, smooth and white above. Juvenile leaves are elliptic to ovate or broadly lance-shaped, and blue-green; adult leaves are lance-shaped, curved, dull, mid-green, and to 20cm (8in) long. Bears umbels of 7–15 white flowers in summer. ↕ 25m (80ft), ↔ 10m (30ft). S.E. Australia. ❄

E. divaricata see *E. gunnii.*

E. ficifolia ▣ ◊ (Red-flowering gum). Dense, spreading tree with rough, dark

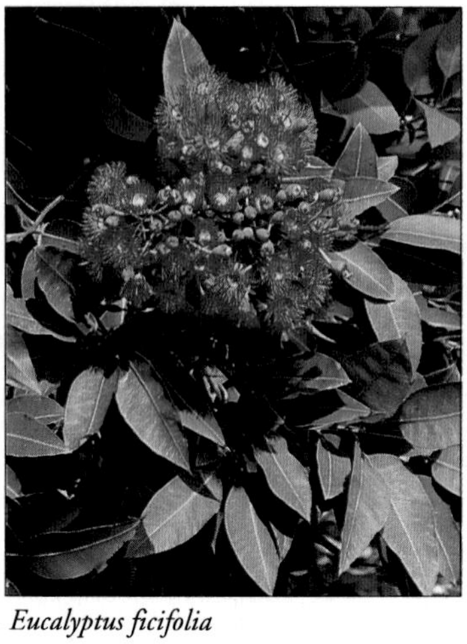

Eucalyptus ficifolia

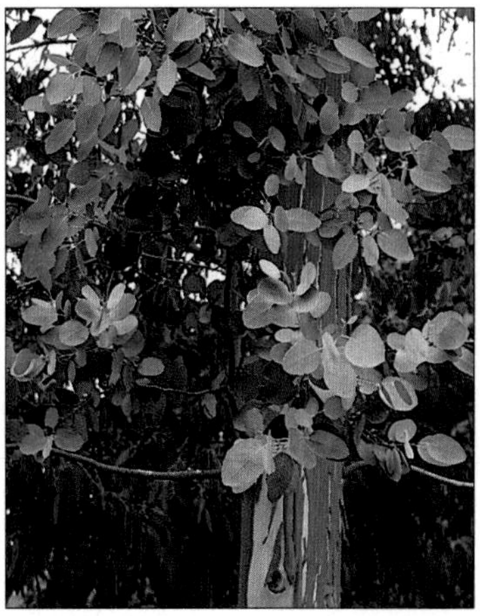

Eucalyptus gunnii

greyish brown bark. Juvenile leaves are ovate to broadly lance-shaped, mid- to deep green above, and paler beneath; adult leaves, 7–15cm (3–6in) long, are similar to the juvenile leaves. From summer to autumn, bears umbels of 3–7 red, occasionally pink or white flowers. Pendent, woody seed capsules, to 3.5cm (1½in) long, are urn-shaped. ↕ 6–15m (20–50ft), ↔ 5–20m (15–70ft). Australia (Western Australia). ❄

E. glaucescens ◊ (Tingiringi gum). Broadly conical tree or shrub with smooth white bark that sheds in red flakes to leave a white surface. Rounded, blue-white juvenile leaves are followed by slender, lance-shaped, blue-grey adult leaves, to 12cm (5in) long. Bears umbels of 3 white flowers in autumn. ↕ 12m (40ft), ↔ 8m (25ft). S.E. Australia. ❄❄

E. globulus ♀ ◊ (Tasmanian blue gum). Spreading, moderately dense tree with smooth, white to cream, yellow, or grey bark that sheds in ribbons to reveal the light green and light brown inner bark. Juvenile plants have square-sectioned or winged stems, and ovate, blue-white, stem-clasping leaves, to 15cm (6in) long. Adult trees have pendent, narrowly lance- to sickle-shaped, mid- to deep green leaves, 10–30cm (4–12in) long, and produce usually solitary, white to cream flowers from spring to summer. Juvenile plants are often used in summer bedding schemes. ↕ 15–50m (50–160ft), ↔ 10–25m (30–80ft). Australia (Victoria, Tasmania). ❄❄

E. gregsoniana, syn. *E. pauciflora* var. *nana* (Wolgan snow gum). Spreading shrub with shoots that are glossy red on the exposed side. Elliptic, bluish green to grey-green juvenile leaves are followed by slender, lance-shaped, curved, red-margined, grey-green adult leaves, to 11cm (4½in) long. In late spring and early summer, produces umbels of 5–12 white flowers. ↕ 2–4m (6–12ft), ↔ 5m (15ft). Australia (New South Wales). ❄❄

E. gunnii ▣ ♀ ◊ syn. *E. divaricata* (Cider gum). Dense, erect then spreading tree with smooth, whitish green bark that is shed annually in late summer to reveal yellowish to greyish green new bark, sometimes flushed pink or orange. Juvenile leaves are ovate to rounded, mid-green, and often glaucous. Adult leaves, 5–8cm (2–3in) long, are elliptic or ovate to broadly lance-shaped, and grey-green. Freely produces umbels of 3 white to cream flowers in summer or autumn. ↕ 10–25m (30–80ft), ↔ 6–15m (20–50ft). Australia (Tasmania). ❄❄❄ (borderline)

E. johnstonii ▣ ◊ (Tasmanian yellow gum). Vigorous, broadly columnar tree with peeling, reddish brown and creamy white bark. Rounded juvenile leaves are followed by lance-shaped or ovate adult leaves, to 12cm (5in) long; all leaves are glossy and dark green. Umbels of 3 white flowers are produced in summer. ↕ 25m (80ft), ↔ 10m (30ft). Australia (Tasmania). ❄❄

E. leucoxylon ◊ (Blue gum, White ironbark, Yellow gum). Erect to spreading, loose to dense tree with rough, fibrous, grey bark, darker at the base, shedding in late summer to reveal paler, smooth, cream, brown, or bluish grey bark. Broadly lance-shaped to ovate or rounded-heart-shaped, dull, dark green or glaucous juvenile leaves are followed by lance-shaped, matt, mid-green or grey-green adult leaves, to 13cm (5in) long. Umbels of 3 white, pink, or red flowers are produced in summer, and sometimes through to autumn or winter. ↕ 15m (50ft), ↔ 6–20m (20–70ft). S.E. Australia. ❄

E. macrocarpa (Mottlecah). Wide-spreading, open shrub with white young stems and smooth grey bark that sheds to reveal pinkish red bark beneath. Juvenile and adult leaves, to 13cm (5in) long, are broadly ovate to elliptic, and silvery grey. Solitary flowers open from white buds as a dense brush of bright red stamens with yellow anthers, mainly from spring to summer. Woody, disc-shaped seed pods are 5cm (2in) across. ↕ 2–4m (6–12ft), ↔ 3–12m (10–40ft). Australia (Western Australia). ⌂ (min. 3–5°C/37–41°F)

E. mannifera* subsp. *maculosa ◊ (Brittle gum). Rounded to spreading, moderately dense tree with smooth white bark covered by a powdery bloom. The bark turns pink then red in summer, and flakes from late summer to autumn to reveal a creamy new surface. Juvenile leaves are elliptic to narrowly lance-shaped, and blue-white to blue-green; adult leaves, to 15cm (6in) long, are lance-shaped and grey-green. Bears umbels of up to 7 white flowers from spring to summer. ↕ 10–20m (30–70ft), ↔ 8–15m (25–50ft). Australia (New South Wales). ❄

E. nicholii ▣ ◊ (Narrow-leaved black peppermint). Wide-spreading, dense tree with a rounded crown and fibrous, grey to reddish brown bark. Narrowly lance-shaped, peppermint-scented leaves, 7–13cm (3–5in) long, are grey- to blue-green on juvenile trees, matt bluish green or light green on adult trees. Bears umbels of 7 white flowers in autumn. ↕ 12–16m (40–52ft), ↔ 5–12m (15–40ft). Australia (Queensland, New South Wales). ❄❄

E. niphophila see *E. pauciflora* subsp. *niphophila.*

E. parvifolia ♀ ◊ (Kybean gum, Small-leaved gum). Spreading tree with peeling, smooth, grey and white bark. Elliptic, mid-green juvenile leaves are followed by lance-shaped, grey-green adult leaves, to 7cm (3in) long. Bears umbels of 7 white flowers in summer. Tolerates chalk soil. ↕ 15m (50ft), ↔ 10m (30ft). Australia (New South Wales). ❄❄

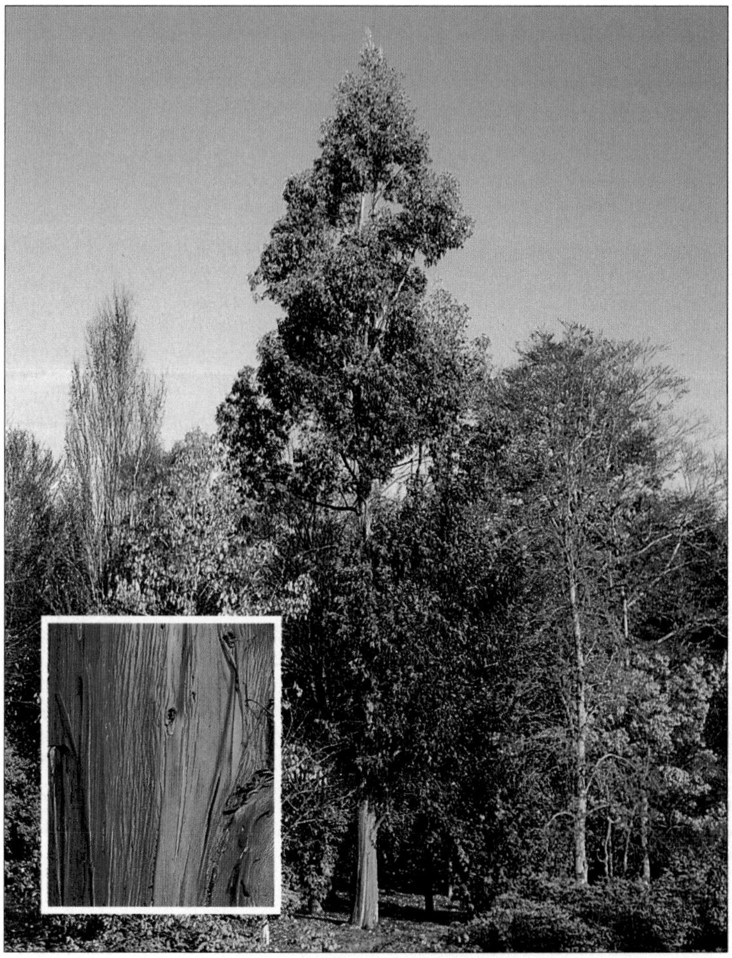

Eucalyptus johnstonii (inset: bark detail)

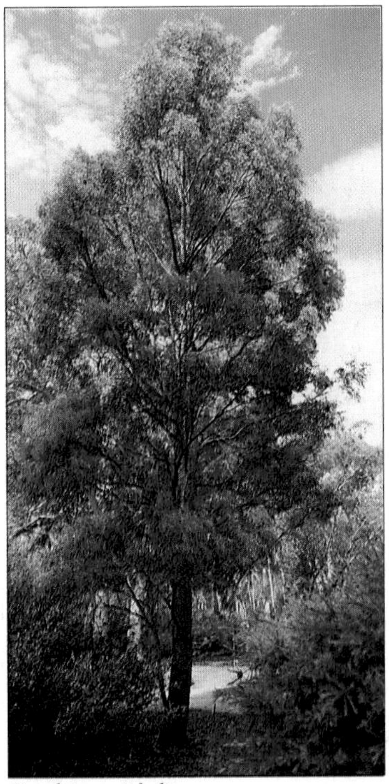
Eucalyptus nicholii

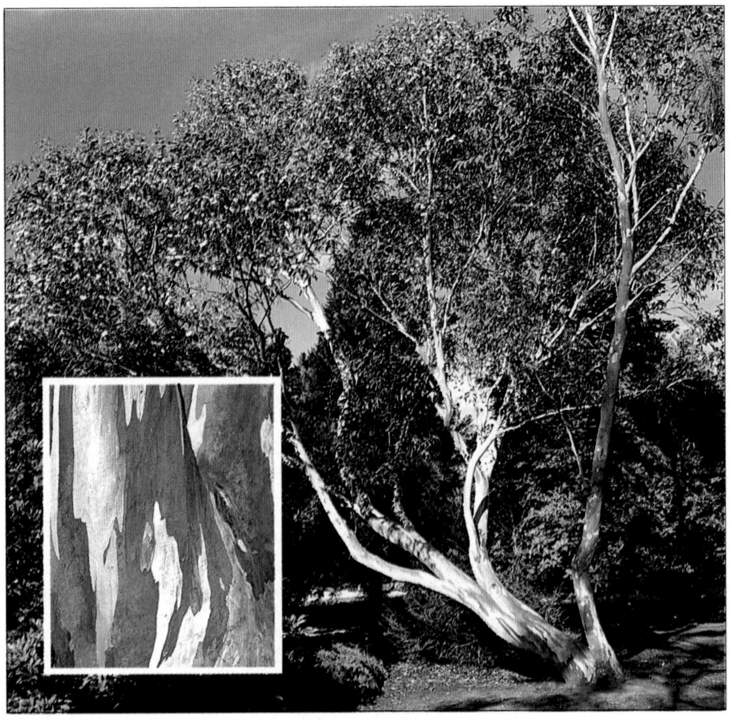
Eucalyptus pauciflora subsp. *niphophila* (inset: bark detail)

E. pauciflora ♀ (Cabbage gum, Weeping gum, White sallee). Usually dense, spreading tree with smooth, whitish grey or pale brown bark that sheds from late summer to autumn to reveal yellow, bronze, or greenish patches; twigs are often yellow or red. Juvenile leaves are ovate to elliptic, and grey-green; adult leaves, to 16cm (6in) long, are lance-shaped to narrowly ovate, pendent, and lustrous, mid- to blue-green. Bears umbels of 7–15 white to cream flowers from late spring to summer. ↕ 8–20m (25–70ft), ↔ 6–15m (20–50ft). Australia (South Australia, New South Wales, Victoria, Tasmania). ✲✲✲. **var. *nana*** see *E. gregsoniana.* **subsp. *niphophila*** ▣ ♀ syn. *E. niphophila* (Alpine snow gum, Snow gum), is very hardy, with twigs covered in a waxy white bloom, glaucous shoots, narrowly lance-shaped leaves, and 3- to 7-flowered umbels; ↕ to 6m (20ft).
E. perriniana ▣ ♀ (Round-leaved snow gum, Spinning gum). Open to moderately dense, small tree or large shrub, branching from the base, with smooth, flaking, off-white, grey, or green bark. Rounded, bluish green juvenile leaves are joined at the bases around the stem; adult leaves, to 12cm (5in) long, are pendent, lance-shaped, and glaucous. Umbels of 3 white or cream flowers are produced in summer. ↕ 4–10m (12–30ft), ↔ 3–8m (10–25ft). Australia (New South Wales, Victoria, Tasmania) ✲✲
E. piperita ♀ (Sydney peppermint). Open to dense tree with bark that is fibrous and grey at the base, and smooth and grey to white above. Ovate, bluish green juvenile leaves are followed by lance- to sickle-shaped, bluish green adult leaves, 8–14cm (3–5½in) long. Leaves are peppermint-scented. Produces umbels of 7–15 white flowers in summer. ↕ 12–30m (40–100ft), ↔ 8–20m (25–70ft). Australia (New South Wales). ✲
E. polyanthemos ♀ (Red box, Silver dollar gum). Broadly conical tree with sometimes fibrous, red-brown bark. Juvenile leaves are rounded, notched, and silvery green; adult leaves, to 9cm (3½in) long, are ovate to broadly lance-shaped, and grey-green. Umbels of up to 7 white flowers are borne in summer. ↕ to 25m (80ft), ↔ 12m (40ft). Australia (New South Wales, Victoria). ✲
E. pulverulenta ♀ (Powdered gum, Silver-leaved mountain gum). Spreading tree with grey to white bark that peels to reveal smooth, grey to bronze or brown bark beneath; twigs are green or white, covered by an intense waxy-white bloom. Heart-shaped, silvery-bloomed juvenile leaves, to 5cm (2in) long, usually persist on mature plants. Umbels of 3 white flowers are produced during winter. ↕ 25m (80ft), ↔ 15m (50ft). Australia (New South Wales). ✲✲
E. sideroxylon ♀ (Mugga, Red ironbark). Tree with a rounded to spreading, open crown and thick, fissured, blackish to reddish brown bark. Linear to lance-shaped, bluish green juvenile leaves are followed by lance-shaped, grey-green adult leaves, to 14cm (5½in) long. Bears umbels of 3–7 red, pink, white, or pale yellow flowers from winter to summer. ↕ 10–30m (30–100ft), ↔ 8–15m (25–50ft). Australia (Queensland to Victoria). ✲
E. urnigera ♀ (Urn-fruited gum, Urn gum). Conical tree with peeling, grey and creamy white bark. Rounded, shiny, mid-green juvenile leaves are followed by ovate to lance-shaped, often slightly glaucous, mid-green adult leaves, to 12cm (5in) long. Bears umbels of 3 white flowers in spring. ↕ 12m (40ft), ↔ 6m (20ft). Australia (Tasmania). ✲✲
E. viminalis ♀ (Manna gum, Ribbon gum, White gum). Erect to spreading, usually open tree with rough grey bark below, and smooth, grey or whitish yellow bark above, which shreds into ribbons during summer. Juvenile leaves, 3.5–6cm (1½–2½in) long, are lance-shaped to narrowly ovate; adult leaves, to 20cm (8in) long, are lance-shaped or narrowly lance-shaped; all are light green. Produces umbels of 3–7 white flowers from summer to autumn. ↕ 10–50m (30–160ft), ↔ 8–15m (25–50ft). Australia (Queensland to Tasmania, South Australia). ✲✲

▷ ***Eucharidium*** see *Clarkia*
E. breweri **'Pink Ribbons'** see *C. breweri* 'Pink Ribbons'

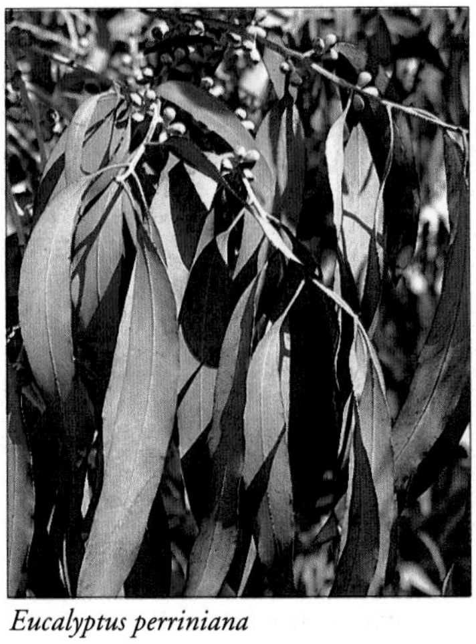
Eucalyptus perriniana

EUCHARIS

AMARYLLIDACEAE

Genus of 17 species of evergreen, summer-flowering, bulbous perennials occurring in moist open forest or forest margins in Central and South America. They are cultivated for their umbels of fragrant, daffodil-like white flowers. Each flower has 6 spreading tepals, arranged in two rows (the outer longer and narrower than the inner), and 6 stamens that fuse to form a cup. The long-stalked, ovate or elliptic to lance-shaped, glossy, basal leaves are often wavy and sometimes folded. In frost-prone climates, grow in a temperate or warm greenhouse or in a conservatory. In warmer areas, grow outdoors in a bed or border.

- **HARDINESS** Frost tender.
- **CULTIVATION** Under glass, grow in loam-based potting compost (JI No.2) with added sharp sand and leaf mould, in bright filtered light. When in active growth, water freely and apply a balanced liquid fertilizer monthly; water sparingly in winter. Pot on every 3 or 4 years in spring. Outdoors, grow in moderately fertile, humus-rich, well-drained soil in light dappled shade.
- **PROPAGATION** Remove offsets after flowering and grow on at 15°C (59°F) until established.
- **PESTS AND DISEASES** Trouble free.

E. amazonica ▣ Bulbous perennial with long-elliptic, wavy, dark green leaves, 40cm (16in) long, that taper to stalks 30cm (12in) long. In late summer, a leafless stem, 70cm (28in) long, produces an umbel of up to 8 fragrant, pure white flowers, 9cm (3½in) across, with the stamens protruding 1.5cm (½in). ↕ 70cm (28in), ↔ 15cm (6in). Colombia, N.E. Peru. ❀ (min. 10°C/50°F)
***E. amazonica* of gardens** see *E.* x *grandiflora.*
***E.* x *grandiflora*,** syn. *E. amazonica* of gardens (Amazon lily). Bulbous perennial with semi-erect, elliptic to ovate, wavy, deep green leaves, 30cm (12in) long, on stalks to 3.5cm (1½in) long. In early summer, a leafless stem, to 50cm (20in) long, produces an umbel of up to 6 fragrant, slightly pendent white flowers, 7cm (3in) across, with long, protruding stamens. ↕ 40–60cm (16–24in), ↔ 30cm (12in). Colombia. ❀ (min. 10°C/50°F)

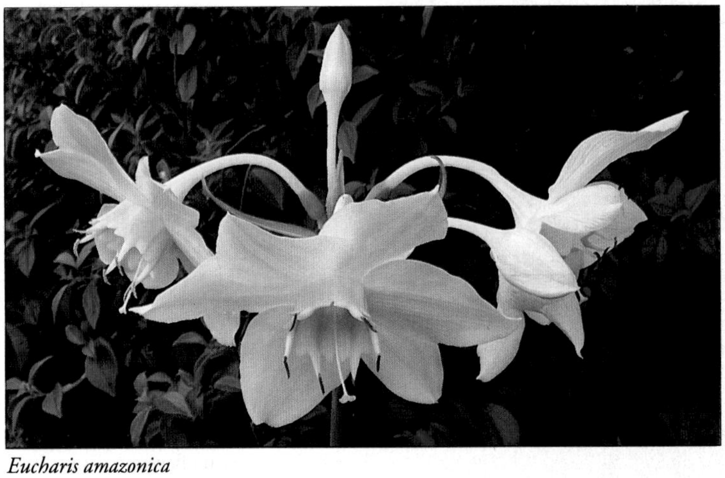
Eucharis amazonica

E

EUCOMIS

Pineapple flower, Pineapple lily

HYACINTHACEAE/LILIACEAE

Genus of about 15 species of bulbous perennials found in habitats ranging from rocky screes to seasonally damp meadows in South Africa and tropical southern Africa. They are cultivated for their unusual racemes of flowers borne in late summer and early autumn. Large bulbs each produce a basal rosette of lance-shaped to strap-shaped, glossy, light green leaves and a stout stem that bears a tight raceme of star-shaped flowers, to 2.5cm (1in) across, topped by a small tuft of leafy bracts, similar to those of a pineapple. Grow in a sunny, sheltered border or at the base of a warm wall. In frost-prone areas, grow less hardy species in a cool greenhouse.

• **HARDINESS** Fully hardy (borderline) to frost tender.
• **CULTIVATION** Plant bulbs 15cm (6in) deep. Grow in fertile, well-drained soil in full sun. Mulch in severe winters. Under glass, grow in loam-based potting compost (JI No.3) with added sharp sand or grit, in full light. Water freely in active growth, sparingly in winter.
• **PROPAGATION** Sow seed at 16°C (61°F) in autumn or spring, or remove offsets in spring.
• **PESTS AND DISEASES** Trouble free.

E. autumnalis, syn. *E. undulata*. Bulbous perennial bearing semi-erect, broadly strap-shaped, light green leaves, 45cm (18in) long, with wavy margins. In late summer and early autumn, bears racemes, 5–15cm (2–6in) long, of pale greenish white flowers that age to darker green. ↕20–30cm (8–12in), ↔20cm (8in). South Africa. ❄❄❄ (borderline)
E. bicolor ▣ Bulbous perennial that produces semi-erect, strap-shaped, wavy-margined, light green leaves, 30–50cm (12–20in) long. In late summer, maroon-flecked stems bear racemes, 15cm (6in) long, of pale green flowers

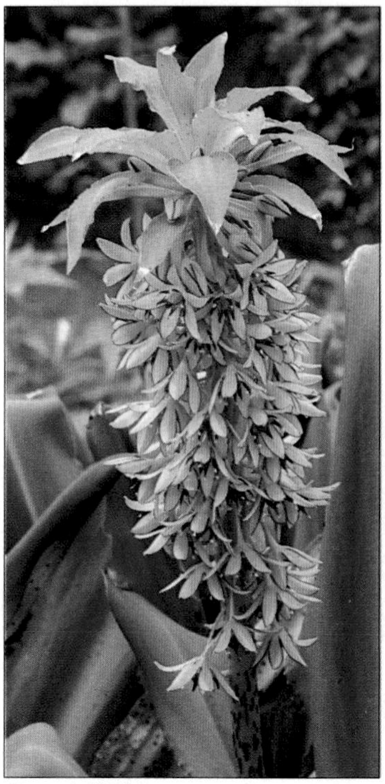

Eucomis bicolor

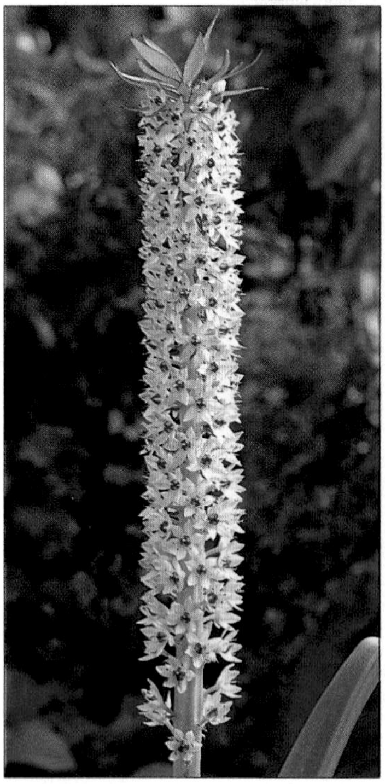

Eucomis comosa

with purple-margined tepals. ↕30–60cm (12–24in), ↔20cm (8in). South Africa. ❄❄❄ (borderline)
E. comosa ▣ syn. *E. punctata*. Bulbous perennial with semi-erect, lance-shaped, wavy-margined, light green leaves, to 70cm (28in) long, with heavy purple spotting beneath. In late summer, purple-striped stems bear racemes, to 30cm (12in) long, of white flowers with conspicuous purple tepal margins and ovaries. ↕75cm (30in), ↔20cm (8in). South Africa. ❄❄❄ (borderline)
E. pallidiflora (Giant pineapple flower). Robust, bulbous perennial with semi-erect, strap-shaped, light green leaves, to 70cm (28in) long, with crinkled margins. In late summer, bears greenish white flowers in racemes 24–45cm (10–18in) long. ↕45–75cm (18–30in), ↔20cm (8in). South Africa. ❄❄
E. punctata see *E. comosa*.
E. undulata see *E. autumnalis*.
E. zambesiaca. Compact, bulbous perennial with semi-erect, strap-shaped, light green leaves, to 15cm (6in) long. In late summer, produces white flowers in racemes 10–20cm (4–8in) long. ↕15–25cm (6–10in), ↔15cm (6in). Malawi. ❄❄

EUCOMMIA

EUCOMMIACEAE

Genus of one species of dioecious, deciduous tree originally from woodland in C. China. It is cultivated for its habit and foliage, and also for a certain curiosity value: the alternate, ovate to elliptic, prominently veined leaves, if torn across, will be held together by rubbery fibres. Grow as a specimen tree.

• **HARDINESS** Fully hardy.
• **CULTIVATION** Grow in fertile, well-drained soil in full sun or partial shade, sheltered from cold, drying winds. Pruning group 1.
• **PROPAGATION** Sow seed in a seedbed in autumn. Insert greenwood cuttings in summer.
• **PESTS AND DISEASES** Trouble free.

E. ulmoides ♀ (Gutta-percha tree). Spreading, broadly domed tree with ovate to elliptic, finely toothed, tapered, glossy, dark green leaves, 7–20cm (3–8in) long. Inconspicuous, axillary, petalless green flowers are usually borne singly, sometimes in clusters, before or with the leaves in spring. Female plants bear groups of winged green fruit. ↕12m (40ft), ↔8m (25ft). C. China. ❄❄❄

EUCRYPHIA

EUCRYPHIACEAE

Genus of 5 or 6 mainly evergreen trees and shrubs from moist woodland in Chile and S.E. Australia, grown for their habit, foliage, and flowers. They have opposite, simple or pinnate, leathery leaves and produce solitary, occasionally paired, cup-shaped to saucer-shaped, fragrant white flowers from the leaf axils. Effective as specimen plants.

• **HARDINESS** Fully hardy to frost hardy.
• **CULTIVATION** Grow in fertile, moist but well-drained, neutral to acid soil (*E. cordifolia* and *E.* x *nymansensis* tolerate alkaline soil). Site so that the roots are shaded and the crown is in full sun. Shelter from cold, drying winds in all but mild, moist areas. Pruning group 1 or 9 for most; group 8 for *E. lucida*.
• **PROPAGATION** Sow seed in containers in a cold frame as soon as ripe or in late winter. Insert semi-ripe cuttings in summer. Overwinter young plants in a cool greenhouse.
• **PESTS AND DISEASES** Trouble free.

E. cordifolia ▣♀ (Ulmo). Columnar, evergreen tree with simple, oblong, wavy-margined leaves, to 8cm (3in) long, dark green above, grey-downy beneath. Saucer-shaped white flowers, 5cm (2in) across, are borne from late summer to autumn. ↕15m (50ft), ↔8m (25ft). Chile. ❄❄
E. glutinosa ▣🏆♀ Upright, deciduous or semi-evergreen tree or shrub with pinnate leaves, to 6cm (2½in) long, composed of 3–5 elliptic-oblong, toothed, glossy, dark green leaflets that turn orange-red in autumn. Produces cup-shaped, sometimes double white flowers, 6cm (2½in) across, in mid- and late summer. The hardiest eucryphia and the most tolerant of exposure. ↕10m (30ft), ↔6m (20ft). Chile. ❄❄❄
***E.* x *intermedia* 'Rostrevor'** ▣🏆♀ Upright, evergreen tree with oblong leaves, to 6cm (2½in) long, either simple or with up to 3 oblong leaflets,

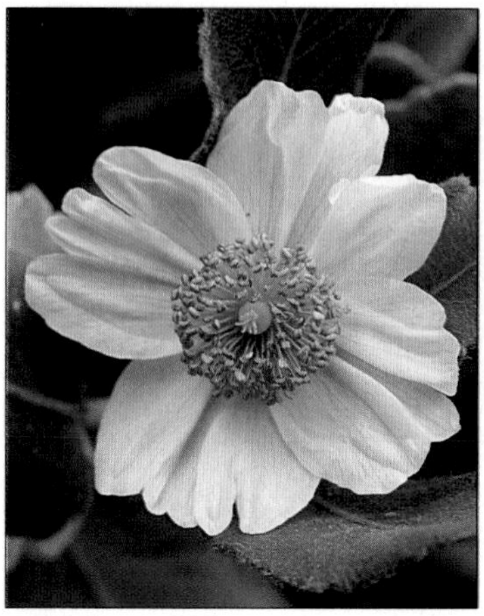

Eucryphia cordifolia

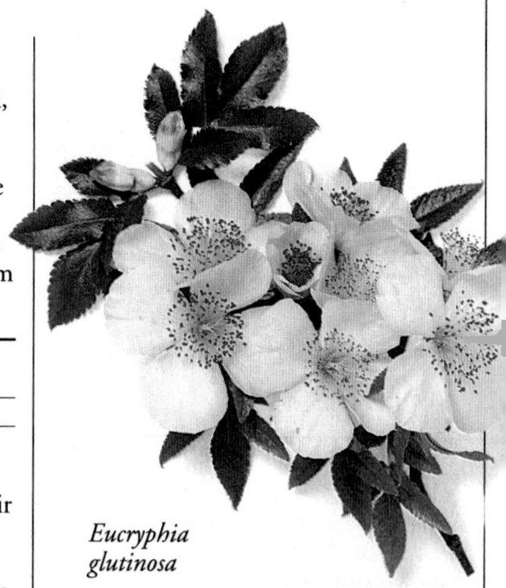

Eucryphia glutinosa

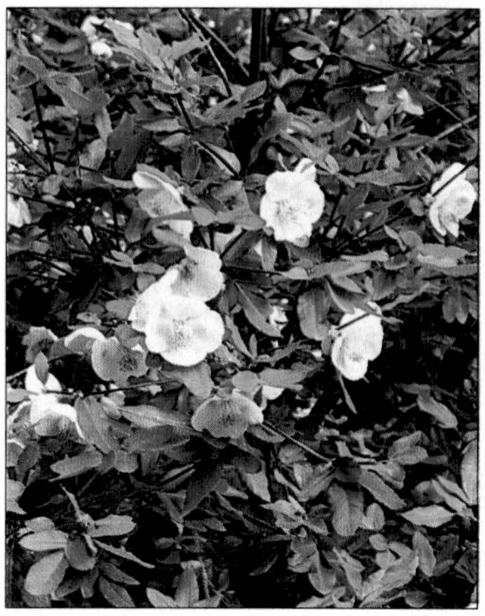

Eucryphia x *intermedia* 'Rostrevor'

glossy, dark green above, pale green and sometimes slightly glaucous beneath, with red shoots. Produces shallowly cup-shaped white flowers, 5cm (2in) across, from late summer to autumn. ↕10m (30ft), ↔6m (20ft). ❄❄❄ (borderline)
E. lucida ▣♀ Columnar, evergreen tree with simple, narrowly oblong to oblong-lance-shaped, glossy, dark green leaves, to 5cm (2in) long, glaucous beneath. Bears saucer-shaped white flowers, to 5cm (2in) across, in early and mid-summer. ↕8m (25ft), ↔4m (12ft). Australia (Tasmania). ❄❄. **'Pink Cloud'** produces pink flowers with crimson centres.
E. milliganii ▣ Slender, upright, evergreen shrub with simple, oblong, glossy, dark green leaves, 1.5–2cm (½–¾in) long, glaucous beneath. Bears shallowly cup-shaped white flowers, 2cm (¾in)

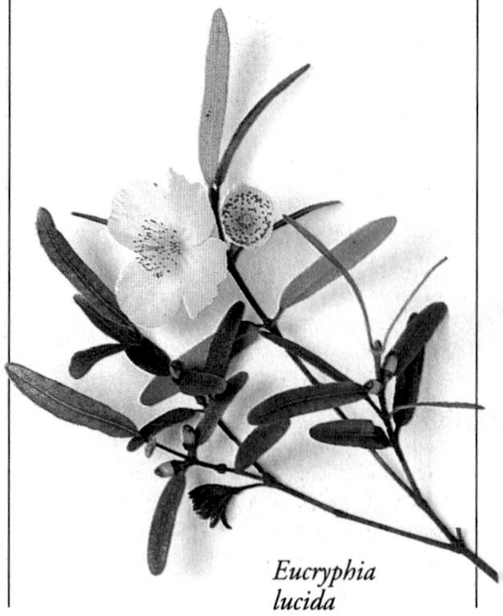

Eucryphia lucida

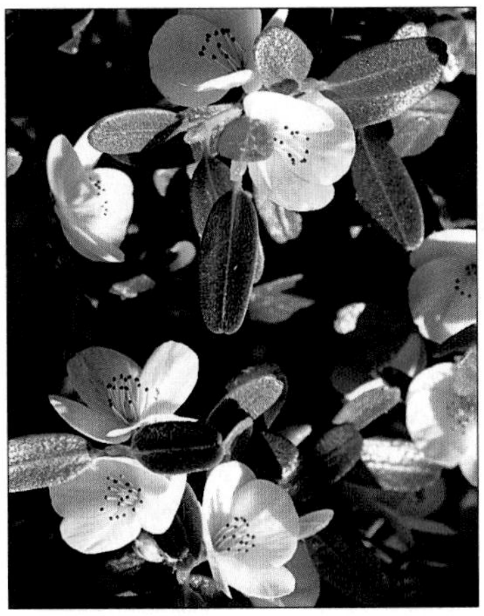
Eucryphia milliganii

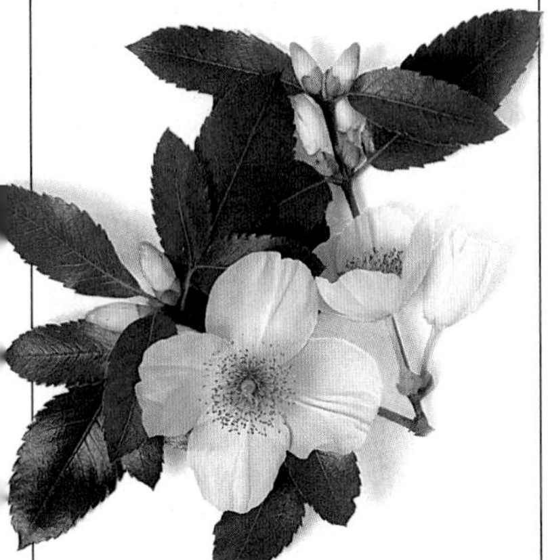
Eucryphia x *nymansensis* 'Nymansay'

across, in midsummer. ↕ 6m (20ft), ↔ 1.5m (5ft). Australia (Tasmania). ❄❄
***E.* x *nymansensis* 'Nymansay'** ▣ 🏆 ◇ Columnar, dense, evergreen tree with elliptic to elliptic-oblong, toothed leaves, to 6cm (2½in) long, dark green above, paler beneath, and simple or composed of 3 oblong leaflets. Bears cup-shaped white flowers, 7cm (3in) or more across, from late summer to autumn. ↕ 15m (50ft), ↔ 5m (15ft). ❄❄❄ (borderline)
***E.* 'Penwith'** ◇ Columnar, evergreen tree with oblong, wavy-margined, dark green leaves, to 7cm (3in) long, glaucous beneath, sometimes with 3 oblong leaflets, and borne on reddish green shoots. From late summer to autumn, bears saucer-shaped white flowers, 5cm (2in) across. ↕ 15m (50ft), ↔ 5m (15ft). ❄❄

▷ ***Eugenia aromatica*** see *Syzygium aromaticum*
▷ ***Eugenia australis* of gardens** see *Syzygium paniculatum*
▷ ***Eugenia paniculata*** see *Syzygium paniculatum*
▷ ***Eugenia smithii*** see *Acmena smithii*
▷ ***Eugenia ugni*** see *Ugni molinae*

EULOPHIA

ORCHIDACEAE

Genus of approximately 300 species of deciduous, mainly terrestrial orchids found in grassland and forest from sea level to almost 2,000m (6,000ft) throughout the tropics, especially in Africa. They have pseudobulbs, tuber-like corms, or fleshy roots, and produce usually 2, sometimes several, lance-shaped to linear, folded or leathery leaves. Flowers are borne in upright racemes from the bases of the plants.
• **HARDINESS** Frost tender.
• **CULTIVATION** Intermediate- or warm-growing orchids. Grow in containers of terrestrial orchid compost. In summer, water freely, applying fertilizer at every third watering, and provide high humidity and bright filtered light. Admit full light and keep dry during winter. See also p.46.
• **PROPAGATION** Divide when the plants fill and overflow their containers.
• **PESTS AND DISEASES** Red spider mites, aphids, whiteflies, and mealybugs may be troublesome.

E. guineensis. Terrestrial orchid with clustered pseudobulbs and narrowly elliptic leaves, 25cm (10in) long. Purplish green or reddish brown flowers, 6cm (2½in) across, with large, pinkish purple lips streaked and spotted with darker purple, are borne in racemes to 35cm (14in) long, in autumn. ↕↔ 30cm (12in). Gambia to Angola, Uganda. ❀ (min. 16°C/61°F; max. 32°C/90°F)

▷ ***Eunomia*** see *Aethionema*
E. oppositifolia see *A. oppositifolium*
▷ ***Euodia*** see *Tetradium*
E. daniellii see *T. daniellii*
E. hupehensis see *T. daniellii*

EUONYMUS

Spindle tree

CELASTRACEAE

Genus of approximately 175 species of deciduous, semi-evergreen, and evergreen shrubs, trees, and climbers found mostly in woodland and thickets, mainly in Asia. They are cultivated for their foliage, autumn colour, and ornamental, often ribbed, winged, or lobed, spherical or almost spherical fruits, borne from autumn to winter, which split to reveal seeds with often colourful arils. Leaves are opposite (rarely alternate), simple, very variable in shape, and toothed or scalloped. Cymes of 3, sometimes 7–15, small, green or white, sometimes purple-red or red-brown flowers are borne in late spring or summer. Uses range from a shrub border to specimen plantings, and from hedging to ground cover. All parts may cause mild stomach upset if ingested.
• **HARDINESS** Fully hardy to frost hardy.
• **CULTIVATION** Grow in any well-drained soil in full sun or light shade. If grown in full sun, they need moister soil, although deciduous species and cultivars are more tolerant of dry soil. Shelter evergreens from cold, drying winds. Variegated cultivars need sun to enhance leaf variegation. Pruning group 1 (deciduous) or group 8 (evergreen).
• **PROPAGATION** Sow seed in containers in a cold frame as soon as ripe. Root greenwood cuttings of deciduous species and cultivars, and semi-ripe cuttings of evergreens, in summer.
• **PESTS AND DISEASES** Caterpillars, vine weevil, powdery mildew, and leaf spot may be troublesome. Scale insects may infest evergreen species.

E. alatus ▣ 🏆 (Winged spindle). Dense, bushy, deciduous shrub with obovate to ovate-elliptic, toothed, dark green leaves, to 7cm (3in) long, that turn brilliant dark red in autumn. Shoots are 4-angled, with broad, corky wings. Almost spherical, reddish purple fruit, 8mm (⅜in) across, are 1–4 lobed; seeds have orange arils. ↕ 2m (6ft), ↔ 3m (10ft). China, Japan. ❄❄❄. **'Compactus'** 🏆 syn. 'Ciliodentatus', is dwarf and very dense; ↕ 1m (3ft).
E. bungeanus ◇ Graceful, deciduous or semi-evergreen shrub or small tree with arching shoots. Produces oval to ovate, finely toothed, sharp-pointed, pale green leaves, to 10cm (4in) long, that turn yellow and pink in autumn. Spherical, 4-lobed, pink-tinged, yellow-white fruit are 1cm (½in) across; seeds have orange arils. ↕ 6m (20ft), ↔ 5m (15ft). China, Korea. ❄❄
***E. cornutus* var. *quinquecornutus*.** Open, evergreen or deciduous shrub with slender, willow-like, narrowly lance-shaped, sharp-pointed, toothed, leathery, mid- to dark green leaves, to 10cm (4in) long. Spherical, strongly 5-winged pink fruit, to 1.5cm (½in) across, have 5 or 6 horns; seeds have orange arils. ↕ 2m (6ft), ↔ 3m (10ft). W. China. ❄❄
***E. europaeus* 'Red Cascade'** ▣ 🏆 ◇ Broadly conical, deciduous shrub or small tree with spreading, somewhat pendent shoots. Bears oval, scalloped, dark green leaves, to 7cm (3in) long, that turn red in autumn. Spherical, 4-lobed, clustered red fruit are 2cm (¾in) across; seeds have orange arils. ↕ 3m (10ft), ↔ 2.5m (8ft). ❄❄❄
E. fortunei* cultivars.** Prostrate to mound-forming, evergreen shrubs with oval, toothed, thinly leathery, dark green leaves, usually to 5cm (2in) long, and often variegated gold or white. Spherical white fruit, 6mm (¼in) across, contain seeds with orange arils. The cultivars described below are best grown in poor soil and full sun; all climb vigorously if supported, and are useful for training against a shady wall or through a tree. ↕ 60cm (24in), or to 5m (15ft) as climbers, ↔ indefinite. ❄❄❄. **'Coloratus'** has dark green leaves that turn purple-red from late autumn to winter in cold weather. **'Dart's Blanket'** has dark green leaves that turn bronze-red in autumn. **'Emerald Cushion'** is compact and mound-forming, with rich green foliage; ↕ 30cm (12in), ↔ 45cm (18in). **'Emerald Gaiety'** 🏆 is compact and bushy, bearing bright green leaves with white margins that are tinged pink in winter; ↕ 1m (3ft), ↔ 1.5m (5ft). **'Emerald 'n' Gold'** ▣ 🏆 is bushy, and bears bright green leaves with broad, bright yellow margins that are tinged pink in winter; ↔ 90cm (36in). **'Golden Prince'**, syn. 'Gold Tip', is small and compact, with deep green leaves that are tipped bright gold when young. **'Gold Tip'** see 'Golden Prince'. **'Kewensis'** forms a dense mat, and bears dark green leaves, to 1cm (½in) long, with pale green veins, on slender shoots; ↕ 10cm (4in). **'Minimus'** is similar to 'Kewensis' but has elliptic to rounded leaves, to 6mm (¼in) long. **var. *radicans has trailing stems and dark green leaves. **'Sarcoxie'** is vigorous and bushy, with glossy, dark green leaves; ↕↔ 1.2m (4ft). **'Silver Queen'** ▣ 🏆 is bushy and upright, with white-margined, dark green leaves, the margins later tinted pink; ↕ 2.5m (8ft), or 6m (20ft) as a climber, ↔ 1.5m (5ft).

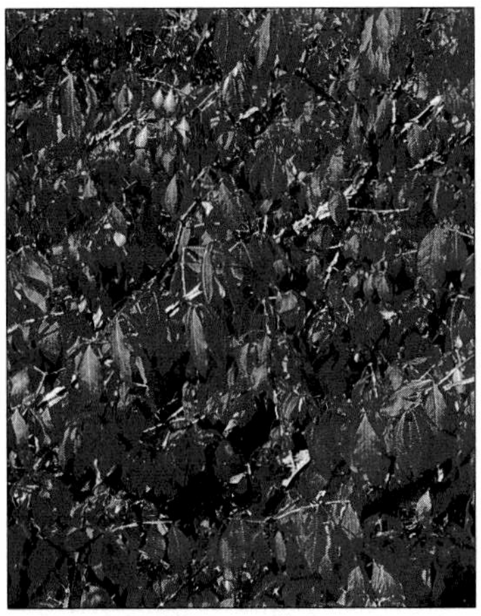
Euonymus alatus

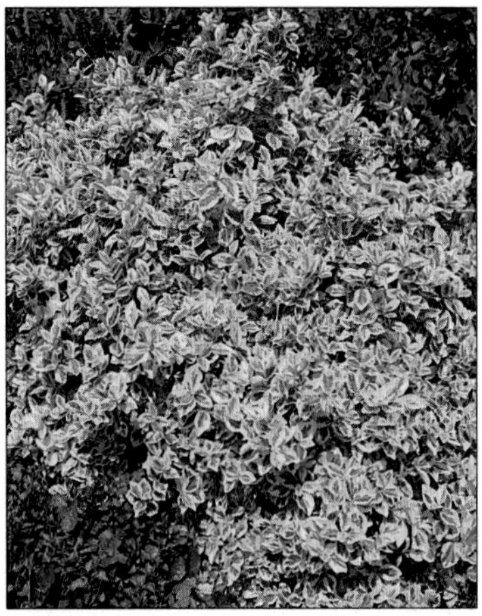
Euonymus fortunei 'Emerald 'n' Gold'

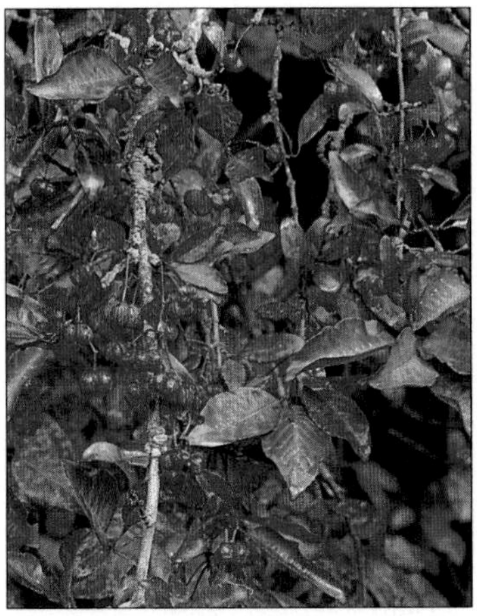
Euonymus europaeus 'Red Cascade'

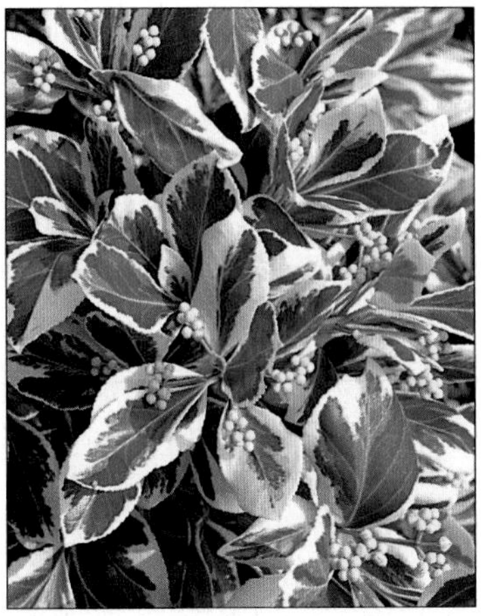
Euonymus fortunei 'Silver Queen'

E

E

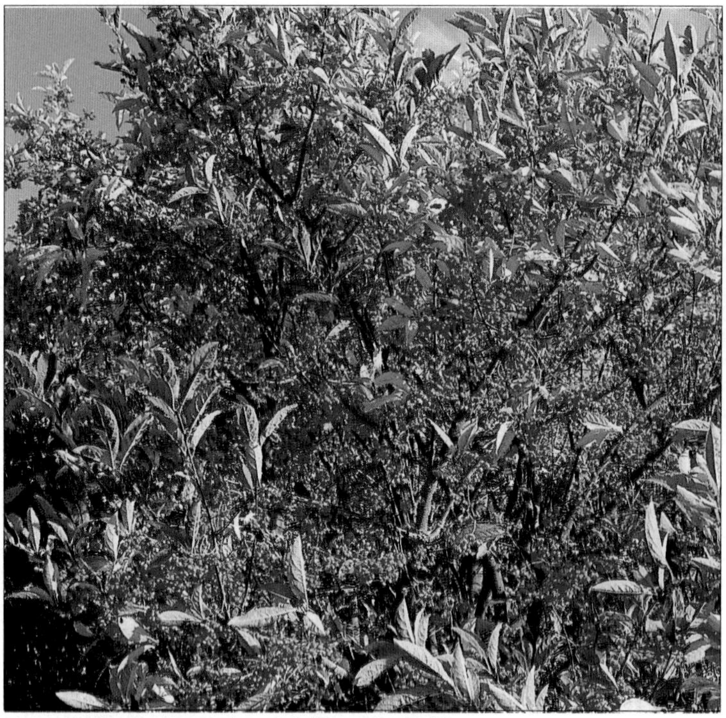

Euonymus hamiltonianus subsp. *sieboldianus* 'Red Elf'

***E. hamiltonianus* subsp. *sieboldianus*,** syn. *E. yedoensis.* Tree-like, deciduous shrub bearing oblong-ovate to elliptic, scalloped, mid-green leaves, to 12cm (5in) long, sometimes with long, sharp points; they turn yellow, pink, or red in autumn. Almost spherical, 4-lobed pink fruit, 0.7–1.5cm (¼–½in) across, contain blood-red seeds with orange arils. ↕↔ 6m (20ft). Korea, Japan. ❄❄❄. **'Red Elf'** ▣ is upright, with profusely borne, dark pink fruit, and seeds with red arils; ↕↔ 3m (10ft).

E. japonicus ♀ (Japanese spindle). Dense, bushy, evergreen shrub or small, erect tree with obovate to narrowly oval, toothed, leathery, glossy, dark green leaves, to 6cm (2½in) long. Spherical fruit, to 8mm (⅜in) long, are pink-tinged white, but are rarely produced; seeds have orange arils. Useful for hedging. Mildew may be a problem. ↕ 4m (12ft), ↔ 2m (6ft). China, Japan, Korea. ❄❄. **'Albomarginatus'** has oval, dark green leaves, 3–5cm (1¼–2in) long, narrowly margined with white. **'Aureopictus'** see 'Aureus'. **'Aureovariegatus'** see 'Ovatus Aureus'. **'Aureus'**, syn. 'Aureopictus', 'Luna', has dark green leaves, each with a central golden mark, often reverting to all-green or all-yellow; ↕ 1.5m (5ft), ↔ 1m (3ft). **'Luna'** see 'Aureus'. **'Macrophyllus'** is vigorous, with leaves to 9cm (3½in) long. **'Microphyllus Aureovariegatus'** has dark green leaves, to 2cm (¾in) long, with narrow yellow margins; ↕↔ 1m (3ft). **'Ovatus Aureus'** 🏆 syn. 'Aureovariegatus', has oval, dark green leaves with broad, golden yellow margins.

E. kiautschovicus. Open, spreading, evergreen or semi-evergreen shrub with oval to obovate, scalloped, bright green leaves, to 7cm (3in) long, that often turn orange-red and pink in autumn. Spherical pink fruit, 1cm (½in) across, containing seeds with orange-red arils, ripen in late autumn. ↕ 3m (10ft), ↔ 5m (15ft). China. ❄❄❄

E. latifolius ▣♀ Open, upright, deciduous shrub or small tree with elliptic to oblong-elliptic, finely scalloped, dark green leaves, to 12cm (5in) long, that turn brilliant red in late autumn. Pendent red fruit, 2.5cm (1in) across, are spherical with 4 or 5 prominent, flattened wings; seeds have orange arils. ↕↔ 3m (10ft). Europe, Turkey. ❄❄❄

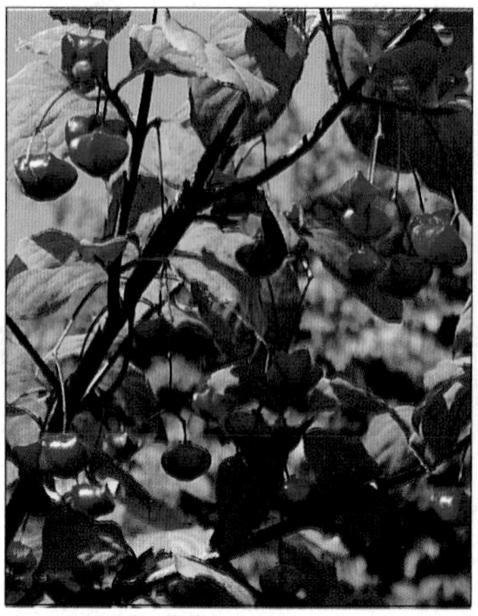

Euonymus latifolius

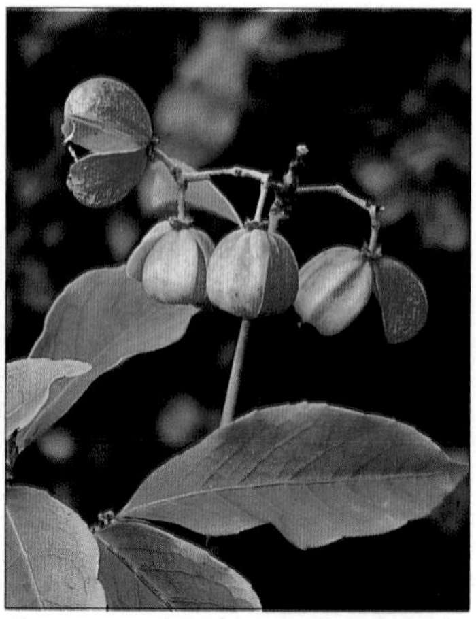

Euonymus myrianthus

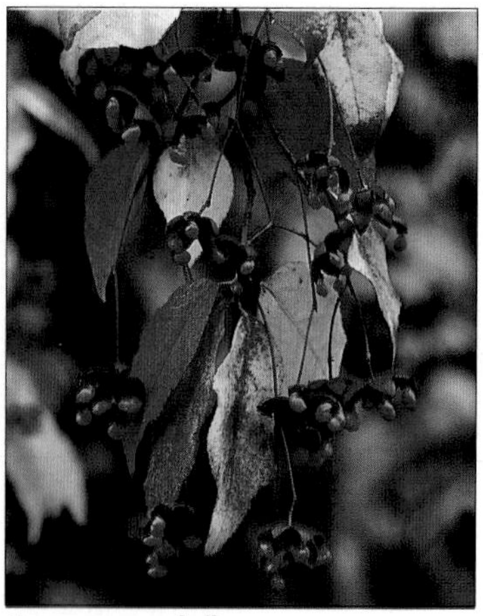

Euonymus oxyphyllus

E. lucidus ♀ syn. *E. pendulus.* Spreading, evergreen tree or shrub with narrowly ovate to lance-shaped, deeply toothed, glossy, deep green leaves, to 12cm (5in) long, bright red when young. Spherical yellow fruit, 1cm (½in) across, are deeply 4-lobed; seeds have orange arils. ↕ 10m (30ft), ↔ 8m (25ft). Himalayas. ❄❄

E. myrianthus ▣ Bushy, upright, evergreen shrub with oval-lance-shaped to oblong-ovate, tapered, sparsely toothed, leathery, dull green leaves, to 10cm (4in) long. Almost spherical, 4-ribbed, bright orange-yellow fruit are 1.5cm (½in) across; seeds have orange-red arils. ↕ 3m (10ft), ↔ 4m (12ft). W. China. ❄❄

E. nanus* var. *turkestanicus. Open, upright, deciduous shrub with alternate or opposite, linear to broadly linear, sparsely toothed, dark green leaves, to 5cm (2in) long, that turn bright red to red-bronze in autumn. Red-brown flowers are followed by spherical, 4-lobed pink fruit, 5–10mm (¼–½in) across; seeds have orange arils. ↕↔ 1m (3ft). C. Asia to China. ❄❄❄

E. oxyphyllus ▣♀ Upright, deciduous shrub or tree with ovate to ovate-oblong, tapered, finely toothed, dull green leaves, to 9cm (3½in) long, that turn purple-red in autumn. Spherical, dark red fruit, 1cm (½in) across, each have 4 or 5 short ribs; seeds have orange-red arils. ↕ 2.5m (8ft) or more, ↔ 2.5m (8ft). Korea, Japan. ❄❄❄

E. pendulus see *E. lucidus.*

E. planipes 🏆 syn. *E. sachalinensis* of gardens. Upright, deciduous shrub with long, pointed leaf-buds opening to elliptic, coarsely toothed, mid-green leaves, to 12cm (5in) long, that turn brilliant red in autumn. Produces 4- or 5-lobed, almost spherical red fruit, 2cm (¾in) across; seeds have bright orange arils. ↕↔ 3m (10ft). N.E. China, Korea, Japan. ❄❄❄

***E. sachalinensis* of gardens** see *E. planipes.*

E. verrucosus. Dense, bushy, rounded, deciduous shrub with rough, warty, dark shoots. Bears ovate to ovate-lance-shaped, tapered, scalloped, mid-green leaves, to 6cm (2½in) long, that turn yellow or red in autumn. Spherical, deeply 4-lobed fruit, 6mm (¼in) across, are red, often tinged with yellow; black seeds have red arils. ↕ 2.5m (8ft), ↔ 3m (10ft). E. Europe, W. Asia. ❄❄❄

E. yedoensis see *E. hamiltonianus* subsp. *sieboldianus.*

EUPATORIUM

Hemp agrimony

ASTERACEAE/COMPOSITAE

Genus of 40 species of annuals, herbaceous perennials, subshrubs, and evergreen shrubs. Originally a genus of over 1,000 species, most have now been transferred by botanists to other genera, including *Ageratina* and *Bartlettina.* They occur in temperate, subtropical, and tropical regions in Europe, Africa, Asia, and North to South America, in habitats ranging from dry, sandy sites in woodland and thickets, to pastureland and swamps. They produce opposite, whorled, or alternate leaves, which are usually toothed and dissected, but sometimes entire. Tubular, bisexual, white, pink, violet, or purple flowerheads are borne in terminal or axillary corymbs or panicles, or occasionally singly. Most eupatoriums have nectar-rich flowerheads that are attractive to bees and butterflies. Many of the hardy species are coarse perennials, useful for a border or a wild or woodland garden. The shrubs and subshrubs are suitable for a mixed or shrub border, but need a warm, sunny site in cool climates. In frost-prone areas, grow tender species in a cool or temperate greenhouse or conservatory.

- **HARDINESS** Fully hardy to frost tender.
- **CULTIVATION** Under glass, grow in loam-based potting compost (JI No.3) with added grit and humus, in full light. Provide good ventilation. When in full growth, water freely and apply a half-strength balanced liquid fertilizer when the flowerheads appear. After flowering, reduce watering and keep just moist in winter. Outdoors, grow in any moist soil in full sun or partial shade. Pruning group 8; may require restrictive pruning under glass.
- **PROPAGATION** Sow seed of hardy species in containers in a cold frame, and seed of tender species at 13–16°C (55–61°F), both in spring. Divide hardy species, and root softwood cuttings of tender species, in spring.
- **PESTS AND DISEASES** Whiteflies and red spider mites may be a problem under glass. Outdoors, slugs and aphids may be troublesome.

E. ageratoides see *E. rugosum.*

E. cannabinum (Hemp agrimony). Robust, clump-forming perennial with erect, red-tinted stems and opposite,

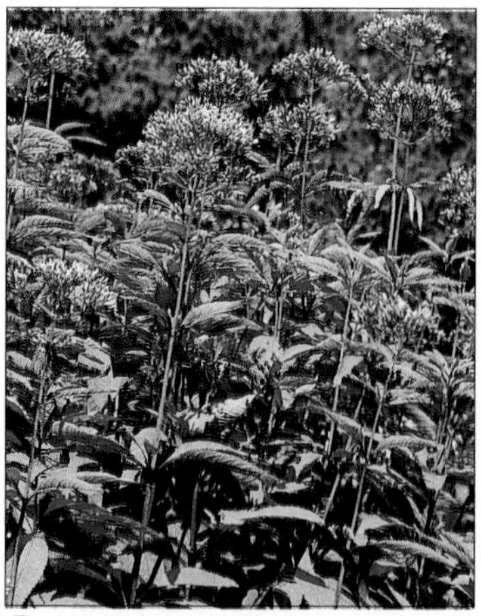

Eupatorium purpureum

palmately lobed, mid- to dark green leaves, 12cm (5in) across, with oblong-lance-shaped, coarsely toothed lobes. From summer to early autumn, bears pink, purple, or white flowerheads in terminal, dense, flat-topped, corymb-like panicles, to 10cm (4in) across. ↕ to 1.5m (5ft), ↔ to 1.2m (4ft). Europe. ❄❄❄

E. ligustrinum, syn. *Ageratina ligustrina*, *E. micranthum*, *E. weinmannianum*. Densely branched, domed shrub with opposite, elliptic to lance-shaped, toothed, long-pointed, light green leaves, to 10cm (4in) long, dotted with glands beneath. Fragrant, creamy white or pink-tinted flowerheads are produced in clustered, terminal corymbs, to 20cm (8in) across, in autumn. ↕↔ 2–5m (6–15ft). Mexico to Costa Rica. ❀ (min. 5°C/41°F)

E. micranthum see *E. ligustrinum*.

E. purpureum ■ (Joe Pye weed). Clump-forming perennial with whorls of lance-shaped-elliptic to ovate, finely toothed, sharp-pointed, coarse, purple-tinged, mid-green leaves, to 25cm (10in) long, borne on stiff, upright stems that are variably suffused purple. Bears terminal, domed, corymb-like panicles, 10–15cm (4–6in) across, of pink, pinkish purple, or creamy white flowerheads from midsummer to early autumn. Prefers alkaline soil. ↕ to 2.2m (7ft), ↔ 1m (3ft). E. USA. ❄❄❄

E. rugosum ■ syn. *Ageratina altissima E. ageratoides*, *E. urticifolium* (White snakeroot). Clump-forming perennial with stiff brown stems bearing opposite, lance-shaped to ovate, nettle-like, grey-green leaves, 4–12cm (1½–5in) long. Long-lasting, pure white flowerheads are produced in terminal corymbs, 6cm (2½in) across, from midsummer to early autumn. Frost may damage new shoots. Prefers alkaline soil in partial shade. ↕ 1.5–1.8m (5–6ft), ↔ 60cm (24in). E. North America. ❄❄❄. **'Braunlaub'** bears brown-flushed young leaves and brown-tinged flowers.

E. sordidum, syn. *Bartlettina sordida*. Bushy, rounded shrub with young stems covered in red woolly hairs. Opposite, broadly ovate, toothed, deep green leaves, 10cm (4in) long, are red-hairy below. Terminal corymbs, to 12cm (5in) across, of fragrant violet flowerheads, are produced mainly in winter. ↕ 2–3m (6–10ft), ↔ 1.5–2.5m (5–8ft). Mexico. ❄

E. urticifolium see *E. rugosum*.

E. weinmannianum see *E. ligustrinum*.

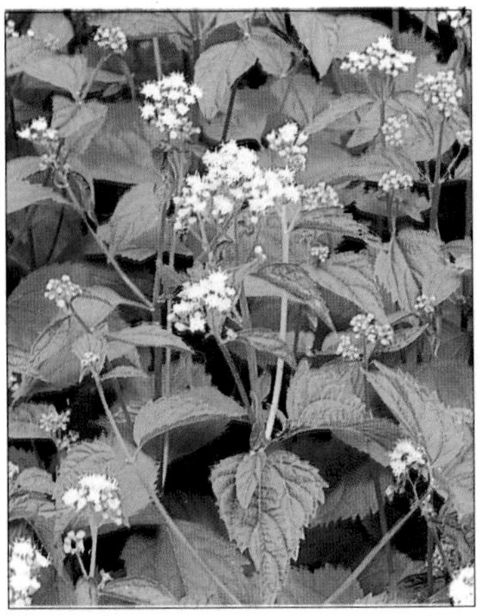

Eupatorium rugosum

EUPHORBIA

Milkweed, Spurge

EUPHORBIACEAE

Very varied genus of about 2,000 species of annuals, biennials, evergreen, semi-evergreen, or herbaceous perennials, deciduous or evergreen subshrubs, shrubs, and trees, and succulents, widely distributed in a range of habitats in temperate, subtropical, and tropical regions. Most have much-reduced, usually male and female floral parts, grouped together into a cyathium; these may be solitary or borne in rounded or pyramidal, terminal or axillary cymes, umbels, or clusters, and are cupped by involucres of long-lasting, yellow, red, purple, brown, or green, fused bracts. Leaves are very variable, and often short-lived. Many euphorbias are suitable for a rock garden, a mixed or shrub border, or a woodland garden. In frost-prone areas, grow tender species in a cool or temperate greenhouse. Succulent species are suitable for a dry, tropical garden, or a warm or temperate greenhouse in frost-prone areas. All parts may cause severe discomfort if ingested; contact with their milky sap may irritate skin.

• **HARDINESS** Fully hardy to frost tender.

• **CULTIVATION** Cultivation requirements have been grouped as below. For pruning, apply group 1 to trees, group 6 to non-succulent shrubs.

1. Well-drained, light soil in full sun.

2. Moist, humus-rich soil in light dappled shade.

3. Permanently moist soil in full sun.

4. Under glass, grow in a mix of 3 parts loam-based potting compost (JI No.2) and 1 part grit, in full light. Ventilate well. When in growth, water sparingly and apply a low-nitrogen liquid fertilizer monthly. Keep dry in winter. Outdoors, apply cultivation group 1. Grow *E. fulgens* and *E. pulcherrima* in loam-based potting compost (JI No.3) with added bark and leaf mould, in full light or bright filtered light. In growth, water moderately and apply a balanced liquid fertilizer every 10–14 days. Keep dry after flowering; resume watering as new growth begins. Re-pot in early summer. *E. pulcherrima* needs 12–14 hours of complete darkness daily for 2 months to initiate flowering. Outdoors, apply cultivation group 2. See also pp.48–49.

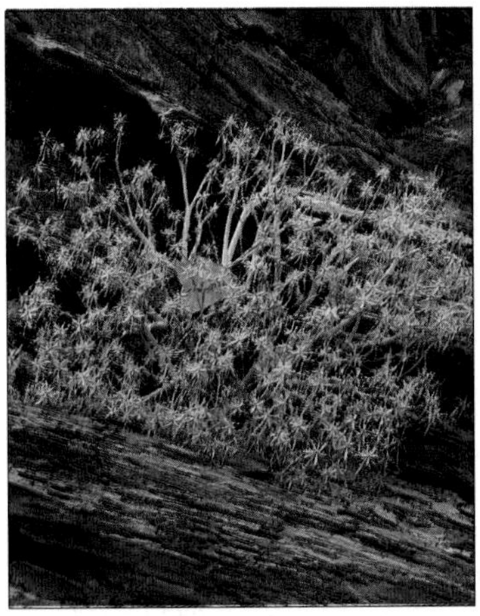

Euphorbia balsamifera

• **PROPAGATION** Sow seed of annuals *in situ* in spring. Sow seed of hardy perennials in containers in a cold frame as soon as ripe or in spring. Divide perennials in early spring, or take basal cuttings in spring or early summer; dip cut surfaces in charcoal or lukewarm water to prevent bleeding. Sow seed of frost-tender succulents as soon as ripe at 15–20°C (59–68°F), or root complete stems, or sections of stems, in spring. Root stem-tip cuttings of shrubby and tree species with bottom heat in spring or early summer.

• **PESTS AND DISEASES** Grey mould (*Botrytis*) may be a problem. Aphids may also be troublesome on herbaceous euphorbias, and mealybugs on succulent ones. *E. cyparissias* is susceptible to rust, and *E. pulcherrima* to whiteflies.

E. amygdaloides (Wood spurge). Bushy, softly hairy, evergreen perennial with reddish green stems and spoon-shaped to obovate, matt, dark green leaves, 2.5–8cm (1–3in) long, red beneath and becoming darker in winter. From mid-spring to early summer, bears terminal cymes, 20cm (8in) tall, of greenish yellow cyathia and involucres. Cultivation group 2. Remove stems immediately after flowering, to encourage new basal growth. ↕ 75–80cm (30–32in), ↔ 30cm (12in). Europe, Turkey, Caucasus. ❄❄❄. **'Purpurea'** has dark reddish purple leaves and acid-yellow cymes. **var. *robbiae*** ♕ syn. *E. robbiae* (Mrs. Robb's bonnet), spreads widely by rhizomes and may become invasive. Leaves are broader, leathery, shiny, darker green, and more closely set. Cymes are to 18cm (7in) tall and less showy. Cultivation group 2 or 3. N.W. Turkey. ↕ 60cm (24in).

E. balsamifera ■ Shrubby, evergreen succulent with gnarled, spineless, grey

E

EUPHORBIA HABITS

Euphorbias are adapted to a wide range of habitats, leading to a great deal of variation in both size and growth habit. They range from impressive, upright, tree-like succulents, up to 20m (70ft) high, to relatively low-growing, spreading plants, which may be as small as 10cm (4in) tall. The 7 types of growth habit shown here are some examples of this diversity.

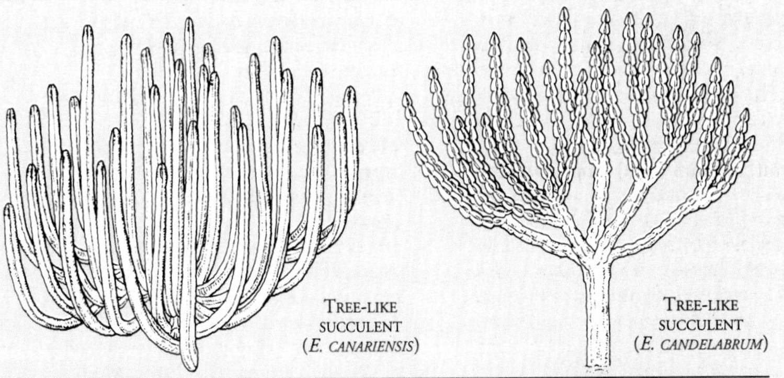

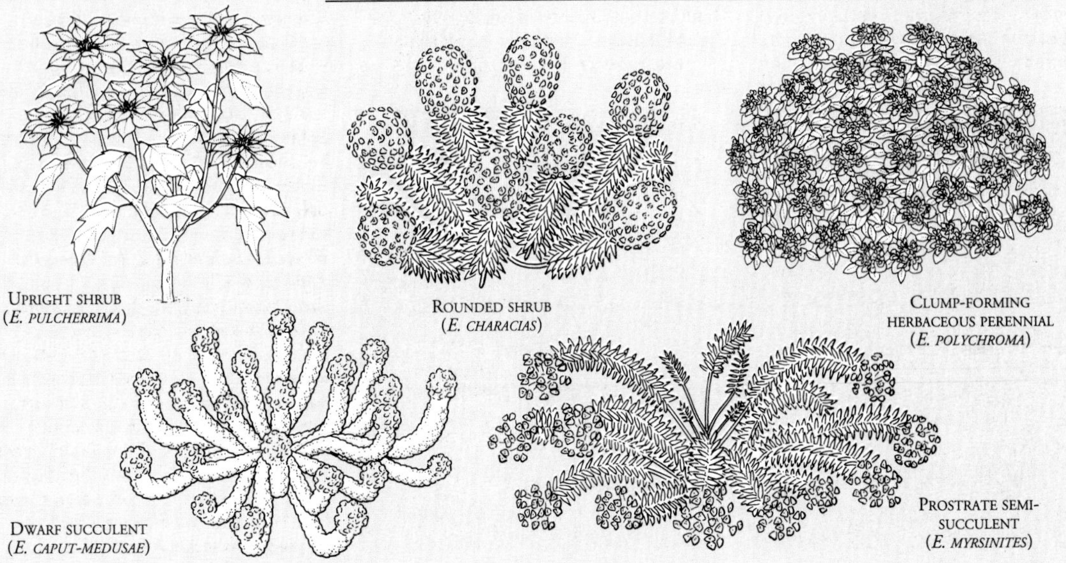

stems, each crowned by a rosette of linear-lance-shaped or oblong-spoon-shaped, slightly fleshy, pale green or bluish green leaves, to 2.5cm (1in) long. Solitary, bell-shaped, pale yellowish white cyathia, cupped by pale yellowish white involucres, are borne on short stalks in late spring. Cultivation group 4. ↕ 2m (6ft), ↔ 1m (3ft). Canary Islands. ❁ (min. 10°C/50°F)

E. biglandulosa see *E. rigida.*

E. bupleurifolia. Dwarf, evergreen succulent with a spherical or ovoid, few-branched, scaly caudex with spirally arranged tubercles. Pale green leaves, to 15cm (6in) long, are lance-shaped, tapering, and fleshy. Solitary, pale green cyathia, cupped by green involucres that become red, are borne in late spring and early summer. Cultivation group 4. ↕ to 20cm (8in) ↔ 8cm (3in). South Africa (Eastern Cape, KwaZulu/Natal). ❁ (min. 10°C/50°F)

E. canariensis ▣ Tree-like succulent, branching freely to form large clumps of 4- to 6-angled, fleshy, sharply ridged, toothed, bright green stems. Curved thorns develop in pairs along the angles. Rudimentary leaves soon fall. Solitary, short-stalked, reddish green cyathia, cupped by reddish green involucres, are borne in summer. Cultivation group 4. ↕ 8–12m (25–40ft) or more, ↔ 2m (6ft). Canary Islands. ❁ (min. 12°C/54°F)

E. candelabrum ▣ Freely branching, tree-like succulent with cracked grey bark and 4- or 5-angled, candelabra-like, fleshy, mid- to deep green stems forming a broad, rounded or angular crown. Stems are constricted into oblong segments, to 15cm (6in) long, and have deeply toothed ridges, paired thorns, and short-lived, spear-shaped leaves, 2–4cm (¾–1½in) long. In spring, bears terminal cymes, 2–6cm (¾–2½in) across, of reddish purple cyathia cupped by yellow involucres. Cultivation group 4. ↕ 20m (60ft), ↔ 3m (10ft). Somalia to South Africa. ❁ (min. 12°C/54°F)

E. caput-medusae (Medusa's head). Freely branching succulent with a caudex-like base, partly subterranean and thickened above. Warty, fleshy, grey-green branches are crowned by linear, fleshy, mid-green leaves, to 2.5cm (1in) long. In spring or early summer, bears solitary, fringed cream cyathia cupped by cream involucres. Cultivation group 4. ↕ 30cm (12in), ↔ 1m (3ft). South Africa (Northern Cape, Western Cape, Eastern Cape). ❁ (min. 15°C/59°F)

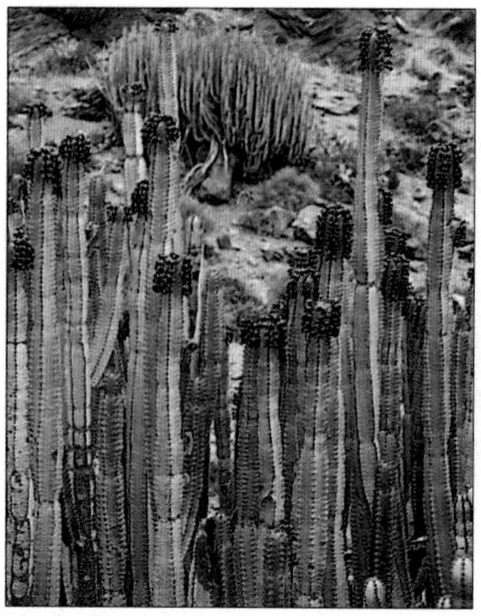

Euphorbia canariensis

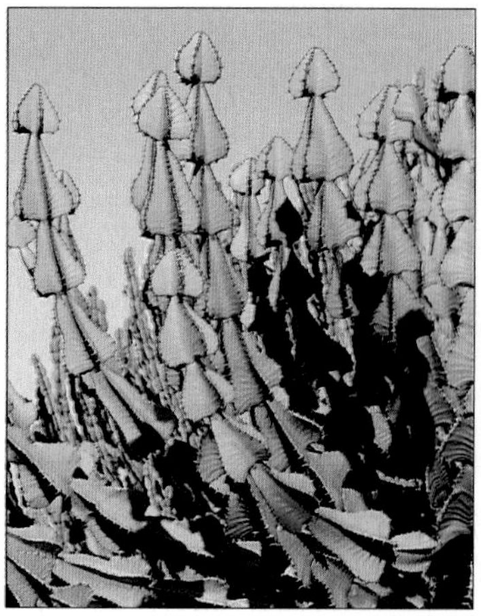

Euphorbia candelabrum

E. characias ▣ Upright, evergreen shrub with biennial shoots and clumps of erect, densely woolly, purple-tinged stems bearing linear to obovate, grey-green leaves, to 13cm (5in) long. Yellow-green cyathia, with purple-black or purple-brown nectar glands, are cupped by green involucres and borne in dense, cylindrical to spherical, terminal cymes, 10–30cm (4–12in) long, from early spring to early summer. Cut out flowered shoots if seed is not required. Cultivation group 1. ↕↔ 1.2m (4ft). Portugal, W. Mediterranean. ✻✻. **subsp. *wulfenii*** ♀ syn. *E. veneta, E. wulfenii,* has yellow-green cyathia with yellow-green nectar glands; S.E. Europe. **subsp. *wulfenii* 'John Tomlinson'** ▣ ♀ has large, nearly spherical cymes, 40cm (16in) long, of bright yellow-green cyathia. **subsp. *wulfenii* 'Lambrook Gold'** ♀ has cylindrical cymes of bright golden green cyathia.

E. clavarioides. Dwarf, freely branching succulent with a partly underground caudex and a dense cushion of cylindrical, fleshy stems with thick tips and 4- or 5-sided tubercles. Ovate to lance-shaped, fleshy, mid-green leaves, 2mm (1/16 in) long, are short-lived. In summer, bears solitary green cyathia cupped by green involucres. Cultivation group 4. ↕↔ 30cm (12in) or more. South Africa (except North West province), Lesotho. ❁ (min. 10°C/50°F)

E. cyathophora, syn. *E. heterophylla* of gardens (Annual poinsettia, Fire-on-the-mountain, Painted leaf). Erect, shrubby annual with whorls of linear to ovate or fiddle-shaped, sinuously lobed, dark green leaves, 5–15cm (2–6in) long,

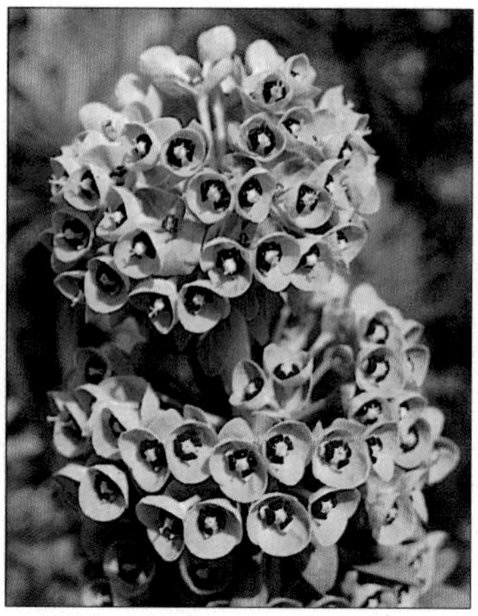

Euphorbia characias

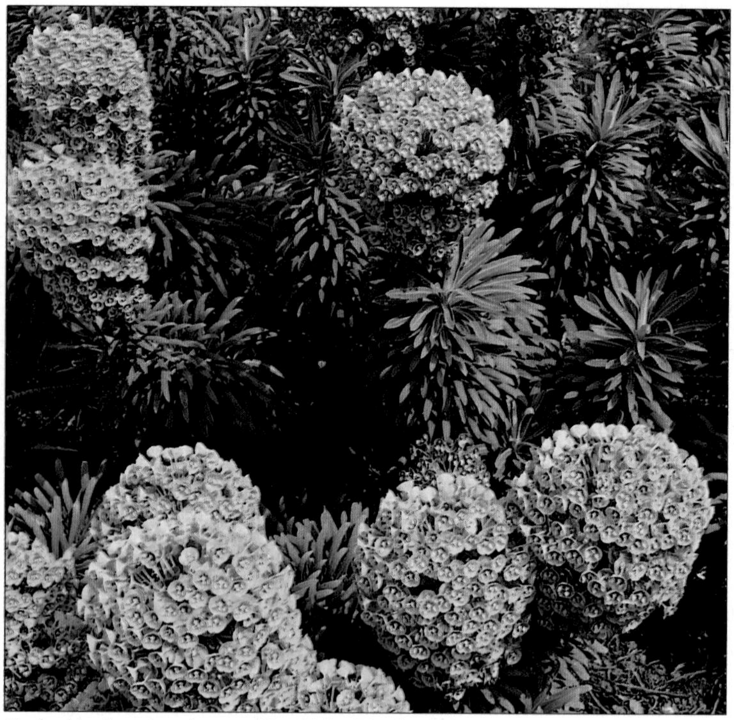

Euphorbia characias subsp. *wulfenii* 'John Tomlinson'

becoming red towards the tops of the stems, slightly downy below. In summer, produces terminal, umbel-like cymes, to 10cm (4in) across, of small, crimson-orange cyathia cupped by leafy, scarlet and green involucres. Cultivation group 1. ↕ 70cm (28in) or more, ↔ to 30cm (12in). USA, E. Mexico. ✻

E. cyparissias (Cypress spurge). Spreading, rhizomatous herbaceous perennial with slender stems, branching above. Crowded, linear, feathery, bluish green leaves, to 4cm (1½in) long, turn yellow in autumn. From late spring to midsummer, bears yellow-green cyathia and involucres, often turning orange in poor soil, in terminal cymes, 2–5cm (¾–2in) across. Invasive. Cultivation group 1. ↕ 20–40cm (8–16in), ↔ indefinite. W., C., and S. Europe. ✻✻✻. **'Orange Man'** has cyathia and involucres that are more orange-shaded, and orange-tinted autumn leaves.

E. dulcis. Rhizomatous herbaceous perennial with erect stems and oblong to inversely lance-shaped, dark or bronze-green leaves, to 7cm (3in) long. In early summer, produces terminal cymes, 5–12cm (2–5in) across, of greenish yellow cyathia and involucres. In autumn, stems turn red, and leaves turn red, gold, and orange. Cultivation group 2, but tolerates dry soil. Self-seeds freely. ↕↔ 30cm (12in). W., C., S., and S.E. Europe. ✻✻✻. **'Chameleon'** ▣ has rich purple leaves and purple-tinted, yellow-green cyathia and involucres.

E. epithymoides see *E. polychroma.*

E. ferox ▣ Clump-forming succulent with 9- to 12-angled, fleshy, partly subterrranean, pale green branches armed with stout thorns. Rudimentary leaves soon fall. In spring, bears solitary, pale yellow cyathia, with brown nectar glands, cupped within white-dotted purple involucres. Cultivation group 4. ↕ 15cm (6in), ↔ 50cm (20in). South Africa (Northern Cape, Western Cape, Eastern Cape). ❁ (min. 10°C/50°F)

E. francoisii. Dwarf, many-branched, thorny, evergreen succulent that spreads by means of stolons. Oblong-linear to ovate, distinctly veined, wavy-margined, fleshy, mid-green leaves, to 6cm (2½in) long, are variegated silvery grey, pink, or white, and often have red midribs. Leaves are arranged in rosettes around the terminal cymes, 2–6cm (¾–2½in) across, of greenish yellow cyathia and involucres borne in summer. Cultivation group 4. ↕ 10cm (4in), ↔ to 30cm (12in). S.E. Madagascar. ❁ (min. 16°C/61°F)

E. fulgens (Scarlet plume). Erect, open, deciduous shrub with slender stems that arch at the tips, and elliptic to lance-shaped, dark green leaves, 5–10cm (2–4in) long. Cyathia contain 5 wide-spreading, petal-like scarlet nectar glands and are produced in cymes, 15–30cm (6–12in) across, from the upper leaf axils in winter. Cultivation group 4. ↕ to 1.2m (4ft), ↔ 45–75cm (18–30in). Mexico. ❁ (min. 13–15°C/55–59°F)

E. gorgonis. Spherical to inversely conical succulent with a mostly underground caudex and radiating, fleshy, spiralled, dark green, sometimes red branches. Rudimentary leaves soon fall. In late spring, the central stem bears a solitary, dark red or brown cyathium,

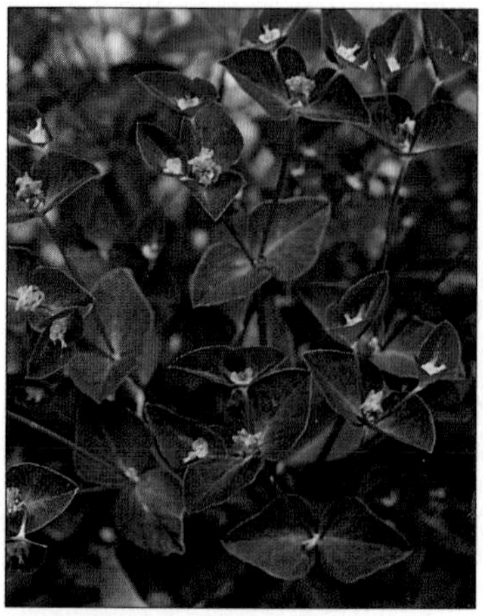

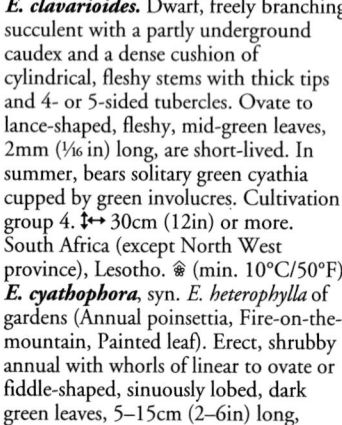

Euphorbia dulcis 'Chameleon'

cupped by a yellow to dull purple involucre. Cultivation group 4. ↕↔ 3cm (1¼in). South Africa (Northern Cape, Western Cape, Eastern Cape). ❁ (min. 12°C/54°F)

E. grandicornis. Shrub-like succulent with a short, fleshy main stem and prominent, 3-angled, erect or projecting, often tiered branches, the angles curved, with horny margins and prominent, paired, light brown thorns. Rudimentary leaves soon fall. In spring or early summer, bears terminal cymes, to 4cm (1½in) across, of yellow-tinged green cyathia within pale yellow involucres, followed by pale red fruit. Cultivation group 4. ↕ 1.5m (5ft), ↔ 1m (3ft) or more. Kenya to South Africa (KwaZulu/Natal). ❁ (min. 16°C/61°F)

E. griffithii. Rhizomatous, sometimes invasive herbaceous perennial with vigorous, erect stems, reddish green when young. Lance-shaped to linear-oblong, dark green leaves, 9–15cm (3½–6in) long, with red midribs, turn red and yellow in autumn. In early summer, bears terminal cymes, 7–12cm (3–5in) across, of yellow cyathia cupped within orange-red to red involucres. Cultivation group 2. ↕ 90cm (36in), ↔ 60cm (24in). Bhutan, Tibet, S.W. China (Yunnan). ❄❄❄. **'Dixter'** 🏆 has copper-tinted, very dark green foliage and dusky orange involucres; ↕ 75cm (30in), ↔ 1m (3ft). **'Fireglow'** ■ has orange-red involucres; ↕ 75cm (30in), ↔ 1m (3ft).

***E. heterophylla* of gardens** see *E. cyathophora.*

E. lathyris (Caper spurge, Mole plant). Erect, unbranched biennial with sparse, strap-shaped, leathery, waxy, grey- to blue-green leaves, to 15cm (6in) long. In summer, produces terminal umbels, to 5cm (2in) across, of yellow cyathia cupped by involucres of triangular to lance-shaped, bright green bracts, followed by caper-like fruit. Cultivation group 1. ↕ 0.3–1.2m (1–4ft), ↔ to 30cm (12in). Europe, N.W. Africa. ❄❄❄

***E. longifolia* of gardens.** Rhizomatous herbaceous perennial with vigorous, erect stems and oblong to linear-lance-shaped, fresh green leaves, 6–11cm (2½–4½in) long, with white midribs. In early summer, produces flat, terminal cymes, 7–12cm (3–5in) across, of yellow cyathia cupped by yellow involucres. Cultivation group 2. ↕ 1m (3ft), ↔ 60cm (24in). Bhutan. ❄❄❄

E. marginata, syn. *E. variegata* (Ghost weed, Snow on the mountain). Erect,

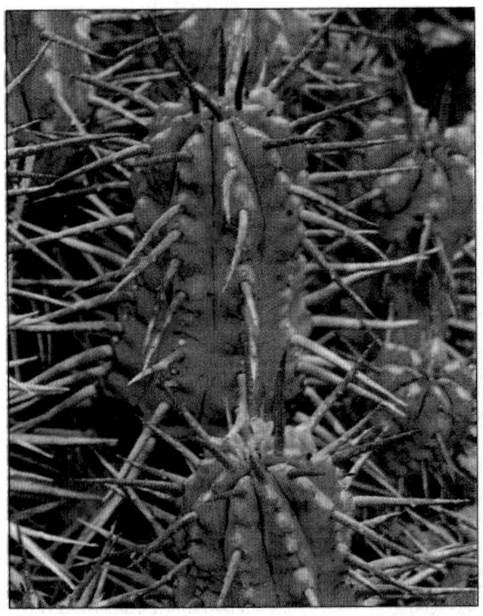

Euphorbia ferox

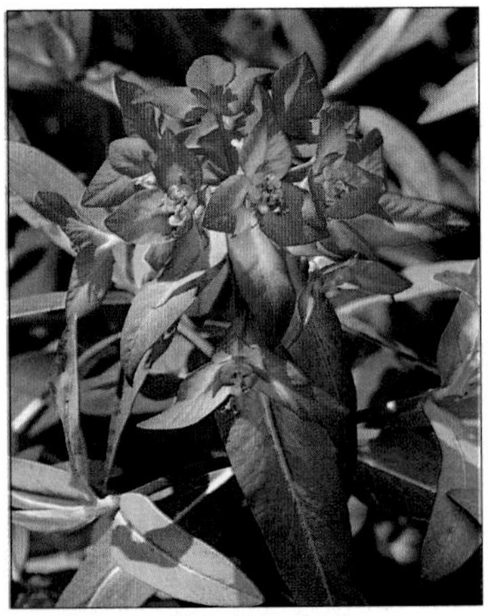

Euphorbia griffithii 'Fireglow'

initially single-stemmed, later branching annual with ovate to obovate, mid-green leaves, to 8cm (3in) long; the margins of the upper leaves are marked and veined white. From late summer to autumn, bears terminal umbels, to 5cm (2in) across, of greenish white cyathia and involucres, both variegated, margined, or spotted white. Cultivation group 1. Good for cutting. ↕ 30–90cm (12–36in), ↔ 30cm (12in). N. America. ❄❄❄

E.* x *martinii ■ 🏆 (*E. amygdaloides* x *E. characias*). Upright, clump-forming, evergreen subshrub. Narrow, inversely lance-shaped, mid-green leaves, to 7cm (3in) long, often tinged purple when young, are borne on red-tinged shoots. From spring to midsummer, produces terminal cymes, 10–12cm (4–5in) across, of yellow-green cyathia with dark red nectar glands; some cyathia are solitary. Cultivation group 1. ↕↔ 1m (3ft). S. France. ❄❄❄

E. mellifera ■ (Honey spurge). Rounded, evergreen shrub with stout shoots and oblong to narrowly lance-shaped, dark green leaves, to 20cm (8in) long. In late spring, honey-scented brown cyathia are produced in terminal cymes, 8–10cm (3–4in) across, followed by pea-like, warty fruit from late summer to autumn. Cultivation group 1. ↕ 2m (6ft) or more, ↔ 2.5m (8ft). Madeira. ❄❄

E. meloformis. Dwarf, almost spherical succulent with a thick tap root. The usually solitary, furrowed, very fleshy, green to greyish green stem, often cross-banded darker green or red, occasionally banded pale green or purple-brown, has 8–12 usually vertical, sometimes spirally

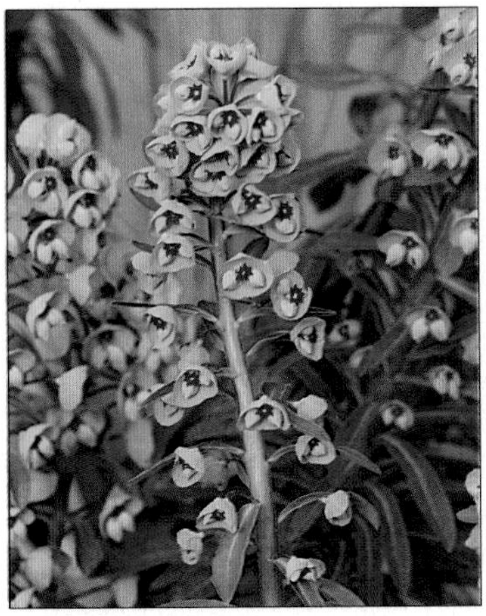

Euphorbia x *martinii*

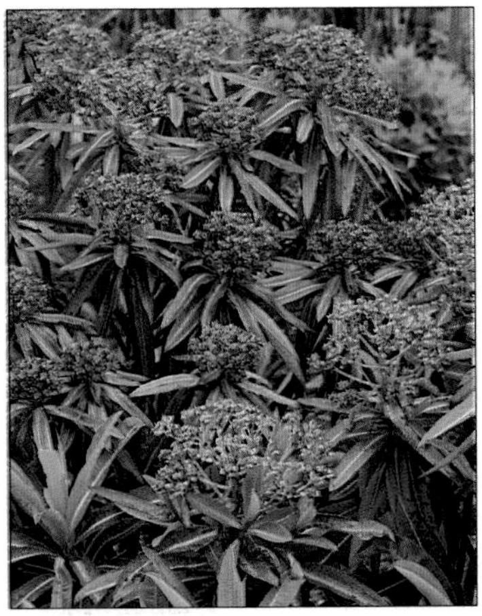

Euphorbia mellifera

arranged ribs. Rudimentary leaves soon fall. In summer, bears terminal clusters, to 4cm (1½in) across, of green or purple cyathia and involucres. Cultivation group 4. ↕↔ 10cm (4in). South Africa (Northern Cape, Western Cape, Eastern Cape). ❁ (min. 10°C/50°F)

E. milii 🏆 (Crown of thorns). Bushy, slow-growing, mainly evergreen, semi-succulent shrub with slender, fleshy, thorny stems and branches; the well-spaced thorns are wider at the bases. Bright green leaves, 3.5cm (1½in) long, are obovate, pointed, and tough. Yellow cyathia, enclosed by very intense red involucres, are borne in axillary cymes in spring or summer. Cultivation group 4. ↕ 1m (3ft) or more, ↔ 45cm (18in). Madagascar. ❁ (min. 12°C/54°F). **var. *splendens***, syn. *E. splendens* (Christ's thorn), is semi-prostrate to scrambling; ↕ 30–90cm (12–36in), ↔ 60–100cm (24–39in); ❁ (min. 7–10°C/45–50°F). **var. *tulearensis*** ■ has pink cyathia.

E. myrsinites ■ 🏆 Evergreen perennial with semi-prostrate stems clothed in spirally arranged, obovate to rounded, pointed, succulent, blue-grey leaves, 5–10cm (2–4in) long. In spring, bears terminal umbels, 5–8cm (2–3in) across, of bright greenish yellow cyathia and involucres. Cultivation group 1. ↕ 10cm (4in), ↔ to 30cm (12in). S. and E. Europe to Turkey, C. Asia. ❄❄❄

E. nicaeensis. Bushy, evergreen or semi-evergreen perennial with lance-shaped to oblong, leathery, glaucous, grey-green leaves, 7cm (3in) long, borne on upright or procumbent, reddish green stems, arising from a woody rootstock. From late spring to midsummer, produces

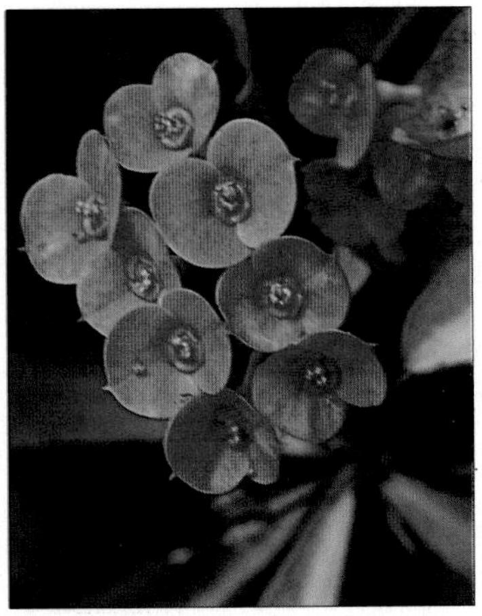

Euphorbia milii var. *tulearensis*

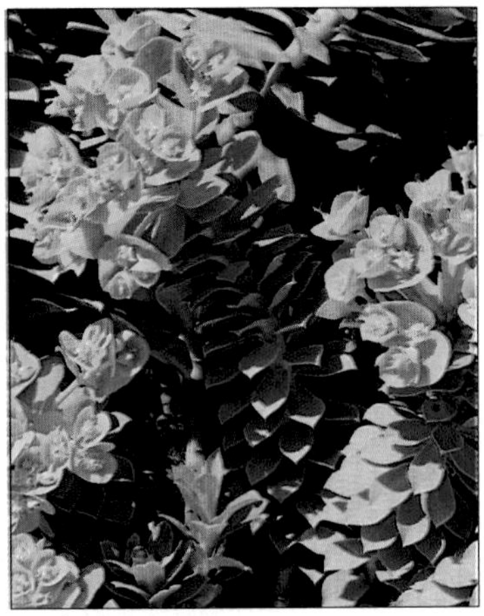

Euphorbia myrsinites

terminal cymes, to 12cm (5in) across, of long-lasting, greenish yellow cyathia and involucres. Cultivation group 1. ↕ 80cm (32in), ↔ 45cm (18in). C. and E. Europe, Turkey, Caucasus. ❄❄❄

E. obesa ■ (Living baseball). Succulent with a spherical to squat-cylindrical, 8-ribbed, blunt-toothed, light greyish green stem, chequered reddish brown or faintly banded purple. In summer, bears rounded, terminal cymes, 4–6cm (1½–2½in) across, of yellow cyathia from the crown. Cultivation group 4. ↕ 15cm (6in), ↔ 12cm (5in). South Africa (Northern Cape, Western Cape, Eastern Cape). ❁ (min. 10°C/50°F)

E. palustris ■ 🏆 Robust, clump-forming herbaceous perennial with erect, pale green stems and elliptic to oblong-lance-shaped, bright green

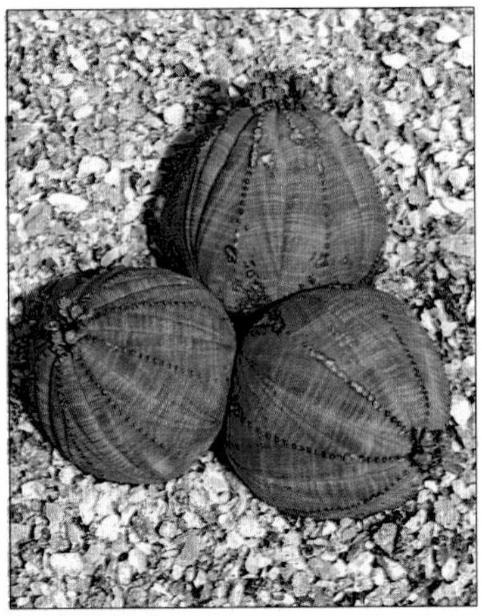

Euphorbia obesa

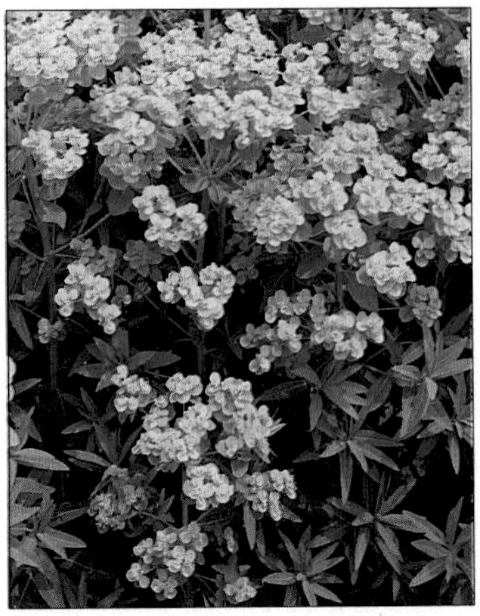

Euphorbia palustris

E

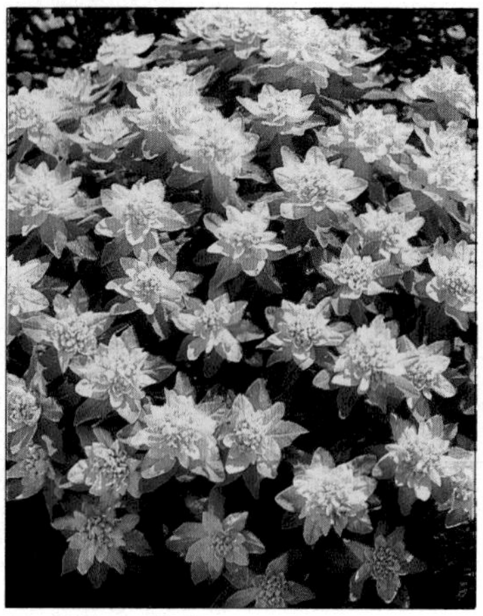
Euphorbia polychroma

leaves, 6cm (2½in) long, turning yellow and orange in autumn. In late spring, produces terminal cymes, to 15cm (6in) across, of large, long-lasting, deep yellow cyathia and involucres. Cultivation group 3. ↕↔ 90cm (36in). S. Scandinavia to Spain to W. Caucasus, W. Asia, Russia (W. Siberia). ❄❄❄
E. pilosa (Hairy spurge). Bushy, rhizomatous herbaceous perennial with numerous erect, branching stems, and linear to oblong, softly hairy, mid-green leaves, 4–10cm (1½–4in) long, sometimes less hairy above. From mid-spring to midsummer, bears terminal cymes, 8–14cm (3–5½in) across, of yellow cyathia and greenish yellow involucres, both becoming greener. Cultivation group 2. ↕ 60–90cm (24–36in), ↔ 30cm (12in). C. Asia, W. Himalayas. ❄❄❄
E. polychroma ▣ 🏆 syn. *E. epithymoides.* Clump-forming herbaceous perennial with robust, softly hairy stems and obovate to elliptic-oblong, dark green leaves, 3.5–5cm (1½–2in) long, sometimes tinged with purple. Long-lasting yellow cyathia, cupped by showy, bright greenish yellow involucres, are borne in terminal cymes, 4–8cm (1½–3in) across, from mid-spring to midsummer. Cultivation group 1 or 2. ↕ 40cm (16in), ↔ 60cm (24in). C. and S. Europe, Turkey. ❄❄❄. **'Candy'**, syn. 'Purpurea', has dark purple-green stems and leaves, and paler yellow cyathia and involucres. **'Emerald Jade'** has very bright green cyathia and involucres that colour well in autumn; ↕ 35cm (14in), ↔ 45cm (18in). **'Purpurea'** see 'Candy'.
E. portlandica (Portland spurge). Bushy, short-lived, evergreen perennial

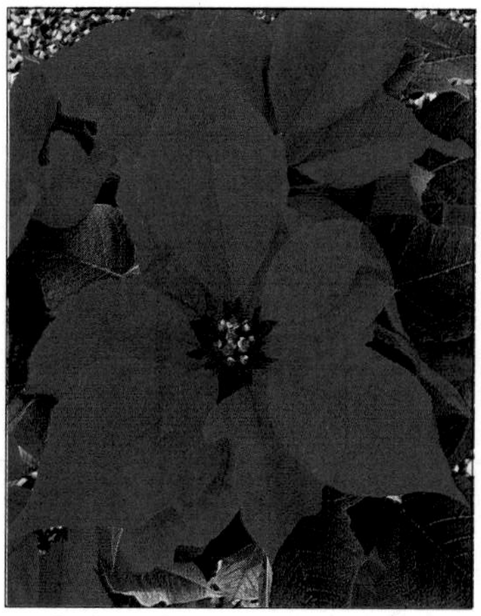
Euphorbia pulcherrima 'Menorca'

with several stems bearing numerous inversely lance-shaped, slightly leathery, grey-tinged, bright green leaves, to 2.5cm (1in) long, with prominent midribs beneath. Throughout summer, bears terminal cymes, 4–7cm (1½–3in) across, of yellow cyathia and involucres. Cultivation group 1. ↕ to 40cm (16in), ↔ 15cm (6in). Coastal W. and S. Europe. ❄❄❄
E. pulcherrima (Mexican flame leaf, Poinsettia). Open, erect to spreading, partially deciduous shrub, usually sparsely branched, with ovate to lance-shaped, sometimes lobed or toothed, mid- to deep green leaves, to 15cm (6in) long. In winter, bears dense, terminal cymes, to 30cm (12in) across, of green cyathia ringed by large, leaf-like, bright red involucral bracts. Cultivation group 4. ↕ 2–4m (6–12ft), ↔ 1–2.5m (3–8ft). Mexico. ❅ (min. 13–15°C/55–59°F). **'Ecke's White'** bears ovate, bright green leaves and cream involucres on slender stems. **'Lilo White'** ▣ branches freely and bears olive-green leaves and upright white involucres and cyathia; ↕ 22cm (9in), ↔ 35cm (14in). **'Menorca'** ▣ is vigorous, with dark olive-green leaves, vivid red involucres, and red-and-white cyathia; ↕ 30cm (12in), ↔ 40cm (16in). **'Paul Mikkelsen'** is freely branching; ↕ to 1m (3ft), ↔ 60cm (24in) or more. **'Plenissima'** bears inflorescences formed from a profusion of very narrow involucral bracts, some of them angled upwards or erect.
E. reflexa see *E. seguieriana* subsp. *niciciana.*
E. rigida ▣ syn. *E. biglandulosa.* Erect then spreading, evergreen perennial with

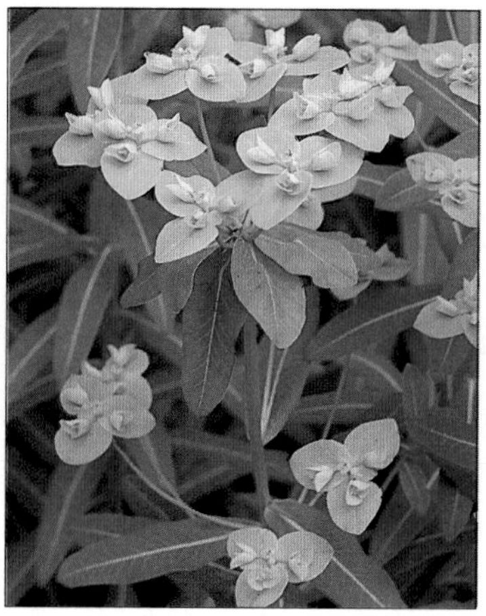
Euphorbia schillingii

lance-shaped, stiff, fleshy, grey-green leaves, 2–7cm (¾–3in) long. From early spring to early summer, bears terminal umbels, 5cm (2in) across, of yellow cyathia cupped by yellow involucres that redden with age. Cultivation group 1. ↕ 30–60cm (12–24in), ↔ to 60cm (24in). Morocco, Mediterranean (Portugal to Turkey), Iran. ❄❄❄
E. robbiae see *E. amygdaloides* var. *robbiae.*
E. schillingii ▣ 🏆 Robust, clump-forming herbaceous perennial with erect stems and elliptic-oblong to inversely lance-shaped, stalkless, dark green leaves, 12cm (5in) long, with pale green or white veins. Each stem branches near its apex, the branches each producing terminal cymes, 8–15cm (3–6in) across, of long-lasting yellow cyathia and rounded, greenish yellow involucral bracts, from midsummer to mid-autumn. Cultivation group 2. ↕ 1m (3ft), ↔ 30cm (12in). E. Nepal. ❄❄❄
E. seguieriana ▣ Clump-forming, woody-based, semi-evergreen perennial with linear to oblong-linear, glaucous, bluish green leaves, 1–4cm (½–1½in) long. In late summer and early autumn, thin stems bear terminal cymes, 8–15cm (3–6in) across, of lime-green cyathia and involucres. Cultivation group 1. ↕ to 50cm (20in), ↔ 45cm (18in). W. Europe to Russia (Siberia), Caucasus. ❄❄❄. **subsp. *niciciana*,** syn. *E. reflexa,* bears more spreading, narrower, lance-shaped leaves on branched stems, and cyathia with many more yellow-green involucres; Balkans to Pakistan.
E. sikkimensis ▣ Spreading, upright herbaceous perennial with bright pink

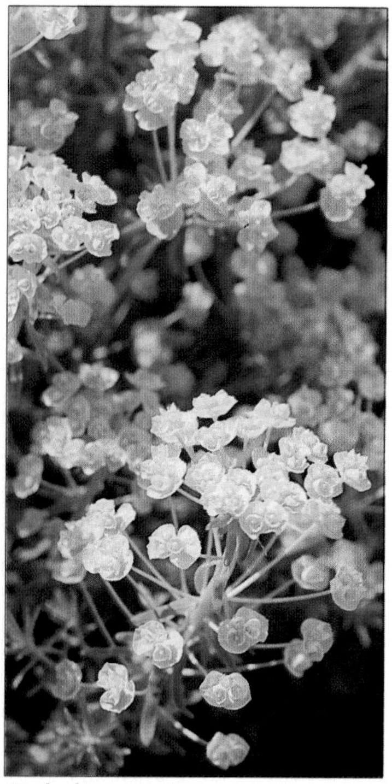
Euphorbia seguieriana

young shoots. Lance-shaped to linear-oblong, red-marked, deep green leaves, 10–12cm (4–5in) long, become soft green, with red margins and ruby-red veins. In mid- and late summer, bears terminal cymes, 6–8cm (2½–3in) across, of yellow cyathia cupped by pale to greenish yellow involucres. Cultivation group 2. ↕ 1.2m (4ft), ↔ 45cm (18in). E. Himalayas. ❄❄❄
E. splendens see *E. milii* var. *splendens.*
E. tirucallii ▣ Bushy, tree-like succulent with fleshy, segmented, bright green stems, with paler vertical lines, and linear to linear-lance-shaped, short-lived leaves, 1.5cm (½in) long. In spring, produces terminal cymes, to 1cm (½in) across, of green cyathia cupped by paler involucres. Cultivation group 4. ↕ to 9m (28ft), ↔ 2m (6ft). Tropical E. and S. Africa. ❅ (min. 10°C/50°F)
E. variegata see *E. marginata.*
E. veneta see *E. characias* subsp. *wulfenii.*
E. villosa. Rhizomatous, semi-evergreen or herbaceous perennial producing numerous pale yellowish green stems with terminal branches, and thin, oblong-lance-shaped to elliptic-oblong, hairless or softly hairy, mid-green leaves,

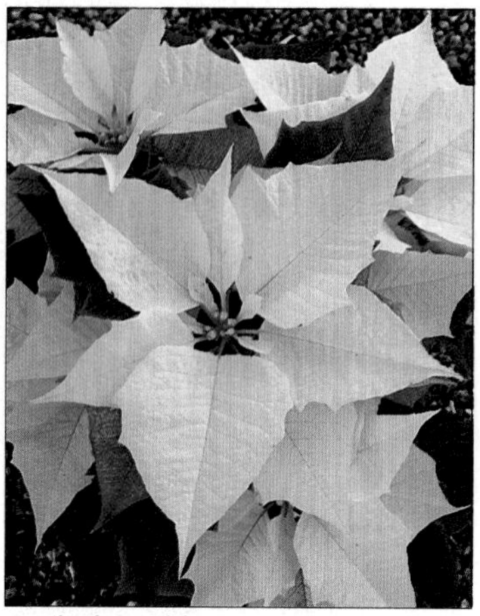
Euphorbia pulcherrima 'Lilo White'

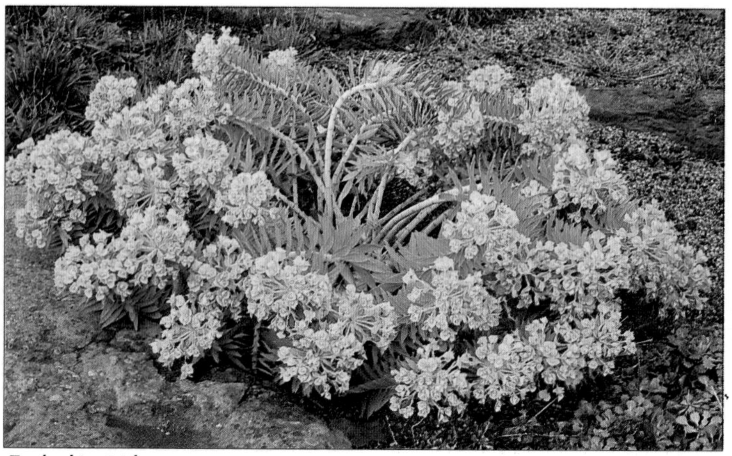
Euphorbia rigida

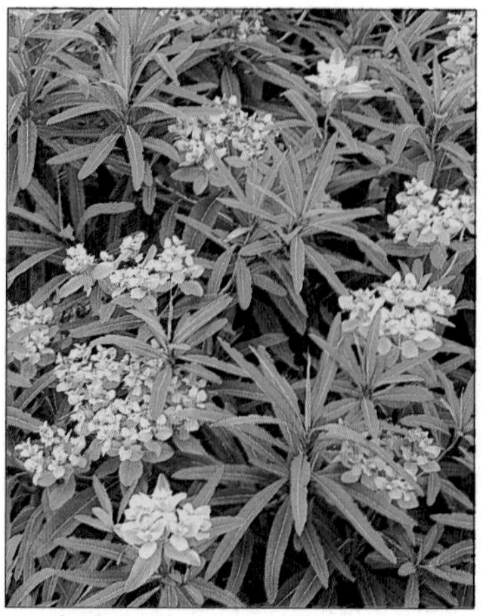
Euphorbia sikkimensis

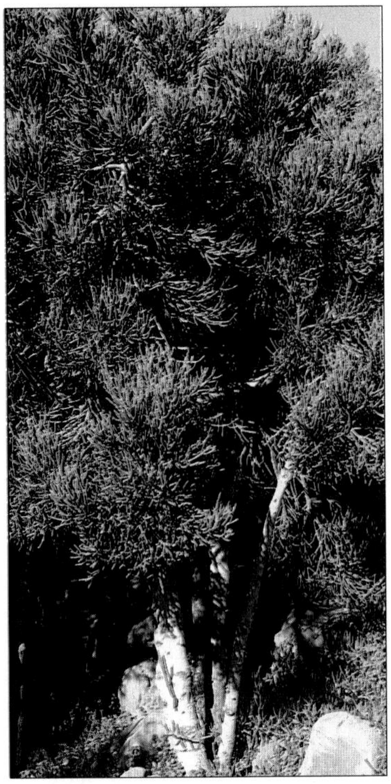

Euphorbia tirucallii

6cm (2½in) long, which turn yellow in autumn. From mid-spring to early summer, bears terminal cymes, 6cm (2½in) across, of greenish yellow cyathia cupped within yellow involucres that mature to greenish yellow. Cultivation group 2. ↕ to 1.2m (4ft), ↔ 45cm (18in). Europe (except S.W.) to C. Russia, Caucasus, W. Siberia. ❄❄❄

E. wallichii. Clump-forming herbaceous perennial with erect stems and linear to elliptic-oblong, dark green leaves, 6–11cm (2½–4½in) long, with white veins and purple-tinted margins. In early summer, produces cymes, eventually 8–15cm (3–6in) across, of umbel-like, orange-yellow cyathia and bright greenish yellow involucres. Cultivation group 2. ↕ 50cm (20in), ↔ 30cm (12in). W. and C. Himalayas. ❄❄❄

E. wulfenii see *E. characias* subsp. *wulfenii.*

EUPTELEA

EUPTELEACEAE

Genus of 2 or 3 species of deciduous trees and shrubs occurring in woodland from the Himalayas to Japan. They are grown mainly for their attractive leaves, which are alternate, simple, rounded to ovate, and often colourful in autumn. The small, petalless, green or reddish green flowers are produced in clusters in spring, before the leaves. Grow in a large shrub border or woodland garden.

• **HARDINESS** Fully hardy, but late frosts may damage young growth.
• **CULTIVATION** Grow in fertile, moist but well-drained soil in full sun or partial shade. Pruning group 1.
• **PROPAGATION** Sow seed in a seedbed as soon as ripe.
• **PESTS AND DISEASES** Trouble free.

E. polyandra ♀ Spreading, suckering shrub or small tree with broadly ovate to rounded, tapered, deeply toothed, glossy, bright green leaves, to 15cm (6in) long, tinged red when young, turning yellow and red in autumn. Bears clusters, 2.5–4cm (1–1½in) across, of inconspicuous, reddish green flowers in spring, before the leaves emerge. ↕ 8m (25ft), ↔ 6m (20ft). Japan. ❄❄❄

EURYA

THEACEAE

Genus of about 70 species of mostly evergreen trees and shrubs from woodland in E. and S.E. Asia and the Pacific islands. They are cultivated for their large, alternate, simple, usually ovate to obovate or elliptic, mid- to dark green leaves with scalloped to toothed margins. The inconspicuous, dioecious flowers are borne singly or in few-flowered clusters from the leaf axils, in spring. Grow in a shrub border, or a peat or woodland garden. In regions that experience long periods below 5°C (41°F), grow half-hardy species in a cool greenhouse.

• **HARDINESS** Frost hardy to half hardy.
• **CULTIVATION** Under glass, grow in loam-based potting compost (JI No.3) in full light. When in full growth, water freely and apply a balanced liquid fertilizer monthly; water sparingly in winter. Outdoors, grow in moist but well-drained, humus-rich soil in full sun or partial shade, sheltered from cold, drying winds. Pruning group 1.
• **PROPAGATION** Sow seed in containers in a cold frame as soon as ripe. Root semi-ripe cuttings in summer with bottom heat.
• **PESTS AND DISEASES** Trouble free.

E. emarginata ♀ Dense, evergreen shrub or small tree with obovate to oblong-obovate, scalloped, leathery, glossy, dark green leaves, to 3.5cm (1½in) long, tinged red in winter. Bears yellow-green flowers in spring. Female plants bear almost spherical, purple-black berries, 5mm (¼in) across, in autumn. ↕↔ 1.5m (5ft). S. Japan. ❄

E. japonica ♀ Dense, evergreen shrub or small tree with elliptic to obovate, toothed, leathery, glossy, dark green leaves, to 8cm (3in) long. In spring, bears greenish white flowers with green or purple-brown sepals. Female plants bear almost spherical black berries, to 5mm (¼in) across, in autumn. ↕↔ 10m (30ft). Korea, Japan, and adjacent islands. ❄❄

EURYALE

Fox nuts, Gorgon plant

NYMPHAEACEAE

Genus of one species of deep-water aquatic perennial, often treated as an annual, that occurs in still and slow-moving water in Asia. One of the world's largest aquatic plants, it has large, floating, rounded, thorny leaves, and shuttlecock-like flowers, each stem and calyx covered with stiff prickles. In all but tropical areas, grow *E. ferox* in a large pool in a warm greenhouse.

• **HARDINESS** Frost tender.
• **CULTIVATION** Grow in a large basket of fertile, loamy soil at a depth of 1m (3ft) in full light (full sun if outdoors). When in growth, insert a proprietary sachet of water-plant food into the soil or compost every 6 weeks. To stimulate the flowers to open, maintain at 20°C (68°F). See also pp.52–53.
• **PROPAGATION** Sow seed singly in 8cm (3in) containers in spring. Submerge in water at 21–23°C (70–73°F), so that the tops of the containers are just under the surface.
• **PESTS AND DISEASES** Trouble free.

E. ferox. Deep-water aquatic perennial with floating, rounded leaves, 0.6–1.5m (2–5ft) across, that are puckered, sparsely spiny, olive-green above and purple underneath, with prominent, prickly veins. Produces shuttlecock-like, red, purple, or lilac flowers, to 6cm (2½in) across, in summer, followed by many-seeded, prickly berries, 5–7cm (2–3in) across. ↔ 1.5m (5ft). N. India, Bangladesh, China, Taiwan, Japan. ❀ (min. 5°C/41°F)

EURYOPS

ASTERACEAE/COMPOSITAE

Genus of approximately 100 species of evergreen shrubs, subshrubs, herbaceous perennials, and annuals found in rocky areas mainly in southern Africa, with one species in the Arabian Peninsula and Socotra, Yemen. They produce attractive, alternate, simple to pinnatisect, linear, or lance-shaped to broadly ovate leaves and showy, daisy-like flowerheads. Grow in a sheltered shrub border, rock garden, or raised bed, or in tufa. In frost-prone areas, grow half-hardy species in a cool greenhouse, conservatory, or alpine house.

• **HARDINESS** Fully hardy to half hardy.
• **CULTIVATION** Under glass, grow in loam-based potting compost (JI No.2) with added sharp sand, in full light. Water freely when in full growth, sparingly in winter. Outdoors, grow in moderately fertile, well-drained soil in full sun. Trim lightly after flowering to restrict growth.
• **PROPAGATION** Sow seed in spring at 10–13°C (50–55°F). Insert softwood cuttings in late spring, or semi-ripe cuttings in summer.
• **PESTS AND DISEASES** Trouble free.

E. acraeus ▣♀ syn. *E. evansii* of gardens. Dense, dome-shaped shrub with branching stems clothed in linear, flattened, leathery, silvery grey leaves, to 3cm (1¼in) long, toothed at the tips. In late spring and early summer, bears deep yellow flowerheads, 2.5cm (1in) across, either singly or in groups of 2 or 3, on strong stems to 4cm (1½in) long. Requires sharp drainage. ↕↔ to 30cm

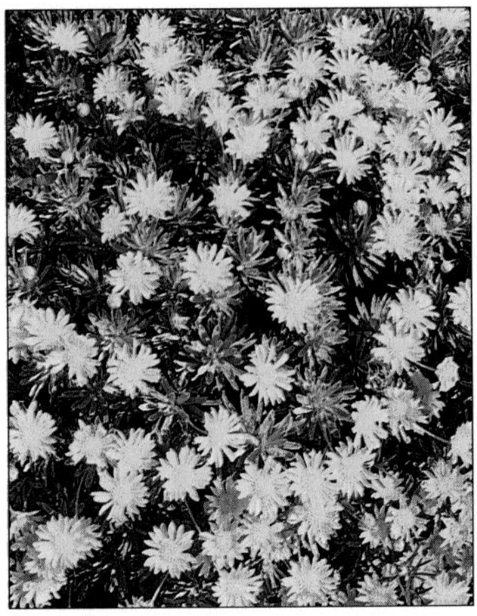

Euryops acraeus

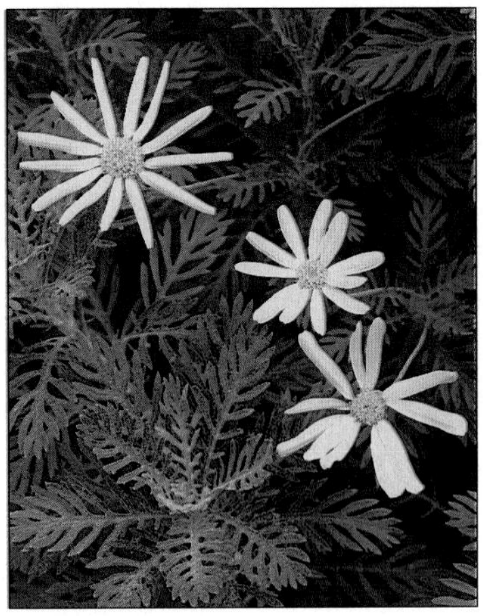

Euryops pectinatus

(12in). South Africa (Drakensberg Mountains, KwaZulu/Natal). ❄❄❄ (borderline)

***E. evansii* of gardens** see *E. acraeus.*

E. pectinatus ▣♀ Vigorous shrub with upright shoots and pinnatifid to pinnatisect, grey-hairy leaves, to 7cm (3in) long, with linear lobes. Bears long-stalked, bright yellow flowerheads, 5cm (2in) across, singly or in small clusters, from early summer to mid-autumn and, under glass, on through winter. ↕↔ 1m (3ft). South Africa. ❄

EUSTOMA *syn.* LISIANTHIUS

GENTIANACEAE

Genus of 3 species of erect, tap-rooted annuals, biennials, and short-lived perennials found in moist prairies and fields from C. and S. USA to N. South America. Leaves are opposite, ovate to oblong-lance-shaped, stalkless, and sometimes stem-clasping. In summer, leafy flowering stems produce showy, deeply cup-shaped or bell-shaped, pastel-coloured flowers, either singly or in clusters, which gradually open from slender, furled buds. In frost-prone areas, grow as flowering container plants in a temperate greenhouse. In warmer areas, grow as annuals in a bed or border. Good for cut flowers.

• **HARDINESS** Frost tender.
• **CULTIVATION** Under glass, grow in loam-based potting compost (JI No.2) in full light, with bright filtered light when in bloom. Ventilate well. In full growth, water freely and apply a balanced liquid fertilizer every 2–3 weeks; water sparingly in winter. Outdoors, grow in well-drained, neutral to alkaline soil in full sun. Support stems.
• **PROPAGATION** Sow seed at 13–16°C (55–61°F) in autumn or late winter.
• **PESTS AND DISEASES** Seedlings are very prone to damping off.

E. grandiflorum, syn. *E. russellianum*, *Lisianthius russellianus* (Texan bluebell). Single-stemmed or branching annual or biennial with slightly fleshy, ovate to oblong, prominently 3- to 5-veined, glaucous, grey-green leaves, to 8cm (3in) long. In summer, broadly bell-shaped, satin-textured, dark-centred, pale purple flowers, to 5cm (2in) across, are produced on long stalks, either singly or in clusters, from the upper leaf axils. ↕ 60–90cm (24–36in), ↔ 30cm (12in). USA (Nebraska, Colorado, Kansas, Texas). ❀ (min. 5–7°C/41–45°F).

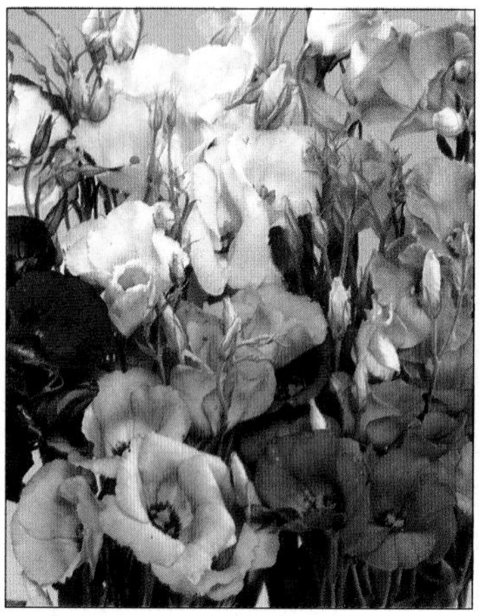

Eustoma grandiflorum Heidi Series

Heidi Series ▣ cultivars bear flowers in shades of blue, rose-pink, white, and bicolours. **Mermaid Series** cultivars have pink, white, or black-centred blue flowers; ↕ to 15cm (6in). **Yodel Series** cultivars are compact, with flowers in white, salmon-pink, or purple-blue with dark centres; ↕ 40–45cm (16–18in).
E. russellianum see *E. grandiflorum.*

EUSTREPHUS
Wombat berry

LILIACEAE/SMILACACEAE

Genus of one species of climbing, evergreen perennial from woodland and forest in New Guinea, E. Australia, and New Caledonia. It is grown for its 6-tepalled, bell-shaped flowers, and glossy orange berries. Leaves are alternate and simple. In frost-prone areas, grow in a cool or temperate greenhouse; elsewhere, train over a support outdoors.
• **HARDINESS** Frost tender.
• **CULTIVATION** Under glass, grow in loam-based potting compost (JI No.2) in bright filtered light. Water freely in full growth, sparingly in winter. Outdoors, grow in fertile, humus-rich soil in partial shade. Pruning group 11, after flowering.
• **PROPAGATION** Sow seed at 13–16°C (55–61°F) in spring. Divide after fruiting.
• **PESTS AND DISEASES** Red spider mites may infest greenhouse plants.

E. latifolius. Tuberous, twining perennial with slender, wiry stems and linear to lance-shaped, sometimes wavy-margined, glossy, bright green leaves, 6–10cm (2½–4in) long. From spring to early summer, bears axillary clusters of usually 2 or 3 pink flowers, 1.5cm (½in) across, with fringed tepals. Glossy, orange berries split to reveal shiny black seeds. ↕ 1.5–4m (5–12ft), ↔ 60–100cm (24–39in). New Guinea, E. Australia, New Caledonia. ❀ (min. 5°C/41°F)

▷ **Evening primrose** see *Oenothera, O. biennis*
  Desert see *O. deltoides*
▷ **Evening trumpet** see *Gelsemium sempervirens*
▷ **Everlasting,**
  Golden see *Bracteantha bracteata*
  Pearl see *Anaphalis*
  Winged see *Ammobium, A. alatum*
▷ **Everlasting pea** see *Lathyrus, L. grandiflorus, L. latifolius*
▷ ***Evodia*** see *Tetradium*

EVOLVULUS

CONVOLVULACEAE

Genus of about 100 species of prostrate to upright annuals, perennials, and evergreen subshrubs found mostly on plains and prairies from N. USA to S. Argentina. Leaves are usually simple, mainly narrowly lance-shaped to broadly ovate, and silky-hairy. Bell- to funnel-shaped, blue, pink, or white flowers are borne singly or in few-flowered, axillary or terminal cymes, usually from spring to autumn. In frost-prone areas, grow in a warm greenhouse. In dry, frost-free areas, grow in a border or for bedding.
• **HARDINESS** Frost tender.
• **CULTIVATION** Under glass, grow in loam-based potting compost (JI No.2), with added sharp sand, in full light. In growth, water moderately and apply a balanced liquid fertilizer monthly; water sparingly in winter, and maintain a dry atmosphere when temperatures are low. Outdoors, grow in poor to moderately fertile, well-drained soil in full sun.
• **PROPAGATION** Sow seed at 13–16°C (55–61°F) in spring, or take softwood cuttings in late spring.
• **PESTS AND DISEASES** Trouble free.

***E. glomeratus* of gardens** see *E. pilosus.*
E. pilosus, syn. *E. glomeratus* of gardens. Slender, trailing, evergreen subshrub or woody-based perennial with spoon-shaped or inversely lance-shaped to ovate-oblong, densely silky-hairy, silvery grey leaves, to 1.5cm (½in) long. In summer, bears solitary, short-tubed, funnel- to bell-shaped, lavender-pink or blue flowers, 1.5–2cm (½–¾in) across. ↕↔ to 50cm (20in). USA (Montana and South Dakota to Arizona and Texas). ❀ (min. 10°C/50°F). **'Blue Daze'** bears elliptic-ovate, white-hairy leaves and powder-blue flowers with white eyes.

EXACUM

GENTIANACEAE

Genus of about 25 species of annuals, biennials, and evergreen perennials occurring near streams from Yemen to India. They have erect, often 4-angled, branched stems and stalkless to short-stalked, lance-shaped to elliptic, simple, entire leaves. They are grown for their saucer-shaped, fragrant, violet to blue, occasionally pink or white flowers, with yellow stamens, borne singly or in leafy cymes. In frost-prone areas, grow in a temperate greenhouse, in a conservatory, or as houseplants. In warmer areas, grow outdoors in a bed or border.
• **HARDINESS** Frost tender.
• **CULTIVATION** Under glass, grow in loam-based potting compost (JI No.2), with added sharp sand, in full light. In full growth, water freely and apply a balanced liquid fertilizer every 2–3 weeks; water sparingly in winter. Outdoors, grow in moderately fertile, well-drained soil in full sun.
• **PROPAGATION** Sow seed at 18°C (64°F) in early spring.
• **PESTS AND DISEASES** Trouble free.

E. affine ▣ (Persian violet). Bushy annual, or short-lived evergreen perennial usually grown as an annual, with 4-angled stems and ovate to elliptic, shiny leaves, to 3cm (1¼) long. In summer, bears scented, lavender-blue, rose-pink, or white flowers, to 2cm (¾in) across, with conspicuous yellow stamens. ↕↔ 23–30cm (9–12in). Yemen (Socotra). ❀ (min. 7–10°C/45–50°F). **'Blue Gem'** is compact, with lavender-blue flowers; ↕ 20cm (8in). **'Blue Midget'** has lavender-blue flowers; ↕ to 12cm (5in). **'White Midget'** has pure white flowers; ↕ to 12cm (5in).

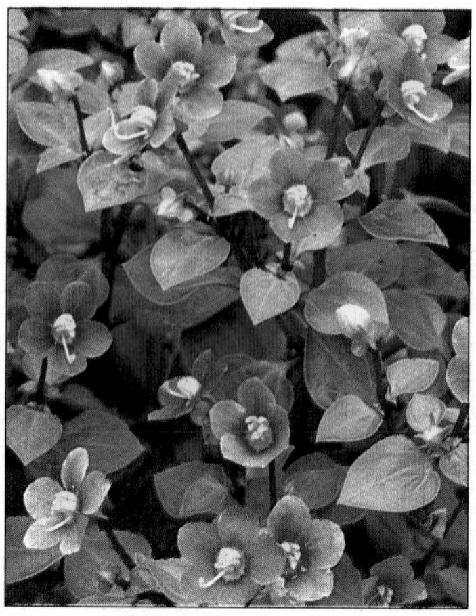

Exacum affine

EXOCHORDA
Pearl bush

ROSACEAE

Genus of 4 species of deciduous shrubs occurring in woodland from C. Asia to China and Korea. They are grown for their habit and abundant, showy, cup- or saucer-shaped white flowers, borne in terminal racemes in spring or summer. Leaves are alternate, simple, oblong or obovate, and entire or toothed. Ideal for a shrub border or as isolated specimens.
• **HARDINESS** Fully hardy.
• **CULTIVATION** Grow in fertile, moist but well-drained soil (most will tolerate all but shallow, chalky soil) in full sun or light dappled shade. *E. racemosa* prefers lime-free soil. Pruning group 2.

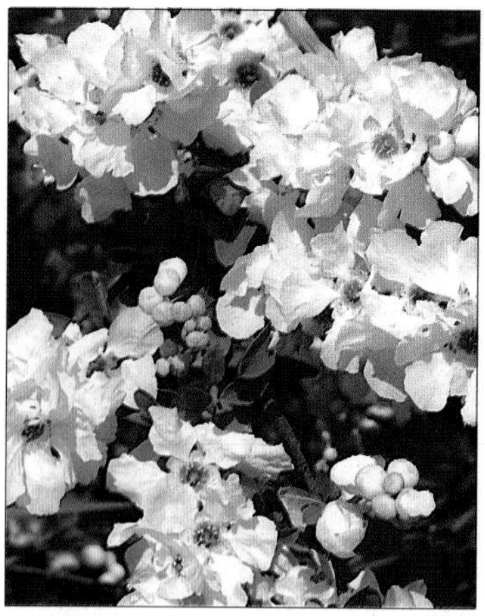

Exochorda × *macrantha* 'The Bride'

• **PROPAGATION** Sow seed in a seedbed in autumn. Insert softwood cuttings in summer.
• **PESTS AND DISEASES** Trouble free.

E. giraldii. Arching shrub with obovate leaves, to 8cm (3in) long, pinkish green when young, later pale green with red-tinged veins and red stalks. Upright racemes of 6–8 white flowers, to 2.5cm (1in) across, are produced in late spring. ↕↔ 3m (10ft). N.W. China. ✻✻✻.
var. *wilsonii* ▣ is more upright, with green-stalked leaves, to 10cm (4in) long, and flowers to 5cm (2in) across.
***E.* x *macrantha* 'The Bride'** ▣ ♀ Compact, arching, mound-forming shrub with obovate, light to mid-green leaves, to 7cm (3in) long. Bears racemes of 6–10 white flowers, to 3cm (1¼in) across, in late spring and early summer. ↕ 2m (6ft), ↔ 3m (10ft). ✻✻✻
E. racemosa. Dense, rounded shrub with arching branches and narrowly obovate leaves, to 7cm (3in) long, light green above, darker beneath. Bears upright racemes of 6–10 pure white flowers, to 4cm (1½in) across, in late spring. ↕↔ 3–4m (10–12ft). N. China. ✻✻✻

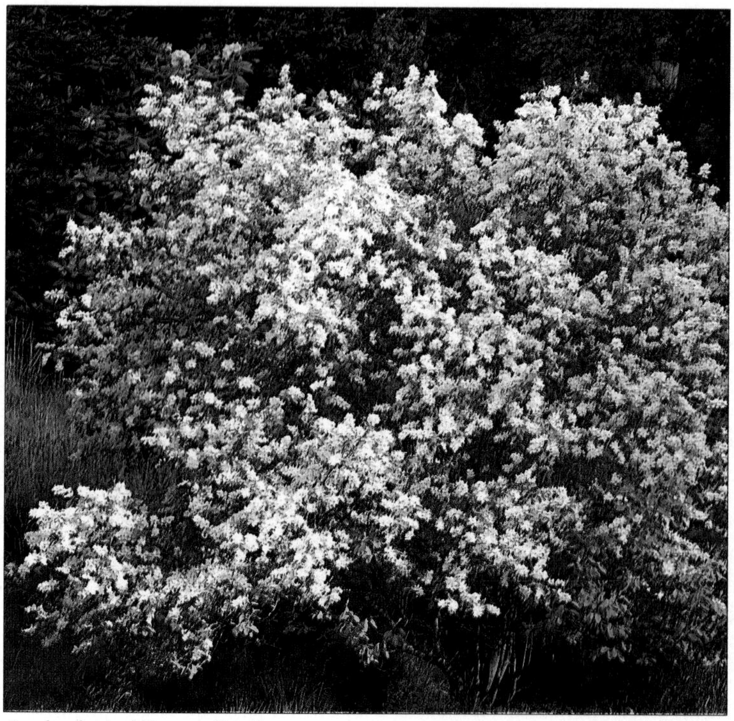

Exochorda giraldii var. *wilsonii*

F

FABIANA

SOLANACEAE

Genus of about 25 species of heath-like, evergreen shrubs from dry, upland slopes in temperate regions of South America. They are cultivated for their small, alternate, overlapping, densely arranged, needle-like leaves and solitary, tubular or bell-shaped flowers, borne terminally or opposite the leaves. Grow in a sheltered, mixed or shrub border, in a rock garden, or against a sunny wall.

• **HARDINESS** Frost hardy.

• **CULTIVATION** Grow in well-drained, poor to moderately fertile, neutral to slightly acid soil in full sun, sheltered from cold, drying winds. They are lime-tolerant, but may become chlorotic on shallow, chalk soils. Pruning group 9.

• **PROPAGATION** Sow seed in containers in a cold frame in autumn or spring. In early summer, take greenwood cuttings. Take semi-ripe cuttings in late summer.

• **PESTS AND DISEASES** Trouble free.

F. imbricata. Dense, mound-forming shrub with plume-like branches densely covered with tiny, needle-like, deep green leaves, to 5mm (¼in) long. In early summer, solitary, tubular, white to pale mauve flowers, 1.5cm (½in) long, are borne opposite the leaves. ↕↔ 2.5m (8ft). Chile. ❄❄. **'Prostrata'** is low-growing, with white flowers; ↕ 1m (3ft), ↔ 2m (6ft). **f. *violacea*** ▣ ♕ is upright, with branches spreading horizontally, and with lavender-mauve flowers.

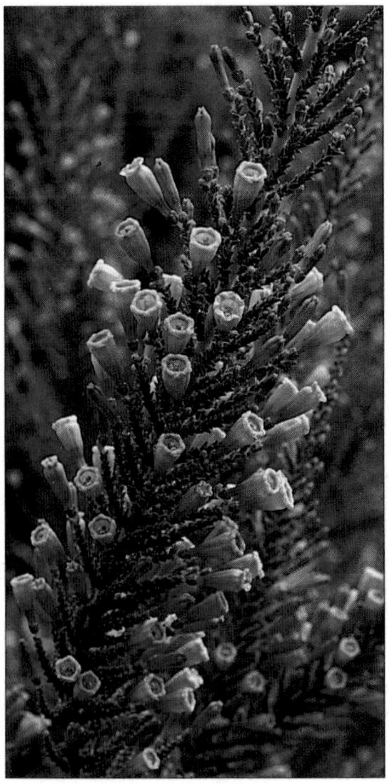

Fabiana imbricata f. *violacea*

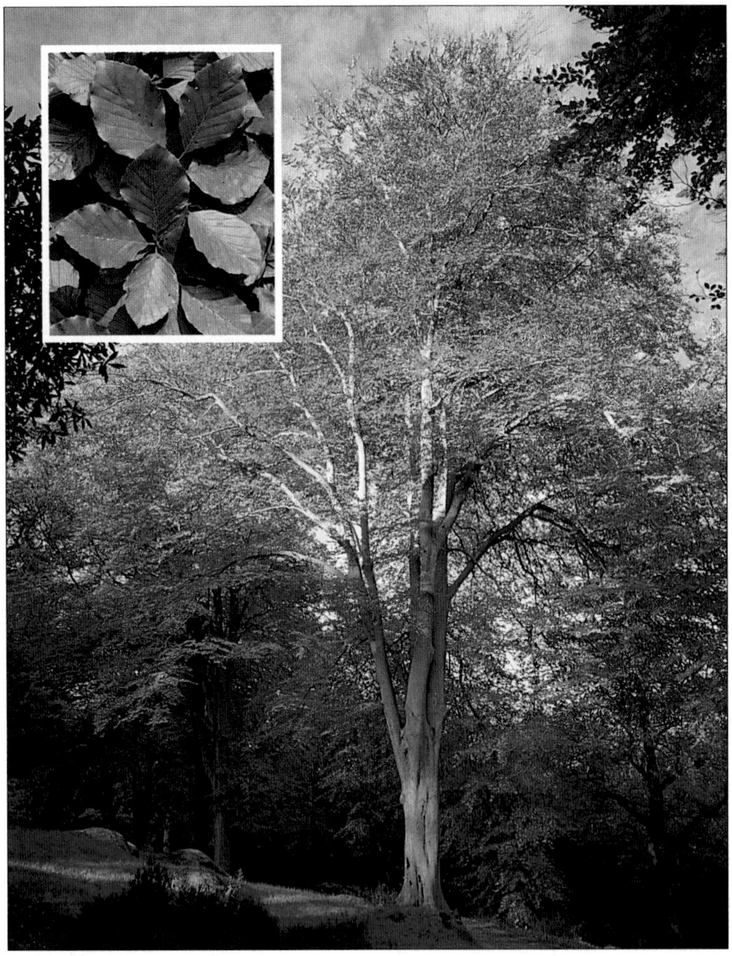

Fagus sylvatica (inset: leaf detail)

FAGUS

Beech

FAGACEAE

Genus of 10 species of deciduous forest trees, widely distributed in temperate regions of the N. hemisphere, valued for their foliage and autumn colour. They have alternate, usually ovate to elliptic-oblong, coarsely to finely toothed, mid- or dark green leaves, and usually smooth grey bark. The monoecious flowers appear with the leaves, the males in spherical heads, the females in pairs within 4-lobed bracts, which develop into smooth or spiny, 4-segmented cupules containing the nuts. Grow in a woodland garden or as specimen trees. Use *F. sylvatica* for hedging or pleaching.

• **HARDINESS** Fully hardy but, except for *F. sylvatica*, they require long, warm summers to thrive.

• **CULTIVATION** Very tolerant of a wide range of well-drained soils, including chalk; grow in full sun or partial shade. For best colour, position purple-leaved beeches in full sun and yellow-leaved ones in partial shade. Pruning group 1.

• **PROPAGATION** Sow seed in a seedbed in autumn, or, after winter stratification, in spring. Graft cultivars in midwinter.

• **PESTS AND DISEASES** Prone to beech bark disease, fungi (particularly bracket fungi), aphids, bark scales, and powdery mildew.

F. americana see *F. grandifolia.*
F. crenata ♀ (Japanese beech). Spreading tree with ovate, glossy, mid-green leaves, 7–13cm (3–5in) long, silky when young, turning yellow in autumn. ↕ 10m (30ft), ↔ 8m (25ft). Japan. ❄❄❄
F. grandifolia ♀ syn. *F. americana* (American beech). Spreading, often shrubby tree. Oval, dark green leaves, 6–15cm (2½–6in) long, with distinctly toothed margins, silky-haired at first, turn golden brown in autumn. ↕↔ 10m (30ft). E. North America. ❄❄❄
F. japonica ♀ Spreading tree with elliptic-ovate to ovate, tapered, blue-green leaves, 5–13cm (2–5in) long, silky-margined, slightly glaucous beneath, turning yellow in autumn. ↕ 10m (30ft), ↔ 8m (25ft). Japan. ❄❄❄
F. orientalis ♀ (Oriental beech). Spreading tree with elliptic to obovate, wavy-margined, toothed, dark green leaves, 8–17cm (3–7in) long, turning yellow-brown in autumn. ↕ 20m (70ft), ↔ 15m (50ft). S.E. Europe, N. Iran, Caucasus, S.W. Asia. ❄❄❄
F. sylvatica ▣ ♕ ♀ (Common beech). Spreading tree with elliptic-ovate, wavy-margined leaves, to 10cm (4in) long, silky-haired and pale green at first, turning glossy dark green, then yellow to orange-brown in autumn. ↕ 25m (80ft), ↔ 15m (50ft). C. Europe to Caucasus. ❄❄❄. **'Aspleniifolia'** ▣ ♕ (Fern-leaved beech) has slender leaves deeply cut into narrow lobes. **'Aurea Pendula'** ◊ is narrow, with pendulous branches and bright yellow young foliage, maturing to green; ↕ 10m (30ft), ↔ 1.5m (5ft). **'Dawyck'** ♕ ◊ is flame-shaped; ↔ 7m (22ft). **'Dawyck Gold'** ♕ ◊ is compact and columnar, with bright yellow young foliage turning green; ↕ 18m (60ft), ↔ 7m (22ft). **'Dawyck Purple'** ▣ ♕ ◊ is narrowly upright, with deep purple foliage; ↕ 20m (70ft), ↔ 5m (15ft). **f. *laciniata*** has deeply cut leaves. **f. *pendula*** ▣ ♕ ♀ (Weeping beech) has pendulous branches that may reach the ground. **f. *purpurea*** (Copper beech) has purple leaves, coppery in autumn. **'Purpurea Pendula'** ♀ is mushroom-headed, with weeping branches and deep blackish purple foliage; ↕↔ 3m

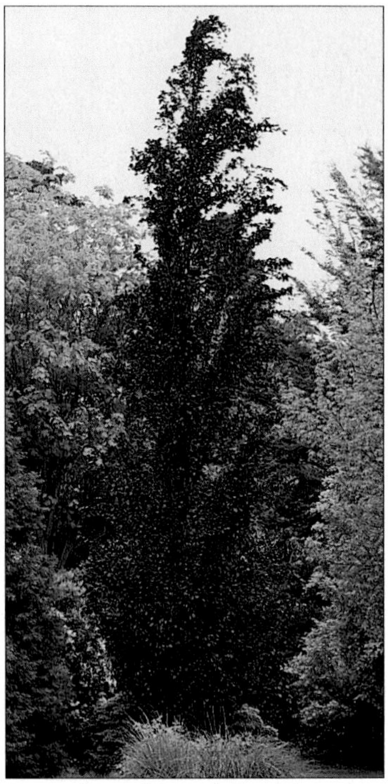

Fagus sylvatica 'Dawyck Purple'

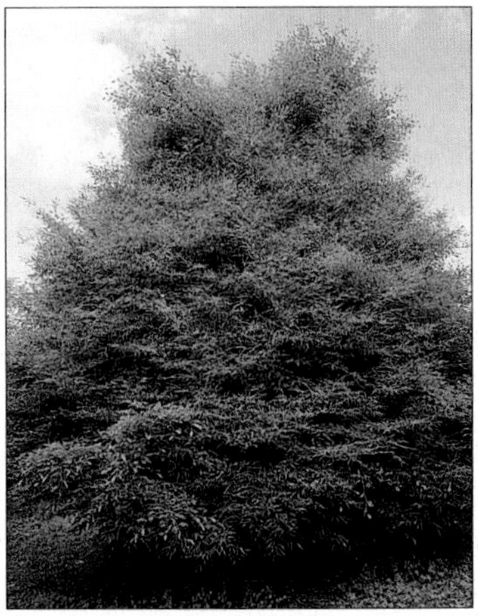

Fagus sylvatica 'Aspleniifolia'

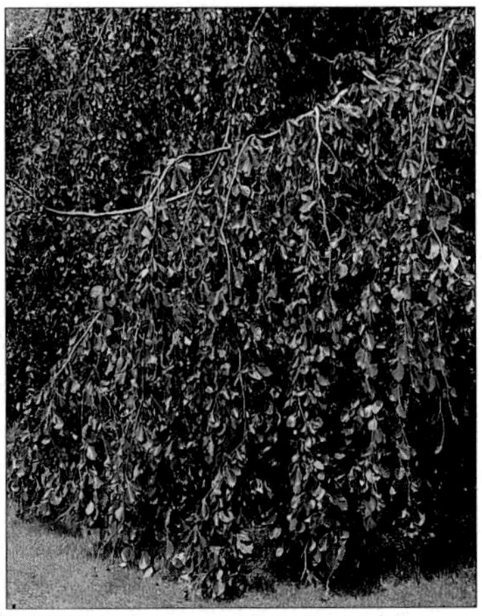

Fagus sylvatica f. *pendula*

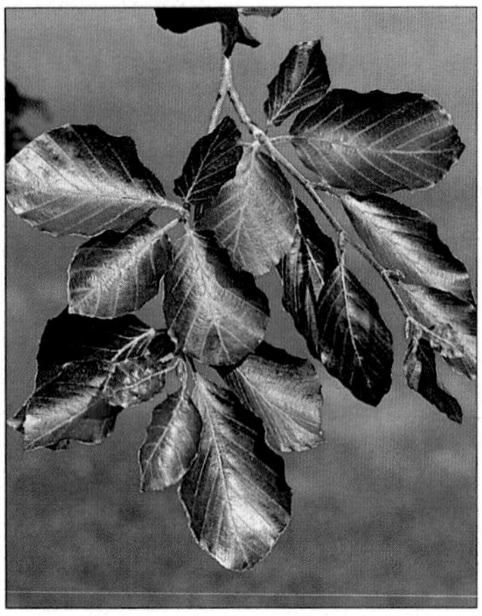
Fagus sylvatica 'Riversii'

(10ft). **'Purpurea Tricolor'** ○ syn. 'Roseomarginata', 'Tricolor' of gardens, has purple leaves edged and striped pink and pinkish white. **'Riversii'** ▣ has very deep purple leaves. **'Rohanii'** has deeply cut purple leaves. **'Roseomarginata'** see 'Purpurea Tricolor'. **'Rotundifolia'** ○ is upright when young, later spreading, bearing small, rounded leaves, to 5cm (2in) long. **'Tricolor' of gardens** see 'Purpurea Tricolor'. **'Zlatia'** has yellow young foliage, maturing to green.

▷ **Fairies' thimbles** see *Campanula cochleariifolia*
▷ **Fair maids of France** see *Ranunculus aconitifolius* 'Flore Pleno', *Saxifraga granulata*
▷ **Fair maids of Kent** see *Ranunculus aconitifolius* 'Flore Pleno'
▷ **Fairy bells** see *Disporum*
▷ **Fairy fan-flower** see *Scaevola aemula*
▷ **Fairy lantern** see *Calochortus*
▷ **Falling stars** see *Campanula isophylla*

FALLOPIA syn. BILDERDYKIA, REYNOUTRIA

POLYGONACEAE

Genus of 7 species of rhizomatous, climbing or scrambling, woody-based perennials found in moist habitats in temperate regions in the N. hemisphere. They have simple, entire, alternate, triangular or narrowly to broadly ovate leaves. In late summer, they produce large panicles of small, funnel-shaped, white, greenish white, or pinkish white flowers. Climbing species are ideal for training on pergolas and deciduous trees, and for covering unsightly structures. *F. aubertii* and *F. baldschuanica* are frequently rampant, and may be difficult to control; the two species are often confused and may be represented in gardens by hybrids between them.
• **HARDINESS** Fully hardy.
• **CULTIVATION** Grow in any poor to moderately fertile, moist but well-drained soil in full sun or partial shade. Provide strong, durable supports. Pruning group 11, in early spring.
• **PROPAGATION** Sow seed in containers in a cold frame in spring, or as soon as ripe. Take heeled, semi-ripe cuttings in summer, hardwood cuttings in autumn.
• **PESTS AND DISEASES** Leaf miners can be a problem.

F. aubertii, syn. *Bilderdykia aubertii*, *Polygonum aubertii* (Mile-a-minute plant). Vigorous, woody, twining,

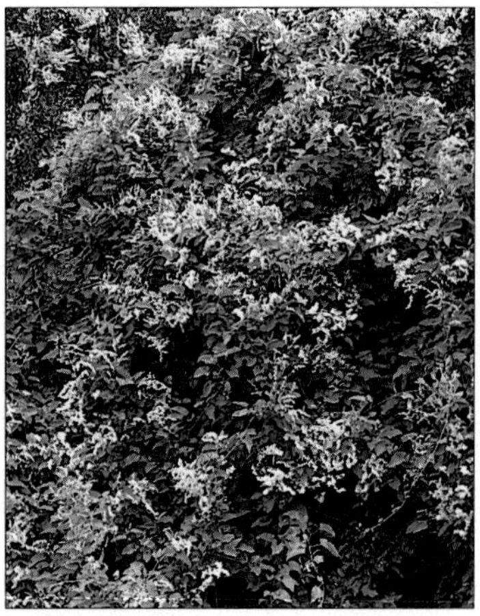
Fallopia baldschuanica

deciduous climber with heart-shaped, mid-green leaves, to 10cm (4in) long, bronze when young. Upright, narrow, minutely hairy, terminal or axillary panicles of tiny, funnel-shaped, white to greenish white flowers, 4–6mm (1/8–1/4in) across, are borne laterally on leafy stems in late summer and autumn, followed by small, angled, pinkish white fruit. ↕ 12m (40ft). China (Gansu, Sichuan, Shaanxi), Tibet. ❄❄❄
F. baldschuanica ▣ syn. *Bilderdykia baldschuanica*, *Polygonum baldschuanicum* (Mile-a-minute plant, Russian vine). Vigorous, woody, twining, deciduous climber with heart-shaped, dark green leaves, to 10cm (4in) long. In late summer and autumn, broad, almost hairless, terminal or axillary panicles of tiny, funnel-shaped, pink-tinged white flowers, 6–8mm (1/4–3/8in) across, are produced towards the ends of the shoots, followed by small, angled, pinkish white fruit. ↕ 12m (40ft). Tajikistan, Afghanistan, W. Pakistan. ❄❄❄

▷ **False acacia** see *Robinia pseudoacacia*
▷ **Fameflower** see *Talinum*

FARFUGIUM

ASTERACEAE/COMPOSITAE

Genus of 2 species of rhizomatous, evergreen perennials found near streams and seashores in E. Asia, grown mainly for their attractive foliage. The large, leathery leaves are borne on long stalks in basal tufts, and the yellow flowerheads are borne in loose corymbs. Variegated cultivars are excellent foliage

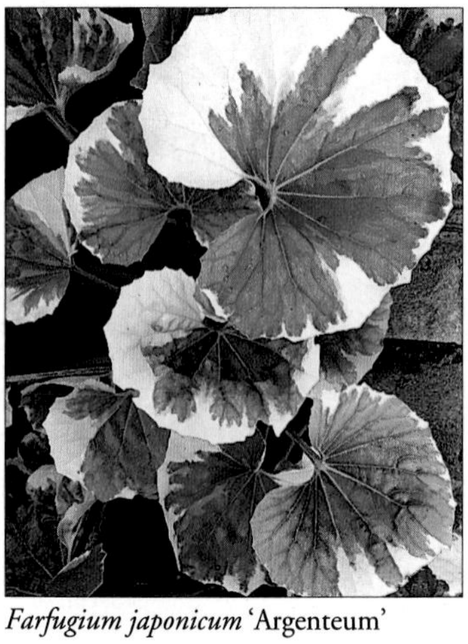
Farfugium japonicum 'Argenteum'

and ground-cover plants near water, in a border, or in containers.
• **HARDINESS** Frost hardy.
• **CULTIVATION** Grow in fertile, moist but well-drained soil in partial shade. Shelter from cold, drying winds. Mulch in winter in heavily frost-prone areas.
• **PROPAGATION** Sow seed of species in containers in a cold frame in winter or spring. Divide variegated cultivars and species in spring.
• **PESTS AND DISEASES** Prone to slugs.

F. japonicum, syn. *F. tussilagineum*, *Ligularia tussilaginea*. Loosely clump-forming perennial with kidney-shaped, long-stalked, shiny leaves, 15–30cm (6–12in) across, with entire or short-toothed margins. Bears yellow flowerheads, 4–6cm (1½–2½in) across, in autumn and winter. ↕↔ 60cm (24in). Japan (Honshu, Shikoku, Kyushu). ❄❄. **'Albovariegatum'** see 'Argenteum'. **'Argenteum'** ▣ syn. 'Albovariegatum', 'Variegatum', has variegated leaves with irregular, creamy white margins. **'Aureomaculatum'** ♀ has conspicuous, irregular yellow markings on its leaves. **'Variegatum'** see 'Argenteum'.
F. tussilagineum see *F. japonicum*.

FARGESIA

GRAMINEAE/POACEAE

Genus of about 4 species of clump-forming, evergreen bamboos from damp woodland in C. China and the N.E. Himalayas. Some species of *Fargesia* were formerly included in *Arundinaria*, *Sinarundinaria*, or *Thamnocalamus*. These often vigorous bamboos are grown for their attractive, linear to lance-shaped, slightly tessellated, bright, mid- or dark green leaves, and erect canes, 2–5m (6–15ft) tall, with yellow, brown, or dark purple-green nodes. The inflorescences are terminal panicles or racemes. Grow as specimen plants. *F. murieliae* is suitable for a hedge or screen. Grow *F. nitida* in a wild garden or in a large container.
• **HARDINESS** Fully hardy to half hardy.
• **CULTIVATION** Grow in fertile, moisture-retentive soil. *F. murieliae* tolerates full sun and wind. *F. nitida* needs partial or light dappled shade with shelter from cold, dry winds.
• **PROPAGATION** Divide established clumps, or take cuttings of sections of young rhizomes, in spring.
• **PESTS AND DISEASES** Slugs may attack young shoots.

F. murieliae ♀ syn. *Arundinaria murieliae*, *F. spathacea* of gardens, *Sinarundinaria murieliae*, *Thamnocalamus spathaceus* of gardens (Umbrella bamboo). Clump-forming bamboo, similar to *F. nitida*, but with white-powdery, yellow-green, then yellow stems, which usually branch in the first year and eventually arch under the weight of lance-shaped, bright green leaves, 6–15cm (2½–6in) long, with long, drawn-out tips. The deciduous leaf sheaths are downy, greenish purple when young, later becoming hairless and pale brown. ↕ to 4m (12ft), ↔ 1.5m (5ft) or more. C. China. ❄❄❄
F. nitida ♀ syn. *Arundinaria nitida*, *Sinarundinaria nitida* (Fountain bamboo). Slow-growing bamboo forming a dense clump of erect, dark purple-green canes, 4–8mm (1/8–3/8in) thick, lined purple-brown, and white-powdery beneath the nodes; canes remain unbranched in their first year. The deciduous leaf sheaths are pale or purple-brown. The upper portions of the canes produce abundant purple-tinted branchlets bearing cascades of alternate, narrow, lance-shaped, finely tapering, dark green leaves, 4–11cm (1½–4½in) long. ↕ to 5m (15ft), ↔ 1.5m (5ft) or more. C. China. ❄❄❄
***F. spathacea* of gardens** see *F. murieliae*.

FASCICULARIA

BROMELIACEAE

Genus of 5 species of stemless or short-stemmed, evergreen, xerophytic, terrestrial or epiphytic perennials (bromeliads) from coastal and central areas, to 400m (1,300ft) high, in Chile. They bear linear, widely spreading leaves in dense rosettes, forming distinct central cups. An inflorescence appears in the centre of each rosette, in summer; it has a very short scape and a spherical, corymb-like flowerhead of tubular blue flowers, and is followed by ovoid, scaly fruits. They are attractive plants for a desert garden, rock garden, or raised bed, by a sunny wall, or in containers. Where temperatures drop below 2–7°C (36–45°F), grow in a cool greenhouse.
• **HARDINESS** Frost tender; frost hardy or half hardy if protected from excessive winter wet.
• **CULTIVATION** Under glass, grow in terrestrial bromeliad compost in full light with good ventilation. During growth, water moderately and apply a nitrogen-based fertilizer monthly. Water sparingly in winter. Outdoors, grow in poor, sharply drained soil in full sun. Protect from winter wet. See also p.47.
• **PROPAGATION** Sow seed at 27°C (81°F) in winter or spring. Divide offsets in spring or summer.
• **PESTS AND DISEASES** Susceptible to greenfly while flowering.

F. andina see *F. bicolor*.
F. bicolor, syn. *F. andina*. Rosetted, terrestrial bromeliad with slender, spiny-toothed, rigid, mid- to deep green leaves, 50cm (20in) long, brown-scaly beneath, the innermost leaves bright crimson at flowering. In summer, each mature rosette bears an inflorescence with dense corymbs of pale blue flowers, 4cm (1½in) long, surrounded by ivory-

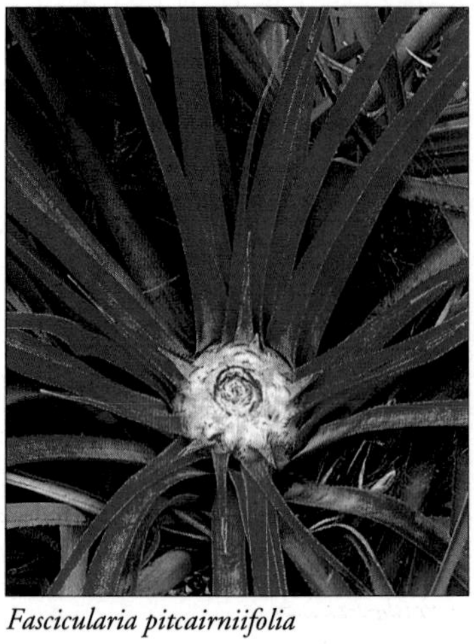
Fascicularia pitcairniifolia

F

white bracts. ↕ to 45cm (18in), ↔ 60cm (24in). Chile. ❄ (min. 2°C/36°F)
F. pitcairniifolia ▣ Rosetted, terrestrial bromeliad with glaucous mid-green leaves, to 1m (3ft) long, edged with short, brown, spreading spines. Leaves become hairless as the plant matures, with undersides white-scaly, and conspicuous sheaths greyish white above, sometimes brown-scaly beneath. In summer at flowering time, the inner rosette leaves turn bright red, forming a "collar" around the inflorescence of blue or bright violet flowers, 4–6cm (1½–2½in) long. ↕↔ to 1m (3ft). Chile. ❄ (min. 7°C/45°F)

x FATSHEDERA

ARALIACEAE

Bigeneric hybrid genus of one loose, spreading, evergreen shrub, derived from *Fatsia* and *Hedera*, grown mainly for its foliage. The leaves are palmately 5- or 7-lobed, dark, lustrous green, 10–24cm (4–10in) long. Umbel-like panicles of small, green-white flowers are borne in autumn. Tolerant of coastal exposure, atmospheric pollution, shade, and a wide range of soils, x *F. lizei* is suitable for a shrub border, a cool conservatory, or as a houseplant. It can also be trained against a wall or pillar.
• **HARDINESS** Frost hardy to half hardy.
• **CULTIVATION** Outdoors, grow in fertile, moist but well-drained soil in full sun or partial shade. Under glass, grow in loam-based potting compost (JI No.3); most light conditions are acceptable, but variegated cultivars need protection from very strong sunlight. During growth, water moderately and apply a balanced liquid fertilizer monthly. Water sparingly in winter. Support container-grown specimens. Pinch young shoots to promote bushiness. Pruning group 1; may need restrictive pruning under glass.
• **PROPAGATION** Root greenwood cuttings in early summer with bottom heat, or heel cuttings at any time of year.

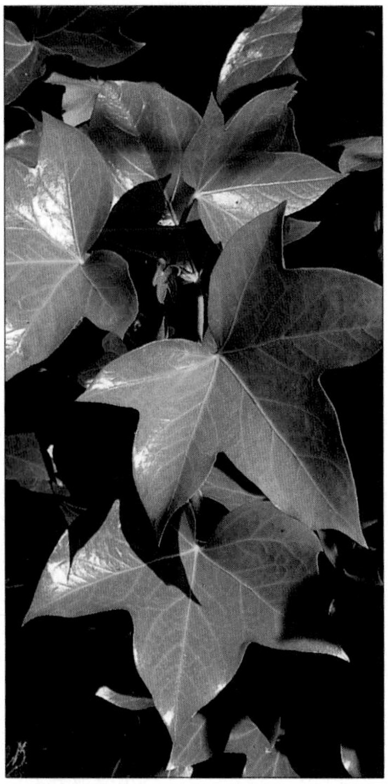

x *Fatshedera lizei*

• **PESTS AND DISEASES** Mealybugs and scale insects may be troublesome under glass.

x *F. lizei* ▣ ♀ (Tree-ivy). Spreading, loosely branched, evergreen shrub with rusty-hairy young growth. The palmate, leathery, dark green leaves are divided into 5, sometimes 7 lobes, deeply cut a third to halfway to the base. In autumn, produces umbel-like panicles of sterile, greenish white flowers, to 1cm (½in) across. ↕ 1.2–2m (4–6ft) or more, ↔ 3m (10ft). Garden origin. ✽✽. **'Anna Mikkels'** ♀ syn. 'Lemon and Lime', bears yellow-variegated leaves; ✽. **'Lemon and Lime'** see 'Anna Mikkels'. **'Pia'** has very wavy leaves; ✽. **'Variegata'** ♀ has leaves that are narrowly margined creamy white; ✽

FATSIA

ARALIACEAE

Genus of 2 or 3 species of evergreen shrubs or small trees from E. Asia. They have large, leathery, palmately 7- to 11-lobed leaves, produced mainly at the branch tips, and compound umbels, to 30cm (12in) or more across, of small, creamy white flowers borne in autumn, followed by clusters of usually spherical black fruits. *F. japonica*, the most widely grown species, occurs wild in coastal woodland in Japan and South Korea. It is tolerant of coastal exposure and atmospheric pollution. Valued for its foliage and architectural habit, and late display of flowers in mid-autumn, *F. japonica* is ideal in a shaded, sheltered courtyard, in a shrub border, or as a container plant in a cool conservatory or greenhouse.
• **HARDINESS** Frost hardy to half hardy.
• **CULTIVATION** Outdoors, grow in fertile, moist but well-drained soil in full sun or light dappled shade, with shelter from cold, drying winds. Variegated cultivars need partial shade. Under glass, grow in loam-based potting compost (JI No.3) in bright filtered light. During growth, water moderately and apply a balanced liquid fertilizer monthly. Water sparingly in winter. Pruning group 9.
• **PROPAGATION** Sow seed at 15–21°C (59–70°F) in autumn or spring. Take greenwood cuttings in early or mid-summer. Air layer in spring or late summer.
• **PESTS AND DISEASES** Mealybugs and scale insects may be troublesome under glass. Outdoors, cold winds may cause die-back and blackening of the shoots and leaves.

F. japonica ▣ ♀ syn. *Aralia japonica, A. sieboldii* (Japanese aralia, Japanese fatsia). Spreading, suckering, rounded, evergreen shrub with thick stems bearing hairless, 7- to 11-lobed, usually toothed, dark green leaves, 15–40cm (6–16in) long. In autumn, produces 5-petalled, creamy white flowers, 6mm (¼in) across, in branching, long-stalked umbels, 2.5–4cm (1–1½in) across, forming large compound umbels, followed by small, spherical black fruit. ↕↔ 1.5–4m (5–12ft). South Korea, Japan. ✽✽. **'Aurea'** is slow-growing, with gold-variegated leaves; ✽. **'Marginata'** has deeply lobed, white-margined, grey-green leaves; ✽.

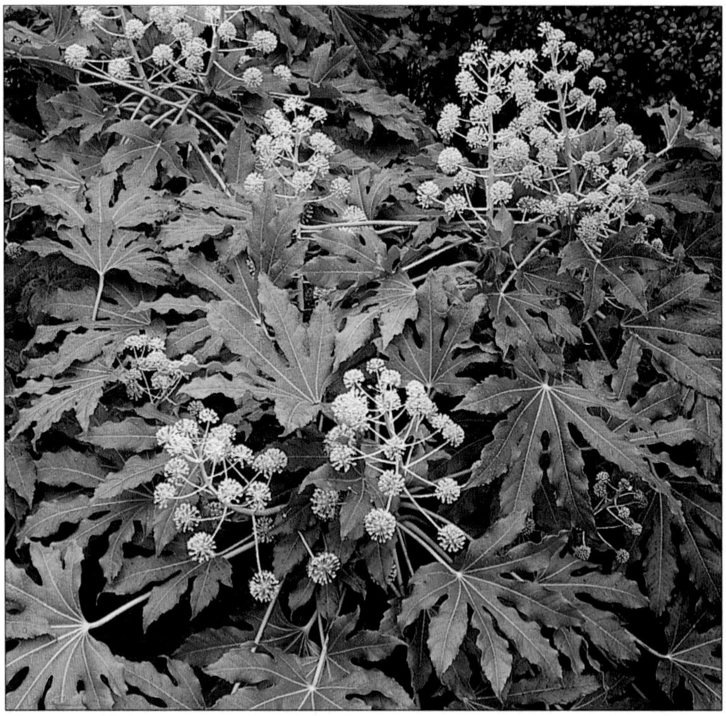

Fatsia japonica

'Moseri' has a compact habit, but with slightly larger leaves. **'Variegata'** ♀ bears leaves that are broadly margined with cream at the tips of the lobes; ✽
F. papyrifera see *Tetrapanax papyrifer.*

▷**Fatsia, Japanese** see *Fatsia japonica*

FAUCARIA

Tiger jaws

AIZOACEAE

Genus of over 30 species of clump-forming, sometimes fleshy-rooted, almost stemless perennial succulents from semi-desert areas in South Africa. The fleshy, spotted leaves are borne 4–8 on each shoot. They usually have stout, soft, marginal teeth, which can resemble gaping jaws. The large, daisy-like, pink, yellow, or white flowers open after mid-day from late summer to mid-autumn. Where temperatures drop below 7°C (45°F), grow in a temperate greenhouse, as houseplants, or with other plants in a bowl garden. In warmer areas, grow in a raised or scree bed, or desert garden.
• **HARDINESS** Frost tender.
• **CULTIVATION** Under glass, grow in standard cactus compost in full light.

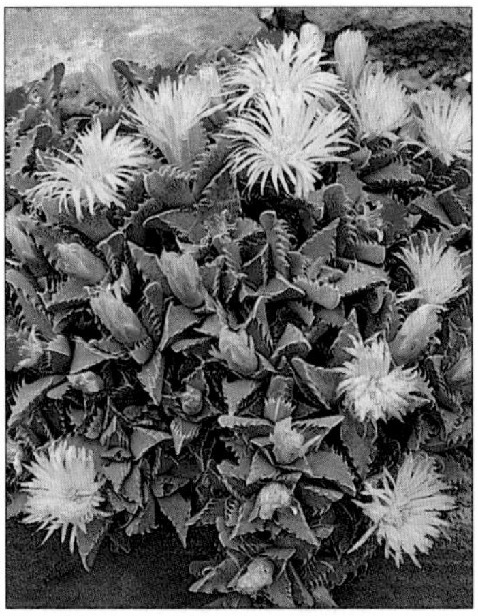

Faucaria tigrina

During growth, water moderately and apply a low-nitrogen fertilizer monthly. Water sparingly in winter. Outdoors, grow in poor soil, with added grit and leaf mould, in full sun. Protect from excessive rain. See also pp.48–49.
• **PROPAGATION** Sow seed at 10–20°C (50–68°F) in autumn or spring. Root stem cuttings in summer in sharply drained compost.
• **PESTS AND DISEASES** Susceptible to greenfly and root mealybugs while flowering.

F. felina. Clump-forming succulent with elongated diamond-shaped or 3-angled, long-pointed, white-spotted leaves, 4–5cm (1½–2in) long, which later turn red. Leaves have slender white keels and 3–5 pointed, recurved, fleshy, marginal teeth. Golden yellow flowers, to 5cm (2in) across, open in autumn. ↕ 7cm (3in), ↔ 21cm (8in). South Africa (Eastern Cape, Western Cape). ❄ (min. 7°C/45°F)
F. tigrina ▣ Clump-forming succulent with diamond-shaped-ovate, pointed, greyish green leaves, 3–5cm (1¼–2in) long, with very rounded, white-spotted undersides and up to 10 recurved, hairy-tipped, marginal teeth. Golden yellow, sometimes red-budded flowers, 5cm (2in) across, are borne in autumn. ↕ 10cm (4in), ↔ 20cm (8in). South Africa (Eastern Cape). ❄ (min. 7°C/45°F)

▷**Feather,**
  Emerald see *Asparagus densiflorus* 'Sprengeri'
  Painted see *Vriesea carinata*
  Prince's see *Persicaria orientale*
  Princess see *Persicaria orientale*
▷**Featherflower** see *Verticordia plumosa*
  Scarlet see *V. grandis*
▷**Featherfoil, American** see *Hottonia inflata*
▷**Feather grass** see *Stipa*
  Giant see *S. gigantea*
▷**Feathertop** see *Pennisetum villosum*
▷***Feijoa*** see *Acca*

FELICIA syn. AGATHAEA

Blue daisy

ASTERACEAE/COMPOSITAE

Genus of about 80 species of annuals, perennials, and evergreen subshrubs and (rarely) shrubs found in open, sunny habitats in the Arabian Peninsula, and tropical and southern Africa. They have alternate or opposite, linear to ovate or obovate leaves, occasionally in basal rosettes. They are grown for their mass of daisy-like, mainly blue flowerheads with yellow disc-florets, often borne over long periods in summer. The annuals, and those treated as annuals, are suitable for bedding and containers; the wind-resistant *F. bergeriana* is especially good for a window-box or balcony. Grow low-growing perennials in a rock garden or raised bed, or at the base of a warm, sunny wall. Blue daisies are attractive container plants for a conservatory or temperate greenhouse.

- **HARDINESS** Frost hardy to frost tender.
- **CULTIVATION** Under glass, grow in loam-based potting compost (JI No.2) in full light, with low humidity and good ventilation. During growth, water moderately and apply a balanced liquid fertilizer monthly. Water sparingly in winter. Outdoors, grow in poor to moderately fertile, well-drained soil in full sun. Intolerant of damp. Pinch back young shoots to encourage bushiness.
- **PROPAGATION** Sow seed of annuals at 10–18°C (50–64°F) in spring. Root stem tip cuttings of tender species in late summer and overwinter under glass.
- **PESTS AND DISEASES** Susceptible to aphids and red spider mites under glass.

F. amelloides, syn. *Aster amelloides*, *A. capensis*, *A. coelestis* (Blue daisy). Rounded, bushy subshrub, often grown as an annual, with ovate to obovate, deep green leaves, to 3cm (1¼in) long. Bears light to deep blue flowerheads, 2–5cm (¾–2in) across, from summer to autumn. ↕↔ 30–60cm (12–24in). South Africa. ❁ (min. 3–5°C/37–41°F). **'Read's Blue'** is compact, with blue flowerheads. **'Read's White'** ▣ is a compact cultivar, with white flowerheads. **'Santa Anita'** ▣🏆 bears large, rich blue flowerheads. **'Santa Anita Variegated'** 🏆 has white-marked leaves.
F. amoena, syn. *Aster pappei*, *F. pappei*. Bushy annual or short-lived perennial with linear to elliptic, downy leaves, 3cm (1¼in) long. Bears solitary, bright

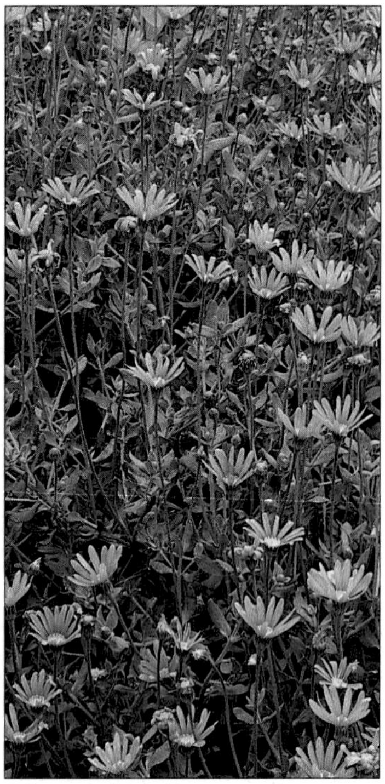
Felicia amelloides 'Santa Anita'

blue flowerheads, 3.5cm (1½in) across, from summer to early autumn. ↕↔ 30–50cm (12–20in). South Africa. ❁ (min. 3–5°C/37–41°F). **'Variegata'** ▣ has cream-splashed leaves.
F. bergeriana ▣ (Kingfisher daisy). Mat-forming annual with lance-shaped, sometimes toothed, softly hairy, grey-green leaves, to 4cm (1½in) long. In summer, bears abundant solitary, brilliant clear blue flowerheads, to 3cm (1¼in) across, with yellow centres. ↕↔ to 25cm (10in). South Africa. ✲
F. heterophylla. Mat-forming annual with inversely lance-shaped, sometimes toothed, grey-green leaves, to 5cm (2in) long. Solitary blue flowerheads, to 2cm (¾in) across, are borne in summer. ↕↔ 50cm (20in). South Africa. ✲. **'Snowmass'** bears white flowerheads. **'The Blues'** has pale blue flowerheads; ↕ to 20cm (8in). **'The Rose'** has pink flowerheads.
F. natalensis see *F. rosulata*.
F. pappei see *F. amoena*.
F. rosulata, syn. *Aster natalensis*, *F. natalensis*. Rhizomatous, rosette-forming perennial with elliptic to obovate, hairy, dark green basal leaves, 7–10cm (3–4in) long, and smaller,

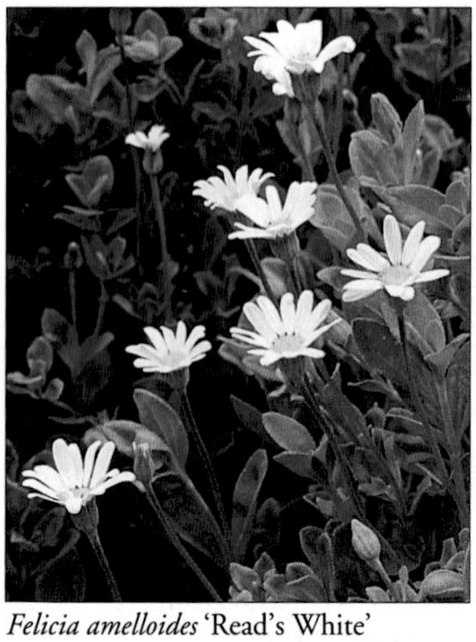
Felicia amelloides 'Read's White'

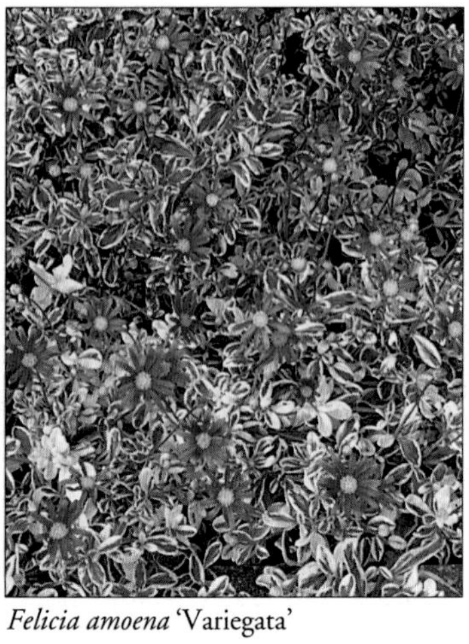
Felicia amoena 'Variegata'

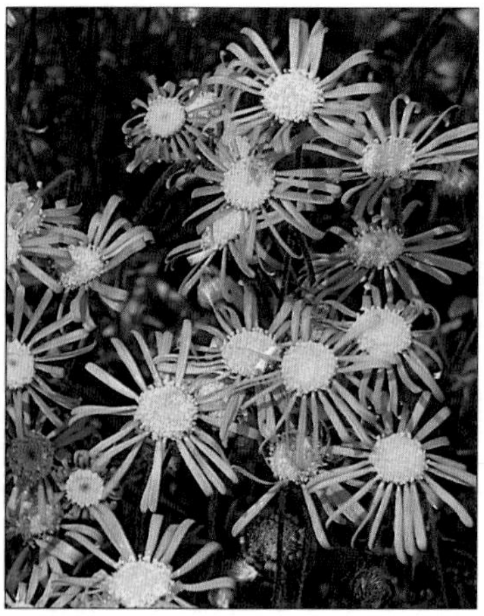
Felicia bergeriana

lance-shaped stem leaves. Solitary, mid-blue flowerheads, to 3cm (1¼in) across, with golden yellow disc-florets, are produced in summer. ↕ 20cm (8in), ↔ 30cm (12in). South Africa. ✲✲

FENDLERA

HYDRANGEACEAE

Genus of 3 or 4 species of deciduous shrubs found on cliffs and rocky ledges in canyons and woodland in S.W. USA and Mexico. They have opposite, entire, lance-shaped to elliptic or ovate, mid-green leaves, to 5cm (2in) long, and are grown for their fragrant, 4-petalled, cup-shaped white flowers, 2½–5cm (1–2in) across, borne singly or in pairs or threes on side branches. Grow in a shrub border or against a warm, sunny wall.

- **HARDINESS** Hardy to -20°C (4°F).
- **CULTIVATION** Grow in moderately fertile, sharply drained soil in full sun. Pruning group 2.
- **PROPAGATION** Sow seed in autumn in a cold frame, or in spring at 13–16°C (55–61°F). Root softwood cuttings in summer with bottom heat.
- **PESTS AND DISEASES** Trouble free.

F. rupicola. Spreading shrub with arching branches and lance-shaped leaves, to 3cm (1¼in) long, white-hairy beneath. In late spring and early summer, fragrant, white, sometimes pink-tinged flowers, to 3cm (1¼in) across, are produced singly or in small clusters. ↕ 1.5m (5ft), ↔ 3m (10ft). S.W. USA, N. Mexico. ✲✲✲

FENESTRARIA

AIZOACEAE

Genus of 1 or 2 species of variable, very dwarf, stemless, cushion-forming, perennial succulents from semi-desert areas of Namibia, grown for their daisy-like, bright yellowish orange or white flowers. Leaves are club-shaped, erect, opposite, hairless, and fleshy, with transparent "windows" in the flattened tips. Where temperatures drop below 7°C (45°F), grow in an indoor garden or temperate greenhouse. In warmer areas, grow in a raised bed or desert garden.

- **HARDINESS** Frost tender.
- **CULTIVATION** Under glass, grow in standard cactus compost in full light with low humidity; ventilate well. During growth, water moderately and apply a low-nitrogen liquid fertilizer monthly. Keep dry in winter. Outdoors,

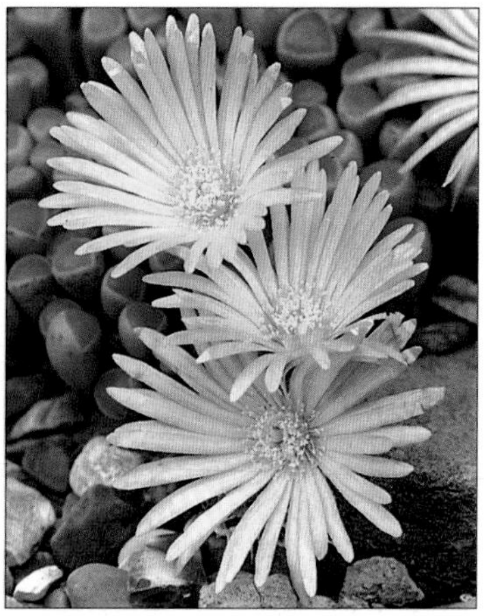
Fenestraria aurantiaca

grow in poor, dry, sharply drained soil, with added grit and leaf mould, in full sun, with shelter from excessive rain. They resent root disturbance. See also pp.48–49.

- **PROPAGATION** Sow seed at 15–21°C (59–70°F) in autumn or spring. Separate offsets in spring or summer.
- **PESTS AND DISEASES** Trouble free.

F. aurantiaca ▣ Succulent that forms dense cushions of club-shaped, erect leaves, 2–3cm (¾–1¼in) long, with "windows" in their slightly flattened tips. From late summer to autumn, golden yellow flowers, 3–7cm (1¼–3in) across, are produced on stalks 4–5cm (1½–2in) long. ↕ 5cm (2in), ↔ 30cm (12in). Namibia. ❁ (min. 7°C/45°F).
f. *rhopalophylla*, syn. *F. rhopalophylla*, forms less dense cushions and has pure white flowers, to 3cm (1¼in) across; ↔ to 20cm (8in).
F. rhopalophylla see *F. aurantiaca* f. *rhopalophylla*.

▷**Fennel** see *Foeniculum*
  Florence see *Foeniculum vulgare* var. *azoricum*
  Giant see *Ferula*
▷**Fern,**
  Asparagus see *Asparagus densiflorus*, *A. setaceus*
  Bamboo see *Coniogramme japonica*
  Barbados maidenhair see *Adiantum tenerum* 'Farleyense'
  Bear's paw see *Aglaomorpha meyeniana*
  Beech see *Phegopteris*, *P. connectilis*
  Bird's nest see *Asplenium australasicum*, *A. nidus*
  Black tree see *Cyathea medullaris*
  Bladder see *Cystopteris*
  Blue see *Phlebodium aureum* 'Mandaianum'
  Boston see *Nephrolepis exaltata* 'Bostoniensis'
  Brittle bladder see *Cystopteris fragilis*
  Broad beech see *Phegopteris hexagonoptera*
  Broad buckler see *Dryopteris dilatata*
  Buckler see *Dryopteris*
  Button see *Pellaea rotundifolia*
  Byfield see *Bowenia spectabilis*
  Cabbage see *Platycerium elephantotis*
  Chain see *Woodwardia*
  Cinnamon see *Osmunda cinnamomea*
  Climbing see *Lygodium*
  Common rasp see *Doodia media*
  Crown see *Blechnum discolor*

▷**Fern cont.**
Dickie's see *Cystopteris dickieana*
Elephant's ear see *Platycerium elephantotis*
Emerald see *Asparagus densiflorus* 'Sprengeri'
Felt see *Pyrrosia*
Flowering see *Osmunda regalis*
Fork see *Psilotum*
Foxtail see *Asparagus densiflorus* 'Myersii'
Glory see *Adiantum tenerum* 'Farleyense'
Goldback see *Pityrogramma triangularis*
Golden male see *Dryopteris affinis*
Goldie's see *Dryopteris goldieana*
Hairy lip see *Cheilanthes tomentosa*
Hard see *Blechnum, B. spicant*
Hard shield see *Polystichum aculeatum*
Hare's foot see *Davallia canariensis, Phlebodium aureum*
Hart's tongue see *Asplenium scolopendrium*
Hawaiian tree see *Cibotium glaucum*
Hen-and-chicken see *Asplenium bulbiferum*
Holly see *Polystichum*
Interrupted see *Osmunda claytoniana*
Japanese climbing see *Lygodium japonicum*
Japanese felt see *Pyrrosia lingua*
Japanese holly see *Cyrtomium falcatum*
Japanese painted see *Athyrium niponicum*
Japanese tassel see *Polystichum polyblepharum*
Korean rock see *Polystichum tsussimense*
Lady see *Athyrium, A. filix-femina*
Large-leaved holly see *Cyrtomium macrophyllum*
Leather see *Rumohra adiantiformis*
Licorice see *Polypodium glycyrrhiza*
Lip see *Cheilanthes*
Maidenhair see *Adiantum*
Male see *Dryopteris filix-mas*
Man see *Dicksonia antarctica*
Marsh see *Thelypteris palustris*
Mrs. Frizell's lady see *Athyrium filix-femina* 'Frizelliae'
Narrow buckler see *Dryopteris carthusiana*
North American hay-scented see *Dennstaedtia punctiloba*
Oak see *Gymnocarpium dryopteris*
Ostrich see *Matteuccia struthiopteris*
Prickly shield see *Polystichum aculeatum*
Queen Victoria's lady see *Athyrium filix-femina* Cruciatum Group 'Victoriae'
Rabbit's foot see *Davallia fejeensis, Phlebodium aureum*
Resurrection see *Polypodium polypodioides*
Rockcap see *Polypodium virginianum*
Royal see *Osmunda regalis*
Rusty-back see *Asplenium ceterach*
Sago see *Cyathea medullaris*
Sensitive see *Onoclea sensibilis*
Shield see *Polystichum*
Shuttlecock see *Matteuccia struthiopteris*
Soft shield see *Polystichum setiferum*
Soft tree see *Dicksonia antarctica*
Squirrel's foot see *Davallia mariesii*
Staghorn see *Platycerium*
Sword see *Nephrolepis, Polystichum munitum*

▷**Fern cont.**
Tatting see *Athyrium filix-femina* 'Frizelliae'
Tongue see *Pyrrosia lingua*
Tree see *Cyathea*
Walking see *Asplenium rhizophyllum*
Wallich's wood see *Dryopteris wallichiana*
Woolly tree see *Dicksonia antarctica*
▷**Fern palm** see *Cycas, C. circinalis*
Mexican see *Dioon edule*
▷**Ferns** see p.51

FEROCACTUS

CACTACEAE

Genus of about 30 species of flattened, spherical to columnar, perennial cacti from lowlands and mountainous areas of S. and S.W. USA, Mexico, and Guatemala. They are usually solitary but some species form thick clumps. The large, prominent ribs have spiny areoles, some hooked. Large, funnel- or bell-shaped flowers are borne from near the crown in summer, followed by ovoid, fleshy fruits. Grow in a desert garden. Where temperatures fall below 7°C (45°F), grow in a temperate greenhouse.

• **HARDINESS** Frost tender.
• **CULTIVATION** Under glass, grow in standard cactus compost in full light with low humidity. During growth, water freely and apply a balanced liquid fertilizer monthly. Keep dry in winter. Mist on warm days in midwinter; keep root zone dry. Outdoors, grow in poor, sharply drained soil in full sun. Protect from excessive rain. See also pp.48–49.
• **PROPAGATION** Sow seed at 10–20°C (50–68°F) in spring.
• **PESTS AND DISEASES** Vulnerable to mealybugs.

***F. acanthodes* of gardens** see *F. cylindraceus.*
F. bicolor see *Thelocactus bicolor.*
F. chrysacanthus. Solitary cactus with a spherical to cylindrical, dark green stem, and 13–22 warty ribs and areoles (4–6 or more white radials and 4–10

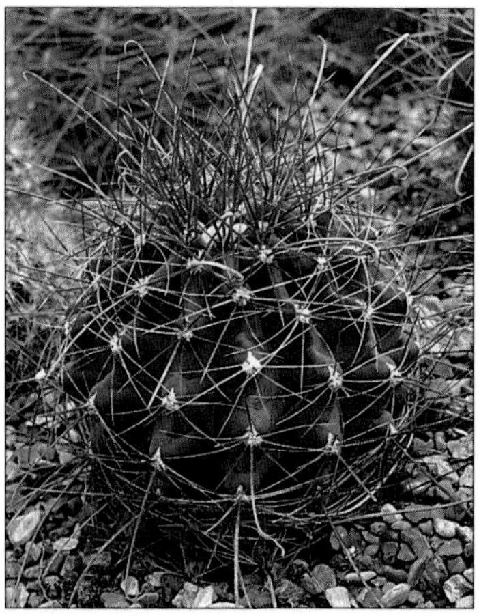
Ferocactus hamatacanthus

flattened and twisted, yellow or reddish yellow centrals). Bell-shaped, yellow or reddish yellow to orange flowers, 4.5cm (1¾in) long, with outer segments striped red-brown or brownish pink, are borne in summer. ↕ to 1m (3ft), ↔ 40cm (16in). Mexico (Baja California). ❄ (min. 7°C/45°F)
F. crassihamatus see *Sclerocactus uncinatus* var. *crassihamatus.*
F. cylindraceus ■ syn. *F. acanthodes* of gardens. Solitary, sometimes offsetting cactus with an ovoid then cylindrical, glaucous green stem with 13–27 warty ribs and red, orange, or buff-yellow spines (9–13 or more radials and 4–7 longer, flat, sometimes hooked, often recurved centrals). Bears bell-shaped, yellow or orange flowers, 3–6cm (1¼–2½in) long, in summer. ↕ 3m (10ft), ↔ 80cm (32in). S.W. USA, N.W. Mexico. ❄ (min. 7°C/45°F)
F. fordii 🏆 Solitary cactus with a slightly depressed-spherical, greyish green stem and about 21 warty ribs and white spines (about 15 spreading, paler radials and 4–7 flattened, hooked or twisted, red or grey centrals). Funnel-shaped, deep pink to purple flowers, to 4cm (1½in) long, are produced in summer. ↕↔ 40cm (16in). Mexico (Baja California). ❄ (min. 7°C/45°F)
F. hamatacanthus ■ syn. *Hamatocactus hamatacanthus.* Solitary or clustering cactus with a spherical to cylindrical, deep green stem, 13–18 prominent, warty ribs, and brownish red spines (6–20 radials and 4–8 centrals). Funnel-shaped yellow flowers, 6–10cm (2½–4in) long, with red throats, are borne in summer. ↕ 60cm (24in), ↔ to 40cm (16in). USA (Texas), N. and N.E. Mexico. ❄ (min. 7°C/45°F)
F. latispinus. Often solitary, depressed-spherical cactus with 15–23 acute, sometimes spiralled, greyish green ribs, notched with large areoles (6–15 yellow radial spines and 4 red centrals, the lowest flattened and hooked). Bears bell-shaped, white, red, purple, or yellow flowers, 4cm (1½in) long, in summer. ↕ 10–40cm (4–16in), ↔ to 40cm (16in). Central S. Mexico. ❄ (min. 7°C/45°F)
F. setispinus see *Thelocactus setispinus.*
F. wislizenii. Solitary cactus with a spherical then cylindrical, dark green to greyish green stem, with 15–25 ribs and areoles (12–30 greyish yellow radial spines and up to 8 longer, flattened, hooked, yellow, brown, or grey centrals with curved, reddish brown tips). Bell-shaped, yellow, orange, or red flowers, 5–8cm (2–3in) long, with green outer segments, are borne in summer. ↕ 1.5m (5ft), ↔ to 80cm (32in). S.W. USA, N.W. Mexico. ❄ (min. 7°C/45°F)

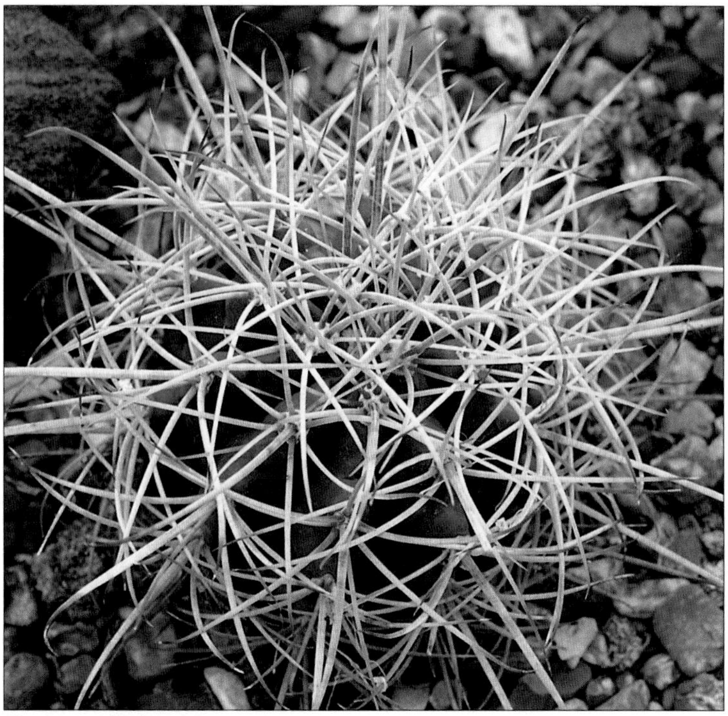
Ferocactus cylindraceus

FERRARIA

IRIDACEAE

Genus of 10 species of cormous perennials from dry, sandy soils, sometimes near the coast, in tropical Africa and South Africa. They are grown for their few-flowered cymes of curious, malodorous, patterned, short-lived flowers, 4–6cm (1½–2½in) across, pollinated by flies. The flowers are iris-shaped with crisped petals, borne in succession on branched stems in late winter and early spring. The basal leaves are lance-shaped; the 2-ranked stem leaves are ovate-lance-shaped. In frost-prone areas, grow in a temperate greenhouse. Elsewhere, use in a rock garden or raised bed, or against a sunny wall.

• **HARDINESS** Half hardy to frost tender.
• **CULTIVATION** Under glass, plant directly into a greenhouse border or in deep containers of loam-based potting compost (JI No.2), with added grit, in full light. In growth (in winter), water moderately and apply a balanced liquid fertilizer monthly. Keep dry in summer. Outdoors, plant 15cm (6in) deep in fertile, well-drained soil in autumn.
• **PROPAGATION** Sow seed in summer or autumn at 6–12°C (43–54°F). Separate offsets from dormant parent corms.
• **PESTS AND DISEASES** Trouble free.

F. crispa, syn. *F. undulata.* Cormous perennial with linear-lance-shaped, stem-clasping leaves, 15–30cm (6–12in) long, forming progressively smaller sheaths around the stem. In spring, bears wavy-petalled, brown or yellowish brown, upward-facing flowers, 2.5cm (1in) across, with 3 outer petals and 3 smaller inner petals, lined and spotted yellow and brown. ↕ 20–40cm (8–16in), ↔ 15cm (6in). South Africa. ✲
F. undulata see *F. crispa.*

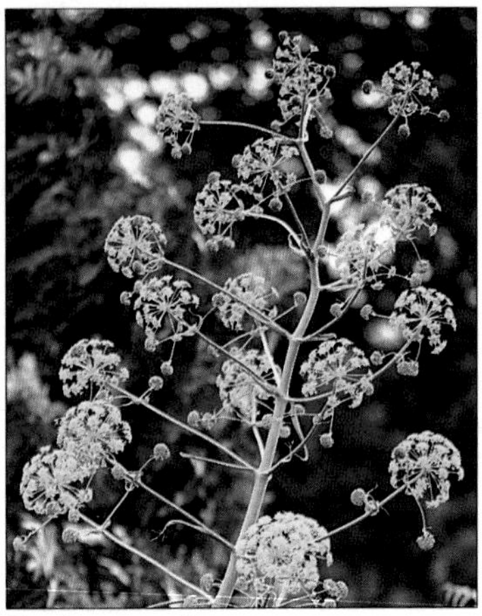

Ferula communis

FERULA

Giant fennel

APIACEAE/UMBELLIFERAE

Genus of 170 species of robust, tap-rooted, usually hairless, aromatic, herbaceous perennials found in rough, grassy places, dry slopes, and gravelly roadsides from the Mediterranean to C. Asia. They bear branching or simple stems, with 2- to 5-pinnate, usually basal, light green leaves, to 80cm (32in) long, the ultimate segments linear to obovate. Usually forming a mound of finely divided leaves, they are effective foliage plants when mature. Giant fennels (which should not be confused with the edible fennels, *Foeniculum*) bear white, greenish white, yellow, or purple flowers in terminal, lateral, compound umbels, to 15cm (6in) across, although they may take several years to flower and often die after seeding. Grow at the back of a border, or as a specimen plant in a sunny, open site in a wild garden.

• **HARDINESS** Hardy to -10°C (14°F).
• **CULTIVATION** Grow in fertile, well-drained soil in full sun. To enhance foliage, remove flowering stems as soon as they show, or immediately after blooming if seed is not required. Protect with a dry, bracken mulch in winter.
• **PROPAGATION** Sow seed as soon as ripe in containers in a cold frame. Prick out seedlings into deep containers to allow tap-root development.
• **PESTS AND DISEASES** Susceptible to aphids, slugs, and mildew.

F. communis ■ Robust perennial bearing 3- or 4-pinnate leaves, 25–45cm (10–18in) long, subdivided into narrow, linear segments. After several years, stout, ridged, branching stems produce clusters of hemispherical, many-branched umbels, 8cm (3in) across, composed of small, 5-petalled yellow flowers, in early and midsummer. May die after seeding. ↕ to 5m (15ft), usually 2–3m (6–10ft), ↔ 60cm (24in). Mediterranean. ❄❄
***F.* 'Giant Bronze'** see *Foeniculum vulgare* 'Giant Bronze'.

▷ **Fescue** see *Festuca*
Blue see *F. glauca*
Grey see *F. glauca*
Ice see *F. glacialis*
Large blue see *F. amethystina*
Tufted see *F. amethystina*

FESTUCA

Fescue

GRAMINEAE/POACEAE

Genus of 300–400 species of deciduous or evergreen, rhizomatous, often tufted, perennial grasses widely distributed in grassland, woodland edges, and stream margins throughout temperate zones. A few have attractive inflorescences, but most are grown for their usually blue-green or blue-grey foliage. Many are grown as turf or pasture grasses. The 5- to 9-veined, lance-shaped leaves are flat, folded, or rolled. Dense or loose, branched panicles of flattened, brownish green, sometimes glaucous spikelets are borne from spring to summer. Grow fescues in a border or rock garden to provide foliage contrast with alpines.

• **HARDINESS** Fully hardy.
• **CULTIVATION** Grow in poor to moderately fertile, dry, well-drained soil in full sun. *F. eskia* will not tolerate alkaline soils. Divide and replant every 2 or 3 years to maintain foliage colour.
• **PROPAGATION** Sow seed from autumn to spring in containers in a cold frame. Divide in spring.
• **PESTS AND DISEASES** Trouble free.

F. amethystina (Large blue fescue, Tufted fescue). Densely tufted, tussock-forming, evergreen, perennial grass with soft, narrowly linear, grey-green leaves, to 25cm (10in) long, the lower halves inrolled and furrowed. In late spring and early summer, bears lax, flexuous, zigzag panicles, 10–20cm (4–8in) long, with paired branches bearing spikelets of 3–7 violet-tinted, greenish to purple or violet flowers. ↕ to 45cm (18in), ↔ 25cm (10in). C. and E. Europe. ❄❄❄. **'Aprilgrün'** has olive-green leaves and purple-tinted flowers. **'Bronzeglanz'** has bronze-tinted leaves.
F. eskia, syn. *F. scoparia*. Compact, rhizomatous, mound- or cushion-forming, evergreen, perennial grass with stiff, narrowly linear, inrolled, rich green leaves, to 20cm (8in) long. In early and midsummer, bears open, pendent, ovoid panicles, to 10cm (4in) long, with spikelets tinted green, orange, or yellow. ↕ to 15cm (6in), ↔ 25cm (10in). Pyrenees. ❄❄❄
F. glacialis (Ice fescue). Densely tufted, hummock-forming, evergreen, perennial grass with erect, narrowly linear, inrolled, grey- to blue-green leaves, to 12cm (5in) long. In mid- and late summer, bears dense, narrow, ovoid, branched panicles, to 2.5cm (1in) long, with spikelets of 3–5 violet flowers. ↕↔ to 10cm (4in). France, Spain, Pyrenees, Alps. ❄❄❄

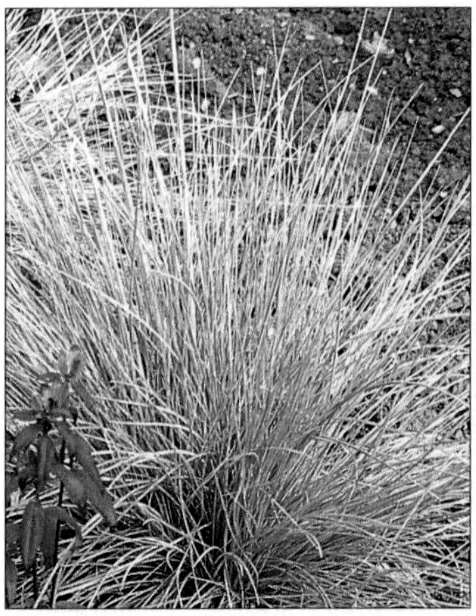

Festuca glauca 'Blaufuchs'

F. glauca (Blue fescue, Grey fescue). Densely tufted, evergreen, perennial grass with erect or arching, narrowly linear, inrolled, 9-ribbed, smooth, blue-green leaves, 7–20cm (3–8in) long. In early and midsummer, bears dense, obovate, shortly branched panicles, to 10cm (4in) long, with spikelets of 4–7 violet-flushed, blue-green flowers. ↕ to 30cm (12in), ↔ 25cm (10in). N. and S. temperate regions. ❄❄❄. **'Blaufuchs'** ■♀ syn. 'Blue Fox', has bright blue leaves. **'Harz'** has purple-tipped, blue-green or dark olive-green leaves. **'Seeigel'**, syn. 'Sea Urchin', has lax, hair-fine, spiky, blue-green leaves in a tight bun, to 15cm (6in) across.
F. scoparia see *F. eskia*.
F. valesiaca. Variable, densely tufted, evergreen, sometimes semi-evergreen, perennial grass with narrowly linear, hair-like, flattened, bluish green leaves, 25cm (10in) or more long. In mid- and late summer, bears dense, oblong or ovate-oblong panicles, 5–10cm (2–4in) long, with spikelets of 3–8 white-frosted, pale green flowers, or purple, violet-tinted flowers. ↕ 50cm (20in), ↔ 45cm (18in). C. Europe. ❄❄❄. **'Silbersee'**, syn. 'Silver Sea', is much more compact, with pale silvery blue leaves; ↕ to 20cm (8in) ↔ 15cm (6in).

▷ **Fetter bush** see *Leucothoe racemosa*
▷ **Feverfew** see *Tanacetum parthenium*

FICUS

Fig

MORACEAE

Genus of about 800 species of mainly evergreen trees, shrubs, and woody climbers, usually found in moist forests in tropical and subtropical regions worldwide. Some behave as stranglers, outgrowing the host tree and eventually killing it, often becoming massive, free-standing trees themselves. They are grown for their foliage, or for their edible fruits (rarely borne on container-grown plants). The alternate leaves are simple, or shallowly to deeply lobed. Minute, petalless flowers are contained in a hollowed-out, inflated stem tip (receptacle) borne in the leaf axils, which enlarges to form the fig fruit, borne sporadically throughout the year. In frost-prone climates, grow in a warm or temperate greenhouse or as houseplants. In warmer areas, use as specimen or shade trees; train climbers against a wall or tree. The foliage may cause mild stomach upset if ingested; the sap may irritate skin or aggravate allergies. The foliage of *F. carica* can cause photodermatitis; its sap may irritate the eyes.

• **HARDINESS** Fully hardy to frost tender.
• **CULTIVATION** Under glass, grow in loam-based potting compost (JI No.3), with added fine bark chippings, in full or filtered light. During growth, water moderately and apply a high-nitrogen fertilizer every 4 weeks. Keep moist in winter. Outdoors, grow in humus-rich, leafy, moist but well-drained soil in full sun or partial shade, with shelter from cold, drying winds. Support figs that have long, lax stems. Mulch annually. Pruning group 1 for shrubs and trees; group 11 for climbers, in late winter.
• **PROPAGATION** Sow seed at 15–21°C (59–70°F) in spring. Root semi-ripe cuttings or leaf-bud cuttings with bottom heat in spring or summer. Air layer *F. elastica* in spring or late summer.
• **PESTS AND DISEASES** Red spider mites, thrips, mealybugs, and scale insects may be troublesome under glass.

F. benghalensis Ϙ (Banyan, Indian fig). Evergreen tree with spreading, often horizontal branches supported by prop roots. Bears elliptic to broadly ovate, leathery, deep green leaves, 13–25cm (5–10in) long, flushed bronze when young and with a distinct pattern of pale veins when mature. Spherical red figs, to 2cm (¾in) across, are borne in pairs. ↕ 20–30m (70–100ft), ↔ to 200m (700ft). S. Asia. ❀ (min. 15°C/59°F)
F. benjamina ♀Ϙ (Weeping fig). Evergreen tree or large shrub, sometimes a strangler, with slender, arching to pendent stems and ovate-elliptic, thinly leathery, glossy leaves, dark green above, lighter beneath, 5–13cm (2–5in) long, each tapering to a slender, twisted point. Spherical to oblong figs, 1cm (½in) long, produced in pairs, mature from green through pink or orange-red to black. ↕ to 30m (100ft) or more, ↔ to 15m (50ft) or more. S. and S.E. Asia, N. Australia, S.W. Pacific. ❀ (min. 15°C/59°F). **'Variegata'** ■ has white-splashed leaves.
F. carica Ϙ (Common fig). Deciduous tree or large shrub with a spreading head and rounded, 3- or 5-lobed leaves, 10–24cm (4–10in) long, heart-shaped at the bases. Pear-shaped receptacles develop into single fruit, to 10cm (4in) long, green when young, maturing to dark green, purple, or dark brown. ↕ 3m (10ft), ↔ 4m (12ft). W. Asia, E. Mediterranean. ❄❄❄
F. deltoidea ■♀Ϙ (Mistletoe fig). Evergreen shrub or small tree, usually bushy, sometimes epiphytic in the wild, with broadly spoon-shaped to obovate,

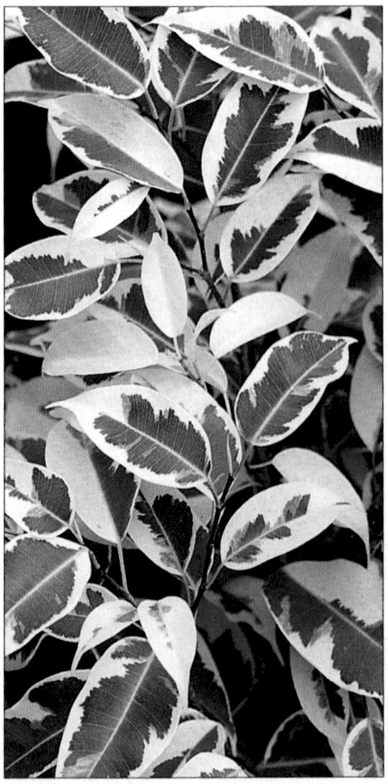

Ficus benjamina 'Variegata'

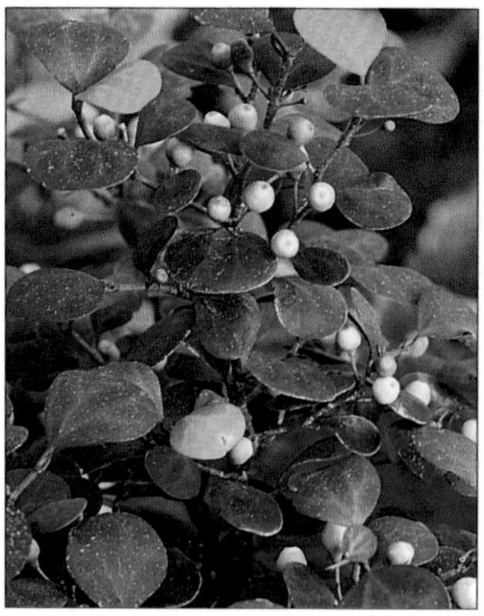

Ficus deltoidea

leathery leaves, 4–8cm (1½–3in) long, bright green above and rust-red to olive-brown beneath. Spherical to ellipsoid figs, to 1cm (½in) across, ripening from dull yellow to orange and red, are freely produced in pairs. ↕ 5–7m (15–22ft), ↔ 1–3m (3–10ft). S.E. Asia to Borneo, Philippines (Palawan). ❀ (min. 15°C/59°F). **var. *diversifolia***, syn. *F. diversifolia*, has rounded or shallowly notched leaves; ↕ to 2m (6ft).

F. diversifolia see *F. deltoidea* var. *diversifolia*.

F. elastica ♀ (India rubber fig, India rubber tree, Rubber plant). Evergreen, many-branched tree with oblong to elliptic, leathery, glossy, dark green, often red-flushed leaves, 30–45cm (12–18in) long. Oblong yellow figs, to 1cm (½in) long, are produced in pairs or clusters on mature trees in the open. ↕ 30–60m (100–200ft), ↔ 20–60m (70–200ft). E. Himalayas, India (Assam), Burma, Malaya, Java. ❀ (min. 15°C/59°F). **'Decora'** 🏆 has broadly elliptic leaves, red flushed beneath, with creamy white midribs when mature. **'Doescheri'** ▣ 🏆 has leaves mottled grey-green, creamy yellow, and white, with pink stalks and midribs.

F. lyrata ▣ 🏆 ♀ (Banjo fig, Fiddle-leaf fig). Open, evergreen tree with leathery, glossy, fiddle-shaped, dark green leaves, 25–45cm (10–18in) long, irregularly corrugated above. Almost spherical figs, to 3cm (1¼in) or more across, ripening green with white dots, are produced singly or in pairs only on mature trees in the open. ↕ 20–30m (70–100ft) or more, ↔ 10–20m (30–70ft). Tropical W. and C. Africa. ❀ (min. 15°C/59°F)

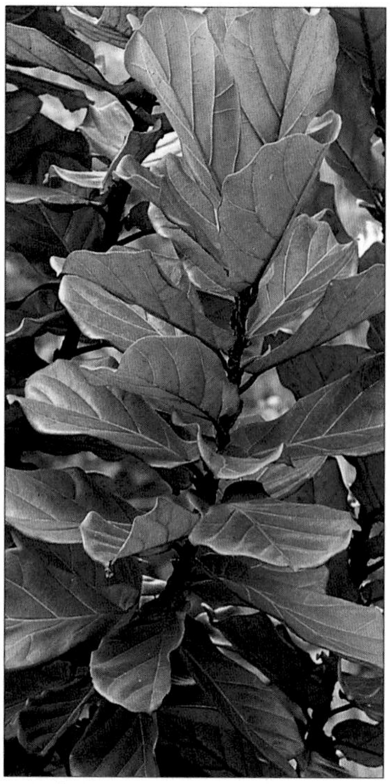

Ficus lyrata

F. macrophylla ▣ ♀ (Australian banyan, Moreton Bay fig). Wide-spreading, evergreen tree with aerial roots (some becoming props). Oblong to elliptic or ovate, leathery leaves, mid-green and hairless above, to 25cm (10in) long, are paler beneath, often with rust-red scales. Ovoid figs, to 2cm (¾in) long, ripening from green to purple with yellow-green flecks, are produced only on mature trees in the open, usually in pairs. ↕ 30–55m (100–180ft), ↔ 20–40m (70–130ft). Australia (Queensland, New South Wales). ❀ (min. 7–10°C/45–50°F)

F. microcarpa ♀ syn. *F. retusa* of gardens (Curtain fig, Indian laurel, Malay banyan). Wide-spreading, evergreen tree with curtains of aerial roots (some root on touching the soil). Bears narrowly to broadly elliptic to obovate, leathery, dark green leaves, 6–12cm (2½–5in) long. Spherical purple figs, 1cm (½in) long, are produced in pairs on mature trees, ripening black. ↕ to 25m (80ft), ↔ to 30m (100ft). Japan (Ryukyu Islands), S. China, S. Malaysia, Australia (Queensland), New Caledonia. ❀ (min. 13°C/55°F). **'Hawaii'** has shiny grey-green and white-splashed leaves.

F. pumila, syn. *F. repens* (Climbing fig, Creeping fig). Root-clinging, evergreen, perennial climber. The leaves of the climbing shoots are asymmetrically ovate, thinly leathery, dark green, to 5cm (2in) long. At the end of its support, leaves on non-climbing stems are oblong to elliptic or ovate, leathery, dark green and very glossy, to 10cm (4in) long. Pear-shaped, mostly solitary, oblong to cylindrical, densely hairy figs, to 6cm (2½in) long, are green with white dots, ripening purple. ↕ 3–5m (10–15ft) or more. China, Vietnam, Japan. ❀ (min. 5–7°C/41–45°F). **'Minima'** has slender stems and juvenile leaves, 1cm (½in) long; ↕ 1–2m (3–6ft).

F. religiosa ♀ (Bo tree, Peepul, Sacred fig). Small tree, or taller strangling climber, with wide-spreading branches, semi- or fully deciduous in monsoon climates, and broadly ovate, glossy, leathery, dark green leaves, 12–18cm (5–7in) long, with unusual tail-like tips. Bears pairs of rounded, flat-topped green figs, to 1.5cm (½in) across, ripening to purple with red dots. ↕↔ 8m (25ft). Himalayas, S.W. China, N. Thailand, Vietnam. ❀ (min. 15°C/59°F)

F. repens see *F. pumila*.

***F. retusa* of gardens** see *F. microcarpa*.

F. rubiginosa 🏆 ♀ (Port Jackson fig). Wide-spreading, evergreen tree, sometimes with aerial roots, a few of which become props. Leaves are oblong to elliptic or ovate, 8–17cm (3–7in) long, rusty-hairy when young, then smooth, leathery, dark green above, paler beneath. Bears pairs of spherical figs, to 1.5cm (½in) across, ripening to greenish brown with soft, rusty brown hairs. ↕↔ 15m (50ft). Australia (New South Wales). ❀ (min. 10–13°C/50–55°F)

▷**Fiddleleaf** see *Philodendron bipennifolium*
▷**Fiery costus** see *Costus igneus*
▷**Fig** see *Ficus*
  Banjo see *Ficus lyrata*
  Climbing see *Ficus pumila*
  Common see *Ficus carica*
  Creeping see *Ficus pumila*
  Curtain see *Ficus microcarpa*
  Devil's see *Argemone mexicana*
  Fiddle-leaf see *Ficus lyrata*
  Hottentot see *Carpobrotus edulis*
  Indian see *Ficus benghalensis*, *Opuntia ficus-indica*
  India rubber see *Ficus elastica*
  Kaffir see *Carpobrotus edulis*
  Mistletoe see *Ficus deltoidea*
  Moreton Bay see *Ficus macrophylla*
▷**Fig cont.**
  Port Jackson see *Ficus rubiginosa*
  Sacred see *Ficus religiosa*
  Weeping see *Ficus benjamina*
▷**Figwort** see *Scrophularia*
  Cape see *Phygelius capensis*
  Water see *Scrophularia auriculata*
▷**Filbert** see *Corylus maxima*

FILIPENDULA

ROSACEAE

Genus of 10 or more species of rhizomatous perennials from damp habitats, such as streamsides and wet ditches, in N. temperate regions, except *F. vulgaris*, which thrives on dry, chalky grassland. The pinnate, alternate leaves have shallowly or palmately lobed terminal leaflets and smaller lateral leaflets, hairless or softly hairy beneath. Plumes of tiny, fluffy, red, pink, or white flowers are borne from late spring to late summer, mainly in dense, cyme-like corymbs, on single or branched stems well above the foliage. Most are suitable for naturalizing in a woodland garden, or for moist sites. Grow *F. vulgaris* in a sunny site in a border.

• **HARDINESS** Fully hardy.

• **CULTIVATION** Grow all but *F. vulgaris* in moderately fertile, leafy, moist but well-drained soil in full sun or partial shade. *F. rubra* and *F. ulmaria* will also thrive in boggy conditions. Gold-leaved forms colour best in shade. Grow *F. vulgaris* in drier, alkaline soil in full sun. Mulch in spring.

• **PROPAGATION** Sow seed in autumn in containers in a cold frame, or in spring at 10–13°C (50–55°C). Divide in autumn or spring. Take root cuttings and place horizontally in seed trays, from late winter to early spring.

• **PESTS AND DISEASES** Prone to fungal leaf spot. May be affected by mildew if malnourished or dry, particularly *F. ulmaria* 'Flore Pleno'.

F. hexapetala see *F. vulgaris*.

F. kamtschatica. Clump-forming perennial with pinnate, toothed leaves, 15–45cm (6–18in) long, softly hairy beneath. The 3- to 5-lobed terminal leaflets, 15–25cm (6–10in) across, are rounded to obovate, the lateral ones smaller or absent. From midsummer to early autumn, bears corymbs, to 25cm (10in) across, of fragrant, white or pale pink flowers, 6–8mm (¼–⅜in) across, on branched stems. ↕ 2–3m (6–10ft), ↔ 1.2m (4ft). Russia (Kamchatka), China (Manchuria), Japan. ❄❄❄

F. palmata, syn. *Spiraea palmata*. Clump-forming perennial with pinnate, sometimes palmate leaves, to 30cm (12in) long, densely white-woolly beneath. The small, toothed lateral leaflets are 2- to 5-lobed, the terminal ones rounded to obovate, 7- to 9-lobed, and 5–10cm (2–4in) across. In midsummer, produces pale to deep pink flowers in feathery corymbs, to 20cm (8in) across, on simple or branching stems. ↕ 1.2m (4ft), ↔ 60cm (24in). Russia (Kamchatka, Siberia), Mongolia, China, Japan. ❄❄❄. **f. *alba*** has white flowers. **'Digitata Nana'**, see 'Nana'. **'Elegantissima'**, syn. 'Elegans', has deep rose-pink flowers and very small, erect, lance-shaped, bronze-red seed heads; ↕ 1m (3ft). **'Nana'**, syn. 'Digitata Nana', has fern-like leaves; deep rose-pink

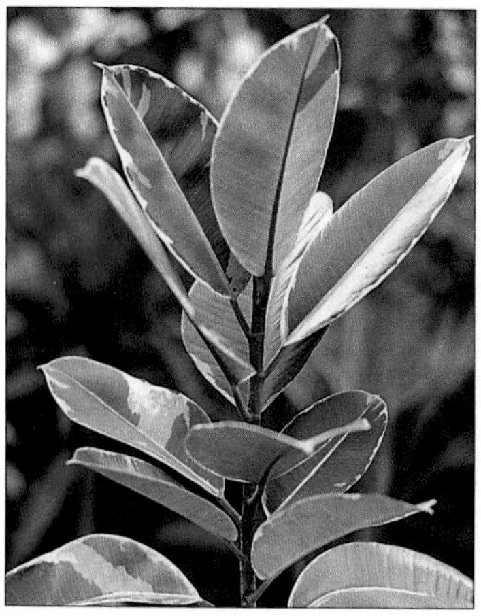

Ficus elastica 'Doescheri'

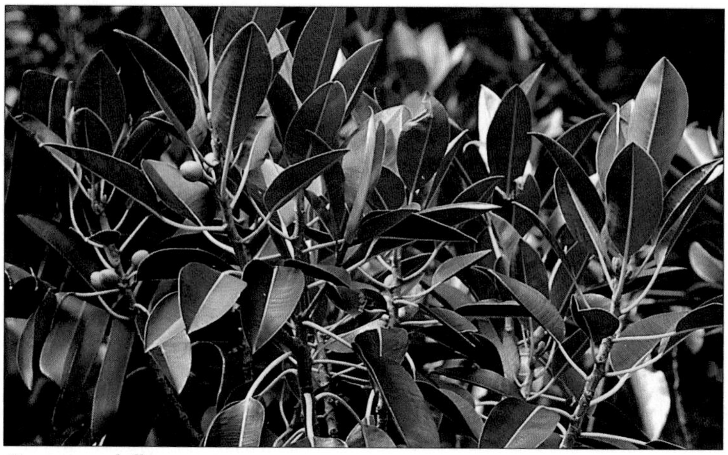

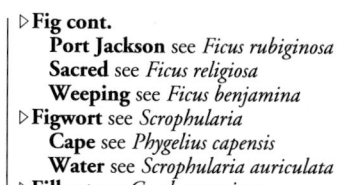

Ficus macrophylla

F

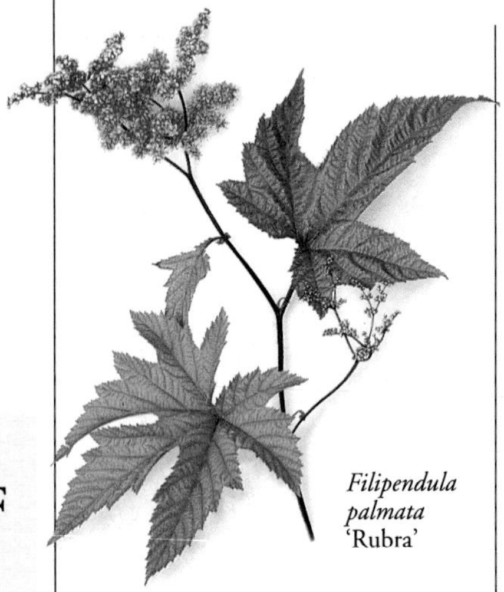

Filipendula palmata 'Rubra'

flowers become paler as they age; ↕ 60cm (24in). **'Rubra'** ▣ has red-pink flowers.
F. purpurea ▣ ♕ Clump-forming perennial bearing pinnate, toothed leaves, with irregularly 5- to 7-lobed, rounded to obovate terminal leaflets, to 25cm (10in) across, and few, if any, small lateral leaflets. In mid- and late summer, branching, crimson-purple stems bear dense corymbs, 5cm (2in) across, of carmine-red flowers, becoming paler as they age. ↕ 1.2m (4ft), ↔ 60cm (24in). Japan. ❄❄❄. **f. *albiflora*** ▣ syn. f. *alba*, has white flowers. **'Purpurascens'** has purple-tinted leaves.
F. rubra (Queen of the prairies). Spreading perennial forming large clumps in moist soil. Produces pinnate, vine-like, irregularly cut leaves, with toothed, 3-lobed, terminal leaflets, to 20cm (8in) across. In early and midsummer, branching red stems bear crowded corymbs, to 15cm (6in) across, of fragrant, deep peach-pink flowers. ↕ 1.8–2.5m (6–8ft), ↔ 1.2m (4ft). E. USA. ❄❄❄. **'Magnifica'** see 'Venusta'. **'Venusta'** ▣ ♕ syn. 'Magnifica', 'Venusta Magnifica', has deep rose-pink flowers, becoming paler pink as they age.

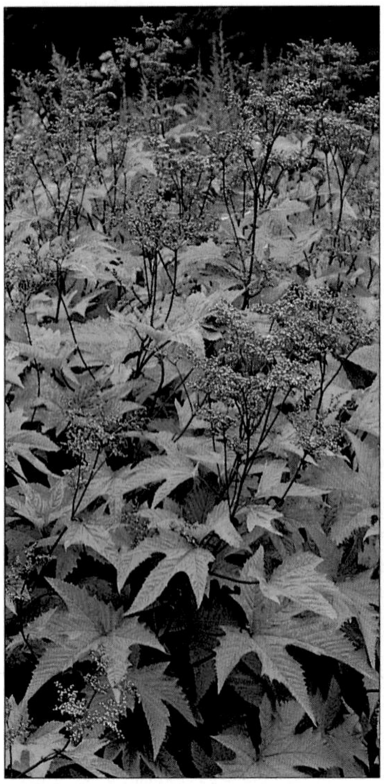

Filipendula purpurea

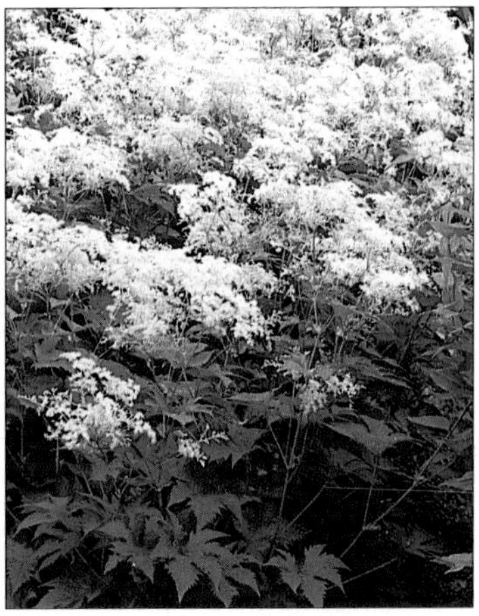

Filipendula purpurea f. *albiflora*

F. ulmaria, syn. *Spiraea ulmaria* (Meadowsweet, Queen of the meadows). Clump-forming perennial with leafy stems bearing irregularly pinnate, strongly veined, inversely lance-shaped leaves, white-downy beneath. The terminal leaflets are 5–10cm (2–4in) across. In summer, branching stems bear dense corymbs, to 25cm (10in) across, of creamy white flowers. ↕ 60–90cm (24–36in), ↔ 60cm (24in). Europe, W. Asia. ❄❄❄. **'Aurea'** has warm yellow, then creamy yellow leaves in spring, later becoming pale green. **'Flore Pleno'** has double flowers. **'Variegata'** has leaves striped and marked yellow.
F. vulgaris, syn. *F. hexapetala* (Dropwort). Rosette-forming perennial producing swollen rhizomes and pinnate, fern-like, finely divided, toothed, hairless, dark green leaves, each leaflet 2cm (¾in) long. In early and midsummer, slender, branching stems bear loose corymbs, to 15cm (6in) across, of white, often red-tinged flowers. ↕ 60cm (24in), ↔ 45cm (18in). Europe, N. and C. Asia. ❄❄❄. **'Flore Pleno'** see 'Multiplex'. **'Multiplex'**, syn. 'Flore Pleno', 'Plena', has bronze buds and double, sometimes pendent, creamy white flowers. **'Plena'** see 'Multiplex'. **'Rosea'** has pink flowers.

▷ **Fingernail plant** see *Neoregelia spectabilis*
▷ **Fir,**
Balsam see *Abies balsamea*
Beautiful see *Abies amabilis*
Blue Douglas see *Pseudotsuga menziesii* var. *glauca*

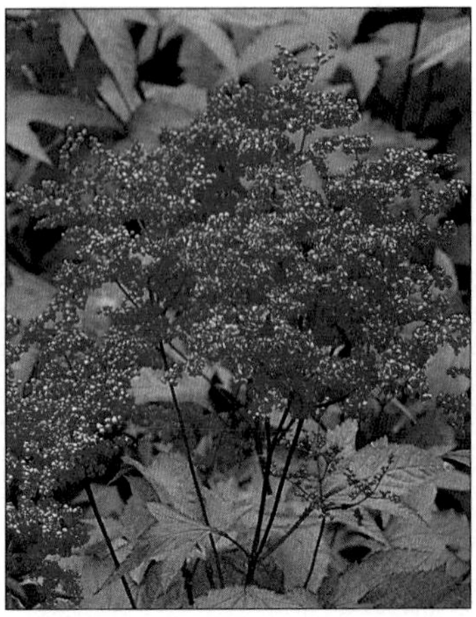

Filipendula rubra 'Venusta'

▷ **Fir cont.**
Bristlecone see *Abies bracteata*
California red see *Abies magnifica*
Caucasian see *Abies nordmanniana*
China see *Cunninghamia, C. lanceolata*
Cilician see *Abies cilicica*
Corkbark see *Abies lasiocarpa* var. *arizonica*
Douglas see *Pseudotsuga menziesii*
European silver see *Abies alba*
Farges see *Abies fargesii*
Forrest see *Abies forrestii*
Giant see *Abies grandis*
Grand see *Abies grandis*
Greek see *Abies cephalonica*
Hedgehog see *Abies pinsapo*
Korean see *Abies koreana*
Nikko see *Abies homolepis*
Noble see *Abies procera*
Nordmann see *Abies nordmanniana*
Pacific see *Abies amabilis*
Santa Lucia see *Abies bracteata*
Silver see *Abies, A. alba*
Spanish see *Abies pinsapo*
Veitch see *Abies veitchii*
Vejar see *Abies vejarii*
White see *Abies concolor*
▷ **Fire bush, Chilean** see *Embothrium, E. coccineum*
▷ **Firecracker,**
Brazilian see *Manettia luteorubra*
Californian see *Dichelostemma ida-maia*
Eaton's see *Penstemon eatonii*
Mexican see *Echeveria setosa*
▷ **Firecracker flower** see *Crossandra infundibuliformis*
▷ **Firecracker plant** see *Russelia equisetiformis*
▷ **Fire-on-the-mountain** see *Euphorbia cyathophora*
▷ **Fire plant, Norse** see *Columnea* 'Stavanger'
▷ **Firethorn** see *Pyracantha*
▷ **Firewheel tree** see *Stenocarpus sinuatus*

FIRMIANA

STERCULIACEAE

Genus of 9 species of deciduous trees and shrubs found in woodland in E. Africa, and E. and S.E. Asia, grown for their handsome foliage. The leaves are alternate, entire, or palmately lobed, and the petalless flowers are unisexual, with bell-shaped, yellow or yellow-green calyces, borne in terminal panicles or racemes. Grow in a woodland garden. In frost-prone areas, grow in containers and overwinter in a cool greenhouse.
• **HARDINESS** Half hardy; may be hardier with prolonged exposure to temperatures over 24°C (75°F).
• **CULTIVATION** Under glass, grow in loam-based potting compost (JI No.3) in full light with shade from the hottest sun, or in bright filtered light. During growth, water freely and apply a balanced liquid fertilizer monthly. Keep just moist in winter. Outdoors, grow in moist but well-drained, moderately fertile soil in full sun or partial shade, sheltered from cold, drying winds. Pruning group 1; may need restrictive pruning under glass.
• **PROPAGATION** Sow seed at 10–13°C (50–55°F) as soon as ripe.
• **PESTS AND DISEASES** Trouble free.

F. platanifolia see *F. simplex*.
F. simplex ▣ ♀ syn. *F. platanifolia, Sterculia platanifolia* (Chinese parasol

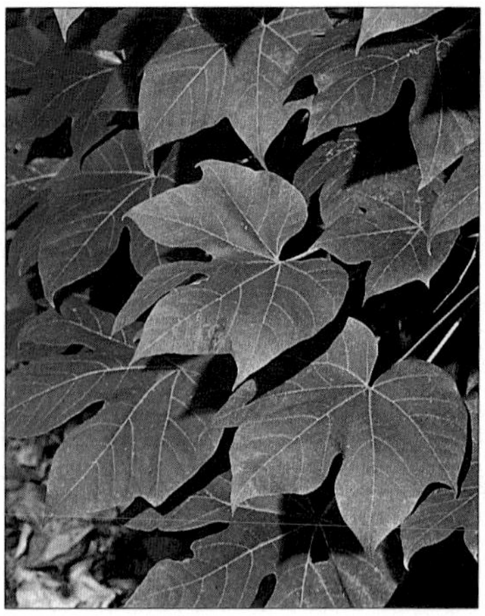

Firmiana simplex

tree). Rounded tree with smooth green bark and alternate, deeply 3- to 7-lobed, dark green leaves, 25–45cm (10–18in) long, turning yellow in autumn. Bears terminal panicles, 20–30cm (8–12in) long, of small, yellow-green flowers, in summer. In autumn, bears unusual papery fruit, which split open when ripe revealing the seeds. ↕ 15m (50ft), ↔ 10m (30ft). Vietnam to Japan (Ryukyu Islands). ❄

▷ **Fish-tail palm** see *Caryota*
Burmese see *Caryota mitis*
Clustered see *Caryota mitis*
Miniature see *Chamaedorea metallica*

FITTONIA

Nerve plant, Painted net leaf

ACANTHACEAE

Genus of 2 species of evergreen perennials, with freely rooting, mat-forming stems, from tropical rainforest in South America, mainly Peru. The leaves are opposite, with short stems and colourful veins. Thin spikes of insignificant white to reddish white flowers are borne rarely and irregularly. Where temperatures drop below 15°C (59°F), grow in a terrarium or hanging basket indoors or in a warm greenhouse. In tropical or subtropical areas, grow as ground cover in semi-shaded sites.
• **HARDINESS** Frost tender.
• **CULTIVATION** Under glass, grow in loamless potting compost in shallow containers, in indirect light with high humidity. Water moderately, keeping the compost just moist; if kept too wet,

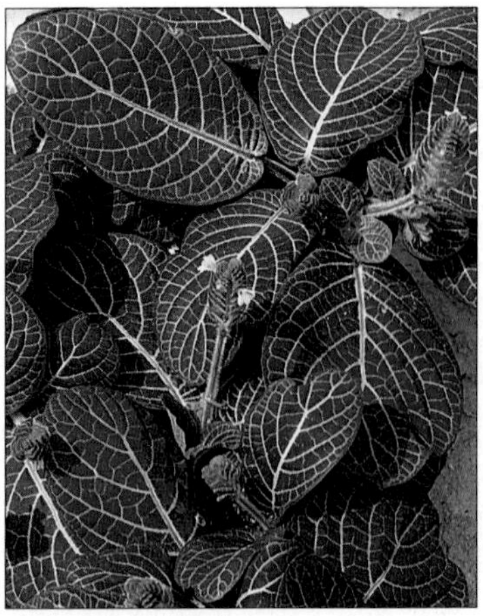

Fittonia verschaffeltii

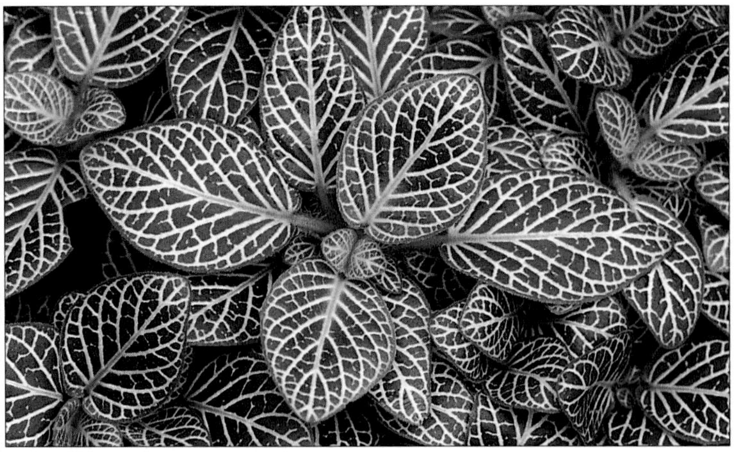

Fittonia verschaffeltii var. *argyroneura*

stem rotting occurs. During growth, apply a balanced liquid fertilizer every 3–4 weeks. Outdoors, grow in humus-rich to leafy, moist but well-drained soil in partial shade.
• **PROPAGATION** Take tip cuttings with 3 or 4 pairs of leaves in spring, or layer stems in spring or summer.
• **PESTS AND DISEASES** Trouble free.

F. argyroneura see *F. verschaffeltii* var. *argyroneura*.
F. verschaffeltii ▣ ♀ Creeping perennial bearing oval to elliptic, olive-green leaves, 6–10cm (2–4in) long, with slightly sunken, carmine-red veins. ↕15cm (6in), ↔ indefinite. Peru. ❀ (min. 15°C/59°F, best at a constant temperature of about 18°C/64°F). **var. *argyroneura*** ▣ ♀ syn. *F. argyroneura* (Silver net leaf) has paler leaves with narrower, silvery white veins. **'Nana'** is compact, with leaves 2–3.5cm (¾–1½in) long; ↕ to 10cm (4in).

FITZROYA

CUPRESSACEAE

Genus of one species of evergreen, monoecious or dioecious, coniferous tree or shrub found only in limited areas of forest in Chile and Argentina, where it is now rare because of overfelling and habitat loss. Although similar to junipers in general appearance, and in having whorls of 3 short, blunt leaves, the cones of *F. cupressoides* differ in having 3 whorls on each of 3 scales, and the seeds are winged. Grow as a specimen tree or shrub in open woodland.
• **HARDINESS** Fully hardy.
• **CULTIVATION** Grow in moderately fertile, moist but well-drained soil in full sun, with shelter from cold, dry winds.
• **PROPAGATION** Sow seed *in situ*, or in containers in a cold frame, in spring. Root semi-ripe cuttings in late summer or autumn, under mist or with gentle bottom heat.
• **PESTS AND DISEASES** Trouble free.

F. cupressoides ▣ ◊ syn. *F. patagonica*. Coniferous, conical tree or spreading shrub with red-brown bark that peels in strips, and oblong, dark green leaves, to 5mm (¼in) long. Produces cylindrical male cones and solitary, spherical, terminal, pale brown female cones, 1cm (½in) across, which ripen in autumn. ↕ to 15m (50ft), ↔ to 6m (20ft). Chile, S. Argentina. ✱✱✱
F. patagonica see *F. cupressoides*.

▷**Fivecorner, Pink** see *Styphelia triflora*
▷**Five finger** see *Pseudopanax arboreus*
▷**Five fingers** see *Syngonium auritum*
▷**Five-spot** see *Nemophila maculata*
▷**Flag,**
Blue see *Iris versicolor*
Soft see *Typha angustifolia*
Southern blue see *Iris virginica*
Spanish see *Ipomoea lobata*
Yellow see *Iris pseudacorus*
▷**Flamboyant tree** see *Delonix regia*
Yellow see *Peltophorum pterocarpum*
▷**Flame bush** see *Templetonia retusa*
Mexican see *Calliandra tweedii*
▷**Flame creeper** see *Tropaeolum speciosum*
▷**Flame flower** see *Embothrium coccineum*
▷**Flame leaf, Mexican** see *Euphorbia pulcherrima*
▷**Flame of the forest** see *Butea monosperma*
▷**Flame of the woods** see *Ixora coccinea*
▷**Flame pea,**
Heart-leaved see *Chorizema cordatum*
Holly see *Chorizema ilicifolium*
▷**Flame tree** see *Brachychiton acerifolius, Delonix regia, Peltophorum pterocarpum*

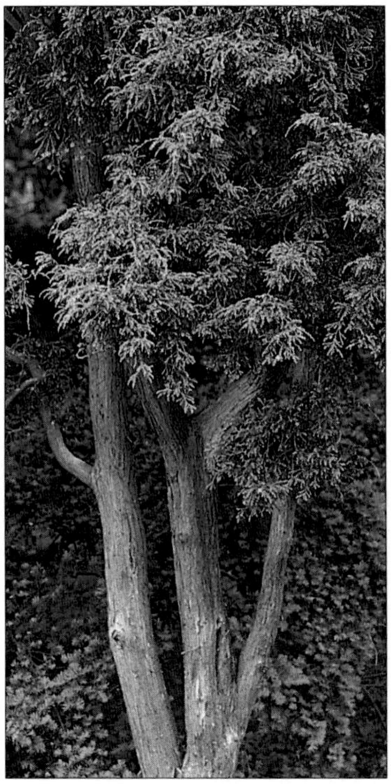

Fitzroya cupressoides

▷**Flamingo flower** see *Anthurium, A. andraeanum*
▷**Flamingo plant** see *Justicia carnea*
▷**Flaming sword** see *Vriesea splendens*
▷**Flannel bush** see *Fremontodendron*
▷**Flax** see *Linum*
Flowering see *Linum grandiflorum*
Golden see *Linum flavum*
Mountain see *Phormium cookianum*
New Zealand see *Phormium tenax*
Perennial see *Linum perenne*
Yellow see *Linum flavum, Reinwardtia indica*
▷**Fleabane** see *Erigeron*
▷**Floating heart** see *Nymphoides*
Yellow see *N. peltata*
▷**Floradora** see *Stephanotis floribunda*
▷**Flora's paintbrush** see *Emilia coccinea*
▷**Floss flower** see *Ageratum*
▷**Floss silk tree** see *Chorisia speciosa*
▷**Flowering currant** see *Ribes, R. sanguineum*
▷**Flower-of-an-hour** see *Hibiscus trionum*
▷**Flower of Jove** see *Lychnis flos-jovis*
▷**Flower of Jupiter** see *Lychnis flos-jovis*
▷**Foam flower** see *Tiarella, T. cordifolia*
Japanese see *Tanakaea*
▷**Foam of May** see *Spiraea* 'Arguta'

FOCKEA

ASCLEPIADACEAE

Genus of about 10 species of dioecious, caudex-forming, mainly deciduous, perennial succulents from open grassland and arid regions of Angola to South Africa (Northern Cape, Eastern Cape, Western Cape), and Zimbabwe. They have thick, fleshy stems, sometimes up to 3m (10ft) thick. The branches are twining or semi-erect, usually with white, milky sap. The leaves are opposite, oblong to oval, sharp-pointed, flat or wavy-edged. In late summer or autumn, starfish-shaped flowers are borne singly, or several in dense clusters, in the leaf axils. Where temperatures drop below 10°C (50°F), grow in a warm greenhouse. In warmer climates, grow in a desert garden or rock garden.
• **HARDINESS** Frost tender.
• **CULTIVATION** Under glass, grow in standard cactus compost in full or bright filtered light with low humidity, in a deep container to accommodate the caudex. When in full leaf, water moderately, allowing soil to dry between waterings, and apply a low-nitrogen liquid fertilizer monthly. Keep dry when dormant. Outdoors, grow in dry, sharply drained, moderately fertile soil, with added leaf mould, in full sun or light dappled shade. See also pp.48–49.
• **PROPAGATION** Sow seed at 19–24°C (66–75°F) as soon as ripe.
• **PESTS AND DISEASES** Vulnerable to greenfly while flowering.

F. capensis see *F. crispa*.
F. crispa, syn. *F. capensis*. Twining or prostrate, deciduous, minutely hairy succulent with a partly subterranean, rough-surfaced, spherical-obovoid caudex bearing many slender branches. Oval, glossy, dark green leaves, 2–3cm (¾–1¼in) long, have wavy margins. Starfish-shaped, greenish grey flowers, 4cm (1½in) across, with small brown marks, are borne in groups of 3–5 in the leaf axils, in autumn. ↕ to 1m (3ft), ↔ to 60cm (24in). South Africa (Western Cape). ❀ (min. 10–12°C/50–54°F)

FOENICULUM

Fennel

APIACEAE/UMBELLIFERAE

Genus of one species of aromatic perennial or biennial, native to rich, well-drained soils in sunny, coastal areas in Europe, especially the Mediterranean. The perennial *F. vulgare* is used to flavour foods; the biennial *F. vulgare* var. *azoricum* is grown for its edible, swollen stem base. Both forms have slender stems and finely cut, aniseed-flavoured leaves. They bear flat umbels of yellow flowers, followed by aromatic seeds. Grow as foliage plants in a herb or wild garden; darker-leaved cultivars provide contrast in a perennial border.
• **HARDINESS** Fully hardy, although young growth may be damaged by frost.
• **CULTIVATION** Grow in fertile, moist but well-drained soil in full sun. Detach flowered stems before they shed seeds.
• **PROPAGATION** In spring, sow seed at 13–18°C (55–64°F), or *in situ*, and thin to space 45–60cm (18–24in) apart.
• **PESTS AND DISEASES** Susceptible to aphids, slugs, and mildew.

F. vulgare. Deep-rooting perennial with airy clumps of triangular, very finely cut, 3- or 4-pinnate, hair-like, aniseed-flavoured, mid-green, sometimes glaucous leaves, to 30cm (12in) long. Slender, smooth, branching stems bear flat, compound umbels, to 10cm (4in) across, of tiny yellow flowers, in mid- and late summer, followed by aromatic seeds. The leaves and seeds are used in cooking and medicinally. ↕1.8m (6ft), ↔ 45cm (18in). S. Europe. ✱✱✱. **var. *azoricum*** (Florence fennel) is biennial, and has swollen, bulb-like stem bases that are eaten as a vegetable. **'Bronze'** see 'Purpureum'. **'Giant Bronze'**, syn. *Ferula* 'Giant Bronze', has copper foliage, becoming dark brownish bronze. **'Purpureum'** ▣ syn. 'Bronze', has bronze-purple foliage when young, becoming glaucous with age.

▷**Footed adder's tongue** see *Scoliopus bigelovii*
▷**Forget-me-not** see *Myosotis*
Alpine see *Eritrichium, Myosotis alpestris*
Chatham Island see *Myosotidium hortensia*
Chinese see *Cynoglossum amabile*
Creeping see *Omphalodes verna*
Water see *Myosotis scorpioides*

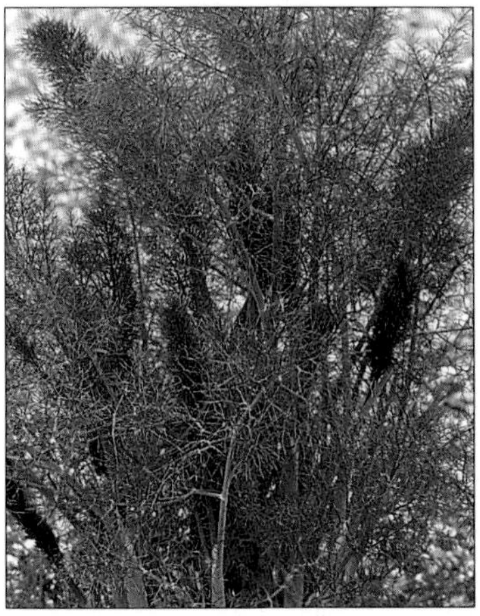

Foeniculum vulgare 'Purpureum'

F

FORSYTHIA

OLEACEAE

Genus of about 7 species of mainly deciduous, sometimes semi-evergreen shrubs found in open woodland in E. Asia, with a single species from S.E. Europe. They bear opposite, simple, toothed or entire, sometimes 3-palmate leaves. The 4-petalled yellow flowers are salverform with narrow tubes, and produce long or short styles on different plants. They are borne before the leaves in early and mid-spring, often profusely. Grow in a shrub border, on a bank, against a wall, or as a specimen plant; they are also useful for hedging.

- **HARDINESS** Fully hardy.
- **CULTIVATION** Grow in moderately fertile, moist but well-drained soil in full sun or light dappled shade. Pruning group 2.
- **PROPAGATION** Root greenwood cuttings in late spring or early summer, or semi-ripe cuttings in late summer.
- **PESTS AND DISEASES** Honey fungus and forsythia gall may be a problem; birds may eat the flower buds.

***F.* 'Beatrix Farrand'.** Vigorous, bushy, deciduous shrub with arching shoots bearing oblong, sharply toothed leaves, to 10cm (4in) long. Usually solitary, deep yellow flowers, to 3cm (1¼in) across, are profusely borne in early and mid-spring. ↕↔ 2m (6ft). ✻✻✻
F. giraldiana ■ Open, deciduous shrub with slender, arching shoots, purple when young, and narrowly ovate leaves, 5–12cm (2–5in) long, grey-green to mid-green above, slightly downy beneath. Produces solitary, pale yellow flowers, 2.5–3cm (1–1¼in) across, in late winter and early spring. ↕↔ 4m (12ft). China (Gansu, Shaanxi, Hubei). ✻✻✻
***F.* 'Golden Nugget'.** Bushy, deciduous shrub with oval to lance-shaped, sharply toothed leaves, to 10cm (4in) long. Bears golden yellow flowers, 2–3.5cm (¾–1½in) across, in early and mid-spring. ↕↔ 1.5m (5ft). ✻✻✻
F. x intermedia (*F. suspensa* x *F. viridissima*). Bushy, deciduous shrub bearing ovate to lance-shaped, simple, occasionally 3-lobed leaves, to 10cm (4in) long, with sharp teeth. Deep, bright yellow flowers, 2.5–3.5cm (1¼–1½in) across, are borne in groups of 2 or 3 in early and mid-spring. ↕↔ 1.5m (5ft). Garden origin. ✻✻✻.

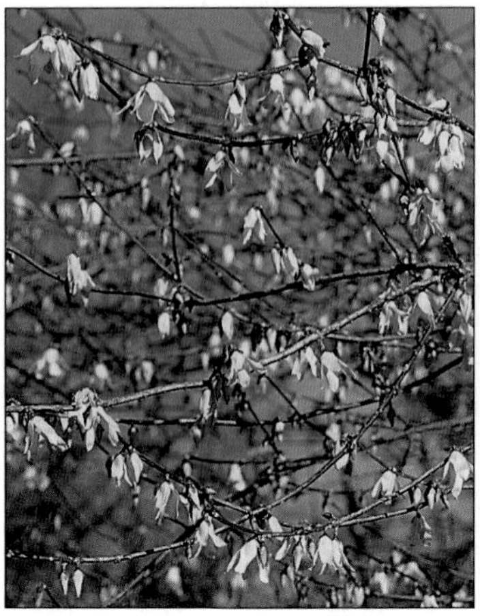
Forsythia giraldiana

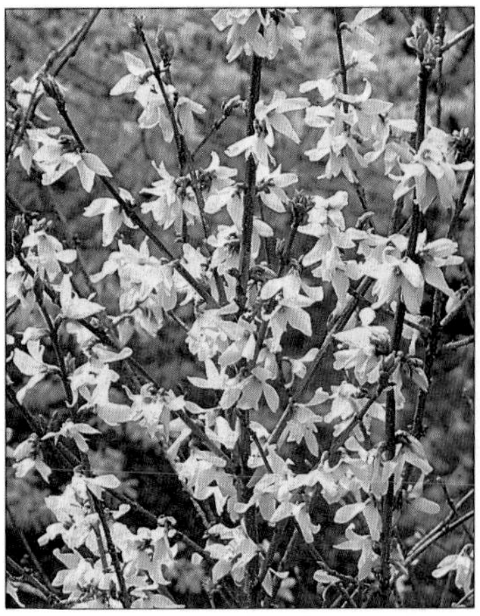
Forsythia x *intermedia* 'Arnold Giant'

'Arnold Giant' ■ has sparsely borne, deep yellow flowers. **'Karl Sax'** is dense, with deep yellow flowers. Some leaves turn red or purple in autumn; ↕↔ 2.5m (8ft). **'Lynwood'** ■♀ has rich yellow flowers; ↕↔ 3m (10ft). **'Spectabilis'** is vigorous, and bears deep yellow flowers, 2–3cm (¾–1¼in) across; ↕ 3m (10ft). ↕ 2m (6ft).
***F.* 'Northern Gold'** ■ Upright, deciduous shrub bearing grey-yellow branches and oval, dark green leaves, 4.5–5cm (1¾–2in) across. Golden yellow flowers, to 3.5cm (1½in) across, are borne at the tips of the branches in spring. ↕ 2–2.5m (6–8ft), ↔ 1.5–2.2m (5–7ft). ✻✻✻
F. ovata (Korean forsythia). Bushy, compact, deciduous shrub with broadly ovate, toothed, dark green leaves, to 9cm (3½in) long. Bears bright yellow flowers, 2cm (¾in) across, singly in the leaf axils, in early spring. ↕ 1.5m (5ft) ↔ 3m (10ft). Korea. ✻✻✻. **'Tetragold'** bears flowers 2–3cm (¾–1¼in) across, in early spring.
***F.* 'Spring Glory'.** Upright shrub with ovate to lance-shaped leaves, to 12cm (5in) long, and pale yellow flowers, 3cm (1¼in) across; ↕ 2m (6ft). ✻✻✻

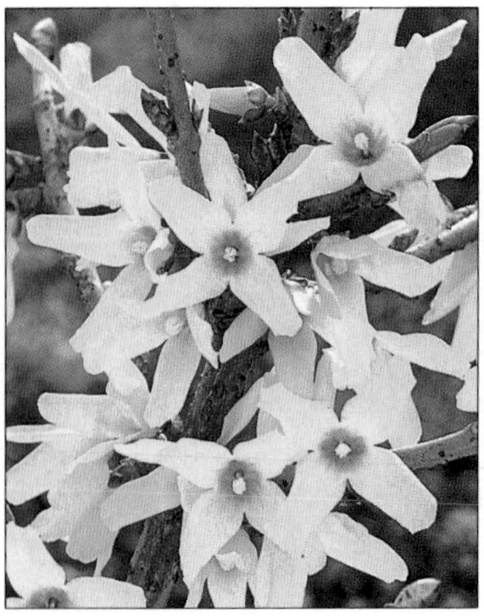
Forsythia 'Northern Gold'

F. suspensa ■♀ (Golden bell). Upright or arching, deciduous shrub with ovate, sometimes 3-palmate, mid- to dark green leaves, to 10cm (4in) long. In early and mid-spring, bears clusters of up to 6 yellow flowers, 2–3cm (1–1¼in) across, in the leaf axils. ↕↔ 3m (10ft). China. ✻✻✻. **f. *atrocaulis*** has purple young shoots and leaves, and pale lemon-yellow flowers, 3.5cm (1½in) across. **'Nymans'** has bronze-purple young shoots and soft yellow flowers. **var. *sieboldii*** has slender, pendent shoots and nodding flowers.
***F.* 'Vermont Sun'.** Upright, deciduous shrub with oval, deep green leaves, 8–12cm (3–5in) long. Deep yellow flowers, to 3.5cm (1½in) across, are produced in early spring. Extremely hardy; useful in areas with prolonged periods of below -32°C (-26°F). ↕ 2.5m (8ft), ↔ 2m (6ft). ✻✻✻
F. viridissima. Erect, deciduous or semi-evergreen shrub with upright shoots, which remain green in the second year, and lance-shaped leaves, to 15cm (6in) long. Bright yellow flowers, 3cm (1¼in) across, are produced singly, or occasionally in pairs or threes, in early and mid-spring. ↕ 2m (6ft), ↔ 1.5m (5ft). China. ✻✻✻. **'Bronxensis'** is spreading, with leaves to 4.5cm (1¾in) long, and primrose-yellow flowers, 2.5cm (1in) across; ↕ 30cm (12in), ↔ 90cm (36in).

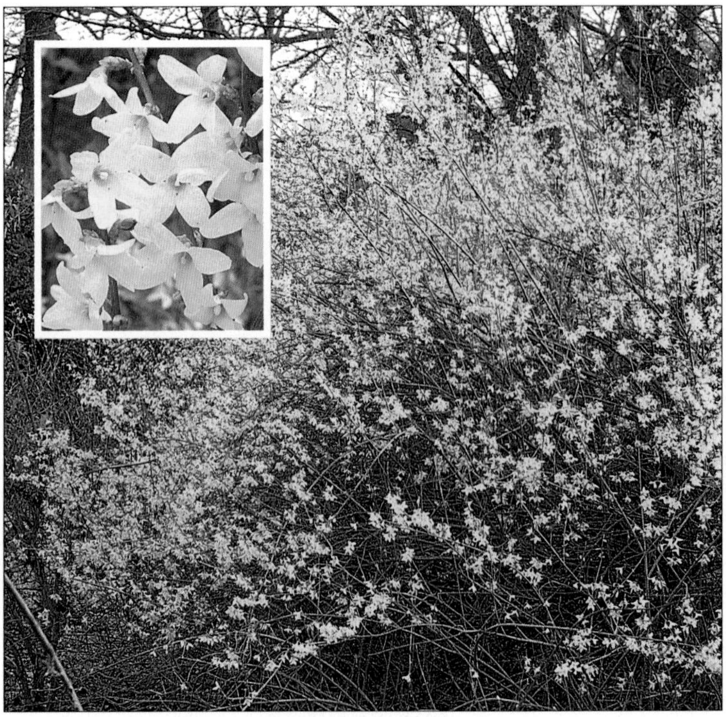
Forsythia x *intermedia* 'Lynwood' (inset: flower detail)

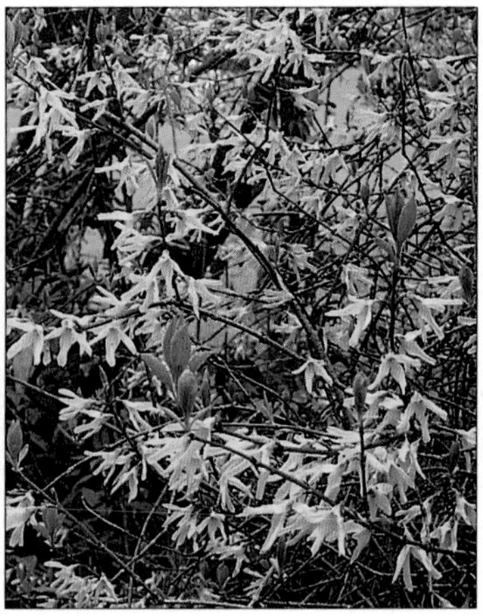
Forsythia suspensa

▷ **Forsythia,**
Korean see *Forsythia ovata*
White see *Abeliophyllum*

FORTUNELLA

Kumquat

RUTACEAE

Genus of about 5 species of sometimes spiny, evergreen shrubs and small trees found in moist woodland from S. China to Malaysia. The simple, leathery, glandular leaves are alternate. Waxy, fragrant, 5-petalled white flowers are borne singly or in few-flowered, axillary clusters, followed by edible, ovoid to spherical, orange-yellow fruits, which resemble miniature oranges. In frost-prone areas, grow in a conservatory, or cool or temperate greenhouse. In warmer regions, use in a mixed or shrub border or courtyard, at the base of a sunny wall, or as a specimen plant.

- **HARDINESS** Frost tender.
- **CULTIVATION** Under glass, grow in loam-based potting compost (JI No.3) in full light. During growth, water freely and apply a balanced liquid fertilizer monthly. Water sparingly in winter. Top-dress or pot on in spring. Outdoors, grow in moderately fertile, moist but well-drained soil in full sun. Pruning group 1; may need restrictive pruning under glass.
- **PROPAGATION** Sow seed at 15–24°C (59–75°F) in spring. Root semi-ripe cuttings in summer with bottom heat.
- **PESTS AND DISEASES** Red spider mites, whiteflies, and scale insects may be troublesome under glass.

F. japonica ○ (Round kumquat). Large shrub or small tree, usually many-branched, with spines in the leaf axils. Bears lance-shaped, glossy, mid- to light green leaves, to 10cm (4in) long, with distinctive vein patterns. Axillary clusters of fragrant flowers, each 1cm (½in) across, are borne from spring to summer, followed by spherical to ovoid, edible, golden yellow fruit, 3–4cm (1¼–1½in) long. ↕ 3–4m (10–12ft), ↔ 1.5–2.5m (5–8ft). S. China, Hong Kong. ❀ (min. 7°C/45°F). **'Sun Stripe'** has variegated, creamy yellow leaves and green-striped yellow fruit.

FOTHERGILLA

HAMAMELIDACEAE

Genus of 2 species of deciduous, low-growing shrubs found in woodland and swamps in S.E. USA. They are grown for their bottlebrush-like flowers, borne before the leaves, and attractive autumn colour. The leaves are alternate, with coarsely toothed margins. The fragrant, petalless flowers have conspicuously long white stamens and are produced in terminal heads or spikes. Grow in a woodland garden or shrub border.
• **HARDINESS** Fully hardy.
• **CULTIVATION** Grow in humus-rich or leafy, moist but well-drained acid soil in full sun or partial shade (full sun encourages more flowers and richer autumn colour). Pruning group 1.
• **PROPAGATION** Sow seed in containers in a cold frame, or in a seedbed, in autumn or winter. Seed germinates in the second spring after sowing. Root softwood cuttings in summer under mist. Air layer in summer.
• **PESTS AND DISEASES** Trouble free.

F. gardenii ■ (Witch alder). Dense, bushy shrub with alternate, oval to obovate, dark green leaves, to 6cm (2½in) long, with toothed margins, turning bright red, orange, and yellow in autumn. Cylindrical, terminal, fragrant spikes, to 4cm (1½in) long, of small white flowers, with filaments 2.5cm (1in) long, are borne in spring before the leaves. ↕↔ 1m (3ft). S.E. USA. ❄❄❄. **'Blue Mist'** has blue-green foliage.
F. major ■🏆 syn. *F. monticola.* Upright shrub with obovate to nearly rounded, alternate, glossy, dark green leaves, 7–12cm (3–5in) long, with toothed margins, turning brilliant red, orange, and yellow in autumn. Erect, terminal spikes, 2.5–5cm (1–2in) long, of fragrant, white, occasionally pink-tinged flowers are borne in late spring and early summer, before or as the leaves

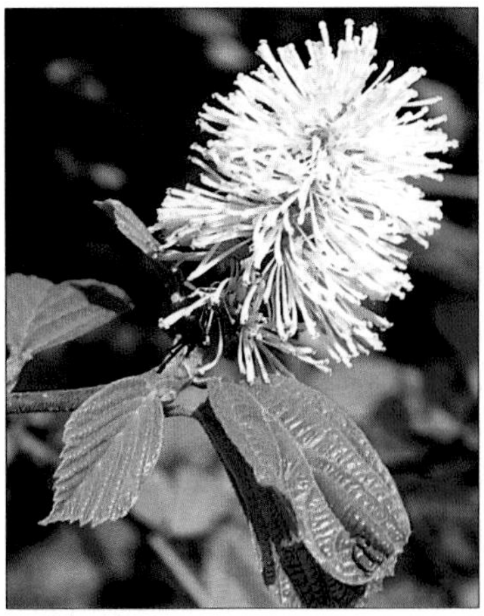

Fothergilla major

unfold. ↕ 2.5m (8ft), ↔ 2m (6ft). USA (Allegheny Mountains, Virginia to South Carolina). ❄❄❄
F. monticola see *F. major.*

▷ **Fountain flower** see *Ceropegia sandersonii*
▷ **Fountain grass** see *Pennisetum alopecuroides, P. setaceum*

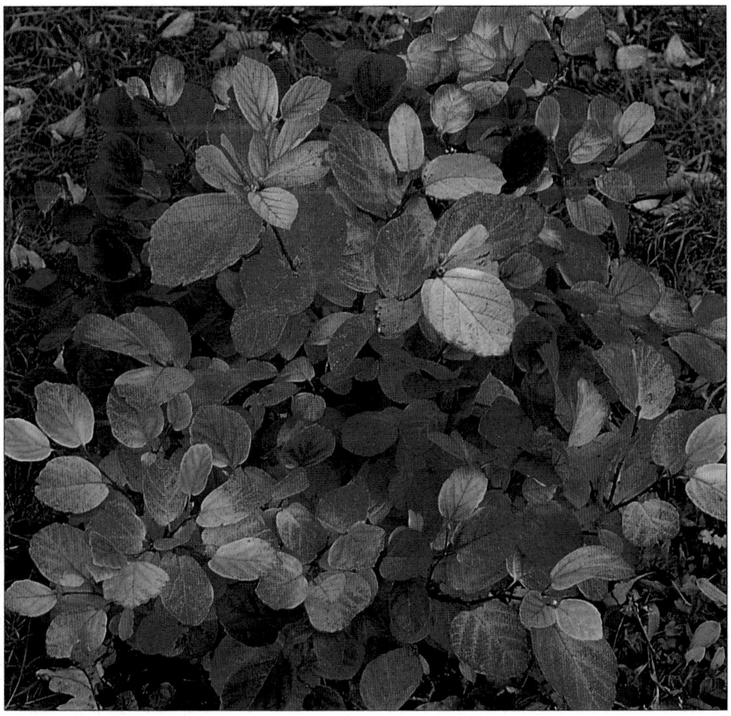

Fothergilla gardenii

FOUQUIERIA

FOUQUIERIACEAE

Genus of about 10 species of mainly bushy or tree-like, small, deciduous, columnar-stemmed succulents and spiny shrubs or trees occurring in low, arid hillsides in S.W. USA and Mexico. They have grooved, swollen, spiny stems and branches, and alternately arranged, simple leaves. The showy, bell-shaped or tubular, red, pale purple, creamy yellow, or white flowers are borne in racemes or panicles. Capsule-like fruits contain winged seeds. Where temperatures drop below 15°C (59°F), grow in a warm greenhouse. In warmer climates, grow in a desert garden or as an informal, spiny hedge.
• **HARDINESS** Frost tender.

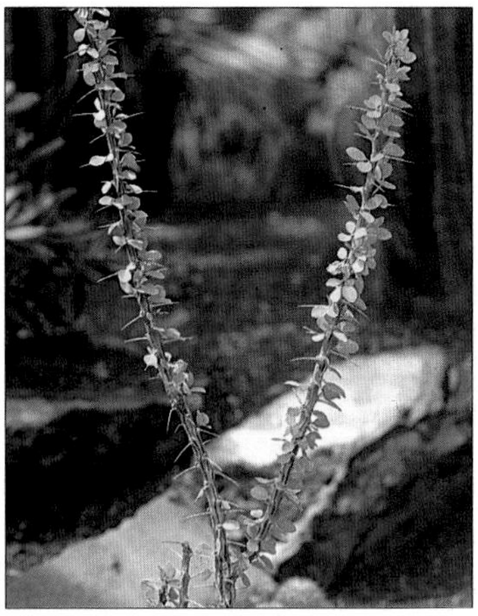

Fouquieria splendens

• **CULTIVATION** Under glass, grow in standard cactus compost in full light with low humidity. From late spring to autumn, water moderately and apply a balanced liquid fertilizer monthly. Keep dry in winter. Outdoors, grow in sharply drained, moderately fertile soil in full sun. See also pp.48–49. Pruning group 1; may need restrictive pruning under glass.
• **PROPAGATION** Sow seed at 19–24°C (66–75°F) in spring. Root softwood cuttings in spring or summer.
• **PESTS AND DISEASES** Susceptible to scale insects.

F. columnaris, syn. *Idria columnaris* (Boojum tree). Spiny tree with a white-barked, caudex-like stem, to 60cm (24in) thick, and simple branches at right angles to the main stem. Bears axillary groups of 2 or 3 elliptic to oval or spoon-shaped leaves, to 1.5–4cm (½–1½in) long. In summer and autumn, bears short racemes of diurnal, narrowly bell-shaped, honey-scented, creamy yellow flowers, to 7mm (¼in) long. ↕ 20m (70ft), ↔ 2.5m (8ft). N.W. Mexico, USA (S.W. California). ⌂ (min. 15°C/59°F)
F. splendens ■ (Ocotillo). Spiny, free-branching shrub with erect, cylindrical, white-striped, dark green stems, 4–5cm (1½–2in) thick, and branches covered with leaf scars and spines. Bears elliptic to inversely lance-shaped leaves, 1.5–5cm (½–2in) long, and shorter, narrowly spoon-shaped leaves, to 3.5cm (1½in) long. Narrowly bell-shaped, diurnal, bright red flowers, 10–28cm (4–11in) long, are borne from early spring to summer. Source of medicinal ocotilla wax. ↕ 10m (30ft), ↔ 2m (6ft). USA (S. California, New Mexico, Texas), N. Mexico (including Baja California). ⌂ (min. 15°C/59°F)

▷ **Four corners** see *Grewia occidentalis*
▷ **Four o'clock flower** see *Mirabilis jalapa*
▷ **Fox and cubs** see *Pilosella aurantiaca*
▷ **Foxglove** see *Digitalis*
Chinese see *Rehmannia elata*
Common see *Digitalis purpurea*
Fairy see *Erinus*
Mexican see *Tetranema roseum*
Rusty see *Digitalis ferruginea*
Yellow see *Digitalis grandiflora*
▷ **Foxglove tree** see *Paulownia tomentosa*
▷ **Fox nuts** see *Euryale*
▷ **Foxtail grass** see *Alopecurus*
Woolly see *A. lanatus*

FRAGARIA

Strawberry

ROSACEAE

Genus of 12 species of stoloniferous perennials from open woodland, hedgerows, and grassy places in Europe, Asia (as far as S. India), North America, and temperate areas of Chile. *F. vesca* is usually found in limy soils. The leaves are 3-palmate and radical, with toothed leaflets. The white, sometimes pink flowers have numerous stamens and carpels, usually 5 rounded petals, and are borne in 2- to 10-flowered cymes, followed by succulent strawberries. Grown mainly for their edible, fleshy fruit, some species and cultivars are useful ground cover, remaining in leaf in all but the severest winters. Grow in a herb garden, as border edging, or in a window-box, container, hanging basket, or specially made "strawberry tower".
• **HARDINESS** Fully hardy.
• **CULTIVATION** Grow in fertile, moist but well-drained, neutral to alkaline soil in full sun or light dappled shade. Strawberries tolerate acid soils, but will thrive in alkaline soils, particularly *F. vesca.* Protect the fruit of *F. vesca* 'Variegata' with a straw mulch underneath. *F.* 'Pink Panda' may become invasive.
• **PROPAGATION** Sow seed at 13–18°C (55–64°F) in spring. Remove and transplant plantlets.
• **PESTS AND DISEASES** Susceptible to leaf spot, powdery mildew, honey fungus and various fungal wilts, red spider mites, and vine weevil grubs.

F. indica see *Duchesnea indica.*
***F.* 'Pink Panda'** ■ Stoloniferous perennial bearing 3-palmate leaves, with broad, ovate, toothed leaflets, 2.5–4cm (1–1½in) long, and reddish green leaf-stalks. Cymes of bright pink flowers, to 2.5cm (1in) across, with 5–7 rounded petals, appear from late spring to mid-autumn. Rarely bears fruit. ↕ 10–15cm (4–6in), ↔ indefinite. ❄❄❄
F. vesca. Stoloniferous perennial forming rosettes of 3-palmate, bright green leaves with ovate, toothed leaflets, 5–7cm (2–3in) long. In late spring, bears cymes of white flowers, to 2cm (¾in) across, with 5 rounded petals, followed by red fruit, 1cm (½in) long. ↕ to 30cm (12in), ↔ indefinite. Europe. ❄❄❄. **'Variegata'** produces variegated, grey-green and cream leaves.

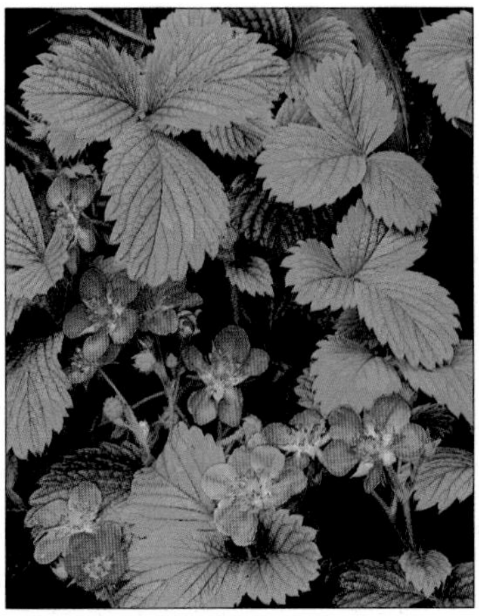

Fragaria 'Pink Panda'

FRAILEA

CACTACEAE

Genus of about 10–15 species of dwarf, flattened spherical or columnar, usually offsetting, perennial cacti from scrub and grassland in E. Bolivia, S. Brazil, Paraguay, Uruguay, and N. Argentina. The ribs are divided into tubercles with finely spined areoles. The diurnal, funnel-shaped yellow flowers develop on or close to the crown in summer, and are followed by thin-walled black fruits with numerous small, glossy, black or brown seeds. In areas where temperatures drop below 7°C (45°F), grow as houseplants or in a temperate greenhouse. In warmer climates, grow in a desert garden, at the base of a sunny wall, or in a container on a patio.

• **HARDINESS** Frost tender.
• **CULTIVATION** Under glass, grow in standard cactus compost (acid mix) in low humidity with good ventilation, and in full light to ensure that flower buds open. During growth, water moderately and apply a balanced liquid fertilizer monthly. Keep just moist in spring and autumn. Keep dry in winter, watering occasionally to prevent shrivelling. Outdoors, grow in sharply drained, moderately fertile, neutral to acid soil, with added grit and leaf mould, in dappled shade. Protect from excessive winter wet. See also pp.48–49.
• **PROPAGATION** Sow seed at 15–21°C (59–70°F) in spring.
• **PESTS AND DISEASES** Trouble free.

F. asterioides see *F. castanea.*
F. castanea, syn. *F. asterioides.* Solitary cactus with a flattened spherical, dark reddish brown or chocolate-brown, occasionally bluish green stem with 10–15 shallow, flat to slightly convex ribs. Conspicuous brown or almost white areoles bear about 8 minute brown spines. Pale to golden yellow flowers, 3–5cm (1¼–2in) across, are produced in small groups from the areoles, in summer. ↕ 1–2cm (½–¾in), ↔ to 5cm (2in). N.E. Argentina, S. Brazil, N. Uruguay. ❀ (min. 7°C/45°F)
F. pulcherrima see *F. pygmaea.*
F. pygmaea ▣ syn. *F. pulcherrima.* Solitary, sometimes offsetting cactus with a spherical to shortly cylindrical, light to dark green or grey-green stem with about 16 shallow ribs. Small grey areoles, with white, grey, or brown wool, each bear 6–9 or more, white, yellow, or pale brown spines. Pale yellow flowers, 3–5cm (1¼–2in) across, are produced in summer. ↕ 1–2cm (½–¾in), ↔ to 7cm (3in). S. Brazil, Argentina, Uruguay. ❀ (min. 7°C/45°F)

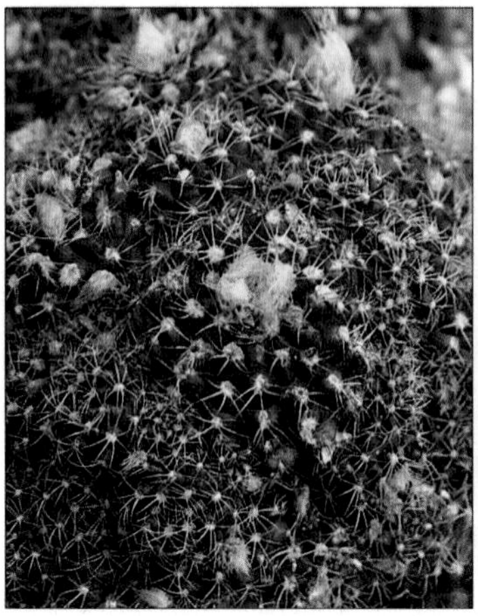

Frailea pygmaea

FRANCOA

Bridal wreath

SAXIFRAGACEAE

Genus of 5 species (or 1 very variable species) of evergreen perennials from semi-shady, rocky crevices in Chile. The leaves are obovate to broadly lance-shaped, wavy-margined, softly hairy, usually pinnatisect, with several small, often rounded lobes and one large terminal lobe, 6–13cm (2½–5in) long, borne in basal rosettes. Cross-shaped, 4-, occasionally 5-petalled, delicate-looking, white or pink flowers, with darker markings, are borne in long-stalked, terminal, spike-like racemes, some with basal branches. Cultivated for use in floral arrangements, bridal wreaths can be grown as edging for a border, or in a woodland or courtyard garden. In frost-prone areas, grow in a cool greenhouse or as houseplants.
• **HARDINESS** Frost hardy; may survive temperatures down to -10°C (14°F).
• **CULTIVATION** Outdoors, grow in humus-rich, moist but well-drained soil in full sun or partial shade. Protect from winter wet. Under glass, grow in loamless or loam-based potting compost (JI No.3) in full light, with shade from the hottest sun. During growth, water freely and apply a balanced liquid fertilizer every 4 weeks. Water sparingly in winter.
• **PROPAGATION** Sow seed at 15–24°C (59–75°F) in spring. Divide in spring.
• **PESTS AND DISEASES** Trouble free.

F. appendiculata ▣ Rosette-forming perennial with broadly lance-shaped, variably lobed, basal leaves. In mid-summer, sparsely branched stems bear wand-like racemes of pale pink flowers, 2cm (¾in) across, with darker pink markings within. ↕ 60–90cm (24–36in), ↔ 30cm (12in). Chile. ✽✽
F. glabrata see *F. ramosa.*
F. ramosa, syn. *F. glabrata.* Rosette-forming perennial with stalked, broadly lance-shaped, variably lobed, basal leaves. In summer, branched flowering stems bear spike-like racemes of white flowers, 2cm (¾in) across, with dark pink markings. ↕ 60–90cm (24–36in), ↔ 30cm (12in). Chile. ✽✽

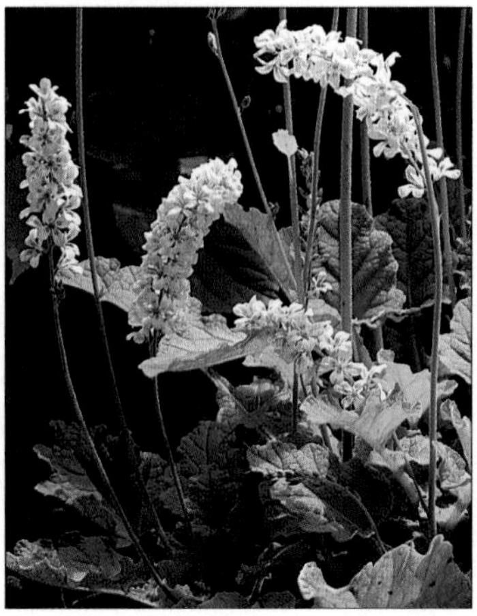

Francoa appendiculata

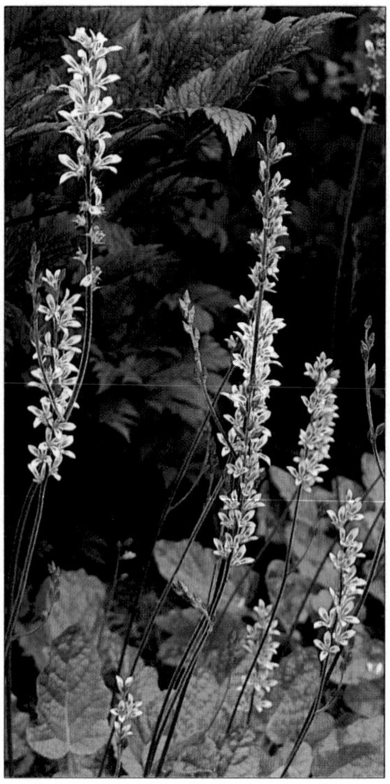

Francoa sonchifolia

F. sonchifolia ▣ Rosette-forming perennial with broadly lance-shaped, variably and deeply lobed, basal leaves. In midsummer, unbranched stems bear compact racemes of pink flowers, 2cm (¾in) across, with darker pink markings, opening from deep pink buds. May survive below -10°C (14°F) for short periods. ↕ 60–90cm (24–36in), ↔ 45cm (18in). Chile. ✽✽

▷ **Frangipani** see *Plumeria*
Australian see *Hymenosporum, H. flavum*
Common see *Plumeria rubra*

FRANKLINIA

THEACEAE

Genus of one species of deciduous tree or shrub from woodland in Georgia, USA, now thought to be extinct in the wild. Grown for its showy, solitary, axillary, fragrant, camellia-like white flowers and colourful autumn foliage, *F. alatamaha* is suitable for open glades in a woodland garden.
• **HARDINESS** Fully hardy, but flowers more freely with prolonged exposure to temperatures over 24°C (75°F).
• **CULTIVATION** Grow in humus-rich, moist but well-drained, acid to neutral soil in full sun. Shelter from cold, drying winds. Pruning group 1.
• **PROPAGATION** Sow seed as soon as ripe at 10–18°C (50–64°F). Root hardwood cuttings in early winter, or softwood cuttings in summer with bottom heat.
• **PESTS AND DISEASES** Trouble free.

F. alatamaha ♀ Upright tree bearing alternate, obovate-oblong, sparsely toothed, glossy, dark green leaves, to 15cm (6in) long, turning red in autumn. Shallowly cup-shaped, fragrant white flowers, to 8cm (3in) across, with yellow stamens, are produced from late summer to early autumn. The fruit are woody, spherical capsules, to 2cm (¾in) across. ↕ 5m (15ft) or more, ↔ 5m (15ft). USA (Georgia). ✽✽✽

FRAXINUS

Ash

OLEACEAE

Genus of about 65 species of deciduous, rarely evergreen trees usually found in woodland, mainly in Europe, Asia, and North America. The leaves are opposite and pinnate, light to dark green, and 5–50cm (2–20in) long. The flowers are borne in terminal or axillary panicles or racemes, from spring to early summer. Ashes are grown for their habit and foliage. Most have inconspicuous, petalless flowers, although some species, including *F. ornus* and *F. sieboldiana*, are grown for their ornamental flowers. *F. americana*, *F. pennsylvanica* and *F. uhdei* usually produce male and female flowers on separate plants; both are needed to produce the single-seeded, winged fruits. Ashes are excellent specimen trees for woodland or coastal gardens. Grow non-fruiting cultivars in areas with long periods of over 24°C (75°F), where self-sown seedlings can cause problems. Contact with lichens on the bark may aggravate skin allergies.
• **HARDINESS** Fully hardy to frost hardy.
• **CULTIVATION** Grow in fertile, moist but well-drained, neutral to alkaline soil in full sun. *F. angustifolia*, *F. ornus*, and *F. texensis* tolerate reasonably dry, acid to alkaline soils. *F. nigra* 'Fallgold' prefers moist soil. Pruning group 1.
• **PROPAGATION** Stratify seed over winter, or chill for 2–3 months in a refrigerator before sowing. Sow seed in autumn or spring in containers in an open frame. Graft cultivars in spring on to seedling stock of the same species.
• **PESTS AND DISEASES** Generally trouble free, although susceptible to a range of pests and diseases in the USA.

F. americana ♀ (White ash). Fast-growing, broadly columnar, deciduous tree bearing pinnate, dark green leaves, to 35cm (14in) long, with 5–9 oblong-lance-shaped to ovate, tapered leaflets, turning yellow or purple in autumn. ↕ 25m (80ft), ↔ 15m (50ft). E. North America. ✽✽✽. **'Autumn Blaze'** ◊ has an oval crown and purple autumn foliage; ↕ 18m (60ft), ↔ 10m (30ft). **'Autumn Purple'** ♤ is broadly conical, with glossy leaves turning red to red-purple in autumn; ↕ 18m (60ft), ↔ 12m (40ft). **'Champaign County'** is very dense, with glossy leaves and little autumn colour; ↕ 14m (46ft), ↔ 10m (30ft). **'Rose Hill'** has dark green leaves turning bronze-red in autumn; ↕ 15m (50ft), ↔ 10m (30ft). **'Skyline'** ◊ is oval-headed, with glossy leaves turning orange-red in autumn; ↕ 15m (50ft), ↔ 12m (40ft).
F. angustifolia ▣ ♀ syn. *F. oxycarpa* (Narrow-leaved ash). Spreading, deciduous tree bearing pinnate, glossy leaves, to 25cm (10in) long, dark green above, paler beneath, often in whorls of 3, each with up to 13 slender, lance-shaped, tapered leaflets, turning yellow-gold in autumn. ↕ 25m (80ft), ↔ 12m (40ft). S.W. Europe, N. Africa. ✽✽✽. **'Raywood'** ♀ (Claret ash) is very vigorous, with dark green leaves turning reddish purple in autumn; ↕ 20m (70ft).
F. excelsior ♀ ♀ (Common ash). Vigorous, spreading, deciduous tree with conspicuous black buds in winter.

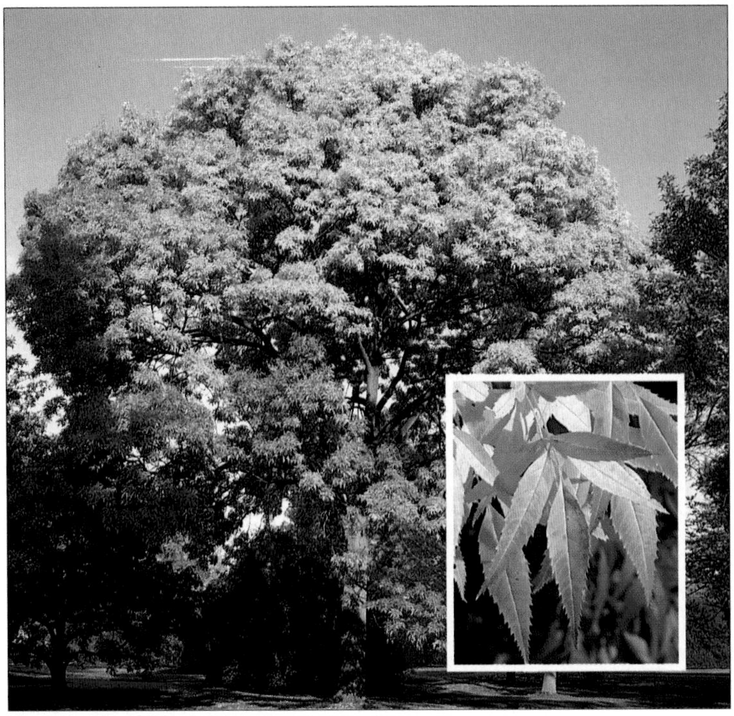
Fraxinus angustifolia (inset: autumn leaf detail)

Pinnate, dark green leaves, to 30cm (12in) long, with 9–11 or 13 oval leaflets, turn yellow in autumn. ↕30m (100ft), ↔20m (70ft). Europe. ❄❄❄. **f. *diversifolia*** (One-leaved ash) has leaves with 1, rarely 3 leaflets. **'Jaspidea'** ▣Y has yellow winter shoots and yellow leaves in spring and autumn. **'Pendula'** ▣YQ (Weeping ash) has branches that weep, often to the ground; ↕15m (50ft), ↔8–10m (25–30ft). **'Westhof's Glorie'** Y0 is narrow, later spreading. Leaves emerge late in spring, bronze at first, then dark green.
F. holotricha Q Rounded, deciduous tree bearing velvety shoots and pinnate, grey-green leaves, to 25cm (10in) long, maturing to glossy, dark green, each with 5–13, usually 11, elliptic to lance-shaped leaflets. ↕12m (40ft), ↔12m (40ft). ❄❄❄. **'Moraine'** has an even, rounded crown and is fast-growing.
F. latifolia Q syn. *F. oregona* (Oregon ash). Spreading, deciduous tree bearing pinnate, dark green leaves, 15–30cm (6–12in) long, with 7–9 oval, tapered leaflets, turning yellow in autumn. ↕25m (80ft), ↔15m (50ft). W. North America. ❄❄❄
F. mariesii see *F. sieboldiana*.
F. nigra 0 Upright, deciduous tree bearing pinnate, dark green leaves, to 12cm (5in) long, with up to 11 oblong, tapered leaflets, turning golden yellow in autumn. ↕15m (50ft), ↔8m (25ft). ❄❄❄. **'Fallgold'** is vigorous, produces no fruit, and has long-lasting, golden yellow colour in autumn.
F. oregona see *F. latifolia*.
F. ornus ▣YQ (Manna ash). Bushy-headed, rounded, deciduous tree bearing pinnate, dark green leaves, to 20cm (8in) long, with 5–9 oval leaflets, turning purple-red in autumn. In late spring and early summer, produces large terminal and axillary panicles of fragrant, creamy white flowers. ↕↔15m (50ft). S. Europe, S.W. Asia. ❄❄❄
F. oxycarpa see *F. angustifolia*.

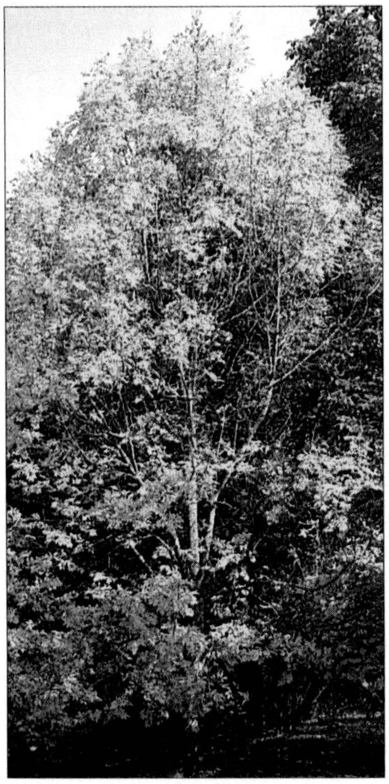
Fraxinus excelsior 'Jaspidea'

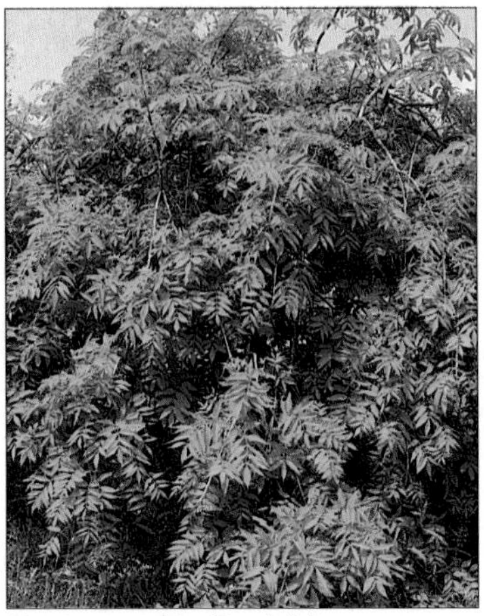
Fraxinus excelsior 'Pendula'

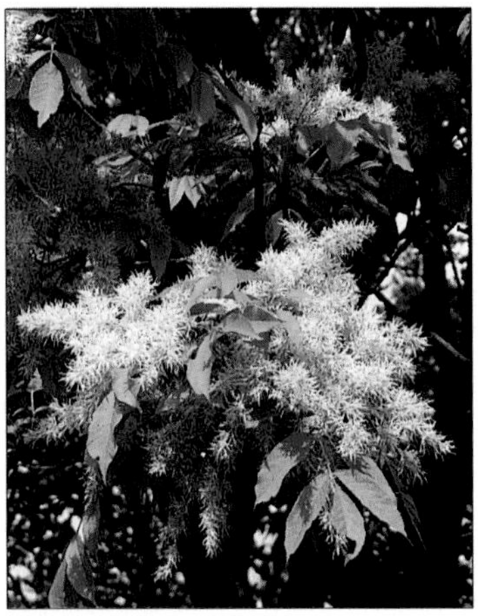
Fraxinus ornus

F. pennsylvanica Q (Green ash, Red ash). Vigorous, spreading, deciduous tree producing pinnate, olive-green leaves, to 30cm (12in) long, composed of 7–9, sometimes 5, ovate to lance-shaped, tapered leaflets, turning yellow in autumn. ↕↔20m (70ft). North America. ❄❄❄. **'Emerald'** has a rounded crown and glossy, dark green leaves, and does not bear fruit; ↕15m (50ft), ↔12m (40ft). **'Marshall's Seedless'** ◊ is vigorous, broadly oval, with glossy, dark green leaves. Does not bear fruit; ↕15m (50ft), ↔12m (40ft). **'Patmore'** ◊ has an oval crown and glossy leaves. Disease-resistant; does not bear fruit; ↕14m (46ft), ↔11m (35ft). **'Summit'** ▣0 is upright with glossy leaves turning yellow in autumn; ↕14m (46ft), ↔8m (25ft).
F. sieboldiana ▣Q syn. *F. mariesii*. Slow-growing, compact, deciduous tree or shrub bearing pinnate, dark green leaves, to 20cm (8in) long, with up to 7 ovate, tapered leaflets. In late spring and early summer, bears axillary, terminal panicles of small, fragrant, creamy white flowers, followed by winged, purple-tinged fruit. ↕6m (20ft), ↔5m (15ft). C. China. ❄❄❄

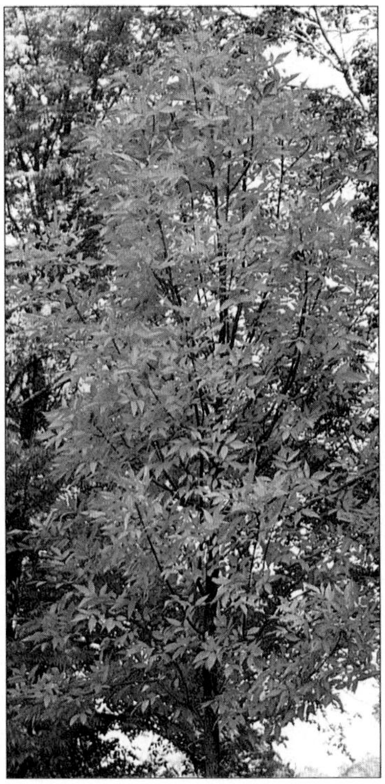
Fraxinus pennsylvanica 'Summit'

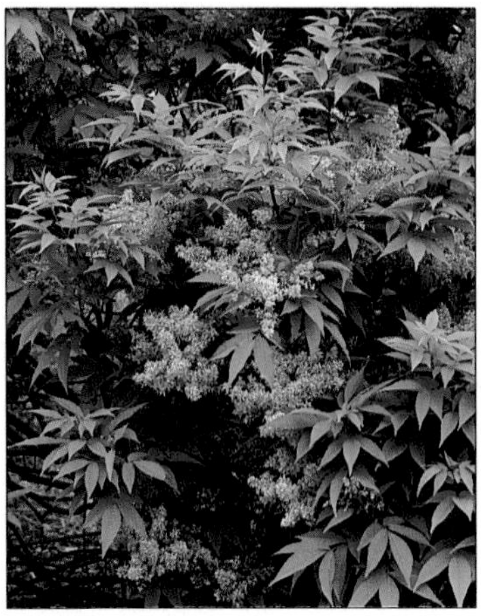
Fraxinus sieboldiana

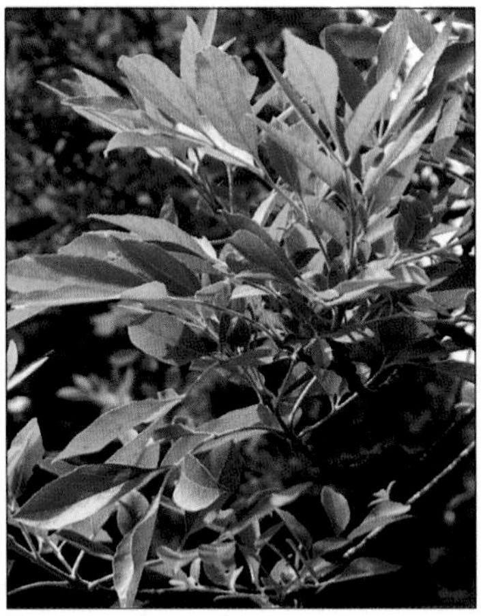
Fraxinus velutina

F. texensis Q Spreading, deciduous tree bearing pinnate, leathery, dark green leaves, to 20cm (8in) long, with 5, sometimes 7 ovate leaflets, 3–8cm (1¼–3in) long. ↕↔15m (50ft). USA (Texas). ❄❄❄
F. uhdei Q Upright to rounded, semi-evergreen or evergreen tree with pinnate, glossy, dark green leaves, to 15cm (6in) long, with up to 7 oval, tapered leaflets. ↕8m (25ft), ↔5m (15ft). Central America. ❄❄ (borderline). **'Tomlinson'** is smaller, with upright branches and leathery leaves. ↕3–4m (10–12ft).
F. velutina ▣Q (Arizona ash, Velvet ash). Spreading, deciduous tree bearing pinnate, leathery, velvety, grey-green leaves, to 15cm (6in) long, with 3–5, sometimes 7, lance-shaped, tapered leaflets, turning yellow in autumn. ↕↔10m (30ft). S.W. USA. ❄❄❄. **'Fan Tex'** is very heat-tolerant, vigorous, and non-fruiting, with dark green leaves.

▷**Freckle face** see *Hypoestes phyllostachya*

FREESIA

IRIDACEAE

Genus of 6 or more species of cormous perennials from sandy, lowland soils to rocky upland slopes in South Africa. Over 300 cultivars have been developed for use as cut flowers. The large, funnel-shaped, usually scented, brightly coloured flowers, held erect in dense racemes at the end of arching, frequently branched stems, are produced in late winter and early spring. Narrowly sword-shaped to linear-lance-shaped leaves, 5–40cm (2–16in) long, develop

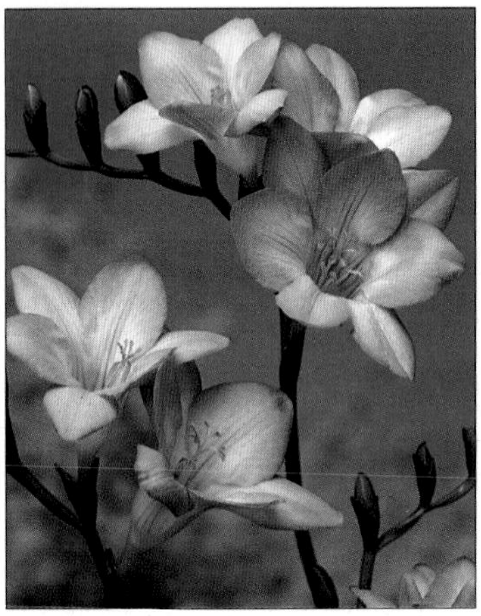

Freesia 'Blue Heaven'

in basal fans. In frost-prone areas, grow freesias in a cool greenhouse. Specially prepared corms may be used outdoors for summer flowering. In warmer areas, grow in groups in a mixed border.

• **HARDINESS** Half hardy.

• **CULTIVATION** Under glass, grow in loam-based potting compost (JI No.2) with added grit. Shade from sun and keep moist until established, then grow in full light with good ventilation, and water freely. Keep temperature below 13°C (55°F). After flower buds appear, apply a balanced liquid fertilizer weekly. After flowering, gradually reduce water until dry, then store corms for re-planting in containers in late summer or autumn. Outdoors, plant 8cm (3in) deep, in moderately fertile, moist but well-drained soil in full sun. Plant in spring for summer flowering; in frost-free areas, plant in autumn for spring flowers.

• **PROPAGATION** Sow seed at 13–18°C (55–64°F) in autumn or winter. Remove small offsets in autumn.

• **PESTS AND DISEASES** Susceptible to red spider mites, aphids, dry rot, and *Fusarium* wilt.

***F. alba* of gardens** see *F. lactea.*
F. armstrongii see *F. corymbosa.*
***F.* 'Ballerina'.** Cormous perennial with white flowers, 5cm (2in) long, borne on robust stems. ↕ to 40cm (16in). ✻
***F.* 'Blue Heaven'** ■ Cormous perennial bearing bluish mauve flowers with yellow throats, to 5cm (2in) long. ↕ to 40cm (16in). ✻
F. corymbosa, syn. *F. armstrongii.* Cormous perennial with linear, acute leaves, 10–20cm (4–8in) long. Bears scented or unscented flowers, 2.5–3.5cm (1–1½in) long, that are creamy white, or pale yellow with bright yellow lower tepals, or pale pink with yellow throats. ↕ to 50cm (20in). South Africa (Eastern Cape, Western Cape). ✻
***F.* 'Elan'.** Cormous perennial with semi-double, lilac-purple flowers, 5cm (2in) long, with white throats. ↕ to 40cm (16in). ✻
***F.* 'Golden Melody'.** Vigorous, cormous perennial with yellow flowers, 5cm (2in) long. ↕ to 40cm (16in). ✻
F. lactea, syn. *F. alba* of gardens, *F. refracta* var. *alba*. Cormous perennial with linear leaves, 12–40cm (5–16in) long. Bears white flowers, 2.5–6cm (1–2½in) long, strongly scented, occasionally flushed purple outside. ↕ 20–40cm (8–16in). South Africa (Western Cape). ✻
***F.* 'Oberon'** ■ Cormous perennial with yellow flowers, 4–5cm, (1½–2in) long, light blood-red inside; the throats are lemon-yellow with small red veins. ↕ to 40cm (16in). ✻
***F.* 'Red Lion'.** Cormous perennial with yellow-centred, orange-red flowers, 5cm (2in) long. ↕ to 40cm (16in). ✻
F. refracta* var. *alba see *F. lactea.*
***F.* 'Rosalinde'.** Cormous perennial with semi-double, dark rose-pink flowers, to 5cm (2in) long, with yellow throats. ↕ to 40cm (16in). ✻
***F.* 'Uchida'.** Cormous perennial with semi-double, lilac-blue flowers, 4–5cm (1½–2in) long. ↕ to 40cm (16in). ✻

▷ ***Fremontia*** see *Fremontodendron*

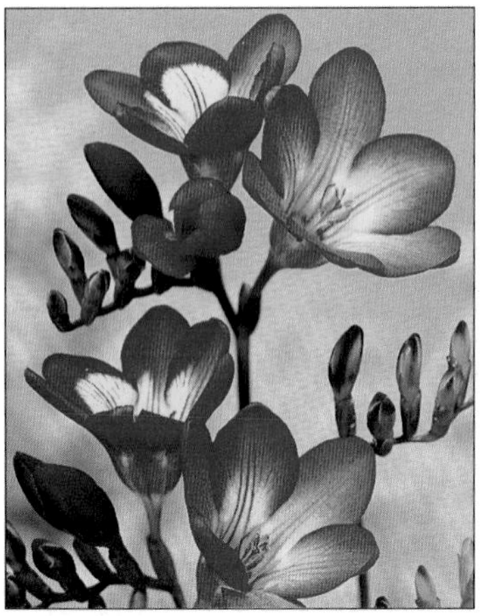

Freesia 'Oberon'

FREMONTODENDRON

syn. FREMONTIA
Flannel bush
STERCULIACEAE

Genus of 2 species of evergreen or semi-evergreen shrubs or trees from dry woodland, canyons, and mountain slopes in the USA and N. Mexico. They have alternate, rounded, 3-, 5-, or 7-lobed, dark green leaves, and densely hairy young shoots covered in scales. Large and very showy yellow flowers are produced over a long period, usually in spring and autumn. Grow flannel bushes against a warm, sunny wall, or as specimen plants at the back of a shrub or mixed border. Contact with the foliage and shoots may irritate the skin.

• **HARDINESS** Frost hardy; may tolerate occasional low temperatures to -15°C (5°F) when trained against a warm, sunny wall.

• **CULTIVATION** Grow in poor to moderately fertile, dry to moist but well-drained, neutral to alkaline soil in full sun, with shelter from cold, drying winds. Pruning group 1, or group 13 if wall-trained.

• **PROPAGATION** Sow seed at 13–18°C (55–64°F) in spring. Root greenwood cuttings in early summer, or semi-ripe cuttings in late summer.

• **PESTS AND DISEASES** *Phytophthora* root rot may be a problem.

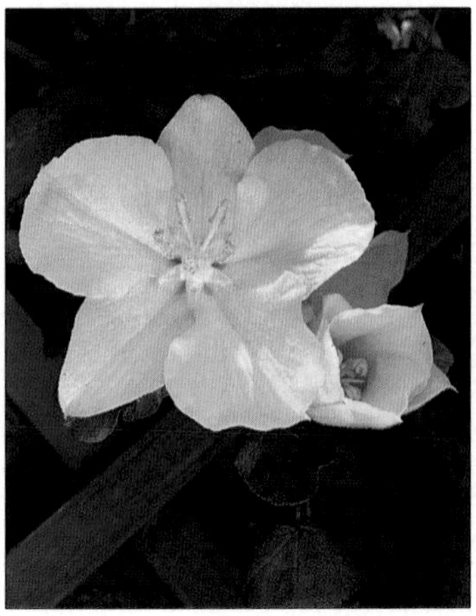

Fremontodendron 'California Glory'

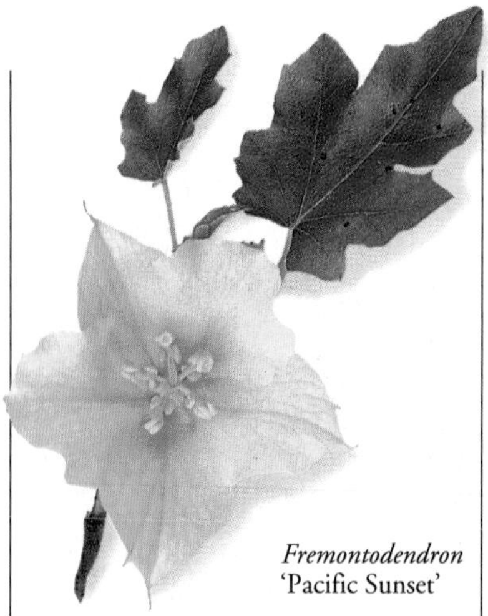

Fremontodendron 'Pacific Sunset'

***F.* 'California Glory'** ■ ♀ Vigorous, upright then spreading, evergreen shrub with rounded, 5-lobed, dark green leaves, to 7cm (3in) long. From late spring to mid-autumn, angled buds open to shallowly saucer-shaped, deep yellow flowers, 4–6cm (1½–2½in) across. ↕ 6m (20ft), ↔ 4m (12ft). ✻✻
F. californicum. Vigorous, upright, evergreen or semi-evergreen shrub with rounded, 3-, 5-, or 7-lobed, dark green leaves, 5–10cm (2–4in) long. Shallowly saucer-shaped yellow flowers, to 6cm (2½in) across, are borne from late spring to mid-autumn. ↕ 6m (20ft), ↔ 4m (12ft). USA (California, Arizona). ✻✻
***F.* 'Ken Taylor'.** Spreading, evergreen shrub with rounded, 3- or 5-lobed, dark green leaves, to 7cm (3in) long. Shallowly saucer-shaped, orange-yellow flowers, 4–6cm (1½–2½in) across, are borne from spring to autumn. ↕ 2m (6ft), ↔ 3m (10ft). ✻✻
F. mexicanum. Upright, vigorous, evergreen or semi-evergreen shrub with rounded, 5- or 7-lobed, dark green leaves, to 7cm (3in) long. From late spring to mid-autumn, bears shallowly saucer-shaped, deep golden yellow flowers, 6–9cm (2½–3½in) across, tinged red on the exterior. ↕ 6m (20ft), ↔ 4m (12ft). USA (S. California), N. Mexico. ✻✻
***F.* 'Pacific Sunset'** ■ Upright, ever-green shrub with rounded, dark green leaves, 5–8cm (2–3in) long, with 3 or 5 angular lobes. In summer, produces saucer-shaped, bright yellow flowers, to 6cm (2½in) across, with long, slender-pointed lobes. ✻✻

▷ ***Frerea*** see *Caralluma*
F. indica see *C. frerei*
▷ **Friendship plant** see *Bilbergia nutans, Pilea involucrata*
▷ **Fringe cups** see *Tellima*
▷ **Fringe tree** see *Chionanthus, C. virginicus*
Chinese see *C. retusus*

FRITILLARIA

Fritillary
LILIACEAE

Genus of about 100 species of bulbous perennials found in a range of habitats from woodland to open meadows and high screes, distributed throughout the temperate regions of the N. hemisphere, particularly the Mediterranean, S.W. Asia, and W. North America. Each bulb has 2 or more scales, and sometimes abundant basal bulblets ("rice-grains"). The leaves are usually lance-shaped or linear, with 1, rarely 2, wider basal leaves, and several alternate, opposite, or whorled stem leaves. In some species, there is an involucre of 2 or 3 leaf-like bracts above the flowers. The flowers, borne in spring or early summer, are usually pendulous and solitary, or in terminal racemes or umbels, and have 6 tepals. They are bell-shaped, tubular, or saucer-shaped, frequently tessellated, and have conspicuous nectaries at the base of the tepals. The fruits are capsules, often angular or winged.

Grow in a rock garden, in a raised bed or border, or in a woodland garden, depending on the cultivation needs (see below). Smaller species, 5–15cm (2–6in) high, often need the protection of a bulb frame or alpine house.

• **HARDINESS** Fully hardy to frost hardy.

• **CULTIVATION** Handle the fragile bulbs carefully and plant at 4 times their own depth. Large, hollow-crowned bulbs, such as *F. imperialis*, are very prone to rot in poorly drained conditions.

Under glass, grow in loam-based potting compost (JI No.2), with added grit and leaf mould, in full light. Water moderately during growth and keep almost dry when dormant. During the second year, apply a half-strength balanced liquid fertilizer monthly or repot into fresh compost.

For ease of reference, the varying cultivation requirements of the different groups have been classified as follows. All except group 3 need a continental climate: ideally a dry winter and summer, and a damp spring.

1. Toughest, most tolerant species, suitable for a sunny border or rock garden. Need fertile, well-drained soil and full sun.

2. Fairly robust species but intolerant of rainfall while dormant. Need sharply drained, moderately fertile soil and full sun. Suitable for a rock garden or raised bed; can be grown in a bulb frame or alpine house.

3. Damp meadow or woodland species, needing humus-rich, moisture-retentive soil with added leaf mould, and full sun to light shade. Grow best in areas with cool, damp summers.

4. Wet-intolerant species, usually small, needing fertile, well-drained soil and full sun, with shelter from rain. Grow in a bulb frame or cold greenhouse, to keep bulbs almost dry when dormant.

• **PROPAGATION** Sow seed in autumn in a cold frame. Expose to winter cold until germination in spring, then transfer to a cold greenhouse. Small species should be grown on for 2 years in containers. Divide offsets, or collect and sow "rice-grain" bulbils, in late summer.

• **PESTS AND DISEASES** Prone to attack by slugs and lily beetles.

FRITILLARIA

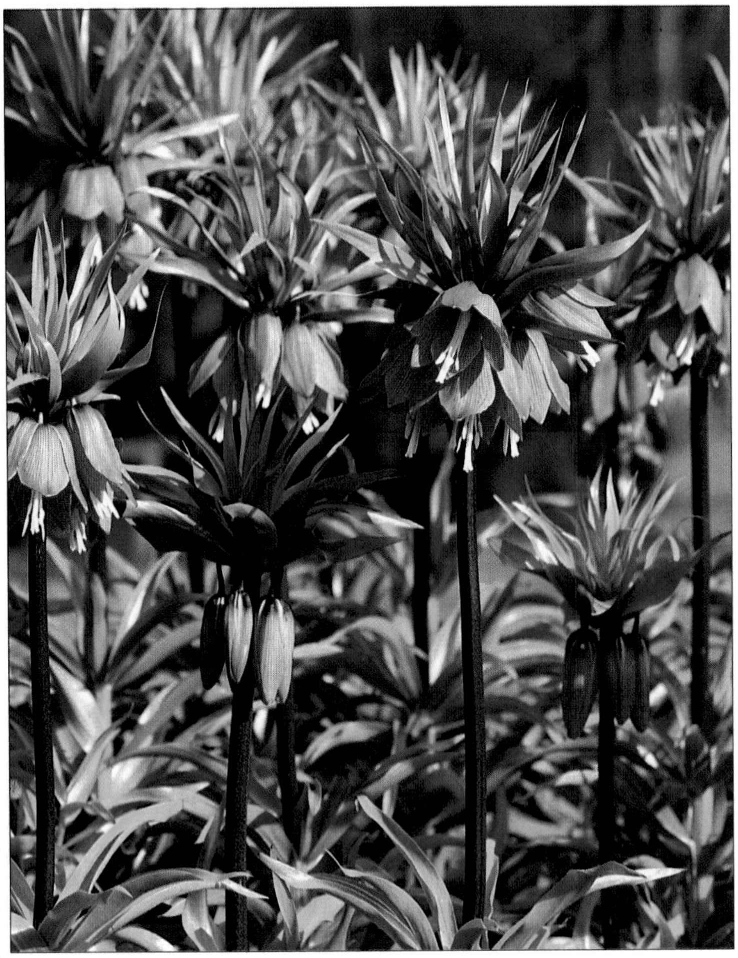

Fritillaria imperialis

F. acmopetala ■ ♡ Bulbous perennial bearing alternate, linear, bluish green leaves, to 20cm (8in) long. In late spring, usually solitary flowers are produced in the uppermost leaf axils, or sometimes in pairs or threes in the lower leaf axils. Flowers are bell-shaped, pendent, pale green, to 4cm (1½in) long, with reflexed tepals; the inner tepals are stained reddish brown. Cultivation group 1. ↕ to 40cm (16in), ↔ 5–8cm (2–3in). Cyprus, S.W. Turkey, Syria, Lebanon. ❄❄❄

F. affinis, syn. *F. lanceolata* (Rice-grain fritillary). Bulbous perennial bearing whorls of broadly lance-shaped to linear, blue-green leaves, 4–16cm (1½–6in) long. From early spring to early summer, bears racemes of 3 or 4, occasionally up to 12, cup-shaped, pendent, greenish white flowers, to 4cm (1½in) long, with reddish purple stains or speckles. Cultivation group 2 or 3. ↕ to 60cm (24in), ↔ 12cm (5in). N.W. North America. ❄❄❄

F. armena. Bulbous perennial with alternate, stem-clasping, lance-shaped, mid-green lower leaves, 2.5–10cm (1–4in) long, and linear upper leaves. Solitary, narrowly bell-shaped, pendent, tessellated, dark purple-brown flowers, to 2cm (¾in) long, with slightly incurved, fringed tepals, are borne in spring. Cultivation group 4. ↕ 8–15cm (3–6in), ↔ 5–8cm (2–3in). N.E. Turkey. ❄❄❄

***F. assyriaca* of gardens** see *F. uva-vulpis.*

F. biflora (Black fritillary, Mission bells). Bulbous perennial with ovate-lance-shaped, very glossy, mid-green leaves, 5–12cm (2–5in) long, usually produced in basal clusters. In early and mid-spring, bears up to 6, occasionally up to 12, bell-shaped, pendent brown flowers, to 3.5cm (1½in) long, tinged black to purple, flushed green, and with ridges on the inner tepals. Cultivation group 4. ↕ 15–30cm (6–12in), ↔ 5–8cm (2–3in). W. USA (California). ❄❄❄. **'Martha Roderick'** ■ syn. *F. roderickii*, produces deep red-purple flowers; the outer two-thirds of the tepals are white.

F. bucharica. Bulbous perennial with broadly lance-shaped, or lance-shaped to ovate, grey-green leaves, to 8cm (3in) long, the lower ones opposite, the upper ones alternate. Racemes of up to 10 widely cup-shaped, nodding flowers, to 2cm (¾in) long, with pointed, green-based, green-veined white tepals and indented green nectaries, are borne in spring. Cultivation group 4. ↕ to 30cm (12in), ↔ 5cm (2in). Uzbekistan, Turkmenistan, N. Afghanistan, Tajikistan. ❄❄❄

F. camschatcensis ■ (Black sarana). Variable, bulbous perennial with lance-shaped, glossy, light green leaves, to 12cm (5in) long, the lower ones in whorls, the upper ones alternate. Up to 8 broadly bell- to cup-shaped, pendent, dark black-purple, sometimes green or yellow flowers, to 3cm (1¼in) long, are borne in early summer. Cultivation group 3. ↕ to 45cm (18in), ↔ 8–10cm (3–4in). N.E. Asia, Alaska to N.W. USA. ❄❄❄

F. chitralensis ■ Upright, bulbous perennial producing loose whorls of ovate, mid- to light green leaves, to 15cm (6in) long. Open umbels of 4 or 5 conical, pendent, bright yellow flowers, 3–4cm (1¼–1½in) long, are borne in early and mid-spring. Similar to *F. imperialis* and often included under it. Cultivation group 1. ↕ 50–80cm (20–32in), ↔ 10cm (4in). N.E. Afghanistan, Pakistan (Chitral). ❄❄❄

F. cirrhosa ■ Bulbous perennial with whorls of linear, greyish green leaves, to 8cm (3in) long, the uppermost leaves with tendril-like tips. In late spring, produces usually solitary, occasionally 2 or 3 broadly bell-shaped, pendent, pale green, sometimes purple-tinged flowers, to 5cm (2in) long, with brownish purple tessellations. Cultivation group 3. ↕ to 45cm (18in), ↔ 5–8cm (2–3in). E. Himalayas, S.W. China. ❄❄❄

F. crassifolia. Variable, bulbous perennial with alternate, lance-shaped, grey-green leaves, 2.5–7cm (1–3in) long. In spring, bears 1–3 broadly bell-shaped, pendent, pale green flowers, to 2.5cm (1in) long, usually with faint brown chequering. Cultivation group 2 or 4. ↕ 7–20cm (3–8in) or more, ↔ 5cm (2in). Turkey (Anatolia), Lebanon, Iran. ❄❄❄

F. davisii. Bulbous perennial with opposite, broadly lance-shaped, grey-green, mainly basal leaves, 3.5–11cm (1½–4½in) long. In spring, bears 1–3 broadly bell-shaped, pendent green flowers, to 2.5cm (1in) long, often with yellow-margined tepals and brown or black tessellation. Cultivation group 4. ↕ to 15cm (6in), ↔ 5cm (2in). S. Greece. ❄❄❄

F. delphinensis see *F. tubiformis.*

F. eduardii. Bulbous perennial with whorls of narrowly lance-shaped, glossy, bright mid-green leaves, to 18cm (7in) long. Crowded umbels of broadly bell-shaped, bright orange-red flowers, to 5cm (2in) long, with a tuft of upright, leaf-like bracts above the flowers, are produced in spring. Very similar to *F. imperialis*, but without the unpleasant smell. Cultivation group 1. ↕ to 1.2m (4ft), ↔ to 30cm (12in). Tajikistan. ❄❄❄

F. graeca ■ Variable, bulbous perennial with usually alternate, broadly lance-shaped, glaucous, grey-green leaves, to 11cm (4½in) long, with narrower upper leaves. In late spring and early summer, bears solitary, rarely 2 or 3, broadly bell-shaped, deep green flowers, strongly chequered brownish purple, to 2.5cm (1in) long; each tepal usually has a green central stripe. Cultivation group 2 or 4. ↕ 5–20cm (2–8in), ↔ 5cm (2in). S. Greece (Peloponnese, Crete). ❄❄❄. **subsp. *thessala***, syn. *F. ionica*, is more robust and easier to grow, with broader, mid-green, not glaucous leaves, and pale greenish brown, lightly chequered flowers, to 3–4cm (1¼–1½in) long. Cultivation group 1. Croatia, Bosnia, Macedonia, S. Albania, N.W. Greece, Corfu.

F. hermonis* subsp. *amana. Very variable, bulbous perennial, usually with alternate, lance-shaped or oblong, very glaucous, sometimes glossy, grey- to mid-green leaves, 4–9cm (1½–3½in) long. In spring, produces broadly bell-shaped, light green, faintly brown- or purple-tessellated flowers, to 3.5cm (1½in) long, with inner tepals margined dark brown-purple, borne singly or in pairs. Cultivation group 2 or 4. ↕ 15–30cm (6–12in), ↔ 7cm (3in). S. Turkey to Lebanon. ❄❄❄

F. imperialis ■ (Crown imperial). Bulbous perennial bearing whorls of lance-shaped, light green leaves, 7–18cm (3–7in) long. Umbels of 3–6, sometimes up to 8, bell-shaped, pendent, orange, yellow, or red flowers, to 6cm (2½in) long, crowned by a cluster of upright, leaf-like bracts, are produced in early summer. The bulbs have an unpleasant foxy odour. Cultivation group 1. ↕ to 1.5m (5ft), ↔ 25–30cm (10–12in). S. Turkey to Kashmir. ❄❄❄. **'Aureomarginata'** has variegated leaves with deep yellow margins, and orange flowers. **'Crown upon Crown'** see 'Prolifera'. **'Lutea'** has bright yellow flowers. **'Prolifera'**, syn. 'Crown upon Crown', produces orange-red flowers in 2 whorls, one above the other. **'The Premier'** bears yellow-tinted, orange flowers, with purple veins.

F. involucrata. Bulbous perennial bearing opposite, linear-lance-shaped, mid-green leaves, 5–11cm (2–4½in) long. Solitary, broadly bell-shaped, pale green flowers, to 4cm (1½in) long, sometimes faintly chequered purple, topped with an involucre of 3 leaf-like bracts, are produced in spring. Cultivation group 1 or 2. ↕ to 30cm (12in), ↔ 5–8cm (2–3in). S.E. France, N.W. Italy. ❄❄❄

F. ionica see *F. graeca* subsp. *thessala.*

F. lanceolata see *F. affinis.*

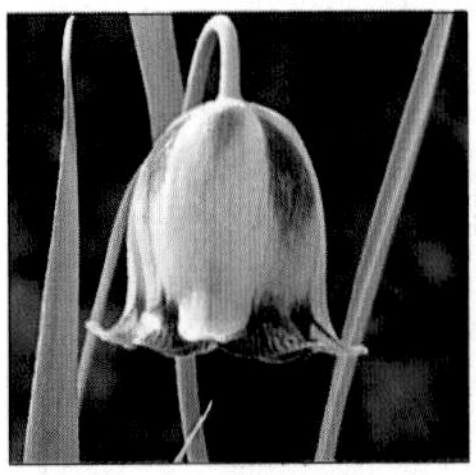

Fritillaria acmopetala

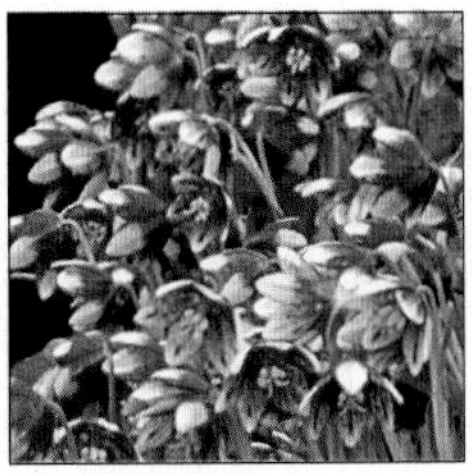

Fritillaria biflora 'Martha Roderick'

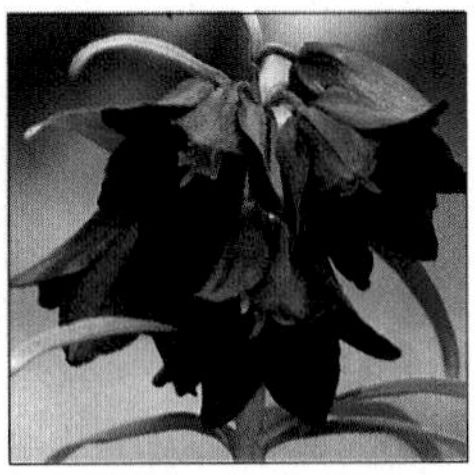

Fritillaria camschatcensis

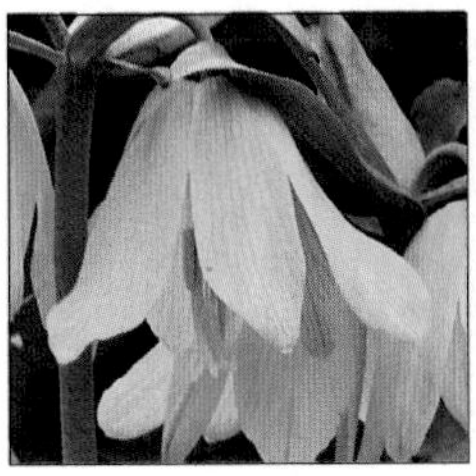

Fritillaria chitralensis

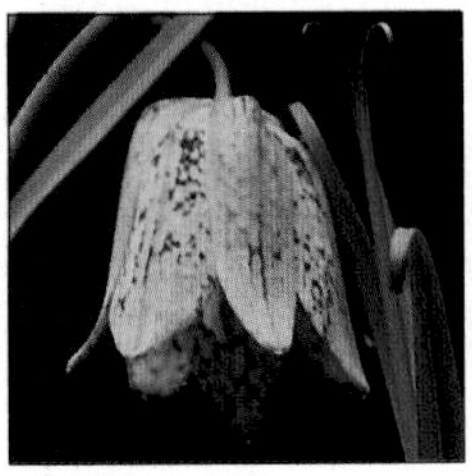

Fritillaria cirrhosa

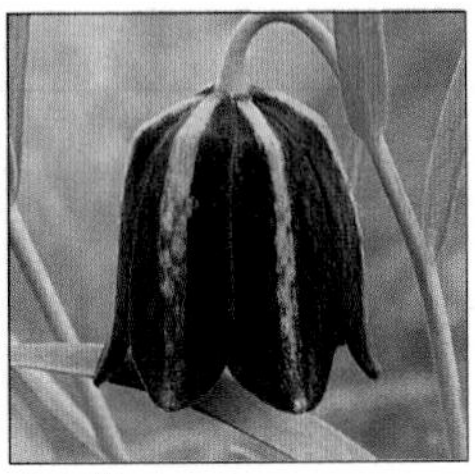

Fritillaria graeca

F

FRITILLARIA

F. latifolia ■ Bulbous perennial with alternate, ovate to lance-shaped, glossy, grey-green leaves, 3.5–8cm (1½–3in) long. In early summer, bears solitary, broadly bell-shaped, dark maroon to purple flowers, to 5cm (2in) long, broad at the shoulders, chequered with yellow tessellations within, and slightly glaucous without. (A colour variant from S. Caucasus, with greenish cream flowers, has been called *F. lagodechiana.*) Cultivation group 2 or 4. ↕ 10–20cm (4–8in), ↔ 5cm (2in). N.E. Turkey, Caucasus, Iran. ✲✲✲. **var. *nobilis*** is a Turkish variant with shorter stems and red-purple flowers, chequered olive-yellow. Cultivation group 4. ↕ to 10cm (4in). Turkish Armenia, Caucasus.

F. meleagris ■ ♀ (Snake's head fritillary). Bulbous perennial bearing alternate, linear, grey-green leaves, 6–13cm (2½–5in) long. In spring, produces solitary, sometimes paired, broadly bell-shaped, pendent, purple, pinkish purple, and white flowers, to 4.5cm (1¾in) long, with strong, purple-pink tessellations. Cultivation group 1 or 3; good for naturalizing in grass. ↕ to 30cm (12in), ↔ 5–8cm (2–3in). S. England to N. Balkans, W. Russia. ✲✲✲. **f. *alba*** ♀ has white flowers.

F. messanensis, syn. *F. oranensis.* Bulbous perennial producing usually opposite, linear, mid-green leaves, 4–9cm (1½–3½in) long. In early spring, bears 1–3 broadly bell-shaped green flowers, to 4cm (1½in) long, chequered brown-purple towards the margins and with a whorl of 3 narrow leaves beneath. Cultivation group 1. ↕ to 30cm (12in), ↔ 5cm (2in). C. Mediterranean. ✲✲✲. **subsp. *gracilis***, syn. *F. neglecta*, has purple-brown and obscurely chequered flowers with the tepals incurved at the tips, and without the whorl of 3 leaves below. Croatia, Macedonia, Albania.

F. michailovskyi ♀ Bulbous perennial with mostly alternate, lance-shaped, mid-green leaves, 5–9cm (2–3½in) long. In early summer, bears umbels of 1–4, or up to 7, broadly bell-shaped, pendent flowers, deep brown-purple, tinged green without, with distinctive yellow tepal tips, to 3cm (1¼in) long. Cultivation group 2 or 4. ↕ 10–20cm (4–8in), ↔ 5cm (2in). N.E. Turkey. ✲✲✲

F. neglecta see *F. messanensis* subsp. *gracilis.*

***F. nigra* of gardens** see *F. pyrenaica.*

F. oranensis see *F. messanensis.*

F. pallidiflora ■ ♀ Robust, bulbous perennial with opposite or alternate, broadly lance-shaped, glaucous, grey-green leaves, to 15cm (6in) long. In late spring and early summer, bears up to 6, rarely 9 or 10, very broadly bell-shaped, nodding, faintly malodorous, green-based, pale creamy yellow flowers, to 4.5cm (1¾in) long, often with faint red-brown tessellations. Cultivation group 1 or 3. ↕ to 40cm (16in), ↔ 5–8cm (2–3in). N.W. China, E. Siberia. ✲✲✲

F. persica. Robust, bulbous perennial with sturdy, upright stems bearing alternate, lance-shaped, glaucous, grey-green leaves, 10–25cm (4–10in) long. Racemes of up to 30 conical, narrowly bell-shaped, pendent, greenish brown to deep purple flowers, to 2cm (¾in) long, are produced in spring. Cultivation group 1, in a hot site. ↕ to 1m (3ft) ↔ 10cm (4in). S. Turkey. ✲✲✲. **'Adiyaman'** is taller and more free-flowering, with brown-purple flowers. ↕ to 1.5m (5ft).

F. pontica. Bulbous perennial with opposite or subopposite, lance-shaped to ovate-lance-shaped, glaucous, grey-green leaves, 5–10cm (2–4in) long. The topmost leaves are in a whorl of 3 above the solitary, sometimes paired, broadly bell-shaped, pendent, pale green flowers, to 4.5cm (1¾in) long, stained maroon at the base, borne in spring. Cultivation group 1 or 2. ↕ 15–20cm (6–8in), ↔ 5cm (2in). N. Greece to N.W. Turkey. ✲✲✲

F. pudica ■ (Yellow fritillary). Bulbous perennial with linear to narrowly lance-shaped, mid-green, sometimes slightly glaucous leaves, 6–20cm (2½–8in) long, the lower ones opposite, the upper ones alternate. In early spring, bears narrowly bell-shaped, pendent, golden to orange-yellow flowers, sometimes tinted red, to 2.5cm (1in) long, singly or in pairs. Cultivation group 4. ↕ to 15cm (6in), ↔ 5cm (2in). W. North America. ✲✲✲

F. pyrenaica ♀ syn. *F. nigra* of gardens. Bulbous perennial with alternate, lance-shaped, glaucous, grey-green leaves, 4.5–11cm (1¾–4½in) long. In late spring, bears solitary, rarely 2, broadly bell-shaped, deep brownish purple, occasionally yellow flowers, strongly tessellated, to 3.5cm (1½in) long, with recurved tepal tips, yellow-green within. Cultivation group 1. ↕ to 45cm (18in), ↔ 5–8cm (2–3in). Pyrenees. ✲✲✲

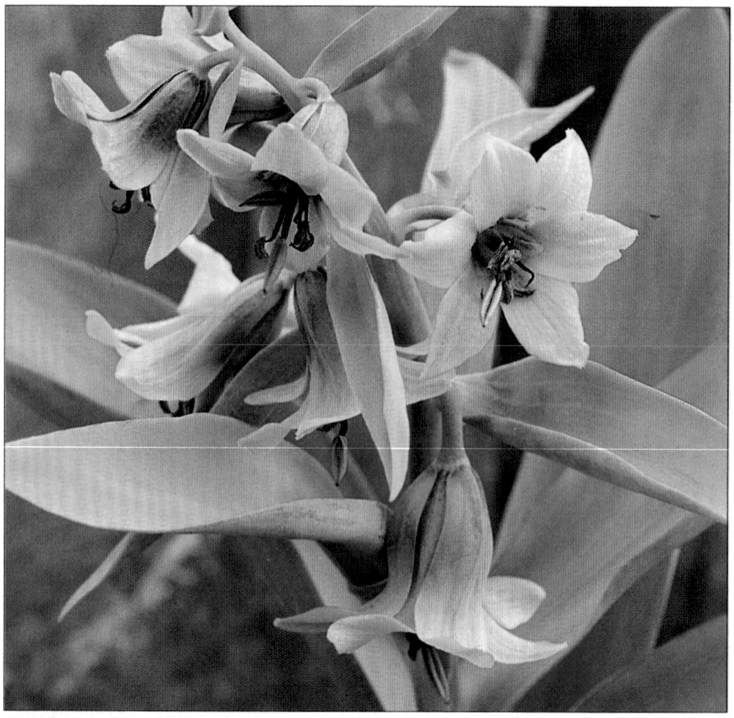

Fritillaria sewerzowii

F. raddeana ■ Robust, bulbous perennial with alternate or whorled, lance-shaped, lustrous, pale green leaves, to 15cm (6in) long. In early spring, bears umbels of 5 or 6, occasionally to 20, broadly bell-shaped, nodding, greenish cream or pale yellow flowers, to 6cm (2½in) long; each umbel is crowned by a tuft of 10–20 leaf-like bracts. Cultivation group 1 or 3. ↕ 60cm (24in), ↔ 8–20cm (3–8in). N.E. Iran, Turkmenistan. ✲✲✲

F. recurva (Scarlet fritillary). Bulbous perennial with whorls of linear-lance-shaped, grey-green, often glaucous leaves, 3–10cm (1¼–4in) long. In spring, bears spike-like racemes of 3–12 narrowly bell-shaped, pendent, faintly yellow-chequered, bright orange-red to scarlet flowers, to 3.5cm (1½in) long, recurved at the mouth. Cultivation group 4. Produces numerous "rice-grain" bulblets that take several years to reach flowering size. ↕ to 60cm (24in), ↔ 8–10cm (3–4in). USA (S. Oregon, California). ✲✲✲

F. roderickii see *F. biflora* 'Martha Roderick'.

F. sewerzowii ■ syn. *Korolkowia sewerzowii.* Variable, stout-stemmed, bulbous perennial with mostly alternate, broadly lance-shaped, grey-green leaves, to 15cm (6in) long, the lowest opposite. In spring, produces elongated racemes of up to 12, rarely solitary, narrowly bell-shaped, nodding, often glaucous, greenish yellow to vivid purple flowers; each flower is yellow to brick-red at the base and within, to 3.5cm (1½in) long, flared at the mouth and stained purple at the throat. Cultivation group 2 or 4. ↕ to 30cm (12in), ↔ 8–10cm (3–4in). Uzbekistan, Tajikistan (Pamirs), N.W. China (Tien Shan Mountains). ✲✲✲

F. stenanthera. Bulbous perennial with a pair of opposite, ovate, mid-green basal leaves, and alternate, lance-shaped to linear stem leaves, to 16cm (6in) long. In early spring, bears racemes of 4–8 narrowly bell-shaped, nodding pink flowers, to 2cm (¾in) long, flared at the mouths, with dark purple centres. Cultivation group 4. ↕ to 20cm (8in), ↔ 5cm (2in). Uzbekistan. ✲✲✲

F. thunbergii ■ syn. *F. verticillata* var. *thunbergii.* Bulbous perennial with opposite, alternate or whorled, linear, glossy, mid-green leaves, to 15cm (6in) long. In spring, bears loose racemes of 2–6 broadly bell-shaped or cup-shaped, nodding, creamy white flowers, to 3.5cm (1½in) long, faintly tessellated or veined green. Cultivation group 1. ↕ to 60cm (24in), ↔ 10–12cm (4–5in). C. China. ✲✲✲

F. tubiformis, syn. *F. delphinensis.* Bulbous perennial with alternate, linear-lance-shaped, glaucous, grey-green leaves, to 5–9cm (2–3½in) long. In late spring, bears solitary, broadly bell-shaped flowers, to 5cm (2in) long, grey-purple externally and white within, with purplish brown tessellations. Cultivation group 2 or 4. ↕ to 15cm (6in), ↔ 5cm (2in). French and Italian Alps. ✲✲✲. **subsp. *moggridgei*** has bright yellow flowers with black chequering.

F. uva-vulpis, syn. *F. assyriaca* of gardens. Bulbous perennial with alternate, lance-shaped, glossy, mid-green leaves, 5–12cm (2–5in) long. In spring, produces solitary, occasionally 2, narrowly bell-shaped, pendent, glaucous, dark brownish purple flowers, tinged yellow within, to 2.5cm (1in) long, with deep yellow, recurving tepal tips. Cultivation group 2 or 4. ↕ to 20cm (8in), ↔ 5cm (2in). S.E. Turkey, N. Iraq, W. Iran. ✲✲✲

F. verticillata* var. *thunbergii see *F. thunbergii.*

▷ **Fritillary** see *Fritillaria*
  Black see *F. biflora*
  Rice-grain see *F. affinis*
  Scarlet see *F. recurva*
  Snake's head see *F. meleagris*
  Yellow see *F. pudica*

▷ **Frogbit** see *Hydrocharis, H. morsus-ranae*

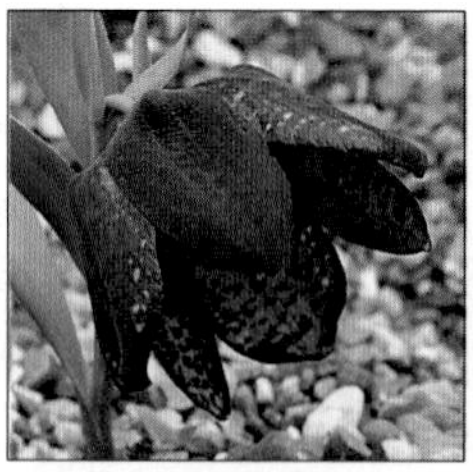

Fritillaria latifolia

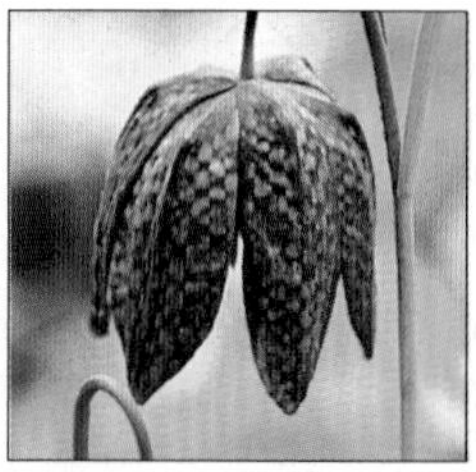

Fritillaria meleagris

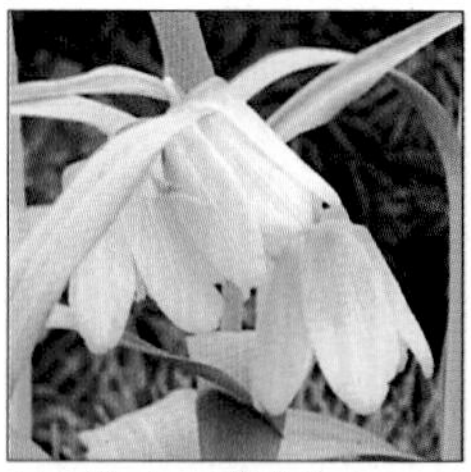

Fritillaria pallidiflora

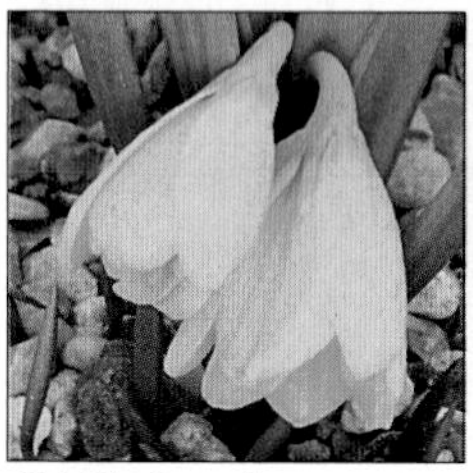

Fritillaria pudica

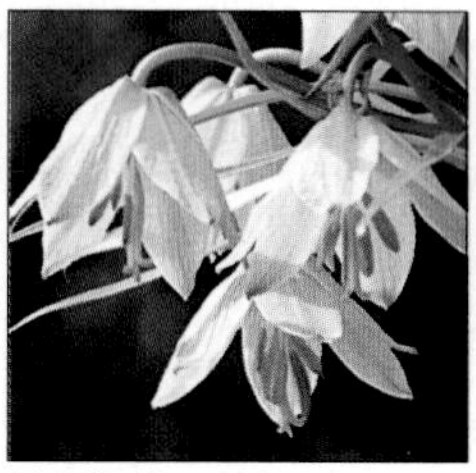

Fritillaria raddeana

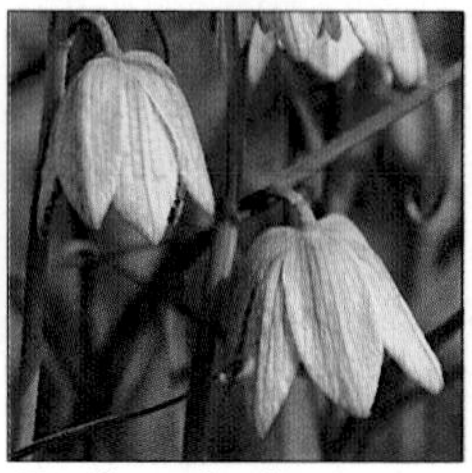

Fritillaria thunbergii

FUCHSIA

FUCHSIA

ONAGRACEAE

Genus of approximately 100 species of deciduous or evergreen trees and shrubs, and a few perennials, from mountainous areas of Central and South America and New Zealand. There are more than 8,000 hybrids and cultivars, which have been developed for their attractive and distinctive flowers, usually borne more or less continuously from summer to autumn. *F. magellanica* is the hardiest species and has been used extensively to produce the modern hardy fuchsias; hybrids of *F. triphylla* have produced the Triphylla Group fuchsias (see panel).

Fuchsia flowers are axillary and usually pendulous, in terminal clusters, with short to long perianth tubes, each topped by far-spreading, coloured sepals and 4 erect, broad petals forming a cup or bell. In some species, the petals are very small or absent. In the following entries, flowers described as "very small" are 0.5–2cm (¼–¾in) across the sepals; "small" are 2–4cm (¾–1½in) across; "medium" are 4–6cm (1½–2½in) across; and "large" are 6cm (2½in) or more across. Fuchsia leaves are opposite or whorled, rarely alternate, simple, lance-shaped to very broadly ovate, mid-green, 0.5–25cm (¼–10in) long, occasionally to 40cm (16in). They are frequently toothed, grow in pairs (sometimes in whorls of 3), and are deciduous unless stated otherwise below. The fruits are berries, usually with many seeds.

In frost-prone areas, treat most fuchsias as half-hardy perennials and grow or overwinter them in a cool or temperate greenhouse. Frost-hardy fuchsias can be left in the open garden throughout winter if correctly planted and mulched (see below). In warmer climates, plant fuchsias in the open garden in a border: grow those with strong, erect stems as bushes, standards, pillars, espaliers, or fans, while those with a trailing habit may be used as weeping standards or grown in a hanging basket, window-box, or trough. *F. procumbens* can be grown in a rock garden in frost-free or mild climates.

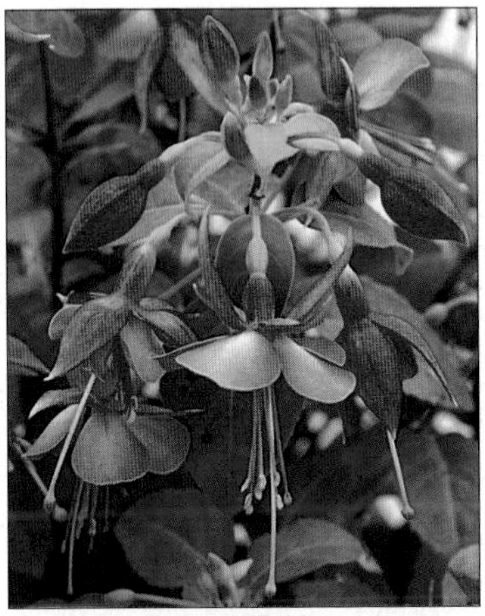

Fuchsia 'Andrew Hadfield'

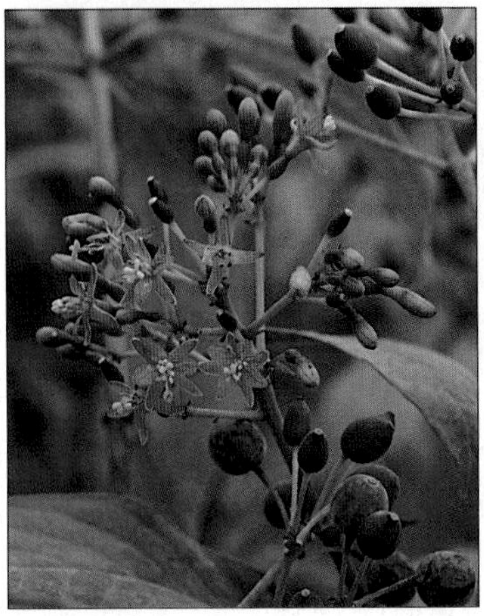

Fuchsia arborescens

FUCHSIA FLOWERS

Fuchsia flowers are usually tubular and pendent, often bicoloured, with a corolla of one hue, and a tube and 4 sepals of another. Single flowers have 4 petals; semi-double flowers 5–7 petals; double flowers 8 or more petals; fully double flowers have more than 8 petals. Triphylla Group fuchsias have long-tubed, single flowers and usually purple-backed foliage. Flowers of *F. procumbens* are erect.

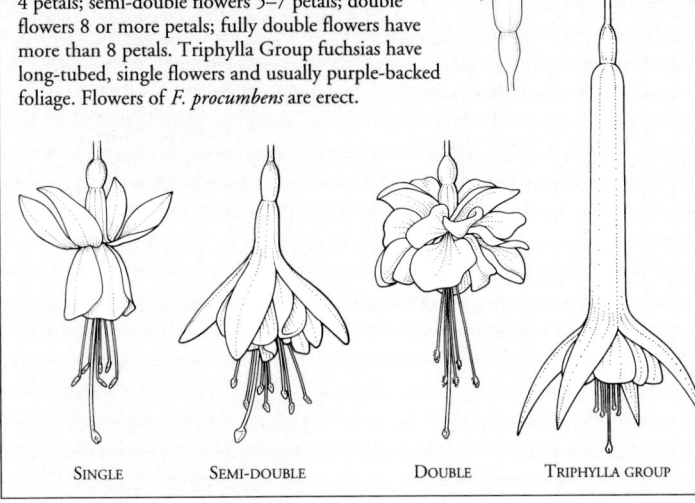

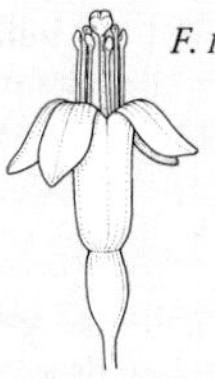

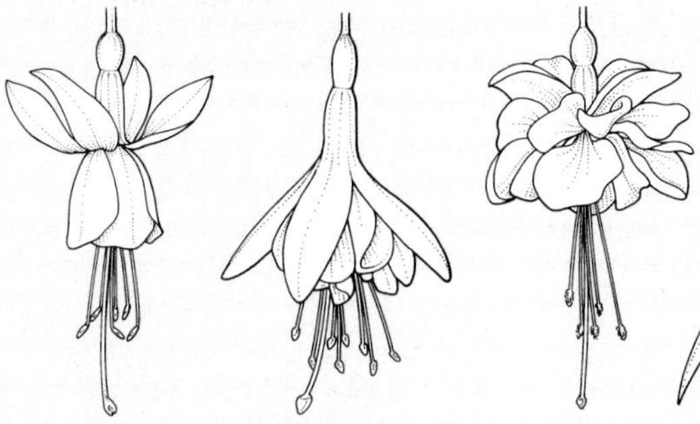

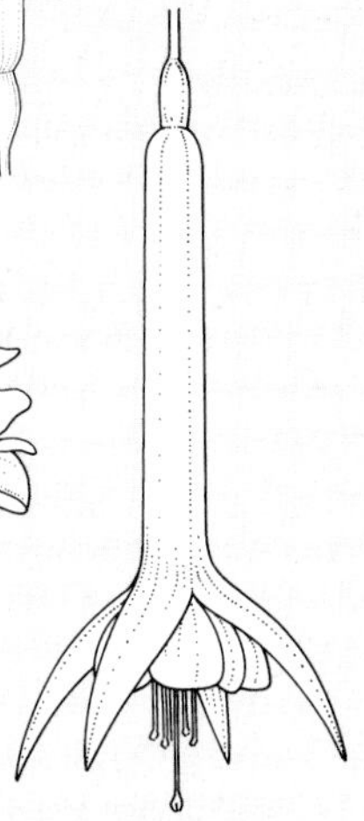

• **HARDINESS** Fully hardy to frost tender, but even fully hardy plants may lose some of their upper growth after severe frosts. If temperatures remain above 4°C (39°F), many fuchsias are more or less evergreen.

• **CULTIVATION** Outdoors, grow in fertile, moist but well-drained soil in full sun or partial shade. For all but the hardiest fuchsias, plant the base of the stem 5cm (2in) below the soil surface and provide a deep, winter mulch. Shelter from cold, drying winds. Under glass, grow in loam-based potting compost (JI No.3) or loamless potting compost, in bright filtered light with moderate to high humidity; ventilate well. During growth, water freely and apply a balanced liquid fertilizer monthly, or every 2 weeks in loamless composts. Keep just moist in winter. Pruning group 6; cut back to base in frost-prone areas.

• **PROPAGATION** Sow seed at 15–24°C (59–75°F) in spring. Root softwood cuttings in spring, or semi-ripe cuttings in late summer with bottom heat.

• **PESTS AND DISEASES** Susceptible to whiteflies, vine weevil, capsid bugs, aphids, red spider mites, grey mould (*Botrytis*), and rust.

***F.* 'Alice Hoffman'.** Free-flowering, upright shrub with densely clustered, purple-tinged, bronze-green foliage. Small, semi-double flowers have rose-pink tubes and sepals, and white corollas veined rose-pink. ↕↔ 45–60cm (18–24in). ❄❄ (borderline)

***F.* 'Andrew Hadfield'** ▣ Very free-flowering, upright shrub bearing medium, single flowers with carmine-red tubes and sepals, and white-based, pink-veined, bright lilac-blue corollas. ↕ 20–45cm (8–18in), ↔ 20–30cm (8–12in). ❀ (min. 5°C/41°F)

***F.* 'Annabel'** ▣ 𝕐 Very free-flowering, upright bush with mid- to light green foliage. Medium, fully double flowers have pink-striped white tubes, white sepals with a slight pink flush, and pink-veined white corollas. Flowers bruise readily. ↕↔ 30–60cm (12–24in). ❄

F. arborea see *F. arborescens*.

F. arborescens ▣ syn. *F. arborea* (Lilac fuchsia). Erect, evergreen shrub or small tree with opposite or whorled, elliptic to inversely lance-shaped, thin, dark green leaves, 10–20cm (4–8in) long. Erect, corymb-like panicles of very small flowers, with rose to magenta or purple-pink tubes, rose-purple sepals, and pale mauve corollas, to 1.5cm (½in) across, appear in one flush in summer. The purple fruit are almost spherical, to 1.5cm (½in) long. ↕ to 2m (6ft), ↔ to 1.7m (5½ft). Mexico, Central America. ❀ (min. 5°C/41°F)

***F.* 'Auntie Jinks'** ▣ Very free-flowering, trailing shrub bearing small, single flowers with pink-red tubes, cerise-margined white sepals, and white-shaded purple corollas. ↕ 15–20cm (6–8in), ↔ 20–40cm (8–16in). ❄

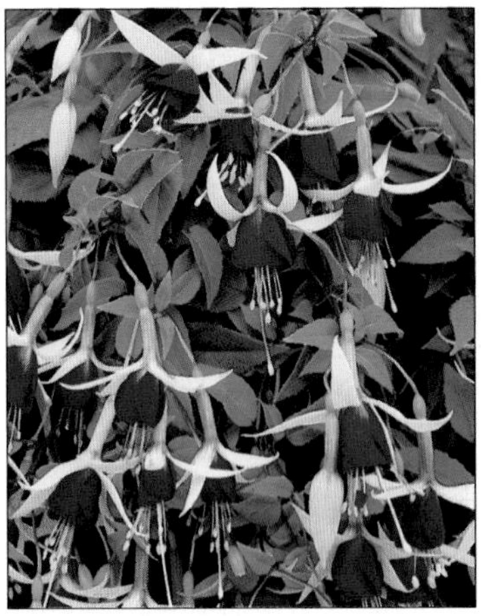

Fuchsia 'Auntie Jinks'

***F.* 'Autumnale'** ▣ syn. *F.* 'Burning Bush'. Prostrate shrub with green and yellow foliage that matures to dark red and salmon with splashes of yellow. Medium, single flowers, with scarlet-rose tubes and sepals, and purple corollas, are produced in late summer. ↕ 15–30cm (6–12in), ↔ 30–60cm (12–24in). ❄

F.* x *bacillaris ▣ (*F. microphylla* x *F. thymifolia*) syn. *F. parviflora* of gardens. Erect or spreading shrub with thin, wiry stems and lance-shaped to ovate, hairy-margined leaves, 0.5–2.5cm (¼–1in) long. Bears very small pink to deep red flowers, 5–8mm (¼–⅜in) across, and almost spherical, glossy, purple-brown fruit. ↕↔ 60–120cm (2–4ft). Natural hybrid from Mexico. ❄❄

***F.* 'Ballet Girl'** ▣ Very free-flowering, upright shrub bearing large, double flowers, each with bright cerise tubes and sepals, and white corollas with cerise veins at the bases. ↕ 30–45cm (12–18in), ↔ 45–75cm (18–30in). ❄

***F.* 'Bicentennial'** ▣ Free-flowering, lax shrub producing medium, double flowers with thin white tubes, orange sepals, and double corollas with magenta centres surrounded by orange petals. ↕ 30–45cm (12–18in), ↔ 45–60cm (18–24in). ❄

***F.* 'Billy Green'** ▣ 𝕐 Extremely free-flowering, upright Triphylla Group shrub with light olive-green foliage. Small flowers, with long, tapering tubes,

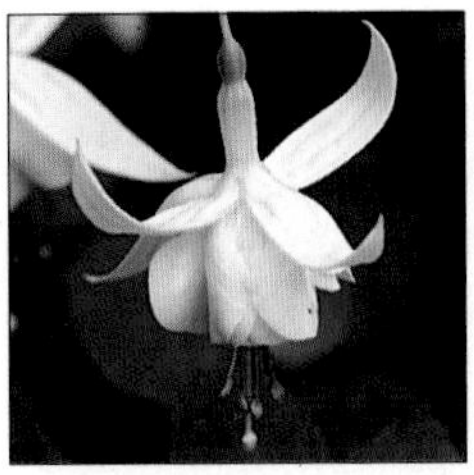

Fuchsia 'Annabel'

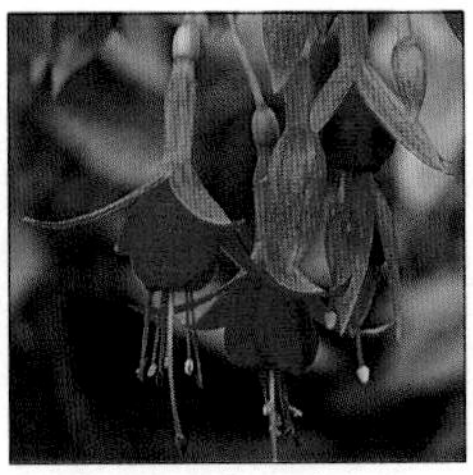

Fuchsia 'Autumnale'

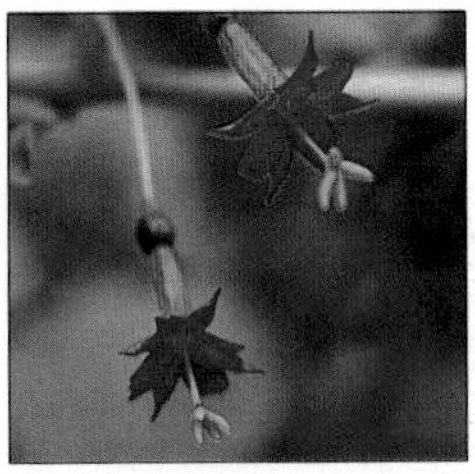

Fuchsia x *bacillaris*

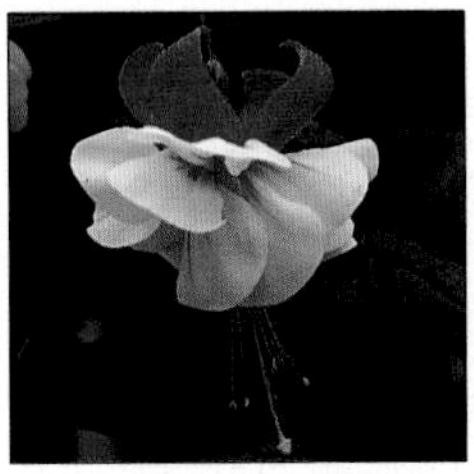

Fuchsia 'Ballet Girl'

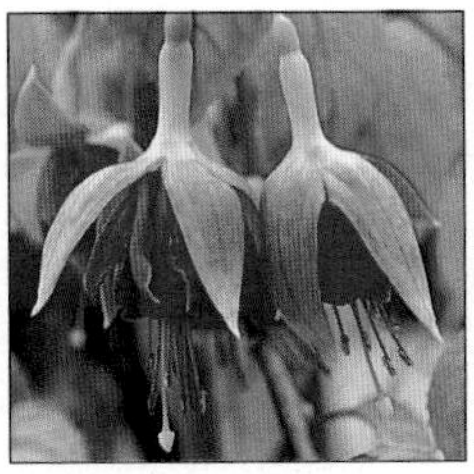

Fuchsia 'Bicentennial'

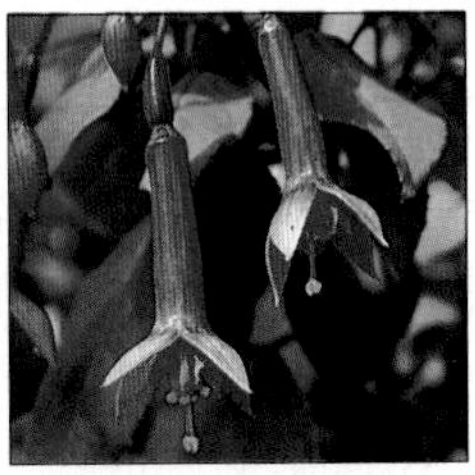

Fuchsia 'Billy Green'

F

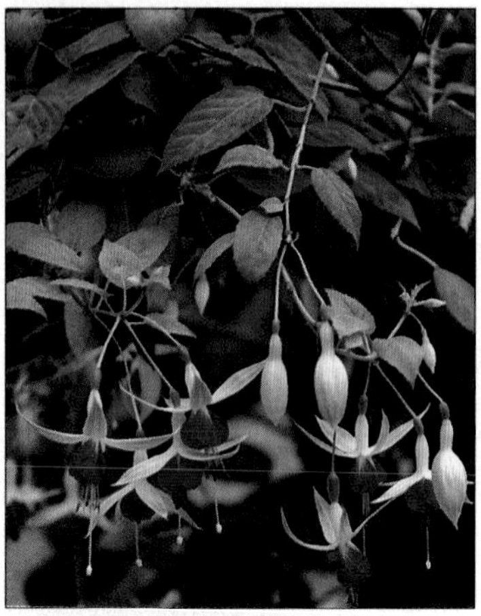

Fuchsia 'Celia Smedley'

salmon-pink sepals, and finely pointed, salmon-pink corollas, are borne at each leaf axil on strong stems. ↕45–60cm (18–24in), ↔ 30–45cm (12–18in). ✲
F. boliviana. Shrub or small tree with lax, arching shoots, and opposite or 3-whorled, narrowly elliptic to broadly ovate, finely glandular-toothed, hairless to softly hairy leaves, 20cm (8in) long, sometimes with reddish veins. Bears large, pendent, terminal racemes or panicles, 5cm (2in) long, of small flowers with pale pink to vermilion tubes, reflexed pale pink to red sepals, and scarlet petals. ↕ to 4m (12ft), ↔ 1–1.2m (3–4ft). S. Peru to N. Argentina. ❀ (min. 5°C/41°F). **var. *alba*** ■ ♀ syn. var. *luxurians*, has white tubes, and white sepals with light red marks at the bases.
***F.* 'Bon Accorde'.** Free-flowering, upright shrub with strong stems. Bears small, erect, single flowers with waxy, ivory-white tubes and sepals, and pale purple corollas suffused white. ↕45–60cm (18–24in), ↔ 30–45cm (12–18in). ✲
***F.* 'Brookwood Belle'** ♀ Lax, bushy shrub with strong, short-jointed stems. Medium, double flowers have deep cerise tubes and sepals, and white corollas flushed pink and veined deep rose-pink. ↕↔ 45–60cm (18–24in). ✲✲
***F.* 'Burning Bush'** see *F.* 'Autumnale'.
***F.* 'Cascade'.** Free-flowering, trailing shrub bearing medium, single flowers with long, thin white tubes and sepals, heavily flushed carmine-red, and deep carmine-red corollas. ↕15–30cm (6–12in), ↔ 30–45cm (12–18in). ✲
***F.* 'Celia Smedley'** ■ ♀ Very free-flowering, upright shrub bearing large, single flowers with dark pink tubes and sepals, and vivid currant-red corollas. ↕↔ 45–75cm (18–30in). ✲
***F.* 'Charming'.** Free-flowering, upright shrub with strong stems and light yellowish green foliage. Medium, single flowers have carmine-red tubes, strongly reflexed, reddish cerise sepals, and cerise-based, rose-purple corollas. ↕45–75cm (18–30in), ↔ 60–75cm (24–30in). ✲✲ (borderline)
***F.* 'Checkerboard'** ■ ♀ Very free-flowering, vigorous, upright shrub with strong stems. Produces medium, single flowers with slightly recurved, long red tubes, red sepals turning white, and white-based, dark red corollas. ↕75–90cm (30–36in), ↔ 45–75cm (18–30in). ✲
***F.* 'Coralle'** ■ ♀ syn. *F.* 'Koralle'. Upright Triphylla Group shrub with strong stems and velvety, olive-green leaves. Bears terminal clusters of very small flowers with tapering, orange-red tubes, pointed, salmon-pink sepals, and orange-red or salmon-pink corollas. ↕45–90cm (18–36in), ↔ 45–60cm (18–24in). ❀ (min. 5°C/41°F)
***F.* 'Dark Eyes'** ♀ Bushy, upright shrub bearing medium, double flowers that hold their shape for a long period. The tubes and upturned sepals are deep red, and the corollas deep violet-blue. ↕45–60cm (18–24in), ↔ 60–75cm (24–30in). ✲
***F.* 'Display'** ♀ Upright, vigorous, freely branching shrub with strong stems and medium, single flowers with carmine-red sepals and rose-pink corollas. ↕60–75cm (24–30in), ↔ 45–60cm (18–24in). ✲✲ (borderline)
***F.* 'Dollar Princess'** ♀ syn. *F.* 'Princess Dollar'. Vigorous, early-flowering, upright shrub producing abundant small to medium, double flowers with cerise tubes and sepals, and rich purple corollas turning deep pink at the base. ↕30–45cm (12–18in), ↔ 45–60cm (18–24in). ✲✲ (borderline)
***F.* 'Elfriede Ott'.** Lax Triphylla Group shrub with dark green leaves. Very small flowers have long, salmon-pink tubes, pointed, salmon-pink sepals, and deeper salmon-pink corollas with curly, rose-red petal margins. ↕45–60cm (18–24in), ↔ 30–45cm (12–18in). ❀ (min. 5°C/41°F)
***F.* 'Estelle Marie'.** Upright shrub with ovate, dark green leaves. Small to medium, semi-erect, single flowers have greenish white tubes, green-tipped, white sepals, and blue-violet corollas that mature to violet with white at the bases. ↕↔ 30–45cm (12–18in). ✲
***F.* 'Flirtation Waltz'.** Vigorous, upright, bushy, freely branching shrub with pale, toothed leaves. Medium, double flowers have pink-flushed, creamy white tubes, wide-spreading, creamy white sepals, and pale pink corollas. ↕45–60cm (18–24in), ↔ 30–45cm (12–18in). ✲
F. fulgens ■ ♀ Upright shrub with spreading branches and ovate to heart-shaped, pale green leaves, 9–23cm (3½–9in) long, with fine, gland-tipped red teeth, flushed red beneath. Pendent terminal racemes of very small flowers, 4–5cm (1½–2in) long, have pink to dull red tubes, pale red sepals tinged yellow-green towards the margins, and bright red corollas. The fruit are oblong-ellipsoid and deep purple. ↕1.5m (5ft) or more, ↔ to 80cm (32in). Mexico. ❀ (min. 5°C/41°F)
***F.* 'Garden News'** ■ ♀ Upright shrub with strong stems producing multiple blooms in each leaf axil. Medium, double flowers have short, thick pink tubes, frost-pink sepals, and magenta-rose corollas becoming rose-pink at the petal bases. ↕↔ 45–60cm (18–24in). ✲✲ (borderline)
***F.* 'Gartenmeister Bonstedt'** ♀ Vigorous, very free-flowering, upright Triphylla Group shrub, similar to *F.* 'Thalia', bearing dark bronze-red leaves with purple undersides and very small, very long-tubed, brick-red flowers. ↕60–75cm (24–30in), ↔ 45–60cm (18–24in). ❀ (min. 5°C/41°F)
***F.* 'Genii'** ■ ♀ Upright, free-flowering shrub with red shoots and lime-yellow foliage. Small, single flowers have cerise tubes and sepals, and violet corollas turning purple-red. ↕↔ 75–90cm (30–36in). ✲✲ (borderline)
***F.* 'Golden Marinka'** ■ ♀ Trailing shrub with variegated leaves of green and yellow. Produces an abundance of medium, single, rich red flowers with slightly darker red corollas. ↕15–30cm (6–12in), ↔ 30–45cm (12–18in). ✲

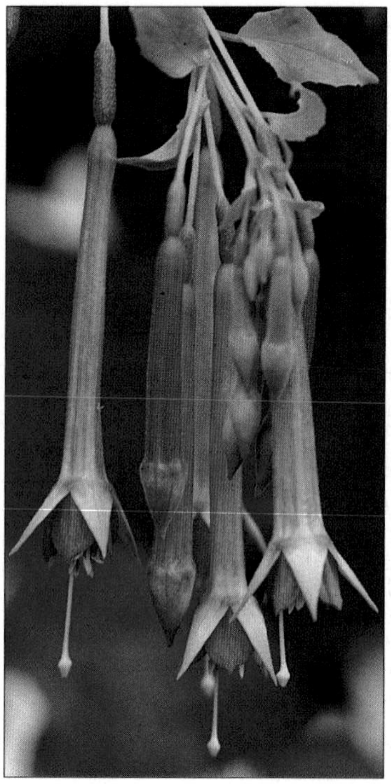

Fuchsia fulgens

***F.* 'Gruss aus dem Bodethal'** ■ (Black fuchsia). Freely branching shrub bearing medium, single flowers with crimson tubes and sepals, and very dark purple corollas. ↕30–45cm (12–18in), ↔ 45–60cm (18–24in). ✲
***F.* 'Heidi Weiss'** see *F.* 'White Ann'.
***F.* 'Herald'** ♀ Vigorous, free-flowering, upright shrub. Medium, single flowers have scarlet tubes and sepals, and deep purple corollas. ↕↔ 60–90cm (24–36in). ✲✲ (borderline)
***F.* 'Hermiena'.** Trailing shrub bearing small to medium, single blooms with white tubes, narrow white sepals, and violet-purple corollas. ↕15–30cm (6–12in), ↔ 30–45cm (12–18in). ✲
***F.* 'Hidcote Beauty'** ■ Free-flowering, upright shrub with light green foliage. Medium, single flowers have waxy cream tubes and sepals, and pale salmon-pink corollas shaded with light rose-pink. ↕45–60cm (18–24in), ↔ 30–60cm (12–24in). ✲
***F.* 'Jack Shahan'** ■ ♀ Free-flowering, trailing shrub bearing large, single flowers with pale rose-pink tubes

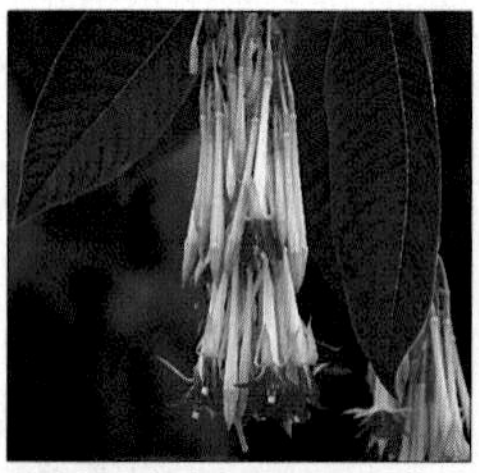

Fuchsia boliviana var. *alba*

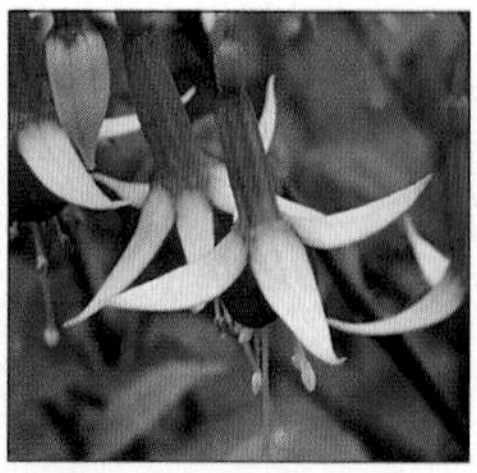

Fuchsia 'Checkerboard'

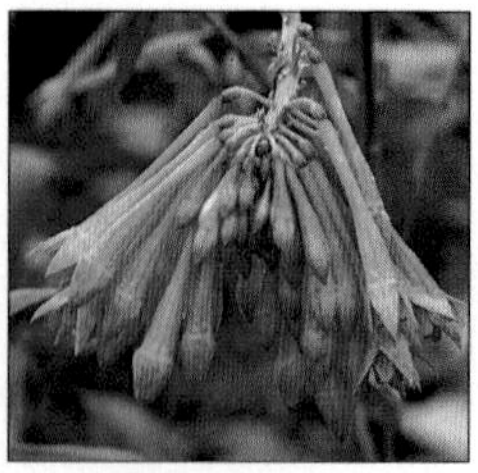

Fuchsia 'Coralle'

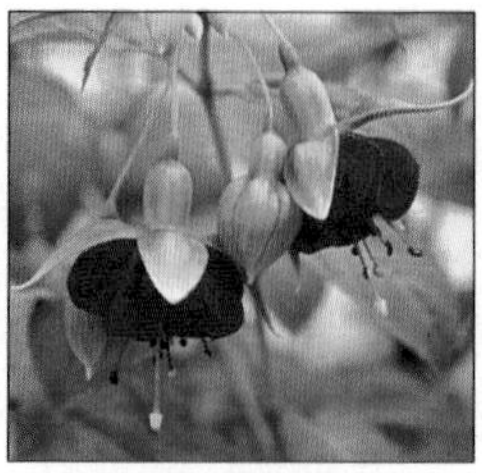

Fuchsia 'Garden News'

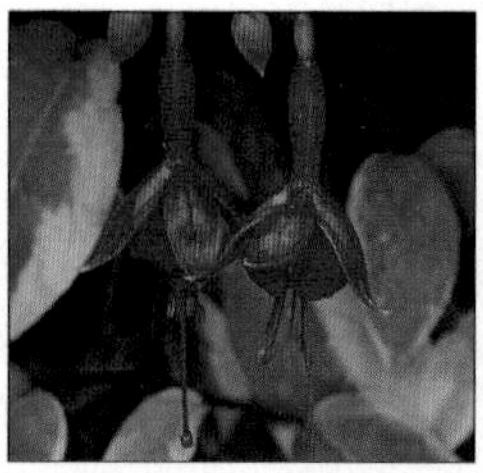

Fuchsia 'Golden Marinka'

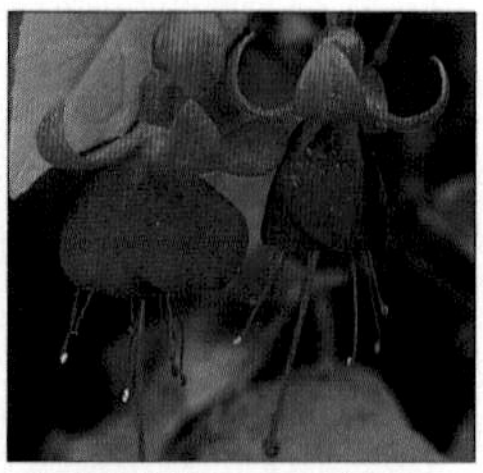

Fuchsia 'Gruss aus dem Bodethal'

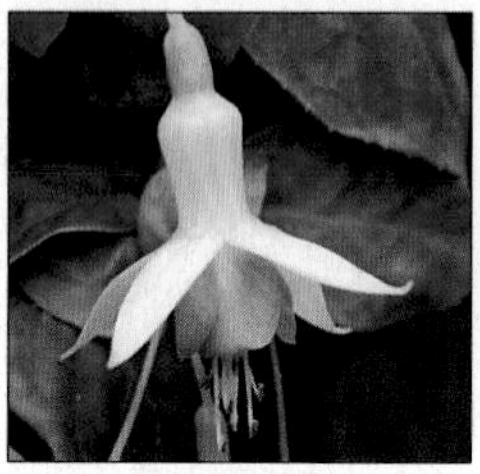

Fuchsia 'Hidcote Beauty'

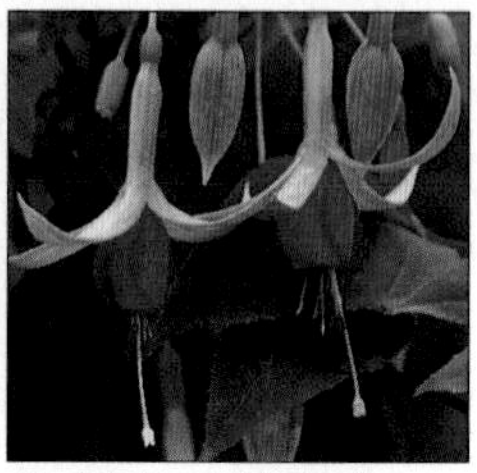

Fuchsia 'Jack Shahan'

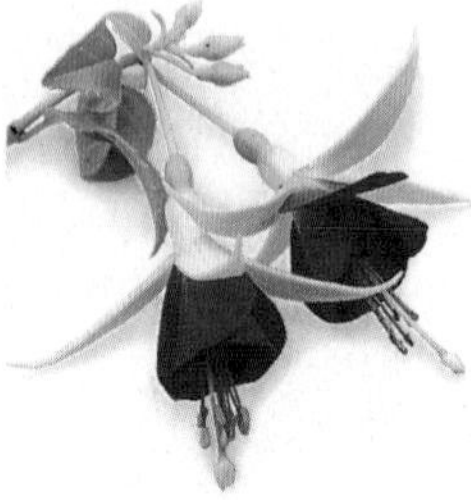

Fuchsia 'Joy Patmore'

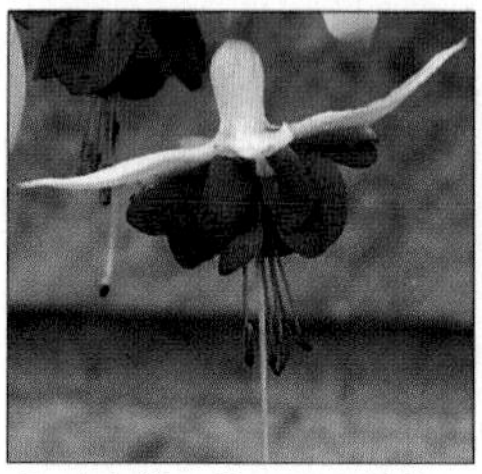

Fuchsia 'La Campanella'

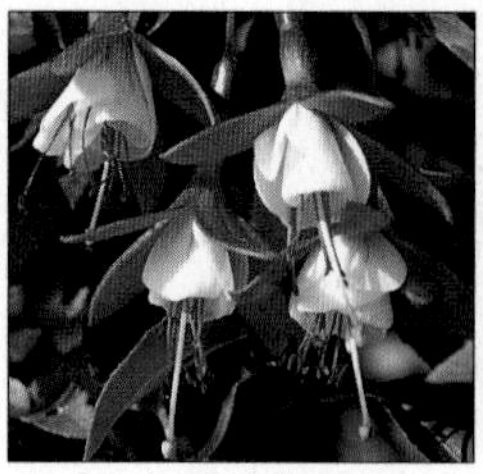

Fuchsia 'Lady Thumb'

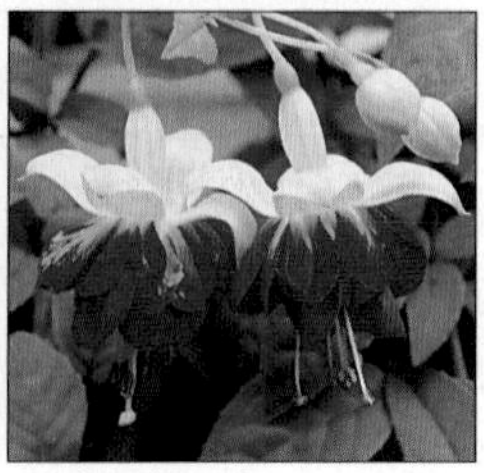

Fuchsia 'Lena'

FUCHSIA

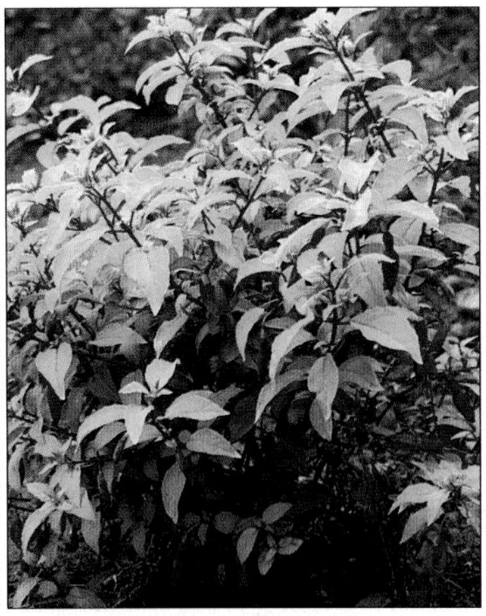

Fuchsia 'Genii'

and sepals, and rose-pink corollas. ↕30–45cm (12–18in), ↔45–60cm (18–24in). ✻

***F.* 'Joy Patmore'** ■ 🏆 Vigorous, upright shrub bearing medium, single flowers with white tubes, and rich carmine-red corollas; the waxy white sepals are tinged pink on the undersides. ↕30–45cm (12–18in), ↔45–60cm (18–24in). ✻

***F.* 'Koralle'** see *F.* 'Coralle'.

***F.* 'La Campanella'** ■ 🏆 Very free-flowering, lax shrub, with sparse growth initially, then rapidly filling out. Small, semi-double flowers have white tubes, white sepals with a slight pink flush, and purple corollas. ↕15–30cm (6–12in), ↔30–45cm (12–18in). ✻

***F.* 'Lady Thumb'** ■ 🏆 Free-flowering, upright shrub bearing small, semi-double flowers with light carmine-red tubes and sepals, and white corollas with slight carmine-red veining. A sport of *F.* 'Tom Thumb'. ↕15–30cm (6–12in), ↔30–45cm (12–18in). ✻✻ (borderline)

***F.* 'Lena'** ■ 🏆 Vigorous, free-flowering, very hardy, lax shrub bearing toothed, pale to mid-green leaves and medium, single to semi-double flowers with flesh-pink, almost white tubes and sepals, the tubes half-reflexed; the rose-magenta corollas are paler pink at the bases. ↕30–60cm (12–24in), ↔60–75cm (24–30in). ✻✻ (borderline)

***F.* 'Leonora'** ■ 🏆 Vigorous, upright, freely branching shrub with medium, bell-shaped, single, soft pink flowers. ↕60–75cm (24–30in), ↔30–60cm (12–24in). ✻

***F.* 'Little Jewel'.** Upright shrub bearing medium, single flowers with carmine-red tubes, star-shaped, carmine-red sepals, and light purple corollas with faint carmine-red markings at the bases. ↕45–60cm (18–24in), ↔30–45cm (12–18in). ✻

***F.* 'Love's Reward'** ■ Upright, short-jointed shrub bearing small to medium, single flowers with white to pale pink tubes and sepals, and violet-blue corollas. ↕↔30–45cm (12–18in). ✻

***F.* 'Lye's Unique'** ■ Free-flowering, upright shrub with strong stems. Medium, single flowers have waxy white tubes and sepals, and salmon-orange corollas. ↕45–60cm (18–24in), ↔30–45cm (12–18in). ✻

***F.* 'Machu Picchu'** ■ Very free-flowering, lax, trailing shrub. Small, single flowers have pale salmon-pink tubes and sepals (with pink undersides to the sepals), and salmon-pink corollas. ↕↔30–60cm (12–24in). ✻

F. magellanica ■ Erect shrub with ovate-elliptic, scalloped to toothed, hairless leaves, 1.5–6cm (½–2½in) long, occasionally with minute stiff hairs, sometimes tinted red beneath. Throughout summer, freely produces small flowers with red tubes, deep red, rarely white or pale pink, wide-spreading sepals, and purple corollas. The fruit are oblong and red-purple. Suitable for hedging in frost-free areas. ↕to 3m (10ft), ↔2–3m (6–10ft). Chile, Argentina. ✻✻ (borderline).

'Riccartonii' see *F.* 'Riccartonii'.

***F.* 'Margaret'** 🏆 Very vigorous, upright shrub bearing abundant small, double flowers with carmine-scarlet tubes and sepals, and violet-purple corollas. Suitable for hedging in frost-free areas. ↕↔to 1.2m (4ft). ✻✻ (borderline)

***F.* 'Margaret Brown'** ■ 🏆 Free-flowering, upright shrub with strong stems and light green foliage. Bears small, single, 2-tone pink flowers in summer. ↕↔60–90cm (24–36in). ✻✻ (borderline)

***F.* 'Marinka'** ■ 🏆 Extremely free-flowering, trailing shrub with dark green leaves veined red beneath. Medium, single flowers have red tubes and sepals, and slightly darker red corollas. ↕15–30cm (6–12in), ↔45–60cm (18–24in). ✻

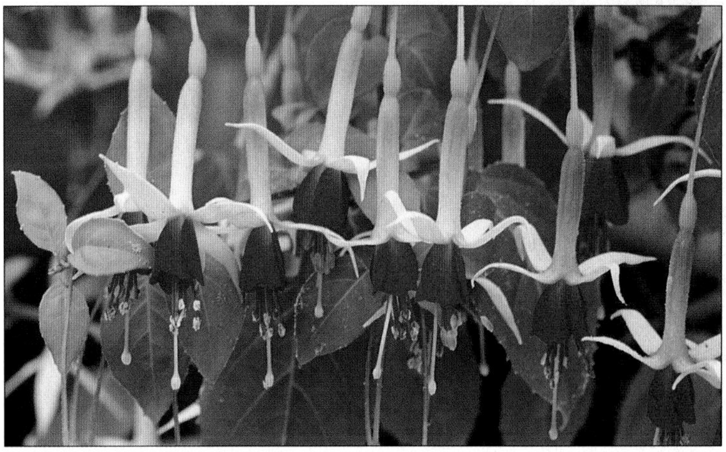

Fuchsia 'Mrs. Lovell Swisher'

***F.* 'Mary'** ■ 🏆 Upright Triphylla Group shrub bearing elliptic, dark green leaves, veined red-purple. Very small, vivid crimson flowers have long tubes and reflexed sepals. ↕↔30–60cm (12–24in). ❀ (min 5°C/41°F)

***F.* 'Micky Gault'** ■ Free-flowering, upright shrub with light green foliage. Small, semi-erect, single flowers have white tubes flushed pink, white sepals with very pale pink undersides, and pink-purple corollas. ↕30–45cm (12–18in), ↔45–60cm (18–24in). ✻

***F.* 'Mieke Meursing'.** Upright, bushy, freely branching shrub bearing medium, single or semi-double flowers with red tubes and sepals, and pale pink corollas veined deeper pink. ↕↔30–60cm (12–24in). ✻

***F.* 'Mrs. Lovell Swisher'** ■ Very vigorous, upright shrub bearing masses of small, single flowers with flesh-pink tubes, pinkish white sepals, and deep rose corollas. ↕45–60cm (18–24in), ↔30–60cm (12–24in). ✻

***F.* 'Mrs. Popple'** ■ 🏆 Upright, bushy, vigorous shrub with deep green leaves. Medium, single flowers have scarlet tubes and sepals, and cerise-centred, purple-violet corollas. ↕↔1–1.1m (3–3½ft). ✻✻✻ (borderline)

***F.* 'Nellie Nuttall'** ■ 🏆 Vigorous, very free-flowering, early-blooming, upright shrub bearing small, upward-looking, single flowers with bright red tubes and sepals, and red-veined white corollas. ↕15–45cm (6–18in), ↔30–45cm (12–18in). ✻

***F.* 'Neopolitan'.** Upright shrub with wiry stems bearing separate, very small, single flowers of red, pink, or white on the same plant. The sepals of each flower reflex back to the tube, and each corolla opens flat. ↕45–60cm (18–24in), ↔60–90cm (24–36in). ✻✻

***F.* 'Other Fellow'** ■ Very free-flowering, upright shrub bearing small, single flowers with waxy white tubes, green-tipped white sepals, and white-based, coral-pink corollas. ↕↔30–45cm (12–18in). ✻

***F.* 'Pacquesa'** 🏆 Upright shrub with foliage borne on freely branching, short-jointed stems. Large, single flowers have deep red tubes, reflexed, glowing, deep red sepals, and pure white corollas veined deep red. ↕45–60cm (18–24in), ↔30–45cm (12–18in). ✻

***F. parviflora* of gardens** see *F.* x *bacillaris*.

***F.* 'Peppermint Stick'.** Upright shrub bearing medium to large, double flowers with carmine-red tubes and upturned, carmine-red sepals, each with a distinct white stripe down the middle. The corollas have rich, royal-purple petals in the centre, and light carmine-rose petals with purple outer margins. ↕↔45–75cm (18–30in). ✻

***F.* 'Phyllis'** 🏆 Very hardy, vigorous, upright shrub bearing masses of small to medium, semi-double flowers with cerise-flushed, waxy, rose-red tubes and sepals, and rose-cerise corollas. Use for hedging. ↕1–1.5m (3–5ft), ↔75–90cm (30–36in). ✻✻ (borderline)

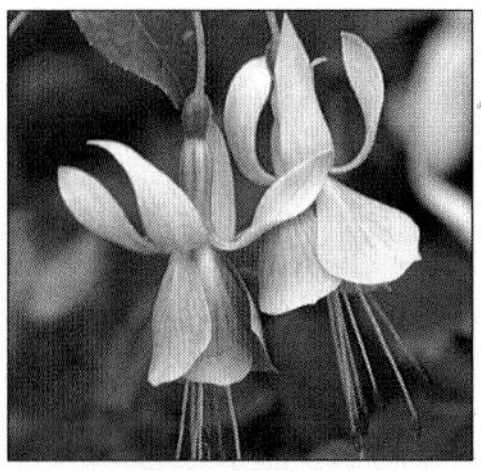

Fuchsia 'Leonora'

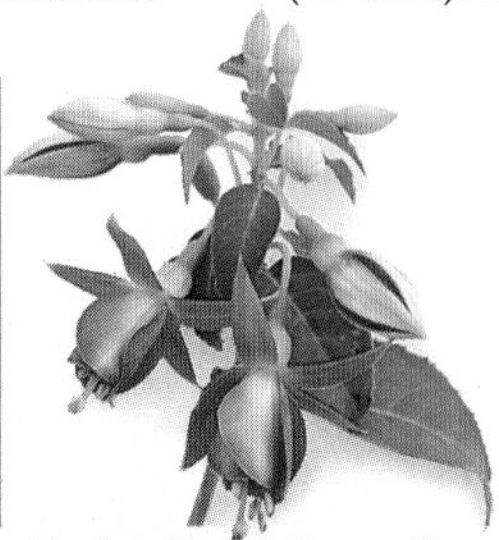

Fuchsia 'Love's Reward'

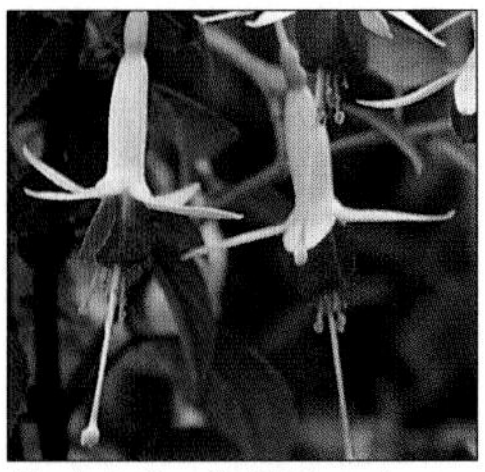

Fuchsia 'Lye's Unique'

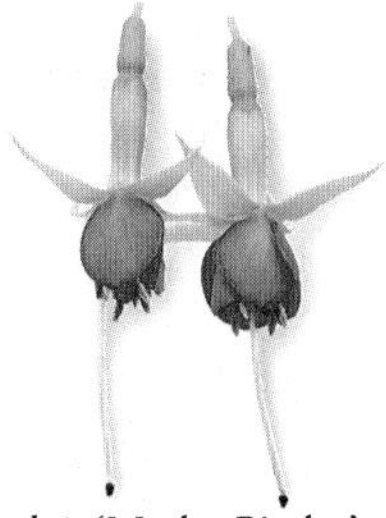

Fuchsia 'Machu Picchu'

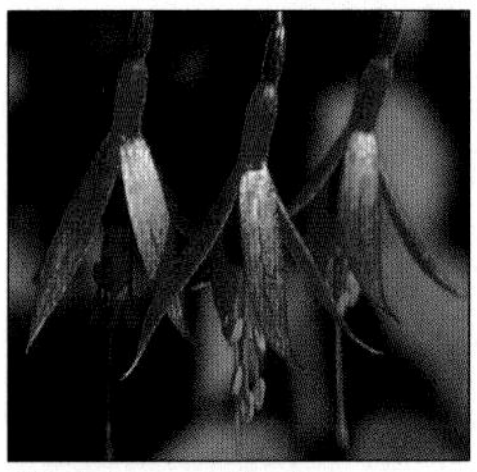

Fuchsia magellanica

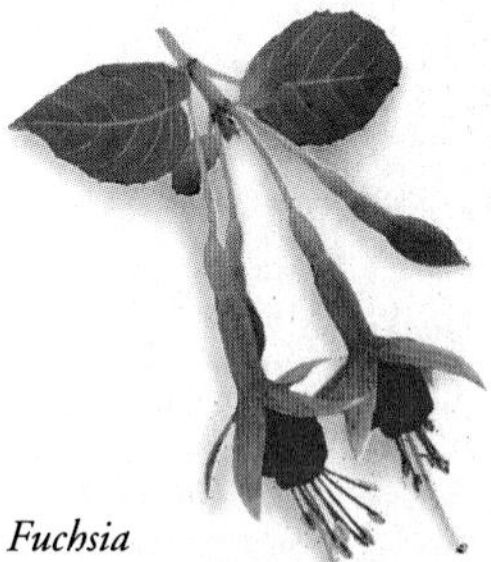

Fuchsia 'Margaret Brown'

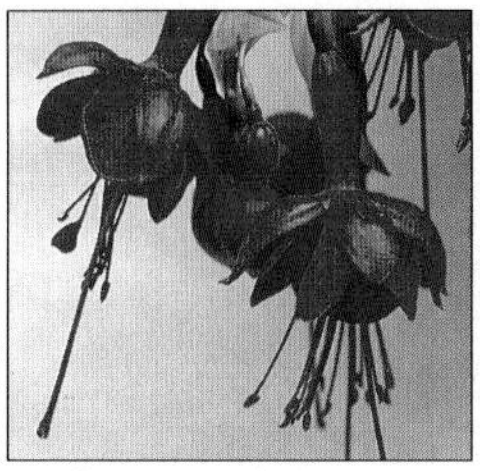

Fuchsia 'Marinka'

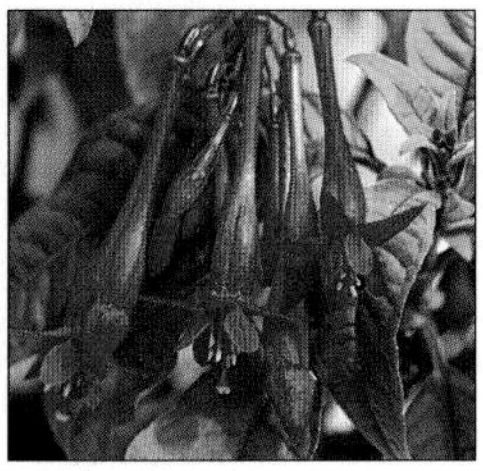

Fuchsia 'Mary'

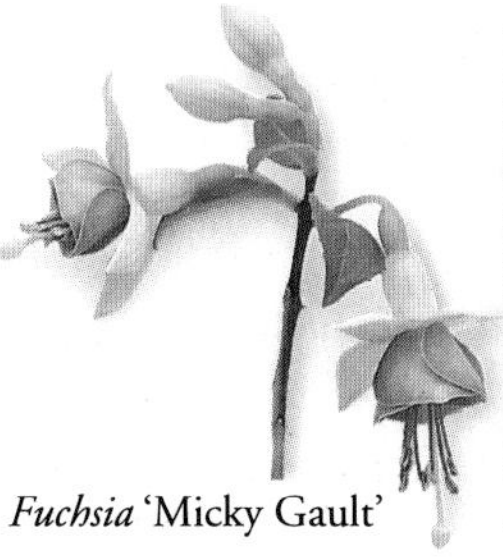

Fuchsia 'Micky Gault'

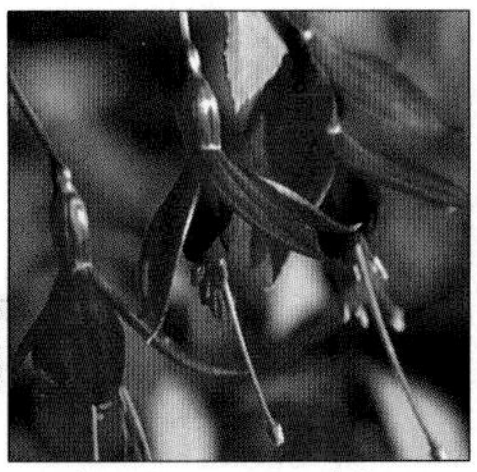

Fuchsia 'Mrs. Popple'

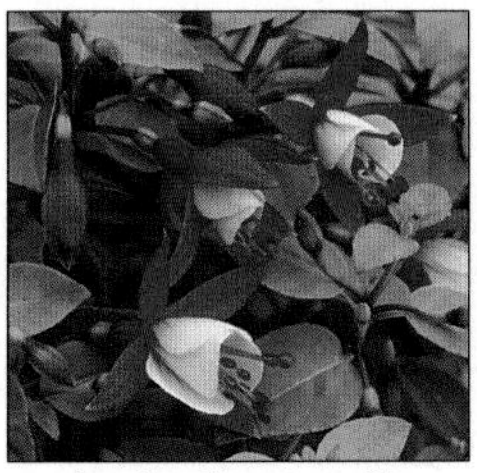

Fuchsia 'Nellie Nuttall'

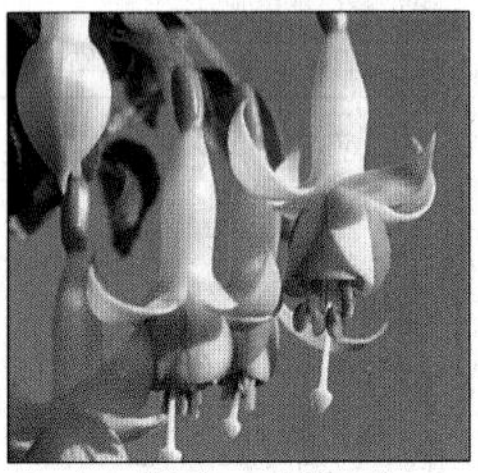

Fuchsia 'Other Fellow'

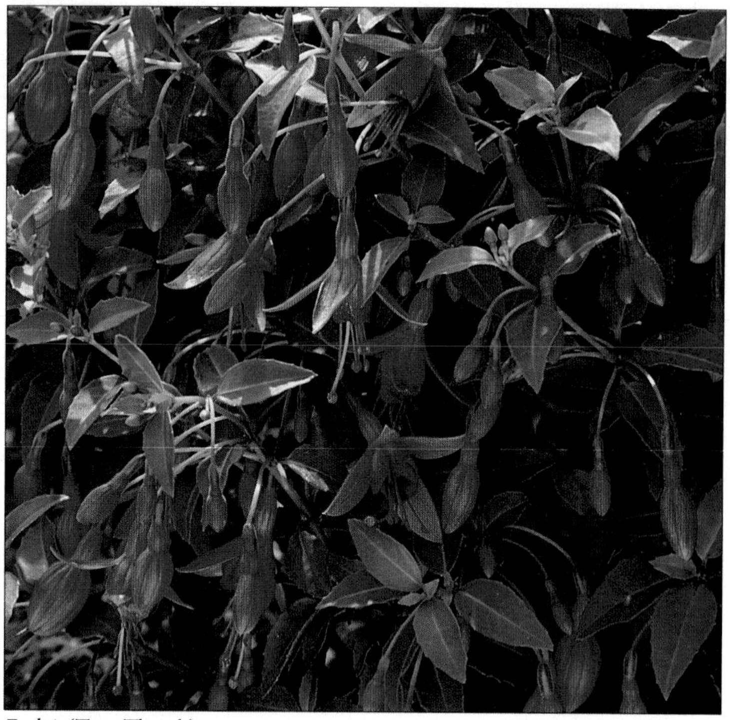

Fuchsia 'Tom Thumb'

***F.* 'Postiljon'.** Trailing shrub bearing small, single flowers. The tubes are creamy white flushed pale pink, the sepals are creamy white flushed rose-pink beneath, and the magenta corollas turn dark mauve-purple when mature. ↕↔ 30–45cm (12–18in). ❄

***F.* 'President Margaret Slater'.** Free-flowering, trailing shrub bearing medium, single flowers with long, thin white tubes and slightly twisted white sepals, flushed salmon-pink on the insides and deep salmon-pink beneath, and mauve-pink corollas. ↕ 30–45cm (12–18in), ↔ 45–75cm (18–30in). ❄

***F.* 'Princess Dollar'** see *F.* 'Dollar Princess'.

F. procumbens ■ (Trailing fuchsia). Prostrate shrub with rounded, heart-shaped leaves, 6–20mm (¼–¾in) long. In summer, produces small, upward-facing flowers, with greenish yellow to pale orange tubes (red-based when mature), and purple-tipped green sepals. There are no corollas, and the stamens bear bright blue pollen. The spherical, glaucous, bright red fruit, to 1.5cm (½in) long, resemble miniature plums. ↕ 10–15cm (4–6in), ↔ 1–1.2m (3–4ft). New Zealand. ❄❄ (borderline)

***F.* 'Red Spider'.** Vigorous, trailing shrub bearing medium, single flowers with deep crimson tubes, narrow, recurved crimson sepals, and deep rose-red corollas. ↕ 15–30cm (6–12in), ↔ 30–60cm (12–24in). ❄

***F.* 'Riccartonii'** ■ ♀ syn. *F. magellanica* 'Riccartonii'. Extremely hardy, upright shrub bearing dark green leaves with a slight bronze sheen. Small, single flowers have scarlet tubes and sepals, and dark purple corollas. Suitable for hedging in frost-free areas. ↕ 2–3m (6–10ft), ↔ 1–2m (3–6ft). ❄❄❄ (borderline)

***F.* 'Rough Silk'.** Trailing shrub with light green foliage. Large, single flowers have pale carmine-pink tubes, upward-sweeping, pale carmine-pink sepals, and crimson-red corollas becoming paler at the bases. ↕ 15–30cm (6–12in), ↔ 30–60cm (12–24in). ❄

***F.* 'Royal Velvet'** ♀ Vigorous, very free-flowering, upright shrub. Medium, double flowers have crimson-red tubes, upturned, crimson-red sepals, and deep purple corollas. ↕ 45–75cm (18–30in), ↔ 30–60cm (12–24in). ❄

***F.* 'Rufus'** ■ syn. *F.* 'Rufus the Red'. Vigorous, early-flowering, upright shrub producing medium, single flowers with bright red tubes, sepals, and corollas. ↕ 45–75cm (18–30in), ↔ 30–60cm (12–24in). ❄❄ (borderline)

***F.* 'Rufus the Red'** see *F.* 'Rufus'.

***F.* 'Swingtime'** ■ ♀ Vigorous, free-flowering, lax, upright shrub bearing red-veined, dark green leaves with finely toothed edges. Large, double blooms have shiny, rich red tubes and sepals, and bright white corollas. ↕ 30–60cm (12–24in), ↔ 45–75cm (18–30in). ❄

***F.* 'Thalia'** ■ ♀ Vigorous, upright Triphylla Group shrub bearing dark olive-green leaves with purple-tinged undersides, and abundant, very small, rich orange-scarlet flowers with very long tubes. ↕↔ 45–90cm (18–36in). ❁ (min. 5°C/41°F)

***F.* 'Tom Thumb'** ■ ♀ Extremely free-flowering, early-flowering, upright shrub bearing small, single flowers with carmine-red tubes and sepals, and mauve corollas veined carmine-red. ↕↔ 15–30cm (6–12in). ❄❄ (borderline)

***F.* 'Tom West'** ■ Upright, lax shrub with green-and-cream-variegated, cerise-veined foliage. Small, single flowers have red tubes and sepals, and purple corollas. ↕↔ 30–60cm (12–24in). ❄

***F.* 'Walsingham'.** Lax, upright shrub with toothed, emerald-green leaves. Medium, semi-double flowers have pale pink tubes, upward-sweeping, pale pink sepals, pale lavender-lilac corollas, and very distinctive, crimped petal margins. ↕ 30–45cm (12–18in), ↔ 45–60cm (18–24in). ❄

***F.* 'White Ann'**, syn. *F.* 'Heidi Weiss'. Vigorous, free-flowering, upright shrub bearing dark green leaves with crimson midribs. Medium, double flowers have crimson-cerise tubes and sepals, and white corollas with scarlet veins. ↕↔ 30–60cm (12–24in). ❄❄

***F.* 'Winston Churchill'** ♀ Extremely free-flowering, bushy, upright shrub bearing medium, fully double flowers with green-tipped pink tubes, broad, reflexed, green-tipped pink sepals, and lavender-blue corollas, maturing to pale purple. ↕↔ 45–75cm (18–30in). ❄

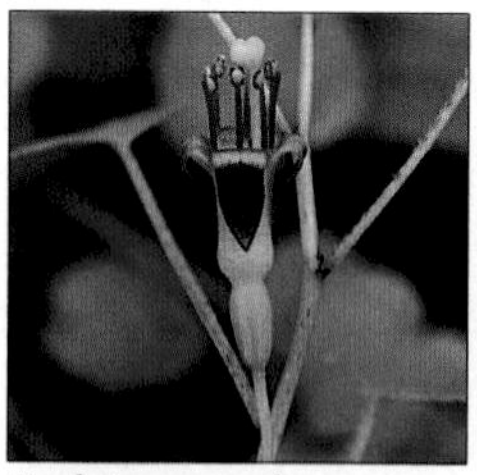

Fuchsia procumbens

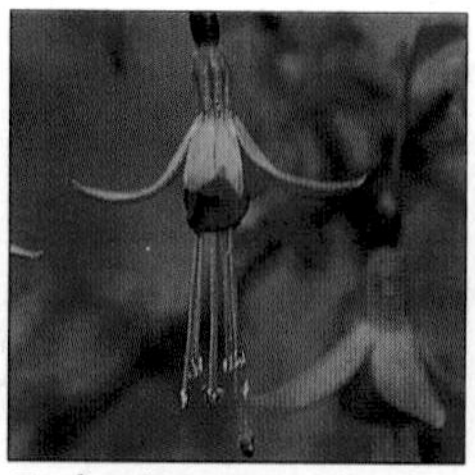

Fuchsia 'Riccartonii'

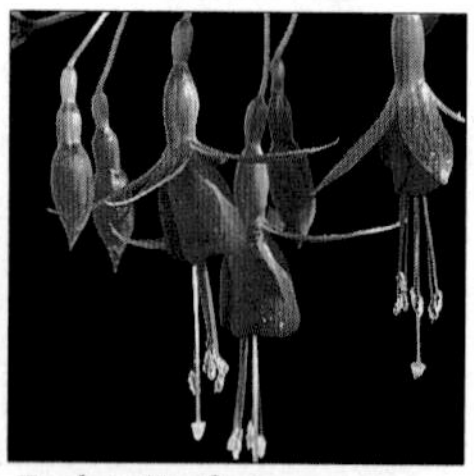

Fuchsia 'Rufus'

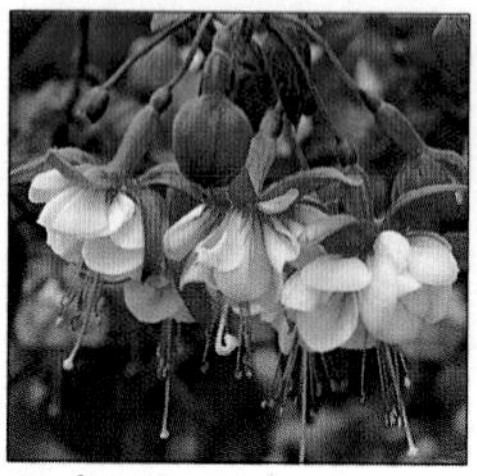

Fuchsia 'Swingtime'

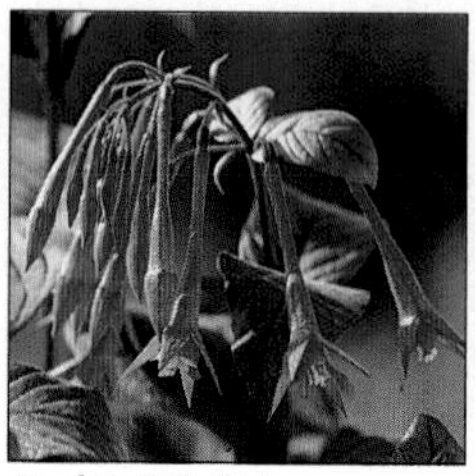

Fuchsia 'Thalia'

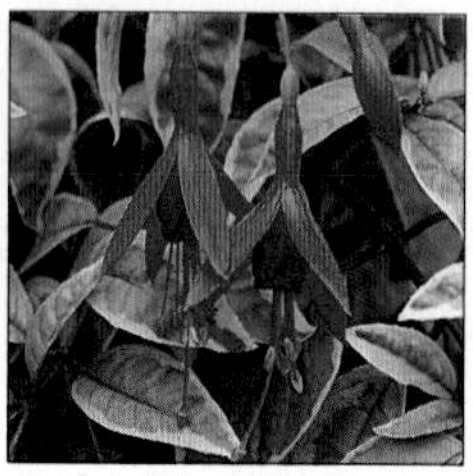

Fuchsia 'Tom West'

▷**Fuchsia,**
Australian see *Correa*
Black see *Fuchsia* 'Gruss aus dem Bodethal'
Californian see *Zauschneria*
Lilac see *Fuchsia arborescens*
Trailing see *Fuchsia procumbens*
Tree see *Schotia brachypetala*

▷**Fuchsia bush** see *Eremophila glabra*

▷**Fukanoki** see *Schefflera heptaphylla*

▷**Fumewort** see *Corydalis solida*

▷**Fumitory, Climbing** see *Adlumia fungosa*

FURCRAEA

AGAVACEAE

Genus of 12 or more species of perennial succulents from desert-like areas of the West Indies, Central America, and N. South America. Dense clusters of long, fleshy leaves are borne in terminal or basal rosettes. In summer, each rosette produces a large, terminal, pyramidal panicle bearing broadly bell-shaped, pendulous, diurnal flowers. Small, adventitious plantlets often form between the flowers. Where temperatures drop below 7°C (45°F), grow in a temperate greenhouse; in warmer climates, use in a desert garden or as specimen plants.

- **HARDINESS** Frost tender.
- **CULTIVATION** Under glass, grow in standard cactus compost in full light with low humidity. During growth, water moderately and apply a low-nitrogen fertilizer monthly. Keep just moist in autumn and winter. Outdoors, grow in poor to moderately fertile, sharply drained soil in full sun. Protect from winter wet. See also pp.48–49.
- **PROPAGATION** Sow seed at 15–24°C (59–75°F) in spring. Divide offsets or pot up plantlets in summer.
- **PESTS AND DISEASES** Susceptible to scale insects.

***F. foetida* 'Mediopicta'** ■ syn. *F. foetida* 'Variegata', *F. gigantea* 'Mediopicta'. Succulent, sometimes clump-forming, with a stem 80–90cm (32–36in) long, and terminal rosettes of broadly inversely lance-shaped to lance-shaped, bright, glossy, mid-green leaves, to 2.5m (8ft) long, with creamy white longitudinal lines; the margins are smooth or bear a few hooked spines. In summer, bears inflorescences, 6–12m (20–40ft) high, of strongly scented white flowers, 5–6cm (2–2½in) long, with green outer petals. Produces plantlets freely. ↕ 1–1.2m (3–4ft), ↔ 2.5m (8ft). Probably West Indies, possibly S. Brazil. ❁ (min. 7°C/45°F)

***F. foetida* 'Variegata'** see *F. foetida* 'Mediopicta'.

***F. gigantea* 'Mediopicta'** see *F. foetida* 'Mediopicta'.

F. selloa. Variable succulent, sometimes clump-forming, with stems to 1.5m (5ft) long. Bears spreading terminal rosettes of narrowly lance-shaped to sword-shaped, rough, glossy, mid-green leaves, 1.2m (4ft) or more long, with large, brown, marginal, hooked spines. Lax-branched inflorescences, to 5m (15ft) high, of faintly scented white flowers, 6–7cm (2½–3in) long, with green outer petals, develop in summer. Produces plantlets freely. ↕ 1.5m (5ft), ↔ 2m (6ft). Mexico, Guatemala, Colombia. ❁ (min. 7°C/45°F). **'Marginata'** has pale, green-white leaf margins.

▷**Furze** see *Ulex, U. europaeus*

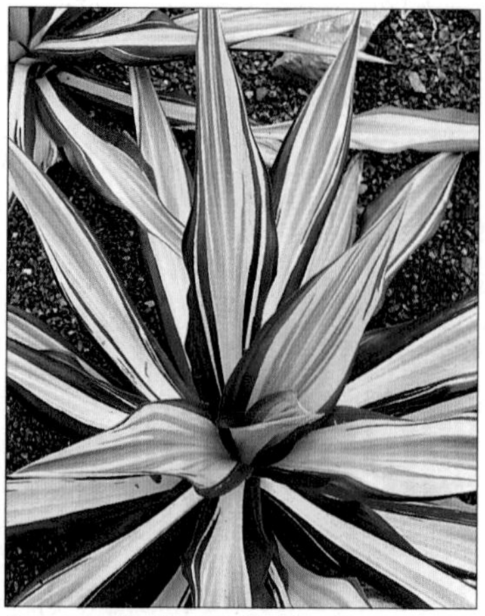

Furcraea foetida 'Mediopicta'

G

GAGEA

LILIACEAE

Genus of about 50 species of small, bulbous perennials from Europe, N. Africa, and W. and C. Asia. They are grown for their star-shaped to cup- or funnel-shaped, yellow or white flowers, borne in umbels or racemes, with prominent leaf-like bracts, from spring to early summer. The leaves are basal, long, and linear or linear-lance-shaped. Some species produce bulbils in the axils of basal leaves and in the inflorescences. Most are suitable for a rock garden; in wet climates, *G. graeca* is best grown in an alpine house or bulb frame.

- **HARDINESS** Fully hardy to half hardy.
- **CULTIVATION** Plant bulbs 3.5cm (1½in) deep. Under glass, grow in a mix of equal parts loam-based potting compost (JI No.2) and grit in full light. Water freely in growth; keep just moist when dormant. Outdoors, grow in well-drained, humus-rich soil in full sun.
- **PROPAGATION** Sow seed in containers in a cold frame in autumn. Separate bulbs when dormant and pot up bulbils after flowering.
- **PESTS AND DISEASES** Trouble free.

G. arvensis see *G. villosa*.
G. graeca, syn. *Lloydia graeca*. Delicate, bulbous perennial with very narrow, linear leaves, 4–12cm (1½–5in) long. In spring, bears umbels of up to 5 pendent, funnel-shaped, purple-veined white flowers, to 1.5cm (½in) long. Keep dry when dormant. ↕ 5–10cm (2–4in), ↔ 5cm (2in). Greece (including Crete), S. Turkey. ❄❄
G. peduncularis. Bulbous perennial with narrow, linear leaves, 6–30cm (2½–12in) long, taller than the flower stems. Loose racemes of up to 7 funnel-shaped yellow flowers, 1.5–3cm (½–1¼in) across, with central green stripes on the outsides, are produced in spring. ↕ 5–15cm (2–6in), ↔ 5cm (2in). Balkans, N. Africa. ❄❄❄ (borderline)
G. villosa, syn. *G. arvensis*. Bulbous perennial with linear leaves, 16cm (6in) long. In spring, bears loose umbels of up to 15 star-shaped yellow flowers, 2cm (¾in) across. Increases rapidly by bulbils borne from the basal leaf axils. ↕ 5–10cm (2–4in), ↔ 5cm (2in). Europe, N. Africa, Turkey, Iran. ❄❄❄

GAILLARDIA

Blanket flower

ASTERACEAE/COMPOSITAE

Genus of 30 species of annuals, perennials, and biennials found in open, sunny habitats on prairies and hillsides in W., C., and S. North America and South America. They bear entire, toothed, lobed, or pinnatifid, hairy leaves, produced in basal rosettes and alternately on the stems. Red, orange, or yellow, daisy-like flowerheads, with dark purple, brown, red, or yellow disc-florets, are borne on long stems. The numerous cultivars are bushy, leafy plants with brightly coloured flowerheads and a long flowering period. They are effective in a sunny border and are also good for cutting.

- **HARDINESS** Fully hardy to frost hardy.
- **CULTIVATION** Grow in fertile, well-drained soil in full sun; poor soil is tolerated. Dead-head regularly. In cool climates, cut perennials back to about 15cm (6in) in late summer, before frosts, to encourage new basal growth, which usually overwinters well.
- **PROPAGATION** Sow seed of annual and perennial species at 13–18°C (55–64°F) in early spring; annual seed may also be sown *in situ* in late spring or early summer. Most perennials flower in their first year from seed. Divide perennials in spring or take root cuttings in winter.
- **PESTS AND DISEASES** Susceptible to downy mildew and to slug damage on young growth.

G. aristata ▣ Erect but often spreading perennial with inversely lance-shaped to lance-shaped, entire or toothed, shallowly lobed or pinnatifid, greyish green leaves, to 20cm (8in) long. From summer to autumn, produces flowerheads, to 10cm (4in) across, with yellow ray-florets, sometimes tinged red at the base, and reddish orange disc-florets. Requires staking. ↕ 75cm (30in), ↔ 60cm (24in). W. Canada (British Columbia, Saskatchewan) to W. USA (Arizona, New Mexico). ❄❄❄

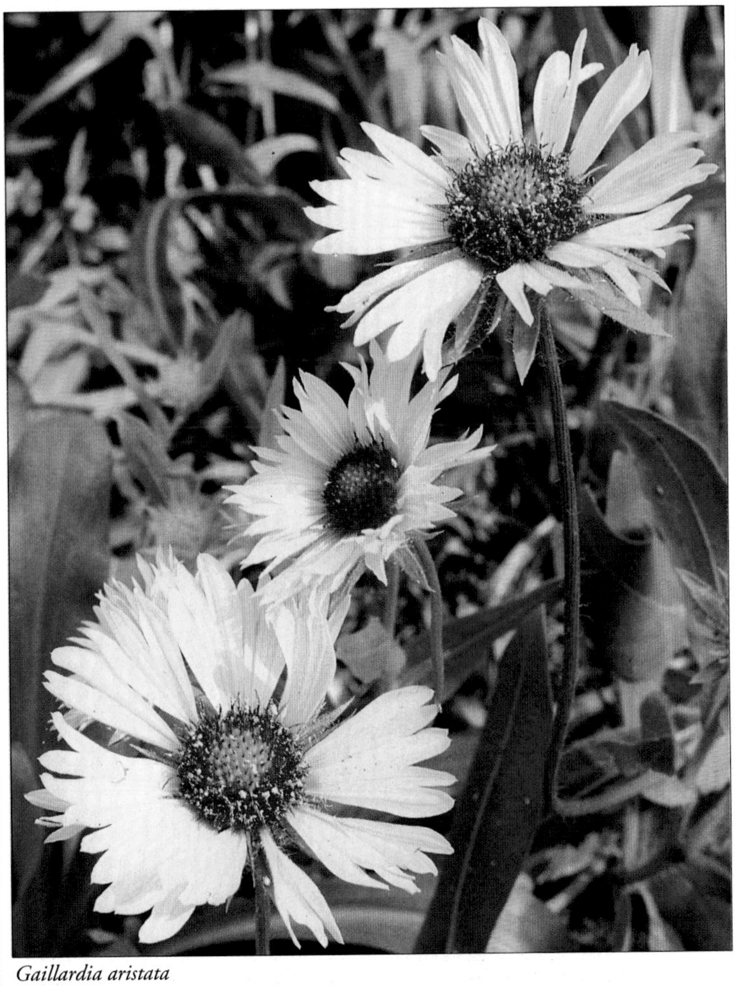

Gaillardia aristata

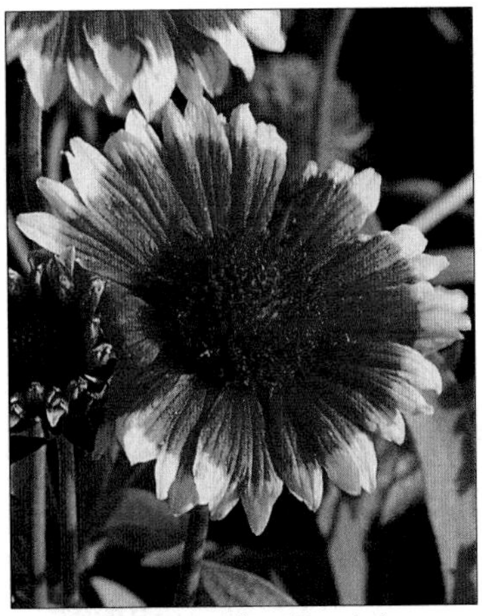

Gaillardia x *grandiflora* 'Dazzler'

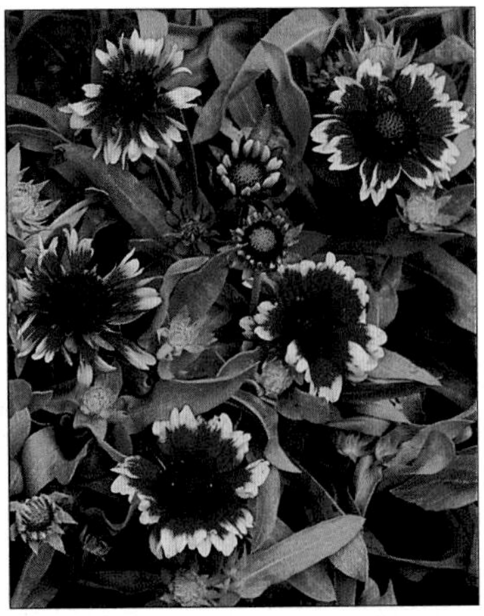

Gaillardia x *grandiflora* 'Kobold'

G.* x *grandiflora (*G. aristata* x *G. pulchella*). Bushy, often short-lived perennial with inversely lance-shaped, entire or lobed, sometimes pinnatifid, grey to mid-green leaves, to 30cm (12in) long. Flowerheads, 7–14cm (3–5½in) across, with yellow ray-florets, touched red at the bases, and yellow-brown disc-florets, are produced from early summer to early autumn. ↕ to 90cm (36in), ↔ 45cm (18in). Garden origin. ❄❄❄. **'Burgunder'**, syn. 'Burgundy', has deep wine-red flowerheads; ↕ 50–60cm (20–24in). **'Dazzler'** ▣♡ is short-lived and has bright orange-red, yellow-tipped ray-florets and maroon disc-florets; ↕ 60–85cm (24–34in). **'Goblin'** see 'Kobold'. **'Golden Goblin'** see 'Goldkobold'. **'Goldkobold'**, syn. 'Golden Goblin', has deep golden yellow ray-florets and darker yellow disc-florets; ↕ 25cm (10in). **'Kobold'** ▣ syn. 'Goblin', has rich red, yellow-tipped ray-florets and red disc-florets; ↕ 30cm (12in). **'Wirral Flame'** has yellow-tipped, deep orange-red flowerheads; ↕ to 75cm (30in).
G. pulchella (Blanket flower, Indian blanket). Upright, bushy annual with spoon-shaped to inversely lance-shaped, entire or coarsely toothed, grey-green leaves, to 8cm (3in) long. From summer to autumn, produces red-tipped yellow, or entirely red or yellow flowerheads, to 5cm (2in) across, with purple disc-florets. ↕ 45cm (18in), ↔ 30cm (12in). C. and S. USA, Mexico. ❄❄❄. **Plume Series** cultivars have double, red or yellow flowerheads; ↕ 30cm (12in). **'Portola Giants'** have bronzed scarlet, gold-tipped flowerheads, to 6cm (2½in) across.

GALANTHUS

Snowdrop

AMARYLLIDACEAE

Genus of about 19 species of bulbous perennials found from Europe to W. Asia, mostly in upland woodland but also in rocky sites. They bloom mainly from late winter to mid-spring, each bulb usually producing a single, pendent bloom with an arching flower-stalk on a slender stem, above 2, rarely 3, semi-erect, strap-shaped to inversely lance-shaped, basal leaves. The pear-shaped flowers are white, with 3 small inner tepals variably marked green, and 3 larger, spreading outer tepals. They are sometimes scented. Most snowdrops are vigorous and easily grown; some are suitable for naturalizing in grass or light woodland, and grow well in borders and rock gardens. All parts may cause mild stomach upset if ingested; contact with the bulbs may irritate skin.

- **HARDINESS** Fully hardy to frost hardy.
- **CULTIVATION** Grow in humus-rich, moist but well-drained soil that does not dry out in summer, in partial shade.
- **PROPAGATION** Sow seed of species as soon as ripe in containers in an open frame; keep shaded in summer. *Galanthus* species hybridize readily in gardens and seed may not come true. Lift and divide clumps of bulbs as soon as the leaves begin to die down after flowering.
- **PESTS AND DISEASES** Prone to narcissus bulb fly and grey mould (*Botrytis galanthina*).

GALANTHUS

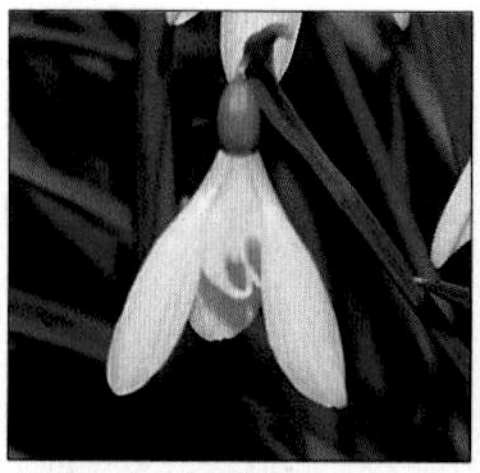
Galanthus 'Atkinsii'

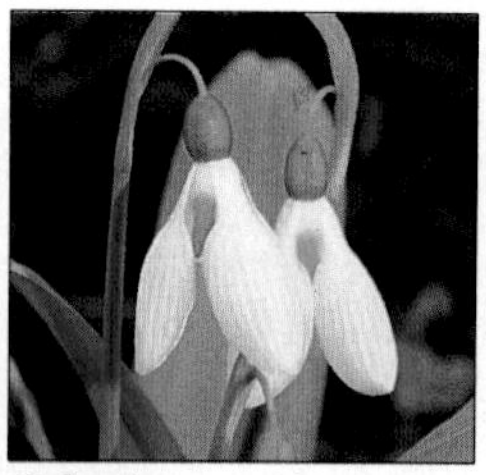
Galanthus caucasicus of gardens

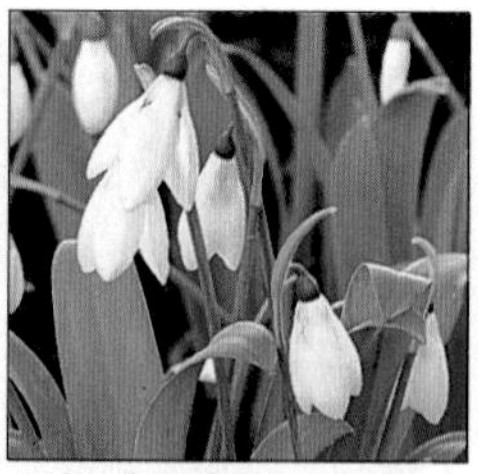
Galanthus elwesii

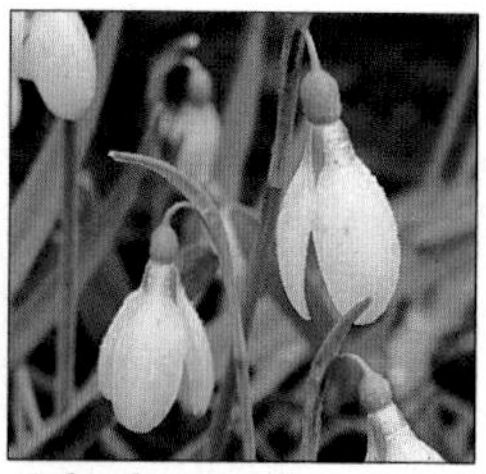
Galanthus gracilis

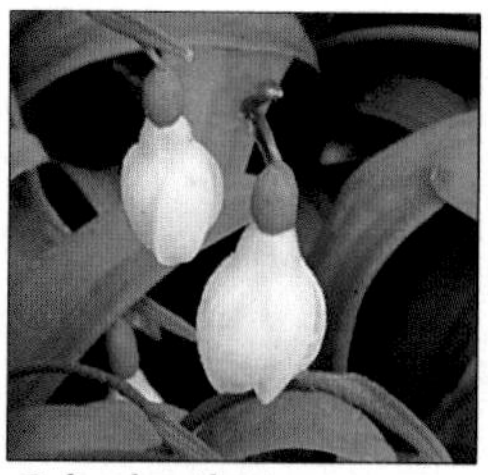
Galanthus ikariae

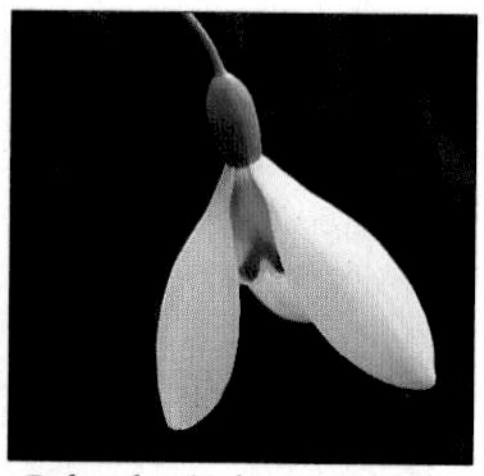
Galanthus 'John Gray'

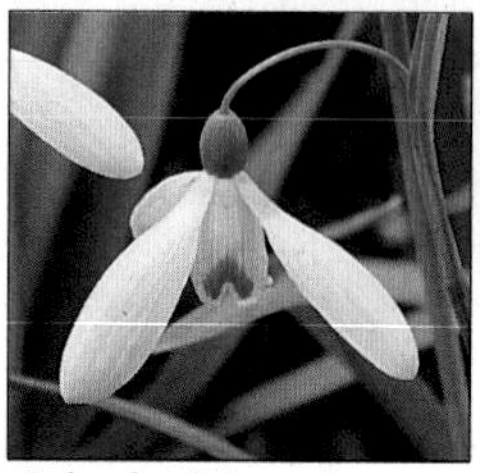
Galanthus 'Magnet'

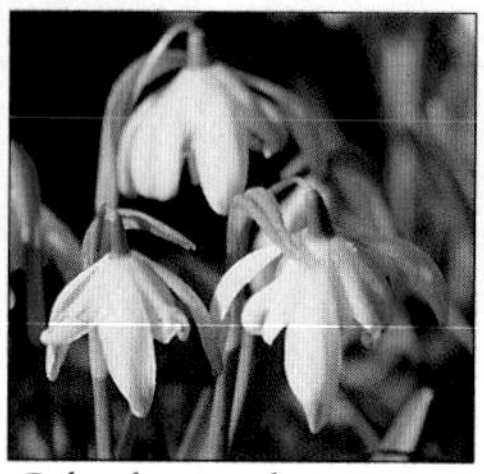
Galanthus nivalis 'Pusey Green Tip'

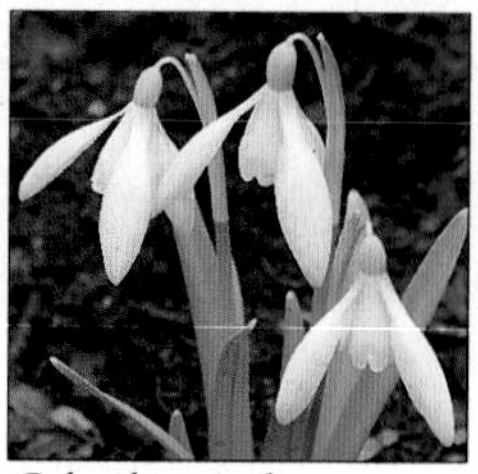
Galanthus nivalis 'Sandersii'

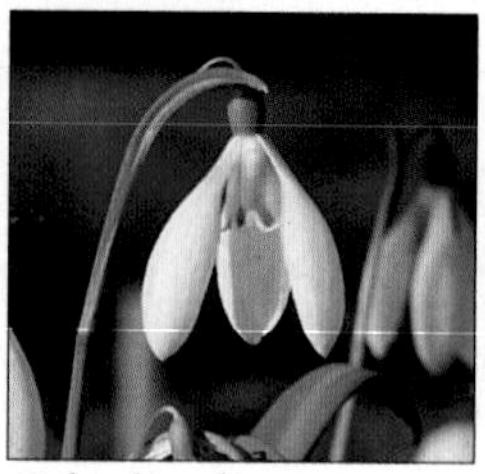
Galanthus plicatus subsp. *byzantinus*

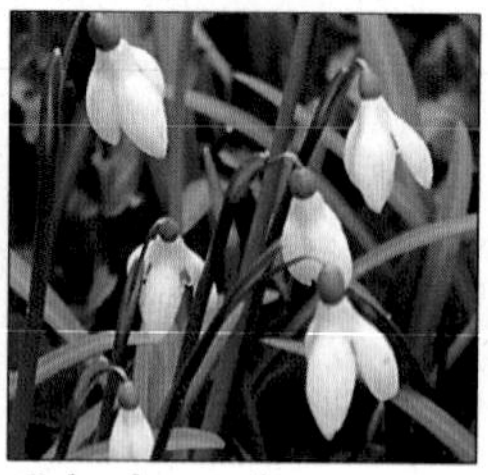
Galanthus rizehensis

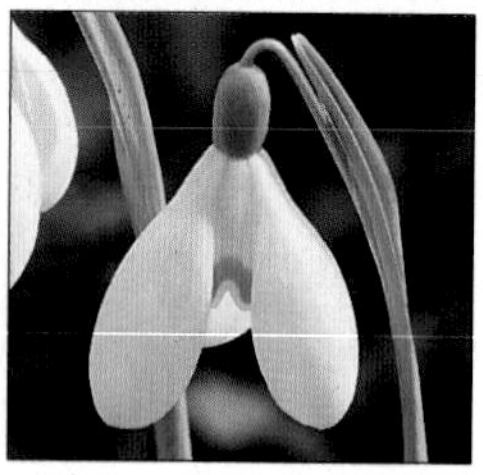
Galanthus 'S. Arnott'

G

G. allenii. Bulbous perennial with broad, dull, somewhat glaucous leaves, 6cm (2½in) long. In late winter and early spring, bears rounded, almond-scented flowers, 2cm (¾in) long, with a large green mark at the tip of each inner tepal. May be difficult to establish. ↕12cm (5in), ↔ 8cm (3in). Unknown origin; probably hybrid from the Caucasus. ❄❄❄

***G.* 'Arnott's Seedling'** see *G.* 'S. Arnott'.

***G.* 'Atkinsii'** ■ ♀ Vigorous, bulbous perennial with narrow, glaucous leaves, to 10cm (4in) long. In late winter, bears slender, elongated flowers, 3cm (1¼in) long, with a heart-shaped green mark at the tip of each inner tepal. May produce malformed tepals. ↕20cm (8in), ↔ 8cm (3in). ❄❄❄

***G.* 'Augustus'.** Robust, bulbous perennial producing broad, pale green leaves, 8–10cm (3–4in) long, each with a glaucous central channel and recurved or folded margins. In late winter and early spring, bears flowers, 1.5–2cm (½–¾in) long, with an H-shaped green mark on each inner tepal. ↕15cm (6in), ↔ 8cm (3in). ❄❄❄

***G.* 'Brenda Troyle'.** Vigorous, bulbous perennial with narrow, glaucous, grey-green leaves, 8–15cm (3–6in) long. In late winter, produces flowers 2–3cm (¾–1¼in) long, with an inverted V-shaped green mark at the tip of each inner tepal. ↕20cm (8in), ↔ 8cm (3in). ❄❄❄

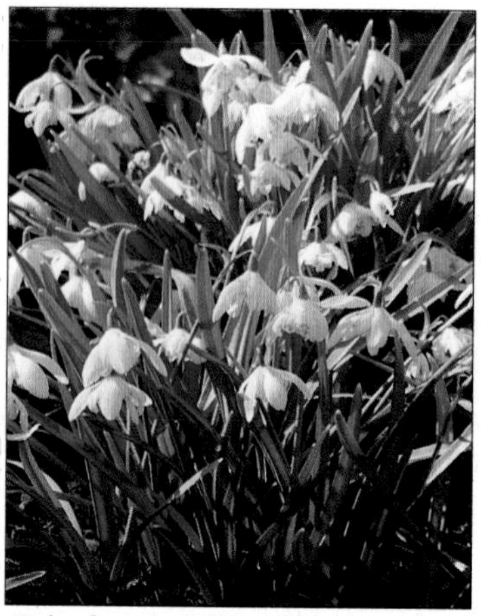
Galanthus nivalis 'Flore Pleno'

***G. caucasicus* of gardens** ■ ♀ Variable, bulbous perennial with broad, glaucous leaves, to 12cm (5in) long, recurving with age. From late autumn to early spring, produces flowers to 3cm (1¼in) long, with a green mark at the tip of each inner tepal. Now considered a variant of *G. elwesii.* ↕10–15cm (4–6in), ↔ 8cm (3in). Probably Turkey. ❄❄❄.

'Double' see *G.* 'Lady Beatrix Stanley'.

G. corcyrensis see *G. reginae-olgae.*

G. elwesii ■ ♀ Robust, bulbous perennial with broad, sometimes twisted, glaucous leaves, 10–15cm (4–6in) long. In late winter, bears slender, honey-scented flowers, 2–3cm (¾–1¼in) long, with 2 green markings, which sometimes merge, on each inner tepal. ↕12–22cm (5–9in), ↔ 8cm (3in). Balkans, W. Turkey. ❄❄❄. **var. *minor*** see *G. gracilis.*

G. fosteri. Slender, bulbous perennial with narrow, bright, deep green leaves, 8–14cm (3–5½in) long. In late winter, bears flowers 1.5–2.5cm (½–1in) long, with inner tepals marked green at the bases and apexes. Needs a dry site. Plant bulbs 10cm (4in) deep to minimize development of non-flowering bulbs. ↕to 8–20cm (3–8in), ↔ 5cm (2in). S. Turkey, Lebanon. ❄❄❄ (borderline)

G. gracilis ■ syn. *G. elwesii* var. *minor*, *G. graecus* of gardens. Slender, bulbous perennial with linear, twisted, glaucous leaves, 5–15cm (2–6in) long. In late winter and early spring, produces scented flowers, to 1.5–2.5cm (½–1in) long, each with 2 green markings on the flared inner tepals, and with long, pale green ovaries. ↕10cm (4in), ↔ 5cm (2in). Bulgaria, Greece, Turkey. ❄❄❄

***G. graecus* of gardens** see *G. gracilis.*

G. ikariae ■ syn. *G. latifolius* of gardens. Bulbous perennial with broad, glossy, bright green leaves, 6–16cm (2½–6in) long. In late winter and early spring, bears flowers, 1–3cm (½–1¼in) long, with a large green mark at the tip of each inner tepal. Much confused with *G. woronowii.* ↕10–15cm (4–6in), ↔ 5cm (2in). Aegean Islands, Turkey. ❄❄❄

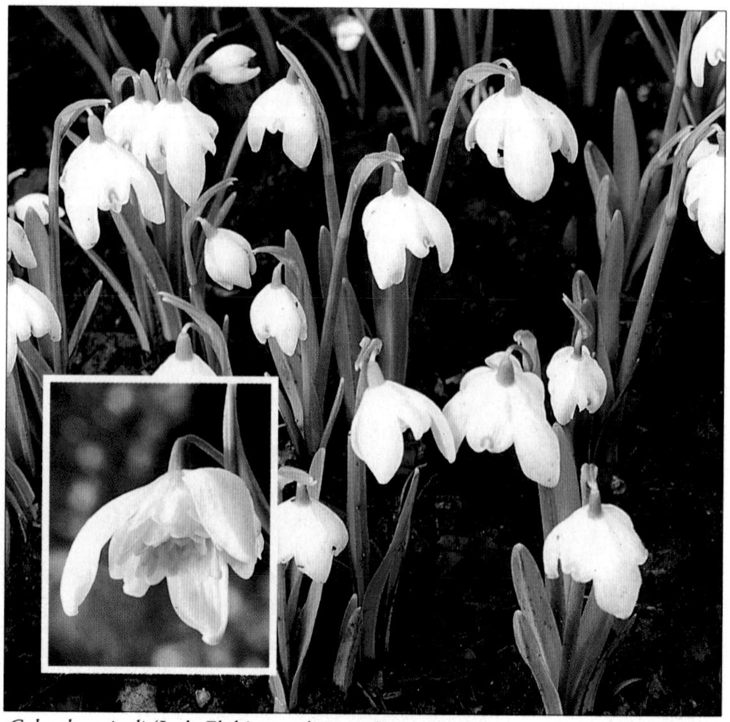
Galanthus nivalis 'Lady Elphinstone' (inset: flower detail)

***G.* 'Jacquenetta'.** Robust, bulbous perennial producing narrow leaves, 10cm (4in) long, each with a somewhat glaucous central stripe and slightly folded margins. In late winter, bears large, double flowers to 2.5cm (1in) across, occasionally with a few irregular tepals; the inner tepals are strongly marked green at the tips, the outer tepals sometimes each have a faint green mark. ↕20cm (8in), ↔ 8cm (3in). ❄❄

***G.* 'John Gray'** ■ Robust, bulbous perennial with narrow, grey-green leaves, 8–18cm (3–7in) long. Very large flowers, 3–3.5cm (1¼–1½in) long, are borne on arching stems in early winter, the inner tepals each with an X-shaped, dark green mark. ↕15cm (6in), ↔ 8cm (3in). ❄❄❄

***G.* 'Ketton'.** Robust, bulbous perennial with narrow, glaucous leaves, 7–15cm (3–6in) long. In late winter, produces large flowers, 3cm (1¼in) or more long, with a pair of green marks, sometimes joined, at the tip of each inner tepal. ↕18cm (7in), ↔ 8cm (3in). ❄❄❄

***G.* 'Lady Beatrix Stanley'**, syn. *G. caucasicus* 'Double'. Bulbous perennial with glaucous leaves, 8–15cm (3–6in) long, erect then recurved. Bears double flowers, to 2.5cm (1in) across, with a tiny green mark at the tip of each inner tepal, in late winter and early spring. ↕12cm (5in), ↔ 5cm (2in). ❄❄❄

***G. latifolius* of gardens** see *G. ikariae.*

***G.* 'Magnet'** ■ ♀ Vigorous, bulbous perennial producing narrow, grey-green leaves, 8–16cm (3–6in) long, with slightly folded margins. In late winter and early spring, bears large flowers, 2–2.5cm (¾–1in) long, on very long flower-stalks; the inner tepals each have an inverted V-shaped green mark at the tip. ↕20cm (8in), ↔ 8cm (3in). ❄❄❄

***G.* 'Merlin'.** Robust, bulbous perennial with narrow, grey-green leaves, 8–15cm (3–6in) or more long. In late winter and early spring, produces large flowers, 2–3cm (¾–1¼in) long, the inner tepals mostly covered with deep green marks. ↕18cm (7in), ↔ 8cm (3in). ❄❄❄

***G.* 'Mighty Atom'.** Bulbous perennial producing narrow, glaucous leaves, 5–12cm (2–5in) long. In late winter, bears large flowers, 3–3.5cm (1¼–1½in) long, with an inverted V-shaped, deep green mark at the tip of each inner tepal. ↕12cm (5in), ↔ 8cm (3in). ❄❄❄

G. nivalis 🏆 (Common snowdrop). Bulbous perennial with narrow, glaucous leaves, 5–16cm (2–6in) long. Small flowers, 1.5–2cm (½–¾in) long, with an inverted V-shaped green mark at the tip of each inner tepal, are honey-scented and produced in winter. ↕↔ 10cm (4in). Pyrenees to Ukraine. ❄❄❄. **'Flore Pleno'** ▣🏆 is robust, with irregular, double flowers. It is sterile, but increases rapidly from offsets. **'Howick Yellow'** see 'Sandersii'. **'Lady Elphinstone'** ▣ has grey-green leaves and double flowers in late winter and early spring. The inner tepal markings are yellow on established plants; ↕ 12cm (5in), ↔ 8cm (3in). **'Lutescens'** see 'Sandersii'. **'Pusey Green Tip'** ▣ has irregularly double flowers with pale green markings on the outer tepals. **'Sandersii'** ▣ syn. 'Howick Yellow', 'Lutescens', is slender with yellow markings on the inner tepals and ovary. **'Scharlokii'**, syn. 'Scharlockii', has slender flowers, with green markings on the outer tepals, overtopped by spathes split in 2. **'Viridapicis'** has a very long spathe, sometimes split in 2, and green marks on the outer tepal tips.

***G.* 'Ophelia'.** Vigorous, bulbous perennial with narrow, glaucous leaves, 10–14cm (4–5½in) long. In late winter, neat, double flowers, to 2cm (¾in) across, the outer tepals marked green, are borne on tall stems. ↕ 20cm (8in), ↔ 8cm (3in). ❄❄❄

G. plicatus 🏆 Bulbous perennial producing broad, dull green leaves, 8–18cm (3–7in) long, with glaucous central bands and recurved margins. In late winter and early spring, bears flowers 2–3cm (¾–1¼in) long, with a single green mark at the tip of each inner tepal. ↕ to 20cm (8in), ↔ 8cm (3in). Ukraine (Crimea), Romania, N. Turkey. ❄❄❄. **subsp. *byzantinus*** ▣🏆 has green markings at the base and apex of each inner tepal. Turkey (N.W. Anatolia).

G. reginae-olgae, syn. *G. corcyrensis.* Slender, bulbous perennial with narrow, recurving, grey-green leaves, to 6cm (2½in) long, each with a narrow, glaucous central stripe. In autumn, bears faintly scented flowers, to 2.5cm (1in) long, the inner tepal tips marked green. Needs a dry site. ↕ 10cm (4in), ↔ 5cm (2in). Italy (Sicily), Greece, former Yugoslavia. ❄❄. **subsp. *vernalis*** blooms in late winter and early spring.

G. rizehensis ▣ Slender, bulbous perennial with linear, recurved, deep green leaves, 6–12cm (2½–5in) long. In late winter and early spring, bears small flowers, 1.5–2cm (½–¾in) long, marked with green at the tips of the inner tepals. ↕ 12cm (5in), ↔ 5cm (2in). N.E. Turkey. ❄❄

***G.* 'Robin Hood'.** Bulbous perennial with narrow, glaucous leaves, 8–14cm (3–5½in) long. In late winter and early spring, bears slender flowers, 2.5–3cm (1–1¼in) long, with an X-shaped green mark on each inner tepal. ↕ 15cm (6in), ↔ 8cm (3in). ❄❄❄

***G.* 'Sam Arnott'** see *G.* 'S. Arnott'.

***G.* 'S. Arnott'** ▣🏆 syn. *G.* 'Arnott's Seedling', *G.* 'Sam Arnott'. Vigorous, bulbous perennial with grey-green leaves, 7–16cm (3–6in) long. In late winter and early spring, bears large, strongly honey-scented, well-rounded flowers, 2.5–3.5cm (1–1½in) long, with an inverted V-shaped green mark at the tip of each inner tepal. ↕ 20cm (8in), ↔ 8cm (3in). ❄❄❄

***G.* 'Straffan'.** Vigorous, bulbous perennial producing narrow, glaucous leaves, 8–16cm (3–6in) long. In mid-spring, bears flowers, 2.5cm (1in) long, with a small, inverted V-shaped green mark on each inner tepal. Each bulb may produce 2 flower stems. ↕ 12cm (5in), ↔ 8cm (3in). ❄❄❄

GALAX

Wandflower

DIAPENSIACEAE

Genus of one species of tufted, evergreen perennial from open woodland in the mountains of S.E. USA. It has a creeping rootstock, rounded leaves, and spike-like racemes of small white flowers. Grown for its flowers and autumn foliage colour, *G. urceolata* is suitable for underplanting in a shaded shrub border, for a large rock garden, or as ground cover in a woodland garden.

- **HARDINESS** Fully hardy.
- **CULTIVATION** Grow in moist, acid, humus-rich soil in partial shade; ensure that the roots do not dry out. Mulch annually in spring with pine needles or other acidic organic matter.
- **PROPAGATION** Sow seed in containers of lime-free (ericaceous) seed compost in an open frame outdoors in autumn. Separate rooted runners in early spring.
- **PESTS AND DISEASES** May be damaged by slugs and snails.

G. aphylla see *G. urceolata.*

G. urceolata ▣ syn. *G. aphylla.* Tufted, evergreen perennial with rounded, toothed, glossy, dark green leaves, to 8cm (3in) across, which are heart-shaped at the bases. The leaves turn red-bronze in autumn. In late spring and early summer, produces narrow, upright, spike-like racemes, to 25cm (10in) long, of tiny, 5-lobed white flowers. ↕ to 30cm (12in), ↔ to 1m (3ft). S.E. USA. ❄❄❄

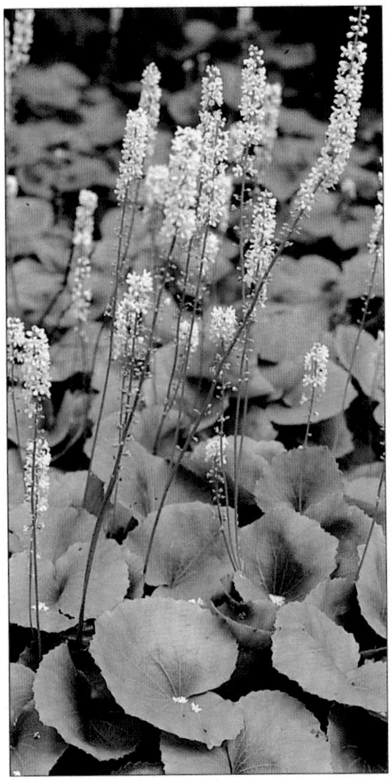

Galax urceolata

GALEGA

Goat's rue

LEGUMINOSAE/PAPILIONACEAE

Genus of about 6 species of tall, bushy perennials from sunny but damp meadows, slopes, and banks in C. and S. Europe, W. Asia, and the mountains of tropical E. Africa. They have alternate, pinnate, soft green or blue-tinged leaves, 8–20cm (3–8in) long, and produce erect, axillary racemes of pea-like, white, blue, mauve, or bicoloured flowers. *Galega* species and cultivars naturalize well, and are effective in a border from midsummer onwards; some are also good for cutting.

- **HARDINESS** Fully hardy.
- **CULTIVATION** Grow in any, preferably moist soil in full sun or partial shade. They need staking, and may spread rapidly in rich soil. Cut back flowered stems to prevent self-seeding.
- **PROPAGATION** Sow seed of species, soaked overnight, in containers in a cold frame in spring. Divide cultivars between late autumn and spring.
- **PESTS AND DISEASES** Pea and bean weevils may be a problem.

***G.* 'Candida'**, syn. *G.* x *hartlandii* 'Candida'. Erect, clump-forming perennial producing pinnate, soft green leaves, with oval leaflets, 5cm (2in) long. Pure white flowers, the standard petals 1.5–2cm (½–¾in) across, are borne in racemes to 15cm (6in) long, from early summer to early autumn. ↕ to 1.5m (5ft), ↔ 90cm (36in). ❄❄❄

***G.* x *hartlandii* 'Candida'** see *G.* 'Candida'.

***G.* 'Her Majesty'** see *G.* 'His Majesty'.

***G.* 'His Majesty'** ▣ syn. *G.* 'Her Majesty'. Erect, clump-forming perennial with pinnate, soft green leaves comprised of oval leaflets, 5cm (2in) long. Bicoloured mauve-pink and white flowers, the standard petals 1.5–2cm (½–¾in) across, are borne in racemes to 15cm (6in) long, from early summer to early autumn. ↕ to 1.5m (5ft), ↔ 90cm (36in). ❄❄❄

***G.* 'Lady Wilson'.** Erect, clump-forming perennial with pinnate, soft green leaves comprised of oval leaflets, 5cm (2in) long. From early summer to early autumn, produces racemes, to 15cm (6in) long, of bicoloured mauve-blue and white flowers, the standard petals 2cm (¾in) across. ↕ to 1.5m (5ft), ↔ 90cm (36in). ❄❄❄

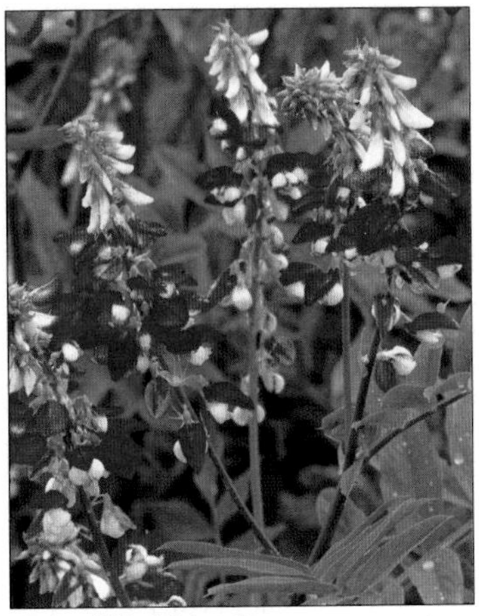

Galega 'His Majesty'

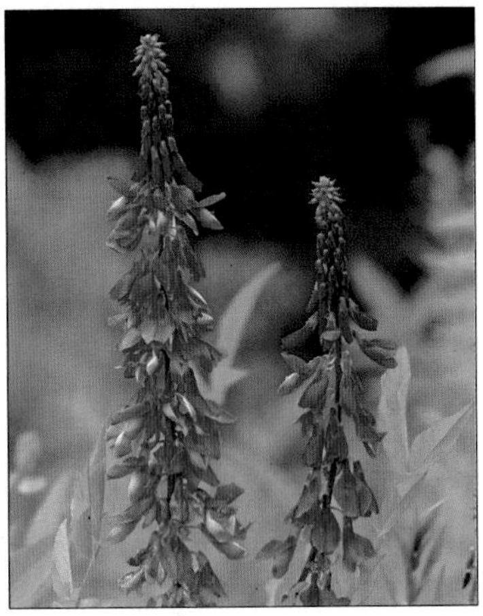

Galega orientalis

G

G. officinalis. Vigorous, clump-forming perennial with lax, sometimes spreading stems and pinnate, soft green leaves, each with 9–17 oblong, elliptic, or lance-shaped, pointed leaflets, 1.5–5cm (½–2in) long. 30–50 white or mauve, sometimes bicoloured flowers, 1.5cm (½in) long, are produced in racemes to 18cm (7in) long, from early summer to early autumn. ↕ 0.3–1.5m (1–5ft), ↔ 90cm (36in). C. and S. Europe, Turkey to Pakistan. ❄❄❄

G. orientalis ▣ Rhizomatous, upright to somewhat lax perennial with pinnate, soft green leaves comprised of 13–25 ovate-lance-shaped leaflets, 6cm (2½in) long, with long, sharp-pointed tips. In late spring and early summer, produces racemes, to 15cm (6in) long, of blue-violet flowers, to 2cm (¾in) long. Spreads rapidly. ↕ 1.2m (4ft), ↔ 60cm (24in). Caucasus. ❄❄❄

▷**Gale, Sweet** see *Myrica gale*
▷***Galeobdolon*** see *Lamium*
G. luteum see *L. galeobdolon*
▷**Galingale** see *Cyperus longus*
American see *C. eragrostis*

GALIUM

Bedstraw

RUBIACEAE

Genus of about 400 species of annuals and perennials, widely distributed in woodland, hedgerows, meadows, and wasteland, mainly in temperate regions. Most have whorls of linear leaves, produced on weak stems that may be scrambling and rough, with recurved bristles, or shorter and smooth. The flowers are white, pinkish white, or yellow, and are borne singly or in terminal or axillary panicles or cymes; they are tubular, with usually 4 or 5 corolla-lobes, which are often recurved. Many *Galium* species are invasive, but a few are good garden plants, including *G. odoratum*, which is useful as ground cover in woodland and is attractive to bees. Alpine species from dry regions are best grown in a scree bed or alpine house.

- **HARDINESS** Fully hardy to frost hardy.
- **CULTIVATION** Grow in almost any, preferably moist, humus-rich soil in sun or partial shade.
- **PROPAGATION** Sow seed in containers in a shaded cold frame as soon as ripe. Separate rhizomes in autumn or early spring.
- **PEST AND DISEASES** Trouble free.

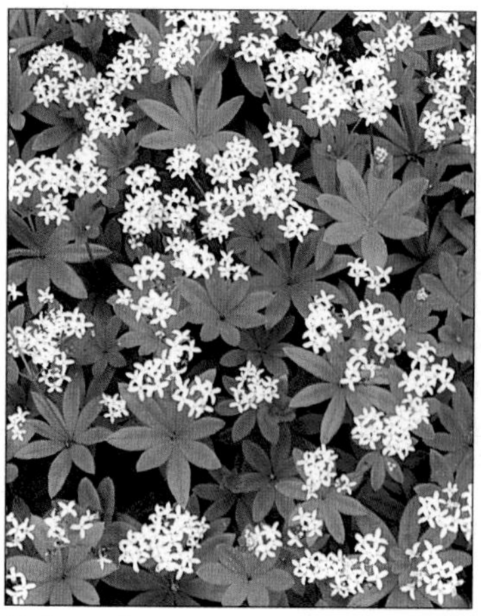

Galium odoratum

G

G. odoratum ▣ syn. *Asperula odorata* (Sweet woodruff). Rhizomatous perennial with erect, square, almost hairless stems, and whorls of 6–9 lance-shaped to elliptic, emerald-green leaves, 2.5–5cm (1–2in) long, with tiny, marginal prickles. Bears star-shaped, scented white flowers, 4–6mm (⅛–¼in) across, in umbel-like cymes, 8cm (3in) across, from late spring to midsummer. Leaves may scorch in strong sun. Hay-scented when dried. ↕45cm (18in), ↔ indefinite. Europe, N. Africa, Russia (Siberia). ✲✲✲

▷**Gallberry** see *Ilex glabra*

GALTONIA

HYACINTHACEAE/LILIACEAE

Genus of 4 species of bulbous perennials from moist grassland in South Africa, grown for their cylindrical to conical racemes of pendent or nodding, tubular to trumpet-shaped, green or white flowers. Leaves are basal, semi-erect, broadly lance-shaped to linear-lance-shaped, and fleshy. Good for a sunny border, *Galtonia* species are particularly useful as they flower late in summer.

• **HARDINESS** Fully hardy to frost hardy.

• **CULTIVATION** Grow in fertile, well-drained soil that is reliably moist from spring to summer, in full sun. In areas with severe winters, lift and pot up in late autumn and overwinter in a cool greenhouse, or protect *in situ* with a deep winter mulch.

• **PROPAGATION** Sow seed in containers in a cold frame as soon as ripe, keeping the seedlings frost-free for the first 2 years. Offsets can be removed in early spring.

• **PESTS AND DISEASES** Trouble free.

G. candicans ▣ Bulbous perennial with linear-lance-shaped, grey-green leaves, 50–100cm (20–39in) long. Slender racemes of up to 30 pendent, tubular, slightly fragrant white flowers, to 5cm (2in) long, faintly tinged green at the bases, are produced on long, leafless stems in late summer. ↕1–1.2m (3–4ft), ↔ 10cm (4in). South Africa (Northern Transvaal, Eastern Transvaal, Orange Free State, KwaZulu/Natal, Eastern Cape), Lesotho. ✲✲✲

G. viridiflora ♀ Bulbous perennial producing broad, lance-shaped, grey-green leaves, to 60cm (24in) long. In late summer, arching stems bear compact racemes of 15–30 nodding,

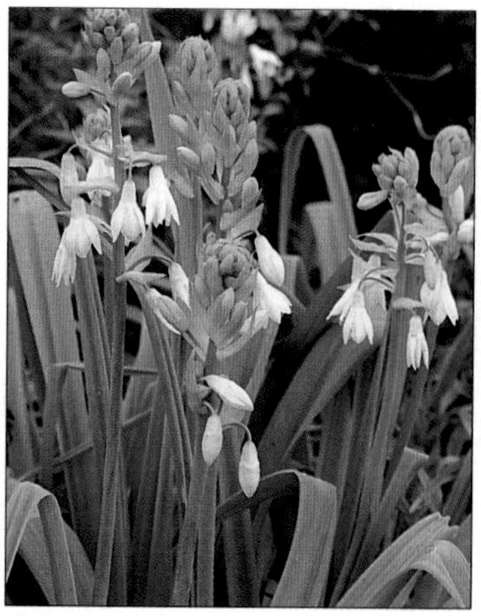

Galtonia candicans

trumpet-shaped, pale green flowers, 2–5cm (¾–2in) long. ↕to 1m (3ft), ↔ 10cm (4in). South Africa (Orange Free State, Eastern Cape), Lesotho. ✲✲

▷**Gardeners' garters** see *Phalaris arundinacea* var. *picta*

GARDENIA

RUBIACEAE

Genus of about 200 species of evergreen trees and shrubs from open woodland or savannah in tropical regions of Africa and Asia. They are grown for their attractive foliage and fragrant, showy flowers. The opposite or whorled leaves are simple and leathery. The terminal or axillary, tubular to funnel-shaped flowers each have 5–12 spreading petal lobes, and are solitary or borne in few-flowered cymes. In cold climates, grow in a temperate or warm greenhouse. In warmer areas, grow in a shrub border.

• **HARDINESS** Frost tender.

• **CULTIVATION** Under glass, grow in lime-free (ericaceous) potting compost in bright filtered light, with moderate humidity. Top-dress or pot on in spring. In growth, water freely with soft water and apply a balanced liquid fertilizer every 4 weeks. Keep barely moist in winter. Outdoors, grow in neutral to acid, fertile, humus-rich, moist but well-drained soil in partial or light dappled shade. Pruning group 1 for trees; group 8 for early-flowering shrubs; group 9 for late-flowering shrubs. May need restrictive pruning under glass.

• **PROPAGATION** Sow seed at 19–24°C (66–75°F) in spring. Take greenwood

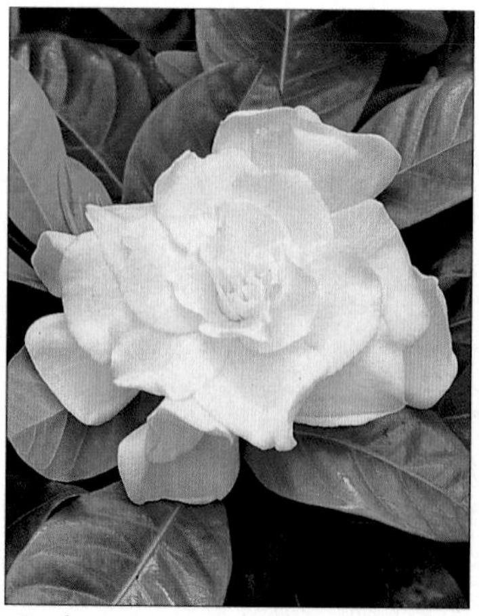

Gardenia augusta 'Veitchii'

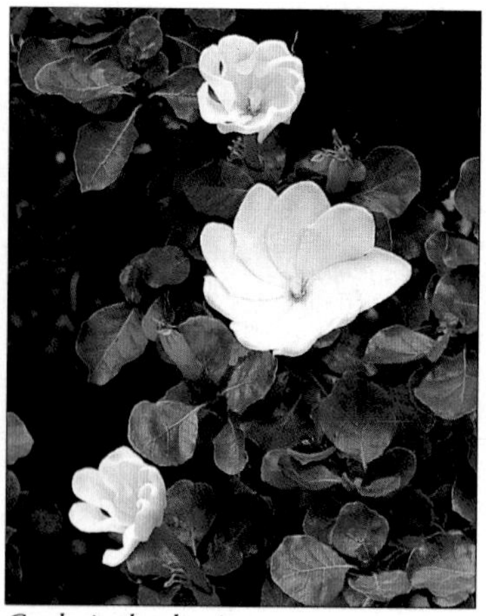

Gardenia thunbergia

cuttings in late spring or early summer, or semi-ripe cuttings in late summer.

• **PESTS AND DISEASES** Whiteflies, stem and root mealybugs, and grey mould (*Botrytis*) may be a problem under glass.

G. augusta ○ syn. *G. florida*, *G. grandiflora*, *G. jasminoides* (Cape jasmine, Common gardenia). Medium to large shrub, or sometimes small tree, frequently bushy, with ovate, elliptic, or lance-shaped, glossy, deep green leaves, 10cm (4in) or more long, usually borne in whorls of 3. From summer to autumn, produces 5- to 12-lobed, salverform, strongly fragrant, white to ivory flowers, to 8cm (3in) across, either singly or in few-flowered cymes. Usually grown in its double-flowered variants. ↕2–12m (6–40ft), ↔ 1–3m (3–10ft). China, Taiwan, Japan. ❀ (min. 10°C/50°F). **'Belmont'**, syn. 'Hadley', is a vigorous, freely branching clone with large leaves, to 15cm (6in) long, and double flowers that age from creamy white to yellow. **'Hadley'** see 'Belmont'. **'Mystery'** is compact, with very deep green leaves, and semi-double flowers; ↕to 1m (3ft). **'Veitchii'** ▣ syn. 'Veitchiana', is upright, with small green leaves, to 7cm (3in) long, and fully double, pure white flowers.

G. capensis see *Rothmannia capensis*.

G. florida see *G. augusta*.

G. globosa see *Rothmannia globosa*.

G. grandiflora see *G. augusta*.

G. jasminoides see *G. augusta*.

G. rothmannia see *Rothmannia capensis*.

G. thunbergia ▣○ (White gardenia). Open, erect shrub or small tree with rigid branches and opposite pairs of elliptic, glossy, dark green leaves, 8–14cm (3–5½in) long, with wavy margins. From winter to spring, bears solitary, tubular, fragrant, white or cream flowers, to 6cm (2½in) across, with 8 spreading petal lobes. ↕2–5m (6–15ft), ↔ 1.5–2.5m (5–8ft). South Africa. ❀ (min. 7°C/45°F)

▷**Gardenia,**
Common see *Gardenia augusta*
Paper see *Tabernaemontana divaricata*
White see *Gardenia thunbergia*

▷**Garland flower** see *Daphne cneorum*, *Hedychium coronarium*

▷**Garlic** see *Allium sativum*
False see *Nothoscordum*
Golden see *Allium moly*
Rosy see *Allium roseum*

GARRYA

GARRYACEAE

Genus of about 13 species of evergreen shrubs or small trees, occurring in woodland and scrub from W. USA to Central America and the West Indies. They are cultivated for their opposite pairs of narrowly ovate to broadly elliptic, leathery leaves, and for their pendent catkins, comprised of dioecious, petalless flowers. Male and female catkins are borne on separate plants: the males are generally more attractive; females produce spherical, purple-brown berries. Grow in a shrub border, against a wall, or as a windbreak in coastal areas.

• **HARDINESS** Frost hardy to half hardy; frost-hardy species may tolerate temperatures to -10°C (14°F).

• **CULTIVATION** Grow in moderately fertile, well-drained soil in full sun or partial shade. Shelter from cold winds in frost-prone areas. Pruning group 8.

• **PROPAGATION** Sow seed in containers in a cold frame in autumn or spring, or take semi-ripe cuttings in summer.

• **PESTS AND DISEASES** Susceptible to fungal leaf spot.

G. elliptica ▣○ (Silk-tassel bush). Dense, upright, evergreen shrub or small tree with ovate to oblong-elliptic, wavy-margined leaves, to 8cm (3in) long, varying from glossy, grey-green to matt, dark green. Pendent, grey-green catkins, the males 15–20cm (6–8in) long, with yellow anthers, are produced from mid-winter to early spring. ↕↔ 4m (12ft).

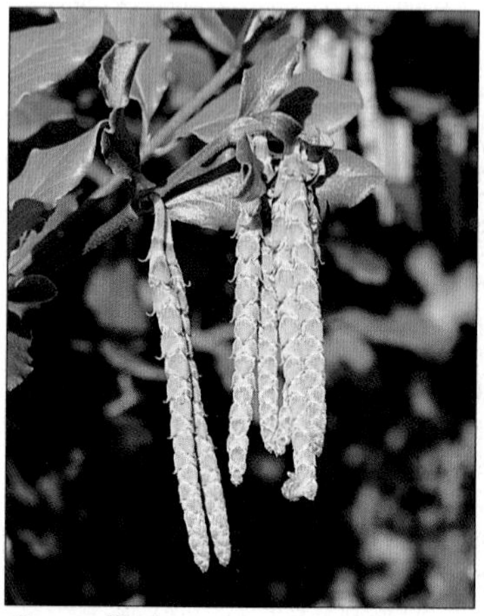

Garrya elliptica

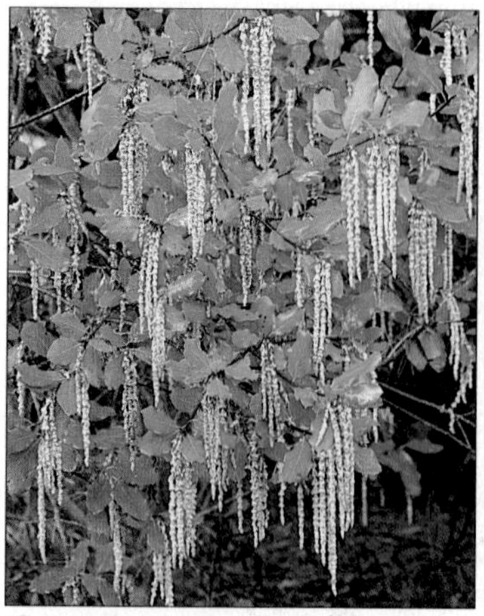

Garrya x *issaquahensis* 'Pat Ballard'

W. USA. ❄❄. **'Evie'** is male, with strongly wavy-margined leaves and very long catkins, to 30cm (12in). **'James Roof'** 🏆 is male, with dark sea-green leaves and dense clusters of silver-grey catkins, to 20cm (8in) or more long.
***G. x issaquahensis* 'Pat Ballard'** ■ Bushy, upright, evergreen shrub with red-purple shoots and ovate, slightly wavy-margined, glossy, mid-green leaves, to 7cm (3in) long. In midwinter, bears pendent, purple-tinged male catkins, to 20cm (8in) long. ↕ 4m (12ft), ↔ 3m (10ft). Garden origin. ❄❄

GASTERIA

ALOEACEAE/LILIACEAE

Genus of 50–80 species of stemless or very short-stemmed, perennial succulents, usually offsetting freely to form clumps, found in the lowlands, and sometimes hillsides, of Namibia and South Africa. They are grown for their flowers and foliage: the firm, dark or greyish green leaves, occasionally slightly suffused red, have white tubercles, and are frequently arranged in 2 ranks, later often forming rosettes and elongating; the usually pendulous, tubular flowers, swollen at the bases and sometimes green-tipped, are borne in lax racemes or few-branched panicles. Where temperatures drop below 7°C (45°F), grow in a temperate greenhouse, or as houseplants. In warm, dry climates, grow in a desert garden.

• **HARDINESS** Frost tender.

• **CULTIVATION** Under glass, grow in standard cactus compost in bright filtered light. During growth, water moderately and apply a low-nitrogen liquid fertilizer every 4 or 5 weeks. Keep dry when dormant. Outdoors, grow in sharply drained, loamy soil, with added leaf mould, in full sun or dappled shade. See also pp.48–49.

• **PROPAGATION** Sow seed at 19–24°C (66–75°F) in spring or summer. Separate offsets, or take leaf cuttings, during the growing season.

• **PESTS AND DISEASES** Trouble free.

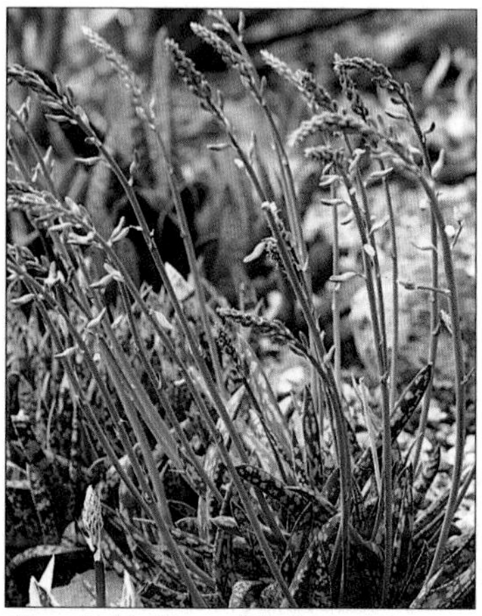

Gasteria bicolor var. *liliputana*

G. bicolor* var. *liliputana ■ syn. *G. liliputana.* Clump-forming succulent with rosettes of lance-shaped to linear, toothed, conspicuously white-spotted, glossy, dark green leaves, to 6cm (2½in) long, rounded and keeled below, with tubercles towards the bases. Racemes of narrow, tubular, orange-green flowers, 1.5cm (½in) long, are produced from late spring to summer. ↕ 7cm (3in), ↔ 10cm (4in). South Africa (Western Cape, Eastern Cape). ❀ (min. 7°C/45°F)
G. carinata* var. *verrucosa ■ syn. *G. verrucosa.* Clump-forming succulent with 2 ranks of 3-angled, linear-lance-shaped, greyish green leaves, 10–15cm (4–6in) long, grooved above, convex below; they are tapering and flat towards the blunt tips, and have thickened margins and white tubercles. Bears racemes of reddish orange flowers, to 1.5cm (½in) long, from late spring to summer. ↕ 15cm (6in), ↔ 30cm (12in). South Africa (Western Cape, Eastern Cape). ❀ (min. 7°C/45°F)
G. liliputana see *G. bicolor* var. *liliputana.*
G. obliqua, syn. *G. pulchra.* Clump-forming succulent with slender, 3-angled, linear, semi-triangular, sometimes sickle-shaped, usually tapering, greyish green leaves, 15–30cm (6–12in) long; they are cross-banded with white marks and have finely toothed, horny white margins. Racemes of red flowers, 2cm (¾in) long, are borne on long, reddish orange stalks from late spring to summer. ↕ 30cm (12in), ↔ 45cm (18in). South Africa (Eastern Cape). ❀ (min. 7°C/45°F)
G. pulchra see *G. obliqua.*
G. verrucosa see *G. carinata* var. *verrucosa.*

▷**x *Gaulnettya*** see *Gaultheria*
x *G.* 'Pink Pixie' see *G.* x *wisleyensis* 'Pink Pixie'
x *G.* 'Wisley Pearl' see *G.* x *wisleyensis* 'Wisley Pearl'

GAULTHERIA

syn. x GAULNETTYA, PERNETTYA

ERICACEAE

Genus of approximately 170 species of evergreen shrubs, some rhizomatous, widely distributed in woodland and open, moist, rocky places in the Himalayas, E. Asia, Australasia, and North, Central, and South America. They are grown for their simple, alternate, usually leathery leaves; for their small, bell- or urn-shaped flowers, 4–7mm (⅛–¼in) long, borne singly in the leaf axils or in racemes or panicles; and for their fleshy, usually spherical fruits. Suitable for woodland plantings, they can also be grown in a rock garden, a heather garden, or a peat garden or peat bank. All parts may cause mild stomach upset if ingested, except the fruits, which are edible.

• **HARDINESS** Fully hardy to half hardy.

• **CULTIVATION** Grow in acid to neutral, peaty, moist soil in partial shade; full sun is tolerated where the soil is permanently moist. Pruning group 8; remove suckers to restrict growth.

• **PROPAGATION** Sow seed in containers outdoors in a cold frame in autumn. Take semi-ripe cuttings in summer or remove rooted suckers (if produced) in spring.

• **PESTS AND DISEASES** Trouble free.

G. cuneata 🏆 Dwarf, densely branched shrub with pointed, ovate-oblong to obovate, toothed, mid-green leaves, to 3cm (1¼in) long. Produces white flowers in racemes, 2.5–3.5cm (1–1½in) long, in late spring and early summer, followed by white fruit, to 6mm (¼in) across, in autumn. ↕ to 30cm (12in), ↔ to 1m (3ft). W. China. ❄❄❄
G. forrestii. Spreading, rounded shrub with arching shoots and narrowly ovate to oblong, sharp-pointed, bristly toothed, glossy, dark green leaves, to 9cm (3½in) long. In late spring and early summer, produces broadly urn-shaped, fragrant white flowers in racemes, 2.5–5cm (1–2in) long, followed by black fruit, 6mm (¼in) across. ↕↔ 1.5m (5ft). S.W. China. ❄❄
G. miqueliana ■ Compact, stiff-stemmed shrub with ovate to obovate, rounded to acute, toothed, dark green leaves, net-veined below, to 4cm (1½in) long. Short racemes, 2.5–5cm (1–2in) long, of urn- to bell-shaped white flowers, are produced in late spring and early summer, followed by white, sometimes pink-flushed white fruit, to 1cm (½in) across, in autumn. ↕ to 30cm (12in), ↔ to 1m (3ft) or more. Japan. ❄❄❄
G. mucronata 🏆 syn. *Pernettya mucronata.* Compact, bushy, suckering shrub with oval-elliptic to oblong-elliptic, toothed, spine-tipped, glossy, dark green leaves, to 2cm (¾in) long. Produces nodding, urn-shaped, solitary, white, sometimes pink-flushed flowers, in late spring and early summer; they are followed by fruit to 1.5cm (½in) across, variously coloured from purple-red to white. Grow male and female plants together to ensure fruiting. ↕↔ 1.2m (4ft). Chile, Argentina. ❄❄❄. **'Cherry Ripe'** has bright cerise fruit. **'Edward Balls'** is male, with upright red shoots and broadly oval, bright green leaves. **'Lilian'** has lilac-pink fruit. **'Mother of Pearl'** see 'Parelmoer'. **'Mulberry Wine'** ■ 🏆 has magenta fruit, ripening to dark purple. **'Parelmoer'**, syn. 'Mother of Pearl', has light pink fruit. **'Sneeuwwitje'**, syn. 'Snow White', has white fruit slightly spotted with pink. **'Snow White'** see 'Sneeuwwitje'. **'Wintertime'** ■ 🏆 has pure white fruit.
G. myrsinoides, syn. *G. prostrata, Pernettya prostrata.* Prostrate, creeping, rhizomatous shrub with elliptic to oblong-elliptic, bristly scalloped, sharp-pointed, dark green leaves, to 7mm (¼in) long. Solitary, urn-shaped white flowers are borne in early summer and followed by deep purple fruit, to 1.5cm (½in) across, with persistent, enlarged calyces. ↕ to 20cm (8in), ↔ to 40cm (16in). Costa Rica to C. Chile. ❄❄❄.

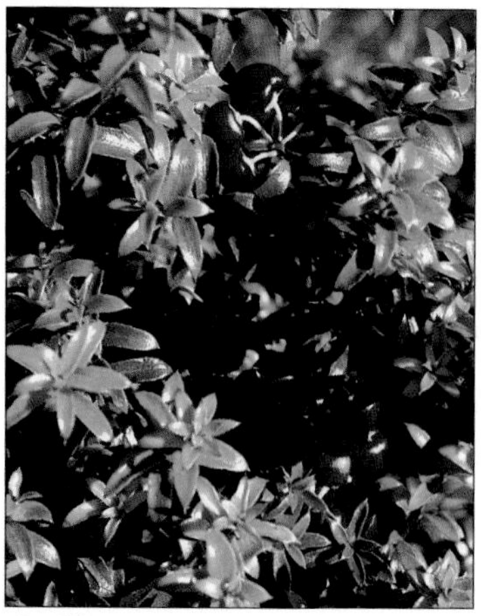

Gaultheria mucronata 'Mulberry Wine'

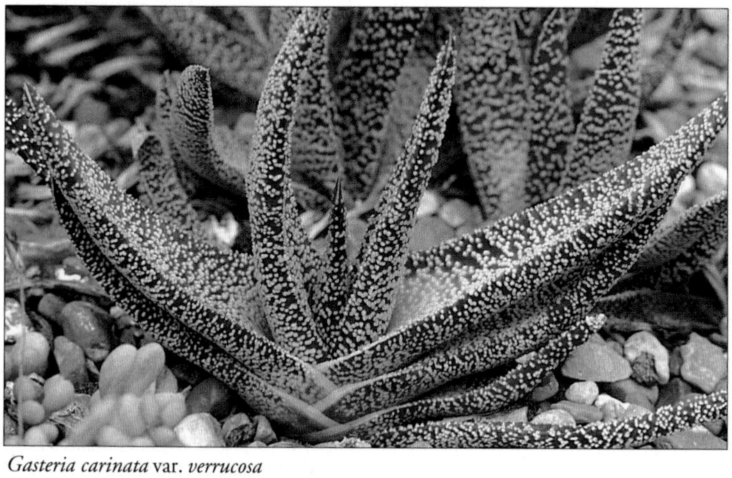

Gasteria carinata var. *verrucosa*

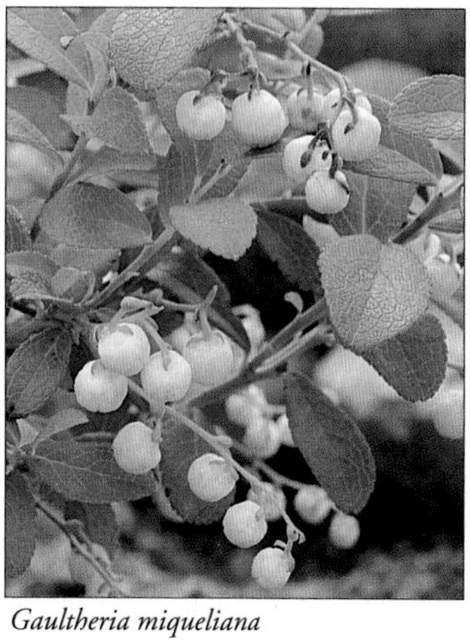

Gaultheria miqueliana

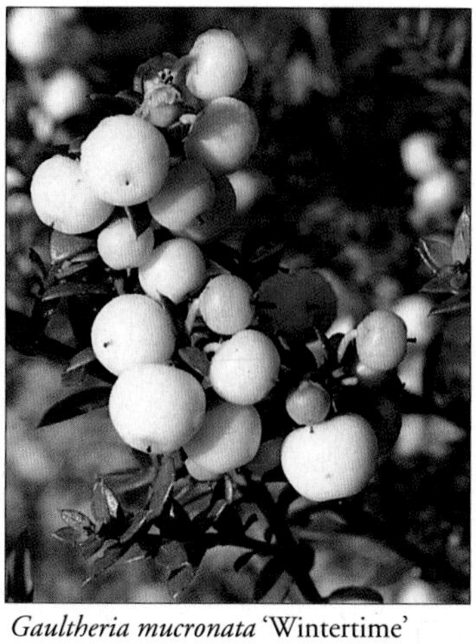

Gaultheria mucronata 'Wintertime'

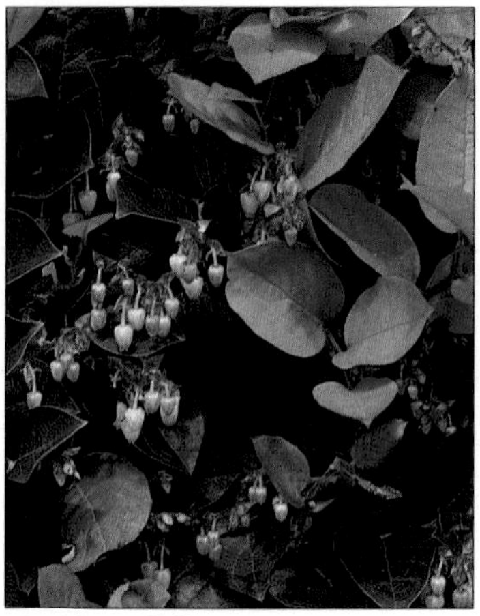
Gaultheria shallon

G

subsp. *pentlandii*, syn. *Pernettya prostrata* subsp. *pentlandii*, is more upright, with oblong-ovate leaves, to 3cm (1¼in) long, and paler fruit; ↕↔ to 40cm (16in).

G. nummularioides. Dense, hairy-stemmed, prostrate shrub with rounded, ovate-elliptic, gland-tipped, bristly toothed, dull green leaves, to 1.5cm (½in) long, becoming smaller towards the stem tips. In late spring and early summer, bears solitary, urn-shaped, pink-flushed white or white-tinged red-brown flowers; these are followed by ovoid, purple-black fruit, to 8mm (⅜in) long. ↕ 10cm (4in), ↔ 30cm (12in). Himalayas, China. ❄❄❄

G. procumbens 🏆 (Checkerberry, Wintergreen). Creeping, rhizomatous shrub producing elliptic to elliptic-oblong, pointed or glandular-tipped, scalloped or bristly toothed, glossy, dark green leaves, to 5cm (2in) long. The leaves have a strong fragrance of wintergreen when crushed. In summer, produces urn-shaped, white or pale pink flowers, either singly or in small racemes, 1–2.5cm (½–1in) long; these are followed by aromatic scarlet fruit, 0.8–1.5cm (⅜–½in) across, which frequently persist until spring. Provides good ground cover in shade. ↕ 15cm (6in), ↔ to 1m (3ft) or more. E. North America. ❄❄❄

G. prostrata see *G. myrsinoides.*

G. pyroloides. Rhizomatous, ground-covering shrublet with obovate to almost rounded, minutely spine-tipped, toothed, dark green leaves, to 3.5cm (1½in) long. In late spring, produces short racemes, to 2.5cm (1in) long, of

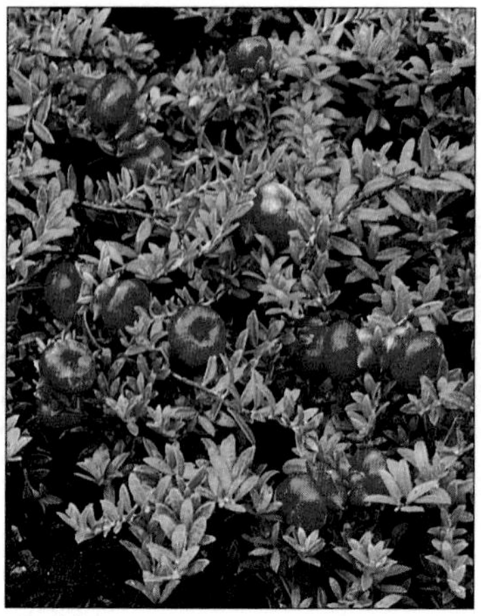
Gaultheria tasmanica

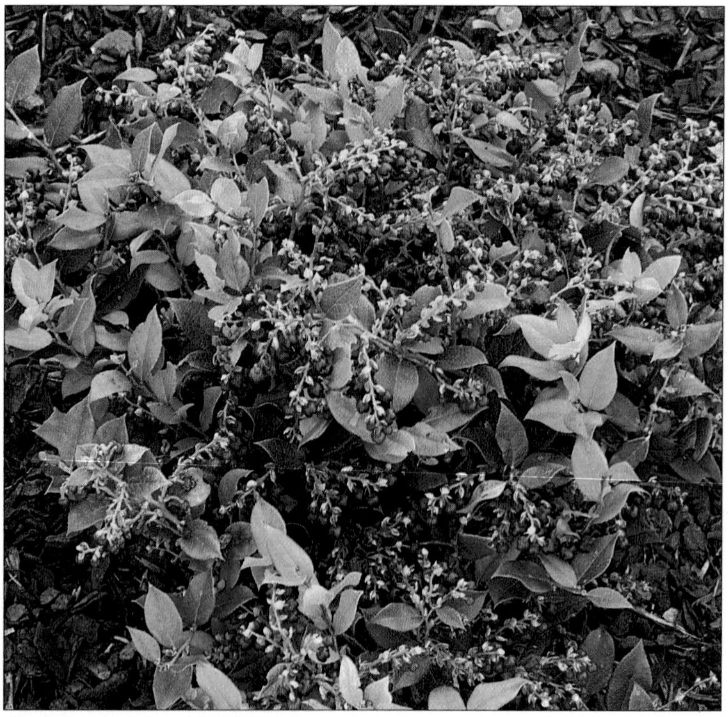
Gaultheria x *wisleyensis* 'Pink Pixie'

ovoid-urn-shaped, pink-flushed white flowers, which are followed by ellipsoid, blue-black fruit, to 8mm (⅜in) long. ↕ 15cm (6in), ↔ to 50cm (20in). Himalayas. ❄❄❄

G. shallon ▣ (Salal, Shallon). Compact, bushy shrub, spreading vigorously by suckers, with red shoots and broadly ovate, sharp-pointed, bristly toothed, glossy, dark green leaves, to 10cm (4in) long. Bears arching racemes, to 10cm (4in) long, of broadly urn-shaped, pink-suffused white flowers, in late spring and early summer; they are followed by purple fruit, to 1cm (½in) across. ↕ 1.2m (4ft), ↔ 1.5m (5ft). W. North America. ❄❄❄

G. tasmanica ▣ syn. *Pernettya tasmanica.* Mat-forming shrublet with narrowly elliptic to oval, scalloped, lustrous, mid-green leaves, to 8mm (⅜in) long, and axillary, solitary, bell-shaped white flowers borne in spring. Produces bright orange-red, occasionally white or yellow fruit, 6–8mm (¼–⅜in) across. Fruits freely, even in shade. ↕ 7cm (3in), ↔ to 25cm (10in). Australia (Tasmania). ❄❄❄

G. trichophylla. Prostrate, mat-forming, slender-stemmed, suckering shrub with elliptic, bristly toothed, glossy, dark green leaves, to 1cm (½in) long. In late spring, bears axillary, solitary, bell-shaped, white or pink flowers, the white sometimes pink-flushed, followed by pale greenish blue fruit, to 1cm (½in) across. Ideal for a rock garden or peat bank. ↕ to 10cm (4in), ↔ to 30cm (12in). Himalayas, W. China. ❄❄❄

G. x wisleyensis (*G. mucronata* x *G. shallon*). Upright, suckering shrub with elliptic to elliptic-oblong, dark green leaves, to 4cm (1½in) long. Urn-shaped white flowers are produced in racemes, to 5cm (2in) long, in late spring and early summer, followed by purple-red fruit, 6mm (¼in) across. ↕↔ 1m (3ft). Garden origin. ❄❄❄. **'Pink Pixie'** ▣ syn. x *Gaulnettya* 'Pink Pixie', is dwarf but vigorous, spreading by suckers, and has pink-tinged white flowers, followed by purple-red fruit; ↕ to 30cm (12in), ↔ 45cm (18in). **'Wisley Pearl'**, syn. x *Gaulnettya* 'Wisley Pearl', has white flowers and dark purple-red fruit.

GAURA

ONAGRACEAE

Genus of about 20 species of annuals, biennials, perennials, and subshrubs from moist places and prairies in North America. They have alternate, simple, rosetted, lance-shaped to elliptic or spoon-shaped, pinnatifid, mainly basal leaves, and airy racemes or panicles of short-lived, flat, irregularly star-shaped, pink or white flowers, usually 4-petalled. They are graceful plants for a border.

- **HARDINESS** Fully hardy.
- **CULTIVATION** Grow in fertile, moist but well-drained soil in full sun, but drought and partial shade are tolerated.
- **PROPAGATION** Sow seed of annuals *in situ* in spring, and seed of perennials in containers in a cold frame from spring to early summer. Perennials may also be divided in spring, or increased by basal or softwood cuttings in spring or semi-ripe heel cuttings in summer.
- **PESTS AND DISEASES** Trouble free.

G. biennis. Subshrubby, hairy annual or biennial with stem leaves to 12cm (5in) long and basal leaves to 40cm (16in) long; both are narrowly elliptic with irregular margins. Racemes, 10–50cm (4–20in) long, of white flowers, to 3.5cm (1½in) across, fading to reddish pink, open at dusk in summer. Stems and foliage are flushed coral-red in late summer. ↕ 1.8m (6ft) or more, ↔ to 1.2m (4ft). USA (Texas, Louisiana). ❄❄❄

G. lindheimeri ▣ 🏆 Bushy, clump-forming perennial with slender stems bearing spoon-shaped to lance-shaped, toothed leaves, 2.5–8cm (1–3in) long. From late spring to early autumn, produces loose panicles, 20–60cm (8–24in) long, of pinkish white buds,

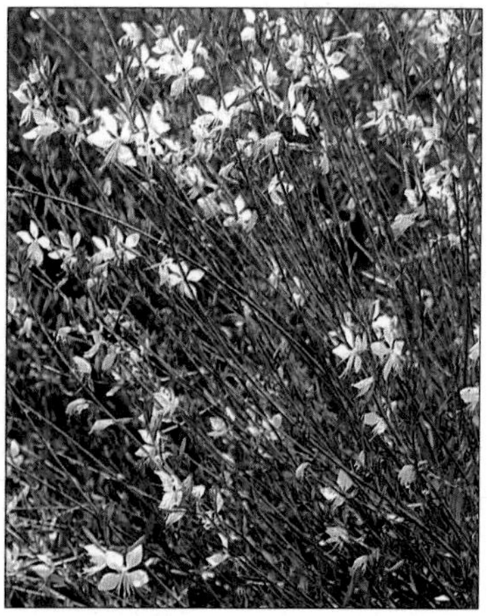
Gaura lindheimeri

opening at dawn to white flowers, 2.5cm (1in) across, fading to pink. ↕ to 1.5m (5ft), ↔ 90cm (36in). USA (Texas, Louisiana). ❄❄❄. **'Corrie's Gold'** has gold-margined leaves. **'Whirling Butterflies'** has grey-green leaves, and is very free-flowering, with red sepals; ↕ 60–75cm (24–30in).

▷ **Gayfeather** see *Liatris, L. spicata*

GAYLUSSACIA

Huckleberry

ERICACEAE

Genus of about 40 species of deciduous and evergreen shrubs from woodland and thickets in North and South America, cultivated mainly for their flowers and edible fruits. They have alternate, simple, entire or toothed leaves, and axillary racemes of urn- or bell-shaped flowers in spring. Excellent for a shrub border or open woodland.

- **HARDINESS** Fully hardy.
- **CULTIVATION** Grow in acid, peaty, moist but well-drained soil in full sun or partial shade. Pruning group 1 if deciduous; group 8 if evergreen.
- **PROPAGATION** Sow seed in containers in an open frame in autumn, or take softwood cuttings in summer.
- **PESTS AND DISEASES** Trouble free.

G. baccata (Black huckleberry). Upright, deciduous shrub with elliptic-oblong, mid- to dark green leaves, to 5cm (2in) long, sticky when young, turning red in autumn. Small, urn-shaped, dull red flowers, to 5mm (¼in) long, are produced in pendent racemes, to 4cm (1½in) long, in late spring; they are followed by edible, spherical, glossy black fruit, to 8mm (⅜in) across. ↕↔ 1m (3ft). E. North America. ❄❄❄

GAZANIA

ASTERACEAE/COMPOSITAE

Genus of about 16 species of low-growing annuals or evergreen perennials from low altitude sands to alpine meadows in tropical Africa. They have mostly lance-shaped, basal leaves, often covered with grey, felted hairs on one or both surfaces, and varying from deeply lobed to pinnatifid, and from entire to toothed. Large, daisy-like, very brightly coloured, dark-centred flowerheads, which close in dull or cool weather, are produced over a long period in summer. Hybrid selections are the most

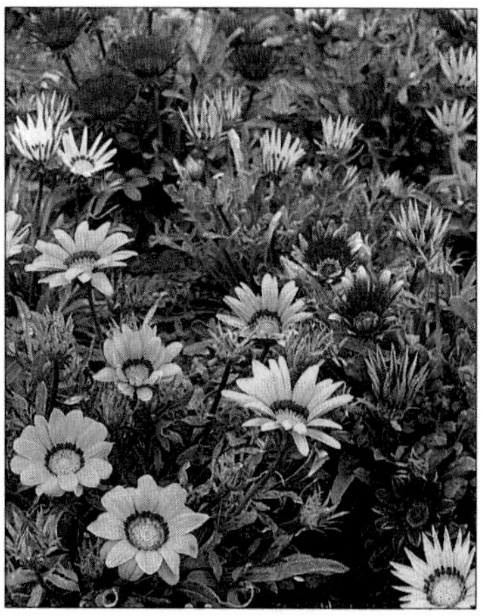

Gazania Chansonette Series

commonly cultivated, and are grown as annuals or half-hardy perennials, with leafy stems bearing spoon-shaped to oblong, often lobed leaves and variously coloured flowerheads. They are useful as summer bedding or in patio containers, and tolerate coastal conditions.

• **HARDINESS** Half hardy to frost tender; most can survive short periods at or below 0°C (32°F).

• **CULTIVATION** Under glass, grow in loam-based potting compost (JI No.1), with added sharp sand, in full light. Water freely when in growth; keep just moist in winter. Outdoors, grow in light, sandy, well-drained soil in full sun. Dead-head to prolong flowering.

• **PROPAGATION** Sow seed at 18–20°C (64–68°F) in late winter or early spring. Take basal cuttings in late summer or early autumn, to overwinter under glass.

• **PESTS AND DISEASES** Plants over-wintered under glass may suffer from grey mould (*Botrytis*) and aphids.

***G.* Chansonette Series** ■ ♀ Vigorous, spreading, evergreen perennials with glossy leaves, to 15cm (6in) long, dark green above, covered with silky white hairs beneath. In summer, bear solitary flowerheads in a mix of bronze, orange, rose-pink, salmon-pink, red-orange, or yellow, zoned in a contrasting colour. ↕ to 20cm (8in), ↔ to 25cm (10in). ❄

***G.* Daybreak Series.** Spreading, evergreen perennials with glossy leaves, to 15cm (6in) long, dark green above, with silky white hairs below. In early summer, bear solitary flowerheads in bronze, orange, yellow, bright pink, or white, usually zoned in a contrasting colour. ↕ to 20cm (8in), ↔ to 25cm (10in). ❄. **'Daybreak Bronze'** is a single-colour selection.

***G.* Mini-star Series** ♀ Compact, tuft-forming, evergreen perennials with glossy leaves, to 15cm (6in) long, dark green above, white silky-hairy beneath. Produce solitary, orange, white, golden yellow, beige, bronze, or bright pink flowerheads in summer, some zoned in a contrasting colour. ↕ to 20cm (8in), ↔ to 25cm (10in). ❄. **'Mini-star Tangerine'** and **'Mini-star Yellow'** are popular single-colour selections.

***G.* Talent Series** ♀ Vigorous, evergreen perennials with highly ornamental, mid-green leaves, to 15cm (6in) long, grey-felted on both surfaces. In summer, produce solitary, yellow, orange, pink, or brown flowerheads on short stems just above the leaves. ↕↔ to 25cm (10in). ❄. **'Talent Yellow'** ■ has bright, deep yellow flowers.

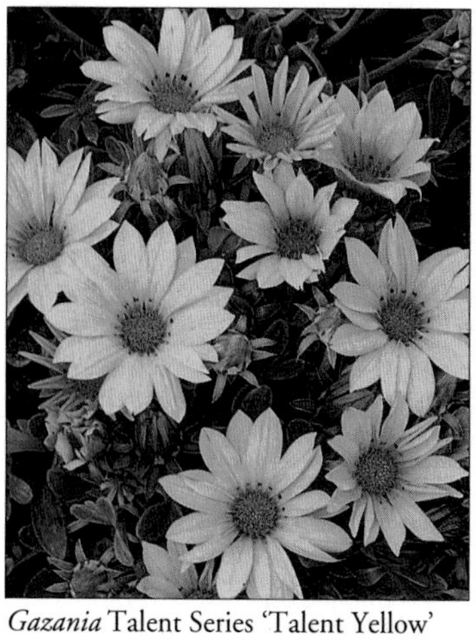

Gazania Talent Series 'Talent Yellow'

▷ **Gean** see *Prunus avium*

GEISSORHIZA

IRIDACEAE

Genus of 60–70 species of erect, cormous perennials from dry lowland sand to moist upland areas in southern Africa. Leaves are basal, lance-shaped, linear, or thread-like, and often curled. Flowers are usually funnel-shaped, and are borne in 1- or 2-sided spikes, with leaf-like bracts, in spring. In frost-prone areas, grow at the base of a warm wall with winter protection, or in a temperate greenhouse. In warmer climates, grow in a bed or border.

• **HARDINESS** Frost hardy to frost tender.

• **CULTIVATION** Under glass, grow in loam-based potting compost (JI No.2), with added grit, in full sun. Water freely during the growing season, but keep dry when dormant. Outdoors, grow in well-drained, sandy loam in full sun. Protect from winter wet.

• **PROPAGATION** Sow seed in containers in a cold frame when ripe; separate offset corms when dormant.

• **PESTS AND DISEASES** Trouble free.

G. radians, syn. *G. rochensis* (Winecups). Upright perennial with thread-like, sometimes 4-angled, basal leaves, to 15cm (6in) long. Bears funnel-shaped, red-centred, white-ringed purple flowers, 1–2cm (½–¾in) long, in spring. ↕ 15cm (6in), ↔ 5cm (2in). South Africa (Western Cape). ❄❄

G. rochensis see *G. radians.*

GELSEMIUM

LOGANIACEAE

Genus of 3 species of evergreen, twining, perennial climbers from S.E. Asia, S. North America, and Central America, usually found in woodland. They are grown for their funnel-shaped, sweetly fragrant flowers, which have 5 petal lobes, borne singly or in small, terminal and axillary clusters. Leaves are simple, entire, and arranged in opposite pairs. In frost-prone areas, grow in a cool or temperate greenhouse. In warmer climates, train over an arbour, pergola or arch, or against a wall.

• **HARDINESS** Frost tender; but *G. sempervirens* will withstand short periods down to 0°C (32°F).

• **CULTIVATION** Under glass, grow in loam-based potting compost (JI No.2) in full or bright filtered light. Top-dress or pot on in spring. During the growing season, water freely and apply a balanced liquid fertilizer monthly. Outdoors, grow in moderately fertile, moist but well-drained soil in full sun or partial shade, with shelter from cold, drying winds. Pruning group 12, after flowering.

• **PROPAGATION** Sow seed at 13–18°C (55–64°F) in spring, or take semi-ripe cuttings with bottom heat in summer.

• **PESTS AND DISEASES** Scale insects and whiteflies may infest greenhouse plants.

G. sempervirens ♀ (Carolina jasmine, Evening trumpet, False yellow jasmine). Vigorous, slender, twining perennial with stems that spiral anti-clockwise, and oblong to narrowly ovate, glossy leaves, to 5cm (2in) long. Bears clusters, 5–8cm (2–3in) across, of fragrant, bright, pale to deep yellow flowers, 3cm (1¼in) long, with darker, orange throats, mainly in spring and summer. ↕ 3–6m (10–20ft). S.E. USA, Mexico, Guatemala. ❄ (borderline)

GENISTA

syn. CHAMAESPARTIUM, ECHINOSPARTUM

Broom

LEGUMINOSAE/PAPILIONACEAE

Genus, similar to *Cytisus*, of about 90 species of mainly deciduous, sometimes spiny shrubs and occasionally trees, found in habitats ranging from pasture and moorland to cliffs and rocky places in Europe, the Mediterranean, and W. Asia. They have alternate, simple or 3-palmate leaves, usually 3–10mm (⅛–½in) long, sometimes more, but may be nearly leafless. They are cultivated for their small, pea-like yellow flowers, borne singly or in terminal racemes or dense heads. Grow as specimen plants, or in a shrub border or rock garden. In frost-prone areas, grow half-hardy species in a cool greenhouse.

• **HARDINESS** Fully hardy to half hardy.

• **CULTIVATION** Grow in light, poor to moderately fertile, well-drained soil in full sun. Pruning group 1; group 3 for *G. cinerea*. Do not cut into old wood.

• **PROPAGATION** Sow seed in containers outdoors in a cold frame in autumn or spring, or take semi-ripe cuttings in summer.

• **PESTS AND DISEASES** Prone to aphids.

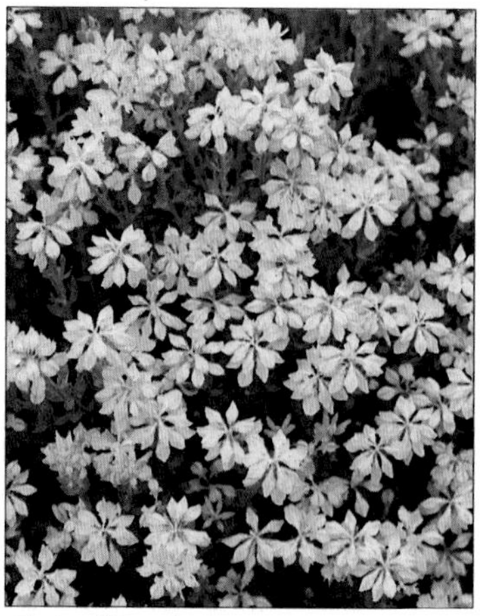

Genista hispanica

G. aetnensis ■ ♀ ♀–♠ (Mount Etna broom). Upright, deciduous tree or large shrub with weeping branches bearing slender, bright green shoots. Linear leaves are produced on young stems only and soon fall. Fragrant, golden yellow flowers, to 1.5cm (½in) long, are freely borne at the ends of pendent shoots in mid- and late summer. ↕↔ 8m (25ft). Italy (Sardinia, Sicily). ❄❄

G. cinerea. Erect, deciduous shrub with arching branches, silky when young, and narrow, lance-shaped to elliptic, grey-green leaves. Pairs of fragrant yellow flowers, to 1.5cm (½in) long, are produced profusely in irregular racemes, to 20cm (8in) long, in early and midsummer. ↕ 3m (10ft), ↔ 4m (12ft). S.W. Europe. ❄❄

G. decumbens see *Cytisus decumbens.*

G. delphinensis ♀ syn. *Chamaespartium sagittale* subsp. *delphinense, G. sagittalis* subsp. *delphinensis.* Low, prostrate, deciduous subshrub with a few lance-shaped, mid-green leaves, softly hairy beneath, and winged green stems that give the plant a leafy, evergreen appearance. Small, golden yellow flowers, to 1.5cm (½in) long, are borne in spike-like, axillary and terminal racemes, to 4cm (1½in) long, in late spring and early summer. ↕ to 15cm (6in), ↔ to 30cm (12in). Pyrenees. ❄❄❄

***G. fragrans* of gardens** see *Cytisus* x *spachianus.*

G. hispanica ■ (Spanish gorse). Dense, mound-forming, spiny, deciduous shrub with ovate-oblong, mid-green leaves, hairy or silky beneath, only present on flowering branches. Bears almost

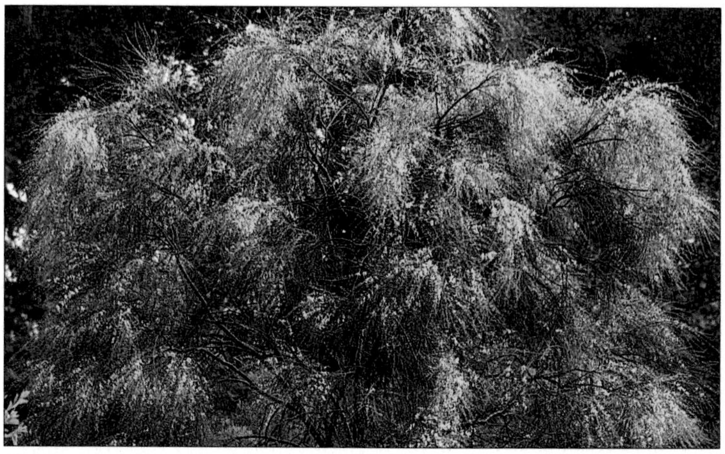

Genista aetnensis

G

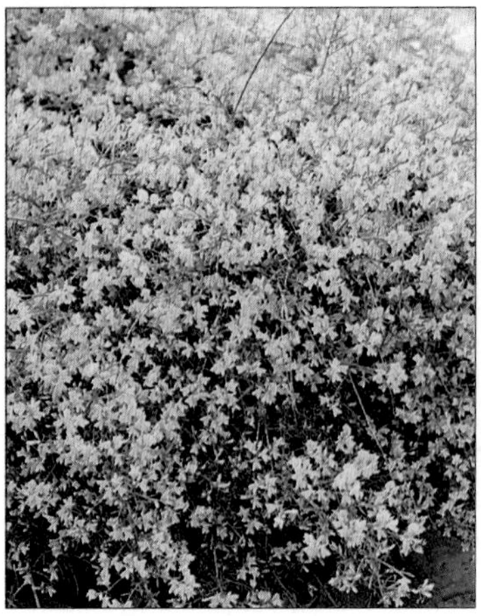
Genista lydia

terminal racemes, 2.5cm (1in) across, of 2–12 golden yellow flowers, 1cm (½in) long, in late spring and early summer. ↕75cm (30in), ↔ 1.5m (5ft). S.W. Europe. ❄❄❄ (borderline). **'Compacta'** is of very dense habit.
G. lydia ■ 🏆 Deciduous, domed shrub bearing slender, arching, prickle-tipped, grey-green branches, with linear-elliptic, blue-green leaves. In early summer, produces a profusion of yellow flowers, to 1.5cm (½in) long, in short racemes, 5cm (2in) long. ↕ to 60cm (24in), ↔ to 1m (3ft). E. Balkans. ❄❄❄
G. monosperma see *Retama monosperma.*
G. pilosa. Deciduous, prostrate or semi-erect shrub, with downy, ascending branches bearing inversely lance-shaped, dark green leaves, to 1.5cm (½in) long,

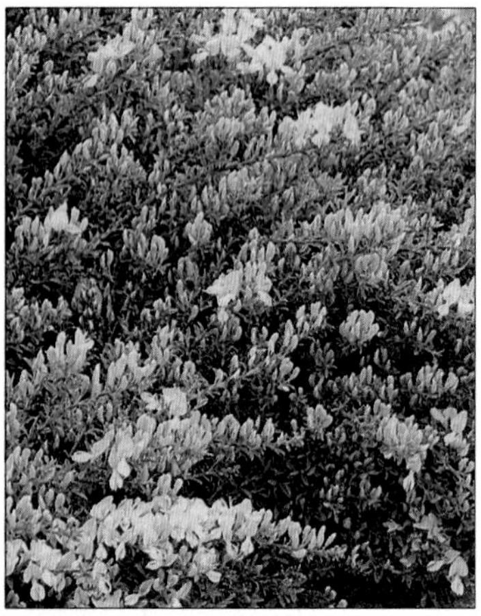
Genista pilosa 'Procumbens'

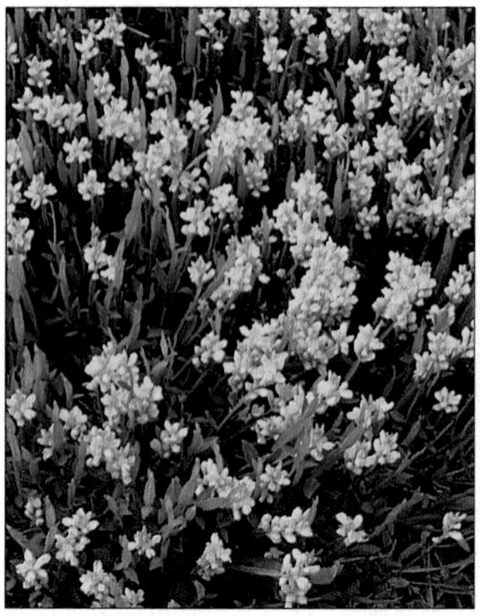
Genista sagittalis

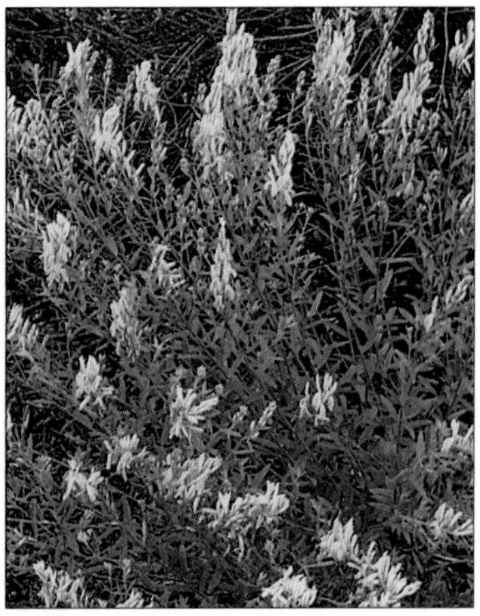
Genista tinctoria

silky-hairy beneath. In late spring and early summer, produces bright yellow flowers, to 1cm (½in) long, in racemes to 14cm (5½in) long. ↕ to 40cm (16in), ↔ to 1m (3ft). W. and C. Europe. ❄❄❄. **'Lemon Spreader'** see 'Yellow Spreader'. **'Procumbens'** ■ has prostrate stems; ↕ to 20cm (8in). **'Vancouver Gold'** is spreading and mound-forming, with golden yellow flowers; ↕45cm (18in). **'Yellow Spreader'**, syn. 'Lemon Spreader', is low-growing and spreading, with lemon-yellow flowers; ↕ to 30cm (12in).
G. sagittalis ■ syn. *Chamaespartium sagittale.* Low-growing, deciduous shrub with upright, broadly winged green stems that give the plant an evergreen appearance; they bear a few lance-shaped, mid-green leaves, to 2cm (¾in) long. In early summer, produces dense, spike-like racemes, to 4cm (1½in) long, of deep yellow flowers, 1cm (½in) long. ↕15cm (6in), ↔ to 1m (3ft). C. and S. Europe. ❄❄❄. **subsp. *delphinensis*** see *G. delphinensis.*
G.* x *spachiana see *Cytisus* x *spachianus.*
***G. tenera* 'Golden Shower'** 🏆 Graceful, deciduous shrub with slender, arching shoots and narrowly oblong, grey-green leaves. In early and midsummer, bears dense racemes, to 5cm (2in) long, of fragrant, brilliant yellow flowers, to 1.5cm (½in) long, towards the ends of short, lateral branches. ↕3m (10ft), ↔ 5m (15ft). ❄❄
G. tinctoria ■ (Dyer's greenweed). Variable, upright, deciduous shrub with narrow, elliptic-lance-shaped or inversely lance-shaped, bright, deep green leaves, to 5cm (2in) long. From spring to early summer, bears golden yellow flowers in upright racemes, 6cm (2½in) long. ↕60–90cm (24–36in), ↔ 1m (3ft). Europe, Turkey. ❄❄❄. **'Flore Pleno'** 🏆 syn. 'Plena', is dwarf and spreading, with double flowers; ↕35cm (14in). **'Plena'** see 'Flore Pleno'. **'Royal Gold'** 🏆 is upright, with flowers in long, conical panicles, to 8cm (3in) long; ↕ 1m (3ft).

▷**Gentian** see *Gentiana*
Bottle see *Gentiana andrewsii*
Fringed see *Gentianopsis crinita*
Spotted see *Gentiana punctata*
Spring see *Gentiana verna*
Star see *Gentiana verna*
Trumpet see *Gentiana acaulis, G. clusii*
Willow see *Gentiana asclepiadea*
Yellow see *Gentiana lutea*

GENTIANA

Gentian

GENTIANACEAE

Genus of about 400 species of hardy annuals, biennials, and deciduous, semi-evergreen, and evergreen perennials. They are widely distributed throughout temperate zones, most occurring in alpine habitats, with some, mainly North American and Japanese species, in woodland. They bear large, usually trumpet-shaped, sometimes bell- or almost urn-shaped flowers from spring to autumn, mainly in shades of intense blue, but also in white, yellow, or occasionally red. Leaves are simple and borne along the stems in opposite pairs or whorls, or produced in basal rosettes. Many autumn-flowering species have overwintering rosettes and are classed as semi-evergreen; the flowered stems die back each year to the rosettes.

Small species, to about 15cm (6in) high, are suitable for a rock garden or peat terrace; more robust species are suitable for borders. Woodland natives, like *G. asclepiadea*, thrive in partially shaded sites, associating well with ferns and grasses. *G. sceptrum* is suitable for a bog garden; *G. lutea* is effective beside water. Autumn-flowering gentians associate well with small, late-flowering bulbs.

- **HARDINESS** Fully hardy.
- **CULTIVATION** Grow in light, humus-rich, reliably moist but well-drained soil. Autumn-flowering species, unless otherwise stated, need neutral to acid soil. Site gentians in full sun only where summers are cool and damp; in areas with warm, dry summers, provide shade from hot sun.
- **PROPAGATION** Sow seed of species in containers in an open frame as soon as ripe. Divide or root offsets in spring.
- **PESTS AND DISEASES** Slugs and snails may cause damage; aphids and red spider mites may be a problem under glass. Susceptible to gentian rust fungus (*Puccinia gentianae*). Various soil fungi may cause stem rots.

G. acaulis ■ 🏆 syn. *G. excisa, G. kochiana* (Trumpet gentian). Evergreen, mat-forming perennial with basal rosettes of elliptic to lance-shaped, pointed, glossy, dark green leaves, to 3.5cm (1½in) long. In late spring and early summer, produces solitary, trumpet-shaped flowers, to 5cm (2in)

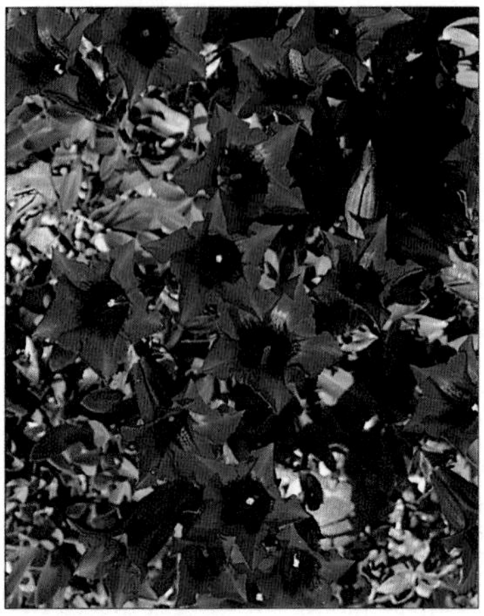
Gentiana acaulis

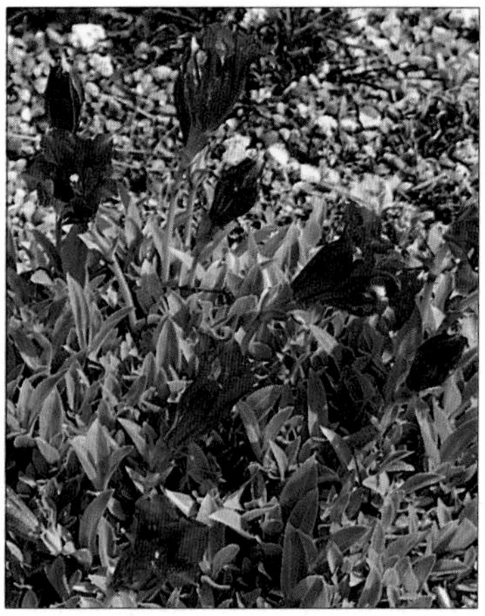
Gentiana alpina

long, deep blue and spotted green inside, on short stems. ↕8cm (3in), ↔ to 30cm (12in). N.E. Spain, Alps, Italy, former Yugoslavia, Carpathians. ❄❄❄. **'Alba'** has white flowers, spotted green inside.
G. alpina ■ Mat-forming, evergreen perennial with basal rosettes of elliptic to rounded, leathery, mid-green leaves, to 2cm (¾in) long. In early summer, bears solitary, often stalkless, trumpet-shaped flowers, to 4.5cm (1¾in) long, deep blue and spotted green inside. ↕ to 5cm (2in), ↔ to 20cm (8in). Spain (Sierra Nevada), Pyrenees, Alps. ❄❄❄
G. andrewsii (Bottle gentian). Erect, tufted, deciduous perennial with pairs of lance-shaped to oblong-ovate, deep green, stem leaves, 5–8cm (2–3in) long. In late summer, bears terminal clusters of 5 or more cylindrical to urn-shaped flowers, to 4cm (1½in) long, white, or dark blue with white on the lobes. ↕30–60cm (12–24in), ↔ 15cm (6in). E. North America. ❄❄❄
G. angustifolia ■ Evergreen, clump-forming perennial with basal rosettes of linear-lance-shaped to inversely lance-shaped, dull green leaves, to 5cm (2in) long. In early summer, produces single, short-stalked, trumpet-shaped flowers, to 5cm (2in) long, deep sky-blue outside, paler and spotted green inside. ↕ to 10cm (4in), ↔ to 30cm (12in). Pyrenees, Jura Mountains, S.W. Alps. ❄❄❄
G. asclepiadea ■ 🏆 (Willow gentian). Clump-forming herbaceous perennial with erect, then arching stems bearing opposite pairs, or whorls of 3, willow-like, lance-shaped to narrowly ovate, pointed, mid-green leaves, 5–8cm (2–3in) long. From mid- or late summer to early autumn, bears axillary clusters of 2 or 3 trumpet-shaped, dark to light blue flowers, to 5cm (2in) long, the throats rarely purple-spotted, or sometimes all white. ↕60–90cm (24–36in), ↔ 45cm (18in). Mountains of C. and S. Europe, Turkey. ❄❄❄. **var. *alba*** has green-tinged white flowers. **'Knightshayes'** has white-throated, deep blue flowers; ↕ to 60cm (24in).
G. cachemirica, syn. *G. cashmeriana.* Rosette-forming herbaceous perennial with purple-tinged, procumbent stems, narrowly ovate, glaucous, mid-green basal leaves, 2.5–5cm (1–2in) long, and shorter, broader stem leaves. In late summer, bears 1–3 terminal, narrowly trumpet-shaped flowers, to 4cm (1½in) long, bright to pale blue, striped yellow

and darker blue. ↕ to 15cm (6in), ↔ to 25cm (10in). Pakistan to India (Kashmir). ❄❄❄

G. cashmeriana see *G. cachemirica.*

G. clusii (Trumpet gentian). Evergreen, tufted perennial with basal rosettes of elliptic to oblong-lance-shaped, leathery, bright green leaves, to 2.5cm (1in) long. Solitary, trumpet-shaped, deep azure-blue flowers, to 5cm (2in) long, are paler and spotted olive-green inside; they appear in early summer. Lime-tolerant. ↕ to 8cm (3in), ↔ to 30cm (12in). C. and S. Alps. ❄❄❄

G. crinita see *Gentianopsis crinita.*

***G.* 'Devonhall'.** Robust, rosette-forming, semi-evergreen perennial, similar to *G. ornata* but more compact and vigorous, with linear, mid-green basal leaves, to 2.5cm (1in) long. Stem leaves are smaller and sharply acute. In autumn, produces prostrate stems with solitary, widely trumpet-shaped, pale blue flowers, about 5cm (2in) long, paler at the throats and spotted green inside. ↕ 5cm (2in), ↔ to 20cm (8in). ❄❄❄

G. excisa see *G. acaulis.*

G. farreri. Slender, trailing, semi-evergreen perennial with basal rosettes of linear-lance-shaped, bright green leaves, to 3.5cm (1½in) long, and paired, recurved stem leaves. In early autumn, bears solitary, narrowly trumpet-shaped, pale blue flowers, to 6cm (2½in) long, the tubes white with greenish blue spots and lines, on prostrate stems. ↕ to 7cm (3in), ↔ to 30cm (12in). N.W. China. ❄❄❄

G. gracilipes, syn. *G. purdomii.* Semi-evergreen, rosette-forming perennial with narrowly lance-shaped, dark green basal leaves, to 15cm (6in) long, and decumbent, branching stems with shorter leaves. In summer, produces solitary, long-stalked, narrowly trumpet-shaped, deep purplish blue flowers, to 3.5cm (1½in) long, stained green outside. Tolerates shade. ↕ 15cm (6in), ↔ 20cm (8in). N.W. China. ❄❄❄

***G.* 'Inverleith'** 🏆 Vigorous, procumbent, semi-evergreen, rosette-forming perennial, producing linear-lance-shaped, recurved, mid-green, basal leaves, to 2.5cm (1in) long. In autumn, bears solitary, trumpet-shaped flowers, to 6cm (2½in) long, of an intense pale blue with darker stripes on the outside, on prostrate stems. ↕ to 10cm (4in), ↔ to 30cm (12in). ❄❄❄

***G.* 'Kingfisher'** ▣ Rosette-forming, semi-evergreen perennial, similar to

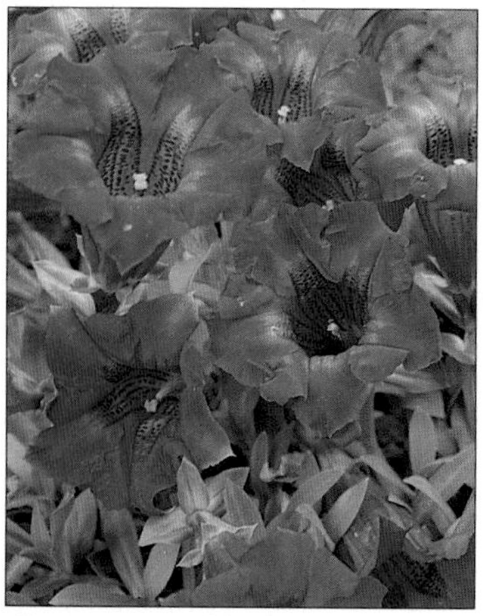

Gentiana angustifolia

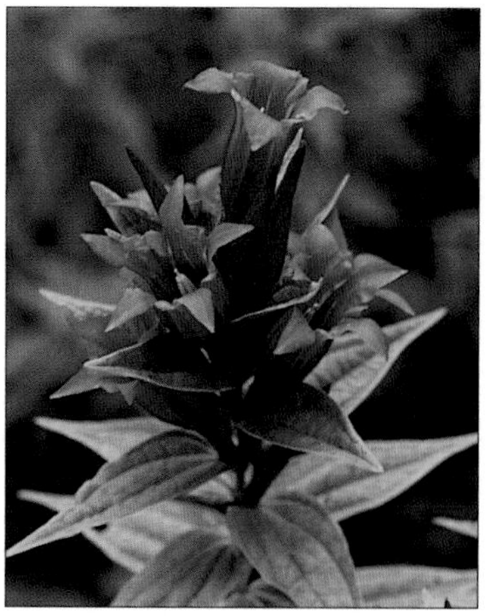

Gentiana asclepiadea

G. sino-ornata but more compact, with linear-lance-shaped, mid- to dark green, basal leaves, to 2.5cm (1in) long. In autumn, bears solitary, trumpet-shaped, vivid blue flowers, to 4cm (1½in) long, on prostrate stems. ↕ 5cm (2in), ↔ to 30cm (12in). ❄❄❄

G. kochiana see *G. acaulis.*

G. lagodechiana see *G. septemfida* var. *lagodechiana.*

G. lutea ▣ (Bitterwort, Yellow gentian). Erect, clump-forming herbaceous perennial with fleshy roots and elliptic to ovate, pleated, strongly ribbed, bluish green basal leaves, to 30cm (12in) long. Stem leaves are in pairs, fused at the base. Terminal and upper axillary clusters of 3–10 star-shaped yellow flowers, 2.5cm (1in) across, with very short tubes, are borne in midsummer. ↕ to 1.5m (5ft), ↔ 60cm (24in). Pyrenees, Alps, Apennines, Carpathians. ❄❄❄

***G.* x *macaulayi* 'Wells's Variety'** ▣ syn. *G.* 'Wellsii'. Semi-evergreen, rosette-forming perennial, with linear-lance-shaped, dark green, basal leaves, to 3.5cm (1½in) long. Solitary, trumpet-shaped, pale blue flowers, to 5cm (2in) long, sometimes mauve-flushed, with

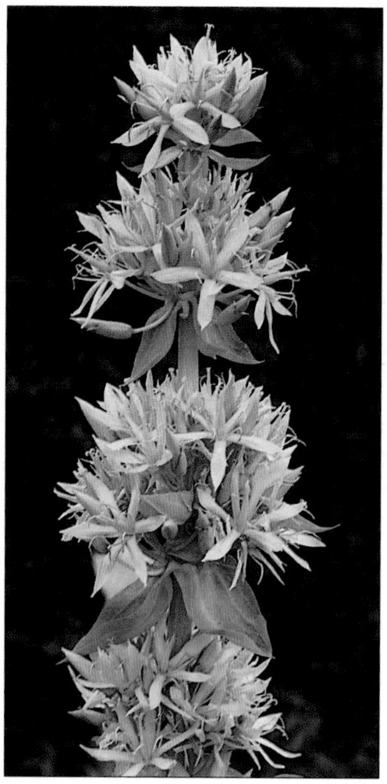

Gentiana lutea

pale stripes outside, appear on prostrate stems from late summer to autumn. ↕ 5cm (2in), ↔ to 30cm (12in). ❄❄❄

G. makinoi. Erect herbaceous perennial with leafy stems bearing pairs of lance-shaped to narrowly ovate, somewhat bluish green leaves, the upper leaf to 5cm (2in) long, the lower 2.5cm (1in). In late summer, bears terminal and axillary clusters of up to 7 tubular-bell-shaped, pale blue flowers, 3–4cm (1¼–1½in) long, heavily spotted dark blue, with unequal sepals. ↕ to 50cm (20in), ↔ 15cm (6in). Japan. ❄❄❄

G. menziesii see *G. sceptrum.*

G. ornata. Semi-evergreen perennial with tufted rosettes of linear, mid-green, basal leaves, to 2.5cm (1in) long. In autumn, prostrate flowering stems bear

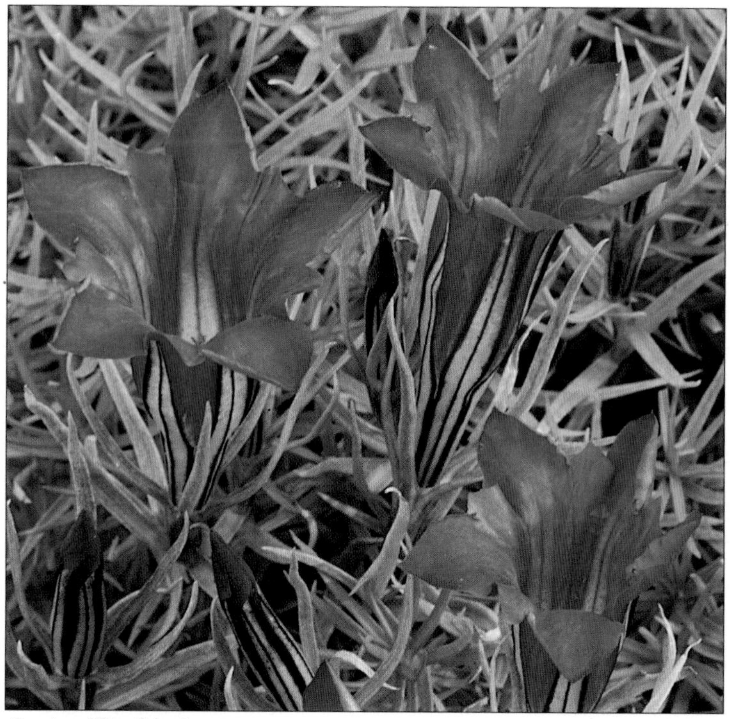

Gentiana 'Kingfisher'

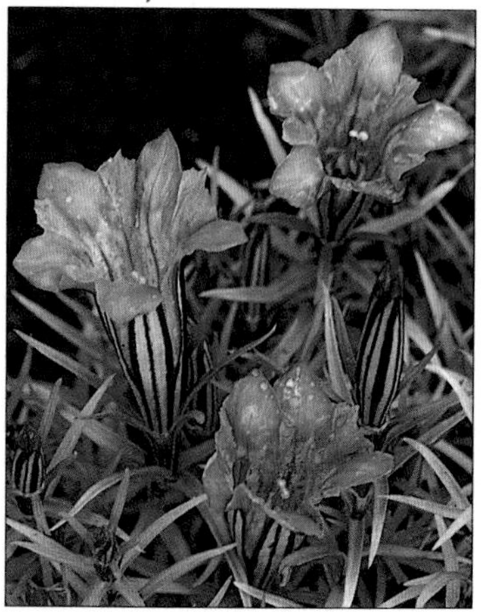

Gentiana x *macaulayi* 'Wells's Variety'

solitary, broadly bell-shaped flowers, to 3.5cm (1½in) long, light pale blue, striped purplish blue and cream outside. ↕ 5cm (2in), ↔ to 15cm (6in). Mountains of Nepal. ❄❄❄

G. punctata (Spotted gentian). Erect, clump-forming herbaceous perennial with broadly lance-shaped to elliptic, glossy, mid-green basal leaves, to 10cm (4in) long. Stem leaves are narrower. All leaves are strongly veined. In late summer, bears terminal and axillary whorls of numerous stalkless, bell-shaped, purple- or maroon-spotted, pale greenish yellow flowers, to 3.5cm (1½in) long. ↕ 30–60cm (12–24in), ↔ 22cm (9in). C. Europe. ❄❄❄

G. purdomii see *G. gracilipes.*

G. saxosa ▣ Evergreen perennial with basal rosettes of spoon-shaped to linear-spoon-shaped, fleshy, dark green leaves, to 3.5cm (1½in) long, often tinged brown-purple. In summer, short, leafy stems bear 1–5 upright, bell-shaped white flowers, to 2cm (¾in) long, with faint green or purple-brown veining. ↕ to 7cm (3in), ↔ to 10cm (4in). New Zealand. ❄❄❄

G. sceptrum, syn. *G. menziesii.* Erect, clump-forming herbaceous perennial with paired, ovate to lance-shaped, mid-green basal and stem leaves, 3–8cm (1¼–3in) long. In late summer, broadly trumpet-shaped, green-spotted, bluish purple flowers, 4–5cm (1½–2in) long, with erect corolla lobes, are produced in terminal clusters or in twos or threes from the upper axils. ↕ 45–90cm (18–36in), ↔ 20cm (8in). W. Canada (British Columbia) to W. USA (California). ❄❄❄

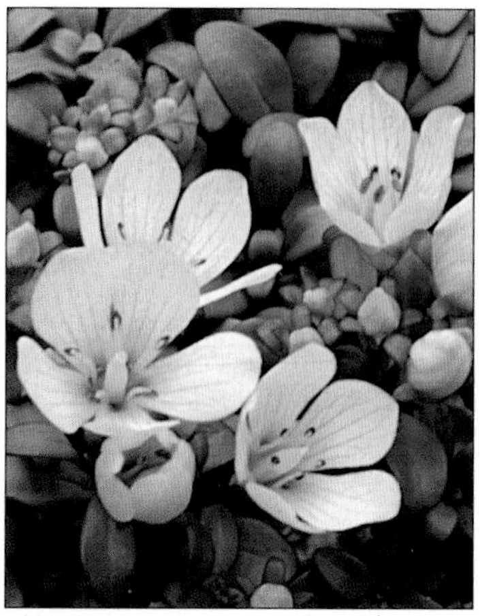

Gentiana saxosa

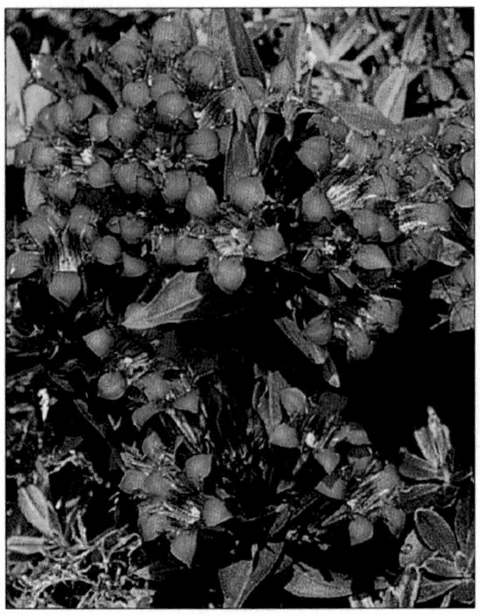

Gentiana septemfida

G

G. septemfida ■ 🏆 Spreading herbaceous perennial with prostrate or ascending stems bearing paired, ovate, pointed, mid-green leaves, to 3.5cm (1½in) long. In late summer, produces terminal clusters of 1–8 narrowly bell-shaped, bright blue or purplish blue flowers, 3.5cm (1½in) long, with white throats and darker stripes. Best in sun. ↕ to 15–20cm (6–8in), ↔ to 30cm (12in). Caucasus, Turkey, Iran to C. Asia. ❄❄❄. **var. *lagodechiana***, syn. *G. lagodechiana*, has branched, almost prostrate stems and a single flower, rarely 2 or 3, per stem.

G. sino-ornata ■ 🏆 Rosette-forming, semi-evergreen perennial with many prostrate shoots bearing paired, linear-lance-shaped, finely pointed, dark green, basal leaves, to 3.5cm (1½in) long. Solitary, stalkless, terminal, trumpet-shaped flowers, to 6cm (2½in) long, usually deep bright blue, striped deep purple-blue and greenish white outside, are borne in autumn. ↕ 5–7cm (2–3in), ↔ 15–30cm (6–12in). W. China, Tibet. ❄❄❄. **'Alba'** has white flowers. **'Angel's Wings'** has blue flowers splashed with white, occasionally all-blue or all-white.

G. speciosa, syn. *Crawfurdia speciosa*. Climbing or trailing herbaceous perennial with slender stems bearing elliptic to ovate, pointed, toothed, mid-green leaves, 5–8cm (2–3in) long, in opposite pairs. In late summer, bears axillary clusters of 1–3 narrowly tubular-bell-shaped, deep blue to blue-purple or white flowers, to 5cm (2in) long, green-tinted outside. Prefers acid soil in shade. ↕ to 1m (3ft). Himalayas, China. ❄❄❄

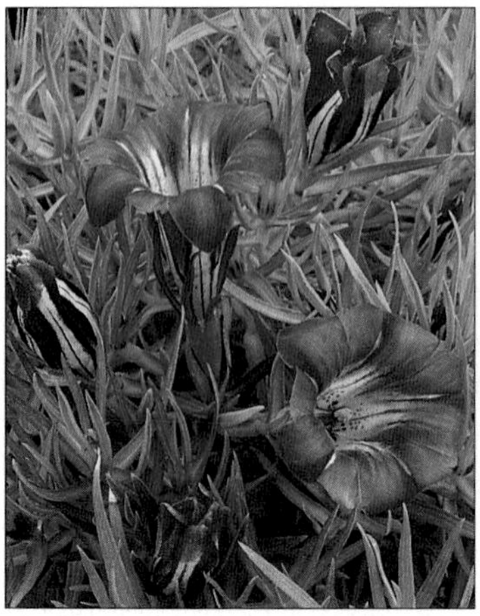

Gentiana sino-ornata

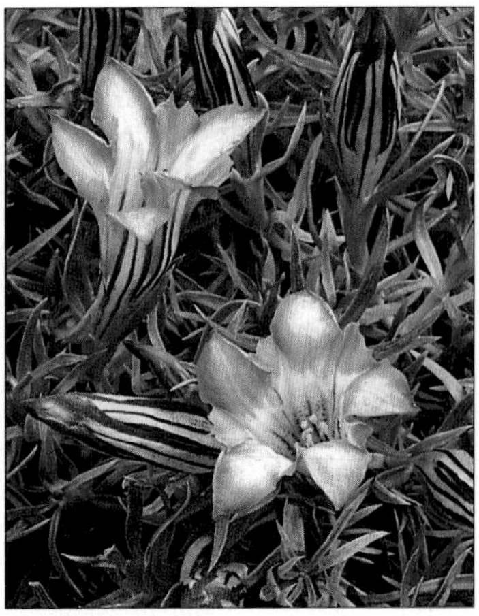

Gentiana ternifolia

G. stylophora see *Megacodon stylophorus*.

G. 'Susan Jane'. Procumbent, rosette-forming, semi-evergreen perennial with linear-lance-shaped, dark green, basal leaves, to 3cm (1¼in) long. In autumn, bears solitary, trumpet-shaped, bright azure-blue flowers, to 5cm (2in) long, with white throats and notched petals, on prostrate stems. ↕ to 8cm (3in), ↔ to 30cm (12in). ❄❄❄

G. ternifolia ■ Vigorous, trailing, semi-evergreen perennial with loose rosettes of linear-lance-shaped, greyish green basal leaves, to 1.5cm (½in) long; stem leaves are similar, in whorls of 2 or 3. In autumn, solitary, trumpet- to bell-shaped, sky-blue flowers, 4cm (1½in) long, striped darker blue and spotted white and green outside, paler inside, are borne on prostrate stems. ↕ to 8cm (3in), ↔ to 30cm (12in). W. China. ❄❄❄

G. triflora ■ Erect herbaceous perennial with slender, leafy stems bearing paired, narrow, lance-shaped, glossy, mid-green leaves, 5–10cm (2–4in) long. Narrowly bell-shaped, deep blue to purple-blue flowers, 3–5cm (1¼–2in) long, with white bands outside, are borne in small, upright, terminal or upper axillary clusters in late summer and early autumn. ↕ 22–60cm (9–24in), ↔ 25cm (10in). Russia (E. Siberia, Sakhalin), China (Manchuria), Japan, Korea. ❄❄❄

G. veitchiorum. Trailing, semi-evergreen perennial with many-branched stems, and rosettes of linear-oblong, mid-green basal leaves, to 3.5cm (1½in) long. Stem leaves are borne in pairs, and are usually fused at the bases. In autumn, bears solitary, dark blue flowers, narrowly trumpet-shaped and to 5cm (2in) long, with very narrow tubes and striped outside with greenish yellow, on prostrate shoots. ↕ 5cm (2in), ↔ to 20cm (8in). W. China. ❄❄❄

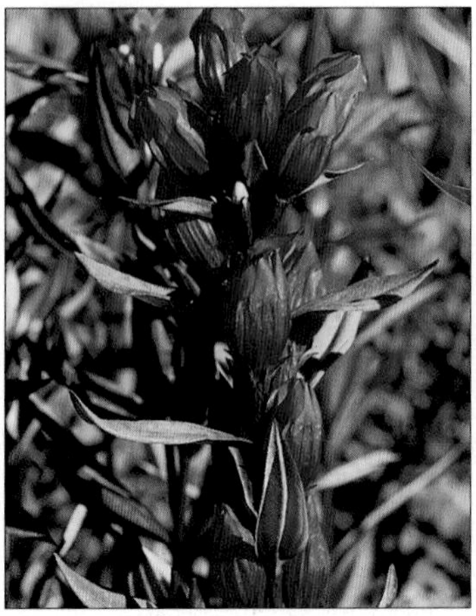

Gentiana triflora

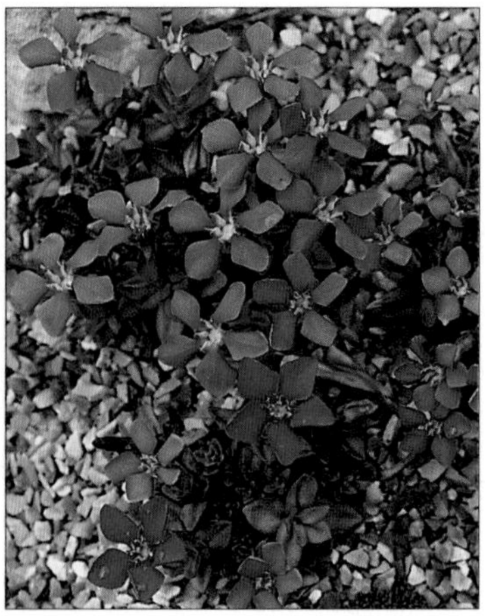

Gentiana verna

G. verna ■ (Spring gentian, Star gentian). Often short-lived, mat-forming, evergreen perennial with basal rosettes of elliptic-lance-shaped, dark green leaves, to 3cm (1¼in) long, and 1–3 pairs of stem leaves. In spring or early summer, bears solitary, short-stemmed, narrowly tubular, usually white-throated, pure sky-blue flowers, to 3cm (1¼in) across, with wide-spreading lobes. ↕ 4cm (1½in), ↔ to 10cm (4in). Mountains in Europe, from Ireland to Russia. ❄❄❄. **subsp. *balcanica*** 🏆 syn. subsp. *pontica*, subsp. *tergestina*, is more vigorous, with usually ovate leaves and larger flowers, to 3.5cm (1½in) across; ↕ to 6cm (2½in).

G. 'Wellsii' see *G.* x *macaulayi* 'Wells's Variety'.

GENTIANOPSIS

GENTIANACEAE

Genus of 20–25 species of erect annuals and biennials, sometimes included in the genus *Gentiana*, found in moist grassland throughout North America and Eurasia. They form basal tufts of simple, glossy leaves, and bear tubular-bell-shaped, 4-petalled, fringed blue flowers on long stems from late summer to autumn. They are suitable for a wild garden or a partially shaded border.

- **HARDINESS** Fully hardy.
- **CULTIVATION** Grow in humus-rich, moist but well-drained soil in a site shaded from hot sun.
- **PROPAGATION** Sow *in situ*, or surface-sow in containers outdoors, in autumn.
- **PESTS AND DISEASES** Slugs and snails may damage young seedlings.

G. crinita, syn. *Gentiana crinita* (Fringed gentian). Tuft-forming annual or biennial with ovate to lance-shaped, glossy, dark green leaves, 2–3cm (¾–1¼in) long. Produces long, branching, hairy stems that terminate in single or clustered, 4-lobed, tubular-bell-shaped, fringed, bright blue flowers, 5cm (2in) long, from late summer to autumn. ↕ 30–90cm (12–36in), ↔ to 23cm (9in). E. North America. ❄❄❄

▷ **Geraldton wax** see *Chamelaucium uncinatum*

GERANIUM

Cranesbill

GERANIACEAE

Genus of about 300 species of annuals, biennials, and herbaceous, semi-evergreen, and evergreen, sometimes tuberous perennials, often confused with the genus *Pelargonium* (which is commonly, though incorrectly, known as geranium). Cranesbills are found in all except very wet habitats throughout temperate regions. The leaves, usually rounded or 5-pointed, are palmately lobed, the divisions often further lobed and toothed; they are frequently aromatic or interestingly marked, textured, or coloured, sometimes also colouring well in autumn. The basal leaves are often arranged in loose, sometimes overwintering or semi-evergreen rosettes; the stem leaves are usually smaller, with fewer lobes. Flowers are white, pink, purple, or blue, usually saucer-shaped, sometimes flat or star-shaped, with petals sometimes reflexed and often contrastingly veined or marked; they are mostly borne in diffuse or dense cymes or umbel- or panicle-like inflorescences.

Cranesbills are generally long-lived, versatile, and undemanding plants. Compact perennials, to about 15cm (6in) tall, are good for a rock garden; trailing, spreading, or mat-forming plants are effective as ground cover in a woodland or wild garden. Taller, clump-forming species and hybrids are suitable for a border or among shrubs.

- **HARDINESS** Fully hardy to half hardy.
- **CULTIVATION** Outdoors, grow larger species and hybrids in any moderately fertile, well-drained soil in full sun or partial shade, but most soils (unless waterlogged), in either sun or shade, are tolerated. Grow small species and hybrids in humus-rich, sharply drained soil in full sun. Under glass, grow half hardy species in loam-based potting compost (JI No.2), with added sharp sand, in bright filtered light. During the growing season, water freely and apply a balanced liquid fertilizer monthly. Water sparingly in winter. For all cranesbills, remove flowered stems and old leaves to encourage the production of fresh leaves and flowers.
- **PROPAGATION** Sow seed of hardy species in containers outdoors as soon as ripe or in spring. Sow seed of half-hardy species at 13–18°C (55–64°F) in spring. Divide in spring. Increase by basal cuttings, taken in early or mid-spring, and root with bottom heat.
- **PESTS AND DISEASES** May be damaged by vine weevil larvae, sawfly larvae, slugs, and snails. Viruses and downy mildew may also be troublesome. In dry conditions, powdery mildew may be a problem.

G. anemonifolium see *G. palmatum*.

G. 'Ann Folkard' ■ Spreading herbaceous perennial producing many long, procumbent or scrambling stems and numerous 5-lobed, toothed, yellowish green leaves, 5–20cm (2–8in) long, becoming greener with age. A profusion of saucer-shaped magenta flowers, 4cm (1½in) across, with black centres and veins, are produced continuously from midsummer to mid-

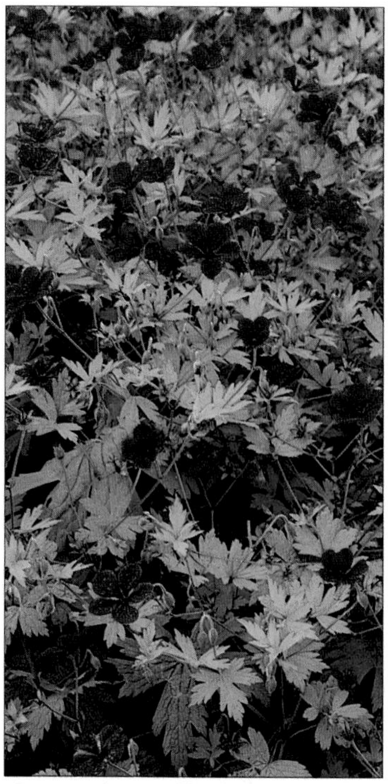

Geranium 'Ann Folkard'

autumn. ↕ to 60cm (24in), ↔ 1m (3ft) or more. ❄❄❄

G. argenteum. Compact, semi-evergreen perennial with silky-hairy, silver, basal leaves, to 5cm (2in) long, deeply 7-lobed, each lobe with 3 segments. In summer, bears short-stalked cymes of pale pink flowers, to 2.5cm (1in) wide, with magenta veins and notched petals. Needs sharp drainage. ↕ to 10cm (4in), ↔ to 15cm (6in). Mountains of C. and E. Europe. ❄❄❄

G. armenum see *G. psilostemon.*

G. asphodeloides ▣ Variable, evergreen perennial, forming a loose mound of 5- to 7-lobed, mid-green, basal leaves, to 8cm (3in) long. Loose cymes of numerous star-shaped, narrow-petalled, pink or white flowers, 2.5–3.5cm (1–1½in) across, with darker veins, are produced in early summer. ↕ 30–45cm (12–18in), ↔ 30cm (12in). Italy (Sicily) to Turkey, Caucasus, N. Iran. ❄❄❄

***G. atlanticum* of gardens** see *G. malviflorum.*

***G.* 'Buxton's Blue'** see *G. wallichianum* 'Buxton's Variety'.

***G. candicans* of gardens** see *G. lambertii.*

G. x cantabrigiense ▣ (*G. dalmaticum* x *G. macrorrhizum*). Compact, evergreen perennial, spreading slowly by runners, with 7-lobed, toothed, aromatic, glossy, light green, basal leaves, 3–9cm (1¼–3½in) long. In early and midsummer, produces dense cymes of numerous flat, bright purplish pink or white flowers, 2.5cm (1in) across, the petals somewhat reflexed. ↕ 30cm (12in), ↔ 60cm (24in). Garden origin. ❄❄❄. **'Biokovo'** ▣ is compact, with long runners and pink-tinged white flowers; ↔ 75–90cm (30–36in). **'Cambridge'** forms compact mats of foliage and is very free-flowering, bearing pinkish mauve flowers; ↕ 15cm (6in), ↔ 45cm (18in).

G. cinereum. Dwarf, rosette-forming, evergreen perennial with grey-green, basal leaves, to 5cm (2in) across, deeply 5- to 7-lobed, with each division itself usually 3-lobed. In late spring and early summer, produces short-stalked cymes of 1–4 upward-facing, cup-shaped, translucent, white or pale pink flowers, to 2.5cm (1in) across, usually veined purple. Needs good drainage. ↕ to 15cm (6in), ↔ to 30cm (12in). Pyrenees. ❄❄❄. The following are excellent rock plants with long flowering seasons: **'Ballerina'** ▣ 🏆 has greyer leaves and purplish red flowers, dark red-veined, with dark eyes. **'Lawrence Flatman'** resembles 'Ballerina' but is more vigorous, with darker eyes and usually darker petals. **subsp. *subcaulescens*** ▣ 🏆 syn. *G. subcaulescens,* is more vigorous than the species, with darker green leaves, longer stems, and brilliant magenta flowers with black centres; Balkans, N.E. Turkey.

***G.* 'Claridge Druce'** see *G.* x *oxonianum* 'Claridge Druce'.

G. clarkei. Spreading, rhizomatous herbaceous perennial with 7-lobed, mid-green, basal leaves, 4.5–15cm (1¾–6in) long, each lobe deeply cut into narrow, pointed segments. Saucer- to cup-shaped flowers, 4–5cm (1½–2in) across, purple-violet or white with mauve-pink veins, are produced in loose cymes from early to late summer. ↕ to 50cm (20in), ↔ indefinite. India (Kashmir). ❄❄❄. **'Kashmir Blue'** bears soft pale blue flowers in early and midsummer; ↕ to 60cm (24in). **'Kashmir Pink'** has pink flowers. **'Kashmir Purple'**, syn. *G. pratense* 'Kashmir Purple', has rich lilac-blue flowers with red veins; it spreads rapidly. **'Kashmir White'** ▣ syn. *G. pratense* 'Kashmir White', is less vigorous than 'Kashmir Purple' and bears white flowers, 2.5–4cm (1–1½in) across, with pale lilac-pink veins, appearing greyish pink overall; ↕ to 45cm (18in).

G. dalmaticum ▣ 🏆 Dwarf, rhizomatous, woody-stemmed, creeping perennial, evergreen in all but the severest winters, with rosettes of glossy, light green, basal leaves, to 4cm (1½in) long, each deeply divided into 5–7 segments. In summer, bears long-stalked, umbel-like clusters of pale to bright pink flowers, 2.5–3.5cm (1–1½in) across, with red anthers and inflated calyces. ↕ to 15cm (6in), ↔ to 50cm (20in) or more. Yugoslavia (Montenegro), Albania. ❄❄❄

G. delavayi. Clump-forming herbaceous perennial with 7-lobed, toothed, mid-green, basal leaves, 5–20cm (2–8in) long, similar to those of *G. sinense* but with broader and overlapping lobes. Saucer-shaped, maroon or blackish red to pale pink flowers, to 2cm (¾in) across, with reflexed petals and white bases, are produced in loose cymes in late summer. ↕↔ 60cm (24in). S.W. China (Sichuan, Yunnan). ❄❄❄

G. endressii ▣ 🏆 Rhizomatous, hairy, evergreen perennial forming clumps of 5-lobed, toothed, wrinkled, light green, basal leaves, 5–15cm (2–6in) long, each lobe divided into pointed segments. Erect, trumpet-shaped, bright pink flowers, 3–4cm (1¼–1½in) across, with notched petals and a silvery sheen, becoming darker with age, are borne in dense cymes from early summer to early autumn. ↕ 45cm (18in), ↔ 60cm (24in). Pyrenees (mainly France). ❄❄❄.

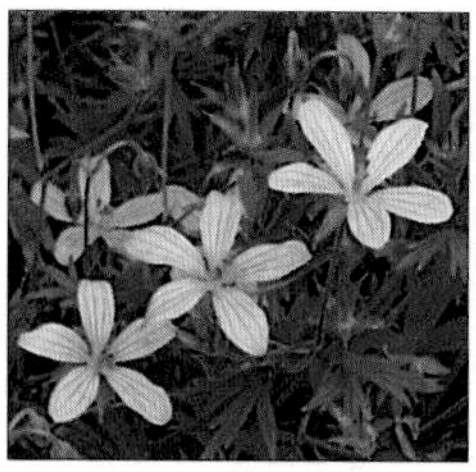

Geranium asphodeloides

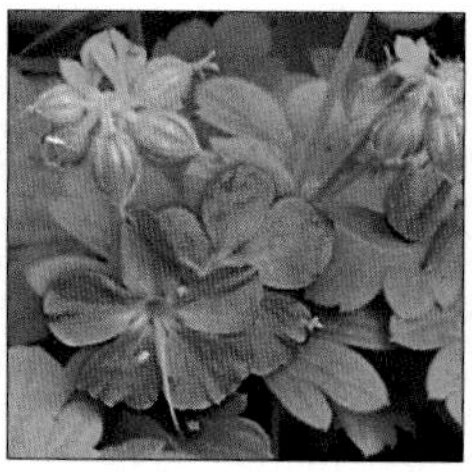

Geranium x *cantabrigiense*

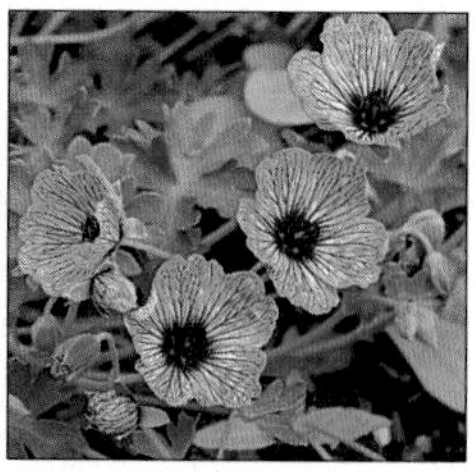

Geranium cinereum 'Ballerina'

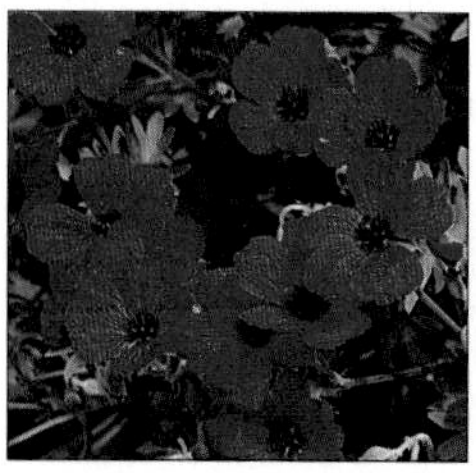

Geranium cinereum subsp. *subcaulescens*

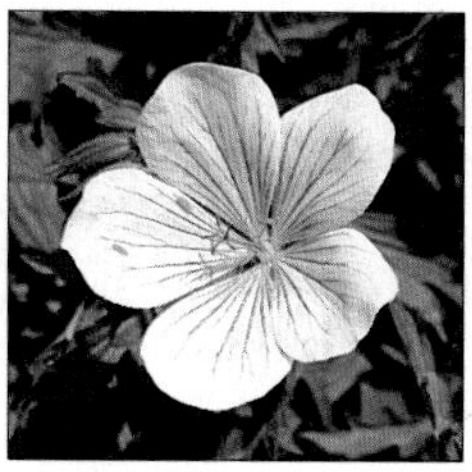

Geranium clarkei 'Kashmir White'

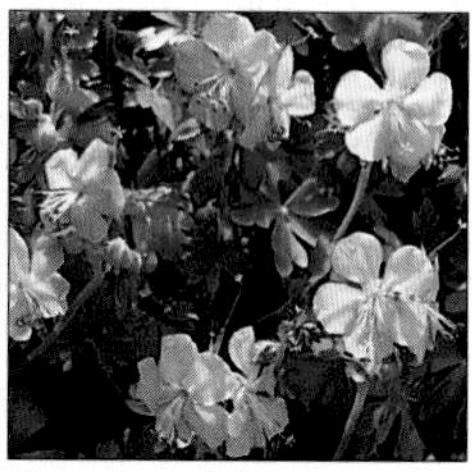

Geranium dalmaticum

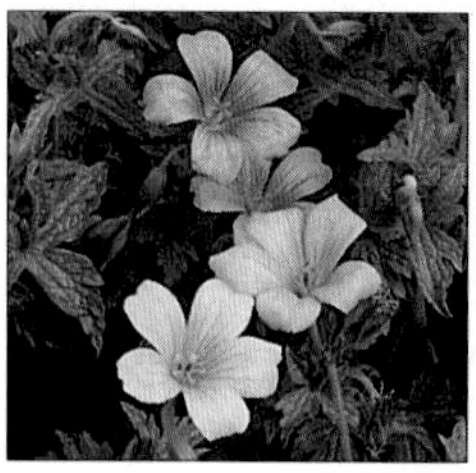

Geranium endressii

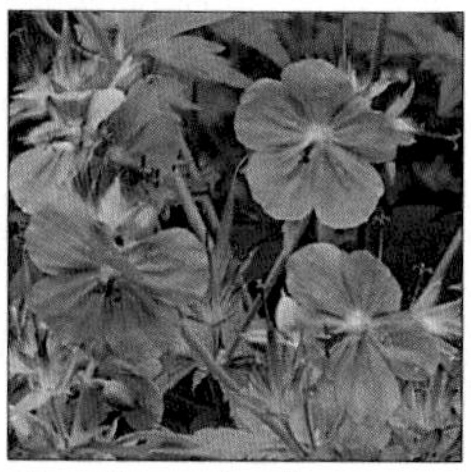

Geranium erianthum

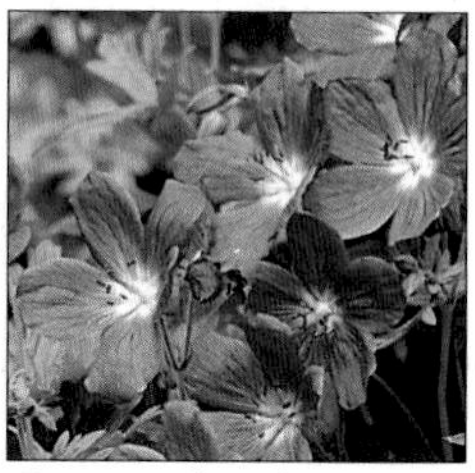

Geranium himalayense

G

'Wargrave Pink' see *G.* x *oxonianum* 'Wargrave Pink'.

G. erianthum ▣ Clump-forming, hairy herbaceous perennial, similar to *G. eriostemon,* with upright stems and 7- to 9-lobed, light green, basal leaves, 5–20cm (2–8in) long, the lobes overlapping and prominently toothed. Bears dense, umbel-like clusters of saucer-shaped to almost flat, violet-blue flowers, 2.5–4cm (1–1½in) across, from late spring to midsummer. Good autumn leaf colour. ↕ 45–60cm (18–24in), ↔ 30cm (12in). Russia (E. Siberia, Sakhalin), Japan, North America (Alaska, Aleutian Islands to N. British Columbia). ❄❄❄

G. eriostemon, syn. *G. platyanthum.* Clump-forming, hairy herbaceous perennial with upright stems and 5- or 7-lobed, shallowly toothed, basal leaves, 5–20cm (2–8in) long, crinkly above. In late spring and early summer, bears umbel-like clusters of horizontal or nodding, flat, pale violet to violet-pink flowers, 3cm (1¼in) across, shaded darker towards the centres, with small white bases to the petals. Good autumn colour. ↕ 30–50cm (12–20in), ↔ 45cm (18in). Russia (E. Siberia), E. Tibet, W. China, Korea, Japan. ❄❄❄

G. farreri 🏆 Dwarf, tap-rooted, rosette-forming herbaceous perennial with somewhat spreading or erect red stems and kidney-shaped, red-margined, matt, mid-green, basal leaves, to 5cm (2in) across, each deeply cut into 7 sparsely toothed divisions, which are 3-lobed at the tips. In early summer, bears loose cymes of shallowly cup-shaped, very pale pink, wavy-margined flowers, to 3.5cm (1½in) wide, with conspicuous black anthers. Best in a scree bed or alpine house. ↕ to 12cm (5in), ↔ to 15cm (6in). W. China. ❄❄❄

G. fremontii. Clump-forming herbaceous perennial with 5- to 7-lobed, light green, basal leaves, 5–10cm (2–4in) long, sticky-hairy beneath, the divisions broadly toothed and lobed at the tips. Bears upward-facing, flat, pale to deep pink flowers, to 4cm (1½in) across, in open, branched cymes from early summer to early autumn. ↕ 30–45cm (12–18in), ↔ 45cm (18in). W. USA (Wyoming to Arizona and New Mexico). ❄❄❄

G. grandiflorum see *G. himalayense.*

G. grandiflorum* var. *alpinum see *G. himalayense* 'Gravetye'.

G. grevilleanum see *G. lambertii.*

G. himalayense ▣ syn. *G. grandiflorum, G. himalayense* var. *meeboldii, G. meeboldii.* Rhizomatous, mat-forming herbaceous perennial bearing 7-lobed, prominently veined, mid-green, basal leaves, 5–20cm (2–8in) long, with broad, blunt-toothed lobes, colouring well in autumn. Loose cymes of saucer-shaped, veined, violet-blue to deep mid-blue flowers, 4–6cm (1½–2½in) across, touched with reddish pink and with white centres, are produced in a main

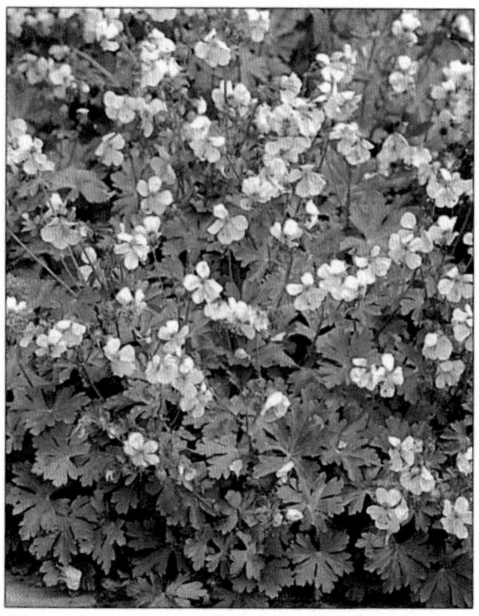

Geranium x *cantabrigiense* 'Biokovo'

flush in early summer and then spasmodically to early autumn. Good ground cover, even in full shade. ↕30–45cm (12–18in), ↔ 60cm (24in). Himalayas. ❄❄❄. **var. *alpinum*** see 'Gravetye'. **'Birch Double'** see 'Plenum'. **'Gravetye'** ■🏆 syn. *G. grandiflorum* var. *alpinum*, *G. himalayense* var. *alpinum*, has smaller leaves, 5–12cm (2–5in) long, and larger flowers, to 7cm (3in) across, with more markedly red zones around the white centres; ↕30cm (12in). **'Irish Blue'** has paler blue flowers, 3.5cm (1½in) across, with larger, purplish red central zones, and is very free-flowering. **var. *meeboldii*** see *G. himalayense*. **'Plenum'**, syn. 'Birch Double', has smaller leaves, 5–12cm (2–5in) long, and double, purplish pink flowers, 2.5cm (1in) across, shaded blue, with darker veins; ↕25cm (10in).

G. ibericum ■ Clump-forming, hairy herbaceous perennial with 9- to 11-lobed, basal leaves, 10–20cm (4–8in) long, the lobes toothed and overlapping. Upward-facing, shallowly cup-shaped, violet-blue flowers, 4–5cm (1½–2in) across, with feathered, darker veins, and petals notched at the tips, are borne in dense cymes in early summer. ↕to 50cm (20in), ↔ 60cm (24in). Caucasus, N.E. Turkey, N. Iran. ❄❄❄

G. incanum. Mounded, bushy, evergreen perennial with branching stems and aromatic, filigree, grey-green, basal leaves, to 8cm (3in) long, each deeply cut into 5 segments, which in turn are lobed and toothed. From summer to autumn, bears loose cymes of deep pink flowers, to about 3.5cm (1½in) across, with dark veins and a V-shaped white mark at the base of each petal. Needs a warm, sunny position. ↕40cm (16in), ↔ to 60cm (24in) or more. South Africa. ❄❄

***G.* 'Johnson's Blue'** 🏆 Rhizomatous, spreading herbaceous perennial, forming a dense mat of 7-lobed, mid-green, basal leaves, 5–20cm (2–8in) long, each lobe itself lobed and toothed. Saucer-shaped, mid- to lavender-blue flowers, 5cm (2in) across, tinged pink at the centres, are produced in loose cymes during summer. ↕30–45cm (12–18in), ↔ 60–75cm (24–30in). ❄❄❄

***G.* 'Kate'**, syn. *G.* 'Kate Folkard'. Dwarf, carpeting, semi-evergreen perennial with rounded, deeply 5- to 7-lobed, dark bronze-green leaves, 1.5–3.5cm (½–1½in) long, each lobe obovate and further lobed. Bears cymes of funnel-shaped, pale pink flowers, 1.5cm (½in) across, with almost translucent bases and dark veins, from late spring to summer. ↕10–15cm (4–6in), ↔ 30cm (12in). ❄❄❄

***G.* 'Kate Folkard'** see *G.* 'Kate'.

G. kishtvariense. Rhizomatous, rounded, bristly-hairy herbaceous perennial with 5-lobed, finely toothed, wrinkled, bright green, basal leaves, 10–23cm (4–9in) long. Loose cymes of upward-facing, shallowly cup-shaped, deep pinkish purple flowers, 4cm (1½in) across, with purple veins and small white centres, and a white V at each base, are produced throughout summer. ↕30cm (12in), ↔ 60cm (24in). India (Kashmir). ❄❄❄

G. lambertii, syn. *G. candicans* of gardens, *G. grevilleanum.* Trailing herbaceous perennial with long, procumbent, non-rooting stems bearing rounded or kidney-shaped, wrinkled, mid-green leaves, 10cm (4in) long, each with 5 lobes and a 3-lobed point. In late summer, bears diffuse cymes of nodding, saucer-shaped, pale pink or white flowers, 3–4cm (1¼–1½in) across, marked purple at the bases, and with crimson centres and veins. ↕30–45cm (12–18in), ↔ 90cm (36in). Himalayas. ❄❄❄

G. libani, syn. *G. libanoticum.* Clump-forming perennial, dormant in summer, but with new foliage in autumn, with rounded, deeply 5- or 7-lobed, glossy, mid-green leaves, 10–20cm (4–8in) long, each ovate lobe toothed and further lobed. In spring, violet or violet-blue flowers, with notched, disc-shaped petals, 3cm (1¼in) across, are borne in umbel-like clusters. ↕40cm (16in), ↔ 45cm (18in). Lebanon, W. Syria, central S. Turkey. ❄❄❄ (borderline)

G. libanoticum see *G. libani.*

***G.* x *lindavicum* 'Alanah'**, syn. *G.* x *lindavicum* 'Purpureum'. Dwarf, rosette-forming, evergreen perennial, similar to *G. cinereum*, with deeply 7-lobed, silky, silvery green, basal leaves, to 7cm (3in) long. In late spring and early summer, bears loose cymes of deep crimson-purple flowers, 3–5cm (1¼–2in) across, with a network of darker veins. ↕to 15cm (6in), ↔ to 20cm (8in). ❄❄❄

***G.* x *lindavicum* 'Purpureum'** see *G.* x *lindavicum* 'Alanah'.

G. macrorrhizum ■ Rhizomatous, semi-evergreen perennial with 7-lobed, toothed, sticky, strongly aromatic, light green, basal leaves, 10–20cm (4–8in) long, colouring well in autumn. Umbel-like clusters of erect, flat, pink to purplish pink or white flowers, 2–2.5cm (¾–1in) across, with inflated red calyces, slightly reflexed petals, and protruding stamens and styles, are produced in early summer. Effective ground cover in shade. ↕50cm (20in), ↔ 60cm (24in). S. Europe. ❄❄❄. **'Bevan's Variety'** has crimson-purple flowers. **'Czakor'** has magenta flowers and purple-tinted foliage in autumn; ↕to 30cm (12in). **'Ingwersen's Variety'** ■🏆 has glossy, light green leaves and soft pink flowers. **'Variegatum'** has greyish green leaves with cream variegation, and purplish pink flowers. It is less vigorous than the species, requiring richer soil and more sun; ↕30cm (12in), ↔ 45cm (18in).

G. maculatum ■ Erect, clump-forming herbaceous perennial with 5- to 7-lobed, glossy, mid-green, basal leaves, 10–20cm (4–8in) long, with narrow, toothed, widely spaced lobes. Slightly upward-facing, saucer-shaped, lilac-pink to bright pink flowers, 3cm (1¼in) across, usually white near the base of each petal, are produced in loose cymes from late spring to midsummer. Prefers moist soil. ↕60–75cm (24–30in), ↔ 45cm (18in). E. North America. ❄❄❄. **f. *albiflorum*** has white flowers and is less robust than the species.

G. maderense ■🏆 Robust, evergreen perennial, usually short-lived or behaving as a biennial, with short, erect stems bearing rosettes of 5- to 7-lobed, deeply toothed, bright green leaves, to 60cm (24in) long, with brownish red stalks. From late winter to late summer, produces numerous flat, pinkish magenta flowers, 4cm (1½in) across, with paler pink veins, darkening towards dark magenta centres, and with red anthers; they are borne in imposing, panicle-like inflorescences, the upper parts of the flower-stalks thickly covered with purple, glandular hairs. ↕↔ 1.2–1.5m (4–5ft). Madeira. ❄

G.* x *magnificum ■🏆 (*G. ibericum* x *G. platypetalum*). Vigorous, clump-forming herbaceous perennial with mid-green, basal leaves, 10–20cm (4–8in) long, that colour well in autumn. Each leaf is divided into 9–11 broad lobes, the lobes themselves lobed, toothed, and overlapping. Dense cymes of numerous saucer-shaped, rich violet flowers, 5cm (2in) across, heavily veined in a darker shade, are produced in one burst in

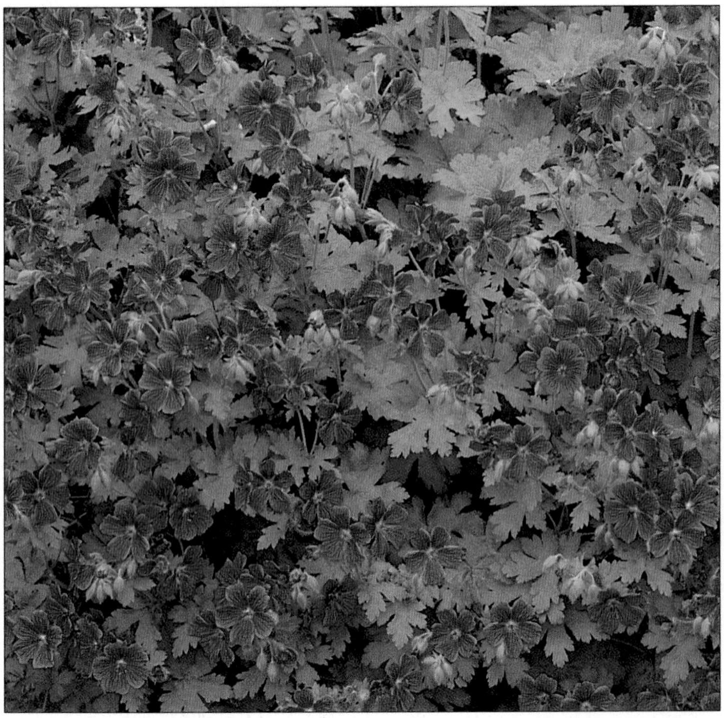

Geranium ibericum

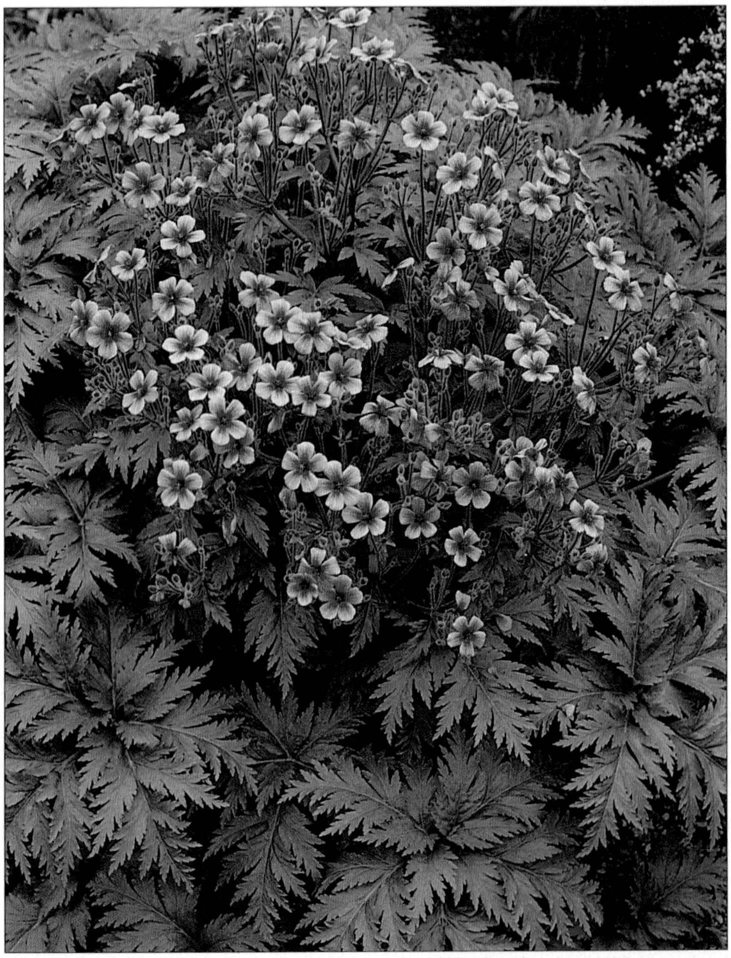

Geranium maderense

midsummer. Prefers a sunny site. ↕↔ 60cm (24in). Garden origin. ✲✲✲
G. malviflorum, syn. *G. atlanticum* of gardens. Tuberous perennial with underground runners, dormant in summer, but with new foliage produced in autumn. Dark green, basal leaves, 6–10cm (2½–4in) long, are deeply cut into 7 pinnatifid divisions. Loose cymes of saucer-shaped, red-veined, pinkish violet-blue flowers, 4cm (1½in) across, with deeply notched, heart-shaped petals, are borne in early and mid-spring. Requires poor soil in full sun. ↕ 22–30cm (9–12in), ↔ 45cm (18in). S. Spain, Morocco, Algeria. ✲✲✲
G. meeboldii see *G. himalayense.*
G. x monacense (*G. phaeum* x *G. reflexum*) syn. *G. punctatum* of gardens. Clump-forming herbaceous perennial with 5- to 7-lobed, basal leaves, 10–20cm (4–8in) long, usually with brown marks at the lobe bases. In late spring and early summer, bears loose cymes of saucer-shaped, purplish red flowers, 2cm (¾in) across, with white and violet zones at the bases of the reflexed petals. ↕ 45cm (18in), ↔ 60cm (24in). Garden origin. ✲✲✲. **'Muldoon'** has dark green leaves heavily spotted with purple, and flowers with protruding stamens and styles; ↕ 60cm (24in).
G. nodosum ▣ Rhizomatous herbaceous perennial forming a clump of 3- or 5-lobed, shallow-toothed, glossy, bright green, basal leaves, 5–20cm (2–8in) long, the stems swollen above the nodes. From late spring to early or mid-autumn, red-tinted stems bear loose cymes of erect, open funnel-shaped, purplish-pink flowers, 2.5–3cm (1–1¼in) across, with paler pink centres, darker veins, and notched petals. Effective ground cover in dry soil in full shade. ↕ 30–50cm (12–20in), ↔ 50cm (20in). Pyrenees, C. Italy, Yugoslavia (Serbia). ✲✲✲
G. orientalitibeticum ▣ syn. *G. stapfianum* var. *roseum* of gardens. Dwarf herbaceous perennial with tuberous, underground runners, and basal leaves, to 10cm (4in) across, cut into narrowly lobed, toothed divisions, marbled dark and pale green. In summer, bears loose cymes of shallowly cup-shaped, deep purplish pink flowers, to 2.5cm (1in) across, the centres white. Spreads rapidly. ↕ to 30cm (12in), ↔ to 1m (3ft) or more. S.W. China. ✲✲✲
G. x oxonianum ▣ (*G. endressii* x *G. versicolor*). Vigorous, clump-forming, evergreen perennial with 5-lobed, light green, basal leaves, 5–20cm (2–8in) long, each lobe with 5 toothed, wrinkled, conspicuously veined divisions. From late spring to mid-autumn, bears loose cymes of broadly funnel-shaped pink flowers, to 4cm (1½in) across, with darker veins and notched petals. ↕ to 80cm (32in), ↔ 60cm (24in). Garden origin. ✲✲✲. **'A.T. Johnson'** ♀ has silvery pink flowers and is very free-flowering; ↕ 30cm (12in). **'Claridge Druce'**, syn. *G.* 'Claridge Druce', is very vigorous, forming strong clumps of greyish green, somewhat glossy leaves, with dark-veined, rose-pink flowers, 4–4.5cm (1½–1¾in) across. Self-seeds freely and usually comes true. Good ground cover; ↕ 45–75cm (18–30in). **'Hollywood'** has pale pink flowers with almost maroon veins; ↕ 45cm (18in). **'Rose Clair'** has red-purple flowers with paler veins and is free-flowering; ↕ 35cm (14in). **'Southcombe Double'** has usually double, warm pink flowers, 2cm (¾in) across; ↕ 40cm (16in). **'Southcombe Star'** ▣ is more spreading, with star-shaped, deep purplish pink flowers, 2–2.5cm (¾–1in) across. **'Wargrave Pink'** ♀ syn. *G. endressii* 'Wargrave Pink', is very vigorous and has bright salmon-pink flowers; ↕ 60cm (24in), ↔ 90cm (36in). **'Winscombe'** ▣ forms a leafy clump, with very pale pink flowers becoming bright pink with darker veins, several shades present on the plant at one time; ↕ 45cm (18in).
G. palmatum ♀ syn. *G. anemonifolium.* Tap-rooted, evergreen, rosetted perennial, sometimes self-seeding as a biennial. Similar to *G. maderense*, it has basal rosettes of 5-lobed, light green leaves, to 35cm (14in) across; each lobe is cut into 6–9 toothed segments, the central segment stalked. Flowering stems with purple glandular hairs bear large, panicle-like inflorescences, to 1.2m (4ft) across, of saucer-shaped, crimson-centred, purple-pink flowers, 3–4cm (1¼–1½in) across, throughout summer. Transplant seedlings while small. ↕↔ to 1.2m (4ft). Madeira. ✲✲
G. phaeum ▣ (Dusky cranesbill, Mourning widow). Clump-forming herbaceous perennial bearing 7- or 9-lobed, soft green, basal leaves, 10–20cm (4–8in) long, often with purplish brown marks; each lobe is itself shallowly lobed. In late spring and early summer, bears branched, almost one-sided cymes of pendent, white-centred, deep purple-

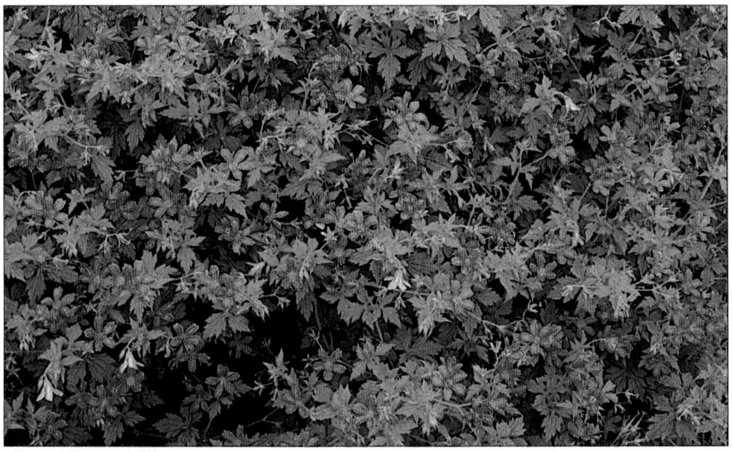
Geranium x *oxonianum*

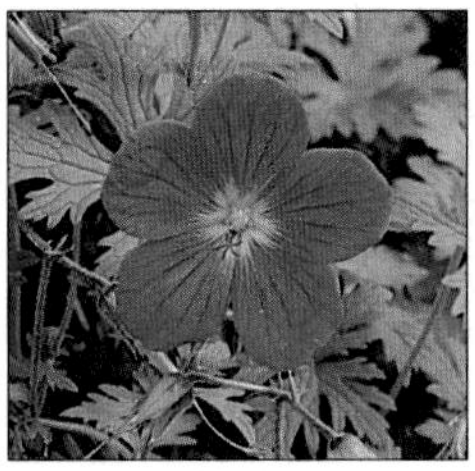
Geranium himalayense 'Gravetye'

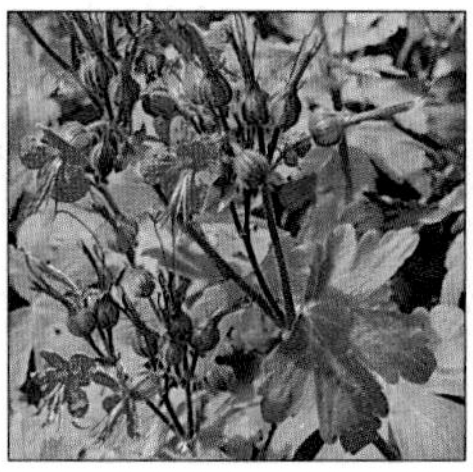
Geranium macrorrhizum

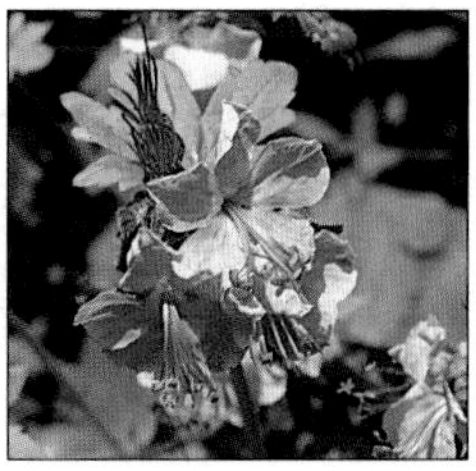
Geranium macrorrhizum 'Ingwersen's Variety'

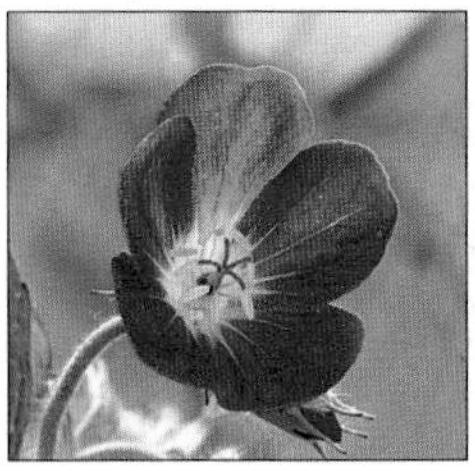
Geranium maculatum

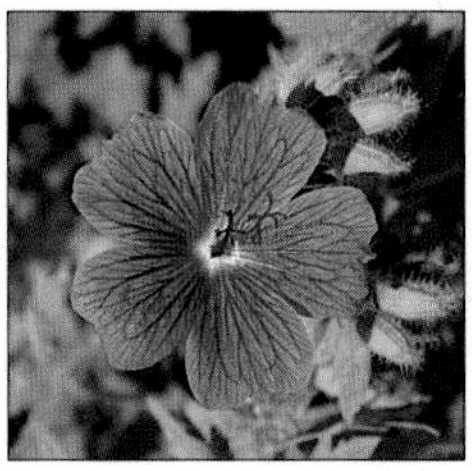
Geranium x *magnificum*

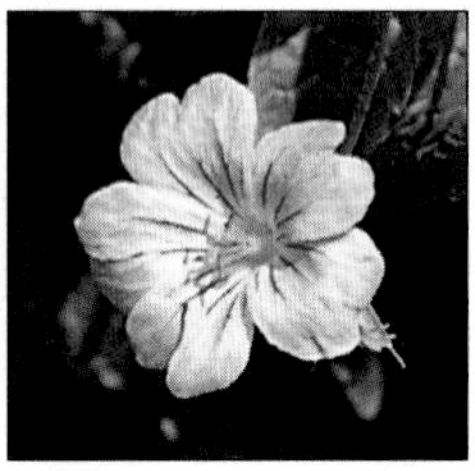
Geranium nodosum

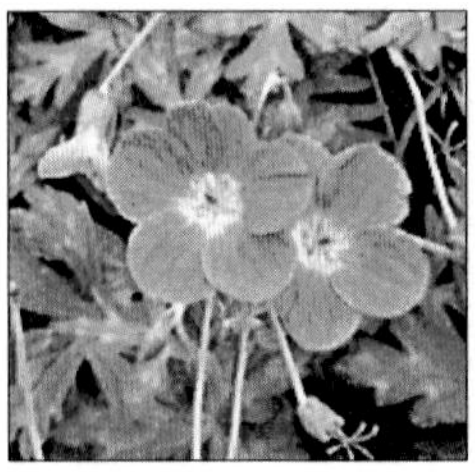
Geranium orientalitibeticum

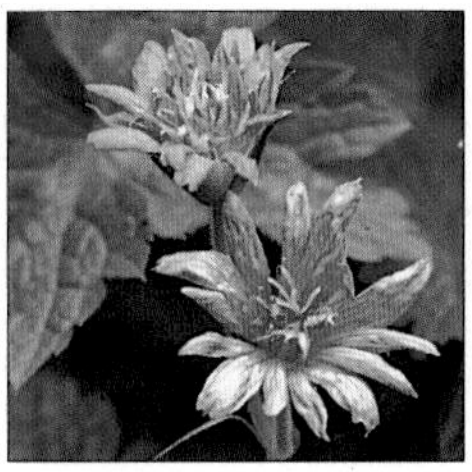
Geranium x *oxonianum* 'Southcombe Star'

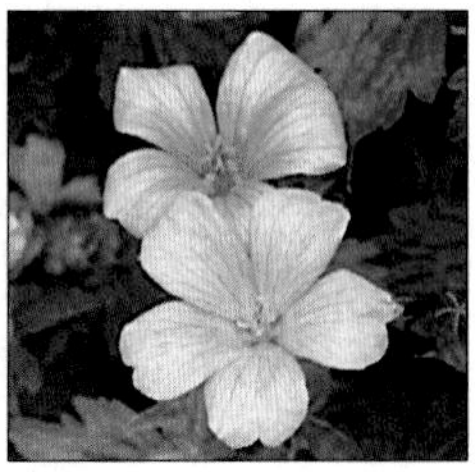
Geranium x *oxonianum* 'Winscombe'

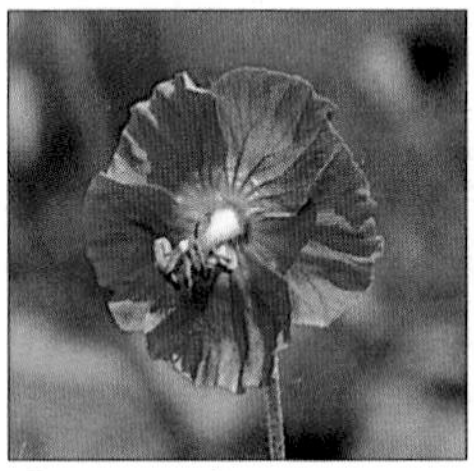
Geranium phaeum

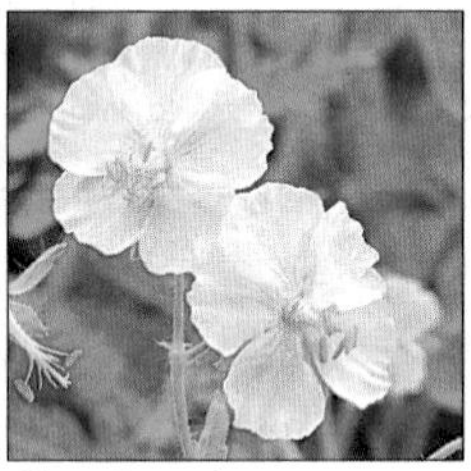
Geranium phaeum f. *album*

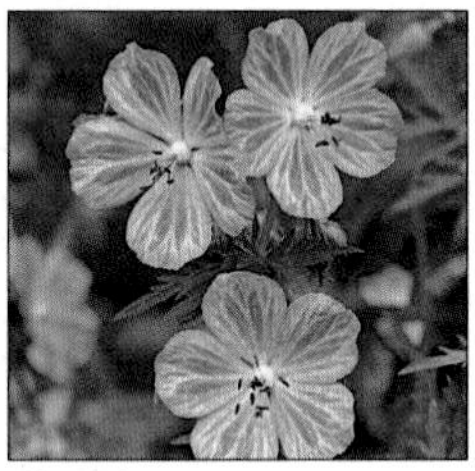
Geranium pratense 'Mrs. Kendall Clark'

black, deep maroon, violet-blue, light mauve, or white flowers, 2–2.5cm (¾–1in) across, with reflexed petals. Good in damp shade. ↕ 80cm (32in), ↔ 45cm (18in). Mountainous regions from Pyrenees to Balkans, S.E. Germany, Czech Republic, W. Russia. ✲✲✲. **f. *album*** ▣ has white flowers. **'Langthorn's Blue'** has violet-blue flowers; ↕ 60–90cm (24–36in). **'Lily Lovell'** has large flowers, 3–4cm (1¼–1½in) across, in rich purple-mauve. **var. *lividum*** has very pale lilac or pink flowers with white bases, and unmarked leaves. **'Variegatum'** has foliage with irregular yellow margins and splashes of reddish pink.
G. platyanthum see *G. eriostemon.*
G. platypetalum. Clump-forming, hairy herbaceous perennial with wrinkled, mid-green, basal leaves, 10–20cm (4–8in) long, each deeply divided into 7 or 9 broadly toothed lobes. During early and midsummer, bears dense cymes of flat, saucer-shaped, deep violet-blue flowers, 3–4.5cm (1¼–1¾in) across, with darker veins. ↕ 30–45cm (12–18in), ↔ 45cm (18in). Caucasus, N.E. Turkey, N.W. Iran. ✲✲✲
G. polyanthes. Clump-forming, often short-lived herbaceous perennial with short stems and kidney-shaped, 7- to 9-lobed, fleshy, mid-green, basal leaves, to 5cm (2in) long. In midsummer, bears clusters of funnel-shaped, shiny, deep pink flowers, 2.5cm (1in) across, with numerous fine veins. ↕ 30–45cm (12–18in), ↔ 30cm (12in). Himalayas, S.W. China. ✲✲✲
G. pratense (Meadow cranesbill). Clump-forming herbaceous perennial with hairy stems and 7- to 9-lobed, basal leaves, 20cm (8in) long, the lobes often deeply divided and toothed. Bears erect, saucer-shaped, variously veined, white, blue, or violet flowers, 3.5–4.5cm (1½–1¾in) across, in dense cymes in early and midsummer. ↕ 60–90cm (24–36in), ↔ 60cm (24in). Europe, C. Asia (Altai Mountains), W. China. ✲✲✲. All except double-flowered cultivars self-seed freely, bearing varying offspring. Double-flowered cultivars have longer-lasting flowers, but require rich soil and regular division, and are more prone to mildew in dry conditions. **f. *albiflorum*** bears white flowers over a long period, sometimes to early autumn; ↕ 1m (3ft). **'Bicolor'** see 'Striatum'. **'Flore Pleno'** see 'Plenum Violaceum'. **'Galactic'** has dark green leaves and milk-white flowers, to 5cm (2in) across; ↕ 75cm (30in). **'Kashmir Purple'** see *G. clarkei* 'Kashmir Purple'. **'Kashmir White'** see *G. clarkei* 'Kashmir White'. **'Mrs. Kendall Clark'** ▣♀ has pearl-grey flowers flushed with pale rose-pink,

G

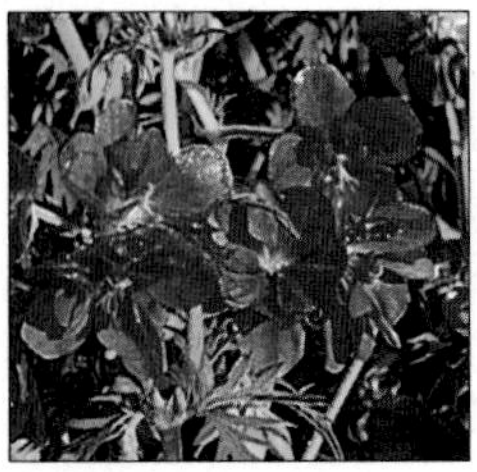
Geranium pratense 'Plenum Caeruleum'

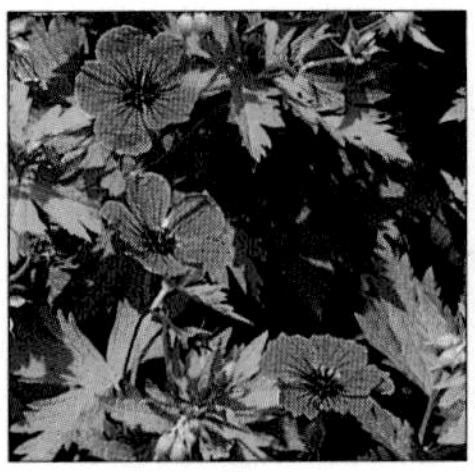
Geranium psilostemon

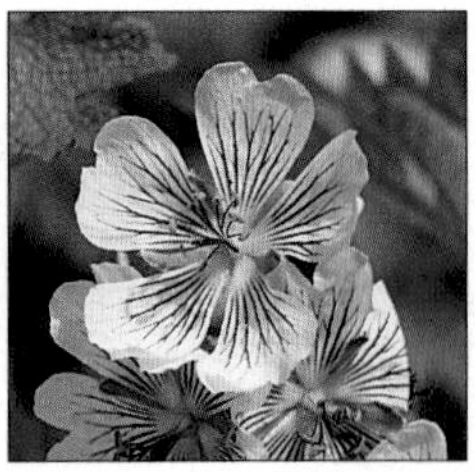
Geranium renardii

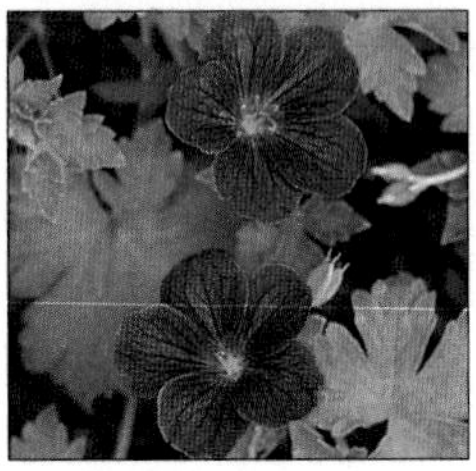
Geranium x *riversleaianum* 'Russell Prichard'

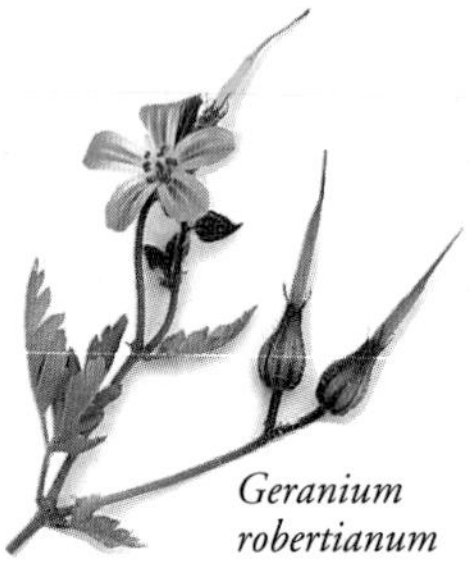
Geranium robertianum

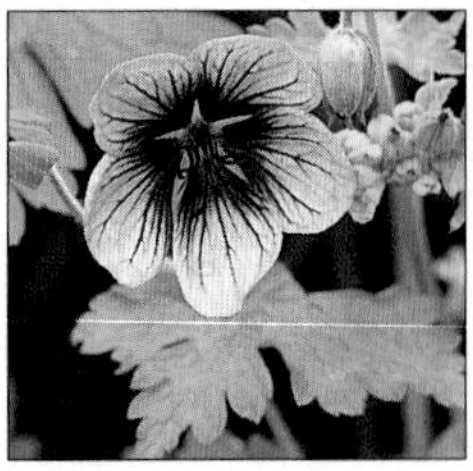
Geranium 'Salome'

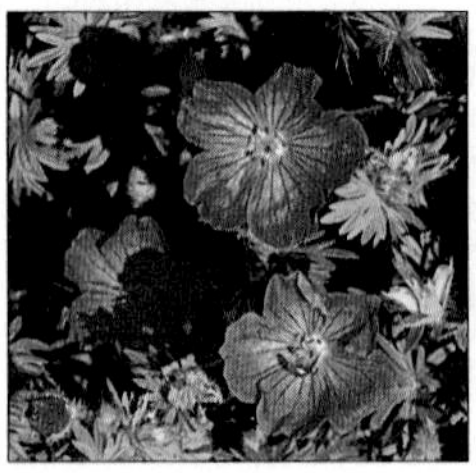
Geranium sanguineum

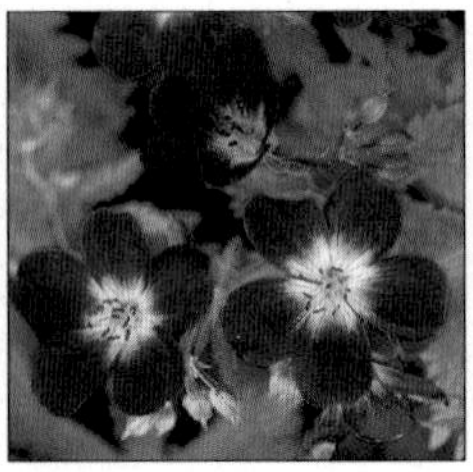
Geranium sylvaticum 'Mayflower'

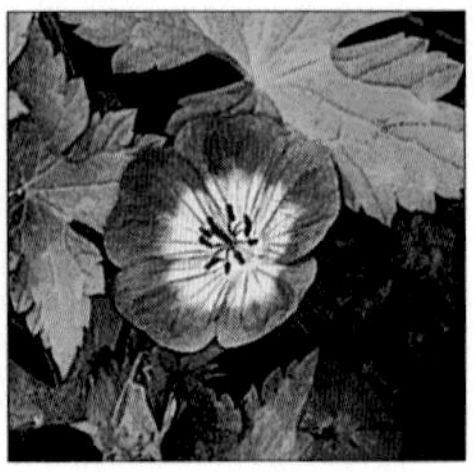
Geranium wallichianum 'Buxton's Variety'

although plants offered often have violet-blue flowers with white veining. **'Plenum Album'** produces loosely double, violet-tinged white flowers, 2–3cm (¾–1¼in) across. **'Plenum Caeruleum'** ▣ has loosely double, lavender-blue flowers, sometimes tinged pink. **'Plenum Purpureum'** see 'Plenum Violaceum'. **'Plenum Violaceum'** 🏆 syn. 'Flore Pleno', 'Plenum Purpureum', has double, deep violet-blue flowers, purple-blue in the centres. **'Silver Queen'** has white flowers touched with very pale violet; ↕ 1.3m (4½ft). **'Striatum'**, syn. 'Bicolor', has white flowers streaked violet-blue; may come true from seed.

G. procurrens. Spreading herbaceous perennial with procumbent red stems that may root at the nodes. Bears 5-lobed, coarsely toothed, mid-green, basal leaves, 5–10cm (2–4in) long, each division 3-lobed at the tip; leaves are wrinkled above. From midsummer to early autumn, bears loose cymes of somewhat star-shaped, dark purple-pink flowers, 2.5–3cm (1–1¼in) across. Each petal has a V-shaped black mark at the base, and black centres and veins. Ideal in dry soil under shrubs. ↕ 45cm (18in), ↔ 1m (3ft) or more. Himalayas. ✽✽✽

G. psilostemon ▣ 🏆 syn. *G. armenum* (Armenian cranesbill). Upright, clump-forming herbaceous perennial with 7-lobed, toothed, mid-green, basal leaves, 20cm (8in) long, crimson-tinted in spring and red in autumn. From early to late summer, bears loose, upright cymes of numerous erect, shallowly bowl-shaped, brilliant magenta flowers, 4cm (1½in) across, with black centres and veins. ↕ 60–120cm (2–4ft), ↔ 60cm (24in). S.W. Caucasus, N.E. Turkey. ✽✽✽. **'Bressingham Flair'** has somewhat crumpled, less vivid magenta flowers with a hint of pink.

***G. punctatum* of gardens** see *G.* x *monacense.*

G. pylzowianum. Spreading herbaceous perennial with tuberous, underground runners and dark green, kidney-shaped or semi-circular, basal leaves, to 5cm (2in) across, each deeply cut into 5–7 narrowly lobed, toothed divisions. In early summer, bears cymes of broadly trumpet-shaped, deep rose-pink flowers, 3–4.5cm (1¼–1¾in) wide, white at the bases and with darker veins. Similar to *G. orientalitibeticum*, but less invasive. ↕ 15–25cm (6–10in), ↔ 25cm (10in) or more. W. China. ✽✽✽

G. pyrenaicum. Clump-forming, hairy, evergreen perennial. Bears scalloped, mid-green, basal leaves, 5–10cm (2–4in) long, with 7 or 9 ill-defined, sometimes toothed lobes. Somewhat star-shaped, violet-pink flowers, 1–2cm (½–¾in) across, white at the bases, with darker veins and notched petals, are borne in loose cymes from spring to autumn. Self-seeds freely. ↕ 30–60cm (12–24in), ↔ 30cm (12in). W. and S. Europe to Caucasus. ✽✽✽. **f. *albiflorum*** has white flowers. **'Bill Wallis'** has rich purple flowers. Comes true from seed.

G. reflexum. Clump-forming herbaceous perennial, similar to *G. phaeum*, with 7-lobed, mid-green, basal leaves, 10–20cm (4–8in) long, with dark blotches. In late spring and early summer, bears branched, one-sided cymes of bright rose-pink flowers, 1.5cm (½in) across; they have narrow, very reflexed petals with white bases and red-shaded sepals showing behind. ↕ 45–60cm (18–24in), ↔ 60cm (24in). Italy to N. Greece. ✽✽✽

G. renardii ▣ 🏆 Clump-forming herbaceous perennial with wrinkled, veined, velvety, grey-green, basal leaves, to 10cm (4in) across, each cut into 5 or 7 broad lobes with scalloped margins. Dense, umbel-like clusters of saucer-shaped, white to pale lavender flowers, 3cm (1¼in) across, with notched petals and bold violet veins, are borne intermittently in early summer. Often shy-flowering, but an effective foliage plant. Best in poor soil. ↕↔ 30cm (12in). Caucasus. ✽✽✽. **'Whiteknights'** has white flowers, with pale lilac-blue ground colour and darker veins.

G. richardsonii. Variable, clump-forming herbaceous perennial with 5- or 7-lobed, broadly toothed, slightly glossy, bright green, basal leaves, 5–10cm (2–4in) long. Bears loose cymes of flat, very lightly veined, pink-tinged white flowers, to 3cm (1¼in) across, from late spring to late summer. Prefers damp soil in sun. ↕ 30–60cm (12–24in), ↔ 30cm (12in). W. North America (British Columbia and Saskatchewan to Mexico). ✽✽✽

G.* x *riversleaianum (*G. endressii* x *G. traversii*). Trailing, hairy herbaceous perennial with long, branching stems bearing grey-green leaves, 5–10cm (2–4in) across, each deeply divided into 7 blunt-toothed lobes. In summer, produces loose cymes of erect, broadly funnel-shaped, light pink to dark magenta flowers, to 3.5cm (1½in) wide, with darker veins. Good ground cover. ↕ to 30cm (12in), ↔ to 1m (3ft). Garden origin. ✽✽✽. **'Mavis Simpson'** bears clear, light pink flowers with paler centres. **'Russell Prichard'** ▣ 🏆 has more sharply toothed leaves, and produces deep magenta flowers over long periods in summer.

G. robertianum ▣ (Herb Robert). Rosette-forming, hairy, strongly aromatic annual or biennial with bright green, basal leaves, to 11cm (4½in) across, cut to the bases into 5 lobes, each in turn very deeply lobed. Produces erect, diffuse, panicle-like clusters of star-shaped pink flowers, to 1cm (½in) across, from summer to autumn. ↕↔ 25cm (10in). Europe, Canary Islands, N.W. Africa, W. Asia, Himalayas, S.W. China. ✽✽✽.

'Celtic White' has white flowers; ↕ 10–40cm (4–16in), ↔ to 30cm (12in).

***G.* 'Salome'** ▣ Trailing herbaceous perennial with branching stems bearing 5-lobed, toothed, pale green, basal leaves, 5–15cm (2–6in) long. In summer, produces loose cymes of flowers to 3cm (1¼in) wide, with widely spaced, purplish pink petals, veined and basally marked deep violet, with almost black styles and stamens. ↕ 30cm (12in), ↔ to 1.2m (4ft). ✽✽✽

G. sanguineum ▣ (Bloody cranesbill). Dense, clump-forming herbaceous perennial with spreading rhizomes. Dark green stem leaves, 5–10cm (2–4in) long, are deeply cut into 5–7 sparsely toothed lobes, each with 3 segments. Has few basal leaves. During summer, bears a profusion of upright, cup-shaped, deep magenta-pink flowers, to 4cm (1½in) wide, with darker veins, white eyes, and usually notched petals, in loose cymes. ↕ 20cm (8in), ↔ to 30cm (12in) or more. Europe, N. Turkey. ✽✽✽. **'Album'** 🏆 is taller, more lax, with pure white flowers borne over many weeks in summer; ↕ 30cm (12in), ↔ 40cm (16in). **var. *lancastriense*** see var. *striatum*. **var. *prostratum*** see var. *striatum*. **'Shepherd's Warning'** 🏆 is compact, with deep red-pink flowers; ↕↔ 15cm (6in). **'Splendens'** see var. *striatum* 'Splendens'. **var. *striatum*** ▣ 🏆 syn. var. *lancastriense*, var. *prostratum*, is compact, with pale flesh-pink flowers, veined darker pink; ↕ 10cm (4in); UK (Walney Island, Cumbria). **var. *striatum* 'Splendens'**, syn. 'Splendens', is taller, with larger, dark-veined pink flowers, to 4.5cm (1¾in) across; ↕ to 45cm (18in).

***G. sessiliflorum* subsp. *novae-zelandiae* 'Nigricans'**, syn. *G. sessiliflorum* subsp. *novae-zelandiae* 'Nigrescens'. Rosette-forming herbaceous perennial with tufts of olive-bronze, basal leaves, 1.5–3cm (½–1¼in) across, divided into 5–7 shallowly 3-lobed segments. In summer, bears loose cymes of erect, funnel-shaped, greyish white flowers, about 7mm (¼in) across.

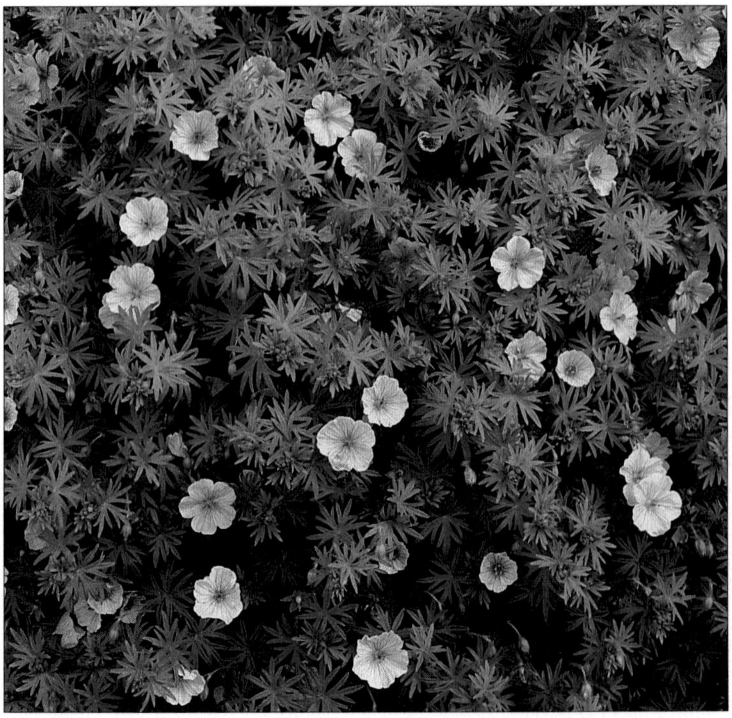
Geranium sanguineum var. *striatum*

Self-seeds freely. ↕ to 8cm (3in), ↔ to 15cm (6in). ❄❄❄

***G. sessiliflorum* subsp. *novae-zelandiae* 'Nigrescens'** see *G. sessiliflorum* subsp. *novae-zelandiae* 'Nigricans'.

G. shikokianum. Bushy, clump-forming herbaceous perennial with 5- to 7-lobed, light green, basal leaves, 5–10cm (2–4in) long, grey-marbled above and shiny beneath, each lobe itself divided and toothed. Funnel-shaped pink flowers, 2.5cm (1in) across, with large white centres and netted, red-purple veins, are borne in loose cymes from midsummer to early autumn. Good autumn colour. Prefers moist soil in light shade. ↕ 20–45cm (8–18in), ↔ 45cm (18in). Korea, S. Japan. ❄❄❄

G. sinense. Slow-growing, clump-forming herbaceous perennial, with red-tinged stems bearing 7-lobed, many-toothed, mid-green, basal leaves, 5–16cm (2–6in) long. Loose cymes of velvety, deep maroon flowers, to 2cm (¾in) across, with reflexed petals revealing red bases, protruding stamen filaments with black anthers, and red stigmas, are produced from late summer to mid-autumn. ↕ 60cm (24in), ↔ 45cm (18in). S.W. China. ❄❄❄

***G. stapfianum* var. *roseum* of gardens** see *G. orientalitibeticum.*

G. striatum see *G. versicolor.*

G. subcaulescens see *G. cinereum* subsp. *subcaulescens.*

G. sylvaticum (Wood cranesbill). Clump-forming herbaceous perennial with 7-lobed, mid-green, basal leaves, 10–20cm (4–8in) long, the lobes deeply cut and toothed. In late spring and early summer, bears dense cymes of erect or upward-facing, saucer-shaped, white-centred, lightly veined, blue-purple, pinkish purple, pink, or white flowers, 2–3cm (¾–1¼in) across. Best in moist soil. ↕ to 75cm (30in), ↔ 60cm (24in). Europe, N. Turkey. ❄❄❄.

'Mayflower' ■ ♀ has larger, rich violet-blue flowers, to 3.5cm (1½in) across, with smaller white centres. **var. *wanneri*** has purplish pink flowers with red veins.

G. traversii* var. *elegans. Low-growing, clump-forming, evergreen perennial with branching stems bearing silver-hairy, grey-green, basal leaves, to 10cm (4in) across, each deeply cut into 7 lobes, further divided into 3 lobes and with a few teeth. During summer, bears loose cymes of cup-shaped, pale pink flowers, to 3cm (1¼in) across, with dark veins. Needs shelter and well-drained soil to overwinter; usually self-seeds. ↕ to 10cm (4in), ↔ to 30cm (12in). New Zealand (Chatham Islands). ❄❄

G. tuberosum. Upright, gently spreading, tuberous perennial, dormant in summer, but with new foliage produced in autumn. The mid-green, basal leaves, 5–10cm (2–4in) long, are deeply cut into 7 narrow, lobed, toothed divisions. Cymes of shallowly cup-shaped flowers, 2–3cm (¾–1¼in) across, with purple-shaded sepals and deeply notched, bright purple-pink petals with darker veins, are produced in mid-spring. ↕ 20–25cm (8–10in), ↔ 30cm (12in). Mediterranean. ❄❄❄

G. versicolor, syn. *G. striatum.* Clump-forming, semi-evergreen perennial with mounds of 5-lobed, toothed, usually brown-marked, light green, basal leaves, 5–20cm (2–8in) long. Loose cymes of funnel-shaped white flowers, 2.5–3cm (1–1¼in) across, with deeply notched petals and netted magenta veins, are produced in late spring, then sporadically into mid-autumn. ↕↔ 45cm (18in). Italy (including Sicily), Balkans. ❄❄❄

G. wallichianum. Tap-rooted herbaceous perennial with long, trailing, branching but non-rooting stems, with distinctive pairs of fused stipules and paired, 3- to 5-lobed, toothed, mid-green leaves, 5–15cm (2–6in) long, wrinkled and marbled above. Loose, leafy cymes of upward-facing, saucer-shaped, lilac or deep pinkish purple flowers, 2.5–3.5cm (1–1½in) across, with darker veins, white centres, and notched petals, are produced from midsummer to mid-autumn. ↕ 30cm (12in), ↔ 1.2m (4ft). N.E. Afghanistan to N. India (Kashmir). ❄❄❄.

'Buxton's Variety' ■ ♀ syn. *G.* 'Buxton's Blue', is dense, compact, and spreading; the flowers, to 3cm (1¼in) across, have sky-blue petals, large, strongly veined white centres, and dark stamens and stigmas. Often comes true from seed. **'Syabru'** has magenta-pink flowers with longer, darker veins and a touch of white at the centres.

G. wlassovianum. Clump-forming, softly hairy herbaceous perennial with 7-lobed, dark green, basal leaves, 5–15cm (2–6in) long, each lobe usually cut into 3 toothed segments, shaded brown and deepening to red in autumn. From midsummer to early autumn, bears loose cymes of long-lasting, broadly funnel-shaped, purple-pink or pink flowers, 3cm (1¼in) across, with darker veins. Prefers moist soil. ↕↔ 60cm (24in). Russia (E. Siberia), Mongolia, N. China. ❄❄❄

G. yesoense. Bushy herbaceous perennial with thin, spreading stems and deeply 7-lobed, mid-green, basal leaves, 5–10cm (2–4in) long, each lobe sharply toothed. In mid- and late summer, produces loose cymes of saucer-shaped, pink or white flowers, 2.5cm (1in) across, with darker veins, and green sepals showing between the petals. Needs moist soil. ↕↔ 30–45cm (12in–18in). N. and C. Japan (including Kurile Islands). ❄❄❄

▷**Geranium,**
Jungle see *Ixora coccinea*
Peppermint-scented see *Pelargonium tomentosum*
Rose see *Pelargonium* 'Graveolens' of gardens
Sweet-scented see *Pelargonium* 'Graveolens' of gardens

GERBERA

ASTERACEAE/COMPOSITAE

Genus of about 40 species of hairy perennials from grassland in temperate and mountainous regions of Africa (except N. Africa), Madagascar, Asia, and Indonesia. Most form spreading, basal rosettes of lobed or pinnate, entire or toothed leaves, and bear long-lasting, solitary, single or double, daisy-like flowerheads in red, pink, purple, orange, or yellow, sometimes with yellow or white centres. In frost-prone climates, grow in a temperate greenhouse. Elsewhere, grow in a sunny border. Gerberas are also good for cutting.

• **HARDINESS** Half hardy to frost tender.
• **CULTIVATION** Under glass, grow in loam-based potting compost (JI No.2) in bright filtered light. During the growing season, water freely and apply a balanced liquid fertilizer every 4 weeks. Keep moist in winter. Pot on annually in spring. Outdoors, grow in moderately fertile, well-drained soil in full sun.
• **PROPAGATION** Sow seed at 13–18°C (55–64°F) in autumn or early spring; divide in early spring, or take basal cuttings in summer.
• **PESTS AND DISEASES** Leaf spot, leaf miners, root rot, aphids, whiteflies, and tarsonemid mites may be a problem.

G. jamesonii ■ (Barberton daisy, Transvaal daisy). Clump-forming, deep-rooting perennial with inversely lance-shaped, deeply lobed to pinnatifid leaves, 15–45cm (6–18in) long, dark green above, paler and sparsely to densely woolly beneath. Solitary, daisy-like, orange-scarlet flowerheads, 8–12cm (3–5in) across, with yellow centres, appear from late spring to late summer. Resents transplanting. ↕ 30–45cm (12–18in), ↔ 60cm (24in). South Africa (Northern Transvaal, Eastern Transvaal, KwaZulu/Natal), Swaziland. ❁ (min. 5°C/41°F). Seed-raised selections are available in mixed colours. **'Californian Giants'** have single flowers in shades of yellow, apricot, orange, red and pink; ↕ to 60cm (24in). **Pandora Series** cultivars are free-flowering, in shades of cream, apricot, crimson-red, scarlet, pink, or lavender, with mid-green leaves; ↕ 25cm (10in). **Parade Series** cultivars have single or double, yellow, orange, red or pink flowerheads. **Sunburst Series** cultivars have flowerheads to 10cm (4in) across, in shades of yellow, orange, red or pink. **Tempo Series** cultivars bloom in shades of red, orange, pink, salmon-pink, cream, and yellow.

▷**Germander,**
Shrubby see *Teucrium fruticans*
Tree see *Teucrium fruticans*

GESNERIA

GESNERIACEAE

Genus of about 50 species of mostly tuberous, usually evergreen perennials, subshrubs, and small trees, often epiphytic or rock-dwelling, found in tropical America and the West Indies. Tubular or bell-shaped flowers, usually 5-lobed, are white, red, orange, yellow, green, or brown, and borne singly or in cymes, with bracts at the bases of the flowering stems. The leaves are ovate, elliptic, or heart- or lance-shaped, and borne alternately or in opposite pairs. In frost-prone areas, grow in a warm greenhouse. Elsewhere, grow in shaded borders or as epiphytes on rocks or trees.

• **HARDINESS** Frost tender.
• **CULTIVATION** Under glass, grow in loam-based potting compost (JI No.2), with added sharp sand and leaf mould, in bright filtered or indirect light. In growth, maintain at 18°C (64°F), with high humidity, and water freely with soft water; keep leaves dry but compost always moist. Apply a quarter-strength balanced liquid fertilizer every 4 weeks. Keep dry in winter. Outdoors, grow in moist, humus-rich soil in deep shade.
• **PROPAGATION** Sow seed at 19–24°C (66–75°F) in spring, or take stem or leaf cuttings in late spring.
• **PESTS AND DISEASES** Flower thrips and *Fusarium* wilt may be a problem.

G. cuneifolia. Erect or decumbent, woody-based perennial with hairless or slightly hairy, inversely lance-shaped or obovate, scalloped or toothed leaves, 2–14cm (¾–5½in) long, clustered at the branch tips. In summer, bears few-flowered, pendent, arching cymes of tubular, pink or deep red flowers, to 2.5cm (1in) long, and yellow or pink inside. ↕↔ 15cm (6in). Puerto Rico. ❁ (min. 14°C/57°F)

G. zebrina see *Smithiantha zebrina.*

▷**Gesneriads** see p.40

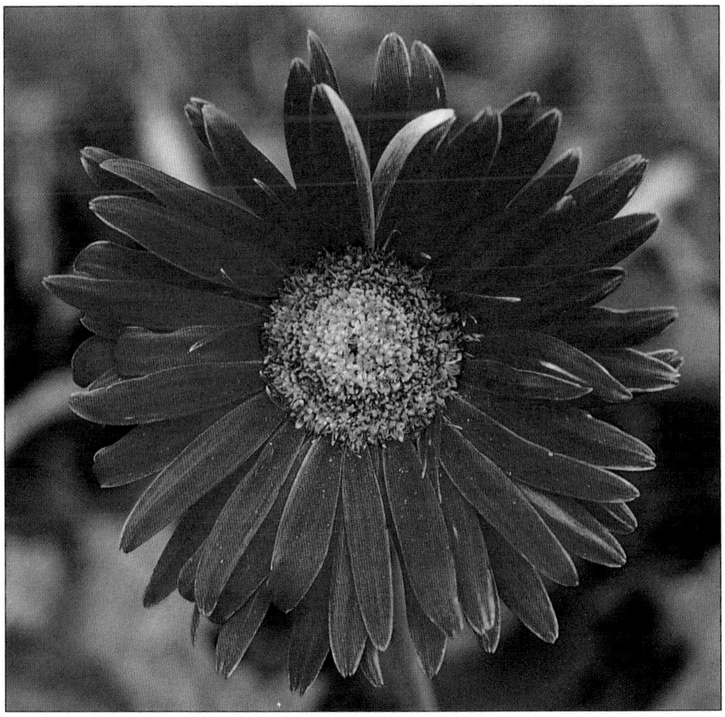

Gerbera jamesonii

G

GEUM

Avens

ROSACEAE

Genus of about 50 species of rhizomatous, occasionally stoloniferous perennials from mountainous habitats, streamsides, moist meadows, and woodland in arctic and temperate regions of Europe, Asia, New Zealand, North and South America, and Africa. They have unequally pinnate to pinnatisect, wrinkled leaves, the leaflets with toothed or scalloped margins; the leaves are mainly borne in basal rosettes. The erect, open, 5-petalled, saucer- to bowl-shaped, usually upright but occasionally pendent flowers, in shades of cream, yellow, orange, pink, or red, are solitary or borne in cymes, and bloom from late spring to summer. The stems of *G. chiloense* hybrids tend to be more branched than those of *G. coccineum* hybrids. The smaller geums are suitable for growing in a rock garden; the larger can be grown at the front of a border.

• **HARDINESS** Fully hardy.

• **CULTIVATION** Grow in fertile, well-drained soil in full sun; *G. rivale* and its cultivars prefer humus-rich, moist soil. Avoid soil that is waterlogged in winter.

• **PROPAGATION** Sow seed in containers in a cold frame, or divide, in autumn or spring. *G.* 'Lady Stratheden' and *G.* 'Mrs. J. Bradshaw' come virtually true from seed, but most of the larger geums hybridize readily in gardens.

• **PESTS AND DISEASES** Sawfly larvae may cause damage to leaves.

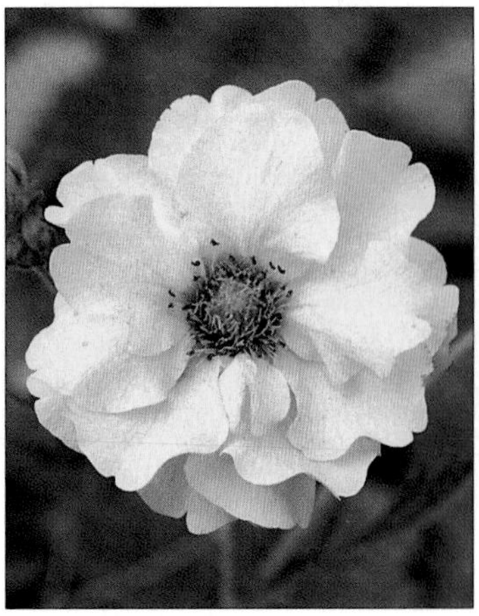

Geum 'Lady Stratheden'

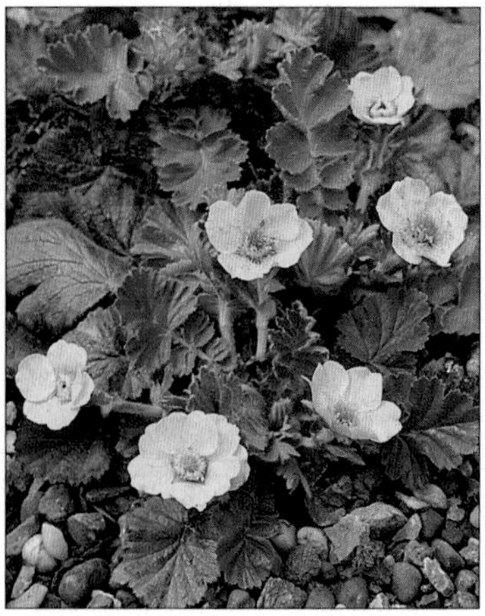

Geum montanum

***G.* x *borisii* of gardens** see *G. coccineum.*

G. chiloense, syn. *G. coccineum* of gardens. Clump-forming, densely woolly perennial. Basal leaves, 10–30cm (4–12in) long, are pinnate; the heart- to kidney-shaped terminal leaflets, 2.5cm (1in) long, are scarcely larger than the lateral leaflets. Stem leaves are deeply 3-lobed and toothed. Branched stems bear cymes of saucer-shaped scarlet flowers, to 4cm (1½in) across, from early to late summer. ↕ 40–60cm (16–24in), ↔ 60cm (24in). Chile. ❄❄❄. **'Dolly North'** produces glowing, deep orange flowers. **'Fire Opal'** 🏆 produces semi-double, reddish orange flowers on purple stems; ↕ to 75cm (30in).

G. coccineum ▣ syn. *G.* x *borisii* of gardens. Clump-forming perennial with upright, pinnate, softly hairy, basal leaves, to 20cm (8in) long, the kidney-shaped terminal leaflets, 5–15cm (2–6in) long, much larger than the lateral leaflets. Stem leaves are deeply toothed but unlobed. From late spring to late summer, bears cymes of 2–4 brick-red flowers, to 4cm (1½in) across, with spreading petals and conspicuous yellow stamens. ↕ 30–50cm (12–20in), ↔ 30cm (12in). Balkans. ❄❄❄

***G. coccineum* of gardens** see *G. chiloense.*

***G.* 'Feuerball'** see *G.* 'Mrs. J. Bradshaw'.

***G.* 'Georgenberg'.** *G. chiloense* hybrid with pinnate, bright green leaves, 10–15cm (4–6in) long. The terminal leaflets are kidney-shaped and to 8cm (3in) long; the other leaflets are much smaller. Branched stems bear saucer-shaped, orange-yellow flowers, to 4cm (1½in) across, from late spring to midsummer. ↕ 25cm (10in), ↔ 30cm (12in). ❄❄❄

***G.* 'Goldball'** see *G.* 'Lady Stratheden'.

***G.* 'Lady Stratheden'** ▣ 🏆 syn. *G.* 'Goldball'. *G. chiloense* hybrid bearing pinnate, hairy leaves, to 20cm (8in) long, comprised of kidney-shaped terminal leaflets, the remainder ovate. Semi-double, rich yellow flowers, 4.5cm (1¾in) across, are produced in cymes of 1–5 throughout summer. ↕ 40–60cm (16–24in), ↔ 60cm (24in). ❄❄❄

G. montanum ▣ 🏆 Clump-forming perennial with thick, spreading rhizomes and dense clusters of radical, pinnate, dark green leaves, to 10cm (4in) long, each with a large, rounded or kidney-shaped, terminal lobe. From spring to early summer, bears solitary, cup-shaped, deep golden yellow flowers, to 4cm (1½in) across, on short stems, occasionally in cymes of 2 or 3. ↕ 15cm (6in), ↔ to 30cm (12in). Mountains of C. and S. Europe. ❄❄❄

***G.* 'Mrs. Bradshaw'** see *G.* 'Mrs. J. Bradshaw'.

***G.* 'Mrs. J. Bradshaw'** 🏆 syn. *G.* 'Feuerball', *G.* 'Mrs. Bradshaw'. Hybrid of *G. chiloense* bearing pinnate, hairy leaves, 15–20cm (6–8in) long, with kidney-shaped terminal leaflets, the remainder ovate. Semi-double scarlet flowers, 4.5cm (1¾in) across, are produced in cymes of 1–5 from early to late summer. ↕ 40–60cm (16–24in), ↔ 60cm (24in). ❄❄❄

***G.* 'Prince of Orange'.** *G. coccineum* hybrid producing pinnate, hairy leaves, to 30cm (12in) long, with kidney-shaped terminal leaflets, the remainder ovate. Bears cymes of 1–4 brilliant orange flowers, 4.5cm (1¾in) across, with slightly cupped petals, in early and midsummer. ↕↔ to 60cm (24in). ❄❄❄

***G.* 'Princess Juliana'** see *G.* 'Prinses Juliana'.

***G.* 'Prinses Juliana'**, syn. *G.* 'Princess Juliana'. *G. chiloense* hybrid bearing pinnate, hairy leaves, 10–20cm (4–8in) long, with heart- to kidney-shaped terminal leaflets, the remainder smaller and ovate. Semi-double, red-flushed, bright yellow flowers, 4.5cm (1¾in) across, are produced in cymes of 1–5 in early and midsummer. ↕↔ 40–60cm (16–24in). ❄❄❄

***G.* 'Red Wings'** ▣ *G. coccineum* hybrid bearing pinnate, hairy leaves, to 25cm (10in) long, with heart- to kidney-shaped terminal leaflets, the remainder

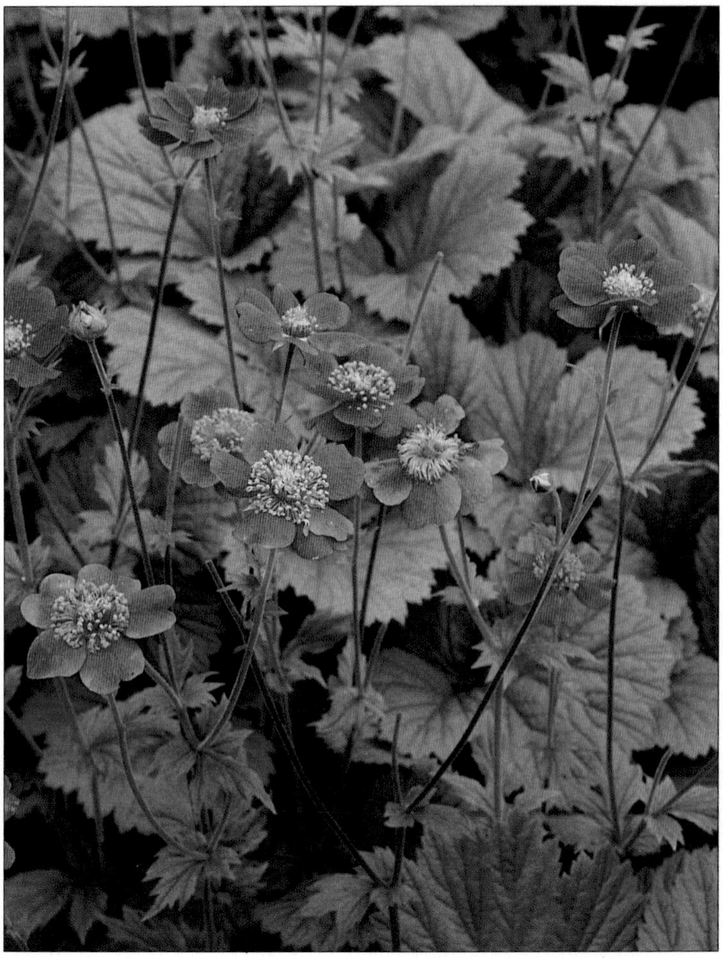

Geum coccineum

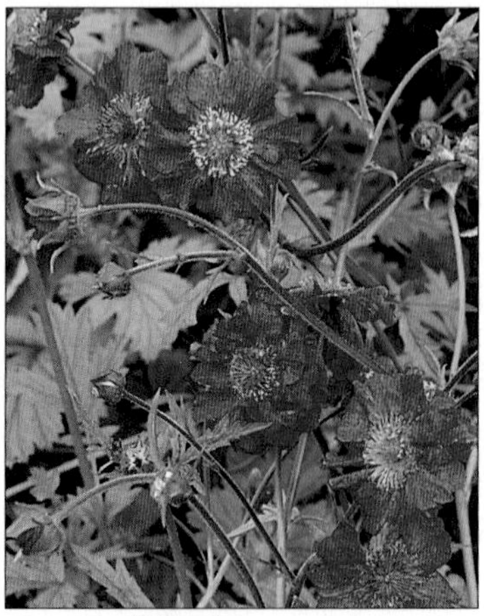

Geum 'Red Wings'

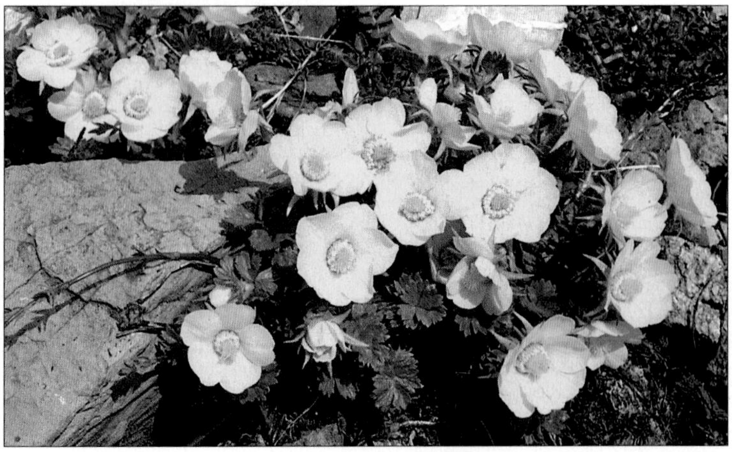

Geum reptans

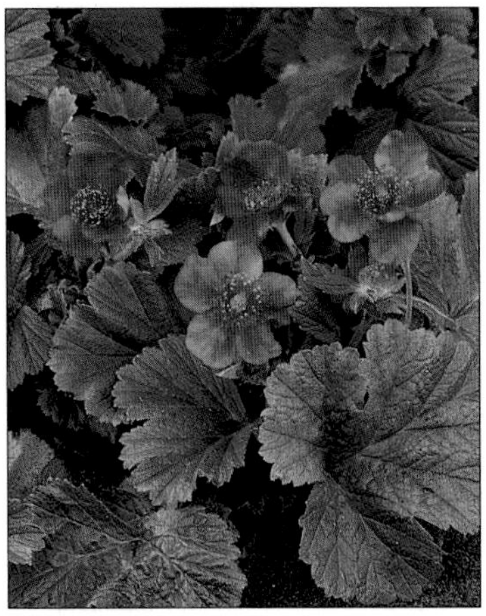

Geum 'Tangerine'

smaller and ovate. Bears semi-double, bright scarlet flowers, 4.5cm (1¾in) across, in cymes of 1–3, in early and midsummer. Very free-flowering. ↕ to 60cm (24in), ↔ to 40cm (16in). ❄❄❄
G. reptans ■ syn. *Sieversia reptans.* Rhizomatous perennial, spreading by stolons, bearing rosettes of radical, pinnate leaves, to 15cm (6in) long, with deeply toothed, rounded leaflets. Produces usually solitary, shallowly cup-shaped, bright yellow flowers, to 4cm (1½in) across, in early summer. Best grown in a scree bed or alpine house. ↕ to 15cm (6in), ↔ to 20cm (8in). Alps, Carpathians, Balkans. ❄❄❄
G. rivale. Upright perennial with pinnate, basal leaves, to 15cm (6in) or more long. The terminal and upper pair of leaflets are obovate or wedge-shaped, coarsely scalloped or toothed, and to 5cm (2in) long; the rest are very small. From late spring to midsummer, bears cymes of 2–5 pendent, bell-shaped, dusky pink to dark orange-red flowers, to 2cm (¾in) across, with conspicuous, red-brown sepals that are almost as long as the petals. ↕↔ 20–60cm (8–24in). Europe. ❄❄❄. **'Coppertone'**, probably a hybrid of *G. rivale*, has toothed leaves, brown flower stems, and slightly pendent, copper-apricot flowers, to 5cm (2in) across, with wavy petals and reddish brown sepals; ↕↔ to 30cm (12in). **'Lemon Drops'**, probably a hybrid of *G. rivale*, has slender brown stems bearing long-stalked, open, lemon-yellow flowers, pendent at first, with brownish green sepals; ↕↔ to 25cm (10in). **'Leonard's Variety'**, syn. 'Leonardii', is very free-flowering, with pendent, copper-pink, orange-tinged flowers, to 4cm (1½in) across, on mahogany stems, borne in mid- and late summer; ↕ to 45cm (18in). **'Lionel Cox'**, probably a hybrid of *G. rivale*, forms large clumps of soft green leaves, and produces pendent, open bell-shaped, creamy apricot flowers with wavy petals; ↕ 30cm (12in). **'Sigiswang'**, probably a hybrid of *G. rivale*, is mound-forming, bearing bright green leaves, 13–15cm (5–6in) long, with kidney-shaped terminal leaflets, the rest smaller, and cymes of red-shaded orange flowers, 3cm (1¼in) across.
***G.* 'Tangerine'** ■ is a hybrid of *G. rivale*, with similar foliage. From late spring to midsummer, produces cymes of 1–3 bright orange, slightly nodding, saucer-shaped flowers, to 2.5cm (1in) across. ↕↔ 30cm (12in). ❄❄❄

GEVUINA

PROTEACEAE

Genus of one species of evergreen tree or shrub found in moist forests in the mountains of Chile. Grown for its attractive, alternate, pinnate or 2-pinnate leaves and its white summer flowers, it thrives outdoors only in relatively mild, moist climates, where it is best planted in sheltered woodland. Elsewhere, grow in a cool greenhouse.
• **HARDINESS** Frost hardy.
• **CULTIVATION** Under glass, grow in lime-free (ericaceous) compost in bright filtered light. Outdoors, grow in fertile, acid to neutral, moist but well-drained soil in partial shade; protect from cold, drying winds. Pruning group 1.
• **PROPAGATION** Sow seed in containers in a cold frame in autumn, or root semi-ripe cuttings with bottom heat in late summer.
• **PESTS AND DISEASES** Trouble free.

G. avellana ♢ (Chilean hazel, Chile nut). Conical, evergreen tree or large shrub with pinnate or 2-pinnate, glossy, dark green leaves, to 40cm (16in) long, each with up to 30 coarsely toothed, ovate-elliptic, leathery leaflets. Slender racemes, to 12cm (5in) long, of spider-like, white, occasionally red- or green-tinged flowers, 2.5cm (1in) long, are produced in late summer, sometimes followed by ovoid red fruit, 1cm (½in) or more long, ripening black. ↕↔ 10m (30ft). Chile. ❄❄

▷**Ghost tree** see *Davidia*
▷**Ghost weed** see *Euphorbia marginata*
▷**Giant Spaniard** see *Aciphylla scott-thomsonii*

GIBBAEUM

AIZOACEAE

Genus of about 20 species of fleshy, perennial succulents found in semi-desert areas of South Africa. Pairs of thick, fleshy leaves, often of different sizes, unite to form an almost spherical or elongated body. Solitary, daisy-like flowers are borne from early autumn to early winter. The plants offset freely, producing large colonies. Where temperatures drop below 7°C (45°F), grow as houseplants or in a temperate greenhouse. In warm, dry climates, grow in a desert garden or mixed border with other succulents.

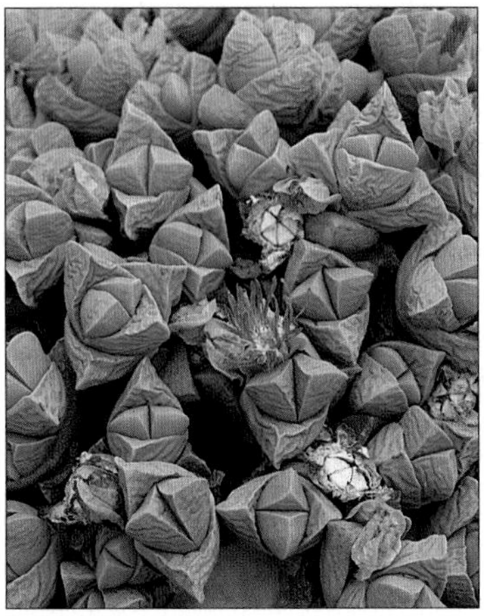

Gibbaeum petrense

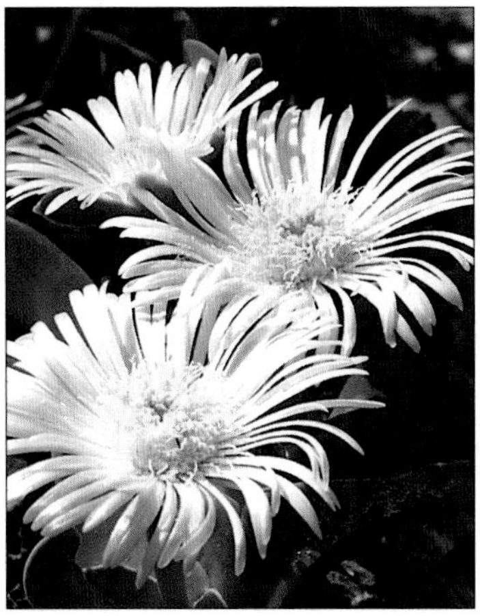

Gibbaeum velutinum

• **HARDINESS** Frost tender.
• **CULTIVATION** Under glass, grow in standard cactus compost in full light. From mid-autumn (when new growth appears) to early spring, water sparingly and apply a low-nitrogen liquid fertilizer every 6–8 weeks. Keep dry during the rest of the year. Outdoors, grow in poor, sharply drained soil in full sun. See also pp.48–49.
• **PROPAGATION** Sow seed at 19–24°C (66–75°F), or divide offsets, in spring or summer.
• **PESTS AND DISEASES** Trouble free.

G. album. Clump-forming succulent with whitish to pale grey, paired leaves of different sizes, each pair united to form an obliquely ovoid body, to 2.5cm (1in) long, densely covered with tiny white hairs and with a cleft below the tip. Bears white or pink flowers, 2.5cm (1in) across, from early autumn to early winter. ↕ 2.5cm (1in) or more, ↔ 24cm (10in) or more. South Africa (Northern Cape, Western Cape). ❁ (min. 7°C/45°F)
G. petrense ■ Mat-forming succulent with fleshy roots and small stems bearing paired, greyish green leaves, 1cm (½in) long, keeled above, rounded below, each pair united for one-third of their length. Bears terminal to axillary, magenta to red or pink flowers, 1.5cm (½in) across, from early autumn to early winter. ↕ to 3cm (1¼in), ↔ 15cm (6in) or more. South Africa (Western Cape). ❁ (min. 7°C/45°F)
G. velutinum ■ Mat-forming succulent with small stems bearing paired, slender, differently sized, bluish grey-green leaves, 4–6cm (1½–2½in) long, each pair united towards the base, the longer leaf with an incurved, hooked tip. Bears lilac, pink, or white flowers, 4–5cm (1½–2in) across, from early autumn to early winter. ↕ 8cm (3in), ↔ 30cm (12in). South Africa (Western Cape). ❁ (min. 7°C/45°F)

GILIA

POLEMONIACEAE

Genus of 25–30 species of erect annuals, occasionally perennials, from grassland and chaparral in S.W. North America and W. and S. South America. The leaves are mostly basal, entire to finely divided, pinnate or 2-pinnate, and often with soft, sticky hairs above. The flowers are small, showy, salverform to tubular-funnel-shaped, violet-blue, pink, or red,

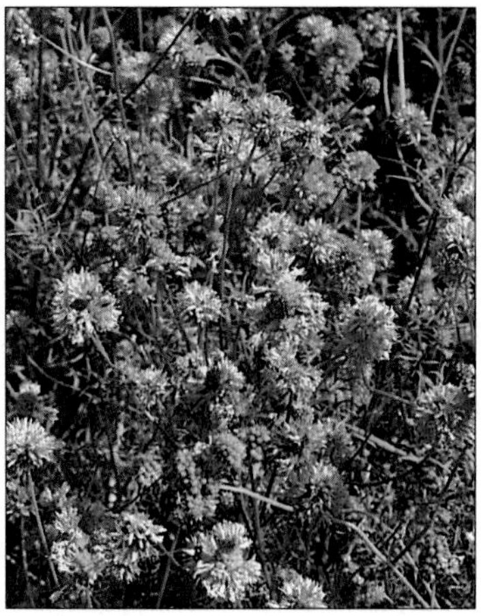

Gilia capitata

produced singly in the leaf axils, in terminal panicles, or in compact clusters borne terminally and in the upper leaf axils, from late spring to late summer. Grow in an annual or mixed border.
• **HARDINESS** Fully hardy.
• **CULTIVATION** Grow in light, well-drained soil in full sun.
• **PROPAGATION** Sow seed *in situ* in autumn or mid-spring, or at 10–13°C (50–55°F) in early spring.
• **PESTS AND DISEASES** Trouble free.

G. achilleifolia. Erect annual with 2-pinnate leaves, 4–10cm (1½–4in) long, and sickle-shaped leaflets. In summer, bears mid-blue to blue-violet flowers, to 2.5cm (1in) long, in dense, fan-shaped, terminal or axillary cymes, 3–8cm (1¼–3in) across. ↕ to 70cm (28in), ↔ 20–23cm (8–9in). USA (California), Mexico (Baja California). ❄❄❄
G. capitata ■ (Queen Anne's thimbles). Erect annual with feathery, 2-pinnate leaves, 4–10cm (1½–4in) long, with linear leaflets. In summer, bears terminal and axillary, pincushion-like heads, 1.5–4cm (½–1½in) across, of many lavender-blue flowers, 6–8mm (¼–⅜in) long, with protruding stamens. ↕ 45–60cm (18–24in), ↔ 20–23cm (8–9in). E. North America. ❄❄❄
G. tricolor (Bird's eyes). Mound-forming annual with pinnate to 2-pinnate leaves, 1–4cm (½–1½in) long, with very narrow leaflets. From late spring to late summer, saucer-shaped, pale to dark violet-blue flowers, 1.5cm (½in) long, with pale violet-blue spots around the orange or yellow centres, are borne on slender, very leafy stalks, either singly or in clusters of 2–5. ↕ 30–45cm (12–18in), ↔ 23cm (9in). USA (California). ❄❄❄

GILLENIA

ROSACEAE

Genus of 2 species of rhizomatous perennials from open woodland in C., E., and S.E. North America. They have 3-palmate, bronze-green leaves and loose, few-flowered panicles of white or pink flowers, with slightly unequal, inversely lance-shaped to linear-lance-shaped petals, the sepals enlarging when in fruit. Gillenias are graceful plants for light woodland or a shady border, and are good for cutting.
• **HARDINESS** Fully hardy.
• **CULTIVATION** Grow in fertile, slightly acid to neutral, moist but well-drained

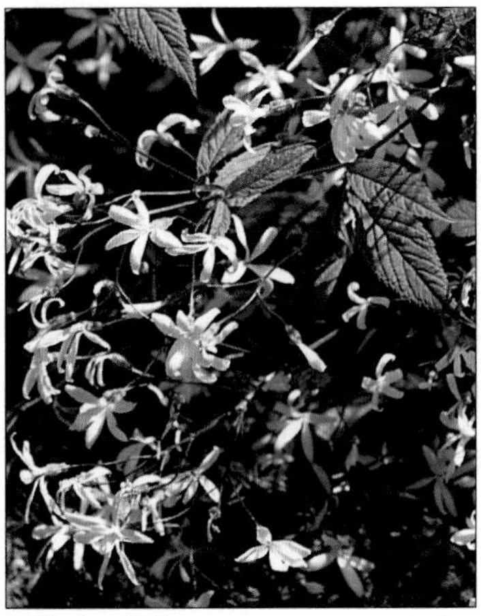

Gillenia trifoliata

soil in partial shade, or full sun with shade during the hottest part of the day.
• **PROPAGATION** Sow seed in containers in a cold frame, or divide, in spring or autumn.
• **PESTS AND DISEASES** Slugs may eat young shoots.

G. trifoliata ■ ♀ (Bowman's root, Indian physic). Erect perennial with branched, red-tinted stems and alternate, 3-palmate, coarsely toothed, conspicuously veined, bronze-green leaves, with ovate-oblong leaflets, each 8cm (3in) long. Bears irregularly star-shaped, white to pinkish white flowers, 2.5–4cm (1–1½in) across, with narrow petals and red-tinted calyces, from late spring to late summer. ↕ to 1m (3ft), ↔ 60cm (24in). E. North America (Ontario to Georgia). ❄❄❄

▷**Gillyflower** see *Matthiola, M. incana*
▷**Ginger,**
Crepe see *Costus speciosus*
Indian see *Alpinia calcarata*
Kahili see *Hedychium gardnerianum*
Red see *Alpinia purpurata*
Shell see *Alpinia zerumbet*
Spiral see *Costus malortieanus*

▷**Ginger cont.**
Torch see *Etlingera elatior*
Variegated see *Alpinia vittata*
Wild see *Asarum*
▷**Ginger lily** see *Alpinia, Hedychium*
Dwarf see *Kaempferia roscoeana*
Red see *Hedychium coccineum*
Scarlet see *Hedychium coccineum*
White see *Hedychium coronarium*

GINKGO

Maidenhair tree

GINKGOACEAE

Genus of one species of deciduous, dioecious tree from S. China, extinct in the wild but preserved and still grown in temple gardens and as a specimen tree. Long shoots bear alternate leaves, while woody spur shoots bear densely clustered leaves and flowers. The fan-shaped, divided, mid- to yellow-green leaves turn golden yellow in autumn. The fleshy fruit smell unpleasant as they decay; they contain large, edible nuts. *G. biloba* tolerates atmospheric pollution and is an excellent landscape tree.
• **HARDINESS** Fully hardy.
• **CULTIVATION** Grow in any fertile, well-drained soil in full sun. Pruning group 1.
• **PROPAGATION** Sow seed in containers in an open frame as soon as ripe, or take semi-ripe cuttings in summer. Graft in winter.
• **PESTS AND DISEASES** Trouble free.

G. biloba ■ ♀ ○ (Maidenhair tree). Upright tree, columnar then wide-spreading, with furrowed, dull grey bark. Flat, fan-shaped, mid- to yellow-green leaves, to 12cm (5in) across, are tapered into the stalks and usually lobed at the tips. Catkin-like, pendulous, cylindrical yellow male flowers, 8cm (3in) long, are borne in clusters. Round, solitary female flowers produce plum-like, yellow-green fruit, 3cm (1¼in) long, in autumn. ↕ to 30m (100ft), ↔ to 8m (25ft). S. China. ❄❄❄. **'Princeton Sentry'** ○ is narrow, upright, and male.

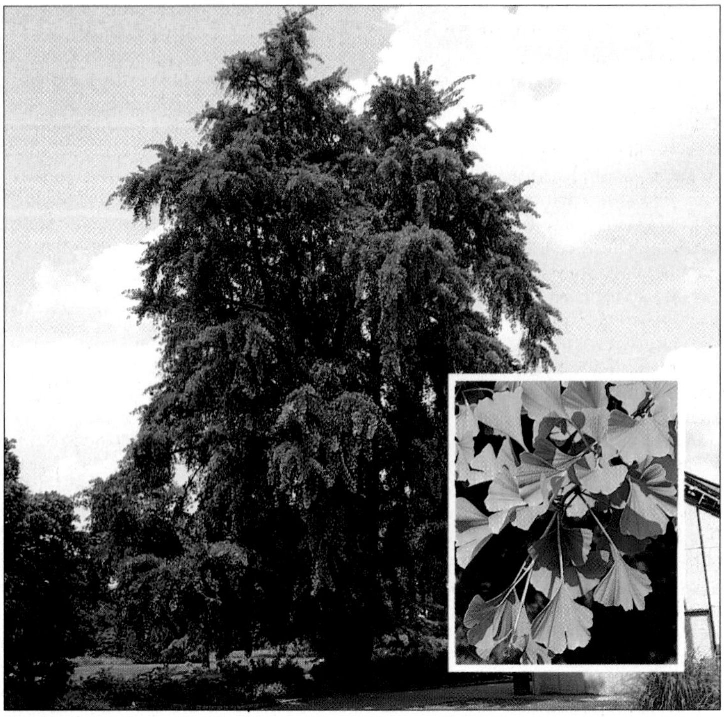

Ginkgo biloba (inset: leaf detail)

GLADIOLUS

syn. ACIDANTHERA, HOMOGLOSSUM

IRIDACEAE

Genus of about 180 species of cormous perennials from rocky slopes, seasonally dry grasslands, and marshy areas, mainly in South Africa, but also from the Mediterranean, the Arabian Peninsula, N.W. and E. Africa, Madagascar, and W. Asia. They are grown for their showy spikes of usually open, funnel-shaped flowers, borne mainly from spring to early autumn. The flowers each have 6 tepals: usually 1 central upper tepal, 3 often quite small lower or lip tepals, and 2 side or wing tepals. They open from the bottom of the spikes upwards, older blooms dying off as new ones develop (the number of buds open at any one time is given in brackets in each hybrid and cultivar description below). Erect leaves, borne in basal fans, are narrow, linear or sword-shaped, mid- to dark green, and 24–60cm (10–24in) long.

Plant gladioli in clumps in a mixed border, or in rows for cutting. In frost-prone climates, grow frost-hardy gladioli by a sheltered, sunny wall; winter-flowering South African gladioli require a cool greenhouse. In warmer areas, plant in open, sunny, well-drained sites.

Over 10,000 hybrids and cultivars have been developed for garden cultivation, exhibiting, and cutting. They are classified into three main groups: Grandiflorus, Nanus, and Primulinus (see below). Flowers may be borne either in a formal arrangement, side by side on the stem, so when open there is no daylight visible between them, or less formally, with one bloom above another, like a step-ladder.

Grandiflorus Group
Hybrids and cultivars in this group flower from early to late summer. Each corm produces one closely packed spike, 50–90cm (20–36in) long, with as many as 28 buds, up to 12 open at a time, usually formally arranged. Tepals may be plain, usually denoting Dutch origin, or ruffled, indicating American origin. The texture of the tepals varies from paper thin to much thicker. Grandiflorus gladioli are classified into 5 sizes, determined by the diameter of the bottom flower on the spike, as follows:

GIANT	14cm (5½in) or more
LARGE	11–14cm (4½–5½in)
MEDIUM	9–11cm (3½–4½in)
SMALL	6–9cm (2½–3½in)
MINIATURE	3.5–6cm (1½–2½in)

Nanus Group
Nanus hybrids and cultivars flower in early summer, and are ideal for cutting and corsages. Each corm produces 2 or 3 slender spikes, 22–35cm (9–14in) long, with loosely arranged flowers, 4–5cm (1½–2in) across. Each spike bears up to 7 buds, 3–5 open at a time. The tepals are moderately thick.
Primulinus Group
Hybrids and cultivars in this group flower from early to late summer. Each corm produces one thin, whip-like stem, 30–60cm (12–24in) long, which bears as many as 23 buds, up to 7 open at a time, mainly in a semi-formal, step-ladder arrangement. The triangular flowers are usually 3.5–7cm (1½–3in) across, with paper thin to moderately thick tepals. The top central tepal is hooded and held at right-angles to the stem, covering the stigma and anthers.

• **HARDINESS** Fully hardy to frost tender.
• **CULTIVATION** Grow in fertile, well-drained soil in full sun, planting the corms 10–16cm (4–6in) deep in spring, on a bed of sharp sand to aid drainage. For frost-hardy to half-hardy gladioli, apply a high-potash liquid fertilizer when the flower spikes reach one-third to half their final height; repeat every 10–14 days until 3 weeks after flowering. In frost-prone areas, lift them when the leaves turn yellow-brown; snap the corms from the stems, dip in fungicide, and dry for 14 days. Separate new corms from old, and discard the old. Keep dry and frost-free until planted. Under glass, grow winter-flowering South African gladioli in loam-based potting compost (JI No.1), with additional sharp sand, in full light. Water moderately in growth.
• **PROPAGATION** Sow seed of hardy species in containers in a cold frame in spring; sow seed of half-hardy to tender species at 15°C (59°F) in spring. Separate cormlets when dormant.
• **PESTS AND DISEASES** Prone to gladiolus corm rot, various types of grey mould (*Botrytis*), thrips, aphids, and slugs.

G. alatus. Short-lived, cormous perennial with linear leaves, 8–40cm (3–16in) long. Bears up to 10 hooded, funnel-shaped, scented flowers, 4.5cm (1¾in) across, from late winter to spring (late spring to summer in cool climates). Upper tepals are salmon-pink to orange or red; lip tepals are lime-green, tipped with salmon-pink to orange or red. Best grown regularly from seed. ↕ 8–35cm (3–14in), ↔ 5cm (2in). South Africa (Northern Cape, Eastern Cape, Western Cape). ❄
G. 'Amanda Mahy' ■ Nanus gladiolus bearing salmon-pink flowers, 5cm (2in)

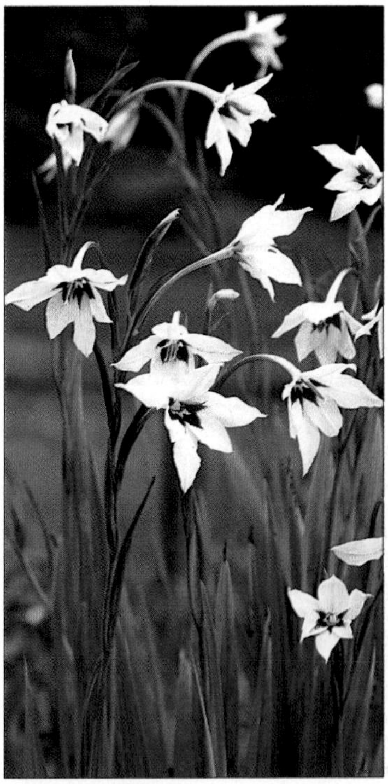

Gladiolus callianthus

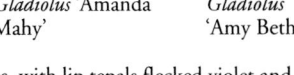

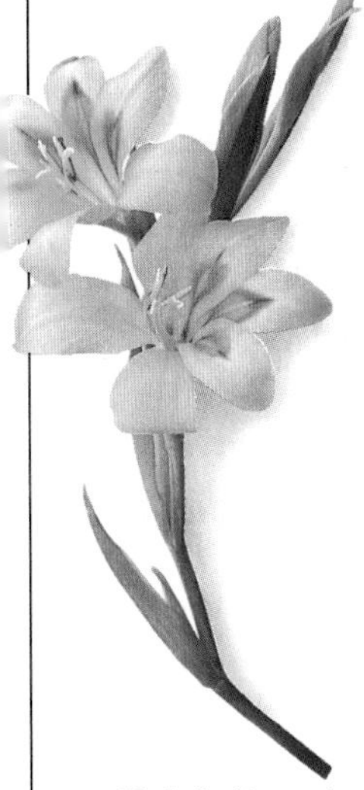
Gladiolus 'Amanda Mahy'

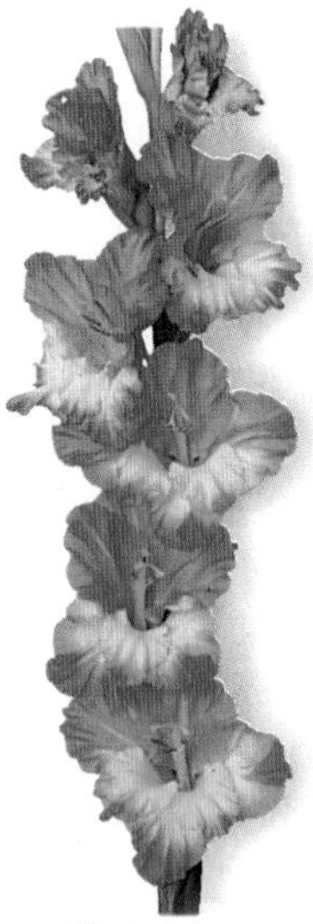
Gladiolus 'Amy Beth'

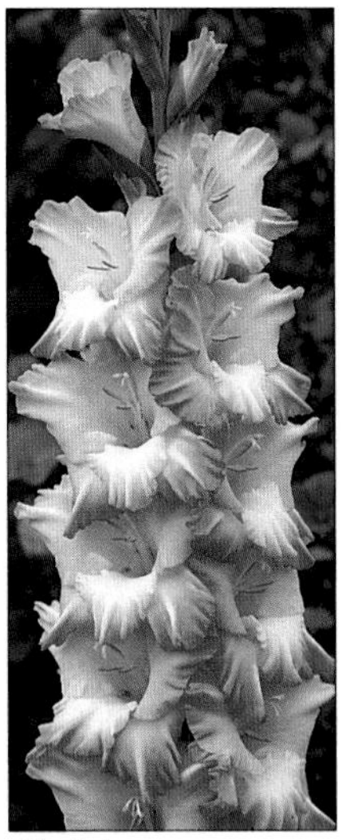
Gladiolus 'Anna Leorah'

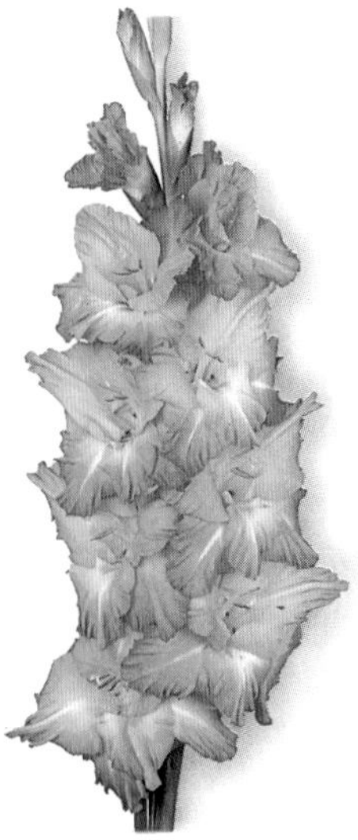
Gladiolus 'Beau Rivage'

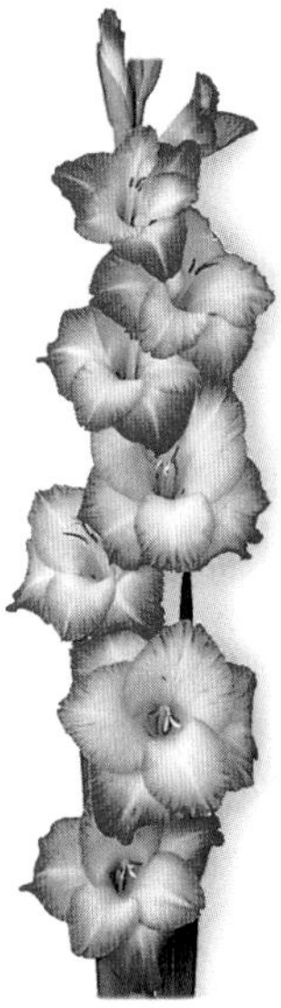
Gladiolus 'Beauty of Holland'

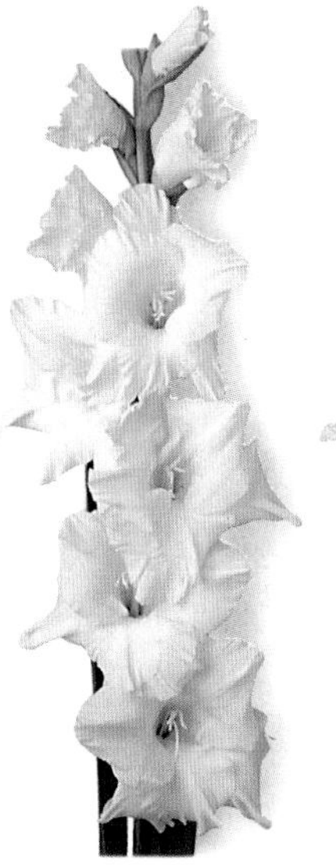
Gladiolus 'Carrara'

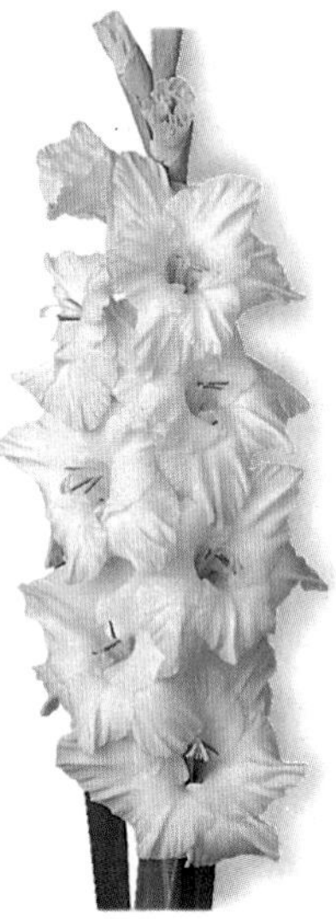
Gladiolus 'Charmer'

across, with lip tepals flecked violet and white, in early summer. Flower spike is 30cm (12in) long, with 7 buds (3 or 4 open). ↕80cm (32in), ↔ 8–10cm (3–4in). ❄

***G.* 'Amsterdam'.** Giant-flowered Grandiflorus gladiolus bearing slightly upward-facing white flowers, with gently ruffled tepals, in late summer. Flower spike is 70–80cm (28–32in) long, with 24–27 buds (10 open). ↕1.7m (5½ft), ↔ 15cm (6in). ❄

***G.* 'Amy Beth'** ■ Small-flowered Grandiflorus gladiolus. In midsummer, bears strongly ruffled, lilac-pink flowers, with cream lip tepals. Flower spike is 55–60cm (22–24in) long, with 22 buds (7 open). ↕1.2m (4ft), ↔ 8–10cm (3–4in). ❄

***G.* 'Anitra'.** Primulinus gladiolus producing blood-red flowers, 4–6cm (1½–2½in) across, in midsummer. Flower spike is 45cm (18in) long, with 17 buds (6 or 7 open). ↕1m (3ft), ↔ 8–10cm (3–4in). ❄

***G.* 'Anna Leorah'** ■ Large-flowered Grandiflorus gladiolus producing strongly ruffled, mid-pink flowers, with large white throats, in midsummer. Flower spike is 70–80cm (28–32in) long, with 25 buds (10 open). ↕1.6m (5½ft), ↔ 15cm (6in). ❄

***G.* 'Antique Rose'.** Medium-flowered Grandiflorus gladiolus. In late summer, produces slightly ruffled, old rose-pink flowers with lavender-blue throats marked with deep rose-pink flashes. Flower spike is 70–80cm (28–32in) long, with 26 buds (10 open). ↕1.5m (5ft), ↔ 12cm (5in). ❄

***G.* 'Award'.** Large-flowered Grandiflorus gladiolus. In midsummer, bears rose-pink flowers, fading to white in the throats, with slightly ruffled tepals. Flower spike is 75cm (30in) long, with 26 buds (8 or 9 open). ↕1.5m (5ft), ↔ 15cm (6in). ❄

***G.* 'Babette'.** Large-flowered Grandiflorus gladiolus producing soft salmon-pink flowers, with small cream throats and slightly ruffled tepals, in midsummer. Flower spike is 80cm (32in) long, with 26 buds (9 open). ↕1.7m (5½ft), ↔ 15cm (6in). ❄

***G.* 'Beau Rivage'** ■ Large-flowered Grandiflorus gladiolus producing ruffled, deep coral-pink flowers in summer. Flower spike is 50cm (20in) long, with 15 buds (5–9 open). ↕to 1.2m (4ft), ↔ 30cm (12in). ❄

***G.* 'Beauty of Holland'** ■ Large-flowered Grandiflorus gladiolus bearing ruffled, pink-margined white flowers in midsummer. Flower spike is 70–75cm (28–30in) long, with 27 buds (9 open). ↕1.7m (5½ft), ↔ 15cm (6in). ❄

G. blandus see *G. carneus.*

G. blandus* var. *carneus see *G. carneus.*

***G.* 'Blue Delight'.** Large-flowered Grandiflorus gladiolus that produces slightly ruffled, mid-blue flowers, with blue-peppered white throats, in midsummer. Flower spike is 70–80cm (28–32in) long, with 25 buds (9 open). ↕1.5m (5ft), ↔ 15cm (6in). ❄

***G.* 'Blue Heaven'.** Large-flowered Grandiflorus gladiolus. In midsummer, produces strongly ruffled, mid-blue flowers, with very large, pure white throats. Flower spike is 70–75cm (28–30in) long, with 25 buds (8 open). ↕1.5m (5ft), ↔ 15cm (6in). ❄

G. byzantinus see *G. communis* subsp. *byzantinus.*

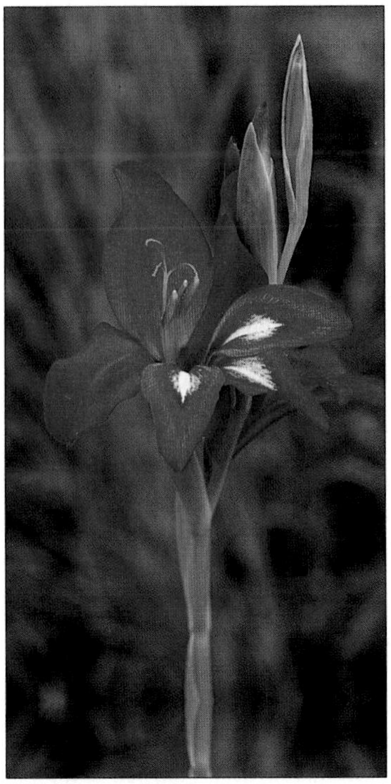
Gladiolus cardinalis

G. callianthus ■ 🏆 syn. *Acidanthera bicolor* var. *murieliae, A. murieliae.* Cormous perennial with linear leaves 15–45cm (6–18in) long. In late summer and early autumn, bears loose spikes of up to 10 hooded, funnel-shaped, strongly scented, pure white flowers, 5cm (2in) across, each with a prominent purple-red mark in the throat. Blooms curve downwards on very long, thin tubes. ↕70–100cm (28–39in), ↔ 5cm (2in). Eritrea to Mozambique. ❄

***G.* 'Caravan'.** Large-flowered Grandiflorus gladiolus. In midsummer, bears strongly ruffled, chocolate-brown flowers with small cream throats marked with maroon flashes. Flower spike is 70cm (28in) long, with 22–24 buds (9 open). ↕1.5m (5ft), ↔ 15cm (6in). ❄

G. cardinalis ■ Cormous perennial with sword-shaped leaves, 40–90cm (16–36in) long. In summer, arching stems bear up to 12 widely funnel-shaped, bright red flowers, 5cm (2in) across, a white flash on each of the lip tepals. ↕60–90cm (24–36in), ↔ 8cm (3in). South Africa (Western Cape). ❄

G. carneus, syn. *G. blandus, G. blandus* var. *carneus.* Slender, cormous perennial with linear or sword-shaped leaves, to 60cm (24in) long. Lax, sometimes branched spikes of 3–12 funnel-shaped flowers, 5cm (2in) across, are produced in late spring and early summer. Flowers are usually cream but may be white or pink; they have a well-defined, usually dark red, sometimes yellow mark on the lip tepals. ↕20–100cm (8–39in), ↔ 5cm (2in). South Africa (Western Cape). ❄

***G.* 'Carrara'** ■ Large-flowered Grandiflorus gladiolus. In late summer, bears ruffled, creamy white flowers. Flower spike is 75–85cm (30–34in) long, with 24–27 buds (9 or 10 open). ↕1.7m (5½ft), ↔ 15cm (6in). ❄

G. caryophyllaceus, syn. *G. hirsutus.* Cormous perennial with linear, hairy leaves, 20–60cm (8–24in) long. From late winter to spring, bears one-sided or 2-ranked spikes of 2–8 bell- or funnel-shaped, hawthorn-scented, pink or mauve flowers, 2–4cm (¾–1½in) across, the lip tepals spotted or streaked red or pink. ↕50–75cm (20–30in), ↔ 15cm (6in). South Africa (Western Cape). ❄

***G.* 'Charm'** ■ Nanus gladiolus producing purple-red flowers, 4cm (1½in) across, with ivory throats, in early summer. Flower spike is 22cm (9in) long, with 7 buds (4 or 5 open). ↕70cm (28in), ↔ 8–10cm (3–4in). ❄

***G.* 'Charmer'** ■ Large-flowered Grandiflorus gladiolus with strongly ruffled, almost translucent, light pink flowers, borne in early and midsummer. Flower spike is 85cm (34in) long, with 27 buds (10 open). ↕1.7m (5½ft), ↔ 15cm (6in). ❄

***G.* 'Cherry Pie'.** Large-flowered Grandiflorus gladiolus. Ruffled, cherry-red flowers, with pure white midribs and throats, are borne in late summer. Flower spike is 75–80cm (30–32in) long, with 27 buds (9 open). ↕1.7m (5½ft), ↔ 15cm (6in). ❄

***G.* 'Chinese Wax'.** Medium-flowered Grandiflorus gladiolus producing strongly ruffled, deep cream flowers in early summer. Flower spike is 65–70cm (26–28in) long, with 24 buds (7 open). ↕1.5m (5ft), ↔ 12cm (5in). ❄

***G.* 'Chiquita'.** Large-flowered Grandiflorus gladiolus bearing strongly ruffled, light yellow flowers in early and

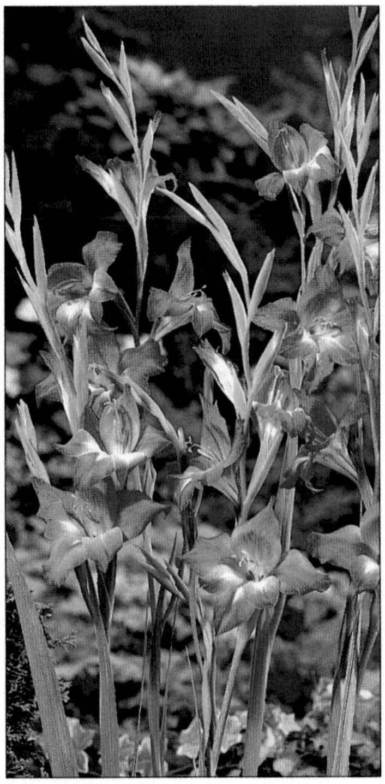
Gladiolus 'Charm'

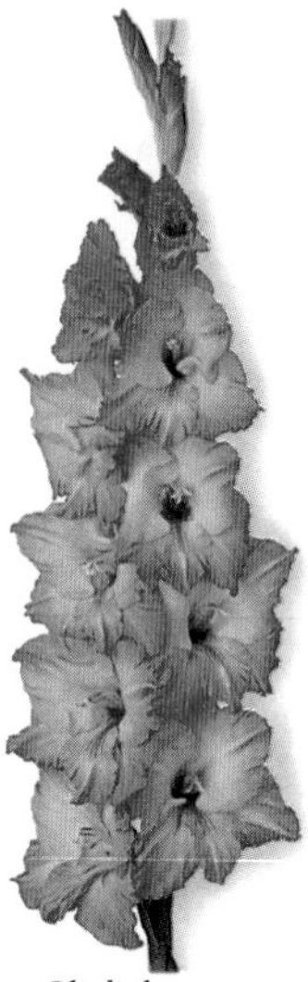

Gladiolus 'Chloe'

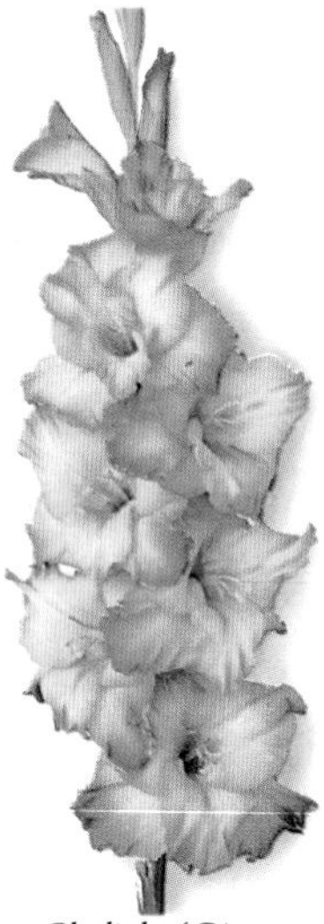

Gladiolus 'Côte d'Azur'

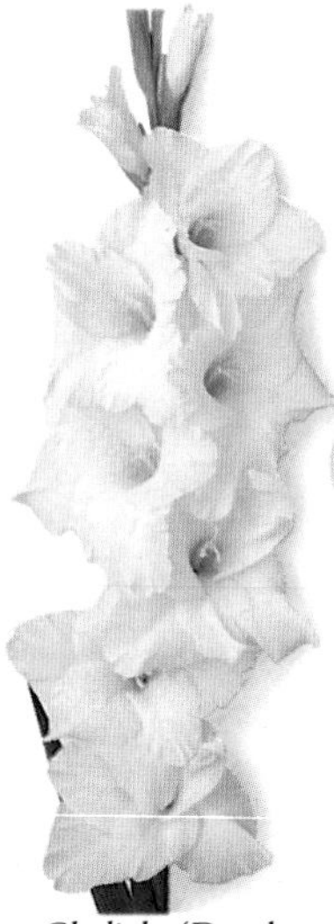

Gladiolus 'Dutch Mountain'

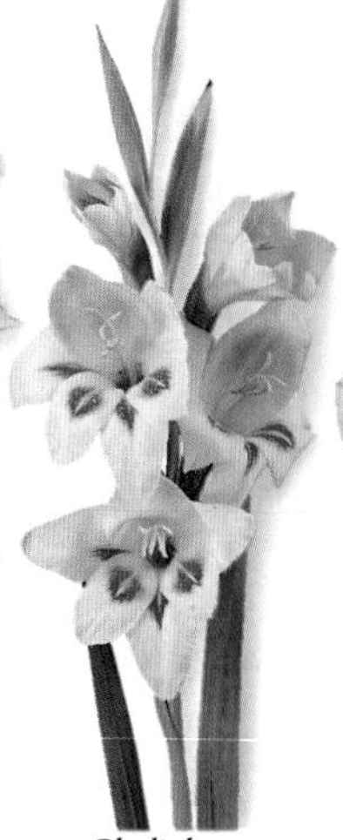

Gladiolus 'Elvira'

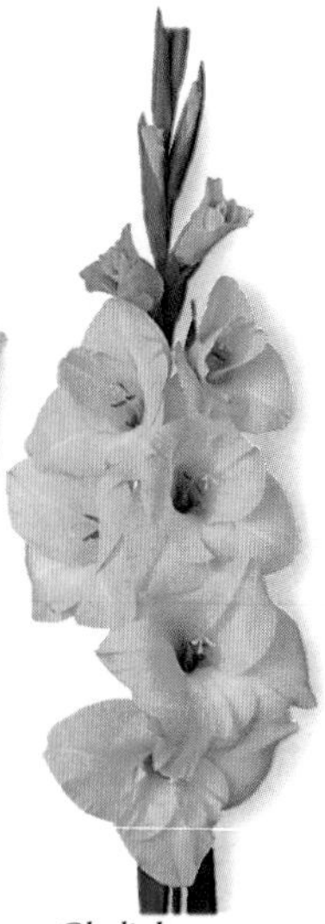

Gladiolus 'Esta Bonita'

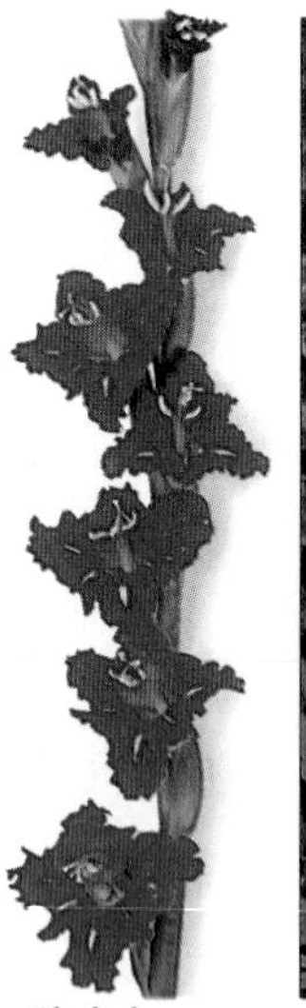

Gladiolus 'Firestorm'

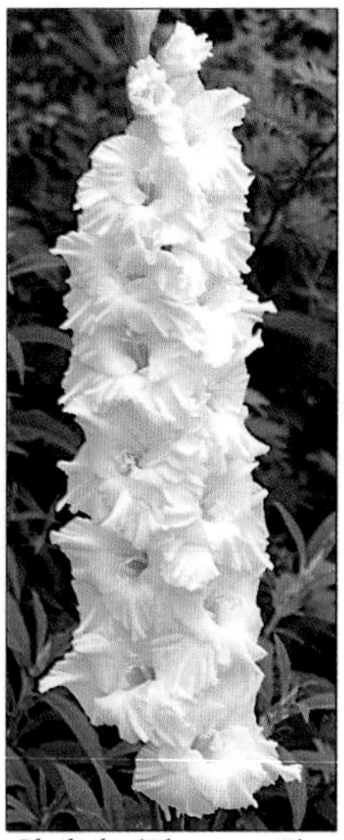

Gladiolus 'Florence C'

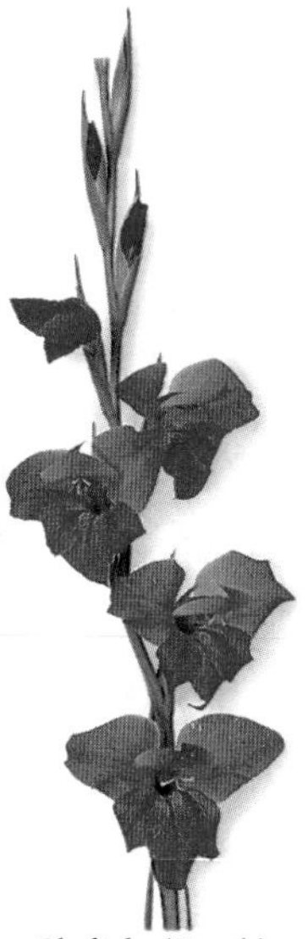

Gladiolus 'Frank's Perfection'

G

midsummer. Flower spike is 70–75cm (28–30in) long, with 24 buds (9 open). ↕1.7m (5½ft), ↔ 15cm (6in). *

G. 'Chloe' ■ Medium-flowered Grandiflorus gladiolus. In early and midsummer, produces slightly ruffled, deep orange flowers with lighter throats. Flower spike is 65–75cm (26–30in) long, with 25 buds (9 open). ↕1.5m (5ft), ↔ 12cm (5in). *

G. 'Christabel'. *G. tristis* hybrid with loose spikes of 6–10 flared, scented, primrose-yellow flowers, 8–10cm (3–4in) across, in spring. Upper tepals are primrose-yellow, marked with purple. ↕45cm (18in), ↔ 5cm (2in). *

G. 'Columbine'. Primulinus gladiolus producing rose-pink flowers, 6cm (2½in) across, with white lip tepals, in midsummer. Flower spike is 50cm (20in) long, with 18 buds (6 or 7 open). ↕1.1m (3½ft), ↔ 8–10cm (3–4in). *

G. x *colvilei* 'The Bride' see *G.* 'The Bride'.

G. 'Comet'. Nanus gladiolus bearing cherry-red flowers, 5cm (2in) across, in early summer. Flower spike is 30cm (12in) long, with 5 buds (3 or 4 open). ↕75cm (30in), ↔ 8–10cm (3–4in). *

G. communis* subsp. *byzantinus ■ ♀ syn. *G. byzantinus.* Vigorous perennial producing linear leaves, 10–70cm (4–28in) long. From late spring to early summer, bears spikes of up to 20 funnel-shaped, deep magenta flowers, 5cm (2in) across, with paler marks on the lip tepals. Spreads freely from cormlets. ↕to 1m (3ft), ↔ 8cm (3in). Spain, N.W. Africa, Sicily. *** (borderline)

G. 'Connie Jean'. Large-flowered Grandiflorus gladiolus producing strongly ruffled, mid-pink flowers, with cream throats, in late summer. Flower spike is 70–75cm (28–30in) long, with 27 buds (10 open). ↕1.7m (5½ft), ↔ 15cm (6in). *

G. 'Coral Embers'. Large-flowered Grandiflorus gladiolus. Ruffled, soft rose-pink flowers, the throats coloured white, are produced in midsummer. Flower spike is 75–80cm (30–32in) long, with 26 buds (9 open). ↕1.7m (5½ft), ↔ 15cm (6in). *

G. 'Côte d'Azur' ■ Giant-flowered Grandiflorus gladiolus bearing ruffled, mid-blue flowers, with pale blue throats, in early summer. Flower spike is 75cm (30in) long, with 23 or 24 buds (9 open). ↕1.7m (5½ft), ↔ 15cm (6in). *

G. 'Crimson Fire'. Giant-flowered Grandiflorus gladiolus. In midsummer, produces strongly ruffled, deep rose-red flowers, with deeper rose-red "thumb prints" on the lip tepals. Flower spike is 80cm (32in) long, with 26 buds (9 open). ↕1.7m (5½ft), ↔ 15cm (6in). *

G. dalenii, syn. *G. natalensis, G. psittacinus, G. quartinianus.* Robust, cormous perennial, spreading freely by underground runners, with linear or sword-shaped leaves, to 60cm (24in) long. In summer, bears one-sided spikes of few to many hooded, funnel-shaped flowers, 5cm (2in) across, which are red, orange, or yellow, sometimes spotted green or brown. ↕1–1.5m (3–5ft), ↔ 8cm (3in). South Africa (Eastern Cape) and through tropical Africa to Ethiopia and W. Arabian Peninsula. *

G. 'Déjà Vu'. Giant-flowered Grandiflorus gladiolus producing ruffled, light pink flowers, with darker margins, in late summer. Flower spike is 80–85cm (32–34in) long, with 25 buds (9 open). ↕1.8m (6ft), ↔ 15cm (6in). *

G. 'Drama' ■ Large-flowered Grandiflorus gladiolus bearing slightly ruffled, deep rose-pink flowers, with red-speckled yellow throats, in late summer. Flower spike is 70–80cm (28–32in) long, with 26 buds (10 open). ↕1.7m (5½ft), ↔ 15cm (6in). *

G. 'Dress Parade'. Large-flowered Grandiflorus gladiolus bearing slightly ruffled, deep salmon-pink flowers in late summer. Flower spike is 80–85cm (32–34in) long, with 26 buds (10 open). ↕1.7m (5½ft), ↔ 15cm (6in). *

G. 'Dutch Mountain' ■ Large-flowered Grandiflorus gladiolus bearing slightly ruffled white flowers, with small green marks in the throats, in midsummer. Flower spike is 80cm (32in) long, with 25 buds (9 open). ↕1.7m (5½ft), ↔ 15cm (6in). *

G. 'Elvira' ■ Nanus gladiolus bearing pale pink flowers, 5cm (2in) across, with red marks on the lip tepals, in early summer. Flower spike is 30cm (12in) long, with 6 buds (3 or 4 open). ↕80cm (32in), ↔ 8–10cm (3–4in). *

G. 'Ermal'. Giant-flowered Grandiflorus gladiolus. Ruffled, glowing red flowers, with small white throats, are produced in late summer. Flower spike is 80–85cm (32–34in) long, with 27 buds (9 open). ↕1.7m (5½ft), ↔ 15cm (6in). *

G. 'Ermine'. Medium-flowered Grandiflorus gladiolus producing strongly ruffled white flowers, with creamy throats, in mid- and late summer. Flower spike is 70–75cm (28–30in) long, with 25 buds (9 open). ↕1.5m (5ft), ↔ 12cm (5in). *

G. 'Esta Bonita' ■ Giant-flowered Grandiflorus gladiolus producing pale orange flowers, with light yellow throats, in late summer. Flower spike is 75–80cm (30–32in) long, with 24 buds (8 open). ↕1.8m (6ft), ↔ 15cm (6in). *

G. 'Eternal Beauty'. Large-flowered Grandiflorus gladiolus bearing ruffled, light blue flowers, with chalk-white throats, in midsummer. Flower spike is

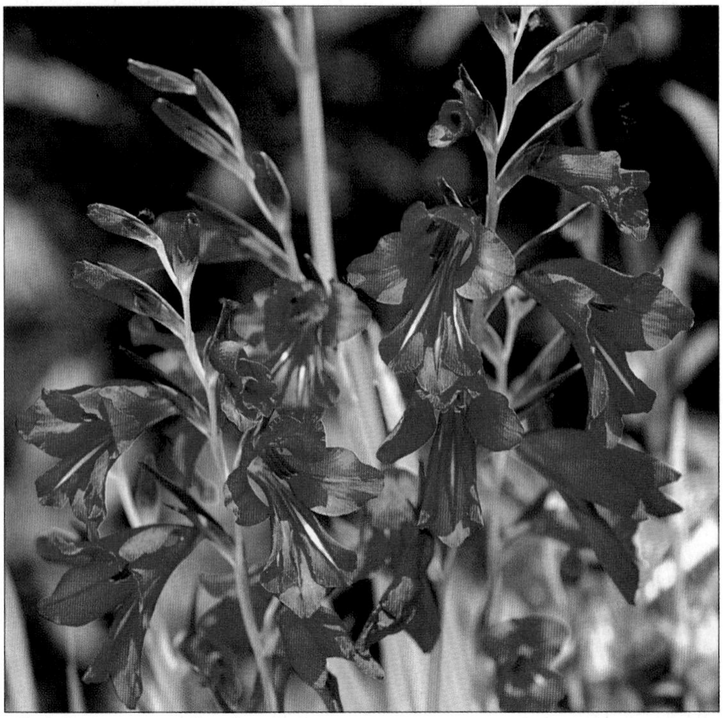

Gladiolus communis subsp. *byzantinus*

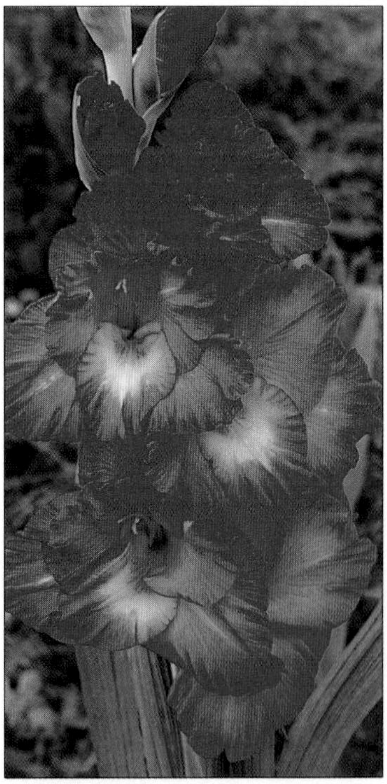

Gladiolus 'Drama'

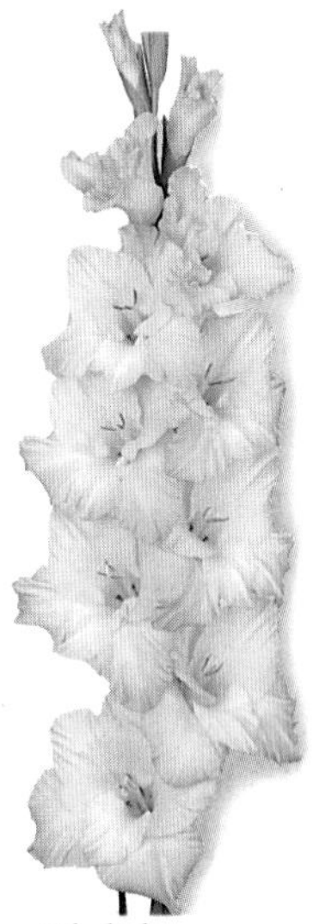

Gladiolus 'Full House'

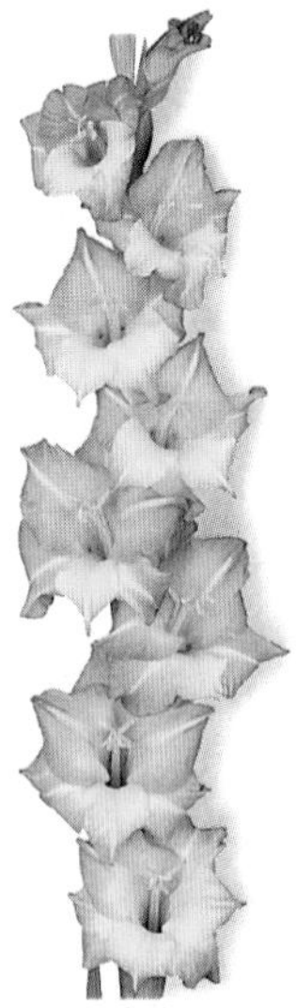

Gladiolus 'Georgette'

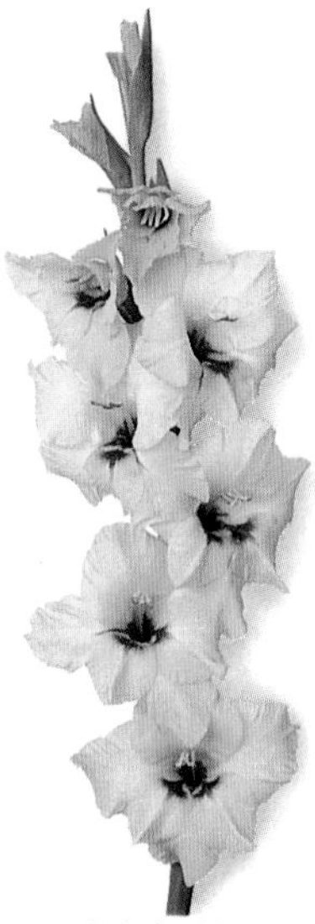

Gladiolus 'Green Woodpecker'

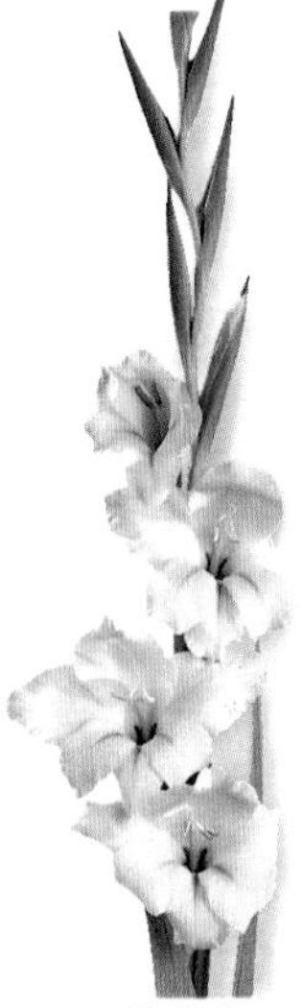

Gladiolus 'Halley'

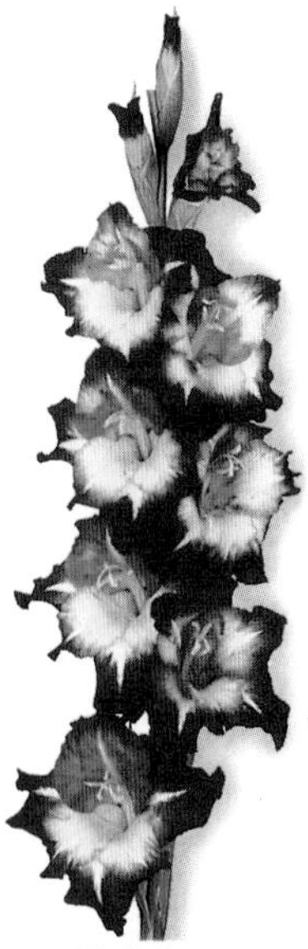

Gladiolus 'Happy Time'

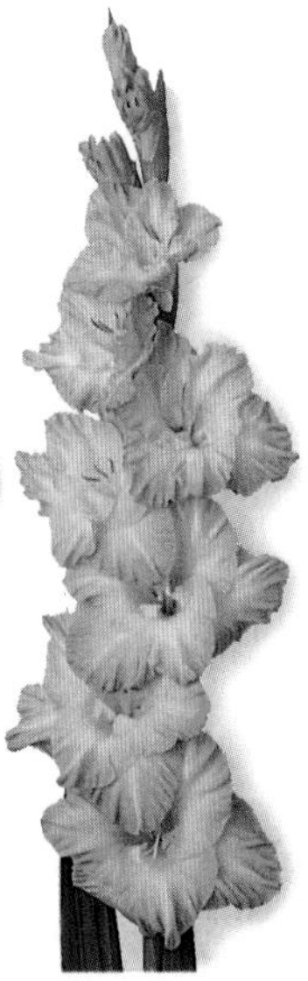

Gladiolus 'Jo Ann'

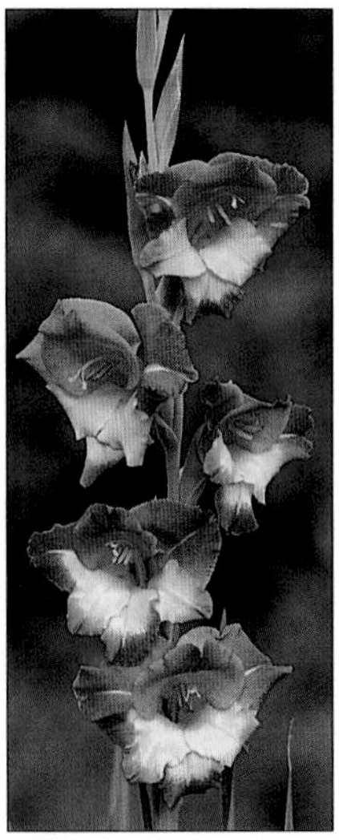

Gladiolus 'Little Darling'

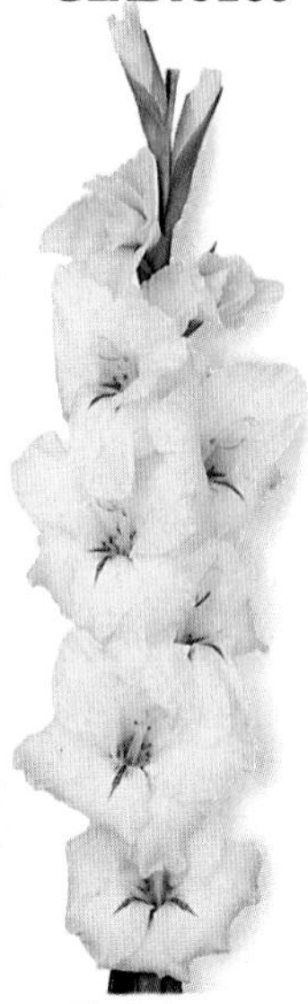

Gladiolus 'Magistral'

70–75 cm (28–30in) long, with 24 buds (8 open). ↕ 1.5m (5ft), ↔ 15cm (6in). ❄

***G.* 'Falling Snow'.** Giant-flowered Grandiflorus gladiolus producing ruffled white flowers in late summer. Flower spike is 80–85cm (32–34in) long, with 27 buds (10 open). ↕ 1.8m (6ft), ↔ 15cm (6in). ❄

***G.* 'Finesse'.** Large-flowered Grandiflorus gladiolus producing strongly ruffled, salmon-pink flowers, with yellow throats, in late summer. Flower spike is 80cm (32in) long, with 27 buds (10 open). ↕ 1.7m (5½ft), ↔ 15cm (6in). ❄

***G.* 'Fire and Ice'.** Large-flowered Grandiflorus gladiolus. In late summer, produces strongly ruffled white flowers, flushed pale pink, with rose-red marks on each tepal. Flower spike is 80–85cm (32–34in) long, with 28 buds (11 open). ↕ 1.7m (5½ft), ↔ 15cm (6in). ❄

***G.* 'Firestorm'** ▣ Miniature-flowered Grandiflorus gladiolus producing ruffled, loosely spaced, vivid scarlet flowers, with yellowish white flecks on the outer tepals, in early summer. Flower spike is 60cm (24in) long, with 22 buds (7 open). ↕ 1.1m (3½ft), ↔ 8–10cm (3–4in). ❄

***G.* 'Flamenco'.** Large-flowered Grandiflorus gladiolus. Ruffled orange flowers, with light yellow throats, are borne in late summer. Flower spike is 80–85cm (32–34in) long, with 27 buds (9 open). ↕ 1.8m (6ft), ↔ 15cm (6in). ❄

***G.* 'Florence C'** ▣ Large-flowered Grandiflorus gladiolus bearing strongly ruffled white flowers in late summer. Flower spike is 75–80cm (30–32in) long, with 26 buds (10 open). ↕ 1.7m (5½ft), ↔ 15cm (6in). ❄

***G.* 'Frank's Perfection'** ▣ Primulinus gladiolus producing loosely spaced, bright red flowers, 5cm (2in) across, in early summer. Flower spike is 60cm (24in) long, with 23 buds (7 open). ↕ 1.1m (3½ft), ↔ 8–10cm (3–4in). ❄

***G.* 'Frizzled Coral Lace'.** Medium-flowered Grandiflorus gladiolus bearing strongly ruffled, coral- to salmon-pink flowers in early summer. Flower spike is 65cm (26in) long, with 18 buds (7 open). ↕ 1.2m (4ft), ↔ 12cm (5in). ❄

***G.* 'Full House'** ▣ Large-flowered Grandiflorus gladiolus bearing slightly ruffled, light rose-pink flowers, with white throats, in midsummer. Flower spike is 80–85cm (32–34in) long, with 27 buds (9 open). ↕ 1.7m (5½ft), ↔ 15cm (6in). ❄

***G.* 'Georgette'** ▣ Small-flowered Grandiflorus gladiolus. In midsummer, bears slightly ruffled, yellow-suffused orange flowers with large, lemon-yellow throats. Flower spike is 60cm (24in) long, with 22 buds (10 open). ↕ 1.2m (4ft), ↔ 8–10cm (3–4in). ❄

***G.* 'Globestar'.** Large-flowered Grandiflorus gladiolus. Ruffled, light orange-buff flowers, with cerise-marked throats, are produced in midsummer. Flower spike is 70cm (28in) long, with 24 buds (7 open). ↕ 1.5m (5ft), ↔ 15cm (6in). ❄

***G.* 'Golden Melody'.** Medium-flowered Grandiflorus gladiolus. Bears ruffled, rich golden yellow flowers in late summer. Flower spike is 75–80cm (30–32in) long, with 26 buds (9 open). ↕ 1.5m (5ft), ↔ 12cm (5in). ❄

***G.* 'Golden Princess'.** Small-flowered Grandiflorus gladiolus. In midsummer, bears slightly ruffled yellow flowers with golden throats. Flower spike is 50cm (20in) long, with 21 buds (7 open). ↕ 1.1m (3½ft), ↔ 8–10cm (3–4in). ❄

***G.* 'Grand Finale'.** Large-flowered Grandiflorus gladiolus bearing strongly ruffled, salmon-pink flowers, with white throats, in midsummer. Flower spike is 85cm (34in) long, with 27 buds (9 open). ↕ 1.7m (5½ft), ↔ 15cm (6in). ❄

***G.* 'Green Jeans'.** Small-flowered Grandiflorus gladiolus producing ruffled green flowers, with ivory throats, in late summer. Flower spike is 60cm (24in) long, with 24 buds (7 open). ↕ 1.3m (4½ft), ↔ 8–10cm (3–4in). ❄

***G.* 'Green Woodpecker'** ▣🏆 Medium-flowered Grandiflorus gladiolus. In mid- and late summer, bears ruffled, greenish yellow flowers with wine-red marks at the throats. Flower spike is 70–75cm (28–30in) long, with 25 buds (10 open). ↕ 1.5m (5ft), ↔ 12cm (5in). ❄

***G.* 'Halley'** ▣ Nanus gladiolus bearing white-flushed, pale yellow flowers, 5cm (2in) across, with bright red marks in the throats, in early summer. Flower spike is 35cm (14in) long, with 7 buds (3 or 4 open). ↕ 1m (3ft), ↔ 8–10cm (3–4in). ❄

***G.* 'Happy Time'** ▣ Small-flowered Grandiflorus gladiolus. In midsummer, produces slightly ruffled, mid-red flowers with ivory throats. Flower spike is 60cm (24in) long, with 21 buds (7 open). ↕ 1.1m (3½ft), ↔ 8–10cm (3–4in). ❄

***G.* 'Hastings'.** Primulinus gladiolus producing pale coffee-coloured flowers, pale cream-throated, 5cm (2in) across, in midsummer. Flower spike is 55cm (22in) long, with 21 buds (6 open). ↕ 1.1m (3½ft), ↔ 8–10cm (3–4in). ❄

***G.* 'Heavenly Sunshine'.** Giant-flowered Grandiflorus gladiolus. In midsummer, bears strongly ruffled, light yellow flowers. Flower spike is 80–85cm (32–34in) long, with 28 buds (9 open). ↕ 1.7m (5½ft), ↔ 15cm (6in). ❄

***G.* 'High Brow'.** Giant-flowered Grandiflorus gladiolus bearing ruffled white flowers, with blush-pink margins, in late summer. Flower spike is 85cm (34in) long, with 27 buds (9 open). ↕ 1.7m (5½ft), ↔ 15cm (6in). ❄

***G.* 'Hi-Lite'.** Large-flowered Grandiflorus gladiolus. Slightly ruffled orange flowers, with small lemon throats, are produced in midsummer. Flower spike is 75–80cm (30–32in) long, with 26 buds (9 open). ↕ 1.7m (5½ft), ↔ 15cm (6in). ❄

G. hirsutus see *G. caryophyllaceus*.

***G.* 'Ice Cap'.** Large-flowered Grandiflorus gladiolus bearing ruffled white flowers in late summer. Flower spike is 80–85cm (32–34in) long, with 27 buds (10 open). ↕ 1.7m (5½ft), ↔ 15cm (6in). ❄

***G.* 'Ice Princess'.** Small-flowered Grandiflorus gladiolus bearing ruffled, snow-white flowers in midsummer. Flower spike is 60cm (24in) long, with 24 buds (8 open). ↕ 1.2m (4ft), ↔ 8–10cm (3–4in). ❄

G. imbricatus. Upright, cormous perennial with sword-shaped leaves, 15–35cm (6–14in) long. Loose spikes of 4–12 funnel-shaped, pinkish red to reddish purple flowers, 3cm (1¼in) across, are produced in late spring. ↕ 30–80cm (12–32in), ↔ 8–10cm (3–4in). C. and E. Europe, Latvia, Estonia. ❄❄❄

***G.* 'Impressive'.** Nanus gladiolus producing rose-pink flowers, 5cm (2in) across, with diamond-shaped, deep rose-pink markings on the lip tepals, in early summer. Flower spike is 25cm (10in) long, with 7 buds (4 or 5 open). ↕ 70cm (28in), ↔ 8–10cm (3–4in). ❄

G. italicus, syn. *G. segetum*. Slender, cormous perennial with sword-shaped leaves, 5–50cm (2–20in) long. Bears loose spikes of 5–15 narrowly funnel-shaped, purplish pink to magenta flowers, 4cm (1½in) across, with paler marks on the lip tepals, in early summer. Flowers best with dry, hot summer dormancy. ↕ 40–90cm (16–36in), ↔ 8cm (3in). S. Europe. ❄❄

***G.* 'Jo Ann'** ▣ Large-flowered Grandiflorus gladiolus producing slightly ruffled, light salmon-pink flowers, with pale yellow throats, in early summer. Flower spike is 80–85cm (32–34in) long, with 25 buds (9 open). ↕ 1.7m (5½ft), ↔ 15cm (6in). ❄

***G.* 'Krakatoa'.** Giant-flowered Grandiflorus gladiolus. Bears slightly ruffled, smoky plum-purple flowers, with large white throats, in midsummer. Flower spike is 70–75cm (28–30in) long, with 23 buds (7 open). ↕ 1.5m (5ft), ↔ 15cm (6in). ❄

***G.* 'Kristin'.** Large-flowered Grandiflorus gladiolus bearing strongly ruffled white flowers in late summer. Flower spike is 80–85cm (32–34in) long, with 27 buds (10 open). ↕ 1.7m (5½ft), ↔ 15cm (6in). ❄

***G.* 'Legend'.** Giant-flowered Grandiflorus gladiolus. In midsummer, bears ruffled, deep pink flowers with small white throats. Flower spike is 80cm (32in) long, with 24 buds (9 open). ↕ 1.7m (5½ft), ↔ 15cm (6in). ❄

***G.* 'Leonore'.** Primulinus gladiolus bearing buttercup-yellow flowers, 6cm (2½in) across, in midsummer. Flower spike is 55cm (22in) long, with 19 buds (5–7 open). ↕ 1.1m (3½ft), ↔ 8–10cm (3–4in). ❄

***G.* 'Little Darling'** ▣ Primulinus gladiolus producing loosely spaced, salmon- to rose-pink flowers, 3.5cm (1½in) across, with lemon lip tepals, in midsummer. Flower spike is 40cm (16in) long, with 16 buds (5 or 6 open). ↕ 1.1m (3½ft), ↔ 8–10cm (3–4in). ❄

***G.* 'Lowland Queen'.** Large-flowered Grandiflorus gladiolus. In midsummer, produces slightly ruffled, blush-pink flowers with large, cerise-red blotches on the lip tepals. Flower spike is 80–85cm (32–34in) long, with 28 buds (10 open). ↕ 1.7m (5½ft), ↔ 15cm (6in). ❄

***G.* 'Magistral'** ▣ Large-flowered Grandiflorus gladiolus bearing ruffled,

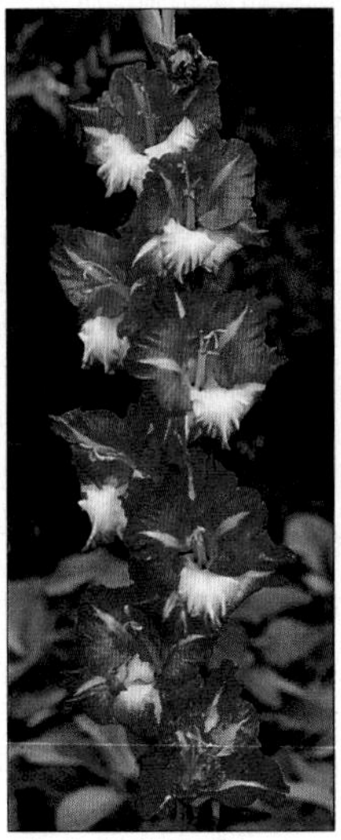
Gladiolus 'Mi Mi'

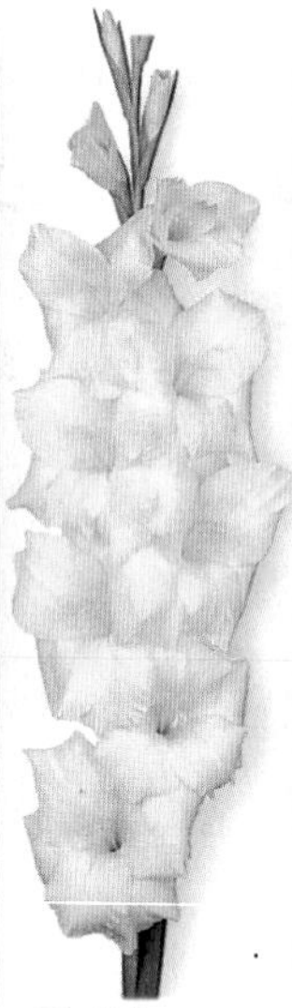
Gladiolus 'Mont Blanc'

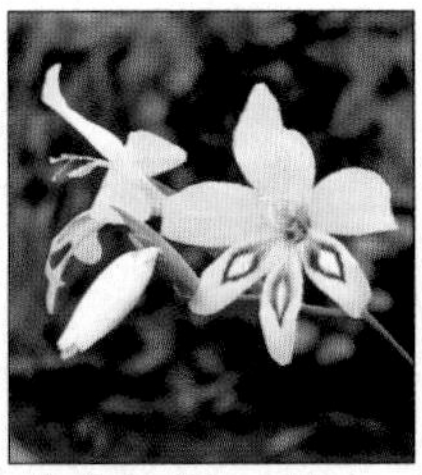
Gladiolus 'Nymph'

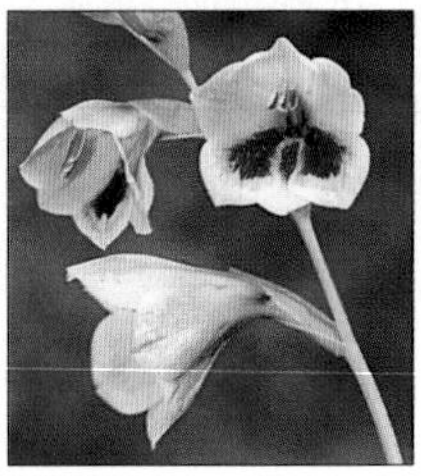
Gladiolus papilio

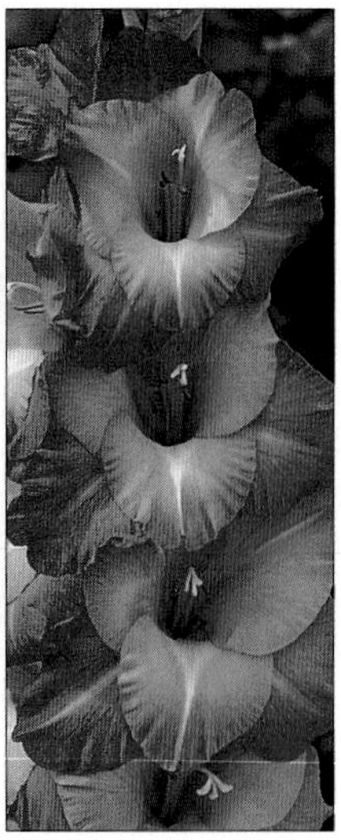
Gladiolus 'Parade'

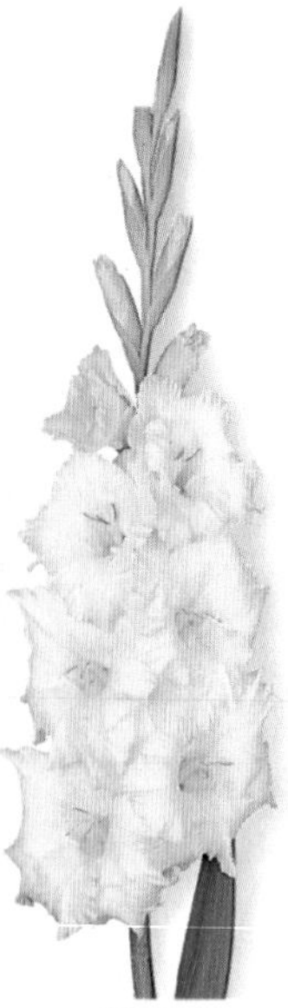
Gladiolus 'Peace'

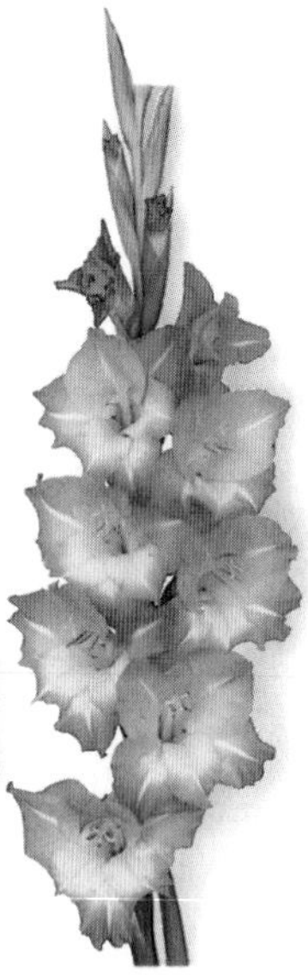
Gladiolus 'Pink Flare'

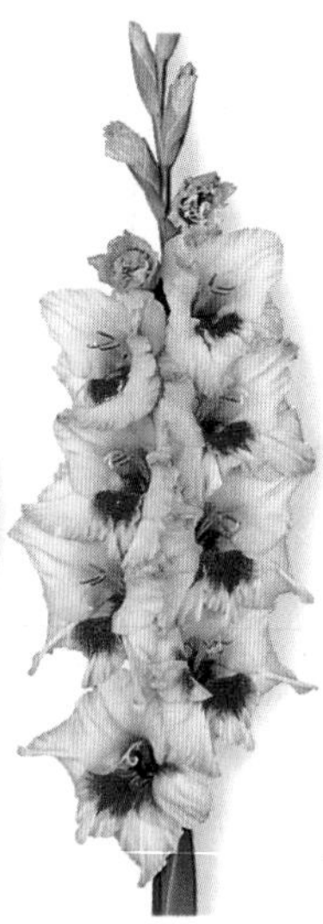
Gladiolus 'Pulchritude'

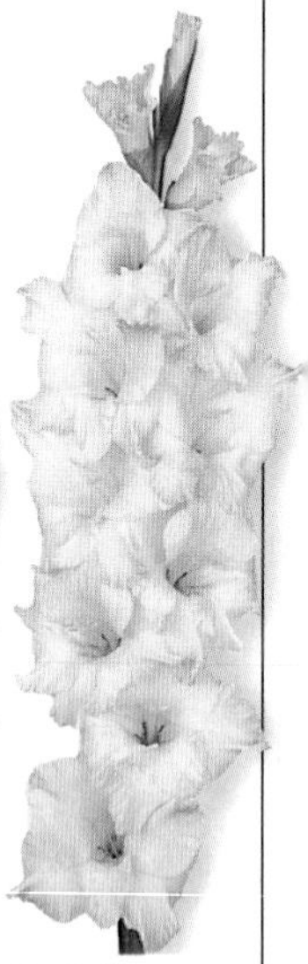
Gladiolus 'Queen's Blush'

G

oyster-white flowers, with magenta lines, in midsummer. Flower spike is 85cm (34in) long, with 24 buds (8 open). ↕ 1.8m (6ft), ↔ 15cm (6in). ✻
***G.* 'Magnolia'.** Large-flowered Grandiflorus gladiolus. Ruffled, light lavender-pink to rose-pink flowers, with creamy throats, are produced in midsummer. Flower spike is 75cm (30in) long, with 25 buds (9 open). ↕ 1.7m (5½ft), ↔ 15cm (6in). ✻
***G.* 'Major League'.** Large-flowered Grandiflorus gladiolus. Slightly ruffled, deep salmon-pink flowers, with cream throats, are produced in late summer. Flower spike is 80–85cm (32–34in) long, with 26 buds (9 open). ↕ 1.8m (6ft), ↔ 15cm (6in). ✻
***G.* 'Margaret Lyall'.** Large-flowered Grandiflorus gladiolus bearing strongly ruffled pink flowers, with small white throats, in late summer. Flower spike is 80cm (32in) long, with 27 buds (8 open). ↕ 1.7m (5½ft), ↔ 15cm (6in). ✻
***G.* 'Michael B'.** Large-flowered Grandiflorus gladiolus bearing ruffled, deep purple flowers, with darker throats, in late summer. Flower spike is 80cm (32in) long, with 26 buds (9 open). ↕ 1.7m (5½ft), ↔ 15cm (6in). ✻
***G.* 'Mileesh'.** Large-flowered Grandiflorus gladiolus. Strongly ruffled, chocolate-tan flowers, with white throats, are borne in midsummer. Flower spike is 75cm (30in) long, with 25 buds (9 open). ↕ 1.7m (5½ft), ↔ 15cm (6in). ✻

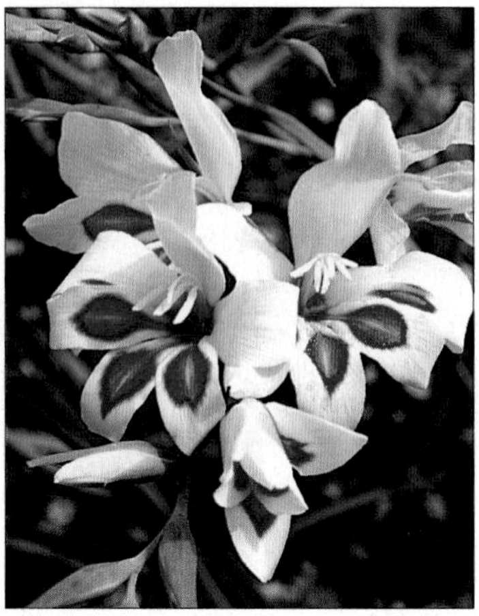
Gladiolus 'Prins Claus'

***G.* 'Mi Mi'** ■ Small-flowered Grandiflorus gladiolus. In midsummer, bears strongly ruffled, deep lavender-pink flowers with white throats. Flower spike is 65cm (26in) long, with 24 buds (7 or 8 open). ↕ 1.3m (4½ft), ↔ 8–10cm (3–4in). ✻
***G.* 'Mondiale'.** Giant-flowered Grandiflorus gladiolus. In midsummer, bears ruffled, light rose-pink flowers with white throats. Flower spike is 80cm (32in) long, with 27 buds (9 or 10 open). ↕ 1.8m (6ft), ↔ 15cm (6in). ✻
***G.* 'Mont Blanc'** ■ Large-flowered Grandiflorus gladiolus bearing slightly ruffled white flowers in midsummer. Flower spike is 80cm (32in) long, with 28 buds (10 open). ↕ 1.7m (5½ft), ↔ 15cm (6in). ✻
***G.* 'Moon Mirage'.** Giant-flowered Grandiflorus gladiolus bearing ruffled, canary-yellow flowers, marked deeper yellow on the lip tepals, in late summer. Flower spike is 80–85cm (32–34in) long, with 29 buds (9–11 open). ↕ 1.7m (5½ft), ↔ 15cm (6in). ✻
***G.* 'Mother's Day'.** Large-flowered Grandiflorus gladiolus bearing ruffled, blue-pink flowers, with white throats, in late summer. Flower spike is 80cm (32in) long, with 25 buds (10 open). ↕ 1.7m (5½ft), ↔ 15cm (6in). ✻
G. natalensis see *G. dalenii.*
***G.* 'Norma J'.** Medium-flowered Grandiflorus gladiolus producing heavily ruffled, deep pink flowers in late summer. Flower spike is 80cm (32in) long, with 26 buds (9–11 open). ↕ 1.5m (5ft), ↔ 30cm (12in). ✻
***G.* 'Nymph'** ■ Nanus gladiolus bearing white flowers, 5cm (2in) across, in early summer. The lip tepals have creamy white markings edged with cerise-red. Flower spike is 25cm (10in) long, with 6 buds (4 or 5 open). ↕ 70cm (28in), ↔ 8–10cm (3–4in). ✻
***G.* 'Obelisk'.** Primulinus gladiolus producing orange-red flowers, 7cm (3in) across, in midsummer. Flower spike is 40cm (16in) long, with 19 buds (6 or 7 open). ↕ 1.1m (3½ft), ↔ 8–10cm (3–4in). ✻
G. papilio ■ syn. *G. purpureoauratus.* Cormous perennial, spreading freely by underground runners, with sword-shaped leaves, 5–45cm (2–18in) long. From summer to autumn, arching stems each bear 5–10 hooded, funnel- or bell-shaped flowers, to 5cm (2in) long, varying from bright yellow to yellowish green, heavily suffused purple. The plant illustrated above is usually grown as *G. purpureoauratus.* ↕ 50–90cm (20–36in), ↔ 8cm (3in). South Africa (Northern Transvaal, Eastern Transvaal). ✻✻
***G.* 'Parade'** ■ Giant-flowered Grandiflorus gladiolus. In late summer, produces strongly ruffled, deep salmon-pink flowers with cream throats. Flower spike is 80–85cm (32–34in) long, with 27 buds (10 open). ↕ 1.7m (5½ft), ↔ 15cm (6in). ✻
***G.* 'Peace'** ■ Giant-flowered Grandiflorus gladiolus producing strongly ruffled cream flowers, with pale lemon throats and pale pink margins, in midsummer. Flower spike is 80cm (32in) long, with 26 buds (9 open). ↕ 1.7m (5½ft), ↔ 15cm (6in). ✻
***G.* 'Pink Flare'** ■ Small-flowered Grandiflorus gladiolus bearing ruffled, mid-pink flowers, with small white throats, in midsummer. Flower spike is 65cm (26in) long, with 25 buds (7 or 8 open). ↕ 1.3m (4½ft), ↔ 8–10cm (3–4in). ✻
***G.* 'Piquant'.** Primulinus gladiolus bearing black-red flowers, 6cm (2½in) across, in midsummer. Flower spike is 35cm (14in) long, with 16 buds (5 or 6 open). ↕ 1m (3ft), ↔ 8–10cm (3–4in). ✻
***G.* 'Portia'.** Giant-flowered Grandiflorus gladiolus. Slightly ruffled, soft pink flowers, the throats coloured pale yellow, are produced in late summer. Flower spike is 85cm (34in) long, with 26 buds (9 open). ↕ 1.7m (5½ft), ↔ 15cm (6in). ✻
***G.* 'Prince Indigo'.** Large-flowered Grandiflorus gladiolus. In midsummer, produces slightly ruffled purple flowers, the white throats marked with wine-red flashes. Flower spike is 85–90cm (34–36in) long, with 26 buds (10 open). ↕ 2m (6ft), ↔ 15cm (6in). ✻
***G.* 'Prins Claus'** ■ Nanus gladiolus bearing pure white flowers, 5cm (2in) across, with cerise markings on the lip tepals, in early summer. Flower spike is 25cm (10in) long, usually curved and with 6 buds (4 or 5 open). ↕ 70cm (28in), ↔ 8–10cm (3–4in). ✻
G. psittacinus see *G. dalenii.*
***G.* 'Pulchritude'** ■ Medium-flowered Grandiflorus gladiolus. Ruffled, light lavender-pink flowers, deepening at the tepal margins and with a magenta-red mark on each lip tepal, are borne in midsummer. Flower spike is 70–75cm (28–30in) long, with 27 buds (9 open). ↕ 1.3m (4½ft), ↔ 12cm (5in). ✻
***G.* 'Purple Star'.** Small-flowered Grandiflorus gladiolus. Slightly ruffled, mid-purple flowers are borne in early summer, inner tepals whorled in a star-like formation. Flower spike is 60cm (24in) long, with 22 buds (6 or 7 open). ↕ 1.3m (4½ft), ↔ 8–10cm (3–4in). ✻
G. purpureoauratus see *G. papilio.*
G. quartinianus see *G. dalenii.*
***G.* 'Queen's Blush'** ■ Large-flowered Grandiflorus gladiolus. In midsummer,

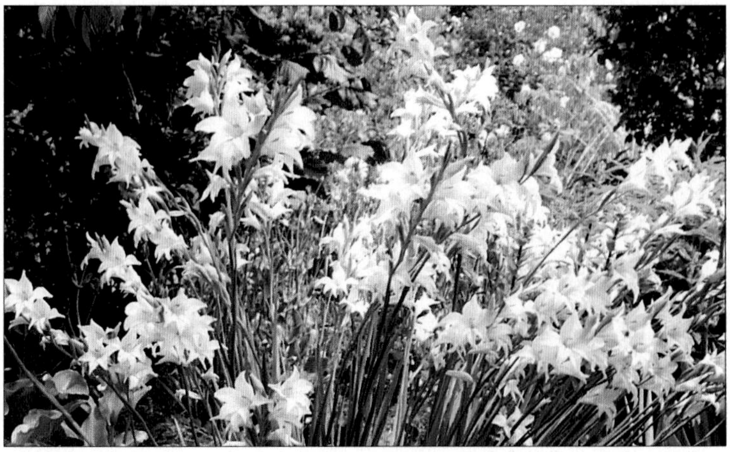
Gladiolus 'The Bride'

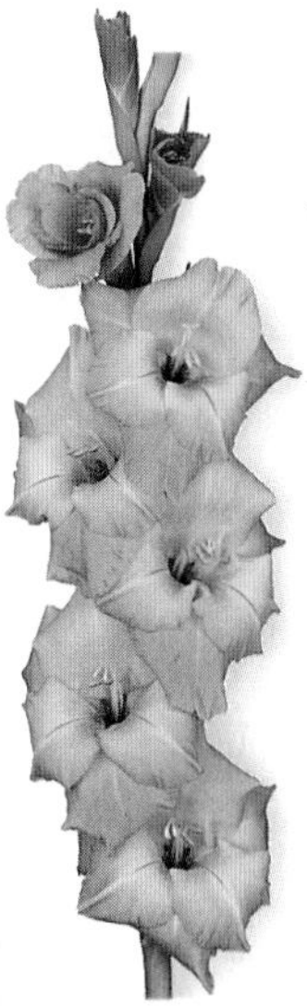

Gladiolus 'Rinette Snoek'

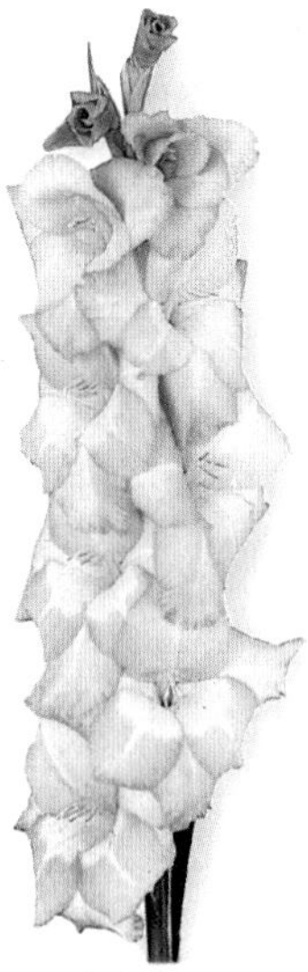

Gladiolus 'Royal Dutch'

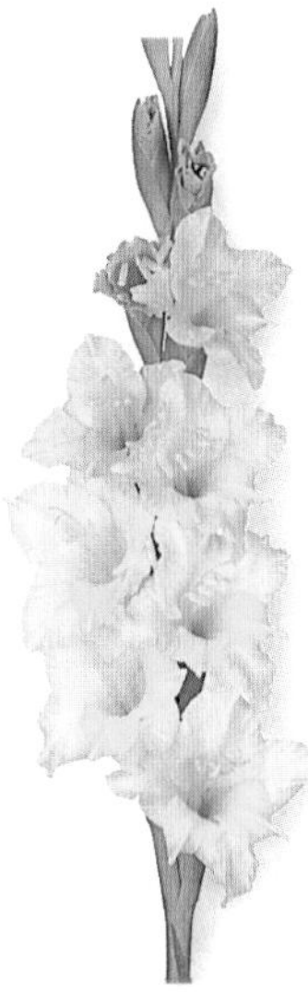

Gladiolus 'Stardust'

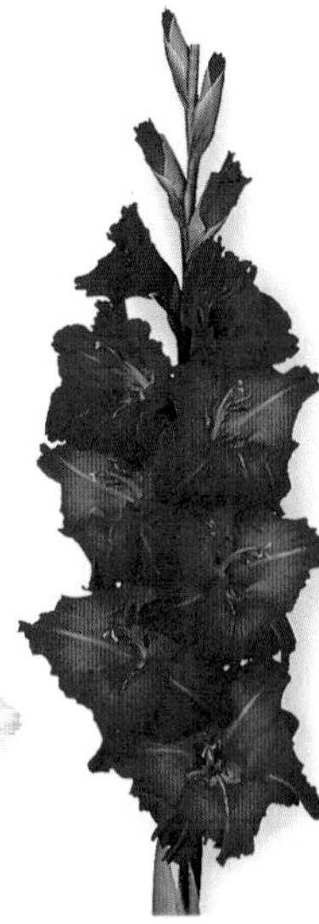

Gladiolus 'Stromboli'

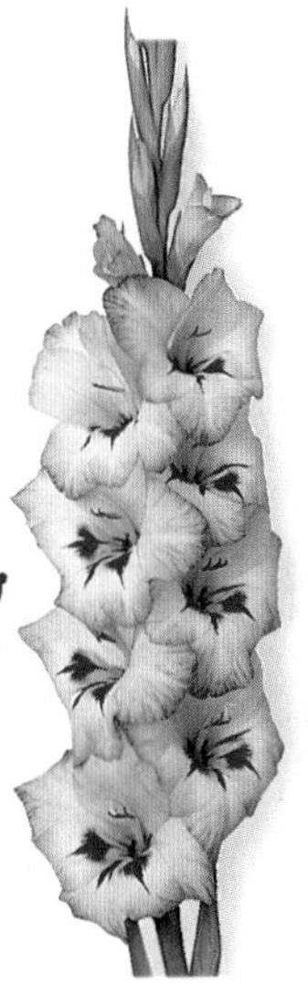

Gladiolus 'Sweet Dreams'

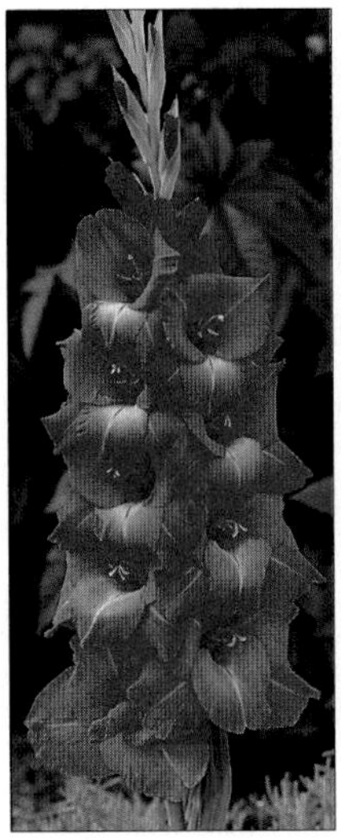

Gladiolus 'Vaucluse'

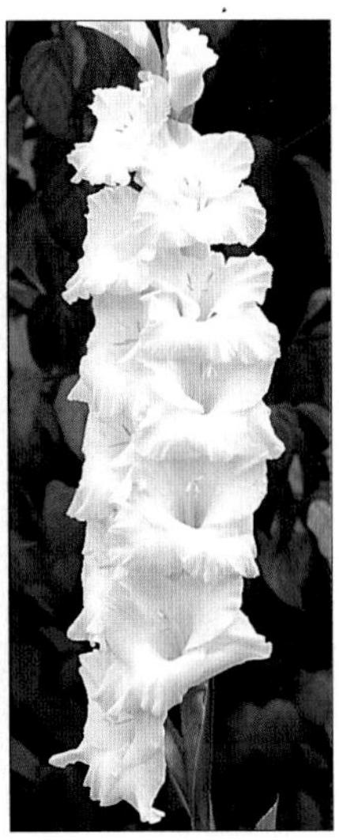

Gladiolus 'White Ice'

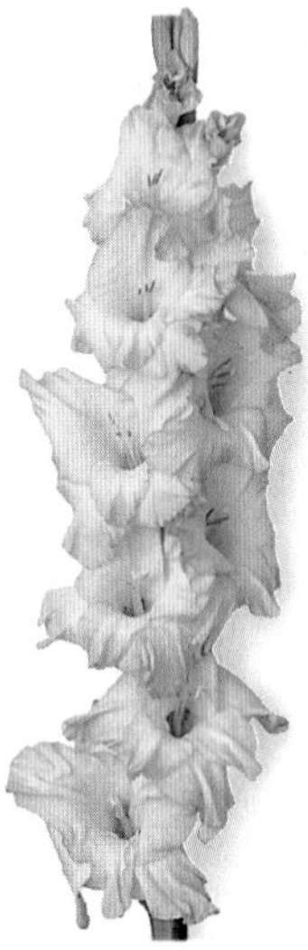

Gladiolus 'Zephyr'

bears slightly ruffled white flowers, blush-pink at the tepal margins. Flower spike is 80cm (32in) long, with 26 buds (10 open). ↕ 1.7m (5½ft), ↔ 15cm (6in). ✲

***G.* 'Rajah's Rose'.** Large-flowered Grandiflorus gladiolus producing slightly ruffled, deep rose-red flowers, with small white throats, in midsummer. Flower spike is 80cm (32in) long, with 27 buds (9 open). ↕ 1.7m (5½ft), ↔ 15cm (6in). ✲

***G.* 'Ravenna'.** Giant-flowered Grandiflorus gladiolus producing slightly ruffled, orange-scarlet flowers, with small buff throats, in early summer. Flower spike is 75cm (30in) long, with 26 buds (10 open). ↕ 1.7m (5½ft), ↔ 15cm (6in). ✲

***G.* 'Rinette Snoek'** ■ Large-flowered Grandiflorus gladiolus. In midsummer, produces ruffled, coral-pink flowers with cream throats. Flower spike is 80cm (32in) long, with 28 buds (9 open). ↕ 1.7m (5½ft), ↔ 15cm (6in). ✲

***G.* 'Rose Elf'.** Small-flowered Grandiflorus gladiolus producing slightly ruffled, light rose-pink flowers, with large, pale cream throats, in midsummer. Flower spike is 70cm (28in) long, with 24 buds (8 or 9 open). ↕ 1.4m (4½ft), ↔ 15cm (6in). ✲

***G.* 'Royal Dutch'** ■ Large-flowered Grandiflorus gladiolus bearing very slightly ruffled, pale lavender-blue flowers, with white throats, in midsummer. Flower spike is 80cm (32in) long, with 27 buds (9 open). ↕ 1.7m (5½ft), ↔ 15cm (6in). ✲

***G.* 'Sailor's Delight'.** Large-flowered Grandiflorus gladiolus bearing strongly ruffled, white-throated pink flowers in late summer. Flower spike is 80–85cm (32–34in) long, with 27 buds (9 open). ↕ 1.7m (5½ft), ↔ 15cm (6in). ✲

***G.* 'San Remo'.** Large-flowered Grandiflorus gladiolus. Ruffled, light pink flowers, with small white throats, are borne in midsummer. Flower spike is 75–80cm (30–32in) long, with 25 buds (10 open). ↕ 1.5m (5ft), ↔ 15cm (6in). ✲

G. segetum see *G. italicus*.

***G.* 'Shiloh'.** Medium-flowered Grandiflorus gladiolus. In midsummer, produces strongly ruffled yellow flowers, each with a bright red mark spreading from the throat. Flower spike is 70–75cm (28–30in) long, with 25 buds (9 open). ↕ 1.5m (5ft), ↔ 12cm (5in). ✲

***G.* 'Spitfire'.** Nanus gladiolus producing blood-red flowers, 5cm (2in) across, with white darts on the lip tepals, in early summer. Flower spike is 22cm (9in) long, with 6 buds (3 or 4 open). ↕ 70cm (28in), ↔ 8–10cm (3–4in). ✲

***G.* 'Stardust'** ■ Miniature-flowered Grandiflorus gladiolus. Ruffled, pale yellow flowers, with lighter yellow throats, are produced in midsummer. Flower spike is 50cm (20in) long, with 21 buds (6 or 7 open). ↕ 1.2m (4ft), ↔ 8–10cm (3–4in). ✲

***G.* 'Stromboli'** ■ Large-flowered Grandiflorus gladiolus. In midsummer, bears slightly ruffled, deep red flowers, with paler throats. Flower spike is 75–80cm (30–32in) long, with 25 buds (9 open). ↕ 1.5m (5ft), ↔ 15cm (6in). ✲

***G.* 'Sumatra'.** Large-flowered Grandiflorus gladiolus. In midsummer, produces gently ruffled, light brown flowers, slightly reflexed towards the stem. Flower spike is 75cm (30in) long, with 25 buds (8 open) in a slightly informal arrangement. ↕ 1.5m (5ft), ↔ 15cm (6in). ✲

***G.* 'Sweet Dreams'** ■ Medium-flowered Grandiflorus gladiolus. In midsummer, produces slightly ruffled, creamy white flowers, tinted deep rose-red at the margins and with deep rose-red lip tepals. Flower spike is 75cm (30in) long, with 27 buds (9 open). ↕ 1.5m (5ft), ↔ 12cm (5in). ✲

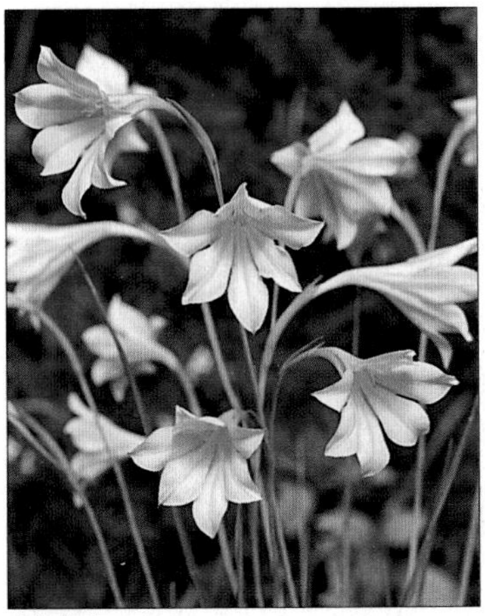

Gladiolus tristis

***G.* 'Tesoro'.** Medium-flowered Grandiflorus gladiolus bearing slightly ruffled yellow flowers in late summer. Flower spike is 70–75cm (28–30in) long, with 26 buds (10 open). ↕ 1.5m (5ft), ↔ 12cm (5in). ✲

***G.* 'The Bride'** ■♀ syn. *G.* x *colvilei* 'The Bride'. Slender *G. cardinalis* hybrid producing small spikes of 3–6 white flowers, 5cm (2in) across, marked with yellow on the lower tepals, from early spring to early summer. ↕ to 60cm (24in), ↔ 5cm (2in). ✲

G. tristis ■ Cormous perennial with very narrow leaves, the lower 40–120cm (16–48in) long and often twisted near the tips. In spring, bears spikes of up to 20 open funnel-shaped, pale yellow or creamy white flowers, 6cm (2½in) long, often green-tinged, usually flushed or dotted mauve, red, brown, or purple, on wiry stems. Strongly scented in the evening. ↕ 45–150cm (1½–5ft), ↔ 5cm (2in). South Africa (Western Cape). ✲

***G.* 'Vaucluse'** ■ Giant-flowered Grandiflorus gladiolus. Slightly ruffled, vermilion-red flowers, with small, creamy white throats, are produced in late summer. Flower spike is 80–85cm (32–34in) long, with 27 buds (10 open). ↕ 1.9m (6ft), ↔ 15cm (6in). ✲

***G.* 'White City'.** Primulinus gladiolus producing white flowers in late summer. Flower spike is 55cm (22in) long, with 18 buds (6 or 7 open). ↕ 1.1m (3½ft), ↔ 8–10cm (3–4in). ✲

***G.* 'White Ice'** ■ Medium-flowered Grandiflorus gladiolus bearing ruffled white flowers in late summer. Flower spike is 75–80cm (30–32in) long, with 25 buds (10 open). ↕ 1.5m (5ft), ↔ 12cm (5in). ✲

***G.* 'Zephyr'** ■ Large-flowered Grandiflorus gladiolus. Ruffled, light lavender-pink flowers, with small ivory throats, are produced in midsummer. Flower spike is 75–80cm (30–32in) long, with 26 buds (9 open). ↕ 1.7m (5½ft), ↔ 15cm (6in). ✲

▷ **Gladiolus, Water** see *Butomus*
▷ **Gladwyn, Stinking** see *Iris foetidissima*
▷ ***Glandularia*** see *Verbena*
▷ ***Glandulicactus crassihamatus*** see *Sclerocactus uncinatus* var. *crassihamatus*
▷ ***Glandulicactus uncinatus*** see *Sclerocactus uncinatus*

GLAUCIDIUM

GLAUCIDIACEAE/PAEONIACEAE

Genus of one species of rhizomatous, clump-forming perennial from mountainous woodland in N. Japan. It has palmately lobed leaves and large, peony- or poppy-like flowers. A very effective plant for a woodland garden, peat bed, or border, *G. palmatum* grows best in cool, moist climates.

- **HARDINESS** Fully hardy.
- **CULTIVATION** Grow in humus-rich, leafy, moist soil in partial to deep shade, sheltered from cold, drying winds.
- **PROPAGATION** Sow seed in containers in an open frame in spring, or divide mature clumps with care in early spring.
- **PESTS AND DISEASES** Susceptible to slug damage.

G. palmatum ■♀ Slow-growing, rhizomatous perennial, softly hairy when young, with unbranched stems, each bearing 2 or 3 palmately 5- to 11-lobed, many-veined, toothed, light green leaves, 20–30cm (8–12in) long, heart-shaped at the bases, with crinkly leaf surfaces. In late spring and early summer, produces solitary, terminal flowers, 5–8cm (2–3in) across, with 4 soft pinkish lilac or mauve tepals, no petals, and numerous gold stamens. ↕↔ 45cm (18in). N. Japan. ✲✲✲. **var. *leucanthum***, syn. 'Album', has white flowers.

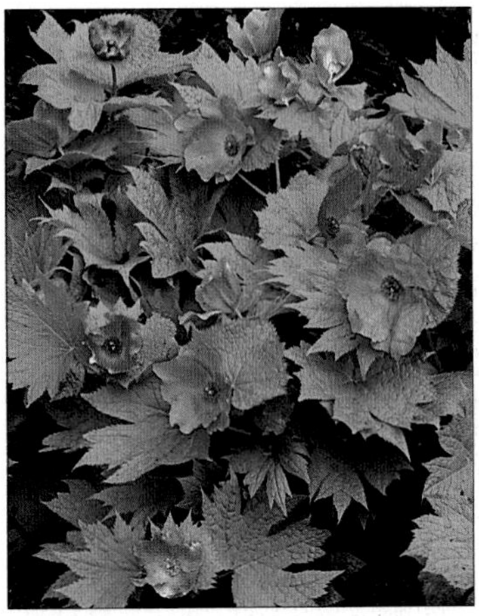

Glaucidium palmatum

GLAUCIUM

Horned poppy

PAPAVERACEAE

Genus of 25 species of erect, often rosette-forming annuals, biennials, and short-lived perennials from disturbed or waste ground in Europe, the Middle East, N. Africa, and C. and S.W. Asia. They have pinnatifid, hairless to softly hairy, narrowly ovate to nearly rounded, glaucous leaves with large terminal lobes and orange-yellow sap. Showy, solitary, terminal and axillary, poppy-like, paper-thin flowers, borne mainly in summer, are followed by long, curved, decorative seed heads. Grow in a border or gravel garden. Roots are toxic if ingested.

- **HARDINESS** Fully hardy.
- **CULTIVATION** Grow in poor to moderately fertile, well-drained soil in full sun. Resent root disturbance.
- **PROPAGATION** Sow seed *in situ* in spring or autumn.
- **PESTS AND DISEASES** Trouble free.

G. corniculatum, syn. *G. phoenicium* (Red horned poppy). Rosette-forming, slightly hairy biennial, with pinnatifid, glaucous, silver-grey leaves, 15–30cm (6–12in) long. Crimson-red to orange flowers, to 5cm (2in) across, usually with a black spot at the base of each petal, are produced freely at the tips of the branched stems from summer to early autumn. ↕↔ 30–40cm (12–16in). Europe, S.W. Asia. ❄❄❄

G. flavum ▣ (Yellow horned poppy). Rosette-forming, slightly hairy, short-lived perennial, usually grown as a biennial, with pinnatifid, glaucous, hairless, rough, blue-green leaves, 15–30cm (6–12in) long, the lobes incised or toothed. Produces branched grey stems of bright golden yellow or orange flowers, to 5cm (2in) across, in summer. ↕ 30–90cm (12–36in), ↔ to 45cm (18in). Europe, Canary Islands, N. Africa, W. Asia. ❄❄❄

G. grandiflorum. Rosette-forming perennial with alternate, pinnatifid or pinnatisect, glaucous, bluish green leaves, to 20cm (8in) long, consisting of obovate-oblong segments. Poppy-like, bowl-shaped, dark orange to crimson flowers, to 6cm (2½in) across, each with a dark spot at the base, are freely borne in summer. ↕↔ 30–50cm (12–20in). Greece, N.E. Egypt (Sinai), Turkey, Syria, Caucasus, Iran. ❄❄❄

G. phoenicium see *G. corniculatum.*

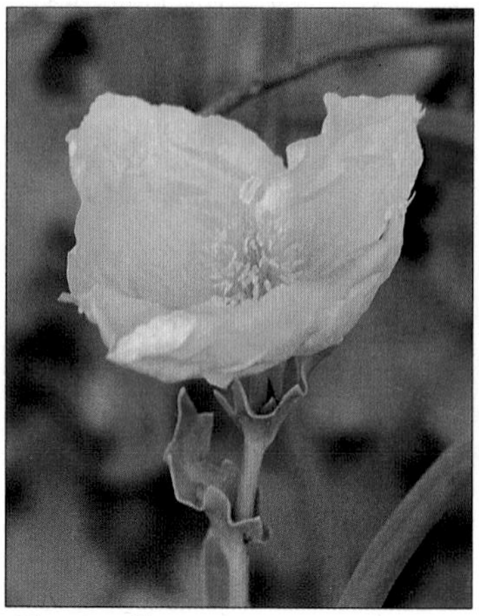

Glaucium flavum

G

GLECHOMA

Ground ivy

LABIATAE/LAMIACEAE

Genus of about 12 species of creeping, rhizomatous and stoloniferous perennials found in woodland and hedgerows throughout Europe. The variable, coarsely toothed leaves are borne in opposite pairs on long, slender, rooting stems and provide good ground cover, but may become invasive. Small, 2-lipped, tubular, usually violet-blue flowers are borne in summer. *G. hederacea* 'Variegata' is most often grown; its handsome foliage is ideal for window-boxes or hanging baskets.

- **HARDINESS** Fully hardy.
- **CULTIVATION** Grow in moderately fertile, moist but well-drained soil in full sun or partial shade.
- **PROPAGATION** Divide in spring or autumn, or take softwood cuttings in late spring.
- **PESTS AND DISEASES** May be damaged by slugs and snails.

***G. hederacea* 'Variegata'**, syn. *Nepeta glechoma* 'Variegata', *N. hederacea* 'Variegata' (Variegated ground ivy). Stoloniferous, evergreen or semi-evergreen perennial with trailing stems bearing kidney-shaped leaves, to 3cm (1¼in) across, heart-shaped at the bases, and soft pale green, marbled pure white, especially around the scalloped margins. Bears whorls of 4–6 lilac-mauve, dead nettle-like flowers in summer. ↕ to 15cm (6in), ↔ to 2m (6ft) or more. ❄❄❄

GLEDITSIA

CAESALPINIACEAE/LEGUMINOSAE

Genus of about 14 species of deciduous, usually spiny trees from woodland in Asia, North and South America, and tropical Africa. They are cultivated for their elegant form and pinnate or 2-pinnate, fern-like leaves, which are borne alternately. The inconspicuous

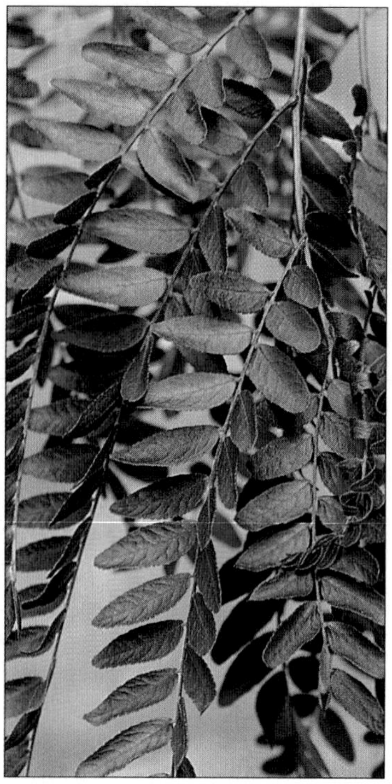

Gleditsia triacanthos 'Rubylace'

racemes of small, greenish white flowers often produce unusual, large, pendent seed pods, particularly after a hot summer. The trunks and branches of most species are armed with simple or branched spines. Grow gleditsias as specimen trees.

- **HARDINESS** Fully hardy, although susceptible to frost damage when young.
- **CULTIVATION** Grow in any fertile, well-drained soil in full sun. Pruning group 1.
- **PROPAGATION** Sow scarified seed in containers in an open frame in autumn. Bud cultivars in summer or graft them in late winter.
- **PESTS AND DISEASES** Gall midges on foliage, especially that of *G. triacanthos* 'Sunburst', may be a problem.

G. caspica (Caspian locust). Spreading, deciduous tree, the trunk armed with branched spines to 15cm (6in) or more long. Glossy, mid-green leaves, to 25cm (10in) long, turning yellow in autumn, are usually pinnate, occasionally 2-pinnate, with 12–20 ovate to oval leaflets. Pendent, curved, twisted seed pods, to 25cm (10in) long, are produced in autumn. ↕ 12m (40ft), ↔ 10m (30ft). Caucasus, N. Iran. ❄❄❄

G. japonica Conical, deciduous tree with a spiny trunk and very spiny shoots (purple when young). Glossy, mid-green leaves, to 30cm (12in) long, turn yellow in autumn. They are either pinnate with 14–24 ovate to lance-shaped leaflets, or 2-pinnate with 2–12 leaflets. Bears pendent, curved, twisted seed pods, to 30cm (12in) long, in autumn. ↕ 20m (70ft), ↔ 12m (40ft). Japan. ❄❄❄

G. triacanthos (Honey locust). Spreading, deciduous tree with a spiny trunk and shoots, the spines branched and 8–15cm (3–6in) long. Glossy, dark green leaves, to 25cm (10in) long, turn yellow in autumn, and are pinnate with 14–24 leaflets or 2-pinnate with 4–16 pairs of oblong-lance-shaped leaflets. Pendent, sickle-shaped, twisted seed pods, to 45cm (18in) long, are borne in autumn. ↕ 30m (100ft) or more, ↔ 20m (70ft). C. and E. North America. ❄❄❄. **'Elegantissima'** ▣ is dense, shrubby, slow-growing, and thornless; ↕ 5–8m (15–25ft), ↔ 5m (15ft). **'Imperial'** is a wide-spreading tree with rounded, bright green leaves and few seed pods; ↕ to 10m (30ft). **f. *inermis*** is thornless. **'Rubylace'** ▣ has dark bronze-red young leaves turning dark bronze-green by midsummer. **'Skyline'** is compact and broadly conical, with ascending upper branches and dark green leaves turning golden yellow in autumn; ↕ to 15m (50ft). **'Sunburst'** ▣ is fast-growing and broadly conical, with spreading, thornless branches, and golden yellow young foliage, pale green at maturity, yellow in autumn. Does not fruit; ↕ 12m (40ft), ↔ 10m (30ft).

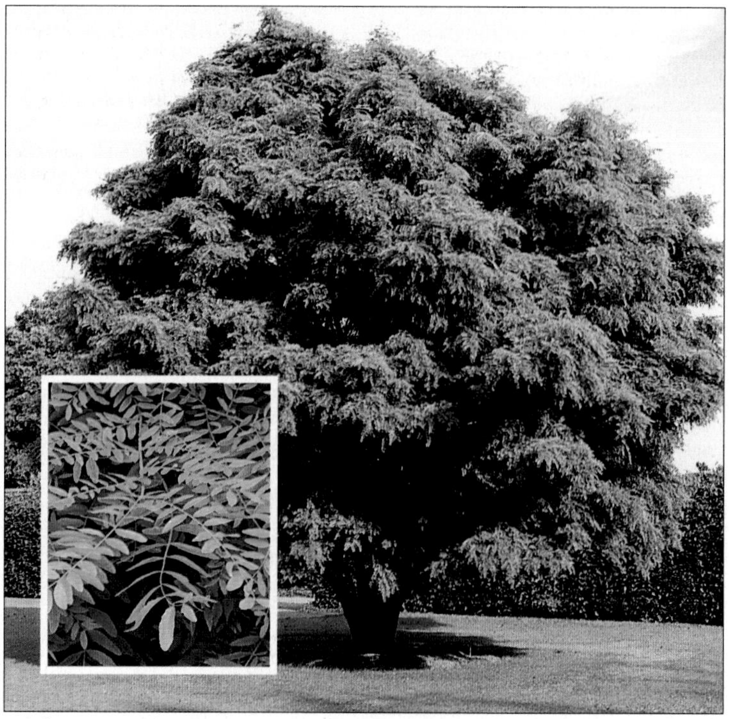

Gleditsia triacanthos 'Elegantissima' (inset: leaf detail)

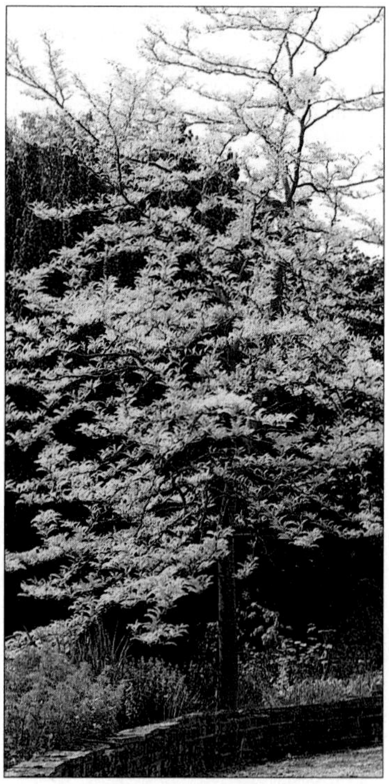

Gleditsia triacanthos 'Sunburst'

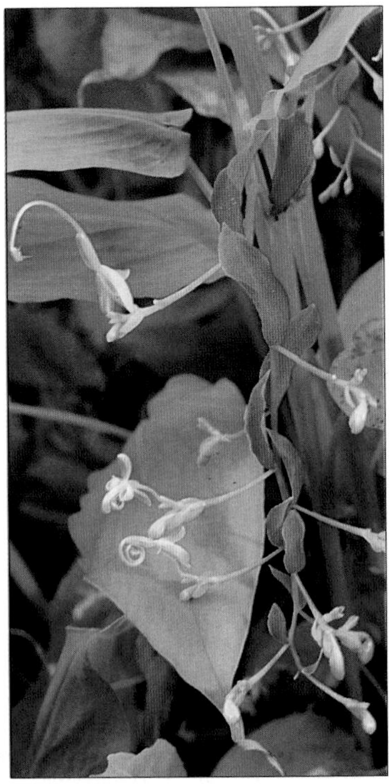

Globba winitii

GLOBBA

ZINGIBERACEAE

Genus of about 70 species of rhizomatous herbaceous perennials from forest in S.E. Asia. Reed-like stems have alternate, 2-ranked, oblong or lance-shaped leaves. They bear 3-petalled, tubular flowers on slender, branched stalks, in terminal, pendent racemes with conspicuous bracts, from autumn to early winter. Among the lower bracts, bulbils may form instead of flowers. Grow as ground cover in warm climates; elsewhere, grow in a warm greenhouse.

• **HARDINESS** Frost tender.
• **CULTIVATION** Under glass, grow in loam-based potting compost (JI No.2) in bright filtered or indirect light. During the growing season, maintain high humidity, water freely, and apply a balanced liquid fertilizer every 2 or 3 weeks. Allow to become dormant in late winter and keep just moist. Outdoors, grow in humus-rich, moist but well-drained soil in partial shade.
• **PROPAGATION** Divide in spring, or plant bulbils in summer.
• **PESTS AND DISEASES** Mealybugs may be troublesome.

G. winitii ▣ Rhizomatous perennial with lance-shaped leaves, 20cm (8in) long, heart-shaped at the bases, lower leaves sheathing the stems; leaf-stalks are 10cm (4in) long. From autumn to early winter, bears nodding or pendent racemes, 15cm (6in) long, of slender, tubular yellow flowers, to 4cm (1½in) long, with reflexed, pink, mauve, or deep purple bracts. ↕ 1m (3ft), ↔ 60cm (24in). Thailand. ❀ (min. 16°C/61°F)

▷ **Globe amaranth** see *Gomphrena globosa*
▷ **Globe artichoke** see *Cynara scolymus*
▷ **Globe daisy** see *Globularia*
▷ **Globeflower** see *Trollius*
Common European see *T. europaeus*
▷ **Globe thistle** see *Echinops*

GLOBULARIA

Globe daisy

GLOBULARIACEAE

Genus of about 20 species of mat- or hummock-forming, mainly evergreen perennials or subshrubs, mostly found in open, rocky habitats around the Mediterranean, often at high altitudes. They produce leathery, simple, entire or sharply toothed leaves and tiny, 2-lipped flowers in dense, spherical heads. Globe daisies are suitable for a rock garden, trough, or alpine house; the more robust are also useful in wall plantings.

• **HARDINESS** Fully hardy.
• **CULTIVATION** Grow in neutral to alkaline, sharply drained soil in full sun. Protect from winter wet.
• **PROPAGATION** Sow seed in containers in an open frame in autumn. Root individual rosettes in spring or early summer.
• **PESTS AND DISEASES** May be damaged by slugs and snails.

G. bellidifolia see *G. meridionalis.*
G. cordifolia 🏆 Dwarf, evergreen, mat-forming, woody-based perennial with rooting stems bearing rosettes of spoon-shaped, glossy, dark green leaves, to 2.5cm (1in) long, with notched tips. In summer, produces lavender-blue flowers in stemless, spherical heads, to 2cm (¾in) across. ↕ 5cm (2in), ↔ to 20cm (8in). Mountains of C. and S. Europe, W. Turkey. ✻✻✻. **subsp. *bellidifolia*** see *G. meridionalis.* **subsp. *meridionalis*** see *G. meridionalis.*
G. meridionalis ▣ syn. *G. bellidifolia, G. cordifolia* subsp. *bellidifolia, G. cordifolia* subsp. *meridionalis, G. pygmaea.* Evergreen, dome-shaped, mat-forming subshrub with lance-shaped to inversely lance-shaped, glossy, dark green leaves, 2–9cm (¾–3½in) long. In summer, produces lavender-purple flowers in spherical heads, to 2cm (¾in) across, just above the foliage. More robust than *G. cordifolia.* ↕ to 10cm (4in), ↔ to 30cm (12in). S.E. Alps, C. and S. Apennines, Balkan Peninsula. ✻✻✻
G. nana see *G. repens.*
G. pygmaea see *G. meridionalis.*
G. repens, syn. *G. nana.* Very compact, mat-forming, evergreen perennial with folded, spoon-shaped, glossy, dark green leaves, 1–2cm (½–¾in) long. Lavender-blue flowers in stemless or short-stemmed, spherical heads, 1–2cm (½–¾in) across, are borne immediately above the leaves in summer. Similar to *G. cordifolia,* but smaller. Suitable for a trough. ↕ 2.5cm (1in), ↔ to 15cm (6in). Pyrenees, S.W. Alps. ✻✻✻

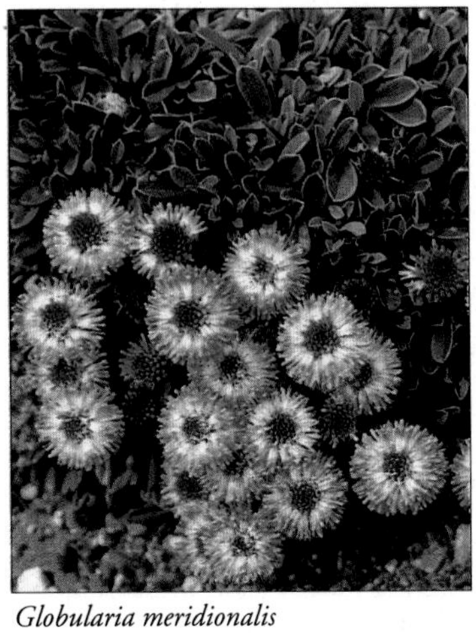

Globularia meridionalis

GLORIOSA

COLCHICACEAE/LILIACEAE

Genus of one very variable species of climbing, tuberous perennial from woodland and forest, often by rivers, in tropical Africa and India. It is cultivated for its brightly coloured flowers, and is effective when scrambling through other plants. In frost-prone climates, grow in a temperate greenhouse or conservatory. Highly toxic if ingested; handling tubers may irritate the skin.

• **HARDINESS** Frost tender.
• **CULTIVATION** Plant tubers 7–10cm (3–4in) deep in early spring. Under glass, grow in loam-based potting compost (JI No.2), with added grit, in full light. Water freely when growth begins and apply a balanced liquid fertilizer every 2 weeks. Keep tubers dry in winter. Pot on only when congested, in late winter. Outdoors, grow in fertile, well-drained soil in full sun.
• **PROPAGATION** Sow seed at 19–24°C (66–75°F), or separate the finger-like tubers, in spring.
• **PESTS AND DISEASES** Prone to aphids.

G. carsonii see *G. superba.*
G. minor see *G. superba.*
G. rothschildiana see *G. superba* 'Rothschildiana'.
G. simplex see *G. superba.*
G. superba 🏆 syn. *G. carsonii, G. minor, G. simplex.* Climbing perennial with ovate-lance-shaped to oblong, glossy, bright green leaves, 5–8cm (2–3in) long, which narrow to form terminal tendrils, 3–5cm (1¼–2in) long. From summer to autumn, nodding flowers, 5–10cm (2–4in) across, are borne from the upper leaf axils. Flowers have 6 reflexed, wavy-margined, red or purple petals, often yellow-margined, sometimes entirely yellow, with long, protruding stamens. ↕ to 2m (6ft), ↔ 30cm (12in). Africa, India. ❀ (min. 8–10°C/46–50°F). **'Citrina'** has citrus-yellow flowers, tinted or striped with deep purple-red. **'Rothschildiana'** ▣ syn. *G. rothschildiana,* has flowers 7–10cm (3–4in) across, with bright red or scarlet tepals fading to ruby or garnet, and yellow near the bases and on the margins.

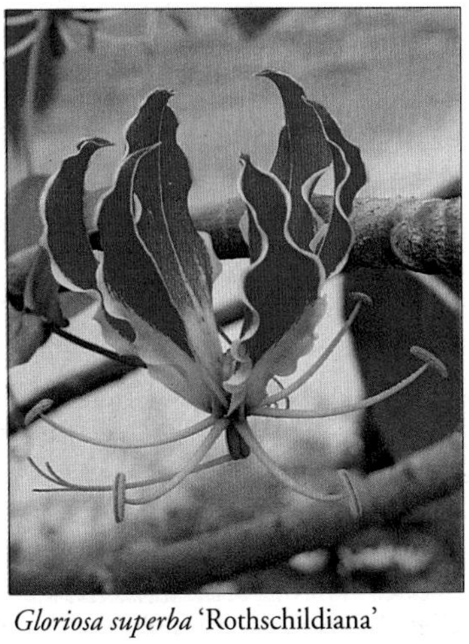

Gloriosa superba 'Rothschildiana'

▷ **Glorybean, Java** see *Clerodendrum speciosissimum*
▷ **Glory bower** see *Clerodendrum philippinum, C. speciosissimum, C. thomsoniae*
Blue see *Clerodendrum ugandense*
▷ **Glory bush** see *Tibouchina organensis, T. urvilleana*
▷ **Glory flower** see *Clerodendrum bungei*
Chilean see *Eccremocarpus, E. scaber*
▷ **Glory of the snow** see *Chionodoxa*
▷ **Glory of the sun** see *Leucocoryne ixioides*
▷ **Glory plant, Purple** see *Sutera grandiflora*

GLOTTIPHYLLUM

AIZOACEAE

Genus of about 60 species of low-growing, branching, perennial succulents from semi-desert areas of South Africa. They have semi-cylindrical or strap-shaped, fleshy, glossy, bright green or pale green leaves, arranged in opposite pairs or alternately along the stems, with 4 or more leaves on a single shoot. Large, daisy-like, bright yellow, rarely white flowerheads are borne singly in the leaf axils, mainly from summer to late winter. Below 10°C (50°F), grow in a warm greenhouse; in warmer areas, grow in a desert garden.

• **HARDINESS** Frost tender.
• **CULTIVATION** Under glass, grow in standard cactus compost in full light. Water sparingly from midsummer to late winter and apply a half-strength low-nitrogen liquid fertilizer once during the growing season. Keep barely moist when dormant. Outdoors, grow in poor, sharply drained soil in full sun. See also pp.48–49.
• **PROPAGATION** Sow seed at 19–24°C (66–75°F), or root basal stem cuttings, in late summer.
• **PESTS AND DISEASES** Trouble free.

G. linguiforme. Succulent, often offsetting, with opposite pairs of strap-shaped, glossy, bright green leaves, 5–6cm (2–2½in) long, which are incurved above and obliquely thickened below, with rounded tips. Bears golden yellow flowerheads, 7cm (3in) across, from autumn to late winter. ↕ 6cm (2½in), ↔ 30cm (12in). South Africa (Northern Cape, Eastern Cape, Western Cape). ❀ (min. 10°C/50°F)
G. nelii. Succulent, forming compact clumps, with thick, strap-shaped, pale green leaves, 4–5cm (1½–2in) long, in uneven, opposite pairs. The shorter leaf of each pair is incurved with rounded margins and tip; the longer is incurved like a hook, flat above, keeled below, with a rounded tip. Bears bright yellow flowerheads, 4cm (1½in) across, from autumn to late winter. ↕ 5cm (2in), ↔ 30cm (12in). South Africa (Northern Cape, Eastern Cape, Western Cape). ❀ (min. 10°C/50°F)

GLOXINIA

GESNERIACEAE

Genus of 8 species of rhizomatous, soft-stemmed perennials or shrubs from forest in Central and South America. The fleshy, creeping rhizomes give rise to erect stems bearing opposite pairs of ovate to elliptic leaves. Bell- or funnel-shaped, blue or pink flowers, finely hairy

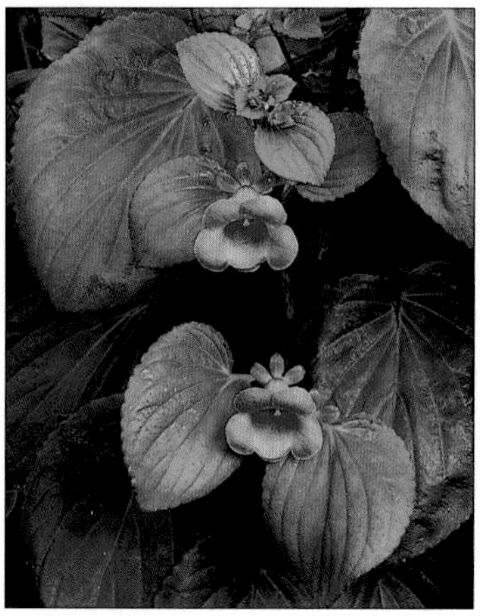

Gloxinia perennis

on the outside, are borne singly or in pairs from the leaf axils from summer to mid-autumn. In frost-prone areas, grow in a warm greenhouse. Elsewhere, grow in a shady border or woodland setting.

- **HARDINESS** Frost tender.
- **CULTIVATION** Under glass, grow in loamless potting compost in bright indirect light and high humidity. During the growing season, water freely and apply a balanced liquid fertilizer every 2 or 3 weeks. Dry off after flowering; resume watering, sparingly at first, in spring. Outdoors, grow in moist, humus-rich soil in dappled shade.
- **PROPAGATION** Sow seed at 19–24°C (66–75°F) in early spring. Divide rhizomes in spring. Root basal cuttings with bottom heat in summer.
- **PESTS AND DISEASES** Prone to vine weevil, tarsonemid mites, western flower thrips, and powdery mildew.

G. gymnostoma, syn. *Seemannia gymnostoma.* Rhizomatous perennial with ovate, softly hairy leaves, 7cm (3in) long, and solitary, funnel-shaped, rose-pink flowers, to 3.5cm (1½in) long, borne in summer. ↕60cm (24in), ↔45cm (18in). Argentina. ❁ (min. 13°C/55°F)
G. perennis ■ Bushy, rhizomatous perennial bearing toothed, ovate leaves with heart-shaped bases, to 20cm (8in) long, glossy, mid-green above, paler and suffused red below. Bears solitary, bell-shaped, lavender- to purple-blue flowers, 2.5–3.5cm (1–1½in) long, marked dark violet at the bases, from early summer to mid-autumn. ↕1.2m (4ft), ↔1m (3ft). Panama to Peru. ❁ (min. 10°C/50°F)
G. speciosa see *Sinningia speciosa.*

▷**Gloxinia,**
Creeping see *Lophospermum erubescens*
Florists' see *Sinningia speciosa*

GLYCERIA

GRAMINEAE/POACEAE

Genus of 16 species of marsh or marginal, aquatic, perennial grasses, mainly from N. temperate regions, but also found in Australia, New Zealand, and South America. Occurring naturally in water to 75cm (30in) deep, they are vigorous, dense, and spreading plants. Use as cover for a large pool.

- **HARDINESS** Fully hardy to frost tender.
- **CULTIVATION** Grow in water to 15cm (6in) deep in full sun; grow in a basket of loamy soil in order to restrict spread. Alternatively, grow in any garden soil that is reliably moist in full sun.
- **PROPAGATION** Divide in spring.
- **PESTS AND DISEASES** Trouble free.

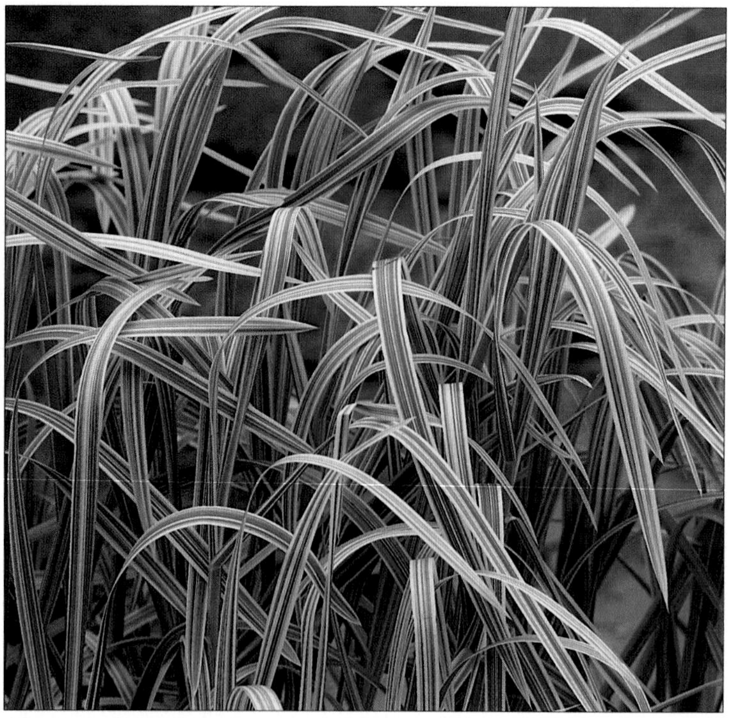

Glyceria maxima 'Variegata'

G. aquatica see *G. maxima.*
G. maxima, syn. *G. aquatica.* Aquatic, rhizomatous, perennial grass, producing narrowly strap-shaped, keeled, deep green leaves, 30–60cm (12–24in) long, flushed pink as they emerge. Panicles of green to purplish green spikelets, to 45cm (18in) long, are borne in mid- and late summer. ↕80cm (32in), ↔ indefinite. Temperate Eurasia. ✻✻✻
'Variegata' ■ is more commonly grown, for its attractive cream, green, and white striped foliage.

GLYCYRRHIZA

LEGUMINOSAE/PAPILIONACEAE

Genus of about 20 species of perennials from a range of moist or dry habitats in the Mediterranean, tropical Asia, and North and South America, occurring in diverse habitats from dry scrub to swampland. They have pinnate, rarely 3-palmate, sticky-glandular leaves, and

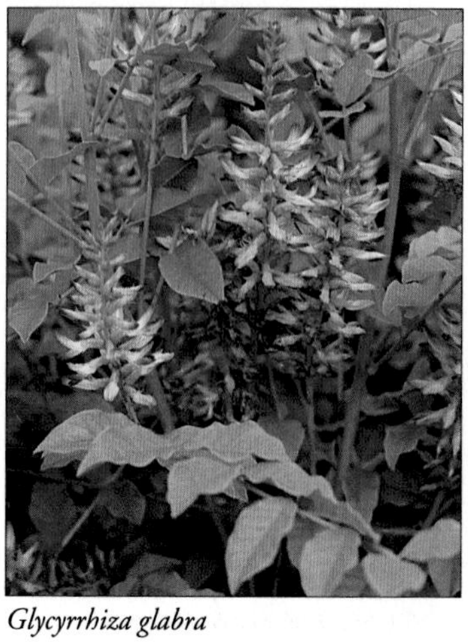

Glycyrrhiza glabra

pea-like flowers borne in axillary racemes or spikes. *G. glabra* is a coarse but interesting plant suitable for a wild garden or informal border; its roots are the source of liquorice.

- **HARDINESS** Fully hardy.
- **CULTIVATION** Grow in deep, fertile, moist soil in full sun. The roots of *G. glabra* are harvested in autumn.
- **PROPAGATION** Sow seed in containers outdoors in spring or autumn. Divide roots, each with one or more growth buds, in early spring.
- **PESTS AND DISEASES** Trouble free.

G. glabra ■ syn. *G. glandulifera* (Liquorice, Sweetwood). Tap-rooted perennial bearing pinnate, sticky-glandular leaves, 5–20cm (2–8in) long, each with 9–17 oblong to elliptic or ovate leaflets. Pea-like, blue or pale violet and white flowers, 1cm (½in) long, are borne in loose racemes, usually 5–8cm (2–3in) long, in late summer. ↕1.2m (4ft), ↔90cm (36in). Mediterranean to S.W. Asia. ✻✻✻
G. glandulifera see *G. glabra.*

▷**Goatsbeard** see *Aruncus dioicus*
▷**Goat's rue** see *Galega*
▷***Godetia*** see *Clarkia*
G. amoena see *C. amoena*
G. grandiflora see *C. amoena*
▷**Gold dust** see *Aurinia saxatilis*
▷**Golden bell** see *Forsythia suspensa*
▷**Golden club** see *Orontium*
▷**Golden eardrops** see *Dicentra chrysantha*
▷**Golden everlasting** see *Bracteantha bracteata*
▷**Golden fleece** see *Thymophylla tenuiloba*
▷**Golden larch** see *Pseudolarix amabilis*
▷**Golden pothos** see *Epipremnum aureum*
▷**Golden rain** see *Laburnum*
▷**Golden-rain tree** see *Koelreuteria paniculata*
▷**Golden rod** see *Solidago*
▷**Golden shower** see *Pyrostegia venusta*
▷**Golden top** see *Lamarckia aurea*
▷**Golden trumpet** see *Allamanda cathartica*
▷**Goldilocks** see *Aster linosyris*
▷**Gold thread** see *Coptis*

GOMPHOCARPUS

ASCLEPIADACEAE

Genus of 50 species of evergreen and deciduous subshrubs and perennials found on dry slopes and in scrub in tropical and southern Africa. They have variable, opposite, alternate, or whorled leaves. Curious, hooded, cup-shaped flowers are produced in terminal or axillary cymes, followed by seed pods that are usually inflated. In frost-prone areas, they are best grown in a cool greenhouse. In warmer climates, plant in a shrub border. Some species exude a milky sap, which may aggravate skin allergies.

- **HARDINESS** Half hardy to frost tender.
- **CULTIVATION** Under glass, grow in loam-based potting compost (JI No.2), with added leaf mould, in full light or bright filtered light. During the growing season, water freely and apply a balanced liquid fertilizer every 4–6 weeks; keep almost dry in winter. Outdoors, grow in any well-drained soil in full sun or partial shade.
- **PROPAGATION** Sow seed at 13–18°C (55–64°F) in spring, or take softwood cuttings in spring.
- **PESTS AND DISEASES** Trouble free.

G. fruticosus, syn. *Asclepias fruticosa* (Milk bush). Upright, deciduous subshrub with linear-lance-shaped, mid-green leaves, 5–10cm (2–4in) long, borne in opposite pairs. Produces axillary clusters, 5cm (2in) across, of cup-shaped, creamy white flowers, 7mm (¼in) long, in early summer, followed by ovoid, inflated, softly spiny, silver-green fruit, to 8cm (3in) long. ↕1–1.5m (3–5ft), ↔1m (3ft). Southern Africa. ✻
G. physocarpus, syn. *Asclepias physocarpa* (Swan plant). Deciduous subshrub, often grown as an annual, with sticky, hairy stems and opposite, sometimes alternate, narrowly lance-shaped, grey-green leaves, to 10cm (4in) long. In summer, bears many-flowered cymes, 5cm (2in) across, of creamy white or greenish white flowers, to 7mm (¼in) across; they are followed by spherical to ovoid, inflated, softly spiny, pale green fruit, to 6cm (2½in) across. ↕2m (6ft), ↔60cm (24in). South Africa (Eastern Transvaal to Eastern Cape). ✻

GOMPHRENA

AMARANTHACEAE

Genus of 90 species of erect or prostrate, often many-branched, softly hairy annuals, occasionally perennials, found in a variety of habitats from open, sandy soils to moist woodland, in Australia and tropical Central and South America. Lance-shaped to ovate leaves are produced in opposite pairs. Upright spikes of clover-like flowerheads, with prominent colourful bracts, are borne from summer to early autumn. In frost-prone areas, use as summer bedding or in an annual border. The flowerheads are good for cutting and drying.

- **HARDINESS** Half hardy to frost tender.
- **CULTIVATION** Grow in moderately fertile, well-drained soil in full sun.

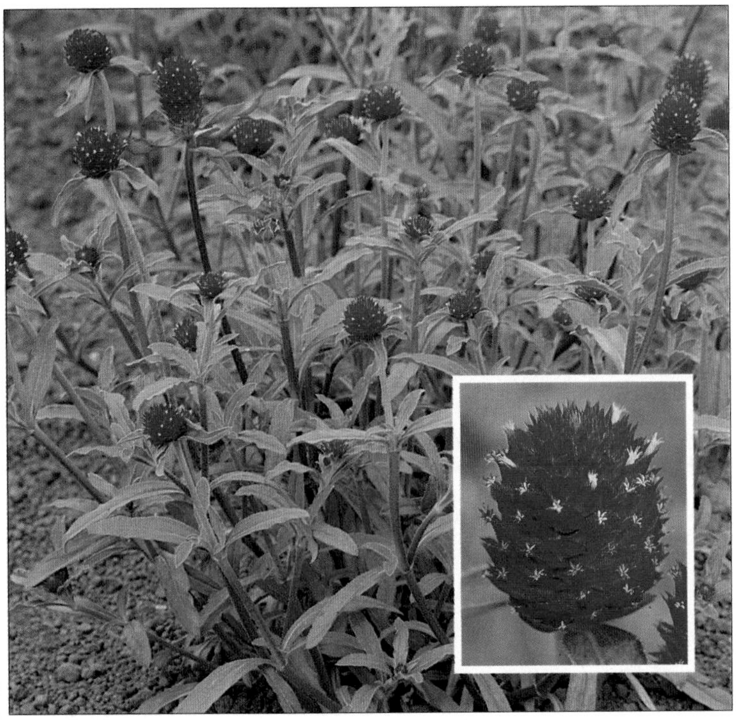

Gomphrena 'Strawberry Fields' (inset: flowerhead detail)

• **PROPAGATION** Sow seed at 15–18°C (59–64°F) in early spring.
• **PESTS AND DISEASES** Trouble free.

G. globosa (Globe amaranth). Upright, bushy annual with ovate to oblong leaves, to 15cm (6in) long, densely white-hairy when young, later sparsely hairy. Bears ovoid-oblong flowerheads, to 3.5cm (1½in) long, of pink, purple, or white flower bracts, from summer to early autumn. ↕ 30–60cm (12–24in), ↔ to 30cm (12in). Guatemala, Panama. ❄. **'Buddy'** has vivid, deep purple flowerheads; ↕ 15cm (6in).
***G.* 'Strawberry Fields'** ▣ Similar in growth and habit to *G. globosa*, but has brilliant red flowerheads, to 5cm (2in) long. ↕ 75–80cm (30–32in), ↔ to 30cm (12in). ❄

GONIOLIMON

PLUMBAGINACEAE

Genus of about 20 species of perennials found in hot, dry habitats from S.E. Europe to Mongolia, and in N.W. Africa. They are grown for their panicles or spike-like corymbs of tubular-trumpet-shaped, "everlasting", white, pink, purple, or red flowers, borne on compressed and flanged, branched stems. Large, smooth, leathery or fleshy leaves are arranged in basal rosettes. They flower best in hot, dry summers or in warm areas. Grow in paving.
• **HARDINESS** Fully hardy.
• **CULTIVATION** Grow in sandy, well-drained soil in full sun.
• **PROPAGATION** Sow seed in containers in a cold frame in mid-spring. Take root cuttings in winter.
• **PESTS AND DISEASES** Trouble free.

G. tataricum, syn. *Limonium tataricum* (Tatarian statice). Rosetted perennial with oblong to obovate or inversely lance-shaped, pale green leaves, 2–15cm (¾–6in) long, with white spots. In mid- and late summer, bears wide-spreading panicles, to 12cm (5in) or more long, of tubular flowers with white sepals and spreading, purple-red to ruby-red petals. Good for cutting and drying. ↕↔ 30cm (12in). S.E. Europe, Caucasus, steppes of S. Russia. ❄❄❄

▷**Good luck plant** see *Oxalis tetraphylla*
▷**Good luck tree** see *Cordyline fruticosa*

GOODYERA

Jewel orchid

ORCHIDACEAE

Genus of about 40 species of evergreen, rarely deciduous, terrestrial, rhizomatous orchids, widely distributed in temperate areas except Africa, occurring in forest leaf litter. They produce basal rosettes of ovate to lance-shaped, veined leaves, usually more attractive than the small white flowers that are borne in erect, narrow spikes or racemes on upright stems, mainly in summer. Grow hardy species in woodland or on a peat bank. Tender species can be grown in an alpine house or cool greenhouse.
• **HARDINESS** Fully hardy to frost tender.
• **CULTIVATION** Outdoors, grow in sandy, humus-rich, well-drained, acid soil in a sheltered site in partial shade. See also p.46.
• **PROPAGATION** Divide rhizomes in spring.
• **PESTS AND DISEASES** Aphids, red spider mites, and mealybugs can be a problem.

G. pubescens. Terrestrial, evergreen orchid with rosettes of ovate to broadly lance-shaped, dark bluish green leaves, to 9cm (3½in) long, with conspicuous white veins. Small white flowers, to 5mm (¼in) long, are produced in dense, cylindrical racemes, 20–40cm (8–16in) tall, from late summer to autumn. ↕ to 40cm (16in) (in flower), ↔ 23cm (9in). E. North America. ❄❄

▷**Gooseberry,**
Barbados see *Pereskia aculeata*
Chinese see *Actinidia deliciosa*
▷**Goosefoot** see *Syngonium podophyllum*

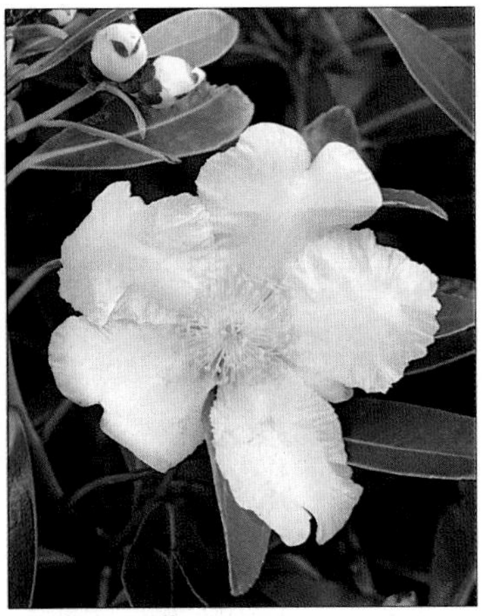

Gordonia axillaris

GORDONIA

THEACEAE

Genus of about 70 species of evergreen trees and shrubs, occurring in moist forest in S.E. Asia, with one species in S.E. USA. They are cultivated for their simple, elliptic, oblong or inversely lance-shaped, alternate, leathery, hairless leaves, and for their camellia-like flowers, each with 5–7 petals. In frost-prone areas, grow in a cool greenhouse. In milder regions, plant in woodland.
• **HARDINESS** Half hardy to frost tender.
• **CULTIVATION** Under glass, grow in lime-free (ericaceous) potting compost in bright filtered light. Water freely when in growth, applying a balanced liquid fertilizer monthly; water sparingly in winter. Outdoors, grow in acid to neutral, moist but well-drained soil in full sun or dappled shade; shelter from cold, drying winds. Pruning group 1; may need restrictive pruning under glass.
• **PROPAGATION** Sow seed in containers as soon as ripe. Take semi-ripe cuttings in summer.
• **PESTS AND DISEASES** Trouble free.

G. axillaris ▣ ♀ Bushy shrub or tree with elliptic-oblong to inversely lance-shaped, glossy, dark green leaves, to 15cm (6in) long. Large, saucer-shaped white flowers, 8–13cm (3–5in) across, with orange-yellow anthers, are borne from winter to spring. ↕↔ 7–10m (22–30ft) or more. China, Vietnam, Taiwan. ❄
G. lasianthus ♀ (Loblolly bay). Upright tree with narrowly elliptic to inversely lance-shaped, glossy, dark green leaves, to 15cm (6in) long. In summer, produces saucer-shaped, wavy-petalled, fragrant white flowers, 6–8cm (2½–3in) across, with yellow anthers. ↕ 20m (70ft) or more, ↔ 10m (30ft). S.E. USA. ❄

▷**Gorgon plant** see *Euryale*
▷**Gorse** see *Ulex, U. europaeus*
Dwarf see *Ulex gallii*
Irish see *Ulex europaeus* 'Strictus'
Spanish see *Genista hispanica*
▷**Gourd, Snake** see *Trichosanthes cucumerina* var. *anguina*
▷**Goutweed, Variegated** see *Aegopodium podagraria* 'Variegatum'
▷**Grama, Blue** see *Bouteloua gracilis*
▷**Granadilla** see *Passiflora*
Giant see *P. quadrangularis*
▷**Granadilla cont.**
Purple see *P. edulis*
Red see *P. coccinea*
▷**Granny's bonnet** see *Aquilegia vulgaris*
▷**Grape,**
Amur see *Vitis amurensis*
Cape see *Rhoicissus capensis*
Oregon see *Mahonia aquifolium*
▷**Grape ivy** see *Cissus rhombifolia*
▷**Grape vine** see *Vitis*

GRAPTOPETALUM

CRASSULACEAE

Genus of about 12 species of rosette-forming, perennial succulents from rocky grasslands to 2,000m (6,500ft) high, in S. USA and Mexico. Bell- or star-shaped flowers, each with 5–7 outward-spreading petals, are produced in axillary cymes, mainly in spring or summer. Where temperatures drop below 5°C (41°F), grow in a temperate greenhouse or as houseplants; elsewhere, plant in a desert garden.
• **HARDINESS** Frost tender.
• **CULTIVATION** Under glass, grow in loam-based potting compost (JI No.2), with added grit, in full light or bright filtered light. Water freely in spring and summer and apply a low-nitrogen liquid fertilizer every 6–8 weeks. Keep barely moist in autumn and winter. Outdoors, grow in moderately fertile, sharply drained soil in full sun or partial shade. See also pp.48–49.
• **PROPAGATION** Sow seed at 19–24°C (66–75°F), or take rosette or leaf cuttings, both in spring or summer.
• **PESTS AND DISEASES** Susceptible to mealybugs and, if in containers, root mealybugs.

G. bellum ▣ syn. *Tacitus bellus.* Compact, perennial succulent with basal rosettes, 3–8cm (1¼–3in) across, of triangular to oval, abruptly pointed, fleshy grey leaves, 2–3.5cm (¾–1½in) long. Short-stalked, star-shaped, pink to deep red flowers, 2–3cm (¾–1¼in) across, are produced in cymes from the centre of the rosettes from late spring to summer. ↕ 5–7cm (2–3in), ↔ to 15cm (6in). Mexico. ⌂ (min. 5°C/41°F)
G. filiferum. Perennial succulent forming clumps of compact, basal rosettes, 5–6cm (2–2½in) across, of wedge- to spoon-shaped, rich green leaves, 1–5cm (½–2in) long. The leaves are white towards the winged margins and have minute papillae near the thin, bristly brown tips. Short-stalked, star-

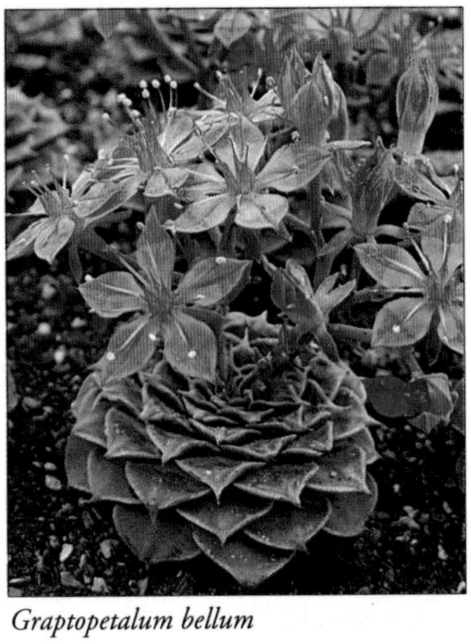

Graptopetalum bellum

G

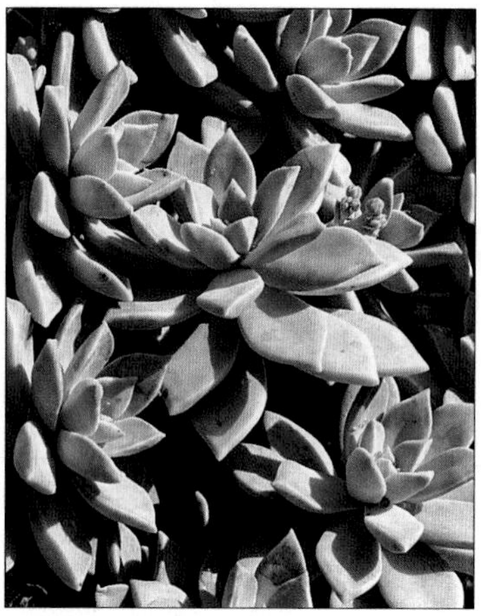

Graptopetalum paraguayense

G

shaped, red-spotted white flowers, 2cm (¾in) across, are produced in 2–5 branched cymes from spring to early summer. ↕ 12cm (5in), ↔ indefinite. N.W. Mexico. ❀ (min. 5°C/41°F)

G. paraguayense ■ syn. *Sedum weinbergii* (Mother of pearl plant). Prostrate, clump-forming, perennial succulent. Forms basal rosettes, to 15cm (6in) across, of spoon-shaped to obovate-lance-shaped, blunt, pink-tinged, grey-green leaves, 2–8cm (¾–3in) long; the young leaves are pale mauve-grey. Large cymes of star-shaped, red-spotted white flowers, 1–2cm (½–¾in) across, are borne in late winter and early spring. ↕ to 20cm (8in), ↔ indefinite. Mexico. ❀ (min. 5°C/41°F)

GRAPTOPHYLLUM

ACANTHACEAE

Genus of 10 species of evergreen shrubs from Australasia and the S.W. Pacific, often found on rainforest margins, and also on seasonally dry, rocky hillsides or beside rivers. They are cultivated mainly for their foliage: the leaves are simple, usually entire, spotted, mottled, or banded with various colours, and borne in opposite pairs. Tubular, 2-lipped flowers are produced in racemes or panicles at the ends of the shoots. Where temperatures fall below 13°C (55°F), grow in a temperate or warm greenhouse, or as houseplants. In warmer climates, use to brighten shady borders; they are effective with ferns.

• **HARDINESS** Frost tender.

• **CULTIVATION** Under glass, grow in loam-based potting compost (JI No.2), with added grit, in full light or bright filtered light. Top-dress or pot on in spring. Water freely from spring to autumn, applying a balanced liquid fertilizer monthly. Water sparingly in winter. Outdoors, grow in fertile, moist but well-drained soil in semi-shade. Pruning group 8; may need restrictive pruning under glass.

• **PROPAGATION** Sow seed at 19–24°C (66–75°F) in spring, root semi-ripe cuttings with bottom heat in summer, or layer in summer.

• **PESTS AND DISEASES** Whiteflies, red spider mites, and scale insects may infest greenhouse plants.

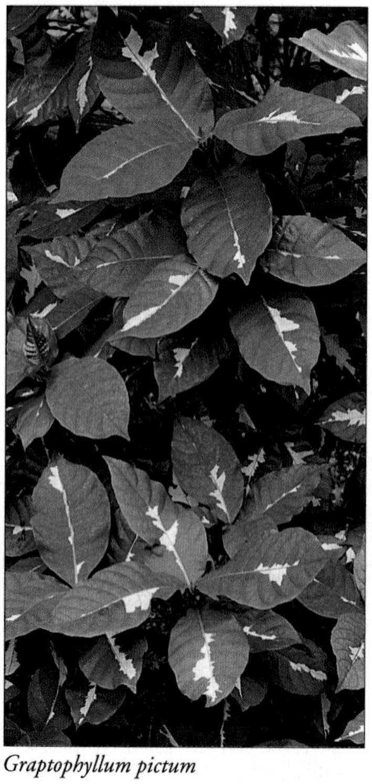

Graptophyllum pictum

G. pictum ■ (Caricature plant). Erect shrub, sparsely branched unless regularly pinched out when young. The elliptic-ovate, glossy, deep green leaves, 10–15cm (4–6in) long, are variously veined and marked yellow, or entirely suffused dark purple. In summer, bears short racemes, to 8cm (3in) long, of crimson to purple flowers with inflated throats. ↕ 1–2m (3–6ft), ↔ 60–90cm (24–36in). Probably New Guinea. ❀ (min. 13°C/55°F). **'Tricolor'** has oval, purplish green leaves, mottled yellow and rose-pink, with red stalks and midribs.

▷**Grass,**
Alpine meadow see *Poa alpina*
Balkan moor see *Sesleria heufleriana*
Blue-eyed see *Sisyrinchium graminoides*
Blue moor see *Sesleria albicans*
Blue oat see *Helictotrichon sempervirens*
Bowles' golden see *Milium effusum* 'Aureum'
Broad-leaved cotton see *Eriophorum latifolium*
Buffalo see *Stenotaphrum secundatum*
Bulbous oat see *Arrhenatherum elatius* subsp. *bulbosum* 'Variegatum'
Common cotton see *Eriophorum angustifolium*
Common quaking see *Briza media*
Cotton see *Eriophorum*
Crab see *Panicum*
Feather see *Stipa*
Feather reed see *Calamagrostis* x *acutiflora*
Fountain see *Pennisetum alopecuroides, P. setaceum*
Foxtail see *Alopecurus*
Giant feather see *Stipa gigantea*
Glaucous hair see *Koeleria glauca*
Greater quaking see *Briza maxima*
Hair see *Aira, A. elegantissima, Deschampsia*
Indian see *Sorghastrum nutans*
Lemon see *Cymbopogon citratus*
Lesser quaking see *Briza minor*
Love see *Eragrostis*

▷**Grass cont.**
Maiden see *Miscanthus sinensis* 'Gracillimus'
Meadow see *Poa*
Mosquito see *Bouteloua gracilis*
Natal see *Melinis repens*
Needle see *Stipa*
Nest moor see *Sesleria nitida*
Oat see *Arrhenatherum*
Pampas see *Cortaderia, C. selloana*
Pheasant's tail see *Stipa arundinacea*
Plume see *Saccharum*
Plumed tussock see *Chionochloa conspicua*
Quaking see *Briza*
Reed see *Calamagrostis*
Reed canary see *Phalaris arundinacea*
Ribbon see *Phalaris arundinacea*
St. Augustine see *Stenotaphrum secundatum*
Signal-arm see *Bouteloua gracilis*
Silver banner see *Miscanthus sacchariflorus*
Silver beard see *Bothriochloa saccharoides*
Spangle see *Chasmanthium latifolium*
Spear see *Poa, Stipa*
Squirrel tail see *Hordeum jubatum*
Switch see *Panicum virgatum*
Toothbrush see *Lamarckia aurea*
Trembling see *Briza media*
Tufted hair see *Deschampsia cespitosa*
Tussock see *Cortaderia, Deschampsia cespitosa*
Umbrella see *Cyperus involucratus*
Wavy hair see *Deschampsia flexuosa*
Whitlow see *Draba*
Witch see *Panicum capillare*
Wood see *Sorghastrum nutans*
Woolly foxtail see *Alopecurus lanatus*
Yellow whitlow see *Draba aizoides*
Zebra see *Miscanthus sinensis* 'Zebrinus'

▷**Grasses** see p.54
▷**Grass of Parnassus** see *Parnassia, P. palustris*
▷**Grass plant, Mexican** see *Dasylirion longissimum*
▷**Grass widow** see *Olsynium douglasii*
▷**Grassy bells** see *Edraianthus*

GREVILLEA

PROTEACEAE

Genus of at least 250 species of evergreen shrubs and trees, most native to Australia, a few native to Indonesia, New Guinea, and New Caledonia, found in woodland, rainforest, and more open habitats. The alternate leaves vary greatly and may be needle-like or broader, pinnatifid, pinnatisect, or pinnate, and boldly toothed. The petalless flowers, 0.5–2cm (¼–¾in) long, each consist of a coloured calyx tube that splits into 4 narrow, rolled-back, petal-like lobes, and long, straight or curved styles. The flowers are produced in simple or branched, terminal racemes or panicles, some one-sided, others cylindrical or feathery. In frost-prone areas, grow in a cool or temperate greenhouse, or conservatory. Elsewhere, use as specimen plants or in a shrub border. All parts may aggravate skin allergies.

• **HARDINESS** Frost hardy to frost tender; some will survive to -7°C (19°F) if wood is well ripened in summer.

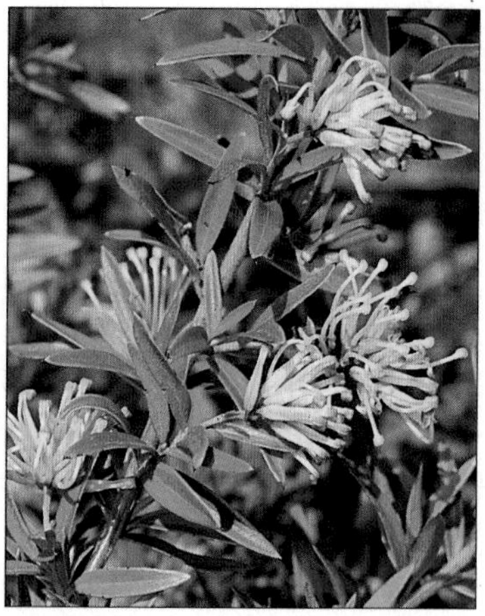

Grevillea 'Austraflora Canterbury Gold'

• **CULTIVATION** Under glass, grow in lime-free (ericaceous) compost, with added grit, in full light. Top-dress or pot on in spring. During the growing season, water freely and apply a low-phosphate liquid fertilizer monthly. Water sparingly in winter. Outdoors, grow in acid to neutral, moderately fertile soil in full sun. Pruning group 1; may need restrictive pruning under glass.

• **PROPAGATION** Sow scarified or pre-soaked seed at 13–18°C (55–64°F) in spring (only *G. robusta* germinates easily). Take semi-ripe cuttings in summer. Graft in winter under glass, or in late summer outdoors.

• **PESTS AND DISEASES** Trouble free.

G. acanthifolia. Sometimes untidy shrub with wide-spreading, prostrate and ascending branches. The oblong-elliptic, glossy, deep green leaves, to 12cm (5in) long, are pinnatisect, with each segment divided into 3–5 spine-tipped lobes. Purplish pink flowers are borne in one-sided, toothbrush-like racemes, 5–10cm (2–4in) long, mainly from spring to autumn. ↕ 0.3–3m (1–10ft), ↔ 2–5m (6–15ft). Australia (New South Wales). ✻

G. alpestris see *G. alpina.*

G. alpina, syn. *G. alpestris.* Prostrate to erect shrub of open habit with linear to broadly elliptic leaves, 1–3cm (½–1¼in) long, deep green to grey-green, sometimes glossy above, paler and hairy beneath. The flowers, borne in short, dense racemes, to 3cm (1¼in) long, range from pink, red, orange, or yellow to cream or pale green, and are borne

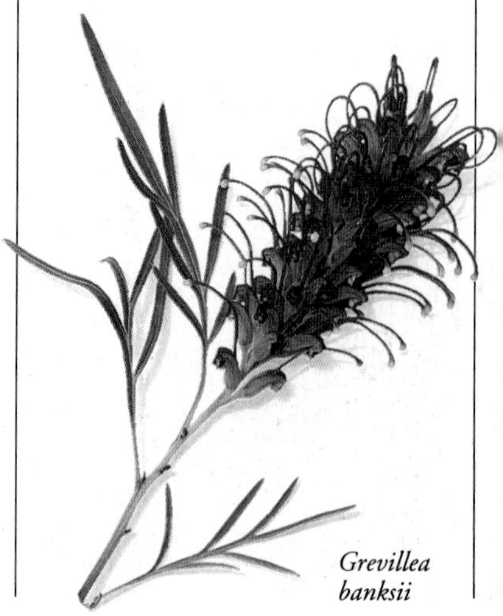

Grevillea banksii

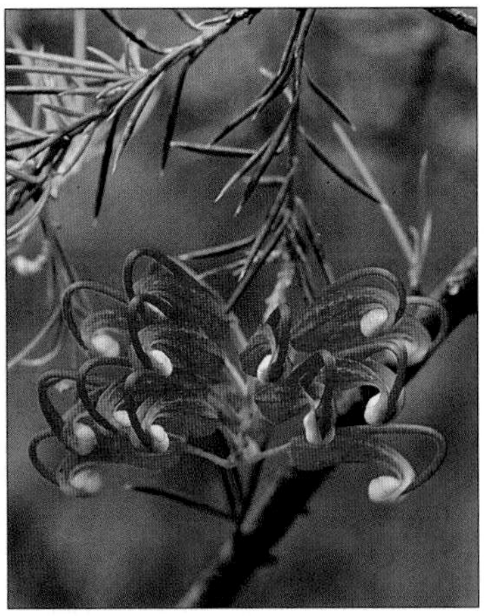

Grevillea 'Canberra Gem'

almost all year round. ↕ to 2m (6ft), ↔ 0.6–2m (2–6ft). Australia (mountain slopes and heathland in New South Wales and Victoria). ✻✻. **'Olympic Flame'** is compact and rounded, with small, sharply pointed, deep green leaves, to 2cm (¾in) long; it produces an abundance of slightly pendulous, dense racemes, 6cm (2½in) long, of bicoloured, red-pink and cream flowers; ↕↔ 1–2m (3–6ft).

G. aspleniifolia. Erect to spreading shrub with reddish green young growth, and linear-lance-shaped, usually entire leaves, 18–30cm (7–12in) long, deep green above and greenish white or sometimes fawn-felted beneath. Deep red and green flowers are produced in one-sided, toothbrush-like racemes, 5cm (2in) long, from the upper leaf axils and shoot tips, mainly from late winter to early summer and again in autumn. ↕ 3–5m (10–15ft), ↔ 6m (20ft). Australia (New South Wales). ✻

***G.* 'Austraflora Canterbury Gold'** ▣ Prostrate to low-arching or more upright shrub with lance-shaped, divided leaves, 4–6cm (1½–2½in) long, light green above, with dense, silky hairs beneath. Pale yellow flowers in pendent, one-sided racemes, to 6cm (2½in) long, are produced mainly from late winter to late summer. ↕ 0.6–2m (2–6ft), ↔ 2–4m (6–12ft). ✻✻

G. banksii ▣ ♀ Large, open, strongly branched shrub or small tree, sometimes prostrate and mat-forming. Ovate, pinnate, or deeply pinnatifid leaves, 15–25cm (6–10in) long, with long, narrow lobes, are deep green above, silky-hairy or rust-red-hairy beneath.

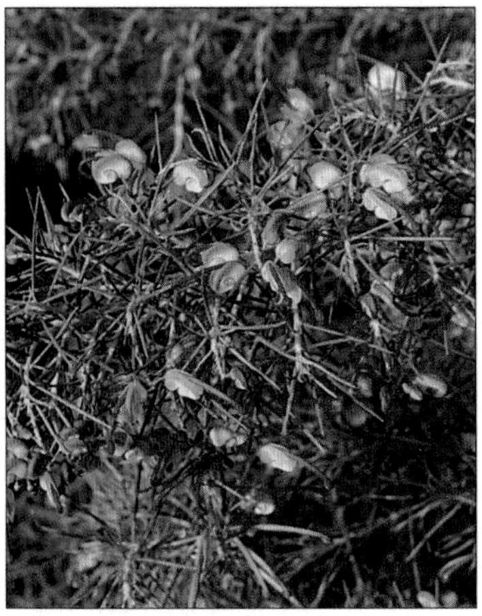

Grevillea juniperina

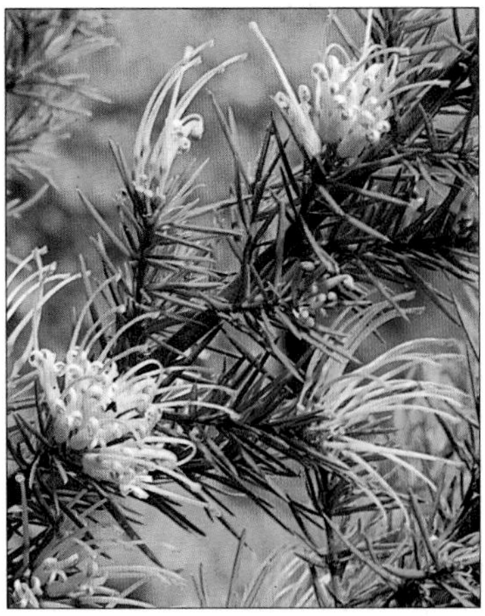

Grevillea juniperina f. *sulphurea*

Bears red, pink, or creamy white flowers in erect, cylindrical racemes, 8–18cm (3–7in) long, mostly from late winter to spring, but also at other times. ↕ 1–10m (3–30ft), ↔ 2–5m (6–15ft). Australia (Queensland). ✻

***G.* 'Canberra Gem'** ▣ 🏆 Vigorous, bushy shrub with densely silky-hairy stems, and crowded, linear leaves, 3cm (1¼in) long, each tipped with a hard point, and rich green above, silky-hairy beneath. Produces short, dense racemes, to 5cm (2in) long, of waxy, pinkish red flowers, mainly from late winter to late summer, but also at other times. ↕ 2–4m (6–12ft), ↔ 2–5m (6–15ft). ✻✻

***G.* 'Clearview David'.** Fast-growing, bushy shrub with densely borne, often clustered, linear leaves, 3cm (1¼in) long, each tipped with a hard point, and deep green above, silky-hairy below. At any time of the year, bears large, spider-like racemes, to 7cm (3in) long, of deep red flowers at the tips of all short lateral shoots. ↕ 2–3m (6–10ft), ↔ 2–4m (6–12ft). ✻✻

G. juniperina ▣ Prostrate to upright-branched, dense, rounded shrub with crowded, often clustered, narrowly lance-shaped to narrowly linear, mid-green to grey-green leaves, 1–2cm (½–¾in) long. Greenish yellow to red flowers are borne in pendent racemes, to 6cm (2½in) long, from late spring to midsummer. ↕ 2m (6ft), ↔ 1m (3ft). Australia (New South Wales). ✻✻. **'Molonglo'** has apricot flowers, and is vigorous and low-spreading; ↕ to 1m (3ft). **'Prostrate Yellow'** is mat-forming, with very dark foliage and lemon-yellow flowers; ↕ 30–60m (12–24in), ↔ 3–5m (10–15ft). ✻. **f. *sulphurea*** ▣ 🏆 syn. *G. sulphurea*, has many-branched, arching stems, and yellow flowers; ↕ 1.5–2m (5–6ft), ↔ 2–3m (6–10ft).

***G.* 'Kentlyn'** see *G.* 'Mason's Hybrid'.

G. lanigera. Usually dwarf to medium-sized, many-branched, rounded shrub, sometimes mat-forming. Bears crowded, linear to narrowly oblong, hairy, mid-green to greyish green leaves, 1–3cm (½–1¼in) long, with margins rolled under. Produces umbel-like, semi-erect racemes, to 6cm (2½in) wide, of light red and cream or green and cream flowers from autumn to summer. ↕ prostrate to 3m (10ft), ↔ 1.5–5m (5–15ft). Australia (New South Wales, Victoria). ✻✻. **'Clearview John'** has lime-green and cream flowers; ↕ 60–90cm (24–36in), ↔ 0.9–1.5m (3–5ft). **'Compacta'**, syn. 'Mt. Tamboritha', 'Prostrate', is spreading, dwarf, and bushy, with pinkish red and cream flowers; ↕ 60–100cm (24–39in). **'Mt. Tamboritha'** see 'Compacta'. **'Prostrate'** see 'Compacta'.

G. lavandulacea. Very variable, sometimes suckering, many-branched, spreading to erect or arching to cascading shrub. Linear to elliptic, sometimes clustered, mid-green to grey-green leaves, to 3.5cm (1½in) long, are prickle-tipped, with recurved margins. Bears many umbel-like racemes, to 6cm (2½in) long, of red to pale pink, red and cream, pink and cream or, more rarely, entirely cream flowers; they appear from late winter to early summer and late summer to autumn. ↕ prostrate to 2m (6ft), ↔ 1–3m (3–10ft). Australia (New South Wales, Victoria). ✻✻. **'Adelaide Hills'** is dwarf, with elliptic leaves and light red flowers; ↕ to 1.2m (4ft). **'Tanunda'** is low and spreading, with greyish green leaves and bright reddish pink flowers; ↕ 60–100cm (24–39in).

***G.* 'Mason's Hybrid'**, syn. *G.* 'Kentlyn', *G.* 'Ned Kelly'. Spreading shrub, tending to open out from the centre, with 2-pinnate, stiffly arching leaves, 12–18cm (5–7in) long, deep green and semi-lustrous above, paler and matt beneath. Cylindrical to almost one-sided racemes, 12–15cm (5–6in) long, of orange-red flowers, becoming pink-tinged with age, with deep pink styles and yellow stigmas, are produced intermittently through the year. ↕ 1–2m (2–6ft), ↔ 50–150cm (20–60in). ✻✻

***G.* 'Ned Kelly'** see *G.* 'Mason's Hybrid'.

***G.* 'Poorinda Constance'** ▣ Erect to spreading, bushy shrub bearing oblong to elliptic, sharp-tipped leaves, 3cm (1¼in) long, deep green above, paler and silky-hairy beneath, the margins rolled under. Short, dense, spider-like racemes, to 8cm (3in) long, of bright orange-red flowers with darker styles, are produced mainly from late autumn to summer. ↕ 2–3m (6–10ft), ↔ 2–5m (6–15ft). ✻✻

***G.* 'Poorinda Golden Lyre'.** Bushy, slow-growing shrub with silky-hairy shoots. Produces narrowly oblong to elliptic leaves, 3cm (1¼in) long, glossy, deep green above, paler and silky-hairy beneath, with margins rolled under. Red, orange, or yellow flowers are borne in pendent, spider-like racemes, to 4cm (1½in) across, from autumn to summer. ↕↔ 1–2m (3–6ft). ✻

***G.* 'Poorinda Queen'.** Freely branching shrub, the stems ascending to spreading. The elliptic leaves, 3–4cm (1¼–1½in) long, with firm, pointed tips, are glossy, deep green above, densely silky-hairy beneath. Bears pendent, congested racemes, 7cm (3in) across, of apricot-pink flowers with deep pink styles, mainly from late summer to late autumn. ↕ 3–4m (10–12ft), ↔ 3–5m (10–15ft). ✻

G. robusta 🏆 ♀ (Silky oak). Fast-growing, upright to conical tree, usually developing an open, elongated crown, but sometimes becoming more spreading. The fern-like leaves, 15–30cm (6–12in) long, are ovate and deeply pinnate or 2-pinnate, and bronze to deep green above, paler with silky hairs beneath. Erect, bright orange-yellow or golden yellow flowers are produced in horizontal, one-sided racemes, 10–15cm (4–6in) long, from late spring to summer. ↕ 15–35m (50–120ft), ↔ 5–20m (15–70ft). Australia (Queensland, New South Wales). ❀ (min. 5°C/41°F)

***G.* 'Robyn Gordon'.** Many-branched, spreading shrub, thinning out from the centre with age. Stiffly arching, 2-pinnate leaves, 15–20cm (6–8in) long, are deep green and semi-lustrous above, paler and matt beneath. Cylindrical to almost one-sided racemes, 10–13cm (4–5in) long, of rich reddish pink flowers, ageing to a lighter pink, with bright red styles and stigmas, are produced intermittently throughout the year. Foliage may cause skin rashes. ↕ 1–1.5m (3–5ft), ↔ 50–150cm (20–60in). ✻

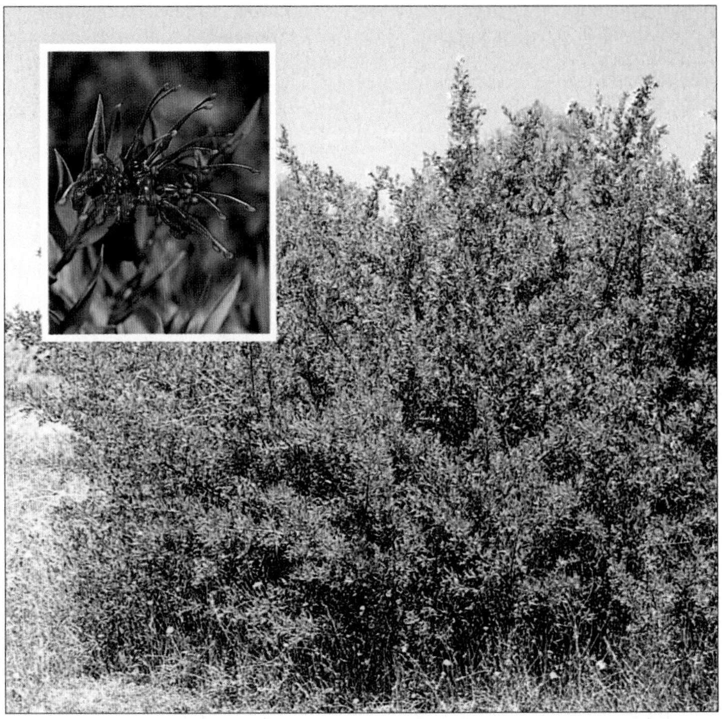

Grevillea 'Poorinda Constance' (inset: flower detail)

G

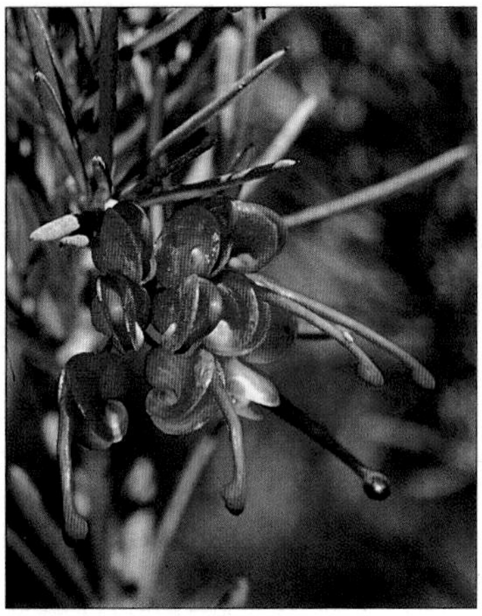
Grevillea rosmarinifolia

G. rosmarinifolia ■ ♀ Many-branched shrub with ascending to spreading, sometimes arching stems, and silky-hairy young growth. Crowded or clustered leaves, 1–4cm (½–1½in) long, are linear to narrowly elliptic or lance-shaped, with margins rolled under, often prickle-tipped, and greyish green to deep green above, paler and silky-downy beneath. Bears spider-like racemes, 4–7cm (1½–3in) long, of pink to light red or cream flowers, mainly from late autumn to early summer. Good for hedging. ↕ 0.5–3m (20–120in), ↔ 1–5m (3–15ft). Australia (New South Wales, Victoria). **
G. 'Sandra Gordon' ◊ Strong-growing, large shrub or small tree, becoming spreading and open unless pruned regularly. The pinnate, ovate leaves, 16–25cm (6–10in) long, with linear leaflets, to 7cm (3in) long, are bronze to silvery when young, maturing to deep green above, and silver-hairy beneath. Bright yellow flowers are produced in one-sided to almost cylindrical racemes, 8–14cm (3–5½in) long, throughout the year, mainly from summer to autumn (winter to spring in Australia). ↕ 3–6m (10–20ft), ↔ 2–3.5m (6–11ft). *
G. sulphurea see *G. juniperina* f. *sulphurea*.
G. 'White Wings'. Strong-growing, dense shrub with spreading to ascending, sometimes arching branches. Bears broadly ovate to rounded, pinnate, light green leaves, 4cm (1½in) long, with numerous slender, linear leaflets with recurved margins and prickle points. Produces terminal and axillary, erect, loose racemes, to 2.5cm (1in) long, of fragrant white flowers, intermittently throughout the year. ↕ 2–3.5m (6–11ft), ↔ 3–5m (10–15ft). *

GREWIA

TILIACEAE

Genus of approximately 150 species of deciduous and evergreen trees, shrubs, and climbers from Africa, S. and E. Asia, and Australia, found in habitats ranging from tropical woodland to dry, open savannah. The alternate leaves are simple and entire or toothed, with persistent stipules. The small, 5-petalled flowers have central bosses of many stamens, and may be borne singly or in small, terminal or axillary cymes. In frost-prone areas, grow half-hardy and frost-tender species in a temperate greenhouse. In warmer climates, grewias are suitable for growing as specimens or in shrub plantings.
• **HARDINESS** Frost hardy to frost tender.
• **CULTIVATION** Under glass, grow in loam-based potting compost (JI No.3) in full light. Top-dress or pot on in spring. Water freely from spring to autumn, applying a balanced liquid fertilizer monthly. Water sparingly in winter. Outdoors, grow in fertile, moist but well-drained soil in full sun. Pruning group 1; may need restrictive pruning under glass.
• **PROPAGATION** Sow seed at 16–18°C (61–64°F), or layer, in spring.
• **PESTS AND DISEASES** Whiteflies and red spider mites may infest plants under glass.

G. occidentalis ◊ (Four corners). Evergreen shrub, scandent climber, or small tree with slender, erect to spreading branches and shoots covered with soft, star-like hairs. The leaves are ovate-diamond-shaped to lance-shaped, 2–8cm (¾–3in) long, with rounded teeth, and hairless or softly hairy. In summer, bears small, stalked, axillary cymes of flowers, 3cm (1¼in) across, with pink sepals and mauve to purple or white petals; they are followed by fleshy, 4-lobed, yellowish orange, then purple fruit, 2.5cm (1in) across. ↕ 2–6m (6–20ft), ↔ 1.5–4m (5–12ft). Southern Africa. ❁ (min. 7°C/45°F)

GREYIA

GREYIACEAE

Genus of 3 species of evergreen shrubs or small trees from South Africa, found in habitats ranging from slopes and rocky places to savannah. They are grown for their showy, 5-petalled flowers, which are borne in terminal racemes. The simple leaves are broadly ovate to rounded, alternate or spiralling, and generally clustered at the stem tips. In frost-prone areas, grow in a cool greenhouse. In warm climates, plant at the base of a house wall or in a shrub border.
• **HARDINESS** Frost tender, although *G. sutherlandii* will withstand very short periods near 0°C (32°F).
• **CULTIVATION** Under glass, grow in loam-based potting compost (JI No.3), with added sharp sand, in full light. Top-dress or pot on in spring. Water freely from spring to autumn, applying a balanced liquid fertilizer monthly. Water sparingly in winter. Outdoors, grow in fertile, moist but well-drained soil in full sun. Pruning group 8; may need restrictive pruning under glass.
• **PROPAGATION** Sow seed at 13–16°C (55–61°F), or air layer, in spring.
• **PESTS AND DISEASES** Red spider mites may be troublesome under glass.

G. sutherlandii ■ ◊ (Natal bottlebrush). Evergreen, large shrub or small tree of open, stiff habit, with rounded to heart-shaped, irregularly toothed, leathery, mid-green leaves, 5–10cm (2–4in) long. Old leaves often turn bright red before falling. Tubular-bell-shaped, crimson to brick-red flowers, 2cm (¾in) long, with long stamens, are borne in racemes, 10–15cm (4–6in) long, in spring, just before or with the newly expanding leaves. ↕ 2–5m (6–15ft), ↔ 1.5–3m (5–10ft). South Africa (KwaZulu/Natal). * (borderline)

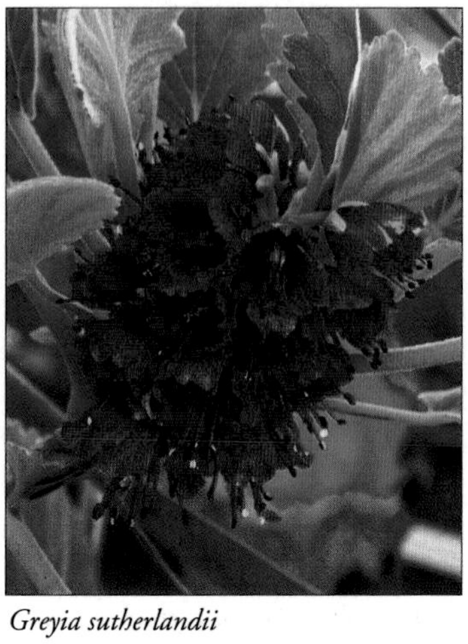
Greyia sutherlandii

GRINDELIA

Gum plant, Rosinweed, Tarweed

ASTERACEAE/COMPOSITAE

Genus of about 60 species of annuals, evergreen, frequently woody-based perennials, and some subshrubs from sunny, dry, often rocky habitats in North, Central, and South America. They are cultivated for their daisy-like, bright yellow flowerheads, borne singly or in corymbs, which often glisten with sticky white resin in bud. The stems and the simple, alternate, entire or toothed, sometimes stalkless leaves are also usually sticky. Suitable for a sunny border, wild garden, or hot, dry bank.
• **HARDINESS** Fully hardy to frost hardy.
• **CULTIVATION** Grow in full sun in poor to moderately fertile, well-drained soil. Remove frost-damaged growth in spring.
• **PROPAGATION** Sow seed in containers in a cold frame in spring. Root semi-ripe cuttings in summer.
• **PESTS AND DISEASES** Trouble free.

G. chiloensis ■ syn. *G. speciosa*. Bushy, evergreen subshrub with stout, upright shoots and mostly basal, inversely lance-shaped to obovate, entire or toothed, greyish green leaves, to 12cm (5in) long. Bears large, bright yellow flowerheads, 7cm (3in) across, singly on long stalks, throughout summer. ↕↔ 1m (3ft). Argentina, Chile. *** (borderline)
G. integrifolia. Erect, woody-based perennial producing several stems with stalkless, lance-shaped to inversely lance-shaped, usually toothed leaves, 35cm (14in) long. Bright yellow flowerheads, 2.5–4cm (1–1½in) across, are borne singly or in corymbs to 12cm (5in) across, from midsummer to early autumn. ↕ to 80cm (32in), ↔ 60cm (24in). W. North America. ***
G. speciosa see *G. chiloensis*.
G. stricta (Pacific grindelia). Clump-forming perennial with both decumbent and upright stems, producing oblong to inversely lance-shaped, entire to minutely toothed leaves, to 25cm (10in) long. Bears solitary, bright yellow flowerheads, to 5cm (2in) across, from midsummer to early autumn. ↕ to 90cm (36in), ↔ 60cm (24in). W. North America. ***

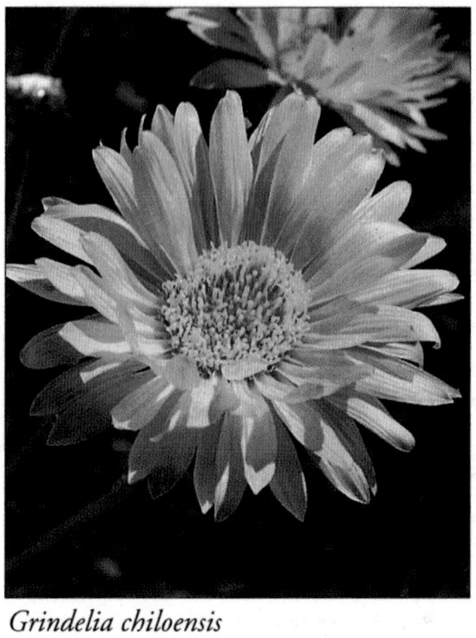
Grindelia chiloensis

GRISELINIA

CORNACEAE/GRISELINIACEAE

Genus of 6 species of dioecious, evergreen shrubs and trees from the forests and coasts of New Zealand and South America. Grown for their handsome, simple, alternate, leathery leaves, they also bear inconspicuous, yellow-green flowers in late spring. In autumn, they produce purple fruits if plants of both sexes are present. Grow as specimen plants for a shrub border or as hedging; ideal as windbreaks in coastal regions. In frost-prone areas, grow half-hardy plants in a cool greenhouse.
• **HARDINESS** Mostly frost hardy or half hardy; *G. littoralis* will withstand temperatures down to -12°C (10°F).
• **CULTIVATION** Under glass, grow in loam-based potting compost (JI No.3), with added sharp sand, in full light. In growth, water moderately and apply a balanced liquid fertilizer monthly; water sparingly in winter. Outdoors, grow in light, fertile, well-drained soil in full sun, with shelter from cold, drying winds. Pruning group 9; may need restrictive pruning under glass.
• **PROPAGATION** Sow seed at 13–18°C (55–64°F) in spring. Take semi-ripe cuttings in summer.
• **PESTS AND DISEASES** Susceptible to fungal leaf spot.

G. littoralis ♀ ◊ (Broadleaf). Vigorous, dense, upright shrub (or tree in very mild areas) producing broadly ovate to ovate-oblong, glossy, leathery, bright apple-green leaves, to 10cm (4in) long. ↕ to 8m (25ft), ↔ 5m (15ft). New Zealand. *** (borderline). **'Dixon's Cream'** ■ bears leaves boldly marked in the centre with creamy white; ↕ 3m

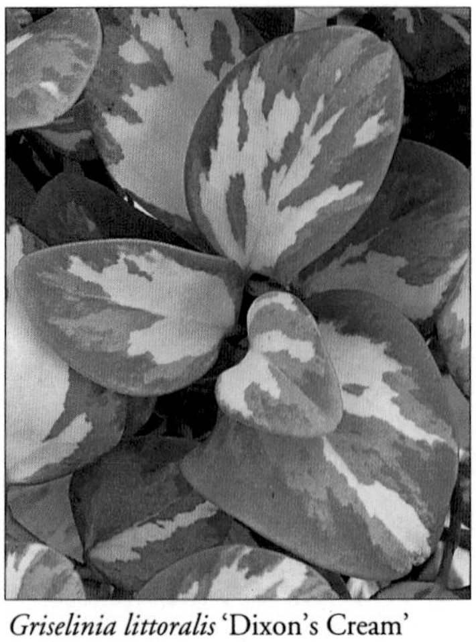
Griselinia littoralis 'Dixon's Cream'

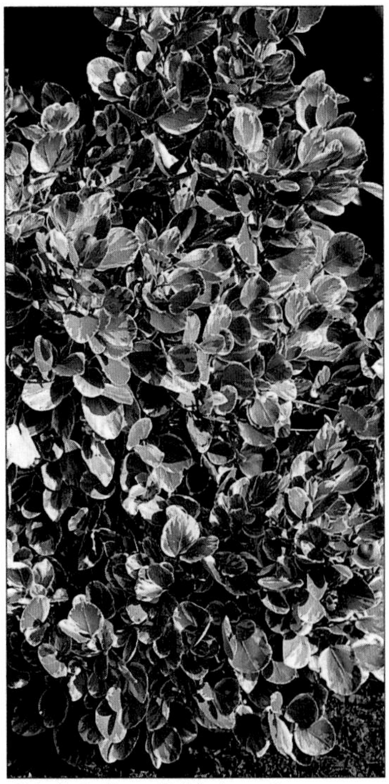

Griselinia littoralis 'Variegata'

(10ft), ↔ 2m (6ft). **'Variegata'** ■ produces leaves irregularly margined creamy white and streaked grey-green; ↕ 3m (10ft), ↔ 2m (6ft).
G. lucida. Vigorous, upright shrub with broadly ovate, leathery, glossy, mid-green leaves, very unequal at the bases, to 18cm (7in) long. ↕ 6m (20ft), ↔ 5m (15ft). New Zealand. ✻

▷**Ground elder** see *Aegopodium*, *A. podagraria* 'Variegatum'
▷**Ground ivy, Variegated** see *Glechoma hederacea* 'Variegata'
▷**Groundsel,**
Bush see *Baccharis halimifolia*
Chinese see *Senecio tanguticus*
Golden see *Ligularia dentata*
▷**Guava,**
Chilean see *Ugni molinae*
Pineapple see *Acca sellowiana*
▷**Guayiga** see *Zamia pumila*
▷**Guelder rose** see *Viburnum opulus*
▷***Guillauminia albiflora*** see *Aloe albiflora*
▷**Gum** see *Eucalyptus*
Alpine snow see *Eucalyptus pauciflora* subsp. *niphophila*
Black see *Nyssa sylvatica*
Blue see *Eucalyptus leucoxylon*
Brittle see *Eucalyptus mannifera* subsp. *maculosa*
Cabbage see *Eucalyptus pauciflora*
Cider see *Eucalyptus gunnii*
Kybean see *Eucalyptus parvifolia*
Manna see *Eucalyptus viminalis*
Mountain see *Eucalyptus dalrympleana*
Oriental sweet see *Liquidambar orientalis*
Powdered see *Eucalyptus pulverulenta*
Red-flowering see *Eucalyptus ficifolia*
Red river see *Eucalyptus camaldulensis*
Ribbon see *Eucalyptus viminalis*
Round-leaved snow see *Eucalyptus perriniana*
Silver dollar see *Eucalyptus polyanthemos*

▷**Gum cont.**
Silver-leaved mountain see *Eucalyptus pulverulenta*
Small-leaved see *Eucalyptus parviflora*
Snow see *Eucalyptus pauciflora* subsp. *niphophila*
Sour see *Nyssa sylvatica*
Spinning see *Eucalyptus perriniana*
Sweet see *Liquidambar styraciflua*
Tasmanian blue see *Eucalyptus globulus*
Tasmanian snow see *Eucalyptus coccifera*
Tasmanian yellow see *Eucalyptus johnstonii*
Tingiringi see *Eucalyptus glaucescens*
Urn see *Eucalyptus urnigera*
Urn-fruited see *Eucalyptus urnigera*
Weeping see *Eucalyptus pauciflora*
White see *Eucalyptus viminalis*
Wolgan snow see *Eucalyptus gregsoniana*
Yellow see *Eucalyptus leucoxylon*
▷**Gum plant** see *Grindelia*

GUNNERA

GUNNERACEAE/HALORAGIDACEAE

Genus of about 45 species of summer-flowering, rhizomatous, herbaceous or evergreen perennials from moist areas in southern Africa, Australasia, and South America. Gunneras vary in size from diminutive and mat-forming to extremely large and clump-forming with massive leaves. They are cultivated primarily for their handsome foliage, although in some species the flower spikes and fruits are also attractive.

The leaves are rounded to ovate, often heart-shaped, lobed, and usually toothed. The tiny, usually greenish yellow flowers are produced in dense, upright, brush-like spikes or panicles; the basal flowers are normally female, the uppermost male, with those in between sometimes bisexual. A few species are dioecious. Large species are excellent architectural plants for the edge of a pond or stream, or a bog garden, while smaller ones are suitable for a rock garden or an alpine house.

• **HARDINESS** Fully hardy to frost hardy. Most fully hardy species are not reliably cold-tolerant below about -12°C (10°F).

• **CULTIVATION** Grow in deep, permanently moist, humus-rich soil in sun or partial shade. Large species need shelter from cold, drying winds. Small species prefer partial shade, but are best in full sun in areas with cool summers.

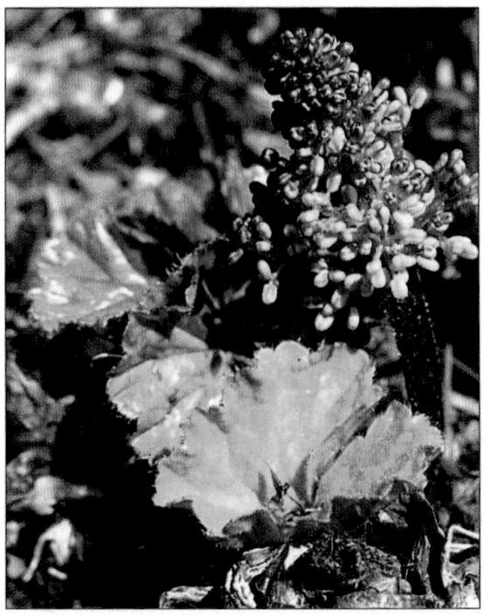

Gunnera magellanica

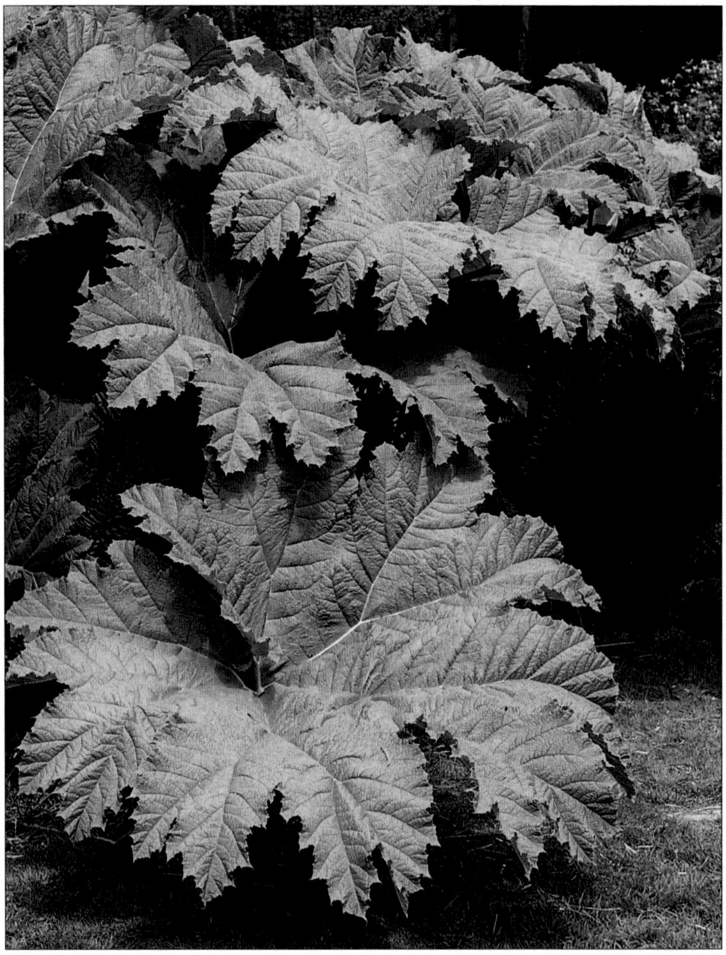

Gunnera manicata

In frost-prone climates, protect the crowns of large species in winter with a dry mulch.

• **PROPAGATION** Sow seed in containers as soon as ripe, and keep cool but frost-free through the winter; germination is slow. Seed quickly loses viability. Large species may also be increased by taking cuttings of leafy, basal buds in spring. Divide small species in spring.

• **PESTS AND DISEASES** Prone to slug and snail damage outdoors; under glass, may be susceptible to aphids and whiteflies.

G. brasiliensis see *G. manicata.*
G. chilensis see *G. tinctoria.*
G. hamiltonii. Compact, cushion-forming, evergreen perennial with triangular-ovate, scalloped, grey-green leaves, to 3cm (1¼in) long. In summer, produces insignificant green flowers in spikes to 5cm (2in) long, followed by ellipsoid red fruit, to 3mm (⅛in) long. ↕ 10cm (4in), ↔ 20cm (8in). New Zealand (coastal dunes on Stewart Island). ✻✻
G. magellanica ■ Mat-forming herbaceous perennial with cupped, kidney-shaped, scalloped, dark green leaves, 5–9cm (2–3½in) across, borne on upright stalks, 8–15cm (3–6in) long. In summer, bears compact panicles, 1.5–12cm (½–5in) long, of tiny green flowers, followed by ovoid to spherical, orange-red fruit, 5mm (¼in) across. ↕ 15cm (6in), ↔ 30cm (12in) or more. S. South America, Falkland Islands. ✻✻
G. manicata ■ ♀ syn. *G. brasiliensis.* Very large, clump-forming herbaceous perennial with rounded to kidney-shaped, palmately lobed, prominently veined, sharply toothed, deep green leaves, to 2m (6ft) long, borne on prickly stalks, to 2.5m (8ft) long. In early summer, branches 15cm (6in) long bear numerous tiny, greenish red flowers in conical, branched panicles, to 1m (3ft) or more tall; these are followed by spherical, red-green fruit, to 3mm (⅛in) long. ↕ 2.5m (8ft), ↔ 3–4m (10–12ft) or more. Colombia to Brazil. ✻✻✻ (borderline)
G. prorepens. Mat-forming herbaceous perennial with ovate, scalloped, short-stalked, purple-green leaves, to 3cm (1¼in) long. In summer, bears compact spikes, to 6cm (2½in) long, of insignificant green flowers, followed by dense, mulberry-like clusters of almost spherical, dark red fruit, to 4mm (⅛in) across. ↕ 10cm (4in), ↔ to 20cm (8in). Bogs and damp grassland in New Zealand. ✻✻✻ (borderline)
G. scabra see *G. tinctoria.*
G. tinctoria, syn. *G. chilensis*, *G. scabra.* Large, slowly spreading herbaceous perennial, forming a denser clump than *G. manicata.* Heart-shaped to rounded, deeply lobed, sharply toothed, deep green leaves, 1–2m (3–6ft) long, are borne on prickly stalks, to 1.5m (5ft) long. Cylindrical panicles, to 50cm (20in) tall, of numerous tiny, rusty red flowers, borne on straight branches, 10cm (4in) long, are produced from early to late summer. Spherical fruit, to 3mm (⅛in) long, are green, strongly suffused red. ↕ 1.5m (5ft), ↔ 2m (6ft). Chile. ✻✻

▷**Gutta-percha tree** see *Eucommia ulmoides*

GUZMANIA

BROMELIACEAE

Genus of over 120 species of virtually stemless, evergreen, mainly epiphytic perennials (bromeliads), found in the USA (S. Florida), Central America, the West Indies, and N. and W. South America. They occur mainly in the Andean rainforest, to 3,500m (11,500ft) high. The lance-shaped leaves form funnel-shaped rosettes, above or within which flowerheads of tubular, white or yellow flowers, usually surrounded by colourful floral bracts, are borne on conspicuous, yellow, orange, or bright red stems, in summer. Where temperatures drop below 15°C (59°F), grow in a warm greenhouse or as houseplants. In warmer areas, grow in shady, humid, moist areas of the garden.

• **HARDINESS** Frost tender.

• **CULTIVATION** Under glass, grow in epiphytic bromeliad compost in bright filtered or indirect light, or grow epiphytically on artificial tree branches. When in growth, mist daily with soft water, preferably in the early morning. In winter, keep barely moist and do not mist. Outdoors, attach to the branches of trees in partial shade. See also p.47.

• **PROPAGATION** Sow seed at 27°C (81°F), or remove offsets, in mid-spring.

• **PESTS AND DISEASES** Vulnerable to mealybugs.

G. dissitiflora. Stemless, stoloniferous, epiphytic bromeliad with rosettes of lance-shaped, mid-green leaves, 30–90cm (12–36in) long, with red-striped, pale green sheaths with dark brown bases. In summer, erect inflorescences of 7–15 flowers, to 3–4cm (1¼–1½in) long, with bright yellow sepals fused to form a tube, and flared white petals, are borne on short, erect stems among overlapping, bright red bracts. ↕↔ to 90cm (36in). Costa Rica, Panama, Colombia. ❀ (min. 15°C/59°F)

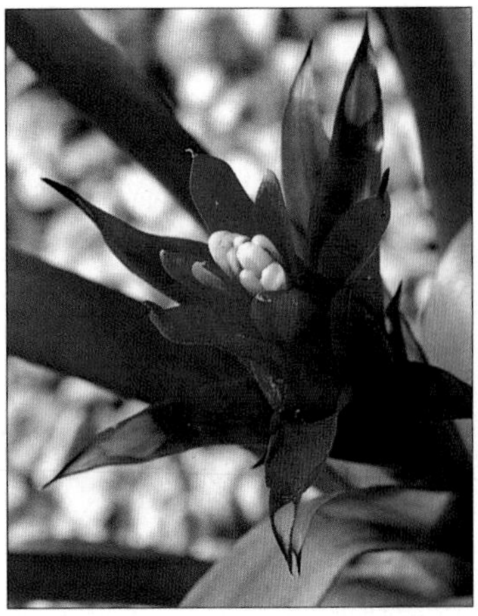

Guzmania lingulata var. *minor*

G. lingulata ▣ ♀ Variable, epiphytic bromeliad with rosettes of narrowly lance-shaped, sometimes red-violet-striped, deep green leaves, 45cm (18in) long, with sheaths brown-scaly beneath. In summer, erect stems produce overlapping, bright red, orange, or pink bracts, around loose corymbs of tubular, yellow-white flowers, 4.5cm (1¾in) long. ↕↔ 30–45cm (12–18in). N. Central America, West Indies to Brazil. ❀ (min. 15°C/59°F). **var. *minor*** ▣ ♀ has dark green sheaths and few-flowered inflorescences with bright red bracts; ↕↔ 23–30cm (9–12in); Central America (Guatemala), N. South America (Colombia to N.E. Brazil).

G. monostachia ▣ ♀ syn. *G. monostachya, G. tricolor.* Stemless, epiphytic bromeliad with dense rosettes of lance-shaped to strap-shaped, pale green or yellowish green leaves, to 40cm (16in) long. In summer, produces cylindrical inflorescences, to 15cm (6in) long, with pale green stem bracts and brown-black-striped green basal bracts. Tubular white flowers, 2.5–3cm (1–1¼in) long, are surrounded by bright red or white bracts. ↕↔ to 40cm (16in). USA (Florida), Central America, West Indies, W. and N. South America. ❀ (min. 15°C/59°F). **'Variegata'** has green- and white-striped leaves.

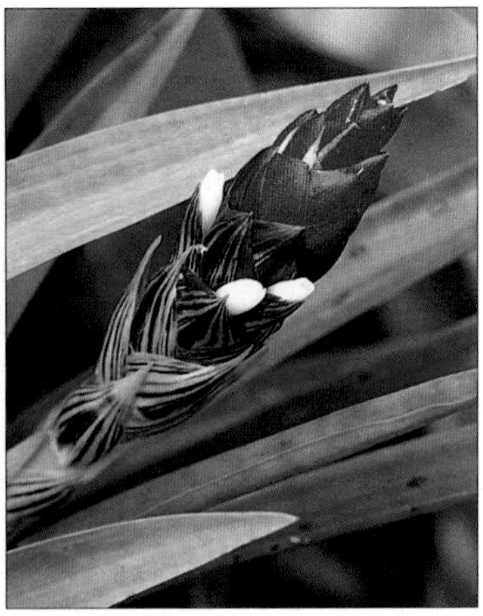

Guzmania monostachia

G. monostachya see *G. monostachia.*

G. musaica ▣ ♀ Stemless, epiphytic bromeliad with rosettes of broadly linear, outward-spreading, brown-sheathed, dark green leaves, to 70cm (28in) long; they are thinly banded with pale green, deep green, or reddish brown, and often flushed purple beneath. In summer, erect stems with overlapping, bright red or pink bracts produce almost spherical heads of rose-pink floral bracts and flowers, to 4.5cm (1¾in) long, with yellow sepals and yellowish white petals. ↕ to 50cm (20in), ↔ 70cm (28in). Panama, Colombia. ❀ (min. 15°C/59°F)

G. sanguinea ♀ Stemless, epiphytic bromeliad with almost flat rosettes of broadly lance-shaped, arching leaves, to 40cm (16in) long, sometimes spotted dark green, becoming suffused with yellow, red, and orange at flowering time. In summer, corymbs of tubular, yellow, greenish yellow, or white flowers, to 8cm (3in) long, with spreading petals and surrounded by red bracts, are borne within the leaf rosettes. Offsets freely. ↕ 20cm (8in), ↔ to 35cm (14in). Costa Rica, Trinidad, Tobago, Venezuela, Colombia, Ecuador. ❀ (min. 15°C/59°F)

G. tricolor see *G. monostachia.*

G. vittata. Stemless, epiphytic bromeliad with loose rosettes of erect, lance-shaped, deep green leaves, 40–60cm (16–24in) long, cross-banded with paler green and sometimes banded purple beneath. In summer, erect stems with overlapping, purple-spotted, pale green basal bracts produce compact, ovoid, branched inflorescences with short spikes of tubular white flowers, 2cm (¾in) or more long. ↕↔ 35–60cm (14–24in). S. and E. Colombia, N.W. Brazil. ❀ (min. 15°C/59°F)

G. wittmackii. Stemless, epiphytic bromeliad with rosettes of lance-shaped, dark green leaves, to 85cm (34in) long, with brown-scaly sheaths and minute scales. In summer, arching stems produce branched inflorescences with densely overlapping red bracts and few-flowered clusters of tubular white flowers, to 9cm (3½in) long. ↕ to 50cm (20in), ↔ 1.2m (4ft). S. Colombia, Ecuador. ❀ (min. 15°C/59°F)

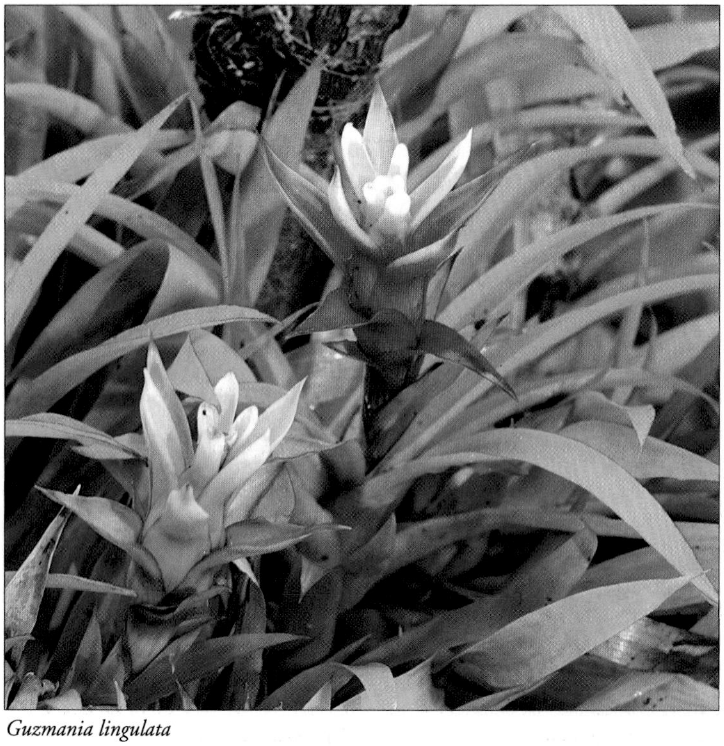

Guzmania lingulata

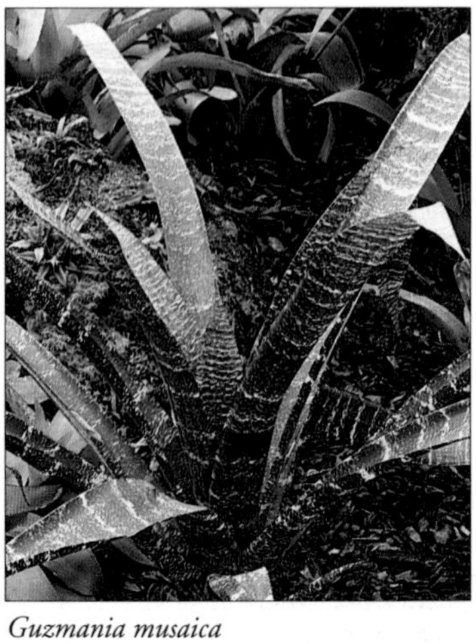

Guzmania musaica

GYMNOCALYCIUM

CACTACEAE

Genus of 50 or more species of spherical to cylindrical, perennial cacti from rocky scrub, hillsides, and grassland in Brazil, Bolivia, Paraguay, Argentina, and Uruguay. Most have prominently rounded, sometimes spiralling ribs, separated by diagonal grooves. Diurnal, funnel- to bell-shaped flowers are produced in early summer, usually from near the crowns or from the side areoles. Where temperatures drop below 10°C (50°F), grow in a warm greenhouse. In warmer climates, grow in a desert garden.

• **HARDINESS** Frost tender.

• **CULTIVATION** Under glass, grow in standard cactus compost in full light with shade from hot sun. Water freely in spring and summer, applying a low-nitrogen liquid fertilizer every 4 or 5 weeks. Keep dry in winter. Outdoors, grow in poor, sharply drained soil in full sun or partial shade. See also pp.48–49.

• **PROPAGATION** Sow seed at 19–24°C (66–75°F) in late winter or early spring. Remove offsets in spring.

• **PESTS AND DISEASES** Susceptible to mealybugs.

G. andreae ▣ ♀ Clustering cactus with spherical, glossy, dark blue-green or black-green stems, each with about 8 nearly flat, warty ribs. Tubercles are rounded, with a central areole bearing 7 thin, straight, spreading, brown-based white radial spines and 1–3 curved, dark brown centrals. Broadly funnel-shaped, bright yellow flowers, 4.5cm (1¾in) across, with yellow-green, darker-striped outer tepals, are borne in early summer. ↕ to 6cm (2½in), ↔ to 15cm (6in). N. Argentina. ❀ (min. 10°C/50°F)

G. bruchii. Clustering cactus with almost spherical, dark green stems, each with 12 low ribs with rounded, indistinct tubercles. Areoles each produce 10–17 white radial spines, sometimes brown at the base, and 1, occasionally 3, longer white to brown central spines. In early summer, bears funnel-shaped, sometimes faintly scented, pale pink flowers, to 4.5cm (1¾in) across, with dark pink mid-stripes outside. ↕ to 4cm (1½in), ↔ to 10cm (4in). N. Argentina. ❀ (min. 10°C/50°F)

G. gibbosum. Simple or offsetting cactus with spherical, later cylindrical, dark bluish green or brownish green stems, each with 12–19 rounded, notched ribs, small, prominent

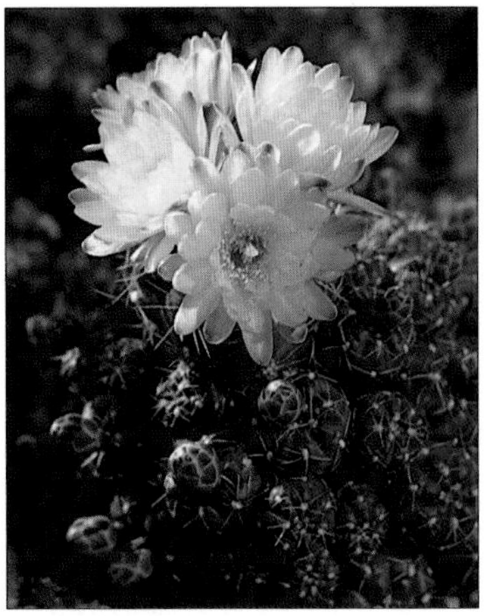

Gymnocalycium andreae

tubercules, and areoles producing pale brown, later grey spines (7–14 radials and up to 3 centrals). Funnel-shaped flowers, to 7cm (3in) across, pure white or with pale pink mid-stripes on the outsides of the outer tepals, are borne in early summer. ↕ 20cm (8in), ↔ 15cm (6in). Argentina. ❄ (min. 10°C/50°F)
***G. mihanovichii* 'Red Head'** ■ syn. *G. mihanovichii* 'Hibotan', *G. mihanovichii* 'Red Cap'. Perennial cactus producing spherical, flat-topped red stems, each with about 8 prominent, scarcely warty ribs. Areoles bear curved, pinkish white spines (3–5 radials and no centrals). Funnel-shaped pink flowers, to 5cm (2in) across, are borne in early summer. Lacks chlorophyll and survives only by being grafted on to robust stock plants of *Hylocereus*. ↕ to 12cm (5in) (grafted), ↔ 6cm (2½in). ❄ (min. 10°C/50°F)
G. quehlianum 🏆 Variable cactus with flat-topped, spherical, greyish green stems, bronzing in sun, each with 8–15 ribs divided into prominent, rounded tubercles. Areoles bear pale brown spines (2–5 or more radials and no centrals). Funnel-shaped white flowers, 3–5cm (1¼–2in) across, often pinkish red in the throats, are borne in early summer. ↕ 5cm (2in), ↔ 7cm (3in). N. Argentina. ❄ (min. 10°C/50°F)
G. saglionis ■ Perennial cactus with flat-topped, spherical, green or bluish green stems with 10–30 or more ribs bearing prominent, rounded tubercles. Areoles produce red-brown to yellow spines (7–15 radials and about 3 centrals). Broadly funnel-shaped flowers, 2cm (¾in) across, with pinkish white inner tepals and pale green, pink-flushed

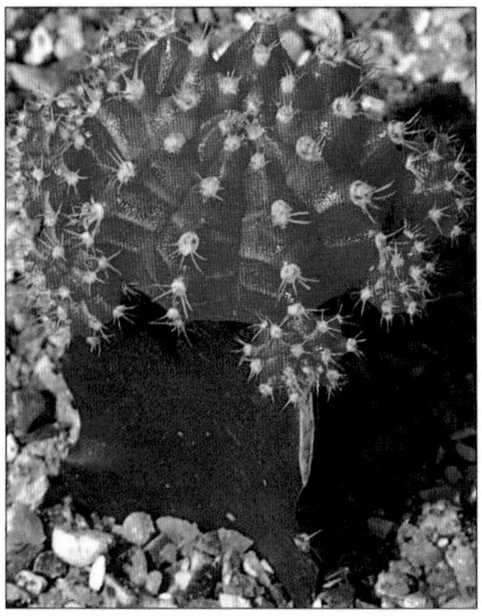

Gymnocalycium mihanovichii 'Red Head'

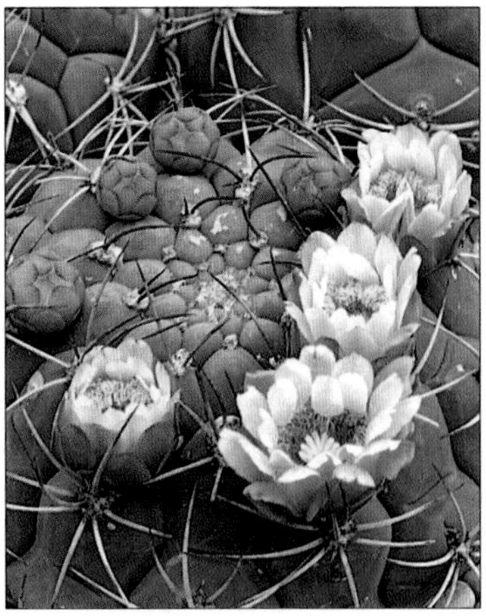

Gymnocalycium saglionis

outer tepals, are borne in early summer. ↕ 10cm (4in), ↔ to 30cm (12in). N.W. Argentina. ❄ (min. 10°C/50°F)
G. schickendantzii. Flat-topped, spherical cactus with 7- to 14-ribbed, dark green stems, bronzing in full sun. Areoles bear grey-red to pale brown, often darker tipped spines (5–7 radials and no centrals). Funnel-shaped, white to red flowers, to 2cm (¾in) across, with olive-green, often red-tinged outer tepals, are borne in early summer. ↕↔ 10cm (4in). N. Argentina. ❄ (min. 10°C/50°F)

GYMNOCARPIUM

DRYOPTERIDACEAE/WOODSIACEAE

Genus of about 5 species of deciduous, rhizomatous, terrestrial ferns found in moist woodland throughout the N. hemisphere. Fronds, arising singly from long, creeping rhizomes in spring, are triangular and 2- or 3-pinnate or pinnatifid, with leaf-blades that tilt at right-angles to the light. Small, rounded sori form on the undersides of the fronds, without protective indusia. Ideal for ground cover in moist, shady places.
- **HARDINESS** Fully hardy.
- **CULTIVATION** Grow in preferably neutral to acid, leafy, moist soil, enriched with garden compost before planting, in deep shade.
- **PROPAGATION** Sow spores at 15°C (59°F) when ripe, or divide in spring. See also p.51.
- **PESTS AND DISEASES** Trouble free.

G. dryopteris 🏆 (Oak fern). Deciduous fern bearing very distinctive, triangular, 3-pinnate fronds, each with a leaf-blade 10–18cm (4–7in) long and across, on a stem 10cm (4in) long. Pinnae are triangular, divided into oblong to ovate, toothed and scalloped segments. Pale yellowish green when young, the fronds darken to vivid rich green with age. ↕ 20cm (8in), ↔ indefinite. Europe, Turkey, N. Asia, China, Japan, Canada, USA. ❄❄❄. **'Plumosum'** has broader, overlapping pinnae.
G. robertianum (Limestone polypody). Rhizomatous, deciduous, spreading fern with dull, dark green, broadly triangular, 3-pinnate fronds, to 35cm (14in) long, on stems to 15cm (6in) long. Pinnae are oblong to narrowly triangular, divided into oblong, entire or finely toothed segments. ↕ to 35cm (14in), ↔ indefinite. Eurasia, North America. ❄❄❄

GYMNOCLADUS

CAESALPINACEAE/LEGUMINOSAE

Genus of 4 species of dioecious, deciduous trees from rich woodland in E. Asia and North America. They are cultivated for their spreading habit and for their large, 2-pinnate leaves, borne alternately. The small, greenish white flowers, borne in terminal panicles, are likely to be produced only in areas with prolonged temperatures above 24°C (75°F). They are best grown as specimen trees.
- **HARDINESS** Fully hardy to frost tender.
- **CULTIVATION** Grow in deep, fertile, moist but well-drained soil in full sun. Pruning group 1.
- **PROPAGATION** Sow seed in containers in a cold frame in autumn, after nicking or soaking. Take root cuttings in winter.
- **PESTS AND DISEASES** Trouble free.

G. dioica 🌳 (Kentucky coffee tree). Slow-growing, spreading, deciduous tree with large, 2-pinnate leaves, to 1m (3ft) long, each leaflet divided again into 8–14 ovate, softly hairy, dark green leaflets, pink-tinged when young, yellow in autumn. Large panicles of small, star-shaped, greenish white or creamy white flowers, to 30cm (12in) long on female trees, 10–13cm (4–5in) long on males, are borne in early summer, followed on female plants by pendent pods, to 25cm (10in) long. Seeds are toxic if ingested. ↕ 20m (70ft) or more, ↔ 15m (50ft). C. and E. North America. ❄❄❄

▷ ***Gymnogramma triangularis*** see *Pityrogramma triangularis*

GYNANDRIRIS

IRIDACEAE

Genus of 9 species of small, cormous perennials occurring in garigue, grassy pastures, and stony slopes in South Africa and from the Mediterranean to Pakistan. In spring, they bear narrow, channelled, basal leaves and a succession of small, short-lived, iris-like flowers, each with 3 large, pendent outer petals and 3 usually smaller inner petals. Plant on a warm, sunny bank or by a warm wall. In wet, frost-prone areas, grow in an alpine house or bulb frame.
- **HARDINESS** Frost hardy.
- **CULTIVATION** Grow in moderately fertile, well-drained soil that is moist in winter and spring but dries out in summer, in full sun. In frost-prone climates, grow in loam-based potting compost (JI No.2), with added sharp sand, in a bulb frame or alpine house.
- **PROPAGATION** Sow seed in containers in a cold frame as soon as ripe, and overwinter seedlings in frost-free conditions. Remove offsets in summer.
- **PESTS AND DISEASES** Trouble free.

G. sisyrinchium ■ syn. *Iris sisyrinchium.* Cormous perennial with 1 or 2 semi-erect or prostrate, narrow, basal leaves, 2–8cm (¾–3in) long. In spring, bears a succession of small, iris-like flowers, 2–4cm (¾–1½in) across; opening in the afternoon, they vary from pale lavender-blue to violet-blue, with a white, yellow, or orange mark on the 3 larger petals. ↕ 10–20cm (4–8in), ↔ 5cm (2in). Mediterranean to S.W. Asia. ❄❄

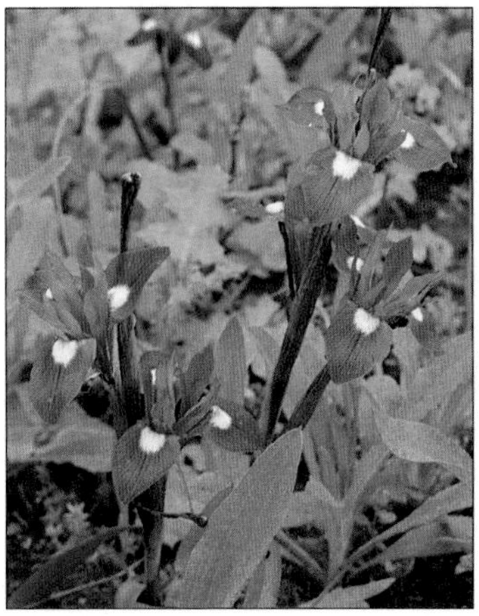

Gynandriris sisyrinchium

G

GYNURA

ASTERACEAE/COMPOSITAE

Genus of about 50 species of evergreen perennials and subshrubs, some scandent and trailing, from tropical woodland in Africa and Asia. The toothed leaves are alternate, simple, and pinnate or pinnatifid. The flowerheads, usually borne singly or in corymbs at the tips of the branches, lack ray-florets; they resemble groundsel (*Senecio*) flowerheads, but are larger and more colourful. Where temperatures fall below 13°C (55°F), grow as houseplants or in a temperate or warm greenhouse. Elsewhere, use in a shady, moist border.
- **HARDINESS** Frost tender.
- **CULTIVATION** Under glass, grow in loam-based potting compost (JI No.2) in bright filtered light. Pot on or top-dress in spring. During the growing season, water freely and apply a balanced liquid fertilizer monthly. Provide scandent species with light support. Pinch out tips to stop plants becoming too leggy and to encourage young shoots. Outdoors, grow in fertile, moist but well-drained soil in partial shade.
- **PROPAGATION** Root softwood cuttings in late spring or semi-ripe cuttings in summer, both with bottom heat.
- **PESTS AND DISEASES** Aphids and red spider mites may be troublesome under glass.

G. aurantiaca ■ (Purple velvet plant, Royal velvet plant, Velvet plant). Woody-based perennial or subshrub,

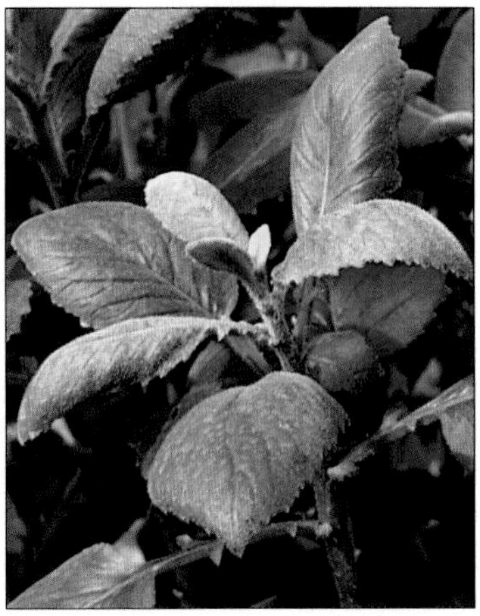

Gynura aurantiaca

erect at first then semi-scandent, densely covered in velvety, violet-purple hairs. Simple, ovate to broadly elliptic leaves, 10–20cm (4–8in) long, are coarsely toothed, semi-lustrous, deep green, and overlaid with purple hairs. Orange-yellow flowerheads, 1.5–2cm (½–¾in) across, tinted purple with age, are borne in loose, terminal corymbs, to 3cm (1¼in) across, mainly in winter. ↕ to 60cm (24in), or 2–3m (6–10ft) with support; ↔ 45–120cm (18–48in). Indonesia (Java). ❀ (min. 13°C/55°F).
'Purple Passion' 🏆 syn. *G. sarmentosa* of gardens, is trailing or semi-twining, with purple-haired stems and lance-shaped, lobed leaves, 6–14cm (2½–5½in) long, densely covered with red-purple hairs beneath, more lightly above; ↕ 1–3m (3–10ft), ↔ 1m (3ft) or more.

G

***G. sarmentosa* of gardens** see *G. aurantiaca* 'Purple Passion'.

GYPSOPHILA

CARYOPHYLLACEAE

Genus of over 100 species of annuals and herbaceous, semi-evergreen, or evergreen perennials, sometimes woody-based, some cushion- or mat-forming. They occur in alpine habitats, dry, stony slopes, or sandy steppes, usually on alkaline soils, from the E. Mediterranean to the Caucasus, C. Asia, and N.W. China. They are valued particularly for their small, 5-petalled, star-shaped to shallowly trumpet-shaped, white or pink flowers, borne singly or in spreading panicles. They have usually lance-shaped to linear-lance-shaped, glaucous leaves, borne in opposite pairs. Larger species are useful annual or border plants and provide good cut flowers. The alpine species are excellent for a raised bed, dry-stone wall, or rock garden, as well as for an alpine house or scree bed.

- **HARDINESS** Fully hardy to frost hardy.
- **CULTIVATION** Grow in deep, light, preferably alkaline, sharply drained soil in full sun. Most dislike winter wet, although *G.* 'Rosenschleier' tolerates moist soil.
- **PROPAGATION** Sow seed of annuals *in situ* in spring. Sow seed of perennials at 13–18°C (55–64°F) in winter, or in a cold frame in spring. Perennials may also be increased by root cuttings (species only) or by grafting (for named cultivars), both in late winter.
- **PESTS AND DISEASES** Stem rots may be a problem.

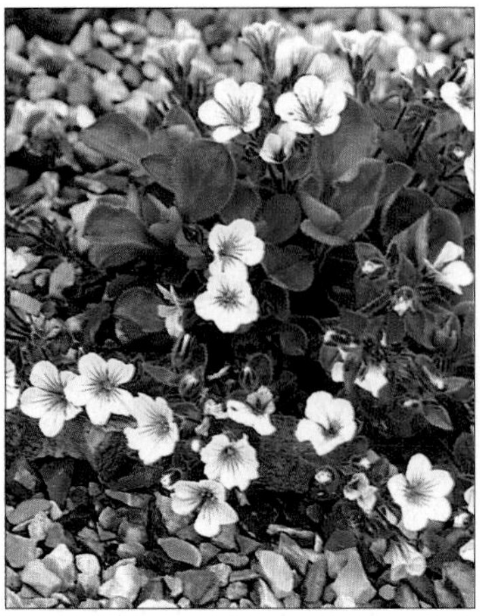

Gypsophila cerastioides

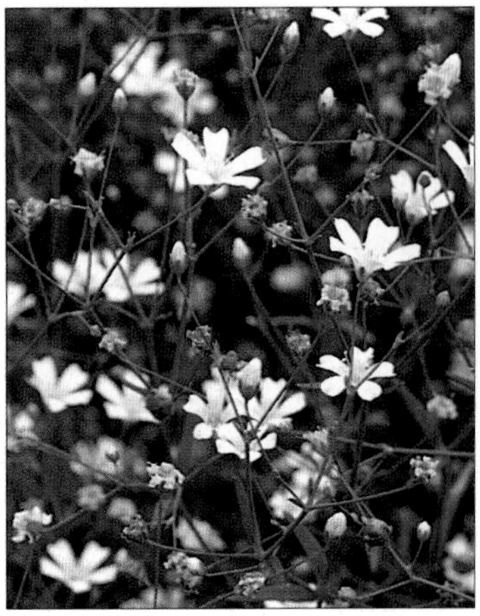

Gypsophila elegans

G. acutifolia. Deep-rooting herbaceous perennial with many-branched stems bearing lance-shaped, pointed, greyish green leaves, 2–8cm (¾–3in) long. From midsummer to early autumn, bears spreading panicles, 5cm (2in) across, of star-shaped, pale pink flowers, to 2cm (¾in) across. ↕ 1m (3ft), ↔ 1.5m (5ft). N. Caucasus, S. Russia. ❄❄❄
G. aretioides. Very dense, hard, cushion-forming, evergreen perennial with tiny, oblong, fleshy, grey-green leaves, 2–5mm (1/16–¼in) long. Bears small, usually solitary, stemless, star-shaped white flowers in summer. Ideal for an alpine house or scree bed. ↕ 5cm (2in), ↔ to 15cm (6in). Caucasus, mountains of N. Iran. ❄❄❄
G. cerastioides ▣ Loose, mat-forming, semi-evergreen perennial with tufts of grey-hairy leaves, 6–10mm (¼–½in) long, that are long-stalked and spoon-shaped, or almost stalkless and broadly obovate. Loose panicles of shallowly trumpet-shaped white flowers, to 1.5cm (½in) across, veined and faintly tinged pink, are borne over long periods from late spring to summer. ↕ 5cm (2in), ↔ to 15cm (6in). Himalayas. ❄❄❄
G. elegans ▣ Erect, branching annual with narrow, oblong-lance-shaped to linear-lance-shaped, grey-green leaves, 2–4cm (¾–1½in) long. Loosely branched panicles, to 10cm (4in) or more across, of 4-petalled, star-shaped, white or carmine-pink, sometimes pink- or purple-veined flowers, to 1cm (½in) across, are produced on long, slender stalks in summer. Good for cut flowers. ↕ to 60cm (24in), ↔ 30cm (12in). S. Ukraine, Turkey. ❄❄❄. **'Bright Rose'**

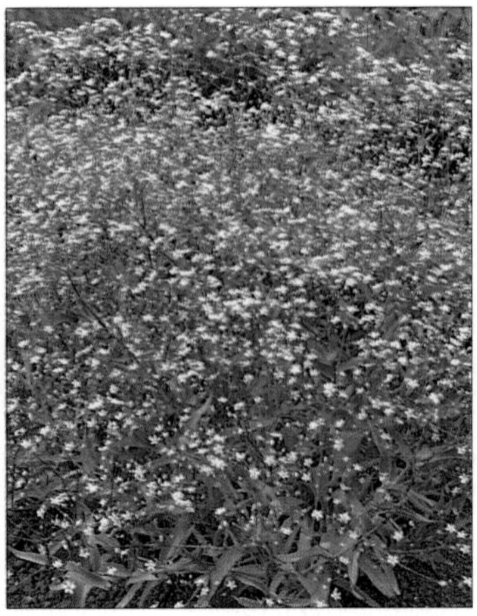

Gypsophila elegans 'Rosea'

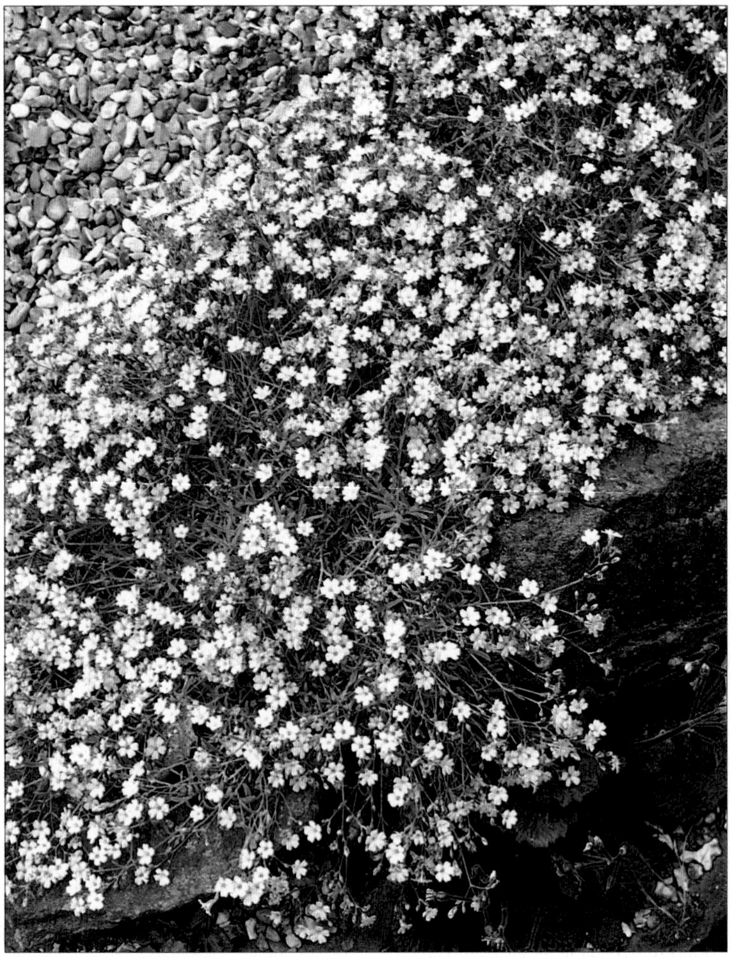

Gypsophila repens 'Dorothy Teacher'

produces bright rose-pink flowers. **'Carminea'** has deep carmine-pink flowers. **'Covent Garden'** bears large, white flowers, to 1.5cm (½in) across. **'Giant White'** has large white flowers, to 2cm (¾in) across. **'Red Cloud'** flowers very profusely, bearing deep carmine-pink blooms. **'Rosea'** ▣ has pale rose-pink flowers.
G. paniculata (Baby's breath). Tap-rooted herbaceous perennial with branching stems forming an airy mound of linear-lance-shaped, usually hairless, glaucous leaves, 5–7cm (2–3in) long. In mid- and late summer, bears numerous loose, many-flowered panicles of shallowly trumpet-shaped white flowers, to 8mm (3/8in) across, forming mounds to 45cm (18in) or more across. ↕↔ to 1.2m (4ft). C. and E. Europe. ❄❄❄.

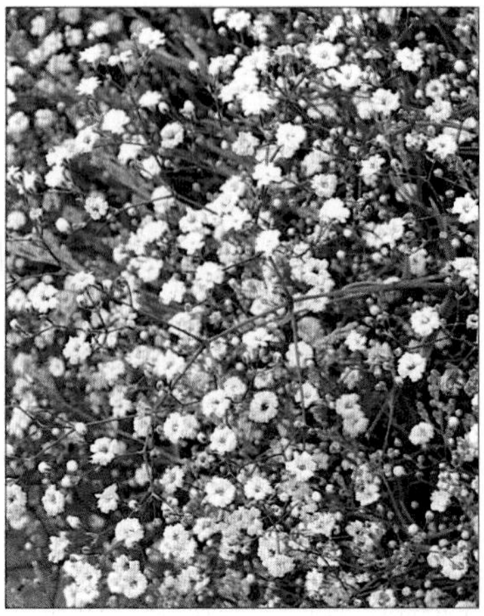

Gypsophila 'Rosenschleier'

'Bristol Fairy' 🏆 has large, double white flowers, to 1.5cm (½in) across, but is less robust, and liable to be short-lived. **'Compacta Plena'** has double, soft pink to white flowers; ↕ 20–30cm (8–12in), ↔ to 60cm (24in). **'Flamingo'** is less robust than the species, with larger, double, pale pink flowers, to 1cm (½in) across; ↕ 75–90cm (30–36in), ↔ 90cm (36in).
G. repens. Mat-forming, semi-evergreen perennial with linear, often sickle-shaped, mid- or slightly bluish green leaves, 1.5–3cm (½–1¼in) long. Over long periods in summer, bears loose, corymb-like panicles, 4–8cm (1½–3in) across, of star-shaped, white, pink, or pink-purple flowers, to 1.5cm (½in) across. ↕ 20cm (8in), ↔ 30–50cm (12–20in). Mountains of C. and S. Europe. ❄❄❄. **'Dorothy Teacher'** ▣🏆 has a neat habit, blue-green leaves, and pale pink flowers that darken with age; ↕ 5cm (2in), ↔ to 40cm (16in). **'Fratensis'** has grey-green leaves and pale pink flowers; ↕ 5–7cm (2–3in), ↔ to 30cm (12in).
***G.* 'Rosenschleier'** ▣🏆 syn. *G.* 'Rosy Veil'. Vigorous, dense, mound-forming, semi-evergreen perennial with branching stems that produce linear-lance-shaped, usually hairless, bluish green leaves, 2.5–4cm (1–1½in) long. In mid- and late summer, bears numerous loose, many-flowered panicles of double flowers, 1cm (½in) across, opening white and becoming very pale pink; they form dense clouds of bloom, 45cm (18in) wide. ↕ 40–50cm (16–20in), ↔ 1m (3ft). ❄❄❄
***G.* 'Rosy Veil'** see *G.* 'Rosenschleier'.

H

HAAGEOCEREUS

CACTACEAE

Genus of 40–50 species (some authorities accept only 5–10) of shrubby or tree-like, columnar, solitary or clump-forming, perennial cacti from dry coastal to mountainous areas, to 2,500m (8,000ft) high, in Peru and Chile. They have ribbed, densely spiny stems and, in summer, bear tubular-funnel-shaped flowers near the tops of the stems; these open from late afternoon until well into the following morning. The green, yellow, or reddish pink fruits, 3–4cm (1¼–1½in) long, are spherical to ovoid, sparsely scaly, hairy, and fleshy. In temperate regions, grow in a temperate greenhouse. In warmer climates, use in a desert garden.

- **HARDINESS** Frost tender.
- **CULTIVATION** Under glass, grow in standard cactus compost in full light. Provide low humidity and good ventilation. In growth, water moderately and apply a low-nitrogen liquid fertilizer monthly; keep completely dry in winter. Outdoors, grow in poor, sharply drained soil in full sun. Protect from excessive winter wet. See also pp.48–49.
- **PROPAGATION** Sow seed at 19–24°C (66–75°F) in spring, or root stem cuttings in spring or summer.
- **PESTS AND DISEASES** Susceptible to aphids while flowering.

H. acranthus see *H. limensis.*
H. aureispinus. Erect, clump-forming cactus with 18- to 20-ribbed, bright green stems. Yellow areoles each bear 30–40 yellow radial spines and 1 or 2 longer, brownish yellow centrals. Pure white flowers, 6–7cm (2½–3in) long, are borne on scaly, woolly tubes in summer. ↕ 80cm (32in), ↔ 8cm (3in) or more. Peru. ❁ (min. 11°C/52°F)
H. australis see *H. decumbens.*
H. decumbens, syn. *H. australis.* Semi-prostrate, clump-forming cactus with 15- to 22-ribbed, often jointed and branching, mid-green stems. White-woolly areoles bear 20–30 thin, red-tipped yellow radial spines and 1–5 longer, erect, black-tipped red centrals. In summer, bears white flowers, to 8cm (3in) long, with reddish brown outer segments and brown- or red-green tubes. ↕ 30cm (12in), ↔ to 1m (3ft). S.W. Peru, N.W. Chile. ❁ (min. 11°C/52°F)
H. limensis, syn. *H. acranthus.* Erect, thickly clustering cactus producing mid-green stems with 10–14 slightly warty, low ribs. White areoles bear 20–30 yellow radial spines and 1–3 longer, downward-pointing brown centrals. Greenish white or pinkish white flowers, 6–8cm (2½–3in) long, with green tubes, are produced in summer. ↕ 2m (6ft), ↔ to 1m (3ft). C. Peru. ❁ (min. 11°C/52°F)

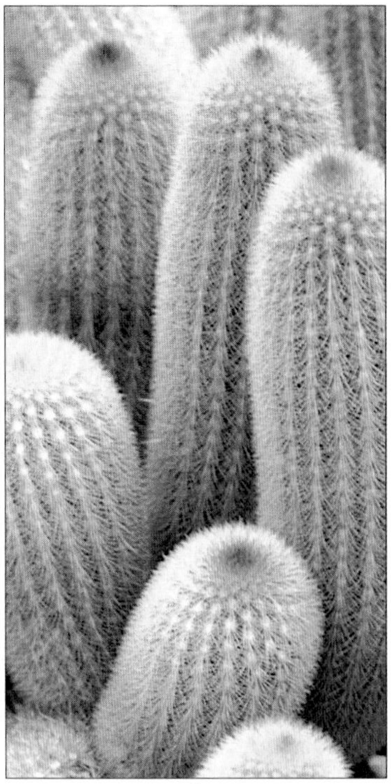

Haageocereus versicolor

H. versicolor ■ Erect, clump-forming cactus, often branching from the base, with 16- to 22-ribbed, dark green stems. Brown-felted areoles bear yellow to reddish brown spines, which comprise 25–30 radials and 1–4 longer centrals. White flowers, 6–8cm (2½–3in) long, with pinkish green outer segments and light green tubes, are borne in summer. ↕ 2m (6ft), ↔ 1m (3ft). N. Peru. ❁ (min. 11°C/52°F)

HAASTIA

Vegetable sheep

ASTERACEAE/COMPOSITAE

Genus of 3 species of cushion-forming or clump-forming, occasionally trailing perennials or subshrubs from high-altitude scree and rocky sites, to 2,000m (6,500ft), in the mountains of New Zealand. They have variably shaped, small, usually densely hairy, overlapping leaves, 1–3.5cm (½–1½in) long, and tiny, daisy-like flowerheads. Vegetable sheep are fascinating foliage plants but difficult to cultivate. Grow in an alpine house, as they must have protection from winter wet.

- **HARDINESS** Fully hardy.
- **CULTIVATION** In an alpine house, grow in loam-based potting compost (JI No.1) with 1 part added leaf mould and 2 parts grit; apply a top-dressing of grit and wedges of small stones to keep the cushion of leaves clear of the soil surface. Provide moderate humidity and good ventilation. When in growth, water moderately but avoid wetting the foliage; keep just moist in winter.
- **PROPAGATION** Sow seed in containers in an open frame as soon as ripe; water seedlings from below. Root rosette cuttings in early summer.
- **PESTS AND DISEASES** Prone to aphids and red spider mites in dry conditions.

H. pulvinaris (Vegetable sheep). Extremely dense, cushion-forming perennial with tightly packed branches concealed by rosetted, overlapping, broadly wedge-shaped, grey, tawny-hairy leaves, to 1cm (½in) long. In summer, produces insignificant white flowerheads, which are hidden within the cushions. ↕ 5cm (2in), ↔ to 10cm (4in) or more. New Zealand. ❄❄❄

HABENARIA

ORCHIDACEAE

Genus of 500–600 species of evergreen and deciduous, terrestrial orchids found in grassland in both tropical and temperate regions, especially in tropical South America, temperate North America, Africa, and Asia. They have fleshy, underground tubers and produce basal tufts of smooth, dark green leaves. Smaller, sheathing leaves are produced on leafy stems, which bear terminal racemes, 12–22cm (5–9in) long, of mostly green or white, hooded flowers with brightly coloured lips. Grow hardy species in humus-rich soil in a woodland garden.

- **HARDINESS** Fully hardy to frost tender.
- **CULTIVATION** Cool- to intermediate-growing orchids. Grow in terrestrial orchid compost in bright filtered light. Pot on in spring. In growth, water freely and apply a dilute balanced liquid fertilizer at every third watering; keep just moist in winter. See also p.46.
- **PROPAGATION** Divide tubers when the plants have died down.
- **PESTS AND DISEASES** Prone to red spider mites, aphids, and mealybugs.

H. rhodocheila. Deciduous, terrestrial orchid with fleshy tubers and an erect stem bearing 4–6 linear to lance-shaped, dark green leaves, 6–12cm (2½–5in) long. Upright racemes of green flowers, 2.5cm (1in) across, with deeply 3-lobed, bold, scarlet, orange, or yellow lips, are borne in summer. ↕ 30cm (12in), ↔ 20cm (8in). S. China to Malaysia and the Philippines. ❁ (min. 13–16°C/55–61°F; max. 30°C/86°F)

HABERLEA

GESNERIACEAE

Genus of 2 species of stemless, evergreen perennials from shaded, rocky habitats in the Balkans. They have basal rosettes of obovate, scalloped, dark green leaves, and loose umbels of up to 6 nodding, trumpet-shaped, 2-lipped flowers, borne from spring to early summer. They are attractive plants for a wall, rock crevice, rock garden, or alpine house.

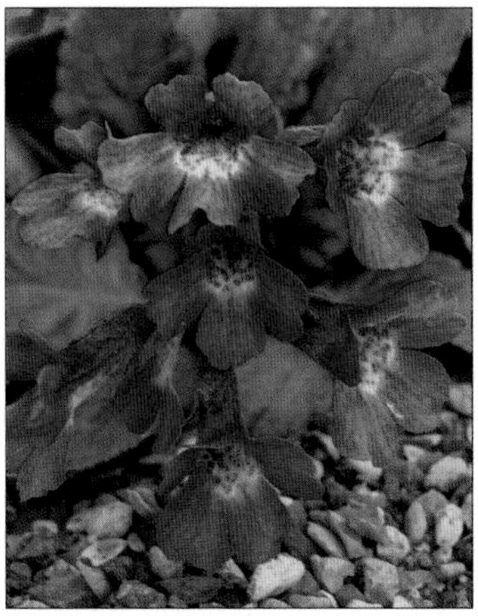

Haberlea ferdinandi-coburgii

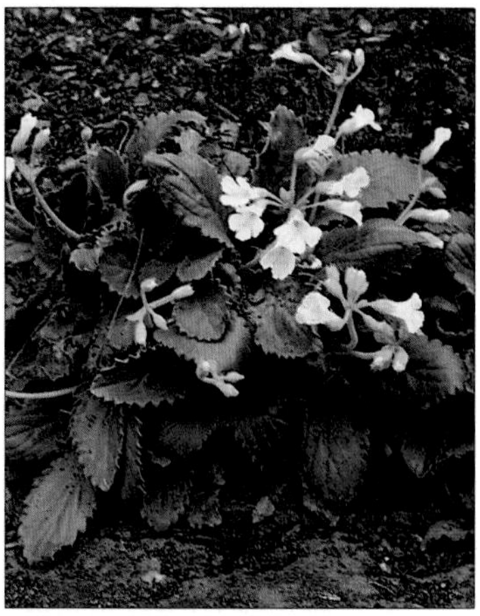

Haberlea rhodopensis 'Virginalis'

- **HARDINESS** Fully hardy.
- **CULTIVATION** In an alpine house, grow in loam-based potting compost (JI No.2) with added grit or sharp sand and leaf mould, in bright indirect light. In the growing season, water freely and apply a half-strength balanced liquid fertilizer monthly. Outdoors, grow in moist but well-drained, acid to neutral, gritty, humus-rich soil in full or partial shade, preferably planted on their sides in vertical rock crevices to avoid an accumulation of moisture in the foliage rosettes. Protect from excessive winter wet and cold, drying winds. Root disturbance is resented.
- **PROPAGATION** Sow seed at 13–18°C (55–64°F) in spring. Divide, or root leaf cuttings, in early summer.
- **PESTS AND DISEASES** Slugs and snails may be a problem.

H. ferdinandi-coburgii ■ syn. *H. rhodopensis* var. *ferdinandi-coburgii.* Dense, rosette-forming perennial with obovate to oblong-ovate, coarsely scalloped leaves, 3–8cm (1¼–3in) long, smooth and almost hairless above, finely hairy beneath. From spring to early summer, produces umbels of violet-blue to lavender-blue flowers, 1.5–2.5cm (½–1in) across, with yellowish white throats speckled dark violet-blue. ↕ to 15cm (6in), ↔ to 25cm (10in). Bulgaria. ❄❄❄
H. rhodopensis 🏆 Dense, rosette-forming perennial with obovate to ovate-oblong, coarsely scalloped leaves, 3–8cm (1¼–3in) long, softly hairy above and beneath. Umbels of pale blue-violet flowers, to 2.5cm (1in) across, are borne from spring to early summer. ↕ to 15cm (6in), ↔ to 25cm (10in). Bulgaria, N.E. Greece. ❄❄❄. **var. *ferdinandi-coburgii*** see *H. ferdinandi-coburgii.* **'Virginalis'** ■ has pure white flowers.

HABRANTHUS

AMARYLLIDACEAE

Genus of 10 species of bulbous perennials from dry, upland slopes in temperate South America. They have semi-erect, narrow, linear, basal leaves, evergreen in some species, deciduous or developing after the flowers in others. Solitary, funnel-shaped flowers, held at an angle to the stems, are borne from summer to autumn. They are followed by seed capsules, which quickly ripen and open to reveal conspicuous black seeds; seed capsules are sometimes

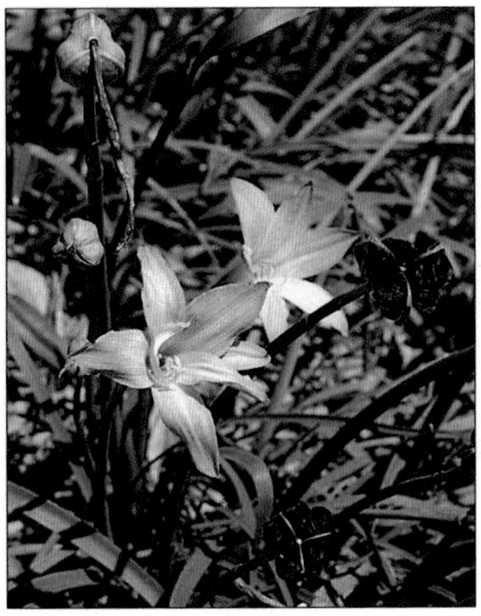
Habranthus robustus

produced at the same time as the flowers. In frost-prone areas, grow in a cool greenhouse or conservatory, or at the base of a warm, sunny wall. In frost-free regions, grow at the front of a bed or border.
• **HARDINESS** Half hardy.
• **CULTIVATION** Under glass, plant bulbs 7–10cm (3–4in) deep, in loam-based potting compost (JI No.2) with added grit and leaf mould, in full light. Water moderately as growth begins, freely in leaf; reduce water as foliage dies back and keep barely moist when dormant. Apply a balanced liquid fertilizer weekly when in bud. Outdoors, plant bulbs in spring with the necks above the soil surface. Grow in fertile, well-drained, neutral to alkaline soil in full sun. Protect from excessive winter wet.
• **PROPAGATION** Sow seed at 16°C (61°F) as soon as ripe. Remove offsets in winter and pot up separately.
• **PESTS AND DISEASES** Trouble free.

H. andersonii see *H. tubispathus.*
H. brachyandrus. Showy, bulbous perennial producing mid-green, basal leaves, 30cm (12in) long, in summer or early autumn, at the same time as leafless stems bear solitary, open funnel-shaped, bright pinkish red flowers, 7–10cm (3–4in) across. ↕ 30cm (12in), ↔ 5cm (2in). Brazil, Paraguay. ✻
H. robustus ▣ syn. *Zephyranthes robusta.* Robust, bulbous perennial with deep green, basal leaves, 15–20cm (6–8in) long, emerging in summer at the same time as, or just before, leafless stems bear solitary, open funnel-shaped, pale pink flowers, 6cm (2½in) across. ↕ 20–30cm (8–12in), ↔ 5cm (2in). Brazil. ✻
H. texanus see *H. tubispathus.*
H. tubispathus, syn. *H. andersonii, H. texanus, Zephyranthes andersonii.* Upright, bulbous perennial producing a succession of solitary flowering stems, each bearing a small, funnel-shaped, coppery red, orange, or yellow flower, 2.5cm (1in) across, in summer. The deep green, basal leaves, 13–15cm (5–6in) long, emerge after the flowers. ↕ 10–15cm (4–6in), ↔ 2.5cm (1in). USA (Texas), S. Brazil, Uruguay, E. Argentina, S. Chile. ✻

▷ **Hackberry** see *Celtis, C. occidentalis*
Common see *C. laevigata*
Mississippi see *C. laevigata*
Sugar see *C. laevigata*
Western see *C. reticulata*

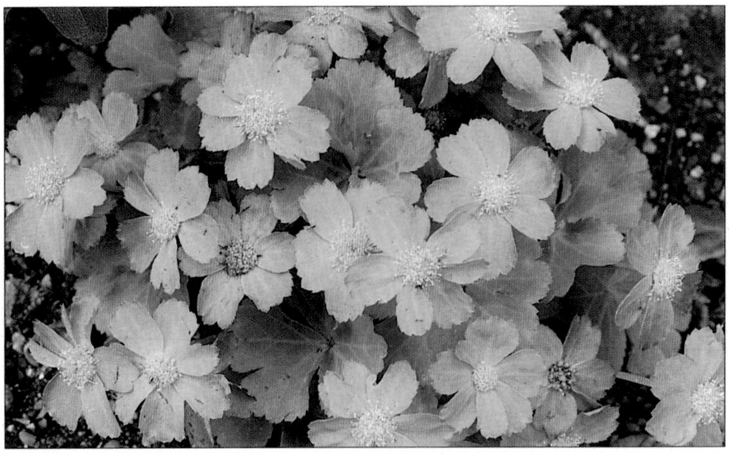
Hacquetia epipactis

HACQUETIA syn. DONDIA

APIACEAE/UMBELLIFERAE

Genus of a single species of small, clump-forming, rhizomatous perennial found in lowland and upland woodland in Europe. Grown for its foliage and early, long-lasting, tiny yellow flowers surrounded by bright green bracts, it is suitable for moist, shady sites, such as a rock or woodland garden, or a peat bed.
• **HARDINESS** Fully hardy.
• **CULTIVATION** Grow in humus-rich, moist but well-drained, neutral to acid soil in partial shade.
• **PROPAGATION** Sow seed in containers in a cold frame as soon as ripe, or in autumn. Divide in spring. Insert root cuttings in winter.
• **PESTS AND DISEASES** Slugs and snails may damage young growth in spring.

H. epipactis ▣ ♀ syn. *Dondia epipactis.* Rhizomatous, clump-forming perennial with glossy, emerald-green leaves that develop fully only after flowering. The leaves, to 7cm (3in) long, are rounded, with 3 wedge-shaped, toothed lobes. Tiny yellow flowers, surrounded by bright green bracts, are borne in dense umbels, to 4cm (1½in) across, in late winter and early spring. ↕ 5cm (2in), to 15cm (6in) after flowering, ↔ 15–30cm (6–12in). Europe. ✻✻✻

HAEMANTHUS

Blood lily

AMARYLLIDACEAE

Genus of 21 species of bulbous perennials, some of them evergreen, from grassy, rocky hillsides in South Africa. From summer to autumn, and occasionally in winter, they bear tiny flowers in showy umbels that resemble shaving brushes. These are borne above erect, or semi-erect to spreading, strap-shaped to lance-shaped, broadly elliptic, or rounded, mid- to dark green, basal leaves. In frost-prone areas, grow in a temperate greenhouse or as houseplants. In frost-free areas, grow in semi-shaded or sunny sites between shrubs. All parts of blood lilies may cause mild stomach upset if ingested; contact with the sap may irritate skin.
• **HARDINESS** Frost tender.
• **CULTIVATION** Plant bulbs with the necks just above the soil surface, in autumn or winter. Under glass, grow in loam-based potting compost (JI No.2) with added leaf mould and grit, in full light. Provide bright filtered light when buds open, to prolong flowering. In growth, water freely and apply a dilute, balanced liquid fertilizer monthly; keep evergreen species just moist when dormant, and deciduous species dry after flowering. Blood lilies flower best when pot-bound; if necessary, pot on as growth begins. Outdoors, grow in well-drained, moderately fertile, neutral to alkaline soil in sun or dappled shade.
• **PROPAGATION** Sow seed at 16–18°C (61–64°F) as soon as ripe. Remove and pot up offsets in early spring.
• **PESTS AND DISEASES** Trouble free.

H. albiflos (Shaving brush plant, White paint brush). Evergreen, bulbous perennial producing pairs of semi-erect then spreading, broadly strap-shaped, mid-green leaves, to 40cm (16in) long, sometimes spotted white, with hairy margins. From autumn to winter, stout stems bear brush-like heads, to 3–7cm (1¼–3in) across, of up to 50 tiny white flowers with protruding stamens; these are followed by ovoid, fleshy, white to red fruit. ↕ 20–30cm (8–12in), ↔ 15cm (6in). South Africa (Eastern Cape, Western Cape) ❀ (min. 10°C/50°F)
H. coccineus ▣ (Cape tulip). Deciduous, bulbous perennial with 2, occasionally 3, semi-erect to prostrate, elliptic to strap-shaped, mid-green, sometimes purple-marked leaves, to 45cm (18in) long, developing soon after flowering. From summer to autumn, leafless, dark red-streaked stems bear up to 100 tiny red flowers, with prominent yellow stamens, surrounded by large

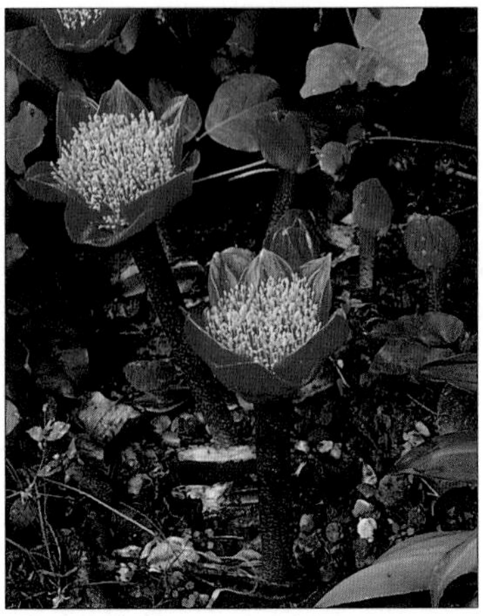
Haemanthus coccineus

scarlet bracts, in umbels to 5–10cm (2–4in) across. Flowers are followed by ovoid, fleshy, white to pink fruit. ↕ to 35cm (14in), ↔ 15cm (6in). South Africa (Eastern Cape, Northern Cape, Western Cape). ❀ (min. 10°C/50°F)
H. katherinae see *Scadoxus multiflorus* subsp. *katherinae.*
H. magnificus see *Scadoxus puniceus.*
H. multiflorus see *Scadoxus multiflorus.*
H. natalensis see *Scadoxus puniceus.*
H. puniceus see *Scadoxus puniceus.*
H. sanguineus. Deciduous, bulbous perennial with pairs of prostrate, broadly elliptic to oblong, dark green leaves, to 40cm (16in) long, hairy beneath, developing soon after flowering. From summer to autumn, leafless, dark red stems bear dense umbels, to 3–8cm (1¼–3in) across, of up to 100 small, red, salmon-pink, or pale pink flowers, with white markings and prominent stamens, followed by spherical to ovoid, fleshy, cream to dark red fruit. ↕ 30cm (12in), ↔ 15cm (6in). South Africa (Eastern Cape, Northern Cape, Western Cape). ❀ (min. 10°C/50°F)

▷ **Hair grass** see *Aira, A. elegantissima, Deschampsia*
Glaucous see *Koeleria glauca*
Tufted see *Deschampsia cespitosa*
Wavy see *Deschampsia flexuosa*

HAKEA

PROTEACEAE

Genus of at least 130 species of evergreen trees and shrubs found in acid soils from coastal to mountainous areas in Australia, where they grow in woodland, on hillsides, and on heathland. The alternate, leathery leaves are often linear and needle-like, but vary greatly within the genus, and may be toothed or lobed. Small, tubular flowers, borne in short, axillary racemes, have prominent, often brightly coloured styles, and are followed by woody seed pods, 2–3cm (¾–1¼in) long, each containing only 1 or 2 seeds. In frost-prone areas, grow in a cool or temperate greenhouse. In mild areas, grow at the base of a sunny wall, in a shrub border, as specimens, or as informal hedging. Long, hot summers are needed for good flowering.
• **HARDINESS** Half hardy to frost tender; *H. lissosperma* will tolerate short spells at -5°C (23°F).
• **CULTIVATION** Under glass, grow in a mix of equal parts loam, peat or leaf mould, and sharp sand, in full light. In growth, water moderately, applying a phosphate-free liquid fertilizer monthly; keep just moist in winter. Pot on or top-dress in spring. Outdoors, grow in fertile, well-drained, sandy, slightly acid soil in full sun, although partial shade is tolerated. Pruning group 1; plants under glass may need restrictive pruning.
• **PROPAGATION** Sow seed at 16–18°C (61–64°F) as soon as ripe; sow seed singly in containers to avoid root disturbance. Root semi-ripe cuttings with bottom heat in summer.
• **PESTS AND DISEASES** *Phytophthora* root rot may be a problem in moist soil.

H. lissosperma ▣ ♀ syn. *H. sericea* of gardens (Mountain hakea). Erect, open to bushy shrub or small tree with linear, stiffly leathery, often upward-curving, grey-green leaves, to 15cm (6in) long,

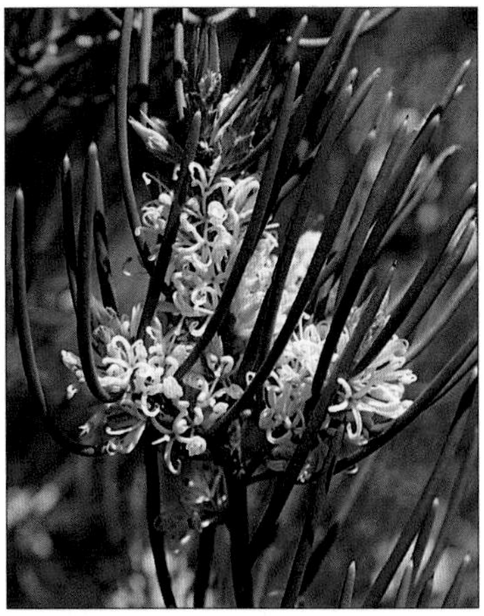

Hakea lissosperma

with prickly tips. From spring to summer, bears small white flowers in axillary racemes, 2.5cm (1in) long, from the upper leaf axils; they are followed by ovoid, smooth or warty, dark brown seed pods. ↕ 3–6m (10–20ft), ↔ 1–4m (3–12ft). Australia (New South Wales, Victoria, Tasmania). ✲
H. salicifolia ○ syn. *H. saligna* (Willow-leaved hakea). Large shrub or small tree with spreading to pendent branches and narrowly lance-shaped to oblong-elliptic leaves, 10–15cm (4–6in) long. Leaves are purple when young, thin, leathery, and dark green when mature. In spring, bears axillary racemes, 2cm (¾in) long, of 4–9 tiny, creamy white flowers, sometimes followed by ovoid, warty, dark brown seed pods. ↕ 3–8m (10–25ft), ↔ 1–6m (3–20ft). Australia (Queensland, New South Wales). ❀ (min. 5–7°C/41–45°F). **'Gold Medal'** has pinkish green young leaves, yellow-variegated when mature.
H. saligna see *H. salicifolia*.
H. sericea of gardens see *H. lissosperma*.

▷ **Hakea,**
Mountain see *Hakea lissosperma*
Willow-leaved see *Hakea salicifolia*

HAKONECHLOA

GRAMINEAE/POACEAE

Genus of one species of deciduous, rhizomatous, clump-forming, perennial grass occurring in wooded and often mountainous areas of Japan. *H. macra* has smooth leaves and loose, nodding panicles of 3- to 5-flowered spikelets. Its variegated cultivars, among the most attractive of ornamental grasses, are useful in a woodland or rock garden, or at the front of a mixed or herbaceous border. They are also ideal for patio containers or a courtyard garden.
• **HARDINESS** Fully hardy.
• **CULTIVATION** Grow in fertile, humus-rich, moist but well-drained soil in full sun or partial shade. Variegated cultivars produce best leaf colour in partial shade.
• **PROPAGATION** Divide in spring.
• **PESTS AND DISEASES** Trouble free.

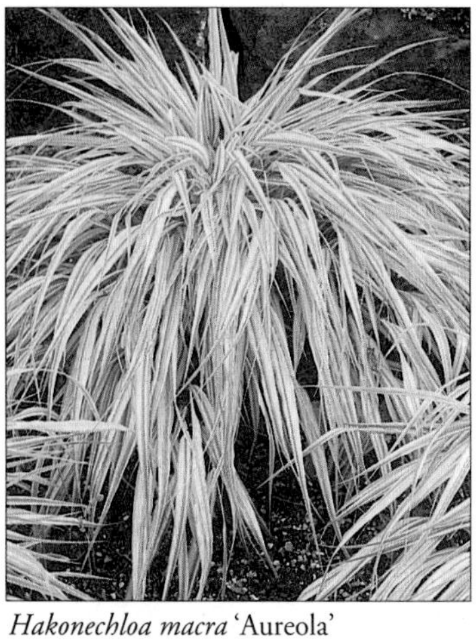

Hakonechloa macra 'Aureola'

H. macra 'Aureola' ▣ 🏆 Perennial grass, spreading slowly to form mounds of arching, linear leaves, to 25cm (10in) long. Leaves are bright yellow with narrow green stripes, becoming red-flushed in autumn, the colour often persisting into winter. From late summer to mid-autumn, bears needle-like, pale green spikelets in open panicles, to 18cm (7in) long. ↕ 35cm (14in), ↔ 40cm (16in). ✲✲✲

HALESIA

Silver bell, Snowdrop tree

STYRACACEAE

Genus of 5 species of deciduous trees and shrubs found in woodland, at woodland margins, and on riverbanks in E. China and S.E. USA. They have alternate, ovate to elliptic, or oblong leaves, and are cultivated for their pendent, bell-shaped flowers, curious winged fruits, and autumn colour. Ideal specimen plants for the back of a shrub border or for a woodland garden.
• **HARDINESS** Fully hardy.
• **CULTIVATION** Grow in fertile, humus-rich, moist but well-drained, neutral to acid soil in sun or partial shade; shelter from cold winds. Pruning group 1.
• **PROPAGATION** Sow seed at 14–25°C (57–77°F) in autumn, moving the containers to a cold frame after 60 days. Root softwood cuttings in summer, or layer in spring.
• **PESTS AND DISEASES** Trouble free.

H. carolina ○ syn. *H. tetraptera*. Spreading tree or shrub with ovate to elliptic, minutely toothed, mid-green leaves, to 16cm (6in) long, turning yellow in autumn. Axillary clusters of 2–6 pendent, bell-shaped white flowers, to 2cm (¾in) long, hang in profusion from the branches in late spring, just before the leaves emerge. They are followed by 4-winged green fruit. ↕ 8m (25ft), ↔ 10m (30ft). S.E. USA. ✲✲✲

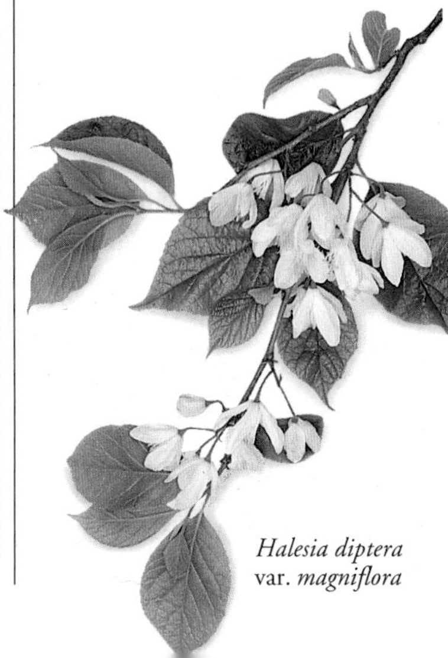

Halesia diptera var. *magniflora*

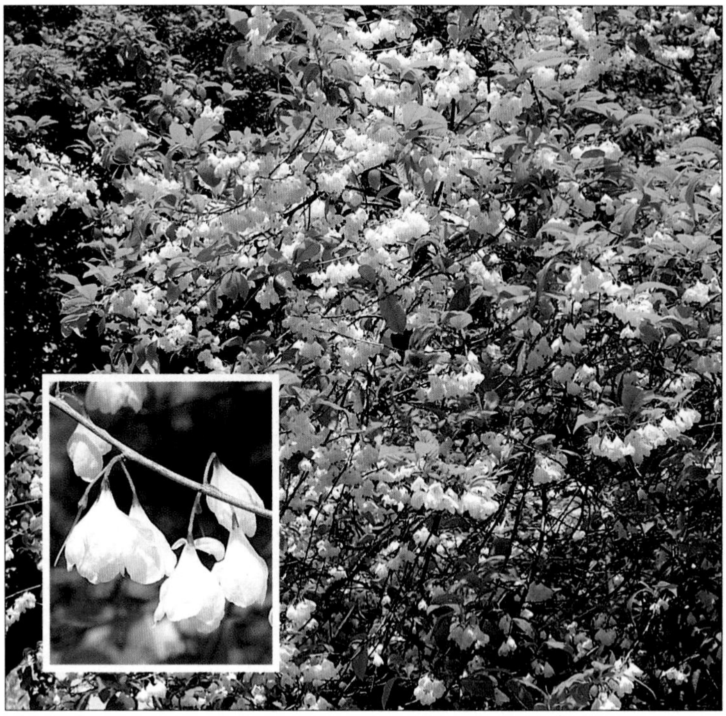

Halesia monticola (inset: flower detail)

H. diptera ○ Spreading shrub or small tree with elliptic to obovate, mid-green leaves, to 14cm (5½in) long, turning yellow in autumn. Axillary clusters or short racemes of 3–6, deeply 4-lobed white flowers, to 2cm (¾in) long, are borne in early summer, after the leaves; they are followed by 2-winged green fruit. ↕ 6m (20ft), ↔ 10m (30ft). S.E. USA. ✲✲✲. **var. magniflora** ▣ has larger flowers, to 3cm (1¼in) long.
H. monticola ▣ △ Vigorous, usually conical tree with ovate, tapered, downy, mid-green leaves, to 20cm (8in) long, becoming hairless with age, and turning yellow in autumn. Axillary clusters of 2–5 wide, bell-shaped white flowers, to 2.5cm (1in) long, are borne in late spring, before or with the leaves; flowers are followed by 4-winged green fruit. ↕ 12m (40ft), ↔ 8m (25ft). USA (N. Carolina, Arkansas). ✲✲✲. **f. rosea** bears pink-tinged white flowers.
f. vestita 🏆 has hairless leaves and bears larger white, occasionally pink-tinged flowers.
H. tetraptera see *H. carolina*.

x HALIMIOCISTUS

CISTACEAE

Hybrid genus of evergreen shrubs derived from crosses between *Cistus* and *Halimium*, some of which are found in hot, dry soils from Portugal to France (Cevennes), where the parent species overlap. They have opposite, linear-lance-shaped to elliptic-lance-shaped or ovate leaves, and are cultivated for their flowers, which resemble rock roses (*Cistus* and *Helianthemum*). Grow at the front of a shrub or mixed border, at the base of a sunny wall, or in a raised bed or large rock garden.
• **HARDINESS** Fully hardy to frost hardy.
• **CULTIVATION** Grow in well-drained, sandy, poor to moderately fertile soil in full sun; they are less hardy if grown in shade or very fertile soil. Shelter from cold, drying winds. Pruning group 9; but pruning is rarely needed.
• **PROPAGATION** Root semi-ripe cuttings in late summer.
• **PESTS AND DISEASES** Trouble free.

x **H. 'Ingwersenii'**, syn. *Cistus ingwerseniana*, x *H. ingwersenii*. Dense, spreading shrub with linear-lance-shaped, dark green leaves, to 3.5cm (1½in) long. From late spring to late summer, bears umbel-like cymes of saucer-shaped white flowers, 2–2.5cm (¾–1in) across. ↕ 45cm (18in), ↔ 90cm (36in). Portugal. ✲✲✲ (borderline)
x **H. sahucii** ▣ 🏆 (*Cistus salviifolius* x *Halimium umbellatum*) syn. *Cistus revolii* of gardens. Compact, mound-forming or spreading shrub with linear to inversely lance-shaped, dark green leaves, to 4cm (1½in) long. Umbel-like cymes of saucer-shaped white flowers, 3cm (1¼in) across, are borne in summer. ↕ 45cm (18in), ↔ 90cm (36in). S. France. ✲✲✲
x **H. wintonensis** 🏆 (*Cistus salviifolius* x *Halimium ocymoides*) syn. *Cistus wintonensis, Halimium wintonense.* Spreading shrub with ovate or elliptic-lance-shaped, white-woolly, grey-green leaves, to 5cm (2in) long. In late spring and early summer, bears umbel-like

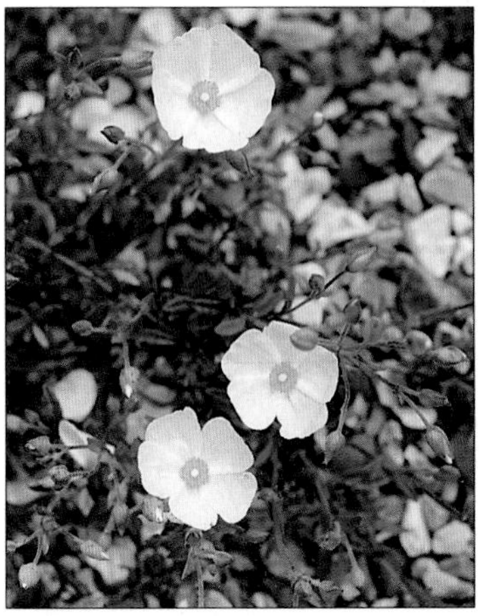

x *Halimiocistus sahucii*

H

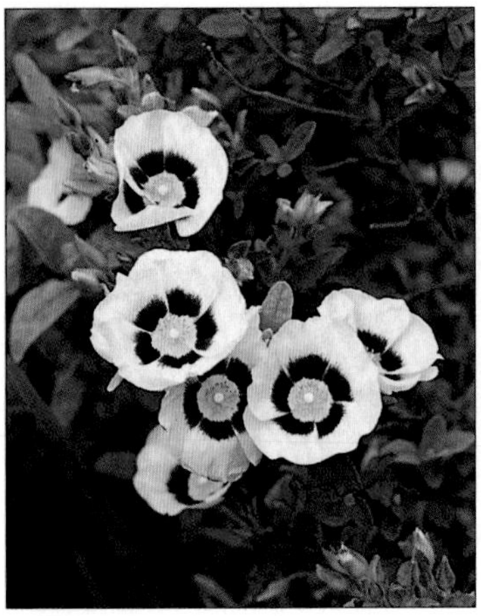
x *Halimiocistus wintonensis* 'Merrist Wood Cream'

cymes of saucer-shaped white flowers, 5cm (2in) across, with yellow stamens and dark crimson-maroon bands. ↕60cm (24in), ↔90cm (36in). Garden origin. ❄❄❄ (borderline). **'Merrist Wood Cream'** ■ ♀ has creamy yellow, red-banded flowers, with yellow centres.

HALIMIUM

CISTACEAE

Genus of 9–12 species of evergreen shrubs found in thickets, rocky and sandy places, and dry woodland in the Mediterranean, Turkey, and N. Africa. They have opposite, variably shaped, light to grey-green leaves and are grown for their showy, saucer-shaped flowers, which resemble rock roses (*Cistus* and *Helianthemum*). Grow at the front of a mixed or shrub border, in a large rock garden, or in containers on a patio or in a courtyard garden. Halimiums flower best in regions with long, hot summers.

- **HARDINESS** Frost hardy.
- **CULTIVATION** Grow in well-drained, moderately fertile, sandy soil in full sun with shelter from cold, drying winds. Established plants dislike transplanting. Pruning group 9.
- **PROPAGATION** Sow seed at 19–24°C (66–75°F) in spring, or root semi-ripe cuttings in late summer.
- **PESTS AND DISEASES** Trouble free.

H. atriplicifolium. Upright shrub with elliptic to broadly elliptic, silver-scaly leaves, to 5cm (2in) long. Bright yellow flowers, 4–4.5cm (1½–1¾in) across, unmarked or with a dark red-brown

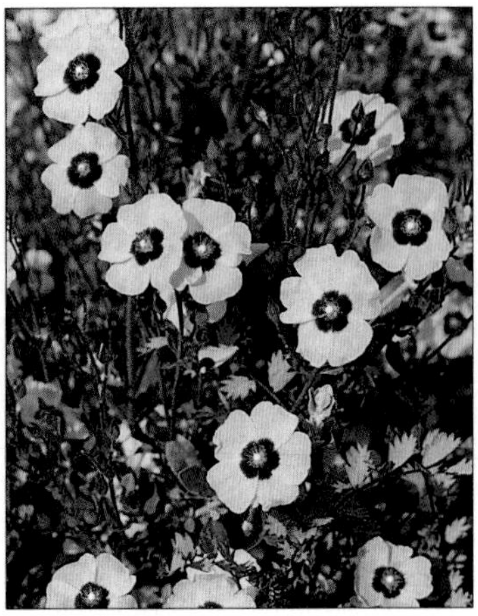
Halimium 'Susan'

spot at the base of each petal, are borne in panicle-like cymes in late spring and early summer. ↕1.5m (5ft), ↔1m (3ft). Spain, Morocco. ❄❄
H. formosum see *H. lasianthum.*
H. halimifolium. Upright shrub with narrowly obovate to elliptic leaves, to 4.5cm (1¾in) long, whitish and hairy at first, later grey-green. Yellow flowers, 3–3.5cm (1¼–1½in) across, sometimes with a dark red-brown spot at the base of each petal, open in panicle-like cymes in late spring and early summer. ↕↔1m (3ft). S.W. Europe, N. Africa. ❄❄
H. lasianthum ♀ syn. *H. formosum.* Spreading, bushy shrub with ovate to oblong, grey-green leaves, 4cm (1½in) long. Axillary clusters of golden yellow flowers, to 3cm (1¼in) across, with or without a brownish red mark at the base of each petal, open in late spring and early summer. ↕1m (3ft), ↔1.5m (5ft). S. Portugal, S. Spain. ❄❄. **subsp. *formosum*** ■ has flowers to 4cm (1½in) across, with bold brownish red marks at the bases of the petals; S. Portugal.
H. ocymoides ♀ syn. *Cistus algarvensis.* Bushy, usually erect shrub with obovate to inversely lance-shaped, white-downy, grey-green leaves, to 3cm (1¼in) long. In early summer, golden yellow flowers, to 3cm (1¼in) across, with black-purple centres, are borne in erect, terminal panicles. ↕60cm (24in), ↔1m (3ft). Portugal, Spain. ❄❄
***H.* 'Susan'** ■ ♀ Spreading shrub with oval, grey-green leaves, to 4cm (1½in) long. In summer, bears terminal panicles of bright yellow, often semi-double flowers, 2–2.5cm (¾–1in) across, with bold red-purple centres. ↕45cm (18in), ↔60cm (24in). ❄❄
H. umbellatum ■ syn. *Helianthemum umbellatum.* Upright shrub with linear, glossy, dark green leaves, to 3cm (1¼in) long, white-hairy beneath. Terminal racemes of up to 8 white flowers, to 2cm (¾in) across, each petal stained yellow at the base, open from red buds in early summer. ↕45cm (18in), ↔60cm (24in). S.W. Europe. ❄❄
H. wintonense see x *Halimiocistus wintonensis.*

HALIMODENDRON

LEGUMINOSAE/PAPILIONACEAE

Genus of one species of deciduous, spiny shrub found on salt-rich flood plains from Ukraine to N. and E. Asia. Valued for its silvery foliage and pea-like flowers, it is useful for a shrub border, and is ideal for coastal areas, where it is an effective windbreak.

- **HARDINESS** Fully hardy.
- **CULTIVATION** Grow in poor, sharply drained, neutral to alkaline soil in full sun. Will tolerate salty soil, but not winter wet. Pruning group 1.
- **PROPAGATION** Sow seed in containers in a cold frame in autumn or spring. Take root cuttings in winter, or layer in summer or autumn. Seedlings grown on their own roots are prone to rot in wet soils or humid climates; graft them on to *Caragana* or *Laburnum* in late winter.
- **PESTS AND DISEASES** Trouble free.

H. halodendron (Salt tree). Open-branched, spiny shrub with alternate, pinnate, silver-grey leaves, 2–3.5cm (¾–1½in) long, each ending in a spine and having 1 or 2 pairs of inversely lance-shaped leaflets. Axillary racemes, to 4cm (1½in) long, of pea-like, violet to purple-pink flowers, to 2cm (¾in) long, are borne in early and mid-summer. ↕↔2m (6ft). Ukraine, Georgia, N.E. Turkey, Iran, C. and E. Asia, and Russia (S.E. Russia, Siberia). ❄❄❄

HAMAMELIS

Witch hazel

HAMAMELIDACEAE

Genus of 5 or 6 species of deciduous shrubs occurring in woodland, at woodland margins, and on riverbanks in E. Asia and North America. They have alternate, broadly ovate to obovate leaves, and are grown for their autumn colour and their frost-resistant, fragrant,

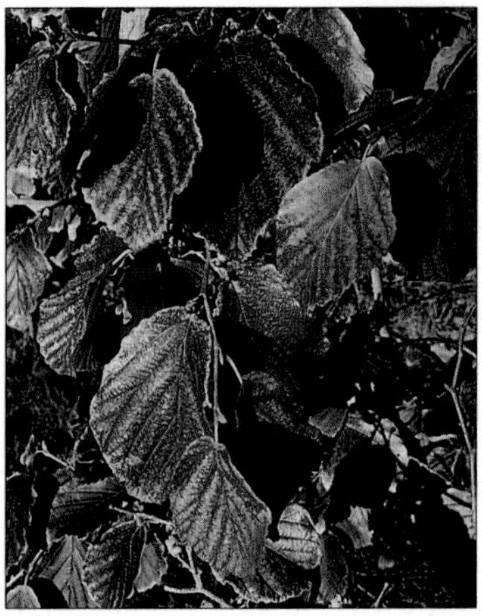
Hamamelis x *intermedia* 'Diane'

spider-shaped flowers. The flowers, 2–3cm (¾–1¼in) across, with 4 narrow petals, are borne in dense, axillary clusters, mainly from winter to autumn. Witch hazels are good specimen plants, and are also effective planted in groups in a shrub border or woodland garden.

- **HARDINESS** Fully hardy.
- **CULTIVATION** Grow in moderately fertile, moist but well-drained, acid to neutral soil in full sun or partial shade, in an open but not exposed site. Witch hazels will also tolerate deep, humus-rich soils over chalk. Pruning group 1.
- **PROPAGATION** Sow seed in containers in a cold frame as soon as ripe. Graft cultivars in late winter, or bud in late summer.
- **PESTS AND DISEASES** Honey fungus and coral spot may be a problem.

H.* x *intermedia (*H. japonica* x *H. mollis*). Vase-shaped shrub with ascending branches and broadly oval to obovate, bright green leaves, to 15cm (6in) long, turning yellow in autumn. In early and midwinter, bears fragrant, yellow, dark red, or orange flowers, with crimped petals, on the bare branches. ↕↔4m (12ft). Garden origin. ❄❄❄. **'Advent'** bears bright yellow flowers in early winter. **'Allgold'** bears small, dark yellow flowers in mid- and late winter. **'Arnold Promise'** ■ ♀ produces large yellow flowers in mid- and late winter. **'Diane'** ■ ♀ has dark red flowers in mid- and late winter, and orange to yellow and red autumn foliage. **'Jelena'** ■ ♀ bears large, coppery orange flowers in early and midwinter, and has orange and red autumn foliage. **'Moonlight'** bears

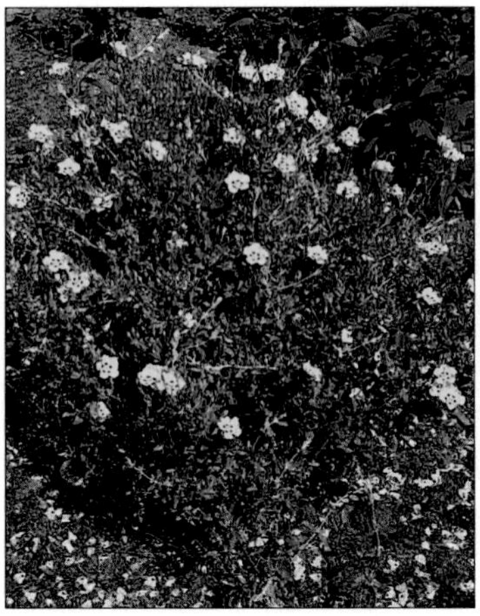
Halimium lasianthum subsp. *formosum*

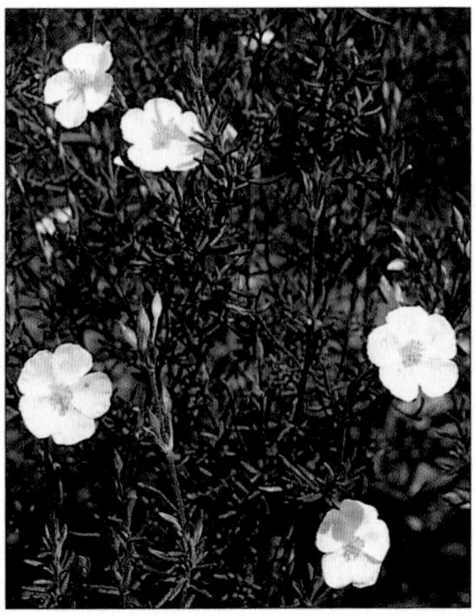
Halimium umbellatum

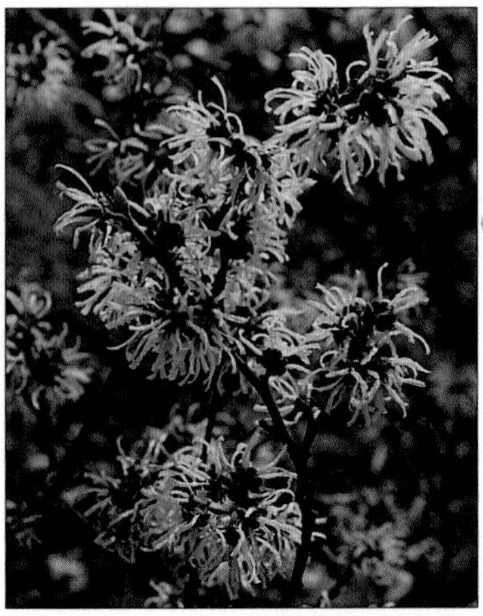
Hamamelis x *intermedia* 'Arnold Promise'

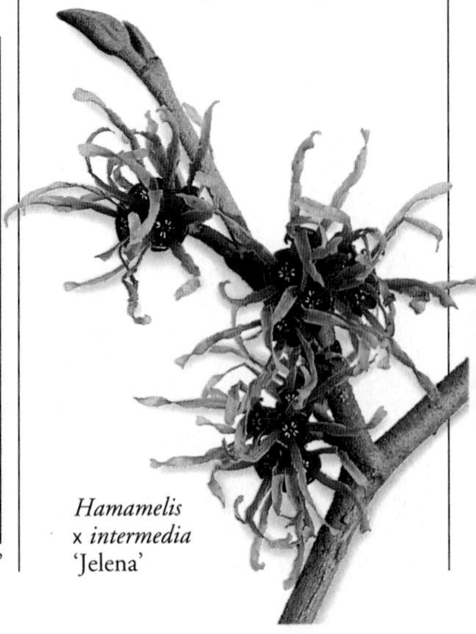
Hamamelis x *intermedia* 'Jelena'

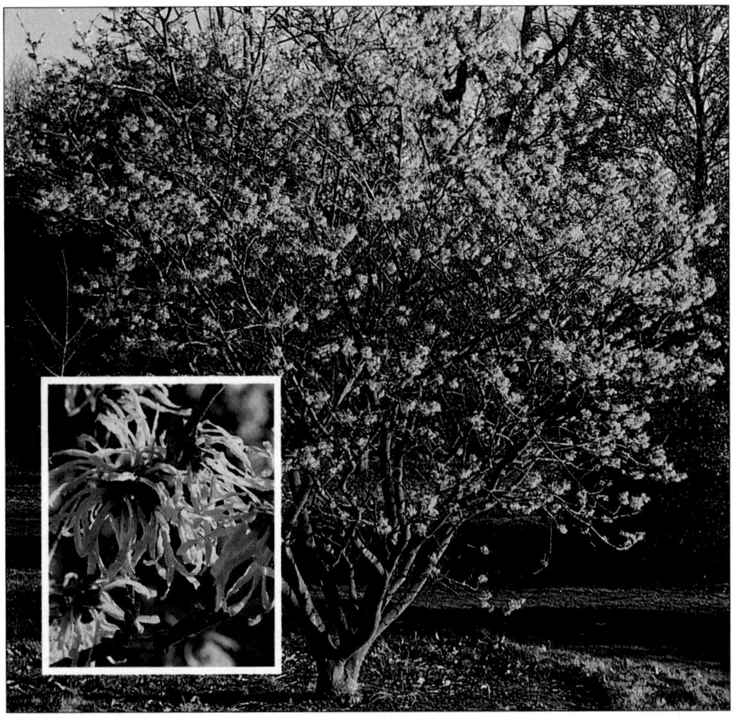

Hamamelis x *intermedia* 'Pallida' (inset: flower detail)

large, pale yellow flowers in mid- and late winter. **'Pallida'** ■♀ syn. *H. mollis* 'Pallida', has clusters of large, sulphur-yellow flowers in mid- and late winter. **'Sunburst'** is narrowly upright, with large, pale yellow flowers in mid- and late winter; ↔ 2.5m (8ft). **'Vezna'** ■ has large, dark orange-yellow flowers with pendent petals, flushed red at the bases, in mid- and late winter.
H. japonica (Japanese witch hazel). Upright, open-branched shrub with broadly oval to obovate, glossy mid-green leaves, to 10cm (4in) long, which turn yellow in autumn. Yellow flowers, with crimped petals, open on bare branches in mid- and late winter. ↕↔ 4m (12ft). Japan. ✼✼✼. **'Sulphurea'** ■ bears a profusion of small, pale sulphur-yellow flowers in mid- and late winter. **'Zuccariniana'** bears pale lemon-yellow flowers in late winter and early spring, and has orange-yellow autumn foliage.
H. mollis (Chinese witch hazel). Erect shrub with broadly oval to obovate, softly hairy, mid-green leaves, to 15cm (6in) long, turning yellow in autumn. Very fragrant, golden yellow flowers are borne on bare branches in mid- and late winter. ↕↔ 4m (12ft). W. and W. central China. ✼✼✼. **'Brevipetala'** ■ has dense clusters of short-petalled, golden yellow flowers, to 1.5cm (½in) across; it is possibly of hybrid origin. **'Coombe Wood'** is spreading, with large, strongly scented flowers; ↕ 4m (12ft), ↔ 5m (15ft). **'Goldcrest'** bears large flowers, flushed red at the bases of the petals, from midwinter to spring. **'Pallida'** see *H.* x *intermedia* 'Pallida'.
H. vernalis (Ozark witch hazel). Erect shrub with obovate, mid-green leaves, to 12cm (5in) long, turning yellow in autumn. Bears small, yellow to orange, sometimes red-tinged flowers on bare shoots in late winter and early spring. ↕↔ 5m (15ft). S. central USA. ✼✼✼. **'Lombart's Weeping'** has spreading, pendent branches; ↕ 2m (6ft), ↔ 3m (10ft). **'Sandra'** ♀ has purple young leaves, turning yellow, orange, red, and purple in autumn, and bears dark yellow flowers.
H. virginiana (Virginian witch hazel). Erect shrub with broadly oval, obovate, or nearly rounded leaves, to 15cm (6in) long, turning yellow in autumn. Small yellow flowers are borne in autumn, as the leaves begin to fall. ↕↔ 4m (12ft). E. North America. ✼✼✼

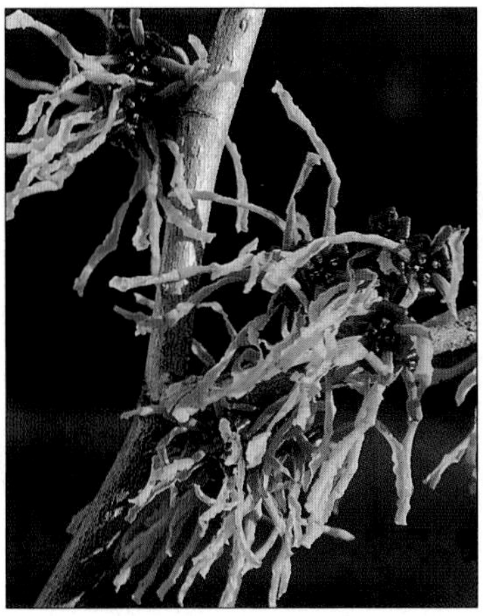

Hamamelis x *intermedia* 'Vezna'

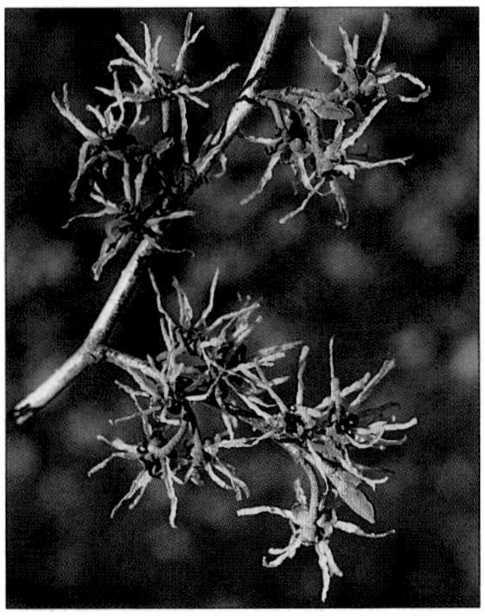

Hamamelis japonica 'Sulphurea'

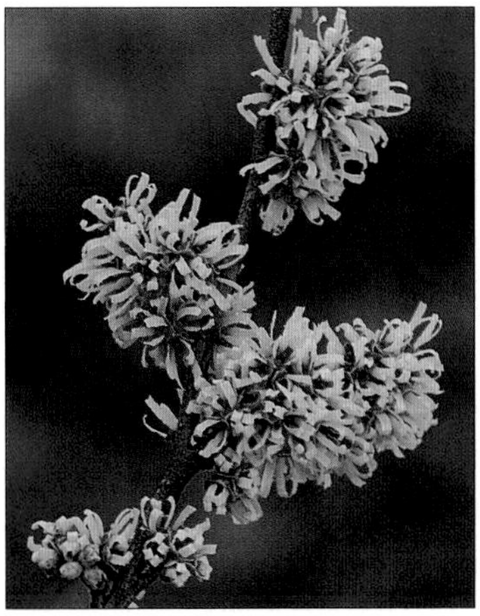

Hamamelis mollis 'Brevipetala'

▷ ***Hamatocactus crassihamatus*** see *Sclerocactus uncinatus* var. *crassihamatus*
▷ ***Hamatocactus hamatacanthus*** see *Ferocactus hamatacanthus*
▷ ***Hamatocactus setispinus*** see *Thelocactus setispinus*
▷ ***Hamatocactus uncinatus*** see *Sclerocactus uncinatus*
▷ **Handkerchief tree** see *Davidia*

HAPLOPAPPUS

ASTERACEAE/COMPOSITAE

Genus of 160 species of annuals, perennials, subshrubs, and shrubs found in open, sunny habitats in North and South America. Cultivated for their usually opposite, entire or lobed leaves, and yellow, sometimes purple, daisy-like flowerheads, they are suitable for a rock garden, trough, or raised bed.
• **HARDINESS** Fully hardy.
• **CULTIVATION** Grow in neutral to slightly alkaline, poor to moderately fertile, sharply drained soil in full sun; protect from excessive winter wet. Trim back untidy plants after flowering.
• **PROPAGATION** Sow seed in containers in a cold frame as soon as ripe or in spring. Root softwood cuttings in spring.
• **PESTS AND DISEASES** Trouble free.

H. acaulis see *Stenotus acaulis*.
H. coronopifolius see *H. glutinosus*.
H. glutinosus, syn. *H. coronopifolius*. Tufted, evergreen perennial, usually forming dense cushions of spreading or erect stems clothed in oblong or elliptic, lobed or pinnatisect, sticky leaves, to 4cm (1½in) long. Solitary, daisy-like yellow flowerheads, to 2.5cm (1in) across, are borne in summer. ↕ 15cm (6in), ↔ to 30cm (12in). Chile, Argentina. ✼✼✼

HARDENBERGIA

Coral pea

LEGUMINOSAE/PAPILIONACEAE

Genus of 3 species of evergreen, twining or trailing climbers occurring in Australia in a diverse range of habitats, from coastal plains to rocky scree in mountainous areas. They have alternate, ovate to lance-shaped leaves, which may be 3-palmate (rarely 5-palmate) or may consist of only 1 leaflet, with the 2 lateral leaflets suppressed. Colourful, small, pea-like flowers are borne, often in profusion, in axillary racemes or

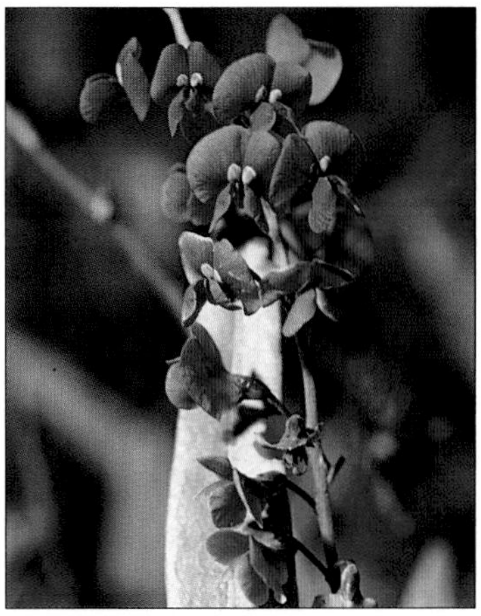

Hardenbergia comptoniana

occasionally in panicles. In frost-prone areas, grow in a temperate greenhouse or conservatory. In milder climates, use to cover an arbour, pergola, or wall, or grow through large shrubs or small trees.
• **HARDINESS** Half hardy to frost tender; *H. comptoniana* may survive short spells down to 0°C (32°F) and *H. violacea* to -4°C (25°F).
• **CULTIVATION** Under glass, grow in a mix of equal parts loam-based potting compost (JI No.2), sharp sand, and leaf mould, in full light with shade from hot sun; provide low to moderate humidity. In the growing season, water moderately and apply a balanced liquid fertilizer monthly; keep just moist in winter. Pot on or top-dress in spring. Provide with support. Outdoors, grow in moderately fertile, moist but well-drained, acid to neutral soil in full sun or partial shade. Pruning group 11, after flowering.
• **PROPAGATION** Sow seed at 20°C (68°F) in spring; pre-soak for 24 hours to aid germination. Root softwood cuttings in spring.
• **PESTS AND DISEASES** Prone to red spider mites and aphids under glass.

H. comptoniana ■♀ Vigorous climber with 3-palmate, occasionally 5-palmate, dark green leaves, composed of narrowly lance-shaped to broadly ovate leaflets, to 15cm (6in) long. From early spring to midsummer, bears pendent racemes, to 13cm (5in) long, of mauve to purple-blue flowers, to 1.5cm (½in) across, the standards with green-spotted white marks at the bases. ↕ 3m (10ft) or more. Australia (Western Australia). (min. 3–5°C/37–41°F)
H. monophylla see *H. violacea*.
H. violacea ♀ syn. *H. monophylla* (Purple coral pea). Strong-growing climber, sometimes trailing in habit. Each leaf has 1 ovate to lance-shaped, leathery, rich green leaflet, to 12cm (5in) long; the other 2 leaflets are suppressed. Purple to violet, sometimes white, pink, or lilac flowers, 1cm (½in) across, the standards spotted yellow or green, are borne in pendent racemes, 10–13cm (4–5in) long, from late winter to early summer. ↕ 2m (6ft) or more. Australia (South Australia, Queensland to Tasmania). ✼. **'Alba'** see 'White Crystal'. **'Happy Wanderer'** is very vigorous, bearing panicles of mauve-purple flowers. **'Pink Cascade'** bears pink flowers. **'White Crystal'**, syn. 'Alba', produces pure white flowers in late winter.

▷ **Hardheads** see *Centaurea*
▷ **Harebell** see *Campanula rotundifolia*
▷ **Hare's ear, Shrubby** see *Bupleurum fruticosum*
▷ **Hare's tail** see *Lagurus, L. ovatus*
▷ **Harlequin flower** see *Sparaxis*

HARRISIA

CACTACEAE

Genus of 10–20 species of tree-like, perennial cacti closely allied to *Eriocereus*, with which they are often confused. They are found in hilly and low mountainous areas of S.E. USA, the Bahamas, the West Indies, and South America. The slender, erect or spreading, occasionally decumbent stems usually have 9–11 rounded ribs. The large, narrowly or widely funnel-shaped flowers open at night in summer. In frost-prone regions, grow in a warm greenhouse or conservatory. In warm, dry climates, use in a desert garden.

• **HARDINESS** Frost tender.
• **CULTIVATION** Under glass, grow in standard cactus compost in full light, with shade from hot sun. In growth, water moderately and apply a low-nitrogen liquid fertilizer monthly; keep dry in winter. Provide good ventilation but keep clear of draughts. Outdoors, grow in poor, sharply drained, acid to neutral soil in full sun. Protect from excessive winter wet. See also pp.48–49.
• **PROPAGATION** Sow seed at 21–24°C (70–75°F) in spring. Root stem cuttings, or remove and pot up offsets, in spring or summer.
• **PESTS AND DISEASES** Prone to scale insects, especially on young growth.

H. bonplandii, syn. *Eriocereus pomanensis, H. pomanensis.* Erect to prostrate cactus with bluish green stems bearing 4 or 5 obtuse or rounded ribs with low, broad grooves between. Grey areoles bear white- or pink-tinged, later black-tipped spines (6–8 radials and 1 longer central). White flowers, 15cm (6in) or more long, with green outer segments, are borne in summer. ↕↔ 2m (6ft). S. Brazil, Paraguay, N. and W. Argentina. ❀ (min. 13°C/55°F)

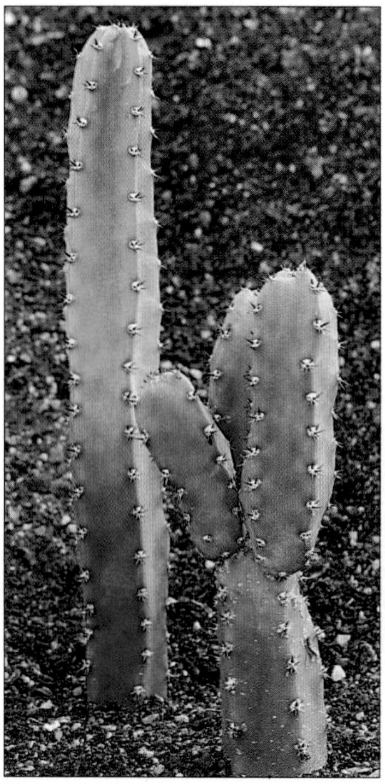

Harrisia jusbertii

H. gracilis. Spreading or erect, tree-like cactus producing branching, dark green stems with 8–12 ribs, white areoles, and black-tipped white spines (10–16 radials and 1 central). In summer, bears white flowers, 20cm (8in) long, with toothed inner tepals and pale brown outer segments. ↕ to 5m (15ft) or more, ↔ 2m (6ft). S.E. USA (Florida), Jamaica. ❀ (min. 13°C/55°F)

H. jusbertii ■ syn. *Eriocereus jusbertii.* Erect, occasionally branching cactus producing dark green stems with 4–6 broad ribs, yellowish grey areoles, and brown or black spines (about 7 radials and 1–4 slightly longer centrals). In summer, bears flowers to 18cm (7in) long, with white inner petals and brownish green outer segments. Origin unknown. ↕↔ 1m (3ft) or more. ❀ (min. 13°C/55°F)

H. pomanensis see *H. bonplandii.*

▷ **Harry Lauder's walking stick** see *Corylus avellana* 'Contorta'

HATIORA syn. RHIPSALIDOPSIS

CACTACEAE

Genus of about 6 species of epiphytic or terrestrial, freely branching, perennial cacti, now incorporating the Easter cacti (*Rhipsalidopsis*), from forest or rocky areas in Brazil. They have slender, generally segmented, erect or pendent stems. New growth and the trumpet- to funnel-shaped, diurnal flowers are produced only from the areoles, which form at the apex of each segment. The flowers are followed by spherical to obovoid, white or yellow fruits, 3–5mm (⅛–¼in) across. Where temperatures fall below 13°C (55°F), grow as house-plants, or in a warm greenhouse, in containers or hanging baskets, or with air plants (*Tillandsia* species) on a bromeliad "tree". In warmer climates, grow in containers on a patio or in a courtyard garden.
• **HARDINESS** Frost tender.
• **CULTIVATION** Under glass, grow epiphytically or in epiphytic cactus compost in bright filtered or indirect light, with high humidity. In growth, water moderately, mist daily with soft water, and apply a half-strength, low-nitrogen liquid fertilizer monthly. Keep just moist in winter until buds develop, then increase water slightly. Outdoors,

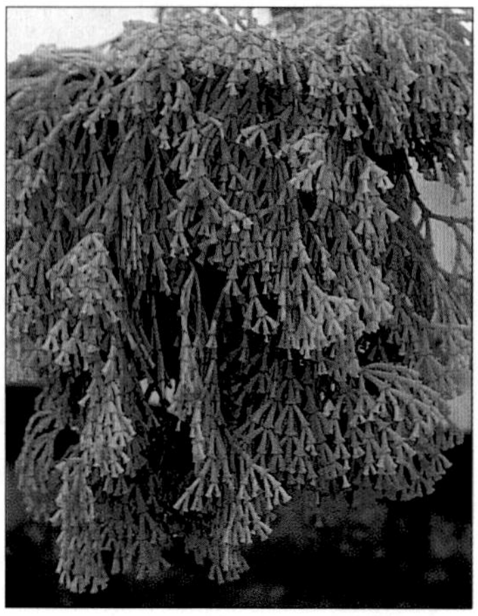

Hatiora epiphylloides

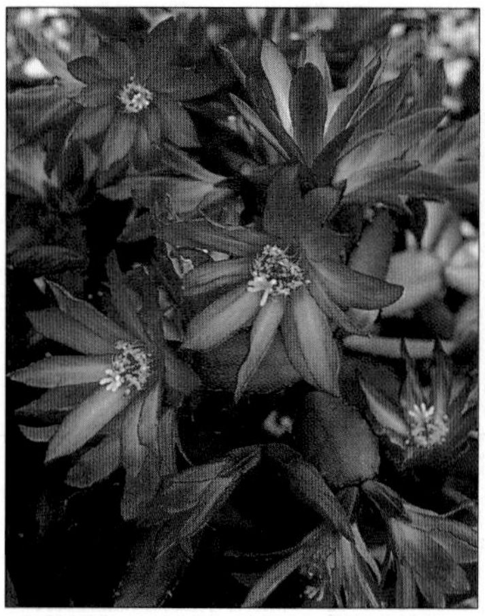

Hatiora gaertneri

grow in containers or in poor, humus-rich, moist but well-drained, acid to neutral soil in full sun or dappled shade. See also pp.48–49.
• **PROPAGATION** Sow seed at 21–24°C (70–75°F) in spring. Root cuttings in spring or summer.
• **PESTS AND DISEASES** Susceptible to mealybugs.

H. epiphylloides ■ syn. *Pseudozygocactus epiphylloides.* Pendent cactus producing stems with cylindrical to wedge-shaped, fleshy, bright green segments, to 2.5cm (1in) long, and minute, spineless areoles. In early spring, bears funnel-shaped yellow flowers, 1cm (½in) long. ↕ 45cm (18in), ↔ 20cm (8in). Brazil. ❀ (min. 13°C/55°F)

H. gaertneri ■ syn. *Rhipsalidopsis gaertneri.* Bushy, semi-pendent cactus producing stems with flat, oblong or elliptic, shallowly scalloped, mid-green segments, 4–7cm (1½–3in) long. Each segment has 3–5 tubercles, with areoles on each side bearing 1 or 2 yellow-brown bristles. Funnel-shaped scarlet flowers, 4–8cm (1½–3in) long, are produced from the newer segments in spring. ↕ 15cm (6in), ↔ 25cm (10in). E. Brazil. ❀ (min. 13°C/55°F)

H. rosea ■ syn. *Rhipsalidopsis rosea* (Easter cactus). Shrubby, pendent or erect cactus producing stems with flat, sometimes 3- to 5-angled, mid-green segments, 2–4cm (¾–1½in) long, usually with thin red margins and minute areoles bearing a few hairy, pale brown bristles. In early spring, trumpet-shaped, rose-pink flowers, 3–4cm (1¼–1½in) long, open on longer areoles

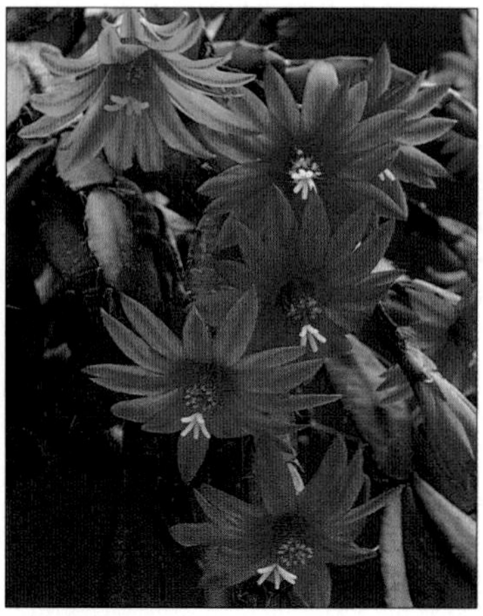

Hatiora rosea

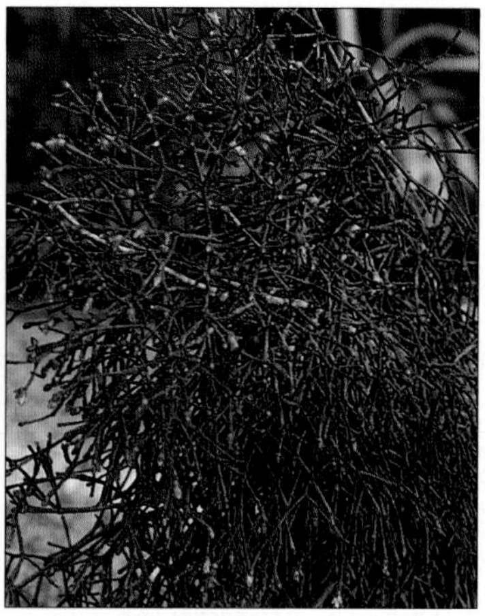

Hatiora salicornioides

at the tops of the segments. ↕↔ to 15cm (6in). S.E. Brazil. ❀ (min. 13°C/55°F)

H. salicornioides ■ 🏆 (Drunkard's dream). Bushy, erect or pendent cactus producing stems with club-shaped, mid-green to bronze-green segments, 1–5cm (½–2in) long, usually arranged in whorls of 2–5. In spring, bears funnel-shaped, golden yellow or orange flowers, 1cm (½in) long, from the areoles of new segments. ↕↔ 40cm (16in). S.E. Brazil. ❀ (min. 13°C/55°F)

▷ **Hat plant, Mexican** see *Kalanchoe daigremontiana*
▷ **Hattie's pincushion** see *Astrantia*
▷ **Haw,**
Possum see *Ilex decidua*
Yellow see *Crataegus flava*
▷ **Hawk's beard** see *Crepis*
▷ **Hawkweed** see *Hieracium*
Leafy see *Hieracium umbellatum*
Orange see *Pilosella aurantiaca*

HAWORTHIA

ALOEACEAE/LILIACEAE

Genus of over 150 species of dwarf, basal-rosetted, more or less stemless, perennial succulents from lowland and sometimes hillsides of Namibia, Swaziland, Mozambique, and South Africa. They generally offset to form clumps. The linear to broadly ovate or triangular, fleshy, variably coloured leaves are often covered with minute, bright tubercles, which are sometimes almost transparent. The small, tubular to funnel-shaped flowers are borne in loose racemes from spring to autumn. In frost-prone areas, grow as foliage plants in a temperate or warm greenhouse or conservatory. In warmer regions, grow in a trough or raised bed, or in containers outdoors.
• **HARDINESS** Frost tender.
• **CULTIVATION** Under glass, grow in standard cactus compost in bright filtered light, with low humidity and good ventilation. In growth, water moderately and apply a low-nitrogen liquid fertilizer monthly; keep dry in winter. Pot on in spring. Outdoors, grow in poor, sharply drained, neutral to slightly alkaline soil in sun or partial shade; protect from excessive winter wet.
• **PROPAGATION** Sow seed at 21–24°C (70–75°F) in spring. Pot up offsets, or divide, in spring. Root leaf cuttings from soft-leaved species in spring or summer.
• **PESTS AND DISEASES** Susceptible to mealybugs.

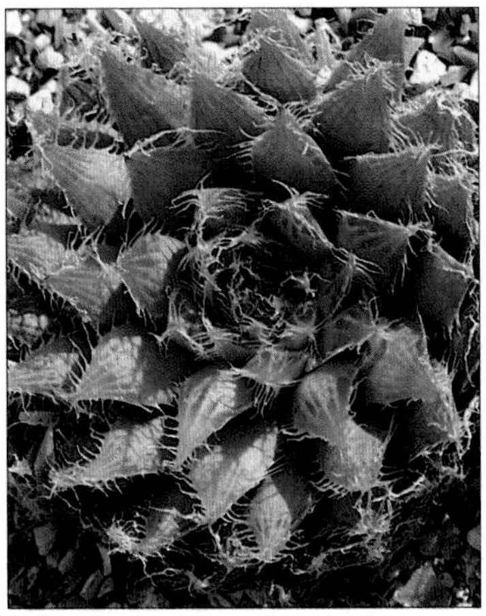

Haworthia arachnoidea

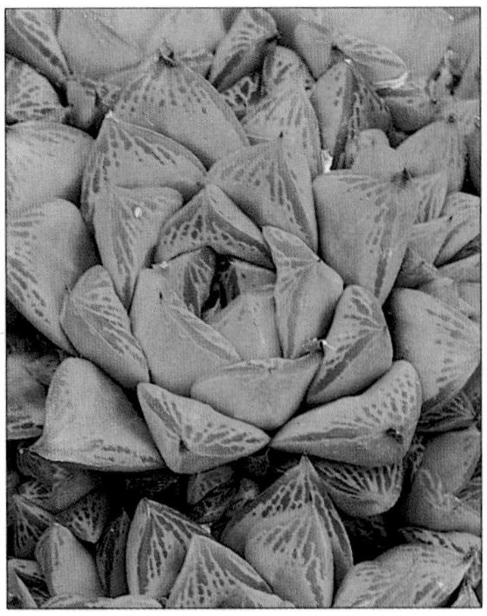

Haworthia cymbiformis

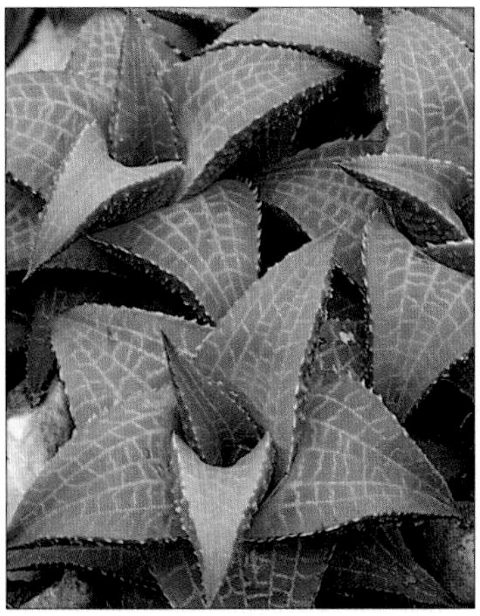

Haworthia tessellata

H. arachnoidea ▣ syn. *Aprica arachnoidea, H. setata.* Clump-forming succulent producing oblong or lance-shaped, dark green leaves, 2–7cm (¾–3in) long, margined and tipped with white to pale brown teeth; leaf surfaces are transparent with continuous darker lines. In spring, stems to 30cm (12in) tall bear tubular to funnel-shaped white flowers, to 1.5cm (½in) long, in racemes 8cm (3in) long. ↕ to 5cm (2in), ↔ 10cm (4in). South Africa (Northern Cape, Western Cape, Eastern Cape). ❄ (min. 10°C/50°F)
H. attenuata. Extremely variable, clump-forming succulent, which is either stemless or has a short stem. Narrowly triangular, dark green leaves, 3–8cm (1¼–3in) long, are covered with a median line of white tubercles above, and a transverse band of white tubercles beneath. In summer, stems to 40cm (16in) long bear tubular to funnel-shaped, green-keeled white flowers, to 1.5cm (½in) long, in racemes to 18cm (7in) long. ↕↔ to 12cm (5in). South Africa (Northern Cape, Eastern Cape). ❄ (min. 10°C/50°F). **f. *clariperla*** ▣ has triangular leaves to 6cm (2½in) long, the upper surfaces covered with small white tubercles, the undersides with rows of larger tubercles.
H. cymbiformis ▣ syn. *H. planifolia.* Variable, clump-forming succulent with obovate to ovate, tapering, smooth or finely toothed leaves, 3–5cm (1¼–2in) long. They are bright pale green, sometimes flushed pink, concave above, convex beneath, and have translucent tips with thin, longitudinal, pale green or greenish white stripes. In spring, stems to 20cm (8in) long bear funnel-shaped, pinkish white flowers, to 1.5cm (½in) long, with brownish green keels, in racemes to 10cm (4in) long. ↕ 8cm (3in), ↔ 25cm (10in). South Africa (Eastern Cape). ❄ (min. 10°C/50°F)
H. fasciata ▣ Very variable, clump-forming, stemless succulent producing triangular-lance-shaped, dark green leaves, to 8cm (3in) long, smooth above, convex and cross-banded with white tubercles beneath. In summer, stems to 40cm (16in) long bear tubular to funnel-shaped white flowers, to 1.5cm (½in) long, with red-brown keels, in racemes 11cm (4½in) long. ↕ to 10cm (4in), ↔ 30cm (12in). South Africa (Eastern Cape). ❄ (min. 10°C/50°F)
H. margaritifera see *H. pumila.*
H. maughanii. Clustering succulent with erect, conical to cylindrical, blunt-tipped, thick, rough, greyish green to reddish brown leaves, to 2.5cm (1in) long; most of the plant is below soil level, with only the flat, translucent, window-tip of each leaf exposed. From autumn to winter, stems to 21cm (8in) long bear brown-keeled white flowers, to 1.5cm (½in) long, in racemes to 7cm (3in) long. ↕ 2cm (¾in), ↔ 10cm (4in). South Africa (Western Cape). ❄ (min. 10°C/50°F)
H. planifolia see *H. cymbiformis.*
H. pumila, syn. *H. margaritifera* (Pearl plant). Very variable, clump-forming succulent with incurved to erect, triangular-ovate, dark green or purple-green leaves, to 10cm (4in) long, with small, silver tubercles on both surfaces and sharp, red-brown tips. In summer, branched stems, to 40cm (16in) long, bear tubular to funnel-shaped, brownish or yellowish green flowers, to 1.5cm (½in) long, in racemes 14cm (5½in) long. ↕ to 12cm (5in), ↔ 45cm (18in). South Africa (Western Cape). ❄ (min. 10°C/50°F)
H. reinwardtii. Variable, freely off-setting succulent with dense rosettes of spirally arranged, ovate to lance-shaped, dark green to yellow-green leaves, 2–5cm (¾–2in) long. The leaves have small, green or white tubercles in 1–3 longitudinal rows above; the undersides have tubercles in longitudinal rows or cross-bands. In spring, stems to 35cm (14in) long bear lax racemes, 9–17cm (3½–7in) long, of tubular, pinkish white flowers, 2cm (¾in) long, with greenish brown keels. ↕ 20cm (8in), ↔ indefinite. South Africa (Western Cape, Eastern Cape). ❄ (min. 10°C/50°F)
H. retusa. Variable, clump-forming succulent with ovate-triangular leaves, 3–8cm (1¼–3in) long, recurved horizontally on the upper surfaces, with rounded, sometimes rough or almost translucent tips. The leaves are pale or deep green, and often have minute tubercles, pale lines, and sometimes numerous isolated soft teeth. In late winter and early spring, stems to 70cm (28in) long bear narrowly tubular, green-keeled white flowers, to 1.5cm (½in) long, in racemes to 50cm (20in) long. ↕ 6cm (2½in), ↔ 20cm (8in). South Africa (Western Cape, Eastern Cape). ❄ (min. 10°C/50°F)
H. setata see *H. arachnoidea.*
H. tessellata ▣ 🏆 syn. *H. venosa* subsp. *tessellata.* Mat-forming succulent spreading by subterranean branches. The triangular-ovate, tapering, usually recurved, bluish grey-green leaves, 5–7cm (2–3in) long, are convex above, roughly warty beneath and on the margins; the upper surfaces are chequered with pale lines. In spring, stems to 50cm (20in) long bear tubular, greenish white flowers, to 2cm (¾in) long, in racemes to 15cm (6in) long. ↕ 10cm (4in), ↔ 30cm (12in). Namibia, South Africa. ❄ (min. 10°C/50°F)
H. truncata ▣ Clustering succulent producing 2 rows of erect, incurved, oblong, thick, bluish grey leaves, 2cm (¾in) long, with grey lines, rough, warty surfaces, and very blunt tips forming flat ends, which are slightly translucent when young. The plant body is below soil level, with only the window-tip of each leaf exposed. From summer to autumn, stems 23cm (9in) long bear tubular, green-keeled white flowers, to 1.5cm (½in) long, in racemes to 7cm (3in) long. ↕ 2cm (¾in), ↔ 10cm (4in). South Africa (Western Cape). ❄ (min. 10°C/50°F)
H. venosa* subsp. *tessellata see *H. tessellata.*

▷**Hawthorn** see *Crataegus*
Common see *Crataegus monogyna*
Indian see *Rhaphiolepis indica*
Midland see *Crataegus laevigata*
Water see *Aponogeton distachyos*
▷**Hazel** see *Corylus*
Chilean see *Gevuina avellana*
Corkscrew see *Corylus avellana* 'Contorta'
Turkish see *Corylus colurna*
▷**Headache tree** see *Umbellularia californica*
▷**Heart leaf** see *Philodendron cordatum, P. scandens*
▷**Heart of flame** see *Bromelia balansae*
▷**Heart of Jesus** see *Caladium bicolor*
▷**Heart pea** see *Cardiospermum halicacabum*
▷**Heartsease** see *Viola tricolor*
▷**Heart seed** see *Cardiospermum*
▷**Hearts on a string** see *Ceropegia linearis* subsp. *woodii*
▷**Heath** see *Erica*
Alpine see *Erica carnea*
Azores see *Daboecia azorica*
Besom see *Erica scoparia*
Blood-red see *Erica cruenta*
Cantabrian see *Daboecia cantabrica*
Channelled see *Erica canaliculata*
Common Australian see *Epacris impressa*
Cornish see *Erica vagans*
Corsican see *Erica terminalis*
Cross-leaved see *Erica tetralix*
Darley Dale see *Erica* x *darleyensis*
Dorset see *Erica ciliaris*
Dwarf Spanish see *Erica umbellata*
Erica see *Erica cerinthoides*
Fire see *Erica cerinthoides*
Irish see *Erica erigena*
Kapokkie see *Erica peziza*
Mackay's see *Erica mackaiana*
Mealie see *Erica patersonia*
Mediterranean see *Erica erigena*
Portuguese see *Erica lusitanica*
Prince of Wales see *Erica perspicua*
St. Dabeoc's see *Daboecia cantabrica*
Spanish see *Erica australis*
Spike see *Bruckenthalia spiculifolia*
Tree see *Erica arborea*
Veitch's see *Erica* x *veitchii*
Wandering see *Erica vagans*
Water see *Erica curviflora*
Watson's see *Erica* x *watsonii*

H

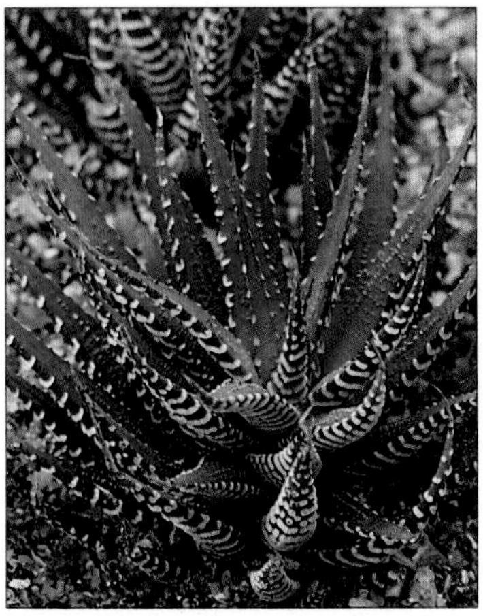

Haworthia attenuata f. *clariperla*

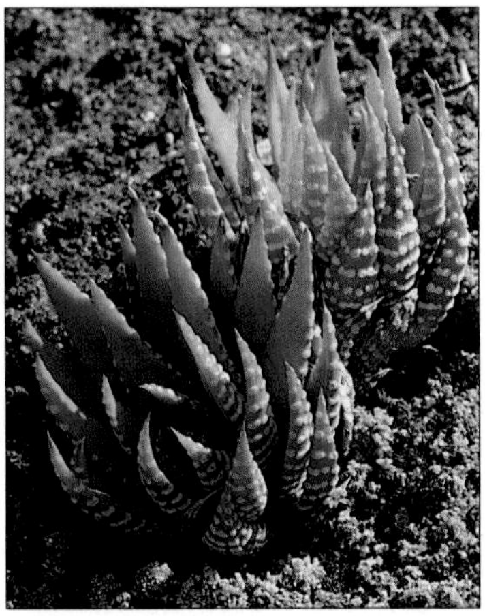

Haworthia fasciata

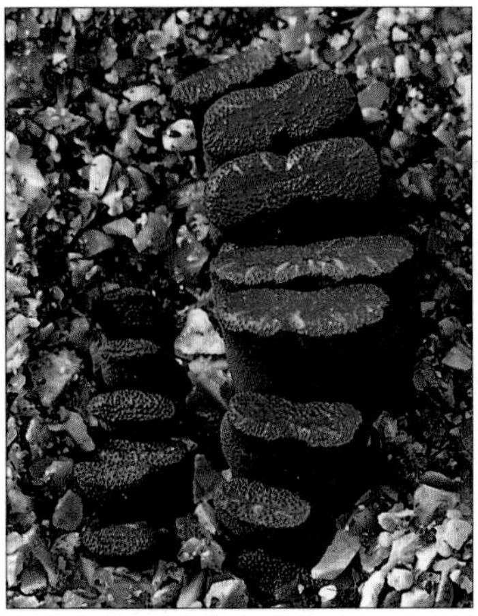

Haworthia truncata

▷**Heath cont.**
Whorled see *Erica manipuliflora*
Williams' see *Erica* x *williamsii*
Winter see *Erica carnea*
▷**Heather** see *Calluna*
Bell see *Erica cinerea*
False see *Cuphea hyssopifolia*
Golden see *Cassinia leptophylla* subsp. *fulvida*
Scots see *Calluna vulgaris*
Silver see *Cassinia leptophylla* subsp. *vauvilliersii* var. *albida*

HEBE

SCROPHULARIACEAE

Genus of approximately 100 species of evergreen shrubs, rarely trees, from a wide variety of habitats, ranging from rocky sites and cliffs to scrub and grassland; they are found from coastal areas to mountain regions, mainly in New Zealand, but also in S.E. Australia, New Guinea, and South America. The dense, opposite, sometimes 2- or 4-ranked leaves are scale-like to lance-shaped, rounded or ovate. Tubular flowers, expanding into 4 spreading lobes, are borne in terminal or axillary racemes, spikes, or small heads; they vary in colour from white to pink, blue, purple, or red. Most flowers range in size from 1–12mm (⅛–½in), and are described below as: small, 1–5mm (⅛–¼in) across; medium, 6–8mm (¼–⅜in) across; and large, 9–12mm (⅜–½in) across.

Hebes are suitable for a wide range of sites, including a mixed or shrub border, or a rock garden. In mild areas, particularly on the coast, they are useful as hedging and ground cover. Grow the less hardy species in an alpine house or cool greenhouse. Hebes are also good container plants and will tolerate some pollution. Those with small, scale-like leaves lying flat against the stems are known as "whipcord hebes", and are excellent plants for growing in a rock garden.

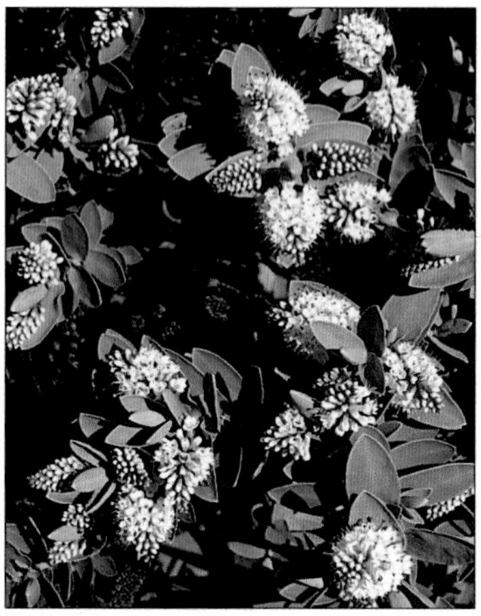
Hebe albicans

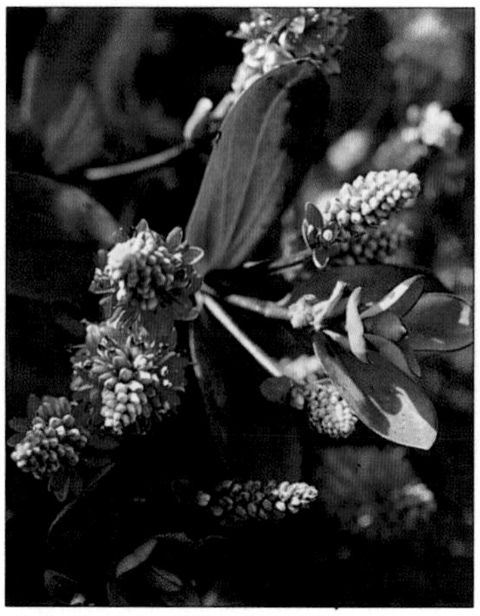
Hebe 'Autumn Glory'

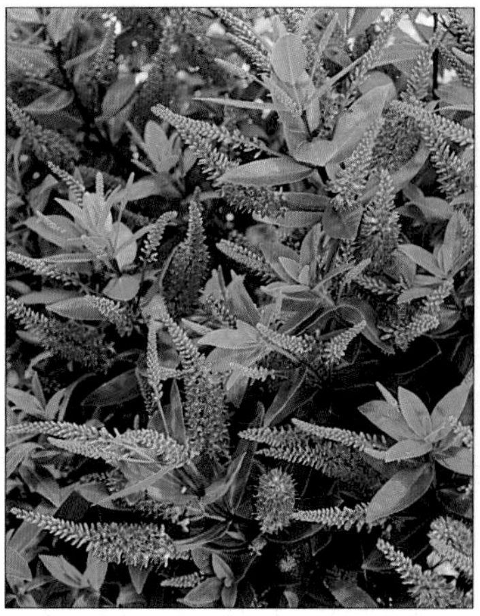
Hebe 'Bowles' Variety'

• **HARDINESS** Fully hardy to half hardy.
• **CULTIVATION** Under glass, grow in loam-based potting compost (JI No.2) in full light, with shade from hot sun. Provide low to moderate humidity and good ventilation. During the growing season, water moderately and apply a balanced liquid fertilizer monthly; water more sparingly in winter. Outdoors, grow in poor or moderately fertile, moist but well-drained, neutral to slightly alkaline soil in sun or partial shade, with shelter from cold, drying winds. Pruning group 9; most hebes need little or no pruning.
• **PROPAGATION** Sow seed in containers in a cold frame as soon as ripe; hebes hybridize freely. Root semi-ripe cuttings with bottom heat in late summer or autumn.
• **PESTS AND DISEASES** Leaf spot, *Phytophthora* root rot, downy mildew, and aphids may be a problem.

H. albicans ■ 🏆 Compact, mound-forming, spreading shrub with ovate, grey-green leaves, to 3cm (1¼in) long. In early and midsummer, bears medium-sized white flowers in short, terminal racemes, 3–6cm (1¼–2½in) long. ↕60cm (24in), ↔ 90cm (36in). New Zealand (South Island). ✻✻.

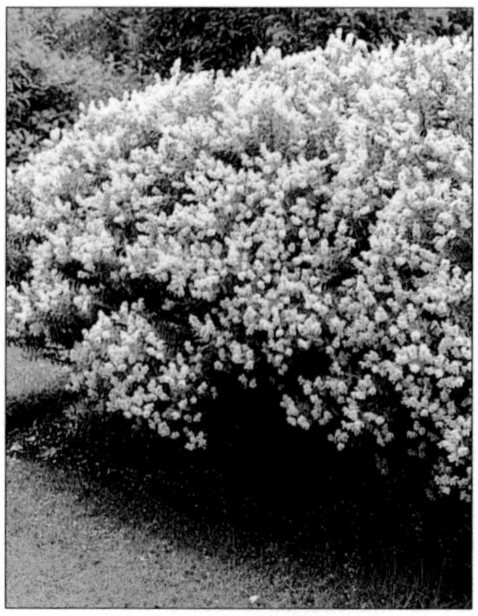
Hebe brachysiphon 'White Gem'

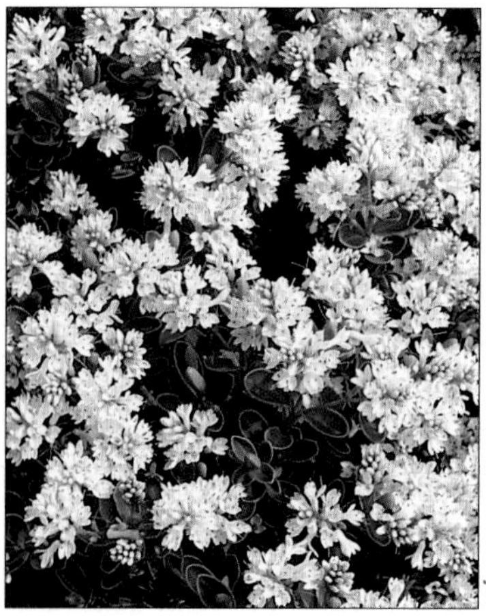
Hebe canterburiensis

'Pewter Dome' see *H.* 'Pewter Dome'.
'Red Edge' see *H.* 'Red Edge'.
***H.* 'Alicia Amherst'** 🏆 syn. *H.* 'Veitchii'. Vigorous, upright shrub producing elliptic to elliptic-ovate, glossy, dark green leaves, to 11cm (4½in) long. Medium-sized, dark violet-purple flowers are borne in axillary spikes, 7–9cm (3–3½in) long, from late summer to autumn. ↕↔ 1.2m (4ft). ✻✻
***H.* 'Amy'**, syn. *H.* 'Lady Ardilaun', *H.* 'Purple Queen'. Rounded, evergreen shrub with elliptic, dark green leaves, to 8cm (3in) long, dark bronze-purple when young and in winter. In late summer, bears large, violet-purple flowers in short, axillary spikes, to 5cm (2in) long. ↕↔ 1.5m (5ft). ✻
***H.* x *andersonii* 'Argenteovariegata'** see *H.* x *andersonii* 'Variegata'.
***H.* x *andersonii* 'Variegata'**, syn. *H.* x *andersonii* 'Argenteovariegata'. Bushy shrub with elliptic to inversely lance-shaped, dark green leaves, to 10cm (4in) long, streaked with grey-green in the centres and margined creamy white. From midsummer to autumn, bears medium-sized, pale violet flowers in axillary spikes, 6–9cm (2½–3½in) long. ↕↔ 2m (6ft). ✻
H. anomala see *H. odora.*
H. armstrongii, syn. *H. lycopodioides* 'Aurea'. Rounded, whipcord hebe with broadly ovate, yellow-green leaves, 1mm (1/16in) long, turning light green in winter. Small white flowers are borne in terminal spikes, 1–2cm (½–¾in) long, in late spring and early summer. ↕↔ 90cm (36in). New Zealand (South Island). ✻✻✻
***H.* 'Autumn Glory'** ■ Erect then spreading shrub with bronze shoots and broadly elliptic to obovate, dark green leaves, to 2.5cm (1in) long, with red margins. Small, dark purple-blue flowers, with white tubes, open in dense, axillary and terminal, sometimes branched racemes, 3–4.5cm (1¼–1¾in) long, from midsummer to early winter. ↕60cm (24in), ↔ 90cm (36in). ✻✻
***H.* 'Bowles' Hybrid'.** Rounded shrub with elliptic, slightly glossy, pale green leaves, to 2.5cm (1in) long. Medium-sized, lavender-purple flowers are borne in axillary racemes, 8–10cm (3–4in) long, from midsummer to autumn. ↕50cm (20in), ↔ 60cm (24in). ✻
***H.* 'Bowles' Variety'** ■ Compact shrub with ovate-oblong, slightly glossy, mid-green leaves, to 4cm (1½in) long. In summer, bears medium-sized, mauve-blue flowers in compact, tapered, terminal racemes, to 8cm (3in) long. ↕45cm (18in), ↔ 60cm (24in). ✻✻
H. brachysiphon. Dense, rounded shrub with elliptic to lance-shaped, mid- to dark green leaves, to 2.5cm (1in) long. In midsummer, bears small white flowers in dense, axillary racemes, to 2.5cm (1in) long. ↕↔ 2m (6ft). New Zealand (South Island). ✻✻✻. **'White Gem'** ■ is a compact hybrid of *H. brachysiphon*, bearing flowers in early and midsummer; ↕75–100cm (30–39in), ↔ 1m (3ft).
H. buchananii. Compact, much-branched, spreading shrub with broadly ovate, leathery, dark green leaves, to 7mm (¼in) long. In summer, small white flowers are borne in erect, axillary spikes, to 2cm (¾in) long, mainly towards the shoot tips. ↕20cm (8in), ↔ to 90cm (36in). New Zealand (Canterbury Alps, South Island). ✻✻✻. **'Minor'** is more compact, with smaller leaves, and is suitable for a trough; ↕to 10cm (4in), ↔ to 15cm (6in).
***H. buxifolia* of gardens** see *H. odora.*
H. canterburiensis ■ syn. *H.* 'Tom Marshall'. Spreading shrub with oval to obovate, dark green leaves, to 1.5cm (½in) long, loosely overlapping and in 2 ranks. In summer, bears a profusion of medium-sized white flowers, to 8mm (⅜in) across, in dense, axillary racemes, to 2.5cm (1in) long. ↕60cm (24in), ↔ to 90cm (36in). New Zealand. ✻✻✻. **'Prostrata'** is procumbent and lower-growing; ↕30cm (12in).
***H.* 'Carl Teschner'** see *H.* 'Youngii'.
H. carnosula. Low or nearly prostrate, spreading shrub with broadly obovate, slightly convex, glaucous, greyish green leaves, to 1cm (½in) long. Medium-sized white flowers, purplish pink in bud, are borne in dense, subterminal racemes, 1cm (½in) long, in early summer. ↕15–30cm (6–12in), ↔ 30cm (12in) or more. New Zealand (South Island). ✻✻
H. chathamica ■ Prostrate shrub with elliptic to ovate-oblong, fleshy, glossy, mid- to deep green leaves, to 3cm (1¼in) long. In early summer, bears medium-sized white flowers, tinged violet at first, in dense, axillary racemes, to 4cm (1½in) long. Good ground cover in mild areas. ↕15cm (6in), ↔ 90cm (36in). New Zealand (Chatham Islands). ✻✻
***H.* 'County Park'.** Wide-spreading, decumbent shrub with ovate, red-margined, grey-green leaves, to 1cm (½in) long. Small violet flowers are

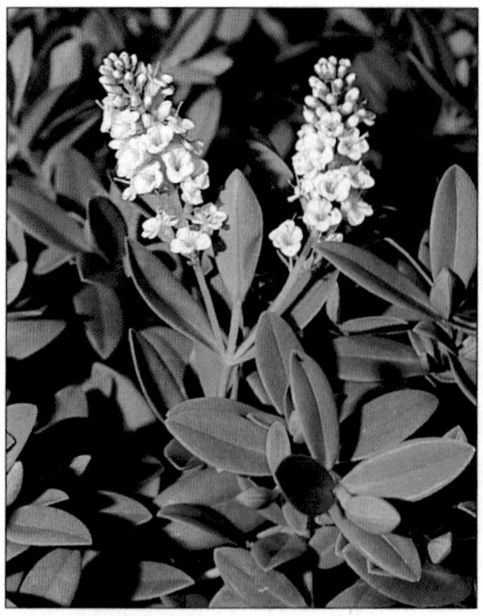
Hebe chathamica

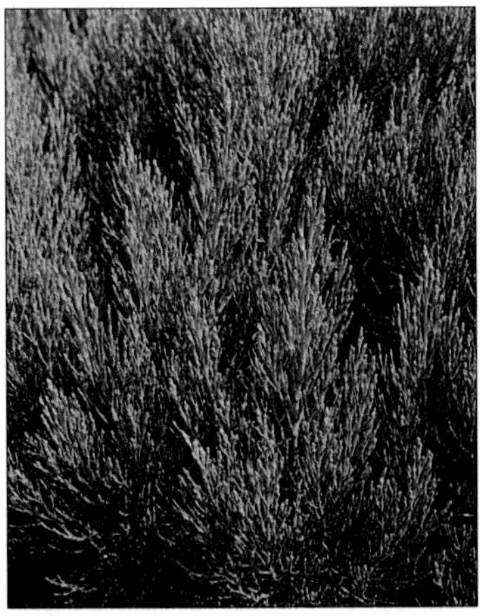
Hebe cupressoides

produced in short, axillary spikes, 2.5cm (1in) long, in early and midsummer. Suitable for ground cover. ↕ 20cm (8in), ↔ 45cm (18in). ❄❄

H. cupressoides ■ Dense, upright, whipcord hebe with cypress-like branches of scale-like, narrowly ovate to triangular, glaucous, mid-green leaves, to 1.5cm (½in) long. In early and midsummer, mature plants bear masses of small, pale lilac-blue flowers in axillary racemes, to 2.5cm (1in) long. ↕↔ 1.2m (4ft). New Zealand (South Island). ❄❄. **'Boughton Dome'** ■ ♀ is a dwarf, domed shrub with congested, slender, grey-green branchlets bearing scale-like, pale green leaves, to 6mm (¼in) long, pressed close to the stems but not hiding them. It seldom flowers. Suitable for a rock garden; ↕ 30cm (12in), ↔ 60cm (24in); ❄❄❄

***H.* 'Edinensis'.** Low, spreading shrub with ascending branches and whipcord-like, narrowly lance-shaped to oblong-ovate, glossy, mid-green leaves, to 6mm (¼in) long. Occasionally bears small, bluish white flowers in summer, but blooms infrequently. ↕ 30cm (12in), ↔ 75cm (30in). ❄❄❄

***H. elliptica* 'Variegata'** see *H.* x *franciscana* 'Variegata'.

***H. epacridea*.** Mat-forming shrub with prostrate and ascending branches clothed in dense, ovate, rigid, dull mid-green leaves, 5–8mm (¼–⅜in) long. Small, fragrant white flowers open in ovoid, terminal heads, to 1.5cm (½in) long, in late spring. ↕ 45cm (18in), ↔ 60cm (24in). New Zealand (South Island). ❄❄❄

***H.* 'Eveline'** see *H.* 'Gauntlettii'.

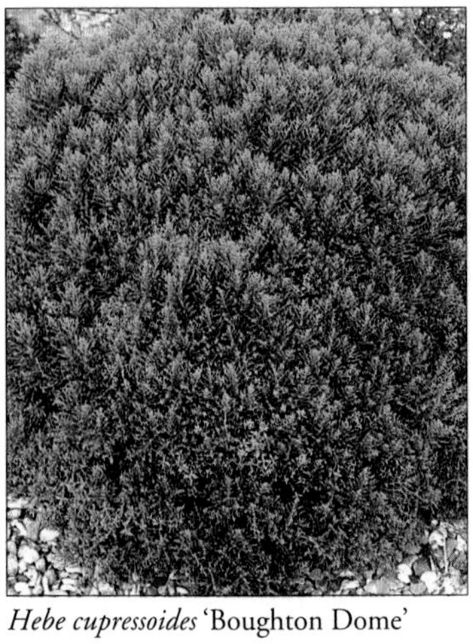
Hebe cupressoides 'Boughton Dome'

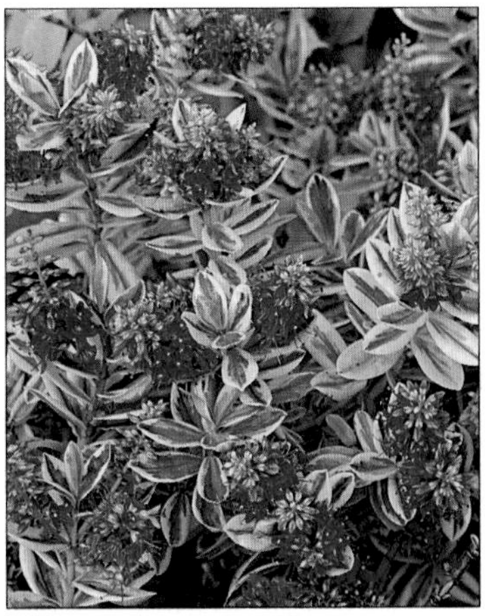
Hebe x *franciscana* 'Variegata'

***H.* 'Fairfieldii'.** Upright shrub with broadly ovate, coarsely toothed, glossy, mid- to dark green, red-margined leaves, 2–3cm (¾–1¼in) long. Medium-sized, lavender-violet flowers are borne in large, open, freely branched, terminal panicles, to 23cm (9in) long, in late spring and early summer. Dead-head after flowering. ↕↔ 60cm (24in). ❄❄

H.* x *franciscana (*H. elliptica* x *H. speciosa*). Dense, rounded shrub with 4-ranked, obovate to elliptic, fleshy, dull dark green leaves, 4–6cm (1½–2½in) long. From summer to autumn, bears pink-tinged purple flowers, to 1cm (½in) across, in dense, axillary racemes, 5–8cm (2–3in) long. ↕↔ 60–120cm (2–4ft). Garden origin. ❄❄. **'Blue Gem'** ♀ syn. *H. latifolia*, is spreading, with elliptic to inversely lance-shaped, light to mid-green leaves, 2.5–7cm (1–3in) long, and light mauve flowers; ↕↔ 1.3m (4½ft). **'Variegata'** ■ ♀ syn. *H. elliptica* 'Variegata', has leaves broadly margined creamy white.

***H.* 'Gauntlettii'** ■ syn. *H.* 'Eveline'. Upright, bushy shrub with elliptic to inversely lance-shaped, glossy, rich green leaves, to 8cm (3in) or more long. Medium-sized pink flowers, 15cm (6in) across, with purple tubes, are borne in pendent, axillary racemes, 12–15cm (5–6in) long, from late summer to late autumn. ↕↔ 1m (3ft). ❄

***H. glaucophylla* 'Variegata'.** Rounded shrub (probably of hybrid origin) with slender shoots and lance-shaped, cream-margined, grey-green leaves, 9–15mm (⅜–½in) long. In summer, bears large, pale lilac-blue flowers in short, terminal racemes, 2–3cm (¾–1¼in) long. ↕↔ 1m (3ft). ❄❄

***H.* 'Great Orme'** ■ ♀ Open, rounded shrub with dark purple shoots and oblong to lance-shaped, glossy, mid-green leaves, to 6cm (2½in) long. Large, bright pink flowers, fading to white, are borne in dense, slender, axillary spikes, 5–10cm (2–4in) long, over a long period from midsummer to mid-autumn. ↕↔ 1.2m (4ft). ❄❄

***H.* 'Hagley Park'** ■ Erect to slightly spreading shrub with upright shoots and oblong-elliptic to obovate, blunt-toothed, glossy, mid-green leaves, to 5cm (2in) long, margined with red. Medium-sized, rose-purple flowers are borne in large, terminal panicles, to 15cm (6in) or more long, in summer. ↕ 45cm (18in), ↔ 60cm (24in). ❄❄

***H. hulkeana*.** Open, upright shrub producing oblong-elliptic to broadly

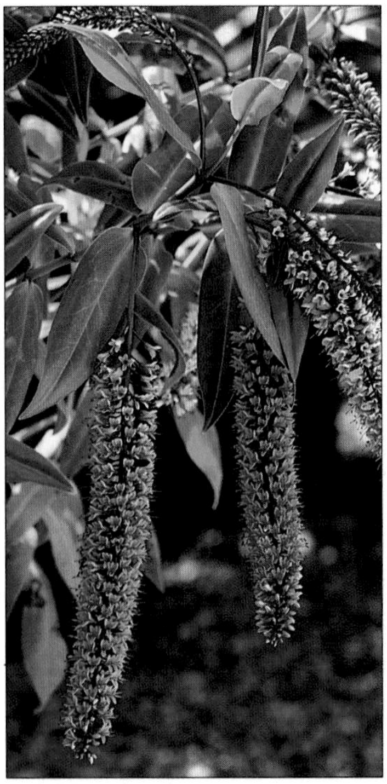
Hebe 'Gauntlettii'

ovate, toothed, glossy, mid-green leaves, to 4cm (1½in) long, with red margins. Bears large, lavender-blue, lilac, or white flowers in terminal panicles, 20–30cm (8–12in) long, in late spring and early summer. ↕↔ 60cm (24in). ❄❄. **'Lilac Hint'** ■ has pale green leaves without red margins, and pale lilac flowers.

***H.* 'Lady Ardilaun'** see *H.* 'Amy'.

***H.* 'La Séduisante'** ♀ syn. *H. speciosa* 'Ruddigore'. Upright shrub with purple-tinged shoots and broadly elliptic, glossy, dark green leaves, to 10cm (4in) long, purple beneath when young. From late summer to autumn, produces medium-sized, dark purple-red flowers in axillary racemes, 8cm (3in) long. ↕↔ 1m (3ft). ❄❄

H. latifolia see *H.* x *franciscana* 'Blue Gem'.

***H.* 'Loganioides'**, syn. *H. selaginoides* of gardens. Whipcord hebe with slender, yellow-green shoots and tiny, ovate to lance-shaped, finely hairy, bright green leaves, 5mm (¼in) long. Small white flowers are borne in axillary or terminal racemes, 2.5–5cm (1–2in) long, in summer. ↕↔ 25cm (10in). ❄❄❄

***H. lycopodioides*.** Whipcord hebe with rigid, angled, yellow-green shoots and

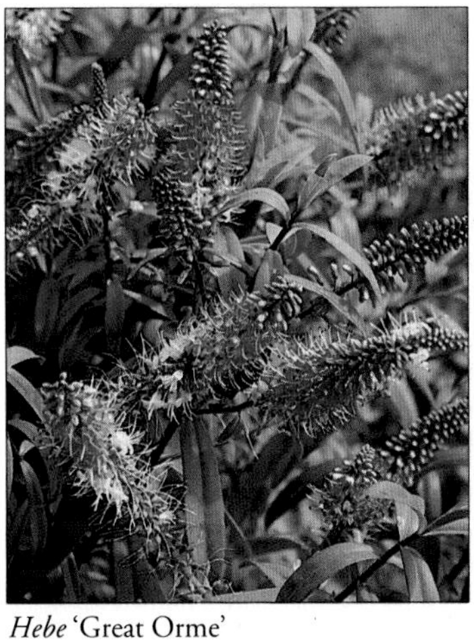
Hebe 'Great Orme'

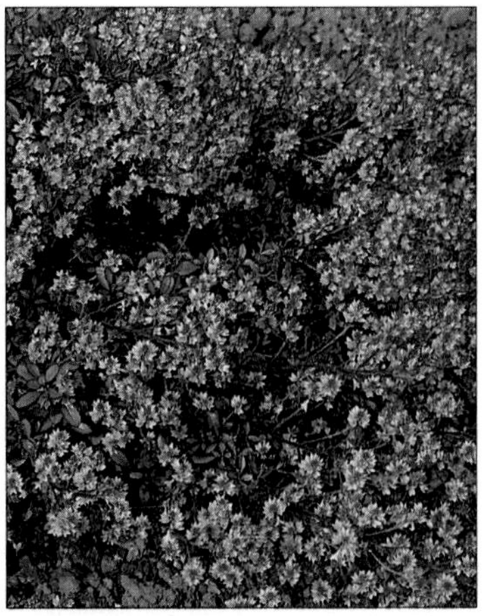
Hebe 'Hagley Park'

triangular to rounded, yellow-margined, mid-green leaves, to 2mm (1/16in) long. Small white flowers are borne in small, terminal racemes, 1–2cm (½–¾in) long, in summer. ↕ 60cm (24in), ↔ 90cm (36in). New Zealand (South Island). ❄❄❄. **'Aurea'** see *H. armstrongii.*

H. macrantha ■ ♀ Erect, open-branched, then spreading shrub with obovate to elliptic, blunt-toothed, leathery, bright green leaves, to 2.5cm (1in) long. Large white flowers, to 2cm (¾in) across, are produced in clusters of 3 from the upper leaf axils in early summer. ↕ 60cm (24in), ↔ 90cm (36in). New Zealand (South Island). ❄❄

***H.* 'Marjorie'.** Compact, rounded shrub with elliptic, glossy, mid-green leaves, to 5cm (2in) long. From midsummer to early autumn, bears axillary racemes,

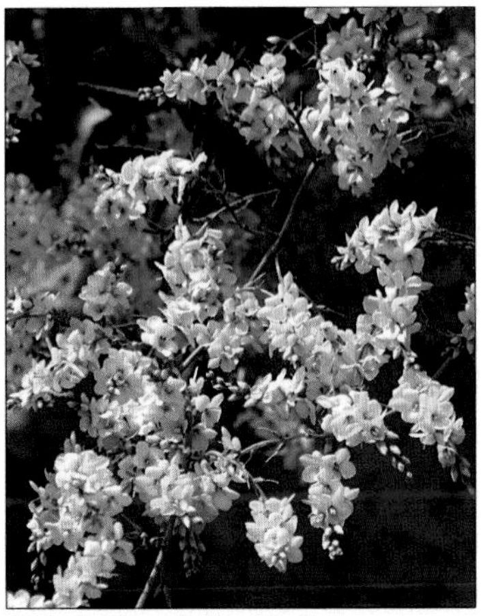
Hebe hulkeana 'Lilac Hint'

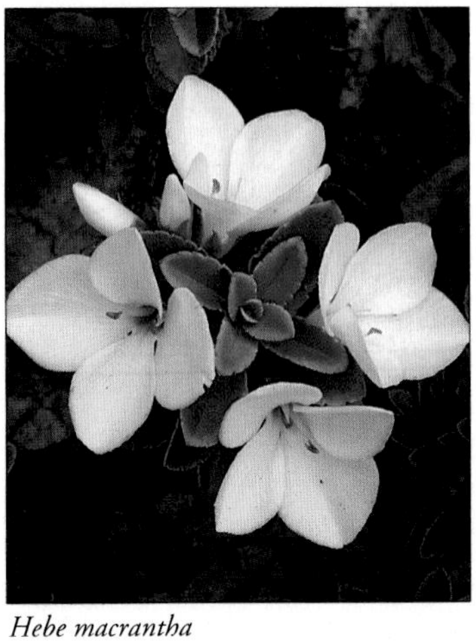
Hebe macrantha

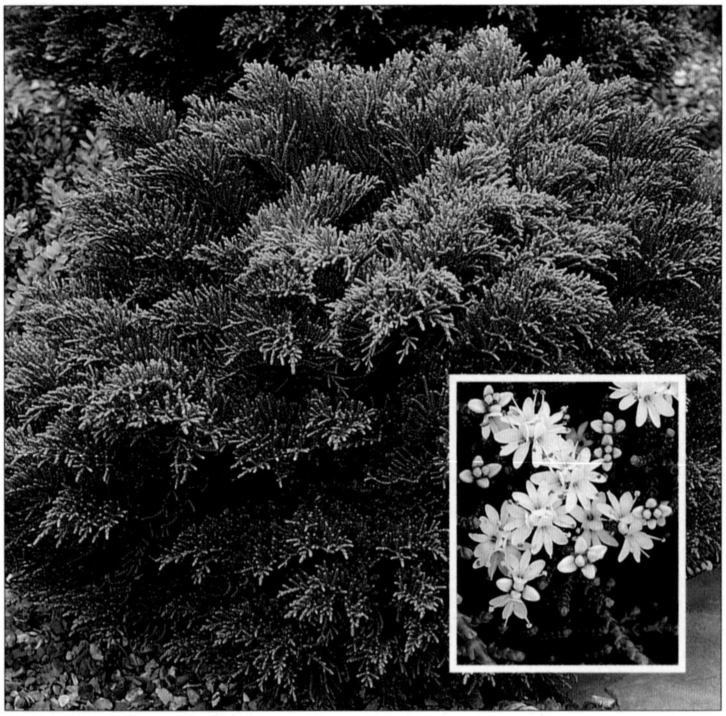

Hebe ochracea 'James Stirling' (inset: flower detail)

to 12cm (5in) long, of medium-sized, mauve-blue flowers, fading to white. ↕ 1.2m (4ft), ↔ 1.5m (5ft). ❄❄

***H.* 'Midsummer Beauty'** 🏆 Upright, rounded shrub with purplish brown stems and oblong to lance-shaped, bright green leaves, 9–11cm (3½–4½in) long, flushed red-purple beneath when young. Medium-sized, lilac-purple flowers, fading to white, are borne in axillary racemes, 12–15cm (5–6in) long, from midsummer to late autumn. ↕ 2m (6ft), ↔ 1.5m (5ft). ❄❄

***H.* 'Mrs. Winder'** 🏆 syn. *H.* 'Waikiki', *H.* 'Warleyensis'. Compact, rounded shrub with purplish brown shoots and oblong-elliptic, dark green leaves, dark red-purple when young, to 4cm (1½in) long, with brown-purple midribs. In late summer, bears medium-sized, violet-blue flowers in axillary racemes, 6–8cm (2½–3in) long. ↕ 1m (3ft), ↔ 1.2m (4ft). ❄❄

***H. ochracea* 'James Stirling'** ■ 🏆 Compact, erect then arching, whipcord hebe with triangular, rich ochre-yellow leaves, to 2–3mm (1/16–⅛in) long, particularly attractive in winter. Small to medium-sized white flowers are borne in small, axillary racemes, 1–2cm (½–¾in) long, in late spring and early summer. ↕ 45cm (18in), ↔ 60cm (24in). ❄❄❄

***H. odora*,** syn. *H. anomala*, *H. buxifolia* of gardens. Bushy shrub with upright shoots and elliptic-ovate, glossy, dark green leaves, 1–2cm (½–¾in) long. In early and midsummer, bears small to medium-sized white flowers in dense, terminal racemes, 1–2cm (½–¾in) long. ↕ 1m (3ft), ↔ 1.5m (5ft). New Zealand. ❄❄❄

***H.* 'Pewter Dome'** ■ syn. *H. albicans* 'Pewter Dome'. Dense, dome-shaped shrub producing ovate, grey-green leaves, to 2cm (¾in) long. In late spring and early summer, bears small white flowers in dense, axillary racemes, 2.5cm (1in) long. ↕ 40cm (16in), ↔ 60cm (24in). ❄❄

H. pimeleoides*.** Rounded shrub with upright, purple-tinged shoots and ovate to narrowly lance-shaped, leathery, glaucous, grey-green leaves, to 1cm (½in) long, with narrow red margins. Small, purple-blue flowers are borne in axillary spikes, 1.5cm (½in) long, in summer. ↕ 45cm (18in), ↔ 60cm (24in). New Zealand (South Island). ❄❄. **var. *glaucocaerulea has very glaucous foliage. **'Quicksilver'** 🏆 is spreading,

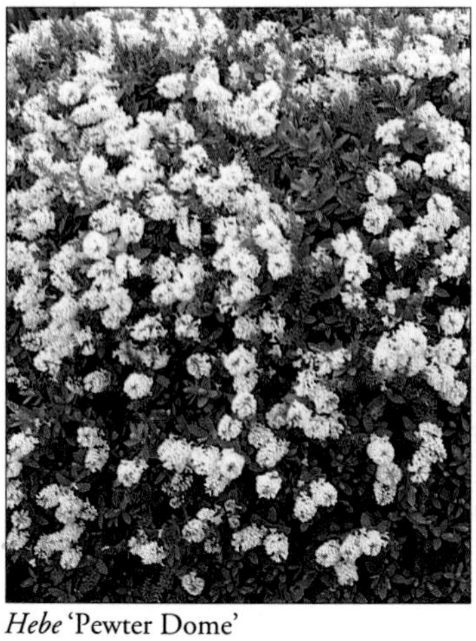

Hebe 'Pewter Dome'

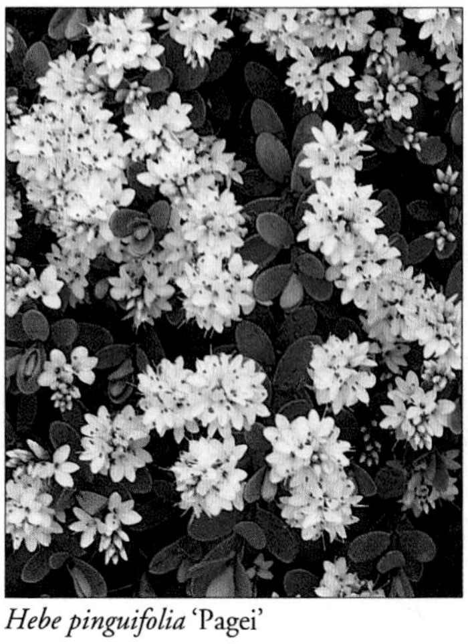

Hebe pinguifolia 'Pagei'

with small, silver-grey leaves and pale lilac-blue flowers; ↕ 30cm (12in).

***H. pinguifolia* 'Pagei'** ■ 🏆 Erect then semi-prostrate shrub with 4-ranked, obovate-elliptic, leathery, blue-green leaves, to 1.5cm (½in) long, borne on purple stems. In late spring and early summer, bears a profusion of medium-sized white flowers, to 8mm (⅜in) across, in dense, axillary spikes, to 2.5cm (1in) long. Good ground cover. ↕ 30cm (12in), ↔ 90cm (36in). ❄❄❄

***H.* 'Purple Queen'** see *H.* 'Amy'.

***H.* 'Purple Tips' of gardens** see *H. speciosa* 'Tricolor'.

H. rakaiensis ■ 🏆 Rounded shrub with dense, elliptic to obovate, glossy, bright green leaves, to 2cm (¾in) long. Bears large white flowers in axillary racemes, to 4cm (1½in) long, in early and mid-summer. ↕ 1m (3ft), ↔ 1.2m (4ft). New Zealand (South Island). ❄❄❄

***H. recurva*.** Compact, spreading shrub with slender, narrowly lance-shaped, curved, blue-grey leaves, to 5cm (2in) long. Small to medium-sized white flowers are borne in narrow, axillary spikes, to 6cm (2½in) long, in summer. ↕ 60cm (24in), ↔ 75cm (30in). New Zealand (South Island). ❄❄

***H.* 'Red Edge'** 🏆 syn. *H. albicans* 'Red Edge'. Spreading shrub producing ovate, grey-green leaves, to 2cm (¾in) long, narrowly margined and veined red when young. Medium-sized, lilac-blue flowers, fading to white, are borne in terminal spikes, to 3cm (1¼in) long, in summer. ↕ 45cm (18in), ↔ 60cm (24in). ❄❄

***H. salicifolia*.** Erect to spreading shrub with narrow, pointed, willow-like, lance-shaped to oblong-lance-shaped, mid-green leaves, to 12cm (5in) or more long. Small, white or pale lilac-blue flowers are borne in slender, axillary, often pendent racemes, to 20cm (8in) long, in summer. ↕↔ 2.5m (8ft). New Zealand (South Island). ❄❄❄

***H. selaginoides* of gardens** see *H.* 'Loganioides'.

***H.* 'Simon Delaux'** 🏆 Rounded shrub with ovate, dark green leaves, to 5cm (2in) long, conspicuously flushed dark red-purple when young. Medium-sized crimson flowers are borne in dense, axillary spikes, to 10cm (4in) long, in summer. ↕↔ 1.2m (4ft). ❄

***H. speciosa* 'Ruddigore'** see *H.* 'La Séduisante'.

***H. speciosa* 'Tricolor'** syn. *H.* 'Purple Tips' of gardens. Rounded shrub with upright shoots and elliptic, grey-green leaves, to 5cm (2in) long, margined creamy white and flushed purple beneath, particularly when young and in winter. In summer, bears medium-sized, violet-purple flowers in axillary spikes, to 8cm (3in) long. ↕↔ 1.2m (4ft). ❄

***H. tetragona*.** Whipcord hebe with stout, upright, 4-angled shoots and tiny, densely set, triangular to awl-shaped, leathery, glossy, yellow-green leaves, 2mm (1/16in) long. Small to medium-sized white flowers are borne in terminal spikes, 4cm (1½in) long, in early summer. ↕ 45cm (18in), ↔ 60cm (24in). New Zealand (North Island). ❄❄❄

***H. tetrasticha*.** Dwarf, whipcord hebe with procumbent then erect, tetragonal stems covered with triangular, scale-like, dark green leaves, to 2mm (1/16in) long. In summer, produces 1–3 pairs of large white flowers from the leaf axils at the stem tips. Seldom blooms in cultivation.

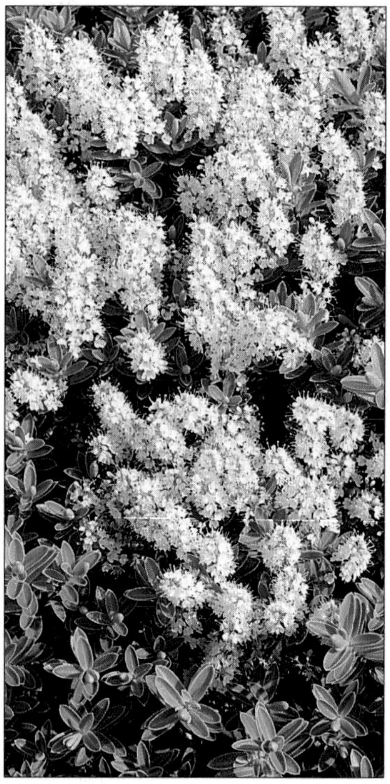

Hebe rakaiensis

Needs cool conditions and humus-rich, gritty soil. ↕ 10cm (4in), ↔ 20cm (8in). New Zealand (Canterbury Alps, South Island). ❄❄❄

***H.* 'Tom Marshall'** see *H. canterburiensis*.

***H. topiaria*.** Dense, dome-shaped shrub with broadly elliptic to obovate, glossy, grey-green leaves, to 1.5cm (½in) long. Medium-sized white flowers are borne in short, dense, terminal racemes, 1–2cm (½–¾in) long, in summer. ↕ 60cm (24in), ↔ 80–90cm (32–36in). New Zealand (South Island). ❄❄❄

***H.* 'Veitchii'** see *H.* 'Alicia Amherst'.

***H. vernicosa*.** Compact, rounded shrub with dense, elliptic, glossy, dark green leaves, to 1cm (½in) long. Medium-sized white flowers, sometimes pale lilac-blue at first, are borne in axillary racemes, to 5cm (2in) long, in early and midsummer. ↕ 60cm (24in), ↔ 1.2m (4ft). New Zealand (South Island). ❄❄

***H.* 'Waikiki'** see *H.* 'Mrs. Winder'.

***H.* 'Warleyensis'** see *H.* 'Mrs. Winder'.

***H.* 'Wingletye'.** Low, spreading shrub with obovate, glaucous, grey-green leaves, to 1cm (½in) long. Small, lilac-blue flowers are borne in axillary racemes, 2.5cm (1in) long, in summer. ↕ 15cm (6in), ↔ 30cm (12in). ❄❄

***H.* 'Youngii'**, syn. *H.* 'Carl Teschner'. Compact, mat-forming, dark-stemmed shrub with elliptic to broadly obovate, dark green leaves, to 7mm (¼in) long, sometimes red-margined. Large violet flowers with white throats are borne in axillary racemes, to 3cm (1¼in) long, in summer. ↕ 20cm (8in), ↔ to 60cm (24in). ❄❄❄

HECHTIA

BROMELIACEAE

Genus of over 40 species of short-stemmed or stemless, dioecious, evergreen, terrestrial perennials (bromeliads) found in rocky terrain and forest, up to altitudes of 2,000m (6,500ft), in S.W. USA, Mexico, Guatemala, Honduras, and Nicaragua. They have dense rosettes of narrowly triangular, fleshy, coarsely spiny leaves. In summer, inconspicuous, funnel-shaped, green, yellow, or white flowers are produced in long, branching racemes or panicles among the foliage rosettes. Plants of both sexes are needed in order to obtain fruits. In frost-prone climates, grow in a temperate greenhouse or conservatory. In frost-free regions, grow outdoors in a desert garden.

- **HARDINESS** Frost tender.
- **CULTIVATION** Under glass, grow in terrestrial bromeliad compost in full light. During the growing season, water moderately and apply a half-strength, low-nitrogen liquid fertilizer monthly; keep plants completely dry in winter. Outdoors, grow in sharply drained, poor to moderately fertile soil in full sun. Provide protection from winter wet. See also p.47.
- **PROPAGATION** Sow seed at 21–24°C (70–75°F) as soon as ripe. Remove and pot up offsets in spring.
- **PESTS AND DISEASES** Susceptible to mealybugs and scale insects.

H. argentea ■ syn. *Dyckia argentea.* Rosetted perennial with about 100 narrowly triangular-linear, densely scaly, silvery green leaves, to 60cm (24in) long, with jagged, marginal spines. Lax panicles of white flowers, with brown bracts and white-hairy sepals, are produced from the rosettes in summer. ↕↔ 1m (3ft) or more. Mexico. ✿ (min. 10°C/50°F)
H. glomerata. Rosetted perennial producing about 40 narrowly triangular, spreading, often red-tipped, mid-green leaves, 25–40cm (10–16in) long, covered on the undersides with fine, white or brown scales. Narrowly ovoid white flowers, with brown bracts and sepals, are borne in branched, lateral racemes, to 50cm (20in) long, in summer. ↕↔ 40cm (16in) or more. USA (Texas), Mexico, Guatemala. ✿ (min. 10°C/50°F)
H. montana. Rosette-forming perennial with numerous, narrowly triangular, shiny, mid-green leaves, 15–45cm (6–18in) long, densely white-scaly beneath, with slender brown, marginal teeth and brown sheaths. Narrowly ovoid, pale yellow flowers are borne in pyramidal, 2-branched, white-woolly racemes, to 50cm (20in) long, in summer. ↕↔ to 50cm (20in). USA (S. California), N.W. Mexico. ✿ (min. 10°C/50°F)

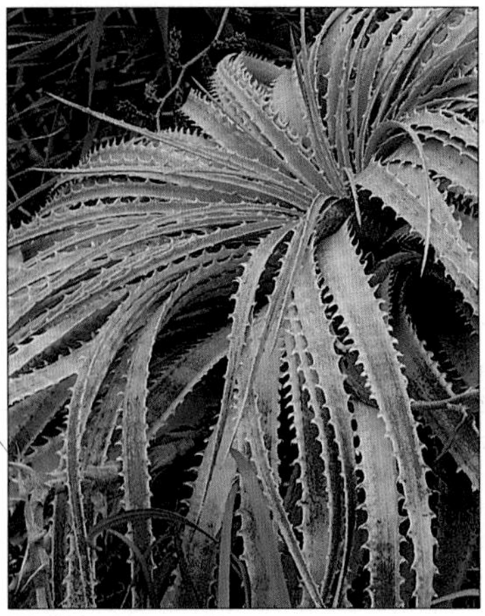
Hechtia argentea

HEDERA
Ivy

ARALIACEAE

Genus of 9–11 species of evergreen, woody-stemmed, trailing or self-clinging climbers. They are found in light woodland or on trees or rocks in N. Africa, the Canary Islands, the Azores, and Madeira, and from Europe to the Himalayas, China, Korea, and Japan. They have alternate, 3- to 5-lobed or entire leaves (see panel right), which are sometimes attractively variegated. Ivies show 2 distinct stages of growth. In the creeping or climbing juvenile stage, ivies have adventitious rootlets, lobed leaves, and minutely hairy young shoots. In the adult stage, they produce aerial "bushes" with entire, usually broadly ovate leaves and, in autumn, spherical umbels of tiny, 5-lobed, yellowish green, bisexual flowers; these are followed by spherical, black, sometimes orange or yellow fruits, 4–7mm (1/8–1/4in) across, which are a valuable winter food source for birds.

Ivies vary greatly in size and vigour and should be selected to suit the space available. They are ideal as a backdrop for other plantings, or for covering a wall. Variegated ivies are useful for lightening a dark corner. If wall-grown, ivies will not damage sound brickwork, but they may dislodge loose mortar and damage paintwork. Dense-growing ivies are excellent ground cover, thriving even in dry shade. *H. helix* has produced numerous variants and cultivars, many of which are easily grown as houseplants in hanging baskets or containers. Ivies may also be trained on wire forms to produce topiary features. All parts of ivy may cause severe discomfort if ingested; contact with the sap may aggravate skin allergies or irritate skin.

- **HARDINESS** Fully hardy to half hardy.
- **CULTIVATION** Under glass, grow in loam-based potting compost (JI No.3) in bright indirect to low light. Water freely in growth, applying a balanced liquid fertilizer monthly; keep moist in winter. Outdoors, ivies tolerate a range of conditions, but grow best in fertile, humus-rich, preferably alkaline, moist but well-drained soil. Green-leaved ivies are shade-tolerant, but variegated ones prefer more light, with shelter from cold wind. Some ivies, especially variegated ones, may be damaged in severe winters, but will usually recover in spring. To encourage rapid establishment of self-clinging growth, peg young stems down to the soil; they will quickly produce lateral, climbing shoots. Pruning group 11, at any time.
- **PROPAGATION** In summer, root semi-ripe cuttings of juvenile growth to obtain plants with a trailing habit; use adult growth to obtain plants with a bushy, "tree-ivy" habit. If standards are required, graft small-leaved ivies on to single-stemmed x *Fatshedera lizei* specimens, 45–90cm (18–36in) above soil level.
- **PESTS AND DISEASES** Red spider mites, scale insects, aphids, and leaf spot may be a problem.

H. algeriensis see *H. canariensis* var. *algeriensis.*
H. azorica, syn. *H. canariensis* 'Azorica'. Vigorous climber with slightly hairy stems producing 5- to 7-lobed, ovate-triangular, matt, light green leaves, to 8cm (3in) long. Excellent for a wall. ↕ 6m (20ft). Azores. ❄❄
H. canariensis (Canary Island ivy, North African ivy). Vigorous climber with 3-lobed, ovate-triangular, glossy, bright green leaves, 10–12cm (4–5in) long, borne on smooth, wine-red leaf-stalks. May be damaged in severe winters. Suitable for a sheltered wall. ↕ 4m (12ft). Algeria, Tunisia. ❄❄. **var. *algeriensis***, syn. *H. algeriensis,* has yellow-green leaves, becoming dark green with age. The stems and undersides of the leaves are red-hairy. **'Azorica'** see *H. azorica.* **'Gloire de Marengo'** ■🏆 has light silvery green leaves, variegated creamy white. An excellent houseplant; also suitable for a sheltered wall. **var. *maderensis***, syn. *H. maderensis,* is slow-growing, with small, dark green leaves, 4cm (1½in) long. Ideal ground cover. Madeira. ↕ 2m (6ft). **'Ravensholst'** ■ is vigorous, with shallowly 3- to 5-lobed, glossy, dark green leaves, 10–14cm (4–5½in) long. Best for a wall or as ground cover. ↕ 5m (15ft).
H. cinerea see *H. nepalensis.*
H. colchica 🏆 (Bullock's heart ivy, Persian ivy). Vigorous climber with entire, ovate, leathery, dark green leaves, 8–12cm (3–5in) long. Suitable for ground cover or for a large wall. ↕ 10m (30ft). Caucasus, N. Iran. ❄❄❄. **'Dentata'** ■🏆 has arching, bright green leaves, 25cm (10in) long, slightly toothed at the margins, with purple-flushed stems and leaf-stalks. Good for ground cover or for a large wall. **'Dentata Variegata'** 🏆 has light green leaves, 15cm (6in) long, mottled grey-green, and broadly margined creamy white. Suitable for a wall or as ground cover. ↕ 5m (15ft). **'Paddy's Pride'** see 'Sulphur Heart'. **'Sulphur Heart'** ■🏆 syn. 'Paddy's Pride', is similar to 'Dentata Variegata' but grows more rapidly and has more elongated, mid-green leaves, suffused with creamy yellow. Good for a wall. ↕ 5m (15ft).
H. helix (Common ivy, English ivy). Vigorous, variable, self-clinging climber or trailing perennial with 3- to 5-lobed, broadly ovate to triangular, glossy, dark green leaves, 4–6cm (1½–2½in) long. Seldom cultivated, but suitable for a wildlife garden. ↕ 10m (30ft). Europe. ❄❄❄. *H. helix* has given rise to many attractive variants and cultivars, which are more commonly grown than the species. In the descriptions below, leaf sizes have been grouped as follows: small, 2–4cm (¾–1½in) long; medium-sized, 4–6cm (1½–2½in) long; large, 6cm (2½in) or more long. **'Adam'** ■ has small, 3-lobed, light to dark grey-green leaves, heart-shaped at the bases, with creamy white variegation; the leaves become suffused and variegated with yellow as they mature. Moderately vigorous; excellent as a houseplant or for growing on a wall. ↕ 5m (15ft). **'Angularis Aurea'** ■🏆 has medium-sized, slightly angular, shallowly lobed, glossy, mid-green leaves; as the leaves mature, they become suffused and variegated with yellow. Moderately vigorous; ideal for a wall. ↕ 5m (15ft).

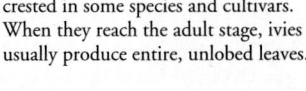

IVY LEAF SHAPES

Ivies produce leaves in a variety of shapes: when young, they are usually 3- to 5-lobed, but may be unlobed or crested in some species and cultivars. When they reach the adult stage, ivies usually produce entire, unlobed leaves.

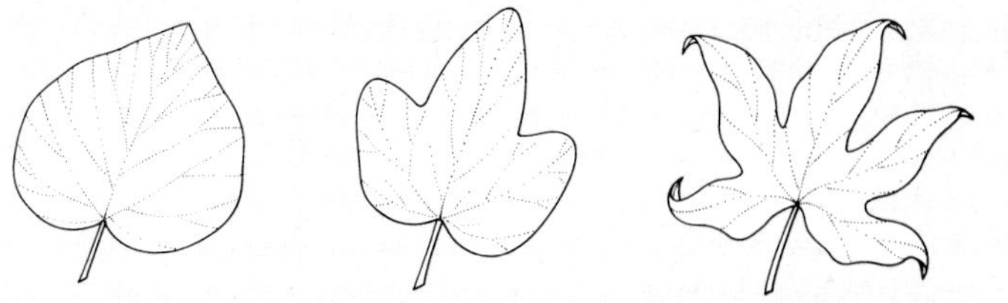

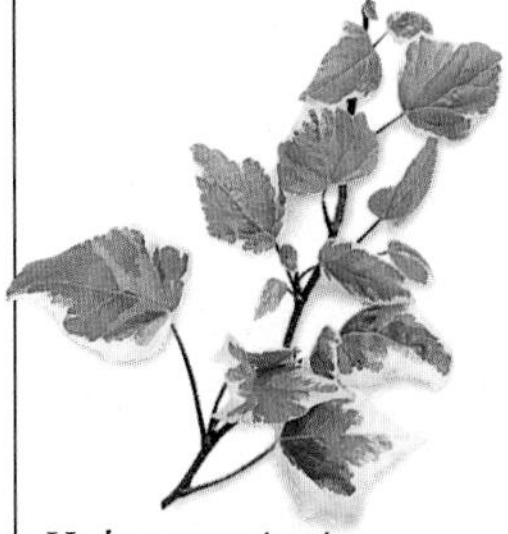
Hedera canariensis 'Gloire de Marengo'

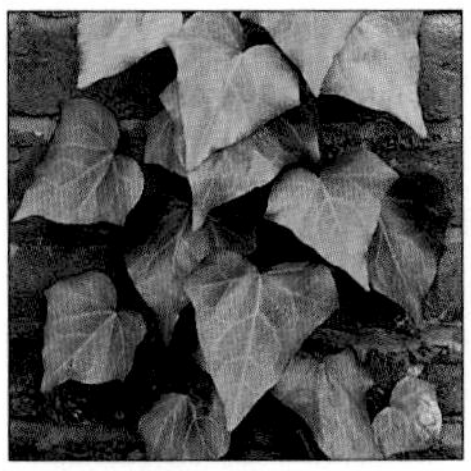
Hedera canariensis 'Ravensholst'

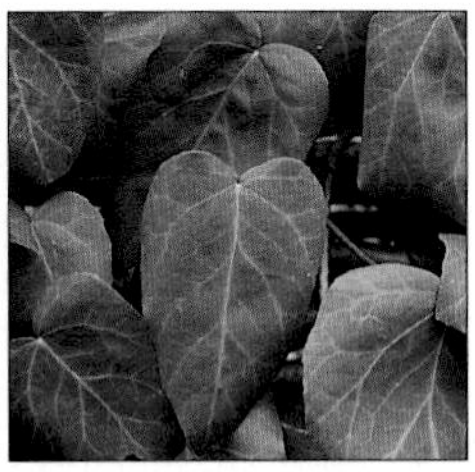
Hedera colchica 'Dentata'

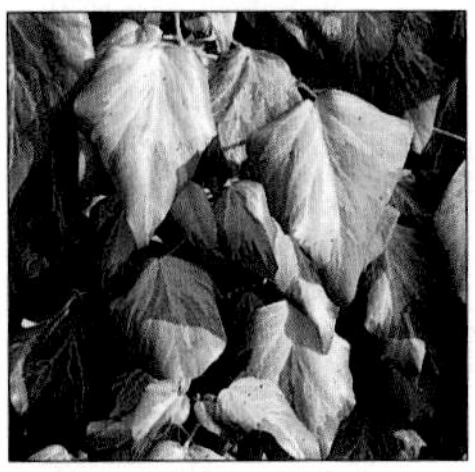
Hedera colchica 'Sulphur Heart'

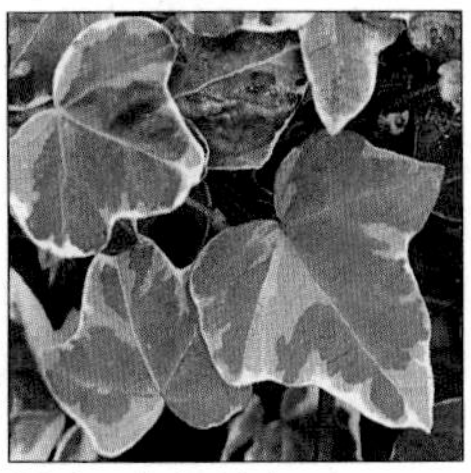
Hedera helix 'Adam'

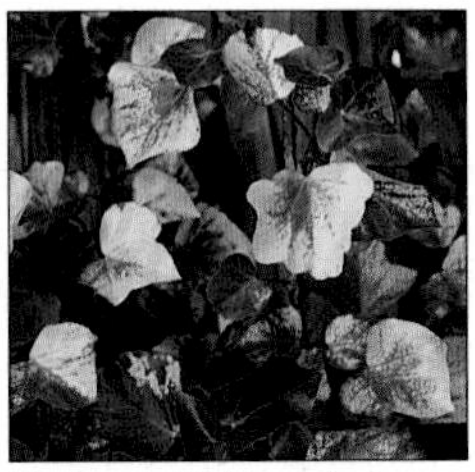
Hedera helix 'Angularis Aurea'

H

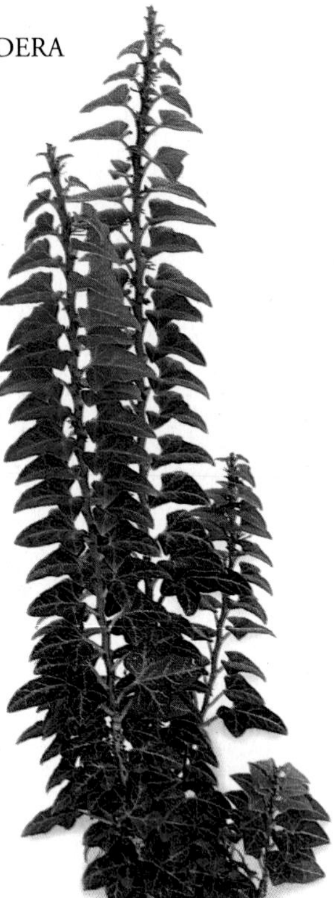

Hedera helix 'Congesta'

'Anne Borch' see 'Anne Marie'. **'Anne Marie'** ▣ syn. 'Anne Borch', produces medium-sized, mid-grey-green leaves with 5 rounded lobes that are cream-variegated mostly on the margins. Use as a houseplant or on a sheltered wall. ↕1.2m (4ft). ❄❄. **'Asterisk'** is a short-jointed climber or trailer, with small, deeply lobed, light green leaves. Use as a houseplant or in a hanging basket. ↕1m (3ft). ❄❄. **'Atropurpurea'** ▣♀ syn. 'Purpurea' (Purple-leaved ivy), has large, 5-lobed, dark green leaves that turn deep purple in cold weather. Use on a wall. ↕8m (25ft). **'Aureovariegata'** has medium-sized, entire, triangular, mid-green leaves with central markings in lime-green and creamy yellow. Use on a wall. ↕2m (6ft). ❄❄. **'Boskoop'** is similar to 'Green Ripple', having large, 5-lobed, mid-green leaves, but the leaves are more curled and have less distinctive veining. ↕1m (3ft). ❄❄. **'Bruder Ingobert'** has small, irregularly shaped, 3- to 5-lobed, grey-green leaves with dark green markings, often margined with creamy white. A good houseplant. ↕1m (3ft). ❄❄. **'Buttercup'** ▣♀ has large, 5-lobed leaves that are pale green when grown in shade but bright yellow in full sun. Ideal for a wall. ↕2m (6ft). **'Caecilia'**, usually grown as a houseplant, has small, 5-lobed, light green leaves with cream variegation and frilled margins. ↕1m (3ft). ❄❄. **'Caenwoodiana'** see 'Pedata'. **'California Fan'** has small, light green leaves with 5–7 boldly veined, fan-shaped lobes. Use as a houseplant. ↕1m (3ft). ❄❄. **'Cavendishii'** ♀ syn. 'Marginata Minor', has medium-sized, mid-green leaves with mostly marginal, creamy yellow variegation. An excellent wall ivy. ↕8m (25ft). **'Chester'** produces small, almost triangular, 3-lobed leaves, variegated lime-green and cream with dark green central blotches. Grow on a low wall or as a houseplant. ↕1m (3ft). ❄❄. **'Congesta'** ▣♀ is non-climbing, forming a neat bush with spire-like shoots. It has small, 3-lobed, dark green leaves borne in 2 opposite ranks along the stems. Use in a rock garden. ↕45cm (18in). **'Conglomerata'** is a scrambling or climbing ivy with medium-sized, entire or shallowly 3-lobed, thick, dark green leaves with wavy margins. Use in a rock garden or as a houseplant. ↕to 1m (3ft). ❄❄. **'Cristata'** see 'Parsley Crested'. **'Curley-Q'** see 'Dragon Claw'. **'Curly Locks'** see 'Manda's Crested'. **'Dealbata'** has small, 3-lobed, triangular to arrow-shaped, dark green leaves, spotted and splashed creamy white. Best grown on a wall. ↕2m (6ft). **'Deltoidea'** see *H. hibernica* 'Deltoidea'. **'Diana'** is trailing, and has variable, medium-sized, 3-lobed, dark green leaves, with the apex of each lobe drawn out to a wisp. Good in a hanging basket. ↕1m (3ft). ❄❄. **'Dragon Claw'** ▣ syn. 'Curley-Q', is a vigorous, climbing ivy with medium-sized, 3- to 5-lobed, strongly curled, dark green leaves. ↕2m (6ft). **'Duckfoot'**, usually grown as a houseplant, has small, light green leaves with 3 shallow lobes and wedge-shaped bases; each leaf resembles a duck's foot. ↕45cm (18in). ❄❄. **'Erecta'** ▣♀ is a stiffly upright ivy, similar to, but more vigorous than 'Congesta', with medium-sized, more rounded leaves. Use in a shrub border or large rock garden. ↕1m (3ft). **'Eva'** ▣♀ has small, 3-lobed, grey-green leaves with creamy white margins; each central lobe is twice as long as the lateral lobes. Similar to 'Adam', but with wedge-shaped leaf bases. Ideal as a houseplant. ↕1.2m (4ft). ❄❄. **'Flamenco'** has variable, small, dark green leaves, usually 5-lobed but often entire, with flattened leaf-stalks. Use as a houseplant. ↕45cm (18in). ❄❄. **'Fluffy Ruffles'** ▣ is usually grown as a houseplant, and has small, wavy, 5-lobed, mid-green leaves with frilled margins. ↕45cm (18in). ❄❄. **'Glacier'** ▣♀ has small, almost triangular, 3- to 5-lobed, grey-green leaves variegated with silver-grey and cream. Use on a wall, as ground cover, or as a houseplant. ↕2m (6ft) or more. **'Glymii'** ▣ syn. 'Scutifolia', has medium-sized, entire to 3-lobed, glossy, dark green leaves that turn deep red-purple in cold weather. Ideal for a wall. ↕2m (6ft). **'Goldchild'** ▣♀ syn. 'Gold Harald', has small, 3- to 5-lobed, grey-green leaves with broad yellow margins. Ideal as a houseplant or on a low wall. ↕1m (3ft). ❄❄. **'Golden Ingot'** is similar to 'Goldchild', but has more pointed leaf lobes. ↕1m (3ft). ❄❄. **'Golden Kolibri'** see 'Midas Touch'. **'Gold Harald'** see 'Goldchild'. **'Goldheart'** ▣ syn. 'Jubiläum Goldherz', 'Jubilee Goldheart', 'Oro di Bogliasco', has medium-sized, 3-lobed, dark green leaves, each with a central splash of bright yellow. An excellent wall ivy, slow to establish but then fast-growing; tends to lose its variegation if grown as ground cover. ↕8m (25ft). **'Green Feather'** see 'Triton'. **'Green Finger'** see 'Très Coupé'. **'Green Ripple'** ▣ has large, mid-green leaves with 5 jagged, forward-pointing, prominently veined lobes. Use on a wall. ↕2m (6ft). **'Hahn's Self-branching'** see 'Pittsburgh'. **'Helena'** has small, 5-lobed, mid-green leaves with creamy white margins. Each leaf has a central lobe, twice as long as the lateral lobes, that is curved and downward-pointing. A good houseplant. ↕45cm (18in). ❄❄. **'Helvig'** see 'White Knight'. **subsp. *hibernica*** see *H. hibernica*. **'Ingelise'** see 'Sagittifolia Variegata'. **'Ivalace'** ▣♀ syn. 'Mini Green', has medium-sized, 5-lobed, lustrous, dark green leaves with wavy, curled, and crimped margins. Excellent, all-round ivy for a low wall,

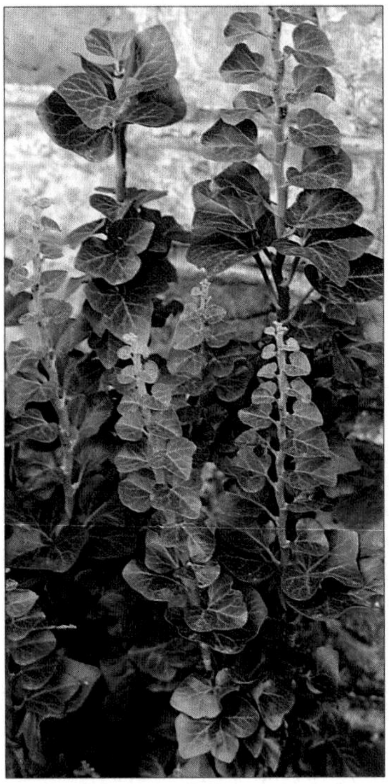

Hedera helix 'Erecta'

as ground cover, or as a houseplant. ↕1m (3ft). **'Jubiläum Goldherz'** see 'Goldheart'. **'Jubilee'** is a compact, slow-growing ivy with small, entire or 3- to 5-lobed, grey-green leaves, marked darker green, and margined with cream. Mostly used as a houseplant. ↕45cm (18in). ❄❄. **'Jubilee Goldheart'** see 'Goldheart'. **'Kolibri'** ♀ has small, neat, 5-lobed, creamy white-variegated, mid-green leaves, with long-pointed central lobes and short-pointed lateral lobes. Very variable but a good houseplant. ↕45cm (18in). ❄❄. **'Königer'** ▣ is a vigorous wall ivy producing large, mid-green leaves with 5 narrow, elongated lobes; the central lobes are often twice as long as the lateral lobes. ↕2m (6ft). ❄❄. **'Lalla Rookh'** is trailing, with medium-sized, light green leaves, the 5 irregularly toothed lobes cut almost to the central veins. Use in hanging basket. ↕1m (3ft). ❄❄. **'Leo Swicegood'** is an unusual houseplant ivy with small, entire, linear, mid-green leaves. ↕45cm (18in). ❄❄. **'Little Diamond'** ▣♀ is compact and

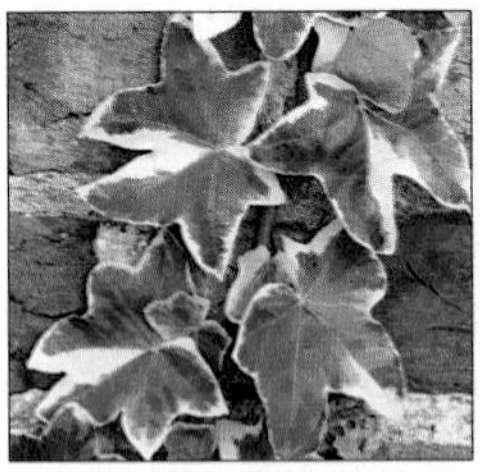

Hedera helix 'Anne Marie'

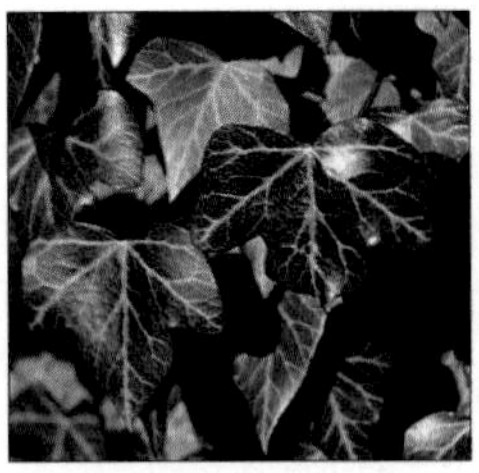

Hedera helix 'Atropurpurea'

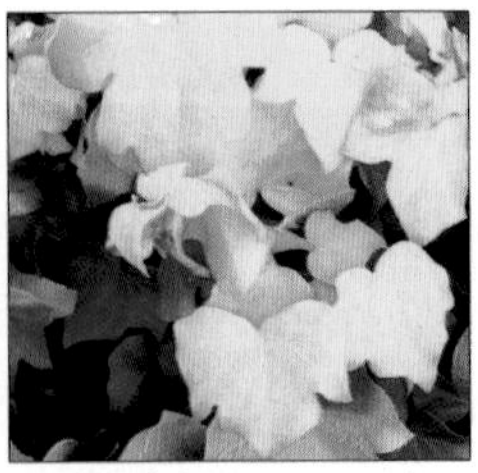

Hedera helix 'Buttercup'

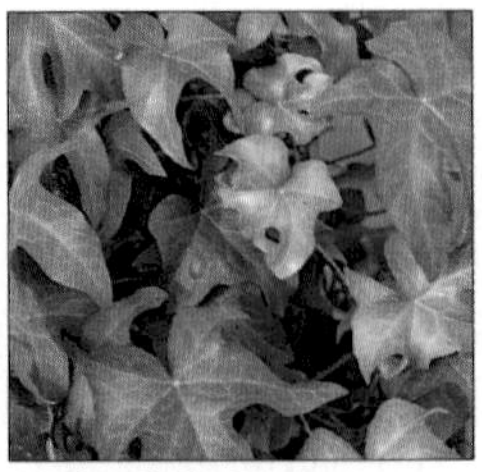

Hedera helix 'Dragon Claw'

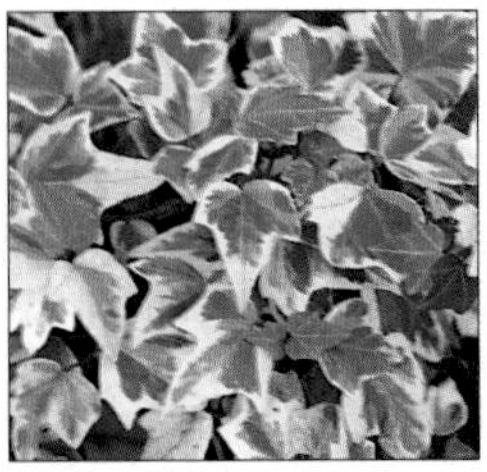

Hedera helix 'Eva'

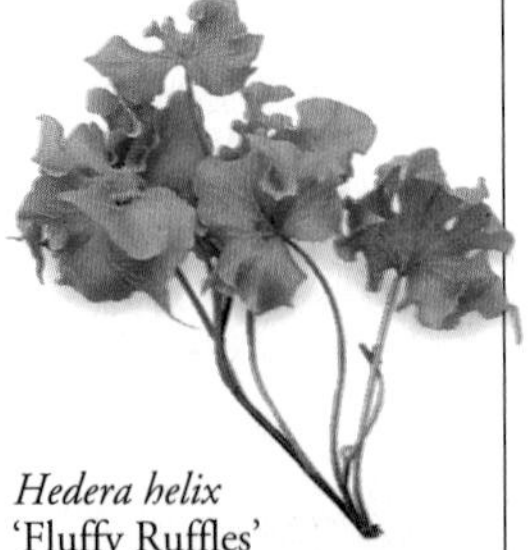

Hedera helix 'Fluffy Ruffles'

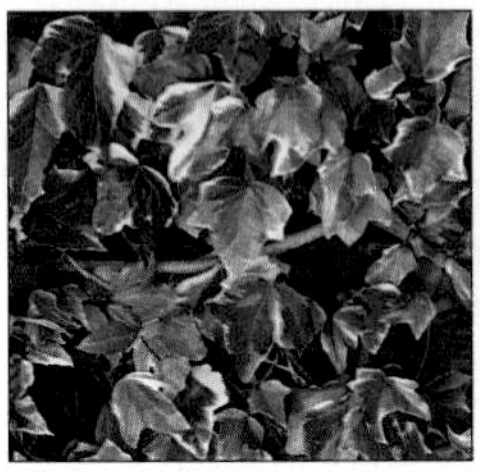

Hedera helix 'Glacier'

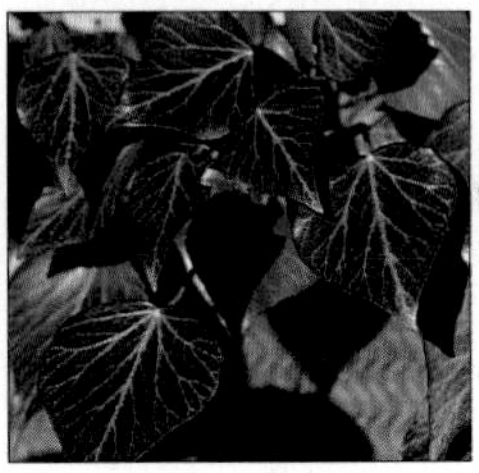

Hedera helix 'Glymii'

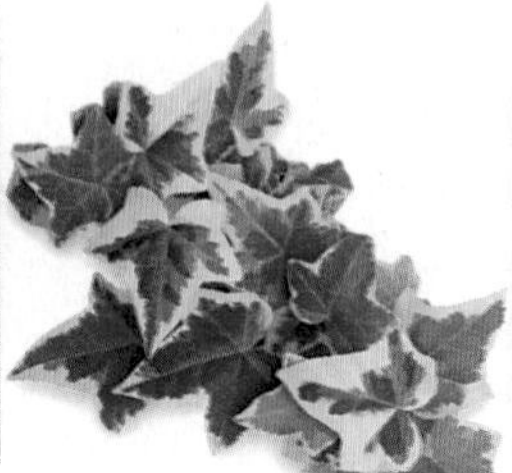

Hedera helix 'Goldchild'

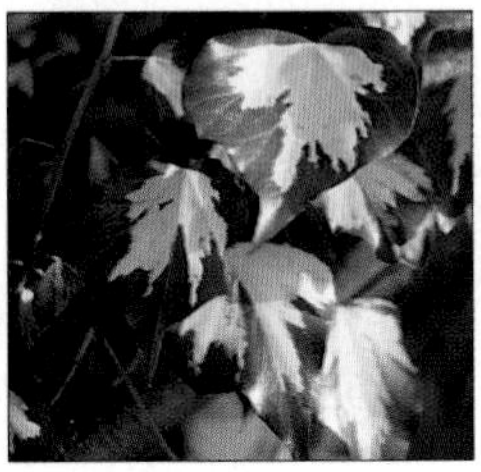

Hedera helix 'Goldheart'

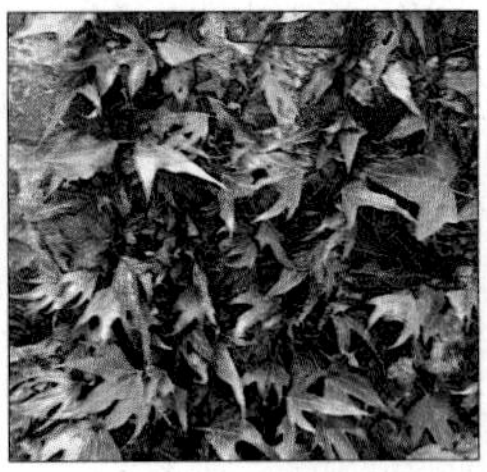

Hedera helix 'Green Ripple'

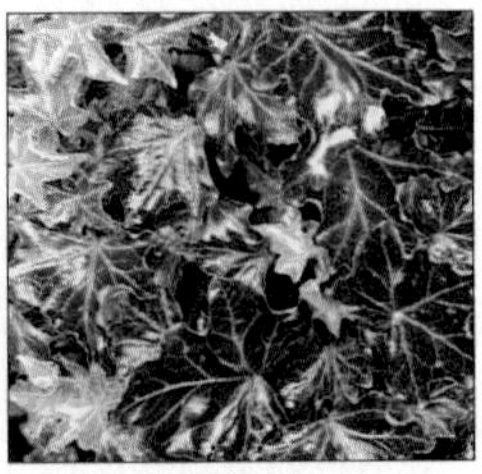

Hedera helix 'Ivalace'

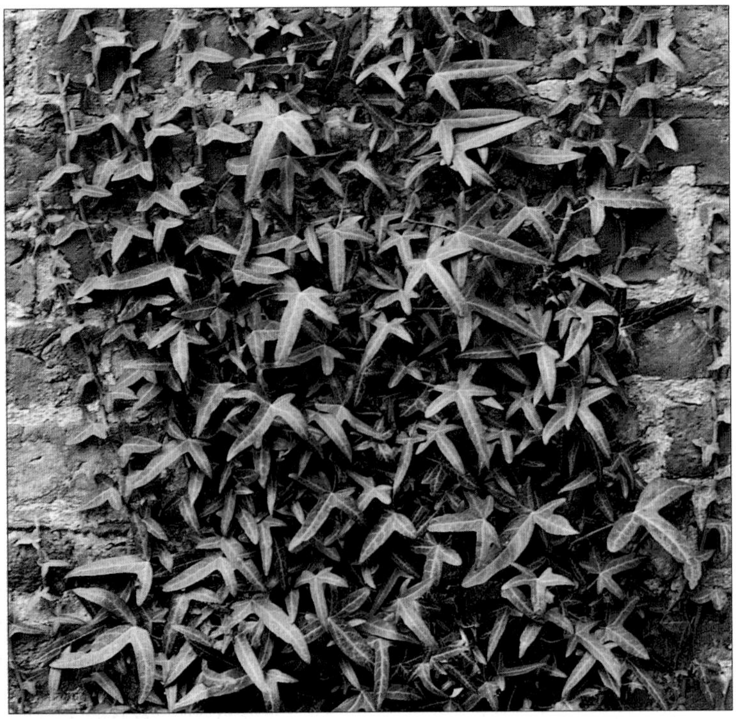

Hedera helix 'Pedata'

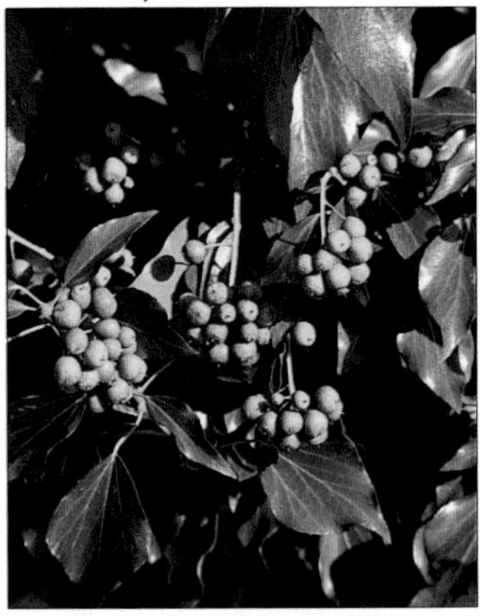

Hedera helix f. *poetarum*

slow-growing, with medium-sized, entire, diamond-shaped, grey-green leaves, variegated creamy white. Use as a houseplant or in a rock garden. ↕30cm (12in). ❄❄. **'Luzii'** ■ has medium-sized, shallowly 5-lobed, mid-green leaves, heavily speckled and spotted yellow-cream. A good houseplant. ↕1m (3ft). ❄❄. **'Manda's Crested'** ■ 𝕐 syn. 'Curly Locks', has large, curled, 5-lobed, mid-green leaves with downward-pointing tips. The leaves become copper-tinted in cold weather. Good for a wall and as ground cover. ↕2m (6ft). ❄❄. **'Maple Leaf'** ■ has medium-sized, 5-lobed, mid-green leaves with irregularly indented margins; each central lobe is almost twice as long as the lateral lobes. Suitable for a wall. ↕2m (6ft). ❄❄. **'Marginata Major'** will cover a high wall with its large, 3-lobed, mid-green leaves, variegated yellow-cream, mainly at the leaf margins. ↕5m (15ft). **'Marginata Minor'** see 'Cavendishii'. **'Melanie'** is similar to 'Parsley Crested', but has leaves with light purple, crested margins. An unusual houseplant ivy, but prone to leaf browning if grown outside. ↕45cm (18in). ❄❄. **'Midas Touch'** 𝕐 syn. 'Golden Kolibri', has small, ovate, usually entire, dark green leaves with irregular, bright yellow variegation. Use as a houseplant or on a low wall. ↕1m (3ft). ❄❄. **'Mini Green'** see 'Ivalace'. **'Minor Marmorata'** (Salt-and-pepper ivy) has small, 3-lobed, dark green leaves, spotted and splashed with creamy white. Use on a wall. ↕2m (6ft). **'Misty'** is a neat houseplant ivy, with small, 3-lobed, grey-green leaves, variegated creamy yellow at the leaf margins, and with arching central lobes. ↕45cm (18in). ❄❄. **'Mrs. Pollock'** has medium-sized, mid-green leaves with 5–7 forward-pointing lobes, suffused with yellow. A good variegated climber for a wall, but totally green when young. ↕3m (10ft). **'Oro di Bogliasco'** see 'Goldheart'. **'Parsley Crested'** ■ syn. 'Cristata', has medium-sized, entire, ovate to almost rounded, mid- to dark green leaves with waved and crested margins. Use on a wall. ↕2m (6ft). ❄❄. **'Pedata'** ■ 𝕐 syn. 'Caenwoodiana' (Bird's foot ivy), is an excellent wall ivy, with medium-sized, 5-lobed, grey-green leaves. Each leaf has an elongated central lobe and backward-pointing lateral lobes, resembling the shape of a bird's foot. ↕4m (12ft). **'Perkeo'** ■ is a short-jointed ivy, with medium-sized, almost rounded, thickened, dark green leaves, streaked mid-green, with purple-tinted veins. Usually grown as a houseplant. ↕45cm (18in). ❄❄. **'Pin Oak'** has small, 3-lobed, light green leaves, with the central lobes twice the length of the lateral lobes; usually grown as a houseplant. ↕1m (3ft). ❄❄. **'Pittsburgh'** ■ syn. 'Hahn's Self-branching', is a short-jointed ivy with medium-sized, mid-green leaves, heart-shaped at the bases, with 5 pointed lobes. Use as a houseplant, on a low wall, or as ground cover. ↕1m (3ft). ❄❄. **f. *poetarum*** ■ syn. 'Poetica Arborea' (Italian ivy, Poet's ivy), has large, 5-lobed, shiny mid-green leaves. It is often grown as a "bush ivy", as it bears distinctive, orange-yellow fruit, even on comparatively young plants. Good for a wall. ↕3m (10ft). **'Poetica Arborea'** see f. *poetarum*. **'Professor Friedrich Tobler'** has small, 3- to 5-lobed, mid-green leaves, the lobes sometimes cut almost to the central veins, giving the impression of separate leaflets. Excellent for a hanging basket. ↕45cm (18in). ❄❄. **'Purpurea'** see 'Atropurpurea'. **'Romanze'** has small, 5-lobed, light green leaves, the margins waved and curled so that the lobing is indistinct. Young leaves are clothed with velvety hairs. An attractive houseplant. ↕45cm (18in). ❄❄. **'Sagittifolia Variegata'**, syn. 'Ingelise', is similar to 'Pedata' but has medium-sized, 5-lobed, creamy white-variegated leaves. A good wall ivy. ↕2m (6ft). **'Schäfer Three'** is a short-jointed houseplant ivy with small, entire or shallowly 3-lobed, dark green leaves, marked grey-green with creamy white variegation. ↕1m (3ft). ❄❄. **'Scutifolia'** see 'Glymii'. **'Shamrock'** 𝕐 (Clover-leaf ivy) has small, 3-lobed, dark green leaves with wedge-shaped central lobes; the lateral lobes are cut almost to the central veins. Use for topiary, on a low wall, or in a hanging basket. ↕1m (3ft). **'Silver Queen'** see 'Tricolor'. **'Spectre'** ■ has medium-sized, 3- to 5-lobed, mid-green, creamy yellow-streaked leaves; each lobe is curled and twisted, with pointed, downward-curling tips. Ideal as a houseplant or for ground cover. ↕1m (3ft). **'Spetchley'** ■ 𝕐 has variable, tiny, dark green leaves, 5–15mm (¼–½in) long, usually 3-lobed, but often with a single elliptic or triangular lobe. It occasionally reverts to leaves similar to those of the species. Ideal for ground cover or as a houseplant. ↕15cm (6in). **'Telecurl'** ■ is an elegant houseplant ivy with small, 5-lobed, slightly folded, bright dark green leaves, with leaf-blades that curl between the lobes. ↕1m (3ft). ❄❄. **'Très Coupé'**, syn. 'Green Finger', has small, dark green leaves with 3 deep lobes. Use as a houseplant or on a low wall. ↕1m (3ft). **'Tricolor'**, syn. 'Silver Queen', has small, entire, triangular, grey-green leaves with irregular cream-yellow margins, the edges of which are pink, becoming more intensely coloured in cold weather. Suitable for a wall. ↕1.5m (5ft). **'Triton'**, syn. 'Green Feather', is a non-climbing, spreading ivy with medium-sized, deeply 5-lobed, prominently veined, dark green leaves; the lobes are slender, pointed, and twisted. Use as ground cover or in a hanging basket. ↕45cm (18in). **'Walthamensis'** has small, matt, dark green leaves with 3 blunt-tipped lobes. Useful for ground cover. ↕1.2m (4ft). **'White Knight'** ■ syn. 'Helvig', is

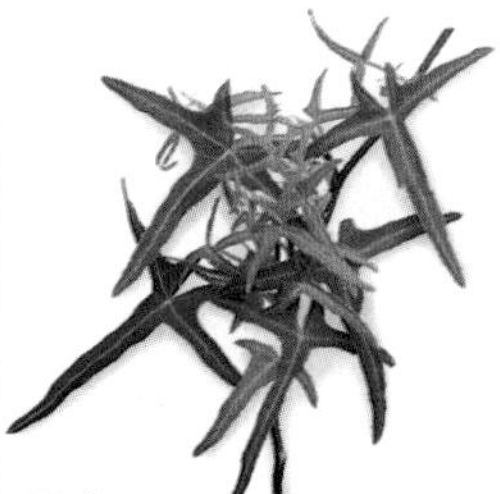

Hedera helix 'Königer'

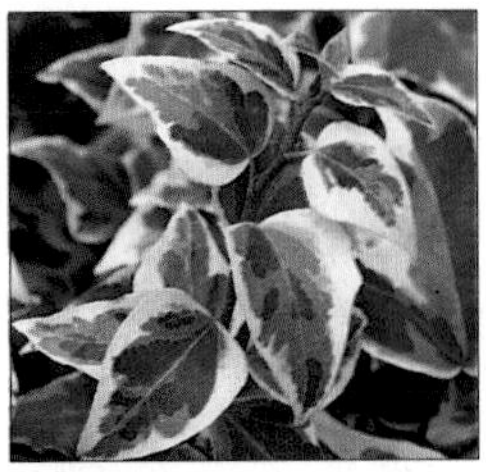

Hedera helix 'Little Diamond'

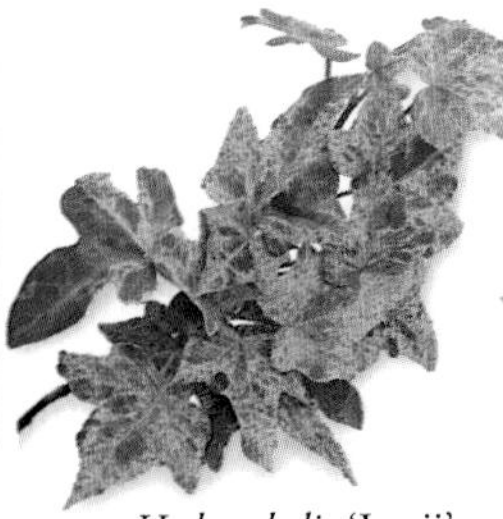

Hedera helix 'Luzii'

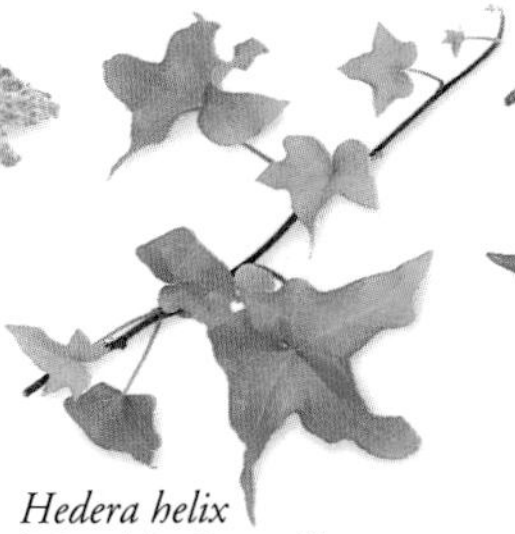

Hedera helix 'Manda's Crested'

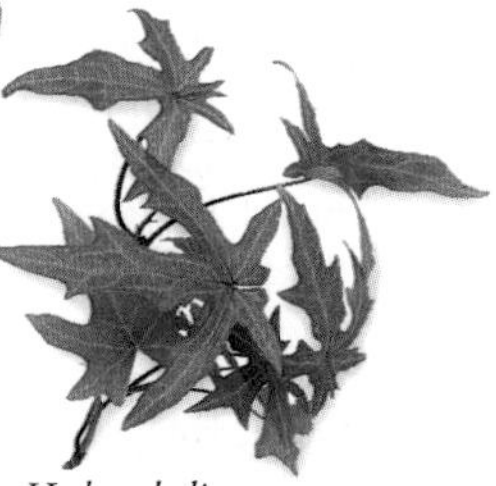

Hedera helix 'Maple Leaf'

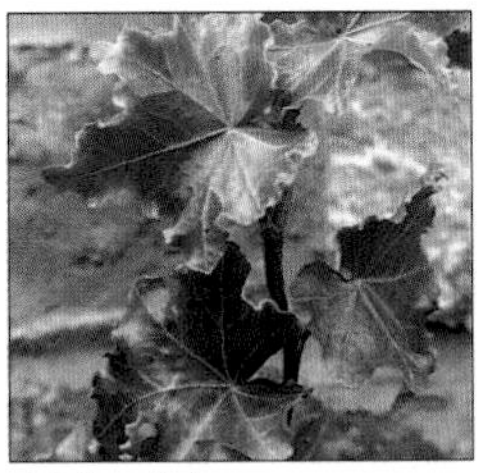

Hedera helix 'Parsley Crested'

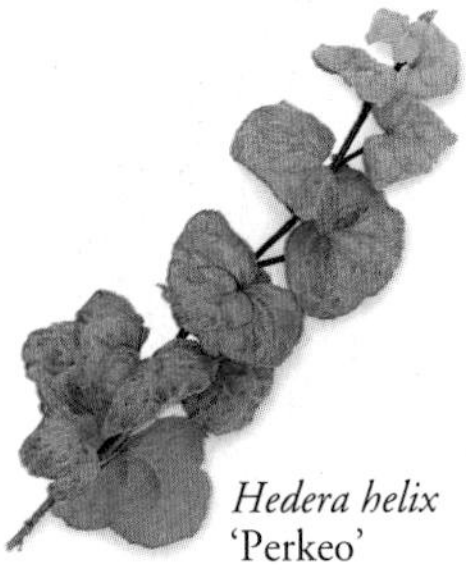

Hedera helix 'Perkeo'

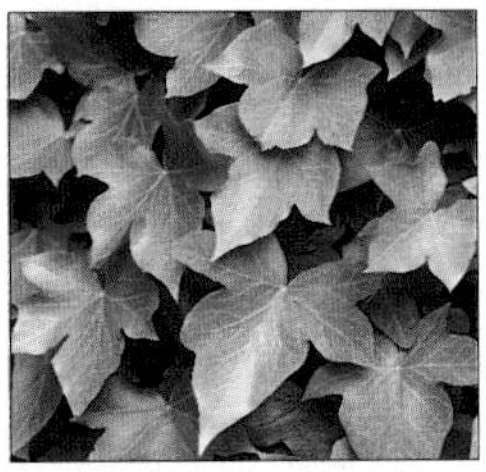

Hedera helix 'Pittsburgh'

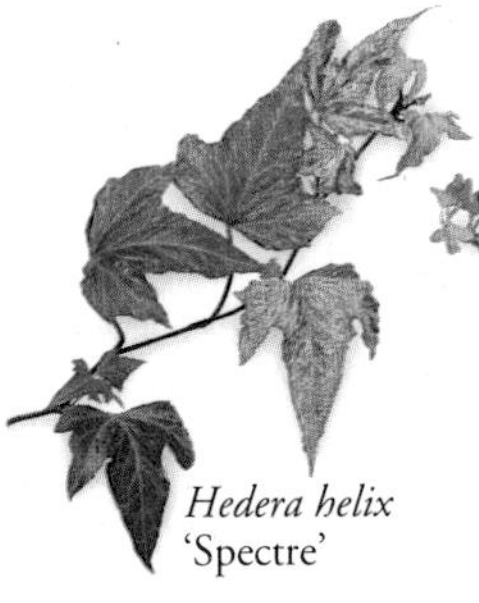

Hedera helix 'Spectre'

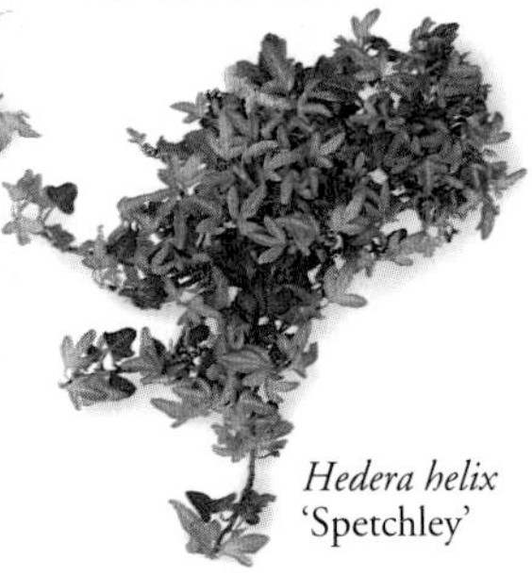

Hedera helix 'Spetchley'

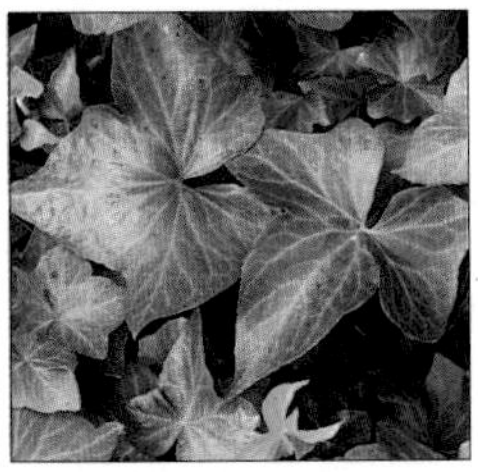

Hedera helix 'Telecurl'

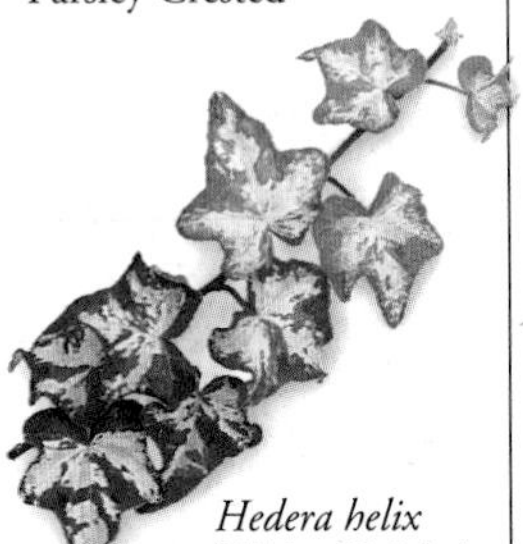

Hedera helix 'White Knight'

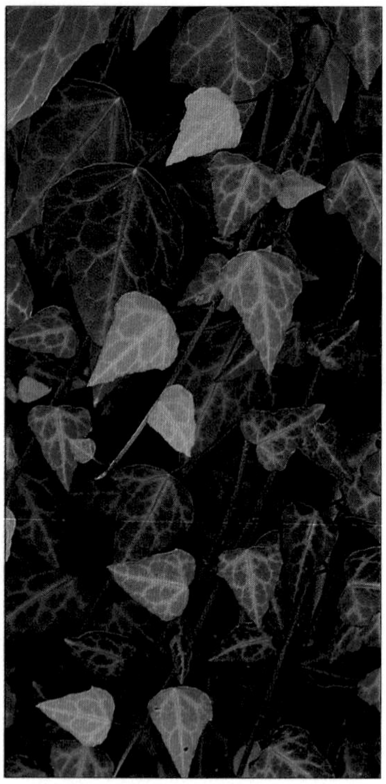

Hedera pastuchovii var. *cypria*

slow-growing, and is usually grown as a houseplant. It has small, 3-lobed, mid-green leaves with white variegation, mostly confined to the centre of each leaf. ↕30cm (12in). ✼✼. **'William Kennedy'** ■ is compact and slow-growing, producing small, usually 3-lobed, but sometimes entire, grey-green leaves with creamy yellow variegation. ↕45cm (18in). ✼✼. **'Wingertsberg'** has large, 5-lobed, dark green leaves that colour purple-green in cold weather. Suitable for growing on a wall or as ground cover. ↕4m (12ft). **'Woerneri'**, syn. 'Woerner', is vigorous and similar to 'Wingertsberg', but has large, 3-lobed, dark green leaves, colouring deep purple in cold weather. ↕4m (12ft).

H. hibernica ■♀ syn. *H. helix* subsp. *hibernica* (Irish ivy). Vigorous climber producing broadly ovate to triangular, dark green leaves, 5–8cm (2–3in) long, with 5 triangular lobes. The leaves are slightly upward-folded. Useful for a wall or as fast-growing ground cover. ↕to 10m (30ft). W. Europe. ✼✼✼.

'Deltoidea' ■ syn. *H. helix* 'Deltoidea' (Sweetheart ivy), is slow-growing, producing neat, densely arranged, entire or very shallowly 3-lobed, dark green leaves, 6–10cm (2½–4in) long. The basal lobes are overlapping, giving each leaf a heart shape. ↕5m (15ft). **'Rona'** is less hardy, and has leaves with extensive, yellow-freckled variegation. ↕3m (10ft). ✼✼. **'Sulphurea'** ■ has irregularly 3-lobed, mid-green to grey-green leaves, 5–7cm (2–3in) long, margined and splashed with sulphur-yellow. Suitable for growing on a wall or as ground cover. ↕3m (10ft). **'Variegata'** produces leaves with sharply defined, yellow-cream variegation, but it sometimes also has totally green, non-variegated leaves. ↕to 10m (30ft).

H. himalaica see *H. nepalensis.*

H. maderensis see *H. canariensis* var. *maderensis.*

H. nepalensis, syn. *H. cinerea, H. himalaica* (Nepal ivy). Strong-growing, self-clinging climber producing usually entire, elliptic, olive-green leaves, 6–10cm (2½–4in) long; the leaves sometimes have 3–6 toothed, projecting lobes, giving the leaf margins a "stepped" appearance. An interesting climber for a sheltered wall. ↕3m (10ft). Himalayas. ✼✼. **var. *sinensis*** is more vigorous than the species, with unlobed or only very shallowly lobed, mid-green leaves, 7–9cm (3–3½in) long. Suitable for covering a tree. ↕4m (12ft). China. **'Suzanne'** ■ is similar to, but less vigorous than, the species. It has 5-lobed, olive-green leaves with backward-pointing basal lobes, resembling the shape of a bird's foot. ↕2m (6ft).

H. pastuchovii. Moderately vigorous, self-clinging climber producing entire, narrowly ovate, dark green leaves, 4–9cm (1½–3½in) long. Suitable only for a wall. ↕2m (6ft). Caucasus, N. Iran. ✼✼✼. **var. *cypria*** ■ has leaves with prominent, grey-green veins. A vigorous wall ivy. ↕3m (10ft). Cyprus (Troodos Mountains).

H. rhombea (Japanese ivy). Self-clinging climber producing unlobed, ovate to triangular, mid-green leaves, 2–4cm (¾–1½in) long. ↕to 3m (10ft). Korea, Japan. ✼✼✼. **'Variegata'** ■ is slower-growing, and produces leaves with attractive creamy white margins. ↕2m (6ft).

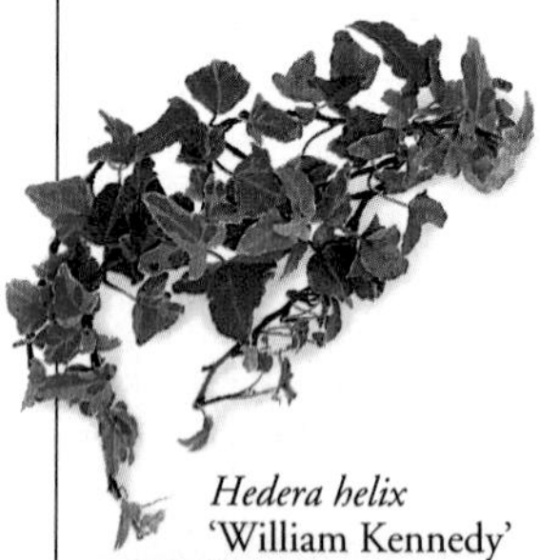

Hedera helix 'William Kennedy'

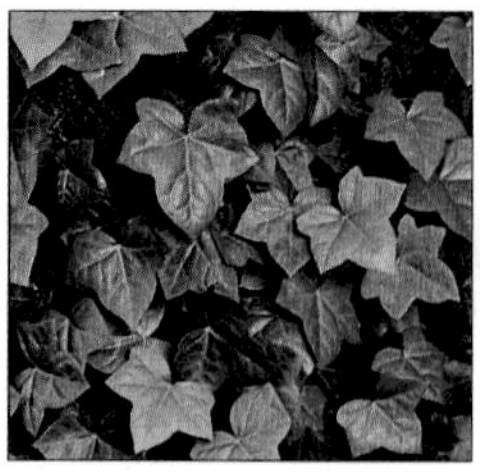

Hedera hibernica

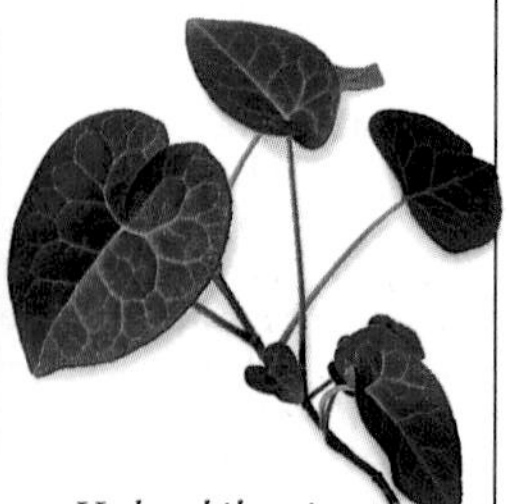

Hedera hibernica 'Deltoidea'

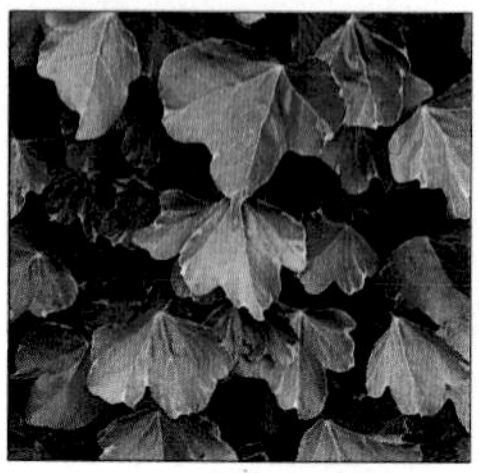

Hedera hibernica 'Sulphurea'

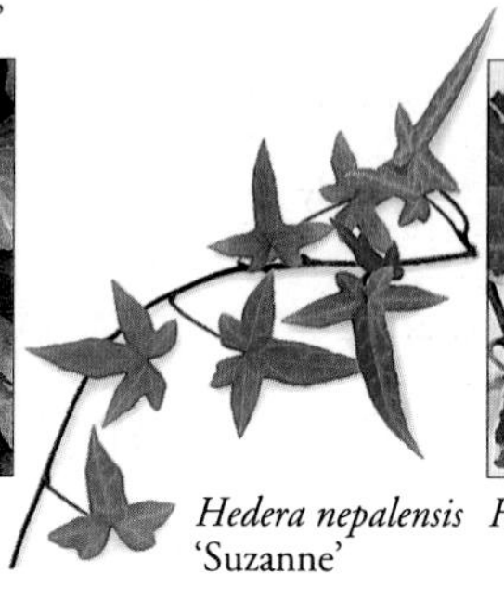

Hedera nepalensis 'Suzanne'

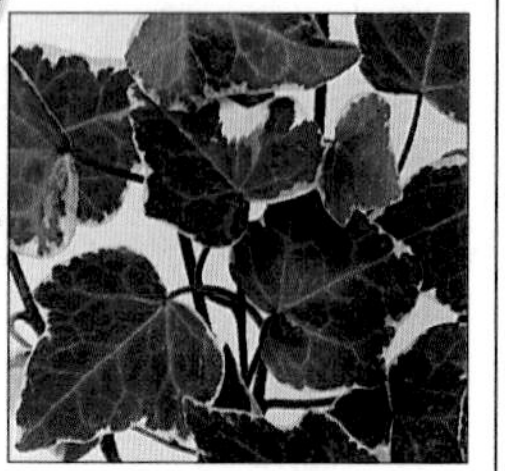

Hedera rhombea 'Variegata'

HEDYCHIUM

syn. BRACHYCHILUM

Garland lily, Ginger lily

ZINGIBERACEAE

Genus of about 40 species of rhizomatous perennials from moist, lightly wooded areas of Asia. They have stout, fleshy rhizomes and usually lance-shaped leaves, borne in 2 parallel ranks on unbranched, reed-like stems. Hedychiums are grown for their foliage and for their exotic, 2-lipped, tubular or almost trumpet-shaped, often fragrant, white, yellow, or orange-red flowers, with large bracts, borne in congested, spike-like racemes. The flowers are followed by ovoid, capsular fruits with sometimes colourful seeds. Hedychiums are most effective when planted in groups next to still water, or in a mixed or herbaceous border. In frost-prone areas, grow tender species in a warm greenhouse and hardier species in a cold one; in summer, they may be placed outdoors or planted out.

- **HARDINESS** Frost hardy to frost tender.
- **CULTIVATION** Under glass, grow in loam-based potting compost (JI No.3) in bright indirect light. Provide moderate to high humidity and good ventilation. In the growing season, water freely and apply a balanced liquid fertilizer monthly. In winter, keep just moist and remove old stems as they deteriorate. Outdoors, grow in humus-rich, moist but well-drained soil in sun or partial shade, with shelter from cold winds. In frost-prone areas, frost-hardy hedychiums may survive in a warm position if given a deep winter mulch.
- **PROPAGATION** Sow seed at 21–24°C (70–75°F) as soon as ripe. Divide rhizomes in spring. Sow bulbils of *H. greenei* when ripe.
- **PESTS AND DISEASES** Prone to red spider mites and aphids under glass.

H. coccineum ♀ (Red ginger lily, Scarlet ginger lily). Erect, rhizomatous perennial with long, sharp-pointed, lance-shaped, mid-green leaves, 30–50cm (12–20in) long. Tubular, scented, pale to deep red, orange, pink, or white flowers, with prominent red stamens, are borne in terminal, cylindrical racemes, to 25cm (10in) long, from late summer to autumn. ↕to 3m (10ft), ↔1m (3ft). Himalayas. ✼. **'Tara'** ♀ has orange flowers with slightly redder stamens and styles; ✼✼

H. coronarium (Garland flower, White ginger lily). Upright, rhizomatous perennial with long, sharp-pointed, lance-shaped, mid-green leaves, 60cm (24in) long, downy beneath. Very fragrant, butterfly-like white flowers, with yellow basal marks, are borne in terminal, elliptic racemes, 20cm (8in) long, in mid- and late summer. ↕to 3m (10ft), ↔1m (3ft) or more. India. ✼

H. densiflorum ■ Clump-forming perennial with oblong to lance-shaped, pointed, glossy, mid-green leaves, 30–40cm (12–16in) long. In late summer, bears tubular, fragrant, orange or yellow flowers in dense, terminal, cylindrical racemes, 20cm (8in) long. ↕to 5m (15ft), ↔2m (6ft) or more. Himalayas. ✼✼. **'Assam Orange'** bears deep orange flowers in very dense, bottlebrush-like racemes. **'Stephen'** ■

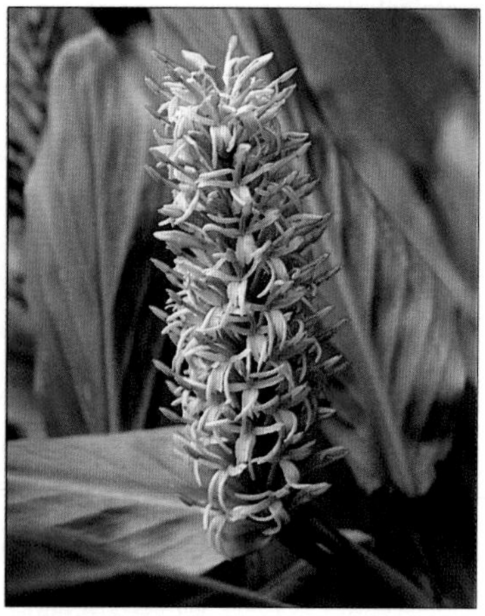

Hedychium densiflorum

has larger, laxer racemes of flowers with more protruding, pale orange-yellow corolla lobes and deep orange stamens.

H. forrestii. Rhizomatous perennial with leafy stems bearing narrow, lance-shaped, stalkless, strongly veined, mid-green leaves, 30–50cm (12–20in) long. In late summer and early autumn, bears narrow-lobed white flowers in dense, cylindrical racemes, to 50cm (20in) long. ↕to 1.5m (5ft), ↔60cm (24in). China (Yunnan). ✼✼

H. gardnerianum ■♀ (Kahili ginger). Upright, rhizomatous perennial with lance-shaped, greyish green leaves, 25–40cm (10–16in) long. Butterfly-like, fragrant, lemon-yellow flowers, with bright red stamens, are borne in dense, broadly cylindrical, terminal racemes, 25–35cm (10–14in) long, in late summer and early autumn. ↕to 2–2.2m (6–7ft) or more, ↔to 1m (3ft). N. India, Himalayas. ✼

H. greenei. Rhizomatous, clump-forming perennial with long, oblong, sharp-pointed, mid-green leaves, 20–25cm (8–10in) long. Butterfly-like, bright red flowers are borne in terminal, cylindrical racemes, 12cm (5in) long, in summer. Sometimes produces bulbils

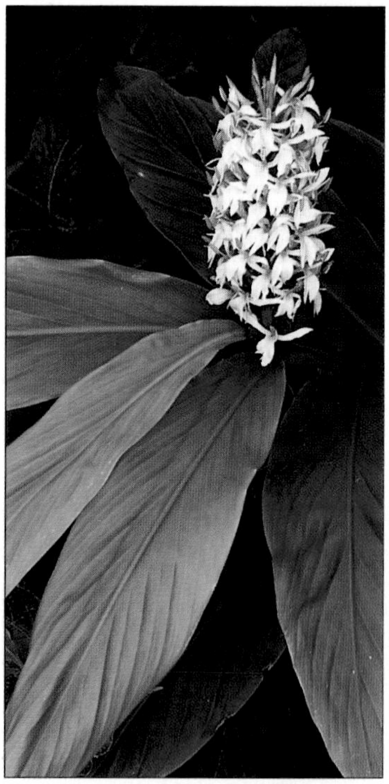

Hedychium densiflorum 'Stephen'

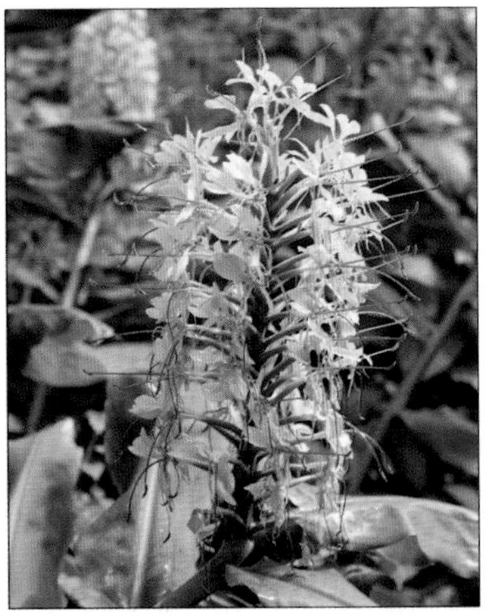

Hedychium gardnerianum

from which it can be propagated. ↕ to 2m (6ft), ↔ 60cm (24in) or more. W. Bhutan. ❄
H. horsfieldii, syn. *Brachychilum horsfieldii.* Slender-stemmed perennial with stalkless, lance-shaped to linear, leathery, glossy, mid-green leaves, 30cm (12in) long. From summer to autumn, bears showy, tubular, greenish white flowers in terminal racemes, 6–17cm (2½–7in) long. ↕ 1–1.5m (3–5ft), ↔ 1m (3ft). Indonesia (Java). ⌂ (min. 16°C/61°F)

HEDYOTIS
Bluets

RUBIACEAE

Genus of about 50 species of upright or prostrate, often stem-rooting perennials, from moist habitats in North America. They are attractive, sometimes short-lived plants valued for their 4-petalled, salverform or funnel-shaped, blue or white flowers, borne in profusion from spring to summer. The small, shiny, ovate or oval leaves, 0.5–5cm (¼–2in) long, are opposite or occasionally clustered. Grow in a woodland or rock garden, ideally in shady rock crevices.
• **HARDINESS** Fully hardy.
• **CULTIVATION** Grow in humus-rich, moist but well-drained, preferably acid soil in dappled to full shade. Mulch in autumn and spring.
• **PROPAGATION** Sow seed in containers in a cold frame in spring. Divide in spring or autumn. Root stem-tip cuttings in early summer.
• **PESTS AND DISEASES** Very susceptible to damage by slugs and snails.

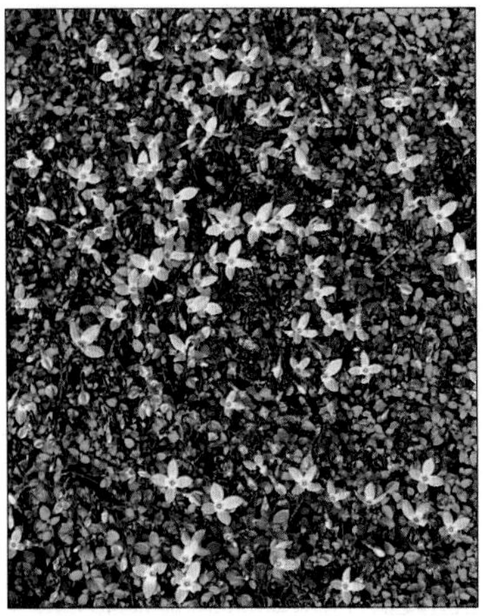

Hedyotis michauxii

H. michauxii ■ syn. *Houstonia serpyllifolia* (Creeping bluets). Mat-forming perennial with rooting stems and rounded, ovate or oval, glossy, mid-green leaves, to 7mm (¼in) long. In late spring and early summer, short, erect stems bear usually solitary, axillary and terminal, salverform, light blue flowers, to 1cm (½in) across, with white eyes. ↕ 7cm (3in), ↔ to 30cm (12in). USA (Virginia, S. Carolina to W. Tennessee). ❄❄❄

HEDYSARUM
LEGUMINOSAE/PAPILIONACEAE

Genus of 100 species of perennials and subshrubs widespread in mountains and prairies throughout the N. hemisphere. They have alternate, pinnate, mid-green leaves and bear axillary racemes of pea-like flowers in violet, purple, red, or pink, occasionally white or yellow. They are attractive to bees. Tall species, such as *H. coronarium*, are suitable for the back of a mixed or herbaceous border, and provide sweet-smelling cut flowers. Small species are ideal for a rock garden.
• **HARDINESS** Fully hardy.
• **CULTIVATION** Grow in well-drained, preferably stony or sandy, poor to moderately fertile, alkaline soil in full sun.
• **PROPAGATION** Sow seed in containers in a cold frame as soon as ripe or in spring. Divide with care in spring, as the roots resent disturbance.
• **PESTS AND DISEASES** Trouble free.

H. coronarium ■ (French honeysuckle). Upright, bushy perennial, sometimes biennial, with pinnate leaves comprising 7–15 paired, elliptic to obovate or rounded, entire leaflets, 3.5cm (1½in) long. Racemes of very fragrant, pea-like, deep red flowers, to 2cm (¾in) long, are borne on erect, angular stems throughout spring. ↕ to 1m (3ft), ↔ 60cm (24in). W. Mediterranean to Italy (Sicily). ❄❄❄. **'Album'** has white flowers.
H. hedysaroides. Rhizomatous, hairless perennial forming spreading clumps of erect, angular, unbranched stems. The numerous pinnate leaves have 7–21 obovate leaflets, 2.5cm (1in) long. Loose, conical racemes of pea-like, red-violet or white flowers, to 2.5cm (1in) long, are borne in mid- and late summer. ↕ to 60cm (24in), ↔ 90cm (36in). Arctic Russia to S. central Europe. ❄❄❄

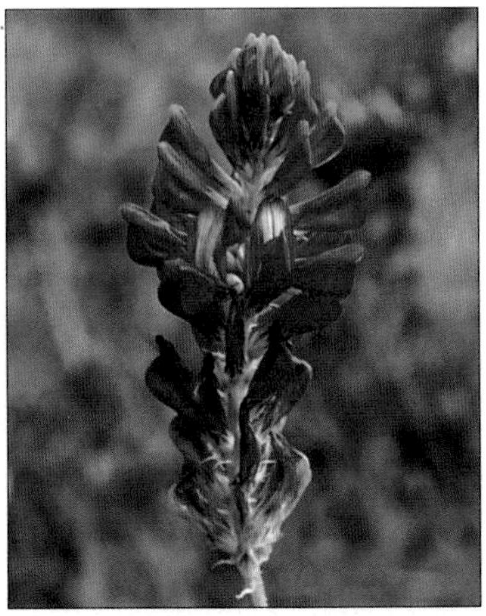

Hedysarum coronarium

HEDYSCEPE
Umbrella palm

ARECACEAE/PALMAE

Genus of one species of single-stemmed palm from the upper mountain slopes of Lord Howe Island, Australia. Pinnate leaves with up to 80 leaflets are carried in terminal tufts above a distinct crownshaft. Panicles of bowl-shaped, 3-petalled flowers are produced one at a time, just below the leaves. Where temperatures fall below 15°C (59°F), grow in a warm conservatory or greenhouse. In tropical areas, use as specimen trees, either singly or in small groups.
• **HARDINESS** Frost tender.
• **CULTIVATION** Under glass, grow in loam-based potting compost (JI No.3), with added leaf mould, in bright filtered or indirect light. Provide moderate to high humidity and good ventilation. In growth, water moderately and apply a balanced liquid fertilizer monthly; keep just moist in winter. Outdoors, grow in fertile, humus-rich, moist but well-drained soil in full sun or partial shade, with shelter from wind.
• **PROPAGATION** Sow seed at 21–24°C (70–75°F) in spring.
• **PESTS AND DISEASES** Trouble free.

H. canterburyana 🌴 syn. *Kentia canterburyana.* Small to medium-sized palm with a slender stem topped by a prominent crownshaft, tinted silvery blue-white. Rigidly curved leaves, to 1.5m (5ft) long, have 40–80 lance-shaped, erect to ascending, rich green leaflets, smooth above, downy beneath. In summer, bears deep yellow to orange-yellow flowers, to 1cm (½in) across, in horizontal panicles, to 45cm (18in) across. ↕ to 10m (30ft), ↔ to 5m (15ft). Australia (Lord Howe Island). ⌂ (min. 15°C/59°F)

▷ ***Heeria*** see *Heterocentron*
▷ ***Heimerliodendron*** see *Pisonia*
H. brunonianum see *P. umbellifera*

HELENIUM
Helen's flower

ASTERACEAE/COMPOSITAE

Genus of about 40 species of annuals, biennials, and perennials found in damp, swampy meadows or at woodland margins in North and Central America. They are mostly clump-forming plants with sturdy, branching stems and ovate to inversely lance-shaped, mid-green leaves, 15–20cm (6–8in) long. The daisy-like flowerheads have prominent yellow or brown disc-florets, and ray-florets in yellow, bronze, orange, or red. Heleniums flower over a long period and are suitable for a sunny, mixed or herbaceous border. The flowerheads are useful for cutting and are attractive to bees. All parts may cause severe discomfort if ingested; contact with the foliage may aggravate skin allergies.
• **HARDINESS** Fully hardy to frost hardy.
• **CULTIVATION** Grow in any fertile, moist but well-drained soil in full sun. Provide support for taller species and cultivars. Dead-head to prolong flowering. Divide every 2–3 years to maintain vigour.
• **PROPAGATION** Sow seed of species, or root basal cuttings of cultivars, in containers in a cold frame in spring. Divide in autumn or spring.
• **PESTS AND DISEASES** Leaf spot may be a problem.

H. autumnale (Sneezeweed). Upright, clump-forming perennial with branched, winged stems and ovate to lance-shaped, toothed leaves, 10–15cm (4–6in) long. From late summer to mid-autumn, bears flowerheads, to 5cm (2in) long, with yellow ray-florets that reflex as the brown disc-florets open. ↕ to 1.5m (5ft), ↔ 45cm (18in). Canada, E. USA. ❄❄❄
***H.* 'Baudirektor Linne'.** Clump-forming perennial bearing large, long-lasting flowerheads, to 7cm (3in) across, with velvety, brownish red ray-florets and brown disc-florets, in late summer and early autumn. ↕ 1.2m (4ft), ↔ 60cm (24in). ❄❄❄
H. bigelovii. Clump-forming perennial with sparsely branched stems and lance-shaped to inversely lance-shaped leaves, 15–23cm (6–9in) long. In early and midsummer, bears flowerheads, 6cm (2½in) across, with brownish yellow disc-florets, and yellow ray-florets that reflex as the disc-florets open. ↕ 60cm (24in), ↔ 30cm (12in). USA (California to Oregon). ❄❄❄. **'Aurantiacum'** has golden yellow flowerheads.
***H.* 'Blütentisch'.** Stout perennial with branched upper stems bearing flowerheads 7cm (3in) across, with golden yellow, brown-flecked ray-florets and brown disc-florets, from midsummer to early autumn. ↕ 80–90cm (32–36in), ↔ 60cm (24in). ❄❄❄
***H.* 'Bressingham Gold'.** Vigorous perennial bearing flowerheads 6–9cm (2½–3½in) across, with deep gold ray-florets, shaded crimson, and brown disc-florets, in mid- and late summer. ↕ 90cm (36in), ↔ 60cm (24in). ❄❄❄
***H.* 'Bruno'** ■ Erect perennial bearing flowerheads 6–9cm (2½–3½in) across, with deep crimson or reddish brown ray-florets and brown disc-florets, in late summer and early autumn. ↕ 1.2m (4ft), ↔ 60cm (24in). ❄❄❄

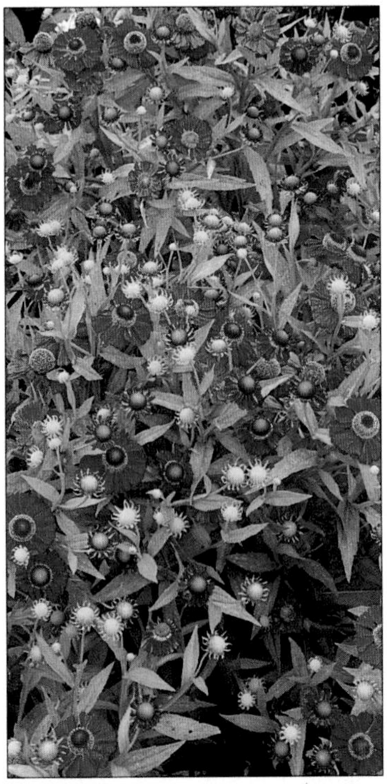

Helenium 'Bruno'

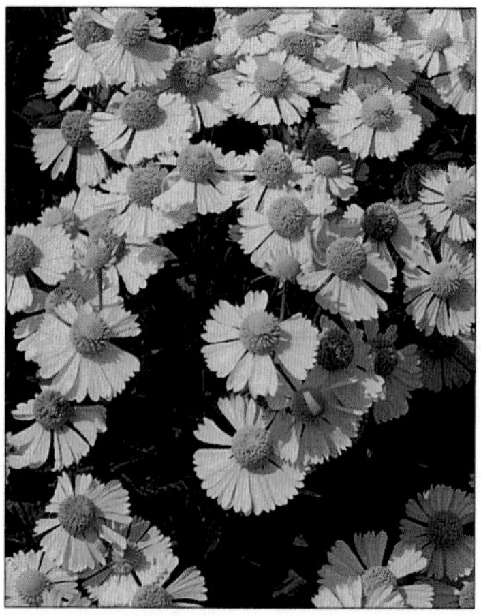

Helenium 'Butterpat'

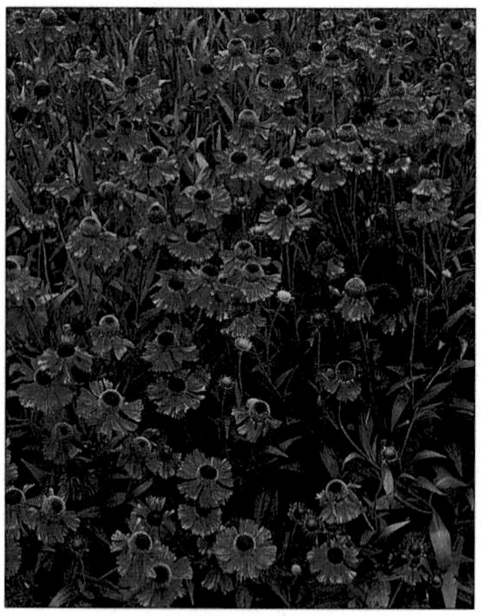

Helenium 'Moerheim Beauty'

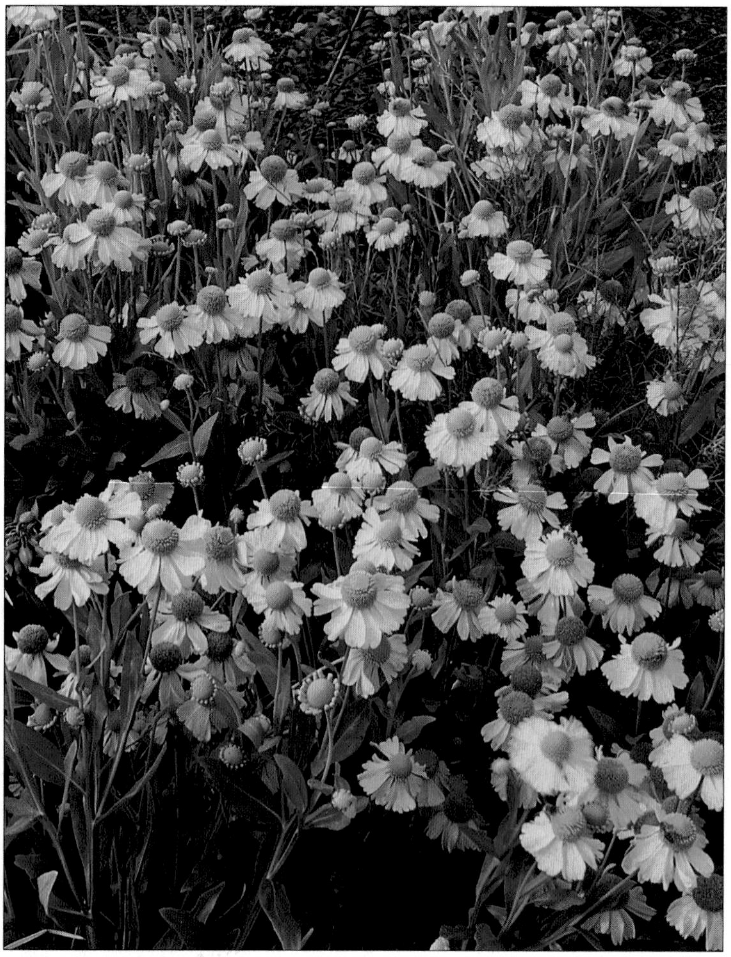

Helenium 'Pumilum Magnificum'

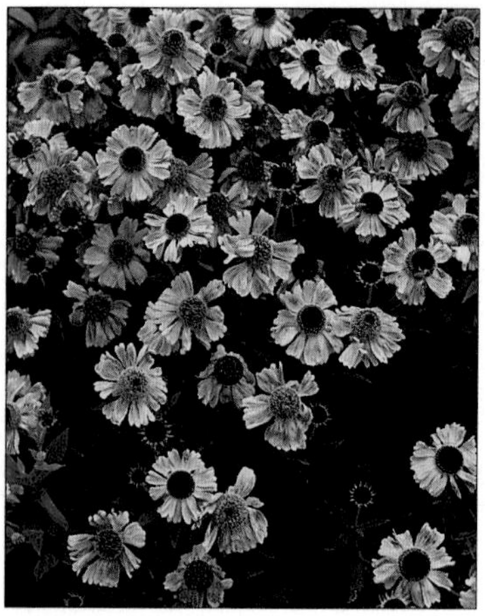

Helenium 'Wyndley'

H

***H.* 'Butterpat'** ■ Upright perennial bearing flowerheads 5–8cm (2–3in) across, with rich yellow ray-florets and yellow-brown disc-florets, from midsummer to early autumn. ↕ 90cm (36in), ↔ 60cm (24in). ✲✲✲

***H.* 'Coppelia'.** Erect perennial bearing flowerheads 5–8cm (2–3in) across, with warm copper-orange ray-florets and brown disc-florets, from midsummer to early autumn. ↕ 90cm (36in), ↔ 60cm (24in). ✲✲✲

***H.* 'Feuersiegel'.** Upright perennial bearing flowerheads 5–8cm (2–3in) across, with golden brown to red ray-florets and brown disc-florets, in late summer and early autumn. ↕ 1.5m (5ft), ↔ 60cm (24in). ✲✲✲

***H.* 'Goldene Jugend'**, syn. *H.* 'Golden Youth'. Upright perennial producing flowerheads to 8cm (3in) across, with golden yellow ray-florets and yellow disc-florets, in early and midsummer. ↕ 80cm (32in), ↔ 60cm (24in). ✲✲✲

***H.* 'Golden Youth'** see *H.* 'Goldene Jugend'.

***H.* 'Gold Fox'.** Erect perennial bearing flowerheads to 8cm (3in) across, with tawny-orange ray-florets and brown disc-florets, from midsummer to early autumn. ↕ 90cm (36in), ↔ 60cm (24in). ✲✲✲

***H.* 'Goldrausch'.** Upright perennial bearing flowerheads to 7cm (3in) across, with golden yellow, brown-marked ray-florets and brown disc-florets, in late summer and early autumn. ↕ to 1.5m (5ft), ↔ 60cm (24in). ✲✲✲

H. hoopesii. Erect, clump-forming perennial with basal rosettes of inversely lance-shaped, greyish green leaves, 25–30cm (10–12in) long, becoming smaller towards the tops of the stems. In early summer, bears branched, lax, terminal corymbs of 3–8 flowerheads to 8cm (3in) across, the bright yellow to orange ray-florets reflexing as the yellow-brown disc-florets open. Will tolerate dry soil. ↕ to 1m (3ft), ↔ 45cm (18in). Mountains of USA (California to Oregon, Wyoming, New Mexico). ✲✲✲

***H.* 'Kupferzwerg'.** Upright perennial bearing flowerheads 5–8cm (2–3in) across, with brownish red ray-florets and brown disc-florets, in mid- and late summer. ↕ 70cm (28in), ↔ 60cm (24in). ✲✲✲

***H.* 'Margot'.** Upright perennial producing flowerheads 5–8cm (2–3in) across, with brownish red, yellow-tipped ray-florets and brown disc-florets, from midsummer to early autumn. ↕ 90cm (36in), ↔ 60cm (24in). ✲✲✲

***H.* 'Moerheim Beauty'** ■ Upright perennial bearing flowerheads 5–8cm (2–3in) across, with dark copper-red ray-florets and dark brown disc-florets, from early to late summer. ↕ 90cm (36in), ↔ 60cm (24in). ✲✲✲

***H.* 'Pumilum Magnificum'** ■ Erect perennial bearing flowerheads to 7cm (3in) across, with golden yellow ray-florets and yellow-brown disc-florets, from late summer to mid-autumn. ↕ 90cm (36in), ↔ 60cm (24in). ✲✲✲

***H.* 'Red and Gold'** see *H.* 'Rotgold'.

***H.* 'Riverton Gem'.** Upright perennial producing flowerheads 5–7cm (2–3in) across, with deep crimson, yellow-streaked ray-florets and brown disc-florets, in late summer and early autumn. ↕ 1.2m (4ft), ↔ 60cm (24in). ✲✲✲

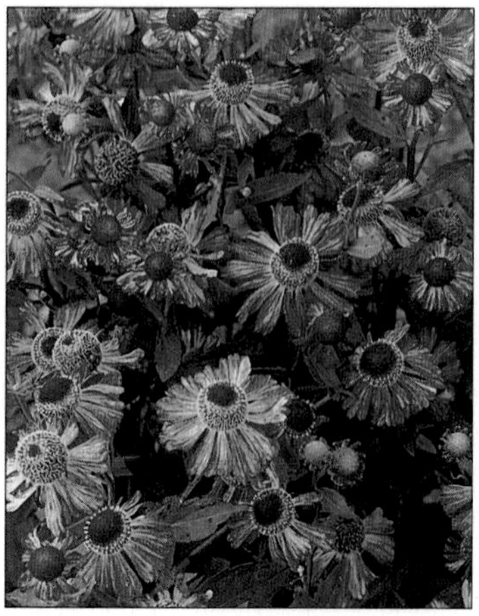

Helenium 'Septemberfuchs'

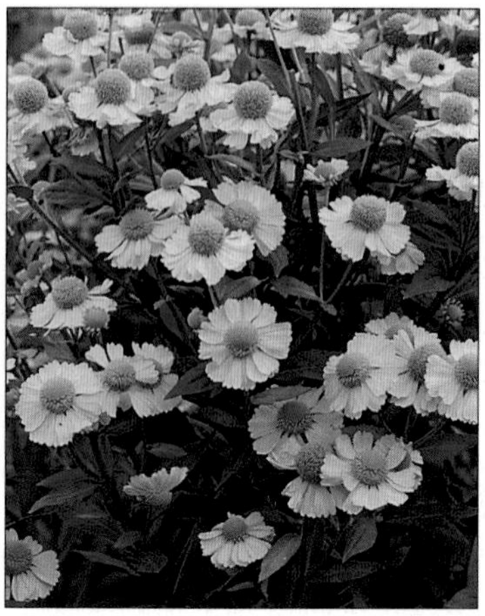

Helenium 'Sonnenwunder'

***H.* 'Rotgold'**, syn. *H.* 'Red and Gold'. Upright perennial bearing flowerheads to 8cm (3in) across, with ray-florets in varying shades or combinations of red and yellow, and brown disc-florets, in late summer and early autumn. ↕ 1.2m (4ft), ↔ 60cm (24in). ✲✲✲

***H.* 'Septemberfuchs'** ■ Upright perennial bearing flowerheads 5–8cm (2–3in) across, with bright orange-brown ray-florets, suffused yellow, and brown disc-florets, from late summer to mid-autumn. ↕ 1.5m (5ft), ↔ 60cm (24in). ✲✲✲

***H.* 'Sonnenwunder'** ■ Erect perennial bearing flowerheads 5–8cm (2–3in) across, with yellow ray-florets and green, then pale brownish yellow disc-florets, from late summer to mid-autumn. ↕ 1.5m (5ft), ↔ 60cm (24in). ✲✲✲

***H.* 'Waldtraut'.** Upright, sturdy perennial bearing flowerheads 5–8cm (2–3in) across, with golden brown ray-florets and brown disc-florets, in late summer and early autumn. ↕ 80–100cm (32–39in), ↔ 60cm (24in). ✲✲✲

***H.* 'Wyndley'** ■ Erect perennial bearing flowerheads 5–8cm (2–3in) across, with yellow ray-florets, overlaid dark orange, and with darker orange-brown disc-florets, from midsummer to early autumn. ↕ 80cm (32in), ↔ 60cm (24in). ✲✲✲

***H.* 'Zimbelstern'.** Upright perennial producing flowerheads 5–8cm (2–3in) across, with golden brown, wavy-margined ray-florets and brown disc-florets, in mid- and late summer. ↕ to 1.2m (4ft), ↔ 60cm (24in). ✲✲✲

▷ **Helen's flower** see *Helenium*

HELIANTHEMUM

Rock rose, Sun rose

CISTACEAE

Genus of about 110 species of evergreen or semi-evergreen shrubs occurring in alpine meadows or open scrub in North and South America, Asia, Europe, and North Africa, particularly around the Mediterranean. They have opposite, oblong to linear, silver- to grey-green or light to mid-green leaves, and are grown for their raceme-like cymes of saucer-shaped, 5-petalled, brightly coloured flowers, which are borne over a long period from late spring to midsummer. They are ideal for a rock garden, a raised

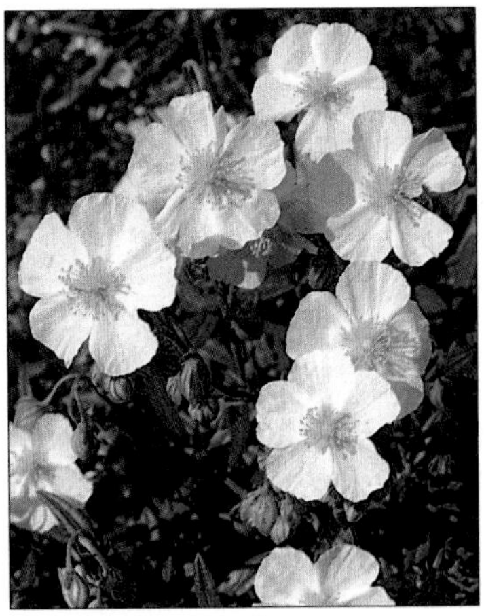

Helianthemum apenninum

bed, or the front of a herbaceous or mixed border, or as ground cover on a sunny bank. The hybrids most often grown are crosses involving *H. apenninum*, *H. nummularium*, and *H. croceum*; those described below are evergreen shrubs of similar habit and appearance to *H. apenninum*, with silver, mid-green, or grey-green leaves and saucer-shaped flowers.

- **HARDINESS** Fully hardy to frost hardy.
- **CULTIVATION** Grow in moderately fertile, well-drained, neutral to alkaline soil in full sun. Pruning group 10, after flowering.
- **PROPAGATION** Sow seed of species in containers in a cold frame as soon as ripe or in spring. Root softwood cuttings in late spring or early summer.
- **PESTS AND DISEASES** Trouble free.

H. apenninum ■ Spreading, loosely mat-forming, evergreen shrub with elliptic-oblong to linear, downy, grey-green leaves, to 3cm (1¼in) long, on branching, downy stems. From late spring to midsummer, bears few-flowered cymes of white flowers, 2.5cm (1in) across, with conspicuous, deep yellow anthers. ↕ to 40cm (16in), ↔ to 60cm (24in). Europe, Turkey. ❄❄❄
***H.* 'Ben Hope'.** Spreading shrub with downy, pale grey-green leaves, 1–4cm (½–1½in) long. Bears carmine-red flowers, to 2.5cm (1in) across, with deep orange centres. ↕ 20–30cm (8–12in), ↔ 30cm (12in). ❄❄❄
***H.* 'Ben Nevis'.** Spreading shrub, more compact than *H. apenninum*, with dark green leaves, 1–4cm (½–1½in) long. Produces rich orange-yellow flowers, to 2.5cm (1in) across, with bronze-crimson centres. ↕↔ to 20cm (8in). ❄❄❄
***H.* 'Chocolate Blotch'.** Spreading shrub producing grey-green leaves, 1–4cm (½–1½in) long, and buff-coloured flowers, to 2.5cm (1in) across, marked chocolate-brown at the petal bases. ↕ 20–30cm (8–12in), ↔ 30cm (12in). ❄❄❄
***H.* 'Fire Dragon'** ■♕ syn. *H.* 'Mrs. Clay'. Spreading shrub with grey-green leaves, 1–4cm (½–1½in) long. Produces vivid orange-red flowers, to 2.5cm (1in) across. ↕ 20–30cm (8–12in), ↔ 30cm (12in). ❄❄❄
H. guttatum see *Tuberaria guttata*.
***H.* 'Henfield Brilliant'** ♕ Spreading shrub producing grey-green leaves, 1–4cm (½–1½in) long, and brick-red flowers, 2.5cm (1in) across. ↕ 20–30cm (8–12in), ↔ 30cm (12in). ❄❄❄
H. lunulatum ■ Dwarf, initially erect then spreading, evergreen shrub with elliptic to lance-shaped, hairy, grey-green leaves, to 1cm (½in) long. In late spring and early summer, clear yellow flowers, to 1.5cm (½in) across, with prominent, orange-yellow anthers, are borne singly or in cymes. ↕ 15cm (6in), ↔ 25cm (10in). S. Europe. ❄❄❄
***H.* 'Mrs. Clay'** see *H.* 'Fire Dragon'.
***H. nummularium* 'Amy Baring'** ♕ Dwarf shrub producing erect then procumbent branches and ovate or lance-shaped to elliptic, grey-green leaves, 0.5–5cm (¼–2in) long. Bears deep yellow flowers, to 2.5cm (1in) across, with orange centres. ↕ 15cm (6in), ↔ to 20cm (8in). ❄❄❄
***H. oelandicum* subsp. *alpestre*.** Neat, mat-forming shrub with lance-shaped, downy, grey-green leaves, to 2cm (¾in) long. Terminal cymes of up to 5 yellow flowers, each to 1.5cm (½in) across, are borne from late spring to midsummer. ↕ 12cm (5in), ↔ to 20cm (8in). S. Europe. ❄❄❄
***H.* 'Raspberry Ripple'** ■ Spreading shrub with dark greyish green leaves, 1–4cm (½–1½in) long. White flowers, to 2.5cm (1in) across, have purplish pink centres, the colour spreading irregularly into the petal margins. ↕ 20cm (8in), ↔ to 30cm (12in). ❄❄❄
***H.* 'Rhodanthe Carneum'** ■♕ syn. *H.* 'Wisley Pink'. Long-flowering, spreading shrub, more robust than *H. apenninum*. It has silver-grey leaves, 2.5–3.5cm (1–1½in) long, and bears pale pink flowers, to 2.5cm (1in) across, flushed yellow at the centres. ↕ to 30cm (12in), ↔ to 45cm (18in). ❄❄❄
H. tuberaria see *Tuberaria lignosa*.
H. umbellatum see *Halimium umbellatum*.
***H.* 'Wisley Pink'** see *H.* 'Rhodanthe Carneum'.
***H.* 'Wisley Primrose'** ♕ Spreading shrub with grey-green leaves, to 4cm (1½in) long. Bears pale primrose-yellow flowers, 2–2.5cm (¾–1in) across, with deep golden yellow centres. ↕ to 30cm (12in), ↔ to 45cm (18in). ❄❄❄
***H.* 'Wisley White'** ■ Spreading shrub with grey leaves, to 4cm (1½in) long. Bears creamy white flowers, 2–2.5cm (¾–1in) across, with mid- to deep yellow centres and yellow stamens. ↕ to 30cm (12in), ↔ to 45cm (18in). ❄❄❄

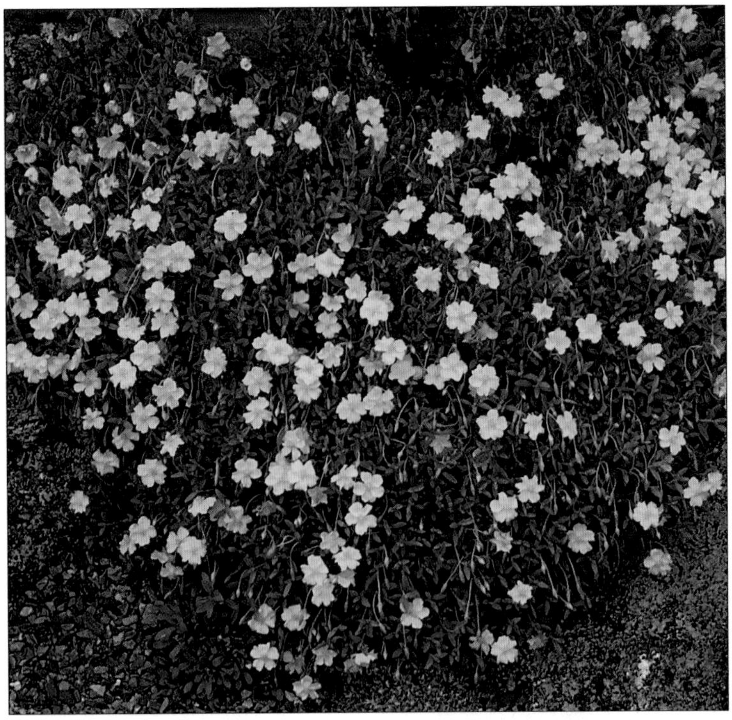

Helianthemum lunulatum

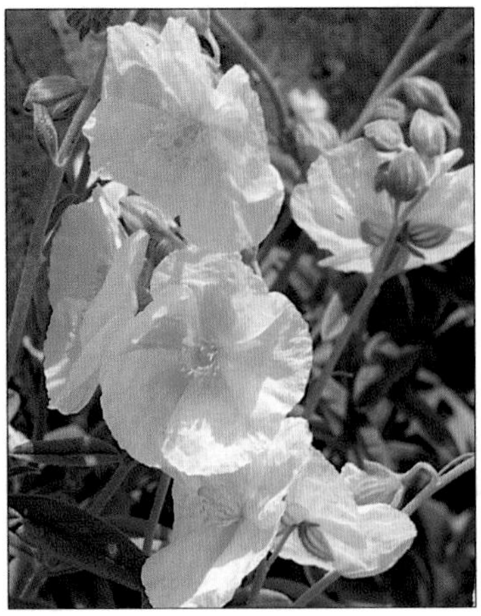

Helianthemum 'Wisley White'

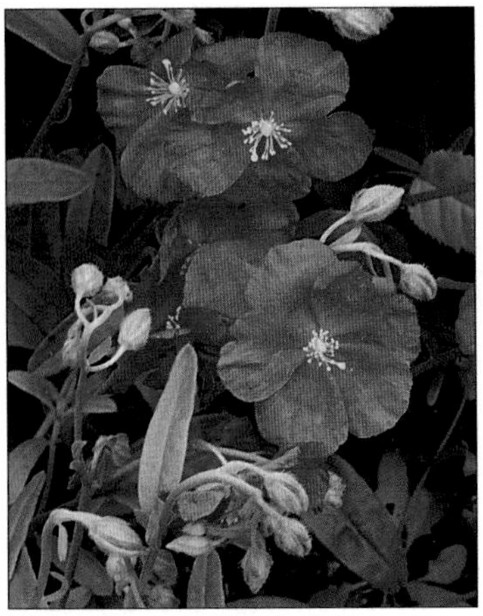

Helianthemum 'Fire Dragon'

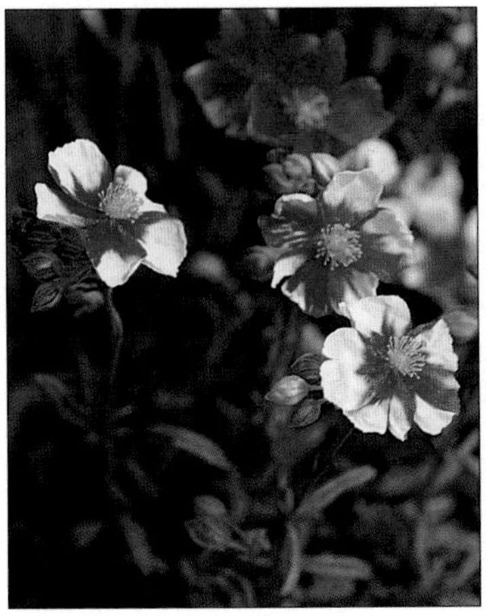

Helianthemum 'Raspberry Ripple'

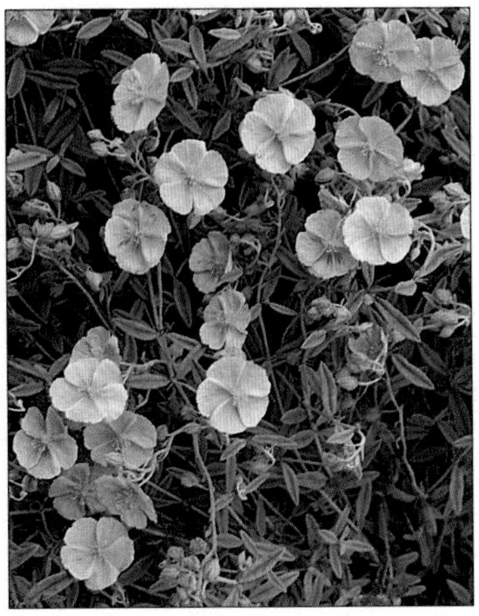

Helianthemum 'Rhodanthe Carneum'

HELIANTHUS

Sunflower

ASTERACEAE/COMPOSITAE

Genus of about 70–80 species of annuals and perennials, some occurring in dry woodland and prairies, others in damp, swampy habitats, in North America, Central America, Peru, and Chile. Usually tall, coarse plants, they have creeping or tuberous roots and large, simple, bristly, alternate or opposite leaves. The showy, daisy-like flowerheads, with sterile ray-florets, are usually 5–10cm (2–4in) across, but up to 30cm (12in) in the giant annuals; they are borne singly or in loose corymbs and have yellow, occasionally red, or very rarely violet, ray-florets, and yellow, brown, or purple disc-florets. As the nomenclature of many cultivars and hybrids is confused, some names used here may be amended in the future.

Sunflowers are effective in an annual, herbaceous, or mixed border. The taller, spreading species and hybrids, such as *H.* x *laetiflorus* and *H. salicifolius*, are suitable for a wild garden; small annuals, such as *H. annuus* 'Teddy Bear', are ideal for containers. Sunflowers provide good cut flowers and many are attractive to bees. Contact with the foliage of sunflowers may aggravate skin allergies.

- **HARDINESS** Fully hardy to frost hardy.
- **CULTIVATION** Grow in moderately fertile, humus-rich, moist but well-drained, neutral to alkaline soil in full sun. Sunflowers need long, hot summers to flower well. Most will tolerate dry soil, *H. pauciflorus* and *H. salicifolius* prefer it. *H. decapetalus*, *H.* x *laetiflorus*, and *H.* x *multiflorus* thrive in moist soil,

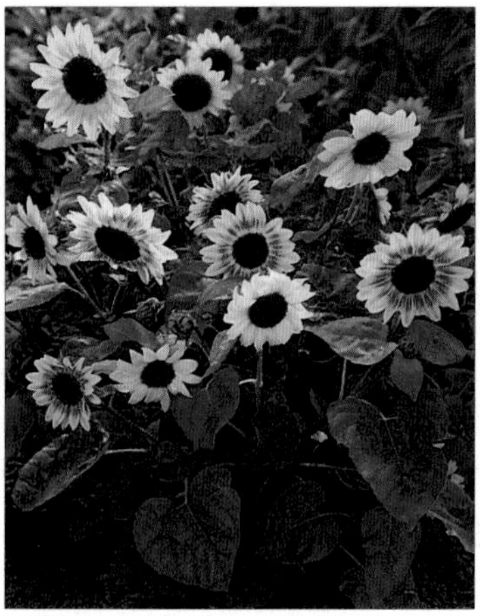
Helianthus annuus 'Music Box'

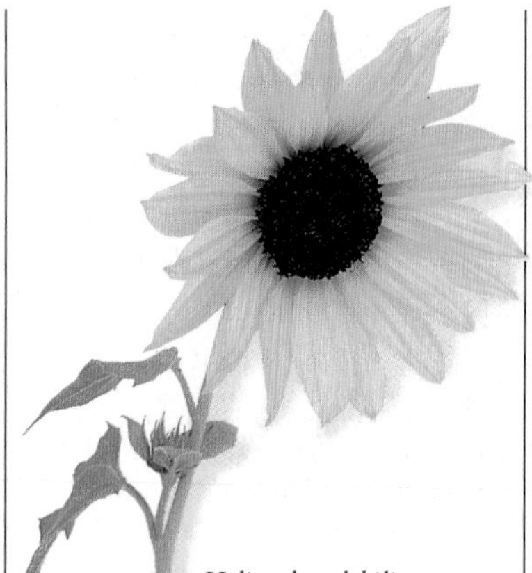
Helianthus debilis subsp. *cucumerifolius* 'Italian White'

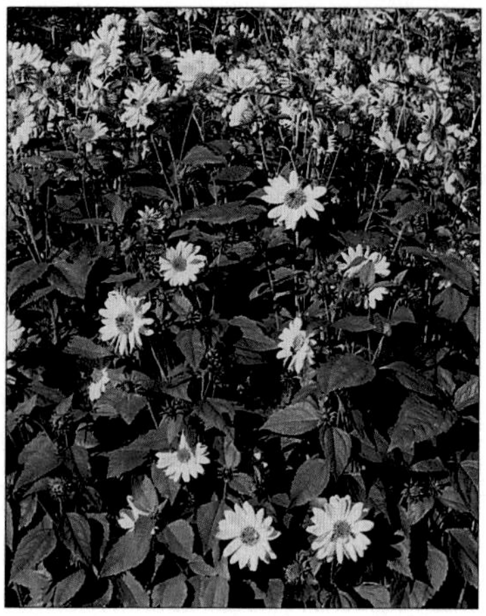
Helianthus x *multiflorus*

particularly near water. Tall species and cultivars require support. Top-dress perennials annually with garden compost or well-rotted manure. Divide and transplant perennials every 2–4 years to maintain vigour.

• **PROPAGATION** Sow seed of perennials in containers in a cold frame in spring; sow annuals at 16°C (61°F) in late winter, or *in situ* in spring. Cultivars may not come true from seed, and hybridize freely. Divide perennials in spring or autumn. Root basal cuttings in spring.

• **PESTS AND DISEASES** Susceptible to slugs, powdery mildew, and *Sclerotinia.*

H. annuus (Sunflower). Fast-growing, tall, branched to unbranched, hairy-stemmed annual with broadly oval to heart-shaped, toothed, roughly hairy, mid- to dark green leaves, 10–40cm (4–16in) long. In summer, bears large, daisy-like flowerheads, to 30cm (12in) wide, with yellow ray-florets and brown or purple disc-florets, sometimes tinged red or purple. ↕ to 5m (15ft), ↔ to 60cm (24in). USA to Central America. ❄❄❄. **'Autumn Beauty'** has flowerheads to 15cm (6in) across, with dark mahogany-red, lemon-yellow, golden yellow, or bronze-red ray-florets, sometimes zoned with additional shades; ↕ 1.5m (5ft) or more. **'Big Smile'** bears flowerheads to 10cm (4in) across, with yellow ray-florets and darker yellow disc-florets; ↕ 40cm (16in). **'Music Box'** ■ is free-flowering and many-branched; it bears flowerheads 10–12cm (4–5in) across, with ray-florets in colours ranging from creamy yellow to dark red, including some bicolours, and black disc-florets; ↕ 70cm (28in). **'Russian Giant'** is tall, with large yellow flowerheads, to 25cm (10in) across; ↕ 3.5m (11ft). **'Sunspot'** produces large yellow flowerheads, to 25cm (10in) across; ↕ 60cm (24in). **'Teddy Bear'** ■ is compact, bearing double, deep yellow flowerheads, to 13cm (5in) across; ↕ 90cm (36in).

H. atrorubens, syn. *H. sparsifolius* (Dark-eye sunflower). Clump-forming perennial with hairy, purple-green stems and ovate to lance-shaped, toothed to scalloped, hairy, mid-green, mainly basal leaves, 20–30cm (8–12in) long. In late summer, bears flowerheads 5–9cm (2–3½in) across, with deep yellow ray-florets and purplish maroon disc-florets. ↕ to 1.5m (5ft), ↔ 1.2m (4ft). S.E. USA. ❄❄❄. **'Gullick's Variety'** is vigorous, wide-spreading, and free-blooming; it produces narrow, pointed leaves, and from late summer to mid-autumn, bears flowerheads with yellow ray-florets and brownish purple disc-florets; ↕ 1.2–1.7m (4–5½ft). **'Monarch'** ■🏆 is vigorous, bearing semi-double flowerheads, to 15cm (6in) across when disbudded, with yellow-brown disc-florets, in early and mid-autumn; ↕ to 2m (6ft); ❄❄

H. cucumerifolius see *H. debilis* subsp. *cucumerifolius.*

H. debilis. Tall, smooth to hairy annual with stout, strongly branched stems, occasionally mottled purple, and ovate to lance-shaped, sometimes toothed, glossy, mid-green leaves, 5–14cm (2–5½in) long. Slightly nodding flowerheads, 6cm (2½in) or more across, with bright yellow, sometimes red-flushed ray-florets and deep purple-red disc-florets, are borne in summer. ↕ 2m (6ft), ↔ 45–60cm (18–24in). USA (Florida, Texas). ❄❄❄. **subsp. *cucumerifolius***, syn. *H. cucumerifolius*, is shorter, with purple-mottled stems, coarsely hairy, sharply toothed leaves, to 10cm (4in) long, and larger flowerheads, to 15cm (6in) across, from summer to autumn; ↕ 1m (3ft); USA (S.E. Texas). **subsp. *cucumerifolius* 'Italian White'** ■ has flowerheads to 10cm (4in) across, with creamy white to pale primrose-yellow ray-florets and black disc-florets; ↕ 1.5m (5ft). **subsp. *cucumerifolius* 'Vanilla Ice'** has creamy yellow ray-florets.

H. decapetalus (Thin-leaved sunflower). Rhizomatous perennial with tall stems, hairless at the bases and bristly towards the flowerheads. Thin, lance-shaped to broadly ovate, mid-green leaves, to 20cm (8in) long, are smooth above and rough-hairy beneath. Flowerheads 5–8cm (2–3in) across, with yellow ray-florets and yellow-brown disc-florets, are borne from late summer to mid-autumn. ↕ 1.5m (5ft), ↔ 1.1m (3½ft). C. and S.E. USA. ❄❄❄

H. x laetiflorus (*H. pauciflorus* x *H. tuberosus*). Spreading, rhizomatous perennial with rough stems and thin, ovate, coarsely toothed, dark green leaves, to 30cm (12in) long. Flowerheads 10–12cm (4–5in) across, with bright yellow ray-florets and yellow disc-florets, open from late summer to mid-autumn. ↕ 1.5–2.2m (5–7ft), ↔ 1.2m (4ft) or more. Garden origin. ❄❄❄. **'Miss Mellish'** spreads vigorously, and bears semi-double flowerheads with orange-yellow ray-florets. **'Morning Sun'** ■ bears large, semi-double flower-

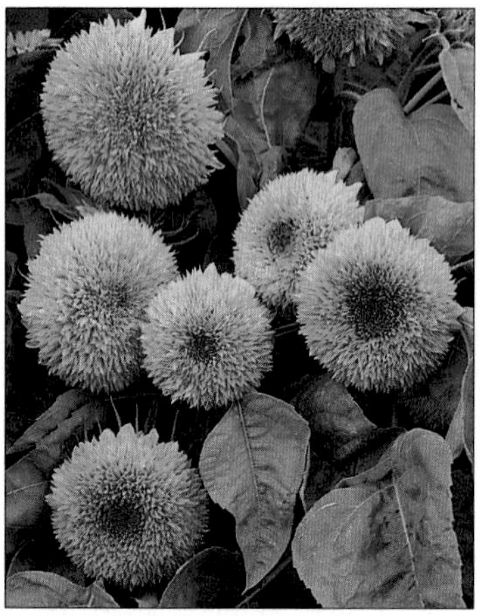
Helianthus annuus 'Teddy Bear'

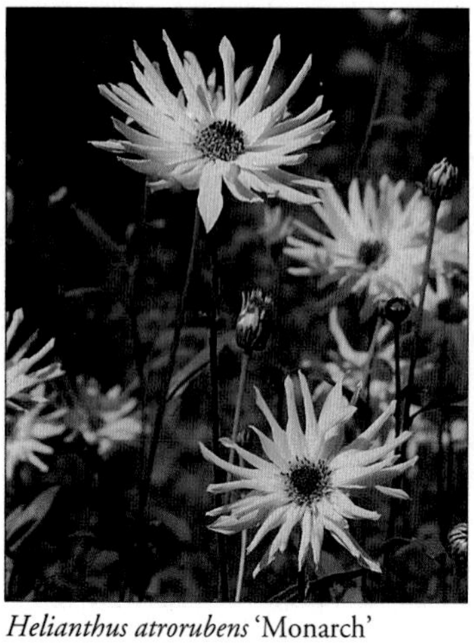
Helianthus atrorubens 'Monarch'

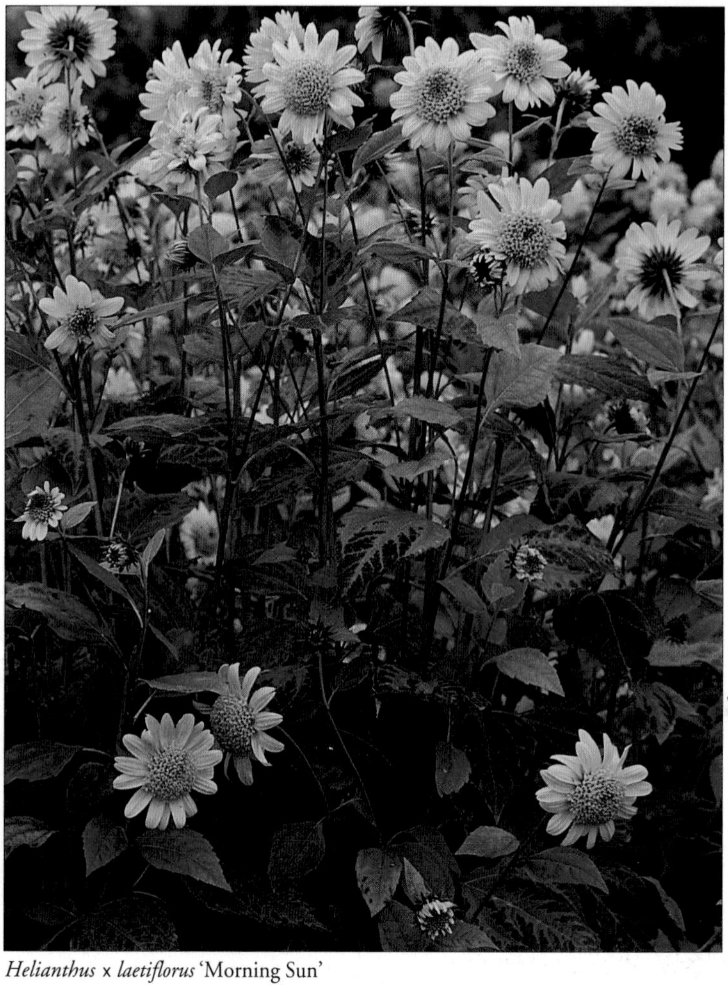
Helianthus x *laetiflorus* 'Morning Sun'

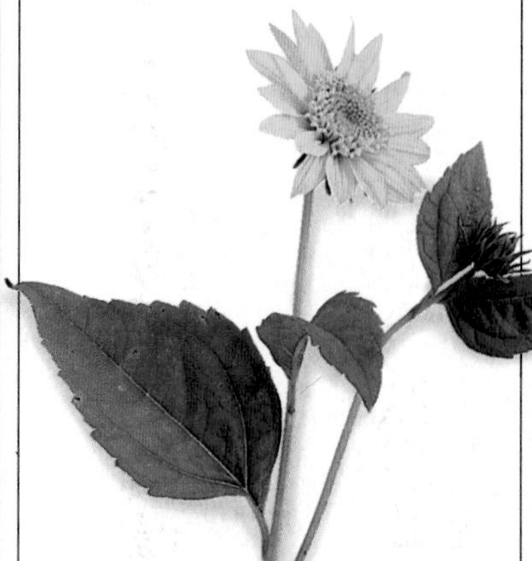
Helianthus x *multiflorus* 'Capenoch Star'

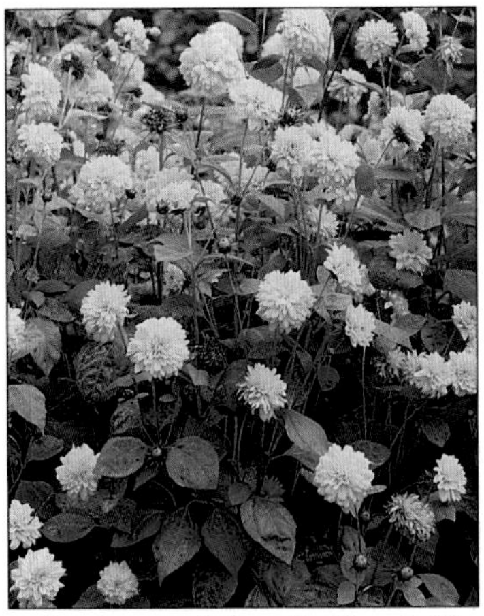
Helianthus x *multiflorus* 'Loddon Gold'

heads with golden yellow ray-florets and quilled disc-florets, from midsummer to autumn; ↕ 1.2m (4ft), ↔ 60cm (24in).
***H.* 'Lemon Queen'.** Rhizomatous perennial with ovate, conspicuously veined, dark green leaves, to 12cm (5in) long. Flowerheads 8–12cm (3–5in) across, with pale yellow ray-florets and slightly darker yellow disc-florets, open from late summer to mid-autumn. ↕ 1.7m (5½ft), ↔ 1.2m (4ft). ❄❄❄
H.* x *multiflorus ▣ (*H. annuus* x *H. decapetalus*). Clump-forming perennial with lance-shaped to ovate, slightly hairy, dark green leaves, to 20cm (8in) long. Flowerheads to 12cm (5in) across, with domed, yellow-brown disc-florets, and golden yellow ray-florets, open from late summer to mid-autumn. ↕ to 2m (6ft), ↔ 90cm (36in). Garden origin. ❄❄❄. **'Capenoch Star'** ▣🏆 has single flowerheads with lemon-yellow ray-florets and quilled, slightly darker yellow disc-florets; good for cutting; ↕ to 1.5m (5ft). **'Loddon Gold'** ▣🏆 has double, rich yellow flowerheads; ↕ to 1.5m (5ft). **'Soleil d'Or'** ▣ has large, double yellow flowerheads. **'Triomphe de Gand'** ▣ bears large flowerheads with deep golden yellow ray-florets and quilled disc-florets; ↔ 1.2m (4ft).
H. orgyalis see *H. salicifolius.*
H. pauciflorus, syn. *H. rigidus.* Vigorous, rhizomatous perennial with roughly hairy stems and coarsely hairy, broadly lance-shaped to narrowly ovate, entire or toothed, dark green leaves, to 25cm (10in) long. Flowerheads 8cm (3in) across, with yellow ray-florets and reddish purple disc-florets, are borne in

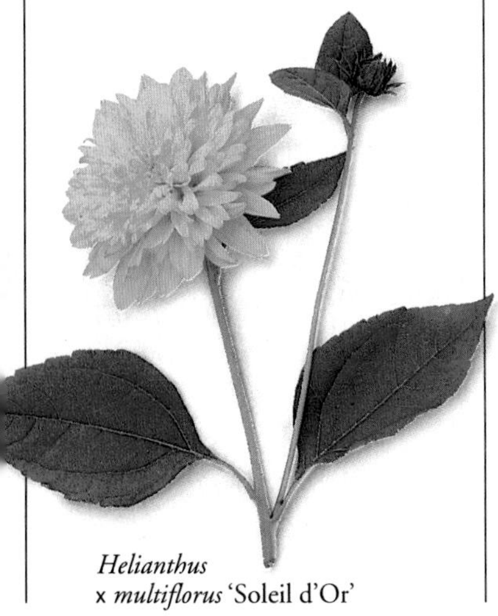
Helianthus x *multiflorus* 'Soleil d'Or'

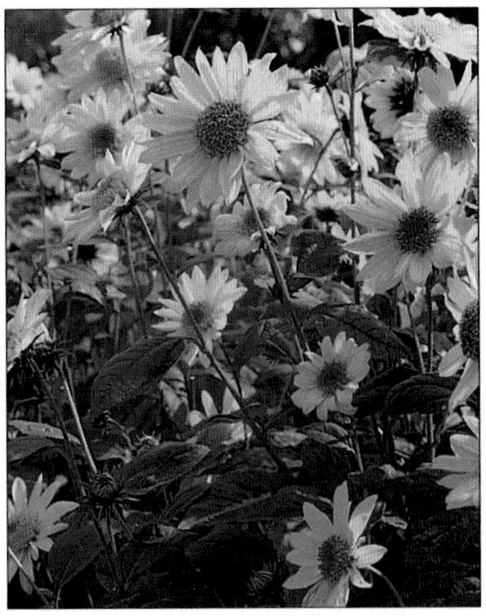
Helianthus x *multiflorus* 'Triomphe de Gand'

late summer. ↕ to 2m (6ft), ↔ 60cm (24in). W. to C. USA. ❄❄❄
H. rigidus see *H. pauciflorus.*
H. salicifolius, syn. *H. orgyalis* (Willow-leaved sunflower). Rhizomatous, clump-forming perennial with linear to lance-shaped, slightly hairy, dark green leaves, to 20cm (8in) long, arching outwards from stout stems. Flowerheads 5–7cm (2–3in) across, with golden yellow ray-florets and brown disc-florets, open in early and mid-autumn. ↕ 2.5m (8ft), ↔ 90cm (36in). S. central USA. ❄❄❄
H. sparsifolius see *H. atrorubens.*

HELICHRYSUM

ASTERACEAE/COMPOSITAE

Genus of about 500 species of annuals, herbaceous or evergreen perennials, and evergreen shrubs and subshrubs, widely distributed in Europe, Asia, Africa, and particularly in Australasia and South Africa, where they usually occur in dry, sunny sites. They have woolly or hairy stems and alternate leaves, sometimes opposite or in basal rosettes, which are aromatic in some species. The flowerheads are daisy-like or shaving-brush-like, either borne singly or in corymbs, and "everlasting" when dried. Grow small, prostrate, or cushion-forming helichrysums in a rock garden, scree bed, or alpine house; taller perennials and subshrubs are suitable for a mixed or herbaceous border. In frost-prone climates, tender species, such as *H. petiolare*, are excellent in hanging baskets or containers; in warmer areas, use as annuals in borders or beds.
- **HARDINESS** Fully hardy to frost tender.
- **CULTIVATION** Grow in well-drained, poor to moderately fertile, neutral to alkaline soil in full sun. Low-growing alpines need gritty, sharply drained soil. Protect from excessive winter wet and cold, drying winds. Pruning group 10, in spring, for larger subshrubs and shrubs, including *H. italicum*, *H. splendidum*, and *H. stoechas.*
- **PROPAGATION** Sow seed at 13–16°C (55–61°F), or in containers in a cold frame, in spring; sow seed of alpines in containers in an open frame as soon as ripe or in spring. Divide perennials in spring. Root heel or semi-ripe cuttings of shrubby species in summer and over-winter in frost-free conditions.
- **PESTS AND DISEASES** Powdery mildew may be a problem.

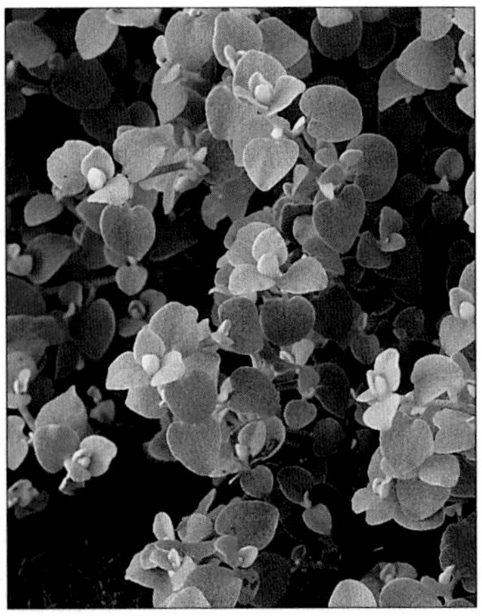
Helichrysum petiolare

H. alveolatum see *H. splendidum.*
H. angustifolium see *H. italicum.*
H. arwae. Prostrate to low mound-forming, evergreen subshrub producing branched, woody stems and alternate, crowded, oblong to lance-shaped, silvery grey leaves, to 1cm (½in) long. Solitary, daisy-like white flowerheads, 1.5–3cm (½–1¼in) across, with incurving white bracts, are borne in summer. ↕ 5cm (2in), ↔ to 30cm (12in). Yemen. ❄❄
H. bellidioides. Mat-forming, evergreen perennial with white-hairy stems when young, later smooth and reddish brown. The obovate to narrowly obovate leaves, 5–10mm (¼–½in) long, are mid-green above and white-felted beneath. From late spring to summer, erect, leafy stems bear solitary, papery, daisy-like white flowerheads, 1.5–3cm (½–1¼in) across. ↕ 15cm (6in) in flower, ↔ 60cm (24in). New Zealand. ❄❄❄ (borderline)
H. bracteatum see *Bracteantha bracteata.*
H. coralloides see *Ozothamnus coralloides.*
H. italicum 🏆 syn. *H. angustifolium.* Bushy, evergreen subshrub with woolly stems and linear, aromatic, silver-grey to yellowish green leaves, to 3cm (1¼in) long. Dark yellow flowerheads, 2–4mm ($\frac{1}{16}$–⅛in) across, are borne in corymbs to 8cm (3in) across, from summer to autumn. ↕ 60cm (24in), ↔ 1m (3ft). S. Europe. ❄❄. **subsp. *serotinum***, syn. *H. serotinum* (Curry plant), is compact, with leaves to 4cm (1½in) long; the foliage is intensely aromatic; ↕ 40cm (16in), ↔ 75cm (30in).
H. lanatum see *H. thianschanicum.*

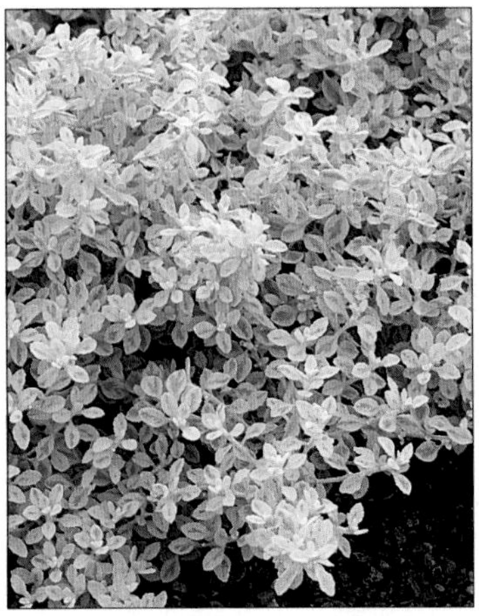
Helichrysum petiolare 'Roundabout'

H. ledifolium see *Ozothamnus ledifolius.*
***H. marginatum* of gardens** see *H. milfordiae.*
H. milfordiae, syn. *H. marginatum* of gardens. Cushion-forming, evergreen perennial with rosettes of alternate, obovate to oblong, densely silvery-hairy, mid-green leaves, to 1.5cm (½in) long. Solitary, "everlasting", daisy-like white flowerheads, 2.5–3cm (1–1¼in) across, with glossy, white, crimson-backed bracts, are borne in spring. ↕ 5–10cm (2–4in) in flower, ↔ 15–30cm (6–12in). South Africa (KwaZulu/Natal), Lesotho, at 3,000m (10,000ft) and above. ❄❄ (borderline)
H. milliganii. Clump-forming, evergreen subshrub or herbaceous perennial with tufted, often woolly stems and ovate-oblong to narrowly spoon-shaped, fleshy, mid-green leaves, to 2.5cm (1in) long. In summer, white-downy stems bear solitary, papery flowerheads, 4cm (1½in) across, white inside and yellowish white or red on the reverse of the bracts. ↕ 15–20cm (6–8in), ↔ 20cm (8in). Australia (Tasmania). ❄❄
H. orientale. Subshrubby, bushy, evergreen perennial with white-woolly, leafy stems and oblong-spoon-shaped, white-woolly leaves, 2–6cm (¾–2½in) long, becoming narrower and shorter higher up the stems. Hemispherical, shiny, light yellow flowerheads, 7–10mm (¼–½in) across, are borne in terminal corymbs, to 8cm (3in) across, in midsummer. ↕ 20–30cm (8–12in), ↔ 30cm (12in). E. Mediterranean (including Greece and the Aegean islands). ❄❄❄
H. petiolare ▣🏆 syn. *H. petiolatum* of gardens. Mound-forming or trailing, evergreen shrub with branching stems and broadly ovate to heart-shaped leaves, 3.5cm (1½in) long, densely grey-woolly above, lighter beneath. In late summer and autumn, bears hemispherical, off-white flowerheads, to 1.5cm (½in) across, in loose, terminal corymbs, 2.5–5cm (1–2in) across. ↕ to 50cm (20in), ↔ 2m (6ft) or more. South Africa. ❄. **'Aurea'** see 'Limelight'. **'Limelight'**, syn. 'Aurea', has bright lime-green leaves. **'Roundabout'** ▣ is a miniature sport of 'Variegatum', and occasionally reverts; ↕ 15cm (6in), ↔ 30cm (12in). **'Sky Net'** has pink-flushed, creamy white flowerheads in corymbs to 2cm (¾in) across, in summer. ↕ 1m (3ft). **'Variegatum'** ▣🏆 has grey leaves, variegated cream.
***H. petiolatum* of gardens** see *H. petiolare.*

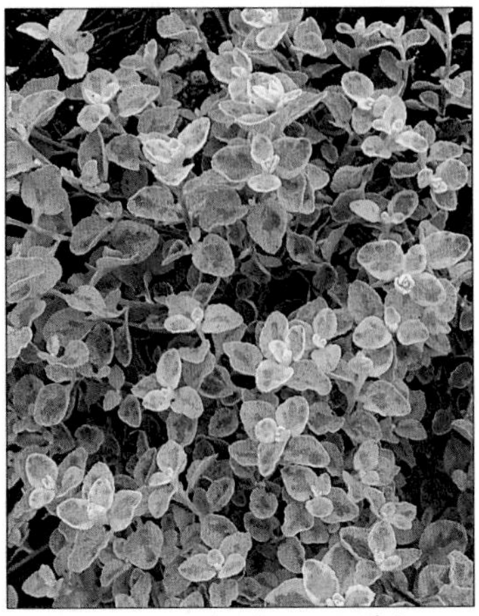
Helichrysum petiolare 'Variegatum'

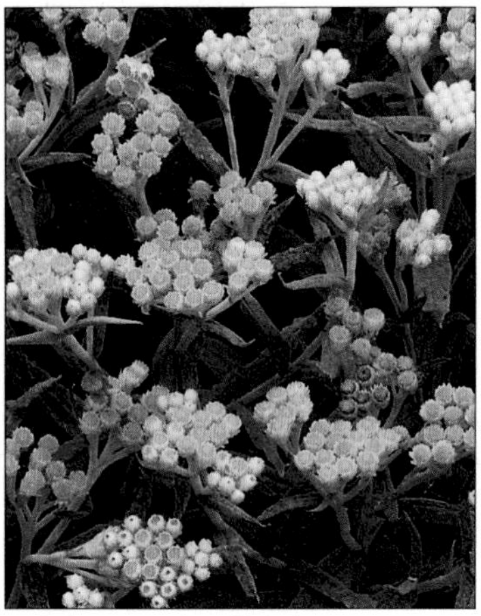
Helichrysum 'Schweffellicht'

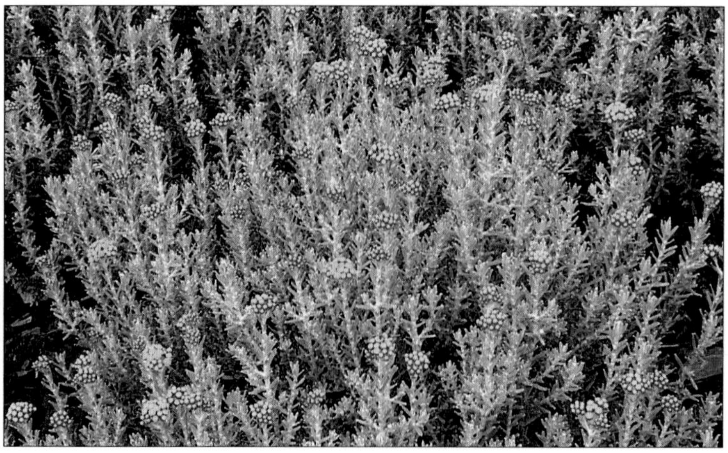
Helichrysum splendidum

H. rosmarinifolium see *Ozothamnus rosmarinifolius.*
***H.* 'Schweffellicht'** ■ syn. *H.* 'Sulphur Light'. Clump-forming herbaceous perennial with erect to spreading, white-woolly stems and narrow, lance-shaped, woolly, silvery white leaves, to 10cm (4in) long. Fluffy, hemispherical, sulphur-yellow flowerheads, 8–15mm (3/8–1/2in) across, becoming orange-yellow with age, are borne in tight, branched corymbs, to 5–8cm (2–3in) across, in late summer. ↕40cm (16in), ↔ 30cm (12in). ❄❄❄
H. selago see *Ozothamnus selago.*
H. serotinum see *H. italicum* subsp. *serotinum.*
H. sibthorpii ■ syn. *H. virgineum.* Cushion-forming, evergreen perennial bearing densely white-woolly stems and alternate, oblong, strongly 3-veined, white-woolly, mid-green leaves, 1.5–6cm (1/2–2 1/2in) long. In summer, bears hemispherical yellow flowerheads, to 1.5cm (1/2in) across, with white bracts, singly or in corymbs of 2 or 3. ↕ to 10cm (4in), ↔ 20cm (8in). N.E. Greece. ❄❄
H. siculum see *H. stoechas* subsp. *barrelieri.*
H. splendidum ■♀ syn. *H. alveolatum, H. trilineatum.* Compact, bushy, evergreen shrub with white-woolly stems and linear-oblong, strongly 3-veined, silver-grey leaves, 2–4cm (3/4–1 1/2in) long. Ovoid-oblong, dark yellow flowerheads, 4–6mm (1/8–1/4in) across, open in hemispherical corymbs, 3cm (1 1/4in) across, from late summer to autumn. ↕↔ 1.2m (4ft). South Africa. ❄❄❄
H. stoechas. Bushy, evergreen subshrub or woody-based, aromatic perennial producing branched or unbranched, white-woolly stems and alternate, linear to linear-spoon-shaped, white-woolly, grey-green leaves, 2–3cm (3/4–1 1/4in) long. In late spring, bears spherical to ovoid yellow flowerheads, 4–6mm (1/8–1/4in) across, in corymbs 3cm (1 1/4in) or more across. ↕20–50cm (8–20in), ↔ 1m (3ft). W. and S. Europe to Balkans. ❄❄. **subsp. *barrelieri*,** syn. *H. siculum*, is shorter-growing, and has broadly linear, non-aromatic leaves, to 2cm (3/4in) long; it bears small clusters of ovoid yellow flowerheads in summer; ↕15–30cm (6–12in); Italy, Greece, Balkans, Turkey, Lebanon, N.W. North Africa. **'White Barn'** has densely white-felted leaves, and bears sulphur-yellow flowerheads.
***H.* 'Sulphur Light'** see *H.* 'Schweffellicht'.
H. thianschanicum, syn. *H. lanatum.* Mound-forming, woolly-hairy herbaceous perennial with erect stems, lance-shaped, silvery grey basal leaves, to 10cm (4in) long, and stalkless, linear stem leaves. Hemispherical to ovoid yellow flowerheads, to 1cm (1/2in) across, are borne in dense, lateral or terminal corymbs, to 8cm (3in) across, in early and midsummer. ↕↔ to 40cm (16in). C. Asia. ❄❄❄. **'Goldkind'**, syn. 'Golden Baby', bears papery, golden yellow flowerheads with a lovage-like scent; ↕30cm (12in).
H. thyrsoideum see *Ozothamnus thyrsoideus.*
H. trilineatum see *H. splendidum.*
H. virgineum see *H. sibthorpii.*

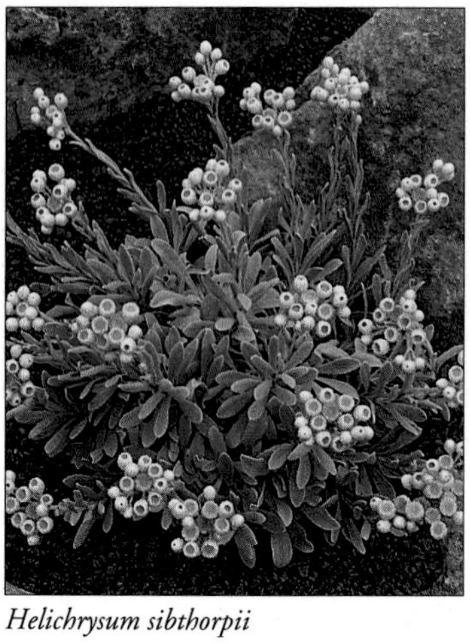
Helichrysum sibthorpii

HELICONIA

HELICONIACEAE/MUSACEAE

Genus of about 100 species of evergreen perennials found in habitats ranging from tropical forest to open scrub in tropical and subtropical Central and South America, and the S.W. Pacific. They have short rhizomes and long-stalked, paddle- or spoon-shaped, mid- to dark green leaves, to 2m (6ft) long, similar to those of the closely related banana (*Musa*) and *Strelitzia.* From spring to summer, they produce large, exotic, erect or pendent flower spikes, made up of brilliantly coloured bracts, arranged spirally or in 2 opposite rows. The bracts enclose the true flowers, which have 3 petals and 3 showy sepals, often in contrasting colours. In frost-prone areas, grow in a warm greenhouse or conservatory; in warmer regions, use as specimen plants for borders or containers outdoors. All last well as cut flowers.

- **HARDINESS** Frost tender.
- **CULTIVATION** Under glass, grow in a mix of equal parts pulverized pine bark, moss peat, and coarse sand or grit, in bright filtered to indirect light. In the growing season, water freely and apply a balanced liquid fertilizer monthly; water moderately in winter. Outdoors, grow in humus-rich, moist but well-drained, neutral to slightly acid soil, enriched with garden compost, in partial shade. Shelter from strong winds, which will damage foliage.
- **PROPAGATION** Sow seed at 19–24°C (66–75°F) in spring. Divide rhizomes in spring.
- **PESTS AND DISEASES** Susceptible to red spider mites, mealybugs, and snails. *Phytophthora* root rot and *Pythium* stem rot may also be a problem.

H. acuminata. Rhizomatous perennial with elliptic to narrowly elliptic or oblong, smooth, leathery, dark green leaf-blades, 15–70cm (6–28in) long. Erect inflorescences, 50–90cm (20–36in) long, each bear 2 ranks of 4–6 slender, clustered, red, orange, or yellow, green-tipped bracts. The red-, orange-, or yellow-stalked flowers have white to orange-yellow sepals with dark green-banded tips. ↕0.6–3m (2–10ft), ↔ indefinite. Brazil to S.E. Peru. ❀ (min. 15°C/59°F)
H. angusta. Rhizomatous perennial with elliptic or oblong, mid- to deep green leaf-blades, 25–90cm (10–36in) long, usually brown-woolly beneath. Erect inflorescences, 70cm (28in) long, each bear 4–8 red or yellow bracts in 2 ranks, and flowers with white sepals. ↕60–120cm (24–48in), ↔ indefinite. S.E. Brazil. ❀ (min. 15°C/59°F)
H. aurantiaca ■ Rhizomatous perennial with oblong or narrowly elliptic, dark green leaf-blades, 17–40cm (7–16in) long. Produces erect, dense inflorescences, to 20cm (8in) long, each with 3–5 broad, clustered, red or yellow, green-tipped bracts arranged in 2 ranks. Flowers have pale yellow to orange sepals, often with paler tips, becoming dark green with age. ↕0.6–2m (2–6ft), ↔ indefinite. S. Mexico to Costa Rica. ❀ (min. 15°C/59°F)
H. bihai, syn. *H. humilis.* Variable, rhizomatous perennial with oblong or oblong-oval, dark green leaf-blades, to 2m (6ft) long, with pale midribs. Erect inflorescences, to 1.1m (3 1/2ft) long, each have 3–15 broad red bracts in 2 ranks, with yellow keels and green margins. Flowers have green-tipped white sepals. ↕0.6–5m (2–15ft), ↔ indefinite. Central America, West Indies (Dominica to Grenada). ❀ (min. 15°C/59°F). **'Aurea'** has inflorescences of 6–12 red-centred bracts with broad, golden yellow margins and green tips; flowers have green and white sepals; ↕3–6m (10–20ft). **'Chocolate Dancer'** has inflorescences of 6–9 brown-red bracts, with gold-edged upper margins, and flowers with green and white sepals; ↕2–3m (6–10ft). **'Purple Throat'** has maroon leaf-stalks, and inflorescences of 7–10 deep red bracts with purple bases and green upper margins; flowers have green sepals; ↕5–6m (15–20ft). **'Yellow Dancer'** has inflorescences of 5–12 green-tipped yellow bracts and flowers with green and white sepals; ↕1.5–5m (5–15ft).
***H. caribaea* 'Chartreuse'.** Rhizomatous perennial with oblong, glaucous, mid-green leaf-blades, 0.6–1.3m (2–4 1/2ft) long. Erect inflorescences, 20–40cm (8–16in) long, have 11 or 12 bright lime-green bracts, arranged in 2 ranks, with yellow bases; the flowers have green and white sepals. ↕4–6m (12–20ft), ↔ indefinite. ❀ (min. 15°C/59°F)
H. humilis see *H. bihai.*
***H. humilis* of gardens** see *H. stricta* 'Dwarf Jamaican'.
H. nutans. Rhizomatous perennial producing oblong, dark green leaf-blades, 50–90cm (20–36in) long. Pendent inflorescences, 60–100cm (24–39in) long, each have 3–12 spirally

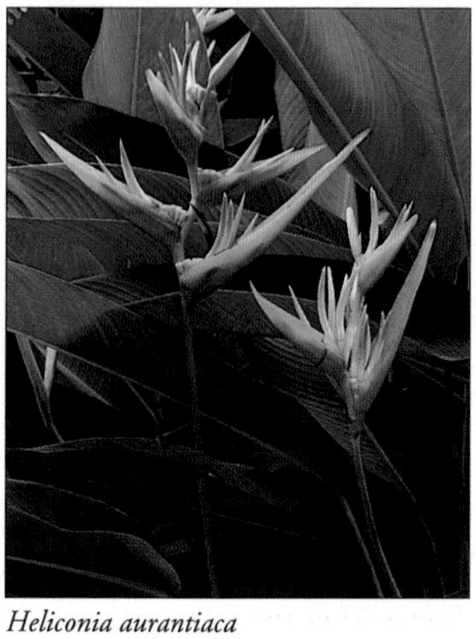
Heliconia aurantiaca

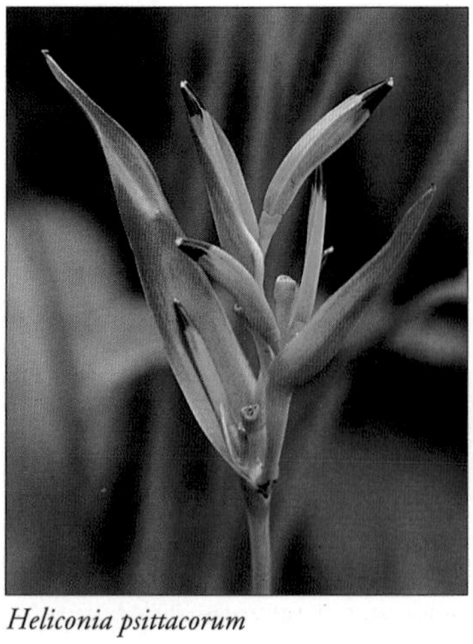
Heliconia psittacorum

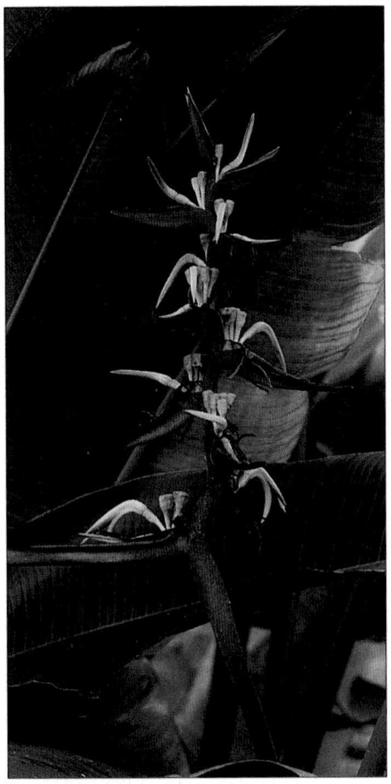

Heliconia schiedeana

arranged or 2-ranked, orange-red bracts; flowers have yellow sepals. ↕ 1–2m (3–6ft), ↔ indefinite. Costa Rica, Panama. ❄ (min. 15°C/59°F)
H. psittacorum ■ (Parrot's flower, Parrot's plantain). Variable, rhizomatous perennial with elliptic or oblong to linear, leathery, rich dark green leaf-blades, 10–50cm (4–20in) long, on red leaf-stalks. Bears erect inflorescences, 12–70cm (5–28in) long, of 2–7 slender, upcurved, orange-red bracts in 2 ranks; flowers have orange-red sepals with green-banded tips. ↕ 0.6–2m (2–6ft), ↔ indefinite. Lesser Antilles to E. Brazil. ❄ (min. 15°C/59°F)
H. rostrata. Rhizomatous perennial producing ovate-oblong, mid-green leaf-blades, 60–120cm (24–48in) long. Pendent inflorescences, 30–60cm (12–24in) long, each have 4–35 red bracts, in 2 ranks, with yellow-green tips and green margins; the flowers have yellowish white sepals. ↕ 1–6m (3–20ft), ↔ indefinite. Ecuador, Peru. ❄ (min. 15°C/59°F).
H. schiedeana ■ Upright, rhizomatous perennial with opposite, oblong, mid-green leaf-blades, to 1.5m (5ft) long. Produces erect, sparsely to densely hairy inflorescences, 30–70cm (12–28in) long, comprising 7–10 spirally arranged, slender red bracts, and flowers with yellow sepals. ↕ 1–3m (3–10ft), ↔ 1m (3ft). S. Mexico. ❄ (min. 15°C/59°F).
H. stricta. Variable, rhizomatous perennial with maroon leaf-stalks bearing oblong, mid- to dark green leaf-blades, 40–150cm (16–66in) long. The upright inflorescences, 20–30cm (8–12in) long, each have 2 ranks of 3–10 red or orange, green-tipped bracts, with yellow upper margins and keels. The flowers have white-tipped green sepals. ↕ 0.6–4m (2–12ft), ↔ indefinite. Venezuela, Surinam, Ecuador, Bolivia. ❄ (min. 15°C/59°F). **'Bucky'** has inflorescences comprising 3–6 bright red bracts with narrow green margins; ↕ 1–2m (3–6ft). **'Dorado Gold'** produces inflorescences of 5 or 6 peach-yellow bracts with small, elongated, central pink marks; ↕ 1–2m (3–6ft). **'Dwarf Jamaican'**, syn. *H. humilis* of gardens, has inflorescences bearing 3–5 peach-red bracts with narrow green upper margins; ↕ 30–100cm (1–3ft). **'Fire Bird'** has leaves with maroon midribs and leaf-stalks, and produces inflorescences comprising 6 or 7 dark red bracts with narrow green margins; ↕ 1–1.5m (3–5ft).

HELICTOTRICHON

GRAMINEAE/POACEAE

Genus of about 50 species of tussock-forming, deciduous and evergreen, perennial grasses from rocky slopes, wasteland, or field margins in temperate Europe, W. Asia, and North America. The linear, mid- to light green, or grey-blue leaves are flat, ribbed, or folded, or have rolled margins. Oblong, flattened, glistening spikelets are borne in erect or nodding panicles. Use in a herbaceous or mixed border, or for gravel plantings, where they associate well with purple- or silver-leaved plants.
• **HARDINESS** Fully hardy.
• **CULTIVATION** Grow in well-drained, poor to moderately fertile, preferably alkaline soil in full sun. Remove dead leaves and old flowering stems in spring.
• **PROPAGATION** Sow seed in containers in a cold frame in spring, or divide in spring.
• **PESTS AND DISEASES** Rust may be a problem.

H. sempervirens ■ 🏆 syn. *Avena candida, A. sempervirens* (Blue oat grass). Densely tufted, evergreen, perennial grass, forming a hemispherical mound of flat or tightly rolled, linear, grey-blue leaves, to 23cm (9in) long. In early and midsummer, stiff, upright stems bear glistening, straw-coloured, purple-marked spikelets in open panicles, to 18cm (7in) long, nodding at the tips. ↕ to 1.4m (4½ft), ↔ 60cm (24in). C. and S.W. Europe. ✻✻✻

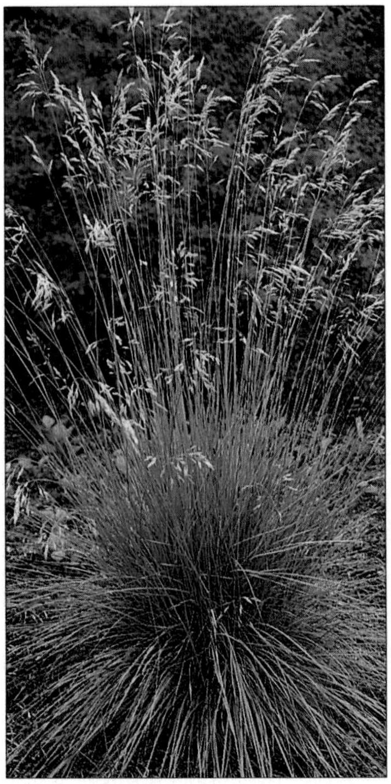

Helictotrichon sempervirens

HELIOCEREUS

CACTACEAE

Genus, closely related to *Disocactus*, of about 6 species of perennial, epiphytic or terrestrial, free-flowering cacti found in a range of shaded habitats in the lowlands of Mexico, Guatemala, and El Salvador. They produce succulent, sometimes spreading, angular-ribbed stems, which bear spiny, white or pale yellow areoles, later becoming brown. Long-lasting, large, trumpet-shaped, colourful flowers open in early summer. Some species have been cross-pollinated with *Epiphyllum* to produce many outstanding cultivars. In frost-prone regions, grow as houseplants or in a warm greenhouse. In humid, tropical gardens, use in a shady border, or in containers on a patio.
• **HARDINESS** Frost tender.
• **CULTIVATION** Under glass, grow in epiphytic cactus compost in bright filtered light, shaded from hot sun; provide high humidity. During the growing season, water freely and apply a half-strength, balanced liquid fertilizer monthly; keep just moist in winter. Outdoors, grow in poor to moderately fertile, sharply drained, acid soil in partial shade. See also pp.48–49.
• **PROPAGATION** Sow seed at 19–21°C (66–70°F) in spring. Root cuttings of stem segments in spring or summer.
• **PESTS AND DISEASES** Susceptible to mealybugs.

H. cinnabarinus. Trailing cactus with 3-ribbed, toothed, dark green stems, 3- or 4-angled above, 5- or 6-angled beneath, bearing short, bristly, white or yellowish brown spines. Trumpet-shaped, glossy red flowers, 12–16cm (5–6in) long, with greenish yellow outer segments, often yellow towards the bases, are produced in early summer. ↕ 60cm (24in), ↔ 45cm (18in). Mexico, Guatemala, El Salvador. ❄ (min. 13°C/55°F)
H. speciosus. Semi-pendent to erect cactus producing cylindrical, unevenly toothed, mid-green stems. The stems have 3–5 prominent, acute ribs, and areoles and spines that are yellow at first, later becoming pale brown. Trumpet-shaped red flowers, 11–17cm (4½–7in) long, with purple-tinged sepals, are borne in early summer. ↕↔ to 45cm (18in). Mexico. ❄ (min. 13°C/55°F). **var. *amecamensis*** ■ produces pure white flowers. **var. *superbus*** has 3- to 7-ribbed stems with yellowish brown spines that often fall quickly; the flowers are rich, glossy, purplish red, with red outer segments.

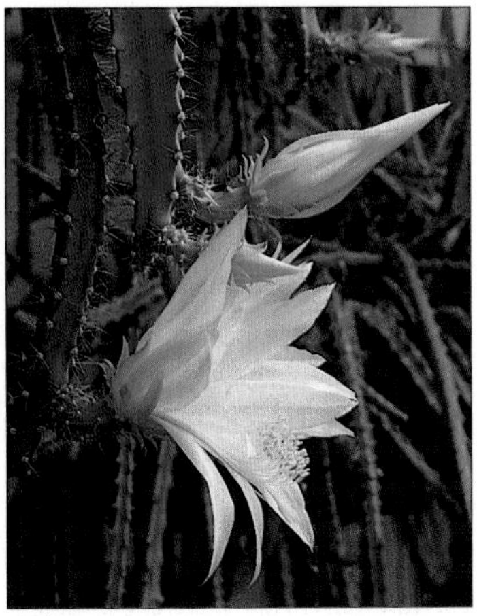

Heliocereus speciosus var. *amecamensis*

HELIOPHILA

BRASSICACEAE/CRUCIFERAE

Genus of about 75 species of erect, spreading, or occasionally climbing annuals, biennials, perennials, and subshrubs found in a range of habitats, including rocky sites, sandy soils, and coastal areas, in South Africa. The leaves are entire, lobed, or finely divided. Heliophilas are grown for their loose racemes of cross-shaped, 4-petalled, often scented flowers in white, blue, or pink, borne from spring to summer. For short-lived summer colour, grow in an annual or mixed border; alternatively, use in a cool greenhouse or conservatory to flower in late winter and spring. The long, pendent, chain-like seedpods of *H. leptophylla* are useful for dried flower arrangements.
• **HARDINESS** Frost hardy.
• **CULTIVATION** Under glass, grow in loam-based potting compost (JI No.2) in bright filtered light. Water plants moderately at all times. Outdoors, grow in fertile, well-drained soil in full sun, providing shelter from strong winds.
• **PROPAGATION** Sow seed *in situ* in spring or, for winter-flowering container plants, at 16–19°C (61–66°F) in early spring or in autumn. Sow seed in succession to obtain a long display of flowers.
• **PESTS AND DISEASES** Trouble free.

H. coronopifolia ■ syn. *H. longifolia.* Slender-stemmed, many-branched, occasionally hairy annual producing simple or pinnate, mid-green leaves, 6–15cm (2½–6in) long, with linear leaflets. From spring to summer, bears pale to bright blue or blue-violet, occasionally pink or white, sometimes purple-spotted flowers, to 1cm (½in) across, with green-yellow centres. ↕ 10cm (4in), ↔ to 30cm (12in). South Africa (Western Cape). ✻✻. **'Atlantis'** produces bright blue flowers with white eyes, which are followed by attractive seed pods in autumn.
H. leptophylla. Slender-stemmed, basally branching annual with pinnate, blue-green leaves, 2.5–5cm (1–2in) long, composed of narrow leaflets. Slightly pendent spikes of clear blue

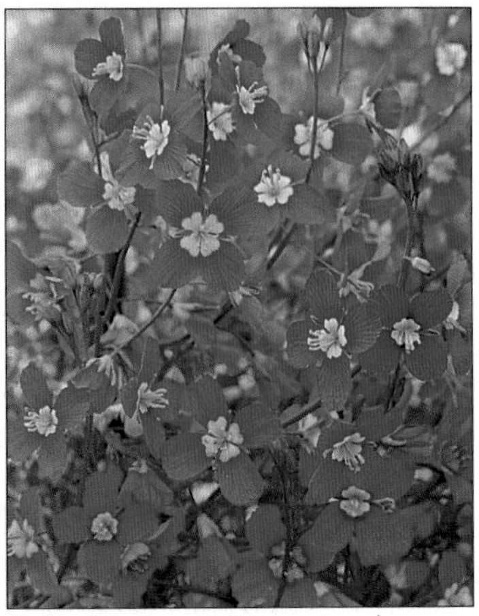

Heliophila coronopifolia

H

flowers, to 1cm (½in) across, with a yellow base to each petal, are produced from spring to summer. ↕45cm (18in), ↔23cm (9in). South Africa (Western Cape). ✻✻
H. longifolia see *H. coronopifolia.*

HELIOPSIS
Ox eye
ASTERACEAE/COMPOSITAE

Genus of 12 or 13 species of perennials found in dry prairies and open woodland in North America. They have stiff, branching stems with opposite, ovate to lance-shaped, toothed, 3-veined, mid- or dark green leaves. The solitary, terminal, sunflower-like flowerheads are usually yellow and to 8cm (3in) across. Unlike the ray-florets of sunflowers (*Helianthus*), those of *Heliopsis* are fertile. Use in a herbaceous or mixed border, or in informal plantings. Ox eyes also provide long-lasting cut flowers.

- **HARDINESS** Fully hardy.
- **CULTIVATION** Grow in moderately fertile, humus-rich, moist but well-drained soil in full sun. Divide every 2–3 years to maintain vigour. Taller species and cultivars may need support.
- **PROPAGATION** Sow seed in containers in a cold frame in spring. Divide in spring or autumn. Root basal cuttings in spring.
- **PESTS AND DISEASES** Young shoots are prone to slug damage.

H. helianthoides. Clump-forming perennial with ovate to lance-shaped, toothed, almost hairless, 3-veined, mid-green leaves, to 15cm (6in) long. Numerous long-stalked, single to double flowerheads, 4–8cm (1½–3in) across, with yellow ray-florets and disc-florets, are borne on branched stems from mid-summer to early autumn. ↕1–1.8m (3–6ft), ↔60cm (24in). E. North America (Ontario to Florida and Missouri). ✻✻✻. **'Ballerina'** has semi-double flowerheads with golden yellow ray-florets and slightly darker disc-florets; ↕1m (3ft). **'Gigantea'** has large, semi-double, golden yellow flowerheads; ↕to 1.2m (4ft). **'Incomparabilis'** ■ has double, zinnia-like, orange-yellow flowerheads, to 8cm (3in) across; ↕90cm (36in). **'Mars'** has large, single, yellow-orange flowerheads; ↕to 1.5m (5ft). **'Patula'** has large, flattish, semi-double, golden yellow flowerheads, with 3 rows of frilled or toothed ray-florets; ↕to 1.2m (4ft). **subsp. *scabra*** has coarsely

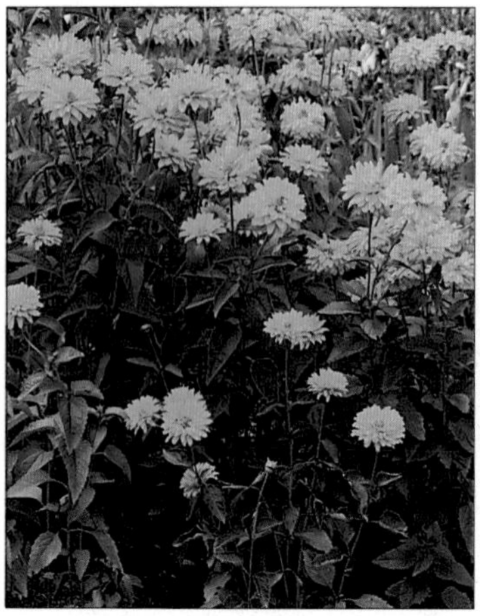
Heliopsis helianthoides 'Incomparabilis'

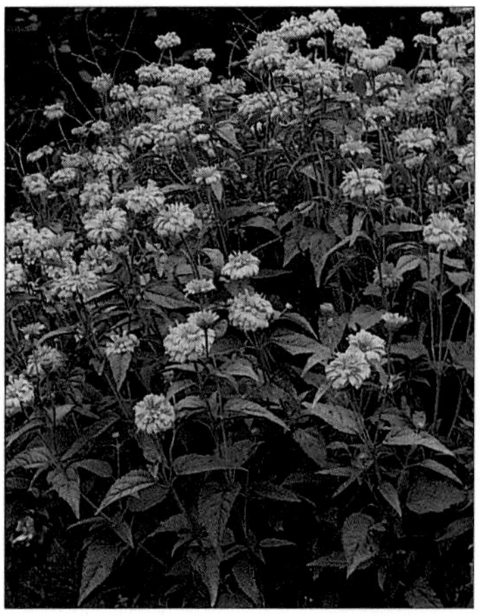
Heliopsis helianthoides subsp. *scabra* 'Light of Loddon'

hairy leaves, and bears only 1–4 yellow flowerheads; ↕to 1m (3ft); USA (New Jersey to Arkansas), Mexico. **subsp. *scabra* 'Goldgefieder'** 𝕍 syn. subsp. *scabra* 'Golden Plume' bears double flowerheads with golden yellow ray-florets and green disc-florets; ↕to 1.4m (4½ft). **subsp. *scabra* 'Goldgrünherz'**, syn. subsp. *scabra* 'Goldgreenheart', has double, lemon-yellow flowerheads, shaded green in the centres until fully open; ↕90cm (36in). **subsp. *scabra* 'Light of Loddon'** ■ has dark green leaves, to 20cm (8in) long, and bears semi-double, bright yellow flowerheads with raised centres; ↕to 1.1m (3½ft); **subsp. *scabra* 'Sommersonne'** ■ syn. subsp. *scabra* 'Summer Sun', bears single, occasionally semi-double flowerheads with deep golden yellow ray-florets, sometimes flushed orange-yellow, and brownish yellow disc-florets; ↕90cm (36in). ✻✻✻

▷ ***Heliosperma alpestris*** see *Silene alpestris*
▷ **Heliotrope** see *Heliotropium, H. arborescens*
Winter see *Petasites fragrans*

HELIOTROPIUM
Heliotrope
BORAGINACEAE

Genus of about 250 species of erect, bushy annuals, perennials, subshrubs, and shrubs from dry, open, and sandy habitats, including scrub, in S.W. and E. USA, Mexico, South America, Hawaii, Pacific islands, and the Canary Islands. They have simple, mostly entire, roughly hairy, and usually alternate leaves. Heliotropes are cultivated mainly for their tiny, sweetly scented, tubular flowers, which are produced in summer in clusters of coiled cymes, each forming a slightly domed or flattened flower-head. They are attractive to butterflies. Contact with the foliage may irritate both skin and eyes. In frost-prone climates, grow in a cool or temperate greenhouse, or use as summer bedding or in containers or window-boxes. In warmer regions, grow heliotropes at the front of a border or in containers outdoors.

- **HARDINESS** Half hardy.
- **CULTIVATION** Under glass, grow in loamless or loam-based potting compost (JI No.3) in full light with shade from hot sun; provide moderate humidity. In the growing season, water moderately and apply a balanced liquid fertilizer monthly; keep just moist in winter. Outdoors, grow in any fertile, moist but well-drained soil in full sun.
- **PROPAGATION** Sow seed at 16–18°C (61–64°F) in spring. Root stem-tip cuttings, or semi-ripe cuttings of named cultivars, in summer.
- **PESTS AND DISEASES** Whiteflies may be a problem under glass.

H. arborescens ■ syn. *H. peruvianum* (Cherry pie, Heliotrope). Bushy, short-lived shrub, often grown as an annual, with broadly oval to lance-shaped, wrinkled, mid- to dark green, sometimes purple-tinged leaves, to 8cm (3in) long. Deep violet-blue or lavender-blue

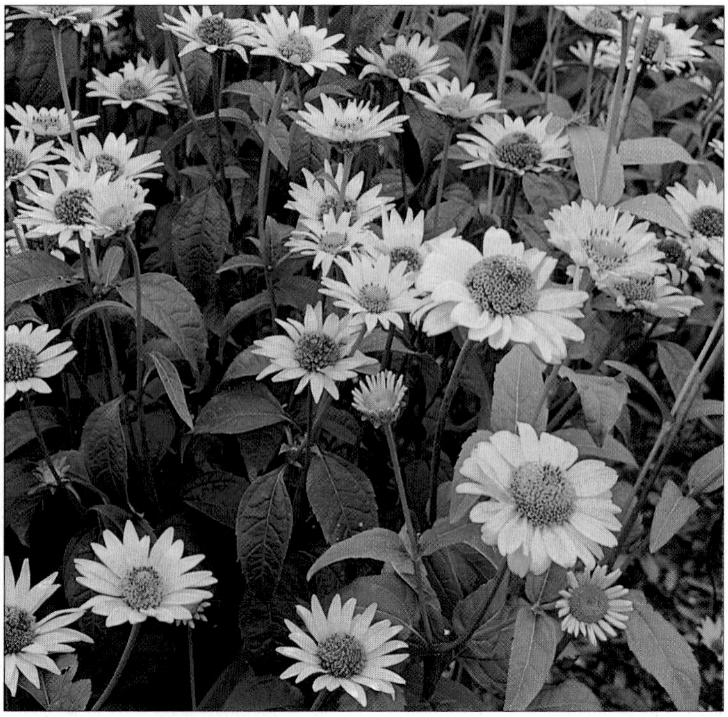
Heliopsis helianthoides subsp. *scabra* 'Sommersonne'

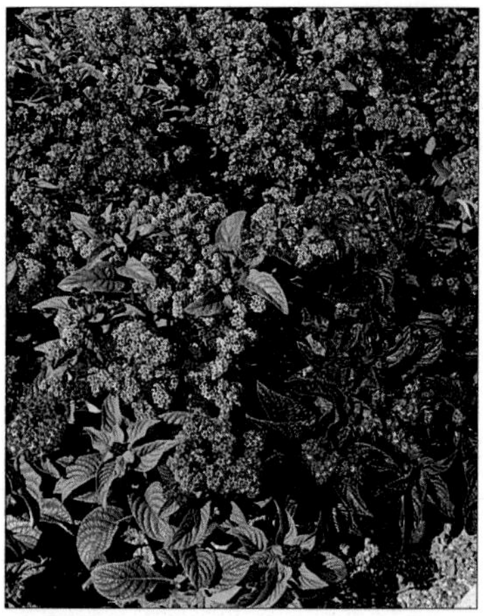
Heliotropium arborescens

flowers are borne in dense flowerheads, 8–10cm (3–4in) across, in summer. ↕1.2m (4ft) in open ground, to 45cm (18in) in containers, ↔30–45cm (12–18in). Peru. ✻. Numerous hybrids and cultivars of *H. arborescens* are used for summer bedding: **'Chatsworth'** 𝕍 is vigorous and strongly scented, bearing bright, deep purple flowerheads. **'Iowa'** is compact, producing deep green, blue-tinged leaves and dark purple flower-heads. **'Lord Roberts'** is compact, bearing light violet-blue flowerheads. **'Marine'** ■𝕍 is compact, with deep violet-blue flowerheads, to 15cm (6in) across; ↕to 45cm (18in). **'Mini Marine'** is dwarf, and has deep violet-blue flowerheads; ↕to 40cm (16in). **'Princess Marina'** is compact, bearing deep violet-blue, highly scented flowerheads; ↕to 30cm (12in). **'Regal Dwarf'** is very compact, and has large, fragrant, dark blue flowerheads. **'White Lady'** is compact, producing white flowerheads tinged pink in bud; ↕to 30cm (12in).
H. peruvianum see *H. arborescens.*

▷ ***Helipterum humboldtianum*** see *Pteropogon humboldtianus*
▷ ***Helipterum manglesii*** see *Rhodanthe manglesii*
▷ ***Helipterum roseum*** see *Rhodanthe chlorocephala* subsp. *rosea*
▷ **Hellebore** see *Helleborus*
Corsican see *Helleborus argutifolius*
False see *Veratrum album*
Green see *Helleborus viridis*
Stinking see *Helleborus foetidus*
White see *Veratrum album*
▷ **Helleborine** see *Epipactis*
Giant see *E. gigantea*

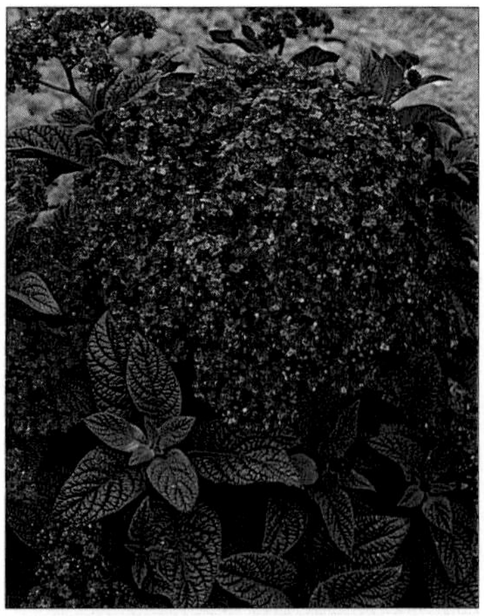
Heliotropium arborescens 'Marine'

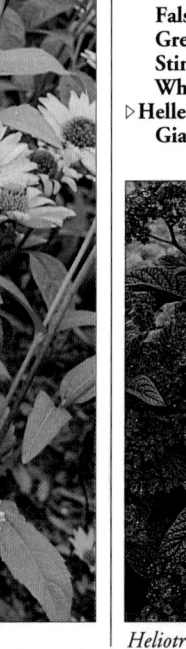

HELLEBORUS

HELLEBORUS

Hellebore

RANUNCULACEAE

Genus of 15 species of perennials found in scrub, woodland, and grassy and rocky sites, usually on chalk or limestone soils, from C., E., and S. Europe to W. Asia. They are rhizomatous, and either clump-forming with deciduous, basal leaves or almost shrub-like, with leafy, biennial stems. The leaves are lobed or fully divided into leaflets, and often pedate (the lateral leaflets or lobes further subdivided or lobed); they are generally toothed, leathery, and light to dark green. The loose, usually few-flowered cymes, to 45cm (18in) tall in most species, have leafy bracts and are borne from late winter to mid-spring. The flowers are white, cream, pink, purple, or green, sometimes spotted, and are pendent or outward-facing, saucer- to cup-shaped, or tubular-bell-shaped. Each has 5 tepals, numerous stamens, and 2–10 free carpels. Hellebores are effective when grown in groups in a mixed or shrub border, or naturalized in a woodland garden. Smaller species are ideal for a rock garden. All parts may cause severe discomfort if ingested, and the sap may irritate skin on contact.

• **HARDINESS** Fully hardy to frost hardy.

• **CULTIVATION** Hellebores tolerate a range of moist, fertile, humus-rich soils, but have varying "ideal" cultivation requirements. For ease of reference, these have been grouped as follows:

1. Neutral to alkaline soil in dappled shade.

2. Heavy, neutral to alkaline soil in dappled shade.

3. Neutral to alkaline soil in full sun or dappled shade.

4. Any soil, but preferably acid, in partial shade.

Incorporate leaf mould or organic matter at planting, and mulch annually in autumn. For all groups, avoid dry or waterlogged soils, and provide shelter from strong, cold winds.

• **PROPAGATION** Sow seed in containers in a cold frame as soon as ripe; named cultivars do not come true from seed. Divide all species and named cultivars after flowering, in early spring or late summer. *H. foetidus* and *H. argutifolius* are best raised from seed as they are not suitable for division.

• **PESTS AND DISEASES** Susceptible to snails, aphids, leaf spot, and black rot.

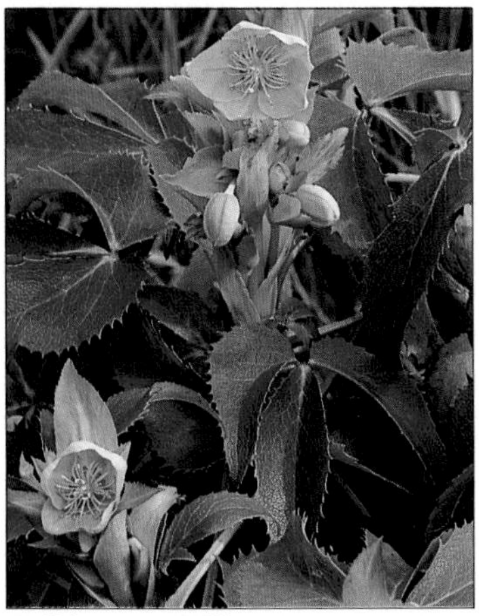

Helleborus argutifolius

H. argutifolius ■ 🏆 syn. *H. corsicus*, *H. lividus* subsp. *corsicus* (Corsican hellebore). Hairless perennial producing overwintering, leafy, biennial flowering stems and leathery, dark green leaves, 8–23cm (3–9in) long, comprising 3 elliptic to broadly elliptic, spiny-toothed leaflets, paler green beneath. Pendent, shallow bowl-shaped, pale green flowers, 2.5–5cm (1–2in) across, open in many-flowered, terminal cymes in late winter and early spring. Cultivation group 1, 2, or 3. ↕ to 1.2m (4ft), ↔ 90cm (36in). Corsica, Sardinia. ❄❄❄

H. atrorubens. Hairless perennial with deciduous, pedate, dark green, basal leaves, to 25cm (10in) long, composed of 7–11 leaflets; the 2 lateral leaflets each have 3–5 narrowly elliptic, toothed lobes. Stems and leaves may be suffused purple. Cymes of 2 or 3 outward-facing, saucer-shaped, deep purple flowers, 4–5cm (1½–2in) across, green-shaded within, open before the leaves, from late winter to spring. Cultivation group 1. ↕ 30cm (12in), ↔ 45cm (18in). N.W. Balkans. ❄❄❄

***H. atrorubens* of gardens** see *H. orientalis* subsp. *abchasicus.*

H. x ballardiae (*H. lividus* x *H. niger*). Clump-forming perennial with short, overwintering, leafy, biennial stems. The pedate, deep bluish green leaves, to 25cm (10in) long, each have 3–5 elliptic to inversely lance-shaped-oblong, toothed leaflets, boldly veined silvery cream. From midwinter to early spring, bears cymes of 3 or 4 saucer-shaped white flowers, 5–9cm (2–3½in) across, flushed pink inside, becoming purplish pink with age. Cultivation group 1. ↕ to 35cm (14in), ↔ 30cm (12in). Garden origin. ❄❄❄. **'December Dawn'** ■ has saucer-shaped white flowers, 6–8cm (2½–3in) across, flushed pinkish purple, maturing to a dull metallic purple.

H. corsicus see *H. argutifolius.*

H. cyclophyllus ■ Deciduous perennial with pedate, toothed, pale green, basal leaves, to 30cm (12in) long, hairy beneath with bold veins; each central leaflet is divided or entire, the 2 lateral leaflets deeply 5- to 7-lobed. From midwinter to early spring, bears cymes of up to 7 outward-facing or pendent, saucer-shaped, scented, yellowish green flowers, 5–7cm (2–3in) across. Cultivation group 1. ↕ to 40cm (16in), ↔ 45cm (18in). S. Balkans. ❄❄❄

H. foetidus ■ 🏆 (Bear's foot, Dungwort, Stinking hellebore, Stinkwort). Erect perennial with hairless, leafy, biennial stems. The pedate, dark green leaves, 23cm (9in) long, smell unpleasant when crushed, and each has 7–10 narrowly lance-shaped or elliptic, coarsely toothed or nearly entire lobes. From midwinter to mid-spring, bears many-flowered cymes of pendent, bell-shaped green flowers, 1.5–2.5cm (½–1in) across, usually purple-margined and sometimes pleasantly scented, above large, pale green bracts. Cultivation group 1, 2, or 3. ↕ to 80cm (32in), ↔ 45cm (18in). W. and C. Europe. ❄❄❄. **'Wester Flisk'** has reddish green stems, leaf-stalks, and flower-stalks, the colour diffusing into the leaf bases; the leaves are dark grey-green. Comes true from seed if isolated from other variants of the species.

H. x hybridus. Group of variable, clump-forming, perennial hybrids of *H. orientalis* and other species. The deciduous or overwintering, pedate, leathery, mid- to dark green leaves, to 40cm (16in) long, each have 7–11 elliptic to inversely lance-shaped, toothed lobes or leaflets. From mid-winter to mid-spring, stout stems bear loose cymes of up to 4 pendent to outward-facing, saucer-shaped flowers, 5–8cm (2–3in) across, in a range of colours including white, purple, yellow, green, and pink. Cultivation group 2, but tolerant of all but very poorly drained or dry soils. ↕↔ to 45cm (18in). Garden origin. ❄❄❄. **'Ballard's Black'** has large, rich, dark purple flowers. **'Citron'** ■ produces bowl-shaped, primrose-yellow flowers. **'Peggy Ballard'** ■ bears large flowers, to 8cm (3in) across, deep reddish pink outside, dusky purple-pink with darker veins inside. **'Pluto'** ■ bears small flowers that are purple outside, green-shaded purple within, with purple nectaries. **'Yellow Button'** bears small, deep yellow flowers that are initially cup-shaped, becoming saucer-shaped.

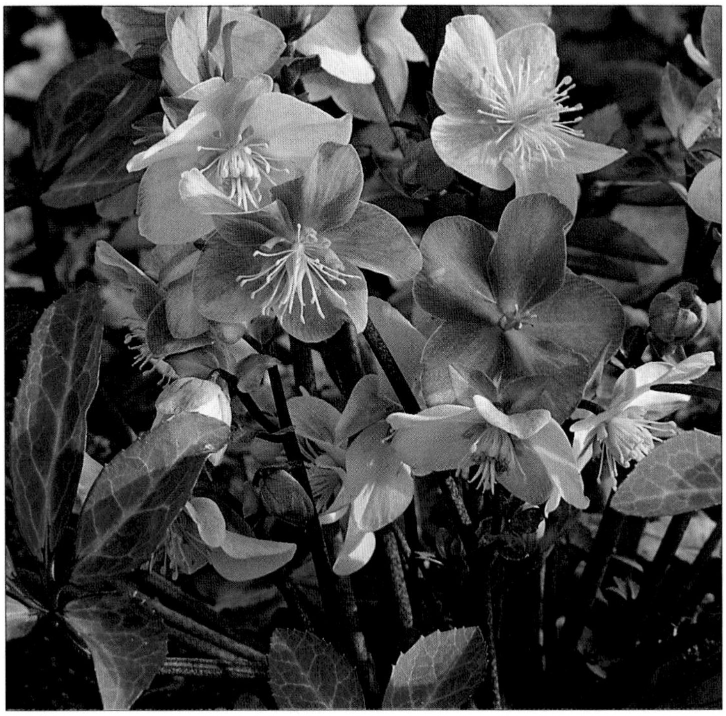

Helleborus x *ballardiae* 'December Dawn'

H. lividus 🏆 Erect or spreading perennial with overwintering, hairless, biennial stems. The leathery, glossy, dark green or bluish green leaves, to 23cm (9in) long, each have 3 elliptic or oblong-elliptic leaflets, entire or with a few shallow teeth; they have creamy silver veins, and pinkish purple leaf-stalks and main veins beneath. From midwinter to early spring, long, purplish green stalks bear cymes of up to 10 bowl-shaped, creamy green flowers, 3–5cm (1¼–2in) across, suffused pinkish purple. Cultivation group 1. In frost-prone areas, best grown in a cold greenhouse. ↕ to 45cm (18in), ↔ 30cm (12in). Majorca. ❄❄. **subsp. *corsicus*** see *H. argutifolius.*

H. multifidus* subsp. *hercegovinus ■ Erect, clump-forming perennial producing deciduous, pedate, mid-green, basal leaves, to 23cm (9in) long, each with 45–70 linear, toothed, prominently veined segments, hairy beneath, often brown-tinted when young. Cymes of 3–8 pendent, conical

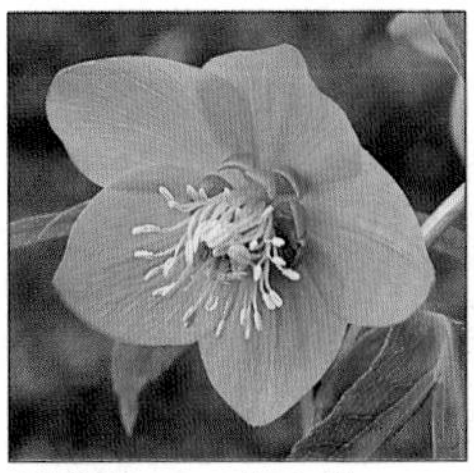

Helleborus cyclophyllus

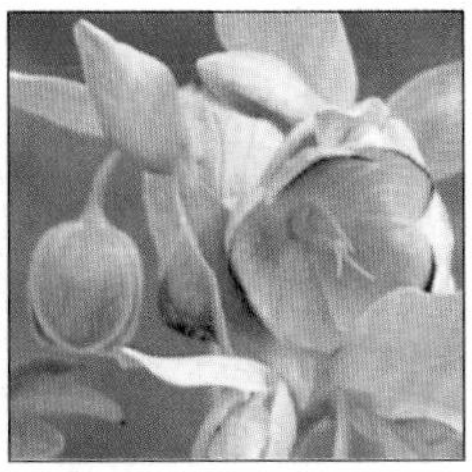

Helleborus foetidus

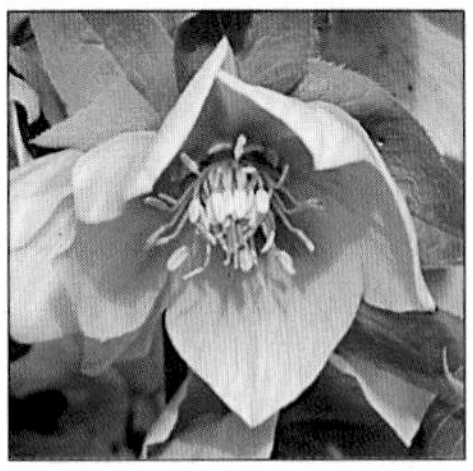

Helleborus x *hybridus* 'Citron'

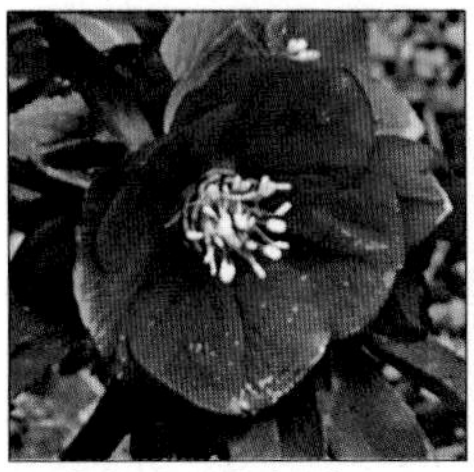

Helleborus x *hybridus* 'Peggy Ballard'

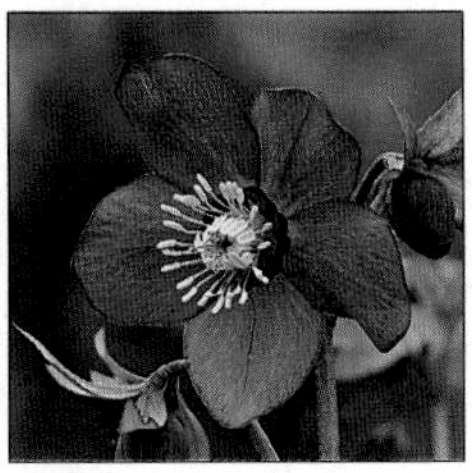

Helleborus x *hybridus* 'Pluto'

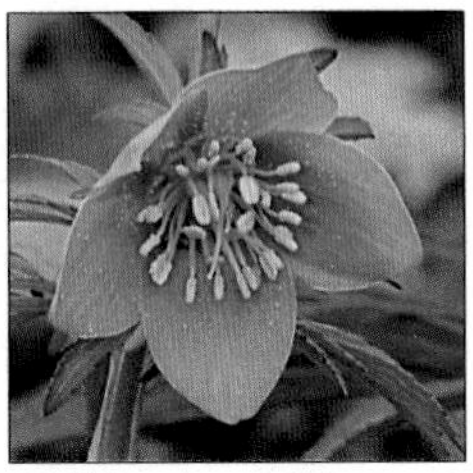

Helleborus multifidus subsp. *hercegovinus*

H

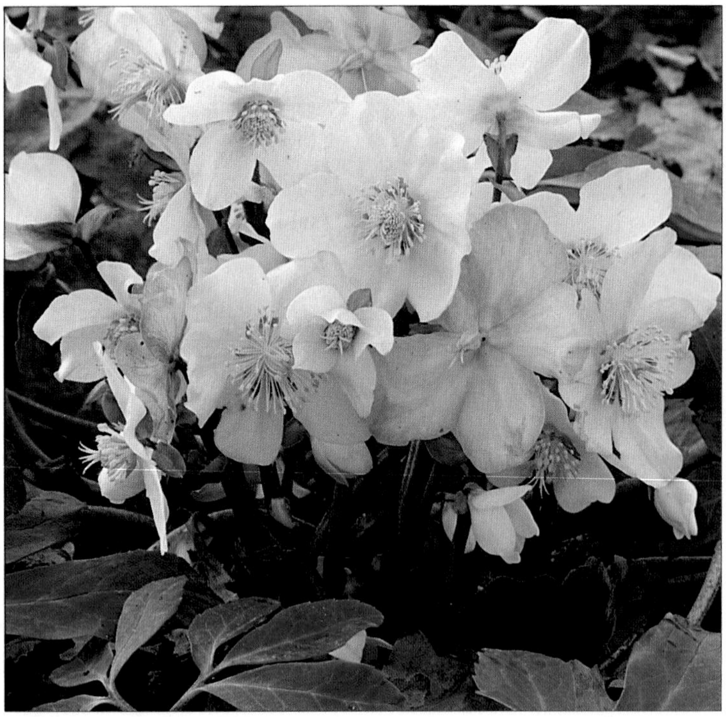

Helleborus niger 'Potter's Wheel'

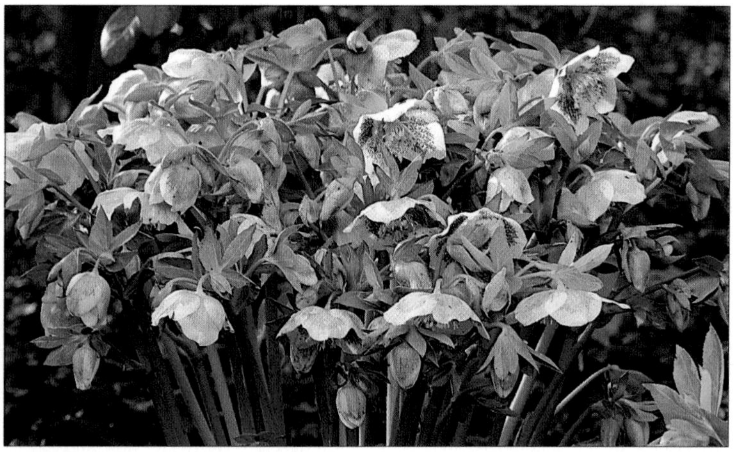

Helleborus orientalis subsp. *guttatus*

to cup-shaped green flowers, 4–5cm (1½–2in) across, are borne in late winter and early spring. Cultivation group 1 or 3. ↕ to 30cm (12in), ↔ 45cm (18in). Bosnia & Herzegovina (Adriatic coastal mountains). ✻✻✻
H. niger ■ ♀ (Christmas rose). Clump-forming, hairless perennial with over-wintering, pedate, leathery, dark green, basal leaves, 5–20cm (2–8in) long, comprising 7–9 oblong to inversely lance-shaped leaflets, toothed towards the apexes. From early winter to early spring, stout, purple-marked stems bear shallowly saucer-shaped flowers, 4.5–8cm (1¾–3in) across, singly, or occasionally in cymes of 2 or 3 blooms; the flowers are white, sometimes strongly pink-flushed, with greenish white centres, ageing to pinkish white. Cultivation group 2. ↕ to 30cm (12in), ↔ 45cm (18in). Germany, Austria, Switzerland, Italy, Slovenia. ✻✻✻.
subsp. *macranthus* has spiny-toothed, bluish or grey-green leaves with broadly lance-shaped lobes, and white flowers, 8–11cm (3–4½in) across; Italy, Slovenia.
'Potter's Wheel' ■ has large, bowl-shaped white flowers with green eyes.
H. x nigercors ♀ (*H. argutifolius* x *H. niger*). Clump-forming perennial with short, overwintering, leafy, biennial stems. Variable, pedate, mid-green basal and stem leaves, 10–30cm (4–12in) long, have 3–5 coarsely toothed lobes. From midwinter to early spring, short stems bear clustered cymes of numerous flattish, white, sometimes pink-flushed flowers, 7–10cm (3–4in) across. Cultivation group 1. ↕ 30cm (12in), ↔ 90cm (36in). Garden origin. ✻✻✻.
'Alabaster' is very vigorous, and bears creamy white flowers, 6–7cm (2½–3in) across, with green shading.
H. odorus. Clump-forming perennial with overwintering, pedate, leathery, deep green, basal leaves, 40cm (16in) long, hairy beneath. Each central leaflet is entire; the lateral leaflets are divided into 3–5 elliptic to inversely lance-shaped, toothed lobes. Cymes of 3–5 saucer-shaped, outward-facing, fragrant green flowers, 5–7cm (2–3in) across, open from midwinter to early spring. Cultivation group 1 or 3. ↕↔ 30–50cm (12–20in). S. Hungary, N. Balkans (including Romania). ✻✻✻
H. orientalis (Lenten rose). Hairless or slightly hairy perennial producing over-wintering, pedate, leathery, deep green, basal leaves, to 40cm (16in) long, each with 7–9 elliptic or inversely lance-shaped leaflets. From midwinter to mid-spring, stout, usually branched stems bear pendent or almost outward-facing, saucer-shaped, white or greenish cream flowers, 5–7cm (2–3in) across, becoming pinker with age. Cultivation group 2, but tolerant of most garden conditions. ↕↔ to 45cm (18in). N.E. Greece, N. Turkey, C. and W. Caucasus. ✻✻✻.
subsp. *abchasicus*, syn. *H. atrorubens* of gardens, has pale green flowers, deeply tinted reddish purple outside, sometimes almost masking the green, and sometimes with deeper purple spots. Reliably early-flowering; W. Caucasus.
subsp. *guttatus* ■ has creamy white flowers, variably spotted maroon within, with green centres; W. Caucasus.
H. purpurascens ■ Clump-forming perennial producing deciduous, leathery, mid-green, basal leaves, to 27cm (11in) long, hairy beneath, usually comprising 5 leaflets, each with 2–6 lance-shaped, toothed lobes. Cymes of 2–4 pendent, cup-shaped flowers, 4–7cm (1½–3in) across, are borne before the leaves, from midwinter to early or mid-spring. The flowers are purplish or slate grey, often pink- or purple-flushed, light green within. Cultivation group 3 or 4. ↕ 5–30cm (2–12in), ↔ 30cm (12in). S.E. Poland, W. Ukraine, Slovakia, C. and N. Hungary, Romania. ✻✻✻
H. x sternii ■ (*H. argutifolius* x *H. lividus*). Clump-forming hybrid perennial, sometimes resembling one parent more than the other, with over-wintering, leafy, biennial stems. Entire to spiny leaves, 10–28cm (4–11in) long, have 3 broadly elliptic leaflets or lobes, creamy veins, and pinkish purple leaf-stalks and main veins. Creamy green flowers, 2.5–5cm (1–2in) across, suffused pinkish purple, are borne in many-flowered cymes from late winter to mid-spring. Cultivation group 3. ↕ 30–35cm (12–14in), ↔ 30cm (12in). Garden origin. ✻✻✻ (borderline).
'Blackthorn' ♀ syn. Blackthorn Group, has purple stems, and boldly veined, greyish green leaves. Produces purplish or pink-stained green flowers; ✻✻.
'Boughton Beauty' ■ has purple-pink stems and veined, mid-green leaves. The flowers are pinkish purple outside, greener within; ↕ 50–60cm (20–24in); ✻✻
H. torquatus. Very variable, clump-forming perennial producing pedate, deciduous, mid-green leaves, to 45cm (18in) long, each with 10–30 tapered, lance-shaped, toothed lobes, hairy beneath. Outward-facing to pendent, saucer-shaped, violet-purple flowers, often green within, with dark veins, are borne before the leaves, from midwinter to early spring; they are 3–6cm (1¼–2½in) across, and borne singly or in cymes of 2–5 (occasionally up to 7) flowers. Cultivation group 2 or 3. ↕ 20–40cm (8–16in), ↔ 30cm (12in). Montenegro, Bosnia & Herzegovina, W. Serbia, Croatia. **'Dido'** ■ produces double flowers, 4–5cm (1½–2in) across, suffused brown or purple-brown on the outsides, green within, with green margins; ↕ 25–30cm (10–12in). ✻✻✻
H. viridis ■ (Green hellebore). Clump-forming perennial with deciduous, pedate, slightly hairy or hairless, dark green, basal leaves, to 30cm (12in) long, each with 7–13 narrowly oblong to lance-shaped or elliptic, toothed lobes. In late winter and early spring, bears cymes of 2–4 saucer-shaped, pendent green flowers, 3–5cm (1¼–2in) across. Cultivation group 2. ↕ 20–40cm (8–16in). ↔ 45cm (18in). Spain, UK to Austria, Germany. ✻✻✻

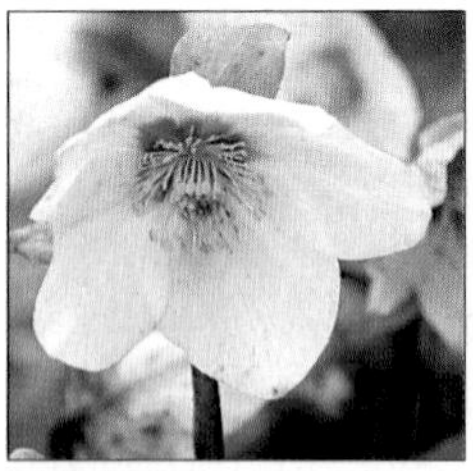

Helleborus niger

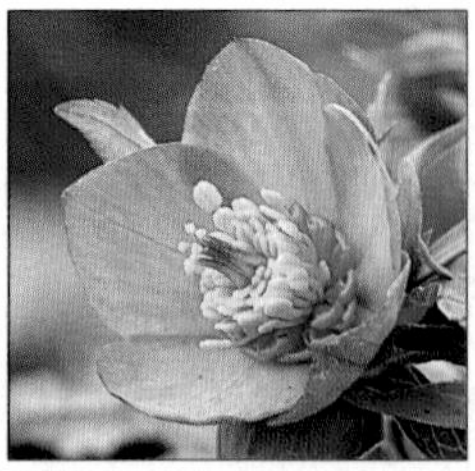

Helleborus purpurascens

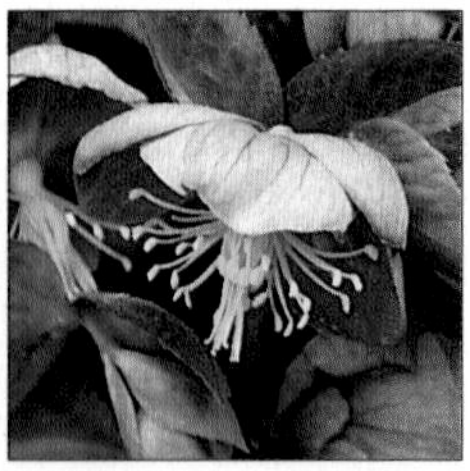

Helleborus x *sternii*

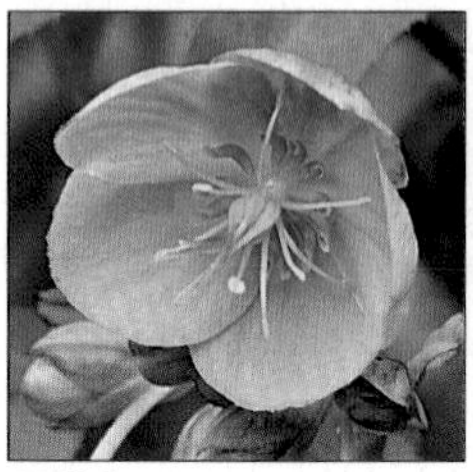

Helleborus x *sternii* 'Boughton Beauty'

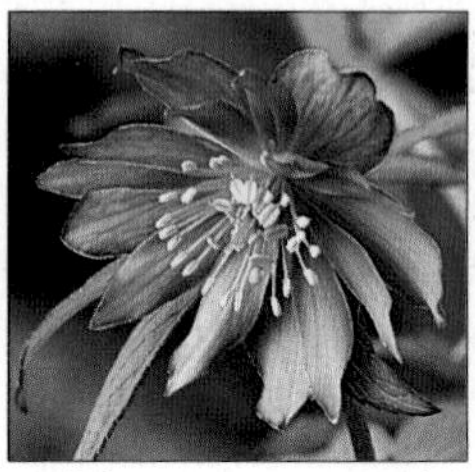

Helleborus torquatus 'Dido'

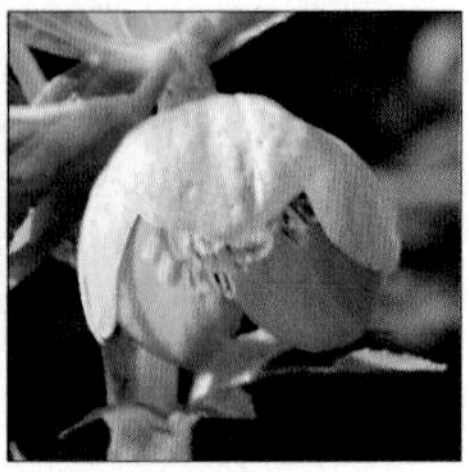

Helleborus viridis

▷ **Helmet flower** see *Scutellaria, Sinningia cardinalis*

HELONIAS

LILIACEAE/MELANTHIACEAE

Genus of one species of evergreen, rhizomatous perennial found in bogs and swampland in the USA. It has rosettes of strap-shaped leaves, and is grown for its dense racemes of many fragrant, star-shaped, pinkish purple flowers, borne in spring. Ideal for a bog garden or for growing beside a pond or stream. May also be grown in a cold greenhouse for early flowering.

- **HARDINESS** Fully hardy.
- **CULTIVATION** Grow in moderately fertile, humus-rich, moist, preferably acid soil in sun or dappled shade.
- **PROPAGATION** Sow seed in containers in an open frame in autumn, or divide in spring.
- **PESTS AND DISEASES** Trouble free.

H. bullata (Swamp pink). Clump-forming, rhizomatous perennial with basal rosettes of strap-shaped, glossy, bright green leaves, 15–45cm (6–18in) long. In spring, 25–30 tiny, fragrant, 6-tepalled, pinkish purple flowers are borne in dense, terminal, conical racemes, 3–10cm (1¼–4in) long, on erect stems above the leaves. ↕ 35–45cm (14–18in), ↔ 30cm (12in). USA (New York to North Carolina). ❄❄❄

HELONIOPSIS

LILIACEAE/MELANTHIACEAE

Genus of 4 species of rhizomatous, evergreen, rosette-forming perennials found in scrub, woodland, and meadows in the mountains of Japan, Korea, Taiwan, and Sakhalin, Russia. They have oblong or lance-shaped, pale to mid-green leaves. From late spring to summer, erect stems bear one-sided racemes of nodding, funnel-shaped flowers, each with 6 spreading tepals. Grow in a shady rock garden or woodland garden; best suited to areas with cool, damp summers.

- **HARDINESS** Fully hardy.
- **CULTIVATION** Grow in humus-rich, neutral to slightly acid, moist but well-drained soil in partial shade. Provide shelter from cold, drying winds.
- **PROPAGATION** Sow seed in containers in a cold frame in autumn or spring, or divide after flowering in spring.
- **PESTS AND DISEASES** Young growth is prone to slug and snail damage.

H. breviscapa see *H. orientalis* var. *breviscapa*.
H. grandiflora see *H. orientalis* var. *breviscapa*.
H. orientalis ▣ Rosetted perennial with broadly lance-shaped, leathery, pale green leaves, 7–15cm (3–6in) long. In late spring and early summer, dark red stems bear dense, umbel-like racemes of 3–10 nodding, narrowly funnel-shaped, rose-pink flowers, 1.5cm (½in) across, with protruding styles and stamens. The stems usually elongate after flowering. ↕↔ 15–20cm (6–8in). Japan, Korea, Russia (Sakhalin). ❄❄❄. **var. *breviscapa***, syn. *H. breviscapa*, *H. grandiflora*, has sharp-pointed, leathery, mid-green leaves, 8–10cm (3–4in) long, shorter flower stems, and smaller, but more widely funnel-shaped, white or very pale pink flowers.

▷ ***Helxine*** see *Soleirolia*
H. soleirolii see *S. soleirolii*

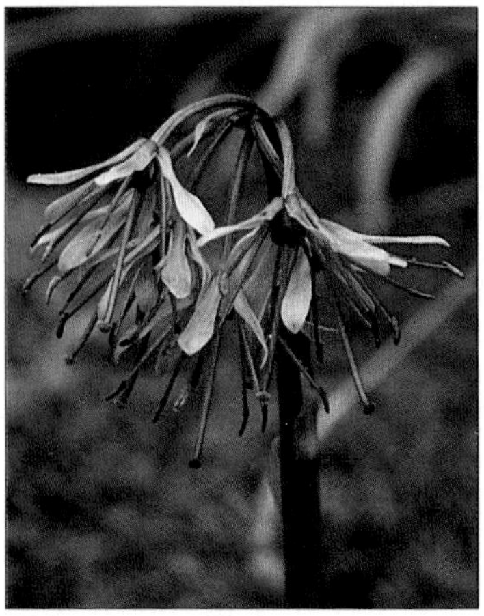

Heloniopsis orientalis

HEMEROCALLIS

Daylily

HEMEROCALLIDACEAE/LILIACEAE

Genus of about 13–15 species of evergreen, semi-evergreen, and herbaceous perennials from which over 30,000 named cultivars have been raised. Daylilies are found at forest margins, in mountainous areas, marshy river valleys, and meadowland in China, Korea, and Japan. They are mostly clump-forming, and occasionally rhizomatous, with arching, strap-shaped, dark green leaves, usually 75–120cm (30–48in) long, but often only 23–35cm (9–14in) long in dwarf or compact species and cultivars. Flowers, in a variety of forms (see panel right), are borne on erect, sometimes branching scapes over a long period, mainly from late spring to late summer. Many daylilies are remontant, flowering repeatedly during the season. The flowers range in colour from almost white through yellow and orange to dark purple and deepest red-black. Most flowers last for only one day; in nocturnal daylilies the flowers open in late afternoon and last throughout the night. The flowers of extended-blooming daylilies remain open for at least 16 hours.

Grow daylilies in a mixed or herbaceous border; some are effective planted in drifts in a wild garden. Dwarf daylilies are ideal for a small garden or for containers.

- **HARDINESS** Fully hardy except for a few evergreen daylilies that are frost hardy only, and may be weakened and killed by alternating frost and thaw.
- **CULTIVATION** Grow in fertile, moist but well-drained soil; all those described here prefer full sun, unless otherwise stated. Mulch in late autumn or spring. From spring until buds develop, water freely and apply a balanced liquid fertilizer every 2–3 weeks. Dry conditions and excessive shade will reduce flowering; some red- and purple-flowered cultivars are intolerant of heavy rainfall and very hot sun. Divide every 2 or 3 years to maintain vigour. Plant evergreen species and cultivars in spring rather than autumn.
- **PROPAGATION** Sow seed in containers in a cold frame in autumn or spring; seed from hybrids and cultivars do not come true. Divide hardy daylilies in spring or autumn; divide all evergreen daylilies in spring.
- **PESTS AND DISEASES** Susceptible to rust, hemerocallis gall midge, aphids, red spider mites, and thrips. Slugs and snails may damage young leaves. Crown rot is usually a problem only in high humidity and temperatures over 32°C (90°F). In climates with alternating winter frosts and thaws, bacterial leaf and stem rot (spring sickness) may be a problem.

HEMEROCALLIS FLOWER FORMS

Daylilies produce shallowly to deeply trumpet-shaped flowers in a variety of forms. The species and older cultivars bear flowers with tapered tepals, while modern hybrids and newer cultivars usually have flowers with thicker, rounded, ruffled-margined, clearer-coloured tepals. The flowers may be **circular**, with mostly rounded, flat or sometimes recurved, ruffled-margined tepals; **star-shaped**, with tapered or sometimes rounded, flat or ruffled-margined tepals; **spider-shaped**, with mostly narrow, tapered tepals; **triangular**, with triangular to rounded, flat or ruffled-margined tepals; or **double**, with rounded or tapered, flat or ruffled-margined tepals. Most daylilies have single flowers, but some hybrids and cultivars bear semi- to fully double flowers; hot weather, in particular, may cause some daylilies to bear flowers with extra petals and stamens.

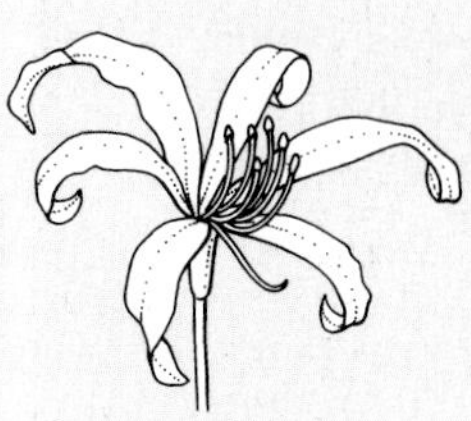

SPIDER-SHAPED

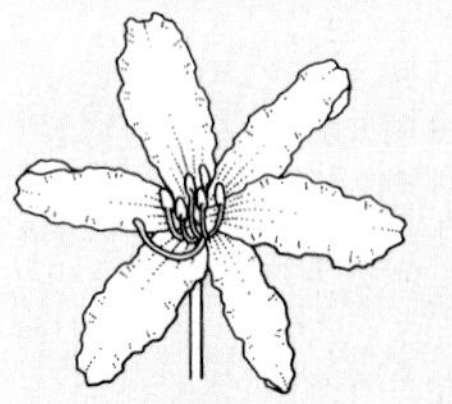

STAR-SHAPED

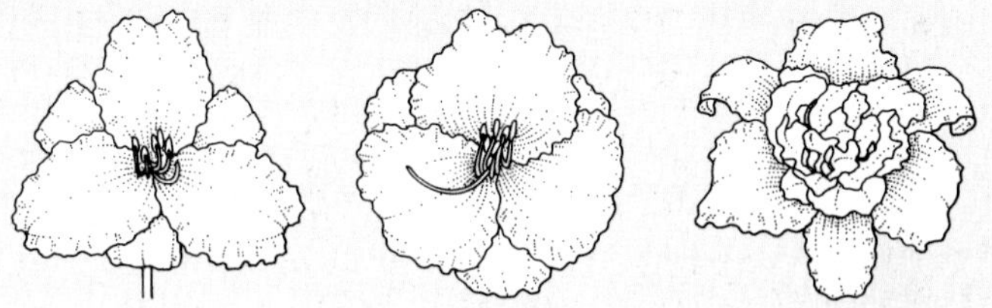

TRIANGULAR CIRCULAR DOUBLE

***H.* 'Amadeus'.** Vigorous, semi-evergreen perennial with sturdy scapes bearing remontant, circular, rich scarlet flowers, 14cm (5½in) across, with thick tepals and yellow throats, in early and midsummer. ↕ 60cm (24in), ↔ 1m (3ft). ❄❄❄
***H.* 'American Revolution'.** Free-flowering, evergreen perennial with narrow leaves and slender scapes. In early and midsummer, black-red buds open to remontant, star-shaped, velvety black to deep red flowers, 10cm (4in) across, with recurved tepals and green throats. ↕ 70cm (28in), ↔ 60cm (24in). ❄❄❄
***H.* 'Ann Kelley'.** Extended-blooming, free-flowering, semi-evergreen perennial with sturdy, branched scapes. In midsummer, bears upward-facing, circular, deep rose-pink flowers, 14cm (5½in) across, with lighter pink midribs and black anthers. ↕ 65cm (26in), ↔ 1m (3ft). ❄❄❄
***H.* 'Apple Court Champagne'.** Very free-flowering, semi-evergreen perennial with well-branched scapes. In mid- and late summer, these bear circular, glistening, creamy lemon flowers, 17cm (7in) across, with recurved, ruffled-margined petals, ivory-pink midribs, and green throats. ↕ 70cm (28in), ↔ 75cm (30in). ❄❄
***H.* 'Apple Tart'** ▣ Semi-evergreen perennial with sturdy scapes bearing nocturnal, triangular to star-shaped, bright red flowers, 15cm (6in) across, in mid- and late summer; they have rounded tepals with yellow midribs and yellow throats. ↕ 70cm (28in), ↔ 75cm (30in). ❄❄❄
***H.* 'Aquamarine'.** Evergreen perennial with slender scapes bearing spider- to star-shaped, lavender-blue flowers, 17cm (7in) across, in early summer. ↕ 70cm (28in), ↔ 60cm (24in). ❄❄❄
***H.* 'Atlanta Full House'.** Evergreen perennial with branched scapes bearing

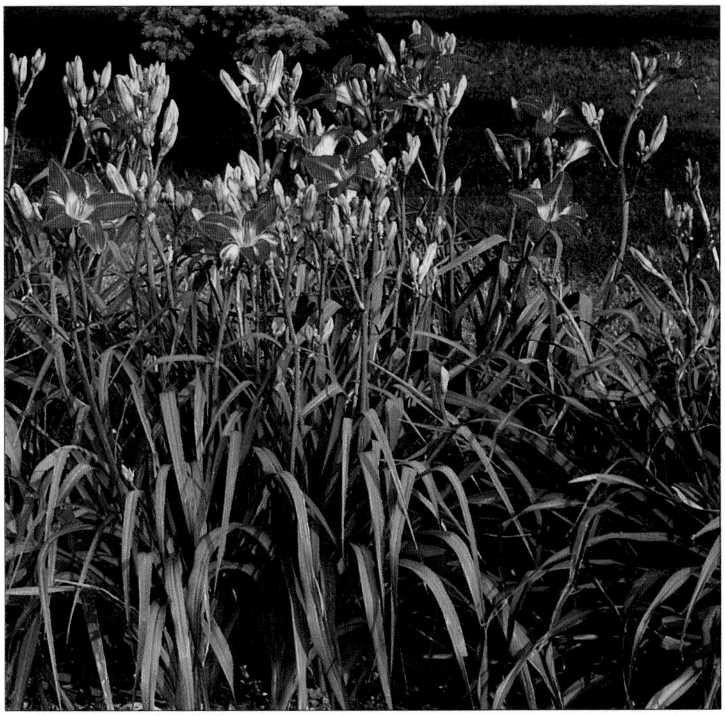

Hemerocallis 'Apple Tart'

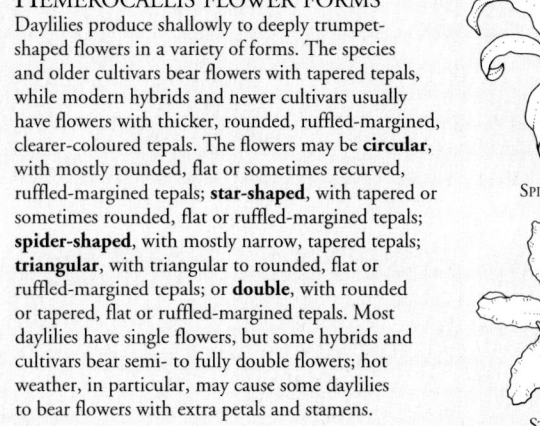

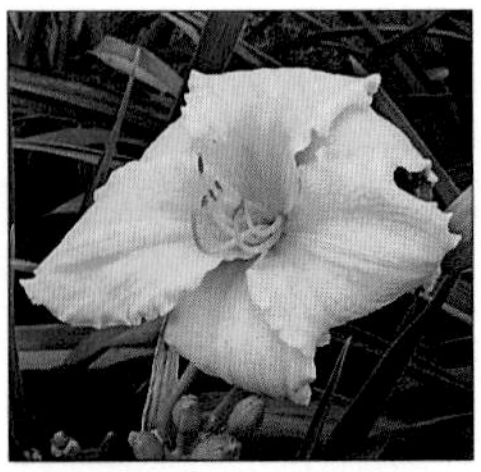
Hemerocallis 'Beauty to Behold'

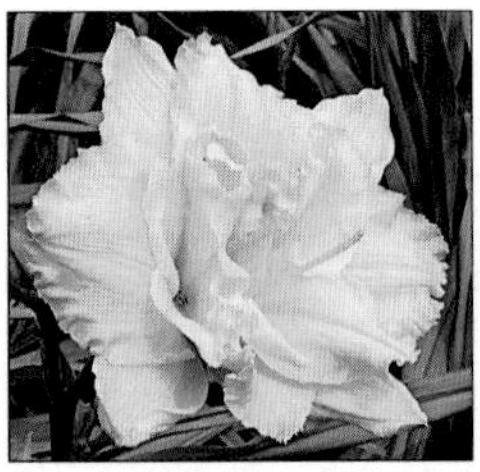
Hemerocallis 'Betty Woods'

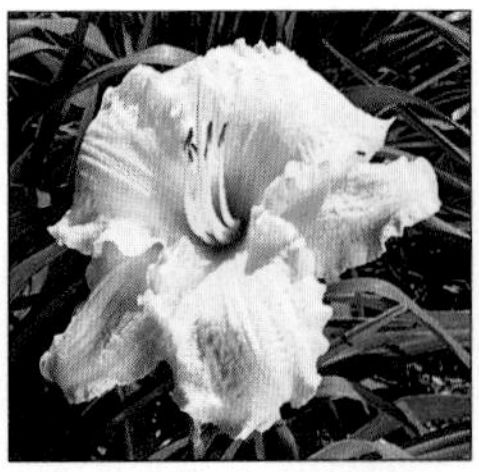
Hemerocallis 'Brocaded Gown'

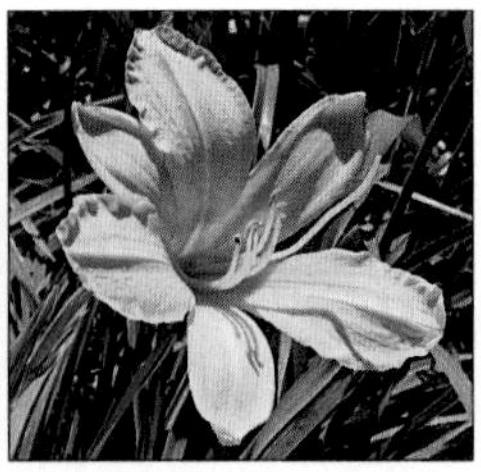
Hemerocallis 'Cartwheels'

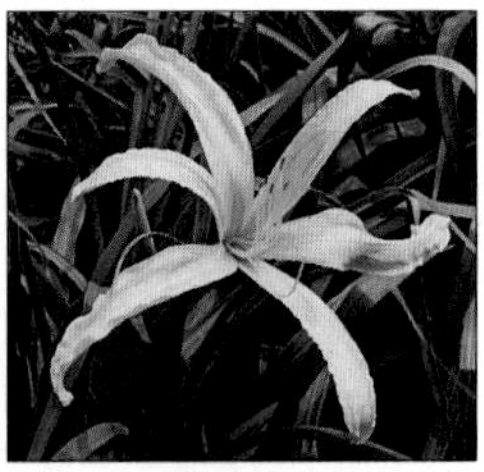
Hemerocallis 'Cat's Cradle'

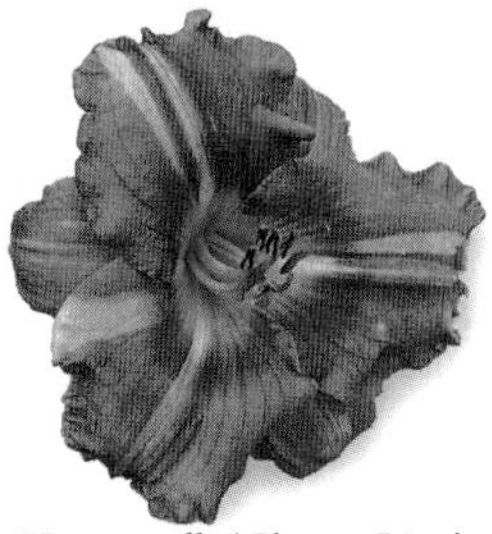
Hemerocallis 'Chorus Line'

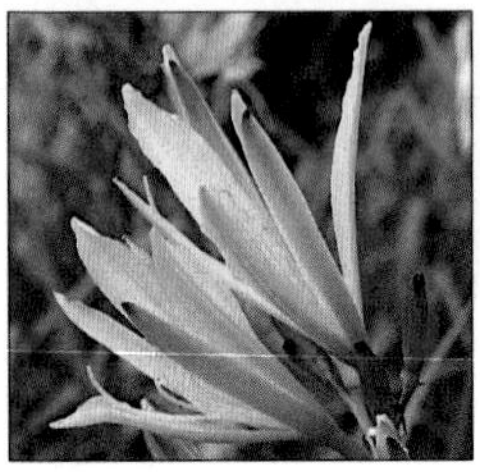
Hemerocallis citrina

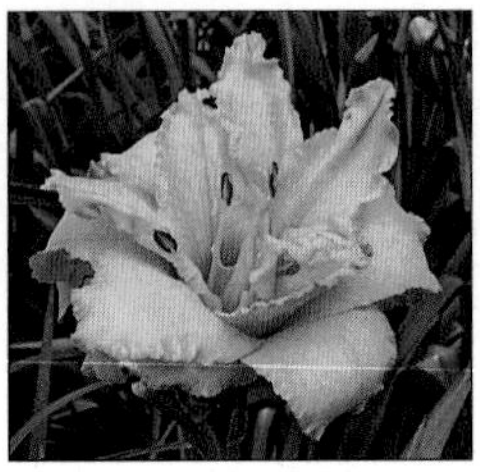
Hemerocallis 'Condilla'

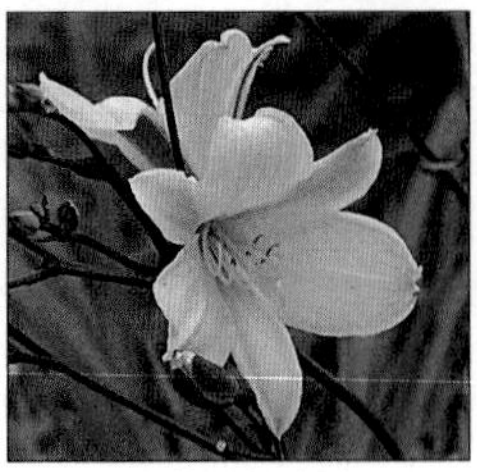
Hemerocallis 'Corky'

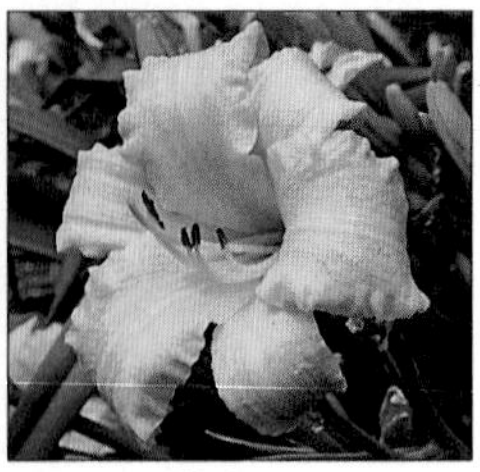
Hemerocallis 'Eenie Weenie'

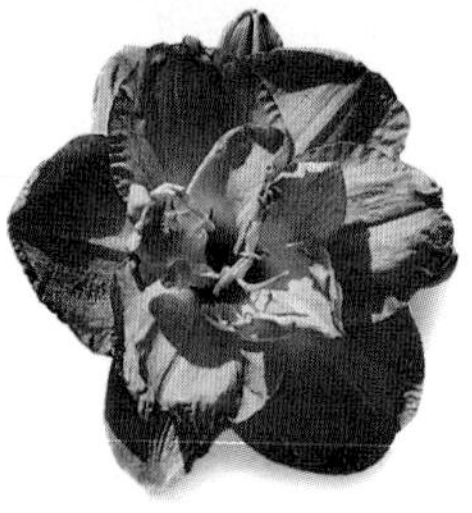
Hemerocallis 'Francis Joiner'

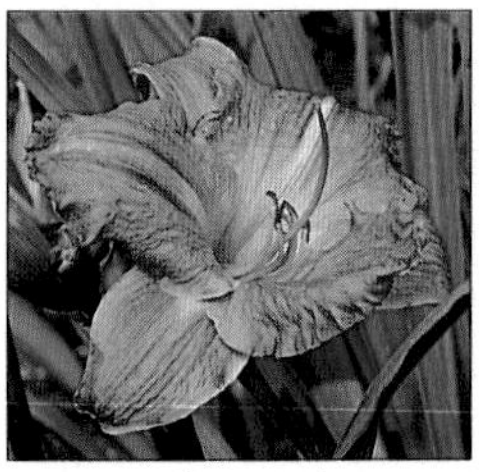
Hemerocallis 'Frank Gladney'

circular yellow flowers, 15cm (6in) across, with flat, ruffled-margined tepals, recurved at the tips, in midsummer. ↕65cm (26in), ↔ 1m (3ft). ***

***H.* 'Attribution'.** Semi-evergreen perennial with slender scapes. In early and midsummer, bears circular, deep rose-pink flowers, 18cm (7in) across, with darker rose-pink eyes, white midribs, green throats, and lighter pink sepals. ↕60cm (24in), ↔ 75cm (30in). ***

***H.* 'Barbara Mitchell'.** Semi-evergreen perennial with relatively few, narrow leaves. Branched scapes bear circular, soft pink flowers, 15cm (6in) wide, with recurved tepals, sometimes tinted beige, in midsummer. ↕50cm (20in), ↔ 75cm (30in). ***

***H.* 'Beauty To Behold'** ■ Vigorous, extended-blooming, free-flowering, semi-evergreen perennial with abundant foliage. Nocturnal, circular, glistening, lemon-yellow flowers, 14cm (5½in) across, are borne on sturdy scapes in mid- or late summer. ↕60cm (24in), ↔ 75cm (30in). ***

***H.* 'Bertie Ferris'** ■ Extended-blooming, compact, herbaceous perennial. Star-shaped, peach-orange flowers, 6cm (2½in) across, with rounded tepals, are borne on slender scapes in early summer. ↕50cm (20in), ↔ 45cm (18in). ***

***H.* 'Bess Ross'.** Evergreen perennial with slender leaves. Narrowly star-shaped, velvety, rich bright red flowers, 12cm (5in) across, with slightly recurved tepals and yellow throats, are produced on slender scapes in midsummer. ↕80cm (32in), ↔ 75cm (30in). **

***H.* 'Betty Woods'** ■ Evergreen perennial with well-branched scapes. From midsummer to late autumn, these bear nocturnal, remontant, double, deep yellow flowers, 14cm (5½in) across, with rounded, ruffled-margined tepals and green throats. ↕65cm (26in), ↔ 60cm (24in). ***

***H.* 'Bitsy'.** Compact, semi-evergreen perennial with narrow, yellowish green leaves. Slender scapes bear remontant, star-shaped, lemon-yellow flowers, 4cm (1½in) across, with slightly ruffled-margined tepals and black-tipped sepals, from early summer to late autumn. Tolerates sun or shade. ↕45cm (18in), ↔ 40cm (16in). ***

***H.* 'Brocaded Gown'** ■ Extended-blooming, semi-evergreen perennial with branched scapes. In midsummer, these bear nocturnal, circular, glistening, creamy yellow flowers, 15cm (6in) across, with green throats and recurved, crêpe-textured tepals. ↕65cm (26in), ↔ 75cm (30in). ***

***H.* 'Butterscotch Ruffles'.** Compact, free-flowering, semi-evergreen perennial with narrow leaves. Well-branched scapes bear remontant, circular, orange-buff flowers, 7cm (3in) across, with crêpe-textured tepals, yellow midribs, and small green throats, from early summer to late autumn. ↕60cm (24in), ↔ 40cm (16in). ***

***H.* 'Camden Gold Dollar'.** Compact, evergreen perennial with narrow, mid- to dark green leaves. Slender scapes bear remontant, circular, deep golden yellow flowers, 7cm (3in) across, with very ruffled-margined tepals, from mid-summer to late autumn. ↕↔ 45cm (18in). ***

***H.* 'Cartwheels'** ■🏆 Free-flowering, evergreen perennial with slender scapes bearing nocturnal, star-shaped, orange-gold flowers, 15cm (6in) across, in mid-summer. ↕↔ 75cm (30in). ***

***H.* 'Catherine Woodbery'.** Extended-blooming, evergreen perennial with narrow leaves. Branched scapes bear star-shaped, light lavender-pink flowers, 12cm (5in) across, with broad, slightly ruffled-margined tepals, light green throats, and recurved sepals, in mid-

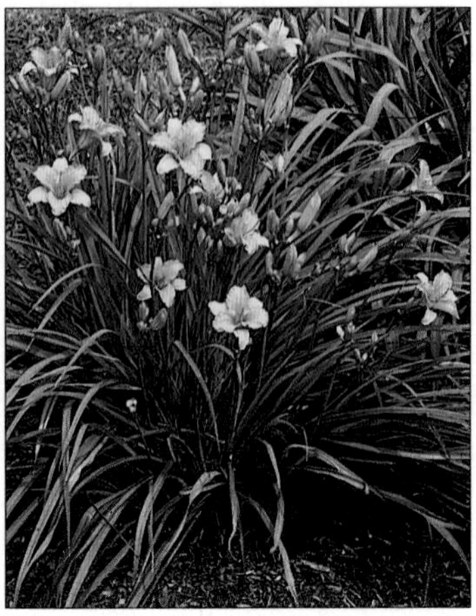
Hemerocallis 'Bertie Ferris'

and late summer. ↕75cm (30in), ↔ 60cm (24in). ***

***H.* 'Cat's Cradle'** ■ Evergreen perennial producing narrow leaves and slender, well-branched scapes. In mid-summer, these bear nocturnal, spider-shaped, bright yellow flowers, 20cm (8in) across. ↕90cm (36in), ↔ 75cm (30in). ***

***H.* 'Charles Johnston'.** Free-flowering, semi-evergreen perennial with sturdy scapes bearing circular, bright cherry-red to bluish red flowers, 15cm (6in) across, with green throats, in early and mid-summer. ↕60cm (24in), ↔ 1m (3ft). ***

***H.* 'Cherry Cheeks'.** Evergreen perennial with sturdy scapes. In mid- and late summer, these bear circular, bright pink-tinted, deep pink flowers, 15cm (6in) across, with white midribs, yellow throats, and black anthers. ↕70cm (28in), ↔ 1m (3ft). ***

***H.* 'Chestnut Lane'.** Free-flowering, semi-evergreen perennial with sturdy scapes bearing circular, light golden brown flowers, 15cm (6in) across, with fluted tepals, chestnut-brown eyes, and yellow throats, in midsummer. ↕75cm (30in), ↔ 1m (3ft). ***

***H.* 'Chicago Apache'.** Vigorous, free-flowering, evergreen perennial with masses of stiff leaves. In late summer, sturdy scapes bear circular, velvety, rich scarlet flowers, 12cm (5in) across, the tepals with ruffled, deeper red margins and white midribs. ↕70cm (28in), ↔ 1m (3ft). ***

***H.* 'Chicago Sunrise'.** Vigorous, free-flowering, evergreen perennial with sturdy scapes bearing circular, deep to golden yellow flowers, 12cm (5in) across, in midsummer. ↕65cm (26in), ↔ 1m (3ft). ***

***H.* 'Chorus Line'** ■ Extended-blooming, semi-evergreen perennial with stiff, wide-branching scapes. From early to late summer, these produce remontant, triangular, slightly fragrant, bright pink flowers, 9cm (3½in) across, with pink- and yellow-marked tepals and dark green throats. ↕50cm (20in), ↔ 60cm (24in). ***

H. citrina ■ Herbaceous perennial with coarse, recurved leaves, 70–80cm (28–32in) long, which die down in late summer. In midsummer, stiff scapes bear nocturnal, star-shaped, fragrant, greenish yellow to pale lemon-yellow flowers, 9–12cm (3½–5in) across, with brown-tipped sepals. China. ↕1.2m (4ft), ↔ 75cm (30in). ***

***H.* 'Condilla'** ■ Slow-growing, ever-green perennial with erect scapes bearing double, deep yellow flowers, 11cm (4½in) across, with broad tepals, in early and midsummer. ↕50cm (20in), ↔ 75cm (30in). ***

***H.* 'Cool Jazz'.** Semi-evergreen perennial with sturdy scapes bearing remontant, circular, clear pink flowers, 14cm (5½in) across, with overlapping, gold-margined tepals, in early summer. ↕70cm (28in), ↔ 75cm (30in). ***

***H.* 'Corky'** ■🏆 Compact, free-flowering, evergreen perennial with narrow leaves. Slender, wiry scapes bear reddish brown buds that open to star-shaped, clear yellow flowers, 6cm (2½in) across, with reddish brown sepals, in midsummer. Prefers a sunny site, but tolerates some shade. ↕70cm (28in), ↔ 40cm (16in). ***

***H.* 'Curly Ripples'.** Free-flowering, evergreen perennial with sturdy scapes. In midsummer, these bear nocturnal, triangular, slightly scented, golden cream to soft apricot flowers, 17cm (7in) across, with rounded, very ruffled-margined tepals. ↕65cm (26in), ↔ 60cm (24in). ***

***H.* 'Dominic'.** Vigorous, evergreen perennial with sturdy scapes bearing circular, very dark black-red flowers, 14cm (5½in) across, in early and mid-summer. ↕↔ 75cm (30in). ***

***H.* 'Dorethe Louise'.** Free-flowering, evergreen perennial with erect scapes bearing nocturnal, circular, very fragrant, greenish yellow flowers, 17cm (7in) across, with green throats, in midsummer. ↕45cm (18in), ↔ 75cm (30in). ***

H. dumortieri. Compact, herbaceous perennial with early-produced, stiff, narrow leaves, to 35cm (14in) long. Slender, arching, reddish brown scapes bear star-shaped, orange-yellow flowers, 5–7cm (2–3in) across, which open from reddish brown buds in early summer. Grow in full sun or partial shade. ↕50cm (20in), ↔ 45cm (18in). Korea, E. Russia, Japan. ***

***H.* 'Edna Spalding'.** Free-flowering, evergreen perennial with slender scapes. In early summer, bears nocturnal, star-

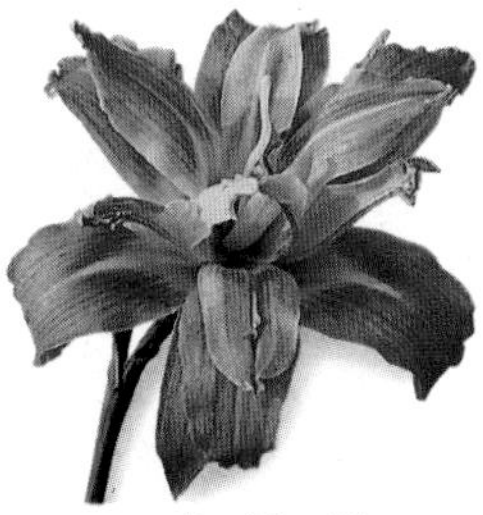
Hemerocallis fulva 'Flore Pleno'

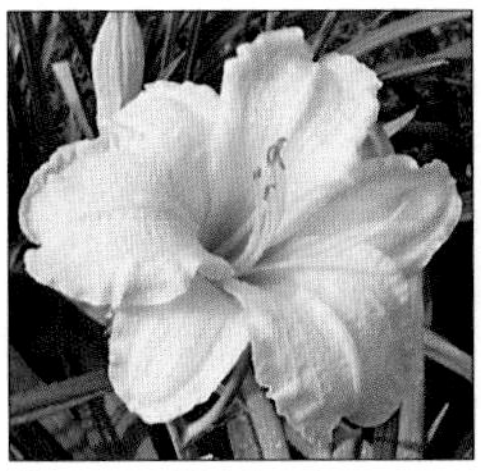
Hemerocallis 'Gentle Shepherd'

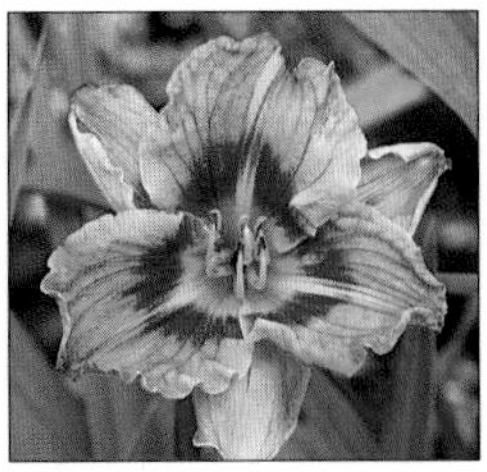
Hemerocallis 'Gingerbread Man'

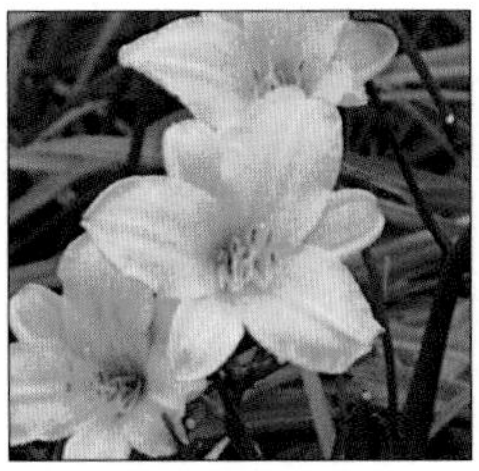
Hemerocallis 'Golden Chimes'

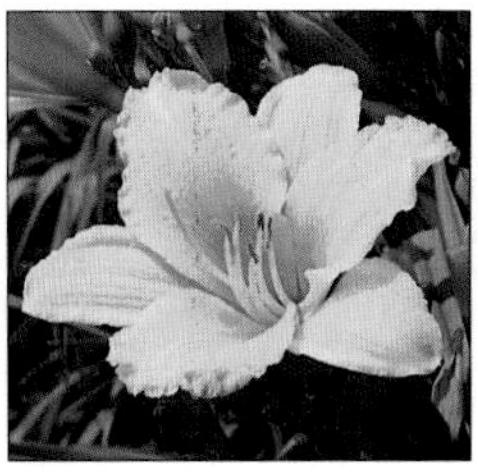
Hemerocallis 'Green Flutter'

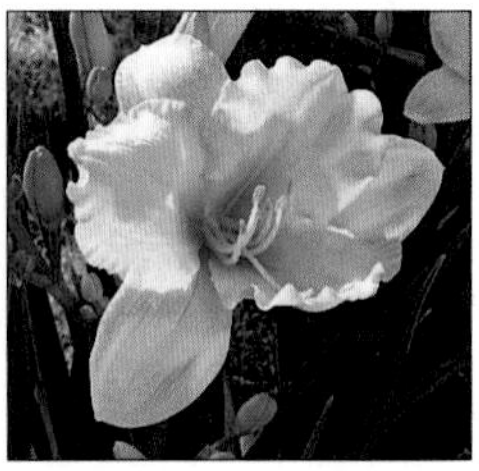
Hemerocallis 'Hope Diamond'

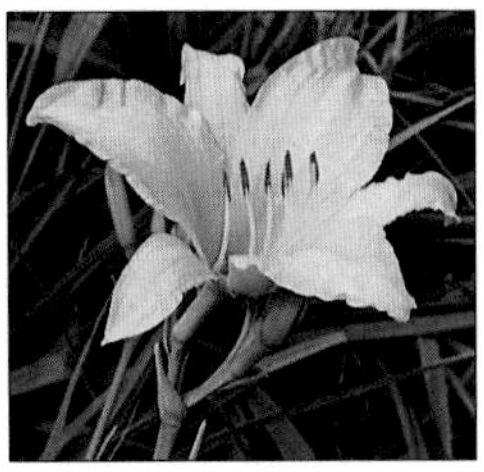
Hemerocallis 'Hyperion'

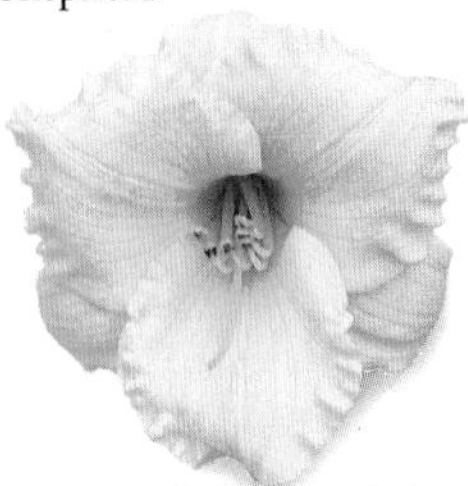
Hemerocallis 'Ice Castles'

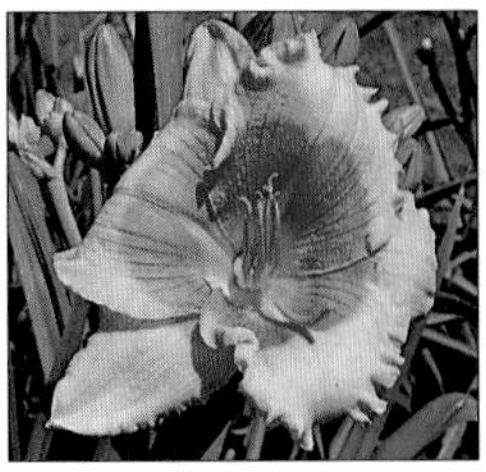
Hemerocallis 'Janice Brown'

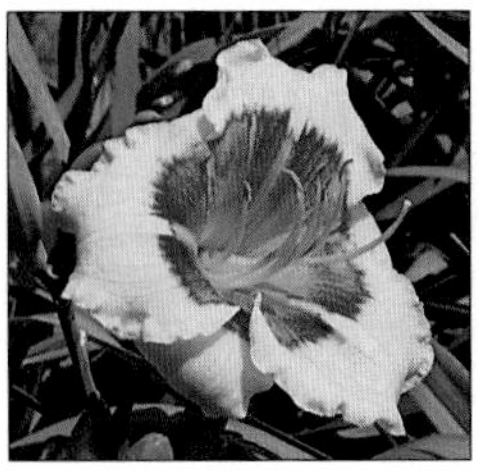
Hemerocallis 'Jason Salter'

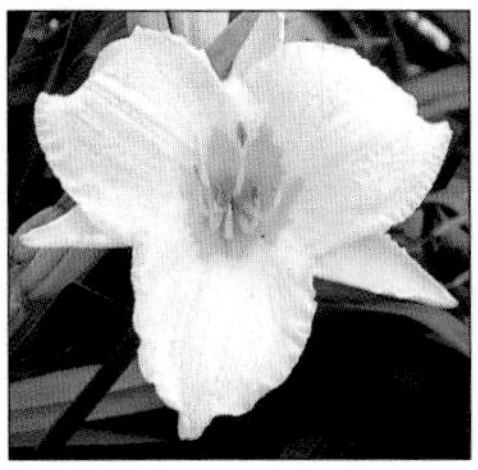
Hemerocallis 'Joan Senior'

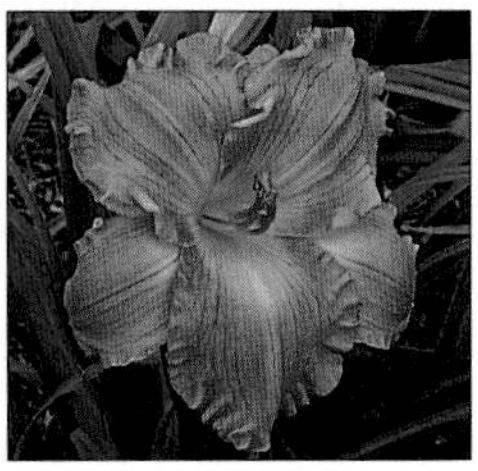
Hemerocallis 'Jolyene Nichole'

shaped, pure pink flowers, 11cm (4½in) across, with yellow-green throats. Grow in partial shade. ↕60cm (24in), ↔75cm (30in). ❄❄❄

***H.* 'Eenie Weenie'** ■ Compact, free-flowering, evergreen perennial with neat, mounded foliage. Erect scapes bear remontant, circular yellow flowers, 5cm (2in) across, with tapered tepals in early and midsummer. ↕25cm (10in), ↔40cm (16in). ❄❄❄

***H.* 'Erin Prairie'.** Free-flowering, evergreen perennial with erect scapes bearing star-shaped, deep lemon-yellow flowers, 17cm (7in) across, with bright green throats, in midsummer. ↕70cm (28in), ↔75cm (30in). ❄❄❄

***H.* 'Fairy Tale Pink'.** Semi-evergreen perennial with narrow, wispy, mid-green leaves hidden by profuse blooms. In midsummer, erect scapes bear circular, glistening, pale orange-pink to beige-pink flowers, 14cm (5½in) across, with ruffled-margined tepals. ↕60cm (24in), ↔1m (3ft). ❄❄❄

H. flava see *H. lilioasphodelus.*

***H.* 'Francis Joiner'** ■ Evergreen perennial with sturdy, well-branched scapes bearing remontant, double, pink-orange flowers, 14cm (5½in) across, with rounded tepals and greenish yellow throats, in midsummer. ↕↔60cm (24in). ❄❄❄

***H.* 'Frank Gladney'** ■ Semi-evergreen perennial with erect scapes bearing circular, coral-pink flowers, 17cm (7in) across, with recurved tepals and gold throats, from early summer to late autumn. ↕65cm (26in), ↔1m (3ft). ❄❄❄

H. fulva. Semi-evergreen, rhizomatous perennial with wide, dark bluish green leaves, 30–90cm (12–36in) long. Branched scapes bear trumpet-shaped, orange-brown flowers, 6–10cm (2½–4in) across, with recurved tepals, in mid- and late summer. ↕to 1m (3ft), ↔1.2m (4ft). China or Japan. ❄❄❄. **'Europa'** ■ is a robust cultivar bearing tawny-orange flowers with yellow tepal bases. **'Flore Pleno'** ■ has strong, erect scapes bearing double flowers with dark red eyes; ↕75cm (30in). **'Kwanzo Variegata'** is similar to 'Flore Pleno', with strong, erect scapes bearing double, red-eyed flowers, 12cm (5in) across, but it has narrow, white-margined leaves; ↕75cm (30in).

***H.* 'Gentle Shepherd'** ■ Semi-evergreen perennial with wispy leaves. Circular, ivory-white flowers, 14cm (5½in) across, with oval tepals and green throats, are borne on slender scapes in midsummer. ↕65cm (26in), ↔1.2m (4ft). ❄❄❄

***H.* 'Gingerbread Man'** ■ Semi-evergreen perennial with sturdy scapes bearing remontant, circular, orange-brown flowers, 17cm (7in) across, with dark red-brown eyes, in early summer. ↕70cm (28in), ↔1m (3ft). ❄❄

***H.* 'Gleber's Top Cream'.** Semi-evergreen perennial with sturdy scapes bearing circular ivory flowers, 15cm (6in) across, with recurved, pale peach-tinted tepals and green throats, in midsummer. ↕45cm (18in), ↔1m (3ft). ❄❄❄

***H.* 'Golden Chimes'** ■🏆 Free-flowering, evergreen perennial with narrow leaves and slender, well-branched, reddish brown scapes. Star-shaped, deep yellow flowers, 5cm (2in) across, with reddish brown backs to the

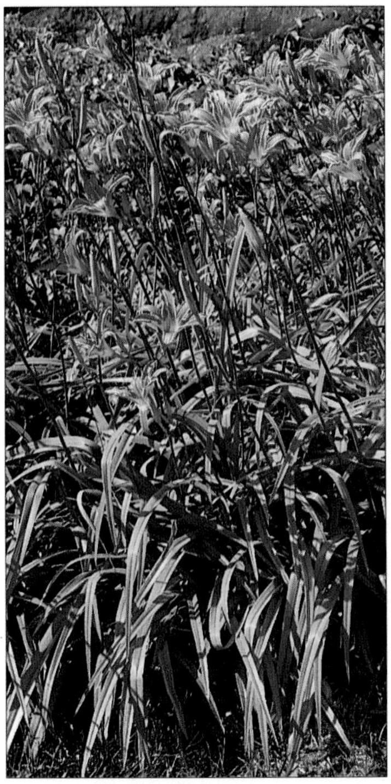
Hemerocallis fulva 'Europa'

outer tepals, open from reddish brown buds in early summer. Grow in full sun or partial shade. ↕90cm (36in), ↔45cm (18in). ❄❄❄

***H.* 'Golden Prize'.** Evergreen perennial with triangular, golden yellow flowers, 17cm (7in) across, borne on sturdy, well-branched scapes in late summer. ↕65cm (26in), ↔1m (3ft). ❄❄❄

***H.* 'Grape Velvet'.** Evergreen perennial with erect scapes. In midsummer, these bear triangular, deep purple flowers, 11cm (4½in) across, with lighter purple midribs, green throats, and recurved tepals. ↕60cm (24in), ↔75cm (30in). ❄❄

***H.* 'Green Flutter'** ■🏆 Extended-blooming, free-flowering, evergreen perennial with narrow leaves. In midsummer, slender scapes bear nocturnal, triangular to star-shaped, light yellow flowers, 9cm (3½in) across, with thick, rounded, slightly ruffled-margined tepals and green-tinted throats. ↕50cm (20in), ↔1m (3ft). ❄❄❄

***H.* 'Green Glitter'.** Vigorous, evergreen perennial with bright green leaves. In early summer, sturdy scapes bear circular, fragrant, creamy yellow flowers, 16cm (6in) across, with thick tepals, deeper yellow eyes, and green throats. ↕↔75cm (30in). ❄❄❄

***H.* 'Happy Returns'.** Free-flowering, evergreen perennial with narrow leaves. In early summer, erect scapes bear nocturnal, remontant, circular, light yellow flowers, 6cm (2½in) across. Good for containers. ↕40cm (16in), ↔60cm (24in). ❄❄❄

***H.* 'Helle Berlinerin'** 🏆 Evergreen perennial with sturdy scapes bearing circular cream flowers, 13cm (5in) across, in midsummer. ↕70cm (28in), ↔1m (3ft). ❄❄❄

***H.* 'Hope Diamond'** ■ Evergreen perennial with erect scapes. Nocturnal, triangular to circular, cream to very pale yellow flowers, 11cm (4½in) across, with rounded, crinkly, slightly ruffled-margined tepals, are borne in midsummer. ↕55cm (28in), ↔1m (3ft). ❄❄❄

***H.* 'Hyperion'** ■ Evergreen perennial with narrow leaves. In midsummer, slender scapes bear nocturnal, triangular to star-shaped, fragrant, lemon-yellow flowers, 10cm (4in) across. ↕90cm (36in), ↔75cm (30in). ❄❄❄

***H.* 'Ice Castles'** ■ Vigorous, evergreen perennial with erect scapes bearing circular, pale ivory flowers, 6cm (2½in) across, with yellow-suffused throats, in midsummer. ↕45cm (18in), ↔75cm (30in). ❄❄❄

***H.* 'Janice Brown'** ■ Semi-evergreen perennial with well-branched scapes bearing circular flowers, 11cm (4½in) across, with flat tepals, strongly recurved at the tips, in midsummer. Flowers are light pink with wide, rose-pink eyes and green throats. ↕55cm (22in), ↔75cm (30in). ❄❄❄

***H.* 'Jason Salter'** ■ Semi-evergreen perennial with erect scapes bearing triangular flowers, 6cm (2½in) across, with flat tepals, recurved at the tips, in midsummer. Flowers are deep yellow with deep purple-red eyes, and lime-green throats. ↕↔45cm (18in). ❄❄❄

***H.* 'Joan Senior'** ■ Vigorous, free-flowering, semi-evergreen perennial with erect scapes bearing circular, off-white, pink-flushed flowers, 15cm (6in) across, with recurved tepals and yellowish green throats, in mid- and late summer. ↕60cm (24in), ↔75cm (30in). ❄❄❄

***H.* 'Jolyene Nichole'** ■ Vigorous, semi-evergreen perennial with abundant blue-green leaves. Sturdy scapes produce nocturnal, circular, rose-pink flowers, 14cm (5½in) across, the tepals veined deep pink, in midsummer. ↕45cm (18in), ↔1m (3ft). ❄❄❄

***H.* 'Journey's End'.** Semi-evergreen perennial with erect scapes bearing circular, off-white flowers, 13cm (5in) across, with crêpe-textured tepals and lemon-yellow throats, in midsummer. ↕40cm (16in), ↔75cm (30in). ❄❄❄

***H.* 'Judah'.** Evergreen perennial with sturdy scapes bearing circular, deep gold flowers, 15cm (6in) across, with yellow throats and rounded, bronze-margined tepals, in midsummer. ↕75cm (30in), ↔1m (3ft). ❄❄❄

***H.* 'Kecia'.** Vigorous, free-flowering, semi-evergreen perennial with branched scapes bearing circular, creamy yellow flowers, 15cm (6in) across, with green throats, and flat tepals with ruffled margins, in midsummer. ↕70cm (28in), ↔60cm (24in). ❄❄❄

***H.* 'Kindly Light'.** Evergreen perennial with narrow leaves. In midsummer, slender scapes bear nocturnal, spider-shaped, bright yellow flowers, 22cm

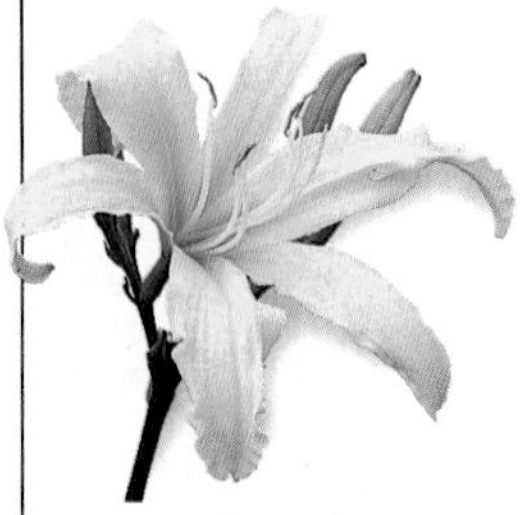
Hemerocallis 'Lady Fingers'

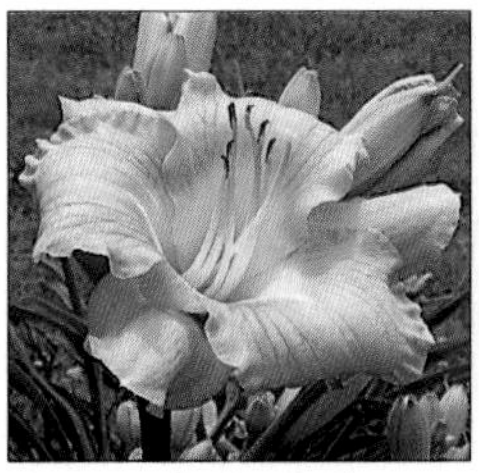
Hemerocallis 'Lavender Tonic'

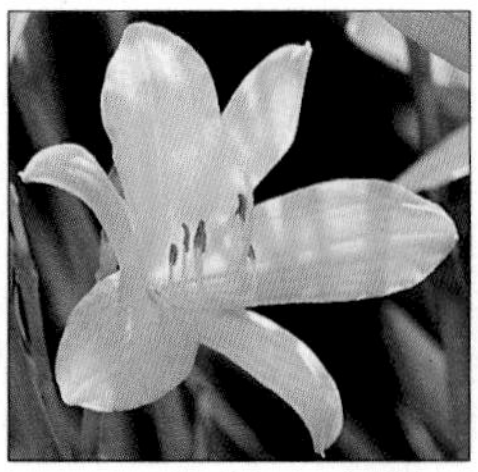
Hemerocallis lilioasphodelus

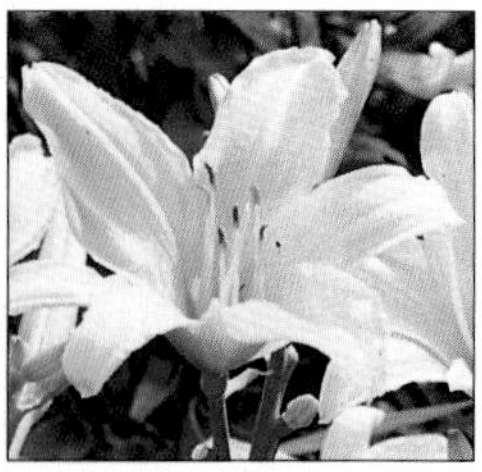
Hemerocallis 'Marion Vaughn'

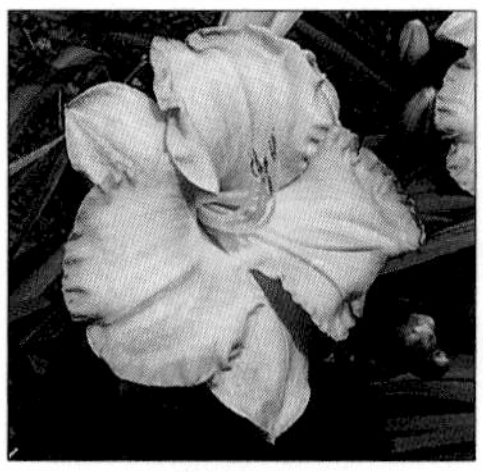
Hemerocallis 'Martha Adams'

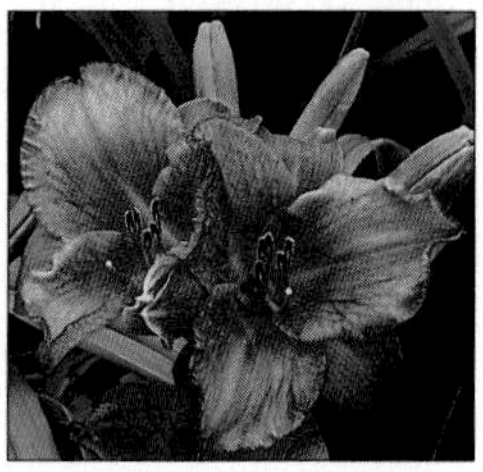
Hemerocallis 'Mauna Loa'

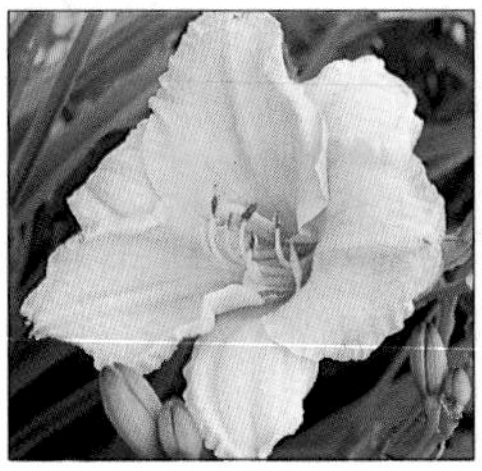
Hemerocallis 'Michele Coe'

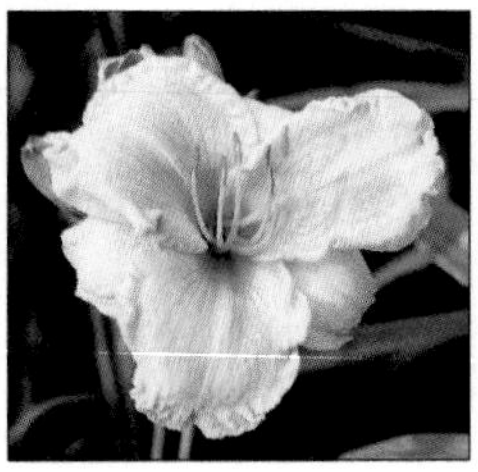
Hemerocallis 'Millie Schlumpf'

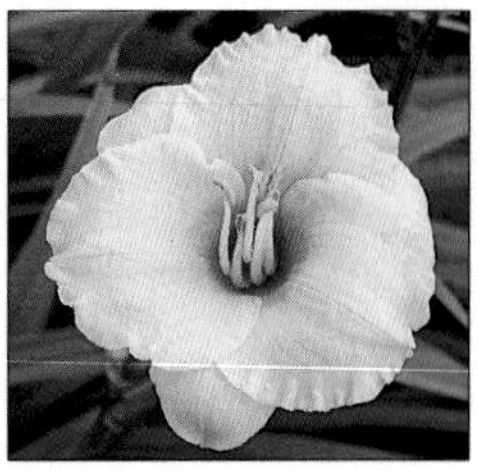
Hemerocallis 'Moonlight Mist'

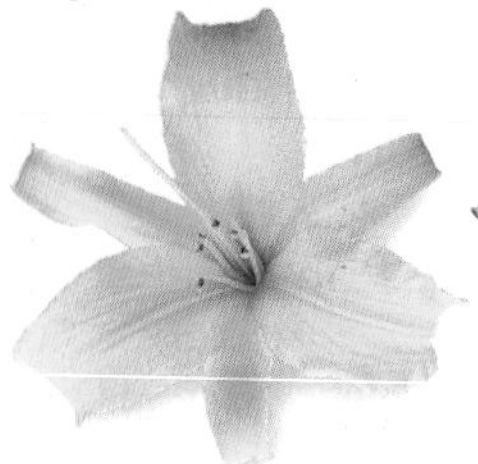
Hemerocallis 'Nova'

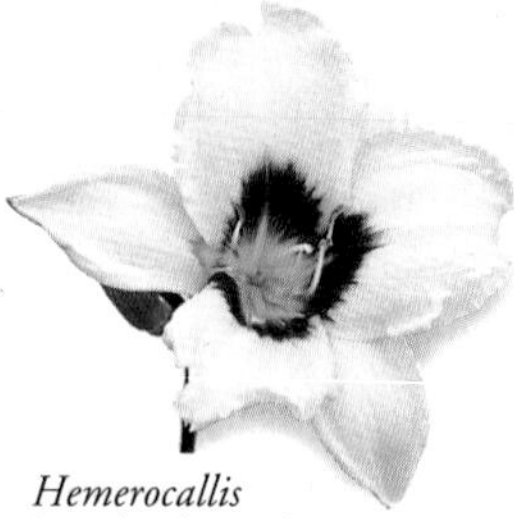
Hemerocallis 'Pandora's Box'

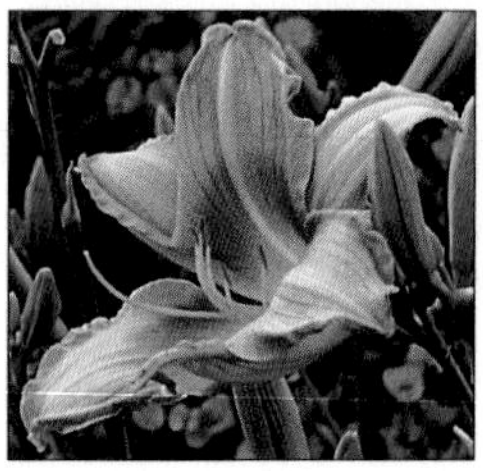
Hemerocallis 'Penelope Vestey'

H

(9in) across, with – in cool conditions – faint salmon-pink eyes. ↕70cm (28in), ↔75cm (30in). ***

***H.* 'Lady Fingers'** ■ Semi-evergreen perennial with narrow leaves. In midsummer, slender scapes bear spider-shaped, pale yellow-green flowers with green throats, 16cm (6in) across, with spoon-shaped tepals. ↕80cm (32in), ↔75cm (30in). ***

***H.* 'Lavender Tonic'** ■ Evergreen perennial with sturdy, well-branched scapes bearing circular, soft lavender-pink flowers, 13cm (5in) across, with yellow throats, in midsummer. ↕↔45cm (18in). ***

H. lilioasphodelus ■🏆 syn. *H. flava*. Rhizomatous, extended-blooming, semi-evergreen perennial with narrow leaves, 50–65cm (20–26in) long. In early summer, slender scapes bear nocturnal, star-shaped, fragrant, clear bright lemon-yellow flowers, to 9cm (3½in) across. China. ↕↔1m (3ft). ***

***H.* 'Little Business'.** Compact, free-flowering, semi-evergreen perennial with abundant mounded leaves. Sturdy scapes bear remontant, triangular, strawberry-crimson flowers, 7cm (3in) across, with velvety tepals and yellow-green throats, in mid- and late summer. ↕40cm (16in), ↔60cm (24in). ***

***H.* 'Little Deeke'.** Vigorous, evergreen perennial with sturdy scapes. In early summer, produces circular, orange-gold flowers, 11cm (4½in) across, with flat, crêpe-textured, ruffled-margined, bronze-veined tepals, recurved at the tips, and green throats. ↕50cm (20in), ↔75cm (30in). ***

***H.* 'Little Fat Dazzler'.** Compact, free-flowering, evergreen perennial with narrow leaves. Circular, deep rose-red flowers, 7cm (3in) across, are borne on erect scapes in early and midsummer. ↕40cm (16in), ↔40cm (16in). ***

***H.* 'Little Grapette'.** Vigorous, free-flowering, compact, semi-evergreen perennial with narrow leaves. In midsummer, slender scapes bear star-shaped, deep purple flowers, 5cm (2in) across, with rounded, ruffled-margined tepals, darker purple eyes, and green throats. ↕30cm (12in), ↔45cm (18in). ***

***H.* 'Little Gypsy Vagabond'.** Semi-evergreen, compact perennial with narrow, arching leaves. In midsummer, slender scapes bear circular, light yellow flowers, 7cm (3in) across, with rounded, flat tepals and black-purple eyes. ↕30cm (12in), ↔35cm (14in). ***

***H.* 'Little Maggie'.** Free-flowering, compact, evergreen perennial with narrow leaves. In early summer, erect scapes bear remontant, circular, deep rose-pink flowers, 8cm (3in) across, with burgundy-red eyes. ↕30cm (12in), ↔45cm (18in). ***

***H.* 'Little Rainbow'** ■ Evergreen perennial with slender scapes bearing multi-coloured, creamy yellow, beige-pink, and mauve-pink flowers, 9cm (3½in) across, with rounded tepals and orange throats, in midsummer. ↕60cm (24in), ↔45cm (18in). ***

***H.* 'Lullaby Baby'.** Evergreen perennial with branched scapes bearing nocturnal, circular, very pale ice-pink flowers, 9cm (3½in) wide, with green throats, in mid- and late summer. ↕45cm (18in), ↔1m (3ft). ***

***H.* 'Lusty Leland'** ■ Extended-blooming, free-flowering, evergreen perennial with bluish green leaves. Sturdy scapes bear nocturnal, circular scarlet flowers, 12cm (5in) across, with velvety, yellow-backed tepals and yellow throats, in midsummer. ↕70cm (28in), ↔1m (3ft). ***

***H.* 'Luxury Lace'.** Evergreen perennial with narrow leaves and slender scapes. These bear star-shaped, pink-tinted, lavender-pink flowers, 10cm (4in) across, with rounded, ruffled-margined tepals and green throats, in midsummer. ↕80cm (32in), ↔75cm (30in). ***

***H.* 'Marion Vaughn'** ■🏆 Free-flowering, evergreen perennial with narrow leaves. Nocturnal, star-shaped, very fragrant, clear lemon-yellow flowers, 10cm (4in) across, are borne on slender scapes in mid- and late summer. ↕85cm (34in), ↔75cm (30in). ***

***H.* 'Martha Adams'** ■ Extended-blooming, evergreen perennial with erect scapes bearing circular, pale pink, beige-tinted flowers, 17cm (7in) across, with yellow-green throats, in early summer. ↕45cm (18in), ↔75cm (30in). ***

***H.* 'Mauna Loa'** ■ Evergreen perennial with sturdy scapes bearing circular, very bright tangerine-orange flowers, 13cm (5in) across, with crimped tepals, green throats, and black anthers, in summer. ↕55cm (22in), ↔1m (3ft). ***

***H.* 'Meadow Sprite'.** Free-flowering, vigorous, compact, evergreen perennial with neatly mounded leaves. Nocturnal, circular, magenta-lilac flowers, 9cm (3½in) across, with purple eyes, bright green throats, and black anthers, are borne on erect scapes in early and midsummer. ↕35cm (14in), ↔45cm (18in). ***

***H.* 'Melon Balls'.** Evergreen perennial with narrow leaves. In midsummer, slender scapes bear star-shaped, glowing, beige-pink flowers, 9cm (3½in) across, tinted mauve-pink, with crêpe-textured tepals, gold throats, and recurved sepals. ↕80cm (32in), ↔75cm (30in). ***

***H.* 'Michele Coe'** ■ Evergreen perennial with sturdy scapes bearing circular, pale apricot flowers, 13cm (5in) across, with light lavender-pink midribs, in midsummer. ↕1m (3ft), ↔75cm (30in). ***

***H. middendorffii*.** Semi-evergreen perennial with narrow, stiff leaves, to 30cm (12in) long. In early summer, slender, reddish brown scapes bear ridged, reddish brown buds that open to star-shaped, deep orange flowers, 6–8cm (2½–3in) across. ↕90cm (36in), ↔45cm (18in). E. Russia, N. China, Korea, Japan. ***

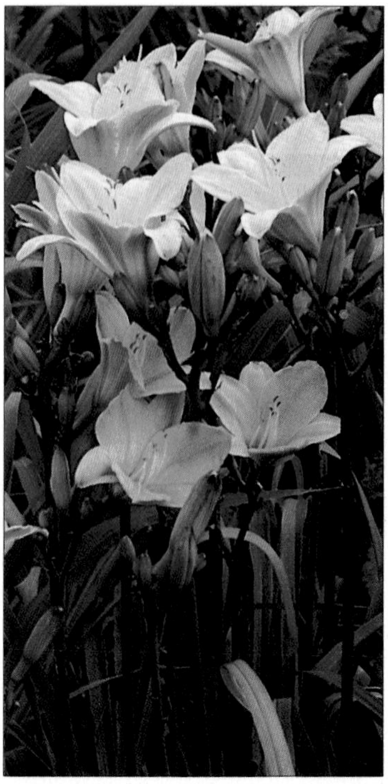
Hemerocallis 'Little Rainbow'

***H.* 'Millie Schlumpf'** ■ Vigorous, free-flowering, evergreen perennial. In midsummer, erect scapes bear nocturnal, remontant, triangular, glistening, pale pink flowers, 13cm (5in) across, with darker pink eyes and bright light green throats. ↕50cm (20in), ↔60cm (24in). ***

***H.* 'Mini Pearl'.** Compact, free-flowering, evergreen perennial with glossy leaves. Remontant, circular, pink-flushed white flowers, 8cm (3in) across, with rounded petals, are borne on erect scapes in early and midsummer. ↕40cm (16in), ↔40cm (16in). ***

***H.* 'Moonlight Mist'** ■ Compact, evergreen perennial with erect scapes bearing circular, pale ivory to pale peach flowers, 8cm (3in) across, in midsummer. ↕45cm (18in), ↔40cm (16in). ***

***H.* 'Night Raider'.** Vigorous, free-flowering, evergreen perennial with well-branched scapes. Nocturnal, circular, bright to dark red flowers, 12cm (5in) across, with slightly recurved tepals and yellow throats, are borne in midsummer. ↕70cm (28in), ↔60cm (24in). ***

***H.* 'Nile Plum'.** Evergreen perennial with sturdy scapes. In late summer, produces nocturnal, circular, rich purple flowers, 11cm (4½in) across, with recurved tepals and large, lemon-ivory eyes. ↕55cm (22in), ↔1m (3ft). ***

***H.* 'Nova'** ■🏆 Free-flowering, evergreen perennial with slender scapes bearing star-shaped, fragrant, lemon-yellow flowers, 14cm (5½in) across, in early and midsummer. ↕60cm (24in), ↔1m (3ft). ***

***H.* 'Olive Bailey Langdon'.** Free-flowering, evergreen perennial. Sturdy scapes bear remontant, circular, violet-purple flowers, 13cm (5in) across, with yellow-green throats, in early and midsummer. ↕70cm (28in), ↔1m (3ft). ***

***H.* 'Outrageous'.** Evergreen perennial with sturdy scapes bearing circular, light copper-orange flowers, 11cm (4½in) across, with large, dark brownish red eyes, in midsummer. ↕55cm (22in), ↔1m (3ft). ***

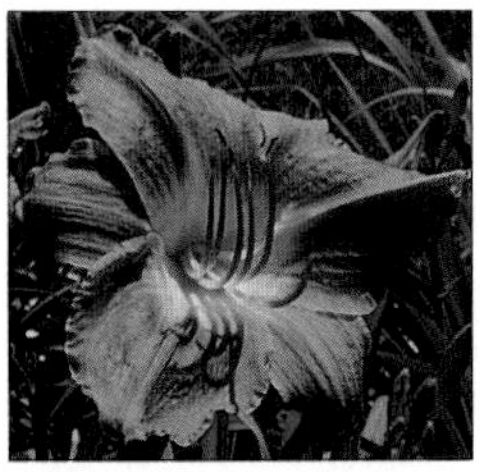
Hemerocallis 'Prairie Blue Eyes'

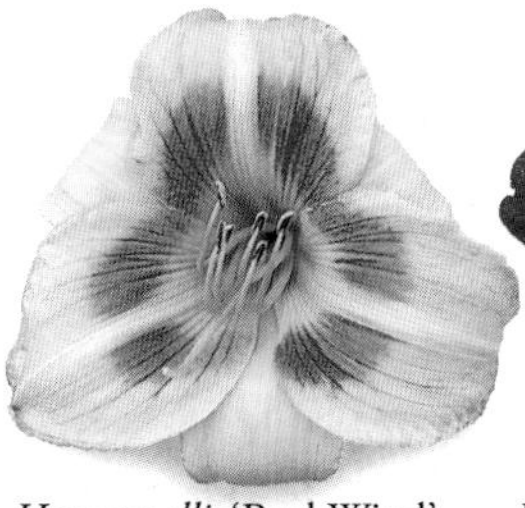
Hemerocallis 'Real Wind'

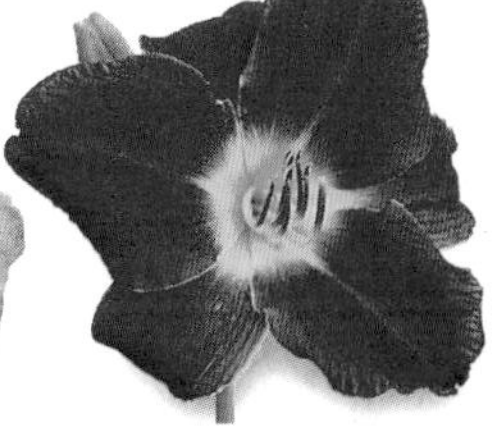
Hemerocallis 'Red Joy'

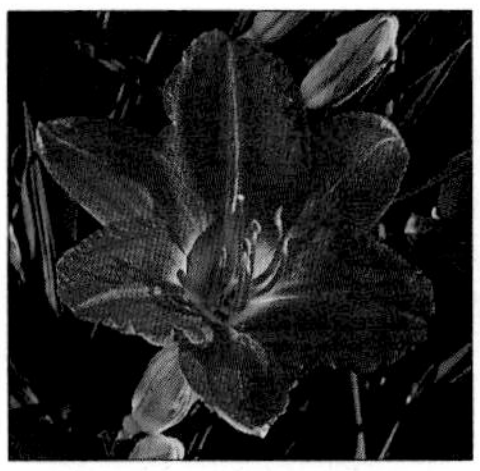
Hemerocallis 'Red Rum'

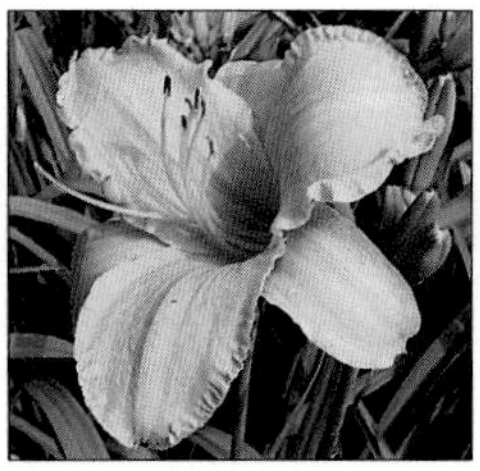
Hemerocallis 'Ruffled Apricot'

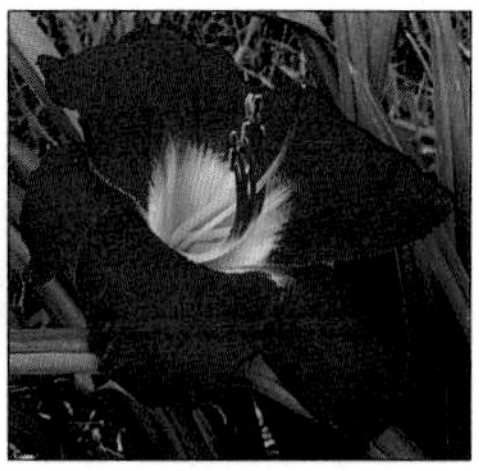
Hemerocallis 'Scarlet Orbit'

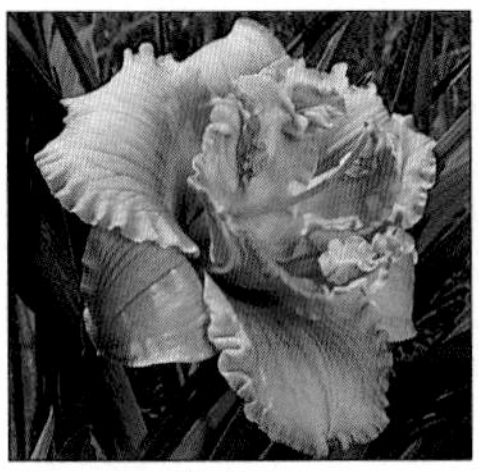
Hemerocallis 'Siloam Double Classic'

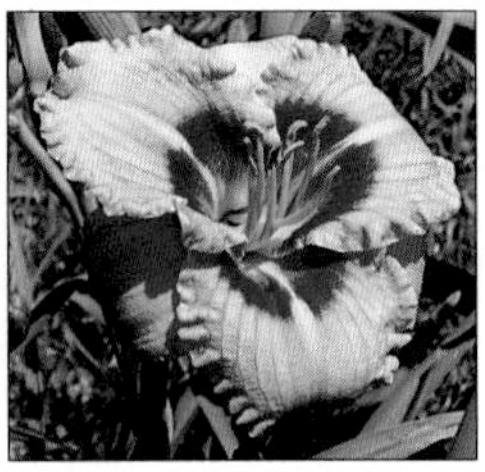
Hemerocallis 'Siloam Merle Kent'

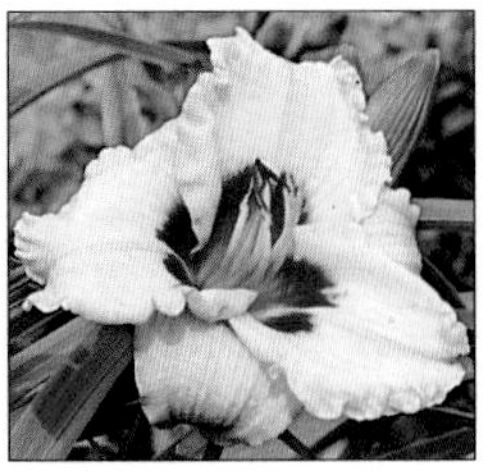
Hemerocallis 'Siloam Ury Winniford'

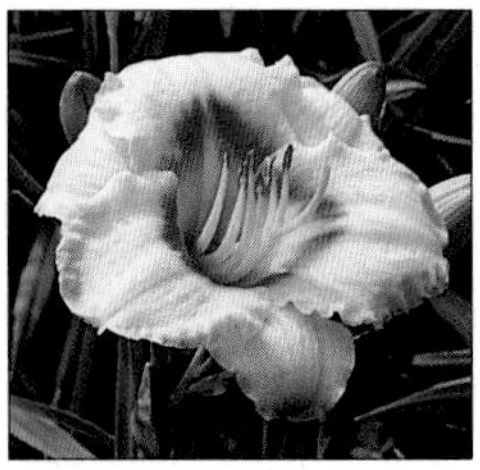
Hemerocallis 'Siloam Virginia Henson'

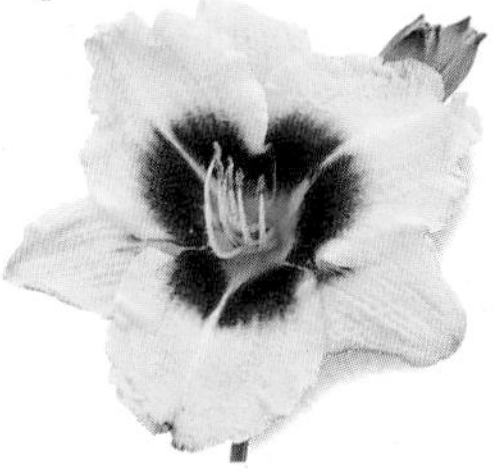
Hemerocallis 'Solano Bulls Eye'

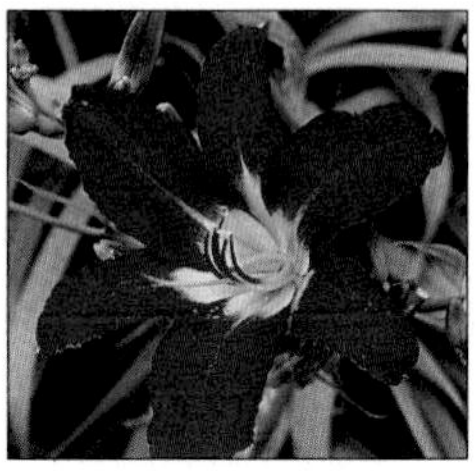
Hemerocallis 'Stafford'

***H.* 'Pandora's Box'** ■ Free-flowering, vigorous, compact, evergreen perennial with narrow leaves. In midsummer, erect scapes bear remontant, star-shaped, pale cream flowers, 11cm (4½in) across, with bright purple eyes and green throats. ↕50cm (20in), ↔60cm (24in). ❄❄❄

***H.* 'Pardon Me'.** Free-flowering, compact, evergreen perennial producing narrow leaves. Slender, well-branched, stiff scapes bear remontant, circular, rich red flowers, 6cm (2½in) across, with green throats, in midsummer. ↕↔45cm (18in). ❄❄❄

***H.* 'Penelope Vestey'** ■ Free-flowering, semi-evergreen perennial producing narrow leaves. In midsummer, slender scapes bear star-shaped to triangular, bright pink flowers, 13cm (5in) across, the tepals marked with darker pink, and with orange throats. ↕85cm (34in), ↔1m (3ft). ❄❄❄

***H.* 'Penny's Worth'.** Compact, evergreen perennial with arching, grass-like leaves. In early summer, slender scapes bear circular, pale yellow flowers, 4cm (1½in) across. ↕24cm (10in), ↔30cm (12in). ❄❄❄

***H.* 'Prairie Blue Eyes'** ■ Free-flowering, semi-evergreen perennial with narrow leaves. In midsummer, slender scapes bear star-shaped, lavender-blue flowers, 13cm (5in) across, with wide, darker blue eyes. ↕70cm (28in), ↔75cm (30in). ❄❄❄

***H.* 'Purple Rain'.** Compact, evergreen perennial with narrow leaves. In early and midsummer, erect scapes bear nocturnal, remontant, circular, bright deep purple flowers, 8cm (3in) across, with large, near-black eyes. ↕40cm (16in), ↔45cm (18in). ❄❄❄

***H.* 'Real Wind'** ■ Free-flowering, evergreen perennial with dense foliage. Sturdy scapes bear triangular, pale salmon-pink flowers, 17cm (7in) across, with recurved tepals and large, rose-pink eyes, in mid- and late summer. ↕65cm (26in), ↔1m (3ft). ❄❄❄

***H.* 'Red Joy'** ■ Evergreen perennial with erect scapes bearing triangular, bright red flowers, 15cm (6in) across, with velvety tepals and wide, yellow-green throats, in midsummer. ↕85cm (34in), ↔1m (3ft). ❄❄❄

***H.* 'Red Rum'** ■ Semi-evergreen perennial with erect, bright green leaves. In midsummer, slender scapes bear remontant, star-shaped, deep brick-red flowers, 11cm (4½in) across, with thick, crêpe-textured tepals and yellow-green throats. ↕40cm (16in), ↔75cm (30in). ❄❄❄

***H.* 'Rose Emily'.** Semi-evergreen perennial with slender scapes bearing circular, rose-pink flowers, 13cm (5in) across, with recurved, ruffled-margined petals and pale green throats, in midsummer. ↕↔45cm (18in). ❄❄❄

***H.* 'Ruffled Apricot'** ■ Slow-growing, evergreen perennial with dense foliage. Star-shaped, rich apricot flowers, 18cm (7in) across, are borne on slender scapes in early and midsummer. ↕70cm (28in), ↔1m (3ft). ❄❄❄

***H.* 'Sari'.** Vigorous, evergreen perennial with erect scapes bearing circular, bright coral-pink flowers, 15cm (6in) across, with thick tepals, in midsummer. ↕50cm (20in), ↔1m (3ft). ❄❄❄

***H.* 'Scarlet Orbit'** ■ Free-flowering, semi-evergreen perennial with sturdy scapes bearing nocturnal, circular, bright red flowers, 16cm (6in) across, with yellow-green throats, in midsummer. ↕50cm (20in), ↔1m (3ft). ❄❄❄

***H.* 'Scarlock'.** Evergreen perennial with sturdy scapes. In early and midsummer, these bear, nocturnal, remontant, circular, rich cherry-red flowers, 17cm (7in) across, with thick, crimped tepals and green throats. ↕80cm (32in), ↔1m (3ft). ❄❄❄

***H.* 'Sebastian'.** Evergreen perennial with sturdy scapes bearing circular, vivid violet-purple flowers, 14cm (5½in) across, with ruffled-margined tepals and lime-green throats, in early and midsummer. ↕50cm (20in), ↔45cm (18in). ❄❄❄

***H.* 'Seductor'.** Evergreen perennial with abundant foliage and erect scapes. Remontant, circular, cranberry-red flowers, 16cm (6in) across, with ruffled-margined, overlapping tepals and lime-green throats, are borne in early and midsummer. ↕↔45cm (18in). ❄❄❄

***H.* 'Selma Timmons'.** Semi-evergreen perennial. In midsummer, well-branched scapes bear circular, orange-pink flowers, 11cm (4½in) across, highlighted deeper pink; they have thick, very ruffled-margined tepals and tiny, rounded, greenish gold throats. ↕45cm (18in), ↔60cm (24in). ❄❄❄

***H.* 'Show Amber'.** Very free-flowering, semi-evergreen perennial. In midsummer, sturdy scapes bear circular, bright, light bronze-orange flowers, 14cm (5½in) across, with deeper bronze eyes, lighter orange midribs, and tangerine-orange throats. ↕↔1m (3ft). ❄❄❄

***H.* 'Siloam Baby Talk'.** Vigorous, compact, free-flowering, evergreen perennial with neatly mounded foliage. Erect scapes bear circular, buff-pink flowers, 6cm (2½in) across, with deep rose-pink eyes and green throats, in midsummer. ↕40cm (16in), ↔60cm (24in). ❄❄❄

***H.* 'Siloam Bo Peep'.** Vigorous, compact, evergreen perennial with erect leaves. In early and midsummer, erect scapes bear circular, buff- to mauve-pink flowers, 11cm (4½in) across, with purple eyes and green throats. ↕↔45cm (18in). ❄❄❄

***H.* 'Siloam Double Classic'** ■ Evergreen perennial with erect scapes bearing double, peach-pink flowers, 11cm (4½in) across, with rounded, recurved, ruffled-margined tepals, in early and mid-summer. ↕50cm (20in), ↔45cm (18in). ❄❄❄

***H.* 'Siloam Ethel Smith'.** Compact, evergreen perennial, free-flowering once established. Circular, creamy beige flowers, 9cm (3½in) across, with flat tepals, recurved at the tips, and large, triangular, red, yellow, and olive-green eyes, are produced on erect scapes in midsummer. ↕50cm (20cm), ↔45cm (18in). ❄❄❄

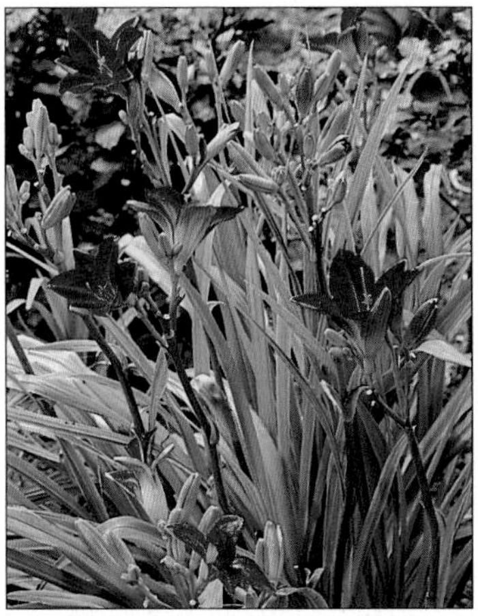
Hemerocallis 'Lusty Leland'

***H.* 'Siloam Grace Stamile'.** Compact, evergreen perennial. In midsummer, erect scapes bear circular, deep red flowers, 6cm (2½in) across, with deeper red eyes and green throats. ↕↔40cm (16in). ❄❄❄

***H.* 'Siloam Merle Kent'** ■ Compact, evergreen perennial with erect scapes. In midsummer, bears circular, bright mauve-pink flowers, 9cm (3½in) across, with deep purple eyes and green throats. ↕↔45cm (18in). ❄❄❄

***H.* 'Siloam Tiny Mite'.** Compact, free-flowering, evergreen perennial with circular, deep gold flowers, 6cm (2½in) across, which have recurved tepals and dark burgundy-red eyes; they are borne on erect scapes in midsummer. ↕↔40cm (16in). ❄❄❄

***H.* 'Siloam Ury Winniford'** ■ Vigorous, free-flowering, compact, evergreen perennial with well-branched scapes. In early and midsummer, these bear remontant, circular to triangular, deep cream flowers, 10cm (4in) across, with red-purple or rich purple eyes and green throats. ↕50cm (20in), ↔60cm (24in). ❄❄❄

***H.* 'Siloam Virginia Henson'** ■ Free-flowering, compact, evergreen perennial. In early and midsummer, well-branched scapes bear remontant, circular, pink-tinted cream flowers, 10cm (4in) across, with flat tepals, recurved at the tips, and ruby-red eyes. ↕↔40cm (16in). ❄❄❄

***H.* 'Smoky Mountain Autumn'.** Free-flowering, evergreen perennial with narrow leaves. Circular, copper-pink flowers, 14cm (5½in) across, with recurved tepals, lavender-pink haloes, and yellow-green throats, are borne on slender scapes in midsummer. ↕45cm (18in), ↔60cm (24in). ❄❄❄

***H.* 'Solano Bulls Eye'** ■ Vigorous, free-flowering, evergreen perennial with erect scapes. These bear circular, bright yellow flowers, 16cm (6in) across, with deep brownish purple eyes, over a long period from early to late summer. ↕50cm (20in), ↔75cm (30in). ❄❄❄

***H.* 'Stafford'** ■ Free-flowering, evergreen perennial with narrow leaves. In midsummer, slender scapes bear star-shaped scarlet flowers, 10cm (4in) across, with yellow midribs and throats. ↕70cm (28in), ↔1m (3ft). ❄❄❄

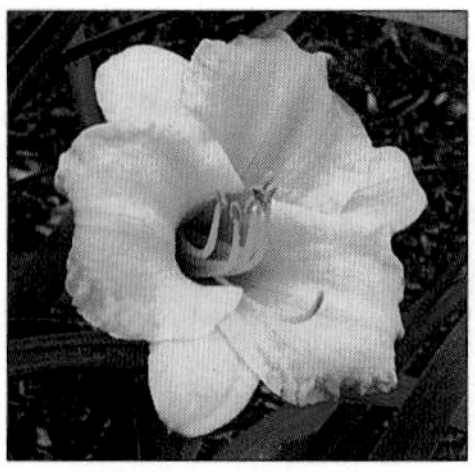
Hemerocallis 'Stella de Oro'

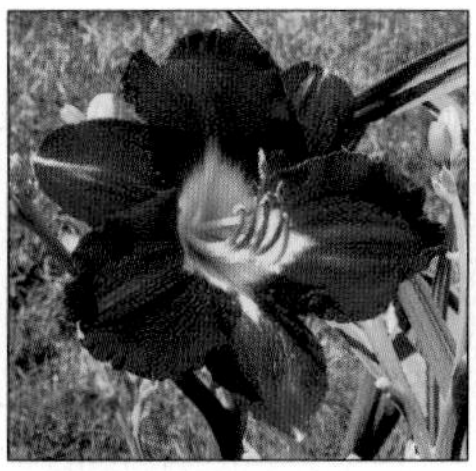
Hemerocallis 'Super Purple'

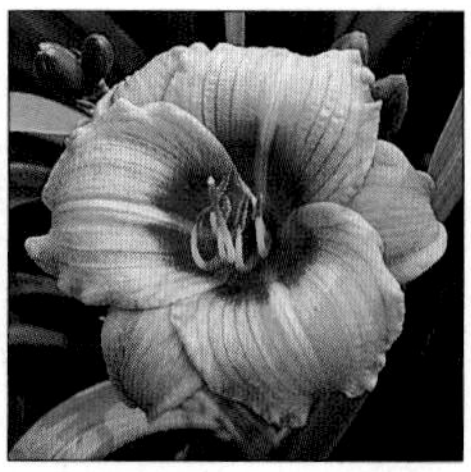
Hemerocallis 'Taffy Tot'

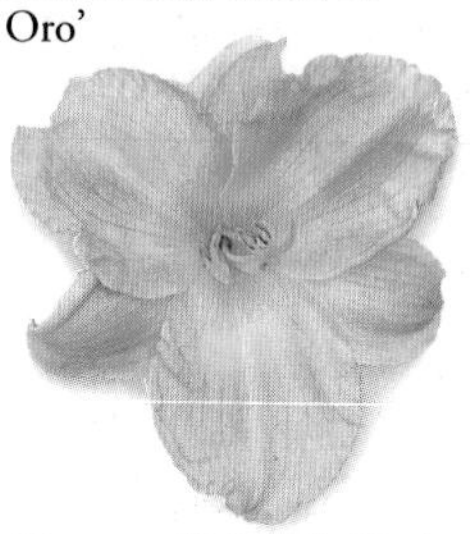
Hemerocallis 'Tonia Gay'

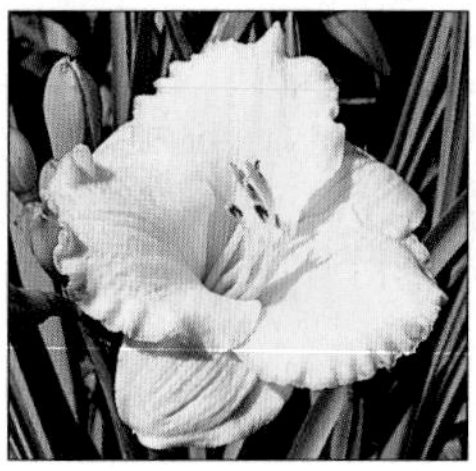
Hemerocallis 'Unique Style'

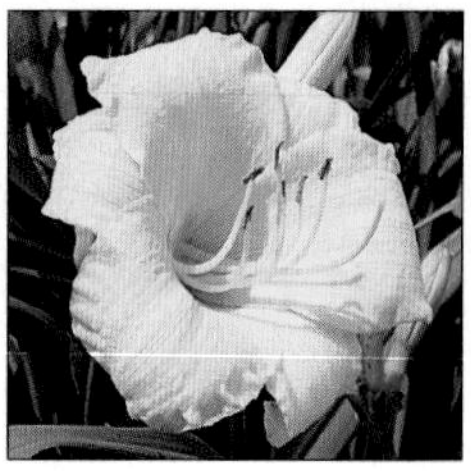
Hemerocallis 'Yellow Lollipop'

***H.* 'Stella de Oro'** ■ ♕ Vigorous, free-flowering, evergreen perennial bearing remontant, circular, bright yellow flowers, 6cm (2½in) across, on slender scapes in early summer. ↕ 30cm (12in), ↔ 45cm (18in). ❄❄❄

***H.* 'Strutter's Ball'.** Free-flowering, evergreen perennial with dense foliage. Erect scapes bear triangular, rich deep blue-purple flowers, 15cm (6in) across, in midsummer. ↕ 70cm (28in), ↔ 60cm (24in). ❄❄❄

***H.* 'Sugar Cookie'.** Evergreen perennial with erect scapes bearing circular, ivory flowers, 9cm (3½in) across, with recurved tepals and green throats, in midsummer. ↕ 50cm (20in), ↔ 45cm (18in). ❄❄❄

***H.* 'Superlative'.** Vigorous, evergreen, free-flowering perennial with slender, semi-erect leaves. In midsummer, erect scapes bear circular, deep red flowers, 14cm (5½in) across, with deep green throats. ↕↔ 60cm (24in). ❄❄❄

***H.* 'Super Purple'** ■ Semi-evergreen, extended-blooming perennial. In midsummer, erect scapes bear circular, deep purple flowers, 14cm (5½in) across, with lime-green and yellow throats. ↕ 65cm (26in), ↔ 75cm (30in). ❄❄

***H.* 'Taffy Tot'** ■ Compact, evergreen perennial with erect scapes bearing circular, light orange-buff flowers, 7cm (3in) across, with brown eyes and yellow throats, in midsummer. ↕↔ 45cm (18in). ❄❄❄

***H. thunbergii*,** syn. *H. vespertina*. Semi-evergreen, robust perennial with narrow leaves. In late summer, well-branched, slender scapes bear nocturnal, star-shaped, fragrant, lemon-yellow flowers, 9–11cm (3½–4½in) across, with green throats and green-backed outer tepals. ↕ 1.1m (3½ft), ↔ 1m (3ft). China, Korea. ❄❄❄

***H.* 'Timeless Fire'.** Evergreen perennial with wide leaves. Nocturnal, triangular, bright red flowers, 13cm (5in) across, later becoming deep orange-red, with wide, yellow-green throats, are produced on erect scapes in midsummer. ↕↔ 45cm (18in). ❄❄❄

***H.* 'Tobacco Road'.** Semi-evergreen perennial with light green leaves. In midsummer, sturdy scapes bear circular, wide-open, bright orange flowers, 18cm (7in) across, with wide, rounded, brownish pink eyes and green throats. ↕ 70cm (28in), ↔ 75cm (30in). ❄❄❄

***H.* 'Tonia Gay'** ■ Free-flowering, evergreen perennial, vigorous once established. In midsummer, erect scapes bear triangular, glistening, light pink flowers, 14cm (5½in) across, with light yellow and green throats. ↕ 40cm (16in), ↔ 75cm (30in). ❄❄❄

***H.* 'Unique Style'** ■ Evergreen perennial with erect scapes bearing circular, greenish yellow flowers, 9cm (3½in) across, in midsummer. The rounded, ruffled yellow tepals have amber margins. ↕ 55cm (22in), ↔ 75cm (30in). ❄❄❄

H. vespertina see *H. thunbergii*.

***H.* 'White Temptation'** ■ Semi-evergreen perennial with slender scapes bearing circular, off-white flowers, 13cm (5in) across, with green throats and lightly ruffled-margined tepals, in midsummer. ↕ 80cm (32in), ↔ 75cm (30in). ❄❄❄

***H.* 'Wind Song'.** Semi-evergreen perennial with abundant wide leaves. Nocturnal, circular, creamy yellow flowers, 15cm (6in) across, are produced on sturdy scapes in early and midsummer. ↕ 70cm (28in), ↔ 1m (3ft). ❄❄❄

***H.* 'Yellow Lollipop'** ■ Compact, free-flowering, evergreen perennial with very narrow leaves. Remontant, circular, bright yellow flowers, 6cm (2½in) across, are produced on erect scapes in early summer. ↕ 28cm (11in), ↔ 60cm (24in). ❄❄❄

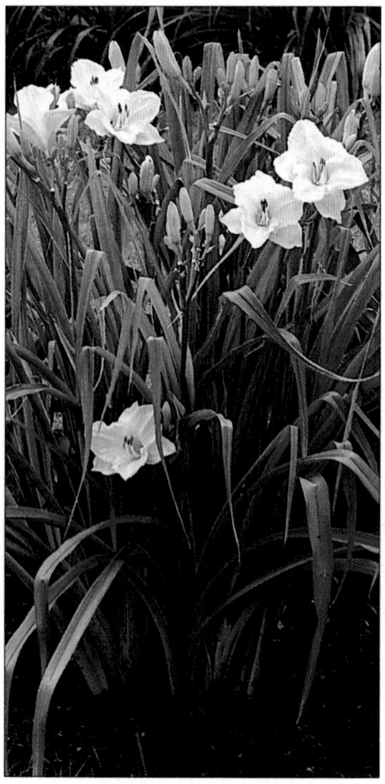
Hemerocallis 'White Temptation'

HEMIGRAPHIS

ACANTHACEAE

Genus of 90 species of low-growing, slender-stemmed annuals, perennials, and subshrubs from woodland margins in tropical Asia. They are grown mainly for their colourful, opposite, toothed or scalloped leaves, which are useful for ground cover. From spring to summer, small, tubular, 5-lobed, usually white flowers are borne in terminal spikes. In frost-prone areas, grow in a temperate greenhouse or conservatory; some species are suitable for use in hanging baskets. In warmer climates, grow in a border or as edging.

- **HARDINESS** Frost tender.
- **CULTIVATION** Under glass, grow in loamless or loam-based potting compost (JI No.3) in bright filtered light, with moderate to high humidity. In growth, water freely and apply a balanced liquid fertilizer monthly; keep moist in winter. Outdoors, grow in any fertile, moist but well-drained soil in partial shade. Shelter from strong winds. Cut back established plants in spring.
- **PROPAGATION** Root softwood or stem-tip cuttings in summer or autumn. Separate rooted stems in spring.
- **PESTS AND DISEASES** Whiteflies may be a problem.

***H. alternata*,** syn. *H. colorata* (Red flame ivy). Slightly hairy, evergreen perennial with prostrate stems that root down freely. The heart-shaped to ovate, scalloped leaves, 9cm (3½in) long, are silver-grey above and purple beneath. White flowers, 1.5cm (½in) across, are produced in terminal spikes, 2.5cm (1in) long, from spring to summer. ↕ 15cm (6in), ↔ 45cm (18in). India, Indonesia (Java). ❁ (min. 10°C/50°F)

H. colorata see *H. alternata*.

***H.* 'Exotica'** (Purple waffle plant). Compact, evergreen perennial producing ovate, hairless, purplish green leaves, 9cm (3½in) long, puckered between the veins, with a purple sheen and deep red beneath. White flowers, 1cm (½in) across, are borne in terminal spikes, 6cm (2½in) long, from spring to summer. ↕ 23cm (9in), ↔ 50cm (20in). ❁ (min. 10°C/50°F)

H. repanda ■ Creeping, evergreen perennial with slender, maroon or red stems that root down freely. The narrowly lance-shaped, toothed leaves, to 5cm (2in) long, are red-flushed greyish green, shading to purple above, and darker purple beneath. White flowers, 1.5cm (½in) across, are borne in dense spikes, 5cm (2in) long, from spring to summer. ↕ 23cm (9in), ↔ 45cm (18in). Malaysia. ❁ (min. 10°C/50°F)

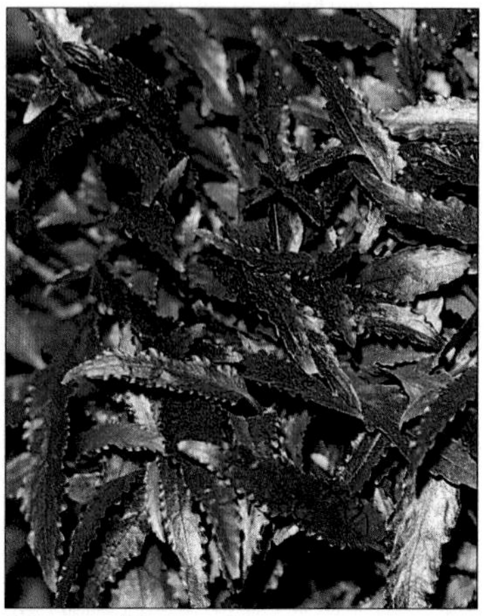
Hemigraphis repanda

HEMIONITIS

PTERIDACEAE

Genus of 7 or 8 species of evergreen ferns, with short rhizomes, mainly from moist, shaded sites in tropical Asia and America. The crowded, rounded, heart-shaped or palmate fronds are usually borne on shining black stalks. Sori form a network of lines on the lower surfaces of fertile fronds, which are narrower than sterile ones. Small plantlets often develop on the main veins of the fronds, near the bases. In temperate regions, grow in a warm greenhouse or as houseplants. In warmer areas, grow as edging or at the front of a border, in containers outdoors, or in a raised bed.

- **HARDINESS** Frost tender.
- **CULTIVATION** Under glass, grow in 1 part each of loam, medium-grade bark, and charcoal, 2 parts sharp sand, and 3 parts coarse leaf mould. Provide bright filtered light. Water moderately in the growing season and keep fairly dry in winter; avoid overwatering, as plants are prone to root rot when waterlogged. Outdoors, grow in fertile, moist but well-drained soil in partial shade. Protect from strong winds. Will tolerate dry conditions.
- **PROPAGATION** Sow spores at 19–24°C (66–75°F) as soon as ripe, or detach and pot up plantlets or bulbils. See also p.51.
- **PESTS AND DISEASES** Trouble free.

***H. arifolia*.** Rhizomatous fern with tufted, simple fronds that have heart- or spear-shaped, glossy, mid-green blades, 5–15cm (2–6in) long, on shining black stalks. Sterile fronds are ovate to oblong, deeply heart- or spear-shaped at the bases, leathery above, hairy and scaly beneath. Fertile fronds are long-stalked and oblong to triangular. ↕ 15cm (6in), ↔ to 20cm (8in). S.E. Asia. ❁ (min. 6°C/43°F)

***H. elegans*,** syn. *Doryopteris elegans*. Rhizomatous fern producing tufted, palmately lobed, dull, dark green fronds, to 18cm (7in) long, with lance-shaped to triangular segments. Sterile fronds are broad; fertile fronds are more deeply lobed. ↕ 25cm (10in), ↔ to 30cm (12in). Mexico. ❁ (min. 6°C/43°F)

▷**Hemlock** see *Tsuga*
Carolina see *T. caroliniana*
Eastern see *T. canadensis*
Mountain see *T. mertensiana*
Northern Japanese see *T. diversifolia*
Southern Japanese see *T. sieboldii*
Western see *T. heterophylla*

▷ **Hemp,**
African see *Sparrmannia africana*
Bowstring see *Sansevieria*
Indian see *Hibiscus cannabinus*
▷ **Hemp agrimony** see *Eupatorium, E. cannabinum*
▷ **Hempweed, Climbing** see *Mikania scandens*
▷ **Hen and chickens houseleek** see *Jovibarba sobolifera*
▷ **Henbane** see *Hyoscyamus, H. niger*
Black see *H. niger*
▷ **Henna tree** see *Lawsonia*

HEPATICA

RANUNCULACEAE

Genus, allied to *Anemone*, of about 10 species of spring-flowering perennials from woodland in N. temperate regions. They have usually kidney-shaped, 3- to 5-lobed, simple or toothed, dark green, basal leaves, often purple beneath, and sometimes marbled silver or white. The solitary, bowl- to star-shaped flowers usually open before the leaves have fully developed. They have brightly coloured, petal-like sepals with an involucre of 3 leaf-like bracts immediately beneath them. Suitable for a shady site in a rock or woodland garden.

• **HARDINESS** Fully hardy.
• **CULTIVATION** Grow in humus-rich, moist but well-drained, neutral to alkaline soil in partial shade; hepaticas thrive in heavy soils. Top-dress each year with leaf mould or garden compost in autumn, or in late spring after flowering. Hepaticas do not transplant easily.
• **PROPAGATION** Sow seed in an open frame as soon as ripe. Divide in spring; divisions are slow to re-establish.
• **PESTS AND DISEASES** Young growth is vulnerable to slug and snail damage.

H. acutiloba. Slow-growing perennial producing rounded or kidney-shaped, 3- to 7-lobed, mid-green leaves, 4–8cm (1½–3in) long, the lobes deeply cut and sharply pointed. In early spring, bears cup-shaped, blue, pink, or white

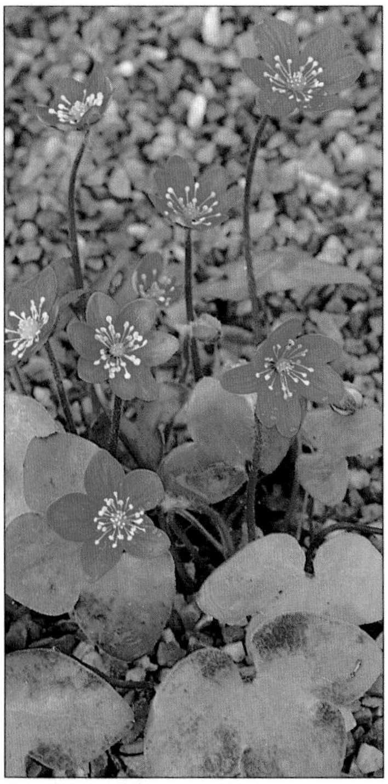

Hepatica nobilis

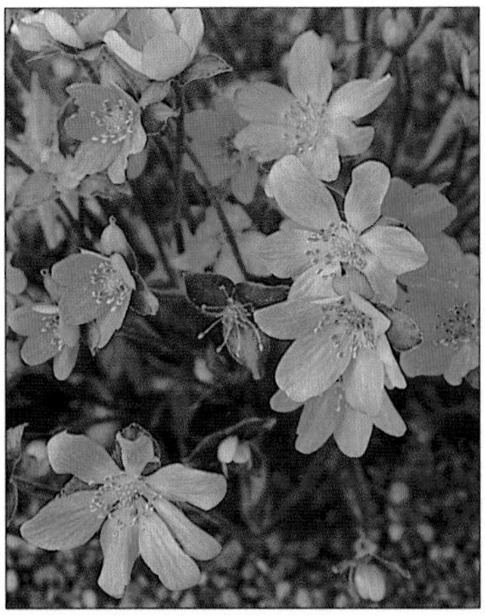

Hepatica nobilis var. *japonica*

flowers, 1–2.5cm (½–1in) across. ↕ 8cm (3in), ↔ to 15cm (6in). E. USA. ❄❄❄
H. angulosa see *H. transsilvanica.*
***H. x media* 'Ballardii'** ♀ Dome-shaped, slow-growing perennial with rounded, 3-lobed, long-stalked, soft, mid-green leaves, to 10cm (4in) long. Cup-shaped, semi-double, deep blue flowers, to 3cm (1¼in) across, are borne in early spring. ↕ 15cm (6in), ↔ to 20cm (8in). ❄❄❄
H. nobilis ■ ♀ syn. *Anemone hepatica, H. triloba.* Slow-growing, semi-evergreen, dome-shaped perennial producing rounded or kidney-shaped, mid-green leaves, 3–6cm (1¼–2½in) long, with 3 ovate, entire lobes, silky-hairy and purple-tinted beneath. Open bowl-shaped, white, pink, blue, or blue-purple flowers, to 2.5cm (1in) across, each with 6 or 7 sepals, are borne in early spring, mainly before the leaves. ↕ 10cm (4in) ↔ 15cm (6in). Europe. ❄❄❄. **var. *japonica*** ■ is smaller, producing dark green leaves with pointed lobes and flowers that are more star-shaped, each with 6–9 white, pink, or blue tepals; ↕ to 8cm (3in); Japan. **'Rubra Plena'** bears fully double, deep purplish red flowers. ❄❄❄
H. transsilvanica ♀ syn. *H. angulosa.* Semi-evergreen, slow-spreading perennial producing hairy, pale green leaves, 6–10cm (2½–4in) long, with 3 ovate, scalloped lobes. In early spring, bears many-petalled, open bowl-shaped, blue, white, or very pale pink flowers, to 4cm (1½in) across. ↕ to 15cm (6in), ↔ to 20cm (8in). Romania. ❄❄❄
H. triloba see *H. nobilis.*

▷ **Herald's trumpet** see *Beaumontia grandiflora*
▷ **Herb Christopher** see *Actaea spicata*

HERBERTIA

IRIDACEAE

Genus of 6 species of cormous perennials from dry slopes and rocky areas of temperate South America. They have lance-shaped, pleated, mid- to deep green, basal leaves. A succession of short-lived, iris-like flowers, 2–4cm (¾–1½in) across, is borne for several weeks from winter to spring. In frost-prone areas, grow in a cool greenhouse; elsewhere, grow at the front of a border or in a sheltered site in a rock garden.

• **HARDINESS** Half hardy, but tolerates occasional temperatures to -5°C (23°F).
• **CULTIVATION** Plant corms 10cm (4in) deep in autumn for spring flowering, or

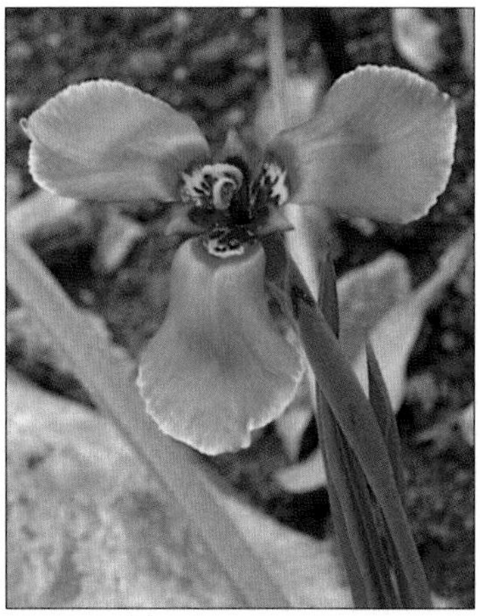

Herbertia lahue

in spring for summer flowering. Under glass, grow in loam-based potting compost (JI No.2) with additional sharp sand and leaf mould, in full light. When in leaf, water freely and apply a balanced liquid fertilizer monthly; keep plants dry when dormant. Outdoors, grow in well-drained, humus-rich soil in full sun. Protect from excessive summer and winter wet; apply a winter mulch in frost-prone areas.
• **PROPAGATION** Sow seed in containers in a cold frame as soon as ripe. Remove offsets in late summer or autumn.
• **PESTS AND DISEASES** Trouble free.

H. lahue ■ syn. *Alophia lahue.* Bulbous perennial with erect, linear, basal leaves, 5–20cm (2–8in) long. In spring, bears a succession of pale blue and violet flowers, 2–3cm (¾–1¼in) across, each with a reflexed, cup-like centre. ↕ 15cm (6in), ↔ 5cm (2in). Chile, Argentina. ❄
H. pulchella. Bulbous perennial with erect, linear, basal leaves, to 20cm (8in) long. In spring, bears a succession of blue or lilac flowers, 5–5.5cm (2–2¼in) across, often streaked deep purple; each flower has a white central stripe, and a partially reflexed, bowl-like centre. ↕ 10–15cm (4–6in), ↔ 5cm (2in). S. Brazil, Chile. ❄

▷ **Herb Robert** see *Geranium robertianum*
▷ **Herbs** see p.39
▷ **Hercules' club** see *Aralia spinosa*

HEREROA

AIZOACEAE

Genus of about 30 species of dwarf, short-stemmed, mat-forming, perennial succulents, mostly from low, dry, hilly terrain in Namibia and South Africa. The opposite, fleshy leaves are joined at the bases, and are wedge-shaped and expanded towards the tips. The scented, daisy-like, usually yellow flowers open mainly by day, in summer. In frost-prone areas, grow as houseplants or in a warm greenhouse. In warmer regions, use in a raised bed, in containers, or in a rock garden or desert garden.

• **HARDINESS** Frost tender.
• **CULTIVATION** Under glass, grow in standard cactus compost in full light with low humidity. When in growth, water moderately and apply a low-nitrogen liquid fertilizer monthly; keep almost dry in winter. Outdoors, grow in poor to moderately fertile, sharply drained, neutral to slightly alkaline soil in full sun. Protect from excessive winter and summer wet. See also pp.48–49.
• **PROPAGATION** Sow seed in spring at 21–24°C (70–75°F). Divide, or separate offsets, in spring or summer.
• **PESTS AND DISEASES** Prone to aphids.

H. dyeri. Compact succulent with short stems bearing cylindrical, bluish green leaves, 5cm (2in) long, keeled beneath, tapering towards the hatchet-shaped tips, and marked with raised dots. In summer, bears open bowl-shaped, golden yellow flowers, 2.5cm (1in) across. ↕ 8cm (3in), ↔ indefinite. South Africa (Eastern Cape, Western Cape, KwaZulu/Natal). ⌂ (min. 10°C/50°F)
H. hesperantha. Erect, stiff, branching succulent with almost columnar to spherical, 3-angled, fleshy, grey-green leaves, 3–5cm (1¼–2in) long, expanded at the tips and covered with dark dots. Open bowl-shaped, golden yellow flowers, to 2cm (¾in) across, are produced in summer. ↕↔ 20cm (8in). Namibia, South Africa (Northern Cape, Western Cape). ⌂ (min. 10°C/50°F)

HERMANNIA

STERCULIACEAE

Genus of at least 100 species of evergreen perennials, subshrubs, and shrubs from open, sandy sites in Africa. The leaves are alternate, and may be simple and entire, or toothed, incised, or lobed, usually with soft, star-shaped hairs. Bell-shaped flowers, each with 5 often overlapping and spirally twisted petals, are borne singly or in terminal or axillary cymes. In frost-prone areas, grow in a cool or temperate conservatory or greenhouse. In warmer areas, grow at the base of a warm, sunny wall or in a border.

• **HARDINESS** Frost tender.
• **CULTIVATION** Under glass, grow in loam-based potting compost (JI No.2) with additional sharp sand, in full light shaded from hot sun; provide low to moderate humidity. When in growth, water moderately and apply a balanced liquid fertilizer monthly; keep just moist in winter. Pot on or top-dress in spring. Outdoors, grow in fertile, moist but well-drained soil in full sun, shaded from midday sun. Protect from excessive winter wet. Pinch out the growing tips of young plants to promote bushiness. Pruning group 8; plants under glass may need restrictive pruning.
• **PROPAGATION** Sow seed at 16–19°C (61–66°F) in spring. Root softwood cuttings in late spring or semi-ripe cuttings in summer.
• **PESTS AND DISEASES** Prone to whiteflies and red spider mites under glass.

H. candicans see *H. incana.*
H. incana, syn. *H. candicans.* Bushy shrub or subshrub, becoming untidy with age unless regularly pruned. Ovate-oblong to oblong, mid-green leaves, to 3.5cm (1½in) long, have scalloped, wavy margins, and grey-white undersides covered in star-shaped, soft white hairs. From spring to summer, produces pendent yellow flowers, 1cm (½in) long, in terminal cymes, 8–15cm (3–6in) long, or sometimes singly from the leaf axils. ↕ 1m (3ft) (more if unpruned), ↔ 45–90cm (18–36in). South Africa (Western Cape). ⌂ (min. 7°C/45°F)

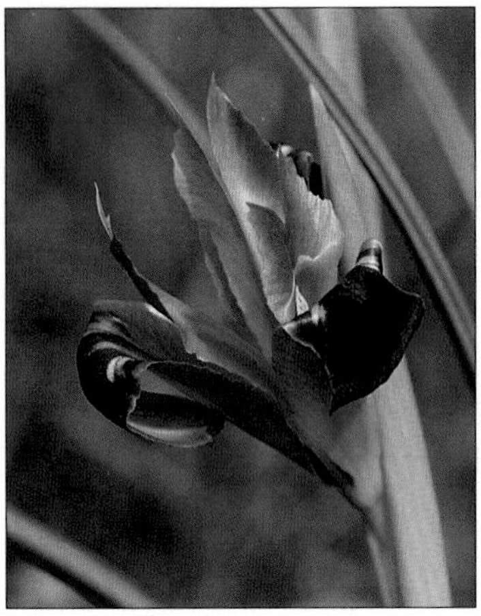

Hermodactylus tuberosus

H

HERMODACTYLUS

IRIDACEAE

Genus of one species of tuberous perennial found on dry slopes and in rocky areas from S. Europe to N. Africa, Israel, and Turkey. It has irregularly shaped, long, finger-like tubers and linear leaves. Grown for its solitary, iris-like, fragrant flowers borne in spring, *H. tuberosus* will thrive in a dry, sunny, mixed or herbaceous border, and is good for naturalizing in grass. It is also suitable for the base of a warm, sunny wall, or as an early-flowering container plant. In frost-prone areas, grow in an alpine house or bulb frame to protect the early flowers.

- **HARDINESS** Fully hardy.
- **CULTIVATION** Plant tubers 10cm (4in) deep in autumn, in moderately fertile, sharply drained, alkaline soil in full sun. Protect from excessive summer rain; needs dry summers to flower well.
- **PROPAGATION** Divide as soon as the leaves have died back in early summer.
- **PESTS AND DISEASES** Slugs and snails may be a problem.

H. tuberosus ■ syn. *Iris tuberosa* (Widow iris). Tuberous perennial with linear, bluish green or greyish green leaves, to 50cm (20in) long, and square in cross-section. In spring, bears solitary, scented, greenish yellow flowers, 5cm (2in) across, with velvety, blackish brown outer segments. ↕ 20–40cm (8–16in), ↔ 5cm (2in). S.E. France to N. Africa, Israel, and Turkey. ✲✲✲

▷**Heron's bill** see *Erodium*
▷**Herringbone plant** see *Maranta leuconeura* 'Erythroneura'

HESPERALOE

AGAVACEAE

Genus of about 3 species of perennial succulents, closely related to *Yucca*, although the flowers are more similar to those of *Aloe*. They occur in semi-arid regions of Texas, USA, and N. Mexico. Short, fleshy stems bear basal rosettes of tough, elongating, linear leaves with fibrous margins. The tall inflorescences of tubular-bell-shaped flowers are often curved and branching. In frost-prone areas, grow in a temperate greenhouse or conservatory. In warmer climates, grow in a desert garden or in containers.

- **HARDINESS** Frost tender.

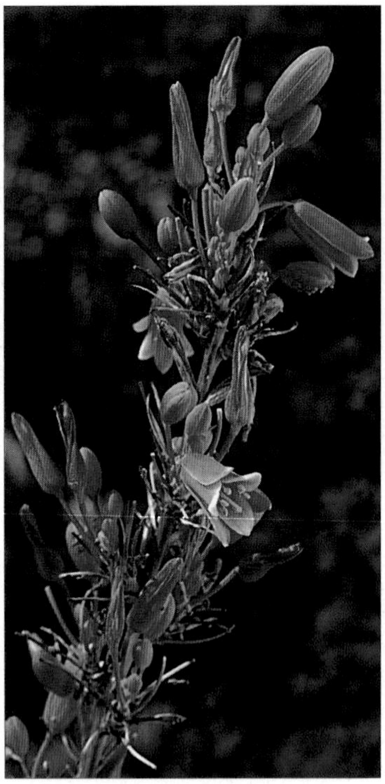

Hesperaloe parviflora

- **CULTIVATION** Under glass, grow in standard cactus compost in full light. When in growth, water moderately and apply a low-nitrogen liquid fertilizer monthly; keep completely dry in winter. Outdoors, grow in poor to moderately fertile, sharply drained, neutral to acid soil in full sun. Protect from excessive winter wet. See also pp.48–49.
- **PROPAGATION** Sow seed at 16–18°C (61–64°F), or pot up offsets, in spring.
- **PESTS AND DISEASES** Prone to scale insects and, while flowering, aphids.

H. parviflora ■ syn. *Yucca parviflora*. Clump-forming succulent with arching, linear, leathery, bright dark green leaves, 60–90cm (24–36in) long, often with peeling, fibrous margins. In summer, the upper part of the panicle-like inflorescence, 1m (3ft) or more long, bears crowded, pendent, dark to bright red flowers, to 3.5cm (1½in) long, with golden yellow throats. ↕ 1m (3ft), ↔ 2m (6ft). USA (S.W. Texas). ❀ (min. 7°C/45°F)

HESPERANTHA

IRIDACEAE

Genus of 55 species of cormous perennials from rocky and sandy areas in Africa. Those in cultivation have linear to lance-shaped, mostly mid-green, basal leaves, and bear spikes or racemes of cup- or star-shaped flowers on wiry stems in spring. In frost-prone climates, grow in a cold greenhouse. In warmer regions, grow at the front of a border, in a rock garden or trough, or at the base of a warm, sunny wall.

- **HARDINESS** Half hardy.
- **CULTIVATION** Plant corms 10–15cm (4–6in) deep in autumn. Under glass, grow in loam-based potting compost (JI No.2) with added leaf mould and grit, in full light. Provide moderate humidity and good ventilation. Water sparingly until flowering, then freely. After flowering, reduce water; keep plants dry while dormant. Outdoors, grow in fertile, well-drained soil in full sun. Protect with a dry mulch in winter.
- **PROPAGATION** Sow seed at 16–18°C (61–64°F) in autumn or spring. Separate offsets when dormant.
- **PESTS AND DISEASES** Trouble free.

H. buhrii see *H. cucullata*.
H. cucullata, syn. *H. buhrii*. Cormous perennial with 3 linear leaves, 14–21cm (5½–8in) long. Single or branched stems of up to 10 star-shaped, scented, white, pink-backed flowers, 4cm (1½in) across, are borne in spring. Flowers open during the afternoon. ↕ to 30cm (12in), ↔ 5cm (2in). South Africa. ✲
H. falcata, syn. *H. lutea*. Cormous perennial with 2–4 linear leaves, 4–8cm (1½–3in) long. In spring, branched stems bear up to 10 star-shaped flowers, 2cm (¾in) across. Flowers are usually white with red-flushed backs, but yellow variants are also known; the white flowers are scented and open at night, the yellow variants are unscented and open during the day. ↕ to 30cm (12in), ↔ 8cm (3in). South Africa. ✲
H. inflexa see *H. vaginata*.
H. lutea see *H. falcata*.
H. vaginata, syn. *H. inflexa*. Cormous perennial with 3 linear leaves, 23cm (9in) long. In spring, bears single or branched stems of up to 4 cup-shaped, clear yellow or purple-striped yellow flowers, 6cm (2½in) across, opening in the late afternoon. ↕ to 18cm (7in), ↔ 8cm (3in). South Africa. ✲

HESPERIS

BRASSICACEAE/CRUCIFERAE

Genus of about 30 species of biennials and perennials found in stony sites, wasteland, and woodland from Europe to China and Siberia. Most have ovate to spoon-shaped, entire to pinnatifid, pale to mid-green leaves. They are grown for their loose racemes or panicles of cross-shaped, 4-petalled, fragrant, purple, yellowish white, or white flowers. Cultivars with double flowers are good for cutting. Use in a mixed or herbaceous border, or in a wild garden.

- **HARDINESS** Fully hardy.
- **CULTIVATION** Grow in fertile, moist but well-drained, neutral to alkaline soil in sun or partial shade. Add leaf mould or organic matter when planting double-flowered cultivars. Replace every 2–3 years, as flowering diminishes with age.
- **PROPAGATION** Sow seed *in situ* in spring. Root basal cuttings in spring.

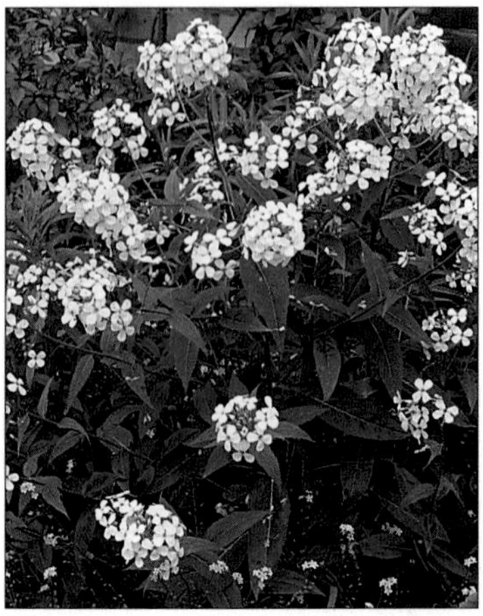

Hesperis matronalis var. *albiflora*

- **PESTS AND DISEASES** Viruses, mildew, slugs, snails, flea beetles, and caterpillars may be a problem.

H. matronalis (Dame's violet, Sweet rocket). Rosette-forming biennial or short-lived perennial with leafy stems and ovate to elliptic or oblong, toothed, hairy, dark green leaves, 10–20cm (4–8in) long. From late spring to mid-summer, bears racemes or panicles of usually lilac or purple, sometimes white or very pale lilac flowers, 3–4cm (1¼–1½in) across. Very attractive to insects. ↕ to 90cm (36in), ↔ 45cm (18in). S. Europe, Russia (Siberia), W. and C. Asia. ✲✲✲. **var. *albiflora*** ■ has white flowers, and comes true from seed if it is isolated from other colour variants. **var. *albiflora* 'Alba Plena'** bears double white flowers. **subsp. *candida*** has hairless leaves and white flowers. **'Lilacina Flore Pleno'** bears double lilac flowers. **'Purpurea Plena'** has double, dark lilac or purple flowers with neatly arranged petals.

HESPEROCALLIS

LILIACEAE

Genus of one species of bulbous perennial occurring in desert areas in S.W. USA. It has linear, wavy-margined bluish green leaves, and is valued for its terminal racemes of funnel-shaped, fragrant white flowers borne from spring to summer. In frost-prone regions, grow in a cool greenhouse. In dry, frost-free areas, use in a desert garden or at the base of a warm, sunny wall.

- **HARDINESS** Half hardy.
- **CULTIVATION** Plant in autumn with the necks of the bulbs at the soil surface. Under glass, grow in standard cactus compost in full light. In the growing season, water sparingly and apply a balanced liquid fertilizer monthly; keep completely dry in winter. Outdoors, grow in gritty, dry, neutral to slightly alkaline soil in full sun. Protect from excessive winter or summer wet.
- **PROPAGATION** Sow seed at 16–18°C (61–64°F), or remove offsets, in spring.
- **PESTS AND DISEASES** Trouble free.

H. undulata (Desert lily). Bulbous perennial with a basal cluster of linear, wavy-margined, blue-green leaves, to 30cm (12in) long. From spring to summer, produces terminal racemes of upward-facing, funnel-shaped, 6-lobed white flowers, to 7cm (3in) long, with a green central stripe on the outside of each tepal. ↕ to 30cm (12in), ↔ 15cm (6in). S.W. USA. ✲

▷***Hesperoyucca*** see *Yucca*
▷**Hesper palm** see *Brahea*
Blue see *B. armata*
San Jose see *B. brandegeei*

HETEROCENTRON

syn. HEERIA

MELASTOMATACEAE

Genus of 27 species of herbaceous perennials and low-growing, evergreen shrubs or subshrubs from open bush in Mexico and Central and South America. They have heart-shaped to lance-shaped, pale to dark green leaves, and bear open funnel-shaped, 4-petalled, white, pink, or mauve flowers singly or in panicles,

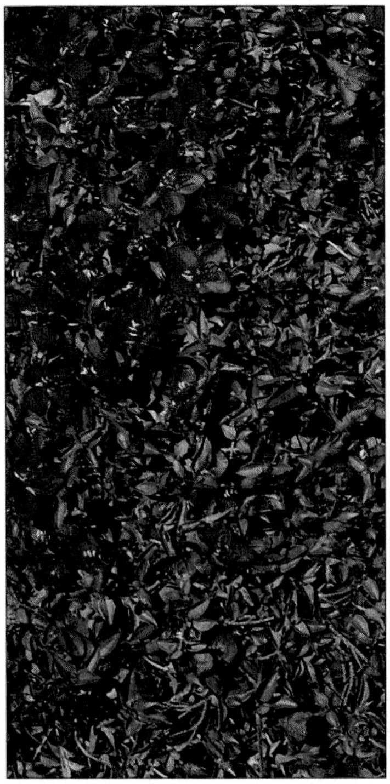

Heterocentron elegans

from summer into autumn and winter. In frost-prone areas, grow as houseplants or in a temperate greenhouse; elsewhere, use as ground cover on a sunny bank or in a rock garden.
• **HARDINESS** Frost tender.
• **CULTIVATION** Under glass, grow in loam-based potting compost (JI No.2) in full light. In growth, water freely and apply a balanced liquid fertilizer every month; keep moist in winter. Outdoors, grow in moderately fertile, well-drained soil in full sun. Pinch out the growing tips to encourage a bushy habit.
• **PROPAGATION** Sow seed at 19–24°C (66–75°F) in spring. Divide in spring, or root softwood cuttings in spring or early summer.
• **PESTS AND DISEASES** Trouble free.

H. elegans ■ (Spanish shawl). Carpet-forming, evergreen subshrub with dense, ovate to oblong-ovate, bristly to downy, mid-green leaves, to 2.5cm (1in) long. From summer to autumn, bears solitary, open funnel-shaped magenta flowers, to 5cm (2in) across. ↕10cm (4in), ↔45cm (18in). Mexico, Guatemala, Honduras. ❀ (min. 7°C/45°F)

▷ ***Heteromeles*** see *Photinia*

HETEROTHECA
syn. CHRYSOPSIS

ASTERACEAE/COMPOSITAE

Genus of about 20 species of clump-forming, erect annuals and perennials from dry, sunny sites, usually in well-drained, sandy soil, in North America. The alternate, simple, ovate to inversely lance-shaped leaves are toothed or entire, sometimes softly silver-hairy, and usually mid-green. Branched stems bear corymbs of daisy-like yellow flowerheads. Grow in a mixed or herbaceous border or in a large rock garden.
• **HARDINESS** Fully hardy to frost hardy.
• **CULTIVATION** Grow in well-drained, poor to moderately fertile soil in full sun. Protect from excessive winter wet.
• **PROPAGATION** Sow seed in containers in a cold frame in spring; if sown early, perennials may flower the same year. Divide perennials in spring.
• **PESTS AND DISEASES** Trouble free.

H. mariana, syn. *Chrysopsis mariana*. Softly grey-hairy perennial with short stolons and both decumbent and erect stems. Basal leaves are spoon-shaped to inversely lance-shaped, shallowly toothed, and to 20cm (8in) long; stem leaves are rounded to elliptic-oblong, entire, and to 3cm (1¼in) long. From midsummer to early autumn, bears corymbs of yellow flowerheads, each 4.5cm (1¾in) across. ↕to 90cm (36in), ↔50cm (20in). USA (New York State south to Florida, Texas). ❄❄❄
H. villosa, syn. *Chrysopsis villosa* (Hairy golden aster). Softly grey-hairy, sometimes rhizomatous perennial with erect to decumbent stems. Basal leaves are oblong-elliptic to lance-shaped, usually entire, occasionally toothed, and 2–4cm (¾–1½in) long; stem leaves are linear-lance-shaped and 1–3cm (½–1¼in) long. From midsummer to early autumn, bears corymbs of yellow flowerheads, each 2–4cm (¾–1½in) across. Needs a very well-drained, sunny site. ↕20–80cm (8–32in), ↔20cm (8in). W. and S. central USA. ❄❄❄

▷ ***Heterotropa*** see *Asarum*

HEUCHERA
Coral flower

SAXIFRAGACEAE

Genus of about 55 species of evergreen and semi-evergreen perennials from woodland and rocky sites in North America, chiefly the Rocky Mountains, with a few from Mexico. They have woody rootstocks and form clumps or mounds of rounded to heart-shaped, lobed, and often toothed, long-stalked, boldly veined leaves. Those with darker or paler shading or variegation are excellent foliage plants. Hybrids of *H. cylindrica*, *H. sanguinea*, and *H. micrantha* share their parents' habits and leaf characteristics. The small, sometimes petalless, tubular flowers, 2–6mm ($^1/_{16}$–¼in) long, occasionally to 10mm (½in), have conspicuous, colourful calyces, and are borne in narrow, loose racemes or panicles. Use as ground cover or in a herbaceous, mixed, or shrub border; the flowers are good for cutting and are attractive to bees.
• **HARDINESS** Fully hardy to frost hardy.
• **CULTIVATION** Grow in fertile, moist but well-drained, neutral soil in sun or partial shade; full shade may be tolerated in a moist site. The woody rootstock tends to push upwards, so mulch annually; eventually lift and replant in late summer or early autumn, with just the crown above the soil surface, or replace with new plants.
• **PROPAGATION** Sow seed of species in containers in a cold frame in spring. Divide species and cultivars in autumn.
• **PESTS AND DISEASES** Leaf eelworms, vine weevil larvae, and a gall-causing infection may be a problem.

H. americana. Mound-forming perennial with rosettes of broadly ovate to heart-shaped, 5- to 9-lobed, glossy, leathery leaves, 5–14cm (2–5½in) long.

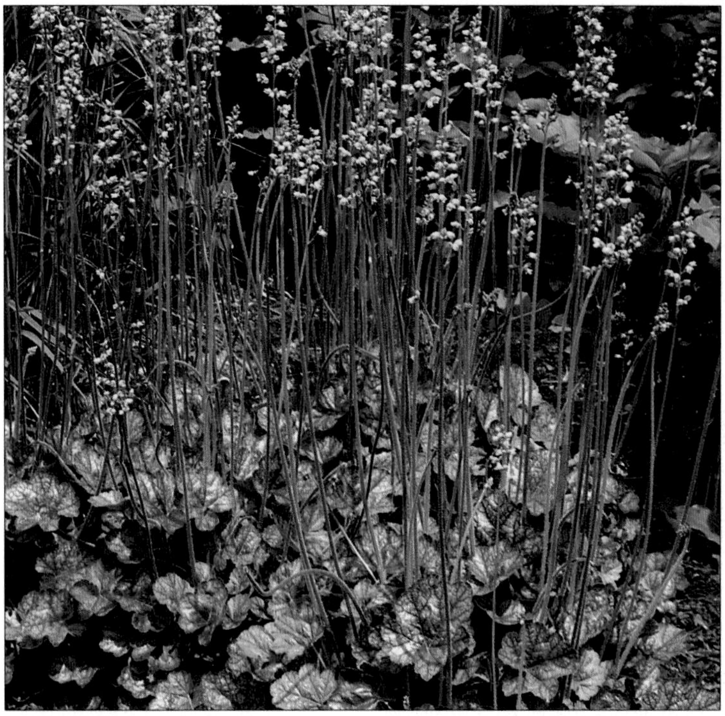

Heuchera cylindrica 'Greenfinch'

Young foliage is marbled and veined brown, maturing to deep green with copper-green shading. In early summer, bears panicles of brownish green flowers, 30cm (12in) or more long. ↕45cm (18in), ↔30cm (12in). C. and E. North America. ❄❄❄
***H.* 'Apple Blossom'.** Clump-forming perennial with leaves similar to those of *H. sanguinea*. Short-branched panicles of pale pink flowers open from rose pink buds in early summer. ↕60cm (24in), ↔30–45cm (12–18in). ❄❄❄
***H.* 'Coral Cloud'.** Clump-forming perennial producing crinkled, glistening leaves, similar to those of *H. sanguinea*. Bears wide panicles of coral-red flowers in early summer. ↕75cm (30in), ↔30cm (12in). ❄❄❄
***H. cylindrica*.** Mound-forming perennial with rounded to broadly ovate, deeply round-lobed, often hairy, dark green leaves, 2.5–8cm (1–3in) long; they have scalloped margins and metallic, paler green mottling. From mid-spring to midsummer, leafless stems bear yellowish green or cream flowers in very short-branched, spike-like panicles, to 15cm (6in) long. Good foliage plant. ↕30–50cm (12–20in), ↔30cm (12in). N.W. North America. ❄❄❄. **'Chartreuse'** has pink buds opening to large, lime-green flowers in early summer. **'Greenfinch'** ■ bears green flowers in tall, stiff, very short-branched panicles; ↕to 90cm (36in), ↔60cm (24in). **'Hyperion'** bears stiff spikes of deep pink, green-tinged flowers; ↕75cm (30in), ↔45cm (18in).
***H.* 'Dennis Davidson'** see *H.* 'Huntsman'.
***H.* 'Feuerregen'** see *H.* 'Pluie de Feu'.
***H.* 'Firebird'.** Compact, free-blooming perennial with leaves similar to those of *H. sanguinea*. In early summer, bears panicles of glowing, crimson-scarlet flowers on erect stems. ↕60cm (24in), ↔30cm (12in). ❄❄❄
***H.* 'Firefly'** ■ syn. *H.* 'Leuchtkäfer'. Clump-forming perennial with leaves similar to those of *H. sanguinea*. Bears fragrant vermilion flowers in short-branched panicles in early summer. ↕75cm (30in), ↔30cm (12in). ❄❄❄
***H.* 'Green Ivory'** ■ Clump-forming perennial with leaves similar to those of *H. cylindrica*. Strong, erect stems bear short-branched panicles of numerous green flowers in early summer. ↕↔75cm (30in). ❄❄❄

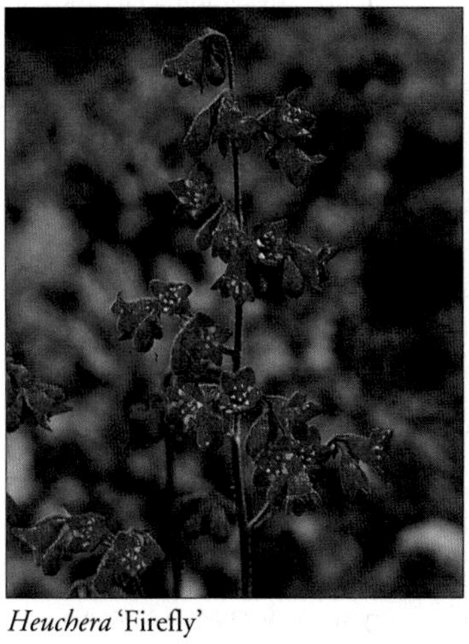

Heuchera 'Firefly'

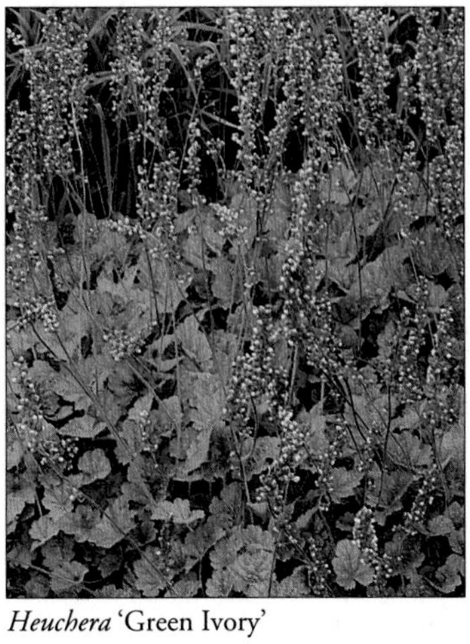

Heuchera 'Green Ivory'

H

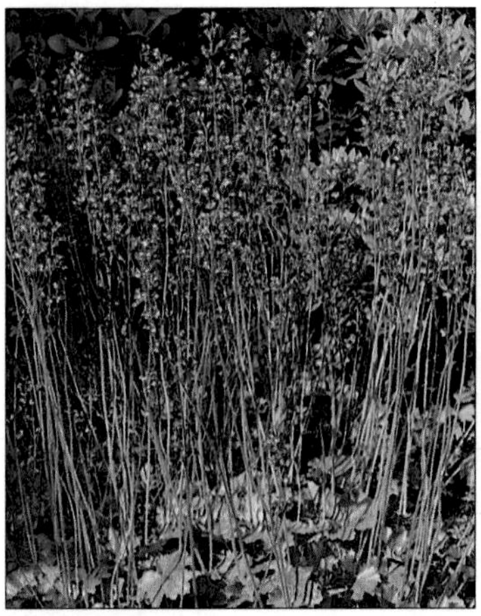

Heuchera 'Huntsman'

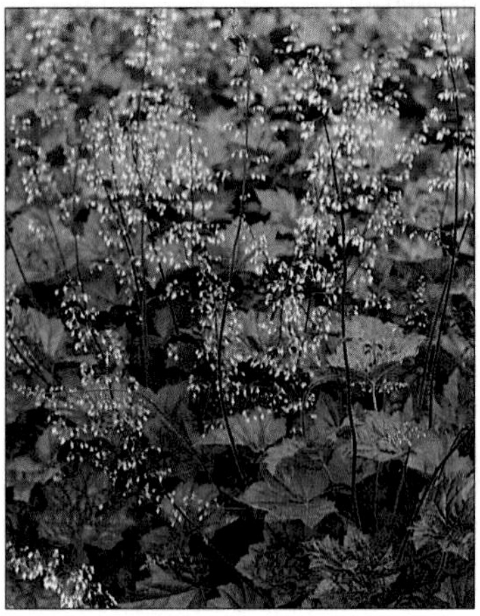

Heuchera micrantha var. *diversifolia* 'Palace Purple'

H. grossulariifolia. Clump-forming perennial producing rounded to kidney-shaped, toothed, mid-green leaves, to 6cm (2½in) long. In early summer, bears bell-shaped, pure white flowers in panicles 1–6cm (½–2½in) long. ↕10cm (4in), ↔ to 15cm (6in). W. USA. ❄❄❄
***H.* 'Huntsman'** ■ syn. *H.* 'Dennis Davidson'. Clump-forming perennial with leaves similar to those of *H. sanguinea.* Short-branched panicles of bright red flowers open in early summer. ↕↔ 30–45cm (12–18in). ❄❄❄
***H.* 'Leuchtkäfer'** see *H.* 'Firefly'.
H. micrantha. Mound- or clump-forming perennial with ovate to heart-shaped, shallowly 5- to 7-lobed, hairy, grey-marbled leaves, 2–8cm (¾–3in) long. In early summer, bears loose panicles, to 30cm (12in) or more long, of numerous tiny, tubular, pink-flushed white flowers with red anthers. ↕90cm (36in), ↔ 45cm (18in). W. North America (British Columbia to Sierra Nevada). ❄❄❄. **var. *diversifolia* 'Palace Purple'** ■𝕐 has large, jagged, glistening, almost metallic, bronze-red leaves, to 15cm (6in) long. Bears loose panicles of numerous greenish cream flowers with red anthers, which give them a salmon-pink appearance; flowers are followed by rose-pink seed heads. Many seed-raised plants do not retain the deep bronze-red leaf colour. ↕↔ 45–60cm (18–24in).
***H.* 'Mother of Pearl'.** Clump-forming perennial with leaves similar to those of *H. sanguinea.* Panicles of pink-flushed white flowers are borne in early summer. ↕60cm (24in), ↔ 30cm (12in). ❄❄❄

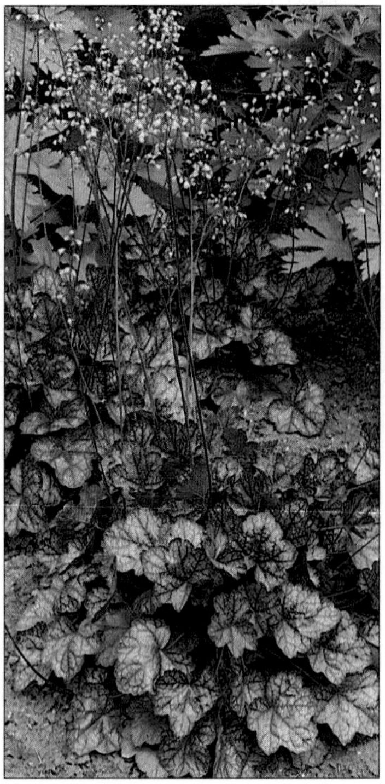

Heuchera 'Pewter Moon'

***H.* 'Pearl Drops'.** Clump-forming perennial with leaves similar to those of *H. sanguinea.* Bears dainty, arching panicles of pink-tinged white flowers in early summer. ↕60cm (24in), ↔ 30cm (12in). ❄❄❄
***H.* 'Pewter Moon'** ■ Clump-forming perennial with leaves similar to those of *H. micrantha.* In early summer, bears panicles of large, pale pink flowers. ↕ to 40cm (16in), ↔ 30cm (12in). ❄❄❄
***H.* 'Pluie de Feu'** ■ syn. *H.* 'Feuerregen', *H.* 'Rain of Fire'. Clump-forming perennial with leaves similar to those of *H. sanguinea.* Bears narrow panicles of bright red flowers from early to late summer. ↕50cm (20in), ↔ 30cm (12in). ❄❄❄
***H.* 'Rachel'.** Clump-forming perennial with leaves similar to those of *H. sanguinea.* In early summer, bears erect panicles of large, pale pink flowers. ↕↔ 30cm (12in). ❄❄❄
***H.* 'Rain of Fire'** see *H.* 'Pluie de Feu'.
***H.* 'Red Spangles'** ■𝕐 Clump-forming perennial with leaves similar to those of *H. sanguinea.* Bears short-branched, open panicles of large, scarlet-crimson flowers throughout summer. ↕50cm (20in), ↔ 25cm (10in). ❄❄❄

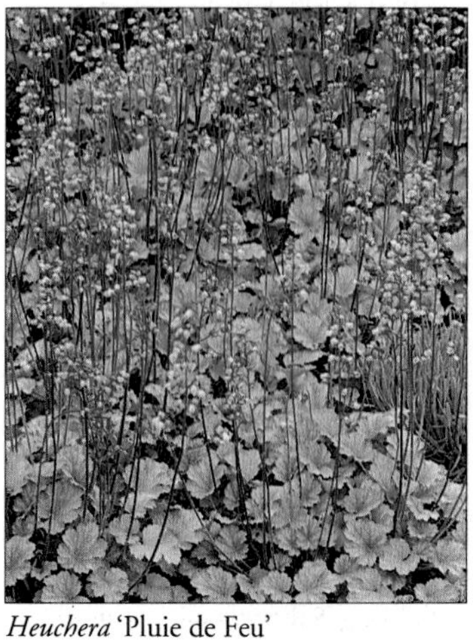

Heuchera 'Pluie de Feu'

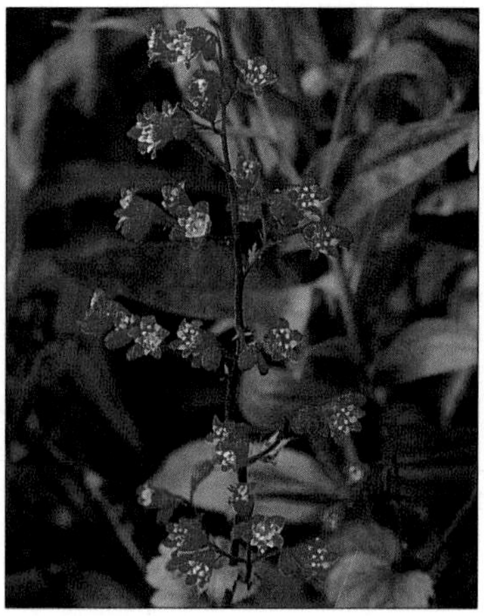

Heuchera 'Red Spangles'

H. rubescens. Clump-forming, tufted perennial with rounded to broadly ovate, deeply 3- to 7-lobed, sharp-toothed, mid-green leaves, to 5cm (2in) long. In summer, bears loose, spike-like panicles, to 15cm (6in) long, of bell-shaped, white to pale pink flowers, becoming reddish pink with age. ↕↔ to 15cm (6in). W. USA. ❄❄❄
H. sanguinea (Coral bells). Mat- or clump-forming perennial with rounded to kidney-shaped, shallowly lobed, toothed, glandular-hairy, dark green leaves, 2–8cm (¾–3in) long, marbled with pale green. In summer, bears large, tubular, red, rarely pink or white flowers in open panicles, to 15cm (6in) long. ↕↔ 30cm (12in). S.W. USA. ❄❄❄
***H.* 'Schneewittchen'.** Clump-forming perennial with leaves similar to those of *H. sanguinea.* Bears short-branched panicles of white flowers in early and midsummer. ↕50cm (20in), ↔ 25cm (10in). ❄❄❄
***H.* 'Scintillation'** 𝕐 Clump-forming perennial with leaves similar to those of *H. sanguinea.* Bears panicles of deep pink, coral-pink-rimmed flowers in early summer. ↕60cm (24in), ↔ 30cm (12in). ❄❄❄
***H.* 'Snow Storm'.** Clump- or mound-forming perennial with leaves similar to those of *H. sanguinea,* but marbled silvery white. Panicles of cerise-red flowers are borne in early summer. ↕↔ 30cm (12in). ❄❄❄
***H.* 'Taff's Joy'.** Clump-forming perennial with leaves similar to those of *H. sanguinea,* but variegated cream and tinged pink. Panicles of pink flowers are produced in early summer. ↕25–30cm (10–12in), ↔ 20cm (8in). ❄❄❄

x HEUCHERELLA

SAXIFRAGACEAE

Hybrid genus, resulting from crosses between *Heuchera* and *Tiarella,* of evergreen, mat- or clump-forming, occasionally stoloniferous perennials. They have heart-shaped or broadly ovate, lobed, boldly veined, sometimes hairy leaves, shaded brown when young and turning reddish brown in autumn. Short, loose panicles of tubular-bell-shaped, pink or white flowers, to 6mm (¼in) long, are borne over a long period from spring to autumn. They are excellent as ground cover or edging in a herbaceous, mixed, or shrub border, or for a woodland garden.
• **HARDINESS** Fully hardy.

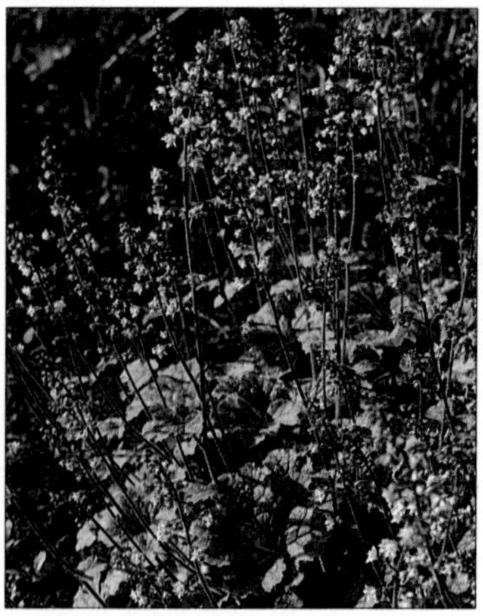

x *Heucherella tiarelloides*

• **CULTIVATION** Grow in light, fertile, moist but well-drained, neutral to slightly acid soil; sun or partial shade is best, but full shade is tolerated.
• **PROPAGATION** Divide in autumn or spring. Separate plantlets from rooted stolons in autumn.
• **PESTS AND DISEASES** Trouble free.

x *H. alba* 'Bridget Bloom'. Clump-forming perennial, lacking stolons, with broadly ovate, shallowly 7- to 9-lobed, toothed, mid-green leaves, 4–10cm (1½–4in) long, heart-shaped at the bases and marked brown along the veins. From late spring to mid-autumn, produces erect panicles of tiny white flowers, 3–5mm (⅛–¼in) long, with pink calyces. ↕ to 40cm (16in), ↔ 30cm (12in). ❄❄❄
x *H. tiarelloides* ■𝕐 (*Heuchera* x *brizoides* x *Tiarella cordifolia*). Stoloniferous, hairless perennial with rounded, shallowly lobed, toothed, light green leaves, 7–9cm (3–3½in) long, heart-shaped at the bases, and often with brown markings when young. Brownish red stems bear narrow, short-branched panicles of tiny pink flowers, to 3mm (⅛in) long, from mid-spring to early summer. ↕↔ 45cm (18in). ❄❄❄

▷ ***Hexastylis*** see *Asarum*
▷ ***Heyderia decurrens*** see *Calocedrus decurrens*
▷ **Hiba** see *Thujopsis dolabrata*

HIBBERTIA syn. CANDOLLEA

DILLENIACEAE

Genus of about 120 species of evergreen trees, shrubs, and climbers mainly from scrub, heathland, and sandy areas of Australia, but also found in Madagascar, New Guinea, New Caledonia, and Fiji. The alternate, simple, variably shaped, sometimes stem-clasping leaves have entire, wavy, or toothed margins. The saucer- to bowl-shaped, yellow, occasionally pink or white flowers each have 5 spreading, shallowly to deeply notched petals and are borne singly or in terminal or axillary, raceme-like cymes. In frost-prone areas, grow in a cool greenhouse. Elsewhere, use the shrubs in a shrub border or at the base of a warm, sunny wall; train the climbers over a pergola, arch, or arbour.
• **HARDINESS** Half hardy to frost tender.
• **CULTIVATION** Under glass, grow in loam-based potting compost (JI No.2) in bright filtered light, with moderate

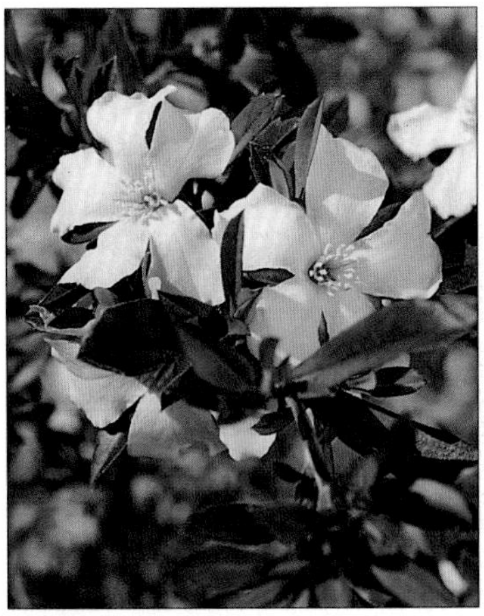
Hibbertia cuneiformis

humidity. In growth, water freely and apply a balanced liquid fertilizer monthly; keep moist in winter. Provide support for climbers. Outdoors, grow in fertile, moist but well-drained soil in partial shade, or in sun with midday shade. Pruning group 8 for shrubs; group 11 for climbers, after flowering.

• **PROPAGATION** Sow seed at 19–24°C (66–75°F) in spring. Root semi-ripe cuttings in late summer.

• **PESTS AND DISEASES** In winter, hairy species are susceptible to grey mould (*Botrytis*). Vulnerable to scale insects under glass.

H. cuneiformis ▣ syn. *Candollea cuneiformis.* Erect, freely branching, sometimes spreading and twining shrub with oblong to narrowly obovate, bright green leaves, 2.5–5cm (1–2in) long, often toothed at the tips. From late winter to spring, short, lateral shoots bear solitary, rich yellow flowers, 1.5–4.5cm (½–1¾in) across, with shallowly notched petals. Tolerates full shade and desert conditions. ↕ 1–2m (3–6ft), ↔ 1–1.5m (3–5ft). Australia (coast of Western Australia). ❀ (min. 5°C/41°F)

H. dentata. Trailing or twining shrub or subshrub with red-flushed green stems. Elliptic-oblong to oblong, sparsely toothed, sometimes wavy-margined leaves, 5–9cm (2–3½in) long, are bronze-red or purple-tinted when young, becoming glossy, deep green when mature. From late winter to summer, bears solitary, terminal flowers, 3–5cm (1¼–2in) across, with shallowly notched, bright yellow petals. Good for a hanging basket. ↕↔ 1–2m (3–6ft). Australia (New South Wales, Victoria). ❀ (min. 3–5°C/37–41°F)

H. scandens ▣ 🏆 syn. *H. volubilis.* Vigorous shrub with procumbent or twining, reddish brown stems and silky-hairy shoots. Elliptic or oblong-elliptic to obovate, leathery leaves, to 10cm (4in) long, are entire or shallowly toothed near the tips; they are usually glossy, rich green above, paler and silky-hairy beneath. Solitary, terminal, pale to bright yellow flowers, 5–7cm (2–3in) across, with slightly notched petals, are borne mainly in summer. Suitable as ground cover. Thrives in coastal sites. ↕ 3–6m (10–20ft), ↔ 1.5–2.5m (5–8ft). Australia (Northern Territory, Queensland, New South Wales, often coastal). ❀ (min. 5°C/41°F)

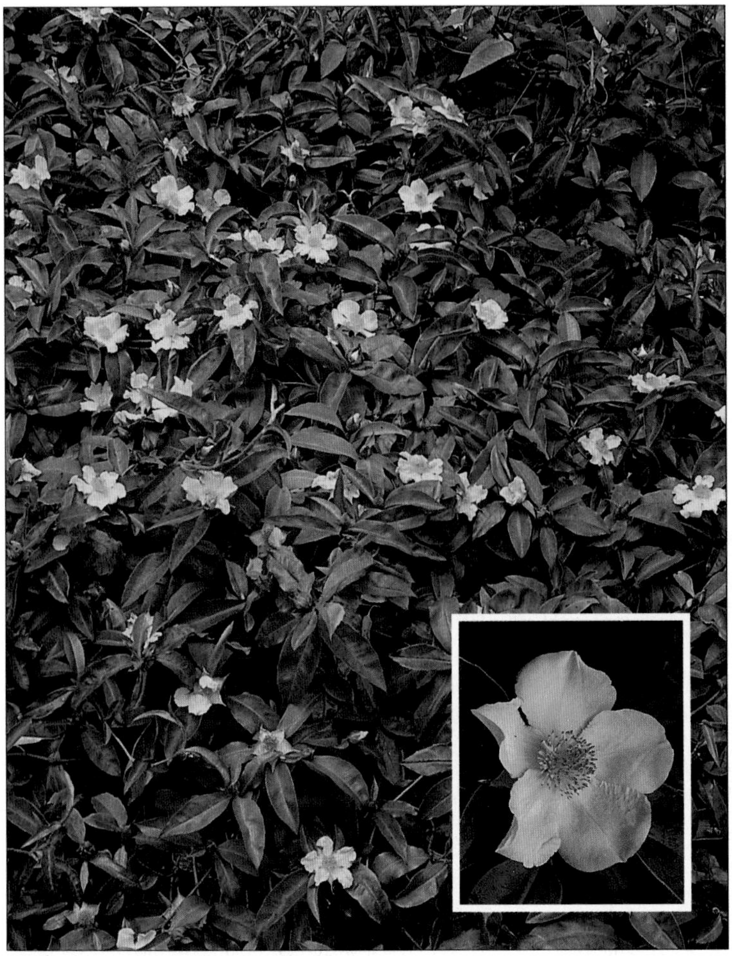
Hibbertia scandens (inset: flower detail)

H. sericea. Dwarf to small shrub, usually erect but sometimes spreading with age, producing grey, silky hairy young shoots. Narrowly linear-lance-shaped to broadly lance-shaped leaves, to 1.5cm (½in) long, are softly hairy and grey- to mid-green, the upper surfaces rough, and the margins rolled under. Pale to rich yellow flowers, 1.5–3cm (½–1¼in) across, with deeply notched, wavy-margined petals, are borne singly or in small, terminal clusters from late winter to summer. ↕ 30–120cm (12–48in), ↔ 30–90cm (12–36in). Australia (New South Wales, Victoria, Tasmania). ✲

H. volubilis see *H. scandens.*

HIBISCUS

MALVACEAE

Genus of more than 200 species of deciduous and evergreen shrubs, trees, annuals, and herbaceous perennials widely distributed in warm-temperate, subtropical, and tropical regions, where they occur in a variety of habitats including streamsides, moist woodland, and dry, rocky sites. They have alternate, entire or shallowly to palmately lobed, sometimes toothed leaves, and are grown for their showy, mainly funnel-shaped, solitary or clustered flowers, borne over a long period from spring to autumn. The flowers are red, pink, purple, blue, yellow, or white, and sometimes have contrasting marks at the bases of the petals, and prominent, colourful stamens. Grow in a sunny mixed, herbaceous, or shrub border; in frost-prone areas, grow tender species and cultivars in a temperate or warm greenhouse. Some perennials may be grown as annuals.

• **HARDINESS** Fully hardy to frost tender.

• **CULTIVATION** Under glass, grow in loamless or loam-based potting compost (JI No.2) in bright filtered light. Provide moderate humidity and good ventilation. In the growing season, water freely and apply a balanced liquid fertilizer monthly; water sparingly in winter. Outdoors, grow in humus-rich, moist but well-drained, neutral to slightly alkaline soil in full sun. Hibiscus need long, hot summers to flower well. Those grown at the limits of their hardiness level need mulching in winter. *H. mutabilis* will regenerate from its woody base if cut back by frost. Pruning group 1 for deciduous hibiscus, group 9 for evergreens; however, little or no pruning is usually necessary.

• **PROPAGATION** Sow seed at 13–18°C (55–64°F) in spring. Divide perennials in spring. Root greenwood cuttings of shrubs in late spring, or semi-ripe cuttings in summer. Layer in spring or summer.

• **PESTS AND DISEASES** Aphids, scale insects, mealybugs, whiteflies, and powdery mildew may be a problem, especially under glass.

H. abelmoschus see *Abelmoschus moschatus.*

H. acetosella, syn. *H. eetveldeanus.* Upright, bushy, fast-growing annual or short-lived, woody-based perennial producing long-stalked, broadly ovate, unlobed or 3- to 5-lobed, often red-flushed, mid-green leaves, to 30cm (12in) long. Solitary, axillary, funnel-shaped, yellow or purple-red flowers, 6–10cm (2½–4in) across, with deep purple centres, are borne from late summer to autumn. ↕ 0.6–1.5m (2–5ft), ↔ to 1m (3ft). C. and E. Africa. ✲. **'Coppertone'** ▣ syn. *H.* 'Red Shield', has brilliant maroon-purple leaves.

H. arnottianus ⚲ Rounded, usually fairly open, evergreen, large shrub or small tree with ovate, entire or toothed, leathery, dark green leaves, to 25cm (10in) long. Solitary, lightly scented, funnel-shaped white flowers, 10–18cm (4–7in) across, with pink veins and central sheaves of red stamens, are produced from the leaf axils in summer. ↕ 3–8m (10–25ft), ↔ 2–6m (6–20ft). Hawaii. ❀ (min. 15°C/59°F). **'Wilder's White'** has pure white flowers.

H. calyphyllus. Woody-based, evergreen perennial or shrub producing leaves and young shoots covered with soft, star-shaped hairs. The broadly ovate, entire or shallowly 3-lobed, occasionally 5-lobed, rich green leaves, to 12cm (5in) long, have pointed to rounded teeth. Axillary, solitary, funnel-shaped, sulphur-yellow flowers, 7–13cm (3–5in) across, with maroon or brownish red eyes, are produced from spring to autumn. ↕ to 3m (10ft), ↔ 1.5–2m (5–6ft). Tropical to southern Africa, Madagascar, Mascarene Islands. ❀ (min. 15°C/59°F)

H. cannabinus (Indian hemp, Kenaf). Erect, almost unbranched, fast-growing, minutely spiny-stemmed annual or short-lived, woody-based perennial. Long-stalked, ovate, dark green upper leaves, to 15cm (6in) long, are palmately 3- to 7-lobed; leaves lower down the stems are unlobed. Axillary, funnel-shaped, pale yellow, occasionally purple-red flowers, 8–15cm (3–6in) across, with crimson-red centres, are borne singly or in few-flowered racemes from summer to autumn. ↕ 1–3.5m (3–11ft), ↔ to 1.5m (5ft). Origin uncertain, possibly Indonesia. ✲

H. eetveldeanus see *H. acetosella.*

H. huegelii see *Alyogyne huegelii.*

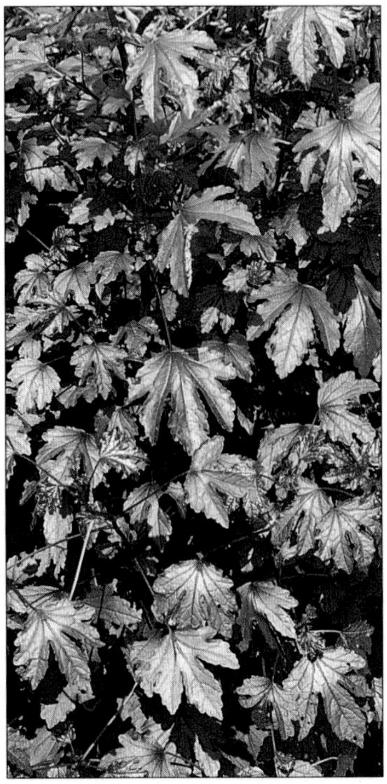
Hibiscus acetosella 'Coppertone'

H

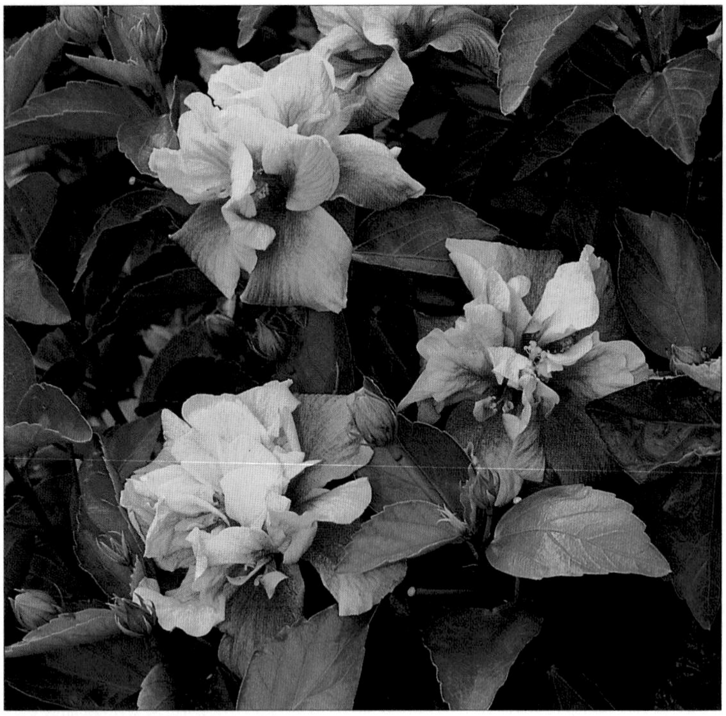

Hibiscus rosa-sinensis 'Crown of Bohemia'

H. moscheutos ■ (Common rose mallow, Swamp rose mallow). Strong-growing, woody-based perennial with erect stems. Produces broadly ovate to lance-shaped, unlobed or shallowly 3- to 5-lobed, toothed, mid-green leaves, 8–23cm (3–9in) long, white-hairy beneath. Widely funnel-shaped flowers, to 20cm (8in) across, with spreading petals, are white, pink, or crimson, sometimes with crimson petal bases, and borne singly from the leaf axils in summer. ↕2.5m (8ft), ↔ 1m (3ft). S. USA. ❀ (min. 5°C/41°F). **Disco Belle Series** cultivars are compact perennials, usually treated as annuals for greenhouse display, with red, pink, or white flowers, to 23cm (9in) across; ↕to 50cm (20in). **'Southern Belle'** has toothed leaves and dark red flowers, 20cm (8in) across, with paler red margins; ↕to 1m (3ft).
H. mutabilis ⚠ (Confederate rose mallow, Cotton rose). Erect to spreading, usually freely branching, evergreen, large shrub or small tree with stems covered in soft, star-shaped hairs. Broadly ovate to rounded, palmately 3- to 7-lobed, toothed leaves, to 17cm (7in) long, are rich green above, and covered with star-shaped hairs beneath. Funnel-shaped, white or pink flowers, 8–12cm (3–5in) across, sometimes with darker pink bases, are produced singly or in few-flowered, terminal clusters from the leaf axils from spring to autumn. ↕2–5m (6–15ft), ↔ 1.5–2.5m (5–8ft). China. ❀ (min. 13°C/55°F)
***H.* 'Red Shield'** see *H. acetosella* 'Coppertone'.
H. rosa-sinensis ⚠ (Chinese hibiscus, Hawaiian hibiscus, Rose of China). Rounded, bushy, evergreen, large shrub or small tree with hairless or slightly hairy shoots and ovate to broadly lance-shaped, glossy, dark green leaves, to 15cm (6in) long, with toothed margins. Solitary, 5-petalled, bright crimson flowers, 10cm (4in) across, with yellow-anthered red stamens, are produced from the leaf axils from summer to autumn. Flower colour is very variable in cultivation, ranging from crimson to orange, yellow, or white. ↕2.5m–5m (8–15ft), ↔ 1.5m–3m (5–10ft). Origin unknown, probably tropical Asia. ❀ (min. 10–13°C/50–55°F). Numerous cultivars have been raised, some with semi-double or double flowers. **'Agnes Galt'** ■ is upright, bushy, and very free-flowering; it bears pink flowers, 12–17cm (5–7in) across, lighter red on the petal margins, with deep rose-pink veins and stamens, and yellow anthers. **'Cooperi'** ■ is compact, with lance-shaped leaves marbled olive-green and white, sometimes tinted pink, and bearing red flowers; ↕1–2m (3–6ft). **'Crown of Bohemia'** ■ bears double, golden yellow flowers, flushed bright reddish orange in the centres, with reddish orange stamens. **'Dainty Pink'** see 'Fantasia'. **'Dainty White'**, syn. *H.* 'Swan Lake', *H.* 'White La France', has white flowers, 10cm (4in) across, with petals margined creamy pale yellow, and white stamens. **'Fantasia'**, syn. 'Dainty Pink', 'Pink La France', is free-flowering, bearing strongly veined, reddish pink flowers, 10cm (4in) across, with pink or white stamens; the outer petals are slightly fringed, margined white, and have creamy-white central zones. **'Fiesta'** has large, deep apricot-orange flowers, 18cm (7in) across, with finely waved petals, bright red and white centres, and cream stamens. **'Full Moon'** see 'Mrs. James E. Hendry'. **'Kinchen's Yellow'** ■ has yellow flowers, 12–15cm (5–6in) across, with white centres and yellow stamens. **'Mrs. James E. Hendry'**, syn. 'Full Moon', has double, lemon-yellow flowers, 15cm (6in) across, with white eyes and white veins, and deep yellow stigmas. **'Pink La France'** see 'Fantasia'. **'Scarlet Giant'** ■ has scarlet flowers, 12–17cm (5–7in) across, with red- and yellow-anthered stamens. **'The President'** ■ is erect and bushy, bearing rich red flowers, 16–18cm (6–7in) across, with darker red centres, stamens, and veins; the petals have slightly ruffled margins, and cream markings at the bases.
H. schizopetalus ■🏆 (Japanese lantern). Tall, slender, evergreen shrub with arching or pendent branches and ovate, toothed, mid- to deep green leaves, to 12cm (5in) long. Long-stalked, pendent, pink or red flowers, to 8cm (3in) across, each with a long staminal

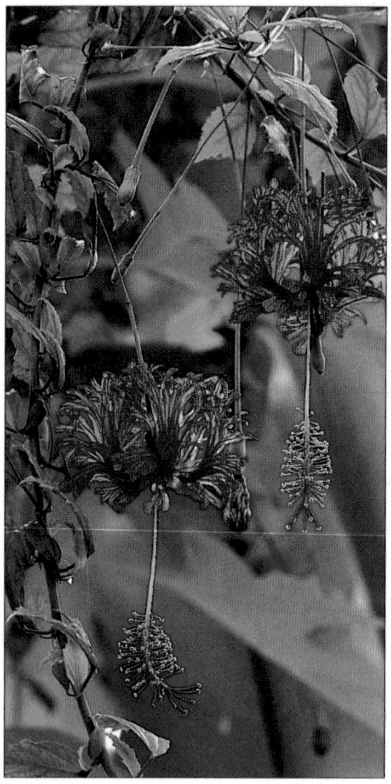

Hibiscus schizopetalus

column, pink stamens, and deeply and irregularly fringed, reflexed petals, are produced singly from the upper leaf axils in summer. ↕to 3m (10ft) or more, ↔ 1–1.5m (3–5ft). Kenya, Tanzania, Mozambique. ❀ (min. 13°C/55°F)
H. sinosyriacus. Spreading, deciduous shrub of open habit with broadly ovate, shallowly 3-lobed, mid-green leaves, to 10cm (4in) long. From late summer to mid-autumn, bears solitary, trumpet-shaped white flowers, 8–9cm (3–3½in) across, with red centres and yellow-anthered white stamens. ↕2.5m (8ft), ↔ 3m (10ft). C. China. ✲✲✲. **'Autumn Surprise'** has white flowers with petal bases feathered cherry pink. **'Lilac Queen'** ■ bears pale lilac-mauve flowers with red centres.
***H.* 'Swan Lake'** see *H. rosa-sinensis* 'Dainty White'.
H. syriacus. Erect, deciduous shrub with ovate to diamond-shaped, shallowly to palmately 3-lobed, coarsely toothed, dark green leaves, to 10cm (4in) long. Large, trumpet-shaped, dark

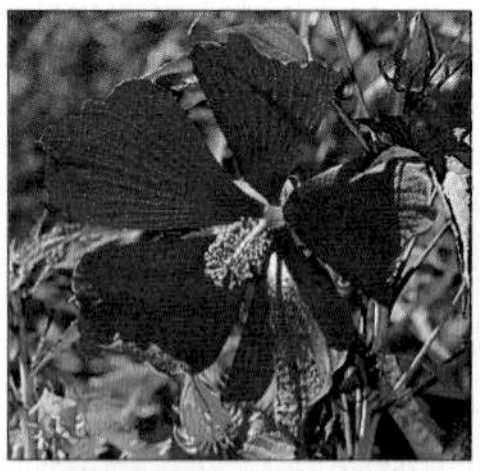

Hibiscus moscheutos

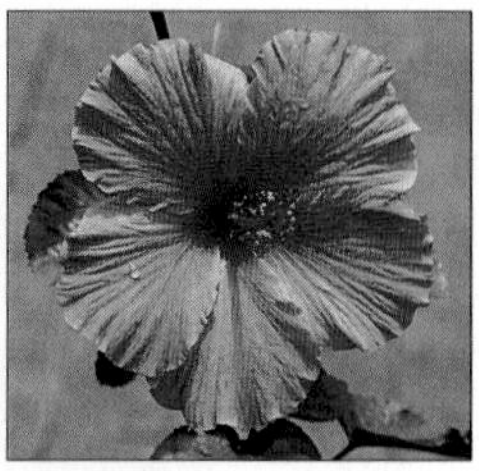

Hibiscus rosa-sinensis 'Agnes Galt'

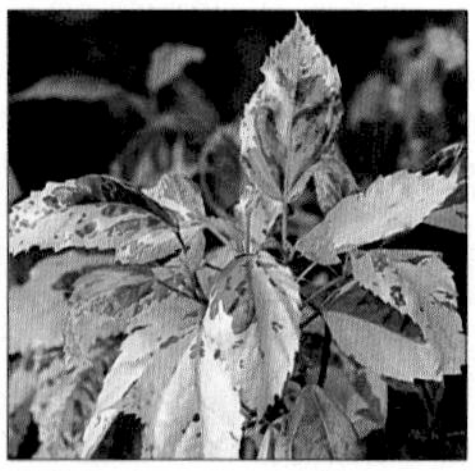

Hibiscus rosa-sinensis 'Cooperi'

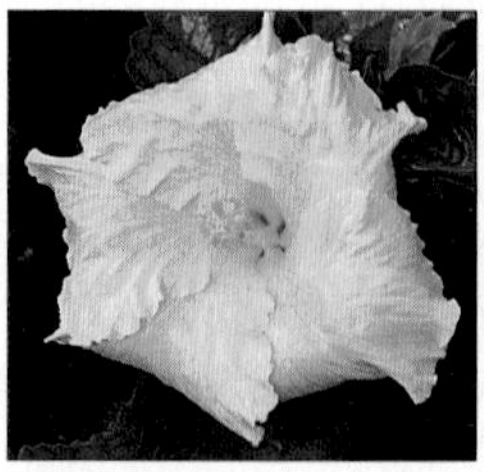

Hibiscus rosa-sinensis 'Kinchen's Yellow'

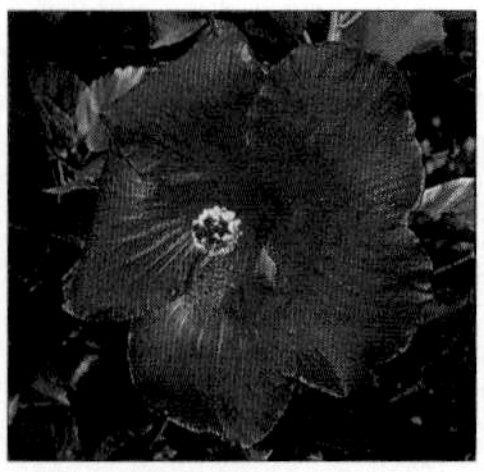

Hibiscus rosa-sinensis 'Scarlet Giant'

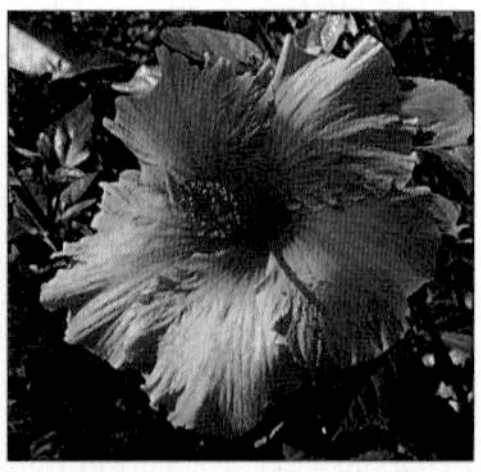

Hibiscus rosa-sinensis 'The President'

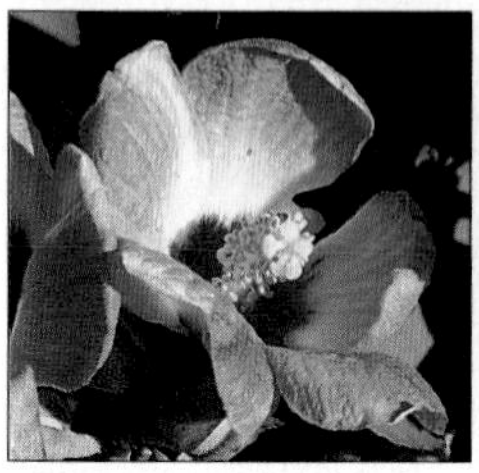

Hibiscus sinosyriacus 'Lilac Queen'

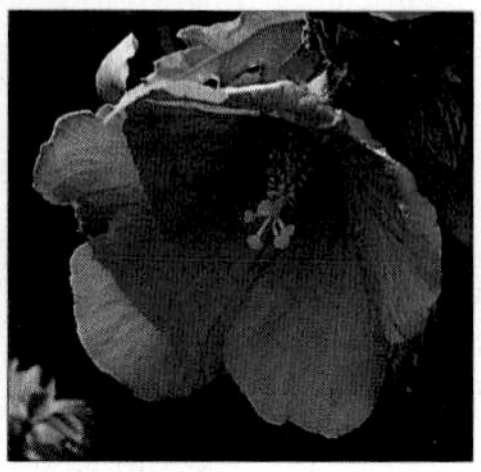

Hibiscus syriacus 'Blue Bird'

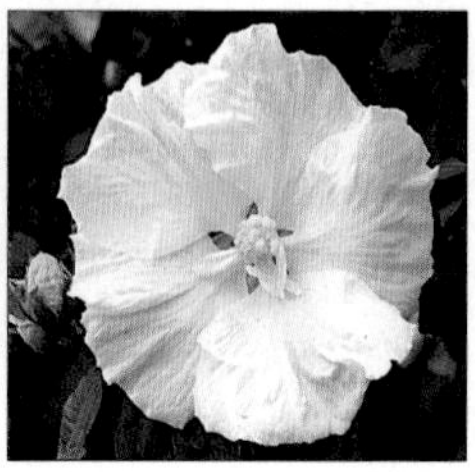

Hibiscus syriacus 'Diana'

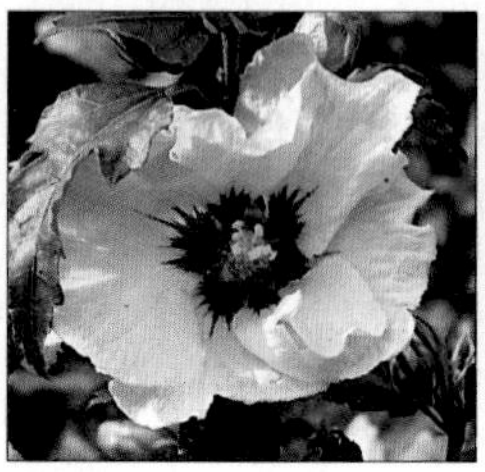

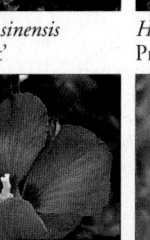

Hibiscus syriacus 'Red Heart'

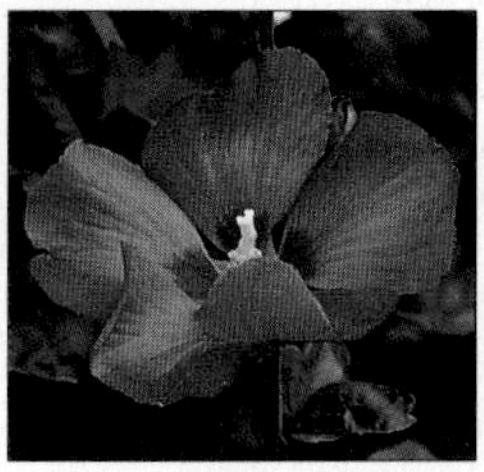

Hibiscus syriacus 'Woodbridge'

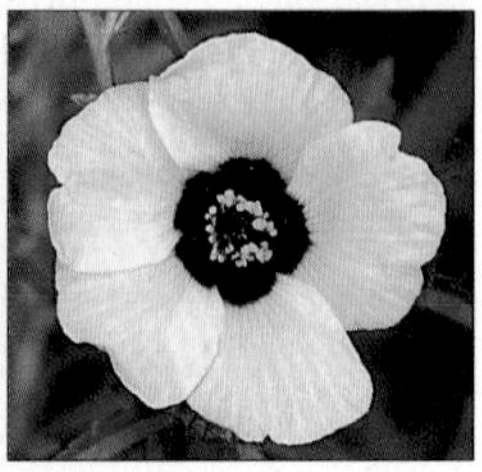

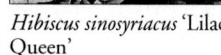

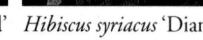

Hibiscus trionum

pink flowers, to 6cm (2½in) across, with dark red centres and yellow-anthered white stamens, are produced singly or in pairs from the leaf axils, from late summer to mid-autumn. ↕ 3m (10ft), ↔ 2m (6ft). China to India. ***.
'Blue Bird' ■ syn. 'Oiseau Bleu', has bright blue flowers, to 8cm (3in) across, with small red centres. **'Diana'** ■ ♀ bears very large white flowers, to 12cm (5in) across, with wavy-margined petals. **'Elegantissimus'** see 'Lady Stanley'. **'Lady Stanley'**, syn. 'Elegantissimus', has double white flowers, flushed pink and dark red in the centres. **'Meehanii'**, syn. 'Variegatus', has leaves margined creamy white, and lilac-mauve, maroon-centred flowers. **'Oiseau Bleu'** see 'Blue Bird'. **'Pink Giant'** ♀ has large, clear pink flowers with dark red eyes. **'Red Heart'** ■ ♀ bears white flowers with dark red centres. **'Variegatus'** see 'Meehanii'. **'William R. Smith'** has large white flowers, to 10cm (4in) across. **'Woodbridge'** ■ ♀ bears large, rich pink flowers, to 10cm (4in) across, with dark pink centres.
H. trionum ■ (Flower-of-an-hour). Fast-growing, erect to spreading, hairy annual or short-lived perennial with ovate, palmately 3- to 5-lobed, toothed, dark green leaves, to 7cm (3in) long, the central lobes longest; leaves lower down the stems are unlobed. From summer to early autumn, trumpet-shaped, creamy yellow flowers, to 8cm (3in) across, with brown centres and dark purple stamens, are produced singly from the leaf axils; they are followed by inflated, bladder-like seed capsules. ↕ 75cm (30in), ↔ to 60cm (24in). Origin uncertain. *
H. waimeae ♀ Evergreen, spreading, small tree with shoots clothed in soft, star-shaped hairs. Broadly ovate to rounded, toothed leaves, to 18cm (7in) long, are rich green above, grey-downy beneath. From late spring to late summer, bears solitary, richly fragrant, funnel-shaped flowers, 12–20cm (5–8in) across, opening white, then fading to pink, with crimson stamens. ↕ 3–5m (10–15ft), ↔ 2–3m (6–10ft). Hawaii. ❀ (min. 15°C/59°F)
***H.* 'White La France'** see *H. rosa-sinensis* 'Dainty White'.

▷**Hibiscus,**
Chinese see *Hibiscus rosa-sinensis*
Hawaiian see *Hibiscus rosa-sinensis*
Norfolk Island see *Lagunaria*
▷**Hickory** see *Carya*
Bitternut see *C. cordiformis*
Pignut see *C. glabra*
Shagbark see *C. ovata*
Swamp see *C. cordiformis*

HIERACIUM
Hawkweed

ASTERACEAE/COMPOSITAE

Genus of 250–260 species (often sub-divided into about 10,000 microspecies) of perennials, many of which are weeds. They are widespread over the N. hemisphere, occurring in diverse habitats, including grassland, dry, stony slopes, cultivated fields, and alpine meadows. They have basal rosettes of lance-shaped to linear or obovate, entire to deeply toothed, pale to dark green leaves, and dandelion-like flowerheads with strap-shaped ray-florets. Those described below are grown mainly for their downy

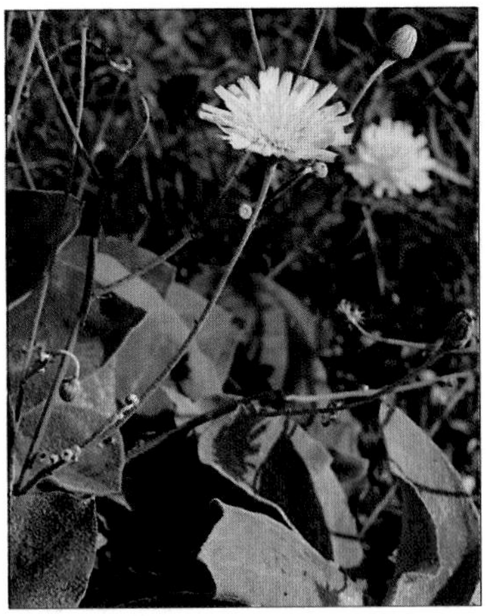

Hieracium lanatum

foliage and loose panicles of yellow flowerheads borne in summer. They are suitable for a large rock garden or wild garden, but may self-seed freely.
• **HARDINESS** Fully hardy.
• **CULTIVATION** Grow in poor, well-drained soil in full sun. The flowerheads may be removed for best foliage effects, but if retained should be dead-headed to prevent excessive self-seeding.
• **PROPAGATION** Sow seed in containers in an open frame in autumn or spring. Divide in spring.
• **PESTS AND DISEASES** Caterpillars, slugs, and snails may be a problem.

H. aurantiacum see *Pilosella aurantiaca.*
H. brunneocroceum see *Pilosella aurantiaca.*
H. lanatum ■ syn. *H. welwitschii.* Clump-forming perennial with lance-shaped to ovate, grey-green, white-margined leaves, to 10cm (4in) long, densely clothed in long white hairs. Loose panicles of 3–7 deep yellow flowerheads, to 2.5cm (1in) across, are borne on wiry, branching stems in summer. ↕ 45cm (18in), ↔ 20cm (8in). S. Europe. ***
H. umbellatum (Leafy hawkweed). Variable, softly hairy perennial with linear to lance-shaped, slightly toothed, dark green leaves, 1.5cm (½in) long. Lax panicles of up to 10 yellow flower-heads, 2–3cm (¾–1¼in) across, with black-brown bracts, are borne on robust stems in summer. ↕ 40–60cm (16–24in), ↔ 25–40cm (10–16in). Europe, W. Asia. ***
H. villosum. Clump-forming perennial with oblong to lance-shaped, grey-green, basal leaves, to 10cm (4in) long, densely clothed in long white hairs. In summer, clear, pale yellow flowerheads, 4–5cm (1½–2in) across, are borne singly or in 2- to 4-flowered panicles on wiry, hairy stems. ↕ to 40cm (16in), ↔ to 20cm (8in). Mountains of Europe. ***
H. welwitschii see *H. lanatum.*

HIMALAYACALAMUS

GRAMINEAE/POACEAE

Genus of 15 species of perennial bamboos from cool forest in India and the Himalayas. They are valued for their dense clumps of hollow, glossy canes, sometimes attractively striped or stained, and their linear, bluish green leaves. They thrive in areas with cool, damp summers, but are intolerant of winter wet and temperatures below -6°C (21°F). In frost-prone areas, grow in a cool greenhouse. In warmer areas, grow as specimen plants in a woodland or wild garden, or in containers.
• **HARDINESS** Frost hardy.
• **CULTIVATION** Under glass, grow in loam-based potting compost (JI No.2) with added leaf mould and sharp sand or grit, in bright filtered light. Provide moderate to high humidity. When in growth, water moderately and apply a balanced liquid fertilizer monthly; water sparingly in winter. Outdoors, grow in moist but well-drained, humus-rich soil in sun or dappled shade, with protection from excessive winter wet.
• **PROPAGATION** Divide in early spring.
• **PESTS AND DISEASES** Trouble free.

H. falconeri, syn. *Arundinaria falconeri, Drepanostachyum falconeri, Thamnocalamus falconeri* (Noble bamboo). Dense, clump-forming bamboo with smooth, olive-green canes, stained purple at the nodes, and linear, blue-green leaves, to 15cm (6in) long. Inner canes are stiffly erect, outer ones arch gently to form a distinctive and graceful clump. ↕ to 9m (28ft) (much smaller in containers), ↔ 3m (10ft). C. Himalayas, India. **

HIPPEASTRUM

AMARYLLIDACEAE

Genus of about 80 species of bulbous perennials found in Central and South America, in habitats ranging from streambanks to rocky hillsides, from sea level to subalpine regions. Umbels of showy, funnel-shaped flowers are borne on leafless stems, mainly from winter to spring. Semi-erect, strap-shaped, light to mid-green or grey-green, basal leaves develop with or just after the flowers. Many large-flowered, colourful hybrids (incorrectly known as *Amaryllis*, a separate South African genus), have been bred for cultivation in containers. These usually produce 4–6 bold, open funnel-shaped flowers, 10–15cm (4–6in) across, and strap-shaped, deep green leaves, 45cm (18in) long. In frost-prone areas, grow as houseplants or in a warm greenhouse or conservatory. In warmer areas, grow in a border or in containers outdoors. All parts may cause mild stomach upset if ingested.
• **HARDINESS** Mainly frost tender; *H.* x *acramannii* may survive short spells outdoors at 0°C (32°F).
• **CULTIVATION** Plant bulbs in autumn with the neck and shoulders above the soil surface. Under glass, grow in loam-based potting compost (JI No.2). Place in bright filtered or full light and water sparingly until in active growth, then water freely and apply a dilute, balanced liquid fertilizer every 2 weeks. After flowering, reduce water as the leaves die off; keep dry when dormant. Root disturbance is resented; pot on every 3–5 years, in autumn. Outdoors, grow in fertile, well-drained soil in sun or dappled shade. Protect *H.* x *acramannii* and tender species grown outdoors with a deep winter mulch in cooler areas.
• **PROPAGATION** Sow seed at 16–18°C (61–64°F) as soon as ripe; keep seedlings growing without a dormant period to encourage early flowering. Remove offsets in autumn.

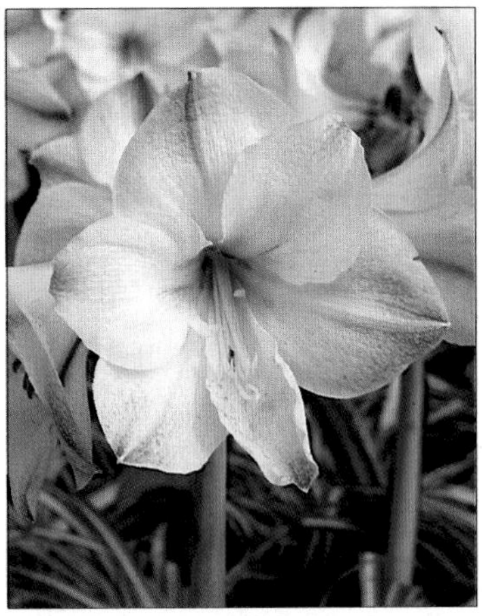

Hippeastrum 'Apple Blossom'

• **PESTS AND DISEASES** Susceptible to bulb scale mite, large narcissus bulb fly, and various fungal diseases.

H.* x *acramannii (*H. aulicum* x *H. psittacinum*). Bulbous perennial with bright green leaves, 30–60cm (12–24in) long, emerging with or just after the flowers. In winter or spring, bears an umbel of up to 3 funnel-shaped scarlet flowers, 15cm (6in) long, with white petal margins and green-and-white centres. ↕ 60cm (24in), ↔ 30cm (12in). Garden origin. * (borderline)
H. advenum see *Rhodophiala advena.*
***H.* 'Apple Blossom'** ■ Robust, large-flowered, bulbous perennial bearing white flowers, 10–15cm (4–6in) across, with pink-tinged petal tips, in winter. ↕ 30–50cm (12–20in), ↔ 30cm (12in). ❀ (min. 13°C/55°F)
H. aulicum ■ syn. *H. morelianum.* Bulbous perennial with mid-green leaves, 30–50cm (12–20in) long, produced with the flowers. In winter or spring, a stout stem bears 2 funnel-shaped crimson flowers, 15cm (6in) across, with green throats. ↕ 30–50cm (12–20in), ↔ 30cm (12in). Brazil, Paraguay. ❀ (min. 13°C/55°F)
H. bifidum see *Rhodophiala bifida.*
***H.* 'Christmas Gift'.** Early-flowering, bulbous perennial bearing pure white flowers, 10–15cm (4–6in) across, in early winter. ↕ 30–50cm (12–20in), ↔ 30cm (12in). ❀ (min. 13°C/55°F)
***H.* 'Liberty'.** Large-flowered, bulbous perennial producing deep red flowers, 10–15cm (4–6in) across, in winter. ↕ 30–50cm (12–20in), ↔ 30cm (12in). ❀ (min. 13°C/55°F)

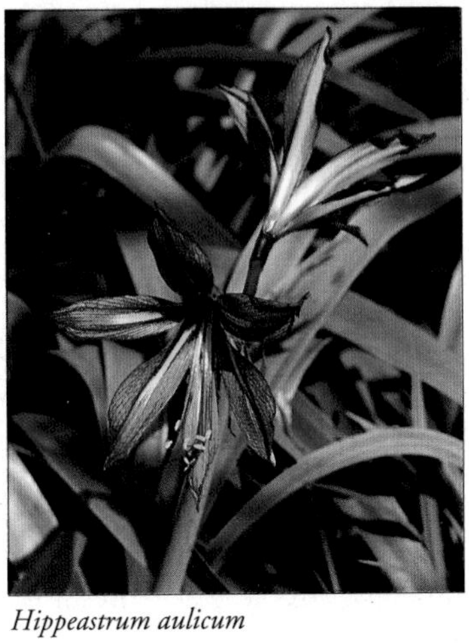

Hippeastrum aulicum

H

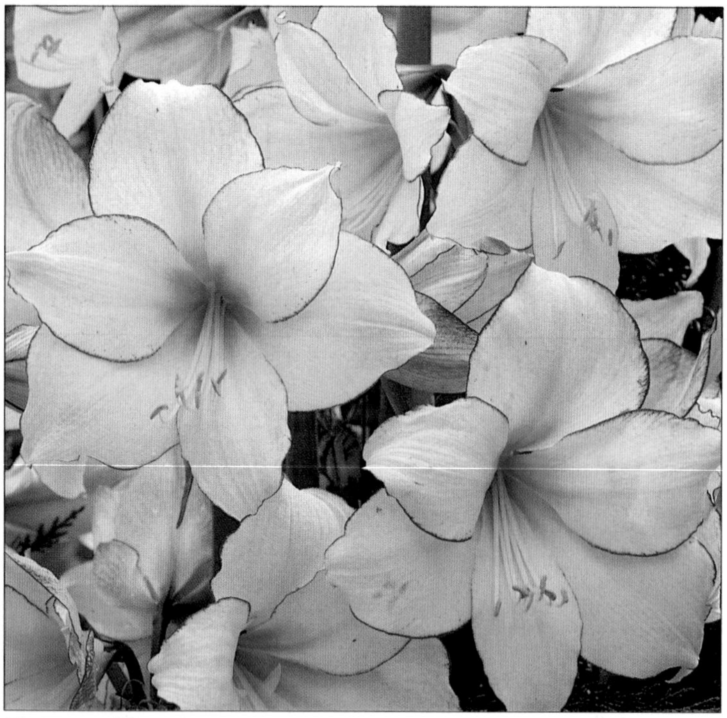

Hippeastrum 'Picotee'

***H.* 'Ludwig's Dazzler'.** Large-flowered, bulbous perennial bearing pure white flowers, 10–15cm (4–6in) across, in winter. ↕ 30–50cm (12–20in), ↔ 30cm (12in). ❀ (min. 13°C/55°F)
***H.* 'Minerva'.** Large-flowered, bulbous perennial with white-centred red flowers, 10–15cm (4–6in) across, in winter. ↕ 30–50cm (12–20in), ↔ 30cm (12in). ❀ (min. 13°C/55°F)
H. morelianum see *H. aulicum.*
***H.* 'Orange Sovereign'** 🏆 Large-flowered, bulbous perennial with orange-red flowers, 10–15cm (4–6in) across, in winter. ↕ 30–50cm (12–20in), ↔ 30cm (12in). ❀ (min. 13°C/55°F)
***H.* 'Picotee'** ▣ Large-flowered, bulbous perennial with red-margined white flowers, 12cm (5in) across, in winter. ↕ 30–50cm (12–20in), ↔ 30cm (12in). ❀ (min. 13°C/55°F)
H. pratense see *Rhodophiala pratensis.*
H. procerum see *Worsleya rayneri.*
***H.* 'Red Lion'** ▣ Large-flowered, bulbous perennial bearing scarlet flowers, 15cm (6in) across, in winter. ↕ 30–50cm (12–20in), ↔ 30cm (12in). ❀ (min. 13°C/55°F)
H. reginae (Mexican lily). Bulbous perennial with mid-green leaves, to 60cm (24in) long, produced after the flowers. In summer, stout stems bear umbels of 2–4 nodding, funnel-shaped scarlet flowers, 10–15cm (4–6in) across, each with a star-shaped green mark in the throat. ↕ 50cm (20in), ↔ 30cm (12in). Mexico, West Indies, Brazil, Peru. ❀ (min. 13°C/55°F)
H. reticulatum* var. *striatifolium ▣ Upright, bulbous perennial producing dark green leaves, 20–30cm (8–12in) long, with prominent white midribs. In summer, bears an umbel of up to 5 funnel-shaped, rose-pink flowers, 8–10cm (3–4in) across, veined darker pink inside. ↕ 25–35cm (10–14in), ↔ 30cm (12in). ❀ (min. 13°C/55°F)
H. rutilum see *H. striatum.*
***H.* 'Star of Holland'** 🏆 Bulbous perennial bearing very large red flowers, 10–15cm (4–6in) across, each with a star-shaped white mark in the throat, in winter. ↕ 30–50cm (12–20in), ↔ 30cm (12in). ❀ (min. 13°C/55°F)
H. striatum, syn. *H. rutilum.* Bulbous perennial with bright green leaves, 30–50cm (12–20in) long, emerging with the flowers. In spring or summer, a stout stem bears an umbel of up to 4 funnel-shaped, coral-red flowers, 10–15cm (4–6in) across, each petal with a central green stripe. ↕↔ 30cm (12in). Brazil. ❀ (min. 13°C/55°F)
H. vittatum (St. Joseph's lily). Robust, bulbous perennial producing stout stems with umbels of 3–6 funnel-shaped, red-striped white flowers, 12cm (5in) across, in spring. Bright green leaves, to 60cm (24in) long, develop after the flowers. ↕ to 90cm (36in), ↔ 30cm (12in). Peru. ❀ (min. 13°C/55°F)

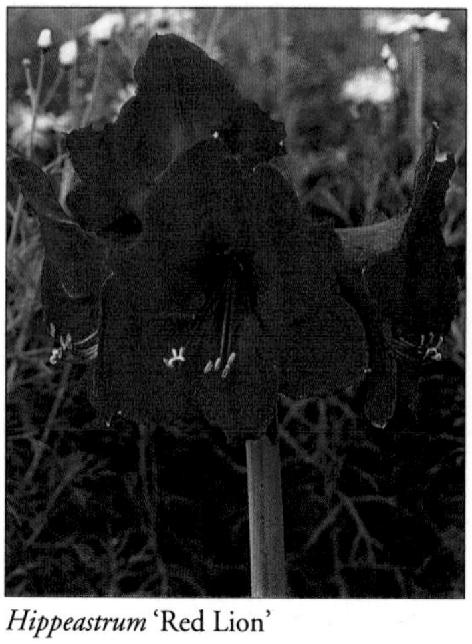

Hippeastrum 'Red Lion'

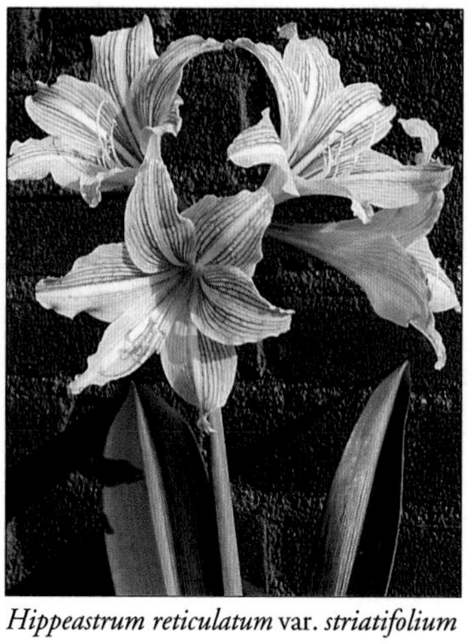

Hippeastrum reticulatum var. *striatifolium*

HIPPOCREPIS

Horseshoe vetch, Vetch

LEGUMINOSAE/PAPILIONACEAE

Genus of about 20 species of annuals and perennials from Europe, N. Africa, and W. Asia, occurring in scree, among alpine rocks, and in short turf on chalk downland. They usually have woody, creeping stems, alternate, pinnate, light to mid-green leaves, and small, pea-like flowers in raceme-like heads, which are attractive to butterflies. Some may be invasive, but others are suitable for a wild garden or rock garden, scree bed, trough, or raised bed. *H. comosa* 'E.R. Janes' is excellent for crevices in a wall, rock, or paving.

- **HARDINESS** Fully hardy.
- **CULTIVATION** Grow in poor, well-drained, alkaline soil in full sun.
- **PROPAGATION** Sow scarified seed in containers in a cold frame in spring or autumn. Root cuttings of non-flowering shoots in summer.
- **PESTS AND DISEASES** Trouble free.

H. comosa. Vigorous, creeping, woody-based perennial with mid-green leaves, 3–10cm (1¼–4in) long, each divided into 3–8 pairs of linear to obovate leaflets. From late spring to late summer, bears raceme-like heads of up to 12 lemon-yellow flowers, 1cm (½in) across. ↕↔ to 40cm (16in). C. and S. Europe, N. Africa. ✻✻✻. **'E.R. Janes'** is compact, and spreads less vigorously; ↕ to 8cm (3in), ↔ indefinite.
H. emerus see *Coronilla emerus.*

HIPPOPHAE

ELAEAGNACEAE

Genus of 3 species of deciduous, dioecious shrubs and trees from Europe and Asia, occurring on coastal dunes, and in screes and on riverbanks in the mountains. They are cultivated for their linear or linear-oblong, silvery, grey-green or mid-green leaves, and for their spherical, usually orange fruits. Both male and female plants are needed to produce fruit. Inconspicuous flowers are borne in racemes in spring. Grow in a mixed or shrub border, in a wild garden, or as specimen plants. In coastal areas, *H. rhamnoides* is used for windbreaks, hedging, and for stabilizing sand dunes.

- **HARDINESS** Fully hardy.
- **CULTIVATION** Grow in full sun in moist but well-drained, neutral to alkaline, preferably sandy soil. Pruning group 1, in late summer; pruning is seldom necessary.
- **PROPAGATION** Sow seed in containers in an open frame as soon as ripe or in spring. Stratify spring-sown seed for 3 months at 4°C (39°F). Root semi-ripe cuttings in summer, hardwood cuttings in late autumn. Layer in autumn.
- **PESTS AND DISEASES** Trouble free.

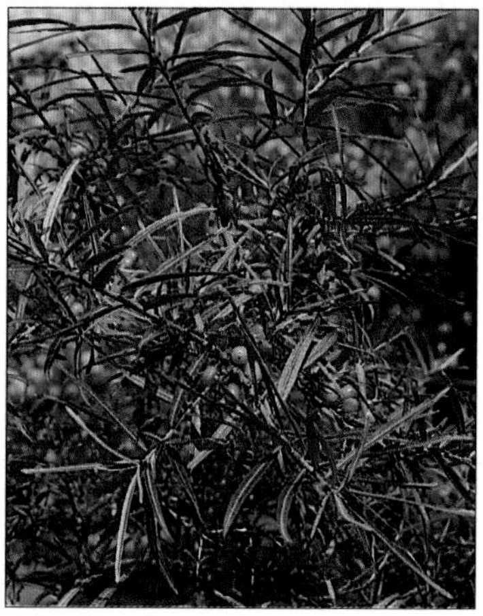

Hippophae rhamnoides

H. rhamnoides ▣ 🏆 ♂–♀ (Sea buckthorn). Bushy, deciduous, large shrub or small tree with spiny shoots bearing linear, grey-green leaves, to 6cm (2½in) long, silver-scaly to bronze-scaly on both surfaces. Tiny, yellow-green flowers are borne in racemes to 2cm (¾in) long, in spring. On female plants, flowers are followed by persistent, spherical, bright orange fruit, to 8mm (⅜in) across. ↕↔ 6m (20ft). Europe, Asia. ✻✻✻

▷**Hobble bush** see *Viburnum lantanoides*
▷**Hognut** see *Carya glabra*

HOHENBERGIA

BROMELIACEAE

Genus of over 40 species of stemless, evergreen, terrestrial or epiphytic perennials (bromeliads) from scrub, rainforest, and rocky terrain up to altitudes of 1,600m (5,000ft) in South America and the West Indies. They produce rosettes of mainly triangular or strap-shaped leaves with spiny tips and margins, and unusually large sheaths. In summer, prominent scapes bear compound spikes of colourful, tubular flowers. Where temperatures fall below 15°C (59°F), grow as houseplants or in a warm green-house. In warmer regions, grow in a humid, moist area of the garden, or in containers or a raised bed.

- **HARDINESS** Frost tender.
- **CULTIVATION** Under glass, grow in terrestrial bromeliad compost in bright indirect to moderate light. Keep just moist at all times. Apply a half-strength, low-nitrogen fertilizer monthly from spring to autumn. Outdoors, grow in fertile, moist but very well-drained soil in partial shade; use terrestrial bromeliad compost for container-grown plants outdoors. Protect from strong winds. See also p.47.
- **PROPAGATION** Sow seed at 24°C (75°F) as soon as ripe. Divide offsets in spring or summer.
- **PESTS AND DISEASES** Young growth is susceptible to scale insects.

H. edmundoi. Rosette-forming, terrestrial perennial producing strap-shaped, grey-scaly, mid-green leaves, to 45cm (18in) long, the rounded tips with sharp brown spines. Branched, spike-like inflorescences, to 70cm (28in) long, have broadly ovate, white-woolly stem bracts, each with 2–4 tiny purple flowers. ↕↔ 45–50cm (18–20in). E. Brazil. ❀ (min. 15°C/59°F)

H. stellata. Rosette-forming, terrestrial or epiphytic perennial producing strap-shaped, silver-scaly, dark green leaves, 60–90cm (24–36in) long, the tips and margins with brown spines. Branched, spike-like inflorescences have white-woolly, red or yellow stem bracts and 2–8 bright blue or purple flowers, each surrounded by triangular, red or purple bracts. ↕↔ 1m (3ft). Trinidad, Tobago, Venezuela, N.E. Brazil. ❀ (min. 15°C/59°F)

HOHENBERGIOPSIS

BROMELIACEAE

Genus of a single species of evergreen, epiphytic perennial (bromeliad), closely related to *Hohenbergia*, from rainforest at altitudes up to 1,800m (6,000ft) in Guatemala. It produces rosettes of strap-shaped, spiny-toothed leaves, and stout, woolly scapes bearing cylindrical, densely flowered inflorescences in summer. Where temperatures fall below 18°C (64°F), grow as a houseplant or in a warm greenhouse. In warmer areas, grow in containers, or in a raised bed in a humid, moist area of the garden.

- **HARDINESS** Frost tender.
- **CULTIVATION** Under glass, grow in epiphytic bromeliad compost in bright filtered light, away from all draughts. Provide moderate to high humidity. Keep just moist and mist daily at all times. Apply a half-strength, low-nitrogen fertilizer monthly from spring to autumn. Outdoors, grow in fertile, moist but well-drained soil in partial shade; use terrestrial bromeliad compost for container-grown plants. Protect from cold, drying winds. See also p.47.
- **PROPAGATION** Sow seed at 24°C (75°F) as soon as ripe. Remove offsets in spring.
- **PESTS AND DISEASES** Scale insects may be a problem.

H. guatemalensis. Epiphytic perennial producing strap-shaped, mid-green leaves, 50–60cm (20–24in) long, each tipped with a spine 1cm (½in) long. In summer, bears a 2- or 3-branched, cylindrical inflorescence, 20cm (8in) long, with brown floral bracts and deep purple flowers, to 8mm (⅜in) long. ↕↔ 1m (3ft) or more. Guatemala. ❀ (min. 18°C/64°F)

HOHERIA

MALVACEAE

Genus of 5 species of deciduous and evergreen trees and shrubs from New Zealand, where they occur from the coast to the mountains in forest, at forest margins, and on streambanks. The alternate leaves are lance-shaped to broadly ovate, toothed, sometimes hairy, and grey- to dark green when mature. Juvenile foliage, which is present for several years on young seedlings, may be lobed and have a metallic cast. Hoherias are grown mainly for their graceful habit and their cup-shaped, fragrant white flowers, attractive to butterflies, borne singly or in cymes. They prefer maritime climates. Grow in a shrub border, in a woodland garden, as specimen plants, or against a sunny wall.

- **HARDINESS** Frost hardy.
- **CULTIVATION** Grow in moderately fertile, well-drained, neutral to alkaline soil in full sun or partial shade, sheltered from cold, drying winds. The deciduous species are more reliably hardy than the evergreens and may regenerate from their woody bases if cut back by frost in winter; protect the roots of evergreens with a winter mulch. Pruning group 1, in spring or after flowering; pruning is seldom necessary.
- **PROPAGATION** Sow seed in containers in a cold frame in autumn. Root semi-ripe cuttings in late summer or autumn.
- **PESTS AND DISEASES** Prone to coral spot, particularly in damp, shady sites.

H. angustifolia 🏆 syn. *H. microphylla.* Columnar, evergreen tree with oblong to inversely lance-shaped, toothed, glossy, dark green leaves, to 3cm (1¼in) long. In mid- and late summer, bears white flowers, to 2cm (¾in) across, often singly from the leaf axils. ↕ 7m (22ft), ↔ 3m (10ft). New Zealand. ❄❄

H. glabrata ▣ 🏆 ◯ Deciduous, spreading tree with hairless, broadly ovate, tapered, dark green leaves, to 10cm (4in) long, turning yellow in autumn. In midsummer, bears small cymes of white flowers, to 4cm (1½in) across, with purple anthers. Often confused with *H. lyallii.* ↕↔ 7m (22ft). New Zealand (South Island). ❄❄

H. 'Glory of Amlwch' 🏆 ◯ Spreading, semi-evergreen tree with narrowly ovate, toothed, glossy, bright green leaves, to 10cm (4in) long. Cymes of large white flowers, to 4cm (1½in) across, are borne in mid- and late summer. ↕ 7m (22ft), ↔ 6m (20ft). ❄❄

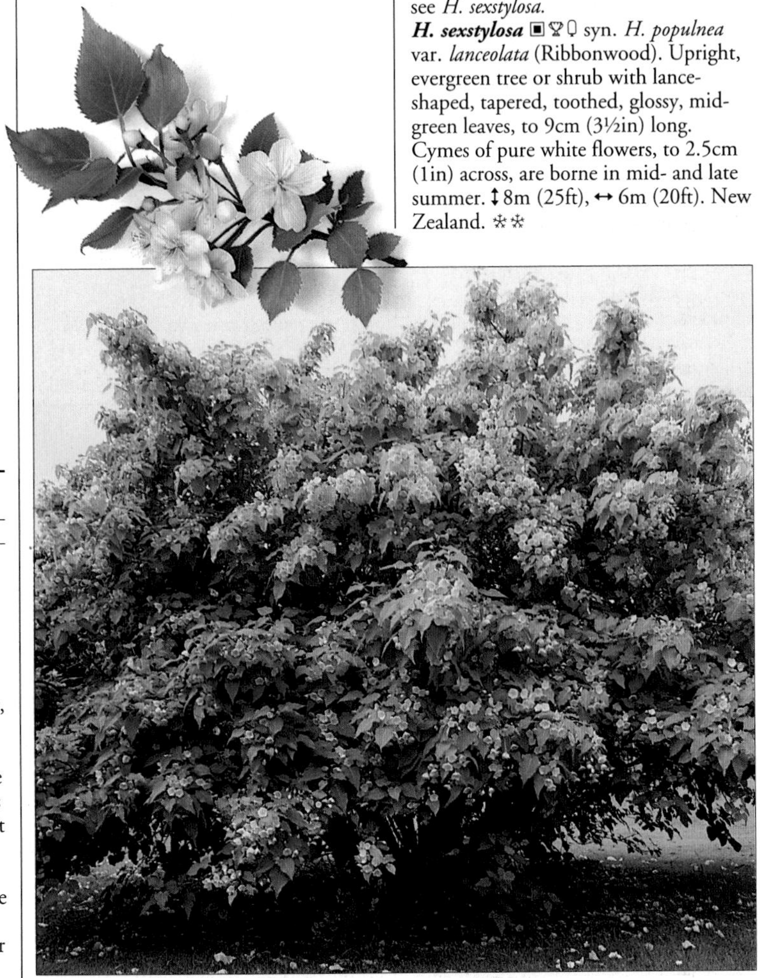

Hoheria glabrata (inset: flower detail)

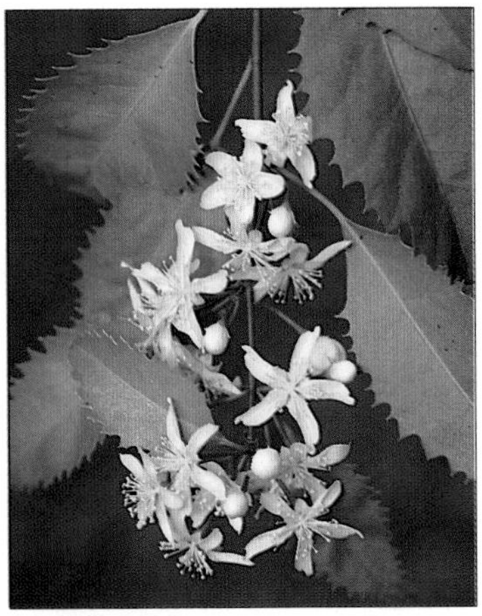

Hoheria sexstylosa

H. lyallii 🏆 ◯ syn. *Plagianthus lyallii.* Spreading, deciduous tree with ovate, deeply toothed, densely hairy, grey-green leaves, to 10cm (4in) long. Cymes of white flowers, to 3cm (1¼in) across, with purple anthers, are borne in mid-summer. Often confused with *H. glabrata.* ↕↔ 7m (22ft). New Zealand (South Island). ❄❄

H. microphylla see *H. angustifolia.*

H. populnea ◯ (Lace-bark). Spreading, evergreen tree, often with flaky, pale brown and white bark when mature. The elliptic to broadly ovate, toothed leaves, to 15cm (6in) long, are glossy, dark green. Dense cymes of pure white flowers, 3cm (1¼in) across, are borne in late summer and early autumn. ↕ 12m (40ft), ↔ 10m (30ft). New Zealand (North Island). ❄❄. **var. *lanceolata*** see *H. sexstylosa.*

H. sexstylosa ▣ 🏆 🏆 syn. *H. populnea* var. *lanceolata* (Ribbonwood). Upright, evergreen tree or shrub with lance-shaped, tapered, toothed, glossy, mid-green leaves, to 9cm (3½in) long. Cymes of pure white flowers, to 2.5cm (1in) across, are borne in mid- and late summer. ↕ 8m (25ft), ↔ 6m (20ft). New Zealand. ❄❄

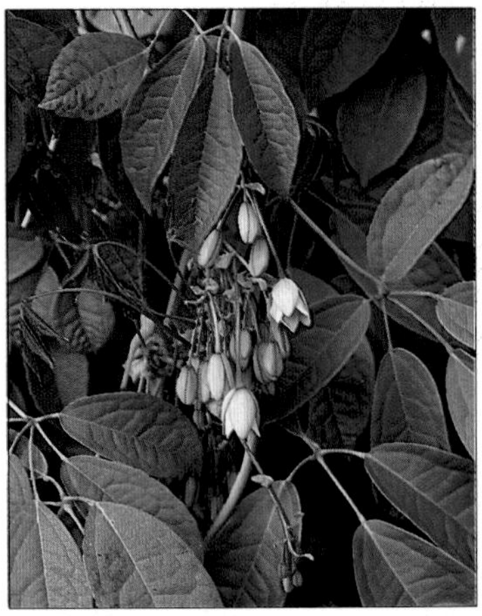

Holboellia coriacea

HOLBOELLIA

LARDIZABALACEAE

Genus of 5 species of twining, evergreen climbers from thickets and shady woodland in the Himalayas and China. They are cultivated mainly for their alternate, 3- to 9-palmate, dark green leaves. Small male and female flowers, to 1.5cm (½in) long, are borne in axillary corymbs or racemes, separately on the same plant; fruits are produced only irregularly. Train on a support, grow through a small tree, or use to clothe a pergola, arch, or trellis.

- **HARDINESS** Frost hardy.
- **CULTIVATION** Grow in well-drained, moderately fertile, humus-rich soil in full sun or partial shade, sheltered from cold, drying winds. Pruning group 11, in spring.
- **PROPAGATION** Sow seed in containers in a cold frame in spring. Root semi-ripe cuttings in late summer or autumn. Layer in autumn.
- **PESTS AND DISEASES** Trouble free.

H. coriacea ▣ Vigorous climber with dark green leaves, to 15cm (6in) long, composed of 3 oblong leaflets. In spring, bears small, mauve male flowers and purple-tinged, greenish white female flowers in dense corymbs, to 15cm (6in) across. Flowers are sometimes followed by sausage-shaped purple fruit, to 6cm (2½in) long. ↕ 7m (22ft). C. China. ❄❄

H. latifolia. Vigorous climber with dark green leaves, to 12cm (5in) long, composed of 3–7 oblong leaflets. Small, greenish white male flowers and purple female flowers are borne in racemes to 12cm (5in) across, in spring. Flowers are sometimes followed by sausage-shaped, red to purple fruit, to 10cm (4in) long. ↕ 5m (15ft). Himalayas. ❄❄

HOLCUS

GRAMINEAE/POACEAE

Genus of 8 species of often invasive, annual or perennial grasses from woodland and grassland in Europe, N. Africa, and W. Asia. They have linear, flat or folded, mid-green or bluish green leaves, and dense or open, spike-like panicles of flattened, 2-flowered spikelets borne in summer. Only *H. mollis* 'Albovariegatus' is usually cultivated; it is an attractive carpeting plant for the front of a herbaceous border or rock garden.

- **HARDINESS** Fully hardy.

H

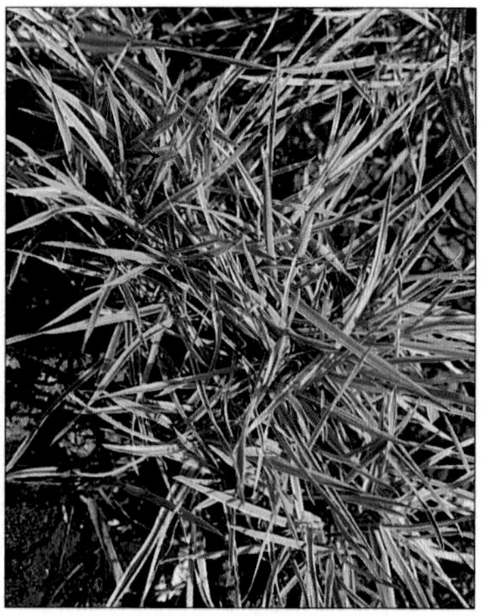

Holcus mollis 'Albovariegatus'

• **CULTIVATION** Grow in any moist but well-drained, poor to moderately fertile soil in sun or partial shade; avoid full sun on poor, dry soil. Trim *H. mollis* 'Albovariegatus' lightly after flowering and dead-head to avoid self-seeding, as offspring will be green-leaved and invasive. Avoid planting too close to less vigorous plants.
• **PROPAGATION** Divide *H. mollis* 'Albovariegatus' in spring; it will not come true from seed.
• **PESTS AND DISEASES** Trouble free.

***H. mollis* 'Albovariegatus'** ■ Loosely tufted, mat-forming, perennial grass producing linear, flat, soft, blue-green leaves, 15–45cm (6–18in) long, with wide, creamy white margins. In summer, erect stems bear pale green spikelets in relatively few, narrowly oblong to ovate panicles, to 12cm (5in) long. ↕ to 30cm (12in), ↔ 45cm (18in) or more. ❄❄❄

▷**Holly** see *Ilex*
American see *Ilex opaca*
Blue see *Ilex* × *meserveae*
Box-leaved see *Ilex crenata*
Common see *Ilex aquifolium*
English see *Ilex aquifolium*
Hedgehog see *Ilex aquifolium* 'Ferox'
Himalayan see *Ilex dipyrena*
Horned see *Ilex cornuta*
Japanese see *Ilex crenata*
Miniature see *Malpighia coccigera*
Moonlight see *Ilex aquifolium* 'Flavescens'
Mountain see *Olearia ilicifolia*
Sea see *Eryngium*
Singapore see *Malpighia coccigera*
Summer see *Arctostaphylos diversifolia*
Topel see *Ilex* × *attenuata*
West Indian see *Leea coccinea*
▷**Hollyhock** see *Alcea*, *A. rosea*

HOLMSKIOLDIA

VERBENACEAE

Genus of 10 species of evergreen shrubs or scandent climbers from tropical woodland in Africa, Madagascar, and the Himalayas. They are valued for their terminal panicles or axillary racemes of tubular to salverform or trumpet-shaped flowers with conspicuous, saucer-shaped, brightly coloured calyces. The opposite leaves are simple and usually ovate to obovate. Where temperatures fall below 16°C (61°F), grow in a warm greenhouse or conservatory. In tropical climates, use as specimen plants or grow in a border.

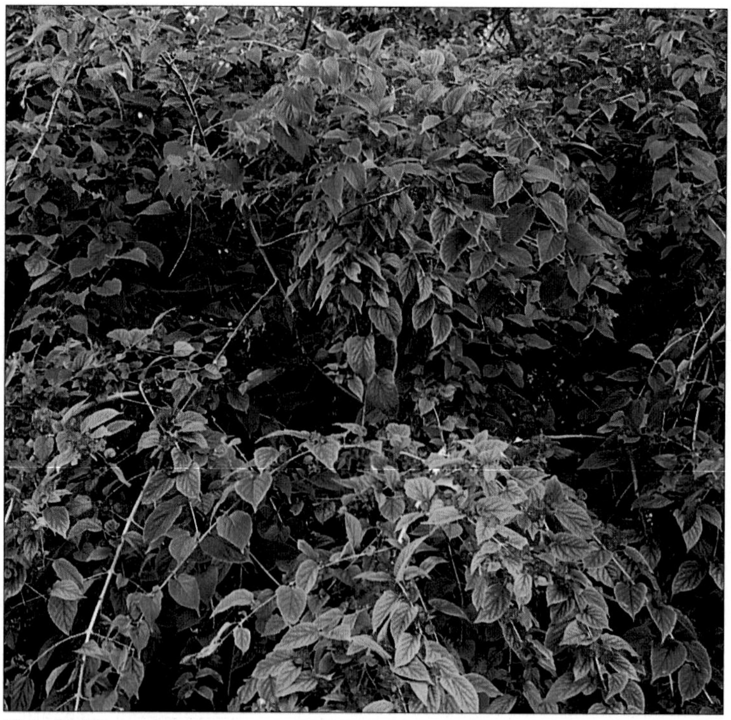

Holmskioldia sanguinea

• **HARDINESS** Frost tender.
• **CULTIVATION** Under glass, grow in loam-based potting compost (JI No.2) in full light, with shade from hot sun. Top-dress in late winter or early spring, and pot on in spring. In summer, water freely and apply a balanced liquid fertilizer monthly; keep moist in winter. Outdoors, grow in moist but well-drained, moderately fertile soil in full sun, with some midday shade and shelter from strong winds. Established plants are drought tolerant and useful in poor, sandy soils. Provide support for climbers. Pruning group 9 for shrubs; group 11 for climbers, after flowering.
• **PROPAGATION** Sow seed at 19–24°C (66–75°F) in spring. Root semi-ripe cuttings with bottom heat in late summer.
• **PESTS AND DISEASES** Whiteflies, red spider mites, and mealybugs may be a problem under glass.

H. sanguinea ■ (Chinese-hat plant). Erect, then scandent shrub with ovate or ovate-elliptic, slender-pointed, slightly toothed leaves, 5–10cm (2–4in) long. From summer to autumn, bears curved, narrowly trumpet-shaped flowers, to 2.5cm (1in) long, with crimson petals and orange-red calyces, 2.5cm (1in) across, in racemes to 12cm (5in) long. ↕ 3–10m (10–30ft), ↔ 1.5–3m (5–10ft). Himalayas. ❀ (min. 15°C/59°F).
var. *citrina* bears yellow flowers.

HOLODISCUS

ROSACEAE

Genus of 8 species of deciduous shrubs found in dry woodland from W. North America to N. South America. They produce alternate, oblong to rounded, lobed to pinnatifid, usually softly hairy leaves, and are valued for their attractive, airy panicles of numerous small, cup-shaped flowers. Suitable for a mixed or shrub border, or for growing in light woodland, or as specimen plants.
• **HARDINESS** Fully hardy.
• **CULTIVATION** Grow in moist but well-drained, fertile, humus-rich soil in sun or partial shade. Pruning group 1 or 2; remove only a few older shoots each year, after flowering.
• **PROPAGATION** Sow seed in containers in an open frame as soon as ripe. Root semi-ripe cuttings in summer. Layer in summer or autumn.
• **PESTS AND DISEASES** Trouble free.

H. discolor ■ (Ocean spray). Vigorous, upright shrub with arching branches and broadly ovate, shallowly to deeply 4- to 8-lobed, grey-green leaves, to 8cm (3in) long, white-hairy beneath. Tiny, cup-shaped, creamy-white flowers are borne in large, pendent, plume-like panicles, to 30cm (12in) long, in mid-summer. ↕↔ 4m (12ft). W. North America. ❄❄❄

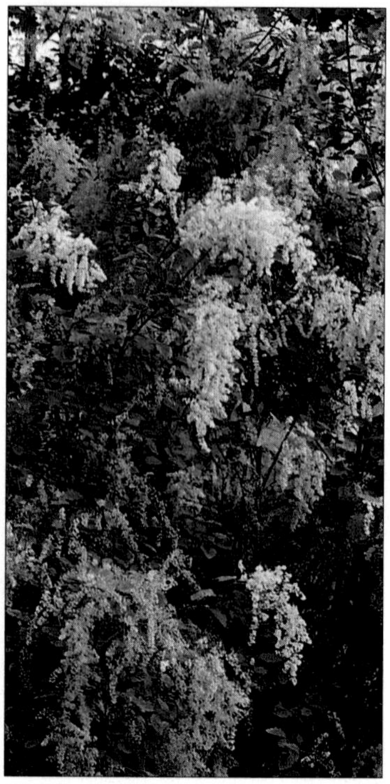

Holodiscus discolor

▷***Homalocephala texensis*** see *Echinocactus texensis*

HOMALOCLADIUM

Ribbon bush

POLYGONACEAE

Genus of one species of evergreen shrub from tropical forest in the Solomon Islands. It is grown for its ornamental, flattened, jointed green stems with alternate, lance- or arrow-shaped leaves, which are usually short-lived or may be absent. The small, petalless, whitish green flowers have 5-lobed calyces that later turn red or red-purple, enlarging and becoming fleshy as the seeds form. In frost-prone areas, grow in a warm greenhouse or as a houseplant (plants in containers rarely flower or fruit). In warmer regions, grow in a shrub border or courtyard garden, or at the base of a warm, sunny wall.
• **HARDINESS** Frost tender.
• **CULTIVATION** Under glass, grow in loam-based potting compost (JI No.2) in bright filtered or full light. Water moderately in growth, more sparingly in winter. Apply a balanced liquid fertilizer once in spring. Pot on or top-dress in spring. Outdoors, grow in moist but well-drained, fertile, humus-rich soil in full sun; partial shade is tolerated. Pruning group 8, if necessary, in spring.
• **PROPAGATION** Sow seed at 16–18°C (61–64°F) in spring. Root stem section cuttings with bottom heat in summer.
• **PESTS AND DISEASES** Scale insects may be a problem under glass.

H. platycladum, syn. *Muehlenbeckia platyclados*. Spreading, erect shrub or scrambling climber producing ribbon-like, jointed, glossy, mid-green stems, to 2cm (¾in) wide, with raised veins running lengthways. Compact flower clusters, to 1.5cm (½in) across, and usually short-lived, lance-shaped, bright green leaves, 1.5–6cm (½–2½in) long, are borne on the margins or at the joints of the stems in spring. ↕ 60–120cm (2–4ft), ↔ 45–90cm (18–36in) in a container or greenhouse border; ↕ to 3m (10ft), ↔ 2m (6ft) outdoors in warm climates. Solomon Islands. ❀ (min. 5–7°C/41–45°F)

HOMERIA

IRIDACEAE

Genus of 31 species of cormous perennials, often found on sandy slopes from low to high altitudes in South Africa. They are cultivated for their scented, showy flowers, borne several in succession from pairs of bracts on branched stems, from spring to summer. They have erect, linear to strap-shaped basal leaves, and 1 or 2 narrow leaves on the lower part of the flowering stems. In frost-prone climates, grow in a sheltered site, at the base of a warm, sunny wall, or in a cool greenhouse. In warmer areas, grow at the front of a border. *H. collina* is toxic to livestock.
• **HARDINESS** Half hardy, but may withstand occasional falls to -5°C (23°F).

• **CULTIVATION** Plant corms 10cm (4in) deep in autumn or spring. Under glass, grow in loam-based potting compost (JI No.2) with equal parts additional sand and leaf mould, in full light with good ventilation. Water freely in growth; dry off gradually as the flowers fade and keep completely dry when dormant. Store corms in a cool, dry place until autumn planting. Outdoors, grow in well-drained, fertile, humus-rich soil in full sun. Where temperatures regularly fall below -5°C (23°F), provide a deep mulch or grow under glass.
• **PROPAGATION** Sow seed at 16–18°C (61–64°F) in autumn. Separate offsets when dormant.
• **PESTS AND DISEASES** Trouble free.

H. collina ▣ Cormous perennial with wiry, unbranched or rarely branched stems and linear, mid-green leaves, to 55cm (22in) long. Cup-shaped, scented, yellow, peach, or pink flowers, to 7cm (3in) across, are borne in succession from spring to summer. ↕16–40cm (6–16in), ↔5cm (2in). South Africa. ✻
H. ochroleuca. Upright, cormous perennial with branched stems and erect, linear, mid-green leaves, to 30cm (12in) long. Cup-shaped, musk-scented, pale yellow flowers, to 8cm (3in) across, sometimes with orange central stains, are borne from spring to summer. ↕40–60cm (16–24in), ↔8cm (3in). South Africa. ✻

▷***Homoglossum*** see *Gladiolus*
▷**Honesty** see *Lunaria, L. annua*
Perennial see *L. rediviva*
▷**Honey-balls** see *Cephalanthus occidentalis*
▷**Honey bush** see *Melianthus major*
▷**Honey locust** see *Gleditsia triacanthos*
▷**Honeysuckle** see *Lonicera*
Bush see *Diervilla*
Cape see *Tecoma capensis*
Common see *Lonicera periclymenum*
Coral see *Lonicera sempervirens*
Early Dutch see *Lonicera periclymenum* 'Belgica'
Etruscan see *Lonicera etrusca*
Fly see *Lonicera xylosteum*
French see *Hedysarum coronarium*
Giant Burmese see *Lonicera hildebrandiana*
Himalayan see *Leycesteria formosa*
Italian see *Lonicera caprifolium*
Japanese see *Lonicera japonica*
Late Dutch see *Lonicera periclymenum* 'Serotina'
New Zealand see *Knightia excelsa*

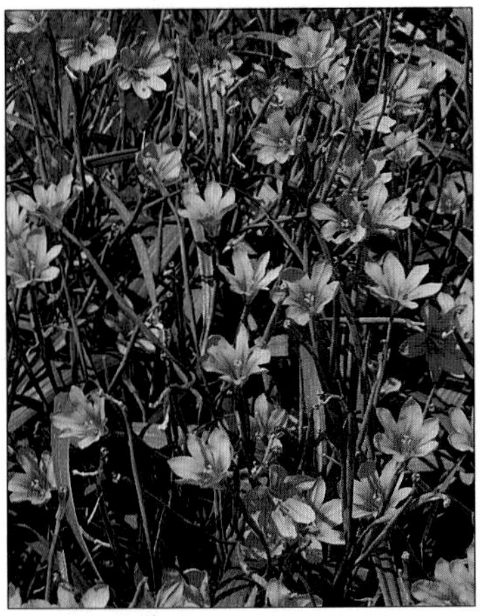
Homeria collina

▷**Honeysuckle cont.**
Scarlet trumpet see *Lonicera* x *brownii*
Trumpet see *Lonicera sempervirens*

HOODIA

ASCLEPIADACEAE

Genus, closely related to *Trichocaulon*, of about 20 species of branching, leafless, perennial succulents found in periodically very dry areas of Angola, Namibia, Botswana, and South Africa. The many-angled, fleshy, greyish green stems have hard, thorn-like tubercles, and produce large, saucer- to cup-shaped or shallowly trumpet-shaped, unpleasantly scented flowers in the stem grooves towards the tips. Where temperatures fall below 10°C (50°F), grow in a warm greenhouse; in warm, dry areas, grow in a desert garden, trough, or raised bed.
• **HARDINESS** Frost tender.
• **CULTIVATION** Under glass, grow in standard cactus compost with additional leaf mould, in full light; shade from hot sun, and provide low humidity. From spring to summer, water moderately and apply a low-nitrogen liquid fertilizer monthly; keep just moist in winter. Outdoors, grow in moderately fertile, sharply drained soil with additional leaf mould and sharp sand, in full sun with some midday shade. Protect from excessive winter wet. See also pp.48–49.
• **PROPAGATION** Sow seed at 19–24°C (66–75°F), or graft stems on to *Stapelia* or *Ceropegia linearis*, both in spring.
• **PESTS AND DISEASES** Trouble free.

H. bainii ▣ Erect succulent with fleshy stems branching from or near the base, with 12–15 angular ribs, each bearing tubercles with a brown spine. From summer to early autumn, cup-shaped to shallowly trumpet-shaped, beige-pink to dull yellow flowers, 2–7cm (¾–3in) across, with dark red-brown coronas, are borne singly, occasionally in clusters of 2 or 3. The 5 shallow petal lobes have outward-curved margins and small red dots at the centres. ↕20cm (8in), ↔10cm (4in). Namibia, South Africa (Western Cape, Northern Cape, Eastern Cape). ❁ (min. 10°C/50°F)
H. currorii. Erect succulent with thick, pale greyish green stems branching freely from the base. The stems have 15–25 angular ribs, each bearing tubercles with sharp, downward-pointing spines. From summer to early autumn, bears cup-shaped or shallowly trumpet-shaped, thick-stalked flowers, to 12cm (5in) across, singly or in clusters of up to 5. The flowers are green to ivory or pink, later becoming yellowish pink, and each has 5 rounded, violet-hairy lobes and a hairy, pale orange-red corolla. ↕60cm (24in), ↔20cm (8in). S.W. Angola, N.W. Namibia. ❁ (min. 10°C/50°F)
H. gordonii. Clump-forming succulent with erect stems branching from the base, each with 12–14 longitudinal ribs and short tubercles tipped with woody spines. Saucer-shaped flowers, 7–10cm (3–4in) across, are borne singly or in clusters of up to 3 blooms, from summer to early autumn. The flowers are pale brownish pink to maroon, with coronas of the same colour, and each has 5 shallow petal lobes with outward-curved margins and small red dots at the

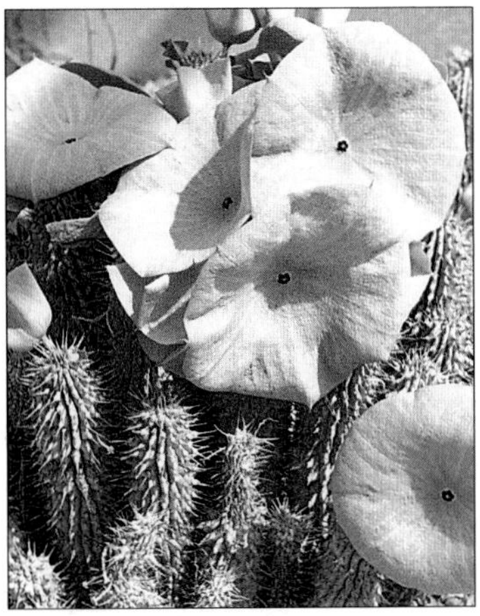
Hoodia bainii

centres. ↕45cm (18in) or more, ↔30cm (12in). S. Namibia, South Africa (Western Cape). ❁ (min. 10°C/50°F)

▷**Hop** see *Humulus, H. lupulus*
False see *Justicia brandegeeana*
▷**Hop bush** see *Dodonaea viscosa*
▷**Hop tree** see *Ptelea trifoliata*

HORDEUM

Barley

GRAMINEAE/POACEAE

Genus of about 20 species of annual and perennial grasses (including the cereal crop, barley) from disturbed ground in the temperate regions of both hemispheres. They have linear, flat or rolled, light to mid-green or blue-green leaves. Dense, narrow, cylindrical, occasionally flattened, spike-like panicles, with long-bristled spikelets, are borne in 2 ranks. The flowerheads of many species are useful for dried flower arrangements. Use in an annual, mixed, or herbaceous border, or in a wild garden.
• **HARDINESS** Fully hardy.
• **CULTIVATION** Grow in well-drained, moderately fertile soil in full sun. Cut flowerheads for drying before fully mature.
• **PROPAGATION** Sow seed *in situ* in spring or autumn.
• **PESTS AND DISEASES** Trouble free.

H. jubatum ▣ (Squirrel tail grass). Densely tufted, annual or perennial grass with erect or arching, linear, light green leaves, to 15cm (6in) long. In early and midsummer, erect stems bear dense, broad, nodding panicles, to 13cm (5in) long, of silky, long-bristled, pale green spikelets, flushed red or purple, which turn beige with age. ↕50cm (20in), ↔30cm (12in). N.E. Asia, North America. ✻✻✻

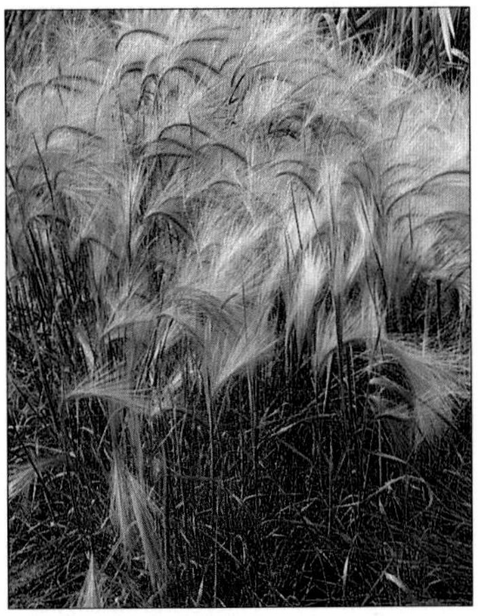
Hordeum jubatum

▷**Horehound** see *Marrubium*

HORMINUM

LABIATAE/LAMIACEAE

Genus of one species of low-growing, rhizomatous perennial from rocks, screes, and meadows in subalpine areas of the Pyrenees and European Alps. It has basal rosettes of dark green leaves, and is grown for its spikes of tubular-bell-shaped, usually violet flowers, borne in summer. Grow at the front of a herbaceous border or in a rock garden.
• **HARDINESS** Fully hardy.
• **CULTIVATION** Grow in moderately fertile, well-drained soil in full sun.
• **PROPAGATION** Sow seed in autumn in containers in an open frame. Divide in spring.
• **PESTS AND DISEASES** Prone to slug and snail damage.

H. pyrenaicum ▣ (Dragon's mouth, Pyrenean dead nettle). Perennial with rosettes of ovate, toothed, glossy, dark green leaves, to 7cm (3in) long. In summer, bears a succession of tubular-bell-shaped, 2-lipped flowers, to 2cm (¾in) long, in axillary whorls. The flowers have prominent stamens, and are usually dark violet-blue, occasionally pink or white. ↕20cm (8in), ↔to 30cm (12in). Pyrenees, Alps. ✻✻✻

▷**Hornbeam** see *Carpinus*
American see *Carpinus caroliniana*
American hop see *Ostrya virginiana*
Common see *Carpinus betulus*
Hop see *Ostrya carpinifolia*
▷**Horncone, Mexican** see *Ceratozamia mexicana*
▷**Hornwort** see *Ceratophyllum, C. demersum*
▷**Horse chestnut** see *Aesculus, A. hippocastanum*
Chinese see *A. chinensis*
Indian see *A. indica*
Japanese see *A. turbinata*
Red see *A.* x *carnea*
Sunrise see *A.* x *neglecta* 'Erythroblastos'
▷**Horsemint** see *Mentha longifolia*
▷**Horseradish** see *Armoracia rusticana*
▷**Horsetail tree** see *Casuarina equisetifolia*

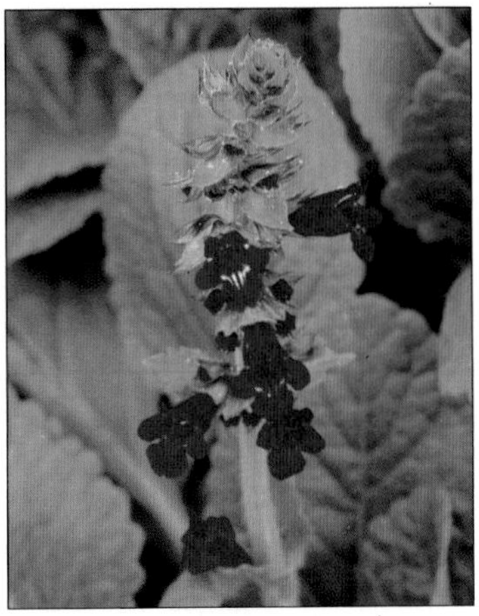
Horminum pyrenaicum

H

HOSTA

Plantain lily

HOSTACEAE/LILIACEAE

Genus of about 70 species of mostly clump-forming, occasionally rhizomatous or stoloniferous perennials from sun-baked volcanic cliffs, rocky streamsides, woodland, and alpine meadows in China, Korea, Japan, and E. Russia. Numerous hybrids have also been raised, mainly in the USA. Hostas are grown primarily for their bold foliage, produced in dense mounds of overlapping, ovate to heart-shaped or lance-shaped leaves (see panel below). The leaves may be green, yellow, grey-blue, or variegated, and are often glaucous. One-sided racemes of bell- or funnel-shaped flowers, to 3cm (1¼in) long, are borne on usually leafless, sometimes leafy scapes, mainly in summer. They are followed by oblong, green, later pale brown seed capsules. Plant heights given in the descriptions below refer to the mounds of foliage; flower (scape) heights are given separately.

Hostas may be grown as ground cover under deep-rooted, deciduous trees, in a mixed or herbaceous border, or near water. Smaller hostas are excellent for a rock garden, a peat bed, or containers.

• **HARDINESS** Fully hardy.

• **CULTIVATION** Grow in fertile, moist but well-drained soil with shelter from cold, drying winds. Most hostas prefer a site in full or partial shade (fewer flowers will be produced in full shade), but yellow-leaved hostas colour better in a sunny position with some midday shade. Hostas will not tolerate drought and should be mulched annually in spring to conserve moisture.

• **PROPAGATION** Although easily raised from seed sown in containers in a cold frame in spring, only seedlings of *H. ventricosa* will come reliably true in cultivation. Divide in late summer or early spring. Many new hostas are propagated through tissue culture.

• **PESTS AND DISEASES** Particularly susceptible to damage from slugs and snails. Container-grown plants are vulnerable to vine weevil. Virus infections may also be a problem.

HOSTA LEAF SHAPES

Hostas are grown for their bold leaves, which may be ovate, lance-shaped, rounded, or heart-shaped.

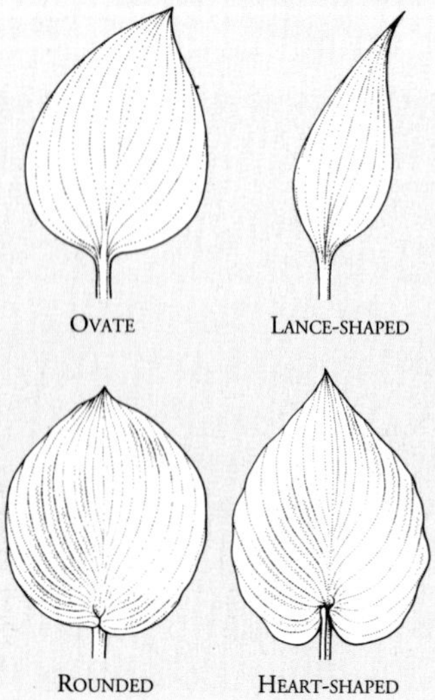

H. albomarginata see *H. sieboldii*.

***H.* 'Allan P. McConnell'** ▣ Clump-forming perennial producing broadly to narrowly ovate, olive-green leaves, 8cm (3in) long, with narrow white margins. In midsummer, bears bell-shaped purple flowers on ridged scapes, 35–40cm (14–16in) long. ↕ 15–20cm (6–8in), ↔ 30–45cm (12–18in). ❄❄❄

***H.* 'Antioch'** ▣ Robust, clump-forming perennial with broadly ovate, tapered, arching, matt, dark green leaves, 25cm (10in) long, irregularly margined grey-green and creamy yellow, fading to white. In midsummer, arching, leafy scapes, 90cm (36in) long, bear funnel-shaped, lavender-blue flowers. ↕ 50cm (20in), ↔ 90cm (36in). ❄❄❄

***H.* 'Argentea Variegata'** see *H. undulata* var. *undulata*.

***H.* 'August Moon'** ▣ Vigorous, clump-forming perennial with rounded to heart-shaped, cupped, puckered, pale green leaves, 15cm (6in) long, becoming golden yellow with a faint glaucous bloom. In summer, glaucous scapes, 70cm (28in) long, bear bell-shaped, greyish white flowers. ↕ 50cm (20in), ↔ 75cm (30in). ❄❄❄

***H.* 'Aureomaculata'** see *H. fortunei* 'Albopicta'.

***H.* 'Big Daddy'.** Clump-forming perennial with rounded to heart-shaped, cupped, deeply puckered, glaucous, grey-blue leaves, 28cm (11in) long. In early summer, bears bell-shaped, greyish white flowers on leafy, glaucous scapes, 80cm (32in) long. ↕ 60cm (24in), ↔ 1m (3ft). ❄❄❄

***H.* 'Birchwood Parky's Gold'** ▣ syn. *H.* 'Golden', *H.* 'Golden Nakaiana'. Vigorous, clump-forming perennial with heart-shaped, matt, yellow-green leaves, 13cm (5in) long, becoming rich yellow with age. In midsummer, scapes 70cm (28in) long bear bell-shaped, pale lavender-blue flowers. ↕ 35–40cm (14–16in), ↔ indefinite. ❄❄❄

***H.* 'Blue Angel'** 🏆 Slow-growing, clump-forming perennial with ovate to heart-shaped, wavy, glaucous, bluish grey leaves, 40cm (16in) long. In midsummer, bears bell-shaped white flowers on glaucous scapes, 1m (3ft) long. ↕ 1m (3ft), ↔ 1.2m (4ft). ❄❄❄

***H.* 'Blue Blush'** ▣ Clump-forming perennial with lance-shaped, glaucous, deep blue-green leaves, 10cm (4in) long. Bell-shaped, lavender-blue flowers are borne on glaucous scapes, 24cm (10in) long, in midsummer. ↕ 20cm (8in), ↔ 35–40cm (14–16in). ❄❄❄

***H.* 'Blue Dimples'.** Clump-forming perennial with ovate to heart-shaped, thick, glaucous, blue-green leaves, 18cm (7in) long, becoming dimpled with wavy margins when mature. In midsummer, bears bell-shaped lilac flowers on glaucous scapes, 50cm (20in) long. ↕ 35cm (14in), ↔ 50cm (20in). ❄❄❄

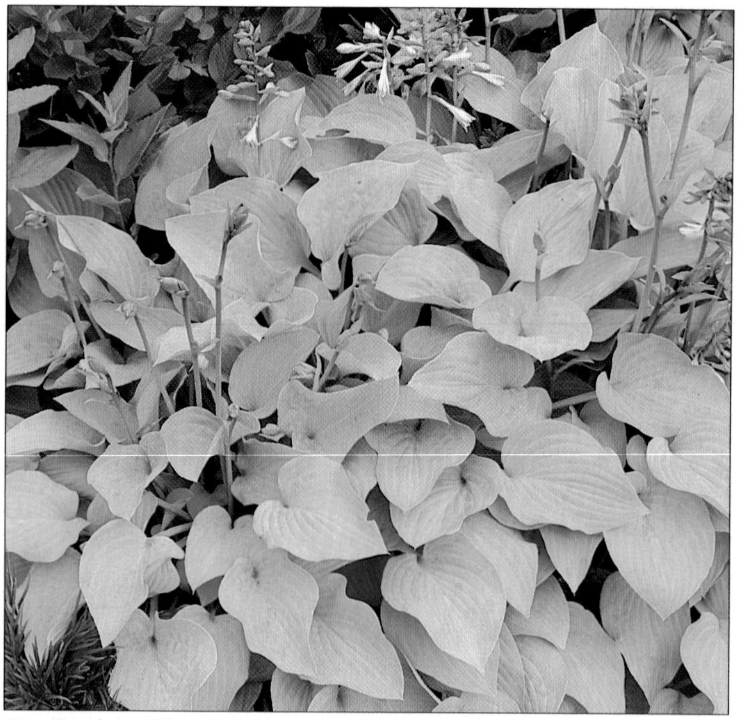

Hosta 'Birchwood Parky's Gold'

***H.* 'Blue Moon'** ▣ Slow-growing, clump-forming perennial producing broadly heart-shaped, pointed, glaucous, deep blue-green leaves, 8cm (3in) long, becoming slightly puckered with age. In midsummer, glaucous scapes, 30cm (12in) long, bear dense racemes of bell-shaped, pale mauve-grey flowers. ↕ 10cm (4in), ↔ 30cm (12in). ❄❄❄

***H.* 'Blue Skies'.** Clump-forming perennial with heart-shaped, pointed, flat, smooth, glaucous, blue-green leaves, 13cm (5in) long. In midsummer, bears bell-shaped, lavender-blue flowers on glaucous scapes, 40cm (16in) long. ↕ 20cm (8in), ↔ 40cm (16in). ❄❄❄

***H.* 'Blue Umbrellas'.** Clump-forming perennial with ovate to heart-shaped, cupped, stiff, puckered, thick, glaucous, blue-green leaves, 33cm (13in) long. Bell-shaped, greyish white flowers are borne on scapes 1m (3ft) long, in midsummer. Will tolerate sun or partial shade. ↕↔ 1m (3ft). ❄❄❄

***H.* 'Blue Wedgwood'.** Clump-forming perennial with ovate to lance-shaped, pointed, wavy, glaucous, grey-blue leaves, 15cm (6in) long, dimpled when mature. Bell-shaped, pale lavender-blue flowers are borne on glaucous scapes, 40cm (16in) long, in midsummer. ↕ 25cm (10in), ↔ 55cm (22in). ❄❄❄

HOSTA LEAF VARIEGATION

Many hostas have attractively variegated foliage. The leaves may be widely or narrowly margined in a paler colour, or have a wide, pale, central marking and darker margins.

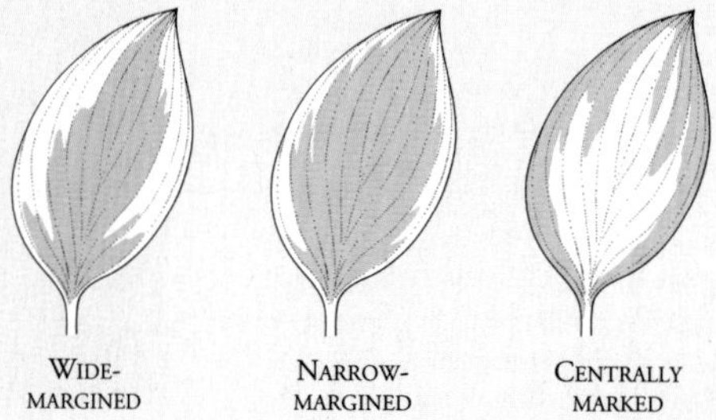

***H.* 'Bold Ribbons'.** Stoloniferous perennial with spoon-shaped, arching, matt, olive-green leaves, 15cm (6in) long, margined with yellow that fades to creamy white. In summer, bears funnel-shaped violet flowers on scapes 60cm (24in) long. ↕ 25cm (10in), ↔ 60cm (24in). ❄❄❄

***H.* 'Brim Cup'.** Slow-growing, clump-forming perennial with erect, heart-shaped, slightly cupped, thick, dark green leaves, 15cm (6in) long, puckered between the veins. The irregular, creamy yellow leaf margins turn white with age. In midsummer, scapes 45cm (18in) long bear bell-shaped, pale lavender-blue flowers, fading to white. ↕ 30cm (12in), ↔ 35–40cm (14–16in). ❄❄❄

***H.* 'Buckshaw Blue'.** Slow-growing, clump-forming perennial with short leaf-stalks bearing ovate to heart-shaped, concave, puckered, glaucous, deep blue-green leaves, 15cm (6in) long. In early summer, bears bell-shaped, greyish white flowers on glaucous scapes, 45cm (18in) long. ↕ 35cm (14in), ↔ 60cm (24in). ❄❄❄

***H.* 'Candy Hearts'.** Vigorous, clump-forming perennial with heart-shaped, pointed, greenish grey-blue leaves, 15cm (6in) long. Bell-shaped, pale lavender-blue to off-white flowers are borne on scapes 50cm (20in) long, in summer. ↕ 35–40cm (14–16in), ↔ 55cm (22in). ❄❄❄

H. capitata. Clump-forming perennial producing ovate to heart-shaped, thin, ruffled leaves, to 13cm (5in) long, with wavy margins. They are deep olive-green with sunken veins, glossy beneath. In midsummer, bell-shaped purple flowers with darker purple veins, open from spherical buds on straight, ridged, leafy scapes, 30–40cm (12–16in) long. Well-established plants are sometimes remontant. ↕ 18cm (7in), ↔ 45cm (18in). Korea, Japan. ❄❄❄

***H.* 'Carol'** ▣ Vigorous, clump-forming perennial with ovate to heart-shaped, slightly concave, puckered, olive-green to dark green leaves, 23cm (9in) long,

H

irregularly margined white, and splashed grey-green. In summer, funnel-shaped, lavender-blue flowers are produced on arching, leafy, glaucous, purple-tinted scapes, 75cm (30in) long. ↕ 50cm (20in), ↔ 1m (3ft). ❄❄❄

***H.* 'Chinese Sunrise'.** Stoloniferous perennial with lance-shaped, pointed, thin, glossy, yellow-green leaves, 15cm (6in) long, fading to pale green, and narrowly margined dark green. In late summer, arching, leafy scapes, 70cm (28in) long, bear bell-shaped purple flowers. ↕ 35cm (14in), ↔ 70cm (28in). ❄❄❄

***H.* 'Christmas Tree'.** Clump-forming perennial whose outline, when in flower, resembles a Norway spruce (*Picea abies*). Heart-shaped, deeply puckered, glaucous, mid- to dark green leaves, 20cm (8in) long, have irregular, creamy white margins. In midsummer, bears funnel-shaped, very pale lavender-white flowers on arching, leafy scapes, 60cm (24in) long. ↕ 45cm (18in), ↔ 1m (3ft). ❄❄❄

***H.* 'Cream Delight'** see *H. undulata* var. *undulata*.

H. crispula 🏆 syn. *H.* 'Crispula', *H.* 'Sazanami'. Clump-forming perennial with deeply channelled leaf-stalks bearing broadly lance-shaped to heart-shaped, wavy-margined, mid- to deep green leaves, 20–30cm (8–12in) long, tapering to long, twisted tips, and irregularly margined white. In early summer, produces funnel-shaped, lavender-white flowers on erect, leafy scapes, 75–90cm (30–36in) long. ↕ 50cm (20in), ↔ 1m (3ft). Probably Japan. ❄❄❄

***H.* 'Crispula'** see *H. crispula*.

***H. decorata*,** syn. *H.* 'Decorata'. Stoloniferous perennial producing broadly ovate to rounded, blunt-tipped, slightly wavy-margined, leathery, matt, dark green leaves, 10–16cm (4–6in) long, margined white. In midsummer, bears funnel-shaped, deep violet or sometimes white flowers, with pale purple stripes, on leafy scapes, 50cm (20in) long. ↕ 30cm (12in), ↔ 45cm (18in). Probably Japan. ❄❄❄.
f. *normalis* has dark green leaves with no variegation.

***H.* 'Decorata'** see *H. decorata*.

***H.* 'Devon Blue'.** Vigorous, clump-forming perennial with ovate to heart-shaped, pointed, glaucous, grey-blue leaves, 18cm (7in) long. Bell-shaped, deep lavender-blue flowers are borne on glaucous scapes, 50cm (20in) long, in midsummer. ↕ 50cm (20in), ↔ 1m (3ft). ❄❄❄

***H.* 'Diamond Tiara'.** Vigorous perennial forming a compact mound of ovate to heart-shaped, slightly wavy-margined, thin, pale olive-green leaves, 10cm (4in) long, irregularly margined cream to white and splashed grey-green. In midsummer, bears bell-shaped, sometimes remontant violet flowers on scapes 70cm (28in) long. ↕ 35cm (14in), ↔ 65cm (26in). ❄❄❄

***H.* 'Dorset Blue'.** Slow-growing, clump-forming perennial with ovate to heart-shaped, slightly cupped, puckered, thick, dark blue-green leaves, 8cm (3in) long, very glaucous beneath. In midsummer, bears bell-shaped, lavender-white flowers on stout, leafy, glaucous, greyish mauve scapes, 25cm (10in) long. ↕ 20cm (8in), ↔ 45cm (18in). ❄❄❄

***H.* 'Eldorado'** see *H.* 'Frances Williams'.

***H.* 'Emerald Tiara'** ▣ Vigorous perennial forming a compact mound of broadly lance-shaped to ovate or heart-shaped, slightly wavy, bright green leaves, 10cm (4in) long. Bell-shaped violet flowers, sometimes remontant, are borne on scapes 70cm (28in) long, in midsummer. ↕ 35cm (14in), ↔ 65cm (26in). ❄❄❄

***H.* 'Fair Maiden'.** Clump-forming perennial with erect leaf-stalks bearing heart-shaped, pointed, flat, dark green leaves, 10cm (4in) long, with irregular cream margins, turning white with age. In midsummer, glaucous scapes, 65cm (26in) long, bear bell-shaped, lavender-blue, sometimes remontant flowers. ↕ 35cm (14in), ↔ 40cm (16in). ❄❄❄

***H. fluctuans* 'Sagae'** 🏆 syn. *H. fluctuans* 'Variegated', *H.* 'Sagae'. Clump-forming perennial with erect leaf-stalks bearing ovate to lance-shaped, horizontal, wavy-margined leaves, 20–30cm (8–12in) long, glaucous, dull olive-green above, glaucous, mid-green beneath, and boldly margined creamy yellow. In mid- and late summer, thick, semi-erect, leafy, glaucous scapes, 1.5m (5ft) long, bear long racemes of bell-shaped white flowers, 5–6cm (2–2½in) long, suffused violet to pale purple. ↕↔ 1m (3ft). Garden origin. ❄❄❄

***H. fluctuans* 'Variegated'** see *H. fluctuans* 'Sagae'.

***H. fortunei*.** Vigorous, clump-forming perennial with ovate, pointed, matt, dark green leaves, 20–30cm (8–12in) long. In midsummer, leafy scapes, 80cm (32in) long, bear funnel-shaped mauve flowers. ↕ 55cm (22in), ↔ 80cm (32in). Probably garden origin. ❄❄❄.
'Albomarginata', syn. *H.* 'Fortunei Albomarginata', has large, dull mid- to deep green leaves, to 30cm (12in) long, the irregular cream margins turning white with age. The amount of variegation may vary from year to year.
'Albopicta' ▣🏆 syn. *H.* 'Aureomaculata', var. *albopicta*, *H.* 'Fortunei Albopicta', produces narrowly heart-shaped, thin, creamy yellow leaves, 20–25cm (8–10in) long, irregularly margined dark green, fading slowly to dull mid-green; ↔ 1m (3ft).
'Aureomarginata' ▣🏆 syn. var. *aureomarginata*, *H.* 'Fortunei Aureomarginata', *H.* 'Obscura Marginata', has ovate to heart-shaped, leathery, distinctly veined, deep olive-green leaves, 20–25cm (8–10in) long, irregularly margined yellow. The flowers are borne freely on scapes 85cm (34in) long, in summer. Tolerates sun or partial shade; ↔ 1m (3ft). **'Gloriosa'**, syn. *H.* 'Fortunei Gloriosa', is slow-growing, producing narrowly elliptic, cupped, slightly puckered, glossy, dark olive-green leaves, 15cm (6in) long, with regular, very narrow white margins. In summer, lavender-blue flowers are borne on scapes 1m (3ft) long; ↕ 45cm (18in), ↔ 60cm (24in). **var. *hyacinthina*** 🏆 syn. 'Hyacinthina', *H.* 'Fortunei Hyacinthina', produces ovate to heart-shaped, wavy, slightly puckered, thick, glaucous, grey-green leaves, finely margined white and blue-grey beneath. In summer, violet flowers are borne freely on slightly arching, glaucous scapes, 1m (3ft) long; ↕ 60cm (24in), ↔ 1m (3ft).

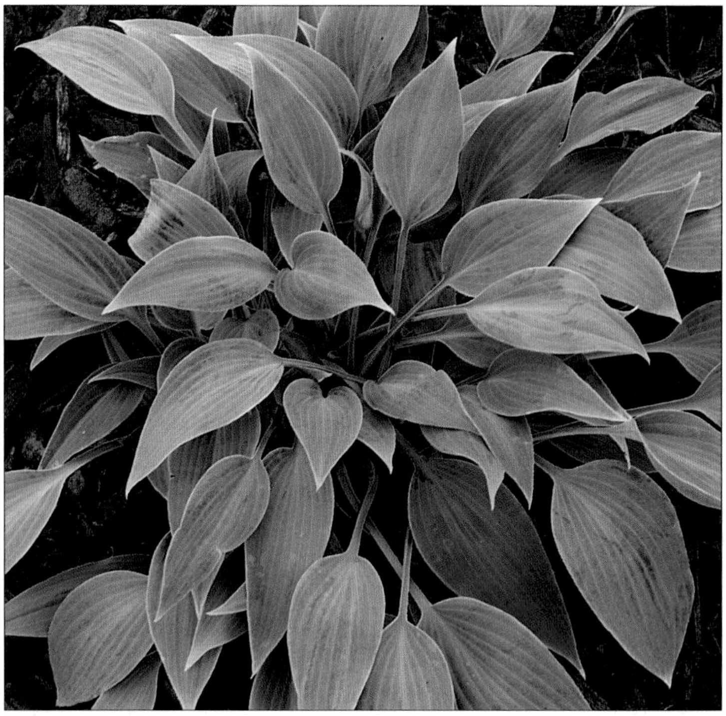
Hosta 'Blue Blush'

H

***H.* 'Fortunei Albomarginata'** see *H. fortunei* 'Albomarginata'.

***H.* 'Fortunei Albopicta'** see *H. fortunei* 'Albopicta'.

***H.* 'Fortunei Aureomarginata'** see *H. fortunei* 'Aureomarginata'.

***H.* 'Fortunei Gloriosa'** see *H. fortunei* 'Gloriosa'.

***H.* 'Fortunei Hyacinthina'** see *H. fortunei* var. *hyacinthina*.

***H.* 'Fragrant Bouquet'.** Clump-forming perennial producing ovate to heart-shaped, slightly wavy-margined, glossy, pale green leaves, 20cm (8in) long, with irregular, creamy yellow margins. In late summer, funnel-shaped, fragrant, mauvish white flowers are borne on scapes 90cm (36in) long. Tolerates sun or partial shade. ↕ 45cm (18in), ↔ 65cm (26in). ❄❄❄

***H.* 'Fragrant Gold'** ▣ Clump-forming perennial with ovate, pointed, wavy, thick, glaucous, pale yellow-green leaves, 18cm (7in) long, turning yellow with age. In summer, scapes 60cm (24in) long bear funnel-shaped, lavender-blue flowers. Thrives in sun or partial shade. ↕ 45cm (18in), ↔ 65cm (26in). ❄❄❄

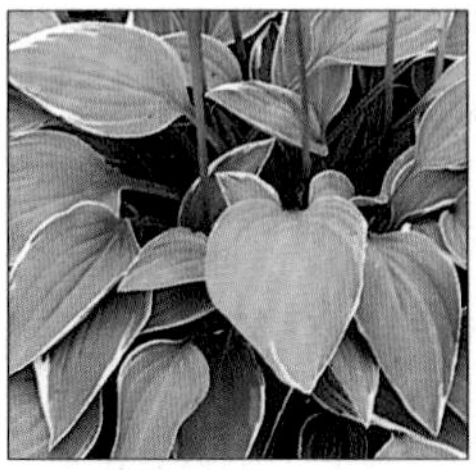
Hosta 'Allan P. McConnell'

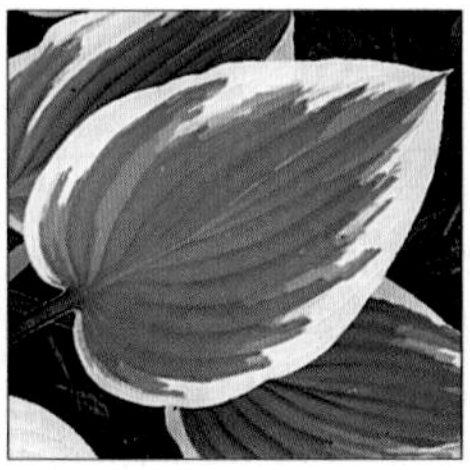
Hosta 'Antioch'

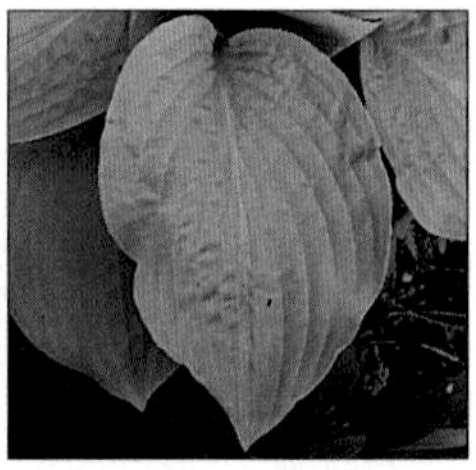
Hosta 'August Moon'

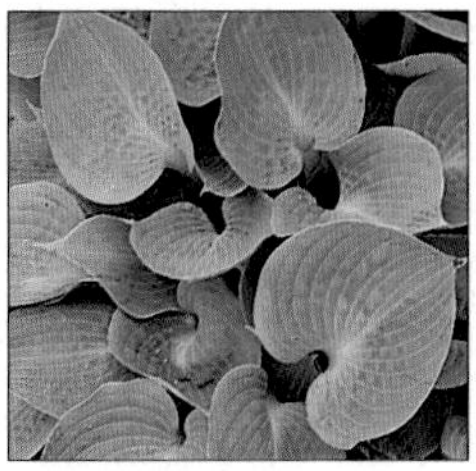
Hosta 'Blue Moon'

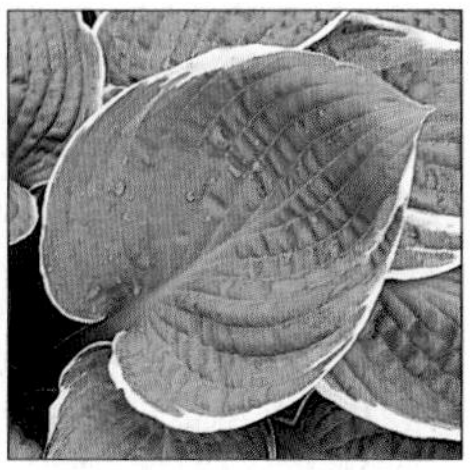
Hosta 'Carol'

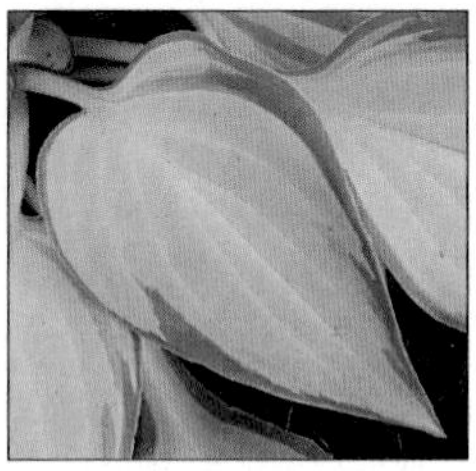
Hosta 'Emerald Tiara'

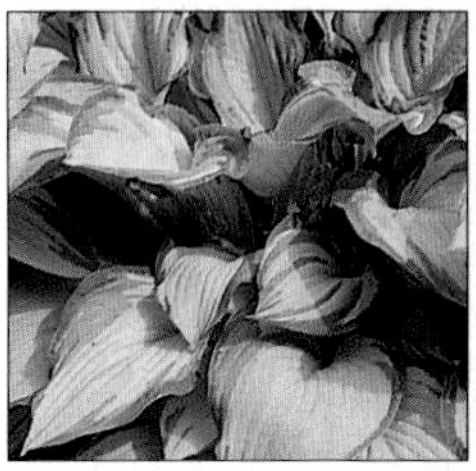
Hosta fortunei 'Albopicta'

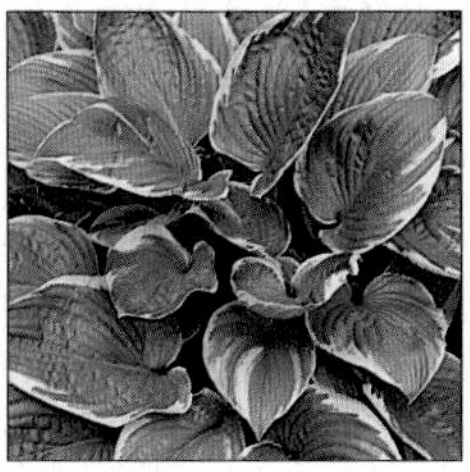
Hosta fortunei 'Aureomarginata'

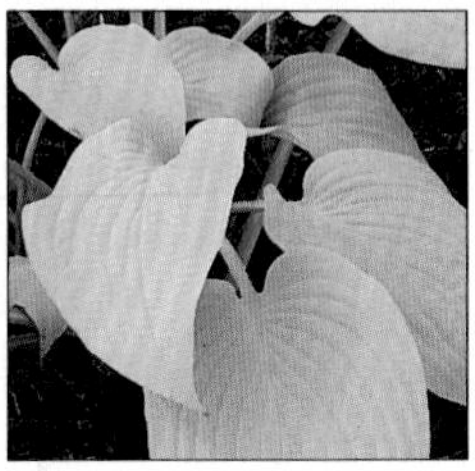
Hosta 'Fragrant Gold'

***H.* 'Francee'** ■ 🏆 Vigorous, clump-forming perennial producing ovate to heart-shaped, slightly cupped, puckered, olive-green leaves, 18cm (7in) long, with irregular white margins. Arching, leafy scapes, 75cm (30in) long, bear funnel-shaped, lavender-blue flowers in summer. ↕ 55 cm (22in), ↔ 1m (3ft). ❄❄❄
***H.* 'Frances Williams'** ■ 🏆 syn. *H.* 'Eldorado', *H.* 'Golden Circles', *H. sieboldiana* 'Frances Williams', *H. sieboldiana* 'Yellow Edge'. Clump-forming perennial producing heart-shaped, cupped, very puckered, thick, glaucous, blue-green leaves, 20cm (8in) long, with wide, irregular, green-yellow margins. In early summer, bears bell-shaped, greyish white flowers on glaucous scapes, 65cm (26in) long. ↕ 60cm (24in), ↔ 1m (3ft). ❄❄❄
***H.* 'Frosted Jade'** ■ Clump-forming perennial with ovate, pointed, glaucous, dark green leaves, 30cm (12in) long, with narrow white margins and splashed grey-green, giving the appearance of 'frosting'. Funnel-shaped, very pale lavender-blue, almost white flowers are borne on arching, leafy scapes, to 1.1m (3½ft) long, in early summer. ↕ 80cm (32in), ↔ 1m (3ft). ❄❄❄
***H.* 'Ginko Craig'.** Clump-forming perennial with lance-shaped, flat, dark green leaves, 8cm (3in) long, margined clear white. Mature plants (after about 4 years if not divided) have broader leaves with wider margins. In summer, bare scapes, 45cm (18in) long, bear funnel-shaped, deep purple to violet flowers. ↕ 25cm (10in), ↔ 45cm (18in). ❄❄❄
H. glauca see *H. sieboldiana* var. *elegans*.
***H.* 'Gold Edger'.** Vigorous perennial with heart-shaped, smooth, pale green-yellow leaves, 10cm (4in) long. Bell-shaped, very pale lavender-blue flowers are borne on scapes 40cm (16in) long, in summer. ↕ 30cm (12in), ↔ 45cm (18in). ❄❄❄
***H.* 'Golden'** see *H.* 'Birchwood Parky's Gold'.
***H.* 'Golden Circles'** see *H.* 'Frances Williams'.
***H.* 'Golden Medallion'.** Slow-growing, clump-forming perennial with rounded to heart-shaped, cupped, puckered yellow leaves, 15cm (6in) long. In mid-summer, bell-shaped, greyish white flowers are borne on scapes 45cm (18in) long. Prefers a sunny site. ↕ 35–40cm (14–16in), ↔ 60cm (24in). ❄❄❄
***H.* 'Golden Nakaiana'** see *H.* 'Birchwood Parky's Gold'.

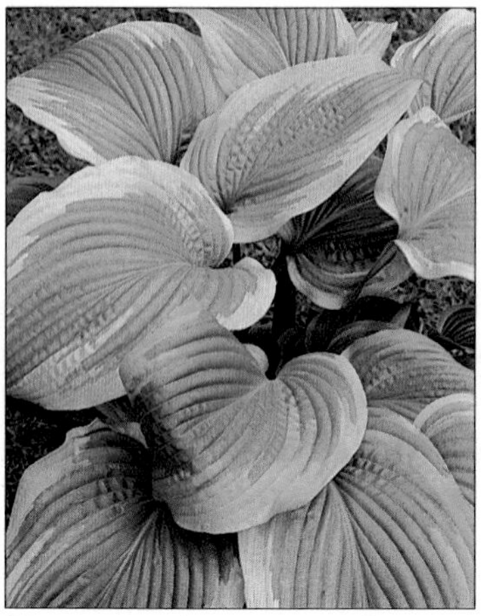
Hosta montana 'Aureomarginata'

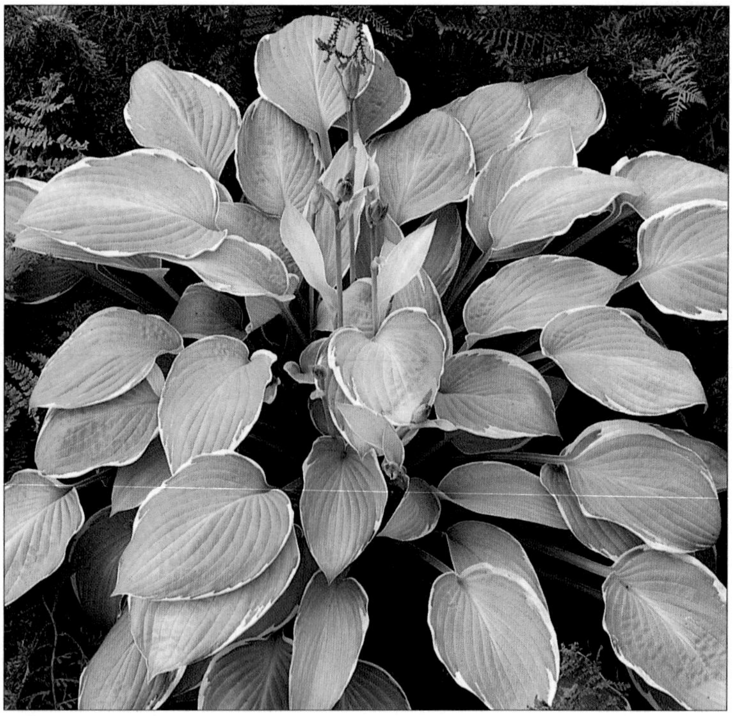
Hosta 'Moonlight'

***H.* 'Golden Prayers'** ■ Erect, clump-forming perennial with heart-shaped, cupped, close-veined, slightly puckered, deep yellow leaves, 10cm (4in) long. In summer, scapes 45cm (18in) long bear bell-shaped, pale lavender-blue flowers. ↕ 35cm (14in), ↔ 60cm (24in). ❄❄❄
***H.* 'Golden Tiara'** ■ 🏆 Vigorous perennial forming a mound of ovate to heart-shaped, mid-green leaves, 10cm (4in) long, irregularly margined with yellow. In summer, scapes 60cm (24in) long bear bell-shaped, deep purple, sometimes remontant flowers, striped lavender-purple. ↕ 30cm (12in), ↔ 50cm (20in). ❄❄❄
***H.* 'Gold Regal'.** Clump-forming perennial with erect leaf-stalks bearing ovate, slightly concave, erect, flat, thick, pale green-yellow leaves, 18cm (7in) long; they only colour well in full sun. Dense racemes of bell-shaped, greyish purple flowers, 2.5–8cm (1–3in) long, are borne on glaucous scapes, 70cm (28in) long, in summer. ↕ 60cm (24in), ↔ 1m (3ft). ❄❄❄
***H.* 'Gold Standard'** ■ Clump-forming perennial with ovate to heart-shaped, green-yellow leaves, 18cm (7in) long, fading through yellow to cream, and narrowly and irregularly margined dark green. In midsummer, funnel-shaped, lavender-blue flowers are borne on scapes to 1.1m (3½ft) long. ↕ 65cm (26in), ↔ 1m (3ft). ❄❄❄
H. gracillima. Clump-forming perennial with lance-shaped, wavy-margined leaves, 2–6cm (¾–2½in) long, glossy, deep green above, paler beneath. From summer to autumn, arching, leafless, purple-dotted scapes, 20–25cm (8–10in) long, bear widely funnel-shaped, lavender-blue flowers, purple-striped inside. ↕ 5cm (2in), ↔ 18cm (7in). Japan. ❄❄❄
***H.* 'Granary Gold'.** Clump-forming perennial with ovate to heart-shaped, wavy, slightly puckered, green- to light yellow leaves, 13cm (5in) long, fading to greenish white. In summer, leafy, glaucous scapes, 75cm (30in) long, bear funnel-shaped, lavender-blue flowers. ↕ 50cm (20in), ↔ 75cm (30in). ❄❄❄
***H.* 'Grand Tiara'** ■ Vigorous perennial forming a compact mound of ovate to heart-shaped, mid-green leaves, 10cm (4in) long, with irregular, wide yellow margins. In summer, bell-shaped, sometimes remontant, deep purple flowers, striped lavender-blue within, are produced on scapes 60cm (24in) long. ↕ 30cm (12in), ↔ 50cm (20in). ❄❄❄
***H.* 'Great Expectations'** ■ Clump-forming perennial with green-margined white leaf-stalks bearing heart-shaped, stiff, puckered, thick leaves, 15cm (6in) long; they are glaucous, blue-green, and irregularly but widely splashed with yellow, fading to white in the centres. In early summer, bell-shaped, greyish white flowers are borne on leafy scapes, 85cm (34in) long. ↕ 55cm (22in), ↔ 85cm (34in). ❄❄❄
***H.* 'Green Acres'.** Clump-forming perennial with ovate to heart-shaped, tapered, furrowed, thick, coarse, mid-green leaves, 45cm (18in) long, with rough undersides. Funnel-shaped, whitish mauve flowers are borne on straight, leafy scapes, 1m (3ft) long, in early summer. ↕↔ 1m (3ft). ❄❄❄
***H.* 'Green Fountain'** ■ Clump-forming perennial with red-dotted leaf-stalks bearing lance-shaped, tapering, arching, wavy-margined, glossy, mid-green leaves, 25cm (10in) long. In summer, bears funnel-shaped, widely spaced, pale mauve flowers on arching, leafy, red-dotted scapes, 60cm (24in) long. ↕ 45cm (18in), ↔ 1m (3ft). ❄❄❄
***H.* 'Green Sheen'.** Vigorous, clump-forming perennial with ovate to heart-shaped, thick, leathery, shiny, pale green leaves, 30cm (12in) long, glaucous beneath. In summer, bears bell-shaped, pale lavender-blue, white-striped flowers on leafless scapes, 1.5m (5ft) long. ↕ 75cm (30in) tall. ↔ 1m (3ft). ❄❄❄
***H.* 'Ground Master'** ■ Vigorous, stoloniferous, prostrate perennial with ovate to lance-shaped, matt, olive-green leaves, 13cm (5in) long, with wavy, irregular cream margins, fading to white. Mature plants (after about 4 years if not divided) have broader leaves with wider margins. In summer, produces funnel-shaped purple flowers on straight, leafy scapes, 50cm (20in) long. ↕ 25cm (10in), ↔ 55cm (22in). ❄❄❄
***H.* 'Hadspen Blue'** ■ Slow-growing, clump-forming perennial with ovate to heart-shaped, thick, glaucous, close-veined, grey-blue leaves, 13cm (5in) long. In summer, purple-dotted scapes, 35cm (14in) long, bear dense racemes of bell-shaped, pale grey-mauve flowers. ↕ 25cm (10in), ↔ 60cm (24in). ❄❄❄
***H.* 'Hadspen Heron'.** Clump-forming perennial with narrowly lance-shaped, slightly wavy-margined, glaucous, grey-blue leaves, 10cm (4in) long. In summer, bears bell-shaped, grey-mauve flowers on scapes 12in (30cm) long. ↕ 23cm (9in), ↔ 55cm (22in). ❄❄❄
***H.* 'Halcyon'** ■ 🏆 syn. *H.* 'Holstein'. Clump-forming perennial with heart-shaped, smooth, thick, glaucous, bright grey-blue leaves, 20cm (8in) long. In summer, bears dense racemes of bell-shaped, lavender-grey flowers on scapes 45cm (18in) long. ↕ 35–40cm (14–16in), ↔ 70cm (28in). ❄❄❄
H. helonioides* f. *albopicta see *H. rohdeifolia*.
***H.* 'Holstein'** see *H.* 'Halcyon'.
***H.* 'Honeybells'** ■ 🏆 Vigorous perennial forming a lax, open mound of ovate to heart-shaped, slightly wavy-margined, strongly veined, lustrous, pale green leaves, 28cm (11in) long. Fragrant, bell-shaped, white, sometimes lavender-blue-striped flowers are borne on leafy scapes, 1m (3ft) long, in late summer. ↕ 75cm (30in), ↔ 1.2m (4ft). ❄❄❄
H. hypoleuca. Clump-forming perennial with broadly ovate to heart-shaped, slightly wavy-margined, glaucous, pale green leaves, 25–45cm (10–18in) long, intensely white-coated beneath. In summer, bears bell-shaped, very pale lavender-blue flowers on arching, leafy, glaucous, red-dotted scapes, 35cm (14in) long. Thrives in sun or partial shade. ↕ 45cm (18in), ↔ 1m (3ft). Japan. ❄❄❄
***H.* 'Invincible'** ■ Vigorous, clump-forming perennial with ovate-oblong to lance-shaped, tapered, wavy-margined, thick, glossy, dark olive-green leaves, 13cm (5in) long. In late summer, bears funnel-shaped, fragrant, pale lavender-blue to white flowers on arching, leafy scapes, 50cm (20in) long. Grow in sun or partial shade. ↕ 30cm (12in), ↔ 60cm (24in). ❄❄❄
***H.* 'June'.** Clump-forming perennial, a variegated sport of *H.* 'Halcyon', with heart-shaped, smooth, glaucous, grey-blue leaves, 20cm (8in) long, centrally and irregularly variegated yellow and yellow-green. Racemes of bell-shaped, lavender-grey flowers are borne on glaucous scapes, 45cm (18in) long, in summer. ↕ 35–40cm (14–16in), ↔ 70cm (28in). ❄❄❄
***H.* 'Kabitan'** ■ syn. *H. sieboldii* 'Kabitan'. Clump-forming perennial producing lance-shaped, thin, bright yellow leaves, 25cm (10in) long, with rippled, dark green margins. In late summer, bears narrow, later flaring, funnel-shaped, deep violet flowers on leafy scapes, 30cm (12in) long. ↕ 20cm (8in), ↔ 25cm (10in). ❄❄❄

H

H. kikutii. Clump-forming perennial with ovate to lance-shaped or elliptic, tapered, prominently veined, arching, glossy, dark green leaves, 18–23cm (7–9in) long, lustrous beneath. In summer, bears dense racemes of funnel-shaped, white, sometimes faintly purple-flushed flowers on arching, leafy, red-dotted scapes, 60cm (24in) long. ↕40cm (16in), ↔ 60cm (24in). Japan. ❄❄❄
***H.* 'Krossa Regal'** 🏆 Clump-forming perennial with semi-erect, ovate to lance-shaped, deeply veined, glaucous, bluish green leaves, 23cm (9in) long. In summer, glaucous scapes, 1.4m (4½ft) long, bear bell-shaped, pale lilac flowers. ↕70cm (28in), ↔ 75cm (30in). ❄❄❄
H. lancifolia ▣🏆 syn. *H. lancifolia* var. *fortis.* Perennial forming a dense mound of arching, narrowly lance-shaped, thin, glossy, dark green leaves, 10–17cm (4–7in) long. In late summer, slender, very leafy, red-dotted scapes, 65cm (26in) long, bear narrowly funnel-shaped, deep purple flowers. ↕45cm (18in), ↔ 75cm (30in). Korea, Japan. ❄❄❄. **var. *fortis*** see *H. lancifolia.*
***H.* 'Lemon Lime'** ▣ Vigorous, clump-forming perennial with lance-shaped, wavy, thin, yellow-green to yellow leaves, 8cm (3in) long. In summer, produces remontant, bell-shaped, white-striped purple flowers on scapes 30cm (12in) long. ↕15cm (6in), ↔ 45cm (18in). ❄❄❄
H. longipes. Vigorous, clump-forming perennial with ovate to heart-shaped, sometimes rounded, slightly wavy-margined, mid- to deep green leaves, 9–13cm (3½–5in) long, glossy beneath, and spotted purple at the bases of the midribs and on the leaf-stalks. In late summer and autumn, leafy, purple-dotted scapes, 40cm (16in) long, bear bell-shaped, wide-tubed, pale purple to chalky white flowers. ↕30cm (12in), ↔ 50cm (20in). Korea, Japan. ❄❄❄
H. longissima ▣ Moisture-loving, upright, clump-forming perennial with narrowly lance-shaped, erect to arching, dark green leaves, 15–20cm (6–8in) long, glossy beneath. In late summer, bears long racemes of funnel-shaped, purple-striped mauve flowers on leafy scapes, 55cm (22in) long. ↕25cm (10in), ↔ 50cm (20in). Japan. ❄❄❄
***H.* 'Love Pat'** ▣🏆 Slow-growing, clump-forming perennial with upright, heart-shaped, cupped, very puckered, thick, glaucous, deep blue leaves, 15cm (6in) long. In midsummer, bell-shaped, off-white flowers are borne on scapes 55cm (22in) long. ↕45cm (18in), ↔ 1m (3ft). ❄❄❄
***H.* 'Mediovariegata'** see *H. undulata* var. *undulata.*
***H.* 'Midas Touch'.** Very slow-growing, clump-forming perennial with ovate to heart-shaped, cupped, very dimpled yellow leaves, 23cm (9in) long. Scapes 50cm (20in) long bear bell-shaped, pale lavender-white flowers in midsummer. Thrives in sun or partial shade. ↕50cm (20in), ↔ 65cm (26in). ❄❄❄
***H. minor* f. *alba* of gardens** see *H. sieboldii* var. *alba.*
H. montana. Clump-forming perennial with ovate to heart-shaped, thick, boldly veined leaves, 20–30cm (8–12in) long, varying from shiny, mid- to dark green to glaucous, pale green, with rough undersides. Leafy, purple-dotted scapes, 1m (3ft) long, bear funnel-shaped, grey-mauve to white flowers in early summer. ↕75cm (30in), ↔ 1m (3ft). Japan. ❄❄❄. **'Aureomarginata'** ▣ has narrower, tapering, wavy-margined, glossy, dark green leaves, 30cm (12in) long, with irregular yellow margins, turning cream; the leaves emerge early in spring. Scapes are 90cm (36in) long; ↕70cm (28in), ↔ 90cm (36in).
***H.* 'Moonlight'** ▣ Clump-forming perennial with ovate to heart-shaped, cupped, olive-green leaves, 18cm (7in) long, fading to yellow, and irregularly margined white. In midsummer, bears funnel-shaped, lavender-blue flowers on straight, leafy scapes, 65cm (26in) long. ↕50cm (20in), ↔ 70cm (28in). ❄❄❄
***H.* 'Neat Splash Rim'.** Stoloniferous perennial with broadly lance-shaped, olive-green leaves, 18cm (7in) long, boldly margined with cream, fading to white. Funnel-shaped purple flowers are borne on leafy scapes, 50cm (20in) long, in late summer. ↕35cm (14in), ↔ 60cm (24in). ❄❄❄
H. nigrescens ▣ Clump-forming perennial with ovate-heart-shaped, concave, partly wrinkled, glaucous, grey-green leaves, 25–45cm (10–18in) long. In late summer, leafy, glaucous scapes, 1.4m (4½ft) long, bear funnel-shaped white flowers. ↕70cm (28in), ↔ 65cm (26in). Japan. ❄❄❄
***H.* 'Obscura Marginata'** see *H. fortunei* 'Aureomarginata'.
***H.* 'On Stage'.** Clump-forming perennial with ovate to heart-shaped, tapered, light yellow leaves, 20cm (8in) long, irregularly margined and splashed dark and light green. In early summer, bears funnel-shaped, pale lavender-blue flowers on scapes 50cm (20in) long. ↕35cm (14in), ↔ 60cm (24in). ❄❄❄
H. opipara, syn. *H.* 'Opipara'. Clump-forming perennial with flattened, wide leaf-stalks and rounded to heart-shaped, leathery, glossy, bright green leaves, 18–23cm (7–9in) long, with broad, wavy, yellow margins, turning cream. In late summer, arching, leafy scapes, 75cm (30in) long, bear bell-shaped, purple-striped mauve flowers. ↕70cm (28in), ↔ 1.5m (5ft). Japan. ❄❄❄
***H.* 'Opipara'** see *H. opipara.*
***H.* 'Patriot'.** Vigorous, clump-forming perennial with ovate to heart-shaped, slightly cupped, puckered, olive-green leaves, 20cm (8in) long, very widely and irregularly margined white, and with grey-green splashes. In summer, bears funnel-shaped, lavender-blue flowers on leafy, glaucous scapes, 75cm (30in) long. ↕55cm (22in), ↔ 1m (3ft). ❄❄❄
***H.* 'Paul's Glory'.** Clump-forming perennial with heart-shaped, puckered yellow leaves, 15cm (6in) long, irregularly margined glaucous, grey-blue and yellow-green. In midsummer, leafy, arching, glaucous scapes, 60cm (24in) long, bear bell-shaped, lavender-grey flowers. ↕45cm (18in), ↔ 65cm (26in). ❄❄❄
***H.* 'Paxton's Original'** see *H. sieboldii.*
***H.* 'Pearl Lake'.** Vigorous perennial forming a mound of heart-shaped, flat, glaucous, grey-green leaves, 10cm (4in) long. Bell-shaped, opalescent, lavender-blue, sometimes remontant flowers open on glaucous scapes, 60–80cm (24–32in) long, in midsummer. ↕35–40cm (14–16in), ↔ 1m (3ft). ❄❄❄
***H.* 'Piedmont Gold'** ▣ Robust, clump-forming perennial with narrowly heart-

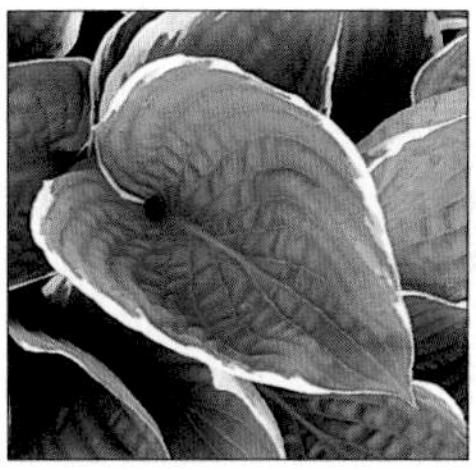
Hosta 'Francee'

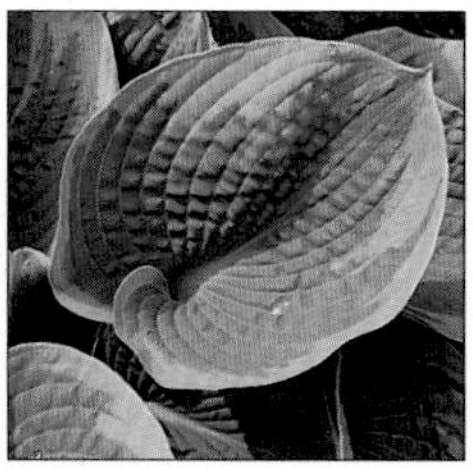
Hosta 'Frances Williams'

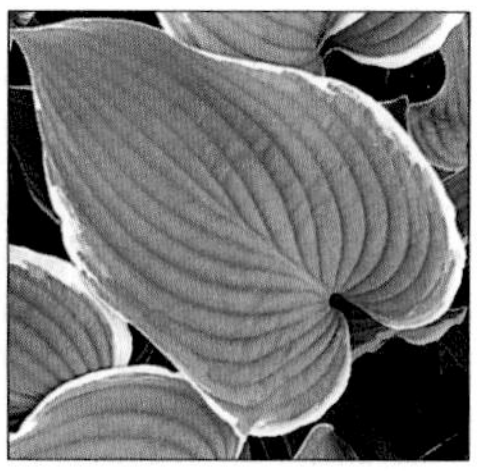
Hosta 'Frosted Jade'

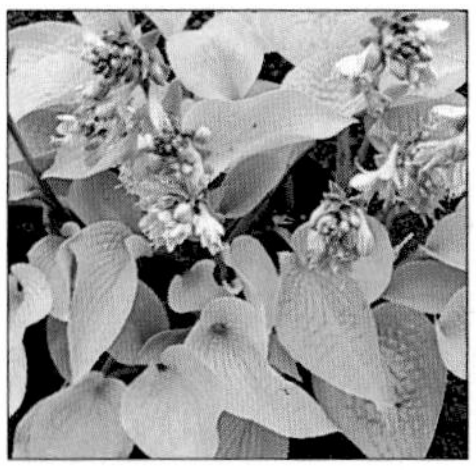
Hosta 'Golden Prayers'

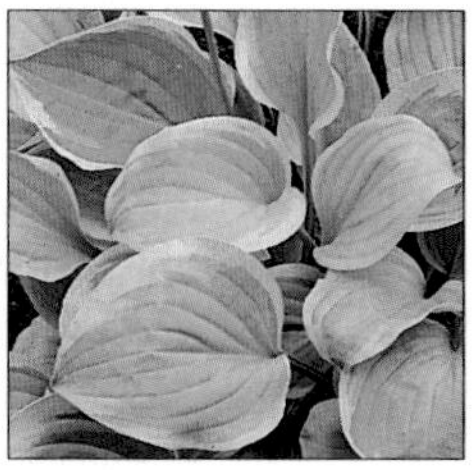
Hosta 'Golden Tiara'

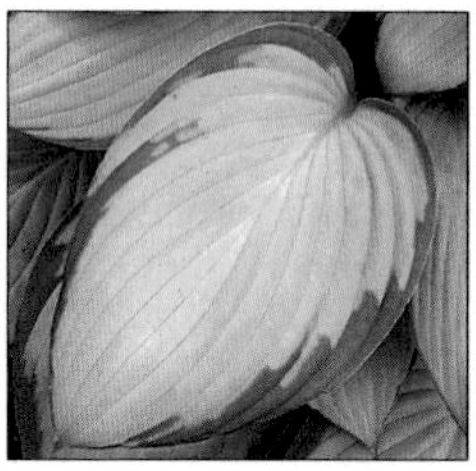
Hosta 'Gold Standard'

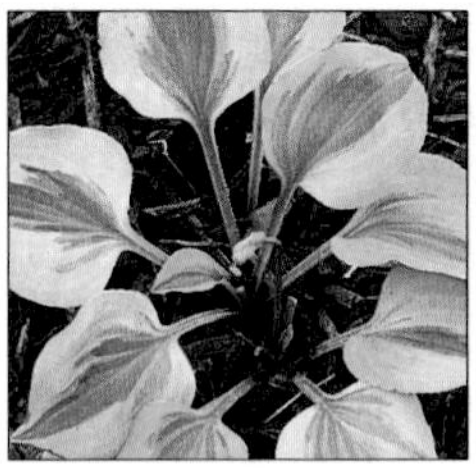
Hosta 'Grand Tiara'

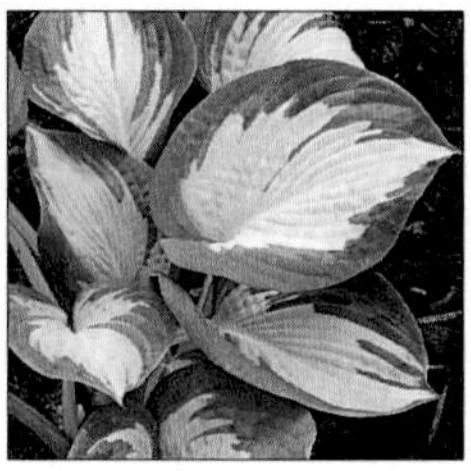
Hosta 'Great Expectations'

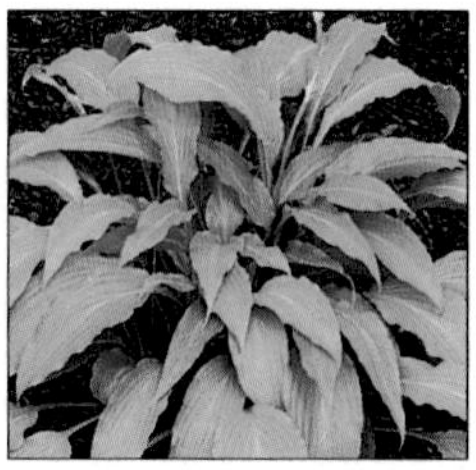
Hosta 'Green Fountain'

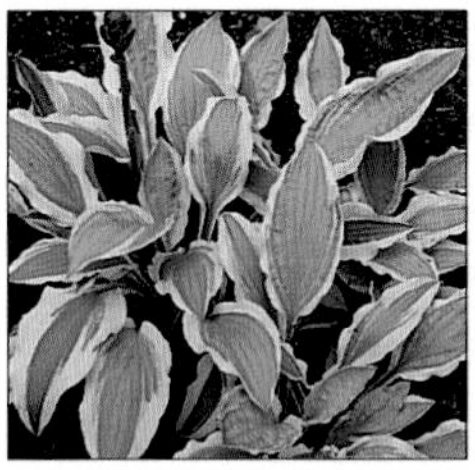
Hosta 'Ground Master'

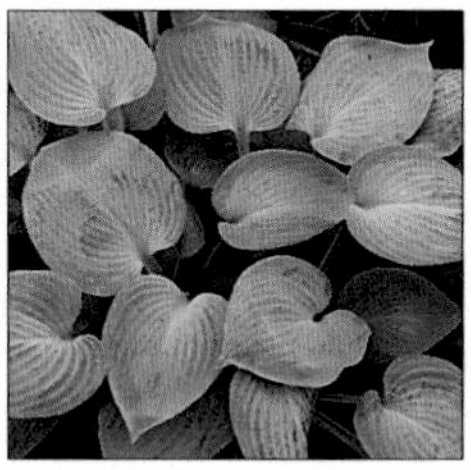
Hosta 'Hadspen Blue'

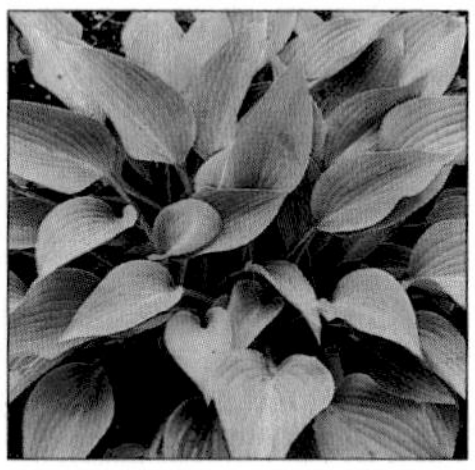
Hosta 'Halcyon'

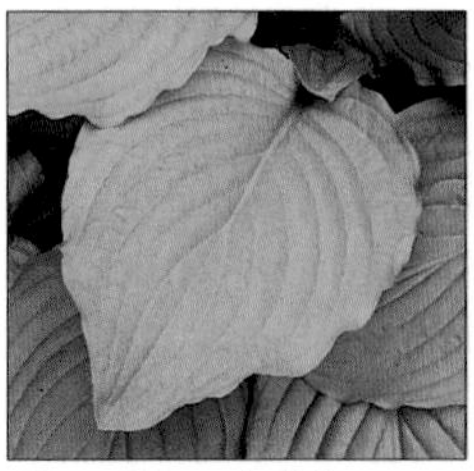
Hosta 'Honeybells'

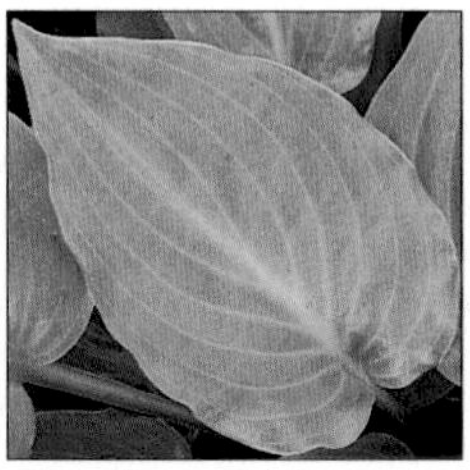
Hosta 'Invincible'

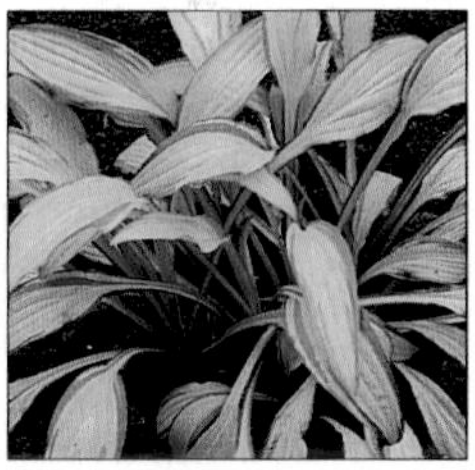
Hosta 'Kabitan'

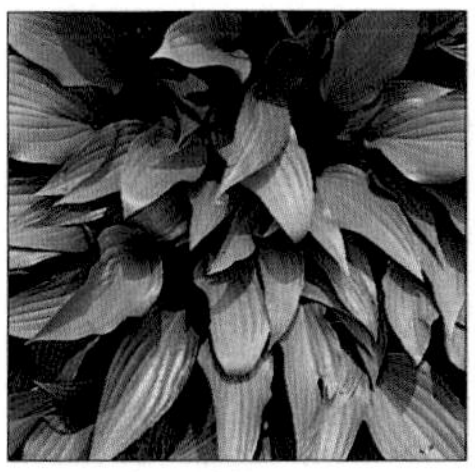
Hosta lancifolia

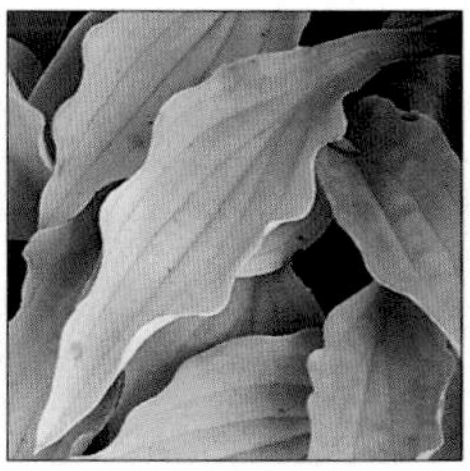
Hosta 'Lemon Lime'

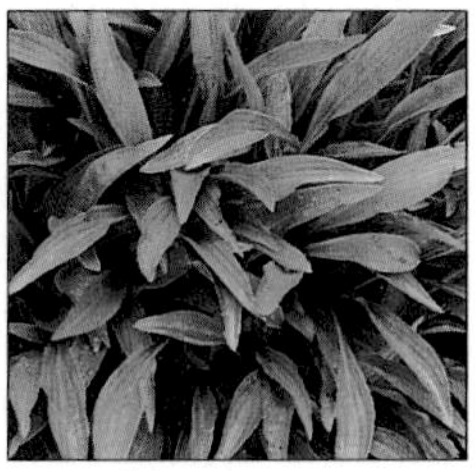
Hosta longissima

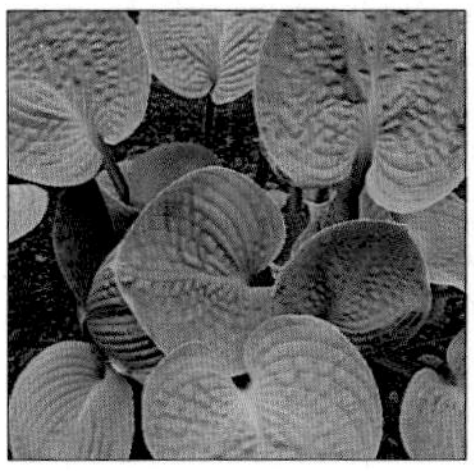
Hosta 'Love Pat'

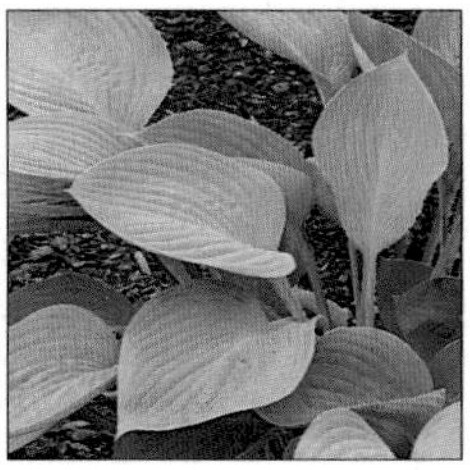
Hosta nigrescens

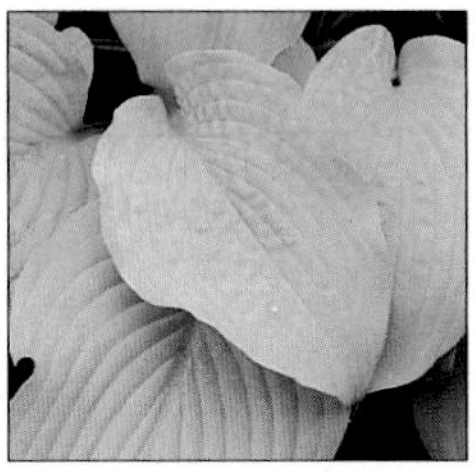
Hosta 'Piedmont Gold'

shaped, wavy-margined, matt, glaucous yellow leaves, 28cm (11in) long. In summer, bears funnel-shaped, greyish white flowers on scapes 65cm (26in) long. ↕ 50cm (20in), ↔ 1m (3ft). ***
***H.* 'Pizzazz'.** Clump-forming perennial producing ovate to heart-shaped, puckered, glaucous, mid-green leaves, 18cm (7in) long, splashed blue-green and irregularly margined cream. Bell-shaped, pale lavender-blue flowers are freely borne on leafy, glaucous scapes, 45cm (18in) long, in summer. ↕ 35cm (14in), ↔ 60cm (24in). ***
H. plantaginea*.** Clump-forming perennial producing ovate to heart-shaped, slightly wavy, glossy, light green leaves, 16–28cm (6–11in) long, with prominent, widely spaced, raised veins. Trumpet-shaped, long-tubed, very fragrant white flowers, 10cm (4in) long, are borne on leafy, bright green scapes, 65–75cm (26–30in) long, in late summer and early autumn. Prefers a sunny site. ↕ 60cm (24in), ↔ 1m (3ft). China. ***. **'Aphrodite'** bears double flowers that hardly ever open. **'Grandiflora'** 🏆 syn. var. *japonica*, has ovate to lance-shaped, wavy leaves, 23cm (9in) long, and bears flowers 13cm (5in) long. **var. *japonica see 'Grandiflora'.

***H. pycnophylla*.** Slow-growing, clump-forming perennial with ovate to heart-shaped, very wavy-margined, glaucous, dull light green leaves, 20–25cm (8–10in) long, coated white beneath. In late summer, bears funnel-shaped, purple to dark purple flowers on arching, leafy, glaucous, purple-dotted scapes, 35cm (14in) long. ↕ 30cm (12in), ↔ 70cm (28in). Japan. ***
***H. rectifolia*.** Sturdy, clump-forming perennial with ovate, shallowly cupped, dull to dark green leaves, to 30cm (12in) long. In late summer, bears widely spaced racemes of bell-shaped, deep-purple-striped purple flowers on stout, leafy scapes, 60–75cm (24–30in) long. ↕ 45cm (18in), ↔ 75cm (30in). Japan, Russia (Kurile Islands). ***
***H.* 'Regal Splendor'** ▣ Clump-forming perennial with long, arching leaf-stalks bearing ovate to lance-shaped, semi-erect, deeply veined, thick, glaucous, grey-green leaves, 30cm (12in) long, irregularly margined white to yellow. In summer, bears bell-shaped, greyish pink flowers on glaucous scapes, 1.4m (4½ft) long. ↕ 75cm (30in), ↔ 1m (3ft). ***
***H.* 'Robusta'** see *H. sieboldiana* var. *elegans*.
***H. rohdeifolia*,** syn. *H. helonioides* f. *albopicta*, *H.* 'Rohdeifolia'. Erect, clump-forming perennial with lance-shaped to inversely lance-shaped, blunt-tipped, flat, olive-green leaves, 13–18cm (5–7in) long, often with yellow margins, fading to cream. Funnel-shaped, dark-purple-striped purple flowers are borne on leafy scapes, 50–100cm (20–39in) long, in summer. ↕ 30cm (12in), ↔ 45cm (18in). Probably Japan. ***
***H.* 'Rohdeifolia'** see *H. rohdeifolia*.
***H.* 'Royal Standard'** ▣🏆 Vigorous, clump-forming perennial with ovate to heart-shaped, ribbed, glossy, bright pale green leaves, 20cm (8in) long. Funnel-shaped, fragrant white flowers, 2.5–8cm (1–3in) long, are borne on leafy scapes, 1m (3ft) long, in late summer. Tolerates sun or partial shade. ↕ 60cm (24in), ↔ 1.2m (4ft). ***

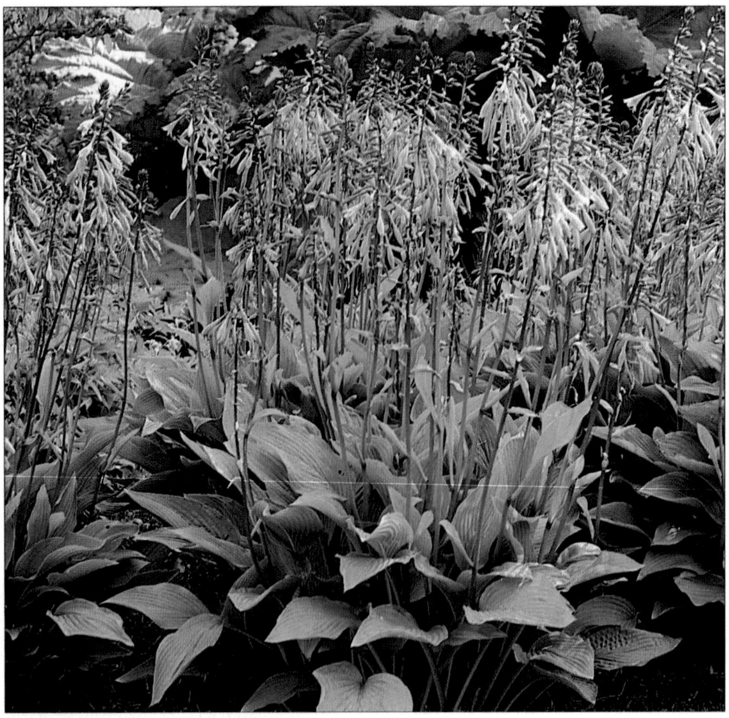

Hosta 'Tall Boy'

***H. rupifraga*.** Clump-forming perennial with broadly ovate-heart-shaped, wavy-margined, smooth, thick, glossy, dark green leaves, 12–15cm (5–6in) long, mid-green beneath. In early autumn, arching, leafy, glaucous, purple-dotted scapes, 30–40cm (12–16in) long, bear dense racemes of bell-shaped, light mauve flowers. ↕ 20cm (8in), ↔ 60cm (24in). Japan. ***
***H.* 'Sagae'** see *H. fluctuans* 'Sagae'.
***H.* 'Saishu Jima'.** Vigorous perennial with narrowly lance-shaped, wavy-margined, dark green leaves, 10cm (4in) long. In mid- and late summer, bears bell-shaped, dark purple-striped purple flowers on scapes 23cm (9in) long. ↕ 20cm (8in), ↔ 35–40cm (14–16in). ***
***H.* 'Sazanami'** see *H. crispula*.
***H.* 'Sea Drift'.** Slow-growing, clump-forming perennial with heart-shaped, pointed, wavy-margined, dark green leaves, 35cm (14in) long. In summer, funnel-shaped, lavender-blue flowers are borne on scapes 70cm (28in) long. ↕ 60cm (24in), ↔ 1m (3ft). ***
***H.* 'Sea Octopus'.** Slow-growing, clump-forming perennial with heart-shaped, pointed, very wavy-margined, dark green leaves, 15cm (6in) long. In summer, funnel-shaped, lavender-blue flowers are borne on scapes 70cm (28in) long. ↕ 20cm (8in), ↔ 1m (3ft). ***
***H.* 'September Sun'** ▣ Vigorous, clump-forming perennial with ovate to heart-shaped, flat, lime-green to yellow leaves, 15cm (6in) long, irregularly margined dark green, the variegation developing as the leaves mature. In summer, scapes 75cm (30in) long bear bell-shaped, very pale lavender-blue flowers. Thrives in sun or partial shade. ↕ 65cm (26in), ↔ 1m (3ft). ***
***H.* 'Shade Fanfare'** ▣🏆 Clump-forming perennial with heart-shaped, wavy-margined, light to mid-green leaves, 18cm (7in) long, irregularly margined cream, turning white with age. Funnel-shaped, lavender-blue flowers are borne freely on leafy scapes, 60cm (24in) long, in summer. ↕ 45cm (18in), ↔ 60cm (24in). ***
***H.* 'Shining Tot'.** Clump-forming perennial with heart-shaped, flat, thick, glossy, dark green leaves, 3cm (1¼in) long. Funnel-shaped, lavender-blue flowers are borne on arching, bare scapes, 15cm (6in) long, in summer. ↕ 5cm (2in), ↔ 20cm (8in). ***
H. sieboldiana*.** Clump-forming perennial with ovate-heart-shaped to rounded, cupped, puckered, thick leaves, 25–50cm (10–20in) long, glaucous, grey-green to blue above, paler, sometimes glaucous beneath. In early summer, leafy, glaucous scapes, 1m (3ft) long, bear bell-shaped, pale lilac-grey flowers, fading to lilac-tinted white or pure white. ↕ 1m (3ft), ↔ 1.2m (4ft). Japan. ***. **var. *elegans ▣🏆 syn. 'Elegans', *H. glauca*, *H.* 'Robusta', has rounded-heart-shaped, heavily and deeply puckered, very thickly glaucous, grey-blue leaves, 20–30cm (8–12in) long. **'Frances Williams'** see *H.* 'Frances Williams'. **'Yellow Edge'** see *H.* 'Frances Williams'.
H. sieboldii 🏆 syn. *H. albomarginata*, *H.* 'Paxton's Original'. Vigorous, clump-forming perennial with broadly lance-shaped, blunt-tipped, flat, matt, olive-green leaves, 10–15cm (4–6in) long, narrowly and irregularly margined white. Racemes of funnel-shaped, deep violet flowers, purple-and-white-striped within, are borne on leafy scapes, 50cm (20in) long, in late summer and early autumn. ↕ 30cm (12in), ↔ 60cm (24in). Japan. ***. **var. *alba*,** syn. *H. minor* f. *alba* of gardens, has mid-green leaves and white flowers. **'Kabitan'** see *H.* 'Kabitan'.
***H.* 'Snow Cap'.** Clump-forming perennial with heart-shaped, slightly cupped, puckered, glaucous, blue-green leaves, 20cm (8in) long, irregularly margined creamy white. In summer, bears large, fragrant, funnel-shaped, purple-striped white flowers on scapes 55cm (22in) long. ↕ 40cm (16in), ↔ 60cm (24in). ***

***H.* 'Snowden'** ▣ Slow-growing, clump-forming perennial with ovate to heart-shaped, pointed, flat, thick, glaucous, grey-green leaves, 35cm (14in) long. Funnel-shaped, greyish white flowers are borne on thick scapes, 1m (3ft) long, in midsummer. ↕↔ 1m (3ft). ***
***H.* 'Snowflakes'.** Clump-forming perennial with ovate to heart-shaped, pointed, flat, thick, glaucous, grey-green leaves, 35cm (14in) long. In midsummer, scapes 35cm (14in) long bear funnel-shaped, greyish white flowers. ↕ 20cm (8in), ↔ 30cm (12in). ***
***H.* 'So Sweet'** ▣ Clump-forming perennial with ovate to lance-shaped, flat, glossy, mid-green leaves, 18cm (7in) long, margined creamy white. In mid- and late summer, lavender-blue buds open to funnel-shaped, fragrant, purple-striped white flowers on scapes 60cm (24in) long. ↕ 35cm (14in), ↔ 55cm (22in). ***
***H.* 'Stiletto'.** Vigorous, erect, clump-forming perennial with lance-shaped, rippled, mid-green leaves, 18cm (7in) long, margined creamy white. Funnel-shaped, purple-striped, lavender-blue flowers are borne on leafy scapes, 30cm (12in) long, in summer. ↕ 15cm (6in), ↔ 20cm (8in). ***
***H.* 'Sugar and Cream'** ▣ Vigorous perennial forming a lax, open mound of ovate to heart-shaped, mid-green leaves, 25cm (10in) long, with slightly wavy, irregular cream margins. Fragrant, bell-shaped white flowers, striped lavender-blue, are borne on leafy scapes, 1m (3ft) long, in late summer. Thrives in sun or partial shade. ↕↔ 75cm (30in). ***
***H.* 'Sum and Substance'** ▣🏆 Clump-forming perennial with heart-shaped, flat, glossy, yellow-green to yellow leaves, 50cm (20in) long, glaucous beneath, becoming puckered when mature. In mid- and late summer, bears dense racemes of bell-shaped, very pale lilac flowers on leaning, glaucous scapes, 1m (3ft) long. Thrives in sun or partial shade. ↕ 75cm (30in), ↔ 1.2m (4ft). ***
***H.* 'Summer Fragrance'.** Clump-forming perennial with ovate to heart-shaped, pointed, flat, mid-green leaves, 20cm (8in) long, irregularly and narrowly margined creamy white. Bell-shaped, fragrant, deep lavender-purple flowers are borne on leafy scapes, 85cm (34in) long, in late summer. ↕ 60cm (24in), ↔ 1.2m (4ft). ***
***H.* 'Sun Power'.** Clump-forming perennial with ovate to heart-shaped, wavy, yellow-green to bright yellow leaves, 25cm (10in) long. Funnel-shaped, pale lavender-blue to white flowers are borne on arching, leafy scapes, to 1.2m (4ft) long, in summer. ↕ 60cm (24in), ↔ 1m (3ft). ***
***H.* 'Tall Boy'** ▣ Erect, clump-forming perennial with short, straight leaf-stalks bearing ovate, mid-green leaves, 23cm (9in) long. Dense racemes of funnel-shaped purple flowers are produced on leafy scapes, 1m (3ft) long, in late summer. ↕ 50cm (20in), ↔ 1m (3ft). ***
H. tardiflora ▣ Clump-forming perennial producing lance-shaped, thick, glossy, dark green leaves, 8–15cm (3–6in) long, matt, dark green beneath. Funnel-shaped mauve flowers are borne on slightly arching, leafy, glaucous, purple-tinted scapes, to 35cm (14in)

long, in autumn. ↕ 25cm (10in), ↔ 60cm (24in). Probably Japan. ❄❄❄
***H.* 'Thomas Hogg'** see *H. undulata* var. *undulata* 'Albomarginata'.
***H.* 'Tiny Tears'.** Clump-forming perennial with narrowly heart-shaped, flat, dark green leaves, 8cm (3in) long. In summer, dense racemes of bell-shaped purple flowers are borne on scapes 25cm (10in) long. ↕ 8cm (3in), ↔ 15cm (6in). ❄❄❄
***H. tokudama*,** syn. *H.* 'Tokudama'. Slow-growing, clump-forming perennial with heart-shaped to rounded, cupped, puckered, vividly glaucous, deep blue-green leaves, 20–30cm (8–12in) long. From early to late summer, bears widely bell-shaped, greyish white flowers on leafy, glaucous scapes, 40cm (16in) long. ↕ 35cm (14in), ↔ 1m (3ft). Japan. ❄❄❄. **'Aureonebulosa'** ■ syn. f. *aureonebulosa*, *H.* 'Tokudama Aureonebulosa', has green-yellow leaves, 20–25cm (8–10in) long, irregularly margined and splashed deep blue-green. **'Flavocircinalis'** ■ syn. f. *flavocircinalis*, *H.* 'Tokudama Flavocircinalis', has ovate to heart-shaped blue leaves, irregularly margined creamy yellow; it bears flowers on scapes 45cm (18in) long, in midsummer; ↕ 40cm (16in), ↔ 75cm (30in).
***H.* 'Tokudama'** see *H. tokudama*.
***H.* 'Tokudama Aureonebulosa'** see *H. tokudama* 'Aureonebulosa'.
***H.* 'Tokudama Flavocircinalis'** see *H. tokudama* 'Flavocircinalis'.
***H.* 'True Blue'.** Clump-forming perennial with ovate to heart-shaped, pointed, puckered, thick, glaucous, grey-blue leaves, 30cm (12in) long. In midsummer, bears bell-shaped, off-white flowers on scapes 70cm (28in) long. ↕ 60cm (24in), ↔ 1m (3ft). ❄❄❄
***H.* 'Undulata'** see *H. undulata* var. *undulata*.
***H.* 'Undulata Erromena'** see *H. undulata* var. *erromena*.
H. undulata* var. *undulata 🏆 syn. *H.* 'Argentea Variegata', *H.* 'Cream Delight', *H.* 'Mediovariegata', *H.* 'Undulata', *H.* 'Variegata'. Clump-forming perennial, the type of the species *H. undulata*, with twisted, deeply channelled, lance-shaped to elliptic or narrowly ovate, slightly pointed, mid-green leaves, 13–18cm (5–7in) long; they are thin but leathery, and strongly wavy-margined, with central white or pale yellow-white markings. Arching, leafy white scapes, 50–80cm (20–32in) long, bear funnel-shaped mauve flowers in early and midsummer. ↕ to 1m (3ft), ↔ 45m (18in). Probably Japan. ❄❄❄. **'Albomarginata'** ■ syn. var. *albomarginata*, *H.* 'Thomas Hogg', produces broadly ovate, flat or only slightly wavy-margined leaves, dark green with irregular cream or pale yellow margins; ↕ 55cm (22in), ↔ 60cm (24in). **var. *erromena*** 🏆 syn. *H.* 'Undulata Erromena', is vigorous, and has broadly ovate, tapering, matt, mid-green leaves, 13–23cm (5–9in) long. **var. *univittata*** ■ 🏆 syn. *H.* 'Undulata Univittata', has ovate, twisted, matt, olive-green leaves, 13–18cm (5–7in) long, each with a central cream zone; ↕ 45cm (18in), ↔ 70cm (28in).
***H.* 'Undulata Univittata'** see *H. undulata* var. *univittata*.
***H.* 'Vanilla Cream'.** Clump-forming perennial with slightly red-dotted leaf-stalks bearing ovate to heart-shaped, cupped, slightly puckered, thick, creamy yellow-green leaves, 8cm (3in) long. Funnel-shaped, pale lavender-blue flowers are produced on scapes 30cm (12in) long, in midsummer. ↕ 12cm (5in), ↔ 25cm (10in). ❄❄❄
***H.* 'Variegata'** see *H. undulata* var. *undulata*.
H. ventricosa ■ 🏆 syn. *H.* 'Ventricosa'. Clump-forming perennial with broadly ovate to heart-shaped, slightly wavy, wide-veined, thin, glossy, dark green leaves, 20–30cm (8–12in) long. In late summer, bears tubular-bell-shaped, deep purple flowers, white-striped within, on leafy, leaning scapes, 80–100cm (32–39in) long. ↕ 50cm (20in), ↔ 1m (3ft). China, N. Korea. ❄❄❄. **'Aureomaculata'**, syn. var. *aureomaculata*, *H.* 'Ventricosa Aureomaculata', is slow-growing, and has leaves centrally splashed yellow, fading to yellow-green. **'Variegata'** ■ 🏆 syn. *H.* 'Ventricosa Aureomarginata', has leaves irregularly margined with yellow, turning creamy white.
***H.* 'Ventricosa'** see *H. ventricosa*.
***H.* 'Ventricosa Aureomaculata'** see *H. ventricosa* 'Aureomaculata'.
***H.* 'Ventricosa Aureomarginata'** see *H. ventricosa* 'Variegata'.
H. venusta ■ 🏆 Clump-forming perennial producing ovate to heart-shaped, flat, wavy-margined, dark green leaves, 3–5cm (1¼–2in) long, glossy beneath. Trumpet-shaped violet flowers are borne freely on ridged, leafy scapes, 25–35cm (10–14in) long, from midsummer to mid-autumn. ↕ 5cm (2in), ↔ 25cm (10in). Korea, Japan. ❄❄❄
***H.* 'Vera Verde'** ■ Stoloniferous perennial with lance-shaped, flat, olive-green leaves, 9cm (3½in) long, narrowly margined cream. In summer, bears funnel-shaped, purple-striped, pale mauve flowers on scapes 30cm (12in) long. ↕ 15cm (6in), ↔ 35–40cm (14–16in). ❄❄❄
***H.* 'Wide Brim'** ■ 🏆 Clump-forming perennial with heart-shaped, slightly cupped, heavily puckered, glaucous, dark green leaves, 18cm (7in) long, irregularly and widely margined cream, fading to white. Funnel-shaped, pale lavender-blue flowers are borne on scapes 55cm (22in) long in summer. ↕ 45cm (18in), ↔ 1m (3ft). ❄❄❄
***H.* 'Wind River Gold'.** Clump-forming perennial with red-dotted leaf-stalks bearing ovate to lance-shaped, tapered, wavy, thin, deep yellow leaves, 10cm (4in) long, fading to yellow-green. In midsummer, produces funnel-shaped purple flowers on scapes 24cm (10in) long. ↕ 13cm (5in), ↔ 25cm (10in). ❄❄❄
***H.* 'Yellow River'** ■ Clump-forming perennial with ovate to heart-shaped, pointed, thick, dark green leaves, 35cm (14in) long, irregularly margined yellow. Leafy scapes, 1m (3ft) long, bear funnel-shaped, very pale lavender-blue flowers in early summer. ↕ 55cm (22in), ↔ 1m (3ft). ❄❄❄
***H.* 'Zounds'** ■ Clump-forming perennial with heart-shaped, puckered, thick yellow leaves, 28cm (11in) long, with a metallic sheen. In summer, leafy scapes, 60cm (24in) long, bear funnel-shaped, pale lavender-blue flowers. ↕ 55cm (22in), ↔ 1m (3ft). ❄❄❄

▷ **Hottentot fig** see *Carpobrotus edulis*

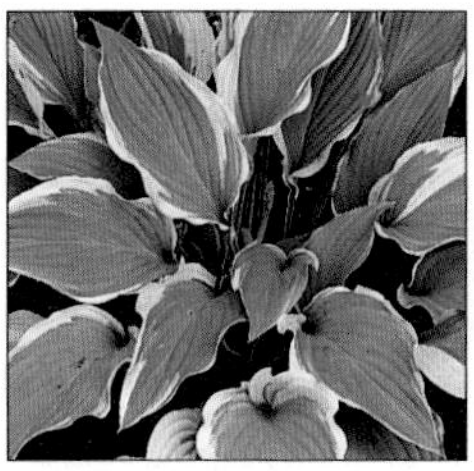
Hosta 'Regal Splendor'

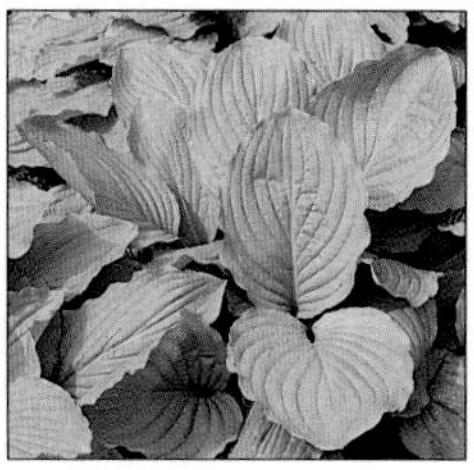
Hosta 'Royal Standard'

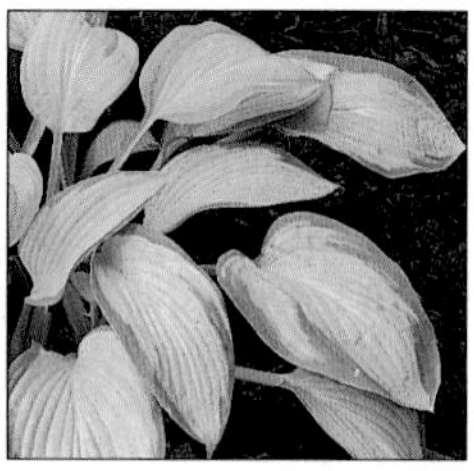
Hosta 'September Sun'

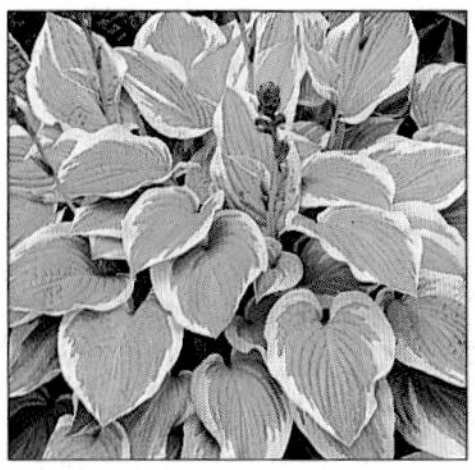
Hosta 'Shade Fanfare'

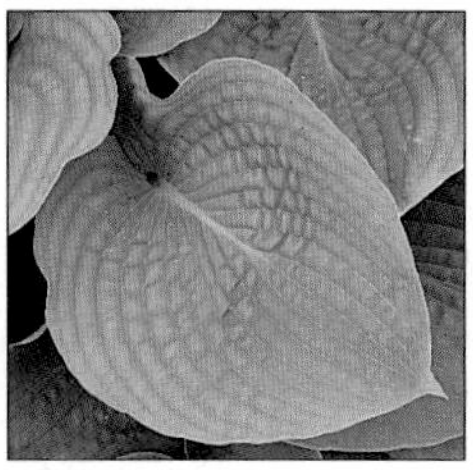
Hosta sieboldiana var. *elegans*

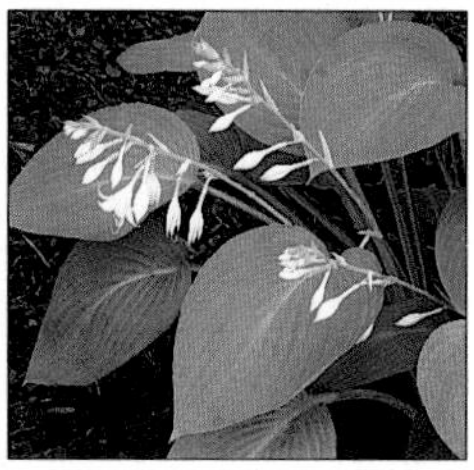
Hosta 'Snowden'

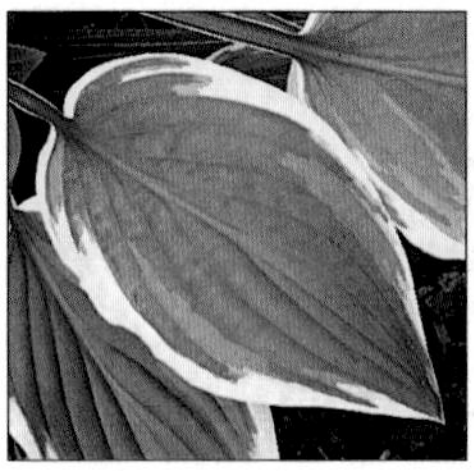
Hosta 'So Sweet'

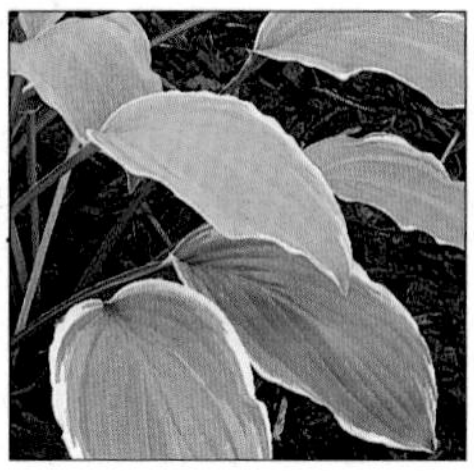
Hosta 'Sugar and Cream'

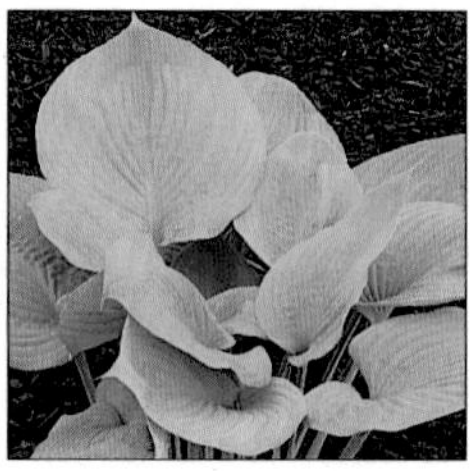
Hosta 'Sum and Substance'

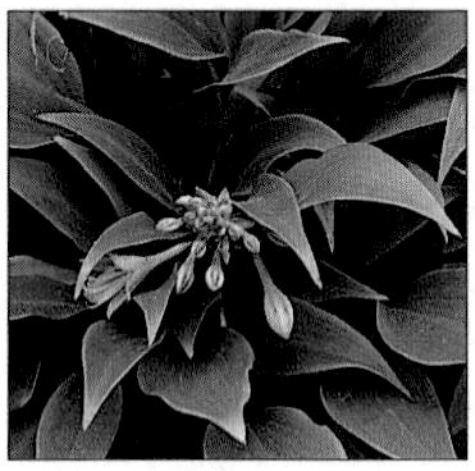
Hosta tardiflora

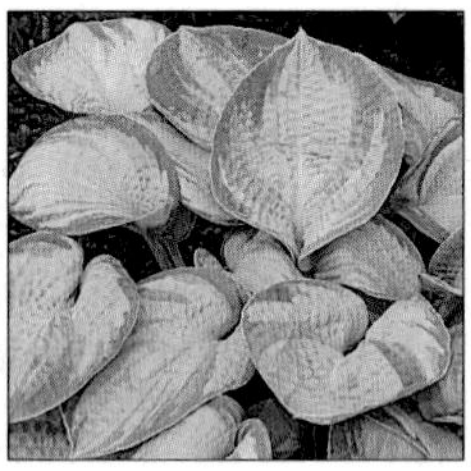
Hosta tokudama 'Aureonebulosa'

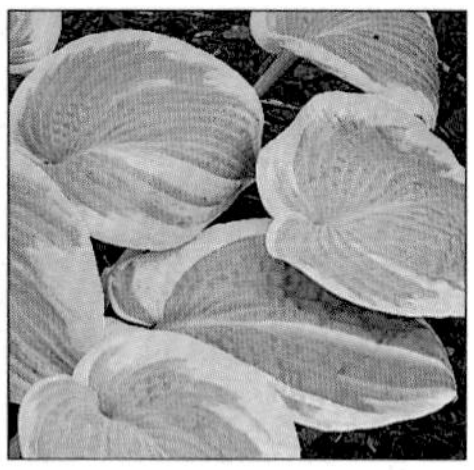
Hosta tokudama 'Flavocircinalis'

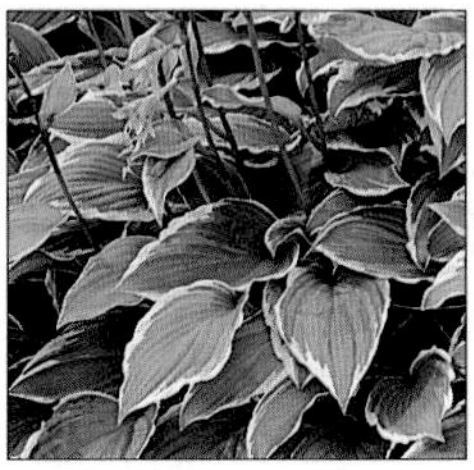
Hosta undulata var. *undulata* 'Albomarginata'

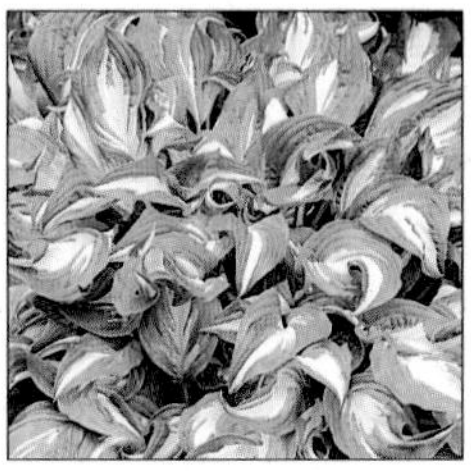
Hosta undulata var. *univittata*

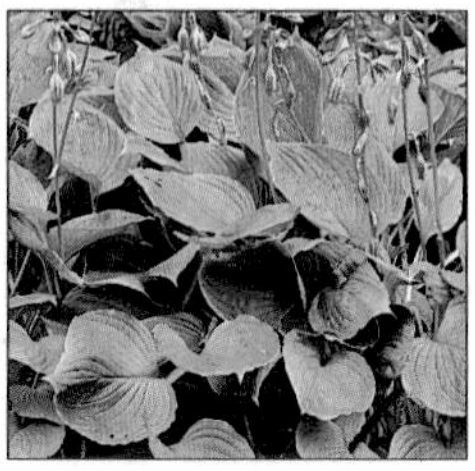
Hosta ventricosa

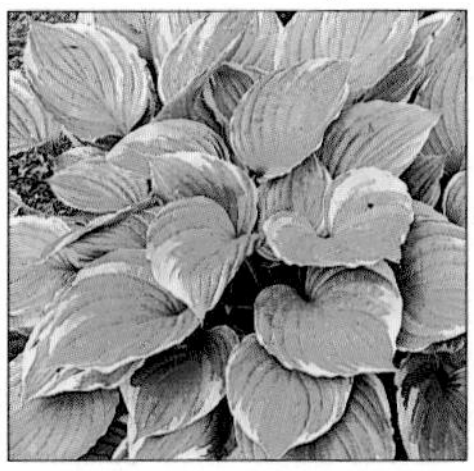
Hosta ventricosa 'Variegata'

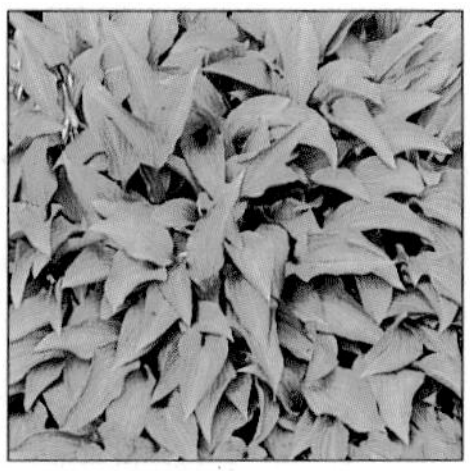
Hosta venusta

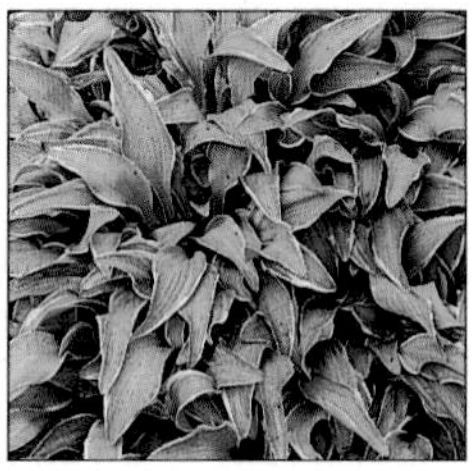
Hosta 'Vera Verde'

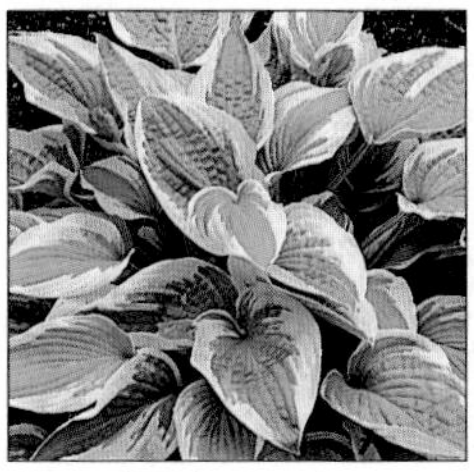
Hosta 'Wide Brim'

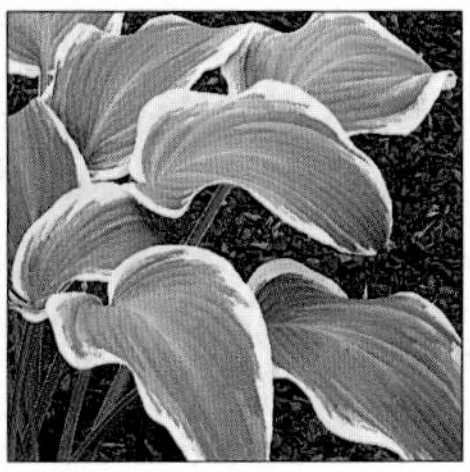
Hosta 'Yellow River'

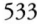

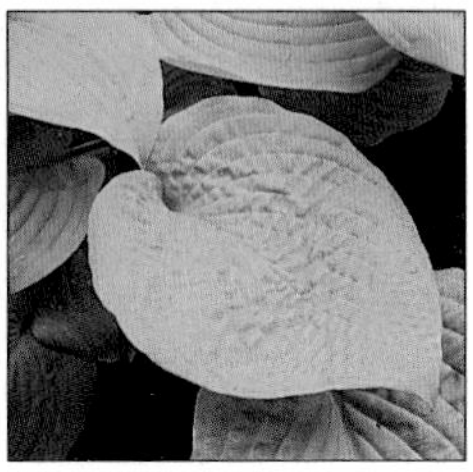
Hosta 'Zounds'

H

HOTTONIA

PRIMULACEAE

Genus of 2 species of submerged aquatic perennials, widely distributed in temperate Eurasia and E. USA, usually found in slow-moving water in ditches and in shallow water where silting has occurred. They have delicate, primula-like, white to lilac flowers, borne in terminal racemes, and attractive, whorled or alternate, feathery, pinnate, light green leaves. Hottonias are good oxygenators, and are suitable for a small decorative pool or a larger wildlife pool.

• **HARDINESS** Fully hardy to half hardy.

• **CULTIVATION** Grow in the muddy bottom of a shallow pond in clear, still water in full sun. Hottonias may be difficult to establish, particularly in a recently constructed pool. Winter-resting buds will sink to the bottom of the pond, usually rising again and producing new growth in spring. See also pp.52–53.

• **PROPAGATION** Sow seed in trays submerged to their rims in water in spring. Divide, or take cuttings of established plants, in spring, and either throw into the water or plant into the submerged, muddy margins of a pond.

• **PESTS AND DISEASES** Filamentous algae may smother the delicate foliage.

H. inflata (American featherfoil). Submerged perennial with branched, spongy stems bearing whorls of stalkless, pinnate to 2-pinnate, oblong, light green leaves, 1–5cm (½–2in) long, composed of linear leaflets. Salverform white flowers, 5–8mm (¼–⅜in) across, are borne in 2- to 10-flowered racemes, 15–20cm (6–8in) tall, above the water in spring. ↕ 60cm (24in), ↔ 45cm (18in). E. USA. ❄❄

H. palustris (Water violet). Submerged perennial with spreading and erect stems bearing whorled or alternate, pinnate to 2-pinnate, comb-like, light green leaves, 2–13cm (¾–5in) long, with linear leaflets. In spring, produces salverform, pale violet, lilac, or white flowers, 2–2.5cm (¾–1in) across, with yellow throats; they are borne above the water in 3–9 whorls on flower-stalks 30–40cm (12–16in) tall. ↕ 30–90cm (12–36in), ↔ indefinite. Eurasia. ❄❄❄

▷ **Hot water plant** see *Achimenes*
▷ **Hound's tongue** see *Cynoglossum, C. nervosum, C. officinale*
▷ **Houpara** see *Pseudopanax lessonii*
▷ **Houseleek** see *Sempervivum*
Cobweb see *Sempervivum arachnoideum*
Common see *Sempervivum tectorum*
▷ ***Houstonia serpyllifolia*** see *Hedyotis michauxii*

HOUTTUYNIA

SAURURACEAE

Genus of one species of perennial found in damp, shady sites in woodland, scrub, and marshy habitats in E. Asia. It has widely spreading rhizomes and is grown mainly for its foliage. Use as ground cover in a damp, mixed or herbaceous border, at a pond- or streamside, or for plantings in shallow water. *H. cordata* may be invasive, especially in moist soils; cultivars are generally less vigorous.

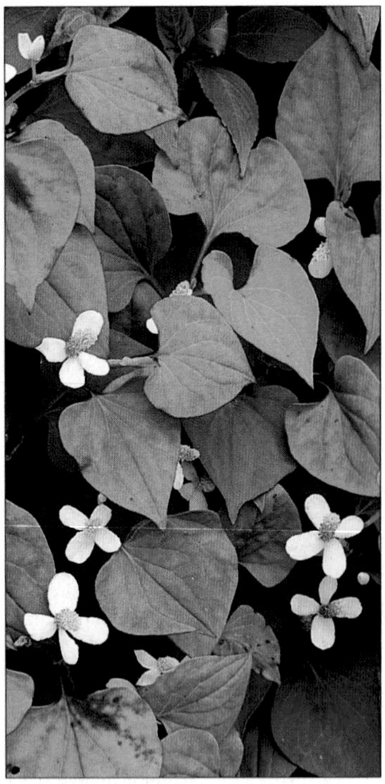

Houttuynia cordata

• **HARDINESS** Fully hardy.

• **CULTIVATION** Grow in moderately fertile, humus-rich, moist soil in full sun or dappled shade; variegated cultivars produce greener leaves in shade. On wet soils in frost-prone areas, apply a winter mulch to protect the roots. At the water's edge, grow in 8–10cm (3–4in) of water; in shallow ponds, spread may be limited by planting in a basket.

• **PROPAGATION** Sow seed in containers in a cold frame as soon as ripe. Divide rhizomes in spring. Root softwood cuttings in late spring.

• **PESTS AND DISEASES** Slugs and snails may be a problem.

H. cordata ■ Rapidly spreading perennial with simple, ovate to heart-shaped, dull bluish or greyish green leaves, 3–9cm (1¼–3½in) long, with red-tinted margins. The leaves have an unusual, orange-like scent when bruised. In spring, bears dense spikes, to 3cm (1¼in) long, of tiny, yellowish green flowers, surrounded at the bases by 4–6 green-white, later pure white, obovate, petal-like bracts, 6–10mm (¼–½in) across. ↕ to 15–30cm (6–12in) or more, ↔ indefinite. China, Japan. ❄❄❄.

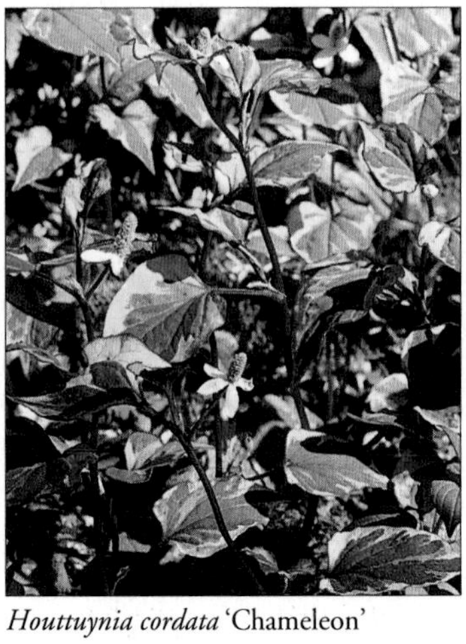

Houttuynia cordata 'Chameleon'

'Chameleon' ■ syn. 'Tricolor', has brightly variegated leaves in shades of green, pale yellow, and red, and is less spreading than the species. The small flowers of **'Flore Pleno'**, syn. 'Plena', are surrounded by 8 or more pure white bracts. **'Tricolor'** see 'Chameleon'.

HOVEA

LEGUMINOSAE/PAPILIONACEAE

Genus of about 20 species of evergreen, sometimes spiny shrubs from Australia, found in sheltered woodland, moist gulleys, on exposed rocky outcrops, and on heathland, from sea level to above the snow line. They produce usually showy, pea-like flowers from the leaf axils, either in short racemes or clusters. The alternate, linear, lance-shaped, oblong-elliptic, or ovate leaves are simple and entire or toothed. In frost-prone areas, grow in a cool or temperate greenhouse; elsewhere, grow at the base of a warm, sunny wall, in a shrub border, or in a courtyard garden.

• **HARDINESS** Half hardy to frost tender.

• **CULTIVATION** Under glass, grow in loam-based potting compost (JI No.2) in bright filtered or full light, with good ventilation and moderate humidity. Water moderately in growth, applying a balanced liquid fertilizer monthly; keep just moist in winter. Outdoors, grow in well-drained, humus-rich, moderately fertile soil in full sun; woodland species will tolerate dappled shade. Chlorosis may occur in low-nitrogen soils. Shelter from cold, drying winds. Pruning group 8; plants under glass may need restrictive pruning.

• **PROPAGATION** Sow scarified or pre-soaked seed at 13–18°C (55–64°F) in spring. Root semi-ripe cuttings with bottom heat in summer.

• **PESTS AND DISEASES** Trouble free.

H. chorizemifolia (Holly-leaved hovea). Open, upright shrub, often with rust-red-hairy stems. The lance-shaped to ovate, prickle-toothed leaves, 2.5–8cm (1–3in) long, are matt, dark green, with prominent veins. In spring, bears short racemes or clusters of 2–8 pea-like flowers, 1cm (½in) across; they are light blue-purple to violet, and have broad standard petals, each with a white patch at the base. ↕ 50–150cm (20–60in), ↔ 30–80cm (12–32in). Australia (Western Australia). ❀ (min. 5°C/41°F)

H. longifolia* var. *montana see *H. montana*.

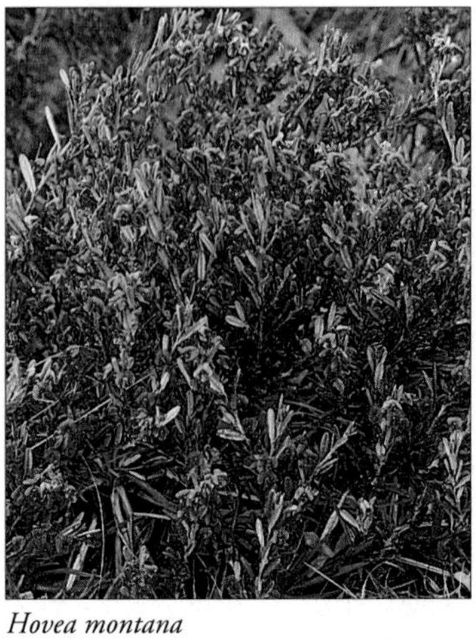

Hovea montana

H. montana ■ syn. *H. longifolia* var. *montana, H. purpurea* var. *montana*. Dwarf, spreading shrub with rust-red-hairy stems. Oblong to linear leaves, 1–3cm (½–1¼in) long, are glossy, deep green above, red-brown-hairy beneath. In spring, bears axillary clusters of 2 or 3 pea-like, deep purple to bluish purple flowers, 8–10mm (⅜–½in) across, with a white patch at the base of each standard petal. ↕ 20–40cm (8–16in), sometimes more, ↔ 50–100cm (20–39in). Australia (New South Wales, Victoria, Tasmania). ❄

H. purpurea* var. *montana see *H. montana*.

▷ **Hovea, Holly-leaved** see *Hovea chorizemifolia*

HOVENIA

RHAMNACEAE

Genus of 2 species of deciduous trees found in woodland or forest, cultivated and naturalized in E. and S.E. Asia (their exact country of origin is unknown). The leaves are alternate, heart-shaped to oval, and toothed. They are grown mainly for their fragrant flowers and small, spherical fruits. The shallowly cup-shaped, yellow or greenish yellow flowers, to 6mm (¼in) across, are produced in terminal and axillary, forked cymes. Hovenias are attractive specimen trees and will thrive in regions with long, hot summers where the shoots can thoroughly ripen. In areas with cool summers, flowers and fruits are not always freely borne.

• **HARDINESS** Fully hardy.

• **CULTIVATION** Grow in moderately fertile, humus-rich, neutral to slightly alkaline soil in full sun, with shelter from cold, drying winds. Unripened wood is liable to frost damage, but regrowth usually occurs from undamaged shoots. Pruning group 1.

• **PROPAGATION** Sow seed in containers in a cold frame in autumn, or scarify seed and sow in spring. Root greenwood

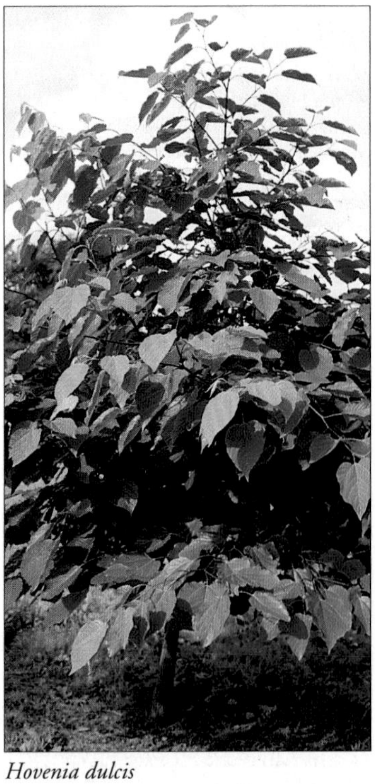

Hovenia dulcis

cuttings in early summer, and hardwood cuttings in late autumn.
• **PESTS AND DISEASES** Prone to coral spot, if wood is not fully ripened.

H. dulcis ■ ⚲ (Raisin-tree). Upright then spreading tree with heart-shaped to oval, toothed, glossy, dark green leaves, 10–20cm (4–8in) long, downy beneath. In summer, bears cymes 5–7cm (2–3in) across of tiny, greenish yellow flowers. After flowering, the flower-stalks swell, becoming red, fleshy, sweet, and edible; they later bear spherical black fruit, to 5mm (¼in) across. ↕ 12m (40ft), ↔ 10m (30ft). E. and S.E. Asia. ❄❄❄

HOWEA

Sentry palm

ARECACEAE/PALMAE

Genus of 2 species of single-stemmed palms found at low altitudes, to 300m (1,000ft), usually on basalt soils, on Lord Howe Island, Australia. The long-stalked, pinnate leaves are arranged in terminal clusters with no crownshaft, and star-shaped, 3-petalled flowers are borne on long spikes between them. In frost-prone areas, grow young specimens as houseplants, or in a conservatory or warm greenhouse. In warmer areas, use as free-standing specimens on a lawn or in a courtyard garden.
• **HARDINESS** Frost tender.
• **CULTIVATION** Under glass, grow in loam-based potting compost (JI No.2) with equal parts added pulverized bark and leaf mould, in full light. Shade from hot sun and provide moderate humidity. In growth, water moderately and apply a balanced liquid fertilizer monthly; water sparingly in winter. Top-dress or pot on in spring; howeas are slow-growing and need repotting infrequently. Outdoors, grow in fertile, moist but well-drained soil in full sun, although they will tolerate dappled shade. Shelter from strong, drying winds.
• **PROPAGATION** Sow seed at 26°C (79°F) as soon as ripe.
• **PESTS AND DISEASES** Prone to scale insects and red spider mites under glass.

H. forsteriana ■ 🏆 ♆ syn. *Kentia forsteriana* (Kentia palm, Thatch leaf palm). Moderately slow-growing palm with a slender stem, ringed with old leaf scars. Long-stalked, pinnate, mid- to dark green leaves, 2–3m (6–10ft) long, are borne almost horizontally. The leaves comprise numerous, narrowly lance-shaped, semi-lustrous leaflets with pendent tips. In summer, bears star-shaped, green female and pale brown male flowers, in erect, later pendent, axillary clusters of spikes to 1m (3ft) long. They are followed by ellipsoid, orange-red fruit, to 2cm (¾in) long. ↕ to 18m (60ft), ↔ to 6m (20ft). Australia (Lord Howe Island). ❀ (min. 15°C/59°F)

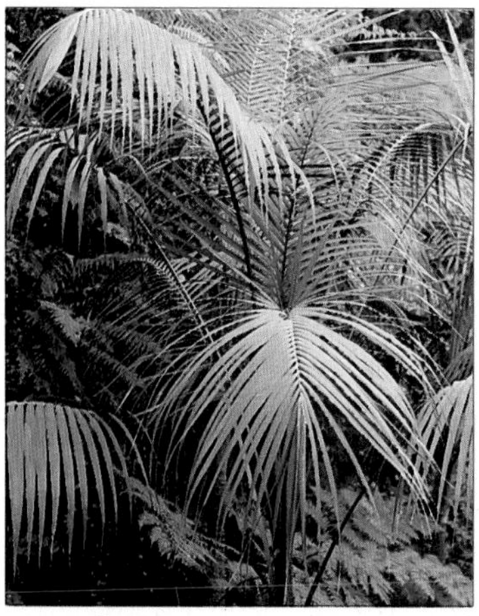
Howea forsteriana

HOYA

Wax flower

ASCLEPIADACEAE

Genus of over 200 species of evergreen, climbing and shrubby perennials, some epiphytic, from coastal bluffs, stream margins, escarpments, and rainforest in the warmer regions of Asia, Australia, and the Pacific islands. They produce opposite pairs of simple, often fleshy or succulent, sometimes leathery, variably shaped leaves. The often colourful and fragrant flowers are borne in stalked umbels or cymes from the upper leaf axils. They each have 5 waxy, usually fleshy, spreading petals, and a central crown or corona of hooded, white, pale yellow, red, pink, or purple stamens. Flowers are followed by long, cylindrical pods containing seeds with tufts of hair. In frost-prone areas, a warm greenhouse is best for all hoyas except *H. carnosa*, which should be grown in a temperate greenhouse or as a houseplant. In warmer areas, grow climbing hoyas through shrubs or trees, or over an arch, arbour, or pergola. Shrubby species may be grown epiphytically on large shrubs or trees, or in hanging baskets.
• **HARDINESS** Frost tender.
• **CULTIVATION** Under glass, grow in loam-based potting compost (JI No.2) with equal parts added leaf mould, sharp sand, pulverized bark, and charcoal, in indirect or bright filtered light. Maintain moderate to high humidity. In growth, water freely and apply a balanced liquid fertilizer monthly; keep moist in winter. Provide support for climbers. Outdoors, grow in fertile, moist but well-drained soil in full sun, with some midday shade. Shelter from strong, drying winds. Pruning group 9 for shrubs; group 11 for climbers, after flowering.
• **PROPAGATION** Sow seed at 19–24°C (66–75°F) in spring. Root semi-ripe cuttings with bottom heat in late summer. Layer in spring or summer.
• **PESTS AND DISEASES** Mealybugs may be a problem under glass.

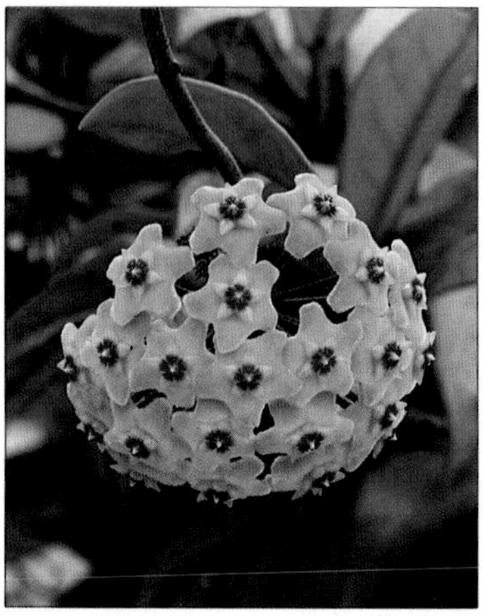
Hoya carnosa

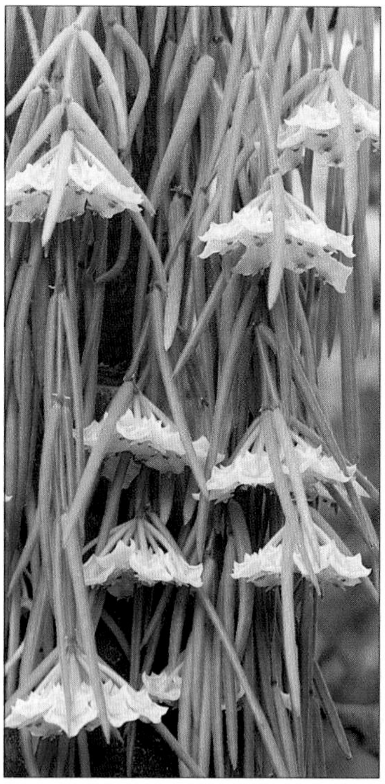
Hoya linearis

H. australis, syn. *H. darwinii* of gardens. Vigorous, twining, succulent climber with broadly ovate to elliptic or obovate, fleshy, dark green leaves, to 12cm (5in) long, smooth above and densely hairy beneath. In summer, bears umbels, 6cm (2½in) across, of 12–40 star-shaped, fragrant white flowers, to 4cm (1½in) across, with a red spot at the base of each petal, and red-purple coronas. ↕ 4–10m (12–30ft). Australia (Queensland, New South Wales). ❀ (min. 10°C/50°F)
H. bella see *H. lanceolata* subsp. *bella*.
H. carnosa ■ 🏆 (Wax plant). Vigorous, stem-rooting, succulent, often epiphytic climber with ovate, rigid, very fleshy leaves, to 8cm (3in) long, usually smooth and dark green. From late spring to autumn, bears dense, convex umbels, to 6cm (2½in) across, of up to 20 star-shaped, waxy, night-scented, pure white flowers, 1.5cm (½in) across, with red coronas; sometimes produces 2 or more umbels per stem. ↕ to 6m (20ft) or more. India, S. China, Burma. ❀ (min. 5–7°C/41–45°F). **'Exotica'** 🏆 has yellow-flushed, pink-variegated foliage. **'Picta'** has leaves with creamy white margins.
H. coronaria. Slow-growing, thick-stemmed climber with broadly oval to oblong, leathery, fleshy, mid-green leaves, to 10cm (4in) long, downy beneath, with prominent midribs. From summer to autumn, produces umbels, 8–10cm (3–4in) across, of up to 10 shallowly bell-shaped, night-scented, creamy yellow to greenish white flowers, to 2.5cm (1in) across; they have a red spot at the base of each petal and crimson-spotted coronas. ↕ to 3m (10ft). Thailand, Philippines, Malaysia, Indonesia, New Guinea. ❀ (min. 10°C/50°F)
***H. darwinii* of gardens** see *H. australis.*
H. imperialis. Strong-growing, twining climber producing thickly downy stems and narrowly oblong to elliptic, leathery, fleshy, mid-green leaves, 15–23cm (6–9in) long, with wavy margins. Umbels, to 20cm (8in) across, of 7–12 star-shaped, reddish brown to purple-brown flowers, to 7cm (3in) across, with white coronas, are borne mainly in summer. ↕ 6m (20ft) or more. Malaysia, Indonesia. ❀ (min. 10°C/50°F)
H. lanceolata* subsp. *bella 🏆 syn. *H. bella.* Spreading to pendent, epiphytic shrub with arching, densely downy, soft stems and narrowly ovate or ovate to lance-shaped, fleshy, rich green leaves, to 3cm (1¼in) long. Bears umbels, 3–4cm (1¼–1½in) across, of 7–9 star-shaped, very sweetly scented white flowers, 1.5cm (½in) across; they have red-violet coronas and are borne mainly in summer. ↕↔ to 45cm (18in). Himalayas to N. Burma. ❀ (min. 10°C/50°F)
H. linearis ■ Pendent, epiphytic, succulent perennial with slender, soft, greyish green stems bearing linear, hairy, dark green leaves, 2.5–5cm (1–2in) long, deeply grooved beneath. From late summer to autumn, produces lax umbels, to 3–4cm (1¼–1½in) across, of 10–13 star-shaped, scented, pure white flowers, to 1cm (½in) across, with pink-tinged, yellowish white coronas. ↕↔ 60–90cm (24–36in). Himalayas. ❀ (min. 13°C/55°F)
H. macgillivrayi ■ Strong-growing, twining climber with thick stems and ovate to broadly ovate, rigid, thickly fleshy, lustrous, dark green leaves, 7–20cm (3–8in) long, tinted red-purple when young. From spring to summer, bears umbels, 20–25cm (8–10in) across, of 5–15 cup-shaped, red, red-purple, purple, or brownish red flowers, each 4–8cm (1½–3in) across, with dark red, occasionally white-centred coronas. ↕ 5–8m (15–25ft). Australia (Queensland). ❀ (min. 7°C/45°F).
H. nepalensis see *H. polyneura.*
H. polyneura, syn. *H. nepalensis.* Pendent, epiphytic shrub with short-stalked, ovate to lance-shaped, fleshy, glossy, dark green leaves, 6–10cm (2½–4in) long, with slightly pointed tips, and prominent, paler green veins. Up to 15 star-shaped, waxy, white to cream flowers, 1cm (½in) across, with purplish brown or bronze-red coronas, are borne in umbels to 4–5cm (1½–2in) across, in summer. ↕↔ to 1m (3ft). Himalayas to S. China. ❀ (min. 13°C/55°F)

▷ **Huckleberry** see *Gaylussacia*
Black see *Gaylussacia baccata*
Fool's see *Menziesia ferruginea*

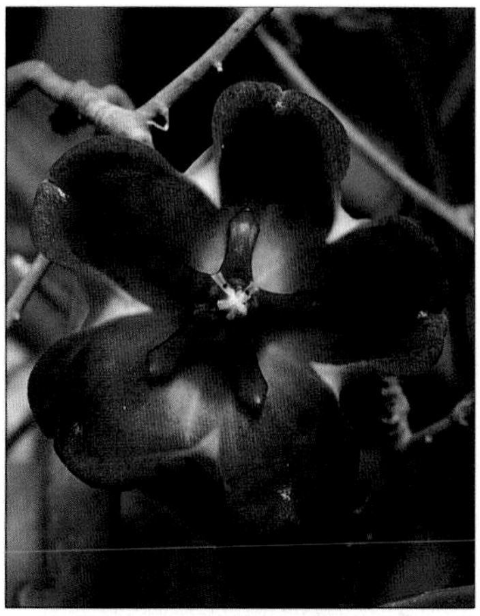
Hoya macgillivrayi

H

H

HUERNIA

ASCLEPIADACEAE

Genus of about 60–70 species of low-growing, perennial succulents from South Africa to Ethiopia and the Arabian Peninsula (with one species from W. Africa), occurring in hilly, semi-desert areas. They branch freely from the bases and often form large clumps of short, angled, fleshy stems; the prominent margins have greyish green or red teeth. The leaves are reduced to scales and are lost soon after they develop. Tubular or cup-shaped to shallowly saucer-shaped, warty, fleshy, unpleasantly scented flowers, with 5 pointed lobes, are borne in short-stalked umbels from summer to early autumn. Where temperatures fall below 11°C (52°F), grow in a warm greenhouse. In warmer areas, grow in a trough, raised bed, or desert garden.

• **HARDINESS** Frost tender.

• **CULTIVATION** Under glass, grow in standard cactus compost with added leaf mould in bright filtered or indirect light; provide low humidity. In growth, water moderately and apply a half-strength, low-nitrogen liquid fertilizer monthly. Keep almost dry in winter; overwatering may cause black rot. Outdoors, grow in poor to moderately fertile, preferably sandy, sharply drained soil; incorporate sharp sand and leaf mould at planting. Grow in dappled shade or in full sun with midday shade. Protect from excessive winter wet.

• **PROPAGATION** Sow seed at 19–24°C (66–75°F) in spring. Root cuttings of stem sections in spring or summer.

• **PESTS AND DISEASES** Trouble free.

H. macrocarpa* var. *arabica ■ Clump-forming succulent producing slender, 4-angled, glossy, mid-green stems with slightly toothed tubercles. Short-lobed, fleshy, white-hairy flowers, 1cm (½in) across, are borne in early autumn; the lobes are pale yellow with concentric purple bands, or unmarked, purple-crimson outside, and roughly warty inside. ↕↔ 10cm (4in). South Yemen. ❀ (min. 11°C/52°F)

H. pillansii ■ Variable succulent with almost spherical, then finger-like, grey-green stems bearing dense, bristly, hairy-tipped tubercles in longitudinal, spiralling rows. Fleshy, densely red-warty and red-spotted, cream to red or pink flowers, 3–4cm (1¼–1½in) across,

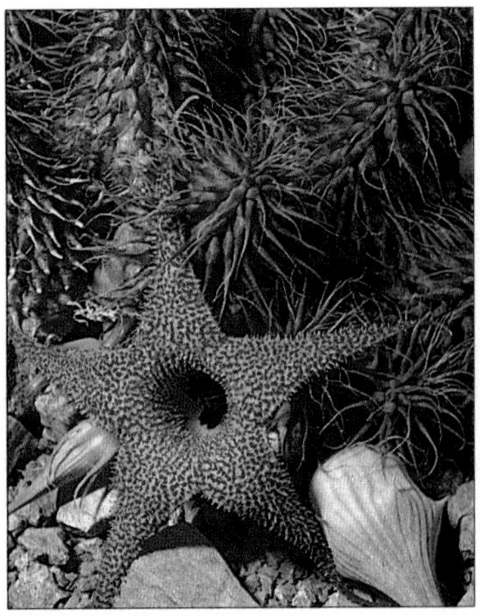

Huernia pillansii

pale yellow inside with crimson spots, are borne from the base of new growth from summer to early autumn. ↕ 4cm (1½in), ↔ 10cm (4in). South Africa (Western Cape). ❀ (min. 11°C/52°F)

H. primulina see *H. thuretii* var. *primulina.*

H. procumbens. Prostrate or semi-pendent succulent with 5- or 6-angled, dull purplish green stems. In late summer, bears fleshy, pale yellowish brown flowers, to 3cm (1¼in) across, margined with brownish red; the narrowly lance-shaped white lobes are covered with short, dark purple-red hairs. ↕↔ to 15cm (6in). South Africa (Northern Transvaal, Eastern Transvaal). ❀ (min. 11°C/52°F)

H. quinta ■ Clump-forming succulent producing 4-angled, greyish purple stems with horned teeth. In summer, bears shallowly 5-lobed, fleshy, white or yellow flowers, to 3cm (1¼in) across, the cup-shaped tubes banded dark red with papillae at the mouths. ↕↔ to 7cm (3in). South Africa (Northern Transvaal, Eastern Transvaal). ❀ (min. 11°C/52°F)

H. thuretii. Clump-forming succulent with 4- or 5-angled, prominently toothed, greyish green stems. From summer to early autumn, bears 5-lobed, fleshy, red-spotted yellow flowers, to 2.5cm (1in) across, with red-banded tubes. ↕ 5cm (2in), ↔ indefinite. South Africa (Eastern Cape). ❀ (min. 11°C/52°F). **var. *primulina*** ■ syn. *H. primulina*, has tufts of acutely angled, greyish green stems, and bears waxy, fleshy, pale red flowers, creamy yellow with red spots on the lobes, and with blackish brown coronas; ↕↔ 8cm (3in).

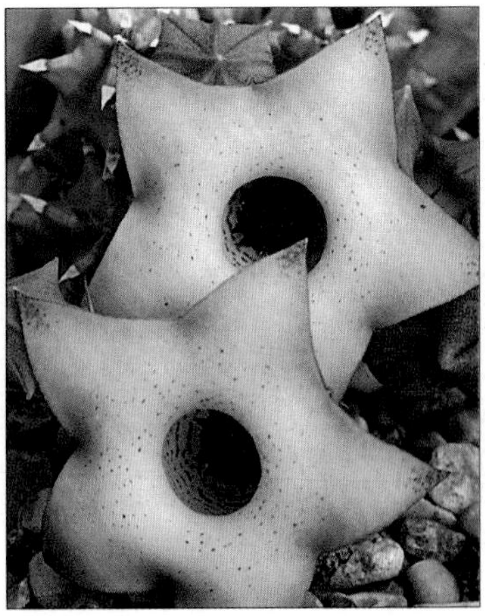

Huernia thuretii var. *primulina*

H. zebrina (Owl's eyes). Variable, clump-forming succulent producing 4- or 5-angled, greyish green stems with stout, conical teeth. From summer to early autumn, bears fleshy, creamy yellow flowers, 3–4cm (1¼–1½in) across, with shallow, maroon-purple tubes, and 5 triangular lobes strongly cross-banded and heavily suffused maroon-purple. ↕ 6–8cm (2½–3in), ↔ 15cm (6in) or more. Namibia, Botswana, South Africa (Northern Transvaal, Eastern Transvaal, KwaZulu/Natal), Swaziland, Zimbabwe. ❀ (min. 11°C/52°F)

▷ **Humble plant** see *Mimosa pudica*
▷ ***Humea*** see *Calomeria*
H. elegans see *C. amaranthoides*

HUMULUS

Hop

CANNABIDACEAE

Genus of 2 species of herbaceous perennials, with twining stems, widely distributed and naturalized in woodland and hedgerows in N. temperate regions (their exact country of origin is unknown). The cultivars are grown for their brightly coloured foliage, which may be golden or attractively variegated. The leaves are opposite and palmately 3- to 7-lobed, with large, broadly ovate to rounded lobes. Small male and female flowers are borne on separate plants in mid- and late summer: the males in axillary panicles, the females in cone-like spikes. The female inflorescences of *H. lupulus* ("hops") are used in brewing. Train over a fence or trellis, or into a

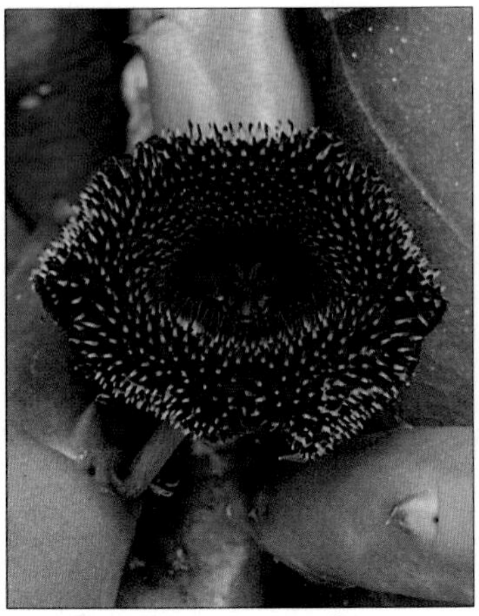

Huernia macrocarpa var. *arabica*

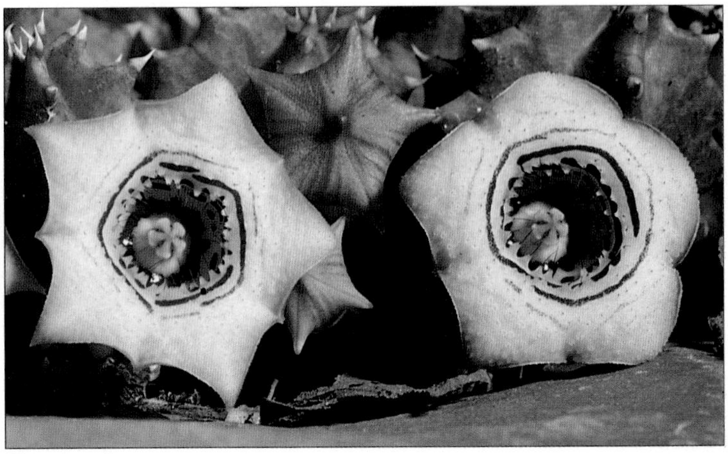

Huernia quinta

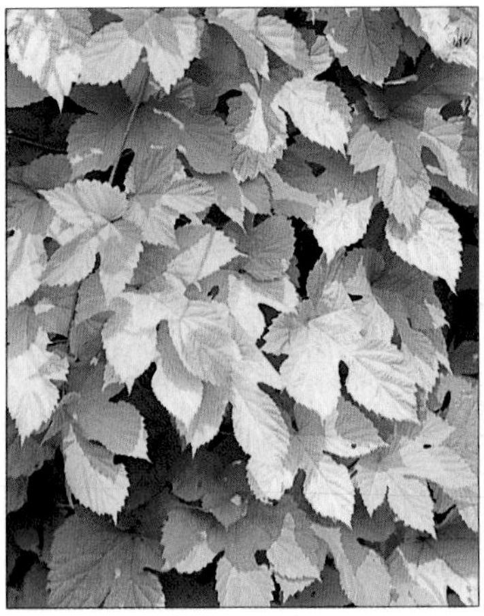

Humulus lupulus 'Aureus'

large shrub or small tree. The flowers are useful for dried flower arrangements.

• **HARDINESS** Fully hardy to half hardy.

• **CULTIVATION** Grow in moist but well-drained, moderately fertile, humus-rich soil in sun or partial shade. For best leaf colour, grow *H. lupulus* 'Aureus' in a sunny position.

• **PROPAGATION** Sow seed at 15–18°C (59–64°F) in spring; seed of *H. japonicus* and its cultivars may be sown *in situ* in late spring. Variegated and golden-leaved cultivars other than *H. japonicus* 'Variegatus' do not often come true from seed. Root softwood cuttings in spring, or greenwood and leaf-bud cuttings with bottom heat in summer.

• **PESTS AND DISEASES** Susceptible to *Verticillium* wilt.

***H. japonicus* 'Variegatus'.** Twining perennial with roughly hairy shoots and deeply 5- to 7-lobed, sharply toothed, dark green leaves, to 13–15cm (5–6in) long, heavily mottled and streaked with white. Ovoid spikes of green female flowers, to 2cm (¾in) long, are borne in mid- and late summer. Usually treated as a half-hardy annual. ↕ 3m (10ft). ✽

H. lupulus (Hop). Rhizomatous, twining perennial with roughly hairy shoots and deeply 3- to 5-lobed, coarsely toothed, light green leaves, to 15cm (6in) long. In summer, bears broadly ovoid, fragrant, green, then straw-coloured spikes of female flowers, to 2cm (¾in) long. ↕ 6m (20ft). Europe, W. Asia, North America. ✽✽✽. **'Aureus'** ■ 🏆 has golden yellow foliage.

HUNNEMANNIA

PAPAVERACEAE

Genus of one species of perennial, closely related to *Eschscholzia*, from rocky and stony areas in the highlands of Mexico. It has deeply divided leaves, with 3 narrow lobes, and glossy, saucer- to cup-shaped flowers that are good for cutting. Grow at the base of a warm, sunny wall, or in a herbaceous or mixed border. In frost-prone areas, grow as an annual or, for winter flowers, in a temperate greenhouse or conservatory.

• **HARDINESS** Half hardy.

• **CULTIVATION** Under glass, grow in loam-based potting compost (JI No.2) in full light with low humidity. In the growing season, water moderately and apply a dilute, balanced liquid fertilizer monthly. Outdoors, grow in moderately fertile, well-drained soil in full sun, with

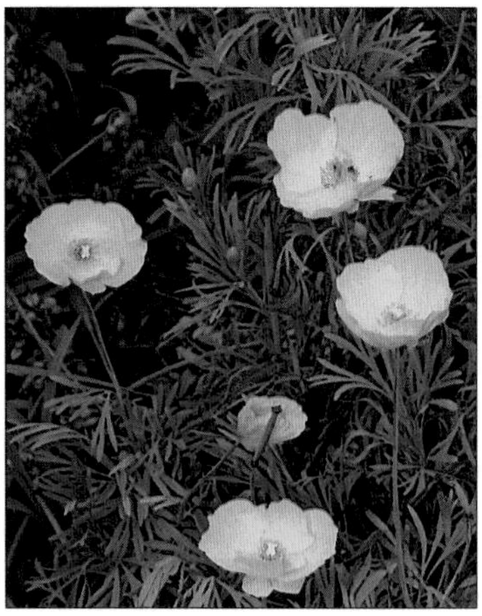

Hunnemannia fumariifolia

protection from winter wet. Avoid disturbing the roots.
• **PROPAGATION** Sow seed *in situ* in early spring, or in autumn in frost-free areas. For winter-flowering container plants, sow seed at 13–16°C (55–61°F) in autumn.
• **PESTS AND DISEASES** Susceptible to slugs, snails, and aphids.

H. fumariifolia ■ (Mexican tulip poppy). Woody-based, hairless perennial producing glaucous, blue-green leaves, 5–10cm (2–4in) long, with 3 linear lobes. From midsummer to late autumn, bears poppy-like, solitary, glossy, golden yellow flowers, to 5–8cm (2–3in) across, with 4 rounded, overlapping petals, later spreading to reveal deeper yellow stamens. ↕ 60–90cm (24–36in), ↔ 25cm (10in). Mexico. ❄. **'Sunlite'** is fast-growing and mostly grown as an annual; it has lax stems and clear yellow flowers; ↕ to 60cm (24in), ↔ 20cm (8in).

HUNTLEYA

ORCHIDACEAE

Genus of about 10 species of evergreen, rhizomatous, epiphytic orchids, without pseudobulbs, from Central and South America, and Trinidad. *H. meleagris*, the only species generally cultivated, grows in cloud forest up to 1,200m (4,000ft). The folded, lance-shaped to ovate, soft-textured leaves are arranged in 2 ranks in a broad fan shape. In summer, scapes arising between the lower leaves bear solitary, star-shaped, waxy flowers with prominent lips.
• **HARDINESS** Frost tender.
• **CULTIVATION** Intermediate-growing orchids. Grow in containers of epiphytic orchid compost or on slabs of bark in bright indirect light, with high humidity. Water freely in growth, and apply fertilizer monthly; water sparingly in winter. Keep foliage dry at all times. See also p.46.
• **PROPAGATION** Pot up offset rhizomes in spring.
• **PESTS AND DISEASES** Prone to red spider mites, aphids, and mealybugs.

H. burtii see *H. meleagris.*
H. meleagris ■ syn. *H. burtii.* Epiphytic orchid with a fan of tufted, lance-shaped to ovate, pale green leaves, 20–40cm (8–16in) long; new growth develops from the base on extending rhizomes. In summer, scapes to 17cm (7in) long bear solitary, star-shaped,

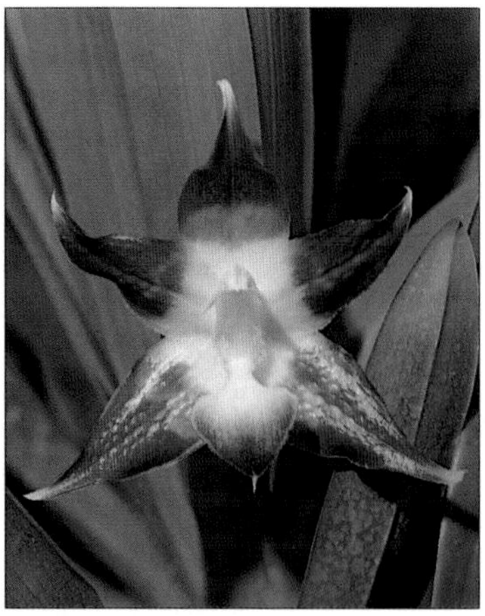

Huntleya meleagris

waxy, very glossy, chestnut-brown flowers, 8–13cm (3–5in) across, with white or cream centres, often flecked with yellow. ↕↔ 30cm (12in). Trinidad, Central America, N.W. South America. ❀ (min. 13°C/55°F; max. 30°C/86°F)

▷ **Huntsman's cup** see *Sarracenia purpurea*
▷ **Hyacinth** see *Hyacinthus*
Grape see *Muscari*
Tassel Grape see *Muscari comosum*
Water see *Eichhornia, E. crassipes*
Wild see *Camassia scilloides*

HYACINTHELLA

HYACINTHACEAE/LILIACEAE

Genus, closely related to *Muscari*, of about 16 species of small, bulbous perennials from E. and S.E. Europe to W. Asia, found on scree and stony, often limestone hillsides and in open pine forest. They have linear to elliptic-ovate, mostly mid-green, basal leaves and are cultivated for their racemes of bell-shaped flowers, 6–15mm (¼–½in) long, borne in spring. In regions with wet summers, they are best grown in an alpine house or bulb frame. In climates with low summer rainfall, grow in a trough, raised bed, or rock garden, or at the base of a warm, sunny wall.
• **HARDINESS** Fully hardy to frost hardy.
• **CULTIVATION** Plant bulbs 5–8cm (2–3in) deep in autumn. Under glass, grow in loam-based potting compost (JI No.2) with added grit, in full light. Maintain low humidity and good ventilation. Water moderately from autumn to spring; keep dry in summer.

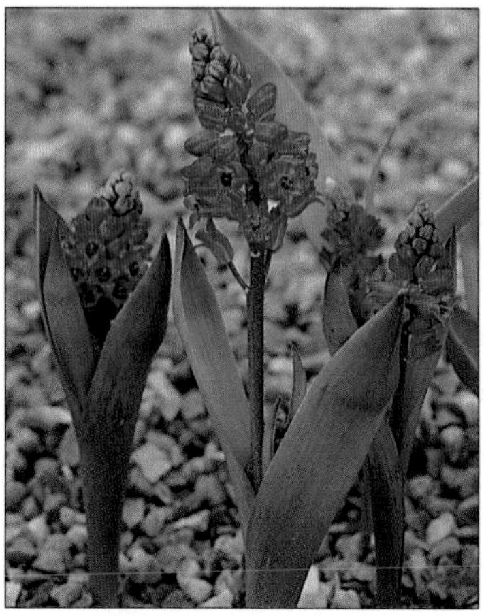

Hyacinthella glabrescens

Apply a high-potash liquid fertilizer once after flowering. Outdoors, grow in moderately fertile, well-drained soil in full sun; protect from summer rain.
• **PROPAGATION** Sow seed in containers in a cold frame in autumn. Remove offsets in summer, when dormant.
• **PESTS AND DISEASES** Trouble free.

H. dalmatica see *H. pallens.*
H. glabrescens ■ Bulbous perennial with 2 wide, strap-shaped leaves, to 12cm (5in) long. In spring, bears loose, erect racemes, 5–15cm (2–6in) long, of 10–25 tubular-bell-shaped, violet-blue flowers. ↕ 5–15cm (2–6in), ↔ 8cm (3in). Turkey (S. Anatolia). ❄❄
H. pallens, syn. *H. dalmatica.* Bulbous perennial with narrow, linear leaves, to 8cm (3in) long. Dense racemes, to 10cm (4in) long, of 6–20 narrowly bell-shaped, mid-blue flowers are borne in spring. ↕ 10cm (4in), ↔ 5cm (2in). Croatia (Dalmatia). ❄❄❄

HYACINTHOIDES

syn. ENDYMION
Bluebell

HYACINTHACEAE/LILIACEAE

Genus, closely related to *Scilla*, of 3 or 4 species of vigorous, bulbous perennials from deciduous woodland and moist meadows in W. Europe and N. Africa. They have strap-shaped to lance-shaped or linear, basal leaves, and bear racemes of bell- or tubular-bell-shaped, blue or white, sometimes pink flowers in spring. Bluebells are ideal for naturalizing in grass, for a wild or woodland garden, or for underplanting in a shrub border. All parts may irritate skin on contact, and may cause severe discomfort if ingested.
• **HARDINESS** Fully hardy.
• **CULTIVATION** Plant bulbs 8cm (3in) deep in autumn, in moderately fertile, humus-rich, moist but well-drained soil in dappled shade. *H. hispanica* tolerates a wide range of soils. Remove flowers as they fade to prevent self-seeding, except in wild plantings.

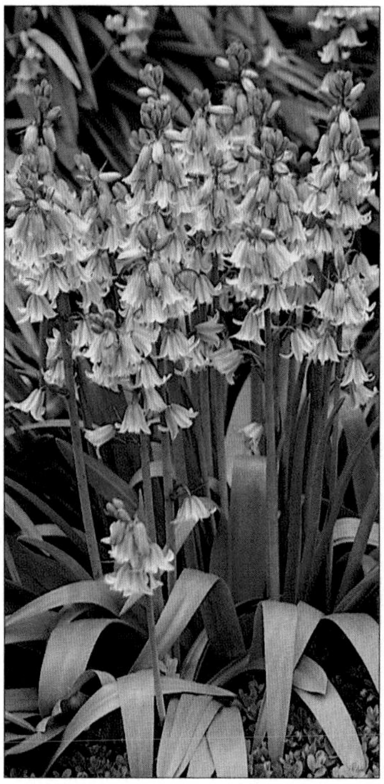

Hyacinthoides hispanica 'Excelsior'

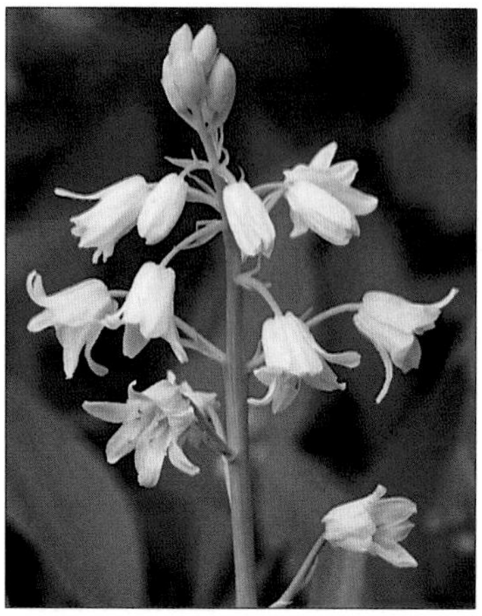

Hyacinthoides hispanica 'La Grandesse'

• **PROPAGATION** Sow seed in containers in a cold frame as soon as ripe; keep shaded and do not allow to dry out. Remove offsets in summer.
• **PESTS AND DISEASES** Trouble free.

H. hispanica, syn. *Endymion hispanicus, Scilla campanulata, S. hispanica* (Spanish bluebell). Robust, bulbous perennial, quickly forming large clumps of erect, strap-shaped, glossy, dark green leaves, 20–60cm (8–24in) long. In spring, bears racemes of up to 15 upright, bell-shaped, unscented blue flowers, 2cm (¾in) long, with reflexed tips and blue anthers. ↕ 40cm (16in), ↔ 10cm (4in). Portugal, Spain, N. Africa. ❄❄❄. Most cultivars offered are hybrids with *H. non-scripta*, and have pendent flowers intermediate between those of the 2 parents. **'Excelsior'** ■ has violet-blue flowers, striped paler blue; ↕ 50–55cm (20–22in). **'La Grandesse'** ■ has nodding, pure white flowers, 2.5cm (1in) long. **'Rosabella'** has racemes of violet-pink flowers.
H. italica. Bulbous perennial with semi-erect, linear to lance-shaped, dull dark green leaves, 10–25cm (4–10in) long. Dense racemes of 6–30 upward-facing, bell-shaped, mid-blue flowers, 1cm (½in) long, are borne in spring. ↕ 10–20cm (4–8in), ↔ 5cm (2in). Portugal, Spain, S.E. France, N.W. Italy. ❄❄❄
H. non-scripta ■ syn. *Endymion non-scriptus, Scilla non-scripta, S. nutans* (English bluebell). Vigorous, clump-forming, bulbous perennial with spreading, linear to lance-shaped, glossy, dark green leaves, 20–45cm (8–18in)

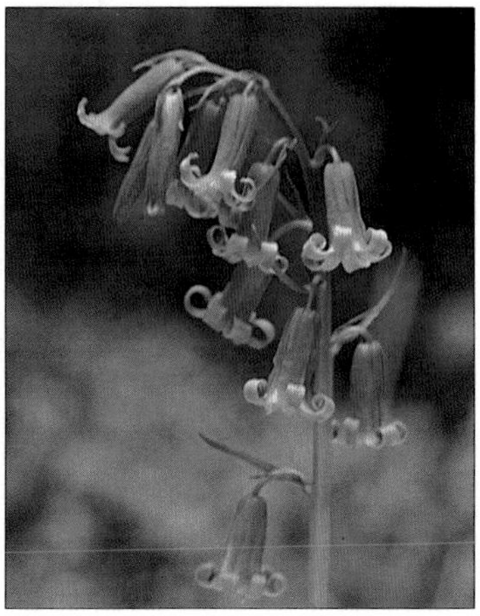

Hyacinthoides non-scripta

H

long. In spring, bears 6–12 pendent, narrowly bell-shaped, scented, mid-blue, sometimes white flowers, 1.5–2cm (½–¾in) long, with cream anthers, in a one-sided raceme that bends over at the top. ↕20–40cm (8–16in), ↔ 8cm (3in). W. Europe. ❄❄❄

HYACINTHUS

Hyacinth

HYACINTHACEAE/LILIACEAE

Genus of 3 species of bulbous perennials from rocky, limestone slopes and cliffs, to 2,600m (8,200ft) high, in W. and C. Asia. They are cultivated for their loose to dense racemes of strongly fragrant flowers, borne in spring. The semi-erect, basal leaves, 15–35cm (6–14in) long, are strap-shaped, channelled, and glossy, dark green. All cultivars are derived from *H. orientalis*, and usually have racemes to 20cm (8in) long, packed with up to 40 tubular-bell-shaped, single or double flowers, 2–3.5cm (¾–1½in) long. Closer in character to the wild species are the Multiflora and Roman cultivars, which produce several smaller, loosely flowered racemes, to 12cm (5in) long. They are now rarely grown.

Hyacinths are excellent for spring bedding displays in an annual, mixed, or herbaceous border, or for growing in containers; some are specially prepared for early flowering indoors. All parts may cause stomach upset if ingested; contact with the bulbs may aggravate skin allergies.

- **HARDINESS** Fully hardy in the ground, but liable to frost damage in containers outdoors.
- **CULTIVATION** Outdoors, plant bulbs 10cm (4in) deep, a minimum of 8cm (3in) apart, in autumn. Grow in any well-drained, moderately fertile soil in sun or partial shade. Protect container-grown plants from excessive winter wet. Specially prepared bulbs may be forced into early growth for indoor display in winter. Plant them with the tips of the bulbs just showing, in loam-based potting compost (JI No.2) in containers with drainage holes; use bulb fibre if planting in bowls. Keep in a cool, dark place at a temperature no higher than 7°C (45°F), for at least 6 weeks to allow roots to develop. When the shoots are about 2.5cm (1in) long, increase light and temperature gradually. Water carefully, avoiding wetting the shoots or waterlogging the compost; damp conditions and poor drainage may cause rot and fungal diseases. After flowering, forced hyacinths may be planted in the garden, where they will flower in spring in subsequent years.
- **PROPAGATION** Remove offsets when dormant in summer.
- **PESTS AND DISEASES** Trouble free.

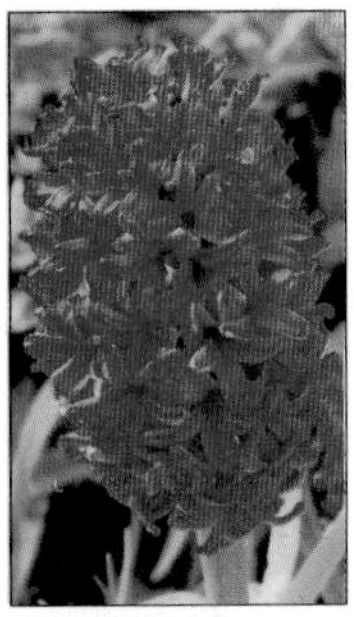
Hyacinthus orientalis 'Amethyst'

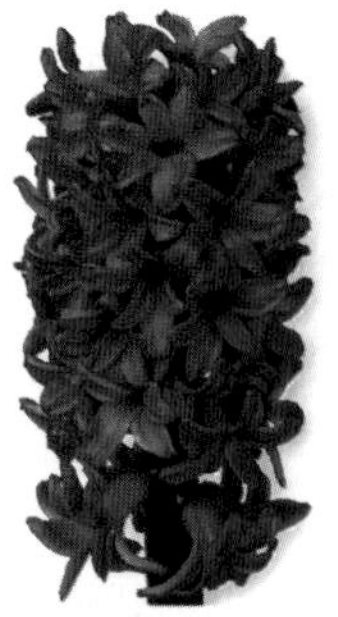
Hyacinthus orientalis 'Blue Jacket'

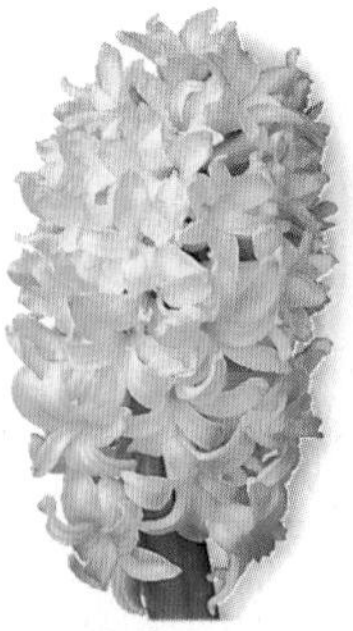
Hyacinthus orientalis 'City of Haarlem'

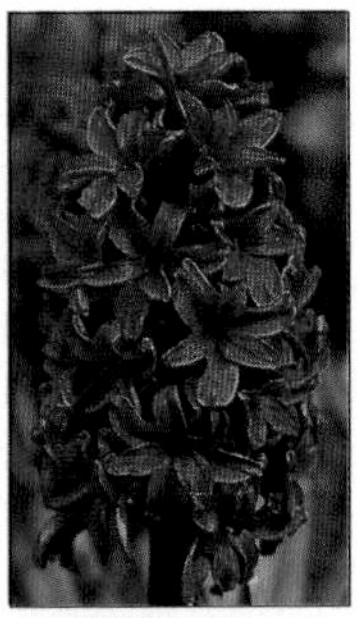
Hyacinthus orientalis 'Distinction'

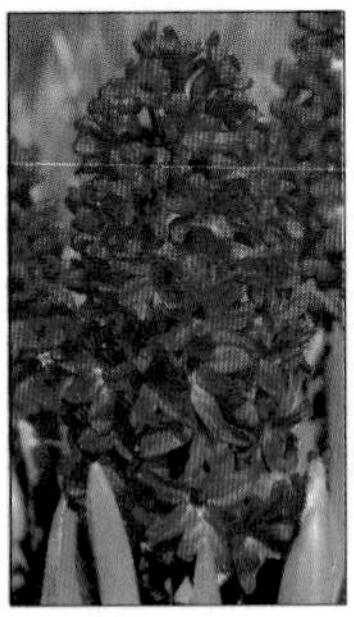
Hyacinthus orientalis 'Jan Bos'

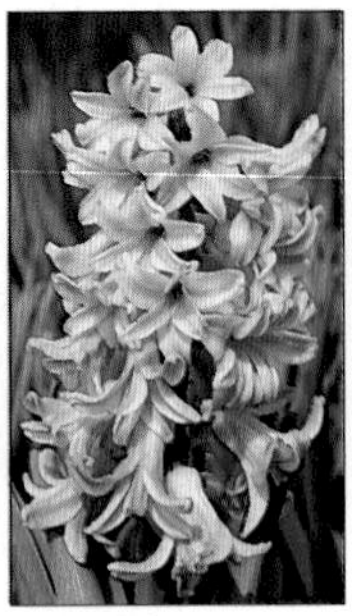
Hyacinthus orientalis 'Lady Derby'

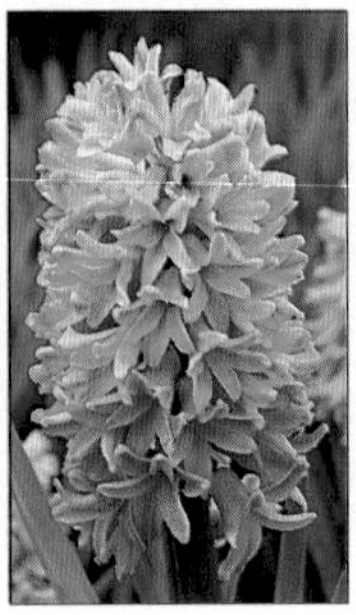
Hyacinthus orientalis 'Princess Maria Christina'

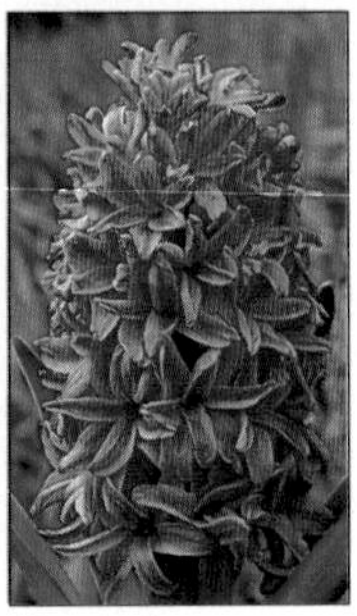
Hyacinthus orientalis 'Queen of the Pinks'

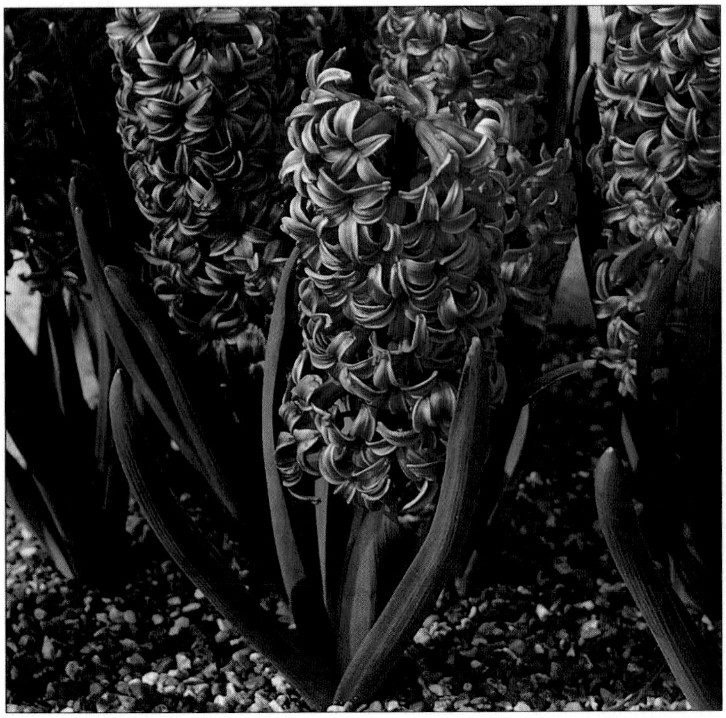
Hyacinthus orientalis 'Ostara'

H. amethystinus see *Brimeura amethystina.*
H. azureus see *Muscari azureum.*
H. orientalis. Bulbous perennial with linear to lance-shaped, channelled, bright green leaves, 15–35cm (6–14in) long. In early spring, bears erect racemes of up to 40 tubular-bell-shaped, waxy, very fragrant, single flowers, 2–3.5cm (¾–1½in) long, pale violet-blue at the bases and almost white above, with spreading, then recurved lobes. ↕20–30cm (8–12in), ↔ 8cm (3in). C. and S. Turkey, N.W. Syria, Lebanon. ❄❄❄. **'Amethyst'** ■ bears strongly scented, single, violet-lilac flowers. **'Amsterdam'** bears single, bright rose-red flowers. **'Anna Liza'** produces single, pale purple flowers with darker veins. **'Anna Marie'** 🏆 bears racemes of single, pale pink flowers; good for forcing. **'Ben Nevis'** bears compact racemes of double, ivory-white flowers. **'Blue Jacket'** ■🏆 produces racemes of single, navy-blue flowers with purple veins. **'Carnegie'** bears compact racemes of single, pure white flowers in late spring. **'City of Haarlem'** ■🏆 bears racemes of single, soft primrose-yellow flowers in late spring. **'Delft Blue'** 🏆 produces single, soft blue flowers. **'Distinction'** ■ bears slender, open racemes of single, beetroot-purple flowers. **'Gipsy Queen'** 🏆 bears single, salmon-orange flowers. **'Hollyhock'** produces double, bright crimson-red flowers in late spring. **'Jan Bos'** ■ produces racemes of single, cerise-red flowers. **'Lady Derby'** ■ has single, rose-pink flowers. **'Ostara'** ■🏆 bears single flowers in violet-blue. **'Pink Pearl'** 🏆 bears single, deep pink flowers with paler edges. **'Princess Maria Christina'** ■ has single apricot flowers. **'Queen of the Pinks'** ■ bears single, deep pink flowers in late spring. **'Sheila'** produces single, pale pink flowers in mid-spring. **'White Pearl'** bears single, pure white flowers in mid-spring.
H. romanus see *Bellevalia romana.*

HYDRANGEA

HYDRANGEACEAE

Genus of 80 or more species of deciduous and evergreen shrubs and climbers, rarely trees, found in woodland in E. Asia and North and South America. Grown mainly for their large, showy flowerheads, many hydrangeas also have ornamental, flaky, peeling bark when mature, and attractive foliage with good autumn colour. The leaves are broadly to narrowly ovate, or lance-shaped, toothed, and either opposite or in whorls of 3. The flat, domed, or conical, terminal flowerheads comprise corymbs or panicles of both tiny fertile flowers and larger sterile flowers with showy, petal-like sepals.

Cultivars of *H. macrophylla* are divided into 2 groups: "Lacecaps" have flattened flowerheads with small fertile flowers in the centres, surrounded by larger sterile flowers; "Hortensias" (mophead hydrangeas) have spherical flowerheads of large sterile flowers. Some cultivars of *H. serrata* are also described as Lacecaps.

Flower colour is affected by the relative availability of aluminium ions in the soil. Acid soils with a pH of less than 5.5 produce blue flowers; soils with a pH greater than this produce pink flowers. In more or less neutral soils, flower colour can be influenced by the addition of a blueing compound. White flowers are not affected by pH.

Hydrangeas are useful for a range of garden sites: they are excellent as specimen plants or in group plantings, in a shrub border, or in containers. Use the climbers to clothe a shaded wall or fence. The flowerheads may be dried for use in arrangements. All parts of hydrangeas may cause mild stomach upset if ingested; contact with the foliage may aggravate skin allergies.

- **HARDINESS** Fully hardy to frost hardy.
- **CULTIVATION** Grow in moist but well-drained, moderately fertile, humus-rich soil in sun or partial shade; provide shelter from cold, drying winds. Some hydrangeas become chlorotic in shallow chalk soil. Pruning group 1 for most species; group 4 for *H. macrophylla*, *H.* 'Preziosa', and *H. serrata*; group 1 or 6 for *H. paniculata*; and group 11 for climbers, after flowering.
- **PROPAGATION** Sow seed in containers in a cold frame in spring. Root softwood cuttings of deciduous hydrangeas in early summer, or hardwood cuttings in winter. Root semi-ripe cuttings of non-flowering shoots of evergreens with bottom heat in summer.
- **PESTS AND DISEASES** Prone to grey mould (*Botrytis*), *Hydrangea* virus, powdery mildew, leaf spot, honey fungus, aphids, red spider mites, scale insects, vine weevil, and capsid bugs.

H. anomala* subsp. *petiolaris see *H. petiolaris.*
H. arborescens (Sevenbark). Rounded, deciduous shrub with long-stalked, broadly ovate leaves, to 18cm (7in) long, dark green above and paler beneath. Domed or flattened corymbs, to 15cm (6in) across, of crowded, dull white, mainly fertile flowers are borne in summer. ↕↔ 2.5m (8ft). E. USA. ❄❄❄. **'Annabelle'** ■🏆 bears large, spherical flowerheads, 20cm (8in) across,

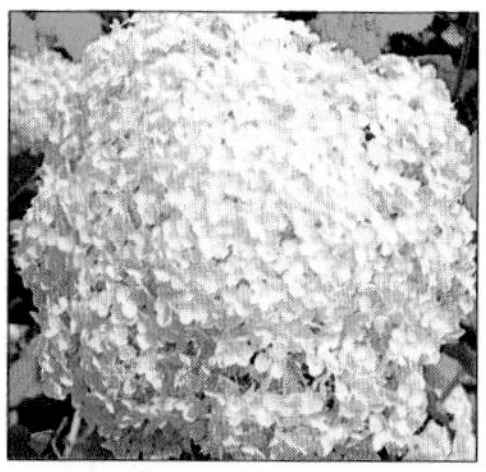
Hydrangea arborescens 'Annabelle'

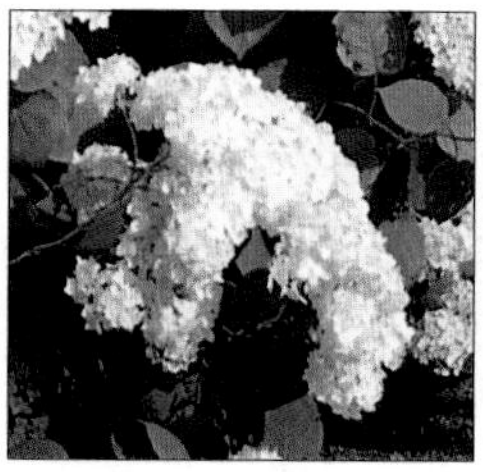
Hydrangea arborescens 'Grandiflora'

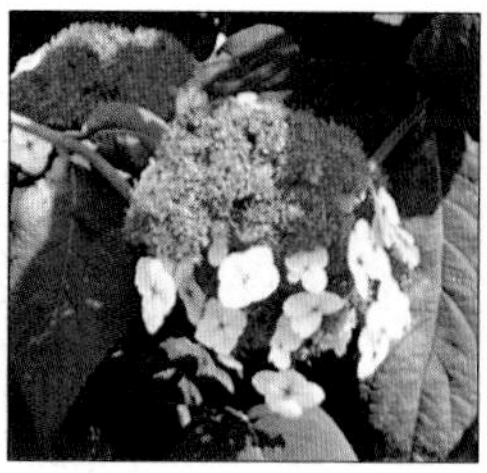
Hydrangea aspera

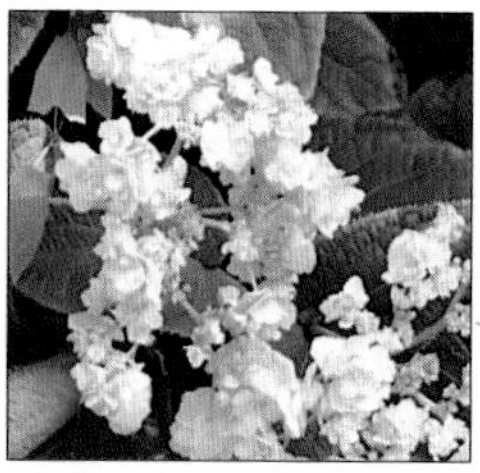
Hydrangea involucrata 'Hortensis'

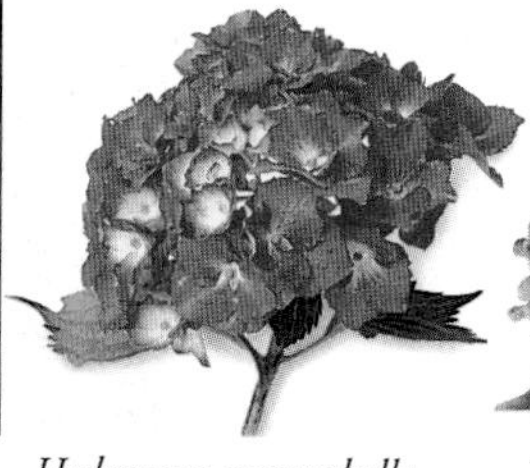
Hydrangea macrophylla 'Altona'

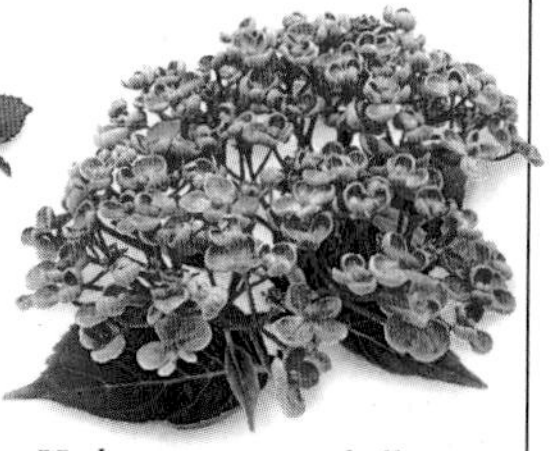
Hydrangea macrophylla 'Ayesha'

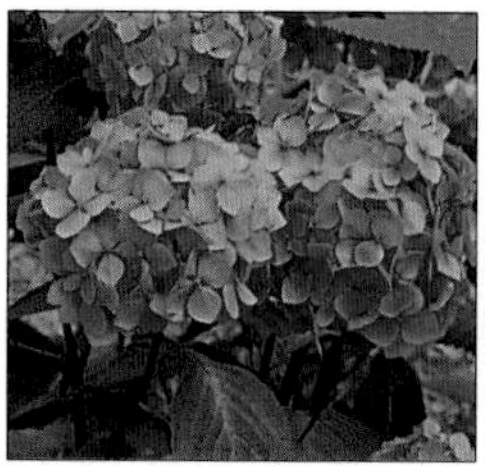
Hydrangea macrophylla 'Blue Bonnet'

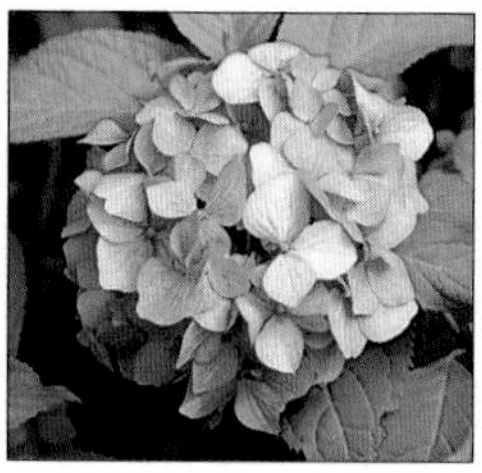
Hydrangea macrophylla 'Bouquet Rose'

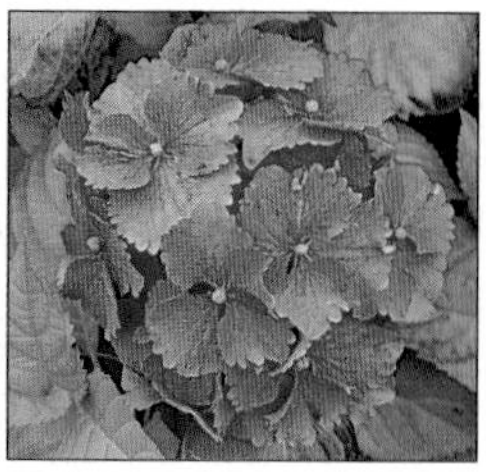
Hydrangea macrophylla 'Hamburg'

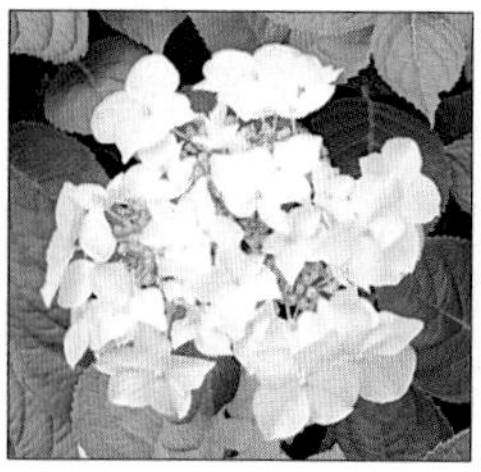
Hydrangea macrophylla 'Lanarth White'

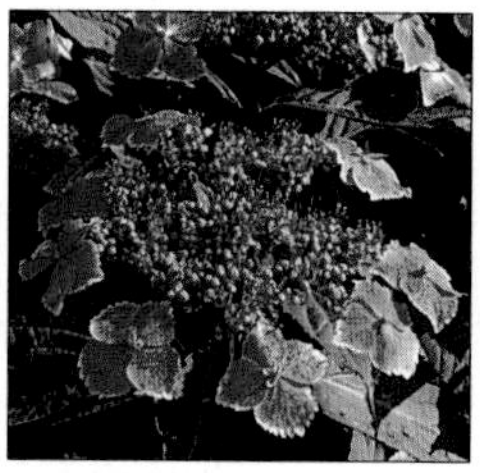
Hydrangea macrophylla 'Lilacina'

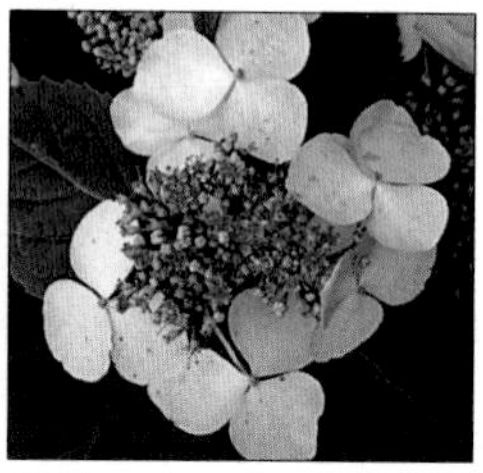
Hydrangea macrophylla 'Veitchii'

H

comprising mainly sterile flowers. **subsp. *discolor* 'Sterilis'**, syn. 'Sterilis', *H. cinerea* 'Sterilis', is similar to 'Grandiflora', but the leaves are grey-hairy beneath, and it has fewer sterile flowers. **'Grandiflora'** ▣ 🏆 has smaller flowerheads than 'Annabelle', but larger sterile flowers. **'Sterilis'** see subsp. *discolor* 'Sterilis'.
H. aspera ▣ Upright, deciduous shrub with large, lance-shaped to narrowly ovate, dark green leaves, to 25cm (10in) long, downy beneath. From late summer to autumn, bears flattened corymbs, to 25cm (10in) across, of blue to purple fertile flowers, surrounded by white, sometimes pink- to mauve-tinged sterile flowers. ↕↔ 3m (10ft). E. Asia. ✲✲✲. **subsp. *sargentiana*** see *H. sargentiana*. **subsp. *strigosa*** has narrower leaves, with short, stiff hairs beneath, and often flowers very late in summer. C. China. **Villosa Group** see *H. villosa*.
***H. cinerea* 'Sterilis'** see *H. arborescens* subsp. *discolor* 'Sterilis'.
H. integerrima see *H. serratifolia*.
H. involucrata. Spreading, deciduous shrub with broadly ovate-oblong, bristly, dark green leaves, to 15cm (6in) long. In late summer, bears domed corymbs, to 12cm (5in) across, of small, blue fertile flowers, surrounded by white to pale blue or pink sterile flowers. ↕ 1m (3ft), ↔ 2m (6ft). Japan, Taiwan. ✲✲. **'Hortensis'** ▣ bears flowerheads of double, pinkish white sterile flowers.
H. macrophylla (Common hydrangea). Rounded, deciduous shrub with broadly ovate, coarsely toothed, glossy, dark green leaves, to 20cm (8in) long. In mid- and late summer, bears flattened corymbs, 15–20cm (6–8in) across, of a few pink sterile flowers and numerous blue or pink fertile flowers. ↕ 2m (6ft), ↔ 2.5m (8ft). Japan. ✲✲✲. Cultivars of *H. macrophylla* are divided into 2 groups: Lacecaps and Hortensias (see introduction). **'Altona'** ▣ 🏆 (Hortensia) has large flowerheads of rich pink to dark purple-blue flowers; ↕ 1m (3ft), ↔ 1.5m (5ft). **'Ami Pasquier'** 🏆 (Hortensia) is slow-growing, with dark crimson or blue-purple flowers; may be grown as a houseplant when young; ↕ 1.5m (5ft), ↔ 2m (6ft). **'Ayesha'** ▣ 🏆 (Hortensia) has unusual, lilac-like flowers with small, cupped, pale pink to pale blue sepals; ↕ 1.5m (5ft), ↔ 2m (6ft). **'Blue Bonnet'** ▣ (Hortensia) has dense flowerheads of rich blue to pink flowers. **'Blue Wave'** ▣ syn. 'Mariesii Perfecta' (Lacecap), produces rich blue to mauve, or lilac-blue to pink sterile flowers, and darker fertile flowers. **'Bouquet Rose'** ▣ (Hortensia) has pink to mauve flowers borne in large flowerheads on slender, arching stems. **'Deutschland'** (Hortensia) bears large flowerheads of dark pink flowers, mauve on acid soil. **'Domotoi'** (Hortensia) has conical flowerheads of large, light blue to mauve or pink flowers with sharply toothed sepals; ↕ 1m (3ft), ↔ 1.5m (5ft). **'Enziandom'**, syn. 'Gentian Dome' (Hortensia), bears deep pink to dark gentian-blue flowers. **'Europa'** 🏆 (Hortensia) is vigorous, with large flowerheads of dark pink to purple-blue flowers. **'Générale Vicomtesse de Vibraye'** ▣ 🏆 (Hortensia) has pale blue or pink flowers in large flowerheads; use as a houseplant when young. **'Gentian Dome'** see 'Enziandom'. **'Geoffrey Chadbund'** 🏆 (Lacecap) has dark brick-red flowers. **'Goliath'** (Hortensia) is vigorous, with large flowerheads of soft pink or pale blue flowers. **'Hamburg'** ▣ (Hortensia) is vigorous, bearing large flowerheads of dark pink to dark blue flowers with toothed sepals. **'Kluis Superba'** (Hortensia) has flowerheads of dark purple-blue to dark pink flowers. **'La France'** (Hortensia) is vigorous, with very large flowerheads of pink to mid-blue flowers. **'Lanarth White'** ▣ 🏆 (Lacecap) has pink to blue fertile flowers surrounded by pure white sterile flowers; ↕↔ 1.5m (5ft). **'Lilacina'** ▣ (Lacecap) has mauve-pink to blue fertile and sterile flowers. **'Maréchal Foch'** (Hortensia) has rich pink to purple, or dark vivid blue flowers; suitable for growing as a houseplant when young. **'Mariesii'** 🏆 (Lacecap) produces domed flowerheads of numerous pale pink to pale blue sterile flowers; ↕↔ 1.2m (4ft). **'Mariesii Perfecta'** see 'Blue Wave'. **'Masja'** (Hortensia) is compact, with dense flowerheads of vivid red flowers and very dark green foliage; ↕ 1m (3ft), ↔ 1.5m (5ft). **'Mme Emile Mouillère'** 🏆 (Hortensia) has white flowers becoming pink-tinged with age; use as a houseplant when young. **'Pia'**, syn. 'Pink Elf' (Hortensia), is compact, producing bright red flowers with white centres; ↕ 60cm (24in), ↔ 1m (3ft). **'Pink Elf'** see 'Pia'. **'Preziosa'** see *H.* 'Preziosa'. **'Quadricolor'** (Lacecap) has leaves boldly variegated with pale and dark green, cream, and yellow, and has pale pink flowers; often confused with 'Tricolor', which is weaker-growing; ↕ 1.5m (5ft), ↔ 1.2m (4ft). **subsp. *serrata*** see *H. serrata*. **'Veitchii'** ▣ 🏆 (Lacecap) has large flowerheads with

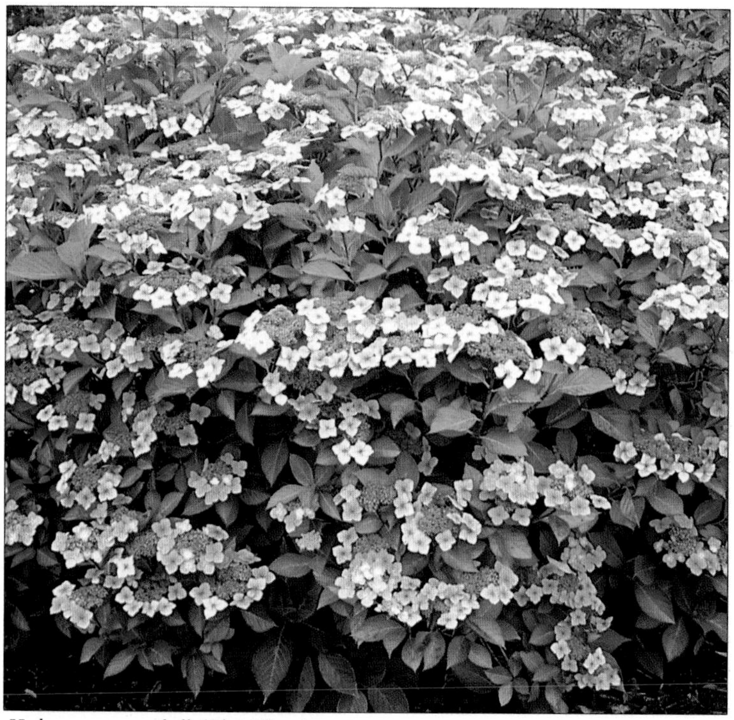
Hydrangea macrophylla 'Blue Wave'

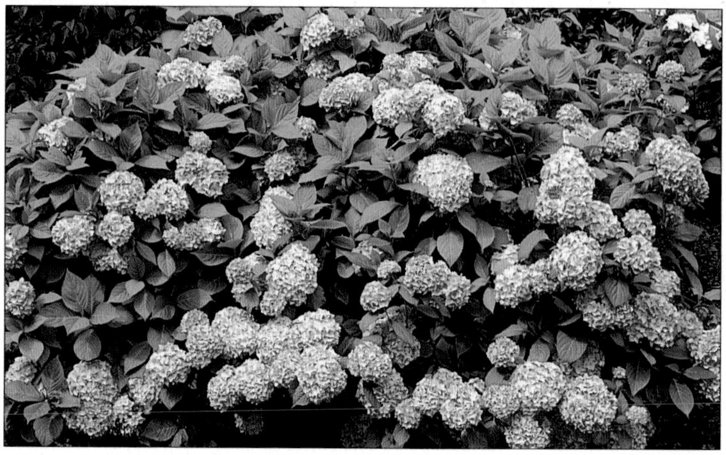
Hydrangea macrophylla 'Générale Vicomtesse de Vibraye'

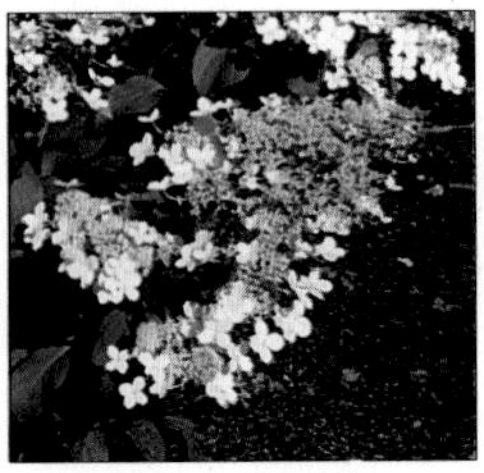
Hydrangea paniculata 'Brussels Lace'

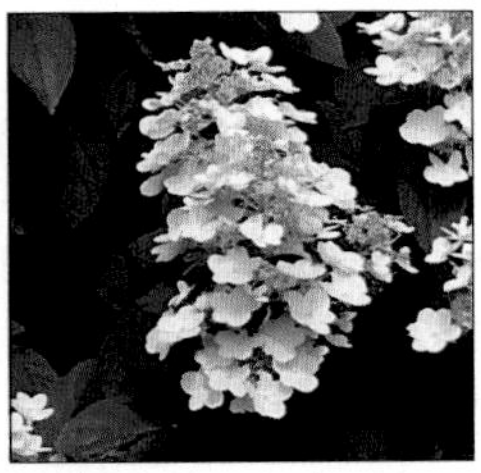
Hydrangea paniculata 'Floribunda'

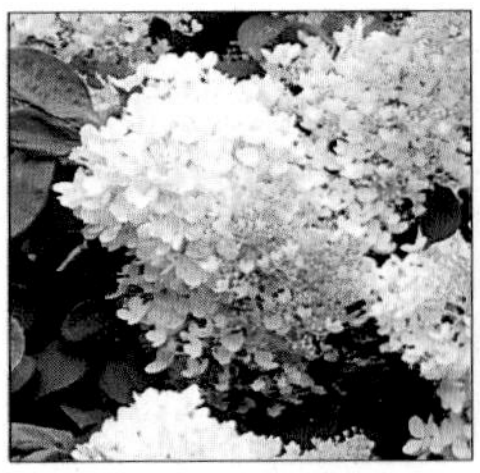
Hydrangea paniculata 'Grandiflora'

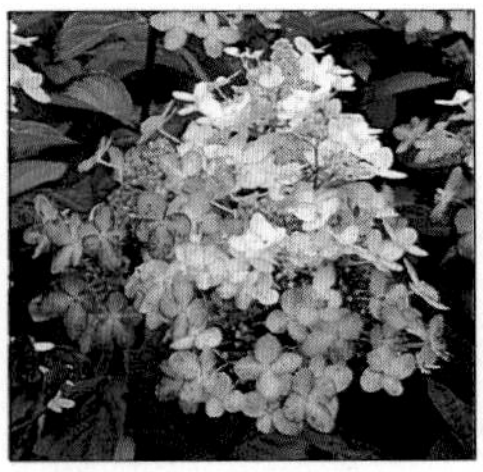
Hydrangea paniculata 'Pink Diamond'

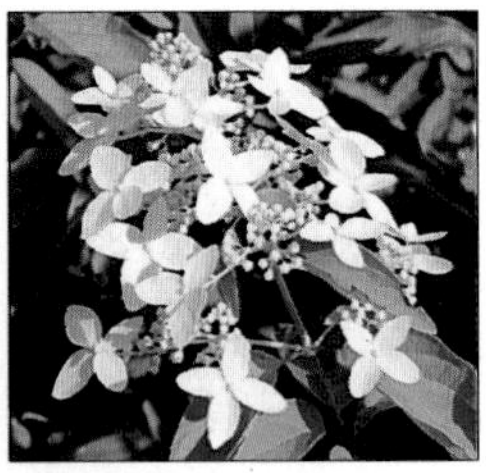
Hydrangea paniculata 'Praecox'

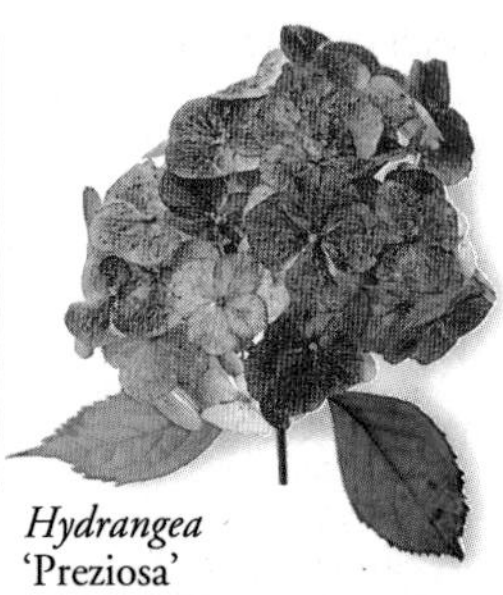
Hydrangea 'Preziosa'

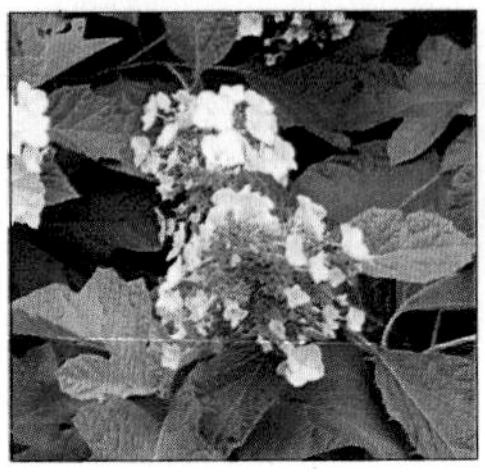
Hydrangea quercifolia

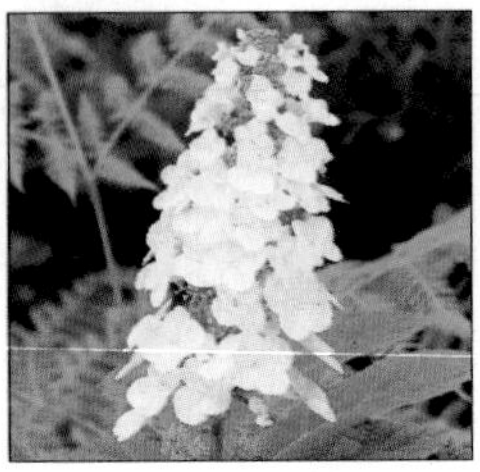
Hydrangea quercifolia 'Snow Queen'

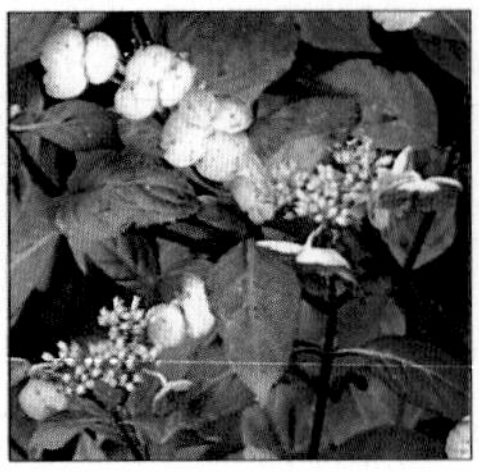
Hydrangea serrata

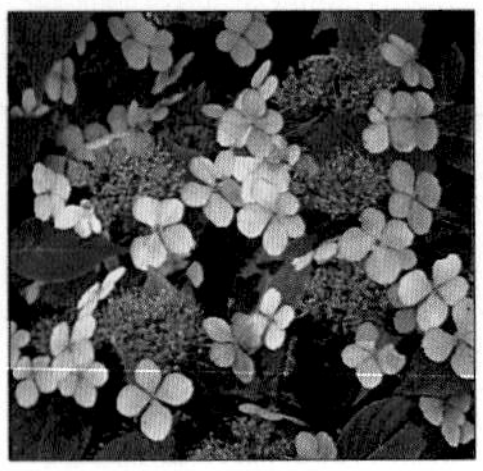
Hydrangea serrata 'Bluebird'

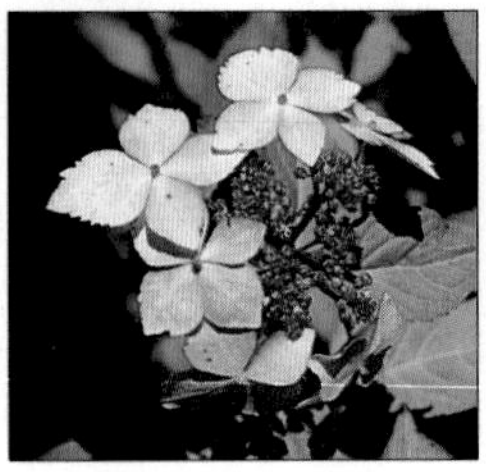
Hydrangea serrata 'Rosalba'

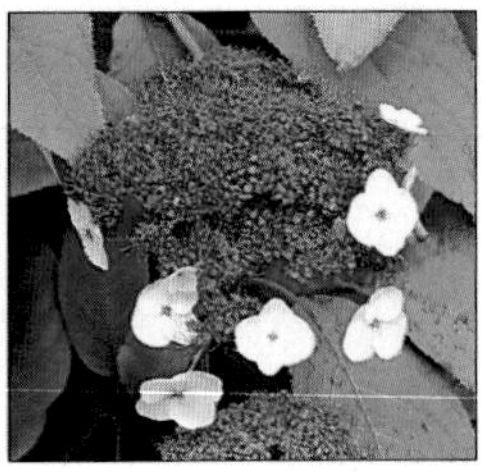
Hydrangea villosa

H

white sterile flowers turning pink to red with age. **'White Wave'** 🏆 (Lacecap) has pink to blue fertile flowers and large white sterile flowers; ↕↔ 1.5m (5ft).
H. paniculata. Vigorous, spreading to upright, deciduous shrub with ovate, pointed, toothed, mid- to dark green leaves, 7–15cm (3–6in) long. Large, conical panicles, 7–20cm (3–8in) tall, of creamy white fertile flowers and large, pinkish white sterile flowers are borne in late summer and early autumn. To obtain larger flowerheads on cultivars, cut back previous season's shoots to within a few buds of the woody framework in spring. ↕ 3–7m (10–22ft), ↔ 2.5m (8ft). Russia (Sakhalin), China, Japan. ❄❄❄. **'Brussels Lace'** ■ bears a profusion of small panicles of mainly fertile flowers and a few sterile flowers. **'Floribunda'** ■🏆 has large flowerheads of white sterile flowers, becoming pink-tinged as they age. **'Grandiflora'** ■ has large flowerheads, 20–30cm (8–12in) tall, sometimes more, of mainly sterile white flowers that turn pinkish white with age. **'Kyushu'** 🏆 is erect, with glossy leaves. **'Pink Diamond'** ■ has broad, open panicles, to 30cm (12in) tall, of fertile and sterile flowers, creamy white at first, becoming deep pink with a red reverse to the petals as they age. **'Praecox'** ■🏆 flowers early, from midsummer onwards. **'Tardiva'** is late-flowering, in early and mid-autumn. **'Unique'** ■🏆 is similar to 'Grandiflora' but more vigorous, with large sterile flowers in flowerheads 20cm (8in) across. **'White Moth'** has spherical flowerheads with large sterile flowers, attractive over a long period in autumn.
H. petiolaris ■🏆 syn. *H. anomala* subsp. *petiolaris* (Climbing hydrangea). Vigorous, woody, deciduous climber, clinging by aerial roots. Ovate-rounded leaves, to 11cm (4½in) long, have heart-shaped bases and are dark green, turning yellow in autumn. In summer, bears domed corymbs, to 25cm (10in) across, of white fertile and sterile flowers. ↕ 15m (50ft). Russia (Sakhalin), Korea, Taiwan, Japan. ❄❄❄

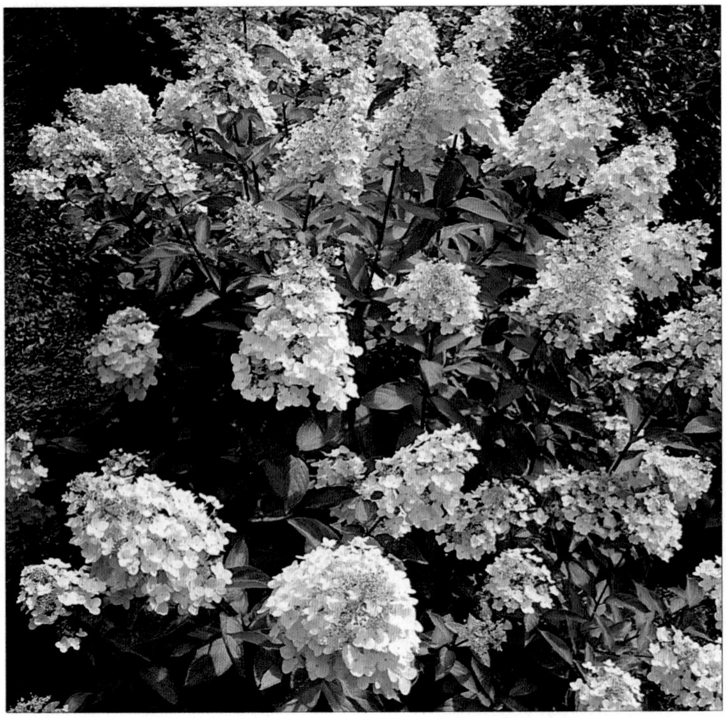
Hydrangea paniculata 'Unique'

***H.* 'Preziosa'** ■🏆 syn. *H. macrophylla* 'Preziosa', *H. serrata* 'Preziosa'. Upright, deciduous shrub with broadly ovate, glossy, mid-green leaves, to 15cm (6in) long. Small, spherical corymbs of white sterile flowers, 10–13cm (4–5in) across, turning to rich red, blue, or mauve on acid soil, are borne on dark stems in late summer. ↕↔ 1.5m (5ft). ❄❄
H. quercifolia ■🏆 (Oak-leaved hydrangea). Deciduous, mound-forming shrub with deeply 5- to 7-lobed, mid-green leaves, to 20cm (8in) long, turning bronze-purple in autumn. From midsummer to autumn, bears conical panicles, to 25cm (10in) tall, of white fertile and sterile flowers; the sterile flowers become pink-tinged with age. ↕ 2m (6ft), ↔ 2.5m (8ft). S.E. USA. ❄❄❄. **'Snow Flake'** has arching panicles of long-lasting, sterile, double white flowers, later turning pink. **'Snow Queen'** ■ has profuse, large sterile flowers in dense, upright flowerheads.
H. sargentiana 🏆 syn. *H. aspera* subsp. *sargentiana*. Upright, deciduous shrub with stout, bristly shoots and large, broadly ovate, very bristly, dark green leaves, to 25cm (10in) long. Flattened corymbs, to 23cm (9in) across, of blue to purple fertile flowers, surrounded by white sterile flowers, sometimes tinged purple, are produced from late summer to autumn. ↕ 3m (10ft) or more, ↔ 2.2–2.5m (7–8ft). China. ❄❄❄
H. seemannii. Woody, evergreen climber, clinging by aerial roots, with elliptic to lance-shaped, leathery, mid-green leaves, to 15cm (6in) long. In summer, bears greenish white fertile flowers surrounded by white sterile flowers, in domed corymbs, to 15cm (6in) across. ↕ 10m (30ft). Mexico. ❄❄
H. serrata ■ syn. *H. macrophylla* subsp. *serrata*. Compact, erect, deciduous shrub with narrowly ovate, pointed, mid-green leaves, to 15cm (6in) long. Flattened corymbs, 5–10cm (2–4in) across, with a few pink or blue sterile flowers and numerous blue or pink fertile flowers, open from summer to autumn. Some *H. serrata* cultivars are also described as Lacecaps (see introduction). ↕↔ 1.2m (4ft). Korea, Japan. ❄❄. **'Acuminata'** see 'Bluebird'. **'Bluebird'** ■🏆 syn. 'Acuminata' (Lacecap), bears rich blue fertile flowers surrounded by pale blue sterile flowers over a very long period. Leaves turn red in autumn. **'Diadem'** (Lacecap) has domed flowerheads of pale pink or blue flowers in early summer; ↕ 80cm (32in), ↔ 1m (3ft). **'Grayswood'** 🏆 (Lacecap) is vigorous, bearing broad flowerheads of small, mauve fertile flowers; the white sterile flowers turn dark red as they age; ↕↔ 2m (6ft). **'Preziosa'** see *H.* 'Preziosa'. **'Rosalba'** ■🏆 (Lacecap) has flowerheads with small, pink fertile flowers and white sterile flowers, becoming red-marked with age.
H. serratifolia, syn. *H. integerrima.* Vigorous, woody, evergreen climber, similar to *H. seemannii*, but with elliptic, leathery, dark green leaves, to 15cm (6in) long, sharply toothed on young plants. In summer, clustered, corymb-like flowerheads, to 15cm (6in) across, with white fertile flowers and usually no sterile flowers, open from large, spherical buds. ↕ 15m (50ft). Chile, Argentina. ❄❄
H. villosa ■🏆 syn. *H. aspera* Villosa Group. Spreading to erect, deciduous

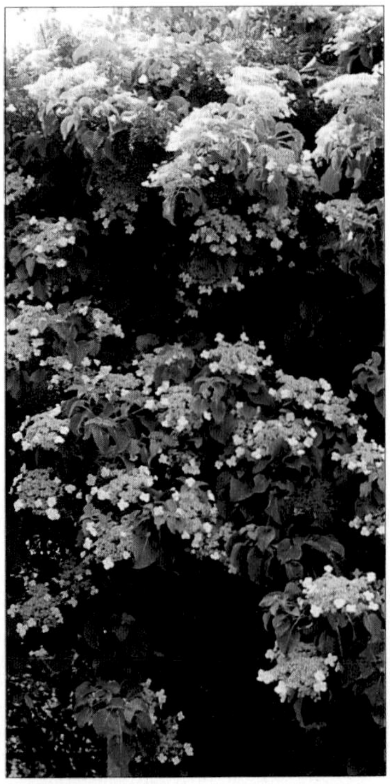
Hydrangea petiolaris

shrub or small tree with lance-shaped to narrowly ovate, velvety, dark green leaves, 9–24cm (3½–10in) long. In late summer, bears flattened corymbs, 15cm (6in) across (often more), of blue-purple or rich blue fertile flowers and lilac-white or rose-lilac sterile flowers. ↕↔ 1–4m (4–12ft). Tibet, China, Burma, Taiwan. ✻✻✻

▷ **Hydrangea,**
Climbing see *Hydrangea petiolaris*
Common see *Hydrangea macrophylla*
Oak-leaved see *Hydrangea quercifolia*

HYDROCHARIS

Frogbit

HYDROCHARITACEAE

Genus of 2 species of submerged or floating aquatic perennials, inhabiting shallow water and marshes in Europe, Asia, and Africa. They have short, stolon-like stems that form mats just below the water surface or root into the mud. Resembling small water lilies, frogbits are cultivated for their foliage and their attractive, 3-petalled white flowers; the male flowers are borne in clusters of up to 4 blooms, the females are solitary. The small, basal leaves are stalked, kidney-shaped to rounded, and mid- to dark green. Use as surface cover for a large wildlife pool.

• **HARDINESS** Fully hardy.
• **CULTIVATION** Grow in still, alkaline, preferably shallow water in full sun. Strongest growth occurs in water shallow enough for the leaves to float and the stolons to root into the mud at the bottom of the pool; in deep water, the plants float on the surface and are less vigorous. Winter water levels must be sufficient to prevent freezing at the bottom of the pool, as this is where the overwintering buds hibernate; they rise to the surface and produce new growth in spring. See also pp.52–53.
• **PROPAGATION** Sow seed in shallow trays of water as soon as ripe, or separate stolons and place them on the water surface in spring.
• **PESTS AND DISEASES** Leaves may be eaten or disfigured by water snails and larvae of the brown china-mark moth.

H. morsus-ranae (Frogbit). Floating perennial with horizontal, floating stolons, which form new plants at their tips, and with rosettes of rounded, glossy, mid-green leaves, 3cm (1¼in) long. Bowl-shaped flowers, 2cm (¾in) across, with 3 broadly ovate, papery white petals, each with a yellow spot at the base, open in summer. ↔ indefinite. Europe, W. Asia, N. Africa. ✻✻✻

HYDROCLEYS

LIMNOCHARITACEAE

Genus of 9 species of stoloniferous, evergreen and deciduous, submerged aquatic annuals or perennials, found in slow-moving or still water in South America. They are cultivated for their attractive, bowl-shaped flowers, borne singly or sometimes in umbels, and their water-lily-like, ovate to rounded, mid- to dark green leaves. In frost-prone areas, grow at the margins of a pond in a cool greenhouse. In warmer climates, grow in submerged containers, or rooted

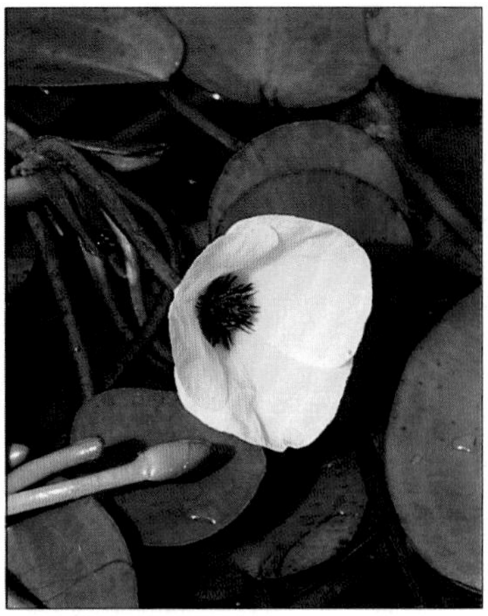

Hydrocleys nymphoides

in the mud at the margins of a sunny pond outdoors.

• **HARDINESS** Frost tender.
• **CULTIVATION** Grow in soft, acid water to 22cm (9in) deep. Under glass, grow in aquatic planting baskets or containers at the pool margins, in bright filtered light. Provide a water temperature of up to 25°C (77°F). Outdoors, grow in containers or at pond margins, in full sun. *H. nymphoides* hibernates below 18°C (64°F). See also pp.52–53.
• **PROPAGATION** Sow seed in pans at 20°C (68°F) as soon as ripe; cover the seed with silver sand, and place the pans in water up to the rims. On germination, immerse, so that the surfaces of the pans are covered by 1cm (½in) of water. Divide young plantlets in spring.
• **PESTS AND DISEASES** Trouble free.

H. nymphoides ▣ (Water poppy). Deciduous, submerged perennial with prostrate, stoloniferous shoots and long-stalked, thick, broadly-ovate to rounded, floating leaves, 5–8cm (2–3in) long, heart-shaped at the bases. Short-lived, solitary, poppy-like, 3-petalled yellow flowers, 5–8cm (2–3in) across, with purple centres, are borne just above the water surface in summer. ↔ indefinite. Tropical S. America. ❀ (min. 1°C/34°F)

HYDROCOTYLE

Pennywort

APIACEAE/UMBELLIFERAE

Genus of 75 species of moisture-loving herbaceous perennials and marginal aquatic perennials from Eurasia, North America, and New Zealand, found at stream or lake margins, in swamps, or in moist woodland. They have a low, creeping habit, rounded, light to dark green leaves, and inconspicuous, rounded flowers in small umbels. Grow as ground cover in a bog garden, in damp sites in a rock garden, or at pond margins. In frost-prone areas, grow tender species at the margins of an indoor pool or in an aquarium.

• **HARDINESS** Fully hardy to frost tender.
• **CULTIVATION** Grow in moderately fertile, humus-rich, moist soil in sun or partial shade. To grow pennyworts as marginal aquatics, plant in the muddy margins of a pond, or in baskets of loamy soil to confine their spread. In an aquarium, grow in an inert medium in bright filtered light or full light, with a water temperature of 5–24°C (41–75°F). See also pp.52–53.
• **PROPAGATION** Sow seed in containers in a cold frame from autumn to spring. Divide in spring.
• **PESTS AND DISEASES** Trouble free.

H. americana, syn. *H. ranunculoides.* Creeping, marginal aquatic perennial with rounded, mid-green leaves, to 5cm (2in) long, borne on leaf-stalks 1–11cm (½–4½in) long. Stalkless umbels of 3–5 inconspicuous, rounded, greenish white flowers are produced in summer. ↔ indefinite. North America, New Zealand. ✻✻✻ (borderline)
H. ranunculoides see *H. americana.*

HYGROPHILA

ACANTHACEAE

Genus of 100 species of evergreen and deciduous, marginal and submerged aquatic perennials found in lakes, rivers, streams, bogs, and marshes in tropical regions, particularly in Africa and S.E. Asia. They have opposite, entire to finely pinnatifid or pinnate, ovate or lance-shaped leaves, and produce tight racemes or panicles of whorled, tubular, 2-lipped flowers from the leaf axils in summer. In tropical areas, hygrophilas are attractive foliage plants for growing at pond margins; elsewhere, grow in a pond in a warm greenhouse, or in an aquarium.

• **HARDINESS** Frost tender.
• **CULTIVATION** Outdoors, grow either at pond margins or in the mud at the base of a pond, in full light. Under glass, grow either in baskets at the margins of a pool or submerged in an aquarium, in bright filtered light and with a water temperature of 20–24°C (68–75°F). See also pp.52–53.
• **PROPAGATION** Divide in summer. Root stem-tip or softwood cuttings in summer. Detached floating leaves will also form roots.
• **PESTS AND DISEASES** Soft young growth may be damaged by water snails.

H. difformis (Water wisteria). Evergreen, marginal or submerged aquatic perennial with slender, soft stems, to 60cm (24in) long, clothed in pinnate, pinnatifid, or comb-like, mid-green, submerged leaves, to 10cm (4in) long. In summer, whorls of tubular, lilac to violet flowers, 10–15mm (½in) long, streaked red-violet within, are produced in leafy racemes, to 45cm (18in) long, from the axils of the thicker, lance-shaped, scalloped, dark green aerial leaves. ↔ indefinite. India to Thailand. ❀ (min. 20°C/68°F)

HYLOCEREUS

CACTACEAE

Genus of about 20 species of robust, climbing, sometimes scrambling, epiphytic, perennial cacti from forest in S. Mexico, the West Indies, and Central and tropical South America. They have prominent aerial roots and 3-ribbed stems, which may grow to 5m (15ft) long. The stems often have scalloped ribs with areoles bearing a few short spines or bristles. Large, funnel-shaped flowers open by night in summer; they are followed by spherical to ovoid, scaly red fruits, to 10cm (4in) across, containing kidney-shaped black seeds. Where temperatures fall below 15°C (59°F), grow in a warm greenhouse. In warmer areas, grow against a wall, or over a fence or tree-trunk.

• **HARDINESS** Frost tender.
• **CULTIVATION** Under glass, grow in loamless, epiphytic cactus compost in bright indirect light; provide high humidity. In growth, water freely and apply a half-strength, balanced liquid fertilizer monthly; keep moist in winter. Outdoors, grow in sharply drained, poor to moderately fertile, acid soil in partial or dappled shade. See also pp.48–49.
• **PROPAGATION** Sow seed at 19–24°C (66–75°F) in spring. Root cuttings of stem segments in spring or summer.
• **PESTS AND DISEASES** Scale insects may be a problem.

H. calcaratus. Semi-epiphytic cactus with ribbed, bright green stems, 4–7cm (1½–3in) thick. Rib margins are divided into prominent, rounded lobes with small areoles, either spineless or bearing 2–4 white bristles. In summer, bears very fragrant, white or creamy white flowers, 20–30cm (8–12in) across, with long, greenish white outer segments. ↕↔ 2m (6ft) or more. Costa Rica. ❀ (min. 15°C/59°F)
H. ocamponis. Climbing cactus with slightly wavy, glaucous, blue-green stems, 6cm (2½in) thick, and areoles bearing 3–8 yellow spines. In summer, bears fragrant flowers, to 30cm (12in) across, with wide, pure white inner petals and narrower, pale yellowish green outer segments. ↕↔ 2m (6ft) or more. S. Mexico. ❀ (min. 15°C/59°F)
H. polyrhizus. Scrambling, epiphytic cactus with slender, low-ribbed greenish white stems, 3–4cm (1¼–1½in) thick, soon becoming green; the areoles bear 2–4 brown spines. In summer, purple buds open to fragrant flowers, 25–30cm (10–12in) across, with off-white inner petals and red outer segments. ↕ 4m (12ft), ↔ 60cm (24in). Panama to Ecuador. ❀ (min. 15°C/59°F)
H. undatus ▣ Fast-growing, free-branching, epiphytic or climbing cactus

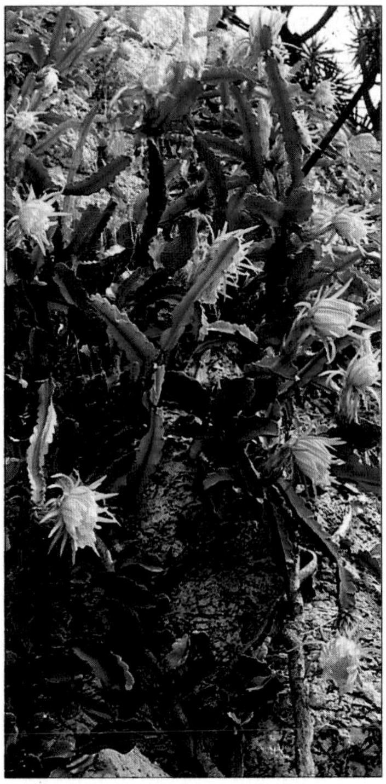

Hylocereus undatus

with jointed, scalloped, horny stems, 5–8cm (2–3in) thick, and areoles bearing up to 3 conical, dark brown or grey-brown spines. In summer, bears fragrant white flowers, 30cm (12in) across, with yellowish green outer segments. ↕↔ 2–4m (6–12ft). West Indies; widely naturalized in tropical America. ❀ (min. 15°C/59°F)

HYLOMECON

PAPAVERACEAE

Genus of one species of rhizomatous herbaceous perennial from woodland in E. Asia. It has mostly basal, pinnate leaves, and is grown for its poppy-like flowers, produced over long periods from late spring to summer. Excellent as a woodland or wild garden plant, or for shady pockets in a large rock garden, but may spread quickly and smother small plants nearby.

- **HARDINESS** Fully hardy.
- **CULTIVATION** Grow in moist but well-drained, moderately fertile, humus-rich, neutral to slightly acid soil in partial to deep shade. Add organic matter at planting.
- **PROPAGATION** Sow seed in containers in a cold frame as soon as ripe or in autumn. Divide in spring.
- **PESTS AND DISEASES** Prone to damage by slugs and snails, especially in spring.

H. japonica ■ Clump-forming perennial with pinnate, pale green leaves, to 20cm (8in) long, consisting of 5- to 7-toothed, ovate or obovate leaflets. Solitary, saucer- to cup-shaped, 4-petalled, deep yellow flowers, to 5cm (2in) across, are borne from late spring to summer. ↕ 30cm (12in), ↔ 30cm (12in) or more. E. China, Korea, Japan. ***

▷ ***Hylotelephium*** see *Sedum*
H. roseum see *S. erythrostictum*
▷ ***Hymenanthera*** see *Melicytus*
H. crassifolia see *M. crassifolius*
H. dentata see *M. dentatus*

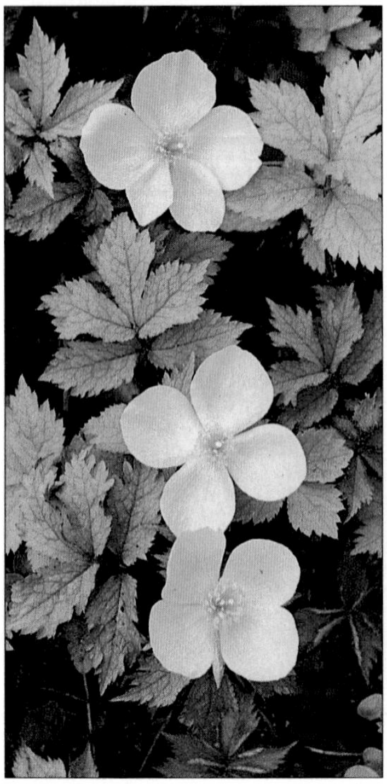
Hylomecon japonica

HYMENOCALLIS

syn. ISMENE
Spider lily

AMARYLLIDACEAE

Genus of about 40 species of bulbous perennials, some evergreen, found in grassland and rocky habitats from S. USA to South America. In spring, summer, or winter, they bear terminal umbels of fragrant flowers resembling spidery daffodils (*Narcissus*), each with 6 narrow petals (tepals), and a large cup, formed from the fused lower parts of the stamens. The anthers are attached to the cup and face inwards. The leaves are basal, strap-shaped or oblong, and mid- to dark green. In frost-prone areas, grow in a warm greenhouse (except for *H. narcissiflora*, which is best in a cool greenhouse); in warmer areas, grow in a bed or border, at the base of a warm, sunny wall, or in containers.

- **HARDINESS** Frost tender; *H. narcissiflora* may withstand short spells around 0°C (32°F).
- **CULTIVATION** Plant bulbs in autumn with the neck and shoulders above soil level. Under glass, grow in loam-based potting compost (JI No.2) with added leaf mould and grit, in bright filtered or full light. Provide low humidity for deciduous species, and moderate to high humidity for evergreens. Water freely in growth, and apply a dilute, balanced liquid fertilizer every 2 or 3 weeks. Keep deciduous species dry and evergreens just moist when dormant. Outdoors, grow in moderately fertile, moist but well-drained soil in sun or partial shade; when dormant, protect from excessive wet. In frost-prone areas, plant *H. narcissiflora* in spring and lift for winter.
- **PROPAGATION** Sow seed at 19–24°C (66–75°F) as soon as ripe. Remove offsets in spring.
- **PESTS AND DISEASES** Trouble free.

H. amancaes. Bulbous perennial with semi-erect, strap-shaped, dark green, basal leaves, to 45cm (18in) long, fused at their bases to form a false stem around the bottom of the flower stems. In summer, these bear loose umbels of 2–6 scented, deep yellow flowers, 9cm (3½in) across. ↕ 30cm (12in), ↔ 25cm (10in). Peru. ❀ (min. 15°C/59°F)
H. calathina see *H. narcissiflora.*
H. caribaea. Evergreen, bulbous perennial with semi-erect, strap-shaped, glossy, mid-green, basal leaves, to 60cm (24in) long. From summer to autumn, bears umbels of 8–10 scented white flowers, 15cm (6in) across. ↕ to 60cm (24in), ↔ 30cm (12in). West Indies. ❀ (min. 15°C/59°F)
H. x festalis ■ (*H. longipetala* x *H. narcissiflora*). Evergreen, bulbous perennial with semi-erect, oblong, mid-green, basal leaves, to 90cm (36in) long. From spring to summer, bears umbels of 2–5 scented white flowers, 8–12cm (3–5in) across, with long, narrow petals and wide cups; the upper 3 stamens of each flower curve downwards, the lower 3 are straight. ↕ 80cm (32in), ↔ 30cm (12in). Garden origin. ❀ (min. 15°C/59°F)
H. x macrostephana ♀ (*H. narcissiflora* x *H. speciosa*). Bulbous perennial with semi-erect, inversely lance-shaped, bright mid-green, basal leaves, 50–90cm (20–36in) long. Umbels of up to 10 fragrant flowers, 15cm (6in) across, varying from white to cream or greenish yellow, are borne in spring or summer. ↕ 80cm (32in), ↔ 30cm (12in). Garden origin. ❀ (min. 15°C/59°F)
H. narcissiflora, syn. *H. calathina*, *Ismene calathina* (Peruvian daffodil). Bulbous perennial with strap-shaped, semi-erect, dark green, basal leaves, to 60cm (24in) long, sheathing at the bases to form a false stem. In summer, bears umbels of up to 5 strongly scented white flowers, 10cm (4in) across, sometimes with green-striped tubes; all the stamens curve upwards across the cup. ↕ 60cm (24in), ↔ 30cm (12in). Peruvian Andes. ❀ (min. 5°C/41°F)
H. speciosa. Evergreen, bulbous perennial producing semi-erect, broadly elliptic to oblong, mid-green, basal leaves, to 65cm (26in) long. Umbels of up to 12 scented, greenish white flowers, 23cm (9in) across, open from autumn to winter. ↕ to 45cm (18in), ↔ 30cm (12in). West Indies. ❀ (min. 15°C/59°F)
H. 'Sulphur Queen'. Bulbous perennial with semi-erect, strap-shaped, dark green, basal leaves, 25–60cm (10–24in) long. Umbels of up to 6 scented, soft sulphur-yellow flowers, 15cm (6in) across, with green-striped, paler yellow tubes, are borne from spring to summer. ↕ 60cm (24in), ↔ 30cm (12in). ❀ (min. 15°C/59°F)

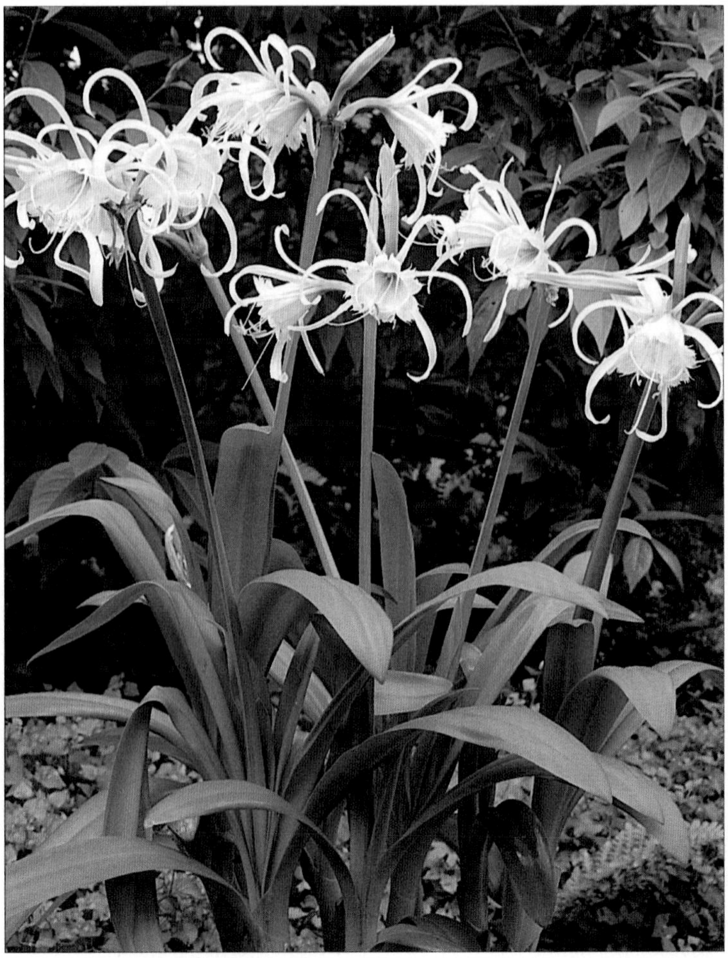
Hymenocallis x *festalis*

HYMENOSPORUM

Australian frangipani

PITTOSPORACEAE

Genus of one species of evergreen, flowering shrub or tree from rainforest or temperate forest in E. Australia and New Guinea. It is valued for its showy, umbel-like panicles of tubular flowers, with 5 spreading lobes, and its alternate, lance-shaped to obovate or oval-oblong, glossy leaves. In frost-prone areas, grow in a conservatory or temperate greenhouse; in warmer regions, grow as a handsome specimen tree.

- **HARDINESS** Frost tender, but may survive short spells around 0°C (32°F), if the shoots are well ripened in summer.
- **CULTIVATION** Under glass, grow in loam-based potting compost (JI No.2) in full light, with shade from hot sun and low to moderate humidity. In growth, water moderately and apply a balanced liquid fertilizer monthly; keep moist in winter. Outdoors, grow in humus-rich, moist but well-drained soil in full sun. Pruning group 1 or 8; hard pruning is tolerated.
- **PROPAGATION** Sow seed at 16–18°C (61–64°F) in spring. Root semi-ripe cuttings with bottom heat in summer. Layer, or air layer, in spring or autumn.
- **PESTS AND DISEASES** Trouble free.

H. flavum ♀ (Australian frangipani). Large shrub or small to medium-sized tree, usually with a single main stem and well-spaced but bushy branches. Lance-shaped to obovate or oval-oblong leaves, 6–15cm (2½–6in) long, are glossy, dark green above, paler green beneath. From spring to summer, bears loose, umbel-like panicles, to 20cm (8in) across, of tubular, fragrant flowers, 3cm (1¼in) across, with 5 spreading lobes; they open pale cream and rapidly age to orange-yellow. ↕ 4–20m (12–70ft), ↔ 3–7m (10–22ft). Australia (Queensland, New South Wales), New Guinea. ❀ (min. 5°C/41°F)

▷ ***Hymenoxys acaulis*** see *Tetraneuris acaulis*

HYOPHORBE

Bottle palm

ARECACEAE/PALMAE

Genus of 5 species of single-stemmed palms from volcanic or limestone soils in forest, from sea level to 700m (2,300ft), on the Mascarene Islands, E. of Madagascar. They have erect trunks, swollen at the base or middle, topped by a cluster of pinnate leaves above a prominent crownshaft. Bowl-shaped, 3-petalled flowers are borne in solitary panicles beneath the lowest leaf. In frost-prone areas, grow in a warm greenhouse or conservatory; elsewhere, use in a courtyard garden or as lawn specimens.

• **HARDINESS** Frost tender.

• **CULTIVATION** Under glass, grow in loam-based potting compost (JI No.2) in full light, shaded from hot sun, with moderate humidity. Water moderately all year. Apply a dilute, balanced liquid fertilizer monthly in growth. Outdoors, grow in moderately fertile, moist but well-drained soil in sun or partial shade.

• **PROPAGATION** Sow seed at 27°C (81°F) in spring.

• **PESTS AND DISEASES** Red spider mites may be a problem under glass.

H. lagenicaulis ▣ ♈ syn. *Mascarena lagenicaulis* (Bottle palm). Small palm with a flask-shaped grey trunk, swollen at ground level, with vertical fissures in the bark. The narrowly ovate, pinnate leaves, 1.3–1.8m (4½–6ft) long, have many linear, mid- to deep green leaflets. In summer, bears tiny, green to cream flowers in panicles to 80cm (32in) long. ↕ to 6m (20ft), ↔ to 3m (10ft). Mascarene Islands (Round Island). ❀ (min. 15–16°C/59–61°C)

HYOSCYAMUS

Henbane

SOLANACEAE

Genus of 15 species of tap-rooted, often strong-smelling, hairy, sticky annuals, biennials, and perennials found on banks, cliffs, wasteland, and shingle beaches in Europe, N. Africa, and Asia. They have lance-shaped to rounded, thick, coarse, felted, usually toothed leaves, and bear branching, leafy racemes of funnel- to bell-shaped flowers from late spring to autumn. They are grown for their unusual flowers and interesting seed heads, which are useful in dried flower arrangements. Grow in poor stony soils, on a dry bank, or in wall crevices. Henbanes will tolerate coastal conditions. All parts of henbanes are highly toxic if ingested, and may irritate the skin on contact.

• **HARDINESS** Fully hardy.

• **CULTIVATION** Grow in well-drained, preferably alkaline soil in full sun.

• **PROPAGATION** Sow seed *in situ* in spring; henbanes often self-seed freely.

• **PESTS AND DISEASES** Trouble free.

H. albus. Erect annual or biennial with broadly ovate, sticky, pale mid-green leaves, to 10cm (4in) long. In spring, bears long racemes of unevenly lobed, 2-lipped, veined, pale yellow-green flowers, 3cm (1¼in) long. ↕ 30–90cm (12–36in), ↔ to 45cm (18in). S. Europe. ❄❄❄

H. niger (Black henbane, Henbane, Stinking nightshade). Sticky, strong-smelling annual or biennial producing oval to lance-shaped, entire or toothed, thickly felted, grey-green leaves, to 20cm (8in) long, mostly in basal rosettes. From summer to autumn, 5-lobed flowers, to 2.5cm (1in) across, dull yellow with purple centres and narrow purple veins, are borne singly or in pairs at the tips of forked, arching racemes. ↕ 0.6–1.2m (2–4ft), ↔ to 1m (3ft). Europe, W. Asia. ❄❄❄

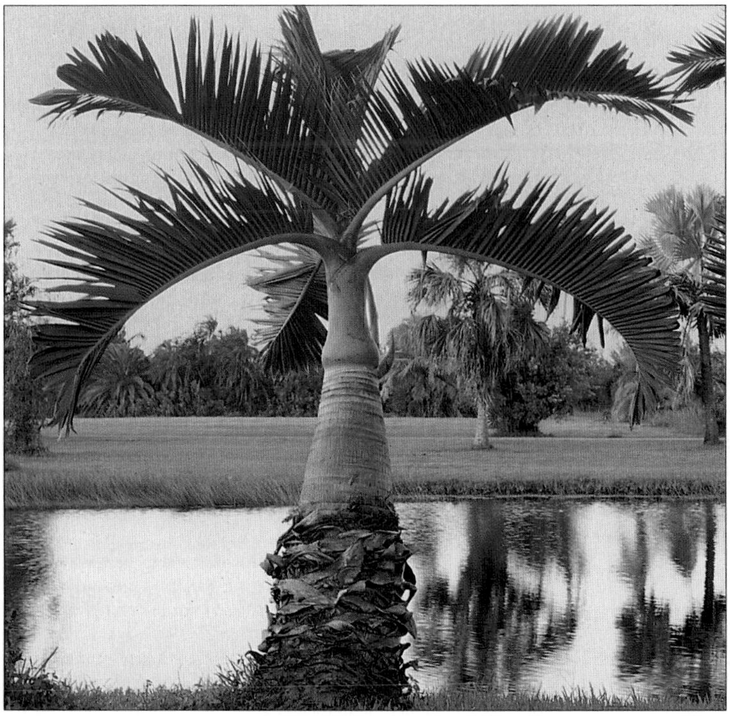

Hyophorbe lagenicaulis

HYPERICUM

St. John's wort

CLUSIACEAE/GUTTIFERAE

Genus of more than 400 species of deciduous, evergreen, and semi-evergreen shrubs and trees, annuals, and herbaceous perennials, occurring worldwide in a wide range of habitats, from woodland and scrub to mountains and cliffs. They have variably shaped, opposite, or occasionally whorled leaves, some with attractive autumn colour. Showy yellow flowers with prominent stamens are borne singly in terminal, occasionally axillary cymes, usually over a long period. The fruits, ornamental in a few species, are usually 3- to 5-valved capsules, or occasionally berry-like. Depending on size, hypericums are suitable for a variety of situations, from a shrub or mixed border to a rock garden; *H. elodes* grows well in boggy ground or as a marginal aquatic. Grow tender species in a cool or temperate greenhouse in frost-prone areas, and in a shrub border in warmer regions.

• **HARDINESS** Fully hardy to frost tender.

• **CULTIVATION** Grow in moderately fertile, moist but well-drained soil, the larger species in sun or partial shade, the dwarf species in full sun and in sharply drained soil. *H. androsaemum* and *H. calycinum* thrive in partial to deep shade. Grow *H. elodes* along the margins of a muddy-bottomed pool, in no more than 2.5cm (1in) of water, in dappled shade. Protect small rock garden species from excessive winter wet; shelter evergreen hypericums from cold, drying winds. Pruning group 1; or group 6 for deciduous species, and group 8 for evergreens. Cut *H. calycinum* to ground level in spring.

• **PROPAGATION** Sow seed in containers in a cold frame in autumn (species may hybridize). Divide perennials in spring or autumn (*H. elodes* in spring only). Root softwood cuttings of perennials in late spring; root greenwood or semi-ripe cuttings of shrubs in summer.

• **PESTS AND DISEASES** *H. calycinum* and *H.* x *inodorum* are susceptible to rust.

H. acmosepalum. Upright, bushy, semi-evergreen shrub with arching branches and oblong to elliptic-oblong, dark green leaves, to 6cm (2½in) long, bluish green or glaucous beneath, turning orange and red in autumn. In summer, bears terminal cymes of up to 6 star-shaped, deep yellow, sometimes red-tinged flowers, to 5cm (2in) across, followed by conical red capsules. ↕↔ 1–2m (3–6ft). China (Yunnan, Sichuan, Guizhou, Guangxi). ❄❄

H. aegypticum. Low, spreading, evergreen shrub with densely arranged, oblong, glaucous, mid-green leaves, to 1.5cm (½in) long. From late spring to summer, bears small, solitary, star-shaped, pale yellow flowers, to 1cm (½in) across, clustered at the ends of leafy shoots. ↕ 50cm (20in), ↔ 90cm (36in). Mediterranean. ❄❄ (borderline)

H. androsaemum (Tutsan). Bushy, deciduous shrub with erect branches and broadly ovate to oblong, mid-green leaves, to 15cm (6in) long, paler green beneath. In midsummer, bears cymes of up to 11 star-shaped or cupped, yellow flowers, to 2cm (¾in) across, followed

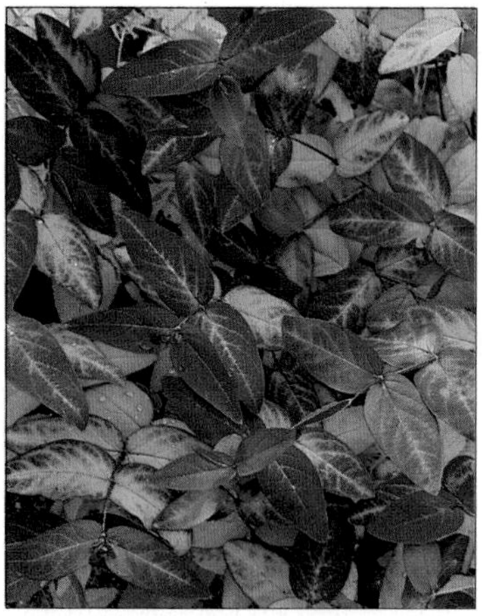

Hypericum androsaemum 'Albury Purple'

by spherical red, berry-like fruit that ripen to black. ↕ 75cm (30in), ↔ 90cm (36in). W. Europe, Mediterranean to N. Iran. ❄❄❄. **'Albury Purple'** ▣ produces purple-flushed leaves, and is often considered to be a cultivar of *H.* x *inodorum.*

H. augustinii. Upright, sparsely branched, evergreen to semi-evergreen shrub with broadly ovate to oblong-lance-shaped, leathery, pale green leaves, to 8cm (3in) long. Cymes of 3–13 saucer-shaped, pale to golden yellow flowers, to 6cm (2½in) across, are borne from late summer to autumn. ↕↔ 1.2m (4ft). S.W. China (Yunnan). ❄❄

H. balearicum. Densely branched, evergreen shrub producing ovate-oblong, leathery, dark green leaves, to 1.5cm (½in) long, with wavy margins and warty glands. From early to late summer, bears solitary, star-shaped, bright yellow flowers, to 4cm (1½in) across. Needs well-drained soil; ideal for a rock garden. ↕↔ to 25cm (10in). Spain (Balearic Islands). ❄❄❄ (borderline)

***H. beanii* 'Gold Cup'** see *H.* x *cyathiflorum* 'Gold Cup'.

H. bellum. Bushy, erect to arching, deciduous shrub producing oblong-lance-shaped to broadly ovate, mid-green leaves, to 8cm (3in) long, with wavy margins. In summer, bears cymes of up to 7 cup-shaped, pale to golden yellow flowers, to 2.5–6cm (1–2½in) across. ↕↔ 1m (3ft). W. and S.W. China, Himalayas, N. India, Burma. ❄❄

H. calycinum ▣ (Aaron's beard, Rose of Sharon). Dwarf, evergreen or semi-evergreen shrub, spreading by runners,

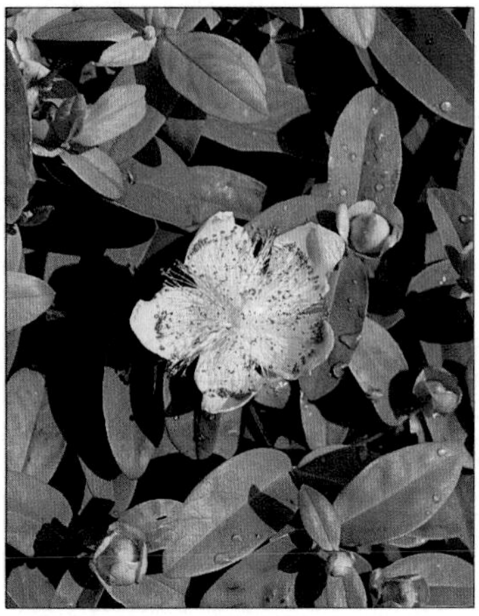

Hypericum calycinum

H

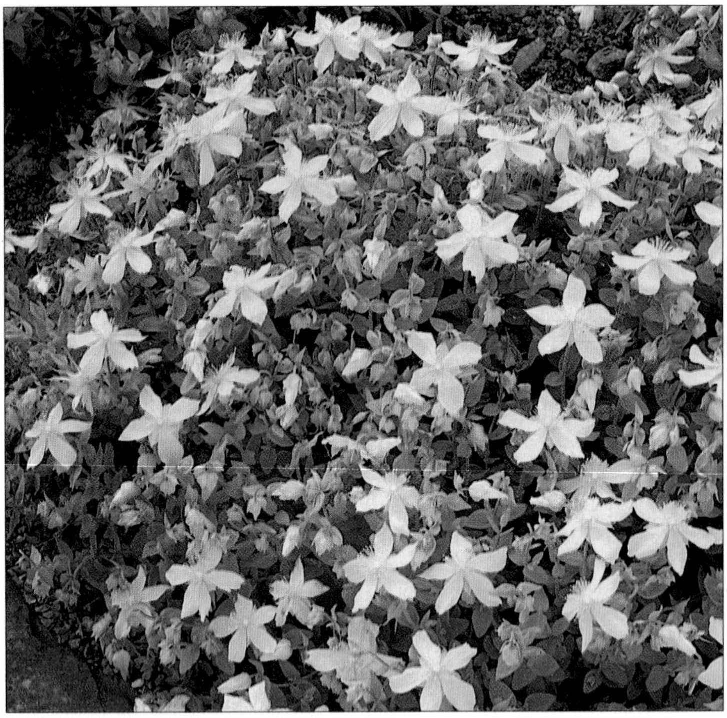

Hypericum cerastioides

with oblong to elliptic or narrowly ovate, dark green leaves, to 10cm (4in) long, paler green beneath. From midsummer to mid-autumn, saucer-shaped, bright yellow flowers, to 10cm (4in) across, are borne singly, or occasionally in small cymes of 2 or 3. Good ground cover in shade. ↕60cm (24in), ↔ indefinite. S.E. Bulgaria, N.W. and N.E. Turkey. ✻✻✻

H. cerastioides ▣ syn. *H. rhodoppeum.* Perennial with upright and arching stems bearing ovate, oblong, or elliptic, downy, grey-green leaves, to 3cm (1¼in) long. Cymes of up to 5 star-shaped, deep yellow flowers, 2–4.5cm (¾–1¾in) across, are borne in profusion in late spring and early summer. ↕15cm (6in), ↔ 40cm (16in) or more. S. Bulgaria, N.E. Greece, N.W. Turkey. ✻✻✻

H. coris. Dome-shaped, evergreen subshrub or herbaceous perennial with erect, wiry stems bearing whorls of linear, mid-green leaves, to 1.5cm (½in) long, glaucous beneath. In summer, bears an abundance of pyramidal cymes of up to 20 shallowly cup-shaped, golden yellow, sometimes red-veined flowers, 1.5–2cm (½–¾in) across, with conspicuous stamens. ↕20cm (8in), ↔ to 30cm (12in). S.E. France, Switzerland, Italy. ✻✻✻

H. cuneatum see *H. pallens.*

***H.* x *cyathiflorum* 'Gold Cup'**, syn. *H. beanii* 'Gold Cup'. Bushy, deciduous shrub with arching branches and lance-shaped, mid-green leaves, to 8cm (3in) long. Pyramidal cymes of up to 9 cup-shaped, golden yellow flowers, 5cm (2in) across, are produced in summer. ↕1.5m (5ft), ↔ 2m (6ft). ✻✻

***H.* 'Eastleigh Gold'.** Semi-evergreen shrub with arching branches and elliptic-oblong to lance-shaped, mid-green leaves, to 5cm (2in) long. In summer, bears cymes of up to 4 large, shallowly cup-shaped, golden yellow flowers, to 6cm (2½in) across. ↕1m (3ft), ↔ 1.5m (5ft). ✻✻✻

H. elodes ▣ (Marsh hypericum). Marsh or submerged aquatic perennial with creeping stolons, 10–30cm (4–12in) long, and broadly ovate to elliptic, soft, densely woolly, grey-green leaves, to 1.5cm (½in) long. Saucer-shaped, bright yellow flowers, to 1cm (½in) across, are borne singly or in cymes of 3–10 in summer. ↕7–15cm (3–6in), ↔ indefinite. W. Europe. ✻✻✻

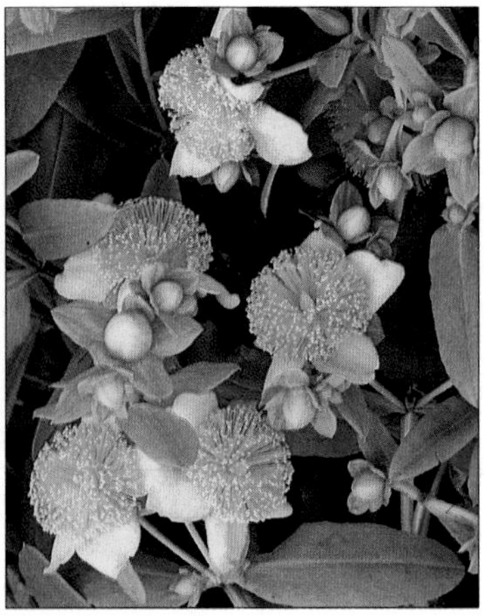

Hypericum frondosum

H. empetrifolium ▣ Dwarf, evergreen, stiffly erect to decumbent and cushion-forming shrub producing linear, mid-green leaves, to 1.5cm (½in) long, usually in whorls of 3. In summer, bears cylindrical to narrowly pyramidal cymes of up to 40 star-shaped, golden yellow flowers, to 2cm (¾in) across. ↕45cm (18in), ↔ 90cm (36in). S.E. Europe, S.W. Asia. ✻✻. **subsp. *oliganthum***, syn. var. *prostratum* of gardens, is prostrate, with branching stems clothed in whorls of stalkless, linear, or sometimes narrowly elliptic, dark green leaves, to 6mm (¼in) long, with rolled margins. In summer, bears cymes of 4–7 deep yellow flowers. Suitable for a sunny wall or rock garden; needs good drainage; ↕5cm (2in), ↔ to 30cm (12in); Greece (Crete); ✻✻✻ (borderline). **var. *prostratum* of gardens** see subsp. *oliganthum.*

H. forrestii 🏆 syn. *H. patulum* var. *forrestii.* Upright, spreading, deciduous shrub with triangular-ovate to broadly ovate or lance-shaped, mid-green leaves, to 6cm (2½in) long, turning red in late autumn and early winter. Cymes of up to 20 large, cup- to saucer-shaped, golden yellow flowers, to 6cm (2½in) across, are borne from summer to autumn. ↕1.2m (4ft), ↔ 1.5m (5ft). China (Yunnan, Sichuan), N.E. Burma. ✻✻✻

H. frondosum ▣ Erect, deciduous shrub with stout, flaking stems and oblong, bluish green leaves, to 6cm (2½in) long. In mid- and late summer, bears cymes of up to 7 saucer-shaped, golden yellow flowers, to 4.5cm (1¾in) across, with prominent, central bosses of yellow stamens. ↕↔ 60–120cm (2–4ft). S.E. USA. ✻✻✻

H. henryi. Variable, bushy, deciduous shrub with upright to arching branches clothed in narrowly elliptic or lance-shaped to ovate, mid-green leaves, to 4cm (1½in) long, glaucous beneath. Cymes of up to 5, occasionally 7, cup-shaped, golden yellow flowers, to 5cm (2in) across, are produced from late summer to autumn. ↕↔ 2m (6ft). S.W. China, E. Burma, North Vietnam, Indonesia. ✻✻

***H.* 'Hidcote'** 🏆 Dense, bushy, evergreen or semi-evergreen shrub with lance-shaped, dark green leaves, to 6cm (2½in) long. From midsummer to early autumn, bears corymb-like cymes of up to 6, sometimes more, large, cup-shaped, golden yellow flowers, to 6cm (2½in) across. ↕1.2m (4ft), ↔ 1.5m (5ft). ✻✻✻

H.* x *inodorum (*H. androsaemum* x *H. hircinum*). Upright, bushy, deciduous or semi-evergreen shrub producing oblong-lance-shaped to broadly ovate, aromatic, dark green leaves, to 11cm (4½in) long. Cymes of 3–23 small, star-shaped yellow flowers, 1.5–3cm (½–1¼in) across, are borne from midsummer to mid-autumn, followed by dark cerise, conical capsules. ↕↔ 1.2m (4ft). ✻✻✻. **'Elstead'** ▣ has large fruit, which flush pinkish red on ripening. **'Ysella'** has golden yellow leaves.

H. kalmianum. Erect, bushy, evergreen shrub producing narrowly oblong to inversely lance-shaped, bluish green leaves, to 5cm (2in) long. In mid- and late summer, bears cymes of up to 7 saucer-shaped, golden yellow flowers, to 3.5cm (1½in) across. ↕↔ 75cm (30in). E. North America (Great Lakes area of Canada and USA). ✻✻✻

H. kouytchense 🏆 syn. *H. patulum* var. *grandiflorum, H.* 'Sungold'. Rounded, bushy, semi-evergreen shrub with arching shoots and elliptic to ovate or lance-shaped, dark bluish green leaves, to 6cm (2½in) long, paler beneath. Cymes of up to 11 star-shaped, golden yellow flowers, to 6cm (2½in) across, with partially reflexed petals, are borne from summer to autumn, followed by conical, bright red fruit. ↕1m (3ft), ↔ 1.5m (5ft). China (Guizhou). ✻✻✻

H. lancasteri ▣ Spreading, deciduous shrub with triangular-lance-shaped to oblong leaves, to 6cm (2½in) long, bronze when young, maturing to mid-green, glaucous beneath. In summer, bears cymes of up to 11 star-shaped to shallowly cup-shaped, golden yellow flowers, to 6cm (2½in) across, with star-shaped calyces with red-margined sepals, conspicuous before they open. ↕↔ 1m (3ft). China (N. Yunnan, S. Sichuan). ✻✻✻

***H.* x *moserianum* 'Tricolor'**, syn. *H.* 'Variegatum'. Spreading, semi-evergreen shrub with arching, red-flushed shoots and ovate, mid-green leaves, to 6cm (2½in) long, attractively variegated with cream, pink, and green. From summer to autumn, bears cymes of up to 8 cup-shaped yellow flowers, to 5cm (2in) across. Needs a sheltered position. ↕30cm (12in), ↔ 60cm (24in). ✻✻✻

H. olympicum 🏆 Deciduous shrub with erect stems clothed in oblong, elliptic, or linear-lance-shaped, pointed, grey-green leaves, to 4cm (1½in) long, glaucous beneath. In summer, bears cymes of up

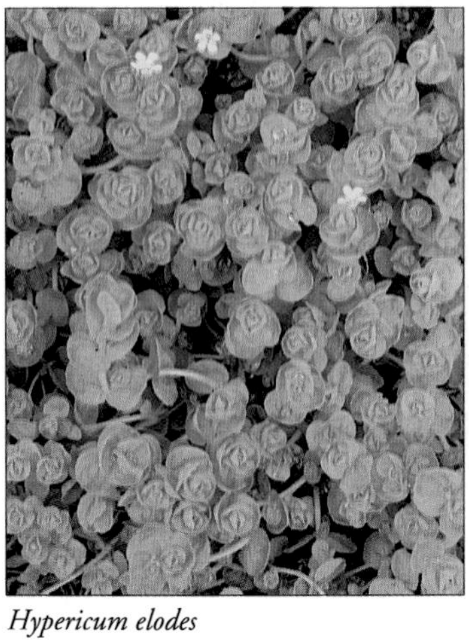

Hypericum elodes

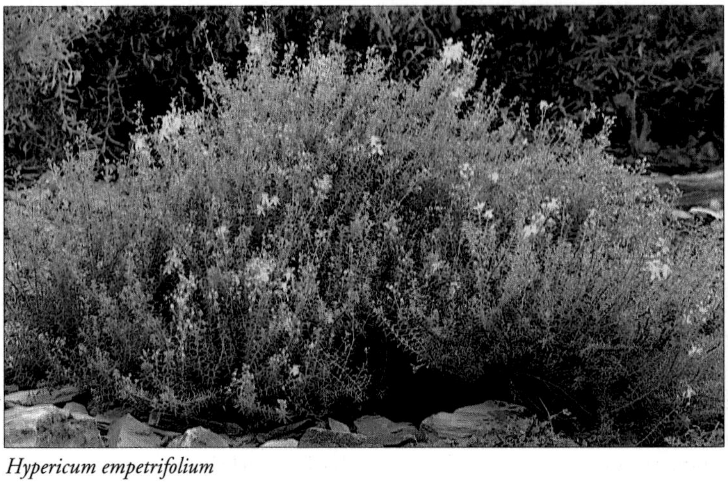

Hypericum empetrifolium

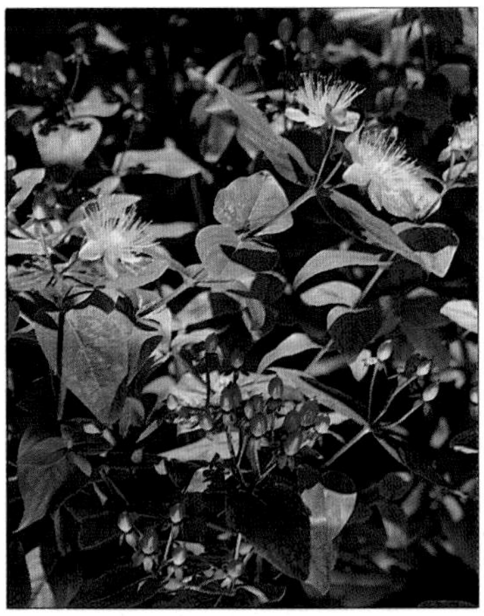

Hypericum x *inodorum* 'Elstead'

to 5 star-shaped, deep yellow flowers, each to 6cm (2½in) across. ↕25cm (10in), ↔ 30cm (12in). N. Greece, N.W. Turkey. ❄❄❄. **f. *uniflorum* 'Citrinum'** 𝕐 syn. 'Citrinum', produces broadly elliptic to obovate leaves, to 2–3cm (¾–1¼in) long, and pale lemon-yellow flowers; ideal for a rock garden.
H. orientale. Erect or decumbent perennial with elliptic, oblong, linear, or inversely lance-shaped, dark green leaves, 1–4cm (½–1½in) long. Dense cymes of up to 17 star-shaped, deep golden yellow flowers, to 3cm (1¼in) across, are borne in summer. ↕30cm (12in), ↔ to 30cm (12in). Turkey, Georgia, Azerbaijan. ❄❄❄
H. pallens, syn. *H. cuneatum.* Dwarf, evergreen shrub with stalkless, elliptic, oblong, inversely lance-shaped, or obovate, mid-green leaves, to 2.5cm (1in) long, borne on brittle, branching, red-tinted stems. Cymes of up to 3 star-shaped, pale yellow flowers, 1.5–2.5cm (½–1in) across, open from red-tipped buds in summer. Excellent for a rock garden or alpine house; requires good drainage. ↕15cm (6in), ↔ to 20cm (8in). S. Turkey, W. Syria. ❄❄❄ (borderline)
H. patulum. Bushy, evergreen or semi-evergreen shrub with spreading branches and lance-shaped to oblong-lance-shaped or oblong-ovate, dark green leaves, to 6cm (2½in) long. Cymes of up to 15 cup-shaped, golden yellow flowers, to 4cm (1½in) across, are borne from summer to early autumn. ↕1.2m (4ft), ↔ 1.5m (5ft). China (Guizhou, Sichuan). ❄❄. **var. *forrestii*** see *H. forrestii.* **var. *grandiflorum*** see *H. kouytchense.* **var. *henryi* of gardens** see *H. pseudohenryi.*
H. perforatum (Perforate St. John's wort). Tufted perennial with stiff, 2-ridged stems bearing opposite, ovate to elliptic-oblong or linear, mid-green leaves, 3cm (1¼in) long, with large, translucent dots. Numerous star-shaped, bright yellow flowers, to 1.5cm (½in) across, are borne in cylindrical cymes in summer. Ideal for a wildflower garden. ↕60–110cm (24–42in), ↔ to 60cm (24in). Europe, W. Asia. ❄❄❄
H. pseudohenryi, syn. *H. patulum* var. *henryi* of gardens. Bushy, semi-evergreen shrub with erect shoots and ovate-oblong to lance-shaped, dark green leaves, to 8cm (3in) long. In summer, bears cymes of up to 7, sometimes up to 25, shallowly cup-shaped to star-shaped, golden yellow flowers, to 6cm (2½in) across, followed by conical, red-tinged green fruit. ↕1.7m (5½ft), ↔ 2m (6ft). China (Yunnan, Sichuan). ❄❄❄
H. reptans ■ Deciduous, prostrate, mat-forming shrub with rooting stems and elliptic, leathery, mid-green leaves, 0.7–2cm (¼–¾in) long, turning red or yellow in autumn. Solitary, deeply cup-shaped, golden yellow flowers, to 3cm (1¼in) across, often crimson-flushed in bud, are borne in summer. Excellent for a sunny wall or rock garden. ↕5cm (2in), ↔ to 20cm (8in). Himalayas (Nepal to Yunnan). ❄❄❄
H. rhodoppeum see *H. cerastioides.*
***H.* 'Rowallane'** 𝕐 Semi-evergreen shrub with upright, arching branches and oblong-ovate to oblong-lance-shaped, dark green leaves, to 7cm (3in) long. Cymes of up to 3 shallowly cupped, dark golden yellow flowers, to 8cm (3in) across, are borne from late summer to autumn. ↕to 1.8m (6ft), ↔ to 1m (3ft). ❄❄
***H.* 'Sungold'** see *H. kouytchense.*
H. trichocaulon. Deciduous subshrub or herbaceous perennial with prostrate branches and ovate-oblong to elliptic or linear, pale grey-green leaves, to 1.5cm (½in) long. In summer, red-tinged buds open to 2 or 3 star-shaped, golden yellow flowers, to 2.5cm (1in) across, borne singly or in cymes. Suitable for an alpine house. ↕10cm (4in), ↔ to 20cm (8in). Greece (Crete). ❄❄❄ (borderline)
***H.* 'Variegatum'** see *H.* x *moserianum* 'Tricolor'.

▷ **Hypericum, Marsh** see *Hypericum elodes*

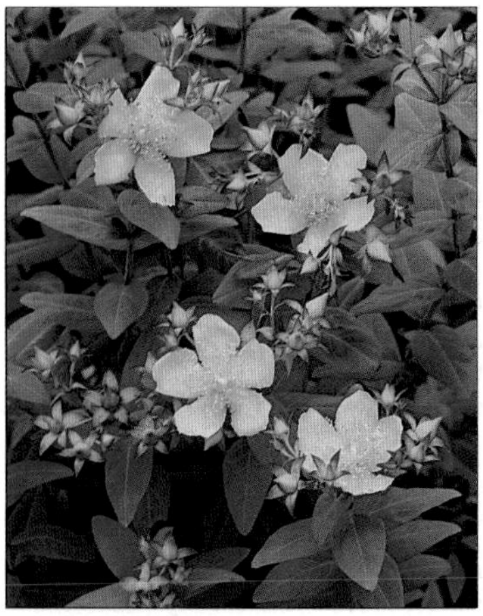

Hypericum lancasteri

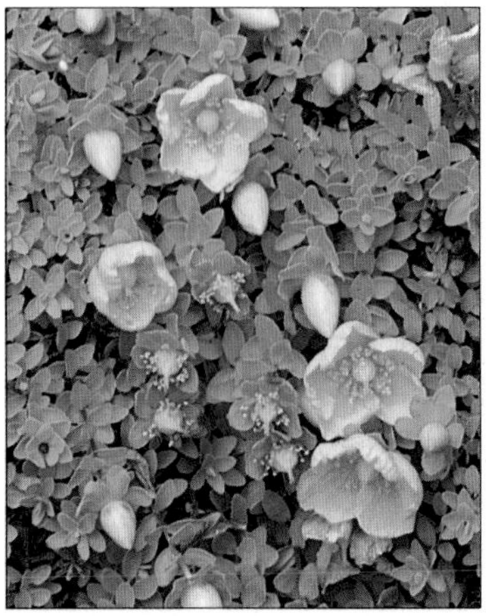

Hypericum reptans

HYPHAENE

Doum palm

ARECACEAE/PALMAE

Genus of about 10 species of palms from Africa, Madagascar, the Arabian Peninsula, India, and Sri Lanka, occurring on poor or exhausted soils, often poorly drained, usually in hot, dry areas. Some doum palms are stemless, some have creeping stems; others are tree-like with branching trunks. The leaves are fan-shaped, and tiny, bowl-shaped, 3-petalled flowers are borne in panicles between them. In frost-prone climates, grow doum palms in a warm greenhouse (they require very dry heat to thrive under glass). In dry, frost-free regions, grow the creeping and stemless species as ground cover and the tree-like ones as specimen trees.

- **HARDINESS** Frost tender.
- **CULTIVATION** Under glass, grow in loam-based potting compost (JI No.2) with additional grit, in full light. Provide low humidity. Water sparingly at all times. Apply a balanced liquid fertilizer every 6–8 weeks, when in growth. Outdoors, grow in poor to moderately fertile, sharply drained soil in full sun. Protect from winter and summer wet.
- **PROPAGATION** Sow seed at 19–24°C (66–75°F) in spring; seed may be difficult to germinate.
- **PESTS AND DISEASES** Red spider mites may be a problem under glass.

H. coriacea 🌴 (Doum palm). Small palm with a single stem, or sometimes suckering to form a clump. Each stem forks several times to form a head of branches all on one plane. Long-stalked, waxy, fan-shaped leaves have many fan-shaped blades, 30–80cm (12–32in) long, grey- to blue-green with scale-like black hairs. Tiny, bowl-shaped, green to white flowers are borne in panicles, to 1m (3ft) long, mainly in summer. ↕to 5m (15ft), ↔ 1.2–4m (4–12ft). E. Africa, South Africa, Madagascar. ❀ (min. 13–15°C/55–59°F)
H. thebaica ■🌴 (Gingerbread palm). Medium-sized palm with a single stem that forks at regular intervals. The fan-shaped, grey-green leaves have long, spiny stalks and numerous rounded leaf-blades, 60–75cm (24–30in) long. Tiny, bowl-shaped yellow flowers are borne in panicles, to 1m (3ft) long, usually in summer. ↕6–10m (20–30ft), ↔ 3–6m (10–20ft). N. Africa. ❀ (min. 13–15°C/55–59°F)

HYPOCALYMMA

MYRTACEAE

Genus, related to *Leptospermum*, of 13 species of evergreen shrubs found on sandy or gravelly soils from sea level to 900m (3,000ft) in Australia. They have opposite, simple, linear to broadly ovate, grey-green to light or dark green leaves, with entire or fringed margins. Cup-shaped, 5-petalled, many-stamened flowers are produced singly, in pairs, or occasionally in small clusters from the leaf axils. Where temperatures fall below 7°C (45°F), grow in a cool greenhouse. In warmer regions, grow at the base of a warm, sunny wall, in a shrub border, in a courtyard garden, or as a hedge.

- **HARDINESS** Half hardy to frost tender.
- **CULTIVATION** Under glass, grow in loam-based potting compost (JI No.2) with additional sharp sand, in full light or bright filtered light; provide low humidity. When in growth, water freely and apply a balanced liquid fertilizer monthly; keep just moist in winter. Outdoors, grow in moderately fertile, moist but well-drained, light, sandy, neutral to slightly alkaline soil in full sun or dappled shade. Pruning group 8; plants grown under glass may need restrictive pruning.
- **PROPAGATION** Surface-sow seed on to permanently moist seed compost at 16–18°C (61–64°F) in spring. Root semi-ripe cuttings with bottom heat in late summer.

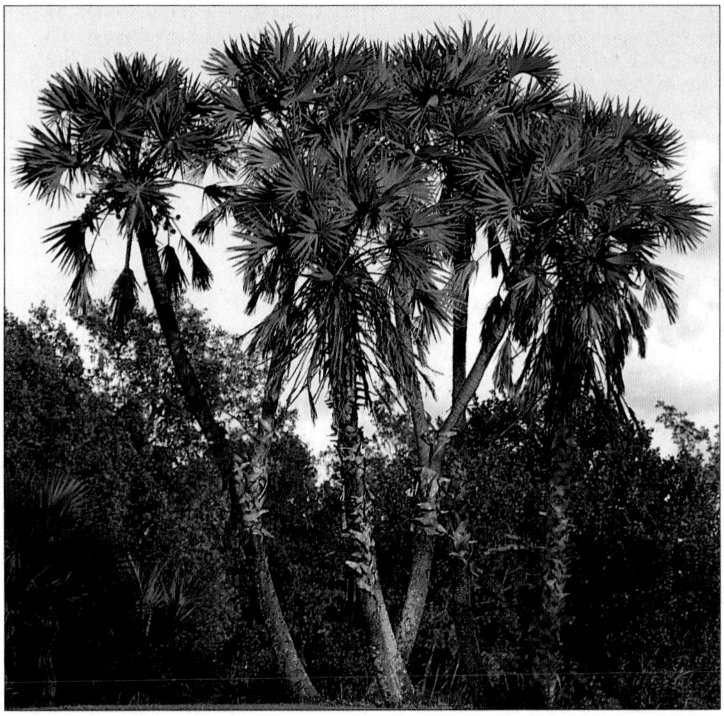

Hyphaene thebaica

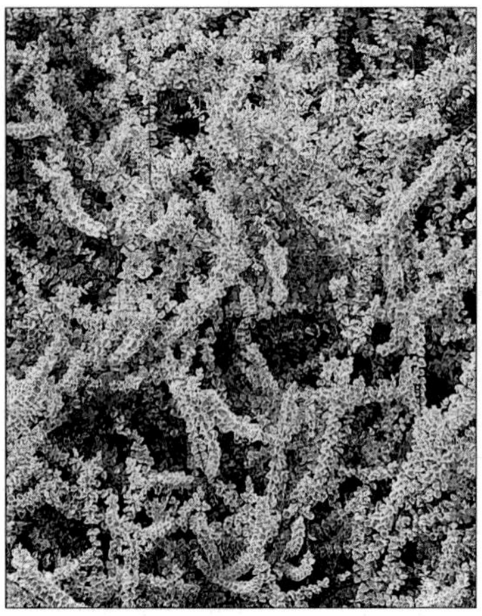

Hypocalymma cordifolium 'Golden Veil'

• **PESTS AND DISEASES** Prone to grey mould (*Botrytis*) under glass, and to *Phytophthora* root rot outdoors.

***H. cordifolium* 'Golden Veil'** ▣ Dwarf to small shrub with branching, 4-angled or 4-winged stems, often bunched or twisted together. Broadly ovate, bright green, cream-variegated leaves, to 1.5cm (½in) long, have heart-shaped bases and recurved, wavy, fringed margins. From early spring to midsummer, white flowers, to 1cm (½in) across, are borne singly or in twos or threes from the leaf axils. ↕0.3–1.5m (1–5ft), ↔ 0.3–2.5m (1–8ft). Australia (Western Australia). ✻

▷ ***Hypocyrta radicans*** see *Nematanthus gregarius*
▷ ***Hypocyrta strigillosa*** see *Nematanthus strigillosus*

HYPOESTES

Polka dot plant

ACANTHACEAE

Genus of 40 species of woody-based, evergreen perennials, subshrubs, and shrubs from open woodland in South Africa, Madagascar, and S.E. Asia. Some polka dot plants are grown for their foliage and some for their flowers. The leaves are opposite, usually ovate, entire or toothed, and smooth or slightly velvety. Terminal or lateral racemes of solitary or clustered, tubular, 2-lipped flowers, with twisted corolla tubes, are borne from late summer to winter. In frost-prone areas, grow in a warm greenhouse. *H. phyllostachya* and its cultivars are good houseplants; they may also be grown as annuals and used as bedding or in patio containers. In warmer regions, grow in a shrub border or in containers.
• **HARDINESS** Frost tender.
• **CULTIVATION** Under glass, grow in loam-based potting compost (JI No.2) in bright filtered light, with moderate to high humidity. Water freely in growth, sparingly in winter. Apply a balanced liquid fertilizer every 2–3 weeks in summer. Outdoors, grow in moist but well-drained, moderately fertile, humus-rich soil in partial shade, sheltered from cold winds. Pinch out the growing tips to promote a bushy habit.
• **PROPAGATION** Sow seed at 15–18°C (59–64°F) in spring. Root softwood or tip cuttings in late spring, or semi-ripe cuttings in summer.
• **PESTS AND DISEASES** Powdery mildew may be a problem.

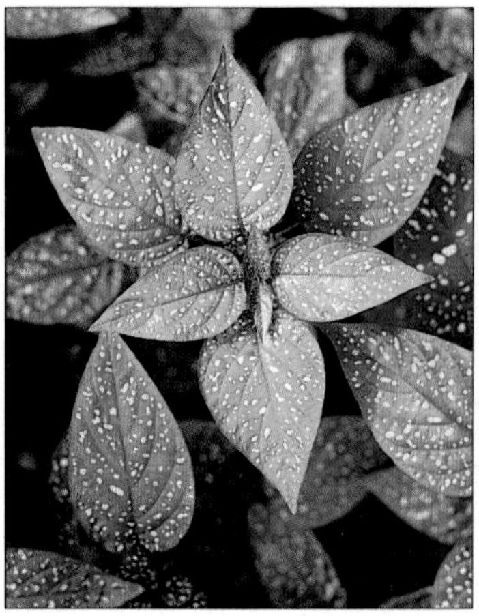

Hypoestes phyllostachya

H. aristata (Ribbon bush). Erect, evergreen, woody-based perennial with ovate, entire, dull mid-green leaves, to 8cm (3in) long, with velvety surfaces. Racemes of pale magenta to purple flowers, 3cm (1¼in) long, sometimes spotted or lined with white or mauve within, are produced from the leaf axils over a long period from summer to winter. ↕1.2m (4ft), ↔ 45cm (18in). South Africa. ⊛ (min. 13°C/55°F)
H. phyllostachya ▣ ♀ syn. *H. sanguinolenta* of gardens (Freckle face, Polka dot plant). Subshrub with ovate, downy, dark green leaves, 5cm (2in) long, spotted with reddish or bluish pink. From late summer to winter, bears terminal, spike-like racemes, 16cm (6in) long, of tiny, magenta to lilac flowers. ↕30cm (12in), ↔ 23cm (9in). Madagascar. ⊛ (min. 10°C/50°F). **'Carmina'** has bright red foliage. **'Purpuriana'** has purple leaves. **'Splash'** has showy leaves splashed with pink.
***H. sanguinolenta* of gardens** see *H. phyllostachya.*

HYPOXIS

Starflower

HYPOXIDACEAE

Genus of about 150 species of cormous perennials widespread in woodland in Africa, S.E. Asia, Australia, and North, Central, and South America. Species in cultivation have linear to lance-shaped, light to mid-green, basal leaves, and bear small, star-shaped flowers from spring to summer. In frost-prone areas, grow in an alpine house or cool greenhouse. In warmer climates, grow in a sheltered rock garden.
• **HARDINESS** Frost hardy to frost tender.
• **CULTIVATION** Plant corms 3cm (1¼in) deep when dormant. Under glass, grow in loam-based potting compost (JI No.2) with added sharp sand and leaf mould; move from a shaded position at planting to full light or bright filtered light as shoots appear. When in growth, water moderately and apply a balanced liquid fertilizer monthly; dry off after flowering and keep dry in winter. Outdoors, grow in humus-rich, moist but well-drained soil in full sun with midday shade, or in dappled shade. Protect from excessive winter and summer wet, and shelter from cold, drying winds. Starflowers resent transplanting once established.
• **PROPAGATION** Sow seed at 13–16°C (55–61°F) in spring. Remove offsets in summer or autumn.

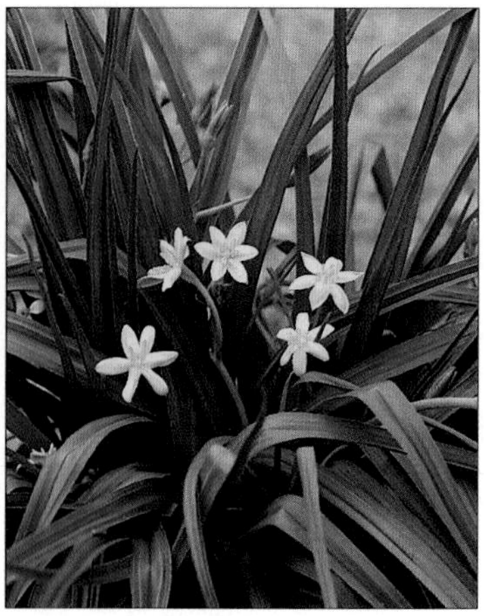

Hypoxis angustifolia

• **PESTS AND DISEASES** Mice may damage clumps outdoors during winter.

H. angustifolia ▣ Small, cormous perennial with erect, grass-like, linear to lance-shaped, hairy, mid-green, basal leaves, 10–15cm (4–6in) long. In summer, bears stems of up to 7 upward-facing yellow flowers, to 1cm (½in) across. ↕10–20cm (4–8in), ↔ 5cm (2in). Widespread in South Africa. ✻
H. capensis, syn. *H. stellata, Spiloxene capensis.* Cormous perennial with erect, narrowly linear, finely toothed, folded, mid-green, basal leaves, 10–30cm (4–12in) long. In spring, bears solitary, upward-facing, white or yellow flowers, 2–6cm (¾–2½in) across, with bright purple or green basal spots. ↕10–20cm (4–8in), ↔ 5cm (2in). South Africa (Western Cape, Northern Cape, Eastern Cape). ✻
H. hemerocallidea, syn. *H. rooperi.* Cormous perennial with arching, lance-shaped, hairy, mid-green, basal leaves 30–45cm (12–18in) long. Branched stems of up to 8 yellow, green-backed flowers, 3–4cm (1¼–1½in) across, are produced from spring to summer. ↕15–20cm (6–8in), ↔ 5cm (2in). Widespread in South Africa. ✻
H. hirsuta. Cormous perennial with semi-erect, narrowly linear, ribbed, hairy, mid-green, basal leaves, to 30cm (12in) long. From spring to summer, bears stems of up to 7 upward-facing, yellow, green-backed flowers, to 2.5cm (1in) across. ↕10–20cm (4–8in), ↔ 5cm (2in). E. North America. ✻✻
H. rooperi see *H. hemerocallidea.*
H. stellata see *H. capensis.*

HYPSELA

CAMPANULACEAE

Genus of 4 species of prostrate perennials found in moist sites at mid- to high altitudes in Australia, New Zealand, and South America. They are cultivated for their alternate, variably shaped, entire or toothed, mid- to dark green leaves, and their tubular, 5-lobed flowers. They are suitable for a large rock garden, but are too invasive for a small area.
• **HARDINESS** Fully hardy to frost hardy.
• **CULTIVATION** Grow in gritty, humus-rich, moist but well-drained soil in sun or shade. Hypselas spread freely in moist soils and warm conditions.
• **PROPAGATION** Sow seed at 6–12°C (43–54°F), or divide, in spring.
• **PESTS AND DISEASES** Slugs and snails may be a problem.

H. longiflora see *H. reniformis.*
H. reniformis, syn. *H. longiflora.* Vigorous, creeping perennial with rooting stems and elliptic or rounded to kidney-shaped, fleshy, bright mid-green leaves, to 1cm (½in) long. Solitary, almost stemless, white to pale pink flowers, to 8mm (⅜in) long, with crimson veins, open from late spring to summer. ↕2cm (¾in), ↔ indefinite. South America. ✻✻✻ (borderline)

▷ **Hyssop** see *Hyssopus, H. officinalis*
Anise see *Agastache foeniculum*

HYSSOPUS

Hyssop

LABIATAE/LAMIACEAE

Genus of about 5 often variable species of aromatic herbaceous perennials and evergreen or semi-evergreen shrubs, occurring in dry, sandy, and rocky sites from the Mediterranean to C. Asia. The linear to lance-shaped, ovate, or oblong leaves are mid- or blue-green. Tubular, violet-blue to pink flowers are borne in whorls on narrow, spike-like, terminal inflorescences. *H. officinalis* and its cultivars are grown for their aromatic foliage and flowers, and are excellent for a rock garden or herb garden. They are also suitable for low hedging, and for growing at the base of a warm, sunny wall or in containers. The flowers are attractive to bees and butterflies; the foliage has culinary and medicinal uses.
• **HARDINESS** Fully hardy.
• **CULTIVATION** Grow in fertile, well-drained, neutral to alkaline soil in full sun. Pruning group 10, in mid-spring.
• **PROPAGATION** Sow seed in containers in a cold frame in autumn. Root softwood cuttings in summer.
• **PESTS AND DISEASES** Trouble free.

H. officinalis ▣ (Hyssop). Dwarf, semi-evergreen, aromatic shrub with erect shoots and linear to narrowly lance-shaped, or oblong, mid-green leaves, to 5cm (2in) long. Slender spikes of whorled, funnel-shaped, 2-lipped, dark blue flowers, 1.5cm (½in) long, are produced from midsummer to early autumn. ↕60cm (24in), ↔ 1m (3ft). S. Europe. ✻✻✻. **f. *albus*** has white flowers. **subsp. *aristatus*** has a dense, upright habit, and produces bright green leaves. **f. *roseus*** has pink flowers.

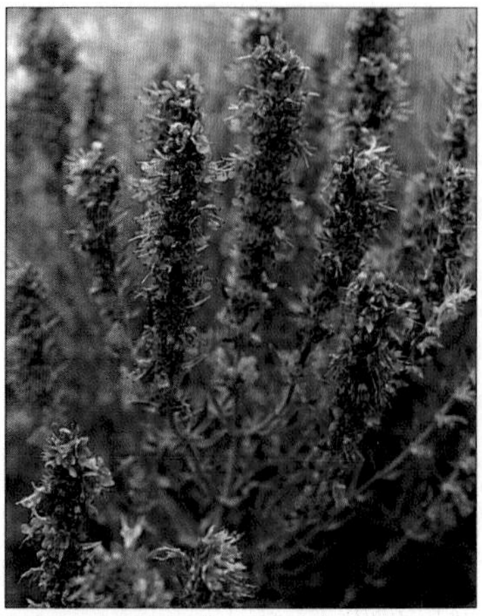

Hyssopus officinalis

I

IBERIS

Candytuft

BRASSICACEAE/CRUCIFERAE

Genus of about 40 species of annuals, perennials, and evergreen subshrubs from open sites in free-draining, calcareous soil in Crimea, S. Europe, N. Africa, Cyprus, Syria, N. Iraq, Turkey, and Caucasus. They have alternate, linear to obovate, entire to pinnatisect leaves. The inflorescences are corymbs or racemes of sometimes fragrant, white, occasionally purple, pink, or red flowers, 1cm (½in) across, each with 4 petals, one pair usually larger than the other. Grow perennials and subshrubs, which may be short-lived, in a rock garden or in walls. Grow annual candytufts, which flower profusely over long periods, mainly in summer, as bedding, at the front of borders, or in containers.

• **HARDINESS** Fully hardy to frost hardy.
• **CULTIVATION** Grow in poor to moderately fertile, moist but well-drained, neutral to alkaline soil in full sun. *I. pruitii* requires sharply drained soil. Pruning group 10, after flowering. Trim perennials and subshrubs lightly after flowering to maintain compactness.
• **PROPAGATION** Sow seed of annuals *in situ* in spring or autumn. Sow seed of perennials and subshrubs in containers in a cold frame in autumn. Root softwood cuttings in late spring or semi-ripe cuttings in summer.
• **PESTS AND DISEASES** Susceptible to clubroot. May be attacked by slugs and snails and occasionally by caterpillars.

I. amara. Variable, erect, branched annual with lance-shaped to spoon-shaped leaves, to 8cm (3in) long, toothed towards the tips. Small, lightly scented, purplish white or white flowers are borne in large, domed racemes, 10–15cm (4–6in) long, in summer. ↕15–45cm (6–18in), ↔ to 15cm (6in). W. Europe. ✻✻✻. **'Giant Hyacinth-flowered'** bears large racemes of white flowers. **'Iceberg'** ■ produces pure white flowers. **'Pinnacle'** has very fragrant, pure white flowers.

I. candolleana see *I. pruitii.*

I. commutata see *I. sempervirens.*

I. jordanii see *I. pruitii.*

I. pruitii, syn. *I. candolleana*, *I. jordanii.* Short-lived, evergreen, procumbent to erect annual or perennial with rosettes of spoon-shaped, fleshy, dark green leaves, to 2cm (¾in) long. In summer, bears dense corymbs, to 4cm (1½in) across, of white, occasionally lilac flowers. ↕ to 15cm (6in), ↔ to 20cm (8in). Spain, France, Italy, Greece. ✻✻

I. saxatilis ■ Evergreen subshrub with linear, almost cylindrical, fleshy, dark green leaves, to 2cm (¾in) long, on upright stems. From late spring to summer, bears flattened corymbs, 3–4cm (1¼–1½in) across, of small white flowers, often purple-tinged with age. Leaves on flowering shoots are flat, linear, and acute. ↕ to 15cm (6in), ↔ to 30cm (12in). Spain, France, Italy, Greece, Romania, Crimea. ✻✻✻

I. semperflorens. Evergreen subshrub with broadly spoon-shaped, slightly fleshy, dark green leaves, 2–6cm (¾–2½in) long. Produces fragrant white flowers borne in crowded corymbs, to 5cm (2in) across, from winter to early spring. ↕ to 30cm (12in), ↔ 60cm (24in) or more. S. Italy (including Sicily). ✻✻

I. sempervirens ■ syn. *I. commutata.* Spreading, evergreen subshrub with oblong-spoon-shaped, dark green leaves, 2.5–3.5cm (1–1½in) long. In late spring and early summer, bears corymb-like racemes, to 5cm (2in) across, of small white flowers, occasionally flushed lilac. ↕ to 30cm (12in), ↔ to 40cm (16in). S. Europe. ✻✻✻. **'Little Gem'** see 'Weisser Zwerg'. **'Schneeflocke'** ♀ syn. 'Snowflake', is mound-forming, and bears dense, corymb-like racemes of snow-white flowers; ↕ to 25cm (10cm), ↔ to 60cm (24in). **'Snowflake'** see 'Schneeflocke'. **'Weisser Zwerg'**, syn. 'Little Gem', is very compact, with short, linear leaves, to 1cm (½in) long. Bears abundant white flowers in spring; ↕15cm (6in), ↔ to 25cm (10in).

I. umbellata (Common candytuft). Bushy, mound-forming annual with linear-lance-shaped leaves, to 10cm (4in) long, the lower leaves toothed. The abundant small, scented flowers are white, lavender, purple, pink, crimson, or occasionally bicoloured, and are borne in flattened corymbs, to 5cm (2in) across, from spring to summer; ↕15–30cm (6–12in), ↔ to 23cm (9in). S. Europe. ✻✻✻. **Fairy Series** ■ cultivars have white, pink, lilac-purple, or red-pink flowers. **Flash Series** cultivars have vibrant pink, purple, or carmine-red flowers.

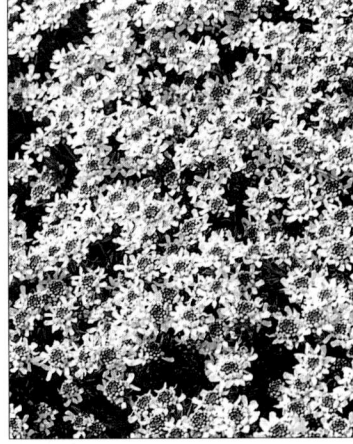

Iberis saxatilis

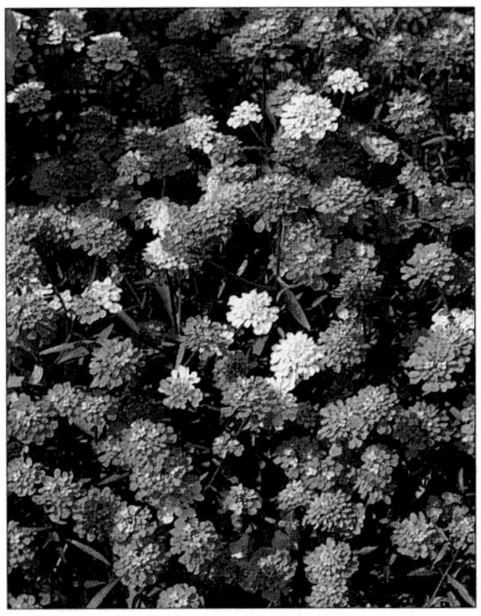

Iberis umbellata Fairy Series

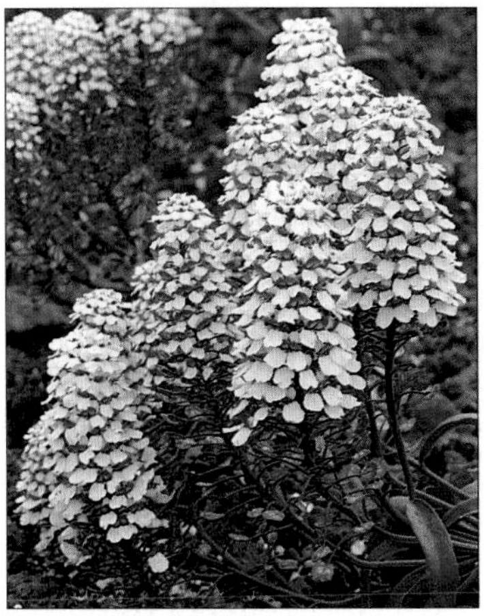

Iberis amara 'Iceberg'

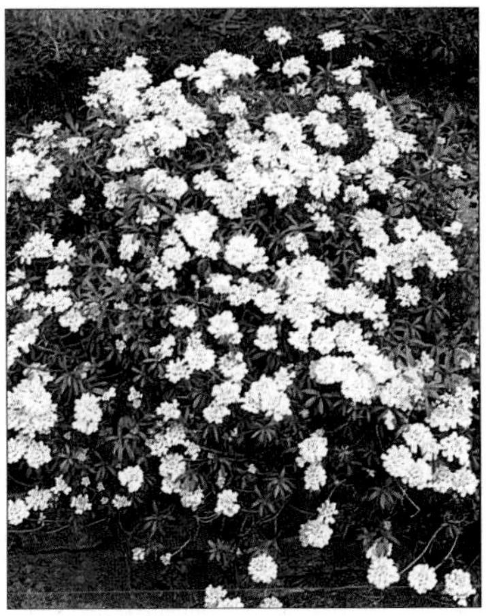

Iberis sempervirens

IBERVILLEA

CUCURBITACEAE

Genus of 3 or 4 species of climbing, perennial, dioecious succulents from semi-desert regions of Texas and Arizona, USA, and N. Mexico. They have swollen, caudex-like stems that are partly underground, and very slender branches bearing ovate to kidney-shaped, deeply 3- to 5-lobed leaves with simple tendrils. In summer, bell-shaped, usually hairy flowers, with pointed lobes, are borne in racemes or clusters on male plants, or singly on female plants. Where temperatures drop below 10°C (50°F), grow in a warm greenhouse. In warmer climates, grow in a desert garden, or on a trellis in a dry, sunny position.

• **HARDINESS** Frost tender.
• **CULTIVATION** Under glass, grow in loam-based potting compost (JI No.2), with added sharp sand or grit, in full light with low humidity. During the growing season, water moderately and apply a balanced liquid fertilizer monthly. Keep totally dry at other times. Outdoors, grow in moderately fertile, sharply drained soil in full sun, and mulch with a layer of limestone chippings, 5cm (2in) deep. Protect from excessive winter wet. See also pp.48–49.
• **PROPAGATION** Sow seed at 20°C (68°F) in early spring. Root softwood cuttings in late spring and early summer with gentle bottom heat.
• **PESTS AND DISEASES** Vulnerable to scale insects.

I. sonorae. Climbing, free-branching succulent with a bottle-shaped caudex and fissured, corky, greyish white bark. Produces bluish green tendrils and fan-shaped, deeply 3-lobed, bluish green leaves, 4–12cm (1½–5in) long, often with rough hairs beneath. Small, hairy, greenish yellow flowers, 1cm (½in) across, are borne in summer. ↕2–3m (6–10ft), ↔ 30cm (12in). N. Mexico. ❀ (min. 10°C/50°F)

▷**Ice plant** see *Dorotheanthus, Sedum spectabile*

IDESIA

FLACOURTIACEAE

Genus of one species of deciduous tree from woodland in China, Korea, Japan, and Taiwan. Leaves are alternate and slightly toothed. Male and female flowers are borne on separate plants; both are needed to produce fruit. Grown for its bold foliage and clusters of red berries, it is a fine specimen tree, or is suitable for a woodland garden.

• **HARDINESS** Fully hardy.
• **CULTIVATION** Grow in moderately fertile, moist but well-drained, neutral to acid soil in full sun or light shade, with shelter from other trees. Pruning group 1.
• **PROPAGATION** Sow seed in containers in a cold frame in autumn. Root greenwood cuttings in late spring or semi-ripe cuttings in midsummer.
• **PESTS AND DISEASES** Trouble free.

I. polycarpa ■ ♀ Spreading, deciduous tree with open, tiered branches and ovate-heart-shaped, sharply pointed, glossy, mid- to dark green leaves, to 20cm (8in) long, often purple-tinged when young. Large, pendulous panicles, to 30cm (12in) long, of small, fragrant, yellow-green flowers, lacking petals, are borne in midsummer, followed by spherical red berries on female plants. ↕↔ 12m (40ft). China (Sichuan), Korea, Japan, Taiwan. ✻✻✻

▷***Idria columnaris*** see *Fouquieria columnaris*

▷**Ilang-ilang** see *Cananga odorata*

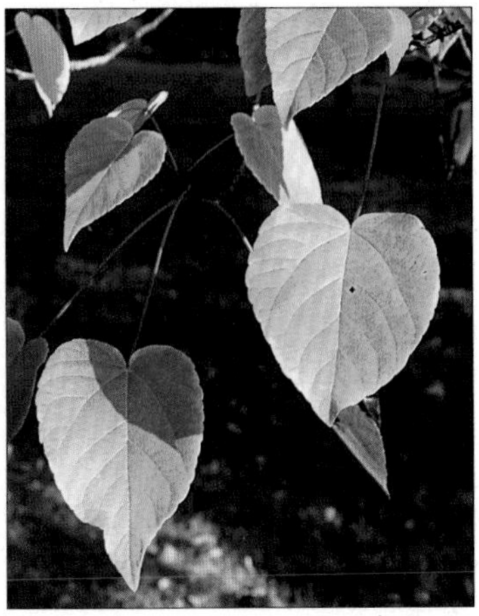

Idesia polycarpa

I

ILEX

Holly

AQUIFOLIACEAE

Genus of over 400 species of evergreen and deciduous trees, shrubs, and climbers from woodland in tropical, subtropical, and temperate regions, grown for their foliage and berries. The leaves may have entire, spine-toothed, spiny, or rarely scalloped margins, and are usually simple and alternate, sometimes in opposite pairs. Flowers, borne from spring to early summer, are produced singly or in clusters or cymes in the leaf axils. They are small, cup-shaped, up to 8mm (3/8in) across, each with 3–8 petals, usually white or cream, but may be pink, green, or lavender-blue. Male and female flowers are usually borne on separate plants; both sexes are needed to obtain fruits. In temperate climates, hollies bear fruits in autumn. The red or black, occasionally white, orange, or yellow berries are spherical, sometimes ellipsoid, and may cause mild stomach upset if ingested.

Grow hollies in a woodland garden or as specimen trees; some make good hedges or windbreaks, particularly *I. aquifolium* and *I.* x *altaclerensis* cultivars; several *I. crenata* cultivars are useful in a rock garden. In cold areas, grow frost-tender species in a cool greenhouse.

I

- **HARDINESS** Fully hardy to frost tender.
- **CULTIVATION** Grow in moist but well-drained, moderately fertile, humus-rich soil in full sun (which produces the best leaf colour in variegated hollies) or in partial shade. Planting or transplanting is best done in late winter or early spring. Pruning group 1. Prune free-standing specimens to shape in the early years only; clip formally grown plants in summer; trim hedges in early spring.
- **PROPAGATION** Sow seed in containers in a cold frame in autumn. Germination may take 2 or 3 years. Take semi-ripe cuttings in late summer or early autumn.

ILEX LEAVES

Most holly leaves are simple and alternate, with spine-toothed, spiny, or entire margins.

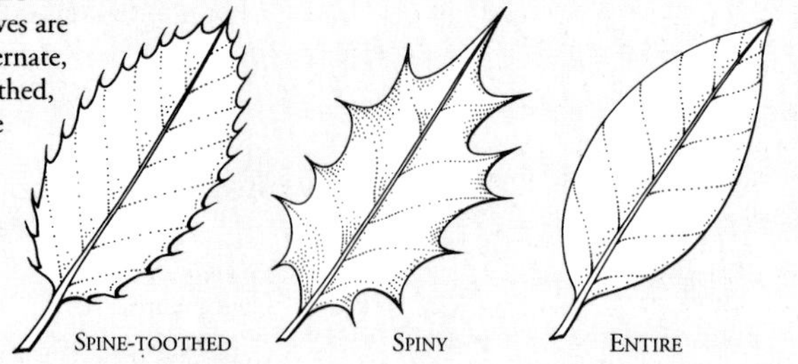

- **PESTS AND DISEASES** Young shoots are susceptible to aphids; scale insects and leaf miners may be a problem on evergreen species. Sometimes suffers from *Phytophthora* root rot.

***I.* 'Accent'** ◊ Narrowly conical, evergreen male tree, spindly when mature, with brittle branches. Bears elliptic, dark green leaves, 2–4cm (3/4–1½in) long. Sometimes short-lived. Pollinating male for *I.* 'Elegance'. ↕ 6m (20ft), ↔ 3m (10ft). ❄❄

I. altaclarensis see *I.* x *altaclerensis.*

I.* x *altaclerensis ⌂ (*I. aquifolium* x *I. perado*) syn. *I. altaclarensis.* Vigorous, evergreen tree or shrub of variable habit, with grey bark. Leaves are elliptic, elliptic-lance-shaped or broadly ovate, glossy, dark green, 6–13cm (2½–5in) long, with spine-toothed or entire margins. Berries are red, 6–8mm (¼–3/8in) across. Similar to *I. aquifolium* but more vigorous, and usually with less spiny, broader, larger leaves. Tolerates pollution and coastal exposure. Excellent for tall hedges and windbreaks. ↕ to 20m (70ft), ↔ 12–15m (40–50ft). Garden origin. ❄❄. **'Belgica Aurea'** ■ ♀ ◯ syn. 'Silver Sentinel', *I. perado* 'Aurea'. An erect female shrub with yellow-streaked green stems, bearing elliptic-lance-shaped, sparsely spine-toothed leaves, to 11cm (4½in) long, mottled grey-green in the centre and with irregular, golden yellow margins. Produces few berries. ↕ 12m (40ft), ↔ 5m (15ft). **'Camelliifolia'** ■ ♀ ◊ is a large, conical female shrub with purple-tinged stems, elliptic-oblong, usually entire, deep green leaves, to 13cm (5in) long, and scarlet berries. ↕ 14m (46ft). **'Golden King'** ■ ♀ is a compact female shrub, a sport of 'Hendersonii', with oblong to ovate, spine-toothed or entire leaves, to 10cm (4in) long, mottled grey-green in the centre, with broad, bright gold margins. Reddish brown berries, ripening to red, are sparsely produced. ↕ 6m (20ft). **'Hendersonii'** ◯ is a compact female tree with oblong-elliptic, dull green leaves, to 11cm (4½in) long. Long-lasting, brown-red berries, ripening to red, are sparsely produced. ↕ to 15m (50ft), ↔ to 4m (12ft). **'Hodginsii'** ♀ ◯ is a magnificent, robust male tree bearing dark purple stems and broadly ovate, glossy, black-green leaves, 5–8cm (2–3in) long, spine-toothed when young. ↕ 14m (46ft), ↔ 10m (30ft). **'Lawsoniana'** ■ ♀ ◯ is a compact female shrub, a sport of 'Hendersonii'. Yellow-streaked green stems bear oblong to ovate leaves, to 11cm (4½in) long, irregularly splashed gold and light green in the centres. Bears reddish brown berries, ripening to red. ↕ to 6m (20ft). **'Silver Sentinel'** see 'Belgica Aurea'. **'Wilsonii'** ♀ ◊ is a vigorous, dense, oblong female tree, well-furnished to the base with purple-green branches. Bears broadly ovate, glossy, bright green, spiny leaves, to 10cm (4in) long, with prominent veins. Large scarlet fruit are produced in abundance. ↕ 8m (25ft).

I. aquifolium ■ ♀ ◊–◯ (Common holly, English holly). Usually erect, dense, pyramidal or oblong, evergreen shrub or tree with grey bark. Bears elliptic or ovate, glossy, dark green leaves, 5–10cm (2–4in) long, with entire, wavy, spine-toothed or spiny margins, and long-lasting, red or rarely yellow or orange berries, 4–6mm (1/8–¼in) across. ↕ to 25m (80ft), ↔ 8m (25ft). W. and S. Europe, North Africa, W. Asia. ❄❄. **'Amber'** ■ is a female tree with mid-green stems. Bears elliptic, usually entire, bright green leaves, to 8cm (3in) long, and abundant amber-yellow fruit. ↕ to 6m (20ft), ↔ 2.5m (8ft). **'Argentea Marginata'** ♀ syn. 'Argentea Variegata', is a columnar female tree with cream-streaked green stems and large, broadly ovate, spiny leaves, to 7cm (3in) long, with wide white margins. Leaves are purplish pink when young. Bears abundant bright red berries. ↕ to 15m (50ft), ↔ 4m (12ft). **'Argentea Marginata Pendula'** ■ ⌂ syn. 'Argentea Pendula', is a weeping female tree with purple stems and elliptic, spiny, cream-margined leaves, to 8cm (3in) long, purple-pink when young. Sparsely produces red fruit. ↕ to 4m (12ft), ↔ 3m (10ft). **'Argentea Pendula'** see 'Argentea Marginata Pendula'. **'Argentea Variegata'** see 'Argentea Marginata'. **'Aurea Regina'** see 'Golden Queen'. **'Bacciflava'** is a female tree with ovate, spiny, dark green leaves, to 8cm (3in) long. Bears yellow berries. ↕ to 15m (50ft), ↔ 4m (12ft). **'Ferox'** (Hedgehog holly) is a large, upright male shrub with purple stems and ovate, thick, leathery leaves, 3–4cm (1¼–1½in) long, covered in spines. ↕ to 15m (50ft). **'Ferox Argentea'** ■ ♀ is a sport of 'Ferox', also male but slower-growing, with cream-margined leaves, 3–4cm (1¼–1½in) long, covered in spines. ↕ to 8m (25ft), ↔ 4m (12ft). **'Flavescens'** (Moonlight holly) is a broadly columnar female shrub with purplish red stems. Bears elliptic to ovate, spine-toothed leaves, 8cm (3in) long, yellow flushed when young, turning mid-green in shade. Yellow leaf colour lasts all year if grown in good light. Produces red berries. ↕ 6m (20ft), ↔ 3m (10ft). **'Golden Milkboy'** ■ ♀ is a dense, upright male shrub with purplish green stems. Bears elliptic, spiny leaves, 6–8cm (2½–3in) long, with irregular gold central markings. ↕ 6m (20ft), ↔ 4m (12ft). **'Golden Queen'** ♀ syn. 'Aurea Regina', is a male tree bearing cream-streaked green stems and large, broadly ovate, spine-toothed leaves, 6–8cm (2½–3in) long, broadly margined with gold. ↕ 10m (30ft), ↔ 6m (20ft). **'Golden van Tol'** ■ is a broad, upright female shrub bearing purple branches and ovate, puckered, dull green leaves, 3–7cm (1¼–3in) long, with golden yellow margins and few marginal spiny teeth. Sparsely produces red fruit. ↕ 4m (12ft), ↔ 3m (10ft). **'Handsworth New Silver'** ■ ♀ is a dense, columnar female shrub with dark purple stems bearing oblong-elliptic, mid-green, spiny leaves, 6–9cm (2½–3½in) long, with creamy margins. Produces bright red berries. ↕ 8m (25ft), ↔ 5m (15ft).

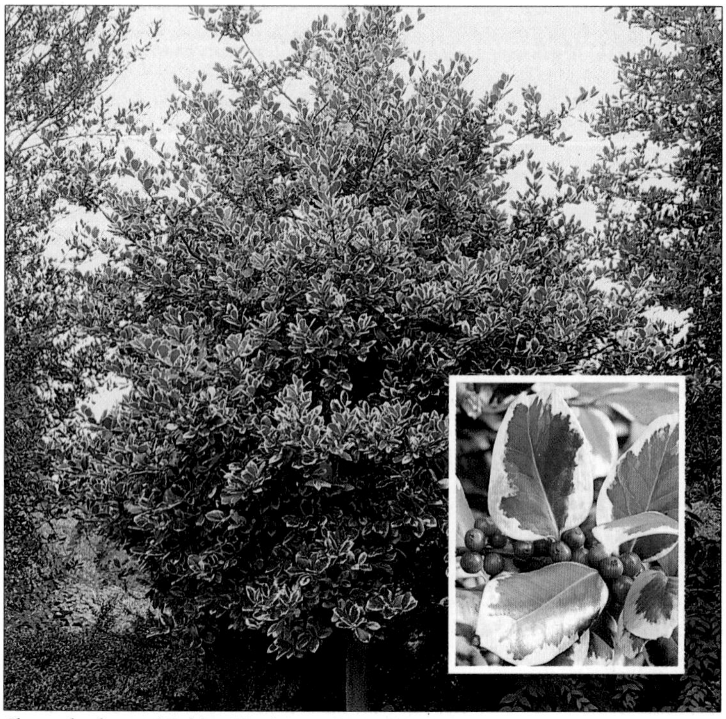

Ilex x *altaclerensis* 'Golden King' (inset: leaf and fruit detail)

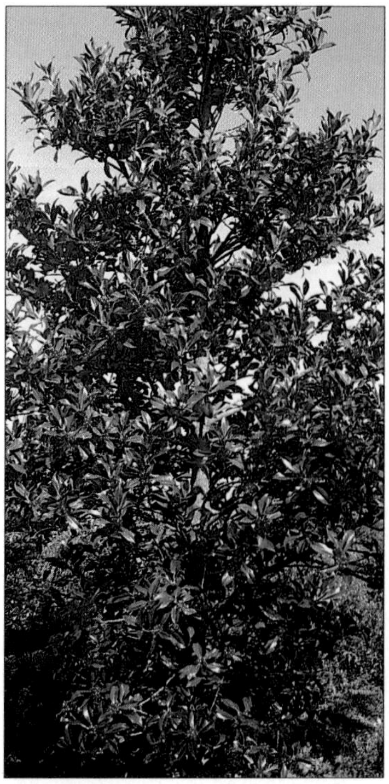

Ilex aquifolium

'J.C. van Tol' ■♀ is a broad female tree with dark purple stems and elliptic, puckered, almost entire, dark green leaves, to 8cm (3in) long. Bears abundant bright red berries. Self-fertile. ↕6m (20ft), ↔4m (12ft). ❄❄❄. **'Mme Briot'** ■♀ is a vigorous, bushy female tree or large shrub with purplish stems. Bears broadly ovate, dark green leaves, 8–10cm (3–4in) long, with spiny, bright gold margins and scarlet fruit. ↕10m (30ft), ↔5m (15ft). **'Pyramidalis'** ♀ is a narrowly conical, upright female shrub or small tree with yellow-green stems bearing narrowly elliptic, entire to few-spined, bright green leaves, 6–8cm (2½–3in) long. Produces abundant bright red berries. Self-fertile. ↕6m (20ft), ↔5m (15ft). **'Pyramidalis Aurea Marginata'** ■ is an upright female shrub or small tree bearing mid-green stems with narrowly elliptic, mid-green leaves, with few to many spines and gold margins. Produces red berries freely. ↕6m (20ft), ↔5m (15ft). ❄❄❄. **'Pyramidalis Fructu Luteo'** ■♀ is a conical female shrub or small tree bearing green stems when young, with oval, usually entire, mid-green leaves. Very freely produces yellow berries. ↕6m (20ft), ↔4m (12ft). **'Silver King'** see 'Silver Queen'. **'Silver Milkboy'** is a dense male shrub bearing greenish yellow stems and elliptic, spiny, mid-green leaves, 5–6cm (2–2½in) long, with irregular silver central markings. Shy flowering, but when it does bear fruit, produces abundant scarlet berries. ↕6m (20ft), ↔4m (12ft). **'Silver Milkmaid'** ■♀ is similar to 'Silver Milkboy', with an open habit, spreading when mature. Produces elliptic-ovate, sharply spined, dark green leaves, 3.5–5cm (1½–2in) long, with irregular, silvery white markings in the centres. Bears abundant scarlet berries. ↕6m (20ft), ↔4m (12ft). **'Silver Queen'** ■♀ syn. 'Silver King', is a dense, upright, slow-growing male tree with purple stems. Bears broadly ovate, spiny leaves, 4.5–7cm (1¾–3in) long, with broad, creamy white margins. ↕10m (30ft), ↔4m (12ft).

I.* x *aquipernyi ◊ (*I. aquifolium* x *I. pernyi*). Conical, evergreen shrub or small tree with diamond-shaped to oblong, spiny, glossy, dark green leaves, to 3.5cm (1½in) long, with long tips. Bears red fruit, 6–8mm (¼–⅜in) across. ↕6m (20ft), ↔4m (12ft). Garden origin. ❄❄❄

I.* x *attenuata (*I. cassine* x *I. opaca*) (Topel holly). Conical, evergreen shrub with obovate-lance-shaped, light green leaves, 3–8cm (1¼–3in) long, spine-toothed near the tip. Produces dark red berries, 6mm (¼in) across. ↕4m (12ft), ↔2m (6ft). Natural hybrid from S. USA. ❄❄

***I.* 'Brilliant'** ■◊ (*I. aquifolium* x *I. ciliospinosa*). Pyramidal, evergreen female shrub with oblong, spiny, bright green leaves, 3.5–4.5cm (1½–1¾in) long. Bears red fruit, 6mm (¼in) across. ↕3m (10ft), ↔2m (6ft). ❄❄

***I. chinensis* of gardens** see *I. purpurea*.

I. ciliospinosa ■◊ Upright, usually multi-stemmed, evergreen shrub bearing elliptic-ovate, dull, dark green leaves, 4–6cm (1½–2½in) long, with short, fine spines. Produces red fruit, 6mm (¼in) across. ↕6m (20ft), ↔4m (12ft). W. China. ❄❄

***I.* 'Clusterberry'** ◊ Upright, evergreen female shrub with oblong or obovate-oblong, few-spined, glossy, dark green leaves, 8–15cm (3–6in) long. Bears large red berries, 8–10mm (⅜–½in) across. ↕to 5m (15ft), ↔to 2.5m (8ft). ❄❄

I. cornuta ♀ (Horned holly). Dense, rounded, evergreen shrub with rectangular, glossy, dark green leaves 5–8cm (2–3in) long, usually with prominent spines. Bears long-lasting, large red berries, 10mm (½in) across. ↕↔2–4m (6–12ft). China, Korea. ❄❄❄. **'Burfordii'** ■ has leaves with a spine at each apex, and bears red berries very freely; ↔4–5m (12–15ft). **'Dwarf Burford'** has a dense, compact habit and produces dark red berries; ↕↔to 2.5m (8ft).

I. crenata ◊ (Box-leaved holly, Japanese holly). Evergreen, very variable shrub or small tree, usually with ovate to elliptic, minutely scalloped, glossy, dark green leaves, 2–3cm (¾–1¼in) long, often pitted beneath. Produces glossy black, sometimes white or yellow fruit, 6mm (¼in) across. ↕5m (15ft), ↔4m (12ft). Russia (Sakhalin), Japan, Korea. ❄❄❄. **'Aureovariegata'** see 'Variegata'. **'Bruns'** ◊ is a compact male shrub with greyish green leaves. ↕1m (3ft), ↔1.5m (5ft). **'Bullata'** see 'Convexa'. **'Convexa'** ■♀◊ syn. 'Bullata', is a dense, broad female shrub with purple-green stems bearing elliptic, curved, glossy, mid- to dark green leaves, 1–2cm (½–¾in) long. Produces abundant glossy black fruit. ↕to 2.5m (8ft), ↔2m (6ft). **'Fukarin'** see 'Shiro-Fukurin'. **'Golden Gem'** ♀ is a compact, low-growing, shy-flowering female shrub with golden yellow leaves, 1–2cm (½–¾in) long, turning yellow-green in summer. Bears black berries. Best grown in full sun. ↕1.1m (3½ft), ↔1.2–1.5m (4–5ft). **'Ivory Tower'** is a fast-growing, upright female shrub with late-ripening, ivory-white fruit. ↕4m (12ft), ↔3m (10ft). **f. *latifolia*** ■ syn. 'Latifolia', is a shrub or small tree with oval, minutely scalloped leaves, 2–4cm (¾–1½in) long; female plants produce black berries. ↕to 1.5m (5ft). **'Luteovariegata'** see 'Variegata'. **'Mariesii'** ■ syn. var. *nummularioides*, *I. mariesii*, is a very slow-growing, erect female shrub with tiny, broadly ovate to rounded, entire, dark green leaves, to 6mm (¼in) long. Produces black fruit. ↕60–100cm (24–36in) after many years. **var. *nummularioides*** see 'Mariesii'. **'Shiro-Fukurin'** syn. 'Fukarin', *I.* 'Snow Flake', is an upright female shrub bearing ovate, grey-green leaves with cream markings. Produces black fruit. ↕↔4m (12ft). **'Variegata'**, syn. 'Aureovariegata', 'Luteovariegata', is a shy-flowering male shrub with elliptic leaves, spotted or marked yellow. Frequently reverts to green-leaved form. ↕to 4m (12ft). **'Wiesmoor Silber'** ◊ is a female sport of 'Convexa', with elliptic, silver-margined, greyish green leaves and black berries. ↕2.5m (8ft), ↔2m (6ft).

I. decidua ◊ (Possum haw). Upright, deciduous shrub, late to come into leaf in spring. Oval or narrowly obovate, scalloped, bright green leaves, 2.5–4cm (1–1½in) long, are crowded on short lateral spurs. Bears red or orange, occasionally yellow fruit, 4–9mm (⅛–⅜in) across. ↕↔2–6m (6–20ft). C. and S.E. USA. ❄❄❄

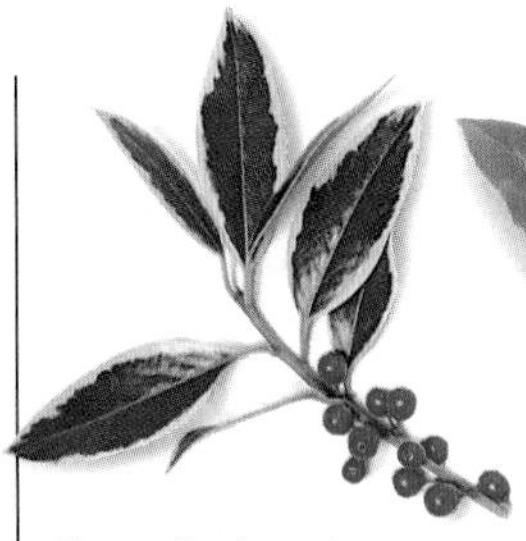
Ilex x *altaclerensis* 'Belgica Aurea'

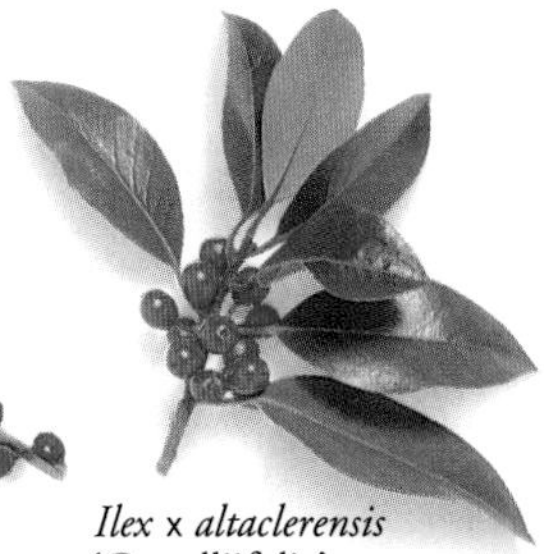
Ilex x *altaclerensis* 'Camelliifolia'

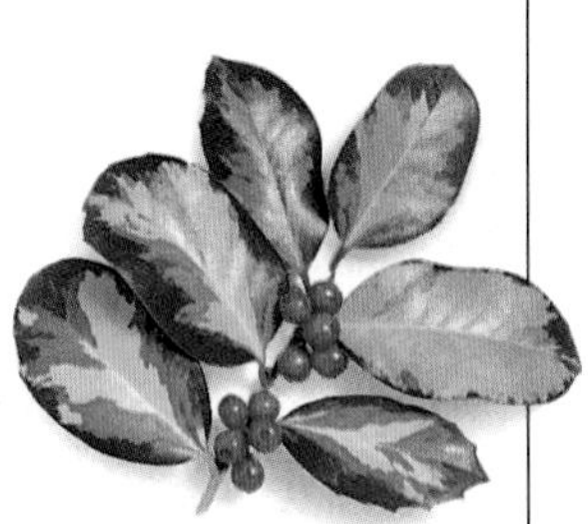
Ilex x *altaclerensis* 'Lawsoniana'

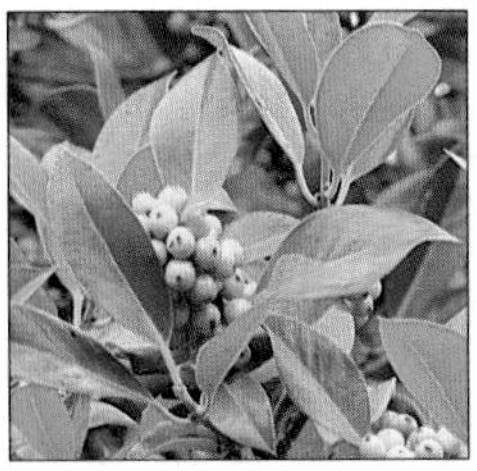
Ilex aquifolium 'Amber'

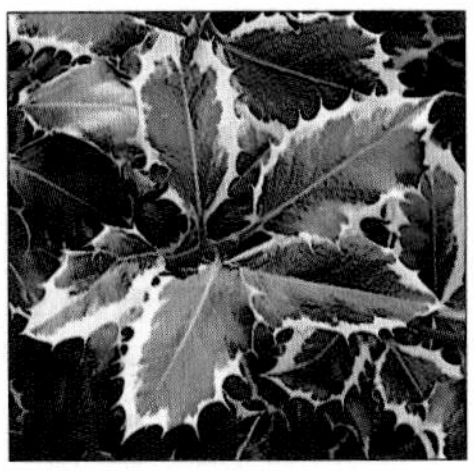
Ilex aquifolium 'Argentea Marginata Pendula'

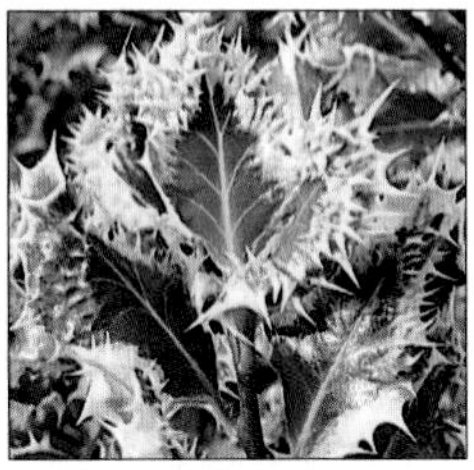
Ilex aquifolium 'Ferox Argentea'

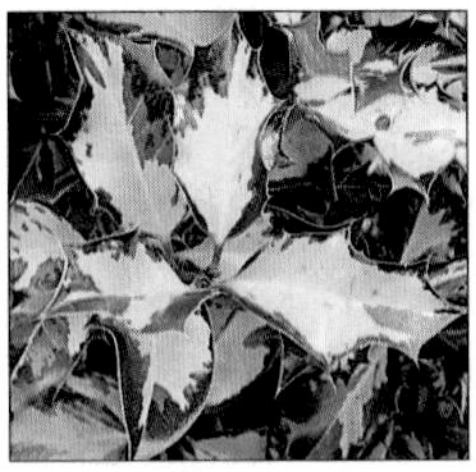
Ilex aquifolium 'Golden Milkboy'

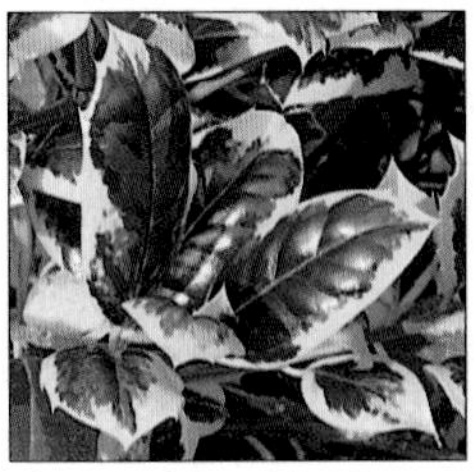
Ilex aquifolium 'Golden van Tol'

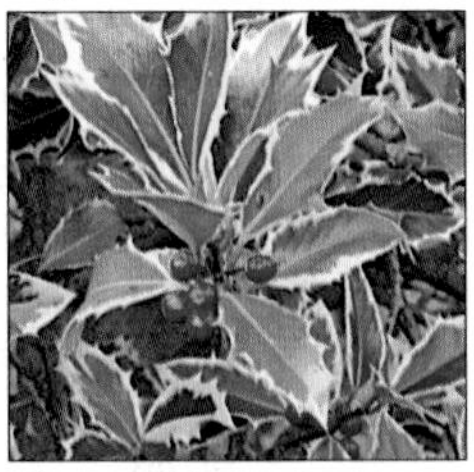
Ilex aquifolium 'Handsworth New Silver'

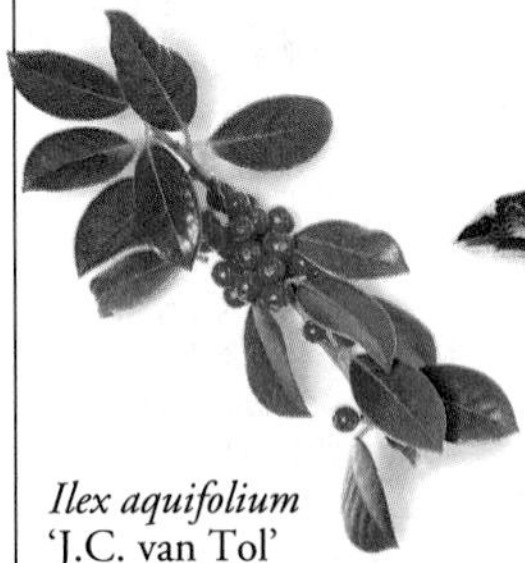
Ilex aquifolium 'J.C. van Tol'

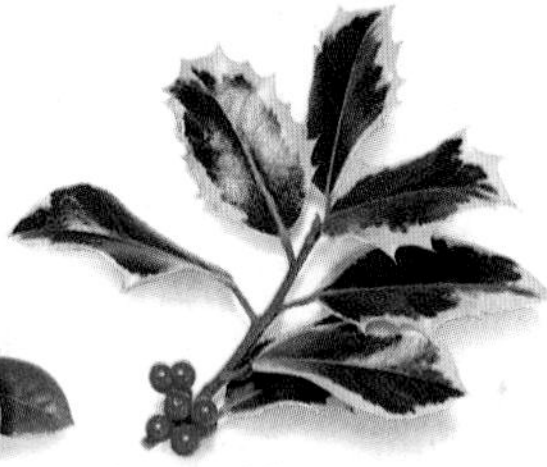
Ilex aquifolium 'Mme Briot'

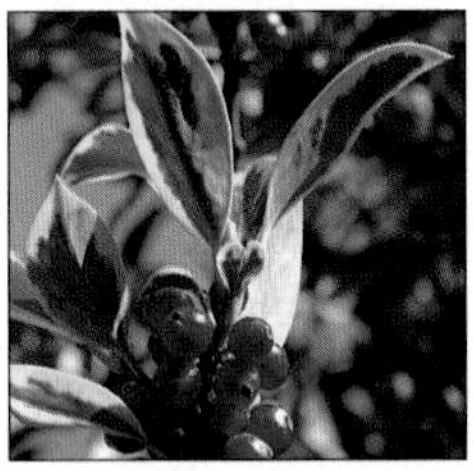
Ilex aquifolium 'Pyramidalis Aurea Marginata'

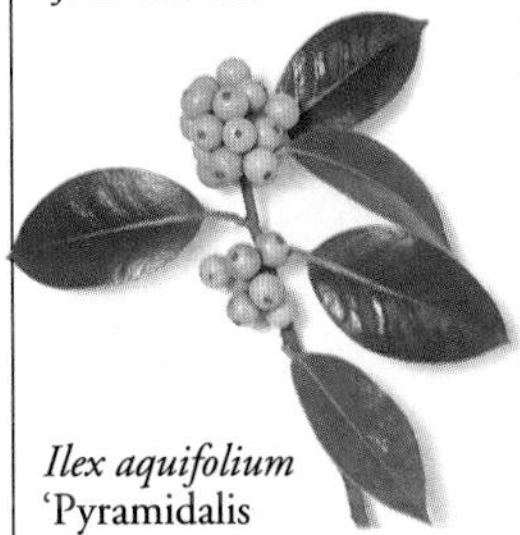
Ilex aquifolium 'Pyramidalis Fructu Luteo'

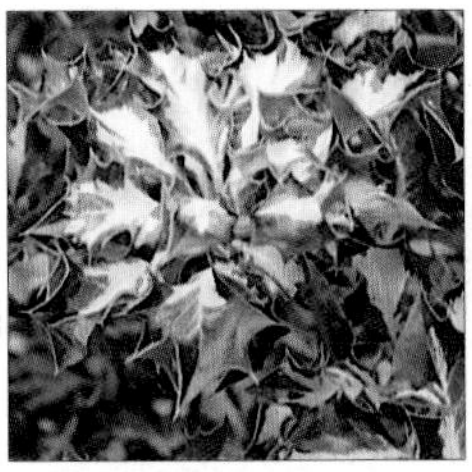
Ilex aquifolium 'Silver Milkmaid'

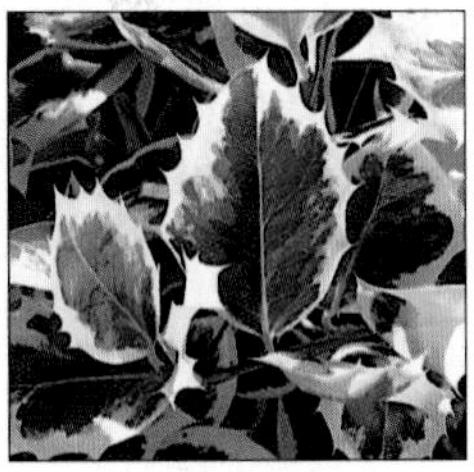
Ilex aquifolium 'Silver Queen'

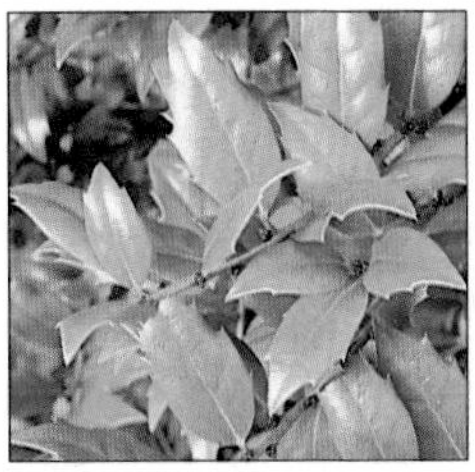
Ilex 'Brilliant'

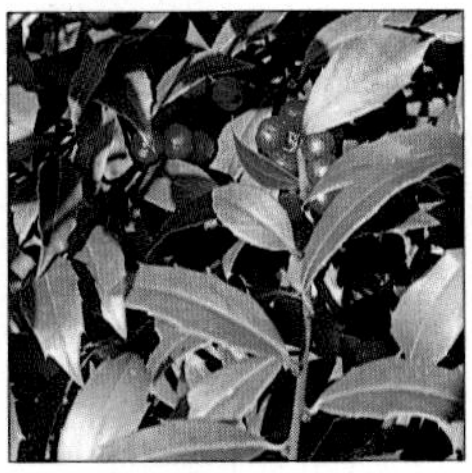
Ilex ciliospinosa

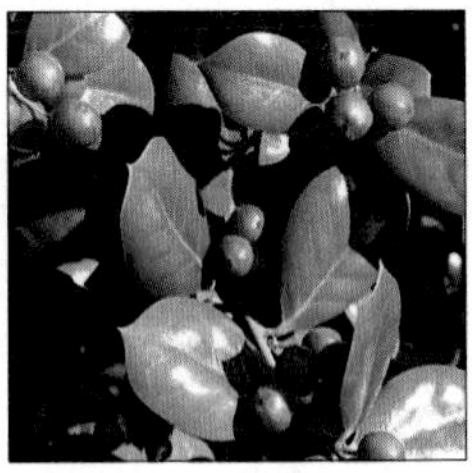
Ilex cornuta 'Burfordii'

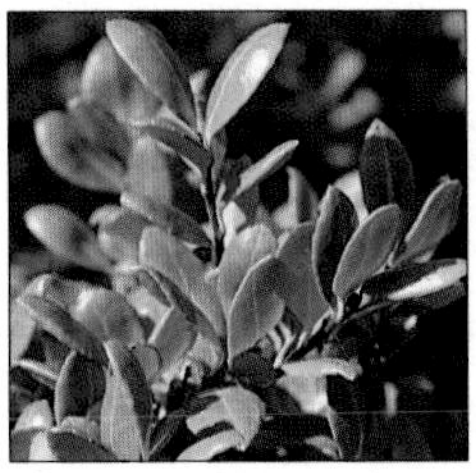
Ilex crenata 'Convexa'

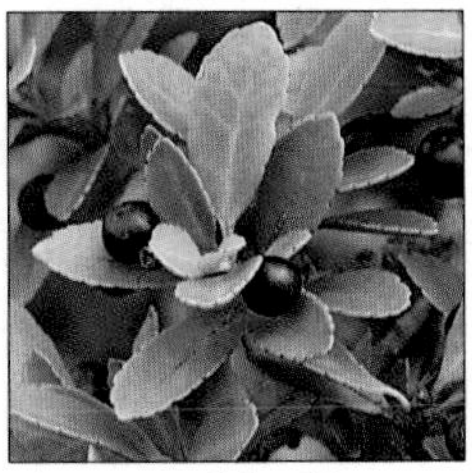
Ilex crenata f. *latifolia*

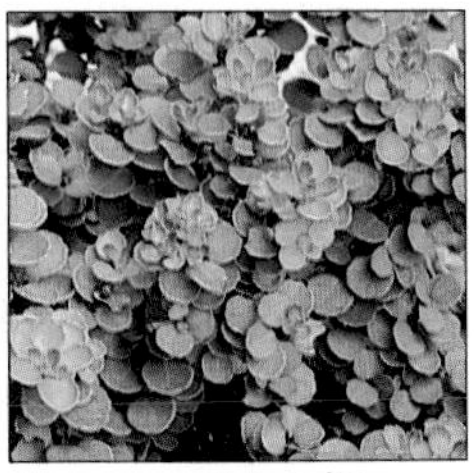
Ilex crenata 'Mariesii'

I

I. dimorphophylla. Evergreen, rounded shrub with ovate, entire, spine-tipped, glossy, dark green leaves, 2–3cm (¾–1¼in) long, elliptic and very spiny when young. Bears small red fruit, 3mm (⅛in) across. ↕1.5m (5ft), ↔1m (3ft). Japan (Liukiu Islands). ❄

I. dipyrena ◊ (Himalayan holly). Dense, upright, evergreen tree bearing oblong or elliptic, leathery, dull green leaves, 5–11cm (2–4½in) long, with abundant spines when young, fewer when mature. Bears red fruit, 6–8mm (¼–⅜in) across. ↕15m (50ft), ↔12m (40ft). E. Himalayas, W. China. ❄❄❄

***I.* 'Elegance'** ■◊ Narrowly conical, evergreen female tree, sometimes spindly when mature, with brittle branches and elliptic, spiny, dark green leaves, 2–5cm (¾–2in) long. Bears red fruit, to 10mm (½in) across. May be short-lived. *I.* 'Accent' is the pollinating male. ↕6m (20ft), ↔3m (10ft). ❄❄

I. fargesii ■◊ Broadly conical, evergreen shrub or tree with oblong to linear-lance-shaped, leathery, dull, dark green leaves, 6–12cm (2½–5in) long. Bears scarlet fruit, 4–7mm (⅛–¼in) across. ↕12m (40ft), ↔6m (20ft). Tibet, China (Hubei, Sichuan, Yunnan), Burma. ❄❄

I. glabra (Gallberry, Inkberry). Erect, evergreen shrub with narrowly obovate to inversely lance-shaped, glossy, dark green leaves, 2–5cm (¾–2in) long, pitted beneath. Bears black, occasionally white fruit, 4–8mm (⅛–⅜in) across. ↕↔3m (10ft). E. North America. ❄❄❄

***I.* 'Indian Chief'** ◊ (*I. cornuta* x *I. pernyi*). Compact, upright, evergreen female shrub with almost stalkless, diamond-shaped to nearly rectangular, glossy, dark green leaves, to 10cm (4in) long, with 5 prominent spines. Bears red fruit, 8mm (¾in) across. ↕2–3m (6–10ft), ↔1.5–2.5m (5–8ft). ❄❄❄

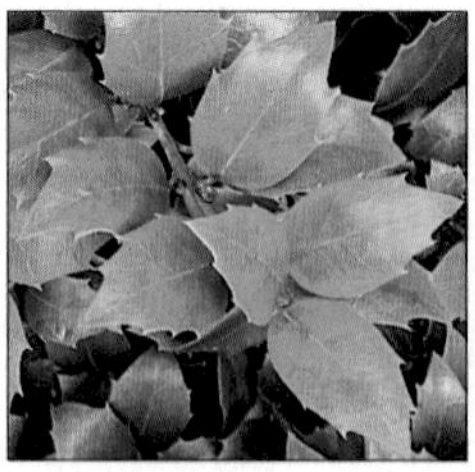

Ilex 'Elegance'

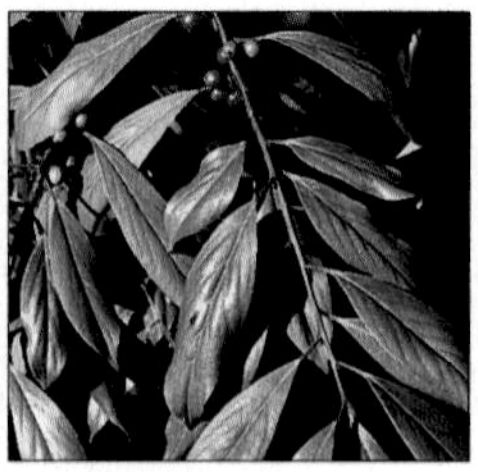

Ilex fargesii

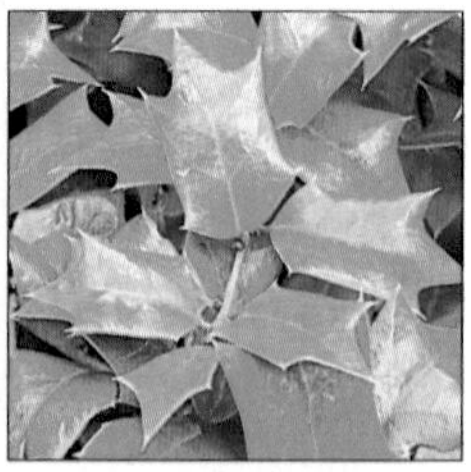

Ilex 'John T. Morris'

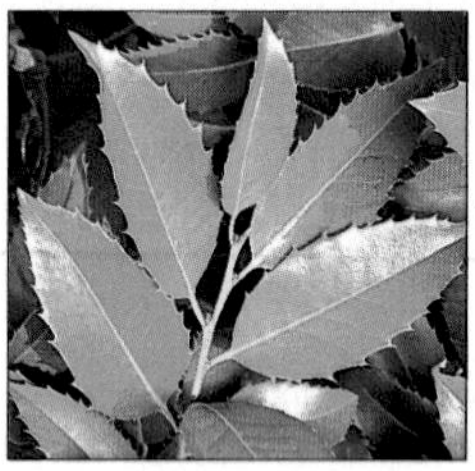

Ilex x *koehneana* 'Chestnut Leaf'

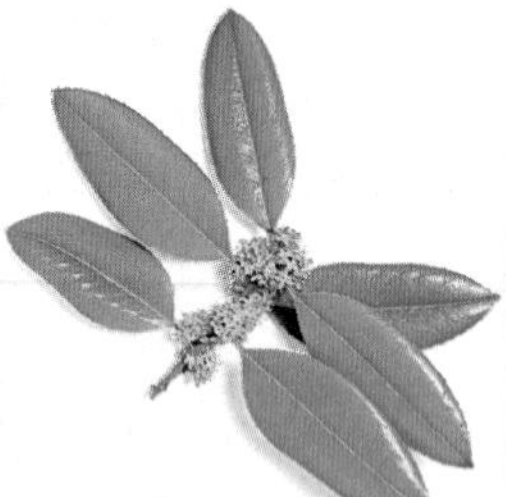

Ilex latifolia

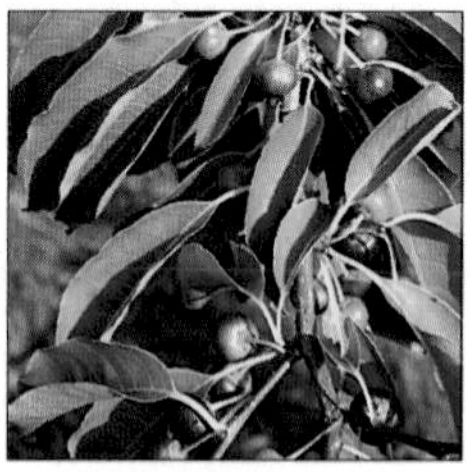

Ilex macrocarpa

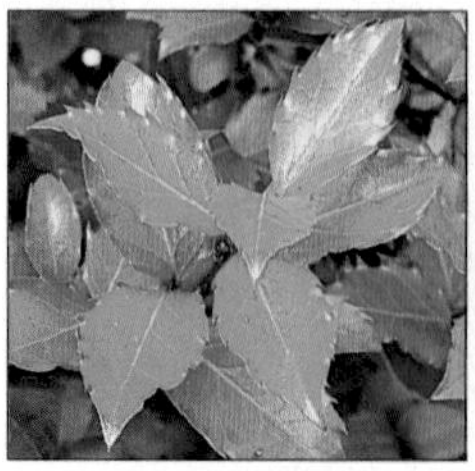

Ilex x *meserveae* 'Blue Prince'

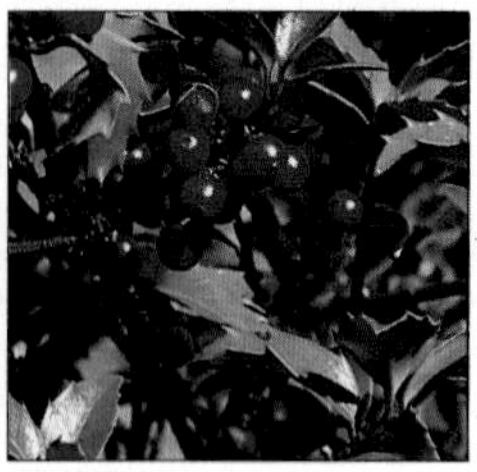

Ilex x *meserveae* 'Blue Princess'

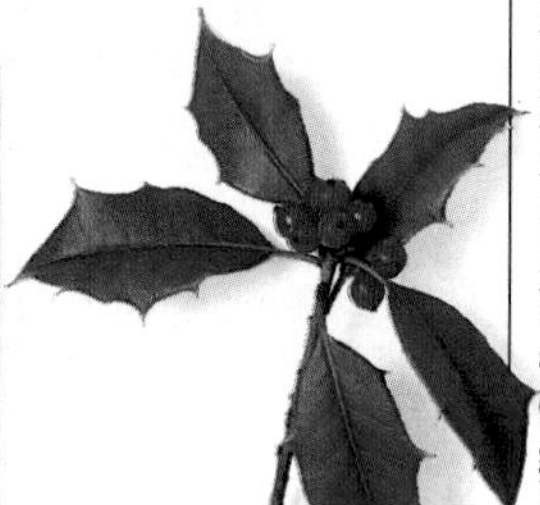

Ilex opaca

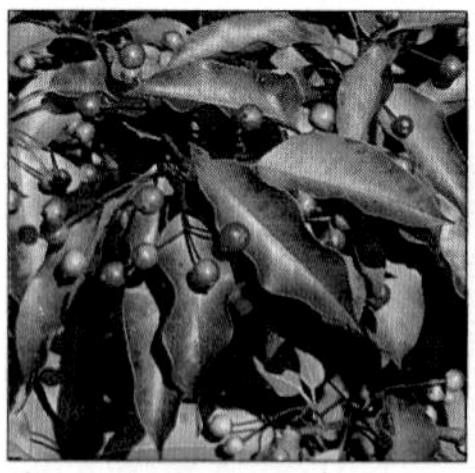

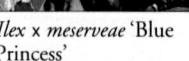

Ilex pedunculosa

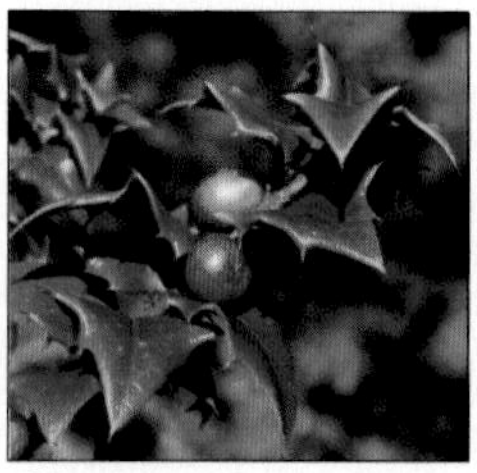

Ilex pernyi

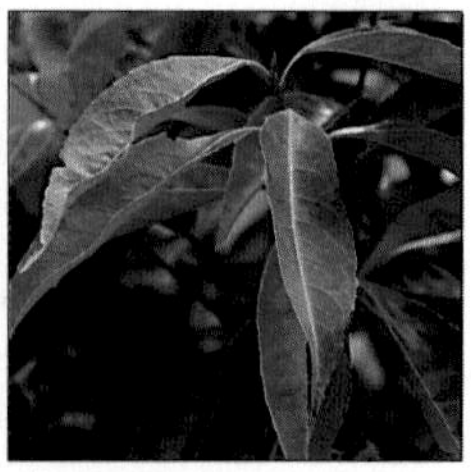

Ilex purpurea

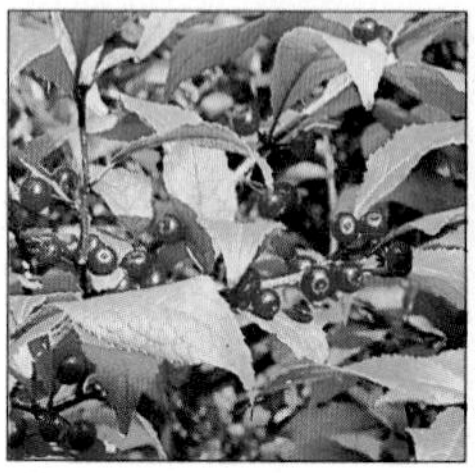

Ilex 'Sparkleberry'

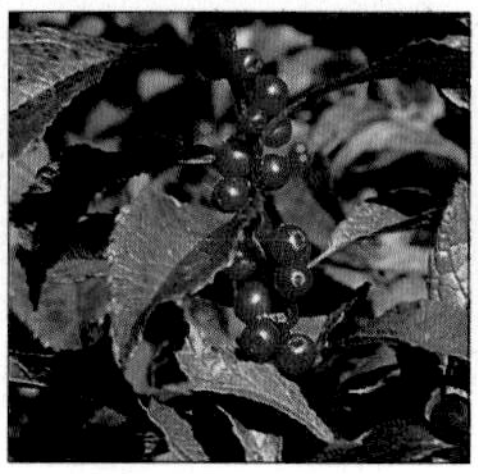

Ilex verticillata

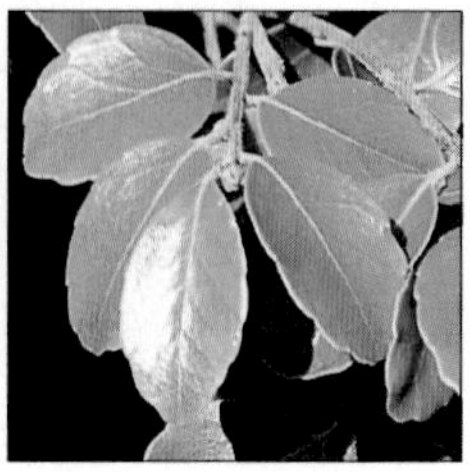

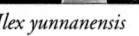

Ilex yunnanensis

I. insignis see *I. kingiana.*

***I.* 'John T. Morris'** ■◊ (*I. cornuta* x *I. pernyi*). Dense, conical, evergreen male shrub. Bears almost stalkless, glossy, diamond-shaped to nearly rectangular, dark green leaves, 4–6cm (1½–2½in) long, with 5 spines. Pollinating male for *I.* 'Lydia Morris'. ↕7m (22ft), ↔5m (15ft). ❄❄❄

I. kingiana ■◊ syn. *I. insignis.* Upright, evergreen tree with stout, silvery grey branches. Bears elliptic-lance-shaped to ovate, leathery, glossy, mid- to dark green leaves, 15–20cm (6–8in) long, very spiny when young, slightly toothed or entire when mature. Young seedlings have waxy leaves, 6–8mm (¼–⅜in) long, with marginal spines pointing in all directions. Bears large clusters of bright red berries, 5mm (¼in) across. ↕5m (15ft), ↔4m (12ft). E. Himalayas, China (Yunnan). ❄❄

I.* x *koehneana ◊ (*I. aquifolium* x *I. latifolia*). Narrowly conical, evergreen shrub with olive-green twigs. Large, glossy, mid-green leaves are oblong to elliptic, 8–12cm (3–5in) long, with large marginal spines. Produces red fruit, 8mm (⅜in) across. ↕7m (22ft), ↔5m (15ft). Garden origin. ❄❄❄. **'Chestnut Leaf'** ■🏆 is female, with light or yellowish green leaves and red berries.

I. latifolia ■ ◊ Narrowly conical, evergreen shrub with stout, olive-green twigs and oblong or oblong-ovate, entire or spine-toothed, leathery, glossy, dark green leaves, 8–18cm (3–7in) long. Yellowish green flowers are borne in late spring and early summer, followed by abundant orange-red berries, 7mm (¼in) across. ↕7m (22ft), ↔5m (15ft). China, Japan. ❄❄

***I.* 'Lydia Morris'** ◊ (*I. cornuta* x *I. pernyi*). Dense, conical, evergreen female shrub with almost stalkless, diamond-shaped to nearly rectangular, glossy, black-green leaves, 4–8cm (1½–3in) long, with 5 spines. Produces red fruit, 8mm (⅜in) across, which is often hidden by the foliage. *I.* 'John T. Morris' is the pollinating male. ↕7m (22ft), ↔5m (15ft). ❄❄❄

I. macrocarpa ■◊ Rounded to broadly spreading, deciduous tree with spur-like branchlets and elliptic or ovate-elliptic, shallowly toothed, bright green leaves, 7–11cm (3–4½in) long. In late spring, bears greenish white flowers, followed by flattened, spherical, mid-green berries, 1–2cm (½–¾in) across, maturing to black. ↕17m (56ft), ↔12m (40ft). S. and S.W. China. ❄❄❄

I. mariesii see *I. crenata* 'Mariesii'.

I.* x *meserveae (*I. aquifolium* x *I. rugosa*) (Blue holly). Dense, vigorous, erect to spreading, evergreen shrub, resembling *I. aquifolium.* Bears usually small, elliptic to ovate, spiny, glossy, bluish green leaves, 2–5cm (¾–2in) long. White to pinkish white flowers appear in late spring, followed on female plants by glossy red fruit, to 7mm (¼in) across. ↕5m (15ft), ↔3m (10ft). Garden origin. ❄❄❄. **'Blue Angel'** 🏆 is a slow-growing, compact female shrub with dark purple stems and elliptic, glossy, dark bluish green leaves, 4.5cm (1¾in) long. Least hardy of the blue hollies. ↕4m (12ft), ↔2m (6ft). **'Blue Boy'** is a spreading male shrub with purplish green stems and ovate, glossy, dark greenish blue leaves, 4–4.5cm (1½–1¾in) long. ↕3m (10ft). **'Blue Girl'** is the female counterpart of 'Blue Boy', with abundant red berries. ↕3m (10ft). **'Blue Maid'** is a dense female shrub producing an abundance of fruit. Probably the hardiest of the blue hollies. ↔4m (12ft). **'Blue Prince'** ■ is similar to 'Blue Boy', with purplish green stems bearing glossy, bright green leaves. ↔4m (12ft). **'Blue Princess'** ■🏆 is similar to 'Blue Girl', with larger, glossier leaves, 4.5–6cm (1¾–2½in) long, and more abundant fruit. ↕3m (10ft).

***I.* 'Nellie R. Stevens'** ◊ (*I. aquifolium* x *I. cornuta*). Vigorous, conical, evergreen female tree with oblong-ovate, sparsely spiny, highly glossy, dark green leaves, 5–8cm (2–3in) long. Produces abundant shiny scarlet fruit, 8–10mm (⅜–½in) across. ↕7m (22ft), ↔4m (12ft). ❄❄❄

I. opaca ■◊ (American holly). Erect, evergreen, large shrub or tree with oblong-elliptic, spine-toothed or entire, leathery, matt, dark green leaves, 5–10cm (2–4in) long. Bears crimson, or occasionally yellow or orange fruit, 6mm (¼in) across. ↕15m (50ft), ↔7m (22ft). C. and E. USA. ❄❄❄. **'Morgan Gold'** is compact and free fruiting, with bright yellow berries.

I. pedunculosa ■◊ Upright, evergreen tree or shrub with elliptic to ovate, spineless, glossy, dark green leaves, 4–8cm (1½–3in) long, bronze-tinted when young. Bears bright red fruit, 8mm (⅜in) across, on long stalks. ↕10m (30ft), ↔7m (22ft). China, Taiwan, Japan. ❄❄❄

I. perado ◊ Upright, evergreen shrub or small tree with ovate to oblong or lance-shaped, toothed or entire, leathery, thorny, glossy, dark green leaves, 6–10cm (2½–4in) long. Bears red fruit, 8mm (⅜in) across. ↕6–10m (20–30ft), ↔7m (22ft). Canary Islands (Gomera, Tenerife), Azores. ❄❄❄. **'Aurea'** see *I.* x *altaclerensis* 'Belgica Aurea'. **subsp. *platyphylla*,** syn. *I. platyphylla*, has broadly ovate leaves, 10–15cm (4–6in) long.

I. pernyi ■◊ Upright, evergreen shrub with almost stalkless, diamond-shaped to nearly rectangular, glossy, dark green leaves, 2–3cm (¾–1¼in) long, with 5 spines. Bears yellowish flowers in late spring, followed by bright red fruit, 6–8mm (¼–⅜in) across. ↕9m (28ft), ↔3m (10ft). W. and C. China (Gansu, Hubei). ❄❄❄. **var. *veitchii*** has larger and broader leaves, 4–5cm (1½–2in) long, with 3–5 spines on each side. China (Hubei).

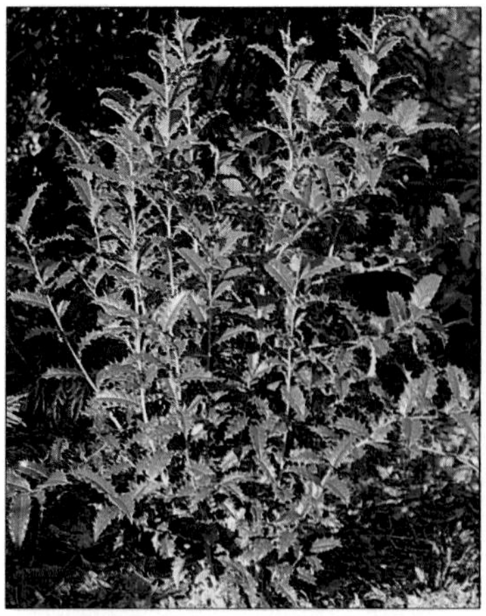

Ilex kingiana

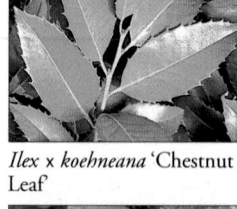

I. platyphylla see *I. perado* subsp. *platyphylla*.
I. purpurea ■ syn. *I. chinensis* of gardens. Conical, evergreen tree with elliptic-lance-shaped, occasionally ovate, mid- to dark green leaves, 5–11cm (2–4½in) long, purplish green when young. Bears ellipsoid, glossy red fruit, to 12mm (½in) across. ↕ to 13m (43ft), ↔ 4m (12ft). China, Japan. ✽✽✽
***I.* 'September Gem'** (*I.* x *aquipernyi* x *I. ciliospinosa*). Conical, evergreen female shrub bearing ovate, glossy, dark green leaves, 4–5cm (1½–2in) long, with insignificant spiny teeth. Bears bright red berries, 6–8mm (¼–⅜in) across. ↕ 3m (10ft), ↔ 2m (6ft). ✽✽
I. serrata (Japanese winterberry). Deciduous, bushy shrub with slender, purple twigs and elliptic, finely toothed, dull green leaves, 4–8cm (1½–3in) long, downy on both surfaces. Bears bright pink flowers, followed by bright red, occasionally yellow or white fruit, 4–5mm (⅛–¼in) across. Often used for bonsai. ↕ to 5m (15ft), ↔ 3m (10ft). China (Sichuan), Japan. ✽✽
***I.* 'Snow Flake'** see *I. crenata* 'Shiro-Fukurin'.
***I.* 'Sparkleberry'** ■ (*I. serrata* x *I. verticillata*). Vigorous (especially when young), deciduous, upright female shrub or small tree. Bears ovate, toothed, dark green leaves, 4–10cm (1½–4in) long, which persist until early winter. Produces glossy red berries, 6mm (¼in) across. *I.* 'Apollo' is the male pollinator. ↕ 5m (15ft), ↔ 4m (12ft). ✽✽✽
I. verticillata ■ (Black alder, Winterberry). Deciduous tree, usually a suckering shrub in cultivation. Leaves are obovate or lance-shaped, toothed, bright green, 4–10cm (1½–4in) long, with long, sharp-pointed tips, softly hairy beneath. In mid-spring, produces white flowers, followed by stalkless, spherical, dark red to scarlet, sometimes orange or yellow fruit, 4–5mm (⅛–¼in) across. ↕↔ 5m (15ft). E. North America. ✽✽✽. Dwarf male selections are available for pollinating cultivars that flower in early to mid-spring, such as 'Nana'. Late male selections are also available to pollinate late-flowering cultivars, such as 'Winter Red'. **'Nana'**, syn. 'Red Sprite', is a small, rounded female shrub with ovate, mid-green leaves, 3–6cm (1¼–2½in) long. Bears abundant large, bright red fruit, to 12mm (½in) across. ↕ 60–120cm (2–4ft), ↔ 1–1.5m (3–5ft). **'Red Sprite'** see 'Nana'. **'Winter Red'** is a robust, broad female shrub with dark green leaves. Produces long-lasting, intensely red berries, 8mm (⅜in) across, which persist until spring. ↕ 2.5–3m (8–10ft). ↔ 3m (10ft).
***I.* 'Washington'** (*I. ciliospinosa* x *I. cornuta*). Erect, conical, evergreen female shrub with ovate to oblong, spiny, glossy, light green leaves, 4–5cm (1½–2in) long. Bears red fruit. ↕ 4m (12ft), ↔ 2m (6ft). ✽✽✽
I. yunnanensis ■ Evergreen, upright to rounded shrub with downy branchlets and ovate or ovate-lance-shaped, scalloped to toothed, glossy, dark green leaves, 2–3.5cm (¾–1½in) long. Bears red fruit, 6mm (¼in) across. ↕↔ 4m (12ft). N. Burma, China (Sichuan, Hubei). ✽✽

▷ ***Iliamna*** see *Sphaeralcea*

ILLICIUM

ILLICIACEAE

Genus of about 40 species of aromatic, evergreen shrubs and trees from woodland in S.E. Asia, S.E. USA, and the West Indies. They are cultivated for their thick, glossy leaves, borne alternately or in near-whorls, their unusual flowers, which are composed of numerous tepals, and their woody, star-shaped fruits. Where temperatures fall below -5°C (23°F), grow in a cool greenhouse. Elsewhere, grow in a woodland garden or shrub border.
• **HARDINESS** Frost hardy to frost tender.
• **CULTIVATION** Under glass, grow in lime-free (ericaceous) potting compost in full light, shaded from the hottest sun, or in bright filtered light. During growth, water moderately and apply a balanced liquid fertilizer monthly. Water sparingly in winter. Outdoors, grow in moist but well-drained, humus-rich, lime-free soil, in full sun or partial shade. Shelter from cold, drying winds. Pruning group 1.
• **PROPAGATION** Take semi-ripe cuttings in summer. Layer in summer.
• **PESTS AND DISEASES** Trouble free.

I. anisatum ■ syn. *I. religiosum* (Chinese anise). Conical, evergreen shrub or small tree bearing oval to lance-shaped, blunt-tipped, glossy, dark green leaves, to 12cm (5in) long. Star-shaped, fragrant, yellow-green, later creamy white flowers, to 2.5cm (1in) across, are produced in mid-spring. ↕ to 8m (25ft), ↔ 6m (20ft). China, Japan, Taiwan. ✽✽
I. floridanum (Purple anise). Bushy, evergreen shrub bearing narrowly oval to lance-shaped, glossy, dark green leaves, to 10cm (4in) long. Nodding, star-shaped, fragrant, red to red-purple flowers, to 5cm (2in) across, are borne in late spring and early summer. ↕↔ 2.5m (8ft). S.E. USA. ✽✽
I. religiosum see *I. anisatum*.
I. verum (Chinese anise, Star anise). Small, rounded, evergreen tree with inversely lance-shaped to narrowly elliptic, sharply tapered, glossy, dark green leaves, to 15cm (6in) long. Star-shaped flowers, 1.5cm (½in) across, with pink- or red-flushed yellow tepals, are borne in early summer, followed by glossy, red-brown fruit. ↕ 18m (60ft), ↔ 6m (20ft). China, Vietnam. ✽✽

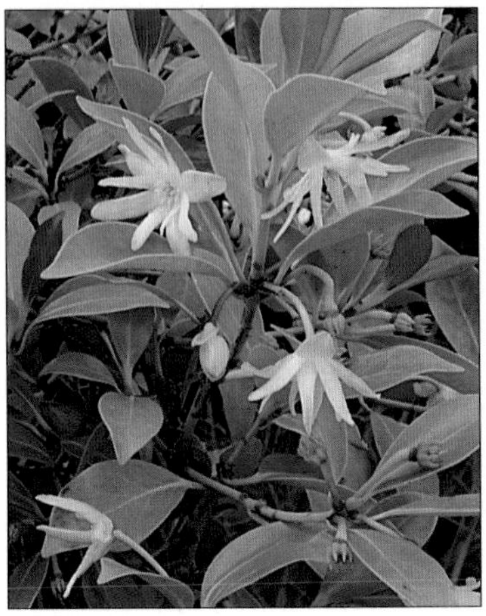

Illicium anisatum

IMPATIENS

Balsam, Busy Lizzie

BALSAMINACEAE

Genus of about 850 species of erect annuals, and evergreen perennials and subshrubs, found in a great variety of often damp habitats, near streams, lakes, or in woodland, throughout tropical and warm-temperate regions (except Australia, New Zealand, and South America). All have brittle, almost succulent stems and lush, fleshy, semi-translucent foliage; leaves vary from alternate to opposite or whorled. Flowers are asymmetrical, spurred and sometimes hooded, 5-petalled, borne singly or in clusters or racemes, and are followed by explosive seed capsules. Most are excellent as houseplants and summer bedding plants, particularly in light shade, and provide long-lasting summer colour in a window-box or container on a patio. *I. walleriana* cultivars and *I. balsamina* are free-flowering and tolerate shade. Many, including some New Guinea Group hybrids, are also grown for their bronze- or yellow-flushed or variegated foliage. Grow hardy perennials in a woodland garden. In frost-prone areas, grow tender perennials in a temperate or warm greenhouse, or as houseplants. All will self-seed in favourable conditions.
• **HARDINESS** Fully hardy to frost tender.
• **CULTIVATION** Under glass, grow in loamless or loam-based potting compost (JI No.2) in full to bright filtered light, with moderate to high humidity. During growth, water moderately and apply a balanced liquid fertilizer monthly. Water sparingly in winter. Outdoors, grow in humus-rich, moist but well-drained soil in partial shade, with shelter from wind.
• **PROPAGATION** Sow seed at 16–18°C (61–64°F) in early spring. For hardy species, sow seed *in situ* in late spring. Root softwood cuttings of *I. walleriana* and New Guinea Group cultivars in spring or early summer.
• **PESTS AND DISEASES** Seedlings are prone to damping off. Grey mould (*Botrytis*) may affect flower buds if conditions are too damp. Red spider mites, whiteflies, vine weevil, and aphids may be troublesome under glass.

I. balsamina. Sparsely branched, slightly hairy annual with alternate, narrowly lance-shaped to narrowly elliptic, deeply toothed, pale green leaves, 2.5–9cm (1–3½in) long. From summer to early autumn, cup-shaped, hooded, pink, red, purple, or white flowers, 2.5–5cm (1–2in) across, are produced either singly in the leaf axils or in small clusters of 2 or 3. ↕ to 75cm (30in), ↔ 45cm (18in). India, China, Malaysia. ⊛ (min. 5°C/41°F). **'Blackberry Ice'** produces abundant double purple flowers, splashed white; ↕ to 70cm (28in). **Camellia-flowered Series** ■ cultivars have large, double, white-mottled, pink or red flowers; ↕ to 70cm (28in). **Tom Thumb Series** ■ cultivars are dwarf, with large, double, pink, scarlet, violet, or white flowers, 5–6cm (2–2½in) across; ↕ to 30cm (12in).
I. glandulifera, syn. *I. roylei* (Policeman's helmet). Tall, fast-growing annual with thick, sparsely branched, red-tinged stems and whorls of ovate to lance-shaped, toothed, light green leaves, to 23cm (9in) long. Long-stalked racemes of 3–15 nodding, hooded, scented, purple, rose-pink, or white flowers, to 5cm (2in) long, spotted yellow or brown inside, are borne in summer, followed by explosive seed capsules. ↕ 1–2m (3–6ft), ↔ to 1m (3ft). Himalayas. ✽✽✽
***I.* New Guinea Group.** Subshrubby, hybrid perennials, derived from *I. hawkeri* and other species, usually grown as annuals, valued for their foliage and brightly coloured flowers. ⊛ (min. 10°C/50°F). **'Spectra'** ■ is a seed-raised cultivar with opposite or whorled, lance-shaped, toothed, mid-green leaves, 8–15cm (3–6in) long.

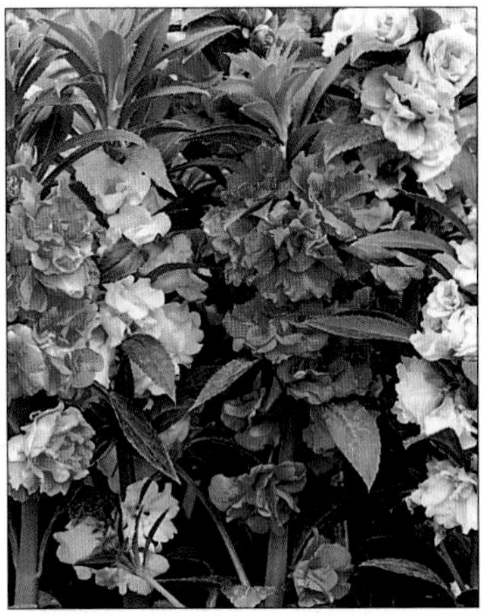

Impatiens balsamina Camellia-flowered Series

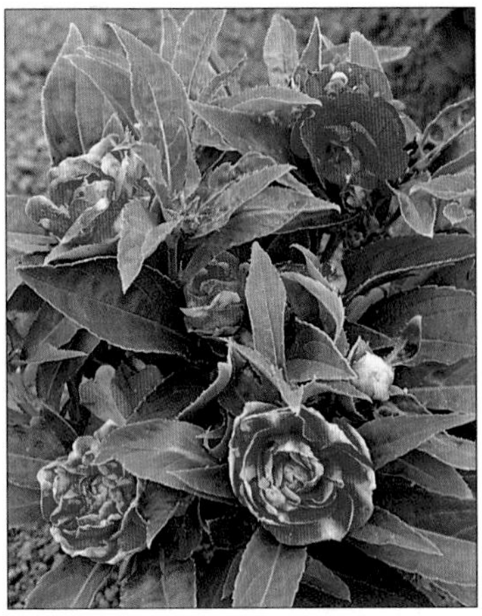

Impatiens balsamina Tom Thumb Series

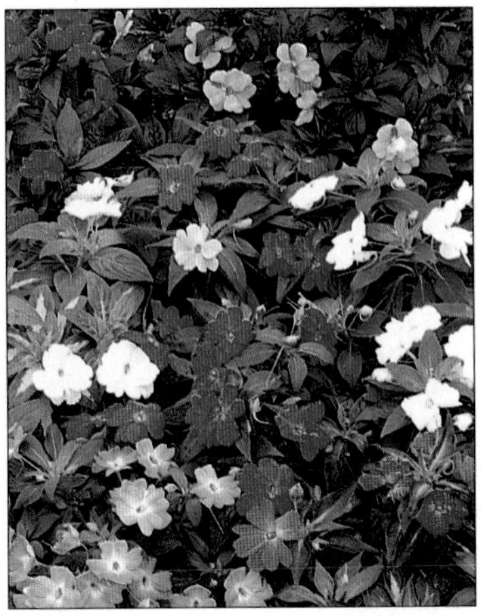

Impatiens New Guinea Group 'Spectra'

I

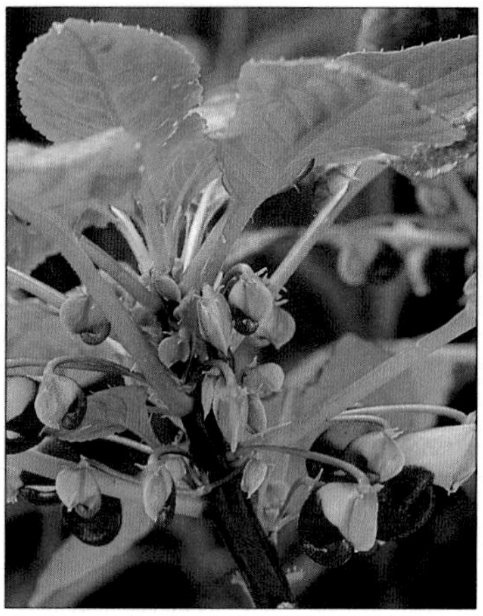
Impatiens niamniamensis 'Congo Cockatoo'

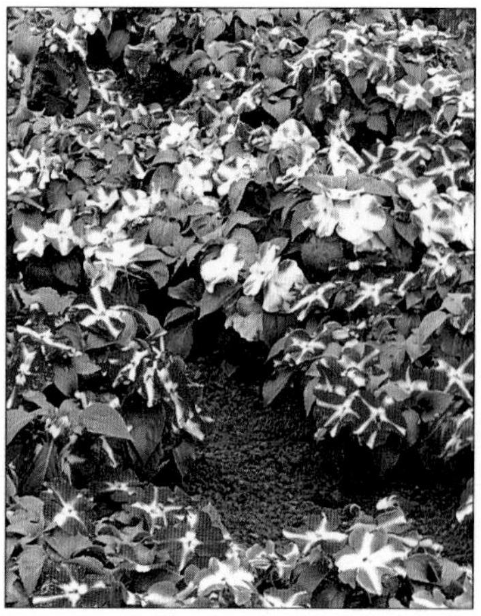
Impatiens walleriana 'Starbright'

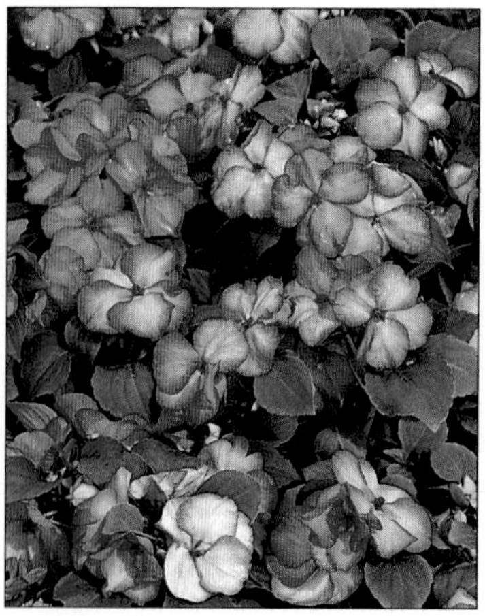
Impatiens walleriana Swirl Series

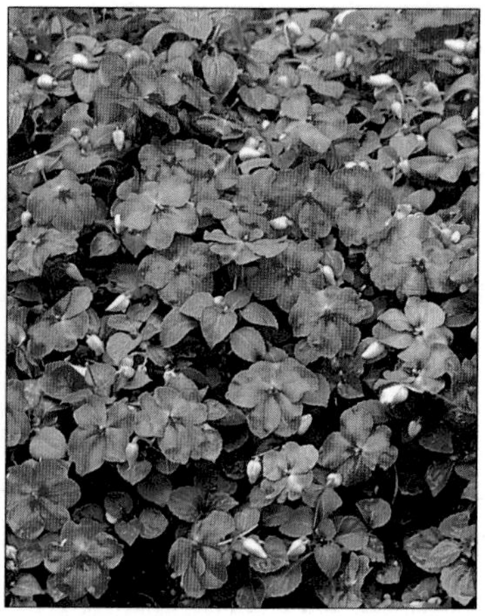
Impatiens walleriana Tempo Series 'Tempo Lavender'

I

From summer to autumn, bears abundant flattened, deep rose-pink, scarlet-red, salmon-pink, lavender, or white flowers, with some bicolours, to 6cm (2½in) across. ↕ 35cm (14in), ↔ 30cm (12in). **'Tango'** is a seed-raised cultivar with opposite or whorled, lance-shaped, toothed, dark bronze-green leaves, 8–15cm (3–6in) long. Bears abundant flattened, 5-petalled, tangerine-orange flowers, to 5cm (2in) across, from summer to autumn. ↕ 35cm (14in), ↔ 30cm (12in).

***I. niamniamensis* 'Congo Cockatoo'** ■ Erect, short-lived perennial with spirally arranged, ovate or elliptic, scalloped, dark green leaves, 5–22cm (2–9in) long. Narrow, hooded, bright red and yellow flowers, 4cm (1½in) long, each with a distinctive hooked spur, are borne singly or in small clusters of 2–8 in the leaf axils at any time of year. ↕ 90cm (36in), ↔ 35cm (14in). ❁ (min. 15°C/59°F)

I. oliveri see *I. sodenii.*

I. repens ♀ Creeping or trailing perennial with alternate, kidney-shaped, scalloped leaves, to 2.5cm (1in) long. Solitary, hooded, clear yellow flowers, 4cm (1½in) long, are borne in the leaf axils from summer to autumn. Good for hanging baskets. ↕ 19cm (7in), ↔ 30cm (12in). India, Sri Lanka. ❁ (min. 13°C/55°F)

I. roylei see *I. glandulifera.*

I. sodenii, syn. *I. oliveri.* Erect, shrubby perennial with whorls of 6–8 inversely lance-shaped, toothed leaves, 20cm (8in) long, with pale green midribs. Long-stalked, pale lilac, pink, or sometimes white flowers, 6cm (2½in) across, are borne mainly in summer. ↕ 3m (10ft), ↔ 1.4m (4½ft). E. tropical Africa. ❁ (min. 10°C/50°F)

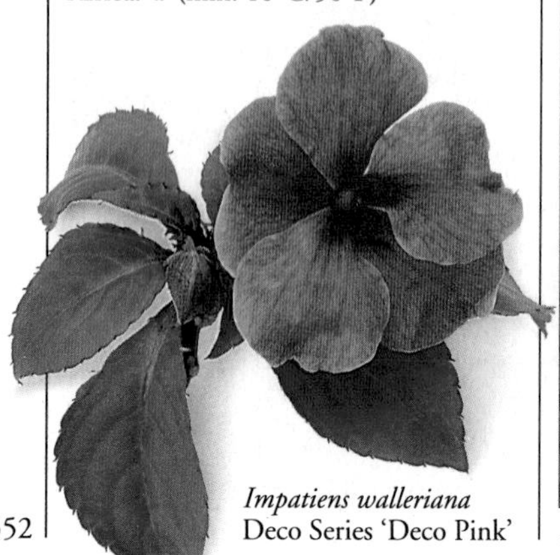
Impatiens walleriana Deco Series 'Deco Pink'

I. tinctoria. Vigorous, erect, tuberous perennial with spirally arranged, oblong, ovate, or oblong-lance-shaped, scalloped or toothed leaves, 8–23cm (3–9in) long. Racemes of long-stalked, scented white flowers, 6cm (2½in) across, the throats marked with pink or magenta, and each with a slender spur, are borne freely from summer to autumn. ↕ 2.2m (7ft), ↔ 1m (3ft). E. Africa. ❄

I. walleriana (Busy Lizzie). Variable subshrubby perennial, usually grown as an annual, with light green to red-flushed stems and spirally arranged, elliptic to lance-shaped, slightly toothed, scalloped, light to bronze-green or red-flushed leaves, to 12cm (5in) long. In summer, the many cultivars from the species produce flattened, slender-spurred flowers, 2.5–6cm (1–2½in) across, in white, many shades of orange, pink, scarlet, red, crimson, violet, purple, and lavender-blue, as well as bicolours. ↕↔ to 60cm (24in). ❁ (min. 10°C/50°F). **Accent Series** ♀ cultivars are compact, with flowers in white and a very wide range of colours, including shades of orange, pink, crimson, wine-red, lilac, violet and lavender-blue, some with central stars; ↕ to 20cm (8in). **Blitz 2000 Series** cultivars are tall and many-branched, with dark green foliage and flowers to 6cm (2½in) across, in white and shades of orange, pink, red, and violet; ↕ to 35cm (14in). **Confection Series** cultivars bear mostly double and semi-double flowers in shades of orange, pink, and red, and have deep green foliage. **Deco Series** cultivars have bronze-green leaves and flowers in shades of orange, pink, red, and violet; ↕ to 20cm (8in). **Deco Series 'Deco Pink'** ■ has mid-pink flowers, each with a deep pink eye. **Expo Series** cultivars are compact and uniform, with flowers to 6cm (2½in) across, in white and shades of orange, pink, red, and violet, including bicolours; ↕ to 20cm (8in). **Florette Star Series** cultivars are low-growing, and have flowers in shades of orange, pink, red, and violet, or mixtures, each with a central white star; ↕ 15–20cm (6–8in). **Impulse Series** cultivars are in a wide colour range, including pastel colours and shades of violet, lilac, orange, pink, and red, and some bicolours. **'Mega Orange Star'** has orange flowers, to 6cm (2½in) across, each with a central white star; ↕ 20–25cm (8–10in). **'Starbright'** ■ has flowers to 6cm (2½in) across, in rose-pink, red, orange, and violet-blue, each with a central white star; ↕ to 20cm (8in). **Super Elfin Series** ■ ♀ cultivars are spreading and flat, with a wide colour range, including pastel colours and shades of violet, orange, pink and red; ↕ to 25cm (10in). **Swirl Series** ■ cultivars have pink-and-orange flowers margined in rose-red; ↕ 15–20cm (6–8in). **Tempo Series** ♀ cultivars have a wide colour range, including shades of violet, lavender-blue, orange, pink, and red, as well as bicolours and picotees; ↕ to 23cm (9in). **Tempo Series 'Tempo Lavender'** ■ has lavender-pink flowers.

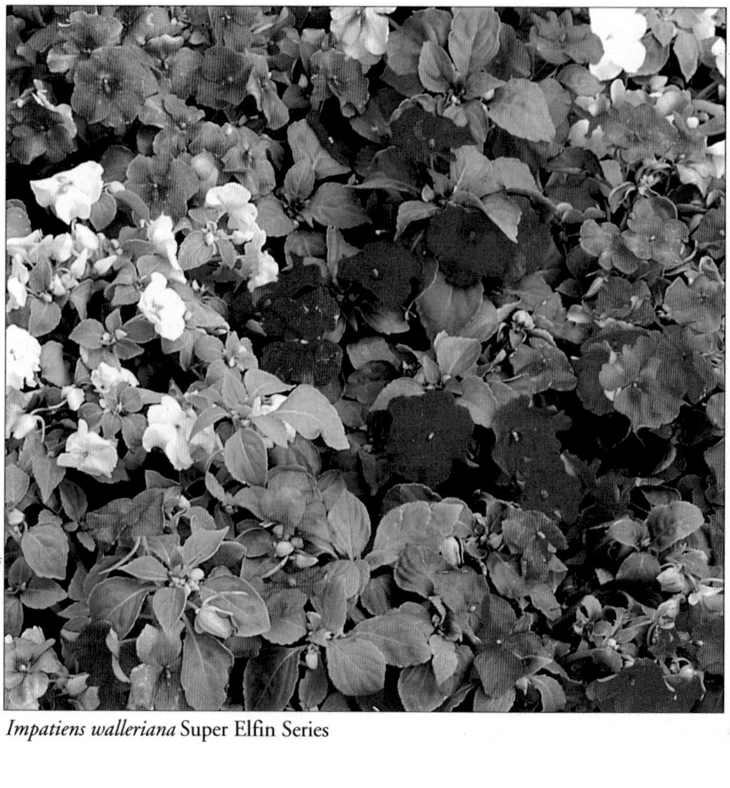
Impatiens walleriana Super Elfin Series

IMPERATA

GRAMINEAE/POACEAE

Genus of 6 species of slender-stemmed, rhizomatous, perennial grasses from tropical and warm-temperate, open grassland in Japan. They have flat, linear, pointed leaves and erect, spike-like panicles of short, silvery spikelets, borne in summer. Variegated cultivars

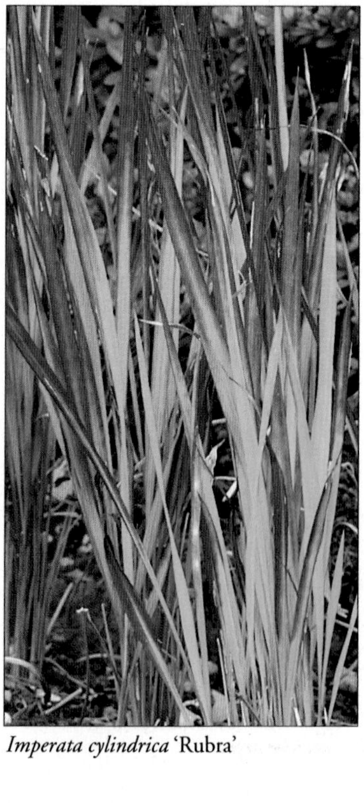
Imperata cylindrica 'Rubra'

are grown for their striking foliage. Grow at the front of a mixed or herbaceous border, in a light woodland garden, or in containers. All need long, warm summers to flower well.

- **HARDINESS** Hardy to -10°C (14°F).
- **CULTIVATION** Grow in moist but well-drained, humus-rich soil in full sun or light dappled shade. In cold climates, provide a winter mulch, especially when plants are young.
- **PROPAGATION** Divide in spring or early summer.
- **PESTS AND DISEASES** Trouble free.

***I. cylindrica* 'Rubra'** ■ syn. *I. cylindrica* 'Red Baron'. Slowly spreading, perennial grass forming loose clumps of flat, linear, mid-green leaves, to 50cm (20in) long, which quickly turn deep blood-red from the tips almost to the bases. Narrow, spike-like panicles, to 20cm (8in) long, of fluffy, silvery white spikelets, to 4.5cm (1¾in) long, are produced in late summer. ↕40cm (16in), ↔ 30cm (12in) or more. ❄❄

INCARVILLEA

syn. AMPHICOME

BIGNONIACEAE

Genus of 14 species of annuals and tap-rooted perennials from mountainous areas, some species in rocky sites, others in open grassland, in C. and E. Asia. They are cultivated for their exotic terminal racemes or panicles of tubular, trumpet-shaped, 2-lipped flowers, with 5 spreading petals. The flowers are supported on strong stems above the usually alternate, pinnate or pinnatisect leaves. Grow in a mixed or herbaceous border, or in a rock garden.

- **HARDINESS** Fully hardy to frost hardy.
- **CULTIVATION** Grow in fertile, moist but well-drained soil in full sun, with some shade in summer. Does not tolerate excessive winter wet. Plant crowns 8–10cm (3–4in) deep; mulch in areas where ground remains frozen for long periods. Avoid damaging thick, fleshy roots.
- **PROPAGATION** Sow seed in containers in a cold frame in spring or autumn. Keep autumn-sown seedlings frost-free over winter. Seedlings take 3 years to flower except *I. arguta*, which usually flowers the same year. In spring, root basal stem cuttings of perennials, or divide with care.
- **PESTS AND DISEASES** May be attacked by slugs.

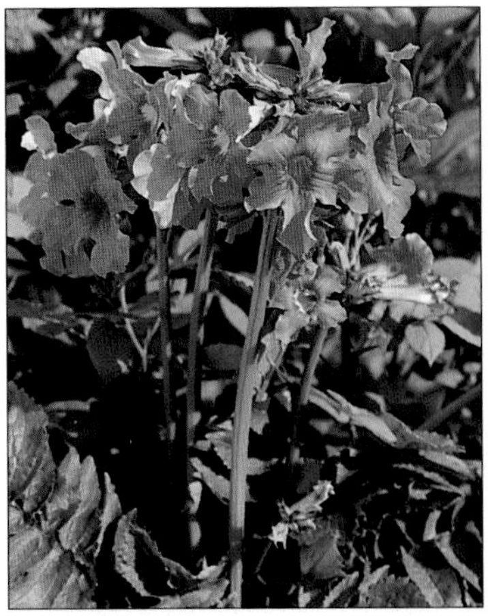

Incarvillea delavayi

I. arguta ■ Erect, woody-based perennial, often grown as an annual, with pinnate, dark green leaves, 5–20cm (2–8in) long, some basal and some arranged alternately on red-tinted stems; the leaflets, in 2–6 opposite pairs, are ovate, lance-shaped, or elliptic, and coarsely toothed. Racemes of 5–20 pendent, tubular, pink or white flowers, to 3.5cm (1½in) long, are produced in early and midsummer. ↕ to 90cm (36in), ↔ 30cm (12in). W. Himalayas to W. China. ❄❄

I. delavayi ■ Tap-rooted perennial with basal rosettes of pinnate, mid-green leaves, to 30cm (12in) long, divided into 6–11 pairs of oblong-lance-shaped, coarsely toothed leaflets, the terminal segment larger. Racemes of up to 10 tubular, widely trumpet-shaped, yellow-throated, deep rose-pink to purple flowers, to 8cm (3in) across, are borne in early and midsummer. ↕60cm (24in), ↔ 30cm (12in). China (Yunnan). ❄❄❄. **'Bee's Pink'** has pale pink flowers, to 10cm (4in) across; ↕30–45cm (12–18in), ↔ 20cm (8in).

I. mairei ■ Tap-rooted perennial with basal rosettes of pinnate, wrinkled, dark green leaves, 12–25cm (5–10in) long, composed of 4–7 pairs of ovate to oblong, finely toothed or scalloped leaflets, the terminal segment larger. In early summer, bears few-flowered racemes of widely trumpet-shaped, yellow-throated, purple-crimson flowers, 4–6cm (1½–2½in) across, with white-striped purple marks on the lower lobes. ↕15–50cm (6–20in), ↔ 30cm (12in). Himalayas to W. Nepal, S.W. China. ❄❄❄. **'Frank Ludlow'** has crimson-pink flowers; ↕10cm (4in), ↔ 15cm (6in). **var. *grandiflora*** has leaves with only 1 or 2 pairs of leaflets. Flowers are usually solitary but slightly larger than the species and deeper crimson-pink; ↕10–15cm (4–6in), ↔ 20cm (8in). **'Nyoto Sama'** has smooth leaves; bears large, bright pink flowers, 8cm (3in) across, in late spring; ↔ 15cm (6in).

I. olgae. Tap-rooted, woody-based, subshrubby perennial, with several sparsely branched stems bearing opposite, pinnate, mid-green leaves, 5–15cm (2–6in) long, with 3 or 4 pairs of elliptic, slightly toothed leaflets. Loose racemes of 3–10 tubular, rose-pink or paler pink, sometimes white flowers, to 3.5cm (1½in) across, are produced in early and midsummer. ↕ to 1.2m (4ft), ↔ 30cm (12in). Turkestan, Afghanistan. ❄❄❄

▷**Incense cedar, Chilean** see *Austrocedrus chilensis*
▷**Incense plant** see *Calomeria, C. amaranthoides, Olearia moschata*
▷**Inch plant, Striped** see *Callisia elegans*
▷**Indian blanket** see *Gaillardia pulchella*
▷**Indian physic** see *Gillenia trifoliata*
▷**Indian root** see *Asclepias curassavica*
▷**Indian shot plant** see *Canna*
▷**India rubber fig** see *Ficus elastica*
▷**India rubber tree** see *Ficus elastica*
▷**Indigo,**
Bastard see *Amorpha fruticosa*
False see *Baptisia*
Wild see *Baptisia*

INDIGOFERA

LEGUMINOSAE/PAPILIONACEAE

Genus of 700 or more species of evergreen or deciduous trees and shrubs, annuals, and herbaceous perennials, widely distributed in mainly tropical and subtropical regions worldwide, in a variety of habitats. They are grown for their small, pea-like flowers and elegant foliage. The flowers are rarely solitary, often borne in loose or dense, terminal or axillary racemes or spikes. The usually pinnate leaves are arranged alternately. Grow in a shrub border or train against a warm, sunny wall; low-growing species are useful in rock gardens.

- **HARDINESS** Fully hardy to frost hardy.
- **CULTIVATION** Grow in moderately fertile, moist but well-drained soil in full sun. Pruning group 1, or 13 if wall-trained; pruning group 6 or 7 in areas with severe winters.

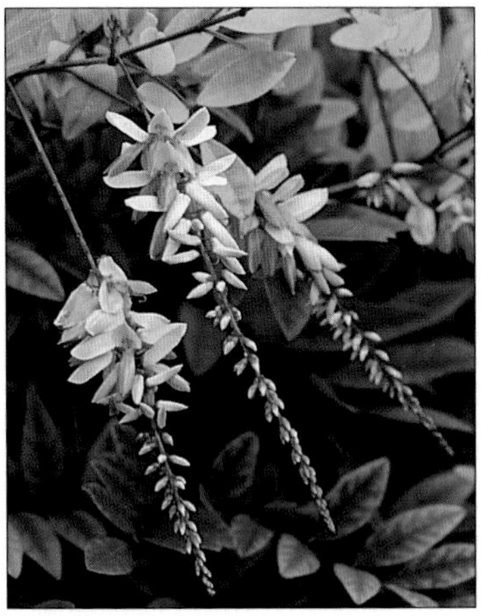

Indigofera decora

- **PROPAGATION** Sow seed in containers in a cold frame in autumn. Root basal cuttings in spring, greenwood cuttings in late spring, and semi-ripe cuttings in early or midsummer.
- **PESTS AND DISEASES** Trouble free.

I. amblyantha ■ 🏆 Deciduous shrub bearing pinnate leaves, to 15cm (6in) long, divided into 7–11 narrowly ovate, bright green leaflets. Produces slender, upright racemes, to 11cm (4½in) long, of small, pea-like pink flowers, to 6mm (¼in) across, from summer to early autumn. ↕2m (6ft), ↔ 2.5m (8ft). China. ❄❄❄

I. decora ■ Spreading deciduous shrub with arching branches bearing pinnate leaves, to 20cm (8in) long, each with 7–13 narrowly oblong, glossy, dark green leaflets. Erect racemes, to 20cm (8in) long, of pea-like white flowers, heavily suffused pale crimson, to 2cm (¾in) across, are produced in mid- and late summer. Suitable for a rock garden. ↕ to 60cm (24in), ↔ 90cm (36in). China, Japan. ❄❄

I. dielsiana ■ Upright, open shrub with pinnate, dark green leaves, to 12cm (5in) long, each with 7–11 pairs of oval leaflets. Bears erect racemes, to 15cm (6in) long, of pea-like, pale pink flowers, 1.5cm (½in) across, from early summer to early autumn. ↕↔ 1.5m (5ft). S.W. China. ❄❄

I. gerardiana see *I. heterantha.*

I. hebepetala. Upright shrub with pinnate, mid-green leaves, 15–20cm (6–8in) long, each with 7–13 elliptic, elliptic-oblong, or rarely ovate leaflets, softly hairy beneath. In late summer

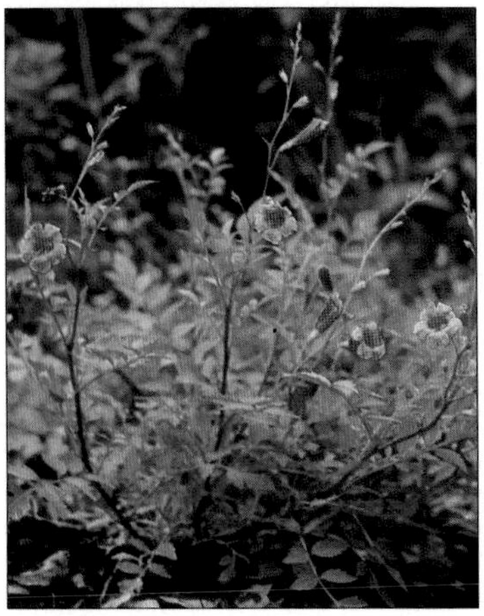

Incarvillea arguta

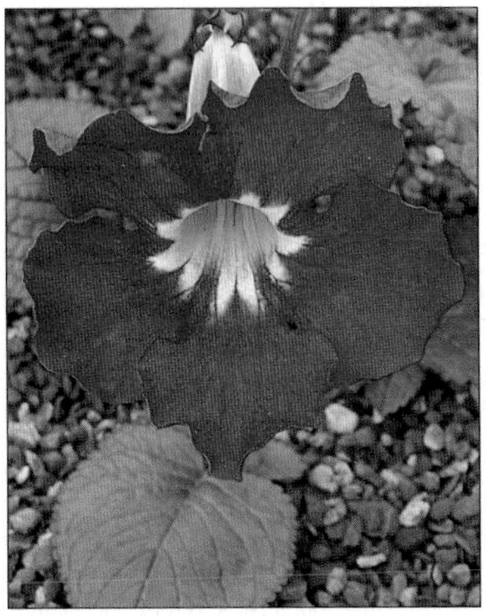

Incarvillea mairei

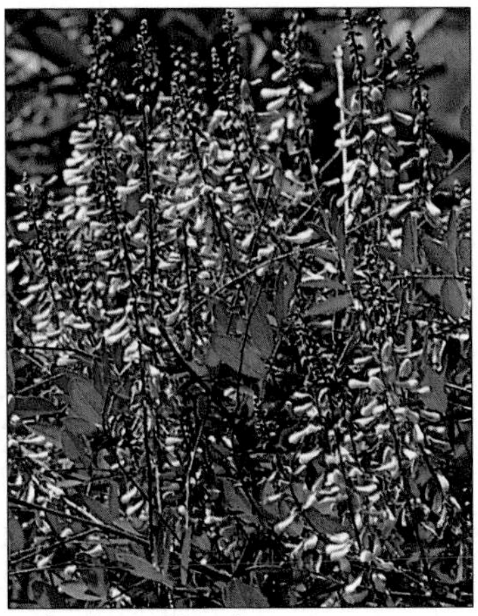

Indigofera amblyantha

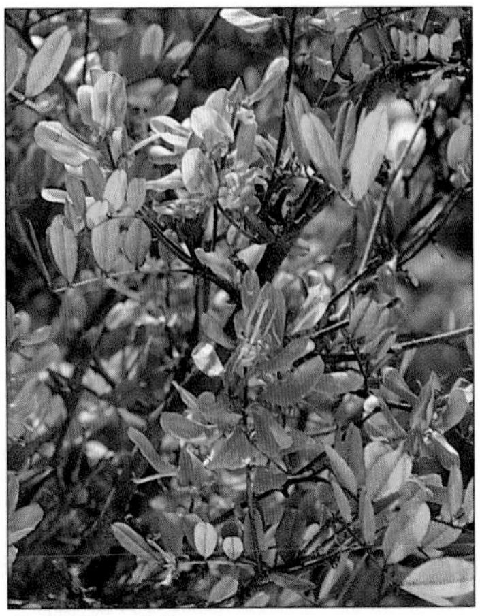

Indigofera dielsiana

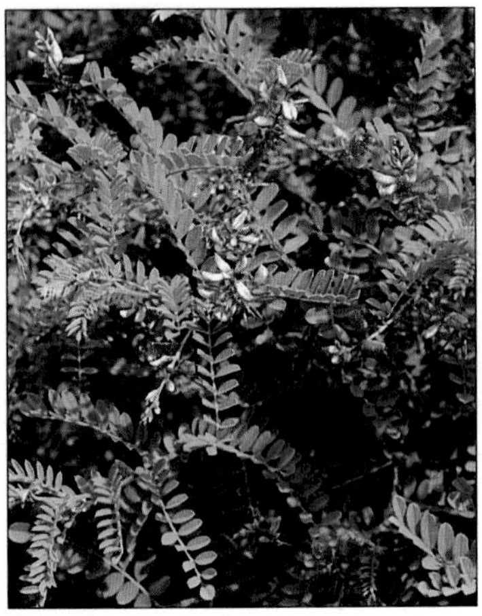

Indigofera heterantha

and early autumn, produces racemes, 7–20cm (3–8in) long, of pea-like, dark carmine-red flowers, 1.5cm (½in) across. ↕ 1.8m (6ft), ↕ 1m (3ft). Himalayas. ❄❄❄

I. heterantha ■ 🏆 syn. *I. gerardiana.* Spreading shrub with arching branches and pinnate, grey-green leaves, to 10cm (4in) long, with up to 21 obovate to oval leaflets. From early summer to early autumn, bears dense, erect racemes, to 15cm (6in) long, of pea-like, purple-pink flowers, 1.5cm (½in) across. ↕↔ 2–3m (6–10ft). N.W. Himalayas. ❄❄❄

I. kirilowii. Spreading shrub or subshrub with upright shoots and pinnate, bright green leaves, to 15cm (6in) long, composed of up to 11 broadly ovate to almost diamond-shaped leaflets. In early and midsummer, produces pea-like, rose-pink flowers, to 2cm (¾in) across, in dense, upright racemes, to 13cm (5in) long. ↕ 75cm (30in), ↔ 1m (3ft). N. China, Korea, S. Japan. ❄❄❄

I. potaninii. Spreading shrub with pinnate leaves, to 8cm (3in) long, with 5–9 elliptic-oblong, grey-green leaflets. Produces slender, upright racemes, to 13cm (5in) long, of small, pea-like pink flowers, to 1cm (½in) across, from summer to early autumn. ↕ 2m (6ft), ↔ 2.5m (8ft). S.W. China. ❄❄❄

▷ **Inkberry** see *Ilex glabra*

INULA

ASTERACEAE / COMPOSITAE

Genus of approximately 100 species of herbaceous perennials, some subshrubby, and a few annuals and biennials, from Europe and temperate and subtropical Africa and Asia. They are found in a wide range of habitats from dry, rocky, montane sites to moist, shady, lowland areas; most grow in well-drained, sunny places. They usually have large basal leaves and progressively smaller stem leaves, arranged alternately. The daisy-like flowerheads are flat, with numerous narrow yellow ray-florets and tubular disc-florets. They are solitary or borne in small panicles or corymbs. Low-growing species, such as *I. ensifolia* 'Compacta', are suitable for a rock garden. Tall, robust species, such as *I. magnifica* and *I. racemosa*, are ideal for a wild garden. Grow *I. helenium* in a herb garden. Rhizomatous species may become invasive.

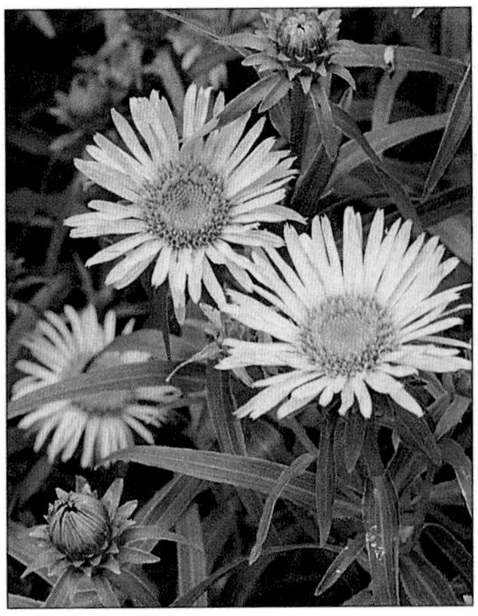

Inula ensifolia

• **HARDINESS** Fully hardy to frost hardy.
• **CULTIVATION** Grow most species in deep, fertile, moist but well-drained soil in full sun. *I. magnifica* will grow in boggy conditions, *I. helenium* tolerates partial shade, and *I. hookeri* prefers partial shade. Taller species may need support.
• **PROPAGATION** Sow seed in containers in a cold frame in spring or autumn. Divide perennials in spring or autumn.
• **PESTS AND DISEASES** Powdery mildew may be a problem if growing conditions are too dry.

***I. afghanica* of gardens** see *I. magnifica.*

I. ensifolia ■ Dense, bushy, slender-stemmed, rhizomatous perennial. Bears stalkless, linear-lance-shaped or lance-shaped, entire, mid-green leaves, to 9cm (3½in) long, with finely hairy margins. In mid- and late summer, abundant golden yellow flowerheads, 2–3cm (¾–1¼in) or more across, are produced singly or in small corymbs. ↕ 25–60cm (10–24in), ↔ 30cm (12in). Caucasus. ❄❄❄. **'Compacta'** is a dwarf cultivar with deep golden yellow flowerheads; suitable for a rock garden; ↕ to 15cm (6in).

I. glandulosa see *I. orientalis.*

I. helenium (Elecampane). Robust, rhizomatous perennial with stout, furrowed, downy stems bearing basal rosettes of ovate or ovate-elliptic, toothed, mid-green leaves, to 80cm (32in) long, densely woolly beneath and with wavy margins. Bright yellow flowerheads, to 8cm (3in) across, are produced singly or in lax corymbs in mid- and late summer. Roots are used

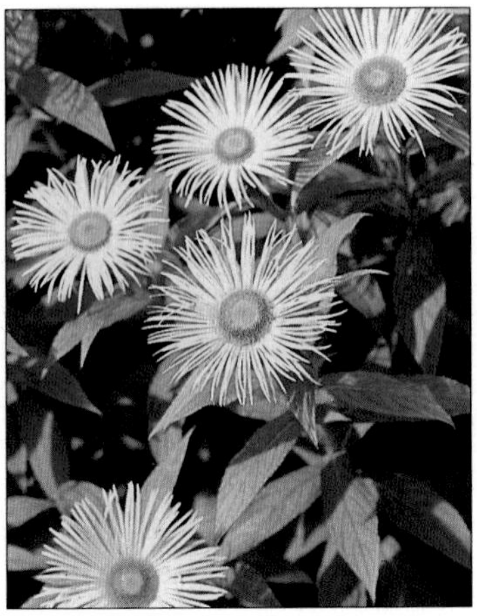

Inula hookeri

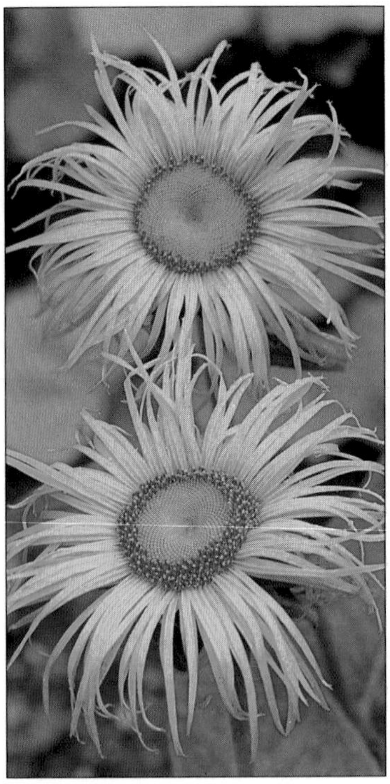

Inula royleana

medicinally as an expectorant. ↕ 0.9–2m (3–6ft), ↔ 90cm (36in). Europe to W. Asia. ❄❄❄

I. hookeri ■ Clump-forming perennial with creeping roots and numerous willowy, softly hairy stems bearing ovate to oblong-lance-shaped, minutely toothed, hairy, mid-green leaves, 8–15cm (3–6in) long. Pale yellow flowerheads, 4–8cm (1½–3in) across, are borne singly or in clusters of 2 or 3, with narrow ray-florets, brownish yellow disc-florets, and broad, very hairy involucral bracts, from late summer to mid-autumn. ↕ 60–75cm (24–30in), ↔ 60cm (24in) or more. Himalayas. ❄❄❄

***I. macrocephala* of gardens** see *I. royleana.*

I. magnifica, syn. *I. afghanica* of gardens. Robust, clump-forming perennial bearing hairy stems, with dark purple streaks along their lengths, and elliptic-ovate, dark green leaves, to 25cm (10in) long, softly hairy beneath. In late summer, bears corymbs of 8–20 bright golden yellow flowerheads, to 15cm (6in) across. ↕ to 1.8m (6ft), ↔ 1m (3ft). E. Caucasus. ❄❄❄

I. oculis-christi. Rhizomatous perennial with erect, hairy stems bearing inversely lance-shaped, entire or toothed, downy, mid-green leaves, to 15cm (6in) long. Corymbs of usually 3–5 bright golden yellow flowerheads, to 7cm (3in) across, with very downy involucres, are produced in mid- and late summer. ↕ to 50cm (20in), ↔ 60cm (24in). E. Europe, Turkey, Caucasus, N. Iraq, Iran. ❄❄❄

I. orientalis, syn. *I. glandulosa.* Rhizomatous perennial producing erect stems, with yellowish brown glandular hairs, bearing ovate-elliptic or inversely lance-shaped, toothed, hairy, mid-green leaves, 12cm (5in) long. Solitary, orange-yellow flowerheads, 9cm (3½in) across, with very woolly buds and wavy ray-florets, are produced in summer. ↕ 60–90cm (24–36in), ↔ 60cm (24in). Caucasus. ❄❄❄

I. racemosa. Robust, clump-forming perennial with red-marked stems and rough, elliptic-lance-shaped to lance-shaped, toothed, mid-green basal leaves, 45cm (18in) or more long, and deeply lobed at the bases. The progressively smaller stem leaves are densely woolly beneath and stalkless near each apex. From late summer to mid-autumn, bears long racemes of usually solitary, light yellow flowerheads, 3.5–6cm (1½–2½in) across, with narrow ray-florets and darker yellow disc-florets. Roots are used medicinally. ↕ to 2.5m (8ft), ↔ 1.5m (5ft). W. Himalayas. ❄❄❄

I. royleana ■ syn. *I. macrocephala* of gardens. Upright, clump-forming perennial with dark green stems and ovate, prominently veined, slightly toothed, hairy, mid-green leaves, 25cm (10in) long, with winged stalks. Solitary, orange-yellow flowerheads, 10–12cm (4–5in) across, with slightly darker orange disc-florets, are borne from midsummer to early autumn, opening from black-brown buds. ↕ 45–60cm (18–24in), ↔ 45cm (18in). W. Himalayas. ❄❄❄

IOCHROMA

SOLANACEAE

Genus of 20 species of evergreen or deciduous shrubs and small trees from moist forest areas, particularly clearings and margins, in tropical Central and South America. Leaves are alternate, simple, and entire. They are grown for their nodding to pendent, trumpet-shaped to tubular, purple, blue, red, white, or yellow flowers, produced in clusters or pairs. The fruits are pulpy berries; each one is enclosed by an enlarged calyx. In frost-prone areas, grow in a temperate greenhouse. In warmer climates, grow in a shrub border or as free-standing specimens.
• **HARDINESS** Frost tender.
• **CULTIVATION** Under glass, grow in loam-based potting compost (JI No.2) in bright to moderate filtered light. During growth, water moderately and apply a balanced liquid fertilizer every month. Keep just moist in winter. Pinch young plants to encourage bushiness. Top-dress mature plants with fresh compost annually in spring. Outdoors, grow in fertile, moist but well-drained soil in full sun or partial shade, with shelter from cold, drying winds. Pruning group 9; group 12 for scandent shrubs,

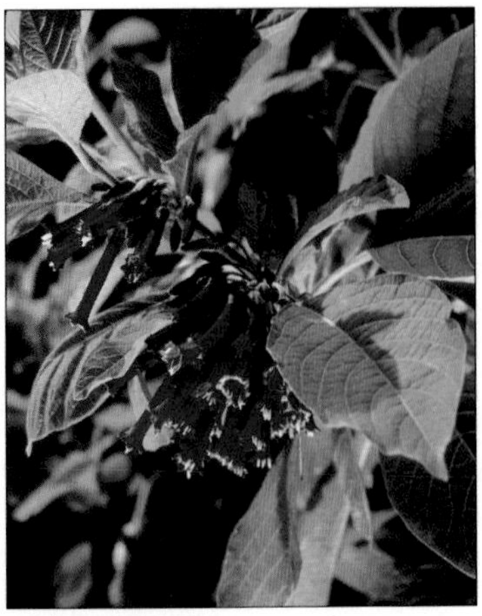

Iochroma cyanea

after flowering; plants under glass may need restrictive pruning in late winter.

• **PROPAGATION** Sow seed at 13–18°C (55–64°F) in spring. Root greenwood cuttings in late spring or semi-ripe cuttings in summer.

• **PESTS AND DISEASES** Red spider mites and whiteflies may be troublesome under glass.

I. coccinea. Lax shrub with downy stems and ovate to oblong, sharp-pointed, prominently veined, lustrous, rich green leaves, 8–13cm (3–5in) long. Clusters of up to 8 tubular scarlet flowers, 4–5cm (1½–2in) long, with light yellow throats, appear mainly during summer. ↕ to 3m (10ft), ↔ 1.5–2m (5–6ft). Central America. ❀ (min. 7°C/45°F)

I. cyanea ▣ syn. *I. tubulosa.* Erect to spreading shrub with downy shoots and narrowly ovate to oblong-lance-shaped or elliptic, softly hairy, grey green leaves, 8–15cm (3–6in) long. Umbel-like trusses of up to 20 tubular, deep purple-blue flowers, 5cm (2in) long, with partly reflexed petal tips, are produced mainly in summer. ↕ to 3m (10ft), ↔ 1.5–2m (5–6ft). Colombia, Ecuador, Peru. ❀ (min. 7°C/45°F)

I. tubulosa see *I. cyanea.*

IPHEION

ALLIACEAE/LILIACEAE

Genus of 10 species of small, bulbous perennials from upland meadows and rocky sites in South America. They are grown for their star-shaped, usually strongly honey-scented flowers borne in spring, singly or in pairs. The grass-like, basal leaves are linear-strap-shaped. Most parts smell of onions when crushed, particularly the leaves. They are useful in a rock garden and for underplanting herbaceous plants such as peonies or hostas. In areas of prolonged frost, grow in a cold greenhouse or alpine house.

• **HARDINESS** Frost hardy to frost tender. *I. uniflorum* is hardy to -10°C (14°F), but may be damaged if exposed to prolonged frost.

• **CULTIVATION** Under glass, grow in loam-based potting compost (JI No.2), with added leaf mould and grit, in bright filtered or indirect light. During growth in spring and early summer, water moderately and apply a balanced liquid fertilizer monthly. Keep just moist while dormant. Outdoors, grow in moderately fertile, humus-rich, moist but well-drained soil in full sun. Provide a protective mulch in winter where temperatures regularly fall below -10°C (14°F). Plant bulbs 8cm (3in) deep, 5cm (2in) apart, in autumn.

• **PROPAGATION** Sow seed in containers in a cold frame as soon as ripe or in spring. Divide in summer when dormant.

• **PESTS AND DISEASES** Slugs and snails can be a problem.

***I.* 'Rolf Fiedler'** 🏆 syn. *Tristagma* 'Rolf Fiedler'. Clump-forming, bulbous perennial with short, narrowly strap-shaped, blunt-tipped, light blue-green leaves, to 15cm (6in) long. In spring, produces solitary, occasionally 2, outward-facing, star-shaped, scented, vivid mid-blue flowers, 3cm (1¼in) across. ↕ 10–12cm (4–5in). ✻✻

I. uniflorum, syn. *Tristagma uniflorum.* Vigorous, clump-forming, bulbous perennial. In late autumn, produces semi-erect, narrowly strap-shaped, light blue-green leaves, to 25cm (10in) long. Flowers are solitary, upward-facing, star-shaped, scented, pale silvery blue, 4cm (1½in) across, frequently with darker midribs, produced mainly in spring. ↕ 15–20cm (6–8in). Argentina, Uruguay. ✻✻. **'Album'** has pure white flowers. **'Froyle Mill'** 🏆 has dusky violet flowers. **'Wisley Blue'** ▣ 🏆 has lilac-blue flowers.

IPOMOEA syn. MINA, PHARBITIS

Morning glory

CONVOLVULACEAE

Genus of about 500 species of annuals and perennials, many of them trailers or twining climbers, and a few evergreen shrubs and trees, native to warm regions worldwide. They are found in a great diversity of habitats from open scrub to dense woodland, seashores and cliffs. Leaves are alternate, and may be simple and entire, or toothed, lobed, or more finely dissected. The funnel-shaped or tubular flowers are solitary or borne in axillary or terminal cymes, racemes, or panicles. Grow annuals in a sunny, sheltered site. Where temperatures drop below 7°C (45°F), grow perennial or shrubby species in a temperate or warm greenhouse. In warmer areas, train climbers over a pergola or arch, or use them as dense ground cover. Seeds are highly toxic if ingested.

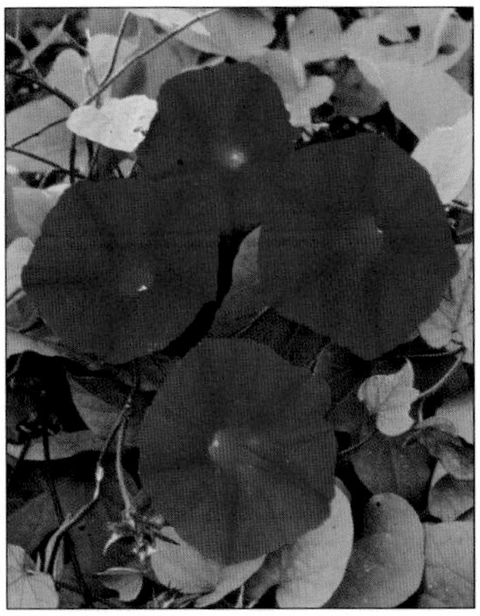

Ipomoea indica

• **HARDINESS** Frost tender.

• **CULTIVATION** Under glass, grow in loam-based potting compost (JI No.2 or 3) in full light, with shade from the hottest sun. During growth, water freely, and apply a balanced liquid fertilizer monthly. Water sparingly in winter. Support climbers and trailing species. Outdoors, grow in moderately fertile, well-drained soil in full sun. Shelter from cold, drying winds. Pruning group 11 for climbing species, in spring.

• **PROPAGATION** Sow seed singly at 18°C (64°F) in spring. Chip seeds or soak for 24 hours before sowing. For perennials and subshrubs, root softwood cuttings in spring or summer, or semi-ripe cuttings in summer.

• **PESTS AND DISEASES** Susceptible to viruses and powdery mildew. Whiteflies and red spider mites may be a problem under glass.

I. acuminata see *I. indica.*

I. alba, syn. *Calonyction aculeatum, I. bona-nox,* (Belle de nuit, Moonflower). Twining perennial, usually grown as an annual, with evergreen, ovate to rounded, sometimes 3-lobed, mid- to deep green leaves, 10–20cm (4–8in) long. Cymes of 1–8 wide-spreading, trumpet-shaped, white flowers, 12–14cm (5–5½in) across, tinted green outside, open at dusk from early summer to autumn. ↕ to 5m (15ft), to 20m (70ft) when grown as a perennial. Tropical regions worldwide. ❀ (min. 7°C/45°F). **'Giant White'** has large white flowers, to 15cm (6in) across.

I. bona-nox see *I. alba.*

I. coccinea ▣ syn. *Quamoclit coccinea* (Red morning glory, Star morning glory). Annual twining climber with entire or boldly toothed, ovate, mid- to deep green leaves, 7–14cm (3–5½in) long. Bears racemes of 3–8 scarlet flowers, to 2cm (¾in) across, with yellow throats, in summer. ↕ 2–4m (6–12ft). S.E. USA. ❀ (min. 7°C/45°F)

I. hederacea, syn. *Pharbitis hederacea.* Annual twining climber with slender, densely hairy stems and ovate to rounded, usually 3-lobed, mid- to deep green leaves, 5–12cm (2–5in) long, with tapering points. In summer, bears cymes of 2–5 funnel-shaped, blue, sometimes purple flowers, 2–3.5cm (¾–1½in) across, with white tubes and prominent, long-tailed, green sepals. Often confused with *I. nil,* which has very narrowly triangular sepals. ↕ 2–3m (6–10ft). S. USA to Argentina. ❀ (min. 7°C/45°F)

I. imperialis see *I. nil.*

I. indica ▣ 🏆 syn. *I. acuminata, I. learii* (Blue dawn flower). Vigorous, perennial climber, bearing evergreen, heart-shaped or 3-lobed, slender-pointed, mid-green leaves, 6–17cm (2½–7in) long. Bears abundant funnel-shaped, rich purple-blue to blue flowers, 6–8cm (2½–3½in) across, in cymes of 3–5, often maturing to purplish red, from late spring to autumn. ↕ 6m (20ft) or more. Tropical regions worldwide. ❀ (min. 7°C/45°F)

I. learii see *I. indica.*

I. lobata ▣ syn. *I. versicolor, Quamoclit lobata* (Spanish flag). Perennial climber, grown as an annual, with crimson-flushed stems and stalks. Bears toothed, mid- to deep green leaves, to 10cm (4in) long, with 3 prominent, finger-like lobes and 2–4 smaller basal lobes. Dense, erect, one-sided racemes, to 30cm (12in) long, of slightly curved, narrow, tubular, scarlet flowers, 1.5–2cm (½–¾in) long, maturing to orange and yellow, then white, with very long stamens and styles, appear from summer to autumn, or throughout the year in warm climates. ↕ 2–5m (6–15ft). Mexico, Central to South America. ❀ (min. 10°C/50°F)

I. x multifida (*I. coccinea* x *I. quamoclit*), syn. *I.* x *sloteri* (Cardinal climber). Slender, twining annual with broadly triangular-ovate, deeply and narrowly 3- to 7-lobed, mid-green leaves, 4–12cm (1½–5in) long, divided into 7–15 narrowly lance-shaped lobes. In summer, bears salverform crimson flowers, to 2.5cm (1in) across, with white throats. ↕ 1–2m (3–6ft). Garden origin. ❀ (min. 7°C/45°F)

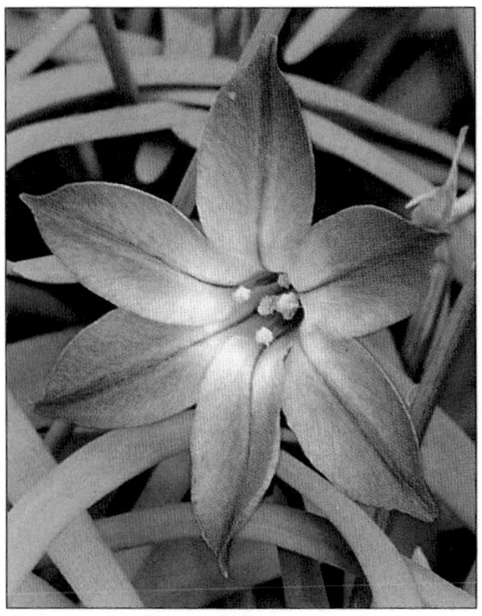

Ipheion uniflorum 'Wisley Blue'

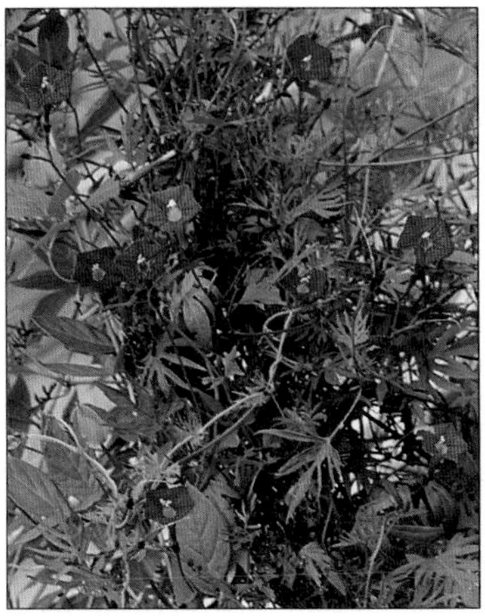

Ipomoea coccinea

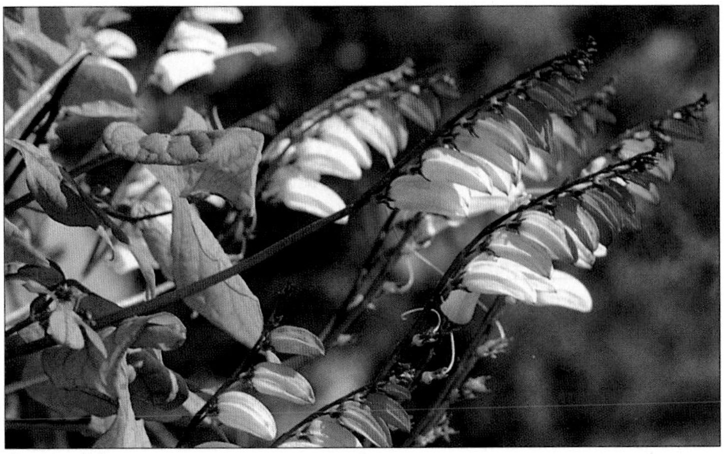

Ipomoea lobata

I

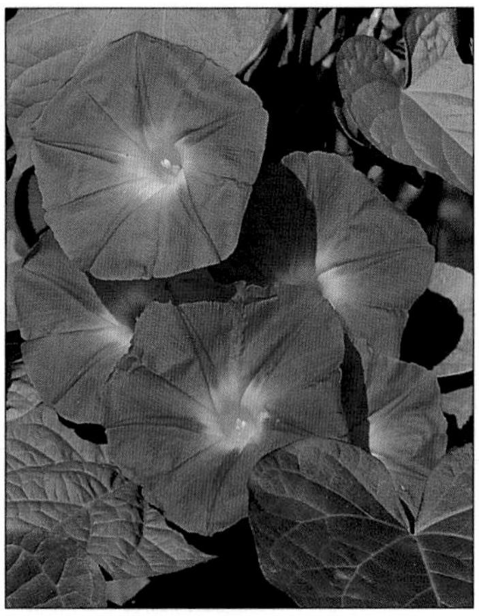

Ipomoea purpurea

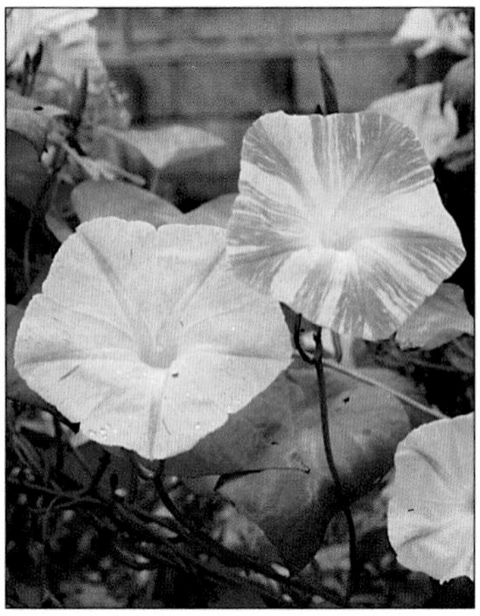

Ipomoea tricolor 'Flying Saucers'

I. nil, syn. *I. imperialis*. Vigorous annual or, in tropical climates, woody-based, short-lived, perennial climber, with bristly yellow-hairy stems. Bears broadly ovate, usually entire, sometimes 3-lobed, mid-green leaves, 5–14cm (2–5½in) long. From summer to autumn, bears solitary, funnel-shaped, white-tubed flowers, 5cm (2in) across, with pale to deep blue, sometimes purple or red petal lobes. ↕ to 5m (15ft) or more. Tropical regions worldwide. ❄ (min. 7°C/45°F). **'Chocolate'** has reddish chocolate-brown flowers, 8cm (3in) across. **'Early Call'** produces white-tubed flowers with scarlet lobes, to 7cm (3in) across. **Platycodon Series** cultivars have single and semi-double, red, purple, or white flowers. **'Scarlet Star'** bears many cerise flowers with central white stars. **'Scarlett O'Hara'** has bright red flowers.
I. purpurea ◼ syn. *Convolvulus purpureus, Pharbitis purpurea* (Common morning glory). Annual twining climber with slender, hairy, and bristly stems. Leaves are broadly ovate, entire or 3-lobed, mid-green, 4–10cm (1½–4in) long. Trumpet-shaped flowers, to 6cm (2½in) across, in pink, purple-blue, magenta, or white (or stripes of these colours on white), with white tubes, are borne in cymes of 3–7, or singly, mainly in summer. ↕ 2–3m (6–10ft). Probably Mexico. ❄ (min. 7°C/45°F)
I. quamoclit, syn. *Quamoclit pennata* (Star glory). Annual twining climber with hairless stems and elliptic to broadly ovate, deeply pinnatisect, deep green leaves, 3–9cm (1¼–3½in) long, composed of 9–19 pairs of linear lobes. Slender-tubed, scarlet, sometimes white

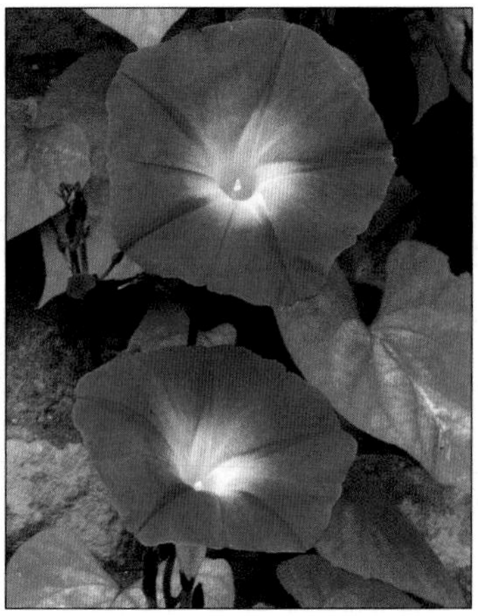

Ipomoea tricolor 'Heavenly Blue'

flowers, to 2cm (¾in) across, with 5 distinct and spreading lobes, are borne in cymes of 2–5, mainly in summer, or for most of the year in the tropics. ↕ 2–6m (6–20ft). Tropical South America. ❄ (min. 7°C/45°F)
I. rubrocaerulea see *I. tricolor*.
I.* x *sloteri see *I.* x *multifida*.
I. tricolor, syn. *I. rubrocaerulea* (Morning glory). Fast-growing, twining annual or short-lived perennial with ovate-heart-shaped, slender-tipped, light to mid-green leaves, 4–10cm (1½–4in) long. Funnel-shaped, bright sky-blue to purple flowers, to 8cm (3in) across, with white tubes, golden yellow inside at the bases, appear singly or in 3- to 5-flowered cymes in summer and throughout the year in the tropics. Tropical Central and South America. ↕ 3–4m (10–12ft). ❄ (min. 7°C/45°F). **'Crimson Rambler'** has red flowers with white throats. **'Flying Saucers'** ◼ has variably marbled, white and purple-blue flowers. **'Heavenly Blue'** ◼♀ has rich azure flowers with white throats. **'Roman Candy'** has cerise and white flowers and white-variegated leaves.
I. tuberosa see *Merremia tuberosa*.
I. versicolor see *I. lobata*.

IRESINE

AMARANTHACEAE

Genus of about 80 species of evergreen, erect or climbing perennials, annuals, and subshrubs from dry, open areas in South America and Australia. They are cultivated for their striking, colourful foliage and are often grown to provide contrast with flowering plants. The leaves are opposite, simple, and entire. The insignificant white or green flowers are borne in terminal or axillary spikes. In frost-prone areas, grow as tender perennials for summer bedding schemes and overwinter in a warm greenhouse. In warmer climates, grow as edging in a bed or mixed border, in a window-box, or in a container on a patio.

- **HARDINESS** Frost tender.
- **CULTIVATION** Under glass, grow in loam-based potting compost (JI No.2) in full light, with shade from the hottest sun. During the growing season, water freely and apply a balanced liquid fertilizer every 4 weeks. Water sparingly in winter. Outdoors, grow in fertile, moist but well-drained soil, in full sun for best leaf colour. Pinch back young plants in spring to encourage bushiness. Cut back mature plants hard in early spring, or propagate each year to maintain bushy specimens, and plant out after all danger of frost has passed.
- **PROPAGATION** Take stem-tip cuttings at any time. In frost-prone areas, take stem-tip cuttings of bedding plants in late summer. Overwinter in a warm greenhouse and pinch out 2 or 3 times to produce strong stock plants, which will provide softwood cuttings in late winter and early spring.
- **PESTS AND DISEASES** Prone to powdery mildew. Susceptible to aphids and red spider mites, particularly under glass.

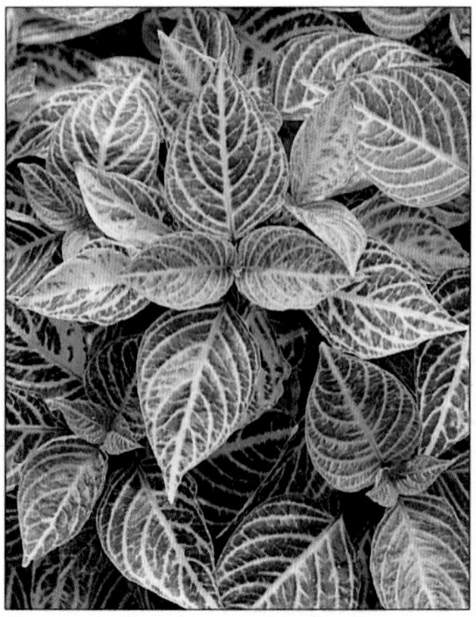

Iresine herbstii 'Aureoreticulata'

I. herbstii (Beefsteak plant). Erect, bushy annual or short-lived perennial with broadly ovate to rounded, waxy, variegated, mid-green, yellow, very deep red, or orange leaves, to 8cm (3in) long, often with vividly contrasting veins and golden hairs beneath, and with notches at the tips. Stems and branches are bright green, purple, or red, and almost translucent when young. ↕ to 1.5m (5ft), ↔ to 90cm (36in). Brazil. ❄ (min. 10°C/50°F). **'Aureoreticulata'** ◼ has mid-green leaves with yellow veins. **'Brilliantissima'** ◼ has rich crimson leaves. **'Wallisii'** is dwarf, with purple-black leaves; ↕ to 60cm (24in), ↔ to 50cm (20in).
I. lindenii ♀ (Blood leaf). Erect, bushy, compact perennial with blood-red stems bearing ovate or oblong-lance-shaped, pointed, glossy, deep blood-red leaves, 5–10cm (2–4in) long, with prominent deep or light red veins. ↕↔ to 1m (3ft). Ecuador. ❄ (min. 10°C/50°F). **'Formosa'** has yellow leaves with crimson veins.

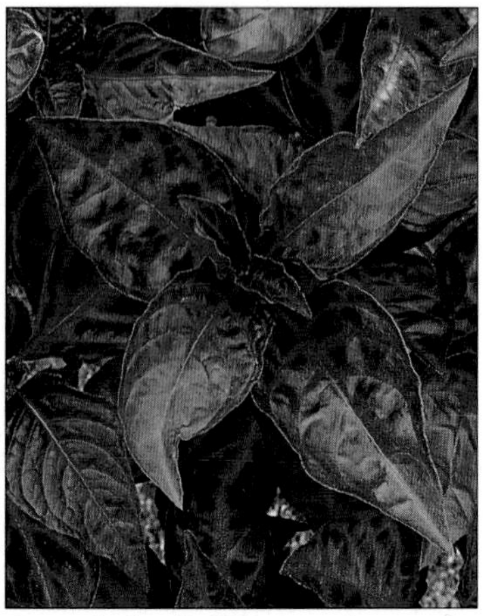

Iresine herbstii 'Brilliantissima'

IRIS

IRIDACEAE

Genus of about 300 species of upright, rhizomatous or bulbous, sometimes fleshy-rooted perennials found in a wide range of habitats in the N. hemisphere. Irises are grown mainly for their colourful, often spectacular flowers. A few are evergreen, but most are deciduous, dying back completely or to a fan of short leaves. Some are dormant in summer. The distinctive iris flowers are illustrated and described in the accompanying panel (see opposite). The seed pods are 3- to 6-angled, either ribbed or smooth, with large seeds.

Most irises flower from spring to summer. Some, mostly bearded hybrids, are "remontant", flowering again in the same year, but they need extra care if they are to succeed reliably in cool climates. Taller irises are suitable for a mixed or herbaceous border. Smaller species and cultivars, and those requiring very free-draining conditions, can be grown in a rock garden, raised bed, or trough. Those requiring a totally dry dormancy period should be grown in a bulb frame or alpine house. A few are not frost hardy and require glass protection. All parts may cause severe discomfort if ingested; contact with the sap may irritate skin.

Botanically, irises are divided into several subgenera and sections. In horticulture, these are often simplified as below and in the table opposite.

Rhizomatous irises
These have rhizomes as rootstocks, close to or on the surface, or just below ground level, which produce linear to strap-shaped, sometimes curved leaves, often in basal fans. Each active rhizome produces several new growths every year and this spread can continue indefinitely. As a rough guide, in 3 years a small iris can attain a spread of 30cm (12in), and a tall one a spread of 60cm (24in). Rhizomatous irises fall into 3 main groups.
Bearded irises – also known as Pogon irises, these have stout, surface rhizomes, giving rise to fans of sword-shaped, usually broad leaves, and simple or branched stems. The flowers, produced in a large range of colours, have well-developed falls and standards, with a prominent "beard" of white or coloured hairs in the centre of each fall petal. Bearded hybrids are the most widely grown group in horticulture. They may be classified for garden use or exhibition according to the blooming season (early spring to early summer) and the height of the flower stem, as follows. Most bear multiple flowers per stem.
Miniature dwarf bearded: ↕ to 20cm (8in); flowers 4–8cm (1½–3in) across.
Standard dwarf bearded: ↕ 20–40cm (8–16in); flowers 5–7cm (2–3in) across.
Intermediate bearded: ↕ 40–70cm (16–28in); flowers 10–13cm (4–5in) across.
Miniature tall bearded: ↕ 40–65cm (16–26in) (zigzag stem); flowers 5–8cm (2–3in) across.
Border bearded: ↕ 40–70cm (16–28in); flowers 10–13cm (4–5in) across.
Tall bearded: ↕ 70cm (28in) or more; flowers 10–20cm (4–8in) across.

Aril irises are so called because of the white protrusion, or aril, on each seed. They become dormant in summer after flowering, and should be kept dry during this period. The main groups are the Oncocyclus and the closely related Regelia irises, and their cultivars and hybrids. **Oncocyclus** irises bear large, brightly coloured flowers with bearded falls. **Regelia** irises have bearded falls and standards. **Regeliocyclus** irises are hybrids between Oncocyclus and Regelia irises. **Arilbred** irises are hybrids between Oncocyclus or Regelia irises and other bearded irises.

Beardless irises **(Limniris)** – also have rhizomes but these are often just below ground. The fall petals on the flowers are smooth. Beardless irises include the following widely differing groups. **Pacific Coast** irises produce flowers in a large range of colours, most with attractive veining. Leaves are usually evergreen. **Siberian** irises bear blue, purple, white, yellow, or deep red flowers, and are suitable for an open border. Leaves are usually deciduous. **Spuria** irises produce flowers in a large range of colours, and have 6-ribbed seed pods with distinctive curved beaks. **Laevigatae** irises, also known as water irises, thrive in damp places. The group includes *I. laevigata* and *I. pseudacorus*, the common yellow flag iris of Europe. Stems are simple or branched, and bear blue, pink, red, purple, white, or yellow flowers. Also included in Laevigatae irises are the numerous cultivars of *I. ensata*, syn. *I. kaempferi*, known as Japanese irises, which flourish at the margins of ponds or streams, or in moist borders. Japanese irises bear large, often flattened, sometimes double flowers, in shades of blue, white, purple, pink, sometimes yellow, or deep red, often in combination. **Louisiana** irises also thrive in damp conditions, often have zigzag stems, and bear flowers in a large range of colours. **Unguiculares** irises are markedly different from other beardless irises: they develop a mass of rhizomes above ground, are evergreen, and bloom from autumn to spring, producing blue, violet, lavender-pink, or white, almost stemless flowers with long perianth tubes.

Irises in the miscellaneous subgroups of the beardless irises not listed here are referred to in their entries simply as "rhizomatous, beardless irises".

Crested irises **(Lophiris)** – also known as Evansia irises, these spread freely by rhizomes, and produce relatively flat flowers in shades of blue, violet, or white. They have a crest or ridge on each fall instead of a beard. Flowers and leaves, which are deciduous to evergreen, may be borne on bamboo-like stems, which vary greatly in height.

IRIS FLOWERS

The flowers have 3 large, pendent, reflexed or spreading outer petals ("falls"), which in some species have conspicuous beards or crests, and 3 frequently smaller, erect, horizontal or sometimes pendent inner petals ("standards"). There are 3 stamens, and the style has 3 usually petal-like branches arching over the falls; these enclose the stigmas and are known as "stigma flaps".

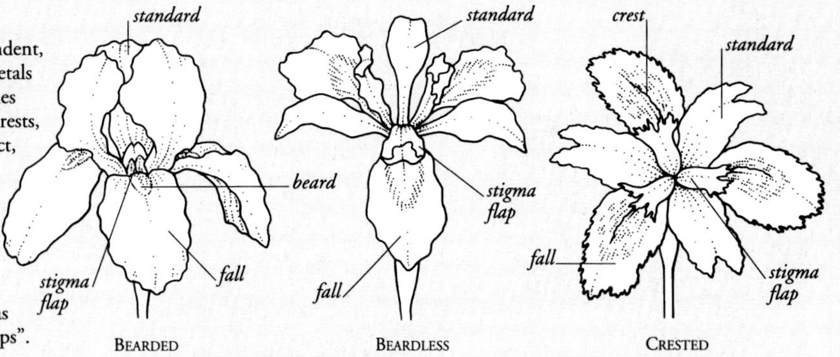

Bulbous irises

These have bulbs as storage organs; Juno irises also have fleshy roots. Leaves are deciduous, and either channelled or quadrangular to almost cylindrical in cross-section. Flowers are beardless and appear from late winter to midsummer. All are summer dormant. Bulbous irises fall into 3 groups. **Reticulata** (Hermodactyloides) irises have netted tunics that cover the bulbs, which produce 1 or 2 long, square-sectioned or cylindrical leaves. The leaf length at flowering is very variable; after flowering, the leaves lengthen to 30cm or more. Flowers are blue, white, or reddish violet. **Juno** (Scorpiris) irises have bulbs with fleshy roots and flat or channelled leaves. The flowers have large, brightly coloured fall petals and very small standards. Some species, such as *I. bucharica*, are good rock garden plants; others, such as *I. magnifica*, do well in a sunny, open border. **Xiphium** irises include the Dutch, English, and Spanish groups, with channelled, linear leaves and blue, lavender-blue, yellow, or white flowers. The English irises prefer more moist soil. Xiphium irises are popular garden plants, widely used as cut flowers; most are easy to grow. Some N. African species are frost tender.

• **HARDINESS** Fully hardy to frost tender. Most irises are hardy, but some thrive only in specific conditions.
• **CULTIVATION** General cultivation advice for irises is outlined here; more specific group requirements are given in the table below. All irises are best

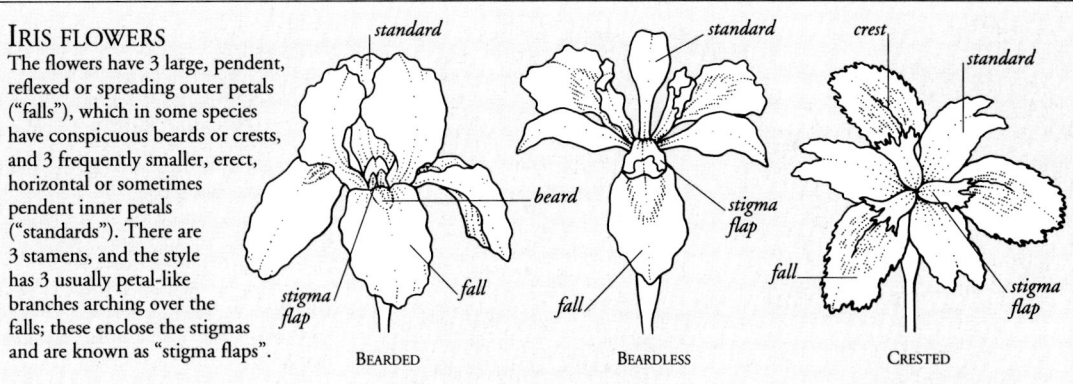

IRIS GROUPS			HEIGHT cm/in	FLOWERS PER STEM	FLOWER SIZE cm/in	FLOWERING TIME	CULTIVATION REQUIREMENTS
RHIZOMATOUS	BEARDED	Species and cultivars	5–50 (2–20)	1 or multiple	2.5–20 (1–8)	mid-spring to early summer	Outdoors, grow in well-drained, fertile, neutral to slightly acid soil in full sun. Under glass, grow in deep containers in loam-based potting compost (JI No.2) with added grit. Provide full light and low humidity. Ventilate freely whenever temperatures rise above freezing. Water moderately when in growth. Keep completely dry during dormancy.
	BEARDED – ARIL	Oncocyclus	10–60 (4–24)	1	5–20 (2–8)	mid- and late spring	
	BEARDED – ARIL	Regelia & Regeliocyclus	10–60 (4–24)	1 or 2	5–10 (2–4)	mid- and late spring	
	BEARDED – ARIL	Arilbred	25–70 (10–28)	2	3 (1¼)	mid-spring to early summer	
	BEARDLESS	Pacific Coast	15–75 (6–30)	multiple	5–10 (2–4)	mid- and late spring	Most beardless irises prefer well-drained, neutral to slightly acid loam in full sun or partial shade. Grow Laevigatae (water irises) in moist to wet, deep, humus-rich, acid soil; they thrive at the margins of ponds or streams. Grow Louisiana irises in damp, humus-rich soil, preferably in areas with high summer temperatures. Grow Unguiculares irises in sharply drained, neutral to alkaline soil in full sun; they are ideal for the base of a sunny wall.
	BEARDLESS	Siberian	30–150 (12–60)	multiple	7–13 (3–5)	mid- and late spring	
	BEARDLESS	Spuria	20–200 (8–72)	multiple	7–15 (3–6)	late spring and early summer	
	BEARDLESS	Laevigatae (water irises)	30–90 (12–36)	multiple	6–25 (2½–10)	late spring and early summer	
	BEARDLESS	Louisiana	40–120 (16–48)	multiple	7–20 (3–8)	mid-spring to early summer	
	BEARDLESS	Unguiculares	5–20 (2–8) (perianth tubes)	1	5–8 (2–3)	autumn to spring	
	CRESTED		5–100 (2–39)	multiple	3–10 (1¼–4)	mid- and late spring	Outdoors, grow in moist, humus-rich soil in full sun or partial shade. Under glass, grow in pans in loam-based potting compost (JI No.2) with added grit and leaf mould. Provide bright filtered light and moderate humidity. Ventilate freely whenever temperatures rise above freezing. Water moderately when in growth. Keep just moist during dormancy.
BULBOUS	Reticulata		5–15 (2–6)	1 or 2	3–8 (1¼–3)	winter to early spring	Outdoors, grow in well-drained, neutral or slightly alkaline soil in full sun. Under glass, grow in deep containers in loam-based potting compost (JI No.2) with added grit. Provide full light and low humidity. Ventilate freely whenever temperatures rise above freezing. Water moderately when in growth. Keep just moist during dormancy. When planting or transplanting, take care not to damage the fleshy roots of Juno irises.
	Juno		5–45 (2–18)	multiple	5–10 (2–4)	early spring	
	Xiphium		25–90 (10–36)	1, 2 or multiple	7–9 (3–3½)	mid-spring to midsummer	

I

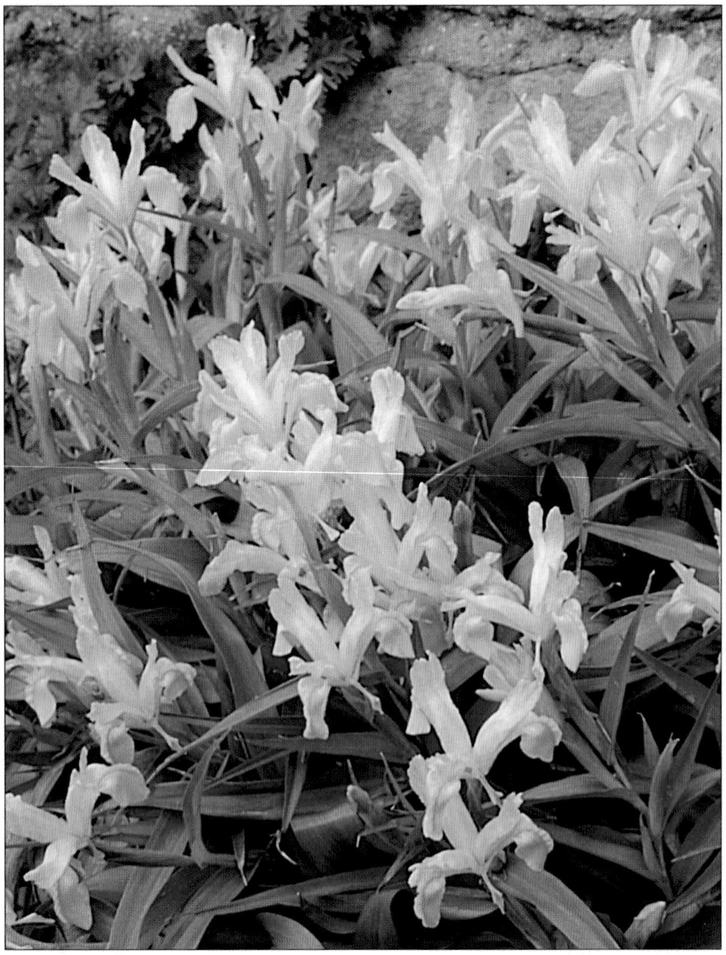

Iris bucharica

planted in late summer and early autumn. Outdoors, grow in well-drained, moderately fertile, neutral or slightly acid or alkaline soil in full sun to light dappled shade. Most irises need long, hot summers to thrive and flower well. Grow irises that require protection from rain or frost under glass.

Rhizomatous irises – Bearded irises have surface rhizomes which should be partially exposed, or thinly covered with soil in hot climates. Plant rhizomes singly or in groups of 3 with the fans outermost, 15–30cm (6–12in) apart, depending on size. They must not be shaded by other plants; many do best in a border on their own. When planting, feed or top-dress with a low-nitrogen fertilizer, and again in early spring. Avoid applying high-nitrogen fertilizers to the surface or mulching with organic matter, which may encourage rhizome rot. After 3–5 years, when clumps become congested or lose vitality, divide and replant active rhizomes in fresh soil.

Beardless irises have rhizomes below the surface of the soil and will benefit from mulching in spring; otherwise follow the feeding instructions for bearded irises. Plant small divisions of beardless and crested rhizomes 8–30cm (3–12in) apart, depending on size.

Bulbous irises – Plant Xiphium and Juno bulbs 10–15cm (4–6in) apart, depending on the size. Plant Reticulata bulbs 5–10cm (2–4in) apart. Plant all bulbs at a depth twice the height of the bulb. After flowering, feed with a high-potash fertilizer to encourage large bulbs to form. Lift and separate bulbs in early autumn.

• **PROPAGATION** Sow seed in containers in a cold frame in autumn or spring. Lift rhizomes or divide clumps, or separate bulb offsets, and plant immediately in the flowering site, usually from midsummer to early autumn.

• **PESTS AND DISEASES** Slugs and snails damage leaves, flowers, bulbs, and rhizomes. Sawfly larvae may damage the leaves of some waterside irises. Many, especially the Oncocyclus irises, are susceptible to aphid-borne viral infection. Bearded irises are particularly prone to bacterial soft rot (which affects the rhizomes) and to leaf spot. Beardless irises, especially Siberians, may suffer from grey mould (*Botrytis*); thrips may eat their leaves. Ink spot fungus can kill Reticulata bulbs.

I. acutiloba. Rhizomatous, bearded Oncocyclus iris with narrow, sickle-shaped leaves, 5–20cm (2–8in) long. In late spring, each stem produces a solitary, brown-veined white flower, 5–7cm (2–3in) across, with pointed petals. Each fall petal has 2 dark brown or black spots and a purple-brown beard. ↕10–25cm (4–10in). Georgia, Azerbaijan, Armenia, Iran. ❄❄. **subsp. *lineolata*** has only one spot on each fall.

***I.* 'Adobe Sunset'** ■ Rhizomatous, beardless Spuria iris with deep orange-yellow flowers, veined and bordered dark brown, borne in early summer. ↕1.5m (5ft). ❄❄❄

I. afghanica ■ Rhizomatous, bearded Regelia iris with curved leaves, 25cm (10in) long. In late spring, each unbranched stem produces 1 or 2 flowers, 8cm (3in) across, with pointed petals. Standards are pale yellow with green beards; falls are cream, veined purple-brown, with purple patches and dark brown beards. ↕15–40cm (6–16in). N.E. Afghanistan, Pakistan. ❄❄

I. albicans. Rhizomatous, bearded iris with broad, lance-shaped, grey-green leaves, 45cm (18in) long. In late spring, each unbranched stem bears 1–3 fragrant white flowers, 9cm (3½in) across, with yellow-tipped white beards. ↕30–60cm (12–24in). Arabian Peninsula. ❄❄❄. **'Madonna'** has blue flowers.

I. albomarginata. Bulbous Juno iris with leaves to 15cm (6in) long. In late spring and early summer, bears 2–5 vivid blue flowers, to 5cm (2in) across, with a white central mark on each fall. ↕20–30cm (8–12in). C. Asia (Kazakhstan to Tajikistan). ❄❄

***I.* 'Ancilla'.** Rhizomatous, bearded Regeliocyclus iris flowering in mid- and late spring. Standards are white with soft blue veins; falls are netted grey-brown with deep purple patches and beards. ↕25cm (10in). ❄❄

***I.* 'Annabel Jane'** ■ Very vigorous, rhizomatous, tall bearded iris. In late spring and early summer, bears flowers with pale lilac standards and mid-lilac falls with pale lilac beards. ↕1.2m (4ft). ❄❄❄

***I.* 'Ann Dasch'.** Rhizomatous, beardless Siberian iris. Bears mottled, light blue-purple flowers with solid, deeper blue-purple margins, and falls with small yellow marks, in mid- and late spring. ↕100cm (39in). ❄❄❄

***I.* 'Anniversary'** ■ Rhizomatous, beardless Siberian iris. Bears white flowers with yellow hafts in mid- and late spring. ↕75cm (30in). ❄❄❄

I. aphylla. Rhizomatous, bearded iris with broadly lance-shaped, grey-green leaves, to 15cm (6in) long, the outer ones curved, the others erect. In mid-spring, each branched stem produces 1–5 purple or blue-violet flowers, 6cm (2½in) across, with yellow-tipped white beards. ↕15–30cm (6–12in). C. and E. Europe to W. Russia, Ukraine, Moldavia, Caucasus. ❄❄❄

***I.* 'Apollo'** ■ Bulbous Dutch Xiphium iris. In late spring and early summer, bears flowers with creamy white standards and primrose-yellow falls. ↕65cm (26in). ❄❄❄

***I.* 'Arctic Fancy'** 🏆 Rhizomatous, intermediate bearded iris. Bears white flowers with deep violet markings and blue beards in early spring. ↕50cm (20in). ❄❄❄

I. arenaria see *I. humilis.*

***I.* 'Arnold Sunrise'** ■🏆 Rhizomatous, beardless Pacific Coast iris. Bears white flowers with a light yellow-orange patch in the centre of each fall in early spring. ↕25cm (10in). ❄❄❄

I. aucheri. Bulbous Juno iris with closely packed leaves, to 25cm (10in) long. In late winter or spring, bears 2 or 3 or more light to dark blue, violet, or white flowers, to 6cm (2½in) across, with a central yellow mark on each fall. ↕10–20cm (4–8in). S.E. Turkey, Iraq, Iran. ❄❄❄ (borderline)

I. aurea see *I. crocea.*

***I.* 'Baby Blessed'.** Remontant, rhizomatous, standard dwarf bearded iris. Bears light yellow blooms, with a small white spot and cream beard on each fall, in late spring and, in favourable conditions, again in early autumn. ↕25cm (10in). ❄❄❄

I. bakeriana. Small, bulbous Reticulata iris with 8-ribbed, cylindrical leaves, 1–10cm (½–4in) long at flowering. In spring, bears solitary flowers with lilac standards and white falls with deep violet tips, heavily marked and veined deep violet. ↕5–7cm (2–3in). S.E. Turkey, Iraq, Iran. ❄❄❄

***I.* 'Banbury Beauty'** ■ Rhizomatous, beardless Pacific Coast iris. Bears light lavender-blue flowers with a purple zone on each fall, in mid- and late spring. ↕55cm (22in). ❄❄❄

I. barnumae. Rhizomatous, bearded Oncocyclus iris with curved, grey-green leaves, to 18cm (7in) long. In late spring, each stem produces one purple-violet flower, 8cm (3in) across, with a yellow beard. ↕10–30cm (4–12in). E. Turkey, Iraq. ❄❄❄ (borderline). **f. *urmiensis*** has bright yellow flowers with orange beards.

***I.* 'Black Watch'.** Rhizomatous, intermediate bearded iris. Velvet-textured, very deep purple flowers with matching beards appear in mid- and late spring. ↕60cm (24in). ❄❄❄

***I.* 'Blue Ballerina'** 🏆 Rhizomatous, beardless Pacific Coast iris. In mid- and late spring, bears near-white flowers; each fall has a violet flash and black markings. ↕40cm (16in). ❄❄❄

***I.* 'Blue Diamond'.** Bulbous Dutch Xiphium iris. Bears deep violet flowers from mid-spring to midsummer. The falls are veined with darker violet and each has a lemon-yellow blotch. ↕65cm (26in). ❄❄❄

***I.* 'Blue-eyed Brunette'** ■🏆 Rhizomatous, tall bearded iris. Brown flowers with a lilac blaze and gold beard on each fall are borne in early summer. ↕90cm (36in). ❄❄❄

***I.* 'Blue Magic'.** Bulbous Dutch Xiphium iris flowering from mid-spring to midsummer. Standards are pale violet; falls are deep violet. ↕65cm (26in). ❄❄❄

***I.* 'Blue Pools'.** Rhizomatous, standard dwarf bearded iris with grey-green leaves. In early spring, bears white flowers with a large, mid-blue spot on each fall. ↕30cm (12in). ❄❄❄

***I.* 'Bold Print'** ■ Rhizomatous, intermediate bearded iris bearing white flowers in mid- and late spring. Standards have a purple border; falls are edged with purple stitching and have

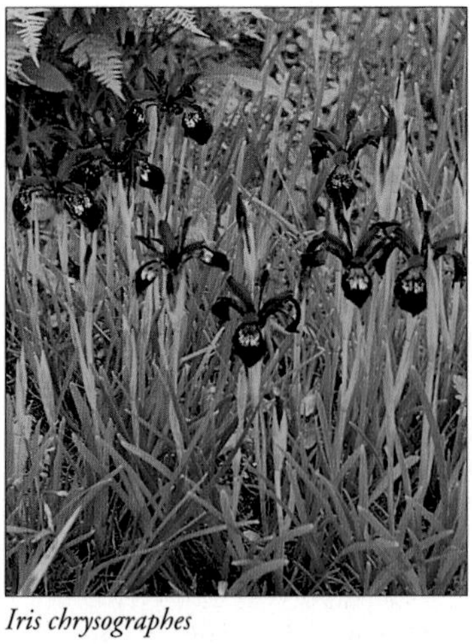

Iris chrysographes

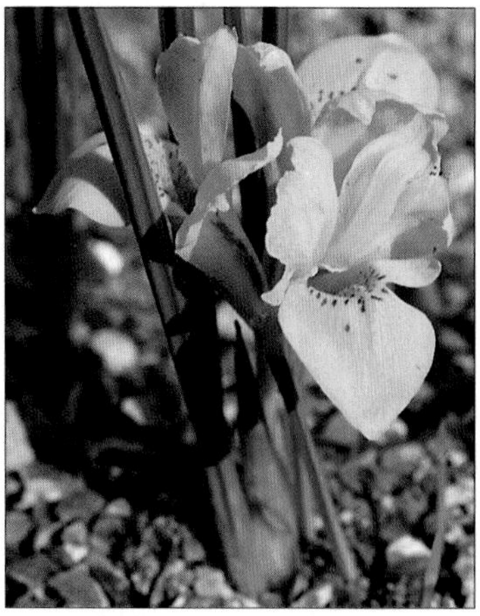

Iris danfordiae

white beards with bronze tips. ‡ 55cm (22in). ❄❄❄

I. brevicaulis, syn. *I. foliosa.* Rhizomatous, beardless Louisiana iris with branched, zigzag stems and large leaves or bracts, to 45cm (18in) long, overtopping the flowers. In early summer, bears terminal and axillary, bright blue-violet flowers, 7–10cm (3–4in) across, with small, spreading standards and broad, ovate falls. ‡ 40–50cm (16–20in). USA (Mississippi valley). ❄❄

***I.* 'Broadleigh Rose'.** Rhizomatous, beardless Pacific Coast iris. Bears pink flowers in mid- and late spring. ‡ 40cm (16in). ❄❄❄

***I.* 'Bromyard'** ▣ Rhizomatous, standard dwarf bearded iris. In early spring, bears flowers with blue-grey standards, blue-purple and ochre falls, and blue-grey beards. ‡ 28cm (11in). ❄❄❄

***I.* 'Bronze Perfection'.** Bulbous Dutch Xiphium iris. Bronze-yellow flowers, stained violet on the standards, are borne from mid-spring to midsummer. ‡ 65cm (26in). ❄❄❄

***I.* 'Bronze Queen'.** Bulbous Dutch Xiphium iris. Brownish yellow flowers are borne from mid-spring to mid-summer. ‡ 65cm (26in). ❄❄❄

***I.* 'Brown Lasso'** ▣ Rhizomatous, intermediate bearded iris flowering in spring. Standards are deep butterscotch-yellow; falls are light violet with brown edging and yellow beards. ‡ 55cm (22in). ❄❄❄

I. bucharica ▣ Vigorous, bulbous Juno iris with glossy leaves, to 20cm (8in) long. Bears up to 6 flowers, 4–6cm (1½–2½in) across, in the upper leaf axils in spring. Flowers vary from golden yellow to white, with a yellow mark on each fall. The white and yellow form is more commonly grown commercially. ‡ 20–40cm (8–16in). N.E. Afghanistan, C. Asia. ❄❄❄

I. bulleyana ▣ Rhizomatous, beardless Siberian iris with linear leaves, to 45cm (18in) long, glossy mid-green above, glaucous beneath. In early summer, hollow, unbranched stems bear 1 or 2 flowers, 6–8cm (2½–3in) across, with violet standards, and spreading white falls streaked violet. ‡ 35–45cm (14–18in). China (Sichuan, Yunnan). ❄❄❄

***I.* 'Butter and Sugar'** ▣ Rhizomatous, beardless Siberian iris flowering in mid- and late spring. Standards are white; falls are yellow; both have greenish yellow veins. ‡ 70cm (28in). ❄❄❄

***I.* 'Butter Pecan'.** Rhizomatous, intermediate bearded iris flowering in mid- and late spring. Standards are pecan-brown over yellow; falls are yellow stitched and bordered in deep pecan-brown, with yellow beards. ‡ 55cm (22in). ❄❄❄

***I.* 'Cambridge'.** Rhizomatous, beardless Siberian iris with narrow, straight leaves, flowering in mid- and late spring. Standards and falls are turquoise-blue, with white and yellow markings at the haft of the falls. ‡ 90cm (36in). ❄❄❄

***I.* 'Canyon Snow'.** Rhizomatous, beardless Pacific Coast iris. In mid- and late spring, bears white flowers with yellow patches. ‡ 45cm (18in). ❄❄❄

***I.* 'Carnaby'** ▣ Rhizomatous, tall bearded iris flowering in late spring and early summer. Standards are pink; falls are rose-pink and slightly ruffled with tangerine beards. ‡ 90cm (36in). ❄❄❄

I. caucasica. Dwarf, bulbous Juno iris bearing sickle-shaped, grey-green leaves, 10–12cm (4–5in) long, with narrow white margins. From late winter to spring, produces up to 4 greenish yellow flowers, 4–6cm (1½–2½in) across. ‡ 15cm (6in). Caucasus, C. and N.E. Turkey, N.E. Iraq, N.W. Iran. ❄❄

I. chamaeiris see *I. lutescens.*

***I.* 'Chance Beauty'.** Rhizomatous, beardless Laevigatae iris. In late spring, each stem bears 6–12 brown-veined, bright yellow flowers, 7–10cm (3–4in) across. ‡ 90cm (36in). ❄❄❄

I. chrysographes ▣ Rhizomatous, beardless Siberian iris with flat, linear, grey-green leaves, 50cm (20in) long. In early summer, each unbranched stem bears 2 fragrant, dark red-violet flowers, 6–7cm (2½–3in) across, with gold streaks on the falls. ‡ 40–50cm (16–20in). China (Sichuan, Yunnan). ❄❄❄. **'Black Knight'** has very dark violet flowers.

***I.* 'Clairette'.** Bulbous Reticulata iris flowering in late winter. Bears pale blue flowers, 6cm (2½in) across, with deep violet falls, each with a white central mark. ‡ 10cm (4in). ❄❄❄

I. clarkei. Rhizomatous, beardless Siberian iris with leaves 50cm (20in) long, and solid, branched stems. In late spring, produces violet, blue, or purple flowers, 8cm (3in) across, with a white patch on each fall. ‡ 60cm (24in). Himalayas: Nepal, India (Sikkim), Bhutan, Tibet. ❄❄❄

***I.* 'Clotho'.** Rhizomatous, bearded Regeliocyclus iris flowering in early summer. Standards are dark violet; falls are black-purple with black beards. ‡ 45cm (18in). ❄❄❄

***I.* 'Clyde Redmond'.** Rhizomatous, beardless Louisiana iris. In mid- and late spring, bears cornflower-blue flowers with yellow patches. ‡ 75cm (30in). ❄❄❄

I. colchica see *I. graminea.*

I. confusa ▣ Rhizomatous Crested iris with erect, bamboo-like stems, topped by fans of broad, evergreen leaves, 20–40cm (8–16in) long. In mid-spring, branching flower stems produce up to 30 short-lived blooms in succession. The flowers are white with yellow or purple spots around the yellow crests, 4–5cm (1½–2in) across. ‡ 1m (3ft) or more. China (Yunnan). ❄❄

***I.* 'Corn Harvest'.** Remontant, rhizomatous, tall bearded iris. Yellow flowers with ruffled falls and yellow beards are borne in early summer and, in warm areas, again in late summer and early autumn. ‡ 75cm (30in). ❄❄❄

I. cristata. Rhizomatous Crested iris with fans of lance-shaped, bright green leaves, to 15cm (6in) long at flowering. Produces 1 or 2 stemless blooms, 3.5cm (1½in) across, on long perianth tubes, 5cm (2in) tall, in late spring. Petals are usually blue-lilac, each with a white patch, and a yellow or orange crest on each fall. ‡ 10cm (4in). E. USA. ❄❄❄. **f. *alba*** has white flowers.

I. crocea, syn. *I. aurea.* Vigorous, rhizomatous, beardless Spuria iris with erect leaves, 75cm (30in) long at flowering. In early summer, each branched stem bears up to 20 golden yellow blooms, 12–18cm (5–7in) across. ‡ to 1.2m (4ft). India (Kashmir). ❄❄❄

***I.* 'Cup Race'.** Rhizomatous, tall bearded iris. Bears all-white flowers in late spring and early summer. ‡ 90cm (36in). ❄❄❄

I. cuprea see *I. fulva.*

***I.* 'Custom Design'.** Rhizomatous, beardless Spuria iris. Produces deep maroon-brown flowers with bright yellow patches in mid- and late spring. ‡ 100cm (39in). ❄❄❄

I. cycloglossa. Vigorous, bulbous Juno iris with leaves to 30cm (12in) long. In spring, bears up to 3 scented, pale violet flowers, 8–10cm (3–4in) across, with yellow-marked white centres, and standards to 4cm (1½in) long. ‡ to 50cm (20in). S.W. Afghanistan. ❄❄❄

I. danfordiae ▣ Bulbous Reticulata iris with 2 erect, narrow, square-sectioned leaves, 10–15cm (4–6in) long at flowering. In late winter and early spring, bears a solitary yellow flower, to 5cm (2in) across, with tiny standards and greenish yellow markings on the falls. ‡ 8–15cm (3–6in). Turkey. ❄❄❄

***I.* 'Dark Vader'.** Rhizomatous, standard dwarf bearded iris. Produces ruffled

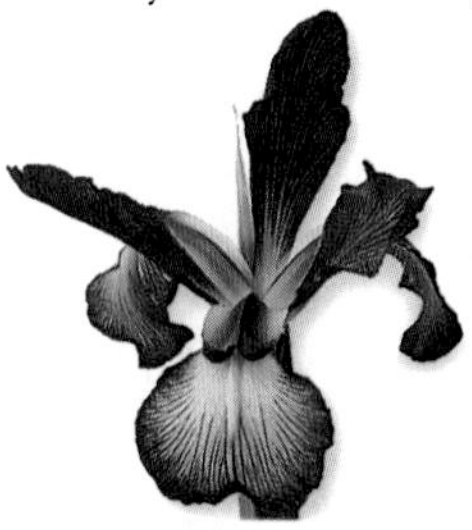

Iris 'Adobe Sunset'

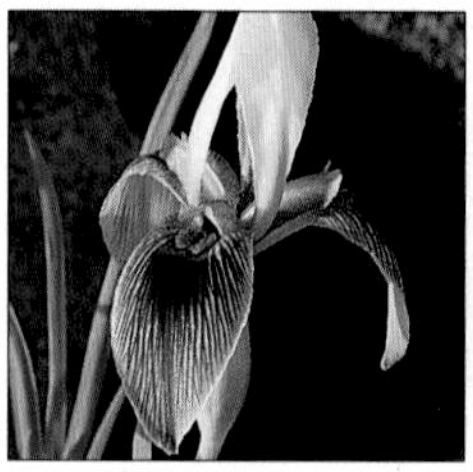

Iris afghanica

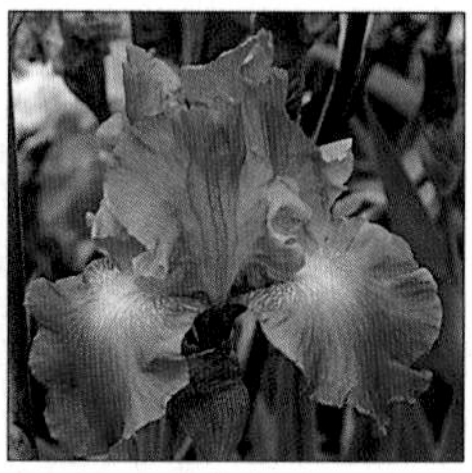

Iris 'Annabel Jane'

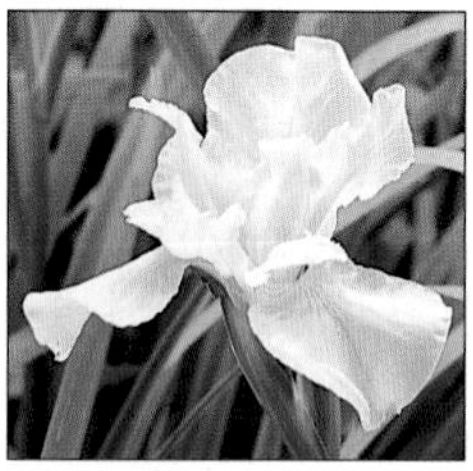

Iris 'Anniversary'

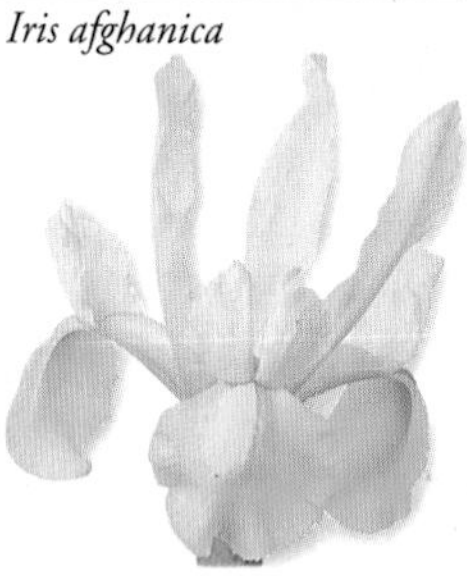

Iris 'Apollo'

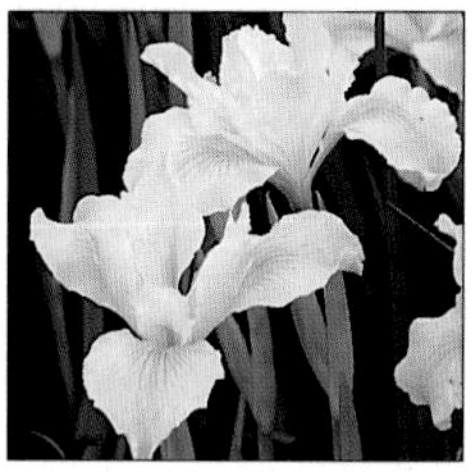

Iris 'Arnold Sunrise'

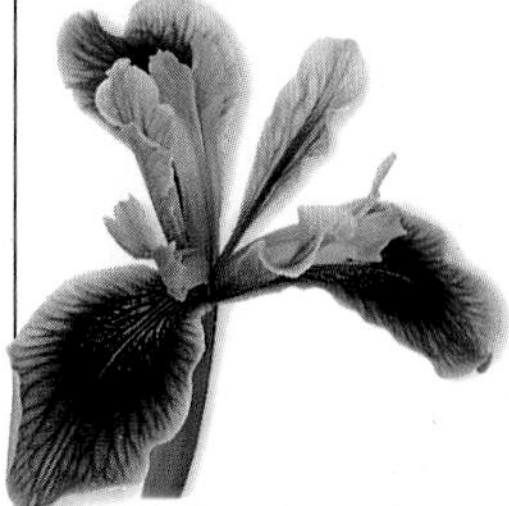

Iris 'Banbury Beauty'

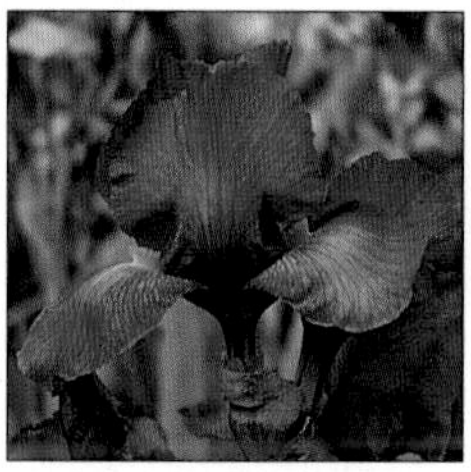

Iris 'Blue-eyed Brunette'

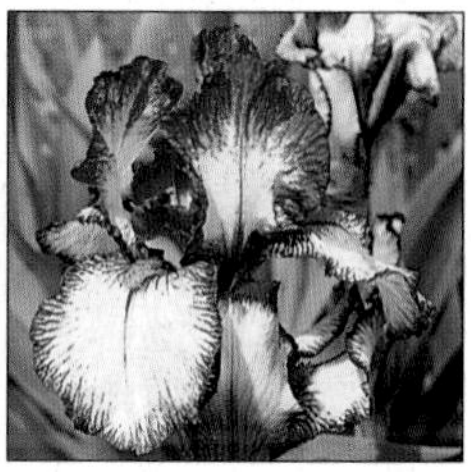

Iris 'Bold Print'

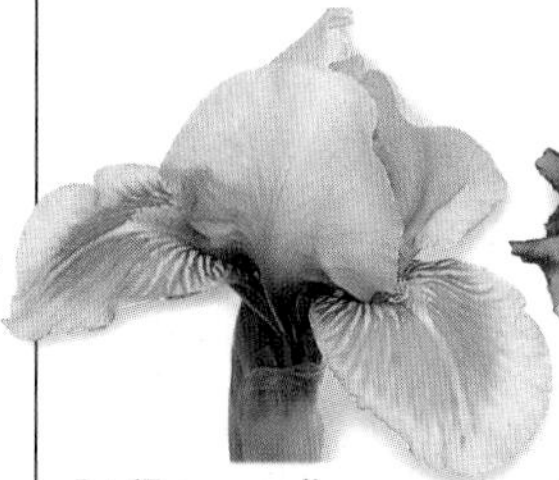

Iris 'Bromyard'

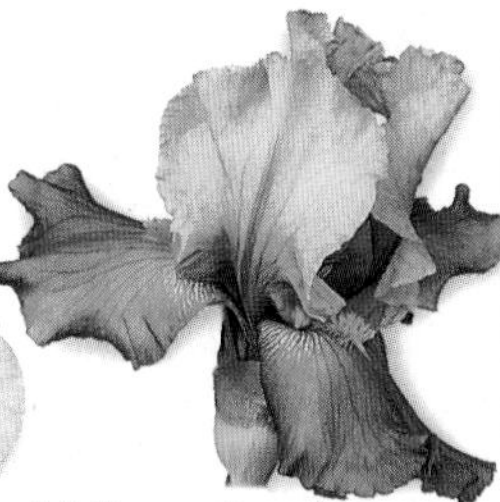

Iris 'Brown Lasso'

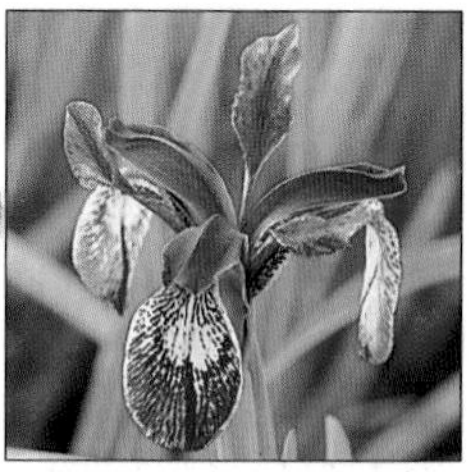

Iris bulleyana

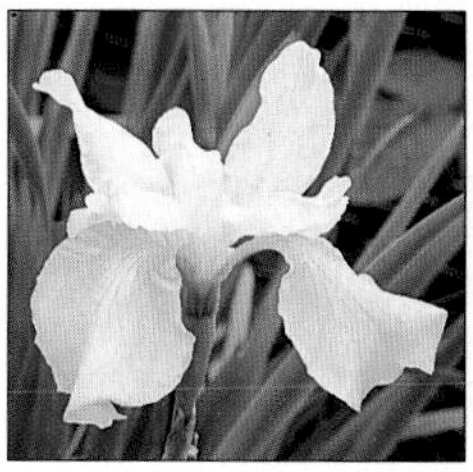

Iris 'Butter and Sugar'

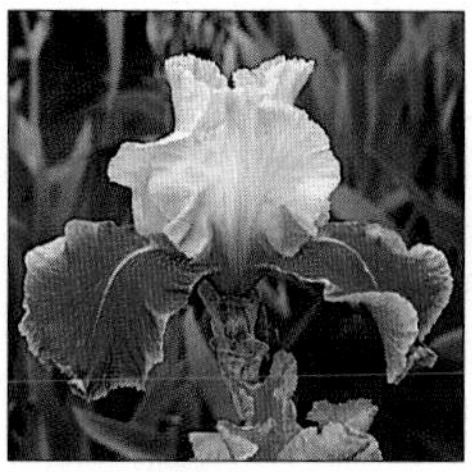

Iris 'Carnaby'

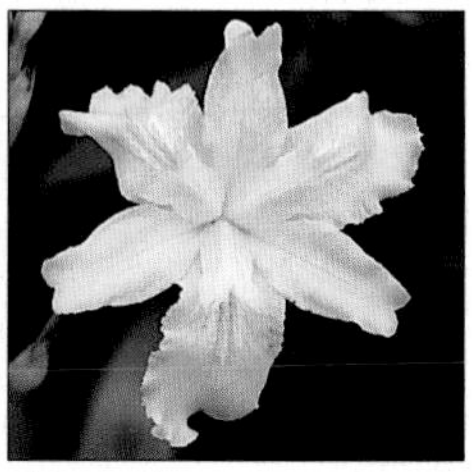

Iris confusa

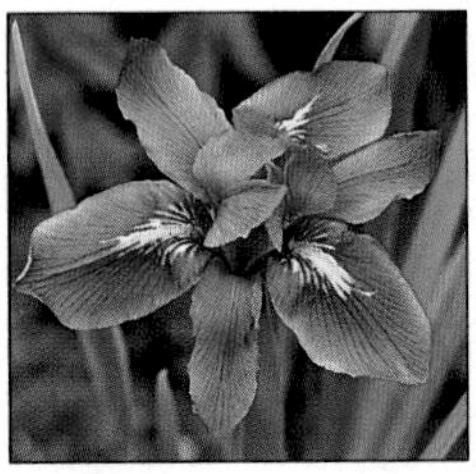
Iris decora

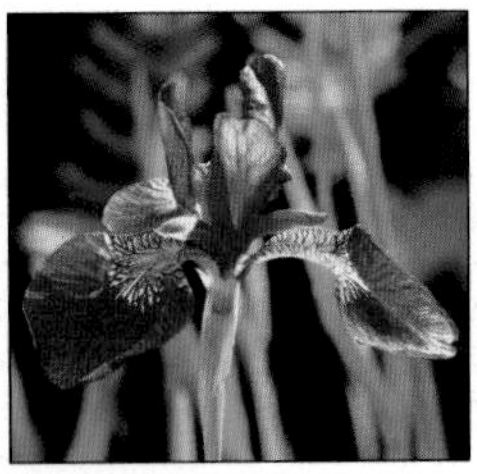
Iris delavayi

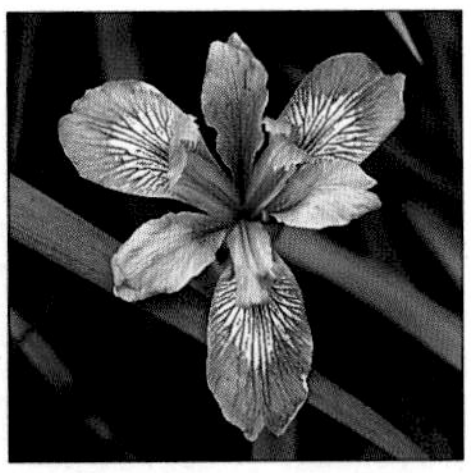
Iris douglasiana

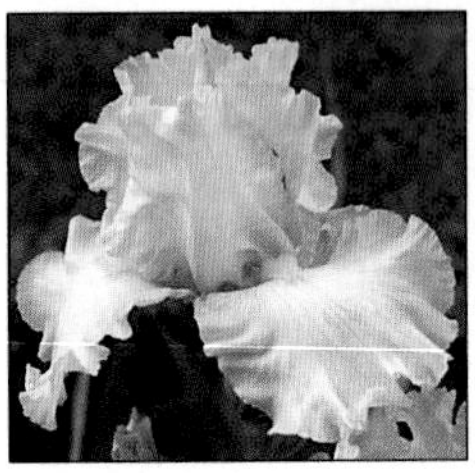
Iris 'Early Light'

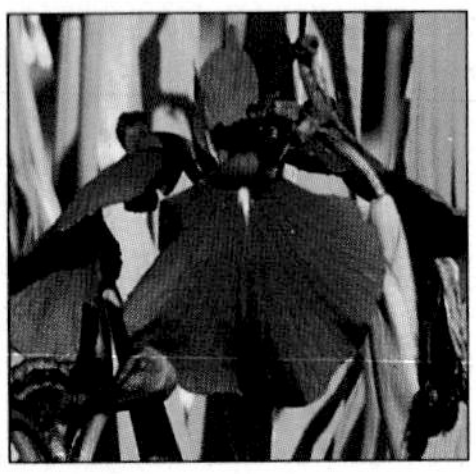
Iris ensata

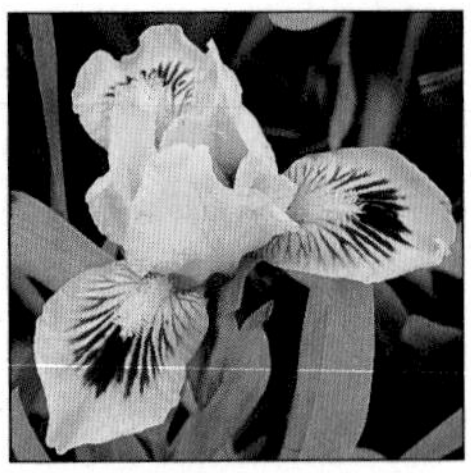
Iris 'Eyebright'

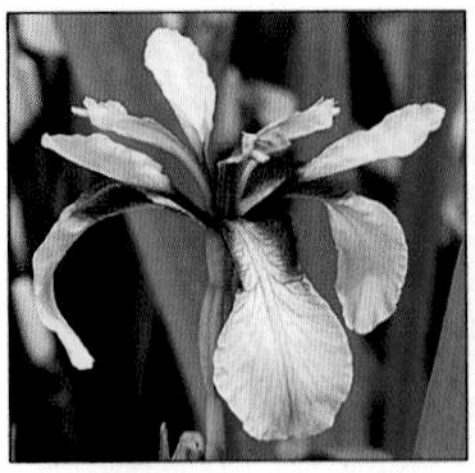
Iris foetidissima var. *citrina*

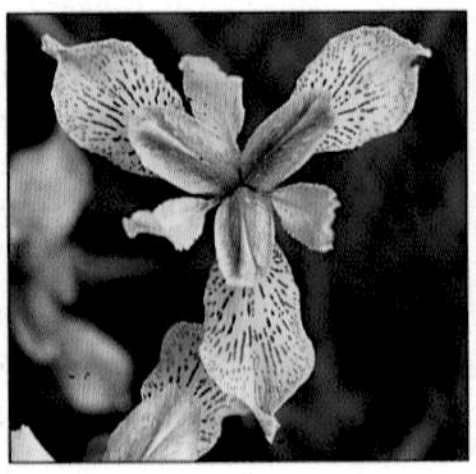
Iris forrestii

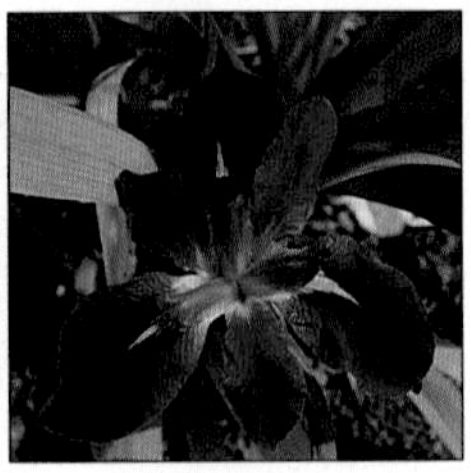
Iris x *fulvala*

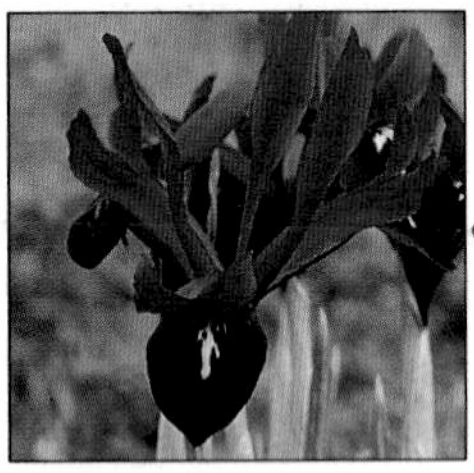
Iris 'George'

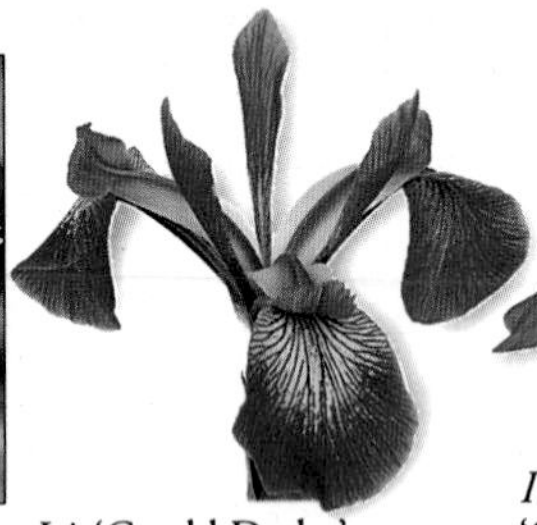
Iris 'Gerald Darby'

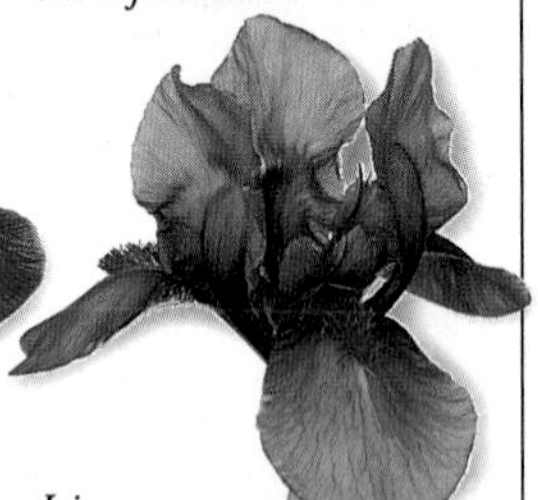
Iris 'Gingerbread Man'

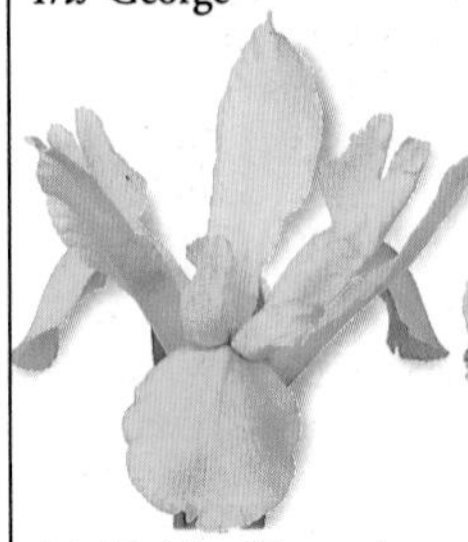
Iris 'Golden Harvest'

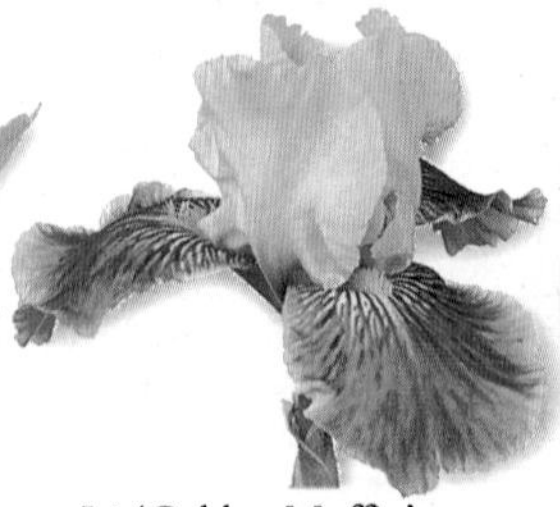
Iris 'Golden Muffin'

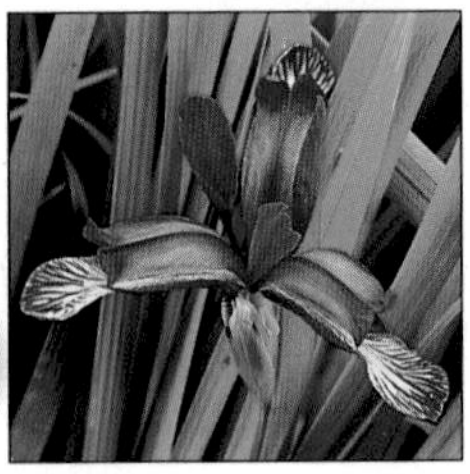
Iris graminea

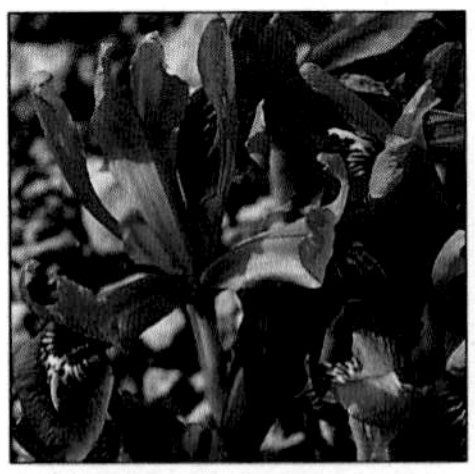
Iris histrioides 'Major'

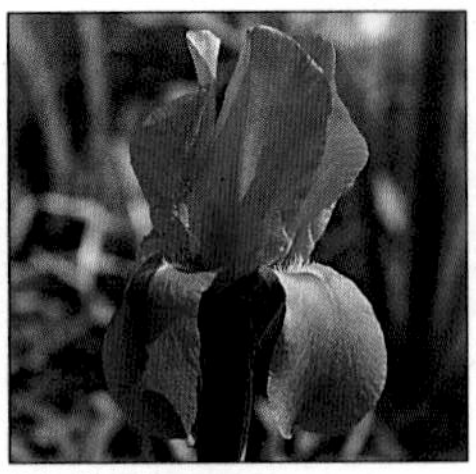
Iris hoogiana

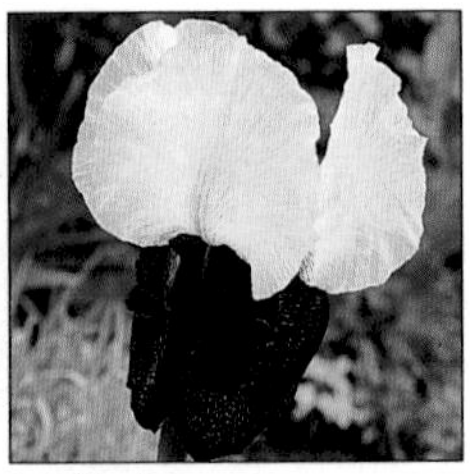
Iris iberica

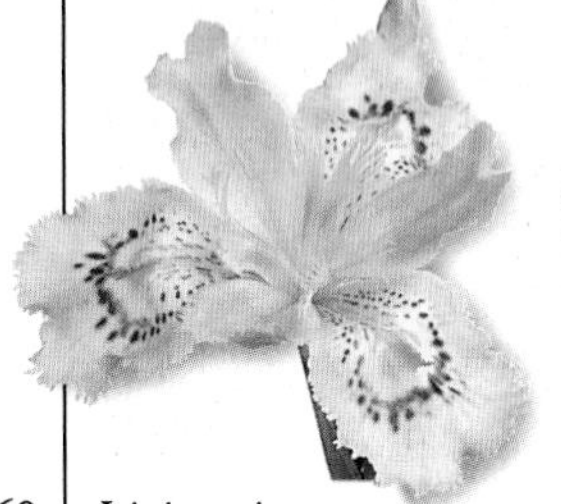
Iris japonica

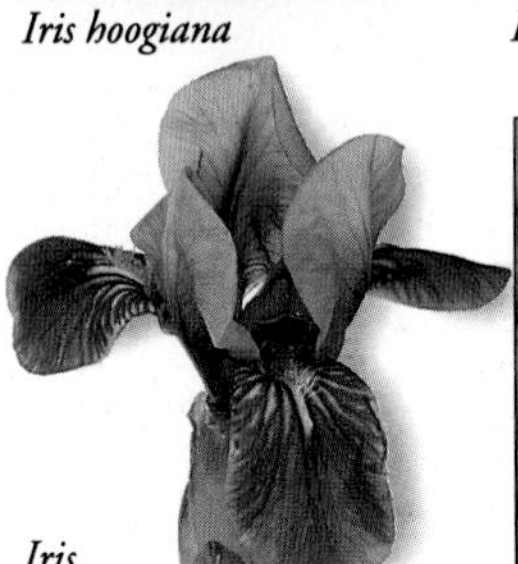
Iris 'Jasper Gem'

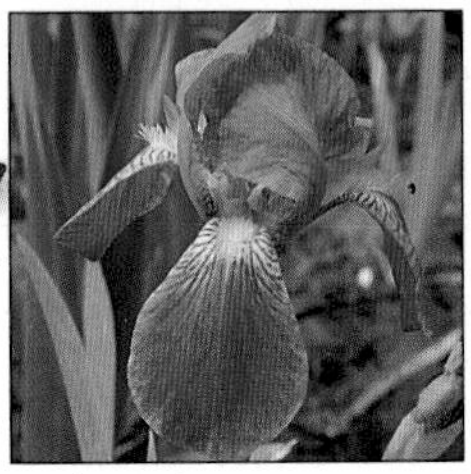
Iris 'Joette'

I

flowers with dark blue-violet standards and black falls with violet beards, in mid- and late spring. ↕28cm (11in). ❄❄❄

I. decora ■ syn. *I. nepalensis.* Rhizomatous, beardless iris with erect, linear, and markedly ribbed leaves, to 40cm (16in) long. In early summer, each branched or unbranched stem produces 1–3 short-lived, slightly flattened, lightly scented, lavender-blue or purple flowers, 5cm (2in) across, with an orange crest on each fall. ↕30cm (12in). Best raised from seed. Himalayas, India (Kashmir) to China (Sichuan, Yunnan). ❄❄

I. delavayi ■ Rhizomatous, beardless Siberian iris with grey-green leaves, 90cm (36in) long, and 3-branched flower stems. In summer, each branch produces 2 light to dark purple-blue flowers, 7–9cm (3–3½in) across, with white and yellow flecks on the rounded falls. ↕to 1.5m (5ft). China (S.W. Sichuan, Yunnan). ❄❄❄

***I.* 'Dorothea K. Williamson'.** Rhizomatous, beardless Louisiana iris with zigzag stems bearing violet flowers in midsummer. ↕45–80cm (18–32in). ❄❄❄

I. douglasiana ■ Vigorous, rhizomatous, beardless Pacific Coast iris bearing evergreen, stiff, glossy, dark green leaves, to 1m (3ft) long, often bright red at the bases. Red-purple, lavender-blue, blue, cream, or white flowers, 7–10cm (3–4in) across, are produced on branched stems, 2 or 3 per branch, in late spring and early summer. ↕15–70cm (6–28in). W. USA. ❄❄❄

***I.* 'Dreaming Yellow'.** Rhizomatous, beardless Siberian iris flowering in mid- and late spring. Produces flowers with white standards and slightly ruffled, creamy yellow falls. ↕80cm (32in). ❄❄❄

***I.* 'Dress Circle'.** Rhizomatous, beardless Spuria iris flowering from mid-spring to early summer. Standards are blue-violet with white veins; falls have yellow patches surrounded by white and violet edging. ↕90cm (36in). ❄❄❄

***I.* 'Dusky Challenger'.** Rhizomatous, tall bearded iris. Bears silky, ruffled, rich purple flowers with deep violet beards in late spring and early summer. ↕100cm (39in). ❄❄❄

I. dykesii. Variable, rhizomatous, beardless Siberian iris with grey-green leaves, to 60cm (24in) long, partly enclosing each stem and overtopping the flowers. In early summer, each unbranched stem bears 2 deep purple-violet flowers, 7–9cm (3–3½in) across, with yellow or white veins on the falls. ↕60cm (24in). Probably a natural hybrid from China. ❄❄❄

***I.* 'Early Light'** ■ 🏆 Rhizomatous, tall bearded iris. In mid- and late spring, produces flowers with lemon-flushed cream standards, slightly darker falls, and yellow beards. ↕100cm (39in). ❄❄❄

***I.* 'Edith Wolford'.** Rhizomatous, tall bearded iris. Ruffled flowers with clear canary-yellow standards, blue-violet falls, and orange-tipped blue beards appear in mid- and late spring. ↕100cm (39in). ❄❄❄

***I.* 'Egret Snow'.** Rhizomatous, miniature dwarf bearded iris flowering in early spring. Produces ruffled, fragrant, pure white flowers; falls are sometimes streaked azure, and have white beards. ↕15cm (6in). ❄❄❄

I. ensata ■ syn. *I. kaempferi.* Rhizomatous, beardless Laevigatae (Japanese) iris with single, occasionally branched stems. Leaves are 20–60cm (8–24in) long, with prominent midribs. In midsummer, each stem bears 3 or 4 purple or red-purple flowers, 8–15cm (3–6in) across. Standards are erect and smaller than the falls. ↕90cm (36in). N. China, Japan, E. Russia. ❄❄❄. **'Alba'** has white flowers. **'Blue Peter'** has mid-blue flowers. **'Moonlight Waves'** bears white flowers with lime-green centres. **'Snowdrift'** has double white flowers.

I. extremorientalis see *I. sanguinea.*

***I.* 'Eyebright'** ■ Rhizomatous, standard dwarf bearded iris. In early spring, bears bright yellow flowers; falls have deep brown lines and deep yellow beards. ↕30cm (12in). ❄❄❄

***I.* 'Feedback'.** Remontant, rhizomatous, tall bearded iris. Bears sweetly fragrant, violet blooms with yellow beards, in early summer and, in warm areas, again in early autumn. ↕90cm (36in). ❄❄❄

I. fernaldii. Rhizomatous, beardless Pacific Coast iris with partly deciduous, slender, grey-green leaves, to 40cm (16in) long, tinged purple at the bases. Each unbranched stem produces 2 pale yellow flowers, 7–9cm (3–3½in) across, with a darker line down the centre of each fall, in late spring. ↕20–45cm (8–18in). W. USA. ❄❄❄

***I.* 'Flamenco'.** Rhizomatous, tall bearded iris. In mid- and late spring, produces flowers with gold standards suffused brown, and white to yellow falls with brown borders. ↕90cm (36in). ❄❄❄

I. flavissima see *I. humilis.*

I. florentina see *I. germanica* 'Florentina'.

I. foetidissima (Stinking gladwyn, Stinking iris). Vigorous, rhizomatous, beardless iris with tufts of tough, evergreen, dark green leaves, to 75cm (30in) long, unpleasantly scented when crushed. In early summer, each branched stem bears up to 5 dull purple flowers, tinged with yellow, 5–7cm (2–3in) across. Large seed capsules split open in autumn, displaying scarlet, yellow, or rarely white seeds. ↕30–90cm (12–36in). S. and W. Europe, Azores, Canary Islands, N. Africa. ❄❄❄. **var. *citrina*** ■ has yellow flowers. **'Fructu-albo'** has white-coated seeds. **'Variegata'** has silver leaves with white variegations. Less susceptible to virus than the species, but flowers less freely.

I. foliosa see *I. brevicaulis.*

I. formosana. Rhizomatous Crested iris with erect fans of leaves, to 35cm (14in) long, borne on cane-like stems, 10cm (4in) high. Bears branched heads of flat, pale lilac flowers, to 8cm (3in) across, with yellow crests, in late spring. ↕10–20cm (4–8in). Taiwan. ❀ (min. 5°C/41°F)

I. forrestii ■ Rhizomatous, beardless Siberian iris with linear leaves, to 25cm (10in) long, glossy, mid-green above, grey-green beneath. In early summer, each unbranched stem produces 1 or 2 scented, clear yellow flowers, 5–6cm (2–2½in) across, with brown lines on the falls. ↕35–40cm (14–16in). China (S. Sichuan, Yunnan), N. Burma. ❄❄❄

***I.* 'Frank Elder'.** Vigorous, bulbous Reticulata iris flowering in late winter. Bears well-rounded, sturdy flowers

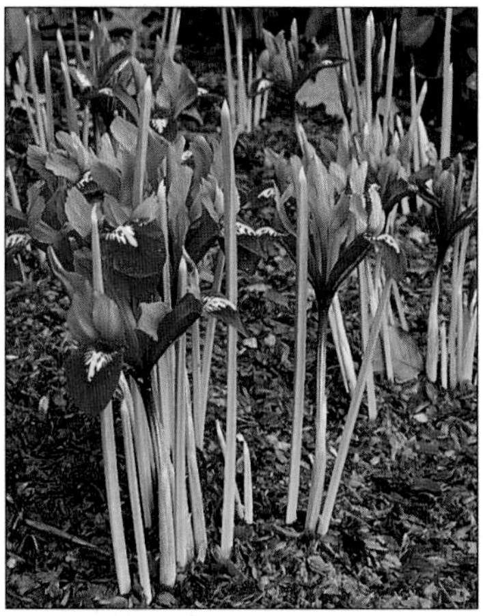

Iris 'Harmony'

in a mixture of blue and yellow-green. ↕15cm (6in) at flowering. ❄❄❄

I. fulva, syn. *I. cuprea*. Rhizomatous, beardless Louisiana iris with strap-shaped, bright green leaves, 30–70cm (12–28in) long, arching at the tips. Each slender, slightly zigzag stem bears 4–6 copper- or orange-red flowers, 6–7cm (2½–3in) across, in late spring; both falls and standards are pendent. ↕45–80cm (18–32in). USA (Mississippi valley). ❄❄❄

I.* x *fulvala ■ (*I. brevicaulis* x *I. fulva*). Robust, rhizomatous, beardless Louisiana iris. In early summer, bears purple-red flowers, 5–6cm (2–2½in) across. ↕45–80cm (18–32in). Garden origin. ❄❄❄

I. gatesii. Rhizomatous, bearded Oncocyclus iris with straight, linear leaves, 10–25cm (4–10in) long. In late spring and early summer, each tall stem produces one large cream flower, 15–20cm (6–8in) across; petals may appear purple, brown, or cream depending on the degree of veining. Falls have yellow or purple beards. ↕45–60cm (18–24in). S.E. Turkey, N.E. Iraq. ❄❄❄ (borderline)

***I.* 'Geisha Gown'**. Rhizomatous, beardless Laevigatae (Japanese) iris. In mid- and late spring, bears single, clear white flowers with deep pinkish purple veins. ↕90cm (36in). ❄❄❄

***I.* 'George'** ■ Vigorous, bulbous Reticulata iris. Well-rounded, sturdy, rich purple flowers are borne in early spring. ↕12cm (5in). ❄❄❄

***I.* 'Gerald Darby'** ■ Rhizomatous, beardless Laevigatae iris with arching leaves spotted purple at the bases, and dark violet stems and spathes. Each unbranched stem produces up to 4 blue-violet flowers in late spring. ↕75cm (30in), sometimes to 1.8m (6ft). ❄❄❄

I. germanica. Rhizomatous, bearded iris with fans of sometimes evergreen, grey-green leaves, 40cm (16in) long. In late spring, sparsely branched stems bear many blue-violet flowers, 10cm (4in) across, with yellow beards. ↕60–120cm (24–48in). Probably Mediterranean. ❄❄❄. **'Amas'** has deep purple falls and rounded, paler blue standards. **'Florentina'**, syn. *I. florentina* (Orris root), produces strongly scented white flowers.

***I.* 'Giant Blue Butterfly'**. Rhizomatous, beardless Laevigatae (Japanese) iris. From mid-spring to early summer, bears double white and mid-blue flowers. ↕1.4m (4½ft). ❄❄❄

***I.* 'Gingerbread Man'** ■ Rhizomatous, standard dwarf bearded iris. Bears deep brown flowers with blue-purple beards in mid- and late spring. ↕35cm (14in). ❄❄❄

***I.* 'Golden Harvest'** ■ Bulbous Dutch Xiphium iris. From mid-spring to midsummer, bears rich golden yellow flowers. ↕to 70cm (28in). ❄❄❄

***I.* 'Golden Muffin'** ■ Rhizomatous, intermediate bearded iris flowering in mid- and late spring. Standards are yellow; falls are deep amber, thinly margined in yellow, with yellow beards. ↕60cm (24in). ❄❄❄

***I.* 'Gordon'**. Bulbous Reticulata iris flowering in early spring. Bears bright blue flowers; falls are darker blue with an orange mark. ↕15cm (6in). ❄❄❄

I. gracilipes. Rhizomatous Crested iris with grass-like leaves, to 30cm (12in) long. In late spring and early summer, each slender, branched stem bears several blue-lilac flowers, 3–4cm (1¼–1½in) across. Each fall has a violet-veined white patch and a yellow-tipped white crest. ↕10–15cm (4–6in). Japan, China. ❄❄❄

I. graeberiana. Robust, bulbous Juno iris bearing glossy, bright green leaves, to 15cm (6in) long, with narrow white margins. In early spring, bears up to 6 blue flowers, 7cm (3in) or more across, with white and deeper blue markings. ↕20–40cm (8–16in). C. Asia (Kazakhstan to Tajikistan). ❄❄❄

I. graminea ■ syn. *I. colchica*. Rhizomatous, beardless Spuria iris with flat, linear, bright green leaves, to 30cm (12in) long. In late spring and early summer, bears 1 or 2 purple-violet flowers, 7cm (3in) across, with a fruity fragrance, often hidden among the foliage. Falls have violet-veined white tips. ↕20–40cm (8–16in). N.E. Spain to W. Russia, N. and W. Caucasus. ❄❄❄

***I.* 'Green Halo'**. Rhizomatous, standard dwarf bearded iris. In early summer, bears pale olive-green flowers. Each fall has a deeper green "halo" and an olive-green beard. ↕30cm (12in). ❄❄❄

***I.* 'Harmony'** ■ Bulbous Reticulata iris flowering in late winter. Bears royal-blue flowers with a yellow central mark on each fall. ↕10–15cm (4–6in) at flowering. ❄❄❄

I. histrio. Small, bulbous Reticulata iris with erect, narrow, square-sectioned leaves, 1–10cm (½–4in) long at flowering. In late winter, bears usually solitary, pale blue and white flowers, 6–8cm (2½–3in) across, with deeper blue markings on the falls. ↕7cm (3in). S. Turkey, Syria, Lebanon. ❄❄❄

I. histrioides. Bulbous Reticulata iris with erect, square-sectioned leaves, 1–10cm (½–4in) long at flowering. In early spring, bears 1 or 2 robust, mid- to dark blue flowers, 6–7cm (2½–3in) across. Each fall is usually spotted deeper blue in the centre with a yellow central ridge. Similar to *I. histrio* but more robust. ↕10–15cm (4–6in). Turkey. ❄❄❄. **'Major'** ■🏆 is vigorous with deep blue flowers.

***I.* 'Holden Clough'**. Rhizomatous, beardless Laevigatae iris with arching, often evergreen, grey-green leaves. In late spring, each branching stem bears 6–12 yellow flowers heavily veined purple, producing a rich brown appearance. ↕50–90cm (20–36in). ❄❄❄

I. hoogiana ■ Rhizomatous, bearded Regelia iris with erect, purple-tinged, mid-green leaves, to 50cm (20in) long. In early summer, each unbranched stem produces 2 or 3 fragrant, silky, pale to mid-blue flowers, 7–10cm (3–4in) across, with yellow beards. ↕40–60cm (16–24in). Tajikistan (Pamir Mountains). ❄❄. **f. *alba*** bears white flowers, faintly overlaid with pale lavender-blue.

I. humilis, syn. *I. arenaria*, *I. flavissima*. Rhizomatous, bearded iris with erect, narrow leaves, to 15cm (6in) long. In mid-spring, each unbranched stem bears 1 or 2 scented yellow flowers, 3–4cm (1¼–1½in) across. Falls are horizontal, longer than the standards, and have orange beards. ↕10–25cm (4–10in). E. Europe to Mongolia. ❄❄❄

I. hyrcana. Bulbous Reticulata iris with square-sectioned leaves, 1–10cm (½–4in) long at flowering. In early spring, bears 1 or 2 flowers, 4–5cm (1½–2in) across, varying from usually clear pale to deep blue, or rarely violet. ↕7cm (3in). Iran. ❄❄❄

I. iberica ■ Rhizomatous, bearded Oncocyclus iris with strongly curved, narrow, grey-green leaves, 15cm (6in) long. In mid- and late spring, each stem produces a solitary, brown-veined, cream or white flower, to 7cm (3in) across. Falls are more heavily veined than the standards, and have black patches and brown-purple beards. ↕15–20cm (6–8in). Caucasus. ❄❄❄ (borderline). **subsp. *elegantissima*** is taller, with larger flowers, 10cm (4in) across; ↕20–30cm (8–12in). N.E. Turkey, N.W. Iran, Armenia.

***I.* 'Immortality'**. Remontant, rhizomatous, tall bearded iris. Bears ruffled, pure white flowers in early summer and, in warm areas, again in late summer and autumn. ↕75cm (30in). ❄❄❄

***I.* 'Imperial Bronze'**. Rhizomatous, beardless Spuria iris flowering in mid- and late spring. Produces deep yellow flowers heavily veined brown, producing a deep bronze appearance. ↕100cm (39in). ❄❄❄

***I.* 'Indeed'**. Rhizomatous, intermediate bearded iris flowering in early spring. Standards are light lemon-yellow; falls are white, margined in lemon, with white beards. ↕55cm (22in). ❄❄❄

I. innominata ■ Rhizomatous, beardless Pacific Coast iris with evergreen, very narrow, deep green leaves, to 30cm (12in) long, purple at the bases. In early summer, each unbranched stem bears 1 or 2 rounded flowers, 7cm (3in) across, ranging from bright yellow to cream, and from purple to pale lavender-blue. ↕15–25cm (6–10in). USA (S.W. Oregon, N.W. California). ❄❄❄

I. japonica ■ Rhizomatous Crested iris, which spreads by surface rhizomes, with fans of strap-shaped, evergreen, glossy, dark green leaves, to 45cm (18in) long. In late spring, each branched stem bears 3 or 4 flattened and frilly, white or pale lavender-blue flowers, 4–5cm (1½–2in) across. Falls have purple patches and orange crests. ↕45cm (18in). C. China, Japan. ❄❄. **'Aphrodite'** see 'Variegata'. **'Ledger's Variety'** is reputed to be hardier with larger flowers; this name is often incorrectly used for variants of the species. **'Variegata'**, syn. 'Aphrodite', has white- and green-striped foliage.

***I.* 'Jasper Gem'** ■ Rhizomatous, miniature dwarf bearded iris. Produces flowers with smoky brown-red standards and yellow-bearded, oxblood-red falls in early spring. ↕20cm (8in). ❄❄❄

***I.* 'Jennifer Rebecca'**. Remontant, rhizomatous, tall bearded iris. Ruffled and laced, rose-pink flowers, lighter around the tangerine beards, appear in early summer and, in warm areas, again in mid-autumn. ↕90cm (36in). ❄❄❄

***I.* 'Joette'** ■ Rhizomatous, miniature tall bearded iris with slender, zigzag stems. Bears lavender flowers with light yellow beards in mid- and late spring. ↕45cm (18in). ❄❄❄

***I.* 'Joyce'** ■ Bulbous Reticulata iris bearing deep sky-blue flowers in early spring. ↕12cm (5in). ❄❄❄

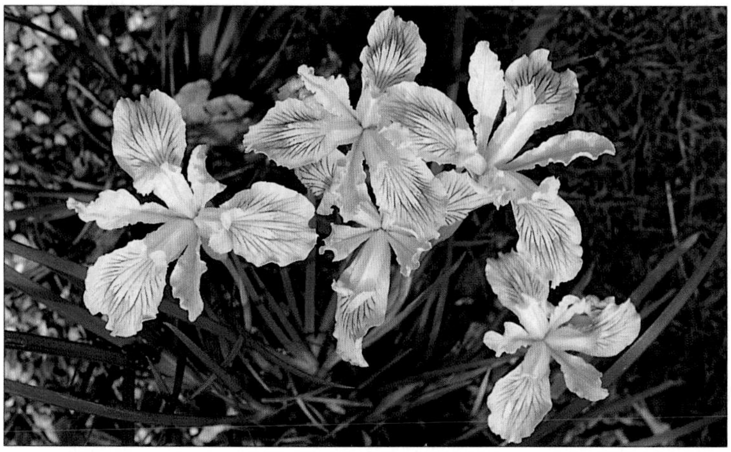

Iris innominata

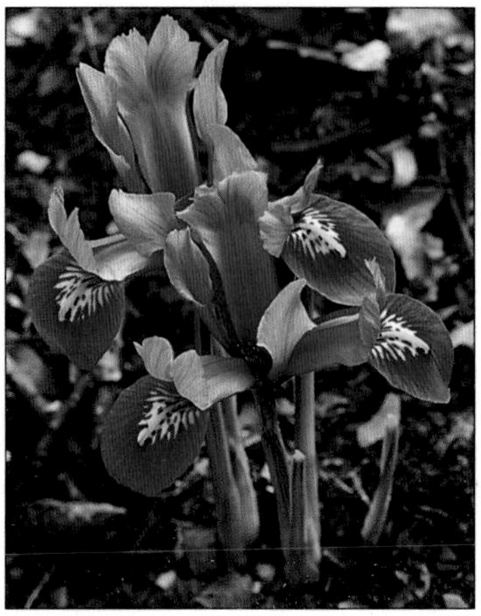

Iris 'Joyce'

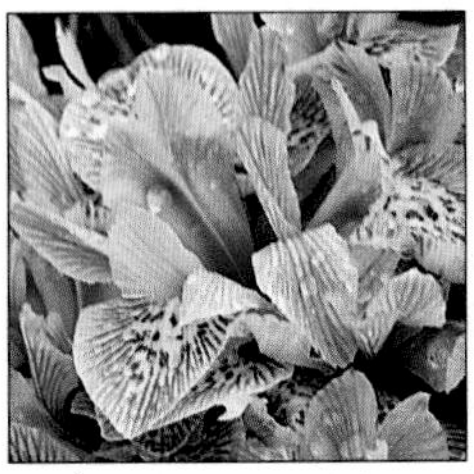
Iris 'Katharine Hodgkin'

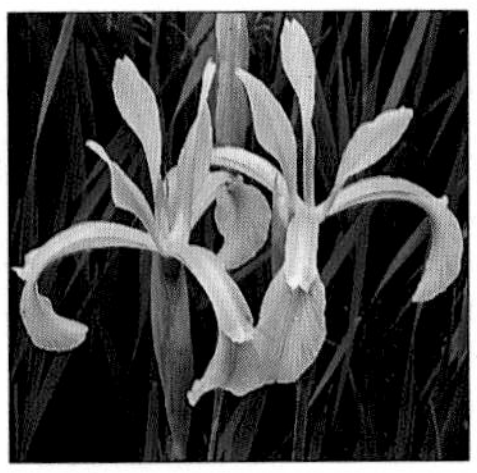
Iris kerneriana

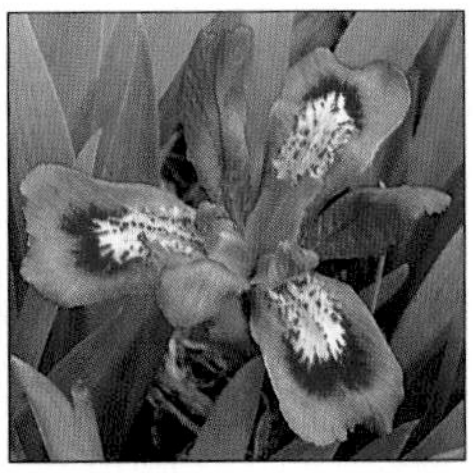
Iris lacustris

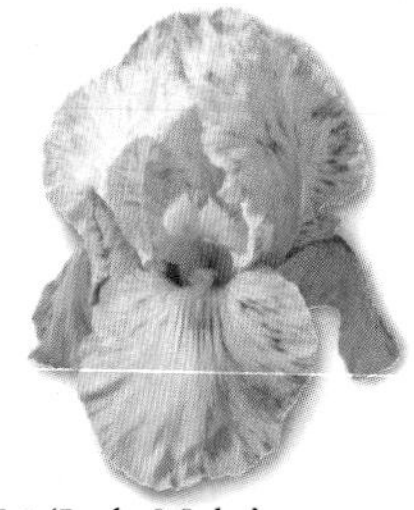
Iris 'Lady Mohr'

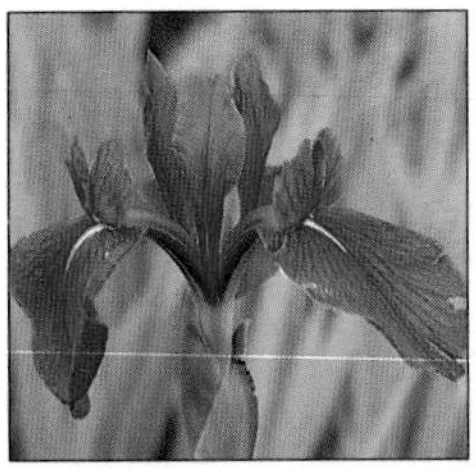
Iris laevigata

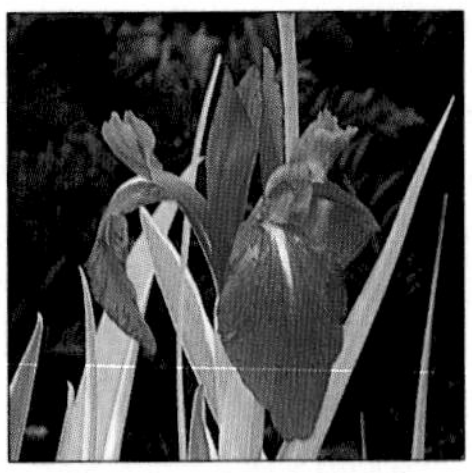
Iris laevigata 'Variegata'

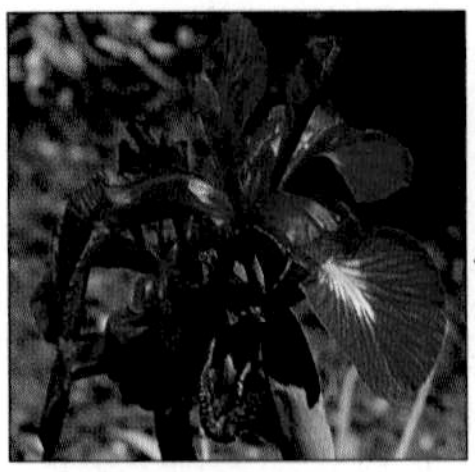
Iris latifolia

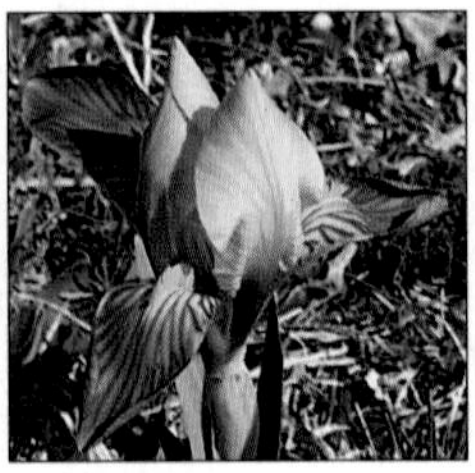
Iris lutescens

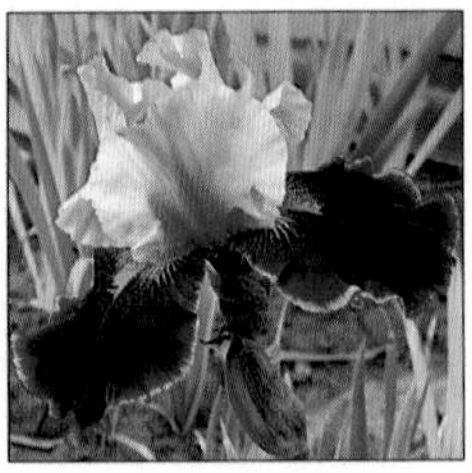
Iris 'Magic Man'

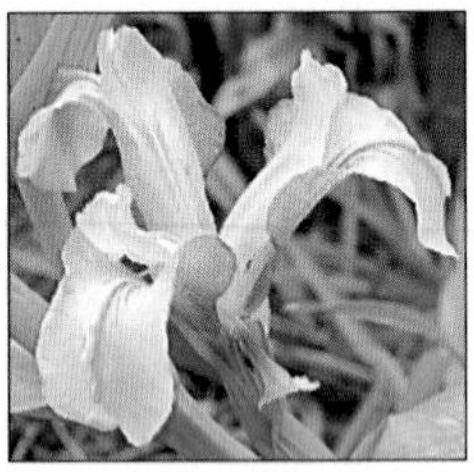
Iris magnifica

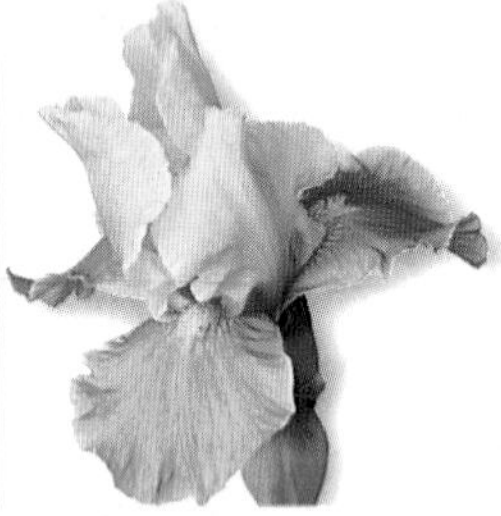
Iris 'Marmalade Skies'

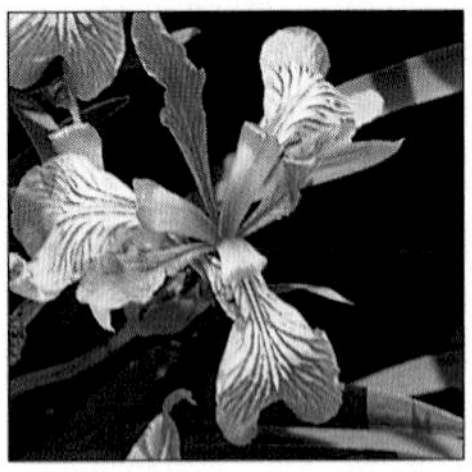
Iris missouriensis

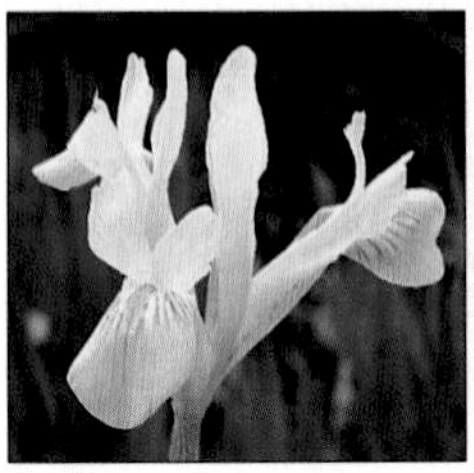
Iris 'Natascha'

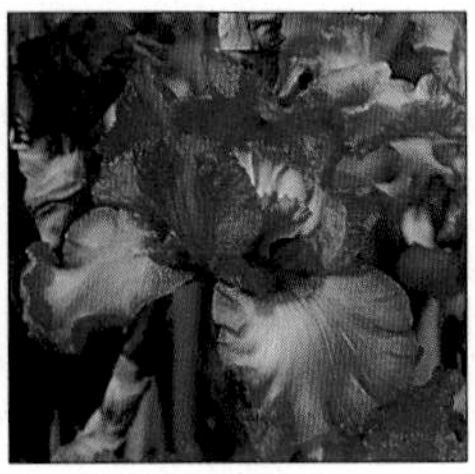
Iris 'Paradise Bird'

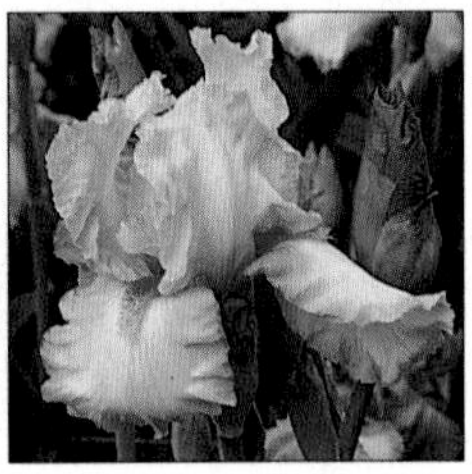
Iris 'Peach Frost'

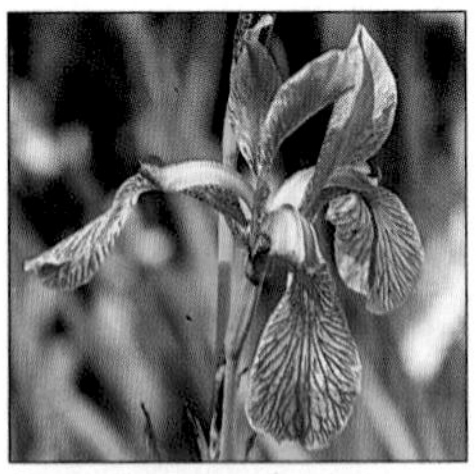
Iris prismatica

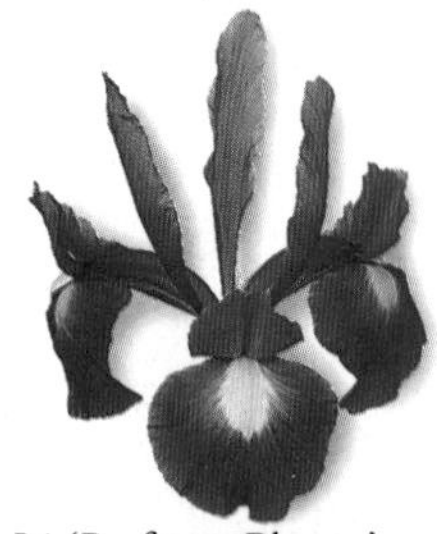
Iris 'Professor Blaauw'

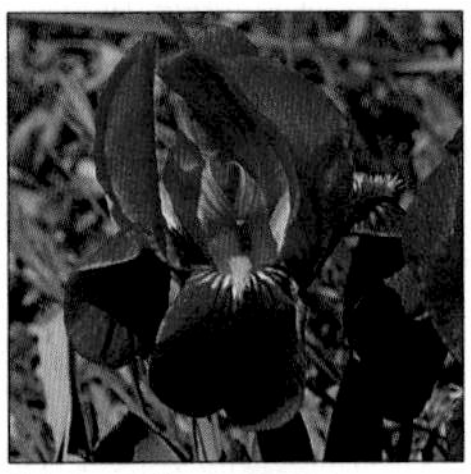
Iris pumila

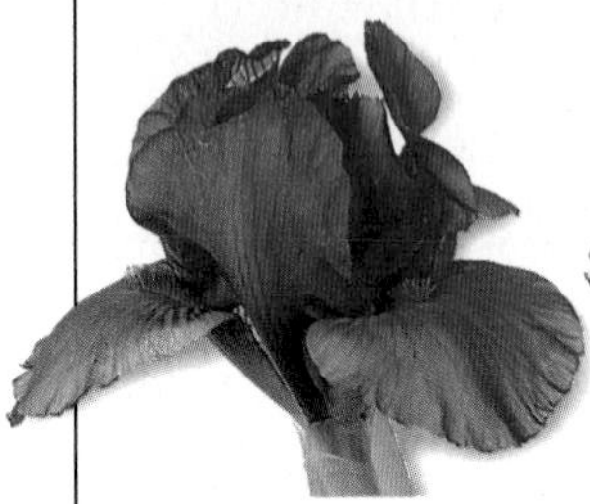
Iris 'Rain Dance'

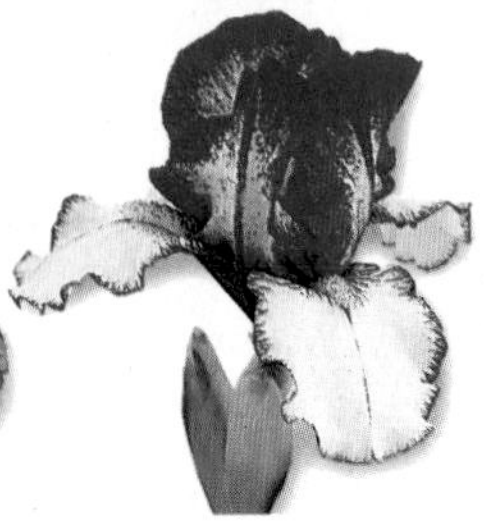
Iris 'Rare Edition'

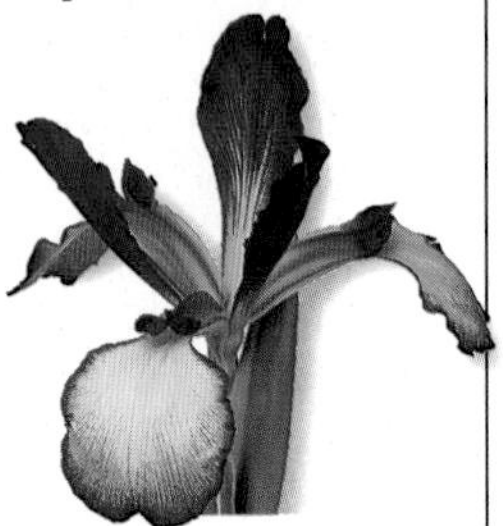
Iris 'Redwood Supreme'

***I.* 'Just Jennifer'.** Rhizomatous, intermediate bearded iris. Produces ruffled white flowers with white-tipped yellow beards in early spring. ↕65cm (26in). ❄❄❄

I. kaempferi see *I. ensata.*

***I.* 'Katharine Hodgkin'** ■ Very vigorous, bulbous Reticulata iris. In late winter, produces delicately patterned blue flowers with yellow and blue marks on the falls. ↕12cm (5in) at flowering. ❄❄❄

I. kerneriana ■ Rhizomatous, beardless Spuria iris with narrow, linear leaves, to 40cm (16in) long. Each erect stem bears 2–4 lemon-yellow flowers, 7–10cm (3–4in) across, in early summer. ↕30–50cm (12–20in). N. Turkey. ❄❄❄

I. korolkowii. Rhizomatous, bearded Regelia iris with linear leaves, to 40cm (16in) long, tinged purple at the bases. In late spring and early summer, each unbranched stem produces 2 or 3 flowers, 8cm (3in) across, with erect standards and pointed falls. All petals are cream with dark maroon veining; beards are small and dark brown. ↕40–60cm (16–24in). N.E. Afghanistan, C. Asia. ❄❄. **f. *violacea*** has violet petals and darker veins.

I. lacustris ■ Rhizomatous Crested iris with fans of narrow leaves, to 10cm (4in) long. In late spring, bears small, purple-blue to sky-blue flowers, 2cm (¾in) across, with a gold crest and a white patch on each fall. Often confused with *I. cristata,* but has narrower leaves and much shorter perianth tubes. ↕5cm (2in). N. USA (Great Lakes area). ❄❄❄

***I.* 'Lady Mohr'** ■ Rhizomatous, bearded Arilbred iris flowering in early spring. Standards are pearly white; falls are pale yellow, veined and spotted brownish purple around the chrome-yellow beards. ↕75cm (30in). ❄❄❄

***I.* 'Lady of Quality'** ■ Rhizomatous, beardless Siberian iris flowering in early summer. Flowers have light blue-violet standards and lighter blue falls, margined with silver. ↕85cm (34in). ❄❄❄

***I.* 'Lady Vanessa'.** Rhizomatous, beardless Siberian iris flowering in mid- and late spring. Standards are light wine-red; falls are darker and ruffled. ↕90cm (36in). ❄❄❄

I. laevigata ■🏆 Rhizomatous, beardless Laevigatae iris with broad leaves, to 40cm (16in) long. In early and midsummer, each unbranched stem bears 2–4 purple-blue flowers, 8–10cm (3–4in) across, the standards much shorter than the falls. Thrives in pond margins and other wet places. ↕80cm (32in). C. Russia to N. China, Korea, Japan. ❄❄❄. **f. *alba*** bears white flowers. **'Mottled Beauty'** has white flowers, with falls spotted pale blue. **'Rosea'** has pink flowers. **'Variegata'** ■ has white- and green-striped leaves and paler purple-blue flowers.

I. latifolia ■🏆 syn. *I. xiphioides* (English iris). Bulbous Xiphium iris with narrowly lance-shaped leaves, to 65cm (26in) long. Bears 1 or 2 broad, blue, violet, or white flowers, 8–10cm (3–4in) across, in early summer. May be naturalized in grass. ↕25–60cm (10–24in). N. Spain. ❄❄❄. **'Aristocrat'** has violet flowers, veined and marked deep violet. **'Duchess of York'** has purple flowers. **'Mont Blanc'** has white flowers, tinged lilac. **'Queen of the Blues'** has blue standards and purple-blue falls.

***I.* 'Lavender Royal'.** Rhizomatous, beardless Pacific Coast iris. In early spring, bears lavender-blue flowers with darker markings. ↕25cm (10in). ❄❄❄

I. lazica. Rhizomatous, beardless Unguiculares iris with arching fans of broad, evergreen, bright green leaves, to 30cm (12in) long. Scentless flowers, 6–8cm (2½–3in) across, are stemless, but have long perianth tubes, to 10cm (4in) tall, and are borne in early spring. Petals are lavender-blue; falls are white in the lower halves, spotted and veined lavender, each with a central yellow stripe. Unlike other Unguiculares, thrives in slight shade in moist soil. ↕15–25cm (6–10in). Black Sea coast, N. Turkey, S.W. Caucasus. ❄❄

***I.* 'Limeheart'.** Rhizomatous, beardless Siberian iris. Bears white flowers with green hafts in mid- and late spring. ↕100cm (39in). ❄❄❄

I. lortetii. Rhizomatous, bearded Oncocyclus iris with straight, linear leaves, to 25cm (10in) long. In late spring, each stem produces a solitary white flower, 9cm (3½in) across. Standards have fine pink veins; each fall has pink or maroon spots, one large deep maroon mark, and a reddish brown beard. ↕30–50cm (12–20in). Lebanon. ❄❄

I. lutescens ■ syn. *I. chamaeiris.* Very variable, rhizomatous, bearded iris with nearly straight leaves, 30cm (12in) long. In early and mid-spring, each erect, often branched stem bears 1 or 2 violet, yellow, bicoloured, or rarely white flowers, 6–7cm (2½–3in) across, with yellow beards. ↕5–30cm (2–12in). N.E. Spain, S. France, Italy. ❄❄❄. **'Nancy Lindsay'** is a dwarf cultivar with strongly scented yellow flowers.

I. macrosiphon. Rhizomatous, beardless Pacific Coast iris with linear, dull, grey-green leaves, to 30cm (12in) long. In late spring, bears violet, lavender,

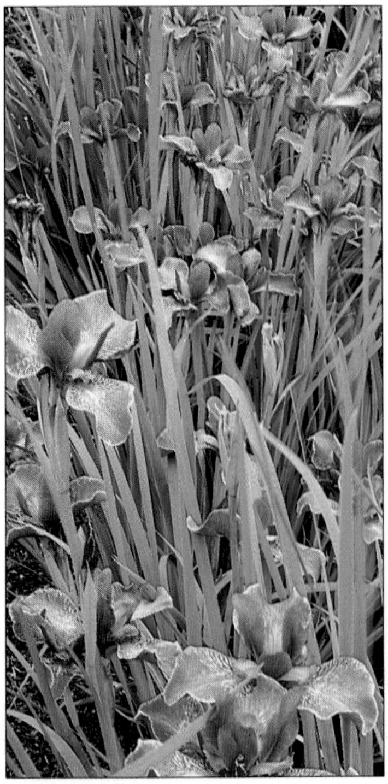
Iris 'Lady of Quality'

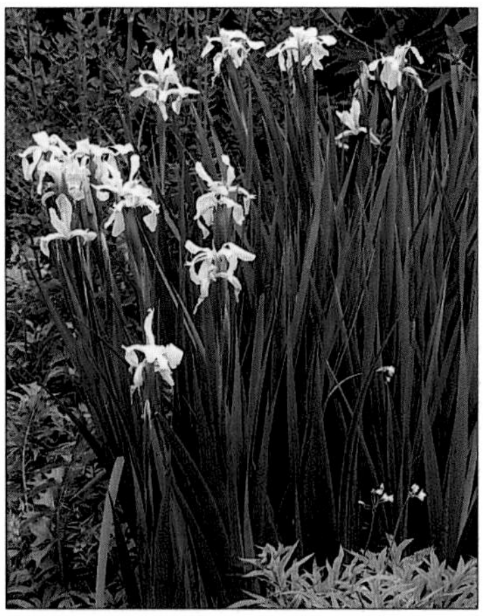
Iris orientalis

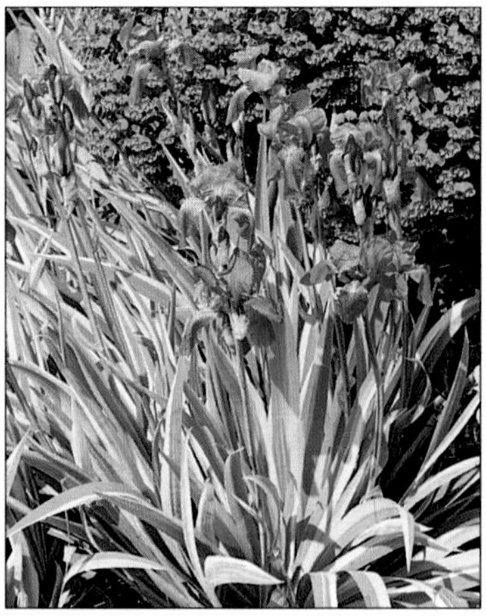
Iris pallida 'Variegata'

or yellow to cream flowers, 3.5–9cm (1½–3½in) across, which may be almost stemless. Some forms are frost tender. ↕ to 15–25cm (6–10in). USA (California). ❄❄
I. 'Magic Man' ■ Rhizomatous, tall bearded iris flowering from mid-spring to early summer. Standards are light purple-blue with darker midribs; falls are velvety purple with light blue edging and tangerine beards. ↕ 100cm (39in). ❄❄❄
I. magnifica ■ Robust, bulbous Juno iris with arching, glossy, mid-green leaves, to 18cm (7in) long. In mid- and late spring, bears up to 7 pale lilac flowers, to 8cm (3in) across, with a pale yellow and white central area on each fall. ↕ 30–60cm (12–24in). Mountains in C. Asia. ❄❄❄. **f. *alba*** has white flowers.
I. 'Marmalade Skies' ■ Vigorous, rhizomatous, intermediate bearded iris flowering in early spring. Standards are orange; falls are deeper orange with tan markings and mandarin-orange beards. ↕ 70cm (28in). ❄❄❄
I. milesii. Rhizomatous Crested iris with large, green, surface rhizomes and large fans of broad, pale green leaves, 30–60cm (12–24in) long. In early and midsummer, tall, branched stems produce many short-lived flowers, 6–8cm (2½–3in) across. Petals are lavender-pink mottled purple, with yellow crests. ↕ 90cm (36in). Himalayas. ❄❄❄
I. missouriensis ■ syn. *I. tolmeiana.* Variable, rhizomatous, beardless iris with narrow leaves, to 50cm (20in) long, overtopping the flowers. In summer, each slender, branched stem bears 2–4 flowers, 6–7cm (2½–3in) across. Standards are short, pale to deep blue or lilac-purple; falls are larger with deep purple veining. ↕ 20–50cm (8–20in). W. and C. North America. ❄❄❄
I. 'Mohr Pretender'. Rhizomatous, bearded Arilbred iris. In mid- and late spring, bears pale blue flowers with blue-tipped brown beards. ↕ 85cm (34in). ❄❄❄
I. 'Natascha' ■ Delicate, bulbous Reticulata iris with leaves 35cm (14in) long at flowering. In early spring, bears very pale blue flowers, which appear grey-white. ↕ 12cm (5in). ❄❄❄
I. nepalensis see *I. decora.*
I. nicolai. Small, bulbous Juno iris with leaves 25cm (10in) long, barely developed at flowering. In early spring, produces 1–3 whitish blue flowers, 5–6cm (2–2½in) across. Falls have rich violet tips and 2 violet stripes beside the orange crests. Similar in shape to, and possibly a colour form of, *I. rosenbachiana.* ↕ 10cm (4in). N.E. Afghanistan, C. Asia. ❄❄❄
I. ochroleuca see *I. orientalis.*
I. 'Orchid Flair'. Rhizomatous, miniature dwarf bearded iris flowering in early spring. The petals are flesh-pink; falls have white beards. ↕ 20cm (8in). ❄❄❄
I. orientalis ■ syn. *I. ochroleuca.* Robust, rhizomatous, beardless Spuria iris with leaves to 90cm (36in), broadest at the bases, often present over winter. In late spring, each strong stem, to 90cm (36in) long, usually with one branch, bears 3–5 flowers, 8–10cm (3–4in) across. Standards are white and erect; falls are white with yellow centres. ↕ to 90cm (36in). N.E. Greece, W. Turkey. ❄❄❄ (borderline)
***I. orientalis* of gardens** see *I. sanguinea.*
I. pallida, syn. *I. pallida* var. *dalmatica.* Rhizomatous, bearded iris with sometimes evergreen, grey-green leaves, 20–60cm (8–24in) long, much shorter than the flower stems, and distinctive, very silvery, papery bracts. In late spring and early summer, each branched stem produces 2–6 large, scented, soft blue flowers, 10cm (4in) across, with yellow beards. ↕ to 1.2m (4ft). Croatia. ❄❄❄. **'Argentea Variegata'** is less vigorous than the species, and has pale green leaves with silver-white stripes. **'Aurea Variegata'** see 'Variegata'. **var. *dalmatica*** see *I. pallida.* **'Variegata'** ■ syn. 'Aurea Variegata', has bright green leaves with light golden yellow stripes.
I. 'Paradise Bird' ■ Rhizomatous, tall bearded iris. In mid- and late spring, bears purple flowers with paler purple falls and orange beards. ↕ 85cm (33in). ❄❄❄
I. 'Pauline'. Bulbous Reticulata iris flowering in early spring. Standards are purple; falls are darker purple with white centres. ↕ 12cm (5in) at flowering. ❄❄❄
I. 'Peach Frost' ■ Rhizomatous, tall bearded iris. Bears ruffled flowers from mid-spring to early summer. Standards are peach-pink; falls are white with peach margins and tangerine beards. ↕ 100cm (39in). ❄❄❄
I. persica. Bulbous, dwarf Juno iris with linear leaves, to 10cm (4in) long, that elongate very little after flowering. From late winter to mid-spring, bears 1–4 flowers, 5–6cm (2–2½in) across. They vary from silvery grey to sand-yellow or pale green, with a darker, contrasting mark at the tip of each fall. ↕ 10cm (4in). S. and S.E. Turkey, N. Syria, N.E. Iraq. ❄❄❄
I. prismatica ■ Rhizomatous, beardless iris with thin, wide-spreading rhizomes, forming large clumps of grass-like leaves, to 70cm (30in) long. In early and mid-summer, bears clusters of 2 or 3 violet-blue flowers, 5–7cm (2–3in) across, veined blue, on slender, angled stems. ↕ 40–80cm (16–32in). North America (Nova Scotia to S. Carolina). ❄❄❄
I. 'Professor Blaauw' ■ Bulbous Dutch Xiphium iris flowering from mid-spring to midsummer. Bears violet-blue flowers with a yellow mark on each fall. ↕ to 60cm (24in). ❄❄❄

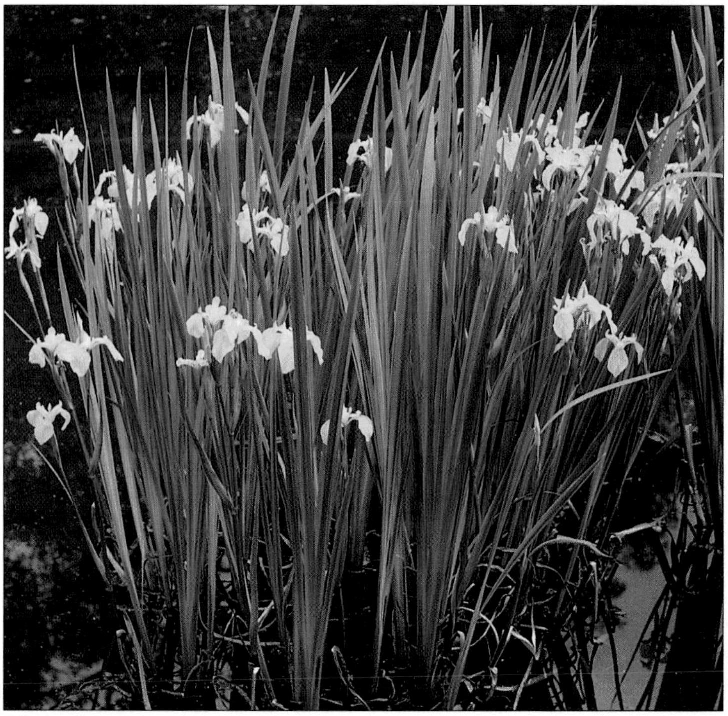
Iris pseudacorus

I. 'Protégé'. Rhizomatous, beardless Spuria iris. In early summer, bears flowers with mid-blue standards and blue-veined white falls. ↕ 90cm (36in). ❄❄❄
I. pseudacorus ■ (Yellow flag). Extremely vigorous, rhizomatous, beardless Laevigatae iris with ribbed, grey-green leaves, 90cm (36in) long. In mid- and late summer, each branched stem bears 4–12 flowers, 7–10cm (3–4in) across. Petals are yellow with brown or violet markings and a darker yellow zone on each fall. Suitable for margins of large ponds, lakes, or other wet places. ↕ 0.9–1.5m (3–5ft). Europe to W. Siberia, Caucasus, Turkey, Iran, N. Africa. ❄❄❄. **'Alba'** has pale cream flowers. **var. *bastardii*** produces clear sulphur-yellow flowers. **'Golden Fleece'** has deep yellow blooms. **'Variegata'** has white- or yellowish white-striped foliage.
I. pumila ■ (Dwarf bearded iris). Variable, rhizomatous, miniature dwarf bearded iris with grey-green leaves, to 15cm (6in) long. In mid-spring, unbranched stems bear usually solitary, scented, blue, purple, or yellow flowers, 5cm (2in) across, with yellow or blue beards. ↕ 10–15cm (4–6in). E. Europe to Urals. ❄❄❄. **'Atroviolacea'** bears purple flowers. **'Aurea'** has yellow blooms.
I. purdyi. Rhizomatous, beardless Pacific Coast iris with fans of evergreen, glossy, dark green leaves, to 35cm (14in) long, pink or red at the base, and with many short leaves on the unbranched flower stems. In late spring, each stem bears 2 lilac-tinted, pale cream flowers, 8cm (3in) across, with spreading petals, making the blooms appear flat. Falls are spotted purple-pink with dark pink margins. ↕ 25–35cm (10–14in). USA (N. California). ❄❄
I. 'Purple Gem'. Bulbous Reticulata iris bearing neat purple flowers in early spring. ↕ 15cm (6in). ❄❄❄
I. 'Rain Dance' ■ Rhizomatous, standard dwarf bearded iris. Bears violet-blue flowers with matching beards in mid- and late spring. ↕ 25cm (10in). ❄❄❄
I. 'Rare Edition' ■ Rhizomatous, intermediate bearded iris flowering in mid- and late spring. Standards are mulberry-purple, lightly speckled in white; falls are white with stitched purple margins and blue-white beards. ↕ 60cm (24in). ❄❄❄
I. 'Raspberry Rimmed'. Rhizomatous, beardless Laevigatae iris producing single flowers in mid- and late spring. Standards and falls are white with narrow, raspberry-red margins and a golden yellow patch on each fall. ↕ 90cm (36in). ❄❄❄
I. 'Redwood Supreme' ■ Rhizomatous, beardless Spuria iris. Bears flowers with dark brown standards, and orange falls with dark brown margins, in mid- and late spring. ↕ 100cm (39in). ❄❄❄
I. reticulata ♀ Bulbous Reticulata iris with square-sectioned leaves, 1–10cm (½–4in) long at flowering. In late winter and early spring, bears a solitary, fragrant flower, 6–8cm (2½–3in) across, varying from pale to deep violet-blue or reddish purple, with a yellow central ridge on each fall. Bulbs often split after blooming and may take some years to reach flowering size again. ↕ 10–15cm (4–6in). Caucasus, N. and E. Turkey,

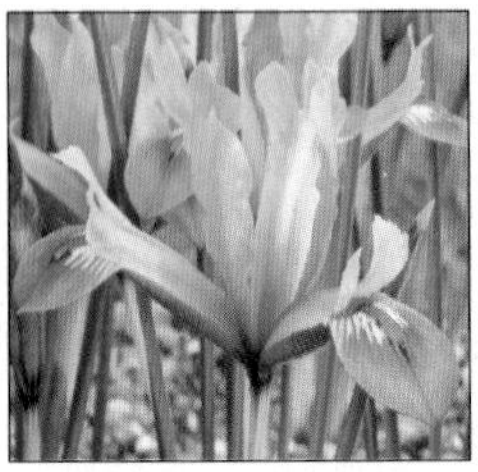
Iris reticulata 'Cantab'

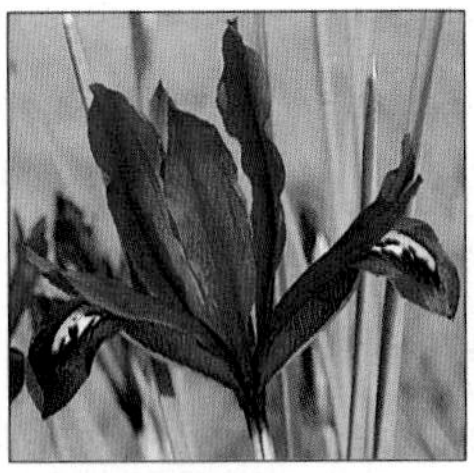
Iris reticulata 'J.S. Dijt'

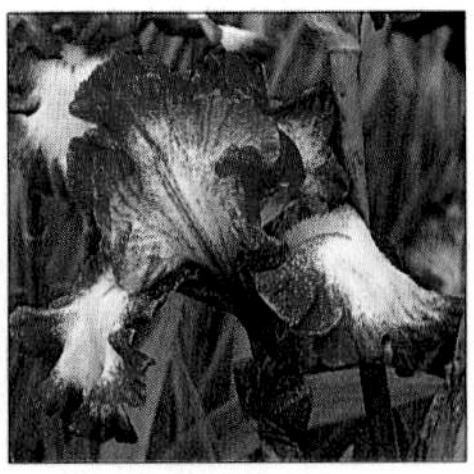
Iris 'Rippling Rose'

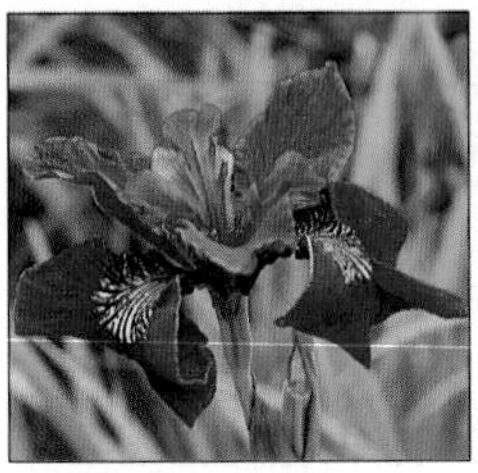
Iris 'Ruffled Velvet'

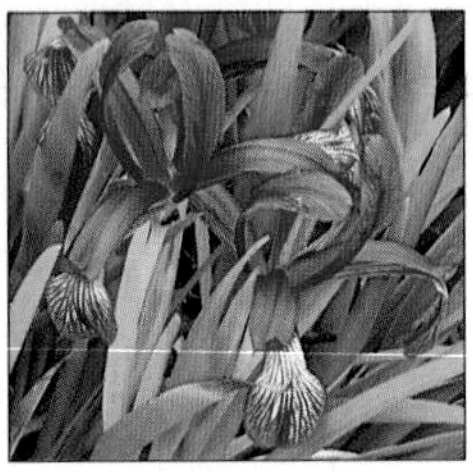
Iris ruthenica

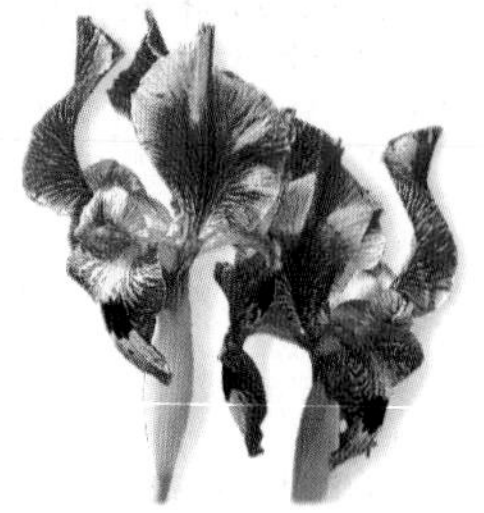
Iris sari

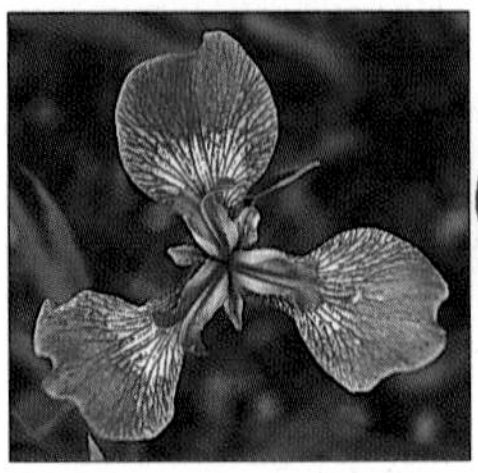
Iris setosa

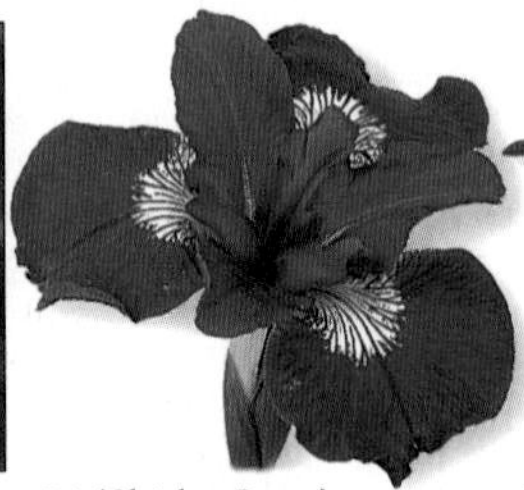
Iris 'Shirley Pope'

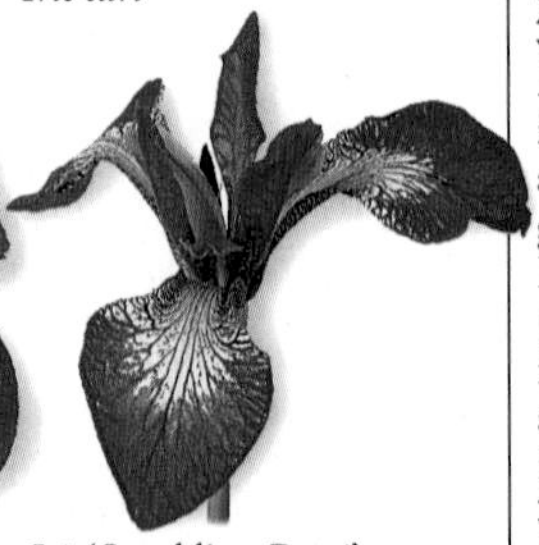
Iris 'Sparkling Rosé'

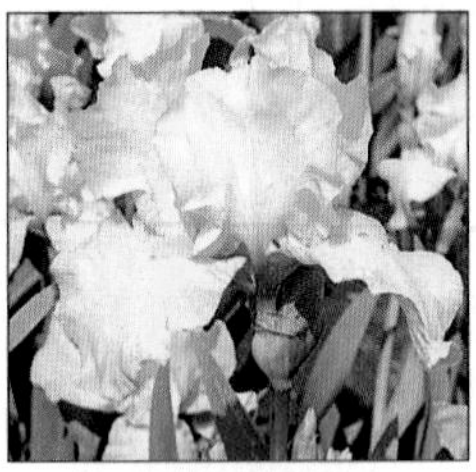
Iris 'Sun Miracle'

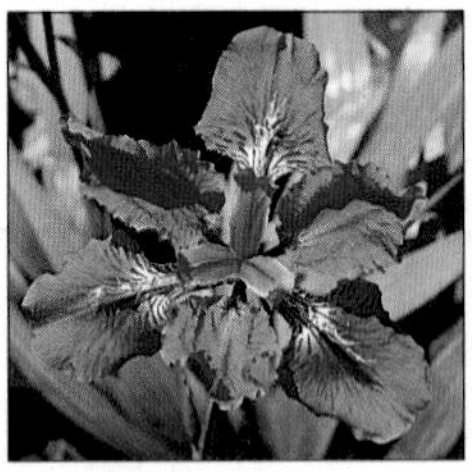
Iris tectorum

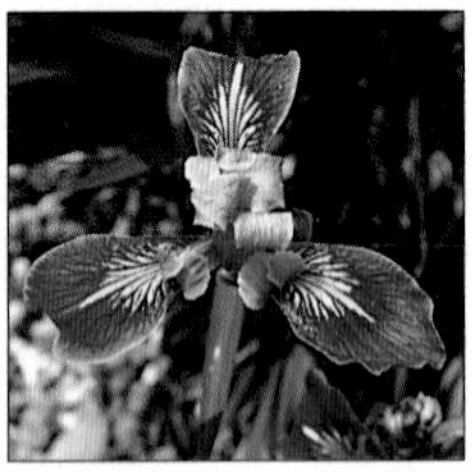
Iris tenax

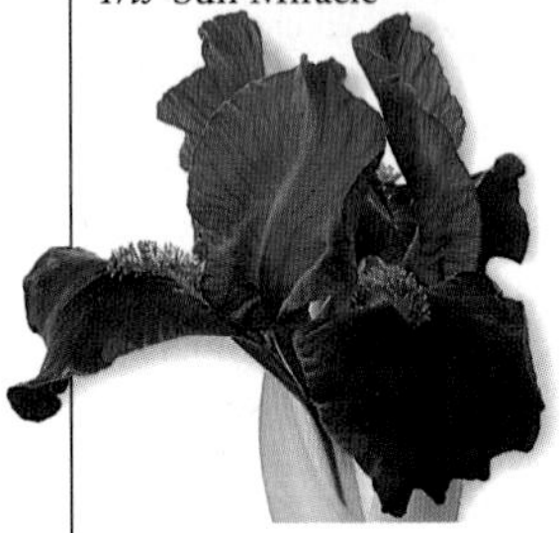
Iris 'Toots'

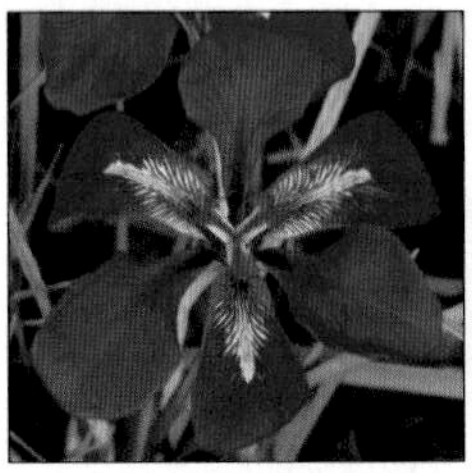
Iris unguicularis 'Mary Barnard'

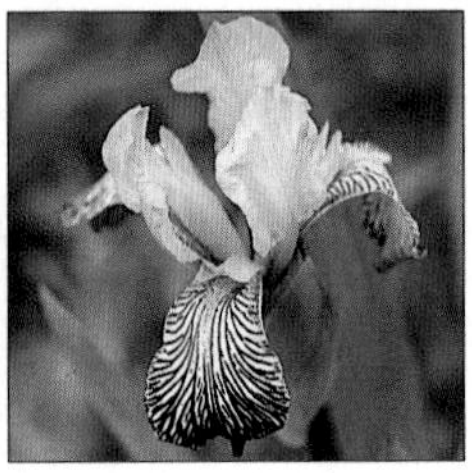
Iris variegata

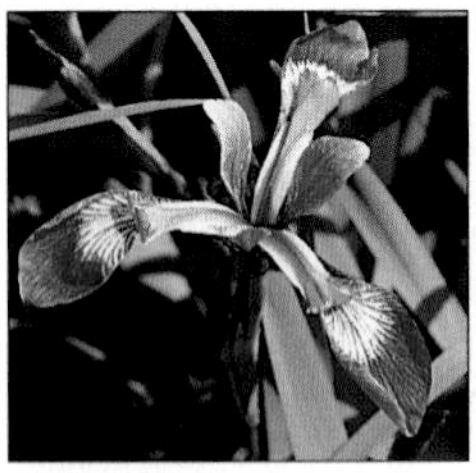
Iris versicolor

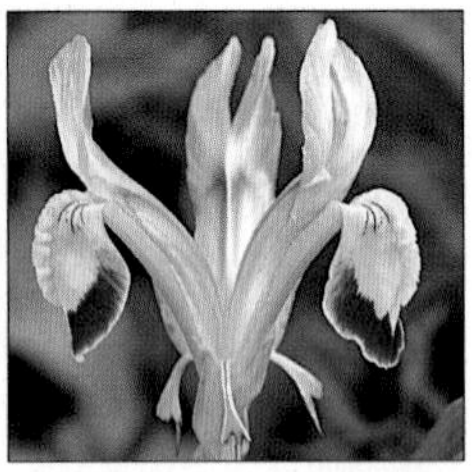
Iris warleyensis

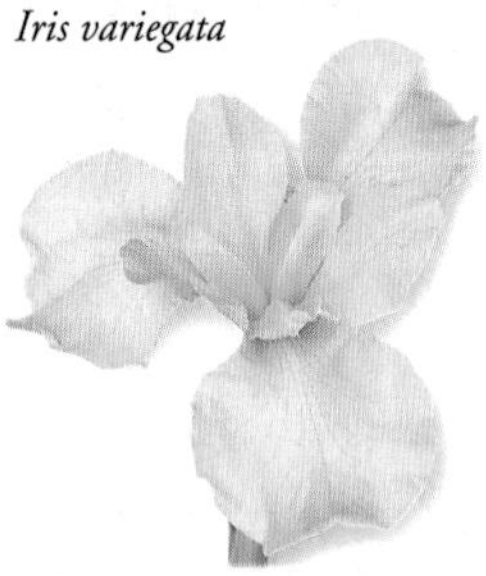
Iris 'White Swirl'

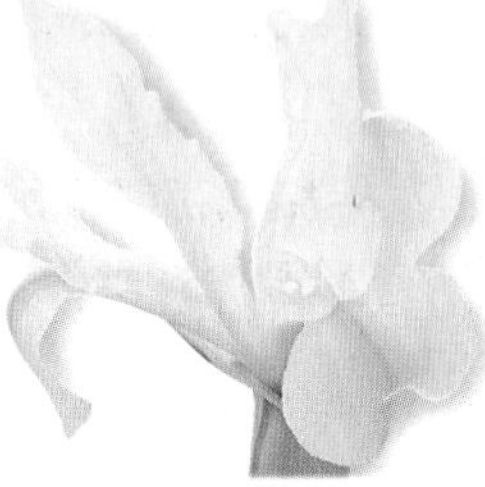
Iris 'White Wedgwood'

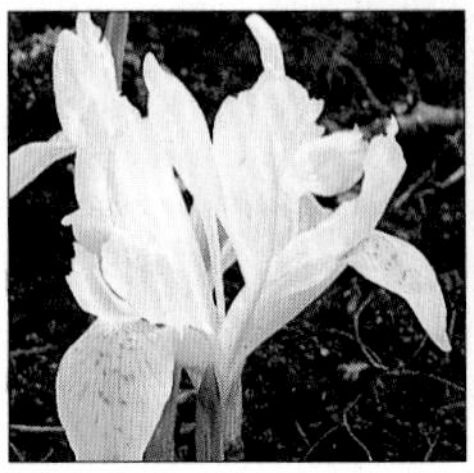
Iris winogradowii

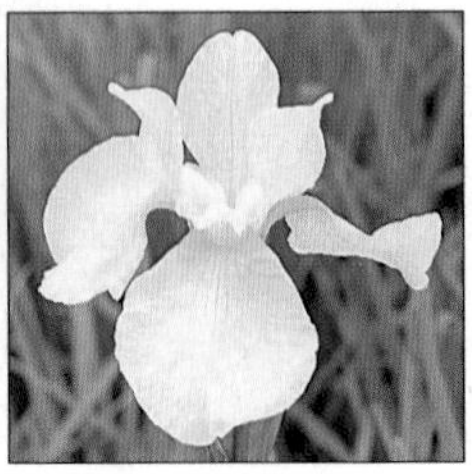
Iris 'Wisley White'

I

N.E. Iraq, N. Iran. ❄❄❄. **'Cantab'** ▣ produces pale blue flowers with deeper blue falls, each with a yellow crest. **'J.S. Dijt'** ▣ has reddish purple flowers with a central orange mark on each fall.

***I.* 'Rippling Rose'** ▣ Rhizomatous, tall bearded iris. In mid- and late spring, bears ruffled white flowers with purple markings and lemon beards. ↕90cm (36in). ❄❄❄

I. rosenbachiana. Small, bulbous Juno iris with glossy, mid-green leaves, eventually to 25cm (10in) long, only slightly developed at flowering. In late winter and early spring, bears solitary, rich purple flowers, 5–6cm (2–2½in) across, with a bright orange-yellow crest on each fall. ↕10cm (4in). C. Asia. ❄❄❄

***I.* 'Ruffled Velvet'** ▣ Rhizomatous, beardless Siberian iris. In early summer, bears flowers with velvety, red-purple standards and darker, ruffled falls. ↕55cm (22in). ❄❄❄

I. ruthenica ▣ Rhizomatous, beardless iris with creeping, branched rhizomes and fans of grass-like, glossy, bright green leaves, to 30cm (12in) long. In late spring, each stem, 3–15cm (1¼–6in) tall, produces 1 or 2 fragrant flowers, 4cm (1½in) across. Erect standards are violet or lavender-blue; falls are white with dark violet markings. ↕to 20cm (8in). E. Europe to China, Korea. ❄❄❄

I. sanguinea, syn. *I. extremorientalis, I. orientalis* of gardens. Rhizomatous, beardless Siberian iris with slightly glaucous, mid-green leaves, to 75cm (30in) long, as tall as or longer than the unbranched flower stems. In late spring and early summer, each stem bears 2 red-purple flowers, 5–8cm (2–3in) across, with small, erect standards, and falls with orange hafts. ↕to 90cm (36in). S.E. Russia, China, Korea, Japan. ❄❄❄. **'Alba'** has white flowers with some purple veining.

I. sari ▣ Rhizomatous, bearded Oncocyclus iris with narrow, curved or nearly straight leaves, 9cm (3½in) long. In late spring, each stem bears one ruffled, crimson-veined, cream flower, 7–10cm (3–4in) across. Each fall has a crimson or brown patch and yellow beard. ↕10–30cm (4–12in). C. and E. Turkey. ❄❄

***I.* 'Scribe'.** Rhizomatous, miniature dwarf bearded iris. In early spring, bears white flowers with blue markings and blue beards. ↕15cm (6in). ❄❄❄

I. setosa ▣ Very variable, rhizomatous, beardless iris with linear, mid-green leaves, to 50cm (20in) long, often red-tinted at the bases. In late spring and early summer, each stem bears 2–12 flowers, 5–9cm (2–3½in) across, with blue or purple-blue falls and bristle-like standards. ↕15–90cm (6–36in). E. Russia (including Sakhalin, Kurile Islands), N. Korea, Japan, Alaska (including Aleutian Islands), N.E. North America. ❄❄❄. **var. *arctica*** is one of several dwarf variants. Each unbranched stem bears 2 purple flowers with white marks.

***I.* 'Shelford Giant'** ▣ Rhizomatous, beardless Spuria iris flowering in early summer. Bears large, lemon-white flowers with a central yellow patch on each fall. ↕1.8m (6ft) or more. ❄❄❄

***I.* 'Shirley Pope'** ▣ Rhizomatous, beardless Siberian iris. In early summer, bears dark red-purple flowers; falls are velvety with white patches. ↕85cm (34in). ❄❄❄

I. sibirica. Rhizomatous, beardless Siberian iris with narrow, grass-like leaves, to 45cm (18in) long. In early summer, each branched stem bears up to 5 flowers, to 7cm (3in) across, well above the foliage. All petals are blue-violet; falls have dark veining, the background colour changing to white near the hafts. A parent of numerous cultivars. ↕50–120cm (20–48in). C. and E. Europe, N.E. Turkey, Russia. ❄❄❄. **f. *alba*** bears white flowers.

I. sisyrinchium see *Gynandriris sisyrinchium.*

***I.* 'Sparkling Rosé'** ▣ Rhizomatous, beardless Siberian iris. In mid- and late spring, bears pinkish mauve flowers. The base of each fall is yellow with purple veins. ↕100cm (39in). ❄❄❄

I. spuria. Robust, very variable, rhizomatous, beardless Spuria iris with tough, broad leaves, 30cm (12in) long. In early and midsummer, each branched stem bears several blue, yellow, or white flowers, 6–8cm (2½–3in) across. ↕to 90cm (36in). S. Europe to C. Asia. ❄❄❄

***I.* 'Stepping Out'** 🏆 Rhizomatous, tall bearded iris. Bears white flowers, with sharply patterned, blue-violet margins and pale blue beards, in mid- and late spring. ↕100cm (39in). ❄❄❄

I. stylosa see *I. unguicularis.*

***I.* 'Sun Miracle'** ▣ Rhizomatous, tall bearded iris. In early summer, bears canary-yellow flowers with yellow beards. ↕90cm (36in). ❄❄❄

***I.* 'Sunrise'.** Bulbous Dutch Xiphium iris flowering from mid-spring to midsummer. Standards are lemon-yellow; falls are golden yellow, each with an orange mark. ↕60cm (24in). ❄❄❄

***I.* 'Superstition'.** Rhizomatous, tall bearded iris. Bears dark purple-brown flowers with blue-black beards in early summer. ↕90cm (36in). ❄❄❄

I. susiana (Mourning iris). Rhizomatous, bearded Oncocyclus iris with slightly curved leaves, 10–15cm (4–6in) long. In late spring, each stem bears a large, solitary flower, 10–15cm (4–6in) across. Petals are grey with deep purple veins, black patches, and purple beards. Very susceptible to virus. ↕30–40cm (12–16in). Probably Lebanon. ❄❄

I. tectorum ▣ (Roof iris). Rhizomatous Crested iris with fans of broad, ribbed, glossy, dark green leaves, to 30cm (12in) long. In early summer, each occasionally branched stem bears 2 or 3 lilac flowers, 3–10cm (1¼–4in) across, with darker veins and a white crest on each fall. ↕25–40cm (10–16in). C., S. and S.W. China. ❄❄❄. **f. *alba*** has white flowers with yellow veins on the crests and falls. **'Variegata'** has green leaves with white stripes.

I. tenax ▣ Rhizomatous, beardless Pacific Coast iris with narrow, deep green leaves, to 30cm (12in) long, tinged red at the bases. From mid-spring to early summer, each stem bears 1 or 2 blue, lavender-blue, yellow, cream, or white flowers, 7–9cm (3–3½in) across. ↕20–35cm (8–14in). USA (Washington, Oregon). ❄❄❄

I. tenuis. Creeping, rhizomatous Crested iris with narrow leaves, 30cm (12in) long. In late spring, each branched stem bears one pale lilac flower, 3–4cm (1¼–1½in) across, with yellow crests. ↕ to 30cm (12in). USA (Oregon). ❄❄❄

***I.* 'Theseus'.** Rhizomatous, bearded Regeliocyclus iris flowering in early spring. Petals are violet: standards have dark violet veins, and falls have ivory veins, dark violet markings, and purple-brown beards. ↕ 45cm (18in). ❄❄❄

I. tingitana. Robust, bulbous Xiphium iris with lance-shaped, silvery grey leaves, 45cm (18in) long, which appear in autumn and are prone to frost damage. In late winter and early spring, bears 1–3 pale to deep blue flowers, 8–12cm (3–5in) across. It is one parent of the Dutch irises. ↕ 60cm (24in). Morocco, Algeria. ❄❄

I. tolmeiana see *I. missouriensis.*

***I.* 'Toots'** ■ Rhizomatous, standard dwarf bearded iris. In mid- and late spring, bears velvety, wine-red flowers with yellow beards. ↕ 30cm (12in). ❄❄❄

I. tuberosa see *Hermodactylus tuberosus.*

I. unguicularis 🏆 syn. *I. stylosa.* Vigorous, rhizomatous, beardless Unguiculares iris with tough, grass-like, evergreen leaves, to 60cm (24in) long. Flowers are large, fragrant, 5–8cm (2–3in) across, pale lavender to deep violet with contrasting veins, and a central band of yellow on the falls, and with perianth tubes 6–20cm (2½–8in) long. They are borne singly on very short stems arising from a branching rhizome in late winter and early spring, occasionally in late autumn. ↕ 30cm (12in). Greece, W. and S. Turkey, W. Syria, Tunisia, Algeria. ❄❄❄. **'Alba'** bears creamy white flowers with a yellow central line on each fall; flowers are more frost tender than on blue forms. **subsp. *cretensis*** ■ is a dwarf variant. Standards are violet or lavender-blue; falls are white or yellow with violet veining at the bases and clear violet tips. ↕ 10cm (4in). Greece (Peloponnese, Crete). ❄❄. **'Mary Barnard'** ■ bears bright violet flowers in midwinter. **'Walter Butt'** has larger, strongly fragrant, pale lavender-blue, almost grey flowers, 8–10cm (3–4in) across; it is one of the earliest to bloom, sometimes in late autumn.

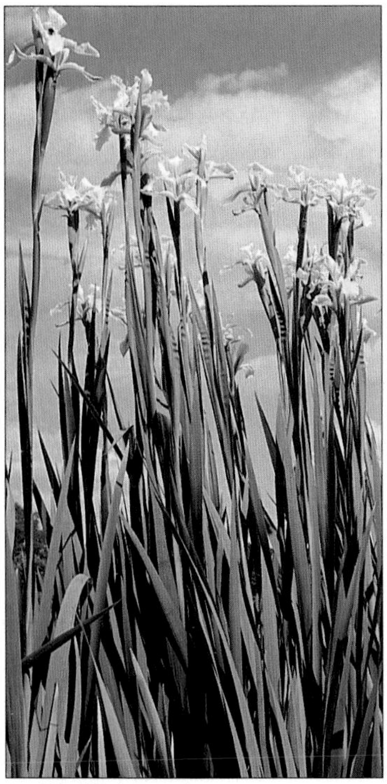

Iris 'Shelford Giant'

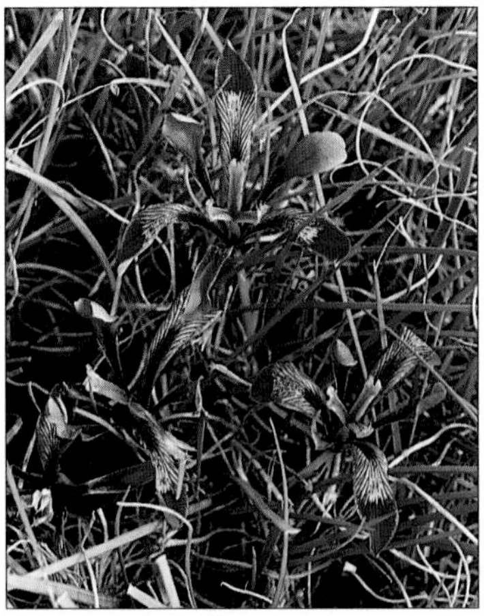

Iris unguicularis subsp. *cretensis*

***I.* 'Vanity'.** Rhizomatous, tall bearded iris. In early summer, bears pink flowers with light coral-pink beards. ↕ 90cm (36in). ❄❄❄

I. variegata ■ Rhizomatous, bearded iris with curved, strongly ribbed, deep green leaves, to 30cm (12in) long. In midsummer, each branched stem bears 3–6 pale yellow flowers, 5–7cm (2–3in) across. Falls have brown or violet veins and yellow beards. Many colour variants are known. ↕ 20–45cm (8–20in). C. and E. Europe. ❄❄❄

I. verna. Small, rhizomatous, beardless iris with fans of deep green leaves, to 6cm (2½in) long, which lengthen after flowering to 10–15cm (4–6in). In early spring, bears solitary, violet or blue flowers, 5cm (2in) across, with a narrow orange stripe on each fall. ↕ 15cm (6in), to 4–6cm (1½–2½in) at flowering. S.E. USA. ❄❄❄

I. versicolor ■ (Blue flag). Rhizomatous, beardless Laevigatae iris with erect or slightly arched leaves, 35–60cm (14–24in) long. In early and midsummer, each branched stem bears 3–5 violet, purple, or lavender-blue flowers, 6–8cm (2½–3in) across, with a white-veined purple area on each fall. ↕ 20–80cm (8–32in). E. North America. ❄❄❄. **'Kermesina'** bears red-purple flowers.

I. virginica (Southern blue flag). Rhizomatous, beardless Laevigatae iris with soft leaves, 50cm (20in) long, arching at the tips. From late spring to summer, each usually unbranched stem bears up to 4 blue to lavender-blue flowers. Falls are spreading and have yellow patches; standards are small and erect. ↕ 50–100cm (20–39in). S.E. USA (Virginia to Florida and E. Texas). ❄❄❄ (borderline)

***I.* 'Virtue'.** Rhizomatous, intermediate bearded iris flowering in mid- and late spring. Standards are rich purple; falls are royal purple with a velvety texture, blue beards, and bronze throats. ↕ 50cm (20in). ❄❄❄

I. warleyensis ■ Vigorous, bulbous Juno iris with curved, glossy leaves, to 20cm (8in) long. In spring, bears up to 5 pale to deep violet or purplish blue flowers, 5–7cm (2–3in) across. Each narrow fall has a white rim, a toothed, cream to yellow crest, and a deep violet patch at the tip. ↕ 20–45cm (8–18in). C. Asia (Altai to Pamir Mountains). ❄❄❄

***I.* 'Warlsind'.** Bulbous Juno iris flowering in early spring. Standards are blue; falls are yellow with blue margins. ↕ 30cm (12in). ❄❄❄

***I.* 'Wedgwood'.** Bulbous Dutch Xiphium iris. Clear blue flowers are borne from mid-spring to midsummer. ↕ 60–70cm (24–28in). ❄❄❄

***I.* 'White Swirl'** ■ Rhizomatous, beardless Siberian iris. In early summer, bears pure white flowers, yellow at the bases, with rounded, flaring petals. ↕ 100cm (39in). ❄❄❄

***I.* 'White Wedgwood'** ■ Bulbous Dutch Xiphium iris. Bears creamy white flowers with a yellow mark on each fall from mid-spring to midsummer. ↕ 65cm (26in). ❄❄❄

***I.* 'Why Not?'.** Rhizomatous, intermediate bearded iris. Bears apricot flowers with orange beards in mid- and late spring. ↕ 55cm (22in). ❄❄❄

I. winogradowii ■ Bulbous Reticulata iris with erect, square-sectioned leaves, 1–10cm (½–4in) long at flowering. In early spring, bears solitary, primrose-yellow flowers, 6–7cm (2½–3in) across, spotted green on the falls. Unlike many other bulbous Reticulata irises, the bulbs do not split up after flowering. ↕ 6–10cm (2½–4in). Caucasus. ❄❄❄

***I.* 'Wisley White'** ■ Rhizomatous, beardless Siberian iris. Bears white flowers with cream veining and bright yellow haft marks in early summer. ↕ 100cm (39in). ❄❄❄

I. xiphioides see *I. latifolia.*

I. xiphium (Spanish iris). Vigorous, bulbous Xiphium iris with lance-shaped leaves, 20–70cm (8–28in) long. In late spring and early summer, produces 2 pale to deep blue or violet, rarely yellow or white flowers, 12cm (5in) across, with an orange or yellow mark on each fall. It is one parent of the Dutch irises. ↕ 40–60cm (16–24in). S. Europe, N. Africa. ❄❄❄

▷ **Iris,**
Dwarf bearded see *Iris pumila*
English see *Iris latifolia*
Mourning see *Iris susiana*
Roof see *Iris tectorum*
Spanish see *Iris xiphium*
Stinking see *Iris foetidissima*
Widow see *Hermodactylus tuberosus*

▷ **Ironbark** see *Eucalyptus*
Red see *E. sideroxylon*
White see *E. leucoxylon*

▷ **Ironweed** see *Vernonia*

▷ **Ironwood** see *Ostrya virginiana*
Catalina see *Lyonothamnus floribundus*
Lemon see *Backhousia citriodora*
Persian see *Parrotia persica*

ISATIS

BRASSICACEAE/CRUCIFERAE

Genus of about 30 species of annuals, biennials, and perennials, growing on waste ground, rocky sites, or as weeds of cultivation, in dry places in C. and S. Europe, and in W. and C. Asia. They have ovate to ovate-oblong, entire or pinnately lobed, stalked basal leaves and smaller, arrow-shaped, stalkless stem leaves. Small, 4-petalled, usually yellow flowers are borne in loose racemes or panicles, and are attractive to bees. They are ideal for a wild garden; *I. tinctoria* is suitable for a herb garden.

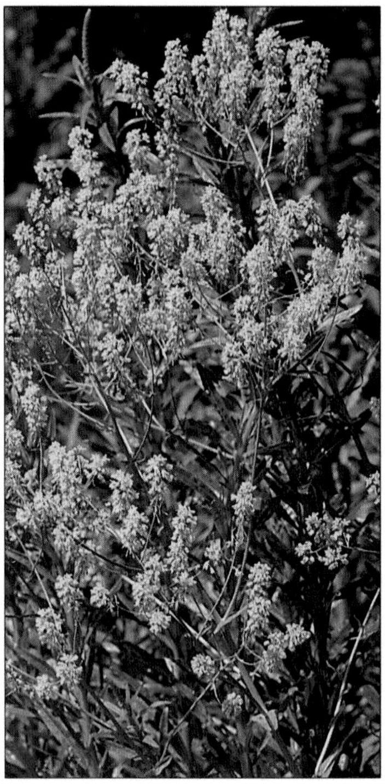

Isatis tinctoria

• **HARDINESS** Fully hardy.

• **CULTIVATION** Grow in moderately fertile, moist but well-drained soil in full sun.

• **PROPAGATION** Sow seed in autumn in containers in a cold frame, or in spring at 13–18°C (55–64°F). Divide in spring.

• **PESTS AND DISEASES** Trouble free.

I. glauca. Upright, clump-forming, almost hairless perennial with glaucous, blue-green leaves: the stalked basal leaves are lance-shaped, to 30cm (12in) long; the smaller, stalkless stem leaves are arrow-shaped, to 12cm (5in) long. Bears abundant 4-petalled yellow flowers, 6mm (¼in) across, in large panicles, 12–30cm (5–12in) across, in early summer. ↕ 60–120cm (24–48in), ↔ 45cm (18in). Turkey, Iran. ❄❄❄

I. tinctoria ■ (Woad). Tap-rooted, hairless or slightly hairy, short-lived perennial or biennial. Produces basal rosettes of oblong-lance-shaped, grey-green stalked leaves, to 10cm (4in) long, and leafy flowering stems bearing arrow-shaped, grey-green stalkless leaves, to 5cm (2in) long. Branched panicles, 3–8cm (1¼–3in) across, of 4-petalled yellow flowers, 8mm (⅜in) across, are borne in early summer. Self-seeds freely. Leaves produce a blue pigment when boiled or fermented with ammonia. ↕ 60–120cm (24–48in), ↔ 45cm (18in). S. Europe. ❄❄❄

▷ ***Ismene*** see *Hymenocallis*
I. calathina see *H. narcissiflora*

ISOPLEXIS

SCROPHULARIACEAE

Genus of 3 species of evergreen subshrubs or shrubs, closely related to *Digitalis*, found in open places in laurel forest and tree heather forest, up to 1,500m (5000ft), in Madeira and the Canary Islands. They are cultivated for their tubular, 5-lobed, colourful flowers,

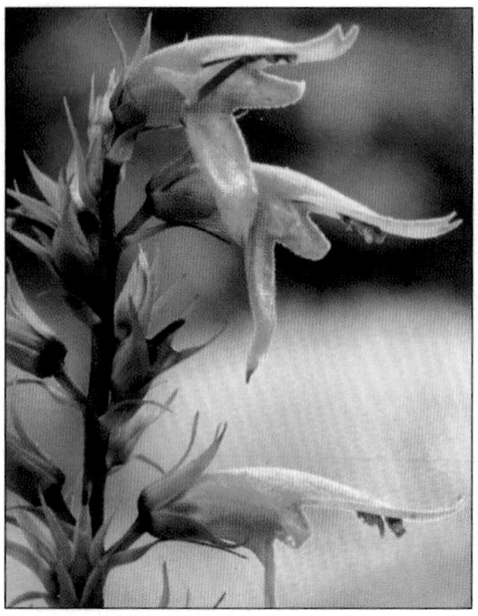

Isoplexis canariensis

which are borne in terminal racemes. Leaves are alternate, narrow, and simple, with toothed margins. Where temperatures fall below 5°C (41°F), grow in a temperate greenhouse or conservatory. In milder climates, grow in a shrub border, small courtyard garden, or as specimen plants.

- **HARDINESS** Frost tender.
- **CULTIVATION** Under glass, grow in loam-based potting compost (JI No.2) in full or bright filtered light, with low to moderate humidity. During growth, water moderately and apply a balanced liquid fertilizer monthly. Water sparingly in winter. Outdoors, grow in fertile, moist but well-drained soil in full sun or partial shade. Shelter from cold, drying winds. Pruning group 9.
- **PROPAGATION** Sow seed at 18–24° (65–75°F) in spring. Root softwood cuttings in spring, or semi-ripe cuttings in summer with bottom heat.
- **PESTS AND DISEASES** Whiteflies and red spider mites may be troublesome under glass.

I. canariensis ■ Erect, bushy shrub when young, spreading with age. Lance-shaped to narrowly ovate, sharply toothed, almost leathery, deep green leaves, to 15cm (6in) long, softly hairy beneath, are borne close together. Produces dense racemes, 30cm (12in) long, of tubular, bright orange-yellow, brownish orange, or yellow-brown flowers, to 3cm (1¼in) long, each with a 2-lobed upper lip, mainly in summer. ↕ to 1.5m (5ft), ↔ to 1m (3ft). Canary Islands (Tenerife). ❂ (min. 5°C/41°F)

ISOPOGON

Cone bush, Drumsticks

PROTEACEAE

Genus of more than 35 species of mainly small, evergreen shrubs from Australia, usually found in heathland, heath woodland and drought-prone forest, from sea level to sub-alpine zones. The alternate or spiralling, leathery leaves are usually pinnately or ternately divided, sometimes simple. They are grown for their firm, cone-like, spherical flowerheads, composed of many bracts and slender florets radiating outwards. Where temperatures regularly fall to 0°C (32°F), grow in a temperate greenhouse. In warm, dry climates grow in a shrub border. The larger species are unusual specimen plants.

- **HARDINESS** Half hardy to frost tender.

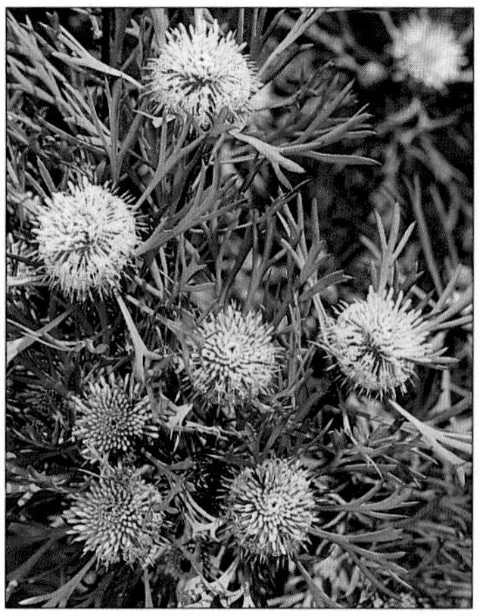

Isopogon anemonifolius

- **CULTIVATION** Under glass, grow in a mix of equal parts of loam-based potting compost (JI No.1), grit, and leaf mould or peat, in full or bright filtered light and low humidity. During the growing season, water sparingly and apply a half-strength, phosphate-free liquid fertilizer monthly. Keep just moist in winter. Outdoors, grow in neutral to acid, poor to moderately fertile soil in full sun, with shelter from cold, drying winds. Pruning group 1.
- **PROPAGATION** In spring, surface-sow seed at 19–24°C (66–75°F) and cover with a fine layer of vermiculite or grit; before sowing, soak seed for 24 hours. Root semi-ripe cuttings in late summer with bottom heat.
- **PESTS AND DISEASES** In moist, humid conditions, *Phytophthora* root rot may kill plants. Scale insects may be a problem under glass.

I. anemonifolius ■ (Broad-leaf drumsticks). Dense, rounded to spreading shrub with hairy, often red-tinted, young shoots. Mid-green leaves, to 10cm (4in) long, vary from simple to 2- or 3-lobed; each slender lobe is deeply cut at the tips into narrow segments. Bears abundant yellow and cream flowerheads, 4cm (1½in) across, each surrounded by a ruff of dissected leaves, from spring to midsummer. ↕ 0.6–2m (2–6ft), ↔ 1–2m (3–6ft). Australia (New South Wales). ❂ (min. 5°C/41°F)

I. dubius (Pin-cushion flower, Rose coneflower). Small, erect to rounded shrub with often densely hairy shoots. Leaves are linear, prickly, bright to greyish green, 3–8cm (1¼–3in) long, deeply dissected 3–4 times into wide-spreading lobes. Produces solitary or clustered, rose-pink flowerheads, to 5cm (2in) across, from late winter to late spring or early summer. ↕ 0.8–1.5m (2½–5ft), ↔ 1–2m (3–6ft). Australia (Western Australia). ❂ (min. 7–10°C/45–50°F)

ISOPYRUM

False rue anemone

RANUNCULACEAE

Genus of 30 species of spring-flowering, rhizomatous, tufted perennials, which grow wild in damp woodland in temperate regions of Europe. They have delicate, deeply divided, ternate to 3-ternate leaves and anemone-like, usually white flowers with 5 petal-like sepals; petals are tiny or absent. These dainty plants are suitable for a peat bed, woodland garden, or rock garden.

- **HARDINESS** Fully hardy.
- **CULTIVATION** Grow in humus-rich, neutral to acid, moist but well-drained soil in partial shade. Shelter from cold, drying winds.
- **PROPAGATION** Sow seed as soon as ripe in containers in an open frame. Divide in autumn.
- **PESTS AND DISEASES** May be badly damaged by slugs and snails.

I. thalictroides. Clump-forming perennial with bluish green leaves, to 5cm (2in) long, each divided into 3 ovate, 3-lobed leaflets. Produces loose, open panicles, to 4cm (1½in) long, of nodding, anemone-like white flowers, to 2cm (¾in) across, from spring to early summer. ↕ 20cm (8in), ↔ 15cm (6in). W. and C. Europe. ❄❄❄

▷ ***Isotoma*** see *Solenopsis*
I. axillaris see *S. axillaris*

ITEA

ESCALLONIACEAE/GROSSULARIACEAE

Genus of about 10 species of evergreen and deciduous shrubs and trees from woodlands and swamps in E. Asia and E. North America. They are cultivated for their holly-like leaves, attractive autumn colour, and their small, white, cream, or green-white flowers. Leaves are toothed and arranged alternately. The flowers are borne in axillary or terminal, catkin-like, many-flowered racemes or panicles. Grow evergreen species in a sheltered position in a shrub border; *I. ilicifolia* and *I. yunnanensis* are suitable for growing against a warm sunny wall; *I. virginica* prefers more moisture, and is best grown in a shrub or mixed border, or as a free-standing specimen.

- **HARDINESS** Fully hardy to frost hardy.
- **CULTIVATION** Grow evergreen species in fertile, moist but well-drained soil in full sun. Shelter from cold, drying winds and mulch young plants in winter. Grow *I. virginica* in moist, slightly acid soil in partial shade. Provide support and tie in long shoots of wall-trained, evergreen species. Pruning group 9 for evergreens; group 2 for deciduous species; group 13 if wall-trained.
- **PROPAGATION** Sow seed as soon as ripe in containers in an open frame. Root greenwood cuttings in spring, or semi-ripe cuttings in summer with bottom heat.
- **PESTS AND DISEASES** Trouble free.

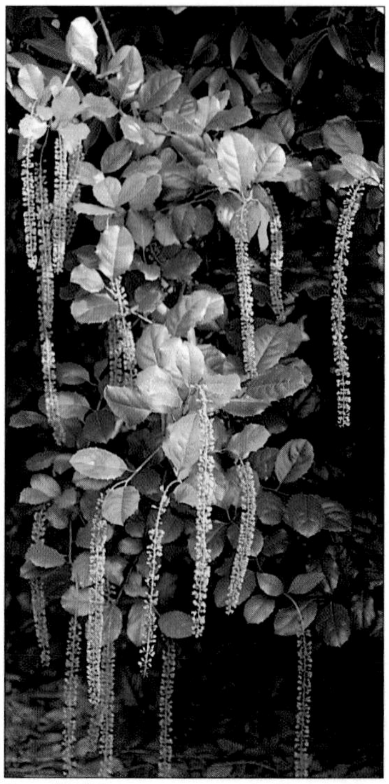

Itea ilicifolia

I. ilicifolia ■ 🏆 Erect then spreading, evergreen shrub with arching shoots and oval to elliptic, spiny-toothed, glossy, dark green leaves, to 10cm (4in) long. Small, greenish white flowers, 7mm (¼in) across, are borne in pendent, catkin-like racemes, to 30cm (12in) long, from midsummer to early autumn. ↕ 3–5m (10–15ft), ↔ 3m (10ft). W. China. ❄❄

I. virginica (Sweetspire, Tassel-white). Upright then arching, deciduous shrub with narrowly elliptic to oblong, finely toothed, dark green leaves, to 10cm (4in) long, turning red to purple in autumn. Fragrant, creamy white flowers, 9mm (⅜in) across, are borne in dense, erect racemes, to 15cm (6in) long, in summer. ↕ 1.5–3m (5–10ft), ↔ 1.5m (5ft). E. USA. ❄❄❄

I. yunnanensis. Erect then spreading, evergreen shrub with arching shoots and narrowly elliptic, spiny-toothed, glossy, dark green leaves, to 10cm (4in) long. Small white flowers, to 6mm (¼in) across, are produced in pendent, catkin-like racemes, to 17cm (7in) long, in late summer and early autumn. ↕ 3–5m (10–15ft), ↔ 3m (10ft). China (Yunnan). ❄❄

▷ **Ivory bells** see *Campanula alliariifolia*
▷ **Ivy** see *Hedera*
Bird's foot see *Hedera helix* 'Pedata'
Boston see *Parthenocissus tricuspidata*
Bullock's heart see *Hedera colchica*
Canary Island see *Hedera canariensis*
Cape see *Senecio macroglossus*
Clover-leaf see *Hedera helix* 'Shamrock'
Common see *Hedera helix*
Devil's see *Epipremnum aureum*
English see *Hedera helix*
German see *Senecio mikanioides*
Grape see *Cissus rhombifolia*
Ground see *Glechoma*
Irish see *Hedera hibernica*
Italian see *Hedera helix* f. *poetarum*
Japanese see *Hedera rhombea*
Natal see *Senecio macroglossus*
Nepal see *Hedera nepalensis*
North African see *Hedera canariensis*
Parlour see *Senecio mikanioides*
Persian see *Hedera colchica*
Poet's see *Hedera helix* f. *poetarum*
Purple-leaved see *Hedera helix* 'Atropurpurea'
Red flame see *Hemigraphis alternata*
Salt-and-pepper see *Hedera helix* 'Minor Marmorata'
Swedish see *Plectranthus australis*
Sweetheart see *Hedera hibernica* 'Deltoidea'
Switch see *Leucothoe fontanesiana*
Variegated ground see *Glechoma hederacea* 'Variegata'
▷ **Ivy of Uruguay** see *Cissus striata*
▷ **Ivy tree** see *Schefflera heptaphylla*

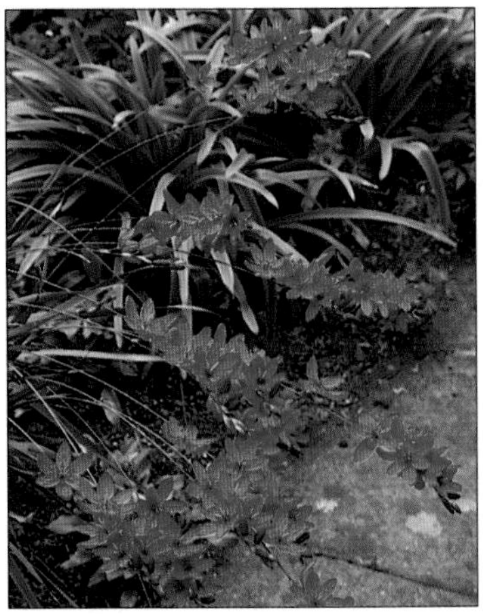

Ixia 'Mabel'

IXIA

Corn lily

IRIDACEAE

Genus of 40–50 species of cormous perennials found in grassland and sandy, sometimes marshy slopes from low to high altitudes in South Africa. They are grown for their open, star-shaped, brightly coloured flowers, which often have conspicuous dark centres, and are borne on wiry stems from early spring to summer. Narrowly linear, usually mid-green leaves are produced from the base of the plant, with shorter leaves on the slender, wiry stems. A large range of cultivars has been developed, with narrow, often branched stems bearing lax or dense spikes of few to many flowers, 3–7cm (1¼–3in) across. In frost-prone areas, grow in a cool greenhouse, or at the front of a border for summer flowering. Elsewhere, grow in a container on a patio or at the base of a warm, sunny wall.

• **HARDINESS** Half hardy.

• **CULTIVATION** Under glass, plant corms 10–15cm (4–6in) deep, 5–8cm (2–3in) apart, in autumn. Grow in loam-based potting compost (JI No.2) with added leaf mould and sharp sand in full light, with low to moderate humidity. Water sparingly until flower spikes appear, then water freely and apply a high potash liquid fertilizer every 2–3 weeks until foliage begins to die back. Lift corms in autumn and store in dry, frost-free conditions while dormant. Outdoors, grow in moderately fertile, well-drained soil in full sun.

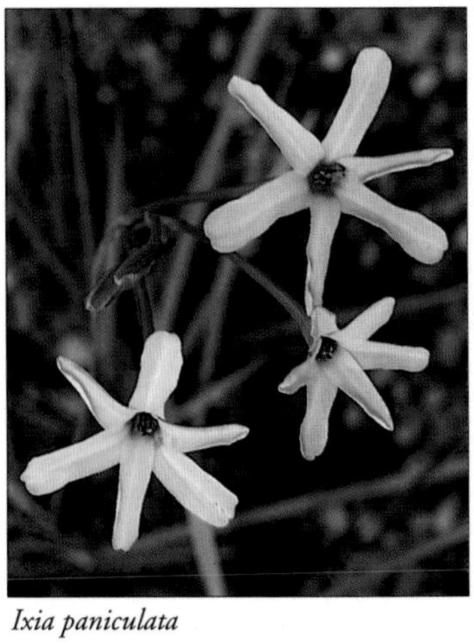

Ixia paniculata

• **PROPAGATION** Sow seed when ripe in containers in a cold frame. Separate offsets when dormant in late summer.

• **PESTS AND DISEASES** Trouble free.

***I.* 'Blauwe Vogel'** see *I.* 'Blue Bird'.

***I.* 'Blue Bird'**, syn. 'Blauwe Vogel'. Cormous perennial producing white flowers with dark purple centres; each outer petal has a broad violet streak and a dark purple tip. ↕40cm (16in). ❄

***I.* 'Hogarth'.** Cormous perennial bearing creamy white flowers with purple centres. ↕40cm (16in). ❄

***I.* 'Hubert'.** Cormous perennial bearing brownish red flowers with black centres. ↕40cm (16in). ❄

***I.* 'Mabel'** ■ Cormous perennial bearing deep pink flowers, paler inside; the outer petals are brownish red. ↕40cm (16in). ❄

I. maculata. Cormous perennial with erect, lance-shaped or awl-shaped, usually twisted leaves, 10–35cm (4–14in) long. From spring to early summer, bears spikes of few to many orange or yellow flowers, 6cm (2½in) across, with dark purple or black centres. ↕18–50cm (7–20in). South Africa (Western Cape). ❄

***I.* 'Marquette'.** Cormous perennial with purple-tipped yellow flowers with dark purple centres. ↕40cm (16in). ❄

I. monadelpha. Cormous perennial with erect, lance-shaped or sword-shaped, twisted leaves, 8–28cm (3–11in) long. From spring to early summer, bears compact spikes of 4–12 white, blue, purple, pink, or white flowers, 4cm (1½in) across, each with a green or brown central mark usually edged with another colour. ↕to 30cm (12in). South Africa (Western Cape). ❄

I. paniculata ■ syn. *Tritonia longiflora.* Cormous perennial with erect, lance-shaped or linear leaves, 15–60cm (6–24in) long. From spring to early summer, branched stems bear spikes of 5–18 pink-suffused, cream or pale yellow flowers, 4–7cm (1½–3in) across, often tinged pink or red on the outside.

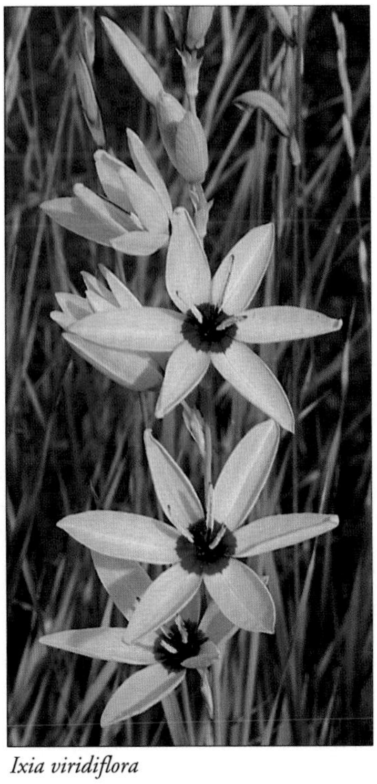

Ixia viridiflora

↕30–90cm (12–36in). South Africa (Western Cape). ❄

I. polystachya. Cormous perennial with erect, grass-like leaves, 15–50cm (6–20in) long, and often branched stems. From spring to early summer, bears spikes or panicles of few to many, lightly fragrant, white, mauve, or blue flowers, 4–5cm (1½–2in) across, often with mauve or purple central marks. ↕30–90cm (12–36in). South Africa. ❄

***I.* 'Rose Emperor'.** Cormous perennial bearing spikes of pink flowers with dark carmine-red centres. ↕40cm (16in). ❄

***I.* 'Uranus'.** Cormous perennial bearing dark lemon-yellow flowers with dark red-black centres. ↕40cm (16in). ❄

***I.* 'Venus'.** Cormous perennial with large, dark-centred magenta flowers, 5–7cm (2–3in) across. ↕40cm (16in). ❄

I. viridiflora ■ Cormous perennial with erect, linear leaves, 40–55cm (16–22in) long. From spring to early summer, bears spikes of 12 or more pale bluish green flowers, 5cm (2in) across, with conspicuous, red-rimmed, black centres. ↕30–60cm (12–24in). South Africa (Western Cape). ❄

IXIOLIRION

AMARYLLIDACEAE/IXIOLIRIACEAE

Genus of 4 species of bulbous perennials from roadsides and grassy places in S.W. and C. Asia. They are cultivated for their racemes or umbels of funnel-shaped, usually deep blue or violet flowers. Linear-lance-shaped leaves are in basal rosettes. They flower best after hot, dry dormant periods in summer. Grow at the base of a sunny wall, or in a raised bed, alpine house, or bulb frame.

• **HARDINESS** Fully hardy.

• **CULTIVATION** Plant bulbs 15cm (6in) deep in autumn. Outdoors, grow in humus-rich, well-drained soil in full sun. Mulch to protect from winter wet. Under glass, grow in loam-based potting compost (JI No.2) in full light. During growth, water freely. Keep just moist in autumn and winter, and completely dry when dormant in summer.

• **PROPAGATION** Sow seed in containers in a cold frame as soon as ripe or in autumn. Separate offsets after flowering.

• **PESTS AND DISEASES** Trouble free.

I. montanum see *I. tataricum.*

I. pallasii see *I. tataricum.*

I. tataricum, syn. *I. montanum, I. pallasii.* Bulbous perennial with erect, linear-lance-shaped, basal leaves, to 60cm (24in) or more long. From spring to early summer, produces loose umbels of up to 10 funnel-shaped, blue or violet-blue flowers, 3–5cm (1¼–2in) long, with a darker central stripe on each petal. ↕24–40cm (10–16in), ↔5cm (2in). Israel, Lebanon, Syria, N. Iraq, N. and N.W. Iran, S.W. and C. Asia to Kashmir and Tien Shan. ❄❄❄

IXORA

RUBIACEAE

Genus of 400 species of evergreen shrubs and trees from tropical woodland and mountains up to 3,000m (10,000ft) worldwide. They are grown for their large, vibrantly coloured, scented, 4-petalled, salverform flowers, produced in terminal panicles or corymb-like cymes. The opposite, occasionally whorled leaves are simple and entire. They grow best in warm, humid climates in a shrub border, or as free-standing specimens. Where temperatures drop below 15°C (69°F), grow as houseplants or in a warm greenhouse.

• **HARDINESS** Frost tender.

• **CULTIVATION** Under glass, grow in loamless potting compost with added leaf mould and grit in bright filtered or indirect light, with moderate to high humidity. Water freely during growth and sparingly in winter. Top-dress annually in spring with fresh compost and a balanced, slow-release fertilizer. Outdoors, grow in fertile, moist but well-drained soil, with shade from the hottest sun and shelter from strong winds. Pruning group 9; may need restrictive pruning under glass.

• **PROPAGATION** Root semi-ripe cuttings in summer with bottom heat.

• **PESTS AND DISEASES** Scale insects may be a problem under glass.

I. chinensis. Bushy, rounded shrub with elliptic, ovate or obovate, semi-lustrous, mid- to deep green leaves, to 6cm (2½in) long. Produces dense, flattened corymb-like cymes, 5–10cm (2–4in) across, of red, orange, pink, or occasionally white flowers, 3.5cm (1½in) long, mainly in summer. ↕2m (6ft) or more, ↔1–2m (3–6ft). S. China, Taiwan. ❀ (min. 15°C/59°F)

I. coccinea ■ (Flame of the woods, Jungle flame, Jungle geranium). Bushy, gently rounded shrub with oblong or obovate to elliptic, glossy, mid- to deep green leaves, 5–10cm (2–4in) long. Freely produces loose, corymb-like cymes, 5–12cm (2–5in) across, of red, orange, pink, or yellow flowers, 2.5–3.5cm (1–1½in) long, from late spring or early summer to autumn. ↕2.5m (8ft) or more, ↔1.5–2m (5–6ft). India, Sri Lanka. ❀ (min. 15°C/59°F). **'Angela Busman'** is compact, with shrimp-pink blooms; ↕1.5m (5ft). **'Frances Perry'** has large trusses of deep yellow flowers. **'Fraseri'** produces bright salmon-pink flowers. **'Gillette's Yellow'** has pale yellow flowers. **'Helen Dunaway'** is tall, and freely produces deep orange blooms. **'Henry Morat'** has fragrant pink flowers. **'Herrera's White'** bears well-formed white flowers. **f. *lutea*** has yellow blooms. **'Orange King'** is compact, and has glowing orange flowers; ↕1.5m (5ft). **'Superkings'** is compact, with red flowers; ↕1m (3ft).

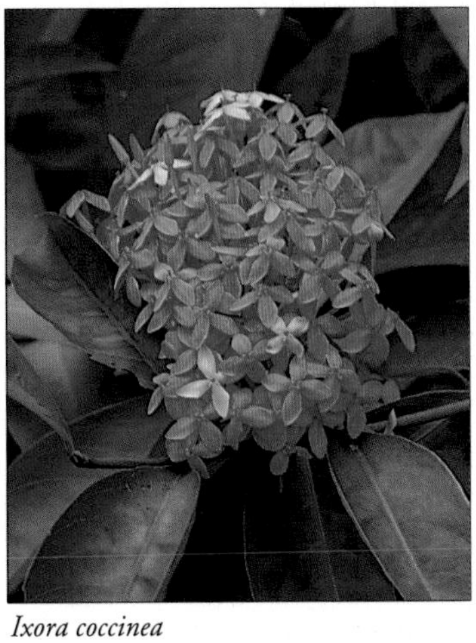

Ixora coccinea

J

JABOROSA

SOLANACEAE

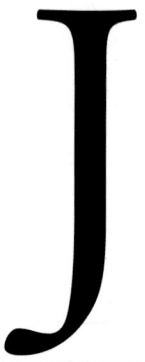

Genus of 20 species of perennials with basal, entire to pinnatifid leaves and axillary, 5- to 6-lobed, tubular or bell-shaped flowers, which are solitary or borne in few-flowered cymes. Most species occur in arid areas of South America. *J. integrifolia*, the only species commonly seen in cultivation, is suitable for a warm, dry site.

• **HARDINESS** Frost hardy to frost tender (*J. integrifolia* is hardy to -10°C/14°F).

• **CULTIVATION** Grow in moderately fertile, light, well-drained soil in a sunny, sheltered spot. *J. integrifolia* is invasive, so site where it will not swamp smaller plants. Provide a dry winter mulch in cold areas.

• **PROPAGATION** Divide, or sow seed at 13–16°C (55–61°F), in spring.

• **PESTS AND DISEASES** May be damaged by slugs and snails.

J

J. integrifolia. Rhizomatous, stemless perennial with basal clusters of oval to elliptic, fleshy, entire, dark green leaves, 20cm (8in) or more long. Bears solitary, tubular, night-scented, greenish white flowers, to 6cm (2½in) across, with star-shaped lobes, in summer. ↕15cm (6in), ↔ indefinite. S. Brazil, Uruguay, Argentina. ✻✻

JACARANDA

BIGNONIACEAE

Genus of 30–45 species of deciduous and evergreen trees from wet rainforests of tropical America. They have opposite, pinnate or 2-pinnate, often elegant, fern-like leaves and terminal panicles of tubular, narrowly bell-shaped, 5-lobed, foxglove-like flowers. In frost-prone areas, grow in a cool greenhouse, mainly as foliage plants, although some flowers may form on container-grown specimens, 2m (6ft) or more tall; young plants of *J. mimosifolia* are suitable for summer bedding. In warmer climates, jacarandas are popular as specimen plants and street trees.

• **HARDINESS** Frost tender.

• **CULTIVATION** Under glass, grow in loam-based potting compost (JI No.3) in full light with good ventilation. In the growing season, water freely and apply a balanced liquid fertilizer every month; water sparingly in winter. Outdoors, grow in fertile, moist, but well-drained soil in full sun. Pruning group 1; plants under glass need restrictive pruning in late winter.

• **PROPAGATION** Sow seed at 16–21°C (61–70°F) in spring. Root semi-ripe cuttings with bottom heat in summer.

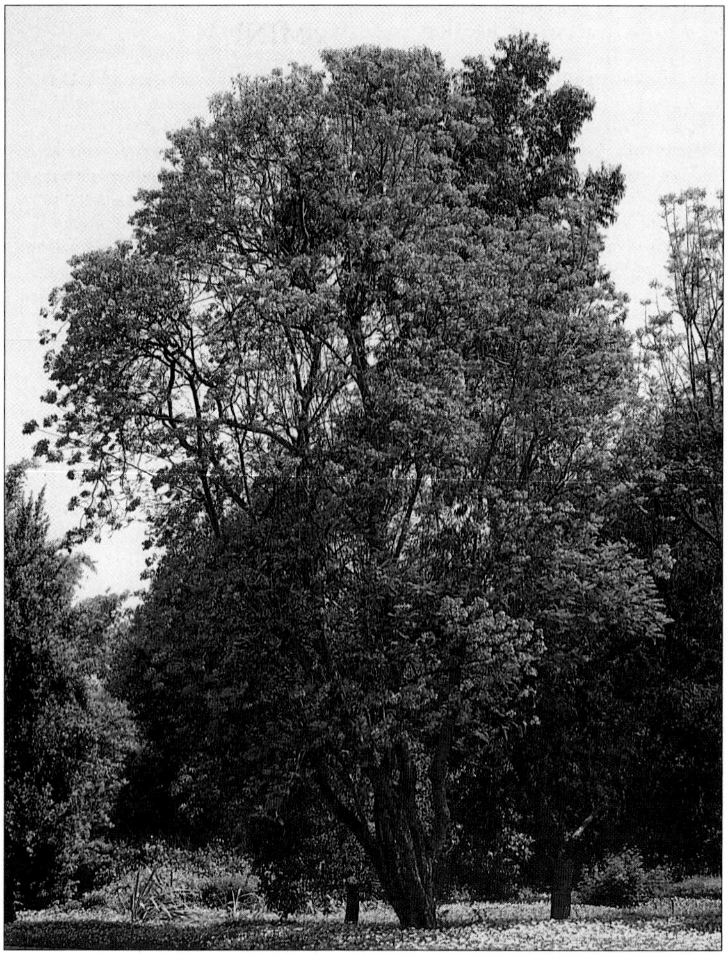

Jacaranda mimosifolia

• **PESTS AND DISEASES** Whiteflies and red spider mites may be troublesome under glass.

***J. acutifolia* of gardens** see *J. mimosifolia.*

J. mimosifolia ■ ⚲ syn. *J. acutifolia* of gardens, *J. ovalifolia, J. ovatifolia.* Spreading, deciduous tree, with broad, 2-pinnate leaves, 25–45cm (10–18in) long, composed of many small, narrowly elliptic, softly hairy, bright mid-green leaflets. From spring to early summer, broadly pyramidal panicles, 20–30cm (8–12in) long, of white-throated, glowing purple-blue flowers, 3.5–5cm (1½–2in) long, are borne on leafless branches or with young foliage. The flowers are followed by woody, disc-shaped seed pods. ↕ to 15m (50ft), ↔ 7–10m (22–30ft). Bolivia, Argentina. ❀ (min. 5–7°C/41–45°F)

J. ovalifolia see *J. mimosifolia.*

J. ovatifolia see *J. mimosifolia.*

▷**Jack-in-the-pulpit** see *Arisaema triphyllum*

▷***Jacobinia carnea*** see *Justicia carnea*

▷***Jacobinia coccinea*** see *Pachystachys coccinea*

▷***Jacobinia pauciflora*** see *Justicia rizzinii*

▷***Jacobinia pohliana*** see *Justicia carnea*

▷***Jacobinia spicigera*** see *Justicia spicigera*

▷***Jacobinia suberecta*** see *Dicliptera suberecta*

▷***Jacobinia velutina*** see *Justicia carnea*

▷**Jacob's ladder** see *Polemonium, P. caeruleum*

▷**Jacob's rod** see *Asphodeline*

JACQUEMONTIA

CONVOLVULACEAE

Genus of 120 species of evergreen perennials and shrubs, many of them scandent or twining climbers, closely related to *Ipomoea* and *Convolvulus.* Most are found in tropical woodland in Central and South America, with a few elsewhere in the tropics. They are grown for their funnel- to bell-shaped flowers, borne in cymes or panicles, and have alternate leaves, which are usually simple and entire, but may be toothed or lobed. Where temperatures drop below 13–16°C (55–61°F), grow in a warm greenhouse. In tropical areas, grow on a trellis, or allow to scramble through other, more vigorous shrubs; they are excellent for a coastal garden.

• **HARDINESS** Frost tender.

• **CULTIVATION** Under glass, grow in loam-based potting compost (JI No.3) in full light with shade from hot sun. In growth, water moderately and apply a balanced liquid fertilizer monthly; water sparingly in winter. Outdoors, grow in moderately fertile, moist, but well-drained soil in full sun. Pruning group 11, to restrict to available space.

• **PROPAGATION** Sow seed at 18°C (64°F) in spring. Root softwood cuttings with bottom heat in summer.

• **PESTS AND DISEASES** Prone to red spider mites and whiteflies under glass.

J. pentantha, syn. *J. violacea.* Fast-growing, twining climber, branching freely from the base, with heart-shaped to ovate, mid- to bright green leaves, 5cm (2in) long, which taper to a slender point. Long-stalked cymes of up to 12 funnel-shaped, white-eyed, violet-blue to blue flowers, 2–4cm (¾–1½in) wide, are produced mainly from summer to late autumn. ↕1.8–2.5m (6–8ft). Tropical America. ❀ (min. 13°C/55°F)

J. violacea see *J. pentantha.*

▷**Jade plant** see *Crassula ovata*
Silver see *C. arborescens*

▷**Jade tree** see *Crassula ovata*

JAMESIA

HYDRANGEACEAE

Genus of one species of deciduous shrub from mountainous, rocky places in W. USA. It has papery bark and simple, toothed, rough-textured leaves, borne in opposite pairs. It is cultivated for its 5-petalled, star-shaped white flowers, produced in small, terminal panicles in late spring and early summer. It is suitable for a shrub border or large rock garden.

• **HARDINESS** Fully hardy.

• **CULTIVATION** Grow in fertile, well-drained soil in full sun. Pruning groups 1 or 2.

• **PROPAGATION** Take greenwood cuttings in early summer, or semi-ripe cuttings in late summer.

• **PESTS AND DISEASES** Trouble free.

J. americana (Cliffbush, Wax flower). Small, spreading, deciduous shrub with peeling, papery bark and ovate, toothed, rough-textured, velvety grey-green leaves, to 7cm (3in) long, sometimes turning red in autumn. Small panicles, to 6cm (2½in) long, of star-shaped, slightly fragrant white flowers, 1cm (½in) across, are produced in late spring and early summer. ↕1.5m (5ft), ↔ 2m (6ft). W. USA. ✻✻✻

JANCAEA syn. JANKAEA

GESNERIACEAE

Genus of one species of evergreen, rosette-forming perennial, grown for its white-hairy, silver-green foliage and bell-shaped, pale lavender-blue flowers. Native to Greece, it grows on the shady cliffs of Mount Olympus. Grow in an alpine house, rock garden, or tufa.

• **HARDINESS** Fully hardy.

• **CULTIVATION** In an alpine house, grow in a mix of equal parts loam, leaf mould and sharp grit, with additional limestone chippings, in bright filtered light. Place a collar of grit at the neck of the plant. When in growth, water moderately, avoiding water on the foliage, and maintain a humid but well-ventilated atmosphere; water sparingly in winter. Outdoors, plant in a vertical cleft and give overhead protection in winter.

• **PROPAGATION** Sow seed in containers in a cold frame in autumn; pot on when seedlings have formed small rosettes. Take leaf cuttings in spring.

• **PESTS AND DISEASES** Susceptible to aphids and red spider mites under glass.

J. heldreichii ■ Evergreen perennial with neat rosettes of thick, corrugated, obovate, densely white-hairy, silver-green leaves, to 4cm (1½in) long. Clusters of 1–2, occasionally 3, broadly bell-shaped, pale lavender-blue flowers, 2cm (¾in) long, with 4, sometimes 5

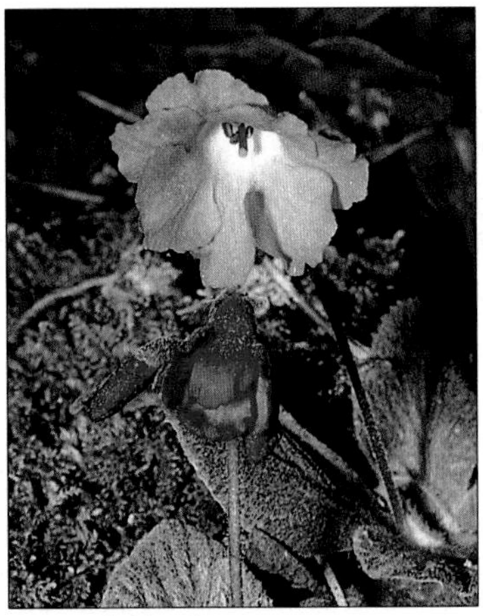

Jancaea heldreichii

spreading lobes, are produced in late spring. ↕ to 5cm (2in), ↔ to 10cm (4in). N.E. Greece. ***

▷***Jankaea*** see *Jancaea*
▷**Japanese anemone** see *Anemone hupehensis* var. *japonica*, *A.* x *hybrida*
▷**Japonica** see *Chaenomeles, C. japonica*

JASIONE
Sheep's bit
CAMPANULACEAE

Genus of about 20 species of summer-flowering annuals, biennials, and perennials with alternate, simple leaves and terminal, scabious-like heads of usually blue flowers. Most species grow in dry, open grassland in temperate Europe and around the Mediterranean. Grow in a rock garden, at the front of a border, or in a wildflower garden.
• **HARDINESS** Fully hardy.
• **CULTIVATION** Grow in moderately fertile, well-drained, preferably sandy soil in full sun.
• **PROPAGATION** Sow seed in containers in a cold frame as soon as ripe or in autumn. Alternatively, divide in spring.
• **PESTS AND DISEASES** Slugs and snails may damage young growth in spring.

J. amethystina see *J. crispa* subsp. *amethystina.*
J. crispa **subsp.** ***amethystina*** syn. *J. amethystina.* Tufted perennial with basal rosettes of toothed, oblong to inversely lance-shaped leaves, to 2.5cm (1in) long. Dense, spiky, purplish blue flowerheads, to 2cm (¾in) across, are produced throughout summer. ↕ 10cm (4in), ↔ to 15cm (6in). S. Spain. ***
J. laevis ■ syn. *J. perennis* (Sheep's bit scabious, Shepherd's scabious). Densely tufted perennial with basal rosettes of entire, narrowly oblong to narrowly obovate or inversely lance-shaped leaves, to 10cm (4in) long. Spiky, almost spherical blue flowerheads, to 2.5–4cm (1–1½in) across, are produced on upright, unbranched stems in summer. ↕ 20–30cm (8–12in), ↔ to 20cm (8in). W. and S. Europe. ***
J. perennis see *J. laevis.*

▷**Jasmine** see *Jasminum*
Arabian see *Jasminum sambac*
Cape see *Gardenia augusta*
Carolina see *Gelsemium sempervirens*
Chilean see *Mandevilla laxa*
Common see *Jasminum officinale*
Confederate see *Trachelospermum jasminoides*
Crepe see *Tabernaemontana divaricata*
False yellow see *Gelsemium sempervirens*
Italian see *Solanum seaforthianum*
Madagascar see *Stephanotis floribunda*
Primrose see *Jasminum mesnyi*
Rock see *Androsace*
Star see *Trachelospermum jasminoides*
West Indian see *Plumeria, P. alba*
Winter see *Jasminum nudiflorum*
Yellow see *Jasminum humile*

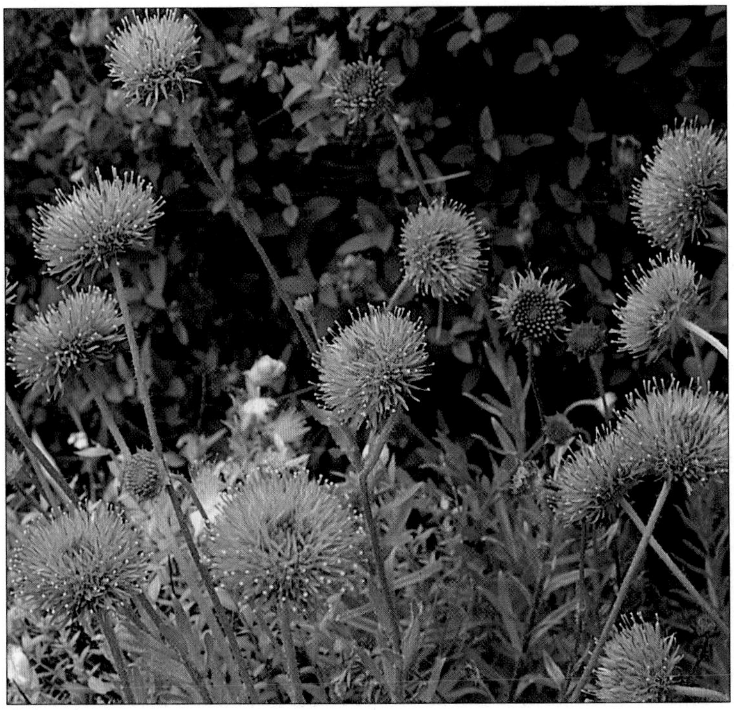

Jasione laevis

JASMINUM
Jasmine, Jessamine
OLEACEAE

Genus of 200 or more species of deciduous and evergreen shrubs and climbers from woodland, scrub, and rocky places in tropical and temperate regions, mainly in Europe, Asia, and Africa. They are cultivated for their terminal or axillary, sometimes umbel- or panicle-like cymes of salverform, often fragrant flowers with broad or narrow, star-shaped segments, and for their opposite or alternate, simple to pinnate leaves (in some species reduced to only one leaflet). Most species have black berries. Climbing jasmines will twine over any suitable support, such as a trellis, fence, arch, or large shrub. Scandent, shrubby jasmines may be trained against a wall, and dwarf species are suitable for a rock garden. In cool areas, grow jasmines in a sheltered position; grow half-hardy species as houseplants in a conservatory or cool greenhouse, and tender species in a warm or temperate greenhouse.
• **HARDINESS** Fully hardy to frost tender.
• **CULTIVATION** Outdoors, grow in fertile, well-drained soil in full sun or partial shade. Under glass, grow in loam-based potting compost (JI No.2) in bright filtered light, or full light with shade from hot sun. In growth, water freely and apply a low-nitrogen liquid fertilizer monthly; water sparingly in winter. Prune *J. mesnyi*, *J. nudiflorum*, and *J. humile* as for shrubs in pruning group 2. Thin old, flowered, and overcrowded shoots of *J. officinale* after flowering. Remaining species need little regular pruning, other than to thin overcrowded growth after flowering.
• **PROPAGATION** Take semi-ripe cuttings in summer, or layer in autumn.
• **PESTS AND DISEASES** Aphids and mealybugs may be a problem.

J. angulare ■ syn. *J. capense.* Scrambling to semi-twining, evergreen climber, usually freely branching when mature, with ridged or angled stems. Leaves are opposite, pinnate, and rich, deep green, with 3, sometimes 5, ovate to lance-shaped, lustrous leaflets, 2–4cm (¾–1½in) long. Bears axillary cymes of 3 salverform, very sweetly scented flowers, to 3cm (1¼in) across, greenish or pale pink then white, from late summer to autumn. ↕ 3–6m (10–20ft).

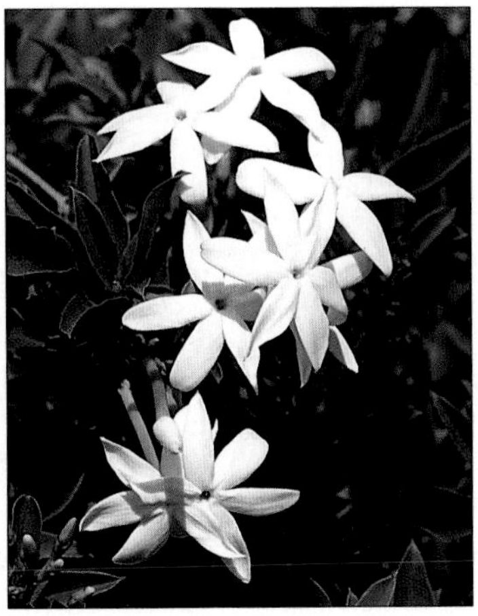

Jasminum angulare

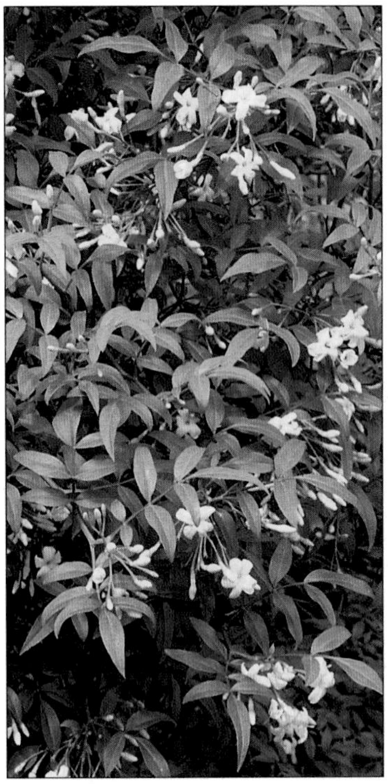

Jasminum humile

South Africa (Northern Transvaal to Eastern Cape, Orange Free State). *
J. azoricum 🏆 syn. *J. fluminense* of gardens. Evergreen, twining climber or sometimes semi-scrambler, branching moderately to freely, with opposite, pinnate, deep green leaves divided into 3 ovate to heart-shaped, wavy-margined leaflets, to 8cm (3in) long. Small, terminal cymes of 3 purple-tinted buds, opening to salverform, fragrant white flowers, to 2.5cm (1in) across, are produced mainly in late summer. ↕ 3–5m (10–15ft). Madeira. *
J. beesianum. Twining, woody, evergreen climber, deciduous in cool areas, with opposite, simple, ovate to lance-shaped, dark green leaves, to 5cm (2in) long. Cymes of 3 small, salverform, fragrant, pinkish red flowers, 1cm (½in) across, are produced in early and mid-summer. ↕ 5m (15ft). S.W. China. **
J. capense see *J. angulare.*
J. dichotomum. Bushy, evergreen scrambler or twining climber with whorls of thick, lustrous, mid-green leaves, each reduced to one ovate to elliptic, boldly veined leaflet, 5–10cm (2–4in) long, with an abrupt, sharp point. Produces loosely branched cymes of up to 60 salverform, sweetly scented white flowers, to 2cm (¾in) across, opening from red-purple or red-tinted buds, intermittently all year round. ↕ to 3m (10ft) or more. Tropical W., C., and E. Africa. ❄ (min. 10–13°C/50–55°F)
J. fluminense **of gardens** see *J. azoricum.*
J. fruticans. Dense, upright, evergreen or semi-evergreen shrub with alternate, pinnate, dark green leaves, each having 3 narrow-oblong or linear-obovate leaflets, to 2cm (¾in) long. Terminal cymes of up to 5 small, salverform, slightly fragrant yellow flowers, 1.5cm (½in) across, are produced in summer. ↕↔ 1.5m (5ft). Portugal, North Africa to Jordan, Turkey to Turkmenistan. **
J. grandiflorum **of gardens** see *J. officinale* f. *affine.*
J. humile ■ (Yellow jasmine). Semi-evergreen or evergreen, erect or arching,

J

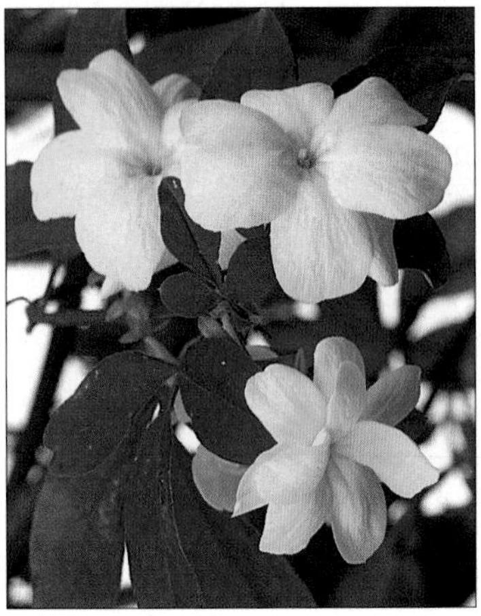

Jasminum mesnyi

bushy shrub with alternate, pinnate, bright green leaves composed of 5–9, occasionally 13, ovate to lance-shaped leaflets, to 5cm (2in) long. Cymes of usually 6, occasionally more, salverform, sometimes fragrant, bright yellow flowers, 1cm (½in) or more across, are produced from late spring to early autumn. ↕ 2.5m (8ft), sometimes to 4m (12ft), ↔ 3m (10ft). Afghanistan to Himalayas and S.W. China. ✻✻. **'Revolutum'** ♀ syn. *J. reevesii* of gardens, is semi-evergreen, with stout shoots, larger leaves, with 5–7 long-pointed leaflets to 1cm (½in) long, and up to 12 large, fragrant flowers, to 2.5cm (1in) across. **f. *wallichianum*** has leaves with 7–13 leaflets and pendulous 3- to 5-flowered cymes; India, Nepal.

J. mesnyi ■ ♀ syn. *J. primulinum* (Primrose jasmine). Tall, open, slender-stemmed, evergreen shrub which acts like a climber when grown against a support. Opposite, pinnate, glossy, deep green leaves have 3 oblong to lance-shaped leaflets, 3–7cm (1¼–3in) long. Salverform, usually semi-double, bright yellow flowers, 3–4.5cm (1¼–1¾in) across, are produced singly or in few-flowered clusters in spring and summer. ↕ to 3m (10ft) or more, ↔ 1–2m (3–6ft). S.W. China. ✻

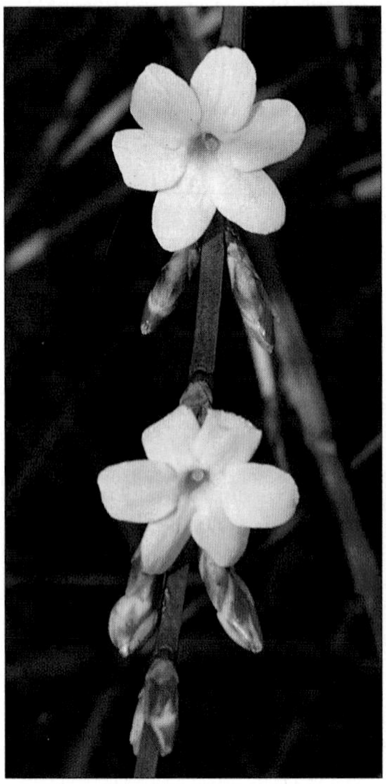

Jasminum nudiflorum

J. nudiflorum ■ ♀ (Winter jasmine). Slender, deciduous shrub with arching to scandent green shoots and opposite, pinnate, dark green leaves, each divided into 3 oval-oblong leaflets, to 3cm (1¼in) long. Solitary, salverform, bright yellow flowers, 1–2cm (½–¾in) across, are produced in the leaf axils, before the leaves, in winter and early spring. ↕↔ 3m (10ft). W. China. ✻✻✻

J. officinale ♀ (Common jasmine). Vigorous, twining, woody, deciduous, occasionally semi-deciduous climber with opposite, pinnate, mid-green leaves composed of 5–9 elliptic leaflets, to 6cm (2½in) long, with long, sharp points. Terminal, umbel-like cymes of up to 5-flowered clusters of salverform, very fragrant white flowers, 2cm (¾in) across, are produced from summer to early autumn. ↕ 12m (40ft). Caucasus, N. Iran, Afghanistan, Himalayas, W. China. ✻✻. **f. *affine***, syn. *J. grandiflorum* of gardens, has pink-tinged white flowers, to 4cm (1½in) across. **'Argenteovariegatum'** ■ ♀ syn. 'Variegatum', has leaves which are grey-green with creamy white margins. **'Aureovariegatum'** syn. 'Aureum', has leaves conspicuously marked yellow.

J. parkeri. Dwarf, dome-forming, evergreen shrub with slender, congested branches bearing alternate, pinnate, dark green leaves with 3–5 sharply pointed, ovate leaflets, to 1cm (½in) long. Terminal or axillary, solitary or paired, salverform yellow flowers, to 1.5cm (½in) across, are produced in early summer, followed by greenish white berries. ↕ to 30cm (12in), ↔ to 40cm (16in). India (Himachal Pradesh). ✻✻✻ (borderline)

J. polyanthum ■ ♀ Vigorous, twining, evergreen climber with opposite, pinnate, deep green leaves made up of 5–7 lance-shaped leaflets, the terminal ones largest, to 8cm (3in) long, with slender points. Bears an abundance of salverform, strongly fragrant, pink-budded white flowers, to 2cm (¾in) wide, in many-flowered, panicle-like cymes, to 10cm (4in) long. Flowers in late winter or early spring in a warm or temperate greenhouse; from spring to summer in warm climates. ↕ to 3m (10ft) or more. W. and S.W. China. ✻

J. primulinum see *J. mesnyi.*

***J. reevesii* of gardens** see *J. humile* 'Revolutum'.

J. rex. Vigorous, twining, evergreen climber with opposite, dark green leaves, each reduced to one broadly ovate leaflet, 12–20cm (5–8in) long. Produces axillary cymes of 2 or 3 salverform, unscented white flowers, 5cm (2in) or more across, mainly in summer. ↕ 3m (10ft) or more. Thailand. ❁ (min. 13°C/55°F)

J. sambac (Arabian jasmine, Pikake). Evergreen, twining climber or scrambler with angular stems and bushy growth. Lustrous, dark green leaves, some in whorls of 3, others opposite, are reduced to one broadly ovate leaflet, to 8cm (3in) long. Produces small cymes of 3–12 salverform, strongly scented white flowers, 2.5cm (1in) across, fading to pink, mainly in summer, but often irregularly throughout the year. ↕ 2–3m (6–10ft). Probably tropical Asia.

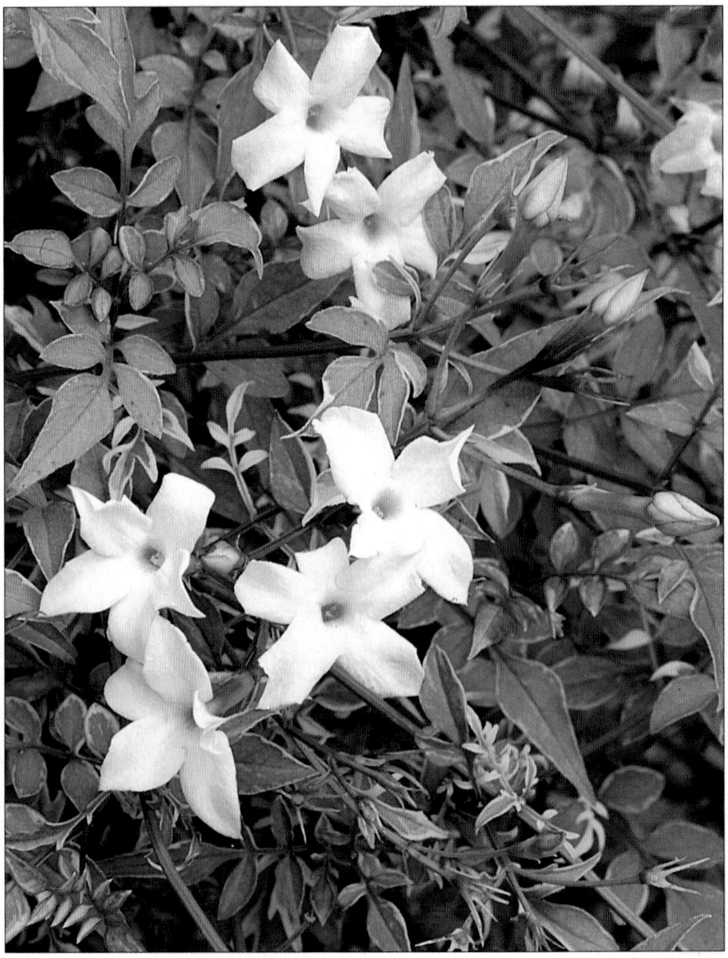

Jasminum officinale 'Argenteovariegatum'

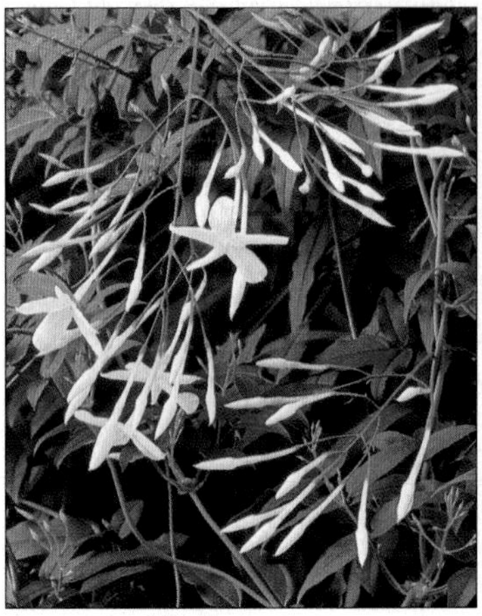

Jasminum polyanthum

❁ (min. 13–15°C/55–59°F). **'Grand Duke of Tuscany'**, syn. 'Flore Pleno', bears double flowers resembling miniature gardenias.

J. x stephanense ♀ (*J. beesianum* x *J. officinale*). Vigorous, twining, woody, deciduous climber with opposite, dull green, sometimes cream-flushed leaves, which may be simple, ovate-lance-shaped, to 5cm (2in) long, or pinnate, with 5 ovate-elliptic leaflets to 5cm (2in) long. Loose cymes of 5 or 6 or more, salverform, fragrant, pale pink flowers, to 1cm (½in) across, appear in early and midsummer. S.W. China (Yunnan). ↕ 5m (15ft). ✻✻

JATROPHA

EUPHORBIACEAE

Genus of about 170 species of succulent perennials and evergreen shrubs, rarely trees, from dry or semi-moist areas of South Africa, Madagascar, tropical North, Central, and South America, and the West Indies. Many are very succulent, often forming a caudex; other species have tuberous rootstocks. Leaves are alternate and simple, palmately lobed, or finely divided. In summer, diurnal flowers with prominent petals appear singly or in flat-topped cymes. In areas where temperatures drop below 10°C (50°F), grow in a warm greenhouse or conservatory; in warmer climates, plant in a shrub border or use as hedging. All parts contain a milky or watery latex, contact with which may irritate skin.

- **HARDINESS** Frost tender.
- **CULTIVATION** Under glass, grow in a mix of 2 parts loam-based potting compost (JI No.2), with 1 part each leaf mould and grit. Provide full light with shade from hot sun. In spring and summer, water moderately and apply a balanced liquid fertilizer monthly; keep completely dry in autumn and winter. Outdoors, grow in moderately fertile, humus-rich, gritty, sharply drained soil in full sun. See also pp.48–49.
- **PROPAGATION** Sow seed in spring or summer at 24°C (75°F).
- **PESTS AND DISEASES** Vulnerable to mealybugs.

J. multifida (Coral plant). Tree-like, evergreen, semi-succulent shrub with rounded, 7- to 15-lobed, finely divided leaves, 4–8cm (1½–3in) across. Numerous long-stalked, small scarlet flowers, 5mm (¼in) across, are borne in

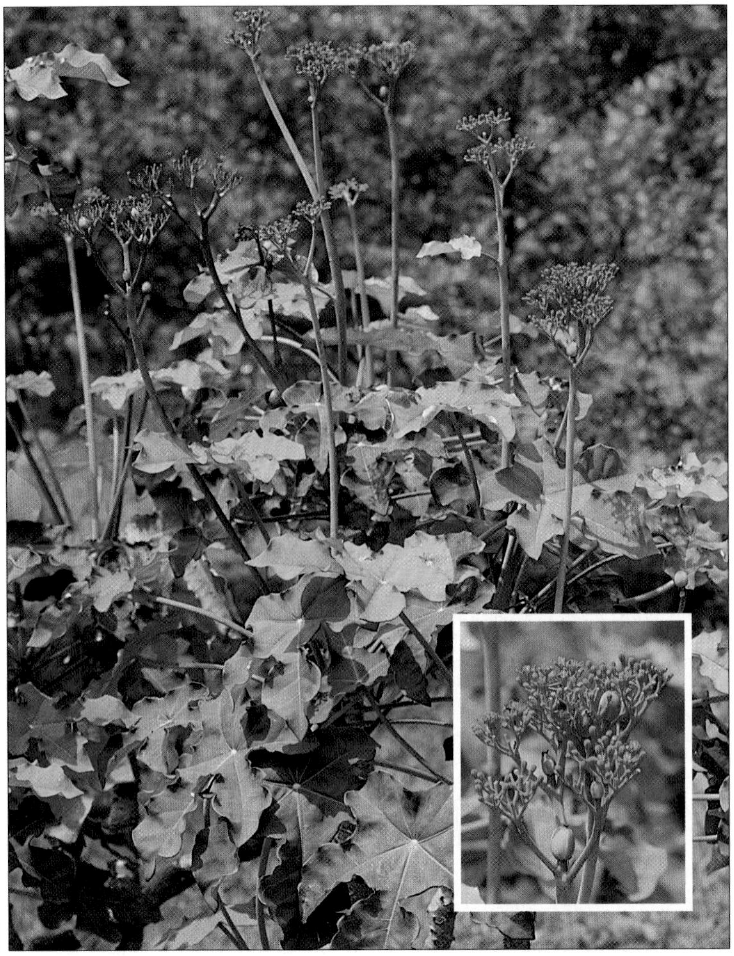

Jatropha podagrica (inset: flower detail)

terminal cymes in summer. ↕ to 7m (22ft), ↔ 4m (12ft). Mexico to Brazil, West Indies. ⊛ (min. 10°C/50°F)
J. podagrica ■ Free-branching, very fleshy, succulent perennial with a short, swollen, caudex-like grey trunk and grey stems covered with spine-like stipules. At the tips, produces rounded-ovate, 3- to 5-lobed, very tough leaves, 18–30cm (7–12in) across, dark green above, glaucous white beneath. Terminal, branched cymes of numerous unisexual, small, brilliant scarlet to coral-red flowers, 1cm (½in) across, are borne on long, green, sometimes red-tinted stalks in summer. ↕ to 50cm (20in) or more, ↔ 25cm (10in). Central America, West Indies. ⊛ (min. 10°C/50°F)

JEFFERSONIA

syn. PLAGIORHEGMA
Twin leaf
BERBERIDACEAE

Genus of 2 species of perennials which grow wild in damp woods and forests in N.E. Asia and North America. They have rounded to kidney-shaped, 2-lobed leaves, and solitary, cup-shaped flowers, with 5–8 petals, borne on long, slender stalks, in late spring or early summer. They are excellent plants for a shaded rock garden or peat bed.
• **HARDINESS** Fully hardy.
• **CULTIVATION** Grow in moist, humus-rich soil in partial or full shade. Top-dress with leaf mould or other humus-rich material in autumn.
• **PROPAGATION** Sow seed in containers in an open frame as soon as ripe. Divide established plants in spring.
• **PESTS AND DISEASES** Prone to slugs and snails, especially in spring.

J. diphylla (Rheumatism root). Tuft-forming perennial with kidney-shaped, deeply cleft leaves, to 15cm (6in) across, pale grey-green above, and glaucous, pale green beneath. Bears solitary, cup-shaped white flowers, 2.5cm (1in) wide, on slender stalks in late spring or early summer. ↕ 20cm (8in), often taller after flowering, ↔ to 15cm (6in). North America (Ontario to Tennessee). ❄❄❄
J. dubia ■ syn. *Plagiorhegma dubia.* Delicate, tufted perennial with kidney-shaped or rounded, 2-lobed, blue-green leaves, to 10cm (4in) across, often purple-tinted, especially when unfolding. In late spring or early summer, bears solitary, cup-shaped, clear lavender-blue, occasionally white flowers, 3cm (1¼in) across, on slender, dark stalks. ↕ 20cm (8in), ↔ to 15cm (6in). N.E. Asia. ❄❄❄

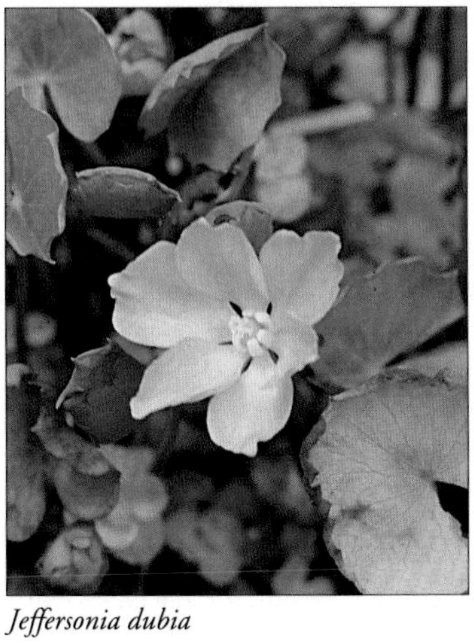

Jeffersonia dubia

▷**Jerusalem cross** see *Lychnis chalcedonica*
▷**Jerusalem thorn** see *Paliurus spina-christi, Parkinsonia aculeata*
▷**Jessamine** see *Jasminum*
Willow-leaved see *Cestrum parqui*
▷**Jesuit's nut** see *Trapa natans*
▷**Jewels of Opar** see *Talinum paniculatum*
▷**Jew's mantle** see *Kerria*
▷**Job's tears** see *Coix lacryma-jobi*
▷**Joe Pye weed** see *Eupatorium purpureum*
▷**Jonquil,**
Campernelle see *Narcissus* x *odorus*
Rush-leaved see *Narcissus assoanus*
Wild see *Narcissus jonquilla*

JOVELLANA

SCROPHULARIACEAE

Genus of 6 species of herbaceous perennials and semi-evergreen sub-shrubs, found on streambanks and at forest margins in New Zealand and Chile. They have simple, toothed or lobed leaves, borne in opposite pairs, and showy, 2-lipped flowers. Grow in a sheltered border or against a wall. In areas prone to heavy frost, grow or overwinter in a cool greenhouse.
• **HARDINESS** Frost hardy.
• **CULTIVATION** Under glass, grow in loamless potting compost in full light, with shade from hot sun and good ventilation. In growth, water moderately and apply a balanced liquid fertilizer monthly; water sparingly in winter. Outdoors, grow in fertile, well-drained soil in full sun. Protect with a dry winter mulch in frost-prone areas. Pruning group 10, in early to mid-spring.
• **PROPAGATION** Take heel cuttings of sideshoots in late summer.
• **PESTS AND DISEASES** Trouble free.

J. sinclairii. Woody-based herbaceous perennial with upright shoots and ovate to ovate-oblong, double-toothed or lobed leaves, to 5cm (2in) long. Terminal panicles, 15cm (6in) long, of 2-lipped, purple-spotted, lilac to white flowers, 8mm (⅜in) across, are borne in summer. ↕ 50cm (20in), ↔ 60cm (24in). New Zealand (North Island). ❄❄
J. violacea ■ 🏆 Upright, suckering, semi-evergreen subshrub with ovate, coarsely toothed or lobed, deep green leaves, 2–3cm (¾–1¼in) long. Bears panicles, 4–8cm (1½–3in) across, of 2-lipped, pale violet-purple flowers, to 1.5cm (½in) across, with purple spots within and yellow throats, in summer. ↕ 60cm (24in), ↔ 1m (3ft). Chile. ❄❄

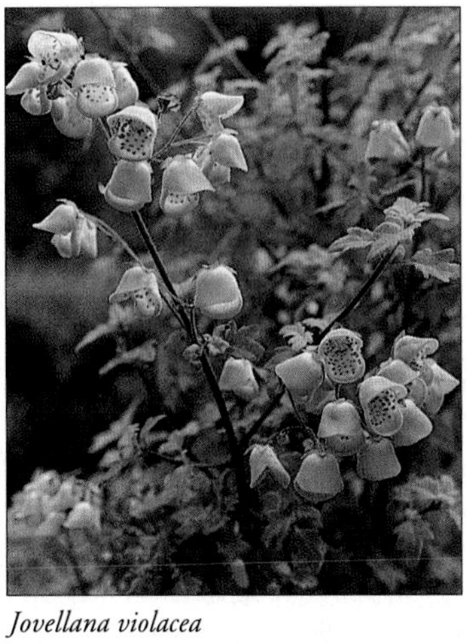

Jovellana violacea

JOVIBARBA

CRASSULACEAE

Genus of 6 species of mat-forming, usually stoloniferous, evergreen perennials, very similar to *Sempervivum*, from the mountains of Europe. They are grown for their symmetrical rosettes of fleshy leaves and terminal cymes of small, 6-petalled, bell-shaped flowers, borne on leafy stems in summer. After flowering, the rosettes are replaced by numerous offsets. Easily cultivated, they are suitable for a rock garden, trough, wall, or alpine house.
• **HARDINESS** Fully hardy.
• **CULTIVATION** Grow in poor, gritty, well-drained soil in full sun. Remove old rosettes after flowering. In an alpine house, grow in equal parts loam-based potting compost (JI No.1) and grit.
• **PROPAGATION** Root offsets in spring or early summer.
• **PESTS AND DISEASES** Trouble free.

J. allionii see *J. hirta* subsp. *allionii.*
J. globifera see *J. sobolifera.*
J. globifera* subsp. *allionii see *J. hirta* subsp. *allionii.*
J. globifera* subsp. *hirta see *J. hirta.*
J. heuffelii, syn. *Sempervivum patens.* Evergreen perennial lacking stolons, with rosettes, 5–7cm (2–3in) across, of lance-shaped, finely hairy or glaucous leaves, to 8mm (⅜in) long, sometimes brown-tipped. Bears bell-shaped, pale yellow flowers in dense, flat cymes, to 5cm (2in) across, in summer. ↕ to 20cm (8in), ↔ to 30cm (12in). E. Carpathians, Balkans. ❄❄❄
J. hirta ■ syn. *J. globifera* subsp. *hirta, Sempervivum hirtum.* Evergreen perennial with lance-shaped to inversely

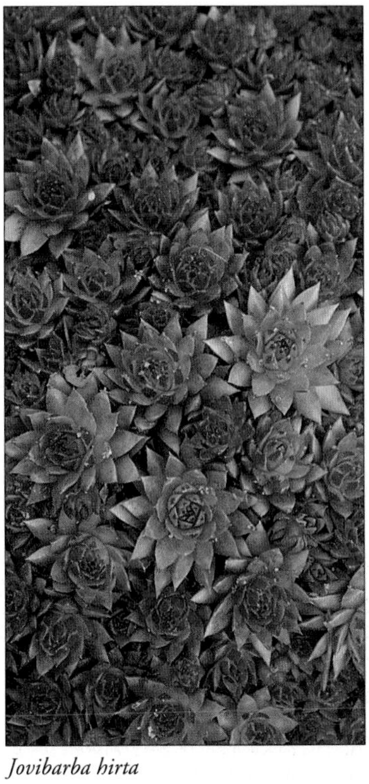

Jovibarba hirta

J

lance-shaped, hairy-margined leaves, to 1cm (½in) long, tipped brownish purple and often red-tinted, borne in rosettes 2.5–7cm (1–3in) across. Bears branching cymes, to 8cm (3in) across, of bell-shaped, pale yellowish brown flowers, in summer. ↕ 15cm (6in), ↔ to 30cm (12in). C. and S.E. Europe. ❄❄❄. **subsp. *allionii***, syn. *J. allionii*, *J. globifera* subsp. *allionii*, has smaller rosettes with glandular-hairy, red-tipped leaves; S.W. and S.E. Alps.

J. sobolifera, syn. *J. globifera*, *Sempervivum soboliferum* (Hen and chickens houseleek). Evergreen perennial with rosettes, 2.5–5cm (1–2in) across, of obovate to oblong, glossy, bright green leaves, to 1cm (½in) long, with fringed margins, and tips that flush red with age. In summer, produces bell-shaped, greenish yellow flowers in cymes to 7cm (3in) across. ↕ 20cm (8in), ↔ to 30cm (12in). S.W., C., and S.E. Europe, N.W. and C. Russia. ❄❄❄

JUANULLOA

SOLANACEAE

Genus of 10 species of epiphytic and terrestrial, scandent, evergreen shrubs from the rainforests of Central America to Peru. They are grown for their 5-lobed, tubular flowers, each with a bell-shaped, deeply ridged calyx, borne in short racemes or panicles. Leaves are alternate, simple, entire, and leathery. Where temperatures fall below about 13°C (55°F), grow in a warm or temperate greenhouse. In tropical or subtropical climates, use to clothe an arch or pillar, or train through a tree.

J

- **HARDINESS** Frost tender.
- **CULTIVATION** Under glass, grow in loam-based potting compost (JI No.2) in full light with shade from hot sun, and moderate to low humidity. In spring and summer, water moderately and apply a balanced liquid fertilizer every month; water sparingly in winter. Outdoors, grow in moderately fertile, humus-rich, moist, but well-drained soil in full sun with some midday shade. Pruning group 9, with restrictive pruning under glass; tip-prune young plants to encourage branching.
- **PROPAGATION** Sow seed at 18°C (64°F) in spring. Root semi-ripe cuttings with bottom heat in spring or summer.
- **PESTS AND DISEASES** Susceptible to red spider mites and mealybugs.

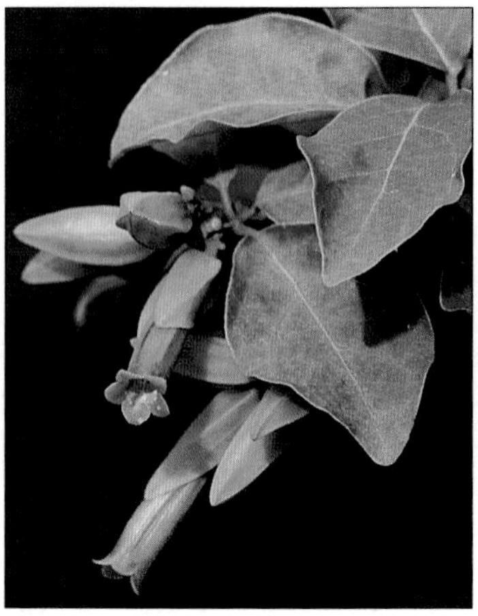

Juanulloa mexicana

J. aurantiaca see *J. mexicana*.
J. mexicana ▣ syn. *J. aurantiaca*. Epiphytic shrub, becoming scandent with age, with elliptic to oblong, mid- to deep green leaves, 8–20cm (3–8in) long, usually densely woolly beneath. Produces short racemes of semi-pendent, tubular, bright orange or orange-yellow flowers, 4–5cm (1½–2in) long, with paler calyces, mainly in summer. ↕ to 2m (6ft) or more, ↔ 60–100cm (24–39in). S. Mexico to Colombia, Peru. ⚘ (min. 13°C/55°F)

JUBAEA

Chilean wine palm

ARECACEAE/PALMAE

Genus of one species of single-stemmed palm from the warm-temperate coastal valleys of Chile. Spreading to arching, pinnate leaves form a dense, terminal, rounded head, and 3-petalled flowers appear in panicles between them. In areas prone to severe frost, grow as a houseplant, or in a cool greenhouse or conservatory. In warm, dry regions, grow as a majestic specimen or avenue palm.

- **HARDINESS** Frost hardy.
- **CULTIVATION** Under glass, grow in loam-based potting compost (JI No.2) in full light. In the growing season, water moderately and apply a balanced liquid fertilizer every month; water sparingly in winter. Outdoors, grow in fertile, moist, but well-drained soil in full sun.
- **PROPAGATION** Sow seed at 25°C (77°F) in spring; germination may take 3–6 months.
- **PESTS AND DISEASES** Red spider mites and scale insects may be troublesome under glass.

J. chilensis ▣ ♆ syn. *J. spectabilis* (Coquito palm, Honey palm). Slow-growing palm with a robust, erect, scarred and cracked grey trunk, occasionally swollen in the middle. Pinnate, oblong-ovate leaves, to 5m (15ft) long, are formed of many linear, rigid, folded, yellow-green to deep green leaflets. Small, bowl-shaped, dull purple or maroon and yellow flowers are produced in panicles to 1.5m (5ft) long, in summer; they are followed by woody, ovoid yellow fruit, to 5cm (2in) long. ↕ to 25m (80ft), ↔ to 9m (28ft). Chile. ❄❄
J. spectabilis see *J. chilensis*.

▷**Judas tree** see *Cercis siliquastrum*

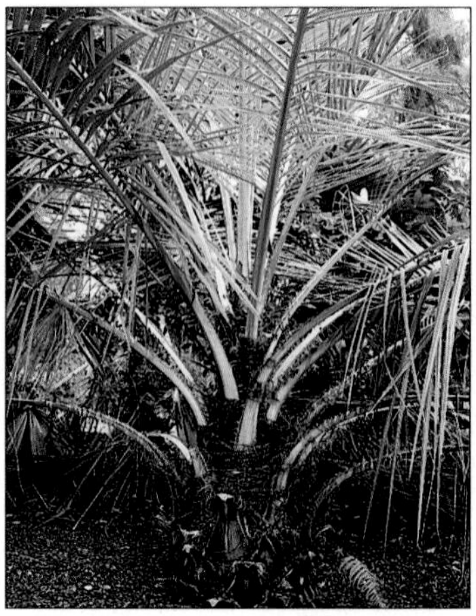

Jubaea chilensis

JUGLANS

Walnut

JUGLANDACEAE

Genus of about 15 species of deciduous trees, sometimes shrubs, occurring in woodland in S.E. Europe, Asia, North America, and N. South America. They have furrowed bark and alternate, pinnate leaves, usually with toothed leaflets. Greenish yellow male and female flowers are borne separately on the same plant in late spring and early summer: males in pendulous catkins and females inconspicuous. Fruits are ovoid or spherical, initially green, ripening to brown, and contain edible nuts with hard, thin or thick, furrowed shells. Cultivated for their habit, foliage, and fruit, walnuts are fine specimen trees.

- **HARDINESS** Fully hardy to frost hardy. Late frosts may cause damage.
- **CULTIVATION** Grow in deep, fertile, well-drained soil, preferably in full sun. In frost-prone areas, provide a sheltered, very sunny site. Plant out as seedlings or young grafted plants when no more than 30–60cm (12–24in) tall. Pruning group 1; formative pruning and removal of damaged branches should be carried out in late summer to prevent bleeding.

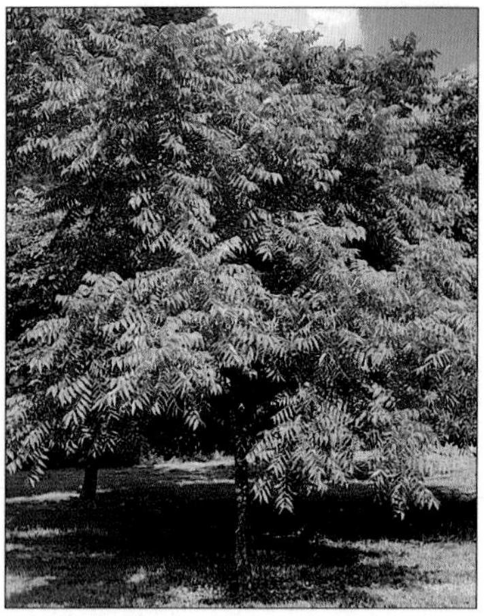

Juglans nigra

- **PROPAGATION** Sow seed in a seedbed as soon as ripe, or stratify and then sow in spring. Named cultivars of *J. regia* and *J. nigra* are usually grafted on to seedling stocks.
- **PESTS AND DISEASES** Aphids, walnut blister mites, honey fungus, coral spot, and leaf spot may be a problem.

J. ailantifolia ▣ ♀ syn. *J. sieboldiana* (Japanese walnut). Spreading tree with stout shoots and pinnate leaves, to 60cm (24in) or more long, with 11–17 oblong to elliptic, glossy, bright green leaflets and sticky, ovoid fruit, to 5cm (2in) long. ↕↔ 15m (50ft). Japan. ❄❄❄. **var. *cordiformis*** syn. *J. cordiformis*, has narrower leaflets.
J. californica ♀ (Californian walnut). Spreading tree or shrub with pinnate

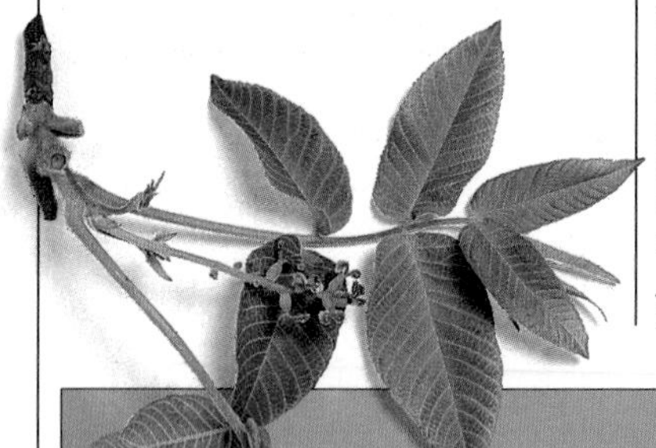

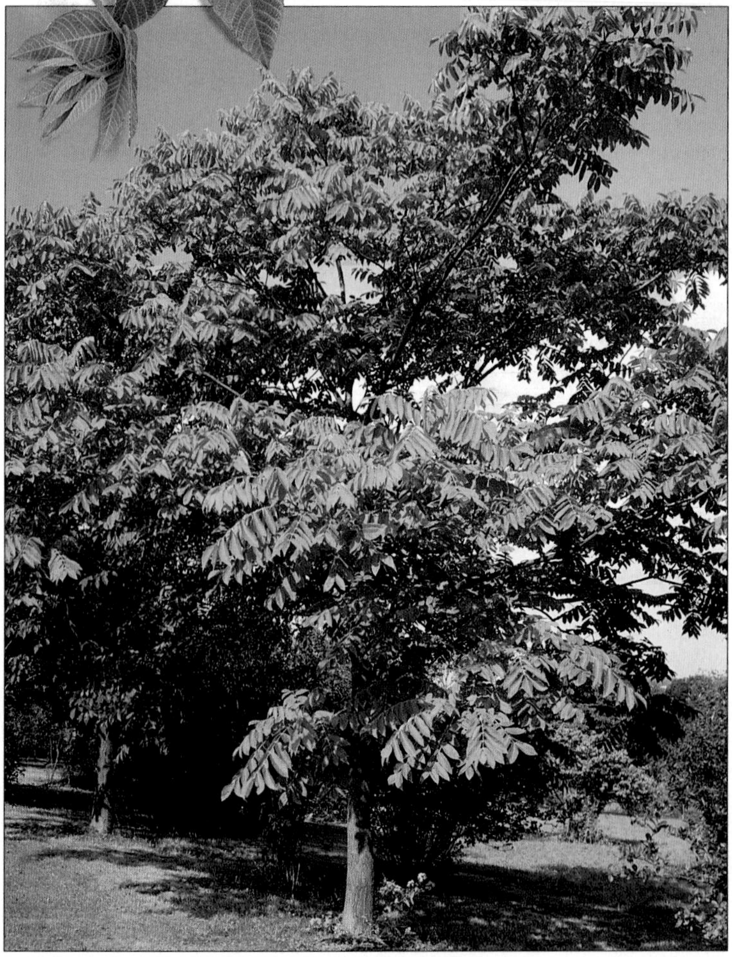

Juglans ailantifolia (inset: leaf and flower detail)

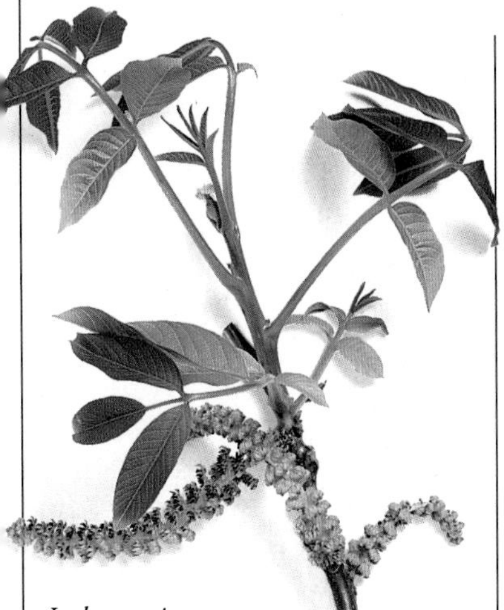

Juglans regia

leaves, to 20cm (8in) long, with 11–15 oblong-lance-shaped leaflets and spherical fruit, to 1.5cm (½in) long. ↕↔ 10m (30ft). USA (S. California). ❄❄

J. cinerea 🌳 (Butternut). Vigorous, spreading tree with pinnate leaves, to 50cm (20in) long, with 7–19 oblong-lance-shaped, aromatic, bright green leaflets. Grown for its sweet, edible nuts, contained within large, clustered, ovoid fruit, to 6cm (2½in) long. ↕ 25m (80ft), ↔ 20m (70ft). E. North America. ❄❄❄

J. cordiformis see *J. ailantifolia* var. *cordiformis.*

J. mandshurica 🌳 (Manchurian walnut). Spreading, suckering tree with stout shoots and pinnate leaves, to 60cm (24in) or more long, with 9–17 oblong, glossy leaflets and sticky, ovoid fruit, to 5cm (2in) long. ↕↔ 20m (70ft). N.E. China, Korea. ❄❄❄

J. microcarpa 🌳 syn. *J. rupestris* (Texan walnut). Bushy-headed, spreading tree or shrub with pinnate, aromatic leaves, to 30cm (12in) long, with 15–23 slender, glossy leaflets, yellow in autumn, and small, spherical fruit, to 2.5cm (1in) long. ↕↔ 10m (30ft). S.W. USA, N. Mexico. ❄❄❄

J. nigra ■ 🏆 🌳 (Black walnut). Vigorous, spreading tree with pinnate, aromatic leaves, to 60cm (24in) long, consisting of 11–23 ovate-oblong, glossy, dark green leaflets. Grown for its edible nuts, contained within spherical fruit, to 5cm (2in) long. ↕ 30m (100ft), ↔ 20m (70ft). E. USA. ❄❄❄

J. regia ■ 🏆 🌳 (Common walnut). Spreading tree with pinnate, aromatic leaves, to 30cm (12in) or more long, consisting of 5–9 elliptic to ovate, entire or serrate, glossy leaflets, bronze-purple when young. Grown for its edible nuts, contained within spherical fruit, to 5cm (2in) long. ↕ 30m (100ft), ↔ 15m (50ft). S.E. Europe to Himalayas, S.W. China, C. Russia. ❄❄❄

J. rupestris see *J. microcarpa.*

J. sieboldiana see *J. ailantifolia.*

JUNCUS

Rush

JUNCACEAE

Genus of about 300 species of grass-like, hairless, evergreen or deciduous, rhizomatous perennials, widely distributed throughout the world, but mostly occurring in cool-temperate regions, particularly in heavy, wet, acid soil. The stems are cylindrical, nodeless, and usually solid, and the leaves, when present, are small and narrow, often reduced to basal sheaths. Unlike grasses and sedges, rushes produce small green or brown flowers with 6 tepals, borne in cymes in midsummer. Ornamental forms include cultivars with twisted or variegated stems. Rushes are suitable for a pond side or bog garden, but some will also thrive in moist garden soil.

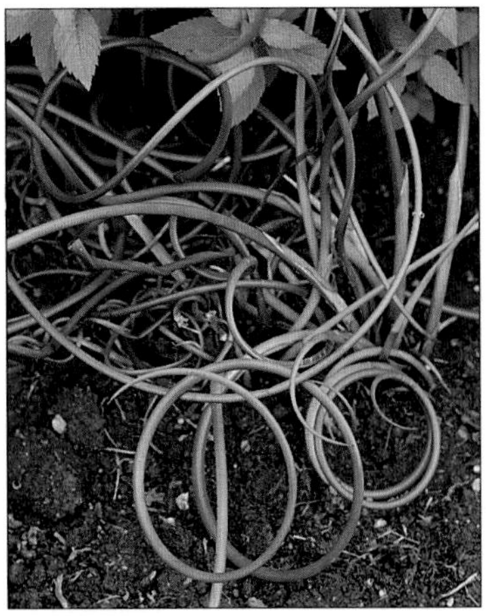

Juncus effusus 'Spiralis'

- **HARDINESS** Fully hardy.
- **CULTIVATION** Grow in permanently moist, acid soil in sun or partial shade. *J. effusus* and *J. inflexus* may also be grown in up to 8cm (3in) of water or in boggy soil. *J. inflexus* thrives in heavy, alkaline soil.
- **PROPAGATION** Sow seed at 6–12°C (43–54°F) in spring, or divide from mid-spring to early summer.
- **PESTS AND DISEASES** Trouble free.

J. articulatus (Jointed rush). Variable, tufted or creeping perennial with slender rhizomes and cylindrical stems bearing alternate, flat, often curved or semi-prostrate, faintly jointed, deep green leaves, 80cm (32in) long. Compound cymes of 5–20 clusters of dark brown flowers, 3mm (⅛in) long, are produced from summer to early autumn. ↕ to 80cm (32in). ↔ to 60cm (24in). W. and S. Europe, Asia, North America. ❄❄❄

***J. effusus* 'Spiralis'** ■ syn. *J. effusus* f. *spiralis, Scirpus lacustris* 'Spiralis' (Corkscrew rush). Densely tufted, leafless perennial with spiralled, shiny, dark green stems, giving a corkscrew effect and forming a rather tangled mass. Small brown flowers, to 3mm (⅛in) long, are produced in loose cymes, to 5cm (2in) long, along the stems throughout summer. ↕ 45cm (18in), ↔ 60cm (24in). ❄❄❄

***J. inflexus* 'Afro'.** Densely tufted, leafless perennial, similar to *J. effusus* 'Spiralis', but with spiralled, matt, blue-green stems, and brown flowers, to 4mm (⅙in) long, produced in small, loose cymes towards the ends of the stems, from late spring to midsummer. ↕↔ 60cm (24in). ❄❄❄

▷**Juneberry** see *Amelanchier*
▷**Jungle flame** see *Ixora coccinea*
▷**Juniper** see *Juniperus*
Alligator see *J. deppeana*
Ashe see *J. ashei*
Bonin Island see *J. procumbens*
Chinese see *J. chinensis*
Coffin see *J. recurva* var. *coxii*
Common see *J. communis*

▷**Juniper cont.**
Creeping see *J. horizontalis*
Flaky see *J. squamata*
Himalayan weeping see *J. recurva*
Rocky Mountain see *J. scopulorum*
Sargent see *J. sargentii*
Shore see *J. conferta*
Syrian see *J. drupacea*
Temple see *J. rigida*

JUNIPERUS syn. SABINA

Juniper

CUPRESSACEAE

Genus of 50–60 species of evergreen, coniferous shrubs and tall trees from dry forests and hillsides throughout the N. hemisphere. Juvenile leaves are usually needle-like or narrowly wedge-shaped, and 0.5–1.5cm (¼–½in) long. Adult leaves are usually scale-like and overlapping, either lying flat along the shoots or spreading, and 2–6mm (1⁄16–¼in) long. In most cases, male and female cones are borne on separate plants: male cones are spherical to ovoid, yellow, and to 5mm (¼in) across; females develop into usually spherical, fleshy, berry-like fruits, 4–10mm (⅛–½in) across, with 1–10 seeds, and are persistent, generally ripening over 2 to 3 years. Junipers tolerate a wide range of soils and conditions, and are useful for hot, sunny sites. Use as specimen plants: the smallest species in a rock garden and the prostrate species as ground cover. Contact with the foliage may aggravate skin allergies.

- **HARDINESS** Fully hardy to frost hardy.
- **CULTIVATION** Grow in any well-drained soil, including dry, chalky, or sandy soils, preferably in full sun or in light dappled shade. Junipers need little, if any, pruning.
- **PROPAGATION** Remove seed from flesh as soon as ripe and sow in containers in a cold frame; germination may take up to 5 years. Root ripewood cuttings in early autumn.
- **PESTS AND DISEASES** Prone to twig blight, aphids, scale insects, webber moth caterpillars, and honey fungus.

J. ashei 🌳 (Ashe juniper). Shrub or spreading tree with an irregular crown, light, ash-grey bark, peeling in strips, and triangular-ovate, scale-like, glaucous, blue-grey leaves in pairs or threes. Produces bluish black fruit with soft, resinous, juicy pulp. ↕↔ to 6m (20ft). S.E. USA. ❄❄❄ (borderline)

J. chinensis △ (Chinese juniper). Ovoid-conical tree to spreading shrub with brown bark, peeling in long strips, and dark green foliage. Narrowly wedge-shaped juvenile leaves have long, sharp points and are borne in pairs or threes; diamond-shaped, scale-like adult leaves are mainly in 4 ranks, lying flat along the stems. Foliage is pungently scented. Bears violet to brown fruit, marked with the outlines of scales. ↕ to 20m (70ft), ↔ to 6m (20ft). China, Mongolia, Japan. ❄❄❄. **'Aurea'** 🏆 ◊ is a columnar tree with golden yellow leaves, and produces numerous cones in mid-spring; ↕ to 11m (35ft), ↔ 5m (15ft). **'Blaauw'** 🏆 syn. *J. x pfitzeriana* 'Blaauw', is a dense, upright shrub with spreading, long-pointed, diamond-shaped, blue-grey leaves; ↕ 1.2m (4ft), ↔ 1m (3ft). **'Blue Alps'** is a vigorous, spreading shrub with shoots arching at the tips, and silver-blue juvenile leaves, to 1.5cm (½in) long; ↕ to 4m (12ft), ↔ 3m (10ft). **'Kaizuka'** 🏆 is a spreading shrub with dense, irregular growth, bright green leaves, and many glaucous berries; ↕ 6m (20ft), ↔ 3–4m (10–12ft). **'Keteleeri'** ◊ is a narrowly conical, dense, regular tree with diamond-shaped, scale-like, dark grey-green leaves; ↕ to 10m (30ft), ↔ 2m (6ft). **'Kuriwao Gold'** is a rounded shrub with bright gold leaves; requires a site in full sun; ↕↔ 2m (6ft). **'Mordigan Gold'**, syn. 'Mordigan Aurea', is a spreading, golden yellow shrub with branches rising at an angle of 30°; ↕ to 1.5m (5ft), ↔ 2.5m (8ft). **'Obelisk'** ■ 🏆 is a slender, erect shrub with long, glaucous, bluish green juvenile leaves, to 1.5cm (½in) long; ↕ to 2.5m (8ft), ↔ 60cm (24in). **'Robusta Green'** see *J. virginiana* 'Robusta Green'. **'Stricta'** is a narrowly conical shrub with a pointed tip, and soft, blue-green leaves; ↕ 2.5m (8ft), ↔ 60cm (24in).

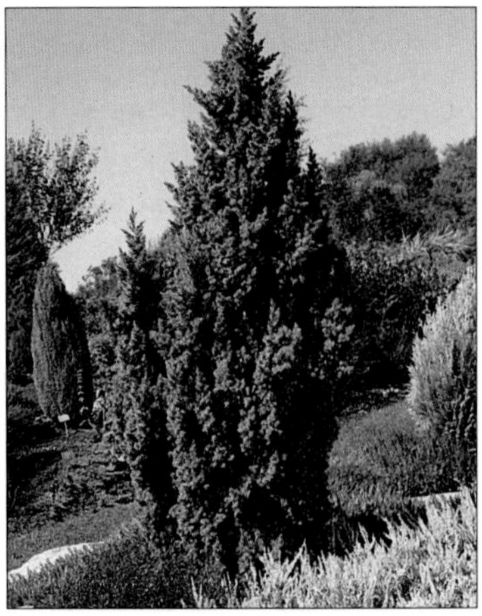

Juniperus chinensis 'Obelisk'

J

J. communis ◊ (Common juniper). Spreading shrub to small, ovoid or columnar tree. Linear, sharply pointed leaves, deep green to blue-green, with single, glaucous white bands on the inner faces, are borne in threes. Ovoid or spherical fruit, green when first produced, ripen to glaucous blue then black over 3 years. ↕ 0.5–6m (1½–20ft) or more, ↔ 1–6m (3–20ft). N. hemisphere. ❄❄❄. **'Compressa'** ■ 🏆 is a dwarf, spindle-shaped shrub, which grows very slowly, at 2–3cm (¾–1¼in) per year. Suitable for growing in a trough; ↕ to 80cm (32in), ↔ 45cm (18in). **var. *depressa*** is prostrate, with

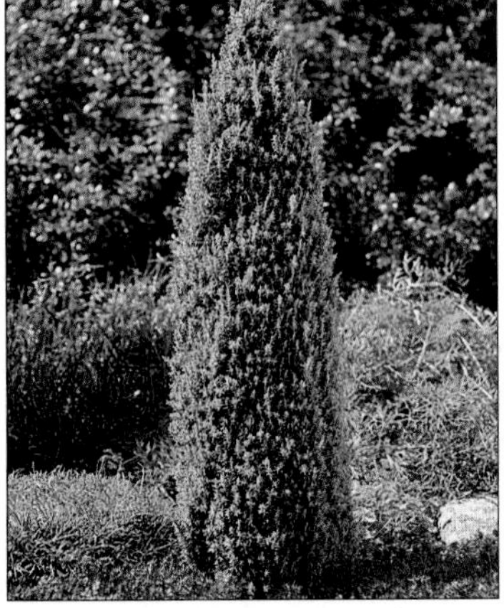

Juniperus communis 'Compressa'

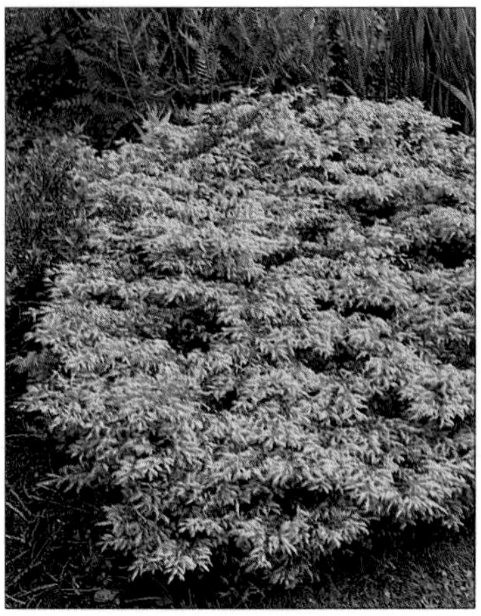

Juniperus communis 'Depressa Aurea'

upturned shoot tips and leaves with narrow white bands; ↕ to 60cm (24in), ↔ 1.5m (5ft). North America, Greenland. **'Depressa Aurea'** ▣ is a spreading shrub with semi-erect branches, and golden yellow leaves in late spring, becoming bronze and almost green over winter; ↕ 60cm (24in), ↔ 1.5m (5ft). **'Hibernica'** ▣🏆 is a spindle-shaped, columnar shrub, similar to 'Compressa' but more vigorous, growing 20cm (8in) per year; ↕ 3–5m (10–15ft), ↔ 30cm (12in). **'Prostrata'** is a very vigorous, prostrate, mat-forming shrub with green foliage; ↕ 20–30cm (8–12in), ↔ 1.5–2m (5–6ft). **'Sentinel'** is an upright, spindle-shaped shrub, similar to 'Compressa' but more vigorous; ↕ to 1.5m (5ft), ↔ to 60cm (24in).

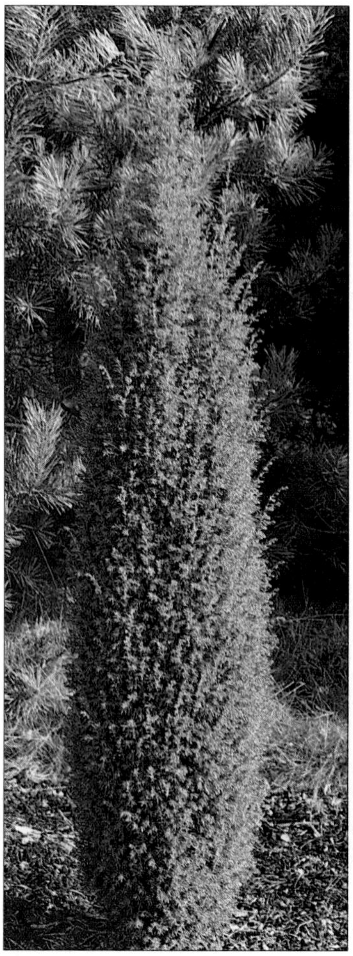

Juniperus communis 'Hibernica'

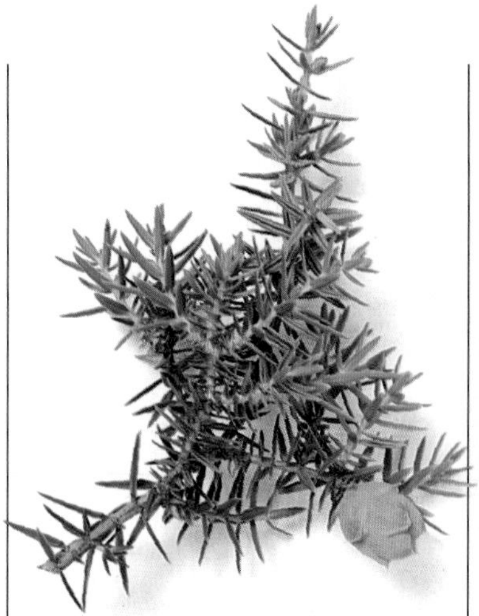

Juniperus drupacea

J. conferta (Shore juniper). Prostrate shrub with dense, sharply pointed, needle-like, bright green or grey-green leaves, borne in groups of 3. The black fruit have a glaucous bloom. ↕ to 30cm (12in), ↔ indefinite. Japan, Russia (Sakhalin). ❄❄❄. **'Blue Pacific'** is a trailing, prostrate shrub with blue-green leaves; ↕ to 30cm (12in), ↔ to 2m (6ft).
J. deppeana △ (Alligator juniper). Broadly conical tree with thick, grooved, grey bark divided up into small, square scales, and needle-like, oval-diamond-shaped, blue-green leaves, to 6mm (¼in) long, lying flat along the branches. Spherical to broadly ellipsoid, red-brown fruit, 1cm (½in) across, are produced in summer, ripening in the second year. ↕ to 20m (70ft), ↔ to 4m (12ft). S.W. USA, Mexico. ❄❄. **'Silver Spire'** ▯ is a narrowly columnar shrub or tree with ash-grey bark and bright silver foliage. Juvenile leaves are borne in whorls of 2 or 3; diamond-shaped adult leaves lie flat along the stems in 4 ranks. Bears reddish brown fruit with dry, fibrous pulp; ↕ to 10m (30ft), rarely 20m (70ft), ↔ 3–5m (10–15ft).
J. drupacea ▣▯ (Syrian juniper). Usually columnar tree with orange-brown bark peeling in strips. Narrowly wedge-shaped leaves, 1–2.5cm (½–1in) long, with long, sharp points, are grey-green with 2 white bands, and borne in whorls of 3. Produces ovoid or spherical green fruit maturing to dark blue, then brown, 2–2.5cm (¾–1in) across. ↕ to 15m (50ft), ↔ to 3m (10ft). S. Greece, Turkey, Syria. ❄❄❄
***J.* 'Grey Owl'** 🏆 syn. *J. virginiana* 'Grey Owl'. Large, spreading shrub with horizontal branches and arching, oval-diamond-shaped, scale-like, soft, silver-grey leaves. Bears ovoid, glaucous, brownish violet fruit which ripen in the first autumn. ↕ 2–3m (6–10ft), ↔ 3–4m (10–12ft). ❄❄❄

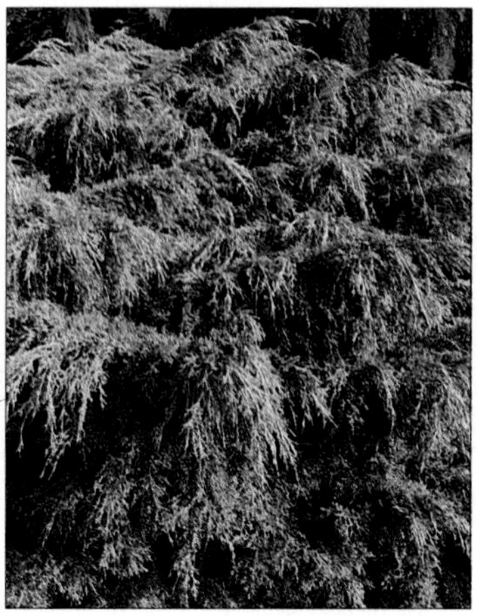

Juniperus x *pfitzeriana* 'Aurea'

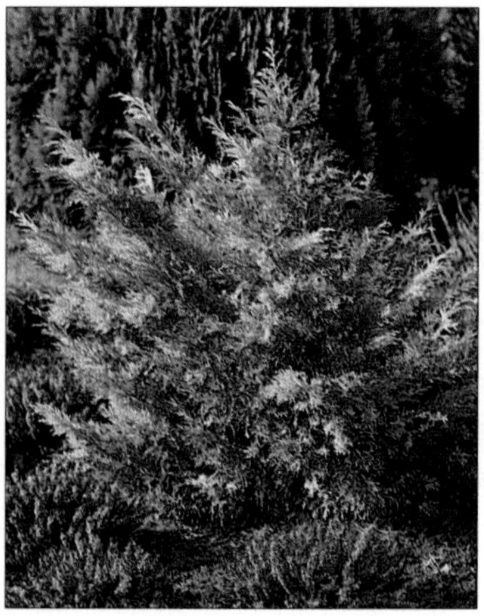

Juniperus x *pfitzeriana* 'Blue and Gold'

***J.* 'Hetz'** see *J. virginiana* 'Hetzii'.
J. horizontalis (Creeping juniper). Prostrate, creeping shrub with grey-green foliage. Needle-like juvenile leaves, with long, sharp points, are borne in pairs or in threes; elliptic, scale-like adult leaves, each with a prominent gland on the back, lie flat along the shoots in 4 rows. Bears ovoid, dark blue fruit. ↕ to 30cm (12in), ↔ indefinite. North America. ❄❄❄. **'Bar Harbor'** has grey-green leaves which become mauve-purple in winter. **'Douglasii'** has a flat, mat-like habit with ascending side branches and glaucous, bright green leaves, purple-bronzed in winter. **'Emerald Spreader'** is a very flat shrub with emerald-green juvenile leaves. **'Turquoise Spreader'** is a flat shrub with greenish blue juvenile leaves. **'Wiltonii'** 🏆 is persistently glaucous with bright blue leaves; it is excellent ground cover. **'Winter Blue'** has bright blue leaves and a less spreading habit.
J.* x *media see *J.* x *pfitzeriana.*
***J.* x *media* 'Hetzii'** see *J. virginiana* 'Hetzii'.
J.* x *pfitzeriana 🏆 (*J. chinensis* x *J. sabina*) syn. *J.* x *media.* Spreading, male shrub with branches ascending at an angle of 45°, gradually forming a flat-topped bush with tiered foliage. Diamond-shaped, scale-like, grey-green leaves, with free tips, lie flat along the shoots. The spherical fruit are initially dark purple, becoming paler later. ↕ 1.2m (4ft), ↔ 3m (10ft). Garden origin. ❄❄❄. **'Armstrongii'** has soft, yellow-green leaves; ↕↔ to 1m (3ft). **'Aurea'** ▣ has golden yellow leaves which become yellowish green over winter; ↕ 90cm (36in), ↔ 2m (6ft). **'Blaauw'** see *J. chinensis* 'Blaauw'. **'Blue and Gold'** ▣ has patches of blue-green foliage intermingled with bright yellow; ↕ 1.5m (5ft), ↔ 2–3m (6–10ft). **'Glauca'** has prickly, silver to greyish blue leaves; ↕ 90cm (36in), ↔ 2m (6ft). **'Gold Coast'** is compact, with deep chrome-yellow leaves which retain their colour in winter; ↕↔ 1m (3ft). **'Golden Saucer'**, has bright golden yellow leaves, especially in winter; ↕ 1–1.5m (3–5ft), ↔ 30cm (12in).

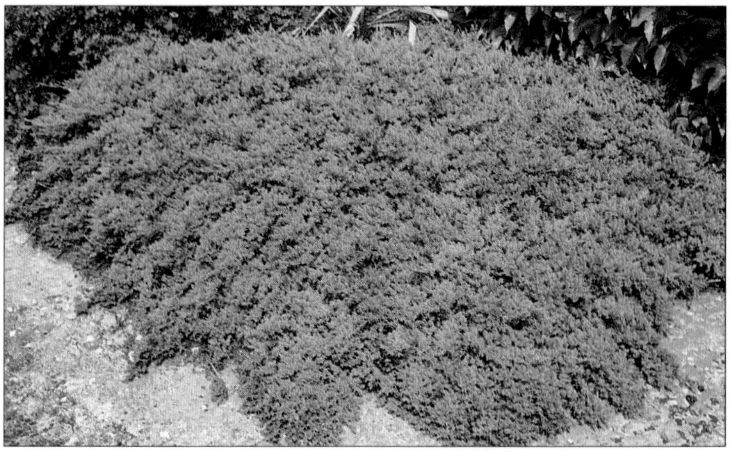

Juniperus procumbens

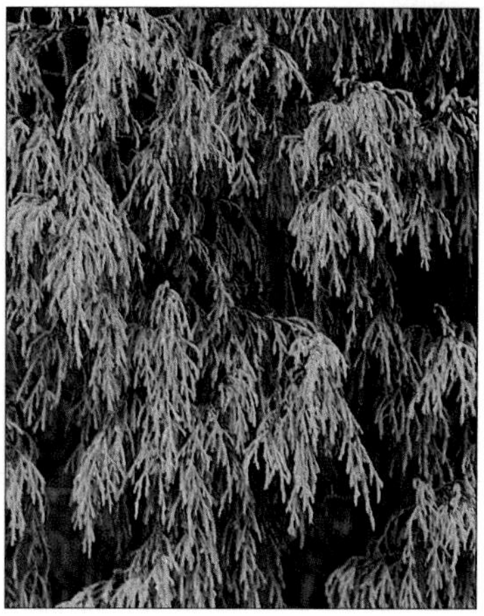

Juniperus recurva

J. procumbens ▣ (Bonin Island juniper). Spreading, procumbent shrub with mostly linear, needle-like, sharply pointed, yellow-green leaves in threes. Bears brown or black fruit. ↕ to 75cm (30in), ↔ to 2m (6ft). S. Japan. ❄❄❄
J. recurva ▣△ (Himalayan weeping juniper). Conical or broadly columnar tree with smooth, orange-brown bark, which peels in strips and is fissured in old trees. Narrowly wedge-shaped, grey-green leaves, 4–7mm (⅛–¼in) long, produced in threes and pointing forwards along the shoots, are borne in pendulous sprays. Produces spherical or ovoid, greenish brown to black fruit, each with a single seed. ↕ to 10m (30ft), ↔ to 5m (15ft). Himalayas to W. China. ❄❄❄. **var. *coxii*** (Coffin juniper) has longer and more widely spaced, rich, dark green leaves, 6–8mm (¼–⅜in) long. N. Burma. **'Densa'**, syn.

J

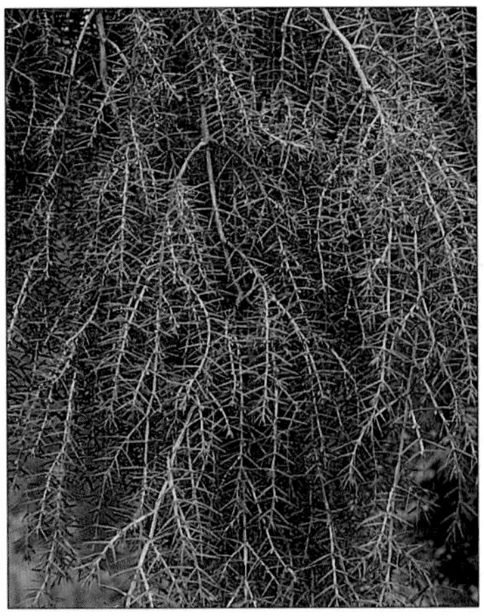
Juniperus rigida

'Nana', is a dwarf, conical, low-growing, spreading shrub with ascending branch tips and dark green leaves; ↕ 60cm (24in), ↔ 1.2m (4ft). **'Nana'** see 'Densa'.

J. rigida ■◊ (Temple juniper). Spreading tree or large shrub with peeling brown to yellow-brown bark and an open crown of pendulous branches bearing groups of 3 needle-like, sharply pointed, bright green leaves, glaucous on the inner face, and 1.5–2.5cm (½–1in) long. Bears purplish black fruit. ↕ to 8m (25ft) or more, ↔ to 6m (20ft). N. China, Korea, Japan. ❄❄❄

J. sabina (Savin). Spreading, occasionally erect shrub with flaking, red-brown bark and slender, 4-sided shoots. Mainly adult leaves, borne in pairs lying flat along the stems, are ovate, scale-like, and dark green to grey-green, each with a small gland on the back, and a foetid smell when crushed. Flattened, spherical fruit, bluish black with white blooms, ripen over the first winter. ↕ 2–5m (6–15ft), ↔ to 6m (20ft). C. Europe to N. China. ❄❄❄. **'Blaue Donau'**, syn. 'Blue Danube', is very hardy, with shoots erect at the tips and light greyish blue leaves; ↕ 60cm (24in), ↔ 2m (6ft). **'Blue Danube'** see 'Blaue Donau'. **'Cupressifolia'** has a compact and horizontal habit with blue-green leaves; ↕ 60cm (24in), ↔ 1.5m (5ft). **'Mas'** is an upright shrub with dark green leaves; ↕ 6m (20ft), ↔ to 1m (3ft). **var. *tamariscifolia*** ■ is low-growing, with horizontal tiers of spreading, short, sharply pointed, mainly juvenile, bright green or bluish

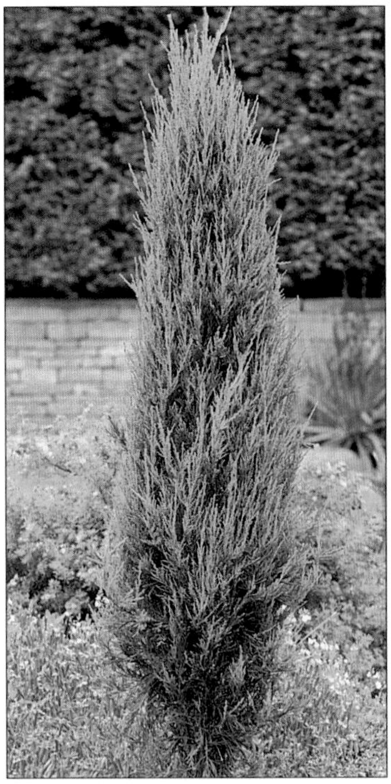
Juniperus scopulorum 'Skyrocket'

green leaves borne in pairs or threes; ↕ to 1–2m (3–6ft), ↔ 1.5–2m (5–6ft).

J. sargentii (Sargent juniper). Creeping shrub with prostrate, flexuous stems, short branchlets, and mostly ovate, camphor-scented, scale-like, bluish green leaves. Other, dark blue-green leaves are paired and lie flat to the branches. Juvenile leaves are needle-like, in whorls of 3. Bears dark blue or black fruit. ↕ to 30cm (12in), ↔ indefinite. N.E. China, N.E. Asia, Japan, Russia (Sakhalin, Kurile Islands). ❄❄❄

J. scopulorum ◊ (Rocky Mountain juniper). Rounded or spreading tree or shrub with red-brown bark, furrowed into strips or square flakes. Paired, ovate, sharply pointed, scale-like, yellow-green to dark green leaves lie flat to the branches. Bears blue-black fruit. ↕ to 15m (50ft), ↔ to 6m (20ft). USA (Rocky Mountains). ❄❄❄. **'Blue Heaven'** 🏆 is a shrub of conical habit and blue-green leaves; ↕ 2m (6ft), ↔ to 60cm (24in). **'Skyrocket'** ■◊ syn. *J. virginiana* 'Skyrocket', is a narrow, pencil-shaped tree with glaucous, grey-green leaves; ↕ to 6m (20ft), ↔ 50–60cm (20–24in). **'Springbank'** ◊ is a narrow, conical tree with pendent branch tips

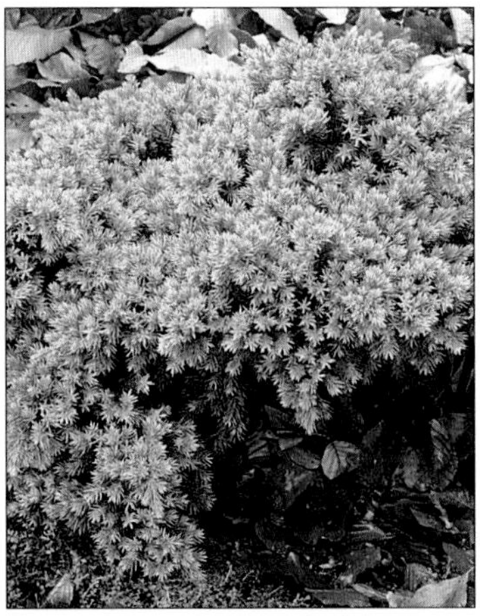
Juniperus squamata 'Blue Star'

and intensely silver-blue leaves; ↕ to 2m (6ft), ↔ to 60cm (24in). **'Table Top'** is a spreading shrub with blue leaves and many berries; ↕ to 2m (6ft), ↔ 5m (15ft). **'Wichita Blue'** ◊ is a broadly conical tree with bright blue-grey leaves; ↕ to 2m (6ft), ↔ 80cm (32in).

J. squamata ◊ (Flaky juniper). Prostrate shrub, spreading bush, or small upright tree with flaky, rusty brown bark. Spreading, narrowly wedge-shaped, sharply pointed, entirely juvenile leaves, dark grey-green to silvery blue-green, each with a bright blue-white band, are borne in whorls of 3. Bears ovoid, glossy black fruit. ↕ to 10m (30ft), ↔ 1–8m (3–25ft). Mountains of N.E. Afghanistan, Himalayas, W. and C. China. ❄❄❄. **'Blue Star'** ■🏆 is a compact, rounded bush, with silvery blue leaves; ↕ to 40cm (16in), ↔ to 1m (3ft). **'Chinese Silver'** is a spreading shrub with vivid silver-blue and silver leaves; ↕↔ to 6m (20ft). **'Holger'** 🏆 is a spreading shrub with sulphur-yellow new growth contrasting with steel-blue older leaves; ↕↔ 2m (6ft). **'Meyeri'** ■ is a spreading shrub with arching and nodding shoot tips and glaucous blue leaves. Dead foliage often persists, marring its appearance; ↕ 4–10m (12–30ft), ↔ 6–8m (20–25ft).

J. virginiana ◊ (Pencil cedar). Conical to columnar tree with a conical crown, spreading branches, and brown bark with narrow, spiral ridges, peeling in shreds. Both the narrowly wedge-shaped, sharply pointed juvenile leaves and the diamond-shaped, scale-like adult leaves are grey-green, borne in pairs on the same shoots, and lie flat along the branches. Ovoid, very glaucous, brown-violet fruit ripen in the first autumn. ↕ 15–30m (50–100ft), ↔ 5–8m (15–25ft). E. USA (Maine to Texas). ❄❄❄. **'Burkii'** ◊ is a dense, upright tree with blue-grey leaves which become purple-tinged over winter; ↕ to 6m (20ft), ↔ 1m (3ft). **'Grey Owl'** see *J.* 'Grey Owl'. **'Hetzii'**, syn. 'Hetz', *J.* 'Hetz', *J.* x *media* 'Hetzii', is an open shrub with tiers of spreading, blue-green leaves on ascending branches. Produces spherical, blue-purple to brown fruit; ↕ 4–5m (12–15ft), ↔ to 3–5m (10–15ft). **'Robusta Green'** ◊ syn. *J. chinensis* 'Robusta Green', is a narrow, columnar tree with blue-green leaves; ↕ to 3m (10ft), ↔ 60cm (24in). **'Skyrocket'** see *J. scopulorum* 'Skyrocket'.

J

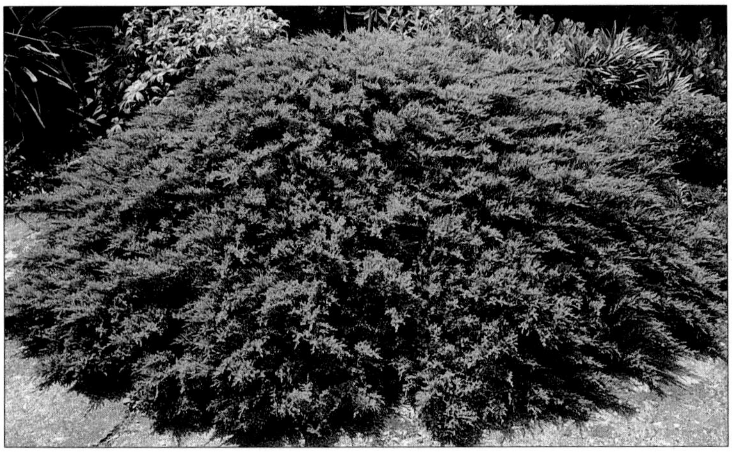
Juniperus sabina var. *tamariscifolia*

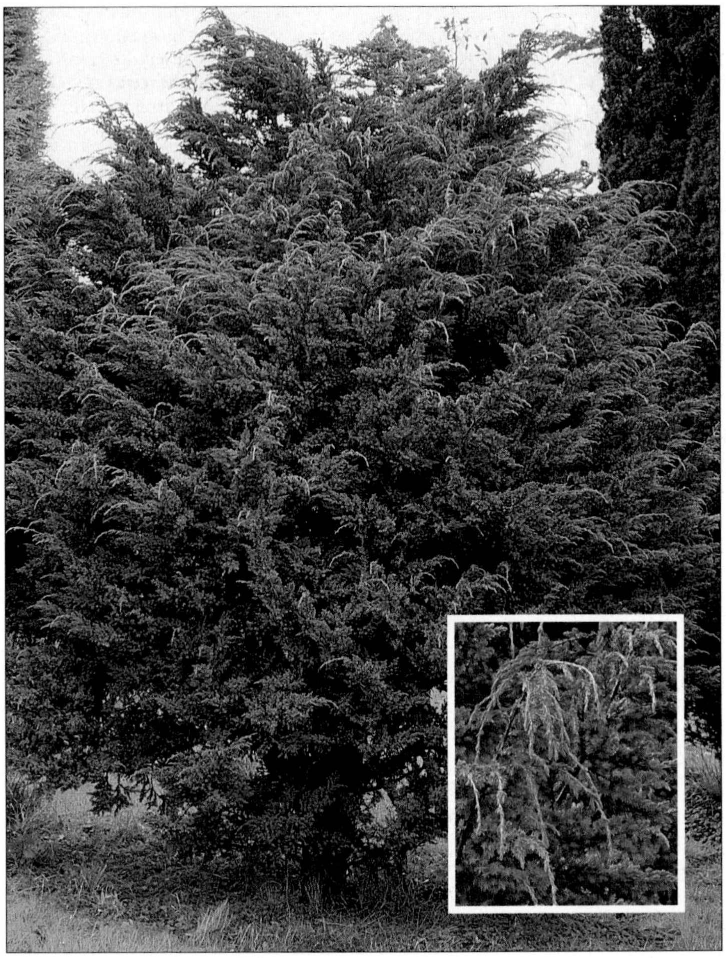
Juniperus squamata 'Meyeri' (inset: leaf detail)

▷ **Jupiter's distaff** see *Salvia glutinosa*
▷ ***Jussiaea longifolia*** see *Ludwigia longifolia*
▷ ***Jussiaea repens*** see *Ludwigia peploides*

JUSTICIA syn. BELOPERONE, DREJERELLA, DUVERNOIA, LIBONIA

ACANTHACEAE

Genus of about 420 species of evergreen perennials, shrubs, and subshrubs from a wide range of habitats in tropical and subtropical regions worldwide and from temperate North America. The opposite, usually simple leaves are ovate to elliptic and often boldly veined. Justicias are grown mainly for their slender, tubular flowers, which have narrow, arching lips and are produced, with conspicuous bracts, in terminal or axillary spikes, cymes, or panicles. Where temperatures fall below 7°C (45°F), grow in a temperate greenhouse, or as houseplants. In milder climates, plant in a mixed border.

• **HARDINESS** Frost tender.

• **CULTIVATION** Under glass, grow in draught-free conditions in loam-based potting compost (JI No.2 or 3) with bright filtered light, or full light with shade from hot sun. Provide high humidity, although *J. brandegeeana* and *J. rizzinii* tolerate lower humidity. In the growing season, water freely and apply a balanced liquid fertilizer every 4 weeks; keep just moist in winter. Pot on in spring. Outdoors, grow in fertile, moist, but well-drained soil in partial shade. Pruning group 9; tip-prune young plants to promote bushiness. Plants under glass need hard restrictive pruning in late winter or early spring; most are best replaced when they become leggy.

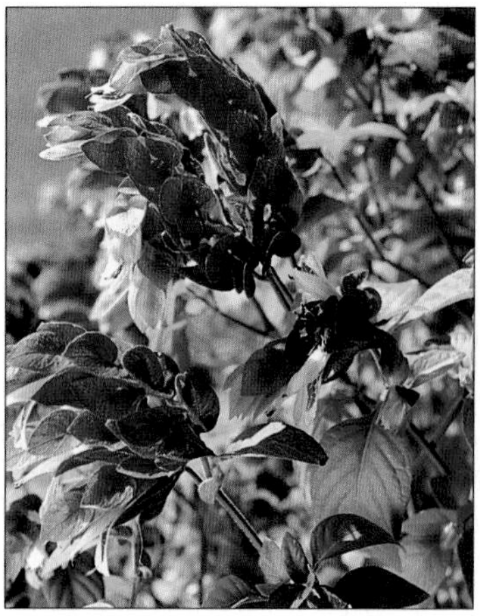

Justicia brandegeeana

• **PROPAGATION** Sow seed at 16°C (61°F) in spring. Root softwood cuttings in late spring, or semi-ripe cuttings in summer, both with bottom heat.

• **PESTS AND DISEASES** Prone to red spider mites and whiteflies under glass.

J. adhatoda ■ syn. *Adhatoda duvernoia, Duvernoia adhatodoides.* Usually erect and sparsely branched, evergreen shrub, spreading with age unless regularly pruned, with ovate-elliptic, mid- to deep green leaves, 10–20cm (4–8in) long. Terminal and axillary spikes, 5cm (2in) or more long, of tubular-bell-shaped, 2-lipped white flowers, 3cm (1¼in) long, appear mainly in summer. The lower lips of the flowers are veined red or rose-purple. ↕ 2–3m (6–10ft), ↔ 1–1.5m (3–5ft). India, Sri Lanka. ❄ (min. 7°C/45°F)

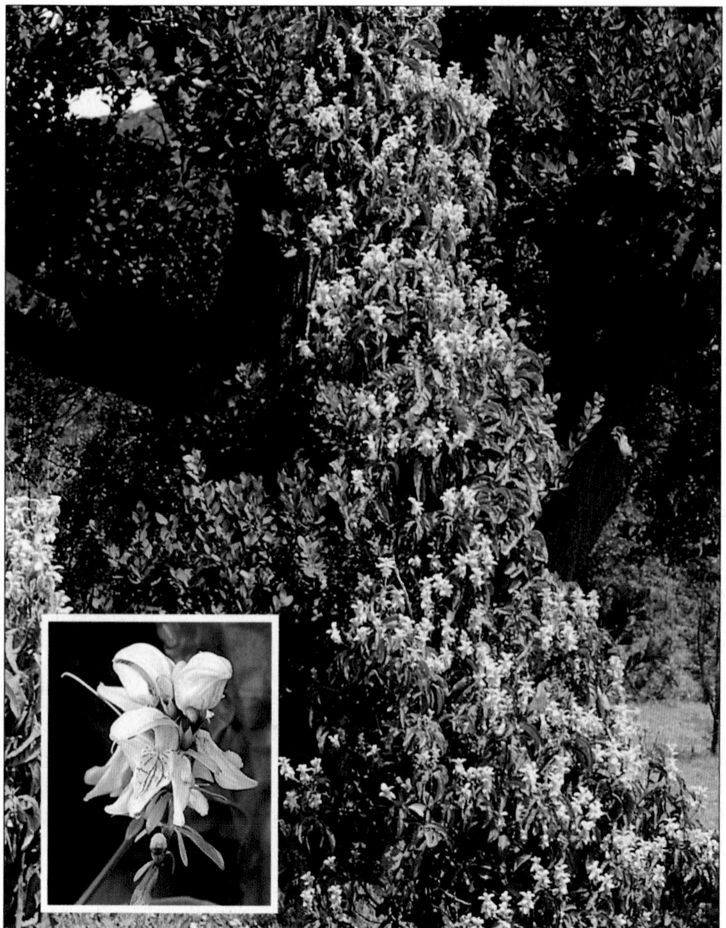

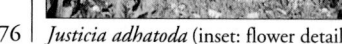

Justicia adhatoda (inset: flower detail)

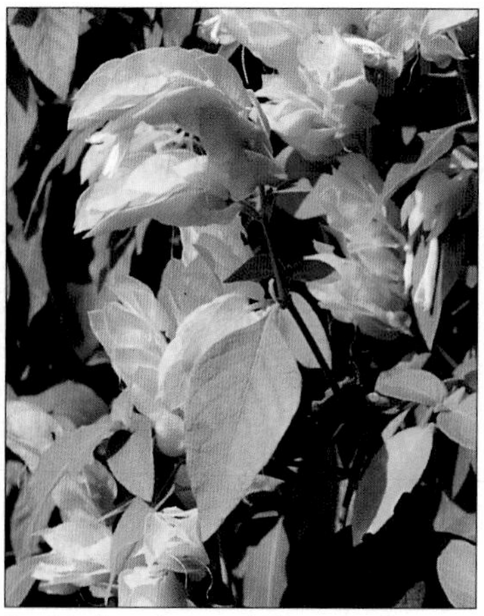

Justicia brandegeeana 'Chartreuse'

J. brandegeeana ■ ♀ syn. *Beloperone guttata, Drejerella guttata, J. guttata* (False hop, Shrimp bush, Shrimp plant). Moderately bushy, soft, evergreen shrub, of rounded habit if regularly tip-pruned, with downy stems and ovate or elliptic leaves, 2.5–8cm (1–3in) long, lustrous mid-green above, downy beneath. Elongated, hop-like, arching to pendent, terminal and axillary spikes, 10cm (4in) or more long, with overlapping, shrimp-pink bracts and slender, tongue-like white flowers, 3cm (1¼in) long, are borne throughout the year. The lower lips of the flowers are marked with purple or red. ↕ to 1m (3ft), ↔ 60–90cm (24–36in). Mexico. ❄ (min. 7°C/45°F). **'Chartreuse'** ■ has bright, lime-green bracts. **var. *lutea*** see 'Yellow Queen'. **'Yellow Queen'**, syn. var. *lutea*, has glowing yellow bracts.

J. carnea ■ syn. *Jacobinia carnea, J. pohliana, J. velutina, Justicia pohliana* (Brazilian plume, Flamingo plant, King's crown). Erect, sparsely branched, evergreen shrub with robust, 4-angled or 4-ridged stems, and oblong to ovate, mid-green leaves, to 25cm (10in) long, sometimes with short, velvety hairs. Dense, terminal and axillary spikes, 10–15cm (4–6in) long, of overlapping green bracts, largely obscured by tubular, 2-lipped, pink to rose- or purple-pink flowers, 5cm (2in) long, are produced during summer and autumn ↕ to 2m (6ft), ↔ to 1m (3ft). N. South America. ❄ (min. 7°C/45°F)

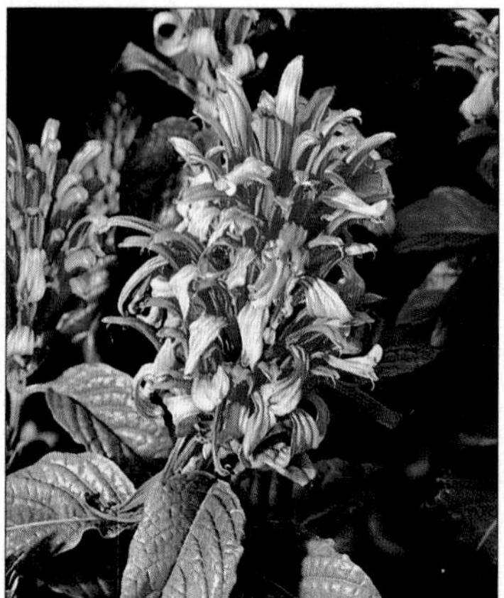

Justicia carnea

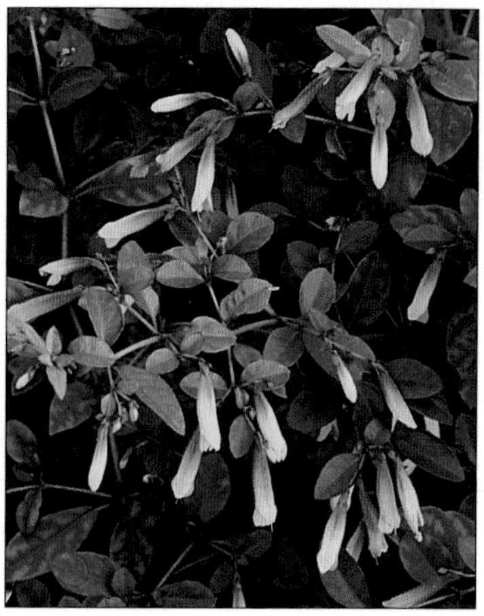

Justicia rizzinii

J. coccinea see *Pachystachys coccinea.*
J. floribunda see *J. rizzinii.*
***J. ghiesbreghtiana* of gardens** see *J. spicigera.*
J. guttata see *J. brandegeeana.*
J. pauciflora see *J. rizzinii.*
J. pohliana see *J. carnea.*

J. rizzinii ■ ♀ syn. *Jacobinia pauciflora, Justicia floribunda, J. pauciflora, Libonia floribunda.* Dwarf, soft, evergreen shrub of rounded habit, with downy stems bearing oblong to broadly obovate, mid-green leaves, to 2cm (¾in) long. One of each pair of leaves is smaller than the other. Small, nodding axillary spikes, 3cm (1¼in) wide, of tubular, yellow and scarlet flowers, 2cm (¾in) long, are produced from autumn to late spring. ↕↔ 30–60cm (12–24in). Brazil. ❄ (min. 7°C/45°F)

J. spicigera ■ syn. *Jacobinia spicigera, Justicia ghiesbreghtiana* of gardens. Freely branching, rounded, pubescent, evergreen shrub, with 4-angled stems and oblong-lance-shaped to ovate, arching, sometimes shallowly toothed, matt green leaves, 8–17cm (3–7in) long. Tubular, crimson to orange flowers, 3–4cm (1¼–1½in) long, are borne in small, forking, one-sided, terminal and axillary spikes, to 12cm (5in) long, from autumn to spring. The lower lips of the flowers are recurved or coiled. ↕ 1–1.8m (3–6ft), ↔ 75–120cm (2½–4ft). Mexico, Central America to Colombia. ❄ (min. 7°C/45°F)

J. suberecta see *Dicliptera suberecta.*

▷ **Justicia, Red** see *Megaskepasma erythrochlamys*

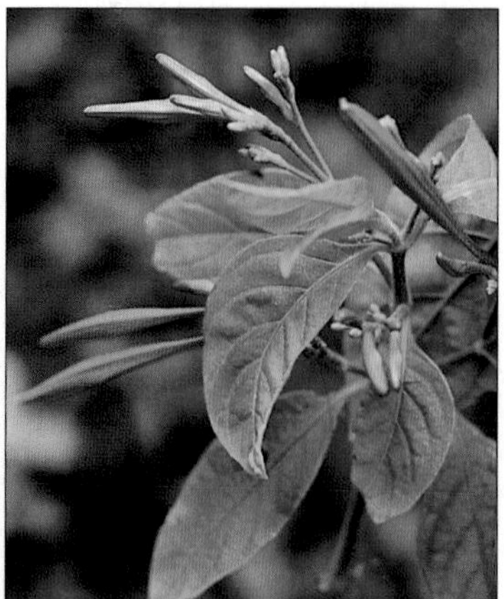

Justicia spicigera

K

KADSURA

SCHISANDRACEAE

Genus of about 20 species of woody, twining, evergreen climbers from forest in E. and S.E. Asia. They are grown for their fleshy fruits and attractive, simple, glossy leaves, arranged alternately. Solitary, cup-shaped flowers are usually produced in the leaf axils; both male and female flowers, borne on separate plants, are required to produce the fruits. *K. japonica*, the only species commonly cultivated, is best grown in a sheltered position where it can be trained against a wall or pillar, or through a large shrub.

• **HARDINESS** Frost hardy.
• **CULTIVATION** Grow in fertile, moist but well-drained soil in full sun or partial shade. Pruning group 12, in winter.
• **PROPAGATION** Take semi-ripe cuttings in summer.
• **PESTS AND DISEASES** Trouble free.

K. japonica. Vigorous, evergreen climber with twining shoots and elliptic to ovate-lance-shaped, slightly toothed, glossy, dark green leaves, to 10cm (4in) long. Small, solitary, cup-shaped, yellowish white flowers, 2cm (¾in) across, are produced from summer to autumn, followed on female plants by red, blackberry-like fruit, 3cm (1¼in) across. ↕ 4m (12ft). China, Korea, Taiwan, Japan. ❄❄. **'Variegata'** has leaves that are broadly margined with creamy yellow and tinged pink, becoming creamy white in winter.

KAEMPFERIA

ZINGIBERACEAE

Genus of about 40 species of aromatic, rhizomatous perennials growing wild in the forests of tropical Asia. The leaves are simple and either 2-ranked on short stems or in basal clusters. White, pink, or lilac, 3-petalled flowers, each with a deeply 2-lobed lip, are borne in terminal spikes on short, leafy or scaly stems and are often fragrant. In frost-prone areas, grow in a warm greenhouse; in tropical and subtropical regions, use outdoors as ground cover.

• **HARDINESS** Frost tender.
• **CULTIVATION** Under glass, grow in loam-based potting compost (JI No.2) in bright filtered light. During the growing season, maintain moderate humidity and water freely, applying a balanced liquid fertilizer every 2–3 weeks. Keep completely dry in winter when dormant. Outdoors, grow in well-drained, humus-rich soil in partial shade.
• **PROPAGATION** Sow seed at 20°C (68°F) as soon as ripe, or divide rhizomes in spring.
• **PESTS AND DISEASES** Trouble free.

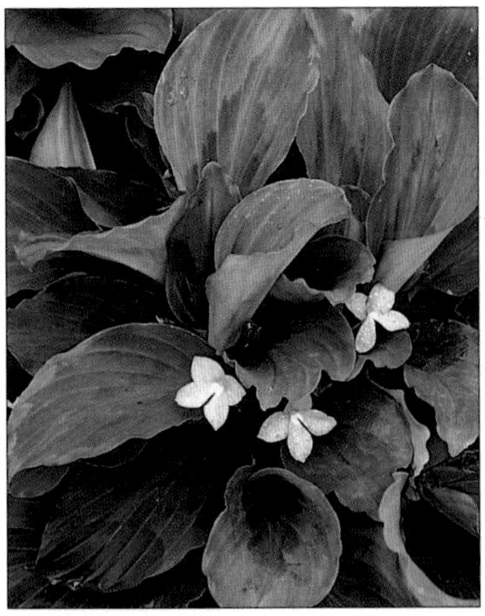

Kaempferia pulchra

K. pulchra ■ Low-growing, rhizomatous perennial with broadly elliptic, dark green leaves, about 15cm (6in) long, sometimes with silver markings. In summer, produces short spikes, to 5cm (2in) long, of 3-petalled, lilac or lilac-pink flowers, 4cm (1½in) across, amid the foliage. ↕ 15cm (6in), ↔ 30cm (12in). Thailand, Malaysia. ❁ (min. 10°C/50°F)
K. roscoeana (Dwarf ginger lily, Peacock lily). Low-growing, rhizomatous perennial with usually 2 rounded leaves, 10cm (4in) across, deep green with lighter green markings above, mid-green, tinged red beneath. From summer to autumn, bears short spikes, 5cm (2in) long, of 3-petalled white flowers, 2.5–5cm (1–2in) across, amid the foliage. ↕ 15cm (6in), ↔ 20cm (8in). Burma. ❁ (min. 10°C/50°F)
K. rotunda (Resurrection lily). Erect, rhizomatous perennial with lance-shaped leaves, to 40cm (16in) long, with long, sharp points, silver-green and unmarked above, purple beneath. In summer, produces spikes, 8cm (3in) long, of up to 6 lilac-lipped, 3-petalled white flowers, 5cm (2in) across, above the foliage. ↕ 15cm (6in), ↔ 45cm (18in). S.E. Asia. ❁ (min. 10°C/50°F)

▷ **Kaffirboom,**
Cape see *Erythrina caffra*
Transvaal see *Erythrina lysistemon*
▷ **Kaffir bread** see *Encephalartos caffer*
▷ **Kaki** see *Diospyros kaki*

KALANCHOE

syn. BRYOPHYLLUM

CRASSULACEAE

Genus of about 130 species of annual, biennial, and perennial succulents, shrubs, climbers, and small trees, occurring in semi-desert or shady areas of Saudi Arabia, Yemen (including Socotra), C. Africa, South Africa, Madagascar, Asia, Australia, and tropical America. Some are tree-like or shrubby, others are more spreading in habit. All have fleshy stems bearing simple to 2-pinnatisect, rarely pinnate, toothed or scalloped, fleshy leaves, arranged in opposite pairs, rarely alternate or whorled. Diurnal, showy, bell-shaped, urn-shaped, or tubular, 4-lobed flowers, often swollen in the middle or at the bases, are borne in terminal, occasionally lateral, cyme-like or corymb-like panicles. Where temperatures drop below 12°C (54°F), grow as houseplants

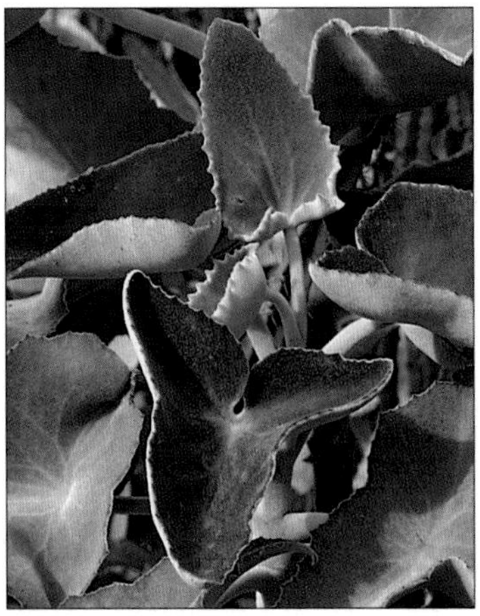

Kalanchoe beharensis

or in a temperate or warm greenhouse; some spreading species are particularly effective in a hanging basket. In warmer climates, grow outdoors in a shrub border or in beds.

• **HARDINESS** Frost tender.
• **CULTIVATION** Under glass, grow in loam-based potting compost (JI No.2) with additional grit, in bright filtered light. During the growing season, water moderately and apply a balanced liquid fertilizer 3 or 4 times; keep just moist in winter. Outdoors, grow in well-drained, humus-rich, moderately fertile soil in partial shade. See also pp.48–49.
• **PROPAGATION** Sow seed at 21°C (70°F) in early spring. Remove offsets and plantlets from leaves or inflorescences, or take stem cuttings, in spring or summer.
• **PESTS AND DISEASES** Susceptible to mealybugs, aphids, downy mildew, and leaf spot.

K. beharensis ■ Bushy, often tree-like, perennial succulent with broadly triangular to lance-shaped, slightly toothed, long-stalked leaves, to 35cm (14in) long, usually concave and brown above, convex and silvery beneath, and

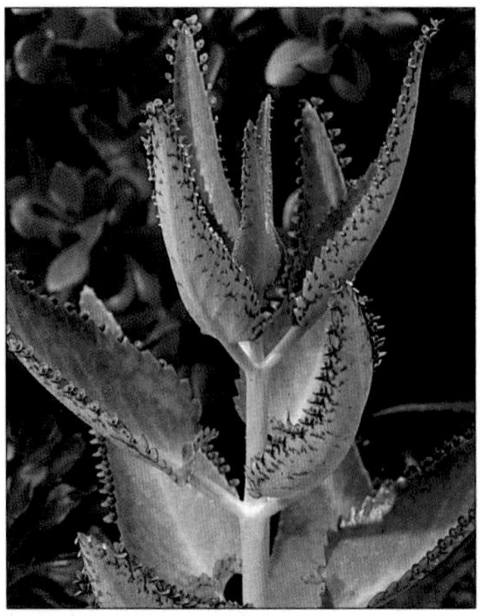

Kalanchoe daigremontiana

covered with minute, fine, silver or golden hairs. In late winter, mature plants bear many lateral, cyme-like panicles of urn-shaped, green-yellow flowers, 7mm (¼in) long, which are violet-veined inside. ↕↔ 1m (3ft) or more. Madagascar. ❁ (min. 10°C/50°F)
K. blossfeldiana ■ Bushy, perennial succulent with oval to oblong-ovate, softly toothed, glossy, dark green leaves, 8cm (3in) long, on long stalks. Tubular scarlet flowers, 1.5cm (½in) long, are produced in early spring, mostly in crowded, corymb-like panicles. ↕↔ to 40cm (16in). Madagascar. ❁ (min. 12°C/54°F). Many hybrids have been developed, with flowers in white, yellow, pink, and other shades.
K. daigremontiana ■ syn. *Bryophyllum daigremontianum* (Mexican hat plant). Erect, perennial succulent with lance-shaped leaves, 15–20cm (6–8in) long, usually spotted reddish brown, that produce adventitious plantlets on the toothed margins. Pendent, broadly tubular, greyish violet flowers, to 2cm (¾in) long, are produced in cyme-like panicles in winter. ↕ 1m (3ft), ↔ 30cm (12in). S.W. Madagascar. ❁ (min. 10°C/50°F)

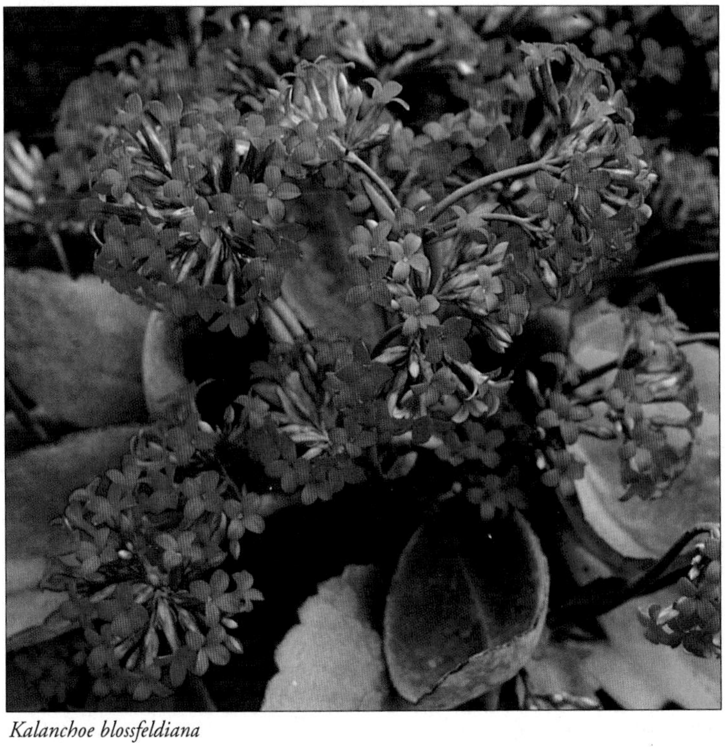

Kalanchoe blossfeldiana

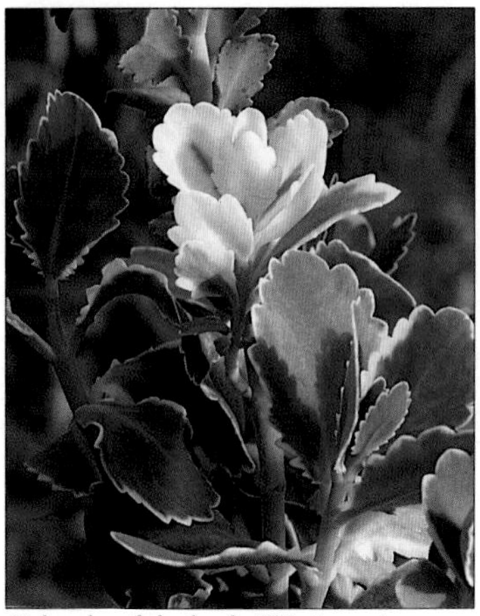
Kalanchoe fedtschenkoi 'Variegata'

K. delagoensis syn. *Bryophyllum tubiflorum, K. tubiflora.* Erect, sparsely branched, perennial succulent with almost cylindrical leaves, to 15cm (6in) long, grey-green, spotted reddish brown; leaves have notched tips that produce adventitious plantlets. In late winter and early spring, produces cyme-like panicles of pendent, tubular-bell-shaped, purple-grey to pale orange-yellow flowers, to 2cm (¾in) or more long. ↕1m (3ft) or more, ↔ 30cm (12in) or more. Madagascar. ❄ (min. 10°C/50°F)

K. eriophylla. Bushy, perennial succulent with slender stems covered with white hairs, except at the bases. Bears ovate-oblong, very thick, white-woolly, mid-green leaves, 3cm (1¼in) long. Young leaves may have red tips. In spring, bears narrowly bell-shaped, blue-violet flowers, 6cm (2½in) long, in more or less erect, corymb-like panicles. ↕↔ 20cm (8in). Madagascar. ❄ (min. 15°C/59°F)

K. fedtschenkoi. Upright to decumbent, perennial succulent bearing hairless, obovate to oblong, blue-green leaves, 1–6cm (½–2½in) long, each with 2–8 prominent teeth. Pendent, bell-shaped, dull red or purple flowers, to 2cm (¾in) long, are produced in small, loose, corymb-like panicles in summer. ↕50cm (20in), ↔ 25cm (10in). Madagascar. ❄ (min. 12°C/54°F). **'Variegata'** ▣ is bushy or semi-erect, with scalloped leaves margined creamy white and often flushed pink and mottled yellow; ↕↔ 50cm (20in).

K. grandiflora. Erect, perennial succulent with ovate to obovate, weakly scalloped, glaucous, mid-green leaves, 4–10cm (1½–4in) long. Tubular, bright yellow flowers, 1cm (½in) long, are borne in compact, cyme-like panicles in summer. ↕80cm (32in), ↔ 40 cm (16in). S. India. ❄ (min. 10°C/50°F)

K. jongmansii. Bushy, woody-stemmed, spreading, perennial succulent with oblong to linear-elliptic, mid-green leaves, to 4.5cm (1¾in) long, rounded above, with entire or partly scalloped margins. In early spring, produces cyme-like panicles of bell-shaped, more or less erect yellow flowers, 3cm (1¼in) long. ↕↔ 30cm (12in). Madagascar. ❄ (min. 12°C/54°F)

K. laciniata, syn. *K. schweinfurthii.* Erect, perennial succulent with pinnatisect, occasionally pinnate, hairless, mid-green leaves, to 20cm (8in) long, each with 3–5 entire or lobed, ovate to elliptic segments. In summer, bears corymb-like panicles of tubular, greenish white to pale orange flowers, 0.8–1.5cm (⅜–½in) long. ↕1.2m (4ft), ↔ 60cm (24in). Namibia to Ethiopia, S. India, Thailand. ❄ (min. 10°C/50°F)

K. manginii. Semi-erect then pendent, free-branching, perennial succulent with obovate to ovate-spoon-shaped, entire or notched, mid-green leaves, 3cm (1¼in) long, minutely hairy when young. In spring, bears few-flowered, cyme-like panicles of tubular, urn-shaped, bright red flowers, 2–3cm (¾–1¼in) or more long. ↕↔ 30cm (12in). Madagascar. ❄ (min. 12°C/54°F)

K. marmorata syn. *K. somaliensis.* Erect or decumbent, perennial succulent, branching from the base, bearing obovate, toothed, grey-frosted leaves, 6–20cm (2½–8in) long, with large, purple-brown marks. In spring, bears cyme-like panicles of narrowly tubular, erect, white, sometimes pink- or yellow-tinged flowers, 6–8cm (2½–3in) long. ↕↔ to 40cm (16in). Sudan to Zaire, Ethiopia, Somalia. ❄ (min. 12°C/54°F)

K. pinnata. Bushy, erect, perennial succulent with ovate, toothed, red-tinged, greyish green leaves, to 20cm (8in) long, which later produce adventitious, marginal plantlets. The lower leaves are simple, the upper ones pinnate, each with 3–5 scalloped, hairless leaflets. Pendent, tubular to bell-shaped, red-tinted, greenish white flowers, to 3.5cm (1½in) long, are produced in cyme-like panicles in late summer. ↕to 1m (3ft) or more, ↔ to 45cm (18in). Widespread in the tropics. ❄ (min. 12°C/54°F)

K. pubescens. Bushy, erect, perennial succulent with hairy stems that are sometimes glandular. Mid-green leaves, to 4cm (1½in) or more long, are ovate-lance-shaped, toothed, and minutely hairy. Cyme-like panicles of pendent, bell-shaped, triangular-lobed, yellow to red flowers, 5mm (¼in) long, are borne in spring. Small, adventitious plantlets form abundantly in the flower clusters as the flowers fade. ↕1m (3ft.), ↔ 45cm (18in). N., C., and E. Madagascar. ❄ (min. 12°C/54°F)

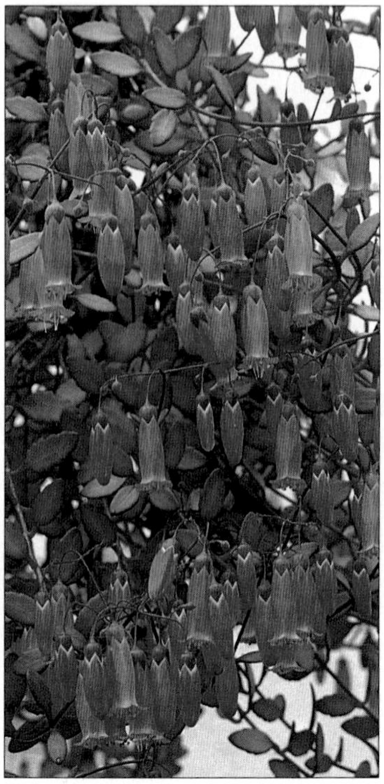
Kalanchoe 'Tessa'

K. pumila 🏆 Semi-pendent, spreading, succulent subshrub with ovate to obovate, chalky, white-frosted, mid-green leaves, to 3.5cm (1½in) long, narrowing towards the bases, and with toothed margins at the tips. Urn-shaped flowers, 1cm (½in) long, pink with purple lines, are borne in few-flowered, corymb-like panicles in spring. ↕20cm (8in), ↔ to 45cm (18in). Madagascar. ❄ (min. 12°C/54°F)

K. schweinfurthii see *K. laciniata.*

K. somaliensis see *K. marmorata.*

***K.* 'Tessa'** ▣🏆 Pendent, perennial succulent bearing narrowly oval, mid-green leaves, 3cm (1¼in) long, with red margins. In late winter and early spring, produces cyme-like panicles of pendent, tubular, orange-red flowers, 2cm (¾in) long. ↕30cm (12in), ↔ 60cm (24in). ❄ (min. 12°C/54°F)

K. thyrsiflora. Bushy, white-frosted, perennial succulent, increasing by offsets. It is densely covered with oval to inversely lance-shaped, red-margined, pale green leaves, 10–15cm (4–6in) long, with blunt, rounded tips and leaf pairs united at the bases. In spring, bears cyme-like panicles of erect to spreading, tubular to urn-shaped, fragrant yellow flowers, 1–2cm (½–¾in) long. ↕60cm (24in), ↔ 30cm (12in). South Africa (Northern Cape, Western Cape, Eastern Cape). ❄ (min. 12°C/54°F)

K. tomentosa 🏆 Erect, bushy, densely white-felted, perennial succulent with thick, oblong, entire grey leaves, 2–9cm (¾–3½in) long, coarsely toothed at the tips, grooved above, and often finely margined reddish brown with furry silver hairs. Bell-shaped, green-yellow flowers, 1.5cm (½in) long, with red glandular hairs and lobes tinged purple, are borne in cyme-like panicles in early spring. ↕to 1m (3ft), ↔ 20cm (8in). Madagascar. ❄ (min. 12°C/54°F)

K. tubiflora see *K. delagoensis.*

K. uniflora syn. *Bryophyllum uniflorum.* Prostrate, perennial succulent with rounded, mid-green leaves, 4–15mm (⅛–½in) long, convex on both sides, and with a few uneven, rounded teeth. Pendent, urn-shaped, red to purple flowers, 1–2cm (½–¾in) long, are borne in few-flowered, corymb-like panicles in summer. ↕15cm (6in), ↔ 60cm (24in). Madagascar. ❄ (min. 10°C/50°F)

***K.* 'Wendy'** ▣🏆 Pendent to semi-erect, perennial succulent with ovate to oblong-ovate, slightly scalloped, glossy, mid-green leaves, to 7cm (3in) long. Corymb-like panicles of bell-shaped, orange- to yellow-tipped, purple-red flowers, 3cm (1¼in) long, are borne in late winter and early spring. ↕↔ 30cm (12in). ❄ (min. 10°C/50°F)

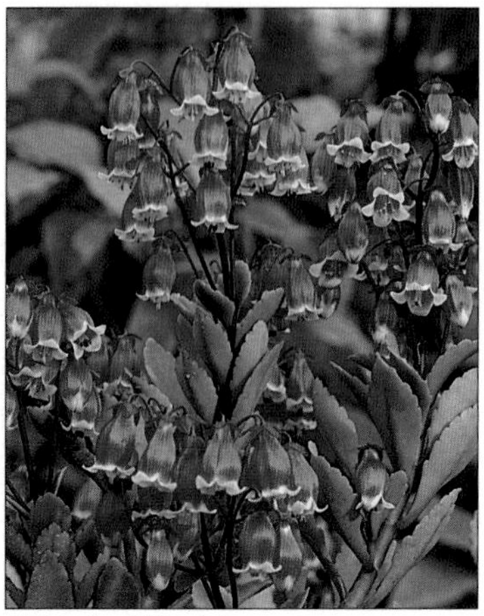
Kalanchoe 'Wendy'

KALMIA

ERICACEAE

Genus of 7 species of evergreen shrubs found in woodland, swamps, and meadows in North America and Cuba. They have leathery leaves, which may be alternate, in opposite pairs, or in whorls, and showy, bowl-, cup-, or saucer-shaped flowers borne in corymbs or racemes. They are useful for a shrub border or woodland garden; the dwarf species and cultivars are suitable for a peat or heather garden. All parts may cause severe discomfort if ingested.

- **HARDINESS** Fully hardy.
- **CULTIVATION** Grow in moist, humus-rich, acid soil in partial shade, or in sun where soils remain reliably moist. Mulch annually in spring with leaf mould or pine needles. Pruning group 8. *K. angustifolia* tolerates hard pruning; renovate all other species over several seasons.
- **PROPAGATION** Sow seed at 6–12°C (43–54°F) in spring. Take greenwood cuttings in late spring and semi-ripe cuttings in midsummer. Layer in late summer.
- **PESTS AND DISEASES** Trouble free.

K. angustifolia ▣ (Sheep laurel). Mound-forming shrub with oblong to elliptic, dark green leaves, to 6cm (2½in) long, in opposite pairs or whorls of 3. Small, bowl- or cup-shaped, pale to deep red, occasionally white flowers, to 1cm (½in) across, are produced in corymbs, 5cm (2in) across, in early summer. ↕60cm (24in), ↔ 1.5m (5ft). E. North America. ❄❄❄. **f. *rubra*** has deep red flowers.

K. latifolia ▣🏆 (Calico bush, Mountain laurel). Dense, bushy shrub with alternate, oval to elliptic-lance-shaped, glossy, dark green leaves, to 12cm (5in) long. From late spring to midsummer, large corymbs, 8–10cm (3–4in) or more across, of bowl- or cup-shaped, pale to deep pink, or occasionally white flowers, 2–2.5cm (¾–1in) across, are produced from distinctively crimped, often dark pink or red buds. May take several years to

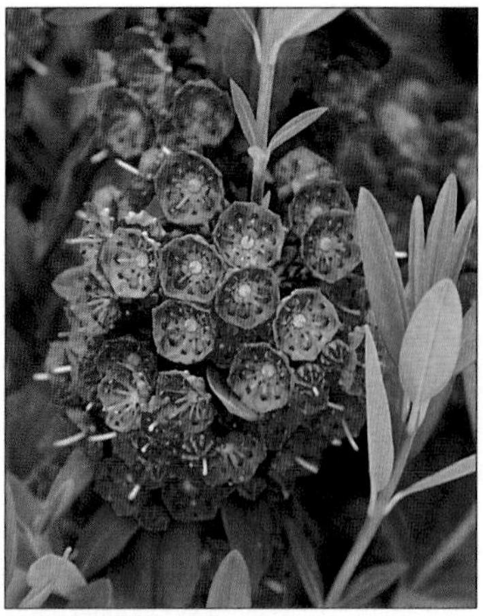
Kalmia angustifolia

K

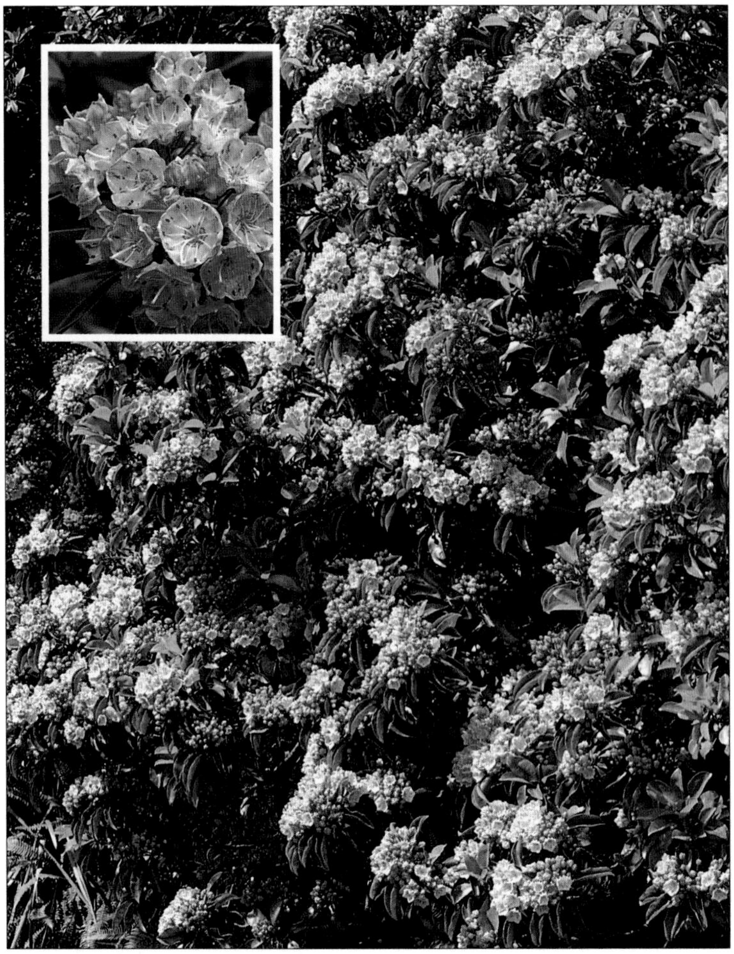

Kalmia latifolia (inset: flower detail)

recover from hard pruning. ↕↔ 3m (10ft). E. USA. ❄❄❄. **'Bullseye'** has white flowers heavily banded red-purple within. **'Carousel'** has white flowers conspicuously banded red and intricately patterned red or white within. **'Clementine Churchill'** ▣ has rich pink flowers opening from dark pink buds. **'Elf'** is compact, with small leaves, 3cm (1¼in) long, and white flowers opening from pale pink buds; ↕↔ 1m (3ft). **'Freckles'** has pale pink flowers ringed with small, red-purple spots just inside the rim. **f. *fuscata*** ▣ has a conspicuous deep maroon, purple, or cinnamon ring inside each of the white flowers. **f. *myrtifolia*** is dense, with small leaves, to 5cm (2in) long, and pale pink flowers; ↕↔ 1.2m (4ft) or more. **'Nipmuck'** has pale green leaves and nearly white flowers opening from dark red buds. **'Olympic Fire'** has wavy-margined leaves and large pink flowers, 2.5cm (1in) across, opening from red buds. **'Ostbo Red'** ▣♀ has pale pink flowers opening from bright red buds. **'Shooting Star'** has unusual white flowers, each deeply cut into 5 lobes that reflex after the blooms open. **'Silver Dollar'** has very large white flowers, to 4cm (1½in) long.

K. microphylla, syn. *K. polifolia* var. *microphylla* (Western laurel). Sparsely branched, dwarf shrub with opposite, leathery, flat, ovate to oval leaves, 0.6–3.5cm (¼–1½in) long. Bears terminal racemes of saucer-shaped, pink to rose-purple flowers, to 3cm (1¼in) across, in late spring and early summer. ↕ to 15cm (6in), occasionally

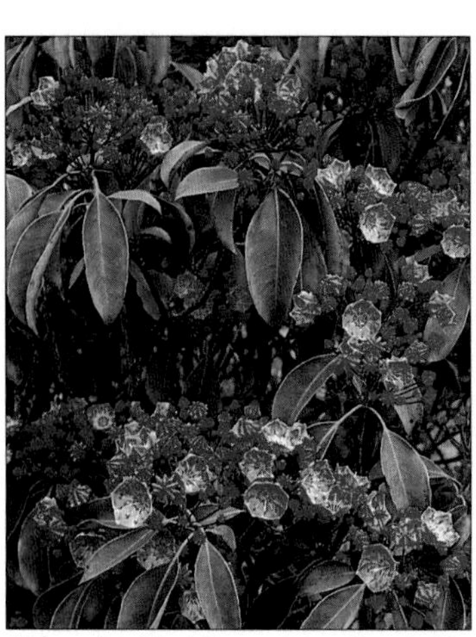

Kalmia latifolia 'Clementine Churchill'

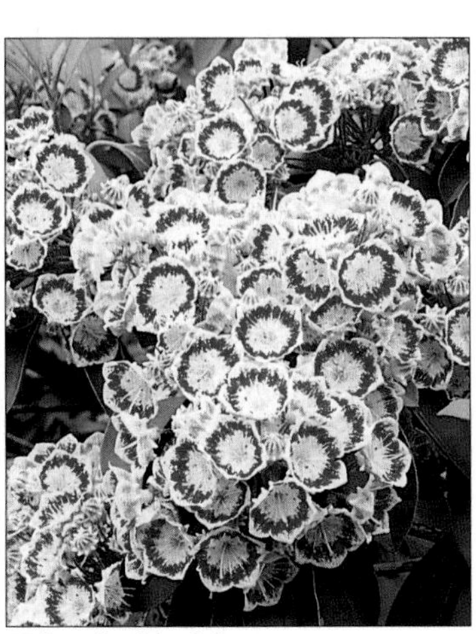

Kalmia latifolia f. *fuscata*

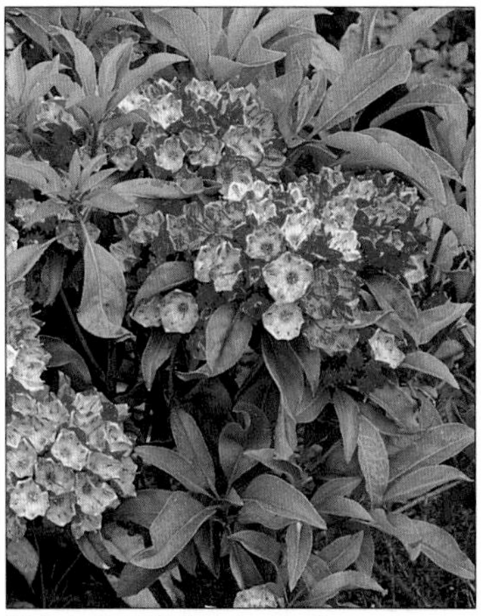

Kalmia latifolia 'Ostbo Red'

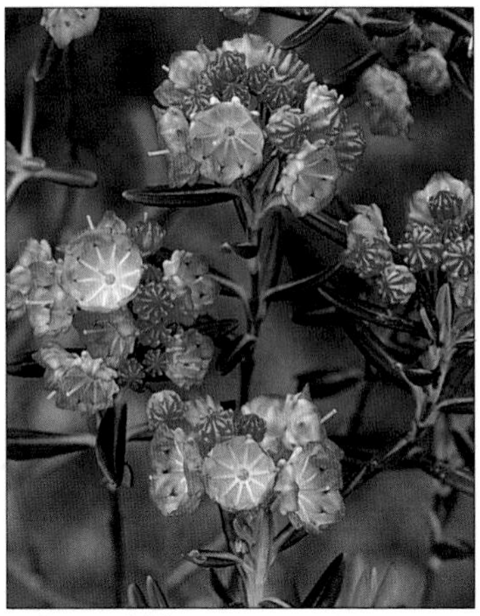

Kalmia polifolia

to 60cm (24in) in very wet, boggy conditions, ↔ 15–30cm (6–12in). USA (Alaska to California). ❄❄❄

K. polifolia ▣ (Eastern bog laurel). Small, sparsely branched shrub with linear to oblong, glossy, dark green leaves, to 4cm (1½in) long, in opposite pairs or whorls of 3, with rolled-back margins and glandular hairs beneath. Bears racemes, 2.5–4cm (1–1½in) across, of up to 12 saucer-shaped, purple-pink flowers, 1–2cm (½–¾in) across, in mid- and late spring. Requires moist soil. ↕ 60cm (24in), ↔ 90cm (36in). Canada, N.E. USA. ❄❄❄. **var. *microphylla*** see *K. microphylla*.

KALMIOPSIS

ERICACEAE

Genus of one species of evergreen shrub from Oregon, USA, where it grows on rocky ledges on mountain cliffs. It has simple leaves, arranged alternately, and is cultivated for its terminal racemes of small, cup-shaped flowers. Suitable for a cool position in a peat garden.

- **HARDINESS** Fully hardy.
- **CULTIVATION** Grow in moist but well-drained, humus-rich, lime-free soil in full sun (provided that the soil remains cool and moist) or in partial shade. Pruning group 8.
- **PROPAGATION** Sow seed at 6–12°C (43–54°F) in spring, or take semi-ripe cuttings in summer.
- **PESTS AND DISEASES** Trouble free.

K. leachiana ♀ Dwarf, evergreen shrub with oval to obovate, bright deep green leaves, to 3cm (1¼in) long, glandular

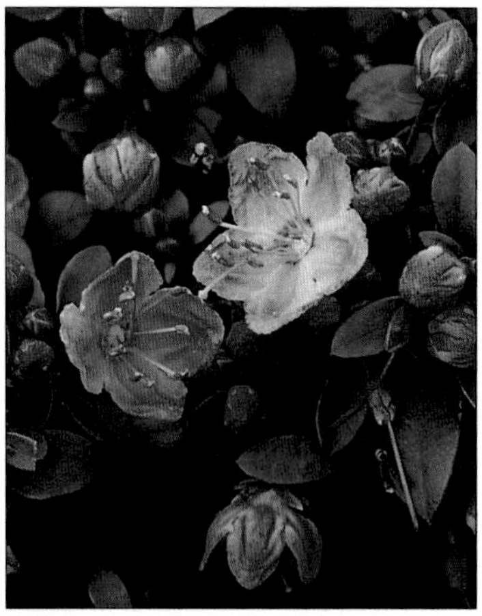

Kalmiopsis leachiana 'La Piniec'

beneath. Cup-shaped, rose-red to purple-pink flowers, to 2cm (¾in) across, are produced in terminal racemes, 2.5–5cm (1–2in) long, from early to late spring. ↕↔ 30cm (12in). USA (Oregon). ❄❄❄. **'La Piniec'** ▣ has glossy, dark green leaves, to 2cm (¾in) long. **'Umpqua Valley'** is compact, vigorous, and free-flowering.

KALOPANAX

ARALIACEAE

Genus of one species of deciduous tree from forest in E. Asia. It has a spreading habit and large, variably shaped, palmately lobed leaves, which are arranged alternately and vary from hairless to very hairy beneath. Large, terminal, umbel-like panicles of usually white, 4- or 5-petalled flowers, are borne in late summer, and are followed by spherical, blue-black fruit. It is a fine specimen tree.

- **HARDINESS** Fully hardy, but young growth may be damaged by late frosts.
- **CULTIVATION** Grow in fertile, moist but well-drained soil in full sun or partial shade, preferably sheltered by other trees and shrubs. Pruning group 1.
- **PROPAGATION** Sow seed in containers in a cold frame in autumn, or take greenwood cuttings in early summer.
- **PESTS AND DISEASES** Trouble free.

K. pictus see *K. septemlobus*.
K. ricinifolius see *K. septemlobus*.
K. septemlobus ▣♀ syn. *Acanthopanax ricinifolius, Eleutherococcus pictus, Kalopanax pictus, K. ricinifolius*. Spreading, deciduous tree with spines

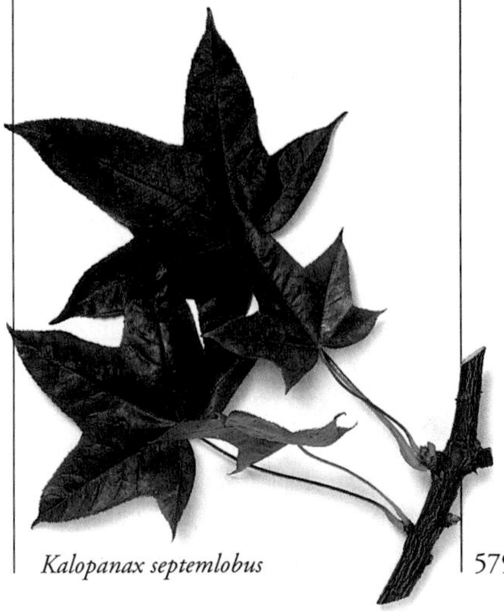

Kalopanax septemlobus

on the trunk and shoots, and variably shaped, shallowly to deeply 5- to 7-lobed, dark green leaves, to 35cm (14in) or more across, which vary from hairless to very hairy beneath. Large, umbel-like panicles, 20–30cm (8–12in) long, of small, 4- or 5-petalled white flowers, 2mm (1/16in) across, are borne in late summer, followed by spherical, blue-black fruit, 4mm (1/8in) across. ↕↔ 10m (30ft). China, Korea, Russia (S. Kurile Islands, Sakhalin), Japan (Ryukyu Islands). ❄❄❄. **var. *magnificus*** has ovate leaves that are shallowly lobed and densely hairy on the lower leaf sides; W. China. **var. *maximowiczii*** is similar to var. *magnificus*, but has deeply lobed, lance-shaped leaves.

▷ **Kangaroo paw** see *Anigozanthos*
 Black see *Macropidia fuliginosa*
 Green see *Anigozanthos viridis*
 Little see *Anigozanthos bicolor*
 Mangles' see *Anigozanthos manglesii*
 Yellow see *Anigozanthos pulcherrimus*
▷ **Kangaroo thorn** see *Acacia paradoxa*
▷ **Kangaroo vine** see *Cissus antarctica*
▷ **Kansas feather** see *Liatris pycnostachya*
▷ **Kapok** see *Ceiba pentandra*
▷ **Karaka** see *Corynocarpus laevigatus*
▷ **Karo** see *Pittosporum crassifolium*
▷ **Kassod tree** see *Senna siamea*
▷ **Katsura tree** see *Cercidiphyllum japonicum*
▷ **Kawaka** see *Libocedrus plumosa*

KELSEYA

ROSACEAE

Genus of one species of evergreen, cushion-forming subshrub found in rock crevices and scree in the Rocky Mountains, USA. Cultivated for its neat rosettes of silvery green foliage, it also has solitary, star-shaped flowers, produced in early summer. It resents winter wet, and is best grown in an alpine house, although it may be grown outdoors in a scree bed, trough, or vertical rock crevice.
• **HARDINESS** Fully hardy.
• **CULTIVATION** In an alpine house, grow in a mix of 3 parts grit and 1 part each of loam and leaf mould. Outdoors, grow in very gritty, humus-rich, moist but sharply drained, preferably alkaline soil, in full sun; provide overhead protection from rain in winter.
• **PROPAGATION** Sow seed in containers in an open frame in autumn, or take soft-tip cuttings in spring.
• **PESTS AND DISEASES** Susceptible to aphids and red spider mites under glass, and to grey mould (*Botrytis*) in damp conditions.

K. uniflora. Slow-growing, cushion-forming subshrub with tight rosettes of overlapping, ovate, leathery, dark green leaves, to 3mm (1/8in) long, clothed in silky silver hairs. Solitary, stemless, star-shaped, white or pink-flushed flowers, 8mm (3/8in) across, are produced from pink buds just above the leaf rosettes in early summer. Does not always flower freely. ↕ to 8cm (3in), ↔ to 15cm (6in). USA (Rocky Mountains). ❄❄❄

▷ **Kenaf** see *Hibiscus cannabinus*

KENNEDIA *syn.* KENNEDYA

Coral pea

LEGUMINOSAE/PAPILIONACEAE

Genus of 16 species of herbaceous and woody-stemmed climbing and trailing perennials from a variety of habitats, including rainforest, open forest, shrubland, heathland, and semi-desert, in Australia and New Guinea. They are grown for their long-keeled, pea-like flowers, produced singly, in pairs, umbels, or racemes in the leaf axils. The leaves, arranged alternately, each have 3 leaflets and a pair of distinctive stipules at the base of the stalk. In frost-prone areas, grow in a cool or temperate greenhouse. In milder regions, train over a pergola or arch. The trailers are also good as ground cover on a bank or between shrubs.
• **HARDINESS** Half hardy to frost tender.
• **CULTIVATION** Under glass, grow in loam-based potting compost (JI No.2) with added sharp sand, in bright filtered light. In growth, water moderately and apply a balanced liquid fertilizer monthly; water sparingly in winter. Provide support for the climbing stems. Outdoors, grow in fertile, moist, but well-drained soil in partial shade. Pruning group 12, after flowering or in late winter.
• **PROPAGATION** Sow seed at 18–21°C (64–70°F) in spring, ideally after soaking in freshly boiled water for 12 hours.
• **PESTS AND DISEASES** Prone to red spider mites and whiteflies under glass.

K. coccinea (Common coral vine). Woody-stemmed, twining climber or trailer, with leaves 3–10cm (1¼–4in) long, each divided into 3 broadly oblong to linear-wedge-shaped, occasionally lobed, slightly leathery, deep green leaflets. From spring to early summer, produces axillary and terminal, umbel-like racemes, 10cm (4in) long, of 4–20 coral-red flowers, 1.5cm (½in) wide, the standard petals marked with yellow and purple-margined at the bases, opening from buds covered with soft red hairs. Tolerates coastal sites and alkaline soil. ↕ 2m (6ft). Australia (Western Australia). ❁ (min. 5–7°C/41–45°F)
K. macrophylla. Woody-stemmed, twining climber or trailer with leaves to 15cm (6in) long, each divided into 3 broadly obovate–rounded, dark green leaflets, mid-green beneath and heart-shaped at the bases. In summer, pea-like, reddish brown or red flowers, to 2cm (1in) long, the standard petals reflexed and boldly splashed yellow, are produced in loose axillary racemes, 8–13cm (3–5in) or more long. Thrives in poor sandy soil; tolerates coastal sites. ↕ to 5m (15ft). Australia (Western Australia). ❄
K. nigricans (Black coral pea). Vigorous, woody, twining climber with leaves 5–15cm (2–6in) long, each divided into 3 ovate, leathery, rich green leaflets, heart-shaped at the bases. From late winter to late spring or early summer, produces one-sided, axillary racemes, 15cm (6in) long, of elongated, velvety, purple-black flowers, to 3cm (1¼in) long, the standard petals reflexed and boldly splashed yellow. Thrives in poor sandy soil; tolerates coastal sites.

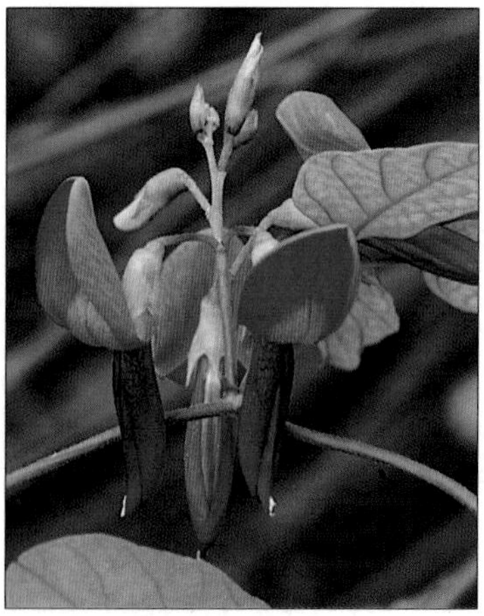

Kennedia rubicunda

↕ 4–6m (12–20ft). Australia (Western Australia). ❁ (min. 5–7°C/41–45°F)
K. prostrata (Running postman, Scarlet runner). Prostrate to mat-forming trailer, with numerous, often sparsely branched, densely softly hairy stems radiating from a woody rootstock. The leaves, to 10cm (4in) long, are each composed of 3 ovate-rounded to rounded, wavy-margined, bright green leaflets. From spring to summer, sometimes also in autumn, scarlet flowers, to 2.5cm (1in) long, the standard petals each with a small, greenish yellow mark at the base, are borne in loose racemes, to 8cm (3in) long. ↔ to 1.5m (5ft). Australia (Western Australia). ❁ (min. 5°C/41°F)
K. rubicunda ▣ (Dusky coral pea). Twining climber or mat-forming perennial with slender, hairy stems, becoming dense and tangled with age. The leaves, to 16cm (6in) long, are each composed of 3 ovate, hairy, mid-green leaflets. From spring to summer, dark red flowers, 3–4cm (1¼–1½in) long, with pointed keel petals and swept-back standards marked pale tan at the bases, are produced in loose, axillary racemes, to 8cm (3in) long. ↕ to 3m (10ft) or more. Australia (New South Wales, Victoria). ❁ (min. 5–7°C/41–45°F)

▷ ***Kennedya*** see *Kennedia*
▷ ***Kentia acuminata*** see *Carpentaria acuminata*
▷ ***Kentia canterburyana*** see *Hedyscepe canterburyana*
▷ ***Kentia forsteriana*** see *Howea forsteriana*
▷ ***Kentia joannis*** see *Veitchia joannis*
▷ **Kerosene bush** see *Ozothamnus ledifolius*

KERRIA

Jew's mantle

ROSACEAE

Genus of one species of deciduous shrub, found in thickets and woodland in China and Japan. It has alternate, simple leaves, and solitary, cup- or saucer-shaped yellow flowers. Kerrias are grown for their foliage and flowers, and are suitable for a shrub border or an open position in a woodland garden.
• **HARDINESS** Fully hardy.
• **CULTIVATION** Grow in fertile, well-drained soil in full sun or partial shade. Pruning group 3.
• **PROPAGATION** Take greenwood cuttings in summer. Divide in autumn.
• **PESTS AND DISEASES** Trouble free.

K. japonica. Suckering shrub with arching green shoots and ovate, pointed, sharply toothed, bright green leaves, to 10cm (4in) long. In mid- and late spring, produces solitary, single or double, golden yellow flowers, 3–5cm (1¼–2in) across. ↕ 2m (6ft), ↔ 2.5m (8ft). China, Japan. ❄❄❄. **'Golden Guinea'** ▣ 🏆 has very large, single flowers, 5–6cm (2–2½in) across. **'Picta'**, syn. 'Variegata', has grey-green leaves margined creamy white; ↕ 1.5m (5ft), ↔ 2m (6ft). **'Pleniflora'** 🏆 is very vigorous and upright, with large, pompon-like, double flowers, 3cm (1¼in) across; ↕↔ 3m (10ft). **'Variegata'** see 'Picta'.

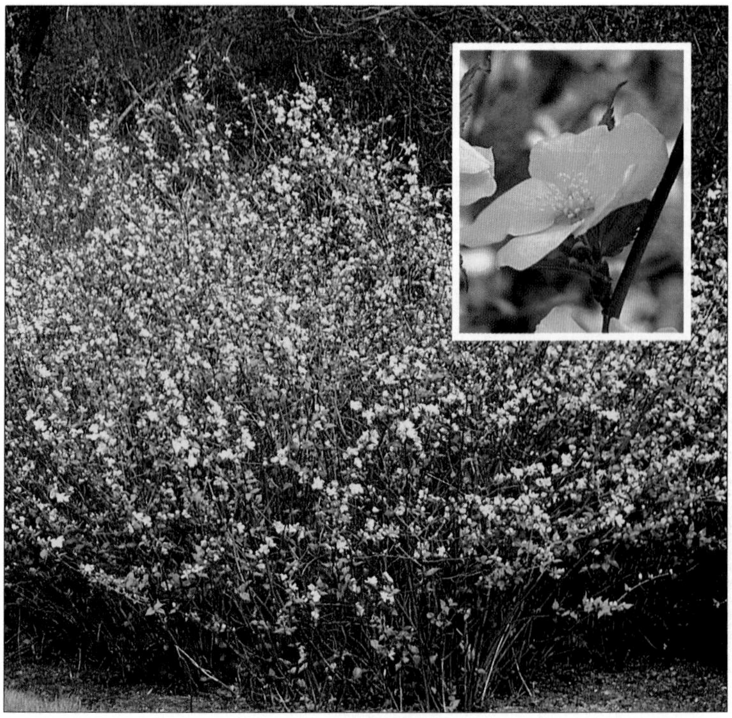

Kerria japonica 'Golden Guinea' (inset: flower detail)

KIGELIA

Sausage tree

BIGNONIACEAE

Genus of one species of variable, evergreen tree from tropical woodland and more open areas in Africa. It has large, pinnate leaves, borne in opposite pairs, and loose, pendent panicles, 1–2m (3–6ft) long, of open, trumpet-shaped flowers, followed by long, woody pods. Where temperatures drop below 16°C (61°F), grow in a warm greenhouse, mainly for its foliage, although flowers may form on specimens reaching 3m (10ft) or more high. In tropical areas, it is an attractive specimen or shade tree.

- **HARDINESS** Frost tender.
- **CULTIVATION** Under glass, grow in loam-based potting compost (JI No.3) in full light but screened from the hottest summer sun, at least during the early years. During the growing season, water moderately and apply a balanced liquid fertilizer monthly; water sparingly in winter. Outdoors, grow in fertile, well-drained soil in full sun. Pruning group 1; plants under glass need restrictive pruning in late winter or after flowering.
- **PROPAGATION** Sow seed at 21–23°C (70–73°F) in spring.
- **PESTS AND DISEASES** Red spider mites, whiteflies, and mealybugs may be troublesome under glass.

K. pinnata ▣ ♀ Rounded to broadly columnar, usually freely branching tree with robust stems. Bears pinnate leaves, to 50cm (20in) long, each composed of 7–11 oblong to obovate, leathery, mid- to deep green leaflets, sometimes notched at the tips. Loose, pendent panicles of bat-pollinated flowers, each 10cm (4in) across, are produced in summer. Yellowish green in bud, they open to rich brownish red at night, when they have an unpleasant smell that is attractive to bats. The cylindrical, woody fruit, to 35–60cm (14–24in) or more long, may weigh 5–7kg (11–15lb), and are pale brown when ripe. They remain on the thickened flowering stems for many months. ↕ 15m (50ft) or more, ↔ 5–10m (15–30ft). Tropical Africa. ❀ (min. 16°C/61°F)

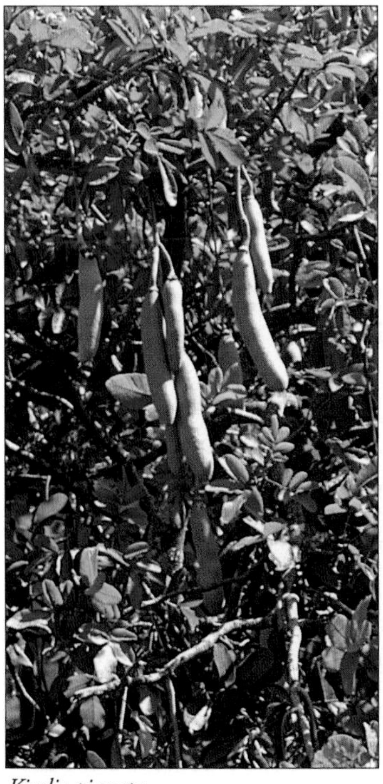

Kigelia pinnata

▷ **Kilmarnock willow** see *Salix caprea* 'Kilmarnock'
▷ **Kindling bark, Broad-leaved** see *Eucalyptus dalrympleana*
▷ **Kingcup** see *Caltha, C. palustris*
▷ **King protea** see *Protea cynaroides*
▷ **King's crown** see *Justicia carnea*
▷ **King's mantle** see *Thunbergia erecta*
▷ **King's spear** see *Asphodeline lutea*
▷ **Kinnikinnick** see *Arctostaphylos uva-ursi*

KIRENGESHOMA

HYDRANGEACEAE

Genus of 2 species of clump-forming perennials, with short rhizomes, from woodland in Korea and Japan. They have broadly tubular, waxy, pale or bright yellow flowers, borne on slender stalks in nodding, terminal cymes above pairs of elegant, sycamore-like leaves. They are suitable for a shady border, peat bed, or woodland garden.

- **HARDINESS** Fully hardy.
- **CULTIVATION** Grow in moist, lime-free soil, enriched with leaf mould, in partial shade sheltered from wind.
- **PROPAGATION** Sow seed in containers in a cold frame as soon as ripe or in spring (germination may be slow and erratic). Divide as growth begins in spring, taking care not to damage tender young shoots.
- **PESTS AND DISEASES** Slugs and snails may attack young growth and leaves.

K. palmata ▣ ♀ Clump-forming perennial with short rhizomes and arching, smooth, reddish purple stems. These bear broadly ovate, palmately lobed, slightly hairy, pale green leaves, 10–20cm (4–8in) long, becoming smaller, simple, and almost stalkless towards the stem tips. Nodding, terminal cymes of 3 broadly tubular, pale yellow flowers, to 3.5cm (1½in) long, with slightly recurved lobes and fleshy petals that overlap at the bases, are borne in late summer and early autumn. ↕ 60–120cm (24–48in), ↔ 75cm (30in). Japan. ❄❄❄

▷ **Kiss-me-over-the-garden-gate** see *Persicaria orientale*

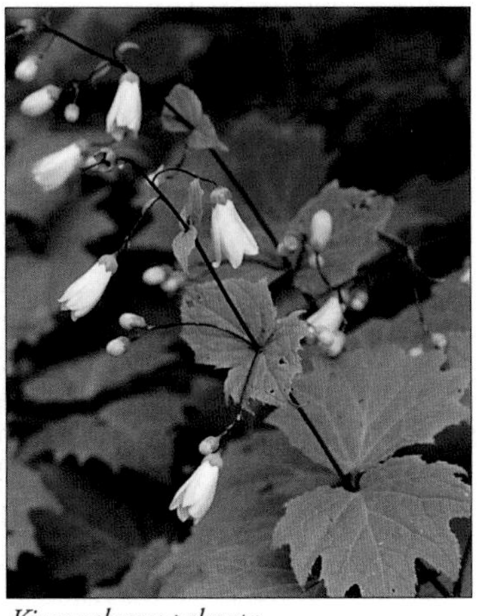

Kirengeshoma palmata

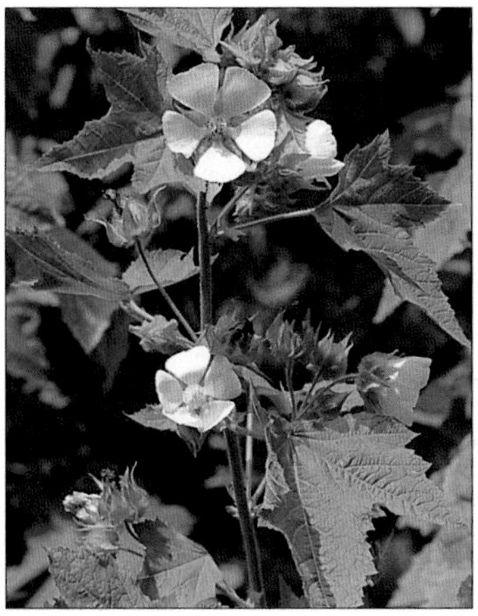

Kitaibela vitifolia

KITAIBELA syn. KITAIBELIA

MALVACEAE

Genus of two species of imposing, often short-lived herbaceous perennials found in damp meadows and scrub from Slovenia to Macedonia. They have palmately lobed, vine-like leaves and showy, mallow-like flowers, produced singly or in axillary cymes. They are suitable for a wild or meadow garden.

- **HARDINESS** Fully hardy.
- **CULTIVATION** Grow in deep, moderately fertile, moist but well-drained soil in full sun or partial shade.
- **PROPAGATION** Sow seed in containers in a cold frame in spring or autumn. Root basal or softwood cuttings in spring.
- **PESTS AND DISEASES** Trouble free.

K. vitifolia ▣ Clump-forming, woody-based, softly white-hairy perennial with erect stems bearing 5- to 7-lobed, coarsely toothed leaves, to 17cm (7in) long. Mallow-like, open cup-shaped, 5-petalled, white to rose-red flowers, 4.5cm (1¾in) across, are produced singly or in few-flowered, axillary cymes from midsummer to early autumn. ↕ to 2.5m (8ft), ↔ 5m (15ft). Slovenia to Macedonia. ❄❄❄

▷ ***Kitaibelia*** see *Kitaibela*
▷ **Kiwi fruit** see *Actinidia deliciosa*
▷ **Klapperbos** see *Nymania capensis*

KLEINIA

ASTERACEAE/COMPOSITAE

Genus of 40 species of succulent perennials, closely related to *Senecio,* from lowlands and mountains in tropical Africa, N.W. Africa, the Canary Islands, southern Africa, Madagascar, and the Arabian Peninsula. Many species have tuberous roots and prostrate to upright, cylindrical to angular stems, with flat or cylindrical, succulent, usually entire leaves. Colourful, thistle-like flowerheads appear singly or in branched, terminal or axillary corymbs in summer. Where temperatures drop below 10°C (50°F), grow as houseplants or in a warm greenhouse. In warmer climates, grow in a desert garden.

- **HARDINESS** Frost tender.
- **CULTIVATION** Under glass, grow in a mix of 2 parts leaf mould and 1 part each loam and gritty sand, in full light. In growth, water moderately and apply a balanced liquid fertilizer 2 or 3 times. Keep dry when dormant. Outdoors, grow in sharply drained, gritty, humus-rich soil in full sun. See also pp.48–49.
- **PROPAGATION** Sow seed at 20°C (68°F), or take cuttings, in spring or summer.
- **PESTS AND DISEASES** Susceptible to scale insects.

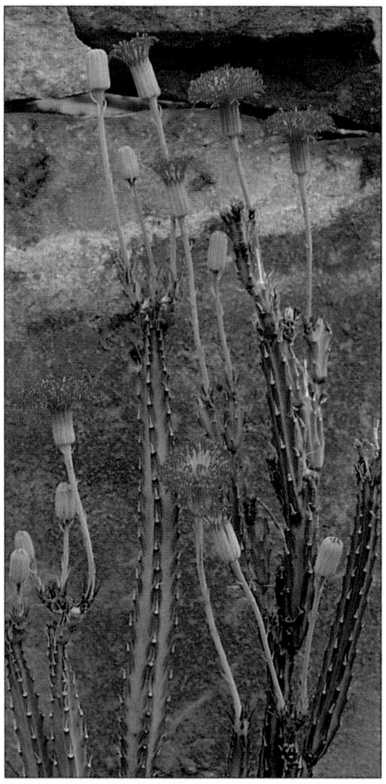

Kleinia stapeliiformis

K. repens see *Senecio serpens.*
K. rowleyana see *Senecio rowleyanus.*
K. stapeliiformis ▣ syn. *Senecio stapeliiformis.* Erect succulent branching from the base, with new shoots growing underground at first. Thick, fleshy, 5- to 7-angled branches, glaucous green with purple staining, bear very slender, oblong, thread-like, fleshy, grey-green leaves, often flushed purple with dark green lines along their lengths. The leaves, 5mm (¼in) long, become thorny as they age. Solitary, thistle-like, red or orange-red flowerheads, to 4cm (1½in) long, are produced in summer. ↕↔ 20–30cm (8–12in). E. South Africa (KwaZulu/Natal). ❀ (min. 10°C/50°F)

▷ **Knapweed** see *Centaurea*

KNAUTIA

DIPSACACEAE

Genus of 40 or more species of scabious-like annuals and perennials from limestone grassland, scrub, and woodland in Europe, Caucasus, Russia (Siberia), and N. Africa. They have overwintering rosettes of simple to pinnatifid basal leaves, and opposite pairs of stem leaves, which are usually deeply pinnatifid, although the uppermost leaves may be simple. Tall stems bear cup-shaped involucres of bracts, with bristly hairs or teeth, surrounding dense, bluish lilac or reddish purple flowerheads. The flowers have unequally lobed corollas and stamens protruding in "pincushion" style. They are attractive to bees. Grow in a herbaceous border, cottage garden, or wild garden.

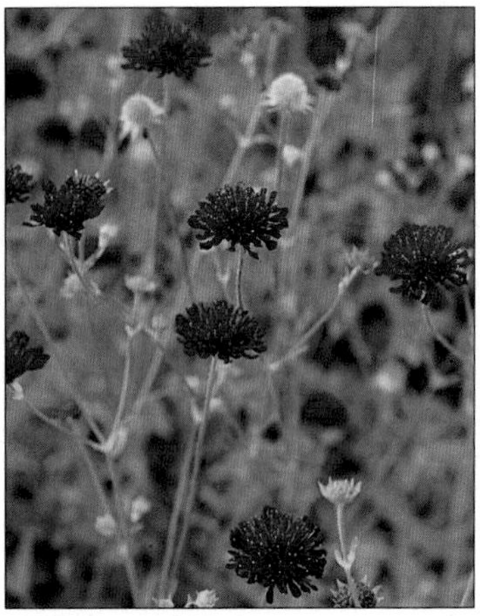
Knautia macedonica

- **HARDINESS** Fully hardy.
- **CULTIVATION** Grow in moderately fertile, well-drained, preferably alkaline soil in full sun.
- **PROPAGATION** Sow seed in containers in a cold frame in spring, or take basal cuttings in spring.
- **PESTS AND DISEASES** Prone to aphids.

K. arvensis, syn. *Scabiosa arvensis* (Field scabious). Clump-forming, deeply tap-rooted perennial with erect but often lax, hairless stems, the lower parts bristly. Produces simple to pinnatifid, hairy, dull green leaves, 5–25cm (2–10in) long, simple or pinnatifid higher up the stem. Flat-topped, bluish lilac flowerheads, 3–4cm (1¼–1½in) across, with softly bristly, involucral bracts, are borne from midsummer to early autumn. ↕ to 1.5m (5ft), ↔ 30cm (12in). Europe, Caucasus, Iran to C. Asia, Russia (Siberia). ❄❄❄
K. macedonica ■ syn. *Scabiosa rumelica.* Clump-forming perennial with slender, branched stems, pinnatifid basal leaves, 8cm (3in) long, each with a large, terminal lobe, and simple or pinnatifid stem leaves, 2–15cm (¾–6in) long. Numerous long-lasting, purple-red flowerheads, 1.5–3cm (½–1¼in) across, with softly bristly, involucral bracts, are produced in mid- and late summer. ↕ 60–80cm (24–32in), ↔ 45cm (18in). C. Balkans into Romania. ❄❄❄

KNIGHTIA

PROTEACEAE

Genus of 3 species of evergreen trees or shrubs from lowland to low mountain forest, one from New Zealand, 2 from New Caledonia. The leathery, entire or toothed leaves are arranged alternately and vary in shape with age: young plants have long, thin leaves; adults have shorter, thicker ones. Tubular flowers, with 4 petal-like tepals that roll up like springs, are borne in dense racemes. In frost-prone areas, grow in a cool or temperate greenhouse. In milder climates, use as a specimen tree.

- **HARDINESS** Frost tender; may survive short periods around 0°C (32°F).
- **CULTIVATION** Under glass, grow in loam-based potting compost (JI No.2) in full light, with shade from hot sun and with good ventilation. During the growing season, water moderately and apply a balanced liquid fertilizer every month; water sparingly in winter. Outdoors, grow in fertile, well-drained, neutral to acid soil, in full sun or partial shade, with shelter from cold winds. Pruning group 1.
- **PROPAGATION** Sow seed at 13–16°C (55–61°F) in spring. Root semi-ripe cuttings with bottom heat in summer (rooting may be slow).
- **PESTS AND DISEASES** Red spider mites may be a problem under glass.

K. excelsa ♀ (New Zealand honeysuckle, Rewarewa). Tall, usually columnar tree, with many short, lateral branches. Adult leaves are narrowly oblong to obovate-oblong, 10–15cm (4–6in) long, blunt-toothed and stiff. From spring to summer, produces few to many tubular red flowers, 2.5–4cm (1–1½in) long, in racemes 10cm (4in) long, covered with short, velvety, red-brown hairs, followed by narrow seed pods, which split open down one side only. ↕ to 30m (100ft), ↔ 7–10m (22–30ft). New Zealand. ❀ (min. 3–7°C/37–45°F)

KNIPHOFIA

Red hot poker, Torch lily

ASPHODELACEAE/LILIACEAE

Genus of about 70 species of evergreen or deciduous, rhizomatous perennials from mountainous or upland areas, often in moist places in rough grass or along streamsides, in southern and tropical Africa. Most are clump-forming, with arching, tufted, linear to strap-shaped, light to mid-green or blue-green leaves. In deciduous species and hybrids these leaves are usually thin, grass-like, and 10–100cm (4–39in) long; in evergreens, they are broader, keeled or strap-shaped, and to 1.5m (5ft) long. Erect, usually dense, spike-like racemes, 5–40cm (2–16in) long, of numerous pendent, occasionally erect, tubular or cylindrical flowers, 0.3–5cm (⅛–2in) long, are borne well above the foliage. They are attractive to bees. The flowers are red, orange, yellow, white, or greenish white; some open red, then turn to yellow, bearing striking, 2-coloured racemes. Numerous cultivars have been raised, ranging in size from dwarf plants, 50cm (20in) high, to tall plants, to 1.8m (6ft) high.
Grow in a herbaceous border; in frost-prone areas, grow tender species in a cool or temperate greenhouse.

- **HARDINESS** Fully hardy to frost tender.
- **CULTIVATION** Grow in deep, fertile, humus-rich, moist but well-drained, preferably sandy soil, in full sun or partial shade. Mulch young plants with straw or leaves for the first winter.
- **PROPAGATION** Sow seed in containers in a cold frame in spring (although cultivars seldom come true from seed). Divide established clumps in late spring. Stimulate offshoots from slow-growing, woody-based, evergreen red hot pokers by cutting off crowns; leave offshoots in place to develop for 2 years before separating from parent plants, or use new shoots as basal cuttings.
- **PESTS AND DISEASES** Thrips may cause mottling of the foliage. Violet root rot may be a problem.

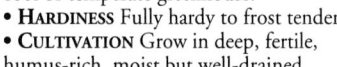

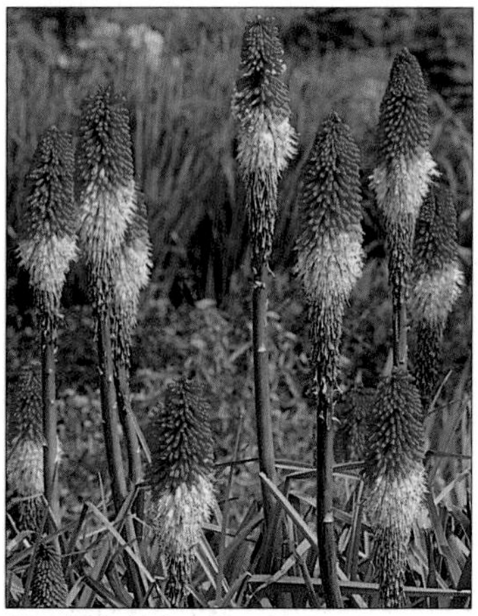
Kniphofia 'Atlanta'

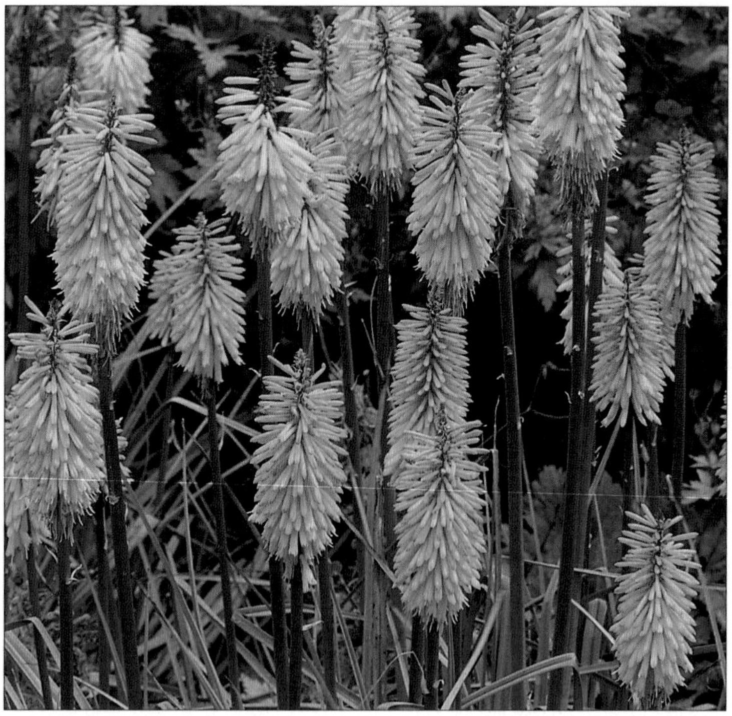
Kniphofia 'Bees' Sunset'

***K.* 'Ada'.** Deciduous perennial with tawny orange-yellow flowers borne in late summer and early autumn. ↕ 90cm (36in), ↔ 60cm (24in). ❄❄❄
***K.* 'Atlanta'** ■ Evergreen perennial with grey-green leaves, and orange-red flowers, fading to pale yellow, borne in late spring and early summer. ↕ 1.2m (4ft), ↔ 75cm (30in). ❄❄❄
***K.* 'Bees' Lemon'.** Deciduous perennial with toothed leaves, and lemon-yellow flowers, green in bud, borne in late summer and early autumn. ↕ 90cm (36in), ↔ 60cm (24in). ❄❄❄
***K.* 'Bees' Sunset'** ■♀ Deciduous perennial with toothed leaves, and soft yellowish orange flowers borne from early to late summer. ↕ 90cm (36in), ↔ 60cm (24in). ❄❄❄
***K.* 'Border Ballet'.** Deciduous perennial with cream to pink flowers borne in late summer and early autumn. ↕↔ 60cm (24in). ❄❄❄
***K.* 'Bressingham Comet'.** Deciduous perennial with red-tipped orange flowers, yellow at the bases, borne in early and mid-autumn. ↕ 45cm (18in), ↔ 22cm (9in). ❄❄❄
***K.* 'Buttercup'** ♀ Deciduous perennial with green buds, opening to clear yellow flowers in early summer. ↕↔ 75cm (30in). ❄❄❄
K. caulescens ■♀ Evergreen perennial with short, thick, woody-based stems and arching, linear, keeled, finely toothed, glaucous leaves, to 1m (3ft) long, purple at the bases. Coral-red flowers, 2.5cm (1in) long, fading to pale yellow, with protruding stamens, are borne in short, oblong-cylindrical racemes from late summer to mid-autumn. ↕ to 1.2m (4ft), ↔ 60cm (24in). South Africa (N. Eastern Cape, Orange Free State, KwaZulu/Natal), Lesotho. ❄❄❄
***K.* 'C.M. Prichard' of gardens** see *K. rooperi.*
***K.* 'Corallina'.** Deciduous perennial with deep green leaves, and coral-red flowers borne in early summer. ↕ 90cm (36in), ↔ 60cm (24in). ❄❄❄
***K.* 'Early Buttercup'.** Deciduous perennial with yellow flowers borne in late spring and early summer. ↕ 90cm (36in), ↔ 60cm (24in). ❄❄❄
K. ensifolia. Robust, evergreen perennial forming clumps of arching, narrowly elliptic, finely toothed, glaucous leaves, to 15cm (6in) long. Bears greenish white flowers, 1.5–2cm (½–¾in) long, often red in bud, in dense, cylindrical racemes from late summer to mid-autumn. ↕ 1.2m (4ft) or more, ↔ 60cm (24in). South Africa (Western Cape, Eastern Cape,

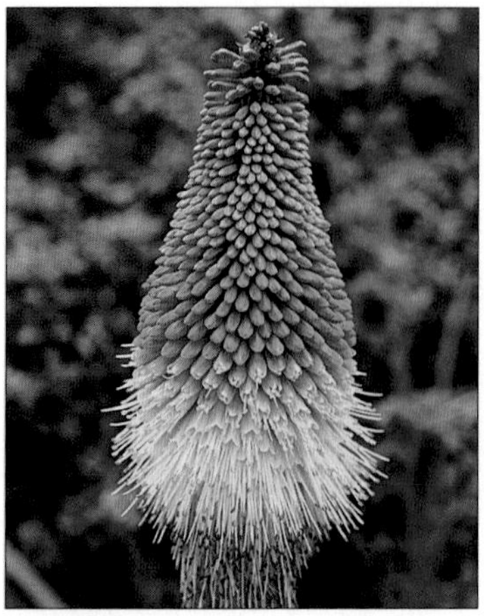
Kniphofia caulescens

K

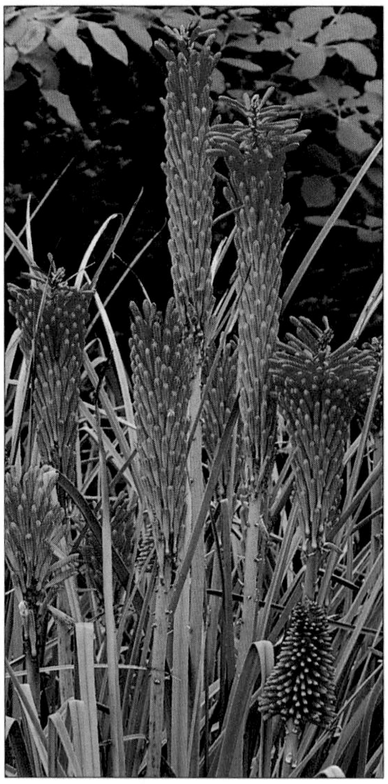

Kniphofia 'Erecta'

KwaZulu/Natal, Eastern Transvaal, Northern Transvaal). ❄❄❄

***K.* 'Erecta'** ■ Deciduous perennial with bright coral-red flowers, turning upwards after opening, borne in late summer and early autumn. ↕90cm (36in), ↔ 60cm (24in). ❄❄❄

***K.* 'Fiery Fred'.** Deciduous perennial with orange-red flowers borne from early to late summer. ↕ to 1.2m (4ft), ↔ 60cm (24in). ❄❄❄

***K. galpinii* of gardens** see *K. triangularis.*

***K.* 'Goldelse'.** Deciduous perennial with grass-like leaves, and yellow flowers borne in racemes in early summer. ↕75cm (30in), ↔ 30cm (12in). ❄❄❄

***K.* 'Green Jade'** ■ Robust, evergreen perennial with keeled leaves, and green flowers, becoming cream and then white, borne in racemes in late summer and early autumn. ↕ to 1.5m (5ft), ↔ 60–75cm (24–30in). ❄❄❄

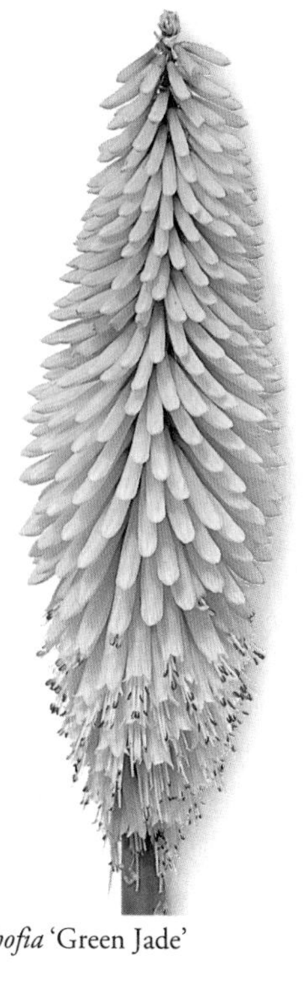

Kniphofia 'Green Jade'

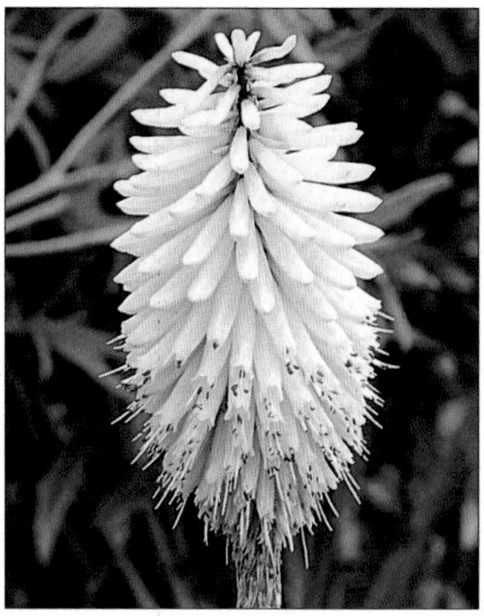

Kniphofia 'Ice Queen'

K. hirsuta. Evergreen perennial with linear, spreading, hairy, dark green leaves, 40–60cm (16–24in) long, red at the bases. Pinkish red flowers, 2–3cm (¾–1¼in) long, becoming yellow, are produced in conical racemes in mid-spring. ↕40cm (16in), ↔ 45cm (18in). Lesotho. ❄❄

***K.* 'Ice Queen'** ■ Robust, deciduous perennial bearing green-budded flowers opening to pale primrose yellow, fading to ivory, in early and mid-autumn. ↕ to 1.5m (5ft), ↔ 75cm (30in). ❄❄❄

***K.* 'Jenny Bloom'.** Deciduous perennial with pink flowers, shading to cream and coral-pink, borne from late summer to mid-autumn. ↕ 1m (3ft), ↔ 30cm (12in). ❄❄❄

***K.* 'Limelight'.** Deciduous perennial with grass-like foliage, and canary-yellow flowers, greenish yellow in bud, borne in early autumn. ↕90cm (36in), ↔ 45cm (18in). ❄❄❄

***K.* 'Little Maid'** ■ ♀ Deciduous perennial with grass-like leaves, and racemes of flowers, pale green in bud, opening to buff-tinted pale yellow and ageing to ivory, borne in late summer and early autumn. ↕60cm (24in), ↔ 45cm (18in). ❄❄❄

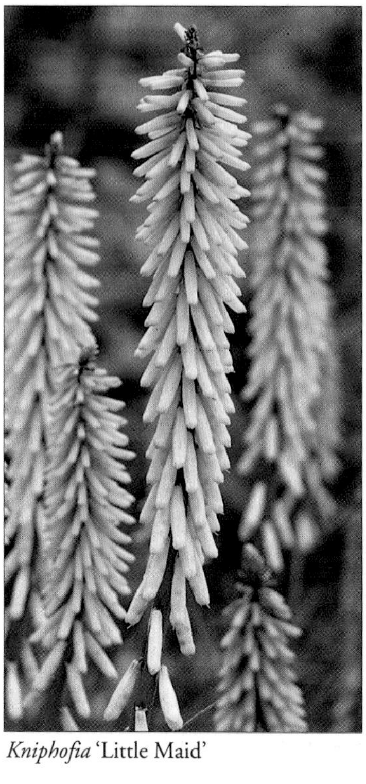

Kniphofia 'Little Maid'

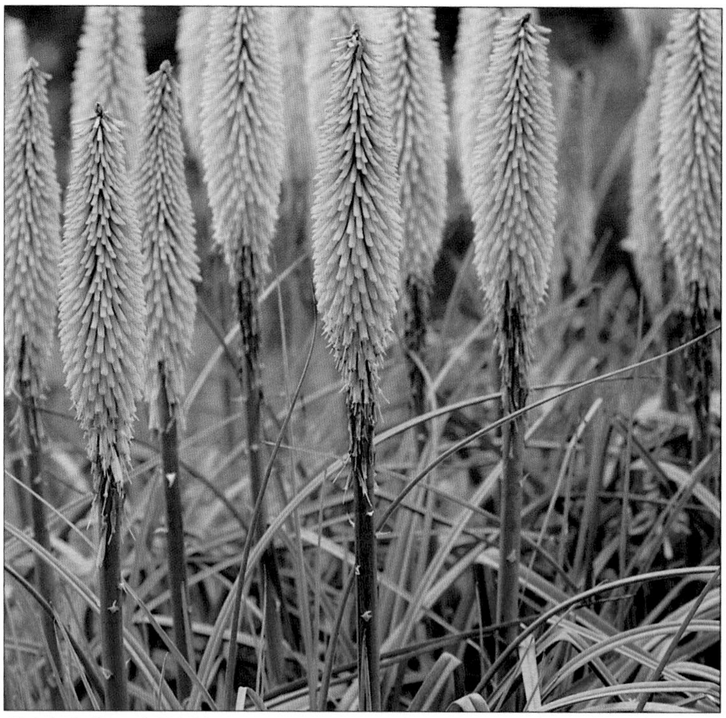

Kniphofia 'Percy's Pride'

K. macowanii see *K. triangularis.*

***K.* 'Maid of Orleans'.** Deciduous perennial bearing long-lasting flowers, pale primrose in bud, opening to deeper yellow, and maturing to ivory, borne in mid- and late summer. ↕ to 1.2m (4ft), ↔ 45cm (18in). ❄❄❄

***K.* 'Mount Etna'.** Deciduous perennial with broad racemes of pale greenish yellow flowers, scarlet in bud, borne in late summer and early autumn. ↕ to 1.2m (4ft), ↔ 90cm (36in). ❄❄❄

K. nelsonii see *K. triangularis.*

K. northiae. Evergreen perennial forming thick-stemmed, solitary plants, not clumps, with arching, linear, broad, unkeeled, glaucous leaves, to 1.5m (5ft) long. Pale yellow flowers, 2.5–3cm (1–1¼in) long, opening from red buds, are produced in oblong, very dense racemes from early to late summer. ↕1.5m (5ft), ↔ 90cm (36in). South Africa (Eastern Cape, KwaZulu/Natal), Lesotho. ❄❄❄

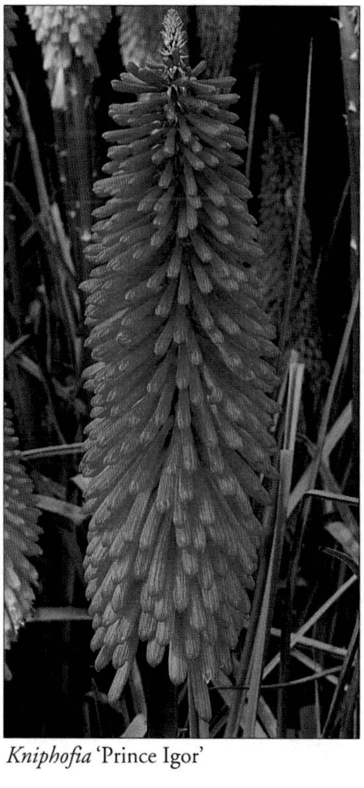

Kniphofia 'Prince Igor'

***K.* 'Percy's Pride'** ■ Deciduous perennial with keeled leaves, and canary-yellow flowers, green-tinted yellow in bud, opening to cream, borne in late summer and early autumn. ↕ 1.2m (4ft), ↔ 60cm (24in). ❄❄❄

***K.* 'Prince Igor'** ■ Deciduous perennial with glowing, deep orange-red flowers borne in racemes in early and mid-autumn. ↕ 1.8m (6ft), ↔ 90cm (36in). ❄❄❄

K. rooperi ■ syn. *K.* 'C.M. Prichard' of gardens. Robust, evergreen perennial with arching, broad, linear, acutely pointed, deeply keeled, dark green leaves. Orange-red flowers, 3.5–4.5cm (1½–1¾in) long, becoming orange-yellow, are borne in broadly ellipsoid, shiny racemes from early to late autumn. ↕ 1.2m (4ft), ↔ 60cm (24in). South Africa (Eastern Cape). ❄❄❄

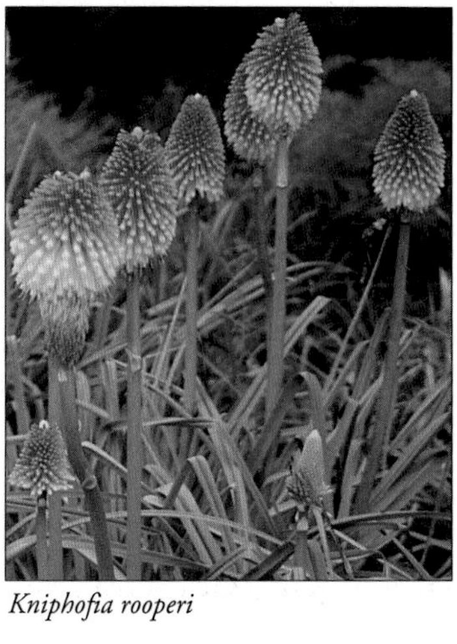

Kniphofia rooperi

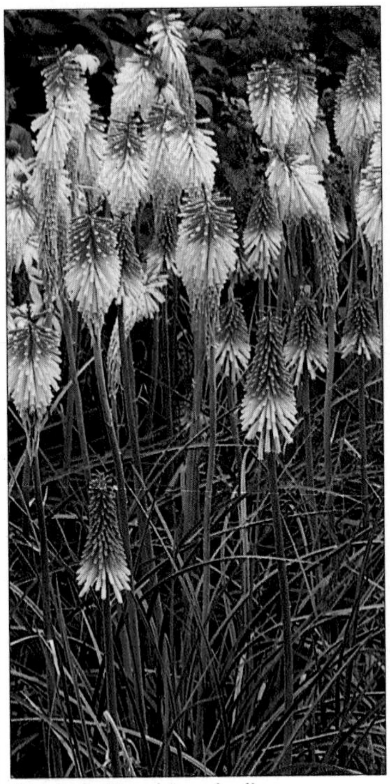
Kniphofia 'Royal Standard'

K

***K.* 'Royal Standard'** ▣ ♀ Deciduous perennial with bright yellow flowers, scarlet in bud, borne on stout stems in mid- and late summer. ↕ 90–100cm (36–39in), ↔ 60cm (24in). ❄❄❄
***K.* 'Samuel's Sensation'** ♀ Deciduous perennial with bright scarlet flowers, tinged with yellow as they fade, borne in racemes in late summer and early autumn. ↕ 1.5m (5ft), ↔ 60–75cm (24–30in). ❄❄❄
***K.* 'Shining Sceptre'.** Deciduous perennial with clear yellow flowers, becoming ivory, borne in midsummer. ↕ 1.2m (4ft), ↔ 60cm (24in). ❄❄❄
***K. snowdenii* of gardens** see *K. thompsonii* var. *snowdenii.*
***K.* 'Strawberries and Cream'** ▣ Deciduous perennial with cream flowers, coral-pink in bud, borne in late summer and early autumn. ↕ 60cm (24in), ↔ 30cm (12in). ❄❄❄
***K.* 'Sunningdale Yellow'** ♀ Deciduous perennial with long-lasting racemes of yellow flowers produced in mid- and late summer. ↕ 90cm (36in), ↔ 45cm (18in). ❄❄❄
***K. thompsonii* var. *snowdenii*,** syn. *K. snowdenii* of gardens. Gently spreading, deciduous, rhizomatous

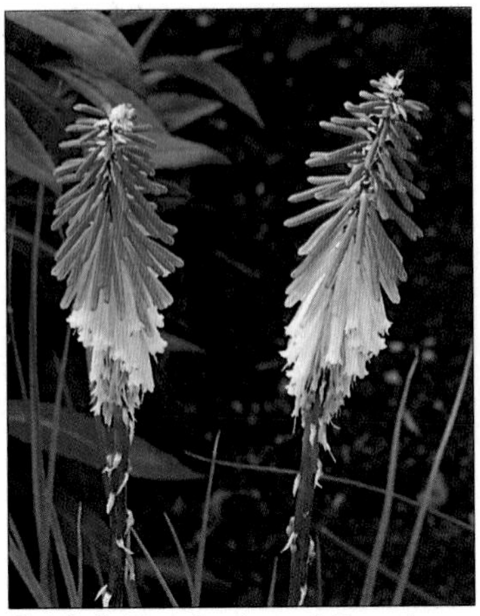
Kniphofia 'Strawberries and Cream'

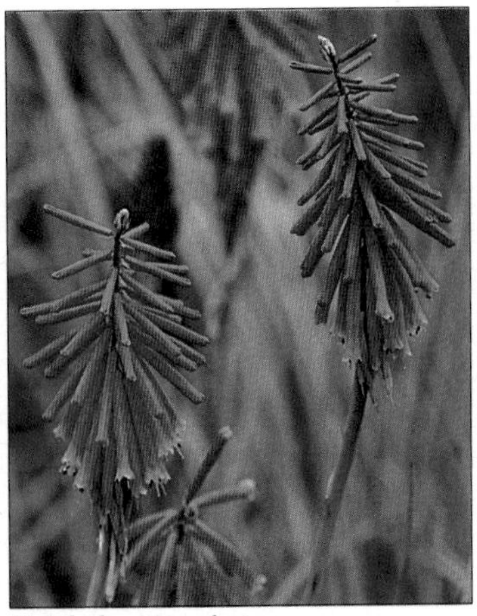
Kniphofia triangularis

perennial forming tufts of upright, linear leaves, to 60cm (24in) long. From midsummer to late autumn, produces a succession of few-flowered, open racemes of curved, yellowish orange or coral-pink flowers, to 3.5cm (1½in) long. ↕ to 90cm (36in), ↔ 45cm (18in). Uganda, Kenya. ❄❄
K. triangularis ▣ ♀ syn. *K. galpinii* of gardens, *K. macowanii, K. nelsonii.* Variable, deciduous perennial with arching, linear, grass-like leaves. Wiry stems, freely borne in moist conditions, produce dense racemes of reddish orange flowers, 2.5–3.5cm (1–1½in) long, becoming slightly yellower around the mouths, in early and mid-autumn. ↕ 60–90cm (24–36in), ↔ 45cm (18in). South Africa (Eastern Cape, Orange Free State, KwaZulu/Natal), Lesotho. ❄❄❄
K. uvaria. Evergreen perennial with lax, linear, keeled, finely toothed, coarse leaves, to 60cm (24in) long. Flowers, 3–4cm (1¼–1½in) long, red in bud, opening to orange, and fading to yellow, are borne in slender, oblong-ovoid racemes in early autumn. ↕ 1.2m (4ft), ↔ 60cm (24in). South Africa (S. Western Cape). ❄❄❄. **'Nobilis'** ♀ has longer racemes of rich orange-red flowers, borne from midsummer to early autumn. ↕ 1.5–2m (5–6ft), ↔ 1m (3ft).
***K.* 'Wrexham Buttercup'** ▣ Deciduous perennial with clear, bright yellow flowers, borne in dense racemes in midsummer. ↕ 1.2m (4ft), ↔ 60cm (24in). ❄❄❄

▷ ***Kochia trichophylla*** see *Bassia scoparia* f. *trichophylla*

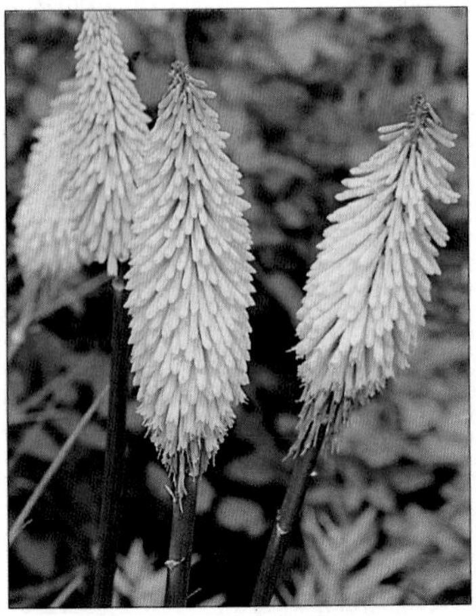
Kniphofia 'Wrexham Buttercup'

KOELERIA

GRAMINEAE/POACEAE

Genus of about 30 species of annual and perennial grasses from chalky and sandy grassland in N. and S. temperate zones and in tropical Africa. Several species are cultivated for their ornamental leaves and narrow panicles of silvery green or blue-green spikelets. They are suitable for a rock garden or the front of a border, either individually or in groups.
• **HARDINESS** Fully hardy.
• **CULTIVATION** Grow in medium to light, not too fertile, well-drained soil in full sun or light dappled shade. Koelerias thrive in alkaline and shallow, chalky soil. Cut back flowering stems either before seeding or in autumn.
• **PROPAGATION** Sow seed *in situ* in spring or autumn, or divide from mid-spring to early summer.
• **PESTS AND DISEASES** *Verticillium* wilt may be a problem.

K. glauca (Glaucous hair grass). Densely tufted, semi-evergreen, perennial grass, forming a compact mound of narrowly linear, glaucous grey-green leaves, to 20cm (8in) long, with inrolled margins. In early and midsummer, produces numerous erect stems bearing cylindrical panicles, to 10cm (4in) long, of shining, silver-green spikelets, which age to buff. ↕ to 40cm (16in) or more, ↔ 30cm (12in). W. and C. Europe to Russia (Siberia). ❄❄❄

KOELREUTERIA

SAPINDACEAE

Genus of 3 species of deciduous trees or shrubs from dry valley woodlands in China, Korea, and Taiwan. They have alternate, pinnate to 2-pinnate leaves, and large, pyramidal panicles, 10–35cm (4–14in) long, of shallowly bowl-shaped flowers, followed by unusual, inflated fruit capsules. They are fine specimen trees, flowering best in areas with hot summers.
• **HARDINESS** Fully hardy to frost hardy, provided the wood has been well ripened in summer.
• **CULTIVATION** Grow in fertile, well-drained soil in full sun. Pruning group 1; prune only to remove damaged or dead wood when dormant in winter.
• **PROPAGATION** Sow seed in containers in a cold frame in autumn. Take root cuttings in late winter.
• **PESTS AND DISEASES** Trouble free.

K. bipinnata Q Spreading tree with large, 2-pinnate, mid-green leaves, to 50cm (20in) long, comprising numerous oval-oblong, finely toothed leaflets. Red-spotted yellow flowers, 1cm (½in) across, are produced in large panicles, to 30cm (12in) long, from summer to autumn, followed by bladder-like fruit capsules, to 5cm (2in) long, red-brown when ripe. ↕ 10m (30ft), ↔ 8m (25ft). S.W. China. ❄❄
K. paniculata ▣ ♀ Q (Golden-rain tree, Pride of India). Spreading tree with pinnate leaves, to 45cm (18in) long, each consisting of 7–15 or more, ovate-oblong, scalloped leaflets. Emerging leaves are pink-red, becoming mid-green, and turning butter-yellow in autumn. Small yellow flowers, 1cm

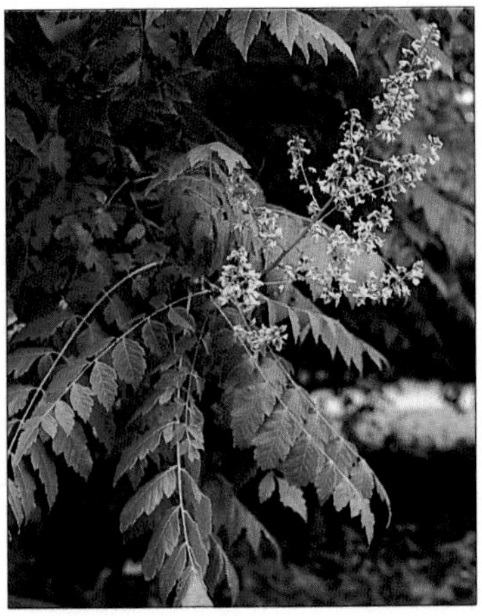
Koelreuteria paniculata

(½in) across, are produced in large, pyramidal panicles, to 30cm (12in) long, in mid- and late summer; they are followed by bladder-like, pink- or red-flushed fruit capsules, to 5cm (2in) long. ↕↔ 10m (30ft) or more. China, Korea. ❄❄❄. **var. *apiculata*** has 2-pinnate leaves and light yellow flowers.

KOHLERIA

GESNERIACEAE

Genus of about 50 species of usually erect, rhizomatous perennials and subshrubs from rainforest of tropical regions of North America, Central America, and South America. They are grown for their foxglove-like flowers, which are bell-shaped or tubular, flaring out into 5 rounded lobes, usually produced from the leaf axils singly, in pairs, or in pendent, umbel-like racemes. Elliptic-lance-shaped to ovate leaves, opposite or in whorls of 3, are usually dark green, sometimes with silver markings, and have toothed or scalloped margins. All parts are hairy, including the flowers. In frost-prone climates, grow taller species in a warm greenhouse or conservatory; use compact species and cultivars as houseplants. In humid, tropical areas, grow in shaded sites in beds or borders.
• **HARDINESS** Frost tender.
• **CULTIVATION** Under glass, start into growth at 21°C (70°F) in early spring. Grow in loamless potting compost in bright filtered light, with high humidity. Using soft water, water moderately at first, then freely when in full growth. When flower buds appear, apply a high potash fertilizer every 2 weeks. In autumn, remove dying top growth and keep almost completely dry. Outdoors, grow in moist, well-drained, humus-rich soil in partial shade.
• **PROPAGATION** Divide in early spring.
• **PESTS AND DISEASES** The growing tips may be infested by aphids. Rhizome rot may occur in winter if conditions are too moist, or in spring if replanted rhizomes are slow to start into growth.

K. amabilis. Erect to prostrate, rhizomatous perennial with ovate, scalloped leaves, 10cm (4in) long, veined silver and purple-brown. In summer, bell-shaped, deep pink flowers, 2.5cm (1in) long, with purple and brick-red bars and stripes on the lobes and throats, are borne singly or in few-flowered, umbel-like racemes. May need

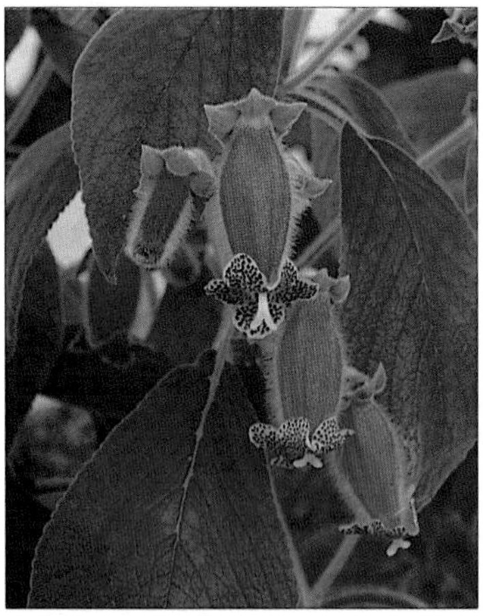

Kohleria digitaliflora

support. ↕↔ 60cm (24in). Colombia. ⊛ (min. 15°C/59°F)
K. bogotensis. Erect, rhizomatous perennial with ovate, toothed, velvety, dark green leaves, 8cm (3in) long, marked paler green or white above. Bell-shaped, red-and-yellow flowers, 2.5cm (1in) long, with mouths spotted red, are borne singly or in pairs, from autumn to early winter. ↕ 60cm (24in), ↕↔ 45cm (18in). Colombia. ⊛ (min. 15°C/59°F)
***K.* 'Connecticut Belle'.** Erect, compact, rhizomatous perennial with lance-shaped, toothed leaves, 7cm (3in) long, red beneath. Bell-shaped flowers, 2.5cm (1in) long, with bright red tubes, purple upper lobes, and purple-spotted, bright pink lower lobes, are produced singly or in pairs in summer. ↕ 40cm (16in), ↔ 20cm (8in). ⊛ (min. 15°C/59°F)
K. digitaliflora ■ ♀ Erect to spreading, rhizomatous perennial with lance-shaped, elliptic-lance-shaped to ovate, scalloped leaves, 20cm (8in) long, marked paler green. From summer to autumn, produces umbel-like racemes of up to 6, occasionally solitary, tubular, purple-pink flowers, 2.5–3cm (1–1¼in) long, white on the inside of the tubes, and with lobes spotted with dark, purplish green. ↕ 60cm (24in), ↔ 40cm (16in). Colombia. ⊛ (min. 15°C/59°F)
K. eriantha ■ ♀ Robust, bushy, rhizomatous perennial with ovate to ovate-lance-shaped, scalloped leaves, 7–13cm (3–5in) long. The leaves have prominent red hairs on the margins, and undersides that are paler and red-veined. In summer, produces tubular, orange-red flowers, 2.5cm (1in) long, with yellow-spotted lower lobes, either singly or in umbel-like racemes. ↕ to 1.2m (4ft), ↔ 30cm (12in) or more. Colombia. ⊛ (min. 15°C/59°F)

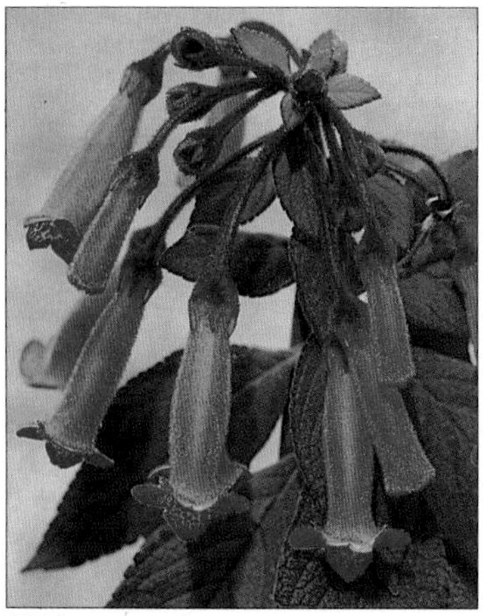

Kohleria eriantha

▷ **Kohuhu** see *Pittosporum tenuifolium*

KOLKWITZIA

Beauty bush

CAPRIFOLIACEAE

Genus of one species of deciduous shrub from rocky, mountainous areas of Hubei, China. It has simple leaves, borne in opposite pairs, and is cultivated for its profusion of bell-shaped flowers borne in dense corymbs. Good for a shrub border or as a specimen plant.

- **HARDINESS** Fully hardy, but foliage may be damaged by late frosts.
- **CULTIVATION** Grow in fertile, well-drained soil, preferably in full sun, although some shade is tolerated. Pruning group 2.
- **PROPAGATION** Take greenwood cuttings in late spring or early summer, or remove suckers in spring.
- **PESTS AND DISEASES** Trouble free.

K. amabilis. Deciduous, suckering shrub with long, arching shoots and broadly ovate, tapered, dark green leaves, to 7cm (3in) long. Masses of bell-shaped, pale to deep pink flowers, to 1.5cm (½in) across, with yellow-flushed throats, are produced in terminal corymbs, 5–8cm (2–3in) across, in late spring and early summer. ↕ 3m (10ft), ↔ 4m (12ft). China (Hubei). ❄❄❄. **'Pink Cloud'** ■ ♀ has bright, deep pink flowers.

▷ **Korokio** see *Corokia buddlejoides*
▷ ***Korolkowia sewerzowii*** see *Fritillaria sewerzowii*
▷ **Kowhai** see *Sophora tetraptera*
▷ **Krauss's spikemoss** see *Selaginella kraussiana*
▷ **Kris plant** see *Alocasia sanderiana*
▷ **Kudzu vine** see *Pueraria lobata*
▷ **Kumquat** see *Fortunella*
Round see *F. japonica*

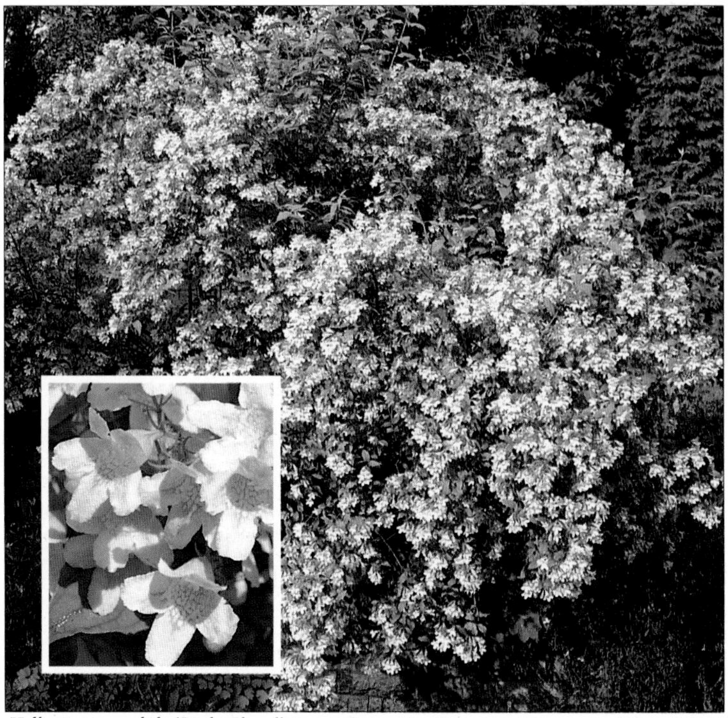

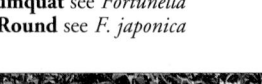

Kolkwitzia amabilis 'Pink Cloud' (inset: flower detail)

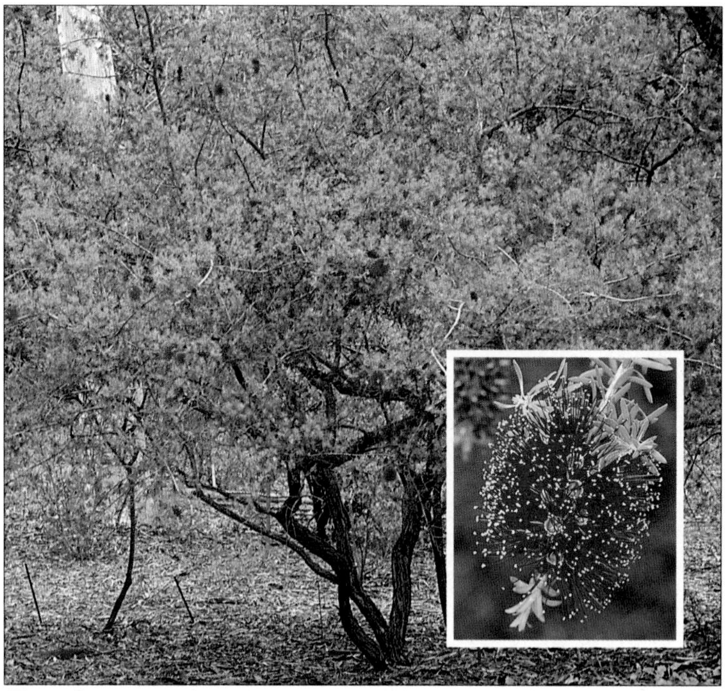

Kunzea baxteri (inset: flower detail)

KUNZEA

MYRTACEAE

Genus of 25 species of evergreen shrubs and small trees from sands or sandy loam areas of mostly coastal habitats in Australia. They have small, often crowded, simple, entire, leathery leaves, and bear terminal "bottlebrush" spikes or heads of flowers. Each flower is composed of 5 small petals and a crown of conspicuous stamens, which in some species give the flowerheads their main colour. Where temperatures drop below 5°C (41°F), grow in a cool greenhouse, moving plants in containers outdoors during the warmer summer months. In milder climates, grow at the base of a house wall or in a shrub border.

- **HARDINESS** Frost tender; *K. baxteri* and *K. capitata* may survive short spells around 0°C (32°F).
- **CULTIVATION** Under glass, grow in lime-free (ericaceous) potting compost in full light, with good ventilation. In growth, water moderately and apply a balanced liquid fertilizer every month; water sparingly in winter. Outdoors, grow in moderately fertile, neutral to acid, well-drained, sandy soil in full sun; shelter from strong and dry winds. Pruning group 1; under glass, may need restrictive pruning after flowering.
- **PROPAGATION** Surface-sow seed at 16°C (61°F) in spring, or root semi-ripe cuttings with bottom heat in summer.
- **PESTS AND DISEASES** Trouble free.

K. baxteri ■ Freely branching shrub, erect at first then spreading to a domed or rounded outline. Bears narrowly oblong, spreading, mid- to deep green leaves, 2cm (¾in) long, with white margins. Scarlet flowers, 2.5cm (1in) across, with long red stamens and yellow anthers, are produced in many short, dense spikes, to 10cm (4in) long, from spring to early summer. Thrives in seaside gardens. ↕↔ 1–2m (3–6ft) or more. Australia (Western Australia). ⊛ (min. 5°C/41°F)
K. capitata. Bushy, rounded, freely branching shrub, erect at first but soon spreading, with upright, narrowly obovate to elliptic, mid-green leaves, 5–10mm (¼–½in) long, with arching tips. From spring to early summer, bears many small, rounded heads, 2cm (¾in) across, of deep mauve-pink flowers, 1cm (½in) long, with long stamens of the same colour tipped with cream anthers. ↕↔ 1–1.5m (3–5ft). Australia (New South Wales, Queensland). ⊛ (min. 5°C/41°F)

▷ **Kurrajong** see *Brachychiton, B. discolor, B. populneus*
Flame see *B. acerifolius*
▷ **Kusamaki** see *Podocarpus macrophyllus*
▷ **Kyo-Chiku** see *Dendrocalamus giganteus*

K

L

LABLAB *syn.* DOLICHOS

LEGUMINOSAE/PAPILIONACEAE

Genus of one species of short-lived, herbaceous, perennial climber found in scrub in tropical Africa. Twining stems bear alternate, 3-palmate leaves and short, axillary racemes of fragrant, pea-like flowers. *L. purpureus* is extensively cultivated in Asia and North Africa for its edible fruit pods. In frost-prone areas, grow as a tender annual, or in a cool or temperate greenhouse. In warmer areas, train over a pergola or wall.

- **HARDINESS** Frost tender.
- **CULTIVATION** Under glass, grow in loam-based potting compost (JI No.2) in full light. When in growth, water freely and apply a balanced liquid fertilizer every 10–14 days until flowering; water sparingly in winter. Outdoors, grow in any well-drained soil in full sun (for the best crop of beans, water and fertilize as for plants under glass). Provide support of netting or trellis. Pruning group 11, in spring.
- **PROPAGATION** In cool climates, sow seed at 19–24°C (66–75°F) in spring. In warm climates, sow *in situ* when warm enough (19–24°C/66–75°F).
- **PESTS AND DISEASES** Trouble free.

L. purpureus ■ syn. *Dolichos lablab, D. niger, D. purpureus* (Egyptian bean, Indian bean). Fast-growing, twining, perennial climber producing 3-palmate, mid- to dark green leaves, composed of ovate to triangular leaflets, 10–15cm (4–6in) long. Bears fragrant, purple or white flowers, 1–2.5cm (½–1in) long, in racemes 20–40cm (8–16in) long, mainly in summer and autumn. Edible green pods, 10–15cm (4–6in) long, are often flushed purple, and contain 3–6 white to buff, reddish brown, brown, or black beans. ↕ 2–6m (6–20ft). Tropical Africa. ❀ (min. 7°C/45°F)

+ LABURNOCYTISUS

LEGUMINOSAE/PAPILIONACEAE

Deciduous tree, a graft hybrid, grown for its colourful, pea-like flowers borne in late spring and early summer. The leaves are alternate and 3-palmate. An ideal specimen tree, + *L. adamii* is also effective planted in small groups.

- **HARDINESS** Fully hardy.
- **CULTIVATION** Grow in moderately fertile, moist but well-drained soil in full sun. Pruning group 1; remove any suckers that arise from the rootstock.
- **PROPAGATION** Graft on to *Laburnum* seedlings in winter.
- **PESTS AND DISEASES** Trouble free.

+ *L. adamii* ■ ♀ (*Chamaecytisus purpureus* + *Laburnum anagyroides*). Spreading, deciduous tree with 3-palmate, dark green leaves, consisting of oval leaflets, to 6cm (2½in) long. Pea-like flowers occur in 3 colours, each borne in separate racemes in late spring and early summer: 2 are single colours, yellow and purple, true to each parent; the third is purple-pink with a yellow flush. ↕ 8m (25ft), ↔ 6m (20ft). Garden origin. ❄❄❄

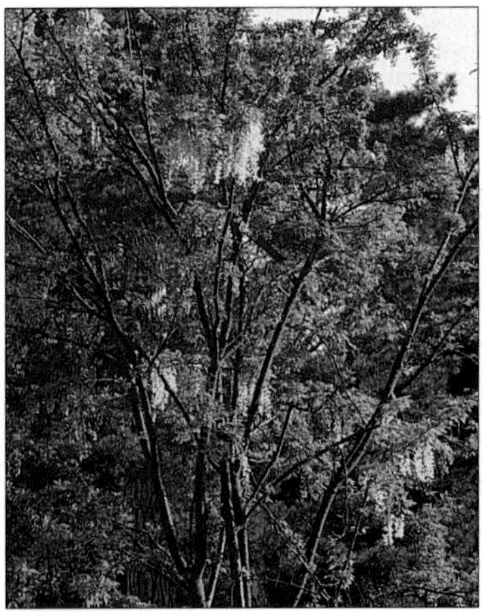

+ *Laburnocytisus adamii*

LABURNUM

Golden rain

LEGUMINOSAE/PAPILIONACEAE

Genus of 2 species of deciduous trees from woodland and thickets in the mountains of S. central Europe, S.E. Europe, and W. Asia. They are grown for their profuse, pendent, usually axillary racemes of pea-like yellow flowers, produced in late spring and early summer. The leaves are alternate and 3-palmate. Useful in a small garden as specimen trees or to form a pergola. All parts are highly toxic if ingested.

- **HARDINESS** Fully hardy.
- **CULTIVATION** Grow in moderately fertile, well-drained soil in full sun. Pruning group 1.
- **PROPAGATION** Sow seed (species only) in containers in a cold frame in autumn. Graft in late winter, or bud in summer.
- **PESTS AND DISEASES** Black fly, leaf miners, honey fungus, powdery mildew, and silver leaf may be troublesome.

L. alpinum ♀ (Scotch laburnum). Spreading tree with almost hairless, glossy, dark green leaves, consisting of 3 elliptic-ovate leaflets, to 8cm (3in) long. In late spring and early summer, bright yellow flowers are produced in slender racemes, 15–40cm (6–16in) long. ↕↔ 8m (25ft). S. central Europe, Italy, W. Balkans. ❄❄❄. **'Pendulum'** has weeping branches; ↕↔ 2m (6ft).
L. anagyroides ♀ syn. *L. vulgare* (Common laburnum). Spreading tree with hairy, grey-green young shoots, and dark green leaves composed of 3 elliptic-obovate leaflets, to 8cm (3in) long, hairy beneath. In late spring and early summer, produces bright yellow flowers in dense racemes, 10–30cm (4–12in) long. ↕↔ 8m (25ft). E. France to Italy, S. central Europe, Slovenia, Croatia. ❄❄❄
L. vulgare see *L. anagyroides.*
L. x watereri ♀ (*L. alpinum* x *L. anagyroides*). Spreading tree with virtually hairless young shoots, and dark green leaves composed of 3 elliptic-obovate leaflets, to 8cm (3in) long. Produces yellow flowers in dense racemes, to 50cm (20in) long, in late spring and early summer. ↕↔ 8m (25ft). Garden origin (also occurs in the wild where parents grow together). ❄❄❄.
'Vossii' ■ ♀ has hairy young shoots, and bears racemes, to 60cm (24in) long, of golden yellow flowers.

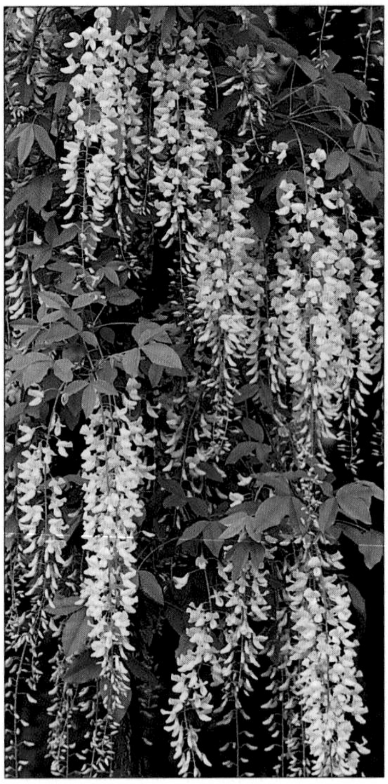

Laburnum x *watereri* 'Vossii'

▷**Laburnum,**
Common see *Laburnum anagyroides*
Dalmatian see *Petteria ramentacea*
East African see *Calpurnia aurea*
Evergreen see *Piptanthus nepalensis*
Indian see *Cassia fistula*
Natal see *Calpurnia aurea*
Scotch see *Laburnum alpinum*

LACCOSPADIX

ARECACEAE/PALMAE

Genus of one species of single- or cluster-stemmed palm from rainforest in N.E. Australia. Arching, pinnate leaves are borne in a terminal cluster and die *in situ*, forming a skirt-like mass below the living crown. Spikes of bowl-shaped, 3-petalled flowers are borne between the leaves. In frost-prone areas, grow in a temperate or warm greenhouse; in warmer areas, grow as a specimen tree.

- **HARDINESS** Frost tender.
- **CULTIVATION** Under glass, grow in loam-based potting compost (JI No.3) in full light. In growth, water freely and apply a balanced liquid fertilizer monthly; water sparingly in winter. Pot on or top-dress in spring. Outdoors, grow in moderately fertile, moist but well-drained soil in full sun.
- **PROPAGATION** Sow seed at 27°C (81°F) in spring.
- **PESTS AND DISEASES** Red spider mites may be troublesome under glass.

L. australasica ↑ Slow-growing palm, usually with a single stem but sometimes with small clusters of stems, ringed with conspicuous leaf scars. Long-stalked, pinnate leaves, 2–3m (6–10ft) long,

L

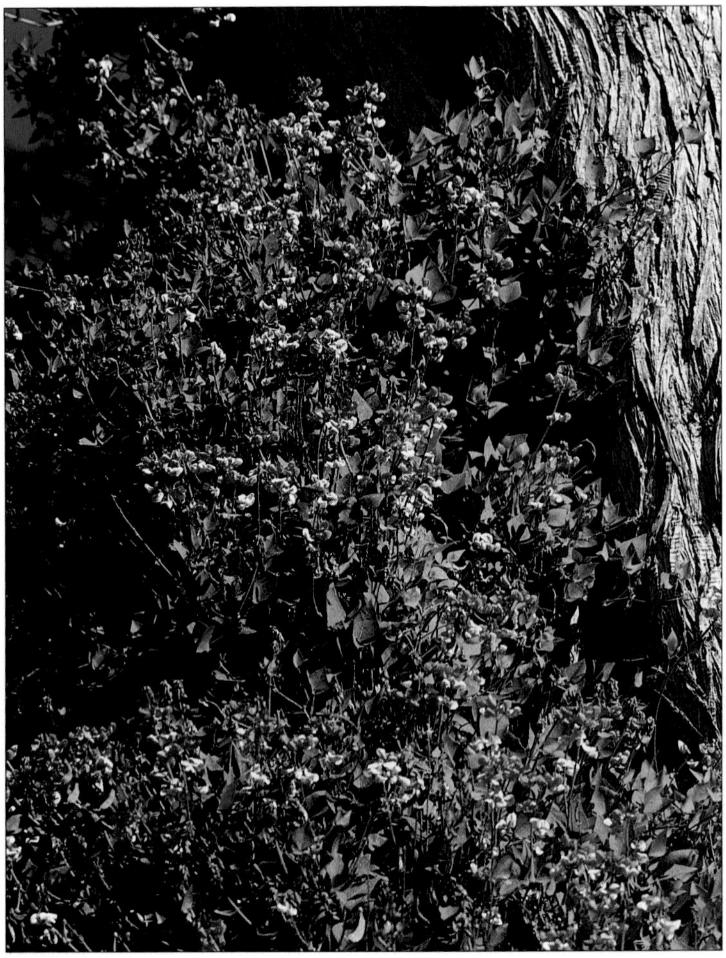

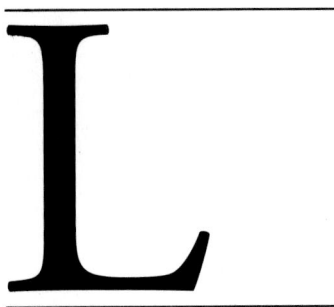

Lablab purpureus

consist of many narrowly linear-lance-shaped, sparsely scaly, mid- to deep green leaflets. Yellow flowers are borne in spikes, 1m (3ft) or more long, usually in summer. ↕ 6m (20ft) occasionally more, ↔ 3–5m (10–15ft). Australia (Queensland). ❁ (min. 13°C/55°F)

▷ **Lace-bark** see *Hoheria populnea*
▷ **Lacebark, Queensland** see *Brachychiton discolor*
▷ **Lace plant** see *Aponogeton madagascariensis*

LACHENALIA

Cape Cowslip

HYACINTHACEAE/LILIACEAE

Genus of 90 species of bulbous perennials from grassland or rocky sites, on often seasonally moist ground, in South Africa. They are grown for their spikes or racemes of showy, tubular, bell-shaped, or cylindrical flowers, borne on often mottled stems from autumn to spring. Leaves are basal, very variably shaped, and frequently attractively spotted. In frost-prone areas, grow in a cool greenhouse or a conservatory. In frost-free areas, grow in a rock garden or in an open site among low shrubs.

• **HARDINESS** Half hardy.

• **CULTIVATION** Plant bulbs 10cm (4in) deep. Under glass, grow in loam-based potting compost (JI No.2) in full light. Water moderately until in full growth, then water freely, adding a balanced liquid fertilizer every 10–14 days. Reduce watering as the leaves fade, then keep dry until fresh growth starts in autumn. Outdoors, grow in light, well-drained soil in full sun.

• **PROPAGATION** Sow seed at 13–18°C (55–64°F) as soon as ripe, or remove bulblets in summer or autumn just before replanting or repotting.

• **PESTS AND DISEASES** Trouble free.

L. aloides ■ syn. *L. tricolor.* Bulbous perennial with semi-erect, broadly lance- to strap-shaped, purple-spotted, slightly

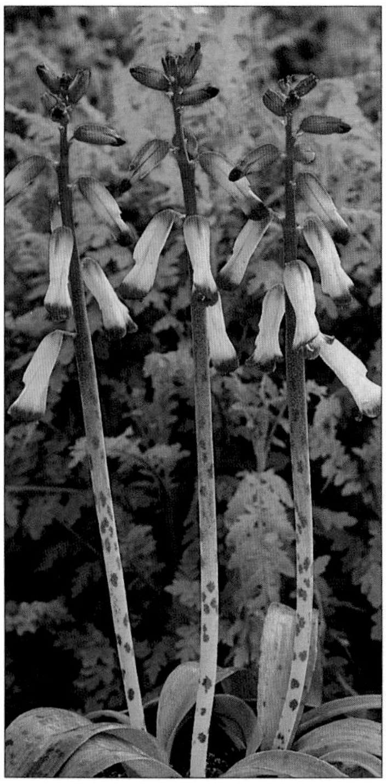

Lachenalia aloides

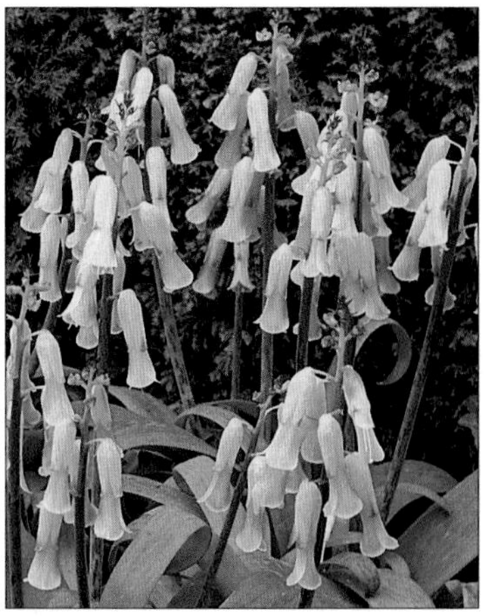

Lachenalia aloides 'Nelsonii'

glaucous, mid-green leaves, 20cm (8in) long. In winter or early spring, produces racemes of up to 20 pendent, tubular yellow flowers, 2–3.5cm (1–1½in) long, that shade to scarlet at the tips. ↕ 15–28cm (6–11in), ↔ 5cm (2in). South Africa (Western Cape). ❄. **'Nelsonii'** ■ has golden yellow flowers and unspotted leaves. **'Pearsonii'** is robust, with semi-erect, strap-shaped, mid-green leaves, to 25cm (10in) long, mottled with brown, and produces apricot flowers, to 3cm (1¼in) long, with the inner tepals tipped red to maroon; ↕ 30–40cm (12–16in). **var. *quadricolor*** ♀ has reddish orange buds opening to reddish orange-based, yellow-and-green flowers, with purple-maroon tips to the inner segments.

L. angustifolia see *L. contaminata.*

L. bulbifera, syn. *L. pendula.* Robust, bulbous perennial with semi-erect, ovate, lance-shaped, or strap-shaped, mid-green leaves, to 30cm (12in) long, usually heavily spotted brown-purple. In winter or spring, produces loose racemes of few to many pendent, cylindrical, red or orange flowers, 3–4cm (1¼–1½in) long, with green and purple tips. ↕ 30cm (12in), ↔ 5cm (2in). South Africa (Western Cape). ❄

L. contaminata, syn. *L. angustifolia.* Bulbous perennial with erect or semi-erect, narrow, grass-like, unmarked, mid- to deep green leaves, to 20cm (8in) long. In spring, bears racemes or spikes of few to many, open bell-shaped, slightly scented white flowers, 5–8mm (¼–⅜in) long, with maroon tips and stripes, held at right-angles to the stems. ↕ 6–25cm (2½–10in), ↔ 5cm (2in). South Africa (Western Cape). ❄

L. glaucina see *L. orchioides* var. *glaucina.*

L. glaucina* var. *pallida see *L. orchioides.*

L. mutabilis. Bulbous perennial with usually one semi-erect, lance-shaped, sometimes glaucous, mid-green leaf, to 20cm (8in) long, occasionally faintly spotted maroon. In winter or spring, produces dense spikes of up to 25 horizontal, stalkless, urn- to bell-shaped flowers, 1cm (½in) long, pale blue and white, with dark yellow inner tepals and dark tips, or rarely entirely greenish white. ↕ 10–45cm (4–18in), ↔ 5cm (2in). South Africa (Northern Cape, Western Cape). ❄

L. orchioides, syn. *L. glaucina* var. *pallida.* Bulbous perennial with 1 or 2 semi-erect, lance- or strap-shaped, mid-green leaves, to 28cm (11in) long, sometimes spotted brown. In late winter or spring, produces dense spikes of many semi-erect, oblong-cylindrical, fragrant, white, greenish yellow, or creamy yellow flowers, 1cm (½in) long, with flared tepals, fading to dull red as they mature. ↕ 15–40cm (6–16in), ↔ 5cm (2in). South Africa (Western Cape). ❄. **var. *glaucina***, syn. *L. glaucina*, has blue- or purple-shaded flowers with a fainter scent.

L. pendula see *L. bulbifera.*

L. rubida. Bulbous perennial with semi-erect, lance- to strap-shaped, mid- to deep green leaves, to 14cm (5½in) long, mottled deep purple. In autumn or early winter, produces racemes of few to many pendent, cylindrical, bright pink or ruby-red flowers, 2–3cm (¾–1¼in) long, shading to purple at the tips. ↕ 6–25cm (2½–10in), ↔ 5cm (2in). South Africa (Western Cape, Eastern Cape). ❄

L. tricolor see *L. aloides.*

L. unicolor. Very variable, bulbous perennial with lance- to strap-shaped, pale to dark green leaves, to 15cm (6in) long, usually with maroon warts above. In spring, bears racemes of many oblong-bell-shaped flowers, 5–8mm (¼–⅜in) long, that vary from cream with green tips, to pink, lilac-pink, magenta, blue, or purple, with darker tips. ↕ 8–30cm (3–12in), ↔ 5cm (2in). South Africa (Western Cape). ❄

▷ ***Lactuca alpina*** see *Cicerbita alpina*
▷ ***Lactuca plumieri*** see *Cicerbita plumieri*
▷ **Ladies' tresses, Nodding** see *Spiranthes cernua*
▷ **Lad's love** see *Artemisia abrotanum*
▷ **Lady of the night** see *Brunfelsia americana*
▷ **Lady palm** see *Rhapis*
▷ **Lady's mantle** see *Alchemilla*
Alpine see *A. alpina*
▷ **Lady's slipper orchid** see *Cypripedium, C. calceolus*
▷ **Lady's smock** see *Cardamine pratensis*

LAELIA

ORCHIDACEAE

Genus of about 50 species of evergreen, epiphytic or terrestrial orchids occurring in coastal regions up to altitudes of 2,600m (8,300ft), often in oak woodland, from Mexico and Central America to Brazil and Argentina. They have robust or slender, elongated pseudobulbs, each bearing 1 or 2 (sometimes 3) semi-rigid, narrowly oval, club-shaped, oblong, strap-shaped, or linear leaves. Brightly coloured flowers are usually produced in racemes from the apex of the pseudobulb. Many intergeneric hybrids derived from crosses with *Cattleya* and other related genera are also available.

• **HARDINESS** Frost tender.

• **CULTIVATION** Cool-growing orchids. Grow large species in epiphytic orchid compost in a slatted basket, and small ones epiphytically on a slab of bark. In summer, provide moist, shady conditions; water freely, adding fertilizer at every third watering, and mist once or twice daily. In winter, provide full light and water sparingly. See also p.46.

• **PROPAGATION** Divide when the plants overflow their containers. Remove

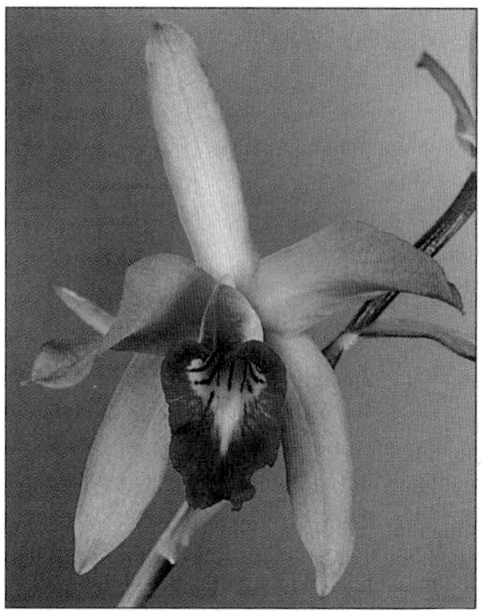

Laelia anceps

backbulbs of the Mexican species and pot up each one separately.

• **PESTS AND DISEASES** Scale insects, red spider mites, aphids, and mealybugs may be troublesome.

L. anceps ■ Epiphytic orchid with ovate-oblong pseudobulbs, each with 1, or occasionally 2, lance-shaped, leathery leaves, 15cm (6in) long. In winter, produces racemes, to 60cm (24in) long, of 2–5 light rose-pink flowers, 6cm (2½in) across, with reddish purple lips and yellow throats with purple veining. ↕ 45–60cm (18–24in), ↔ 30cm (12in). C. Mexico. ❁ (min. 10°C/50°F; max. 30°C/86°F)

L. autumnalis. Epiphytic orchid with ovate-oblong pseudobulbs, each with 2 or 3 oblong to lance-shaped, leathery leaves, 12–20cm (5–8in) long. In winter, bears long-stemmed racemes, 30–100cm (12–39in) long, of 4–10 rose-pink flowers, 6cm (2½in) across, with rose-purple lips. ↕ 30–100cm (12–39in), ↔ 30cm (12in). Mexico. ❁ (min. 10°C/50°F; max. 30°C/86°F)

L. cinnabarina ■ Epiphytic orchid with cylindrical, stem-like pseudobulbs, each with 1 or 2 linear to oblong, dark green leaves, 10–25cm (4–10in) long. Racemes, to 40cm (16in) long, of 5–15 brilliant cinnabar-red flowers, 4.5cm (1¾in) across, are produced in winter. ↕ 40cm (16in), ↔ 15cm (6in). S.E. Brazil. ❁ (min. 13°C/55°F; max. 30°C/86°F)

L. crispa. Epiphytic orchid with slender pseudobulbs, each with one oblong to strap-shaped, leathery leaf, 18cm (7in) long. In summer, bears racemes,

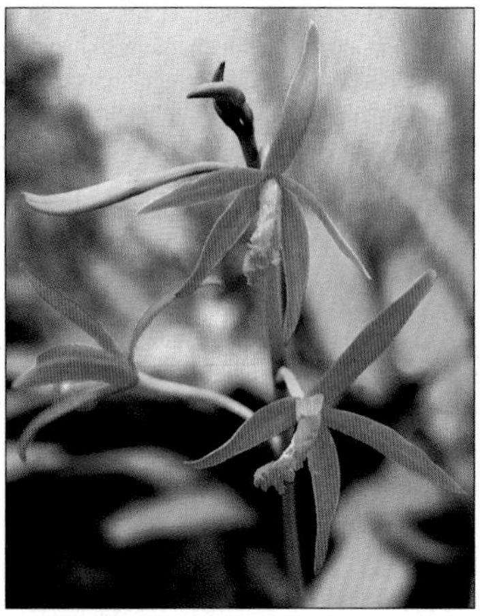

Laelia cinnabarina

L

10–25cm (4–10in) long, of 2 or 3 white flowers, 10cm (4in) across, with deep magenta veining on frilly lips. ↕ 40cm (16in), ↔ 30cm (12in). S. Brazil. ❀ (min. 13°C/55°F; max. 30°C/86°F)

L. flava. Epiphytic orchid with cylindrical, stem-like pseudobulbs, each with one lance-shaped to oblong, dark green leaf, 8–15cm (3–6in) long. In spring, bears upright racemes, 30–45cm (12–18in) long, of 5–10 yellow flowers, 3–4.5cm (1¼–1¾in) across. ↕ 30–45cm (12–18in), ↔ 15cm (6in). S.E. Brazil. ❀ (min. 13°C/55°F; max. 30°C/86°F)

L. majalis see *L. speciosa.*

L. pumila. Epiphytic orchid with ovoid pseudobulbs, each with one linear to oblong leaf, 8–12cm (3–5in) long. In autumn, lilac-rose flowers, 6cm (2½in) across, with rose-purple on the lips, are borne singly, or rarely in twos, on stems 4–10cm (1½–4in) tall, at the apex of each pseudobulb. ↕ 20cm (8in), ↔ 23cm (9in). S.E. Brazil. ❀ (min. 13°C/55°F; max. 30°C/86°F)

L. purpurata ♀ Epiphytic orchid with slender pseudobulbs, each with one oblong, leathery leaf, 20–30cm (8–12in) long. In early summer, bears racemes, to 30cm (12in) long, of 2–7 white flowers, 15cm (6in) across, with purple in the lip centres. ↕ 45cm (18in), ↔ 30cm (12in). Brazil. ❀ (min. 13°C/55°F; max. 30°C/86°F)

L. speciosa, syn. *L. majalis.* Epiphytic orchid with stout, ovoid pseudobulbs, each with one oblong to lance-shaped, stiff leaf, 10–15cm (4–6in) long. In early summer, pale rose-lilac to rich magenta flowers, 9cm (3½in) across, are borne singly or in twos, on slender stems, 10–20cm (4–8in) tall, from the apex of each pseudobulb. ↕↔ 15–20cm (6–8in). C. Mexico. ❀ (min. 10°C/50°F; max. 30°C/86°F)

L

x LAELIOCATTLEYA

ORCHIDACEAE

Bigeneric hybrid genus of evergreen orchids, derived from crosses between *Laelia* and *Cattleya*. Racemes of large, showy flowers, in a range of bright colours, are borne at the tips of the pseudobulbs, above the foliage. They mostly produce a single, lance-shaped, leathery leaf, but may also bear 2 on each elongated pseudobulb, depending on the parentage of the hybrid. Often referred to colloquially as cattleyas.

• **HARDINESS** Frost tender.

• **CULTIVATION** Cool-growing orchids. Grow in epiphytic orchid compost in a slatted basket. In summer, provide high humidity and bright filtered light; water freely, adding fertilizer at every third watering, and mist once or twice daily. In winter, provide full light and water more sparingly. See also p.46.

• **PROPAGATION** Divide when the plants overflow their containers, or remove backbulbs and pot up separately.

• **PESTS AND DISEASES** Scale insects, red spider mites, aphids, and mealybugs may be troublesome.

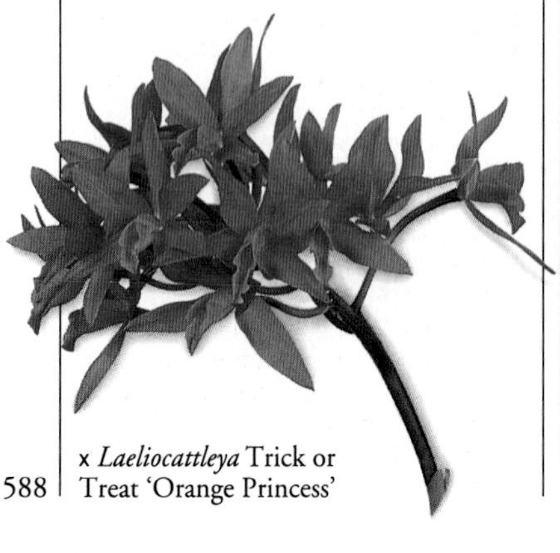

x *Laeliocattleya* Trick or Treat 'Orange Princess'

x *L.* Rojo 'Mont Millais' (*Cattleya aurantiaca* x *Laelia milleri*). Evergreen orchid with cylindrical pseudobulbs and 1 or 2 ovate leaves, 10cm (4in) long. Bears slender, deep cinnabar-red flowers, 6cm (2½in) across, in short racemes in winter. ↕↔ 30cm (12in). ❀ (min. 13°C/55°F; max. 30°C/86°F)

x *L.* Trick or Treat 'Orange Princess' ▣ (x *L.* Icarus x x *L.* Chit Chat). Evergreen orchid with cylindrical pseudobulbs and 2 narrowly oval leaves, 10cm (4in) long. Produces star-shaped, bright orange flowers, 4cm (1½in) across, in short racemes in spring. ↕↔ 30cm (12in). ❀ (min. 13°C/55°F; max. 30°C/86°F)

LAGAROSIPHON

Curly water thyme

HYDROCHARITACEAE

Genus of 9 species of semi-evergreen, submerged aquatic perennials occurring in still or slow-moving water in Africa. Used extensively as oxygenators in aquaria and in outdoor pools, they form dense, submerged masses of branched stems that support numerous linear-lance-shaped, recurved, often spirally arranged leaves and very small, white or pink flowers. In frost-prone climates, grow half-hardy species in a cold-water aquarium.

• **HARDINESS** Fully hardy to half hardy.

• **CULTIVATION** In an aquarium, admit full light, but do not provide additional heat; plants tend to become leggy in temperatures above 20°C (68°F). In an outdoor pond, grow in a submerged basket of loamy soil in full sun. Cut back regularly to restrict spread, and remove dead stems to prevent them from decomposing in the water.

• **PROPAGATION** Take stem-tip cuttings in spring or summer.

• **PESTS AND DISEASES** Trouble free.

L. major ▣ syn. *Elodea crispa* of gardens. Submerged aquatic perennial with branched, fragile stems, to 1m (3ft) long, covered in linear to lance-shaped, recurved, dark green leaves, 0.6–2.5cm (¼–1in) long. Tubular, pink-tinged green flowers, 3mm (⅛in) long, develop inside translucent spathes in summer. ↔ indefinite. Southern Africa. ✼✼✼

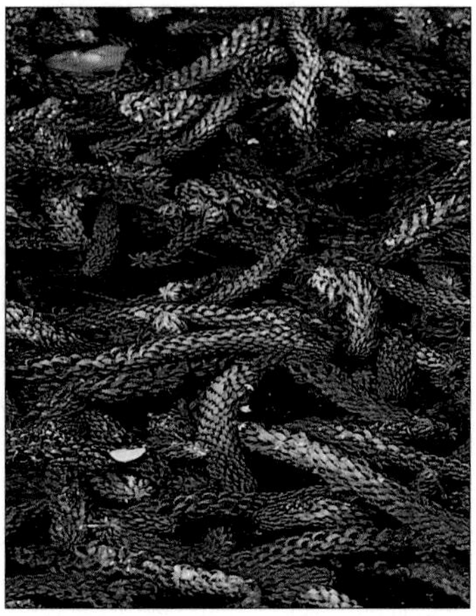

Lagarosiphon major

LAGENOPHORA

ASTERACEAE/COMPOSITAE

Genus of about 15 species of low-growing, herbaceous perennials found mostly in open sites in scrub, grassland, and at forest margins, from lowland to subalpine altitudes, in Asia, Australasia, and Central and South America. They are cultivated for their solitary, daisy-like, white to purple flowerheads, borne over long periods in summer. The mostly basal leaves are oblong to broadly ovate, and may be entire or toothed to pinnatifid. Grow in a rock garden, on a sunny bank, or at the front of a border.

• **HARDINESS** Hardy to about -10°C (14°F).

• **CULTIVATION** Grow in well-drained soil in full sun. Propagate regularly, as they are often short-lived.

• **PROPAGATION** Sow seed in containers in a cold frame as soon as ripe.

• **PESTS AND DISEASES** Slugs and snails may be a probem.

L. pinnatifida. Mat-forming herbaceous perennial with rosettes of obovate to oblong, pinnatifid, sometimes toothed or further lobed, hairy, bronze-tinted, mid-green leaves, to 6cm (2½in) long. In summer, bears solitary, off-white flowerheads, to 1.5cm (½in) across, on stems 5–10cm (2–4in) long, sometimes to 25cm (10in) long. ↕ to 10cm (4in), ↔ to 15cm (6in). Mountain grassland in New Zealand. ✼✼

LAGERSTROEMIA

LYTHRACEAE

Genus of approximately 50 species of deciduous or evergreen shrubs and trees occurring in deciduous woodland, often near rivers, in warm-temperate and tropical regions from Asia to Australia. They are cultivated for their conical, brightly coloured panicles of flowers, with characteristic crinkled petals, and their often peeling bark. The leaves vary greatly in shape within the genus, but are usually opposite. In frost-prone areas, grow against a warm, sunny wall, or overwinter in a cool or temperate greenhouse. In warmer climates, grow as specimens, in group plantings, or as a hedge or screen.

• **HARDINESS** Half hardy, or frost hardy in areas with very hot summers where the wood can ripen fully.

• **CULTIVATION** Under glass, grow in loam-based potting compost (JI No.3) in full light. During the growing season, water freely and apply a balanced liquid fertilizer every 6–8 weeks; water sparingly at other times. Outdoors, grow in moderately fertile, well-drained soil in full sun. Pruning group 1; will withstand hard pruning if renovation is required.

• **PROPAGATION** Sow seed at 10–13°C (50–55°F) in spring. Root softwood cuttings in late spring, or semi-ripe cuttings with bottom heat in summer.

• **PESTS AND DISEASES** Mealybugs, red spider mites, and whiteflies may be a problem under glass.

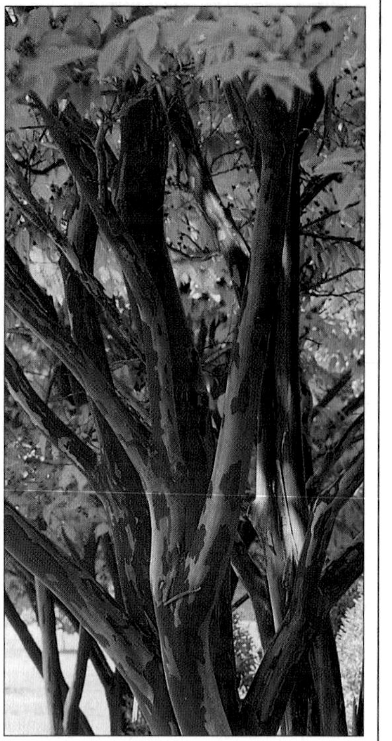

Lagerstroemia fauriei

L. fauriei ▣♀ Upright, many-stemmed, deciduous tree with peeling, red-brown bark and oblong, dark green leaves, to 10cm (4in) long. In summer, white flowers, 1cm (½in) across, are produced in panicles 5–10cm (2–4in) long. ↕↔ 8m (25ft). Japan. ✼✼

L. indica ♀♀ (Crepe flower, Crepe myrtle). Upright, deciduous tree or large shrub with peeling, grey-and-brown bark and obovate to oblong, bronze when young. From summer to autumn, white, pink, red, or purple flowers, 2–2.5cm (¾–1in) across, are produced in panicles to 20cm (8in) long. ↕↔ 8m (25ft). China. ✼✼. Some of the following are thought to be hybrids of *L. indica* and *L. fauriei.* **'Catawba'** produces purple flowers and orange-red autumn leaves; ↕↔ to 2m (6ft); ✼. **'Dallas Red'** is particularly hardy and fast-growing, and produces dark red flowers. **'Lavender Dwarf'** is a spreading shrub, bearing a profusion of light lavender-purple flowers; ↕↔ to 2m (6ft); ✼. **'Miami'** ▣ is of hybrid origin, and bears dark pink flowers from midsummer to early autumn; ↕ 5m (15ft), ↔ 2.5m (8ft). **'Natchez'** ▣ is a vigorous hybrid with

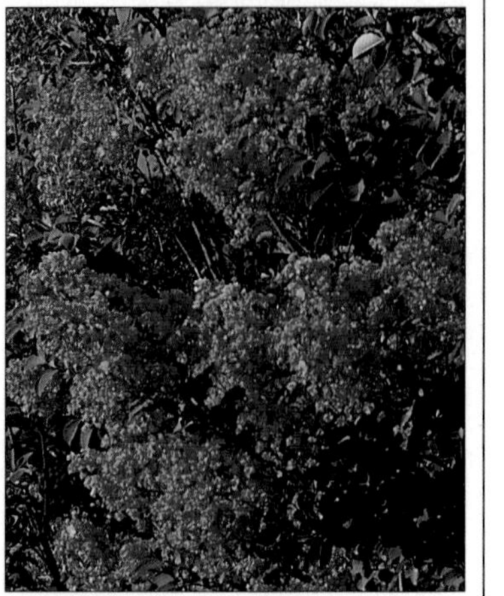

Lagerstroemia indica 'Miami'

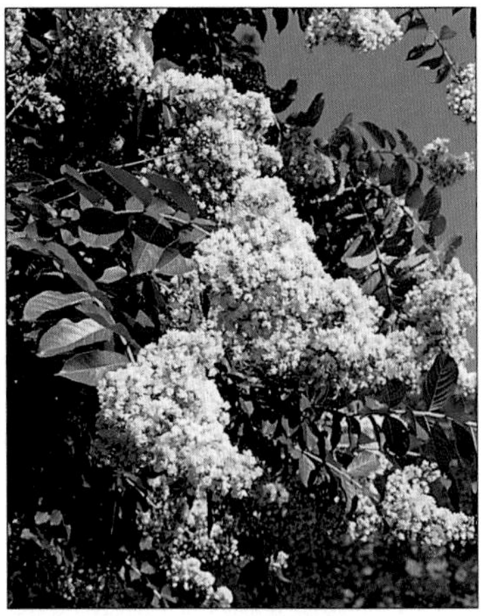

Lagerstroemia indica 'Natchez'

white flowers; ↕↔ to 2m (6ft); ✻. **'Near East'** produces pale pink flowers; ↕↔ 5m (15ft). **'Seminole'** ■ is compact, and produces mid-pink flowers from mid-summer to early autumn; ↕ 2.2–2.5m (7–8ft), ↔ 6–7m (20–22ft). **'Sioux'** is of hybrid origin, with very large pink flowers, 5cm (2in) across; ↕↔ to 2.5m (8ft); ✻. **'Tuskegee'** is a hybrid with spreading branches; it bears large panicles, to 35cm (14in) long, of dark pink flowers; ↕↔ 5m (15ft). **'White Dwarf'** is a low mound-forming shrub, and freely bears white blooms; ↕↔ 1m (3ft); ✻. **'Wichita'** is vase-shaped, sometimes forming a small tree; it bears lavender-blue flowers from summer to late autumn; ↕↔ 3.5m (11ft); ✻

L. speciosa ♀ (Giant crepe myrtle, Pride of India, Queen's crepe myrtle). Spreading, freely branching, evergreen tree with peeling, light brown bark. Ovate to elliptic-oblong leaves, 8–20cm (3–8in) long, are grey-green above, sepia-flushed beneath. From spring to autumn, produces erect, open panicles, to 40cm (16in) long, of many pink, mauve, purple, or white flowers, to 5cm (3in) wide. ↕ 10–24m (30–78ft), ↔ 5–10m (15–30ft). Tropical Asia. ✻

LAGUNARIA

Norfolk Island hibiscus

MALVACEAE

Genus, allied to *Hibiscus,* of one species of evergreen tree from coastal woodland in E. Australia. It is grown for its habit, its alternate, simple, entire, leathery leaves, and its solitary, 5-petalled, hibiscus-like flowers, produced from the upper leaf axils. In frost-prone areas, grow in a cool greenhouse. In warmer areas, grow as a specimen tree, or as a windbreak in a coastal garden. Contact with the seeds may irritate skin.

• **HARDINESS** Frost tender; may survive short periods just below 0°C (32°F) if the wood is well ripened in summer.

• **CULTIVATION** Under glass, grow in loam-based potting compost (JI No.3) in full light. When in full growth, water freely and apply a balanced liquid fertilizer monthly; water sparingly at other times. Outdoors, grow in moderately fertile, well-drained soil in full sun. Pruning group 1; may need restrictive pruning under glass.

• **PROPAGATION** Sow seed at 16°C (61°F) in spring, or root greenwood cuttings with bottom heat in summer.

• **PESTS AND DISEASES** Scale insects may be a problem under glass.

L. patersonii ♤ (Cow itch tree, Queensland pyramid tree). Pyramidal to columnar tree, loosely branched when young, denser when mature, with ovate to broadly lance-shaped, blunt-tipped leaves, 5–10cm (2–4in) long, matt, almost olive-green above, densely whitish grey-scaled beneath. Bears a succession of cup- to trumpet-shaped, pink to rose-pink flowers, 4–6cm (1½–2½in) across, mainly in summer, followed by ovoid seed capsules, 2.5cm (1in) long. More than one plant is needed to produce seed. ↕ to 15m (50ft), ↔ 8–12m (25–40ft). E. Australia (including Lord Howe Island, Norfolk Island). ❀ (min. 3–5°C/37–41°F)

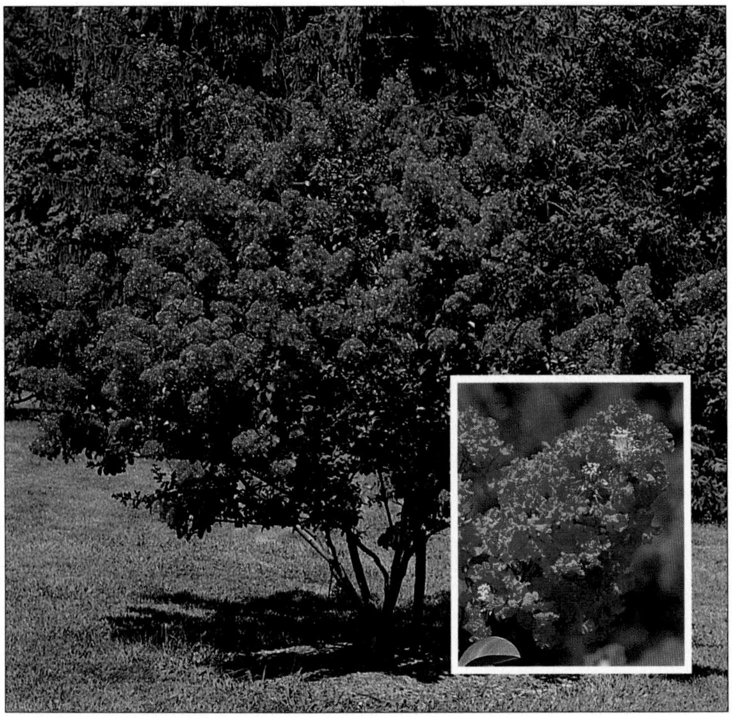

Lagerstroemia indica 'Seminole' (inset: flower detail)

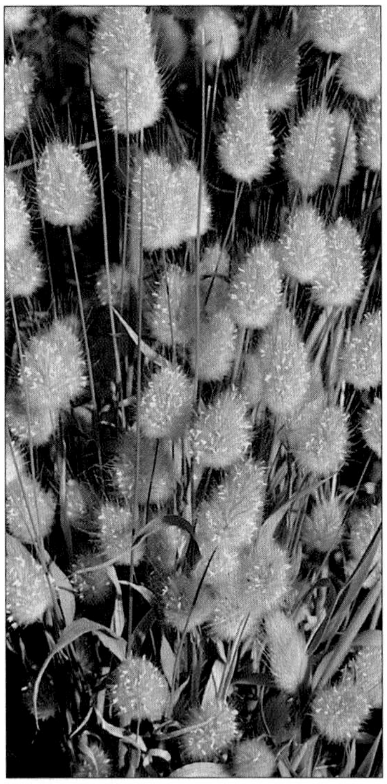

Lagurus ovatus

LAGURUS

Hare's tail

GRAMINEAE/POACEAE

Genus of one species of annual grass occurring on maritime sands on the Mediterranean coast of S. Europe and, more rarely, on dry wasteland inland. Valued for the effect of its ornamental flowerheads in summer, it is effective in groups in a herbaceous or mixed border. The flowerheads are also useful in fresh or dried arrangements; pick them before fully mature for drying.

• **HARDINESS** Fully hardy.

• **CULTIVATION** Grow in light, ideally sandy, moderately fertile, well-drained soil in full sun.

• **PROPAGATION** Sow seed *in situ* in spring, or in containers in a cold frame in autumn.

• **PESTS AND DISEASES** Trouble free.

L. ovatus ■ (Hare's tail). Tufted grass with arching, linear to narrowly lance-shaped, flat, pale green leaves, to 20cm (8in) long. Throughout summer, bears dense, ovoid to oblong-cylindrical, spike-like panicles, to 6cm (2½in) long, of softly hairy, often purple-tinged, pale green spikelets, which mature to pale creamy buff. ↕ to 50cm (20in), ↔ 30cm (12in). Mediterranean. ✻✻✻. **'Nanus'** is much more compact; ↕ to 12cm (5in).

LAMARCKIA

GRAMINEAE/POACEAE

Genus of one species of annual grass occurring in open habitats in the Mediterranean region. It has twisted, linear leaves and one-sided panicles of attractively coloured spikelets. Grow in a herbaceous, mixed, or annual border for its distinctive inflorescences, which are useful in both fresh and dried flower arrangements.

• **HARDINESS** Fully hardy.

• **CULTIVATION** Grow in light, sandy, well-drained soil in full sun.

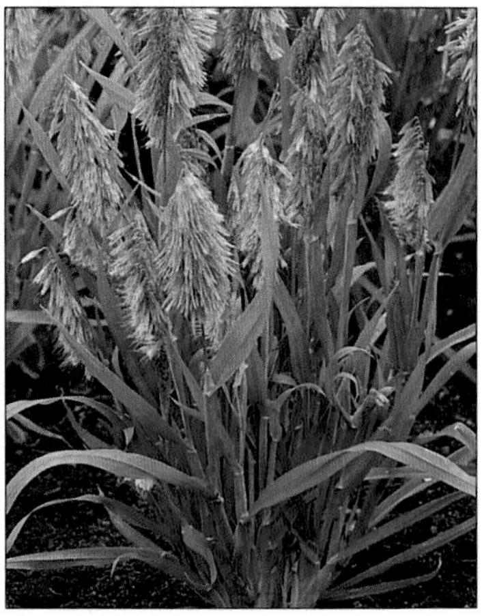

Lamarckia aurea

• **PROPAGATION** Make successional sowings *in situ* from early to late spring. Alternatively, sow in containers in a cold frame in late spring and transfer to the flowering site, to replace earlier sown plants after they have flowered. Plants from early sowings are usually past their best by midsummer.

• **PESTS AND DISEASES** Trouble free.

L. aurea ■ (Golden top, Toothbrush grass). Loosely tufted grass with wiry stems and flat, twisted, broadly linear, pale green leaves, to 12cm (5in) long. From mid-spring to summer, produces one-sided, oblong panicles, to 7cm (3in) long, of densely packed, downswept, bristled spikelets, shimmering golden yellow or whitish green, becoming silvery, and often purple flushed when mature. ↕ 30cm (12in), ↔ 25cm (10in). Mediterranean. ✻✻✻

LAMBERTIA

PROTEACEAE

Genus of 9 or 10 species of evergreen shrubs found on sandy or gravelly soils in heathland and woodland in Australia. They are cultivated for their slender, tubular flowers, which are solitary or borne in terminal clusters of 2–7, and surrounded by often colourful bracts; each flower has 4 narrow tepals that roll back like watch springs on opening. Leaves are usually narrow, simple, and entire, and are borne in pairs or whorls of 3. In frost-prone areas, grow in a cool or temperate greenhouse. In warmer climates, grow outdoors in a border.

• **HARDINESS** Generally frost tender; *L. formosa* may survive short periods near 0°C (32°F), provided the wood has been well ripened in summer.

• **CULTIVATION** Under glass, grow in a mix of 1 part loam and 3 parts each grit (or perlite) and peat, in full light. From spring to summer, water freely and apply a phosphate-free liquid fertilizer monthly; water sparingly in winter. Outdoors, grow in poor to moderately fertile, sharply drained, neutral to acid soil in full sun. Pruning group 1; may need restrictive pruning under glass.

• **PROPAGATION** Sow seed at 18°C (64°F) in spring, ideally singly in small containers. Root softwood cuttings in spring, or semi-ripe cuttings with bottom heat in summer; rooting may be slow and unreliable.

• **PESTS AND DISEASES** *Phytophthora* root rot may be a problem in moist soil.

L

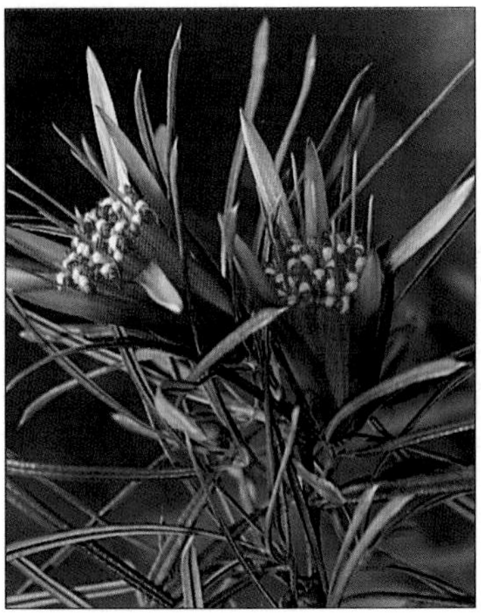

Lambertia formosa

L. formosa ▣ (Mountain devil). Erect shrub of open habit, spreading with age, and growing from a thickened, underground rootstock. Linear, sharp-tipped leaves, to 5cm (2in) long, usually borne in whorls of 3, are glossy, mid- to deep green above, white downy beneath. Bears clusters of up to 7 red flowers, 3–5cm (1¼–2in) long, surrounded by narrow, spreading, pink-flushed green bracts, some shorter than the flowers, some much longer, mainly from spring to summer, but often at other times of year. ↕ to 2m (6ft), ↔ to 1.5m (5ft). Australia (New South Wales). ❄ (borderline)

▷**Lambs' ears** see *Stachys byzantina*
▷**Lambs' lugs** see *Stachys byzantina*
▷**Lambs' tails** see *Stachys byzantina*
▷**Lambs' tongues** see *Stachys byzantina*
▷***Lamiastrum*** see *Lamium*
L. galeobdolon see *L. galeobdolon*

LAMIUM

syn. GALEOBDOLON, LAMIASTRUM
Dead nettle

LABIATAE/LAMIACEAE

Genus of about 50 species of annuals and usually rhizomatous perennials, occurring in habitats ranging from dry, open scrub to moist woodland, from Europe to Asia, and widespread in the Mediterranean and N. Africa. They have square stems and opposite, mainly ovate or kidney-shaped, coarsely toothed, wrinkled leaves, sometimes with coloured markings. The 2-lipped flowers are solitary, or borne in whorls in dense, leafy, spike-like inflorescences ("spikes"), mainly from late spring to summer. Grown mainly for their foliage, they provide good ground cover among shrubs or robust perennials. The larger species can be very invasive in moist, moderately fertile soils, but are less vigorous in poor soils; they may also be used in a border or in light woodland. Grow smaller, non-invasive species in a scree bed, rock garden, or alpine house.

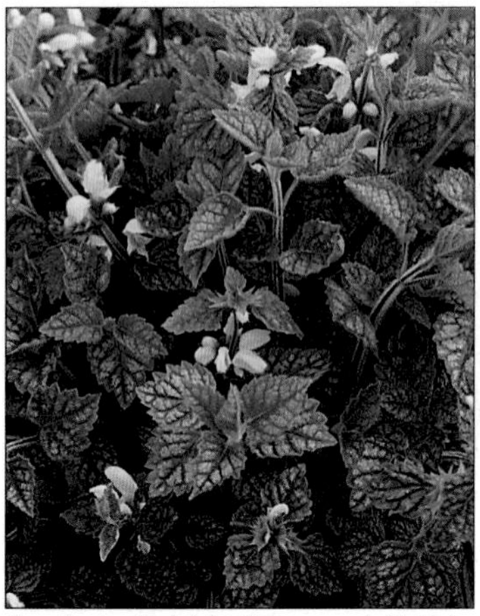

Lamium galeobdolon 'Hermann's Pride'

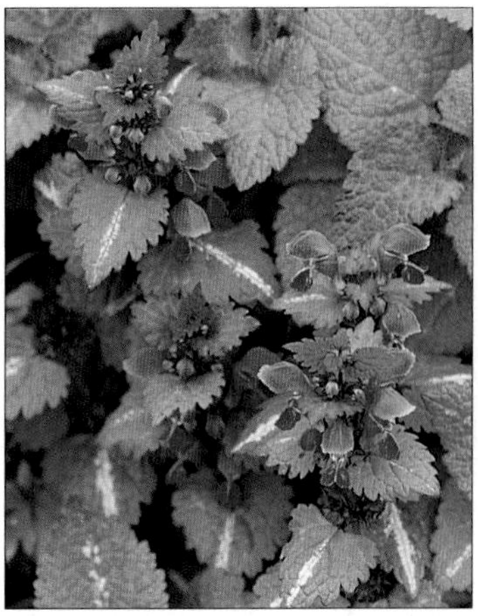

Lamium maculatum

• **HARDINESS** Fully hardy.
• **CULTIVATION** Grow the vigorous, ground-covering species in moist but well-drained soil in deep or partial shade. Site away from other small plants, and dig out rhizomes when necessary to confine spread. Grow *L. armenum* and *L. garganicum* subsp. *striatum* in sharply drained soil in full sun or partial shade. Protect *L. armenum* from excessive winter wet.
• **PROPAGATION** Sow seed in containers in a cold frame in autumn or spring. Divide in autumn or early spring. For small species, take stem-tip cuttings of non-flowering shoots in early summer.
• **PESTS AND DISEASES** Foliage may be damaged by slugs and snails.

L. armenum. Slow-growing, non-invasive, mat-forming or tufted perennial with obovate to diamond-shaped, scalloped, sometimes palmately lobed, mid-green leaves, 1cm (½in) long. In summer, produces solitary, long-tubed and hooded, pale pink to white flowers, to 5cm (2in) long, from the upper leaf axils. ↕ 5cm (2in), ↔ to 10cm (4in). Turkey (Anatolia). ❄❄❄
L. galeobdolon, syn. *Galeobdolon luteum*, *Lamiastrum galeobdolon* (Yellow archangel). Very invasive, rhizomatous and often stoloniferous perennial with erect or creeping stems bearing very broadly ovate or diamond-shaped, sometimes heart-shaped, toothed, mid-green leaves, to 6cm (2½in) long, often marked silver. Spikes of whorled, brown-spotted yellow flowers, to 2cm (¾in) long, are produced in summer. ↕ 60cm (24in), ↔ indefinite. Europe to W. Asia. ❄❄❄. The following cultivars are less invasive, but still require careful siting. **'Hermann's Pride'** ▣ forms a dense mat of small, ovate, heavily silver-streaked leaves, 3cm (1¼in) long. **'Silver Angel'** is more prostrate, with silver leaves; ↕ to 50cm (20in).

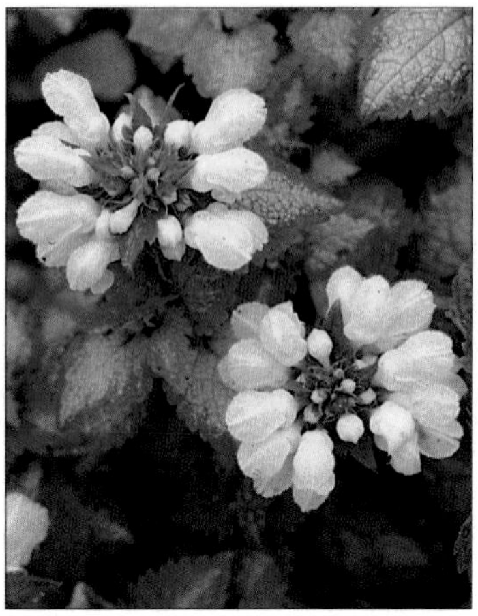

Lamium maculatum f. *album*

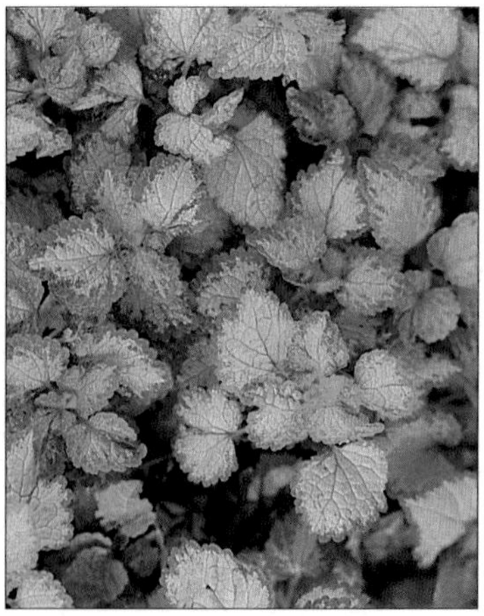

Lamium maculatum 'Beacon Silver'

L. garganicum. Mat- to clump-forming perennial with upright stems that bear heart-shaped, broadly ovate, toothed, mid-green leaves, to 7cm (3in) long. Produces upright spikes of whorled, pale pink flowers, to 3cm (1¼in) long, from the upper leaf axils in early summer. ↕ 45cm (18in), ↔ 50cm (20in). Italy, Greece to Turkey and Iraq. ❄❄❄. **'Golden Carpet'** has mid-green leaves variegated with gold, and produces pink-and-white striped flowers. **subsp. *striatum*** is compact, with abundant spikes of pink flowers, heavily spotted and streaked dark purple; ↕ to 15cm (6in), ↔ to 20cm (8in).
L. maculatum ▣ Low-growing, rhizomatous and stoloniferous perennial with prostrate and ascending stems bearing triangular-ovate, toothed, matt, mid-green leaves, 2–8cm (¾–3in) long, heart-shaped at the bases, and often mottled or zoned silvery white or pink. In summer, bears spikes of whorled, red-purple, sometimes white or pink flowers, to 2cm (¾in) long. Excellent ground cover. ↕ 20cm (8in), ↔ 1m (3ft). Europe and North Africa to W. Asia. ❄❄❄. **f. *album*** ▣ is mat-forming, with matt, mid-green leaves, zoned silvery white; it produces white flowers from mid-spring to midsummer; ↕ 15cm (6in), ↔ 60cm (24in); Europe. **'Aureum'**, syn. 'Gold Leaf', has yellow leaves with paler white centres, and produces pink flowers. **'Beacon Silver'** ▣ has silver leaves, narrowly margined green, and bears clear pale pink flowers. **'Cannon's Gold'** has gold leaves and purple flowers. **'Gold Leaf'** see 'Aureum'. **'Red Nancy'** has silver leaves with narrow, mid-green margins, and bears purplish red flowers. **'Sterling Silver'** has silver leaves and purple flowers. **'White Nancy'** 🏆 produces pure white flowers above silver leaves that are narrowly margined green; ↕ to 15cm (6in), ↔ to 1m (3ft) or more.

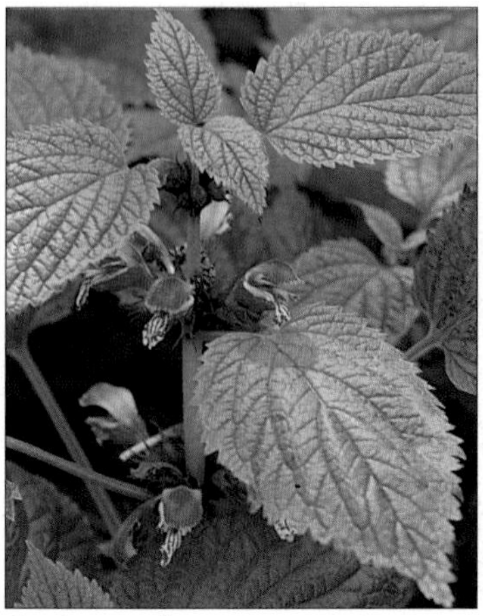

Lamium orvala

L. orvala ▣ Non-invasive, clump-forming perennial with broadly ovate to triangular, toothed, softly hairy, dark green leaves, 10–15cm (4–6in) long. Produces spikes of whorled, pinkish purple flowers, 3–4cm (1¼–1½in) long, from late spring to summer. ↕ to 60cm (24in), usually less, ↔ 30cm (12in). Central S. Europe. ❄❄❄. **f. *album*** bears white flowers.

LAMPRANTHUS

AIZOACEAE

Genus of 180 or more species of erect or prostrate, perennial succulents from semi-desert areas of South Africa, especially the coastal belt. The opposite, cylindrical or 3-angled leaves often redden in full sun. Daisy-like flowers are profusely borne from summer to early autumn. In frost-prone areas, grow in a temperate greenhouse; they may also be used for summer bedding, especially in arid conditions. In warmer areas, grow in a desert garden or in a border with other succulents.
• **HARDINESS** Frost tender.
• **CULTIVATION** Under glass, grow in standard cactus compost in full light. From late spring to late summer, water moderately and apply low-nitrogen fertilizer every 4–6 weeks; water very sparingly at other times. Outdoors, grow in poor, sharply drained soil in full sun. In frost-prone climates, lift in autumn and overwinter under glass. See also pp.48–49.

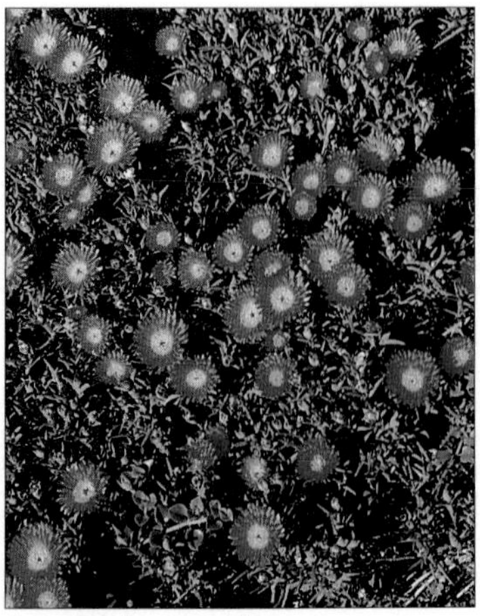

Lampranthus aurantiacus

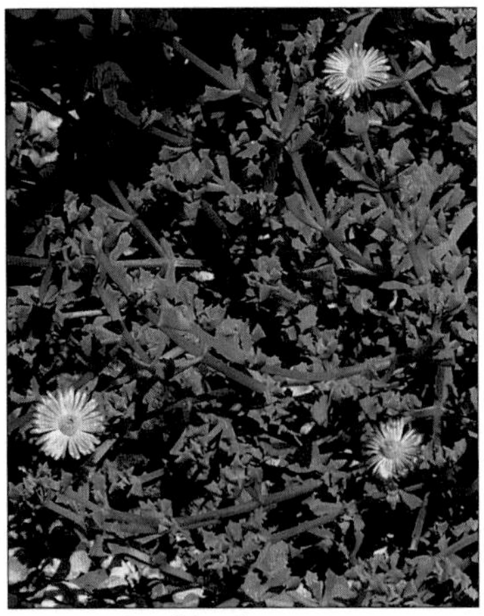

Lampranthus deltoides

• **PROPAGATION** Sow seed at 19–24°C (66–75°F) in spring. Root sections of stem in spring and summer.
• **PESTS AND DISEASES** Susceptible to mealybugs and, in flower, greenfly.

L. aurantiacus ■ Spreading, shrubby, sparsely branched succulent with semi-cylindrical, tapering, minutely spotted, grey-frosted, mid-green leaves, 2–3cm (¾–1¼in) long. Orange flowers, 4–5cm (1¼–2in) across, open in full sun from summer to early autumn. ↕ to 45cm (18in), ↔ indefinite. South Africa (Western Cape, Eastern Cape). ❄ (min. 7°C/45°F)
L. deltoides ■ syn. *Oscularia deltoides.* Spreading succulent with a mass of short stems bearing 3-angled, toothed, bluish grey leaves, 1cm (½in) long. From summer to early autumn, produces sometimes fragrant, pink to red flowers, 1.5–2cm (½–¾in) across. ↕ to 30cm (12in), ↔ indefinite. South Africa (Western Cape). ❄ (min. 7°C/45°F)
L. falcatus. Spreading, prostrate succulent with a mass of slender, tangled stems and 3-angled, curved, spotted, greyish green leaves, 6mm (¼in) long. Fragrant, purplish pink flowers, to 1.5cm (½in) across, are borne from summer to early autumn. ↕ to 30cm (12in), ↔ indefinite. South Africa (Western Cape). ❄ (min. 7°C/45°F)
L. haworthii ■ Trailing or semi-erect, freely branching succulent with semi-cylindrical, tapering, densely grey-frosted, pale green leaves, 2.5–4cm (1–1½in) long. Bright purplish pink flowers, to 7cm (3in) across, are borne from summer to early autumn. ↕ to 50cm (20in), ↔ indefinite. South Africa (Western Cape, Eastern Cape). ❄ (min. 7°C/45°F)

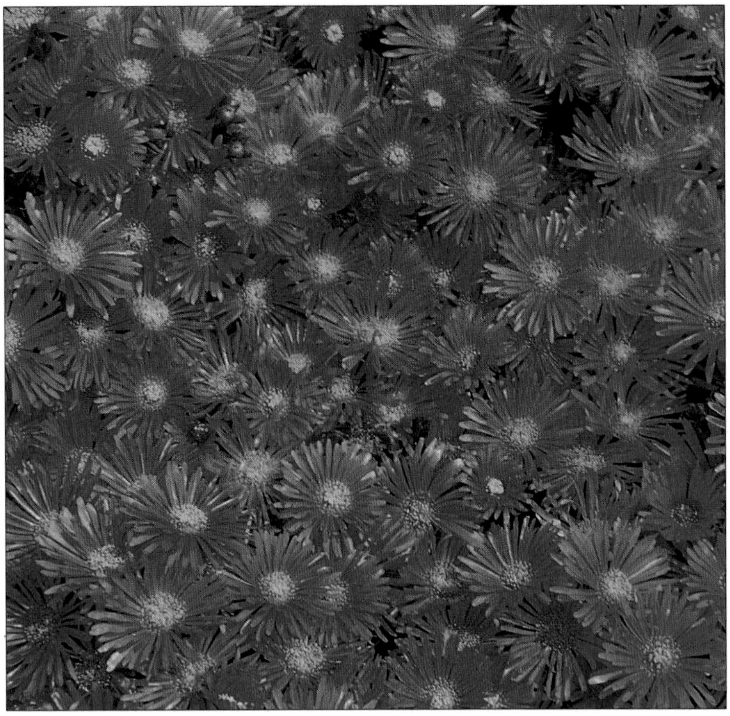

Lampranthus purpureus

L. purpureus ■ Trailing or semi-erect succulent with slender stems and branches bearing rounded, rough, bluish green leaves, to 3.5cm (1½in) long, shortly tapered at the tips. From summer to early autumn, produces pinkish purple flowers, to 3cm (1¼in) across. ↕ to 40cm (16in), ↔ indefinite. South Africa (Western Cape). ❄ (min. 7°C/45°F)
L. roseus, syn. *Mesembryanthemum multiradiatum.* Creeping or semi-erect succulent with 3-angled, mid-green to glaucous, grey-green leaves, 3cm (1¼in) long, covered with prominent, translucent dots. Bears pale rose-pink flowers, 4cm (1½in) across, from summer to early autumn. ↕ to 50cm (20in), ↔ indefinite. South Africa (Western Cape, Eastern Cape). ❄ (min. 7°C/45°F)
L. spectabilis ■ Variable, spreading, prostrate succulent with narrowly 3-angled to cylindrical, keeled, mid-green leaves, 5–8cm (2–3in) long, partly tinged red. Produces reddish purple or, occasionally, white flowers, 5–7cm (2–3in) across, from summer to early autumn. ↕ to 30cm (12in), ↔ indefinite. South Africa (Western Cape). ❄ (min. 7°C/45°F)

▷**Lancewood** see *Pseudopanax crassifolius*
Toothed see *P. ferox*

LANTANA

VERBENACEAE

Genus of 150 species of evergreen shrubs and perennials from tropical North, Central, and South America, and South Africa, usually occurring in pine woodland and on disturbed ground. They are grown for their small, 5-lobed, salverform flowers, grouped tightly into rounded, flattened, or domed, terminal heads. Leaves are simple and toothed, often wrinkled, and borne in opposite pairs or whorls of 3. In frost-prone areas, grow in a temperate greenhouse, or use as summer bedding. In warmer areas, grow in a border; low, spreading species are good ground cover on a bank or between shrubs. All parts may cause severe discomfort if ingested, and contact with foliage may irritate skin.

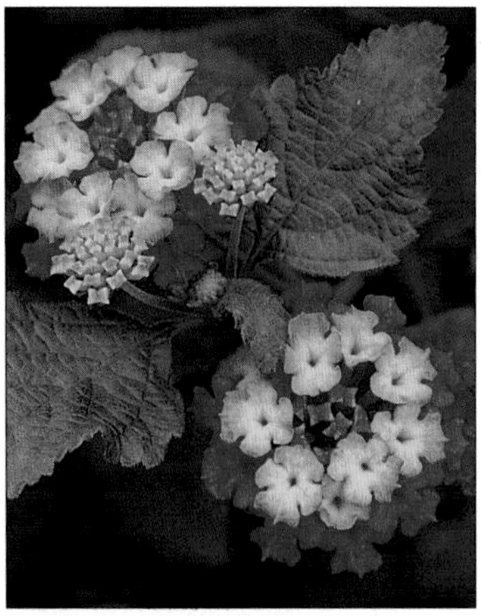

Lantana camara 'Radiation'

• **HARDINESS** Frost tender.
• **CULTIVATION** Under glass, grow in loam-based potting compost (JI No.3) in full light. During the growing season, water freely and apply a balanced liquid fertilizer monthly; keep just moist in winter. Outdoors, grow in fertile, moist but well-drained soil in full sun. Pruning group 9; may need restrictive pruning in late winter under glass.
• **PROPAGATION** Sow seed at 16–18°C (61–64°F) in spring, or root semi-ripe cuttings with bottom heat in summer.
• **PESTS AND DISEASES** Whiteflies, red spider mites, and powdery mildew may be troublesome under glass.

L. aculeata* f. *varia see *L. camara* f. *varia.*
***L. camara* cultivars.** Variable, often prickly-stemmed shrubs with ovate, finely wrinkled, slightly toothed, deep green leaves, 5–10cm (2–4in) long. Flowerheads 2.5–5cm (1–2in) across, in colours ranging from white to yellow and salmon-pink to red or purple, are borne from late spring to late autumn. ↕↔ 1–2m (3–6ft). ❄ (min. 10°C/50°F). **'Cream Carpet'** is low and spreading, with creamy white flowers; ↕ 30cm (12in), ↔ 75cm (30in). **'Fabiola'** bears bicoloured, salmon-pink and yellow flowers. **'Feston Rose'** ■ has bicoloured, pink and yellow flowers. **'Goldmine'** see 'Mine d'Or'. **'Mine d'Or'**, syn. 'Goldmine', produces golden yellow flowers. **'Radiation'** ■ bears bicoloured, orange and red flowers. **'Schloss Ortenburg'** bears bicoloured, brick-red and orange-yellow flowers. **'Snow White'** ■ bears white flowers.

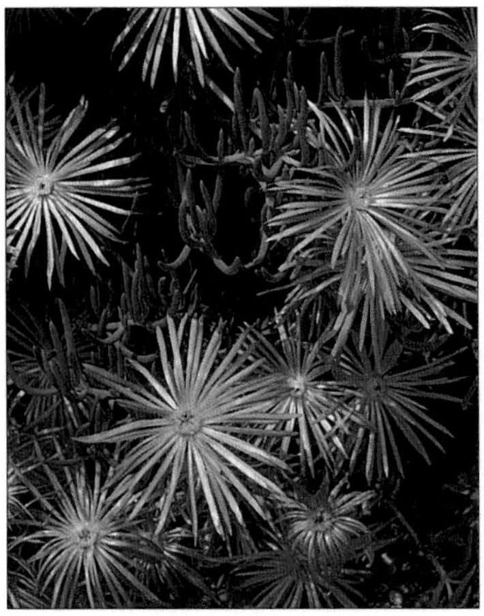

Lampranthus haworthii

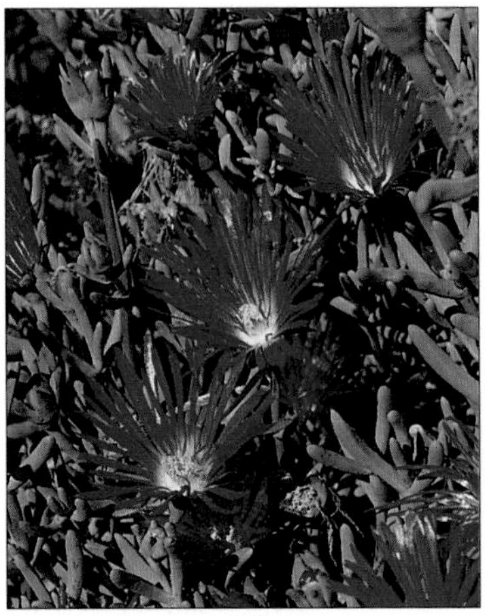

Lampranthus spectabilis

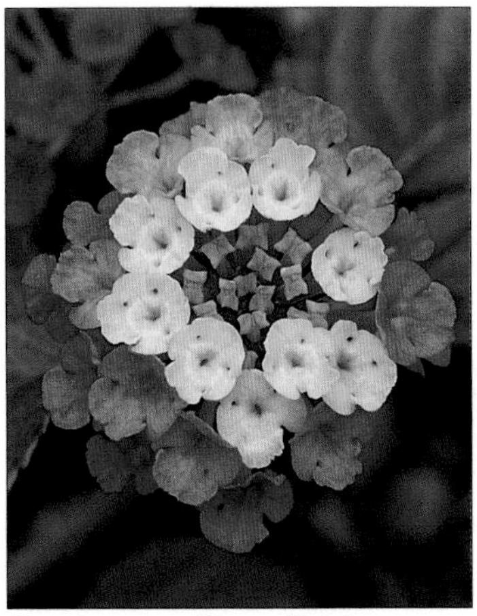

Lantana camara 'Feston Rose'

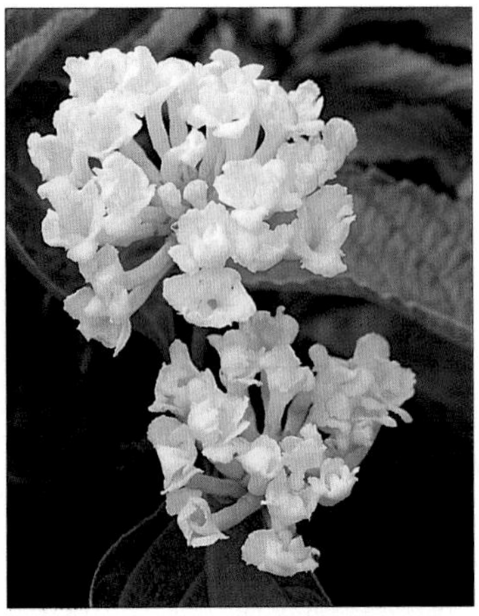

Lantana camara 'Snow White'

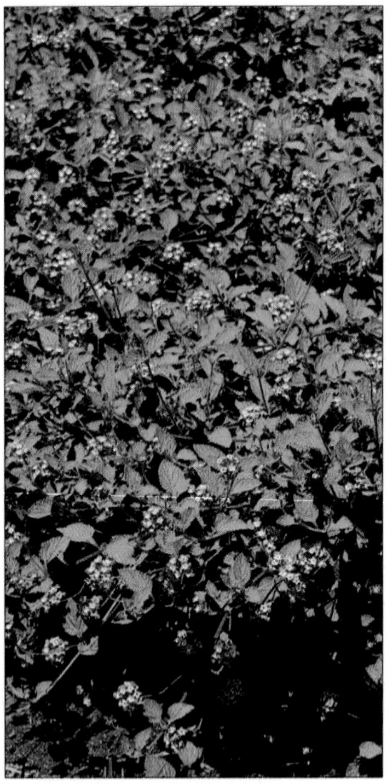

Lantana montevidensis

'Spreading Sunset' produces orange-yellow flowers that take on reddish pink tints with age. **f. *varia***, syn. *L. aculeata* f. *varia*, bears yellow flowers turning purple on the outside, orange inside.
L. delicatissima see *L. montevidensis.*
L. montevidensis ■ syn. *L. delicatissima, L. sellowiana.* Spreading shrub, often forming a dense mat, with slender, flexible stems, usually covered with coarse, short hairs. Ovate to oblong or lance-shaped, coarsely toothed, mid- to deep green leaves are 2.5–3.5cm (1–1½in) long. Bears long-stalked, domed flowerheads, 2–3cm (¾–1¼in) wide, of yellow-eyed, lilac-pink to violet flowers, to 1cm (½in) across, mainly in summer. ‡ 20–100cm (8–39in), ↔ 60–120cm (2–4ft). Tropical South America. ❀ (min. 10°C/50°F)
L. sellowiana see *L. montevidensis.*
***L.* 'Tangerine'** ■ Low, spreading, often prickly stemmed shrub, probably a cultivar of *L. camara*, with ovate to ovate-oblong, finely wrinkled, slightly toothed, deep green leaves, 5–10cm (2–4in) long. Bears orange flowerheads, 2.5–5cm (1–2in) across, from late spring to late autumn. ‡↔ 1–2m (3–6ft). ❀ (min. 10°C/50°F)

L

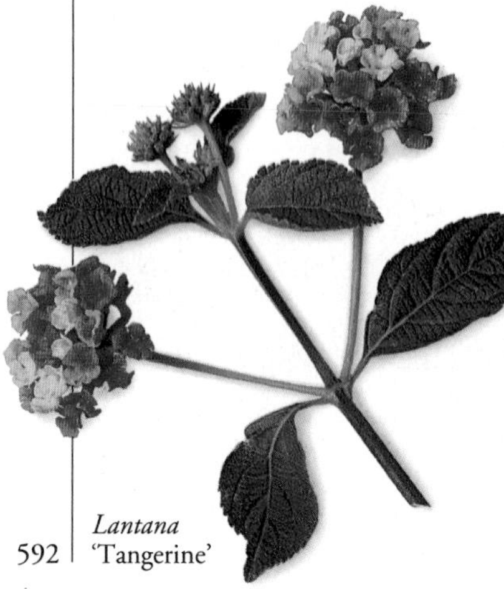

Lantana 'Tangerine'

L. tiliifolia. Coarsely hairy shrub with broadly ovate to elliptic or rounded, wrinkled, scalloped or toothed, mid-green leaves, 10cm (4in) long. Yellow or orange flowers, to 1cm (½in) across, ageing to brick red, are produced in short-stalked, domed flowerheads, to 6cm (2½in) wide, mainly in summer. ‡↔ 1.5m (5ft). Brazil. ❀ (min. 10°C/50°F)

▷**Lantern,**
Chinese see *Physalis alkekengi*
Japanese see *Hibiscus schizopetalus, Physalis alkekengi*
▷**Lanterns, Chinese** see *Nymania capensis*
▷**Lantern tree** see *Crinodendron hookerianum*

LAPAGERIA

LILIACEAE/PHILESIACEAE

Genus of one species of woody, twining, evergreen climber occurring in moist forest habitats in Chile. It is grown for its very showy, pendent, oblong-bell-shaped flowers. The leaves are alternate and ovate. In frost-prone climates, grow in a cool greenhouse; elsewhere, it is best grown against a shady wall.
• **HARDINESS** Frost hardy to half hardy.
• **CULTIVATION** Under glass, grow in lime-free (ericaceous) potting compost with added sharp sand, in bright filtered light. During the growing season, water moderately and apply a balanced liquid fertilizer monthly; water sparingly in winter. Outdoors, grow in humus-rich, moist but well-drained, neutral to acid soil in partial shade. In frost-prone areas, shelter from cold, drying winds and protect with a dry mulch in winter. Provide support. Pruning group 11, after flowering, but best left unpruned.
• **PROPAGATION** Sow seed that has been soaked in water for 48 hours, at 13–18°C (55–64°F) in spring. Take semi-ripe cuttings in late summer, or layer in autumn.
• **PESTS AND DISEASES** Aphids, mealybugs, scale insects, and thrips may be a problem, particularly under glass.

L. rosea ■ ♀ (Chilean bellflower). Twining climber, spreading slowly by suckers, with ovate, dark green leaves, to 12cm (5in) long. From summer to late autumn, oblong-bell-shaped, fleshy, pink to red flowers, to 9cm (3½in) long, are borne singly or in twos or threes in the upper leaf axils. ‡ 5m (15ft). Chile.

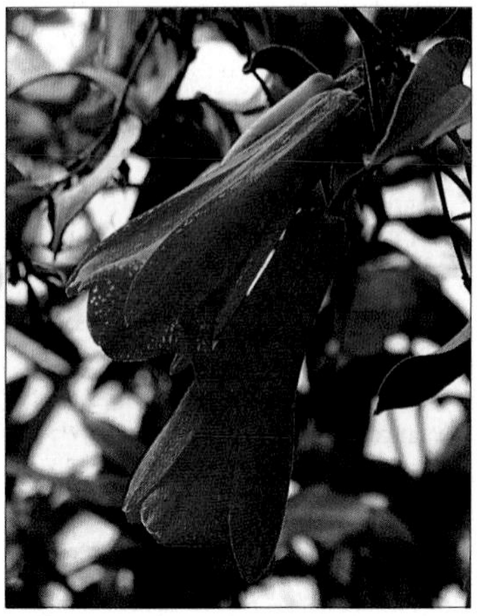

Lapageria rosea

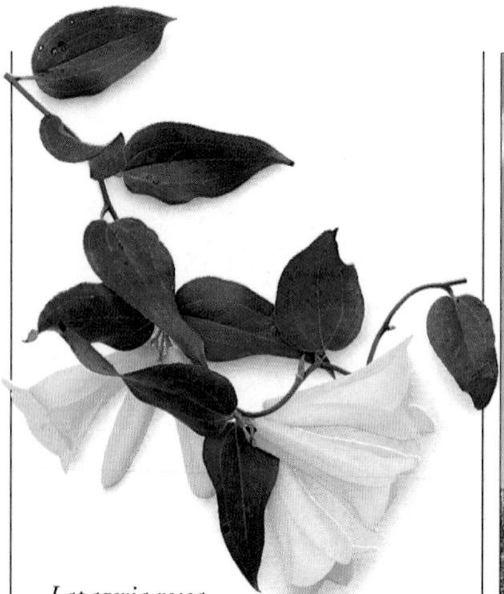

Lapageria rosea var. *albiflora*

❄❄ (borderline). **var. *albiflora*** ■ bears white flowers. **'Nash Court'** has soft pink flowers with deeper mottling.

▷***Lapeirousia cruenta*** see *Anomatheca laxa*
▷***Lapeirousia laxa*** see *Anomatheca laxa*
▷**Larch** see *Larix*
Dunkeld see *Larix* x *marschlinsii*
European see *Larix decidua*
Golden see *Pseudolarix amabilis*
Hybrid see *Larix* x *marschlinsii*
Japanese see *Larix kaempferi*
Siberian see *Larix sibirica*
Western see *Larix occidentalis*

LARDIZABALA

LARDIZABALACEAE

Genus of 2 species of monoecious, woody, twining, evergreen climbers from woodland in Chile. They are grown mainly for their ternate to 3-ternate, dark green leaves and striking flowers with 6 fleshy tepals. Train on a pergola or trellis, or against a wall.
• **HARDINESS** Frost hardy.
• **CULTIVATION** Grow in moderately fertile, well-drained soil in full sun or partial shade. In frost-prone areas, shelter from cold, drying winds. Pruning group 11, after flowering.
• **PROPAGATION** Sow seed in containers in a cold frame in spring, or take semi-ripe cuttings in late summer or autumn.
• **PESTS AND DISEASES** Trouble free.

L. biternata. Monoecious, sometimes dioecious climber. Ternate to 3-ternate, dark green leaves are composed of up to 9 ovate, rigid leaflets, 5–10cm (2–4in) long. From late autumn to winter, bears reflexed, 6-tepalled, purple-brown and white flowers, 2–2.5cm (¾–1in) across. Male flowers are borne in pendent racemes, 8–10cm (3–4in) long; female flowers are borne singly from the leaf axils. Edible, sausage-shaped purple berries are 5–8cm (2–3in) long. ‡ 3–4m (10–12ft). Chile. ❄❄

LARIX

Larch

PINACEAE

Genus of 10–14 species of upright, deciduous, monoecious, coniferous trees from coniferous forests of the N. hemisphere. They have attractive young foliage and normally brilliant, yellow to red autumn colour. The needle-shaped leaves are borne in loose spirals on the long shoots, and near-whorls on the short shoots. Terminal, erect, cylindrical or ovoid to conical, usually purple female cones are produced in spring, and turn woody and brown in the first season, usually persisting on the tree. Male cones are spherical to ovoid, and pink or yellow. Larches are useful as specimen trees, and are tolerant of a wide range of conditions.
• **HARDINESS** Fully hardy.
• **CULTIVATION** Grow in any deep, well-drained soil in full sun.
• **PROPAGATION** Sow seed in a seedbed in early spring, graft in winter, or root semi-ripe cuttings in summer under mist; cuttings are difficult to root.
• **PESTS AND DISEASES** Honey fungus and adelgids may be a problem. Canker may cause dieback.

L. decidua ■ ♀ ♤ syn. *L. europaea* (European larch). Conical, coniferous tree, often with a large, spreading crown when old, and with smooth, scaly grey bark, ridged on old trees. Linear, soft, pale green leaves, to 3.5cm (1½in) long, are borne on hairless shoots, which are straw-yellow during the first winter. Cylindrical to conical female cones, to

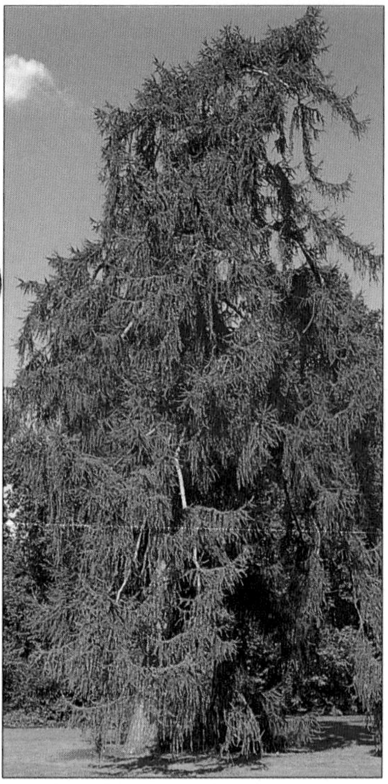

Larix decidua

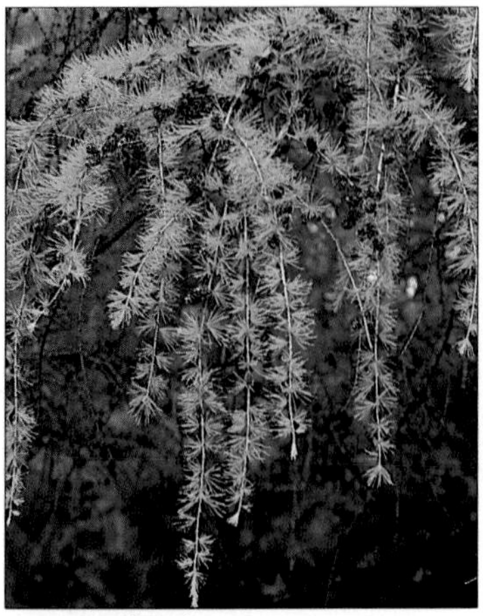

Larix occidentalis

3.5cm (1½in) long, have 40–50 scales, and protruding bracts. ↕30m (100ft) or more, ↔ 4–6m (12–20ft). Mountains of continental Europe. ❄❄❄. **'Corley'** is a dwarf, spreading or rounded shrub. Suitable for a rock garden; ↕↔ 1m (3ft).
L.* x *eurolepis see *L.* x *marschlinsii.*
L. europaea see *L. decidua.*
L. kaempferi 🏆 △ syn. *L. leptolepis* (Japanese larch). Conical, coniferous tree with fissured and scaly, rust-brown to grey bark. Very similar to *L. decidua,* but with purplish red winter shoots covered in a waxy bloom. Hairless shoots bear linear, grey-green or bluish green leaves, to 4cm (1½in) long. Conical female cones, to 3cm (1¼in) long, have reflexed scales and concealed bracts. ↕30m (100ft) or more, ↔ 4–6m (12–20ft). Japan. ❄❄❄. **'Blue Haze'** has brighter foliage.
L. leptolepis see *L. kaempferi.*
L.* x *marschlinsii △ (*L. decidua* x *L. kaempferi*) syn. *L.* x *eurolepis* (Dunkeld larch, Hybrid larch). Fast-growing, conical, coniferous tree with bloomed, slightly hairy yellow shoots, and linear, grey-green leaves, to 4cm (1½in) long. Conical female cones, to 3cm (1¼in) long, have slightly reflexed scales and only a few visible bract scales. ↕to 30m (100ft), ↔ to 6m (20ft). Garden origin. ❄❄❄
L. occidentalis ▣ △ (Western larch). Coniferous tree with a narrowly conical crown and scaly, red-brown to brown bark, becoming furrowed and fissured with age. Pointed, linear, blue-green to grey-green leaves, 2.5–4cm (1–1½in) long, each with 2 white bands beneath, are held on stout, orange-brown shoots, which are hairy when young. Female cones, 2.5–4.5cm (1–1¾in) long, are cylindrical to ovoid, with protruding bracts. ↕to 25m (80ft) or more, ↔ to 5m (15ft). W. North America. ❄❄❄
L. sibirica △ syn. *L. russica* (Siberian larch). Conical, coniferous tree with scaly, rust-brown bark and bright yellow or yellowish grey shoots, which are hairy when young. Narrowly linear leaves, 2–4cm (¾–1½in) long, are bright green, each with 2 white bands beneath. Ovoid female cones, 3–4cm (1¼–1½in) long, have hairy scales. ↕10–30m (30–100ft), ↔ to 5m (15ft). N.E. Europe to Russia (Siberia) and China. ❄❄❄
L. russica see *L. sibirica.*

▷**Larkspur** see *Consolida, C. ajacis*

LATANIA
Latan palm

ARECACEAE/PALMAE

Genus of 3 species of single-stemmed palms from seasonally dry areas, often near the coast, in the Mascarene Islands. Fan-shaped, grey- to light green leaves are borne in terminal clusters, with bowl-shaped, 3-petalled flowers borne on separate male and female panicles between them. Where temperatures fall below 16°C (61°F), grow in a warm greenhouse; in warmer climates, grow as specimen plants.
• **HARDINESS** Frost tender.
• **CULTIVATION** Under glass, grow in loam-based potting compost (JI No.3) with added leaf mould and sharp sand, in full light with shade from the hottest sun. In growth, water freely and apply a balanced liquid fertilizer monthly; water

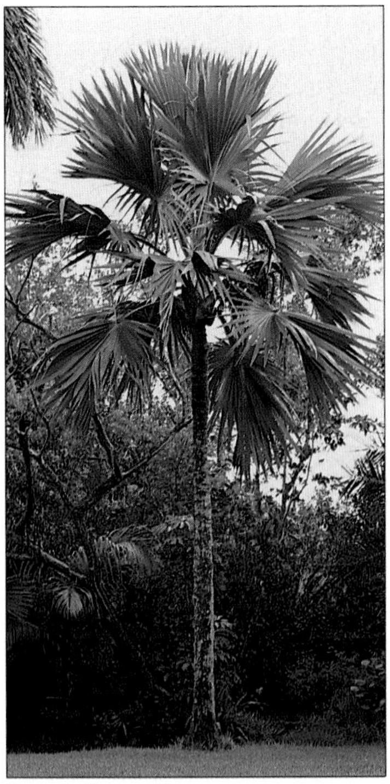
Latania lontaroides

sparingly in winter. Pot on or top-dress in spring. Outdoors, grow in moderately fertile, well-drained soil in full sun.
• **PROPAGATION** Sow seed at 27°C (81°F) in spring.
• **PESTS AND DISEASES** Red spider mites may be troublesome under glass.

L. loddigesii 🌴 Small to medium-sized palm with blue-green leaf-blades, to 1.5m (5ft) across, deeply divided into many narrow lobes. Bears pale green or greenish white flowers in panicles to 1.5m (5ft) long, usually in summer. ↕10–16m (30–52ft), ↔ 3–3.5m (10–11ft). Mascarene Islands (Mauritius). ❁ (min. 16°C/61°F)
L. lontaroides ▣ 🌴 Small to medium-sized palm with deeply lobed, grey-green leaf-blades, to 1.5m (5ft) across, with red-purple-flushed bases and leaf-stalks. Greenish white to cream flowers are borne in panicles to 1.5m (5ft) long, usually in summer. ↕10–16m (30–52ft), ↔ 3–3.5m (10–11ft). Mascarene Islands (Réunion). ❁ (min. 16°C/61°F)
L. verschaffeltii 🌴 Small to medium-sized palm with yellow-margined, light green leaf-blades, to 1.2m (4ft) across, deeply divided into many slender lobes. Bears greenish white to cream flowers, usually in summer; male panicles are up to 3m (10ft) long, females to 1.7m (5½ft) long. ↕12–16m (40–52ft), ↔ 4m (12ft). Mascarene Islands (Rodrigues). ❁ (min. 16°C/61°F)

▷**Latan palm** see *Latania*

LATHRAEA

SCROPHULARIACEAE

Genus of 7 species of leafless, mainly subterranean, parasitic perennials from damp woodland in temperate Europe and Asia. Branching rhizomes bear usually rounded, scale-like, fleshy, ivory to mauve leaves. They are cultivated for their unusual, tubular, 2-lipped, white to mauve flowers, borne in raceme-like inflorescences at ground level in spring.

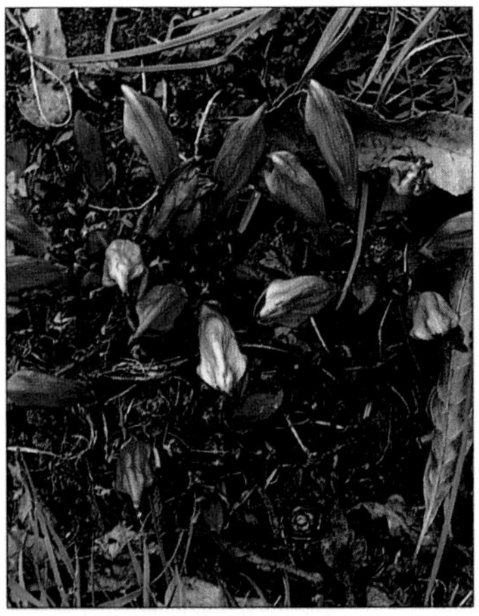
Lathraea clandestina

Grow at the base of a host tree or shrub. *L. clandestina* is parasitic on willow (*Salix*), poplar (*Populus*), and alder (*Alnus*). Other species parasitize other trees and are usually host-specific.
• **HARDINESS** Fully hardy.
• **CULTIVATION** Grow in moist but well-drained soil in partial shade. Mulch with leaf mould in autumn.
• **PROPAGATION** Scatter seed at the base of a suitable host plant as soon as ripe.
• **PESTS AND DISEASES** Trouble free.

L. clandestina ▣ (Purple toothwort). Parasitic, rhizomatous perennial with opposite, kidney-shaped, stem-clasping, scale-like white leaves, 5mm (¼in) long. Racemes of 4–8 tubular, 2-lipped mauve flowers, to 3cm (1¼in) long, are borne just above the ground in early and mid-spring. ↕2cm (¾in), ↔ indefinite. W. Europe. ❄❄❄

LATHYRUS
Everlasting pea

LEGUMINOSAE/PAPILIONACEAE

Genus of 150 species of annuals and herbaceous or evergreen perennials from sunny, sandy or shingle banks, grassy slopes, wasteland, or open woodland in N. temperate regions, N. and E. Africa, and temperate South America. They are grown for their showy, pea-like, often scented flowers, in many colours, which are produced from the leaf axils, either singly or in racemes. Stems are usually winged, and bear alternate, pinnate leaves. Many are climbers (with tendrils); others are clump-forming. The climbers are useful for growing through shrubs or over a bank. Sweet peas (*L. odoratus*) are suitable for a trellis or arch, or an annual border for cut flowers and exhibition. Clump-forming species and cultivars are suitable for a rock garden, woodland garden, or herbaceous border. Seeds may cause mild stomach upset if ingested.
• **HARDINESS** Fully hardy to frost hardy.
• **CULTIVATION** Grow in fertile, humus-rich, well-drained soil in full sun or light dappled shade. Climbers need support. For the best flowers from *L. odoratus,* incorporate well-rotted organic matter in the season before planting, and apply a balanced liquid fertilizer every 2 weeks while in growth. Dead-head regularly. Sweet peas are usually grown on cane pyramids or trellis. Long-stemmed, exhibition-quality blooms are grown as cordons in beds prepared in autumn. Bush sweet peas are dwarf, largely self-supporting, non-climbing cultivars.
• **PROPAGATION** Soak seed and sow in containers in a cold frame in early spring; seed of annuals may also be sown *in situ* in mid-spring. Sweet peas may also be sown in autumn: pre-soak or chip seed and sow *in situ* in mild areas, or in containers in a cold frame where frosts are severe. Divide perennials in early spring, although they sometimes resent disturbance.
• **PESTS AND DISEASES** Aphids, slugs, snails, and thrips may be troublesome. *L. odoratus* may suffer from powdery mildew, *Fusarium* wilt, foot rot, root rot, and viruses.

L. aureus, syn. *L. luteus* of gardens, *L. vernus* var. *aurantiacus, Orobus aureus.* Clump-forming herbaceous perennial with upright, unwinged stems, and dark green leaves divided into 3–5 pairs of elliptic leaflets, 3.5–5cm (1½–2in) long. Bears one-sided racemes of 8–25 yellow-orange flowers, 1.5–2cm (½–¾in) long, from late spring to early summer. ↕to 60cm (24in), ↔ 30cm (12in). Ukraine (Crimea), Caucasus, N. Turkey. ❄❄❄
L. chloranthus. Erect or scrambling, sparsely branched, annual climber with slender, winged stems, and mid-green leaves composed of one pair of elliptic leaflets, 2–6cm (¾–2½in) long. Sulphur- to bright yellow flowers, 1.5–2.5cm (½–1in) long, are produced singly or in pairs in summer. ↕to 70cm (28in), sometimes more. C. and E. Turkey, N. Iraq, Iran, Armenia. ❄
L. gmelinii, syn. *L. luteus.* Clump-forming herbaceous perennial, similar to *L. aureus,* with upright, unwinged stems, and mid-green leaves divided into 3–6 pairs of oval leaflets, to 10cm (4in) long. Produces one-sided racemes of 4–15 brown-striped, orange-yellow flowers, 2.5–3cm (1–1¼in) long, from late spring to midsummer. ↕to 90cm (36in), ↔ 30cm (12in). C. and S. Urals, Mountains of C. Asia. ❄❄❄
L. grandiflorus ▣ (Everlasting pea). Herbaceous, perennial climber,

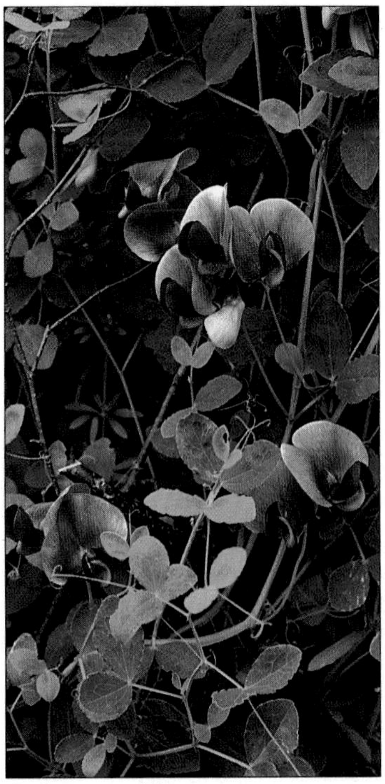
Lathyrus grandiflorus

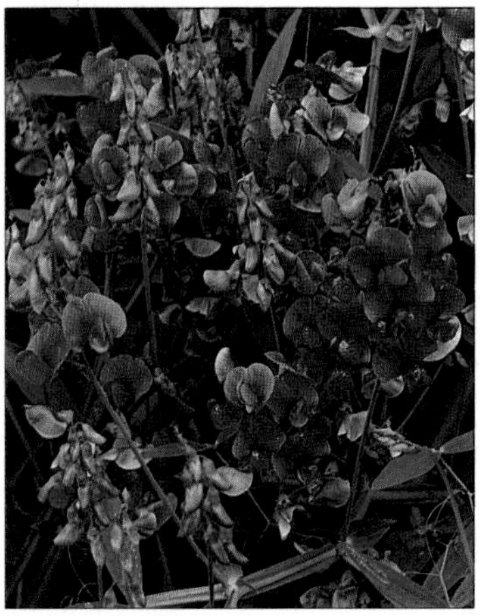

Lathyrus latifolius

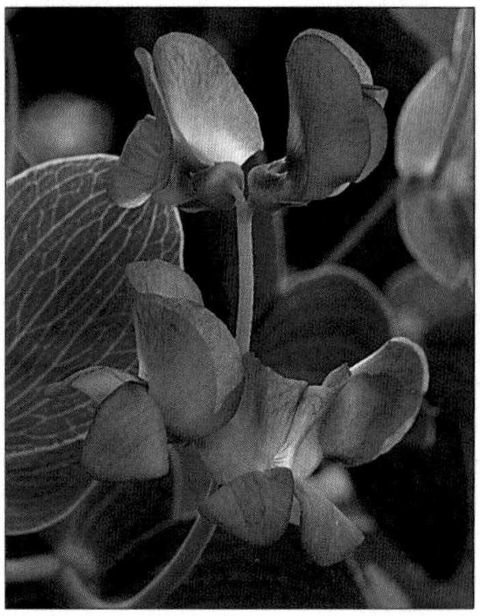

Lathyrus nervosus

spreading by suckers, with unwinged stems. Mid-green leaves usually consist of one pair of ovate to elliptic leaflets, to 5cm (2in) long. Racemes of 1 or 2 (sometimes up to 4) pink-purple and red flowers, to 3cm (1¼in) long, are produced in summer. ↕ 1.5m (5ft). Italy (including Sicily), Slovenia to Albania, Bulgaria. ❄❄❄

L. latifolius ◼ ♕ (Everlasting pea, Perennial pea). Herbaceous, perennial climber with winged stems. Blue-green leaves consist of one pair of oblong-elliptic leaflets, 8–11cm (3–4½in) long, with 2 broad stipules. Racemes of 6–11 pink to purple flowers, 1.5–3cm (½–1¼in) long, are produced from summer to early autumn. ↕ 2m (6ft) or more. S. Europe. ❄❄❄. **'Blushing Bride'** produces pink-flushed white flowers. **'White Pearl'** ♕ bears pure white flowers.

L. linifolius var. montanus, syn. *L. montanus* (Bitter vetch). Tufted herbaceous perennial with upright, winged stems, and blue-green leaves divided into 1–4 pairs of oval to linear leaflets, to 5cm (2in) long. From spring to early summer, produces long-stalked racemes of 2–6 reddish purple flowers, 1.5cm (½in) long. Suitable for a wild-flower garden. ↕ 30–40cm (12–16in), ↔ 20–40cm (8–16in). W. and C. Europe, Asia. ❄❄❄

L. luteus see *L. gmelinii.*

L. luteus of gardens see *L. aureus.*

L. magellanicus of gardens see *L. nervosus.*

L. montanus see *L. linifolius* var. *montanus.*

L. nervosus ◼ syn. *L. magellanicus* of gardens (Lord Anson's blue pea). Herbaceous, perennial climber with unwinged stems. Prominently veined, leathery, grey-green leaves consist of one pair of ovate leaflets, to 4cm (1½in) long, with prominent stipules. Long-stalked racemes of 3 fragrant, purplish blue flowers, to 2cm (¾in) long, are produced in summer. ↕ 5m (15ft). South America. ❄❄

L. odoratus ♕ (Sweet pea). Annual climber with winged stems, and mid- to dark green leaves consisting of one pair of ovate-elliptic leaflets, 5–6cm (2–2½in) long. From summer to early autumn, produces racemes of 2–4 fragrant flowers, to 3.5cm (1½in) long, with wine-red standard petals and purple wings and keels. ↕ to 2m (6ft). Italy (including Sicily). ❄❄❄. Many cultivars have been developed. "Old-fashioned", sweet peas were the earliest, selected mainly for their scent and intense colours; they have prominent stipules, and produce racemes of up to 4 small, highly scented flowers in single or mixed shades of white, red, pink, and blue. They are suitable for growing as a bush and for cutting. ↕ 2–2.5m (6–8ft). Newer developments, of which by far the most widely grown are the Spencer cultivars, have led to greater variety in the colour of the blooms, which occur in most colours except yellow. Spencer cultivars are vigorous, with prominent stipules, and bear racemes of 4 or 5 variably scented flowers, which may be single colours, bicoloured, picotee, or variably marked in contrasting colours, with upright standards and spreading wing petals, both waved. They are excellent for cut flowers. ↕ 2–2.5m (6–8ft), much more as cordons.

Cultivars of **Bijou Group** ◼ are bushy, with prominent stipules; they bear racemes of up to 4 slightly scented flowers, to 3.5cm (1½in) long, with small, wavy petals, in shades of pink, blue, red, or white. Require only limited support. ↕↔ to 45cm (18in). Cultivars of **Continental Group** are semi-climbing and vigorous, with prominent stipules, and bear racemes of up to 5 flowers in shades of red, blue, pink, or white, with flat standards and slightly waved, spreading wing petals. Suitable as a bush and for cutting. Require support. ↕ 1–1.1m (3–3½ft). **Early Multiflora** cultivars are vigorous, with prominent stipules, and bear racemes of 5–8 waved, lightly scented flowers in deep rose-pink, salmon-pink, lavender-blue, mid-blue, scarlet, or white. Suitable as a bush and ideal for cutting. Best in a cool greenhouse. ↕ 2–2.5m (6–8ft). **Explorer Group** ♕ cultivars have prominent stipules, and produce racemes of up to 4 waved flowers in mid-blue, navy blue, crimson, scarlet, rose-pink, light pink, purple, or white. Dead-head to prolong flowering. Grow as a bush, for cut flowers, or as ground cover if sown in autumn and pinched out twice. ↕ 60cm (24in), ↔ to 1m (3ft). Cultivars of **Galaxy Group** are vigorous, with prominent stipules, and bear racemes of up to 8 waved flowers in rose-pink, salmon-pink, scarlet, white, or lavender-blue. Grow as a bush (with support); ideal for cutting. ↕ 2–2.5m (6–8ft). **'Jayne Amanda'** ◼ ♕ (Spencer cultivar) bears racemes of usually 4,

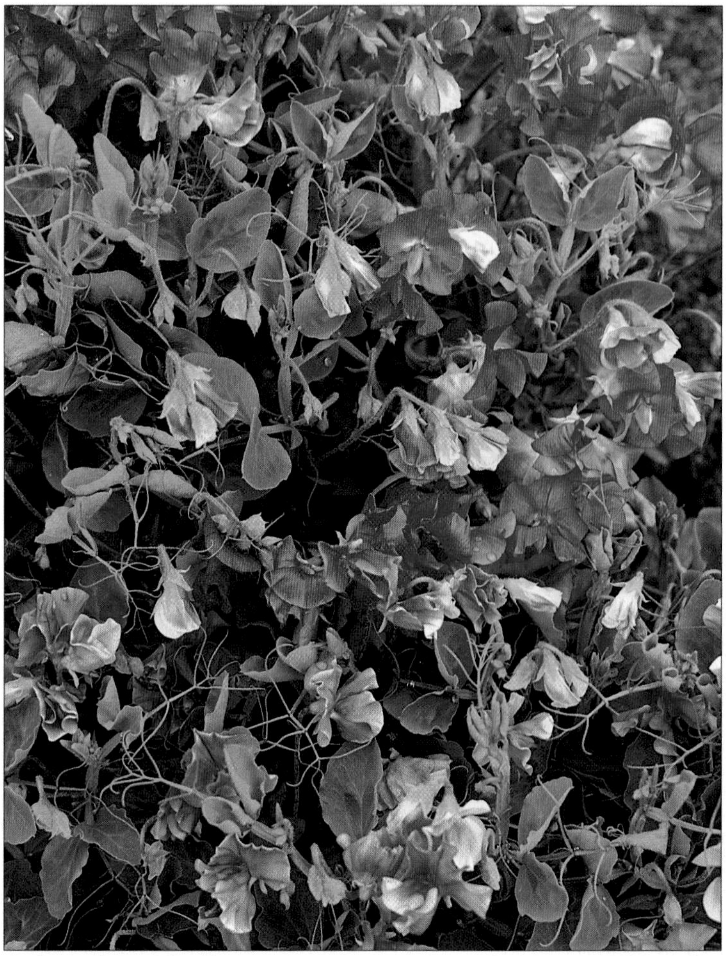

Lathyrus odoratus Bijou Group

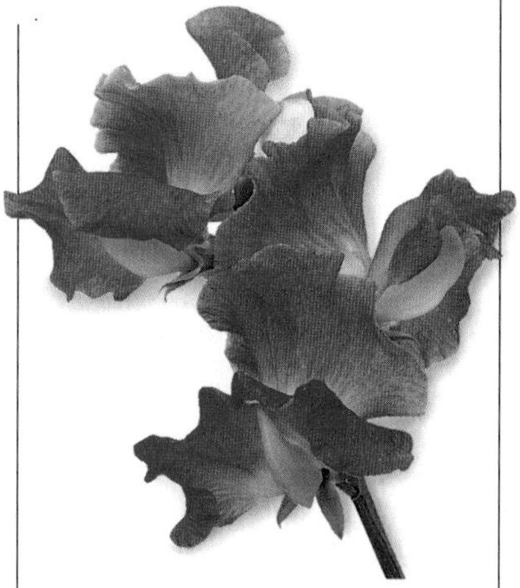

Lathyrus odoratus 'Jayne Amanda'

rarely 5, rose-pink flowers. Suitable as a cordon or bush. Cultivars of **Jet Set Group** are bushy, with prominent stipules, and bear racemes of up to 5 flowers in shades of red, blue, pink, and white; the upright standards and spreading wing petals are both slightly waved. Grow as a bush, or in rows for cutting (with support). ↕ 1–1.2 (3–4ft). Cultivars of **Knee-hi Group** are bushy, with prominent stipules, and bear racemes of up to 4 flowers in shades of red, blue, pink, and white, with the upright standards and spreading wing petals both slightly waved. Suitable as a bush with support. ↕ to 1m (3ft). **'Lady Fairbairn'** (Spencer cultivar) produces racemes of usually 4 lilac-pink flowers. Suitable as a cordon or bush. ↕ 2–2.5m (6–8ft). **'Mrs. Bernard Jones'** ♕ (Spencer cultivar) bears racemes of usually 4, occasionally 5, white-flushed, almond-pink flowers. Suitable as a cordon or bush. **Multiflora** cultivars are vigorous, with prominent stipules, and bear racemes of 5–8 waved, lightly scented flowers in mid-blue, lavender-blue, deep rose-pink, salmon-pink, scarlet, or white. Suitable as a bush and for cutting. Best in a cool greenhouse. ↕ 2–2.5m (6–8ft). **'Noel Sutton'** ◼ ♕ (Spencer cultivar) produces racemes of 4, sometimes 5, heavily scented, mid-blue flowers, tinged mauve. Grow as a cordon or bush. **'Pink Cupid'** has prominent stipules, and bears racemes of 3–6 small, plain, strongly scented flowers, with pink standards and whitish pink wing petals. Ideal for growing in a tub, trough, or hanging basket. ↕ 15cm (6in), ↔ 45cm (18in). **'Quito'** (Old-

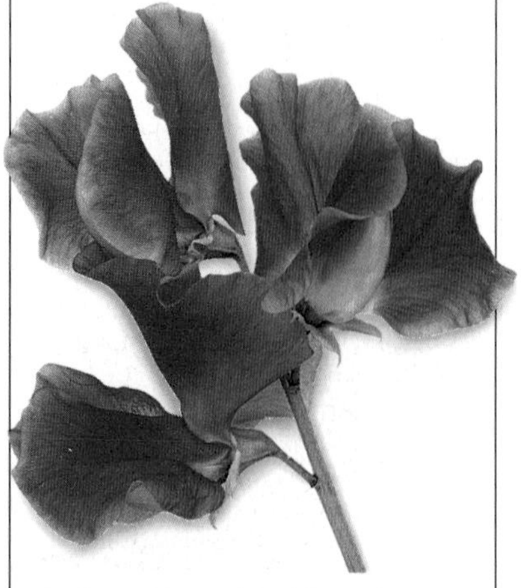

Lathyrus odoratus 'Noel Sutton'

L

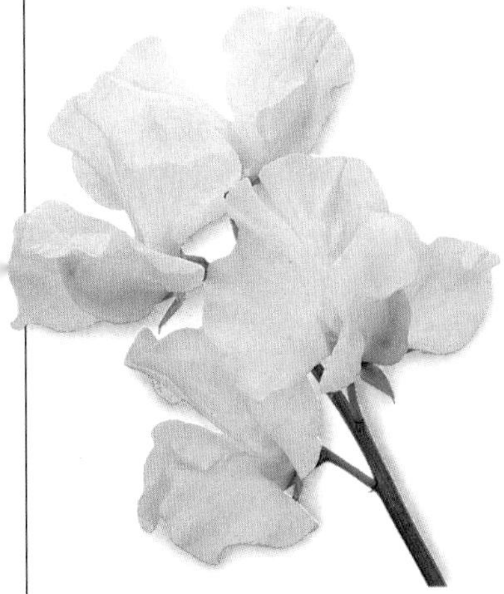

Lathyrus odoratus 'White Supreme'

fashioned) has prominent stipules, and bears racemes of up to 4 small, plain, strongly scented flowers, with maroon standards and variously coloured wing petals. **Snoopea Group** cultivars lack tendrils, have prominent stipules, and bear racemes of up to 4 waved flowers in shades of red, blue, pink, and white. Dead-head to prolong flowering. Grow as a bush, or as ground cover if sown in autumn and pinched out twice. ↕60cm (24in), ↔ to 1m (3ft). Cultivars of **Supersnoop Group** are similar to Snoopea Group, but slightly stronger-growing. **'White Supreme'** ■ ♀ (Spencer cultivar) is vigorous, and bears racemes of usually 4, rarely 5, lightly scented white flowers. Grow as a cordon or bush; ideal for cutting.
L. pratensis (Common vetchling, Meadow vetchling). Variable, herbaceous, perennial climber with unwinged stems. Bluish green leaves are composed of one pair of linear-lance-shaped to elliptic leaflets, to 4cm (1½in) long. From late spring to summer, bears long-stalked racemes of 2–12 yellow flowers, to 1.5cm (½in) long. Suitable for a wildflower garden. ↕70–120cm (28–48in), ↔ to 2m (6ft). Europe, N. Africa to W. Asia. ✽✽✽
L. pubescens ■ Herbaceous, perennial climber with unwinged stems. Mid- to dark green leaves are composed of 1 pair (sometimes 2) of elliptic to lance-shaped leaflets, to 8cm (3in) long, with prominent stipules. In summer, bears long-stalked racemes of 6–16 pale to deep lilac-blue flowers, 0.8–1.5cm (⅜–½in) long. ↕3m (10ft). Chile, Argentina. ✽✽

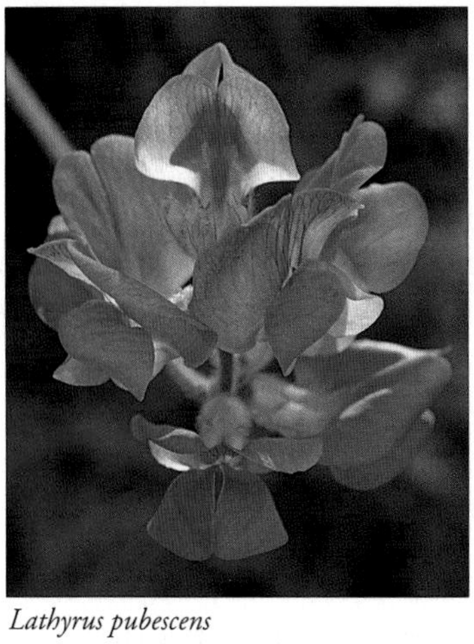

Lathyrus pubescens

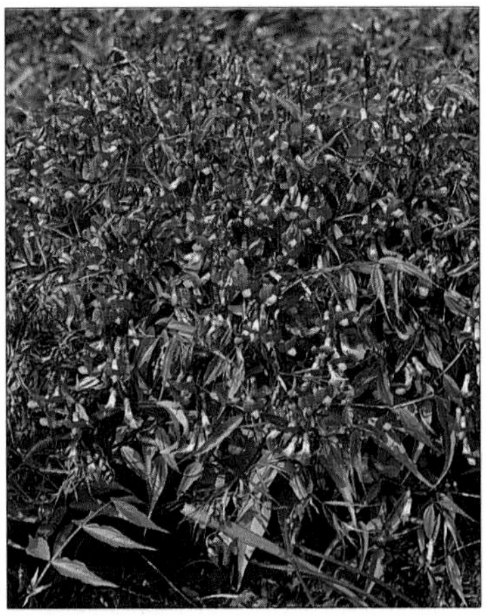

Lathyrus vernus

L. rotundifolius (Persian everlasting pea). Herbaceous, perennial climber with winged stems. Mid-green leaves consist of one pair of ovate to elliptic leaflets, 3–4.5cm (1¼–1¾in) long. Small racemes of 4–11 dark purplish pink to brownish red flowers, 1.5–2cm (½–¾in) long, are produced in summer. ↕1m (3ft). Ukraine (Crimea), Caucasus, E. Turkey, Iraq, Iran. ✽✽✽
L. sativus (Chickling pea). Scrambling, annual climber with angular, winged stems, and mid-green leaves divided into 2 or 3 pairs of narrowly elliptic, pointed leaflets, 4–6cm (1½–2½in) long. In summer, produces solitary, dainty blue flowers, to 1.5cm (½in) long, that fade to white and sometimes have pink veins. Largely grown for animal fodder, but suitable for a mixed or herbaceous border. ↕to 1m (3ft), ↔ to 45cm (18in). C. and S. Europe, N. Africa, S.W. Asia. ✽✽✽
L. sylvestris (Perennial pea). Herbaceous, perennial climber with winged stems. Mid-green leaves consist of one pair of slender, linear-elliptic leaflets, 5–15cm (2–6in) long, with one pair of narrow stipules. Long-stalked racemes of 3–8 pink flowers, to 2cm (¾in) long, with purplish pink wing petals, are produced from summer to early autumn. ↕2m (6ft). Europe, N.W. Africa, Caucasus. ✽✽✽.
L. tingitanus. Herbaceous, perennial climber with slender, winged stems, and mid- to deep green leaves divided into one pair of narrowly elliptic to oblong-elliptic or linear-elliptic leaflets, 4–8cm (1½–3in) long. Pale pink or crimson-magenta flowers, 2–3cm (¾–1¼in) long, are produced singly or in twos or threes, in summer. ↕to 1.5m (5ft). Spain, Portugal, Azores, Canary Islands, Morocco, Algeria, Sardinia. ✽✽
L. vernus ■ ♀ syn. *Orobus vernus* (Spring vetchling). Dense, clump-forming herbaceous perennial with unwinged, upright stems, and mid- to dark green leaves divided into 2–4 pairs of ovate to elliptic, sharp-pointed leaflets, 3–8cm (1¼–3in) long. In spring, bears one-sided racemes of 3–6 purplish blue flowers, to 2cm (¾in) long, that become almost greenish blue. ↕20–45cm (8–18in), ↔ 45cm (18in). Continental Europe, Turkey, Caucasus, Russia (Siberia). ✽✽✽. **'Alboroseus'** ■ bears pink-and-white flowers. **f. *albus*** bears white flowers. **var. *aurantiacus*** see *L. aureus.*

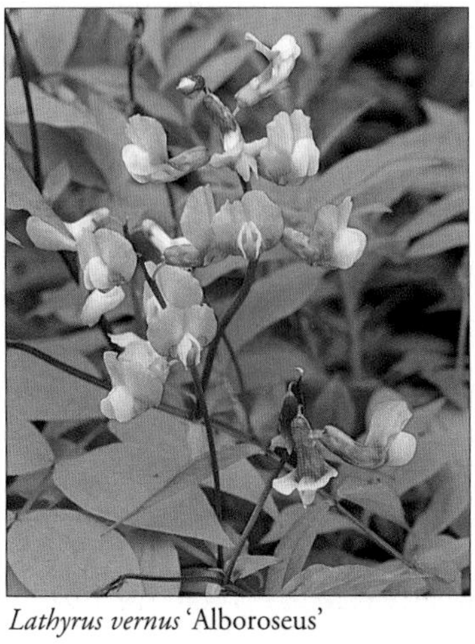

Lathyrus vernus 'Alboroseus'

▷**Lattice leaf plant** see *Aponogeton madagascariensis*
▷**Laudanum** see *Cistus ladanifer*
▷**Laurel** see *Prunus laurocerasus, P. lusitanica*
Alexandrian see *Danae racemosa*
Bay see *Laurus nobilis*
California see *Umbellularia californica*
Cherry see *Prunus laurocerasus*
Diamond-leaved see *Pittosporum rhombifolium*
Eastern bog see *Kalmia polifolia*
Indian see *Ficus microcarpa*
Mountain see *Kalmia latifolia*
Portugal see *Prunus lusitanica*
Sheep see *Kalmia angustifolia*
Sierra see *Leucothoe davisiae*
Spotted see *Aucuba japonica*
Spurge see *Daphne laureola*
Tasmanian see *Anopterus glandulosus*
Western see *Kalmia microphylla*

LAURELIA

ATHEROSPERMATACEAE / MONIMIACEAE

Genus of 3 species of evergreen shrubs and trees occurring in forest and on streambanks in New Zealand, Chile, and Argentina. They are cultivated for their opposite, elliptic, entire or toothed, leathery, aromatic leaves. In summer, inconspicuous, often dioecious flowers are borne in axillary panicles or racemes. Grow in a shrub border, in a woodland garden, or against a warm, sunny wall.
• **HARDINESS** Fully hardy to frost hardy.
• **CULTIVATION** Grow in moist but well-drained, moderately fertile soil in full sun or partial shade, in a site that is sheltered from cold, drying winds. Pruning group 1.
• **PROPAGATION** Take semi-ripe cuttings in summer.
• **PESTS AND DISEASES** Trouble free.

L. sempervirens ◊ syn. *L. serrata* of gardens. Dense, conical shrub or tree with narrowly elliptic to elliptic, very aromatic, bright green leaves, to 10cm (4in) long, with toothed margins, except near the bases. Axillary panicles of tiny, cup-shaped green flowers are produced in early summer. ↕15m (50ft), ↔ 10m (30ft), usually less. Chile, Argentina. ✽✽✽ (borderline)
***L. serrata* of gardens** see *L. sempervivens.*

▷***Laurentia axillaris*** see *Solenopsis axillaris*

LAURUS

LAURACEAE

Genus of 2 species of evergreen shrubs and trees from woodland, scrub, and rocky places in the Azores, the Canary Islands, and the Mediterranean. They are valued for their aromatic, alternate, ovate leaves. Small, greenish yellow male and female flowers are borne on separate plants. In areas with prolonged frosts, grow in a container and move into a cool greenhouse during winter and early spring. In warmer areas, grow as specimen trees, in a woodland garden, against a warm, sunny wall, or as a windbreak. They are effective in a container in a patio, as they tolerate clipping well.
• **HARDINESS** Frost hardy. Foliage may be damaged by strong, cold winds.
• **CULTIVATION** Grow in fertile, moist but well-drained soil in full sun or partial shade, sheltered from cold, drying winds. Pruning group 1; clip topiary specimens twice during summer.
• **PROPAGATION** Sow seed in containers in a cold frame in autumn, or take semi-ripe cuttings in summer.
• **PESTS AND DISEASES** Bay sucker, scale insects, tortrix moth caterpillars, powdery mildew, and leaf spot may be troublesome.

L. nobilis ♀ △ (Bay laurel, Sweet bay). Conical tree or large shrub with aromatic, narrowly ovate, glossy, dark green leaves, to 10cm (4in) long. In spring, bears clusters of greenish yellow flowers, 5mm (¼in) across, followed on female plants by broadly ovoid black berries, to 1.5cm (½in) long. Leaves are often used as a flavouring in cooking. Contact with foliage may aggravate skin allergies. ↕12m (40ft), ↔ 10m (30ft). Mediterranean. ✽✽. **'Aurea'** ■ ♀ has golden yellow foliage.

▷**Laurustinus** see *Viburnum tinus*
▷**Lavandin** see *Lavandula* x *intermedia*

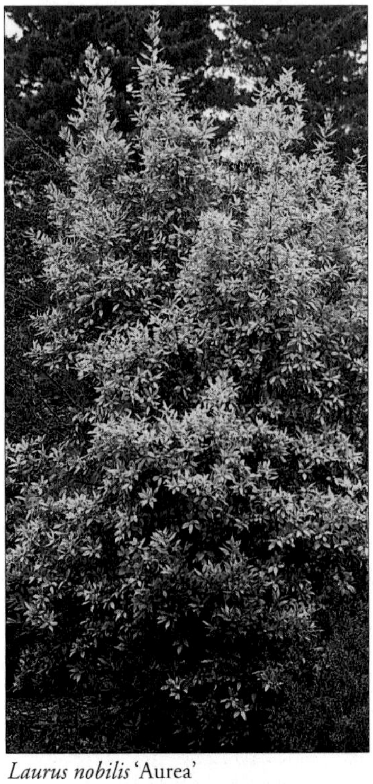

Laurus nobilis 'Aurea'

L

LAVANDULA

Lavender

LABIATAE/LAMIACEAE

Genus of about 25 species of aromatic, evergreen shrubs and subshrubs occurring in dry, sunny, exposed, rocky habitats from the Canary Islands, the Mediterranean, and N.E. Africa to S.W. Asia and India. The leaves are opposite, and may be simple and entire, or toothed to pinnatifid, pinnate, or 2-pinnate, with the margins usually rolled under. They are cultivated for their mainly long-stalked spikes of fragrant, tubular, 2-lipped flowers, which, in many species, have a very high nectar content, making them particularly attractive to bees. In warm areas, lavenders are suitable for a variety of situations, from a shrub border to a rock garden, and are useful for edging and as a low hedge. In frost-prone climates, the half-hardy species should be grown at the base of a warm, sunny wall, or in a container which can be overwintered in a cool greenhouse or conservatory. The leaves and flowerheads are often dried for use in sachets or pot-pourri. If grown for drying, cut the flowerheads before they are fully open.

- **HARDINESS** Fully hardy to half hardy.
- **CULTIVATION** Grow in moderately fertile, well-drained soil in full sun. Pruning group 10, in early or mid-spring.
- **PROPAGATION** Sow seed in containers in a cold frame in spring, or take semi-ripe cuttings in summer.
- **PESTS AND DISEASES** Froghoppers, honey fungus, and grey mould (*Botrytis*) may be troublesome.

L. angustifolia (Lavender). Compact, bushy shrub with linear, grey-green leaves, to 5cm (2in) long. In mid- and late summer, long, unbranched stalks produce fragrant, pale to deep purple flowers in dense spikes, to 8cm (3in) long. ↕ 1m (3ft), ↔ 1.2m (4ft). W. Mediterranean. ❄❄❄. **'Hidcote'** ■♀ is more compact, and produces silvery grey leaves and dark purple flowers; ↕ 60cm (24in), ↔ 75cm (30in). **'Jean Davis'** produces pale pink flowers. **'Loddon Pink'** ■ is more compact, and produces soft pink flowers; ↕ 45cm (18in), ↔ 60cm (24in). **'Munstead'** produces blue-purple flowers; ↕ 45cm (18in), ↔ 60cm (24in). **'Nana Alba'** is very compact, and produces spikes of white

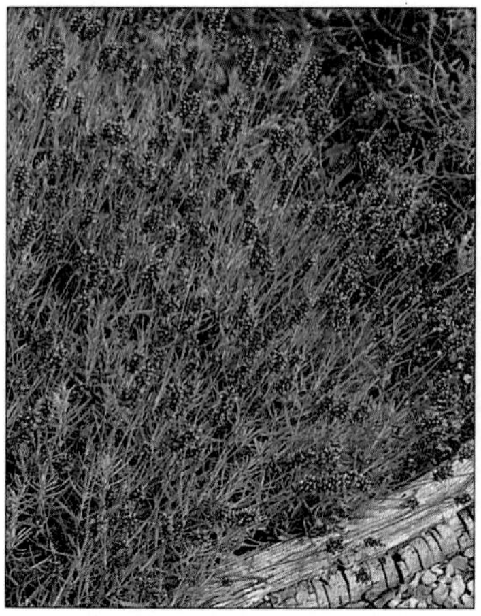

Lavandula angustifolia 'Hidcote'

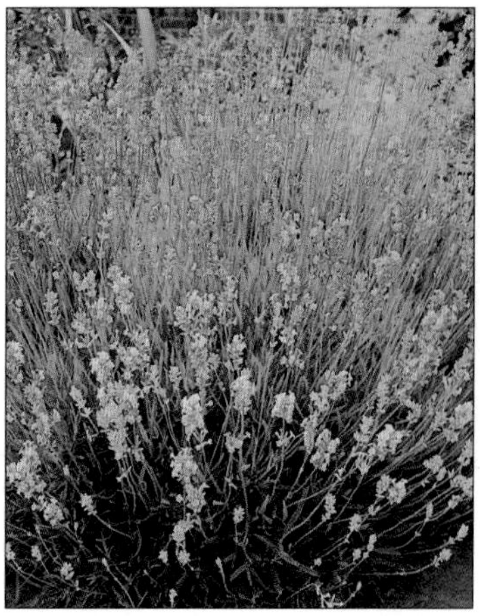

Lavandula angustifolia 'Loddon Pink'

flowers; ↕↔ 30cm (12in). **'Twickel Purple'** ■♀ has narrowly oblong leaves, to 5cm (2in) long, and bears purple flowers in midsummer; ↕ 60cm (24in), ↔ 1m (3ft).

L. dentata ■ Spreading, bushy shrub with linear-oblong, scalloped, dark green leaves, to 4cm (1½in) long. In mid- and late summer, long, unbranched stalks produce dense spikes, to 5cm (2in) long, of slightly fragrant, purple-blue flowers, tipped with purple bracts. ↕ 1m (3ft), ↔ 1.5m (5ft). Atlantic islands, W. Mediterranean, Arabian Peninsula. ❄❄

L. x intermedia (*L. angustifolia* x *L. latifolia*) (English lavender, Lavandin). Rounded shrub with branching stems bearing oblong to lance-shaped to almost spoon-shaped, aromatic, grey-green leaves, 4–6cm (1½–2½in) long, covered in fine, silvery grey hairs. In summer, light blue to violet flowers are produced in spikes 10–20cm (4–8in) long. ↕↔ 30–50cm (12–20in). Garden origin. ❄❄❄. **'Grappenhall'** has narrowly oblong leaves, to 6cm (2½in) long, and bears spikes, to 7cm (3in) long, of slightly fragrant, blue-purple flowers; ↕ 1m (3ft), ↔ 1.5m (5ft); ❄❄. **'Seal'** bears pale purple flowers.

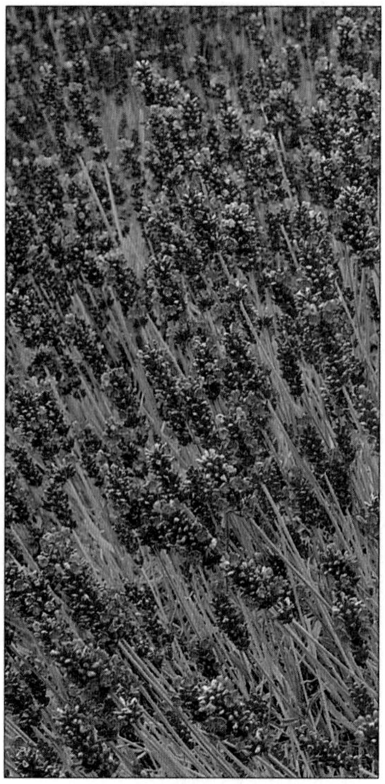

Lavandula angustifolia 'Twickel Purple'

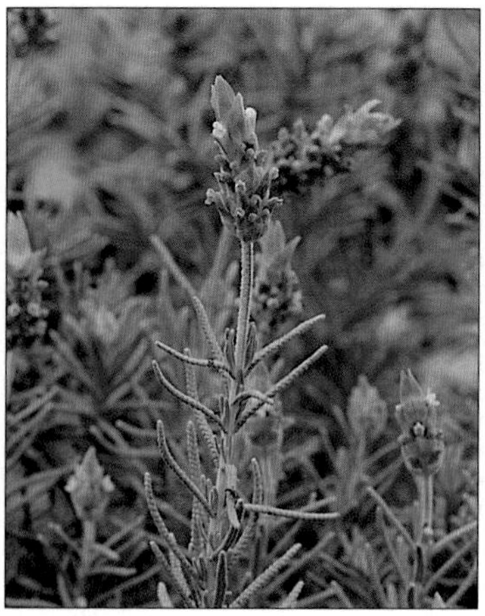

Lavandula dentata

L. lanata ♀ Rounded, bushy shrub with linear to inversely lance-shaped, densely white-woolly leaves, to 5cm (2in) long. Dense spikes, to 10cm (4in) long, of fragrant, dark purple flowers are produced on long, unbranched stalks in late summer. ↕ 75cm (30in), ↔ 90cm (36in). S. Spain. ❄❄

L. latifolia (Spike lavender). Upright, bushy shrub or subshrub with slender, elliptic or spoon-shaped to oblong-lance-shaped, grey-green leaves, to 6cm (2½in) long. In mid- and late summer, long, branched stalks produce fragrant, mauve-blue flowers in narrow, branching spikes, to 20cm (8in) long. ↕ 1m (3ft), ↔ 1.2m (4ft). W. Mediterranean. ❄❄

L. pinnata. Spreading, bushy shrub with pinnate, white-hairy, grey-green leaves, to 8cm (3in) long, consisting of numerous, oblong leaflets. In late summer, long, unbranched stalks bear fragrant, blue-purple flowers in spikes to 9cm (3½in) long. ↕↔ 1m (3ft). Canary Islands. ❄❄

L. stoechas ♀ (French lavender). Compact, bushy shrub with linear, grey-green leaves, to 4cm (1½in) long. Dense, ovoid-oblong spikes, to 3cm (1¼in) long, of fragrant, dark purple flowers, topped by conspicuous, purple bracts, are borne on very short, unbranched stalks from late spring to summer. ↕↔ 60cm (24in). Mediterranean. ❄❄❄ (borderline). **subsp. *pedunculata*** ■♀ has flower spikes borne on long stalks well above the foliage; Portugal, Spain.

L. viridis. Upright, bushy shrub with oblong, pale green leaves, to 5cm (2in) long. In mid- and late summer, small white flowers emerge from short-stemmed, unbranched, dense spikes, 2–3cm (¾–1¼in) long, each with a cluster of green bracts at the tip. ↕ 60cm (24in), ↔ 75cm (30in). Portugal, Spain, Madeira. ❄❄

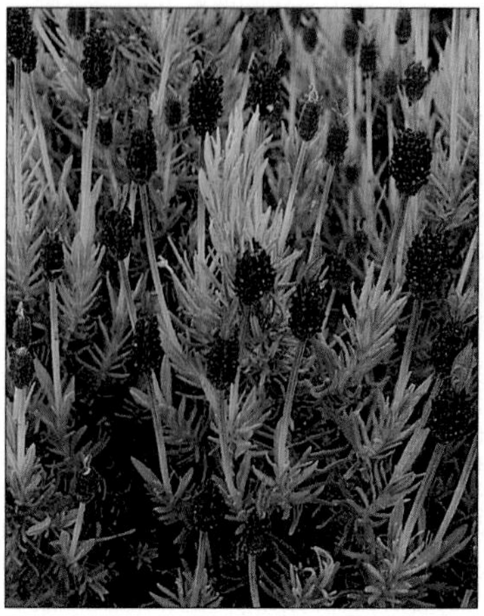

Lavandula stoechas subsp. *pedunculata*

LAVATERA

Mallow

MALVACEAE

Genus of approximately 25 species of annuals, biennials, herbaceous, semi-evergreen, or evergreen perennials, and deciduous, semi-evergreen, or evergreen subshrubs and shrubs. They have a wide distribution, occurring from the Azores, Canary Islands, W. Europe, and the Mediterranean to C. Asia, Russia (E. Siberia), Australia, and California, USA, and usually grow in dry, rocky places, often near coasts. They are cultivated for their showy, 5-petalled, saucer- or funnel-shaped flowers (similar to those of *Malva*), borne singly or in racemes, mainly in summer. Leaves are alternate, variably shaped, long-stalked, and usually palmately lobed. The annual, biennial, and short-lived perennial species are suitable for a herbaceous border or for summer bedding; shrubby lavateras are best grown in a shrub border or, in areas prone to severe frost, against a warm, sunny wall.

- **HARDINESS** Fully hardy to frost hardy.
- **CULTIVATION** Grow in ideally light, moderately fertile, well-drained soil in full sun. Shelter from cold, drying winds in frost-prone areas. Pruning group 6.
- **PROPAGATION** Sow seed of annuals *in situ* in mid- to late spring, or under glass in mid-spring. Sow seed of biennials in a cold frame in midsummer. Take softwood and greenwood cuttings of perennials in spring, and of subshrubs and shrubs in early summer. Propagate regularly as shrubs and perennials are often short-lived.
- **PESTS AND DISEASES** Prone to stem rot, rust, and soil-borne fungal diseases.

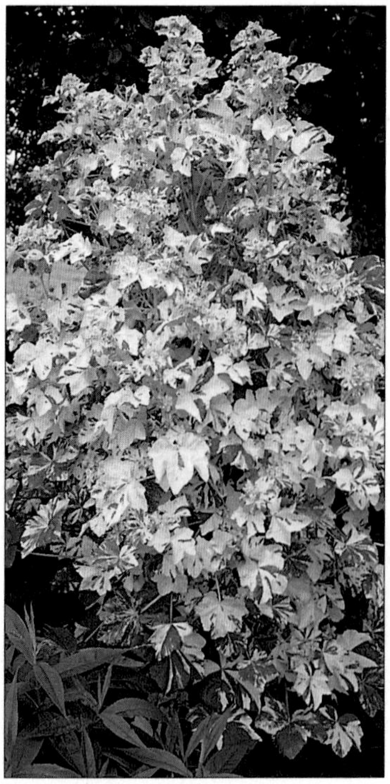

Lavatera arborea 'Variegata'

LAVATERA

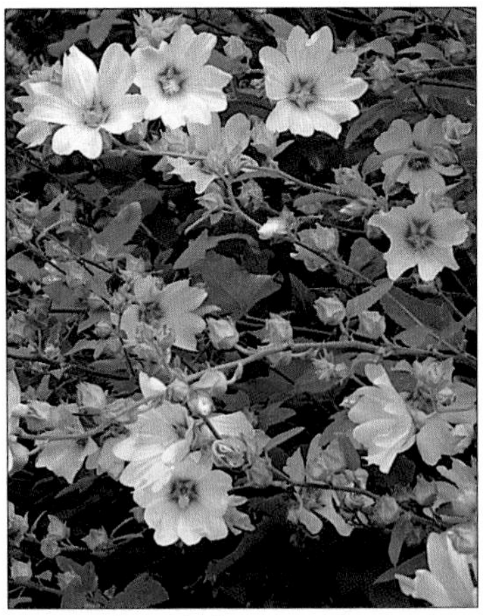
Lavatera 'Barnsley'

L. arborea (Tree mallow). Tree-like, woody-stemmed annual, biennial, or short-lived, evergreen perennial with stout stems and rounded, palmately 5- to 7-lobed, mid-green leaves, to 20cm (8in) long. Racemes of 2–7 funnel-shaped, purple-pink flowers, to 6cm (2½in) across, with darker veins, are profusely borne throughout summer. May be grown as a windbreak in a coastal garden. ↕3m (10ft), ↔1.5m (5ft). W. Europe, Mediterranean. ❄❄. **'Variegata'** ■ has conspicuous white markings on the leaves.
L. assurgentiflora. Deciduous or semi-evergreen shrub with twisted shoots and palmately 5- to 7-lobed, mid-green leaves, to 15cm (6in) long, with heart-shaped bases and white-hairy lower surfaces. In midsummer, produces funnel-shaped, dark cerise-pink flowers, to 8cm (3in) across, with darker veins, singly or in racemes of 2–4. A good windbreak in coastal gardens. ↕2m (6ft), ↔1.5m (5ft). USA (California, Santa Catalina Islands). ❄❄
***L.* 'Barnsley'** ■🏆 Vigorous, semi-evergreen subshrub with palmately 3- to 5-lobed, grey-green leaves, to 12cm (5in) long. Throughout summer, bears profuse racemes of open funnel-shaped, red-eyed white flowers, to 7cm (3in) across, ageing to soft pink, with deeply notched petals. ↕↔2m (6ft). ❄❄❄
L. bicolor see *L. maritima.*
***L.* 'Bredon Springs'** ■ Vigorous, semi-evergreen subshrub with palmately 3- to 5-lobed, grey-green leaves, to 12cm (5in) long. Funnel-shaped, mauve-flushed, dusky pink flowers, to 7cm (3in) across, are borne in profuse

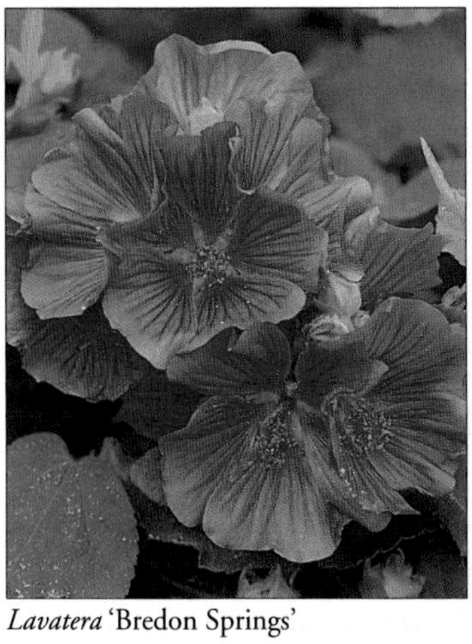
Lavatera 'Bredon Springs'

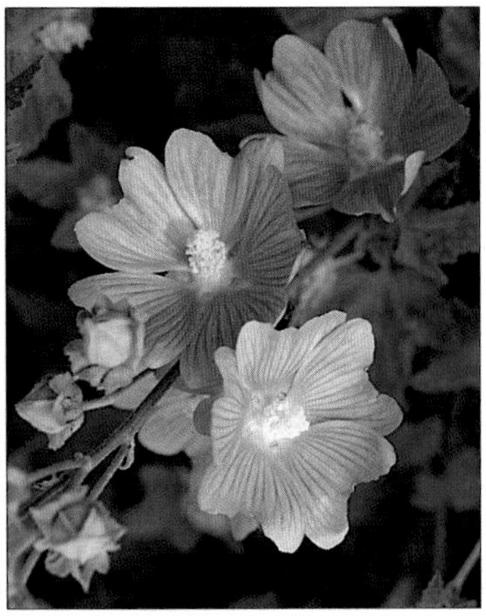
Lavatera cachemiriana

racemes throughout summer. ↕↔2m (6ft). ❄❄❄
***L.* 'Bressingham Pink'.** Upright, shrubby, semi-evergreen perennial with rounded-heart-shaped, shallowly lobed, hairy, pale grey-green leaves, 9cm (3½in) long. From midsummer to early autumn, produces racemes of many saucer-shaped, pale pink flowers, 5–10cm (2–4in) across. ↕1.8m (6ft), ↔1.2m (4ft). ❄❄❄
***L.* 'Burgundy Wine'.** Vigorous, semi-evergreen subshrub with palmately 3- to 5-lobed, grey-green leaves, to 12cm (5in) long. Profuse racemes of funnel-shaped, rich dark pink flowers, to 7cm (3in) across, with darker veins, are produced throughout summer. ↕↔2m (6ft). ❄❄❄
L. cachemiriana ■ syn. *L. cachemirica.* Annual, or short-lived, woody-based, semi-evergreen perennial, with rounded to heart-shaped, palmately 3- to 5-lobed, blunt-toothed leaves, 7–16cm (3–6in) long, mid-green above, downy beneath. Racemes of many open funnel-shaped, silky-textured, clear rose-pink flowers, to 8cm (3in) across, are borne in summer. ↕to 2.5m (8ft), ↔to 1.2m (4ft). India (Kashmir). ❄❄❄

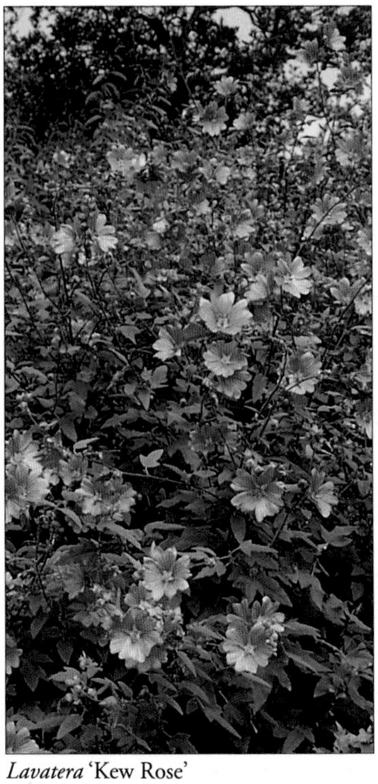
Lavatera 'Kew Rose'

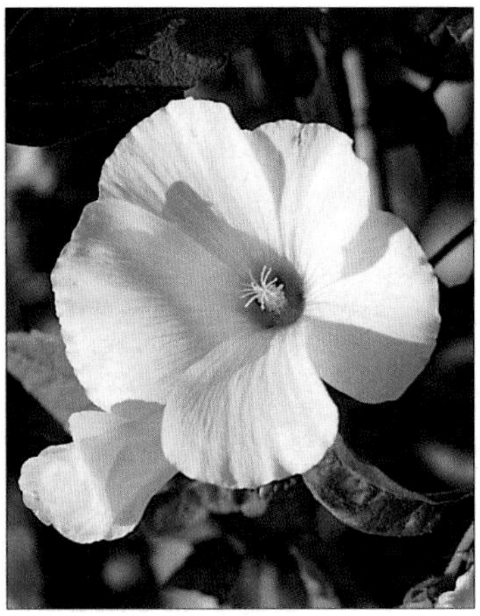
Lavatera trimestris 'Mont Blanc'

L. cachemirica see *L. cachemiriana.*
***L.* 'Candy Floss'.** Vigorous, semi-evergreen subshrub with palmately 3- to 5-lobed, grey-green leaves, to 12cm (5in) long. Profuse racemes of funnel-shaped, pale pink flowers, to 7cm (3in) across, are borne throughout summer. ↕↔2m (6ft). ❄❄
***L.* 'Kew Rose'** ■ Vigorous, semi-evergreen subshrub with purplish green shoots and palmately 3- to 5-lobed, grey-green leaves, to 12cm (5in) long. Profuse racemes of funnel-shaped, bright pink flowers, to 7cm (3in) across, with darker veins, are borne throughout summer. ↕↔2m (6ft). ❄❄
L. maritima 🏆 syn. *L. bicolor, L. maritima* var. *bicolor.* Upright, shrubby, evergreen perennial that bears almost rounded, shallowly lobed, toothed, hairy, grey-green leaves, to 6cm (2½in) long. From late summer to mid-autumn, produces solitary, axillary, saucer-shaped, pink, lilac-pink, or white flowers, 4–8cm (1½–3in) across, with magenta veins, each petal notched and with a magenta basal mark. ↕1.5m (5ft), ↔1m (3ft). W. Mediterranean. ❄❄.
var. *bicolor* see *L. maritima.*
L. mauritanica. Downy annual with rounded to heart-shaped, shallowly 5- to 7-lobed, toothed, mid-green leaves, 3–5cm (1¼–2in) long. Racemes of many funnel-shaped purple flowers, to 3cm (1¼in) across, are produced in summer. ↕80cm (32in), ↔to 30cm (12in). Algeria, Morocco. ❄❄
***L. olbia* 'Rosea'** see *L.* 'Rosea'.
***L.* 'Peppermint Ice'** see *L. thuringiaca* 'Ice Cool'.
***L.* 'Rosea'** 🏆 syn. *L. olbia* 'Rosea'. Vigorous, semi-evergreen subshrub with palmately 3- to 5-lobed, grey-green leaves, to 12cm (5in) long. Produces racemes of many funnel-shaped, dark pink flowers, to 7cm (3in) across, throughout summer. ↕↔2m (6ft). ❄❄❄
***L.* 'Shorty'.** Semi-erect, semi-evergreen perennial with heart-shaped, lobed, hairy, pale green leaves, 5–8cm (2–3in) long. Racemes of many saucer-shaped, white or rose-pink flowers, to 5cm (2in) across, are produced from midsummer to early autumn. ↕↔to 1m (3ft). ❄❄❄
L. thuringiaca (Tree lavatera). Upright herbaceous perennial with finely grey-hairy stems. Mid-green leaves, 9cm (3½in) long, are rounded with heart-shaped bases; basal leaves are unlobed, stem leaves are palmately 3- to 5-lobed. In summer, bears open funnel-shaped,

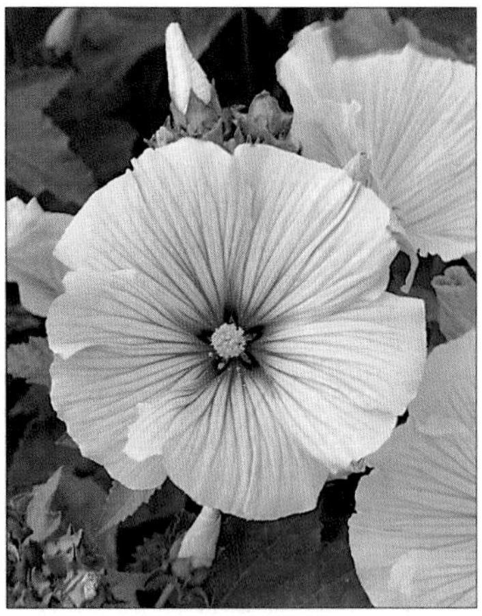
Lavatera trimestris 'Pink Beauty'

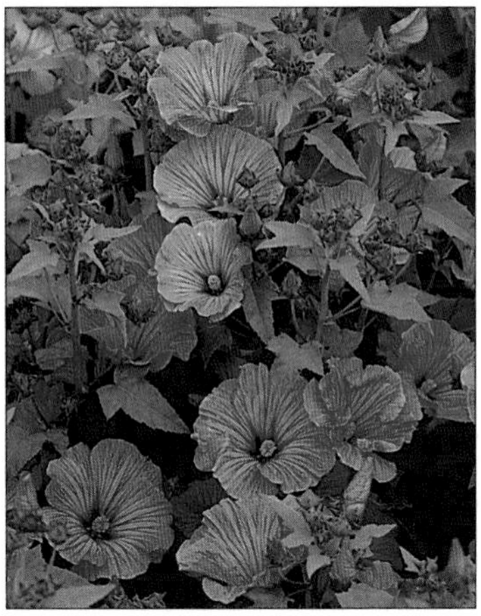
Lavatera trimestris 'Silver Cup'

long-stalked, purple-pink flowers, to 8cm (3in) across, either singly in the leaf axils or in loose racemes. ↕to 2m (6ft), ↔1.8m (6ft). C. and S.E. Europe. ❄❄❄. **'Ice Cool'**, syn. *L.* 'Peppermint Ice', produces pure white flowers; ↕↔1.5m (5ft).
***L. trimestris* cultivars.** Softly hairy annuals bearing rounded, shallowly 3-, 5-, or 7-lobed, mid- to dark green leaves, 3–6cm (1¼–2½in) long, with heart-shaped bases. Open funnel-shaped, pink, reddish pink, or white flowers, 7–10cm (3–4in) across, are produced singly from the upper leaf axils in summer. They provide good cut flowers. ↕to 1.2m (4ft), ↔to 45cm (18in). Mediterranean. ❄❄❄. **'Loveliness'** produces deep rose-pink flowers; ↕0.9–1.2m (3–4ft). **'Mont Blanc'** ■ is compact, with very dark green foliage and white flowers; ↕50cm (20in). **'Pink Beauty'** ■ bears purple-centred, very pale pink flowers, with purple veining; ↕to 60cm (24in). **'Ruby Regis'** bears deep reddish pink flowers; ↕to 60cm (24in). **'Silver Cup'** ■ produces bright rose-pink flowers, to 12cm (5in) across, with darker veining; ↕to 75cm (30in).

▷**Lavatera, Tree** see *Lavatera thuringiaca*
▷**Lavender** see *Lavandula, L. angustifolia*
Cotton see *Santolina chamaecyparissus*
English see *Lavandula* x *intermedia*
French see *Lavandula stoechas*
Sea see *Limonium, L. latifolium*
Spike see *Lavandula latifolia*

L

LAWSONIA

Henna tree, Mignonette tree

LYTHRACEAE

Genus of one species of evergreen shrub or small tree occurring in tropical forest from N. Africa to S.W. Asia and N. Australia. It has opposite, simple, entire leaves and large, terminal panicles of small, 4-petalled, fragrant flowers. In areas where temperatures drop below 13°C (55°F), grow *L. inermis* in a temperate or warm greenhouse. In warmer areas, plant in a shrub border or grow as a hedge. Widely cultivated in the tropics and subtropics, it is a source of the orange-red dye henna.

• **HARDINESS** Frost tender.

• **CULTIVATION** Under glass, grow in loam-based potting compost (JI No.3) with added sharp sand, in full light. When in full growth, water moderately and apply a balanced liquid fertilizer monthly; water sparingly in winter. Outdoors, grow in moderately fertile, well-drained soil in full sun. Pruning group 1; may need restrictive pruning under glass. Clip hedges in early summer.

• **PROPAGATION** Sow seed at 18–21°C (64–70°F) in spring. Take softwood cuttings in spring or hardwood cuttings in autumn.

• **PESTS AND DISEASES** Whiteflies and red spider mites may be troublesome under glass.

L

L. alba see *L. inermis*.

L. inermis 🏆 syn. *L. alba*. Often spiny, large shrub, or sometimes small tree, with an open habit. Elliptic to narrowly obovate or broadly lance-shaped, slender-pointed, mid- to dark green leaves are 2–5cm (¾–2in) long. Many tiny, fragrant flowers, with 4 crumpled, clawed, broadly ovate or spoon-shaped, white, pink, or cinnabar-red petals, are borne in pyramidal panicles, 20–40cm (8–16in) long, mainly in summer. ↕3–6m (10–20ft), ↔ 2–4m (6–12ft). N. Africa to S.W. Asia, N. Australia. ❁ (min. 13°C/55°F)

LAYIA

ASTERACEAE/COMPOSITAE

Genus of 15 species of erect to spreading, well-branched annuals, usually found in moist, grassy meadows, but also on sandy and gravelly soils in woodland or in stream washes, in W. USA. They are cultivated for their daisy-like, single, terminal flowerheads, which are composed of white, yellow, or white-tipped yellow ray-florets (each 3-toothed at the tip), and yellow disc-florets, and are profusely borne, mainly in summer. The alternate leaves are narrowly linear to oblong, and entire to finely divided or pinnatifid. Grow in a hot, dry, herbaceous or mixed border or bed, or on a bank. They provide long-lasting cut flowers.

• **HARDINESS** Fully hardy to half hardy.

• **CULTIVATION** Grow in moist but well-drained, ideally light, sandy, moderately fertile to poor soil in full sun. Very fertile soil encourages lax growth.

• **PROPAGATION** Sow seed *in situ* in early spring or autumn. In frost-prone areas, protect autumn sowings with cloches.

• **PESTS AND DISEASES** Trouble free.

L. elegans see *L. platyglossa*.

L. platyglossa, syn. *L. elegans* (Tidy tips). Almost succulent-stemmed annual with usually linear to narrowly lance-shaped, toothed to pinnatifid, softly hairy, grey-green leaves, to 3cm (1¼in) long. From summer to autumn, bears flowerheads, to 5cm (2in) across, with white-tipped yellow ray-florets and deep golden yellow disc-florets. ↕30–45cm (12–18in), ↔ 24–30cm (10–12in). USA (California). ❄❄❄

▷**Leadwort** see *Plumbago*
Cape see *P. auriculata*
Scarlet see *P. indica*
▷**Leatherleaf** see *Chamaedaphne calyculata*
▷**Leatherwood** see *Cyrilla racemiflora, Dirca palustris*
▷***Lechenaultia*** see *Leschenaultia*

LEDEBOURIA

HYACINTHACEAE/LILIACEAE

Genus of 16 species of semi-evergreen or evergreen, bulbous perennials occurring in seasonally dry, open areas or river valleys in South Africa. They are cultivated for their attractively marked leaves and their racemes of small, bell- or urn-shaped flowers, reminiscent of lily-of-the-valley (*Convallaria*); the flowers are produced in spring or summer. In areas where temperatures drop below 7°C (45°F), they are best grown in a conservatory or cool greenhouse. In warmer areas, grow in open sites in a rock or desert garden.

• **HARDINESS** Half hardy to frost tender.

• **CULTIVATION** Plant bulbs with the necks above soil level. Under glass, grow in loam-based potting compost (JI No.2), with added sharp sand, in full light. When in full growth, water freely and apply a high-potash fertilizer every 4 weeks; keep just moist in winter. Outdoors, grow in moderately fertile, well-drained soil in full sun.

• **PROPAGATION** Sow seed under glass in spring or autumn. Remove offsets in spring.

• **PESTS AND DISEASES** Trouble free.

L. cooperi, syn. *Scilla adlamii, S. cooperi*. Very variable, semi-evergreen, bulbous perennial producing semi-erect, ovate to ovate-oblong or linear, mid- to dark green, basal leaves, 5–25cm (2–10in) long, with bold purple stripes. In summer, bears racemes of up to 50 bell-shaped, purple-pink flowers, 6mm (¼in) long, tipped or striped green. ↕5–10cm (2–4in), ↔ 5cm (2in). South Africa. ❄

L. socialis ■ syn. *Scilla socialis, S. violacea*. Evergreen, bulbous perennial bearing erect, broadly lance-shaped, fleshy, pale silvery green, basal leaves, to 10cm (4in) long, with large, dark green marks above, purple beneath. Racemes of up to 25 bell-shaped, purplish green flowers, 5mm (¼in) long, are produced in late spring or summer. ↕5–10cm (2–4in), ↔ 5cm (2in). South Africa (Northern Cape, Western Cape). ❄

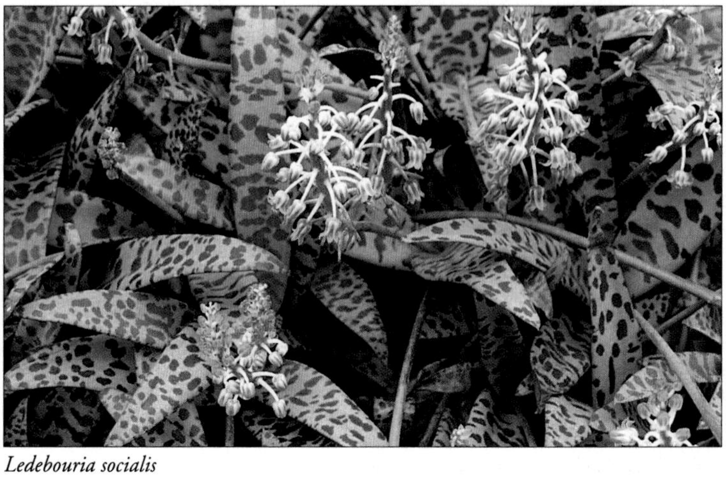

Ledebouria socialis

x LEDODENDRON

ERICACEAE

Bigeneric hybrid genus of one evergreen shrub, a cross between *Rhododendron trichostomum* and *Ledum glandulosum* var. *columbianum*, with characteristics intermediate between those of its parents. It is grown for its lance-shaped, dark green leaves and large, terminal corymbs of tubular flowers. Grow in a woodland garden, or at the front of a shrub border or peat bank; associates well with dwarf rhododendrons.

• **HARDINESS** Fully hardy.

• **CULTIVATION** Grow in humus-rich, moist but well-drained, acid soil in partial shade. Dead-head after flowering. Pinch out the stem tips on young plants to encourage a bushy habit. Pruning group 8.

• **PROPAGATION** Take semi-ripe cuttings in early summer.

• **PESTS AND DISEASES** Trouble free.

x *L.* 'Arctic Tern' 🏆 syn. *Rhododendron* 'Arctic Tern'. Upright to spreading shrub with lance-shaped, hairy, dark green leaves, to 5cm (2in) long. Bears rounded corymbs of tubular, 5-lobed, pure white flowers, to 2cm (¾in) long, in late spring and early summer. ↕↔ to 60cm (24in). ❄❄❄

LEDUM

ERICACEAE

Genus of approximately 4 species of evergreen shrubs widely distributed in bogs, marshes, and moist, often coniferous woodland in cool-temperate regions of the N. hemisphere. They are cultivated for their compact habit, aromatic leaves (which are alternate, and may be linear, ovate, oval, or oblong), and their dense, terminal, umbel-like corymbs of small, 5-petalled white

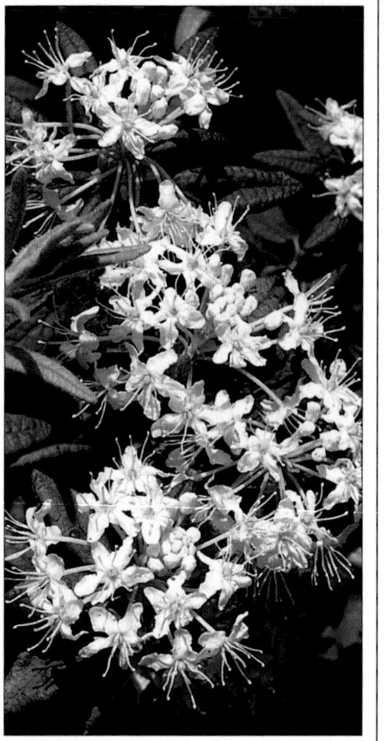

Ledum groenlandicum

flowers, produced in spring or early summer. Suitable for a cool position in a heather garden or peat bed.

• **HARDINESS** Fully hardy.

• **CULTIVATION** Grow in humus-rich, moist but well-drained, acid to neutral soil in full sun or partial shade. Pruning group 8.

• **PROPAGATION** Surface-sow seed in containers under glass in spring or autumn. Take semi-ripe cuttings in late summer. Layer in autumn.

• **PESTS AND DISEASES** Trouble free.

L. glandulosum. Bushy, rounded shrub with smooth shoots and ovate to oval leaves, to 5cm (2in) long, deeply veined and dark green above, white scaly beneath. In late spring, produces white flowers, to 1.5cm (½in) across, in rounded, terminal corymbs, 5cm (2in) across. ↕90cm (36in), ↔ 1.2m (4ft). W. North America. ❄❄❄

L. groenlandicum ■ (Labrador tea). Bushy, rounded shrub with rusty-woolly shoots and narrowly oval to elliptic-oblong leaves, to 5cm (2in) long, dark green above, densely rusty-felted beneath, with recurved margins. White flowers, 1–2cm (½–¾in) across, are borne in rounded, terminal corymbs, 5cm (2in) across, in late spring. ↕90cm (36in), ↔ 1.2m (4ft). Greenland, North America (Alaska, Canada south to N. USA). ❄❄❄

L. palustre (Marsh ledum). Bushy, erect to spreading, usually rounded shrub with rusty-hairy shoots and narrowly oblong to linear leaves, 1–5cm (½–2in) long, dark green above, rusty-hairy beneath, with recurved margins. In late spring, bears white flowers, to 1.5cm (½in) across, in rounded, terminal corymbs, 5cm (2in) across. ↕0.3–1.2m (1–4ft), ↔ to 75cm (30in). N. Europe, N. Asia, North America. ❄❄❄.

f. *decumbens* is more or less mat-forming, with linear leaves, to 2cm (¾in) long; ↕20cm (8in), ↔ 1m (3ft).

▷**Ledum, Marsh** see *Ledum palustre*

LEEA

LEEACEAE

Genus of about 40 species of evergreen shrubs and small trees found in humid forest in tropical Africa, Madagascar, and from India to Malaysia. The alternate or opposite, often velvety leaves are simple to 3-pinnate, and are often flushed red to bronze when young. Small flowers, with tubular bases and 5, sometimes only 4, petal lobes, are borne in flattened, axillary or terminal cymes. Where temperatures drop below 16°C (61°F), grow mainly for their foliage, as houseplants or in a warm greenhouse. In warmer areas, they are distinctive specimens for a small lawn, and are also useful for hedging.

- **HARDINESS** Frost tender.
- **CULTIVATION** Under glass, grow in loam-based potting compost (JI No.3) in bright filtered light and moderate humidity. When in full growth, water freely and apply a balanced liquid fertilizer monthly; water sparingly in winter. Outdoors, grow in moderately fertile, moist but well-drained soil in partial or dappled shade. Pruning group 9; need restrictive pruning under glass. Prune hedges in spring.
- **PROPAGATION** Sow seed at 18°C (64°F) in spring, take semi-ripe cuttings in summer, or air layer in spring or early autumn.
- **PESTS AND DISEASES** Red spider mites may be a problem under glass.

L. coccinea (West Indian holly). Open shrub, becoming denser with age, bearing 2- or 3-pinnate leaves, to 60cm (24in) long, with numerous, oblong-lance-shaped to elliptic or obovate, slender-pointed, toothed leaflets, bronzed when young, maturing to glossy, deep green. Even when young, bears terminal cymes, 8–12cm (3–5in) across, of rounded scarlet buds opening to small pink flowers with yellow anthers, mainly in summer. ↕ 1.5–2.5m (5–8ft), ↔ 1–1.5m (3–5ft). Burma. ❀ (min. 16°C/61°F)

▷ **Leek, Roundheaded** see *Allium sphaerocephalon*

LEGOUSIA

CAMPANULACEAE

Genus of about 15 species of small, erect or spreading, unbranched or bushy annuals occurring on arable or stony ground in N. Africa, from Spain to Greece, and in the Caucasus, Turkey, Cyprus, Syria, Iraq, and Iran. They have ovate, oblong, or lance-shaped, wavy-margined, light to mid-green leaves, and produce small, 5-lobed, saucer- to bell-shaped flowers, singly or in delicate panicles or corymbs. Suitable for an annual border or wildflower garden. They provide unusual cut flowers.

- **HARDINESS** Fully hardy.
- **CULTIVATION** Grow in light, well-drained soil in full sun or partial shade.
- **PROPAGATION** Sow seed *in situ* in autumn or mid-spring.
- **PESTS AND DISEASES** Trouble free.

L. speculum-veneris, syn. *Specularia speculum-veneris* (Venus's looking glass). Erect, bushy annual with oblong to inversely lance-shaped, toothed leaves, 1.5–5cm (½–2in) long. From early summer to autumn, saucer-shaped, white-centred, violet-blue, occasionally white or pale purple flowers, to 2cm (¾in) across, with prominent, reflexed sepals, are profusely borne, either singly or in corymbs of 2 or 3, at the tips of branching stems. ↕ to 30cm (12in), ↔ 10cm (4in). C. and S. Europe, N. Africa, Cyprus, W. Syria, N. Iraq, Caucasus. ❄❄❄

LEIOPHYLLUM

ERICACEAE

Genus of one species of upright to mat-forming, evergreen shrub from acid woodland in E. USA. It is grown for its glossy foliage and abundance of star-shaped white flowers borne in terminal, umbel-like corymbs. Grow in a peat bed, shrub border, or woodland garden. It may spread widely by suckers.

- **HARDINESS** Fully hardy.
- **CULTIVATION** Grow in humus-rich, moist but well-drained, acid soil in partial or deep shade. In frost-prone areas, protect from cold, drying winds. Pruning group 8.
- **PROPAGATION** Surface-sow seed in containers outdoors in spring, take softwood cuttings in early summer, or pot up rooted suckers in spring.
- **PESTS AND DISEASES** Trouble free.

L. buxifolium ▣ ♀ (Sand myrtle). Bushy, usually suckering shrub with upright and spreading stems. Oblong or ovate, glossy, dark green leaves, to 1cm (½in) long, are tinted bronze in winter. In late spring and early summer, bears pink-budded white flowers, 6mm (¼in) across, in dense corymbs, to 2.5cm (1in) across. ↕ 30–60cm (12–24in), ↔ 60cm (24in) or more. USA (New Jersey to Florida). ❄❄❄. **'Nanum'** is compact, with pink flowers; ↕ 5–10cm (2–4in), ↔ 30cm (12in) or more.

LEIPOLDTIA

AIZOACEAE

Genus of about 20 species of erect or prostrate, shrubby, perennial succulents from periodically very dry areas of Namibia and South Africa. Leaves are opposite, often laterally compressed, thicker than wide, and often marked with raised spots. Daisy-like, pink or reddish purple flowers are borne singly or in cymes of 2–5 in summer, followed by ovoid green capsules with rough, papillose seeds. In frost-prone areas, they are best grown in a bowl garden or a warm greenhouse. In frost-free climates, they are effective in a desert garden.

- **HARDINESS** Frost tender.
- **CULTIVATION** Under glass, grow in standard cactus compost in full light. When in full growth, water sparingly and apply low-nitrogen fertilizer every 4–6 weeks; keep dry when dormant. Outdoors, grow in poor, sharply drained soil in full sun. Protect from winter wet. See also pp.48–49.
- **PROPAGATION** Sow seed at 19–24°C (66–75°F) in spring, or take cuttings of stem sections in late spring.
- **PESTS AND DISEASES** Vulnerable to greenfly and other aphids while flowering.

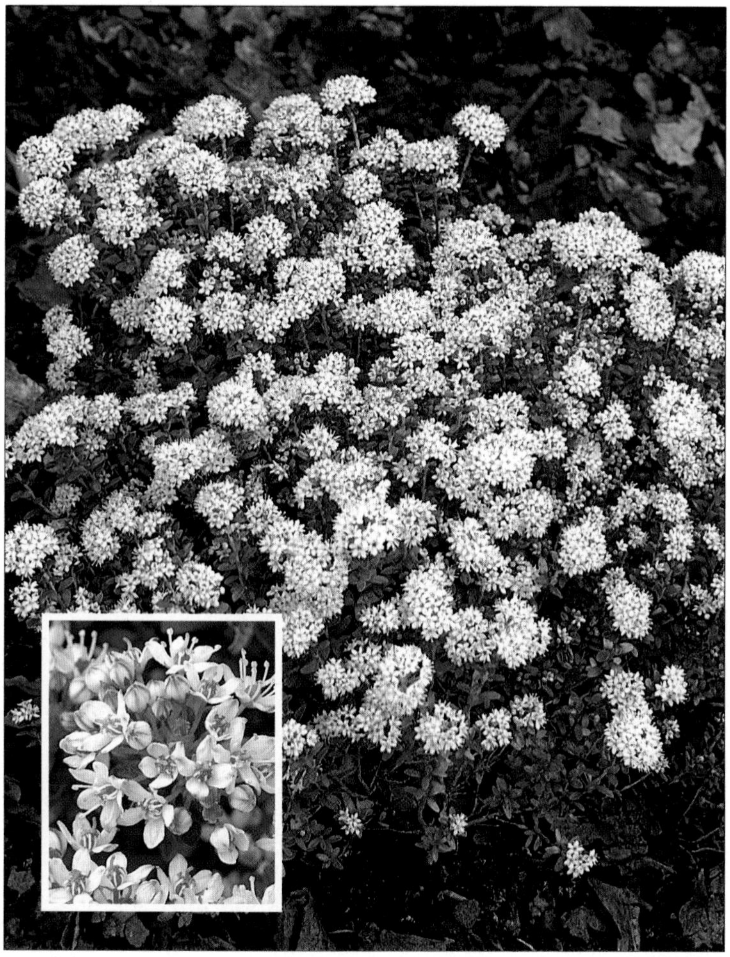

Leiophyllum buxifolium (inset: flower detail)

L. weigangiana. Erect, perennial succulent with woody stems, 3mm (⅛in) thick, and yellowish white bark. Boat-shaped, 3-angled, spotted, bluish green leaves are 1.5cm (½in) long by 5mm (¼in) thick. Produces solitary, violet to pink flowers, 2cm (¾in) across, in summer. ↕ to 50cm (20in), ↔ 25cm (10in). Namibia. ❀ (min. 10°C/50°F)

▷ ***Lemaireocereus euphorbioides*** see *Neobuxbaumia euphorbioides*

▷ ***Lemaireocereus thurberi*** see *Stenocereus thurberi*

LEMBOGLOSSUM

ORCHIDACEAE

Genus of about 14 species of evergreen, mostly epiphytic, rhizomatous orchids (often included within the genus *Odontoglossum*) occurring in humid forests at altitudes of 1,300–3,000m (4,300–10,000ft) in Mexico and Central and South America. They have broadly ovoid to oblong-ovoid, clustered pseudobulbs, each producing up to 3 linear, lance-shaped, ovate, or elliptic leaves. Flowers are produced in racemes from the bases of the pseudobulbs.

- **HARDINESS** Frost tender.
- **CULTIVATION** Cool- to intermediate-growing orchids. Grow in fine-grade epiphytic orchid compost in a container that constricts the roots. In summer, provide high humidity and bright filtered light, water freely, apply fertilizer at every third watering, and mist once or twice daily. In winter, provide full light and water sparingly. See also p.46.
- **PROPAGATION** Divide when the plants fill and overflow their containers.
- **PESTS AND DISEASES** Susceptible to red spider mites, aphids, and mealybugs.

L. bictoniense ▣ ♀ syn. *Odontoglossum bictoniense.* Epiphytic orchid with ovoid, compressed pseudobulbs, each with 2 or 3 elliptic-oblong to linear leaves, 10–45cm (4–18in) long. Light green flowers, 2.5cm (1in) across, heavily barred with brown, with heart-shaped, white or pink lips, are borne in tall, upright racemes from winter to spring. ↕ 60cm (24in), ↔ 30cm (12in). Mexico, Guatemala, El Salvador. ❀ (min. 10°C/50°F; max. 24°C/75°F)

L. cervantesii, syn. *Odontoglossum cervantesii.* Epiphytic orchid with ovoid pseudobulbs, each with one ovate-lance-shaped to elliptic-oblong leaf, 4–30cm (1½–12in) long. From winter to spring,

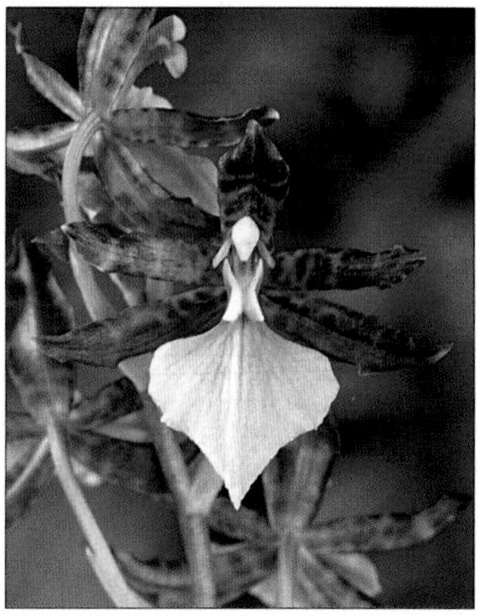

Lemboglossum bictoniense

L

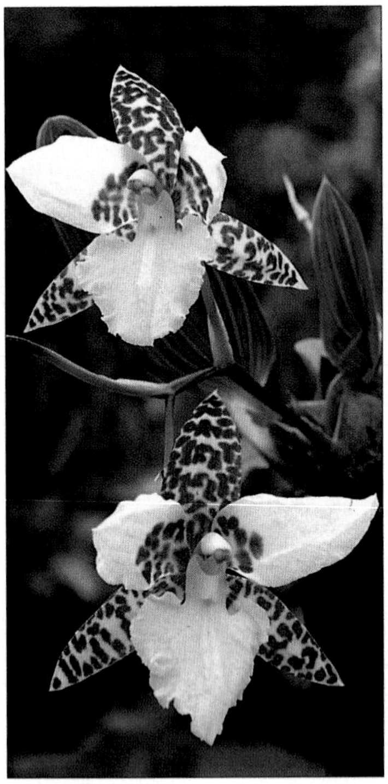

Lemboglossum rossii

bears short, arching racemes of white to pink flowers, 4–6cm (1½–2½in) across, with narrow, central red spots and bands. ↕↔ 15cm (6in). S. Mexico, Guatemala. ⊛ (min. 10°C/50°F; max. 24°C/75°F)
L. cordatum, syn. *Odontoglossum cordatum.* Epiphytic orchid with oblong, compressed, furrowed pseudobulbs, each with one narrowly elliptic, leathery leaf, 9–30cm (3½–12in) long. Brown-marked, green, white, or yellow flowers, to 6cm (2½in) across, are borne in erect racemes in late summer. ↕ 20cm (8in), ↔ 15cm (6in). Central America, Venezuela. ⊛ (min. 10°C/50°F; max. 24°C/75°F)
L. rossii ■ syn. *Odontoglossum rossii.* Epiphytic orchid with ovoid pseudobulbs, each with one elliptic or elliptic-lance-shaped leaf, 5–20cm (2–8in) long. White, pink, or sometimes yellow flowers, 5–7cm (2–3in) across, with brown to pink-brown bars or spots on the sepals and petal bases, are borne in short, arching racemes from late winter to spring. ↕↔ 15cm (6in). Mexico, Guatemala, Honduras, Nicaragua. ⊛ (min. 10°C/50°F; max. 24°C/75°F)
L. stellatum, syn. *Odontoglossum stellatum.* Epiphytic orchid with narrowly oblong pseudobulbs, each with one ovate to elliptic or inversely lance-shaped leaf, 6–15cm (2½–6in) long. From winter to spring, produces short, arching racemes of yellowish white flowers, 4cm (1½in) across, barred with brown (or sometimes entirely brown), with large, pink or white lips spotted deep pink. ↕↔ 15cm (6in). Mexico, Guatemala, El Salvador. ⊛ (min. 10°C/50°F; max. 24°C/75°F)

▷***Lembotropis nigricans*** see *Cytisus nigricans*
▷**Lemon** see *Citrus limon*
Meyer's see *C. limon* 'Meyer'
▷**Lemon balm** see *Melissa officinalis*
▷**Lemon verbena** see *Aloysia triphylla*
▷**Lemonwood** see *Pittosporum eugenioides*

LENOPHYLLUM

CRASSULACEAE

Genus of about 6 species of clustering, perennial succulents from low-lying, often scrub or woodland areas of California, Texas, and New Mexico, USA, and Mexico. Very variably shaped, fleshy leaves are borne mainly in opposite pairs, forming loose, basal rosettes. Sparsely leafy flowering stems produce small, 5-petalled flowers, borne singly or in terminal racemes or panicles, from summer to winter. In areas where temperatures drop below 5°C (41°F), they may be grown outdoors in summer, but need to be protected in a temperate greenhouse at other times. In warmer climates, grow permanently outdoors in a shrub border or a desert garden.
• **HARDINESS** Frost tender.
• **CULTIVATION** Under glass, grow in standard cactus compost in full light. From spring to late summer, water freely and apply a balanced liquid fertilizer every 6–8 weeks. Water moderately in autumn and keep just moist in winter. Outdoors, grow in moderately fertile, sharply drained soil in full sun. See also pp.48–49.
• **PROPAGATION** Sow seed at 19–24°C (66–75°F), or divide offsets, in spring or early summer. Root leaf cuttings in summer.
• **PESTS AND DISEASES** Prone to greenfly while flowering.

L. guttatum. Rosetted, perennial succulent with ovate-elliptic to diamond-shaped, blunt-tipped, grey-green leaves, 2–3.5cm (¾–1½in) long, with purple-black spots, the upper surfaces broadly grooved. Cup-shaped, thick-sepalled, pale yellow flowers, to 1cm (½in) across, later tinged red, are produced in open, sparsely branched panicles from summer to autumn. ↕↔ 10–12cm (4–5in). N.E. Mexico. ⊛ (min. 5°C/41°F)
L. texanum. Perennial succulent with loose rosettes of very thick, lance-shaped to ovate, mid-green leaves, 1.5–3cm (½–1¼in) long. Cup-shaped, fleshy, primrose-yellow flowers, 6–8mm (¼–⅜in) across, with red-tipped petals, are borne in few-branched panicles from late summer to early winter. ↕ to 10cm (4in), ↔ to 20cm (8in). USA (Texas), N.E. Mexico. ⊛ (min. 5°C/41°F)

▷**Lenten rose** see *Helleborus orientalis*
▷**Lentisc** see *Pistacia lentiscus*

LEONOTIS

LABIATAE/LAMIACEAE

Genus of about 30 species of aromatic annuals, perennials, and evergreen to semi-evergreen subshrubs and shrubs (deciduous in cold climates) from upland grassland and rocky areas, mainly in South Africa, with one species widely distributed in tropical regions. They have square stems and opposite, lance-shaped to ovate leaves, and are cultivated for their showy whorls of 2-lipped flowers produced in terminal, leafy, raceme-like inflorescences. In frost-prone climates, they may be treated as tender perennials and grown in a cool greenhouse, or planted outdoors once there is little risk of frost. In warmer areas, grow outdoors in a border or against a warm wall.
• **HARDINESS** Half hardy.
• **CULTIVATION** Under glass, grow in loam-based potting compost (JI No.2) in full light. When in full growth, water freely and apply a balanced liquid fertilizer every 6–8 weeks; water sparingly in winter. Outdoors, grow in moderately fertile, well-drained soil in full sun. Pruning group 10, in spring, if grown permanently outdoors; if grown under glass or as tender perennials, cut to ground level in early spring.
• **PROPAGATION** Sow seed at 13–18°C (55–64°F) in spring, or take greenwood cuttings in late spring or summer.
• **PESTS AND DISEASES** Susceptible to grey mould (*Botrytis*), red spider mites, and whiteflies under glass.

L. leonurus ■ (Lion's ear). Upright, semi-evergreen or deciduous shrub or subshrub with lance-shaped to inversely lance-shaped, entire or scalloped, mid- to deep green leaves, 6–12cm (2½–5in) long. From autumn to early winter, produces whorls of tubular, 2-lipped, orange-red to scarlet flowers, 6cm (2½in) long. ↕ 2m (6ft) or more, ↔ 1m (3ft) or more. South Africa (except PWV and North West province). ❄. **'Harrismith White'** bears white flowers.
L. ocymifolia. Woody-based, herbaceous perennial with ovate, toothed or scalloped, mid-green leaves, to 8cm (3in) long, with very hairy undersides. From late summer to autumn, produces dense whorls of tubular, 2-lipped, velvety-haired orange flowers, to 4cm (1½in) long, with the upper lip twice as long as the lower. ↕ to 3m (10ft), ↔ 1m (3ft). South Africa (except for Orange Free State, PWV, and North West province). ❄

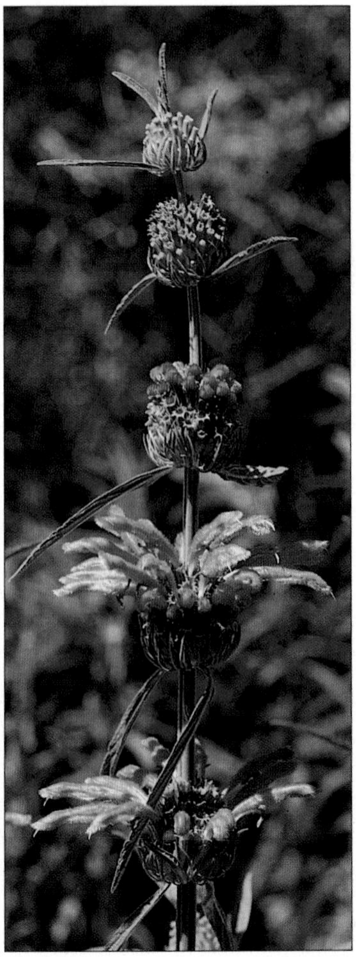

Leonotis leonurus

LEONTICE

BERBERIDACEAE

Genus of 3 species of tuberous perennials occurring on dry hillsides in N. Africa, the E. Mediterranean, the Middle East, and S.W. and C. Asia. They are cultivated for their large, axillary or terminal racemes or panicles of small, cup-shaped flowers held above 3-palmate or pinnate leaves. Grow in an alpine house or bulb frame.
• **HARDINESS** Frost hardy.
• **CULTIVATION** Plant tubers 20cm (8in) deep in autumn. Under glass, grow in loam-based potting compost (JI No.2) with added grit, in full light. When in growth, water moderately and apply a low-nitrogen fertilizer every 6–8 weeks; keep dry when dormant. Outdoors, grow in any well-drained soil in full sun.
• **PROPAGATION** Sow seed in containers in a cold frame as soon as ripe.
• **PESTS AND DISEASES** Trouble free.

L. leontopetalum. Tuberous perennial with grey-green, basal leaves, to 25cm (10in) wide, each usually divided into 3 broadly obovate leaflets. From spring to early summer, produces panicles of cup-shaped yellow flowers, to 1.5cm (½in) across, which open flat. ↕ 20–80cm (8–32in), ↔ 15cm (6in). N. Africa, E. Mediterranean to Iran. ❄❄

LEONTOPODIUM

Edelweiss

ASTERACEAE/COMPOSITAE

Genus of approximately 35 species of perennials found in grassland and stony habitats in the mountains of Europe and Asia. They have simple, entire, hairy, mainly basal leaves. Upright stems bear compact, terminal cymes of small flowerheads consisting only of yellowish white disc-florets, surrounded by leaf-like, usually white-felted bracts. Easily grown, most species are suitable for a rock garden, raised bed, or alpine house.
• **HARDINESS** Fully hardy.
• **CULTIVATION** Grow in sharply drained, neutral to alkaline soil in full sun. Protect from excessive winter wet. In an alpine house, grow in loam-based potting compost (JI No.1) with added grit or sharp sand.
• **PROPAGATION** Sow seed in containers in an open frame as soon as ripe. Divide in early spring, although divisions are slow to establish.
• **PESTS AND DISEASES** Susceptible to slugs and snails outdoors, and to aphids and red spider mites under glass.

L. aloysiodorum see *L. haplophylloides.*
L. alpinum ■ (Edelweiss). Clump-forming perennial with linear to oblong-lance-shaped, grey-green, basal leaves, to 4cm (1½in) long. In spring or early summer, bears conspicuous heads of yellowish white flowers surrounded by stars of flannel-textured, grey-white bracts, 3–10cm (1¼–4in) across. ↕ 20cm (8in) ↔ 10cm (4in). Mountains of Europe. ❄❄❄. **subsp. *nivale***, syn. *L. nivale*, has densely white-hairy leaves,

L

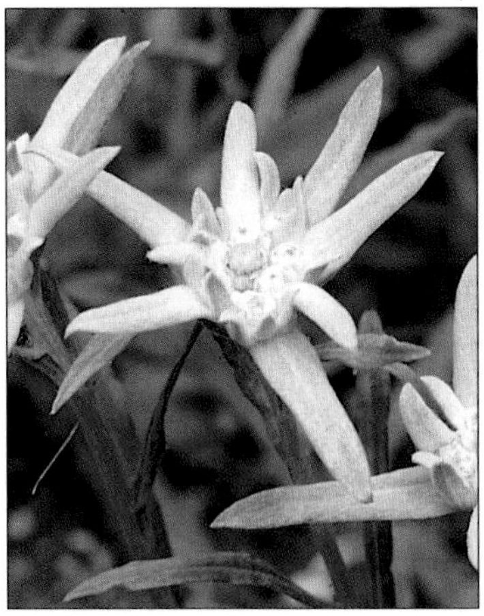
Leontopodium alpinum

and bears woolly, pure white flowerheads and bracts, on short stems; ↕↔ to 15cm (6in); C. Apennines, mountains of Bulgaria and former Yugoslavia.
L. haplophylloides, syn. *L. aloysiodorum.* Upright, clump-forming or tufted perennial with linear-lance-shaped, lemon-scented, hairy, grey-green leaves, 5–7cm (2–3in) long, spotted black beneath. In early summer, bears yellowish white flowers surrounded by stars of many white-hairy, grey-green bracts, 5cm (2in) across. More tolerant of winter wet than *L. alpinum.* ↕ 30cm (12in), ↔ to 20cm (8in). Mountains of C. and S.W. China. ***
L. nivale see *L. alpinum* subsp. *nivale.*
L. stracheyi. Mound-forming perennial with ovate-lance-shaped to linear leaves, to 4.5cm (1¾in) long, sparsely grey-hairy above, grey-downy beneath. In spring, bears short-stemmed heads of glistening, yellowish white flowers surrounded by many white-felted bracts, to 6cm (2½in) across. ↕ to 50cm (20in), ↔ to 30cm (12in). Himalayas, Mountains of India (Uttar Pradesh) to S.W. China. ***

▷ **Leopard's bane** see *Doronicum*
▷ ***Leopoldia comosa*** see *Muscari comosum*
▷ ***Lepachys columnifera*** see *Ratibida columnifera*
▷ ***Lepachys pinnata*** see *Ratibida pinnata*

LEPIDOZAMIA

ZAMIACEAE

Genus of 2 species of palm-like, dioecious cycads from slopes, gullies, and rainforest in E. Australia. The erect trunks are clad in old leaf bases, with the pinnate, light or deep green leaves borne in terminal whorls. Narrow, cone-like, green to brown, male or female flowerheads ("cones") are borne in the centres of the leaf rosettes. In frost-prone climates, grow in a temperate or warm greenhouse or as houseplants. In frost-free climates, grow as specimen plants.
• **HARDINESS** Frost tender.
• **CULTIVATION** Under glass, grow in a mix of equal parts garden compost, loam, and coarse bark, with added slow-release fertilizer, grit, and charcoal, in bright filtered light. Water moderately when in growth, sparingly in winter. Outdoors, grow in moderately fertile, moist but well-drained soil in full sun or partial shade.

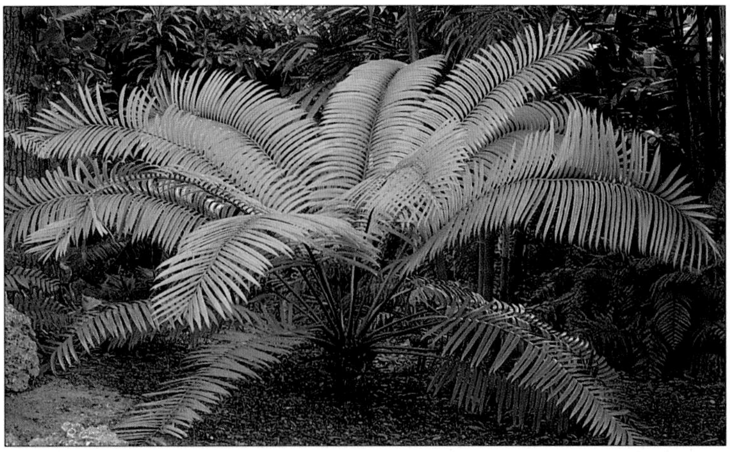
Lepidozamia hopei

• **PROPAGATION** Sow seed at 24°C (75°F) in spring.
• **PESTS AND DISEASES** Red spider mites, mealybugs, and scale insects may be troublesome under glass.

L. hopei ■ ♆ Medium-sized to tall cycad with ascending to arching, pinnate, light green leaves, to 3m (10ft) long, each consisting of many lance-shaped, curved, lustrous leaflets. Green to brown flowering cones are borne usually in summer: the ovoid females to 60cm (24in) long, the cylindrical males to 80cm (32in) long. ↕ to 20m (70ft), ↔ to 6m (20ft). Australia (N.E. Queensland). ❀ (min. 13–15°C/ 55–59°F)
L. peroffskyana ♆ Medium-sized to tall cycad with pinnate, deep green leaves, to 3m (10ft) long, composed of linear to lance-shaped, lustrous leaflets, each with a yellow basal gland. Green to brown flowering cones are borne in summer: the ovoid females to 60cm (24in) long, the cylindrical males to 80cm (32in) long. ↕ to 20m (70ft), ↔ to 6m (20ft). Australia (Queensland, New South Wales). ❀ (min. 13–15°C/55–59°F)

LEPTINELLA

ASTERACEAE/COMPOSITAE

Genus of approximately 30 species of annuals and creeping, tufted, or mat-forming perennials from subalpine grassland and rocky areas in Australasia and South America. They form low carpets of pinnatifid, pinnatisect, or pinnate, often aromatic leaves, and bear solitary, button-like flowerheads on short stalks from late spring to summer.

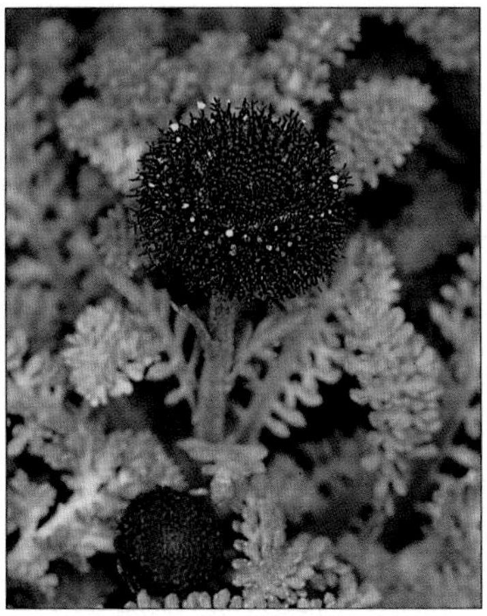
Leptinella atrata

Effective as low ground cover and tolerant of some treading, they are suitable for paving crevices or gravel gardens, but are mostly too invasive for a rock garden. *L. atrata* is suitable for a scree bed or alpine house.
• **HARDINESS** Fully hardy.
• **CULTIVATION** Grow in moderately fertile, sharply drained soil in full sun.
• **PROPAGATION** Sow seed in containers in an open frame as soon as ripe. Divide in spring.
• **PESTS AND DISEASES** Trouble free.

L. atrata ■ syn. *Cotula atrata.* Creeping, tufted perennial with fern-like, broadly elliptic, 2-pinnatifid, purple-tinged, grey-green leaves, to 8cm (3in) long. In late spring and early summer, bears hemispherical, purplish black flowerheads, to 1.5cm (½in) across, with yellow anthers that become prominent as the flowers mature. ↕ to 15cm (6in), ↔ to 20cm (8in). New Zealand. ***. **subsp. *luteola*** has less deeply divided leaves, and bears conical flowerheads with dark red-brown centres and very prominent, creamy white stigmas.
L. pectinata. Tufted or mat-forming perennial with narrowly oblong, hairy or hairless, sometimes toothed, pinnatifid to pinnate leaves, 4cm (1½in) long, with linear to lance-shaped leaflets or lobes. White or pale yellow-red flowerheads, to 8mm (⅜in) across, are produced in late spring and early summer. ↕ to 15cm (6in), ↔ to 45cm (18in). New Zealand. ***

LEPTOSPERMUM

Tea tree

MYRTACEAE

Genus of about 80 species of evergreen shrubs and trees occurring in rainforest and semi-arid areas mainly in Australia, but also from S.E. Asia to New Zealand. They are cultivated for their usually aromatic, neat foliage and their small, sometimes profusely borne flowers. The variably shaped leaves are alternate, entire, and hairless to densely silky-hairy. The flowers are produced from the leaf axils, either singly or in clusters of 2 or 3, and are shallowly cup-shaped to star-shaped, each with 5 white, red, or pink, clawed, usually broadly ovate petals. In frost-prone areas, grow hardy species against a warm, sunny wall, and half-hardy and frost-tender species in a cool greenhouse or conservatory. A few are also suitable for an alpine house. In warmer areas, grow in a shrub border.
• **HARDINESS** Fully hardy (borderline) to frost tender.
• **CULTIVATION** Under glass, grow in loam-based potting compost (JI No.3) in full light or bright filtered light. When in active growth, water freely and apply a balanced liquid fertilizer every 4 weeks; water sparingly in winter. Outdoors, grow in moderately fertile, well-drained soil in full sun or partial shade. Pruning group 8; may need restrictive pruning under glass.
• **PROPAGATION** Sow seed at 13–16°C (55–61°F) in autumn or spring, or root semi-ripe cuttings with bottom heat in summer.
• **PESTS AND DISEASES** Trouble free.

L. flavescens see *L. polygalifolium.*
L. grandiflorum, syn. *L. rodwayanum.* Upright shrub with white-hairy stems and ovate to elliptic, aromatic, silky-hairy, grey-green leaves, to 1.5cm (½in) long. Solitary, saucer-shaped, white or, rarely, pale pink flowers, to 2cm (¾in) across, are produced in mid- and late summer. ↕ 4m (12ft), ↔ 2m (6ft). Australia (Tasmania). **
L. humifusum see *L. rupestre.*
L. lanigerum ■ ♀ ♀ syn. *L. pubescens* (Woolly tea tree). Freely branching, erect shrub or tree with softly hairy and often red-flushed green stems. Crowded, more or less spreading, obovate-oblong to oval, aromatic leaves, 0.5–1.5cm (¼–½in) long, often have recurved points, and are usually grey silky-hairy, at least beneath. From late spring to summer, bears solitary, shallowly cup-

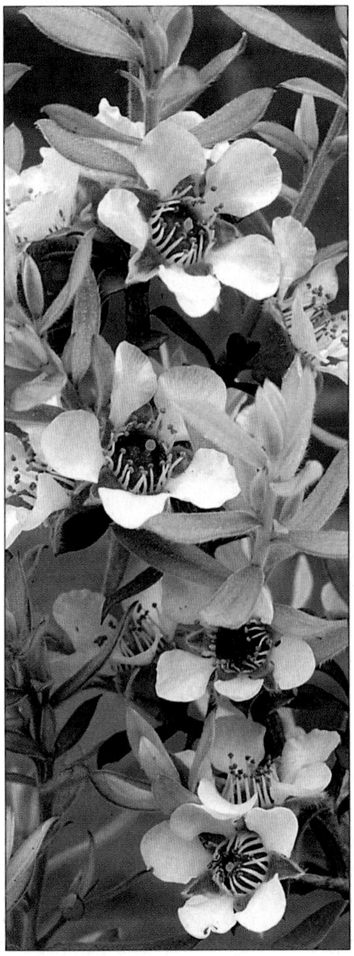
Leptospermum lanigerum

L

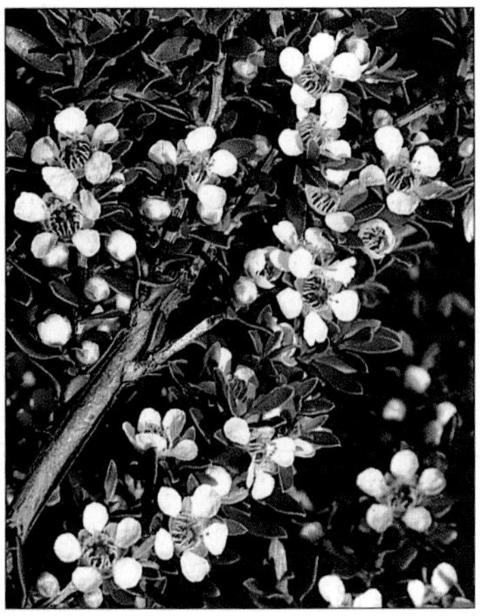
Leptospermum rupestre

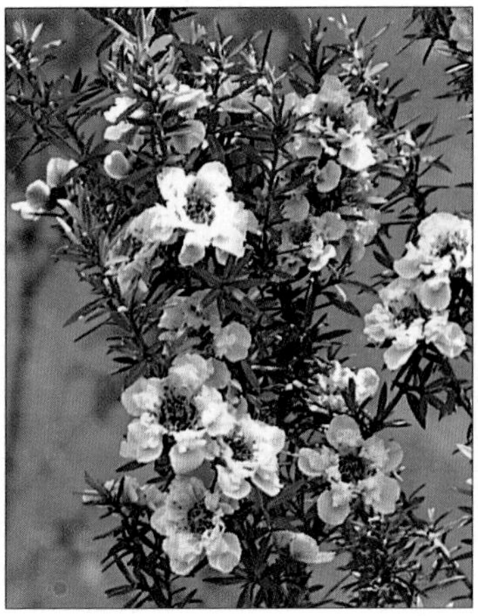
Leptospermum scoparium 'Gaiety Girl'

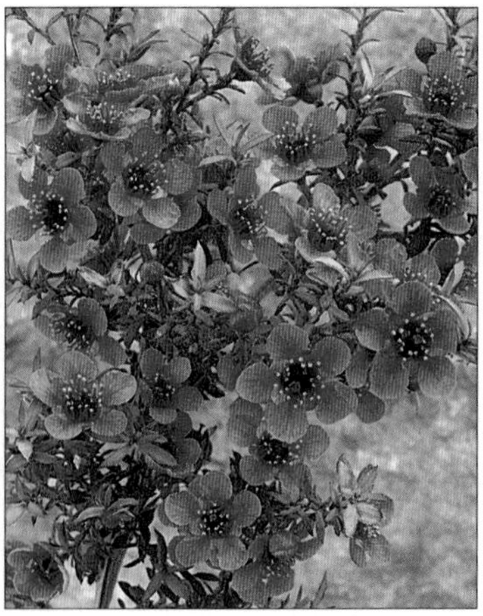
Leptospermum scoparium 'Kiwi'

shaped white flowers, to 1.5cm (½in) across, with prominent red-brown calyces. ↕3–5m (10–15ft), ↔ 1.5–3m (5–10ft). Australia (New South Wales, Victoria, Tasmania). ✻✻
L. polygalifolium Q syn. *L. flavescens.* Erect to spreading, freely branching shrub or tree. Crowded, spreading or occasionally reflexed, mid- to deep green leaves, 0.5–2cm (¼–¾in) long, are linear to inversely lance-shaped-elliptic, with conspicuous oil glands, and sometimes lightly aromatic. From late spring to summer, bears a profusion of solitary, cup-shaped, white or cream, sometimes green- or pink-tinted flowers, 1cm (½in) across. ↕2–7m (6–22ft), ↔ 1–3m (3–10ft). Australia (Queensland, New South Wales, Lord Howe Island). ✻
L. prostratum see *L. rupestre.*

L

L. pubescens see *L. lanigerum.*
L. rodwayanum see *L. grandiflorum.*
L. rupestre ■♀ syn. *L. humifusum, L. prostratum, L. scoparium* var. *prostratum.* Prostrate shrub, sometimes mounded and bushy, with dense foliage. Broadly to narrowly elliptic or obovate, glossy, deep green leaves, 0.7–2cm (¼–¾in) long, are spreading and aromatic. Star-shaped white flowers, to 1cm (½in) across, are borne singly or in pairs from late spring to summer. ↕0.3–1.5m (1–5ft), ↔ 0.9–1.5m (3–5ft). Australia (Tasmania). ✻✻✻ (borderline)
L. scoparium ■ (Manuka, New Zealand tea-tree). Compact shrub, rarely tree-like, with arching shoots and ascending to widely spreading, elliptic, broadly lance-shaped, or inversely lance-shaped, aromatic, mid- to dark green leaves, 0.7–2cm (¼–¾in) long, often silver-hairy when young. Solitary, shallowly cup- to saucer-shaped, white or pink-tinged white flowers, 1.5cm (½in) across, are profusely borne in late spring and early summer. ↕↔ 3m (10ft). S.E. Australia, New Zealand. ✻. **'Apple Blossom'** has white flowers overlaid with pink; ✻✻. **'Gaiety Girl'** ■ bears semi-double flowers, deep pink outside, paler within; ✻✻. **'Huia'** is compact, with dark pink flowers. Suitable for a rock garden or alpine house; ↕30cm (12in), ↔ 45cm (18in). **'Keatleyi'** ♀ has pale pink flowers, 2.5cm (1in) across. **'Kiwi'** ■♀ has purple-tinged young foliage and dark crimson flowers. Suitable for a rock garden or alpine house; ↕↔ 1m (3ft). **'Nicholsii'** ♀ has purple-tinged foliage and crimson flowers. **'Pink Cascade'** has a weeping habit and produces pink flowers; ✻✻. **var. *prostratum*** see *L. rupestre.* **'Red Damask'** ♀ has dark green leaves, and bears double, dark red flowers. **'Snow Flurry'** has double white flowers.

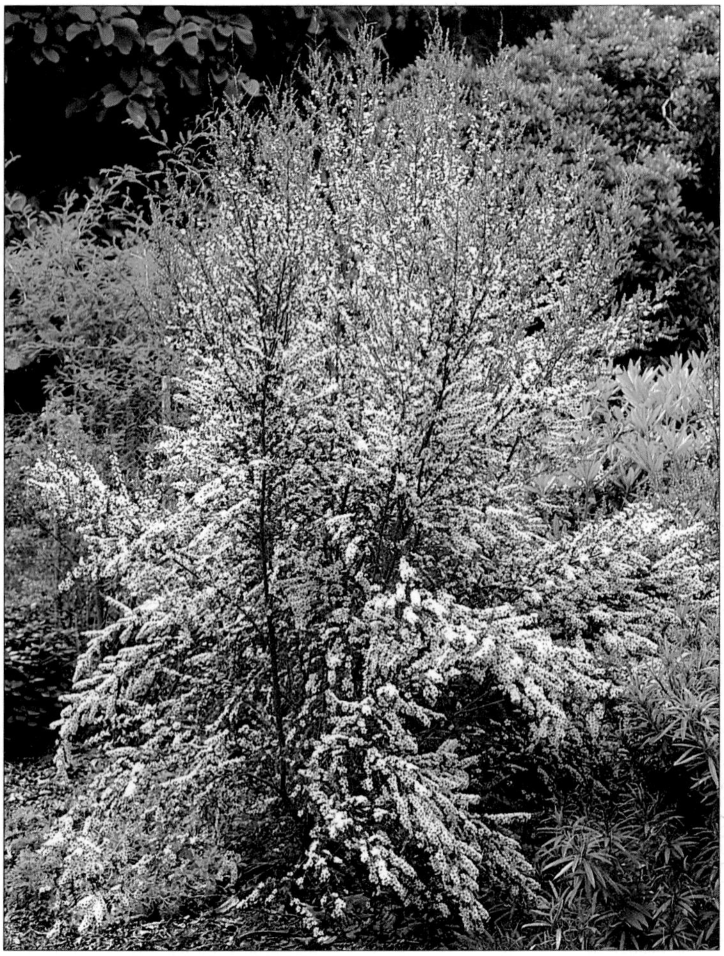
Leptospermum scoparium

LESCHENAULTIA
syn. LECHENAULTIA

GOODENIACEAE

Genus of about 20 species of evergreen shrubs, subshrubs, and perennials from semi-arid or arid areas of Australia. The usually linear leaves are entire, stalkless, and alternate or spiralling on the wiry stems. The showy, terminal flowers are solitary or borne in corymbs; they each have 5 free, often centrally "winged", white, yellow to red, or blue petals, 2 small and 3 large, which form a basal tube. In frost-prone areas, grow in a cool or temperate greenhouse. In frost-free climates, grow in a shrub border or as ground cover.
• **HARDINESS** Frost tender, although *L. biloba* and *L. formosa* may survive temperatures near to 0°C (32°F) if kept almost dry.
• **CULTIVATION** Under glass, grow in a mix of 1 part loam-based potting compost (JI No.1) and 3 parts each grit (or perlite) and peat, in full light with shade from hot sun and with good ventilation. In active growth, water moderately and apply a phosphate-free liquid fertilizer monthly; water sparingly in winter. Outdoors, grow in sharply drained soil that is low in nitrates and phosphates, in full sun with some midday shade. Pruning group 8 for shrubs.
• **PROPAGATION** Sow seed at 13–18°C (55–64°F) in spring, or root softwood cuttings in spring with bottom heat.
• **PESTS AND DISEASES** Under glass, red spider mites may be troublesome, and poor ventilation in winter will encourage grey mould (*Botrytis*).

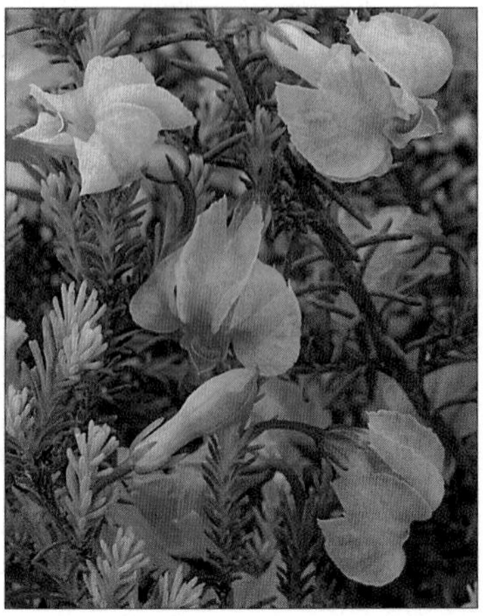
Leschenaultia formosa

L. biloba. Open shrub with linear, soft, mid-green to grey-green leaves, 1cm (½in) long. Bright blue, sometimes white flowers, 3cm (1¼in) across, are borne in leafy corymbs, to 8cm (3in) across, in late spring and early summer. Each petal lobe is roughly the shape of a fish-tail, the "tail fins" having sharp to blunt points. ↕↔ 30–60cm (12–24in). Australia (open eucalyptus forest in Western Australia). ❀ (min. 5–7°C/41–45°F)
L. floribunda. Erect, shrubby, woody-based perennial or short-lived shrub, with alternate, narrowly oblong to linear, mid-green leaves, 3–8mm (⅛–⅜in) long. Blue or white flowers, 1.5cm (½in) across, are borne in loose corymbs, to 10cm (4in) across, from late spring to midsummer. ↕45cm (18in), ↔ 35cm (14in). Australia (coastal plains of Western Australia). ❀ (min. 5–7°C/41–45°F)
L. formosa ■ Suckering, many-branched, spreading shrub with linear, blunt-tipped or pointed, light to grey-green leaves, to 1cm (½in) long. In late spring and early summer, produces solitary flowers, 2cm (¾in) across, in shades of bright red, orange, or orange-yellow. Usually short-lived, especially under glass. ↕↔ 30–60cm (12–24in). Australia (dry heathland in acid, quartzite sand in Western Australia). ❀ (min. 5–7°C/41–45°F)

LESPEDEZA
Bush clover

LEGUMINOSAE/PAPILIONACEAE

Genus of about 40 species of annuals, perennials, and deciduous subshrubs and shrubs found in meadows, grassland, and rocky places in E. Asia, Australia, and North America. They are cultivated for their small, pea-like flowers, profusely borne in axillary or terminal racemes. Leaves are alternate and 3-palmate. Excellent late-flowering plants for a mixed or shrub border.
• **HARDINESS** Fully hardy.
• **CULTIVATION** Grow in light, moderately fertile, well-drained soil in full sun. Pruning group 6 for shrubs;

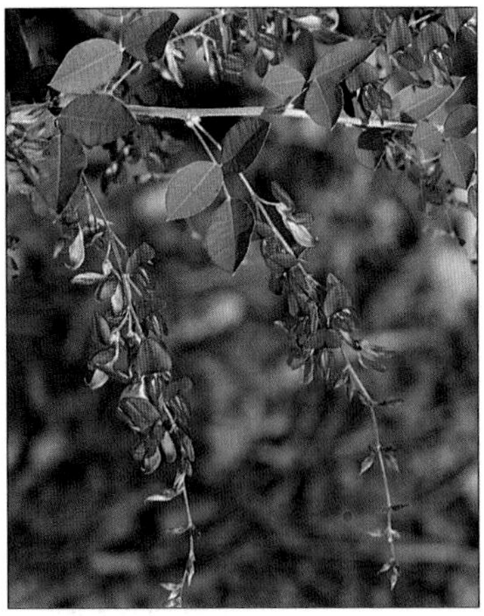

Lespedeza thunbergii

treat as perennials in very cold areas, where shrubby species may be cut to the ground by frost in winter.
• **PROPAGATION** Sow seed in containers outdoors in spring, or take greenwood cuttings in early summer. *L. thunbergii* may also be divided in spring.
• **PESTS AND DISEASES** Trouble free.

L. bicolor. Upright shrub with arching shoots and 3-palmate, mid- to dark green leaves consisting of broadly oval to obovate leaflets, to 5cm (2in) long. In mid- and late summer, purple-pink flowers, to 1cm (½in) long, are borne in slender racemes, 5–12cm (2–5in) or more long, from the upper leaf axils. ↕↔ 2m (6ft). E. Asia. ✻✻✻
L. thunbergii ▣ 🏆 Woody-based perennial or subshrub with long, arching shoots and 3-palmate, blue-green leaves consisting of oval or oval-lance-shaped leaflets, to 5cm (2in) long. In early autumn, purple-pink flowers, to 1.5cm (½in) long, are profusely borne in pendent, terminal racemes, to 15cm (6in) long. ↕ 2m (6ft), ↔ 3m (10ft). N. China, Japan. ✻✻✻

▷**Lettuce, Water** see *Pistia, P. stratiotes*

LEUCADENDRON

PROTEACEAE

Genus of 80 species of small, dioecious, evergreen shrubs and trees from varied habitats, ranging from sea plains to mountain slopes in dry or moist sites, in South Africa. They are grown mainly for their dense, cone-like, terminal clusters of small, tubular flowers, surrounded by large, leaf-like, often coloured or tinted bracts. Leaves are alternate or spiralling, stalkless, entire, leathery, and variably shaped. Both male and female plants are needed for fruiting cones to develop. Where temperatures fall below 5°C (41°F), grow in a cool or temperate greenhouse, although they seldom bear flowers or fruits in the former. In warm, dry areas, grow in a courtyard garden or against a sunny wall; the larger species are spectacular specimen plants.
• **HARDINESS** Frost tender.
• **CULTIVATION** Under glass, grow in a mix of 1 part lime-free (ericaceous) potting compost and 3 parts each grit (or perlite) and peat, in full light and low humidity. During the growing season, water moderately and apply magnesium sulphate and urea at half the recommended strength in spring and autumn; water sparingly in winter. Outdoors, grow in poor, well-drained, neutral to acid soil in full sun. May become chlorotic in magnesium-deficient soil. Pruning group 1.
• **PROPAGATION** Stratify seed below 5°C (41°F), then sow at 13–16°C (55–61°F) in a mix of equal parts peat and grit in spring. Root semi-ripe cuttings with bottom heat in summer.
• **PESTS AND DISEASES** Red spider mites may be a problem under glass.

L. argenteum ♤ (Silver tree). Erect, pyramidal to columnar tree with robust stems densely covered with lance-shaped, sharp-pointed, brilliant, silvery-hairy leaves, 10–15cm (4–6in) long. From spring to summer, bears spherical flowerheads, to 4cm (1½in) across, yellowish green on male trees, greenish silver on females, surrounded by leaf-like but broader and more lustrous bracts, to 2cm (¾in) long. The silvery cones often persist on the tree for several years. ↕ 6–10m (20–30ft), ↔ 2–4m (6–12ft). South Africa (Cape Peninsula). ❁ (min. 5–7°C/41–45°F)
L. discolor. Erect, open shrub with grooved, often purple-red stems and inversely lance-shaped, rigid, leathery, densely short-hairy, greyish green leaves, 2.5–4cm (1–1/½in) long, often tipped and margined purple. From spring to early summer, bears ovoid to spherical flowerheads, 3cm (1¼in) across, purple-red to red on male shrubs, whitish green on females, surrounded by ivory to creamy white bracts, 4–5cm (1½–2in) long, with purple-red tips or margins (usually more boldly coloured in males). Cones are brown. ↕ 1.5–2.5m (5–8ft), ↔ 1–2m (3–6ft). South Africa (Northern Cape, Western Cape, Eastern Cape). ❁ (min. 5–7°C/41–45°F)
L. 'Safari Sunset' ▣ Vigorous, erect, freely branching shrub with narrowly oblong leaves, to 9cm (3½in) long, deep green flushed purple-red, more colourful when young. From summer to autumn, produces ovoid, sterile, yellowish green female flowerheads, 4cm (1½in) across, surrounded by light red bracts, 10–20cm (4–8in) long, maturing to purple-red and fading to golden yellow. ↕ to 2.5m (8ft), ↔ to 1.8m (6ft) or more. ❁ (min. 5–7°C/41–45°F)
L. tinctum. Spreading, freely branching shrub with robust stems, bent towards their bases, and oblong, dark green leaves, 8cm (3in) long, increasing in size towards the stem tips. From spring to summer, bears ovoid, greenish yellow flowerheads, to 3cm (1¼in) across, surrounded by glossy yellow bracts, 8cm (3in) long, which reflex after the flowers have faded. Cones have a sweet, spicy aroma. ↕↔ to 1.2m (4ft). South Africa (Northern Cape, Western Cape, Eastern Cape). ❁ (min. 5–7°C/41–45°F)

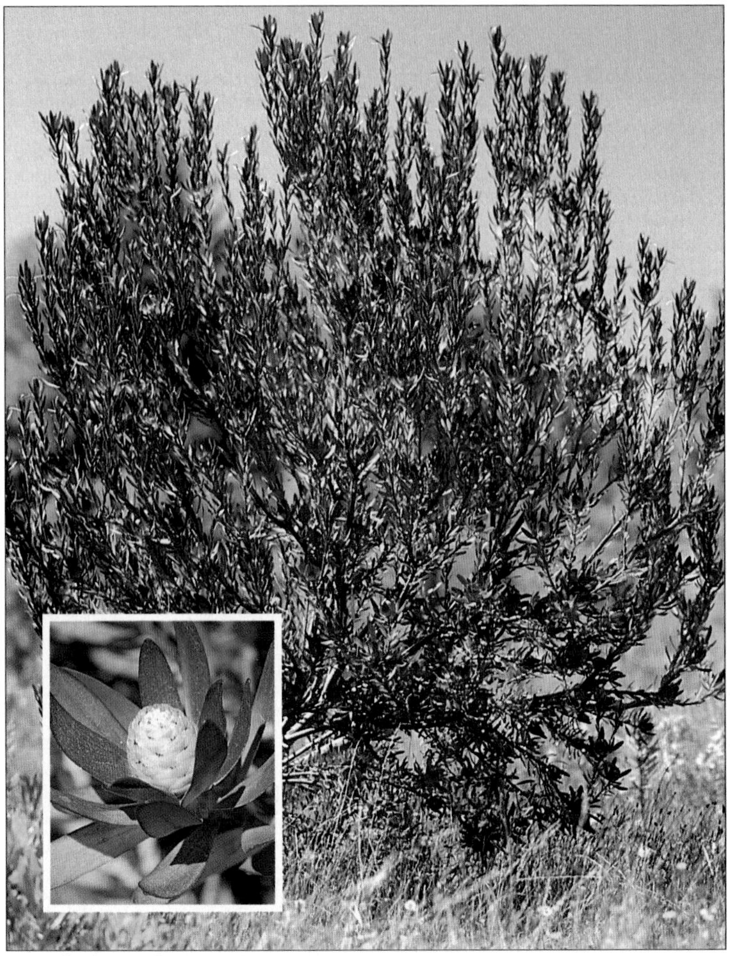

Leucadendron 'Safari Sunset' (inset: flowerhead detail)

LEUCANTHEMELLA

ASTERACEAE/COMPOSITAE

Genus of 2 species of hairy perennials found in wet meadows or marshy places, one species in S.E. Europe, the other in E. Asia. They have tall stems, which bear numerous alternate, lance-shaped to broadly elliptic or oblong, entire to sharply toothed leaves. They are grown mainly for their chrysanthemum-like flowerheads, borne singly or in 2- to 8-flowered corymbs in autumn. Grow in a mixed or herbaceous border. Also good for cutting.

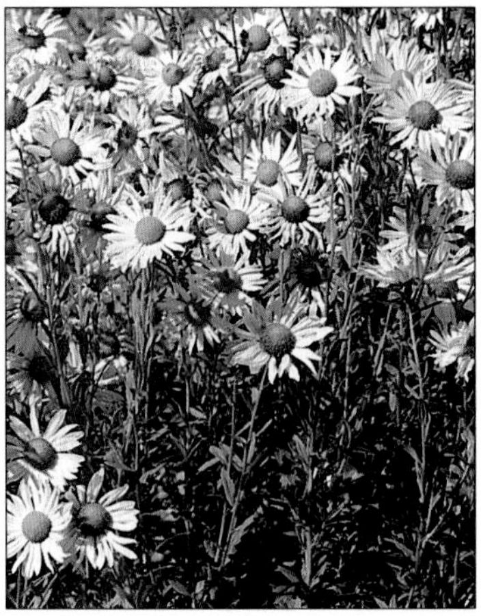

Leucanthemella serotina

• **HARDINESS** Fully hardy.
• **CULTIVATION** Grow in any reliably moist soil in full sun or partial shade.
• **PROPAGATION** Divide, or take basal cuttings, in spring.
• **PESTS AND DISEASES** Susceptible to slugs; thrips may damage leaves.

L. serotina ▣ 🏆 syn. *Chrysanthemum serotinum, C. uliginosum.* Strong-growing, erect perennial with simple, lance-shaped to broadly elliptic or oblong, toothed leaves, 6–12cm (2½–5in) long. From early to late autumn, white flowerheads, to 7cm (3in) across, with greenish yellow centres, are borne singly or in lax corymbs of 2–8. ↕ to 1.5m (5ft), ↔ 90cm (36in). S.E. Europe. ✻✻✻

LEUCANTHEMOPSIS

ASTERACEAE/COMPOSITAE

Genus of 6 species of dwarf, tufted, clump- or mat-forming perennials from mountain habitats in Europe and North Africa. They are grown for their solitary, daisy-like, white or yellow flowerheads, borne in summer. The leaves are pinnatisect, pinnatifid, or palmately lobed. Frequently short-lived, they are suitable for a rock garden, scree bed, or alpine house.
• **HARDINESS** Fully hardy (borderline).
• **CULTIVATION** Grow in any sharply drained soil in full sun. In an alpine house, grow in equal parts loam, leaf mould, and grit.
• **PROPAGATION** Sow seed in containers in an open frame as soon as ripe. Divide, or take basal cuttings, in spring.
• **PESTS AND DISEASES** Susceptible to aphids and red spider mites under glass.

L. alpina, syn. *Chrysanthemum alpinum* (Alpine chrysanthemum). Mat-forming, rhizomatous perennial with variable, ovate to spoon-shaped, pinnatisect, deeply pinnatifid, or palmately lobed, silvery grey leaves, to 4cm (1½in) long. In mid- and late summer, produces short-stemmed flowerheads, to 4cm (1½in) across, with white ray-florets, sometimes turning pink with age, and orange-yellow disc-florets. Best grown in a scree bed. ↕ 10cm (4in), ↔ to 20cm (8in). Pyrenees, Alps, Apennines, Carpathians. ✻✻✻

L

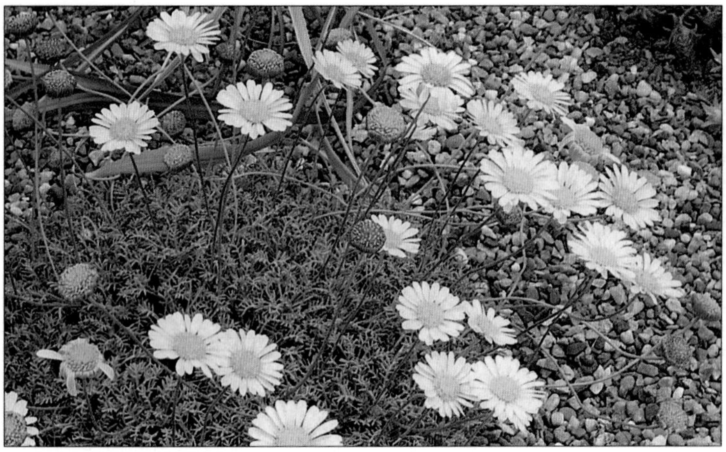

Leucanthemopsis pectinata

L. pectinata ■ syn. *Chrysanthemum pectinata, L. radicans, Pyrethrum radicans.* Densely tufted perennial, spreading by runners, with pinnatifid, grey-green to silvery green leaves, 7–14cm (3–6in) long, with 5–9 lobes. In summer, bears flowerheads to 2cm (¾in) across, with yellow-orange disc-florets, and golden yellow ray-florets that turn orange-red. ↕ 15cm (6in), ↔ to 30cm (12in). Spain (Sierra Nevada). ❄❄❄ (borderline)
L. radicans see *L. pectinata.*

LEUCANTHEMUM

ASTERACEAE/COMPOSITAE

Genus of 26 species of annuals and perennials from rocky alpine slopes and moist meadows, grassland, and waste-land in Europe and temperate Asia. They have alternate, entire, deeply pinnatifid, toothed, scalloped, or lobed leaves, and solitary, daisy-like, terminal flowerheads, which are usually white with yellow disc-florets. Grow alpine species in a scree bed or rock garden, taller perennials in a wild garden. Some hybrids and cultivars are useful in a herbaceous border and for cut flowers.

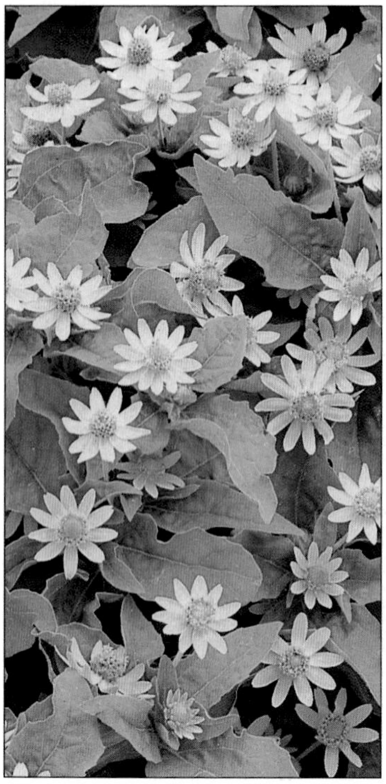

Leucanthemum paludosum 'Show Star'

- **HARDINESS** Fully hardy to frost hardy.
- **CULTIVATION** Grow in moderately fertile, moist but well-drained soil in full sun or partial shade. Alpine species need sharply drained soil in full sun. Many of the taller plants need support.
- **PROPAGATION** Sow seed of annuals *in situ* in spring. Sow seed of perennials in containers in a cold frame in autumn or spring. Divide perennials in early spring or late summer.
- **PESTS AND DISEASES** Aphids, slugs, earwigs, chrysanthemum eelworm, and leaf spots may be troublesome.

L. atratum, syn. *Chrysanthemum atratum.* Variable, clump- or mat-forming perennial with spoon-shaped, scalloped or lobed, dark green basal leaves, to 5cm (2in) long, and shorter, oblong to linear, deeply toothed to pinnatifid stem leaves, with toothed tips. In summer, upright stems bear solitary flowerheads, to 5cm (2in) across, with yellow disc-florets and white ray-florets. ↕↔ to 30cm (12in). Alps, Apennines, mountains of Slovenia, Bosnia & Herzegovina, and Yugoslavia (Serbia and Montenegro). ❄❄❄
L. hosmariense see *Rhodanthemum hosmariense.*
L. paludosum, syn. *Chrysanthemum paludosum.* Hairless, bushy annual with obovate, spoon-shaped, grey-green basal leaves, to 12cm (5in) long, and shorter, oblong-wedge-shaped stem leaves; all leaves are toothed to pinnatifid. In summer, produces solitary flowerheads, 2–3cm (¾–1¼in) across, with yellow or yellowish white ray-florets and deeper yellow disc-florets. ↕ 5–15cm (2–6in),

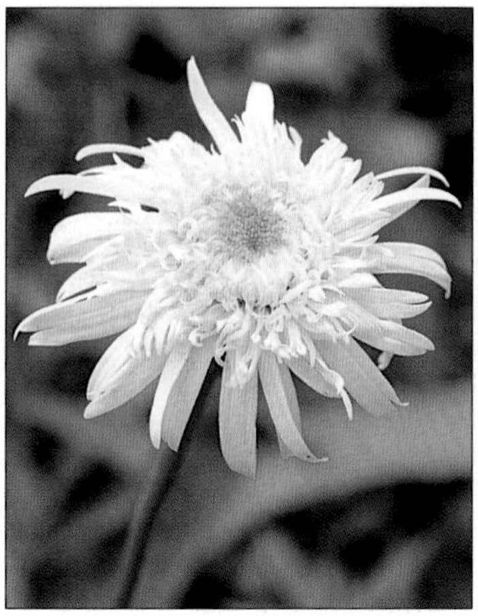

Leucanthemum x *superbum* 'Cobham Gold'

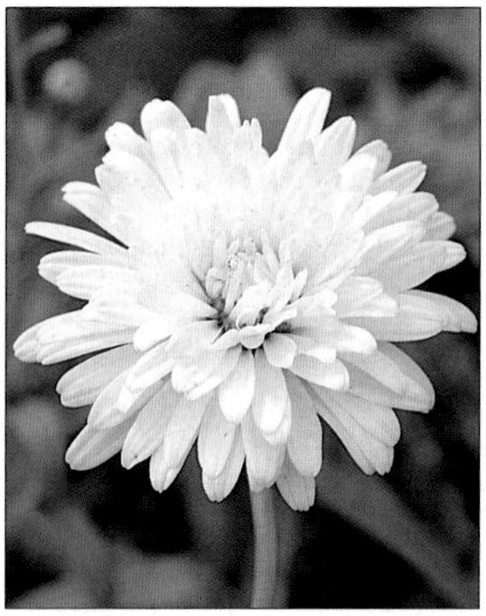

Leucanthemum x *superbum* 'Horace Read'

↔ 20cm (8in). S. Portugal, S. and S.E. Spain, Balearic Islands. ❄❄❄. **'Show Star'** ■ has wavy-margined, toothed, mid-green leaves and bright yellow flowerheads.
L. x superbum (*L. lacustre* x *L. maximum*) syn. *Chrysanthemum maximum* of gardens, *C.* x *superbum* (Shasta daisy). Robust, clump-forming perennial with inversely lance-shaped, toothed, glossy, almost fleshy, dark green basal leaves, to 30cm (12in) long, and shorter, lance-shaped, stalkless stem leaves. From early summer to early autumn, bears solitary, single or double white flowerheads, 10–12cm (4–5in) across, with yellow disc-florets, paler in the double-flowered forms. Good for cutting. ↕ 90cm (36in), ↔ 60cm (24in). Garden origin. ❄❄❄. **'Aglaia'** 🏆 produces fringed, semi-double flower-heads; ↕ 60cm (24in). **'Bishopstone'** has feathery, single flowerheads with narrow, cut ray-florets. **'Cobham Gold'** ■ has double flowerheads; ↕ 60cm (24in). **'Esther Read'** has double, pure white flowerheads; ↕↔ 50–60cm (20–24in). **'Everest'** see 'Mount Everest'. **'Fiona Coghill'** has double flowerheads. **'Horace Read'** ■ has double white flowerheads with incurved disc-florets; ↕ 60cm (24in). **'Little Silver Princess'** see 'Silberprinzesschen'. **'Mount Everest'**, syn. 'Everest', bears single flowerheads, to 10cm (4in) across. **'Phyllis Smith'** ■ has single flower-heads with twisted, recurved ray-florets. **'Silberprinzesschen'**, syn. 'Little Silver Princess', has single flowerheads; ↕↔ 30cm (12in). **'Snowcap'** very freely bears single flowerheads, to 10cm (4in)

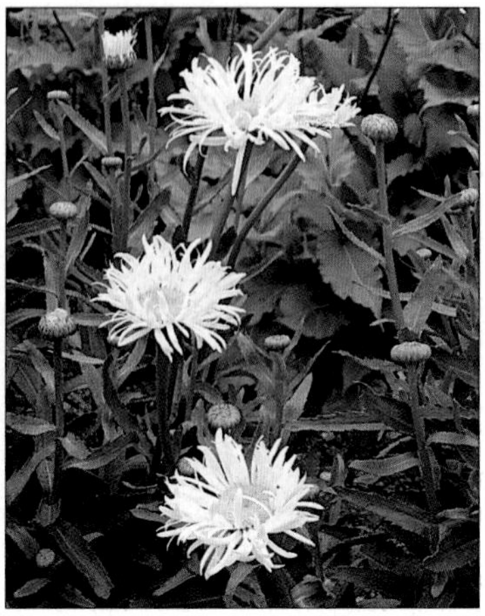

Leucanthemum x *superbum* 'Phyllis Smith'

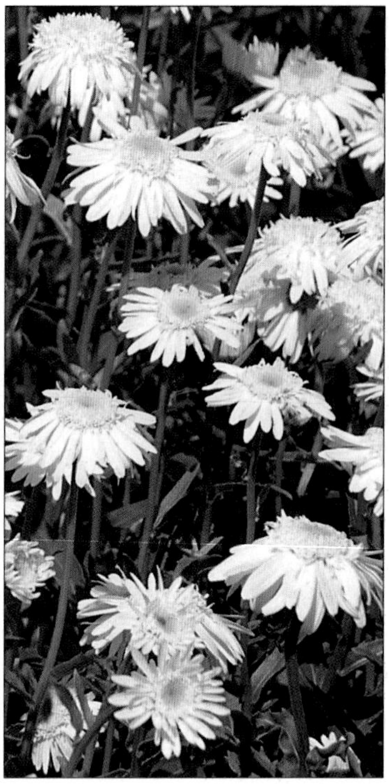

Leucanthemum x *superbum* 'Wirral Pride'

across; ↕↔ 45cm (18in). **'Snow Lady'** is a fast-growing, erect, bushy perennial usually grown as an annual, with oval to lance-shaped, deeply toothed leaves; produces single white flowerheads in summer; ↕ 25–45cm (10–18in), ↔ 30cm (12in). **'T.E. Killin'** 🏆 has double flowerheads, to 10cm (4in) across, with yellow anemone centres. **'Wirral Pride'** ■ has double flower-heads with anemone centres; ↔ 75cm (30in). **'Wirral Supreme'** 🏆 has dense, double flowerheads with slightly shorter centre ray-florets; ↔ 75cm (30in).
L. vulgare, syn. *Chrysanthemum leucanthemum* (Marguerite, Ox-eye daisy). Extremely variable, rhizomatous perennial with obovate-spoon-shaped, toothed, smooth, dark green basal leaves, 2–10cm (¾–4in) long, and shorter, sometimes pinnatifid stem leaves. Solitary flowerheads, 2.5–5cm (1–2in) across, with bright yellow disc-florets and white ray-florets, are borne in late spring and early summer. ↕ 30–90cm (12–36in), ↔ 60cm (24in). Most of Europe, temperate Asia. ❄❄❄

LEUCHTENBERGIA

CACTACEAE

Genus of one species of perennial cactus with a thick, forked, tuberous rootstock, sometimes branching from the base, from hilly regions in central N. Mexico. The plant is covered with narrowly triangular, spirally arranged tubercles, each tipped by an areole bearing papery, twisted spines. The areoles on young tubercles produce fragrant flowers by day from summer to autumn. Where temperatures drop below 10°C (50°F), grow in a warm greenhouse; in warmer climates, grow in a desert garden.

- **HARDINESS** Frost tender.
- **CULTIVATION** Under glass, grow in standard cactus compost in full light. From mid-spring to early autumn, water moderately and apply a balanced liquid fertilizer every 6–8 weeks; keep

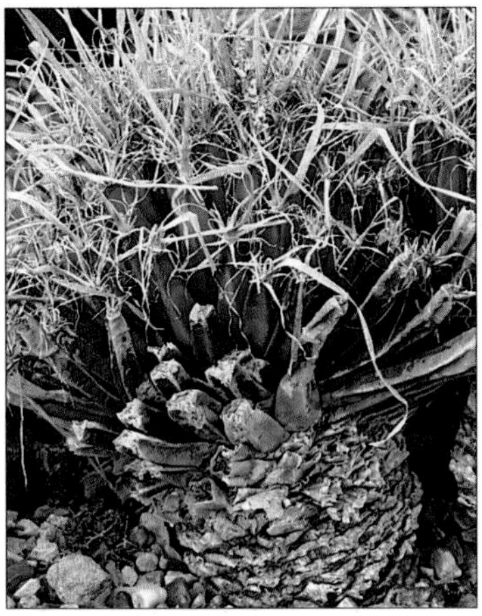

Leuchtenbergia principis

completely dry from mid-autumn to early spring. Outdoors, grow in moderately fertile, sharply drained, ideally alkaline soil, in full sun. Protect from winter wet. See also pp.48–49.
• **PROPAGATION** Sow seed at 19–24°C (66–75°F) in spring.
• **PESTS AND DISEASES** Susceptible to scale insects when in growth.

L. principis ■ Simple or branching cactus with a thick, cylindrical, fleshy root, appearing woody when mature, and spherical to short cylindrical stems. Narrowly triangular, glaucous, bluish green tubercles, 10–12cm (4–5in) long, cover the stems. Large grey areoles bear 8–14 radial spines, to 5cm (2in) long, and 1 or 2 centrals, to 15cm (6in) long. From summer to autumn, bears funnel-shaped, bright yellow flowers, to 8cm (3in) long. ↕30–60cm (12–24in), ↔ 30cm (12in). Central N. Mexico. ❀ (min. 10°C/50°F)

LEUCOCORYNE

ALLIACEAE/LILIACEAE

Genus of 12 species of garlic-scented, bulbous perennials from dry scrub and rocky hillsides in Chile. They are grown for their umbels of large, open funnel-shaped, scented, blue, white, or purple flowers, borne in spring. Each bulb produces 2–5 linear, often channelled, basal leaves, smelling of garlic. In frost-prone areas, grow in a cool greenhouse; in warmer areas, grow in a rock garden.
• **HARDINESS** Frost tender.
• **CULTIVATION** Plant bulbs 10cm (4in) deep. Under glass, grow in loam-based potting compost (JI No.2) with added sharp sand, in full light with good ventilation. When in growth, water moderately and apply a balanced liquid fertilizer monthly when in leaf. Reduce water after flowering and keep almost dry when dormant in summer. Pot on every 2 years in autumn. Outdoors, grow in moderately fertile, sharply drained soil in full sun.
• **PROPAGATION** Sow seed at 19–24°C (66–75°F) as soon as ripe, or remove offsets in autumn before repotting.
• **PESTS AND DISEASES** Trouble free.

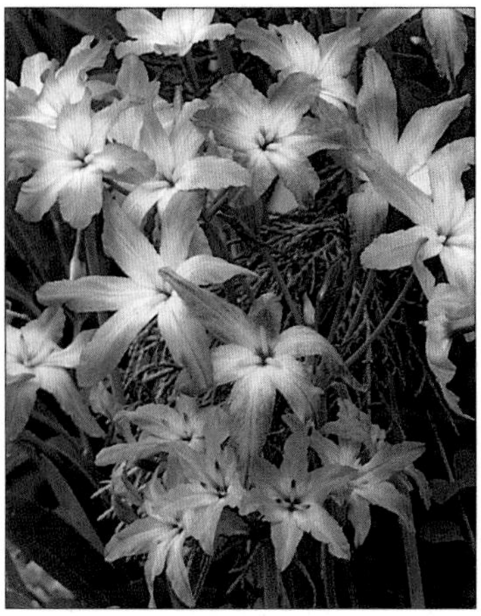

Leucocoryne ixioides

L. ixioides ■ (Glory of the sun). Bulbous perennial with narrow, grass-like, basal leaves, to 45cm (18in) long, which wither as the flowers open. In spring, produces umbels of up to 12 outward-facing, open funnel-shaped, scented flowers, 2cm (¾in) across, white with purple veins, or lilac-blue with white throats. ↕45cm (18in), ↔ 8cm (3in). Chile. ❀ (min. 5–7°C/41–45°F)
L. purpurea. Bulbous perennial with narrow, grass-like, basal leaves, to 30cm (12in) long, which wither as the flowers open. In spring, produces umbels of 2–7 open funnel-shaped, scented, pale lilac flowers, 2.5cm (1in) across, with broad, red-purple centres. ↕45cm (18in), ↔ 8cm (3in). Chile. ❀ (min. 5–7°C/41–45°F)

LEUCOGENES

New Zealand edelweiss

ASTERACEAE/COMPOSITAE

Genus of 3 or 4 species of dwarf, hummock-, mat-, or clump-forming perennials from screes or rocky, fell-fields in the mountains of New Zealand. They have obovate-wedge-shaped or linear to lance-shaped, closely overlapping, intensely silver-hairy leaves and, in summer, bear small, flat yellow flowerheads surrounded by collars of white-woolly bracts. Effective in a peat bed, rock garden, or alpine house, but difficult to grow in dry climates.
• **HARDINESS** Hardy to -10°C (14°F), possibly more.
• **CULTIVATION** Grow in gritty, humus-rich, moist but sharply drained soil in full sun. They grow best in cool, moist climates and resent a dry atmosphere in summer. Protect from winter wet. In an alpine house, grow in a mix of equal parts loam, leaf mould, and coarse sand.
• **PROPAGATION** Sow seed in containers in an open frame as soon as ripe. Take stem-tip cuttings in late summer.
• **PESTS AND DISEASES** Susceptible to red spider mites under glass; may be damaged by slugs and snails outdoors.

L. grandiceps ■ Mat-forming perennial with closely overlapping, obovate-wedge-shaped, silver-downy leaves, to 1cm (½in) long, that obscure the stems. In early summer, bears yellow flowerheads, 0.9–1.5cm (⅜–½in) across, near the shoot tips, each surrounded by a collar, 1cm (½in) across, of densely white-woolly bracts. ↕↔ 10–15cm (4–6in). New Zealand (South Island). ❄❄❄ (borderline)
L. leontopodium, syn. *Raoulia leontopodium.* Hummock-forming perennial with linear to lance-shaped-oblong leaves, to 2cm (¾in) long, clothed in yellowish or greyish silver or silvery white down. In early summer, produces yellow flowerheads, to 2.5cm (1in) across, near the shoot tips, each surrounded by a collar, to 1.5cm (½in) across, of white-woolly bracts. ↕↔ 10–15cm (4–6in). New Zealand. ❄❄❄ (borderline)

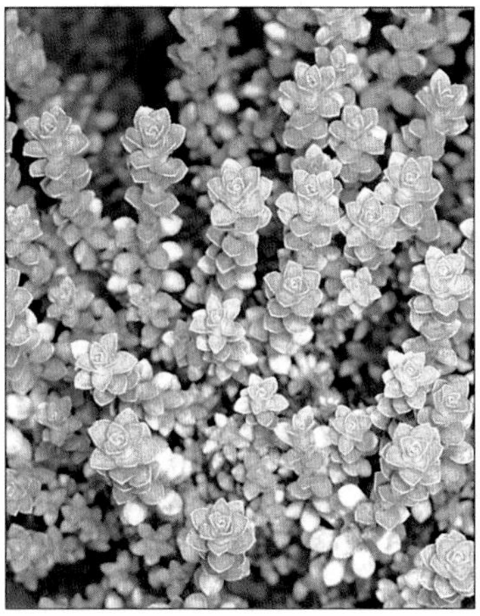

Leucogenes grandiceps

LEUCOJUM

Snowflake

AMARYLLIDACEAE

Genus of about 10 species of mainly spring- or autumn-flowering, bulbous perennials from a variety of habitats, including woodland, shaded hillsides, wet sites, dunes, rocky grassland, and scrub, from W. Europe to the Middle East and N. Africa. They are related and similar to snowdrops (*Galanthus*), with usually 1 or 2, occasionally up to 8 flowers per stem, but the nodding or pendent, bell-shaped, usually white, sometimes pink flowers have 6 equal segments. Leaves are basal and strap-shaped to linear, or occasionally narrowly cylindrical. Small species are suitable for a rock garden, alpine house, or bulb frame, while larger species such as *L. aestivum* and *L. vernum* are excellent in a border, near water, or naturalized in grass.
• **HARDINESS** Fully hardy to frost hardy.
• **CULTIVATION** Plant dry bulbs 8–10cm (3–4in) deep in autumn. Grow in any moist but well-drained soil in full sun, apart from *L. aestivum* and *L. vernum,* which need reliably moist, humus-rich soil. In an alpine house, grow in equal parts loam, leaf mould, and sharp sand.
• **PROPAGATION** Sow seed in containers in a cold frame in autumn, or remove offsets once the leaves have died down.
• **PESTS AND DISEASES** Prone to slugs and narcissus bulb fly.

L. aestivum (Summer snowflake). Robust, bulbous perennial with erect, strap-shaped, glossy, dark green leaves, to 40cm (16in) long. In spring, leafless stems bear up to 8 bell-shaped, faintly chocolate-scented white flowers, 2cm (¾in) long, with green tips. ↕45–60cm (18–24in), ↔ 8cm (3in). Ireland, UK, Belgium, France, C. and E. Europe, N. Turkey, Ukraine (Crimea), Caucasus, N. and N.W. Iran. ❄❄❄.
'Gravetye Giant' ■♀ is more robust; ↕90cm (36in), especially when grown near water.
L. autumnale ■♀ Slender, bulbous perennial with erect, narrow, grass-like leaves, to 16cm (6in) long, produced with or just after the flowers. In late summer and early autumn, each bulb produces up to 4 leafless stems, each bearing 2–4 bell-shaped white flowers, 1cm (½in) long, with red-tinged bases. ↕10–15cm (4–6in), ↔ 5cm (2in). S.W. Europe, N. Africa. ❄❄❄
L. hiemale see *L. nicaeense.*
L. nicaeense ♀ syn. *L. hiemale.* Bulbous perennial with 2–4 almost prostrate, curled, narrowly linear leaves, to 30cm (12in) long. In early spring, leafless stems produce 1 or 2 bell-shaped, waxy white flowers, 1cm (½in) long. Survives outside in a sunny, sheltered site, but is best grown in an alpine house. ↕10cm (4in), ↔ 5cm (2in). S.E. France. ❄❄
L. roseum. Bulbous perennial with leafless stems bearing 1 or 2 bell-shaped, pale pink flowers, 1cm (½in) long, in late summer or autumn. Erect, thread-like, narrowly linear leaves, to 10cm (4in) long, appear just after the flowers. Best in an alpine house, especially in areas that experience prolonged frost. ↕10cm (4in), ↔ 5cm (2in). Corsica, Sardinia. ❄❄
L. trichophyllum. Bulbous perennial with 3 linear leaves, 5–20cm (2–8in)

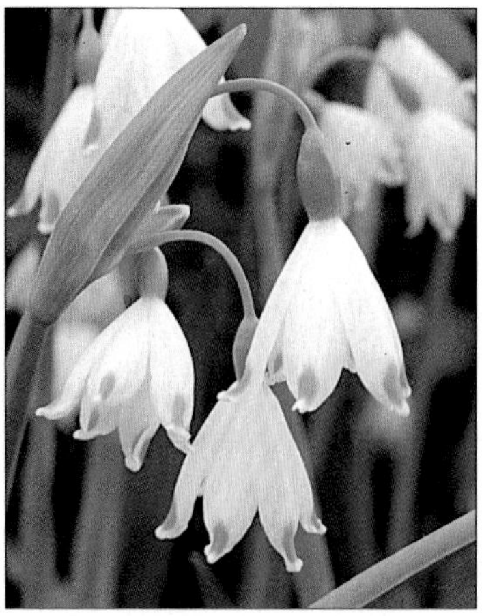

Leucojum aestivum 'Gravetye Giant'

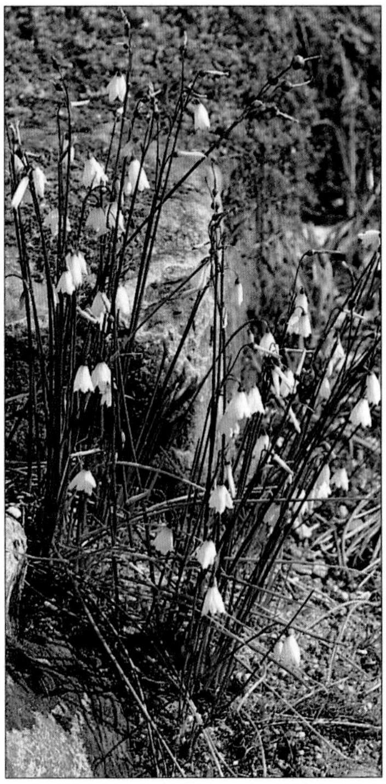

Leucojum autumnale

L

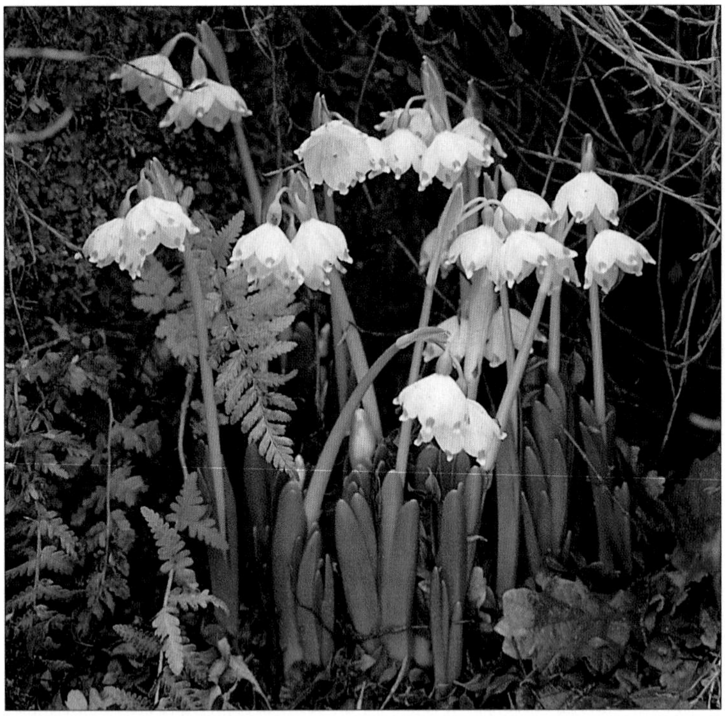

Leucojum vernum var. *vagneri*

long, that appear before or with the flowers. From winter to spring, slender, leafless stems bear 2–4 bell-shaped white flowers, to 2cm (¾in) long, sometimes flushed pink or purple. Best in an alpine house. ↕10–30cm (4–12in), ↔ 5cm (2in). S. Portugal, S.W. Spain, Morocco. ✽✽

L. valentinum. Bulbous perennial with narrowly linear, grey-green leaves, to 25cm (10in) long, produced after the flowers. In autumn, leafless stems bear 1–3 bell-shaped white flowers, 1cm (½in) long. ↕15cm (6in), ↔ 3–5cm (1¼–2in). C. Spain, N.W. Greece, Ionian Islands. ✽✽✽ (borderline)

L. vernum ♕ (Spring snowflake). Bulbous perennial with erect, strap-shaped, glossy, dark green leaves, to 25cm (10in) long. In early spring, produces stout, leafless stems with usually 1, occasionally 2, bell-shaped, green-tipped white flowers, 2.5cm (1in) long. ↕20–30cm (8–12in), ↔ 8cm (3in). S. and E. Europe. ✽✽✽. **var. *carpathicum*** produces 1 or 2 flowers per stem, each with yellow-tipped tepals. **var. *vagneri*** ■ is robust, and flowers in late winter and early spring, bearing 2 flowers per stem; ↕20cm (8in).

L

LEUCOPHYTA

syn. CALOCEPHALUS

Cushion bush

ASTERACEAE/COMPOSITAE

Genus of 18 species of annuals and evergreen perennials and small shrubs from rocky coastal habitats, often exposed to salt spray, in Australia. They are cultivated for their alternate, very narrow, entire, often white-woolly leaves and spherical, rayless flowerheads, which are clustered into terminal corymbs. In frost-prone climates, grow in a cool greenhouse, or as summer bedding or edging foliage plants. In warmer climates, they are useful for adding a silver edging to a shrub border.

• **HARDINESS** Frost tender; may withstand short periods down to 0°C (32°F).

• **CULTIVATION** Under glass, grow in loam-based potting compost (JI No.1) with added grit, in full light. Pot on or top-dress in spring, or plant outside in early summer. When in growth, water moderately and apply a balanced liquid fertilizer monthly; water sparingly in winter. Outdoors, grow in sharply drained, moderately fertile soil in full sun. Pinch out stem tips of young plants to promote bushiness. Pruning group 10, in spring.

• **PROPAGATION** Root semi-ripe cuttings in summer.

• **PESTS AND DISEASES** Prone to grey mould (*Botrytis*) in damp conditions.

L. brownii ■ syn. *Calocephalus brownii.* Bushy shrub with intricately branched, slender, silvery white-downy stems. Scale-like, silvery grey leaves, 5mm (¼in) long, are pressed closely against the stems, so that the bush appears leafless. In summer, produces small, rounded, terminal corymbs of creamy white, rarely purple flowerheads, 1cm (½in) across. ↕40–75cm (16–30in), ↔ 40–90cm (16–36in). Australia (Western Australia to New South Wales, Tasmania). ❁ (min. 5–7°C/41–45°F)

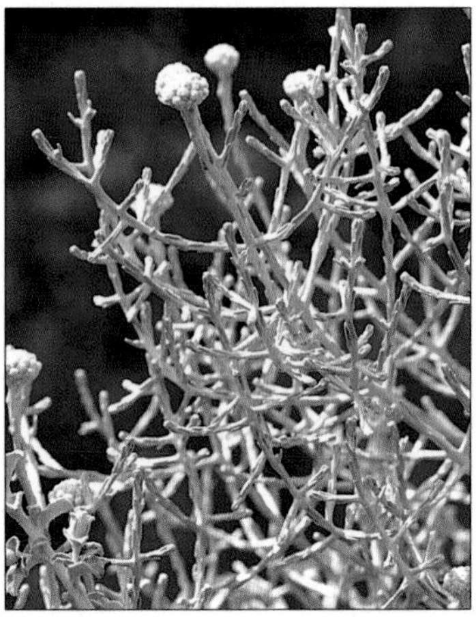

Leucophyta brownii

LEUCOPOGON

EPACRIDACEAE

Genus of about 150 species of erect or spreading, evergreen shrubs and small trees from heathland and forest in S. Asia and Australasia. They have variably shaped, entire leaves, and bear tubular flowers, with reflexed lobes, either singly or in spikes, followed by small, fleshy, berry-like fruits. Grow in a rock garden. In frost-prone areas, grow tender species in a cool greenhouse.

• **HARDINESS** Fully hardy to frost tender.

• **CULTIVATION** Grow in humus-rich, moist but well-drained, acid soil in full sun or partial shade. Pruning group 8 or 9.

• **PROPAGATION** Sow seed in containers outdoors as soon as ripe, or take greenwood cuttings in early summer.

• **PESTS AND DISEASES** Trouble free.

L. colensoi see *Cyathodes colensoi.*

L. fraseri, syn. *Cyathodes fraseri.* Creeping subshrub with densely overlapping, heath-like, obovate, short-stalked, glossy, dark green leaves, 5–10mm (¼–½in) long, often tinted red in autumn, with bristles on the tips and margins. Bears axillary, solitary, 5-lobed, fragrant white flowers, 5–10mm (¼–½in) across, towards the tips of upright shoots in summer. In autumn, produces edible, sweet-tasting, spherical, fleshy, pale orange fruit, 6–9mm (¼–⅜in) across. ↕10–15cm (4–6in), ↔ to 30cm (12in). New Zealand. ✽✽

x LEUCORAOULIA

ASTERACEAE/COMPOSITAE

Bigeneric hybrid genus between *Leucogenes leontopodium* and *Raoulia rubra*, from the Tararua mountains of New Zealand. Grown for its cushions of silvery, rosetted foliage, it is best grown in a scree bed or alpine house.

• **HARDINESS** Fully hardy.

• **CULTIVATION** Grow in gritty, sharply drained soil in full sun. Protect from winter wet. Under glass, grow in a mix of equal parts loam, leaf mould, and grit; top-dress with grit. Water freely from spring to summer; resents a hot, dry atmosphere in summer, so mist in hot weather. Keep just moist in winter.

• **PROPAGATION** Detach individual rosettes and root as cuttings in spring.

• **PESTS AND DISEASES** Susceptible to mildew, especially in dry conditions.

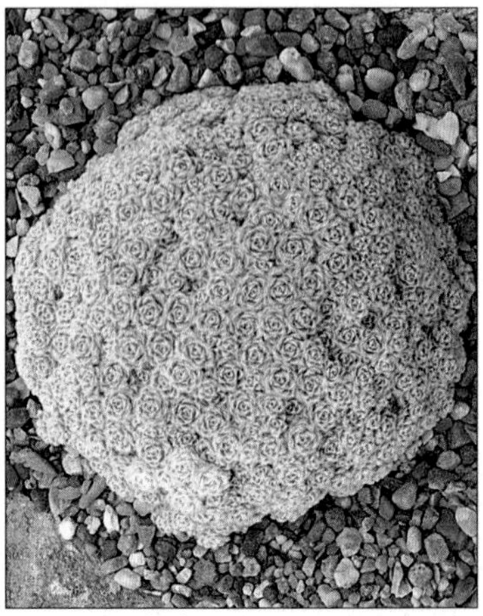

x *Leucoraoulia loganii*

x L. loganii ■ syn. *Raoulia* x *loganii.* Dense, cushion-forming perennial with neat, symmetrical, almost columnar rosettes of tiny, overlapping, densely hairy, silvery white leaves, to 2mm (1/16in) long. Produces insignificant pink flowerheads in summer in the wild, but very seldom in cultivation. ↕8cm (3in), ↔ 10cm (4in). New Zealand. ✽✽✽

LEUCOSPERMUM

Pincushion

PROTEACEAE

Genus of 47 species of evergreen shrubs and small trees from varied habitats, including scrub, subtropical coastal dune forest, evergreen temperate forest, and mountain slopes, in Zimbabwe and South Africa. The alternate, leathery, simple, entire or toothed leaves may be linear to elliptic, inversely lance-shaped, oval, ovate, obovate, oblong, or spoon-shaped. Dense, cone-like, clustered or solitary, terminal flowerheads are borne on short axillary shoots and have very prominent, red, orange, pink, yellow, or white styles. Where temperatures fall below 5°C (41°F), grow in a cool or temperate greenhouse. In warmer, dry areas, plant in a shrub border. The larger species are good specimen plants.

• **HARDINESS** Frost tender.

• **CULTIVATION** Under glass, grow in a mix of 1 part loam-based potting compost (JI No.1) and 3 parts each grit (or perlite) and peat, in full light. In active growth, water moderately and apply magnesium sulphate and urea at half the recommended strength in spring and autumn; water sparingly in winter, never allowing the compost to dry out. Outdoors, grow in well-drained, neutral to acid soil, with low levels of phosphates and nitrates, in full sun. Magnesium deficiency may lead to chlorosis. Pruning group 1; may need restrictive pruning under glass.

• **PROPAGATION** Stratify ripe seed below 5°C (41°F), then sow at 13–16°C (55–61°F) in spring. Root semi-ripe cuttings in summer with bottom heat.

• **PESTS AND DISEASES** Red spider mites may be a problem under glass.

L. catherinae (Catherine's pincushion). Densely bushy, erect shrub with a short, stout trunk. Crowded, inversely lance-shaped to elliptic, stalked, hairless leaves, 9–14cm (3½–5½in) long, each with 3 or 4 teeth at the tip, are usually mid- to deep green, tinted yellow or grey, with often red-flushed tips and margins. From spring to early summer, bears solitary, conical flowerheads, 10–15cm (4–6in) across, with erect, then arching styles that are light orange, tipped mauve-pink, ageing to deep reddish gold. ↕↔ 2.5m (8ft). South Africa (Western Cape). ❁ (min. 5°C/41°F)

L. cordifolium ■ syn. *L. nutans.* Rounded, spreading shrub with ovate to oblong, entire, stalkless, mid-green leaves, to 8cm (3in) long, heart-shaped at the bases, sometimes with 3–6 teeth at the tips, and initially downy, later almost smooth. From early spring to midsummer, horizontal to downward-arching stems, which bend sharply upwards at their tips, produce solitary, spherical flowerheads, 10–12cm (4–5in) wide, with numerous forward-arching, usually orange, but also crimson or

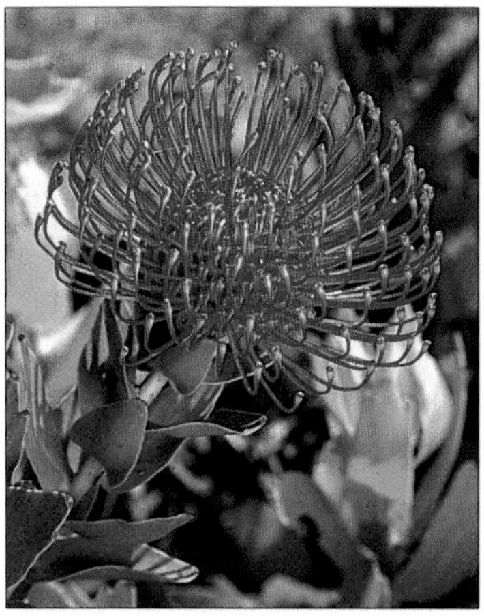
Leucospermum cordifolium

yellow styles. ↕ to 2m (6ft), ↔ 1.5–3.5m (5–11ft). South Africa (Northern Cape, Western Cape, Eastern Cape, on acid soils). ❀ (min. 5°C/41°F)
L. nutans see *L. cordifolium.*
L. reflexum. Rounded, moderately open shrub, thickening with age. Oblong-elliptic to inversely lance-shaped, hairy, grey-green leaves, 2–6cm (¾–2½in) long, sometimes have 2 or 3 teeth at the tips. From early spring to early summer, erect shoots produce solitary or paired, ovoid to spherical flowerheads, 4.5–6cm (1¾–2½in) across, composed of initially outward- and upward-curving orange styles, which are later strongly reflexed and deep crimson. ↕ to 3m (10ft), ↔ 2–4m (6–12ft). South Africa (Cedar Berg mountains in Western Cape). ❀ (min. 5°C/41°F)

LEUCOTHOE

ERICACEAE

Genus of about 50 species of deciduous, semi-evergreen, or evergreen shrubs from woodland, thickets, swamps, and streambanks in Madagascar, the Himalayas, E. Asia, and North and South America. They are cultivated for their handsome leaves, which are alternate, very variably shaped, simple, often glossy, and dark green, and for their cylindrical to urn-shaped, usually white flowers, borne in terminal or axillary racemes or panicles. Effective in a peat bed or acid woodland garden.
• **HARDINESS** Fully hardy to frost hardy.
• **CULTIVATION** Grow in humus-rich, reliably moist, acid soil in deep or partial shade. Pruning group 1.

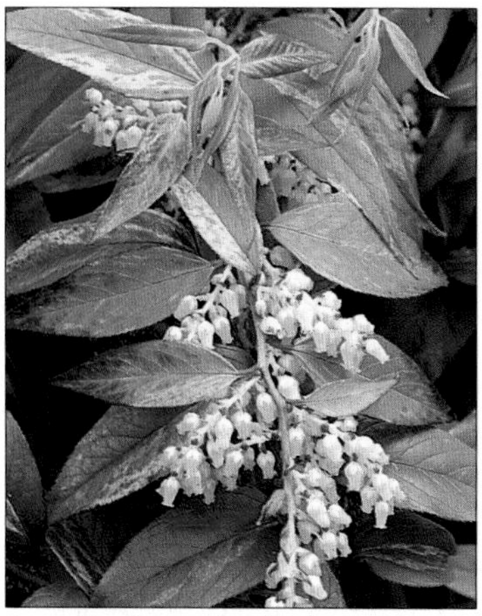
Leucothoe fontanesiana 'Rainbow'

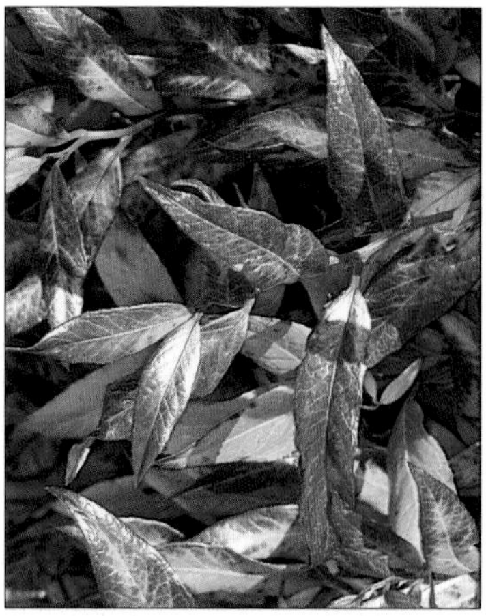
Leucothoe fontanesiana 'Scarletta'

• **PROPAGATION** Sow seed in containers in a cold frame in spring. Root semi-ripe cuttings with bottom heat in summer. Divide suckering species in spring.
• **PESTS AND DISEASES** Trouble free.

***L. catesbaei* of gardens** see *L. fontanesiana.*
L. davisiae (Sierra laurel). Upright, suckering, evergreen shrub with ovate-oblong, glossy, dark green leaves, to 8cm (3in) long. Urn-shaped white flowers, 5mm (¼in) long, are produced in erect, axillary racemes, 5–15cm (2–6in) long, in early summer. ↕ 1m (3ft), ↔ 1.5m (5ft). USA (California, Oregon). ❄❄❄
L. fontanesiana 🏆 syn. *L. catesbaei* of gardens, *L. walteri* (Switch ivy). Upright, evergreen shrub with arching branches and oblong-lance-shaped to ovate-lance-shaped, toothed, leathery, hairless leaves, 6–16cm (2½–6in) long, dark green and glossy above, paler below. In spring, produces almost cylindrical white flowers, 5mm (¼in) long, in axillary racemes, 4–6cm (1½–2½in) long. ↕ 1–2m (3–6ft), ↔ 3m (10ft). S.E. USA. ❄❄❄. **'Rainbow'** ■ is thicket-forming, with lance-shaped, dark green leaves, heavily mottled cream and pink. Flowers are produced in late spring; ↕ 1.5m (5ft), ↔ 2m (6ft). **'Rollissonii'** 🏆 has narrowly elliptic-lance-shaped leaves, to 10cm (4in) long. **'Scarletta'** ■ has dark red-purple young foliage, which turns dark green, then bronze in winter.
L. keiskei. Clump-forming, evergreen shrub with upright to prostrate shoots and narrowly ovate to ovate-lance-shaped, slenderly tapered, glossy, dark green leaves, to 9cm (3½in) long, red when young. Urn-shaped white flowers, to 1cm (½in) long, are borne in nodding racemes, to 5cm (2in) long, at or near the ends of young shoots in midsummer. Suitable for a peat bed. ↕↔ 60cm (24in). Japan. ❄❄❄
L. racemosa (Fetter bush, Sweetbells). Bushy, suckering, deciduous or semi-evergreen shrub with upright shoots and oblong to ovate or elliptic, pointed, glossy, dark green leaves, to 6cm (2½in) long. In early summer, urn-shaped white flowers, 6mm (¼in) long, are profusely borne in upright to spreading, usually terminal racemes, to 10cm (4in) long. ↕↔ 1.5m (5ft). E. USA. ❄❄❄
L. walteri see *L. fontanesiana.*

▷ ***Leuzea centauroides*** see *Centaurea* 'Pulchra Major'

LEVISTICUM

Lovage

APIACEAE/UMBELLIFERAE

Genus of one species of hairless perennial occurring in mountain regions in the E. Mediterranean. It has 2- or 3-pinnate, dark green leaves, and umbels of star-shaped flowers produced in midsummer. The strongly celery-scented roots and shoots are used as a vegetable or in salads, and the seeds for flavouring. Suitable for a herb garden. Contact with the foliage may cause photodermatitis.
• **HARDINESS** Fully hardy.
• **CULTIVATION** Tolerant of most soils, but best in deep, moderately fertile, moist but well-drained soil in full sun.
• **PROPAGATION** Sow seed in a seedbed as soon as ripe, or divide in early spring.
• **PESTS AND DISEASES** Leaf miners may be troublesome.

L. officinale. Robust perennial with stout, hollow, finely ribbed stems and 2- or 3-pinnate, triangular to diamond-shaped, dark green leaves, to 70cm (28in) long, with ovate, toothed leaflets. Star-shaped, greenish yellow flowers are borne in umbels, to 15cm (6in) across, in midsummer, followed by ovoid, slightly winged green fruit. ↕ 2m (6ft), ↔ 1m (3ft). E. Mediterranean. ❄❄❄

LEWISIA

PORTULACACEAE

Genus of approximately 20 species of deciduous or evergreen perennials from W. North America, with fleshy rootstocks, and rosettes or tufts of fleshy leaves that vary greatly in shape. The deciduous species occur in open, stony meadows or grassland, and die down after flowering; evergreens are more commonly found in partial shade among rocks or in crevices. The funnel-shaped to open funnel-shaped flowers, each with 5–9, sometimes up to 19 petals, are produced in shades of pink, magenta, purple, orange, yellow, or white. They are usually borne in cymes or panicles, occasionally singly or in racemes or corymbs, in spring and summer, often over long periods. Grow in an alpine house or rock garden, or in the crevices of a retaining wall.
• **HARDINESS** Fully hardy.
• **CULTIVATION** Grow in moderately fertile, humus-rich, sharply drained, neutral to acid soil: deciduous species and hybrids in full sun, evergreens in light shade. Protect all from winter wet; protect deciduous lewisias from rain in summer, when dormant. In an alpine house, grow in equal parts loam, leaf mould, and sharp sand.
• **PROPAGATION** Sow seed in containers in a cold frame in autumn, or remove offsets (evergreen species only) in early summer. Seed of *L.* Cotyledon Hybrids does not come true to colour, and many species hybridize freely in cultivation.
• **PESTS AND DISEASES** Susceptible to aphids under glass, and to slugs and snails outdoors. Prone to neck rot in wet conditions.

L. brachycalyx ■ 🏆 Dwarf, tufted, deciduous perennial with a basal rosette of inversely lance-shaped, dark green leaves, 3–8cm (1¼–3in) long. In late spring and early summer, numerous solitary, funnel-shaped, white, sometimes pale pink flowers, 2.5–5cm (1–2in) across, are borne on scapes to 6cm (2½in) long. ↕↔ to 8cm (3in). USA (S. California, Arizona). ❄❄❄
L. columbiana. Variable, evergreen perennial with compact, symmetrical or irregular rosettes of inversely lance-shaped or linear, dark green leaves, 2–10cm (¾–4in) long. From spring to summer, bears panicles of many open funnel-shaped, usually deep magenta-pink flowers, to 2.5cm (1in) across, sometimes pale pink with darker veins. ↕↔ to 15cm (6in). Canada (British Columbia), USA (Oregon). ❄❄❄
L. cotyledon 🏆 Evergreen perennial with flat rosettes of spoon-shaped or

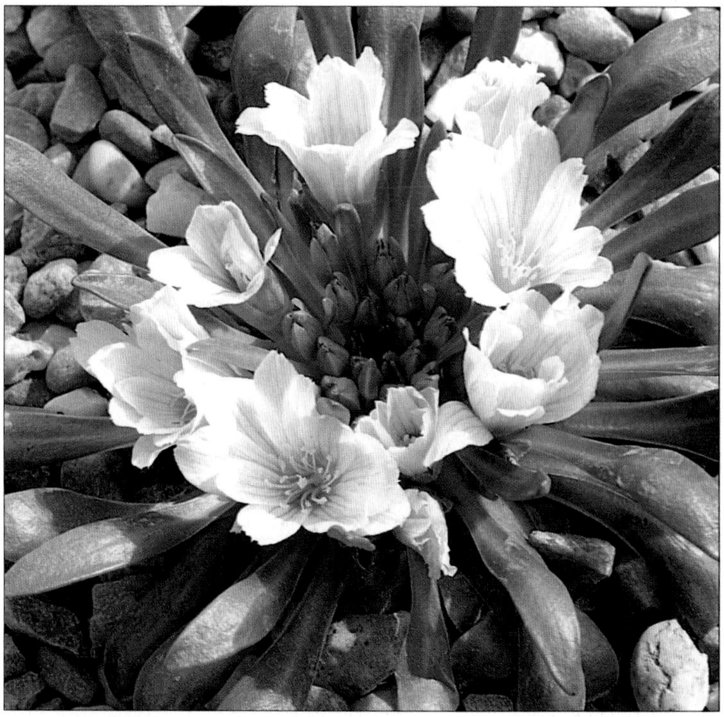
Lewisia brachycalyx

L

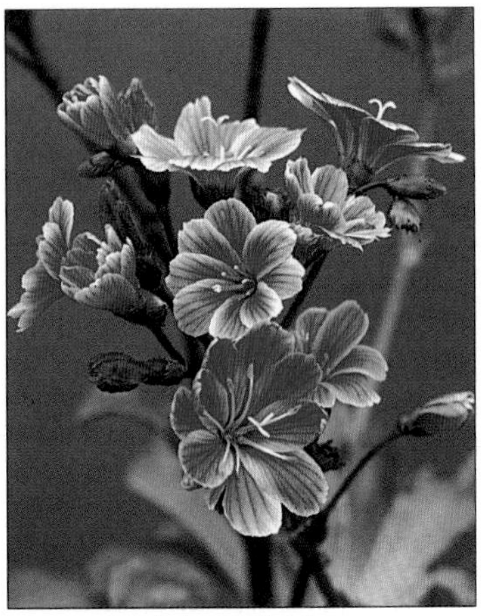
Lewisia Cotyledon Hybrids

inversely lance-shaped or obovate, slightly glaucous, dark green leaves, 3–14cm (1¼–5½in) long. From spring to summer, produces compact panicles of many open funnel-shaped, paler and darker striped, usually pinkish purple, sometimes white, cream, yellow, or apricot flowers, to 2.5cm (1in) across. ‡ 30cm (12in), ↔ to 25cm (10in). USA (N.W. California). ❄❄❄. **f. *alba*** has pure white flowers. **var. *howellii*** has leaves with wavy, toothed margins, and pale pink flowers with darker veining.
***L.* Cotyledon Hybrids** ■ Clump-forming, evergreen perennials that produce rosettes of thick, variably shaped, mid- to dark green leaves, 3–14cm (1¼–5½in) long, with toothed or wavy margins. From late spring to summer, funnel-shaped flowers, 2–4cm (¾–1½in) across, in a range of bright colours, including shades of pink, deep magenta, yellow, and orange, are borne in compact panicles. ‡ 15–30cm (6–12in), ↔ 20–40cm (8–16in). ❄❄❄
***L.* 'George Henley'** ■ Clump-forming, evergreen perennial with rosettes of narrowly spoon-shaped, fleshy, dark green leaves, to 8cm (3in) long. From late spring to late summer, produces many-flowered cymes of funnel-shaped, purplish pink flowers, to 2.5cm (1in) across, with magenta veining. ‡ 10cm (4in) or more, ↔ 10cm (4in). ❄❄❄
L. longipetala, syn. *L. pygmaea* subsp. *longipetala.* Deciduous perennial with basal tufts of narrowly linear or linear-inversely lance-shaped, dark green leaves, 2–5cm (¾–2in) long. In late spring or early summer, produces several scapes, 3–6cm (1¼–2½in) long, bearing

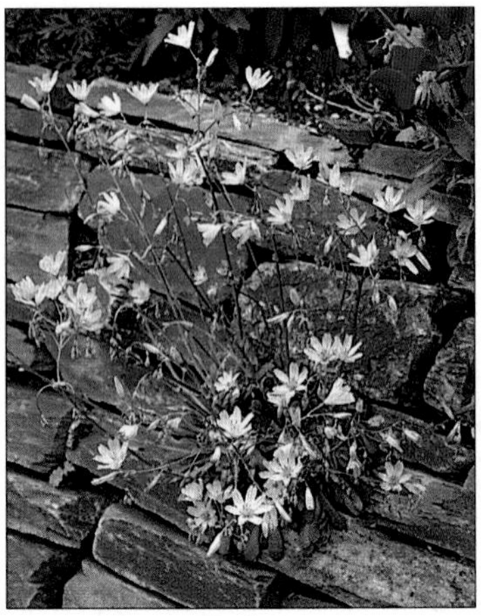
Lewisia 'George Henley'

L

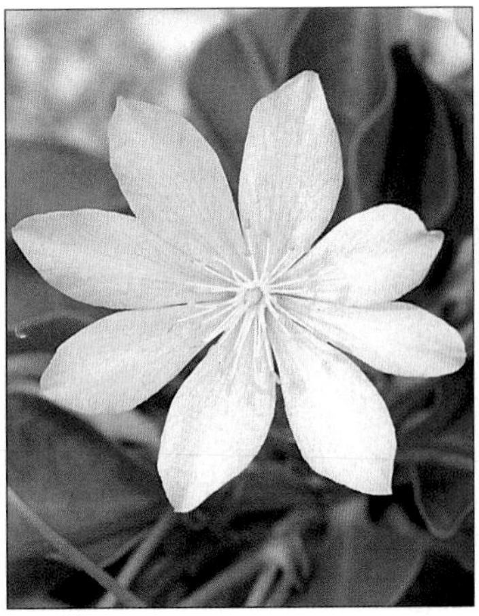
Lewisia tweedyi

cymes of 1–3 open funnel-shaped, star-like, pure white or pink-flushed white flowers, 2.5–4cm (1–1½in) across, with red-tinted sepals. Similar to, but easier to grow than *L. brachycalyx.* ‡↔ to 10cm (4in). USA (California). ❄❄❄
L. nevadensis. Deciduous perennial with loose, basal rosettes of narrowly linear, suberect, dark green leaves, 4–15cm (1½–6in) long. From late spring to summer, bears solitary, broadly funnel-shaped, star-like, white, rarely pink flowers, to 3.5cm (1½in) across, on scapes 10–15cm (4–6in) long. ‡↔ to 10cm (4in). W. USA. ❄❄❄
L. pygmaea. Deciduous perennial with tufts of linear or linear-inversely lance-shaped, erect, dark green leaves, 3–9cm (1¼–3½in) long. In summer, prostrate or semi-erect scapes, 1–6cm (½–2½in) long, bear cymes of 1–7 funnel-shaped, deep purplish pink, occasionally white or pale pink flowers, 1.5–2cm (½–¾in) across. ‡↔ to 8cm (3in). Canada, USA (Alaska to New Mexico). ❄❄❄. **subsp. *longipetala*** see *L. longipetala.*
L. rediviva (Bitterroot). Deciduous perennial with tufts of linear or club-shaped, dark green leaves, 1.5–5cm (½–2in) long, dying back rapidly at or after flowering. From early spring to summer, bears several solitary, broadly funnel-shaped, pink or white flowers, 5cm (2in) across, with 12–19 narrow petals, on scapes 1–3cm (½–1¼in) long. ‡ 5cm (2in), ↔ 10cm (4in). Canada (British Columbia), USA (California, Nevada, Utah). ❄❄❄
L. tweedyi ■ 🏆 Rosette-forming, evergreen perennial with broad, inversely lance-shaped or obovate, purple-tinted, mid-green leaves, to 10cm (4in) long. From spring to early summer, scapes, 10–20cm (4–8in) long, bear open funnel-shaped, white to peach-pink flowers, to 6cm (2½in) across, singly or in cymes of up to 4. ‡ 20cm (8in), ↔ 30cm (12in). N.W. USA. ❄❄❄. **f. *alba*** has pure white to ivory flowers.

LEYCESTERIA

CAPRIFOLIACEAE

Genus of about 6 species of suckering, deciduous shrubs, with hollow, cane-like stems, from cliffs and mountain woodland in India, the Himalayas, China, and Burma. They are cultivated for their terminal or axillary racemes or spikes of whorled, tubular, 5-lobed flowers; *L. formosa* also has long-persistent, claret-red bracts below the blooms. The leaves

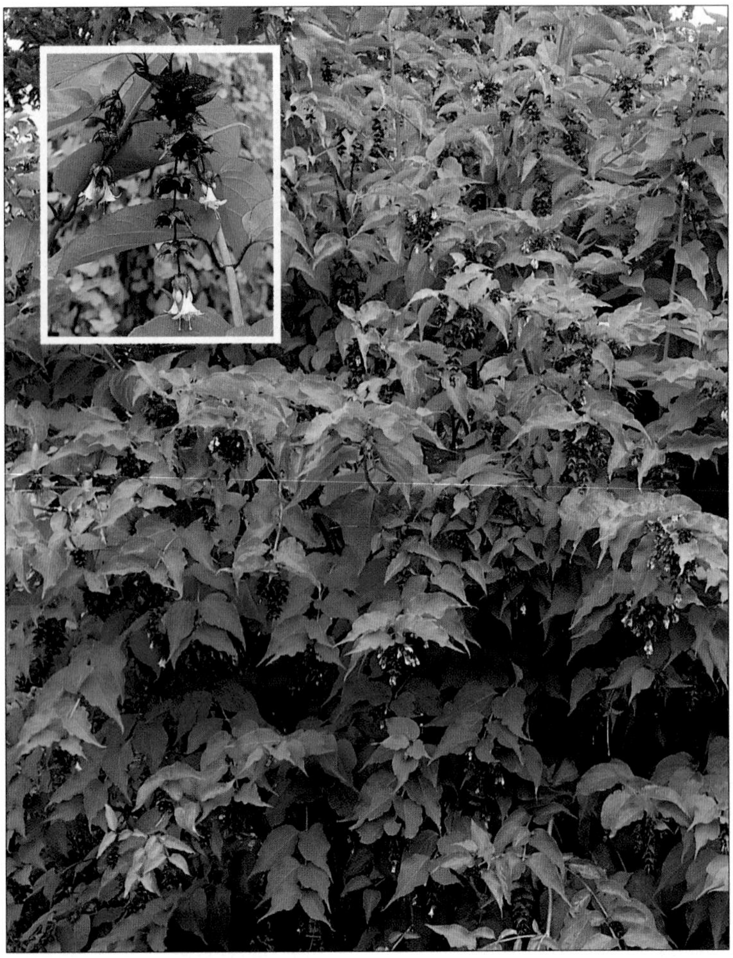
Leycesteria formosa (inset: flower detail)

are opposite, narrowly ovate to ovate, and long-pointed, with entire or toothed margins. Grow in a woodland garden or shrub border. In frost-prone areas, grow half-hardy species in a cool greenhouse.
• **HARDINESS** Fully hardy (borderline) to half hardy.
• **CULTIVATION** Grow in moderately fertile, well-drained soil in full sun or partial shade. Protect from cold, drying winds and mulch deeply in autumn where frosts are severe. Pruning group 3 or 6.
• **PROPAGATION** Sow seed in containers in a cold frame in autumn, or take softwood cuttings in summer.
• **PESTS AND DISEASES** Trouble free.

L. crocothyrsos. Upright shrub with arching shoots and ovate, tapered leaves, to 15cm (6in) long. Golden yellow flowers, to 2cm (¾in) long, with wide-spreading lobes, are produced in arching, terminal racemes, 12–17cm (5–7in) long, from late spring to late summer, followed by small, spherical green berries. ‡↔ 2m (6ft). India (Assam), N. Burma. ❄❄
L. formosa ■ (Himalayan honeysuckle). Upright, thicket-forming shrub with attractive, bamboo-like, blue-green first-year shoots, and ovate, tapered, dark green leaves, to 17cm (7in) long. Pendent spikes, to 10cm (4in) long, of white flowers among dark purple-red bracts, are borne terminally or from the upper leaf axils, from summer to early autumn. Flowers are followed by spherical, red-purple berries. ‡↔ 2m (6ft). Himalayas, W. China. ❄❄❄ (borderline)

LEYMUS

GRAMINEAE/POACEAE

Genus of approximately 40 species of rhizomatous, perennial grasses, formerly included in *Elymus.* They occur mainly in grassland in N. temperate regions, with one species from Argentina. They have linear, flat or rolled, stiff, glaucous leaves, and bear narrowly linear racemes of usually paired, sometimes solitary spikelets in summer. The ornamental species are grown for the architectural value of their blue-green leaves; although invasive, they are also suitable for a mixed or herbaceous border.
• **HARDINESS** Fully hardy.
• **CULTIVATION** Grow in moderately fertile but not heavy, well-drained soil in full sun. Cut down dead growth in autumn.
• **PROPAGATION** Divide from mid-spring to early autumn.
• **PESTS AND DISEASES** Trouble free.

L. arenarius ■ syn. *Elymus arenarius.* Densely tufted grass with long rhizomes, forming loose, spreading clumps of arching, broadly linear, flat, pale blue-grey leaves, to 60cm (24in) long. Throughout summer, stiff, erect stems bear spike-like racemes, to 35cm (14in) long, of paired, blue-grey, then buff spikelets. ‡ to 1.5cm (5ft), ↔ indefinite. N. and W. Europe, Eurasia. ❄❄❄
L. giganteus see *L. racemosus.*
L. racemosus, syn. *Elymus racemosus, L. giganteus.* Rhizomatous grass with arching, broadly linear, flat, blue-green leaves, to 30cm (12in) long, rough

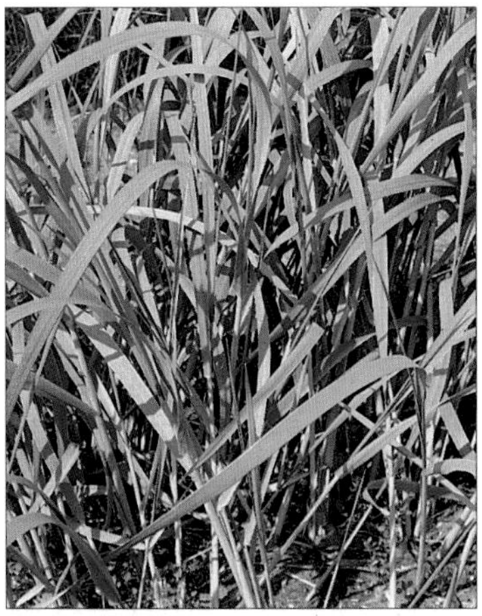

Leymus arenarius

textured above, smooth beneath. Throughout summer, stiff, upright stems produce spike-like racemes, to 35cm (14in) long, of flattened, softly hairy, initially bluish green, later buff spikelets, in clusters of 6. ↕ to 1.2m (4ft), ↔ 75cm (30in) or more. N. Europe, Eurasia. ✽✽✽. **'Glaucus'** is less invasive, and has erect or arching, clear, pale blue-green leaves; ↕ 75cm (30in).

▷ **Liana** see *Semele androgyna*

LIATRIS

Blazing star, Gayfeather

ASTERACEAE/COMPOSITAE

Genus of approximately 40 species of perennials with tuber- or corm-like, swollen, flattened stems. They occur mainly in prairie or open woodland, on dry, stony ground (although *L. spicata* grows in damper sites), in E. and C. North America. Linear to ovate-lance-shaped leaves are borne in basal tufts, and arranged alternately on the stiff stems. The numerous button-like flowerheads, produced in corymb-like spikes or racemes, are composed of dense clusters of tubular, pinkish purple

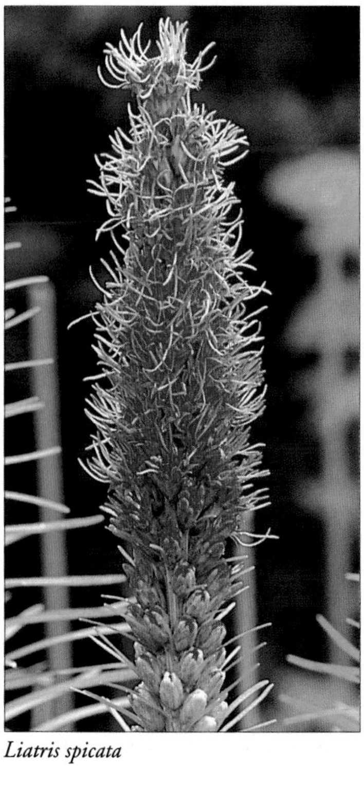

Liatris spicata

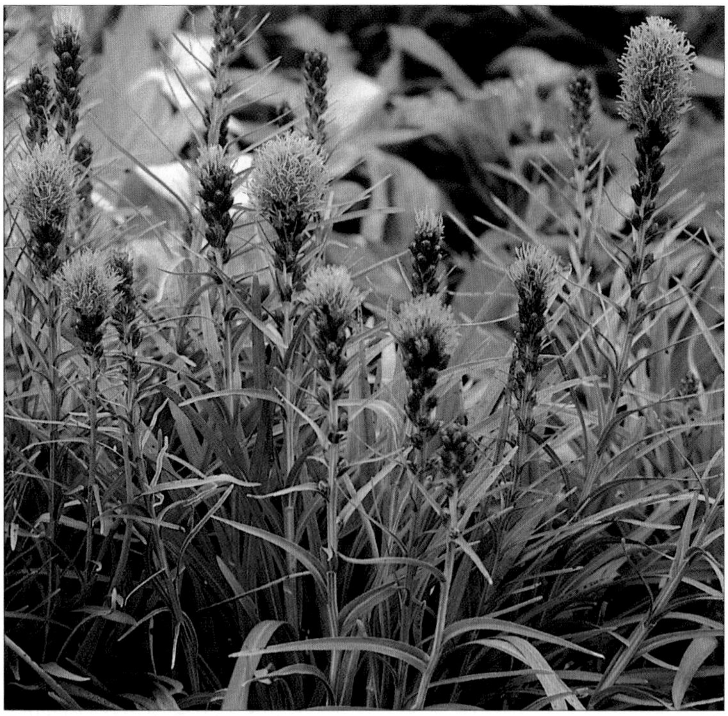

Liatris spicata 'Kobold'

or white disc-florets, and are unusual in that they open from the top of the inflorescence downwards. Suitable for a mixed or herbaceous border, and also good for cutting. The flowerheads are attractive to bees.

• **HARDINESS** Fully hardy.

• **CULTIVATION** Grow in light, moderately fertile, moist but well-drained soil in full sun; *L. spicata* needs reliably moist soil. Liable to rot in wet winters in heavy soils.

• **PROPAGATION** Sow seed in containers in a cold frame in autumn. Divide in spring.

• **PESTS AND DISEASES** Susceptible to slugs, snails, and mice (which eat the rootstocks).

***L. callilepis* of gardens** see *L. spicata.*

L. pycnostachya (Kansas feather). Perennial with densely clustered, linear basal leaves, 10–30cm (4–12in) long, which reduce in size up the robust, hairy stems. Bears dense spikes, 45cm (18in) long, of bright purple flowerheads, 1cm (½in) across, from midsummer to early autumn. ↕ to 1.5m (5ft), ↔ 45cm (18in). C. and S.E. USA. ✽✽✽

L. scariosa. Perennial with densely clustered, lance-shaped to narrowly ovate or obovate, rough basal leaves, to 25cm (10in) long, reducing in size and inversely lance-shaped on the robust, hairy stems. Similar to *L. pycnostachya*, but with less dense spikes, 45cm (18in) long, of reddish purple flowerheads, 2.5cm (1in) across, in early autumn. ↕ 0.6–1.2m (2–4ft), ↔ 45cm (18in). N.E. and S.E. USA. ✽✽✽. **'September Glory'** has deep purple flowerheads; ↕ 1.3m (4½ft).

L. spicata ■ syn. *L. callilepis* of gardens (Gayfeather). Perennial with hairless stems and linear or linear-lance-shaped basal leaves, 30–40cm (12–16in) long; stem leaves are smaller and linear. Long-lasting, pink-purple or white flower-heads, to 1cm (½in) across, are borne in dense spikes, 45–70cm (18–28in) long, in late summer and early autumn. ↕ to 1.5m (5ft), ↔ 45cm (18in). E. and S. USA. ✽✽✽. **'Blue Bird'** has blue-purple flowerheads. **'Floristan Weiss'** has white flowerheads; ↕ to 90cm (36in). **'Goblin'** see 'Kobold'. **'Kobold'** ■ syn. 'Goblin', produces deep purple flower-heads; ↕ 40–50cm (16–20in). **'Snow Queen'** produces white flowerheads; ↕ 75cm (30in).

LIBERTIA

IRIDACEAE

Genus of 20 species of fibrous-rooted, clump-forming, rhizomatous, evergreen perennials occurring in moist, grassy areas and scrub in New Caledonia, New Zealand, and temperate North and South America. They have linear, leathery, 2-ranked, overlapping, mainly basal leaves; leaves on the stiff flowering stems are sparse and smaller. They are cultivated for their saucer-shaped, white or blue flowers, each usually with 3 small outer tepals, 3 broad inner tepals, and sheathing bracts, produced in panicles and followed by glossy, light brown seed heads. Grow the larger libertias in a herbaceous or mixed border, or in a gravel garden; the smaller species are suitable for a rock garden.

• **HARDINESS** Fully hardy (borderline) to frost hardy. *L. ixioides* may survive to -10°C (14°F).

• **CULTIVATION** Grow in moderately fertile, humus-rich, moist but well-drained soil in full sun. In frost-prone areas, protect in winter with a dry mulch.

• **PROPAGATION** Sow seed in containers outdoors as soon as ripe, or divide in spring.

• **PESTS AND DISEASES** Trouble free.

L. caerulescens. Clump-forming, rhizomatous perennial with linear, rigid, leathery leaves, 30–45cm (12–18in) long. In late spring, flowering stems bear 1 or 2 short leaves, and terminal, short-branched panicles consisting of umbel-like clusters of many pale blue flowers,

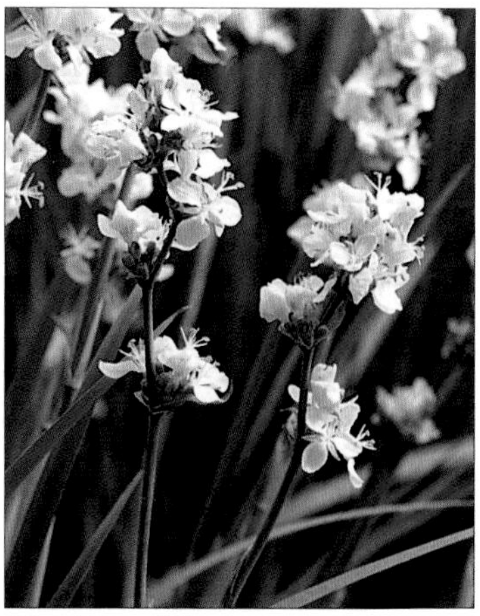

Libertia grandiflora

1cm (½in) across. ↕ to 60cm (24in), ↔ 30cm (12in). Chile. ✽✽

L. chilensis see *L. formosa.*

L. formosa, syn. *L. chilensis.* Rhizomatous perennial forming large clumps of linear, stiff, leathery, deep green leaves, 15–45cm (6–18in) long. Dense panicles composed of umbel-like clusters of 3–8 white or pale yellow-white flowers, 3.5cm (1½in) across, are borne in long succession from late spring to midsummer. ↕ 90cm (36in), ↔ 60cm (24in). Chile. ✽✽✽ (borderline)

L. grandiflora ■ Rhizomatous perennial forming dense clumps of linear, leathery leaves, 30–75cm (12–30in) long. In late spring and early summer, bears long panicles composed of dense, umbel-like clusters of 3–6 white flowers, 3cm (1¼in) across, the outer tepals with olive or bronze keels. ↕ to 90cm (36in), ↔ 60cm (24in). New Zealand. ✽✽✽ (borderline)

L. ixioides. Rhizomatous perennial, similar to *L. grandiflora*, forming dense clumps of linear, leathery leaves, 20–30cm (8–12in) long. Leaves of some variants turn orange-brown in winter. In late spring and early summer, produces dense panicles composed of umbel-like clusters of usually 2–10 white flowers, 7–8mm (¼–⅜in) across, the outer tepals tinted brown or green. ↕↔ 60cm (24in). New Zealand (including Chatham Island). ✽✽

LIBOCEDRUS

CUPRESSACEAE

Genus of 6 species of conical, monoecious, evergreen, coniferous trees and shrubs from forest in New Zealand, New Caledonia, and South America. In the past, species of *Austrocedrus* and *Calocedrus* were included in the genus *Libocedrus.* The linear juvenile leaves and usually scale-like adult leaves are arranged in sets of 2 pairs, one on either side of the shoot (spreading pair), and one above and below (facial pair), forming 4 rows. Female cones are solitary, ovoid, and usually 4-scaled, with 2 pairs of enlarged, bract-like leaves at the bases; male cones are small, oblong, and borne at the tips of short shoots. Grow as specimen trees. In frost-prone areas, grow half-hardy species in a sheltered site or in a cool greenhouse.

• **HARDINESS** Fully hardy to half hardy.

• **CULTIVATION** Grow in any deep, moist but well-drained soil in full sun.

L

L. uvifera tolerates and often prefers a wet site or copious water supply. In frost-prone climates, shelter from cold, drying winds.

• **PROPAGATION** Sow seed in containers in a cold frame in spring, or take semi-ripe cuttings in summer.

• **PESTS AND DISEASES** Trouble free.

L. bidwillii ◊ Conical, coniferous tree at lower elevations, reduced to a shrub at altitudes above 1,000m (3,200ft). It has fibrous bark and scale-like, glossy, yellow-green adult leaves, to 2mm (1/16in) long, lying flat along the shoots. Ovoid female cones, 1cm (½in) long, have a green terminal spine on each scale. ↕ to 15m (50ft), ↔ to 3m (10ft). New Zealand. ❄❄

L. chilensis see *Austrocedrus chilensis.*

L. decurrens see *Calocedrus decurrens.*

L. plumosa ◊ (Kawaka). Conical, coniferous tree with fibrous bark and unequal pairs of scale-like, glossy, bright green adult leaves; the spreading pair, 3–5mm (⅛–¼in) long, is larger than the facial pair. Ovoid female cones are 1–2cm (½–¾in) long. ↕ to 15m (50ft), ↔ to 3m (10ft). New Zealand. ❄❄

L. uvifera ◊ syn. *Pilgerodendron uviferum.* Slow-growing, conical, coniferous shrub or small tree with thin bark, peeling in strips. Green shoots bear narrowly wedge-shaped leaves, to 5mm (¼in) long, with fine, tapered points, whitish green on the inner side, dark green on the outer. Ovoid female cones are 1cm (½in) long. ↕ to 6m (20ft), ↔ to 2m (6ft). S. Chile, S. Argentina (Andes and Tierra del Fuego). ❄❄❄ (borderline)

▷ ***Libonia*** see *Justicia*
L. floribunda see *J. rizzinii*

L

LICUALA

ARECACEAE/PALMAE

Genus of approximately 100 species of single- or cluster-stemmed palms found in rainforest and swamps, in low-lying areas from S.E. Asia to Malaysia, the New Hebrides, and Australia. Rounded, fan-like or palmately lobed leaves are arranged spirally along the upper parts of the stems; fibrous leaf bases remain on the stems after the leaves have withered. Spikes of cup-shaped, 3-petalled flowers are produced from the leaf axils. Where temperatures fall below 15–16°C (59–61°F), grow in a warm greenhouse. In warmer areas, grow the shrubby, suckering species in a border or in plantings against a wall, and the larger, single-stemmed species as lawn specimens or in a courtyard garden.

• **HARDINESS** Frost tender.

• **CULTIVATION** Under glass, grow in loam-based potting compost (JI No.3), with added peat or leaf mould and sharp sand, in bright filtered light and high humidity. When in growth, water freely and apply a balanced liquid fertilizer monthly. Mist twice a day in summer. Water moderately in winter. Pot on or top-dress in spring. Outdoors, grow in moderately fertile, moist but well-drained soil in partial shade.

• **PROPAGATION** In spring, sow seed at 24°C (75°F), or remove suckers.

• **PESTS AND DISEASES** Red spider mites and mealybugs may be troublesome under glass.

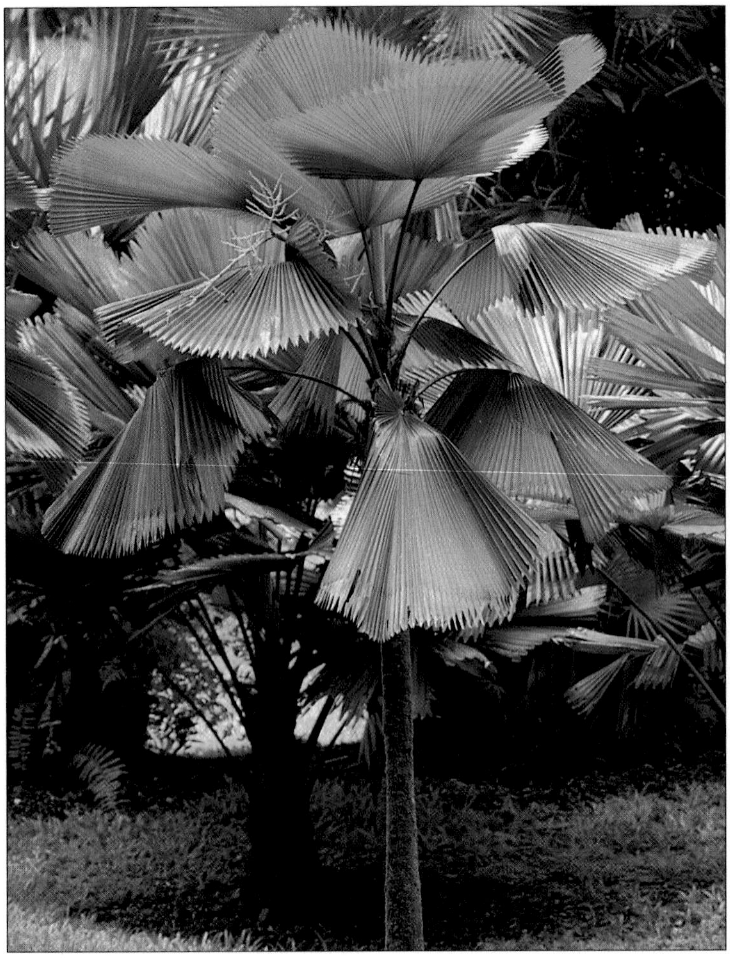

Licuala grandis

L. grandis ▣ ♆ Small palm with a single, slender, erect trunk clad in fibrous leaf bases. Long-stalked, rounded leaf-blades, 1m (3ft) across, are glossy, mid- to pale green with notched margins, and are occasionally divided into 3 broadly wedge-shaped to rounded, wavy-margined segments. Green to greenish white flowers, 1cm (½in) across, are borne in pendent spikes, longer than the leaves, usually in summer. Flowers are followed by spherical, glossy red fruit. ↕ to 3m (10ft), ↔ 1.5–2.5m (5–8ft). New Hebrides. ❁ (min. 15–16°C/59–61°F)

L. muelleri see *L. ramsayi.*

L. ramsayi ♆ syn. *L. muelleri.* Medium-sized palm with a single, erect stem, the upper part clad with fibrous leaf bases, the lower part smooth. Long, spiny leaf-stalks bear rounded leaf-blades, to 1m (3ft) across, divided into many wedge-shaped, radiating, rich green segments, some of which may be joined at the tips. Cream flowers, 1cm (½in) across, are borne in spikes, as long as, or longer than the leaves, usually in summer, and are followed by spherical, orange-red fruit. ↕ to 12m (40ft), ↔ 3–5m (10–15ft). Australia (N.E. Queensland). ❁ (min. 15–16°C/59–61°F)

L. spinosa ✾ Small, cluster-stemmed palm forming clumps of cane-like stems. These bear spirals of leaves, and are clad with fibrous leaf bases in the upper parts. Long, spiny-stalked, rounded leaf-blades, to 1.5m (5ft) across, are divided into 12–20 narrow, deep green, wedge-shaped segments with squared-off tips. Greenish white flowers, 1cm (½in) across, are borne in branched spikes, to 2m (6ft) long, mainly in summer, followed by ovoid red fruit. ↕↔ to 5m (15ft). Thailand, Malaysian peninsula, Indonesia, Philippines. ❁ (min. 15–16°C/59–61°F)

▷ **Lignum, Climbing** see *Muehlenbeckia adpressa*

LIGULARIA

ASTERACEAE/COMPOSITAE

Genus of about 150 species of large, robust, often coarse perennials, mostly from C. and E. Asia, with a few from Europe, found in moist or wet grassland, open, wet scrub and woodland, by mountain streams, and in ditches. They have, ovate-oblong or elliptic to kidney-shaped or rounded, sometimes palmately lobed, often toothed basal leaves, borne on long leaf-stalks, and smaller, alternate stem leaves. Erect stems bear terminal corymbs or racemes of few to many, showy, daisy-like, yellow or orange flowerheads, with yellow or brown disc-florets. Grow in a mixed or herbaceous border, or naturalize in moist soil; they are also imposing waterside plants.

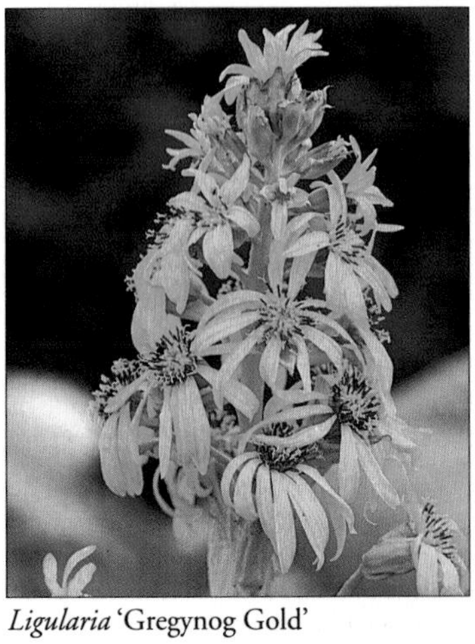

Ligularia 'Gregynog Gold'

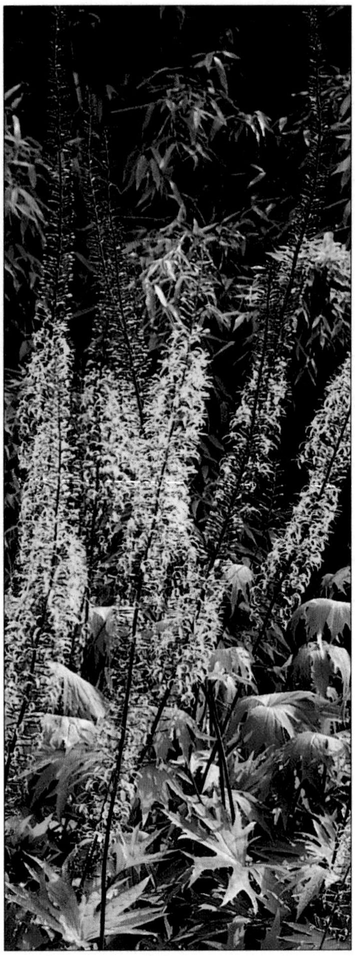

Ligularia przewalskii

• **HARDINESS** Fully hardy.

• **CULTIVATION** Grow in moderately fertile, deep, reliably moist soil, in full sun with some midday shade. Shelter from strong winds.

• **PROPAGATION** Sow seed of species in containers outdoors in autumn or spring, or divide species and cultivars in spring or after flowering. When seed-raised, *L. dentata* 'Desdemona' and *L. dentata* 'Othello' will often produce similar seedlings.

• **PESTS AND DISEASES** Slugs and snails may damage emerging leaves in spring.

L. clivorum see *L. dentata.*

L. dentata, syn. *L. clivorum, Senecio clivorum* (Golden groundsel). Clump-forming perennial with kidney-shaped to rounded, toothed, mid-green leaves, to 30cm (12in) long, deeply heart-shaped at the bases; the basal leaves have red leaf-stalks. Flat corymbs of many red-stalked, brown-centred, orange-yellow flowerheads, 10cm (4in) across, are borne from midsummer to early autumn. ↕ 1–1.5m (3–5ft), ↔ 1m (3ft). China, Japan. ❄❄❄. **'Desdemona'** 🏆 has deep orange flowerheads and rounded, brownish green leaves that are deep maroon-purple beneath; ↕ 1m (3ft).

'Othello' is similar to 'Desdemona', but with deep purplish green leaves, purple-red beneath; ↕ 1m (3ft).
***L.* 'Gregynog Gold'** ■ 🏆 Clump-forming perennial with rounded, toothed leaves, to 35cm (14in) long, heart-shaped at the bases. In late summer and early autumn, bears tall, pyramidal racemes of many brown-centred, golden orange flowerheads, to 10cm (4in) across. ↕ to 1.8m (6ft), ↔ 1m (3ft). ❄❄❄
L. hodgsonii. Clump-forming perennial with kidney-shaped, toothed leaves, to 12cm (5in) across, heart-shaped at the bases. In mid- and late summer, bears corymbs of many yellow-orange flowerheads, 5cm (2in) across, with reddish brown centres, on stems often marked purple towards the bases. ↕ 90cm (36in), ↔ 60cm (24in). Japan. ❄❄❄
L. przewalskii ■ syn. *Senecio przewalskii.* Clump-forming perennial with palmately lobed leaves, to 30cm (12in) long, deeply cut and irregularly lobed and toothed. In mid- and late summer, dark purple-green stems bear slender, dense racemes of yellow flowerheads, 2cm (¾in) across. ↕ to 2m (6ft), ↔ 1m (3ft). N. China. ❄❄❄
L. stenocephala. Clump-forming perennial with triangular, pointed, toothed leaves, to 35cm (14in) long, with heart-shaped bases. In early and late summer, tall, slender racemes of numerous yellow flowerheads, to 4cm (1½in) across, with orange-yellow centres, are borne on black-green stems. ↕ 1.5m (5ft), ↔ 1m (3ft). N. China, Taiwan, Japan. ❄❄❄. **'The Rocket'** 🏆, of hybrid origin, has tall black flower stems and boldly toothed leaves; ↕ 1.8m (6ft). **'Weihenstephan'**, of hybrid origin, has golden yellow flowerheads, 6–7cm (2½–3in) across; ↕ 1.8m (6ft).
L. tangutica see *Senecio tanguticus.*
L. tussilaginea see *Farfugium japonicum.*
L. veitchiana. Clump-forming perennial bearing triangular to heart-shaped leaves, 30–35cm (12–14in) long, with wavy, toothed margins. Pyramidal racemes of numerous brown-centred yellow flowerheads, to 7cm (3in) across, are borne in mid- and late summer, followed by conspicuous, fluffy, purple-brown fruit. ↕ 1.8m (6ft), ↔ 1.2m (4ft). W. China. ❄❄❄

LIGUSTRUM
Privet

OLEACEAE

Genus of about 50 species of deciduous, semi-evergreen, or evergreen shrubs and trees found in woodland and thickets in Europe, N. Africa, the Himalayas, S.W. and E. Asia, and Australia. They bear opposite, variably shaped, often glossy leaves, and terminal panicles of small, tubular, 4-lobed, unpleasantly scented white flowers, followed by spherical or ovoid fruit. Grown for their foliage and flowers, they are good for a shrub border or as specimen plants; most species may be used for hedging. All parts may cause severe discomfort if ingested.

- **HARDINESS** Fully hardy to frost hardy.
- **CULTIVATION** Grow in any well-drained soil in full sun or partial shade; variegated privets colour better in sun. Pruning group 1; clip hedges twice in summer.

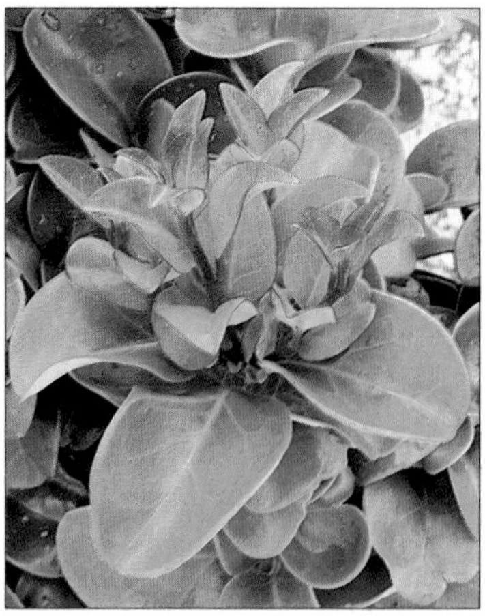

Ligustrum japonicum 'Rotundifolium'

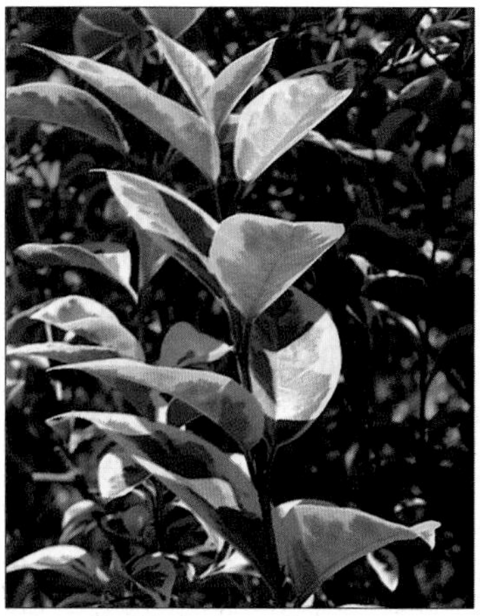

Ligustrum lucidum 'Excelsum Superbum'

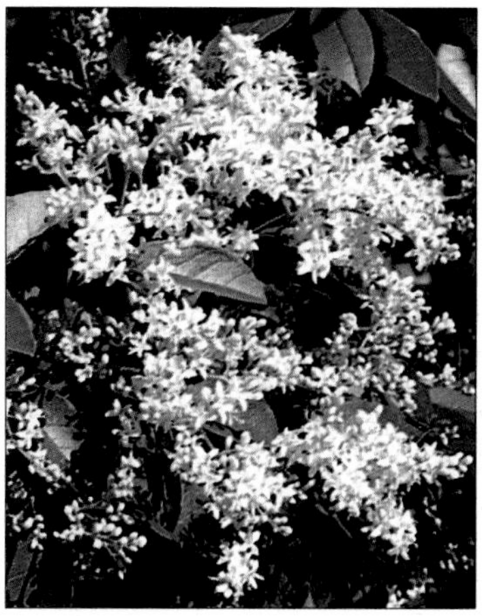

Ligustrum sinense

- **PROPAGATION** Sow seed in containers in a cold frame in autumn or spring. Take semi-ripe cuttings in summer or hardwood cuttings in winter.
- **PESTS AND DISEASES** Susceptible to aphids, leaf spots, scale insects, leaf miners, thrips, honey fungus, and wilt.

L. amurense (Amur privet). Dense, upright, deciduous or semi-evergreen shrub with elliptic, mid-green leaves, to 5cm (2in) long. White flowers are produced in panicles, 4–5cm (1½–2in) long, in late spring and early summer, followed by small, ovoid black fruit. Useful for hedging. ↕↔ 5m (15ft). N. China. ❄❄❄
L. chenaultii △ Vigorous, broadly conical, semi-evergreen tree with lance-shaped, occasionally notched, dark green leaves, 15cm (6in) or more long. White flowers are borne in panicles, 15–18cm (6–7in) long, in midsummer, followed by small, spherical black fruit. ↕ 10m (30ft), ↔ 8m (25ft). S.W. China. ❄❄

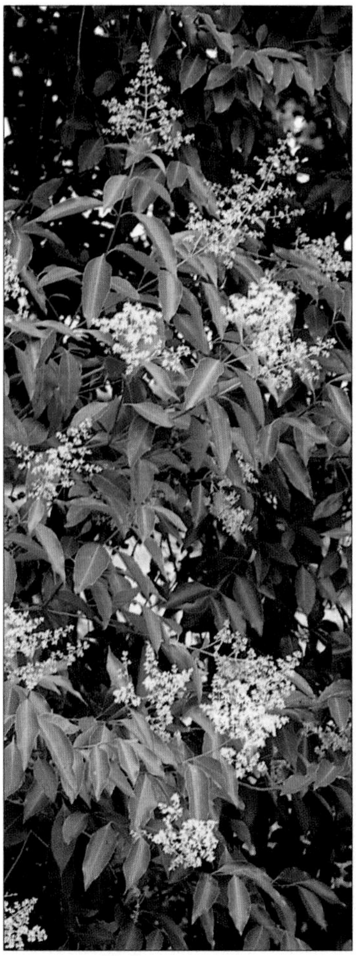

Ligustrum lucidum

L. delavayanum. Compact, spreading, evergreen shrub with ovate, oval, or oblong, dark green leaves, to 3cm (1¼in) long. White flowers are produced in panicles, to 5cm (2in) long, in early summer, followed by spherical to ovoid, blue-black fruit. Useful for hedging. ↕ 2m (6ft), ↔ 3m (10ft). W. China (Sichuan, Yunnan). ❄❄❄
L. x ibolium (*L. obtusifolium* x *L. ovalifolium*). Upright, deciduous to semi-evergreen shrub with oval, glossy, mid-green leaves, to 6cm (2½in) long. White flowers are produced in panicles, 5–8cm (2–3in) long, in midsummer. Useful for hedging. ↕↔ 3m (10ft). Garden origin. ❄❄❄
L. japonicum (Japanese privet). Upright, dense, evergreen shrub with ovate, glossy, very dark green leaves, to 10cm (4in) long. White flowers are produced in panicles, to 15cm (6in) long, from midsummer to early autumn, and are followed by ovoid-oblong black fruit. ↕ 3m (10ft), ↔ 2.5m (8ft). N. China, Korea, Japan. ❄❄❄. **'Rotundifolium'** ■ is slow-growing and stiffly branched, with rounded, very leathery leaves, to 6cm (2½in) long; ↕ 1.5m (5ft), ↔ 1m (3ft).
L. lucidum ■ 🏆 △ (Chinese privet). Conical, evergreen tree or shrub with ovate or oval, tapered, glossy, dark green leaves, to 15cm (6in) long. White flowers are produced in panicles, to 20cm (8in) long, in late summer and early autumn, followed by ovoid-oblong, blue-black fruit. ↕↔ 10m (30ft). China. Korea, Japan. ❄❄❄. **'Excelsum Superbum'** ■ 🏆 has yellow-margined, bright green leaves. **'Tricolor'** has narrow, green and grey-green leaves with white margins (pink when young).
L. obtusifolium. Graceful, spreading, deciduous shrub with oval, dark green leaves, to 5cm (2in) long, often tinged purple in autumn. White flowers are produced in nodding panicles, to 5cm (2in) long, in midsummer, followed by spherical, blue-black fruit. Useful for hedging. ↕ 3m (10ft), ↔ 4m (12ft). Japan. ❄❄❄
L. ovalifolium. Vigorous, upright, evergreen or semi-evergreen shrub with oval, rich green leaves, to 6cm (2½in) long. White flowers are borne in dense panicles, to 10cm (4in) long, in midsummer, followed by spherical, shiny black fruit. Useful for hedging. ↕↔ 4m (12ft). Japan. ❄❄❄. **'Argenteum'** has leaves margined creamy white. **'Aureum'** 🏆 syn. 'Aureomarginatum' (Golden privet), has leaves with broad, bright yellow margins.
L. quihoui 🏆 Upright then rounded, deciduous shrub with slender, arching branches and narrowly oval to obovate, glossy, mid-green leaves, to 5cm (2in) long. Fragrant white flowers are produced in open panicles, 20cm (8in) or more long, in late summer and early autumn, followed by ovoid, glossy, black-purple fruit. Useful for hedging. ↕↔ 2.5m (8ft). China. ❄❄❄
L. sinense ■ Vigorous, bushy, tree-like, deciduous or semi-evergreen shrub with arching branches and elliptic-oblong or lance-shaped, pale green leaves, to 7cm (3in) long. White flowers are profusely borne in panicles, to 10cm (4in) long, in midsummer, and are followed by spherical, purple-black fruit. Useful for hedging. ↕↔ 4m (12ft). China. ❄❄❄. **'Variegatum'** has white-margined, pale green leaves. **'Wimbei'** is compact and slow-growing, with upright leaves, to 1cm (½in) long. Rarely flowers; ↕ 1.5m (5ft), ↔ 1.2m (4ft).
L. 'Vicaryi'. Dense, bushy, semi-evergreen shrub with broadly oval, golden yellow leaves, to 9cm (3½in) long. White flowers are produced in panicles, to 7cm (3in) long, in midsummer, followed by spherical, blue-black fruit. ↕↔ 3m (10ft). ❄❄❄
L. vulgare (Common privet). Bushy, deciduous or semi-evergreen shrub with narrowly oval to lance-shaped, dark green leaves, to 6cm (2½in) long. White flowers are produced in panicles, to 5cm (2in) long, in early and midsummer, followed by spherical to ovoid black fruit. Useful for hedging. ↕↔ 3m (10ft). Europe, N. Africa, S.W. Asia. ❄❄❄. **'Aureum'** has golden yellow foliage; ↕↔ 2m (6ft).

▷**Lilac** see *Syringa*
California see *Ceanothus*
Common see *Syringa vulgaris*
Himalayan see *Syringa emodi*
Persian see *Melia azedarach*, *Syringa* x *persica*
Rouen see *Syringa* x *chinensis*
St. Vincent see *Solanum seaforthianum*

L

LILIUM

Lily

LILIACEAE

Genus of approximately 100 species of bulbous perennials, mainly from wooded habitats and scrub in Europe, Asia south to the Philippines, and North America; there are also innumerable garden hybrids. The bulbs are composed of overlapping, fleshy scales and are sometimes rhizomatous. The stems are unbranched and usually erect; in some lilies, roots develop on the stems just above the bulb. Numerous elliptic to lance-shaped or linear, glossy, mid- to dark green leaves are arranged in whorls or spirals, or are scattered alternately up the stems. Lilies are often tall-growing, attaining a height of up to 3m (10ft), but do not spread (therefore only height measurements are given in the entries below).

The showy, sometimes very fragrant flowers are solitary or borne in racemes, panicles, or umbels, and are followed by 3-parted capsules containing flat, papery seeds. The flowers may be upward-facing, horizontal or outward-facing, nodding, or pendent. They may be cup- to bowl- or bell-shaped, trumpet-shaped, funnel-shaped, turkscap (in which the blooms have strongly reflexed tepals), or occasionally star-shaped; each with 6 stamens and 6 tepals (see panel above). The tepals, occurring in most colours except blue, may be plain or marked with lines, spots, or papillae. Three categories of flower size – small, medium, and large – are used in the descriptions below. For turkscap, bowl-, cup-, and star-shaped flowers: small is up to 5cm (2in) across; medium is 5–7cm (2–3in) across; large is over 7cm (3in) across. For trumpet- and funnel-shaped flowers: small is up to 7cm (3in) long; medium is 7–10cm (3–4in) long; large is over 10cm (4in) long.

Lilies may be grown in many sites, including woodland and wild gardens and among shrubs or herbaceous plants. They are often grown for exhibition and provide excellent cut flowers. A few are suitable for a rock garden. Many also grow well in a large container on a patio. In frost-prone climates, grow half-hardy lilies in a cool greenhouse.

Lilies are classified into 9 divisions:

LILY FLOWERS

Lilies are valued for their very showy, often fragrant flowers. The 6 plain or strikingly marked tepals are variably curved, giving rise to the different shapes shown here, and to forms intermediate between them.

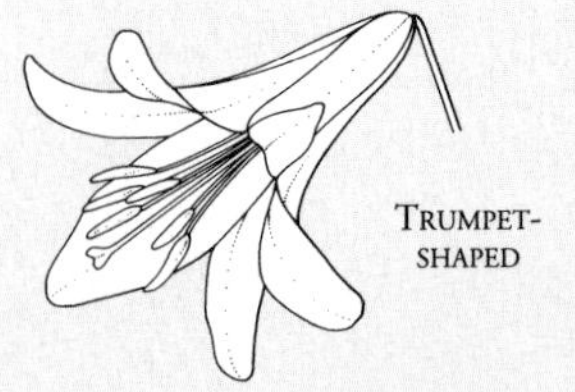

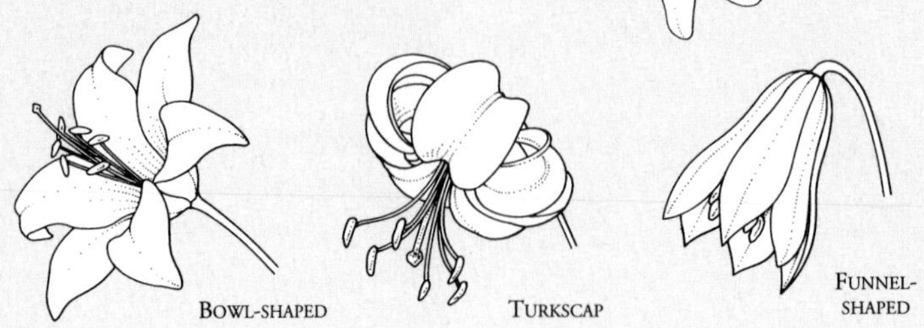

Division 1 (Asiatic hybrids)
These lilies are derived from various Asiatic species, including *L. bulbiferum*, *L. cernuum*, *L. concolor*, *L. davidii*, *L. lancifolium*, and *L. maculatum*. The flowers are borne in racemes or umbels, and are usually unscented. The leaves are narrowly ovate and arranged alternately. There are 3 subdivisions: **1a**) upward-facing flowers; **1b**) outward-facing flowers; **1c**) pendent flowers.

Division 2 (Martagon hybrids)
Derived primarily from *L. hansonii* and *L. martagon*, these lilies produce racemes of turkscap, sometimes scented flowers, and have whorls of elliptic leaves.

Division 3 (Candidum hybrids)
Derived from *L. candidum* and other European species, except *L. martagon*, these lilies produce sometimes scented, mostly turkscap flowers, singly or in umbels or racemes. Leaves are elliptic, and spirally arranged or scattered.

Division 4 (American hybrids)
Derived from American species, these lilies bear racemes of sometimes scented, mostly turkscap, but occasionally funnel-shaped flowers, and have whorls of lance-shaped to elliptic leaves.

Division 5 (Longiflorum hybrids)
Derived from *L. formosanum* and *L. longiflorum*, these lilies bear racemes or umbels of large, often sweetly scented, trumpet- or funnel-shaped flowers, sometimes only 2 or 3 per stem. Leaves are linear to narrowly lance-shaped, and scattered.

Division 6 (Trumpet and Aurelian hybrids)
Derived from Asiatic species, including *L. regale*, *L. henryi*, and *L. sargentiae*, these lilies bear racemes or umbels of usually scented flowers. Leaves are elliptic to linear, and alternate or spirally arranged. There are 4 subdivisions: **6a**) trumpet-shaped flowers; **6b**) bowl-shaped flowers; **6c**) very shallowly bowl-shaped flowers, some almost flat; **6d**) distinctly recurved flowers.

Division 7 (Oriental hybrids)
These lilies are derived from E. Asian species, such as *L. auratum*, *L. japonicum*, and *L. speciosum*, as well as their hybrids with *L. henryi*. Flowers are borne in racemes or panicles, and are often scented. Leaves are lance-shaped and alternate. There are 4 subdivisions: **7a**) trumpet-shaped flowers; **7b**) bowl-shaped flowers; **7c**) flat or very shallowly bowl-shaped flowers; **7d**) turkscap or variously recurved flowers.

Division 8. Other hybrids.
Division 9. All true species.

• **HARDINESS** Fully hardy to half hardy, but young growth may be damaged by frost.

• **CULTIVATION** Grow in well-drained soil enriched with leaf mould or well-rotted organic matter. Most prefer acid to neutral soil, but some are lime-tolerant or prefer alkaline soils. The majority like a position in full sun, with the base of the plant in shade; a few prefer partial shade in light, open woodland. They do not thrive in deep shade. Under glass, grow in loam-based potting compost (JI No.2), with added grit and leaf mould, in full light with shade from hot sun. In active growth, water freely and apply a high-potash liquid fertilizer every 2 weeks. Keep moist in winter. Plant most bulbs (which should be plump) in autumn, at a depth of 2–3 times their height, and with a distance between them equivalent to 3 times the diameter of the bulb; plant bulbs of stem-rooting lilies at a depth of at least 3 times the bulb height. Plant *L. candidum* and *L.* x *testaceum* very close to the soil surface; they also tolerate drier soil than other lilies.

• **PROPAGATION** Sow seed as soon as ripe; sow seed of hardy lilies in containers in a cold frame, and of half-hardy lilies at 13–18°C (55–64°F). Remove scales, offsets, or bulblets from dormant bulbs as soon as the foliage dies down, or detach stem bulbils (where these are produced) in late summer.

• **PESTS AND DISEASES** Lily beetle, aphids, slugs, thrips, leatherjackets, and wireworms, as well as small mammals such as rabbits and voles, may be a problem. Various fungi can infect lilies either below or above ground. Grey mould (*Botrytis*) is sometimes a problem, especially in a wet, cool spring. Viruses may be troublesome, although some cultivars are virus-tolerant and grow well despite infection.

***L.* 'African Queen'** ▣ Vigorous Division 6a lily with erect stems. In mid- and late summer, large, fragrant, outward-facing to nodding, trumpet-shaped flowers, brownish purple outside, yellow or orange-apricot inside, are borne in pyramid-shaped racemes. ↕1.5–2m (5–6ft). ❄❄

L. amabile. Delicate Division 9 lily with slender, downy stems bearing scattered, linear leaves, 9cm (3½in) long, on the upper half of the stem only. In early and midsummer, produces racemes of up to 10 small, unpleasantly scented, turkscap red flowers, 2.5–3cm (1–1¼in) across, with recurved tepals, to 6cm (2½in) long; they have dark purple or black spots and reddish brown anthers. Grow in acid or alkaline soil. ↕40–90cm (16–36in). Korea. ❄❄❄. **var. *luteum*** produces yellow flowers.

***L.* 'Amber Gold'.** Division 1c lily bearing racemes, in early and mid-summer, of medium-sized, unscented, turkscap, bright orange-yellow flowers, spotted maroon in the centres and with reddish brown anthers. ↕1.2–1.5m (4–5ft). ❄❄❄

***L.* 'Angela North'** ▣ Clump-forming, moderately vigorous Division 1c lily. In midsummer, bears racemes of medium-sized, faintly scented, turkscap, deep wine-red flowers, with some darker spotting. ↕70–120cm (28–48in). ❄❄❄

***L.* 'Ariadne'** ▣ Elegant Division 1c lily with slender stems. In midsummer, produces racemes of small, scented, turkscap, pale orange flowers, flushed purple towards the tips of the tepals. ↕0.8–1.4m (2¾–4½ft). ❄❄❄

L. auratum (Golden-rayed lily). Vigorous Division 9 lily with stiff stems bearing scattered, lance-shaped, deep green leaves, 22cm (9in) long. In late summer and early autumn, produces racemes of usually up to 12, sometimes up to 30, sweetly fragrant, open bowl-shaped flowers, to 30cm (12in) across; the white tepals are recurved towards the tips, have a prominent central gold band, and are often crimson-speckled. Susceptible to virus. ↕0.6–1.5m (2–5ft). Japan. ❄❄❄. **'Crimson Beauty'** produces flowers with a crimson band along the centre of each tepal; ↕to 1m (3ft). **'Golden Ray'** produces large

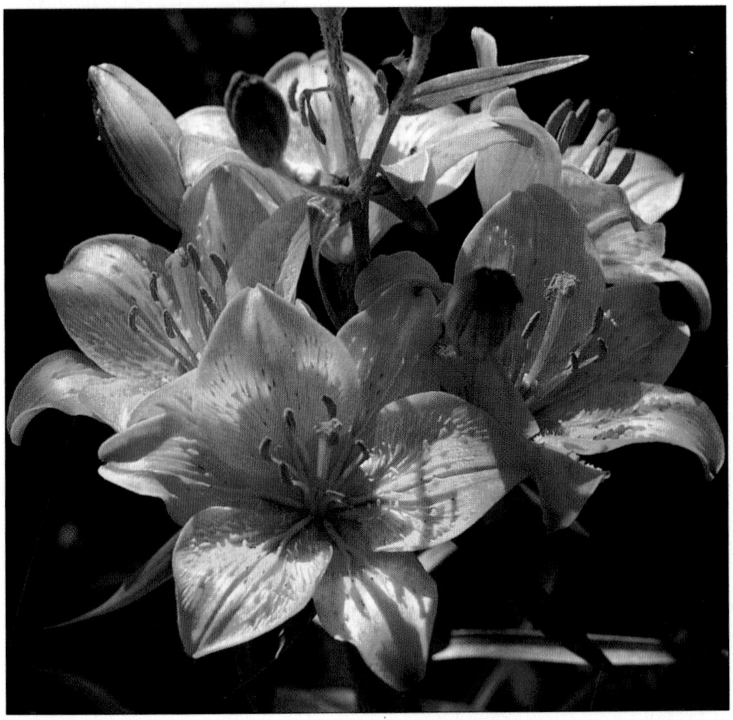

Lilium bulbiferum var. *croceum*

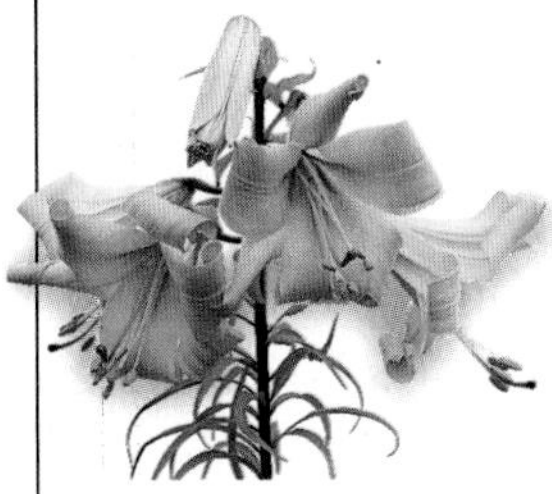
Lilium 'African Queen'

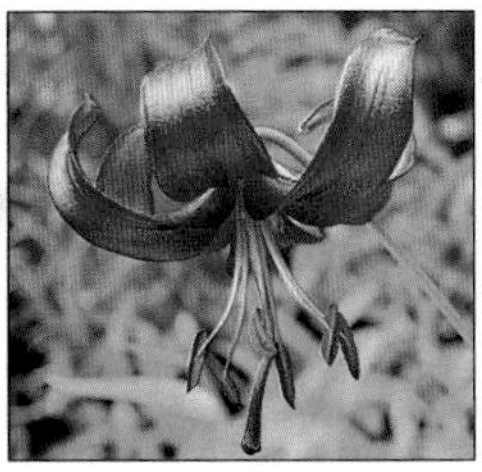
Lilium 'Angela North'

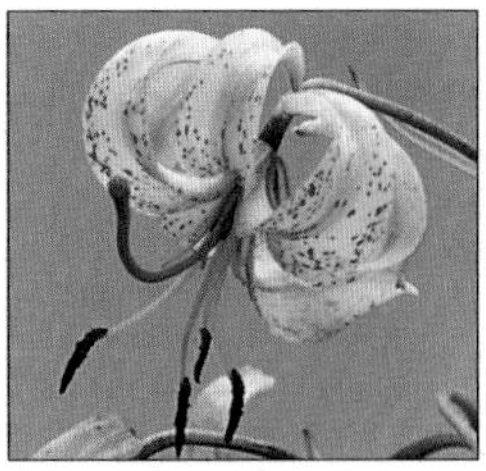
Lilium 'Ariadne'

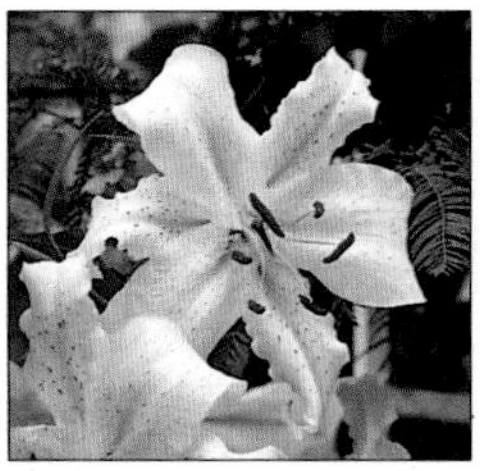
Lilium auratum var. *platyphyllum*

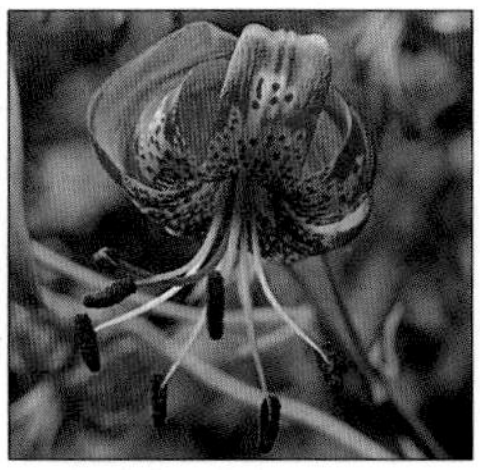
Lilium Bellingham Hybrids

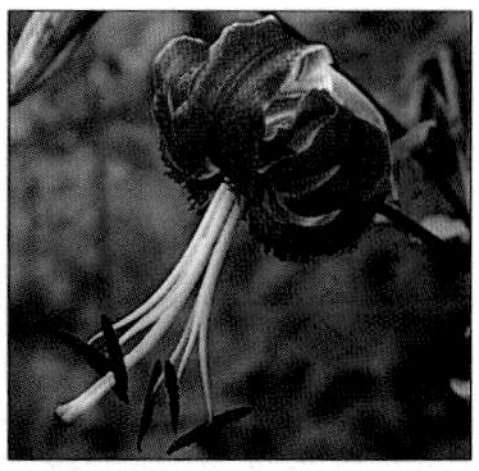
Lilium 'Black Beauty'

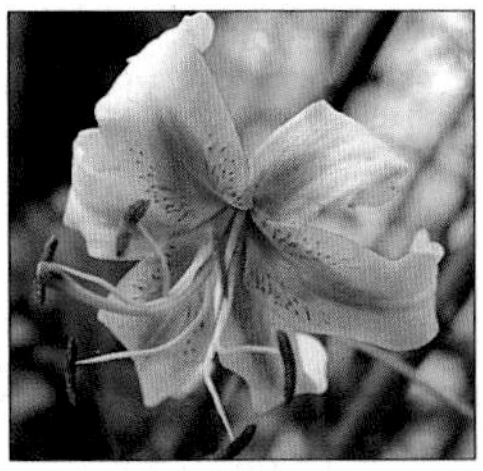
Lilium 'Bright Star'

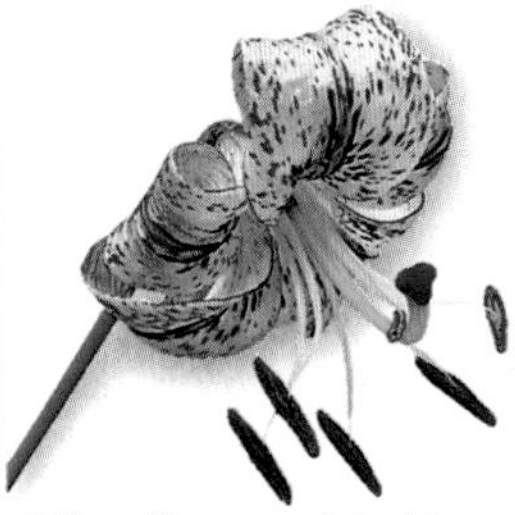
Lilium 'Bronwen North'

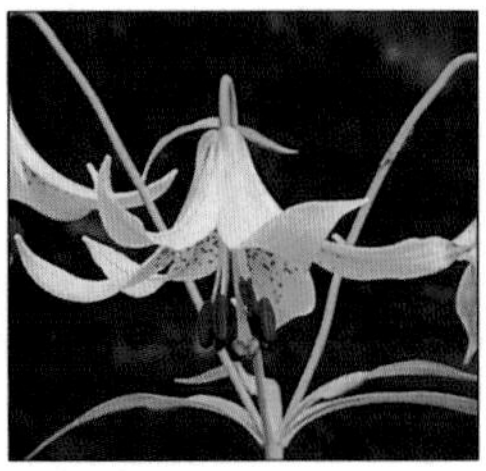
Lilium canadense

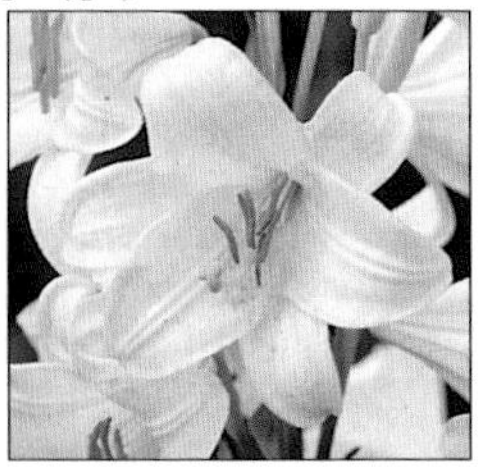
Lilium candidum

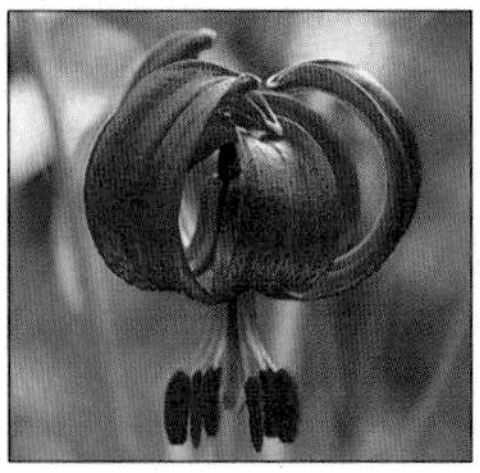
Lilium chalcedonicum

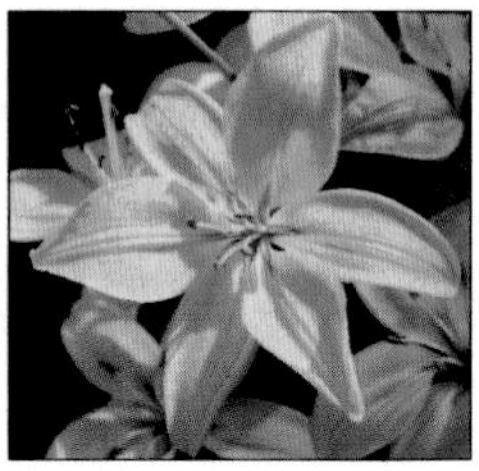
Lilium 'Connecticut King'

flowers, to 35cm (14in) across, with a deep yellow band along each tepal; ↕ to 2m (6ft). **var. *platyphyllum*** ■ ♀ has broadly lance-shaped leaves, and bears flowers with a yellow band along each tepal but few spots; ↕ to 1.5m (5ft).

***L.* 'Barbara North'** ♀ Sturdy, clump-forming Division 1c lily. In midsummer, produces racemes of medium-sized, slightly scented, broad, turkscap, mid-pink flowers, with paler throats and a scattering of small, dark red spots. ↕ 70–120cm (28–48in). ✻✻✻

***L.* Bellingham Hybrids** ■ ♀ (*L. humboldtii* x *L. pardalinum* x *L. parryi*). Vigorous Division 4 lilies with rhizomatous bulbs. In early and midsummer, bear racemes of medium-sized, unscented, turkscap flowers, ranging from yellow to orange and red, spotted with brown or deep red. They increase rapidly but require acid soil and partial shade. ↕ 1.8–2.2m (6–7ft). ✻✻✻

***L.* 'Black Beauty'** ■ Vigorous Division 7d lily. In midsummer, bears racemes of medium-sized, scented, turkscap, dark blackish red flowers, with green centres and white tepal margins. ↕ 1.4–2m (4½–6ft). ✻✻✻

***L.* 'Black Dragon'.** Division 6a lily bearing stout racemes of large, scented, outward-facing, trumpet-shaped flowers, dark purplish red outside, white within, in early summer. ↕ 1.5m (5ft). ✻✻✻

***L.* 'Black Magic'.** Vigorous Division 6a lily bearing racemes of large, fragrant, trumpet-shaped flowers in mid- and late summer; opening from maroon buds, they are glistening white inside, reddish black outside. ↕ 1.5–2m (5–6ft). ✻✻✻

***L.* 'Bright Star'** ■ Division 6d lily bearing racemes of large, scented, outward-facing, ivory-white flowers in mid- and late summer; spreading tepals are recurved at the tips and each has an orange central band, producing a star-like effect. Lime-tolerant. ↕ 1–1.5m (3–5ft). ✻✻✻

***L.* 'Bronwen North'** ■ Division 1c lily bearing racemes of medium-sized, slightly scented, turkscap, pale mauve-pink flowers, the throats pale pink with purple spots and lines, in early summer. ↕ 80–100cm (32–39in). ✻✻✻

***L.* 'Brushmarks'.** Division 1a lily producing racemes of large, upward-facing, cup-shaped orange flowers, with deep red marks and green throats, in early summer. ↕ to 1m (3ft). ✻✻✻

L. bulbiferum (Orange lily). Vigorous, clump-forming Division 9 lily producing scattered, narrowly to broadly lance-shaped leaves, 5–15cm (2–6in) long, with marginal hairs; bulbils are borne in the upper leaf axils. In early and midsummer, bears usually 1- to 5-flowered umbels (sometimes many-flowered, dense racemes) of unscented, erect, bowl-shaped, bright orange-red flowers, 10–15cm (4–6in) across; the tepals are broad, with black or maroon spots and darker bases and tips. Grows well in acid or alkaline soil. ↕ 40–150cm (16–60in). S. Europe. ✻✻✻. **var. *croceum*** ■ ♀ has orange flowers and does not produce bulbils.

L. canadense ■ (Meadow lily). Division 9 lily with rhizomatous bulbs and whorls of lance-shaped to inversely lance-shaped leaves, 15cm (6in) long, each with 5–7 parallel veins. In mid- and late summer, produces umbels, or occasionally racemes, of up to 30 faintly scented, narrowly to broadly trumpet-shaped yellow flowers, 5–8cm (2–3in) long, with recurved tips and maroon spots in the centres. ↕ 1–1.6m (3–5½ft). E. North America. ✻✻✻. **var. *coccineum***, syn. var. *rubrum*, bears bright red flowers with yellow throats. **var. *editorum*** has broader leaves and red flowers. **var. *rubrum*** see var. *coccineum*.

L. candidum ■ ♀ (Madonna lily). Division 9 lily with broad, inversely lance-shaped, shiny, bright green basal leaves, 22cm (9in) long, appearing in autumn. Stiffly erect stems bear smaller, scattered or spirally arranged, often somewhat twisted, lance-shaped leaves, to 8cm (3in) long. In midsummer, produces a raceme of 5–20 sweetly fragrant, broadly trumpet-shaped, pure white flowers, 5–8cm (2–3in) long, with yellowish bases and bright yellow anthers. Produces overwintering basal leaves (the only lily with this character). Requires neutral to alkaline soil. ↕ 1–1.8m (3–6ft). S.E. Europe to E. Mediterranean. ✻✻✻

L. carniolicum see *L. pyrenaicum* subsp. *carniolicum*.

***L.* 'Casa Blanca'** ♀ Division 7b lily, derived from *L. auratum*, with stout, stiff stems. In mid- and late summer, large, sweetly fragrant, bowl-shaped, pure white flowers, with widely spreading tepals that are recurved near the tips, are produced in umbels; they have white papillae near the bases inside, and orange-red anthers. ↕ 1–1.2m (3–4ft). ✻✻✻

L. cernuum (Nodding lily). Small, stem-rooting Division 9 lily. Scattered, linear leaves, 8–18cm (3–7in) long, are mostly concentrated in the middle third of the slender stem. In early and midsummer, bears racemes of usually up to 6 (occasionally up to 15) fragrant, turkscap, pale lilac, pink, or purple flowers, 3–5cm (1¼–2in) across. Lime-tolerant, but prefers moist, peaty soil. ↕ 40–60cm (16–24in). Russia (N.E. Siberia) to Korea. ✻✻✻

L. chalcedonicum ■ ♀ syn. *L. heldreichii* (Scarlet turkscap lily). Relatively small, stem-rooting Division 9 lily with spirally arranged, lance-shaped, deep green leaves, 12cm (5in) long, with silver-hairy margins; the lower leaves are spreading, the upper ones erect. In midsummer, produces racemes of up to 12 small, unpleasantly scented, turkscap, sealing-wax-red flowers, 8cm (3in) across, unspotted, but with self-coloured papillae at the bases. Grow in any soil, in full sun or partial shade. ↕ 0.6–1.5m (2–5ft). N. Greece, Albania. ✻✻✻

***L.* 'Cherrywood'.** Division 4 lily producing racemes of medium-sized, unscented, turkscap, deep red or orange-red flowers, with orange throats speckled magenta-brown, in midsummer. Suitable for full sun or partial shade. ↕ to 2m (6ft). ✻✻✻

***L.* 'Chinook'.** Moderately vigorous Division 1a lily. In early and midsummer, bears umbels of medium-sized, unscented, bowl-shaped, pale apricot-buff flowers. ↕ 1–1.2m (3–4ft). ✻✻✻

***L.* 'Citronella'** ■ Vigorous, clump-forming Division 1c lily. In midsummer, bears racemes or panicles of medium-sized, turkscap, bright yellow to lemon-yellow flowers, speckled with faint black or reddish spots inside. ↕ 1.2–1.5m (4–5ft). ✻✻✻

L. concolor (Morning star lily). Stem-rooting Division 9 lily with reddish green stems bearing scattered, linear to linear-lance-shaped leaves, to 9cm (3½in) long, slightly hairy on the margins and beneath. In early and midsummer, produces racemes or umbels of up to 10 fragrant, upward-facing, star-shaped, glossy scarlet flowers, 3–4cm (1¼–1½in) across. ↕ 30–90cm (12–36in). W. China. ✻✻✻

***L.* 'Connecticut Beauty'.** Moderately vigorous Division 1a lily. In early and midsummer, bears umbels of medium-sized, slightly scented, bowl-shaped yellow flowers, darker along the centre of each tepal and with some darker spotting. ↕ 60–100cm (24–39in). ✻✻✻

***L.* 'Connecticut King'** ■ Vigorous, clump-forming Division 1a lily. In early and midsummer, produces racemes of medium-sized, unscented, long-lasting, star-shaped, rich deep yellow flowers, paling slightly towards the tips of the spreading, somewhat recurved tepals. ↕ 1m (3ft). ✻✻✻

***L.* 'Connecticut Yankee'.** Elegant Division 1c lily bearing racemes of medium-sized, unscented, turkscap, rich orange-red flowers, with a few darker spots within, in midsummer. ↕ 1.2–2m (4–6ft). ✻✻✻

L. cordatum see *Cardiocrinum cordatum*.

***L.* 'Corsage'.** Vigorous Division 1b lily producing racemes of medium-sized, unscented, shallow, star-shaped flowers in midsummer; they are pale pink with white centres, the spreading, recurved tepals flushed cream and yellow outside, finely dotted maroon inside. ↕ 1.2m (4ft). ✻✻✻

***L.* 'Côte d'Azur'.** Early-flowering Division 1a lily. In early and mid-

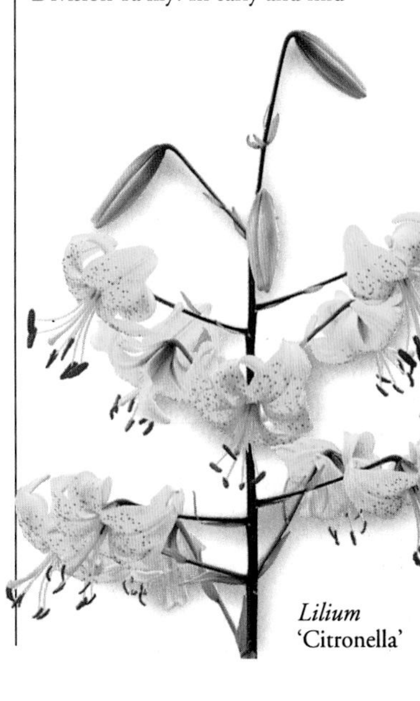
Lilium 'Citronella'

L

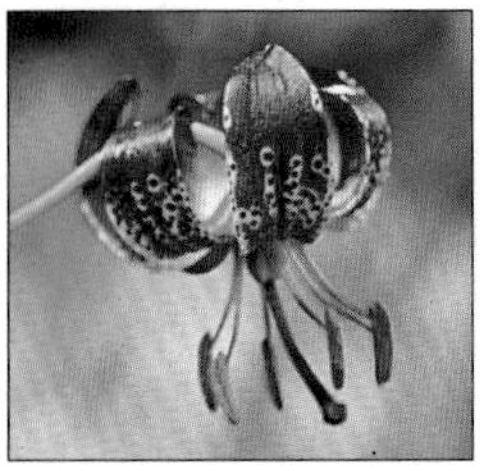
Lilium x *dalhansonii*

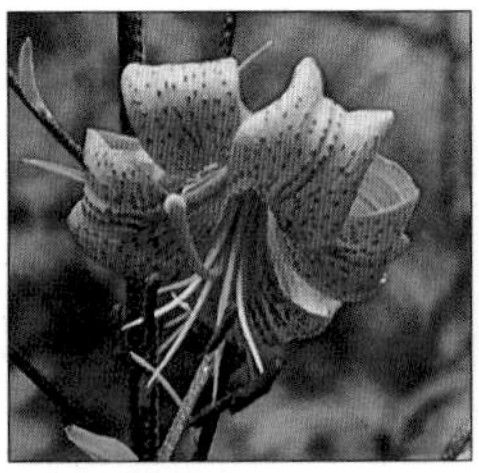
Lilium davidii var. *willmottiae*

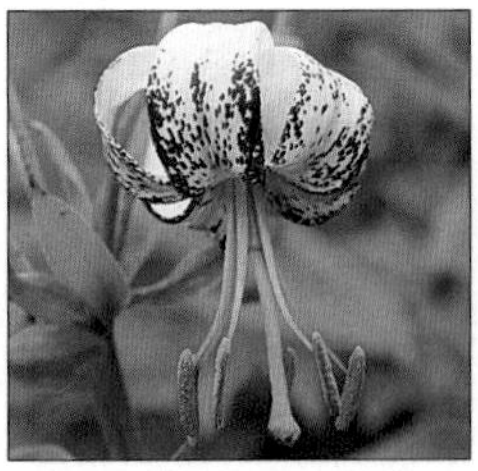
Lilium duchartrei

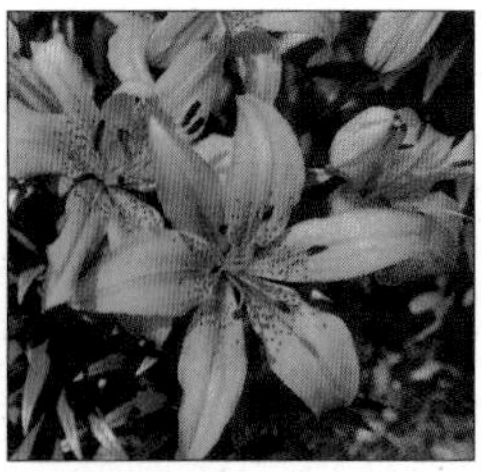
Lilium 'Enchantment'

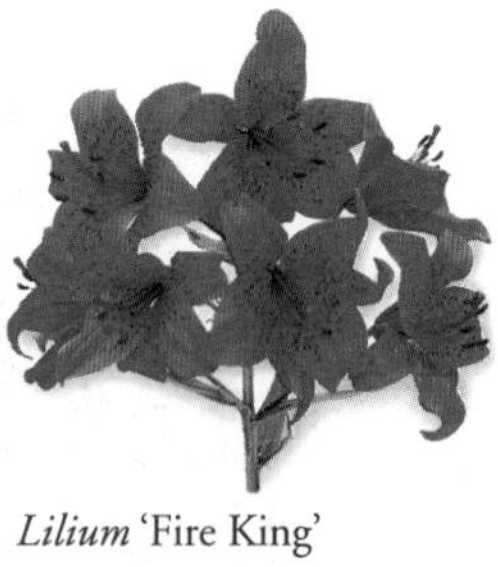
Lilium 'Fire King'

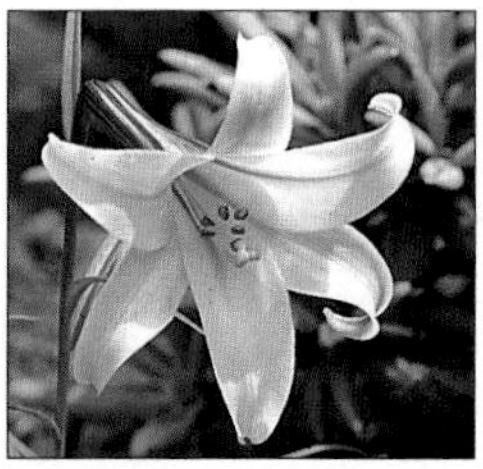
Lilium formosanum var. *pricei*

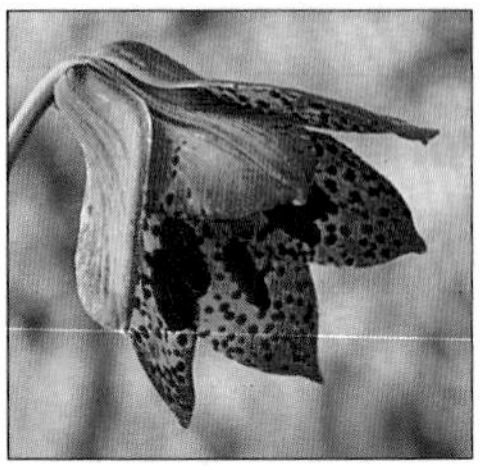
Lilium grayi

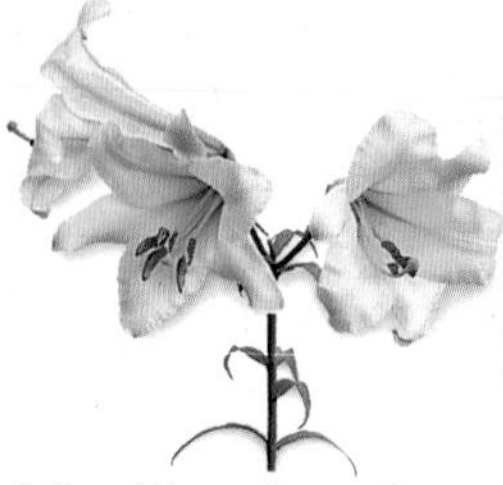
Lilium 'Green Dragon'

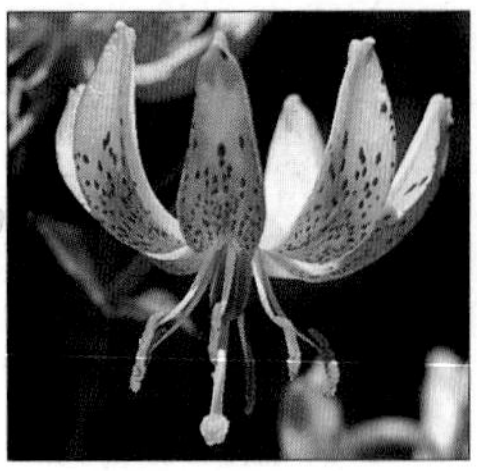
Lilium hansonii

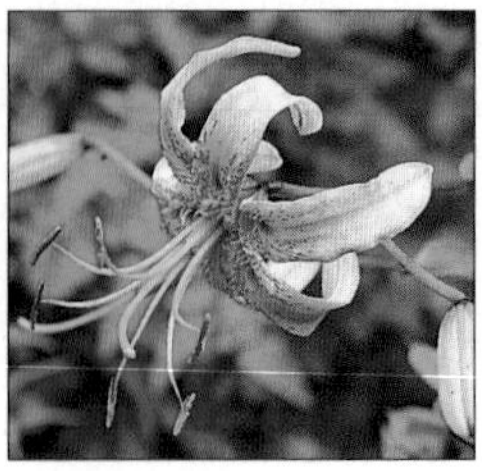
Lilium henryi

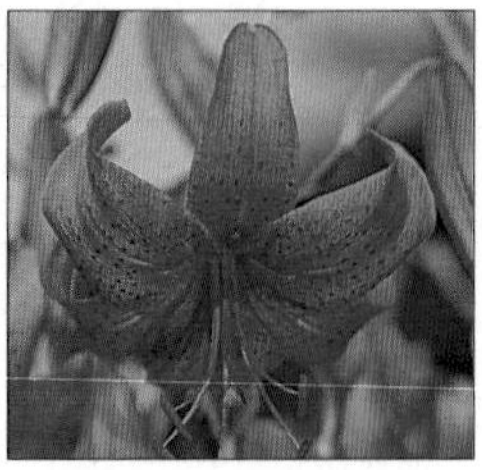
Lilium 'Lady Bowes Lyon'

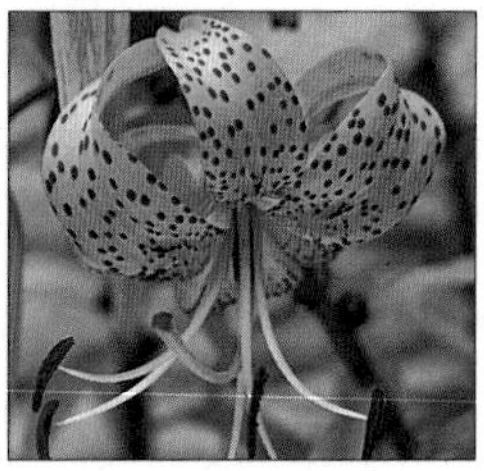
Lilium lancifolium

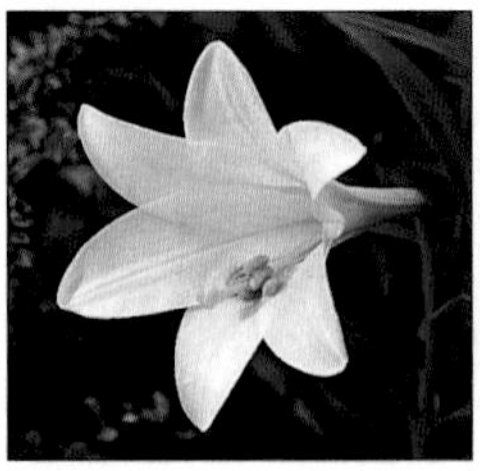
Lilium longiflorum

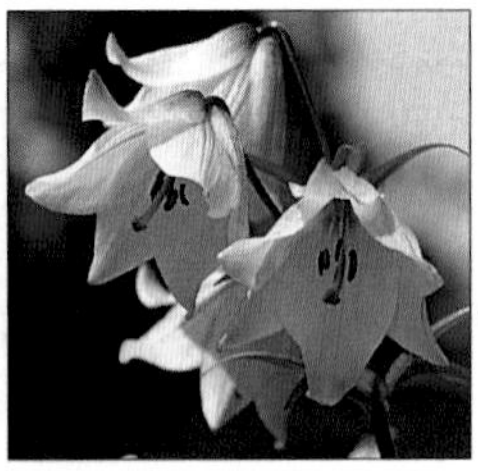
Lilium mackliniae

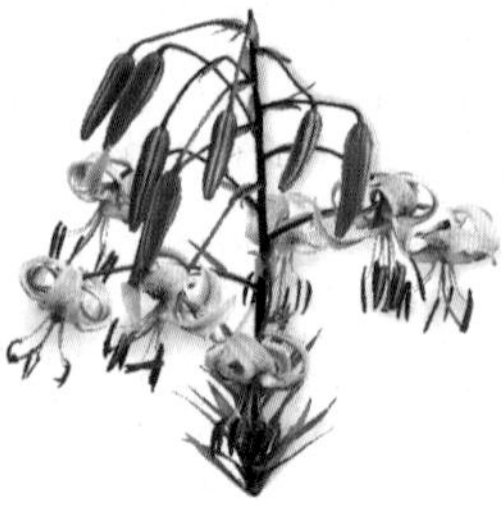
Lilium 'Marie North'

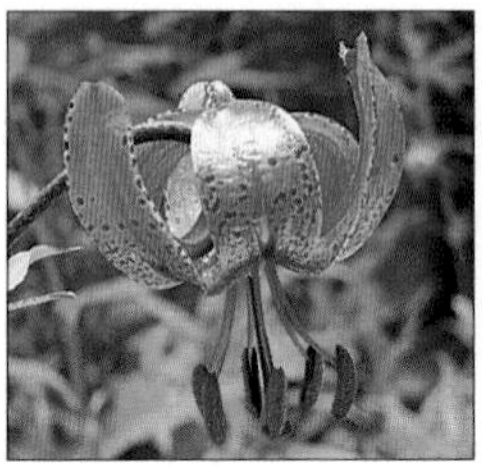
Lilium martagon

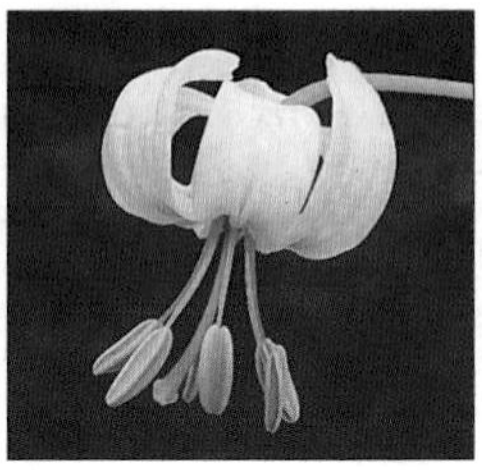
Lilium martagon var. *album*

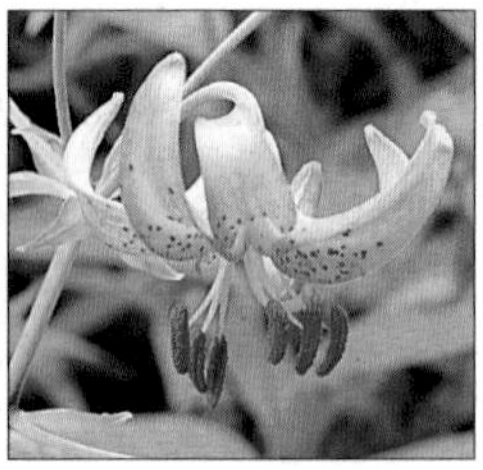
Lilium medeoloides

L

summer, bears umbels of medium-sized, unscented, bowl-shaped, deep pink flowers, with paler centres and tepals recurved towards the tips. ↕70–100cm (28–39in). ❄❄❄

L.* x *dalhansonii ■ (*L. martagon* var. *cattaniae* x *L. hansonii*). Division 8 lily bearing whorls of inversely lance-shaped leaves, 15–18cm (6–7in) long. In early summer, bears racemes of numerous small, unpleasantly scented, turkscap, maroon flowers, 3–5cm (1¼–2in) across, spotted and suffused orange in the centres. ↕1–1.5m (3–5ft). Garden origin. ❄❄❄

L. dauricum. Stem-rooting Division 9 lily with rhizomatous bulbs and brown-spotted green stems. Lance-shaped to linear, hairy-margined leaves, 5cm (2in) long, are scattered, but with the uppermost in a whorl below the flowers. In early and midsummer, produces umbels of up to 6 medium-sized, unscented, upward-facing, bowl-shaped, deep orange-scarlet flowers, to 10cm (4in) across, with yellowish orange centres, brownish red or purple spots, and hairy stalks. Best in acid soil, in full sun or partial shade. ↕50–70cm (20–28in). N.E. Asia. ❄❄❄

L. davidii. Division 9 lily, sometimes rhizomatous, with brown-spotted green stems bearing scattered, linear, finely toothed, dark green leaves, 6–10cm (2½–4in) long, hairy beneath. In summer, produces racemes of 10–20 unscented, long-stalked, turkscap, vermilion-red flowers, to 8cm (3in) across, with purple-black spots. ↕1–1.2m (3–4ft). W. China. ❄❄❄. **var. *willmottiae*** ■ has rhizomatous bulbs, tall, arching stems with broader leaves, and up to 40 flowers per raceme; ↕to 2m (6ft). China.

***L.* 'Destiny'.** Vigorous, clump-forming Division 1a lily. In early summer, bears umbels of medium-sized, unscented, bowl-shaped yellow flowers, with brown spots and tepals recurved towards the tips. ↕1–1.2m (3–4ft). ❄❄❄

L. duchartrei ■ Stem-rooting Division 9 lily with rhizomatous bulbs and ribbed, brown-flushed green stems bearing scattered, lance-shaped, stalkless leaves, to 10cm (4in) long, with rough margins. In summer, bears umbels of up to 12 scented, long-stalked, nodding, turkscap white flowers, 6–8cm (2½–3in) across, deep purple-spotted inside, and purple-flushed, ageing to red outside. ↕60–100cm (24–39in). China (Gansu, Sichuan, Yunnan). ❄❄❄

***L.* 'Enchantment'** ■♀ Very vigorous, clump-forming Division 1a lily. In early summer, produces umbels of medium-sized, unscented, cup-shaped, rich bright orange flowers with black spots inside. Easy to grow and good for cutting. ↕60–100cm (24–39in). ❄❄❄

***L.* 'Festival'.** Early-flowering Division 1a lily producing racemes of medium-sized, unscented, shallowly cup-shaped flowers, with spreading tepals, in early and midsummer. Flowers are pale orange, each with a deep red central star, brown spots, and tepals with red tips and margins; they are often flushed purple-brown on the outside. ↕1m (3ft). ❄❄❄

***L.* 'Fire King'** ■ Vigorous Division 1b lily. In midsummer, produces racemes of large, unscented, shallowly funnel-shaped, bright reddish orange flowers, spotted purple inside and with recurved tepal tips. Excellent in a container. ↕1–1.2m (3–4ft). ❄❄❄

L. formosanum. Elegant, stem-rooting Division 9 lily with rhizomatous bulbs, and green stems that are purplish brown towards the bases. Numerous dark green, linear to narrowly oblong-lance-shaped leaves, 8–20cm (3–8in) long, are scattered, and sparse towards the stem tops. Slender, very fragrant, trumpet-shaped white flowers, 12–20cm (5–8in) long, flushed reddish purple outside, and with flared and somewhat recurved tepal tips, are borne singly, in pairs, or in umbels of up to 10, in late summer and early autumn. Requires moist, acid soil. Suitable for a conservatory. ↕0.6–1.5m (2–5ft). Taiwan. ❄❄. **var. *pricei*** ■♀ produces solitary or clusters of up to 3 flowers, which are more strongly flushed purple on the outside, and borne earlier in the summer; ↕10–30cm (4–12in).

L. giganteum see *Cardiocrinum giganteum.*

***L.* Golden Clarion Group.** Vigorous, variable Division 6a lilies producing large, scented, trumpet-shaped, golden yellow or orange-brown flowers, often flushed red outside, in short racemes in midsummer. ↕1.5–2m (5–6ft). ❄❄❄

***L.* Golden Splendor Group** ■ Vigorous, variable Division 6a lilies. In midsummer, strong, sturdy stems produce umbels of large, scented, outward-facing, shallowly trumpet-shaped, almost bowl-shaped flowers, in shades of yellow with dark burgundy-red bands outside. ↕1.2–2m (4–6ft). ❄❄❄

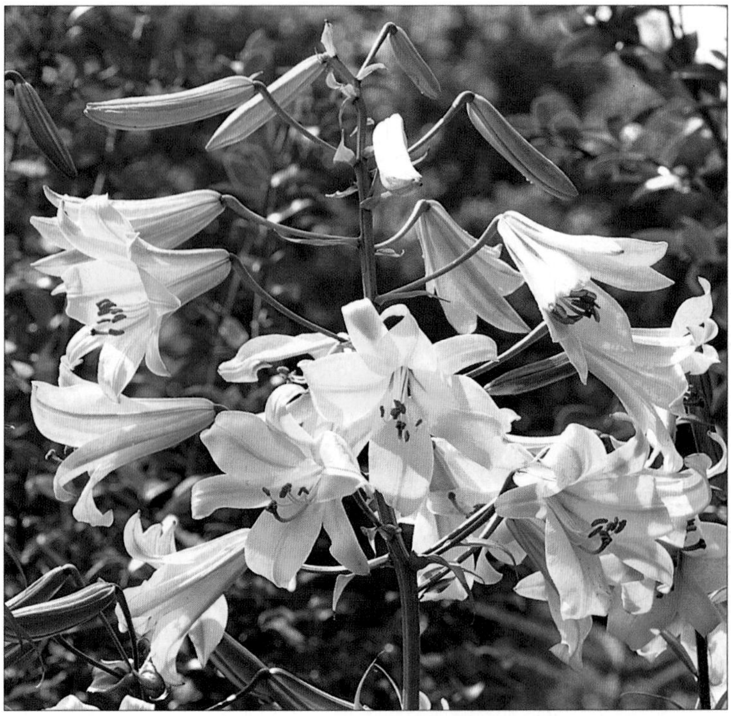
Lilium Golden Splendor Group

L. grayi ■ Division 9 lily with rhizomatous bulbs. Stems bear whorls of lance-shaped to oblong-lance-shaped leaves, 5–10cm (2–4in) long. In midsummer, produces tiered umbels of up to 12 scented, tubular-funnel-shaped, nodding flowers, 6cm (2½in) long, red outside, paler inside, with yellowish centres and purple spots. Requires moist, acid soil. ↕ 1–1.7m (3–5½ft). E. USA. ❄❄❄
***L.* 'Green Dragon'** ■ ♀ Stout Division 6a lily, derived from the Olympic Hybrids. In midsummer, bears short racemes of large, fragrant, trumpet-shaped white flowers flushed greenish brown outside and stained yellow in the centres. ↕ 1.5–2.2m (5–7ft). ❄❄❄
L. hansonii ■ ♀ Vigorous, early-flowering, stem-rooting Division 9 lily. Inversely lance-shaped to elliptic, pale green leaves, to 18cm (7in) long, are borne in dense whorls of 12–20. In early summer, produces racemes of up to 12 small, fragrant, nodding, turkscap, brilliant orange-yellow flowers, 3–4cm (1¼–1½in) across, with thick, recurved tepals spotted purplish brown near the bases. Grow in well-drained soil in partial shade. ↕ 1–1.5m (3–5ft). Russia (E. Siberia), Korea, Japan. ❄❄❄
L. heldreichii see *L. chalcedonicum.*
L. henryi ■ ♀ Vigorous, stem-rooting, clump-forming Division 9 lily with purple-marked green stems. Ovate-lance-shaped to lance-shaped leaves, 8–15cm (3–6in) long, are scattered; the lower leaves have short stalks, the upper ones are crowded below the flowers. In late summer, produces racemes of up to 10 (occasionally up to 20) faintly scented, turkscap, deep orange flowers, 6–8cm (2½–3in) across, spotted black, with deep red anthers. Easy to grow in neutral to alkaline soil in partial shade. ↕ 1–3m (3–10ft). C. China. ❄❄❄
***L.* 'Hornback's Gold'.** Division 1c lily bearing few-flowered umbels of large, unscented, cup-shaped, pale yellow flowers with light brown spotting, in midsummer. ↕ 1–1.2m (3–4ft). ❄❄❄
***L.* 'Imperial Gold'.** Division 7c lily bearing racemes, in late summer, of large, fragrant, star-shaped, glistening white flowers, each tepal with recurved tips and a yellow stripe down the centre. ↕ 1.8–2m (6ft). ❄❄❄
***L.* 'Imperial Silver'.** Division 7c lily with the stems often spotted red. In late summer, produces racemes of large, fragrant, broad, shallowly bowl-shaped white flowers, with wide-spreading, burgundy-spotted tepals with recurved tips, and orange-red anthers. ↕ 1.5–2m (5–6ft). ❄❄❄
***L.* 'Jetfire'.** Early-flowering Division 1a lily bearing umbels of medium-sized, unscented, cup-shaped, rich orange flowers with yellow centres, in early and midsummer. ↕ 80–120cm (32–48in). ❄❄❄
***L.* 'Journey's End'** ■ Stout Division 7d lily producing racemes of large, unscented, broad, turkscap flowers in late summer; the spreading tepals are deep pink, with maroon spots and white margins and tips. ↕ 1–2m (3–6ft). ❄❄❄
***L.* 'Joy'**, syn. *L.* 'Le Rêve'. Division 7b lily bearing racemes of medium-sized, unscented, bowl-shaped, reddish purple flowers with maroon spotting towards the centres, in midsummer. ↕ 60–80cm (24–32in). ❄❄❄

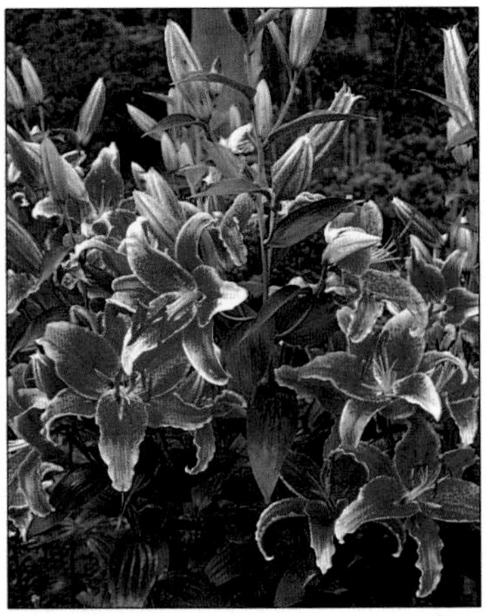

Lilium 'Journey's End'

***L.* 'Karen North'** ♀ Elegant Division 1c lily producing lax racemes of medium-sized, unscented, turkscap, orange-pink flowers with deep pink spots, in midsummer. ↕ 1–1.4m (3–4½ft). ❄❄❄
***L.* 'King Pete'.** Vigorous, clump-forming Division 1b lily. In midsummer, produces umbels of medium-sized, unscented, broad, bowl-shaped cream flowers, marked and spotted orange and with orange-red anthers. Long-lasting in flower and good for cutting. ↕ 90cm (3ft). ❄❄❄
***L.* 'Lady Bowes Lyon'** ■ Division 1c lily bearing racemes of medium-sized, unscented, turkscap, vivid red flowers spotted black, in midsummer. ↕ 1–1.2m (3–4ft). ❄❄❄
***L.* 'Lake Tahoe'.** Division 4 lily bearing racemes of medium-sized, unscented, turkscap flowers in midsummer; the red, pink-spotted tepals have gold bands towards their white bases. ↕ 1.6–2m (5½–6ft). ❄❄❄
L. lancifolium ■ syn. *L. tigrinum* (Tiger lily). Robust, stem-rooting, clump-forming Division 9 lily with dark purple, often white-hairy stems. Scattered, narrowly lance-shaped leaves, 12–20cm (5–8in) long, have rough margins; the upper ones produce dark purplish black bulbils in the axils. Up to 40 unscented, nodding, turkscap, orange-red flowers, 12cm (5in) across, with dark purple spots and papillae, are produced in racemes in late summer and early autumn. Prefers moist, acid soil, but tolerates some lime. ↕ 0.6–1.5m (2–5ft). E. China, Korea, Japan. ❄❄❄. **var. *flaviflorum*** produces yellow flowers; Japan. **'Flore Pleno'** bears double flowers with 24–36 tepals and no stamens. **var. *splendens*** is exceptionally vigorous, with up to 25 large, black-spotted, deep orange-red flowers on downy stems. **'Yellow Tiger'** is a selection from var. *flaviflorum*, with purple-spotted, bright yellow flowers.
***L.* 'Le Rêve'** see *L.* 'Joy'.
***L.* 'Limelight'** ♀ Moderately robust Division 6a lily. In midsummer, bears short racemes of large, fragrant, slightly pendent, trumpet-shaped, lime-yellow flowers that are flushed with green, especially outside. ↕ 1–2m (3–6ft). ❄❄❄
L. longiflorum ■ ♀ (Easter lily). Vigorous, stem-rooting Division 9 lily with scattered, lance-shaped to oblong-lance-shaped, shiny, deep green leaves, to 18cm (7in) long. In midsummer, bears short racemes of 1–6 very fragrant, trumpet-shaped, horizontally placed, pure white flowers, to 18cm (7in) long, with yellow anthers. Widely grown for cut flowers; excellent in a container. Lime-tolerant. Grow in partial shade. ↕ 40–100cm (16–39in). S. Japan, Taiwan. ❄. **'Casa Rosa'** bears white flowers, flushed rose-pink. **'White American'** produces white flowers with green tips and deep yellow anthers.
L. mackliniae ■ ♀ Small, stem-rooting Division 9 lily with slender green stems, sometimes tinged purple, and linear-lance-shaped to narrowly elliptic, deep green leaves, 3–6cm (1¼–2½in) long, scattered or whorled near the tops of the stems. In early and midsummer, bears racemes of up to 6 unscented, semi-pendent, bowl-shaped, purple-flushed, rose-pink flowers, 5cm (2in) across, with purple anthers. ↕ 30–60cm (12–24in). N.E. India (Assam). ❄❄❄
L. maculatum, syn. *L. thunbergianum.* Short, stem-rooting Division 9 lily with ribbed stems and scattered, elliptic to lance-shaped leaves, 5–10cm (2–4in) long. In early and midsummer, produces umbels of faintly scented, bowl-shaped, orange, red, or yellow flowers, 8–10cm (3–4in) across, with varying amounts of darker spotting. Prefers neutral to alkaline soil. ↕ 50–60cm (20–24in). Japan. ❄❄❄. **var. *flavum*** produces yellow flowers.
***L.* 'Magic Pink'** ■ Clump-forming Division 7b lily. In midsummer, produces short racemes of large, slightly scented, half-nodding, bowl-shaped, soft pink flowers, with a darker centre to each tepal. ↕ 1.2m (4ft). ❄❄❄
***L.* 'Marhan'** ♀ Stout Division 2 lily producing racemes, in early summer, of medium-sized, unpleasantly scented, turkscap, orange flowers, with reddish brown spotting. ↕ 1.5–2m (5–6ft). ❄❄❄
***L.* 'Marie North'** ■ Clump-forming Division 1c lily producing racemes of medium-sized, slightly scented, turkscap flowers in midsummer; dark pink in bud, the flowers open white, suffused pinkish mauve with some deeper speckling in the centres. Bulbils are sometimes produced. ↕ 80–120cm (32–48in). ❄❄❄
L. martagon ■ (Common turkscap lily). Vigorous, clump-forming, stem-rooting Division 9 lily producing stiff, purple- or red-flushed green stems. Elliptic to inversely lance-shaped leaves, to 16cm (6in) long, often hairy on the undersides, are mostly borne in dense whorls. In early and midsummer, produces narrow racemes of up to 50 small, somewhat unpleasant-smelling, pendent or nodding, glossy, turkscap, pink to purplish red flowers, to 5cm (2in) across, with some darker coloured spotting or flecking. Grow in almost any well-drained soil in full sun or partial shade. ↕ 0.9–2m (3–6ft). Europe to Mongolia. ❄❄❄. **var. *album*** ■ ♀ has bright green stems bearing small, pure white flowers, to 4cm (1½in) across. **var. *cattaniae*** ♀ syn. var. *dalmaticum*, has hairy stems and buds, and produces deep maroon flowers. **var. *dalmaticum*** see var. *cattaniae.* **'Inshriach Ivory'** bears ivory-white flowers. **'Inshriach Rose'** has stout stems bearing deep rose-purple flowers with darker spots.
***L.* 'Maxwill'.** Striking Division 1c lily. In midsummer, stout stems produce racemes of small, unscented, turkscap, black-spotted, brilliant orange-red flowers, with strongly recurved tepals. ↕ 1.5–2.2m (5–7ft). ❄❄❄
L. medeoloides ■ Stem-rooting Division 9 lily with hollow green stems and stalkless, lance-shaped leaves, 12cm (5in) long, mostly in 1 or 2 whorls on the lower parts of the stems, with a few scattered in the upper parts. In midsummer, produces short racemes or umbels of up to 10 unscented, turkscap, orange-red to apricot flowers, 4.5cm (1¾in) across, with darker spots and purple anthers. Requires acid soil and partial shade. ↕ 40–75cm (16–30in). Russia (E. Siberia), N. China, Korea, Japan. ❄❄❄

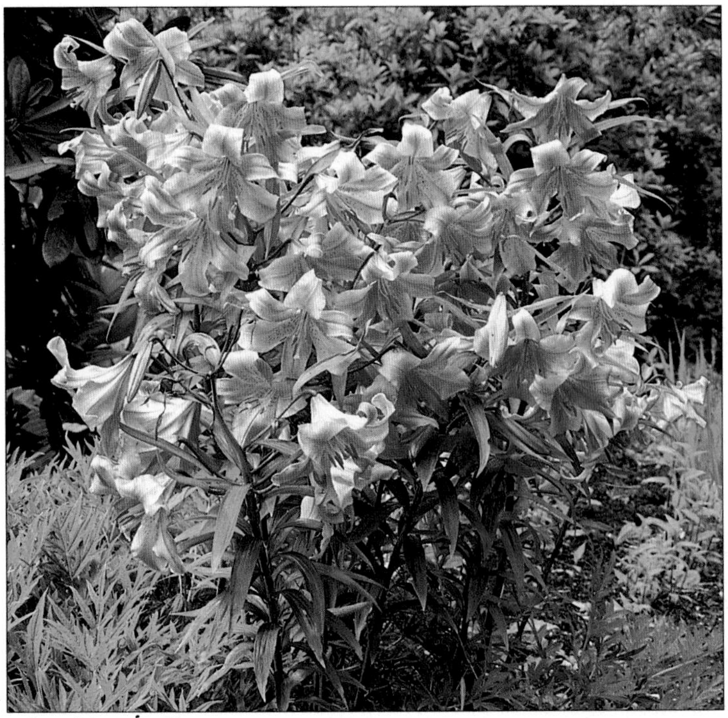

Lilium 'Magic Pink'

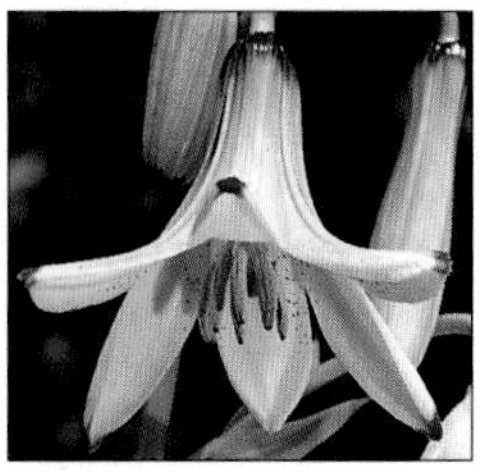
Lilium monadelphum

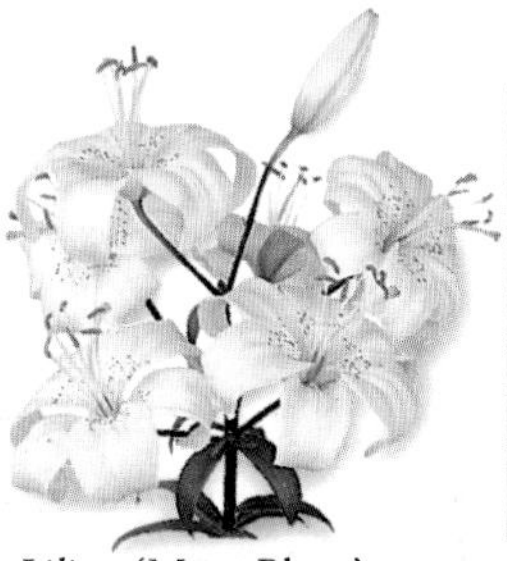
Lilium 'Mont Blanc'

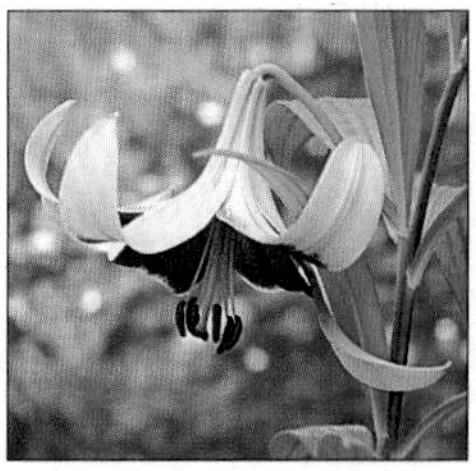
Lilium nepalense

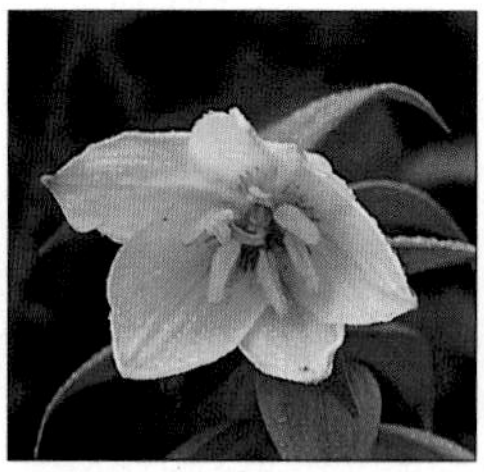
Lilium oxypetalum

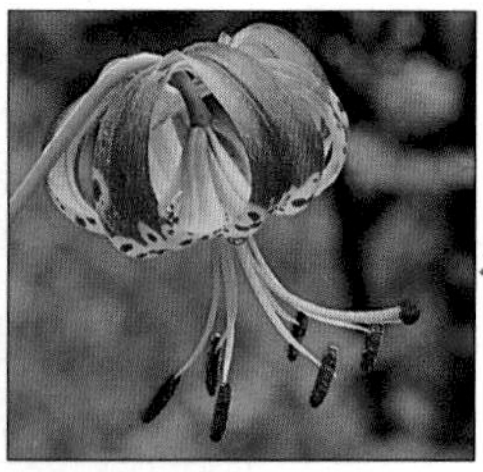
Lilium pardalinum

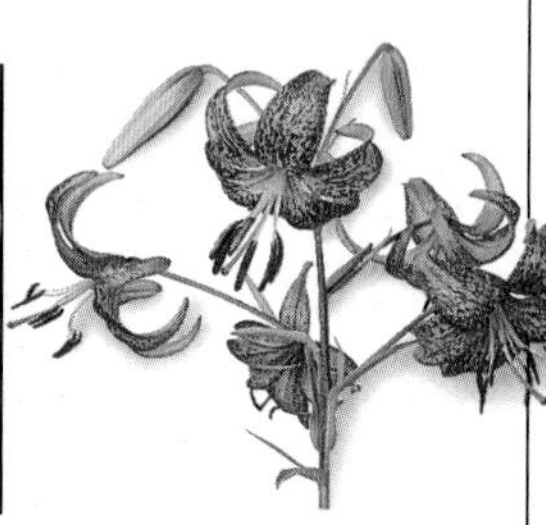
Lilium 'Peggy North'

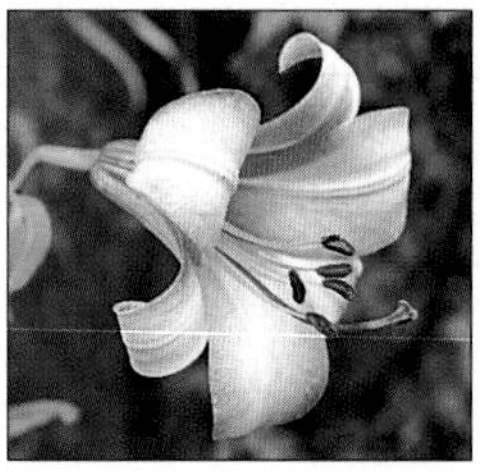
Lilium Pink Perfection Group

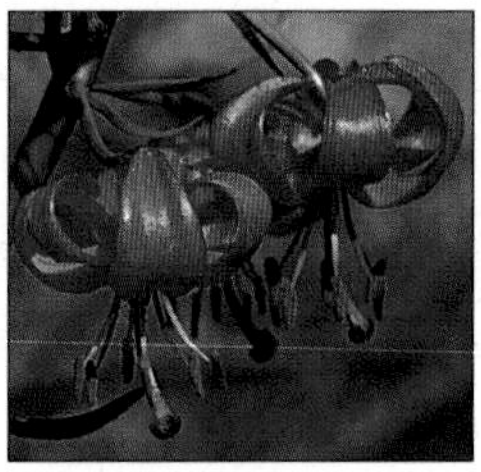
Lilium pomponium

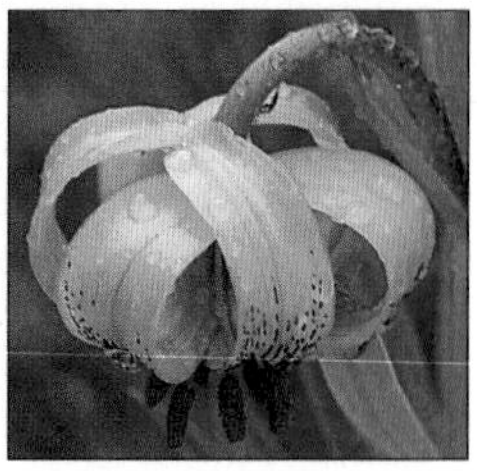
Lilium pyrenaicum

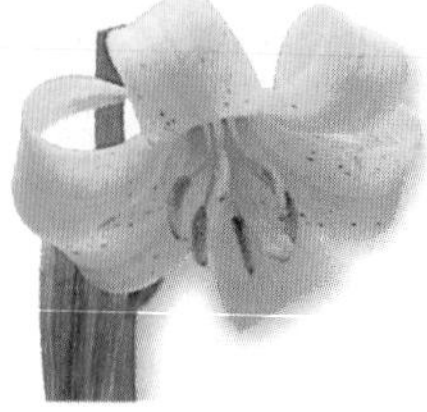
Lilium pyrenaicum subsp. *carniolicum* var. *albanicum*

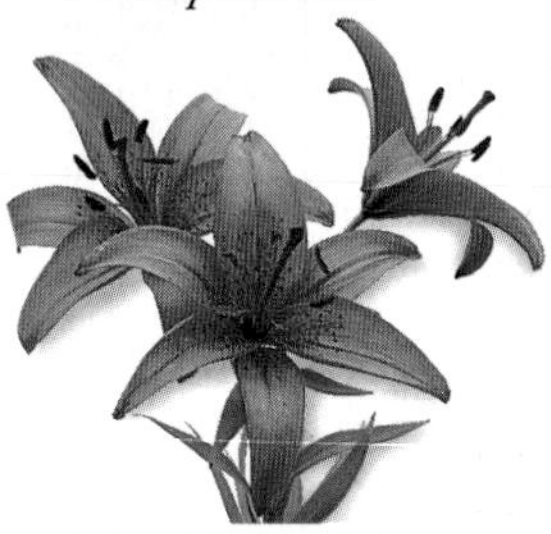
Lilium 'Red Night'

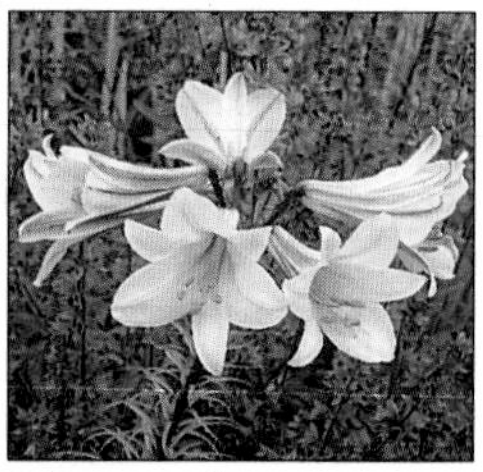
Lilium regale

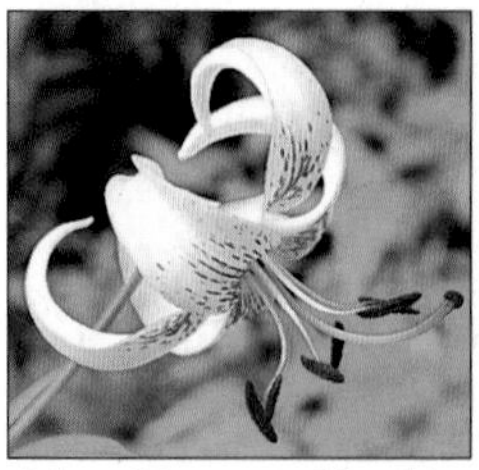
Lilium 'Rosemary North'

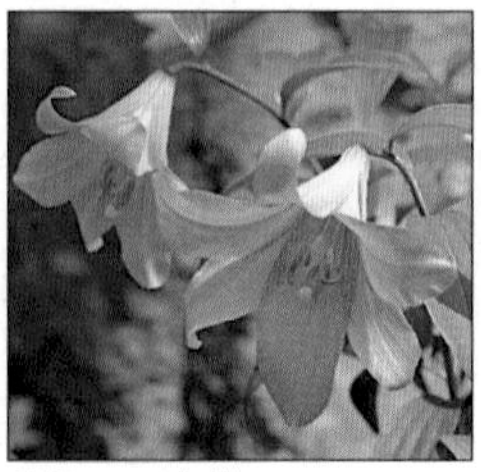
Lilium rubellum

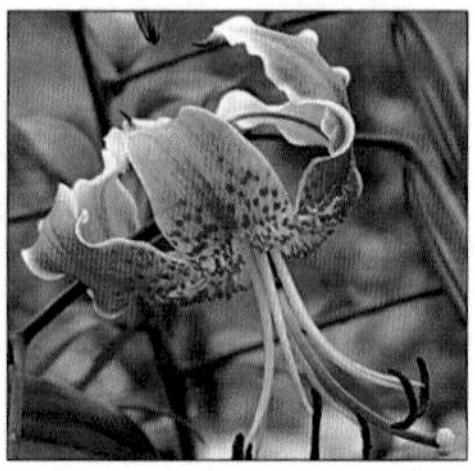
Lilium speciosum var. *rubrum*

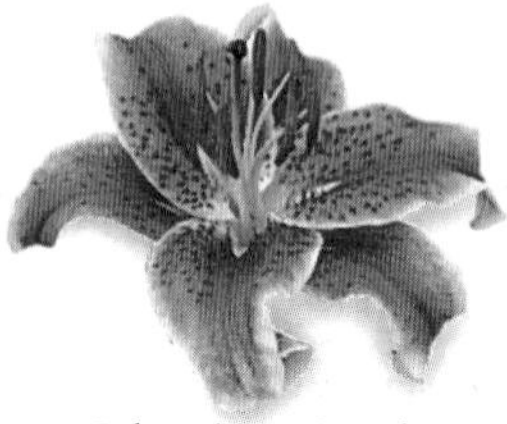
Lilium 'Star Gazer'

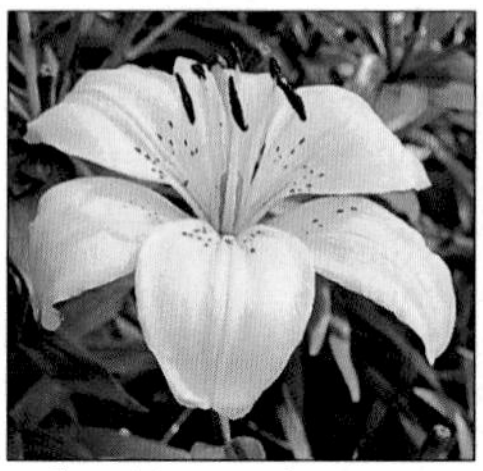
Lilium 'Sun Ray'

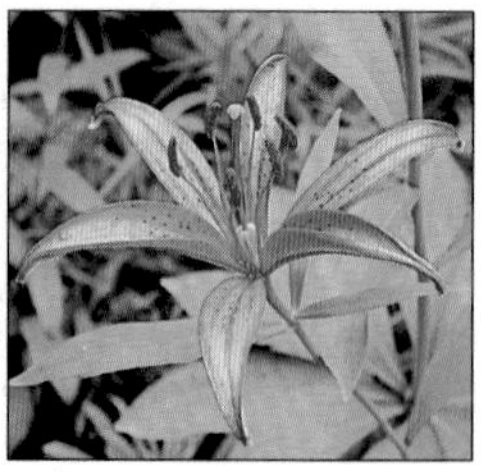
Lilium tsingtauense

L. monadelphum ▣♀ syn. *L. szovitsianum.* Stout, clump-forming, sparsely stem-rooting Division 9 lily with stiff stems and scattered, lance-shaped to inversely lance-shaped or ovate, bright green leaves, to 14cm (5½in) long. In early summer, bears racemes of up to 30 large, nodding, fragrant, broadly trumpet-shaped yellow flowers, to 10cm (4in) across, flecked and spotted maroon or purple inside, flushed purplish brown outside. Tepals are moderately to prominently recurved. Lime-tolerant. Thrives in fairly heavy soil, and survives in drier, sunnier conditions than most lilies. ↕1–1.5m (3–5ft). N.E. Turkey, Caucasus. ❄❄❄

***L.* 'Mont Blanc'** ▣ Short Division 1a lily producing umbels of large, unscented, wide, bowl-shaped white flowers, slightly brown-spotted in the centres, in early and midsummer. ↕60–70cm (24–28in). ❄❄❄

***L.* 'Montreux'.** Short Division 1a lily bearing umbels, in midsummer, of medium-sized, unscented, cup-shaped pink flowers, with brown dots in the centres and buff-yellow anthers. ↕80–100cm (32–39in). ❄❄❄

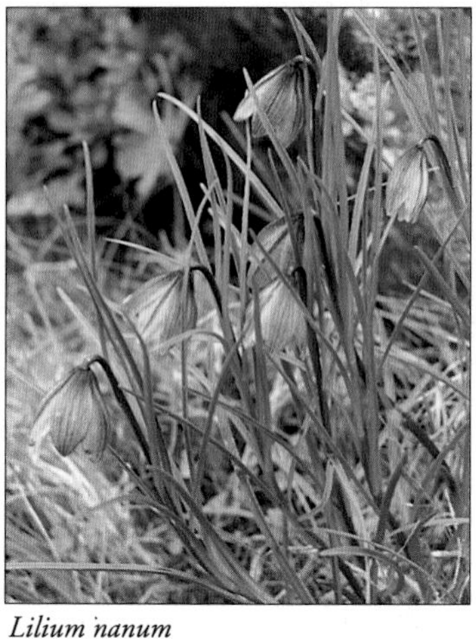
Lilium nanum

L. nanum ▣ syn. *Nomocharis nana.* Small Division 9 lily with slender stems and scattered, linear leaves, to 12cm (5in) long. Bears solitary, scented, bell-shaped, pale pink to rose-purple flowers, 1–4cm (½–1½in) long, often with darker markings or spots, in early summer. Requires cool, moist, acid soil and partial shade. ↕6–30cm (2½–12in). Himalayas, W. China. ❄❄❄. **var. *flavidum*** bears pale yellow flowers.

L. nepalense ▣ Stem-rooting Division 9 lily with rhizomatous bulbs, erect or arching, smooth stems, and scattered, lance-shaped to oblong-lance-shaped, deep green leaves, to 15cm (6in) long. In early and midsummer, produces unscented or unpleasantly scented, funnel-shaped, yellow, greenish yellow, or greenish white flowers, singly or occasionally in groups of 2 or 3 in the upper leaf axils. The tepals later reflex, and are either flecked and spotted reddish purple, or are entirely reddish purple or maroon in the centres. Needs cool, acid soil and partial shade. ↕60–100cm (24–39in). N. India to Nepal and Bhutan (Himalayas). ❄

***L.* Olympic Hybrids.** Vigorous Division 6a lilies. A group of hybrids derived from various Asiatic species, including *L. brownii, L. leucanthum,* and *L. sargentiae.* In mid- and late summer, they bear racemes of up to 15 large, sweetly fragrant, trumpet-shaped flowers, ranging from white, greenish white, cream, and yellow, to pink and purple, often yellow in the throats. Tepals are flushed pink or purplish red on the outside. ↕1.2–2m (4–6ft). ❄❄❄

***L.* 'Omega'.** Division 7d lily with short stems producing short racemes, in late summer, of large, rose-pink flowers, with yellowish centres and sparse red spotting; the tepals are spreading and slightly recurved. ↕60–80cm (24–32in). ❄❄❄

L. oxypetalum ▣ syn. *Nomocharis oxypetala.* Small Division 9 lily with slender stems and scattered, linear to linear-lance-shaped leaves, to 7cm (3in) long, sometimes whorled below the flowers. In early summer, each slender stem produces 1 or 2 small, unscented, semi-pendent, shallowly bowl-shaped yellow flowers, to 5cm (2in) across, usually with some purple dots in the centres. Needs cool, moist, acid soil and partial shade. ↕20–30cm (8–12in). N.W. Himalayas. ❄❄❄. **var. *insigne*** produces purple flowers.

***L.* 'Pan'.** Delicate Division 1c lily bearing racemes of small, pleasantly scented, turkscap white flowers in midsummer. ↕1–1.2m (3–4ft). ❄❄❄

L. pardalinum ▣ Vigorous, clump-forming, rhizomatous Division 9 lily. Strong stems bear dense whorls of elliptic to inversely lance-shaped, dull deep green leaves, to 18cm (7in) long. In midsummer, produces racemes of up to 10 unscented, nodding, turkscap, orange-red to crimson flowers, 9cm (3½in) across, paler towards the bases and with large maroon spots, some spots encircled with yellow. Prefers moist soil in full sun or partial shade; lime-tolerant, but not in dry soil. ↕1.5–2.5m (5–8ft). W. USA. ❄❄❄. **var. *giganteum*** ♀ is particularly vigorous, with as many as 30 flowers per stem; they are crimson, and yellow towards the bases with crimson spots; ↕to 3m (10ft).

***L.* 'Peggy North'** ▣ Moderately vigorous, clump-forming Division 1c lily. In midsummer, bears racemes of medium-sized, faintly scented, turkscap, orange flowers, finely speckled dark brown. ↕1.2–1.5m (4–5ft). ❄❄❄

***L.* Pink Perfection Group** ▣♀ Division 6a lilies with stout stems. In midsummer, bear short racemes or umbels of large, scented, slightly nodding, trumpet-shaped flowers, which are deep purplish red or purple-pink, with bright orange anthers. ↕1.5–2m (5–6ft). ❄❄❄

***L.* 'Pirate'.** Division 1a lily with slender stems bearing umbels of medium-sized, unscented, star-shaped, orange-red flowers in early summer. ↕1–1.2m (3–4ft). ❄❄❄

L. pomponium ▣ Slender, stem-rooting Division 9 lily with green stems that are spotted purple on the lower halves. Scattered, linear leaves, to 15cm (6in) long, have silver-hairy margins. In early and midsummer, bears racemes of up to 6 (rarely up to 10) unpleasantly scented, pendent, turkscap, sealing-wax-red flowers, 5cm (2in) across, generally with black spots and streaks in the throats. Prefers alkaline soil in full sun or partial shade. ↕1m (3ft). French and Italian Alps. ❄❄❄

L. ponticum see *L. pyrenaicum* subsp. *ponticum.*

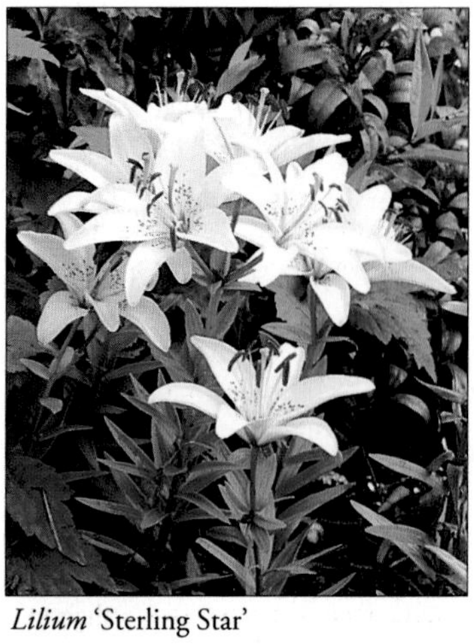
Lilium 'Sterling Star'

L. pumilum ♀ syn. *L. tenuifolium.* Stem-rooting Division 9 lily with slender stems bearing numerous scattered, linear leaves, to 10cm (4in) long. In early summer, bears racemes of up to 30 fragrant, nodding to pendent, turkscap, scarlet flowers, 5cm (2in) across, unspotted or with a few black spots in the centres. Requires acid soil and full sun or partial shade. ↕15–45cm (6–18in). Russia (Siberia) to Mongolia, N. China, and N. Korea. ❄❄❄

L. pyrenaicum ■♀ Stem-rooting, clump-forming Division 9 lily with green stems, sometimes spotted purple, and numerous scattered, linear to linear-lance-shaped, bright green leaves, 15cm (6in) long, often with silver-hairy margins. In early and midsummer, bears racemes of up to 12 unpleasant-smelling, pendent, turkscap, yellow or greenish yellow flowers, 5cm (2in) across, flecked and spotted dark maroon in the throats. Needs neutral to alkaline soil and full sun or partial shade. ↕30–100cm (12–39in). Pyrenees. ❄❄❄. **subsp. *carniolicum*,** syn. *L. carniolicum,* has leaves with densely downy veins on the undersides, and produces orange or red flowers, spotted purple-brown; ↕to 1.2m (4ft); Alps, former Yugoslavia. **subsp. *carniolicum* var. *albanicum*** ■ has leaves that are hairless beneath, and bears plain yellow flowers; ↕rarely more than 40cm (16in); N. Greece, Albania. **subsp. *ponticum*,** syn. *L. ponticum,* bears leaves 3–8cm (1¼–3in) long, with hairs beneath, and deep yellow flowers, flecked and spotted reddish brown or purple; ↕to 90cm (36in); N.E. Turkey. **var. *rubrum*** bears orange-red flowers.

***L.* 'Red Night'** ■ syn. *L.* 'Roter Cardinal'. Division 1a lily. In early and midsummer, produces umbels of medium-sized, unscented, cup-shaped red flowers, lighter on the tepal lobes, spotted black in the centres. ↕70–100cm (28–39in). ❄❄❄

L. regale ■♀ (Regal lily). Vigorous, stem-rooting Division 9 lily with erect or arching, purple-flushed, grey-green stems and numerous scattered, linear, shiny, deep green leaves, 5–13cm (2–5in) long. In midsummer, produces umbels of up to 25, very fragrant, broadly trumpet-shaped white flowers, 12–15cm (5–6in) long, flushed purple or purple-brown outside, with yellow centres and gold anthers. Grow in most well-drained soils, except very alkaline; prefers full sun. ↕0.6–2m (2–6ft). W. China. ❄❄❄. **var. *album*** bears almost pure white flowers with orange anthers.

***L.* 'Rosemary North'** ■♀ Division 1c lily producing racemes, in early and midsummer, of medium-sized, slightly scented, turkscap ochre flowers with a few dark ochre spots on the outside. ↕90–100cm (36–39in). ❄❄❄

***L.* 'Roter Cardinal'** see *L.* 'Red Night'.

L. rubellum ■ Stem-rooting Division 9 lily with scattered, narrowly elliptic or narrowly ovate to lance-shaped leaves, 10cm (4in) long. In early summer, up to 9, but usually 1–4, fragrant, funnel-shaped pink flowers, 8cm (3in) long, often spotted maroon in the centres, are borne from the upper leaf axils. Requires moist, acid soil and partial shade. ↕30–80cm (12–32in). Japan. ❄❄❄

***L.* 'Shuksan'.** Stem-rooting Division 4 lily with stout stems bearing racemes, in midsummer, of medium-sized, slightly scented, turkscap, orange-yellow flowers, with large black or reddish brown spots. Good in partial shade, especially in acid soil. ↕1.4–2m (4½–6ft). ❄❄❄

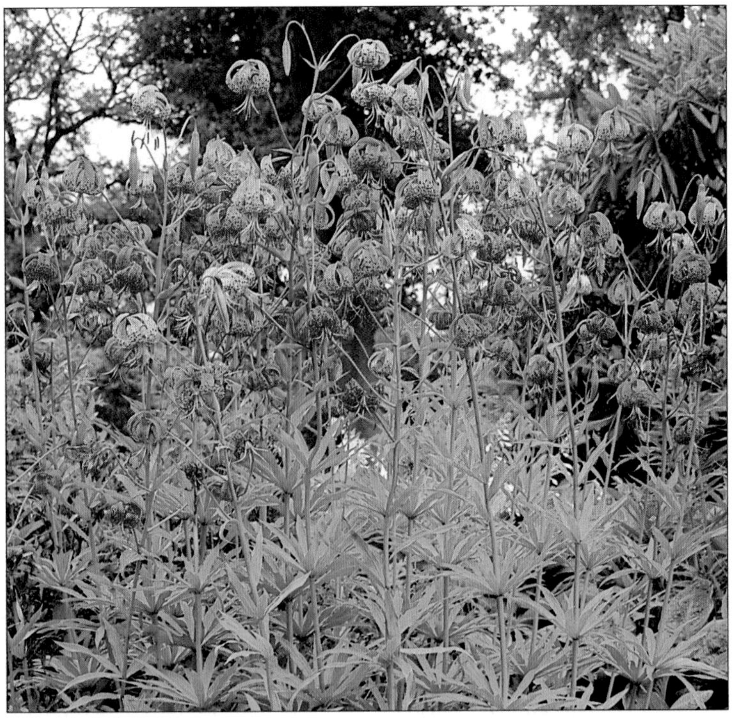

Lilium superbum

L. speciosum ♀ Vigorous, stem-rooting Division 9 lily with erect to ascending, purple-flushed green stems. Short-stalked leaves, to 18cm (7in) long, are scattered and broadly lance-shaped to almost ovate. In late summer and early autumn, produces racemes of usually up to 12, sometimes more, large, fragrant, pendent or outward-facing, turkscap, pale pink or white flowers, to 18cm (7in) across, flushed deeper pink in the centres, and with papillae and pink or crimson spots. Needs moist, acid soil and partial shade. ↕1–1.7m (3–5½ft). E. China, Japan, Taiwan. ❄❄❄. **var. *album*** produces white flowers and purple stems. **'Grand Commander'** has red-spotted, lilac-purple flowers with white-margined tepals. **var. *roseum*** has rose-pink flowers and green stems. **var. *rubrum*** ■ produces purple-brown stems and deep carmine-red flowers. **'Uchida'** bears crimson-red flowers with delicate, darker red spotting.

***L.* 'Star Gazer'** ■ Vigorous Division 7d lily bearing racemes, in midsummer, of large, unscented, star-shaped red flowers with spreading tepals, recurved at the tips and marked with darker spots. Good in a container and for forcing. ↕1–1.5m (3–5ft). ❄❄❄

***L.* 'Sterling Star'** ■ Vigorous Division 1a lily. In early and midsummer, bears short racemes of large, faintly scented, cup-shaped, off-white flowers, flushed cream and speckled brown. ↕1–1.2m (3–4ft). ❄❄❄

***L.* 'Sun Ray'** ■ Division 1a lily producing umbels of medium-sized, unscented, bowl-shaped yellow flowers, with a sparse scattering of brown dots, in early and midsummer. ↕1m (3ft). ❄❄❄

L. superbum ■♀ (American turkscap lily). Vigorous, stem-rooting Division 9 lily with rhizomatous bulbs, purple-mottled green stems, and linear-lance-shaped to elliptic leaves, 3.5–11cm (1½–4½in) long, mostly produced in dense whorls. In late summer and early autumn, bears long racemes of up to 40 unscented, pendent, turkscap flowers, to 7cm (3in) across; tepals are red-flushed orange, with maroon spots, and green towards the bases. Prefers moist, acid soil, and full sun or partial shade. ↕1.5–3m (5–10ft). E. USA. ❄❄❄

L. szovitsianum see *L. monadelphum.*

L. tenuifolium see *L. pumilum.*

L.* x *testaceum ■♀ (*L. candidum* x *L. chalcedonicum*) (Nankeen lily). Division 3 lily with alternate, somewhat twisted, lance-shaped leaves. In early and midsummer, produces racemes of up to 12 scented, nodding, turkscap, pale apricot-orange flowers, to 8cm (3in) across, with faint red markings in the centres and red anthers. Lime-tolerant; grow in full sun or partial shade. ↕1–1.5m (3–5ft). Garden origin. ❄❄❄

L. thunbergianum see *L. maculatum.*

L. tigrinum see *L. lancifolium.*

***L.* 'Trance'.** Relatively short Division 7b lily. In early and midsummer, bears racemes of medium-sized, unscented, outward-facing, bowl-shaped pink flowers, with pale spots in the centres; tepals are dark pink along the centres, fading to almost white at the margins. ↕60–100cm (24–39in). ❄❄❄

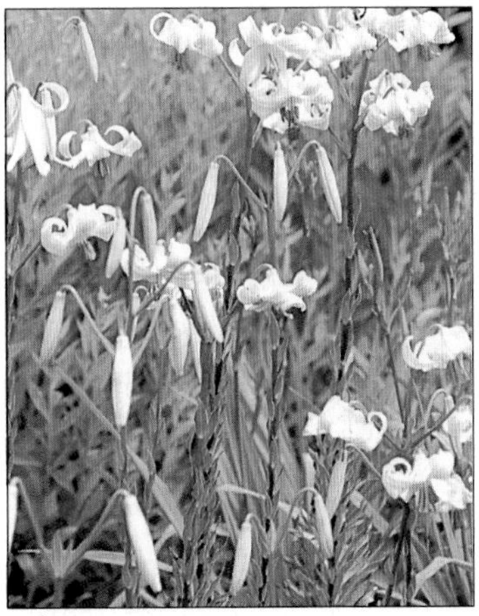

Lilium x *testaceum*

L. tsingtauense ■ Stem-rooting Division 9 lily with hollow stems and inversely lance-shaped, hairless leaves, to 13cm (5in) long, mostly in 2 whorls. In midsummer, bears loose umbels of up to 6 (sometimes up to 15) unscented, upright, shallowly trumpet-shaped, maroon-spotted, orange or orange-red flowers, 5–8cm (2–3in) across, with narrow tepals. Lime-tolerant, but best in moist, acid soil; grow in full sun or partial shade. ↕70–100cm (28–39in). E. China, Korea. ❄❄❄

L. wallichianum. Stem-rooting Division 9 lily with stiff green stems that are tinged purple and bear numerous scattered, linear to lance-shaped, deep green leaves, to 25cm (10in) long. In early autumn, bears umbels of up to 4 large, horizontal, very fragrant, trumpet-shaped, white or cream flowers, tinged yellow or green, to 20cm (8in) across. Prefers moist, acid soil. ↕1–2m (3–6ft). Himalayas. ❄

L. wigginsii. Stem-rooting Division 9 lily with hairless stems and linear-lance-shaped leaves, to 22cm (9in) long, that are scattered and in 2–4 whorls roughly halfway up the stems. In midsummer, produces few-flowered racemes of unscented, pendent, turkscap, deep yellow flowers, 7cm (3in) across, with purple spots. Needs moist, acid soil and partial shade. ↕0.9–1.2m (3–4ft). W. USA. ❄❄❄

***L.* 'Yellow Blaze'.** Moderately vigorous Division 1a lily producing umbels of medium-sized, unscented, bowl-shaped, bright yellow flowers with red-brown spots, in mid- and late summer. ↕1.2–1.5m (4–5ft). ❄❄❄

▷**Lillypilly** see *Acmena smithii*

▷**Lily** see *Lilium*

- **African blue** see *Agapanthus*
- **Amazon** see *Eucharis* x *grandiflora*
- **American trout** see *Erythronium revolutum*
- **American turkscap** see *Lilium superbum*
- **Arum** see *Zantedeschia, Z. aethiopica*
- **Atamasco** see *Zephyranthes atamasco*
- **Aztec** see *Sprekelia formosissima*
- **Blackberry** see *Belamcanda chinensis*
- **Blood** see *Haemanthus, Scadoxus*
- **Common turkscap** see *Lilium martagon*
- **Corn** see *Clintonia borealis, Ixia*
- **Desert** see *Hesperocallis undulata*
- **Dwarf ginger** see *Kaempferia roscoeana*
- **Easter** see *Lilium longiflorum*
- **Fire** see *Cyrtanthus*
- **Florida swamp** see *Crinum americanum*
- **Foxtail** see *Eremurus*
- **Garland** see *Hedychium*
- **Giant** see *Cardiocrinum*
- **Ginger** see *Alpinia, Hedychium*
- **Golden-rayed** see *Lilium auratum*
- **Golden spider** see *Lycoris aurea*
- **Guernsey** see *Nerine sarniensis*
- **Impala** see *Adenium*
- **Jaburan** see *Ophiopogon jaburan*
- **Jacobean** see *Sprekelia formosissima*
- **Japanese pond** see *Nuphar japonica*
- **Kaffir** see *Schizostylis*
- **Lent** see *Narcissus pseudonarcissus*
- **Leopard** see *Belamcanda chinensis*
- **Madonna** see *Lilium candidum*

▷ **Lily cont.**
May see *Maianthemum*
Meadow see *Lilium canadense*
Mexican see *Hippeastrum reginae*
Morning star see *Lilium concolor*
Mount Cook see *Ranunculus lyallii*
Nankeen see *Lilium* x *testaceum*
Nodding see *Lilium cernuum*
Orange see *Lilium bulbiferum*
Painted wood see *Trillium undulatum*
Paradise see *Paradisea*
Peacock see *Kaempferia roscoeana*
Peruvian see *Alstroemeria*
Pineapple see *Eucomis*
Pink porcelain see *Alpinia zerumbet*
Plantain see *Hosta*
Pyjama see *Crinum macowanii*
Queen see *Curcuma petiolata, Phaedranassa*
Red spider see *Lycoris radiata*
Regal see *Lilium regale*
Resurrection see *Kaempferia rotunda, Lycoris squamigera*
St. Bernard's see *Anthericum liliago*
St. Bruno's see *Paradisea*
St. Joseph's see *Hippeastrum vittatum*
Scarborough see *Cyrtanthus elatus*
Scarlet turkscap see *Lilium chalcedonicum*
Sea see *Pancratium*
Snowdon see *Lloydia serotina*
Spear see *Doryanthes*
Spider see *Hymenocallis*
Tiger see *Lilium lancifolium*
Toad see *Tricyrtis*
Torch see *Kniphofia*
Trout see *Erythronium*
Voodoo see *Sauromatum venosum*
Water see *Nymphaea*
Wood see *Trillium*
Yellow pond see *Nuphar, N. lutea*
▷ **Lily-of-the-valley** see *Convallaria*
False see *Maianthemum bifolium*
Wild see *Pyrola rotundifolia*
▷ **Lily of the valley tree** see *Clethra arborea*
▷ **Lily tree** see *Magnolia denudata*
▷ **Lilyturf** see *Liriope, Ophiopogon*
White *Ophiopogon jaburan*
▷ **Lime** see *Tilia*
American see *T. americana*
Common see *T.* x *europaea*
European white see *T. tomentosa*
Japanese see *T. japonica*
Large-leaved see *T. platyphyllos*
Mongolian see *T. mongolica*
Pendulous silver see *T.* 'Petiolaris'
Red-twigged see *T. platyphyllos* 'Rubra'
Silver see *T. tomentosa*
Small-leaved see *T. cordata*
▷ ***Limnanthemum nymphoides*** see *Nymphoides peltata*
▷ ***Limnanthemum peltatum*** see *Nymphoides peltata*

L

LIMNANTHES

Poached egg plant

LIMNANTHACEAE

Genus of about 17 species of low-growing annuals from moist habitats in W. USA. They have 2-pinnatifid, bright green leaves, and produce cup-shaped, 5-petalled flowers from summer to autumn. *L. douglasii*, the only species usually cultivated, is suitable for a rock garden and as path edging. It self-seeds freely. The nectar-rich flowers are attractive to bees and hoverflies.

• **HARDINESS** Fully hardy.

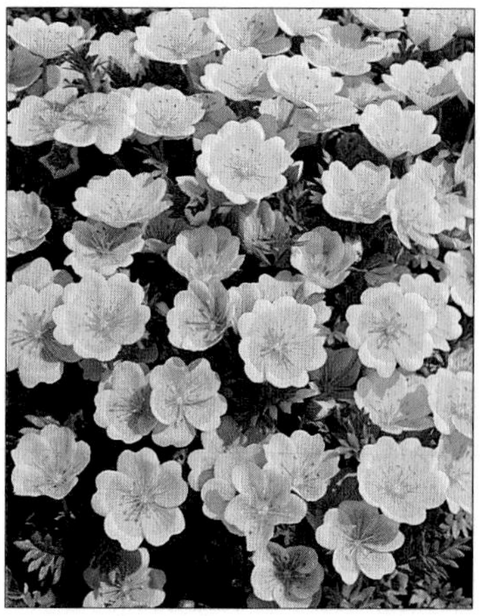

Limnanthes douglasii

• **CULTIVATION** Grow in fertile, moist but well-drained soil in full sun.

• **PROPAGATION** Sow seed *in situ* in spring or autumn. Protect autumn sowings with cloches in frost-prone areas.

• **PESTS AND DISEASES** Trouble free.

L. douglasii ■ ♀ (Poached egg plant). Slender-stemmed, erect to spreading annual with 2-pinnatifid, finely toothed, fleshy, glossy, bright yellow-green leaves, 5–12cm (2–5in) long. Bears numerous shallowly cup-shaped, fragrant, yellow-centred white flowers, to 2.5cm (1in) across, from summer to autumn. ↕↔ to 15cm (6in) or more. USA (California, Oregon). ❄❄❄

LIMNOCHARIS

LIMNOCHARITACEAE

Genus of 2 species of evergreen and deciduous aquatic annuals and perennials, found in the shallow margins of tropical pools in S.E. Asia, South America, and the West Indies. They produce rosettes of lance-shaped to ovate leaves, and umbels of saucer-shaped yellow flowers. In areas where temperatures fall below 10°C (50°F), grow in an indoor pool. In mild, temperate areas, use for temporary summer planting around an outdoor pool; in warmer climates grow permanently outdoors. They self-seed freely, the stems that bear the seed capsules bending over to water level, where each throws up another shoot.

• **HARDINESS** Frost tender.

• **CULTIVATION** Under glass, grow in baskets of heavy loam at the margins of a pool, in slightly acid water, at 20–25°C (68–77°F), in bright filtered light. Outdoors, grow in deep, acid, permanently wet soil in full sun. See also pp.52–53.

• **PROPAGATION** Scatter seed on the water surface as soon as ripe. Divide in summer.

• **PESTS AND DISEASES** Trouble free.

L. flava. Evergreen, marginal aquatic perennial with upright, long-stalked, lance-shaped to ovate leaves, to 20cm (8in) long, with heart-shaped bases. Umbels of 2–12 saucer-shaped yellow flowers, 2.5cm (1in) across, with off-white margins, are produced several times during summer. ↕↔ 60cm (24in). Tropical South America, West Indies. ❀ (min. 10°C/50°F)

LIMONIUM

Sea lavender, Statice

PLUMBAGINACEAE

Genus of 150 species of annuals, biennials, and deciduous and evergreen perennials and subshrubs from coasts, salt marshes, and deserts worldwide. Simple, entire or pinnatifid, tapering leaves, often appearing almost stalkless, are mostly borne in basal rosettes. Spikelets composed of small, stalkless, papery flowers and bracts are borne in more or less one-sided, corymb-like panicles in summer and autumn; the calyces are tubular, the corollas have 5 lobed petals joined only at the bases. The calyces are usually a different colour from the corollas, and persist after the petals have fallen. Long-flowering plants, they are suitable for a sunny herbaceous or annual border, and for naturalizing in a gravel garden. They are also good for cutting and drying. The larger perennials grow well in coastal sites; the dwarf species are effective in a trough or rock garden, the less hardy ones being suitable for an alpine house.

• **HARDINESS** Fully hardy to frost tender.

• **CULTIVATION** Outdoors, grow in preferably sandy, well-drained soil in full sun. Large perennials tolerate dry, stony soil. Protect dwarf species from winter wet. In an alpine house, grow in a mix of equal parts loam-based potting compost (JI No.1) and grit.

• **PROPAGATION** Sow seed in early spring: sow perennials in containers outdoors and annuals at 13–18°C (55–64°F). Divide perennials in spring.

• **PESTS AND DISEASES** Susceptible to powdery mildew.

***L. aureum* 'Supernova'.** Erect perennial, often grown as an annual, with narrowly spoon- to lance-shaped, mostly basal, grey-green leaves, 1–5cm (½–2in) long, tapering gradually to leaf-stalks. In summer, stiff, branched stems bear panicles of small, terminal spikelets, each with tiny, funnel-shaped, orange-yellow flowers, to 5mm (¼in) long, enclosed in hairy white, papery calyces. Good for cut flowers. ↕ to 30cm (12in), ↔ to 23cm (9in). ❄❄❄

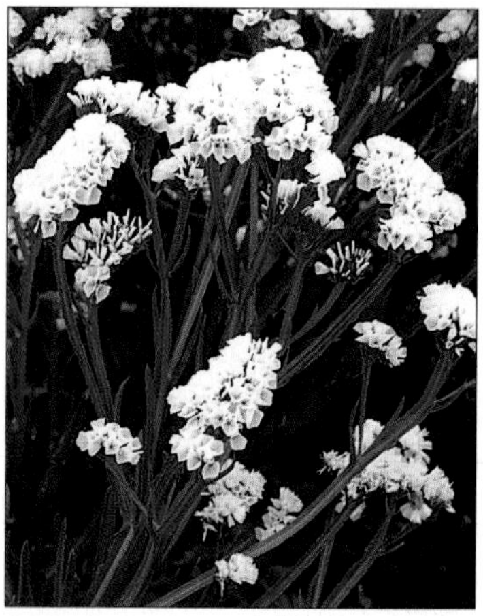

Limonium sinuatum California Series 'Iceberg'

L. bellidifolium, syn. *L. reticulata, Statice bellidifolia.* Compact, dome-forming, evergreen, woody-based perennial with spoon-shaped, dark green leaves, to 5cm (2in) long. Open panicles of dense spikelets that consist of tiny, trumpet-shaped, pale violet or blue-violet flowers, 5mm (¼in) long, with white, papery calyces, are borne on wiry, branched stems in early summer. Suitable for a rock garden, trough, or alpine house. ↕↔ to 15cm (6in). Coasts from E. England to the Mediterranean and the Black Sea. ❄❄❄

L. latifolium ■ syn. *L. platyphyllum* (Sea lavender). Rosette-forming perennial with elliptic to spoon-shaped, mid- to dark green leaves, usually to 30cm (12in) long, occasionally to 60cm (24in). In late summer, branched, wiry stems bear panicles of spikelets that consist of shortly tubular, deep lavender-blue flowers, 6mm (¼in) long, with white calyces. ↕ 60cm (24in) or more,

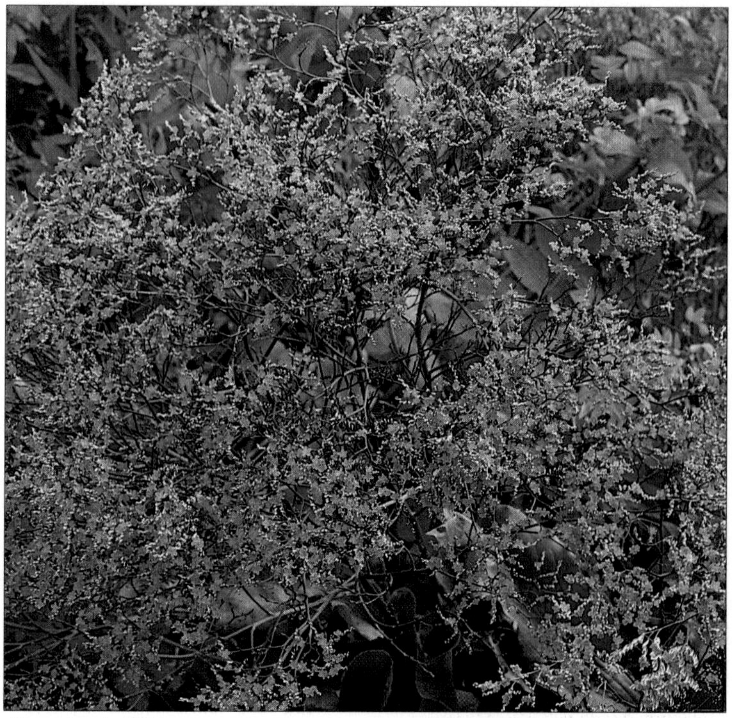

Limonium latifolium

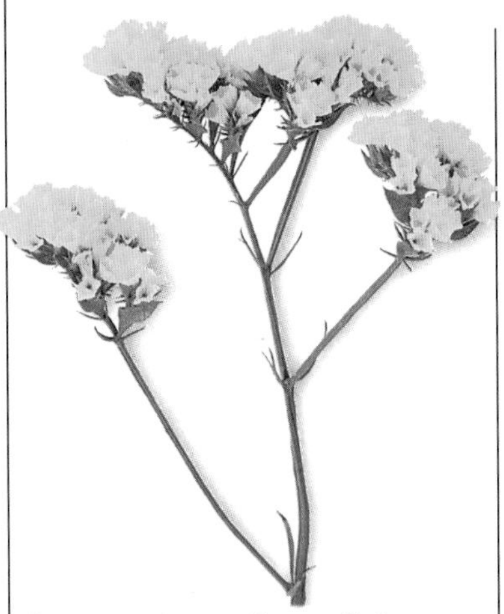

Limonium sinuatum Forever Series 'Forever Gold'

↔ 45cm (18in). E. Bulgaria to S.E. Russia. ✻✻✻. **'Blue Cloud'** produces mauve flowers, 7mm (¼in) across. **'Violetta'** produces deep violet flowers.
L. minutum, syn. *Statice minuta.* Woody-based, evergreen perennial with cushion-like rosettes of spoon-shaped, dark green leaves, to 1cm (½in) long, with incurved margins. In early summer, short, slightly woody, branched stems bear panicles of spikelets with 1–4 tiny purple flowers, 5mm (¼in) long. ↕ 10cm (4in), ↔ 15cm (6in). S.E. France. ✻✻✻
L. platyphyllum see. *L. latifolium.*
L. reticulata see. *L. bellidifolium.*
L. sinuatum (Statice). Erect, densely hairy perennial, usually grown as an annual, with basal rosettes of oblong to lance-shaped, deeply lobed, wavy-margined, dark green leaves, 15cm (6in) long. In summer and early autumn, stiff, branched, winged, slightly leafy, bright green stems bear panicles of clustered spikelets that consist of tiny, funnel-shaped, pink, white, or blue flowers, 0.9–1.5cm (⅜–½in) long, enclosed in hairy, white or pale violet calyces. Good for cut flowers. ↕ to 40cm (16in), ↔ 30cm (12in). Mediterranean. ✻✻. **'Art Shades'** bears flowers in orange, salmon-pink, yellow, rose-pink, red, carmine-red, blue, creamy white, or lavender-blue. **California Series** cultivars have 9 strongly toned colour forms, each coming true from seed, ranging from rich, deep purple to the clear white flowers of **'Iceberg'** ▣. Cultivars of **Forever Series** bear large, tightly packed flower spikes in a mixture of 6 or 7 colours, including blue, pink, and yellow; **'Forever Gold'** ▣ has yellow flowers; ↕ to 60cm (24in). **Fortress Series** ▣ cultivars are freely branched, and bear flowers in about 6 vivid shades, including bright blues, pastels, and unusual apricot-yellows; ↕ to 60cm (24in). Cultivars of **Pacific Series** have flowers in deep rose-pink, apricot, yellow, sky blue, white, deep blue, or lavender blue. Cultivars of **Petite Bouquet Series** are very dwarf, with tightly bunched spikelets in blue, purple, deep salmon-pink, pure white, creamy white, lemon-yellow, or golden yellow; ↕ to 30cm (12in). **Sunburst Series** cultivars have flowers in warm colours, including orange-peach, apricot-yellow, and rose-red; good for cutting; ↕ to 75cm (30in).
L. spicatum see *Psylliostachys spicata.*
L. suworowii see *Psylliostachys suworowii.*
L. tataricum see *Goniolimon tataricum.*
L. tetragonum. Erect biennial with basal rosettes of narrowly spoon-shaped to oblong, leathery leaves, 8–15cm (3–6in) long. In autumn, stiff, branched stems bear panicles of small, terminal spikelets that consist of tiny, funnel-shaped pink flowers, 4–6mm (⅛–¼in) long, with white-hairy calyces. Good for cut flowers. ↕ 45cm (18in), ↔ 30cm (12in). China, Korea, Japan. ✻✻. **'Confetti'** 🏆 has lemon-yellow flowers. **'Stardust'** 🏆 is very tolerant of adverse weather, and bears up to 30 flowering stems per plant; ↕ to 60cm (24in).

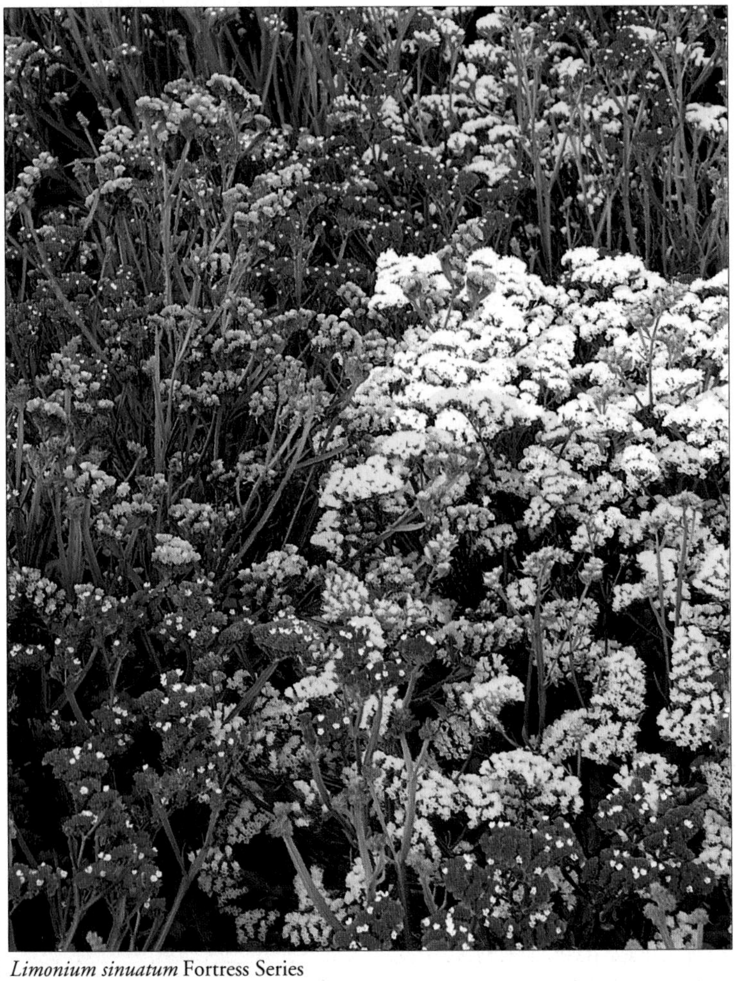

Limonium sinuatum Fortress Series

LINANTHUS

POLEMONIACEAE

Genus of about 35 species of annuals and perennials, usually found in sandy and gravelly sites in grassland or scrub in W. USA, Mexico, and Chile. They have branched stems with alternate or opposite leaves, which are sometimes simple, but usually pinnately or palmately lobed, or fully divided, with linear segments. Bell- or funnel-shaped, white, blue, lilac, pink, or yellow flowers are borne singly or in loose cymes or dense heads, from spring to summer. Grow the perennial species in a rock garden; the annuals are suitable for an annual border or a wild garden.

• **HARDINESS** Fully hardy to frost hardy. The perennials are hardy to -8°C (18°F).
• **CULTIVATION** Grow in any light, well-drained soil in full sun.
• **PROPAGATION** Sow seed *in situ*: perennial species in autumn, annuals in spring. Take stem-tip cuttings of *L. nuttallii* in early summer.
• **PESTS AND DISEASES** Trouble free.

L. dianthiflorus (Ground pink). Erect, slender, branching, downy annual with mostly opposite, narrowly linear leaves, 1–2cm (½–¾in) long. Funnel-shaped then spreading, yellow-throated, white, pink, or lilac-blue flowers, to 2.5cm (1in) across, the petals lobed, toothed, and spotted at the bases, are borne singly or in short, few-flowered, leafy cymes from spring to summer. ↕ 5–12cm (2–5in), ↔ to 5cm (2in). USA (S. California) to Mexico (Baja California). ✻✻✻
L. grandiflorus (Mountain phlox). Erect, slender, branching, downy to almost smooth annual with alternate or opposite, palmately lobed leaves, to 10cm (4in) long, with 5–11 linear lobes, 1–3cm (½–1¼in) long. From spring to summer, bears dense heads of funnel-shaped then spreading, lavender-pink, lilac, or white flowers, to 3cm (1¼in) across, the petals lobed, toothed, and flecked with white. Good for cut flowers. ↕ 30–50cm (12–20in), ↔ to 23cm (9in). USA (S. California). ✻✻✻
L. nuttallii. Compact, bushy perennial with opposite, palmately lobed, pale green leaves, to 8cm (3in) long, with 5–9 pointed, linear lobes, to 1.5cm (½in) long, on densely branched stems. In early summer, bears abundant cymes of funnel-shaped to salverform white flowers, to 1.5cm (½in) across, with spreading lobes. ↕ to 15cm (6in), ↔ to 20cm (8in). USA (Washington State to California). ✻✻

LINARIA

Toadflax

SCROPHULARIACEAE

Genus of approximately 100 species of annuals, biennials, and herbaceous perennials from dry, sunny habitats, including scree, in temperate regions of the N. hemisphere, especially the Mediterranean. They have erect, sometimes trailing, branched stems, with simple, ovate or linear to lance-shaped, stalkless, often grey-green leaves, the lower ones usually whorled or opposite, the upper more or less alternate. They are grown for their irregular, 2-lipped, spurred, white, pink, red, purple, orange, or yellow flowers, resembling snapdragons (*Antirrhinum*), which are borne in terminal racemes from spring to autumn. The taller toadflaxes are useful for a herbaceous border, or for naturalizing in stony soil or a gravel garden. The smaller, alpine species are suitable for a rock garden, scree bed, or wall crevice. In frost-prone areas, grow half-hardy species in a cool greenhouse.

• **HARDINESS** Fully hardy to half hardy.
• **CULTIVATION** Grow in moderately fertile, light, well-drained, preferably sandy soil, in full sun.
• **PROPAGATION** Sow seed of annuals *in situ* in early spring; they self-seed freely. Sow seed of perennials in containers in a cold frame in early spring and plant out with care. Divide perennials, or take basal softwood cuttings, in spring.
• **PESTS AND DISEASES** Aphids and powdery mildew may be a problem.

L. alpina ▣ (Alpine toadflax). Trailing, short-lived perennial with linear-lance-shaped, blue-green leaves, 0.5–1.5cm (¼–½in) long, the lower leaves whorled, the upper ones alternate. Throughout summer, produces 3- to 15-flowered racemes of 2-lipped, bicoloured, violet and deep yellow flowers, 1.5–2.5cm (½–1in) long, sometimes entirely violet, pink, or yellowish white, with spurs 8–10mm (⅜–½in) long. ↕ 8cm (3in), ↔ to 15cm (6in). C. and S. Europe. ✻✻✻
L. dalmatica see *L. genistifolia* subsp. *dalmatica.*
L. x dominii (*L. purpurea* x *L. repens*). Erect to spreading, branching perennial with opposite, simple, linear or linear-lance-shaped, mid-green leaves, 1–5cm (½–2in) long, the upper leaves sometimes whorled. From early summer to

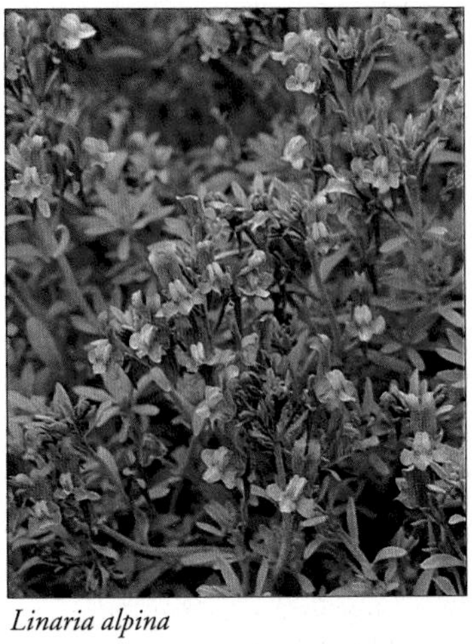

Linaria alpina

L

mid-autumn, produces branching flowerheads of tubular, 2-lipped, pale lilac to purplish violet flowers, 0.8–1.5cm (⅜–½in) long, with spurs to 5mm (¼in) long. ↕ to 1m (3ft), ↔ 60cm (2ft). Europe. ✽✽✽
L. genistifolia. Upright, branching perennial with alternate, semi-erect, linear to ovate, pointed, mid-green leaves, 9–18cm (3½–7in) long. From early to late summer, bears racemes of 2-lipped, lemon-yellow to orange flowers, 1.5–2cm (½–¾in) long, with spurs to 2.5cm (1in) long. ↕ 1m (3ft), ↔ 60cm (24in). Italy to Russia, Turkey. ✽✽✽. **subsp. *dalmatica*** ■ syn. *L. dalmatica*, has shorter, ovate to lance-shaped, glaucous leaves and yellow flowers, 2–5cm (¾–2in) long, in loose racemes; S. Italy, Balkan Peninsula, Romania.
L. glareosum see *Chaenorhinum glareosum.*
L. maroccana. Erect, sticky-hairy annual with alternate, narrowly linear, light green leaves, to 4cm (1½in) long. In summer, bears slender, slightly lax racemes of tiny, 2-lipped, violet-purple, occasionally pink or white flowers, to 1.5cm (½in) long, the lower lips marked orange to yellow, paler at the centres. ↕ 23–45cm (9–18in), ↔ to 15cm (6in). Morocco. ✽✽✽. **'Fairy Bouquet'** freely produces flowers, to 2cm (¾in) long, in yellow, rose-pink, salmon-pink, orange, carmine, lavender, and white; ↕ to 23cm (9in). **'Northern Lights'** ■ occurs in the same colours as 'Fairy Bouquet' but is long-flowering; ↕ to 60cm (24in). **'White Pearl'** has pure white flowers, to 2cm (¾in) long; ↕ to 23cm (9in).
L. purpurea. Erect, slender perennial with linear, mid-green leaves, 2–6cm (¾–2½in) long, the lower whorled, the upper alternate. From early summer to early autumn, 2-lipped, violet-purple flowers, 1.5cm (½in) long, with curved spurs to 5mm (¼in) long, are borne in long, slender, dense racemes. Self-seeds freely. ↕ to 90cm (36in), ↔ 30cm (12in). S. Europe. ✽✽✽. **'Canon J. Went'** ■ syn. 'Canon Went', bears pale pink flowers. Self-seeds true if isolated from the species. **'Springside White'**, syn. 'Radcliffe Innocence', has white flowers.
L. reticulata (Purple-net toadflax). Erect annual with whorls of linear, blue-green leaves, to 1cm (½in) long, deeply channelled at the centres. In late spring and summer, bears short, dense, tapering racemes of 2-lipped, downy, deep purple flowers, to 1.5cm (½in) long, finely veined yellow, each with a large, purple-

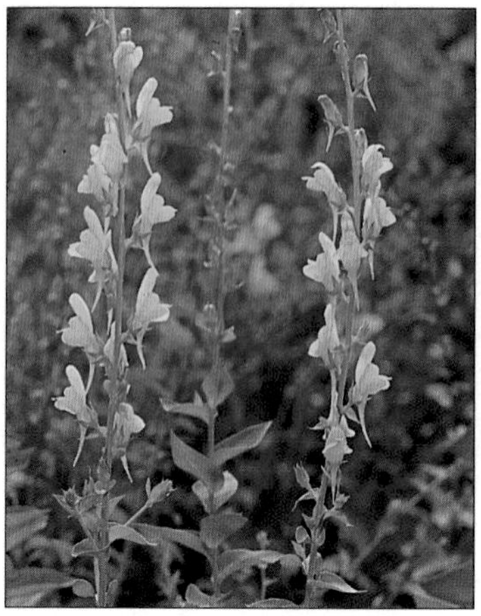
Linaria genistifolia subsp. *dalmatica*

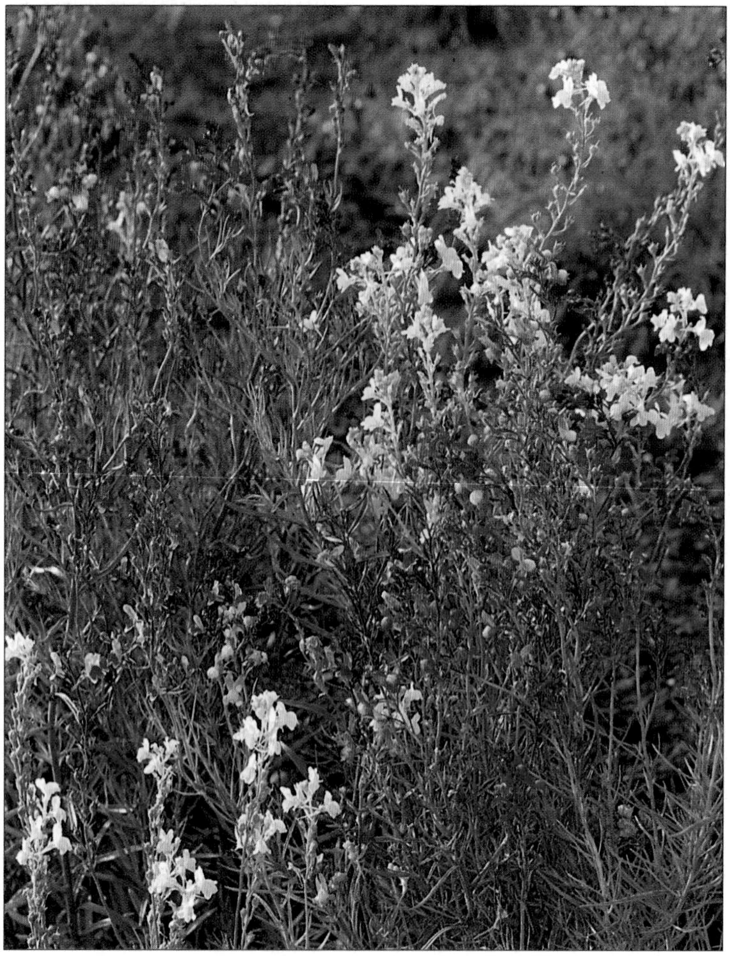
Linaria maroccana 'Northern Lights'

veined, copper-orange or yellow mark on the lower lip, and a spur 5–8mm (¼–⅜in) long. Often confused with *L. aeruginea* in gardens. ↕ 0.6–1.2m (2–4ft), ↔ to 23cm (9in). N. Africa. ✽✽✽.
'Aureo-purpurea' has dark, rich purple flowers, each with a purple-veined, orange or yellow mark on the lower lip. **'Crown Jewels'** has maroon-red, orange, red, or golden yellow flowers; ↕ to 23cm (9in). **'Flamenco'** has purple, maroon-red, red, golden yellow, or orange, often bicoloured flowers, covered in a fine network of dark purple veins; good for cut flowers.
L. triornithophora. Erect perennial bearing whorls of lance-shaped to ovate-lance-shaped, mid-green leaves, 2.5–8cm (1–3in) long. From early or midsummer to early autumn, produces

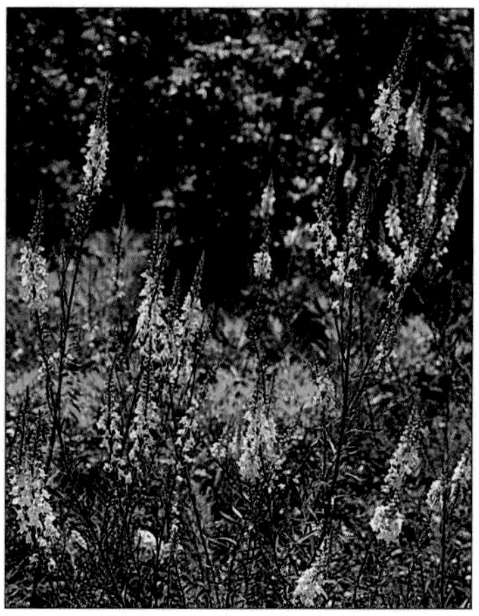
Linaria purpurea 'Canon J. Went'

loose racemes of 2-lipped, purple-and-yellow flowers, 5–8cm (2–3in) long, usually in whorls of 3, with brownish purple spurs, 1.5–2.5cm (½–1in) long. ↕ 90cm (36in) or more, ↔ 60cm (24in). N. and C. Portugal, W. Spain. ✽✽
***L. tristis* 'Toubkal'.** Mound-forming perennial with decumbent stems bearing linear to oblong-lance-shaped, blue-green leaves, 1–4cm (½–1½in) long, the lower leaves in whorls, the upper alternate. In summer, produces racemes of 2-lipped, yellow-green flowers, 2.5cm (1in) long, each with a brown-purple mark on the lower lip and a spur 1cm (½in) long. Self-sterile. ↕ 8cm (3in), ↔ to 15cm (6in). ✽✽✽
L. vulgaris (Toadflax). Erect perennial, spreading by runners, with stiff, branched or unbranched stems bearing linear to narrowly elliptic, pale green leaves, 2–6cm (¾–2½in) long. From late spring to mid-autumn, bears pale yellow flowers, to 4.5cm (1¾in) long, with spurs 1cm (½in) long, in dense racemes. Self-seeds freely. ↕ 30–90cm (12–36in), ↔ 30cm (12in). Europe (except extreme north and much of Mediterranean). ✽✽✽

LINDELOFIA

BORAGINACEAE

Genus of about 12 species of clump-forming, hairy perennials, sometimes with short rhizomes, found on dry, stony slopes or in scrub from C. Asia to the Himalayas. They have lance-shaped, long-stalked basal leaves and alternate, ovate to oblong-lance-shaped, stalkless stem leaves. From spring to autumn, tubular, 2-lipped, brilliant blue to purple flowers, with 5 spreading lobes, are borne in terminal or axillary, one-sided cymes. Suitable for a sunny herbaceous border or gravel garden, or for naturalizing on a dry bank.
• **HARDINESS** Fully hardy.
• **CULTIVATION** Grow in moderately fertile, well-drained soil in full sun.
• **PROPAGATION** Sow seed in containers outdoors in early spring, or divide in spring.
• **PESTS AND DISEASES** Powdery mildew may be a problem.

***L. anchusiflora* of gardens** see *L. longiflora.*
L. longiflora, syn. *Cynoglossum longiflorum, L. anchusiflora* of gardens, *L. spectabilis.* Clump-forming, branched perennial with short rhizomes and long-stalked, lance-shaped, mid-green basal leaves, 7–25cm (3–10in) long; stem leaves are shorter, and clasp the stems. In late spring and early summer, bears deep blue, sometimes purple flowers, to 1.5cm (½in) long, with protruding stamens, in one-sided, terminal cymes. ↕↔ 60cm (24in). W. Himalayas. ✽✽✽. **'Hartington White'** has grey-green leaves and white flowers; ↕↔ to 30cm (12in).
L. spectabilis see *L. longiflora.*

▷**Linden** see *Tilia*

LINDERA

LAURACEAE

Genus of about 80 species of deciduous and evergreen, dioecious trees and shrubs occurring in woodland and on riverbanks in E. Asia and North America. They are cultivated for their aromatic, alternate, entire or 3-lobed leaves, which often colour well in autumn on deciduous species, and for their star-shaped flowers, which are borne in axillary umbels, rarely singly, early in the year. Grow in a woodland garden. In frost-pone areas, grow half-

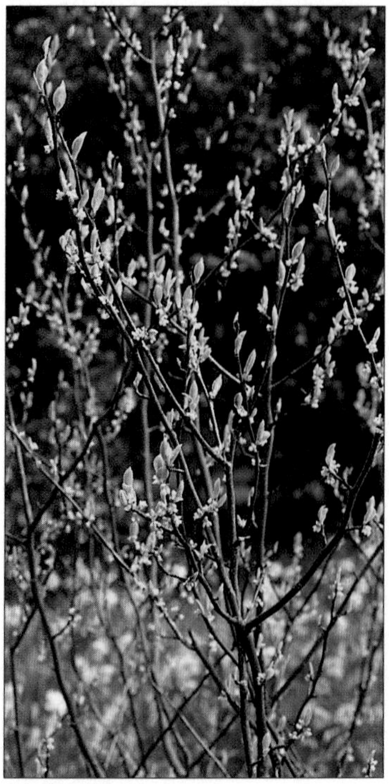
Lindera benzoin

hardy species in a cool greenhouse or against a warm wall. Male and female plants need to be planted together in order to bear fruits.
• **HARDINESS** Fully hardy to frost tender.
• **CULTIVATION** Grow in fertile, moist but well-drained, acid soil in partial shade. Pruning group 1.
• **PROPAGATION** Sow seed in containers in a cold frame in autumn. Take greenwood cuttings in early summer.
• **PESTS AND DISEASES** Trouble free.

L. benzoin ■ (Spice bush). Rounded, deciduous shrub with upright branches and obovate, aromatic, bright green leaves, to 12cm (5in) long, turning yellow in autumn. Umbels of tiny, star-shaped, greenish yellow flowers, 4mm (⅛in) across, are borne in mid-spring, followed by ovoid red berries on female plants. ↕↔ 3m (10ft). S.E. Canada, E. USA. ❄❄❄
L. obtusiloba ♀ ◯ Spreading, deciduous shrub or small tree with ovate to rounded, entire or 3-lobed, aromatic, glossy, dark green leaves, to 12cm (5in) long. Bears umbels of tiny, star-shaped, dark yellow flowers, 3mm (⅛in) across, in early and mid-spring, before the leaves, followed by spherical, glossy, red-brown berries on female plants. ↕↔ 6m (20ft). China, Korea, Japan. ❄❄❄

LINDHEIMERA
Star daisy
ASTERACEAE/COMPOSITAE

Genus of 1, possibly 2 species of erect, branched, roughly hairy annuals from dry, limestone prairies in Texas, USA. They are grown for their small, daisy-like yellow flowerheads, profusely borne in lax, long-stalked corymbs. They have alternate, ovate-lance-shaped, entire to coarsely pinnatifid leaves, which are smaller and finer on the flowering stems. Persistent bright green, bract-like leaves surround the seed heads. Grow in an informal mixed or annual border.
• **HARDINESS** Fully hardy.

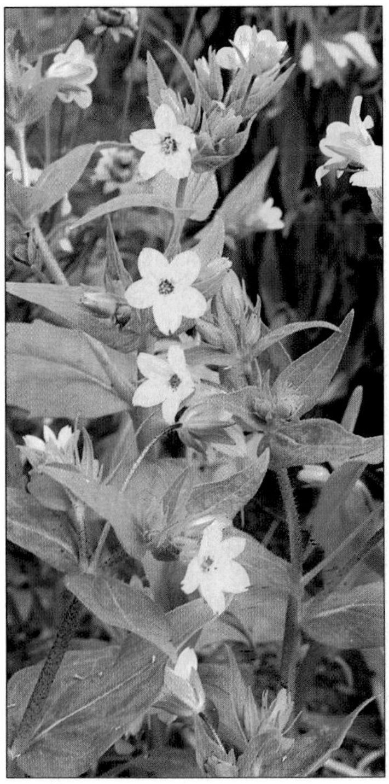
Lindheimera texana

• **CULTIVATION** Grow in moderately fertile, light, well-drained soil in full sun.
• **PROPAGATION** Sow seed in containers in a cold frame in early spring, or *in situ* in mid-spring.
• **PESTS AND DISEASES** Trouble free.

L. texana ■ (Star daisy). Tall, erect annual with branching red stems. Bears ovate-lance-shaped, pinnatifid, often toothed basal leaves, 4cm (1½in) long, and smaller, entire leaves on the upper stems and flower-stalks. Lax corymbs of broad-petalled, yellow-centred, golden yellow to creamy yellow flowerheads, to 2.5cm (1in) across, are borne in late spring and summer. ↕ to 60cm (24in), ↔ to 30cm (12in). USA (Texas). ❄❄❄

▷**Ling** see *Calluna, C. vulgaris*

LINNAEA
Twin-flower
CAPRIFOLIACEAE

Genus of one species of slender, prostrate, mat-forming, evergreen shrub, with stems that root where they touch the soil. It is native to woodland, heaths, and tundra in N. Eurasia and North America. Cultivated for its neat foliage and bell-shaped flowers, it is suitable for ground cover in a peat bed, woodland garden, or large rock garden.
• **HARDINESS** Fully hardy.
• **CULTIVATION** Grow in moderately fertile, humus-rich, reliably moist, acid soil in partial shade.
• **PROPAGATION** Sow seed in containers outdoors in autumn. Take softwood cuttings in early summer. Remove rooted runners between autumn and spring and pot up until established.
• **PESTS AND DISEASES** Trouble free.

L. borealis. Prostrate, mat-forming shrub with opposite, oval to rounded, scalloped leaves, to 1.5cm (½in) long, glossy, dark green above, buff to pale green beneath. In summer, pairs of nodding, narrowly bell- or funnel-shaped, pale pink flowers, to 1cm (½in) long, are produced on stalks, 5cm (2in) long, from the tips of leafy side shoots. ↕ to 8cm (3in), ↔ to 1m (3ft) or more. N. Eurasia, North America. ❄❄❄. **var. *americana*** ■ has rounded, lobed, mid-green leaves, 2.5cm (1in) long, and bears funnel-shaped, white or pale pink flowers, to 1cm (½in) long, in late spring; ↕ 10cm (4in), ↔ to 30cm (12in); North America.

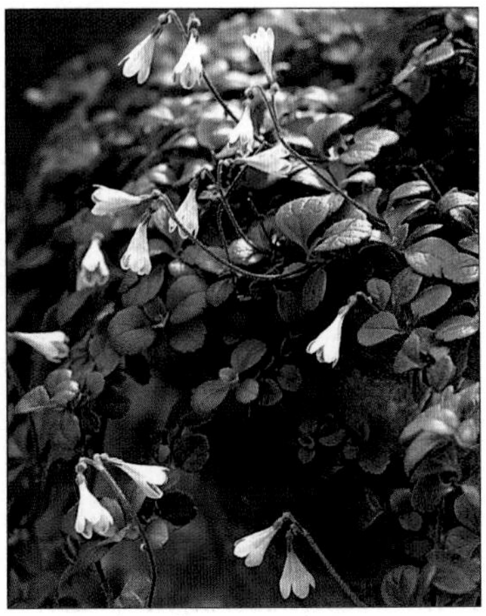
Linnaea borealis var. *americana*

LINOSPADIX
ARECACEAE/PALMAE

Genus of about 11 species of slender, single- or cluster-stemmed palms from rainforest and upland or coastal sands in New Guinea and Australia. Pinnate leaves are loosely clustered at the tops of the stems, and axillary, 3-petalled flowers are borne in slim, erect spikes. Where temperatures drop below 13°C (55°F), grow in a warm greenhouse. In tropical areas, grow as specimen plants;
• **HARDINESS** Frost tender.
• **CULTIVATION** Under glass, grow in loam-based potting compost (JI No.3) in bright filtered light. Pot on or top-dress in spring. In growth, water freely and apply a balanced liquid fertilizer every month. Water moderately in winter. Outdoors, grow in moderately fertile, humus-rich, moist but well-drained, acid soil in partial shade.
• **PROPAGATION** Sow seed at 24°C (75°F) in spring.
• **PESTS AND DISEASES** Red spider mites may be troublesome under glass.

L. monostachya 🌴 (Walking stick palm). Small palm with a slender, erect stem and spreading to arching, pinnate, lustrous, mid- to deep green leaves, to 1m (3ft) long, with irregularly shaped leaflets. Greenish yellow flowers are borne in initially erect, then pendent, catkin-like spikes, to 1m (3ft) long, from spring to summer. ↕ 2–3m (6–10ft), ↔ 1–2m (3–6ft). Australia (Queensland, New South Wales). ❀ (min. 13–15°C/55–59°F)

LINUM
Flax
LINACEAE

Genus of about 200 species of annuals, biennials, and semi-evergreen, evergreen, and deciduous perennials, shrubs, and subshrubs, mainly from grassland, scrub, and dry slopes in temperate areas of the N. hemisphere. They are cultivated for their terminal or axillary racemes, panicles, cymes, or corymbs of colourful, 5-petalled, funnel- to saucer-shaped flowers, which are usually blue, yellow, or white, sometimes pink or red, and are borne over long periods. The simple, mainly alternate, sometimes opposite leaves are usually hairless, and deciduous unless otherwise stated. The smaller species are suitable for a rock garden, the larger ones for a border. Grow annuals in an annual border or as fillers in a herbaceous border.
• **HARDINESS** Fully hardy to frost hardy.
• **CULTIVATION** Grow in light, moderately fertile, humus-rich, well-drained soil (sharply drained for alpines) in full sun. Protect from winter wet.
• **PROPAGATION** Sow seed in spring or autumn: sow annuals *in situ*, perennials and shrubs in containers in a cold frame. Take stem-tip cuttings of perennials in early summer, and semi-ripe cuttings of subshrubs and shrubs in summer.
• **PESTS AND DISEASES** Susceptible to slugs, snails, and occasionally aphids.

L. arboreum ■ ♀ Dwarf, evergreen shrub with elliptic or spoon-shaped, thick, glaucous, bluish green leaves, 2–4cm (¾–1½in) long, often in

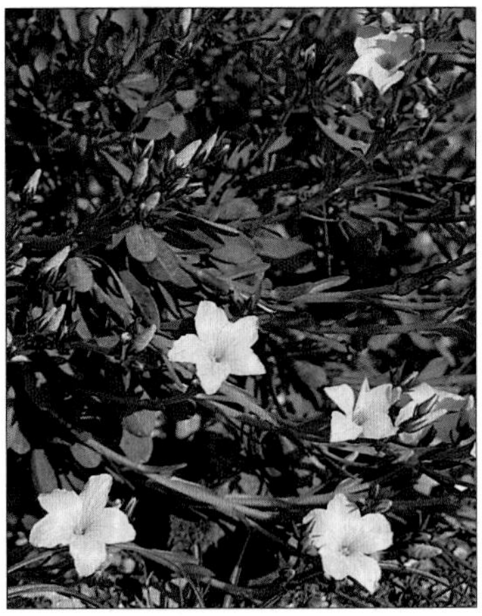
Linum arboreum

crowded rosettes. Compact, few-flowered, terminal cymes of funnel-shaped, deep yellow flowers, 2–3cm (¾–1¼in) across, are produced in succession in late spring and summer. ↕↔ to 30cm (12in). Greece (S. Aegean to Crete), W. Turkey. ❄❄
L. capitatum. Sturdy, rhizomatous perennial, sometimes confused with *L. flavum*, with rosettes of oblong-spoon-shaped basal leaves, and lance-shaped stem leaves, all dark green and 2–3.5cm (¾–1½in) long. During summer, produces compact, terminal cymes of upward-facing, funnel-shaped yellow flowers, to 2.5cm (1in) across. ↕ 40cm (16in), ↔ 25cm (10in). Balkan Peninsula, S. Italy. ❄❄❄
L. flavum (Golden flax, Yellow flax). Upright, woody-based perennial with spoon- to lance-shaped, dark green leaves, 2–3.5cm (¾–1½in) long. Bears dense, many-branched, terminal cymes of upward-facing, funnel-shaped, golden yellow flowers, to 2.5cm (1in) across, which open in sunshine in summer. ↕ 30cm (12in), ↔ to 20cm (8in). C. and S. Europe. ❄❄❄. **'Compactum'** ■ is more compact, and produces bright yellow flowers; ↕↔ 15cm (6in).

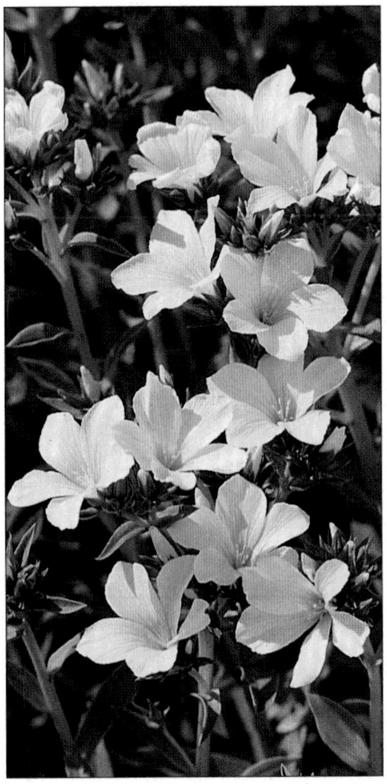
Linum flavum 'Compactum'

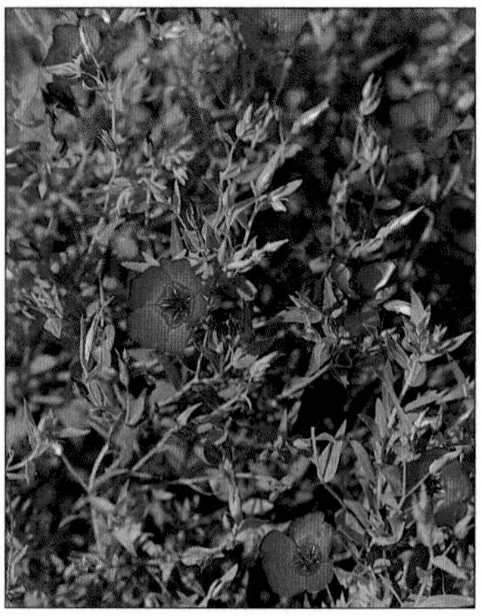
Linum grandiflorum 'Rubrum'

***L.* 'Gemmell's Hybrid'** 🏆 Semi-evergreen, dome-forming perennial that has a woody rootstock and bears ovate, glaucous, bluish green leaves, to 5cm (2in) long. Short-stalked, broadly funnel-shaped, chrome-yellow flowers, 3cm (1¼in) across, are profusely borne in terminal cymes over long periods in summer. ↕ 15cm (6in), ↔ to 20cm (8in). ❄❄

L. grandiflorum 🏆 (Flowering flax). Erect, slender, basally branching, slightly downy annual with narrowly lance-shaped to ovate-lance-shaped, grey-green leaves, to 3cm (1¼in) long. Bears saucer-shaped, clear rose-pink flowers, to 4cm (1½in) across, with darker eyes, in loose, terminal panicles in summer. ↕ 40–75cm (16–30in), ↔ 15cm (6in). N. Africa. ❄❄❄. **'Bright Eyes'** produces ivory-white flowers, to 5cm (2in) across, with brownish red eyes; ↕ to 45cm (18in). **'Caeruleum'** produces blue-purple flowers. **'Rubrum'** ▣ produces brilliant crimson-red flowers; ↕ to 45cm (18in).

L. narbonense ▣ Clump-forming, short-lived perennial with wiry stems that bear erect, narrowly lance-shaped, pointed, glaucous, mid-green leaves, to 2cm (¾in) long. Few-flowered, terminal cymes of saucer-shaped, white-eyed, rich blue flowers, 3–4cm (1¼–1½in) across, individually fading by afternoon, are produced continuously in early and mid-summer. ↕ 30–60cm (12–24in), ↔ 45cm (18in). W. and C. Mediterranean. ❄❄❄ (borderline)

L. perenne (Perennial flax). Variable, clump-forming perennial, similar to *L. narbonense*, with slender stems bearing narrow, linear to lance-shaped, glaucous, bluish green leaves, to 2.5cm (1in) long. Terminal panicles of wide, funnel-shaped, clear blue flowers, 2–3cm (¾–1¼in) across, individually fading by afternoon, are produced continuously in early and midsummer. ↕ 10–60cm (4–24in), ↔ 30cm (12in). Europe to C. Asia. ❄❄❄. **'Blau Saphir'**, syn. 'Blue Sapphire', produces sky-blue flowers; ↕ to 30cm (12in).

L. salsoloides see *L. suffruticosum* subsp. *salsoloides*.

L. suffruticosum* subsp. *salsoloides, syn. *L. salsoloides*. Low-cushion-forming, woody-based perennial with branching stems bearing narrowly linear, greyish green leaves, to 4.5cm (1¾in) long. Loose, terminal cymes of saucer-shaped, pearl-white flowers, 3cm (1¼in) across, sometimes faintly veined purple, are produced in succession during summer. ↕ 10cm (4in), ↔ to 15cm (6in). Spain to N. Italy. ❄❄

▷**Lion's ear** see *Leonotis leonurus*
▷***Lippia citriodora*** see *Aloysia triphylla*
▷**Lipstick plant** see *Aeschynanthus pulcher*
▷**Lipstick tree** see *Bixa orellana*
▷**Lipstick vine** see *Aeschynanthus lobbianus*

LIQUIDAMBAR

HAMAMELIDACEAE

Genus of 4 species of deciduous, monoecious trees occurring in moist woodland in E. and S.W. Asia, North America, and Mexico. They are cultivated particularly for their attractive foliage, which colours well in autumn, and for their upright but open habit. The maple-like leaves are alternate and palmately 3- to 7-lobed. Inconspicuous, yellow-green flowers are produced in rounded heads in late spring; the female flowers are followed by spiky, spherical fruit clusters. Liquidambars are excellent as part of a woodland planting, or as specimen trees isolated in grass.

• **HARDINESS** Fully hardy to frost hardy.

• **CULTIVATION** Grow in moderately fertile, preferably acid or neutral, moist but well-drained soil, in full sun for best autumn colour, or partial shade. Lime-tolerant, given a good depth of soil. Pruning group 1.

• **PROPAGATION** Sow seed in containers in a cold frame in autumn. Take greenwood cuttings in summer.

• **PESTS AND DISEASES** Trouble free.

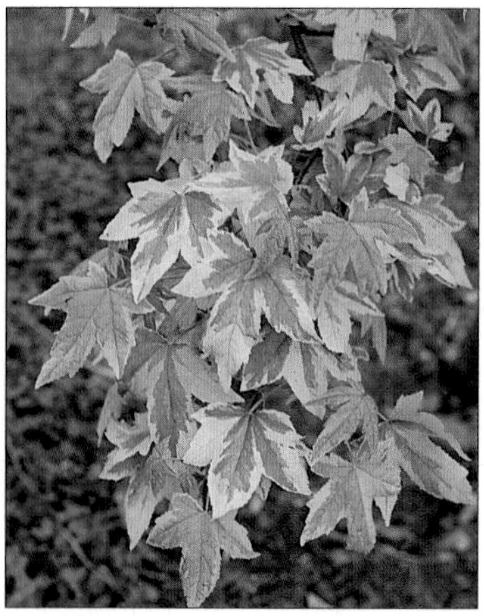
Liquidambar styraciflua 'Golden Treasure'

L. formosana △ syn. *L. formosana* var. *monticola*. Broadly conical tree with palmately 3-lobed leaves, to 12cm (5in) across, purple when young, turning dark green, then orange, red, and purple in autumn. Plants from China grown as var. *monticola* are considered to be hardier than those from Taiwan. ↕ 12m (40ft), ↔ 10m (30ft). China, Taiwan. ❄❄. **var. *monticola*** see *L. formosana*.

L. orientalis ▣ ○ (Oriental sweet gum). Small, slow-growing, bushy tree with palmately 5-lobed, mid-green leaves, to 7–10cm (3–4in) across, turning yellow and orange in autumn. ↕ 6m (20ft), ↔ 4m (12ft). S.W. Asia. ❄❄❄ (borderline)

L. styraciflua △ (Sweet gum). Broadly conical tree with young shoots often with corky wings. Palmately 5- or 7-lobed, glossy, mid-green leaves, to 15cm (6in) across, turn orange, red, and purple in autumn. ↕ 25m (80ft), ↔ 12m (40ft). E. USA, Mexico. ❄❄❄. **'Burgundy'** has dark red-purple autumn colour. **'Golden Treasure'** ▣ is slow-growing, with mid-green leaves margined dark yellow, becoming yellow-margined red-purple in autumn; ↕ 10m (30ft), ↔ 6m (20ft). **'Lane Roberts'** 🏆 has dark blackish red leaves over a long period in autumn. **'Moonbeam'** is slow-growing, with creamy yellow leaves turning red, yellow, and purple in autumn; ↕ 10m (30ft), ↔ 6m (20ft). **'Palo Alto'** has orange-red autumn colour. **'Variegata'** has leaves striped and mottled yellow; ↕ 15m (50ft), ↔ 8m (25ft). **'Worplesdon'** ▣ 🏆 has deeply lobed leaves turning purple then orange-yellow in autumn.

▷**Liquorice** see *Glycyrrhiza glabra*

LIRIODENDRON

Tulip tree

MAGNOLIACEAE

Genus of 2 species of deciduous trees from woodland in China, Vietnam, and North America. They are cultivated for their stately habit and curiously shaped, alternate leaves, which colour well in autumn. The solitary, cup-shaped flowers, inconspicuous from a distance, add interest in summer, but are not produced on young plants; they are followed by cone-like fruits. Excellent grown as specimen trees.

• **HARDINESS** Fully hardy.

L

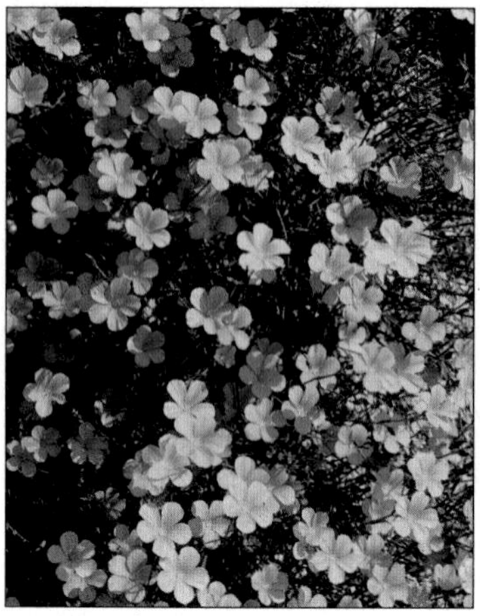
Linum narbonense

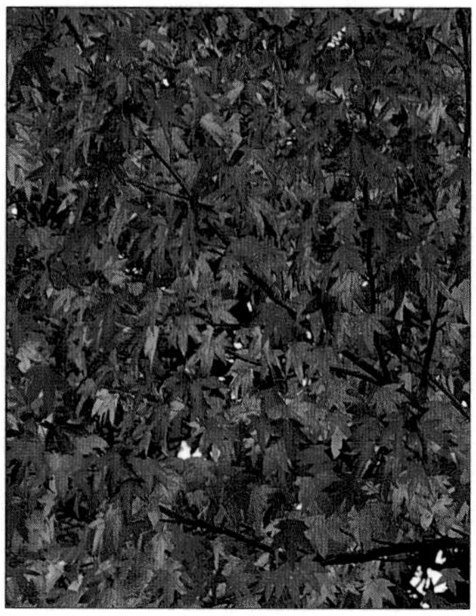
Liquidambar orientalis

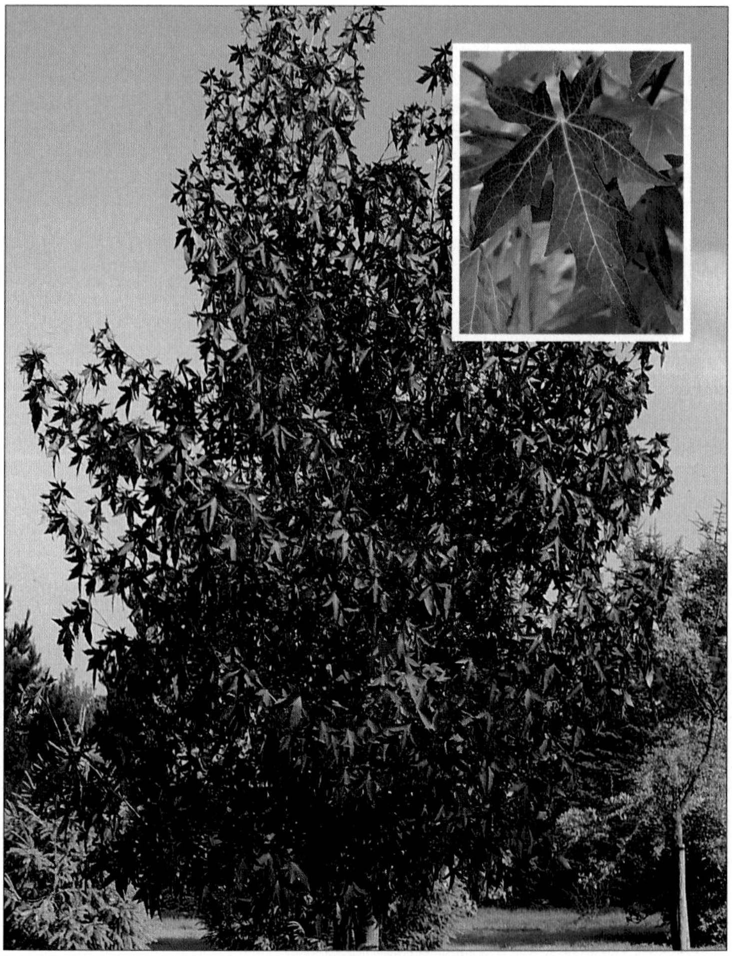
Liquidambar styraciflua 'Worplesdon' (inset: leaf detail)

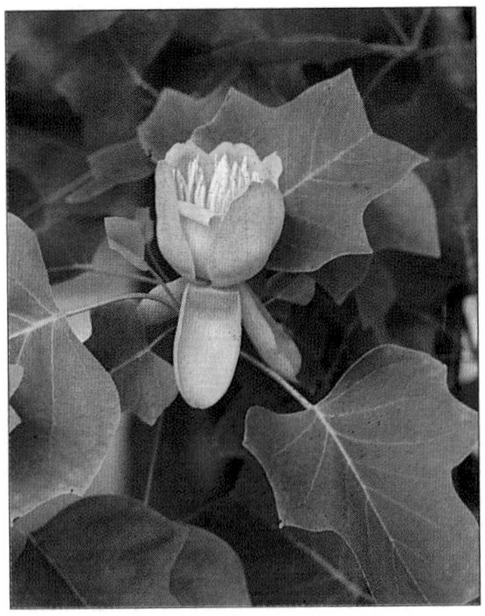

Liriodendron tulipifera

- **CULTIVATION** Grow in moderately fertile, preferably slightly acid, moist but well-drained soil in full sun or partial shade. Pruning group 1.
- **PROPAGATION** Sow seed (of species only) in containers in a cold frame in autumn. Graft in early spring, or bud in late summer.
- **PESTS AND DISEASES** Leaf spot and *Verticillium* wilt may be a problem.

L. chinense ○ (Chinese tulip tree). Vigorous, broadly columnar, deciduous tree with saddle-shaped, dark green leaves, to 15cm (6in) long, turning yellow in autumn; the leaves are more or less square, and indistinctly lobed at the tips, hollowed at the bases, with a pointed lobe at each side. Cup-shaped green flowers, 4cm (1½in) long, with yellow veins, are produced in midsummer. ↕25m (80ft), ↔ 12m (40ft). China, Vietnam. ❄❄❄
L. tulipifera ▣ ♀ ○ (Tulip tree). Vigorous, broadly columnar to conical, deciduous tree with saddle-shaped, dark green leaves, to 15cm (6in) long, that turn yellow in autumn; the leaves are more or less square, and lobed at the tips, hollowed at the bases, with a pointed lobe at each side. Cup-shaped, pale green flowers, 6cm (2½in) long, orange-banded at the bases, are borne in midsummer. ↕30m (100ft), ↔ 15m (50ft). E. North America. ❄❄❄. **'Aureomarginatum'** ▣ ♀ has leaves with broad, golden yellow margins; ↕20m (70ft), ↔ 10m (30ft). **'Fastigiatum'** ♀ ◊ is narrowly conical, with upright branches; ↕20m (70ft), ↔ 8m (25ft).

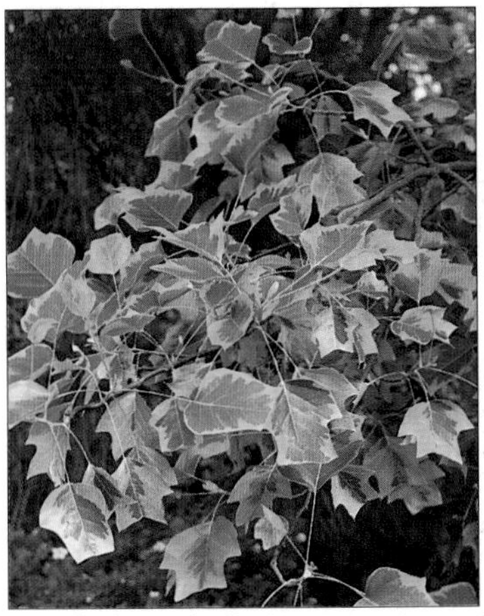

Liriodendron tulipifera 'Aureomarginatum'

LIRIOPE

Lilyturf

CONVALLARIACEAE/LILIACEAE

Genus of 5 or 6 species of tufted, rhizomatous and tuberous, evergreen and semi-evergreen perennials, found in usually acid woodland habitats in China, Vietnam, Taiwan, and Japan. They have arching, linear, grass-like, radical leaves, forming dense clumps or mats. Small, ovoid to spherical flowers, opening only slightly, are clustered in short, dense spikes or racemes, and are followed by black berries. Grow in a border or as ground cover.

- **HARDINESS** Fully hardy.
- **CULTIVATION** Grow in light, moderately fertile, preferably acid, moist but well-drained soil in partial or full shade, sheltered from cold, drying winds. Tolerant of drought.
- **PROPAGATION** Sow seed in containers outdoors, or divide, both in spring.
- **PESTS AND DISEASES** Young growth is susceptible to slug damage.

***L. exiliflora* 'Ariaka-janshige'**, syn. *L. exiliflora* 'Silvery Sunproof'. Clump-forming, evergreen, rhizomatous perennial with linear, mid-green leaves, to 40cm (16in) long, striped white and gold. Lax racemes of pale violet-purple flowers, to 6mm (¼in) across, are borne on violet-brown stems in late summer. ↕22–30cm (9–12in), ↔ 30cm (12in). ❄❄❄
***L. exiliflora* 'Silvery Sunproof'** see *L. exiliflora* 'Ariaka-janshige'.
L. graminifolia* var. *densiflora see *L. muscari.*
L. muscari ▣ ♀ syn. *L. graminifolia* var. *densiflora*, *L. platyphylla.* Stout, tufted, evergreen, tuberous perennial with dense clumps of linear to strap-shaped, dark green leaves, 25–45cm (10–18in) long. From early to late autumn, purple-green stems bear dense spikes of bright violet-mauve flowers, 5–8mm (¼–⅜in) across. ↕30cm (12in), ↔ 45cm (18in). China, Taiwan, Japan. ❄❄❄. **'John Burch'** has gold-variegated foliage, and bears tall spikes of large flowers. **'Majestic'** has narrower leaves, and produces tall, sometimes fused and flattened spikes of rich lavender-blue flowers. **'Monroe White'** produces numerous green-stalked racemes of white flowers, to 9mm (⅜in) across. Requires full shade.
L. platyphylla see *L. muscari.*
L. spicata, syn. *Ophiopogon spicatus.* Rhizomatous, semi-evergreen perennial forming a dense mat of grassy, dark green leaves, 20–40cm (8–16in) long, with tiny marginal teeth. Violet-brown stems bear racemes of pale violet to white flowers, 7–8mm (¼–⅜in) across, in late summer. ↕25cm (10in), ↔ 45cm (18in). China, Vietnam, Japan. ❄❄❄

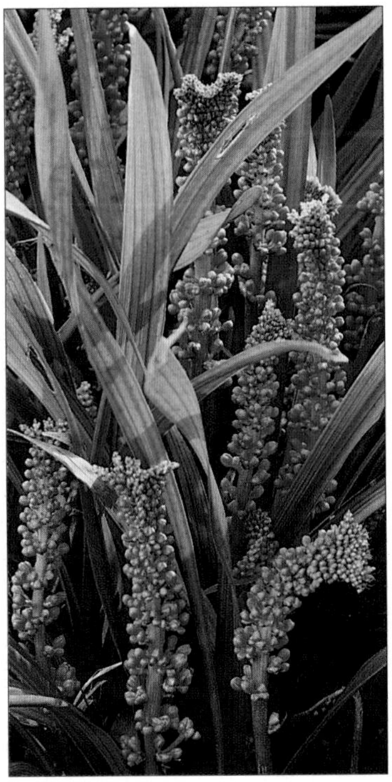

Liriope muscari

▷ ***Lisianthius*** see *Eustoma*
L. russellianus see *E. grandiflorum*

LITHOCARPUS

FAGACEAE

Genus of about 300 species of oak-like, evergreen trees and shrubs from forest and mountain slopes, mainly in E. and S.E. Asia, with one species in the W. USA. Leaves are alternate, leathery, and mostly entire, but occasionally toothed. Cylindrical male and female flowers (either unisexual or bisexual) are borne in erect spikes at or near the ends of the branches, and are followed by clusters of acorns, usually closely packed on the spikes. Cultivated for their handsome foliage, they are effective both as specimen trees and in an open site in a woodland garden.

- **HARDINESS** Fully hardy to frost hardy.
- **CULTIVATION** Grow in moderately fertile, acid to neutral, moist but well-drained soil in full sun or partial shade. In frost-prone areas, shelter from cold, drying winds. Pruning group 1.
- **PROPAGATION** Sow seed in containers in a cold frame in autumn.
- **PESTS AND DISEASES** Trouble free.

L. densiflorus ○ (Tanbark oak). Spreading, evergreen tree with oblong, toothed, prominently veined, leathery, dark green leaves, to 12cm (5in) long, downy at first, becoming hairless and glossy with age. In summer, produces tiny, cylindrical white flowers in upright spikes, to 10cm (4in) long, sometimes followed by solitary or paired acorns, to 2.5cm (1in) long, in autumn. ↕↔ 10m (30ft). USA (Oregon, California). ❄❄❄
L. henryi ▣ ○ Slow-growing, broadly conical, evergreen tree with narrowly oblong to elliptic-oblong, tapered, entire, leathery leaves, to 25cm (10in) long, pale green at first, later dark green. Tiny white flowers are borne in upright spikes, to 15cm (6in) long, in autumn or winter. Bears clustered acorns, to 2.5cm (1in) long, in upright spikes in winter. ↕↔ 10m (30ft). China. ❄❄

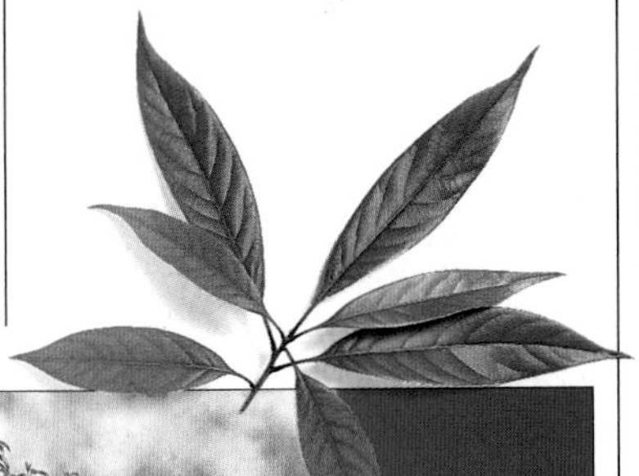

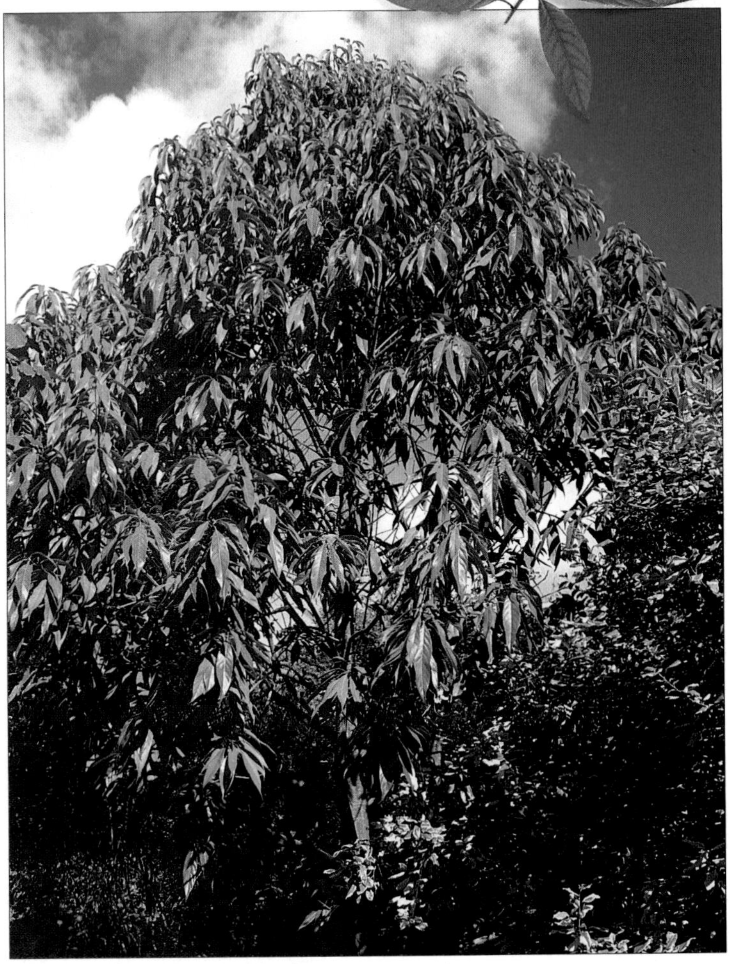

Lithocarpus henryi (inset: leaf detail)

LITHODORA

BORAGINACEAE

Genus of about 7 species of low-growing, spreading or upright, evergreen shrubs and subshrubs, found in scrub, thickets, and woodland margins, and on mountains, from S.W. Europe to S. Greece, Turkey, and Algeria. They are cultivated for their 5-lobed, funnel-shaped, blue or white flowers, produced in leafy, terminal cymes, mainly in summer. Leaves are linear, lance-shaped, elliptic, or obovate, and hairy. The hardiest species are ideal for an open position in a rock garden or raised bed. Where temperatures fall below -5°C (23°F), grow frost-hardy species in an alpine house.

• **HARDINESS** Fully hardy to frost hardy; *L. zahnii* is hardy to at least -7°C (20°F).

• **CULTIVATION** Grow most species in well-drained, ideally alkaline to neutral soil, in full sun; *L. diffusa* 'Heavenly Blue' needs acid, humus-rich soil. In an alpine house, grow in a mix of equal parts loam, leaf mould, and sharp sand. Pruning group 8; or 10, after flowering.

• **PROPAGATION** Take semi-ripe cuttings in summer. Remove rooted suckers of *L. oleifolia* in spring.

• **PESTS AND DISEASES** Prone to aphids and red spider mites under glass.

L

***L. diffusa* 'Heavenly Blue'** ■ 🏆 syn. *Lithospermum diffusum* 'Heavenly Blue'. Prostrate, spreading, many-branched, evergreen shrub with elliptic to narrowly oblong, deep green leaves, 1–3.5cm (½–1½in) long, hairy above and beneath. Bears a profusion of deep azure-blue flowers, 1cm (½in) across, in terminal cymes over long periods in late spring and summer. ↕ 15cm (6in), ↔ to 60cm (24in) or more. ***

L. graminifolia see *Moltkia suffruticosa*.

L.* x *intermedia see *Moltkia* x *intermedia*.

L. oleifolia ■ 🏆 syn. *Lithospermum oleifolium*. Semi-upright, loosely

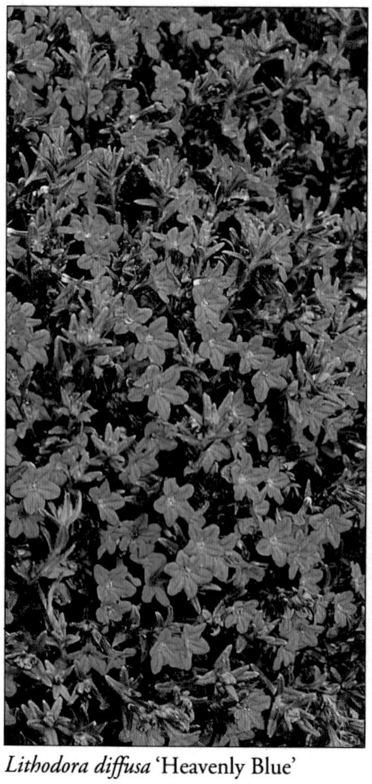

Lithodora diffusa 'Heavenly Blue'

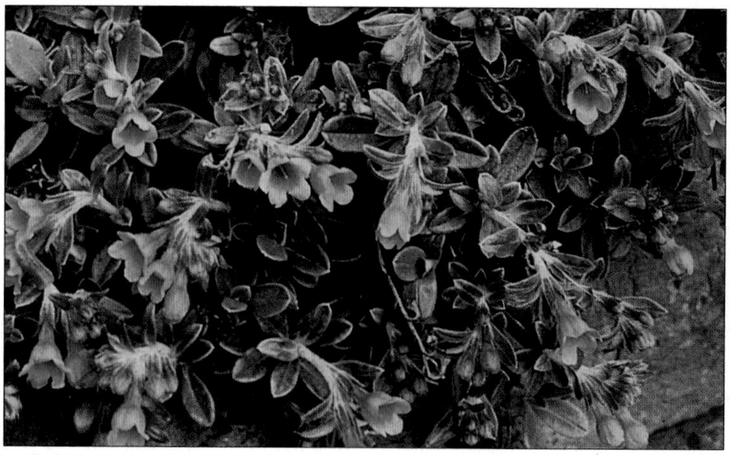

Lithodora oleifolia

branched, suckering, evergreen shrub with obovate to oblong, dull, dark green leaves, 1cm (½in) long, silky-hairy beneath. Bears loose, terminal cymes of 3–7 sky-blue flowers, 9mm (⅜in) across, opening from pink-tinted buds in early summer. ↕ 20cm (8in), ↔ 30cm (12in) or more. E. Pyrenees. ***

L. rosmarinifolia, syn. *Lithospermum rosmarinifolium*. Domed, tufted, evergreen subshrub with upright, branching stems and lance-shaped to linear, dark green leaves, 2.5–6cm (1–2½in) long, grey-bristly beneath. Produces loose, open, terminal cymes of gentian-blue flowers, 2cm (¾in) across, in summer. ↕ 30cm (12in), ↔ 40cm (16in). S. Italy, Algeria. **

L. zahnii, syn. *Lithospermum zahnii*. Upright, many-branched, evergreen shrub with linear or narrowly oblong, leathery, dark grey-green leaves, to 4cm (1½in) long, grey-bristly beneath. Produces few-flowered, terminal cymes of blue or white flowers, 1.5cm (½in) across, in succession during summer, then intermittently until mid-autumn. ↕ 30cm (12in), ↔ 40cm (16in). S. Greece. **

LITHOPHRAGMA

Woodland star

SAXIFRAGACEAE

Genus of about 9 species of rosette-forming perennials from woodland in W. North America. They have fibrous rootstocks with basal bulbils, and kidney-shaped to rounded, palmately 3- to 5-lobed leaves, the lobes often toothed or further lobed. Simple or

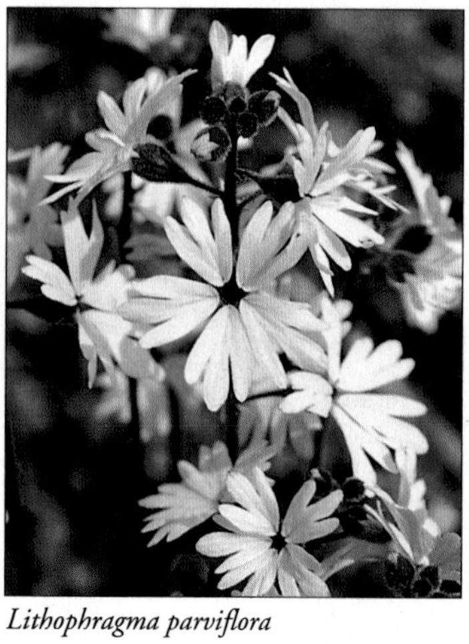

Lithophragma parviflora

branched, upright stems bear racemes of small, campion-like, 5-petalled flowers in late spring. Grow in a peat bed, woodland garden, or rock garden.

• **HARDINESS** Fully hardy.

• **CULTIVATION** Grow in moderately fertile, humus-rich, sharply drained soil in partial or deep shade.

• **PROPAGATION** Sow seed in containers outdoors in autumn. Divide, or separate bulbils, in spring or autumn.

• **PESTS AND DISEASES** New growth may be eaten by slugs in spring.

L. parviflora ■ (Prairie star). Clump-forming perennial producing basal bulbils and rounded, palmately 3- to 5-lobed, hairy, dark green, basal leaves, 1–3cm (½–1¼in) long. In late spring, unbranched stems produce open racemes of 4–14 nodding, white or pale pink flowers, 3cm (1¼in) across, with 3-lobed petals. ↕ 15cm (6in), ↔ to 30cm (12in). USA (California). ***

LITHOPS

Living stones, Stone plant

AIZOACEAE

Genus of about 40 species of dwarf, almost stemless, succulent perennials occurring among rocks and pebbles in semi-desert regions of Namibia and South Africa. They have thick, soft rootstocks that produce usually inversely cone-shaped "bodies", each composed of a pair of very fleshy leaves, 2–3cm (¾–1¼in) across, with a fissure usually running along much of their lengths. On the upper surface of each leaf is a window-like, translucent panel of dots, lines, or patches. Solitary, occasionally 2 or 3, daisy-like flowers, usually 2–3cm (¾–1¼in) across, sometimes larger, emerge from each fissure, mainly from midsummer to mid-autumn. They are followed by small, ovoid, fleshy capsules, containing tiny seeds. In areas where temperatures drop below 12°C (54°F), grow in a warm greenhouse or as houseplants; in warmer climates, grow in a desert garden.

• **HARDINESS** Frost tender.

• **CULTIVATION** Under glass, grow in standard cactus compost with added leaf mould, in full light. From early summer to late autumn, water freely and apply a half-strength balanced liquid fertilizer monthly. Keep dry at other times. Outdoors, grow in moderately fertile, sharply drained soil in full sun. See also pp.48–49.

• **PROPAGATION** Sow seed at 19–24°C (66–75°F) in spring or early summer, or remove offsets in early summer.

• **PESTS AND DISEASES** Susceptible to aphids when flowering.

L. aucampiae. Clump-forming succulent with pairs of reddish to sandy brown or ochre leaves forming inversely cone-shaped bodies, with darker marks on the flat upper surfaces. Yellow flowers are produced from late summer to mid-autumn. ↕ 3cm (1¼in), ↔ to 10cm (4in). South Africa (Northern Cape, Northern Transvaal, Eastern Transvaal). ❁ (min. 12°C/54°F)

L. bella see *L. karasmontana* subsp. *bella*.

L. dinteri ■ Clustering succulent with pairs of reddish or greyish yellow leaves forming inversely cone-shaped bodies with convex upper surfaces. Each leaf has a conspicuous panel with 5–15 red spots. Bears yellow flowers from late summer to mid-autumn. ↕ 3cm (1¼in), ↔ 10cm (4in). Namibia, South Africa (Northern Cape, Western Cape). ❁ (min. 12°C/54°F)

L. dorotheae ■ Clustering succulent with pairs of unequally sized, beige or buff leaves forming inversely cone-shaped bodies with almost flat or convex upper surfaces. Each leaf has a translucent grey-green or olive panel marked with red lines and dots. Yellow flowers are produced in late summer. ↕ 2–3cm (¾–1¼in), ↔ 10cm (4in). South Africa (Northern Cape). ❁ (min. 12°C/54°F)

L. hookeri see *L. turbiniformis*.

L. insularis. Solitary or clump-forming succulent with pairs of greenish brown leaves united into ovoid bodies with flat to concave upper surfaces. Each leaf has a translucent, dark green panel pitted with large red dots or lines. Bears yellow flowers, to 4cm (1½in) across, from late summer to mid-autumn. ↕ 1.5cm (½in), ↔ 3–8cm (1¼–3in) or more. South Africa (Western Cape, Eastern Cape). ❁ (min. 12°C/54°F)

L. julii. Variable, clump-forming succulent producing pairs of faintly red-tinged, whitish grey to dark grey leaves; they form spherical bodies with flat to slightly concave, furrowed upper surfaces and brown-marked fissures. Each leaf has dark brown to pale green panels with broad markings and red dots. White flowers are borne from late summer to mid-autumn. ↕ 3cm (1¼in), ↔ indefinite. Namibia, South Africa (Northern Cape, Western Cape). ❁ (min. 12°C/54°F)

L. karasmontana ■ Variable, clump-forming succulent with pairs of pale red-brown leaves forming inversely cone-shaped bodies, with dark brown markings and wrinkles on the flat to convex upper surfaces. White flowers, 2.5–4cm (1–1½in) across, are borne from late summer to mid-autumn. ↕ to 4cm (1½in), ↔ indefinite. Namibia, South Africa (Northern Cape, Western Cape). ❁ (min. 12°C/54°F). **subsp. *bella***, syn. *L. bella*, has yellowish brown leaves, with dull olive-green marks on the convex, uneven upper surfaces; ↕ to 3cm (1¼in).

L. kuibisensis see *L. schwantesii*.

L. lesliei. Clump-forming succulent with pairs of grey-green to buff to pale terracotta leaves, that form inversely cone-shaped bodies with convex upper

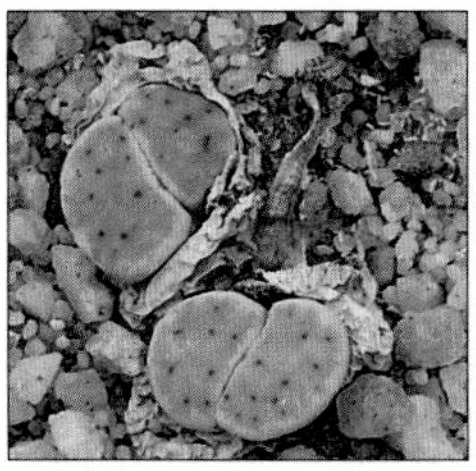
Lithops dinteri

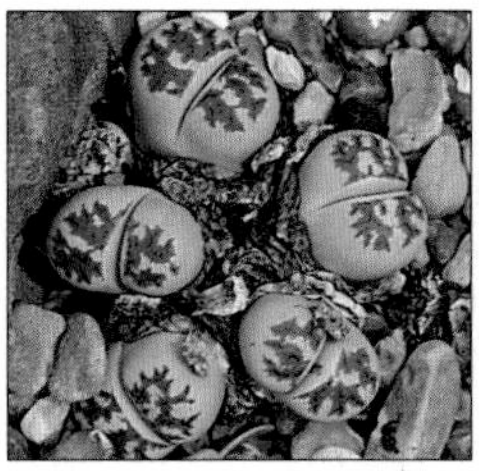
Lithops dorotheae

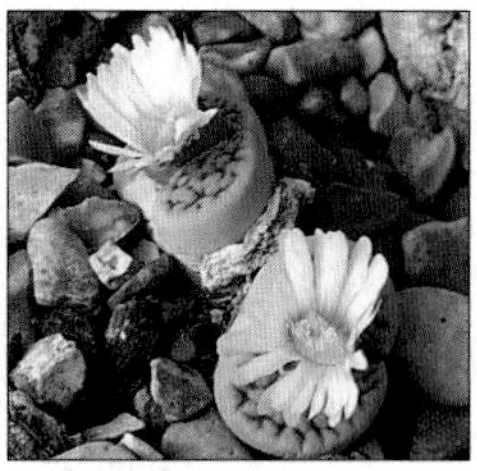
Lithops karasmontana

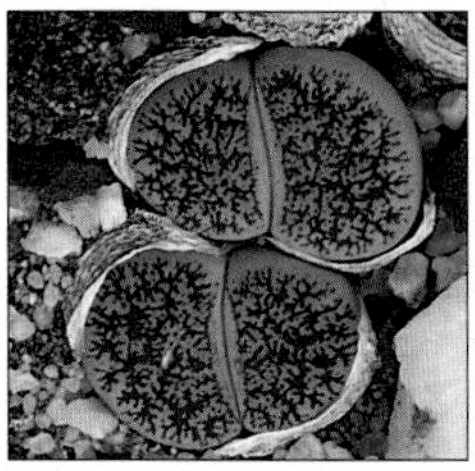
Lithops lesliei var. *hornii*

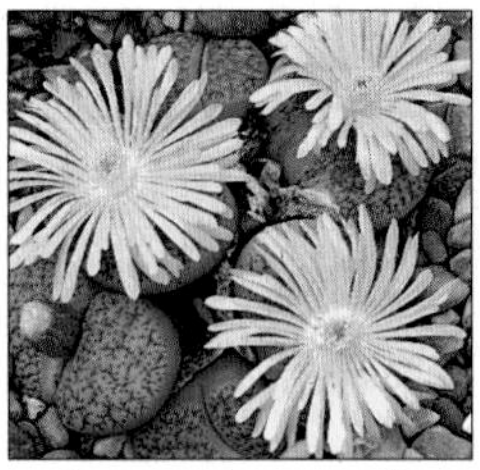
Lithops pseudotruncatella var. *pulmonuncula*

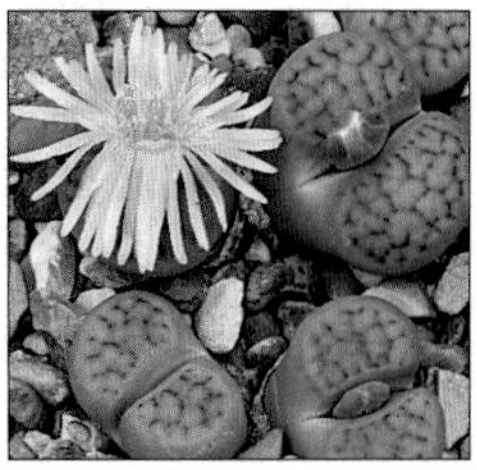
Lithops schwantesii

surfaces. Each leaf has a pale to dark olive-green panel, with transparent dots. Yellow, rarely white flowers are borne from late summer to mid-autumn. ↕ to 1.5cm (½in), ↔ to 4cm (1½in). South Africa (Northern Cape, Orange Free State, Northern Transvaal, Eastern Transvaal). ❄ (min. 12°C/54°F). **var. *hornii*** ■ has light to dark brown or greenish brown leaves, the upper surfaces with tiny panels and irregular channels of opaque, dark greyish brown to reddish brown. Flowers are yellow and up to 4cm (1½in) across. ↕ to 3.5cm (1½in), ↔ 4cm (1½in). South Africa (Northern Cape). **var. *rubrobrunnea*** has reddish brown bodies, with greenish brown panels on flat to slightly convex upper surfaces. ↕ 3cm (1¼in), ↔ 6–8cm (2½–3in). South Africa (Northern Transvaal, Eastern Transvaal).

L. marmorata ■ Mainly solitary succulent with a pair of pale grey or beige, sometimes grey-green or lilac leaves forming an inversely cone-shaped body, with greyish green lines on the slightly convex, deeply fissured upper surface. Scented white flowers are produced from late summer to mid-autumn. ↕ 3cm (1¼in), ↔ 5cm (2in) or more. South Africa (Northern Cape). ❄ (min. 12°C/54°F)

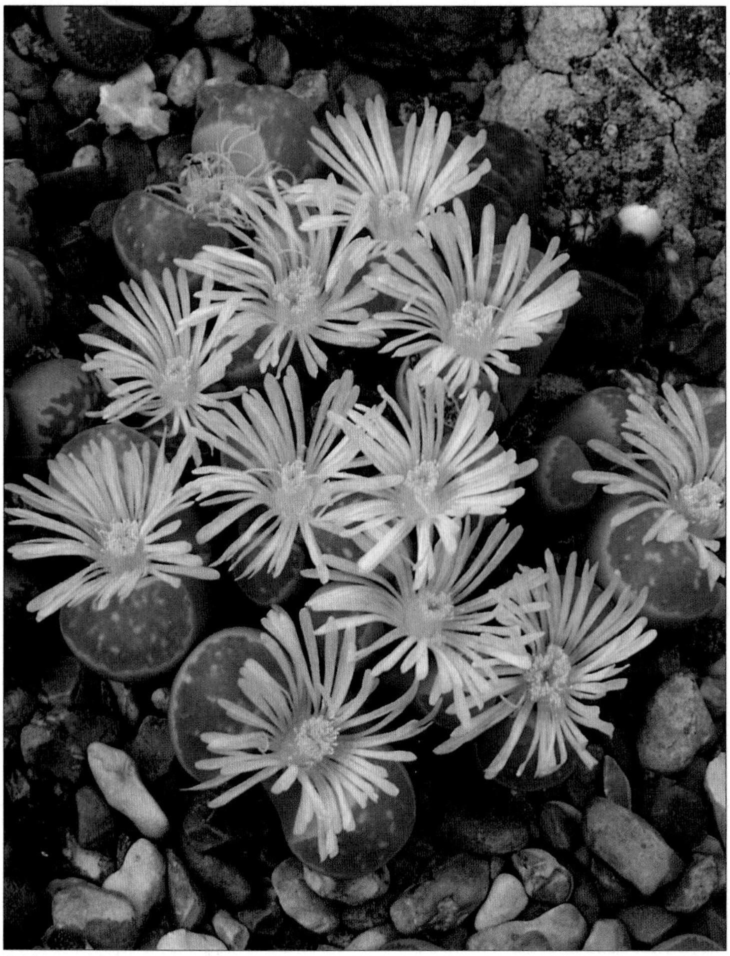
Lithops marmorata

L. optica. Mat-forming succulent with pairs of sometimes uneven, greyish purple to grey-green leaves forming ovoid bodies, with convex, deeply fissured upper surfaces and greenish white panels. From late summer to mid-autumn, bears white, often pink-tipped flowers. ↕ 3cm (1¼in), ↔ indefinite. Namibia, South Africa (Northern Cape, Western Cape). ❄ (min. 12°C/54°F)

L. otzeniana. Clump-forming succulent. Pairs of greyish violet leaves form inversely cone-shaped bodies, with pale green to violet panels on the convex, deep-fissured upper surfaces. From late summer to mid-autumn, bears bright yellow flowers, 2cm (¾in) across. ↕ 3cm (1¼in), ↔ indefinite. South Africa (Northern Cape). ❄ (min. 12°C/54°F)

L. pseudotruncatella* var. *pulmonuncula ■ Usually solitary succulent producing a pair of unequal, brownish grey leaves that form an inversely cone-shaped body, with an indistinct panel lined and dotted with brownish green. From late summer to mid-autumn, produces golden yellow flowers, to 3.5cm (1½in) across. ↕↔ to 3cm (1¼in). Namibia, South Africa (Northern Cape, Western Cape). ❄ (min. 12°C/54°F)

L. schwantesii ■ syn. *L. kuibisensis*, *L. schwantesii* var. *kuibisensis.* Very variable, mat-forming succulent with pairs of leaves forming inversely cone-shaped bodies, varying from light to dark grey, to yellowish green, orange, or reddish brown, with pink margins and dark green or pinkish red dots on the flat to slightly convex, often blue-tinged upper surfaces. Bright yellow flowers are borne from late summer to mid-autumn. The "type" of the species (pictured) has silvery blue-grey bodies, with red or blue-grey marks on the flat upper surfaces. ↕ 4cm (1½in), ↔ 15cm (6in). Namibia, South Africa (Northern Cape, Western Cape). ❄ (min. 12°C/54°F). **var. *kuibisensis*** see *L. schwantesii.*

L. turbiniformis, syn. *L. hookeri.* Variable, clump-forming succulent with pairs of brown, buff, or grey leaves forming ovoid bodies with warty, flat or convex upper surfaces, each with a deeply grooved, rich brown panel. Red-tipped, straw-coloured flowers, 3–4.5cm (1¼–1½in) across, are borne from late summer to mid-autumn. ↕ to 2.5cm (1in), ↔ 15cm (6in) or more. South Africa (Northern Cape, Eastern Cape). ❄ (min. 12°C/54°F)

L. vallis-mariae. Clump-forming succulent with pairs of yellowish green to bluish white leaves forming inversely cone-shaped bodies, with slightly convex or flat upper surfaces marked with a network of grey lines or dots. Produces yellow flowers, 2.5–3.5cm (1–1½in) across, in summer. ↕ to 2–4cm (¾–1½in), ↔ 5–10cm (2–4in). Namibia. ❄ (min. 12°C/54°F)

▷ ***Lithospermum diffusum* 'Heavenly Blue'** see *Lithodora diffusa* 'Heavenly Blue'
▷ ***Lithospermum doerfleri*** see *Moltkia doerfleri*
▷ ***Lithospermum graminifolium*** see *Moltkia suffruticosa*
▷ ***Lithospermum oleifolium*** see *Lithodora oleifolia*
▷ ***Lithospermum purpureocaeruleum*** see *Buglossoides purpurocaerulea*
▷ ***Lithospermum rosmarinifolium*** see *Lithodora rosmarinifolia*
▷ ***Lithospermum zahnii*** see *Lithodora zahnii*
▷ ***Litocarpus cordifolia*** see *Aptenia cordifolia*
▷ ***Litsea glauca*** see *Neolitsea sericea*
▷ **Little pickles** see *Othonna capensis*

LITTONIA

LILIACEAE

Genus of 8 species of tuberous, perennial, tendril climbers occurring in scrub and sandy, often coastal areas in Senegal, South Africa, and the Arabian Peninsula. They are cultivated for their pendent, bell-shaped flowers, which are borne in summer. Ovate-lance-shaped to linear leaves are alternate or opposite on the upper parts of the stems, and often almost whorled on the lower parts; they taper to tendrils at the tips. In frost-prone areas, grow in a temperate greenhouse or conservatory. In warmer areas, grow among low shrubs.

- **HARDINESS** Frost tender.
- **CULTIVATION** Plant tubers 10–15cm (4–6in) deep in autumn or early spring. Under glass, grow in loam-based potting compost (JI No.2) with added grit, in full light. As growth begins, water freely, then apply a half-strength balanced liquid fertilizer every 3–4 weeks. Reduce watering as the leaves fade, then keep just moist in winter. The brittle tubers resent disturbance, so pot on only when necessary. Outdoors, grow in moderately fertile, humus-rich, well-drained soil in full sun. Stems require support.
- **PROPAGATION** Sow seed at 19–24°C (66–75°F) in spring, or divide tubers with care when dormant.
- **PESTS AND DISEASES** Trouble free.

L. modesta ■ Tuberous tendril climber with slender stems bearing whorled or alternate, linear to ovate-lance-shaped, mid-green leaves, to 15cm (6in) long, with tendrils at their tips. Pendent, bell-shaped orange flowers, to 5cm (2in) long, are produced singly from the leaf axils in summer. ↕ 1–2m (3–6ft). South Africa (Northern Transvaal, Eastern Transvaal, KwaZulu/Natal, Orange Free State). ❄ (min. 8°C/46°F)

▷ **Living baseball** see *Euphorbia obesa*
▷ **Living granite** see *Pleiospilos*
▷ **Living rock** see *Ariocarpus fissuratus*
▷ **Living stones** see *Lithops*

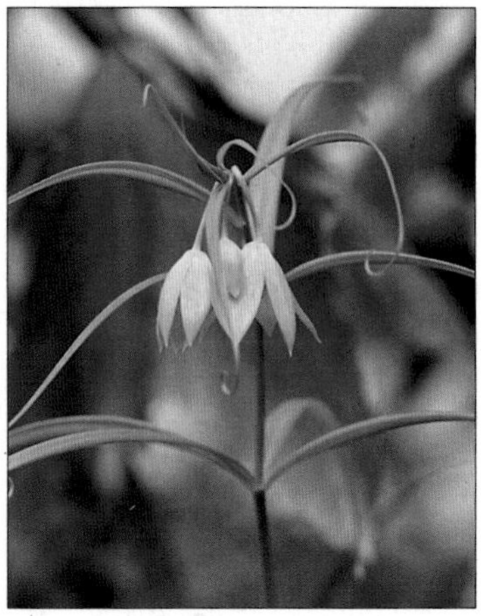
Littonia modesta

LIVISTONA

ARECACEAE/PALMAE

Genus of about 28 species of single-stemmed palms, found in habitats ranging from streambanks and swamps to woodland, rainforest, and inland gorges, in the warmer parts of Asia and Australasia. Fan-shaped leaves are borne in often dense, terminal heads, and bowl-shaped, 3-petalled flowers are produced in panicles between them. In frost-prone climates, grow in a cool or warm greenhouse, or as houseplants. In warmer regions, they are suitable for growing as specimen plants.

• **HARDINESS** Frost tender.

• **CULTIVATION** Under glass, grow in loam-based potting compost (JI No.3) in full or bright indirect light. In the growing season, water freely and apply a balanced liquid fertilizer every month. Water sparingly in winter. Outdoors, grow in fertile, moist but well-drained soil in full sun or partial shade.

• **PROPAGATION** Sow seed at 23°C (73°F) in spring.

• **PESTS AND DISEASES** Red spider mites and scale insects may be troublesome under glass.

L. australis ▣ ♆ (Australian fan palm, Cabbage palm). Large palm with an erect, robust trunk that is initially covered with a skirt of dead leaves and rough or almost prickly fibres. Long, spiny leaf-stalks support longer, lustrous, deep green blades, to 1.7m (5½ft) long, divided for two-thirds of their length into many linear lobes, often arching at the tips. From spring to summer, cream flowers are produced in panicles as long as, or shorter than the leaves; they are followed by spherical, brownish red to black fruit, 2cm (¾in) across. ↕ to 25m (80ft), ↔ to 5m (15ft). Coastal forest in E. Australia. ❄ (min. 3–5°C/37–41°F)

L. chinensis ▣ ♀ ♆ (Chinese fan palm). Medium-sized palm with an erect, robust trunk swollen at the base, the upper part covered with fibrous leaf bases, at least at first. Glossy, rich green leaves, to 2m (6ft) long, with shorter, spiny leaf-stalks, are divided for up to two-thirds of their length into many linear, pendent segments. Cream flowers are borne in panicles to 1m (3ft) or more long, usually in summer, followed by ovoid to spherical, glossy, blue-green to grey-pink fruit, 2–2.5cm (¾–1in) across. ↕ to 12m (40ft), ↔ to 5m (15ft). S. Japan (including Ryukyu and Bonin Islands) to S. Taiwan. ❄ (min. 3–5°C/37–41°F)

L. mariae ♆ (Red fan palm). Tall palm with a slim trunk, swollen at the base, and bearing old leaf bases, at least in the upper part. Spiny leaf-stalks, 2m (6ft) long, support prominently ribbed blades, 2m (6ft) long, divided to about half their length into linear, pendent lobes, initially flushed red to bronze-red, maturing to bluish green. In spring and summer, bears cream to pale yellow flowers in erect panicles, shorter than the leaves, followed by spherical, glossy black fruit, 2cm (¾in) across. ↕ to 30m (100ft), ↔ to 8m (25ft). C. Australia. ❄ (min. 13–15°C/55–59°F)

L. rotundifolia ♆ Medium-sized to large palm with a slim trunk bearing prominent leaf scars. Spiny leaf-stalks, 2m (6ft) long, support shorter, rounded, lustrous, deep green blades, divided for about two-thirds of their length into many linear, rigid, shallowly notched lobes. Cream flowers are produced in panicles shorter than the leaves, usually in summer, and are followed by spherical, scarlet fruit, 2cm (¾in) across, which ripen to black. ↕ to 25m (80ft), ↔ to 8m (25ft). Philippines, Malaysia (Sabah), Indonesia (Sulawesi, Moluccas). ❄ (min. 13–15°C/55–59°F)

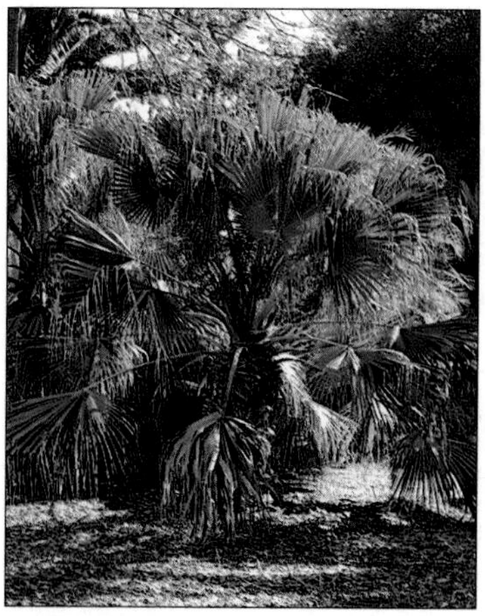

Livistona chinensis

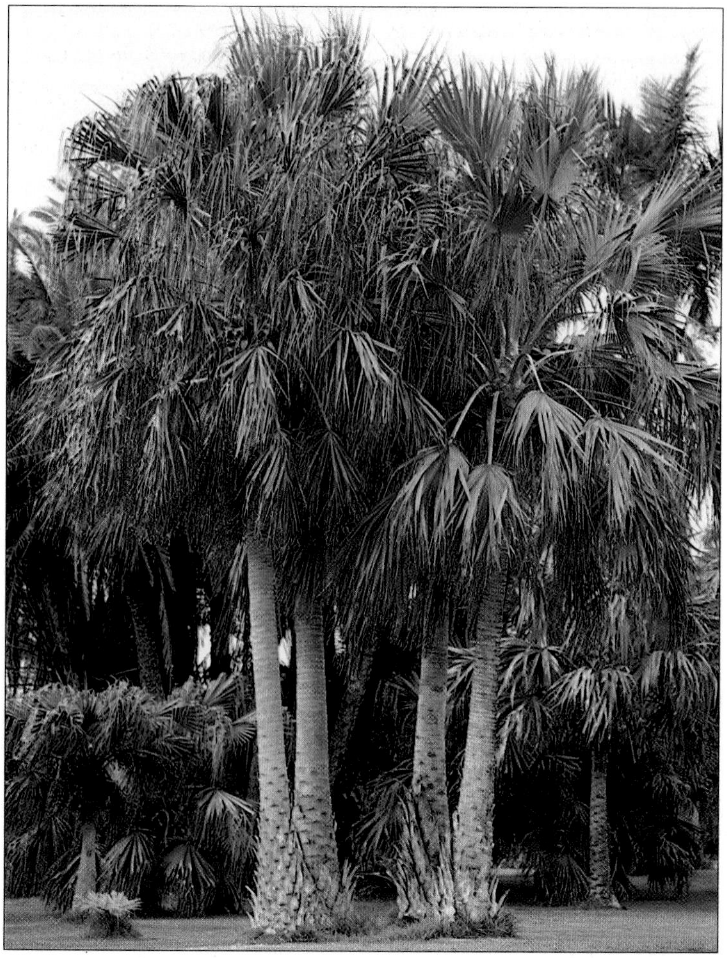

Livistona australis

▷**Lizard plant** see *Tetrastigma voinierianum*

▷**Lizard tail** see *Crassula muscosa*

LLOYDIA

LILIACEAE

Genus of approximately 12 species of bulbous perennials from damp upland meadows and screes in temperate and arctic areas of the N. hemisphere. They have narrowly linear leaves and solitary or paired, bell-shaped flowers borne in spring or summer. Grow in an alpine house, bulb frame, or open rock garden.

• **HARDINESS** Fully hardy.

• **CULTIVATION** Plant bulbs 7cm (3in) deep in autumn. Grow in poor, peaty, humus-rich, moist but sharply drained soil in partial shade. In an alpine house use a mix of 1 part loam, 1 part leaf mould or peat, and 2 parts grit.

• **PROPAGATION** Sow seed in containers in an open frame in spring.

• **PESTS AND DISEASES** Trouble free.

L. graeca see *Gagea graeca*.

L. serotina (Snowdon lily). Bulbous perennial with erect, thread-like leaves, to 20cm (8in) long. In late spring and early summer, upright stems bear solitary or paired, upward-facing, bell-shaped white flowers, to 1.5cm (½in) long, with purple-red veins and pale yellow bases. ↕ 5–15cm (2–6in), ↔ 5cm (2in). Arctic and European mountains, Himalayas, S.W. China. ✲✲✲

LOASA

LOASACEAE

Genus of about 100 species of usually bushy, occasionally spreading or twining annuals, biennials, perennials, and subshrubs from open habitats, often by roads or on gravelly slopes, in Mexico and temperate South America. They have opposite or alternate, entire to palmately lobed, sometimes 3-palmate leaves, and bear nodding, yellow, white, or red flowers singly or in racemes. Each flower has 5 boat-shaped petals, which are inflated in appearance, and nectar scales banded in contrasting colours. Some species are covered in stinging hairs. Best in containers on a patio; grow alpine species in an alpine house.

• **HARDINESS** Frost hardy to half hardy.

• **CULTIVATION** Grow in fertile, reliably moist but well-drained soil in full sun.

• **PROPAGATION** Sow seed at 13–18°C (55–64°F) in mid-spring or *in situ* in late spring.

• **PESTS AND DISEASES** Trouble free.

***L. triphylla* var. *volcanica*.** Erect, bushy to loosely twining, densely glandular-hairy annual, with shallowly to deeply 3- to 5-lobed, coarsely toothed leaves, 7–15cm (3–6in) across, becoming less lobed on the upper parts of the stems. In summer, bears open, leafy racemes of nodding, hooded white flowers, to 5cm (2in) across, each with golden yellow nectar scales, crossbanded red and white, that form a central disc with concentric rings. Covered in stinging hairs. ↕ 60–90cm (24–36in), ↔ to 30cm (12in). Ecuador. ✲✲

▷***Lobeira macdougallii*** see *Nopalxochia macdougallii*

LOBELIA

CAMPANULACEAE/LOBELIACEAE

Genus of about 370 species of annuals, perennials (including some aquatics), and shrubs, found in tropical and temperate areas worldwide, especially in North, Central, and South America. Their habitats range from marshes, wet meadows, and riverbanks, to woodland, well-drained hilly and mountainous slopes, and deserts. Valued for their often brightly coloured flowers, lobelias vary enormously, but all have simple, alternate, often stalkless leaves and 2-lipped, tubular flowers, each with 5 lobes, the upper 2 lobes often erect, the lower 3 often spreading and fan-like; the calyx tubes are sometimes swollen. The flowers are usually borne in terminal racemes or panicles, but may also be solitary. The popular Bowden Hybrids, sometimes grouped under *L.* x *speciosa*, are perennials with ovate-lance-shaped, pointed leaves, 10–15cm (4–6in) long, which are sometimes red-purple with matching stems. Their flowers,

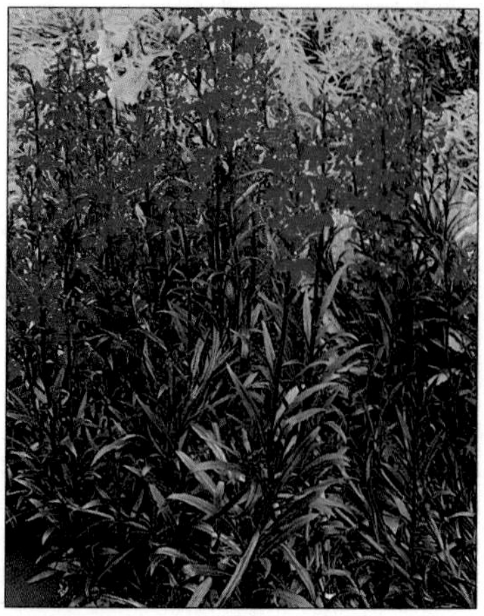

Lobelia 'Bees' Flame'

L

Lobelia 'Cherry Ripe'

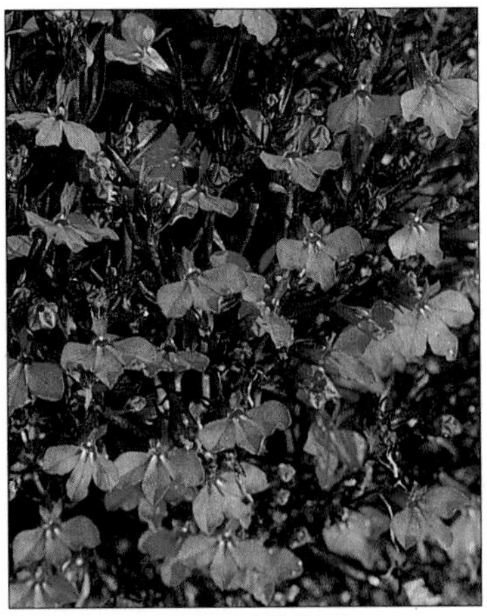

Lobelia erinus 'Crystal Palace'

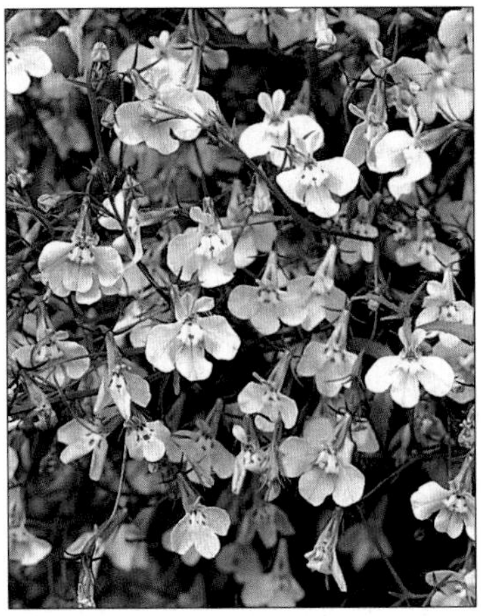

Lobelia erinus 'Lilac Fountain'

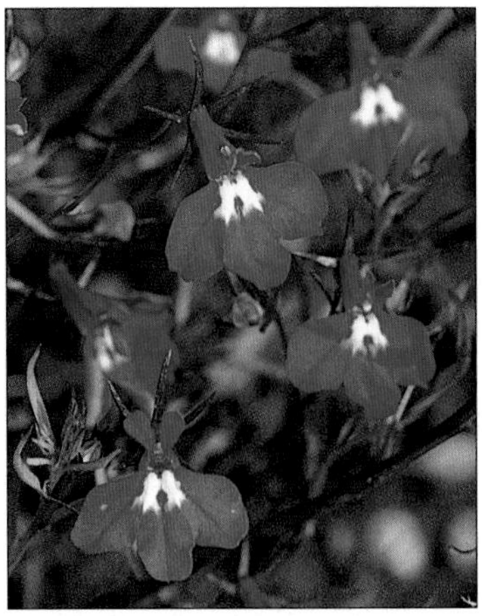

Lobelia erinus 'Sapphire'

2.5–3.5cm (1–1½in) across, are borne in terminal racemes, 15–20cm (6–8in) long, from midsummer to early autumn.

Perennials are effective beside water, or in a mixed border. Annuals are suitable for edging, or for a hanging basket or window-box. Aquatic species are useful in a wildlife pool. The shrubby and tree-like species are seldom grown. Contact with the milky sap may irritate skin.

• **HARDINESS** Fully hardy to frost tender. *L. tupa* is hardy to -10°C (14°F).

• **CULTIVATION** Grow in deep, fertile, reliably moist soil in full sun or partial shade. To improve the flowering performance of annuals, apply a balanced liquid fertilizer every 2 weeks in spring and early summer, then a nitrogen-free fertilizer every 2 weeks from midsummer onwards. In frost-prone areas, protect half-hardy perennials with a dry winter mulch. Grow aquatics in baskets of acid soil at the margins of a pool or stream.

• **PROPAGATION** Sow seed at 13–18°C (55–64°F): sow seed of annuals in late winter, of perennials as soon as ripe. Divide border perennials in spring, aquatics in summer. Take bud cuttings of *L. cardinalis* in midsummer.

• **PESTS AND DISEASES** Susceptible to slugs and leaf blotch, the latter especially on *L. siphilitica*. Crowns may rot in damp, mild conditions. *L. splendens* may be affected by viruses.

L. angulata see *Pratia angulata*.
***L.* 'Bees' Flame'** ▣ Clump-forming, slightly hairy perennial with reddish purple stems and linear-lance-shaped, reddish purple leaves, to 15cm (6in) long. In mid- and late summer, produces racemes, to 45cm (18in) long, of tubular, 2-lipped, bright crimson flowers, 3.5–4.5cm (1½–1¾in) across. ↕75cm (30in), ↔30cm (12in). ❄❄❄
***L.* 'Brightness'.** Bowden Hybrid with mid-green leaves, and blood-red flowers produced from midsummer to early autumn. ↕90cm (36in), ↔30cm (12in). ❄❄❄
L. cardinalis 🏆 (Cardinal flower). Short-lived, clump-forming perennial, with short rhizomes, often reddish purple stems, and narrowly ovate to oblong-lance-shaped, toothed, often glossy, bronze-tinged, bright green leaves, to 10cm (4in) long. In summer and early autumn, bears racemes, 35cm (14in) long, of tubular, 2-lipped,

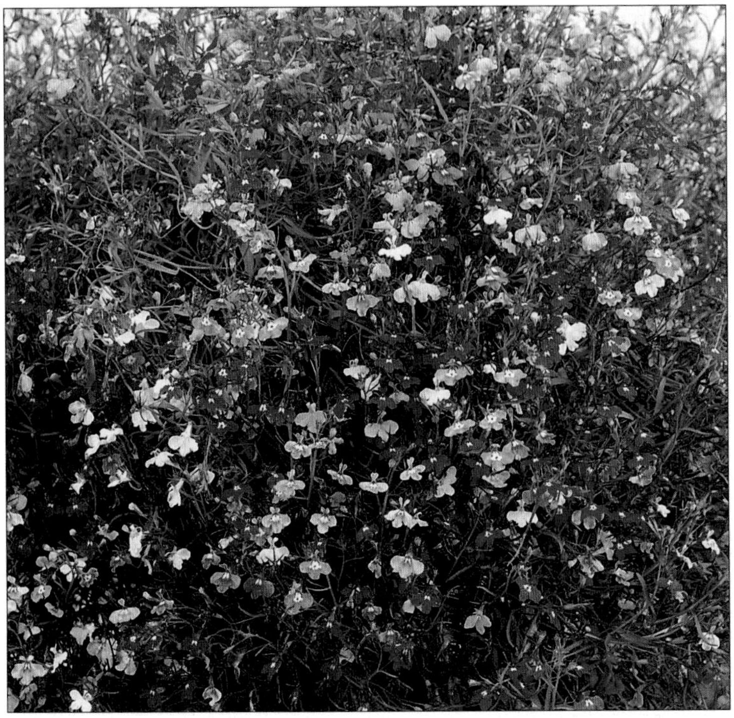

Lobelia erinus Cascade Series

brilliant scarlet-red flowers, 5cm (2in) long, with reddish purple bracts. ↕90cm (36in), ↔30cm (12in). E. Canada (New Brunswick) to USA (Michigan to Florida to Texas). ❄❄❄. **f. *alba*** has white flowers. **f. *rosea*** has pink flowers.
***L.* 'Cherry Ripe'** ▣ Bowden Hybrid with mid-green leaves, often suffused maroon. Bears tubular, 2-lipped, cherry-red flowers in mid- and late summer. ↕90cm (36in), ↔30cm (12in). ❄❄❄
***L.* 'Dark Crusader'.** Bowden Hybrid with maroon stems and leaves. Bears tubular, 2-lipped, velvety, deep red flowers in mid- and late summer. ↕60–90cm (24–36in), ↔30cm (12in). ❄❄❄
L. dortmanna (Water lobelia). Partly submerged aquatic perennial producing hollow, almost leafless stems and a mat of rosette-forming, oblong, dark green leaves, 3–7cm (1¼–3in) long. Pendent, tubular, 2-lipped, pale blue to pale violet flowers, to 2cm (¾in) long, are borne in loose racemes, 5cm (2in) long, above the water in summer. ↕60cm (24in), ↔30cm (12in). W. Europe, North America. ❄❄❄
***L. erinus* cultivars.** Low-growing, bushy, or trailing perennials, grown as annuals, with tiny, ovate to narrowly linear, or linear-obovate, toothed, mid- to dark green or bronze-flushed leaves, 1.5cm (½in) long. From summer to autumn, they bear small, loose racemes, 5cm (2in) long, of tubular, 2-lipped, blue, violet, white, pink, red, or purple flowers, to 1cm (½in) across, with white or yellow eyes and broad, fan-shaped lower lips. ↕10–23cm (4–9in), ↔10–15cm (4–6in). ❄. Cultivars of **Cascade Series** ▣ are trailing, with carmine-red, violet-blue, blue, pink, or white flowers; ↕15cm (6in). **'Cobalt Blue'** is compact, with very early, intensely mid-blue flowers; ↕to 12cm (5in). **'Crystal Palace'** ▣🏆 is compact, and has dark blue flowers and dark green foliage; ↕to 10cm (4in). **'Lilac Fountain'** ▣ is trailing, and profusely bears lilac-pink flowers; ↕15cm (6in). **Moon Series** cultivars are early-flowering, with white, blue-and-white, or deep blue flowers. **'Mrs. Clibran'** 🏆 is compact, with brilliant blue, white-eyed flowers; ↕10–15cm (4–6in). Cultivars of **Palace Series** have neat, blue to dark blue or white flowers, some with white eyes; ↕to 12cm (5in). Cultivars of **Regatta Series** are trailing, and bear blue, pink, crimson, or white flowers over a very long season. They bloom early; ↕to 20cm (8in). **Riviera Series** cultivars bear very early flowers in lilac-blue, sky-blue, or a mottled blue with picotee margins; ↕10–15cm (4–6in). **'Rosamund'** is compact, and produces white-eyed, cherry-red flowers; ↕10–15cm (4–6in). **'Sapphire'** ▣ is trailing, with bright blue, white-eyed flowers; ↕to 15cm (6in).
L. fulgens see *L. splendens*.
***L. x gerardii* 'Vedrariensis'** ▣ Clump-forming perennial with short rhizomes and basal rosettes of broadly lance-shaped to elliptic, dark green leaves, to 10cm (4in) long, often suffused red. Throughout summer, stout stems bear many-flowered racemes, to 45cm (18in) long, of tubular, 2-lipped, violet-purple flowers, 2–3.5cm (¾–1½in) across. ↕75–120cm (30–48in), ↔30cm (12in). ❄❄❄
***L.* 'Illumination'.** Clump-forming perennial with short rhizomes, downy, dark red stems, and linear-lance-shaped, dark green leaves, to 15cm (6in) long. In summer, bears tubular, 2-lipped scarlet flowers, 2.5–3cm (1–1¼in) across, in one-sided racemes, to 35cm (14in) long. ↕90cm (36in), ↔30cm (12in). ❄❄
L. laxiflora. Spreading, hairy, sub-shrubby, rhizomatous perennial with arching, red-tinted stems bearing linear-lance-shaped to elliptic, finely toothed, light green leaves, to 8cm (3in) long, with long, sharp points. In late spring and summer, bears semi-pendent, tubular, 2-lipped, red and yellow flowers, 4cm (1½in) long, usually singly, from the upper leaf axils. ↕to 90cm (36in), ↔2m (6ft) or more. Mexico, Central America. ❄❄ (borderline).

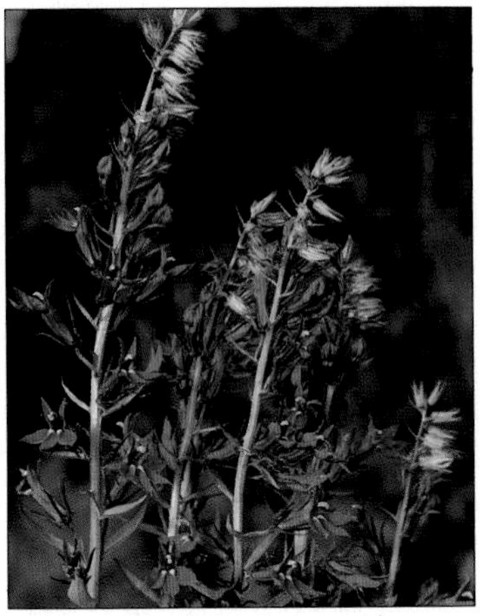

Lobelia x gerardii 'Vedrariensis'

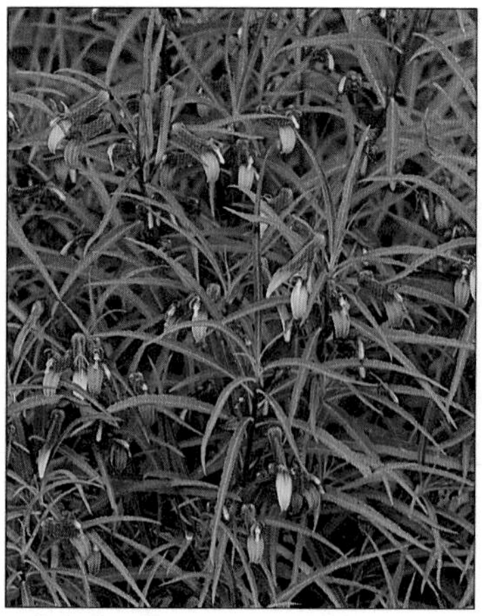

Lobelia laxiflora var. *angustifolia*

var. *angustifolia* ■ bears linear leaves, to 7cm (3in) long; ↕ to 60cm (24in), ↔ 45cm (18in); USA (Arizona).

L. paludosa (Swamp lobelia). Marginal aquatic perennial bearing inversely lance-shaped, bright mid-green leaves, 15–22cm (6–9in) long. In summer, produces tubular, 2-lipped, pale blue flowers, to 1.5cm (½in) long, in racemes to 30cm (12in) long. ↕ 30–120cm (12–48in), ↔ 90cm (36in). USA (Georgia, Florida). ❄❄❄

L. pedunculata see *Pratia pedunculata.*

L. perpusilla see *Pratia perpusilla.*

***L.* 'Queen Victoria'** ♀ Clump-forming, short-lived perennial with deep purple-red stems and lance-shaped, deep purple-red leaves, 10–15cm (4–6in) long. From late summer to mid-autumn, bears tubular, 2-lipped scarlet flowers, 2.5–3.5cm (1–1½in) long, in slightly one-sided racemes, to 45cm (18in) long. ↕ 90cm (36in), ↔ 30cm (12in). ❄❄❄

L. richardsonii. Bushy then trailing, evergreen perennial with pendent shoots clothed with narrowly elliptic, sparsely toothed, mid- to dark green leaves, to 5cm (2in) long. In summer and autumn, bears numerous long-stalked, tubular, 2-lipped, white-throated, bright lilac-blue flowers, to 2cm (¾in) long, singly in the leaf axils. ↕ 10cm (4in), ↔ 30cm (12in). Origin unknown. ❄

L. siphilitica (Blue cardinal flower). Clump-forming perennial with erect, leafy stems and ovate, oblong, or broadly lance-shaped, irregularly toothed, softly hairy, light green leaves, 10–15cm (4–6in) long. From late summer to mid-autumn, long-lasting, tubular, 2-lipped, bright blue flowers, 2.5–3.5cm

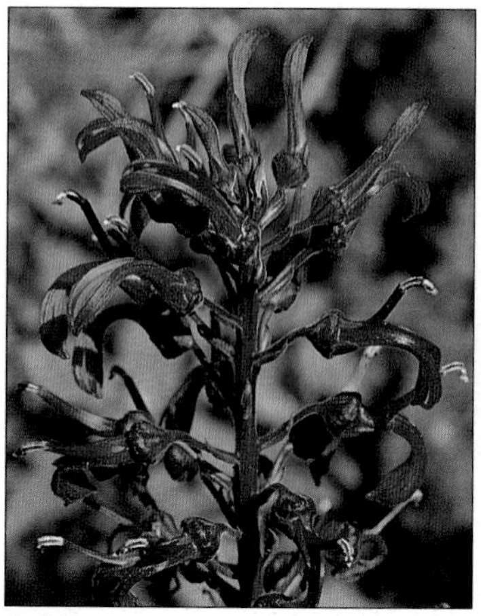

Lobelia tupa

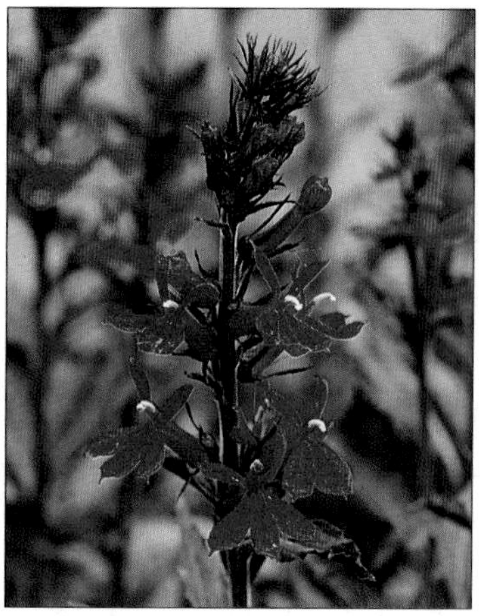

Lobelia 'Will Scarlet'

(1–1½in) across, with leafy green bracts, are borne in dense racemes, 10–50cm (4–20in) long. ↕ 60–120cm (24–48in), ↔ 30cm (12in). E. USA. ❄❄❄. **f. *albiflora*** bears white flowers.

***L.* x *speciosa* cultivars.** Clump-forming, slightly hairy perennials, often grown as annuals or biennials, with basal rosettes of oval to oblong-obovate, pointed, mid-green to red-flushed or ruby-red leaves, to 12cm (5in) long. From summer to autumn, they bear tubular, 2-lipped, red, pink, or mauve-blue flowers, 3–4cm (1¼–1½in) across, in erect, dense, leafy racemes, to 35cm (14in) long. ↕ 1.2m (4ft), ↔ 30cm (12in). ❄❄❄. **Compliment Series** cultivars have dark green foliage and long-stemmed, loose racemes of scarlet, deep red, or blue-purple flowers; ↕ 75cm (30in) or more, ↔ to 23cm (9in). Cultivars of **Fan Series** have bronze-green or dark green leaves and compact, dense racemes, branching at the bases, of narrow-petalled flowers, to 2.5cm (1in) long, in pink, deep carmine-pink, scarlet, or deep red; ↕ 50–60cm (20–24in), ↔ to 23cm (9in).

L. splendens, syn. *L. fulgens* (Scarlet lobelia). Clump-forming, rhizomatous perennial with narrowly lance-shaped to linear-lance-shaped, mid-green leaves, to 15cm (6in) long, sometimes flushed red-purple, on downy, dark red stems. In late summer, bears tubular, 2-lipped scarlet flowers, 2–4cm (¾–1½in) long, in one-sided racemes, to 40cm (16in) long. ↕ 90cm (36in), ↔ 30cm (12in). USA (California, Texas), Mexico. ❄❄ (borderline)

L. tupa ■ Robust, upright, clump-forming perennial with red-purple stems and ovate-lance-shaped to lance-shaped, downy, light grey-green leaves, to 30cm (12in) long. Narrowly tubular, 2-lipped, brick-red to orange-red flowers, 6cm (2½in) long, with red-purple calyces, are borne in racemes, to 45cm (18in) long, from mid- or late summer to mid-autumn. ↕ to 2m (6ft), ↔ 90cm (36in). Chile. ❄❄

***L.* 'Will Scarlet'** ■ Bowden Hybrid with mid-green leaves, suffused maroon and tubular, 2-lipped, bright blood-red flowers, borne from midsummer to early autumn. ↕ 90cm (36in), ↔ 30cm (12in). ❄❄❄

▷ **Lobelia,**
Scarlet see *Lobelia splendens*
Swamp see *Lobelia paludosa*
Water see *Lobelia dortmanna*

▷ ***Lobivia backebergii*** see *Echinopsis backebergii*
▷ ***Lobivia caespitosa*** see *Echinopsis maximiliana*
▷ ***Lobivia cinnabarina*** see *Echinopsis cinnabarina*
▷ ***Lobivia ferox*** see *Echinopsis ferox*
▷ ***Lobivia pentlandii*** see *Echinopsis pentlandii*
▷ ***Lobivia silvestrii*** see *Echinopsis chamaecereus*
▷ **Loblolly bay** see *Gordonia lasianthus*
▷ **Lobster claw** see *Clianthus puniceus, Vriesea carinata*

LOBULARIA

Sweet Alison, Sweet alyssum

BRASSICACEAE/CRUCIFERAE

Genus of 5 species of low, mound-forming or spreading, hairy annuals and perennials from seashores, disturbed ground, and stony slopes in the Canary Islands and Mediterranean. They have narrow, linear-lance-shaped to oblong, light to mid-green leaves. In summer and early autumn, they produce cross-shaped, 4-petalled, often scented white flowers in compact, sometimes corymb-like, terminal racemes that elongate in fruit. Grown for their flowers, they are useful for the edges of a gravel drive or to fill paving cracks, and are very tolerant of maritime conditions. *L. maritima* cultivars are particularly good summer bedding plants.

- **HARDINESS** Fully hardy.
- **CULTIVATION** Grow in light, moderately fertile, well-drained soil in full sun. Clip over after the first flush of bloom to encourage further flowering.
- **PROPAGATION** Sow seed *in situ* in late spring.
- **PESTS AND DISEASES** Downy mildew, slugs, flea beetles, clubroot, and white blister may be troublesome.

L. maritima, syn. *Alyssum maritimum.* Freely branching, usually compact, low-growing annual or short-lived perennial with linear-lance-shaped, slightly hairy,

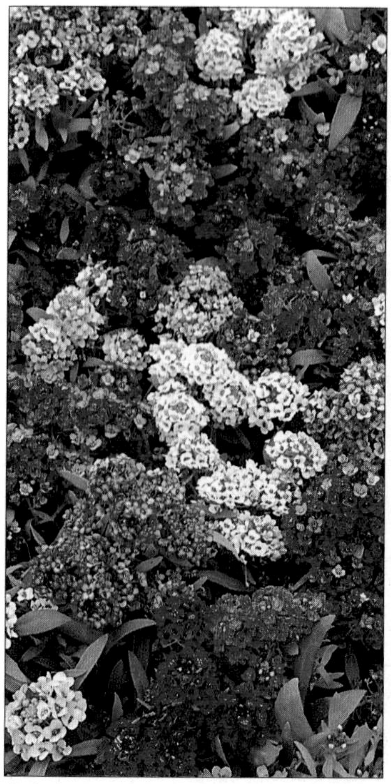

Lobularia maritima Easter Bonnet Series

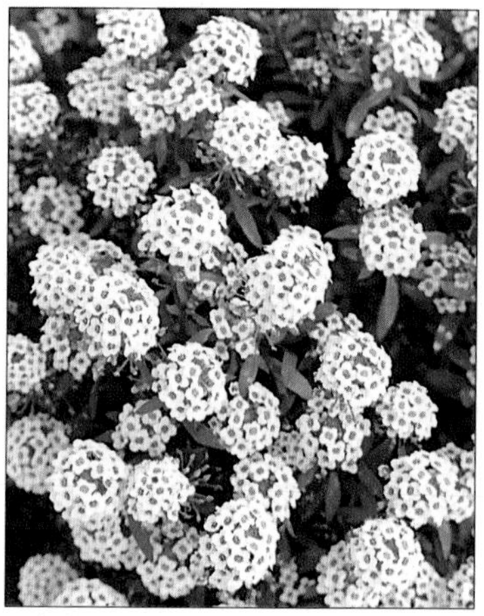

Lobularia maritima 'Little Dorrit'

grey-green leaves, 3cm (1¼in) long. In summer, produces tiny, cross-shaped, slightly cupped, scented, white, occasionally pale purple-pink flowers in rounded, corymb-like racemes, 2.5–8cm (1–3in) across. ↕ 5–30cm (2–12in), ↔ 20–30cm (8–12in). Mediterranean, Canary Islands. ❄❄❄. **Alice Series** cultivars are compact, and bear white, purple, or rose-pink flowers; ↕ 8cm (3in). **'Carpet of Snow'** is loosely branched and ground-hugging, with white flowers; ↕ to 10cm (4in). Cultivars of **Easter Bonnet Series** ■ are very compact, bearing early, white, reddish purple, or pink flowers; ↕ 8–10cm (3–4in). **'Little Dorrit'** ■ is loosely branched and spreading, with white flowers; ↕ to 10cm (4in). **'Navy Blue'** is very compact, with deep purple flowers; ↕ to 10cm (4in). **'New Purple'** is very compact and long-flowering, with purple flowers, shading to a lighter tone at the petal margins; ↕ to 10cm (4in). **'Rosario'** is vigorous and compact, with rose-pink flowers; ↕ 10cm (4in). **'Snowcloth'** is spreading, with white flowers. **'Snow Crystals'** ■ is mound-forming and compact, and bears white flowers; ↕ to 25cm (10in). **'Wonderland Rose'** is less densely branched and more compact than 'Snowcloth', and bears rose-pink flowers; ↕ to 15cm (6in).

▷ **Locust** see *Robinia pseudoacacia*
Black see *Robinia pseudoacacia*
Bristly see *Robinia hispida*
Caspian see *Gleditsia caspica*
Honey see *Gleditsia triacanthos*
New Mexico see *Robinia neomexicana*

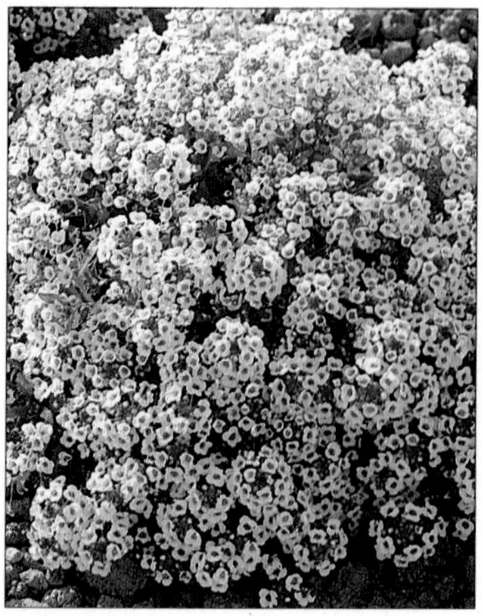

Lobularia maritima 'Snow Crystals'

LODOICEA

Coco-de-mer, Double coconut

ARECACEAE/PALMAE

Genus of one rare species of single-stemmed, dioecious palm found in wooded valleys in the Seychelles. It produces terminal clusters of fan-shaped leaves, and spikes of 3-petalled flowers between the lower leaves, followed by very large, coconut-like fruit. In frost-prone climates, grow in a warm greenhouse. In tropical climates, grow as a specimen plant.

- **HARDINESS** Frost tender.
- **CULTIVATION** Under glass, grow in loam-based potting compost (JI No.3) with added leaf mould, in full light. In the growing season, water freely and apply a balanced liquid fertilizer every month; water sparingly in winter. Outdoors, grow in fertile, moist but well-drained soil in full sun.
- **PROPAGATION** Sow seed at 24°C (75°F) in spring, half-buried in damp sand, in containers at least 1m (3ft) deep to allow room for the roots to develop.
- **PESTS AND DISEASES** Trouble free.

L. maldivica 🌴 syn. *L. seychellarum.* Large palm with a columnar trunk that is slightly swollen at the base and ringed with old leaf scars. Robust leaf-stalks, 3–4m (10–12ft) long, support fan-shaped blades, to 7m (22ft) long, glossy, rich green above, matt and densely woolly beneath, and divided for up to one-third of their length into many narrow, often pendent lobes. Green flowers are borne in spikes, to 2m (6ft) long, at intervals throughout the year, followed on female trees by heavy, woody, broadly heart-shaped, green then brown fruit, to 50cm (20in) across, which take 6 years to mature. ↕ to 30m (100ft), ↔ 15–20m (50–70ft). Seychelles. 🏠 (min. 20°C/68°F)

L. seychellarum see *L. maldivica.*

LOISELEURIA

Alpine azalea, Trailing azalea

ERICACEAE

Genus of one species of mat-forming, evergreen shrub from high alpine and subarctic regions in Europe, Japan, and North America. Cultivated for its foliage and flowers, it is suitable for a rock garden, peat bed, or alpine house, but is difficult to grow in dry climates.

- **HARDINESS** Fully hardy.
- **CULTIVATION** Grow in moderately fertile, humus-rich, moist but well-drained, acid soil in full sun. In an alpine house, use a mix of 4 parts peat or leaf mould and 1 part sharp sand.
- **PROPAGATION** Root softwood cuttings in early summer, or semi-ripe cuttings in midsummer. Layer in spring.
- **PESTS AND DISEASES** Trouble free.

L. procumbens. Prostrate shrub forming tight mats of crowded, oval to oblong, glossy, dark green leaves, to 1cm (½in) long. Terminal, upturned, broadly cup-shaped, rose-pink to white flowers, 6mm (¼in) across, are borne singly or in small umbels in early summer. ↕ 8cm (3in), ↔ to 30cm (12in). Europe, Japan, North America. ❄❄❄

▷ **Lollipop plant** see *Pachystachys lutea*

LOMANDRA

Mat rush

LOMANDRACEAE

Genus of over 50 species of tuft- or tussock-forming, rhizomatous perennials found in a wide range of habitats in Australia, Papua New Guinea, and New Caledonia. They have linear, flat or cylindrical, hairy or hairless leaves. The male and female flowers, borne in spikes, racemes, or panicles, are often inconspicuous and not long-lasting. Some species are aromatic, others have an overpowering smell. Grow for mass planting or as individual accent plants. In damp, frost-prone areas, grow in a cool greenhouse or conservatory.

- **HARDINESS** Frost hardy to frost tender.
- **CULTIVATION** Outdoors, grow in any well-drained soil in full sun, or in partial shade in very hot regions. Rejuvenate old clumps by burning off the foliage. Under glass, grow in well-drained loam-based potting compost (JI No.2) in full light. Water moderately during the growing season, sparingly in winter.
- **PROPAGATION** Sow seed at 13–18°C (55–64°F) as soon as ripe. Divide in spring.
- **PESTS AND DISEASES** Trouble free.

L. glauca (Pale mat rush). Tussock-forming perennial with linear, mainly flat, mid-green leaves, 8–20cm (3–8in) long. In summer, bears cylindrical or tubular, purple-flushed yellow flowers, 5mm (¼in) long: the male flowers clustered in spikes 10–15cm (4–6in) long, the female flowers borne in spherical heads 1.5cm (½in) across. ↕ 20cm (8in), ↔ 35cm (14in). Australia (New South Wales). ❄❄

L. longifolia ▣ (Spiny-headed mat rush). Dense, tussock-forming perennial with linear, flat or nearly flat, yellow-green to dark green leaves, 1m (3ft) long. In summer, cylindrical, often fragrant, yellow or cream, male and female flowers, 4mm (⅛in) long, are borne in racemes or panicles 30–90cm (12–36in) long. ↕ 1m (3ft), ↔ 2m (6ft). Australia (E. South Australia, New South Wales, E. Tasmania). ❄❄

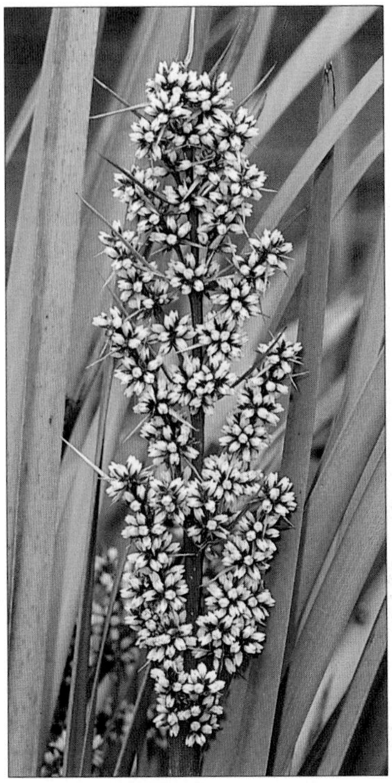

Lomandra longifolia

▷ ***Lomaria gibba*** see *Blechnum gibbum*

LOMATIA

PROTEACEAE

Genus of about 12 species of evergreen trees and shrubs from moist woodland in Australasia and South America. They have opposite or alternate, entire to pinnatifid, or pinnate to 3-pinnate leaves, and racemes of initially tubular, later star-shaped flowers, with 4 narrow, twisted lobes and prominent, curved styles. Grow in a woodland garden or shrub border.

- **HARDINESS** Frost hardy.
- **CULTIVATION** Grow in poor to moderately fertile, moist but well-drained, acid to neutral soil in full sun or in partial shade. Shelter from cold winds in frost-prone areas. Pruning group 1.
- **PROPAGATION** Take softwood cuttings in early summer, or semi-ripe cuttings in midsummer.
- **PESTS AND DISEASES** Trouble free.

L. ferruginea ▣♀ Upright, bushy shrub or small tree with felted brown shoots and oblong to oval, 2-pinnate, dark green leaves, to 50cm (20in) long, the ovate-lance-shaped leaflets sometimes deeply lobed and fawn-felted beneath. In midsummer, bears yellow-and-red flowers, 1.5cm (½in) long, in axillary racemes to 5cm (2in) long. ↕ 10m (30ft), ↔ 5m (15ft). Chile, Argentina. ❄❄

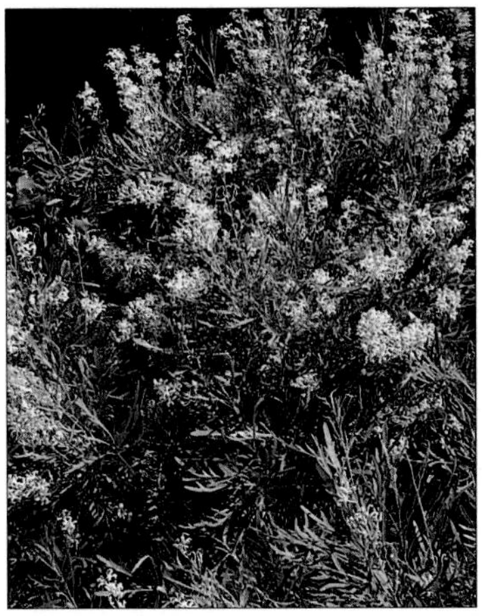

Lomatia silaifolia

L. silaifolia ▣ Bushy shrub with upright branches bearing 2- or 3-pinnate, dark green leaves, to 30cm (12in) long, composed of lance-shaped leaflets with margins rolled under. In mid- and late summer, bears fragrant, creamy white flowers, 1.5cm (½in) long, in erect racemes or panicles, to 30cm (12in) long. ↕↔ 2m (6ft). S.E. Australia. ❄❄

L. tinctoria. Small, bushy, often suckering shrub with ovate to triangular, pinnate or 2-pinnate (rarely simple), dark green leaves, to 8cm (3in) long, deeply and finely cut into linear-lance-shaped leaflets. Fragrant, creamy white flowers, 1cm (½in) long, are borne in racemes to 10cm (4in) or more long, in midsummer. ↕ 1m (3ft), ↔ 1.5m (5ft). Australia (Tasmania). ❄❄

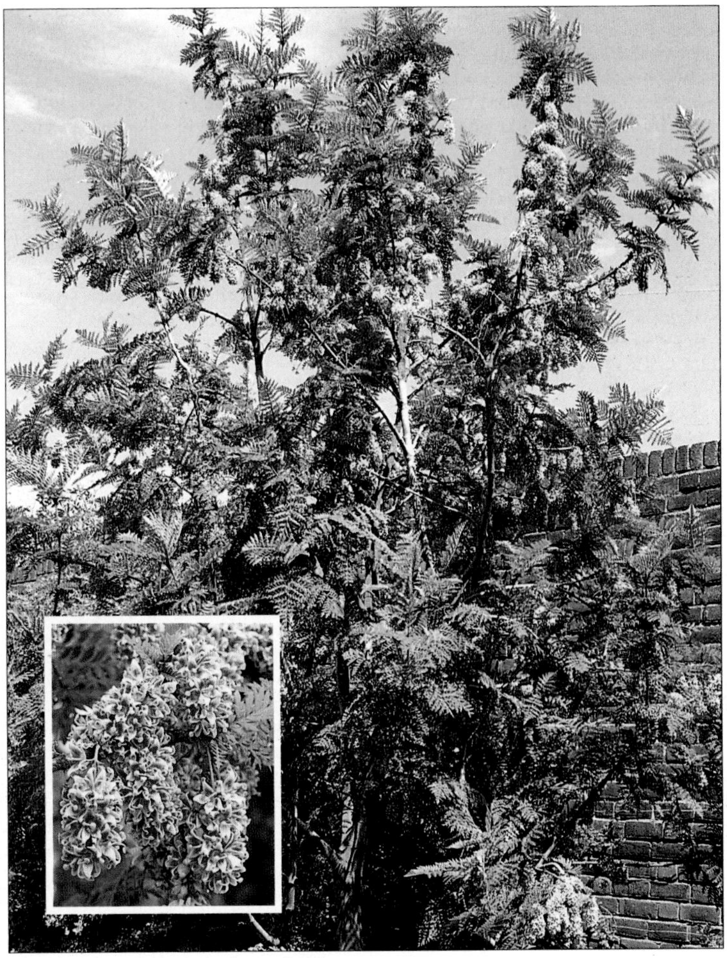

Lomatia ferruginea (inset: flower detail)

LOMATIUM

APIACEAE/UMBELLIFERAE

Genus of approximately 60 species of tap-rooted herbaceous perennials from open areas and rock crevices in W. North America. Cultivated for their foliage and flowers, they have finely divided, pinnate to 4-pinnate, fern-like leaves, and produce compound umbels of tiny, yellow, green, purple, or white flowers in spring and summer. Suitable for a rock garden or raised bed.
• **HARDINESS** Fully hardy to frost hardy.
• **CULTIVATION** Grow in moderately fertile, sharply drained soil in full sun.
• **PROPAGATION** Sow seed in containers in a cold frame as soon as ripe.
• **PESTS AND DISEASES** Trouble free.

L. dissectum. Low-growing perennial with triangular, 2- to 4-pinnate, fresh mid-green leaves, to 15–35cm (6–14in) long, composed of oblong leaflets. Bright yellow or purple flowers are borne in rounded, compound umbels, 3–13cm (1¼–5in) across, very early in spring, as the leaves develop. ↕ 15cm (6in) in flower, to 40cm (16in) or more later, ↔ to 20cm (8in). USA (Rocky Mountains). ❄❄❄

LOMATOPHYLLUM

ALOEACEAE/LILIACEAE

L

Genus of about 11 species of mainly stemless, succulent perennials occurring on low, hilly terrain in Madagascar and Mauritius. They have fleshy leaves forming loose rosettes, similar to those of many *Aloe* species, and bear racemes or panicles of diurnal, bell-shaped or tubular flowers in summer. Where temperatures drop below 12°C (54°F), grow as houseplants or in a warm greenhouse; in warmer climates, grow in a shrub border or desert garden.
• **HARDINESS** Frost tender.
• **CULTIVATION** Under glass, grow in loam-based potting compost (JI No.2) with added leaf mould and grit, in full light. From early spring to early autumn, water freely and apply a half-strength balanced liquid fertilizer every 6–8 weeks. Keep barely moist at other times. Outdoors, grow in moderately fertile, sharply drained soil in full sun. See also pp.48–49.
• **PROPAGATION** Sow seed at 19–24°C (66–75°F), or detach offsets, in spring.
• **PESTS AND DISEASES** Susceptible to scale insects.

L. citreum see *L. occidentale* var. *citreum.*
L. occidentale. Stemless or short-stemmed, succulent perennial forming rosettes of 15–20 stiff, spreading, lance-shaped, mid-green leaves, 80–100cm (32–39in) long, with recurved, toothed or sparsely spiny margins. In summer, produces dense panicles of 50 or more tubular, deep pink flowers, 2–3cm (¾–1¼in) long. ↕ to 1m (3ft), ↔ to 1.5m (5ft). W. Madagascar. ⚘ (min. 12°C/54°F). **var. *citreum*,** syn. *L. citreum*, has a short stem, dark green leaves, 30cm (12in) long, and yellowish green flowers; ↕ 45–50cm (18–20in), ↔ 60cm (24in).

LONICERA

Honeysuckle

CAPRIFOLIACEAE

Genus of about 180 species of deciduous and evergreen shrubs and twining climbers, widely distributed in the N. hemisphere, where they grow in varied habitats ranging from woodland and thickets to rocky places. They are cultivated mainly for their tubular or funnel- to bell-shaped, often fragrant flowers, which are usually 2-lipped or have 5 small, spreading lobes. The leaves are borne in opposite pairs and are usually simple. Honeysuckles may be grown in a variety of situations: train climbers on a wall or fence, or into a large shrub or small tree; grow shrubs in a shrub border, or use for hedging or ground cover. In frost-prone climates, grow half-hardy species in a cool greenhouse. The berries may cause mild stomach upset if ingested.
• **HARDINESS** Fully hardy to half hardy.
• **CULTIVATION** Grow shrubs in any well-drained soil in full sun or partial shade; grow climbers in fertile, humus-rich, moist but well-drained soil. All will tolerate full sun, but are less prone to aphids in partial shade. Under glass, grow in loam-based potting compost (JI No.3) in bright filtered light. When in growth, water freely and apply a balanced liquid fertilizer monthly; water sparingly in winter. Pruning group 2 for shrubs; group 11 for climbers (those flowering on the previous year's shoots, such as *L. periclymenum*, are best pruned back to strong young growth immediately after flowering each year). Trim hedges twice during summer.
• **PROPAGATION** Sow seed of hardy species in containers in a cold frame as soon as ripe; sow *L. hildebrandiana* at 13–18°C (55–64°F) in spring. Take semi-ripe cuttings of evergreens in summer, and greenwood or hardwood cuttings of deciduous honeysuckles in summer or autumn respectively.
• **PESTS AND DISEASES** Aphids may be a problem, particularly on some climbers.

L. x americana ▣ ♀ Vigorous, woody, deciduous, twining climber with paired, oval, dark green leaves, to 8cm (3in) long, the upper pairs united. Large whorls of tubular, 2-lipped, very fragrant yellow flowers, to 5cm (2in) long, strongly flushed red-purple, are borne in the leaf axils in summer and early autumn, followed by red berries. ↕ 7m (22ft). Garden origin. ❄❄❄
L. x bella. Upright, deciduous shrub with paired, ovate, pointed, mid-green leaves, to 5cm (2in) long. Axillary pairs of tubular, 5-lobed, pink or red flowers, 1.5–3cm (½–1¼in) long, becoming yellow, are produced in summer, and are followed by red berries. ↕ 2.5m (8ft), ↔ 3m (10ft). Garden origin. ❄❄❄. **'Atrorosea'** bears dark pink flowers with paler margins, in late spring. **'Candida'** bears white flowers.
L. x brownii (*L. hirsuta* x *L. sempervirens*) (Scarlet trumpet honeysuckle). Deciduous or semi-evergreen, twining climber with paired, ovate, blue-green leaves, to 8cm (3in) long. Bears terminal whorls of tubular, 2-lipped, slightly fragrant, orange to red flowers, 3.5cm (1½in) long, in summer,

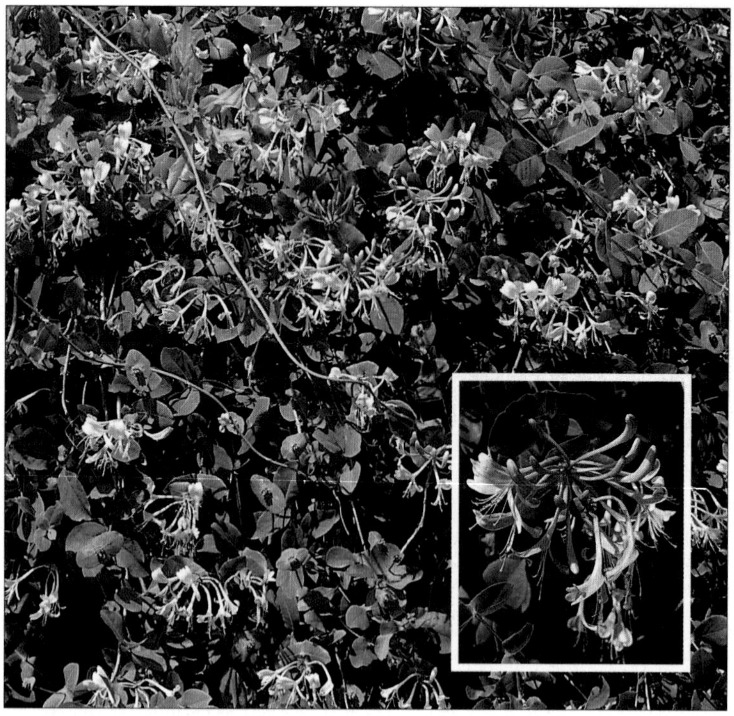

Lonicera x *americana* (inset: flower detail)

sometimes followed by red berries. ↕ 4m (12ft). Garden origin. ❄❄❄. **'Dropmore Scarlet'** ▣ bears long, trumpet-shaped, bright scarlet flowers over a long period. **'Fuchsioides'** has orange-scarlet flowers.
L. caprifolium ♀ (Italian honeysuckle). Woody, deciduous, twining climber with paired, oval to obovate, grey-green leaves, to 10cm (4in) long, the upper pairs united. Whorls of tubular, 2-lipped, very fragrant, pink-flushed, creamy white to yellow flowers, to 5cm (2in) long, are borne from the leaf axils in summer, and are followed by orange-red berries. ↕ 6m (20ft). Europe, W. Asia. ❄❄❄. **'Praecox'** bears creamy white flowers in late spring; they are often tinted light red, and turn yellow.
L. chaetocarpa. Upright, deciduous shrub with bristly shoots and paired, ovate to oblong, bristly, mid-green leaves, to 8cm (3in) long. In early summer, paired, sometimes solitary, funnel-shaped, 5-lobed, primrose-yellow flowers, to 3cm (1¼in) long, with large, leafy, pale green bracts, are borne in the leaf axils; the berries are red and cupped by the persistent, now red-tinted bracts. ↕↔ 2m (6ft). W. China. ❄❄❄

L. etrusca (Etruscan honeysuckle). Vigorous, woody, twining, deciduous or semi-evergreen climber with paired, oval or obovate, mid-green leaves, to 10cm (4in) long, blue-green beneath, the upper pairs united. Tubular, 2-lipped, fragrant yellow flowers, 5cm (2in) long, flushed red and darkening with age, are produced in terminal and axillary whorls from midsummer to autumn, and are followed by red berries. Grows best in full sun. ↕ 4m (12ft). Mediterranean. ❄❄❄ (borderline). **'Donald Waterer'** produces flowers that are red outside, becoming orange-yellow, and white inside. **'Superba'** ▣ is vigorous, and produces large clusters of cream flowers that turn orange.
L. fragrantissima. Bushy, spreading, deciduous or semi-evergreen shrub with paired, oval leaves, to 7cm (3in) long, dull, dark green above, blue-green beneath, with bristly margins when young. Tubular, 2-lipped, very fragrant, creamy white flowers, 1cm (½in) long, are produced in pairs from the leaf axils in winter and early spring, but are often sparsely produced unless grown against a wall. Berries are dull red. ↕ 2m (6ft), ↔ 3m (10ft). China. ❄❄❄

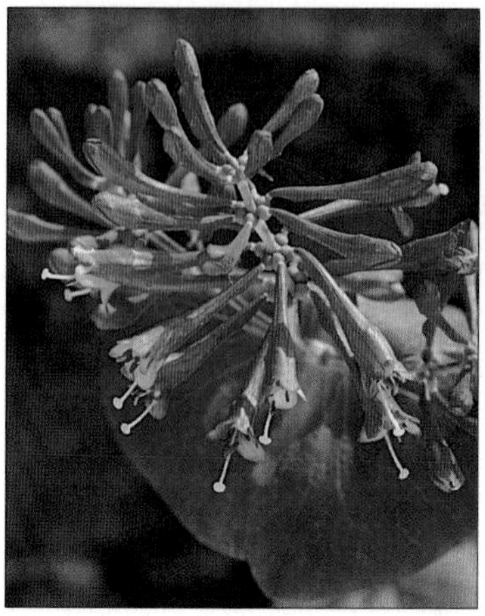

Lonicera x *brownii* 'Dropmore Scarlet'

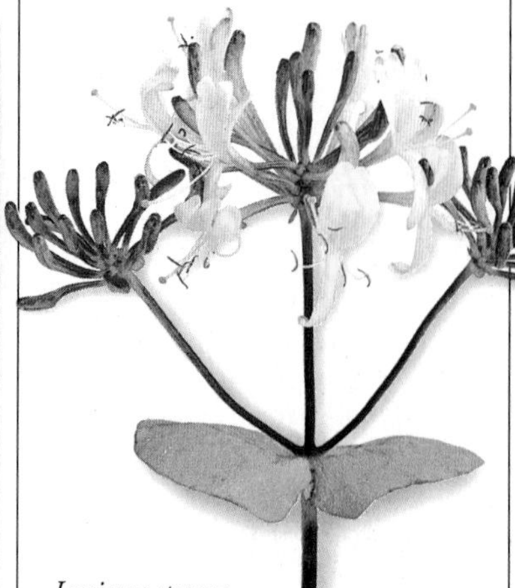

Lonicera etrusca 'Superba'

▷**London pride** see *Saxifraga* x *urbium*

LONICERA

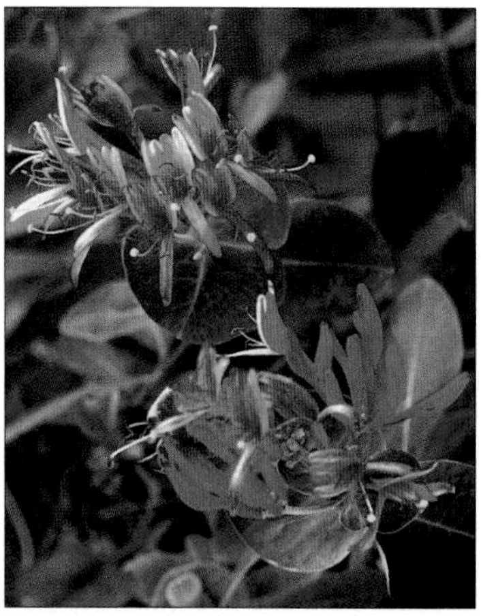

Lonicera x *heckrottii*

L. giraldii. Evergreen, twining climber with densely hairy shoots and paired, narrowly oblong, velvet-textured, dark green leaves, to 8cm (3in) long, with long, sharp points and heart-shaped bases. Dense, terminal whorls of tubular, 2-lipped, purple-red flowers, to 2cm (¾in) long, with yellow stamens, are produced in early and midsummer, followed by white-frosted, purple-black berries. ↕ 5m (15ft). China. ❄❄❄
***L.* 'Gold Flame'** see *L.* x *heckrottii* 'Gold Flame'.
L.* x *heckrottii ■ (*L.* x *americana* x *L. sempervirens*). Deciduous or semi-evergreen, twining climber with paired, oblong to oval or elliptic, dark green leaves, to 6cm (2½in) long, blue-green beneath, with the upper pairs united. Tubular, 2-lipped, fragrant flowers, 4cm (1½in) long, pink outside, orange-yellow inside, are borne in terminal whorls during summer, and are sometimes followed by red berries. ↕ 5m (15ft). Garden origin. ❄❄❄. **'Gold Flame'**, syn. *L.* 'Gold Flame', is more vigorous, with brighter coloured flowers.
L. henryi. Vigorous, woody, evergreen, twining climber with paired, oblong-lance-shaped to oblong-ovate, tapered, glossy, dark green leaves, to 10cm (4in) long. Terminal or axillary whorls of tubular, 2-lipped, yellow-throated, purplish red flowers, to 2cm (¾in) long, are produced in early and midsummer, followed by purple-black berries. ↕ 10m (30ft). W. China. ❄❄❄ (borderline)
L. hildebrandiana ■ (Giant Burmese honeysuckle). Very vigorous, evergreen or semi-evergreen, twining climber with paired, broadly ovate or oval, dark green leaves, to 15cm (6in) long. Tubular, 2-lipped, very fragrant, creamy white flowers, to 8–15cm (3–6in) long, ageing to orange, are borne in pairs in terminal and axillary racemes in summer, and are followed by red berries. ↕ 10m (30ft) or more. China, S.E. Asia. ❄
L. involucrata (Twinberry). Dense, bushy, deciduous shrub with stout shoots and paired, ovate to oblong or lance-shaped, bright mid-green leaves, to 12cm (5in) long. Tubular, dark yellow, often red-suffused flowers, 1cm (½in) long, each with 5 short lobes, are borne in pairs from the leaf axils in late spring; they are surrounded by large green bracts that soon turn red, and are followed by glossy black berries. ↕ 2m (6ft), ↔ 3m (10ft). W. North America, Mexico. ❄❄❄
L. japonica (Japanese honeysuckle). Vigorous, woody, evergreen or semi-evergreen, twining climber with paired, broadly elliptic to ovate, sometimes deeply lobed, dark green leaves, to 8cm (3in) long. Tubular, 2-lipped, very fragrant, often purple-flushed, white flowers, to 4cm (1½in) long, ageing to yellow, are borne in pairs from the leaf axils over a long period from spring to late summer, followed by blue-black berries. ↕ 10m (30ft). E. Asia. ❄❄❄. **'Aureoreticulata'** has leaves attractively veined yellow; ↕ 6m (20ft); ❄❄. **'Dart's World'** is a particularly hardy evergreen cultivar of bushy, spreading habit, with dark green leaves and very fragrant, strongly red-flushed white flowers that turn yellow. **'Halliana'** ■ ♀ is very vigorous, with pure white flowers that age to dark yellow. **var. *repens*** has purple-tinged foliage, and produces white flowers heavily flushed red-purple. **var. *repens* 'Red Coral'** see 'Superba'. **'Superba'**, syn. var. *repens* 'Red Coral', has mid-green leaves, 5cm (2in) long, and bears scarlet flowers, 4–5cm (1½–2in) long.
L. korolkowii ■ Open, spreading, deciduous shrub with arching shoots and paired, ovate or oval leaves, to 3cm (1¼in) long, with long, sharp points, glaucous pale green above, glaucous blue-green beneath. In early summer, bears tubular, 2-lipped, pale rose-pink flowers, 1.5cm (½in) long, in pairs along the shoots, followed by bright red berries. ↕ 3m (10ft), ↔ 5m (15ft). Mountains of C. Asia, Afghanistan, Pakistan. ❄❄❄. **var. *zabelii***, syn. *L. tatarica* 'Zabelii', bears bright pink flowers.

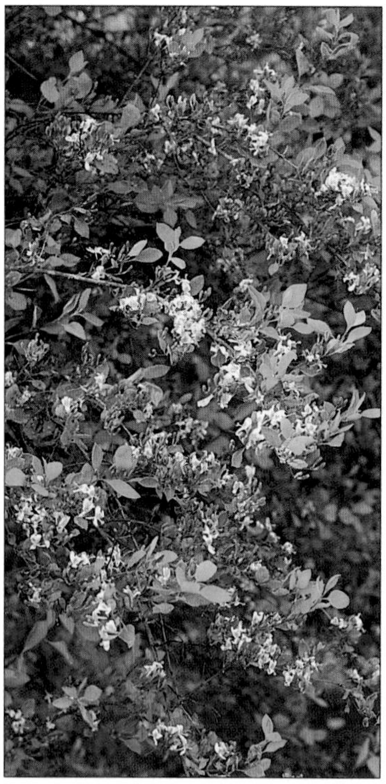

Lonicera korolkowii

L. ledebourii ■ Dense, bushy, deciduous shrub with stout shoots and paired, ovate-oblong, dark green leaves, to 12cm (5in) long. Funnel-shaped, 5-lobed, red-flushed, deep orange-yellow flowers, to 2cm (¾in) long, each with 2 large, persistent red bracts, are borne from the leaf axils in late spring and early summer, followed by glossy black berries. ↕ 3m (10ft), ↔ 4m (12ft). USA (California). ❄❄❄
L. maackii. Vigorous, upright, often tree-like, deciduous shrub with paired, oval-lance-shaped, tapered, dark green leaves, to 8cm (3in) long. Tubular, 2-lipped, fragrant white flowers, to 2cm (¾in) long, ageing to yellow, are borne in axillary pairs along the shoots in early summer, followed by dark red berries. ↕↔ 5m (15ft). China, Korea, Japan. ❄❄❄
L. morrowii. Spreading, deciduous shrub with arching branches and paired, oblong or ovate to elliptic, dull mid-green leaves, to 6cm (2½in) long, purple-tinged when young. Pairs of tubular, creamy white flowers, 1.5cm (½in) long, ageing to yellow, each with 5 short lobes, are borne along the shoots in late spring and early summer,

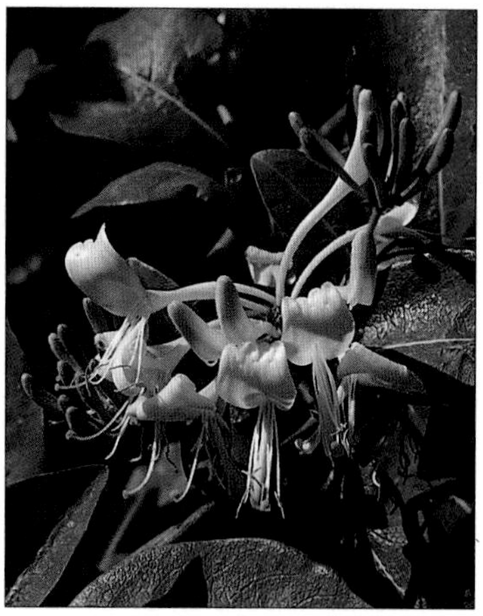

Lonicera periclymenum 'Graham Thomas'

followed by red berries. ↕ 2m (6ft), ↔ 3m (10ft). Japan. ❄❄❄
L. nitida. Bushy, evergreen shrub with paired, ovate to broadly ovate leaves, to 1cm (½in) long, glossy, dark green above, lighter beneath. Produces pairs of tubular, creamy white flowers, to 1cm (½in) long, from the leaf axils in spring, followed by glossy, blue-purple berries. Good for hedging. ↕ to 3.5m (11ft), ↔ 3m (10ft). S.W. China. ❄❄❄. **'Baggesen's Gold'** ♀ has long, arching shoots and ovate, bright yellow leaves; ↕↔ 1.5m (5ft). **'Ernest Wilson'** is vigorous and spreading, with tiny, ovate, dark green leaves, 3–6mm (⅛–¼in) long; ↕ 2m (6ft). **'Yunnan'** is broad and upright, with larger leaves, 2cm (¾in) long, and with abundant flowers and berries; ↕↔ 2m (6ft).
L. periclymenum (Common honey-suckle, Woodbine). Vigorous, woody, deciduous, twining climber with paired, ovate, oval, or obovate, mid-green leaves, to 6cm (2½in) long, glaucous beneath. Terminal whorls of tubular, 2-lipped, very fragrant, white to yellow, often red-flushed flowers, to 5cm (2in) long, are borne in mid- and late summer, followed by bright red berries. ↕ 7m (22ft). Europe, North Africa, Turkey, Caucasus. ❄❄❄. **'Belgica'** ♀ (Early Dutch honeysuckle) produces white flowers that turn yellow, and are richly streaked red outside. **'Graham Thomas'** ■ ♀ has white flowers turning yellow, borne over a long period. **'Serotina'** ■ ♀ (Late Dutch honey-suckle) produces creamy white flowers streaked dark red-purple.

L

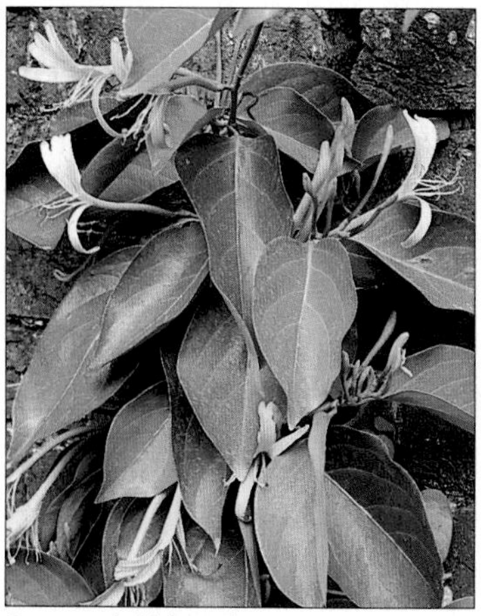

Lonicera hildebrandiana

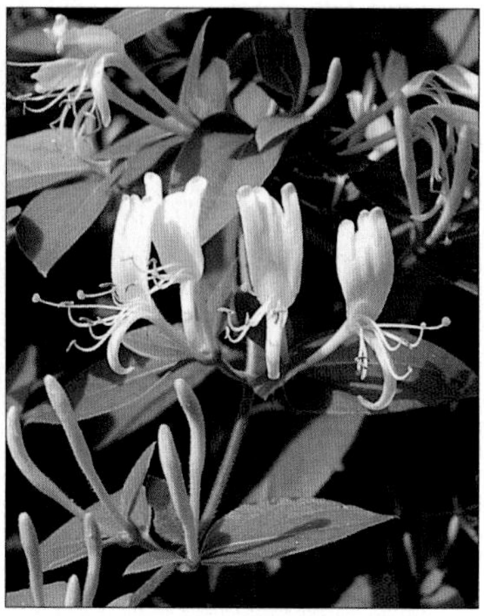

Lonicera japonica 'Halliana'

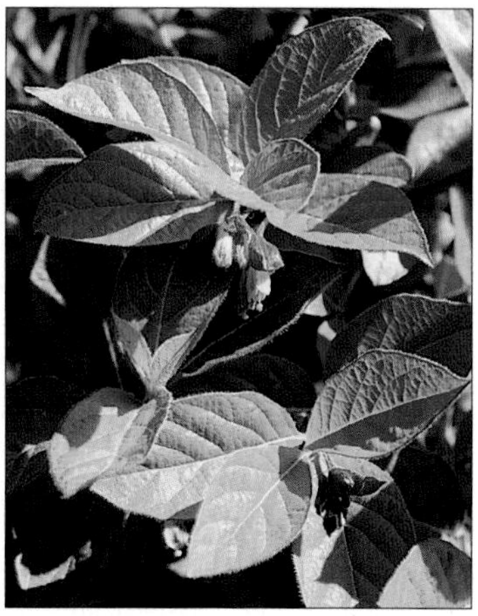

Lonicera ledebourii

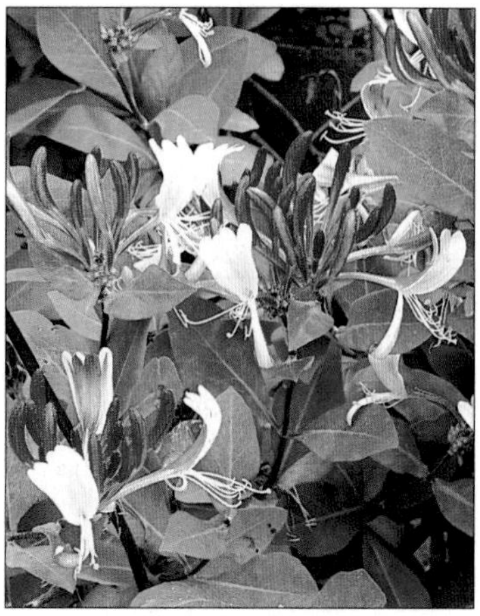

Lonicera periclymenum 'Serotina'

L. pileata. Dense, spreading, evergreen shrub with paired, ovate-oblong to oblong-lance-shaped, glossy, dark green leaves, to 3cm (1¼in) long. Funnel-shaped, 5-lobed, creamy white flowers, to 8mm (⅜in) long, are produced in pairs from the leaf axils in late spring, followed by violet-purple berries. Good ground cover. ↕ 60cm (24in), ↔ 2.5m (8ft). China. ❄❄❄

***L.* x *purpusii* 'Winter Beauty'** ♀ Rounded, deciduous or semi-evergreen shrub with red-purple shoots and paired, ovate, dark green leaves, to 8cm (3in) long. Tubular, 2-lipped, very fragrant white flowers, 2cm (¾in) long, with conspicuous yellow anthers, are produced in small, axillary clusters in winter and early spring. Berries are rarely produced. ↕ 2m (6ft), ↔ 2.5m (8ft). ❄❄❄

L. rupicola* var. *syringantha see *L. syringantha.*

L. sempervirens ■ ♀ (Coral honeysuckle, Trumpet honeysuckle). Woody, deciduous or evergreen, twining climber with paired, oval or obovate leaves, to 7cm (3in) long, dark green above, blue-green beneath, the upper pairs united. Tubular flowers, to 5cm (2in) long, with 2 short lips, rich scarlet-orange outside, yellowish orange inside, are produced in terminal whorls in summer and autumn, and are followed by bright red berries. ↕ 4m (12ft). E. and S. USA. ❄❄❄ (borderline). **f. *sulphurea*** produces yellow flowers.

L

L. standishii. Upright, deciduous or semi-evergreen shrub with paired, oblong-lance-shaped, bristly, dark green leaves, to 10cm (4in) long, with long, slender points. Tubular, 2-lipped, fragrant, creamy white flowers, 3cm (1¼in) long, sometimes tinged very pale pink, are produced in axillary pairs along the shoots from late autumn to early spring, followed by red berries. ↕↔ 2m (6ft). China. ❄❄❄

Lonicera sempervirens

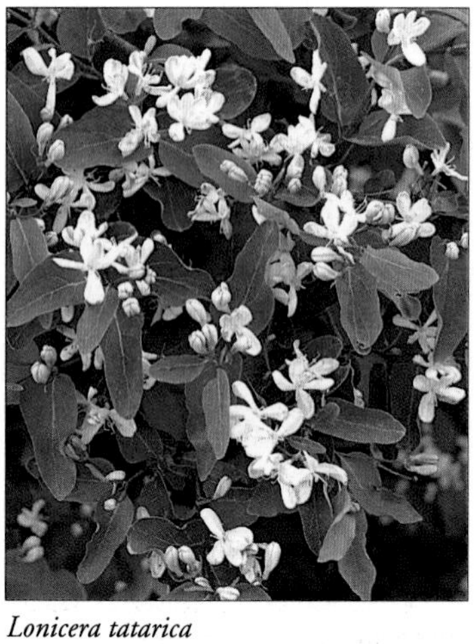

Lonicera tatarica

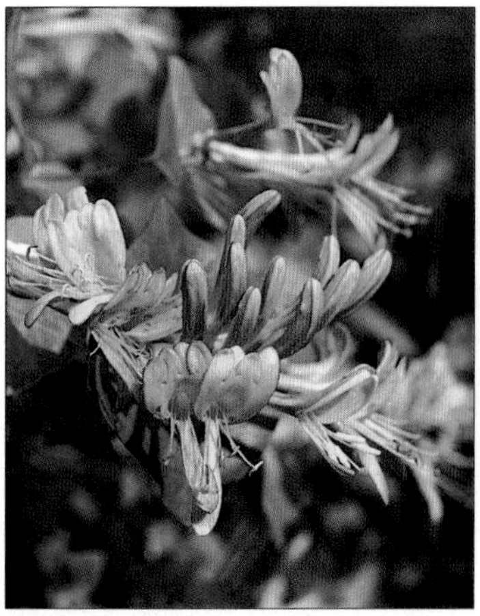

Lonicera x *tellmanniana*

L. syringantha, syn. *L. rupicola* var. *syringantha.* Graceful, rounded, deciduous shrub with oblong-ovate, grey-green leaves, to 2.5cm (1in) long, usually paired, sometimes in threes. Small, tubular-bell-shaped, 5-lobed, very fragrant, lilac-pink flowers, to 1cm (½in) across, are produced in pairs from the leaf axils in late spring and early summer, followed by red berries. ↕ 2–3m (6–10ft), ↔ 2m (6ft). W. China, Tibet. ❄❄❄

L. tatarica ■ Upright, bushy, deciduous shrub with paired, oblong-ovate to lance-shaped, dark green leaves, to 6cm (2½in) long, glaucous beneath. Axillary pairs of tubular, 5-lobed, white to pink or red flowers, to 2.5cm (1in) long, are profusely borne along the shoots in late spring and early summer, followed by scarlet to yellow-orange berries. ↕ 4m (12ft), ↔ 2.5m (8ft). S. Russia to C. Asia. ❄❄❄. **'Arnold Pink'** produces dark rose-pink flowers. **'Hack's Red'** bears very dark purplish red flowers. **'Zabelii'** see *L. korolkowii* var. *zabelii.*

L.* x *tellmanniana ■ ♀ (*L. sempervirens* 'Superba' x *L. tragophylla*). Woody, deciduous, twining climber with paired, elliptic-ovate to oblong, deep green leaves, to 10cm (4in) long, blue-white beneath, the upper pairs united. Terminal whorls of tubular, 2-lipped, bright copper-orange flowers, to 5cm (2in) long, are produced from late spring to midsummer. ↕ 5m (15ft). Garden origin. ❄❄❄

L. tragophylla ♀ Woody, deciduous, twining climber with paired, oval to oblong, mid-green leaves, to 12cm (5in) long, blue-white beneath, the upper pairs united. Long-tubed, 2-lipped, bright yellow or orange-yellow flowers, to 8cm (3in) long, red-tinted above, are produced in large, terminal whorls in mid- and late summer, followed by red berries. ↕ 6m (20ft). C. China. ❄❄❄

***L.* x *xylosteoides* 'Clavey's Dwarf'.** Slow-growing, dense, upright, rounded, deciduous shrub with paired, oval to obovate, grey-green leaves, to 6cm (2½in) long. Pairs of small, tubular, 2-lipped white flowers, 1cm (½in) long, are produced from the leaf axils in late spring and early summer, followed by red berries. Suitable for hedging. ↕ 1.5m (5ft), ↔ 1m (3ft). ❄❄❄

L. xylosteum ■ (Fly honeysuckle). Dense, bushy, deciduous shrub with paired, ovate to obovate or oblong, grey-green leaves, to 6cm (2½in) long. Tubular, 2-lipped, creamy white flowers, to 1cm (½in) long, are produced in pairs along the shoots in late spring and early summer, followed by showy red, rarely yellow berries. ↕↔ 3m (10ft). Europe, Caucasus, Russia (Siberia). ❄❄❄

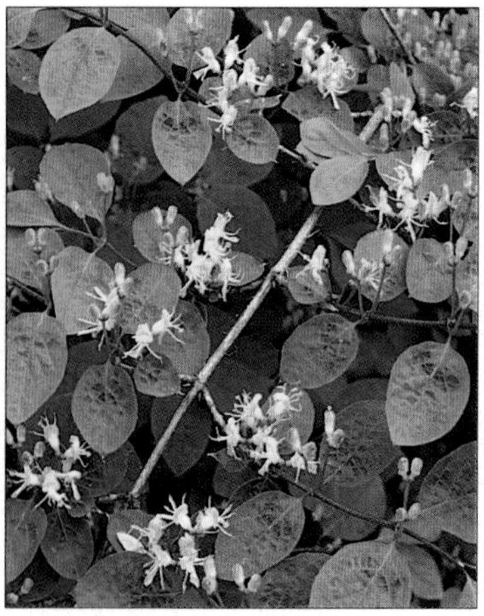

Lonicera xylosteum

▷ **Looking glass plant** see *Coprosma repens*

▷ **Loosestrife** see *Lysimachia, Lythrum*
Purple see *Lythrum salicaria*
Yellow see *Lysimachia vulgaris*

▷ ***Lophocereus*** see *Pachycereus*
L. schottii see *P. schottii*

LOPHOMYRTUS

MYRTACEAE

Genus of 2 species of evergreen shrubs or small trees, closely related to the genus *Myrtus*, occurring in coastal and lowland forest in New Zealand. They are cultivated for their flowers, foliage, and fruits. The leaves are opposite, simple, and leathery. In summer, 4-petalled flowers, each with a boss of prominent stamens, are borne singly from all the upper leaf axils, followed by many-seeded, purple-black to red berries. In frost-prone areas, grow in a cool greenhouse or against a warm wall. In milder areas, plant in a shrub border.

• **HARDINESS** Frost hardy to frost tender.

• **CULTIVATION** Under glass, grow in loam-based potting compost (JI No.2) in bright filtered light. During the growing season, water freely and apply a balanced liquid fertilizer monthly. Water sparingly in winter. Outdoors, grow in fertile, humus-rich, moist but well-drained soil in partial shade. Pruning group 1; may need restrictive pruning under glass.

• **PROPAGATION** Sow seed at 13–18°C (55–64°F) as soon as ripe. Root semi-ripe cuttings, with heels, in summer with bottom heat.

• **PESTS AND DISEASES** Red spider mites may be a problem under glass.

L. bullata ○ syn. *Myrtus bullata.* Rounded, moderately bushy or open, large shrub or small tree with downy stems. Broadly ovate to rounded leaves, 1.5–3cm (½–1¼in) long, sometimes more, are strongly puckered or blistered between the veins, and bronze- to red-tinted when young, maturing to glossy, dark green. In summer, produces open cup-shaped white flowers, 1cm (½in) wide, usually followed by broadly ovoid, deep black-red berries, 7–10mm (¼–½in) long. ↕ 3–8m (10–25ft), ↔ 1–3m (3–10ft). New Zealand. ❄

L.* x *ralphii ○ (*L. bullata* x *L. obcordata*). Large, rounded, vigorous shrub or small tree, of open habit. Broadly oblong-ovate, dark green leaves, usually 1.5–2.5cm (½–1in) long, are flat or slightly blistered between the veins. Mature plants produce open cup-shaped white flowers, 1cm (½in) wide, in summer, followed by dark black-red berries, 4–8mm (⅛–⅜in) long. ↕ 2–5m (6–15ft), ↔ 1.5–2.5m (5–8ft). Garden origin. ❄❄ (borderline). **'Gloriosa'** see 'Variegata'. **'Indian Chief'** has rounded, lustrous, reddish green leaves, to 1cm

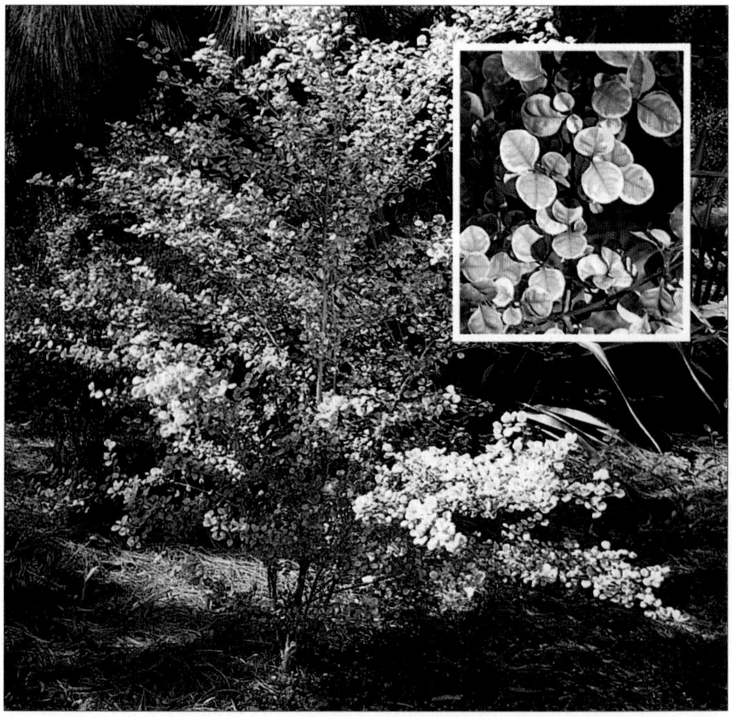

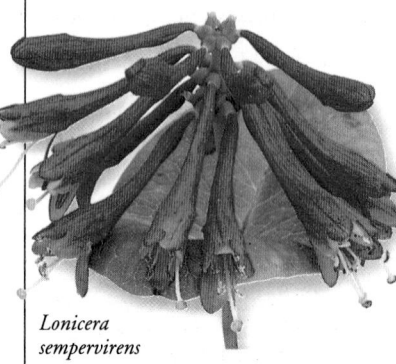

Lophomyrtus x *ralphii* 'Variegata' (inset: leaf detail)

(½in) long. **'Kathryn'** has blistered leaves, flushed rich purple. **'Purpurea'** has slightly blistered, bronze-purple to deep purple-red leaves. **'Sundae'**, syn. 'Tricolor', has almost flat, rich green- and yellow-variegated leaves, with pink or bronze-red overtones, especially in sunny sites. **'Tricolor'** see 'Sundae'. **'Variegata'** ■ syn. 'Gloriosa', *Myrtus bullata* 'Gloriosa', *Myrtus* x *ralphii* 'Variegata', has rounded, lustrous, deep green leaves, barely 1cm (½in) long, with creamy yellow variegation.

LOPHOPHORA

CACTACEAE

Genus of 2 species of variable, perennial cacti occurring in semi-arid areas of S. Texas (USA), and N. and E. Mexico. They have thick, tuberous rootstocks, and flattened-spherical stems that may become more cylindrical with age. Areoles bear a few weak spines when young, later just a few white hairs. Diurnal, solitary, bell-shaped flowers are produced at the tips of the stems and last 2–3 days. Where temperatures drop below 10°C (50°F), grow in a warm greenhouse or as houseplants; in warmer climates, plant outdoors in a desert garden, preferably on sloping ground.

- **HARDINESS** Frost tender.
- **CULTIVATION** Under glass, grow in standard cactus compost with added limestone chippings, in full light. From mid-spring to late summer, water freely and apply a balanced liquid fertilizer every 6–8 weeks. Keep dry at other times. Outdoors, grow in moderately fertile, sharply drained, alkaline soil in full sun. See also pp.48–49.
- **PROPAGATION** Sow seed at 19–24°C (66–75°F) in spring.
- **PESTS AND DISEASES** Trouble free.

L. echinata see *L. williamsii.*
L. lutea see *L. williamsii.*
L. williamsii ■ syn. *L. echinata, L. lutea* (Dumpling cactus). Variable cactus, sometimes solitary, but usually forming large groups. Dark blue-green stems, 5–8cm (2–3in) thick, each have 4–14 low ribs, divided by narrow furrows, with prominent tubercles and white-woolly areoles. Bell-shaped, pink to carmine-red flowers, to 2.5cm (1in) across, sometimes with paler margins, are borne at the crowns from spring to autumn. ↕ to 5cm (2in), ↔ to 30cm (12in), in groups. USA (S. Texas), N. and N.E. Mexico. ❀ (min. 10°C/50°F)

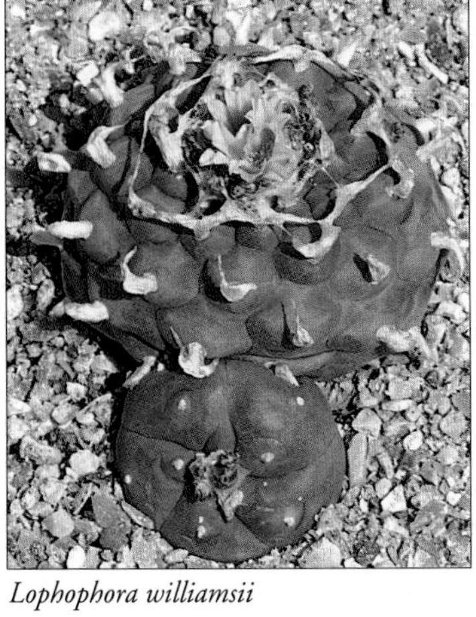

Lophophora williamsii

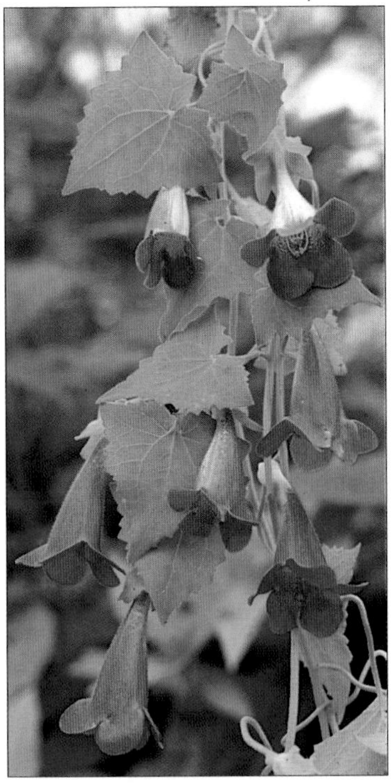

Lophospermum erubescens

LOPHOSPERMUM

SCROPHULARIACEAE

Genus of 8 species of deciduous and evergreen, perennial climbers and shrubs from rocky slopes in North and Central America. They have entire or toothed, triangular to rounded leaves, and bear solitary, axillary, tubular to funnel- or trumpet-shaped, white to purple flowers. In temperate areas, grow in a cool greenhouse. In warmer areas, grow through a shrub or small tree.

- **HARDINESS** Half hardy to frost tender.
- **CULTIVATION** Under glass, grow in loam-based potting compost (JI No.2) with added sharp sand, in full light. In growth, water moderately and apply a balanced liquid fertilizer monthly. Water sparingly in winter. Outdoors, grow in moderately fertile, ideally sandy, moist but well-drained soil in full sun.
- **PROPAGATION** Sow seed at 19–24°C (66–75°F) in spring. Root semi-ripe cuttings in late summer.
- **PESTS AND DISEASES** Trouble free.

L. erubescens ■ 🏆 syn. *Asarina erubescens, Maurandya erubescens* (Creeping gloxinia). Scandent, evergreen, perennial climber (deciduous in cool areas), often grown as an annual, with soft, woody-based stems and triangular, toothed, downy, grey-green leaves, to 7cm (3in) long, with twining leaf-stalks. Bears trumpet-shaped, rose-pink flowers, 7cm (3in) long, in summer and autumn. ↕ 3m (10ft) or more. Mexico. ❀ (min. 3–5°C/27–41°F)

LOPHOSTEMON

MYRTACEAE

Genus of 4–6 species of evergreen trees or tall shrubs, closely related to *Tristania* and *Eucalyptus.* They occur in heavy, moist soil, frequently in rainforest or along the borders of streams, in N. and E. Australia and S. New Guinea. Leaves are simple, usually entire, and borne alternately or in whorls, often more densely towards the stem tips. The flowers have 5 spreading petals and many stamens fused into 5 separate bundles, and are produced in axillary cymes; they are followed by small, woody, cup- or top-shaped, 3-celled seed capsules. In frost-prone areas, grow as foliage plants in a cool or warm greenhouse; flowers are likely to form only on plants 2–3m (6–10ft) tall. In milder areas, lophostemons are good specimen and shade trees, and are effective as a windbreak or hedge.

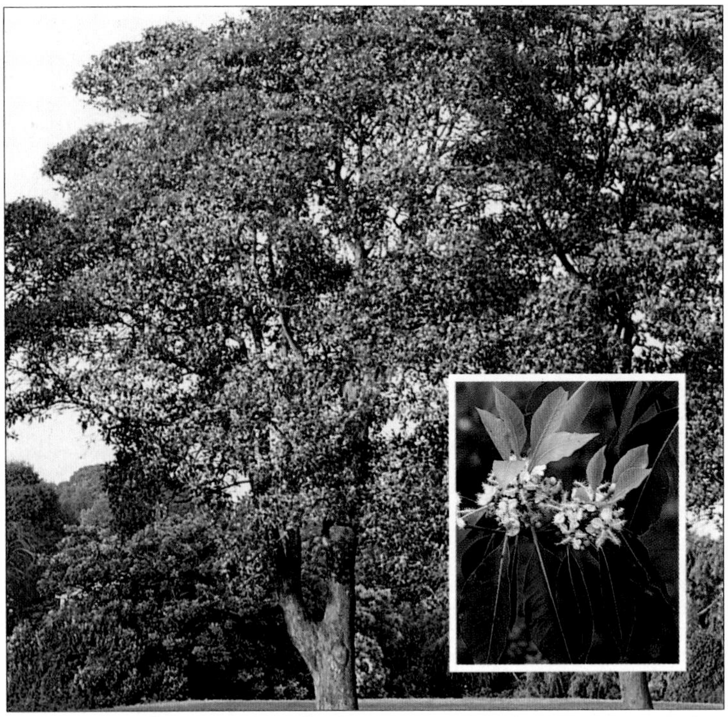

Lophostemon confertus (inset: flower detail)

- **HARDINESS** Half hardy to frost tender.
- **CULTIVATION** Under glass, grow in lime-free (ericaceous) potting compost with added sharp sand, in full or bright filtered light. During the growing season, water freely and apply a half-strength, balanced liquid fertilizer every month; water sparingly in winter. Outdoors, grow in poor to moderately fertile, neutral to acid, moist but well-drained soil in full sun or partial shade. Pruning group 1; trim hedges in late summer.
- **PROPAGATION** Sow seed at 13–18°C (55–64°F) in spring. Root semi-ripe cuttings in summer with bottom heat.
- **PESTS AND DISEASES** Red spider mites may be a problem under glass.

L. confertus ■ ♀ syn. *Tristania conferta* (Brush box). Bushy, round-headed tree with lance-shaped to ovate, smooth, bright green leaves, 7–15cm (3–6in) long, usually in whorls of 3–5. Bears cymes of 3–7 star-shaped white flowers, 2.5–4cm (1–1½in) across, in spring and summer, followed by top-shaped seed capsules, 1.5cm (½in) across. ↕ 10–15m (30–50ft), or to 40m (130ft) in moist, warm climates, ↔ 3–10m (10–30ft) or more. Australia (Queensland, New South Wales). ✲. **'Perth Gold'** has bright green leaves, strongly variegated yellow.

▷**Loquat** see *Eriobotrya japonica*
▷**Lords and ladies** see *Arum*

LOROPETALUM

HAMAMELIDACEAE

Genus of 1, possibly up to 3 species of rounded, evergreen shrubs or small trees found in woodland in the Himalayas, China, and Japan. The alternate leaves are ovate or oval, mid-green and rough above, paler beneath. Clusters of fragrant, spider-like white flowers, with 4 narrow, strap-shaped petals, are borne in terminal cymes in late winter and early spring. Grow in a woodland garden or shrub border.

- **HARDINESS** Frost hardy to half hardy.
- **CULTIVATION** Grow in fertile, humus-rich, moist but well-drained soil in partial shade. Pruning group 8.
- **PROPAGATION** Sow seed in containers in an open frame as soon as ripe. Root semi-ripe cuttings in summer with bottom heat.
- **PESTS AND DISEASES** Trouble free.

L. chinense. Bushy shrub with ovate or oval leaves, 2.5–6cm (1–2½in) long. In late winter or early spring, bears sweetly scented, spider-like white flowers, 2cm (¾in) across, in small, crowded cymes of 3–6. ↕↔ 2m (6ft). China, Burma, Japan. ✲✲ (borderline)

LOTUS syn. DORYCNIUM

LEGUMINOSAE / PAPILIONACEAE

Diverse genus of about 150 species of annuals, short-lived perennials, and deciduous, semi-evergreen, or evergreen subshrubs, found throughout most of the world, some in pasture, others in dryish, rocky areas. The alternate leaves are simple, palmate, or pinnate. Pea-like flowers, in a range of colours, occur either singly from the leaf axils or in terminal or axillary clusters. Suitable for a variety of sites, including a wild garden, rock garden, or shrub border; trailing species are useful for a hanging basket. In frost-prone areas, grow tender species in a cool greenhouse.

• **HARDINESS** Fully hardy to frost tender.
• **CULTIVATION** Under glass, grow in loam-based potting compost (JI No.2) with added grit, in full light. In growth, water freely and apply a balanced liquid fertilizer monthly; water sparingly in winter. Outdoors, grow in moderately fertile, well-drained soil in full sun. Pruning group 9 for shrubs (although most do not need pruning); may need restrictive pruning under glass.
• **PROPAGATION** Sow seed of hardy species in containers outdoors in spring or autumn. Sow seed of half-hardy and frost-tender species at 19–24°C (66–75°F) in spring. Take semi-ripe cuttings of shrubs in summer.
• **PESTS AND DISEASES** Mealybugs, aphids, and red spider mites may be a problem under glass.

L. berthelotii ■ ♀ (Coral gem, Parrot's beak, Pelican's beak). Prostrate or trailing, evergreen subshrub with long stems densely clothed with palmate, silver-grey leaves, each with 3–5 linear leaflets, 1–2cm (½–¾in) long. In spring and early summer, freely bears solitary or paired, orange-red to scarlet, black-centred flowers, 3–4cm (1¼–1½in) long, resembling lobster claws. ↕ 20cm (8in), ↔ indefinite. Canary Islands, Cape Verde Islands. ✲ (borderline)
***L. corniculatus* 'Plenus'** (Double bird's foot trefoil). Spreading perennial with upright or prostrate stems bearing pinnate, mid- to bluish green leaves, each with 5 obovate to rounded leaflets, 0.5–1.5cm (¼–½in) long, the upper 3 separated from the lower 2 by a short stalk. In spring and early summer, produces axillary, umbel-like racemes of 3–8 pea-like, double yellow flowers, 1.5cm (½in) long, orange in bud, and often reddening with age. Less vigorous than the species. Suitable for a rock garden. ↕ 20–30cm (8–12in), ↔ to 30cm (12in) or more. ✲✲✲
L. hirsutus ■ syn. *Dorycnium hirsutum* (Hairy canary clover). Rounded to spreading, evergreen or semi-evergreen,

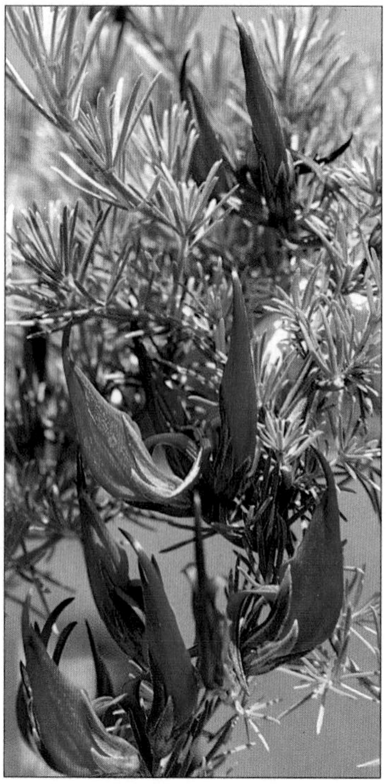

Lotus berthelotii

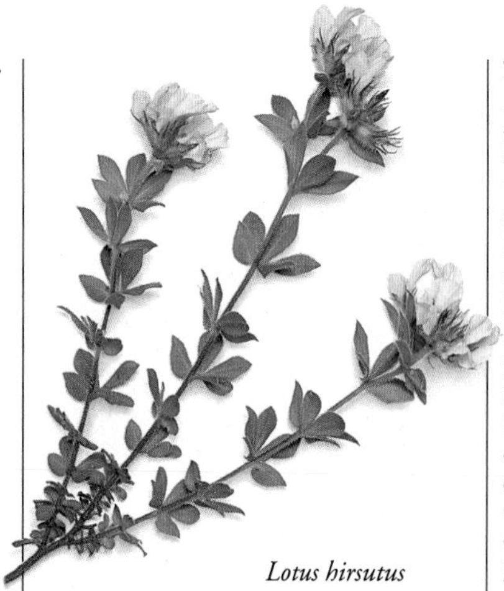

Lotus hirsutus

silver-hairy subshrub with pinnate, densely hairy, grey-green leaves, each consisting of 5 elliptic to narrowly obovate leaflets, to 2cm (¾in) long. In summer and early autumn, produces axillary and terminal umbels of 4–10 pea-like, pink-flushed, creamy white flowers, 2cm (¾in) long, followed by reddish brown seed pods. Dislikes wet soil in winter. ↕ to 60cm (24in), ↔ to 1m (3ft). S. Portugal, Mediterranean. ✲✲✲ (borderline)
L. jacobaeus. Erect perennial with grey-hairy, sometimes pendent stems. Bears pinnate, mid-green leaves, each composed of 5 linear to narrowly obovate leaflets, 4cm (1½in) long, the upper 3 separated from the lower 2 by a short stalk. Pea-like, chocolate- to purple-brown flowers, to 1.5cm (½in) long, with brown-streaked yellow standard petals, are borne in axillary clusters of up to 6, on stalks longer than the leaves, from spring to autumn, but mainly in summer. ↕ 90cm (36in), ↔ 50cm (20in). Cape Verde Islands. ✲
L. maculatus ♀ Trailing perennial, similar to *L. berthelotii,* with palmate, mid-green leaves, each consisting of 3–5 linear leaflets, 1–2cm (½–¾in) long. In spring and early summer, red- or orange-tipped yellow flowers, 2.5cm (1in) long and shaped like lobster claws, are borne singly or in clusters of 2–5 from the leaf axils. ↕ 20cm (8in), ↔ indefinite. Canary Islands (Tenerife). ❀ (min. 5°C/41°F)
***L. mascaensis* of gardens** see *L. sessilifolius.*
L. sessilifolius, syn. *L. mascaensis* of gardens. Low-growing, spreading, shrubby perennial with stalkless, 5-palmate, silver-grey leaves, each with oblong-lance-shaped leaflets, 5–10mm (¼–½in) long. Pea-like, vivid yellow flowers, 7mm (¼in) long, are borne in terminal and axillary clusters of 3–5 for several weeks in spring. ↕ to 60cm (24in), ↔ to 1.5m (5ft). Canary Islands. ❀ (min. 5°C/41°F)

▷ **Lotus** see *Nelumbo*
  American see *Nelumbo lutea*
  Blue see *Nymphaea caerulea*
  Sacred see *Nelumbo nucifera*
▷ **Lovage** see *Levisticum*
▷ **Love-in-a-mist** see *Nigella, N. damascena*
▷ **Love-in-a-puff** see *Cardiospermum halicacabum*
▷ **Love-in-idleness** see *Viola tricolor*
▷ **Love-lies-bleeding** see *Amaranthus caudatus*
▷ **Lucerne** see *Medicago sativa*

LUCULIA

RUBIACEAE

Genus of 5 species of deciduous and evergreen shrubs and small trees from E. Asia, found mostly in upland scrub and woodland and forest margins. They have large, prominently veined leaves, borne in opposite pairs, and terminal panicles or corymbs of salverform, waxy, fragrant flowers with 5 spreading lobes. In frost-prone climates, grow in a cool or temperate greenhouse. In milder climates, grow in a shrub border.
• **HARDINESS** Half hardy to frost tender.
• **CULTIVATION** Under glass, grow in loam-based potting compost (JI No.3) in full light. In spring, pot on or top-dress, and water moderately as growth begins. From summer to autumn, mist daily and water freely, applying a balanced liquid fertilizer monthly; keep just moist in winter. Outdoors, grow in moderately fertile, moist but well-drained soil in full sun. Pruning group 8 or group 9; may need restrictive pruning under glass.
• **PROPAGATION** Sow seed at 13–18°C (55–64°F) in spring. Root greenwood cuttings in summer with bottom heat.
• **PESTS AND DISEASES** Red spider mites, whiteflies, and mealybugs may be troublesome under glass.

L. grandifolia ○ Erect to spreading, bushy, deciduous, large shrub or small tree. Ovate to elliptic, mid-green leaves, 20–35cm (8–14in) long, have red to brownish red stalks, veins, and margins, colouring richly in autumn. In summer, salverform, fragrant, greenish white to pure white flowers, 6–7cm (2½–3in) long, are borne in corymbs 10–20cm (4–8in) wide. ↕ 4–6m (12–20ft), ↔ 2–4m (6–12ft). Bhutan. ❀ (min. 5–7°C/41–45°F)
L. gratissima ♀ ○ Erect then spreading, semi-evergreen or evergreen, large shrub or sometimes small tree, with downy, red-flushed green stems. Lance-shaped to ovate-oblong, long-pointed, prominently veined, mid- to deep green leaves are 10–20cm (4–8in) long, and downy beneath. Salverform, fragrant pink flowers, 2.5–4cm (1–1½in) long, with very slender tubes, are produced in corymbs, 10–20cm (4–8in) wide, from autumn to winter. ↕ 3–6m (10–20ft), ↔ 1.5–3m (5–10ft). Himalayas. ❀ (min. 7–10°C/45–50°F)

LUDWIGIA

ONAGRACEAE

Genus of 75 species of marginal and submerged aquatic perennials, occurring throughout the world, but mainly in warmer regions of North America. They have usually alternate, rarely opposite, simple, mainly stalkless leaves, borne on horizontal or upright, often floating stems. Small, sometimes showy, yellow or white flowers are produced singly from the leaf axils or in terminal clusters. In warm-temperate areas, grow at the margins of a wildlife pool. In cooler climates, grow tender species in an indoor pool or aquarium; *L. peploides* is particularly effective in an aquarium, where it may develop vertical, spongy, white, respiratory roots.
• **HARDINESS** Frost hardy to frost tender.

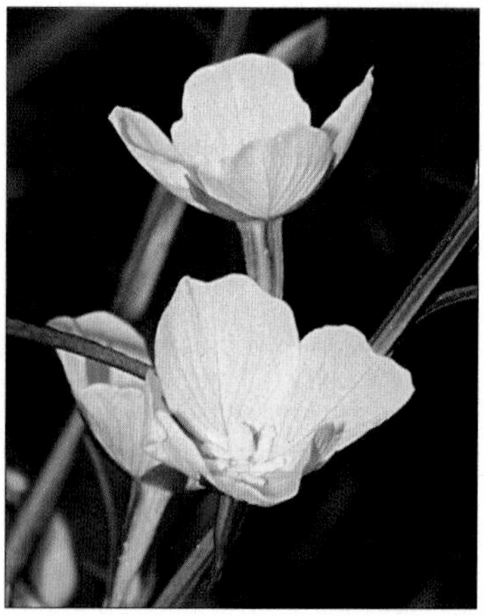

Ludwigia peploides

• **CULTIVATION** Grow in mud at the margins of a pool, in baskets of heavy loam in water 15–30cm (6–12in) deep, or in fertile soil in a bog garden, in full sun or dappled shade. In an aquarium, grow in bunches in an inert medium, at about 20°C (68°F), in full light. See also pp.52–53.
• **PROPAGATION** Divide in early spring. Take softwood cuttings in spring.
• **PESTS AND DISEASES** Trouble free.

L. longifolia, syn. *Jussiaea longifolia.* Upright, marginal aquatic perennial with narrowly winged stems sparsely covered with lance-shaped, mid-green leaves, 10–20cm (4–8in) long. Bears solitary, bell-shaped, pale yellow flowers, 3–5cm (1¼–2in) across, from the upper leaf axils in summer. ↕ 2m (6ft), ↔ 1m (3ft). Brazil to Argentina. ❀ (min. 13°C/55°F)
L. palustris (Water purslane). Marginal aquatic perennial with weak stems: either floating, to 50cm (20in) long, in water; or branched, creeping, and mat-forming on mud. Lance-shaped to elliptic-ovate leaves, 2–5cm (¾–2in) long, shiny, bright green above, dark olive-green to red-purple beneath, have long, sharp points. Axillary, paired, bell-shaped, yellowish green flowers, 2mm ($\frac{1}{16}$in) across, are borne in summer. ↕ 50cm (20in), ↔ indefinite. Europe, Asia, North and South America. ✲✲
L. peploides ■ syn. *Jussiaea repens.* Scrambling, marginal aquatic perennial with horizontal shoots, to 60cm (24in) long, that root at the nodes or float. Elliptic, mid-green leaves, to 6cm (2½in) long, occasionally have vertical, spongy respiratory roots. In summer, bears axillary, solitary, cup-shaped, bright golden yellow flowers, 5cm (2in) across, with darker yellow spots at the bases. ↕ 60cm (24in), ↔ indefinite. North and South America. ✲

LUMA

MYRTACEAE

Genus of 4 species of evergreen shrubs and small trees from woodland in Chile and Argentina. They are mainly grown for their aromatic, leathery leaves, borne in opposite pairs, and their axillary, 4- or 5-petalled, cup-shaped white flowers; *L. apiculata* is also grown for its peeling bark. Grow as lawn specimens or in a small group; in frost-prone areas, grow in a sheltered border or against a wall. They may also be used for hedging.

L

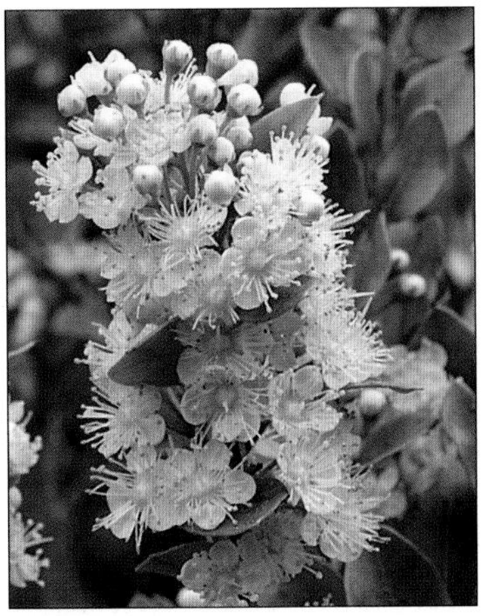

Luma apiculata

• **HARDINESS** Frost hardy.
• **CULTIVATION** Grow in fertile, ideally humus-rich, well-drained soil in full sun or partial shade. Pruning group 1.
• **PROPAGATION** Sow seed in containers in a cold frame in spring. *L. apiculata* may self-seed. Take semi-ripe cuttings in late summer.
• **PESTS AND DISEASES** Trouble free.

L. apiculata ▣ ♀ ◻ syn. *Myrtus luma.* Vigorous, upright, bushy shrub or tree with peeling, cinnamon-brown and creamy white bark, and broadly elliptic, aromatic, glossy, dark green leaves, to 2.5cm (1in) long. Cup-shaped, 5-petalled white flowers, 2cm (¾in) long, are produced singly or in few-flowered cymes from midsummer to mid-autumn, followed by spherical purple berries. ↕↔ 10–15m (30–50ft) or more. Chile, Argentina. ❄❄. **'Glanleam Gold'** is less vigorous, and has leaves with creamy yellow margins, pink-tinged when young; ↕↔ 3m (10ft).
L. chequen ◻ syn. *Myrtus chequen.* Upright shrub or small tree with broadly elliptic or broadly ovate, wavy-margined, aromatic, dark green leaves, to 2.5cm (1in) long. Cup-shaped, 4- or 5-petalled white flowers, 1.5cm (½in) across, are produced singly or in 3-flowered cymes in late summer and early autumn, followed by spherical black berries. ↕ 6m (20ft), ↔ 5m (15ft). Chile. ❄❄

LUNARIA

Honesty, Satin flower

CRUCIFERAE

Genus of 3 species of erect, branching annuals, biennials, and perennials occurring on disturbed ground and in uncultivated fields in Europe and W. Asia. They have alternate, ovate to triangular-heart-shaped, toothed leaves, and bear tall, open, terminal racemes of many 4-petalled, cross-shaped, violet-blue to white flowers in late spring and summer. Valued for their flowers, they may be naturalized in a shrub border, in woodland, or in a wild garden, where they self-seed. *L. annua* and *L. rediviva* have translucent seed pods that are excellent for dried flower arrangements.
• **HARDINESS** Fully hardy.
• **CULTIVATION** Grow in fertile, moist but well-drained soil in full sun or partial shade.
• **PROPAGATION** Sow seed in a seedbed: *L. rediviva* in spring, *L. annua* in early summer. Divide *L. rediviva* in spring.

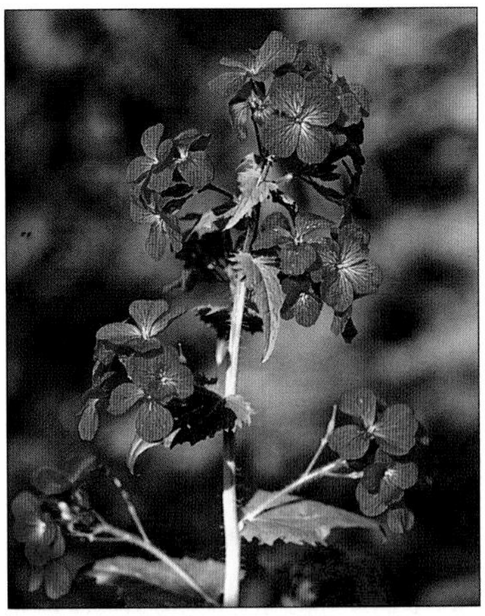

Lunaria annua 'Munstead Purple'

• **PESTS AND DISEASES** Clubroot, white blister, and viruses may cause problems.

L. annua, syn. *L. biennis* (Honesty, Satin flower). Annual or biennial with ovate to heart-shaped, coarsely toothed, light to mid-green leaves, to 15cm (6in) long. In late spring and summer, cross-shaped, white to light purple flowers, to 1cm (½in) across, are borne in broad, leafy racemes, to 18cm (7in) long. Flat seed pods, 2.5–8cm (1–3in) long, are rounded and silvery. ↕ to 90cm (36in), ↔ to 30cm (12in). Europe. ❄❄❄. **'Alba Variegata'** has leaves variegated and margined creamy white, and white flowers. **var. *albiflora*** ♀ bears white flowers. **'Munstead Purple'** ▣ has deep reddish purple flowers. **'Variegata'** ▣ has leaves variegated and margined

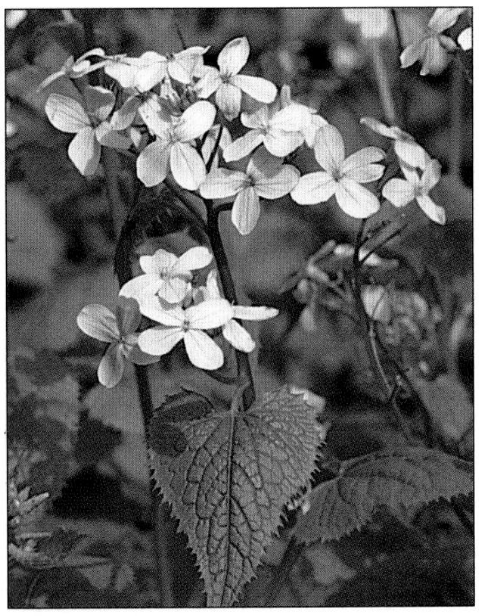

Lunaria rediviva

creamy white, and produces purple or red-purple flowers.
L. biennis see *L. annua.*
L. rediviva ▣ (Perennial honesty). Clump-forming perennial with triangular-heart-shaped, finely toothed, dark green leaves, to 20cm (8in) long. Leafy stems bear loose racemes, to 18cm (7in) long, of fragrant, lilac-white flowers, 2.5cm (1in) across, in late spring and early summer, followed by flat, elliptic seed pods, to 5–8cm (2–3in) long, ripening to beige. ↕ 60–90cm (24–36in), ↔ 30cm (12in). Europe, Russia (W. Siberia). ❄❄❄

▷ **Lungwort** see *Pulmonaria*
▷ **Lupin** see *Lupinus*
Carolina see *Thermopsis villosa*
Tree see *Lupinus arboreus*

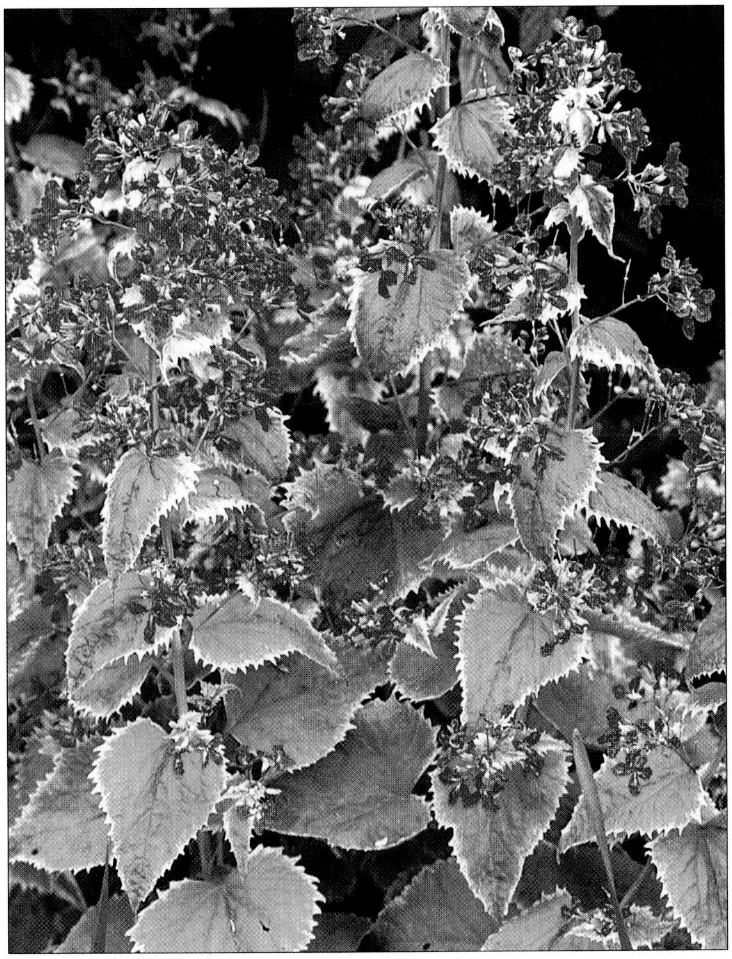

Lunaria annua 'Variegata'

LUPINUS

Lupin

LEGUMINOSAE/PAPILIONACEAE

Genus of about 200 species of annuals, perennials, and semi-evergreen and evergreen subshrubs or shrubs, mostly from the Mediterranean, North Africa, and North, Central, and South America; they are found in dry, hilly grassland and open woodland, on coastal sands or cliffs, and on riverbanks. Most have short-stemmed, palmate, often softly hairy, mid-green, mainly basal leaves, with lance-shaped leaflets; some alpines have silvery green leaves. Long, terminal racemes or spikes of pea-like flowers in many colours, including bicolours, are borne mainly in summer. There are numerous hybrid perennials (including the popular Russell lupins), which form dense clumps of palmate leaves and bear colourful flowers, 2.5cm (1in) long, in racemes or spikes 20–60cm (8–24in) long. Grow larger lupins in a border or wild garden, smaller species in a rock garden or scree bed; where winters are wet, grow the densely silver-hairy species in an alpine house. The seeds may cause severe discomfort if ingested.
• **HARDINESS** Fully hardy to half hardy.
• **CULTIVATION** Grow in moderately fertile, light and slightly acid, well-drained, sandy soil in full sun or partial shade. In an alpine house, grow in equal parts loam, leaf mould, and grit.
• **PROPAGATION** Sow seed in spring or autumn: for annuals and larger species, nick or soak for 24 hours and sow in a seedbed; for alpines and smaller species, sow in containers in a cold frame. Will self-seed. Take basal cuttings of cultivars in mid-spring.
• **PESTS AND DISEASES** Fungal and bacterial rot, gall, mildew, leaf spot, virus, and slugs may be a problem.

L. albifrons ▣ Erect to semi-erect, evergreen subshrub with 7- to 10-palmate, silver silky-hairy leaves,

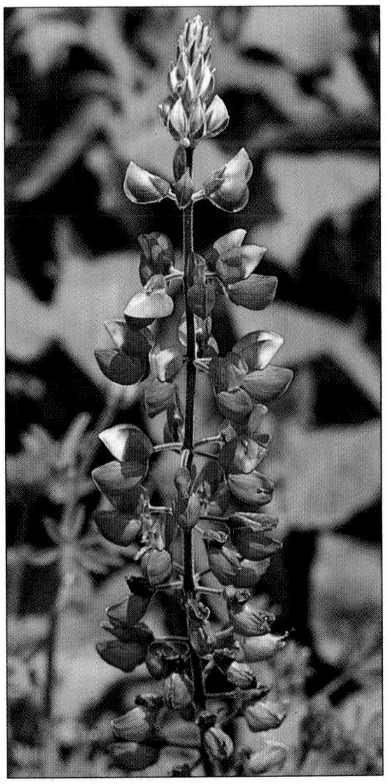

Lupinus albifrons

L

composed of inversely lance-shaped to spoon-shaped leaflets, to 3cm (1¼in) long. In summer, pea-like, pale blue to red-purple flowers, 0.9–1.5cm (⅜–½in) across, with white-marked wing petals, are borne in racemes 10–30cm (4–12in) long. ↕↔ to 75cm (30in) or more. USA (California). ❄❄ (hardy to -7°C/20°F, but needs excellent drainage and full sun). **var. *collinus*** is lower-growing and much more compact; ↕↔ 10cm (4in).

L. arboreus ■ 🏆 (Tree lupin). Bushy, vigorous, evergreen or semi-evergreen shrub or subshrub, with silky shoots and 5- to 12-palmate, grey-green leaves, composed of obovate-oblong leaflets, to 6cm (2½in) long, silky-hairy beneath. Bears pea-like, fragrant, yellow, or rarely blue flowers, to 1.5cm (½in) long, in dense to lax, upright racemes, to 30cm (12in) long, in late spring and summer. ↕↔ 2m (6ft). USA (California). ❄❄. **'Mauve Queen'** has lilac flowers. **'Snow Queen'** has white flowers.

***L.* 'Band of Nobles'.** Clump-forming perennial bearing racemes of flowers in white, yellow, pink, red, blue, or bicolours (usually white or yellow in combination with another colour), in early and midsummer. ↕ to 1.5m (5ft), ↔ 75cm (30in). ❄❄❄

***L.* 'Beryl, Viscountess Cowdray'** ■ Clump-forming perennial bearing dense racemes of bicoloured, rich pink and red flowers in early and midsummer. ↕ 90cm (36in), ↔ 75cm (30in). ❄❄❄

***L.* 'Blushing Bride'.** Clump-forming perennial bearing dense racemes of pink-tinged, ivory-white flowers in early and midsummer. ↕ 90cm (36in), ↔ 75cm (30in). ❄❄❄

***L. breweri*.** Tufted, mat-forming, short-lived, woody-based perennial with 7- to 10-palmate, densely silky-hairy, silver-green leaves, consisting of inversely lance-shaped leaflets, to 2cm (¾in) long. In summer, bears dense racemes, to 5cm (2in) long, of pea-like, white-throated, violet-blue flowers, 6–9mm (¼–⅜in) long. ↕ 10cm (4in), ↔ to 20cm (8in). Stony meadows in W. USA. ❄❄❄

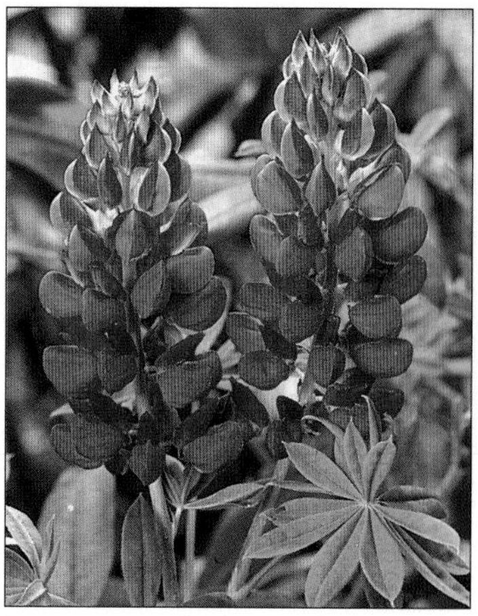

Lupinus 'Beryl, Viscountess Cowdray'

***L.* 'Catherine of York'.** Clump-forming perennial bearing racemes of bicoloured, pure salmon-orange and yellow flowers in early and midsummer. ↕ 90cm (36in), ↔ 75cm (30in). ❄❄❄

***L.* 'Chandelier'** ■ Clump-forming perennial producing racemes of bright yellow flowers in early and midsummer. ↕ 90cm (36in), ↔ 75cm (30in). ❄❄❄

L. cruckshankii see *L. mutabilis.*

***L.* 'Lady Fayre'.** Clump-forming perennial bearing racemes of deep rose-pink flowers in early and midsummer. ↕ 90cm (36in), ↔ 75cm (30in). ❄❄❄

***L. lepidus* var. *lobbii*,** syn. *L. lyallii.* Semi-prostrate to mat-forming, short-lived perennial with 5- to 7-palmate, silky-hairy, silver-green leaves, consisting of inversely lance-shaped leaflets, to 1cm (½in) long. Pea-like, bright blue flowers, 1cm (½in) long, the standard petals each with a white spot, are borne in dense racemes, to 5cm (2in) long, in late summer. ↕ 10cm (4in), ↔ to 20cm (8in). USA (Washington State to California). ❄❄❄

***L. luteus* 'Yellow Javelin'.** Erect, bushy annual with densely hairy stems and 7- to 11-palmate leaves, each with obovate-oblong, round-tipped, softly hairy, mid-

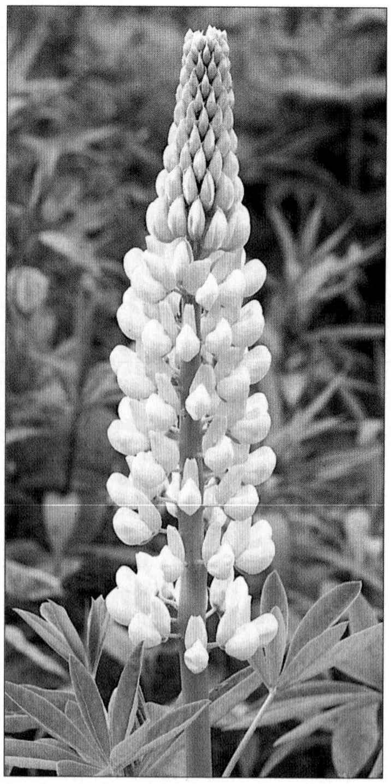

Lupinus 'Chandelier'

green leaflets, 3–6cm (1¼–2½in) long. In summer, bears pea-like, bright golden yellow flowers, to 2cm (¾in) long, in tall racemes, to 25cm (10in) long. ↕ to 60cm (24in), ↔ 30cm (12in). ❄❄❄

L. lyallii see *L. lepidus* var. *lobbii.*

***L.* 'Moonraker'.** Clump-forming perennial bearing racemes of lemon-yellow flowers in early and midsummer. ↕ 90cm (36in), ↔ 75cm (30in). ❄❄❄

***L. mutabilis*,** syn. *L. cruckshankii.* Erect, bushy annual, with 7- to 9-palmate leaves, each with inversely lance-shaped to spoon-shaped, round-tipped, blue-green leaflets, to 5–6cm (2–2½in) long, softly hairy beneath. In summer, bears racemes, 10–20cm (4–8in) long, of pea-like flowers, 2–3cm (¾–1¼in) long, with pale purple-blue keel petals, yellow standard petals, and deep blue wing petals. ↕ 1–1.1m (3–3½ft), ↔ 45–60cm (18–24in). ❄❄

***L.* 'My Castle'.** Clump-forming perennial bearing racemes of deep rose-pink flowers in early and midsummer. ↕ 90cm (36in), ↔ 75cm (30in). ❄❄❄

***L. nanus* 'Pixie Delight'** ■ Erect, single-stemmed to bushy annual with 5- to 7-palmate leaves, composed of linear-lance-shaped, pointed, softly hairy, mid-

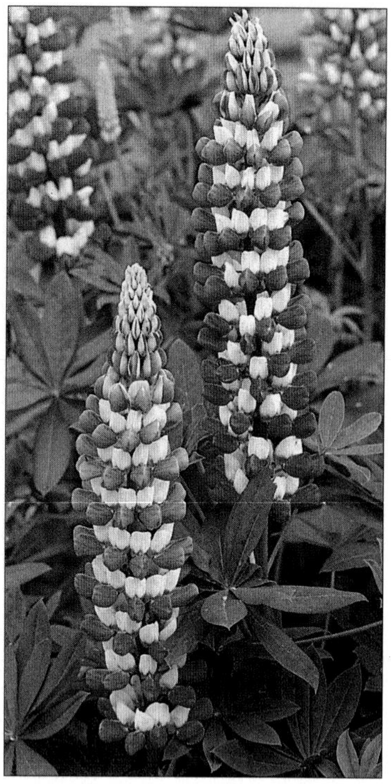

Lupinus 'The Chatelaine'

green leaflets, to 3cm (1¼in) long. In summer, bears racemes, to 20cm (8in) long, of pea-like, pink, blue, lavender-blue, white, or bicoloured flowers, 1.5cm (½in) across, the standard petals often with purple-dotted white marks or yellow spots. ↕ 50cm (20in), ↔ to 23cm (9in). ❄❄❄

***L.* 'Noble Maiden'.** Clump-forming perennial bearing racemes of creamy white flowers in early and midsummer. ↕ 90cm (36in), ↔ 75cm (30in). ❄❄❄

L. texensis (Texas bluebonnet). Erect to spreading, bushy annual with softly hairy stems and 5-palmate, mid-green leaves, each with lance-shaped, pointed leaflets, to 3cm (1¼in) long, hairy beneath and on the margins. Compact, crowded racemes, to 8cm (3in) long, of pea-like, deep blue to blue-purple flowers, 1cm (½in) across, are produced in summer. ↕ 25–30cm (10–12in), ↔ to 23cm (9in). USA (Texas). ❄❄❄

***L.* 'The Chatelaine'** ■ Clump-forming perennial producing racemes of bicoloured, pink and white flowers in early and midsummer. ↕ 90cm (36in), ↔ 75cm (30in). ❄❄❄

***L.* 'The Governor'.** Clump-forming perennial producing racemes of

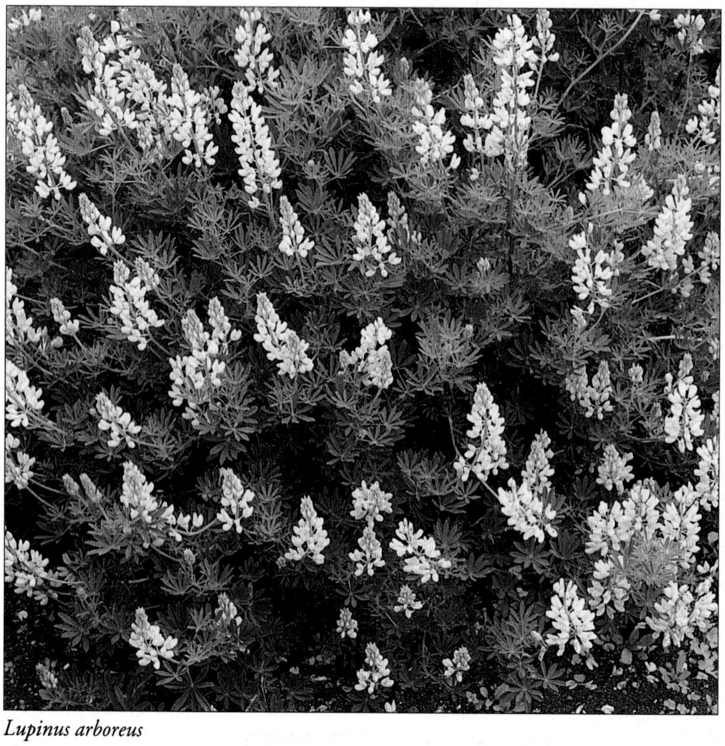

Lupinus arboreus

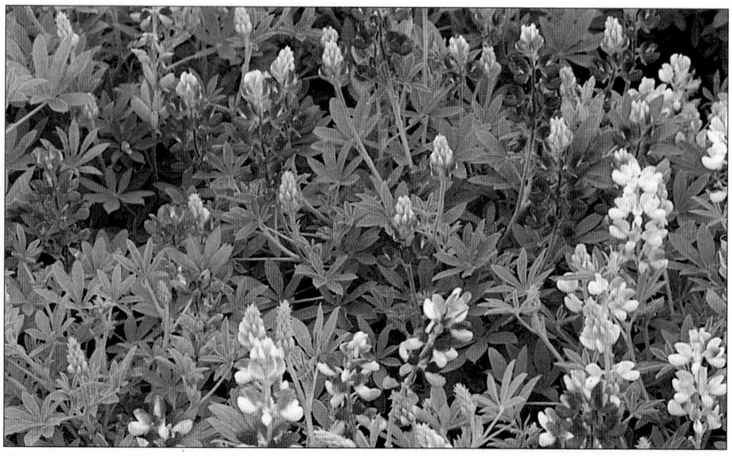

Lupinus nanus 'Pixie Delight'

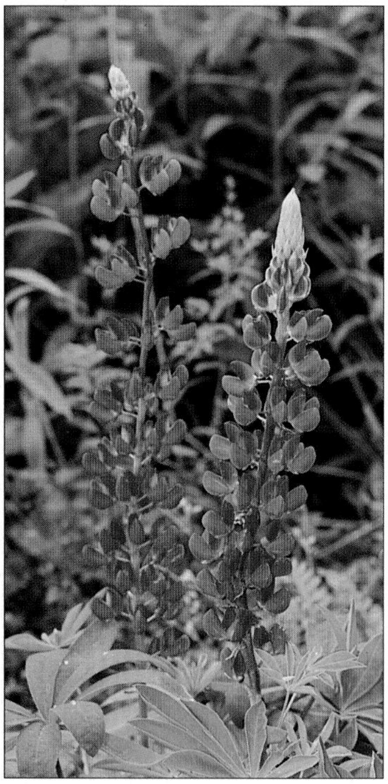

Lupinus 'The Page'

bicoloured, deep blue and white flowers in early and midsummer. ↕ 90cm (36in), ↔ 75cm (30in). ❄❄❄

***L.* 'The Page'** ■ Clump-forming perennial producing racemes of rich carmine-red flowers in early and midsummer. ↕ 90cm (36in), ↔ 75cm (30in). ❄❄❄

***L.* 'Thundercloud'.** Clump-forming perennial producing racemes of deep violet-blue flowers in early and midsummer. ↕ 90cm (36in), ↔ 75cm (30in). ❄❄❄

LUZULA

Woodrush

JUNCACEAE

Genus of approximately 80 species of mostly evergreen, tufted, grass-like perennials (rarely annuals), sometimes with short rhizomes or stolons. Woodrushes are widely distributed on heaths and moors, in fens and bogs, and in scrub, woodland, and mountain grassland throughout the temperate regions of the world. Broadly linear basal and stem leaves are flat or grooved along their lengths, and have fringes of zigzagged white hairs at the margins, which distinguish them from rushes (*Juncus*). Tiny flowers are produced in terminal, panicle-, corymb-, or cyme-like clusters, in spring or summer. Valued for their shade tolerance, woodrushes provide useful ground cover in damp shade, either in a mixed border or in a woodland garden. *L. ulophylla* is also suitable for a trough or rock garden.

• **HARDINESS** Most are fully hardy; *L. ulophylla* is hardy to -8°C (18°F) for short periods.

• **CULTIVATION** Grow in poor to moderately fertile, humus-rich, moist but well-drained soil in partial or deep shade (or in full sun where the soil is reliably moist). *L. nivea* prefers full sun.

• **PROPAGATION** Sow seed in containers outdoors in spring or autumn. Divide between mid-spring and early summer.

• **PESTS AND DISEASES** Trouble free.

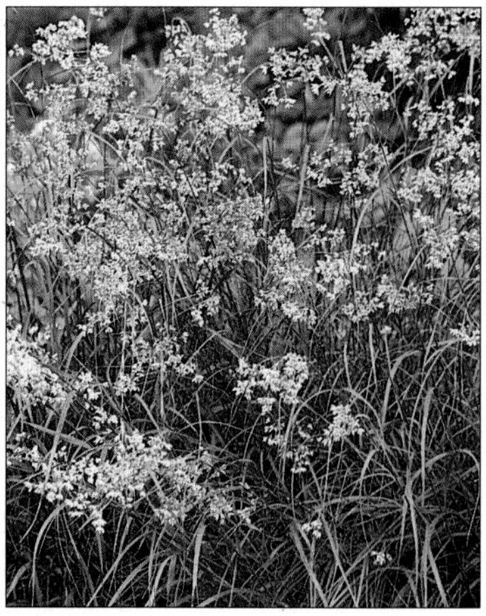

Luzula nivea

L. maxima see *L. sylvatica*.

L. nivea ■ (Snowy woodrush). Slowly spreading, loosely tufted, evergreen perennial forming loose clumps of flat, linear, deep green basal leaves, to 30cm (12in) long; stem leaves are to 20cm (8in) long. In early and midsummer, bears lax panicles, to 5cm (2in) long, of shiny, pure white flowers in tight clusters of up to 20. May be dried. ↕ to 60cm (24in), ↔ 45cm (18in). Spain, France, Italy, Slovenia, C. Europe. ❄❄❄

L. sylvatica, syn. *L. maxima* (Greater woodrush). Densely tufted, tussock-forming, evergreen perennial with linear, channelled, glossy, dark green leaves, to 30cm (12in) long. Groups of 2–5 small, chestnut-brown flowers are produced in open panicles, to 8cm (3in) long, from mid-spring to early summer. ↕ to 70–80cm (28–32in), ↔ 45cm (18in). S., W., and C. Europe, S.W. Asia. ❄❄❄. The following cultivars provide useful, dense ground cover.

'Aurea' ■ syn. *L. maxima* 'Aurea', has broad leaves that are bright, shiny yellow in winter, yellow-green in summer.

'Aureomarginata' see 'Marginata'.

'Marginata', syn. 'Aureomarginata', has

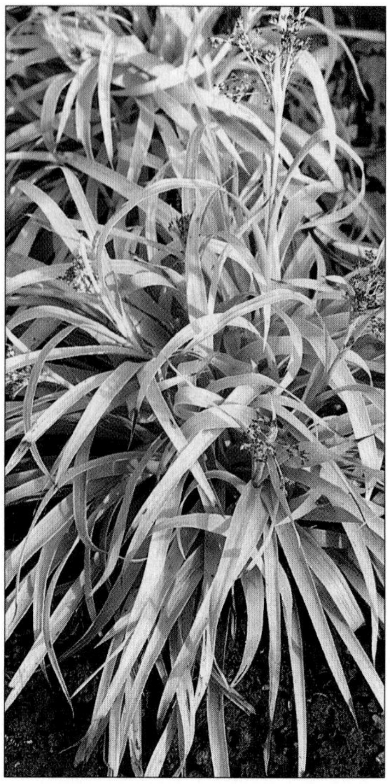

Luzula sylvatica 'Aurea'

a dense habit, rich green leaves with neat cream margins, and pendent, brown and gold spikelets.

L. ulophylla. Dwarf, densely tufted, evergreen perennial forming a low mound of linear, deep green leaves, to 3–7cm (1¼–3in) long, V-shaped in cross-section, with conspicuous silvery hairs beneath and on the margins. In early summer, very dark brown flowers, the tepals with white membranous margins, are produced in short, stubby clusters, to 2cm (¾in) long. ↕ to 15cm (6in), ↔ 30cm (12in). New Zealand. ❄❄

LYCASTE

ORCHIDACEAE

Genus of about 45 species of deciduous, epiphytic or terrestrial orchids found in cloud forest at altitudes of 600–2,200m (2,000–7,700ft) in Mexico, Central and South America, and the West Indies. They produce robust, ovoid or ellipsoid, compressed pseudobulbs, and a number of broad, lance-shaped to oblong-elliptic, often soft, folded leaves. Large, waxy, fragrant flowers, produced singly on leafless stems from the bases, are typically triangular in shape, with the sepals framing the smaller, cupped petals and 3-lobed lips.

• **HARDINESS** Frost tender.

• **CULTIVATION** Cool-growing orchids. Grow in containers of crushed bark or loamless potting compost, or grow epiphytically on bark slabs. In summer, provide high humidity and water freely (keeping the foliage dry); apply a balanced liquid fertilizer at every third watering. In winter, provide bright filtered light and keep dry. See also p.46.

• **PROPAGATION** Divide when plants overflow their containers, or remove and pot up backbulbs.

• **PESTS AND DISEASES** Red spider mites, aphids, whiteflies, and mealybugs may be troublesome.

L. aromatica. Epiphytic orchid with lance-shaped leaves, to 30–40cm (12–16in) long. Cinnamon-scented flowers, 4–6cm (1½–2½in) across, with deep golden to orange-yellow petals, yellowish green sepals, and lips with orange dots, are produced in abundance from spring to summer. ↕↔ 30cm (12in). Mexico, Guatemala, Belize, Honduras. ❀ (min. 11–12°C/52–54°F; max. 30°C/86°F)

L. brevispatha, syn. *L. candida.* Epiphytic orchid with lance-shaped leaves, to 50cm (20in) long. From winter to spring, produces an abundance of flowers, to 10cm (4in) across, with light green sepals with reddish brown spots, brown-spotted white petals, and white lips suffused and spotted pink. ↕↔ 30cm (12in). Guatemala, Nicaragua, Costa Rica, Panama. ❀ (min. 11–12°C/52–54°F; max. 30°C/86°F)

L. candida see *L. brevispatha.*

L. cruenta ■ Epiphytic orchid with lance-shaped leaves, to 35cm (18in) long. From spring to summer, produces an abundance of faintly cinnamon-scented flowers, to 7cm (3in) across, with greenish yellow sepals, yellowish orange petals with red spots near the bases, and orange lips with red spots and red triangular patches at the bases. ↕↔ 45cm (18in). Mexico, Guatemala,

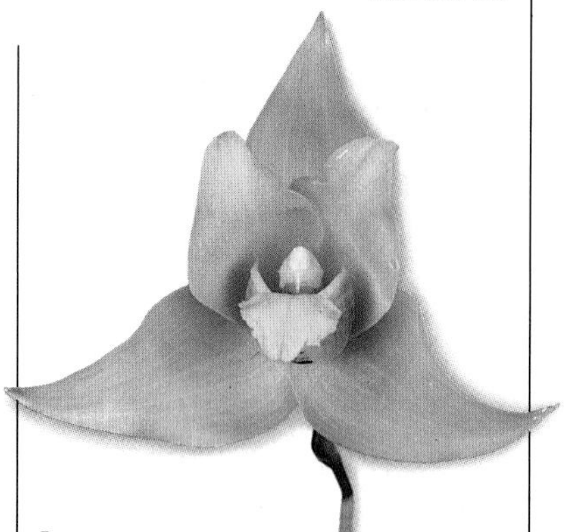

Lycaste cruenta

El Salvador, Costa Rica. ❀ (min. 11–12°C/52–54°F; max. 30°C/86°F)

L. deppei ■ Epiphytic orchid with lance-shaped leaves, 30–50cm (12–20in) long. From spring to summer, produces abundant flowers, 9cm (3½in) across, with green sepals spotted red-brown, white petals flecked red-brown at the bases, and red-spotted, deep yellow lips, striped and dotted red at the bases. ↕↔ 30cm (12in). Mexico, Guatemala. ❀ (min. 11–12°C/52–54°F; max. 30°C/86°F)

L. gigantea see *L. longipetala.*

L. longipetala, syn. *L. gigantea.* Epiphytic orchid with lance-shaped leaves, to 60cm (24in) long. In summer, bears large, fleshy flowers, to 16cm (6in) across, with pale green sepals suffused brown, darker green petals, and red-brown lips with light orange margins; the flowers do not open fully. ↕↔ 45cm (18in). Venezuela, Colombia, Ecuador, Peru. ❀ (min. 11–12°C/52–54°F; max. 30°C/86°F)

L. skinneri, syn. *L. virginalis.* Epiphytic orchid with lance-shaped leaves, 50–60cm (20–24in) long. From winter to spring, produces flowers 12–15cm (5–6in) across, with cream sepals shaded lavender-pink to pink, reddish purple petals, and pink lips sometimes mottled purple. ↕↔ 30cm (12in). Mexico, Guatemala, Honduras, El Salvador. ❀ (min. 11–12°C/52–54°F; max. 30°C/86°F)

L. virginalis see *L. skinneri.*

***L.* Wyldfire** (*L.* Balliae x *L.* Wyld Court). Robust, epiphytic orchid with lance-shaped leaves, 40cm (16in) long. In spring, produces an abundance of deep wine-red flowers, 12cm (5in) across, with darker lips. ↕↔ 45cm (18in). ❀ (min. 11–12°C/52–54°F; max. 30°C/86°F)

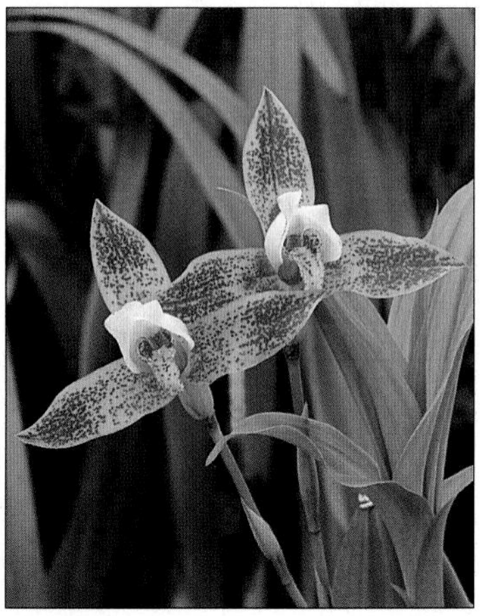

Lycaste deppei

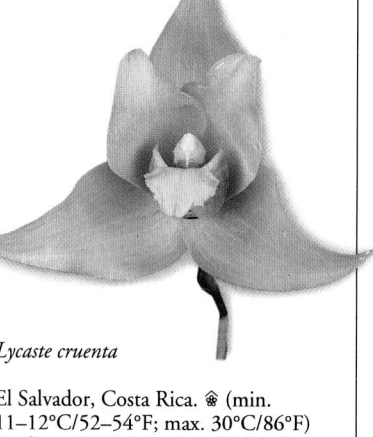

LYCHNIS syn. VISCARIA

Campion, Catchfly

CARYOPHYLLACEAE

Genus of 15–20 species of biennials and perennials found in sites ranging from damp meadows and woodland to alpine habitats, in N. temperate and arctic regions. They have erect, usually branched stems, and simple, often hairy leaves borne in opposite pairs. The 5-petalled, salverform to tubular or star-shaped flowers occur in scarlet, purple, pink, or white, and are either solitary or borne in terminal cymes or occasionally panicles. Grow the larger perennials in a sunny border or a wild garden, the smaller, alpine species in a rock garden, and the biennials in an annual or herbaceous border.

- **HARDINESS** Fully hardy.
- **CULTIVATION** Grow in any moderately fertile, well-drained soil in full sun or partial shade. *L. chalcedonica*, *L.* x *haageana*, and *L. viscaria* prefer moist, fertile soil; grey-leaved species produce their best leaf colour in dry soil in full sun. Dead-head to prolong flowering.
- **PROPAGATION** Sow seed in containers in a cold frame as soon as ripe or in spring; *L.* x *haageana* will flower the same year and may be treated as an annual. Divide or take basal cuttings in early spring.
- **PESTS AND DISEASES** Slugs may be a problem, especially on less woolly species.

L. alpina ■ (Alpine campion, Alpine catchfly). Dwarf, tufted perennial with rosettes of oblong-lance-shaped to elliptic-lance-shaped, dark green leaves,

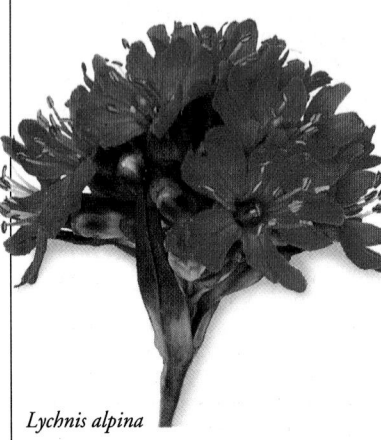

Lychnis alpina

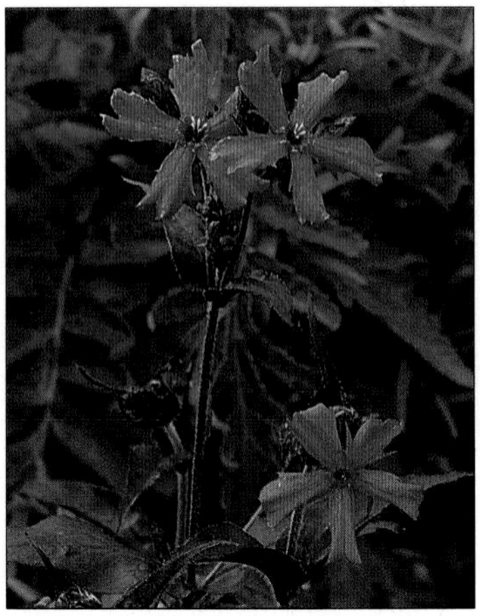

Lychnis x *arkwrightii* 'Vesuvius'

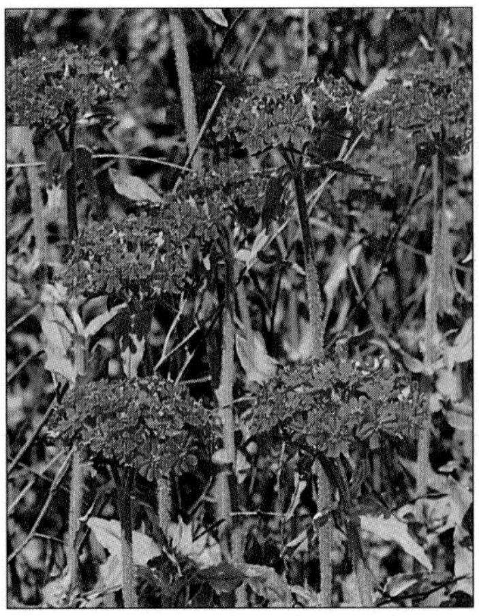

Lychnis chalcedonica

to 4cm (1½in) long. In summer, bears dense, rounded, terminal cymes of 6–20 salverform, purplish pink flowers, to 2cm (¾in) across, with frilled, 2-lobed petals. ↕↔ to 15cm (6in). Mountains of N. hemisphere, subarctic regions. ❄❄❄

***L.* x *arkwrightii* 'Vesuvius'** ■ Short-lived, clump-forming perennial with ovate-lance-shaped, hairy, dark brownish green leaves, 8cm (3in) long. In early and midsummer, bears terminal cymes of 5–10 star-shaped, orange-scarlet flowers, 3–4cm (1¼–1½in) across, with notched petals. ↕45cm (18in), ↔ 30cm (12in). ❄❄❄

L. chalcedonica ■ ♀ (Jerusalem cross, Maltese cross). Erect, stiff perennial with ovate, mid-green basal leaves, and unbranched, hairy stems bearing clasping, ovate leaves, 5–8cm (2–3in) long, with heart-shaped bases. In early and midsummer, produces terminal, rounded, umbel-like cymes of 10–30 star-shaped scarlet flowers, 1.5cm (½in) across, the petals each with 2 deep notches. Requires support. Self-seeds freely. ↕0.9–1.2m (3–4ft), ↔ 30cm (12in). European Russia. ❄❄❄. **'Rosea'** has rose-pink flowers.

L. coeli-rosa see *Silene coeli-rosa.*

L. coronaria ■ (Dusty miller, Rose campion). Erect, woolly, silver-grey biennial or short-lived perennial with ovate-lance-shaped, silver-grey leaves: the basal leaves up to 18cm (7in) long, the stem leaves up to 10cm (4in). In late summer, long-stalked, salverform, rounded, purple-red or pale purple flowers, 3cm (1¼in) across, with slightly reflexed, shallowly 2-lobed petals, are borne in few-flowered, terminal cymes;

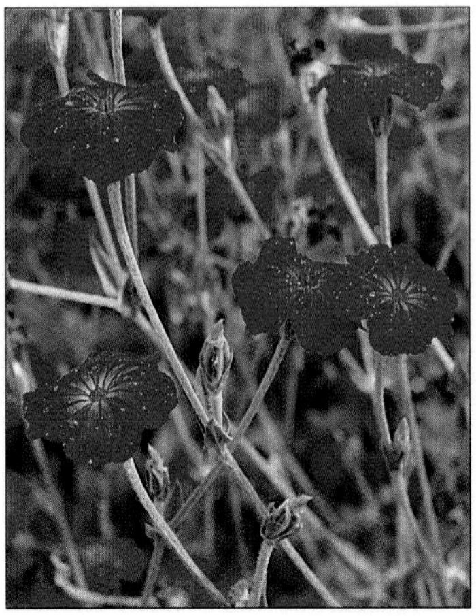

Lychnis coronaria

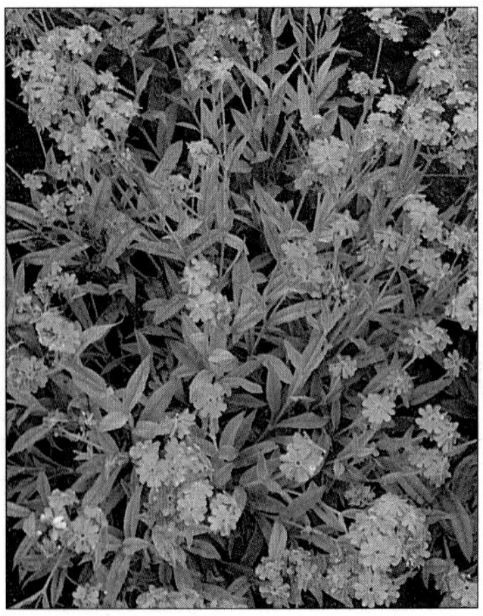

Lychnis flos-jovis

they open singly, but in long succession. Self-seeds freely. ↕80cm (32in), ↔ 45cm (18in). S.E. Europe. ❄❄❄. **'Alba'** ♀ produces white flowers.

L. coronata* var. *sieboldii see *L. sieboldii.*

L. flos-cuculi (Ragged robin). Slender, upright or spreading, sparsely hairy perennial with inversely lance-shaped, mid- to bluish green basal leaves, to 12cm (5in) long, and smaller, oblong-lance-shaped stem-clasping leaves. In late spring and early summer, produces loose, few-flowered, branched, terminal cymes of star-shaped, pale to bright purplish pink, sometimes white flowers, to 4cm (1½in) across, with petals deeply cut into 4 linear segments. Suitable for a wild garden. ↕ to 75cm (30in), ↔ to 80cm (32in). Damp places in Europe, Caucasus, and Russia (Siberia). ❄❄❄

L. flos-jovis ■ (Flower of Jove, Flower of Jupiter). Mat-forming perennial with usually unbranched, erect, white-hairy stems, and lance- to spoon-shaped basal and stem-clasping leaves, to 10cm (4in) long. From early to late summer, bears loosely rounded cymes of 4–10 rounded, pink, white, or scarlet flowers, 2.5cm (1in) across, with slightly reflexed, notched petals. ↕20–60cm (8–24in) or more, ↔ 45cm (18in). C. Alps. ❄❄❄. **'Hort's Variety'** has rose-pink flowers; ↕30cm (12in).

L.* x *haageana (*L. fulgens* x *L. sieboldii*). Short-lived, clump-forming, hairy perennial with lance-shaped, mid-green leaves, 4–8cm (1½–3in) long. In mid- and late summer, salverform, brilliant red or orange flowers, 5cm (2in) across, with notched petals, are borne in few-flowered, loose, terminal cymes. ↕45–60cm (18–24in), ↔ 30cm (12in). Garden origin. ❄❄❄ (borderline)

L. sieboldii, syn. *L. coronata* var. *sieboldii.* Clump-forming, hairy perennial bearing inversely lance-shaped to elliptic, mid-green leaves, 5–8cm (2–3in) long. Clustered, terminal cymes of many flat, rounded, deep red flowers, 5cm (2in) across, the petals with shallowly toothed lobes, are produced in summer and early autumn. ↕60cm (24in), ↔ 30cm (12in). Japan. ❄❄❄

L. viscaria ■ syn. *Viscaria vulgaris* (German catchfly). Mat-forming to tufted perennial with elliptic-lance-shaped to oblong-lance-shaped, hairless, dark green basal leaves, to 8cm (3in) long. The usually unbranched stems are sticky, with a few lance-shaped leaves. In early and midsummer, bears narrow, spike-like panicles of numerous salverform, purplish pink flowers, 2cm (¾in) across, with notched petals. ↕↔ 45cm (18in). Europe to W. Asia. ❄❄❄. **'Flore Pleno'** see 'Splendens Plena'. **'Fontaine'** produces large, double, pale red flowers, 2.5cm (1in) across. **'Snowbird'** produces white flowers. **'Splendens Plena'** ♀ syn. 'Flore Pleno', bears double, bright pinkish magenta flowers, 2.5cm (1in) across.

***L.* x *walkeri* 'Abbotswood Rose'** ♀ Clump-forming, woolly, silver-grey perennial, similar to *L. coronaria* but more spreading and shorter, with ovate, silver-grey basal leaves, to 8cm (3in) long, and smaller stem leaves. From early to late summer, produces terminal cymes of numerous salverform, rose-

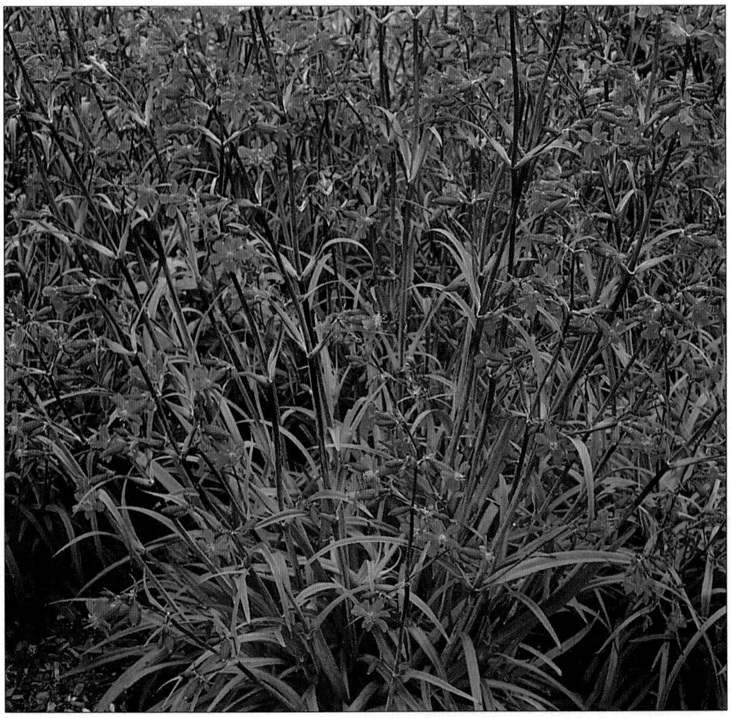

Lychnis viscaria

pink flowers, 3cm (1¼in) across, with slightly reflexed, shallowly notched petals. ↕40cm (16in) or more, ↔ 45cm (18in). ❄❄❄

▷ ***Lycianthes*** see *Solanum*
L. rantonnetii see *S. rantonnetii*

LYCIUM

SOLANACEAE

Genus of about 100 species of sometimes spiny, deciduous and evergreen, often scandent shrubs, occurring throughout temperate and subtropical regions, usually in dry soil. Leaves are entire and alternate, and funnel-shaped or tubular flowers are borne singly or in clusters of up to 4 from the leaf axils. Cultivated for their habit, flowers, and fruits, they are useful for a shrub border or for covering a dry bank; they are particularly effective as a windbreak or hedge in a coastal garden. In frost-prone areas, grow tender species in a cool or temperate greenhouse.

- **HARDINESS** Fully hardy to frost tender.
- **CULTIVATION** Grow in moderately fertile, well-drained soil in full sun. Pruning group 1, or, for scandent species, group 11, in winter or early spring. Cut back hedges hard in spring; trim in early summer.
- **PROPAGATION** Sow seed in containers outdoors in autumn. Take hardwood cuttings in winter, or softwood cuttings in early summer.
- **PESTS AND DISEASES** Trouble free.

L. barbarum, syn. *L. halimifolium* (Chinese box thorn, Duke of Argyll's tea-tree). Variable, vigorous, erect or wide-spreading, sometimes scandent, often spiny, deciduous shrub. Long, arching branches bear narrowly oblong-lance-shaped, elliptic, or ovate, mid-green to grey-green leaves, to 6cm (2½in) long. Small clusters of 1–4 funnel-shaped, purple, lilac, or pink flowers, 9mm (⅜in) long, are produced in late spring and summer, followed by ovoid, orange-red or yellow berries, to 2cm (¾in) long. ↕3.5m (11ft) or more, ↔ 5m (15ft). China. ❄❄❄
L. halimifolium see *L. barbarum.*

LYCOPODIUM

Club moss

LYCOPODIACEAE

Genus of 100 or more species of rhizomatous, evergreen, terrestrial or epiphytic, moss-like perennials, found in most parts of the world in a very wide range of habitats, but mainly in tropical or temperate rainforest or cloud forest. They have erect, pendent, or creeping stems, which are usually repeatedly forked, and bear small, simple, linear-lance-shaped to ovate-triangular leaves, overlapping or in whorls. Spores are produced in the leaf axils, or sometimes in terminal cones on the smaller leaves. Only the epiphytic species are cultivated. In frost-prone areas, grow in a temperate or warm greenhouse. In frost-free climates, grow as epiphytes in shaded, damp sites.

- **HARDINESS** Frost tender.
- **CULTIVATION** Under glass, grow in slatted wooden baskets in equal parts peat, roughly chopped sphagnum moss, charcoal, and broken crocks, in bright

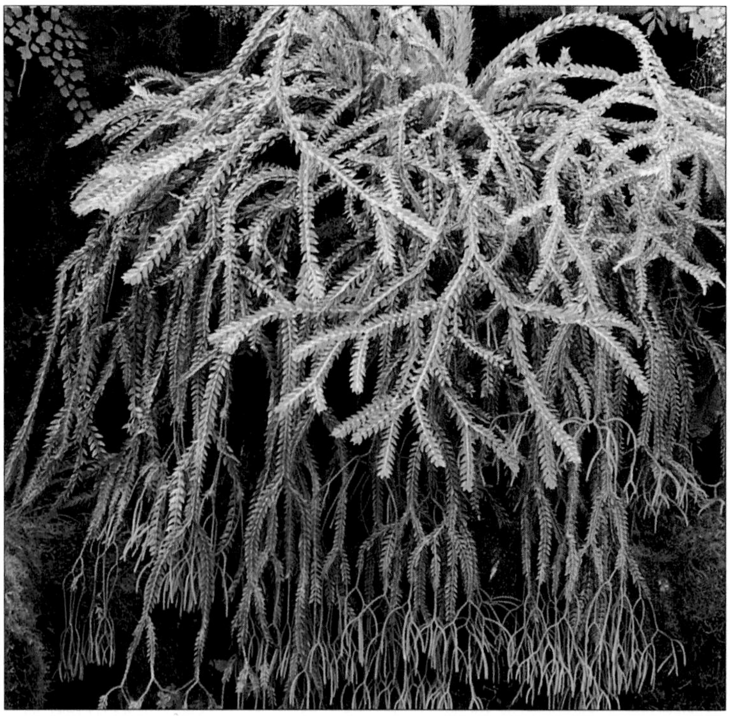

Lycopodium phlegmaria

indirect light. In the growing season, water moderately (avoiding the foliage), mist daily in summer, and apply a half-strength, seaweed-based liquid fertilizer as a foliar spray every month. Reduce watering in winter but do not allow the compost to dry out. Outdoors, grow epiphytically in a permanently damp niche on a tree, in partial shade.

- **PROPAGATION** Layer tips of fertile leaves at any time of year. See also p.51.
- **PESTS AND DISEASES** Slugs, snails, or mites may eat the soft, tender tips of growing stems. Fern scale may be a serious problem.

L. phlegmaria ▣ Epiphytic perennial with initially upright, later pendent stems, to 1m (3ft) long, forked several times. Produces often upright, broadly ovate-triangular, yellow- to olive-green leaves, to 2cm (¾in) long. Spores are formed in branched, terminal cones, to 1.5cm (½in) across, on small leaves. Probably an aggregate of several species. ↕90cm (36in), ↔ 1m (3ft). Asia, Australia, Pacific islands. ❀ (min. 10°C/50°F)

LYCORIS

AMARYLLIDACEAE

Genus of 10–12 species of bulbous perennials from wooded hills or rocky sites in low mountains, and the margins of cultivated fields, in China and Japan. They are grown for their showy umbels of tubular-funnel-shaped flowers, with narrow, spreading, sometimes reflexed tepal lobes, borne on leafless stems from spring to early autumn. The leaves are linear or strap-shaped. In areas with dry summers, grow in a sunny border or rock garden. Where summers are wet, they are best grown as container plants in a conservatory or cool greenhouse, but do not always flower regularly.

- **HARDINESS** Frost hardy to half hardy. *L. aurea*, *L. radiata*, and *L. squamigera* tolerate occasional temperatures to -15°C (5°F).
- **CULTIVATION** Plant in autumn with the necks of the bulbs at the surface. Under glass, grow in loam-based potting compost (JI No.2) in full light. Top-dress when growth begins, then water freely and apply a balanced liquid fertilizer monthly until the leaves die down. Keep dry in summer when dormant. Outdoors, grow in fertile, well-drained soil that dries out in summer, in full sun. In frost-prone areas, protect with a dry winter mulch.
- **PROPAGATION** Sow seed at 6–12°C (45–54°F) as soon as ripe. Remove offsets after flowering.
- **PESTS AND DISEASES** Trouble free.

L. albiflora. Bulbous perennial bearing umbels of 4–6 small, tubular-funnel-shaped white flowers, 4–5cm (1½–2in) long, with strongly reflexed, wavy-margined tepals and protruding stamens, in late summer and early autumn. Semi-erect, strap-shaped, glaucous, mid-green leaves, 30–60cm (12–24in) long, are produced after the flowers. Similar to *L. radiata*, and probably a variety of it. ↕45cm (18in), ↔ 20cm (8in). Japan. ❄
L. aurea ▣ (Golden spider lily). Bulbous perennial producing umbels,

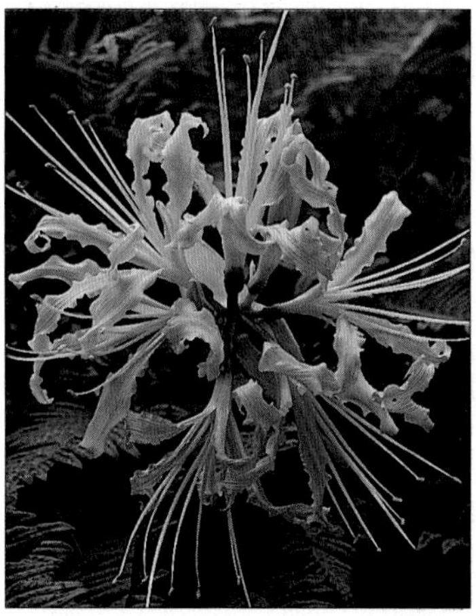

Lycoris aurea

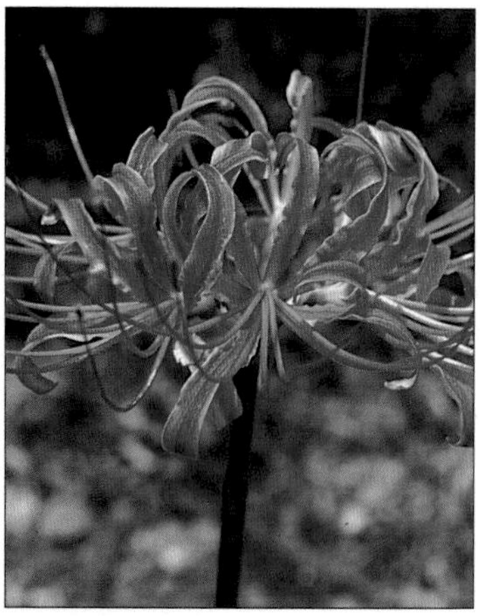

Lycoris radiata

from spring to summer, of 5 or 6 tubular-funnel-shaped, wavy-margined yellow flowers, 10cm (4in) across, with the tepals reflexed at the tips, and protruding stamens. Semi-erect, strap-shaped, fleshy, glaucous, mid-green leaves, to 60cm (24in) long, appear after the flowers. ↕ to 60cm (24in), ↔ 20cm (8in). China, Japan. ❄❄
L. radiata ▣ (Red spider lily). Bulbous perennial with wavy-margined, rose-red or deep red flowers, 4–5cm (1½–2in) long, with strongly reflexed tepals and conspicuous, protruding stamens, borne in umbels of 4–6 in late summer and early autumn. Semi-erect, strap-shaped, dark green leaves, 30–60cm (12–24in) long, appear after the flowers. ↕30–50cm (12–20in), ↔ 20cm (8in). Japan. ❄❄
L. sanguinea. Bulbous perennial producing umbels of up to 6 funnel-shaped, wavy-margined, bright red flowers, 5–6cm (2–2½in) across, the tepals with slightly reflexed tips, in summer and early autumn. Semi-erect, linear, dark green leaves, to 60cm (24in) long, appear after the flowers. ↕ to 50cm (20in), ↔ 20cm (8in). China, Japan. ❄
L. squamigera (Resurrection lily). Bulbous perennial with almost erect, tubular-funnel-shaped, slightly wavy, fragrant, pale rose-red flowers, 9–10cm (3½–4in) across, flushed or veined blue or purple, the tepals with reflexed tips, borne in umbels of up to 8 in summer. Semi-erect, strap-shaped, mid-green leaves, 30cm (12in) long, are produced the following spring. ↕45–70cm (18–28in), ↔ 30cm (12in). Japan. ❄❄

LYGODIUM

Climbing fern

SCHIZAEACEAE

Genus of 40 species of semi-evergreen and deciduous, scrambling or climbing ferns from tropical and subtropical forests worldwide. A single, palmately lobed or pinnate frond arises from the creeping, branching rhizomes. The midrib of the frond continues to grow, producing new pinnae in distant pairs; each pinna has a long, often forked stalk and a varying number of leaf-like segments. Spores are produced in small spikes at the segment margins. In frost-prone areas, grow in a warm greenhouse. In warmer areas, grow in moist woodland.

- **HARDINESS** Half hardy to frost tender. *L. palmatum* will withstand short periods at -5°C (23°F).

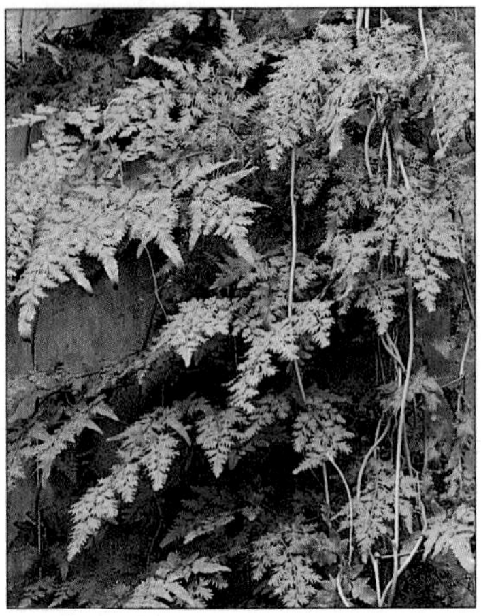

Lygodium japonicum

• **CULTIVATION** Under glass, grow in a mix of equal parts coarse leaf mould or peat, loam-based potting compost (JI No.2), chopped sphagnum moss, and charcoal, in bright filtered light. Support on wires and provide plenty of space to climb. During the growing season, water freely, apply a balanced liquid fertilizer monthly, and mist daily. Reduce watering in winter but do not allow the compost to dry out. Outdoors, grow in moderately fertile, moist, peaty soil in deep or partial shade. *L. palmatum* needs lime-free soil.
• **PROPAGATION** Sow spores at 21°C (70°F) as soon as ripe. Divide plants before the leaves develop. See also p.51.
• **PESTS AND DISEASES** Trouble free.

L. japonicum ■ (Japanese climbing fern). Deciduous, climbing fern producing 2- or 3-pinnate, very finely divided fronds. Sterile pinnae, 5–12cm (2–5in) long, are irregularly and deeply lobed to pinnate; fertile pinnae are similar, or more finely divided. ↕ 2–3m (6–10ft) or more. India, China, Korea, Japan. ⊛ (min. 5°C/41°F)
L. palmatum. Deciduous, climbing fern with palmately 3- to 7-lobed fronds, to 4cm (1½in) long. Fertile pinnae are much more finely divided than sterile ones. ↕ to 2m (6ft) or more. E. USA (N. Carolina to Florida). *

▷**Lygos** see *Retama*

LYONIA

ERICACEAE

Genus of approximately 35 species of deciduous and evergreen shrubs, sometimes small trees, from the Himalayas, E. Asia, USA, Mexico, and the Antilles, generally occurring in woodland. They have simple, glossy, leathery leaves, borne alternately, and are cultivated for their dense, axillary racemes or clusters of often urn-shaped, sometimes bell-shaped, ovoid, or cylindrical flowers, borne on the previous year's shoots. Suitable for a woodland garden or peat garden.
• **HARDINESS** Fully hardy to frost hardy.
• **CULTIVATION** Grow in acid to neutral, moderately fertile, humus-rich, moist but well-drained soil in partial or deep shade. Pruning group 1 or 8.
• **PROPAGATION** Sow seed in containers outdoors in autumn. Take semi-ripe cuttings in summer. Layer in spring.
• **PESTS AND DISEASES** Trouble free.

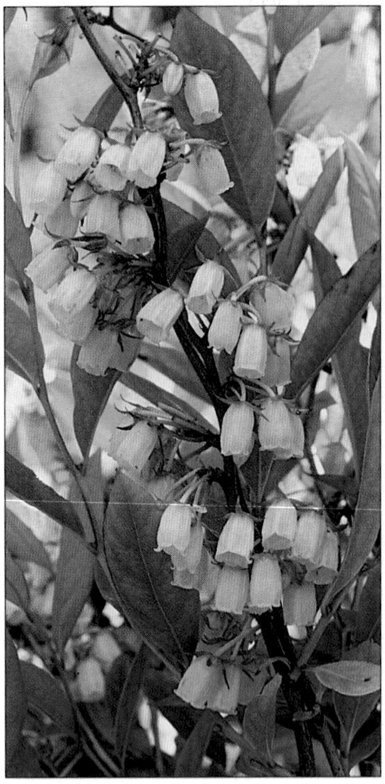

Lyonia mariana

L. ferruginea ♀ (Rusty lyonia). Spreading, bushy, evergreen shrub or small tree with elliptic to ovate or obovate, leathery, dark green leaves, to 9cm (3½in) long, usually with the margins rolled under. The shoots and the undersides of the leaves are covered with red-brown scales. Pendent clusters of up to 10 urn-shaped white flowers, 4mm (⅛in) long, are produced in late winter or spring. ↕ 5m (15ft), usually less, ↔ 2m (6ft). S.E. USA. **
L. mariana ■ (Stagger-bush). Rounded, deciduous shrub with oblong, elliptic, or narrowly obovate, leathery, dark green leaves, to 8cm (3in) long, red in autumn, dotted with brown glands beneath. Pendent, ovoid-cylindrical, white to pale pink flowers, 0.8–1.5cm (⅜–½in) long, are borne in many-flowered, umbel-like racemes in late spring and early summer. ↕ to 2m (6ft), ↔ 1.2m (4ft). E. USA. ***
L. ovalifolia ♀ Bushy, rounded, deciduous or semi-evergreen shrub or small tree with red shoots. Paired, ovate-elliptic, ovate, or ovate-oblong, leathery, dark green leaves, to 15cm (6in) long, are often finely downy beneath. In late spring or summer, bears ovoid white flowers, to 1cm (½in) long, in racemes 5–10cm (2–4in) long. ↕ 3m (10ft), ↔ 2m (6ft) as a shrub; ↕ 12m (40ft), ↔ 8m (25ft) as a tree. Himalayas, China, Japan, Taiwan. ***

▷**Lyonia, Rusty** see *Lyonia ferruginea*

LYONOTHAMNUS

ROSACEAE

Genus of one species of evergreen tree, growing wild in canyons and on dry slopes in California, USA. Cultivated mainly for its habit, attractive bark, and simple to pinnate, thick, glossy leaves, borne in opposite pairs, it is effective as a specimen tree or in woodland.
• **HARDINESS** Frost hardy.
• **CULTIVATION** Grow in fertile, moist but well-drained soil in full sun or partial shade. Shelter from cold, drying winds in frost-prone areas. Pruning group 1.
• **PROPAGATION** Sow seed in containers outdoors in autumn, or take greenwood cuttings in summer.
• **PESTS AND DISEASES** Trouble free.

L. floribundus ◊ (Catalina ironwood). Conical, evergreen tree with peeling, red-brown bark and oblong to lance-shaped, glossy, deep green leaves, to 20cm (8in) long, softly hairy beneath; leaves are simple, or sometimes partially or fully pinnate on the same tree. From spring to summer, bears large, terminal, corymb-like panicles, to 20cm (8in) across, of small, 5-petalled, star-shaped white flowers. ↕ 12m (40ft), ↔ 6m (20ft). USA (California, Santa Catalina Island). **. **var. *aspleniifolius*** has pinnate or 2-pinnate leaves, often with pinnatifid leaflets; USA (islands off the coast of California).

▷**Lyre flower** see *Dicentra spectabilis*

LYSICHITON

Skunk cabbage

ARACEAE

Genus of 2 species of robust, marginal aquatic perennials, with short rhizomes, from N.E. Asia and W. North America. They are grown for their basal clusters of large, ovate-oblong, glossy, mid- to dark green leaves, and yellow or white spathes that surround spadices bearing small, bisexual green flowers. They have a musky smell. Grow beside a stream or pool.
• **HARDINESS** Fully hardy.
• **CULTIVATION** Grow in fertile, humus-rich soil at the margins of a stream or pool, in full sun or partial shade. Allow ample room for the leaves to develop. See also pp.52–53.
• **PROPAGATION** Sow seed on a tray of wet soil in a cold frame as soon as ripe. Remove offsets at the bases of the main stems in spring or summer.
• **PESTS AND DISEASES** Trouble free.

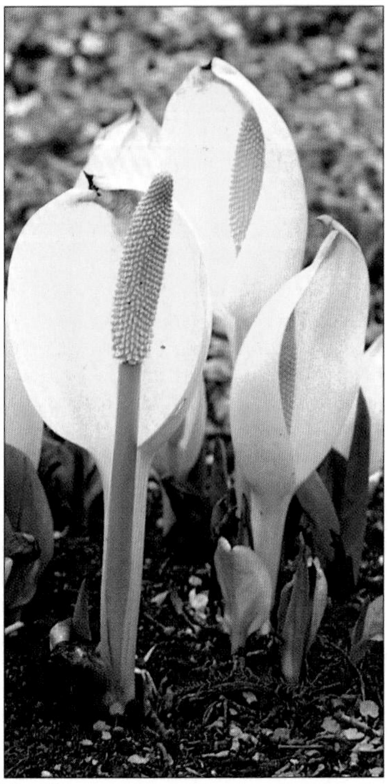

Lysichiton americanus

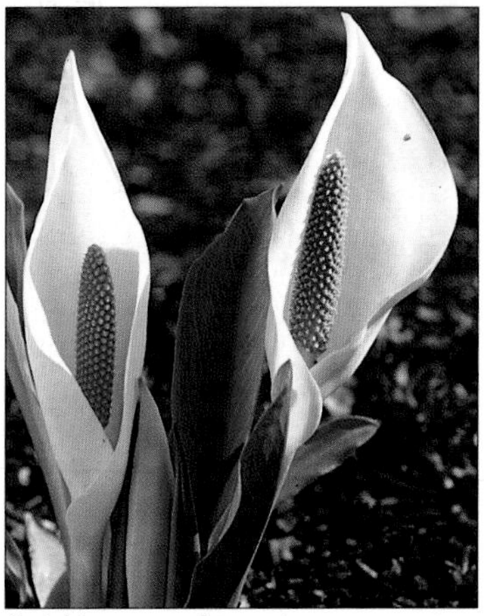

Lysichiton camtschatcensis

L. americanus ■ ♀ (Yellow skunk cabbage). Marginal aquatic perennial with rosettes of ovate-oblong, strongly veined, leathery, glossy, mid- to dark green leaves, 50–120cm (20–48in) long. Ovate to narrowly ovate, bright yellow spathes, to 40cm (16in) long, are borne in early spring. ↕ 1m (3ft), ↔ 1.2m (4ft). W. North America. ***
L. camtschatcensis ■ ♀ (White skunk cabbage). Marginal aquatic perennial with rosettes of ovate-oblong, strongly veined, leathery, glossy, mid- to dark green leaves, 50–100cm (20–39in) long. In early spring, produces ovate to broadly lance-shaped, usually pointed white spathes, to 40cm (16in) long. ↕↔ 75cm (30in). N.E. Asia. ***

LYSIMACHIA

Loosestrife

PRIMULACEAE

Genus of about 150 species of herbaceous and evergreen perennials and shrubs, mainly growing in damp grassland and woodland or by water, in subtropical regions, including South Africa, and N. temperate regions. They have opposite, alternate, or whorled, simple, entire or sometimes toothed or scalloped, often hairy leaves. The 5-petalled flowers vary from star-shaped to saucer- or cup-shaped, and are usually white or yellow, sometimes pink or purple, and either solitary and axillary or borne in terminal racemes or panicles. Larger species are suitable for a moist herbaceous border, bog garden, or pond margin, or for naturalizing in a wild or woodland garden. Low-growing species provide good ground cover. In frost-prone climates, grow tender species in a cool greenhouse.
• **HARDINESS** Fully hardy to frost tender.
• **CULTIVATION** Grow in humus-rich, preferably moist but well-drained soil that does not dry out in summer, in full sun or partial shade. Tall species may need support.
• **PROPAGATION** Sow seed in containers outdoors in spring. Divide in spring or autumn.
• **PESTS AND DISEASES** May be damaged by slugs and snails.

L. barystachys. Erect herbaceous perennial with softly hairy stems and alternate, rarely opposite, linear-oblong to lance-shaped, hairy, mid-green leaves, to 8cm (3in) long, glaucous beneath. Dense, pendent then erect, terminal

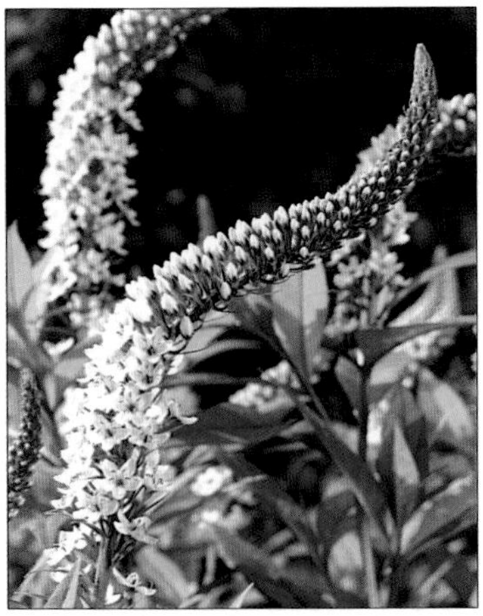
Lysimachia clethroides

racemes, to 30cm (12in) long, of star-shaped white flowers, 7–10mm (¼–½in) across, are borne in mid- and late summer. ↕ 60cm (24in), ↔ 45cm (18in). E. Russia, China, Korea, Japan. ❄❄❄

L. ciliata, syn. *Steironema ciliata.* Erect, rhizomatous herbaceous perennial with opposite or whorled, ovate-lance-shaped to ovate, hairy, mid-green leaves, to 15cm (6in) long, with hairy leaf-stalks. Solitary or paired, slightly pendent, star-shaped yellow flowers, 2.5cm (1in) across, with small, reddish brown centres, are produced on slender stalks from the upper leaf axils in midsummer. ↕ 1.2m (4ft), ↔ 60cm (24in). North America. ❄❄❄

L. clethroides ■ 🏆 Spreading, softly hairy, rhizomatous herbaceous perennial with erect stems bearing alternate, narrowly ovate-lance-shaped, pointed leaves, to 13cm (5in) long, mid-green above, pale green beneath. In mid- and late summer, saucer-shaped white flowers, 1cm (½in) across, are produced in dense, tapering, terminal racemes, 10–20cm (4–8in) long, which are pendent before the flowers open but become upright with arching tips as they

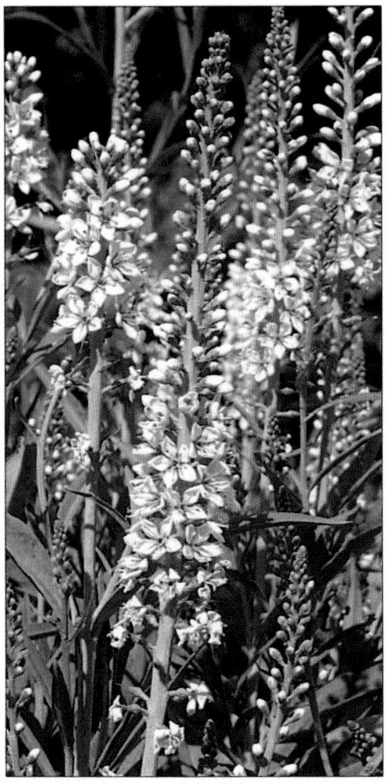
Lysimachia ephemerum

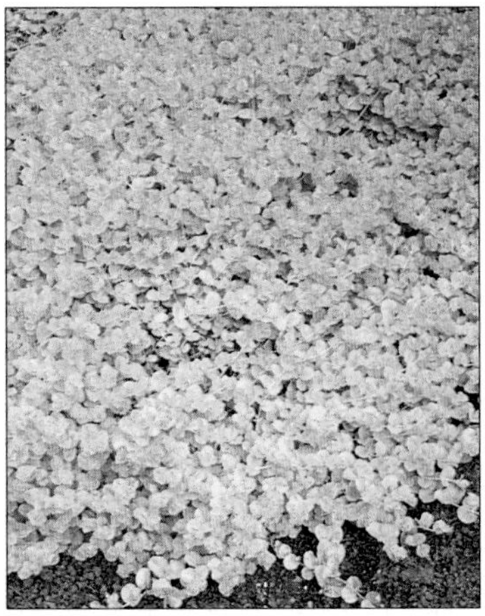
Lysimachia nummularia 'Aurea'

mature. ↕ 90cm (36in), ↔ 60cm (24in). China, Korea, Japan. ❄❄❄

L. ephemerum ■ Clump-forming herbaceous perennial with erect stems and opposite, linear-lance-shaped to linear-spoon-shaped, hairless, glaucous, grey-green, stem-clasping leaves, 15cm (6in) long. Saucer-shaped white flowers, 1cm (½in) across, are borne in slender, upright, dense, terminal racemes, to 40cm (16in) long, in early and mid-summer. Provide protection in severe winters. ↕ 1m (3ft), ↔ 30cm (12in). W. Portugal, S., C., and E. Spain, Pyrenees. ❄❄❄ (borderline)

***L. nummularia* 'Aurea'** ■ 🏆 (Golden creeping Jenny). Rampant, prostrate, stem-rooting, evergreen perennial with opposite, broadly ovate to rounded, golden yellow leaves, to 2cm (¾in) long, heart-shaped at the bases. During summer, produces usually solitary, upturned, cup-shaped, bright yellow flowers, to 2cm (¾in) across. ↕ to 5cm (2in), ↔ indefinite. ❄❄❄

L. punctata ■ Erect, rhizomatous, softly hairy herbaceous perennial with opposite or whorled, elliptic to lance-shaped, dark green leaves, 8cm (3in) long. Whorls of cup-shaped yellow

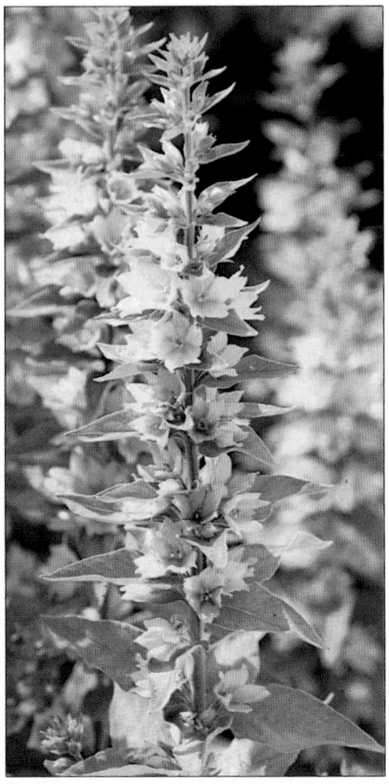
Lysimachia punctata

flowers, 2.5cm (1in) across, are borne on short stalks from the leaf axils in mid- and late summer. May be invasive. ↕ to 1m (3ft), ↔ 60cm (24in). C. and S. Europe to Turkey. ❄❄❄

L. vulgaris (Yellow loosestrife). Stoloniferous, softly hairy herbaceous perennial with erect stems bearing opposite or whorled, ovate to lance-shaped, mid- to bright green leaves, to 9cm (3½in) long. During summer, cupped yellow flowers, to 1.5cm (½in) across, are produced in leafy, terminal panicles, 10–30cm (4–12in) long. ↕ to 1.2m (4ft), ↔ to 1m (3ft). Europe, W. Asia. ❄❄❄

LYTHRUM

Loosestrife

LYTHRACEAE

Genus of 38 species of annuals and perennials found in moist meadows and scrub, and in ditches and riversides, in N. temperate regions. They have 4-angled stems and usually opposite, ovate to lance-shaped or linear, stalkless leaves, which are occasionally softly hairy. Small, star-shaped or shallowly funnel-shaped, purple, pink, or rarely white flowers are produced singly or in groups from the leaf axils, sometimes forming spike-like racemes. Loosestrifes are long-flowering, and effective in a moist border, or bog garden, or naturalized near water. Some provide attractive autumn colour. A few species have become noxious weeds in the USA.

- **HARDINESS** Fully hardy.
- **CULTIVATION** Grow in any (preferably fertile), moist soil in full sun. Remove flowered stems to prevent self-seeding.
- **PROPAGATION** Sow seed at 13–18°C (55–64°F) in spring. Divide in spring. Take basal cuttings in spring or early summer.
- **PESTS AND DISEASES** Slugs and snails may damage young shoots.

***L.* 'Morden Pink'.** Clump-forming perennial with erect, branched stems and linear-lance-shaped, hairless leaves, 10cm (4in) long. From early to late summer, bears star-shaped, clear pink flowers, 1cm (½in) across, in loose, spike-like racemes, to 45cm (18in) long. ↕ to 80cm (32in), ↔ 45cm (18in). ❄❄❄

L. salicaria (Purple loosestrife). Clump-forming perennial with erect, stiff, branched stems bearing lance-shaped, downy leaves, 10cm (4in) long. From midsummer to early autumn, produces star-shaped, bright purple-red to purple-pink flowers, 2cm (¾in) across, in spike-like racemes, to 45cm (18in) long. ↕ 1.2m (4ft), ↔ 45cm (18in). Europe, temperate Asia. ❄❄❄. **'Feuerkerze'** 🏆 syn. 'Firecandle', bears intense rose-red flowers in slender racemes; ↕ to 90cm (36in). **'Firecandle'** see 'Feuerkerze'. **'Happy'** has dark pink flowers; ↕ 45cm (18in). **'Robert'** produces bright pink flowers; ↕ 90cm (36in).

L. virgatum. Clump-forming perennial with erect, branched stems and linear-lance-shaped, hairless leaves, 10cm (4in) long. From early to late summer, star-shaped, purple-red flowers, 1cm (½in) across, are borne in slender, spike-like racemes, to 30cm (12in) long. ↕ 90cm (36in), ↔ 45cm (18in). E. Europe, W. and C. Asia, N.W. China. ❄❄❄. **'Rose Queen'** produces bright rose-pink flowers, purple in bud; ↕ 60cm (24in). **'The Rocket'** ■ produces deep pink flowers; ↕ 80cm (32in).

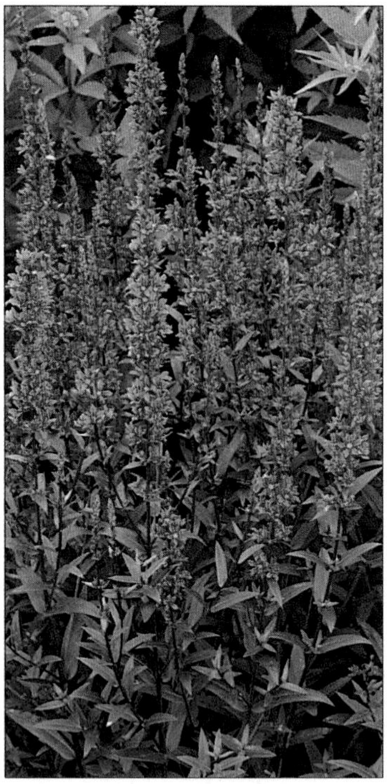
Lythrum virgatum 'The Rocket'

LYTOCARYUM

ARECACEAE/PALMACEAE

Genus of 3 species of single- or multi-stemmed palms occurring in open woodland in seasonally dry areas, or among shrubs on rocky ridges, in southern Brazil. The upright stems each bear a terminal rosette of lance-shaped, pinnate, bright mid-green leaves, with about 60 pairs of linear leaflets. Small, cup-shaped flowers are borne in panicles, to 1.5m (5ft) long, arising from the leaf bases. They are followed by spherical green fruits, which split when ripe to reveal nut-like seeds. In frost-prone areas, grow in a temperate or warm greenhouse. In frost-free areas, grow as specimen trees.

- **HARDINESS** Frost tender.
- **CULTIVATION** Under glass, grow in loam-based potting compost (JI No.2) in full light, with moderate humidity. Water moderately when in growth, sparingly when dormant. Apply a balanced liquid fertilizer monthly when in growth. Outdoors, grow in fertile, well-drained soil in full sun or partial shade; shelter from cold, drying winds.
- **PROPAGATION** Sow seed at 18–24°C (64–75°F) in spring.
- **PESTS AND DISEASES** Trouble free.

L. weddellianum 🏆 🌴 syn. *Microcoelum weddellianum, Syagrus weddelliana* (Weddell palm). Small palm with a slender, erect stem. Pinnate leaves, to 1.2m (4ft) long, have red-black scales along the stalks and midribs, and are composed of many narrowly linear leaflets, bright green above, greyish green beneath. Cup-shaped, 3-petalled green flowers are borne in panicles to 1m (3ft) long, usually in summer. ↕ 2–3m (6–10ft), ↔ 1–2m (3–6ft). Brazil. ❀ (min. 13°C/55°F)

L

M

MAACKIA

LEGUMINOSAE/PAPILIONACEAE

Genus of about 8 species of deciduous trees or shrubs occurring in woodland in E. Asia. Maackias are cultivated both for their foliage and flowers. The leaves are alternate and pinnate, each with up to 17 pairs of leaflets and a single terminal one. The small, pea-like flowers are produced in dense, terminal racemes or panicles in summer, and are followed by compressed, linear-oblong seed pods. Maackias are unusual specimen trees.

- **HARDINESS** Fully hardy.
- **CULTIVATION** Grow in moderately fertile, well-drained, neutral to acid soil in full sun. Pruning group 1.
- **PROPAGATION** Sow seed outdoors in containers or in a seedbed, in autumn. Insert greenwood cuttings in early or midsummer.
- **PESTS AND DISEASES** Trouble free.

M. amurensis ▣ ♀ Open, spreading tree with pinnate, dark green leaves, 20–30cm (8–12in) long, with 7–11 ovate leaflets. In mid- and late summer, white flowers, to 1cm (½in) long, are produced in upright racemes, 10–15cm (4–6in) long, followed by flattened seed pods, to 5cm (2in) long, with ridged seams. ↕ to 15m (50ft), ↔ to 10m (30ft). N.E. China. ❄❄❄

M. chinensis ♀ Rounded, sometimes flat-topped tree bearing pinnate, dark green leaves, to 20cm (8in) long, with 9–13 oblong to elliptic leaflets, silvery grey-blue when they unfold. In mid- and late summer, white flowers, to 1cm (½in) long, are produced in upright panicles, 15–20cm (6–8in) long, followed by oblong to elliptic seed pods, to 7cm (3in) long. ↕↔ 10m (30ft). China (Hubei, Sichuan). ❄❄❄

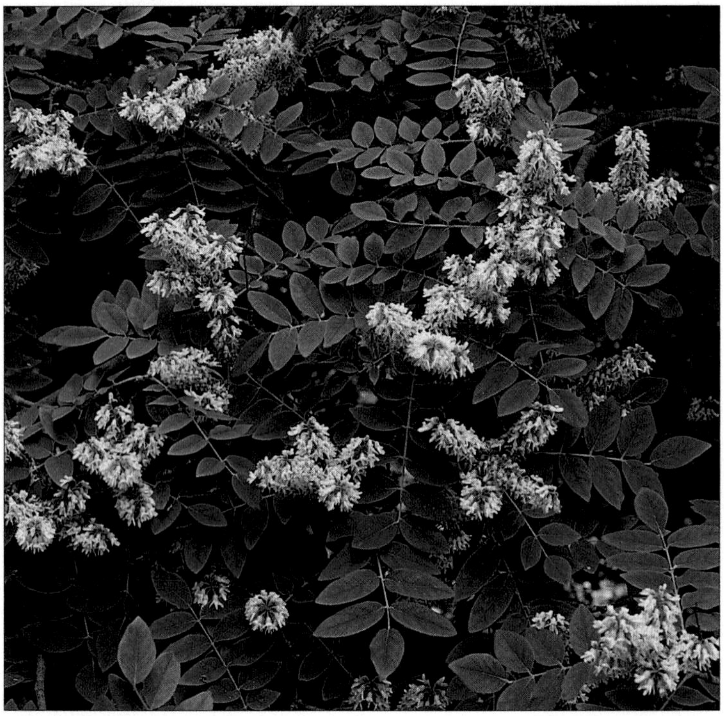

Maackia amurensis

MACFADYENA

syn. DOXANTHA

Cat's claw vine

BIGNONIACEAE

Genus of 3 or 4 species of evergreen climbers found in tropical forest and dry woodland from Mexico and the West Indies to Uruguay and Argentina. The leaves are borne in opposite pairs, each with 2 spreading leaflets and a short, 3-clawed tendril. Tubular-bell-shaped flowers, with 5 spreading lobes, are solitary or produced in axillary cymes from spring to summer. In frost-prone climates, grow these attractive climbers in a temperate greenhouse. In warm areas, grow over a fence, pergola, arch, or trellis, or use for ground cover.

- **HARDINESS** Frost tender.
- **CULTIVATION** Under glass, grow in loam-based potting compost (JI No.2) in bright filtered light, or full light with shade from hot sun. In the growing season, water freely and apply a balanced liquid fertilizer monthly; water sparingly in winter. Outdoors, grow in moderately fertile, moist but well-drained, slightly acid to slightly alkaline soil in full sun. Provide shelter from cold, drying winds. Pruning group 11, after flowering.
- **PROPAGATION** Sow seed at 16–21°C (61–70°F) as soon as ripe or in spring. Root semi-ripe cuttings with bottom heat in summer. Layer in spring.
- **PESTS AND DISEASES** Red spider mites, whiteflies, and mealybugs may prove troublesome under glass.

M. unguis-cati ▣ syn. *Bignonia unguis-cati, Doxantha unguis-cati* (Common cat's claw vine). Slender-stemmed, vigorous climber with lance-shaped to ovate leaflets, 5–10cm (2–4in) or more long. From spring to summer, produces tubular, bright yellow flowers, 10cm (4in) across, usually with orange lines in the throats, followed by slender, bean-like seed pods, 25–90cm (10–36in) long. ↕ 6–10m (20–30ft). Mexico and West Indies to Argentina. ❀ (min. 7°C/45°F)

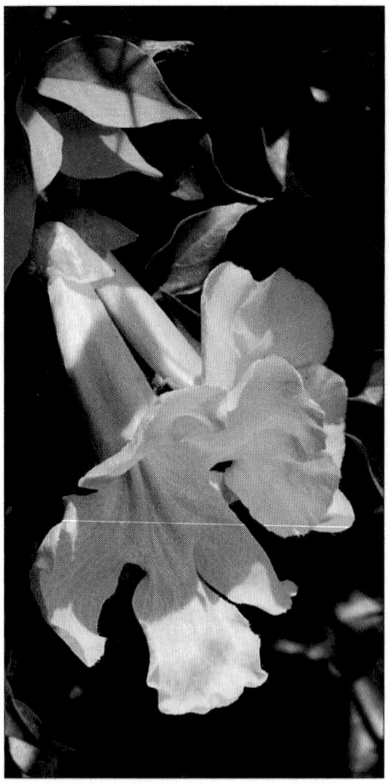

Macfadyena unguis-cati

▷ ***Machaerocereus eruca*** see *Stenocereus eruca*

MACKAYA *syn.* ASYSTASIA

ACANTHACEAE

Genus of one species of evergreen shrub occurring in dry, open, mixed forest in southern Africa. *M. bella* is cultivated for its opposite, slender-pointed, elliptic leaves and its arching, terminal racemes of tubular-funnel-shaped flowers, each with 5 large, flared lobes, usually borne from spring to autumn. In frost-prone areas, grow in a temperate or warm greenhouse. In warmer climates, grow in a shrub border or as a specimen plant.

- **HARDINESS** Frost tender.
- **CULTIVATION** Under glass, grow in loam-based potting compost (JI No.2) in bright filtered light, or full light with shade from hot sun. In growth, water freely and apply a balanced liquid fertilizer monthly; water sparingly in winter. Outdoors, grow in moderately fertile, moist but well-drained, neutral to slightly acid or alkaline soil in full sun or light dappled shade. Pruning group 9; plants under glass need restrictive pruning in late winter.
- **PROPAGATION** Sow seed at 16°C (61°F) in spring. Root semi-ripe cuttings with bottom heat in summer.
- **PESTS AND DISEASES** Red spider mites and whiteflies may be troublesome under glass.

M. bella ▣ ♀ syn. *Asystasia bella.* Erect then spreading shrub, with elliptic, slender-pointed, wavy-margined, lustrous, deep green leaves, 8–12cm (3–5in) long, with prominent veins. Terminal racemes of narrowly funnel-shaped flowers, to 5cm (2in) across, with large, pale lilac petal lobes finely veined dark purple, are mainly produced from spring to autumn. ↕ 1–2m (3–6ft), ↔ 1–1.5m (3–5ft). South Africa (Northern Traansvaal, Eastern Transvaal, E. Northern Cape, KwaZulu/Natal), Swaziland. ❀ (min. 10°C/50°F)

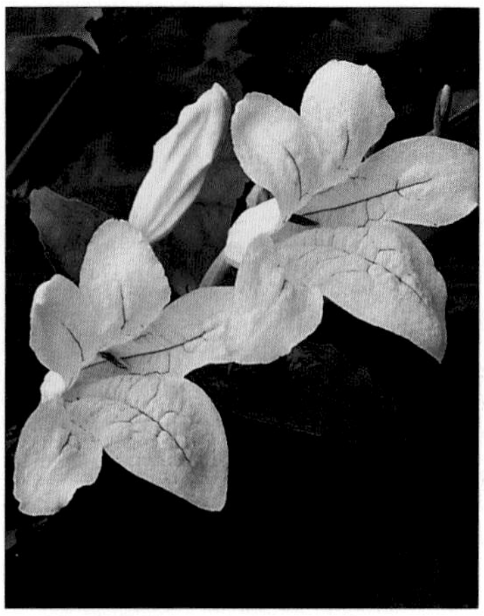

Mackaya bella

MACLEANIA

ERICACEAE

Genus of 40 species of evergreen shrubs and climbers, some scrambling or semi-scandent, and sometimes epiphytic, occurring in tropical forest in Central and South America. They are cultivated for their waxy, tubular flowers, each with 5 short petal lobes, which are produced in pendent racemes from the upper leaf axils. The simple, leathery leaves are arranged alternately. In areas where temperatures fall below 10°C (50°F), grow in a temperate or warm greenhouse. In frost-free climates, train over an arch or pergola, or grow against a wall.

- **HARDINESS** Frost tender.
- **CULTIVATION** Under glass, grow in lime-free (ericaceous) potting compost in bright filtered light. In the growing season, water moderately and apply a balanced liquid fertilizer monthly; water sparingly in winter. Outdoors, grow in moderately fertile, humus-rich, moist but well-drained, acid soil in partial shade. Pruning group 11 for climbers, immediately after flowering; group 8 for shrubs.
- **PROPAGATION** Surface-sow seed at 13–16°C (55–61°F) in spring. Root semi-ripe cuttings with bottom heat in early summer. Air layer in spring.
- **PESTS AND DISEASES** Scale insects may be a problem under glass.

M. insignis. Semi-scandent, sparsely branched shrub with a woody, tuberous base, often epiphytic in the wild. Ovate to elliptic leaves, 5–10cm (2–4in) long, are red-tinted when young, maturing to deep green. Orange to deep scarlet flowers, 2.5–4cm (1–1½in) long, with small, triangular petal lobes and softly hairy mouths, are produced in short, leafy racemes, mainly in summer. ↕ 2–4m (6–12ft), ↔ 1–1.5m (3–5ft). S. Mexico, Honduras, Guatemala. ❀ (min. 10°C/50°F)

MACLEAYA syn. BOCCONIA

Plume poppy

PAPAVERACEAE

Genus of 2 or 3 species of rhizomatous perennials from grassy meadows, scrub, and woodland in China and Japan. They are cultivated for their foliage and graceful inflorescences. Erect, glaucous stems bear alternate, heart-shaped, palmately lobed, glaucous, grey-green to olive-green leaves, to 25cm (10in) long, with rounded, toothed lobes and prominent veins. Numerous petalless, tubular flowers, to 1cm (½in) long, with 2 or 4 sepals and a cluster of stamens, are borne in airy, plume-like panicles. The stems and leaf-stalks produce a yellowish orange latex. Grow in a mixed or herbaceous border or as free-standing specimens; they may also be grown among shrubs or used to form a tall screen. They can be invasive.

• **HARDINESS** Fully hardy, but new growth may be damaged by late frosts.
• **CULTIVATION** Grow in moderately fertile, moist but well-drained soil in full sun, although they will tolerate most soils and partial shade. Provide shelter from cold, drying winds.
• **PROPAGATION** Sow seed in containers in a cold frame in spring. Divide in late autumn or spring. Separate and transplant rooted rhizomes when dormant. Insert root cuttings in winter.
• **PESTS AND DISEASES** Slugs may attack young growth.

M. cordata 🏆 syn. *Bocconia cordata* (Plume poppy). Rhizomatous perennial with 5- to 7-lobed, grey- to olive-green leaves, white-downy beneath. In mid- and late summer, produces large, plume-like panicles of pendent, buff-white flowers, each with 25–40 stamens, on grey-green stems. ↕ to 2.5m (8ft), ↔ 1m (3ft). China, Japan. ❄❄❄
M. x kewensis (*M. cordata* x *M. microcarpa*). Rhizomatous perennial with 5- to 9-lobed, grey-green leaves. Creamy buff flowers, each with 12–18 stamens, are produced in loose, terminal panicles in early and late summer. ↕ 2.5m (8ft), ↔ 1m (3ft) or more. Garden origin. ❄❄❄. **'Flamingo'** has pink buds and buff-pink flowers.
***M. microcarpa* 'Kelway's Coral Plume'** ▣ 🏆 Rhizomatous perennial with 5- to 7-lobed, grey- to olive-green leaves, white-downy beneath. Large, loose panicles of pendent, deep buff- to coral-pink flowers, each with 8–15 stamens, open from pink buds in early and midsummer. ↕ 2.2m (7ft), ↔ 1m (3ft) or more. ❄❄❄

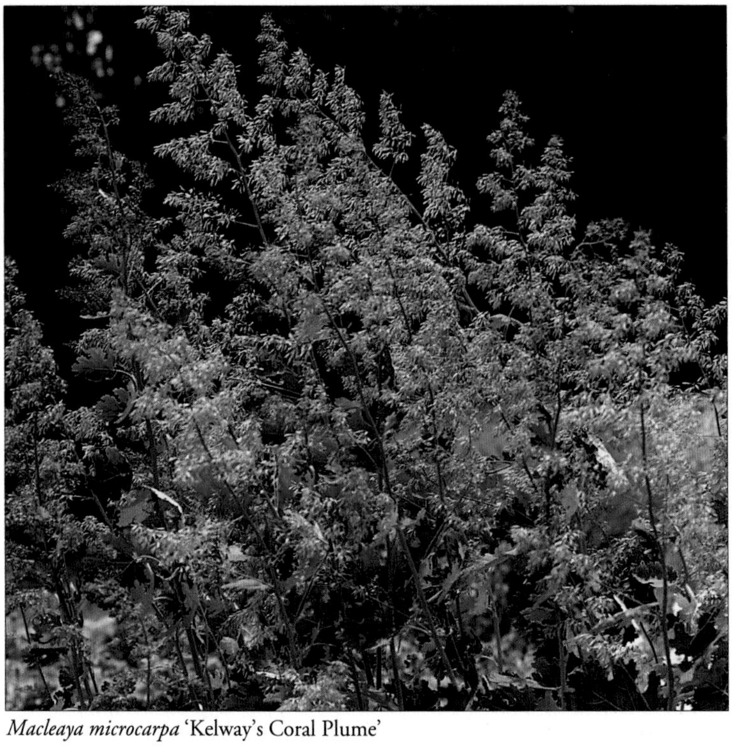
Macleaya microcarpa 'Kelway's Coral Plume'

MACLURA syn. CUDRANIA

MORACEAE

Genus of 15 species of usually thorny, evergreen or deciduous, dioecious trees, shrubs, or climbers, the branches often reduced to spines, found in woodland and clearings, and by roadsides, from E. Asia to Australia, and from S. central USA to South America. The alternate or spiralling leaves are obovate or narrowly to broadly ovate. Racemes or clusters of small, spherical or cup-shaped, usually green flowers are followed by fleshy, spherical fruits, surrounded by enlarged bracts. Grow in a shrub border or as specimens; *M. pomifera* is also used for hedging. They need long, hot summers to grow well and produce fruit.

• **HARDINESS** Fully hardy. Unripened wood, particularly of young plants, may be susceptible to frost damage.
• **CULTIVATION** Grow in moderately fertile, well-drained soil in full sun. Pruning group 1.
• **PROPAGATION** Sow seed in containers in an open frame as soon as ripe. Root semi-ripe cuttings with bottom heat in summer, or take root cuttings in winter.
• **PESTS AND DISEASES** Trouble free.

M. aurantiaca see *M. pomifera*.
M. pomifera 🌳 syn. *M. aurantiaca* (Osage orange). Rounded, deciduous tree, thorny when young, becoming less so with age, with ovate, pointed, dark green leaves, to 10cm (4in) long, turning yellow in autumn. Tiny, cup-shaped, yellow-green flowers – the females in short racemes, the males in dense, spherical clusters – are borne in early summer, followed on female trees by large, wrinkled, yellow-green fruit, to 12cm (5in) across. ↕ 15m (50ft), ↔ 12m (40ft). S. central USA. ❄❄❄
M. tricuspidata 🌳 syn. *Cudrania tricuspidata*. Compact, rounded, deciduous shrub or small tree with ovate or obovate, dark green leaves, to 10cm (4in) long, sometimes 3-lobed at the apexes. In summer, spherical clusters of tiny green flowers are borne singly or in pairs from the leaf axils of the current year's growth, followed on female trees by glossy, edible, orange-red fruit, 2–5cm (¾–2in) across. ↕ 7m (22ft), ↔ 6m (20ft). C. China, Korea. ❄❄❄

▷**Macqui** see *Aristotelia chilensis*

MACROPIDIA

HAEMODORACEAE

Genus of one species of evergreen, rhizomatous perennial from Australia, found in open ground at the edges of scrub. It has fans of sword-shaped, basal leaves, and produces panicles of woolly, swollen, tubular flowers, with sharply reflexed segments often likened to a kangaroo's foot. In frost-prone areas, grow in a cool or temperate greenhouse. In warmer climates, it is an unusual and effective border plant.

• **HARDINESS** Frost tender.
• **CULTIVATION** Under glass, grow in loam-based potting compost (JI No.2), with added grit, in bright filtered light, or full light with shade from hot sun, with low humidity. In the growing season, water moderately and apply a balanced liquid fertilizer monthly; water sparingly in winter. Outdoors, grow in moderately fertile, well-drained, neutral to slightly acid soil in full sun, with shade from midday sun. Protect from excessive winter wet.
• **PROPAGATION** Sow seed at 10°C (50°F) as soon as ripe or in spring. Divide as growth starts in spring.
• **PESTS AND DISEASES** Trouble free.

M. fuliginosa (Black kangaroo paw). Perennial with short rhizomes and fan-shaped tufts of linear to narrowly strap-shaped, bluish green leaves, to 30cm (12in) long. Panicles of yellow flowers, 4.5cm (1¾in) long, covered in plume-like black hairs, are borne on stout, branched stems, to 1.2m (4ft) long, in summer. ↕ 1.2m (4ft), ↔ 60cm (24in). S.W. Australia. ❀ (min. 7°C/45°F)

▷***Macrotomia echioides*** see *Arnebia pulchra*

MACROZAMIA

ZAMIACEAE

Genus of 12 species of dioecious cycads from well-drained sites in open forest in Australia. Some species have a palm-like stem; in others, the stem is short and completely or partly buried. Evergreen, pinnate leaves, with linear to lance-shaped, leathery, light to mid-green leaflets, are borne in terminal whorls or rosettes. Male or female inflorescences

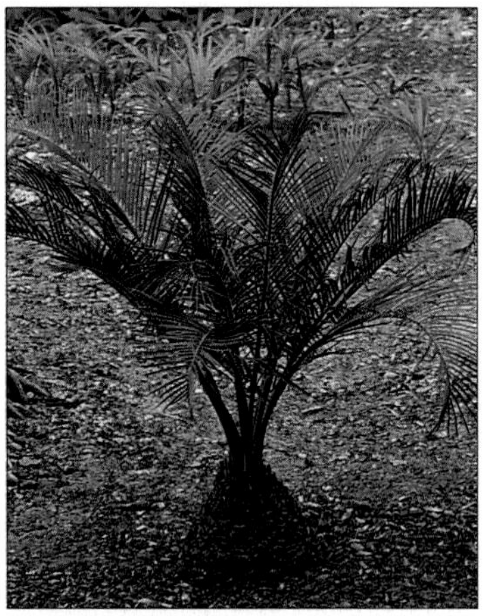
Macrozamia communis

("cones") are borne among the leaves. In frost-prone areas, grow in a temperate or warm greenhouse. In warmer climates, grow as specimen trees.

• **HARDINESS** Frost tender.
• **CULTIVATION** Under glass, grow in loam-based potting compost (JI No.2), with added grit, in full light with shade from hot sun, and with low to moderate humidity. Pot on or top-dress in spring. In growth, water moderately and apply a balanced liquid fertilizer monthly; water sparingly in winter. Outdoors, grow in poor to moderately fertile, well-drained, neutral to slightly acid soil in full sun, with shade from midday sun.
• **PROPAGATION** Sow seed at 21–30°C (70–86°F) as soon as ripe or in spring.
• **PESTS AND DISEASES** Trouble free.

M. communis ▣ (Burrawong). Cycad with a robust stem, buried at first then slowly elongating. Whorled leaves, to 2m (6ft) long, have linear, sharply pointed, lustrous, rich green leaflets. Cylindrical, green to brown flowering cones usually appear in summer: male cones are 20–45cm (8–18in) long, females to 45cm (18in) long. They are followed by ovoid fruit containing large, fleshy red seeds. ↕ 2–3m (6–10ft), ↔ to 4m (12ft). Australia (New South Wales). ❀ (min. 10°C/50°F)
M. corallipes see *M. spiralis*.
M. moorei ✱ Palm-like cycad with a thick, columnar trunk and whorled leaves, to 3m (10ft) long, with narrowly lance-shaped, deep green, often bluish green leaflets. Bears cylindrical, usually green flowering cones in summer: the males to 30cm (12in) long, the females to 90cm (36in) long. Flowers are followed by ovoid fruit with bright red seeds. ↕ to 9m (28ft), ↔ to 6m (20ft). Australia (New South Wales, Queensland). ❀ (min. 10°C/50°F)
M. spiralis, syn. *M. corallipes*. Small cycad with a largely underground stem, with only the growing point above the surface. Leaves, to 90cm (36in) or more long, have stalks with pink, red, or orange bases, and consist of many linear, matt, deep green leaflets that spiral longitudinally, at least when young. Cylindrical to ellipsoid green flowering cones, 15–20cm (6–8in) long, appear in summer, followed by ovoid fruit with orange to scarlet seeds. ↕ 1m (3ft) or more, ↔ to 2m (6ft). Australia (New South Wales). ❀ (min. 10°C/50°F)

▷**Madroño** see *Arbutus menziesii*.

MAGNOLIA

MAGNOLIACEAE

Genus of about 125 species of deciduous and evergreen trees and shrubs, occurring in woodland, in scrub, and on riverbanks from the Himalayas to E. and S.E. Asia, and from E. North America to tropical North and South America. They are grown for their showy, solitary, fragrant, usually erect, sometimes pendent or horizontal, cup-, saucer-, goblet-, or star-shaped flowers (see panel opposite), often borne before the leaves. The flowers have usually 6–9 petals; colours include pure white, white flushed or stained pink or purple, pink, rich purple, creamy yellow, greenish yellow, glaucous green, and light to mid-yellow. The alternate leaves are usually obovate to ovate, oblong, or elliptic. Cone-like fruits, often with red-coated seeds, are attractive in autumn.

Grow magnolias as specimens or among other trees and shrubs. In frost-prone climates, grow tender speices in a cool or temperate greenhouse. Some species take many years to flower: up to 30 years for *M. campbellii* when grown from seed and about 15 years for grafted or budded plants. *M. grandiflora* and *M.* x *soulangeana* may be wall-trained.

• **HARDINESS** Fully hardy to frost tender. Flowers, and sometimes young foliage, of early-flowering magnolias may be damaged by late frosts.

• **CULTIVATION** Grow in moist, well-drained, humus-rich, preferably acid to neutral soil in sun or partial shade, with shelter from strong winds. *M. delavayi* and *M. grandiflora* will tolerate dry, alkaline soil; *M. kobus, M.* x *loebneri, M. sieboldii, M. stellata,* and *M. wilsonii* will grow in moist, alkaline soils. Mulch with manure and leaf mould in early spring, particularly on dry soils. Pruning group 1 for trees and deciduous shrubs; group 9 for evergreen shrubs; group 13 if wall-trained.

• **PROPAGATION** Sow seed in a seedbed in autumn. Stratified seeds germinate freely. For deciduous magnolias, root greenwood cuttings in early summer, or semi-ripe cuttings in late summer. For evergreens, root semi-ripe cuttings from late summer to early autumn. Graft in winter. Bud in summer. Layer in early spring.

• **PESTS AND DISEASES** Prone to honey fungus, coral spot, and scale insects.

M. acuminata ▣ △ (Cucumber tree). Vigorous, conical, deciduous tree with ovate to elliptic or oblong-ovate leaves, dark green above, lighter and softly hairy beneath, to 25cm (10in) long. In late spring and early summer, produces small, cup-shaped, yellow-green or glaucous green flowers, to 9cm (3½in) across, among the leaves, followed by red or brown fruit. ↕ 20m (70ft), ↔ 10m (30ft). E. North America. ❄❄❄. **'Golden Glow'** has yellow flowers. **var. *subcordata*,** syn. *M. cordata,* is shrubby, with smaller leaves, to 15cm (6in) long, and pale yellow to yellow-green flowers; ↕ 8m (25ft), ↔ 6m (20ft); S.E. USA.

M. ashei ▣ ♀ syn. *M. macrophylla* subsp. *ashei.* Spreading, deciduous shrub or small tree with stout shoots and large, obovate leaves, glossy, light green above and glaucous beneath, to 60cm (24in) long. In early summer, produces saucer-shaped white flowers, 20–25cm (8–10in) across, the petals stained maroon at the bases. Differs from *M. macrophylla* in its smaller flowers and cylindrical to ovoid (not spherical) fruit. ↕ 10–20m (30–70ft), ↔ 8–15m (25–50ft). USA (N.W. Florida). ❄❄❄

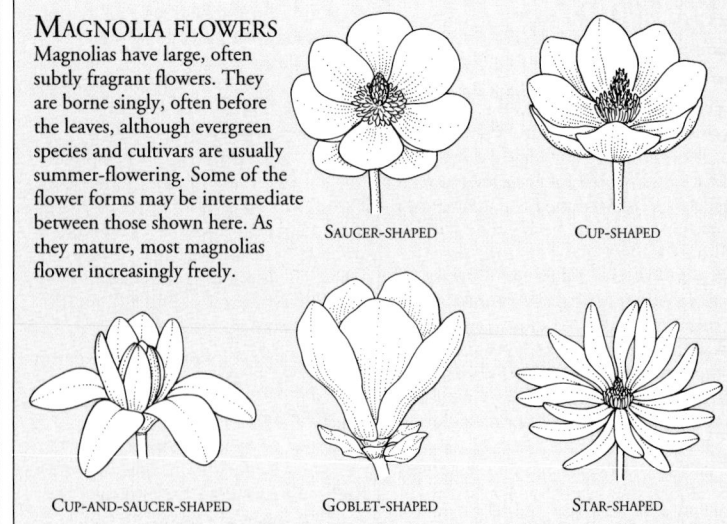

MAGNOLIA FLOWERS

Magnolias have large, often subtly fragrant flowers. They are borne singly, often before the leaves, although evergreen species and cultivars are usually summer-flowering. Some of the flower forms may be intermediate between those shown here. As they mature, most magnolias flower increasingly freely.

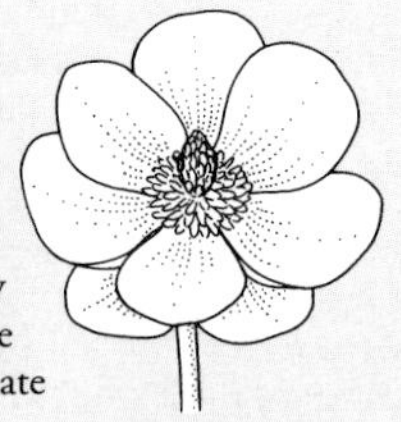

SAUCER-SHAPED

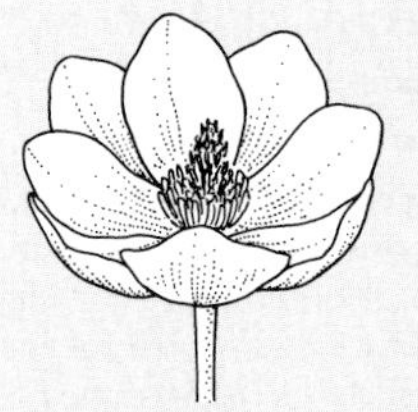

CUP-SHAPED

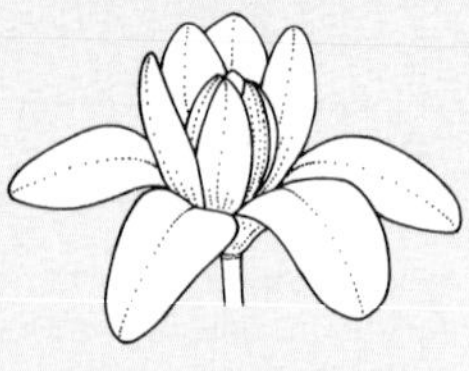

CUP-AND-SAUCER-SHAPED

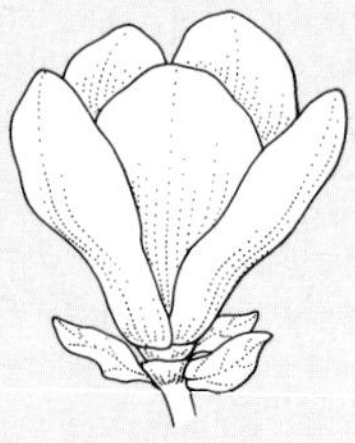

GOBLET-SHAPED

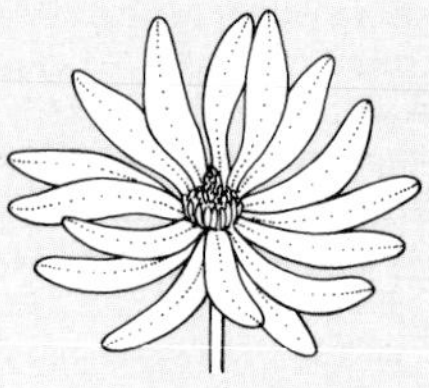

STAR-SHAPED

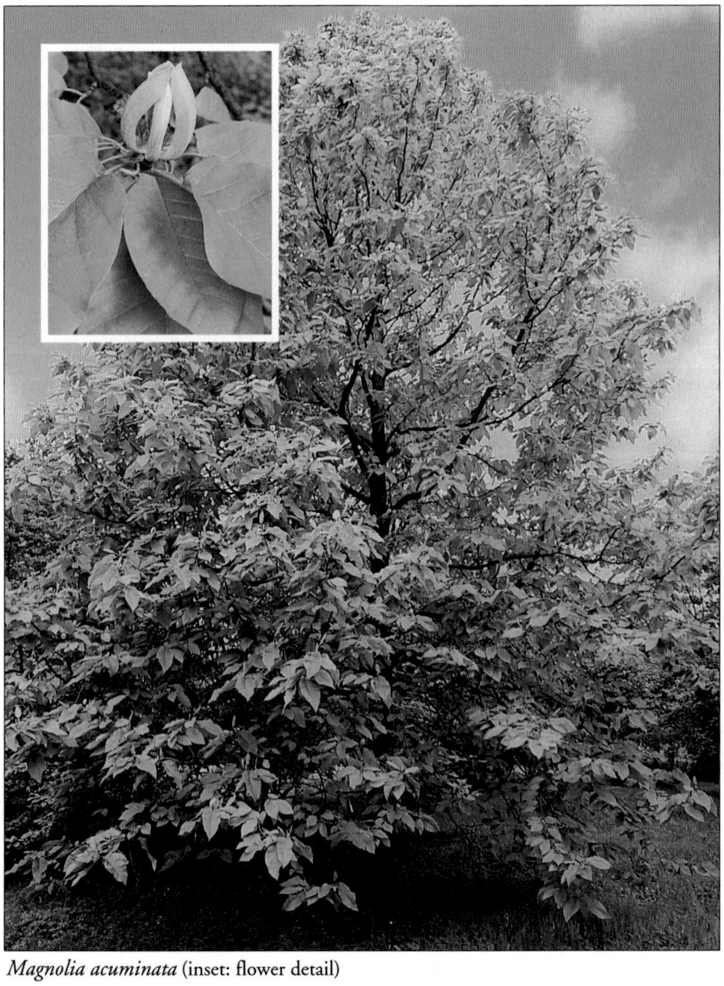

Magnolia acuminata (inset: flower detail)

***M.* 'Betty'** 🏆 Vigorous, rounded, deciduous shrub with broadly ovate, mid-green leaves, to 15cm (6in) long. In mid-spring, bears large, cup-shaped flowers, to 20cm (8in) across, with up to 19 petals, purple-red outside and white inside. ↕↔ 4m (12ft). ❄❄❄

***M.* x *brooklynensis* 'Woodsman'** △ Conical, later spreading, deciduous tree with ovate, mid-green leaves, to 25cm (10in) long. In late spring and early summer, bears narrowly cup-shaped flowers, to 12cm (5in) across, the outer 3 petals green, the middle 3 green-flushed purple, and the central 3 pale pink. ↕ 10m (30ft), ↔ 6m (20ft). ❄❄❄

M. campbellii ▣ △ Vigorous, conical then spreading deciduous tree with elliptic-ovate to oblong-elliptic, mid-green leaves, to 25cm (10in) long. Cup-and-saucer-shaped, white or crimson to rose-pink flowers, to 30cm (12in) across, with up to 16 petals, are borne from late winter to spring, before the leaves. ↕ 15m (50ft), ↔ 10m (30ft). Nepal, India (Sikkim), Bhutan. ❄❄❄. **var. *alba*** has white flowers. **'Charles Raffill'** ▣ 🏆 has purple-pink flowers. **'Darjeeling'** ▣ produces very dark pink flowers. **'Kew's Surprise'** has dark purple-pink flowers. **'Lanarth'** has rich lilac-purple flowers. **'Maharajah'** has large white flowers with purple bases. **subsp. *mollicomata*** ▣ bears pink to purple-pink flowers at an earlier age and slightly later in the year; S.W. Tibet, N. Burma, China (Yunnan). **'Strybing White'** has large white flowers.

***M.* 'Charles Coates'** ▣ Vigorous, open, spreading, deciduous shrub with ovate leaves, clustered at the shoot tips, dark green above and slightly glaucous green beneath, to 25cm (10in) long. In late spring and early summer, produces erect or horizontal, fragrant, saucer-shaped, creamy white flowers, to 10cm (4in) across, with red anthers and 9–12 petals. ↕ 10m (30ft), ↔ 6m (20ft). ❄❄❄

M. cordata see *M. acuminata* var. *subcordata.*

M. cylindrica ▣ 🏆 ♀ Deciduous shrub or small, spreading tree with obovate leaves, to 15cm (6in) long, dark green above and pale green beneath. Cup-shaped, creamy white or yellowish white flowers, to 10cm (4in) long, are borne in spring, before and with the young leaves. ↕↔ 6m (20ft). E. China. ❄❄❄

M. dawsoniana ♀ Broadly oval-headed, deciduous tree, occasionally a large shrub, with obovate, dark green leaves, to 15cm (6in) long, slightly glaucous beneath. Large, horizontal to pendent, saucer-shaped, pale lilac-pink flowers, to 12cm (5in) across, are borne in early spring, before the leaves. ↕ 15m (50ft), ↔ 10m (30ft). China. ❄❄. **'Chyverton'** ▣ has deep purplish pink petals, white or very pale pink at the tips and within, and crimson anthers; ❄❄❄

M. delavayi ▣ ♀ Dense, rounded, evergreen shrub or tree with ovate to oblong, dark green leaves, to 30cm (12in) long. Short-lived, cup-shaped, creamy or yellowish white flowers, to 20cm (8in) across, are borne in late summer. Grows well against a wall. ↕↔ 10m (30ft). China. ❄❄

M. denudata ▣ 🏆 ♀ syn. *M. heptapeta* (Lily tree, Yulan). Spreading, deciduous shrub or tree with obovate, mid-green leaves, to 15cm (6in) long. Cup-shaped, pure white flowers, to 15cm (6in) across, are borne in spring, before the leaves. ↕↔ 10m (30ft). China. ❄❄❄

***M.* 'Elizabeth'** ▣ 🏆 △ Conical, deciduous tree with obovate leaves, to 20cm (8in) long, bronze when young, maturing to dark green. Cup-shaped, clear primrose-yellow flowers, to 15cm (6in) across, are produced in mid- and late spring, before and with the young leaves. ↕ 10m (30ft), ↔ 6m (20ft). ❄❄❄

M. fraseri ▣ ♀ Open, spreading, deciduous tree with obovate leaves, usually to 25cm (10in) long, but occasionally much larger, with distinct auricles, bronze when young, maturing to mid-green. Narrowly cup- or goblet-shaped, green-flushed, creamy white flowers, 15–20cm (6–8in) across, are borne in late spring and early summer. ↕↔ 10m (30ft). S.E. USA. ❄❄❄

***M.* 'Galaxy'** 🏆 △ Fast-growing, broadly conical, deciduous tree with obovate, mid-green leaves, to 20cm (8in) long. Large, goblet-shaped, rich purple-pink flowers, to 12cm (5in) across, are borne

M

in mid-spring, before the leaves. ↕ 12m (40ft), ↔ 8m (25ft). ❄❄❄
M. glauca see *M. virginiana.*
M. globosa ♤ Rounded, deciduous shrub or tree with rust-red young branches and elliptic to obovate, glossy, dark green leaves, to 20cm (8in) long. Pendent, rounded, cup-shaped white flowers, to 12cm (5in) across, with red anthers and 9–12 petals, are produced in early summer. ↕↔ 5m (15ft). Himalayas, W. China. ❄❄
M. grandiflora ♤ (Bull bay). Dense, broadly conical, evergreen tree with narrowly elliptic to broadly ovate, leathery, glossy, dark green leaves, to 20cm (8in) long, with paler green and often rusty-hairy undersides. Large, cup-shaped, creamy white flowers, to 25cm (10in) across, with 9–12 petals, are produced from late summer to autumn. ↕ 6–18m (20–60ft), ↔ to 15m (50ft). S.E. USA. ❄❄. **'Exmouth'** 🏆 is particularly hardy, with narrowly ovate, light green leaves, thinly hairy beneath. **'Ferruginea'** ■ has dark green leaves, rusty-hairy beneath. **'Goliath'** ■ 🏆 has broad, slightly twisted leaves and very large flowers, 20–30cm (8–12in) across. **'Little Gem'** ♤ is compact and upright, with elliptic to oval, dark green leaves, to 12cm (5in) long, rusty-hairy beneath, and small flowers; ↕ 6m (20ft), ↔ 3m (10ft). **'Russet'** has upright, dark green leaves, orange-brown beneath. **'Samuel Sommer'** has glossy, dark green leaves, rusty-hairy beneath, and very large flowers, to 35cm (14in) across.
***M.* 'Heaven Scent'** 🏆 ♤ Spreading, deciduous tree or large shrub with broadly elliptic, glossy, mid-green leaves, to 20cm (8in) long. Goblet-shaped flowers, to 12cm (5in) long, with 9–12 petals, pink outside and white inside, are produced from mid-spring to early summer. ↕↔ 10m (30ft). ❄❄❄

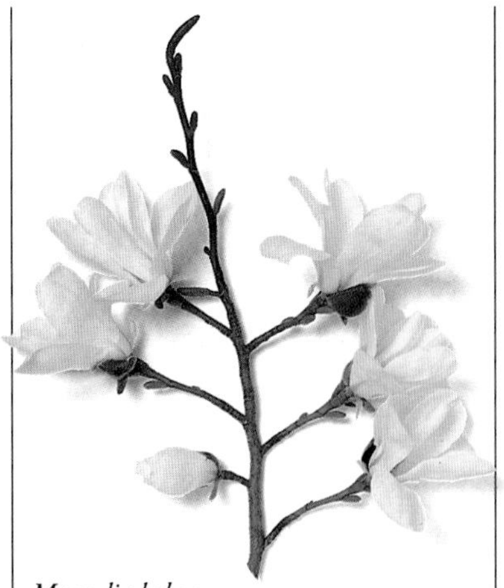
Magnolia kobus

M. heptapeta see *M. denudata.*
M. hypoleuca ■ 🏆 ♤ syn. *M. obovata* (Japanese big-leaf magnolia). Vigorous, conical, deciduous tree with large, obovate, mid-green leaves, to 40cm (16in) long, clustered at the ends of the shoots. Large, cup-shaped, very fragrant, creamy white flowers, to 20cm (8in) across, with 9–12 petals and crimson stamens, are produced in late spring and early summer, after the leaves. ↕ 15m (50ft), ↔ 10m (30ft). Japan. ❄❄❄
M. insignis see *Manglietia insignis.*
***M.* 'Iolanthe'** 🏆 ♤ Vigorous, upright, deciduous tree with obovate, mid-green leaves, to 25cm (10in) long. From an early age, very large, cup-shaped flowers, to 25cm (10in) across, rose-pink outside and creamy white inside, are borne in mid-spring. ↕ 12m (40ft), ↔ 8m (25ft). ❄❄❄
***M.* 'Jane'** 🏆 Upright, deciduous shrub with ovate, glossy, mid-green leaves, to 15cm (6in) long. Cup-shaped, very fragrant flowers, to 10cm (4in) across, with 10 petals, red-purple outside and white inside, are produced from slender, erect, red-purple buds in late spring. ↕ 4m (12ft), ↔ 3m (10ft). ❄❄❄
M. x kewensis ♤ (*M. kobus* x *M. salicifolia*). Deciduous tree or shrub, conical when young, later spreading, with elliptic, mid-green leaves, bluish green below, to 12cm (5in) long. Bears open cup-shaped white flowers, smelling of orange blossom, to 12cm (5in) across, in mid-spring, before the leaves. ↕ 12m (40ft), ↔ 8m (25ft). Garden origin. ❄❄❄
M. kobus ■ ♤ Broadly conical, deciduous tree with narrowly obovate, often puckered, aromatic, mid-green leaves, to 20cm (8in) long. Goblet- to saucer-shaped white flowers, to 10cm (4in) across, occasionally flushed pink at the bases, are borne profusely in mid-spring. ↕ 12m (40ft), ↔ 10m (30ft). Japan. ❄❄❄
M. liliiflora, syn. *M. quinquepeta.* Bushy, deciduous shrub with elliptic to obovate, dark green leaves, to 20cm (8in) long. Goblet-shaped, purplish pink flowers, to 7cm (3in) across, are borne from mid-spring to midsummer. ↕ 3m (10ft), ↔ 4m (12ft). China. ❄❄❄. **'Nigra'** ■ 🏆 is compact and flowers when young, bearing very dark purple-red flowers in early summer and intermittently into autumn; ↔ 2.5m (8ft).
M. x loebneri ♤ (*M. kobus* x *M. stellata*). Small, slender-branched, upright, deciduous tree or large shrub, with narrowly obovate, mid-green leaves, 10–15cm (4–6in) long. Star-shaped flowers, 8–13cm (3–5in) across, with 10–14 slender white petals, sometimes suffused lilac-purple outside and pale pink inside, are produced before the leaves in mid-spring. ↕ 10m (30ft), ↔ 7m (22ft). Garden origin. ❄❄❄. **'Leonard Messel'** ■ 🏆 ♤ is

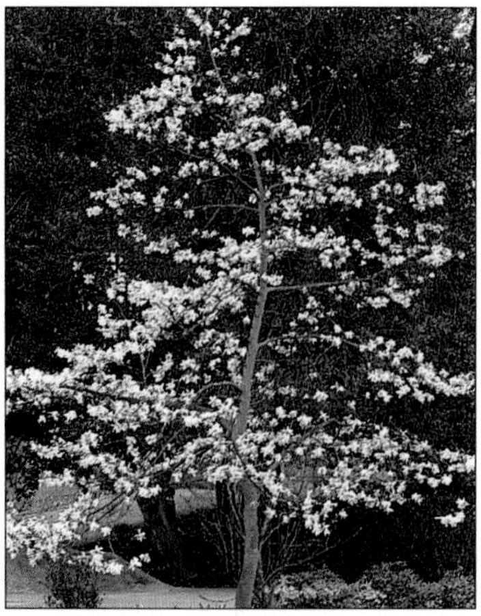
Magnolia x *loebneri* 'Merrill'

more rounded in habit, and produces abundant 12-petalled, pale lilac-pink flowers in mid-spring; ↕ 8m (25ft), ↔ 6m (20ft). **'Merrill'** ■ 🏆 ♤ is vigorous, erect, and compact in habit, with broader leaves; flowers are initially goblet-shaped then star-shaped, with 15 broad white petals; ↔ 8m (25ft). **'Spring Snow'** has pure white flowers with 15 petals; ↕ 9m (28ft).
M. macrophylla ♤–♤ (Great-leaved magnolia, Umbrella tree). Broadly upright, later rounded, deciduous tree with stout, blue-grey shoots and very large, obovate leaves, to 1m (3ft) long, light green above, silvery grey beneath. In early summer, produces open-cup-shaped, fragrant, creamy white flowers, to 30cm (12in) or more across, with 6 petals, the inner 3 marked maroon at the bases. ↕↔ 10m (30ft). S.E. USA. ❄❄. **subsp. *ashei*** see *M. ashei.*
***M.* 'Manchu Fan'** ■ ♤ Spreading, deciduous tree or shrub with obovate, mid-green leaves, to 20cm (8in) long.

M

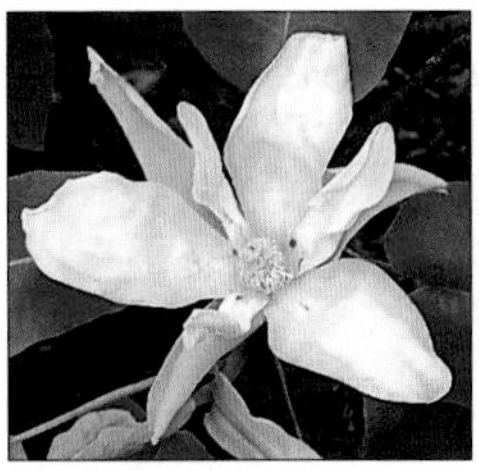
Magnolia ashei

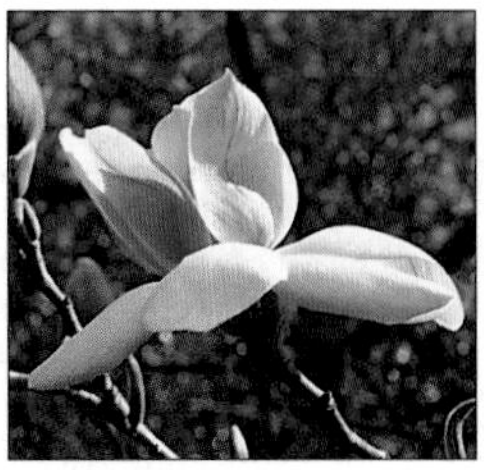
Magnolia campbellii

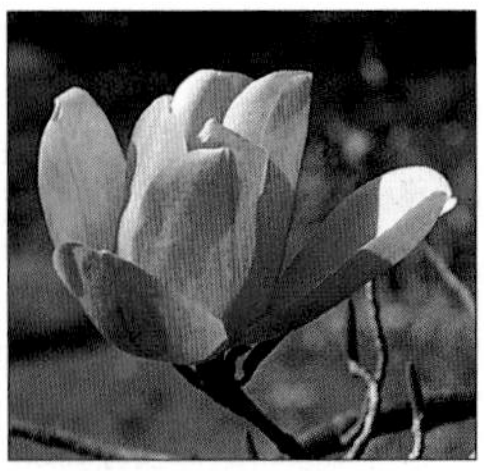
Magnolia campbellii 'Charles Raffill'

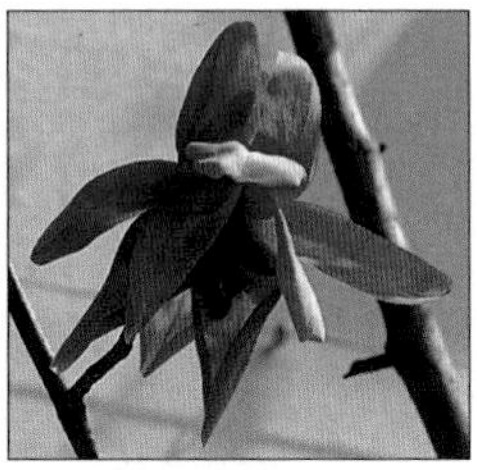
Magnolia campbellii 'Darjeeling'

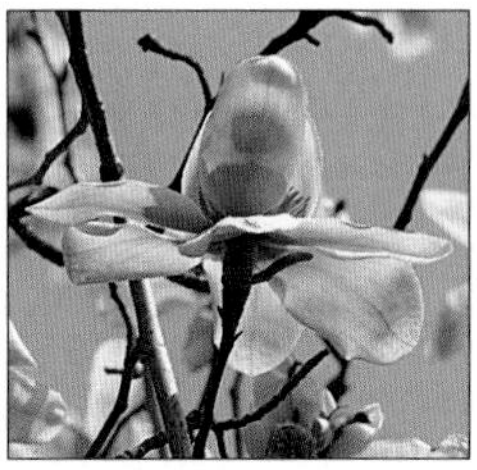
Magnolia campbellii subsp. *mollicomata*

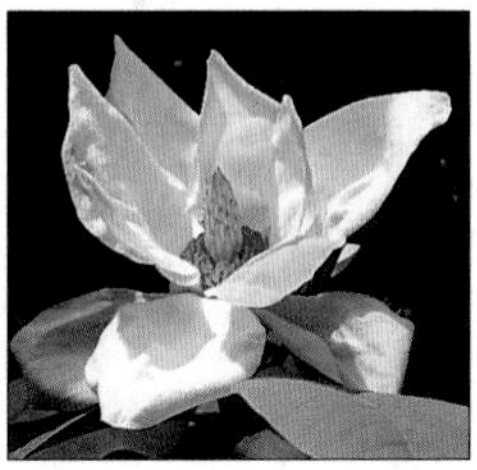
Magnolia 'Charles Coates'

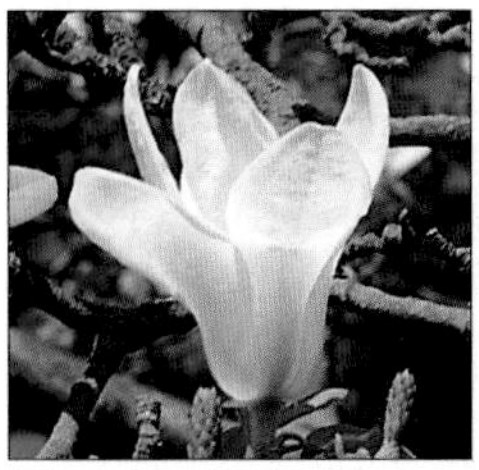
Magnolia cylindrica

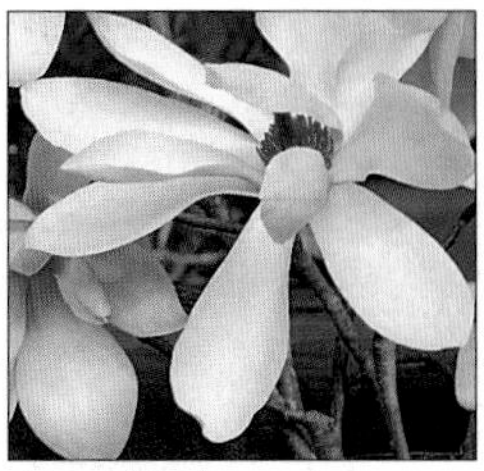
Magnolia dawsoniana 'Chyverton'

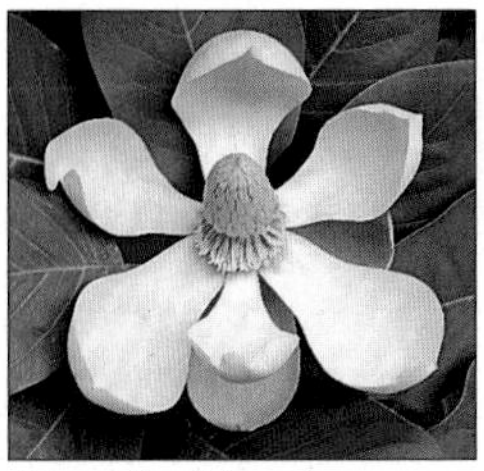
Magnolia delavayi

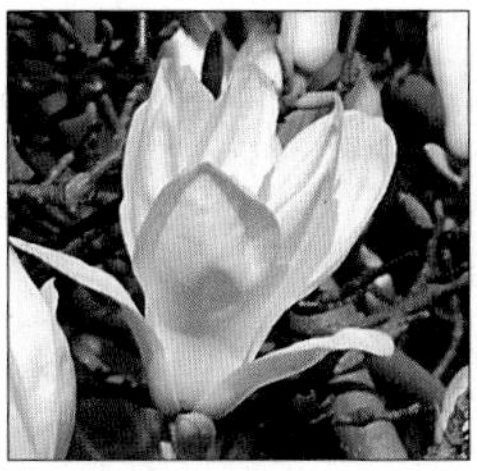
Magnolia denudata

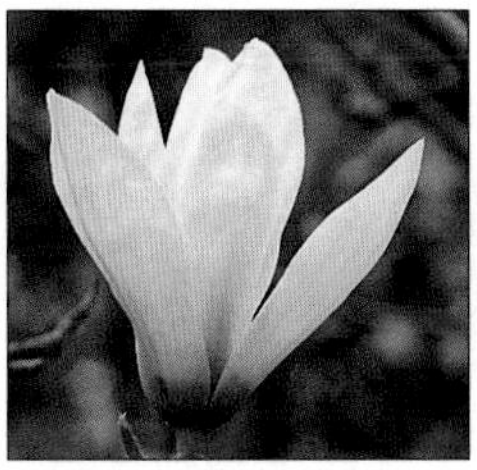
Magnolia 'Elizabeth'

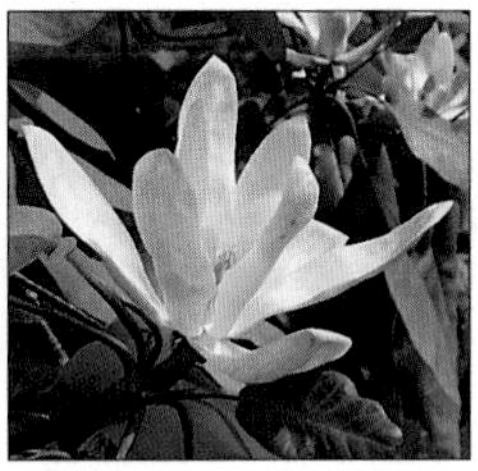
Magnolia fraseri

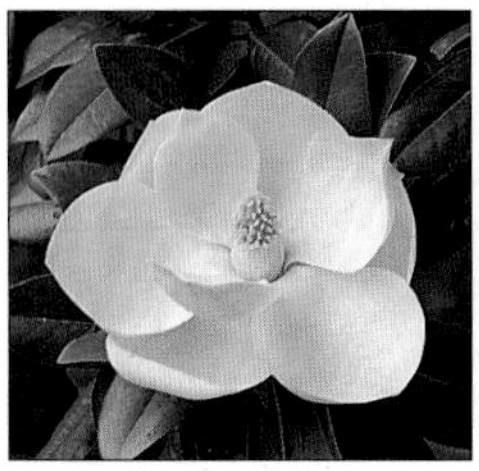
Magnolia grandiflora 'Ferruginea'

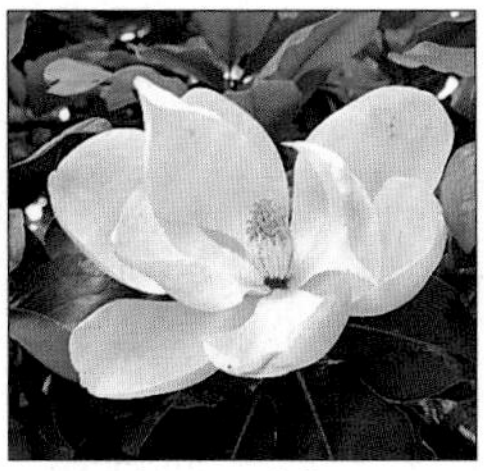
Magnolia grandiflora 'Goliath'

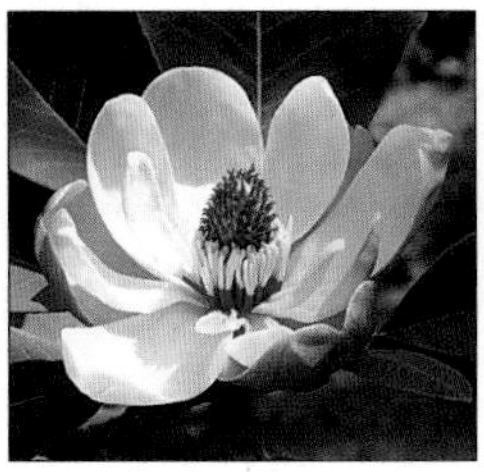
Magnolia hypoleuca

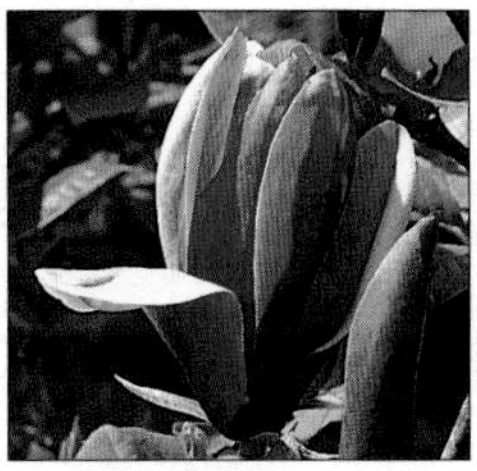
Magnolia liliiflora 'Nigra'

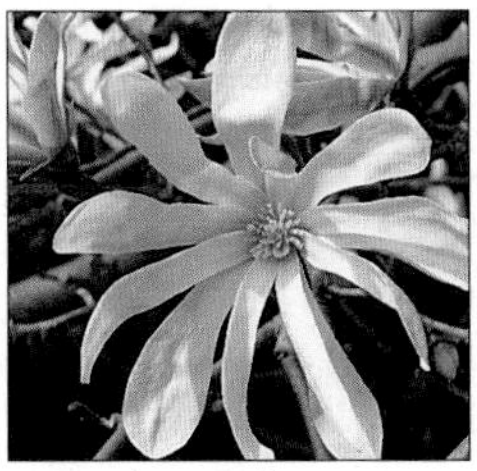
Magnolia x *loebneri* 'Leonard Messel'

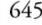

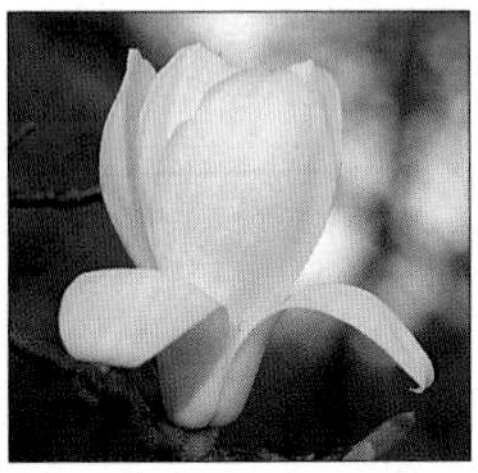
Magnolia 'Manchu Fan'

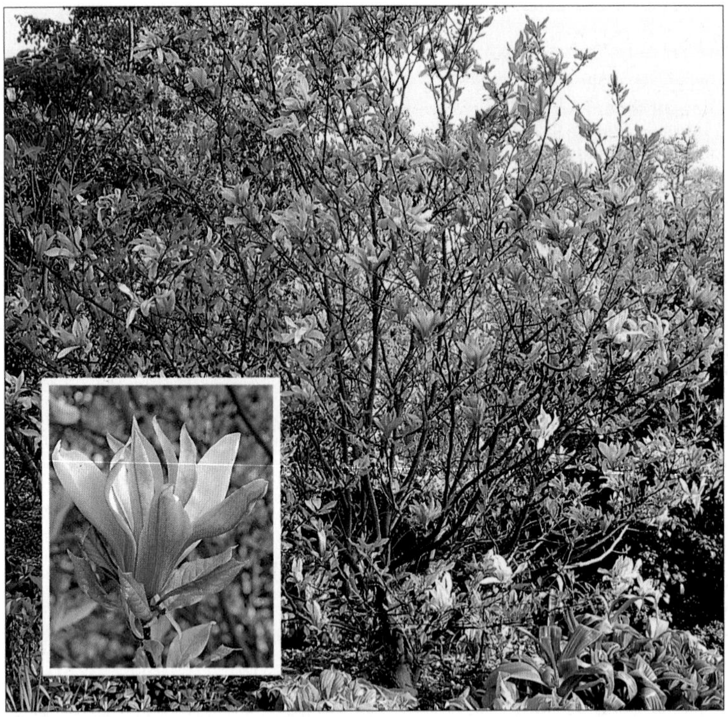

Magnolia 'Ricki' (inset: flower detail)

In late spring, bears large, goblet-shaped, creamy white flowers, to 12cm (5in) across, each with 9 petals, the inner ones flushed purple-pink at the bases. ↕6m (20ft), ↔5m (15ft). ***
***M.* 'Maryland'** ♀⌂ Broadly conical, evergreen shrub or tree with oblong, slightly wavy-margined, glossy, mid-green leaves, to 23cm (9in) long. Bears cup-shaped, strongly fragrant white flowers, to 15cm (6in) across, in late summer. Flowers when young. ↕6m (20ft) or more, ↔5m (15ft). ***
***M.* 'Norman Gould'** ▣♤ Small, open, spreading, deciduous tree with obovate, mid-green leaves, to 12cm (5in) long. Goblet-shaped white flowers, to 12cm (5in) across, with 9–12 broad petals, faintly streaked pink on the outside, are borne horizontally in early and mid-spring. ↕↔5m (15ft). ***
M. obovata see *M. hypoleuca*.
M. parviflora see *M. sieboldii*.
***M.* 'Peppermint Stick'** ♀⌂ Conical, deciduous tree or large shrub, with obovate, mid-green leaves, to 20cm (8in) long. From mid-spring to early summer, large, cup-and-saucer-shaped flowers, to 11cm (4½in) across, with creamy white petals, flushed dark purple-pink at the bases, are produced from long, slender buds. ↕10m (30ft), ↔6m (20ft). ***
***M.* 'Princess Margaret'** ⌂ Deciduous tree, conical when young, spreading when mature, with oblong-elliptic, mid-green leaves, to 25cm (10in) long. In early spring, before the leaves, bears large, cup-and-saucer-shaped flowers, to 28cm (11in) across, with 11 petals, rich rose-pink outside and white inside. ↕15m (50ft), ↔10m (30ft). ***
M.* x *proctoriana ♀⌂ (*M. salicifolia* x *M. stellata*). Conical, deciduous tree with oval, aromatic leaves, to 12cm (5in) long, mid-green above and pale green beneath. Erect or horizontal, star-shaped white flowers, to 10cm (4in) across, with up to 12 petals, are produced in mid-spring. ↕8m (25ft), ↔6m (20ft). Garden origin. ***
M. quinquepeta see *M. liliiflora*.
***M.* 'Randy'** ♀ Upright, almost columnar, free-flowering, deciduous shrub with broadly ovate, mid-green leaves, to 15cm (6in) long. The flowers, to 12cm (5in) across, produced from dark purple-red buds in mid-spring, are initially goblet-shaped, then star-shaped when fully open; each has 10 petals, purple-pink outside and white inside. ↕4m (12ft), ↔2.5m (8ft). ***
***M.* 'Ricki'** ▣♀ Upright, deciduous shrub with broadly ovate, mid-green leaves, to 15cm (6in) long. Goblet-shaped flowers, to 15cm (6in) across, with 15 twisted petals, pink to dark purple-pink at the bases, are produced from dark purple-pink buds in mid-spring. ↕↔4m (12ft). ***
M. salicifolia ▣♀⌂ (Willow-leaved magnolia). Conical, deciduous tree with narrowly elliptic to lance-shaped, lemon-scented leaves, dull green above and grey-white beneath, to 15cm (6in) long. Abundant star-shaped, fragrant, pure white flowers, to 10cm (4in) across, are borne in mid-spring, before the leaves. ↕10m (30ft), ↔6m (20ft). Japan. ***. **'Jermyns'** is shrubby and spreading, with flowers to 13cm (5in) across, and broad leaves; ↕5m (15ft).
M. sargentiana ⌂ Broadly conical, deciduous tree with obovate, light to mid-green leaves, to 18cm (7in) long. Large, horizontal to nodding, goblet- to cup-shaped, 12- to 14-petalled flowers, to 20cm (8in) across, white inside and purple-pink outside, are borne in mid- and late spring, before the leaves. ↕15m (50ft), ↔10m (30ft). W. China. ***. **var. *robusta*** is usually more spreading, with oblong-obovate leaves and large flowers, 22–30cm (9–12in) across.
***M.* 'Sayonara'** ♀♤ Spreading, deciduous tree or shrub with obovate, mid-green leaves, to 20cm (8in) long. Large, broadly goblet-shaped, creamy white flowers, to 12cm (5in) across, the inner petals faintly flushed purple-pink at the bases, are borne in mid- and late spring. ↕6m (20ft), ↔5m (15ft). ***
M. sieboldii, syn. *M. parviflora*. Spreading, deciduous shrub with oblong to ovate-elliptic leaves, to 15cm (6in) long, dark green above, grey-green and downy beneath. From late spring to late summer, bears cup-shaped, erect then horizontal or slightly nodding, fragrant white flowers, to 10cm (4in) across, with 12 petals and crimson anthers. ↕8m (25ft), ↔12m (40ft). China, Korea, Japan. ***. **subsp. *sinensis*** ♀ syn. *M. sinensis*, produces slightly larger, fully pendent flowers and more rounded, oval leaves; W. China.

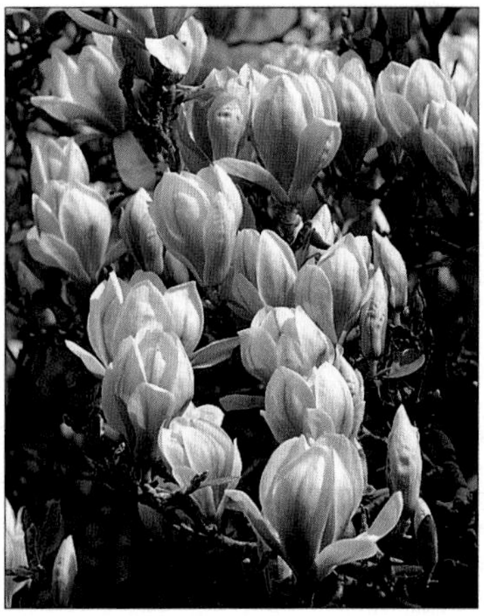

Magnolia x *soulangeana*

M. sinensis see *M. sieboldii* subsp. *sinensis*.
M.* x *soulangeana ▣♤ (*M. denudata* x *M. liliiflora*). Variable, deciduous shrub or spreading tree with obovate, dark green leaves, to 20cm (8in) long. Large, goblet-shaped flowers, 8–30cm (3–6in) across, varying from deep rose-pink to violet-purple or pure white, are borne in mid- and late spring, before and with the young leaves. ↕↔6m (20ft). Garden origin. ***. **'Alba Superba'** ⌂ syn. 'Alba', is upright, with large, fragrant white flowers, slightly purple-flushed at the bases; ↕7m (22ft), ↔5m (15ft). **'Alexandrina'** ♀⌂ is upright, with deeply saucer-shaped white flowers, to 10cm (4in) across, purple-flushed outside. **'Brozzoni'** ♀⌂ is tree-like, with white flowers, to 13cm (5in) across, faintly purple-flushed outside; ↕8m (25ft). **'Burgundy'** bears profuse deep purple-pink flowers, 10cm (4in) across. **'Lennei'** ♀ has dark purple-pink flowers, to 10cm (4in) across, white within. **'Lennei Alba'** ▣♀ bears ivory-white flowers, 10cm (4in) across. **'Picture'** ⌂ is compact and upright, with flowers, 10–13cm (4–5in) across, richly streaked dark reddish purple, white within, and flowering when only

M

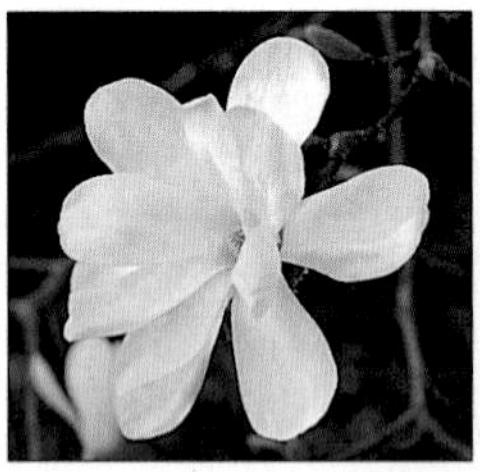

Magnolia 'Norman Gould'

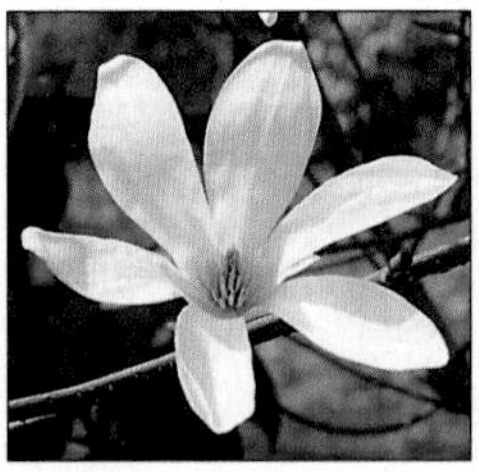

Magnolia salicifolia

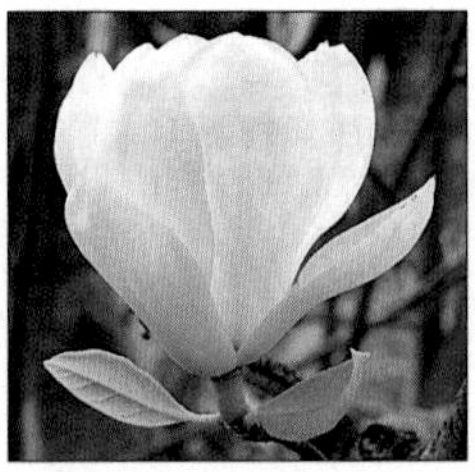

Magnolia x *soulangeana* 'Lennei Alba'

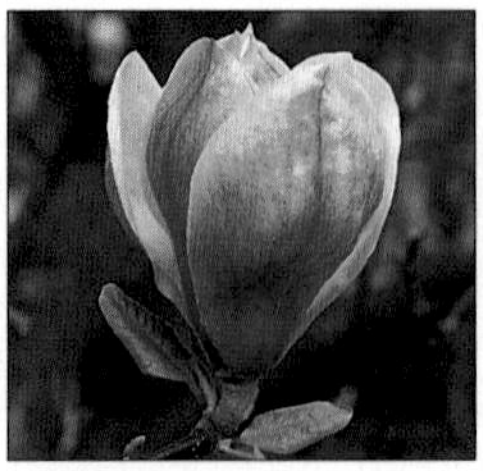

Magnolia x *soulangeana* 'Rustica Rubra'

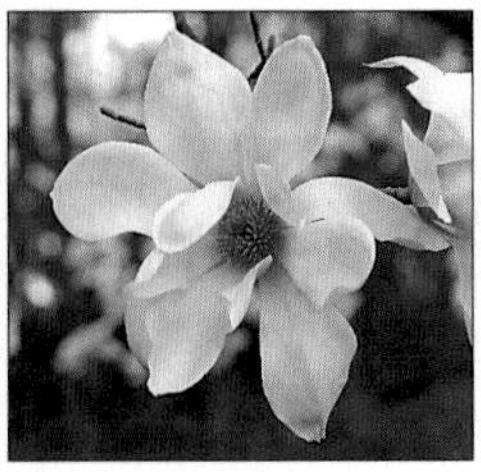

Magnolia sprengeri

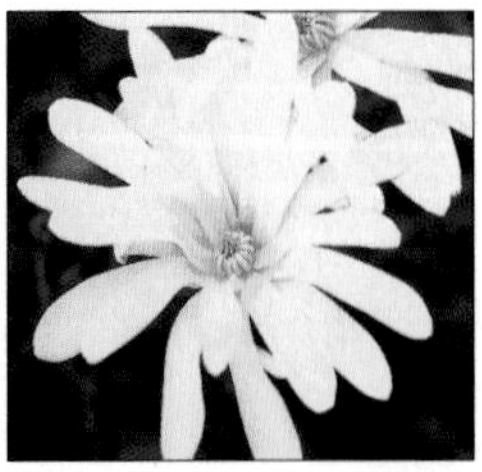

Magnolia stellata 'Royal Star'

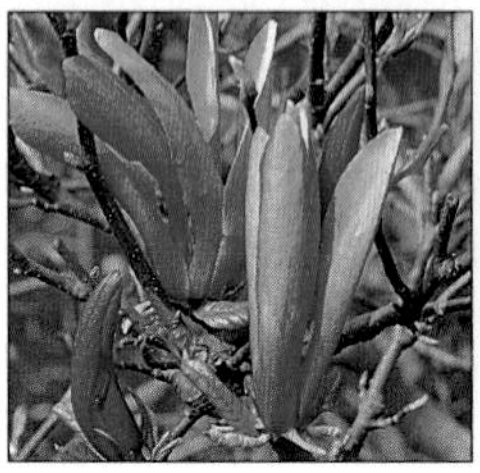

Magnolia 'Susan'

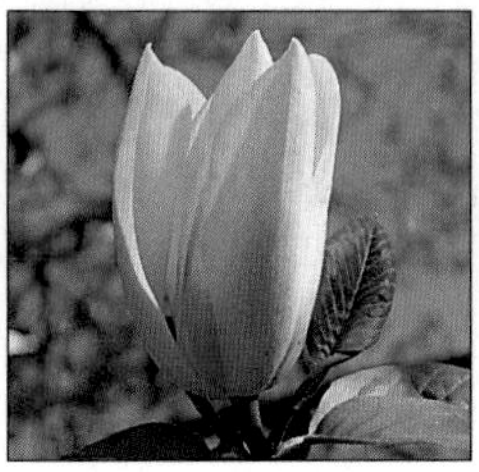

Magnolia x *veitchii* 'Peter Veitch'

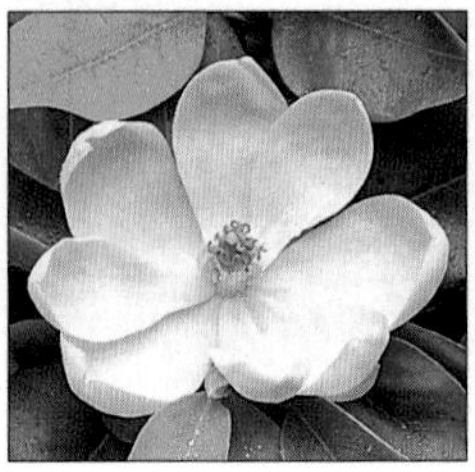

Magnolia virginiana

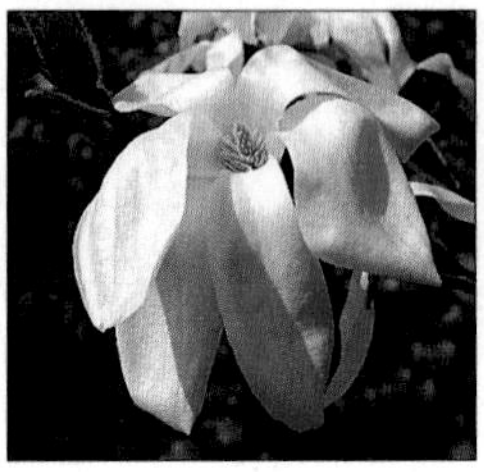

Magnolia 'Wada's Memory'

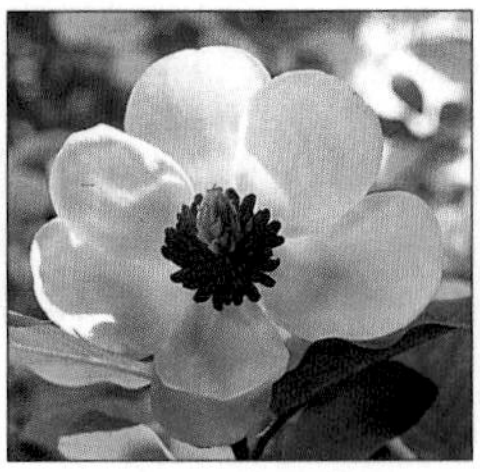

Magnolia x *wieseneri*

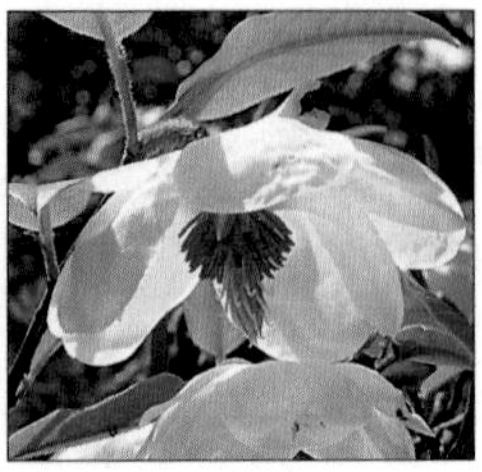

Magnolia wilsonii

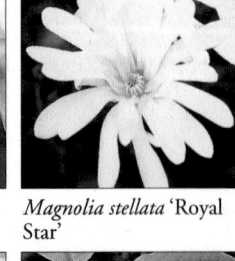

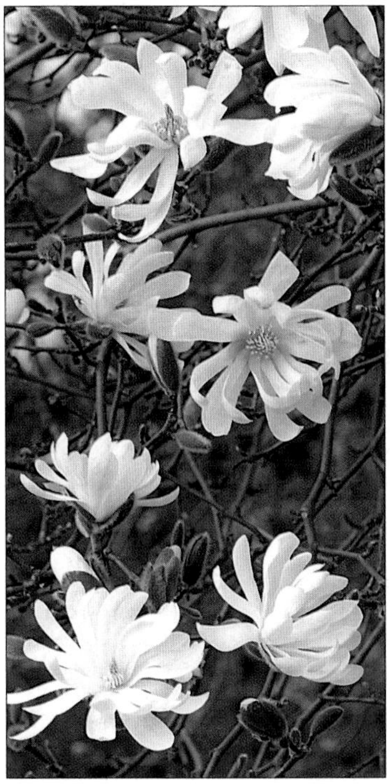

Magnolia stellata

1m (3ft) high; ↕ 8m (25ft). **'Rubra'** see 'Rustica Rubra'. **'Rustica Rubra'** ■ 🏆 syn. 'Rubra', has deeply goblet-shaped, dark purplish red flowers, 10–13cm (4–5in) across, milky white within. **'San José'** bears creamy white flowers, 10–13cm (4–5in) across, heavily flushed dark pink outside.
M. sprengeri ■ Ϙ Spreading, deciduous tree with obovate, dark green leaves, to 15cm (6in) long. Bears large, cup-shaped, white to pink flowers, to 15cm (6in) across, with 12–15 petals, in mid-spring, before the leaves. ↕ 15m (50ft), ↔ 10m (30ft). China. ❄❄❄. **var. *diva*** has rich deep pink flowers, streaked with white and pink inside. **'Wakehurst'** 🏆 has dark purple-pink flowers, rich pink inside.
M. stellata ■ 🏆 (Star magnolia). Compact, bushy then spreading, deciduous shrub with obovate-oblong to inversely lance-shaped, mid-green leaves, to 10cm (4in) long. Silky buds open to star-shaped, mostly erect but sometimes horizontal, pure white, sometimes faintly pink-flushed flowers, 12cm (5in) across, with up to 15 petals; flowers are borne profusely in early and mid-spring, before the leaves. ↕ 3m (10ft), ↔ 4m (12ft). Japan. ❄❄❄. **'Centennial'** bears white flowers, to 14cm (5½in) across, with 28–32 petals. **'Royal Star'** ■ has faintly pink buds and white flowers, 12cm (5in) across, with 25–30 petals. **'Rubra'** has dark pink flowers, to 12cm (5in) across. **'Waterlily'** 🏆 has white flowers, to 12cm (5in) across, with up to 32 petals; it is similar to 'Centennial' but has slightly smaller flowers.
***M.* 'Susan'** ■ 🏆 Upright, deciduous shrub bearing ovate, mid-green leaves, to 15cm (6in) long. In mid-spring, narrowly goblet-shaped, fragrant flowers, to 15cm (6in) across, with usually slightly twisted petals, purple-red outside and paler inside, are produced from slender, dark red-purple buds. ↕ 4m (12ft), ↔ 3m (10ft). ❄❄❄
M. tripetala ⌂ (Elkwood, Umbrella tree). Broadly conical, deciduous tree with obovate to inversely lance-shaped, dark green leaves, to 60cm (24in) long, clustered at the ends of the shoots. Cup-shaped, unpleasantly scented, creamy white flowers, to 15cm (6in) across, with 9–16 petals, are produced in late spring and early summer. ↕↔ 10m (30ft). E. USA. ❄❄❄
M.* x *veitchii Ϙ (*M. campbellii* x *M. denudata*). Large, upright, deciduous tree with purple-green juvenile foliage and branches. Leaves are obovate or oblong, 15–30cm (6–12in) long, mostly rounded at the bases and pointed at the tips, and dark green when mature. Bears goblet-shaped, pink to white flowers, 15cm (6in) long, on bare branches in mid-spring. ↕ 30m (100ft), ↔ 3–10m (10–30ft). Garden origin. ❄❄. **'Isca'** has obovate leaves and satin-textured white flowers, faintly pink-tinged at the petal bases; ↕ 25m (80ft), ↔ 15m (50ft). **'Peter Veitch'** ■ has pale pink flowers, shading to white at the petal tips.
M. virginiana ■ ⌂ syn. *M. glauca* (Sweet bay). Conical, deciduous or semi-evergreen shrub or small tree with elliptic to ovate, glossy, bright green leaves, to 15cm (6in) long, glaucous beneath. From early summer to early autumn, bears almost spherical, deeply cup-shaped, very fragrant flowers, to 6cm (2½in) across, with 8 or 9 creamy white petals and an outer row of up to 6 smaller, greenish white petals. ↕ 9m (28ft), ↔ 6m (20ft). E. USA. ❄❄❄
***M.* 'Wada's Memory'** ■ 🏆 ⌂ Compact, broadly conical, deciduous tree with narrowly ovate, dark green leaves, to 18cm (7in) long, bronze when young. Abundant cup-shaped white flowers, to 15cm (6in) across, are produced in mid- and late spring, before the leaves. ↕ 9m (28ft), ↔ 7m (22ft). ❄❄❄
M.* x *watsonii see *M.* x *wieseneri.*
M.* x *wieseneri ■ Ϙ (*M. hypoleuca* x *M. sieboldii*), syn. *M.* x *watsonii*. Spreading, deciduous shrub or tree with obovate, leathery, bright green leaves, to 20cm (8in) long, glaucous beneath. In early and midsummer, spherical white buds open to deeply cup-shaped, strongly fragrant flowers, 15cm (6in) across, with 6–9 ivory-white inner petals, 3 smaller, pink-flushed outer petals, and rose-crimson anthers. ↕ 6m (20ft), ↔ 5m (15ft). Garden origin. ❄❄❄
M. wilsonii ■ 🏆 Ϙ Spreading, deciduous shrub or small tree with red-purple shoots and elliptic or ovate to lance-shaped, dark green leaves, to 15cm (6in) long, felted red-brown beneath. In late spring and early summer, bears pendent, cup-shaped white flowers, to 10cm (4in) across, with crimson stamens. ↕↔ 6m (20ft). W. China. ❄❄❄
***M.* 'Yellow Bird'** ⌂ Conical, later spreading, deciduous tree with ovate, mid-green leaves, to 25cm (10in) long. Deeply cup-shaped, pure yellow flowers, to 12cm (5in) across, are borne in late spring and early summer. ↕ 10m (30ft), ↔ 6m (20ft). ❄❄❄

▷ **Magnolia,**
Great-leaved see *Magnolia macrophylla*
Japanese big-leaf see *Magnolia hypoleuca*
Star see *Magnolia stellata*
Willow-leaved see *Magnolia salicifolia*

MAHONIA

BERBERIDACEAE

Genus of about 70 species of evergreen shrubs occurring in rocky places and woodland in the Himalayas, E. Asia, and North and Central America. They are grown for their handsome foliage, fragrant flowers, decorative fruits, and, in tall species and cultivars, for their deeply fissured bark. The alternate, pinnate or occasionally 3-palmate, usually spiny-margined leaves are light grey-green to dark green, and sometimes purplish red or orange-red when young. Racemes or panicles (see panel below) of cup-shaped, usually yellow flowers, 0.8–1.5cm (⅜–½in) across, are followed by spherical or ovoid, mainly purple to black berries. Mahonias are useful for a variety of situations: use low-growing species and cultivars as ground cover, and taller ones as specimens in a shrub border or woodland garden.
• **HARDINESS** Fully hardy to frost hardy.
• **CULTIVATION** Grow in moderately fertile, humus-rich, moist but well-drained soil. Most mahonias prefer full or partial shade, but will tolerate sun if the soil is not too dry. *M. fremontii* and *M. nevinii* require very well-drained soil and full sun. Shelter *M. fortunei*, *M. lindsayae*, and *M. lomariifolia* from cold, drying winds. Pruning group 8.
• **PROPAGATION** Sow seed outdoors in a seedbed or containers, in autumn or as soon as ripe. Stratified seeds germinate freely. Root semi-ripe or leaf-bud cuttings from late summer to autumn.
• **PESTS AND DISEASES** Rust and mildew may attack *M. aquifolium.*

M. acanthifolia see *M. napaulensis.*
M. aquifolium (Oregon grape). Open, suckering shrub with pinnate, bright

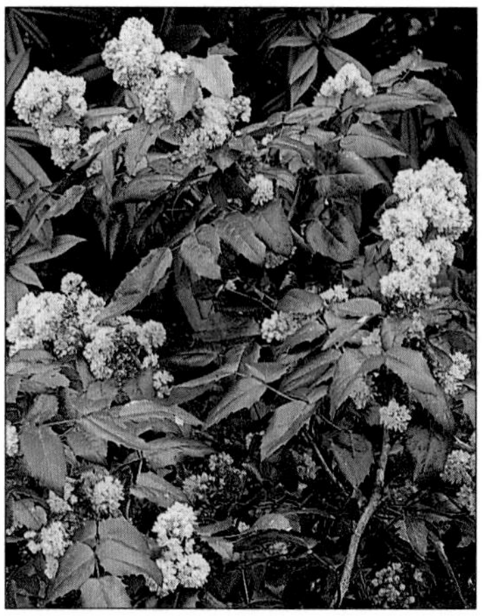

Mahonia aquifolium 'Smaragd'

green leaves, to 30cm (12in) long, with up to 9 obliquely ovate, spiny-toothed leaflets, often turning red-purple in winter. Yellow flowers are borne in densely clustered racemes, to 8cm (3in) long, in spring, followed by spherical blue-black berries. ↕ 1m (3ft), ↔ 1.5m (5ft). W. North America. ❄❄❄. **'Atropurpurea'** has leaves that turn dark red-purple in winter. **'Orange Flame'** has rust-orange young foliage, turning red in winter; ↕ 60cm (24in), ↔ 1m (3ft). **'Smaragd'** ■ is compact, bearing bright yellow flowers in large clusters, to 10cm (4in) long; ↕ to 60cm (24in), ↔ to 1m (3ft).
M. bealei see *M. japonica* 'Bealei'.
M. fortunei. Upright shrub with pinnate, dark green leaves, to 20cm (8in) long, with up to 13 slender, sharply toothed, elliptic-lance-shaped leaflets. Bright yellow flowers are borne in dense, upright racemes, to 7cm (3in) long, in early and mid-autumn; they are followed by ovoid to spherical, white-

MAHONIA INFLORESCENCES

Mahonia flowers are borne from autumn to spring in clustered or spreading, terminal racemes (or panicles). The spreading, often arching racemes may reach 45cm (18in) long; the smaller, more densely flowered, clustered racemes are typically less than 10cm (4in) long. Both forms may be upright.

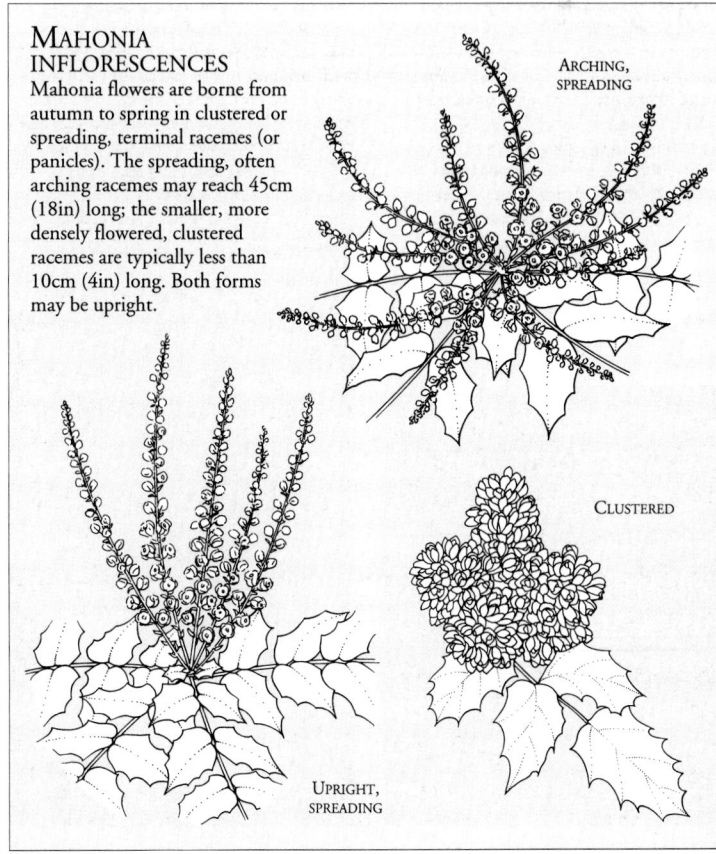

ARCHING, SPREADING

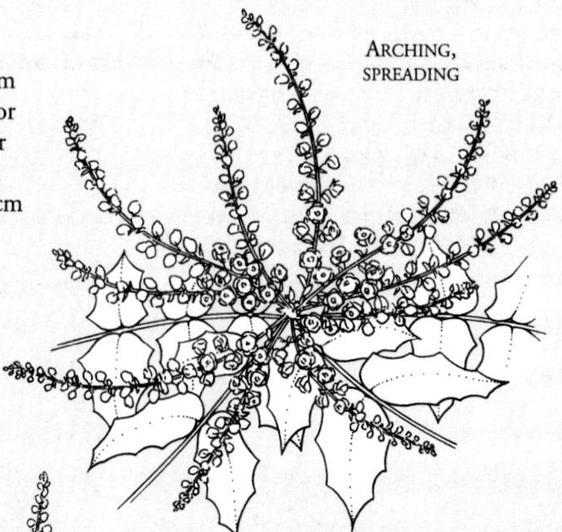

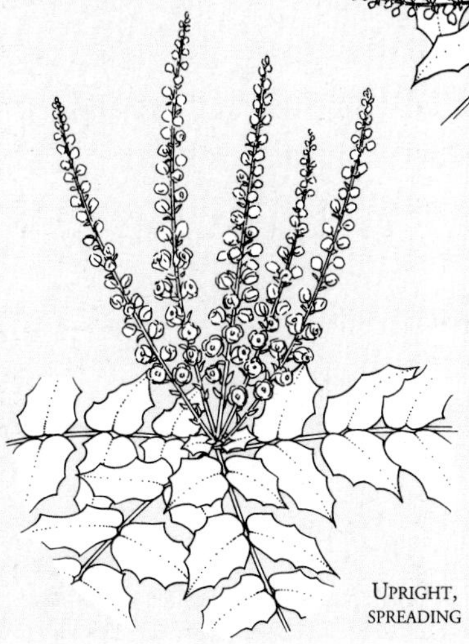

UPRIGHT, SPREADING

CLUSTERED

M

frosted, dark blue berries. ↕ 1.2m (4ft), ↔ 1m (3ft). China. ❄❄
M. fremontii. Upright, stiffly branched shrub bearing pinnate leaves, to 10cm (4in) long, with 3–7 wavy-margined, sharply toothed, oblong-lance-shaped, glaucous, grey-green leaflets. In summer, produces densely clustered racemes, to 5cm (2in) long, of yellow flowers, followed by ovoid, white-frosted, dark blue berries. ↕↔ 2m (6ft). S.W. USA, Mexico. ❄❄
***M.* 'Heterophylla'.** Upright shrub with red-purple shoots and pinnate, glossy, bright green leaves, to 30cm (12in) long, with up to 7 slender, ovate, lance-shaped to narrowly oblong-ovate, twisted leaflets, turning red-purple in winter. Yellow flowers are produced in clustered racemes, to 8cm (3in) long, in spring. Seldom produces fruit. ↕ 1m (3ft), ↔ 1.5m (5ft). ❄❄
M. japonica ♀ Erect shrub with stout, upright branches and pinnate, dark green leaves, to 45cm (18in) long, with up to 19 sharply toothed, ovate-oblong to lance-shaped leaflets. Fragrant, pale yellow flowers are produced in arching, then spreading racemes, to 25cm (10in) long, from late autumn to early spring, followed by ovoid, blue-purple berries. ↕ 2m (6ft), ↔ 3m (10ft). China. ❄❄❄. **'Bealei'**, syn. *M. bealei*, has blue-green leaves divided into broad leaflets, and produces flowers in shorter, upright racemes, to 10cm (4in) long.
***M. x lindsayae* 'Cantab'.** Stoutly branched shrub bearing large, arching, pinnate, glossy, rich, deep green leaves, to 60cm (24in) long, with up to 15 ovate-oblong, sharply toothed leaflets, some turning red in winter. Fragrant, lemon-yellow flowers are produced in spreading racemes, to 30cm (12in) long, in late autumn and early winter. ↕↔ 2.5m (8ft). ❄❄
M. lomariifolia ♀ Erect shrub with stout, upright shoots bearing pinnate, dark green leaves, to 60cm (24in) long, with up to 41 oblong-ovate to oblong-lance-shaped, sharply toothed leaflets. Fragrant yellow flowers are produced in densely clustered, upright racemes, 20cm (8in) long, from late autumn to winter, followed by ovoid, blue-black berries. ↕ 3m (10ft), ↔ 2m (6ft). W. China (S. Sichuan, Yunnan). ❄❄
M. x media (*M. japonica* x *M. lomariifolia*). Erect shrub with pinnate leaves, to 45cm (18in) long, with 17–21 ovate to lance-shaped, sharply toothed, dark green leaflets. Bright yellow to

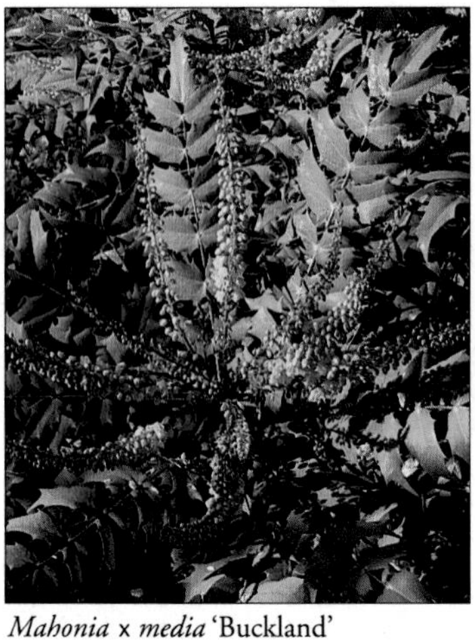
Mahonia x *media* 'Buckland'

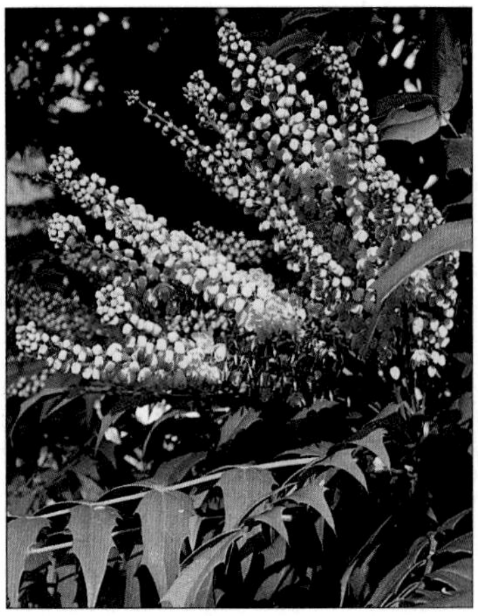
Mahonia x *media* 'Charity'

lemon-yellow flowers are borne in erect then spreading racemes, 25–35cm (10–14in) long, from late autumn to late winter. ↕ to 5m (15ft), ↔ to 4m (12ft). Garden origin. ❄❄❄. **'Arthur Menzies'** produces lemon-yellow flowers in upright, later spreading racemes, to 25cm (10in) long, in late autumn and early winter; ↕ 4m (12ft). **'Buckland'** ■♀ bears bright yellow flowers in arching racemes, to 45cm (18in) long. **'Charity'** ■♀ has densely clustered, upright then spreading racemes. **'Lionel Fortescue'** ♀ bears bright yellow flowers in upright racemes, to 40cm (16in) long. **'Winter Sun'** ♀ bears bright yellow flowers in densely clustered, arching racemes.
M. napaulensis, syn. *M. acanthifolia.* Open, upright shrub with pinnate, glossy, dark green leaves, to 50cm (20in) long, with up to 15 lance-shaped to narrowly ovate, sharply toothed leaflets. In early and mid-spring, bears yellow flowers in spreading racemes, to 20cm (8in) long, followed by ovoid, white-frosted, blue-black berries. ↕ 2.5m (8ft), ↔ 3m (10ft). Himalayas. ❄❄
M. nervosa. Dwarf, suckering shrub with pinnate, glossy, dark green leaves,

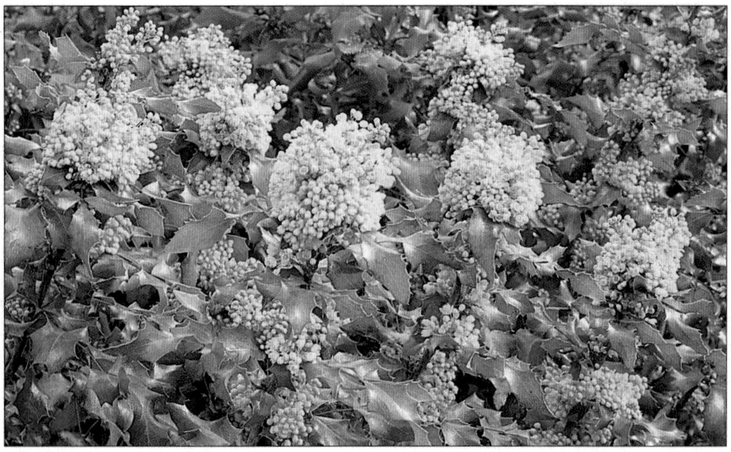
Mahonia x *wagneri* 'Pinnacle'

to 60cm (24in) long, with up to 23 ovate-oblong to lance-shaped leaflets, often red-purple in winter. Bears yellow flowers in dense racemes, to 20cm (8in) long, in late spring and early summer, followed by spherical, blue-black berries. ↕ 45cm (18in), ↔ 1m (3ft). W. North America. ❄❄❄
M. nevinii. Upright shrub with purplish green shoots and pinnate leaves, grey-green to blue-green above, greyish white beneath, to 10cm (4in) long, with 5 lance-shaped, sharply toothed leaflets. Bright yellow flowers are produced in small, dense racemes, to 5cm (2in) long, in early and mid-spring, followed by spherical, dark red berries. ↕↔ 2m (6ft). USA (S. California). ❄❄
***M. pinnata* of gardens** see *M.* x *wagneri* 'Pinnacle'.
M. pumila. Low, dense, suckering shrub bearing pinnate, grey-green leaves, to 15cm (6in) long, with up to 9 ovate-oblong, sharply toothed leaflets, wedge-shaped at the bases, with long, pointed tips. Dark yellow flowers are borne in densely clustered racemes, to 5cm (2in) long, in spring, followed by ellipsoid, blue-black berries. ↕ 30cm (12in), ↔ 1m (3ft). USA (California, Oregon). ❄❄❄

M. repens. Upright, suckering shrub bearing pinnate, matt green leaves, to 25cm (10in) long, with up to 7 pointed, ovate, wavy-margined, sharply toothed leaflets. Dark yellow flowers are borne in dense, upright racemes, to 8cm (3in) long, in mid- and late spring, followed by spherical, blue-black berries. ↕ 30cm (12in), ↔ 1m (3ft). W. North America. ❄❄❄. **'Rotundifolia'** ■ is taller, with broadly ovate, almost entire, rounded leaflets; ↕ 1.5m (5ft), ↔ 2m (6ft).
***M.* 'Undulata'** see *M.* x *wagneri* 'Undulata'.
M. x wagneri (*M. aquifolium* x *M. pinnata*). Upright shrub bearing pinnate leaves, to 20cm (8in) long, with 7–11 ovate, sharply toothed, dull to dark green leaflets. Yellow flowers are borne in dense racemes, to 8cm (3in) long, in spring, followed by spherical, white-frosted, blue-black berries. ↕ 80cm (32in), ↔ 1m (3ft). Garden origin. ❄❄❄. **'Moseri'** has pale green leaves, flushed pink or red. **'Pinnacle'** ■♀ syn. *M. pinnata* of gardens, is upright and taller, with bronze juvenile leaves, maturing to bright green; ↕↔ 1.5m (5ft). **'Undulata'** ♀ syn. *M.* 'Undulata', has leaves with glossy, dark green, wavy-margined leaflets, turning red-purple in winter, and produces rich yellow flowers; ↕↔ 2m (6ft).

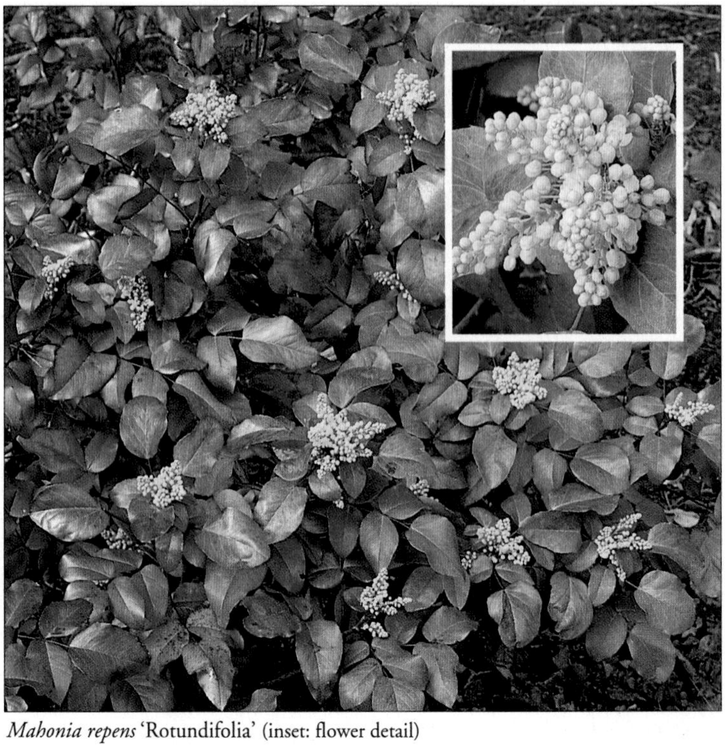
Mahonia repens 'Rotundifolia' (inset: flower detail)

MAIANTHEMUM

May lily

CONVALLARIACEAE/LILIACEAE

Genus of 3 species of creeping, rhizomatous perennials from woodland in the N. hemisphere. They are grown for their dense, terminal racemes of tiny, fluffy, star-shaped, 4-tepalled white flowers, followed by red berries, and for their alternate, heart-shaped leaves, borne on upright stems. Use for ground cover in a wild or woodland garden.
- **HARDINESS** Fully hardy.
- **CULTIVATION** Grow in humus-rich, leafy, moist but well-drained, neutral to acid soil in light dappled or deep shade.
- **PROPAGATION** Sow seed in containers in a cold frame as soon as ripe. Separate rooted runners in spring.
- **PESTS AND DISEASES** Slugs and snails may attack young leaves.

M. bifolium ■ (False lily-of-the-valley). Spreading perennial with 2 broadly heart-shaped to ovate, thin, glossy, dark green leaves, to 8cm (3in) across. In early summer, produces slender-

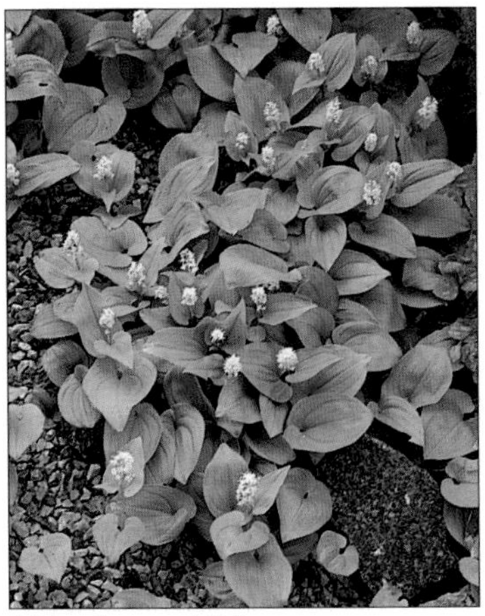
Maianthemum bifolium

stemmed racemes of 8–20 white flowers, followed by small, spherical berries. ↕15cm (6in), ↔ indefinite. W. Europe to Japan. ❄❄❄
M. racemosum see *Smilacina racemosa.*

▷**Maidenhair fern** see *Adiantum*
Aleutian see *A. aleuticum*
Australian see *A. formosum*
Barbados see *A. tenerum* 'Farleyense'
Brittle see *A. tenerum*
Delta see *A. raddianum*
Diamond see *A. trapeziforme*
Dwarf see *A. aleuticum* var. *subpumilum*
Giant see *A. formosum, A. trapeziforme*
Himalayan see *A. venustum*
Northern see *A. aleuticum*
Silver dollar see *A. peruvianum*
Tassel see *A. raddianum* 'Grandiceps'
Trailing see *A. caudatum*
True see *A. capillus-veneris*
Walking see *A. caudatum*
▷**Maidenhair tree** see *Ginkgo, G. biloba*

MAIHUENIA

CACTACEAE

Genus of 3–5 species of dwarf, clustering, perennial cacti found at high altitudes in the Andes of S. Chile and S. Argentina. Cylindrical or spherical, fleshy, jointed stems bear small, ovate, slender, evergreen leaves. Diurnal, cup-shaped flowers are produced from the near-terminal areoles in summer, followed by soft berries, to 5cm (2in) across, containing numerous black-coated seeds. Where temperatures fall below 0°C (32°F), grow in a cool or temperate greenhouse. In warmer areas, grow in a rock or desert garden. Long, hot summers are needed for production of flowers.
• **HARDINESS** Half hardy.
• **CULTIVATION** Under glass, grow in standard cactus compost in bright filtered light, or full light with shade from hot sun, with low humidity. From spring to summer, water moderately and apply a dilute fertilizer monthly; at other times, keep almost dry. Outdoors, grow in moderately fertile, sharply drained soil in dappled shade, or full sun with shade from midday sun. Protect from excessive winter wet. See also pp.48–49.
• **PROPAGATION** Sow seed at 19–24°C (66–75°F) in spring. Root stem cuttings in spring and summer.
• **PESTS AND DISEASES** Mealybugs may cause problems.

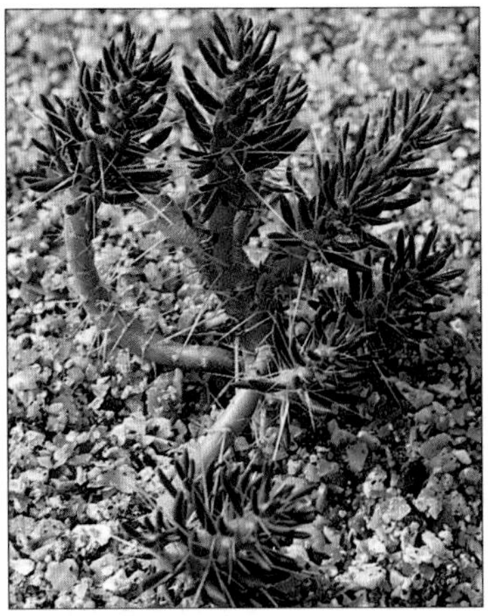
Maihuenia poeppigii

M. poeppigii ▣ Clustering cactus with many short, cylindrical stems and fleshy, evergreen leaves, 5mm (¼in) long. Areoles bear 3 or 4 slender, generally short, stiff spines, one of which grows to 2cm (¾in) long. Produces bright yellow flowers, 3–4.5cm (1¼–1¾in) long, in summer. ↕6cm (2½in), ↔ 30cm (12in). S. Chile, S. Argentina. ❄

▷**Maiten** see *Maytenus boaria*
▷**Maize** see *Zea mays*
▷***Majorana onites*** see *Origanum onites*

MALCOLMIA

BRASSICACEAE/CRUCIFERAE

Genus of 35 species of bushy, sometimes prostrate annuals and perennials found on rocky slopes and as wild species in cultivated and disturbed ground, from the Mediterranean region to Afghanistan. They are grown for their short racemes of narrow, cross-shaped, 4-petalled, white, purple, or red flowers, borne from spring to autumn; they self-seed freely. Leaves are linear-oblong to ovate, spoon-shaped, or pinnatisect with lance-shaped lobes. Suitable for the front of an annual or mixed border, and for paving crevices, edging, or a gravel path; they thrive in coastal gardens.
• **HARDINESS** Fully hardy.
• **CULTIVATION** Grow in moderately fertile, well-drained soil in full sun, with shade from midday sun. Flowering is poor in regions with hot, humid summers, unless seed is sown early.
• **PROPAGATION** Sow seed thinly *in situ* from late spring. For a succession of flowers, repeat at intervals of 4–6 weeks.
• **PESTS AND DISEASES** Downy mildew may be troublesome.

M. maritima (Virginian stock). Low-growing, erect to spreading, basally branching annual, with oval to elliptic, hairy-toothed or entire, blunt-tipped, grey-green leaves, to 5cm (2in) long. From spring to autumn, produces open, many-flowered, slender-stemmed spikes of sweetly fragrant, red or purple flowers, to 1cm (½in) across, each petal notched at the apex. ↕20–40cm (8–16in), ↔ 10–15cm (4–6in). Mediterranean. ❄❄❄. **Compacta Series** ▣ cultivars have white, pink, red, or purple flowers; ↕40cm (16in).

MALEPHORA

AIZOACEAE

Genus of about 15 species of bushy, prostrate to erect, woody-based, perennial succulents from dry, hilly areas of southern Africa. The stems have prominent internodes. The opposite, semi-cylindrical or bluntly 3-angled, soft, fleshy, pale to mid-green leaves are united at the bases and coated with blue or white wax. Short-stalked, star-shaped, terminal or axillary flowers open in daytime from late summer to autumn. In frost-prone climates, grow in a cool or temperate greenhouse. In warmer areas, grow in a rock garden or desert garden.
• **HARDINESS** Frost tender.
• **CULTIVATION** Under glass, grow in standard cactus compost in full light with shade from hot sun, and with low

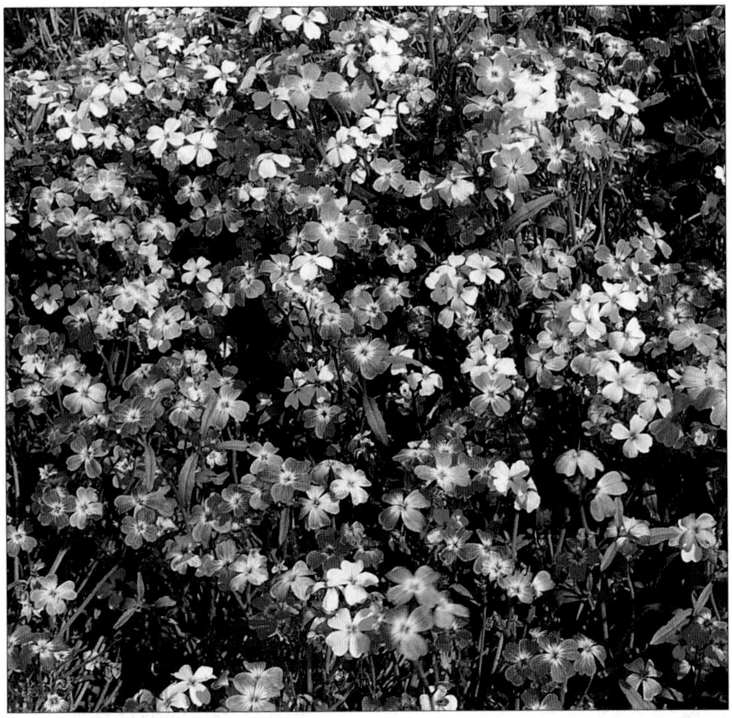
Malcolmia maritima Compacta Series

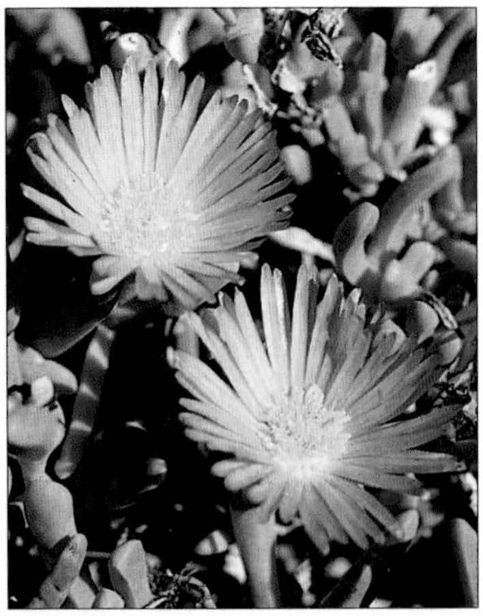
Malephora crocea

humidity. From late spring to early autumn, water freely and apply a balanced liquid fertilizer monthly. Keep just moist at other times. Outdoors, grow in poor or moderately fertile soil in full sun. Provide protection from excessive winter wet. See also pp.48–49.
• **PROPAGATION** Sow seed at 19–24°C (66–75°F) in spring. Root leaf cuttings or stem segments in spring or summer.
• **PESTS AND DISEASES** Susceptible to mealybugs.

M. crocea ▣ Semi-prostrate or erect, woody-based succulent with a thick, gnarled stem and greyish brown branches. Bears clusters of blunt-tipped, white-frosted, mealy, pale green leaves, to 4.5cm (1¾in) long, on short shoots. Solitary, golden yellow flowers, 3cm (1¼in) across, with red-backed petals, are produced in late summer. ↕20cm (8in), ↔ indefinite. South Africa (Western Cape). ❀ (min. 7°C/45°F)

▷**Mallow** see *Lavatera, Malva*
Annual see *Malope, M. trifida*
Common rose see *Hibiscus moscheutos*
Confederate rose see *Hibiscus mutabilis*
False see *Sidalcea, Sphaeralcea*
Globe see *Sphaeralcea*
Hollyhock see *Malva alcea*
Indian see *Abutilon*
Marsh see *Althaea officinalis*
Musk see *Abelmoschus moschatus, Malva moschata*
Poppy see *Callirhoe*
Prairie see *Sidalcea, Sphaeralcea coccinea*
Prairie poppy see *Callirhoe involucrata*
Sleepy see *Malvaviscus*
Swamp rose see *Hibiscus moscheutos*
Tree see *Lavatera arborea*
Wax see *Malvaviscus arboreus*

MALOPE

Annual mallow

MALVACEAE

Genus of 4 species of tall, bushy to almost unbranched annuals and perennials found on rocky limestone slopes, in thickets of prickly shrubs, and growing wild in arable fields, from the Mediterranean region to W. Asia. The ovate leaves are entire or lobed, and the showy, axillary flowers are long-stalked, broadly trumpet-shaped, and paper thin, ranging from pink or violet-blue to

M

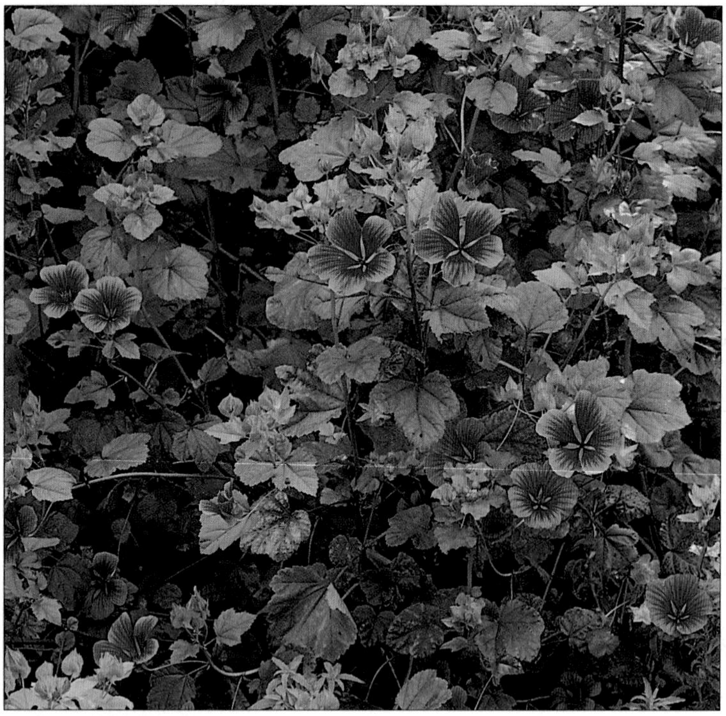

Malope trifida 'Vulcan'

white, often veined in a deeper shade. Grow at the front or middle of an annual or mixed border, where they self-seed freely and provide long-lasting cut flowers. Annual mallows thrive in coastal gardens, although they do poorly in hot, humid summer conditions.
- **HARDINESS** Fully hardy.
- **CULTIVATION** Grow in moderately fertile, moist but well-drained soil in full sun, although partial shade is tolerated. Dead-head to prolong flowering. Give brushwood support in exposed sites.
- **PROPAGATION** Sow seed at 13–18°C (55–64°F) in early spring, or *in situ* in mid-spring.
- **PESTS AND DISEASES** Aphids and rust may be troublesome.

M. trifida (Annual mallow). Erect, branching to almost unbranched, stout-stemmed annual with hairy stems and leaves. Ovate, mid-green leaves, to 10cm (4in) long, are entire near the stem bases but 3- to 5-lobed higher up. From summer to autumn, produces broadly trumpet-shaped, pale to dark purple-red flowers, 5–8cm (2–3in) across, heavily veined dark purple, the petals narrowing at the bases to reveal bright green sepals below. ↕ to 90cm (36in), ↔ 23cm (9in). W. Mediterranean. ❄❄❄. **'Rosea'** has rose-red flowers. **'Vulcan'** ■ bears abundant bright magenta-pink flowers, to 8cm (3in) across. **'White Queen'** has pure white flowers, 5cm (2in) across.

MALPIGHIA

MALPIGHIACEAE

Genus of about 45 species of evergreen shrubs and small trees found in dry woodland in tropical North, Central, and South America, especially the Caribbean. They are grown for their opposite, simple, often toothed and leathery leaves, and their star-shaped to shallowly trumpet-shaped flowers, each with 5 unequally sized, clawed petals, often with crimped, waved, or fringed tips or margins. Flowers are borne singly or in axillary or terminal corymbs, followed by colourful, edible fruits. Where temperatures fall below 16°C (61°F), grow in a temperate or warm greenhouse. Elsewhere, use as specimen trees, in a shrub border, or for hedging.
- **HARDINESS** Frost tender.
- **CULTIVATION** Under glass, grow in loam-based potting compost (JI No.2) in full light, with shade from hot sun. In spring and summer, water moderately and apply a balanced liquid fertilizer monthly; water sparingly in winter. Outdoors, grow in moderately fertile, moist but well-drained soil in full sun with shade from midday sun. Pruning group 9.
- **PROPAGATION** Sow seed at 18–24°C (64–75°F) in spring. Root semi-ripe cuttings with bottom heat in summer.
- **PESTS AND DISEASES** Red spider mites may be troublesome under glass.

M. coccigera (Miniature holly, Singapore holly). Small, bushy shrub, often prostrate unless regularly trimmed. Elliptic to obovate or rounded leaves, 1–2cm (½–¾in) long, are wavy-margined, spiny-toothed, and lustrous, deep green. Shallowly trumpet-shaped, pink or lilac-pink flowers, 1.5cm (½in) across, are produced singly or in pairs from all the upper leaf axils in summer, and usually followed by broadly ovoid red berries, 0.5–1.5cm (¼–½in) across. ↕ 30–150cm (1–5ft), ↔ 1–2m (3–6ft) or more. West Indies. ❀ (min. 16°C/61°F)
M. glabra (Barbados cherry). Upright, bushy shrub with ovate to elliptic-lance-shaped, entire, lustrous, dark green leaves, 2.5–7cm (1–3in) long. In summer, produces star-shaped pink flowers, 1.5cm (½in) across, with fringed margins, in axillary or terminal corymbs of 3–8 flowers, followed by spherical red berries, 1.5cm (½in) across. ↕ 3m (10ft), ↔ 1.5m (5ft). USA (Texas) to West Indies and N. South America. ❀ (min. 16°C/61°F)

▷**Maltese Cross** see *Lychnis chalcedonica*

MALUS

Apple, Crab apple

ROSACEAE

Genus of about 35 species of deciduous trees and shrubs from woodland and thickets in Europe, Asia, and North America. They are grown for their often fragrant flowers, mostly 2–5cm (¾–2in) across, borne singly or in umbel-like corymbs, for their attractive, more or less spherical, edible fruits (although some are unpalatable if uncooked), and sometimes for their purple foliage and autumn colour. The flowers are usually shallowly cup-shaped and 5-petalled; in some cultivars, they may be semi-double or double. The leaves are alternate, oval to ovate or elliptic, mostly toothed, rarely entire, and occasionally lobed. Crab apples are ideal specimen trees, many of them suitable for small gardens. Apples of commerce, *Malus* x *domestica* and its cultivars, are not described here.
- **HARDINESS** Fully hardy.
- **CULTIVATION** Grow in moderately fertile, moist but well-drained soil in full sun, although partial shade is tolerated. Purple-leaved forms colour best in full sun. Pruning group 1.
- **PROPAGATION** Sow seed in a seedbed in autumn. Bud in late summer. Graft in midwinter.
- **PESTS AND DISEASES** Aphids, red spider mites, caterpillars, apple scab, honey fungus, canker, fireblight, and mildew may cause problems.

***M.* 'Aldenhamensis'** ⚲ Spreading tree with ovate to shallowly lobed leaves, to 10cm (4in) long, red-purple when young, later bronze-green. Single or semi-double, dark red flowers are produced in late spring, followed by broadly ovoid, red-purple fruit, to 3cm (1¼in) long. ↕↔ 8m (25ft). ❄❄❄
***M.* 'Almey'** ■ ⚲ Rounded tree with ovate leaves, to 8cm (3in) long, red-purple when young, later dark green. Deep rose-pink flowers, paler at the bases, are produced in late spring, followed by orange-red fruit, to 2.5cm (1in) across. ↕↔ 8m (25ft). ❄❄❄

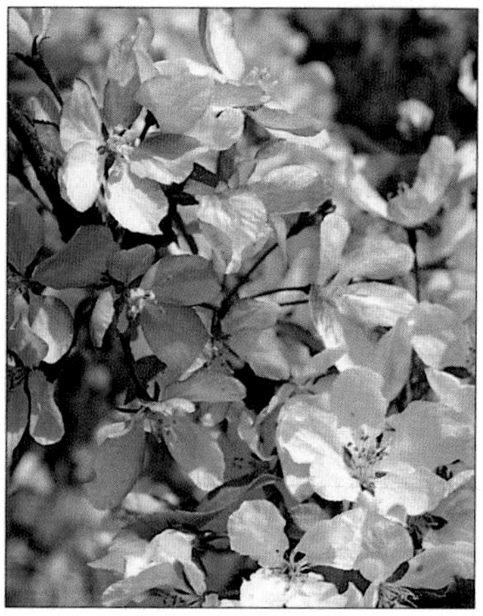

Malus x *arnoldiana*

M.* x *arnoldiana ■ ⚲ (*M. baccata* x *M. floribunda*). Low, spreading tree with long, arching branches and oval, mid-green leaves, to 8cm (3in) long. In mid- and late spring, red buds open to fragrant pink flowers, fading to white, followed by ovoid, red-flushed yellow fruit, to 2cm (¾in) long. ↕ 5m (15ft), ↔ 8m (25ft). Garden origin. ❄❄❄
M.* x *atrosanguinea ⚲ (*M. halliana* x *M. sieboldii*). Spreading tree with oval or slightly lobed, glossy, dark green leaves, to 8cm (3in) long. Rich pink flowers are produced from red buds in mid-spring, followed by long-stalked, yellow-flushed red fruit, to 1cm (½in) across. ↕↔ 6m (20ft). Garden origin. ❄❄❄
M. baccata ⚲ (Siberian crab apple). Vigorous, rounded tree with oval, dark green leaves, paler beneath, to 9cm (3½in) long. Abundant white flowers are produced in mid- and late spring, followed by long-stalked, red or yellow fruit, 1cm (½in) across. ↕↔ 15m (50ft). E. Asia. ❄❄❄. **var. *mandschurica*** ■ (Manchurian crab apple) has more sparsely toothed leaves, downy beneath.

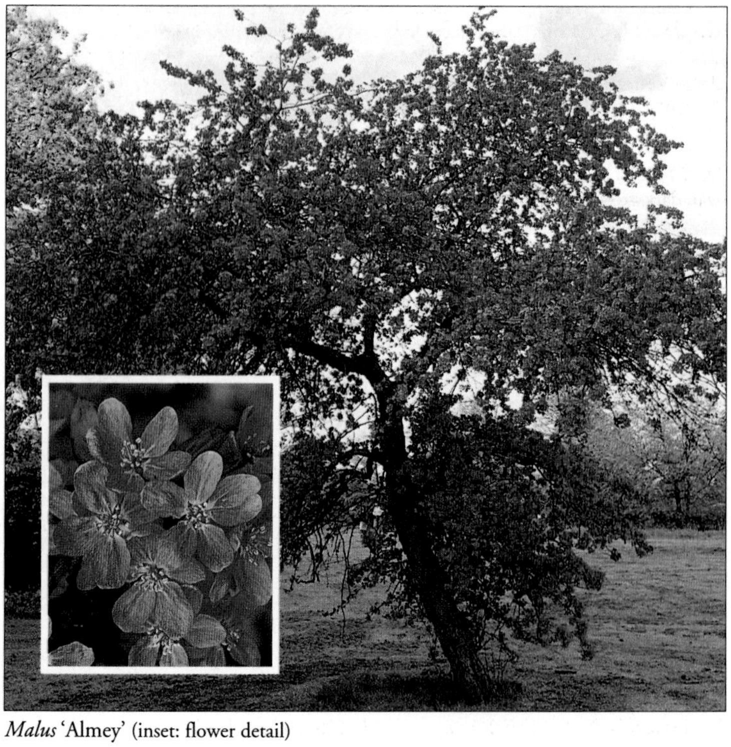

Malus 'Almey' (inset: flower detail)

M

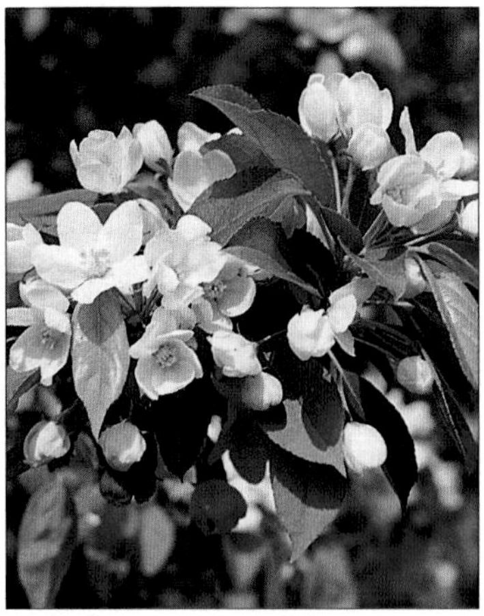
Malus baccata var. *mandschurica*

***M.* 'Baskatong'** Small, rounded tree with oval, dark green leaves, to 8cm (3in) long. Purple-red flowers, with paler centres, are produced from darker buds in late spring, followed by dark purple-red fruit, to 2.5cm (1in) across. ↕↔ 8m (25ft). ❄❄❄
***M.* 'Brandywine'** Rounded tree with ovate, red-flushed, dark green leaves, to 9cm (3½in) long. Abundant fragrant, double pink flowers are produced in late spring, followed by yellow-green fruit, to 2.5cm (1in) across. ↕↔ 6m (20ft). ❄❄❄
***M.* 'Butterball'** ■ Spreading tree with broadly ovate to heart-shaped, bright green leaves, to 8cm (3in) long, grey-green when young. Pink-flushed white flowers are borne in late spring, followed by striking, orange-yellow fruit, red-flushed at first, 3cm (1¼in) across. ↕↔ 8m (25ft). ❄❄❄
***M.* 'Candied Apple'** syn. *M.* 'Weeping Candied Apple'. Small, spreading tree with weeping branches and ovate, red-flushed, dark green leaves, to 8cm (3in) long. Pink flowers are produced from red buds in late spring, followed by long-lasting, bright red fruit, 1cm (½in) across. ↕↔ 5m (15ft). ❄❄❄
***M.* 'Centurion'** Narrowly upright tree, developing an oval head with age. Ovate, bronze-green leaves, to 10cm (4in) long, are red when young. Bears rose-red flowers in late spring, followed by long-lasting cerise fruit, to 1cm (½in) across. ↕ 8m (25ft), ↔ 6m (20ft). ❄❄❄
***M.* 'Chilko'** Spreading tree with oval, dark green leaves, 8–9cm (3–3½in) long, red-purple when young. Dark rose-pink flowers are produced in mid-spring, followed by bright crimson fruit, 5cm (2in) across. ↕↔ 8m (25ft). ❄❄❄
M. coronaria (Wild sweet crab apple). Spreading tree producing ovate, toothed, sometimes shallowly lobed, dark green leaves, to 10cm (4in) long, red-tinged when young, turning scarlet-red and orange in autumn. Violet-scented pink flowers are borne in late spring, followed by acid-tasting, yellow-green fruit, 4cm (1½in) across. ↕↔ 9m (28ft). E. North America. ❄❄❄. **'Charlottae'** has semi-double flowers.
***M.* 'Cowichan'** ■ Spreading tree with oval, glossy, dark green leaves, to 11cm (4½in) long, red-purple when young. Rose-pink, later almost white flowers are produced in mid-spring, followed by bright red-purple fruit, 4cm (1½in) across. ↕↔ 8m (25ft). ❄❄❄

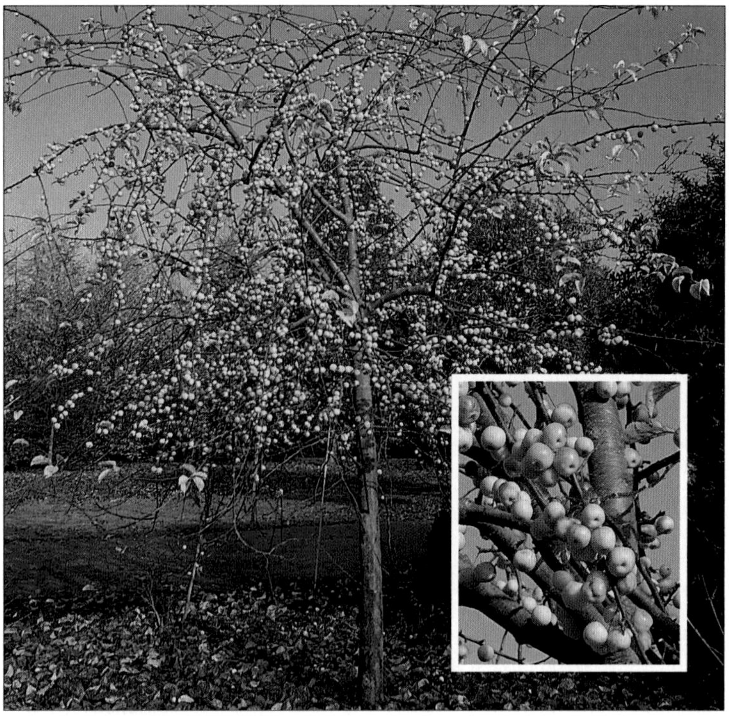
Malus 'Butterball' (inset: fruit detail)

***M.* 'Crittenden'** Compact, spreading tree with oval, dark green leaves, to 9cm (3½in) long. Pink-flushed white flowers are produced in late spring, followed by profuse, glossy, scarlet fruit, 2.5cm (1in) across, which last well into winter. ↕ 7m (22ft), ↔ 8m (25ft). ❄❄❄
***M.* 'Dartmouth'** Vigorous, broadly upright to rounded tree with elliptic to broadly ovate, dark green leaves, to 11cm (4½in) long. White flowers are produced from pink buds in late spring, followed by large, smooth, red-purple fruit, to 5cm (2in) across. ↕ 8m (25ft), ↔ 7m (22ft). ❄❄❄
***M.* 'Dolgo'** Vigorous, spreading tree with ovate, dark green leaves, to 8cm (3in) long. Fragrant white flowers are produced from pink buds in late spring, followed by ovoid-spherical, bright red-purple fruit, 5cm (2in) long. ↕ 11m (35ft), ↔ 10m (30ft). ❄❄❄
***M.* 'Dorothea'** Spreading tree with oval, dark green leaves, to 8cm (3in) long. Semi-double to double, silvery pink flowers are produced from darker buds in late spring, followed by yellow fruit, 1cm (½in) across. Slow-growing and susceptible to scab. ↕↔ 8m (25ft). ❄❄❄

***M.* 'Echtermeyer'** ■ syn. *M.* 'Okonomierat Echtermeyer'. Weeping tree with oval, sometimes slightly lobed, bronze-green leaves, 8–10cm (3–4in) long, bronze-purple when young. Dark red-purple flowers are produced in late spring, followed by ovoid-spherical, purple-red fruit, 2.5cm (1in) long. ↕↔ 5m (15ft). ❄❄❄
***M.* 'Eleyi'** Spreading tree with oval, purple-green leaves, to 10cm (4in) long, bronze-purple when young. Dark red-purple flowers are produced in late spring, followed by obovoid purple fruit, 2.5cm (1in) long. ↕↔ 8m (25ft). ❄❄❄
***M.* 'Evereste'** Conical tree with oval, sometimes lobed, dark green leaves, 8–11cm (3–4½in) long. White flowers are freely produced from red buds in late spring, followed by red-flushed, orange-yellow fruit, 2.5cm (1in) across. ↕ 7m (22ft), ↔ 6m (20ft). ❄❄❄
M. floribunda ■ (Japanese crab apple). Dense, spreading tree with ovate, sometimes lobed, dark green leaves, to 8cm (3in) long. Pale pink flowers are produced in mid- and late spring, from red buds, followed by very small, pea-like yellow fruit, 2cm (¾in) across. ↕↔ 10m (30ft). Japan. ❄❄❄

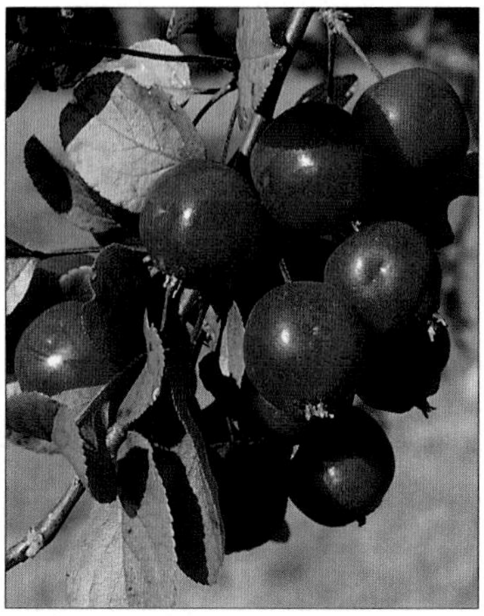
Malus 'Cowichan'

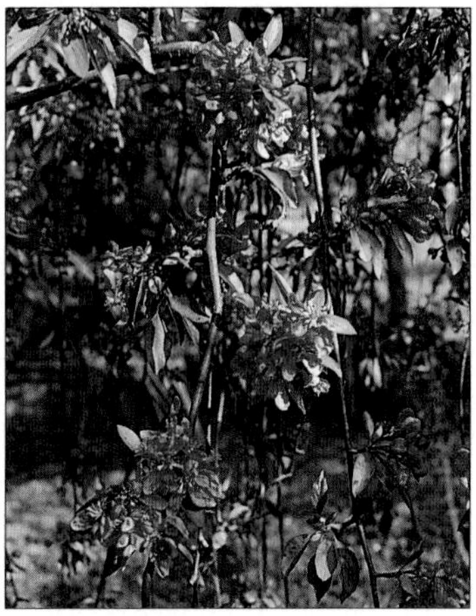
Malus 'Echtermeyer'

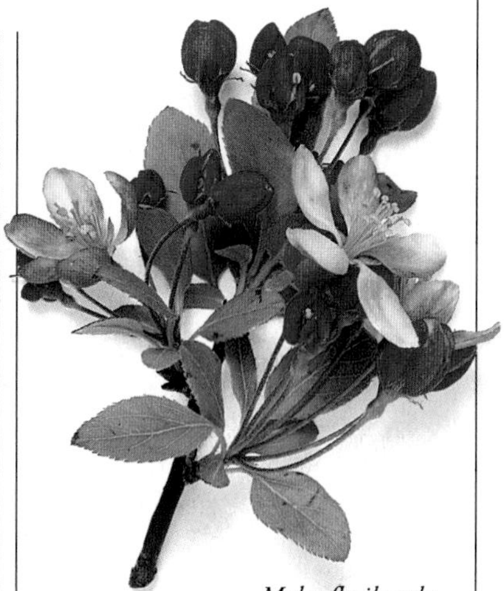
Malus floribunda

***M.* 'Frettingham's Victoria'** Upright tree with oval, dark green leaves, to 8cm (3in) long. White flowers are produced in late spring, followed by red-flushed yellow fruit, 4cm (1½in) across. ↕ 8m (25ft), ↔ 4m (12ft). ❄❄❄
***M.* 'Golden Hornet'** Rounded tree with oval, sharply toothed, bright green leaves, to 9cm (3½in) long. White flowers are produced from pink buds in late spring, followed by long-lasting, ovoid-spherical, golden yellow fruit, 2.5cm (1in) long. ↕ 10m (30ft), ↔ 8m (25ft). ❄❄❄
***M.* 'Hopa'** Spreading tree with oval, dark green leaves, to 10cm (4in) long, red-purple when young. Dark pink flowers, with white centres, open from red-purple buds in mid-spring, followed by bright red fruit, to 2.5cm (1in) across. ↕↔ 10m (30ft). ❄❄❄
M. hupehensis ■ Vigorous, spreading tree with elliptic to ovate, dark green leaves, to 10cm (4in) long. Fragrant white flowers are produced from pink buds in mid- and late spring, followed by cherry-like red fruit, 1cm (½in) across. ↕↔ 12m (40ft). China. ❄❄❄
***M.* 'Indian Magic'** Rounded tree with ovate, dark green leaves, 8–10cm (3–4in) long. Rose-pink flowers open from red buds in late spring, followed by long-lasting, ellipsoid, glossy red, later orange fruit, 1cm (½in) across. ↕↔ 6m (20ft). ❄❄❄
***M.* 'Jewelberry'** Dense, rounded tree or shrub with ovate, dark green leaves,

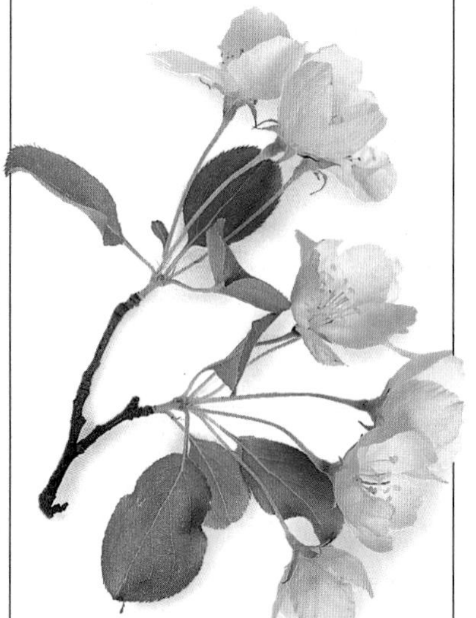
Malus hupehensis

M

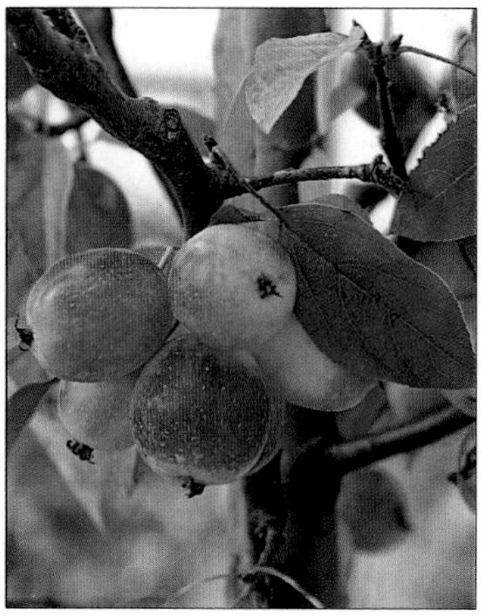
Malus 'John Downie'

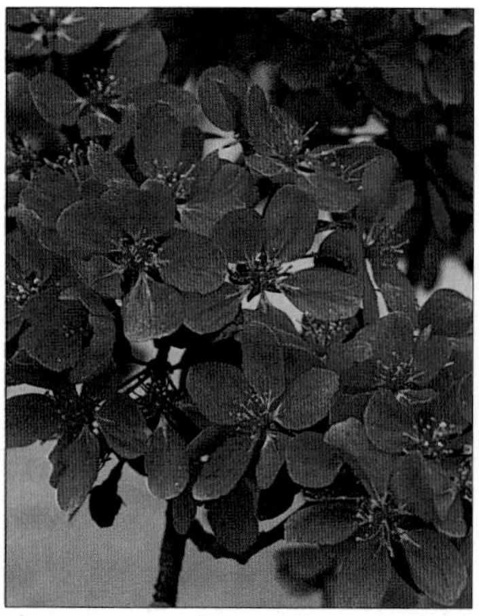
Malus 'Lemoinei'

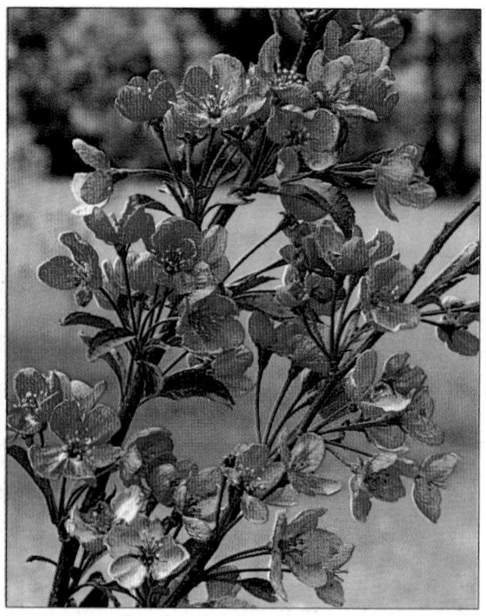
Malus 'Liset'

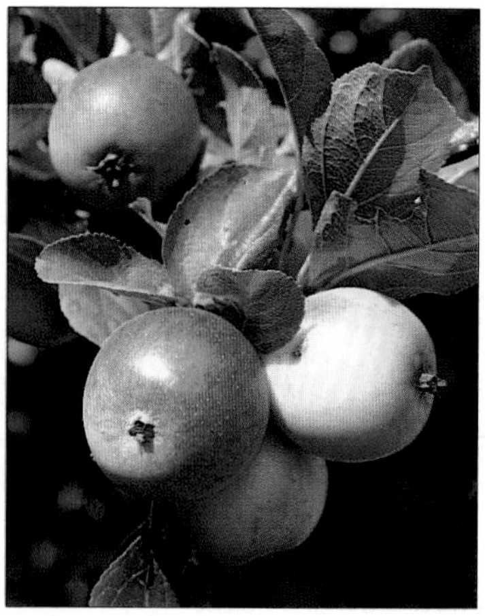
Malus 'Marshall Oyama'

7–9cm (3–3½in) long. White flowers open from pink buds in late spring, followed by glossy red fruit, 1cm (½in) across, profusely borne, even on young trees. ↕↔ 5m (15ft). ❄❄❄
M. 'John Downie' ■ 𝕐 ♢–♤ Narrow, upright tree, broadly conical when mature, with ovate, bright green leaves, to 10cm (4in) long. White flowers open from pale pink buds in late spring, followed by ovoid, orange and red fruit, to 3cm (1¼in) long. ↕ 10m (30ft), ↔ 6m (20ft). ❄❄❄
M. 'Katherine' ■ 𝕐 ♤ Open, rounded tree with oval, dark green leaves, to 8cm (3in) long. Large, double, pale pink flowers, maturing to white, are borne in mid- and late spring, followed by very small, pea-like, red-flushed yellow fruit, 1cm (½in) across. ↕↔ 6m (20ft). ❄❄❄
M. 'Lemoinei' ■ ♤ Spreading tree with ovate or slightly lobed, dark red-purple leaves, to 8cm (3in) long, turning purple-green. Dark wine-red flowers are produced in late spring, followed by cherry-like, dark red-purple fruit, 1.5cm (½in) across. ↕↔ 8m (25ft). ❄❄❄
M. 'Liset' ■ ♤ Rounded tree with ovate, often lobed, bronze-green leaves, to 8cm (3in) long, reddish purple when young. Dark purple-pink flowers open from dark red buds in late spring, followed by cherry-like, dark purple-red fruit, 1cm (½in) across. ↕↔ 6m (20ft). ❄❄❄
M. 'Magdeburgensis' ■ ♤ Spreading tree with ovate, dark green leaves, to 8cm (3in) long. Dense clusters of semi-double, deep pink flowers are produced in late spring, sometimes followed by yellow fruit, 1cm (½in) across. ↕ 6m (20ft), ↔ 6m (20ft). ❄❄❄
M. 'Marshall Oyama' ■ ♤ Broadly conical tree with elliptic, dark green leaves, to 8cm (3in) long. Pink-flushed white flowers are borne in late spring, followed by ovoid-spherical, yellow-flushed red fruit, to 4cm (1½in) long. ↕ 8m (25ft), ↔ 6m (20ft). ❄❄❄
M. 'Molten Lava' ♤ Weeping tree with yellowish green winter bark and ovate, dark green leaves, 6–10cm (2½–4in) long. White flowers open from dark red buds in late spring, followed by orange-red fruit, 1cm (½in) across. ↕ 5m (15ft), ↔ 4m (12ft). ❄❄❄
M. 'Neville Copeman' 𝕐 ♤ Spreading tree with oval, dark green leaves, to 10cm (4in) long, purplish red when young. Dark purple-pink flowers are borne in mid- and late spring, followed by orange-red to crimson fruit, 3.5cm (1½in) across. ↕↔ 9m (28ft). ❄❄❄
M. *niedzwetskyana* ■ ♤ syn. *M. pumila* var. *niedzwetskyana*. Spreading tree with oval, purple-green leaves, red when young, to 12cm (5in) long. Dark red-purple flowers are produced in late spring, followed by conical, red-purple fruit, to 5cm (2in) long. ↕ 6m (20ft), ↔ 8m (25ft). C. Asia. ❄❄❄
M. 'Okonomierat Echtermeyer' see *M.* 'Echtermeyer'.
M. 'Pink Spires' ♢ Narrowly upright tree with ovate, red-purple young leaves, 6–12cm (2½–5in) long, maturing to bronze-green in summer. Lavender-pink flowers are produced from darker buds in mid- and late spring, followed by long-lasting, purple-red fruit, 1cm (½in) across. ↕ 6m (20ft), ↔ 4m (12ft). ❄❄❄
M. *prattii* ♤–♤ Broadly conical, upright tree, spreading with age, with ovate, tapered, mid-green leaves, to 12cm (5in) long, turning orange and red in autumn. Bears white flowers in late spring, followed by spherical to ovoid, white-speckled red fruit, 1cm (½in) across. ↕↔ 10m (30ft). W. China. ❄❄❄
M. 'Professor Sprenger' ■ ♤ Dense, rounded tree with broadly ovate, glossy, bright green leaves, to 8cm (3in) long, turning yellow in late autumn. In mid- and late spring, pink buds open to very fragrant white flowers, followed by long-lasting, orange-red fruit, to 1.5cm (½in) across. ↕↔ 7m (22ft). ❄❄❄
M. 'Profusion' ♤ Spreading tree with elliptic, bronze-green leaves, to 8cm (3in) long, purple-red when young. Dark purple-pink flowers are freely

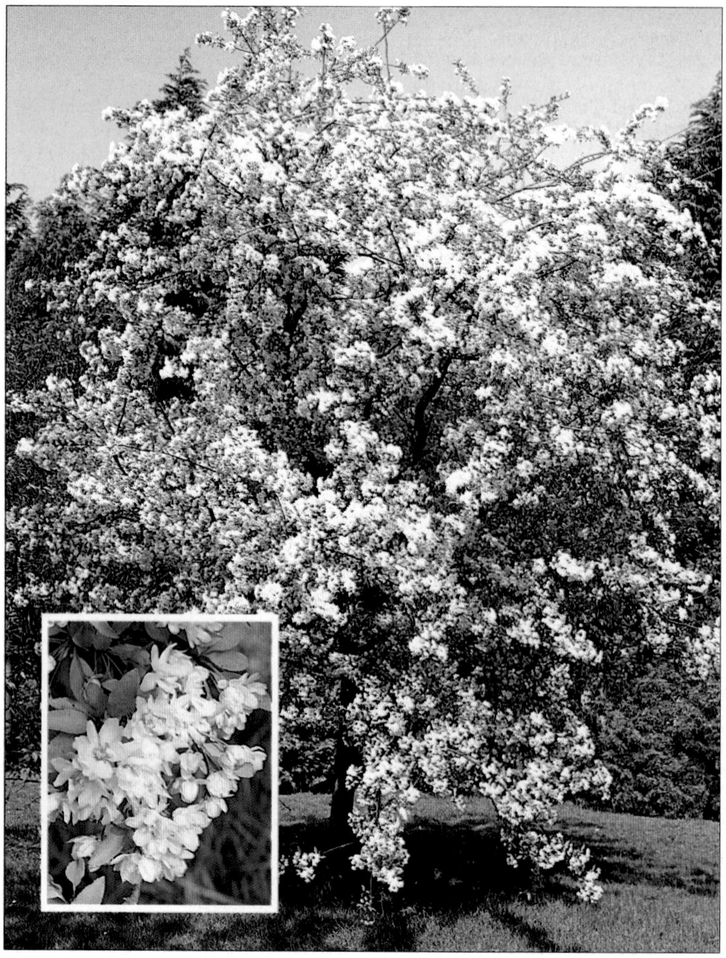
Malus 'Katherine' (inset: flower detail)

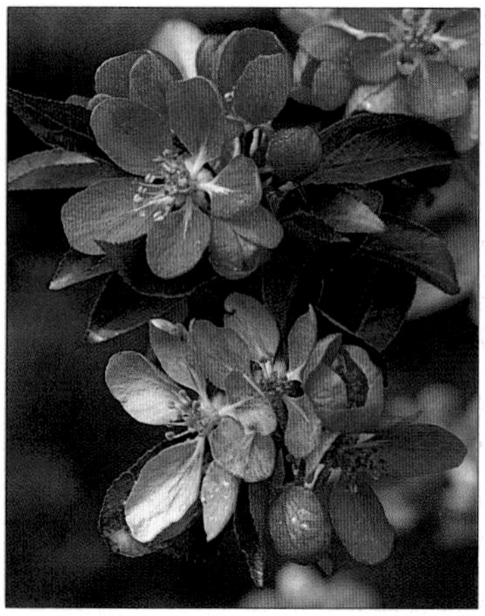
Malus niedzwetskyana

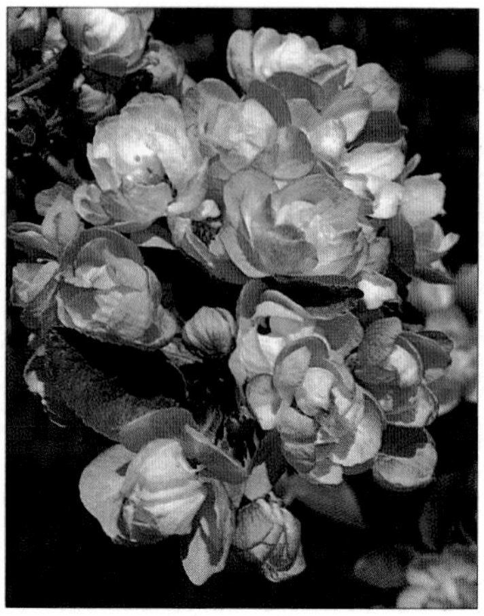
Malus 'Magdeburgensis'

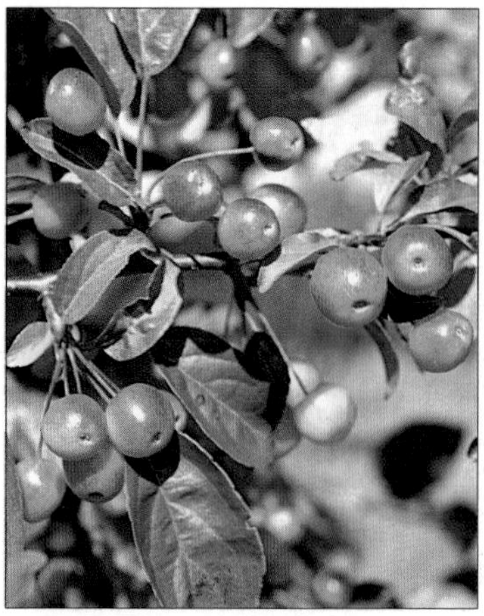
Malus 'Professor Sprenger'

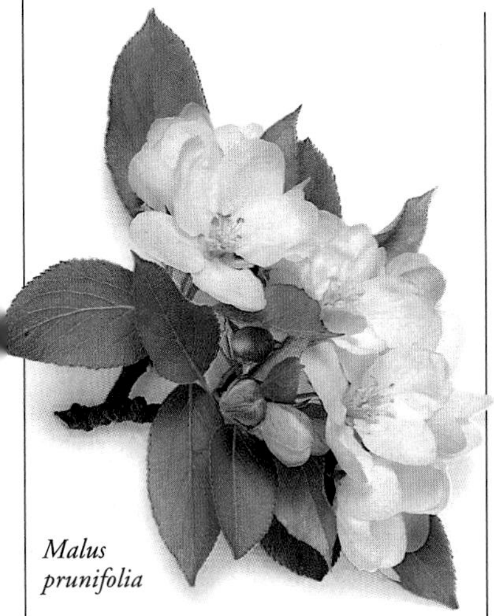

Malus prunifolia

produced in late spring, followed by cherry-like, reddish purple fruit, 1cm (½in) across. ↕↔ 10m (30ft). ❄❄❄

M. prunifolia ▣ ♀ Spreading tree with elliptic to ovate, dark green leaves, to 10cm (4in) long. Fragrant white flowers open from pink buds in mid-spring, followed by long-lasting, spherical to ovoid, red or sometimes yellow fruit, 2.5cm (1in) across. ↕↔ 9m (28ft). Probably China. ❄❄❄

M. pumila* var. *niedzwetskyana see *M. niedzwetskyana.*

M.* x *purpurea ♀ (*M. atrosanguinea* x *M. niedzwetskyana*). Erect, open tree with broadly ovate, sometimes lobed, dark green leaves, to 10cm (4in) long. The young wood and spring foliage are both purplish red. Purplish pink flowers open from ruby-red buds in mid-spring, followed by dark red fruit, 2–2.5cm (¾–1in) across. Several cultivars listed here under their own names, *M.* 'Aldenhamensis', *M.* 'Eleyi', and *M.* 'Lemoinei', are sometimes referred to this hybrid. ↕ 4–7m (12–22ft), ↔ 2–4m (6–12ft). Garden origin. ❄❄❄

***M.* 'Red Barron'** ♀ Broadly upright tree with ovate, bronze-green leaves, 6–10cm (2½–4in) long, purple when young. Dark pink flowers open from dark red buds in late spring, followed by glossy, dark red fruit, 1cm (½in) across. ↕↔ 6m (20ft). ❄❄❄

***M.* 'Red Jade'** ♀ Weeping tree with ovate, tapered, glossy, mid-green leaves, to 9cm (3½in) long. White or pink-flushed flowers are produced from red buds in late spring, followed by ovoid, glossy, bright red fruit, to 1.5cm (½in) long. ↕ 4m (12ft), ↔ 6m (20ft). ❄❄❄

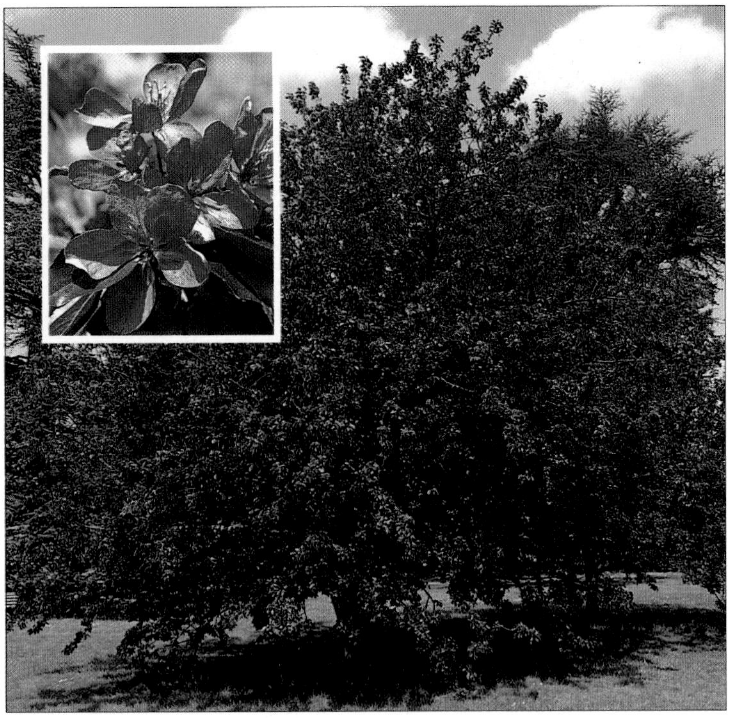

Malus 'Royalty' (inset: flower detail)

***M.* 'Red Sentinel'** ▣ ♀ Broadly upright tree with ovate, dark green leaves, to 8cm (3in) long. White flowers are produced in late spring, followed by long-lasting, yellow-flushed red, later glossy, dark red fruit, 2.5cm (1in) across. ↕↔ 7m (22ft). ❄❄❄

***M.* 'Red Siberian'** see *M.* x *robusta* 'Red Siberian'.

***M.* 'Red Silver'** ♀ Spreading tree with ovate leaves, grey-hairy at first, turning purple-red and hairless, then dark green, to 8cm (3in) long. Dark red-purple flowers are produced in late spring, followed by purple fruit, 2cm (¾in) across. ↕ 6m (20ft), ↔ 7m (22ft). ❄❄❄

***M.* x *robusta* 'Red Siberian'** 🏆 ♀ syn. *M.* 'Red Siberian'. Vigorous, spreading tree with oval, dark green leaves, to 10cm (4in) long. In mid- and late spring, produces abundant pink-tinged white flowers followed by long-lasting red fruit, 2cm (¾in) across. ↕ 12m (40ft), ↔ 10m (30ft). ❄❄❄. **'Yellow Siberian'** 🏆 syn. *M.* 'Yellow Siberian', has yellow fruit.

***M.* 'Royal Beauty'** 🏆 ♀ Small, weeping tree with elliptic, reddish purple leaves, to 6cm (2½in) long, turning dark green, purple beneath. Dark red-purple flowers are produced in late spring, followed by dark red fruit, 1cm (½in) across. ↕ 2m (6ft), ↔ 2.5m (8ft). ❄❄❄

***M.* 'Royalty'** ▣ ♀ Spreading tree with ovate, dark red-purple leaves, to 10cm (4in) long, retaining colour well and turning red in autumn, the larger leaves often slightly lobed. Crimson-purple flowers are produced in mid- and late spring, followed by dark red fruit, 1.5cm (½in) across. ↕↔ 8m (25ft). ❄❄❄

***M.* 'Rudolph'** ♀ Upright tree with ovate, glossy, dark green leaves, to 7cm (3in) long, reddish purple when young. Rose-red flowers open from darker red buds in late spring, followed by long-lasting, orange-yellow fruit, 1.5cm (½in) long. ↕ 7m (22ft), ↔ 4m (12ft). ❄❄❄

M. sargentii ♀ syn. *M. toringo* subsp. *sargentii.* Spreading shrub or tree with ovate or 3-lobed, dark green leaves, to 8cm (3in) long. Abundant white flowers are produced in late spring, followed by long-lasting, dark red fruit, 8mm (⅜in) across. ↕ 4m (12ft), ↔ 5m (15ft). Japan. ❄❄❄

M. sieboldii ▣ syn. *M. toringo.* Spreading shrub with arching branches and ovate to deeply 3- to 5-lobed leaves, to 6cm (2½in) long. Fragrant white flowers open from pink buds in mid-spring, followed by slender-stalked, red or yellow fruit, 1cm (½in) across. ↕ 2.5m (8ft), ↔ 3m (10ft). Japan. ❄❄❄.

'Calocarpa' see *M.* x *zumi* 'Calocarpa'.

***M.* 'Snowdrift'** ♀ Dense, rounded tree with elliptic to ovate, glossy, dark green leaves, to 10cm (4in) long. Abundant white flowers open from pink buds in late spring, followed by long-lasting, glossy, orange-red fruit, 1.5cm (½in) across. ↕↔ 6m (20ft). ❄❄❄

M. spectabilis ♀ Rounded tree with oval, glossy, dark green leaves, to 9cm (3½in) long. Blush-pink flowers are produced from rose-red buds in mid- and late spring, followed by yellow fruit, to 2.5cm (1in) across. ↕↔ 10m (30ft). Probably China. ❄❄❄

***M.* 'Spring Snow'** ♀ Dense, upright tree with oval, bright green leaves, 3–8cm (1¼–3in) long. Abundant fragrant white flowers are borne in late spring. Fruit are seldom produced. ↕ 8m (25ft), ↔ 6m (20ft). ❄❄❄

***M.* 'Striped Beauty'** ▣ ♀ Spreading tree with broadly elliptic, dark green leaves, to 12cm (5in) long. Bears white flowers in late spring, followed by red-striped yellow fruit, 2.5cm (1in) across. ↕↔ 7m (22ft). ❄❄❄

M. sylvestris ♀ (Common crab apple, Wild crab apple). Rounded, sometimes thorny tree with ovate, mid-green leaves, 4–8cm (1½–3in) long. Pink-flushed white flowers are produced in late spring, followed by greenish yellow, red-flushed fruit, to 2.5cm (1in) across. ↕ 9m (28ft), ↔ 7m (22ft). Europe. ❄❄❄

M. toringo see *M. sieboldii.*

M. toringo* subsp. *sargentii see *M. sargentii.*

M. toringoides ♀ Spreading tree with ovate to lance-shaped, usually deeply 3- to 7-lobed, mid-green leaves, to 9cm (3½in) long. Slightly fragrant, creamy white flowers are produced in late spring, followed by spherical to ovoid yellow fruit, to 1.5cm (½in) long. ↕ 8m (25ft), ↔ 10m (30ft). W. China. ❄❄❄

M. transitoria ▣ 🏆 ♀ Elegant, spreading tree with oblong to deeply 3-lobed, bright green leaves, 2–3cm (¾–1¼in) long, turning yellow in autumn. In late spring, white flowers open from pink buds, followed by very small, pea-like yellow fruit, 8mm (⅜in) long, on slender red stalks. ↕ 8m (25ft), ↔ 10m (30ft). N.W. China. ❄❄❄

M. trilobata ♀ Conical tree with maple-like, 3-lobed, glossy, bright green leaves, to 9cm (3½in) long, the lobes

M

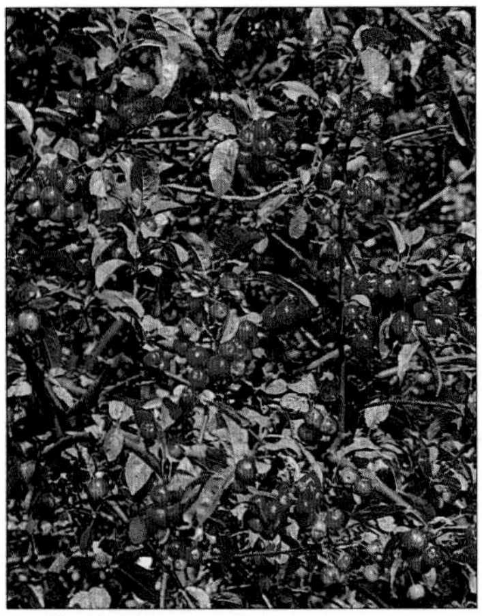

Malus 'Red Sentinel'

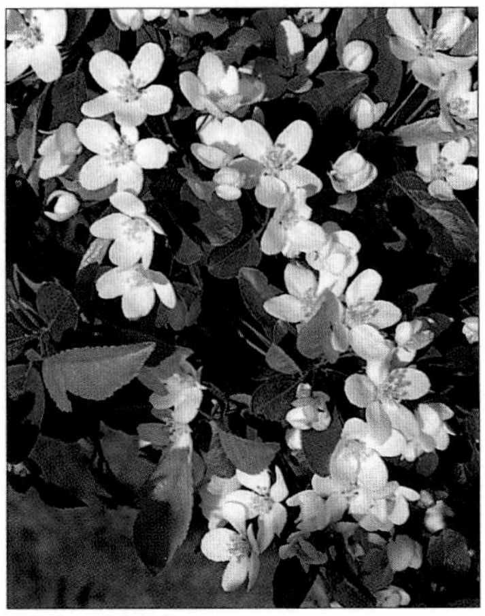

Malus sieboldii

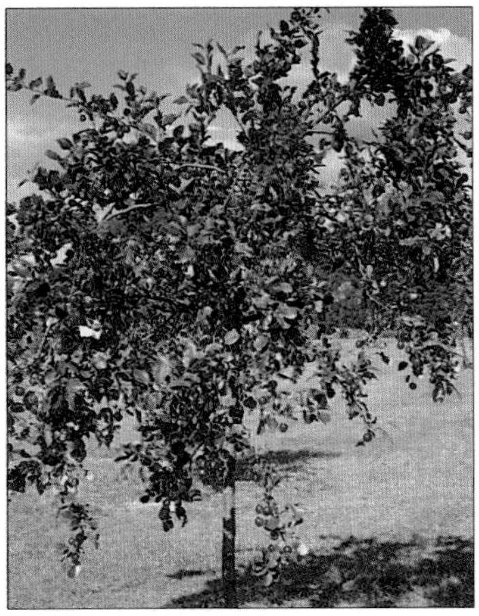

Malus 'Striped Beauty'

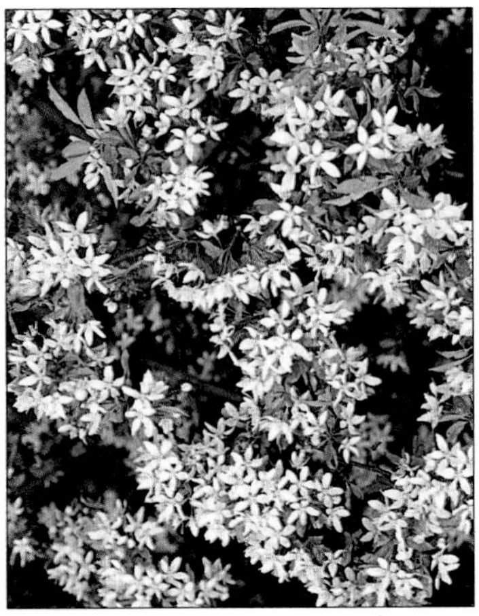

Malus transitoria

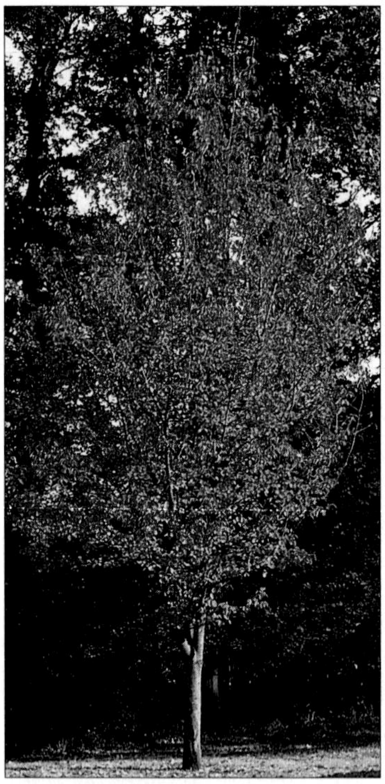

Malus tschonoskii

sometimes further lobed, turning yellow, red, and purple in autumn. White flowers are produced in early summer, followed by ellipsoid, red-flushed green fruit, 2cm (¾in) long. ↕ 15m (50ft), ↔ 7m (22ft). Greece, Syria, Lebanon, Israel. ❄❄❄

M. tschonoskii ■ Erect tree with broadly ovate, glossy, mid-green leaves, to 12cm (5in) long, turning brilliant orange, red, and purple in autumn. In late spring, bears pink-flushed white flowers, followed by red-flushed, yellow-green fruit, 3cm (1¼in) across. ↕ 12m (40ft), ↔ 7m (22ft). Japan. ❄❄❄

***M.* 'Van Eseltine'** Upright tree with ovate, glossy, mid-green leaves, to 9cm (3½in) long. Double pink flowers are produced in late spring, followed by red-flushed yellow fruit, 1.5cm (½in) across, which fall early. ↕ 8m (25ft), ↔ 6m (20ft). ❄❄❄

***M.* 'Veitch's Scarlet'** ■ Upright, spreading tree with ovate to elliptic, dark green leaves, to 8cm (3in) long. White flowers are produced in late spring, followed by ellipsoid, crimson-flushed scarlet fruit, 4.5cm (1¾in) long. ↕↔ 9m (28ft). ❄❄❄

***M.* 'Weeping Candied Apple'** see *M.* 'Candied Apple'.

***M.* 'White Cascade'** Weeping tree with ovate, dark green leaves, 6–10cm (2½–4in) long. Abundant white flowers open from pink buds in late spring, followed by small, greenish yellow fruit, 1cm (½in) across. ↕↔ 5m (15ft). ❄❄❄

***M.* 'Winter Gold'** Rounded tree with elliptic, often slightly lobed leaves, to 7cm (3in) long, bronze-tinged when young. White flowers open from pink buds in mid- and late spring, followed by long-lasting, lemon-yellow fruit, 1cm (½in) across. ↕↔ 6m (20ft). ❄❄❄

***M.* 'Wisley'** Rounded tree with elliptic to obovate leaves, to 10cm (4in) long, bronze-red at first, turning dark green. Lightly fragrant, dark purple-red flowers are produced in late spring, followed by large, conical, dark red fruit, 7cm (3in) long. ↕↔ 6m (20ft). ❄❄❄

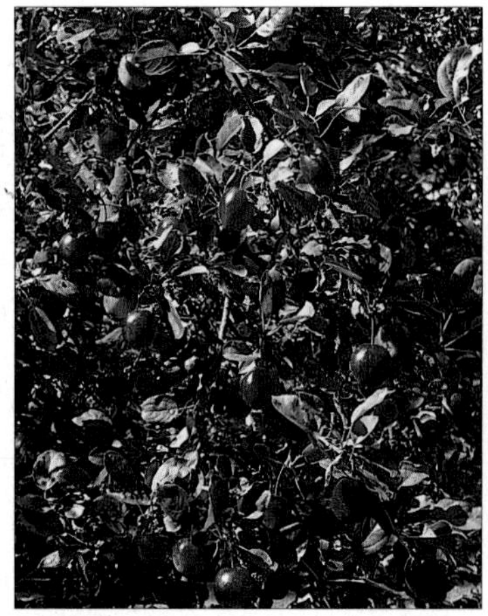

Malus 'Veitch's Scarlet'

***M.* 'Yellow Siberian'** see *M.* x *robusta* 'Yellow Siberian'.

M. yunnanensis Broadly upright tree with ovate, sometimes shallowly lobed, pale green leaves, to 12cm (5in) long, with pale brown, felted hairs beneath, turning orange, red, and purple in autumn. White, sometimes pink-tinged flowers are borne in late spring, followed by speckled red fruit, 1.5cm (½in) across. ↕ 6–12m (20–40ft), ↔ 6m (20ft). S.W. China. ❄❄❄

***M.* x *zumi* 'Calocarpa'** syn. *M. sieboldii* 'Calocarpa'. Upright, pyramidal to rounded tree with ovate, frequently deeply lobed, dark green leaves, to 9cm (3½in) long. White flowers open from pink buds in late spring, followed by long-lasting, cherry-like, bright red fruit, 1cm (½in) across. ↕ 9m (28ft), ↔ 8m (25ft). ❄❄❄

MALVA

Mallow

MALVACEAE

Genus of about 30 species of annuals, biennials, and perennials, sometimes woody-based, occurring in dry, open habitats, waste ground, roadsides, and hedge banks in Europe, N. Africa, and temperate Asia, and widely naturalized elsewhere. The alternate, rounded or heart- or kidney-shaped leaves are entire, toothed, or shallowly 3- to 9-lobed, sometimes pinnatisect. The 5-petalled, shallowly funnel-shaped, or saucer- to cup-shaped, purple, blue, pink, or white flowers are produced singly, in clusters from the leaf axils, or sometimes in leafy, terminal racemes. An involucre of 1–3 distinct bracts is usually produced below the flowers (distinguishing *Malva* species and cultivars from those of the genus *Lavatera*, which have 3–9 joined bracts). Mallows are easily grown and produce long-lasting, often showy flowers; they are suitable for an annual, herbaceous, mixed, or shrub border, or for a wildflower garden.

- **HARDINESS** Fully hardy.
- **CULTIVATION** Grow in moderately fertile, moist but well-drained soil in full sun. Provide support, especially in rich soils. Perennials are often short-lived, but will self-seed.
- **PROPAGATION** Sow seed *in situ* or in containers in early spring or early summer. Root basal cuttings of perennials in spring.
- **PESTS AND DISEASES** Susceptible to rust and leaf spot.

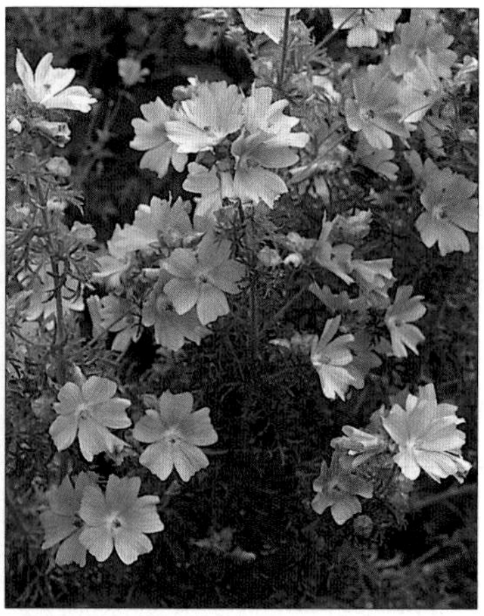

Malva moschata

M. alcea (Hollyhock mallow). Erect, bushy, hairy, woody-based perennial with heart-shaped, scalloped, light green lower leaves, to 30cm (12in) long, and deeply pinnatisect upper leaves, to 15cm (6in) long. From early summer to early autumn, open funnel-shaped, purplish pink flowers, 5–7cm (2–3in) across, the petals slightly notched, are produced in terminal racemes and axillary clusters. ↕ 1.2m (4ft), ↔ 60cm (24in). S. Europe. ❄❄❄. **var. *fastigiata*** is narrow and upright, bearing deep pink flowers well into autumn; ↕ to 80cm (32in).

M. moschata ■ (Musk mallow). Erect, bushy, woody-based perennial with slightly musk-scented leaves, to 10cm (4in) long, the lower ones heart-shaped and the upper ones pinnatisect. From early summer to early autumn, bears saucer-shaped, pale pink or white flowers, 4–6cm (1½–2½in) across, in axillary clusters. ↕ 90cm (36in), ↔ 60cm (24in). Europe, N.W. Africa. ❄❄❄

M. nicaeensis. Erect, slightly hairy annual or biennial with semi-circular, shallowly 3- to 7-lobed, blunt-toothed leaves, to 10cm (4in) long, the leaf-stalks often considerably longer than the leaf-blades. In summer, saucer-shaped

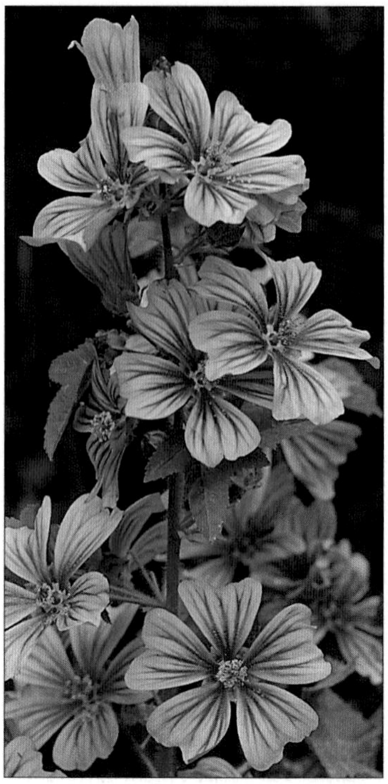

Malva sylvestris 'Primley Blue'

pink or lilac-pink flowers, to 3.5cm (1½in) across, with hairy petal bases, are borne singly or in clusters from the upper leaf axils. ↕ to 50cm (20in), ↔ 23cm (9in). Mediterranean, Arabian Peninsula to Iran, S. Russia. ❄❄❄

M. sylvestris. Erect to spreading, bushy, hairy, woody-based perennial, occasionally biennial. Broadly heart-shaped to rounded, shallowly 3- to 7-lobed leaves are dark green, to 10cm (4in) long. From late spring to mid-autumn, produces axillary clusters of open funnel-shaped, pinkish purple flowers, to 6cm (2½in) across, with notched petals and darker purple veins. ↕ to 1.2m (4ft), ↔ 60cm (24in). N. Europe, N. Africa, S.W. Asia. ❄❄❄. **f. *alba*** has white flowers; ↕ to 80cm (32in). **'Brave Heart'** is upright, with large purple flowers, to 8cm (3in) across, with strong veins and dark purple centres; ↕ to 90cm (36in). **'Cottenham Blue'** is early-flowering, and has pale blue flowers, veined darker blue; ↕ to 75cm (30in). **'Primley Blue'** ■ is prostrate, and produces pale blue-violet flowers, veined darker blue; ↕ to 20cm (8in), ↔ 30–60cm (12–24in).

MALVASTRUM

MALVACEAE

Genus of about 30 species of spreading to erect, evergreen, sometimes semi-evergreen perennials and shrubs, found on rock outcrops, rocky areas of prairies, and alluvial soils in arid and semi-arid areas of North and South America. The alternate, entire or lobed leaves are lance-shaped to rounded, 2.5–11cm (1–4½in) long, often with toothed margins. They are usually cultivated for their attractive, funnel- or cup-shaped, yellow, orange, pink, or red flowers, either solitary and axillary, or borne in terminal or axillary racemes or spikes. Grow in a sunny border or on a bank. In frost-prone areas, grow tender species in a cool greenhouse.

- **HARDINESS** Fully hardy to frost tender.
- **CULTIVATION** Grow in well-drained soil in full sun. Trim back any excess growth or dead shoots in spring.
- **PROPAGATION** Sow seed in containers in spring. Insert softwood cuttings in late spring or summer.
- **PESTS AND DISEASES** Trouble free.

M. capensis see *Anisodontea capensis.*

M. coccineum see *Sphaeralcea coccinea.*

M. lateritium. Prostrate perennial with alternate, rounded leaves, 8cm (3in) long, with 3–5 wedge-shaped to oblong lobes. Solitary, cup-shaped, peach-coloured flowers, 5cm (2in) across, with yellow anthers and deep yellow centres surrounded by deep rose-pink bands, are produced from late spring to summer. ↕ 20cm (8in), ↔ 1.5m (5ft). Argentina, Uruguay. ❄❄❄ (borderline)

MALVAVISCUS

Sleepy mallow

MALVACEAE

Genus of 3 species of evergreen shrubs found in coppices and thickets, often in coastal areas, in tropical North and South America. They have alternate, simple to palmately lobed, toothed, pale to mid-green leaves, and solitary, axillary or terminal racemes of long-stemmed,

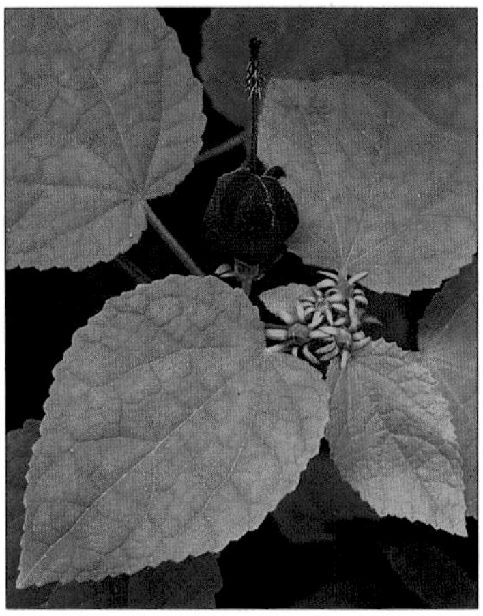

Malvaviscus arboreus

pendent, red, pink, or white flowers. The flowers are similar to those of *Hibiscus*, although the long petals only partially unfurl, producing a narrowly funnel-shaped outline. In frost-prone climates, grow in a temperate or warm greenhouse. In warmer areas, grow in a shrub border or as an informal hedge.
• **HARDINESS** Frost tender.
• **CULTIVATION** Under glass, grow in loam-based potting compost (JI No.2) in bright filtered light, or full light with shade from hot sun. In growth, water freely, and apply a balanced liquid fertilizer monthly; water sparingly in winter. Outdoors, grow in moderately fertile, moist but well-drained soil in full sun; tolerates partial shade. Pruning group 8.
• **PROPAGATION** Sow seed at 15–21°C (59–70°F) in spring. Root softwood cuttings with bottom heat in spring, or semi-ripe cuttings in summer.
• **PESTS AND DISEASES** Susceptible to red spider mites, whiteflies, and mealybugs under glass.

M. arboreus ■ syn. *M. mollis* (Wax mallow). Large, erect to spreading, usually freely branching shrub with densely velvety, downy stems and leaves. Bright green leaves are broadly ovate to heart-shaped, 6–12cm (2½–5in) long, and sometimes 3-lobed. Axillary, bright red flowers, to 5cm (2in) long, are borne mainly in late summer and early autumn. ↕ to 4m (12ft) or more, ↔ 1.5–3m (5–10ft). S.E. USA, Mexico to Colombia, Peru, Brazil. ❄ (min. 10°C/50°F). **var. *drummondii***, syn. *M. conzattii*, *M. grandiflorus*, has rounded, symmetrically lobed leaves, and flowers to 3cm (1¼in) long; S.W. USA, Mexico to Colombia. **var. *mexicanus*** is almost hairless, with lance-shaped to ovate leaves; Mexico to Colombia.
M. candidus. Erect, freely branching shrub with hairy stems. Hairy, mid-green leaves, to 18cm (7in) long, are broadly ovate to rounded, with 5-lobed, heart-shaped bases. Red flowers, 3cm (1¼in) long, are produced in terminal racemes in summer. ↕ to 4m (12ft), ↔ to 2m (6ft). Mexico. ❄ (min. 8°C/46°F).
M. conzattii see *M. arboreus* var. *drummondii*.
M. grandiflorus see *M. arboreus* var. *drummondii*.
M. mollis see *M. arboreus*.

▷ ***Mamillopsis senilis*** see *Mammillaria senilis*

MAMMILLARIA

CACTACEAE

Genus of about 150 species of spherical to cylindrical or columnar, perennial cacti from semi-desert regions, mainly in Mexico, but also in S. USA, the West Indies, Central America, Colombia, and Venezuela. Most offset freely to form clusters. Conical, cylindrical, or somewhat flattened tubercles encircle spined stems. The funnel-shaped, diurnal, white to yellow, orange, red, pink, or purple flowers are mostly borne in a ring around the crown. The berry-like fruits are oblong-ovoid to club-shaped. In frost-prone areas, grow in a temperate greenhouse or as houseplants. In warmer areas, grow on a gentle slope or raised ground in a desert garden.
• **HARDINESS** Frost tender.
• **CULTIVATION** Under glass, grow in standard cactus compost in full light with shade from hot sun. Provide low humidity. From mid-spring to autumn, water freely, applying a balanced liquid fertilizer monthly in late spring and summer; water sparingly in winter. Outdoors, grow in poor or moderately fertile, sharply drained soil in full sun. Protect from excessive winter wet. See also pp.48–49.
• **PROPAGATION** Sow seed at 19–24°C (66–75°F) in late winter or early spring. Remove offsets in early spring.
• **PESTS AND DISEASES** Vulnerable to mealybugs and root mealybugs.

M. armillata. Clustering or solitary cactus with narrowly columnar, dull green stems, 4.5cm (1¾in) thick, and brown or brown-yellow spines (9–15 radials, one or more of which is hooked, and 1–4 centrals). Pale pink, creamy white, or pale yellow flowers, 2cm (¾in) long, are borne in summer. ↕ to 30cm (12in), ↔ indefinite. N.W. Mexico. ❄ (min. 7–10°C/45–50°F)
M. baumii 🏆 syn. *Dolichothele baumii.* Clustering cactus with spherical to ovoid, mid-green stems, 3–6cm (1¼–2½in) thick. The areoles produce 30–35 thread-like white radial spines and 5 or 6 longer, pale yellow centrals. Bright yellow flowers, 3cm (1¼in) long, are produced in summer. ↕ 8cm (3in), ↔ 12cm (5in). N.E. Mexico. ❄ (min. 7–10°C/45–50°F)
M. blossfeldiana, syn. *M. shurliana.* Solitary or clustering cactus with spherical to short, cylindrical, dark green

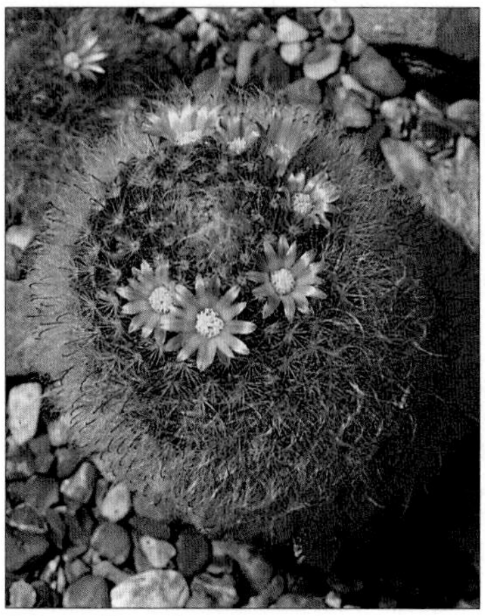

Mammillaria bocasana

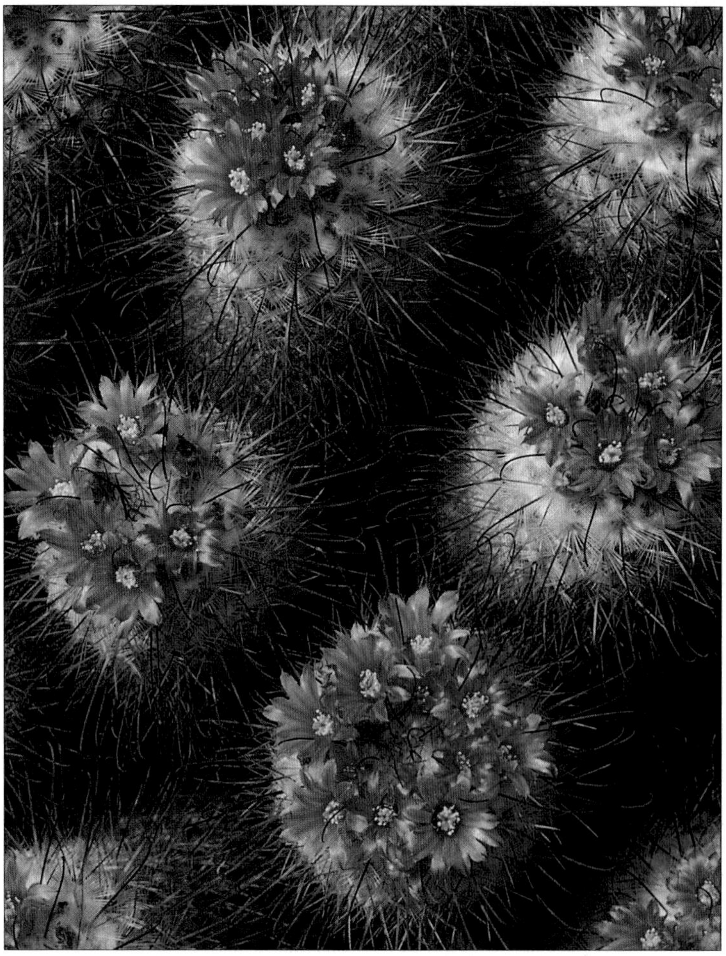

Mammillaria bombycina

stems, 4cm (1½in) thick, bearing close-set areoles with 15–20 black-tipped yellow radial spines and 3 or 4 black centrals, one of which is hooked. In summer, bears pale pink flowers, 3.5cm (1½in) long, with deep carmine-red median lines. ↕↔ 4cm (1½in). N.W. Mexico. ❄ (min. 7–10°C/45–50°F)
M. bocasana ■ 🏆 (Snowball cactus). Clump-forming cactus with spherical, white-hairy, dark bluish green stems, to 5cm (2in) thick. Close-set areoles bear 25–50 spreading white radial spines and 1 or 2 (sometimes up to 5) red or brown-yellow centrals. From spring to summer, bears yellowish white flowers, 1.5cm (½in) long, with red or pink median lines and often red-tipped petals. ↕ 5cm (2in), ↔ indefinite. C. Mexico. ❄ (min. 7–10°C/45–50°F)
M. bombycina ■ 🏆 Densely clustering cactus with spherical to cylindrical, mid-green stems, 5–8cm (2–3in) thick, densely white-woolly in the axils. Areoles bear 30–40 white radial spines and 2–4 longer, white to yellow or red-brown centrals, one of which is hooked and twice as long as the other centrals. Produces reddish purple flowers, 1.5cm (½in) long, from spring to summer. ↕ 20cm (8in), ↔ indefinite. W. central Mexico. ❄ (min. 7–10°C/45–50°F)
M. camptotricha ■ syn. *Dolichothele camptotricha.* Freely clustering cactus with spherical, deep green stems, 7cm (3in) thick, the areoles with 2–8 pale yellow radial spines, but no centrals. Produces scented white flowers, to 2cm (¾in) long, each with a green median line, from summer to autumn. ↕ to 8cm

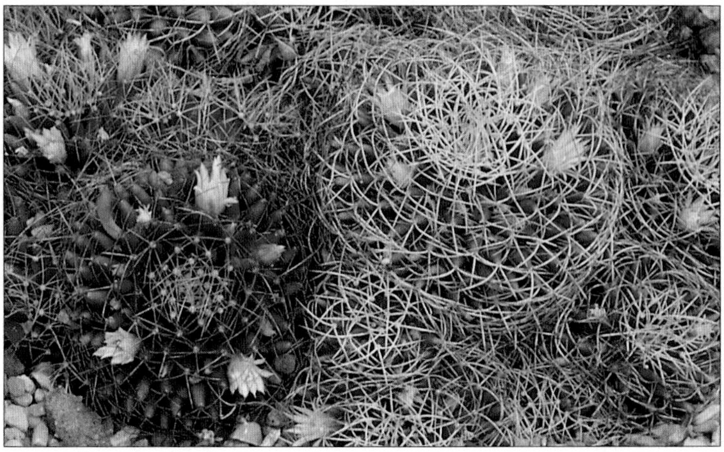

Mammillaria camptotricha

M

(3in), ↔ 20cm (8in). E. central Mexico. ❄ (min. 7–10°C/45–50°F)
M. candida ♀ (Snowball cushion cactus). Slow-growing, solitary or clustering cactus with spherical to cylindrical, mid-green stems, 6–12cm (2½–5in) thick, with 4–7 white bristles in each axil. White-felted areoles bear white, often brown- or pink-tipped spines (50 radials and 8–12 centrals). Bears rose-pink flowers, 2cm (¾in) long, with white margins, from spring to summer. ↕↔ 15cm (6in). N.E. Mexico. ❄ (min. 7–10°C/45–50°F)
M. carmenae ▣ ♀ Clustering cactus with spherical to ovoid, mid-green stems, 3–4cm (1¼–1½in) thick, with white wool and long white bristles in the axils. The areoles bear 100 or more white or cream radial spines but no centrals. Pink- or cream-flushed white flowers, 1cm (½in) long, are produced from spring to summer. ↕ to 8cm (3in), ↔ 15cm (6in). E. central Mexico. ❄ (min. 7–10°C/45–50°F)
M. centricirrha see *M. magnimamma.*
M. conoidea see *Neolloydia conoidea.*
M. crucigera. Clustering, branching cactus with depressed spherical or cylindrical to obovoid, dark brownish green stems, 3–5cm (1¼–2in) thick, with white-woolly axils and areoles. The areoles bear 24 or more needle-like white radial spines and usually 4 longer, thicker, waxy-yellow, brown- or black-tipped centrals. Pinkish purple flowers, 1.5cm (½in) long, are produced in summer. ↕ to 15cm (6in), ↔ indefinite. S. Mexico. ❄ (min. 7–10°C/45–50°F)
M. dealbata see *M. haageana.*
M. densispina. Solitary cactus with spherical or cylindrical, dark green stems, to 10cm (4in) thick, and white-woolly areoles bearing about 25 yellow or pale brown radial spines and 5 or 6 longer, reddish brown, black-tipped centrals. Sulphur-yellow flowers, 2cm (¾in) long, often with red-flushed outer petals, are produced from spring to summer. ↕↔ 10cm (4in). C. Mexico. ❄ (min. 7–10°C/45–50°F)
M. elongata ♀ (Gold lace cactus). Variable, densely clustering cactus with cylindrical, mid-green stems, 1–3cm (½–1¼in) thick, and white, yellow, or dark reddish brown spines (15–20 radials and up to 3 centrals, although the centrals may be absent). Bears white or yellow, sometimes faintly pink-striped flowers, to 1.5cm (½in) long, in summer. ↕ 15cm (6in), ↔ 30cm (12in). C. Mexico. ❄ (min. 7–10°C/45–50°F)

M

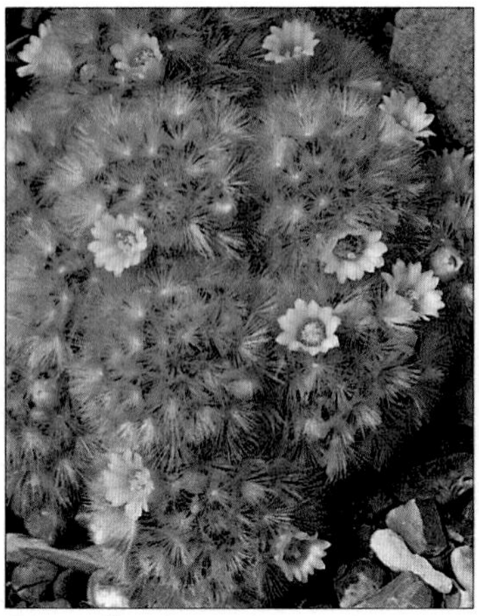
Mammillaria carmenae

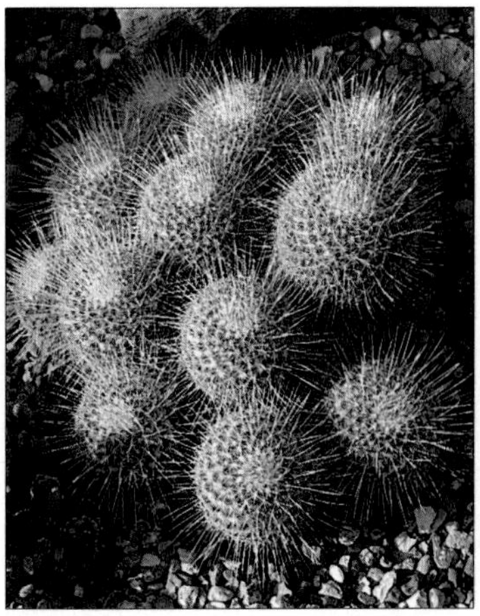
Mammillaria geminispina

M. geminispina ▣ ♀ Solitary cactus, later offsetting and forming mounds, producing spherical, mid-green stems, 8cm (3in) thick, becoming cylindrical. The white-woolly areoles bear white spines (16–20 radials and 2–4 longer, often brown-tipped centrals). White to creamy white flowers, 1.5cm (½in) or more long, with carmine-red stripes, are produced from summer to autumn. ↕ 25cm (10in), ↔ 50cm (20in). C. Mexico. ❄ (min. 7–10°C/45–50°F)
M. gracilis. Freely clustering cactus producing cylindrical, fresh green stems, 3–4.5cm (1¼–1¾in) thick, and slightly woolly areoles with 3–5 brown central spines and 12–17 shorter, yellowish white radials. From spring to summer, bears yellowish white flowers, 1.5cm (½in) long, with pink or white median

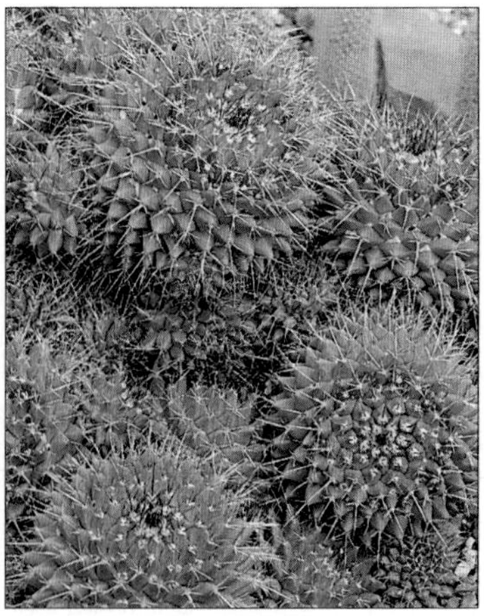
Mammillaria magnimamma

lines. Offsets fall away at the least touch. ↕ 5cm (2in), ↔ 20cm (8in). E. central Mexico. ❄ (min. 7–10°C/45–50°F). **var. *fragilis*** has 2 brown-tipped white central spines per areole; ↕ to 4cm (1½in), ↔ to 12cm (5in).
M. haageana, syn. *M. dealbata.* Cactus offsetting from the base and sides, with spherical or cylindrical, mid-green stems, 10cm (4in) thick, with slightly woolly axils. Areoles bear 18–20 thin white radial spines and 1 or 2 longer, black-tipped, red-brown centrals. Bears carmine-red flowers, 1.5cm (½in) long, from spring to summer. ↕ 15cm (6in), ↔ 24cm (10in). C. and S.E. Mexico. ❄ (min. 7–10°C/45–50°F)
M. hahniana ▣ ♀ (Old lady cactus). Solitary cactus, forming groups when mature, with spherical, mid-green stems,

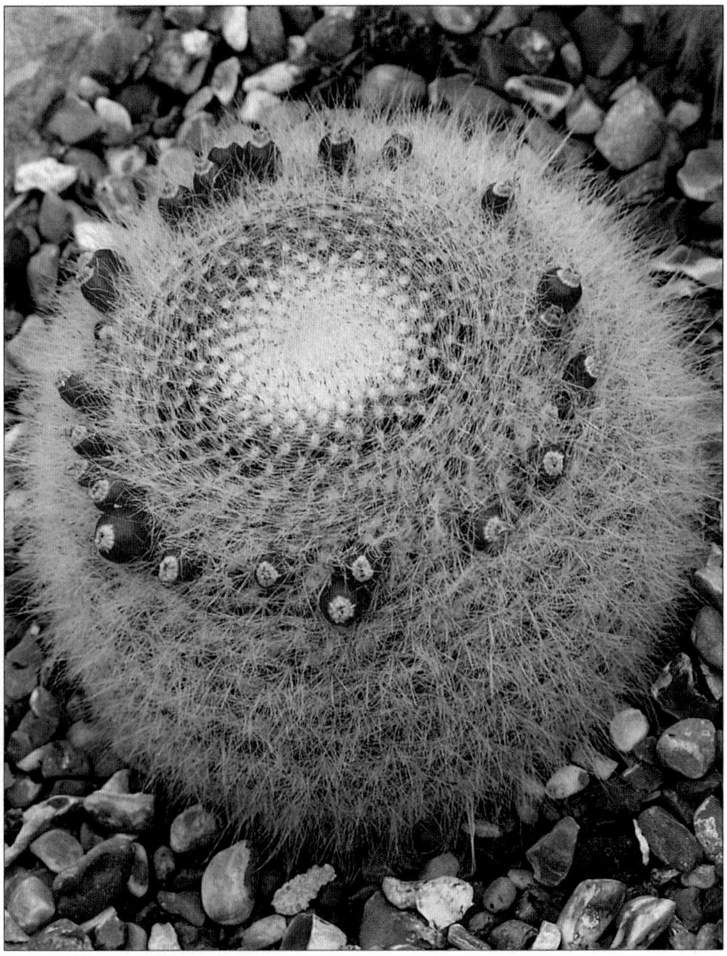
Mammillaria hahniana

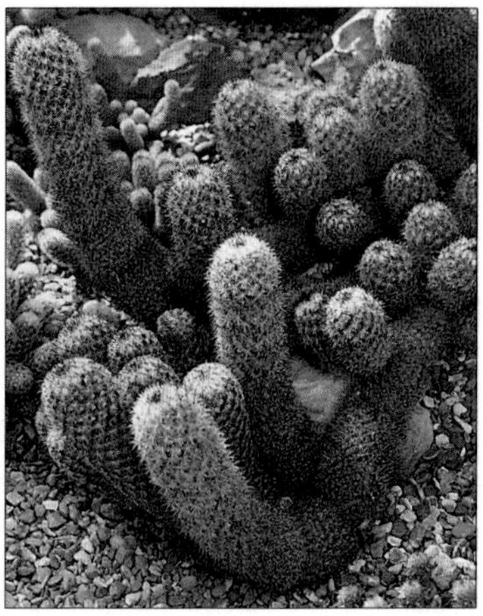
Mammillaria microhelia

12cm (5in) thick, coated with long white hairs, bristles, and spines (20–30 fine, hair-like radials and 1–3 or more shorter, dark-tipped centrals). Purplish red flowers, to 1cm (½in) long, are produced from spring to summer. ↕ to 20cm (8in), ↔ to 40cm (16in). C. Mexico. ❄ (min. 7–10°C/45–50°F)
M. herrerae. Solitary or clustering cactus with spherical, mid-green stems, 2–3cm (¾–1¼in) thick, occasionally elongating slightly with age, and densely coated with about 100 near-white radial spines but no centrals. Pale pink to reddish violet flowers, 2.5cm (1in) long, are produced from spring to summer. ↕↔ 3–4cm (1¼–1½in). C. Mexico. ❄ (min. 7–10°C/45–50°F). **var. *albiflora*** has pure white flowers.
M. magnimamma ▣ syn. *M. centricirrha.* Extremely variable, freely clustering cactus with spherical, greyish green stems, 10–15cm (4–6in) thick, and white-woolly axils and areoles, the latter with 3–6 brown-tipped, yellowish white radial spines of unequal length, but no centrals. From spring to summer, bears purple-red to pink or brownish yellow flowers, 2.5cm (1in) long. ↕ to 30cm (12in), ↔ to 60cm (24in). C. Mexico. ❄ (min. 7–10°C/45–50°F)
M. mazatlanensis. Clustering cactus with cylindrical, greyish green stems, 4cm (1½in) thick. Rounded, woolly areoles bear 12–15 white radial spines and 3 or 4 longer, hooked, glossy, reddish brown centrals with cream bases. Bright carmine-red flowers, 4cm (1½in) long, develop in summer. ↕ 12cm (5in), ↔ 30cm (12in). W. Mexico. ❄ (min. 7–10°C/45–50°F)
M. microhelia ▣ Solitary or clustering cactus with cylindrical, greyish green stems, 3.5–5cm (1½–2in) thick, densely covered with spines (up to 50 golden yellow to pale brown-white radials and up to 8, shorter, dark red-brown centrals, although these may be absent). Bears creamy white, occasionally pink-suffused flowers, to 1.5cm (½in) long, from spring to summer. ↕↔ 15cm (6in). C. Mexico. ❄ (min. 7–10°C/45–50°F)
M. mystax. Clustering or solitary cactus with spherical to cylindrical, grey-green stems, 10cm (4in) thick, with white wool and bristles in the axils. The areoles bear 5–10 brown-tipped white radial spines and 3 or 4 longer, purplish grey centrals. From spring to summer, bears purplish pink flowers, 2.5cm (1in) long. ↕ to 15cm (6in), ↔ 24cm (10in). S. Mexico. ❄ (min. 7–10°C/45–50°F)

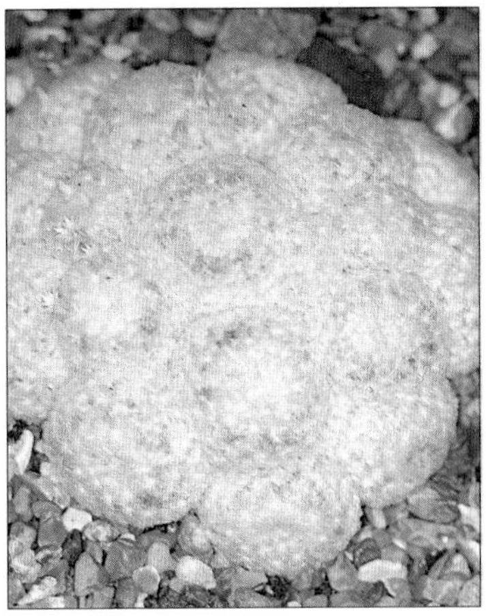

Mammillaria plumosa

M. plumosa ■ ♀ Clustering cactus with spherical, mid-green stems, 7cm (3in) thick, and white-woolly axils. The areoles bear about 40 feathery white radial spines but no centrals. Greenish white or pale yellow flowers, 1.5cm (½in) long, with reddish brown median lines, are borne in late summer. ↕ 12cm (5in), ↔ 40cm (16in). N.E. Mexico. ❁ (min. 7–10°C/45–50°F)
M. rhodantha. Solitary cactus with mostly spherical to cylindrical, mid-green stems, 10–12cm (4–5in) thick, and white-woolly axils. The areoles bear 16–24 straight, glossy, white to yellow radial spines and 4–7 longer, often curved, red-brown, occasionally straw-coloured or golden yellow centrals. Purplish pink flowers, 2cm (¾in) long, are borne in summer. ↕↔ 40cm (16in). C. Mexico. ❁ (min. 7–10°C/45–50°F)
M. schiedeana. Solitary or clustering cactus with slightly depressed spherical, mid-green stems, 4–6cm (1½–2½in) thick, with long, woolly hairs in the axils. The areoles bear 70–80 yellow to white radial spines but no centrals. Cream flowers, 2cm (¾in) long, are produced from summer to autumn. ↕ 10cm (4in), ↔ 30cm (12in). C. Mexico. ❁ (min. 7–10°C/45–50°F)
M. sempervivi. Solitary to clump-forming cactus with depressed spherical to short, cylindrical, dark green stems, to 10cm (4in) thick, often elongating, and densely woolly in the axils. The areoles bear 3–7 white radial spines and 2–4 slightly longer, yellow-brown or red centrals. White or yellowish pink flowers, 1cm (½in) long, with red median lines, are borne from spring to summer. ↕↔ 8cm (3in). C. Mexico. ❁ (min. 7–10°C/45–50°F)
M. senilis, syn. *Mamillopsis senilis.* Slow-growing, solitary cactus, eventually clustering, with spherical to cylindrical, pale green stems, 6–10cm (2½–4in) thick, white-woolly, bristly axils, and white spines (30–40 radials and 4–6 longer centrals, 1 or 2 of which are hooked). Violet-red flowers, 6cm (2½in) long, with slender tubes, are produced from spring to summer. ↕ 15cm (6in), ↔ to 40cm (16in). N.W. Mexico. ❁ (min. 7–10°C/45–50°F)
M. shurliana see *M. blossfeldiana.*
M. zeilmanniana ■ ♀ Clustering cactus with spherical, dark green stems, 4.5cm (1¾in) thick, with bare axils. The areoles bear 15–18 hair-like white radial spines and 4 shorter, reddish brown centrals, 1 of which is hooked. Reddish violet, pink, or white flowers, to 2cm (¾in) long, are produced in summer. ↕ 15cm (6in), ↔ 30cm (12in). C. Mexico. ❁ (min. 7–10°C/45–50°F)

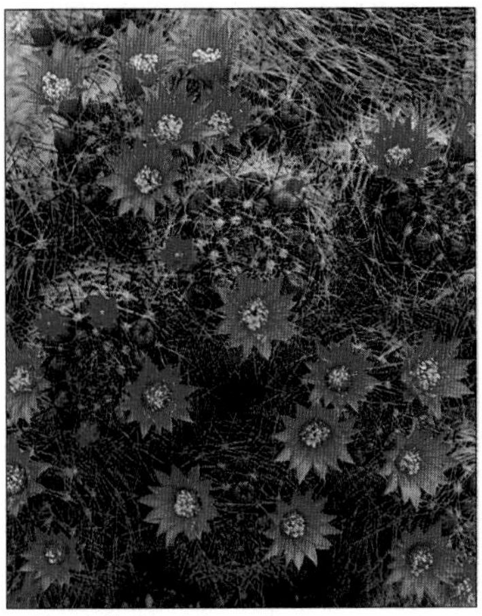

Mammillaria zeilmanniana

▷**Mandarin** see *Citrus reticulata*

MANDEVILLA

syn. DIPLADENIA

APOCYNACEAE

Genus of about 120 species of mainly tuberous-rooted, woody-stemmed, twining climbers, with some perennials, from tropical woodland in Central and South America. Opposite, simple leaves are borne on stems containing a milky latex. They have often showy, funnel-shaped to tubular-salverform flowers, each with 5 broad, spreading petal lobes, borne mainly in axillary racemes. Use to clothe a pergola, arch, or trellis, or grow as a screen. In frost-prone climates, grow in a temperate or warm greenhouse. Contact with the sap may cause skin irritation, and all parts may cause mild stomach upset if ingested.
• **HARDINESS** Frost tender; *M. laxa* may survive temperatures near to 0°C (32°F).
• **CULTIVATION** Under glass, grow in loam-based potting compost (JI No.3), in full light with shade from hot sun. In the growing season, water moderately, and apply a balanced liquid fertilizer monthly; water sparingly in winter. Outdoors, grow in moderately fertile, moist but well-drained soil in full sun with some midday shade. Pruning group 12, in late winter or early spring.
• **PROPAGATION** Sow seed at 18–23°C (64–73°F) in spring. Root softwood cuttings in late spring or semi-ripe cuttings in summer, with bottom heat.
• **PESTS AND DISEASES** Red spider mites, whiteflies, and mealybugs may be troublesome under glass.

***M. x amabilis* 'Alice du Pont'** see *M.* x *amoena* 'Alice du Pont'.
***M. x amoena* 'Alice du Pont'** ■ syn. *M.* x *amabilis* 'Alice du Pont'. Woody-stemmed, twining climber bearing elliptic-oblong to ovate-oblong, slightly wrinkled, mid- to deep green leaves, 9–18cm (3½–7in) long, with short points. Racemes of up to 20 narrowly funnel-shaped, glowing pink flowers, 8–10cm (3–4in) across, are freely produced in summer. ↕ to 7m (22ft). ❁ (min. 10–15°C/50–59°F)
M. boliviensis, syn. *Dipladenia boliviensis.* Slender-stemmed, usually freely branching, woody, twining climber with elliptic to oblong or elliptic-obovate, slender-pointed, shiny, mid-green leaves, 5–10cm (2–4in) long. In mid- and late summer, bears racemes of 3–7 white flowers, 5–7cm (2–3in) across, with yellow eyes and angular petal lobes. ↕ 3–4m (10–12ft). Ecuador, Bolivia. ❁ (min. 10–15°C/50–59°F)

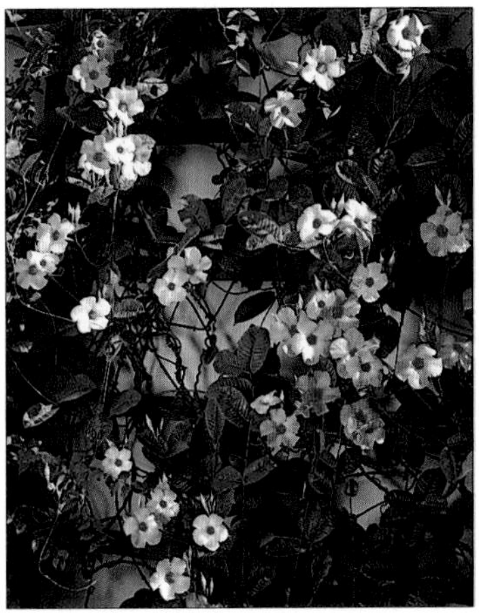

Mandevilla x *amoena* 'Alice du Pont'

M. laxa, syn. *M. suaveolens, M. tweediana* (Chilean jasmine). Vigorous, freely branching, woody-stemmed, twining climber. Ovate to oblong leaves, 5–10cm (2–4in) long, have heart-shaped bases and slender-pointed tips, lustrous, rich green above and purple or grey-green beneath. From summer to early autumn, bears racemes of 5–15 tubular, strongly fragrant, pure white or creamy white flowers, 5–9cm (2–3½in) across, with broad, rounded, often crimped petal lobes. ↕ 3–5m (10–15ft). Peru, Bolivia, Argentina. ❁ (min. 5°C/41°F)
M. splendens ■ syn. *Dipladenia splendens.* Vigorous, moderately to freely branching, woody-stemmed, twining climber with downy young stems and broadly elliptic, lustrous, mid-green leaves, 10–20cm (4–8in) long, with heart-shaped bases and slender-pointed tips. In summer, produces racemes of 3–5 narrowly funnel-shaped flowers, to 10cm (4in) across, with rounded, rose-pink petal lobes and white and yellow throats. ↕ 3–6m (10–20ft). S.E. Brazil. ❁ (min. 10–15°C/50–59°F). **'Rosacea'** has rose-pink flowers, margined and flushed deep purplish pink, with the tops of the throats ringed brighter pink.
M. suaveolens see *M. laxa.*
M. tweediana see *M. laxa.*

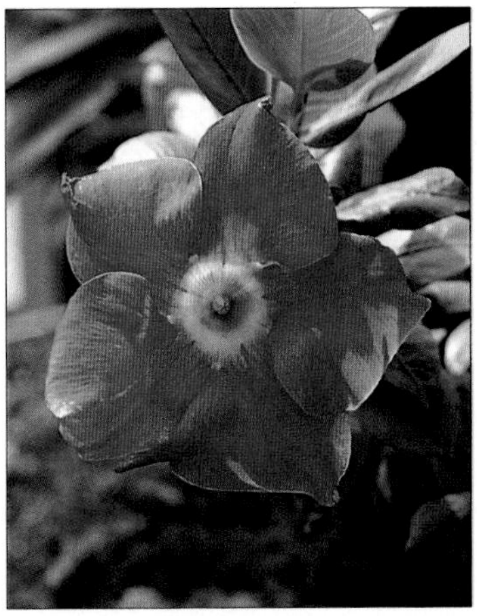

Mandevilla splendens

MANDRAGORA

Mandrake

SOLANACEAE

Genus of 6 species of perennials, with fleshy tap roots, found in dry, stony areas from the Mediterranean region to the Himalayas. They produce large, basal rosettes of ovate to lance-shaped leaves, and are grown for their stemless or short-stemmed, tubular-bell-shaped flowers, with triangular lobes, borne singly or in basal clusters from autumn to early spring. The fleshy fruits are spherical or ellipsoid. Grow in a rock garden or at the base of a warm, sunny wall. Alkaloids in the plant may be harmful if ingested.
• **HARDINESS** Hardy to -10°C (14°F).
• **CULTIVATION** Grow in deep, moderately fertile, well-drained soil in full sun. Shelter from cold, drying winds and protect from excessive winter wet. Avoid disturbance once established.
• **PROPAGATION** Sow seed in containers in an open frame as soon as ripe or in autumn. Insert root cuttings in winter.
• **PESTS AND DISEASES** Slugs and snails may damage leaves and fruits.

M. autumnalis (Autumn mandrake). Perennial with rosettes of oblong to lance-shaped, dark green leaves, to 25cm (10in) long. From autumn to winter, produces basal clusters of tubular-bell-shaped, violet or white flowers, to 3cm (1¼in) across, often with green or white streaks, followed by ellipsoid, orange or yellow fruit, to 3cm (1¼in) long. ↕ 15cm (6in), ↔ to 30cm (12in). Portugal, Spain, E. Mediterranean. ✲✲
M. officinarum ■ (Common mandrake, Devil's apples, Love apple). Perennial with rosettes of ovate to lance-shaped, wavy-margined, dark green leaves, to 30cm (12in) long, upright at first, then lying flat on the ground. In spring, bears basal clusters of upward-facing, tubular-bell-shaped, greenish white flowers, to 2.5cm (1in) across, sometimes stained purple, followed by spherical yellow fruit, to 3cm (1¼in) across. ↕ 15cm (6in), ↔ to 30cm (12in). N. Italy, W. Balkans, Greece, W. Turkey. ✲✲

▷**Mandrake** see *Mandragora*
American see *Podophyllum peltatum*
Autumn see *Mandragora autumnalis*
Common see *Mandragora officinarum*

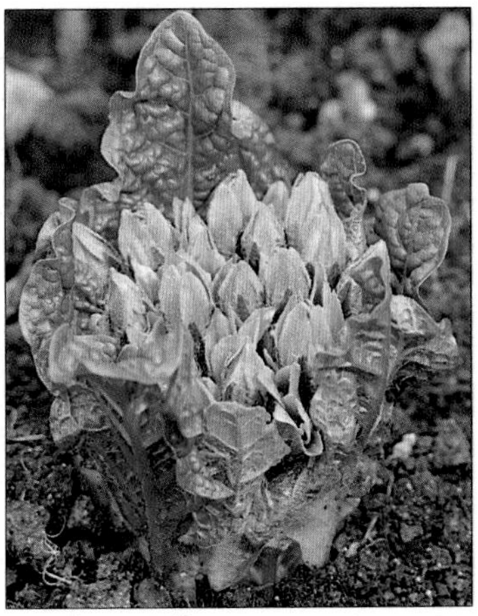

Mandragora officinarum

M

MANETTIA

RUBIACEAE

Genus of about 80 species of evergreen perennials and woody-stemmed, twining climbers from moist woodland or rainforest in tropical North and South America, and the West Indies. They produce opposite pairs of usually simple, sometimes toothed leaves. Tubular to funnel-shaped, often brightly coloured flowers, each with 4 short lobes, are borne singly or in small, axillary panicles or cymes. In frost-prone areas, grow in a cool or temperate greenhouse. In warmer areas, use to clothe an arch, or grow on a wall or through small trees.

• **HARDINESS** Frost tender.

• **CULTIVATION** Under glass, grow in loam-based potting compost (JI No.2) in full light or bright filtered light. In the growing season, water moderately and apply a balanced liquid fertilizer every 3–4 weeks; water sparingly in winter. Outdoors, grow in moderately fertile, moist but well-drained soil in full sun, although they will tolerate partial shade. Pruning group 12, in late winter or early spring.

• **PROPAGATION** Sow seed at 13–18°C (55–64°F) in spring. Root stem-tips of softwood cuttings in late spring or summer.

• **PESTS AND DISEASES** Whiteflies may be a problem under glass.

M. bicolor see *M. luteorubra.*
M. cordifolia (Firecracker vine). Vigorous climber with thin, oblong to lance-shaped, ovate, or heart-shaped leaves, to 8cm (3in) long, lustrous, bright green above, paler and downy or hairless beneath. From late winter to summer, tubular, brilliant red to deep orange flowers, 3–5cm (1¼–2in) long, sometimes yellow-flushed on the lobes, are borne singly or in crowded, leafy panicles. ↕2–4m (6–12ft). Peru, Bolivia, Argentina. ❀ (min. 7°C/45°F)
M. inflata see *M. luteorubra.*

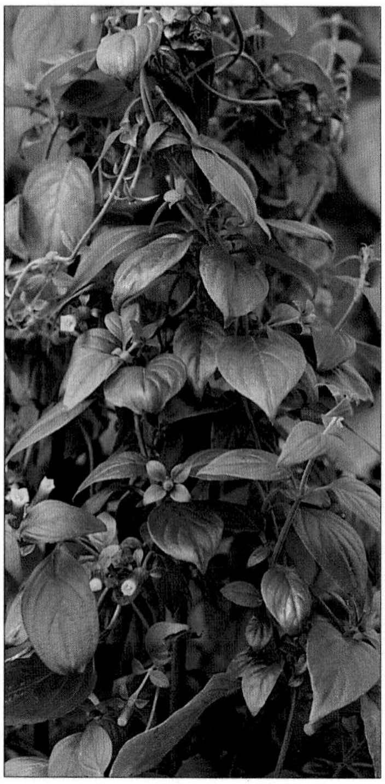

Manettia luteorubra

M. luteorubra ▣ syn. *M. bicolor, M. inflata* (Brazilian firecracker). Fast-growing climber with angular, slightly sticky, hairy stems bearing ovate to lance-shaped, light to dark green leaves, 3.5–15cm (1½–6in) long, semi-leathery when mature. Solitary, occasionally paired, tubular, bright red, yellow-lobed flowers, 2.5–5cm (1–2in) long, inflated at the bases and with dense velvety hairs, are borne in summer. ↕2–4m (6–12ft). Paraguay, Uruguay. ❀ (min. 7°C/45°F)

MANGLIETIA

MAGNOLIACEAE

Genus of 25 species of upright to spreading, evergreen trees and shrubs found in mountain woodland from the Himalayas to S. and W. China and Malaysia. The alternate, mostly oblong-ovate to elliptic or inversely lance-shaped leaves are glossy, light or dark green. *Manglietia* species are usually cultivated for their magnolia-like flowers, borne singly at the tips of the branches. They are followed by cone-like heads containing oblong to ovoid, fleshy-coated seeds. Grow as specimen plants. In frost-prone areas, grow in a cool or temperate greenhouse.

• **HARDINESS** Frost tender, although *M. insignis* may survive short periods near to 0°C (32°F).

• **CULTIVATION** Under glass, grow in loam-based potting compost (JI No.2) in bright filtered or indirect light. In the growing season, water moderately and apply a balanced liquid fertilizer monthly; water sparingly in winter. Outdoors, grow in humus-rich, moist but well-drained soil in partial shade, or in full sun in humid conditions. Pruning group 1; need restrictive pruning under glass, after flowering.

• **PROPAGATION** Sow seed at 5–9°C (41–48°F) as soon as ripe. Root softwood cuttings with bottom heat in spring. Layer or air layer one-year-old stems in spring.

• **PESTS AND DISEASES** Scale insects may be a problem under glass.

M. insignis ⚲ syn. *Magnolia insignis.* Erect then spreading, many-branched tree with grey-downy young shoots. The narrowly oval to inversely lance-shaped, leathery leaves, 10–20cm (4–8in) long, are glossy, rich green above and slightly glaucous beneath. Erect, cup-shaped, cream-tinted, pink to rose-pink or carmine-red flowers, 8cm (3in) across, with 9–12 tepals, are produced from spring to early summer, sometimes followed by elongated, oblong-ovoid purple fruit, 5–10cm (2–4in) long. ↕8–12m (25–40ft), ↔3–5m (10–15ft). C. Himalayas to N. Vietnam and W. China. ❀ (min. 5°C/41°F)

▷**Manuka** see *Leptospermum scoparium*
▷**Manzanita** see *Arbutus, Arctostaphylos, A. manzanita*
Bigberry see *Arctostaphylos glauca*
Dune see *Arctostaphylos pumila*
Eastwood see *Arctostaphylos glandulosa*
Greenleaf see *Arctostaphylos patula*
Parry see *Arctostaphylos manzanita*
Pine-mat see *Arctostaphylos nevadensis*
Stanford see *Arctostaphylos stanfordiana*

▷**Maple** see *Acer*
Amur see *Acer tataricum* subsp. *ginnala*
Ash-leaved see *Acer negundo*
Big-leaf see *Acer macrophyllum*
Canyon see *Acer saccharum* subsp. *grandidentatum*
Cappadocian see *Acer cappadocicum*
Caucasian see *Acer cappadocicum*
Eagle's claw see *Acer platanoides* 'Laciniatum'
Flowering see *Abutilon*
Full-moon see *Acer japonicum*
Greek see *Acer heldreichii* subsp. *trautvetteri*
Hawthorn see *Acer crataegifolium*
Hornbeam see *Acer carpinifolium*
Italian see *Acer opalus*
Japanese see *Acer japonicum, A. palmatum*
Korean see *Acer pseudosieboldianum*
Lobel's see *Acer cappadocicum* subsp. *lobelii*
Montpellier see *Acer monspessulanum*
Mountain see *Acer spicatum*
Nikko see *Acer maximowiczianum*
Norway see *Acer platanoides*
Oregon see *Acer macrophyllum*
Paper-bark see *Acer griseum*
Parlour see *Abutilon*
Père David's see *Acer davidii*
Red see *Acer rubrum*
Red bud see *Acer heldreichii* subsp. *trautvetteri*
Rock see *Acer saccharum*
Scarlet see *Acer rubrum*
Shantung see *Acer truncatum*
Silver see *Acer saccharinum*
Snake-bark see *Acer capillipes, A. davidii, A. rufinerve*
Striped see *Acer pensylvanicum*
Sugar see *Acer saccharum*
Swamp see *Acer rubrum*
Tatarian see *Acer tataricum*
Three-toothed see *Acer buergerianum*
Trident see *Acer buergerianum*
Vine see *Acer circinatum*
▷**Maracuja de refresco** see *Passiflora alata*

MARANTA

MARANTACEAE

Genus of about 20 species of evergreen, rhizomatous perennials from rainforest in tropical Central and South America. They are cultivated for their crowded clumps of blunt-ended, elliptic leaves, spreading by day and raised to an erect position in the evening. Small, tubular, 2-lipped white flowers are produced in pairs in loose racemes. In frost-prone areas, grow as houseplants or in a warm greenhouse, either in hanging baskets or trained up moss poles. In warmer climates, use as ground cover among shrubs in shade.

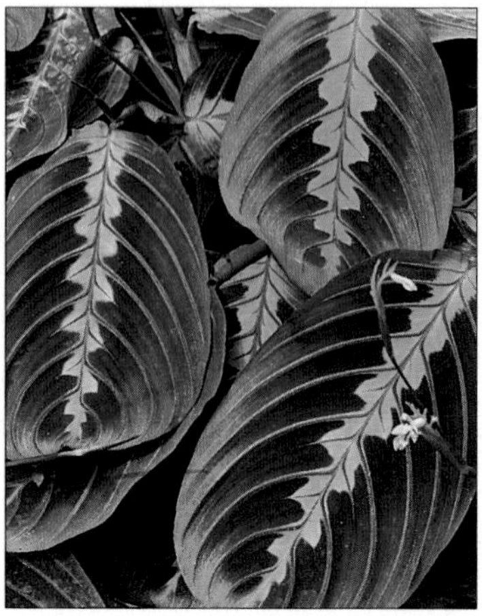

Maranta leuconeura 'Erythroneura'

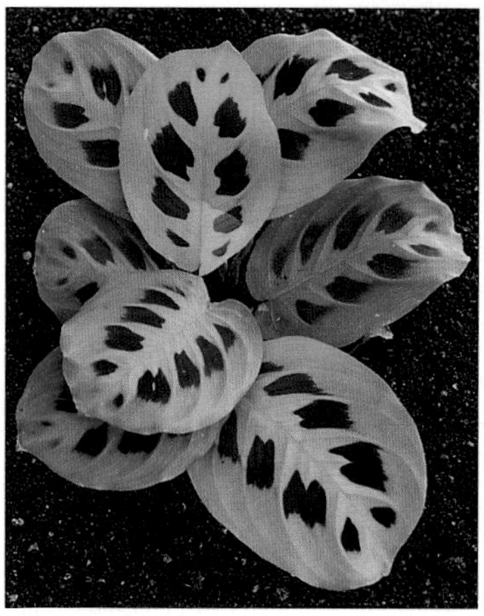

Maranta leuconeura 'Kerchoveana'

• **HARDINESS** Frost tender.

• **CULTIVATION** Under glass, grow in loamless or loam-based potting compost (JI No.2) in bright filtered or bright indirect light, in half-pots or pans to accommodate the shallow root system. Provide high humidity at all times. In the growing season, water moderately and apply a balanced liquid fertilizer monthly; water sparingly in winter. Outdoors, grow in humus-rich, moist but well-drained soil in deep or partial shade.

• **PROPAGATION** Sow seed at 13–18°C (55–64°F) as soon as ripe. Divide in spring. Take basal cuttings, 7–10cm (3–4in) long, and root with bottom heat in spring.

• **PESTS AND DISEASES** Red spider mites may be troublesome under glass.

M. kerchoveana see *M. leuconeura* 'Kerchoveana'.
M. leuconeura (Prayer plant). Very variable, clump-forming perennial with elliptic to obovate, dark green leaves, 12cm (5in) long, with silver lines that fan from the midribs to the margins; the undersides are deep purple or grey-green. ↕↔30cm (12in). Brazil. ❀ (min. 15°C/59°F). **'Erythroneura'** ▣ syn. 'Erythrophylla' (Herringbone plant), bears oblong-obovate to obovate, velvety, olive- and black-green leaves with bright red midribs and veins, and jagged, light yellow-green markings around the midribs; the undersides are deep red. **'Kerchoveana'** ▣♀ syn. *M. kerchoveana* (Rabbit's foot, Rabbit's tracks), bears broadly oblong-elliptic, light grey-green leaves with roughly square brown marks, turning green with age, either side of the pale green midribs; the undersides are pale blue-grey. **'Massangeana'**, syn. var. *massangeana*, produces broadly elliptic, blackish green leaves with silver-grey feathering along the midribs and veins; the undersides are purple.
M. makoyana see *Calathea makoyana.*

▷***Marginatocereus marginatus*** see *Stenocereus marginatus*
▷**Marguerite** see *Leucanthemum vulgare*
Golden see *Anthemis tinctoria*

M

MARGYRICARPUS

ROSACEAE

Genus of one species of dwarf, evergreen shrub from dry, open sites in northern mountains and southern lowlands of the Andes. It produces pinnate leaves and insignificant flowers, and is valued for its long-lasting fruit. Suitable for a scree bed, a rock garden, or an alpine house.
• **HARDINESS** Hardy to -7°C (19°F) in well-drained soil.
• **CULTIVATION** Grow in moderately fertile, acid, moist but well-drained soil in full sun with some midday shade. In an alpine house, grow in lime-free (ericaceous) compost. Shelter from cold, drying winds and protect from excessive winter wet. Pruning group 1.
• **PROPAGATION** Sow seed in containers in a cold frame in autumn or as soon as ripe. Layer or root softwood cuttings in late spring or early summer.
• **PESTS AND DISEASES** Susceptible to aphids and whiteflies under glass.

M. pinnatus, syn. *M. setosus* (Pearl berry). Spreading, densely branched shrub bearing sharply pointed, pinnate leaves, to 2cm (¾in) long, with linear, dark green leaflets with inrolled, silky-hairy margins. In early summer, bears axillary clusters of 1–3 tiny green flowers, followed by spherical, leathery, purple-tinted white fruit, to 7mm (¼in) across. ↕ to 30cm (12in), ↔ to 45cm (18in). Andes. ❄❄
M. setosus see *M. pinnatus*.

▷**Marigold** see *Calendula*
African see *Tagetes* African Group
Afro-French see *Tagetes* Afro-French Group
Corn see *Chrysanthemum segetum*
English see *Calendula*
French see *Tagetes* French Group
Marsh see *Caltha, C. palustris*
Pot see *Calendula*
Signet see *Tagetes* Signet Group
▷**Mariposa, Yellow** see *Calochortus luteus*
▷**Mariposa tulip** see *Calochortus*
▷**Marjoram** see *Origanum*
Compact see *O. vulgare* 'Compactum'
French see *O. onites*
Golden wild see *O. vulgare* 'Aureum'
Hop see *O. dictamnus*
Pot see *O. onites*
Sweet see *O. majorana*
Wild see *O. vulgare*
▷**Marlberry** see *Ardisia japonica*
▷**Marmalade bush** see *Streptosolen jamesonii*
▷***Marniera chrysocardium*** see *Epiphyllum chrysocardium*

MARRUBIUM

Horehound

LABIATAE/LAMIACEAE

Genus of about 40 species of woolly perennials from Mediterranean Europe and temperate Asia, mainly found in sunny, dry, stony wasteland. They have square stems and alternate, opposite pairs of usually ovate or ovate-oblong, often malodorous leaves. Tubular, 2-lipped flowers are borne in axillary whorls. Grow in a large rock garden or a mixed border; they are particularly effective in a Mediterranean garden.
• **HARDINESS** Hardy to -10°C (14°F).
• **CULTIVATION** Grow in poor, well-drained soil in full sun. Provide shelter from cold, drying winds and protection from excessive winter wet.
• **PROPAGATION** Sow seed in containers in a cold frame in late spring, although germination is erratic. Root softwood cuttings in spring.
• **PESTS AND DISEASES** Trouble free.

***M. candidissimum* of gardens** see *M. incanum*.
M. incanum, syn. *M. candidissimum* of gardens. Spreading, silky-hairy perennial with many erect, densely white-hairy shoots bearing oblong-ovate, scalloped or toothed, grey-green leaves, white-felted beneath. In early summer, bears congested whorls of very pale lilac, almost white flowers, to 1.5cm (½in) long, within grey-woolly calyces. ↕ 20–50cm (8–20in), ↔ 60cm (24in). Italy, Sicily, Balkan Peninsula. ❄❄

▷***Marsdenia*** see *Cionura*
M. erecta see *C. erecta*
▷**Marsh mallow** see *Althaea officinalis*
▷**Marsh marigold** see *Caltha, C. palustris*
Giant see *C. palustris* var. *palustris*
▷**Marsh orchid** see *Dactylorhiza*
Robust see *D. elata*

MARSILEA

Pepperwort, Water clover

MARSILEACEAE

Genus of 65 species of rhizomatous, terrestrial, amphibious, and aquatic perennial ferns from warm-temperate Europe, tropical W. Africa, N. Asia, Australia, and E. USA. They grow in large numbers, mainly beside rivers, but also in lakes, where the elongated rhizomes grow upwards, producing a canopy of surface leaves that develop a terrestrial form if the water recedes. Triangular to ovate, 4-lobed leaves each bear a spore case at the base, and close up at night when submerged. Grow at

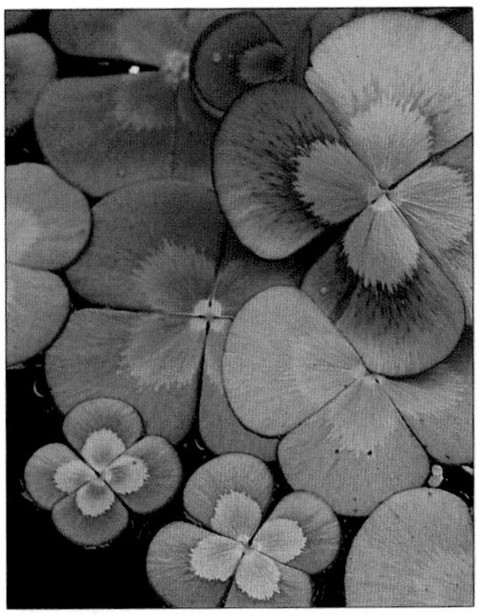

Marsilea quadrifolia

the margins of a pool. In frost-prone areas, grow the tender species in an indoor pool in a warm greenhouse or conservatory, or in a tropical aquarium; *M. quadrifolia* is suitable for a cold-water aquarium.
• **HARDINESS** Fully hardy to frost tender.
• **CULTIVATION** Outdoors, grow in the muddy margins of a pool, or in lattice baskets filled with loamy soil, in full sun, at a depth of 15cm (6in). Under glass, grow in baskets of fertile soil at the pool margins, in slightly acid water at 20–26°C (68–79°F), in full light. In an aquarium, root in containers of fine sand or peat; feed with a proprietary aquatic fertilizer. See also pp.52–53.
• **PROPAGATION** Cut the rhizomes into sections and anchor to the substrate in shallow water.
• **PESTS AND DISEASES** Trouble free.

M. drummondii ■ (Common nardoo). Creeping, terrestrial or aquatic, perennial fern with fan-shaped leaves, 1–4cm (½–1½in) across, with 4 leaflets, and upright stems, to 30cm (12in) long, produced singly from the rhizomes. ↕ to 15cm (6in), ↔ indefinite. Australia. ❁ (min. 18°C/64°F)

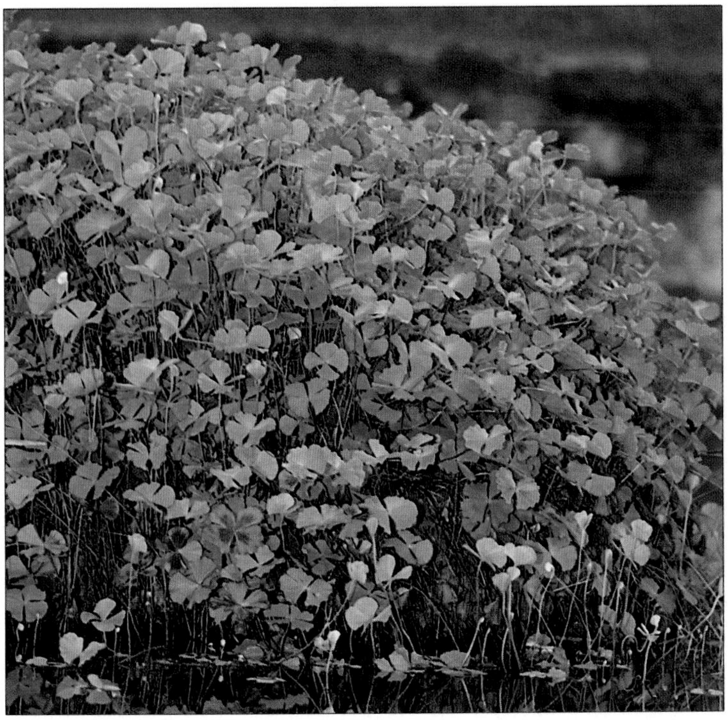

Marsilea drummondii

M. quadrifolia ■ (Water clover). Creeping, aquatic, perennial fern with long rhizomes, and leaves to 3cm (1¼in) across, with 4 soft, triangular, sometimes overlapping leaflets, downy when young; when submerged, they float on the surface, on stalks to 15cm (6in) long. ↕ to 15cm (6in), ↔ indefinite. Europe, N. Asia, E. USA. ❄❄❄

▷***Martynia*** see *Proboscidea*
▷**Marvel of Peru** see *Mirabilis jalapa*
▷***Mascarena lagenicaulis*** see *Hyophorbe lagenicaulis*

MASDEVALLIA

ORCHIDACEAE

Genus of about 340 species of evergreen, epiphytic, terrestrial, or lithophytic orchids, mainly found in cloud forest at 800–4,200m (2,600–13,700ft), from Mexico to Central and South America. They lack pseudobulbs but have short, erect stems, each supporting a single, oblong to ovate or linear to lance-shaped, curved or upright, rigid, fleshy leaf. Flowers are borne singly or in racemes, among or usually above the foliage, mostly from spring to summer. Enlarged, often long-tailed sepals surround the minute petals and lips, giving the flowers a triangular shape.
• **HARDINESS** Frost tender.
• **CULTIVATION** Cool-growing orchids. Grow in small pots of epiphytic orchid compost made with fine-grade bark. Provide full light and ample ventilation. In summer, provide moist shade, water freely, feed at every third watering, and mist once or twice daily. In winter, water more sparingly, but do not allow to dry out. See also p.46.
• **PROPAGATION** Not suitable for division, although cuttings or offshoots may be rooted successfully.
• **PESTS AND DISEASES** Red spider mites, aphids, mealybugs, and yellow bean virus may be troublesome.

***M.* Angel Frost** ■ (*M. strobelii* x *M. veitchiana*). Epiphytic orchid with upright, oblong to narrowly ovate leaves, 15cm (6in) long. Bears racemes of orange flowers, 8cm (3in) long, in spring. ↕ 23cm (9in), ↔ 15cm (6in). ❁ (min. 11°C/52°F; max. 24°C/75°F)
***M.* Angel Heart** (*M. ignea* x *M. infracta*). Epiphytic orchid with upright, linear to lance-shaped leaves, 15cm (6in) long. Red flowers, 8cm (3in) long, are borne singly or in racemes, in spring.

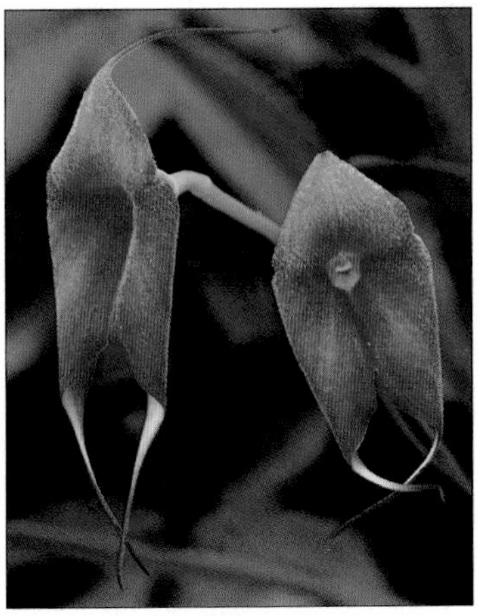

Masdevallia Angel Frost

M

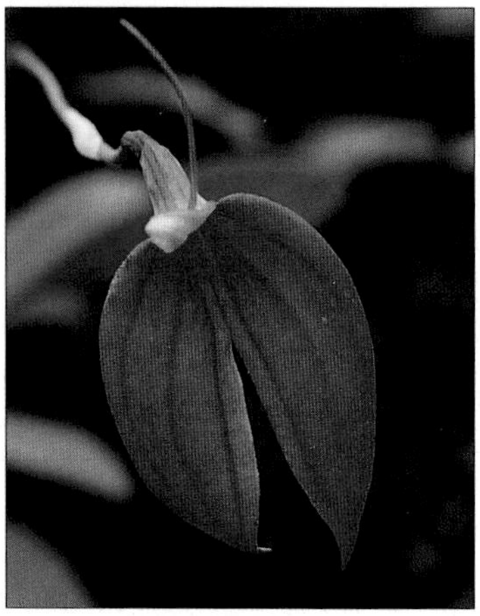

Masdevallia coccinea

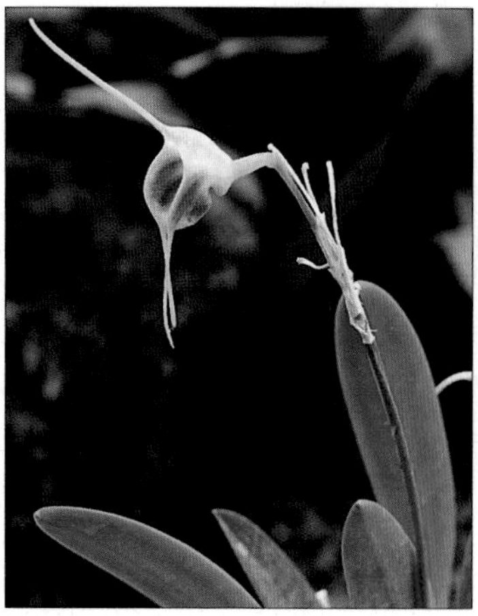

Masdevallia infracta

↕ 23cm (9in), ↔ 15cm (6in). ❀ (min. 11°C/52°F; max. 24°C/75°F)
M. coccinea ▣ Terrestrial orchid with upright, oblong to lance-shaped leaves, 15–20cm (6–8in) long. In summer, bears solitary flowers, 6–10cm (2½–4in) long, with purple-pink, crimson, red-orange, yellow, or white sepals, and white petals. ↕ 40cm (16in), ↔ 30cm (12in). Colombia, Peru. ❀ (min. 11°C/52°F; max. 24°C/75°F)
M. elephanticeps* var. *pachysepala see *M. mooreana.*
***M.* Hugh Rogers** ▣ (*M. amabilis* x *M. yungasensis*). Epiphytic orchid with upright, oblong to lance-shaped leaves, 15cm (6in) long. In spring, bears racemes of orange or red flowers, 8cm (3in) long, with darker veins in the same colour. ↕ 23cm (9in), ↔ 15cm (6in). ❀ (min. 11°C/52°F; max. 24°C/75°F)
M. ignea see *M. militaris.*
M. infracta ▣ Epiphytic orchid with upright, oblong to lance-shaped leaves, 8–14cm (3–5½in). Bears short racemes of cupped, yellow-flushed, dull red to purplish pink flowers, 10–15cm (4–6in) long, with long, pale yellow tails, in summer. ↕↔ 15cm (6in). Peru, Brazil. ❀ (min. 11°C/52°F; max. 24°C/75°F)
***M.* Measuresiana** (*M. amabilis* x *M. tovarensis*). Epiphytic orchid with upright, oblong to lance-shaped leaves, 10–15cm (4–6in) long. Bears racemes of long-tailed white flowers, 8cm (3in) long, flushed pale pink, in succession in winter. ↕ 23cm (9in), ↔ 15cm (6in). ❀ (min. 11°C/52°F; max. 24°C/75°F)

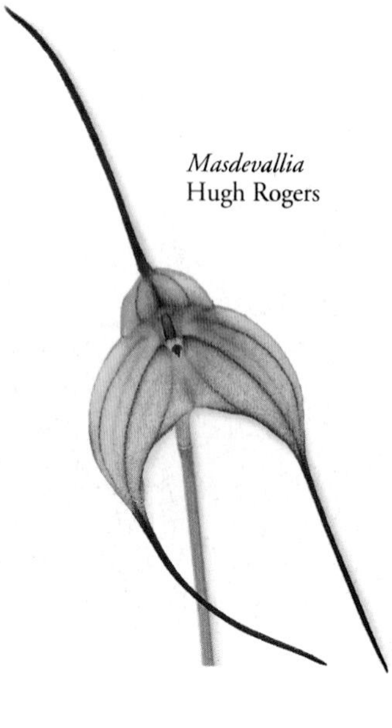

Masdevallia
Hugh Rogers

M. militaris, syn. *M. ignea.* Lithophytic orchid with upright, oblong to lance-shaped leaves, to 15cm (6in) long. Orange-scarlet to red-brown flowers, 4.5cm (1¾in) long, are borne singly in summer. ↕ 30cm (12in), ↔ 23cm (9in). Venezuela, Colombia. ❀ (min. 11°C/52°F; max. 24°C/75°F)
M. mooreana, syn. *M. elephanticeps* var. *pachysepala.* Epiphytic orchid with upright, linear-oblong leaves, to 20cm (8in) long. Greenish yellow flowers, to 9cm (3½in) across, spotted dull purple, with bright yellow tails, are borne singly in summer. ↕↔ 15cm (6in). Venezuela, Colombia. ❀ (min. 11°C/52°F; max. 24°C/75°F)
M. rolfeana. Epiphytic orchid with upright, obovate to elliptic leaves, 11–14cm (4½–5½in) long. Dark reddish purple flowers, 6cm (2½in) long, with short yellow tails, are borne singly from spring to summer. ↕↔ 15cm (6in). Costa Rica. ❀ (min. 11°C/52°F; max. 24°C/75°F)
M. tovarensis ▣ Epiphytic orchid with upright, obovate to lance-shaped leaves, to 15cm (6in) long. Milk-white flowers, 8cm (3in) long, with short tails, are produced in short racemes in winter. ↕↔ 15cm (6in). Venezuela. ❀ (min. 11°C/52°F; max. 24°C/75°F)
M. veitchiana. Lithophytic orchid with upright, oblong to narrowly obovate leaves, 15–25cm (6–10in) long. Bright orange-red, purple-hairy flowers, 10–15cm (4–6in) long, shot with crimson, with short tails, are borne singly from spring to summer. ↕ 30cm (12in), ↔ 23cm (9in). Peru. ❀ (min. 11°C/52°F; max. 24°C/75°F)

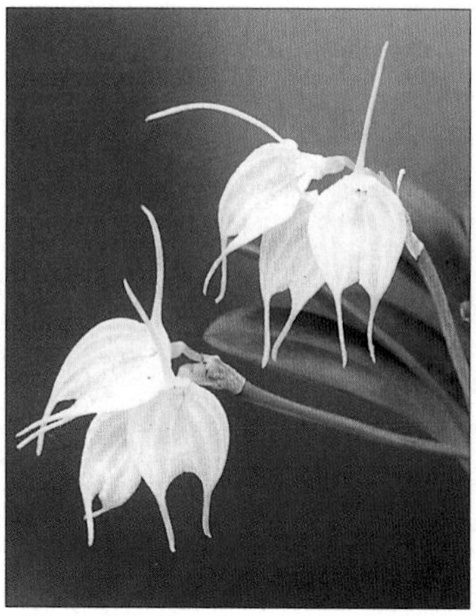

Masdevallia tovarensis

▷ **Mask flower** see *Alonsoa*
▷ **Masterwort** see *Astrantia*
▷ **Mastic, Chinese** see *Pistacia chinensis*
▷ **Mastic tree** see *Pistacia lentiscus*
Peruvian see *Schinus molle*
▷ **Mat rush** see *Lomandra*
Pale see *L. glauca*
Spiny-headed see *L. longifolia*

MATTEUCCIA

DRYOPTERIDACEAE/WOODSIACEAE

Genus of 3 or 4 species of deciduous, terrestrial ferns, commonly occurring in deciduous woodland in Europe, E. Asia, and North America. In spring, the erect or creeping rhizomes produce lance-shaped, pinnate to 2-pinnatifid sterile fronds in regular "shuttlecocks". These are followed in mid- and late summer by distinctive, smaller, more erect, darker, and longer-stalked fertile fronds, which persist over winter. Grow in moist shade in a woodland garden, a damp border, or at the edge of a pond.

- **HARDINESS** Fully hardy.
- **CULTIVATION** Grow in humus-rich, moist but well-drained, neutral to slightly acid soil in partial or light dappled shade.
- **PROPAGATION** Sow spores at 15°C (59°F) as soon as ripe. Divide established clumps in early spring.
- **PESTS AND DISEASES** Trouble free.

M. struthiopteris ▣ 🏆 (Ostrich fern, Shuttlecock fern). Rhizomatous fern with erect "shuttlecocks" of broadly lance-shaped, pinnate, pale green sterile fronds, 1.2m (4ft) or more long, with narrowly lance-shaped, pinnatifid pinnae. Shorter, lance-shaped, dark brown fertile fronds, 30cm (12in) or more long, have linear pinnae with strongly inrolled margins, and appear in late summer. Spreads by horizontal rhizomes, producing separate "shuttlecocks" 10–20cm (4–8in) from the parent plant. ↕ 1.7m (5½ft), ↔ to 1m (3ft). Europe, E. Asia, E. North America. ❄❄❄

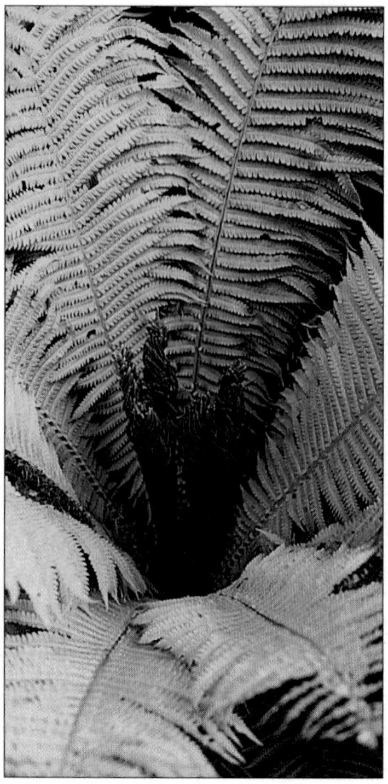

Matteuccia struthiopteris

MATTHIOLA

Gillyflower, Stock

BRASSICACEAE/CRUCIFERAE

Genus of 55 species of bushy, erect annuals and perennials, occasionally subshrubs, from scrub and hilly areas in W. Europe, South Africa, and C. and S.W. Asia. The leaves are simple, usually lance-shaped, sometimes pinnatifid or shallowly lobed, and grey-green to mid-green. *Matthiola* species and cultivars are grown for their usually sweetly scented, pastel pink, purple, or white flowers. The flowers are cross-shaped (double in some cultivar selections), and borne in terminal, spike-like racemes or panicles. Grow in a mixed or annual border.

Cultivars of *M. incana* are useful spring and summer bedding plants, and provide attractive cut flowers. They are often divided by horticulturists into the following 4 groups. Brompton stocks, grown as biennials, bear tall panicles of single or double flowers. East Lothian stocks may be grown as biennials or spring-sown annuals; more compact and smaller-flowered than Brompton Group stocks, they produce spike-like racemes of single or double flowers. Ten Week stocks are grown as annuals, and may be dwarf or tall: dwarf cultivars, suitable for bedding or containers, bear single or double flowers, usually in panicles; tall cultivars bear mostly double flowers in dense, usually unbranched, spike-like racemes. Column stocks are generally grown under glass for cut flowers, and produce long, dense, upright, spike-like racemes of mainly double flowers.

- **HARDINESS** Fully hardy to frost hardy.
- **CULTIVATION** Grow in moderately fertile, moist but well-drained, preferably neutral to slightly alkaline soil in a sheltered position in full sun. Give support to tall cultivars.
- **PROPAGATION** Sow seed of *M. longipetala* subsp. *bicornis in situ* in spring, and repeat for a succession of flowers. For bedding, sow seed of *M. incana* Cinderella Series, Midget Series, and Ten Week Mixed at 10–18°C (50–64°F) in early spring. Sow seed of *M. incana* Legacy Series, Sentinel Series, and Excelsior Mammoth Column Series in a seedbed or in containers in a cold frame in midsummer; overwinter under cloches in cold climates and plant out in spring. Seedlings are prone to "damping off". Sow seed of perennials in containers in a cold frame in spring or summer; overwinter in a cold frame and plant out in the following spring.
- **PESTS AND DISEASES** Susceptible to aphids, flea beetles, cabbage root flies, clubroot, downy mildew, grey mould (*Botrytis*), seed-borne infections of bacterial leaf spot, root and stem rots, and cucumber mosaic virus.

M. bicornis see *M. longipetala* subsp. *bicornis.*
M. fruticulosa. Dwarf, lax or tufted, woody-based, hairy to densely white-woolly perennial with simple or pinnatifid, linear to oblong, grey-green leaves, to 12cm (5in) long. In summer, bears long, upright, spike-like racemes of flowers, 1.5–3cm (½–1¼in) across, varying from yellow to purplish violet. ↕ to 60cm (24in), ↔ to 20cm (8in). C. and S. Europe, Turkey (in Europe

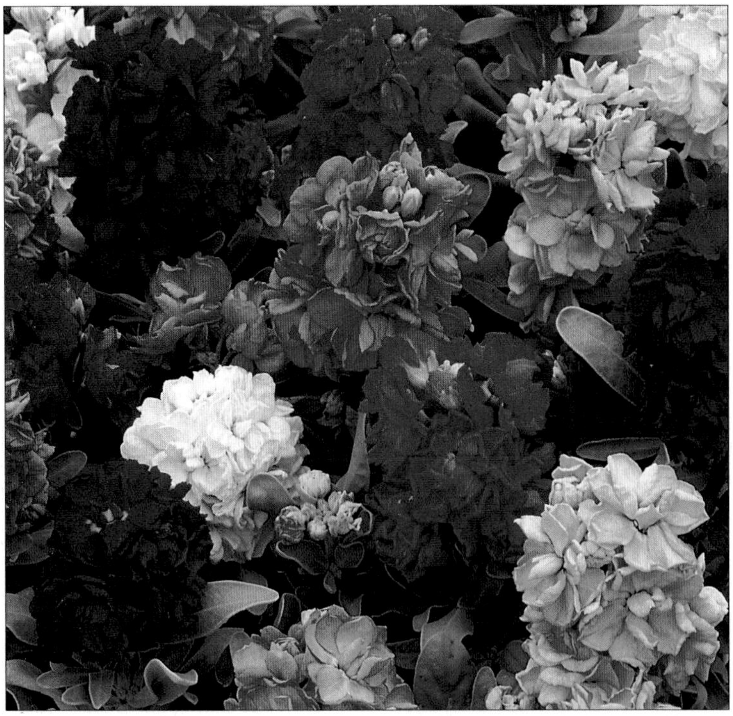
Matthiola incana Cinderella Series

only), Cyprus, Lebanon, N.W. Africa. ✻✻✻. **subsp. *valesiaca*** is tufted, spreads by underground runners, and bears dense racemes of mauve-purple to red-purple flowers; prefers acid soil; ↕25cm (10in), ↔ 30cm (12in); N. and E. Spain, Pyrenees, S. Alps, Balkans.
M. incana (Gillyflower, Stock). Woody-based perennial or subshrub, sometimes short-lived, with entire, occasionally pinnatifid or lobed, inversely lance-shaped to linear-lance-shaped, grey-green to white-hairy leaves, 5–10cm (2–4in) long. Upright racemes of sweet-scented, mauve, purple, violet, pink, or white flowers, to 2.5cm (1in) across, are borne from late spring to summer. ↕to 80cm (32in), ↔ to 40cm (16in). Coastal S. and W. Europe, from Spain to W. Turkey, Cyprus, Arabian Peninsula, Egypt. ✻✻✻ (borderline). The many cultivars of *M. incana*, sometimes resulting from crosses with *M. sinuata*, are grown as annuals or biennials, and produce single or fully double, almost rosette-like, scented flowers in dense, spike-like racemes or panicles, 15–45cm (6–18in) tall, in summer. *M. incana* cultivars are sometimes divided into informal groups (see introduction). **Cinderella Series** ▣ 🏆 cultivars bear double, dark blue-purple, lavender-blue, red, rose-pink, silvery blue, or white flowers in racemes 15cm (6in) long; ↕20–25cm (8–10in), ↔ to 25cm (10in). **Excelsior Mammoth Column Series** cultivars bear mostly double, pink, red, pale blue, or white flowers in spike-like racemes, 30cm (12in) long; ↕ to 75cm (30in), ↔ to 30cm (12in). **Legacy Series** cultivars bear mainly double flowers in scarlet-red, crimson-red, rose-pink, lavender-blue, white, and creamy yellow, in panicles 30cm (12in) long; ↕30–45cm (12–18in) or more, ↔ to 30cm (12in). **Midget Series** cultivars produce double flowers in a range of pastel and deeper tones, including rose-red, red, violet, and white, in spikes 15cm (6in) long; ↕↔ to 25cm (10in). **Sentinel Series** cultivars produce racemes 30cm (12in) long, of double flowers in colours including white, pink, carmine-red, and light to dark blue; ↕ to 75cm (30in), ↔ to 30cm (12in). **Ten Week Mixed** ▣ bears mainly double flowers in shades of crimson, pink, lavender-pink, purple, and white, in racemes 15cm (6in) long; ↕30cm (12in), ↔ to 25cm (10in).

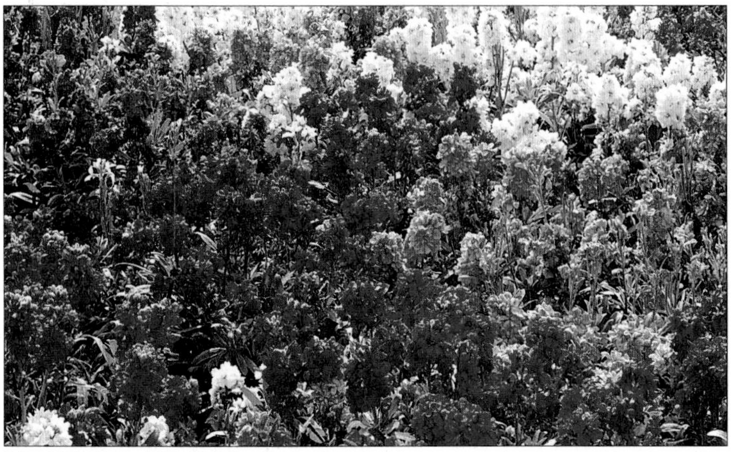
Matthiola incana Ten Week Mixed

M. longipetala* subsp. *bicornis, syn. *M. bicornis* (Night-scented stock). Erect to spreading, single-stemmed to branching annual with narrowly linear, sometimes pinnatifid, grey-green leaves, to 8cm (3in) long. In summer, produces open racemes of pink, mauve, or purple flowers, to 2cm (¾in) across, which are strongly fragrant at night. ↕30–35cm (12–14in), ↔ 23cm (9in). Greece to S.W. Asia. ✻✻✻

▷ ***Matucana aurantiaca*** see *Oreocereus aurantiacus*
▷ ***Matucana haynei*** see *Oreocereus haynei*
▷ ***Matucana intertexta*** see *Oreocereus intertexta*

MAURANDELLA

SCROPHULARIACEAE

Genus of one species of twining, herbaceous, perennial climber from dry desert riverbeds, subject to flooding, in limestone areas of S.W. USA and Mexico. It has hairless, slender, many-branched stems, to 2.2m (7ft) long, and ovate-triangular, lobed leaves. Tubular flowers are borne singly from the leaf axils throughout summer and autumn. In frost-prone climates, grow as a half-hardy annual or in a cool greenhouse. In warmer areas, use to clothe a pergola, arch, or trellis, or grow against a wall.

- **HARDINESS** Half hardy.
- **CULTIVATION** Under glass and when grown as an annual, grow in loam-based potting compost (JI No.2) in full light with shade from hot sun. In growth, water moderately and apply a balanced liquid fertilizer monthly; water sparingly in winter. Outdoors, grow in moderately fertile, moist but well-drained soil in full sun with some midday shade, or in light dappled shade. Shelter from cold, drying winds. Remove dead top growth.
- **PROPAGATION** Sow seed at 13–18°C (55–64°F) in spring. Root softwood cuttings with bottom heat in late spring.
- **PESTS AND DISEASES** Trouble free.

M. antirrhiniflora ▣ syn. *Asarina antirrhiniflora* (Violet twining snapdragon). Wiry-stemmed climber with shallowly lobed, bright to mid-green leaves, 2.5–10cm (1–4in) or more long. Produces snapdragon-like flowers, to 4.5cm (1¾in) long, with white tubes and usually violet or purple, occasionally pink lobes, in summer and autumn. ↕1–2m (3–6ft). S.W. USA, Mexico. ✻

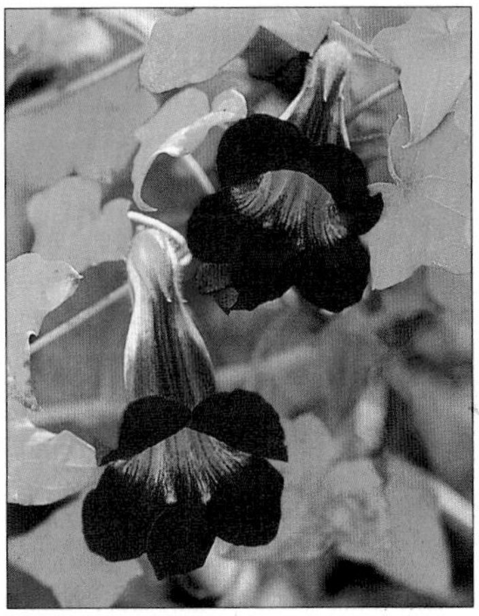
Maurandella antirrhiniflora

MAURANDYA

SCROPHULARIACEAE

Genus of 2 species of twining, woody-based, herbaceous, perennial climbers found in rocky areas and woodland in Mexico and Central America. The leaves are triangular to broadly ovate, sometimes heart-shaped at the bases, and sometimes 5-lobed. Solitary, trumpet-shaped blooms are borne in the leaf axils throughout summer and autumn. Use to clothe a trellis, or grow against a wall. In frost-prone areas, grow in a cool greenhouse or outdoors as annuals.

- **HARDINESS** Half hardy.
- **CULTIVATION** Under glass, grow in loam-based potting compost (JI No.2) in full light with shade from hot sun, or in bright filtered light. In growth, water freely; apply a balanced liquid fertilizer monthly. Keep just moist in winter. Outdoors, grow in moderately fertile, moist but well-drained soil in full sun. Remove dead top growth in autumn.
- **PROPAGATION** Sow seed at 13–18°C (55–64°F) in spring. Root softwood cuttings with bottom heat in late spring.
- **PESTS AND DISEASES** Trouble free.

M. barclayana ▣ syn. *Asarina barclayana.* Medium-sized, erect, free-flowering climber with angular to shallowly lobed, ovate, mid- to light green leaves, 2.5–4.5cm (1–1¾in) long, with heart-shaped bases. From summer to autumn, produces flowers, 4–7cm (1½–3in) long, with white or green-tinted white tubes and white, pink, or deep purple lobes. ↕2–5m (6–15ft). Mexico. ✻
M. erubescens see *Lophospermum erubescens.*
M. purpusii, syn. *Asarina purpusii.* Tuberous climber with triangular-ovate, softly hairy, mid-green leaves, 4–8cm (1½–3in) long, sometimes coarsely toothed. Produces purplish pink flowers, 4cm (1½in) long, throughout summer and autumn. ↕60cm (24in). Mexico. ✻

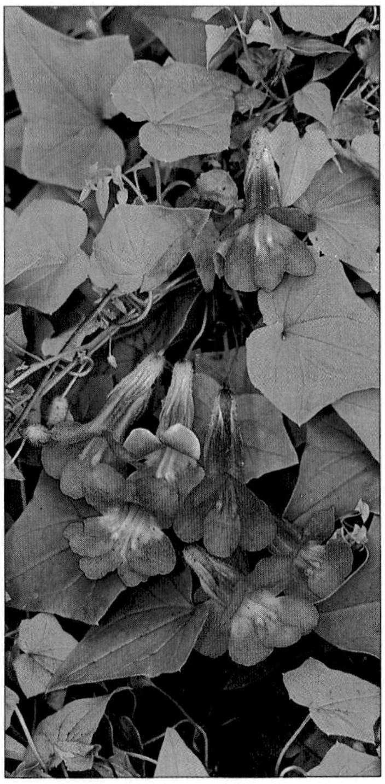
Maurandya barclayana

MAXILLARIA

ORCHIDACEAE

Genus of about 250 species of evergreen, rhizomatous, epiphytic or terrestrial orchids from tropical and subtropical Central and South America, found from sea level to over 3,000m (10,000ft), sometimes in cloud forest. Solitary or clustered, usually laterally compressed, ovoid to spherical, sometimes oblong pseudobulbs produce 1 or 2 thin to leathery, grass-like or broadly oblong, usually mid-green leaves. Flowers are borne singly or in clusters on scapes produced from long or short rhizomes. They range from white to dark red or yellow, and usually appear intermittently throughout summer.

- **HARDINESS** Frost tender.
- **CULTIVATION** Cool- or intermediate-growing orchids. Grow in epiphytic orchid compost in pots or slatted baskets, or epiphytically on slabs of bark. In summer, grow in moist partial shade, water freely, feed at every third watering, and mist once or twice daily. Admit full light in winter; keep moist throughout the year. See also p.46.
- **PROPAGATION** Divide when plants fill the containers and "flow" over the sides.
- **PESTS AND DISEASES** Susceptible to red spider mites, aphids, and mealybugs.

M. cucullata, syn. *M. meleagris*. Very variable, epiphytic orchid with small, ovoid pseudobulbs producing 1, occasionally 2, strap-shaped leaves, to 30cm (12in) long. From summer to autumn, bears deep red, occasionally yellow, pink, or black-maroon flowers with yellow to white lips, heavily spotted and striped dark red, on scapes 12–16cm (5–6in) long. ↕↔ 15cm (6in). Mexico, Guatemala, Panama. ❀ (min. 10°C/50°F; max. 30°C/86°F)

M. grandiflora. Epiphytic orchid with compressed, ovoid pseudobulbs and one strap-shaped, apical leaf, 25–50cm (10–20in) long. White flowers, 6cm (2½in) across, with white or yellow, pink- or purple-margined lips, are borne on scapes 10–30cm (4–12in) long, from spring to early summer. ↕↔ 30cm (12in). N.W. South America. ❀ (min. 10°C/50°F; max. 30°C/86°F)

M. meleagris see *M. cucullata.*

M. picta. Epiphytic orchid with conical pseudobulbs and one narrowly oblong leaf, to 30cm (12in) long. Fragrant, deep yellow to white flowers, spotted purple, dark red, or brown, to 4cm (1½in) across, are borne on scapes 15cm (6in) long, from spring to summer. ↕↔ 23cm (9in). Colombia, Brazil. ❀ (min. 10°C/50°F; max. 30°C/86°F)

M. porphyrostele ▣ Epiphytic orchid with ovoid pseudobulbs and 2 lance-shaped, apical leaves, 20cm (8in) long. From winter to spring, slightly fragrant, light yellow flowers, 2.5cm (1in) across, with purple-striped throats, are borne on scapes 8cm (3in) long. ↕↔ 15cm (6in). Brazil. ❀ (min. 10°C/50°F; max. 30°C/86°F)

M. sanderiana. Epiphytic or terrestrial orchid with compressed, ovoid pseudobulbs, with one narrowly oblong leaf, to 40cm (16in) long. Bears fragrant white flowers, 12cm (5in) across, with heavy red basal spotting, on short, horizontal or erect scapes, to 25cm (10in) long, from summer to early autumn. ↕↔ 45cm (18in). Ecuador, Peru. ❀ (min. 10°C/50°F; max. 30°C/86°F)

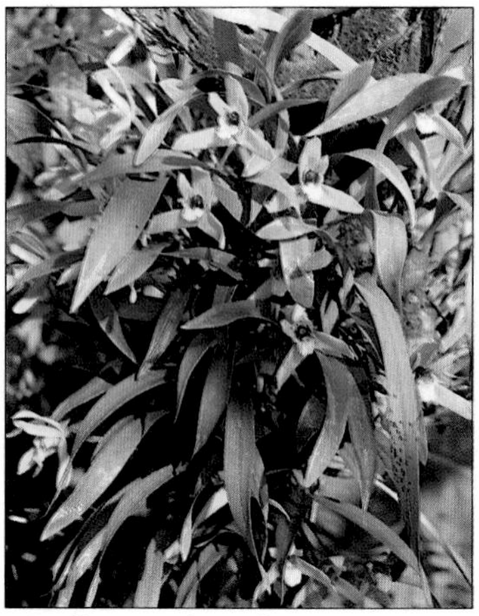

Maxillaria porphyrostele

▷**May** see *Crataegus laevigata, C. monogyna*
▷**May apple** see *Podophyllum peltatum*
Chinese see *P. pleianthum*
▷**Mayflower** see *Epigaea repens*
▷**Maypops** see *Passiflora incarnata*

MAYTENUS

CELASTRACEAE

Genus of about 225 species of evergreen, mainly dioecious trees and shrubs from forest in North and South America and tropical Africa. The variably shaped, alternate leaves are entire or toothed. Tiny, star-shaped to tubular flowers are produced in axillary cymes, racemes, or panicles, or sometimes singly. Grow as specimen trees or in woodland. In frost-prone areas, grow tender species in a cool or temperate greenhouse. Long, hot summers are needed for production of flowers and fruits.

- **HARDINESS** Fully hardy to frost tender.
- **CULTIVATION** Grow in moderately fertile, moist but well-drained soil in full sun with midday shade. Shelter from cold, drying winds. Pruning group 1.
- **PROPAGATION** Sow seed under glass in autumn. Remove suckers, which may appear at some distance from the parent plant, in spring. Root semi-ripe cuttings with bottom heat in summer.
- **PESTS AND DISEASES** Trouble free.

M. boaria ♀–♂ syn. *M. chilensis* (Maiten). Tree or shrub, of variable habit, with pendent or upright branches and narrowly elliptic to lance-shaped, glossy, dark green, finely toothed leaves, to 5cm (2in) long. Bears small clusters of tiny, tubular, pale green flowers, the males with yellow anthers, in mid- and late spring; on the same plant, female flowers produce orange-red capsules, which open to release red seeds. ↕ 20m (70ft), ↔ to 10m (30ft). Chile. ❄❄❄

M. chilensis see *M. boaria.*

MAZUS

SCROPHULARIACEAE

Genus of about 30 species of annuals and creeping, usually mat-forming, prostrate perennials, which root at the nodes. They are found in wet habitats from lowland to mountainous regions of the Himalayas, India, Pakistan, China, Taiwan, Japan, S.E. Asia, and Australasia. The leaves, 1–5cm (½–2in) long, borne in opposite pairs, are mostly linear to spoon-shaped or obovate, toothed, and usually mid-green. Narrowly tubular flowers, with erect upper lips and large, spreading, 3-lobed lower lips, are produced singly or in few-flowered racemes from the leaf axils. *Mazus* species are suitable for ground cover in a sheltered rock garden or in paving crevices, or as pan plants in an alpine house.

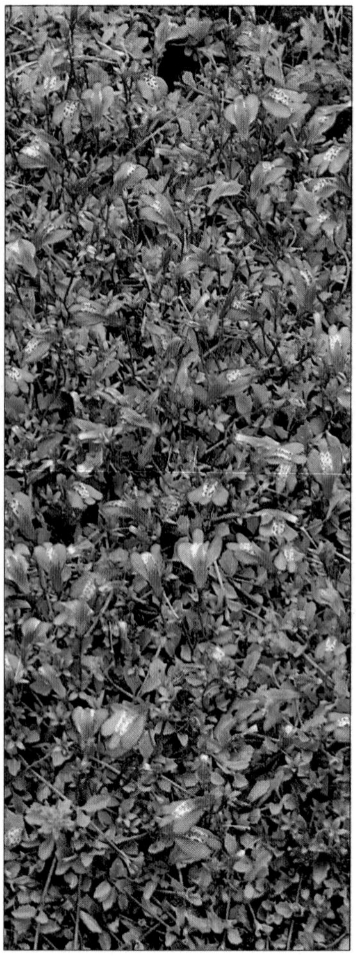

Mazus reptans

- **HARDINESS** Hardy to -10°C (14°F).
- **CULTIVATION** Grow in moderately fertile, moist but well-drained soil in a sheltered site in full sun. In an alpine house, grow in shallow containers of loam-based potting compost (JI No.2).
- **PROPAGATION** Sow seed in containers in a cold frame in spring or autumn. Divide in spring.
- **PESTS AND DISEASES** Slugs and snails may be a problem.

M. reptans ▣ Mat-forming perennial with lance-shaped to elliptic or obovate, coarsely toothed leaves, 1–3cm (½–1¼in) long. From late spring to summer, produces 2- to 5-flowered racemes of purple-blue flowers, 1.5–2cm (½–¾in) long, with yellow- and red-spotted white lower lips. ↕ to 5cm (2in), ↔ to 30cm (12in) or more. Himalayas. ❄❄

▷**Meadow beauty** see *Rhexia, R. virginica*
▷**Meadow rue** see *Thalictrum*
Yellow see *T. flavum*
▷**Meadowsweet** see *Filipendula ulmaria*

MECONOPSIS

PAPAVERACEAE

Genus of about 45 species of annuals, biennials, and deciduous or evergreen, often short-lived or monocarpic perennials. They occur in moist, shady mountainous areas, alpine meadows, woodland, scrub, scree, and rocky slopes in the Himalayas, Burma, and China, with one species from W. Europe. Usually hairy or bristly, they produce basal rosettes of pinnate or simple leaves, which may be entire, toothed, lobed, or pinnatisect. The lower leaves are long-stalked, the upper ones short-stalked or stalkless. The flowering stems, usually one per leaf rosette, are either leafless and unbranched, each bearing a solitary flower, or leafy and branched near the top, bearing flowers singly or in short racemes or panicles, the uppermost opening first. The flowers are generally pendent, saucer- to cup-shaped, poppy-like, and silky, with numerous stamens and usually 4, but sometimes up to 9 petals. The flower-stalks lengthen after flowering as the fruits develop.

Meconopsis species grow best in areas with cool, damp summers. Most are suitable for growing in large groups in a moist, cool woodland garden, but also perform well in a moist peat bed or terrace. *M. cambrica* is suitable for a wildflower garden but will thrive almost anywhere, except in very dry soils.

- **HARDINESS** Fully hardy; young growth may be damaged by late frosts.
- **CULTIVATION** Grow in humus-rich, leafy, moist but well-drained, neutral to slightly acid soil, open enough to prevent stagnation and rot in winter; site in partial shade with shelter from cold, drying winds. Mulch generously, and water in dry spells in summer. Short-lived perennials, e.g. *M. betonicifolia*, are less likely to be monocarpic in moist conditions, and if flowering is prevented until several crowns have been formed.
- **PROPAGATION** Sow seed in containers in a cold frame, preferably as soon as ripe or in spring. Use loamless seed compost, sow thinly, and keep moist; light is needed for germination. Over winter, keep young plants produced from autumn sowings in a cold greenhouse or frame. Seedlings are prone to damping off.

Divide after flowering. Root vegetative buds of *M. chelidoniifolia* when they appear in the upper leaf axils.

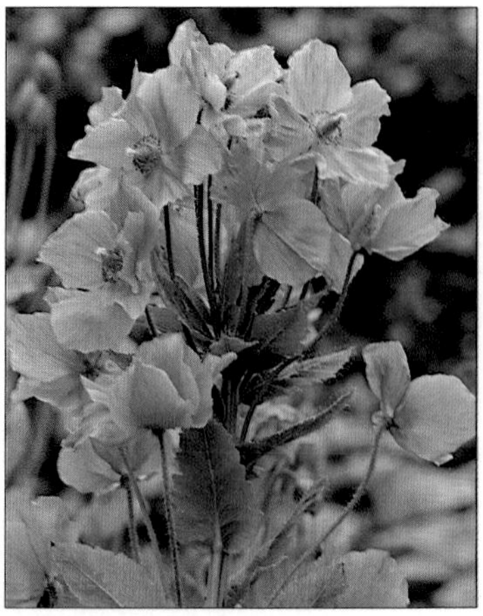

Meconopsis betonicifolia

M

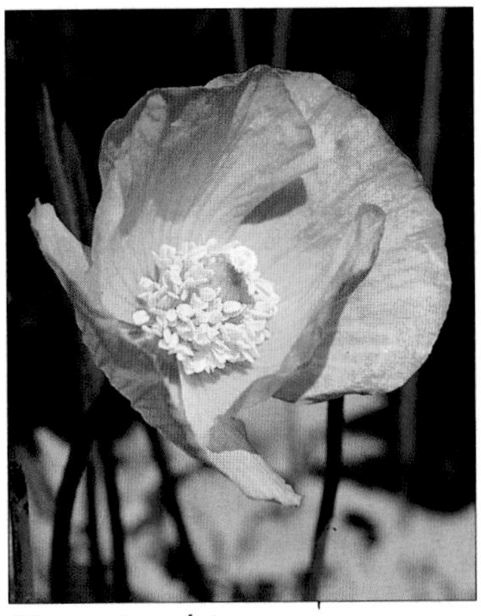

Meconopsis cambrica

• **PESTS AND DISEASES** Susceptible to downy mildew and to damage caused by slugs and snails.

M. betonicifolia ■ 🏆 (Himalayan blue poppy, Tibetan blue poppy). Deciduous perennial, sometimes short-lived, with loose rosettes of oblong to ovate, toothed, light bluish green leaves, 15–30cm (6–12in) long, heart-shaped or truncate at the bases and covered with rust-coloured hairs. In early summer, pendent to horizontal, saucer-shaped, bright blue, sometimes purple-blue or white flowers, 8–10cm (3–4in) across, with yellow stamens, are borne singly on bristly stalks, to 20cm (8in) long, sometimes clustered towards the tops of the stems. ↕1.2m (4ft), occasionally more, ↔ 45cm (18in). Tibet, S.W. China, Burma. ❄❄❄

M. cambrica ■ (Welsh poppy). Tap-rooted, deciduous perennial. Elliptic, pinnatisect to pinnatifid or irregularly lobed, pale to bluish green, hairless to hairy leaves, to 20cm (8in) long, are borne on branched stems and in basal tufts. From mid-spring to mid-autumn, produces solitary, shallowly cup-shaped, lemon-yellow to orange flowers, 5–6cm (2–2½in) across, on slender stalks, to 25cm (10in) long, from the upper leaf axils. ↕45cm (18in) occasionally more, ↔ 25cm (10in). W. Europe. ❄❄❄. **var. *aurantiaca*** has orange flowers. **'Flore Pleno'** has double yellow flowers.

M. chelidoniifolia ■ Deciduous perennial, spreading by offset buds to form clumps of slender, semi-scandent, leafy, branched stems. The hairy, pale green leaves, to 40cm (16in) long at the base and 3–12cm (1¼–5in) on the stems, are pinnatisect with pinnatifid lobes. In mid- and late summer, nodding, saucer-shaped, pale yellow flowers, 2.5–3.5cm (1–1½in) across, are produced from the upper leaf axils, on stalks 4–5cm (1½–2in) long. ↕1m (3ft), ↔ 60cm (24in). China (W. Sichuan). ❄❄❄

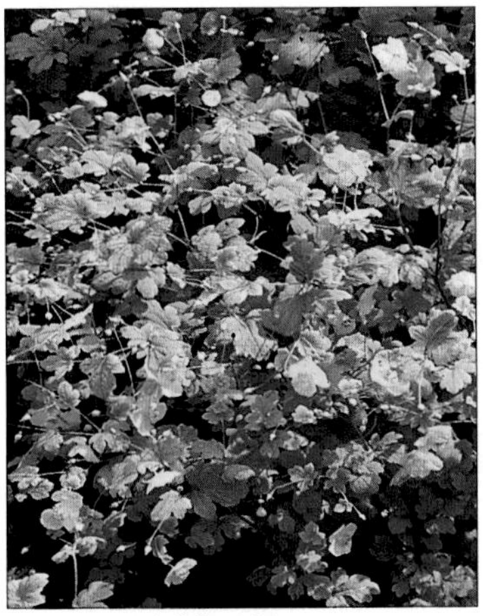

Meconopsis chelidoniifolia

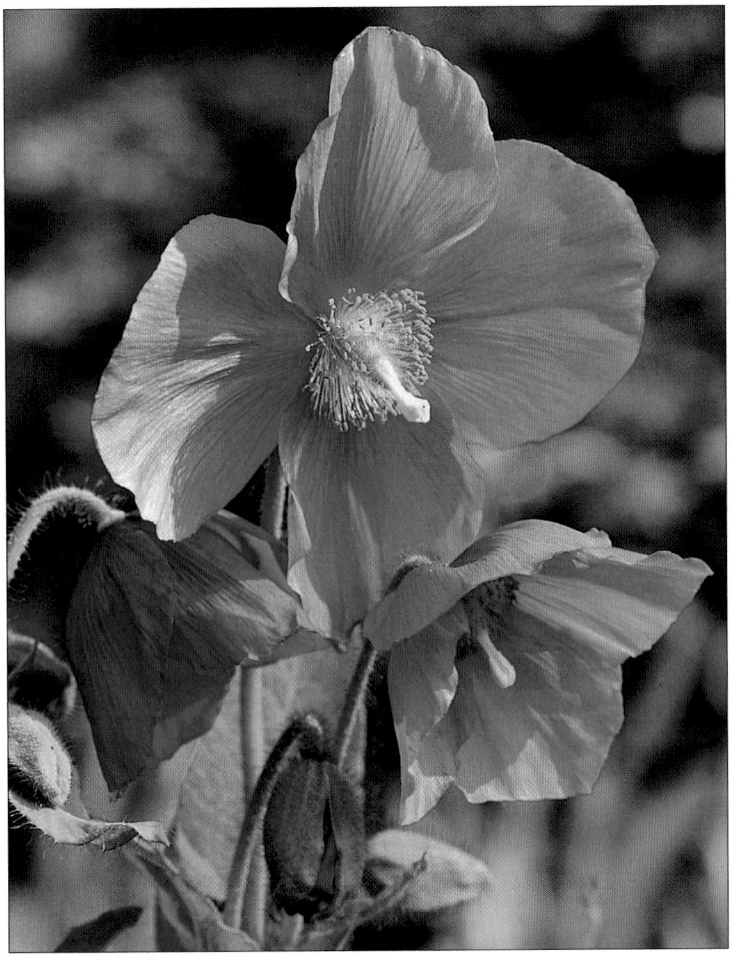

Meconopsis grandis

M. dhwojii. Monocarpic, evergreen perennial forming basal rosettes of pinnatisect leaves, to 30cm (12in) long, with elliptic-oblong or inversely lance-shaped, lobed segments, covered with bristly, black-based yellow hairs. Branched, leafy stems, to 60cm (24in) long, bear numerous nodding, shallowly cup-shaped, pale yellow flowers, 4–5cm (1½–2in) across, with stalks to 15cm (6in) long, in early summer. The upper flowers are solitary; those on the lower branches are in short racemes of up to 5 flowers. ↕to 90cm (36in), ↔ 30cm (12in). E. Nepal. ❄❄❄

M. grandis ■ 🏆 (Himalayan blue poppy). Clump-forming, deciduous perennial with erect, elliptic, irregularly toothed leaves, 15–25cm (6–10in) long, tapered at the bases. The leaves are borne in basal rosettes and on branched stems, the uppermost forming a whorl below the flowers; they are mid-to dark green, with red-brown or rust-coloured hairs. In early summer, nodding, shallowly cup-shaped, rich blue to purplish red flowers, 12–15cm (5–6in) across, each with up to 9 petals and clusters of yellow anthers, are produced singly from the upper leaf axils on stalks to 40cm (16in) long. Monocarpic in dry conditions. ↕1–1.2m (3–4ft), ↔ 60cm (24in). E. Tibet, E. Nepal to India (Sikkim) and Bhutan. ❄❄❄

M. horridula ■ Monocarpic, deciduous perennial with loose rosettes of simple, entire, elliptic to narrowly inversely lance-shaped, wavy-margined, mid- to grey-green leaves, to 25cm (10in) long, covered with yellow to purple spines. In early and midsummer, branched, leafless, spiny stems bear numerous semi-pendent, cup-shaped, pale to deep blue or reddish blue (rarely white) flowers, 5–8cm (2–3in) across, usually in racemes, on stalks to 15cm (6in) long. ↕20–90cm (8–36in), ↔ 45cm (18in). W. Nepal to S.E. Tibet and China (Gansu, Sichuan, Yunnan). ❄❄❄

M. integrifolia ■ Monocarpic, deciduous perennial covered in downy, red-brown or yellow hairs, and forming rosettes of entire, inversely lance-shaped to obovate or linear, pale green, strongly 3-veined leaves, 35cm (14in) long, yellow-hairy when young, almost hairless when mature. From late spring to midsummer, stout, sometimes branched stems bear leaves in a loose whorl below 2–10 erect flowers. The shallowly cup-shaped, 6- to 8-petalled flowers, to 23cm (9in) across, are pale to rich lemon-yellow with dark yellow or orange stamens, and produced on stalks to 45cm (18in) long. ↕to 90cm (36in), ↔ 45–60cm (18–24in). N.E. Tibet, China (Gansu, Sichuan, Yunnan). ❄❄❄

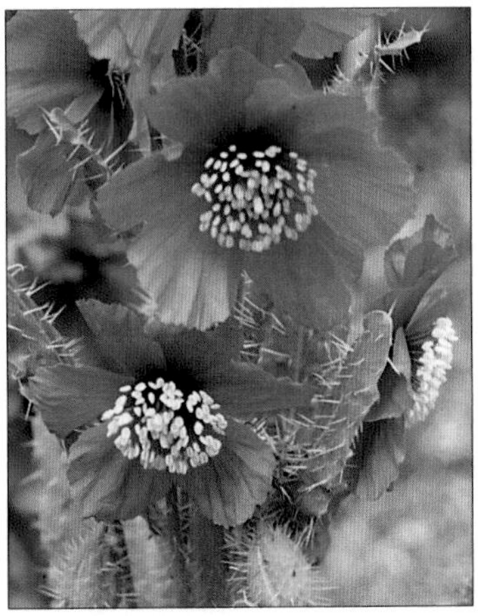

Meconopsis horridula

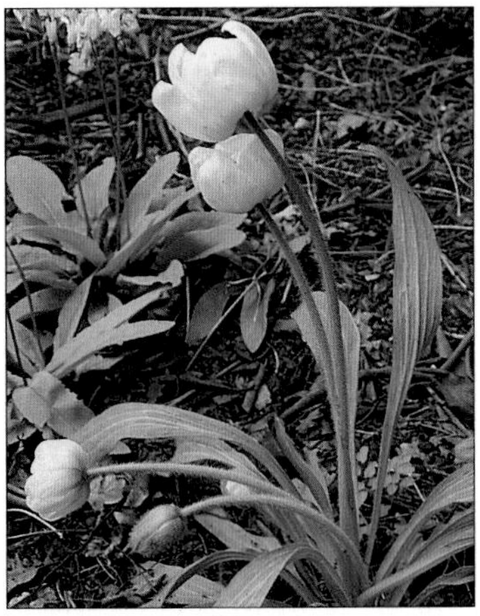

Meconopsis integrifolia

M. napaulensis ■ Monocarpic, evergreen perennial forming rosettes of pinnatisect, yellow-green, red-bristly basal leaves, to 50cm (20in) long, with oblong, lobed segments; the upper stem leaves are pinnatifid or simple. From late spring to midsummer, branching stems bear semi-pendent, bowl-shaped, pink, red, or purple (rarely white) flowers, 6–8cm (2½–3in) across; flowers are borne on stalks to 8cm (3in) long, often in racemes of up to 17 on the lower branches but singly near the stem tops. ↕2.5m (8ft), ↔ 60–90cm (24–36in). C. Nepal to China (W. Sichuan). ❄❄❄

M. paniculata. Monocarpic, evergreen perennial, similar to *M. napaulensis*, with rosettes of pinnatisect or pinnatifid, greyish green leaves, to 60cm (24in) long, covered with rough yellow hairs. From late spring to midsummer, tall, branched stems bear shallowly lobed leaves and many-flowered racemes or panicle-like cymes of pendent, shallowly

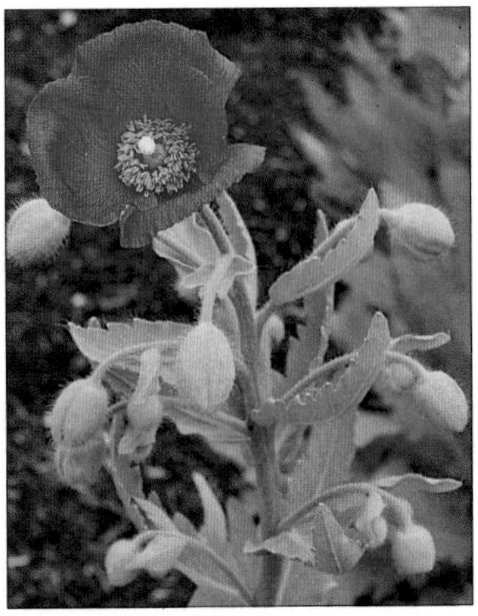

Meconopsis napaulensis

M

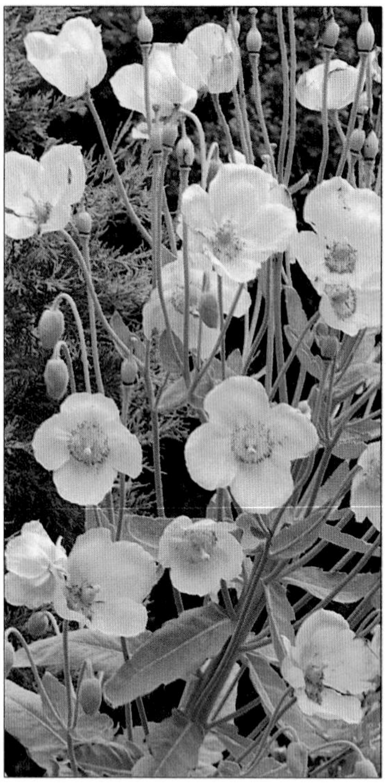

Meconopsis regia

cup-shaped, pale yellow flowers, 5–9cm (2–3½in) across. ↕ to 2m (6ft), ↔ 60cm (24in). E. Nepal to India (Assam). ❄❄❄

M. punicea. Tap-rooted, deciduous perennial with crowded rosettes of entire, inversely lance-shaped, densely grey-hairy, mid-green, basal leaves, 15–35cm (6–14in) long. From mid-summer to early autumn, unbranched scapes, to 45cm (18in) long, up to 6 per rosette, bear solitary, pendent, narrowly funnel-shaped, vivid crimson flowers, to 10cm (4in) long, with 4–6 long, somewhat flared petals. Monocarpic in dry conditions. ↕ to 75cm (30in), ↔ 30cm (12in). N.E. Tibet, W. China. ❄❄❄

M. quintuplinervia ♀ (Harebell poppy). Slowly clump-forming, deciduous perennial forming rosettes of entire, obovate to narrowly inversely lance-shaped or lance-shaped, mid- to dark green, basal leaves, to 25cm (10in) long, with dense golden to rust-coloured bristles. From early to late summer, pendent, cup-shaped, pale lavender-blue or purplish blue (rarely white) flowers, 3.5cm (1½in) across, are produced singly, or rarely in twos or threes, on unbranched, slender scapes, to 35cm (14in) long. ↕ 45cm (18in), ↔ 30cm (12in). N.E. Tibet, W. China (Gansu, N.W. Sichuan to C. Shaanxi). ❄❄❄

M. regia ▣ Monocarpic, evergreen perennial with branched, leafy, hairy stems, and rosettes of simple, narrowly elliptic, finely but deeply toothed, densely silver- or gold-hairy leaves, to 60cm (24in) long. From late spring to midsummer, bears numerous outward-facing, cup-shaped, soft yellow or red flowers, 9–13cm (3½–5in) across, with 4, occasionally 6, overlapping, rounded petals. Upper flowers are solitary; the lower ones are grouped on lateral branches in the upper leaf axils. ↕ to 2m (6ft), ↔ 1m (3ft). C. Nepal. ❄❄❄

M. x sarsonsii (*M. betonicifolia* x *M. integrifolia*). Deciduous, sometimes monocarpic, fertile perennial with ovate, toothed, mid-green leaves, to 15cm (6in) long, covered with rust-coloured hairs and arranged in loose rosettes. In early summer, branched stems produce solitary, pendent to erect, saucer-shaped, pale creamy yellow flowers, 7–10cm (3–4in) across, on stalks to 40cm (16in) long, produced from the axils of loose whorls of stem leaves. ↕ 1.2m (4ft), ↔ 90cm (3ft). Garden origin. ❄❄❄

M. x sheldonii ♀ (*M. betonicifolia* x *M. grandis*). Rosette-forming, hairy perennial with elliptic-oblong to lance-shaped, toothed, dark green basal and stem leaves, 15–30cm (6–12in) long. In late spring and early summer, shallowly cup-shaped, deep rich to pale blue flowers, 6–10cm (2½–4in) across, are borne singly in the upper leaf axils of the branched stems, on stalks 20–50cm (8–20in) long. ↕ 1.2–1.5m (4–5ft), ↔ 60cm (24in). Garden origin. ❄❄❄. **'Branklyn'** has coarsely toothed leaves, and produces vivid blue flowers, to 12cm (5in) across; ↕ to 1.8m (6ft). **'Slieve Donard'** ♀ is vigorous and free-flowering, with entire leaves and brilliant, rich blue flowers with long, pointed petals; ↕ to 1m (3ft).

M. villosa, syn. *Cathcartia villosa.* Rosette-forming, evergreen perennial with ovate to rounded, hairy, light green basal and stem leaves, to 12cm (5in) long, palmately 3- to 5-lobed and sparsely toothed. In late spring and early summer, semi-pendent, saucer-shaped yellow flowers, 4–5cm (1½–2in) across, on stalks to 13cm (5in) long, are borne singly from the upper leaf axils of hairy, branched stems. ↕ 60cm (24in), ↔ 30cm (12in). E. Nepal to Bhutan. ❄❄❄

MEDICAGO
Medick

LEGUMINOSAE/PAPILIONACEAE

Genus of 50–60 species of annuals, perennials, and small shrubs from dry, sunny grassland in Europe and W. and S.W. Asia. They have 3-palmate, light or yellow-green to mid-green or bluish green leaves, sometimes with red spots, and bear short, axillary racemes of pea-like flowers. Grow annuals and perennials in a wild or meadow garden; the shrubby species tolerate coastal conditions, and are best grown in a sunny, open border or against a warm wall. *M. sativa* is grown as a crop plant, as sprouted seeds for salads, and as a "green manure". The flowers attract bees and butterflies.

• **HARDINESS** Fully hardy to frost hardy.
• **CULTIVATION** Grow in poor to moderately fertile, well-drained soil in full sun. Pruning group 1; remove dead wood in spring.
• **PROPAGATION** Sow seed of perennials *in situ* in spring or autumn. Sow seed of shrubs in containers in a cold frame in spring or autumn. Root greenwood cuttings with bottom heat in early summer.
• **PESTS AND DISEASES** Trouble free.

M. arborea (Moon trefoil). Dense, bushy, evergreen shrub with dark green leaves with obovate leaflets, 0.6–2cm (¼–¾in) long, silky-hairy when young. From late spring to early autumn, bears dense racemes of 4–8 yellow flowers, 1.5–2cm (½–¾in) long, followed by flattened, spiralled, green, later brown seed pods. ↕↔ 2m (6ft). Canary Islands, S. Europe and Mediterranean to S.W. Asia. ❄❄ (borderline)

M. sativa (Alfalfa, Lucerne). Erect or spreading, hairy, slender-stemmed perennial bearing bluish green leaves with obovate to linear leaflets, to 3cm (1¼in) long. In summer and early autumn, produces long-stalked racemes of pale mauve to violet flowers, to 1cm (½in) long, followed by small, spiralled or sickle-shaped, deep brown seed pods. ↕ to 80cm (32in), ↔ 30–80cm (12–32in). Europe, W. Asia. ❄❄❄

▷**Medick** see *Medicago*

MEDINILLA

MELASTOMATACEAE

Genus of about 150 species of evergreen shrubs and scandent climbers, some epiphytic, from rainforest in tropical Africa, S.E. Asia, and the Pacific. They have simple, entire, boldly veined leaves, borne in whorls or opposite pairs. Small, star- to bowl-shaped, 4- to 6-petalled flowers, often with large, coloured bracts, are borne in pendent or upright panicles or cymes. Where temperatures fall below 15°C (59°F), grow in a warm greenhouse. In moist, tropical areas, grow climbing species over an arch or pergola; the shrubs are suitable for specimen planting or a shrub border. Long, hot summers are required for production of flowers and fruits.

• **HARDINESS** Frost tender.
• **CULTIVATION** Under glass, grow in loam-based potting compost (JI No.2) in bright filtered light, or full light with shade from hot sun; provide high humidity. In growth, water moderately and apply a balanced liquid fertilizer monthly; water sparingly in winter. Outdoors, grow in moderately fertile, moist but well-drained soil in dappled shade, or full sun with some midday shade. Pruning group 11 for climbers, after flowering; group 8 for shrubs.
• **PROPAGATION** Sow seed at 19–24°C (66–75°F) in spring. Root softwood cuttings in spring or semi-ripe cuttings with bottom heat in summer. Air layer in spring.
• **PESTS AND DISEASES** Scale insects may be troublesome under glass.

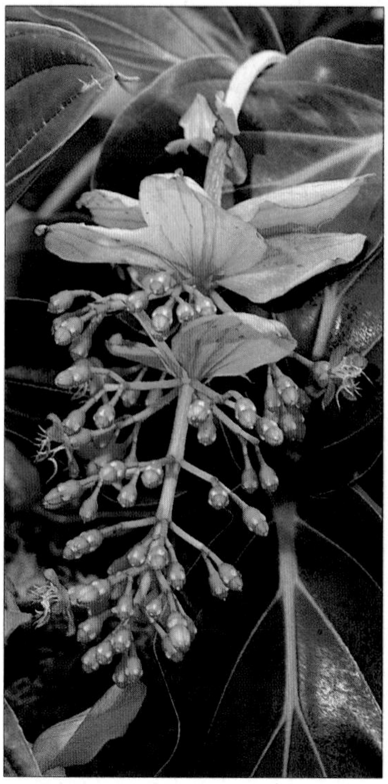

Medinilla magnifica

M. magnifica ▣ Erect, sparsely branched, epiphytic shrub with robust, ribbed to strongly winged stems bearing broadly ovate to obovate, leathery, lustrous, deep green leaves, 20–30cm (8–12in) long, with prominent, pale green veins. From spring to summer, yellow-stamened, pink to coral-red flowers, to 2.5cm (1in) across, are borne in dense, pendent panicles, 25–40cm (10–16in) long, with several pairs of large, cupped pink basal bracts. ↕ 1–2m (3–6ft), ↔ 0.6–1.5m (2–5ft). Philippines. ⚘ (min. 15°C/59°F)

▷**Mediterranean heath** see *Erica erigena*
▷**Medlar** see *Mespilus germanica*
▷**Medusa's head** see *Euphorbia caput-medusae*

MEEHANIA

LABIATAE/LAMIACEAE

Genus of 6 species of stoloniferous, clump-forming perennials found in moist, deciduous woodland in Asia and North America. Square stems bear opposite pairs of ovate to heart-shaped, finely hairy leaves. Tubular, 2-lipped, violet or blue flowers are produced from the leaf axils from late spring to summer. Grow in a shady border or as ground cover in a woodland garden.

• **HARDINESS** Fully hardy.
• **CULTIVATION** Grow in humus-rich, moist but well-drained soil in full to light dappled shade.
• **PROPAGATION** Sow seed in containers in a cold frame in spring. Separate stolons in early spring or autumn. Root stem-tip cuttings in spring.
• **PESTS AND DISEASES** Susceptible to damage by slugs.

M. urticifolia ▣ Stoloniferous, clump-forming perennial, spreading widely, with broadly ovate, heart-shaped, wrinkled, softly hairy leaves, 3–6cm (1¼–2½in) long, with scalloped margins. One-sided spikes of 3–12 deep violet flowers, 4–5cm (1½–2in) long, sometimes with white lines and the lower lips spotted dark purple, are produced in late spring and early summer. ↕ 30–45cm (12–18in), ↔ to 2.5m (8ft). Japan. ❄❄❄

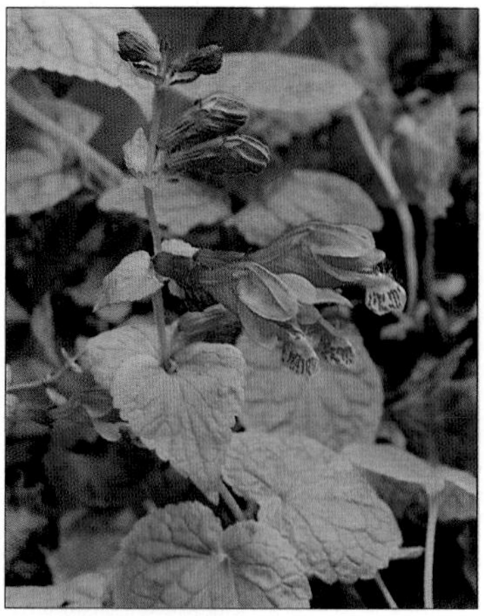

Meehania urticifolia

M

MEGACODON

GENTIANACEAE

Genus of one species of clump-forming perennial found in damp pastures and streamsides from C. Nepal to S.W. China. It has basal rosettes of elliptic to broadly elliptic leaves, and bears smaller leaves on stout, erect stems. Broadly bell-shaped flowers are produced in summer. Grow in a woodland or bog garden, or plant near pools and streams.

- **HARDINESS** Fully hardy.
- **CULTIVATION** Grow in humus-rich, moist but well-drained soil in partial or light dappled shade. Provide a dry winter mulch and shelter from cold, drying winds.
- **PROPAGATION** Sow seed in containers in a cold frame as soon as ripe. Basal shoots can be rooted in spring, although seldom successfully. Like the large herbaceous gentians (*Gentiana*), *M. stylophorus* does not transplant readily.
- **PESTS AND DISEASES** Susceptible to damage by slugs.

M. stylophorus, syn. *Gentiana stylophora*. Upright, clump-forming perennial with basal rosettes of elliptic to broadly elliptic, glossy, dark green leaves, 30cm (12in) long, and pairs of smaller leaves, 10–15cm (4–6in) long, joined at their bases around the stems. In mid- and late summer, pale to mid-yellow flowers, 6–8cm (2½–3in) long, with green lines inside, are borne in pairs from the upper leaf axils. ↕ to 2m (6ft), ↔ 60cm (24in). C. Nepal to China (Yunnan). ✻✻✻

▷ ***Megalonium*** see *Aeonium*
M. nobile see *A. nobile*
▷ ***Megasea*** see *Bergenia*

MEGASKEPASMA

ACANTHACEAE

Genus of one species of evergreen shrub from tropical woodland in Venezuela. It has opposite, simple, entire leaves, and is grown for its colourful, terminal, spike-like cymes of 2-lipped, tubular flowers surrounded by crimson bracts. Where temperatures fall below 15°C (59°F), grow in a temperate or warm greenhouse; in warmer areas, grow in a courtyard garden or a shrub border.

- **HARDINESS** Frost tender.
- **CULTIVATION** Under glass, grow in loam-based potting compost (JI No.2 or No.3) in full light, with high humidity. In the growing season, water freely and apply a balanced liquid fertilizer monthly; water sparingly in winter. Outdoors, grow in moderately fertile, moist, well-drained soil in full sun. Pruning group 8; withstands restrictive pruning and renovation well.
- **PROPAGATION** Sow seed at 18–21°C (64–70°F) in spring. Root greenwood cuttings in early summer, or semi-ripe cuttings with bottom heat in late summer.
- **PESTS AND DISEASES** Red spider mites, whiteflies, and mealybugs may be troublesome under glass.

M. erythrochlamys ▣ (Brazilian red cloak, Red justicia). Erect, robust-stemmed shrub, sparsely branched unless regularly pruned, with ovate to broadly elliptic or lance-shaped, boldly veined, mid-green leaves, 12–30cm (5–12in) long. From early autumn to winter, terminal, columnar to narrowly pyramidal, spike-like cymes, 20–30cm (8–12in) long, of tubular, 2-lipped, white or pink flowers, to 8cm (3in) long, are produced from the axils of broadly ovate crimson bracts, to 4cm (1½in) long. ↕ 2–3m (3–10ft), ↔ 1–2m (3–6ft). Venezuela. ❄ (min. 15°C/59°F)

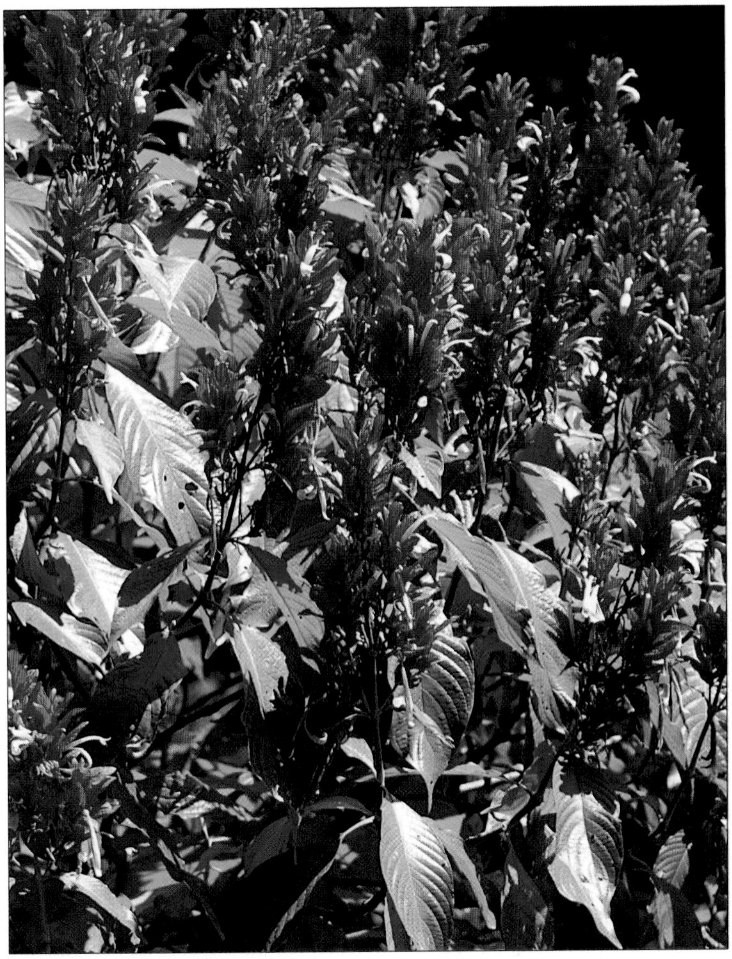

Megaskepasma erythrochlamys

MELALEUCA

Paperbark

MYRTACEAE

Genus of at least 150 species of evergreen shrubs and trees, allied to *Callistemon*, found in habitats ranging from rainforest to semi-arid areas in tropical to cool-temperate zones, mainly in Australia but also in New Caledonia, New Guinea, and Malaysia. Many species have several layers of paper-thin, corky bark, which is shed continuously. The small, flat or cylindrical, often leathery leaves are mainly alternate, or sometimes opposite or whorled. Small flowers, each with 5 short petals and numerous conspicuous, coloured stamens, arranged in 5 fused bundles, are borne in dense, axillary spikes, resembling those of bottlebrushes. In frost-prone areas, grow in a cool or temperate greenhouse. Elsewhere, grow in a shrub border or as specimen trees. Long, hot summers are required for production of flowers and fruits.

- **HARDINESS** Half hardy to frost tender.
- **CULTIVATION** Under glass, grow in loam-based potting compost (JI No.2), with added leaf mould, in full light with shade from hot sun. In the growing season, water moderately and apply a balanced liquid fertilizer monthly; water sparingly in winter. Outdoors, grow in moderately fertile, well-drained soil in full sun with some midday shade. Shelter from cold, drying winds. Pruning group 1; plants under glass need restrictive pruning after flowering.
- **PROPAGATION** Sow seed at 13–24°C (55–75°F) in spring. Root semi-ripe cuttings with bottom heat in summer.
- **PESTS AND DISEASES** Prone to scale insects and red spider mites under glass.

M. elliptica ▣ (Granite bottlebrush). Many-branched shrub, erect at first, then spreading or rounded, with furrowed, peeling bark. The opposite, broadly elliptic to elliptic-oblong leaves, 0.5–1.5cm (¼–¾in) long, are mid- to deep green above and paler beneath. From spring to early summer, small, bright pink to crimson flowers, with stamens of the same colour, are borne in abundant short, dense spikes, to 4cm (1½in) or more long. ↕↔ 1–3m (3–10ft). Australia (Western Australia). ❄ (min. 5–7°C/41–45°F)

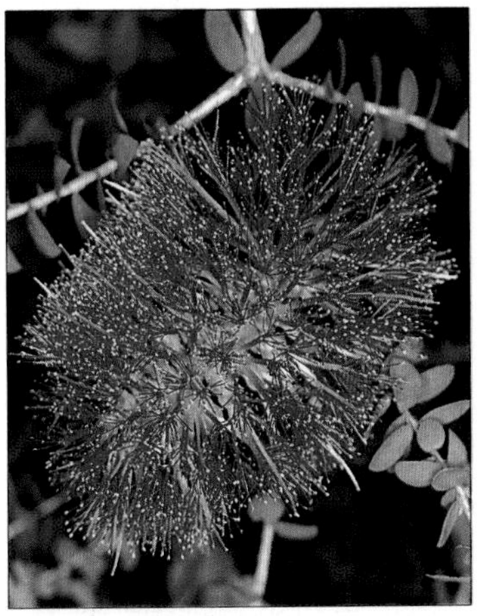

Melaleuca elliptica

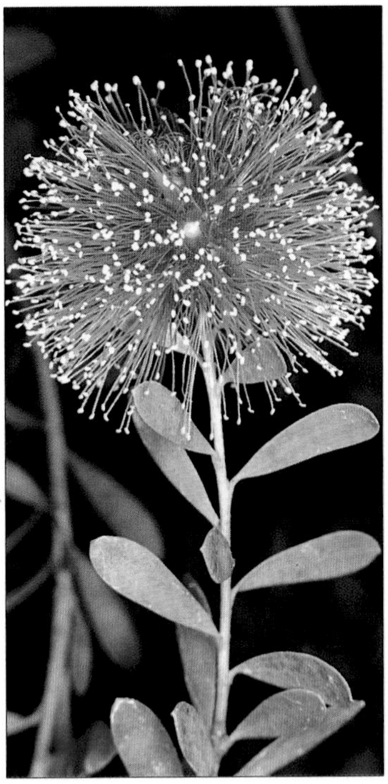

Melaleuca nesophila

M. hypericifolia ♀ Many-branched, large shrub or small tree, erect at first, then spreading, with very firm, papery bark and opposite, sometimes arching, narrowly oblong-elliptic or obovate leaves, 1–4cm (½–1½in) long. From spring to summer, small red flowers, with crimson stamens, are produced in loose, feathery, lateral spikes, 5–8cm (2–3in) long. ↕ 2–5m (6–15ft), ↔ 1.5–2.5m (5–8ft). Australia (New South Wales). ❄ (min. 5–7°C/41–45°F)

M. nesophila ▣ ♀ syn. *M. nesophylla* (Western tea myrtle). Erect to spreading, large shrub or small tree with freely branching stems and spongy, peeling bark. Alternate, mid- to deep green leaves are narrowly obovate, 2–3cm (¾–1¼in) long, with 1–3 faint veins. From spring to summer, bears lavender-pink to rose-pink flowers in dense, spherical spikes, to 2.5cm (1in) or more across. ↕ 3–7m (10–22ft), ↔ 2–4m (6–12ft). Australia (Western Australia). ❄ (min. 5–7°C/41–45°F)

M. nesophylla see *M. nesophila.*

▷ ***Melandrium elisabethae*** see *Silene elisabethae*

MELASPHAERULA

IRIDACEAE

Genus of one species of spring-flowering, cormous perennial from shaded woodland in South Africa. It has narrow, grass-like leaves, and produces spikes of star-shaped flowers. In frost-prone areas, grow in a cool greenhouse or in a bulb frame. In warmer climates, grow at the base of a warm, sunny wall.

M

• **HARDINESS** Half hardy.
• **CULTIVATION** Plant 10–15cm (4–6in) deep. Under glass, grow in loam-based potting compost (JI No.2), with additional sharp sand, in full light. Water sparingly until the flower spikes appear, then water moderately; apply a balanced liquid fertilizer every 6–8 weeks in the growing season; keep just moist in winter. Outdoors, grow in moderately fertile, well-drained soil in full sun. In mild areas, plant in autumn, providing a dry winter mulch; in areas with prolonged frosts, plant in early spring and lift in autumn, after the leaves die down. Protect from excessive winter wet.
• **PROPAGATION** Sow seed at 6–12°C (43–54°F) in autumn. Remove offsets when dormant in autumn.
• **PESTS AND DISEASES** Trouble free.

M. graminea see *M. ramosa.*
M. ramosa, syn. *M. graminea.* Cormous perennial with spreading, branched stems bearing erect, grass-like leaves, 5–25cm (2–10in) long. Spikes of up to 7 star-shaped, creamy white or yellowish flowers, 2–3cm (¾–1¼in) across, often veined purple, are produced in spring. ↕20–50cm (8–20in), ↔ 8cm (3in). South Africa (S. Western Cape). ✲

MELASTOMA

MELASTOMATACEAE

Genus of up to 70 species of evergreen shrubs, small trees, and a few herbaceous perennials from moist woodland, often in hilly areas, in India, S.E. Asia, and adjacent Pacific islands. The opposite leaves are lance-shaped to oblong or elliptic, mostly dark green, and often leathery. Usually 5-petalled, open bowl- to saucer-shaped, purple, red, pink, or white flowers are produced in terminal cymes of 3–7 or, rarely, are borne singly; the flowers are followed by fleshy berries. Where temperatures fall below 13–15°C (55–59°F), grow in a warm greenhouse. In warmer regions, grow as free-standing specimen plants or among other shrubs. Long, hot summers are required for the production of flowers and fruits.
• **HARDINESS** Frost tender.
• **CULTIVATION** Under glass, grow in loam-based potting compost (JI No.2) in full light with shade from hot sun. Provide moderate humidity. In the growing season, water moderately and apply a balanced liquid fertilizer monthly; water sparingly in winter. Outdoors, grow in moderately fertile, moist but well-drained soil in full sun with some midday shade. Shelter from cold, drying winds. Pruning group 1 or 8; need restrictive pruning under glass.
• **PROPAGATION** Sow seed at 6–12°C (43–54°F) in spring. Root semi-ripe cuttings with bottom heat in summer.
• **PESTS AND DISEASES** Scale insects and red spider mites may be troublesome under glass.

M. malabathricum (Indian rhododendron). Many-branched, spreading shrub with densely scaly-hairy stems and ovate to broadly lance-shaped, coarsely hairy, dark green leaves, 7–10cm (3–4in) long, with prominent veins. Produces shallowly bowl-shaped purple flowers, 3cm (1¼in) across, singly or in cymes of 2–5, from spring to summer, sometimes followed by spherical, red-pulped berries, 8mm (⅜in) across. ↕2–3m (6–10ft), ↔ 1.5–2.5m (5–8ft). India, S.E. Asia. ❀ (min. 13°C/55°F)

MELIA

MELIACEAE

Genus of 3–5 species of deciduous or semi-evergreen trees and shrubs from India to China, S.E. Asia, and N. Australia. They have alternate, pinnate or 2-pinnate leaves, and bear small, star-shaped flowers in large, axillary panicles. Each flower has 5 or 6 spreading petals and 10–12 stamens, the filaments of which are fused into a tube with the anthers arranged around the rim. The attractive, bead-like, spherical, single-seeded berries are poisonous. In frost-prone areas, grow in a temperate greenhouse mainly for their foliage, although plants in large containers may flower when 2–3m (6–10ft) tall. In warmer areas, grow as specimen or shade trees.
• **HARDINESS** Frost tender.
• **CULTIVATION** Under glass, grow in loam-based potting compost (JI No.2) in full light. In the growing season, water freely and apply a balanced liquid fertilizer monthly; water sparingly in winter. Outdoors, grow in moderately fertile, well-drained soil in full sun. Provide shelter from cold, drying winds. Pruning group 1; plants under glass may need restrictive pruning.
• **PROPAGATION** Sow seed at 13–18°C (55–64°F) in spring. Root softwood cuttings with bottom heat in summer.
• **PESTS AND DISEASES** Red spider mites may be a problem under glass.

M. azedarach ▣ ♀ (Bead-tree, Persian lilac, Pride of India). Fast-growing, many-branched, spreading, round-headed, deciduous tree with fissured grey bark. Pinnate or 2-pinnate leaves, 30–60cm (12–24in) long, have many ovate to elliptic, sharply toothed, sometimes lobed, mid- to bright green leaflets. Produces a profusion of star-shaped, fragrant lilac flowers, 2cm (¾in) across, in arching to pendent panicles, 10–20cm (4–8in) long, from spring to early summer; they are followed by spherical to broadly ovoid yellow fruit, 1cm (½in) long. Seeds are used as beads in Asia. ↕10–15m (30–50ft), ↔ 5–8m (15–25ft). N. India, China. ❀ (min. 7°C/45°F)

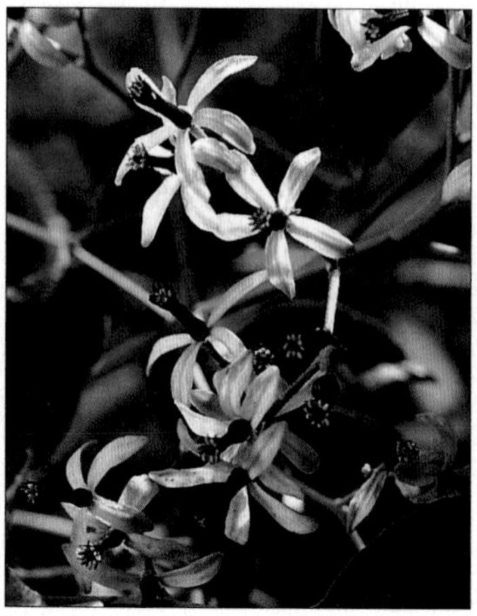
Melia azedarach

MELIANTHUS

MELIANTHACEAE

Genus of 6 species of evergreen shrubs from grassland in hilly areas of southern Africa. The alternate, pinnate, light green, grey-green, or blue-green leaves have prominent stipules. Small flowers, producing profuse quantities of nectar, are borne in erect, terminal and axillary racemes; each has 5 irregular sepals and petals, the upper ones often forming a hood or tube, and the lower ones making a short spur. Grow in a border or as specimen plants; they are particularly suited to a coastal garden. In frost-prone areas, grow tender species as foliage plants in a cold greenhouse, and stand or plant outside in summer. Alternatively, treat them as herbaceous perennials; where temperatures do not fall much below -5°C (23°F), they will usually re-sprout annually from the base.
• **HARDINESS** Frost hardy to frost tender; *M. major* may survive temperatures just below 0°C (32°F), if the wood has been well ripened in summer.
• **CULTIVATION** Under glass, grow in loam-based potting compost (JI No.2) in full light. Provide low humidity. In growth, water freely and apply a balanced liquid fertilizer monthly; water sparingly in winter. Outdoors, grow in moderately fertile, moist but well-drained soil in full sun. Provide a dry winter mulch and protect from excessive winter wet. Shelter from cold, drying winds. Pruning group 7 or 8.
• **PROPAGATION** Sow seed at 13–18°C (55–64°F) in spring. Root basal or softwood cuttings in late spring or early summer. Remove any rooted suckers in spring.
• **PESTS AND DISEASES** Susceptible to red spider mites and whiteflies under glass.

M. major ▣ (Honey bush). Tall, erect to spreading shrub with robust, hollow stems, most of them near ground level and branching sparingly. Spreading, pinnate leaves, 30–50cm (12–20in) long, have 9–17 closely set, ovate, sharply and boldly toothed, grey-green to bright blue-grey leaflets. From late spring to midsummer, produces spike-like racemes, 30–80cm (12–32in) long, of brownish crimson to deep brick-red flowers, 2.5cm (1in) long. ↕2–3m (6–10ft), ↔ 1–3m (3–10ft). South Africa (Northern Cape, Western Cape, Eastern Cape). ✲

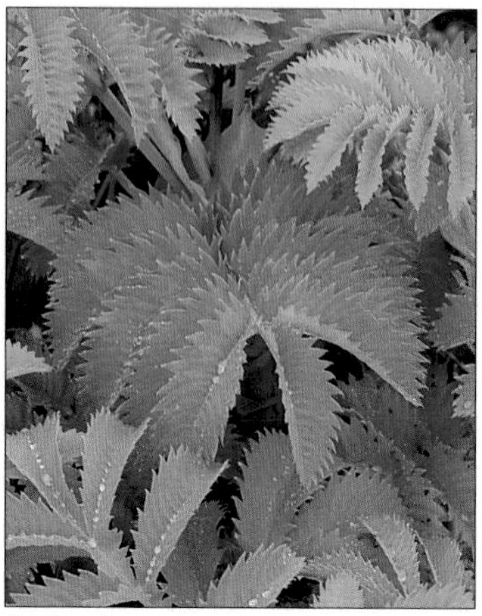
Melianthus major

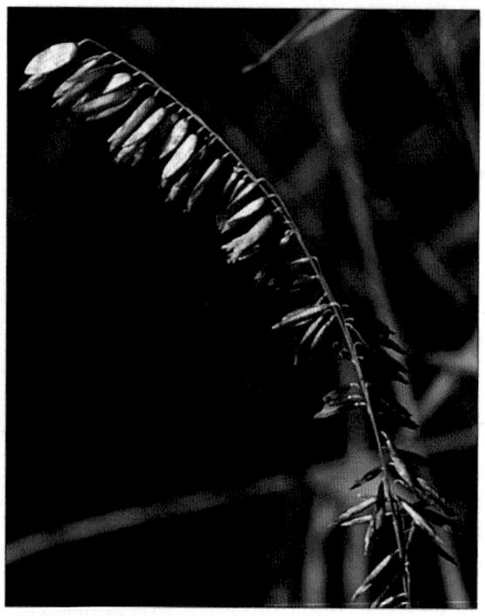
Melica altissima 'Atropurpurea'

MELICA

Melick

GRAMINEAE/POACEAE

Genus of about 75 species of deciduous, rhizomatous, clump-forming, perennial grasses occurring in grasslands of most temperate regions, except Australia. In summer, panicles of laterally compressed spikelets are borne on erect stems among clumps of linear, flat or inrolled, arching leaves. Grow in a mixed or herbaceous border or in a woodland garden.
• **HARDINESS** Fully hardy.
• **CULTIVATION** Grow in moderately fertile, moist but well-drained soil. *M. altissima* thrives in full sun or light dappled shade; *M. nutans* prefers light shade; *M. uniflora* will tolerate full shade and drier conditions. Protect from excessive winter wet.
• **PROPAGATION** Sow seed *in situ* in spring or as soon as ripe. Divide as growth starts in early or mid-spring.
• **PESTS AND DISEASES** Trouble free.

M. altissima (Siberian melick). Tufted, perennial grass with creeping rhizomes and pointed, linear, pale to mid-green leaves, 10–23cm (4–9in) long, with rough surfaces. In summer, green spikelets are produced in erect, one-sided panicles, 10–25cm (4–10in) long, with densely flowered tips. ↕0.6–1.5m (2–5ft), ↔ 40–80cm (16–32in). Europe. ✲✲✲. **'Alba'** has pale green leaves, and produces conspicuous, pale greenish white spikelets from late spring to late summer. **'Atropurpurea'** ▣ has lustrous, deep purple spikelets that become paler with age. Good for drying.
M. nutans (Mountain melick, Wood melick). Slowly creeping, perennial grass forming loose clumps of shiny, fresh green leaves, to 20cm (8in) long. Gracefully arching stems bear one-sided panicles, to 15cm (6in) long, of bead-like, brown and cream spikelets from late spring to midsummer. ↕45cm (18in), ↔ 30cm (12in) or more. Europe, N. and S.W. Asia. ✲✲✲
M. uniflora. Perennial grass with slender, creeping rhizomes forming loose tufts of linear, pointed, bright green leaves, 5–20cm (2–8in) long, with hairy upper surfaces. Purple or brown spikelets are borne in sparsely branched, erect or nodding panicles, 2.5–20cm (1–8in) long, in summer. ↕20–60cm (8–24in), ↔ to 60cm (24in). Europe, S.W. Asia. ✲✲✲. **'Variegata'** has fresh

green leaves with creamy white central stripes and purple-flushed bases, and bears dark purplish brown spikelets from late spring to midsummer.

▷**Melick** see *Melica*
Mountain see *M. nutans*
Siberian see *M. altissima*
Wood see *M. nutans*

MELICYTUS
syn. HYMENANTHERA

VIOLACEAE

Genus of about 7 species of evergreen or semi-evergreen shrubs from Australasia, found in rocky sites from mountains to woodland, dry riverbeds, and coasts. They have alternate, lance-shaped to broadly ovate, elliptic, or oblong, sweetly fragrant leaves. Small male and female flowers, with 5 spreading petals, are usually borne on separate plants. *M. crassifolius* and *M. dentatus* are grown for their attractive habits and their decorative fruits. Grow in an open, sunny site in a shrub border. In frost-prone areas, grow tender species in a cool greenhouse. Need long, hot summers to flower and fruit well.
• **HARDINESS** Fully hardy to frost tender.
• **CULTIVATION** Grow in moderately fertile, moist but well-drained soil in full sun. Protect from cold, drying winds. Pruning group 8 or 9.
• **PROPAGATION** Sow seed in containers in a cold frame in spring. Root semi-ripe cuttings in summer.
• **PESTS AND DISEASES** Trouble free.

M. crassifolius, syn. *Hymenanthera crassifolia*. Densely branched, twiggy, and often slightly spiny shrub with obovate to oblong-elliptic, leathery, dark green leaves, to 2cm (¾in) long. In late spring and early summer, bears tiny yellow flowers, followed by ovoid purple berries, 5mm (¼in) across. ↕↔ 1.2m (4ft). New Zealand. ❄❄❄ (borderline)
M. dentatus, syn. *Hymenanthera dentata*. Dense shrub with oblong, leathery, dark green leaves, to 4cm (1½in) long. Tiny, yellow to greenish white flowers are borne in late spring, followed by spherical purple berries, 5mm (¼in) across. ↕ 1.5m (5ft), ↔ 2m (6ft) or more. S.E. Australia. ❄❄

MELINIS syn. RHYNCHELYTRUM

GRAMINEAE/POACEAE

Genus of about 15 species of clump-forming, annual or perennial grasses from savannah grasslands of tropical Africa and S.E. Asia. They have flat, linear to thread-like leaves, and produce compact or open panicles of spikelets from summer to autumn. *M. repens*, the only species in general cultivation, is grown for its brightly coloured flower-heads, which may be cut for fresh flowers. Grow at the front of a border; in frost-prone areas, treat as an annual, or lift and keep frost-free in winter.
• **HARDINESS** Half hardy to frost tender; *M. repens* may tolerate short periods below 0°C (32°F).
• **CULTIVATION** Grow in moderately fertile, light, well-drained soil in full sun. In areas with light frosts, provide a deep, dry winter mulch. In colder areas, lift in late autumn and pot up in a loam-based potting compost (JI No.1); keep barely moist and frost-free in winter, and plant out again in spring when danger of frost has passed.
• **PROPAGATION** Sow seed at 13–18°C (55–64°F) in late winter, harden off, and plant out after all danger of frost has passed. Divide in spring.
• **PESTS AND DISEASES** Trouble free.

M. repens, syn. *Rhynchelytrum repens*, *R. roseum* (Natal grass). Loosely tufted, annual or short-lived, perennial grass. Upright, ascending stems bear flat, linear, long-pointed leaves, to 30cm (12in) long. From midsummer to early autumn, bears cylindrical to ovoid panicles, to 20cm (8in) long, of keeled, flattened spikelets, densely clothed in silky white hairs and strongly tinted bright purple to rose-red. ↕ 45–120cm (18–48in), ↔ 60–100cm (24–39in). Tropical Africa. ❄

MELIOSMA

MELIOSMACEAE/SABIACEAE

Genus of 20–25 species of evergreen and deciduous trees and shrubs occurring in forests from India and Sri Lanka to Japan, and in Mexico, Central America, and tropical South America. The alternate leaves are simple, sometimes pinnate, and mid- to dark green. Large panicles of tiny, cup- and saucer-shaped, 5-petalled, fragrant flowers are borne in spring or summer. Grow as specimen plants in a shrub border or woodland garden, or against a warm, sunny wall.
• **HARDINESS** Fully hardy to frost hardy; young foliage may be damaged by late frosts.
• **CULTIVATION** Grow in moderately fertile, moist but well-drained, neutral to slightly acid soil, in full sun with some midday shade. Shelter from cold, drying winds. Pruning group 1, or 13 if grown as a wall specimen.
• **PROPAGATION** Sow seed in containers in a cold frame in autumn. Root green-wood cuttings in early summer.
• **PESTS AND DISEASES** Trouble free.

M. myriantha ♀ Spreading, deciduous, small tree or shrub with arching branches and simple, narrowly elliptic to ovate-lance-shaped, sharply toothed, mid-green leaves, to 20cm (8in) long; these have soft, red-brown hairs on the midribs and leaf-stalks. Very fragrant, minute, creamy white flowers are borne in panicles, 30cm (12in) long, in midsummer, followed by small, peppercorn-like, dark red fruit, to 2mm (1/16in) across. ↕ 2.5m (8ft) or more, ↔ 4m (12ft). China, Korea, Japan. ❄❄❄
M. oldhamii see *M. pinnata* var. *oldhamii*.
M. pinnata* var. *oldhamii ♀ syn. *M. oldhamii*. Stoutly branched, deciduous tree, upright when young, later spreading, with pinnate, dark green leaves, to 35cm (14in) long, with up to 13 broadly ovate to obovate leaflets. White flowers are borne in panicles, to 30cm (12in) long, in early summer, followed by small, black or dark red fruit, 5mm (¼in) across. ↕ 10m (30ft), ↔ 6m (20ft). China, Korea. ❄❄❄
M. veitchiorum ▣♀ Slow-growing, deciduous tree, upright when young, later spreading, with pinnate, dark green leaves, to 75cm (30in) long, with up to 11 ovate or oblong leaflets and red stalks. Creamy white flowers are borne in dense panicles, to 45cm (18in) long, in late spring, followed by spherical violet fruit, to 8mm (3/8in) across. ↕ 10m (30ft), ↔ 8m (25ft). W. China. ❄❄❄

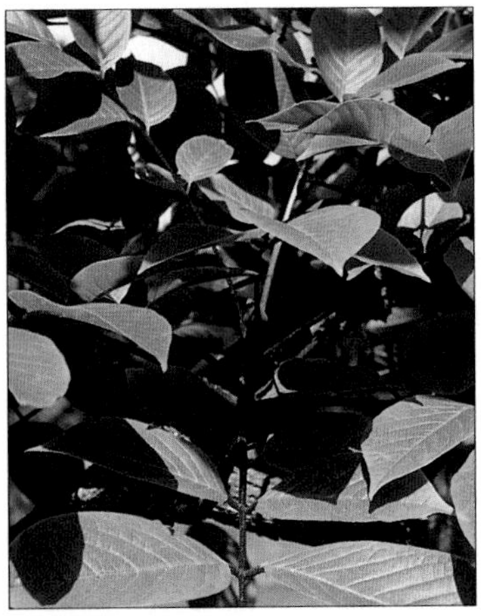
Meliosma veitchiorum

MELISSA
Balm

LABIATAE/LAMIACEAE

Genus of 3 species of herbaceous perennials occurring from Europe to C. Asia on damp wasteland, from sea level to mountains. Toothed, ovate, pale or mid-green leaves, which smell strongly of lemons when bruised, are borne in opposite pairs on square, branching stems. Leafy, whorled spikes of tubular, 2-lipped, pale yellow or white flowers are borne in summer. *M. officinalis* is a decorative, drought-tolerant plant, useful for a herbaceous or mixed border, or a herb garden. The flowers attract bees and other insects, and the leaves may be used in pot-pourri or for herb tea.
• **HARDINESS** Fully hardy.
• **CULTIVATION** Grow in poor, well-drained soil in full sun, with protection from excessive winter wet. In early summer, cut back variegated forms to encourage strongly coloured growth.
• **PROPAGATION** Sow seed in containers in a cold frame in spring. Divide as growth starts in spring, or in autumn.
• **PESTS AND DISEASES** Trouble free.

M. officinalis (Bee balm, Lemon balm). Bushy, upright perennial with hairy, glandular stems and wrinkled, ovate, light green leaves, to 7cm (3in) long. Throughout summer, produces irregular spikes of pale yellow flowers, becoming white or lilac-tinted white, to 1.5cm (½in) long. ↕ 60–120cm (2–4ft), ↔ 30–45cm (12–18in). S. Europe. ❄❄❄. **'All Gold'** has golden yellow leaves and white flowers, tinted pale lilac. **'Aurea'** ▣ syn. 'Variegata' of gardens, has dark green leaves, heavily splashed gold at the margins.

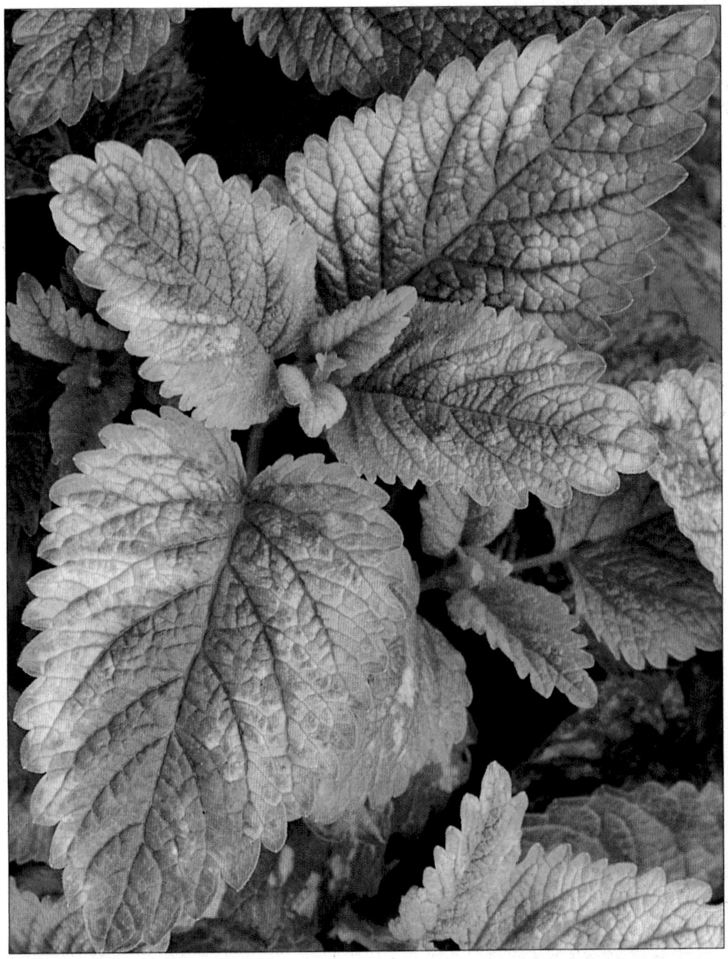
Melissa officinalis 'Aurea'

MELITTIS
Bastard balm

LABIATAE/LAMIACEAE

Genus of one species of clump-forming perennial occurring in light woodland throughout Europe, except the extreme north, as far as the Ukraine. It has leafy, square stems, bearing opposite pairs of leaves, and produces 2-lipped flowers in

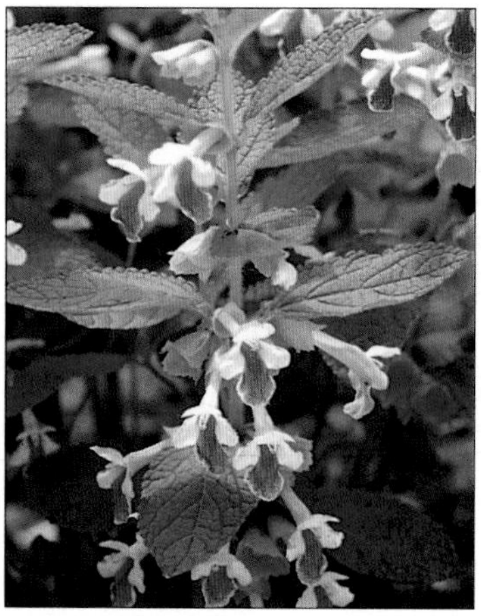

Melittis melissophyllum

white, pink, or purple, or white with pink or purple lips, in whorls from the upper leaf axils. Grow *M. melissophyllum* in a shady, mixed or herbaceous border, or in a woodland garden. The flowers are attractive to bees.
• **HARDINESS** Fully hardy.
• **CULTIVATION** Grow in moderately fertile, moist but well-drained soil in partial shade; avoid excessively dry soil.
• **PROPAGATION** Sow seed in containers in a cold frame as soon as ripe or in spring. Divide as new growth starts in spring.
• **PESTS AND DISEASES** Trouble free.

M. melissophyllum ▣ Herbaceous perennial with erect, hairy or glandular stems. The oval, scalloped, aromatic, honey-scented leaves, to 8cm (3in) long, are hairy and wrinkled, with prominent veins. In late spring and early summer, produces whorls of 2–6 tubular, 2-lipped flowers, 4cm (1½in) long, in pink, purple, or white, or creamy white with pink or purple lips and spots. ↕ 20–70cm (8–28in), ↔ 50cm (20in). Europe to Ukraine. ✲✲✲

MELOCACTUS
Turk's cap cactus
CACTACEAE

Genus of 20 or more species of spherical, rarely elongated, simple, occasionally branching, perennial cacti from coastal areas of Central and South America, Cuba, and the West Indies. They have prominently spined ribs. As plants mature, a cephalium, consisting of a mass of wool and bristles, which in some species gradually elongates to over 1m (3ft) tall, forms on the crown of each stem. The plant body apparently does not develop further once the cephalium appears. Spreading, funnel-shaped, diurnal flowers are borne on the cephalium in summer, followed by berry-like fruits with glossy, black-coated seeds. Where temperatures fall below 16°C (61°F), grow in a warm greenhouse. Elsewhere, grow in a desert garden.
• **HARDINESS** Frost tender.
• **CULTIVATION** Under glass, grow in standard cactus compost in full light and away from draughts. In growth, water sparingly, mist very occasionally, and apply fertilizer monthly. Plants are prone to root rot if overwatered or will rot if too cold. Water very sparingly in winter. Outdoors, grow in moderately fertile, gritty, sharply drained soil in full sun. See also pp.48–49.
• **PROPAGATION** Sow seed at 19–24°C (66–75°F) in spring.
• **PESTS AND DISEASES** Trouble free.

M. actinacanthus see *M. matanzanus.*
M. azureus. Cactus with a spherical to cylindrical, mid- to grey-green, often glaucous stem with 9–12 ribs bearing white spines (1–3 centrals and 7–11 radials). The white-woolly cephalium bears conspicuous red bristles. Pink flowers, 1.5–2cm (½–¾in) across, are borne in summer, followed by white to pale pink fruit. ↕ 14–30cm (5½–12in), ↔ 14–20cm (5½–8in). E. Brazil. ❅ (min. 16°C/61°F)
M. communis see *M. intortus.*
M. curvispinus, syn. *M. oaxacensis.* Cactus with a spherical or ovoid, dull green stem bearing 10–15 furrowed ribs and reddish brown spines (8–12 radials and 1 or 2 longer centrals). The low-set cephalium has dense brown bristles and a white-woolly top. Dark rose-pink flowers, 2–4cm (¾–1½in) across, are produced in summer. ↕↔ 15cm (6in). S. and E. Mexico, Guatemala. ❅ (min. 16°C/61°F)
M. intortus ▣ syn. *M. communis.* Cactus with a flattened-spherical, dark green stem, elongating with age, bearing 12–24 ribs and yellow-brown spines (10–14 radials and 1–3 centrals). Rose-pink flowers, 1.5–2cm (½–¾in) across, are borne from the cylindrical, brown-bristly cephalium in summer. ↕ 1m (3ft) or more, ↔ 25cm (10in). West Indies. ❅ (min. 16°C/61°F)
M. macrodiscus see *M. zehntneri.*
M. matanzanus, syn. *M. actinacanthus.* Cactus with a spherical, dark green stem bearing 8–13 straight ribs and brownish white or grey spines (5–9 radials and 1 longer central). The low-set cephalium has dense, orange-red bristles. Pink flowers, 1.5–2cm (½–¾in) across, are borne in summer. ↕ 8cm (3in), ↔ 9cm (3½in). N. Cuba. ❅ (min. 16°C/61°F)
M. oaxacensis see *M. curvispinus.*
M. zehntneri, syn. *M. macrodiscus.* Cactus with a spherical, bluish green stem with 10 ribs and pale brown spines (6–10 radials and 1 central, although the central one may be absent). The low-set, white-woolly cephalium is often slow to develop. Rose-red flowers, 1.5–2.5cm (½–1in) across, are borne in summer, followed by reddish violet fruit. ↕ 14cm (5½in), ↔ 18cm (7in). E. Brazil. ❅ (min. 16°C/61°F)

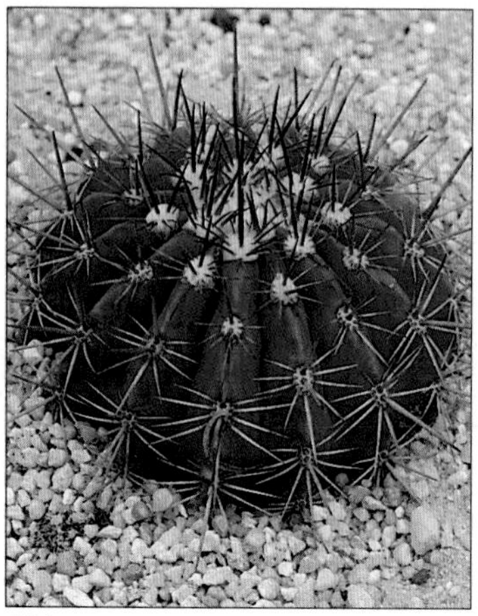

Melocactus intortus

MENISPERMUM
Moonseed
MENISPERMACEAE

Genus of 2 species of twining, suckering, semi-woody, sometimes herbaceous, deciduous, dioecious climbers from woodland in E. Asia and E. North America. They are grown for their long racemes or panicles of grape-like, glossy black fruits. The alternate, peltate leaves are ovate-heart-shaped to almost rounded. Inconspicuous, bowl-shaped, male and female flowers are borne in racemes or panicles. Grow on a trellis, against a wall, or through small trees. The fruits may cause severe discomfort if ingested.
• **HARDINESS** Fully hardy; unripened growth may be damaged by frost.
• **CULTIVATION** Grow in moderately fertile, moist but well-drained soil in full sun or dappled shade. Provide support. Pruning group 11, in early spring.
• **PROPAGATION** Sow seed in containers outdoors in autumn. Transplant suckers in autumn or spring.
• **PESTS AND DISEASES** Trouble free.

M. canadense (Canadian moonseed, Yellow parilla). Usually semi-woody, suckering climber with slender shoots and long-stalked, ovate-heart-shaped to rounded, 3- to 7-angled leaves, 8–15cm (3–6in) long. In summer, produces tiny, yellow-green flowers in axillary racemes or panicles, followed on female plants by grape-like, glossy black fruit, to 1cm (½in) long. ↕ 5m (15ft). E. North America. ✲✲✲

MENTHA
Mint
LABIATAE/LAMIACEAE

Genus of 25 species of aromatic, rhizomatous perennials, rarely annuals, widely distributed in Europe, Africa, and Asia, often found in shallow water or wet or moist soil. Erect, branching stems bear lance-shaped to rounded, light to dark green, purple-, blue-, or grey-green leaves. The tubular to bell-shaped flowers are weakly 2-lipped, each with 4 spreading lobes and leafy bracts. They are borne in summer, in spikes of whorl-like clusters, or occasionally in a single, terminal cluster. Mints are widely used as culinary herbs.

Grow in a herb or vegetable garden; the less invasive species are also suitable for a herbaceous border. *M. aquatica* is useful for stabilizing the muddy edges of a pool, *M. pulegium* can be used as low ground cover, and *M. requienii* is useful for a rock garden. All attract bees; most dry well for use in pot-pourri.
• **HARDINESS** Fully hardy.
• **CULTIVATION** Grow in poor, moist soil in full sun. Restrict spread of invasive species by planting in deep containers and plunging in the soil, or by growing in small beds to restrict root run. *M. aquatica* can be grown in containers submerged in water up to 15cm (6in) deep. See also pp.52–53.
• **PROPAGATION** Sow seed in containers in a cold frame in spring. Divide in spring or autumn. Portions of rhizome will root at any time during the growing season; pot up until established. Root tip cuttings in spring or summer.

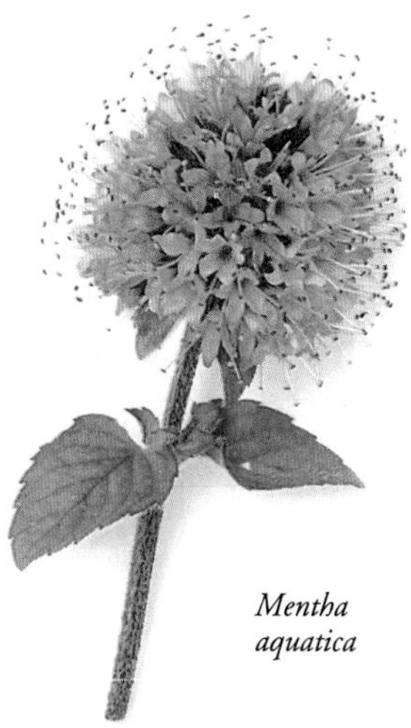

Mentha aquatica

• **PESTS AND DISEASES** Powdery mildew, especially during drought, and rust are troublesome.

M. aquatica ▣ (Watermint). Marginal aquatic or semi-aquatic perennial with long, thin, segmented rhizomes, often reddish purple stems, and ovate to ovate-lance-shaped, toothed, aromatic, sometimes hairy, dark green leaves, to 6cm (2½in) long, occasionally to 9cm (3½in). In summer, produces whorls of shallowly tubular lilac flowers, to 5mm (¼in) long, in dense, spherical, terminal clusters. ↕ 15–90cm (6–36in), ↔ 1m (3ft) or more. Eurasia. ✲✲✲
M. corsica see *M. requienii.*
***M. x gentilis* 'Aurea'** see *M.* x *gracilis* 'Variegata'.
***M. x gentilis* 'Variegata'** see *M.* x *gracilis* 'Variegata'.
***M. x gracilis* 'Variegata'** (*M. arvensis* x *M. spicata*), syn. *M.* x *gentilis* 'Aurea', *M.* x *gentilis* 'Variegata' (Ginger mint, Red mint). Spreading perennial with erect, often red-tinted stems and short-stalked, ovate-lance-shaped to elliptic-oblong leaves, 3–7cm (1¼–3in) long, striped and flecked gold, and strongly aromatic and ginger-flavoured. In summer, bears dense, whorled clusters of tubular lilac flowers, to 4mm (⅛in) long, widely spaced on upright stems. ↕ 30cm (12in) or more, ↔ to 1m (3ft) or more. ✲✲✲
M. longifolia, syn. *M. sylvestris* (Horsemint). Vigorous, creeping perennial with grey-hairy stems and oblong-elliptic, toothed, strongly aromatic, musty-scented, green to silver-grey leaves, 6–9cm (2½–3½in) long, with unbranched hairs. In summer,

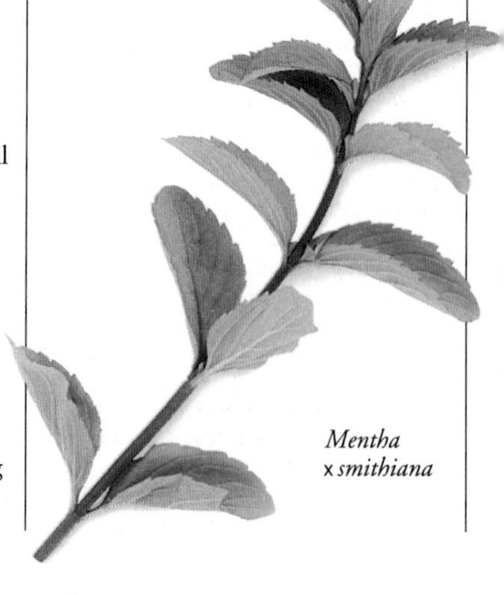

Mentha x *smithiana*

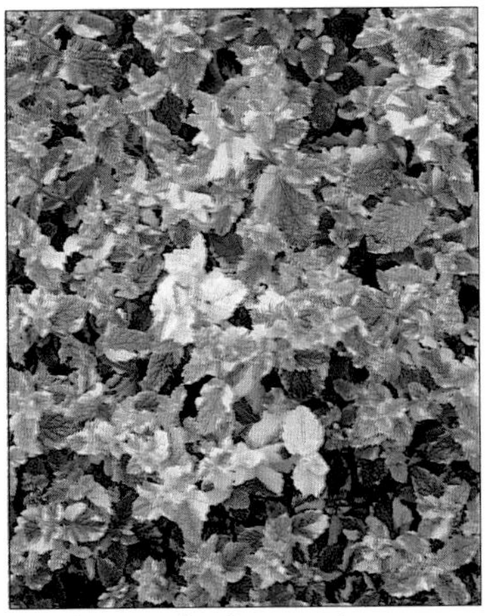

Mentha suaveolens 'Variegata'

tubular, lilac or white flowers, to 5mm (¼in) long, are borne in dense whorls in terminal, tapering spikes. ↕ to 1.2m (4ft), ↔ 1m (3ft) or more. Europe, Turkey, Caucasus, N.W. Iran. ***
M. odorata see *M.* x *piperita* f. *citrata.*
M.* x *piperita* f. *citrata (*M. aquatica* x *M. spicata*), syn. *M. odorata, M. piperita* var. *citriodora* (Eau de Cologne mint, Lemon mint). Vigorous, spreading, eau de Cologne-scented perennial with hairless stems and thin-textured, ovate, dark green leaves, 4–9cm (1½–3½in) long, tinged reddish purple in sun or copper-red in shade. Dense, terminal, oblong spikes of congested whorls of tubular, pinkish purple flowers, 4mm (⅛in) long, are borne in late summer. ↕ 50cm (20in), ↔ 1m (3ft) or more. Garden origin. ***
M. piperita* var. *citriodora see *M.* x *piperita* f. *citrata.*
M. pulegium (Pennyroyal). Spreading perennial with upright and procumbent stems bearing short-stalked, narrowly elliptic to rounded, sharply aromatic, bright green leaves, to 3cm (1¼in) long, hairy beneath. Widely spaced, leafy whorls of tubular lilac flowers, 4–6mm (⅛–¼in) long, are borne in spikes in summer. ↕ 10–40cm (4–16in), ↔ to 50cm (20in). S.W. and C. Europe, Mediterranean to Iran. ***
M. requienii, syn. *M. corsica* (Corsican mint). Procumbent, mat-forming, hairy or hairless perennial with slender, creeping, rooting stems bearing broadly ovate to rounded, peppermint-scented, bright green leaves, to 7mm (¼in) across. In summer, bears whorls of tiny, tubular lilac flowers, 2mm (1/16in) long, in short spikes. Prefers shade. ↕ to 1cm (½in), ↔ indefinite. France (Corsica), Italy (including Sardinia). ***
***M. rotundifolia* of gardens** see *M. suaveolens.*
M. rubra* var. *raripila see *M.* x *smithiana.*
M.* x *smithiana ■ (*M. aquatica* x *M. arvensis* x *M. spicata*), syn. *M. rubra* var. *raripila* (Red raripila). Vigorous, spreading perennial with ovate, toothed, sweet-smelling, sparsely hairy, dark green, red-tinted leaves, 3–9cm (1¼–3½in) long. In summer, produces spikes of dense whorls of tubular lilac flowers, to 5mm (¼in) long, usually well spaced, sometimes clustered at the stem tips. ↕ to 1m (3ft), ↔ 1.2m (4ft) or more. N. and C. Europe. ***
M. spicata, syn. *M. viridis* (Spearmint). Spreading perennial with stalkless, lance-shaped to oblong-ovate, toothed, aromatic (usually sweet-smelling but sometimes pungent), bright green leaves, 5–9cm (2–3½in) long, hairless or with branched and unbranched hairs beneath. Bears dense, cylindrical spikes of usually separated whorls of tubular to bell-shaped, pink, lilac, or white flowers, to 3mm (⅛in) long, in summer. ↕ to 1m (3ft), ↔ indefinite. W. and C. Europe, Mediterranean. ***
M. suaveolens, syn. *M. rotundifolia* of gardens (Apple mint). Vigorous, spreading, apple-scented perennial with often white-hairy stems and toothed, oblong-ovate to rounded, irregularly wrinkled and softly hairy, greyish green leaves, to 3cm (1¼in) long, the margins sometimes rolled under and wavy. In summer, bears tubular, pink or white flowers, to 2mm (1/16 in) long, in dense whorls in terminal, often branched spikes. ↕ to 1m (3ft), ↔ indefinite. W. and S. Europe, Mediterranean. ***.
'Variegata' ■ (Pineapple mint) has leaves with broad cream streaks and margins, and a rich, fruity fragrance.
M. sylvestris see *M. longifolia.*
M.* x *villosa* f. *alopecuroides (*M. spicata* x *M. suaveolens*) (Bowles' mint). Variable, spreading perennial with softly hairy, broadly ovate or rounded, aromatic, toothed, bright green leaves, 4–8cm (1½–3in) long. In summer, whorls of tubular pink flowers, 2–3mm (1/16–⅛in) long, are produced in large, leafy spikes. ↕ 30–90cm (12–36in), ↔ indefinite. Garden origin. ***
M. viridis see *M. spicata.*

MENTZELIA
Starflower

LOASACEAE

Genus of 60 species of spreading to erect, freely branching, densely stiff-haired annuals, biennials, perennials, and subshrubs, mostly from dry, sandy, or rocky scrub in S.W. USA, Mexico, and the West Indies. Alternate, mainly lance-shaped, coarsely toothed, light to mid-green leaves may be simple, lobed, or pinnatifid. The poppy-like, 5- to 10-petalled, bright orange, yellow, or white flowers, often night-scented or opening only in strong sunlight, are borne singly or in loose cymes in summer. Grow in an annual or mixed border, or a wild garden; they need long, hot summers to flower well. In frost-prone areas, grow tender species in a cool greenhouse.
• **HARDINESS** Fully hardy to frost tender.
• **CULTIVATION** Grow in moderately fertile, well-drained soil in a warm, sheltered site in full sun. Water freely in the growing season for repeat flowering. After first flush of bloom, cut annuals back to 5cm (2in).
• **PROPAGATION** Sow seed of annuals *in situ* in spring.
• **PESTS AND DISEASES** Trouble free.

M. lindleyi ■ syn. *Bartonia aurea* (Blazing star). Erect, freely branching annual with lance-shaped to oval, pinnatifid, mid-green to grey leaves, to 15cm (6in) long, the lobes sometimes toothed. In summer, 5-petalled, very fragrant, night-scented, golden yellow blooms, 5–9cm (2–3½in) across, are borne singly from the leaf axils or in 2- or 3-flowered cymes at the stem tips; petals are flushed orange-red at the bases. ↕ 15–70cm (6–28in), ↔ to 23cm (9in). USA (California). ***

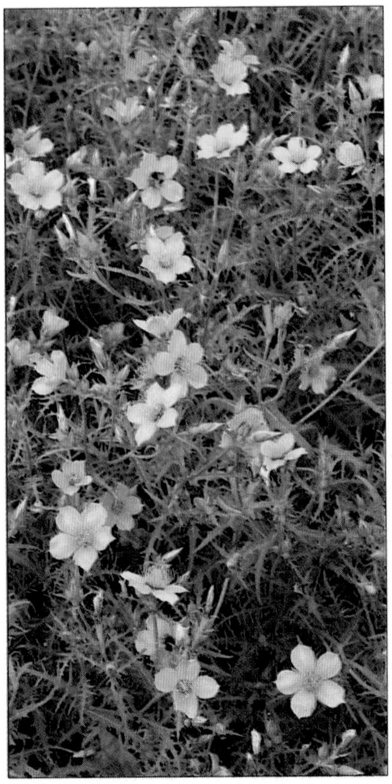

Mentzelia lindleyi

MENYANTHES

MENYANTHACEAE

Genus of one species of rhizomatous, aquatic or semi-aquatic perennial from the N. hemisphere, especially in Europe. It forms large, spreading, floating mats that extend over the shallow, still or slow-moving water of lakes or ponds, and sometimes across the muddy margins. *M. trifoliata* has 3-palmate leaves and bears racemes of star-shaped flowers. It is a decorative plant for ponds and for the margins of a wildlife pool, and is useful for disguising hard edges.
• **HARDINESS** Fully hardy.
• **CULTIVATION** In a large pool, grow in an aquatic planting basket, at a depth of 15–23cm (6–9in), or in muddy pond margins. Provide a site in full sun to encourage production of the short-lived flowers. See also pp.52–53.
• **PROPAGATION** Sow seed in winter in containers standing in water. In summer, divide young rhizomes into pieces, 23–30cm (9–12in) long, and place them horizontally on soft mud in an aquatic planting basket or in shallow water; push in and peg down.
• **PESTS AND DISEASES** Trouble free.

M. trifoliata ■ (Bogbean). Aquatic perennial with extensive, creeping rhizomes, to 1.2m (4ft) long, and 3-palmate leaves with elliptic to ovate or obovate leaflets, to 6cm (2½in) long. In summer, bears erect racemes of 10–20 white flowers, 2.5cm (1in) across, pink outside and in bud, with very finely fringed and bearded petals. ↕ 20–30cm (8–12in), ↔ indefinite. Europe, N. Asia, N.W. India, North America. ***

MENZIESIA

ERICACEAE

Genus of about 7 species of freely branching, spreading to upright, deciduous shrubs, found in woodland in E. Asia and North America. The ovate to elliptic or oblong leaves are arranged alternately and often clustered at the shoot tips. Small, nodding, urn- to bell-shaped, 4- or 5-lobed flowers are borne in umbels in late spring and early summer. Grow *Menziesia* species in a peat bed or woodland garden; they grow best in areas with cool, damp summers.
• **HARDINESS** Fully hardy, although young growth may be damaged by late frosts.
• **CULTIVATION** Grow in moist but well-drained, humus-rich, acid soil in partial shade. Shelter from cold, drying winds. Pruning group 8.
• **PROPAGATION** Sow seed in containers in spring at 13°C (55°F), or in a cold

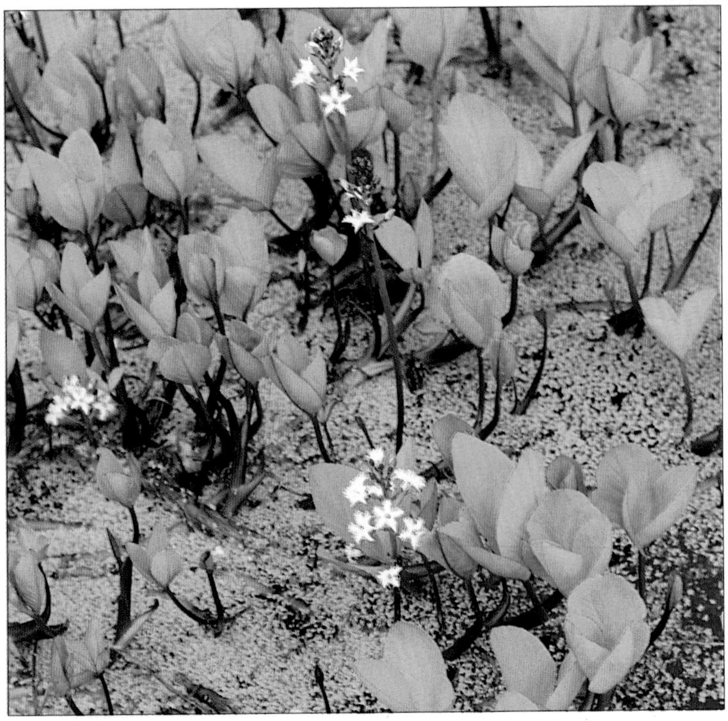

Menyanthes trifoliata

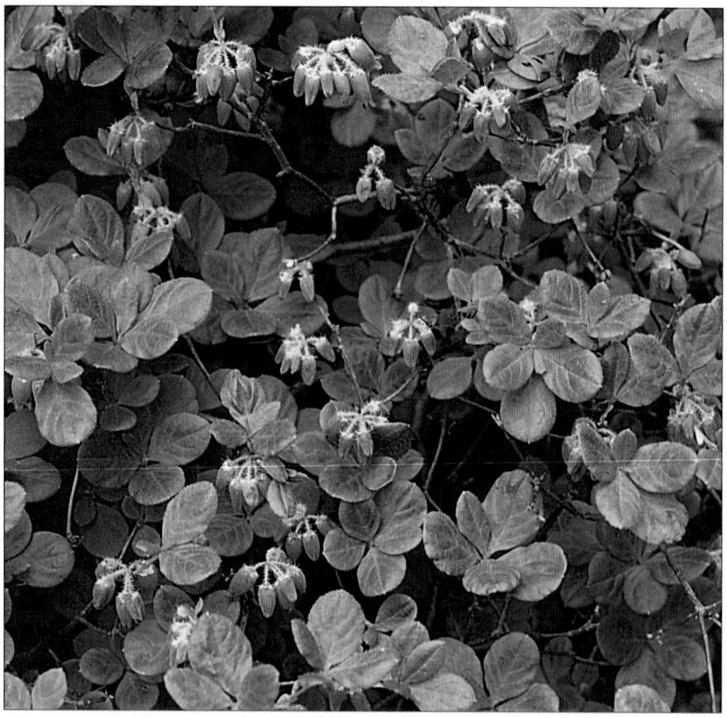
Menziesia ciliicalyx var. *purpurea*

frame outdoors in autumn. Root greenwood cuttings with bottom heat in early summer.
• **PESTS AND DISEASES** Trouble free.

M. ciliicalyx* var. *lasiophylla see *M. ciliicalyx* var. *purpurea.*
M. ciliicalyx* var. *purpurea ■ syn. *M. ciliicalyx* var. *lasiophylla.* Slow-growing, bushy shrub with clustered, obovate to oval, bright green leaves, to 7cm (3in) long. In late spring and early summer, bears umbels of 3–8 urn-shaped, dark purple-pink flowers, 1.5cm (½in) long. ↕↔ 1m (3ft). Japan. ❄❄❄
M. ferruginea (Fool's huckleberry, Rusty leaf). Upright, twiggy shrub with clustered, obovate to elliptic, mid-green leaves, to 6cm (2½in) long, covered in soft, rust-brown hairs and turning red in autumn. From late spring to summer, bears umbels of 2–5 urn-shaped, red-flushed yellow flowers, 7mm (¼in) long. ↕ 2m (6ft), ↔ 1.5m (5ft). N.W. North America (Alaska to N. California). ❄❄❄

MERENDERA

COLCHICACEAE/LILIACEAE

Genus of about 10 species of bulbous perennials from subalpine meadows and dry sites in open woodland in the Mediterranean region, N. Africa, the Middle East, and W. Asia. The basal, semi-erect leaves are linear to linear-lance-shaped, strap-shaped, or inversely lance-shaped, and elongate after flowering. Small, funnel-shaped flowers, with separate, often narrow, star-shaped tepals, are borne at ground level, with or before the leaves in spring or autumn. Grow in a raised bed, alpine house, or bulb frame; *M. montana* is suitable for a sunny rock garden.
• **HARDINESS** Fully hardy to half hardy.
• **CULTIVATION** Plant 5–7cm (2–3in) deep in late summer. Outdoors, grow in moist but well-drained soil in full sun. In a bulb frame, grow in loam-based potting compost (JI No.2) with added sharp sand. Water moderately in the growing season. *Merendera* species require a hot, dry period of summer dormancy. Repot annually in summer.
• **PROPAGATION** Sow seed in containers in a cold frame: in spring for autumn-flowering species, in autumn for spring-flowering species. Remove offsets during summer dormancy.
• **PESTS AND DISEASES** Trouble free.

M. bulbocodium see *M. montana.*
M. caucasica see *M. trigyna.*
M. montana ■ syn. *M. bulbocodium, M. pyrenaica.* Cormous perennial with 3 or 4 linear, channelled leaves, to 22cm (9in) long, borne just with or after the flowers. In autumn, produces 1 or 2 upright, funnel-shaped, purple to red-purple flowers, to 7cm (3in) long, sometimes with white bases. ↕↔ 5cm (2in). C. Pyrenees, Iberian peninsula. ❄❄❄
M. pyrenaica see *M. montana.*
M. raddeana see *M. trigyna.*
M. robusta. Cormous perennial with 3–6 linear to lance-shaped leaves, to 25cm (10in) long, with the flowers. Produces 1–4 upright, funnel-shaped, deep pink to lilac or white flowers, 2–4cm (¾–1½in) long, in spring. ↕ 8cm (3in), ↔ 5cm (2in). Iran, Afghanistan, Turkmenistan, N. India. ❄❄
M. trigyna, syn. *M. caucasica, M. raddeana.* Bulbous perennial with linear to linear-lance-shaped leaves, to 17cm (7in) long, borne with the flowers. In spring, bears 1–3 funnel-shaped, purple-pink to white flowers, 2–3cm (¾–1¼in) long, with narrow, inversely lance-shaped tepals. ↕↔ 5cm (2in). Turkey, Caucasus, Iran. ❄❄

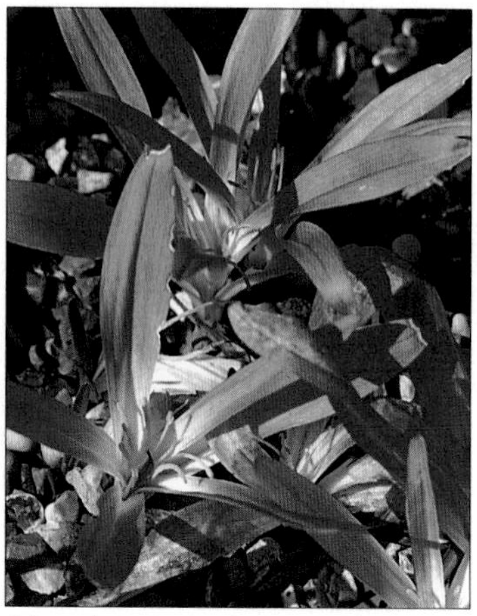
Merendera montana

MERREMIA

CONVOLVULACEAE

Genus of at least 70 species of woody, evergreen and herbaceous, mainly twining climbers found in tropical regions in diverse habitats, including mudflats, grassland, and woodland. The alternate or spiralling leaves are entire or palmately lobed or divided. Funnel- to bell-shaped flowers are borne singly or in small clusters from the upper leaf axils. In frost-prone areas, grow in a temperate greenhouse, or treat as tender annuals and grow outdoors. Elsewhere, grow over a pergola, arch, or trellis.
• **HARDINESS** Frost tender.
• **CULTIVATION** Under glass, grow in loam-based potting compost (JI No.2) in full light with shade from hot sun. In the growing season, water moderately and apply a balanced liquid fertilizer monthly; water sparingly in winter. Outdoors, grow in moderately fertile, moist but well-drained soil in full sun with some midday shade. Shelter from cold, drying winds. Pruning group 11, in late winter or early spring.
• **PROPAGATION** Sow seed at 18–24°C (64–75°F) in spring.
• **PESTS AND DISEASES** Susceptible to red spider mites and whiteflies under glass.

M. tuberosa, syn. *Ipomoea tuberosa, Operculina tuberosa* (Spanish morning glory, Wood rose, Yellow morning glory). Vigorous, woody-stemmed, evergreen twining climber. Palmately 5- to 7-lobed, bright to mid-green leaves have oblong-lance-shaped lobes, to 15cm (6in) long. Bears funnel-shaped yellow flowers, 5–6cm (2–2½in) across, usually in stalked clusters of 3–9, but sometimes also singly, mainly in summer. Spherical fruit, to 4cm (1½in) across, develop from the woody sepals. ↕ 10–20m (30–70ft). Mexico to tropical South America. ❀ (min. 7–10°C/45–50°F)

▷ **Merrybells** see *Uvularia*
Large see *U. grandiflora*

MERTENSIA

BORAGINACEAE

Genus of about 50 species of clump-forming, mound-forming, or prostrate perennials from wet meadows, woodland, and coasts in Europe, Asia, North America, and Greenland. The alternate, lance-shaped to rounded leaves, sometimes with heart-shaped bases, are light to dark green or greyish or bluish green. Pendent, tubular or bell-shaped, 5-lobed blue flowers, with flared, funnel-shaped mouths, are borne in terminal or axillary cymes. Grow the smaller species in a gravel bed, rock garden, or alpine house, the larger ones in a peat bed, herbaceous border, or woodland garden.
• **HARDINESS** Fully hardy.

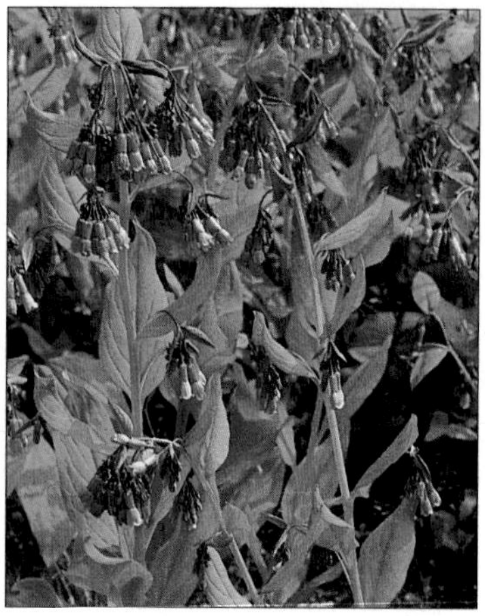
Mertensia ciliata

• **CULTIVATION** Grow in moist but well-drained, humus-rich soil in light dappled shade. Alpine species, such as *M. echioides,* require humus-rich, gritty soil; *M. maritima* and *M. simplicissima* prefer low-fertility, sharply drained, very gritty or sandy soil. All prefer full sun with some midday shade.
• **PROPAGATION** Sow seed in containers in a cold frame in autumn; keep young plants shaded and do not allow the soil to dry out. Divide clumps carefully as new growth commences in spring. Take root cuttings of *M. pulmonarioides* when dormant, in autumn or early winter.
• **PESTS AND DISEASES** Slugs and snails may cause damage.

M. asiatica see *M. simplicissima.*
M. ciliata ■ Upright perennial with stemless, ovate, lance-shaped, or oblong, bluish green basal leaves, to 15cm (6in) long, and ovate to lance-shaped stem leaves. Axillary cymes of bell-shaped, clear blue flowers, to 8mm (⅜in) long, are borne in summer. ↕ to 60cm (24in), ↔ to 30cm (12in). W. USA. ❄❄❄
M. echioides. Clump-forming perennial with spoon-shaped or ovate to lance-shaped or oblong, dark green leaves, to 9cm (3½in) long. Many-flowered, curving cymes, to 12cm (5in) long, of funnel-shaped, deep blue flowers, to 7mm (¼in) long, are borne on upright stems in summer. ↕ 15cm (6in), ↔ to 10cm (4in). Himalayas. ❄❄❄
M. maritima (Oyster plant). Spreading, prostrate perennial with fleshy, spoon-shaped to oblong-ovate, very glaucous, blue-green leaves, to 10cm (4in) long. Bell-shaped, bright blue flowers, to

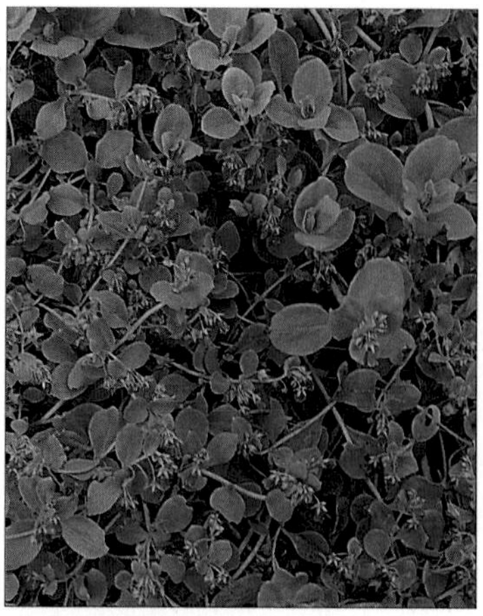
Mertensia simplicissima

M

8mm (3/8in) across, open from pink buds in branching, terminal cymes in early summer. ↕ 10cm (4in), ↔ to 30cm (12in). Coasts of E. North America, Greenland, and N. Europe. ❄❄❄
M. pterocarpa see *M. sibirica.*
M. pulmonarioides ♀ syn. *M. virginica* (Blue bells, Virginia cowslip). Clump-forming perennial with erect, branching stems bearing elliptic to ovate, soft, hairless, bluish green leaves, to 15cm (6in) long. Terminal cymes of flared, long-tubed, violet-blue or white flowers, 2–2.5cm (3/4–1in) long, are borne in mid- and late spring. ↕ 45cm (18in), ↔ 25cm (10in). North America. ❄❄❄
M. sibirica, syn. *M. pterocarpa.* Clump-forming perennial with broadly elliptic, broadly ovate, or heart-shaped, light green basal leaves, 5–10cm (2–4in) long. The erect, unbranched, hairless, light green stems bear more oval, pointed leaves. From late spring to midsummer, terminal cymes of flared, tubular, deep blue or purple-blue flowers, to 1cm (1/2in) long, are borne on long, axillary flower-stalks. ↕ 60cm (24in), ↔ 30cm (12in). E. Siberia, E. Asia. ❄❄❄
M. simplicissima ■ syn. *M. asiatica.* Prostrate perennial with procumbent, leafy shoots and rosettes of obovate to broadly ovate, glaucous, blue-green leaves, 3–8cm (1 1/4–3in) long. From late spring to early autumn, bears terminal cymes of flared, tubular, turquoise-blue flowers, 1cm (1/2in) long, on spreading stems. ↕ to 90cm (36in), ↔ 30cm (12in). Russia (Sakhalin), Korea, Japan. ❄❄❄
M. virginica see *M. pulmonarioides.*

▷ ***Mesembryanthemum cordifolium*** see *Aptenia cordifolia*
▷ ***Mesembryanthemum criniflorum*** see *Dorotheanthus bellidiformis*
▷ ***Mesembryanthemum derenbergianum*** see *Ebracteola derenbergiana*
▷ ***Mesembryanthemum multiradiatum*** see *Lampranthus roseus*
▷ ***Mesembryanthemum tricolor*** see *Dorotheanthus gramineus*

MESPILUS

ROSACEAE

Genus of one species of deciduous tree or large shrub found in woodland and thickets in mountainous regions of S.E. Europe and S.W. Asia. It is grown for its attractive, spreading habit, its colourful autumn foliage, its bowl-shaped flowers, borne singly at the ends of short shoots, and its flattened, apple-like fruit, which have prominent, persistent calyces. Grow as a specimen tree. The fruit are edible following the first frosts in late autumn, when they are well-ripened and partly rotten.
• **HARDINESS** Fully hardy.
• **CULTIVATION** Grow in moderately fertile, moist but well-drained soil in full sun or light shade. Pruning group 1.
• **PROPAGATION** Sow seed in a seedbed in autumn. Bud in late summer.
• **PESTS AND DISEASES** Aphids, brown rot, caterpillars, and powdery mildew may cause problems.

M. germanica ■ Ǫ (Medlar). Spreading tree or large shrub with alternate, lance-shaped to oblong-oval, dark green leaves, to 15cm (6in) long, turning yellow-brown in autumn. Bears white, sometimes pink-tinged flowers, to 5cm (2in) across, in late spring and early summer. Almost spherical, fleshy brown fruit grow up to 5cm (2in) or more across. ↕ 6m (20ft), ↔ 8m (25ft). S.E. Europe, S.W. Asia. ❄❄❄. **'Dutch'** has russet-brown fruit. **'Nottingham'** has brown fruit, 4cm (1 1/2in) across.

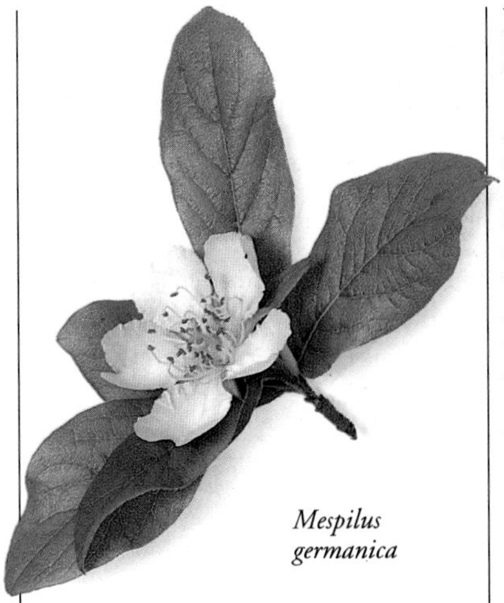

Mespilus germanica

▷ **Mespilus, Snowy** see *Amelanchier*

METASEQUOIA

TAXODIACEAE

Genus of one species of deciduous, monoecious, coniferous tree from valley forests of C. China. It has 2-ranked, linear leaves that turn gold to red-brown in autumn. The shoots, leaves, and cone scales grow in opposite pairs. Tolerant of waterlogged soils, it is an excellent specimen tree, growing quickly to a considerable height.
• **HARDINESS** Fully hardy.
• **CULTIVATION** Grow in humus-rich, moist but well-drained soil in full sun. Initial growth is fast, but on dry sites is slower after plants reach 10m (30ft) tall.
• **PROPAGATION** Sow seed in a seedbed in autumn. Root hardwood cuttings in winter or semi-ripe cuttings with bottom heat in midsummer.
• **PESTS AND DISEASES** Trouble free.

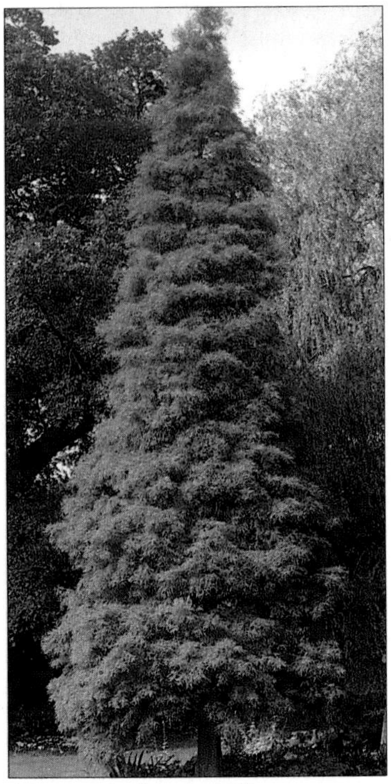

Metasequoia glyptostroboides

M. glyptostroboides ■ ♀ ◊ (Dawn redwood). Conical tree with ascending branches and fibrous, orange-brown bark, often fluted in cultivation. Soft, spreading leaves are bright fresh green, to 1.5cm (1/2in) long on mature trees, 2cm (3/4in) or more on seedlings, with 2 light green bands beneath. Deciduous shoots are green, without growth buds; permanent shoots, bearing growth buds, are pink-brown, later brown. Produces ovoid, light brown female cones, 2cm (3/4in) long, on stalks 2–4cm (3/4–1 1/2in) long, and pendent, spherical brown male cones, 0.5–1.5cm (1/4–1/2in) long, with 15–20 scales, in the upper crown. ↕ 20–40m (70–130ft), ↔ 5m (15ft) or more. China (N.W. Hubei). ❄❄❄

METROSIDEROS

Pohutakawa, Rata

MYRTACEAE

Genus of 50 species of dwarf to tall, upright, evergreen shrubs, trees, and climbers found in rainforest, dry river valleys, and subalpine areas from South Africa to Malaysia, Australasia, and the Pacific islands (including Hawaii). The simple, mostly entire, leathery leaves are borne in opposite pairs. Small, trumpet-shaped flowers, with insignificant petals and conspicuous, brush-like tufts of stamens with coloured filaments, are borne in terminal or axillary cymes or racemes. In frost-prone areas, grow in a cool greenhouse. Elsewhere, grow as specimens or as a hedge or screen.
• **HARDINESS** Frost hardy to frost tender; *M. excelsus* and *M. robustus* survive short spells several degrees below 0°C (32°F).
• **CULTIVATION** Under glass, grow in loam-based potting compost (JI No.2) in full light, with shade from hot sun. In growth, water freely and apply a balanced liquid fertilizer monthly; water sparingly in winter. Outdoors, grow in humus-rich, moderately fertile, moist but well-drained, neutral to acid soil, in full sun. Shelter from cold, drying winds. Pruning group 1; plants under glass need restrictive pruning.
• **PROPAGATION** Surface-sow seed at 13–15°C (55–59°F) in spring. Root semi-ripe cuttings with bottom heat in summer. Air layer in spring.
• **PESTS AND DISEASES** Scale insects may be a problem under glass.

M. excelsus ■ Ǫ syn. *M. tomentosus* (Christmas tree, Common Pohutakawa). Erect, freely branching tree, spreading with age, with elliptic to oblong leaves, 5–10cm (2–4in) long, semi-glossy, dark green above, densely white-felted beneath. Broad, compact, many-flowered, terminal cymes of flowers, 3–4cm (1 1/4–1 1/2in) long, with crimson filaments and golden anthers, are borne in summer. ↕ to 20m (70ft), ↔ 10–20m (30–70ft). New Zealand (North Island). ❄. **'Aureus'** has rich yellow filaments.
M. kermadecensis Ǫ Bushy, rounded to spreading tree with broadly ovate to oblong-elliptic leaves, 2.5–5cm (1–2in) long, with recurved margins, dark green above and densely white-felted beneath. In summer, produces abundant dense, terminal cymes of flowers 2cm (3/4in) long, with crimson filaments and yellow anthers. ↕ to 20m (70ft), ↔ 8–12m (25–40ft). New Zealand, including Raoul Island. ❄. **'Sunninghill'** has variegated leaves, irregularly splashed creamy yellow. **'Variegatus'** has leaves marbled dark green and grey-green, with broad, irregular, creamy white margins.
M. robustus Ǫ (Northern rata, Rata). Erect, freely branching tree, often epiphytic when young, spreading with age. Elliptic to ovate-oblong leaves, 2.5–5cm (1–2in) long, are semi-glossy, dark green above and hairless and paler beneath. In summer, flowers 3cm (1 1/4in) long, with matt crimson filaments and yellow anthers, are borne in dense, terminal cymes on 4-angled stems. ↕ to 30m (100ft), ↔ to 12m (40ft). New Zealand. ❄
M. tomentosus see *M. excelsus.*

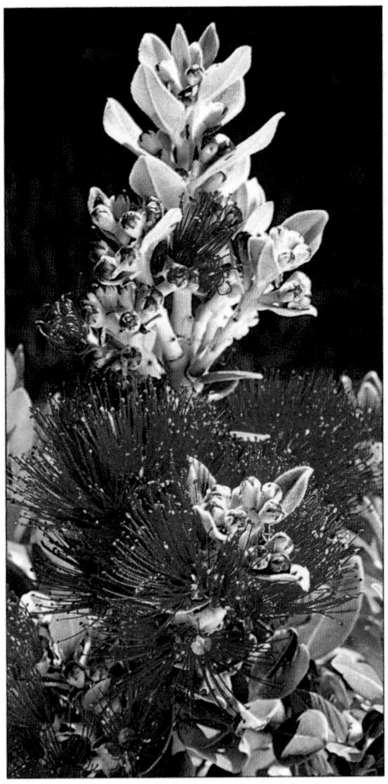

Metrosideros excelsus

MEUM

APIACEAE/UMBELLIFERAE

Genus of one species of clump-forming perennial from mountain slopes, poor grassland, and roadsides in W. and C. Europe. The hairless, aromatic, mainly basal leaves are pinnate with whorled, hair-like segments. Small, star-shaped flowers are borne in compound umbels in summer. Grow as a foliage plant in a mixed or herbaceous border.
• **HARDINESS** Fully hardy.
• **CULTIVATION** Grow in moderately fertile, well-drained, preferably alkaline soil in full sun.
• **PROPAGATION** Sow seed in containers in a cold frame as soon as ripe. Divide in spring; pot up until established.
• **PESTS AND DISEASES** Slugs and snails may damage young growth. Aphids may also be a problem.

M. athamanticum (Baldmoney, Spignel). Perennial with oblong, 3- or 4-pinnate, light to mid-green leaves, with finely cut leaflets 5mm (1/4in) long. In early and midsummer, bears tiny, white or purple-tinged white flowers in small umbels, 3–6cm (1¼–2½in) across, grouped into larger, compound umbels. ↕ 20–60cm (8–24in), ↔ 30cm (12in). W. and C. Europe. ✲✲✲

▷**Mexican bush** see *Salvia leucantha*
▷**Mexican creeper** see *Antigonon leptopus*
▷**Mexican hat** see *Ratibida*
▷**Mexican hat plant** see *Kalanchoe daigremontiana*
▷**Mexican orange blossom** see *Choisya, C. ternata*
▷**Mezereon** see *Daphne mezereum*
▷**Michaelmas daisy** see *Aster novi-belgii*

MICHAUXIA

CAMPANULACEAE

Genus of 7 species of imposing biennials or short-lived, monocarpic perennials from sunny, well-drained, stony sites in the E. Mediterranean region and S.W. Asia. The toothed, hairy, rosette-forming leaves are pinnatisect or pinnatifid, each leaf with a single large, terminal lobe. Racemes or panicles of white or blue flowers, with spreading or reflexed corollas consisting of many narrow petals, are produced on stout, leafy stems. Grow in a mixed border.
• **HARDINESS** Fully hardy.
• **CULTIVATION** Grow in moderately fertile, well-drained, alkaline soil in full sun. Provide a dry winter mulch.
• **PROPAGATION** Sow seed *in situ* in spring. May also self-seed.
• **PESTS AND DISEASES** Trouble free.

M

M. campanuloides. Perennial with robust, branched stems and lance-shaped, pinnatifid leaves, to 20cm (8in) long. Pendent, purple-tinged white flowers, 2–4cm (¾–1½in) across, with narrow, reflexed corolla lobes and protruding, tubular, hairy styles, are borne in panicles in early summer. ↕ to 1.5m (5ft), ↔ 45cm (18in). E. Mediterranean (Turkey, Syria). ✲✲✲
M. tchihatchewii ▣ Perennial with long-stalked, oblong to broadly lance-shaped, coarsely toothed leaves, 15–20cm (6–8in) long. In midsummer, robust, stiff, branching stems, one per rosette, bear dense, spike-like racemes of nodding, initially broadly bell-shaped, white or blue flowers, to 3cm (1¼in) across, with mildly reflexed corollas, the lobes divided only to one-third of their length. ↕ 1.5m (5ft) or more, ↔ 45cm (18in). Turkey. ✲✲✲

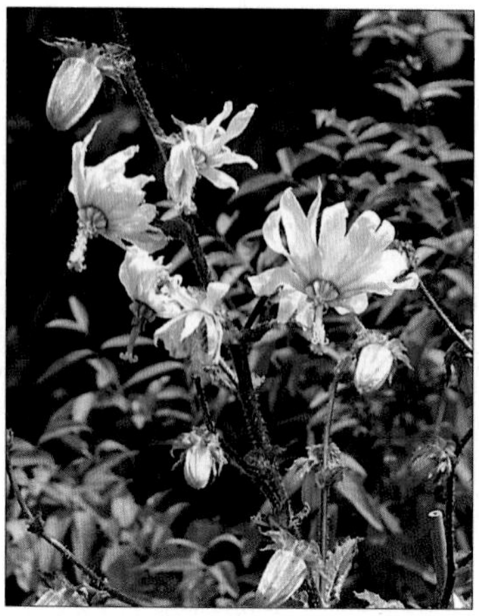
Michauxia tchihatchewii

MICHELIA

MAGNOLIACEAE

Genus of 45 species of deciduous and evergreen, rounded, spreading shrubs and upright trees from broad-leaved woodland in India and Sri Lanka, and from the Himalayas to China and S.E. Asia. They are grown for their usually fragrant, magnolia-like flowers, borne singly from the leaf axils in spring or summer. The oblong, oval-oblong, or elliptic, leathery leaves are alternate or spiralling. In frost-prone areas, grow in a cool greenhouse or conservatory. Elsewhere, grow the shrubs in a border or small courtyard garden and the trees in a woodland garden or as specimen plants.
• **HARDINESS** Half hardy to frost tender; *M. doltsopa* and *M. figo* may survive short spells near to 0°C (32°F).
• **CULTIVATION** Under glass, grow in loam-based potting compost (JI No.2), with added peat or composted bark, in full light with shade from hot sun, and low or moderate humidity. In growth, water moderately and apply a balanced liquid fertilizer monthly; water sparingly in winter. Outdoors, grow in humus-rich, moist but well-drained, neutral to acid soil, in full sun with some midday shade, or in partial shade. Shelter from cold, drying winds. Pruning group 1.
• **PROPAGATION** Sow seed in containers in a cold frame or under glass either in autumn or as soon as ripe. Root greenwood cuttings in early summer or semi-ripe cuttings in mid- or late summer. Layer in spring.
• **PESTS AND DISEASES** Prone to scale insects and red spider mites under glass.

M. doltsopa ▣ ⚲ Small, evergreen tree, sometimes shrubby. It is erect, bushy, and pyramidal when young, with slightly warty stems, spreading with age. Leaves are oval-oblong to lance-shaped, 8–18cm (3–7in) long, lustrous, dark green above, silky, grey-hairy beneath. Bowl-shaped, fragrant, white to very pale yellow flowers, 7–10cm (3–4in) across, are borne from spring to early summer. ↕ 8–15m (25–50ft), ↔ 5–10m (15–30ft). E. Himalayas, Tibet, W. and S.W. China. ❀ (min. 5°C/41°F)
M. figo ▣ Rounded, bushy, freely branching, evergreen shrub with downy, yellowish brown stems and elliptic-oblong to slightly obovate or oval leaves, 5–10cm (2–4in) long, lustrous, dark green above, paler beneath. From spring

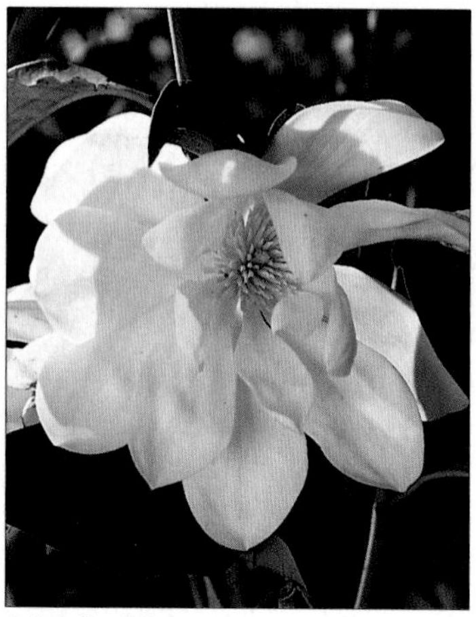
Michelia doltsopa

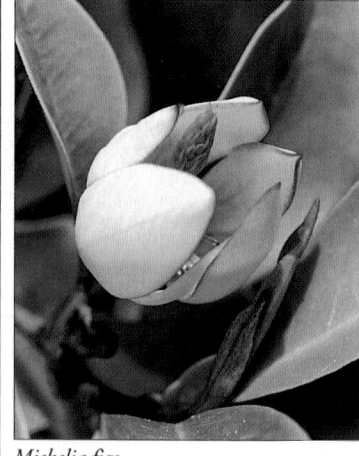
Michelia figo

to summer, bears cup-shaped, banana-scented, yellowish green to ivory-white flowers, 3cm (1¼in) across, with dark red or maroon petal margins. Flowers are initially enclosed in woolly brown bracts. ↕ 3–6m (10–20ft), ↔ 1.5–3.5m (5–11ft). China. ❀ (min. 5°C/41°F)

▷**Mickey Mouse plant** see *Ochna serrulata*

MICROBIOTA

CUPRESSACEAE

Genus of one species of prostrate to low mound-forming, evergreen, dioecious or monoecious, coniferous shrub from open slopes in S.E. Siberia. It has scale-like, broadly triangular, pointed leaves that turn bronze over winter; this can be a striking feature, although it sometimes appears that the plant is dying. The minute, ovoid cones have leathery scales, each one opening to release a single seed. Grow in a shrub border or as a specimen shrub; *M. decussata* is also a useful ground-cover plant, similar to the spreading junipers (*Juniperus*).
• **HARDINESS** Fully hardy.
• **CULTIVATION** Grow in moderately fertile, moist but well-drained soil in full sun. Pruning is not required.
• **PROPAGATION** Sow seed in a seedbed in autumn. Root semi-ripe cuttings in summer.
• **PESTS AND DISEASES** Trouble free.

M. decussata ▣ ♡ Spreading coniferous shrub with green shoots, later turning red-brown, and flat sprays of bright mid-green leaves, to 3mm (⅛in) long, paler below, in symmetrical pairs. Female cones, 3mm (⅛in) long, each have 2–4 scales, one of which is fertile; male cones, 2–4mm (1/16–⅛in) long, are pale yellow. ↕ to 1m (3ft), ↔ indefinite. Russia (S.E. Siberia). ✲✲✲

MICROCACHRYS

PODOCARPACEAE

Genus of one species of monoecious, evergreen, spreading, coniferous shrub, found on 2 mountain summits in W. Tasmania. It is cultivated for its small, scale-like, triangular leaves, borne on procumbent, snake-like branches, and, to a lesser extent, for its small, mulberry-like cones. *M. tetragona* is suitable for a shrub border or rock garden, or for ground cover.

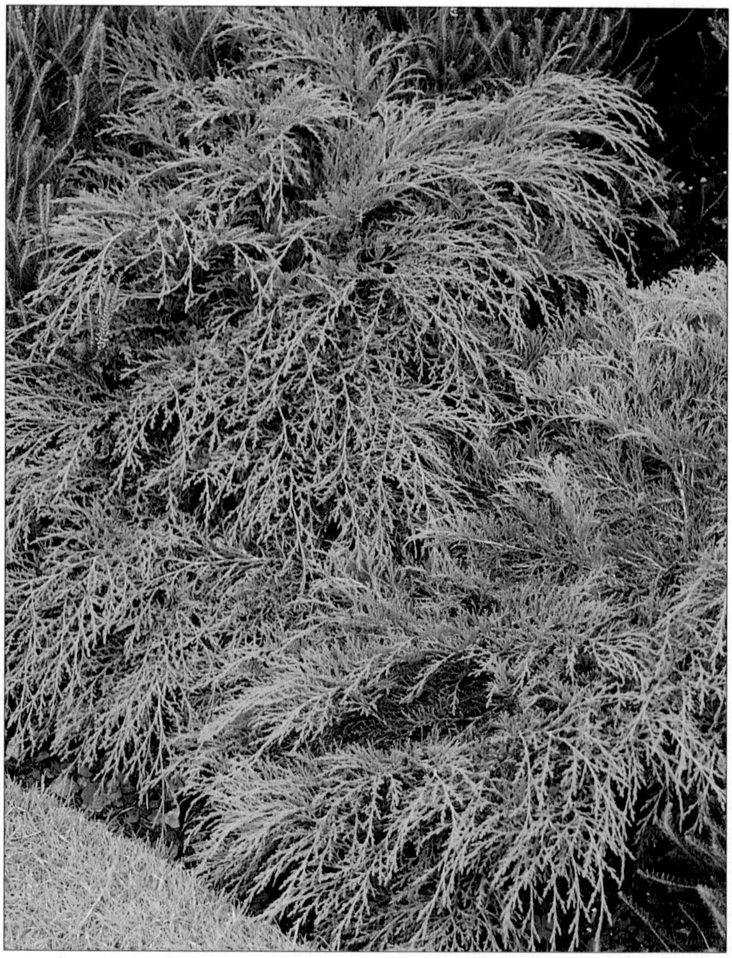
Microbiota decussata

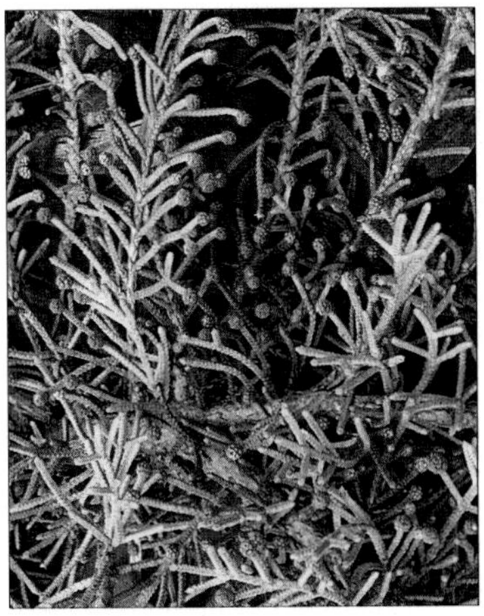

Microcachrys tetragona

• **HARDINESS** Frost hardy.
• **CULTIVATION** Grow in humus-rich, moist but well-drained, neutral to slightly acid soil in full sun, with some midday shade.
• **PROPAGATION** Sow seed as soon as ripe in a seedbed, or in containers in a cold frame. Root semi-ripe cuttings in summer.
• **PESTS AND DISEASES** Trouble free.

M. tetragona ■ Spreading, coniferous shrub with overlapping, dark green leaves, 2–3mm (1/16–1/8in) long, arranged spirally in 4 rows on the shoots. Ovoid female cones, 1cm (1/2in) long, have whorls of 4 rounded scales, becoming fleshy and translucent red, each with a single seed; oblong male cones, 3mm (1/8in) long, are borne at the ends of the shoots. ↕ to 50cm (20in), ↔ 1m (3ft). Australia (W. Tasmania). ❄❄

▷***Microcoelum weddellianum*** see *Lytocaryum weddellianum*
▷***Microglossa*** see *Aster*
M. albescens see *A. albescens*

MICROLEPIA

DENNSTAEDTIACEAE

Genus of about 45 species of terrestrial, evergreen ferns from tropical regions worldwide, mainly found at forest margins. Long-creeping rhizomes produce soft, usually dark green fronds. These are pinnate to 3-pinnate, the pinnae sometimes shallowly to deeply lobed. The round sori are formed within the margins of the leaf-blade. In frost-prone areas, grow in a temperate greenhouse. In warmer climates, *Microlepia* species and cultivars are suitable for a peat bed or woodland garden.
• **HARDINESS** Frost tender.
• **CULTIVATION** Under glass, grow in 1 part coarse leaf mould (or peat) and charcoal, and 2 parts loam-based potting compost (JI No.2), in bright indirect light with high humidity. In the growing season, water freely and apply a balanced liquid fertilizer monthly; water sparingly in winter. Outdoors, grow in humus-rich, moist but well-drained soil in light dappled or partial shade. See also p.51.
• **PROPAGATION** Sow spores in containers at 20°C (68°F) as soon as ripe. Divide rhizomes of well-established plants in spring, before new growth commences.
• **PESTS AND DISEASES** Trouble free.

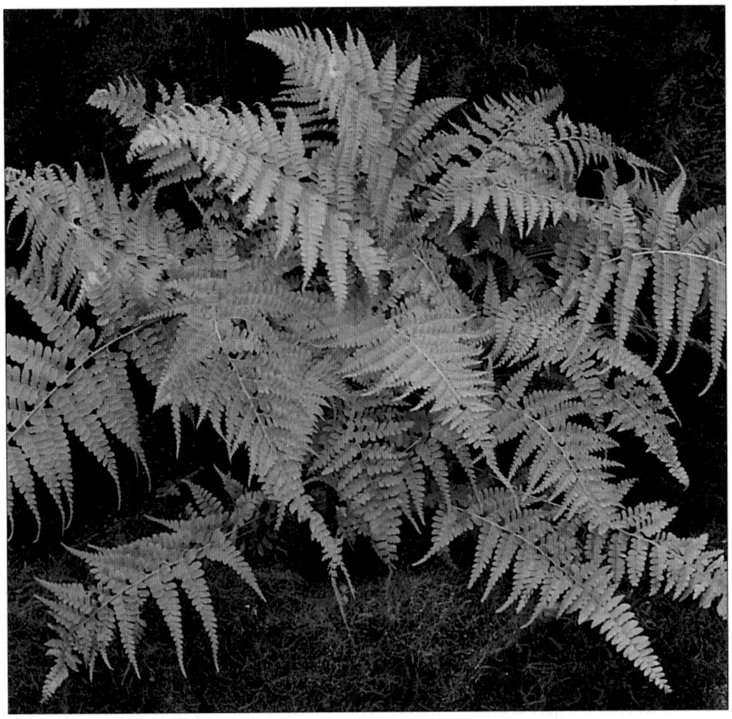

Microlepia speluncae

M. speluncae ■ Large, terrestrial, clump-forming fern producing long-stalked, triangular, 2- or 3-pinnate, dark green fronds, 0.8–1.5m (32–60in) long, which consist of triangular or lance-shaped to oblong pinnae without raised veins. ↕ to 1.5m (5ft), ↔ to 3m (10ft). S.E. Asia to Australia. ⊛ (min. 5–10°C/41–50°F)
M. strigosa. Terrestrial fern producing ovate to lance-shaped, 2- or 3-pinnate, dark green fronds, 70–90cm (28–36in) long, consisting of linear to lance-shaped pinnae. Fronds are small and often arching, and have raised veins on their lower surfaces. ↕ to 1m (3ft), ↔ to 2m (6ft). N. India to Japan and Polynesia. ⊛ (min. 5–10°C/41–50°F). **'Cristata'** produces fronds with lobed pinnae, which are crested at the tips.

MICROMERIA

LABIATAE/LAMIACEAE

Genus of about 70 species of annuals, perennials, and dwarf, evergreen shrubs (which at one time included species now placed in the genus *Acinos*). They occur in dry, rocky sites in the Mediterranean region, the Caucasus, and S.W. China. The ovate, linear, or lance-shaped, often aromatic, light to dark green leaves are arranged in opposite pairs. Spike-like racemes of small, tubular, 2-lipped, white to purple flowers are produced in short-stalked whorls in summer. *Micromeria* species are suitable for a rock garden, or at the front of a mixed border.
• **HARDINESS** Hardy to -10°C (14°F).
• **CULTIVATION** Grow in moderately fertile, well-drained soil in full sun, with protection from excessive winter wet. Pruning group 10, in early spring or after flowering.
• **PROPAGATION** Sow seed of perennials in containers in a cold frame in spring; sow seed of annuals *in situ* in late spring. Divide perennials in spring. Root softwood cuttings in early summer.
• **PESTS AND DISEASES** Trouble free.

M. corsica see *Acinos corsicus.*
M. juliana. Rounded, evergreen, downy shrub with stalkless, ovate to linear or lance-shaped, aromatic, dark green leaves, 5–10mm (1/4–1/2in) long. In summer, upright, spike-like racemes, comprising whorls of up to 20 purplish pink flowers, to 4mm (1/8in) long, are borne at the stem tips. ↕↔ 10–40cm (4–16in). Mediterranean. ❄❄

▷**Mignonette** see *Reseda*
Common see *R. odorata*
▷**Mignonette tree** see *Lawsonia*

MIKANIA

ASTERACEAE/COMPOSITAE

Genus of about 300 species of woody-stemmed and herbaceous, deciduous or evergreen, twining or scandent climbers, allied to *Eupatorium.* They occur in tropical to warm-temperate regions worldwide in a broad range of habitats, from prairies and grassland to deciduous and tropical woodland. The usually opposite leaves are simple, and may be entire, toothed, or shallowly to palmately lobed. Hemispherical flower-heads, similar to those of groundsel (*Senecio*), lack ray-florets, and are borne in spikes, racemes, corymbs, or panicles. In frost-prone areas, grow in a temperate greenhouse. In warmer climates, grow in a woodland garden, use to clothe an arch or pergola, or allow to scramble through shrubs.
• **HARDINESS** Frost tender; *M. scandens* may survive short periods at 0°C (32°F).
• **CULTIVATION** Under glass, grow in loam-based potting compost (JI No.2) in bright filtered light. In the growing season, water freely and apply a balanced liquid fertilizer monthly; water sparingly in winter. Outdoors, grow in moderately fertile, moist but well-drained soil in light dappled shade. Pruning group 11, in early spring.
• **PROPAGATION** Sow seed at 13–15°C (55–59°F) in spring. Insert softwood cuttings in late spring.
• **PESTS AND DISEASES** Red spider mites and whiteflies may prove troublesome under glass.

M. scandens (Climbing hempweed, Hemp vine). Twining climber, often semi- or fully evergreen in tropical areas, with triangular to heart-shaped, glossy, mid- to bright green leaves, 5–10cm (2–4in) long, with entire or irregularly toothed margins. From late summer to late autumn, small but dense corymbs, 2–5cm (3/4–2in) long, of vanilla-scented, usually white to pale flesh-pink, sometimes lilac to purple or yellow-tinted white flowerheads are produced from the upper leaf axils. ↕ 2–5m (6–15ft). Tropical North and South America. ⊛ (min. 5°C/41°F)

▷**Mile-a-minute plant** see *Fallopia aubertii, F. baldschuanica*
▷**Milfoil** see *Myriophyllum*
Diamond see *M. aquaticum*
Western see *M. hippuroides*

MILIUM

GRAMINEAE/POACEAE

Genus of 6 species of annual and tussock-forming, perennial grasses found mainly in woodland in temperate regions of Europe, Asia, and E. North America. They have flat, linear to lance-shaped, light to yellow-green leaves, and produce open, spreading panicles of well-spaced, single-flowered spikelets from late spring to midsummer. Grow in a herbaceous or mixed border, or in woodland.
• **HARDINESS** Fully hardy.
• **CULTIVATION** Grow in humus-rich, moist but well-drained soil in partial shade; will tolerate sun where soils remain reliably moist. May self-seed, but not in profusion.
• **PROPAGATION** Sow seed *in situ* in spring; *M. effusum* 'Aureum' comes true from seed. Divide in early spring and early summer.
• **PESTS AND DISEASES** Trouble free.

***M. effusum* 'Aureum'** (Bowles' golden grass, Golden wood millet). Slowly spreading, loosely tufted, semi-evergreen, perennial grass. Smooth, flat strap-shaped to linear leaves, to 30cm (12in) long, are rich golden yellow, particularly in spring. From late spring to midsummer, tiny golden spikelets are produced in delicate, slender, golden-stemmed, nodding panicles, 30cm (12in) long. ↕ to 60cm (24in), ↔ 30cm (12in). ❄❄❄

▷**Milk bush** see *Gomphocarpus fruticosus*
▷**Milkmaids** see *Burchardia*
▷**Milkweed** see *Asclepias, Euphorbia*
Swamp see *Asclepias incarnata*
▷**Milkwort** see *Polygala, P. calcarea*

MILLA

ALLIACEAE/LILIACEAE

Genus of about 6 species of bulbous perennials, related to *Brodiaea*, often found on dry slopes in S. USA, Mexico, and Central America. They have cylindrical or flat, linear leaves. Umbels of erect, tubular, scented flowers, each with 6 spreading tepals, are produced from summer to autumn. In frost-prone areas, lift and overwinter in frost-free

conditions, or grow in a cool greenhouse or alpine house. In warmer climates, grow in a sheltered bed under a wall, or in a herbaceous border.
• **HARDINESS** Half hardy.
• **CULTIVATION** In frost-prone areas, plant 8cm (3in) deep in well-drained soil in spring. Provide a sheltered site in full sun. Lift after flowering, and keep frost free during winter. Under glass, grow in a mix of equal parts loam, leaf mould, and sharp sand, in full light. Water sparingly until shoots appear, then apply a balanced liquid fertilizer every 4–6 weeks and water moderately. Reduce water as leaves wither and keep dry in winter. In frost-free areas, plant 10cm (4in) deep in autumn, in a well-drained, sheltered site in full sun.
• **PROPAGATION** Sow seed at 13–18°C (55–64°F) in spring. Remove offsets when dormant.
• **PESTS AND DISEASES** Trouble free.

M. biflora. Bulbous perennial with semi-erect, narrowly linear, glaucous, mid-green, basal leaves, 10–50cm (4–20in) long. In summer, bears umbels of 1–6, occasionally 8, white or white-flushed lilac or pink flowers, 1.5–3.5cm (½–1½in) long, with green central veins on the flat, spreading, reflexed tepals. ↕ 30cm (12in), ↔ 5cm (2in). S.W. USA, Mexico, Central America. ✲

▷**Millet** see *Panicum miliaceum*
Golden wood see *Milium effusum* 'Aureum'

M

MILLETTIA

LEGUMINOSAE/PAPILIONACEAE

Genus of about 120 species of deciduous and evergreen trees, shrubs, and woody-stemmed climbers from deciduous and evergreen woodland in Africa, Madagascar, India, and E. Asia. They have pinnate leaves, with lance-shaped to broadly ovate leaflets, borne alternately or in opposite pairs. Pea-like flowers are produced in terminal and lateral racemes or panicles, similar to those of wisterias. In frost-prone areas, grow in a cool or temperate greenhouse. In milder areas, grow as specimen trees or shrubs, and use climbers to clothe a fence, arch, pergola, or trellis.
• **HARDINESS** Half hardy to frost tender; *M. reticulata* will survive short periods at 0°C (32°F).
• **CULTIVATION** Under glass, grow in loam-based potting compost (JI No.2) in full light, with shade from hot sun. In the growing season, water freely and apply a balanced liquid fertilizer monthly; water sparingly in winter. Outdoors, grow in moderately fertile, well-drained soil in full sun. Pruning group 1 for trees and shrubs; group 11 for climbers, after flowering; group 13 for wall-trained plants.
• **PROPAGATION** Sow seed at 6–12°C (43–54°F) as soon as ripe. Root semi-ripe cuttings with bottom heat in summer.
• **PESTS AND DISEASES** Whiteflies, aphids, and red spider mites may be troublesome under glass.

M. reticulata. Twining, woody climber or scandent shrub bearing pinnate leaves with 5–9 lance-shaped to elliptic, semi-leathery leaflets, 3–9cm (1¼–3½in) long. In summer, produces pea-like, rose-pink, red, or blue flowers, to 1cm (½in) long, in dense racemes or panicles, 15–20cm (6–8in) long. ↕ 5m (15ft) or more, ↔ 1–2m (3–6ft). S. China, Taiwan. ❁ (min. 5°C/41°F)

MILTONIA

ORCHIDACEAE

Genus of about 15 species of evergreen, epiphytic orchids (which at one time included species now in *Miltoniopsis*), occurring mainly in warm, moist forests in Brazil. They produce ovoid to cylindrical, compressed pseudobulbs, each with 2 linear, oblong, oblong-linear, or oblong-lance-shaped, apical, usually mid-green leaves. Often star-shaped, sometimes fragrant flowers are produced in usually erect racemes from the bases of the pseudobulbs, at various times of the year.
• **HARDINESS** Frost tender.
• **CULTIVATION** Intermediate-growing orchids. Grow in containers of epiphytic compost, epiphytically on bark, or in slatted baskets. In summer, provide humid conditions with partial shade, water freely, feed at every third watering, and mist once or twice daily. In winter, admit full light and water moderately. See also p.46.
• **PROPAGATION** Divide when the plant fills the pot and "flows" over the sides.
• **PESTS AND DISEASES** Prone to aphids, red spider mites, and mealybugs.

***M.* Bluntii** (*M. clowesii* x *M. spectabilis*). Naturally occurring, epiphytic hybrid orchid with elongated pseudobulbs and linear leaves, 15cm (6in) long. In autumn, produces racemes of 3–7 star-shaped, fragrant, light yellow flowers, 8cm (3in) long, with red-brown markings, white lips, and purplish crimson bases. ↕↔ 23cm (9in). Brazil. ❁ (min. 13°C/55°F; max. 30°C/86°F)
M. candida ♀ syn. *Anneliesia candida*. Epiphytic orchid with oblong-ovoid pseudobulbs and linear-lance-shaped leaves, 30cm (12in) long. In autumn, produces racemes of 2–8 star-shaped, greenish yellow flowers, 8cm (3in) across, spotted chestnut-brown and yellow, with lips sometimes flushed white or pink. ↕↔ 23cm (9in). Brazil. ❁ (min. 13°C/55°F; max. 30°C/86°F)
M. clowesii ▣ Epiphytic orchid with narrowly ovoid pseudobulbs and linear leaves, 30cm (12in) long. In autumn, bears long racemes of 3–7 star-shaped, greenish yellow flowers, 5cm (2in) across, each barred chestnut-brown, with white lips tinted violet-purple at the bases. ↕↔ 23cm (9in). Brazil. ❁ (min. 13°C/55°F; max. 30°C/86°F)
M. phalaenopsis see *Miltoniopsis phalaenopsis*.
M. roezlii see *Miltoniopsis roezlii*.
M. spectabilis ♀ Epiphytic orchid producing elongated pseudobulbs and linear-oblong leaves, 15cm (6in) long. Throughout summer, white, red, or purple flowers, 8cm (3in) across, with red or purple lips, each with 3 yellow ridges at the base, are borne singly or occasionally in pairs. ↕↔ 23cm (9in). Brazil. ❁ (min. 13°C/55°F; max. 30°C/86°F)

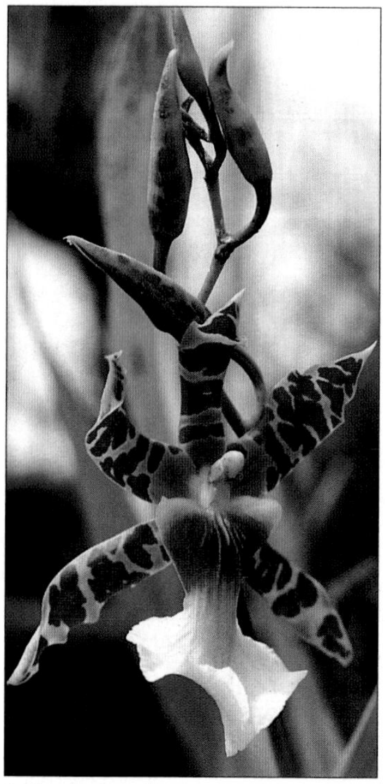

Miltonia clowesii

MILTONIOPSIS

Pansy orchid

ORCHIDACEAE

Genus of 5 species of evergreen, epiphytic or lithophytic orchids (often included in *Miltonia*) from Central and South America, found in mountainous regions from 300m (1,000ft) to over 2,000m (7,000ft). The fleshy, ovoid pseudobulbs are partially covered by soft-textured, linear, grey-green, basal leaves. Decorative, fragrant flowers, with large, flat lips, are produced in racemes from the bases of the pseudobulbs. There are many colourful hybrids, often blooming twice a year, with up to 6 flowers in a raceme.
• **HARDINESS** Frost tender.
• **CULTIVATION** Cool-growing orchids. Grow in containers of epiphytic orchid compost. In summer, provide humid, shady conditions with plenty of fresh air, water freely, and feed at every third watering; water sparingly in winter. Do not spray the foliage, as it may become spotted. See also p.46.
• **PROPAGATION** Divide when the plant fills the pot and "flows" over the sides.
• **PESTS AND DISEASES** Red spider mites, aphids, and mealybugs may prove troublesome.

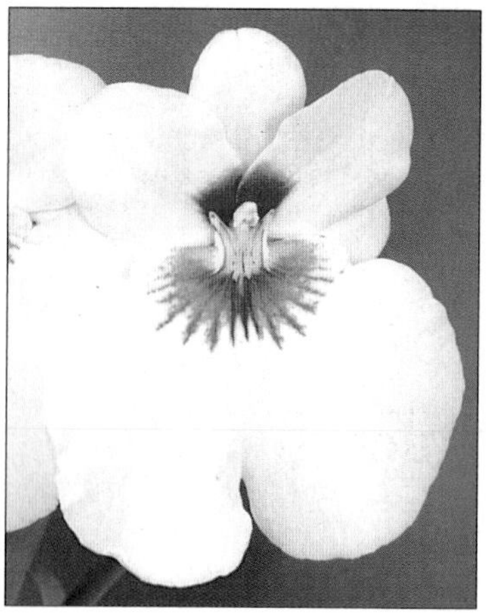

Miltoniopsis Robert Strauss 'Ardingly'

***M.* Anjou 'St. Patrick'** ▣ (*M.* Hoggar x *M.* Piccadilly). Epiphytic orchid with ovoid pseudobulbs and linear leaves, 20cm (8in) long. Deep red flowers, 8cm (3in) across, with white and orange-red marks at the bases of the lips, are borne in racemes, mostly in summer. ↕↔ 23cm (9in). ❁ (min. 11°C/52°F; max. 24°C/75°F)
***M.* Emotion 'Redbreast'** (*M.* Emoi x *M.* Nyasa). Epiphytic orchid with ovoid pseudobulbs and linear leaves, 20cm (8in) long. Bears racemes of bright cream flowers, 8cm (3in) across, with attractive brownish red flushing on the lips, mostly in summer. ↕↔ 23cm (9in). ❁ (min. 11°C/52°F; max. 24°C/75°F)
***M.* Jersey** (*M.* Hamburg x *M.* Hannover). Epiphytic orchid with ovoid pseudobulbs and linear leaves, 20cm (8in) long. Produces racemes of dark red flowers, 8cm (3in) across, with red lips, mostly in summer. ↕↔ 23cm (9in). ❁ (min. 11°C/52°F; max. 24°C/75°F)
M. phalaenopsis, syn. *Miltonia phalaenopsis*. Epiphytic orchid with compressed, ovoid pseudobulbs and narrowly linear leaves, 15–22cm (6–9in) long. Racemes of 2–4 white flowers, 5cm (2in) across, with bold, red-purple splashes on the lips, are produced in autumn. ↕↔ 15cm (6in). Colombia. ❁ (min. 11°C/52°F; max. 24°C/75°F)
***M.* Robert Strauss 'Ardingly'** ▣ (*M.* Augusta x *M.* Gattonensis). Epiphytic orchid with ovoid pseudobulbs and linear leaves, 20cm (8in) long. White flowers, 8cm (3in) across, highlighted with yellow, with red or pink petal bases, and flushed orange at the bases of the lips, are produced in racemes,

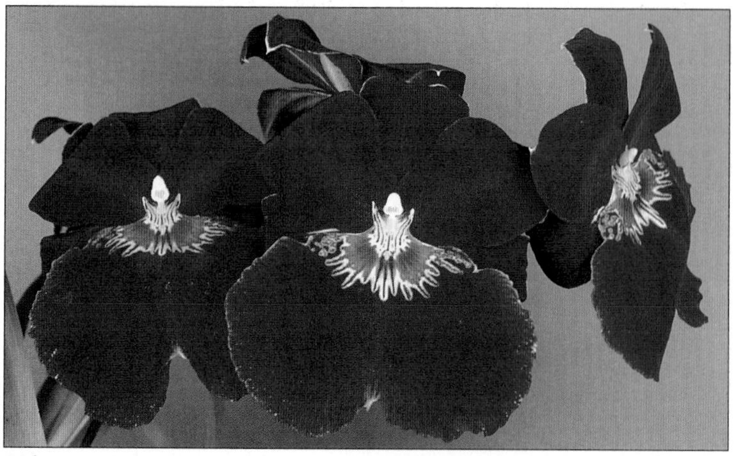

Miltoniopsis Anjou 'St. Patrick'

mostly in summer. ↕↔ 23cm (9in). ❄ (min. 11°C/52°F; max. 24°C/75°F)
M. roezlii, syn. *Miltonia roezlii*. Epiphytic orchid with ovoid pseudobulbs. Linear leaves, 15–25cm (6–10in) long, have dark green longitudinal lines beneath. In autumn and winter, bears 4- to 6-flowered racemes of white flowers, 6cm (2½in) across, with purple or red-mauve patches at the bases of the petals. ↕↔ 15cm (6in). Colombia. ❄ (min. 11°C/52°F; max. 24°C/75°F)

MIMETES

PROTEACEAE

Genus of 11 species of upright, evergreen shrubs or subshrubs from heath and scrub, often exposed, in South Africa. Alternate or spiralling, narrowly to broadly ovate, oblong, or lance-shaped, mid- to blue-green or silvery leaves are usually crowded and overlap to varying degrees. Tubular flowers enclosed in overlapping, leaf-like bracts, often with protruding perianth segments and styles, are borne terminally or in the upper leaf axils. In frost-prone climates, grow in a cool or temperate greenhouse. Elsewhere, grow in a shrub border.

• **HARDINESS** Frost tender; may survive brief spells near 0°C (32°F).

• **CULTIVATION** Under glass, grow in a mix of equal parts loam, leaf mould, and grit or perlite, with added charcoal, in full light and with good ventilation. Water moderately in growth, sparingly in winter. In spring and early autumn, apply a liquid fertilizer of magnesium sulphate and urea. Outdoors, grow in moist but well-drained, neutral to slightly acid, poor or moderately fertile soil with low levels of phosphates and nitrates, in full sun. Pruning group 1.

• **PROPAGATION** Sow seed at 6–12°C (43–54°F) as soon as ripe, in equal parts of grit and peat. Prick out seedlings into individual containers as soon as possible.

• **PESTS AND DISEASES** Red spider mites may be a problem under glass.

M. cucullatus ■ syn. *M. lyrigera* (Rooistompie). Usually erect, sometimes decumbent shrub with densely downy stems that branch from near the base. Spiralling, narrowly oblong, slightly glaucous, mid-green leaves, 3–8cm (1–3in) long, have rounded, irregularly notched, orange-brown tips. In summer, bears axillary, or sometimes terminal flowerheads, 5–7cm (2–3in) long, which consist of overlapping, red and yellow leaf-like bracts and flowers with perianth segments in the same colours but with protruding, feathery, silver-white tips and red styles. Grows on stony slopes. ↕↔ to 1.5m (5ft). South Africa (Western Cape). ❄ (min. 5°C/41°F)
M. hirtus. Erect shrub with stems that branch near the base and spiralling, ovate, very hairy, mid-green leaves, 1–6cm (½–2½in) long, often pinkish brown when young. In summer, bears terminal or axillary flowerheads, 5cm (2in) long, consisting of overlapping green leaf-like bracts, and flowers with prominent, silvery white and red-tipped, bright yellow perianth segments and red styles. Grows in marshy ground. ↕↔ to 1.5m (5ft). South Africa (Western Cape). ❄ (min. 10°C/50°F)
M. lyrigera see *M. cucullatus*.

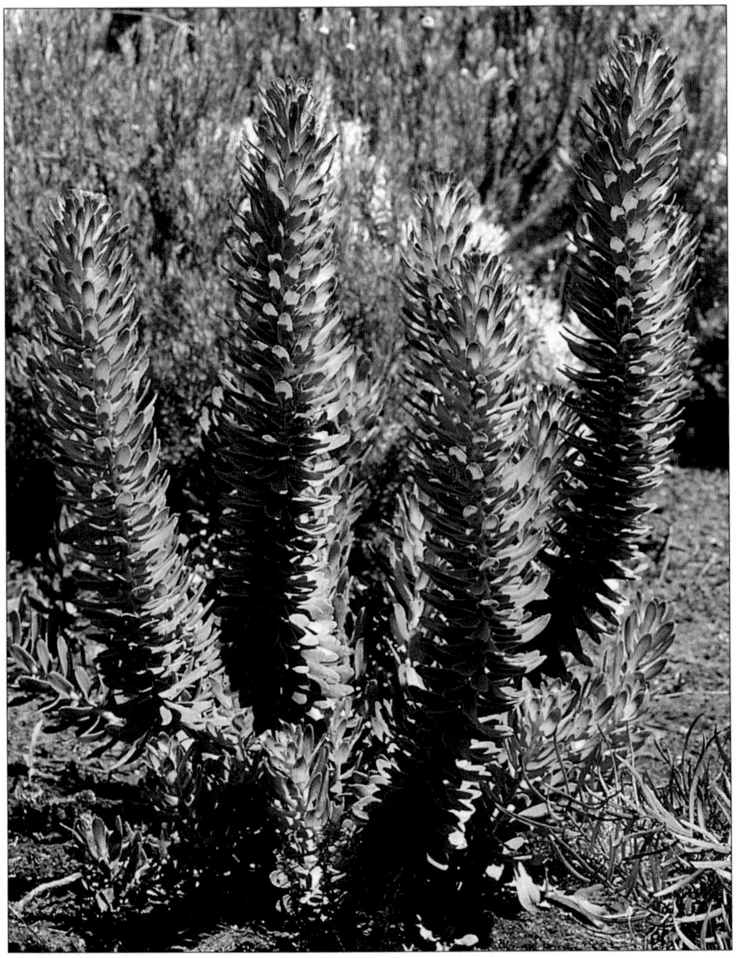

Mimetes cucullatus

MIMOSA

LEGUMINOSAE/MIMOSACEAE

Genus of about 400 species of annuals, evergreen perennials, shrubs (which are sometimes scandent or trailing), and small trees, found in habitats ranging from forest to dry savannah in tropical regions worldwide. The often spiny stems bear alternate, 2-pinnate leaves, which in some species are sensitive to touch. Tiny, pea-like flowers, each with 4 or 5 petals and up to 10 long stamens, are lightly clustered in spherical heads, which are borne singly, or in spikes or panicles. The seed pods are sometimes twisted, curled, or spiny. In climates where temperatures fall below 13–16°C (55–61°F), grow in a warm greenhouse or as houseplants. In warmer areas, grow the annuals and perennials as ground cover, the shrubs in a border, and the trees as specimen plants. Long, hot summers are required for the production of flowers and fruits. (For the yellow-flowered florists' mimosa, see *Acacia dealbata*.)

• **HARDINESS** Frost tender.

• **CULTIVATION** Under glass, grow in loam-based potting compost (JI No.2) in full light, with shade from hot sun. In the growing season, water moderately and apply a balanced liquid fertilizer monthly; water sparingly in winter. Outdoors, grow in moderately fertile, well-drained soil in full sun, although they will tolerate light dappled shade. Pruning group 1.

• **PROPAGATION** Sow seed at 18–24°C (64–75°F) in spring. Alternatively, root softwood cuttings with bottom heat in early summer.

• **PESTS AND DISEASES** Red spider mites may be troublesome under glass.

M. pudica ■ (Humble plant, Sensitive plant). Bushy, mat-forming annual or short-lived, evergreen perennial with slender, prickly, branching stems. Bright green to greyish green leaves, 5–10cm (2–4in) long, each have 4 radiating linear leaflets divided into 10–25 pairs of narrow, oblong segments that fold up when touched. Spherical, light pink to lilac flowerheads, 1–2cm (½–¾in) across, are produced mainly in summer. ↕ 30–75cm (12–30in), ↔ 40–90cm (16–36in). Tropical North and South America. ❄ (min. 13°C/55°F)

▷**Mimosa** see *Acacia dealbata*

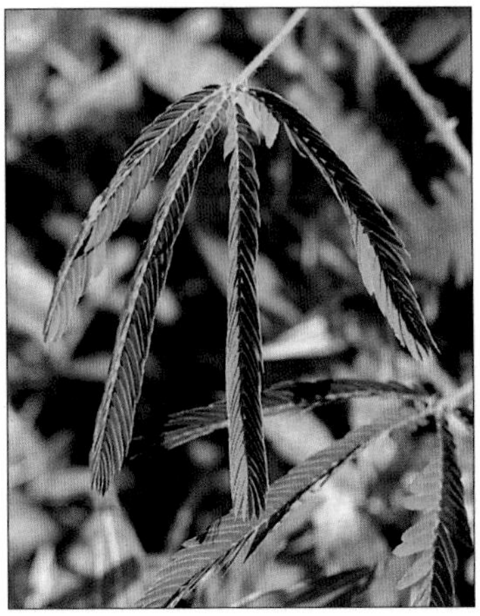

Mimosa pudica

MIMULUS syn. DIPLACUS

Monkey flower, Musk

SCROPHULARIACEAE

Genus of about 150 species of annuals, perennials, and evergreen shrubs found in southern Africa, Asia, Australia, and North, Central, and South America, usually occurring in damp areas but sometimes found in chaparral or deserts. The opposite, entire or toothed leaves are linear to nearly rounded, and mostly pale to dark green. Snapdragon-like, 5-lobed, 2-lipped, tubular or trumpet- or funnel-shaped flowers, often heavily spotted in contrasting colours, are borne from spring to autumn on upright stems, either in the axils or in spike-like racemes. The smaller species and cultivars are suitable for a damp pocket in a rock garden; grow most of the larger ones in a damp border or bog garden. Use the shrubs in a warm border. In frost-prone areas, grow the tender perennials in a cold greenhouse or as bedding annuals, and the tender shrubs in a cool greenhouse or conservatory.

• **HARDINESS** Fully hardy to frost tender.

• **CULTIVATION** Outdoors, grow most species in fertile, humus-rich, very moist soil in full sun or light dappled shade. *M. aurantiacus*, *M. longiflorus*, and *M. puniceus* need well-drained soil and full sun; *M. cardinalis* and *M. lewisii* tolerate drier soils. *M. luteus* can be grown in water to 7cm (3in) deep, *M. ringens* to 15cm (6in). Under glass, grow in loam-based potting compost (JI No.2) in full light, with shade from hot sun and good ventilation. In the growing season, water freely and apply a balanced liquid fertilizer monthly; keep moist in winter. Monkey flowers are often short-lived, so propagate regularly. Pruning group 9 for shrubs.

• **PROPAGATION** Sow seed of hardy species and variants in containers in a cold frame in autumn or early spring; sow seed of tender ones at 6–12°C (43–54°C) in spring; plant out after danger of frost has passed. Divide perennials in spring. Root softwood cuttings in early summer, and semi-ripe cuttings of shrubs in midsummer.

• **PESTS AND DISEASES** Slugs and snails may cause damage. Young plants are susceptible to powdery mildew.

M. 'Andean Nymph' ■ ♀ Spreading perennial with branching rhizomes and narrowly ovate to triangular-ovate,

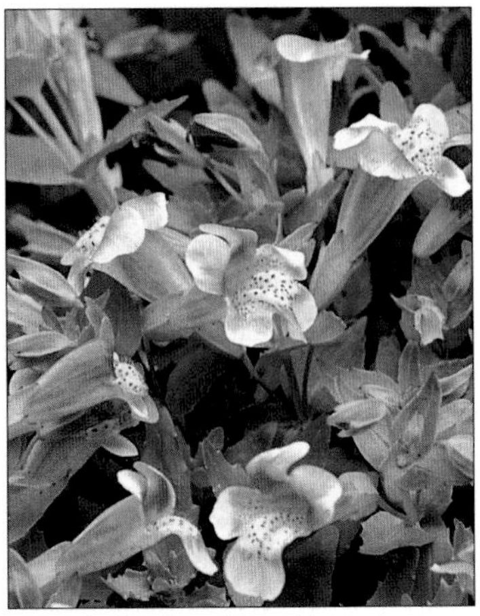

Mimulus 'Andean Nymph'

MIMULUS

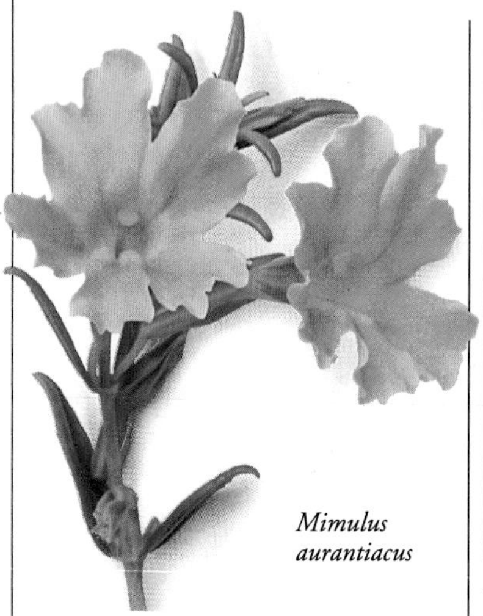

Mimulus aurantiacus

hairy, sparsely toothed, pale green leaves, to 3cm (1¼in) long. Leafy racemes of trumpet-shaped, white to cream flowers, to 2cm (¾in) across, the lobes heavily stained pink-purple, and with pink-spotted cream throats and lower lips, are borne over a long period in summer. ↕ to 20cm (8in), ↔ to 30cm (12in). Andes. ❄❄

M. aurantiacus ■ ♀ syn. *Diplacus glutinosus, M. glutinosus.* Erect, often laxly branched shrub with lance-shaped to oblong, toothed, sticky, glossy, rich green leaves, to 7cm (3in) long. Open trumpet-shaped, orange, yellow, or dark red flowers, to 4.5cm (1¾in) long, with wavy petal margins, are produced in leafy racemes from late summer to autumn. ↕↔ 1m (3ft). USA (Oregon, California). ❄❄

M. x bartonianus (*M. cardinalis* x *M. lewisii*). Upright perennial with elliptic, lobed, toothed, softly hairy, sticky, mid-green leaves, to 7cm (3in) long. From early summer to early autumn, produces solitary, axillary, tubular, bright clear pink to rose-red flowers, to 3cm (1¼in) long, with wide lips and with red-brown spots on the yellow throats. ↕ 60cm (24in), ↔ 45cm (18in). Garden origin. ❄❄

M. cardinalis ■ ♀ (Scarlet monkey flower). Creeping perennial with erect, branching, hairy stems bearing ovate to oblong-elliptic, sharply toothed, downy, light green leaves, to 10cm (4in) long. Throughout summer, produces solitary, axillary, tubular scarlet flowers, 4–5cm (1½–2in) long, sometimes with yellow throat markings; the lips are wide open but the tubular throats pinched. ↕ 90cm

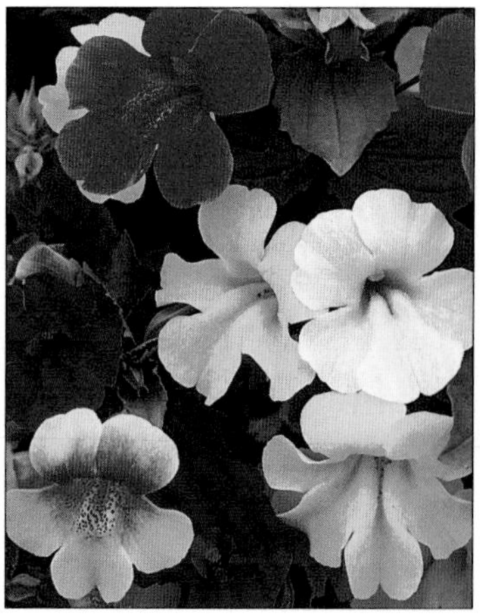

Mimulus x *hybridus* Magic Series

(36in), ↔ 60cm (24in). W. USA to Mexico. ❄❄❄ (borderline)

***M. cupreus* 'Whitecroft Scarlet'** see *M.* 'Whitecroft Scarlet'.

M. glutinosus see *M. aurantiacus.*

M. glutinosus* var. *puniceus see *M. puniceus.*

M. guttatus, syn. *M. langsdorfii.* Upright to spreading, vigorous perennial, producing stolons that root at the nodes. Broadly ovate to oval, mid-green leaves, 1–8cm (½–3in) long, are coarsely or sometimes deeply toothed. In summer, produces racemes of funnel-shaped yellow flowers, 1.5–2.5cm (½–1in) long, often tinged or strongly spotted or marked red at the throats. ↕ to 30cm (12in), ↔ 50–120cm (20–48in). North America (Alaska to California). ❄❄❄

***M.* 'Highland Yellow'.** Upright perennial with branching rhizomes and narrowly ovate, sparsely toothed, hairy, pale green leaves, 3–8cm (1¼–3in) long. Trumpet-shaped, pale creamy yellow flowers, 2 per axil, each to 2.5cm (1in) across, usually with few spots, are produced over a long period in summer. ↕ to 20cm (8in), ↔ to 30cm (12in). ❄❄

***M. x hybridus* cultivars** (*M. guttatus* x *M. luteus*). Erect, basally branching, bushy, tender perennials, often grown as annuals, with oval to elliptic, toothed, mid- to dark green leaves, 3–7cm (1¼–3in) long. In summer, they bear axillary, solitary, tubular then flaring, open-mouthed, brightly coloured, usually spotted flowers, to 5cm (2in) across; the upper lips are 2-lobed, the lower ones 3-lobed. ↕ 12–30cm (5–12in), ↔ to 30cm (12in). ❄❄❄.

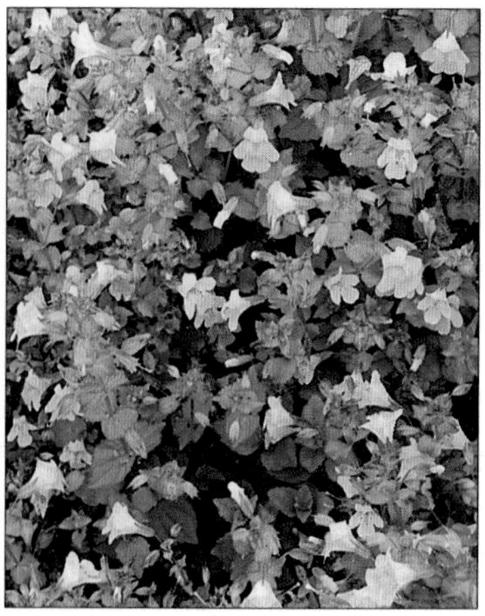

Mimulus luteus

'Calypso' is available as a mixture, and produces self-coloured, bicoloured, and spotted flowers in a wide colour range, including mixtures of orange, yellow, burgundy-red, and pink; ↕ 13–23cm (5–9in). **Magic Series** ■ cultivars are early-flowering, producing small flowers in a broad range of colours, including bright oranges, yellows, and reds, as well as more unusual pastel shades and bicolours; ↕ 15–20cm (6–8in). **Mystic Series** cultivars are compact and early-flowering, producing wine-red or bright red, ivory-white, yellow, rose-pink, or orange flowers, almost entirely without marking or spotting; ↕ 13–23cm (5–9in). **'Viva'** is large and vigorous, with large, bright yellow flowers, with a broad red mark on each lobe; ↕ 20–30cm (8–12in).

M. langsdorfii see *M. guttatus.*

***M.* 'Leopard'.** Spreading perennial with branching rhizomes and narrowly ovate, sparsely toothed, hairy, pale green leaves, 3–8cm (1¼–3in) long. Solitary, axillary, trumpet-shaped yellow flowers, 2.5cm (1in) across, spotted reddish brown, are borne over long periods in summer. ↕ to 20cm (8in), ↔ to 30cm (12in). ❄❄

M. lewisii ■ ♀ Upright perennial with oblong-elliptic, minutely toothed, stalkless, softly hairy, glandular, sticky, mid-green leaves, to 7cm (3in) long. Solitary, axillary, tubular, purple-pink to deep rose-pink, sometimes white flowers, 3–5cm (1¼–2in) long, with yellowish white throats, are produced throughout summer. ↕ 60cm (24in), ↔ 45cm (18in). North America (Alaska to California). ❄❄

M. longiflorus. Variable, erect-branched shrub with lance-shaped to oblong, toothed, sticky, pale green leaves, to 8cm (3in) long, with impressed veins. From spring to summer, bears trumpet-shaped, orange, lemon-yellow to cream, or dark red flowers, to 6cm (2½in) long, with dark orange bands at the mouths, in leafy racemes. ↕↔ 1m (3ft). USA (California), N.W. Mexico. ❄

M. luteus ■ (Monkey musk, Yellow monkey flower). Vigorous, spreading perennial with decumbent or upright stems and toothed, broadly ovate to oblong, mid-green leave^, 2–3cm (¾–1¼in) long. Yellow flowers, 2–5cm (¾–2in) long, 2 per axil, with dark red or purple-red spots on the petal lobes and throats, are borne from late spring to summer. Self-seeds freely. ↕ 30cm (12in), ↔ to 60cm (24in). Chile, widely naturalized elsewhere. ❄❄❄

M. primuloides. Rhizomatous, mat-forming perennial with hairy, oblong to obovate, entire or toothed, light to mid-green leaves, 1–4cm (½–1½in) long. Trumpet-shaped yellow flowers, to 2cm (¾in) long, with red-spotted throats, are produced on short stems, usually 2 per axil, in summer. ↕ to 10cm (4in), ↔ to 20cm (8in). W. USA. ❄❄❄

M. puniceus, syn. *M. glutinosus* var. *puniceus.* Erect-branched shrub with narrowly lance-shaped, toothed, sticky, dark green leaves, to 7cm (3in) long. Funnel-shaped, brick-red to orange-red flowers, 5cm (2in) long, are produced in leafy racemes from spring to late summer. ↕ 1.5m (5ft). USA (California), N.W. Mexico. ❄❄

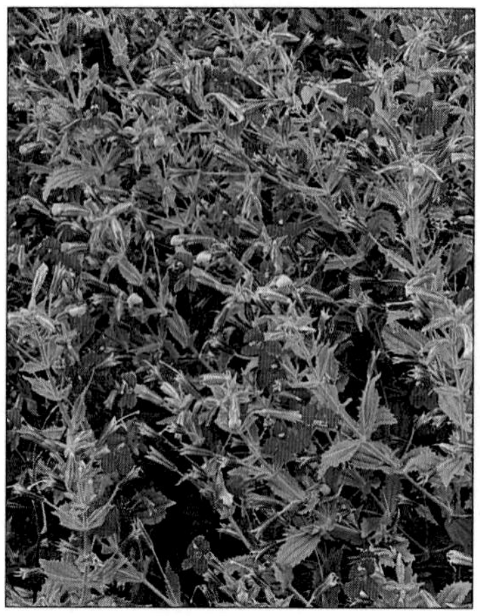

Mimulus cardinalis

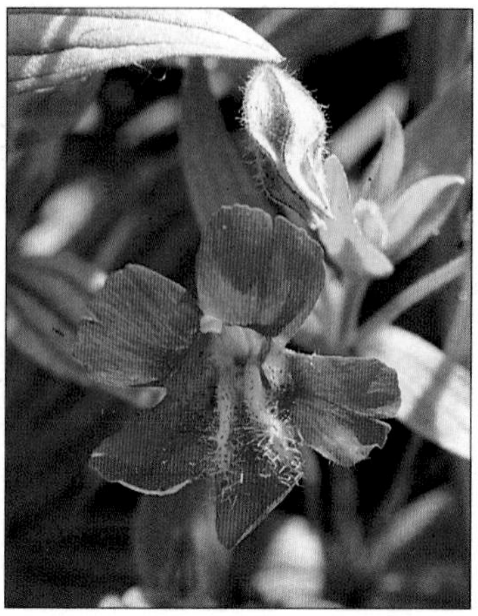

Mimulus lewisii

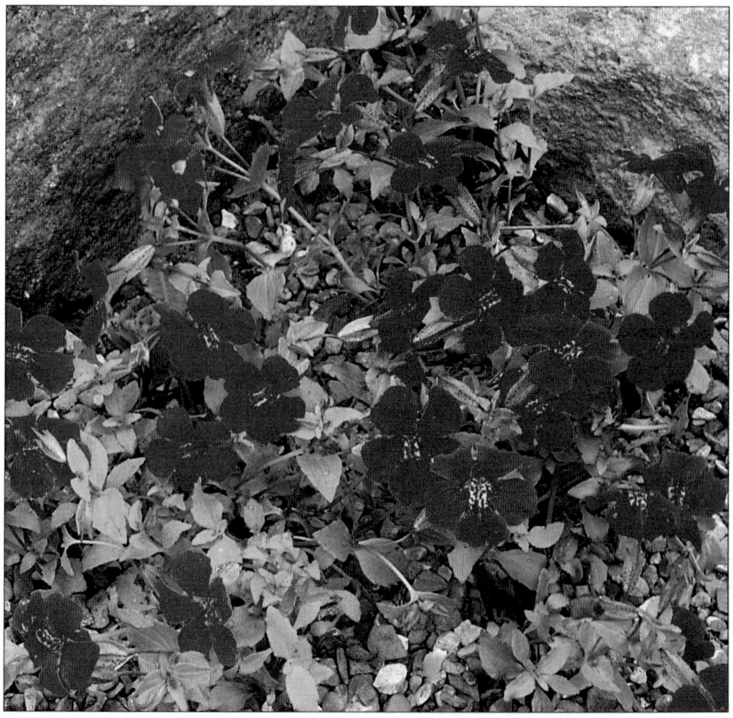

Mimulus 'Whitecroft Scarlet'

M

M. ringens (Allegheny monkey flower). Erect, hairless perennial with square, branching stems and semi-clasping, lance-shaped to narrowly oblong or inversely lance-shaped, toothed, mid-green leaves, 5–10cm (2–4in) long. Solitary, axillary, tubular, violet, violet-blue, white, or rarely pink flowers, 3cm (1¼in) long, with narrow throats, are produced from early to late summer. ↕ to 90cm (36in), ↔ 30cm (12in). E. North America. ❄❄❄

***M.* 'Whitecroft Scarlet'** ■ 🏆 syn. *M. cupreus* 'Whitecroft Scarlet'. Short-lived, spreading perennial bearing ovate, mid-green leaves, 2–8cm (¾–3in) long, with toothed margins. Numerous trumpet-shaped, deep scarlet flowers, 2cm (¾in) across, are produced in many-flowered racemes over a long period from early to late summer. ↕ to 10cm (4in), ↔ to 15cm (6in). ❄❄

***M.* 'Wisley Red'.** Short-lived, spreading perennial with branching rhizomes and narrowly ovate to lance-shaped, hairy, pale green leaves, to 3cm (1¼in) long, with sparsely toothed margins. Solitary, axillary, trumpet-shaped, velvety, blood-red flowers, to 2cm (¾in) across, are produced in summer. ↕ 15cm (6in), ↔ to 20cm (8in). ❄❄

▷***Mina*** see *Ipomoea*
▷**Mind your own business** see *Soleirolia soleirolii*
▷**Mint** see *Mentha*
Apple see *M. suaveolens*
Bowles' see *M.* x *villosa* f. *alopecuroides*
Corsican see *M. requienii*
Eau de Cologne see *M.* x *piperita* f. *citrata*
Ginger see *M.* x *gracilis* 'Variegata'
Lemon see *M.* x *piperita* f. *citrata*
Pineapple see *M. suaveolens* 'Variegata'
Red see *M.* x *gracilis* 'Variegata'
▷**Mint bush** see *Prostanthera*
Alpine see *P. cuneata*
Oval-leaved see *P. ovalifolia*
Round-leaved see *P. rotundifolia*
Snowy see *P. nivea*
▷**Mintleaf** see *Plectranthus madagascariensis*

MIRABILIS

NYCTAGINACEAE

Genus of about 50 species of annuals and tuberous perennials occurring in dry, open habitats in S.W. USA and Central and South America. Branched stems bear opposite, ovate leaves. Large, trumpet-shaped, often fragrant flowers, are borne in axillary corymbs or panicles over a long period in summer. In frost-prone areas, grow most perennial species as annuals, lift after flowering, and overwinter in frost-free conditions; alternatively, grow in a cool greenhouse. In warmer climates, grow in a border.

• **HARDINESS** Frost hardy to frost tender.

• **CULTIVATION** Outdoors, grow in moderately fertile, well-drained soil in full sun, watering freely while in growth. Provide protection from excessive winter wet. In frost-prone areas, protect perennials with a mulch or lift tubers and store in frost-free conditions over winter, and then plant out in late spring. Under glass, grow in loam-based potting compost (JI No.2), with added grit, in full light. In the growing season, water freely and apply a balanced liquid fertilizer monthly; keep dry in winter.

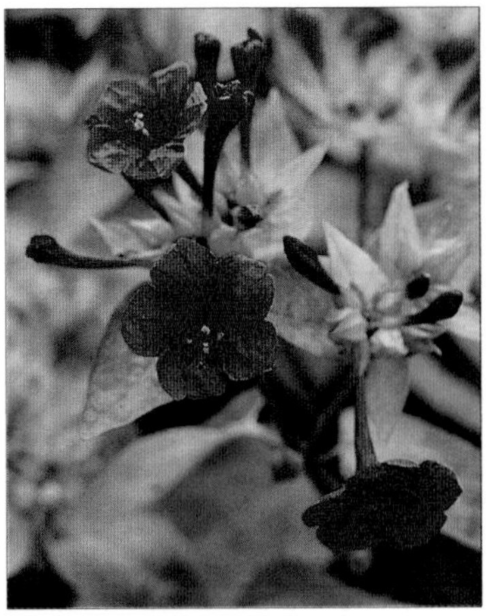

Mirabilis jalapa

• **PROPAGATION** Sow seed at 13–18°C (55–64°F) in early spring, or *in situ* after danger of frost has passed. Divide tubers in spring.

• **PESTS AND DISEASES** Slugs and aphids may be troublesome.

M. jalapa ■ (Four o'clock flower, Marvel of Peru). Bushy perennial with ovate leaves, 5–10cm (2–4in) long. Fragrant, red, pink, magenta, yellow, or white flowers, to 5cm (2in) long, some striped, and often with several colours present on the same plant, are borne from early to late summer. Individual flowers open in late afternoon and die by morning. ↕↔ 60cm (24in) or more. Peru, tropical North, Central, and South America. ❄❄ (borderline)

MISCANTHUS

GRAMINEAE/POACEAE

Genus of 17–20 species of deciduous or evergreen, tufted or rhizomatous, perennial grasses occurring in moist meadows and marshland from Africa to E. Asia. The reed-like stems bear linear or narrowly lance-shaped, folded, arching, light or mid-green, or blue- or purplish green leaves. Dense, terminal, arching panicles of silky-hairy spikelets are borne in late summer and autumn; flowerheads are more numerous following long, hot summers. In many cases, the dying growth provides russet autumn colours, and is sometimes attractive in winter. Grow *Miscanthus* species and cultivars as free-standing specimens, or in a mixed or herbaceous border. They may also be used for waterside planting or temporary summer screening. The flowerheads may be used for cutting.

• **HARDINESS** Fully hardy to frost hardy.

• **CULTIVATION** Tolerant of most conditions but best in moderately fertile, moist but well-drained soil in full sun. Protect from excessive winter wet. Where withered stems are left for winter effect, they should be cut to the ground by early spring; however, *M. floridulus* may lose dead foliage in strong winds.

• **PROPAGATION** Sow seed in containers in a cold frame in early spring. Divide as new growth commences in spring. May be slow to establish; pot on divisions or grow in a cold frame or cold or cool greenhouse until established.

• **PESTS AND DISEASES** Trouble free.

M. floridulus 🏆 Deciduous or evergreen, slowly spreading, clump-forming, perennial grass with sturdy, upright stems and downward-arching, linear, glaucous, pale green leaves, to 90cm (36in) long, with silver midribs. Erect, pyramidal panicles, to 50cm (20in) long, of silvery spikelets, are produced in autumn, although these are rarely borne in cooler regions. Often confused with *M. sacchariflorus*. ↕ 2.5m (9ft), ↔ 1.5m (5ft) or more. S.E. Asia. ❄❄❄

M. sacchariflorus (Silver banner grass). Deciduous, robust, clump-forming, perennial grass bearing stiff, flat, linear, blue-green leaves, to 90cm (36in) long, with pale, silver-green midribs. In late summer and early autumn, produces finely hairy, pyramidal or fan-shaped panicles, to 40cm (16in) long, of numerous silky-hairy, silvery white spikelets. ↕ 1.5–2.2m (5–7ft), ↔ 1.4m (4½ft). S.E. Asia. ❄❄

M. sinensis 🏆 Deciduous, clump-forming, perennial grass with erect stems and mostly basal, flat, erect or arching, linear, blue-green leaves, to 1.2m (4ft) long. Pyramidal panicles, to 40cm (16in) long, of silky-hairy, pale grey spikelets, tinted maroon or purple-brown, are produced in autumn. ↕ to 4m (12ft), ↔ 1.2m (4ft). S.E. Asia. ❄❄❄. **'Cabaret'** has broad, mid-green leaves with conspicuous white stripes; ↕ to 1.8m (6ft). **'Gracillimus'** (Maiden grass) has very narrow, curved leaves with white midribs, becoming bronzed in autumn; ↕ 1.3m (4½ft). **'Kleine Silberspinne'** is lower-growing, bearing open, spidery, white-tinged red panicles, fading to silver, from late summer to autumn; ↕ 1.2m (4ft). **'Morning Light'** resembles 'Gracillimus' but has narrow white leaf margins, giving a silvery effect; ↕ 1.2m (4ft). **'Pünktchen'** is stiffly upright, with creamy yellow horizontal bands on the leaves; ↕ 1.2m (4ft). **var. *purpurascens*** has leaves that turn purplish green, with pink midribs, in summer, and develop red and orange tones in autumn; ↕ 1.2m (4ft).

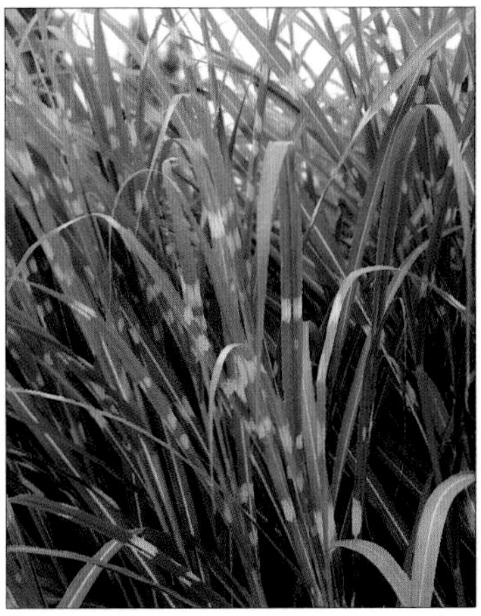

Miscanthus sinensis 'Zebrinus'

'Rotsilber' bears rich red-tinted silver panicles in late summer and early autumn, above narrow leaves with prominent silver midribs; ↕ 1.2m (4ft). **'Silberfeder'** ■ syn. 'Silver Feather', is free-flowering, bearing silvery to pale pinkish brown panicles in early and mid-autumn, remaining through winter; ↕ to 2.5m (8ft). **'Silver Feather'** see 'Silberfeder'. **'Variegatus'** has leaves with creamy white and pale green longitudinal bands; ↕ 1.8m (6ft). **'Zebrinus'** ■ (Zebra grass) is broadly arching, with creamy white or pale yellow horizontal bands on the leaves; ↕ to 1.2m (4ft).

M. yakushimensis. Dense, clump-forming, deciduous, perennial grass with narrowly linear leaves, to 60cm (24in) long; leaves are light green, with silvery pink midribs, and turn yellow in autumn. Slender, open, conical or fan-shaped silvery panicles, to 50cm (20in) long, are produced in late summer and early autumn. ↕ 60–75cm (24–30in), ↔ 75cm (30in). Japan. ❄❄❄

▷**Mission bells** see *Fritillaria biflora*
▷**Miss Willmott's ghost** see *Eryngium giganteum*

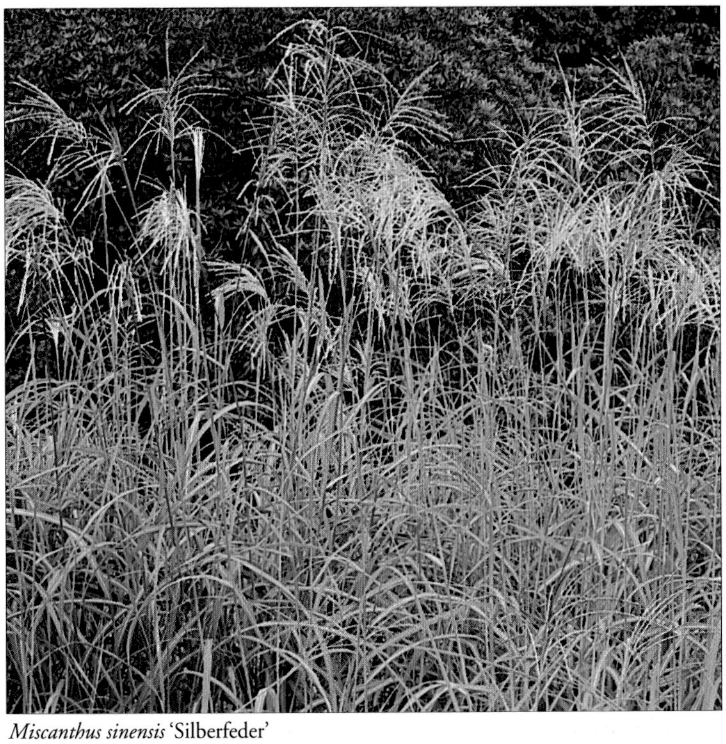

Miscanthus sinensis 'Silberfeder'

MITCHELLA

Partridge berry

RUBIACEAE

Genus of 2 species of trailing, evergreen perennials found in woodland in North America and Japan. The trailing stems root at the nodes and bear opposite, broadly ovate to lance-shaped leaves. Small, funnel-shaped, fragrant white flowers, borne in pairs in summer, are followed by ornamental red berries. Grow in a rock garden or woodland garden, or on a peat terrace.
• **HARDINESS** Fully hardy.
• **CULTIVATION** Grow in moist but well-drained, humus-rich, acid soil in light dappled or partial shade.
• **PROPAGATION** Sow seed in containers in a cold frame in autumn; keep moist after sowing. Separate rooted runners in spring.
• **PESTS AND DISEASES** Trouble free.

M. repens (Creeping box, Partridge berry). Prostrate, mat-forming perennial with broadly ovate, glossy, dark green, white-veined leaves, to 2cm (¾in) long. White, often pink-flushed flowers, 1cm (½in) long, are borne in early summer, followed by spherical, bright red berries, to 1cm (½in) across. ↕5cm (2in), ↔ to 30cm (12in). North America. ❄❄❄

MITELLA

Bishop's cap, Mitrewort

SAXIFRAGACEAE

Genus of 20 species of clump-forming, rhizomatous perennials occurring in woodland in E. Asia and North America. The long-stalked, lobed, ovate, glossy, mid- or dark green, basal leaves are heart-shaped at the bases. Slender, often one-sided, occasionally leafy racemes of tiny, pendent or horizontal, bell-shaped flowers, each with 5 fringed petals, are borne in summer. Use for ground cover in a woodland garden.
• **HARDINESS** Fully hardy.

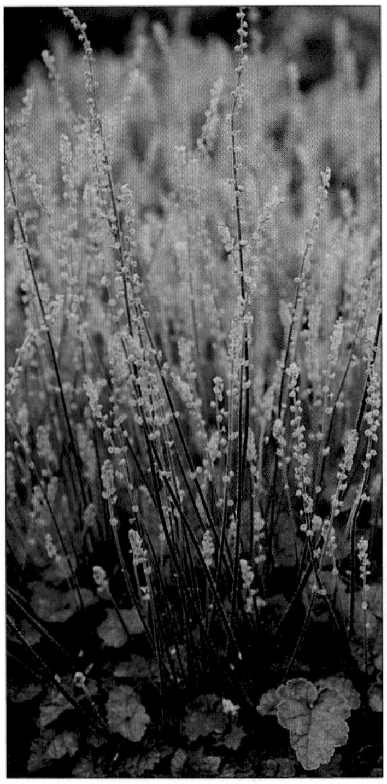

Mitella breweri

• **CULTIVATION** Grow in moist but well-drained, leafy, acid soil in partial or dappled shade. They self-seed freely.
• **PROPAGATION** Sow seed in containers in a cold frame in autumn. Divide in spring.
• **PESTS AND DISEASES** Slugs and snails may be a problem.

M. breweri ▣ Perennial with hairy, indistinctly lobed, broadly ovate, mid-green leaves, 5–10cm (2–4in) long. In late spring and summer, bears racemes of 20–40 yellowish green flowers, 2mm (1⁄16in) long, with fringed, comb-like petals, on stems to 15cm (6in) tall. ↕15cm (6in), ↔ to 20cm (8in). W. to C. North America. ❄❄❄

M. stauropetala. Vigorous perennial with broadly ovate, slightly lobed, often purple-tinged, mid-green leaves, 4–10cm (1½–4in) long. In summer, bears racemes of 10–35 white or purple flowers, to 4mm (⅛in) long, with deeply cut and fringed petals, on stems to 50cm (20in) tall. ↕ to 50cm (20in), ↔ to 30cm (12in). North America (Rocky Mountains). ❄❄❄

MITRARIA

GESNERIACEAE

Genus of one species of woody, evergreen, scandent or spreading shrub from moist woodland in Chile and Argentina. The leaves are opposite and ovate, and the showy flowers are tubular. *M. coccinea* prefers cool, humid climates. Grow in a woodland garden or sheltered shrub border. Where frosts are severe, grow in a cool greenhouse.
• **HARDINESS** Frost hardy borderline.
• **CULTIVATION** Under glass, grow in lime-free (ericaceous) potting compost in bright filtered light, with moderate to high humidity. In growth, water freely and apply a balanced liquid fertilizer monthly; water sparingly in winter but do not allow to dry out. Outdoors, grow in moist but well-drained, humus-rich, acid soil in light dappled shade. Shelter from cold, drying winds. Keep roots cool and shaded, but allow the top to grow into sunlight. Pruning group 9.
• **PROPAGATION** Sow seed in containers in a cold frame in spring. Root semi-ripe cuttings with bottom heat in summer.
• **PESTS AND DISEASES** Trouble free.

M. coccinea ▣ Weakly scandent shrub with opposite, ovate, toothed, leathery, glossy, dark green leaves, to 2.5cm (1in) long. Scarlet flowers, 3cm (1¼in) long, each with 5 small lobes, are borne singly from the leaf axils over a long period from late spring to autumn. ↕ to 2m (6ft). Chile, Argentina. ❄❄ (borderline)

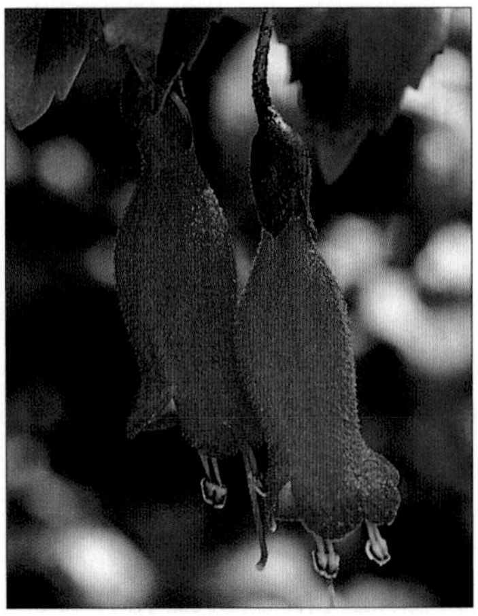

Mitraria coccinea

▷**Mitrewort** see *Mitella*
▷**Mock orange** see *Philadelphus*, *P. coronarius*
Australian see *Pittosporum undulatum*
Japanese see *Pittosporum tobira*
▷***Modecca digitata*** see *Adenia digitata*
▷**Mole plant** see *Euphorbia lathyris*

MOLINIA

GRAMINEAE/POACEAE

Genus of 2 species of loosely or densely tufted, perennial grasses found in damp moorland in Europe and N. and S.W. Asia. They are grown for their attractive habit, autumn foliage, and graceful, dense to open panicles of compressed spikelets, each with 4 florets, held well above the foliage. Grow in a mixed or herbaceous border, or woodland garden.
• **HARDINESS** Fully hardy.
• **CULTIVATION** Grow in any moist but well-drained, preferably acid to neutral soil, in full sun or partial shade.
• **PROPAGATION** Sow seed of species in containers in a cold frame in spring. Divide species and cultivars in spring, and pot up until established.
• **PESTS AND DISEASES** Trouble free.

M. caerulea (Purple moor grass). Tufted perennial with dense clumps of flat, linear-oblong, mid-green leaves, to 45cm (18in) long, with purple bases. From spring to autumn, bears dense, narrow panicles, 40cm (16in) long, of purple spikelets on yellow-tinted stems. ↕ to 1.5m (5ft), ↔ 40cm (6in). Europe, N. and S.W. Asia. ❄❄❄. **subsp. *arundinacea* 'Karl Foerster'** ▣ has leaves to 80cm (32in) long, and open panicles of purple spikelets on arching stems. **subsp. *arundinacea* 'Sky Racer'** has leaves, to 1m (3ft) long, that turn clear gold in autumn; ↕ to 2.2m (7ft). **'Moorhexe'** is very upright, with dark purple spikelets held tightly against erect stems; ↕45cm (18in). **'Variegata'** is tufted and compact, with dark green, cream-striped leaves, ochre stems, and purple spikelets; ↕45–60cm (18–24in).

MOLTKIA

BORAGINACEAE

Genus of about 6 species of perennials or shrubs, some evergreen, found in alkaline soils in rock crevices or on open hillsides from N. Italy and Greece to S.W. Asia. They have alternate, oblong or linear to lance-shaped or inversely lance-shaped, hairy, mid- or dark green leaves. Tubular or funnel-shaped, blue, purple, or yellow flowers are borne in short, one-sided, terminal cymes from late spring to summer. Grow in a Mediterranean or rock garden, or at the front of a mixed or shrub border.
• **HARDINESS** Fully hardy to frost hardy.
• **CULTIVATION** Grow in poor, well-drained, preferably alkaline soil in full sun. Protect from excessive winter wet and shelter from cold, drying winds. Pruning group 10, after flowering, if required.

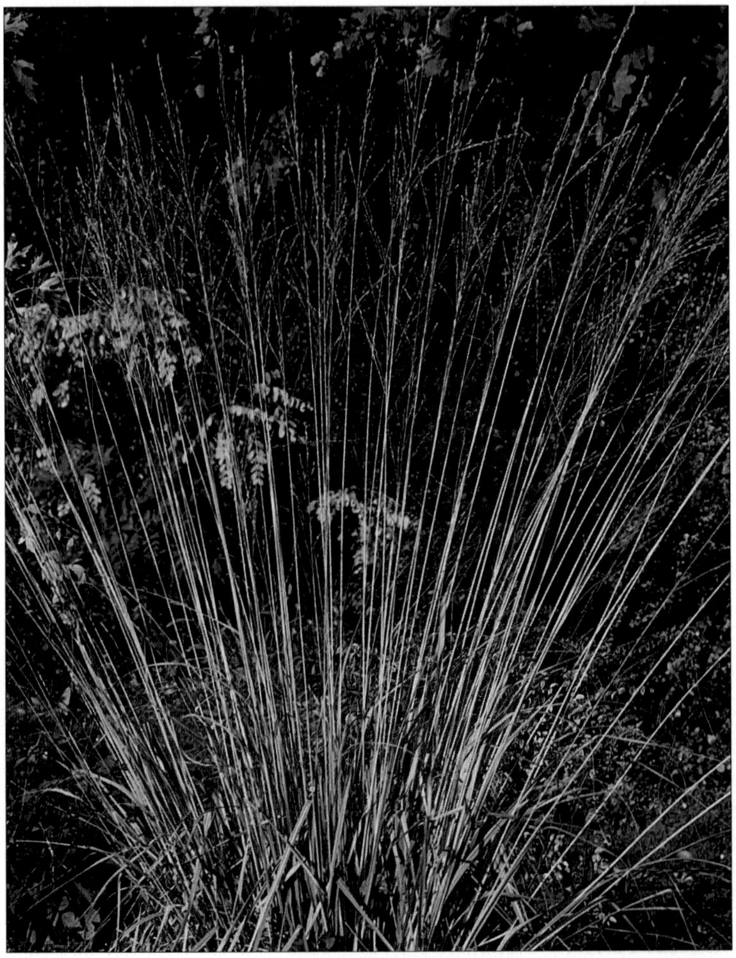

Molinia caerulea subsp. *arundinacea* 'Karl Foerster'

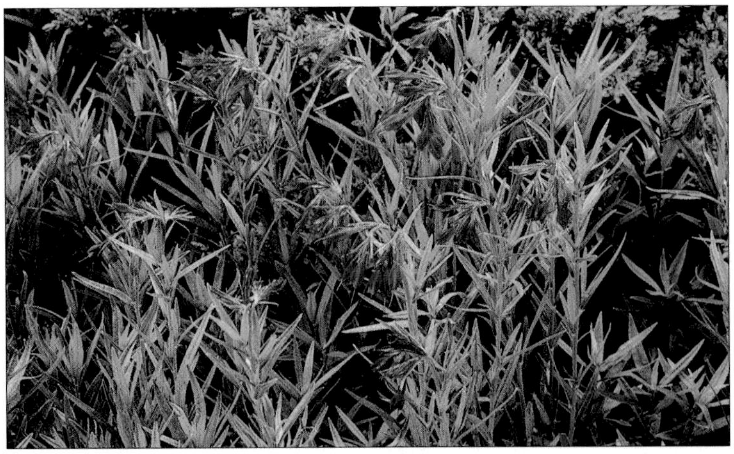

Moltkia doerfleri

- **PROPAGATION** Sow seed under glass or in containers in a cold frame in autumn. Root softwood cuttings in early summer. Layer woody species in spring.
- **PESTS AND DISEASES** Susceptible to aphids and whiteflies under glass.

M. doerfleri ▣ syn. *Lithospermum doerfleri*. Rhizomatous, woody-based perennial with wiry, upright stems and lance-shaped, mid-green leaves, to 5cm (2in) long. Bears cymes of pendent, narrowly tubular, deep purple flowers, to 2.5cm (1in) long, from late spring to midsummer. ↕↔ 30–50cm (12–20in). N.E. Albania. ✼✼✼

M. x intermedia 🏆 (*M. petraea* x *M. suffruticosa*), syn. *Lithodora* x *intermedia*. Evergreen, dome-shaped subshrub with linear or narrowly oblong, dark green leaves, to 10cm (4in) long. In early summer, bears compact cymes of open funnel-shaped, bright blue flowers, 1.5cm (½in) long, often pink-tinged in bud. ↕ 15–30cm (6–12in), ↔ to 30cm (12in). Garden origin. ✼✼✼

M. petraea. Semi-evergreen, dwarf shrub with oblong-lance-shaped to linear, inrolled leaves, to 5cm (2in) long, dark green above and white beneath. In summer, pink-purple buds open to funnel-shaped, deep blue or violet-blue flowers, to 8mm (⅜in) long, with prominent stamens, borne in compact cymes. ↕↔ 20–40cm (8–16in). Former Yugoslavia, Albania, Greece. ✼✼✼

M. suffruticosa ▣ syn. *Lithodora graminifolia, Lithospermum graminifolium*. Deciduous, upright, loosely branched shrub with narrowly linear, bristly, dark green leaves, to 15cm (6in) long. In summer, tubular, bright blue to purple-blue flowers, to 1.5cm (½in) long, are borne in dense, clustered cymes. ↕↔ to 30cm (12in). N. Italy. ✼✼✼

MOLUCCELLA

LABIATAE/LAMIACEAE

Genus of 4 species of erect, branching annuals and short-lived perennials found in fallow fields and on stony slopes from the Mediterranean to N.W. India. The 4-sided stems bear opposite, simple, rounded to ovate, incised or scalloped, mid- to pale green leaves. From summer to autumn, small, tubular, 2-lipped, hooded flowers, with expanded, bell-shaped calyces, are borne in whorls from the upper leaf axils. Grow in a mixed or annual border; the unusual flower spikes are useful for dried flower arrangements.

- **HARDINESS** Half hardy.
- **CULTIVATION** Grow in moderately fertile, moist but well-drained soil in full sun.
- **PROPAGATION** Sow seed at 13–18°C (55–64°F) in early or mid-spring, or *in situ* in late spring.
- **PESTS AND DISEASES** Trouble free.

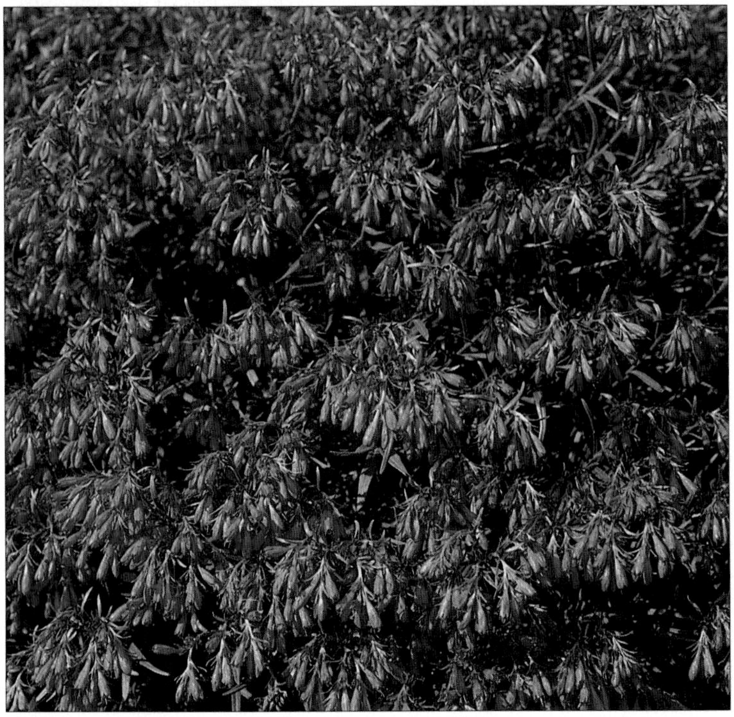

Moltkia suffruticosa

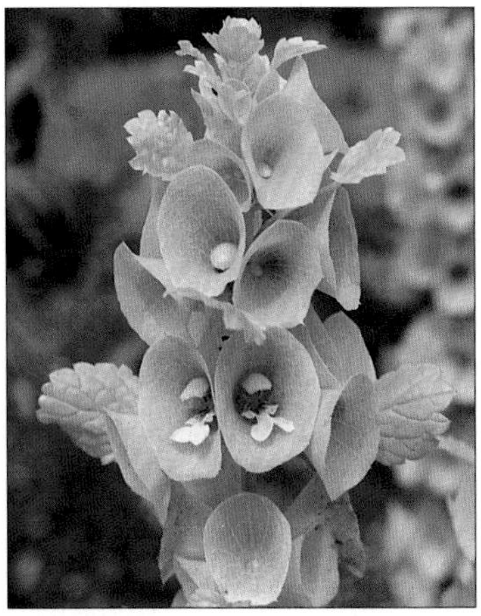

Moluccella laevis

M. laevis ▣ (Bells of Ireland, Shell flower). Annual with very broadly ovate, deeply scalloped, pale green leaves, to 6cm (2½in) long. In late summer, bears whorls of 6–8 fragrant, white to pale purplish pink flowers in spikes 23–30cm (9–12in) tall; each flower is cupped in a pale green calyx, which becomes white-veined and papery in fruit. ↕ 60–90cm (24–36in), ↔ 23cm (9in). Caucasus, Turkey, Syria, Iraq. ✼

MONADENIUM

EUPHORBIACEAE

Genus of about 50 species of bushy, tree-like, or trailing, monoecious, perennial succulents from low to high altitudes in tropical E. Africa, Angola, Namibia, South Africa, and Zimbabwe. Some species produce annual growth from a subterranean, thickened tuber or caudex; others retain fleshy stems all year. The fleshy or scaly leaves may fall quickly. In summer, unusual, small, petalless, diurnal flowers are borne in cup-like bracts within yellow, green, or brown-orange involucres. In areas where temperatures fall below 18°C (64°F), grow in a warm greenhouse. Elsewhere, grow in a rock or desert garden.

- **HARDINESS** Frost tender.
- **CULTIVATION** Under glass, grow in standard cactus compost in full light, with low humidity. From spring to summer, water moderately and apply a low-nitrogen liquid fertilizer monthly; keep dry in winter. Outdoors, grow in poor to moderately fertile, sharply drained soil in full sun. Protect from excessive winter wet. See also pp.48–49.
- **PROPAGATION** Sow seed at 19–24°C (66–75°F) in spring. Root cuttings of stem sections in spring and summer.
- **PESTS AND DISEASES** Trouble free.

M. ellenbeckii. Bushy succulent with thick, fleshy, cylindrical stems, and pitted branches, to 2.5cm (1in) thick, produced at or near the base. A few oval, stiff, fleshy, hairy, mid-green leaves, 1cm (½in) long, are borne at the branch tips and soon fall. Yellow-green involucres, with bract-cups 1cm (½in) across, form in summer. ↕ 1m (3ft), ↔ 45cm (18in). Ethiopia, Kenya. ❀ (min. 18°C/64°F)

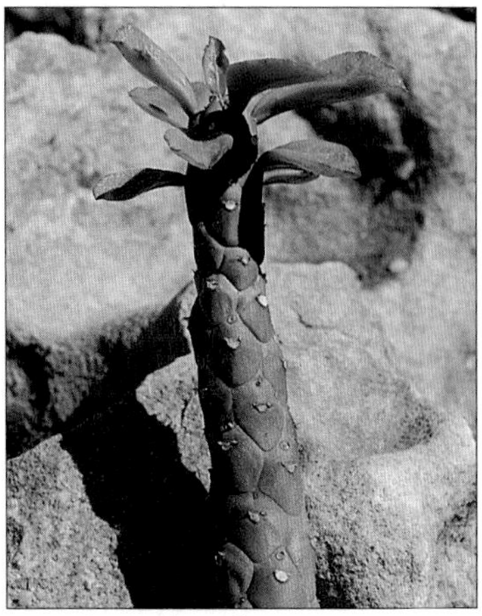

Monadenium lugardiae

M. lugardiae ▣ Erect succulent with a caudiciform base and a spineless stem, to 3cm (1¼in) thick, branching freely at or near the base. Thick, obovate, scalloped to toothed, fleshy leaves, to 9cm (3½in) long, form at the branch tips. Pale green involucres, yellow or orange-brown within, with bract-cups 7mm (¼in) across, are produced in summer. ↕ 60cm (24in), ↔ 45cm (18in). Namibia, South Africa (Northern Transvaal, Eastern Transvaal, KwaZulu/Natal), Zimbabwe. ❀ (min. 18°C/64°F)

MONANTHES

CRASSULACEAE

Genus of about 12 species of mat-forming or shrubby, perennial or annual succulents from rocky, upland areas in N. Africa and the Canary Islands. Rosettes of fleshy, often warty leaves are crowded at the ends of thick, fleshy branches. Small, star-shaped, diurnal flowers, often in compact racemes or branched cymes, are borne from spring to summer. Where temperatures fall below 7°C (45°F), grow in a temperate greenhouse throughout the year, or use for outdoor bedding from spring to summer. In warmer climates, grow in a rock or desert garden.

- **HARDINESS** Frost tender.
- **CULTIVATION** Under glass, grow in standard cactus compost in full light. From spring to autumn, water moderately and apply a low-nitrogen liquid fertilizer monthly; keep dry in winter. Outdoors, grow in poor, sharply drained soil in full sun. Protect from excessive winter wet. See also pp.48–49.
- **PROPAGATION** Sow seed at 19–24°C (66–75°F) in spring. Root stem-tip or leaf cuttings in spring or summer.
- **PESTS AND DISEASES** Trouble free.

M. dasyphylla. Semi-prostrate succulent with thick, inversely lance-shaped, softly hairy, reddish green to dark green leaves, to 2cm (¾in) long, with purple stripes and spots, the inner leaves shorter and incurved. Sub-erect racemes of 2–5 yellow, red-striped flowers, to 5mm (¼in) across, are produced in summer. ↕ to 5cm (2in), ↔ 15cm (6in). Canary Islands (Tenerife). ❀ (min. 7°C/45°F)

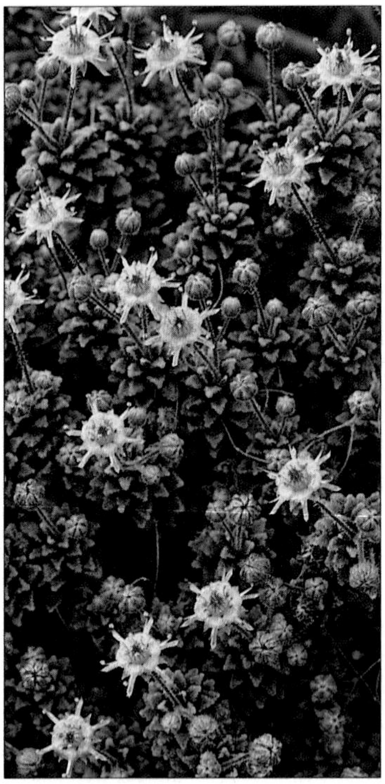
Monanthes muralis

M. laxiflora. Shrubby, slightly pendent succulent with opposite, ovate, wrinkled, dark green leaves, to 1.5cm (½in) long. Suberect racemes of 6–10 yellow, sometimes purple flowers, to 1cm (½in) across, with minute red spots, are produced from spring to summer. ↕↔ 10cm (4in) or more. Canary Islands. ❀ (min. 7°C/45°F)
M. muralis ■ Shrubby succulent with dense rosettes of obovate, warty leaves, to 1cm (½in) long, marked deep greyish purple or red. From spring to summer, produces racemes of 3–7 yellowish white flowers, 1cm (½in) across, with red tufted stamens. ↕ 10cm (4in), ↔ 15cm (6in) or more. Canary Islands (Hierro, Gomera). ❀ (min. 7°C/45°F)
M. polyphylla. Mat- or cushion-forming succulent with cylindrical to club-shaped, pale green leaves, to 1cm (½in) long. From spring to summer, produces erect racemes, usually with 1–4 red flowers, 1cm (½in) across, with white-hairy stalks and calyces. ↕ to 12cm (5in), ↔ indefinite. Canary Islands. ❀ (min. 7°C/45°F)

▷**Monarch of the East** see *Sauromatum venosum*
▷**Monarch of the veldt** see *Arctotis fastuosa*

MONARDA
Bergamot

LABIATAE/LAMIACEAE

Genus of about 15 species of annuals and clump-forming, rhizomatous herbaceous perennials occurring in dry scrub, prairies, and woodland in North America. Simple or sparsely branching, square stems bear alternate, opposite, lance-shaped to oval, usually toothed but sometimes entire, aromatic, mid- to dark green or purple-green leaves with conspicuous veins. From midsummer to early autumn, tubular, sage-like, white, pink, red, or violet flowers, often with coloured bracts, are produced in terminal whorls. Each flower has 2 lips, the upper one hooded and erect, the lower one 3-lobed and more spreading. Most monardas in general cultivation (including those described below) are derived from *M. didyma*, or are hybrids with *M. fistulosa*. They have ovate, toothed, usually dark green leaves, to 14cm (5½in) long, sometimes softly hairy beneath. Flowers, to 5cm (2in) long, are borne in whorls, with usually red-tinged bracts. Long-flowering and colourful, monardas are suitable for a mixed or herbaceous border; the flowers attract bees.

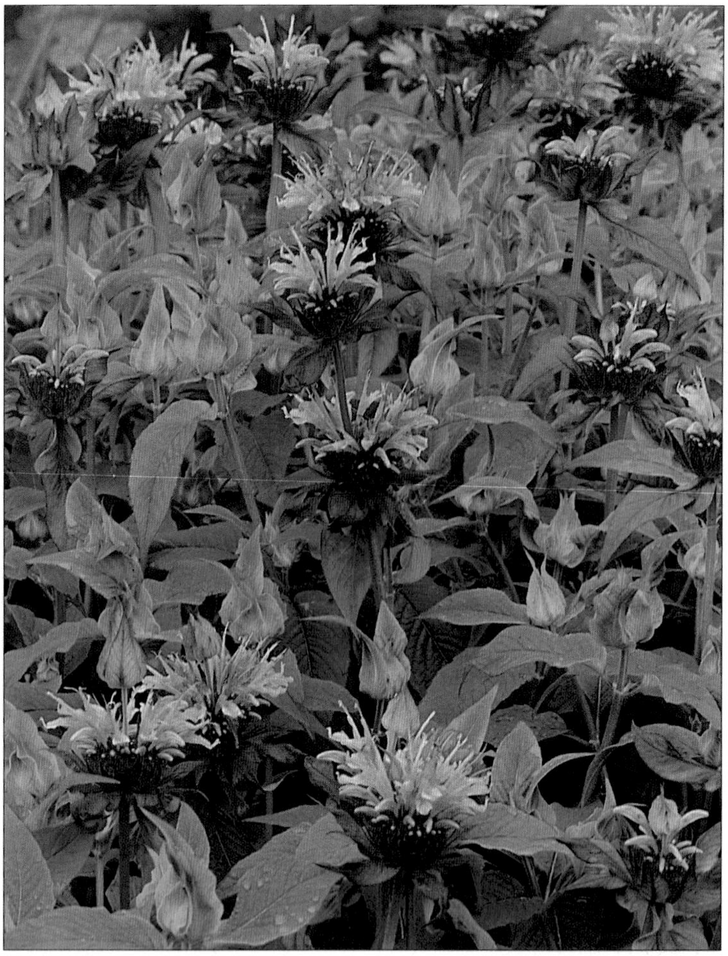
Monarda 'Beauty of Cobham'

• **HARDINESS** Fully hardy.
• **CULTIVATION** Grow in moderately fertile, humus-rich, moist but well-drained soil in full sun or light dappled shade. Protect from excessive winter wet; do not allow to dry out in summer.
• **PROPAGATION** Sow seed in containers in a cold frame in spring or autumn. Divide clumps in spring, before new growth commences. Root basal cuttings in spring.
• **PESTS AND DISEASES** Susceptible to slugs, especially in spring, and to powdery mildew in hot, dry summers. Some cultivars are mildew-resistant.

***M.* 'Adam'.** Clump-forming perennial bearing cherry-red flowers from midsummer to early autumn. ↕ 90cm (36in), ↔ 45cm (18in). ❄❄❄
***M.* 'Beauty of Cobham'** ■ ♀ Clump-forming perennial with purplish green leaves. Pale pink flowers, with purple-pink bracts, are produced from midsummer to early autumn. ↕ 90cm (36in), ↔ 45cm (18in). ❄❄❄
***M.* 'Blaustrumpf'**, syn. *M.* 'Blue Stocking'. Clump-forming perennial bearing deep violet-purple flowers, with purple bracts, from midsummer to early autumn. ↕ 90cm (36in), ↔ 45cm (18in). ❄❄❄
***M.* 'Blue Stocking'** see *M.* 'Blaustrumpf'.
***M.* 'Cambridge Scarlet'** ■ ♀ Clump-forming perennial bearing rich scarlet-red flowers, with brownish red calyces, from midsummer to early autumn. ↕ 90cm (36in), ↔ 45cm (18in). ❄❄❄
***M.* 'Croftway Pink'** ■ ♀ Clump-forming perennial producing clear rose-pink flowers, with pink-tinged bracts, from midsummer to early autumn. ↕ 90cm (36in), ↔ 45cm (18in). ❄❄❄
M. didyma (Bee balm, Bergamot, Oswego tea). Bushy, clump-forming perennial with branching, square stems and ovate to ovate-lance-shaped, dull, mid-green leaves, to 14cm (5½in) long, softly hairy beneath. From mid- to late summer, each flowering stem bears 2 whorls of bright scarlet or pink flowers, 3–4.5cm (1¼–1¾in) long, with red-tinged bracts. ↕ 90cm (36in) or more, ↔ 45cm (18in). E. North America. ❄❄❄
M. fistulosa (Wild bergamot). Bushy, clump-forming perennial with branching stems, more rounded than *M. didyma*. Bears ovate to ovate-lance-shaped, softly hairy, dull, mid-green leaves, 4–10cm (1½–4in) long. From mid- to late summer or early autumn, bears lilac-purple or pale pink flowers, 2–3cm (¾–1¼in) long, with purple-tinged bracts. ↕ 1.2m (4ft), ↔ 45cm (18in). E. North America. ❄❄❄
***M.* 'Loddon Crown'.** Clump-forming perennial bearing rich, dark red-purple flowers, with purplish brown bracts and calyces, from midsummer to early autumn. ↕ 90cm (36in), ↔ 45cm (18in). ❄❄❄
***M.* 'Mahogany'** ■ Clump-forming perennial bearing wine-red flowers, with brownish red bracts, from midsummer to early autumn. ↕ 90cm (36in), ↔ 45cm (18in). ❄❄❄
***M.* 'Prairie Night'** see *M.* 'Prärienacht'.
***M.* 'Prärienacht'** ■ syn. *M.* 'Prairie Night'. Clump-forming perennial bearing purple-lilac flowers, with green, slightly red-tinged bracts, from midsummer to early autumn. ↕ 90cm (36in), ↔ 45cm (18in). ❄❄❄
***M.* 'Schneewittchen'**, syn. *M.* 'Snow Witch'. Clump-forming perennial bearing white flowers, with green bracts,

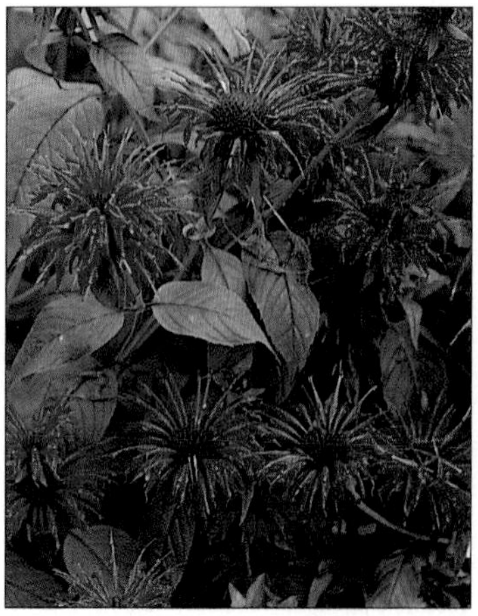
Monarda 'Cambridge Scarlet'

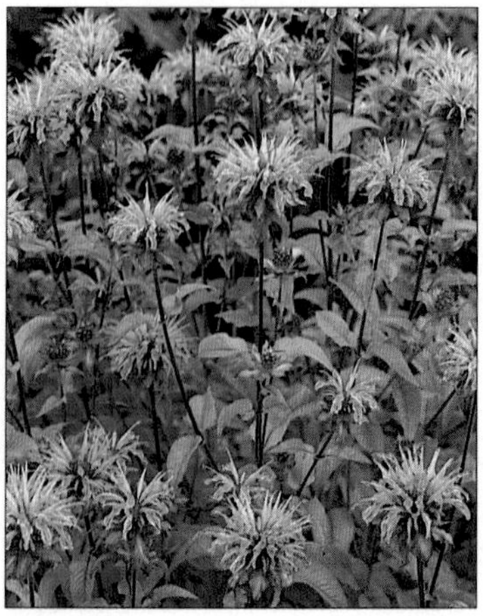
Monarda 'Croftway Pink'

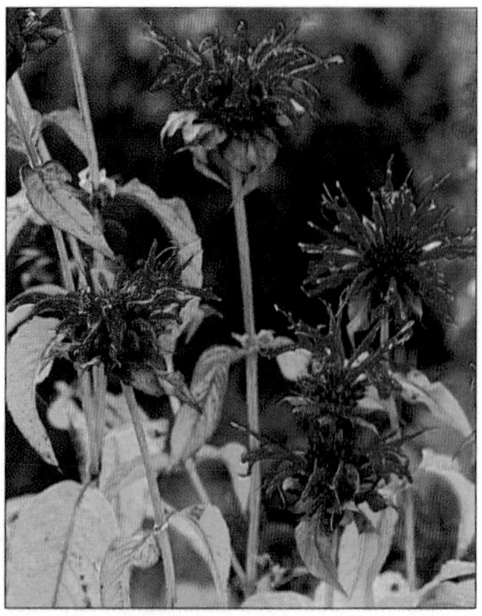
Monarda 'Mahogany'

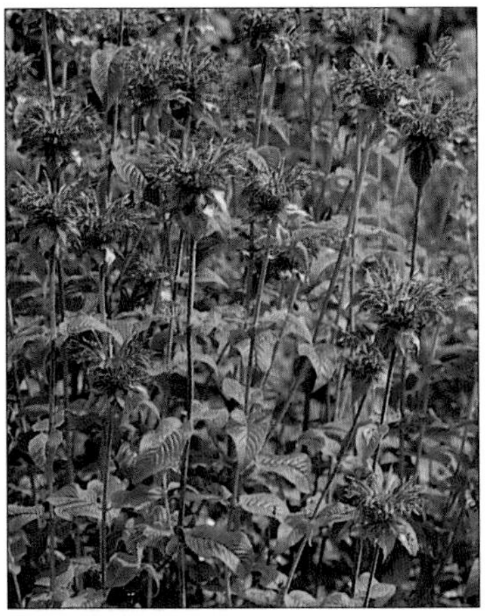

Monarda 'Prärienacht'

from midsummer to early autumn. ↕90cm (36in), ↔45cm (18in). ❄❄❄

***M.* 'Snow Witch'** see *M.* 'Schneewittchen'.

***M.* 'Vintage Wine'.** Clump-forming perennial bearing red-purple flowers, with brownish green bracts and calyces, from midsummer to early autumn. ↕90cm (36in), ↔45cm (18in). ❄❄❄

MONARDELLA

LABIATAE/LAMIACEAE

Genus of about 20 species of annuals and herbaceous perennials, often with creeping stems, occurring mainly on dry, stony slopes in W. North America. The small, opposite, aromatic, entire or toothed leaves are linear to diamond-lance-shaped, oblong, ovate, or elliptic. Terminal, spherical whorls of 2-lipped, tubular flowers (the upper lip 2-lobed and the lower one 3-lobed), often with purplish red, leaf-like bracts, are produced in summer. Suitable for a Mediterranean or rock garden, the front of a mixed border, or an alpine house.

- **HARDINESS** Fully hardy to frost hardy.
- **CULTIVATION** Grow in poor, sharply drained soil in full sun. In an alpine house, grow in shallow containers in a mix of equal parts loam-based potting compost (JI No.2) and grit. Protect from excessive winter wet and shelter from cold, drying winds.
- **PROPAGATION** Sow seed under glass in autumn. Divide, or root basal or softwood cuttings in spring, both with bottom heat.
- **PESTS AND DISEASES** Susceptible to aphids and whiteflies under glass.

M. macrantha. Deciduous, decumbent, woody-based perennial with spreading branches and ovate to elliptic, toothed, hairy, slightly leathery, mid-green leaves, to 3cm (1¼in) long. In mid- and late summer, bears scarlet flowers, 1cm (½in) long, in whorled flowerheads, 3–4cm (1¼–1½in) across, surrounded by purplish red bracts. ↕15cm (6in), ↔ to 20cm (8in). USA (California). ❄❄

▷**Monkey cup** see *Nepenthes*
▷**Monkey flower** see *Mimulus*
Allegheny see *M. ringens*
Scarlet see *M. cardinalis*
Yellow see *M. luteus*
▷**Monkey plant** see *Ruellia makoyana*
▷**Monkey puzzle** see *Araucaria araucana*
▷**Monkshood** see *Aconitum, A. napellus*

MONSTERA

ARACEAE

Genus of 22 species of evergreen, often epiphytic root climbers found in rainforest in tropical North, Central, and South America. The alternate leaves usually differ in size and shape on young and mature plants, but are mainly ovate and entire, lobed, or deeply pinnatifid. On mature plants, arum-like spathes, enclosing tiny, star-shaped, petalless flowers, are produced singly from the leaf axils. Where temperatures fall below 15°C (59°F), grow in a warm greenhouse or as houseplants. In warmer climates, grow up palm trees or on an arch or pergola. The fruit of *M. deliciosa* taste of pineapple when fully ripe. Other parts may cause mild stomach upset if ingested, and contact with the fruit may irritate skin.

- **HARDINESS** Frost tender.
- **CULTIVATION** Under glass, grow in loam-based potting compost (JI No.2), in bright indirect light with moderate to high humidity. In the growing season, water freely and apply a balanced liquid fertilizer monthly; water sparingly in winter. Outdoors, grow in humus-rich, moist but well-drained soil in partial shade. Pruning group 11, in spring; plants grown under glass may require restrictive pruning.
- **PROPAGATION** Sow seed at 18–24°C (64–75°F) as soon as ripe. Root tip or leaf cuttings with bottom heat in summer. Layer in autumn.
- **PESTS AND DISEASES** Scale insects and red spider mites may be troublesome under glass.

M. deliciosa ■ ♀ (Ceriman, Mexican breadfruit, Swiss cheese plant). Robust, strong-growing climber with thick, sparingly branched stems. Mature plants have broadly ovate to heart-shaped, long-stalked, leathery, glossy, mid- to deep green leaves, 30–90cm (12–36in) long. Each leaf is pinnatifid and often perforated with elliptic to oblong holes between the main lateral veins. Juvenile leaves are shorter-stalked, much smaller, and entire. Bears creamy white spathes, 20–30cm (8–12in) long, usually from spring to summer, sometimes followed by edible, cone-shaped cream fruit, to 25cm (10in) long. ↕10–20m (30–70ft). S. Mexico to Panama. ⊛ (min. 15°C/59°F). **'Albovariegata'** produces leaves with irregular, creamy white patches. **'Variegata'** ♀ produces leaves splashed and marbled yellowish cream; very liable to revert to green.

***M. latevaginata* of gardens** see *Rhaphidophora celatocaulis.*

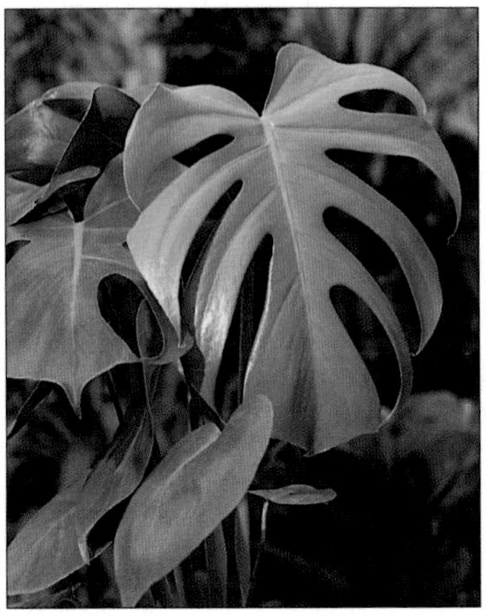

Monstera deliciosa

▷**Montbretia** see *Crocosmia, C.* x *crocosmiiflora*
▷***Montia australasica*** see *Neopaxia australasica*
▷**Moonflower** see *Ipomoea alba*
▷**Moonseed** see *Menispermum*
Canadian see *M. canadense*
▷**Moor grass,**
Balkan see *Sesleria heufleriana*
Blue see *Sesleria albicans*
Nest see *Sesleria nitida*
Purple see *Molinia caerulea*
▷**Moosewood** see *Acer pensylvanicum*

MORAEA

IRIDACEAE

Genus of about 120 species of deciduous or semi-deciduous, cormous perennials, occurring in seasonally moist grassland throughout Africa. The linear or lance-shaped, flat or rolled, often channelled, light to mid-green leaves may be basal or borne on the stems. From spring to summer, a succession of short-lived, colourful, iris-like flowers are produced in clusters within pairs of large bracts. In frost-free climates, some species, such as *M. angusta, M. moggii,* and *M. spathulata,* are evergreen. In frost-prone areas, grow the half-hardy species in a cool greenhouse. In warmer climates, the frost-hardy species are best in a mixed border or at the base of warm, sunny wall; grow the half-hardy species in a mixed border or a rock garden.

- **HARDINESS** Frost hardy to half hardy.
- **CULTIVATION** Plant 7cm (3in) deep in spring or autumn. Outdoors, grow frost-hardy species in well-drained, humus-rich, moderately fertile soil in full sun with some midday shade. Provide protection from excessive winter wet. In areas prone to severe frosts, grow under glass, as for half-hardy species. Under glass, grow half-hardy species in loam-based potting compost (JI No.2), with additional sharp sand, in full light. Water sparingly as growth begins, then freely when in full growth. Dry off as leaves wither, in order to ensure a dry dormancy from midsummer to autumn. In warmer areas, grow outdoors, as for frost-hardy species above.
- **PROPAGATION** Sow seed of frost-hardy species in containers in a cold frame in spring; sow seed of half-hardy species under glass in autumn. Separate offsets when dormant.
- **PESTS AND DISEASES** Trouble free.

M. angusta. Cormous perennial producing a solitary, erect, linear, rolled, stem leaf, to 60cm (24in) long. Brown- or grey-tinged yellow flowers, 6–8cm (2½–3in) across, are produced in spring. ↕20–40cm (8–16in), ↔8cm (3in). South Africa (S. Western Cape). ❄

M. aristata, syn. *M. glaucopis.* Cormous perennial producing a solitary, erect, narrowly linear, flat, basal leaf, to 45cm (18in) long. Produces white flowers, 5–7cm (2–3in) across, with conspicuous, green, blue, or violet central eyes on the outer tepals, on occasionally branched stems in late spring. ↕25–35cm (10–14in), ↔8cm (3in). South Africa. ❄

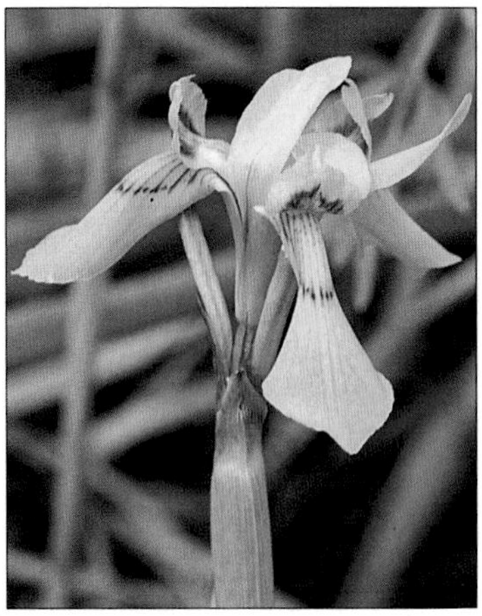

Moraea huttonii

M. glaucopis see *M. aristata.*

M. huttonii ■ Cormous perennial with a solitary, semi-erect, narrowly linear, flat or channelled, basal leaf, to 1m (3ft) long. Scented, golden yellow flowers, to 8cm (3in) across, with brown marks and deeper yellow eyes towards the centres, are produced on occasionally branched stems from spring to early summer. Similar to *M. spathulata,* but with purple-brown marks on the styles. ↕70–90cm (28–36in), ↔8cm (3in). South Africa (KwaZulu/Natal), Lesotho. ❄❄

M. moggii. Robust, cormous perennial with a solitary, erect, narrowly linear, basal leaf, to 60cm (24in) long, channelled at the base and rolled at the tip. Yellow, sometimes cream or white flowers, to 5cm (2in) across, with bright yellow and purple veins on the outer tepals, are borne in late summer. One of the easiest species to grow. ↕70cm (28in), ↔8cm (3in). South Africa (KwaZulu/Natal), Swaziland. ❄❄

M. natalensis. Cormous perennial with a solitary, narrowly linear, channelled leaf, to 20cm (8in) long, borne near the top of the stem. In summer, produces lilac or violet-blue flowers, 2.5–3cm (1–1¼in) across, with a conspicuous yellow central mark, ringed dark mauve, on each of the outer tepals. ↕ to 45cm (18in), ↔8cm (3in). Zaire, Zambia, Malawi, Zimbabwe, Mozambique, South Africa (KwaZulu/Natal, Eastern Transvaal). ❄

M. polystachya ■ Cormous perennial bearing 3–5 erect but later spreading,

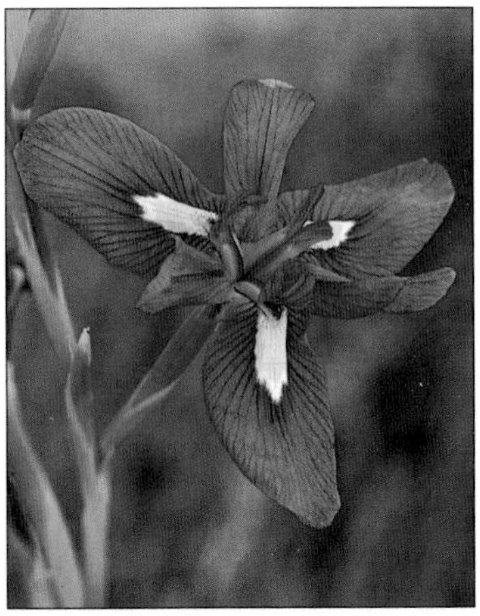

Moraea polystachya

M

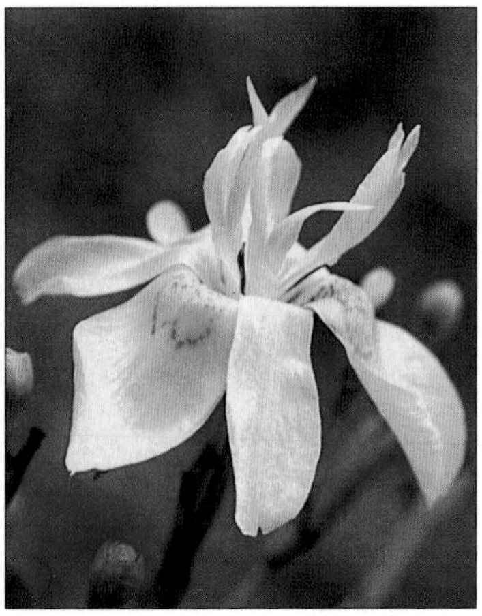

Moraea ramosissima

linear, channelled to almost flat leaves, to 80cm (32in) long, on branching stems. In summer, bears violet to pale blue flowers, 6–8cm (2½–3in) across, with a conspicuous, white-margined yellow mark at the centre of each outer tepal. ↕ to 80cm (32in), ↔ 8cm (3in). Namibia, Botswana, South Africa (Northern Cape, Eastern Cape, W. Northern Transvaal). ❄

M. ramosissima ■ Cormous perennial with numerous semi-erect, narrowly linear, channelled, basal leaves, 30–50cm (12–20in) long. Produces yellow flowers, 4–6cm (1½–2½in) across, with deeper yellow centres, on many-branched stems from spring to early summer. Produces offset corms. ↕ 50–120cm (20–48in), ↔ 10cm (4in). South Africa. ❄

M. spathacea see *M. spathulata.*

M. spathulata, syn. *M. spathacea.* Robust, cormous perennial with a solitary, semi-erect, narrowly linear, flat or channelled, basal leaf, to 80cm (32in) long. Golden yellow flowers, to 9cm (3½in) across, are produced in early and midsummer. The outer tepals each have a deep yellow to orange-yellow central mark and purple-brown margins. Similar to *M. huttonii* but more robust and with larger flowers. ↕ 50–90cm (20–36in), ↔ 8cm (3in). Zimbabwe, Mozambique, Swaziland, Lesotho, South Africa (KwaZulu/Natal, Northern Transvaal, Eastern Transvaal, Eastern Cape). ❄❄

M. tripetala. Cormous perennial with a solitary (occasionally 2), trailing, linear or lance-shaped, channelled, basal leaf, 20–60cm (8–24in) long. In spring, pale or deep blue, purple, pink, or sometimes yellow flowers, 4–5cm (1½–2in) across, are produced on sometimes branched stems; the 3 large outer tepals each have a white or yellow central mark. ↕ 10–50cm (4–20in), ↔ 8cm (3in). South Africa (Northern Cape, Western Cape, Eastern Cape). ❄

M. villosa. Very variable, cormous perennial with a solitary, trailing, narrowly linear, channelled, basal leaf, 20–50cm (8–20in) long. In early spring, branched stems bear white, cream, pink, orange, vivid blue, lilac, or purple flowers, 5–7cm (2–3in) across. The outer tepals each have a yellow central mark, surrounded by 1 or 2 darker yellow, purple, or black bands. ↕ 15–40cm (6–16in), ↔ 5cm (2in). South Africa (Northern Cape, Western Cape, Eastern Cape). ❄

MORINA *syn.* ACANTHOCALYX

MORINACEAE

Genus of 4 or 5 species of evergreen perennials found on open, rocky and grassy slopes and in open woodland in E. Europe, Turkey to C. Asia, the Himalayas, and S.W. China. They have rosettes of lance-shaped, glossy, mid- to dark green leaves with spiny-toothed, wavy margins; the leaves become smaller near the tops of the stems. Whorled, spiny bracts are held immediately below spikes of tubular, red, pink, white, or yellow flowers, borne in whorled clusters. Each flower has a long perianth tube and a wide, 2-lipped mouth. Grow in a mixed or herbaceous border; *M. persica* is useful for a rock or Mediterranean garden. The seed heads are useful for dried flower arrangements.

• **HARDINESS** Fully hardy.

• **CULTIVATION** Grow in poor or moderately fertile, sharply drained soil in full sun. Protect from winter wet.

• **PROPAGATION** Sow seed in a cold frame as soon as ripe, with one seed per container of gritty seed compost. *M. persica* is difficult to germinate. Over-winter young plants in a well-ventilated cold frame. Insert root cuttings in winter.

• **PESTS AND DISEASES** Susceptible to slug damage and rot, especially in shade.

M. longifolia ■ (Whorlflower). Rosette-forming perennial with linear to oblong, pinnatifid, aromatic, glossy, dark green basal leaves, to 25cm (10in) long, with sharp marginal spines. In midsummer, tiered, whorled clusters of waxy white flowers, 3cm (1¼in) long, are produced in spikes; flowers become rose-pink then red after fertilization. ↕ to 90cm (36in) or more, ↔ 30cm (12in). Himalayas. ❄❄❄

M. persica. Rosette-forming perennial with linear to elliptic, deeply lobed to pinnatifid, very spiny, dark green basal leaves, to 20cm (8in) long. In mid- and late summer, numerous flowering stems bear dense whorls of bracts below spikes of whorled clusters of scented flowers, 3–3.5cm (1¼–1½in) long; flowers are white, sometimes with yellow-flushed throats, and become pink or reddish pink after fertilization. ↕ to 1.5m (5ft), ↔ 60cm (24in). S. and E. Balkans, Turkey, Iran. ❄❄❄

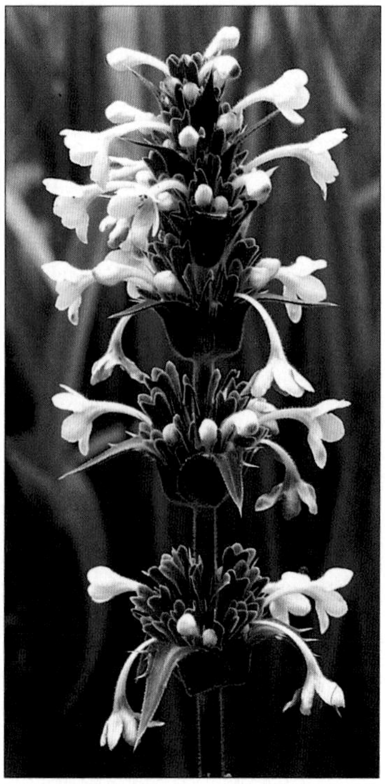

Morina longifolia

MORISIA

BRASSICACEAE/CRUCIFERAE

Genus of one species of compact, rosette-forming, tap-rooted perennial occurring in sandy areas of Corsica and Sardinia. It produces pinnatifid leaves and almost stemless, cross-shaped flowers. Grow in a rock garden, scree bed, trough, or alpine house.

• **HARDINESS** Fully hardy.

• **CULTIVATION** Grow in moderately fertile, sharply drained soil in full sun. Protect from excessive winter wet. In an alpine house, use a mix of equal parts loam-based potting compost (JI No.1) and grit.

• **PROPAGATION** Sow seed in containers in a cold frame in spring. Insert root cuttings in a cold frame in winter.

• **PESTS AND DISEASES** Neck rot may be a problem in very damp conditions.

M. hypogaea see *M. monanthos.*

M. monanthos ■ syn. *M. hypogaea.* Perennial forming neat rosettes of lance-shaped, pinnatifid, slightly fleshy, glossy, dark green leaves, 5–8cm (2–3in) long, with oblong segments. In late spring and early summer, bears almost stemless, golden yellow flowers, to 1.5cm (½in) across. ↕ 5cm (2in), ↔ to 10cm (4in). France (Corsica), Italy (Sardinia). ❄❄❄. **'Fred Hemingway'** has flowers to 2cm (¾in) across.

▷**Morning glory** see *Ipomoea, I. tricolor*
Common see *Ipomoea purpurea*
Red see *Ipomoea coccinea*
Spanish see *Merremia tuberosa*
Star see *Ipomoea coccinea*
Woolly see *Argyreia nervosa*
Yellow see *Merremia tuberosa*

▷**Mortiña** see *Vaccinium floribundum*

MORUS

Mulberry

MORACEAE

Genus of about 10 species of upright to rounded, deciduous shrubs and trees found mainly in woodland in Africa, Asia, and North and South America. The alternate, ovate to rounded, toothed leaves, often lobed and heart-shaped at the bases, are light to dark green. In late spring and early summer, tiny, cup-shaped, pale green male and female flowers are borne in separate catkins on the same plant; each female flower cluster develops into a single, spherical to oblong, edible, raspberry-like fruit. Grow as specimen trees; *M. alba* 'Pendula' is particularly suitable for a small garden; *M. nigra* is the best species for edible fruit. In frost-prone areas, grow tender species in a temperate greenhouse. The leaves of several species are used to feed silkworms.

• **HARDINESS** Fully hardy to frost tender; unripened wood may be damaged by frost.

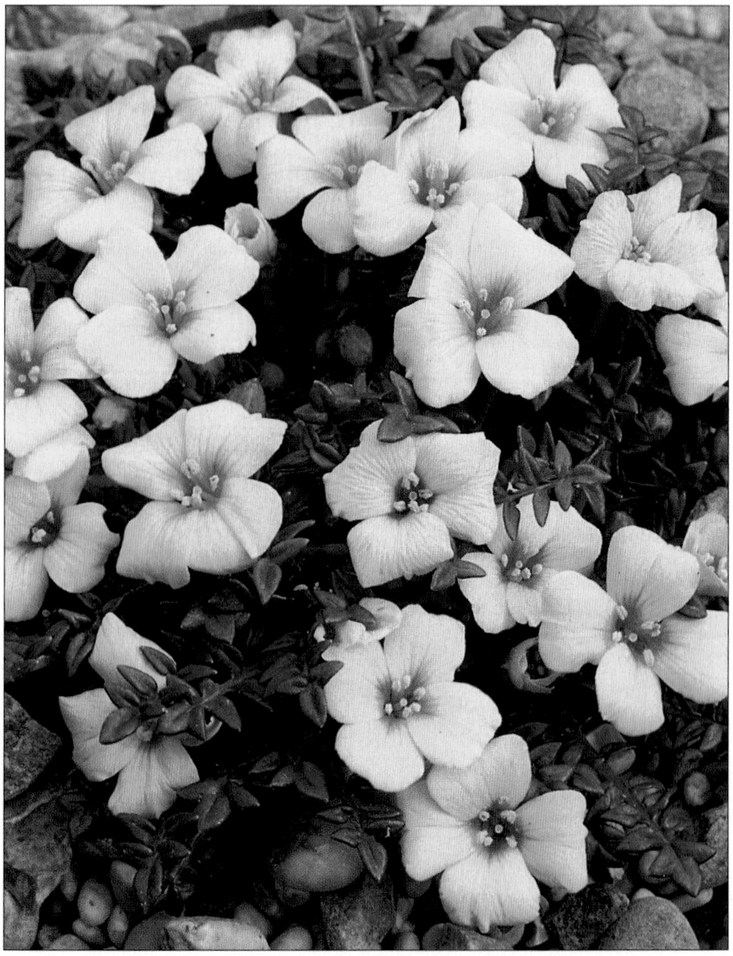

Morisia monanthos

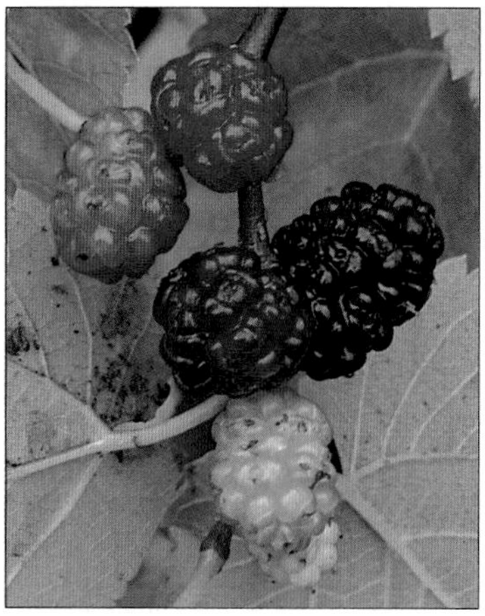
Morus nigra

• **CULTIVATION** Grow in moderately fertile, moist but well-drained soil in full sun. Shelter from cold, drying winds. Pruning group 1, in late autumn or early winter, as trees "bleed" at other times.
• **PROPAGATION** Sow seed in containers outdoors in autumn. Root semi-ripe cuttings in summer. Root hardwood cuttings in a prepared bed in a cold frame in autumn; thick pieces of 2- to 4-year-old wood, known as "truncheons", will also root if treated as hardwood cuttings. Bud cultivars in summer.
• **PESTS AND DISEASES** Susceptible to bacterial blight, canker, coral spot, and powdery mildew.

M. alba ♀ syn. *M. bombycis* (White mulberry). Spreading tree with ovate to heart-shaped, sometimes lobed, glossy, bright green leaves, to 20cm (8in) long, turning yellow in autumn. Ovoid, insipid-tasting white fruit, to 2.5cm (1in) long, ripening to pink and red, are borne in late summer. ↕↔ 10m (30ft). China. ❄❄❄. **'Laciniata'** has deeply lobed leaves. **'Pendula'** ♀ is weeping, and produces pendent shoots; ↕ 3m (10ft), ↔ 5m (15ft).
M. bombycis see *M. alba*.
M. nigra ▣ ♀ ♀ (Black mulberry). Rounded tree with ovate to heart-shaped, often doubly toothed, mid-green leaves, to 15cm (6in) long, rough-textured above. Ovoid, green fruit, to 2.5cm (1in) long, turn red then dark purple in late summer, and have a pleasant, slightly acidic flavour. ↕ 12m (40ft), ↔ 15m (50ft). Origin uncertain (probably S.W. Asia). ❄❄❄
M. rubra ♀ (Red mulberry). Rounded tree with broadly ovate, sometimes lobed leaves, usually to 12cm (5in) long but sometimes more, with heart-shaped bases and abruptly pointed tips; they are dark green, turning yellow in autumn. Cylindrical, sweet-tasting fruit, to 3cm (1¼in) long, ripen to dark purple in late summer. ↕ 12m (40ft), ↔ 15m (50ft). S.E. Canada, E. USA. ❄❄❄

▷**Moses-in-the-cradle** see *Tradescantia spathacea*
▷**Mosquito bills** see *Dodecatheon hendersonii*
▷**Mosquito grass** see *Bouteloua gracilis*
▷**Mosquito plant** see *Azolla filiculoides*
▷**Moss,**
Club see *Lycopodium*
Fairy see *Azolla filiculoides*
Rose see *Portulaca, P. grandiflora*
Spanish see *Tillandsia usneoides*
▷**Moss rose, Common** see *Rosa* x *centifolia* 'Muscosa'
▷**Mother-in-law's cushion** see *Echinocactus grusonii*
▷**Mother-in-law's tongue** see *Dieffenbachia, Sansevieria trifasciata*
▷**Mother of pearl plant** see *Graptopetalum paraguayense*
▷**Mother of thousands** see *Saxifraga stolonifera* 'Tricolor', *Soleirolia soleirolii*
▷**Mother of thyme** see *Acinos arvensis*
▷**Mottlecah** see *Eucalyptus macrocarpa*
▷**Mountain ash** see *Sorbus aucuparia*
American see *S. americana*
Korean see *S. alnifolia*
▷**Mountain devil** see *Lambertia formosa*
▷**Mountain fringe** see *Adlumia fungosa*
▷**Mountain pine** see *Pinus uncinata*
Dwarf see *P. mugo*
▷**Mountain spinach, Red** see *Atriplex hortensis*
▷**Mourning widow** see *Geranium phaeum*
▷**Mouse plant** see *Arisarum proboscideum*
▷**Moutan** see *Paeonia suffruticosa*
▷**Mrs. Robb's bonnet** see *Euphorbia amygdaloides* var. *robbiae*

MUCUNA

LEGUMINOSAE/PAPILIONACEAE

Genus of about 100 species of herbaceous and woody-stemmed, evergreen, twining climbers and shrubs from woodland in tropical regions worldwide. The 3-palmate leaves are alternate or arranged in spirals. *Mucuna* species are grown for their large, pea-like flowers, with prominent, curved and pointed, keeled petals, which are borne in showy, pendent, axillary racemes. Where temperatures fall below the minimum levels given below, grow in a temperate or warm greenhouse. In warmer areas, use to clothe an arch, pergola, or trellis.
• **HARDINESS** Frost tender.
• **CULTIVATION** Under glass, grow in loam-based potting compost (JI No.2) in bright filtered light. In growth, water freely and apply a balanced liquid fertilizer monthly; water sparingly in winter. Outdoors, grow in moderately fertile, moist but well-drained soil in full sun, with some midday shade. Pruning group 11 or 12 outdoors; group 12 under glass. Prune after flowering.
• **PROPAGATION** Sow seed at 18–24°C (64–75°F) in spring.
• **PESTS AND DISEASES** Susceptible to red spider mites and whiteflies under glass.

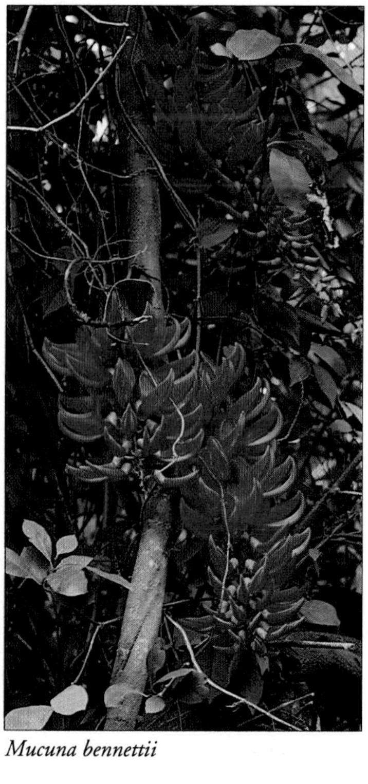
Mucuna bennettii

M. bennettii ▣ (New Guinea creeper). Fast-growing, woody-stemmed climber with sparingly to moderately branched, wrinkled stems, and dark green leaves with elliptic to oblong leaflets, 11–14cm (4½–5½in) long. Short, dense racemes of scarlet to flame-red flowers, 8–13cm (3–5in) long, with downy orange calyces, are borne mainly in summer. ↕ to 20m (70ft) or more. New Guinea. ❁ (min. 15°C/59°F)
M. pruriens. Semi-woody, annual or short-lived perennial climber bearing branched stems with a rough covering of long, bristly hairs when young, eventually becoming hairless. Leaves are mid-green with elliptic to oblong leaflets, 5–16cm (2–6in) long. From late spring to summer, produces racemes of deep blackish purple to lilac or white flowers, 2–4cm (¾–1½in) long, with downy, pale brown calyces. ↕ 4m (12ft). Tropical Asia, widely naturalized elsewhere. ❁ (min. 8°C/46°F)

MUEHLENBECKIA

POLYGONACEAE

Genus of 20 species of dioecious, deciduous and evergreen shrubs (sometimes mat-forming with runners) and twining, woody climbers, from rocky areas and woodland in New Guinea, Australia, New Zealand, and South America. They are cultivated for their intricate habit, their minute, alternate, linear to rounded leaves (absent in some species), and their tiny, cup-shaped, sweet-scented flowers, produced singly or in pairs, in axillary clusters or spikes, or in terminal or axillary racemes or panicles. The shrubs are suitable for a border, the climbing species for clothing an arch, pergola, or trellis. *M. complexa* is also useful as ground cover. In frost-prone climates, grow tender species in containers in a temperate greenhouse.
• **HARDINESS** Frost hardy to frost tender.
• **CULTIVATION** Grow in moderately fertile, moist but well-drained soil in full sun, with some midday shade. Provide shelter from cold, drying winds and suitable support where required. Pruning group 11, after flowering; may need restrictive pruning under glass.
• **PROPAGATION** Sow seed at 19–24°C (66–75°F) as soon as ripe. Root semi-ripe cuttings with bottom heat in summer.
• **PESTS AND DISEASES** Trouble free.

M. adpressa (Climbing lignum, Macquarie vine). Small, deciduous, wiry-stemmed climber with lance-shaped to broadly ovate, glossy, dark green leaves, 1–6cm (½–2½in) long, with crinkly margins and often heart-shaped bases. From spring to summer, whitish green flowers are produced in short, axillary spikes, 2.5–8cm (1–3in) long. ↕ 2m (6ft) or more. Coastal, temperate Australia. ❄
M. axillaris. Small, deciduous, prostrate or spreading, many-branched shrub, often rooting at the nodes, with broadly ovate-oblong to rounded, mid-green leaves, 5–10cm (2–4in) long. Cup-shaped, yellowish green flowers are produced singly or in pairs from the leaf axils, from summer to early autumn. ↕ 20cm (8in), ↔ 80cm (32in). S.E. Australia, New Zealand. ❄❄
***M. axillaris* of gardens** see *M. complexa*.
M. complexa, syn. *M. axillaris* of gardens. Vigorous, deciduous, creeping shrub or twining climber with slender shoots and rounded to violin-shaped, dark green leaves, 0.5–1.5cm (¼–½in) long. Bears greenish white flowers in terminal and axillary racemes, 2.5–3cm (1–1¼in) long, in summer, followed by fleshy white fruit, 5mm (¼in) across. ↕ 3m (10ft). New Zealand. ❄❄
M. platyclados see *Homalocladium platycladum*.

▷**Mugga** see *Eucalyptus sideroxylon*
▷**Mugwort** see *Artemisia*
Western see *A. ludoviciana*
White see *A. lactiflora*

MUKDENIA

syn. ACERIPHYLLUM

SAXIFRAGACEAE

Genus of 2 species of slowly spreading herbaceous perennials from woodland in N.E. Asia. They have short, thick rhizomes and large, long-stalked, palmately 5- to 9-lobed, toothed leaves. Leafless panicles or racemes of small, bell-shaped, 5- to 6-petalled white flowers are borne in spring. *Mukdenia* species are suitable for a woodland garden or peat terrace, and grow best in areas with cool, damp summers.
• **HARDINESS** Fully hardy.
• **CULTIVATION** Grow in leafy, moist but well-drained soil in light dappled or partial shade.
• **PROPAGATION** Sow seed in containers in a cold frame in autumn. Divide in spring, just before buds expand.
• **PESTS AND DISEASES** Slugs and snails may damage young leaves.

M. rossii, syn. *Aceriphyllum rossii*. Perennial with short, thick rhizomes and palmately 5- to 9-lobed, bronze-tinted, mid-green leaves, 15cm (6in) across. Dense, short-branched panicles of creamy white flowers, to 5mm (¼in) across, are borne above the leaves in spring. ↕ to 35cm (14in), ↔ to 40cm (16in) or more. N. China, Korea. ❄❄❄

▷**Mulberry** see *Morus*
Black see *Morus nigra*
Paper see *Broussonetia papyrifera*
Red see *Morus rubra*
White see *Morus alba*
▷***Mulgedium alpinum*** see *Cicerbita alpina*
▷***Mulgedium plumieri*** see *Cicerbita plumieri*
▷**Mulla mulla, Pink** see *Ptilotus exaltatus*
▷**Mullein** see *Verbascum*
Dark see *V. nigrum*
Great see *V. thapsus*
Nettle-leaved see *V. chaixii*
Purple see *V. phoeniceum*

MUSA

Banana, Plantain

MUSACEAE

Genus of 40 species of evergreen, palm-like, suckering perennials found in light woodland and at forest margins, in N.E. India and Bangladesh, and from S.E. Asia to Japan and N. Australia. The leaf-blades are huge and often paddle-shaped (although the shape may vary) and light to mid-green, or grey-green; the leaf-sheaths form false stems. In summer, clusters of tubular flowers are produced from the axils of broad, coloured bracts in erect or pendent spikes. The cylindrical fruits are edible; several different species and cultivars produce the bananas of commerce. In frost-prone areas, grow in a temperate greenhouse (in a border or containers), or plant out in a subtropical, summer bedding scheme. In warmer climates, grow as specimen plants.

• **HARDINESS** Frost hardy to frost tender.

• **CULTIVATION** Under glass, grow in loam-based potting compost (JI No.3) in full light, with shade from hot sun. From spring to summer, water freely and apply a balanced liquid fertilizer monthly; keep just moist in winter. Repot ornamental species annually or every other year, in spring. For bedding, plant out when danger of frost has passed; lift and pot-up in autumn. Outdoors, grow in humus-rich soil in full sun. Provide a sheltered position, as wind causes leaves to shred, especially on soft new growth.

• **PROPAGATION** Sow seed as soon as ripe at 21–24°C (70–75°F). Pre-soak spring-sown seed for 24 hours. Separate suckers in early spring, removing the older leaves to allow better establishment. Divide established clumps every 5 years.

• **PESTS AND DISEASES** Red spider mites, mealybugs, and aphids may be troublesome, particularly under glass.

M. acuminata ✾ syn. *M. cavendishii.* Upright, very variable, suckering perennial with false stems and paddle-shaped, glaucous, mid-green leaf-blades, 2–3m (6–10ft) long, with brown, papery margins. In summer, pendent, pear-shaped, white, cream, or yellow flowers, 2–3cm (¾–1¼in) long, with dull purple bracts, are produced in 2 rows per bract, followed by edible fruit, 15–20cm (6–8in) long, which are yellow when ripe. ↕4–6m (12–20ft),

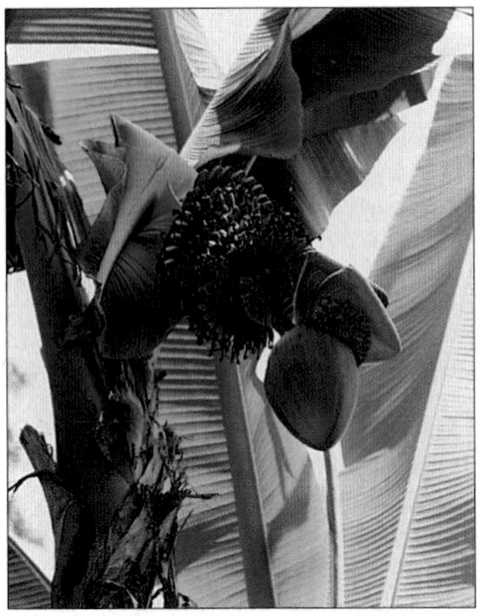

Musa basjoo

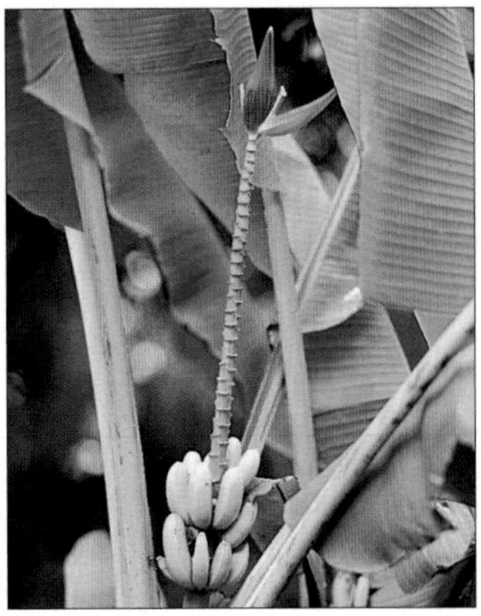

Musa ornata

↔ 2–3m (6–10ft). S.E. Asia to N. Australia. ❁ (min. 7°C/45°F). **'Dwarf Cavendish'** ♀ syn. 'Basrai', *M.* x *paradisiaca* 'Dwarf Cavendish' (Edible banana, French plantain), has oblong, mid-green leaf-blades, to 1.5m (5ft) long. Pendent clusters of yellow flowers, with reddish purple bracts, are produced irregularly throughout the year. Seedless yellow fruit, to 20cm (8in) long, borne in long bunches, have sweet-tasting white pulp. The most suitable cultivar for general garden cultivation; should produce fruit annually if a minimum temperature of 15–18°C (59–64°F) is maintained. ↕↔ to 3m (10ft).

M. arnoldiana see *Ensete ventricosum.*

M. basjoo ▣ ✾ syn. *M. japonica* (Japanese banana). Suckering perennial with slender false stems, green at first, becoming papery with age, and arching, oblong-lance-shaped, bright green leaf-blades, to 3m (10ft) long. In summer, produces pale yellow or cream flowers, 2–3cm (¾–1¼in) long, with large brown bracts, in pendent, terminal spikes, followed by unpalatable, yellowish green fruit, 6cm (2½in) long, with black seeds in white pulp. ↕ to 5m (15ft), ↔ to 4m (12ft). Japan (including Ryukyu Islands). ❄❄

M. cavendishii see *M. acuminata.*

M. coccinea ♀ syn. *M. uranoscopus* (Scarlet banana). Suckering perennial with reddish green false stems, becoming papery with age. Produces oval to elliptic leaf-blades, 1m (3ft) long, glossy, bright green above, paler and waxy beneath. In summer, bears erect spirals of tubular yellow flowers, 2–3cm (¾–1¼in) long, enclosed in bright red bracts, followed by orange-yellow fruit, 5cm (2in) long, with black seeds. Good for containers and cut flowers. ↕↔ 1.5m (5ft). S.E. Asia (S. China, Vietnam, Laos, Cambodia). ❁ (min. 7°C/45°F)

M. ensete see *Ensete ventricosum.*

M. japonica see *M. basjoo.*

M. ornata ▣ ♀ ✾ (Flowering banana). Suckering perennial with oblong to elliptic, waxy, slightly glaucous, blue-green leaf-blades, 2m (6ft) long. Produces yellowish orange flowers, 3cm (1¼in) long, with purplish pink bracts, on short, erect false stems at various times of year, followed by greenish yellow fruit, 6cm (2½in) long, with black seeds. ↕ to 3m (10ft), ↔ to 4m (12ft). Bangladesh. ❁ (min. 7°C/45°F)

M. x paradisiaca 'Dwarf Cavendish' see *M. acuminata* 'Dwarf Cavendish'.

M. uranoscopus see *M. coccinea.*

MUSCARI syn. MUSCARIMIA

Grape hyacinth

HYACINTHACEAE/LILIACEAE

Genus of 30 species of bulbous perennials occurring from sea level to subalpine areas, in woodland and on steppes, stony slopes, and screes, in the Mediterranean region and S.W. Asia. The fleshy leaves, arranged in basal clusters, are linear to inversely lance-shaped, or sickle- or spoon-shaped, mostly channelled, and mid-green, or blue- or grey-green. Flowers are borne in terminal racemes on leafless stems in spring or, occasionally, autumn; the lower fertile flowers are sometimes crowned by smaller, paler sterile ones. They may be tubular, bell-shaped, or spherical, often with constricted mouths, and are 4–8mm (⅛–⅜in) long, occasionally to 1cm (½in) long. Grow in massed displays in a mixed border; they are also suitable for a deciduous woodland garden, a wild garden, or for naturalizing in grassland. Use the smaller species in a rock garden.

• **HARDINESS** Fully hardy to frost hardy.

• **CULTIVATION** Plant 10cm (4in) deep in groups in autumn, in moderately fertile, moist but well-drained soil in full sun. Lift and divide congested clumps to maintain vigour, when dormant in summer.

• **PROPAGATION** Sow seed in containers in a cold frame in autumn. Remove offsets in summer.

• **PESTS AND DISEASES** Prone to viruses.

M. armeniacum ▣ ♀ Vigorous, bulbous perennial producing semi-erect, narrowly linear to linear-inversely lance-shaped, mid-green leaves, 30cm (12in) long, in autumn. Tubular, bright blue flowers with distinct, constricted white mouths, are borne in dense racemes, 2–8cm (¾–3in) long, in spring. May be invasive. ↕ 20cm (8in), ↔ 5cm (2in). S.E. Europe to Caucasus. ❄❄❄. **'Argaei'** has bright blue flowers. **'Blue Spike'** ▣ has large, densely bunched, double, blue flowers.

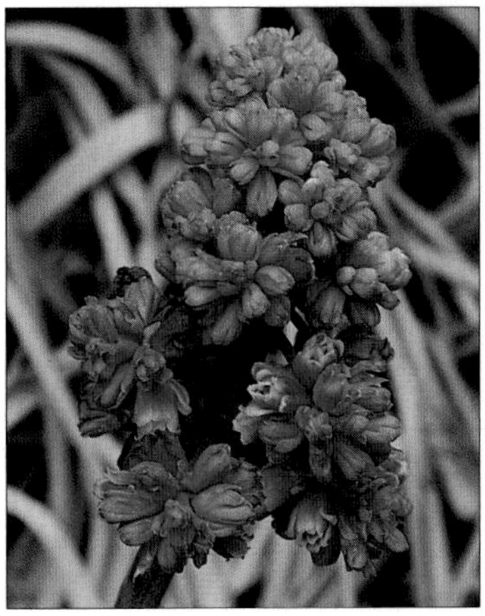

Muscari armeniacum 'Blue Spike'

M. aucheri ▣ ♀ syn. *M. lingulatum.* Bulbous perennial with erect or semi-erect, narrowly sickle- to narrowly spoon-shaped, mid-green leaves, 5–20cm (2–8in) long. In spring, bears tight racemes, 1–4cm (½–1½in) long, of tubular, bright blue flowers with constricted white mouths, usually crowned with paler blue, sterile flowers. ↕ 10–15cm (4–6in), ↔ 5cm (2in). Turkey. ❄❄❄. **'Tubergenianum'**, syn. *M. tubergenianum*, is more robust, with a conspicuous crown of sterile flowers; ↕ 20cm (8in).

M. azureum ♀ syn. *Hyacinthus azureus, Pseudomuscari azureum.* Bulbous perennial with erect, narrowly inversely lance-shaped, greyish green leaves, 6–20cm (2½–8in) long. In spring, bears shortly bell-shaped, bright sky-blue flowers with a darker stripe on each lobe and scarcely constricted mouths, in dense, conical to ovoid racemes, 1–3cm (½–1¼in) long. May self-seed freely. ↕ 10cm (4in), ↔ 5cm (2in). Turkey. ❄❄❄. **f. album** has pure white flowers.

M. botryoides. Slender perennial with semi-erect, narrowly spoon-shaped,

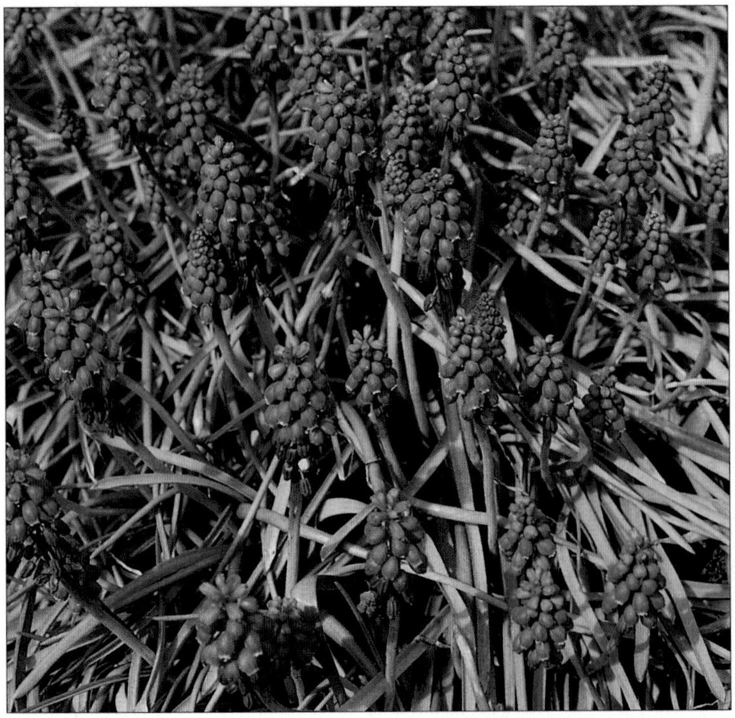

Muscari armeniacum

M

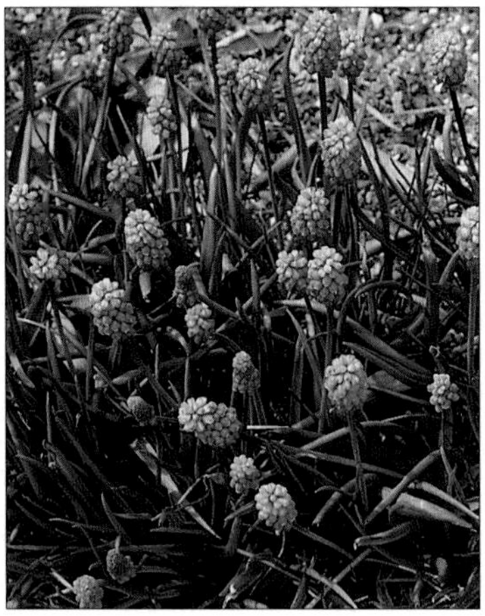
Muscari aucheri

mid-green leaves, 5–25cm (2–10in) long. In spring, bears spherical, bright blue flowers with constricted white mouths, in dense racemes 2–5cm (¾–2in) long. ↕ 15–20cm (6–8in), ↔ 5cm (2in). C. and S.E. Europe. ❄❄❄. **f. *album*** ▣ has slender racemes of fragrant white flowers.
M. comosum, syn. *Leopoldia comosa* (Tassel grape hyacinth). Bulbous perennial with spreading, linear, mid-green leaves, to 15cm (6in) long. In spring, bears oblong-urn-shaped, creamy brown flowers with constricted mouths, in racemes 6–30cm (2½–12in) long. Spherical, bright violet, upper, sterile flowers are borne in tassels on long, upright stalks. ↕ 20–60cm (8–24in), ↔ 5cm (2in). S. Europe, Turkey, Iran. ❄❄. **'Plumosum'**, syn. 'Monstrosum', has feathery heads composed entirely of purple, sterile threads.
M. latifolium. Bulbous perennial with solitary, semi-erect, inversely lance-shaped, mid-green leaves, 7–30cm (3–12in) long. In spring, bears dense racemes, 2–6cm (¾–2½in) long, of oblong-urn-shaped, violet-black flowers, constricted at the mouths, and crowns of paler, sterile flowers. ↕ 20cm (8in), ↔ 5cm (2in). S.W. Asia. ❄❄
M. lingulatum see *M. aucheri.*
M. macrocarpum ▣ syn. *M. moschatum* var. *flavum, M. muscarimi* var. *flavum.* Bulbous perennial with thick, fleshy, persistent roots and semi-erect, linear, greyish green leaves, to 30cm (12in) long. In spring, produces tubular, strongly fragrant yellow flowers, with constricted mouths, opening from purplish brown buds, in racemes 4–6cm

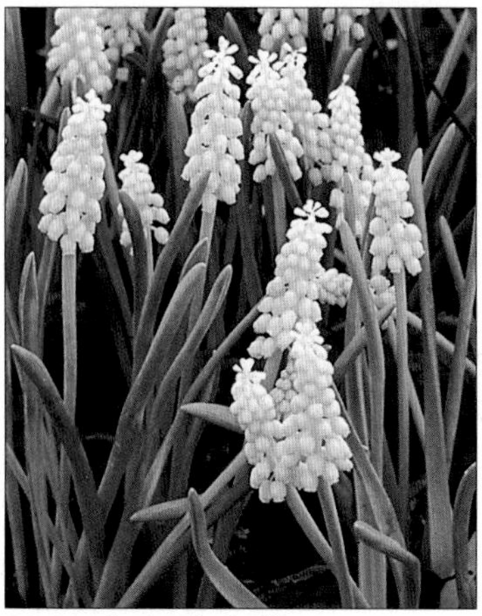
Muscari botryoides f. *album*

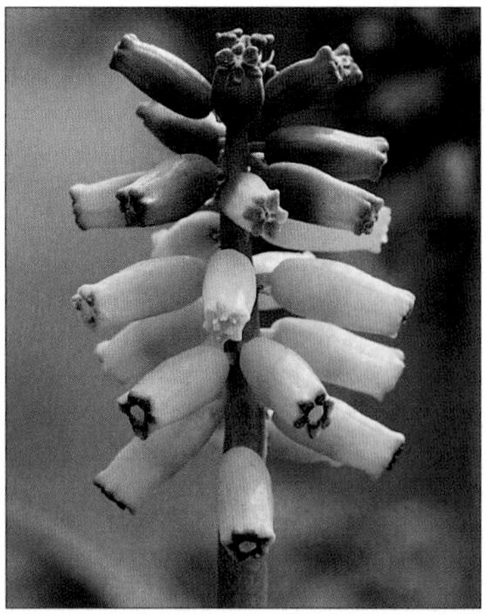
Muscari macrocarpum

(1¾–2½in) long. Requires a hot, dry summer dormancy to flower well. ↕ 10–15cm (4–6in), ↔ 8cm (3in). Greece (Aegean islands), W. Turkey. ❄❄
M. moschatum* var. *flavum see *M. macrocarpum.*
M. muscarimi* var. *flavum see *M. macrocarpum.*
M. neglectum, syn. *M. racemosum.* Bulbous perennial with many semi-erect, linear, channelled to almost cylindrical, bright, mid-green leaves, 6–40cm (2½–16in) long, often produced in autumn. In spring, bears blue-black flowers with constricted white mouths, in dense racemes 1–5cm (½–2in) long. Increases rapidly. ↕ 10–20cm (4–8in), ↔ 5cm (2in). Europe, N. Africa, S.W. Asia. ❄❄❄
***M. paradoxum* of gardens** see *Bellevalia pycnantha.*
M. pycnantha see *Bellevalia pycnantha.*
M. racemosum see *M. neglectum.*
M. tubergenianum see *M. aucheri* 'Tubergenianum'.

▷ ***Muscarimia*** see *Muscari*
▷ **Musk** see *Mimulus*
Monkey see *M. luteus*

MUSSAENDA

RUBIACEAE

Genus of about 100 species of evergreen perennials, shrubs, subshrubs, and twining climbers found in woodland from tropical Africa and Asia to Malaysia. The opposite or whorled, membranous, lance-shaped to elliptic, or ovate or oblong, usually mid-green leaves are often hairy on the lower surfaces. Tubular or funnel-shaped, yellow, red, pink, or white flowers, each with 5 spreading lobes, are borne in often large, terminal or axillary panicles or cymes. One sepal of each flower is often greatly enlarged and colourful. Where temperatures fall below 15°C (59°F), grow in a warm greenhouse. In warmer areas, grow as free-standing specimens or in a shrub border, or use climbers to clothe an arch or pergola.
• **HARDINESS** Frost tender.
• **CULTIVATION** Under glass, grow in loam-based potting compost (JI No.2) in full light, with shade from hot sun. In growth, water freely and apply a balanced liquid fertilizer monthly; water sparingly in winter. Outdoors, grow in moderately fertile, moist but well-drained soil in full sun, with some

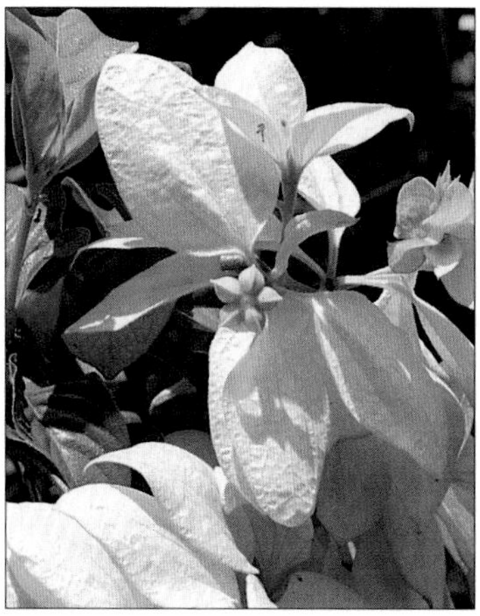
Mussaenda 'Don Leonila'

midday shade. Pruning group 1 for shrubs; group 12, after flowering, for climbers under glass.
• **PROPAGATION** Sow seed at 19–24°C (66–75°F) in spring. Root semi-ripe cuttings with bottom heat in summer.
• **PESTS AND DISEASES** Susceptible to red spider mites and whiteflies under glass.

***M.* 'Aurorae'**, syn. *M. phillippica* 'Aurorae'. Rounded, evergreen shrub with opposite, ovate, prominently veined, downy leaves, 8–15cm (3–6in) long. Narrowly funnel-shaped, deep golden yellow flowers, with pendent, obovate white sepals, to 8cm (3in) long, are borne in terminal cymes, 8cm (3in) long, in summer, or throughout the year in warm regions. ↕↔ 1.5m (5ft). ❀ (min. 12°C/54°F)
***M.* 'Don Leonila'** ▣ Rounded, evergreen shrub with opposite, ovate, downy leaves, 8–15cm (3–6in) long, with prominent veins. In summer, bears narrowly funnel-shaped, deep yellow flowers, with obovate, creamy white sepals, to 8cm (3in) long, in terminal cymes, 8cm (3in) long. ↕ 3m (10ft), ↔ 1.5m (5ft). ❀ (min. 12°C/54°F)
M. erythrophylla ▣ Twining climber, usually grown as a shrub, with ovate or broadly elliptic to broadly ovate, softly hairy, red-veined, dark green leaves, 10–18cm (4–7in) long. In summer, bears small, creamy white, red-centred flowers, each with one broadly ovate sepal, 5–10cm (2–4in) long, in large, dense panicles, 4cm (1½in) long. ↕ 2–3m (6–10ft) (grown as a shrub), 8–10m (25–30ft) (grown as a climber); ↔ 1.5–2.5m (5–8ft). Tropical Africa.

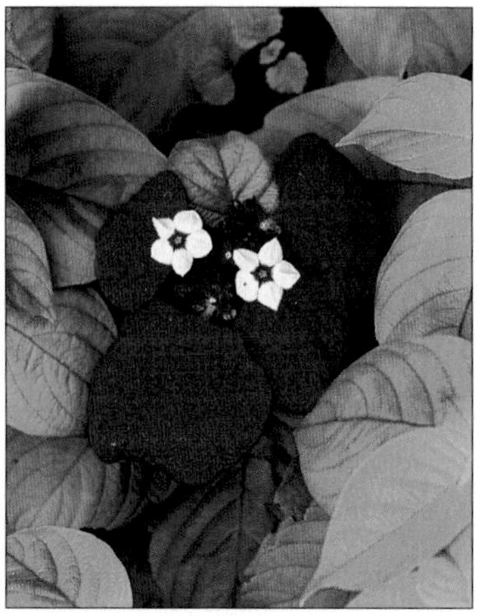
Mussaenda erythrophylla

❀ (min. 15°C/59°F). **'Queen Sirikit'** bears pendent flowers, with numerous large, wavy, deep pink to ivory sepals, on arching branches.
***M. phillippica* 'Aurorae'** see *M.* 'Aurorae'.

MUTISIA

ASTERACEAE/COMPOSITAE

Genus of about 60 species of evergreen shrubs and tendril climbers occurring in woodland and scrub in South America. The leaves are alternate, linear to oblong-ovate, sometimes pinnate, and mid- or dark green. Showy, daisy-like flowerheads are borne singly from the leaf axils from summer to autumn. Grow in a small courtyard garden or through shrubs in a border, or use to clothe a fence or trellis. In frost-prone areas, grow frost-hardy species in a cool or temperate greenhouse.
• **HARDINESS** Frost hardy to half hardy.
• **CULTIVATION** Under glass, grow in loam-based potting compost (JI No.2) in bright filtered light, or full light with shade from hot sun. In growth, water moderately and apply a balanced liquid fertilizer monthly; keep just moist in winter. Outdoors, grow in moderately fertile, moist but well-drained soil in full sun. Protect from excessive winter wet and shelter from cold, dry winds. Keep roots cool and moist. Pruning group 11, in spring, if necessary to restrict size.
• **PROPAGATION** Sow seed in autumn: frost-hardy species in containers in a cold frame; half-hardy species at 13–18°C (55–64°F). Can be difficult to germinate. Root stem-tip cuttings in late spring or summer. Layer in autumn. Separate suckers in spring.
• **PESTS AND DISEASES** Trouble free.

M. decurrens ▣ Suckering climber with winged stems and narrowly oblong, entire or toothed, dark green leaves, to 12cm (5in) long, each ending in a 2-lobed tendril. Bright orange flowerheads, to 12cm (5in) across, are borne in summer. Best propagated from suckers. ↕ 3m (10ft). Chile, Argentina. ❄❄
M. ilicifolia. Climber with winged shoots and holly-like, ovate to ovate-elliptic, bright green leaves, to 6cm (2½in) long, each ending in a long, unbranched tendril. Short-stalked, pale pink flowerheads, to 7cm (3in) across, with yellow centres, are borne from summer to autumn and often irregularly during the year. ↕ 3m (10ft). Chile. ❄❄

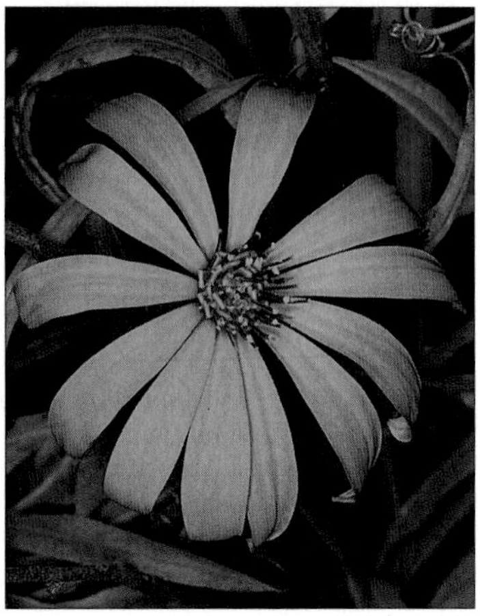
Mutisia decurrens

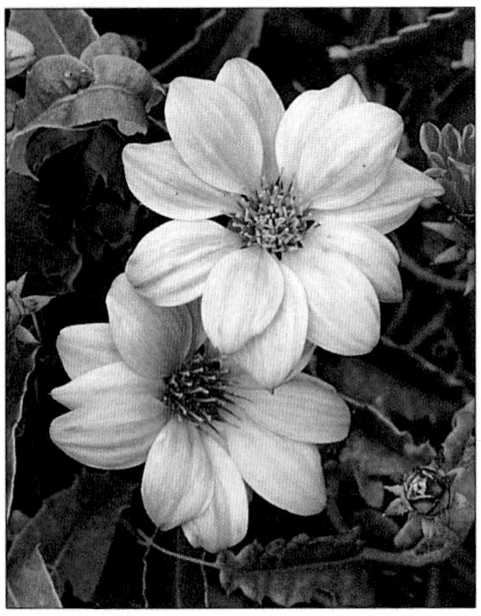

Mutisia oligodon

M. oligodon ■ Climber with oblong, sharply toothed, glossy, dark green leaves, white woolly beneath, to 3.5cm (1½in) long, each ending in a long tendril. Long-stalked pink flowerheads, to 7cm (3in) across, with yellow centres, are produced from summer to autumn. ↕1.5m (5ft). Chile, Argentina. ❄❄

▷**Myall, Weeping** see *Acacia pendula*

MYOPORUM

MYOPORACEAE

Genus of about 30 species of spreading, prostrate to upright, evergreen shrubs and trees from open, dry areas, usually at low altitudes, from E. Asia to Australia, New Zealand, and Hawaii. The alternate, variably shaped, entire or toothed, light to mid-green leaves are dotted with glands. Small, bell-shaped or tubular-bell-shaped flowers, each with 5 spreading lobes, are borne singly or in short cymes from the leaf axils, followed by small, succulent berries. In frost-prone areas, grow in a temperate or warm greenhouse, mainly for foliage. Elsewhere, they are suitable for a shrub border, and are ideal as informal hedges and windbreaks, especially near the sea.

M

- **HARDINESS** Frost tender; may survive brief spells near 0°C (32°F).
- **CULTIVATION** Under glass, grow in loam-based potting compost (JI No.2) in full light, with shade from hot sun, or in bright filtered light. In growth, water freely; apply a balanced liquid fertilizer monthly. Water sparingly in winter. Outdoors, grow in moderately fertile, moist but well-drained soil in full sun, with midday shade. Pruning group 9.
- **PROPAGATION** Sow seed at 6–12°C (45–54°F) as soon as ripe. Root semi-ripe cuttings with bottom heat in summer.
- **PESTS AND DISEASES** Scale insects may be a problem under glass.

M. laetum ○ (Ngaio). Large shrub or small tree of dense habit, with sticky stem tips and thick, furrowed brown bark when mature. Fleshy, bright green leaves are lance-shaped to oblong or obovate, 4–10cm (1½–4in) long. Bears cymes of 2–6 bell-shaped, purple-spotted white flowers, 1cm (½in) across, in summer. Narrowly ovoid berries are pale to deep reddish purple, 6–9mm (¼–⅜in) long. ↕5–10m (15–30ft), ↔2–5m (6–15ft). New Zealand. ❀ (min. 2°C/36°C). **var. *decumbens*** is

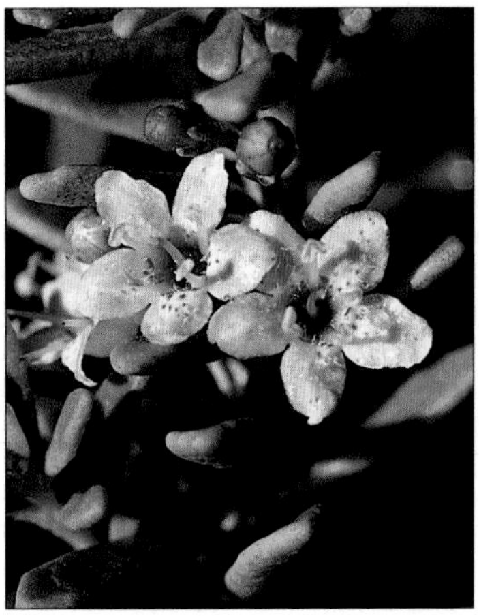

Myoporum parvifolium

spreading or prostrate, and useful for ground cover; ↕to 1m (3ft).
M. parvifolium ■ Small, spreading, bushy shrub with reddish green, sticky stems, and narrowly spoon-shaped to linear, fleshy, bright green leaves, to 3cm (1¼in) long, with prominent glands. In summer, produces bell-shaped, honey-scented, white, occasionally lilac flowers, 1cm (½in) across, usually purple-dotted, singly or in twos or threes, followed by broadly ovoid purple berries, 7mm (¼in) long. ↕to 60cm (24in), ↔60–90cm (24–36in). Australia (South Australia, Victoria, Tasmania). ❀ (min. 2°C/36°C)

MYOSOTIDIUM

BORAGINACEAE

Genus of one species of evergreen perennial from rocky or sandy coasts on Chatham Island, New Zealand. It has thick, fleshy stems and leaves, the latter large, simple, and glossy, and forget-me-not-like flowers. Grow in a peat bed or rock garden; it can be difficult to grow as it needs cool, damp conditions, preferably in a coastal location. In frost-prone areas, grow in a cool greenhouse.

- **HARDINESS** Half hardy, although will survive temperatures just below 0°C (32°F) with some protection.
- **CULTIVATION** Under glass, grow in loam-based potting compost (JI No.2) in bright filtered light. In growth, water freely and apply a seaweed-based fertilizer monthly; keep just moist in winter. Outdoors, grow in humus-rich, gritty, moist but well-drained soil with a seaweed mulch, in light dappled shade. Provide shelter from cold, drying winds.
- **PROPAGATION** Sow seed under glass in autumn or as soon as ripe. Divide in spring.
- **PESTS AND DISEASES** Prone to slugs.

M. hortensia ■ syn. *M. nobile* (Chatham Island forget-me-not). Clump-forming, evergreen perennial with very glossy, ovate to heart-shaped, ribbed, basal leaves, to 30cm (12in) long, with conspicuous veins and wavy margins. In early summer, bears dense, corymb-like cymes of open bell-shaped, pale to dark blue flowers, 1cm (½in) across, sometimes with white-margined lobes. ↕↔ to 60cm (24in). New Zealand (Chatham Island). ❄
M. nobile see *M. hortensia*.

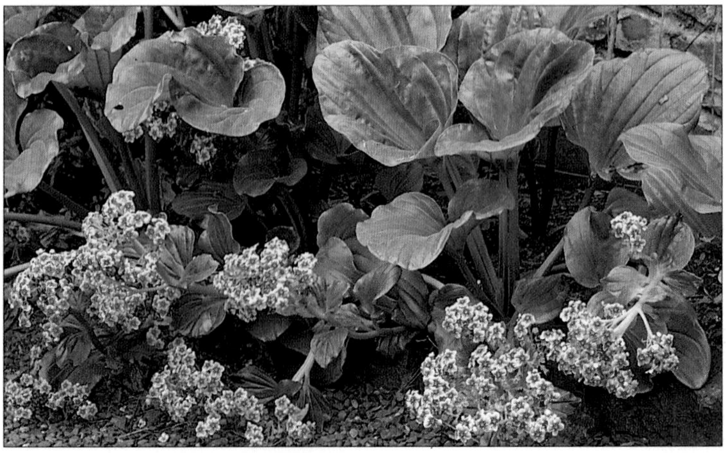

Myosotidium hortensia

MYOSOTIS

Forget-me-not

BORAGINACEAE

Genus of 50 or more species of annuals, biennials, and clump- or mat-forming perennials found in woods, meadows, swampy soils, and at pond margins in Europe, Asia, Australasia, and North and South America. They produce alternate, variably shaped, hairy leaves, and usually paired cymes of 5-lobed, salverform, occasionally funnel-shaped flowers in blue, yellow, or white, mostly with yellow or white eyes. The dwarf perennials are mainly short-lived but self-seed freely; they are useful for a rock garden, bank, scree bed, or alpine house. Grow *M. scorpioides* at the margins of a pond. *M. sylvatica* is suitable for a mixed or wildflower border; its cultivars are useful for spring bedding.

- **HARDINESS** Fully hardy; *M. alpestris* and *M. explanata* need gritty, sharply drained soil to survive wet winters.
- **CULTIVATION** Grow in moderately fertile or poor, moist but well-drained soil in full sun, with some midday shade, or in partial shade. Dwarf perennials need soil that is not too fertile as they may become coarse in rich soils; in an alpine house, grow in a mix of equal parts loam, leaf mould, and grit. Grow *M. scorpioides* in wet soil, or in an aquatic planting basket as a shallow-water marginal, at a maximum depth of 10cm (4in); see also pp.52–53.
- **PROPAGATION** Sow seed of annuals and biennials *in situ* in spring or, for spring bedding, in containers in a cold frame or seedbed in early summer. Sow seed of perennials in containers in a cold frame in spring; divide when dormant,

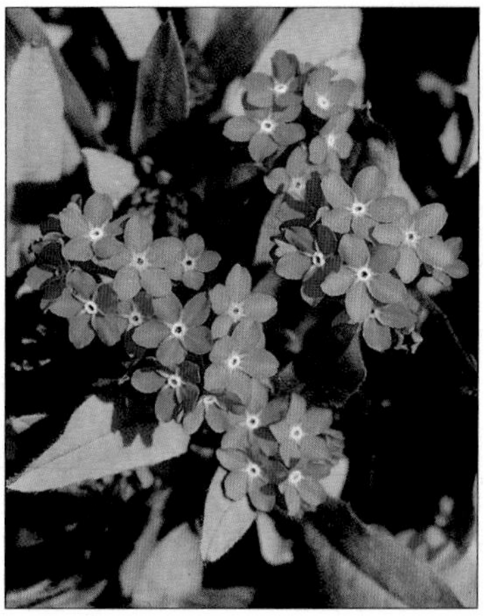

Myosotis alpestris

and propagate regularly as they are often short-lived. Sow seed of *M. scorpioides in situ* in mud at pond margins, or in moist compost in containers in a cold frame, in spring; divide and replant in mud or in baskets in shallow water.

- **PESTS AND DISEASES** Susceptible to powdery and downy mildew. Slugs and snails may cause damage outdoors.

M. alpestris ■ syn. *M. rupicola* (Alpine forget-me-not). Short-lived, clump-forming perennial with oblong-lance-shaped or spoon-shaped, bright green leaves, to 8cm (3in) long. Dense cymes of salverform, bright blue, yellow-eyed flowers, to 9mm (⅜in) across, are borne from spring to early summer. ↕20cm (8in), ↔to 15cm (6in). Europe. ❄❄❄
M. explanata. Clump- to hummock-forming perennial with rosettes of obovate to spoon-shaped, white-hairy, grey-green leaves, to 7cm (3in) long. In early summer, spreading stems bear large cymes of salverform to funnel-shaped white flowers, to 1cm (½in) across. ↕to 20cm (8in), ↔to 15cm (6in). New Zealand (South Island). ❄❄❄
M. palustris see *M. scorpioides*.
M. rupicola see *M. alpestris*.
M. scorpioides, syn. *M. palustris* (Water forget-me-not). Marginal aquatic perennial with creeping rhizomes and upright or semi-upright, angular stems. Leaves are narrowly ovate and mid-green, to 10cm (4in) long at the bases, becoming slightly longer up the stem. In early summer, bears open cymes of salverform, bright blue flowers, to 8mm (⅜in) across, each with a white, pink, or yellow eye. ↕15–30cm (6–12in) or

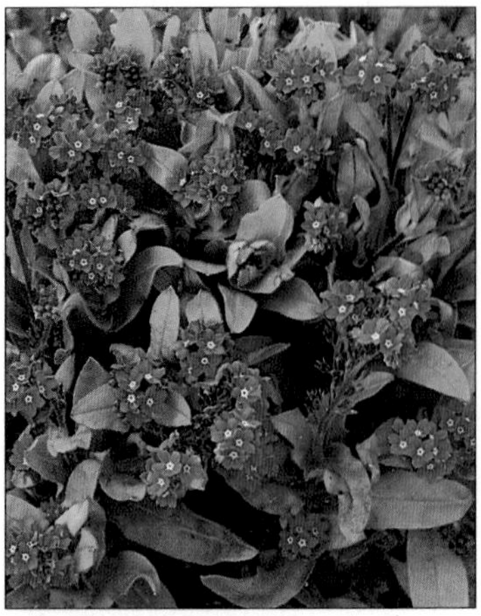

Myosotis sylvatica 'Music'

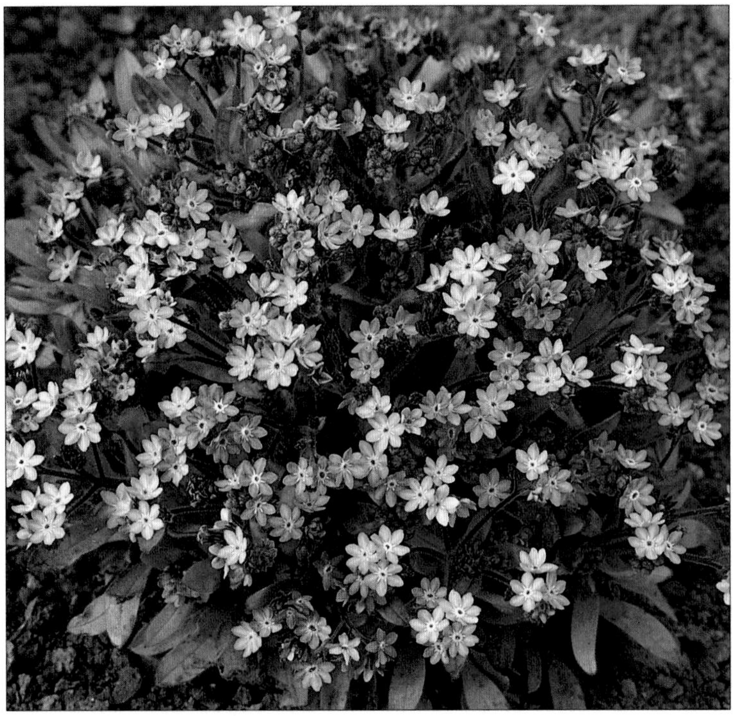

Myosotis sylvatica Victoria Series 'Victoria Rose'

more, ↔ 30cm (12in). Europe, Asia, North America. ❄❄❄. **'Mermaid'** is strong-stemmed and more compact, with dark green leaves, 4–6cm (1½–2½in) long, and bright blue, yellow-eyed flowers; ↕ 15–23cm (6–9in). ***M. sylvatica.*** Tufted, hairy biennial or short-lived perennial, usually grown as a biennial, with ovate to elliptic or lance-shaped, grey-green leaves, to 11cm (4½in) long. From spring to early summer, bears saucer-shaped, yellow-eyed, blue or occasionally white flowers, to 9mm (⅜in) across, in numerous dense cymes. ↕ 12–30cm (5–12in), ↔ to 15cm (6in). Europe. ❄❄❄. Cultivars of **Ball Series** are ball-shaped and compact; ↕ 15cm (6in); the series includes **'Blue Ball'** with azure flowers, and **'Snowball'** with white flowers. **'Blue Basket'** is tall and erect, with deep azure flowers; ↕ 25–30cm (10–12in). **'Music'** ■ is vigorous and erect, with large, very bright blue flowers; ↕ to 25cm (10in). **'Pompadour'** is compact and ball-shaped, with large, deep rose-pink flowers; ↕ 15–20cm (6–8in). **'Ultramarine'** 🏆 is dwarf and compact, with deep indigo-blue flowers; ↕ to 15cm (6in). **Victoria Series** cultivars are dwarf and compact, with white, blue, or pink flowers; the series includes **'Victoria Rose'** ■ with bright rose-pink flowers; ↕ 10cm (4in).

▷**Myriad leaf** see *Myriophyllum verticillatum*

MYRICA

MYRICACEAE

Genus of about 50 species of dioecious or monoecious, deciduous and evergreen, usually suckering shrubs and erect trees, found in moist ground worldwide. They have alternate, lance-shaped to ovate, usually aromatic, dark green leaves. *M. cerifera* and *M. gale* are both effective when grown in groups. *M. cerifera* may also be used as a screening plant; *M. gale* is a useful bog plant.

- **HARDINESS** Fully hardy to frost hardy.
- **CULTIVATION** Grow in humus-rich, moist soil. *M. gale* will also grow in permanently waterlogged, acid soil. Pruning group 1.
- **PROPAGATION** Sow seed in containers outdoors as soon as ripe. Root greenwood cuttings in early to midsummer. Layer in spring.
- **PESTS AND DISEASES** Trouble free.

M. cerifera (Wax myrtle). Rounded, deciduous or evergreen shrub with upright branches and obovate or narrowly inversely lance-shaped, aromatic leaves, to 10cm (4in) long. In spring, bears inconspicuous, yellow-green male catkins, to 2cm (¾in) long. Spherical, waxy, grey-white fruit, 3mm (⅛in) across, are densely clustered along the shoots and persist over winter. ↕↔ 5m (15ft). S.E. USA. ❄❄
M. gale (Bog myrtle, Sweet gale). Thicket-forming, suckering, deciduous shrub with upright branches and inversely lance-shaped, toothed, aromatic leaves, to 6cm (2½in) long. Yellow-brown male catkins, to 1.5cm (½in) long, are borne in mid- and late spring, followed by spherical, yellow-brown fruit, to 3mm (⅛in) across, dotted with resin. ↕↔ 1.5m (5ft). Europe, Asia, North America. ❄❄❄

MYRIOPHYLLUM

Milfoil

HALORAGACEAE

Genus of 45 species of submerged or marginal aquatic annuals and perennials occurring in wet ground, ponds, and streams, widely distributed but mainly found in the S. hemisphere. The foliage is highly decorative, with long, submerged, delicate stems and alternate, opposite, or whorled leaves. The submerged leaves are linear to oblong or rounded, and pinnatifid with fine, hair-like segments; the emergent leaves are entire or toothed, and lance-shaped to ovate or linear. Milfoils provide refuge for fish fry, as well as oxygenating the water. Grow in an outdoor pool, or use *M. aquaticum* in a tropical aquarium and *M. hippuroides* and *M. verticillatum* in a cold-water aquarium.

- **HARDINESS** Fully hardy to frost hardy.
- **CULTIVATION** In an aquarium, grow in an inert medium in full light, preferably in hard water, at 10–15°C (50–59°F) for *M. hippuroides* and *M. verticillatum*, 18–24°C (64–75°F) for *M. aquaticum*. Outdoors, grow in baskets of loamy soil in full sun, at a depth of 1m (3ft) for *M. aquaticum* and *M. verticillatum*, and 45cm (18in) for *M. hippuroides*. Top growth may be damaged by frost but should re-emerge below the surface in spring. See also pp.52–53.
- **PROPAGATION** Root cuttings (young tips, or segments) by inserting in the bottom sand.
- **PESTS AND DISEASES** Young growth may be eaten by fishes. Algae or detritus in the water chokes the leaves.

M. aquaticum ■ syn. *M. brasiliense*, *M. proserpinacoides* (Diamond milfoil, Parrot feather). Aquatic perennial with rarely branched stems, to 2m (6ft) long, becoming woody at the bases and often creeping out of shallow water. Rounded, pinnatifid, bright yellowish green submerged leaves, to 4cm (1½in) long, have 4–8 segments and are arranged in whorls of 4 or 5; rounded, bluish green emergent leaves are shorter. In summer, minute, monoecious, bright yellow-green flowers are borne in spikes from the axils of the submerged leaves. ↔ indefinite. Indonesia (Java), Australia, New Zealand, South America. ❄❄
M. brasiliense see *M. aquaticum*.
M. hippuroides ■ (Western milfoil). Aquatic perennial with thin stems, to 60cm (24in) long. Bears lance-shaped to ovate, pinnatifid, yellow-green submerged leaves, to 2cm (¾in) long, with up to 25 segments. Linear to lance-shaped, finely divided, olive-green to red emergent leaves, 5cm (2in) long, borne in whorls of 4–6, are usually upward-pointing. Bears minute white flowers from the axils of the emergent leaves in summer. ↔ indefinite. S.W. USA. ❄❄
M. proserpinacoides see *M. aquaticum*.
M. verticillatum (Myriad leaf). Aquatic perennial with stems to 1m (3ft) long. Linear, pinnatifid, tightly packed, bright green submerged leaves, to 4cm (1½in) long, are arranged in whorls of 4–6, with 8–16 pairs of opposite segments. Emergent leaves are pinnatifid and

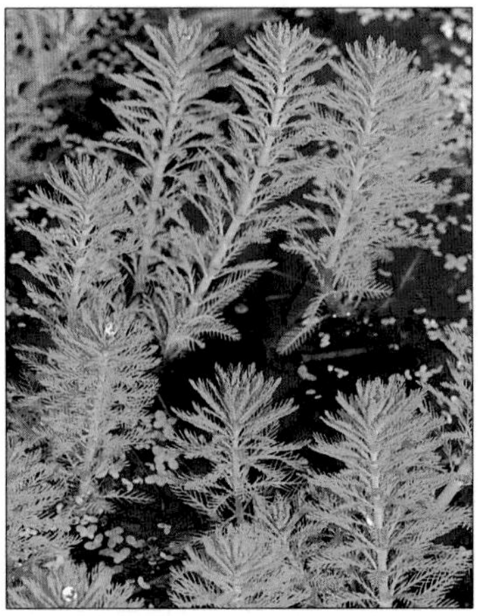

Myriophyllum aquaticum

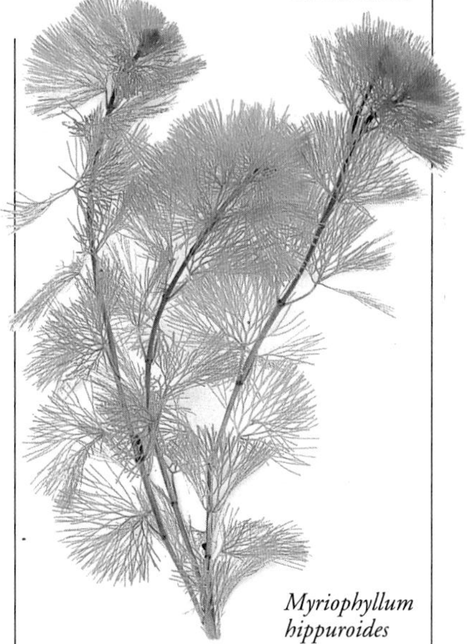

Myriophyllum hippuroides

comb-like, to 2.5cm (1in) long. In summer, bears yellowish flowers in a spike, to 15cm (6in) tall, just above the water surface. ↔ indefinite. Europe, Asia, North America. ❄❄❄

▷***Myrmecophila tibicinis*** see *Schomburgkia tibicinis*
▷**Myrobalan** see *Prunus cerasifera*
▷**Myrrh, Garden** see *Myrrhis odorata*

MYRRHIS

Sweet Cicely

APIACEAE/UMBELLIFERAE

Genus of one species of aromatic herbaceous perennial originally found in mountains of S. Europe, now widespread in damp sites in Europe and Asia. It has compound umbels of small white flowers and delicate, fern-like foliage. Grow in a mixed border, or in a herb or wildflower garden. Self-seeds freely.

- **HARDINESS** Fully hardy.
- **CULTIVATION** Grow in moderately fertile, moist but well-drained soil in dappled shade. Harvest leaves from early spring to late summer. To improve the flavour and quality of the leaves, remove the flowering stems as they develop.
- **PROPAGATION** Sow seed in containers in a cold frame in spring or as soon as ripe. Divide in spring or autumn.
- **PESTS AND DISEASES** Trouble free.

M. odorata ■ (Garden myrrh, Sweet Cicely). Perennial with stout, hairy, hollow stems and soft, 2- or 3-pinnate,

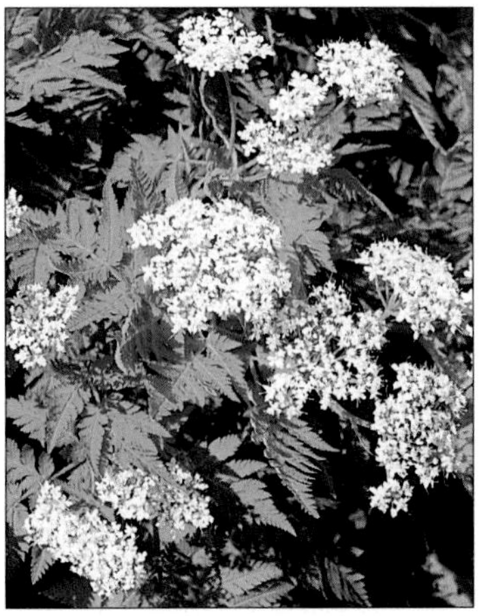

Myrrhis odorata

M

bright green leaves, to 45cm (18in) long, comprising deeply toothed, oblong to lance-shaped pinnae. Compound umbels of small, star-shaped white flowers, are produced in early summer, followed by ridged, beaked, shiny brown fruit, to 2cm (¾in) long. Aniseed-flavoured leaves and young shoots provide sweetness when cooked with fruit. ↕ 2m (6ft), ↔ 1.5m (5ft). S. Europe. ❄❄❄

MYRSINE

MYRSINACEAE

Genus of about 5 species of dioecious, evergreen, many-branched, upright or rounded shrubs and small trees, found in forest and scrub in Africa, the Azores, the Himalayas, China, and New Zealand. They are mainly cultivated for their alternate, linear or lance-shaped to rounded, usually entire, leathery, sometimes glossy, mid- or dark green leaves. Inconspicuous male and female flowers are produced in umbels on separate plants; both are needed to produce fruit. Grow in a shrub border, against a wall, or in a rock, heather, peat, or woodland garden. In frost-prone areas, grow half-hardy and frost-tender species in a temperate greenhouse.

- **HARDINESS** Frost hardy to frost tender.
- **CULTIVATION** Grow in humus-rich, moist but well-drained soil in full sun or light dappled shade. *M. africana* is lime-tolerant, but will not thrive on shallow, dry, chalk soil. Pruning group 1 or 8.
- **PROPAGATION** Sow seed in containers in a cold frame in autumn. Root semi-ripe cuttings with bottom heat in summer.
- **PESTS AND DISEASES** Trouble free.

M. africana (African boxwood, Cape myrtle). Slow-growing, densely leafy, upright shrub with narrowly obovate to elliptic, aromatic, glossy, dark green leaves, to 2cm (¾in) long. In late spring, produces umbels of 3–6 tiny, yellow-brown flowers. Female plants bear spherical, pale blue fruit, 5mm (¼in) across. ↕ 1.2m (4ft), ↔ 75cm (30in). Azores, E. and S. Africa, Himalayas, China. ❄❄

MYRTEOLA

MYRTACEAE

Genus of 12 species of dwarf, evergreen, mat-forming to rounded, bushy shrubs or subshrubs from upland slopes and raised bogs in South America. They are grown for their attractive fruits and glossy foliage. Leaves are opposite, ovate to rounded, and mid- to dark green. Cup-shaped, 4- or 5-petalled, pale yellow to white flowers are borne singly from the leaf axils from late spring to summer, followed by spherical, pink to dark red berries in autumn. Grow in a peat bed, or a rock or woodland garden.

- **HARDINESS** Fully hardy.
- **CULTIVATION** Grow in humus-rich, moist but well-drained, acid soil in full sun, with some midday shade, or in dappled shade. Pruning is not required; trim wayward shoots if necessary.
- **PROPAGATION** Sow seed in containers in an open frame in autumn. Root semi-ripe cuttings, taken with a heel, with bottom heat in summer.
- **PESTS AND DISEASES** Trouble free.

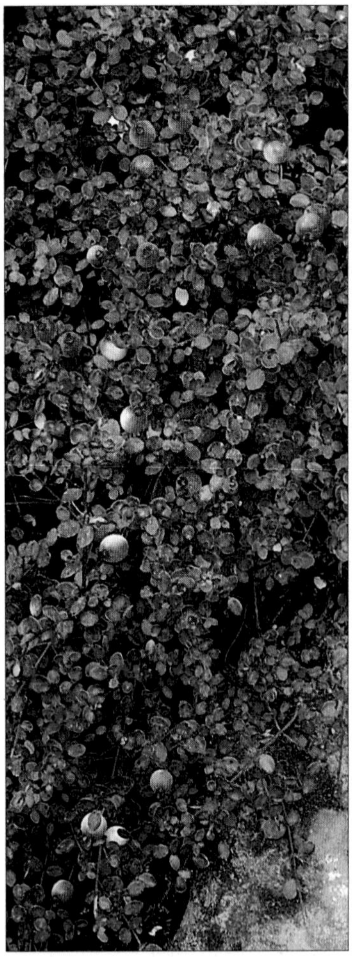

Myrteola nummularia

M. nummularia ■ syn. *Myrtus nummularia*. Mat-forming subshrub with branching stems clothed in tiny, ovate, dark green leaves, to 8mm (⅜in) long. In early summer, bears small white flowers, 8mm (⅜in) across, followed in late summer by spherical to ellipsoid pink berries, 7–10mm (¼–½in) long. ↕ 5cm (2in), ↔ 30cm (12in). S. Chile, S. Argentina, Falkland Islands. ❄❄❄

MYRTILLOCACTUS

CACTACEAE

Genus of 4 species of shrubby or tree-like perennial cacti occurring in semi-arid areas of Mexico and Guatemala. They have short, deep bluish green stems and thick, erect branches with 5–8 ribs and spiny, felted areoles. Open funnel-shaped, short-tubed flowers are borne from the upper lateral areoles in early and midsummer, followed by ovoid, purplish blue fruits. Where temperatures drop below 10°C (50°F), grow in a warm greenhouse. In warmer areas, grow in a rock or desert garden.

- **HARDINESS** Frost tender.
- **CULTIVATION** Under glass, grow in standard cactus compost in full light with low humidity. From mid-spring to early autumn, water moderately and apply a low-nitrogen fertilizer monthly; keep just moist at other times. Outdoors, grow in poor to moderately fertile, sharply drained soil in full sun. Provide protection from excessive winter wet. See also pp.48–49.
- **PROPAGATION** Sow seed at 19–24°C (66–75°F), or take stem cuttings, both in spring.

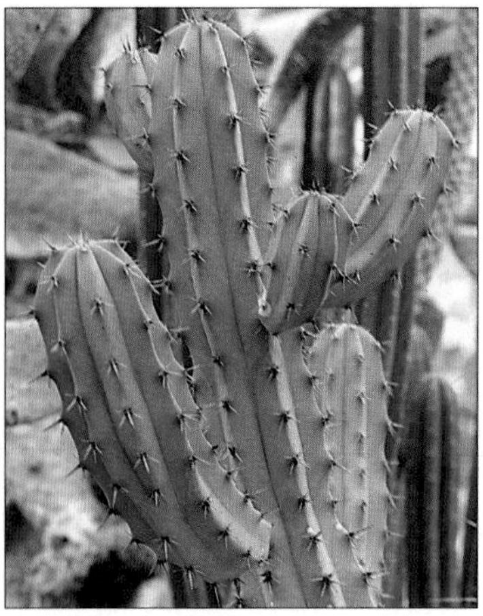

Myrtillocactus geometrizans

- **PESTS AND DISEASES** Susceptible to damage by mealybugs.

M. cochal. Tree-like cactus with mid-green stems, 15cm (6in) or more thick, with 6–8 shallow-grooved ribs and grey or black spines (3–5 radials and sometimes 1 longer central). White or pale yellow flowers, 2.5cm (1in) across, tinged green or purple, are borne both diurnally and nocturnally in early and midsummer. ↕ 1m (3ft), ↔ 45cm (18in). N.W. Mexico. ❀ (min. 10°C/50°F)

M. geometrizans ■ Tree-like cactus with bluish green stems, to 10cm (4in) thick, branching from about 30cm (12in) above ground level. Each has 5–6 smooth, acute ribs with 5–9 red-brown then grey radial spines and 1 longer, almost black central spine. White or cream flowers, 2.5–3.5cm (1–1½in) across, are produced diurnally in early and midsummer. ↕ 4m (12ft), ↔ 2m (6ft). Mexico. ❀ (min. 10°C/50°F)

▷**Myrtle** see *Myrtus*
Bog see *Myrica gale*
Cape see *Myrsine africana, Phylica*
Common see *Myrtus communis*
Crepe see *Lagerstroemia indica*
Giant crepe see *Lagerstroemia speciosa*
Heath see *Thryptomene*
Lemon-scented see *Backhousia citriodora, Darwinia citriodora*
Queen's crepe see *Lagerstroemia speciosa*
Sand see *Leiophyllum buxifolium*
Sea see *Baccharis halimifolia*
Snow see *Calytrix alpestris*
Tarentum see *Myrtus communis* subsp. *tarentina*
Wax see *Myrica cerifera*
Western tea see *Melaleuca nesophila*

MYRTUS

Myrtle

MYRTACEAE

Genus of 2 species of upright or rounded, evergreen trees and shrubs from scrub, woodland, and woodland margins in the Mediterranean region, N. Africa, South America, and the Falkland Islands. They are cultivated for their aromatic leaves and their solitary, bowl-shaped, fragrant white flowers, borne from spring to autumn. Myrtles are suitable for a mixed or shrub border, or for growing against a warm, sunny wall. They may also be grown as free-standing specimen shrubs or as an informal hedge. Long, hot summers are required for the production of flowers and fruits.

- **HARDINESS** Frost hardy.
- **CULTIVATION** Grow in moderately fertile, moist but well-drained soil in full sun, sheltered from cold, drying winds. Pruning group 1 for *M. lechleriana*; group 9 for *M. communis*; group 13 if wall-trained.
- **PROPAGATION** Sow seed in containers in a cold frame in autumn. Root semi-ripe cuttings with bottom heat in late summer.
- **PESTS AND DISEASES** Trouble free.

M. bullata see *Lophomyrtus bullata*.
***M. bullata* 'Gloriosa'** see *Lophomyrtus* x *ralphii* 'Variegata'.
M. chequen see *Luma chequen*.
M. communis ■ ♀ (Common myrtle). Upright, bushy shrub, arching with age, bearing opposite, ovate, glossy, dark green leaves, to 5cm (2in) long. From mid- to late summer or early autumn, produces solitary, 5-petalled flowers, 2cm (¾in) across, with conspicuous central tufts of white stamens; flowers are followed by oblong-ellipsoid, purple-black berries, 1cm (½in) long. ↕↔ 3m (10ft). Mediterranean. ❄❄. **'Jenny Reitenbach'** see subsp. *tarentina*. **'Microphylla'** see subsp. *tarentina*. **'Nana'** see subsp. *tarentina*. **subsp. *tarentina*** ♀ syn. 'Jenny Reitenbach', 'Microphylla', 'Nana' (Tarentum myrtle), is more compact and rounded, with narrowly elliptic leaves, to 2cm (¾in) long, pink-tinted cream flowers, and white berries; ↕↔ 1.5m (5ft). **subsp. *tarentina* 'Microphylla Variegata'** is similar to subsp. *tarentina*, but has white-margined leaves. **'Variegata'** has leaves margined creamy white.
M. lechleriana □ syn. *Amomyrtus luma, M. luma* of gardens. Upright, bushy shrub or many-stemmed tree with ovate, slightly aromatic, dark green leaves, to 2.5cm (1in) long, coppery-brown when young. Compact, axillary racemes of 4–10 fragrant, 5-petalled, creamy white flowers, 1cm (½in) across, are produced in mid- and late spring, followed by edible, spherical, aromatic red berries, ripening to black. ↕ 6m (20ft) or more, ↔ 4m (12ft). Chile. ❄❄
M. luma see *Luma apiculata*.
***M. luma* of gardens** see *M. lechleriana*.
M. nummularia see *Myrteola nummularia*.
***M. x ralphii* 'Variegata'** see *Lophomyrtus* x *ralphii* 'Variegata'.
M. ugni see *Ugni molinae*.

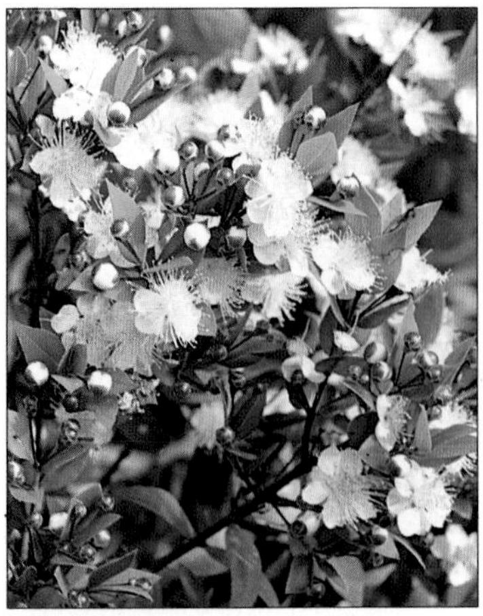

Myrtus communis

N

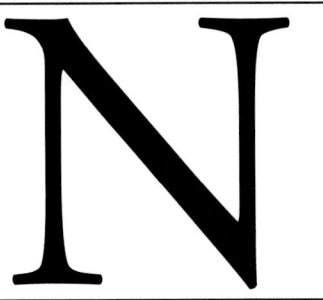

▷ ***Naegelia cinnabarina*** see *Smithiantha cinnabarina*
▷ ***Naegelia zebrina*** see *Smithiantha zebrina*
▷ **Naked ladies** see *Colchicum*
▷ ***Nananthus rubrolineata*** see *Aloinopsis rubrolineata*
▷ ***Nananthus schooneesii*** see *Aloinopsis schooneesii*

NANDINA

BERBERIDACEAE

Genus of one species of evergreen or semi-evergreen shrub, with alternate, pinnate leaves, from mountain valleys in India, China, and Japan. *N. domestica* is grown for its flowers, fruit, and elegant foliage. Grow in a shrub border; low-growing cultivars are fine ground cover.

- **HARDINESS** Frost hardy.
- **CULTIVATION** Grow in a sheltered site in moist but well-drained soil, preferably in full sun. Pruning group 9.
- **PROPAGATION** Sow seed in containers in a cold frame as soon as ripe. Root semi-ripe cuttings in summer.
- **PESTS AND DISEASES** Viruses can cause narrow, distorted leaflets to develop.

N. domestica ▣ ♀ (Heavenly bamboo). Evergreen or semi-evergreen shrub with upright shoots and pinnate to 3-pinnate leaves, to 90cm (36in) long, with lance-shaped leaflets, red to reddish purple when young and in winter. In mid-summer, bears conical panicles, to 40m (16in) long, of small, star-shaped white flowers, to 1cm (½in) across, with large yellow anthers, followed by long-lasting, spherical, bright red fruit, 8mm (⅜in) across. ↕ 2m (6ft), ↔ 1.5m (5ft). India, China, Japan. ✻✻. **'Firepower'** is dwarf and compact, with bright red leaves; ↕ 45cm (18in), ↔ 60cm (24in). **'Harbor Dwarf'** is compact; ↕ 1m (3ft), ↔ 1.2m (4ft). **'Umpqua Chief'** is compact; ↕ 1.5m (5ft), ↔ 1.2m (4ft).

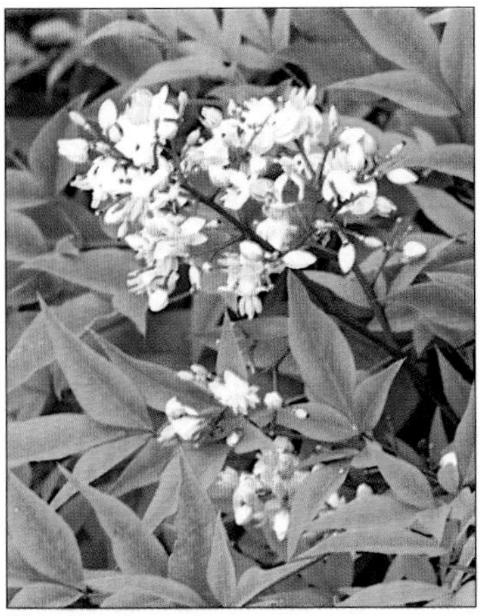

Nandina domestica

NARCISSUS

Daffodil

AMARYLLIDACEAE

Genus of about 50 species of bulbous perennials from a variety of habitats in Europe and N. Africa, usually found in meadows from sea level to subalpine altitudes, and in woodland, river silts, and rock crevices. Many thousands of cultivars have been developed. All are grown for their attractive flowers, borne in spring, sometimes autumn or winter. Leafless stems bear between 1 and 20 flowers, each with 6 spreading perianth segments (petals) surrounding an almost flat or long and narrow corona (the cup or trumpet). The flowers are mostly yellow or white, occasionally green; some have red, orange, or pink coronas. The leaves are basal, often strap-shaped or cylindrical, 15–75cm (6–30in) long, depending on the species.

Most daffodils are suitable for planting between shrubs or in a border, or for growing in containers; many are easily naturalized in grass or in a woodland garden. They are excellent for cutting. Smaller species, hybrids, and cultivars are good rock garden plants; some can be naturalized in fine, short grass. *N. cantabricus*, *N. romieuxii*, *N. rupicola*, and *N. watieri* either need a warm, dry summer dormancy or produce delicate flowers early in the year, and are therefore best grown in an alpine house or bulb frame. In frost-prone areas, grow the less hardy members of Division 8 in a cool greenhouse. Contact with the sap of daffodils may irritate skin or aggravate skin allergies.

For horticultural purposes, daffodils are split into 12 divisions, each with distinct characteristics. All are of garden origin, except for Division 10 species. The spreads given for each division provide a guide to planting distance.

Division 1. Trumpet
Flowers are solitary, each with a trumpet (corona) as long as, or longer than, the perianth segments. Spring-flowering. ↔ 8–16cm (3–6in).

Division 2. Large-cupped
Flowers are solitary, each with a cup (corona) more than one-third the length of, but not as long as, the perianth segments. Usually mid-spring-flowering. ↔ 16cm (6in).

Division 3. Small-cupped
Flowers are solitary, each with a cup (corona) up to one-third the length of the perianth segments. Early and mid-spring-flowering. ↔ 16cm (6in).

Division 4. Double
Each stem has one or more flowers, with doubling of the perianth segments or the corona or both. Some are sweetly scented. Usually early and mid-spring-flowering. ↔ 16cm (6in).

Division 5. Triandrus
Each stem produces 2–6 nodding flowers, usually with reflexed perianth segments and shortish cups (coronas). Mid- and late spring-flowering. ↔ 5–8cm (2–3in).

Division 6. Cyclamineus
Flowers are solitary, each acutely angled to the stem, with significantly reflexed perianth segments and usually a long cup or trumpet (corona). Early- and mid-spring-flowering. ↔ 8cm (3in).

Division 7. Jonquilla
Each stem produces 1–5 usually scented flowers, with spreading perianth segments and small, shallow cups (coronas). The stems are cylindrical; the dark green leaves are very narrow and almost cylindrical. Mid- and late spring-flowering. ↔ 8cm (3in).

Division 8. Tazetta
Small-flowered cultivars produce up to 20 flowers per stem; larger-flowered cultivars bear 3 or 4 flowers per stem. They have stout stems, wide leaves, broad perianth segments, and small cups (coronas). They are usually scented, and are good as cut flowers. Some cultivars are half-hardy and should be grown in a cool greenhouse. Late-autumn- to mid-spring-flowering. ↔ 8cm (3in).

Division 9. Poeticus
Flowers are fragrant, usually solitary, with spreading, pure white perianth segments and small, open, red-rimmed cups (coronas). Mid- to late spring- or early-summer-flowering. ↔ 16cm (6in).

Division 10. Wild species
Includes all wild daffodils and their wild hybrids, such as the tiny hoop-petticoat daffodil, *N. bulbocodium*, the larger, single-flowered *N. pseudonarcissus*, and the multi-headed *N. tazetta*. Some are difficult to grow in an open garden. Autumn- to spring-flowering. ↔ 5–8cm (2–3in), or 16cm (6in) for larger bulbs.

Division 11. Split-corona
Flowers are usually solitary, each with a corona split for more than half its length. Spring-flowering. ↔ 16cm (6in). There are 2 subdivisions:
Division 11a. Collar – The corona segments lie on top of the perianth segments.
Division 11b. Papillon – The flowers have alternating corona segments and perianth segments.

Division 12. Miscellaneous
Includes daffodils not in any other division, such *N. bulbocodium* cultivars, and the twin-headed, cyclamineus cultivars like *N.* 'Jumblie'. ↔ 5–8cm (2–3in) or 16cm (6in), depending on the size of the bulbs.

- **HARDINESS** Fully hardy to half hardy.
- **CULTIVATION** Plant bulbs at one-and-a-half times their own depth in autumn, slightly deeper in light soils and in grass. Most tolerate a range of soils but grow best in moderately fertile, well-drained soil that is moist during the growing season. *N. asturiensis*, *N. bulbocodium*, *N. cyclamineus*, *N. triandrus*, and their

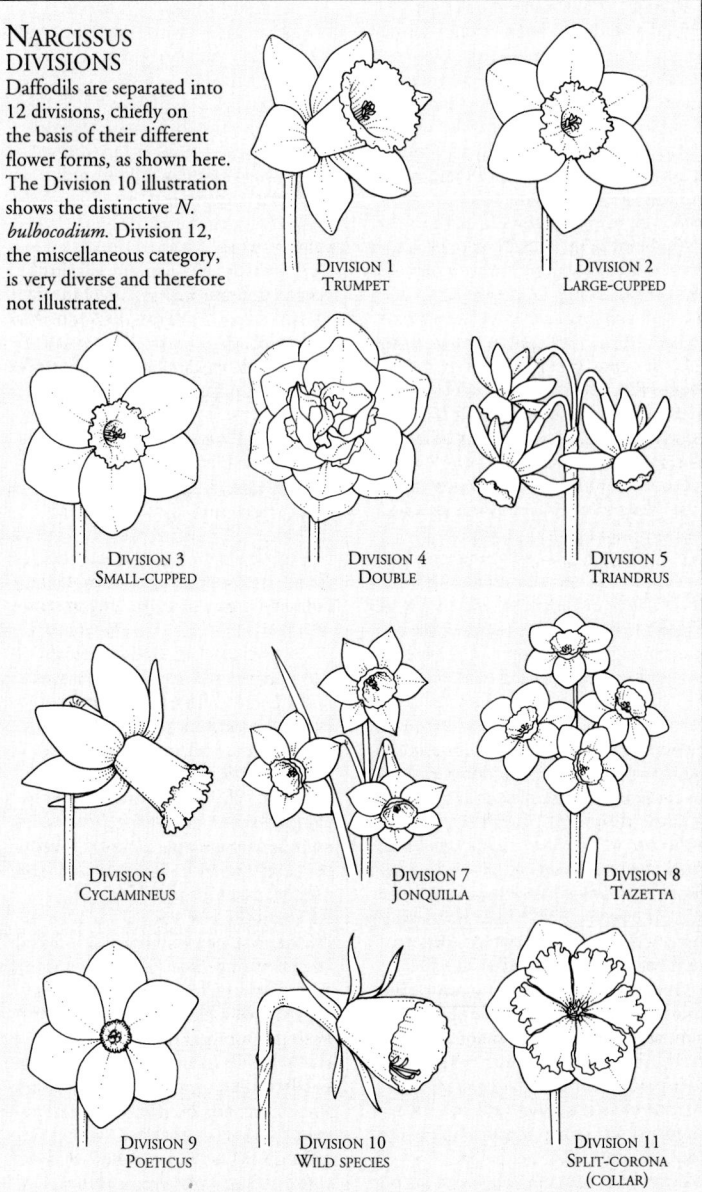

NARCISSUS DIVISIONS

Daffodils are separated into 12 divisions, chiefly on the basis of their different flower forms, as shown here. The Division 10 illustration shows the distinctive *N. bulbocodium*. Division 12, the miscellaneous category, is very diverse and therefore not illustrated.

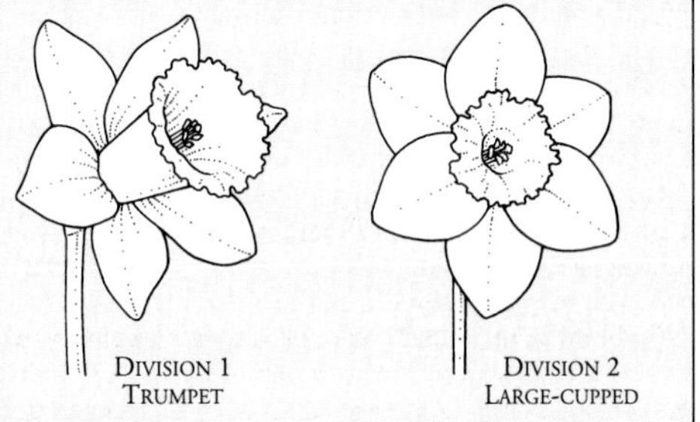

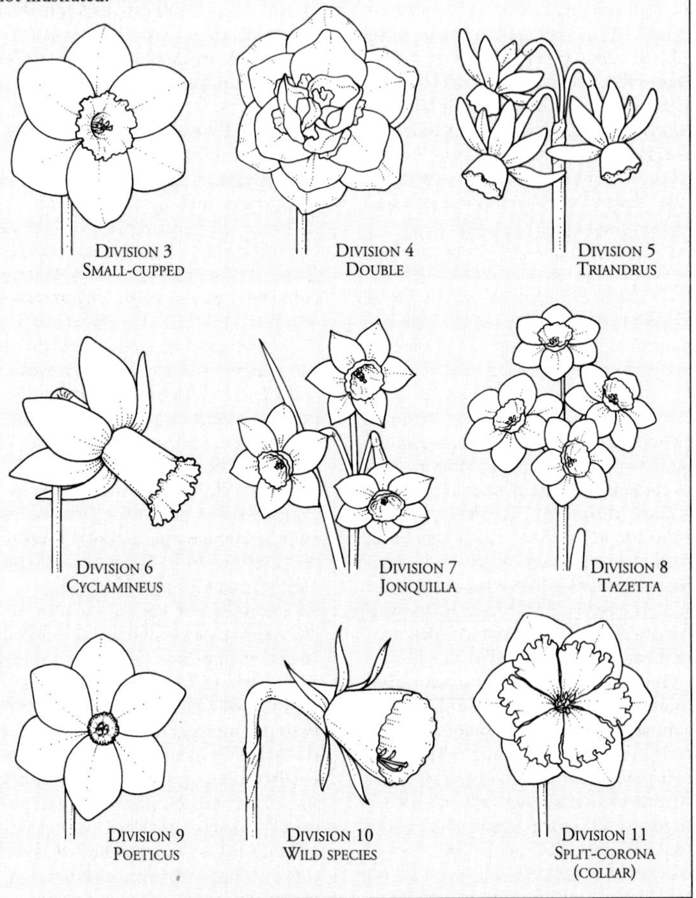

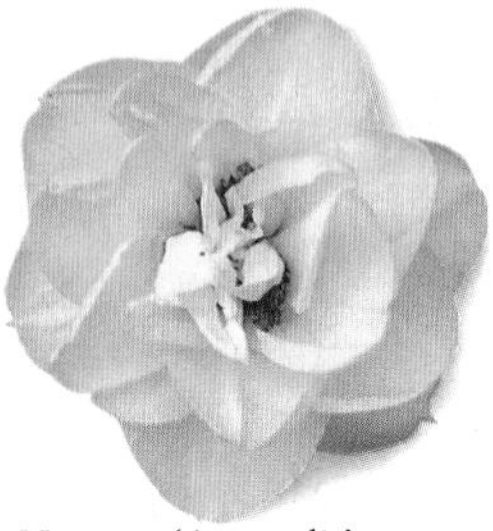
Narcissus 'Acropolis'

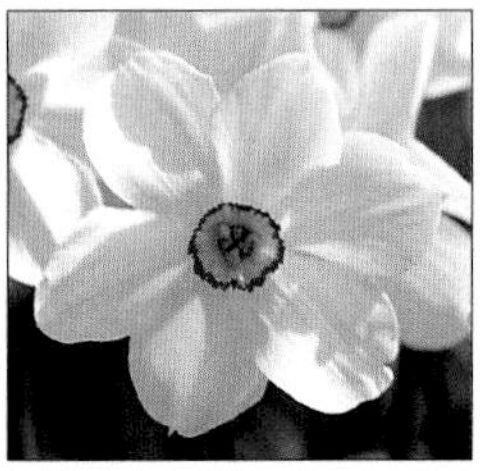
Narcissus 'Actaea'

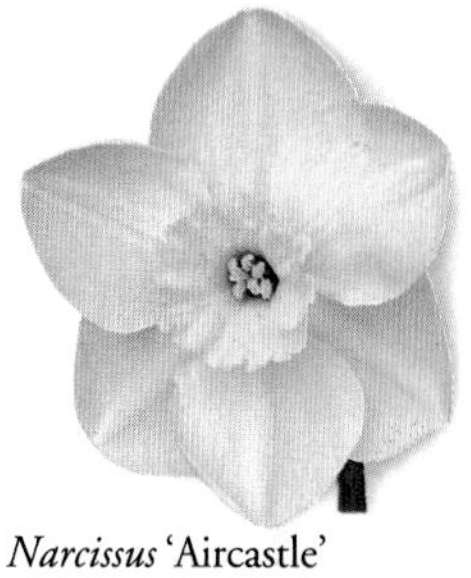
Narcissus 'Aircastle'

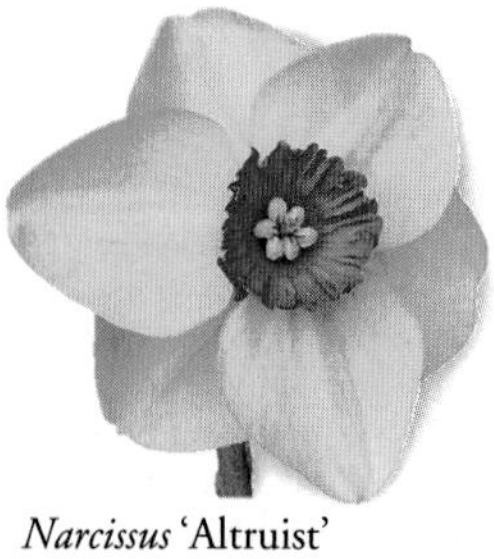
Narcissus 'Altruist'

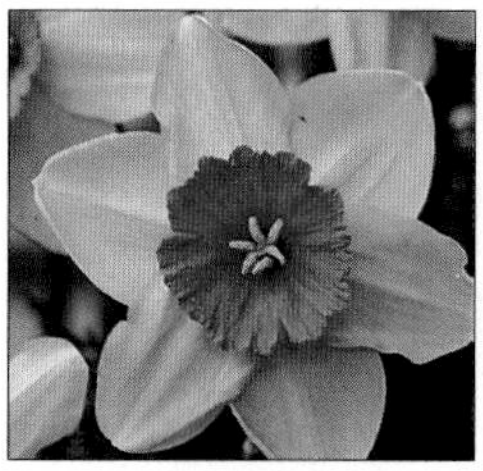
Narcissus 'Ambergate'

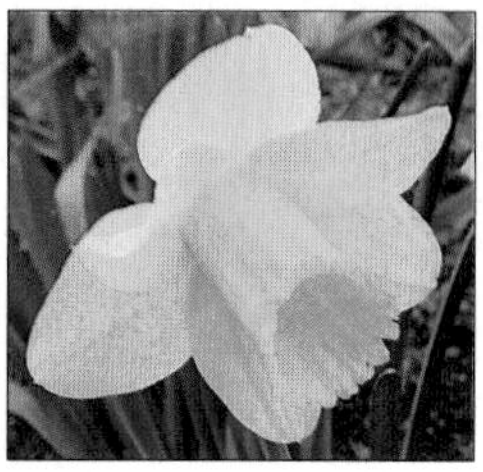
Narcissus 'Arkle'

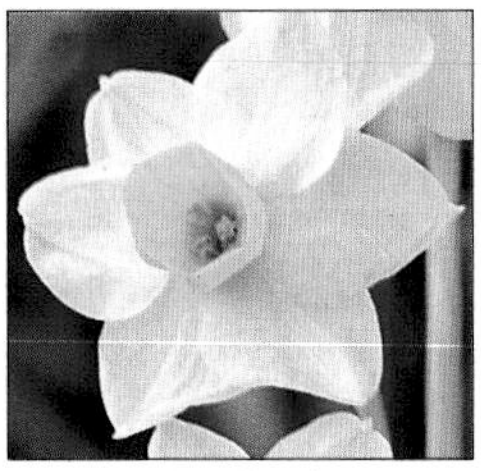
Narcissus 'Avalanche'

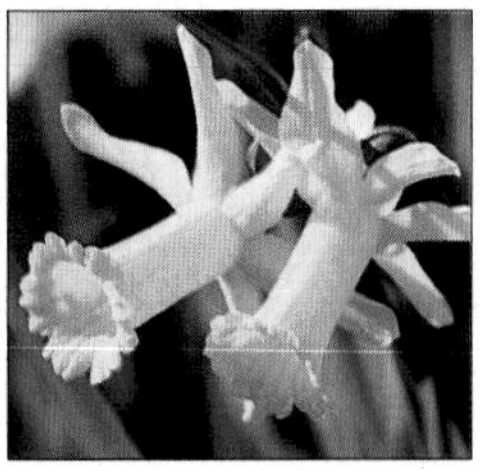
Narcissus 'Bartley'

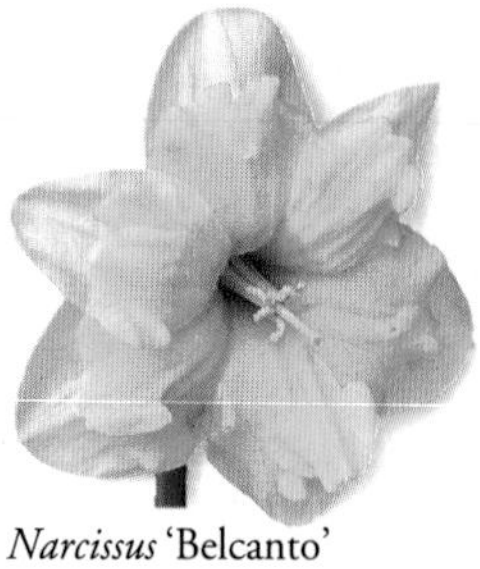
Narcissus 'Belcanto'

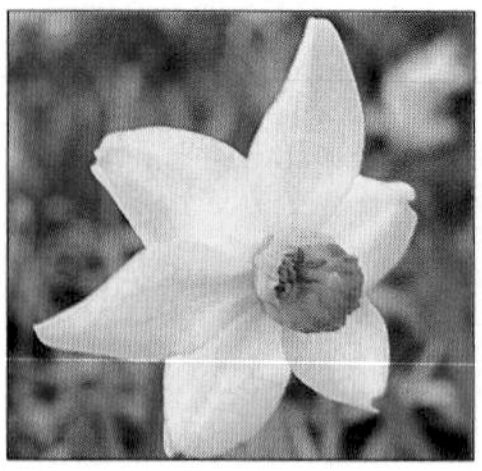
Narcissus 'Beryl'

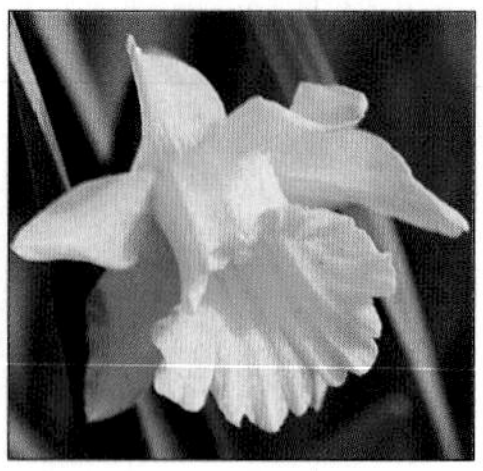
Narcissus 'Bob Minor'

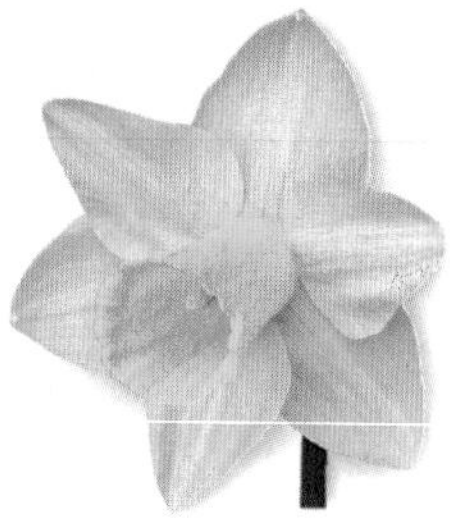
Narcissus 'Bravoure'

cultivars need neutral to acid soils. *N. jonquilla* and *N. tazetta* prefer slightly alkaline soils. Most daffodils thrive in full sun or dappled part-day shade. *N. assoanus* and *N. asturiensis* need full sun. Division 7 and 8 daffodils flower best in full sun and drier soils. Division 6 daffodils like cooler conditions and do well in grass. Water late-flowering daffodils in dry spring weather (flowers may abort in dry conditions). Dead-head plants as flowers fade, and allow leaves to die down naturally for at least 6 weeks. Apply a low-nitrogen, high-potash fertilizer after flowering if bulbs are not performing well. Lift and divide clumps when flowering becomes sparse or the clumps congested. If daffodils are naturalized in grass, delay the first cut until 4–6 weeks after flowers have faded; for species such as *N. pseudonarcissus*, *N. bulbocodium*, and *N. cyclamineus*, delay cutting until seeds have dispersed.

Under glass, grow in a mix of 2 parts loam-based potting compost (JI No.2) and 1 part grit. Plunge outdoors in a cool, shady spot and keep dry when dormant.

For indoor display, plant bulbs 5cm (2in) deep in early autumn in loamless or loam-based potting compost (JI No.2). Plunge in a cold frame outdoors until the roots are well-established and shoots appear. Keep cool and moist, and protect from frost. Move into a cool greenhouse in full light, and gradually increase the temperature to 10°C (50°F), then to no more than 18°C (64°F) when flowering. Water freely and apply a half-strength, high-potash fertilizer weekly. Bring indoors as the buds begin to open. Discard or plant out into the garden after flowering.

• **PROPAGATION** Sow seed of species as soon as ripe in deep containers in a cold frame. Cultivars do not come true from seed, but new cultivars are often selected from seed of crosses between cultivars, or from open-pollinated seed. After germination, keep frost-free, cool, and moist. After 2 years, transfer seedlings to a nursery bed and grow on until they reach flowering size, which may take up to 7 years. Alternatively, separate and replant offsets as leaves fade in early summer, or in early autumn before new roots are produced.

• **PESTS AND DISEASES** The most serious problems include large narcissus bulb fly, narcissus eelworm, slugs, narcissus basal rot and other fungal infections, viruses (including narcissus yellow stripe virus), and bulb scale mite on bulbs forced for early flowering.

***N.* 'Acropolis'** ■ Division 4 daffodil bearing well-formed, double flowers, 11cm (4½in) across, in mid-spring. Numerous snow-white segments are interspersed with bright orange-red ones. ↕45cm (18in). ✻✻✻

***N.* 'Actaea'** ■ 🏆 Division 9 daffodil producing strongly scented flowers, 8.5cm (3¼in) across, in late spring. Open, wavy, pure white perianth segments surround the red ribbon-like margin of each flattened, bowl-shaped yellow corona. ↕45cm (18in). ✻✻✻

***N.* 'Aircastle'** ■ Division 3 daffodil flowering in mid-spring. Flowers, 9cm (3½in) across, have rounded perianth segments, white on opening, green-tinged with age, and small, flat, lemon-yellow cups, darker at the rims. ↕40cm (16in). ✻✻

***N.* 'Albus Plenus Odoratus'** see *N. poeticus* 'Plenus'.

***N.* 'Altruist'** ■ Division 3 daffodil flowering in mid-spring. Flowers, 8–8.5cm (3–3¼in) across, have pointed, pale apricot perianth segments and fluted, bright orange-red cups. Colour fades rapidly in sunlight. ↕45cm (18in). ✻✻✻

***N.* 'Ambergate'** ■ Division 2 daffodil flowering in mid-spring. Flowers, 9.5cm (3¾in) across, have soft tangerine perianth segments and expanded, rich orange cups. ↕40cm (16in). ✻✻✻

***N.* 'April Love'.** Division 1 daffodil producing all-white flowers, 12.5cm (5in) across, in mid-spring. The rim of each slender trumpet is neatly rolled back; the perianth segments are slightly pointed and broadly overlapping. ↕40cm (16in). ✻✻✻

***N.* 'Arctic Gold'** 🏆 Division 1 daffodil. In mid-spring, bears smooth, waxy, rich golden yellow flowers, 9.5cm (3¾in) across, with widely flanged, deeply notched trumpets. ↕40cm (16in). ✻✻✻

***N.* 'Arkle'** ■ Strong, vigorous Division 1 daffodil. Flowers, 12.5cm (5in) across, among the largest of the yellow trumpet daffodils, are borne in mid-spring. The perianth segments are smooth and each corona is slightly flared, with a roll at the mouth. ↕40cm (16in). ✻✻✻

N. assoanus, syn. *N. juncifolius*, *N. requienii* (Rush-leaved jonquil). Tiny Division 10 daffodil with thin, cylindrical leaves, to 20cm (8in) long. In mid-spring, bears circular, scented, golden yellow flowers, 2cm (¾in) across, singly or in pairs. ↕15cm (6in). S. France, S. and E. Spain. ✻✻✻

N. asturiensis, syn. *N. minimus*. Division 10 daffodil with spreading, channelled, glaucous, mid-green leaves, to 15cm (6in) long. In late winter and early spring, bears solitary, pale yellow flowers, 3.5cm (1½in) across, with narrow perianth segments and waisted trumpets. ↕8cm (3in). N. Portugal, N. and C. Spain. ✻✻✻. **subsp. *jacatensis* 'Cedric Morris'** produces larger, lemon-yellow flowers, 8cm (3in) across, in early winter; ↕15cm (6in).

***N.* 'Avalanche'** ■ Division 8 daffodil producing 10 or more sweetly scented flowers, 3.5cm (1½in) across, with pure white perianth segments and lemon-yellow cups, in mid-spring. Long-lasting as cut flowers. ↕35cm (14in). ✻✻

***N.* 'Avenger'.** Division 2 daffodil flowering in mid-spring. Flowers, 9cm (3½in) across, have rounded, smooth, almost pure white perianth segments and slightly flattened, intense orange-red coronas. ↕40cm (16in). ✻✻✻

***N.* 'Ballyrobert'.** Division 1 daffodil producing well-balanced, deep yellow flowers, 10cm (4in) across, in mid-spring. Perianth segments are slightly pointed and waved; trumpets are slender. ↕40cm (16in). ✻✻✻

***N.* 'Balvenie'.** Division 2 daffodil. In mid-spring, bears flowers 10.5cm (4¼in) across, with pure white perianth segments and white cups suffused pink, intensifying in colour at the mouths. Among the largest and most vigorous of the pink daffodils. ↕40cm (16in). ✻✻✻

***N.* 'Bantam'** 🏆 Division 2 daffodil with well-shaped flowers, 5.5cm (2¼in) across, on stiff stems, produced in mid-spring. Short, bright golden yellow perianth segments surround short, flared, intense orange cups with orange-red rims. ↕20–24cm (8–10in). ✻✻✻

***N.* 'Bartley'** ■ Division 6 daffodil producing long-lasting, golden yellow flowers, 6cm (2½in) across, with long, slender, angled trumpets and strongly reflexed perianth segments, borne in early spring. ↕40cm (16in). ✻✻✻

***N.* 'Beige Beauty'.** Division 3 daffodil flowering in mid-spring. Flowers, 10cm (4in) across, have rounded perianth segments, opening white and turning soft lemon-yellow, and pale yellow, almost flat coronas, fading to very pale yellow. ↕40cm (16in). ✻✻✻

***N.* 'Belcanto'** ■ Division 11a daffodil flowering in late spring. Flowers, 8–12cm (3–5in) across, have pure white perianth segments, almost obscured by the flattened, pale yellow coronas. ↕45cm (18in). ✻✻✻

***N.* 'Bell Song'.** Division 7 daffodil. In mid- and late spring, bears 2 or 3 flower stems, each with 1 or 2 nodding white flowers, 4cm (1½in) across, with pale pink cups. ↕30cm (12in). ✻✻✻

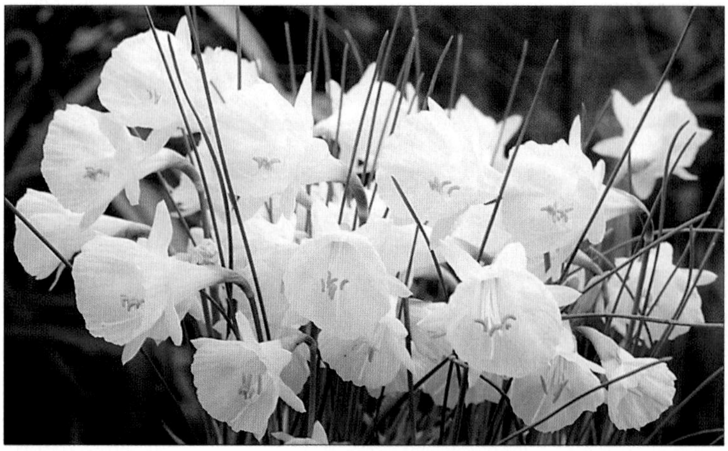
Narcissus cantabricus

N

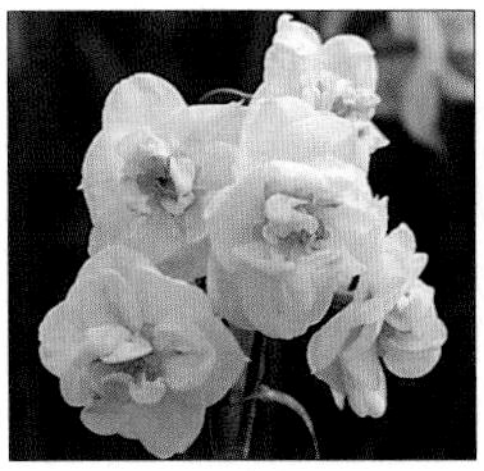
Narcissus 'Bridal Crown'

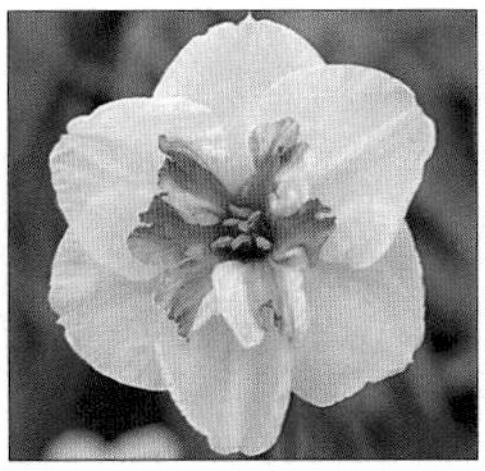
Narcissus 'Broadway Star'

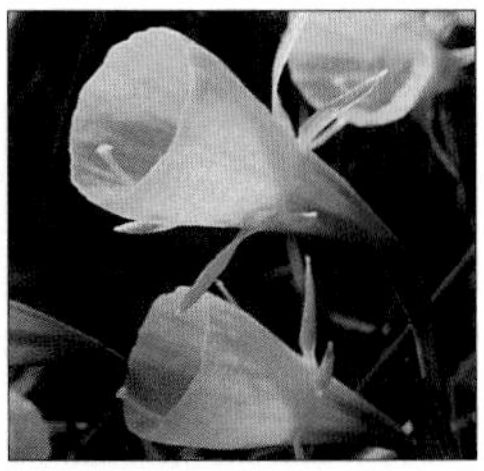
Narcissus bulbocodium

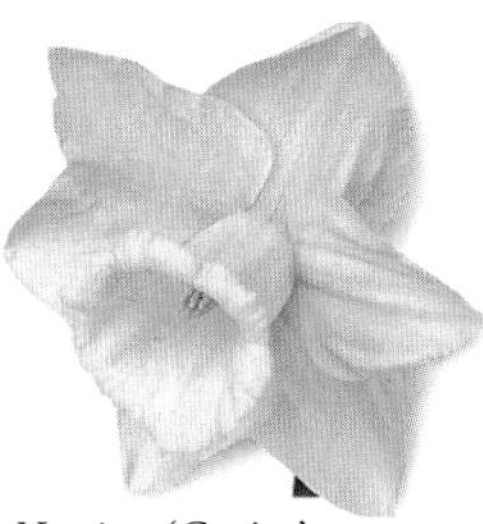
Narcissus 'Canisp'

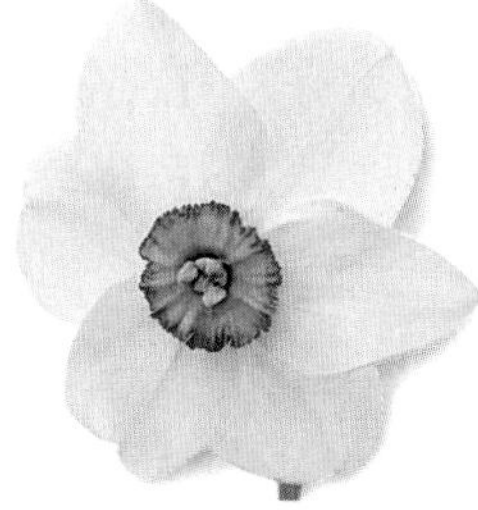
Narcissus 'Cantabile'

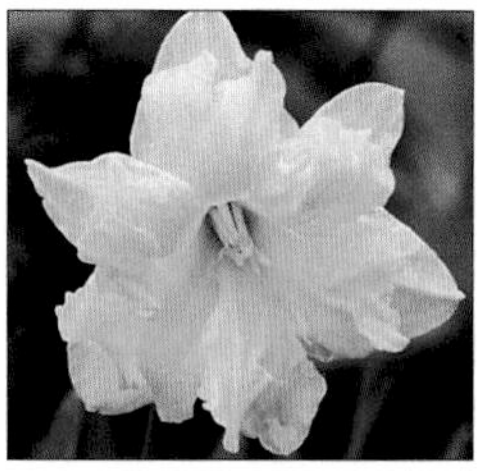
Narcissus 'Cassata'

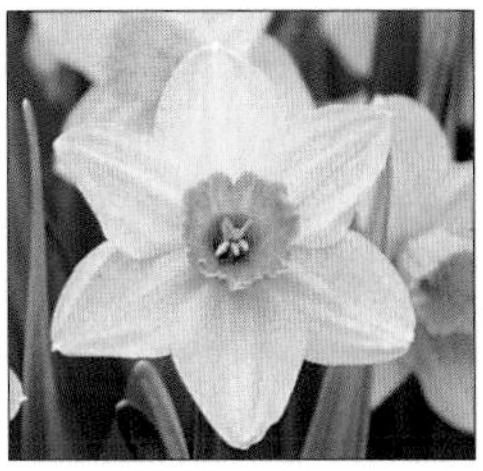
Narcissus 'Ceylon'

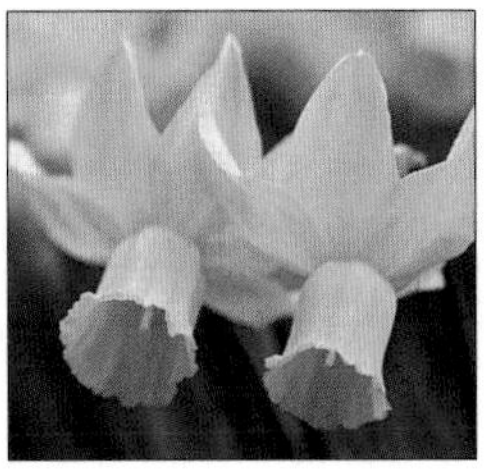
Narcissus 'Charity May'

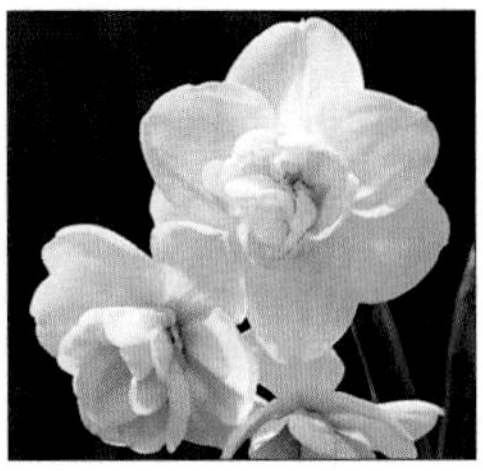
Narcissus 'Cheerfulness'

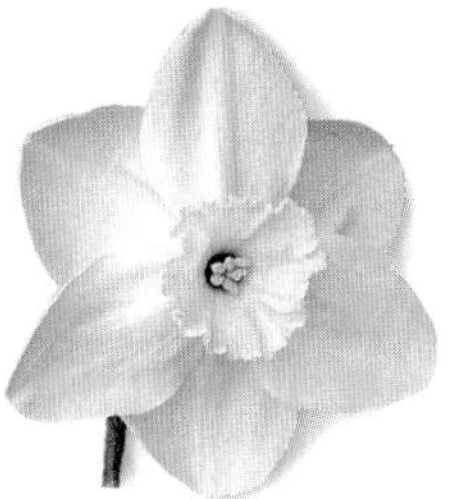
Narcissus 'Cool Crystal'

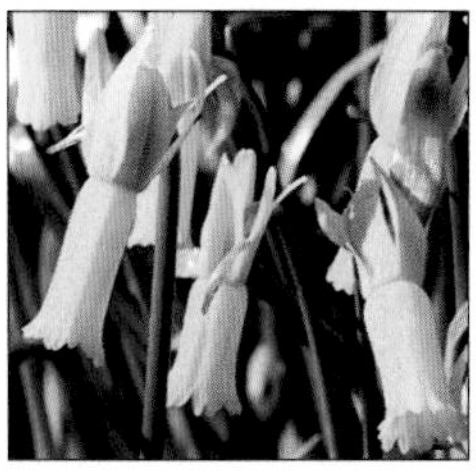
Narcissus cyclamineus

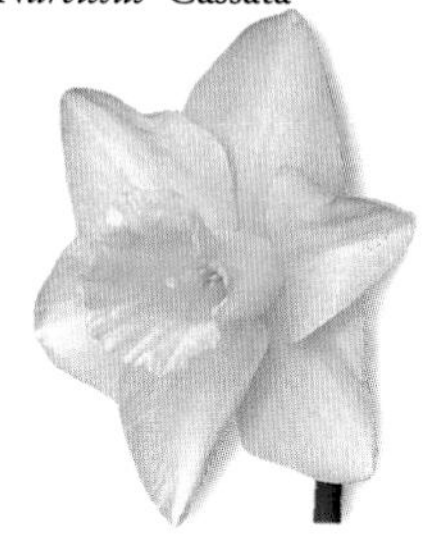
Narcissus 'Dover Cliffs'

***N.* 'Bere Ferrers'.** Division 4 daffodil. In mid-spring, bears fully double flowers, 10cm (4in) across, with evenly arranged, broadly ovate white perianth segments contrasting with bright orange corona segments. ↕40cm (16in). ❄❄❄
***N.* 'Beryl'** ■ Vigorous Division 6 daffodil flowering in early spring Flowers, 7.5cm (3in) across, have reflexed perianth segments, opening yellow but quickly fading to creamy white, and small yellow and orange cups. ↕20cm (8in). ❄❄❄
***N.* 'Binkie'.** Robust Division 2 daffodil producing clear lemon-yellow flowers, 10cm (4in) across, in mid-spring. The long cups gradually fade to cream. ↕35cm (14in). ❄❄❄
***N.* 'Birthright'.** Division 1 daffodil flowering in mid-spring. Bears almost square, crystalline, pure white flowers, 11cm (4½in) across, with narrow, flanged trumpets. ↕40cm (16in). ❄❄❄
***N.* 'Bobbysoxer'.** Division 7 daffodil producing 1 or 2 flowers per stem, in late spring. Flowers, 3cm (1¼in) across, have primrose-yellow perianth segments and yellow and orange cups. ↕18cm (7in). ❄❄❄
***N.* 'Bob Minor'** ■ Division 1 daffodil with stiff stems bearing golden yellow flowers, 6.5cm (2½in) across, in mid-spring. The perianth segments are twisted and the long trumpets slightly flared. ↕20cm (8in). ❄❄❄
***N.* 'Brabazon'** ♀ Vigorous Division 1 daffodil bearing rich golden yellow flowers, 10cm (4in) across, in early spring. Among the earliest-flowering trumpet daffodils. ↕40cm (16in). ❄❄❄
***N.* 'Bravoure'** ■♀ Division 1 daffodil flowering in mid-spring. Flowers, 12cm (5in) across, have unusually long and slender yellow trumpets and overlapping, slightly pointed white perianth segments. ↕45cm (18in). ❄❄❄
***N.* 'Bridal Crown'** ■ Division 4 daffodil producing numerous sweetly scented, double flowers, 4cm (1½in) across, in early spring. Flowers are mostly white, highlighted by short, orange-yellow corona segments in central clusters. ↕40cm (16in). ❄❄❄
***N.* 'Broadway Star'** ■ Division 11b daffodil producing white flowers, 8cm (3in) across, in mid-spring. The expanded segments of the split coronas are flattened against the perianth segments; each has a narrow, orange mid-stripe running lengthways. ↕40cm (16in). ❄❄❄
***N.* 'Broomhill'.** Long-lasting Division 2 daffodil producing robust, well-proportioned, smooth, waxy, pure white flowers, 10cm (4in) across, in mid-spring. ↕40cm (16in). ❄❄❄
***N.* 'Bryanston'.** Vigorous Division 2 daffodil bearing yellow flowers, 9.5–10cm (3¾–4in) across, in mid-spring. The pointed, smooth, wide perianth segments lie very flat; the cups are indented. ↕40cm (16in). ❄❄❄
N. bulbocodium ■ (Hoop-petticoat daffodil). Small Division 10 daffodil with narrow, semi-cylindrical, dark green leaves, 10–40cm (4–16in) long. In mid-spring, bears funnel-shaped, deep yellow flowers, 3.5cm (1½in) across, with expanded trumpets and tiny, pointed perianth segments. Can be naturalized in damp grass that dries out in summer. ↕10–15cm (4–6in). S.W. and W. France, Portugal, Spain, N. Africa. ❄❄❄. **var. *citrinus*** has pale lemon-yellow flowers.
***N.* 'Burntollet'.** Division 1 daffodil. In mid-spring, bears smooth, pure white flowers, 11cm (4½in) across, with long, well-proportioned trumpets, flanged at the mouths. ↕40cm (16in). ❄❄❄
N. campernelli see *N.* x *odorus.*
***N.* 'Canisp'** ■ Division 2 daffodil bearing white flowers, 12cm (5in) across, in mid-spring. Cups are slender and trumpet-like, with a hint of green in the throats; the perianth segments are pointed. ↕40cm (16in). ❄❄❄
***N.* 'Cantabile'** ■ Division 9 daffodil. In late spring, stiff stems bear neat, well-rounded white flowers, 4cm (1½in) across, with tiny, red-rimmed, green and yellow cups. ↕25cm (10in). ❄❄❄
N. cantabricus ■ (White hoop-petticoat daffodil). Division 10 daffodil with narrow, semi-cylindrical, slightly channelled leaves, to 15cm (6in) long. In winter, bears funnel-shaped white flowers, 3.5cm (1½in) across, with tiny, pointed perianth segments and expanded trumpets. ↕15–20cm (6–8in). S. Spain, N. Africa. ❄❄❄
***N.* 'Cantatrice'.** Division 1 daffodil producing pure white flowers, 11cm (4½in) across, in mid-spring. The perianth segments are pointed; the trumpets are smooth and slender. ↕40cm (16in). ❄❄❄
***N.* 'Capax Plenus'** see *N.* 'Eystettensis'.
***N.* 'Cassata'** ■ Division 11a daffodil. In mid-spring, produces flowers 10cm (4in) across, with pure white perianth segments nearly obscured by the flattened corona segments, which open lemon-yellow and become white. ↕40cm (16in). ❄❄❄
***N.* 'Ceylon'** ■ Robust, erect Division 2 daffodil. In mid-spring, bears flowers 10cm (4in) across, with yellow perianth segments and goblet-shaped, fiery orange cups. ↕40cm (16in). ❄❄❄
***N.* 'Charity May'** ■♀ Division 6 daffodil bearing lemon-yellow flowers, 9cm (3½in) across, with broad, reflexed perianth segments and long cups, in early spring. ↕30cm (12in). ❄❄❄
***N.* 'Charter'** ♀ Division 2 daffodil flowering in mid-spring. Flowers, 11cm (4½in) across, open greenish lemon-yellow; the perianth segments retain their colour, the cups fade almost to pure white. ↕40cm (16in). ❄❄❄
***N.* 'Cheerfulness'** ■ Division 4 daffodil flowering in mid-spring. Each stem bears several sweetly scented, double white flowers, 5.5cm (2¼in) across, with clusters of cream segments in the centres. ↕40cm (16in). ❄❄❄
***N.* 'Cherrygardens'.** Division 2 daffodil flowering in mid-spring. Flowers, 10.5cm (4¼in) across, have overlapping, sparkling white perianth segments and intense pink coronas, with darker rims and green eyes. ↕40cm (16in). ❄❄❄
***N.* 'Chiloquin'.** Division 1 daffodil with strong, vigorous stems, each bearing a solitary greenish yellow flower, 8.5cm (3¼in) across, in mid-spring. The trumpets gradually fade almost to white. ↕40cm (16in). ❄❄❄
***N.* 'Cloud Nine'.** Division 2 daffodil bearing lemon-yellow flowers, 8.5cm (3¼in) across, with pointed, smooth perianth segments, in mid-spring. The goblet-shaped cups soon fade almost to white. ↕40cm (16in). ❄❄❄
***N.* 'Como'.** Division 9 daffodil with scented flowers, 5.5cm (2¼in) across, borne in late spring. The rounded, snow-white perianth segments surround small, flattened yellow coronas, with green throats and bright red margins. ↕30cm (12in). ❄❄❄
***N.* 'Cool Crystal'** ■ Division 3 daffodil with white flowers, 10.5cm (4¼in) across, produced in mid-spring. The bowl-shaped coronas have green eyes. ↕50cm (20in). ❄❄❄
***N.* 'Cragford'.** Division 8 daffodil flowering in early spring. Each stem bears several scented white flowers, 5.5cm (2¼in) across, the coronas interspersed with tangerine-orange perianth segments. ↕50cm (20in). ❄❄❄
***N.* 'Cristobal'.** Division 1 daffodil flowering in mid-spring. Flowers, 11cm (4½in) across, have prominent, overlapping, rounded white perianth segments and deep lemon-yellow coronas, evenly indented at the mouths. ↕40cm (16in). ❄❄❄
N. cyclamineus ■♀ Robust, vigorous Division 10 daffodil with spreading, narrow, keeled, bright green leaves, 12–30cm (5–12in) long. Bears solitary, nodding, golden yellow flowers, 4.5cm (1¾in) long, in early spring. Narrow perianth segments are completely reflexed from the long, narrow-waisted trumpets. ↕15–20cm (6–8in). N.W. Portugal, N.W. Spain. ❄❄❄
***N.* 'Dailmanach'.** Division 2 daffodil. In mid-spring, bears flowers 11.5cm (4½in) across, with broad, smooth, glistening white perianth segments; the large, rich bright pink cups, of almost trumpet-like proportions, have darker pink, rolled, indented mouths. ↕40cm (16in). ❄❄❄
***N.* 'Daydream'.** Division 2 daffodil flowering in mid-spring. Flowers, 8cm (3in) across, have greenish yellow perianth segments; each cup has a white halo surrounding the base. At maturity, cups become almost white. ↕35cm (14in). ❄❄❄
***N.* 'Descanso'.** Strong-growing Division 1 daffodil flowering in mid-spring. Flowers, 11.5cm (4½in) across, have triangular, shining white perianth segments and slender, deep lemon-yellow trumpets, fading to clear lemon-yellow, each flanged at the mouth. ↕45cm (18in). ❄❄❄
***N.* 'Doubtful'.** Division 3 daffodil flowering in early spring. Bears flowers 9.5cm (3¾in) across, with smooth, deep yellow perianth segments and goblet-shaped, rich scarlet cups. ↕45cm (18in). ❄❄❄
***N.* 'Dover Cliffs'** ■ Division 2 daffodil producing well-proportioned, pure white flowers, 11cm (4½in) across, in mid-spring. The smooth perianth segments tend to form a hood over each corona. ↕40cm (16in). ❄❄❄

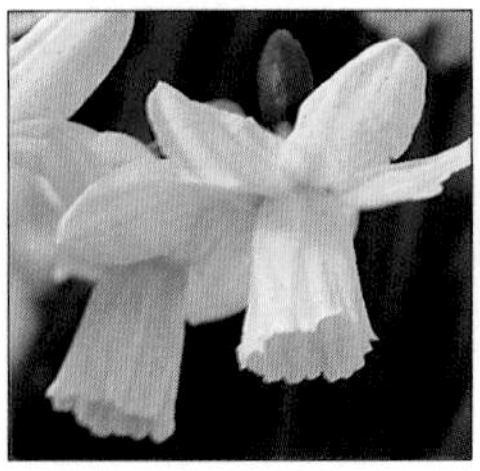
Narcissus 'Dove Wings'

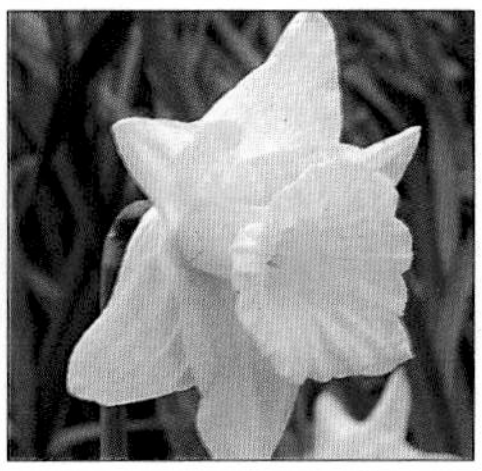
Narcissus 'Empress of Ireland'

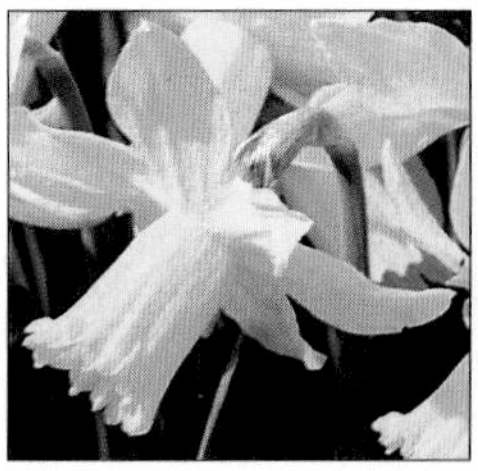
Narcissus 'February Gold'

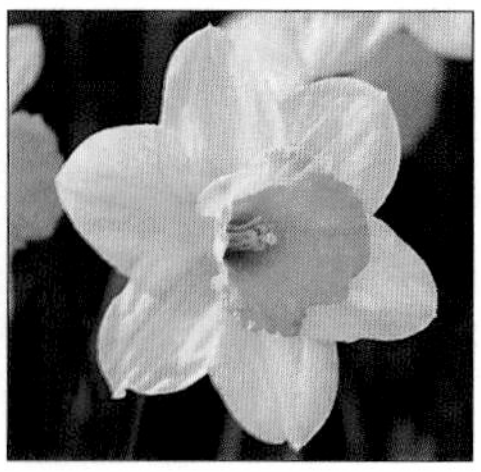
Narcissus 'Fortune'

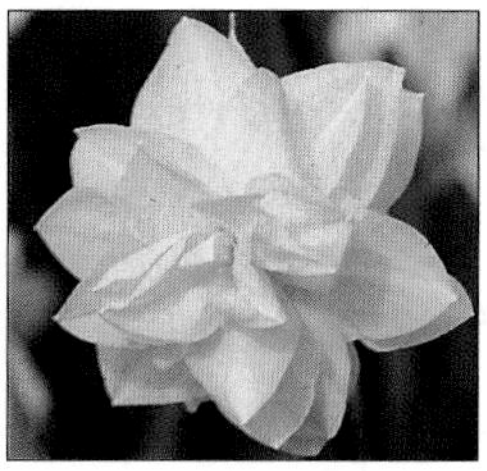
Narcissus 'Golden Ducat'

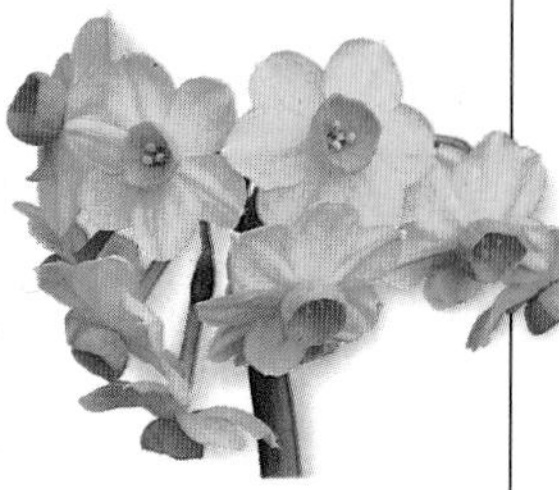
Narcissus 'Grand Soleil d'Or'

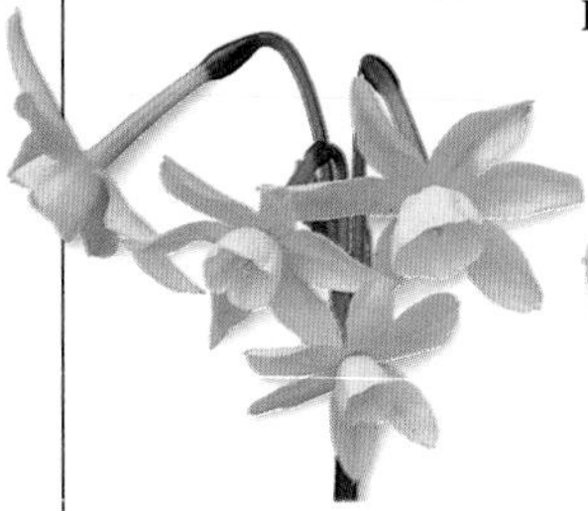
Narcissus 'Hawera'

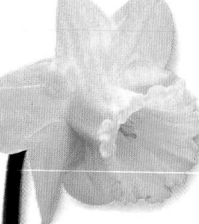
Narcissus 'Honeybird'

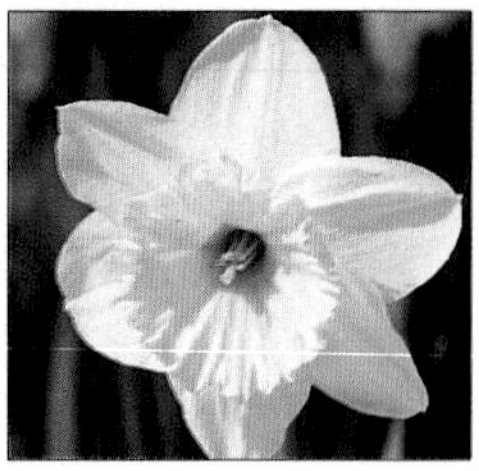
Narcissus 'Ice Follies'

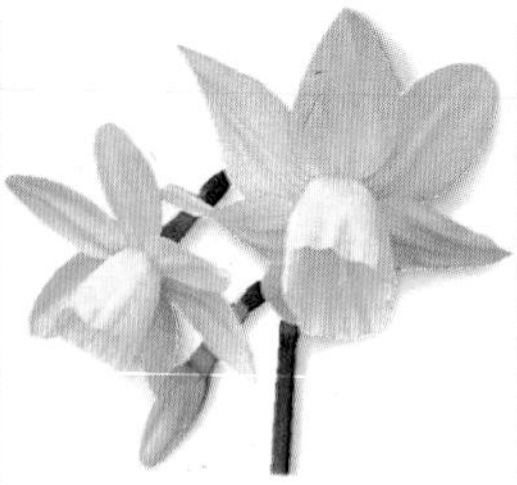
Narcissus 'Ice Wings'

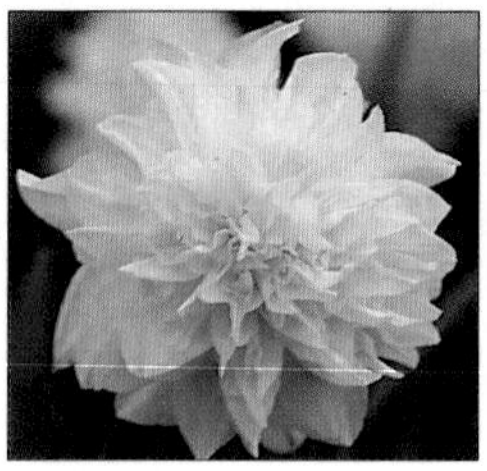
Narcissus 'Irene Copeland'

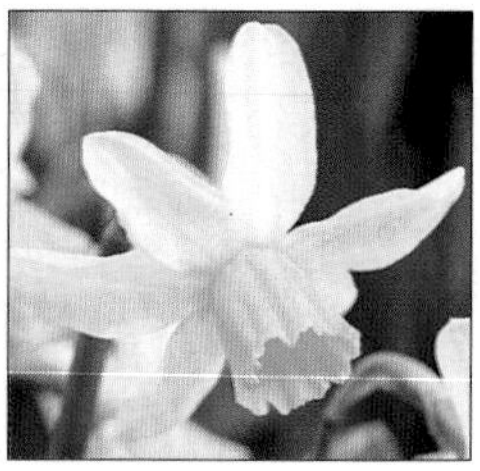
Narcissus 'Jack Snipe'

***N.* 'Dove Wings'** ■ ♀ Division 6 daffodil flowering in early spring. Flowers, 8.5cm (3¼in) across, have broad, creamy white perianth segments swept back from long, clear lemon-yellow cups. ↕30cm (12in). ❄❄❄

***N.* 'Downpatrick'.** Division 1 daffodil bearing consistently good-quality flowers, to 11.5cm (4½in) across, in mid-spring, with smooth, white perianth segments and dark primrose-yellow trumpets. ↕40cm (16in). ❄❄❄

***N.* 'Dr. Hugh'.** Division 3 daffodil flowering in mid-spring. Flowers, 11cm (4½in) across, have smooth white perianth segments surrounding small orange cups with clear green eyes. ↕50cm (20in). ❄❄❄

N

***N.* 'Dunmurry'.** Division 1 daffodil. In mid-spring, bears flowers 11cm (4½in) across, with broad, smooth, waxy white perianth segments overlapping the deep golden yellow coronas, set at right-angles. ↕40cm (16in). ❄❄❄

***N.* 'Dutch Master'.** Prolific Division 1 daffodil. In mid-spring, bears golden yellow flowers, 11cm (4½in) across, with broadly ovate perianth segments, and coronas expanded at the deeply indented mouths. ↕45cm (18in). ❄❄❄

***N.* 'Easter Moon'.** Division 2 daffodil with circular, waxy, pure white flowers, 10cm (4in) across, borne in mid-spring. The short cups have faintly green-tinted throats. ↕40cm (16in). ❄❄❄

***N.* 'Empress of Ireland'** ■ ♀ Division 1 daffodil flowering in mid-spring. Produces large white flowers, 10–11cm (4–4½in) across, with very broad, triangular, overlapping perianth segments and narrow, widely flanged trumpets. Among the largest white trumpet daffodils. ↕40cm (16in). ❄❄❄

***N.* 'Eystettensis'**, syn. *N.* 'Capax Plenus' (Queen Anne's double daffodil). Division 4 daffodil with fully double, lemon-yellow flowers, 6cm (2½in) across, with many rows of evenly overlapping perianth segments, borne in mid-spring. ↕23cm (9in). ❄❄❄

***N.* 'February Gold'** ■ ♀ Vigorous Division 6 daffodil flowering in early spring. Flowers, 7.5cm (3in) across, have reflexed, golden yellow perianth segments and long, slightly darker trumpets. ↕30cm (12in). ❄❄❄

***N.* 'February Silver'** ■ Robust, long-lasting Division 6 daffodil flowering in early spring. Flowers, 5cm (2in) across, have white perianth segments slightly reflexed from the large, lemon-yellow trumpets. ↕30cm (12in). ❄❄❄

***N.* 'Fortune'** ■ Division 2 daffodil. In mid-spring, bears flowers 11cm (4½in) across, with rich butter-yellow perianth segments and expanding warm orange cups, becoming darker towards the mouths. ↕45cm (18in). ❄❄❄

***N.* 'Foundling'.** Division 6 daffodil flowering in mid-spring. Flowers, 7cm (3in) across, have broad white perianth segments, well-reflexed from short, clear rose-pink cups. ↕30cm (12in). ❄❄❄

***N.* 'Foxfire'.** Division 2 daffodil flowering in mid-spring. Flowers, 9.5cm (3¾in) across, have broad, pure white perianth segments and greenish white cups, with a wide band of coral-pink at the mouths and green eyes. ↕40cm (16in). ❄❄❄

***N.* 'Galway'.** Division 2 daffodil flowering in mid-spring. Bears golden yellow flowers, 11.5cm (4½in) across, with well-proportioned, trumpet-like, prominently flanged cups. ↕40cm (16in). ❄❄❄

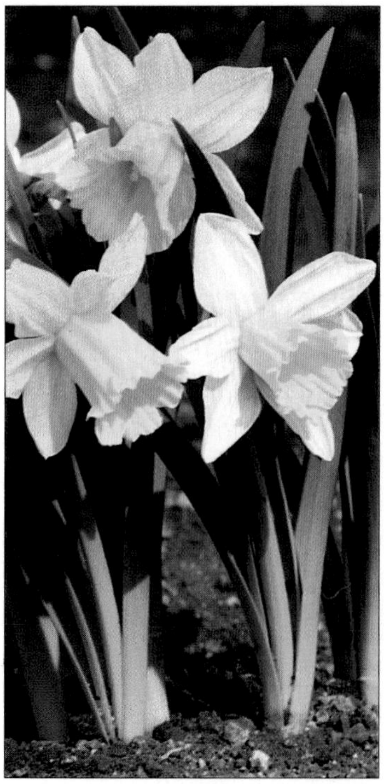
Narcissus 'February Silver'

***N.* 'Gay Kybo'.** Division 4 daffodil producing well-formed, double flowers, 10.5cm (4¼in) across, in mid-spring. The regularly arranged, creamy white perianth segments surround the shorter, rich orange central segments. ↕45cm (18in). ❄❄❄

***N.* 'Geranium'.** Division 8 daffodil bearing up to 6 scented, glistening white flowers, 5.5cm (2¼in) across, with bright orange-red cups, in mid- and late spring. Excellent for cutting. ↕35cm (14in). ❄❄❄

***N.* 'Golden Aura'.** Division 2 daffodil producing rich golden yellow flowers, 9.5cm (3¾in) across, in mid-spring. Flowers have smooth, flat perianth segments and large, well-proportioned, bell-shaped cups. ↕40cm (16in). ❄❄❄

***N.* 'Golden Ducat'** ■ Division 4 daffodil bearing double, golden yellow flowers, 11cm (4½in) across, with many layers of pointed segments, in mid-spring. ↕35cm (14in). ❄❄❄

***N.* 'Golden Jewel'.** Division 2 daffodil flowering in mid-spring. Bears rich golden yellow flowers, 10cm (4in) across, with overlapping, broadly ovate perianth segments; the frilled coronas expand slightly towards the mouths, with a hint of green in the eyes. ↕45cm (18in). ❄❄❄

***N.* 'Golden Vale'.** Division 1 daffodil. In mid-spring, bears large, rich golden yellow flowers, 12cm (5in) across, with the trumpets expanding towards the indented mouths. ↕45cm (18in). ❄❄❄

***N.* 'Grand Soleil d'Or'** ■ Division 8 daffodil with each stem bearing many scented, double gold and tangerine-orange flowers, 4.5cm (1¾in) across, in early spring. ↕45cm (18in). ❄❄

***N.* 'Hawera'** ■ Slender Division 5 daffodil with multiple stems per bulb, each bearing up to 5 canary-yellow flowers, 3–5cm (1¼–2in) across, with slightly reflexed perianth segments, in late spring. ↕18cm (7in). ❄❄

***N.* 'Highfield Beauty'.** Division 8 daffodil producing stems with up to 3 slightly scented, butter-yellow flowers, 6.5cm (2½in) across, in mid-spring. The small cups are several shades darker than the smooth, overlapping perianth segments. ↕50cm (20in). ❄❄❄

***N.* 'Home Fires'.** Division 2 daffodil flowering in mid-spring. Flowers, 11cm (4½in) across, have spreading, distinctly pointed, bright yellow perianth segments and short, brilliant orange coronas. ↕45cm (18in). ❄❄❄

***N.* 'Honeybird'** ■ Division 1 daffodil bearing well-proportioned flowers, 10.5cm (4¼in) across, opening greenish yellow, in mid-spring. The trumpets gradually fade almost to pure white. ↕50cm (20in). ❄❄❄

***N.* 'Ice Follies'** ■ ♀ Division 2 daffodil flowering in mid-spring. Flowers, 9.5cm (3¾in) across, have large, creamy white perianth segments and wide cups, frilled at the mouths, that open lemon-yellow and fade almost to white. Very prolific. ↕40cm (16in). ❄❄❄

***N.* 'Ice Wings'** ■ Division 5 daffodil. In mid-spring, bears 2 or 3 pure white flowers, 4cm (1½in) across, with strongly reflexed perianth segments and relatively long, straight-sided trumpets. ↕35cm (14in). ❄❄❄

***N.* 'Irene Copeland'** ■ Division 4 daffodil. In mid-spring, bears double flowers, 8.5cm (3¼in) across, with pure white perianth segments and sulphur-yellow corona segments. ↕40cm (16in). ❄❄❄

***N.* 'Irish Charm'.** Division 2 daffodil flowering in mid-spring. Flowers, 10cm (4in) across, have well-formed, smooth, snow-white perianth segments and flattish, bowl-shaped, apricot-orange coronas. ↕45cm (18in). ❄❄❄

***N.* 'Jack Snipe'** ■ Vigorous Division 6 daffodil. In early and mid-spring, produces long-lasting flowers, 4cm (1½in) across, with reflexed white perianth segments and short, lemon-yellow trumpets. Increases rapidly. ↕20cm (8in). ❄❄❄

***N.* 'Jenny'** ♀ Division 6 daffodil. In early and mid-spring, bears flowers 5cm (2in) across, with strongly reflexed, pointed, creamy white perianth segments and long, clear lemon-yellow trumpets that fade to cream. Similar to *N.* 'Dove Wings' but perianth segments are more pointed. ↕30cm (12in). ❄❄❄

***N.* 'Jetfire'** ■ Division 6 daffodil. In early spring, bears flowers 7.5cm (3in) across, with strongly reflexed, golden yellow perianth segments and long, bright orange trumpets, which fade in bright sun. ↕20cm (8in). ❄❄❄

N. jonquilla ♀ (Wild jonquil). Division 10 daffodil with erect to spreading, narrow, semi-cylindrical leaves, 40–45cm (16–18in) long. In late spring, bears heads of up to 5 strongly

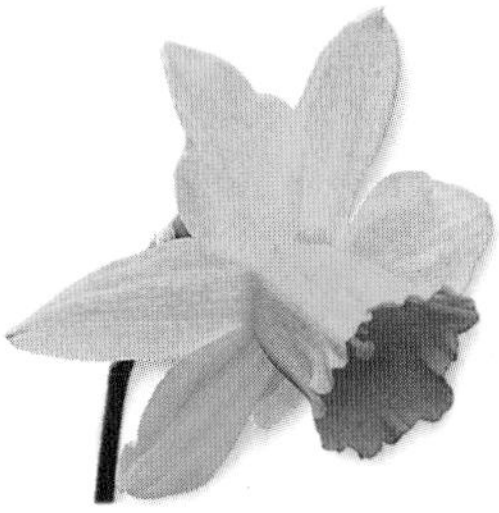
Narcissus 'Jetfire'

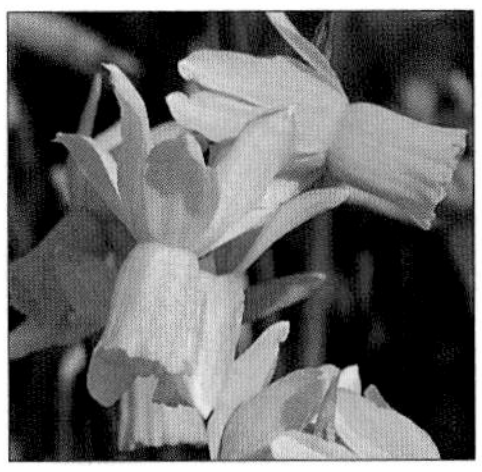
Narcissus 'Jumblie'

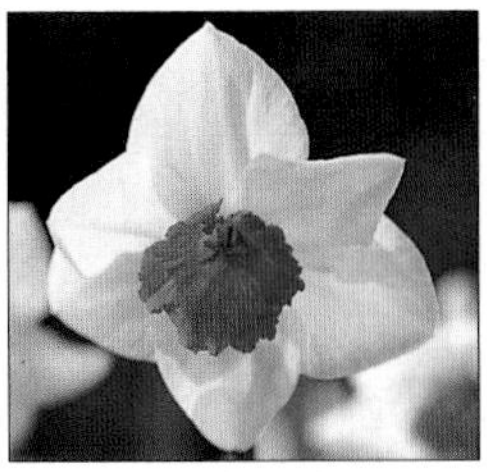
Narcissus 'Kilworth'

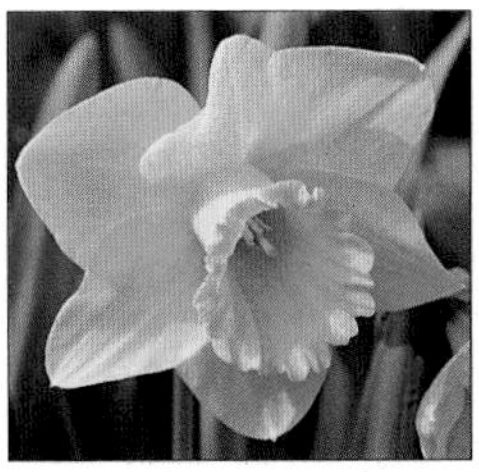
Narcissus 'Kingscourt'

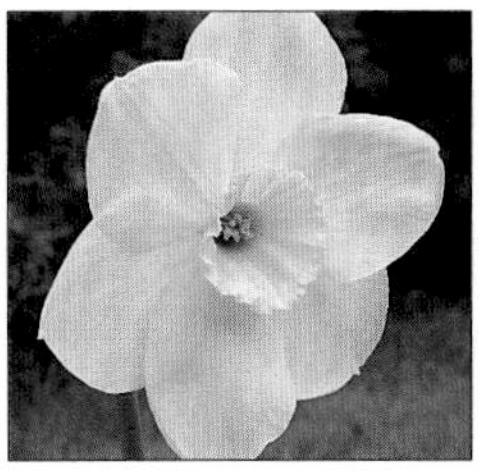
Narcissus 'Lemonade'

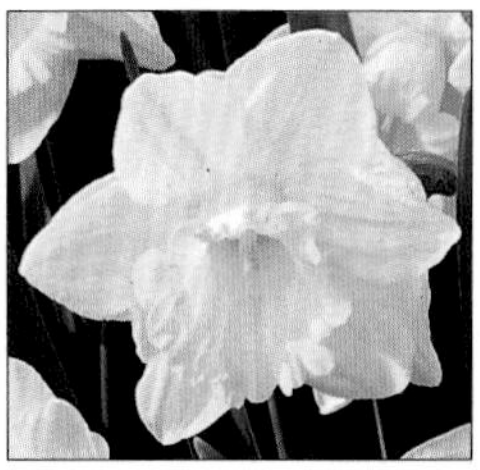
Narcissus 'Lemon Glow'

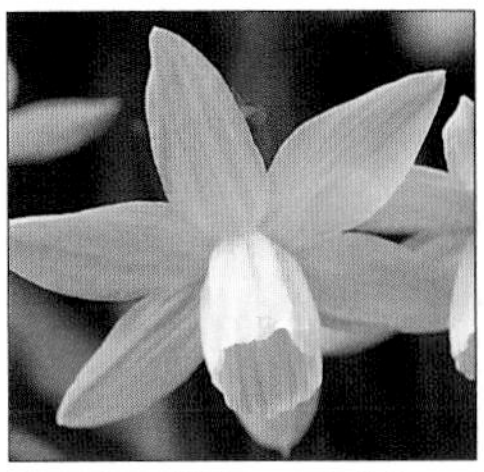
Narcissus 'Liberty Bells'

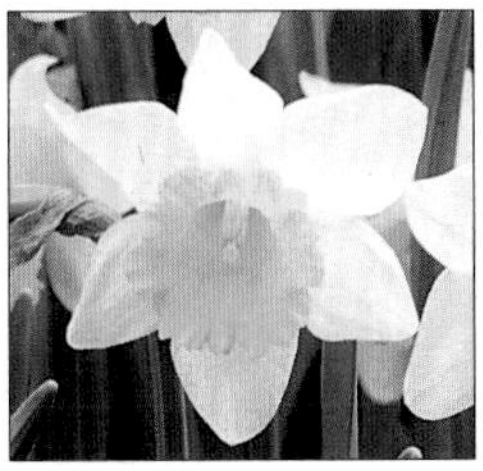
Narcissus 'Little Beauty'

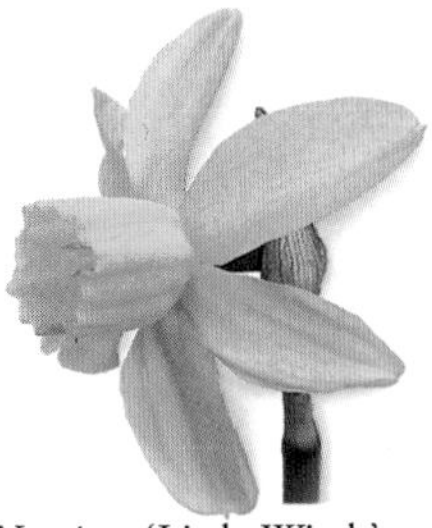
Narcissus 'Little Witch'

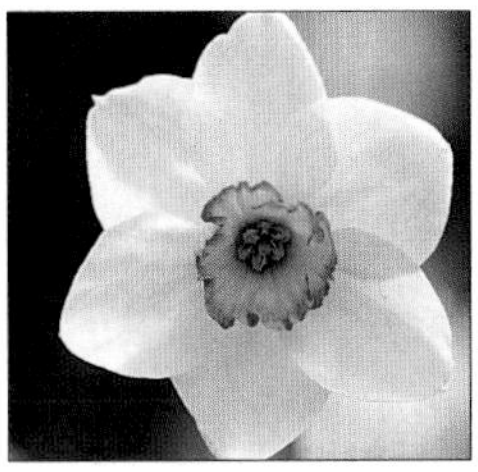
Narcissus 'Merlin'

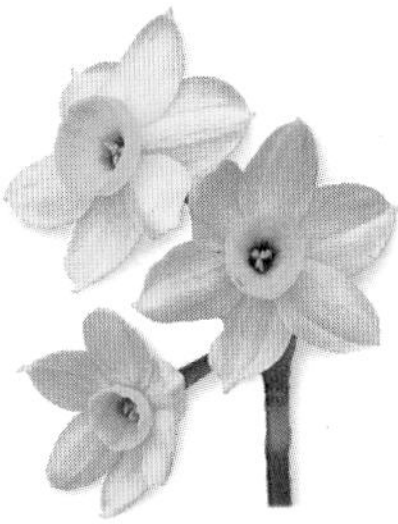
Narcissus 'Minnow'

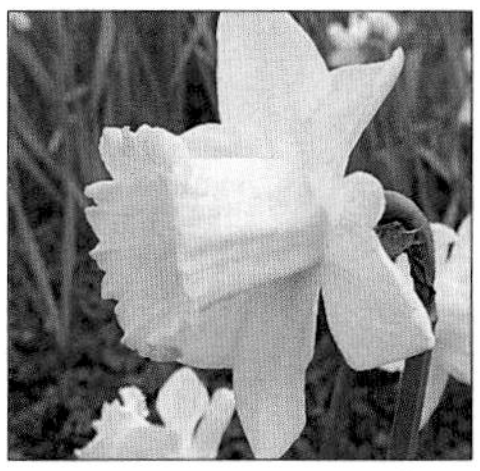
Narcissus 'Mount Hood'

scented, golden yellow flowers, 3cm (1¼in) across, with small, pointed perianth segments and tiny, flat cups. ↕30cm (12in). Spain. ❄❄❄

***N.* 'Jumblie'** ■ Small Division 12 daffodil. In early spring, bears multiple stems per bulb, each with up to 3 nodding flowers, 3cm (1¼in) across, with strongly reflexed, bright golden yellow perianth segments and deeper yellow-orange cups. ↕17cm (7in). ❄❄

N. juncifolius see *N. assoanus.*

***N.* 'Kilworth'** ■ Division 2 daffodil flowering in mid-spring. Flowers, 11cm (4½in) across, have broad white perianth segments and intense red-orange, well-proportioned, bowl-shaped coronas. ↕50cm (20in). ❄❄❄

***N.* 'Kimmeridge'.** Division 3 daffodil flowering in mid-spring. Bears flowers, 9.5cm (3¾in) across, with smooth, flat, pure white perianth segments and small, neat, pale yellow cups with rich orange rims. Fades rapidly in sunlight. ↕40cm (16in). ❄❄❄

***N.* 'Kingscourt'** ■🏆 Division 1 daffodil bearing rich golden yellow flowers, 11cm (4½in) across, in mid-spring. Flowers have large, smooth perianth segments and well-balanced trumpets that broaden gently towards the mouths. ↕45cm (18in). ❄❄❄

***N.* 'Lemonade'** ■ Division 3 daffodil producing white flowers, 8.5cm (3¼in) across, with smooth, rounded perianth segments and small, flattened cups, in mid-spring. The perianth segments gradually become yellow tinged green; the cups are slightly darker. ↕45cm (18in). ❄❄❄

***N.* 'Lemon Glow'** ■ Division 1 daffodil bearing greenish yellow flowers, to 8cm (3in) across, bordering between trumpet and large-cupped, in mid-spring. Each straight corona darkens slightly towards the indented mouth. ↕45cm (18in). ❄❄❄

***N.* 'Liberty Bells'** ■ Sturdy Division 5 daffodil bearing 2 nodding, clear lemon-yellow flowers, 9cm (3½in) across, with spreading perianth segments, in mid-spring. ↕30cm (12in). ❄❄❄

***N.* 'Lintie'.** Division 7 daffodil. In mid-spring, produces 1 or 2 unscented, primrose-yellow flowers, 5.5cm (2¼in) across, with orange cups. Similar to *N.* 'Bobbysoxer' but the flowers are slightly larger and each cup has a distinct green eye. ↕25cm (10in). ❄❄❄

***N.* 'Little Beauty'** ■ Sturdy, dwarf Division 1 daffodil bearing well-formed, creamy white flowers, 3cm (1¼in) across, with clear yellow trumpets, in early spring. ↕14cm (5½in). ❄❄❄

***N.* 'Little Gem'.** Dwarf Division 1 daffodil bearing golden yellow flowers, 4.5cm (1¾in) across, in early spring. Similar to *N. minor* and probably a selection from it. ↕13cm (5in). ❄❄❄

***N.* 'Little Witch'** ■ Vigorous, sturdy Division 6 daffodil. In early and mid-spring, produces long-lasting, golden yellow flowers, 4cm (1½in) across, with strongly reflexed perianth segments and long trumpets. ↕22cm (9in). ❄❄❄

N. lobularis see *N. pseudonarcissus.*

***N.* 'Loch Hope'.** Division 2 daffodil. In mid-spring, bears flowers, 10cm (4in) across, with well-formed, smooth, gold perianth segments and small, tubular, fiery red cups. ↕45cm (18in). ❄❄❄

***N.* 'Meldrum'.** Division 1 daffodil producing among the darkest yellow daffodil flowers, 10cm (4in) across, in spring. The widening trumpets, each neatly indented at the mouth, are several shades deeper than the broadly ovate perianth segments. ↕45cm (18in). ❄❄❄

***N.* 'Merlin'** ■🏆 Division 3 daffodil flowering in mid-spring. Flowers, 7.5cm (3in) across, have rounded, pure white perianth segments and flattened, pale yellow cups, each trimmed with a band of intense red. ↕45cm (18in). ❄❄❄

N. minimus see *N. asturiensis.*

***N.* 'Minnow'** ■ Dwarf Division 8 daffodil. In mid-spring, bears up to 5 flowers, 2.5cm (1in) across, with cream perianth segments and pale yellow cups fading to cream. Increases rapidly but may be shy to flower. ↕18cm (7in). ❄❄❄

N. minor ■🏆 syn. *N. nanus* of gardens. Dwarf Division 10 daffodil with erect, narrow, flat or channelled, grey-green leaves, 8–15cm (3–6in) long, and yellow flowers, 3cm (1¼in) across, borne in early spring. Increases well. ↕10–15cm (4–6in). France, N. Spain. ❄❄❄.
subsp. *pumilus* see *N. pumilus.*
subsp. *pumilus* 'Plenus' see *N.* 'Rip van Winkle'.

***N. minor* of gardens** see *N. pumilus.*

***N.* 'Monksilver'.** Division 3 daffodil bearing pure white flowers, 11cm (4½in) across, in mid-spring. Flowers have overlapping, smooth perianth segments and bowl-shaped coronas. ↕40cm (16in). ❄❄❄

***N.* 'Mount Hood'** ■ Division 1 daffodil flowering in mid-spring. Flowers, 10cm (4in) across, have well-formed, broadly overlapping, off-white perianth segments and creamy white trumpets, soon fading to off-white; each trumpet broadens towards the mouth. ↕45cm (18in). ❄❄❄

***N.* 'Nampa'.** Division 1 daffodil flowering in mid-spring. Flowers, 9cm (3½in) across, have bright yellow perianth segments and trumpets with white bases, which open greenish yellow and soon fade to white. ↕50cm (20in). ❄❄❄

N. nanus. Dwarf Division 10 daffodil with semi-erect, glaucous, grey-green leaves, to 15cm (6in) long. In early spring, bears nodding, sulphur-yellow flowers, 3.5cm (1½in) across, with deep yellow trumpets. Very similar to *N. minor.* ↕15cm (6in). Unknown in the wild. ❄❄❄

***N. nanus* of gardens** see *N. minor.*

***N.* 'Newcastle'.** Division 1 daffodil flowering in mid-spring. Flowers, 12cm (5in) across, have off-white perianth segments, which seldom lie flat, and deep golden yellow trumpets, slightly expanded at the mouths, with indented rolls. ↕45cm (18in). ❄❄❄

***N.* 'Norval'.** Division 2 daffodil flowering in mid-spring. Flowers, 10.5cm (4¼in) across, have overlapping, pointed, pure white perianth segments and large, shallow, bright orange coronas. ↕50cm (20in). ❄❄❄

N. obvallaris 🏆 syn. *N. pseudonarcissus* subsp. *obvallaris* (Tenby daffodil). Sturdy Division 10 daffodil with erect, glaucous, mid-green leaves, 30cm (12in) long, and stiff stems that bear neat, golden yellow flowers, 4cm (1½in) across, in early spring. Excellent for naturalizing. ↕30cm (12in). UK (S. Wales), W. Europe. ❄❄❄

N.* x *odorus (*N. jonquilla* x *N. pseudonarcissus*) syn. *N. campernelli* (Campernelle jonquil). Division 10 daffodil with narrow, strap-shaped, strongly keeled leaves, to 50cm (20in) long. In early spring, bears 1 or 2

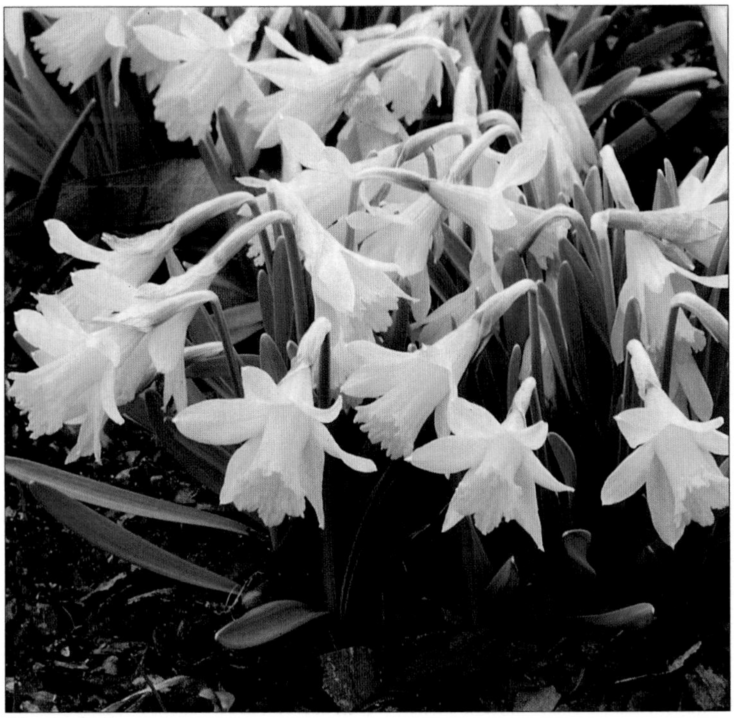
Narcissus minor

N

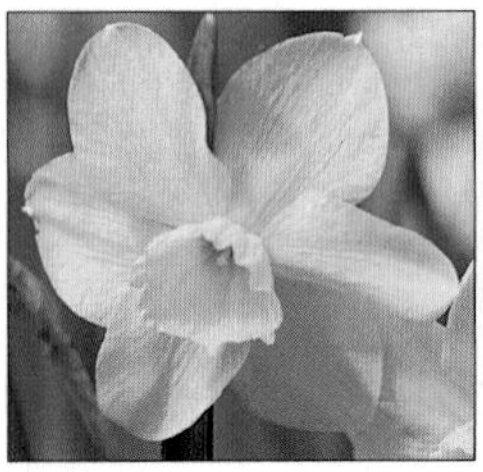
Narcissus x *odorus* 'Rugulosus'

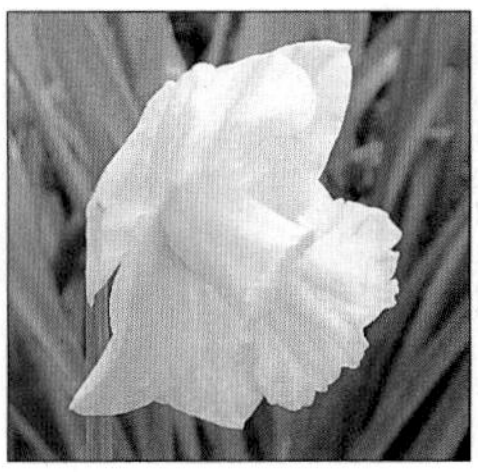
Narcissus 'Panache'

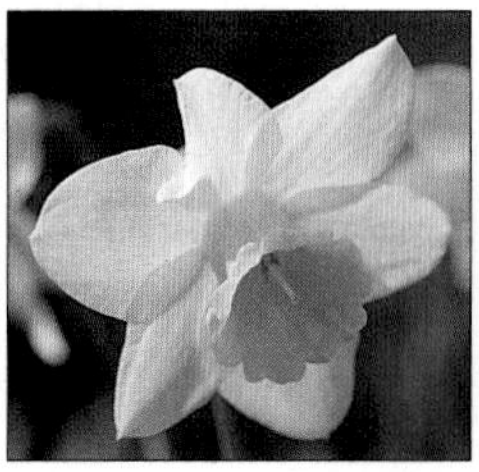
Narcissus 'Passionale'

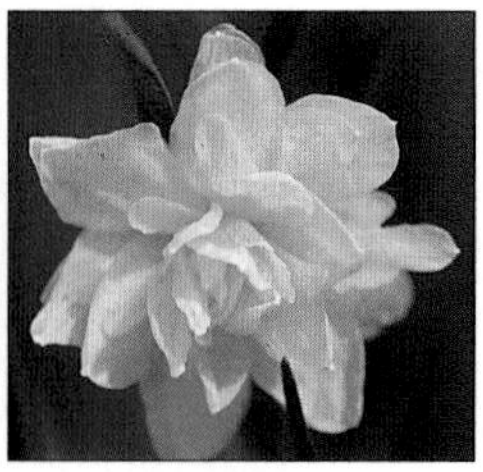
Narcissus 'Pencrebar'

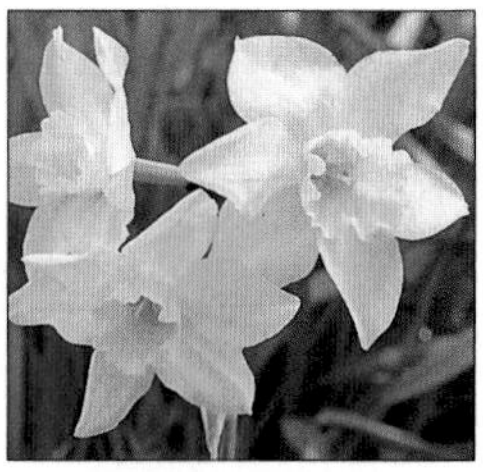
Narcissus 'Pipit'

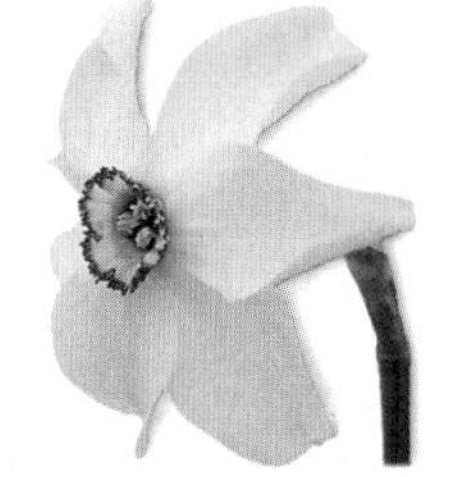
Narcissus poeticus var. *recurvus*

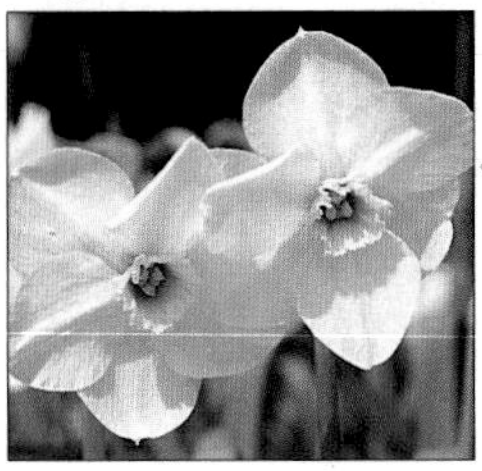
Narcissus 'Portrush'

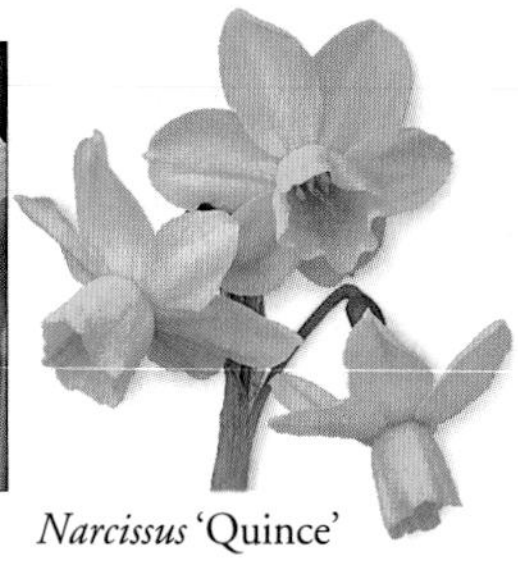
Narcissus 'Quince'

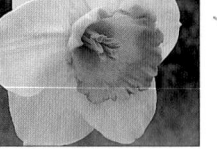

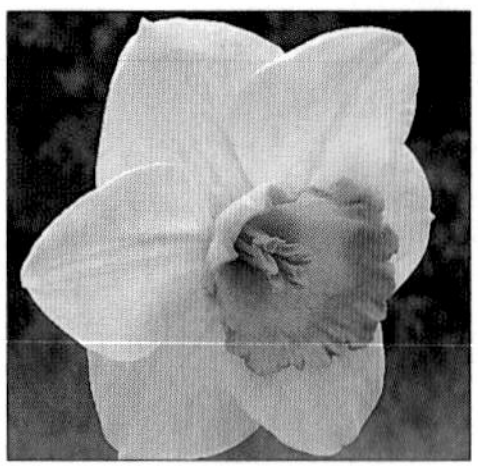
Narcissus 'Rainbow'

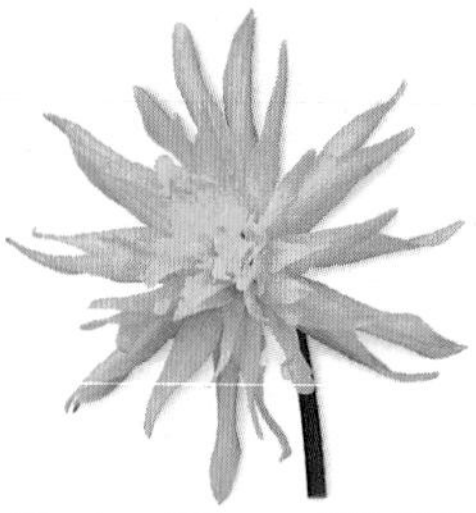
Narcissus 'Rip van Winkle'

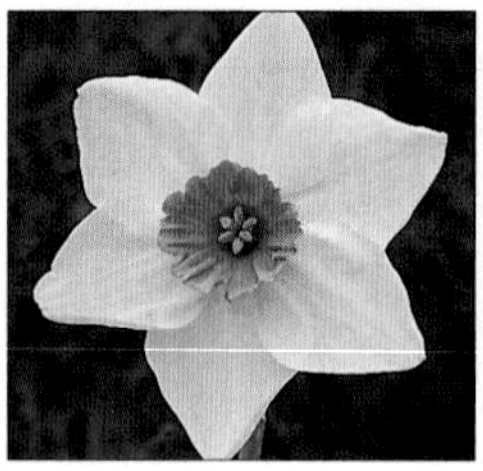
Narcissus 'Rockall'

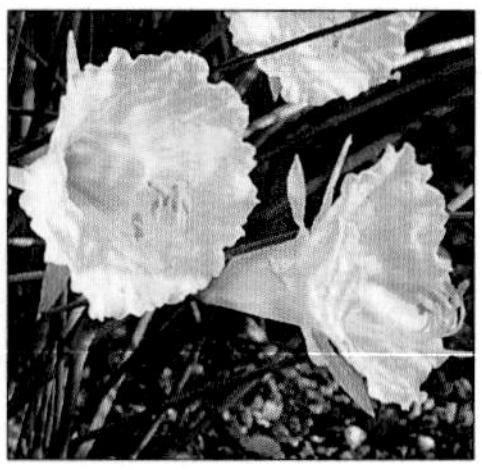
Narcissus romieuxii

strongly scented, golden yellow flowers, 4cm (1½in) across, with large cups and narrow perianth segments. ↕25cm (10in). Garden origin. ❄❄❄. **'Rugulosus'** ■ is more robust with up to 4 flowers, 5.5cm (2¼in) across; ↕30cm (12in).

***N.* 'Olympic Gold'.** Division 1 daffodil bearing golden yellow flowers, 11.5cm (4½in) across, in mid-spring. Smooth, flat perianth segments are at right-angles to the long trumpets, which are rolled at the mouths. ↕45cm (18in). ❄❄❄

***N.* 'Osmington'.** Division 2 daffodil flowering in mid-spring. Flowers, 9.5cm (3¾in) across, have broad, smooth white perianth segments and bright red coronas. ↕40cm (16in). ❄❄❄

N

***N.* 'Panache'** ■ Division 1 daffodil producing among the largest white daffodil flowers, 11.5cm (4½in) across, in mid-spring. Flowers are pure white, with well-balanced trumpets, tinged green at the bases, and broad, overlapping perianth segments. ↕40cm (16in). ❄❄❄

***N.* 'Paper White'** see *N. papyraceus.*

***N.* 'Paper White Grandiflorus'** see *N. papyraceus.*

N. papyraceus, syn. *N.* 'Paper White', *N.* 'Paper White Grandiflorus' (Paperwhite narcissus). Division 8 daffodil with erect, keeled, glaucous, mid-green leaves, 30cm (12in) long. Bears clusters of up to 10 strongly fragrant, glistening white flowers, 1.5cm (½in) across, from winter to early spring. ↕35cm (14in). S. France, S. Spain, N. Africa. ❄❄. **'Ziva'**, syn. *N.* 'Ziva', is a clone of *N. papyraceus* used for forcing and bowl culture.

***N.* 'Park Springs'.** Division 3 daffodil flowering in mid-spring. Flowers, 9.5–10.5cm (3¾–4¼in) across, have rounded, pure white perianth segments and greenish white cups with cream rims. ↕45cm (18in). ❄❄❄

***N.* 'Passionale'** ■🏆 Division 2 daffodil flowering in mid-spring. Flowers, 10cm (4in) across, have overlapping, pure white perianth segments and rose-pink cups that are rolled and slightly frilled at the mouths. ↕40cm (16in). ❄❄❄

***N.* 'Pencrebar'** ■ Small Division 4 daffodil with circular, fragrant, double, golden yellow flowers, 3cm (1¼in) across, often 2 per stem, borne in mid-spring. ↕18cm (7in). ❄❄❄

***N.* 'Pennine Way'.** Division 1 daffodil flowering in mid-spring. Flowers, 9.5cm (3¾in) across, have off-white perianth segments and rich ochre trumpets. ↕40cm (16in). ❄❄❄

***N.* 'Perimeter'.** Division 3 daffodil flowering in mid-spring. Bears lemon-yellow flowers, 9.5cm (3¾in) across, each with a narrow, sharply defined band of orange at the rim of the slightly flattened cup. ↕45cm (18in). ❄❄❄

***N.* 'Petrel'.** Division 5 daffodil producing clusters of up to 7 nodding, pure white flowers, 3cm (1¼in) across, with slightly reflexed perianth segments, in late spring. ↕25cm (10in). ❄❄❄

***N.* 'Pink Champagne'.** Division 4 daffodil. In mid-spring, bears double flowers, 9cm (3½in) across, with broadly overlapping white perianth segments and abundant bright pink corona segments. ↕40cm (16in). ❄❄❄

***N.* 'Pipe Major'.** Division 2 daffodil flowering in mid-spring. Flowers, 10cm (4in) across, have rounded, smooth, deep primrose-yellow perianth segments and bowl-shaped, deep red-orange coronas. ↕45cm (18in). ❄❄❄

***N.* 'Pipit'** ■ Division 7 daffodil bearing 2 or 3 sweetly scented, lemon-yellow flowers, 7cm (3in) across, in mid- and late spring. The cups quickly fade to cream. ↕25cm (10in). ❄❄❄

***N.* 'Pixie's Sister'.** Dwarf Division 7 daffodil producing clusters of up to 5 well-shaped, scented, golden yellow flowers, 2.5cm (1in) across, in late spring. ↕16cm (6in). ❄❄❄

N. poeticus, (Poet's narcissus). Robust, variable Division 10 daffodil with erect, narrow, strap-shaped, channelled leaves, to 45cm (18in) long. In late spring, bears solitary, fragrant flowers, 4.5–7cm (1¾–3in) across, with flat, pure white perianth segments and tiny, red-rimmed yellow cups. ↕20–50cm (8–20in). France, Switzerland, Italy (widely naturalized in S. Europe). ❄❄❄. **'Plenus'**, syn. *N.* 'Albus Plenus Odoratus', has strongly fragrant, untidy, double, pure white flowers, 4cm (1½in) across. Occasionally, the remains of the red cups are visible between the perianth segments. Excellent for cutting; ↕40cm (16in). **var. *recurvus*** ■🏆 (Old pheasant's eye) has flowers 4cm (1½in) across, with recurved, glistening white perianth segments; ↕35cm (14in); Switzerland.

***N.* 'Poet's Way'.** Division 9 daffodil producing scented flowers, 5.5cm (2¼in) across, in mid-spring. Flowers have broad, smooth, pure white perianth segments and bright yellow cups with deep red rims and green eyes. ↕40cm (16in). ❄❄❄

***N.* 'Portrush'** ■ Division 3 daffodil bearing pure white flowers, 8.5cm (3¼in) across, in mid-spring. Broadly overlapping perianth segments surround flat cups with distinctive dark green eyes. ↕45cm (18in). ❄❄❄

***N.* 'Preamble'.** Division 1 daffodil producing long-lasting flowers, 11.5cm (4½in) across, in mid-spring. The perianth segments are pure white; the trumpets open deep canary-yellow and darken with age. ↕40cm (16in). ❄❄❄

***N.* 'Pride of Cornwall'.** Division 8 daffodil producing 2 or 3 scented white flowers, 6cm (2½in) across, with deep orange-yellow cups, margined with red, in mid-spring. Excellent for cutting. ↕40cm (16in). ❄❄

N. pseudonarcissus, syn. *N. lobularis* (Lent lily, Wild daffodil). Very variable Division 10 daffodil with erect, strap-shaped, usually glaucous, mid-green leaves, 8–50cm (3–20in) long. Nodding flowers, 4–7cm (1½–3in) across, with yellow trumpets and narrow, twisted cream perianth segments, are produced in early spring. Good for naturalizing. ↕15–35cm (6–14in). Europe. ❄❄❄. **subsp. *obvallaris*** see *N. obvallaris.*

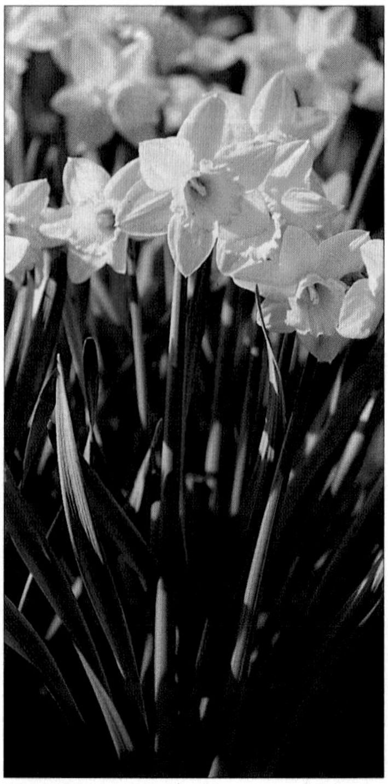
Narcissus 'St. Keverne'

N. pumilus, syn. *N. minor* of gardens, *N. minor* subsp. *pumilus.* Small Division 10 daffodil with erect, channelled or flat, grey-green leaves, 8–15cm (3–6in) long. Bears yellow flowers, 3cm (1¼in) across, with flared, frilled trumpets, in early spring. Similar to *N. minor*, which has straighter trumpets. ↕10–15cm (4–6in). Possibly garden origin. ❄❄❄. **'Plenus'** see *N.* 'Rip van Winkle'.

***N.* 'Purbeck'.** Division 3 daffodil flowering in mid-spring. Flowers, 9.5cm (3¾in) across, have broad, bright white perianth segments and small, goblet-shaped yellow cups, each with a green-tinged throat, fringed with a bright orange band. ↕45cm (18in). ❄❄❄

***N.* 'Quail'.** Robust Division 7 daffodil. In mid-spring, bears 2 or 3 scented, golden yellow flowers, 4cm (1½in) across, with long cups and neat perianth segments. ↕40cm (16in). ❄❄❄

***N.* 'Quince'** ■ Division 12 daffodil producing 1–3 soft yellow flowers, 3cm (1¼in) across, with short, frilled, golden yellow cups, in early and mid-spring. Each bulb bears a succession of flower stems. ↕16cm (6in). ❄❄

***N.* 'Rainbow'** ■ Vigorous Division 2 daffodil flowering in mid-spring. Bears consistently good-quality flowers, 10cm (4in) across, with fine-textured white perianth segments and white cups, each with a broad band of copper-pink at the slightly indented mouth. ↕45cm (18in). ❄❄❄

***N.* 'Rameses'.** Division 2 daffodil flowering in mid-spring. Flowers, 8.5cm (3¼in) across, have broadly ovate white perianth segments contrasting with rich red cups. ↕50cm (20in). ❄❄❄

N. requienii see *N. assoanus.*

***N.* 'Rijnveld's Early Sensation'** 🏆 Division 1 daffodil producing yellow flowers, 9cm (3½in) across, in late winter. Very early-flowering and long-lasting. ↕25–35cm (10–14in). ❄❄❄

***N.* 'Rip van Winkle'** ■ syn. *N. minor* subsp. *pumilus* 'Plenus', *N. pumilus* 'Plenus'. Division 4 daffodil bearing double, greenish yellow flowers, 5cm (2in) across, with irregular, pointed

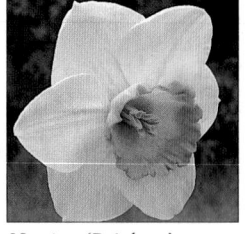

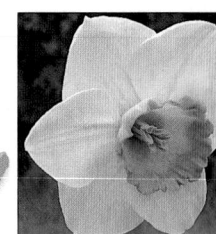

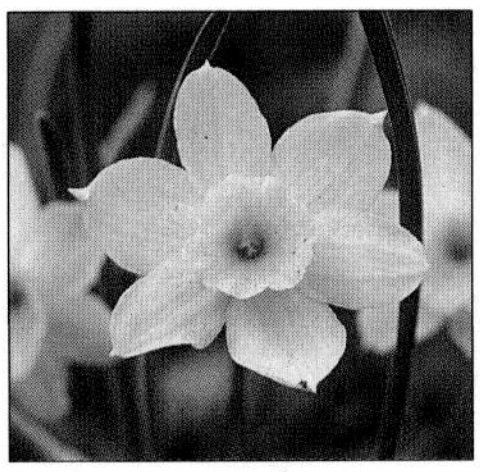
Narcissus rupicola

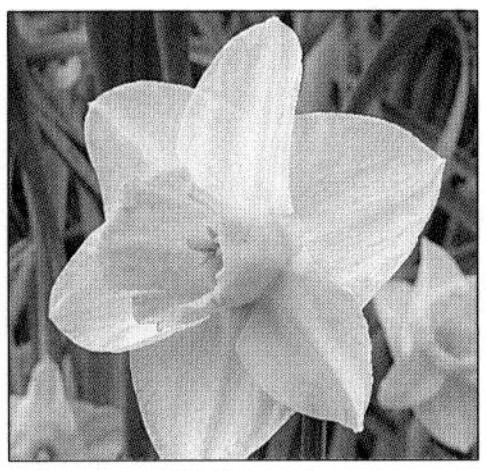
Narcissus 'Salome'

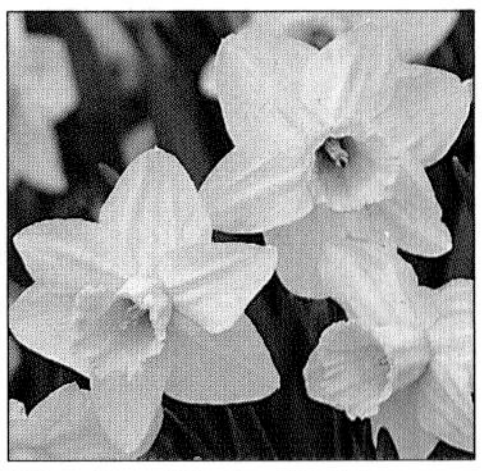
Narcissus 'Satin Pink'

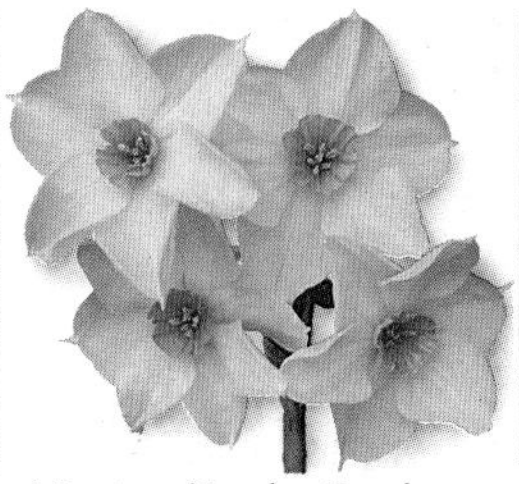
Narcissus 'Scarlet Gem'

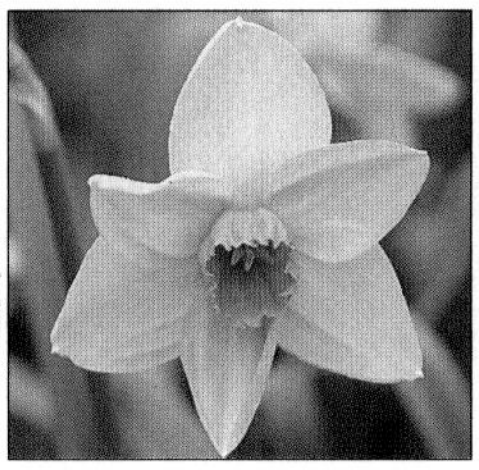
Narcissus 'Sealing Wax'

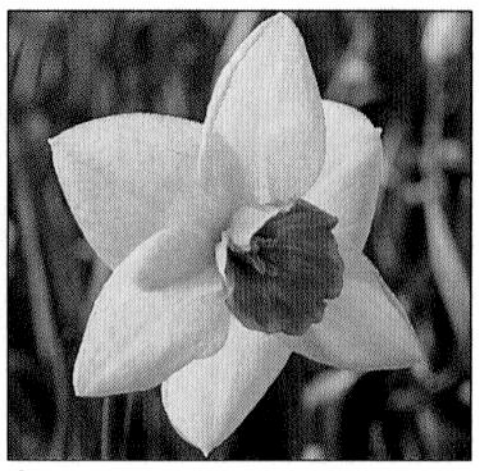
Narcissus 'Shining Light'

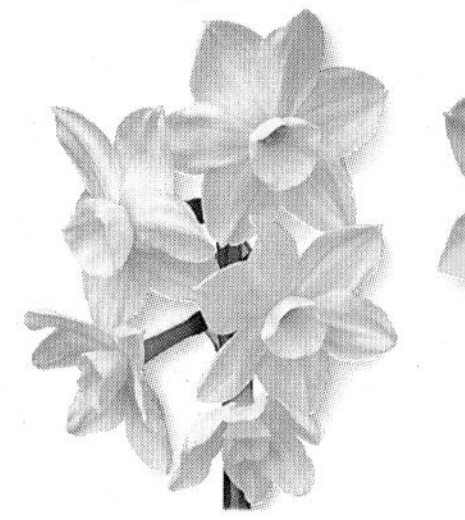
Narcissus 'Silver Chimes'

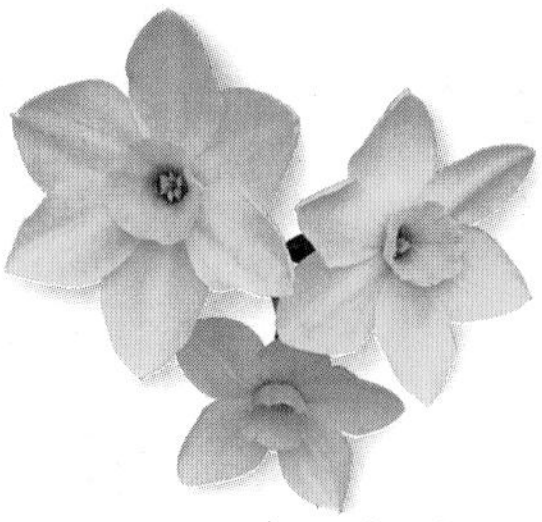
Narcissus 'Stratosphere'

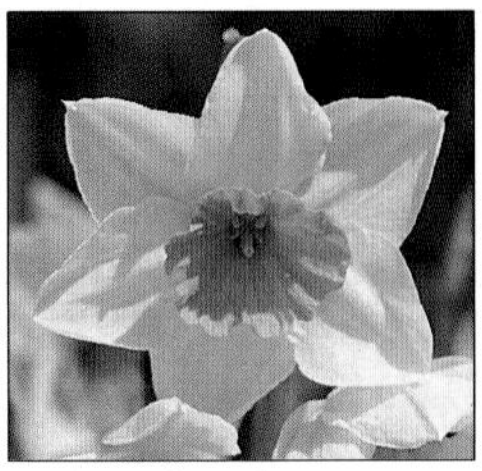
Narcissus 'Suzy'

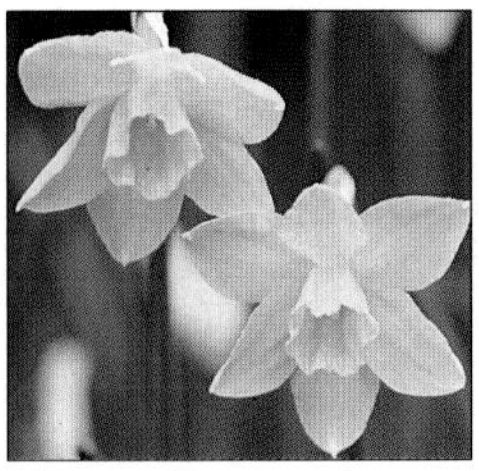
Narcissus 'Sweetness'

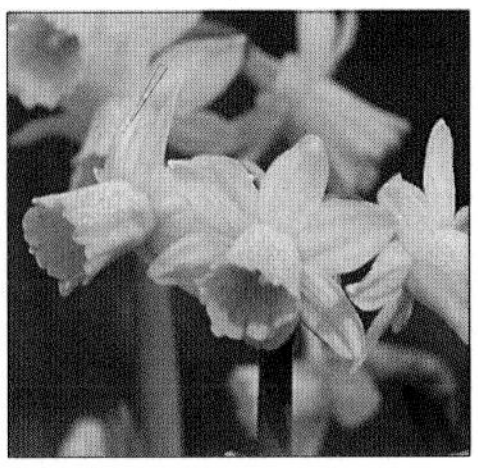
Narcissus 'Tête-à-Tête'

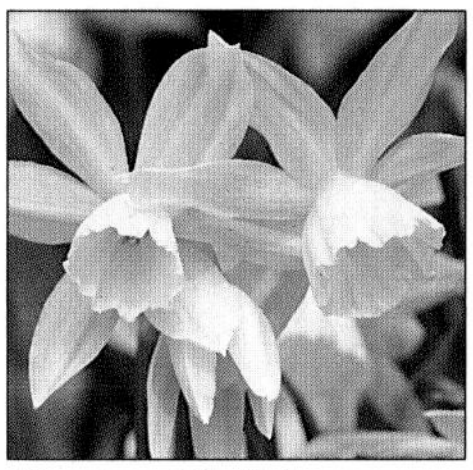
Narcissus 'Thalia'

perianth segments, in early spring. ↕14cm (5½in). ***

***N.* 'Rockall'** ■ Division 3 daffodil flowering in mid-spring. Flowers, 11cm (4½in) across, have large, overlapping, slightly pointed white perianth segments and saucer-shaped, finely fluted, rich orange-red coronas. ↕50cm (20in). ***

N. romieuxii ■ ♀ Small Division 10 daffodil with erect or spreading, narrow, semi-cylindrical, dark green leaves, to 20cm (8in) long. In early spring, bears funnel-shaped flowers, 3.5cm (1½in) across, which vary from pale straw-yellow to pale primrose-yellow. Similar to *N. bulbocodium*, which has deeper yellow flowers. ↕8–10cm (3–4in). N. Africa. **

N. rupicola ■ Division 10 daffodil with erect, thin, cylindrical, keeled, grey-green leaves, 18cm (7in) long. Circular, golden yellow flowers, 3cm (1¼in) across, with shallow, 6-lobed cups, are produced in mid-spring. ↕15cm (6in). Portugal, Spain. ***

***N.* 'St. Keverne'** ■ ♀ Erect Division 2 daffodil bearing rich golden yellow flowers, 10cm (4in) across, in mid-spring. Large cups, occasionally trumpet-sized, are indented at the rims and slightly flared. ↕45cm (18in). ***

***N.* 'Salome'** ■ Division 2 daffodil flowering in mid-spring. Produces consistently good quality flowers, 9cm (3½in) across, with smooth, waxy, pale cream perianth segments and large, almost trumpet-shaped, peach pink cups. ↕45cm (18in). ***

***N.* 'Satin Pink'** ■ Division 2 daffodil flowering in mid-spring. Flowers, 8–12cm (3–5in) across, have neatly overlapping white perianth segments and pale pink cups, deepening slightly at the finely indented mouths and with greenish yellow eyes. ↕45cm (18in). ***

***N.* 'Scarlet Gem'** ■ Division 8 daffodil with clusters of many scented yellow flowers, 5cm (2in) across, with red-orange cups, produced in mid-spring. Good for cutting. ↕35cm (14in). **

***N.* 'Sea Green'.** Division 9 daffodil producing scented flowers, 6cm (2½in) across, in late spring. Rounded, snow-white perianth segments surround white coronas that are rich green at the bases and trimmed with bright red margins. ↕40cm (16in). ***

***N.* 'Sealing Wax'** ■ Division 2 daffodil flowering in mid-spring. Flowers, 9cm (3½in) across, have wide, rounded, rich golden yellow perianth segments and relatively small, goblet-shaped, deep red-orange coronas. ↕50cm (20in). ***

***N.* 'Shining Light'** ■ Division 2 daffodil bearing uniform flowers, 8.5cm (3¼in) across, in mid-spring. They have slightly pointed, smooth, butter-yellow perianth segments and goblet-shaped, bright orange-red cups, slightly indented at the mouths. ↕40cm (16in). ***

***N.* 'Silent Valley'.** Division 1 daffodil bearing snow-white flowers, 11.5cm (4½in) across, in mid-spring. Strongly overlapping, broad, pointed, smooth perianth segments surround trumpets highlighted by striking green eyes. ↕40cm (16in). ***

***N.* 'Silver Chimes'** ■ Sturdy Division 8 daffodil. In mid- and late spring, produces up to 10 nodding, scented, creamy white flowers, 5cm (2in) across, with pale primrose-yellow cups. ↕30cm (12in). ***

***N.* 'Smyrna'.** Division 9 daffodil. In mid-spring, bears scented flowers, 6cm (2½in) across, with rounded, pure white perianth segments and small, flattened, bright orange coronas. ↕40cm (16in). ***

***N.* 'Spellbinder'** ♀ Vigorous Division 1 daffodil bearing sulphur-yellow flowers, 10–11.5cm (4–4½in) across, in mid-spring. Coronas gradually fade to white, with whitish green at the mouths. ↕50cm (20in). ***

***N.* 'Stratosphere'** ■ Division 7 daffodil. In mid-spring, each tall, strong stem bears up to 3 scented blooms, to 6.5cm (2½in) across, with smooth yellow perianth segments and small, rich deep gold cups. ↕65cm (26in). ***

***N.* 'Strines'.** Division 2 daffodil. In mid-spring, produces flowers 12.5cm (5in) across, with well-balanced, deep yellow cups, slightly flared and indented at the mouths and of near trumpet proportions; the overlapping perianth segments are a shade or so deeper. ↕45cm (18in). ***

***N.* 'Sundial'.** Small Division 7 daffodil producing 1 or 2 golden yellow flowers, 3.5cm (1½in) across, in mid-spring. ↕20cm (8in). ***

***N.* 'Sun Disc'.** Neat, dwarf Division 7 daffodil with stiff stems, each bearing a single, perfectly circular, mid-yellow flower, 5cm (2in) across, in mid-spring. The perianth segments fade to cream with age. ↕18cm (7in). ***

***N.* 'Suzy'** ■ ♀ Division 7 daffodil producing 1 or 2 scented flowers, 6cm (2½in) across, with primrose-yellow perianth segments and rich orange cups, in mid-spring. ↕40cm (16in). ***

***N.* 'Sweetness'** ■ ♀ Vigorous Division 7 daffodil with stiff stems bearing solitary, strongly fragrant, golden yellow flowers, 4cm (1½in) across, in mid-spring. Long-lasting as a cut flower. ↕40cm (16in). ***

***N.* 'Tahiti'** ■ Division 4 daffodil with double flowers, 11cm (4½in) across, borne in mid-spring. Regular, rounded, rich golden yellow perianth segments surround a cluster of bright red-orange corona segments. ↕45cm (18in). ***

***N.* 'Tamar Fire'.** Division 4 daffodil bearing well-formed, scented flowers, 7cm (3in) across, with rich yellow outer perianth segments and blood-red inner segments. ↕30cm (12in). ***

***N. tazetta*.** Very variable Division 10 daffodil with erect, broad, twisted, keeled, glaucous, mid-green leaves, 20–50cm (8–20in) long. In winter or spring, bears up to 20 sweetly scented flowers, 4cm (1½in) across, with white perianth segments and yellow cups. ↕15–50cm (6–20in). Mediterranean region. Widely naturalized in many parts of the world. **

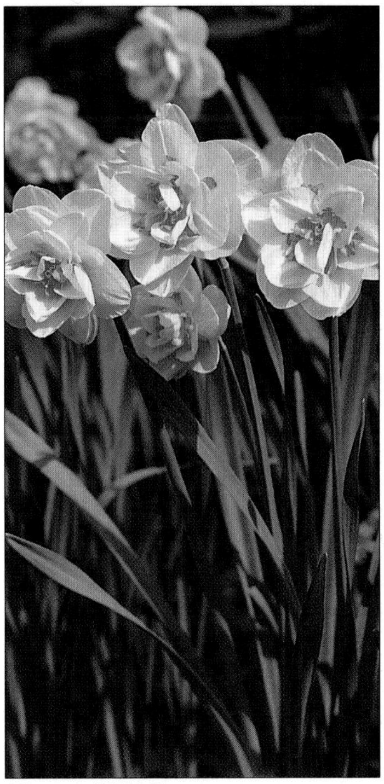
Narcissus 'Tahiti'

***N.* 'Telamonius Plenus'**, syn. *N.* 'Van Sion'. Vigorous Division 4 daffodil producing double, greenish yellow flowers, 10cm (4in) across, in early spring. This very old cultivar is variable in flower shape: it is occasionally fully double; sometimes the trumpet is filled with segments, but the perianth segments remain distinct. Excellent for naturalizing. ↕35cm (14in). ***

***N.* 'Tête-à-Tête'** ■ ♀ Vigorous, dwarf Division 12 daffodil bearing 1–3 flowers, 6.5cm (2½in) across, in early spring. They have deep golden yellow perianth segments, slightly reflexed from deeper yellow cups. ↕15cm (6in). ***

***N.* 'Thalia'** ■ Division 5 daffodil flowering in mid-spring. Bears 2 milk-white flowers, 5cm (2in) across, with narrow, twisted, slightly reflexed perianth segments and open cups. ↕35cm (14in). ***

***N.* 'Tonga'.** Division 4 daffodil bearing well-formed, scented, double flowers, 8cm (3in) across, in mid-spring. Deep primrose yellow perianth segments, becoming paler yellow, are intermingled with short, bright red corona segments. ↕40cm (16in). ***

***N.* 'Torridon'.** Division 2 daffodil bearing long-lasting flowers, 8cm (3in) across, in mid-spring. The well-formed perianth segments are deep yellow and the corona is fiery orange-red. ↕35cm (14in). ***

***N.* 'Tracey'.** Division 6 daffodil flowering in early spring. Bears flowers, 7cm (3in) across, with reflexed white perianth segments and trumpet-shaped, pale yellow coronas. ↕25cm (10in). ***

***N.* 'Tresamble'.** Robust Division 5 daffodil producing 1–3 well-formed flowers, 9cm (3½in) across, in mid-spring. Flowers have spreading, milk-white perianth segments and cream cups. ↕40cm (16in). ***

***N.* 'Trevithian'.** Vigorous Division 7 daffodil bearing 1–3 scented, soft lemon-yellow flowers, 7cm (3in) across, in mid-spring. The perianth segments

N

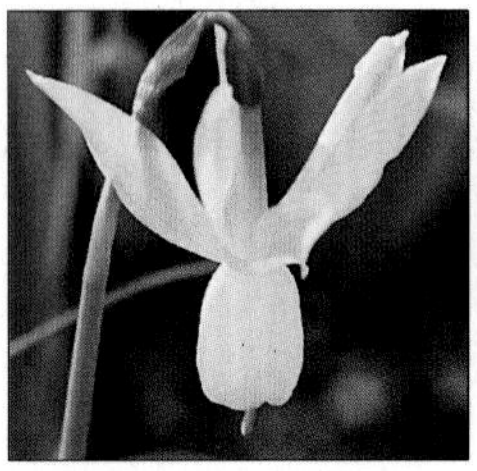
Narcissus triandrus

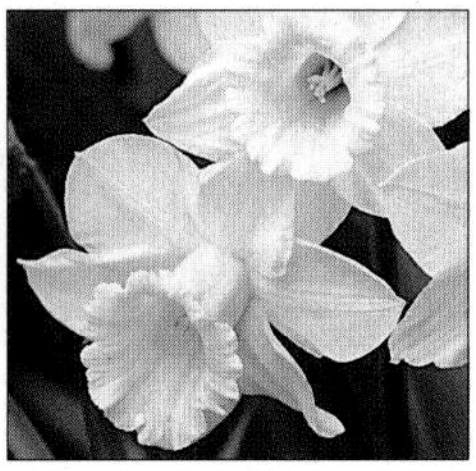
Narcissus 'Trousseau'

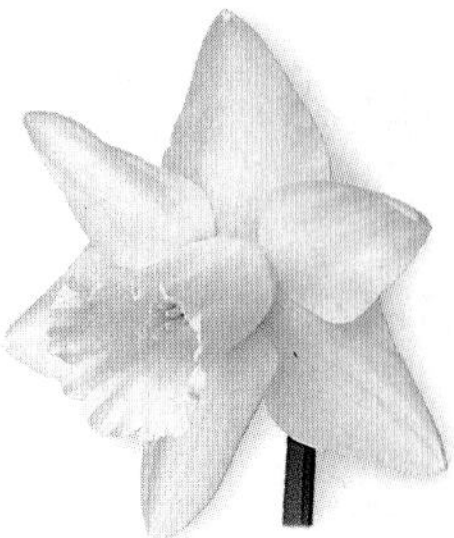
Narcissus 'Vigil'

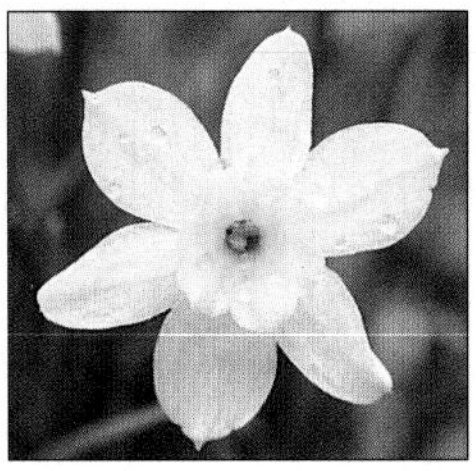
Narcissus watieri

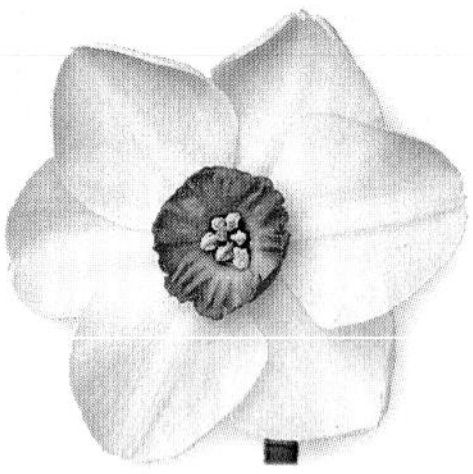
Narcissus 'Woodland Star'

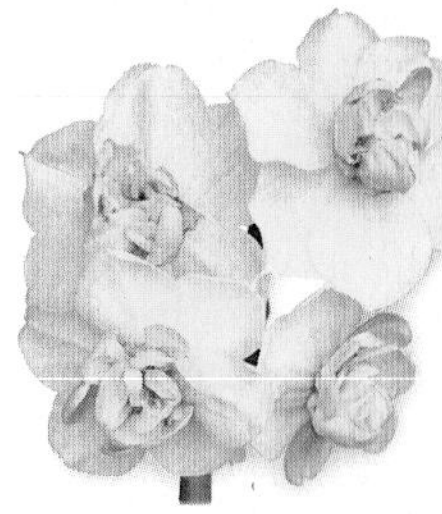
Narcissus 'Yellow Cheerfulness'

are well-rounded; the cups are short and flared. ↕45cm (18in). ❄❄❄
N. triandrus ■ ♀ (Angel's tears). Small Division 10 daffodil with decumbent or erect, narrow, flat or channelled leaves, 20–30cm (8–12in) long. In mid-spring, bears 1–6 nodding cream flowers, 6cm (2½in) across, with reflexed perianth segments and rounded cups. ↕10–25cm (4–10in). Portugal, Spain. ❄❄❄
***N.* 'Tripartite'.** Division 11a daffodil bearing stems of up to 3 golden yellow flowers, 6.5cm (2½in) across, in late spring. Each expanded corona is split into 6 segments that lie flat against the perianth segments. ↕45cm (18in). ❄❄❄
***N.* 'Trousseau'** ■ Division 1 daffodil bearing delicate, satin-like flowers, 12cm (5in) across, in mid-spring. White perianth segments surround flanged trumpets that open soft yellow and turn beige-pink. ↕45cm (18in). ❄❄❄
***N.* 'Tudor Minstrel'.** Division 2 daffodil flowering in mid-spring. Flowers, 11cm (4½in) across, have pointed, slightly hooded white perianth segments and large, slightly expanded, rich golden yellow coronas, frilled at the mouths. ↕50cm (20in). ❄❄❄
***N.* 'Tuesday's Child'.** Division 5 daffodil bearing 1–3 slightly pendent flowers, 6cm (2½in) across, in mid-spring. Pointed white perianth segments are swept back from short, lemon yellow coronas. ↕35cm (14in). ❄❄❄
***N.* 'Tutankhamun'.** Division 2 daffodil. In mid-spring, bears trumpet-shaped, intense white flowers, 10.5cm (4¼in) across, with conspicuous green eyes. ↕40cm (16in). ❄❄❄
***N.* 'Unique'.** Division 4 daffodil producing well-formed, double flowers, 10.5cm (4¼in) across, in mid-spring. They are circular, with broad, rounded white perianth segments, interleaved with rich yellow corona segments in the centres. ↕50cm (20in). ❄❄❄
***N.* 'Van Sion'** see *N.* 'Telamonius Plenus'.
***N.* 'Verona'** ♀ Division 3 daffodil flowering in mid-spring. Bears circular flowers, 9.5–10cm (3¾–4in) across, with broadly overlapping white perianth segments. The flattish, fluted cups open cream and soon fade to white. ↕45cm (18in). ❄❄❄
***N.* 'Vigil'** ■ ♀ Division 1 daffodil bearing pure white flowers, 12.5cm (5in) across, in mid-spring. Flowers have sharply pointed, finely textured perianth segments and long, slender trumpets, slightly rolled at the mouths. ↕40cm (16in). ❄❄❄
***N.* 'Viking'.** Division 1 daffodil. In mid-spring, bears deep golden yellow flowers, 11.5cm (4½in) across, with broad, pointed perianth segments and long, slightly expanded trumpets, frilled at the mouths. ↕45cm (18in). ❄❄❄
***N.* 'Vulcan'** ♀ Division 2 daffodil flowering in mid-spring. Flowers, 9.5cm (3¾in) across, have rounded, smooth, rich golden yellow perianth segments and fiery orange-red cups, each widening slightly to a jagged mouth. ↕50cm (20in). ❄❄❄
N. watieri ■ Tiny Division 10 daffodil with erect, narrow, keeled, grey-green leaves, 18cm (7in) long. In mid-spring, bears solitary flowers, 1.5cm (½in) across, with flat, pure white perianth segments, and widely funnel-shaped coronas. ↕10cm (4in). N. Africa. ❄❄
***N.* 'Woodland Prince'.** Division 3 daffodil producing consistently good quality flowers, 9cm (3½in) across, in mid-spring. The creamy white perianth segments are broad and smooth; the small, lemon-yellow cups have deeper yellow rims. ↕50cm (20in). ❄❄❄
***N.* 'Woodland Star'** ■ Division 3 daffodil. In mid-spring, produces flowers 9.5cm (3¾in) across, with pure white perianth segments contrasting with the small, bowl-shaped, deep orange-red cups. ↕50cm (20in). ❄❄❄
***N.* 'W.P. Milner'.** Sturdy Division 1 daffodil bearing nodding flowers, 6cm (2½in) across, in early and mid-spring. Forward-pointing, cream perianth segments surround the pale, creamy white trumpets. ↕23cm (9in). ❄❄❄
***N.* 'Yellow Cheerfulness'** ■ Division 4 daffodil producing strong stems of 3 or 4 circular, sweetly scented, double, golden yellow flowers, 2cm (¾in) across, in mid-spring. ↕45cm (18in). ❄❄❄
***N.* 'Ziva'** see *N. papyraceus* 'Ziva'.

▷**Narcissus,**
Paper-white see *Narcissus papyraceus*
Poet's see *Narcissus poeticus*
▷**Nardoo, Common** see *Marsilea drummondii*
▷**Nasturtium** see *Tropaeolum majus*
Flame see *T. speciosum*

NAUTILOCALYX

GESNERIACEAE

Genus of 38 species of evergreen perennials, often woody at the bases, from open woodland in the West Indies, Central America and tropical South America. They are grown for their opposite, prominently veined, glossy leaves and tubular, 5-lobed flowers, borne singly or in clustered cymes in the upper leaf axils. In frost-prone areas, grow in a warm greenhouse. In warmer areas, plant among shrubs or trees.
• **HARDINESS** Frost tender.
• **CULTIVATION** Under glass, grow in loamless potting compost in bright filtered light and high humidity. During growth, water freely with soft water and apply a balanced liquid fertilizer monthly. Water moderately in winter. Outdoors, grow in moist but well-drained, humus-rich soil in light shade.
• **PROPAGATION** Root softwood or stem-tip cuttings in spring or summer.
• **PESTS AND DISEASES** Mealybugs and tarsonemid mites may be troublesome.

N. bullatus, syn. *N. tessellatus*. Erect perennial with elliptic, finely toothed, puckered, dark green leaves, to 23cm (9in) long, purple beneath. From spring to summer, bears cymes of up to 10 hairy, pale yellow flowers, 3cm (1¼in) across. ↕60cm (24in), ↔35cm (14in). Peru. ❀ (min. 16°C/61°F)
N. lynchii ■ Erect, branched perennial with elliptic-lance-shaped, toothed, very dark green, sometimes red-purple leaves, 12cm (5in) long, red-purple beneath. In summer, bears cymes of 2 or 3 yellow flowers, to 3cm (1¼in) across, with red hairs outside, purple streaks inside, and maroon sepals. ↕60cm (24in), ↔30cm (12in). Colombia. ❀ (min. 16°C/61°F)
N. tessellatus see *N. bullatus.*

▷**Navelwort** see *Omphalodes*
Venus's see *O. linifolia*
▷***Neanthe bella*** see *Chamaedorea elegans*

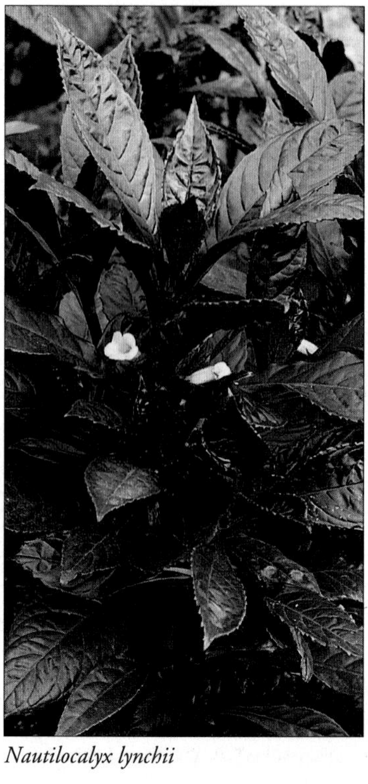
Nautilocalyx lynchii

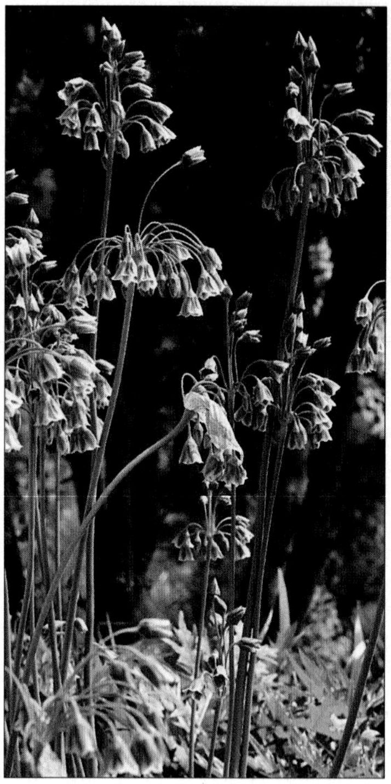
Nectaroscordum siculum subsp. *bulgaricum*

NECTAROSCORDUM

ALLIACEAE/LILIACEAE

Genus of 3 species of bulbous perennials from damp or shady woodland, rocky places, and dry mountain slopes of S. Europe and W. Asia. They have linear, deeply channelled or keeled leaves, which smell of garlic. Loose umbels of bell-shaped flowers, 2–2.5cm (¾–1in) long, are borne in summer. Grow in a wild garden or herbaceous border.
• **HARDINESS** Fully hardy.
• **CULTIVATION** Grow in any moderately fertile, well-drained soil in full sun or partial shade. May self-seed freely.
• **PROPAGATION** Sow seed in containers in a cold frame in autumn or spring. Remove offsets in summer.
• **PESTS AND DISEASES** Trouble free.

N. dioscoridis see *N. siculum* subsp. *bulgaricum.*
N. siculum, syn. *Allium siculum.* Robust, bulbous perennial with linear, sharply keeled, basal leaves, 30–40cm (12–16in) long. In summer, stout stems bear umbels of 10–30 pendulous, open bell-shaped, white or cream flowers, 1.5–2.5cm (½–1in) long, flushed pink or purplish red, and tinted green at the bases. Seed pods become erect as flowers fade. ↕to 1.2m (4ft), ↔10cm (4in). France, Italy. ❄❄❄. **subsp. *bulgaricum*** ■ syn. *Allium bulgaricum, N. dioscoridis*, has off-white flowers, flushed green and purple. S.E. Europe, N.W. Turkey, Ukraine (Crimea).

NEILLIA

ROSACEAE

Genus of 10 species of deciduous shrubs and subshrubs, with branching, zigzag stems, found in scrub and at rocky stream margins in the Himalayas and E. Asia. The dark, glossy leaves are alternate, irregularly toothed, each with up to 5, but usually 3, lobes. They are

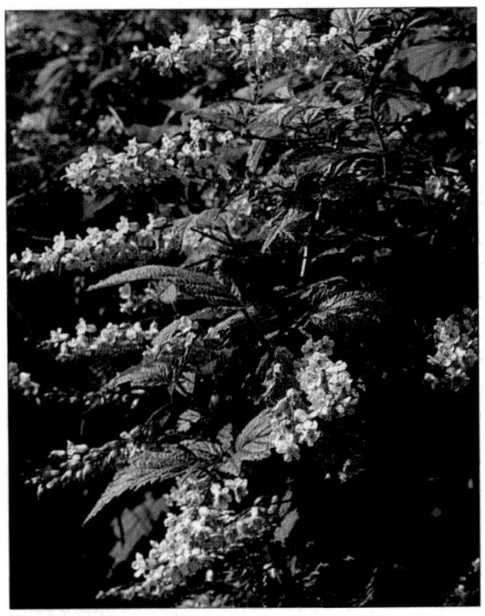

Neillia thibetica

cultivated for their graceful, arching habit and their racemes or panicles of small, bell-shaped or tubular flowers, profusely borne in late spring and early summer. Grow in a shrub border or woodland garden.

- **HARDINESS** Fully hardy.
- **CULTIVATION** Grow in fertile, well-drained soil in full sun or partial shade. Pruning group 2 or 3, after flowering.
- **PROPAGATION** Take greenwood cuttings in early summer. Remove suckers in autumn.
- **PESTS AND DISEASES** Trouble free.

N. longiracemosa see *N. thibetica.*
N. sinensis. Thicket-forming, suckering shrub with arching shoots and peeling brown bark. Leaves are usually 3-lobed, ovate to oblong, sharply toothed, and long-pointed, to 10cm (4in) long. In late spring and early summer, small, tubular, pinkish white flowers, to 12mm (½in) long, are produced in slender, 12- to 20-flowered racemes, to 6cm (2½in) long. ↕↔ 2m (6ft). C. China. ❄❄❄
N. thibetica ■ syn. *N. longiracemosa.* Thicket-forming, suckering shrub with arching shoots and ovate or ovate-oblong, 3-lobed, long-pointed, toothed, bright green leaves, to 10cm (4in) long. In early summer, small, tubular-bell-shaped, rose-pink flowers, to 8mm (⅜in) long, are produced in arching racemes, to 15cm (6in) long. ↕↔ 2m (6ft). W. China. ❄❄❄

NELUMBO

Lotus

NELUMBONACEAE

Genus of 2 species of rhizomatous, marginal aquatic perennials from Asia, N. Australia, and E. North America, found at the shallow margins or on the muddy banks of pools. They are widely cultivated and naturalized in subtropical and tropical areas. The handsome, horizontally held, peltate, waxy-bloomed, almost circular leaves are held well above the water. The showy, solitary, fragrant, water lily-like flowers are borne on long stalks, and develop distinctive, flat-topped seed pods that may be dried for use in flower arrangements. They are excellent as specimen plants in an outdoor pool. In frost-prone areas, grow *N. nucifera* with giant water lilies (*Victoria*) in an indoor tropical pool, or in large, water-filled half-barrels on a patio outdoors; overwinter in frost-free conditions.

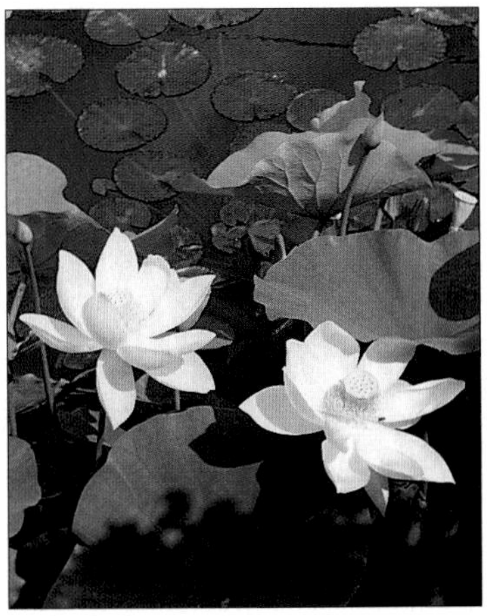

Nelumbo lutea

- **HARDINESS** Half hardy to frost tender; in cold climates, *N. lutea* and some *N. nucifera* cultivars can be overwintered outdoors given sufficient summer warmth to ripen the rhizomatous roots; these will survive if well below any frozen soil or water.
- **CULTIVATION** In an outdoor pool, grow in large containers in heavy loam enriched with well-rotted farmyard manure or compost, in full sun. As growth proceeds, gradually lower the containers to increase the water depth to 40–60cm (16–24in), or 15–22cm (6–9in) for smaller cultivars. Remove fading foliage. In very cold areas, reduce the water level gradually in autumn, remove the containers, and overwinter in frost-free conditions, keeping the rhizomes just moist. Under glass, grow in large containers in an indoor pool in full light. See also pp.52–53.
- **PROPAGATION** Sow seed in spring, preferably scarified before sowing, at a minimum temperature of 25°C (77°F), in small containers of loam covered by 5cm (2in) of water. Increase water depth and container size until plants are large enough to plant in the flowering site.

Carefully divide the fragile rhizomes, which resent disturbance. In spring, plant rootstock horizontally just below the soil surface, and barely submerge until growth starts.

- **PESTS AND DISEASES** Outdoors, leaves may be attacked by corn-borers and woolly-bear caterpillars, and by various leaf-spotting diseases, particularly brown spot and dry brown spot. Red spider mites and whiteflies may be a problem under glass.

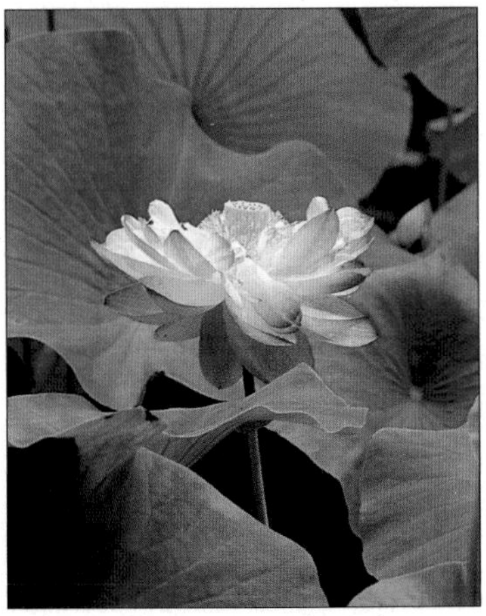

Nelumbo 'Mrs. Perry D. Slocum'

N. lutea ■ (American lotus, Water chinquapin, Yanquapin). Aquatic perennial with radical, concave-circular, bluish green leaves, 50cm (20in) across, prominently veined beneath, held on stalks to 2m (6ft) long. In summer, produces rose-like yellow flowers, to 25cm (10in) across. ↕ 2m (6ft), ↔ indefinite. North America. ✲ (min. 7°C/45°F)
N. 'Mrs. Perry D. Slocum' ■ Aquatic perennial with rounded, flat or wavy-margined, glaucous, grey-green leaves, 80cm (32in) across, on stalks to 1.4m (4½ft) long. In summer, freely produces deep pink flowers, to 30cm (12in) across, turning yellow over a period of several days. ↕ 1.2–1.5m (4–5ft). ↔ indefinite. ✲ (min. 5°C/41°F)
N. nucifera (Sacred lotus). Aquatic perennial with flat or concave-circular, wavy-margined, glaucous, mid-green leaves, 80cm (32in) across, on stalks to 2m (6ft) long. Peony-like, sometimes double, pink or white flowers, to 30cm (12in) across, are produced in summer on long stalks with short, fleshy prickles. ↕ 0.7–1.5m (28–60in), above water level, ↔ indefinite. Asia (Iran to Japan), N. Australia. ✲ (min. 5°C/41°F). **'Alba Grandiflora'** has wavy-margined, dark green leaves and white flowers, 22–25cm (9–10in) across, sometimes hidden in the foliage; ↕ 1.2–1.8m (4–6ft). **'Alba Striata'** has white flowers, with jagged red margins. **'Charles Thomas'** has lavender-pink flowers, 15–20cm (6–8in) across. Grow in a tub or small pool; ↕ 60–90cm (26–36in). **'Kermesina'** has fully double, rose-pink to bright red flowers, 15–20cm (6–8in) across, produced on stiff stems well above the leaves; ↕ 60–90cm (26–36in). **'Momo Botan'** has long-lasting flowers, to 15cm (6in) across, with dark rose-pink petals, yellow towards the bases. Suitable for a small pool or half-barrel. ↕ 60–120cm (2–4ft). **'Rosea Plena'** produces double, dark rose-pink flowers, 25–35cm (10–14in) across, yellowish towards the bases; ↕ 1.2–1.5m (4–5ft).

NEMATANTHUS

GESNERIACEAE

Genus of about 30 species of scandent or trailing, evergreen, usually epiphytic subshrubs, often becoming woody at the bases, from tropical rainforest in South America. They have opposite, sometimes whorled, elliptic to obovate, entire to toothed, fleshy leaves. The colourful flowers, borne singly or in clustered cymes in the leaf axils, are tubular and pouched. In frost-prone areas, grow in a warm greenhouse or as houseplants. Elsewhere, grow epiphytically on trees or shrubs, or underplant among them.

- **HARDINESS** Frost tender.
- **CULTIVATION** Under glass, grow in loamless potting compost in bright filtered light, or full light with shade from hot sun, with moderate humidity. Water moderately with soft water (less in winter), and feed actively growing plants every month with a balanced liquid fertilizer. For sporadic flowering through winter, maintain a minimum temperature of 15–16°C (59–61°F). Tip-prune young plants when young to encourage branching. Outdoors, grow in moist but well-drained, humus-rich soil in partial shade.

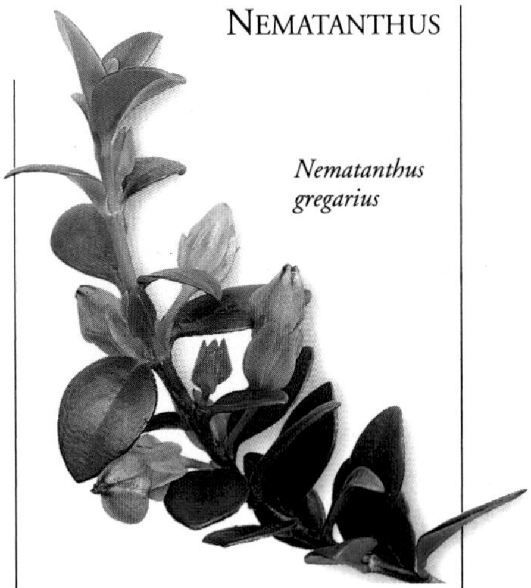

Nematanthus gregarius

- **PROPAGATION** Take stem-tip cuttings in spring.
- **PESTS AND DISEASES** Aphids may infest new growth, including calyces and flowers.

N. gregarius ■ syn. *Hypocyrta radicans, N. radicans.* Trailing to pendent or scandent subshrub with elliptic to obovate, fleshy, glossy, rich green leaves, 2–4cm (¾–1½in) long, borne in opposite pairs or whorls of 3. Clusters of 1–3 tubular, pouched, bright orange flowers, 2.5cm (1in) long, with purple-brown stripes and green, orange-tipped calyces, are borne in summer. ↕ to 80cm (32in), ↔ 90cm (36in) or more. Brazil. ✲ (min. 10–15°C/50–59°F)
N. radicans see *N. gregarius.*
N. strigillosus, syn. *Hypocyrta strigillosa.* Scandent to trailing subshrub, woody at the base, with opposite, elliptic, mid- to deep green leaves, to 3.5cm (1½in) long, sparsely hairy above, pale green and densely downy beneath. Solitary, tubular, orange and yellow flowers, to 2cm (¾in) long, with prominent pouches and green calyces flushed brownish red, are produced mainly in summer. Becomes pendent if grown in a hanging basket. ↕ to 1.5m (5ft), ↔ to 90cm (36in), or more if trailing. Brazil. ✲ (min. 10–15°C/50–59°F)
N. 'Tropicana' ■ 🏆 Erect, freely-branching subshrub with purple stems and opposite, obovate, thick, fleshy, glossy, dark green leaves, 3cm (1¼in) long. Tubular, pouched, glossy, dark yellow flowers, 2.5cm (1in) long, with maroon stripes, enclosed in long-lasting, leafy, bright red calyces, are produced throughout the year. ↕ 30cm (12in), ↔ 45cm (18in). ✲ (min. 13°C/55°F)

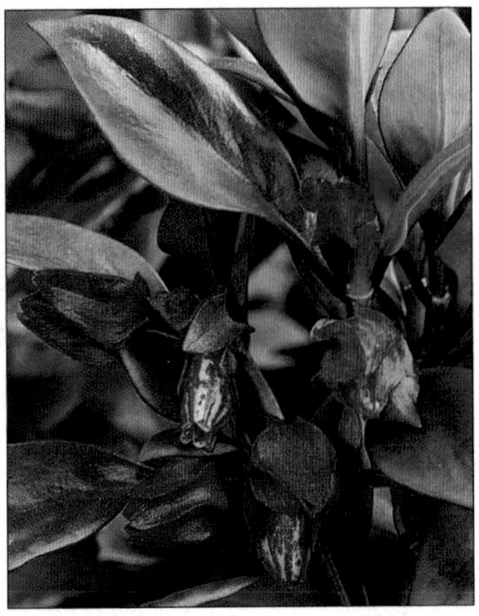

Nematanthus 'Tropicana'

NEMESIA

SCROPHULARIACEAE

Genus of 50 or more species of bushy, erect annuals, perennials, and subshrubs from South Africa, where they grow in sandy soils near the coast or in scrubby, often disturbed soil inland. The leaves are opposite, simple, usually linear to lance-shaped, frequently toothed. The showy, almost trumpet-shaped, 2-lipped flowers (the upper lip 4-lobed, the lower lip unlobed or 2-lobed) are borne singly in the upper leaf axils or in short terminal racemes. Annual cultivars are colourful summer bedding plants outdoors, or may be grown as short-lived, early spring-flowering container plants in a cool greenhouse. They are good for cutting. *N. caerulea* is suitable for a raised bed or herbaceous border, and is often used as a container plant.

- **HARDINESS** Frost hardy to half hardy.
- **CULTIVATION** Grow in moist but well-drained, moderately fertile, slightly acidic soil in full sun. Water annuals freely in dry weather to maintain flower production. Under glass, grow in loam-based potting compost (JI No.2) in full light. Water moderately during growth. Pinch out growing tips to promote bushiness.
- **PROPAGATION** Sow seed at 15°C (59°F) from early to late spring, or in autumn for spring-flowering container plants. Take tip cuttings of unflowered shoots from perennial species in late summer; overwinter young plants in frost-free conditions.
- **PESTS AND DISEASES** Foot rot and root rot may cause problems.

N. caerulea ■ syn. *N. foetens* of gardens, *N. fruticans* of gardens. Woody-based perennial with erect or spreading stems and entire or toothed, linear to lance-shaped leaves, 4cm (1½in) long. Produces terminal racemes of short-tubed, 2-lipped, pink, pale blue, lavender-blue, or white flowers, to

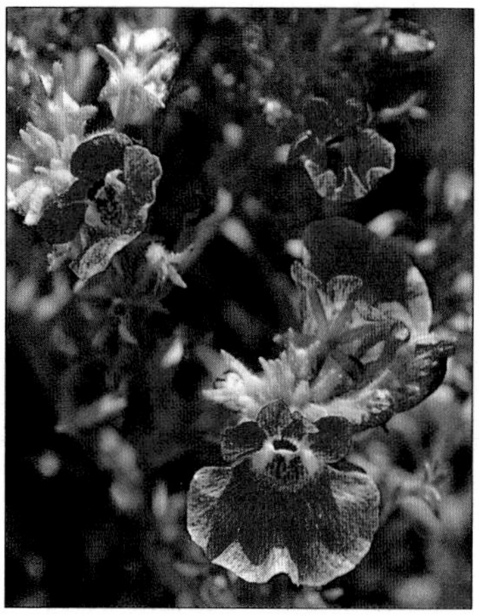

Nemesia strumosa Carnival Series

1.5cm (½in) long, with yellow throats, from early summer to autumn. ↕ to 60cm (24in), ↔ 30cm (12in). South Africa (Northern Transvaal, Eastern Transvaal, Orange Free State, KwaZulu/Natal), Lesotho. ❄❄. **'Innocence'** has white flowers. **'Joan Wilder'** has deep lavender-blue flowers.

***N. foetens* of gardens** see *N. caerulea.*

***N. fruticans* of gardens** see *N. caerulea.*

N. strumosa. Basally branching annual with lance-shaped, entire to coarsely toothed, slightly hairy leaves, to 7cm (3in) long. In mid- and late summer, produces terminal racemes of 2-lipped red, yellow, pink, blue, purple, or white flowers, to 2.5cm (1in) across. The flowers may be in single colours, or bicolours with the upper and lower lips in contrasting colours; they often have external purple veins, and yellow, "bearded" throats with darker marks. ↕ 18–30cm (7–12in), ↔ 10–16cm (4–6in). South Africa. ❄. **'Blue Gem'** bears bright blue flowers. **Carnival Series** ■ cultivars are compact and dwarf, with purple-veined yellow, red, bronze-yellow, orange, pink, or white flowers; ↕ 17–23cm (7–9in). **'Danish Flag'** has bicoloured flowers in red and white. **'KLM'** ■ has bicoloured flowers in blue and white, with yellow throats. **'National Ensign'** is a bicoloured cultivar with deep pink-red and white flowers. **'Prince of Orange'** produces orange flowers with purple veins; ↕ to 20cm (8in).

NEMOPHILA

HYDROPHYLLACEAE

Genus of 11 species of spreading to erect, slender, fleshy-stemmed, sometimes sticky-hairy annuals found in variable habitats in W. North America, from coastal sands to chaparral and redwood forest. The mid-green or grey-green leaves are opposite, lobed or pinnate, ovate to rounded, spoon-shaped, or oblong, and toothed. Small, saucer- or bell-shaped, blue or white flowers are borne singly in the upper leaf axils in summer. Grow as edging in a border, or in a window-box or other container.

- **HARDINESS** Fully hardy.
- **CULTIVATION** Grow in fertile, moist but well-drained soil in full sun or partial shade. May cease flowering in hot, dry weather if not watered.
- **PROPAGATION** Sow seed *in situ* in early spring or autumn; they self-seed freely.
- **PESTS AND DISEASES** Aphids may be troublesome.

N. insignis see *N. menziesii.*

N. maculata ■ (Five-spot). Fleshy-stemmed, sometimes slightly downy annual with 5- to 9-pinnate leaves, oblong to oval in outline and 1–3cm (½–1¼in) long. In summer, produces solitary, saucer-shaped white flowers, to 4.5cm (1¾in) across, borne on long stalks; each petal is tipped with a small, violet-blue mark, and is sometimes faintly veined or tinted mauve-blue. ↕↔ 15–30cm (6–12in). USA (California). ❄❄❄

N. menziesii, syn. *N. insignis* (Baby blue-eyes). Fleshy-stemmed, downy annual with 9- to 11-pinnate, toothed,

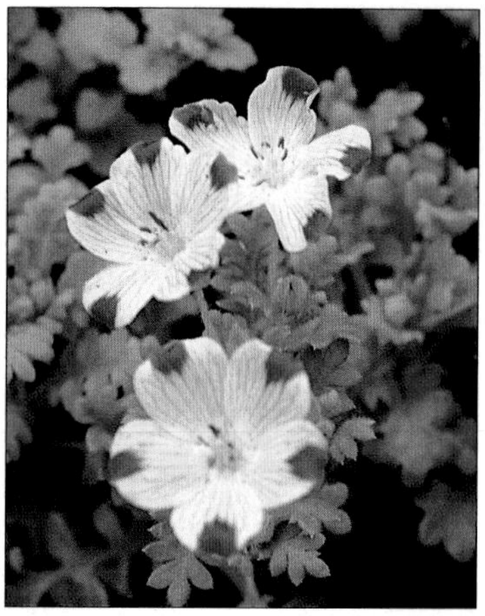

Nemophila maculata

grey-green leaves, oval to oblong in outline, 2–5cm (¾–2in) long. In summer, bears solitary, long-stalked, saucer-shaped, bright blue flowers, to 4cm (1½in) across, with lighter blue centres often stained white or yellow, and with darker blue or deep purple spots or marks on the petals. ↕ 20cm (8in), ↔ 30cm (12in). USA (California). ❄❄❄. **subsp. *atromaria*** has white flowers, to 3cm (1¼in) across, with black or dark purple spots. **'Coelestis'** has white flowers margined sky-blue. **'Oculata'** has pale blue flowers with deep purple centres.

▷ ***Neobesseya asperispina*** see *Escobaria asperispina*

▷ ***Neobesseya macdougallii*** see *Ortegocactus macdougallii*

NEOBUXBAUMIA

CACTACEAE

Genus of about 8 species of columnar or tree-like, perennial cacti from dry to humid areas of Mexico. The stems are cylindrical and the ribs usually low-set; the areoles bear numerous bristles and bristly spines. The nocturnal, white, pink, or red flowers, produced in summer, are followed by angular fruits, which open like stars when ripe. In areas where temperatures drop below 15°C (59°F), grow in a warm greenhouse. In warmer climates, grow in a courtyard or border.

- **HARDINESS** Frost tender.
- **CULTIVATION** Under glass, grow in standard cactus compost with added grit in full light, with shade from hot sun, and with low humidity. From mid-spring to late summer, water freely and apply a dilute liquid fertilizer monthly. Keep completely dry at other times. Outdoors, grow in sharply drained, gritty, poor to moderately fertile, humus-rich soil in full sun. See also pp.48–49.
- **PROPAGATION** Sow seed at 19–24°C (66–75°F) in spring.
- **PESTS AND DISEASES** Susceptible to scale insects.

N. euphorbioides ■ syn. *Cephalocereus euphorbioides, Lemaireocereus euphorbioides, Rooksbya euphorbioides.* Simple, tree-like cactus with a columnar, greyish green, dark green, or blue-green, sometimes red-tinged stem, 10–15cm (4–6in) thick, with 8–10 acute, straight ribs. White-woolly areoles produce

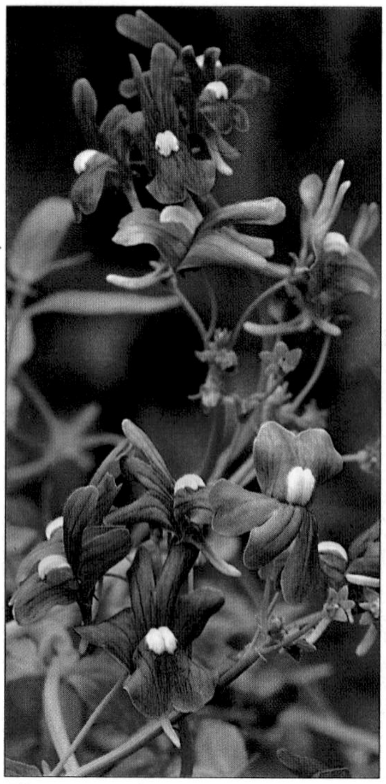

Nemesia caerulea

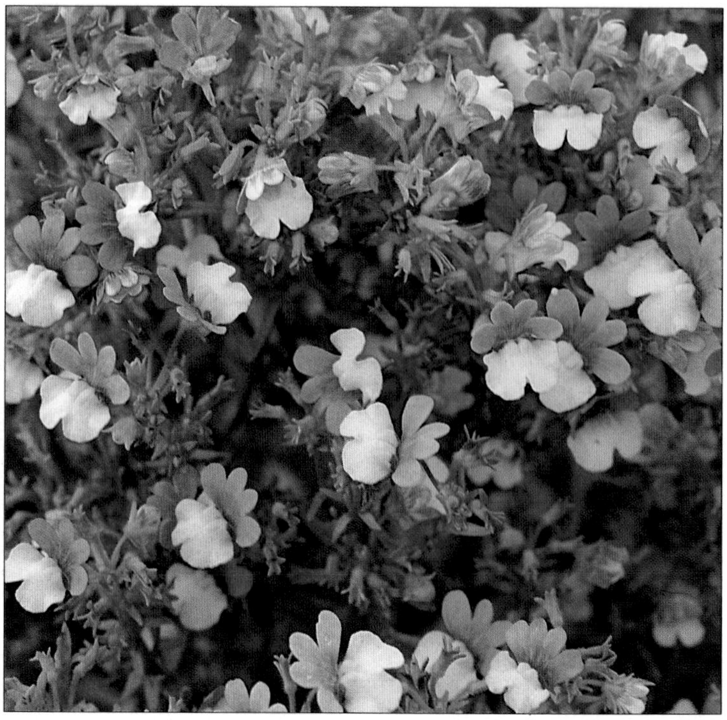

Nemesia strumosa 'KLM'

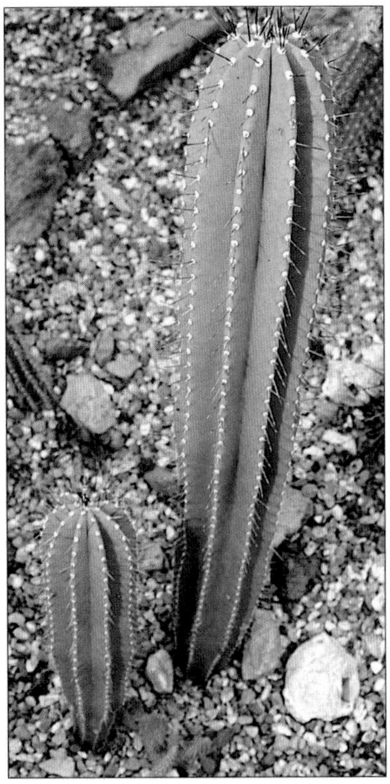

Neobuxbaumia euphorbioides

bristly, black to dark grey spines (1–5 radials and sometimes 1 central), becoming white. Funnel-shaped flowers, 8–10cm (3–4in) long, with reddish pink tubes, wine-red outer tepals, and cream throats, are borne in summer. ↕ 1–2m (3–6ft), ↔ 15cm (6in). E. Mexico. ⊛ (min. 15°C/59°F)

N. polylopha. Usually simple, columnar cactus producing a pale green stem, 35cm (14in) or more thick, bearing 20–50 slightly rounded ribs with white-woolly areoles, yellow bristles, and yellow spines (7–9 radials and 1 shorter central). Funnel-shaped, red or pink flowers, to 5–8cm (2–3in) long, with purple-brown tubes, develop in summer. ↕ 2–3m (6–10ft), ↔ 35cm (14in). C. Mexico. ⊛ (min. 15°C/59°F)

▷ ***Neochilenia chilensis*** see *Neoporteria chilensis*

▷ ***Neochilenia mitis* of gardens** see *Neoporteria napina*

NEOLITSEA

LAURACEAE

Genus of 60 species of evergreen, dioecious shrubs and trees from tropical woodland in E. and S.E. Asia, Malaysia, and Indonesia. Only *N. sericea* is usually cultivated, for its handsome, simple, alternate, leathery leaves. Flowers are insignificant, each having 4 sepals that fall on opening; on female plants these are followed by red or black berries. In very cold areas, grow in a cool greenhouse as foliage plants. In milder climates, grow at the base of a warm, sunny wall, in a woodland garden, or as specimen plants; they also make useful screens or hedges.

- **HARDINESS** Frost hardy to frost tender.
- **CULTIVATION** Under glass, grow in loam-based potting compost (JI No.3) in full light or bright filtered light. During growth, water moderately and apply a balanced liquid fertilizer monthly. Water sparingly in winter. Outdoors, grow in fertile, moist but well-drained soil in full sun or partial shade, with shelter from cold, dry winds. Pruning group 1; may need restrictive pruning under glass.
- **PROPAGATION** Sow seed in containers in a cool greenhouse as soon as ripe. Root semi-ripe cuttings with bottom heat in summer.
- **PESTS AND DISEASES** Scale insects may be a problem under glass.

N. glauca see *N. sericea*.

N. sericea △ syn. *Litsea glauca, N. glauca.* Large shrub or small tree, ovoid to columnar, later spreading, with yellow-brown, silky-hairy shoots. Leaves are ovate to oblong-elliptic, 10–18cm (4–7in) long, with 3 prominent veins; they are softly golden-hairy above when young, becoming deep green above and glaucous beneath. In late summer, produces small, star-shaped yellow flowers in stalkless umbels, followed in autumn by red berries, 1.5cm (½in) long, on female plants. ↕ to 6m (20ft), ↔ to 3m (10ft) or more. China, Taiwan, Korea, Japan. ❄

NEOLLOYDIA

CACTACEAE

Genus of 10–14 species of spherical or cylindrical, perennial cacti found on low hillsides in S.W. Texas, USA, and in E. and N.E. Mexico. They frequently form clumps by offsetting. The ribs bear spined tubercles, often spirally arranged, sometimes with dense hairs or wool in the axils. The wide-spreading, funnel-shaped, diurnal flowers are produced from spring to summer. In areas where temperatures drop below 15°C (59°F), grow in a warm greenhouse. In warmer climates, grow in a border or desert garden.

- **HARDINESS** Frost tender.
- **CULTIVATION** Under glass, grow in standard cactus compost in full light. From mid-spring to early autumn, water moderately and apply a dilute, balanced liquid fertilizer monthly. Keep dry at other times. Outdoors, grow in sharply drained, humus-rich, moderately fertile soil in full sun. See also pp.48–49.
- **PROPAGATION** Sow seed at 19–24°C (66–75°F) in spring.
- **PESTS AND DISEASES** Susceptible to root mealybugs when container-grown.

N. conoidea ▣ syn. *Coryphantha conoidea, Mammillaria conoidea.* Often offsetting, variable cactus with spherical to cylindrical, bluish grey or yellow-green stems, to 7cm (3in) thick. Ovoid tubercles have woolly axils and white-woolly areoles (8–28 white to grey radial spines, 0–6 longer black centrals). In summer, produces reddish violet, magenta, or deep purple flowers, to 6cm (2½in) across. ↕ to 10cm (4in), ↔ 15cm (6in) in clusters. S.W. Texas, E. and N.E. Mexico. ⊛ (min. 15°C/59°F)

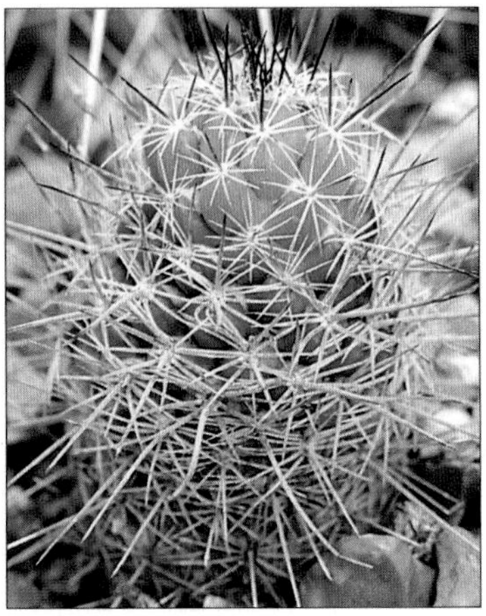

Neolloydia conoidea

N. schmiedickeana, syn. *Turbinicarpus schmiedickeanus.* Variable, simple or clump-forming cactus with spherical or short-cylindrical, dark blue to grey-green stems, to 5cm (2in) thick; they have 10–12 ribs divided into pyramidal, 4-angled tubercles with bare axils. White-woolly areoles, later bare, produce 1–8 incurved grey spines. In spring, bears white, yellow, or pink to magenta flowers, 1–3cm (½–1¼in) across, with violet mid-lines on the inner petals. ↕ to 5cm (2in), ↔ to 15cm (6in). Mexico. ⊛ (min. 15°C/59°F)

NEOMARICA

IRIDACEAE

Genus of about 15 species of rhizomatous, herbaceous perennials from often mountainous habitats in tropical Central and South America. They are cultivated for their short-lived, iris-like flowers, borne in summer on erect stems. The erect, sword-shaped leaves are ribbed or heavily veined, and arranged in basal fans. In frost-prone areas, grow in a temperate or warm greenhouse. In warmer climates, grow in a border or among shrubs.

- **HARDINESS** Frost tender.
- **CULTIVATION** Under glass, grow in loam-based potting compost (JI No.2), with added sharp sand and leaf mould, in bright filtered light, or in full light with shade from the hottest sun. Water moderately in summer, sparingly in winter. Apply a balanced liquid fertilizer monthly when in full growth. Outdoors, grow in well-drained, moderately fertile, humus-rich soil in partial shade.
- **PROPAGATION** Sow seed at 15–18°C (59–64°F) in spring, or divide in spring.
- **PESTS AND DISEASES** Trouble free.

N. caerulea ▣ Rhizomatous perennial with a basal fan of sword-shaped, dark green leaves, to 1.6m (5½ft) long. In summer, bears a succession of flat, scented, mid-blue flowers, 8–10cm (3–4in) across, striped white, yellow, and brown in the centres. ↕↔ 60cm (24in). Brazil. ⊛ (min. 10°C/50°F)

▷ ***Neopanax arboreum*** see *Pseudopanax arboreus*

NEOPAXIA

PORTULACACEAE

Genus of one variable species of prostrate, stoloniferous, mat-forming, herbaceous perennial found in moist habitats, including bogs, swamps, and streams, at high altitudes in Australia and New Zealand. It is grown for its erect, alternate, fleshy leaves and its saucer-shaped, white or pale pink flowers, borne from spring to summer. Grow at the margins of streams and ponds, or in any other moist, boggy soil.

- **HARDINESS** Fully hardy.
- **CULTIVATION** Grow in moderately fertile, moist soil, preferably in full sun.
- **PROPAGATION** Sow seed as soon as ripe in containers in a cold frame. Divide mats in spring.
- **PESTS AND DISEASES** Trouble free.

N. australasica, syn. *Montia australasica.* Prostrate, stoloniferous, mat-forming perennial with alternate, linear to spoon-shaped, fleshy, deep green to bright light green, or grey-green leaves, 3–10cm (1¼–4in) long. From spring to early summer, bears saucer-shaped, white or pink flowers, 1–2cm (½–¾in) across, borne singly or in few-flowered cymes. ↕ 10cm (4in), ↔ 40cm (16in). Australia (Western Australia, South Australia, Victoria, Tasmania), New Zealand. ❄❄❄

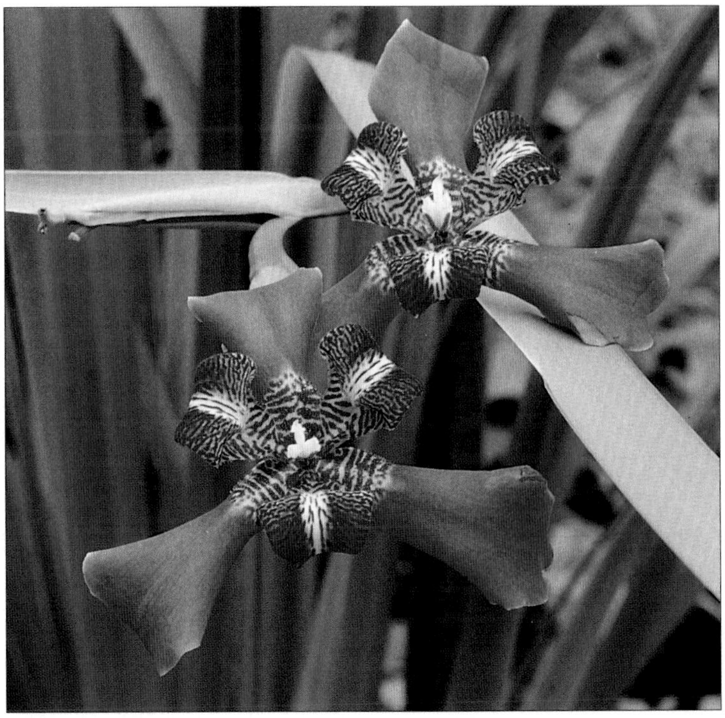

Neomarica caerulea

NEOPORTERIA

CACTACEAE

Genus of 20–30 species of simple, sometimes clustering, perennial cacti, most from rocky, coastal sites in Chile, a few from S. Peru and W. Argentina. They have spherical to short-cylindrical, ribbed, spiny stems and usually solitary, funnel- or bell-shaped flowers produced from or close to the crowns. Where temperatures drop below 10°C (50°F), grow in a warm greenhouse or as houseplants; elsewhere, use in a desert garden.

• **HARDINESS** Frost tender.

• **CULTIVATION** Under glass, grow in standard cactus compost in full light, with low humidity. From mid-spring to early autumn, water moderately and apply a dilute liquid fertilizer monthly. Keep dry at other times. Outdoors, grow in sharply drained, poor to moderately fertile, humus-rich soil in full sun. See also pp.48–49.

• **PROPAGATION** Sow seed at 19–24°C (66–75°F) in spring or summer.

• **PESTS AND DISEASES** Vulnerable to root mealybugs and mealybugs, especially when container-grown.

N. chilensis, syn. *Echinocactus chilensis, Neochilenia chilensis.* Simple or clustering cactus with spherical to short-cylindrical, pale green stems, each with about 20 ribs. Areoles each bear about 20 glassy white radial spines and 6–8 longer, yellowish brown centrals. From late spring to early autumn, bears broadly funnel-shaped, white or pink flowers, 5cm (2in) across, with carmine-red outer petals. ↕ 30cm (12in), ↔ 10cm (4in). Chile. ❄ (min. 10°C/50°F)

N. crispa, syn. *Pyrrhocactus crispus.* Simple cactus with a tuberous rootstock. The spherical, dark green stem has 13–16 ribs, and black or grey spines (6–10 radials, 2–4 longer centrals). Funnel-shaped red flowers, 3.5cm (1½in) across, with a deeper red mid-stripe to each inner petal, are borne from late summer to autumn. ↕↔ 7cm (3in). Chile. ❄ (min. 10°C/50°F)

N. litoralis see *N. subgibbosa.*

N. mitis see *N. napina.*

N. napina ■ syn. *Neochilenia mitis* of gardens, *Neoporteria mitis.* Variable, simple cactus with a spherical, brownish green stem, sometimes tinged red, divided into chin-like tubercles, and with dark brownish black spines (3–9 radials, no centrals). From late spring to early autumn, bell- to funnel-shaped, pale yellow, sometimes pink-flushed flowers, 3–4cm (1¼–1½in) across, open from green-woolly buds. ↕ 2.5cm (1in), ↔ 3.5cm (1½in). Chile. ❄ (min. 10°C/50°F)

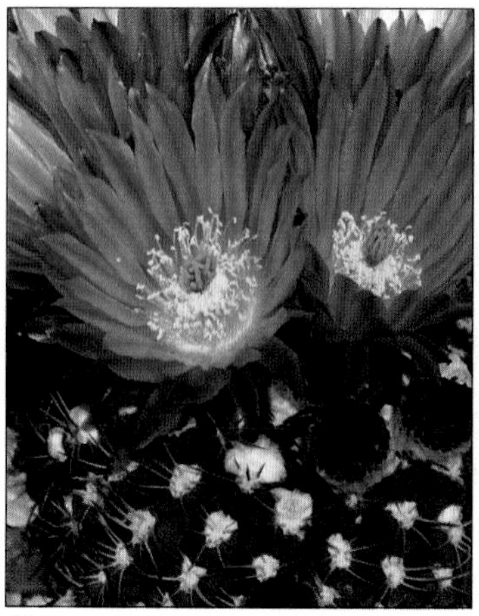

Neoporteria napina

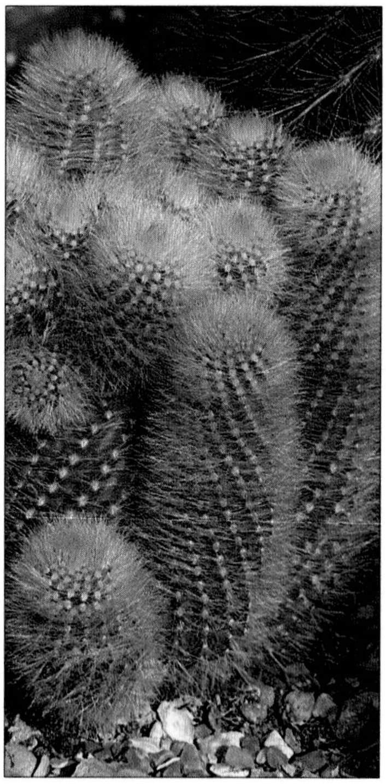

Neoporteria villosa

N. nidus. Simple cactus with a spherical to short-cylindrical, dark green stem, rarely elongating, bearing 16–18 deeply scalloped ribs hidden by about 30 upward-curved, pale grey, cream, or yellow spines per areole. Tubular-funnel-shaped, red or pink flowers, 4cm (1½in) across, with prominently pointed petals, are produced from late spring to early autumn. ↕ to 30cm (12in), ↔ to 10cm (4in). Chile. ❄ (min. 10°C/50°F)

N. subgibbosa, syn. *N. litoralis.* Variable, simple cactus producing a spherical, mid-green to grey-green stem, later elongating and often decumbent; the stem bears 16–20 warty ribs and deep orange-yellow, brown, or black spines (16–30 thin radials, 4–8 much thicker centrals). Funnel-shaped, carmine-pink flowers, 4cm (1½in) across, with paler, almost white throats, develop from late spring to early autumn. ↕ to 30cm (12in), ↔ 10cm (4in). Chile. ❄ (min. 10°C/50°F)

N. taltalensis. Simple cactus with a spherical, dull dark green stem, 10–16 warty ribs, and pale yellowish brown areoles bearing 6–20 curving to twisted, brown, later white radial spines, and up to 6 dark greyish brown to black centrals. Bears funnel-shaped, purplish pink, yellow, or white flowers, 3cm (1¼in) across, in summer. ↕↔ 8cm (3in). Chile. ❄ (min. 10°C/50°F)

N. villosa ■ Simple or clustering cactus with spherical then short-cylindrical, grey-green stems turning black-purple; the stems bear 13–15 ribs covered with upward-curved, hair-like, yellowish grey or pale brown spines (12–16 or more radials, 4 thicker centrals). Funnel-shaped, white-throated pink flowers, to 3cm (1¼in) across, are borne from late spring to summer. ↕ 15cm (6in), ↔ to 10cm (4in). Chile. ❄ (min. 10°C/50°F)

NEOREGELIA syn. AREGELIA

BROMELIACEAE

Genus of about 70 species of evergreen, sometimes rhizomatous or stoloniferous, epiphytic or terrestrial perennials (bromeliads) from coastal scrub, woodland, and rainforest, to 1,600m (5,000ft) high, in South America. They are grown for the striking colouring of their central leaves and bracts when flowering. The variable, usually spiny-margined leaves are borne in rosettes; large sheaths totally enclose the scape and its bracts. An umbel-like, sometimes raceme- or corymb-like, compact inflorescence nestles in the heart of each leaf rosette and, in summer, bears numerous long-lasting, tubular flowers. Offsets form around the flowering rosettes. Where temperatures drop below 10°C (50°F), grow in a temperate greenhouse, or as houseplants. In warm climates, grow in a shady, moist site.

• **HARDINESS** Frost tender.

• **CULTIVATION** Under glass, grow in epiphytic or terrestrial bromeliad compost in bright filtered light. During growth, water freely with soft water. Apply a low-nitrogen liquid fertilizer monthly from spring to late autumn. Keep rosette cups filled with soft water from spring to early autumn. Water sparingly in winter. Sever spent leaf rosettes at the bases. Outdoors, grow in gritty, leafy soil in an open site with partial shade, or grow epiphytically in a tree. See also p.47.

• **PROPAGATION** Sow seed at 27°C (81°F) as soon as ripe. Separate offsets in spring or summer.

• **PESTS AND DISEASES** Susceptible to scale insects.

N. ampullacea. Stoloniferous, terrestrial bromeliad with dense, funnel-shaped rosettes of 6–15 tongue-shaped, sometimes red-banded, mid-green leaves, 15–20cm (6–8in) long. Tubular flowers, to 2.5cm (1in) long, with blue, white-based petals and white-margined green sepals, are borne in summer. Stolons appear from beneath the rosettes; at the tips, further rosettes develop. ↕↔ 40cm (16in). Brazil. ❄ (min. 10°C/50°F)

N. carolinae, syn. *Aregelia carolinae, Nidularium carolinae* (Blushing bromeliad). Epiphytic bromeliad with open rosettes of 12–20 strap-shaped, toothed, copper-suffused, mid-green leaves, 40–60cm (16–24in) long; at

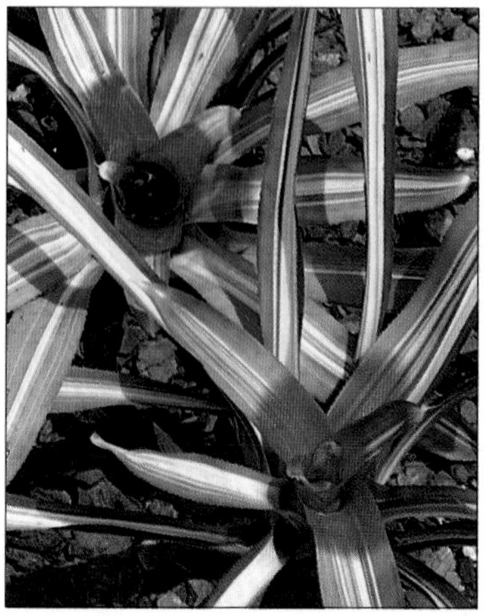

Neoregelia carolinae 'Tricolor'

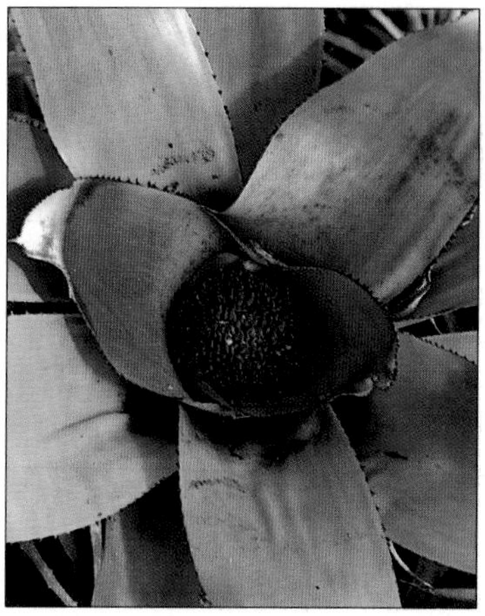

Neoregelia concentrica

flowering time, the central leaves turn crimson. Red bracts surround violet-purple to lavender-blue flowers, to 4cm (1½in) long, produced in summer. ↕ 20–30cm (8–12in), ↔ 40–60cm (16–24in). Brazil. ❄ (min. 10°C/50°F). **'Tricolor'** ■ 🏆 syn. f. *tricolor*, var. *tricolor*, has leaves striped ivory-white, green and rose-red.

N. concentrica ■ Rhizomatous, epiphytic bromeliad with dense rosettes of 7–30 broadly strap-shaped, spreading, glossy, mid- to dark green leaves, 20–40cm (8–16in) long, often marked dark purple at the tips, and with black marginal spines. Yellow-white bracts, suffused violet or purple, turn purple-pink in summer, when the pale blue or white flowers, 4–5cm (1½–2in) long, are produced. ↕ to 30cm (12in), ↔ to 70cm (28in). Brazil. ❄ (min. 10°C/50°F). **var. *plutonis*** ■ syn. 'Plutonis', has spreading rosettes of broad, mid-green, sometimes pale green leaves, which are flushed magenta-red during flowering; the flowers are pale lavender; ↔ 40cm (16in) or more.

N. eleutheropetala ■ Stoloniferous, terrestrial or epiphytic bromeliad with rosettes of about 30 tongue-shaped, mid-green leaves, 50–70cm (20–28in) long, turning reddish green towards the bases, and with sharp marginal spines and brown sheaths. The innermost, purple-brown leaves surround dense, umbel-like inflorescences of white flowers, to 3.5cm (1½in) long, borne in summer and interspersed with long, purple-tipped bracts. ↕↔ to 70cm (28in). Venezuela, Colombia, Peru, Amazonian Brazil. ❄ (min. 10°C/50°F)

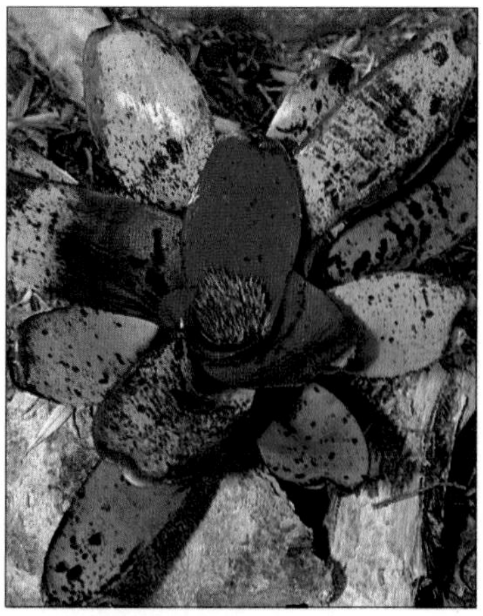

Neoregelia concentrica var. *plutonis*

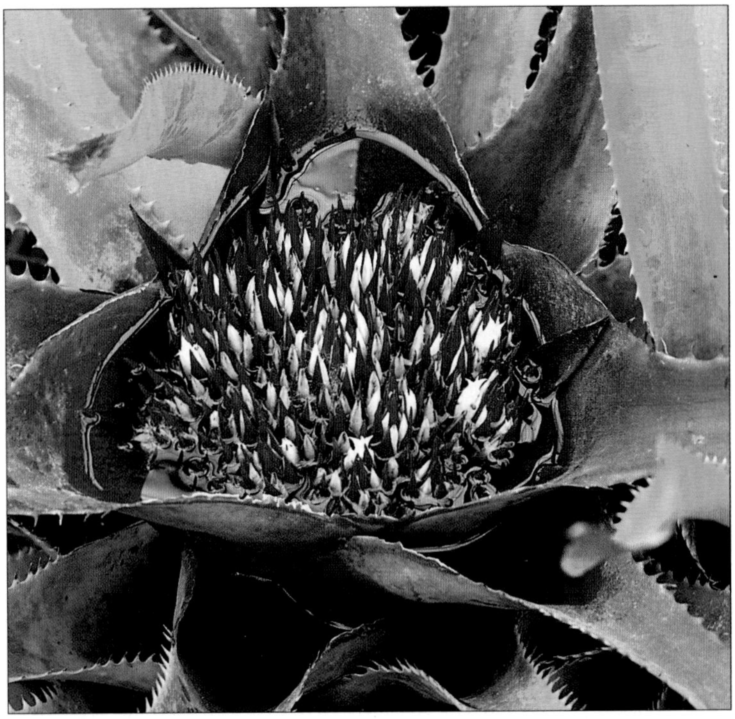

Neoregelia eleutheropetala

N. pineliana. Epiphytic bromeliad with a short stem producing ascending stolons, which bear leaves along their lengths. The rosettes have up to 12 narrowly lance-shaped to linear, mid-green leaves, grey-scaly on both surfaces, to 50cm (20in) long, with minute marginal spines and purple sheaths. In summer, the central leaves turn red, and dense umbels of blue, white-based flowers, to 6cm (2½in) long, darkening towards the tips, are produced. ↕↔ 40cm (16in) or more. Possibly Brazil. ❀ (min. 10°C/50°F)

N. princeps. Epiphytic or terrestrial bromeliad with spreading rosettes of 15–20 strap-shaped, pointed, minutely scaly, laxly toothed, mid-green leaves, 50cm (20in) long, with densely grey-scaly sheaths; the inner leaves are smaller and bright red. White flowers, 3–4cm (1¼–1½in) long, with deep blue tips and red sepals, are produced in summer. ↕↔ 75cm (30in). S. Brazil. ❀ (min. 10°C/50°F)

N. spectabilis 🏆 (Fingernail plant). Terrestrial bromeliad producing broadly funnel-shaped rosettes of 20–30 strap-shaped, arching, red-tipped, grey-scaly, glossy, olive-green leaves, 40–45cm (16–18in) long, with smooth or minutely spiny margins and grey-white cross-banding beneath. The inner leaves are red, often margined purple, with white bases. Blue flowers, 4–4.5cm (1½–1¾in) long, with red or purple bracts, are borne in summer. ↕ to 40cm (16in), ↔ to 80cm (32in). S. Brazil. ❀ (min. 10°C/50°F)

NEPENTHES

Monkey cup, Tropical pitcher plant

NEPENTHACEAE

Genus of over 70 species and numerous hybrids of dioecious, evergreen, carnivorous, climbing, terrestrial or epiphytic perennials from Madagascar, the Seychelles, S.E. Asia, Borneo, and Queensland, Australia. They are found in moist, acid, organic soils in open grassland or forest, and sometimes grow epiphytically on trees. The usually lance-shaped or strap-shaped leaves, 5–65cm (2–26in) long, each have a prolonged midrib, which acts as a tendril and may be terminated by a hanging, hollow "pitcher", 5–35cm (2–14in) long, with 2 vertical ridges, or "wings", at the front. Pitchers vary greatly in shape and colour, from pale yellow to green or purplish red, and are frequently mottled; upper and lower pitchers often differ in colour on the same plant. The colourful, thickened rim of a pitcher secretes nectar to attract insects, small mammals, and even birds, which become trapped inside. Its apex forms a lid to deflect excess rain. The tiny, petalless male and female flowers, with green or brown sepals, are borne in spike-like racemes. In frost-prone areas, grow in a warm greenhouse or conservatory; in tropical climates, grow climbers through trees or attach epiphytes to branches. Heights vary greatly according to conditions and support; in cultivation, most are cut back to encourage young foliage and the development of large pitchers.

• **HARDINESS** Frost tender.

• **CULTIVATION** Lowland species and hybrids from sea level to 1,000m (3,300ft) need daytime temperatures of 24°C (75°F) and night-time temperatures of 15°C (59°F) in winter, 21°C (70°F) in summer. Provide ventilation when over 38°C (100°F). Highland species and hybrids from 1,000–3,000m (3,300–9,900ft) need daytime temperatures of 18°C (64°F), and 10°C (50°F) at night. Ventilate when over 21°C (70°F). Under glass, grow in slatted baskets in a mix of 2 parts bark, 2 parts perlite, and 1 part coarse peat or coconut fibre, or in clean, live sphagnum moss. Provide bright filtered light, or full light with shade from hot sun, and high humidity. In summer, apply a high-nitrogen liquid fertilizer weekly. Prune mature plants in spring, reducing stems by two-thirds of their length, to induce vigorous, pitcher-producing shoots. Outdoors, grow in moist, open, leafy soil in partial shade, or as epiphytes.

• **PROPAGATION** Sow seed as soon as ripe on the surface of moist peat or fine coir compost, and place in a tray of water in a shaded propagator; maintain a temperature of 27°C (81°F). In spring, insert cuttings with 3 or 4 leaves into nepenthes compost (described above) and maintain at 21–27°C (70–81°F). Air layer in spring or summer.

• **PESTS AND DISEASES** Mealybugs may be troublesome. Grey mould (*Botrytis*) may affect leaves.

N. ampullaria. Lowland climber with rounded, squat, deep red or green, sometimes mottled pitchers, to 5cm (2in) long, with round, horizontal mouths, and small, narrow, reflexed lids. Wings are broad, spreading, and toothed. Pitchers are produced only from the basal leaves or in clusters from the rhizomes, not from climbing shoots. ↕ to 20m (70ft). Malaysia to New Guinea. ❀ (min. day: 24°C/75°F; night: 15°C/59°F in winter, 21°C/70°F in summer)

N. x coccinea (*N.* x *dominii* x *N. mirabilis*). Lowland climber with yellow-green pitchers, to 15cm (6in) long, mottled purple-red, with inflated bases and oblique mouths. The green lids have red markings. ↕ to 6m (20ft). Garden origin. ❀ (min. day: 24°C/75°F; night: 15°C/59°F in winter, 21°C/70°F in summer)

***N.* 'Director G.T. Moore'** ▣ Lowland climber with pear-shaped, light green pitchers, to 13cm (5in) long, with dense purple-red mottling, oblique mouths, and fringed, mottled wings. ↕ 3m (10ft). ❀ (min. day: 24°C/75°F; night: 15°C/59°F in winter, 21°C/70°F in summer)

N. gracilis. Slender, lowland climber with linear to elliptic leaves and numerous pitchers. Lower pitchers are small, cylindrical, light green, sometimes suffused pink or maroon, to 7cm (3in) long, with narrow lips, round lids, and narrow wings. Upper pitchers, to 15cm (6in) long, are dark mahogany-red and narrow in the middle. Even young plants bear inflorescences, 15cm (6in) long, of red-brown flowers. ↕ to 2m (6ft). Philippines to Indonesia. ❀ (min. day: 24°C/75°F; night: 15°C/59°F in winter, 21°C/70°F in summer)

N. x hookeriana (*N. ampullaria* x *N. rafflesiana*). Lowland climber producing ovoid lower pitchers with broad wings and rim, and funnel-shaped upper pitchers. Both are pale green with dark red spots, and have oblique mouths. Upper pitchers grow to 13cm (5in) long, lower to 11cm (4¼in). ↕ 3m (10ft). Malaysia to Borneo. ❀ (min. day: 24°C/75°F; night: 15°C/59°F in winter, 21°C/70°F in summer)

N. mirabilis. Lowland climber or terrestrial perennial with cylindrical pitchers, to 18cm (7in) long, red, or pale green with red blotches; each has an oblique, round mouth and an oval lid. ↕ to 10m (30ft). S. China, S.E. Asia to Australia (N. Queensland). ❀ (min. day: 24°C/75°F; night: 15°C/59°F in winter, 21°C/70°F in summer)

N. rafflesiana ▣ Lowland climber with creamy green pitchers, marked chocolate-red, each with a striped rim.

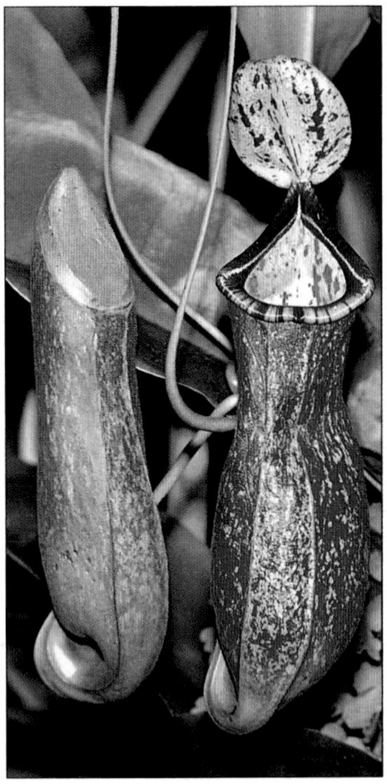

Nepenthes 'Director G.T. Moore'

Lower pitchers, to 13cm (5in) long, each have a rounded base, an oblique, oval mouth with the rim rising vertically at the back to form a stalk for the lid, and large, toothed wings. Upper pitchers, to 30cm (12in) long, with small wings, are tapered at the bases. ↕ to 9m (28ft). Sumatra to Borneo. ❀ (min. day: 24°C/75°F; night: 15°C/59°F in winter, 21°C/70°F in summer)

N. rajah. Rare, highland climber with large green pitchers, to 35cm (14in) long, mottled red to red-purple, each with an elliptic and oblique mouth, a broad, wavy rim, and a large, oval lid. Lower pitchers are ellipsoid, while upper ones are tapered only at the bases. The pitchers have been known to catch rats. Commercial trading in this species is severely regulated. ↕ 2m (6ft). Borneo (Mt. Kinabalu). ❀ (min. day: 18°C/64°F; night: 10°C/50°F)

N. ventricosa. Highland, terrestrial or epiphytic perennial producing numerous cylindrical pitchers, to 18cm (7in) long, each narrower in the middle, with a round to oval mouth and small green lid, suffused red. ↕ 4m (12ft). Philippines. ❀ (min. day: 18°C/64°F; night: 10°C/50°F)

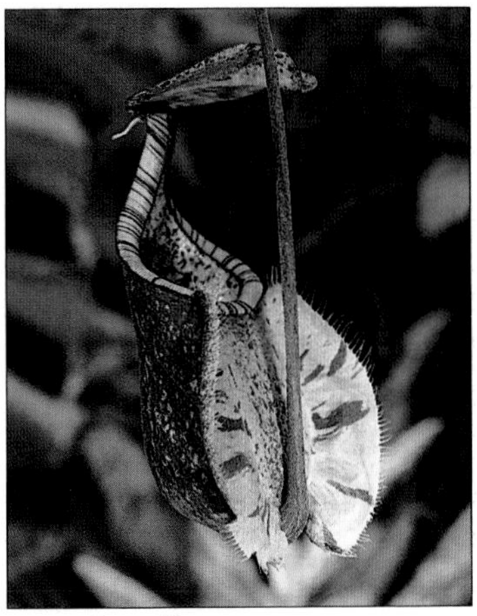

Nepenthes rafflesiana

NEPETA

Catmint

LABIATAE/LAMIACEAE

Genus of approximately 250 species of perennials, rarely annuals, native to a variety of habitats, from cool and moist to hot and dry sites in scrub, on grassy banks and stony slopes, or in high mountains, in non-tropical parts of the N. hemisphere. Ovate to lance-shaped, entire, scalloped, or toothed, often aromatic leaves are borne in opposite pairs; some are hairy, producing a silvery or greyish green effect. The spike-like cymes (sometimes racemes or panicles) of tubular, irregularly 2-lipped flowers, in white and shades of blue and purple, occasionally yellow, are borne in interrupted axillary whorls along the flower stems, often over long periods. Grow taller catmints in a mixed or herbaceous border, the shorter ones in a rock garden. Some species attract cats; most are attractive to bees.

• **HARDINESS** Fully hardy to half hardy.

• **CULTIVATION** Grow in any well-drained soil in full sun or partial shade. *N. govaniana* and *N. subsessilis* prefer moist, cool soils. *N. sibirica* likes fairly dry conditions. Grow *N. phyllochlamys* in a hot, dry rock crevice or in a trough. Provide support for taller catmints; trim *N. nervosa* and *N.* x *faassenii* after flowering to keep plants compact and to induce a second flowering.

• **PROPAGATION** Sow seed in a seedbed, or in containers in a cold frame, in autumn; some catmints self-seed freely. Divide in spring or autumn. Take softwood cuttings in early summer.

• **PESTS AND DISEASES** Slugs may damage young growth. Powdery mildew may be a problem in dry summers.

***N.* 'Blue Beauty'** see *N.* 'Souvenir d'André Chaudron'.

N.* x *faassenii ■ (*N. nepetella* x *N. racemosa*), syn. *N. mussinii* of gardens. Clump-forming perennial with erect to spreading, branched stems and narrowly ovate to lance-shaped, scalloped, wrinkled, hairy, aromatic, silvery grey-green leaves, to 3cm (1¼in) long. From early summer to early autumn, freely bears spike-like, whorled cymes of pale lavender-blue flowers, to 12mm (½in) long, with darker purple spots. ↕↔ to 45cm (18in) Garden origin. ❄❄❄

***N. glechoma* 'Variegata'** see *Glechoma hederacea* 'Variegata'.

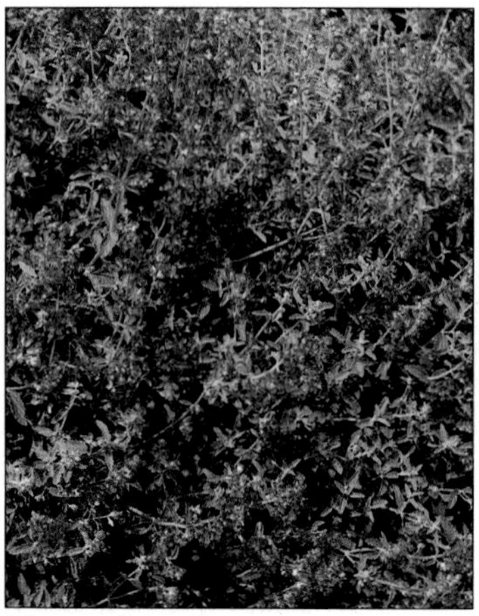

Nepeta x *faassenii*

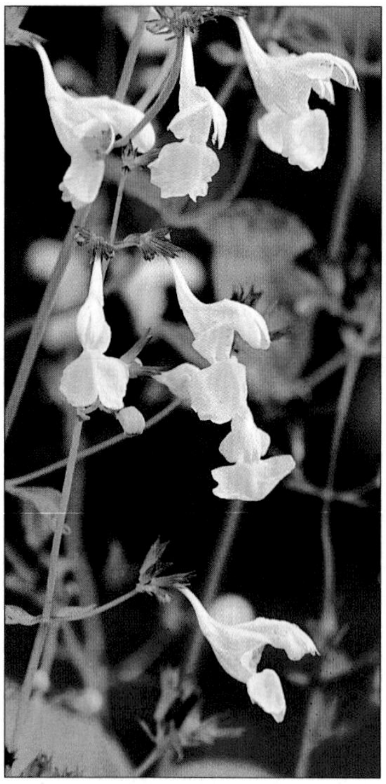

Nepeta govaniana

N. govaniana ■ syn. *Dracocephalum govanianum*. Clump-forming perennial bearing erect, branching, hairy stems and ovate to oblong-elliptic, pointed, scalloped, softly hairy, aromatic leaves, to 10cm (4in) long. From midsummer to early autumn, bears long, lax racemes or panicles of light yellow flowers, to 3cm (1¼in) long. ↕ 90cm (36in), ↔ 60cm (24in). W. Himalayas. ❄❄❄

***N. grandiflora*.** Clump-forming perennial with erect, sparsely branched stems and ovate, scalloped, softly hairy, aromatic leaves, 10cm (4in) long. In early summer, produces spike-like, whorled cymes of violet-blue flowers, to 2cm (¾in) long. ↕ 75cm (30in), ↔ 30cm (12in). Caucasus. ❄❄❄

***N. hederacea* 'Variegata'** see *Glechoma hederacea* 'Variegata'.

N. macrantha see *N. sibirica.*

N. mussinii see *N. racemosa.*

***N. mussinii* of gardens** see *N.* x *faassenii.*

N. nervosa ■ Bushy perennial bearing erect, unbranched stems with narrowly lance-shaped, entire to slightly toothed, conspicuously veined, hairy, faintly aromatic, mid- to grey-green leaves, to 10cm (4in) long. Dense, cylindrical,

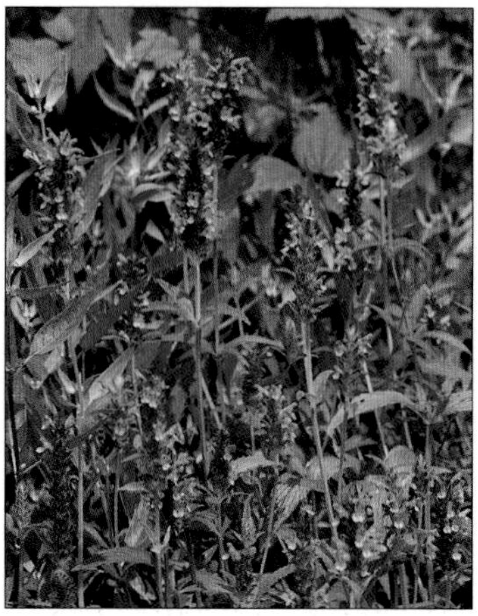

Nepeta nervosa

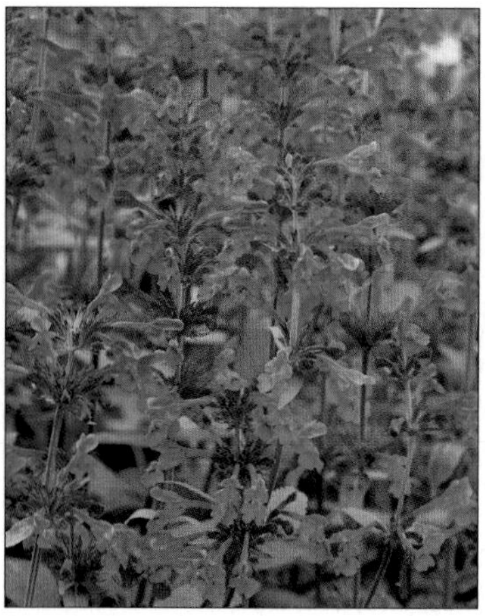

Nepeta sibirica

spike-like, whorled cymes of purplish blue, rarely yellow flowers, to 12mm (½in) long, are borne from midsummer to early autumn. ↕ 45–60cm (18–24in), ↔ 30cm (12in). India (Kashmir). ❄❄❄

***N. phyllochlamys*.** Spreading perennial with decumbent stems and triangular-ovate, scalloped, intensely white-downy, aromatic leaves, to 1.5cm (½in) long. In summer, bears short, spike-like, whorled cymes of lilac-pink flowers, 1cm (½in) long, with white-felted bracts. Requires very sharply drained soil. ↕ to 10cm (4in), ↔ to 20cm (8in). Turkey. ❄❄❄

***N. racemosa*,** syn. *N. mussinii.* Spreading to upright perennial with opposite, ovate, scalloped, finely hairy, aromatic, mid-green leaves, 1–3cm (½–1¼in) long, with heart-shaped bases. In summer, produces raceme-like, whorled cymes of deep violet- to lilac-blue flowers, 1–2cm (½–¾in) long. ↕ to 30cm (12in), ↔ to 45cm (18in). Caucasus, Turkey, N. and N.W. Iran. ❄❄❄. **'Little Titch'** has pale lavender-blue flowers; ↕↔ 15cm (6in).

N. sibirica ■ syn. *Dracocephalum sibiricum, N. macrantha.* Erect, leafy perennial with branching stems bearing oblong-lance-shaped, toothed, aromatic, dark green leaves, to 9cm (3½in) long, minutely hairy at the margins. In mid- and late summer, bears long, raceme-like, whorled cymes of blue to lavender-blue flowers, to 4cm (1½in) long. ↕ 90cm (36in), ↔ 45cm (18in). Russia (Siberia), E. Asia. ❄❄❄

***N.* 'Six Hills Giant'.** Vigorous, clump-forming perennial with narrowly ovate, toothed, hairy, aromatic, light grey-green leaves, to 4cm (1½in) long. In summer, bears abundant spike-like, whorled cymes of lavender-blue flowers, 2cm (¾in) long. ↕ to 90cm (36in), ↔ 60cm (24in). ❄❄❄

***N.* 'Souvenir d'André Chaudron'**, syn. 'Blue Beauty'. Spreading, clump-forming perennial with oval to lance-shaped, toothed, smooth, aromatic, grey-green leaves, to 8cm (3in) long. Throughout summer, bears spike-like, whorled cymes of large, dark lavender-blue flowers, 4cm (1½in) long. ↕↔ 45cm (18in). ❄❄❄

***N. subsessilis*.** Clump-forming perennial with erect, unbranched stems bearing ovate, toothed, hairless, aromatic, dark green leaves, 8–10cm (3–4in) long. Spike-like, whorled cymes of bright blue flowers, 3cm (1¼in) long, appear from midsummer to early autumn. ↕ to 90cm (36in), ↔ 30cm (12in). Japan. ❄❄❄

NEPHROLEPIS

Sword fern

NEPHROLEPIDACEAE/OLEANDRACEAE

Genus of about 30 species of evergreen or semi-evergreen, epiphytic and terrestrial ferns from rainforest or more open habitats in tropical and subtropical regions worldwide. They have short, erect rhizomes, usually with numerous runners. The dense clusters of pinnate fronds may be erect, spreading, or pendent. Pinnae are usually linear and simple, but may be divided, forked, or crisped in cultivars, of which there are many. In frost-prone areas, grow in a temperate greenhouse or as houseplants; in warmer climates, grow in moist, shady sites among shrubs.

• **HARDINESS** Mostly frost tender. *N. cordifolia* is half hardy.

• **CULTIVATION** Under glass, grow in a mix of 1 part loam, 2 parts sharp sand, and 3 parts leaf mould in bright filtered light, with moderate to high humidity and good ventilation. During the growing season, water moderately with soft water and apply a half-strength, balanced liquid fertilizer monthly. Water sparingly in winter. Outdoors, grow in moderately fertile, moist but well-drained, humus-rich soil in partial shade.

• **PROPAGATION** Sow spores at 21°C (70°F) as soon as ripe. Many cultivars are sterile, or do not come true from spores. Separate rooted runners in late winter or early spring. See also p.51.

• **PESTS AND DISEASES** Some cultivars are susceptible to fern scale, as well as rot, when fronds become too wet.

N. cordifolia ■ Tufted fern bearing erect to arching or pendent, lance-shaped to linear fronds, to 80cm (32in) long, with up to 70 pairs of oblong to linear pinnae, sometimes toothed at the tips. ↕ 80cm (32in), ↔ to 1.5m (5ft). Tropical regions. ❄. **'Duffii'** has short, rounded pinnae, and its fronds are often

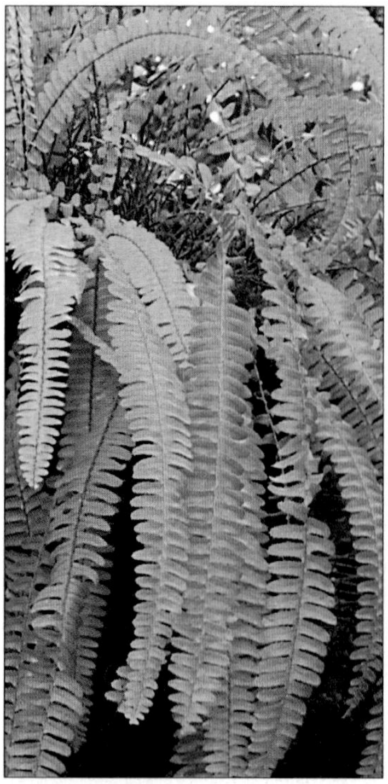

Nephrolepis cordifolia

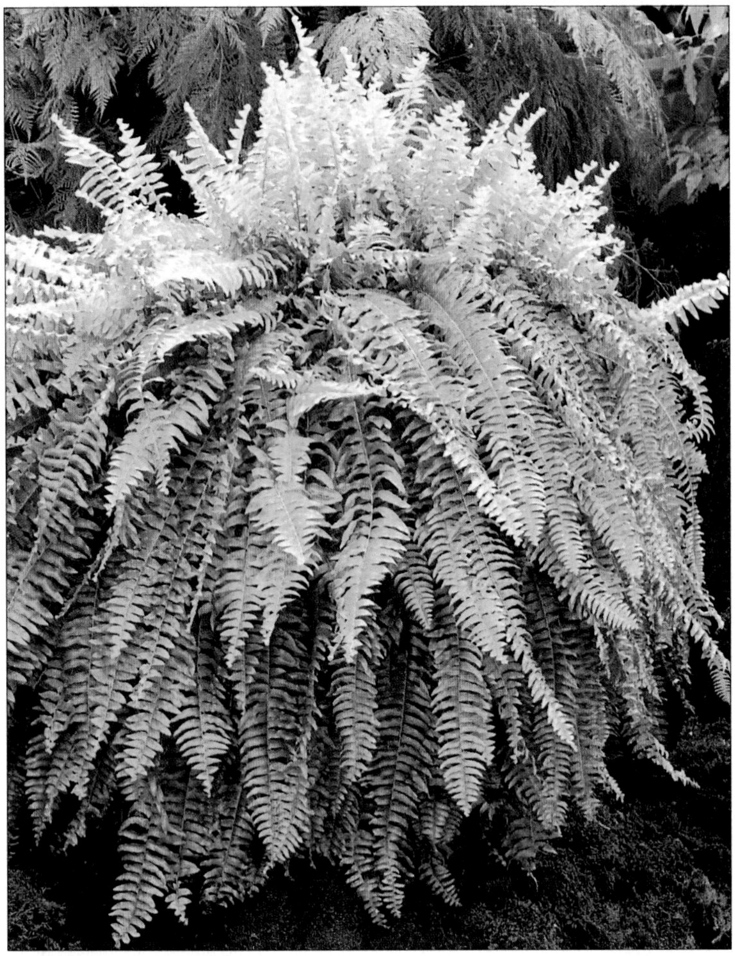
Nephrolepis exaltata 'Bostoniensis'

forked at the tips. **'Plumosa'** is slow-growing, with lobed pinnae.
N. exaltata. Tufted fern with widely arching to erect, linear fronds, to 2m (7ft) long, with shallowly toothed, sickle-shaped pinnae. It is the source of nearly all *Nephrolepis* cultivars. ↕↔ to 2m (7ft). USA (Florida), Mexico, West Indies, Central America, tropical South America, Polynesia, and Africa. ❀ (min. 7–10°C/45–50°F). **'Aurea'** see 'Golden Boston'. **'Bostoniensis'** ■ (Boston fern) has broader, lance-shaped fronds, erect at first, then arching to pendent. A very tolerant houseplant. **'Childsii'** has very broad, 3- or 4-pinnate, closely overlapping fronds. **'Elegantissima'** has 2-pinnate fronds. **'Golden Boston'** ■ syn. 'Aurea', is similar to 'Bostoniensis' but with golden yellow fronds. **'Gracillima'** has lacy, 3-pinnate fronds. **'Hillii'** is very vigorous, with 2-pinnate or 2-pinnatifid fronds, the pinnae variously lobed or crisped; ↕ to 1m (3ft), ↔ to 2m (6ft). **'Mini Ruffle'** is a very compact cultivar with 2- or 3-pinnate fronds; ↕ to 5cm (2in), ↔ 8cm (3in). **'Silver Balls'** has fronds covered with dense, silvery scales as they unfurl. **'Verona'** has dense, pendent, 3- or 4-pinnate fronds.
N. falcata. Tufted fern with arching to pendent, lance-shaped, glossy, dark green fronds, 2.5m (8ft) long, divided into close-set, sickle-shaped pinnae. ↕ to 2.5m (8ft), ↔ to 1m (36in). S.E. Asia. ❀ (min. 7–10°C/45–50°F). **f. *furcans*** ■ has pinnae with 1 or 2 forks at the tips.

▷ ***Nephthytis triphylla* of gardens** see *Syngonium podophyllum*

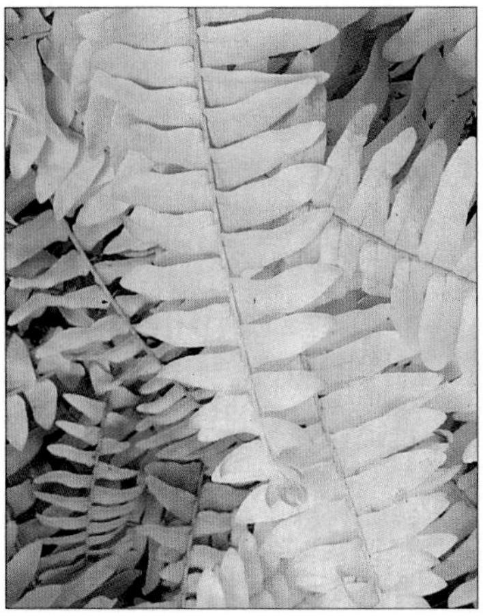
Nephrolepis exaltata 'Golden Boston'

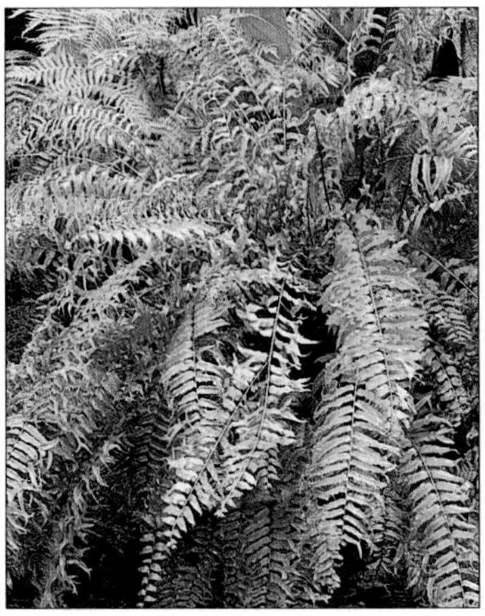
Nephrolepis falcata f. *furcans*

NERINE

AMARYLLIDACEAE

Genus of about 30 species of bulbous perennials, some evergreen, found on mountain screes, on rock ledges, and in other well-drained or arid habitats in southern Africa. They are grown for their spherical umbels of lily-like flowers, with reflexed, often wavy-margined tepals; in herbaceous species, these appear before or with the strap-shaped leaves. Many cultivars with large, colourful flowers have been developed; flowers are borne in umbels, 10–20cm (4–8in) across, of up to 25 flowers, followed by semi-erect, basal leaves. Grow *N. bowdenii* at the base of a sunny wall. *N. sarniensis* and *N. undulata* thrive where frosts are rare. Grow *N. filifolia* and *N. masoniorum* in a rock garden. All are ideal greenhouse plants, and are good as cut flowers. If ingested, all parts may cause mild stomach upset.
• **HARDINESS** Fully hardy to half hardy.
• **CULTIVATION** Under glass, plant in autumn or spring with the tips of the bulbs above the surface of the loam-based potting compost (JI No. 2); they flower best when bulbs are congested. Provide full light. Water freely during active growth. Keep warm and dry when dormant in summer. After flowering, apply a low-nitrogen liquid fertilizer. Outdoors, plant in well-drained soil in full sun in early spring. Provide a deep, dry winter mulch in cold areas.
• **PROPAGATION** Sow seed at 10–13°C (50–55°F) as soon as ripe. Divide clumps after flowering.
• **PESTS AND DISEASES** Prone to attack by slugs.

***N.* 'Baghdad'.** Bulbous perennial bearing loose umbels of crimson flowers with paler centres in autumn. ↕ 60cm (24in), ↔ 8cm (3in). ✻
***N.* 'Blanchefleur'.** Bulbous perennial bearing glistening white flowers in compact umbels in autumn. ↕ 50cm (20in), ↔ 8cm (3in). ✻
N. bowdenii ■ 🏆 Robust, bulbous perennial with broad, strap-shaped leaves, to 30cm (12in) long. In autumn, bears open umbels of up to 7 or more funnel-shaped, faintly scented pink flowers, to 8cm (3in) across, with recurved, wavy-margined tepals. ↕ 45cm (18in), ↔ 8cm (3in). South Africa (Eastern Cape, KwaZulu/Natal, Orange Free State). ✻✻✻. **f. *alba*** ■ has white

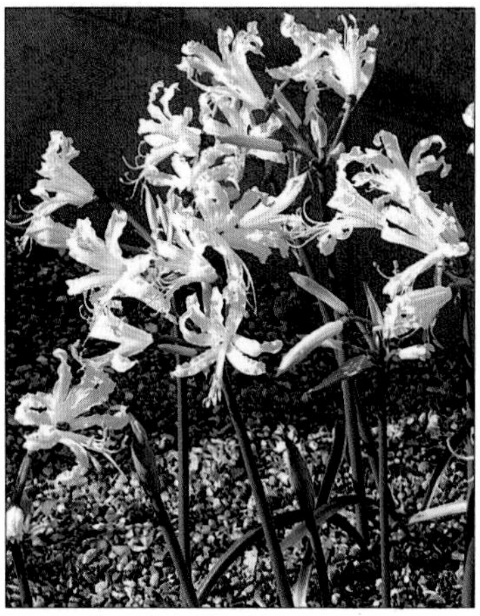
Nerine bowdenii f. *alba*

flowers, sometimes flushed pale pink. **'Mark Fenwick'**, syn. 'Fenwick's Variety', has pink flowers on dark stalks.
***N.* 'Corusca Major'**, syn. *N. sarniensis* var. *corusca* 'Major'. Bulbous perennial bearing compact umbels of scarlet flowers with bold stamens in early autumn. Grown commercially for cutting. ↕ 60cm (24in), ↔ 8cm (3in). ✻
N. crispa see *N. undulata.*
***N.* 'Early Snow'.** Bulbous perennial with compact umbels of pure white flowers, borne in early autumn. ↕ 60cm (24in), ↔ 8cm (3in). ✻
N. filifolia ■ Bulbous perennial with narrow, grass-like leaves, 20cm (8in) long. In autumn, bears compact umbels of 5–10 small, bright pink to white flowers, to 2.5cm (1in) across, with wavy-margined tepals. Bears new leaves as old ones fade, so the plant is virtually evergreen. ↕ 30cm (12in), ↔ 5cm (2in). South Africa (Orange Free State). ✻
N. flexuosa. Bulbous perennial with arching, narrow, strap-shaped leaves, to 30cm (12in) long. In late autumn, bears compact umbels of 10–20 dark-veined pink flowers, to 3cm (1¼in) across, with wavy-margined tepals, the upper ones recurved. ↕ 45cm (18in), ↔ 8cm (3in). South Africa (Eastern Cape, KwaZulu/Natal, Orange Free State). ✻. **'Alba'** has white flowers.
***N.* 'Fothergillii Major'.** Bulbous perennial bearing large, compact umbels of 10–20 bright orange-red flowers, with wavy margined tepals, in late summer and early autumn. ↕ 50cm (20in), ↔ 8cm (3in). ✻
N. masoniorum. Slender, bulbous perennial with narrow, grass-like, almost

N

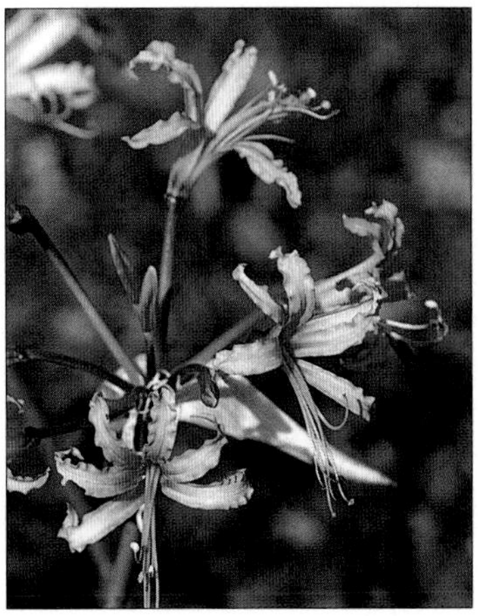
Nerine bowdenii

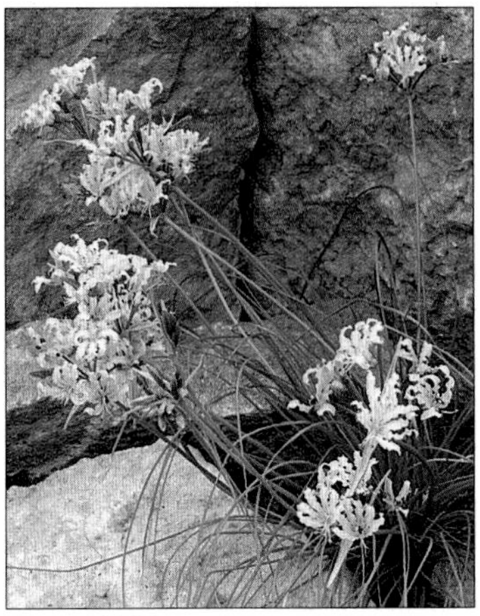
Nerine filifolia

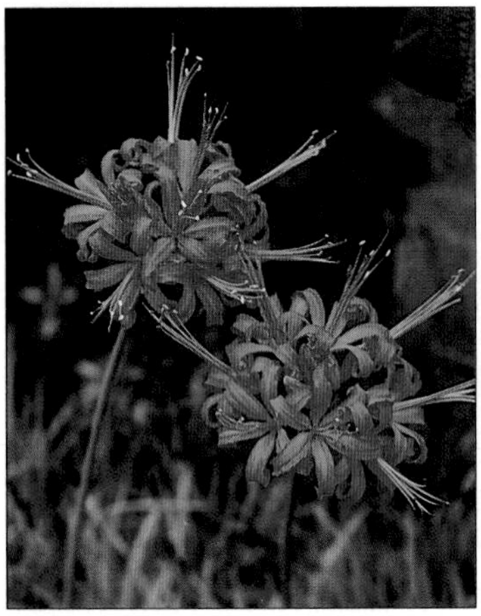

Nerine sarniensis

evergreen leaves, to 20cm (8in) long. In autumn, downy stems bear compact umbels of 4–15 bright pink flowers, to 2cm (¾in) across, with a deep rose-red vein down the centre of each wavy-margined petal. ↕30cm (12in), ↔5cm (2in). South Africa (Eastern Cape). ✻

***N.* 'Radiant Queen'.** Bulbous perennial bearing loose umbels of rose-pink flowers in autumn. ↕60cm (24in), ↔8cm (3in). ✻

***N.* 'Salmon Supreme'.** Bulbous perennial bearing compact umbels of salmon-pink flowers in autumn. ↕60cm (24in), ↔8cm (3in). ✻

N. sarniensis ■ (Guernsey lily). Bulbous perennial with erect, strap-shaped, bright green leaves, to 30cm (12in) long. In early autumn, bears compact umbels of 10–20 crimson to orange-red flowers, 3–4cm (1¼–1½in) across, with wavy-margined tepals and conspicuous stamens. ↕45cm (18in), ↔8cm (3in). South Africa (Northern Cape, Western Cape). ✻. **var. *corusca* 'Major'** see *N.* 'Corusca Major'.

N. undulata, syn. *N. crispa*. Bulbous perennial with strap-shaped leaves, to 45cm (18in) long. In autumn, bears umbels of 8–12 slender, mid-pink flowers, 4–5cm (1½–2in) across, with narrow, crinkled tepals. ↕45cm (18in), ↔8cm (3in). South Africa (Eastern Cape). ✻

NERIUM
Oleander

APOCYNACEAE

Genus of 1 or 2 species of evergreen shrubs or small trees found in seasonally dry stream beds and margins from the Mediterranean to China. They are grown for their often large, terminal cymes of colourful, narrowly funnel-shaped or salverform flowers, which each have 5 broad, spreading, angular petal lobes, and are followed by forked, elongated, bean-like seed pods. Lance-shaped leaves are narrow, leathery, and borne in opposite pairs or whorls of 3. *N. oleander* has been widely naturalized. Numerous cultivars have been raised, both single- and double-flowered, with white, yellow, apricot, pink, red, purple-red, and lilac flowers. In frost-prone areas, grow *N. oleander* in a cool greenhouse and move outdoors in summer; in warmer climates, use as a specimen plant or grow in a shrub border, or as a hedge. All parts are highly toxic if ingested; contact with foliage may irritate skin.

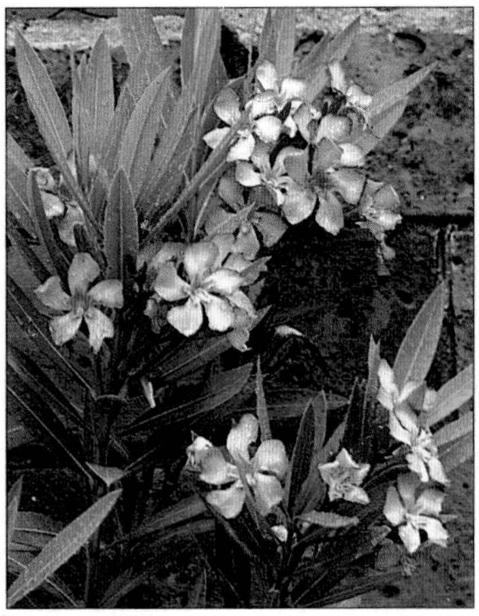

Nerium oleander

• **HARDINESS** Most are frost tender, but may survive short periods at 0°C (32°F). *N. oleander* 'Little Red' is hardy to -12°C (10°F).

• **CULTIVATION** Under glass, grow in loam-based potting compost (JI No.3) in full light; ventilate well. During growth, water moderately and apply a balanced liquid fertilizer monthly. Water sparingly in winter. Outdoors, grow in fertile, moist but well-drained soil in full sun. Pruning group 9; plants under glass may need restrictive pruning in late winter; will tolerate hard pruning.

• **PROPAGATION** Sow seed at 16°C (61°F) in spring. Root semi-ripe cuttings in summer, with bottom heat. Air layer in spring.

• **PESTS AND DISEASES** Scale insects, mealybugs, and red spider mites may be a problem under glass.

N. obesum see *Adenium obesum*.

N. oleander ■ ♀ (Rose bay). Tall, erect to spreading shrub or small tree with lance-shaped, deep green to greyish green leaves, 6–20cm (2½–8in) long. In summer, bears cymes of up to 80 pink, red, or white flowers, 3–5cm (1¼–2in) across. ↕2–6m (6–20ft), ↔1–3m (3–10ft). E. Mediterranean (possibly to W. China); widely naturalized. ❁ (min. 2–5°C/36–41°F). **'Casablanca'** ■ syn. 'Monca', has single white flowers, sometimes suffused pink. **'Little Red'** has single red flowers; ✻✻✻ (borderline). **'Monca'** see 'Casablanca'. **'Monta'** see 'Tangier'. **'Monvis'** see 'Ruby Lace'. **'Mrs. George Roeding'** is dwarf, with double, salmon-pink flowers; ↕1–2m (3–6ft), ↔60–100cm (24–39in). **'Petite Pink'** is dwarf, with single, pale pink flowers; ↕1–2m (3–6ft), ↔60–100cm (24–39in). **'Petite Salmon'** ■ is dwarf, with large, single, salmon-pink flowers; ↕1–2m (3–6ft), ↔60–100cm (24–39in). **'Ruby Lace'**, syn. 'Monvis', has showy clusters of large, single, deep red flowers, 8cm (3in) across, with fringed lips and wavy edges. **'Tangier'**, syn. 'Monta', bears single, light pink flowers. **'Variegatum'** has leaves with white to pale yellow margins, and double pink flowers.

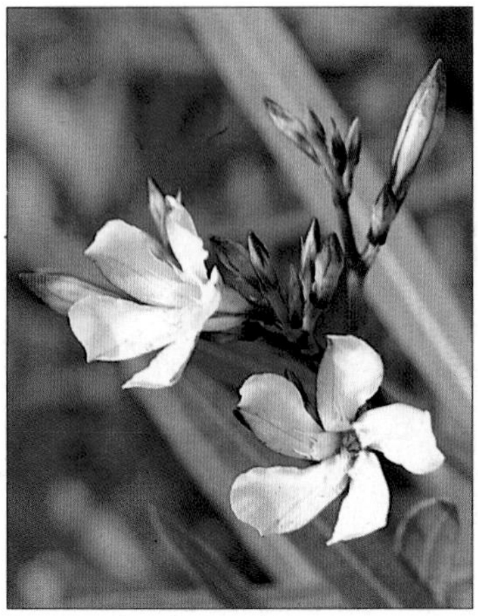

Nerium oleander 'Casablanca'

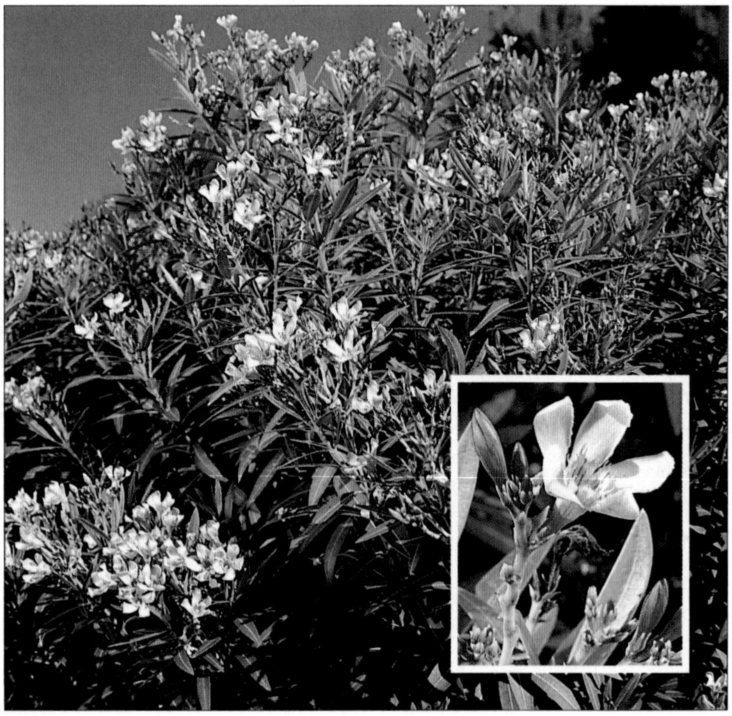

Nerium oleander 'Petite Salmon' (inset: flower detail)

NERTERA

RUBIACEAE

Genus of approximately 6 species of mat-forming perennials from moist lowland to mountainous forest, and moist grassland and scrub, in S. China, S.E. Asia to Australasia, the Antarctic, and Mexico to South America. They have very small, broadly ovate to lance-shaped leaves, tiny funnel- or bell-shaped flowers, and fleshy, spherical to pear-shaped fruits. In frost-prone areas, grow as houseplants, or in an alpine house or cool greenhouse. Elsewhere, grow as ground cover in a rock garden.

• **HARDINESS** Fully hardy to frost tender; *N. granadensis* tolerates temperatures to -3°C (27°F) for short periods.

• **CULTIVATION** Under glass, grow in loamless potting compost in bright filtered light or indirect light. During growth, water freely and apply a balanced liquid fertilizer monthly. Water sparingly in winter. Outdoors, grow in humus-rich, gritty, moist but well-drained soil in partial shade. Protect from excessive winter wet.

• **PROPAGATION** Sow seed at 13–16°C (55–61°F), or divide, in spring.

• **PESTS AND DISEASES** May be infested by aphids or red spider mites.

N. granadensis ■ (Bead plant). Stem-rooting, moss-like perennial with broadly ovate, bright green leaves, to 8mm (⅜in) long. In summer, bears small, stemless, bell-shaped, yellowish green flowers, 3mm (⅛in) across, followed by masses of spherical, shiny, orange or red berries, 5mm (¼in) across. (Populations from South America, New Zealand, and Australia are sometimes considered a distinct species, *N. depressa*.) ↕2cm (¾in), ↔ to 20cm (8in). Mexico, Central America. ✻

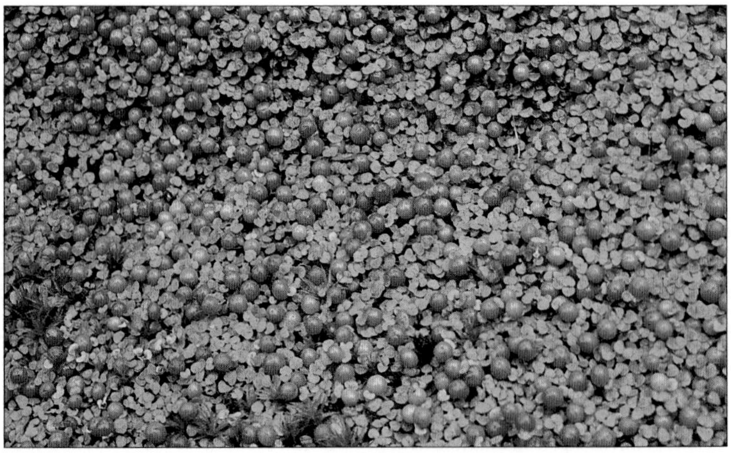

Nertera granadensis

N

▷**Nerve plant** see *Fittonia*
▷**Net bush** see *Calothamnus*
Common see *C. quadrifidus*
▷**Net leaf,**
Painted see *Fittonia*
Silver see *Fittonia verschaffeltii* var. *argyroneura*
▷**Nettle,**
Dead see *Lamium*
Flame see *Solenostemon, S. scutellarioides*
Hedge see *Stachys*
Painted see *Solenostemon, S. scutellarioides*
Pyrenean dead see *Horminum pyrenaicum*
▷**Nettle tree** see *Celtis*
Southern see *C. australis*
▷**Never-never plant** see *Ctenanthe oppenheimiana* 'Tricolor'
▷**New Guinea creeper** see *Mucuna bennettii*
▷**New Zealand daisy** see *Celmisia*
▷**New Zealand flax** see *Phormium tenax*
▷**Ngaio** see *Myoporum laetum*

NICANDRA

Apple of Peru, Shoo-fly

SOLANACEAE

Genus of one species of upright, branching annual from open sites and wasteland in Peru. It has alternate, solitary, oval to elliptic-lance-shaped or ovate, toothed leaves. The short-lived, bell-shaped flowers are followed by brown berries borne in green, lantern-like calyces. Grow in a wild garden or a mixed border. Fruiting branches can be dried for use in winter arrangements.

• **HARDINESS** Fully hardy.
• **CULTIVATION** Grow in fertile, moist but well-drained soil in full sun.
• **PROPAGATION** Sow seed at 15°C (59°F) in early spring, or *in situ* in mid-spring; self-seeds freely.
• **PESTS AND DISEASES** Trouble free.

N. physalodes (Apple of Peru, Shoo-fly). Erect, vigorous annual with wavy-margined leaves, to 10cm (4in) or more long. White-throated, light violet-blue flowers, to 3.5cm (1½in) across, are borne profusely in the upper leaf axils, from summer to autumn, followed by round berries that are enclosed in green calyces, 3–4cm (1¼–1½in) across. Peru. ↕ to 90cm (36in), ↔ 30cm (12in). ❄❄❄. **'Violacea'** has flowers with the upper section of each corolla indigo-blue, the lower part white.

▷***Nicodemia madagascariensis*** see *Buddleja madagascariensis*
▷***Nicolaia elatior*** see *Etlingera elatior*

NICOTIANA

Tobacco plant

SOLANACEAE

Genus of about 67 species of erect, frequently rosette-forming annuals, biennials, perennials, and shrubs from Australia, North America, and tropical South America, where they grow on mountain slopes and valley floors, often in moist soils. They have alternate, linear or oblong-lance-shaped to broadly ovate, glandular-hairy leaves. The flowers are tubular to trumpet-shaped or salverform, occasionally scented, and borne in racemes or panicles, usually over long periods in summer, sometimes

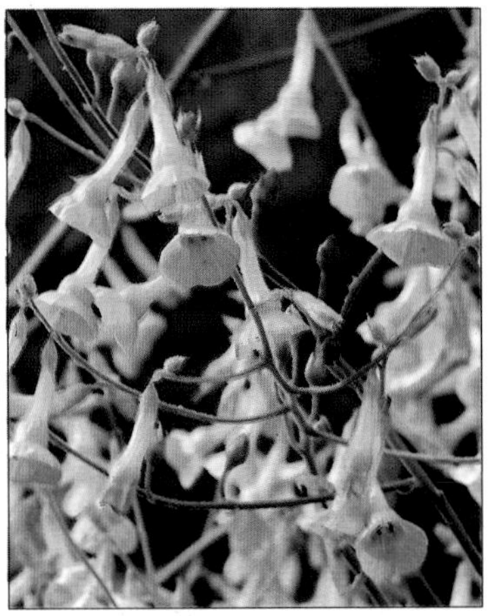

Nicotiana langsdorffii

in autumn. Flowers usually open only in the early evening and at night; flowers of some cultivars remain open during the day if sited in partial shade. Cultivars derived from *N. alata* and *N.* x *sanderae* are ideal summer bedding annuals, their upward- or horizontally-facing blooms remaining open in full sun. Grow *N. sylvestris* in a mixed border or semi-wild garden. Contact with the foliage may irritate skin.

• **HARDINESS** Frost hardy to half hardy.
• **CULTIVATION** Grow in fertile, moist but well-drained soil in full sun or partial shade. Stake tall plants in open positions. Although half hardy, *N. alata* and *N. sylvestris* can be overwintered outdoors where temperatures only occasionally fall to -5°C (23°F); they will resprout from rootstocks the following spring. Provide a dry winter mulch. Pruning group 6 for shrubs.
• **PROPAGATION** Surface-sow seed at 18°C (64°F) in mid-spring.
• **PESTS AND DISEASES** Prone to aphids, whiteflies, leafhoppers, and grey mould (*Botrytis*), particularly under glass. Also prone to viruses, especially mosaic virus.

N. affinis see *N. alata.*
N. alata, syn. *N. affinis.* Short-lived, rosette-forming perennial, grown as an annual, with spoon-shaped to ovate leaves, to 25cm (10in) long, becoming smaller up the stems. Tubular, greenish yellow flowers, to 10cm (4in) long, with funnel-shaped mouths, white within, are produced in open racemes, and are strongly fragrant at night. ↕ to 1.5m (5ft), ↔ 30cm (12in). S. Brazil, N. Argentina. ❄

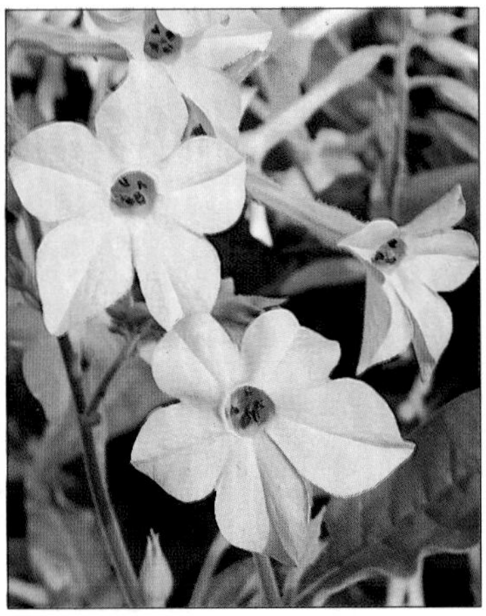

Nicotiana 'Lime Green'

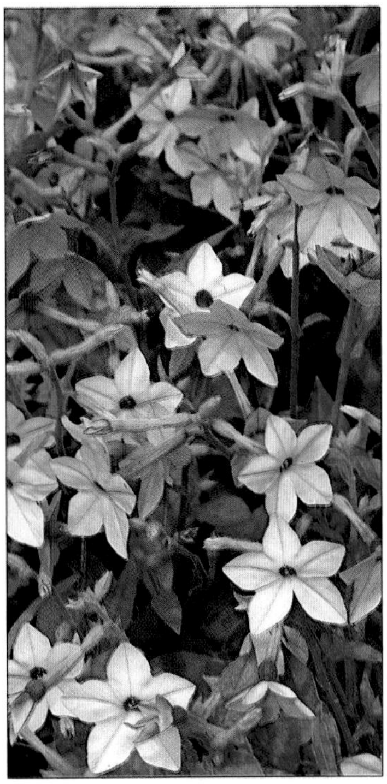

Nicotiana x *sanderae* Domino Series 'Salmon Pink'

N. glauca. Fast-growing, gaunt, semi-evergreen shrub with long, arching, smooth, glaucous shoots and ovate, fleshy, blue-grey leaves, 10cm (4in) or more long. Bears tubular, bright yellow flowers, to 4cm (1½in) long. ↕↔ 2.5–3m (8–10ft). S. Bolivia to N. Argentina. ❄
N. langsdorffii ■ 🏆 Well-branched, sticky annual with a basal rosette of ovate leaves, to 25cm (10in) long. Bears nodding, slender panicles of tubular, apple-green flowers, to 5cm (2in) long, with spreading, 5-lobed mouths. ↕ to 1.5m (5ft), ↔ to 35cm (14in). Brazil. ❄
N. 'Lime Green' ■ 🏆 Upright annual with spoon-shaped leaves, 5–20cm (2–8in) long, the upper leaves oblong-lance-shaped. Produces salverform, lime-green flowers, to 12cm (5in) long, each with an abruptly flattened limb. ↕ 60cm (24in), ↔ 25cm (10in). ❄
N.* x *sanderae (*N. alata* x *N. forgetiana*). Upright, woody-based, sticky annual or short-lived perennial with spoon-shaped to oblong-ovate, wavy-edged basal leaves, 5–25cm (2–10in), the upper leaves oblong-lance-shaped. Bears open racemes or panicles of red, occasionally white, rose-pink, or purple, salverform

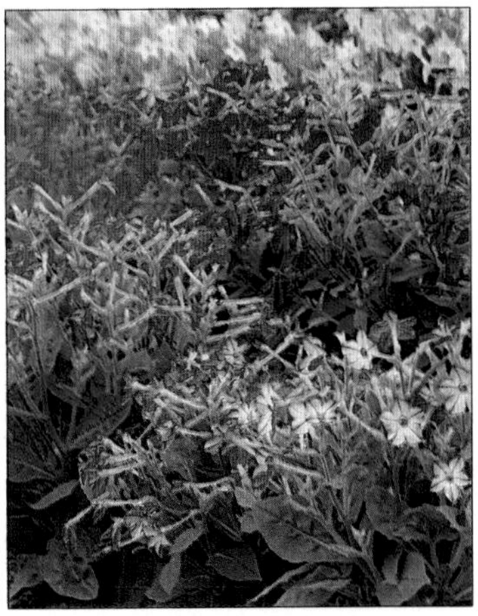

Nicotiana x *sanderae* Starship Series

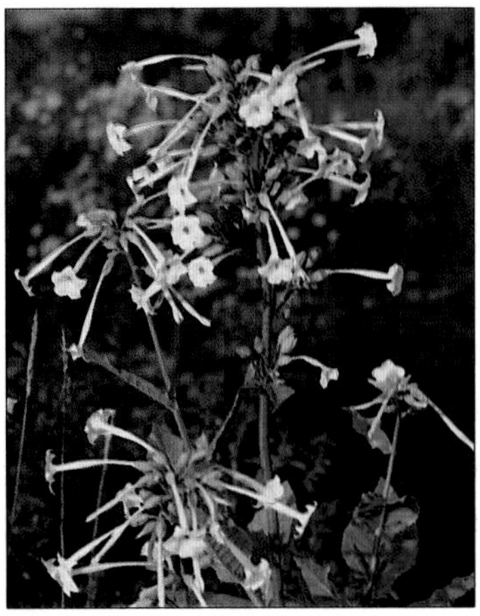

Nicotiana sylvestris

flowers, to 5cm (2in) across. ↕ to 60cm (24in), ↔ 30–40cm (12–16in). Garden origin. ❄. **Domino Series** cultivars have upward-facing flowers in red, white, crimson-pink, lime-green, pink with white eyes, purple, purple with white eyes, salmon-pink, or white with rose-pink margins; ↕ 30–45cm (12–18in). **Domino Series 'Salmon Pink'** ■ has salmon-pink flowers. **Havana Series** cultivars are compact; colours include pale pink with deep rose-pink reverse, and lime-green with rose-pink reverse; ↕ 30–35cm (12–14in). **Merlin Series** cultivars are dwarf, bred for containers; colours include purple, purple with white eyes, crimson-pink, lime-green, and white; ↕ 23–30cm (9–12in). **Metro Series** cultivars have rose-pink, red, lime-green, white, or lilac-pink flowers; ↕ to 35cm (14in). **Starship Series** ■ cultivars have pink, red, rose-pink, white, or lime-green flowers, and good all-weather tolerance; ↕ 30cm (12in).
N. sylvestris ■ 🏆 Many-branched, stout-stemmed biennial or short-lived perennial with a basal rosette of dark green, oblong-elliptic to elliptic-ovate leaves, to 35cm (14in) long. Produces short, densely packed panicles of nodding, sweet-scented, long-tubed, trumpet-shaped white flowers, to 9cm (3½in) long, with 5 spreading lobes. Flowers close in full sun. ↕ to 1.5m (5ft), ↔ to 60cm (24in). Argentina. ❄

NIDULARIUM

Bird's-nest bromeliad

BROMELIACEAE

Genus of about 25 species of rosette-forming, evergreen, usually epiphytic perennials (bromeliads), sometimes rhizomatous, related to *Neoregelia*, from woodland and rainforest, to 2,000m (6,500ft) high, mainly in Brazil. The toothed leaves are narrow to broadly strap-shaped. The conspicuous leaf sheaths surround tubular flowers, usually borne in summer; they nestle in a cluster of large bracts, resembling a bird's nest. Where temperatures drop below 12°C (54°F), grow in a warm greenhouse or as houseplants; in warmer areas, grow in a moist, shady border.

• **HARDINESS** Frost tender.
• **CULTIVATION** Under glass, grow in epiphytic bromeliad compost in bright filtered light with moderate to high humidity. During the growing season, water freely with soft water. Apply a low-nitrogen liquid fertilizer monthly

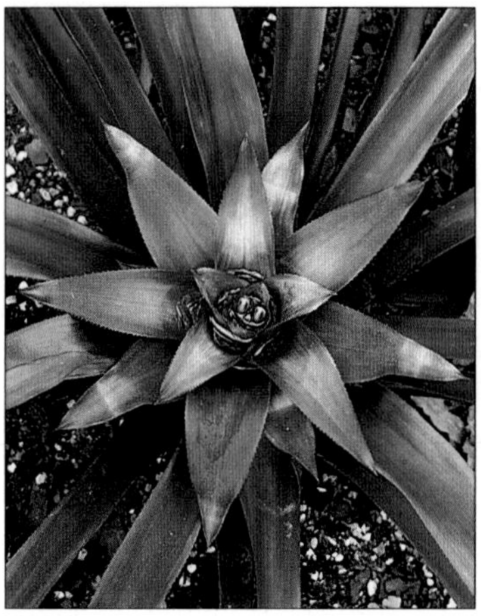

Nidularium procerum var. *kermesianum*

from spring to late autumn. Keep rosette cups filled with soft water from spring to early autumn. Keep just moist in winter. Outdoors, grow in an open site, in gritty, moderately fertile, leafy soil in partial shade, or grow epiphytically on a tree. See also p.47.
- **PROPAGATION** Sow seed at 27°C (81°F) as soon as ripe. Separate offsets in spring or summer.
- **PESTS AND DISEASES** Susceptible to scale insects.

N. carolinae see *Neoregelia carolinae.*
N. fulgens (Blushing bromeliad). Epiphytic, rhizomatous bromeliad with spreading rosettes of 15–20 strap-shaped, sparsely and sharply toothed, pointed, bright pale green leaves, to 40cm (16in) long, slightly scaly beneath. Bears clusters of tubular white flowers, 5cm (2in) long, with purple-blue tips and bright red sepals, among the lance-shaped, brilliant red bracts. ↕ 40cm (16in), ↔ to 60cm (24in). S. Brazil. ❀ (min. 12°C/54°F)
N. innocentii. Very variable, epiphytic bromeliad with funnel-shaped rosettes of 30 or more sword- or strap-shaped, minutely toothed, dark green or reddish green leaves, 20–60cm (8–24in) long, widening towards the tips, with dark red undersides. Produces clusters of tubular, white- or pink-sepalled, green-based white flowers, to 6cm (2½in) long, in rosettes of bright red or green-tipped red bracts. ↕ 20–30cm (8–12in), ↔ 60cm (24in). Brazil. ❀ (min. 12°C/54°F)
N. procerum. Epiphytic bromeliad with erect rosettes of 12–40 sharp-pointed, finely toothed, waxy, copper-suffused, pale green leaves, 40–100cm (16–39in) long. Bears 25–30 or more tubular, blue-tipped vermilion flowers, to 3cm (1¼in) long, among clusters of red floral bracts. ↕ 20–30cm (8–12in), ↔ to 75cm (30in). Brazil. ❀ (min. 12°C/54°F). **var. *kermesianum*** ■ has red-suffused, often narrower, shorter leaves, to 40cm (16in) long; ↔ to 45cm (18in).
N. regelioides ■ Terrestrial or epiphytic bromeliad with tubular rosettes of 12–20 strap-shaped, pointed, toothed, bright green leaves, 35–40cm (14–16in) long, suffused deeper green. Bright red bracts surround clusters of 5–8 tubular red flowers, 4–5cm (1½–2in) long, with purple-tipped white sepals. ↕ 30cm (12in), ↔ 45cm (18in). S. Brazil. ❀ (min. 12°C/54°F)

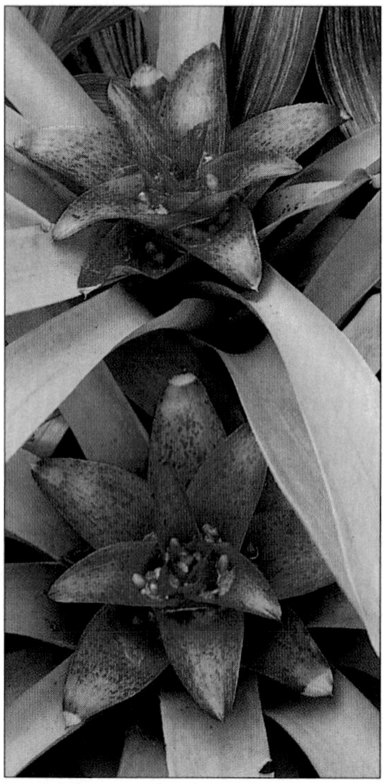

Nidularium regelioides

NIEREMBERGIA

Cup flower

SOLANACEAE

Genus of over 20 species of annuals, perennials, and shrubs from moist, sunny habitats in temperate South America. Slender, spreading or upright stems bear alternate, entire leaves and colourful, open cup- or bell-shaped, sometimes tubular flowers in summer. Most perennial species are frost tender, but are easily propagated and are often grown as annuals; use as bedding, as border edging, or in containers under glass for early spring flowers. In warm areas, grow in open sites among shrubs. Grow *N. repens* in a rock garden or in paving crevices; may become invasive.
- **HARDINESS** Fully hardy to frost tender.
- **CULTIVATION** Outdoors, grow in a sheltered site in moist but well-drained soil in full sun. *N. repens* prefers dry, sandy soils. Under glass, grow in loam-based potting compost (JI No.1) in full light. During growth, water moderately and apply a balanced liquid fertilizer monthly. Water sparingly in winter. Trim lightly after flowering.
- **PROPAGATION** Sow seed in autumn for spring flowering, or in spring at 15°C (59°F). Take stem-tip cuttings of tender perennials at any time during summer. Divide *N. repens* in spring.
- **PESTS AND DISEASES** Susceptible to aphids and whiteflies under glass, and may be damaged by slugs and snails outdoors. May be affected by viruses, especially tobacco mosaic virus.

N. caerulea ♀ syn. *N. hippomanica.* Upright, branching, downy-stemmed perennial with narrowly spoon-shaped, pointed leaves, to 8mm (⅜in) long. Cup-shaped, lavender-blue flowers, to 2cm (¾in) across, with yellow throats, are borne over long periods in summer. ↕↔ to 20cm (8in). Argentina. ✻. **'Mont Blanc'** ■ bears white flowers. **'Purple Robe'** has rich violet-blue flowers; ✻✻✻. **var. *violacea*** has longer leaves and deep violet-blue flowers.

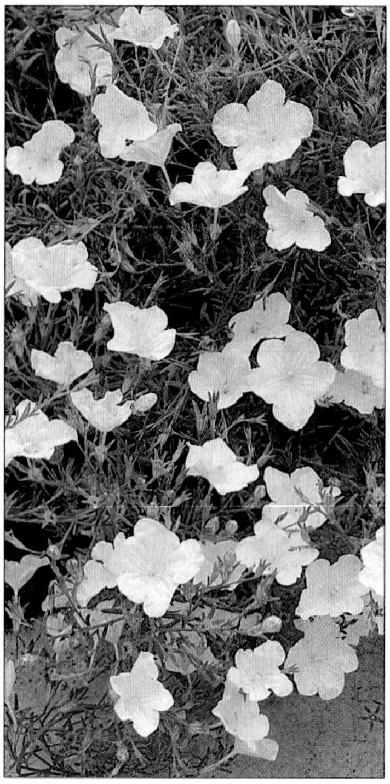

Nierembergia caerulea 'Mont Blanc'

N. frutescens see *N. scoparia.*
N. hippomanica see *N. caerulea.*
N. repens, syn. *N. rivularis* (White cup). Creeping, mat-forming, stem-rooting perennial with rounded, spoon-shaped, light green leaves, to 3cm (1¼in) long. Bears open bell-shaped, yellow-centred white flowers, 2.5–5cm (1–2in) across, over long periods in summer. ↕ 5cm (2in), ↔ 60cm (24in) or more. Andes, warm-temperate South America. ✻✻. **'Violet Queen'** produces rich purple flowers.
N. rivularis see *N. repens.*
N. scoparia, syn. *N. frutescens.* Shrubby perennial with well-branched stems and linear to narrowly spoon-shaped, stalkless leaves, to 5cm (2in) long. Numerous tubular, pale blue flowers, 2.5cm (1in) across, fading to white at the margins, and with wide-spreading mouths, are produced from midsummer to early autumn. ↕ to 45cm (18in) or more, ↔ 30cm (12in). Chile. ✻✻

NIGELLA

Devil-in-a-bush, Love-in-a-mist

RANUNCULACEAE

Genus of 20 species of stiffly erect, bushy annuals found on rocky slopes, wasteland, and in fallow fields in the Mediterranean, Eurasia, and N. Africa. Leaves are alternate, feathery, pinnatisect to 3-pinnatisect. The solitary, sometimes paired, terminal or axillary flowers, borne mainly in summer, are pink, blue, yellow, or white, with 5 petal-like sepals and 5–10 smaller, 2-lipped true petals; they sometimes nestle within a showy, ruff-like surround of strongly veined leaves with hair-like, wispy divisions at each tip. The decorative, sometimes inflated capsules with persistent styles can be dried for flower arrangements. Grow in an informal, mixed or annual border; self-seeding may occur. They also provide long-lasting cut flowers.
- **HARDINESS** Fully hardy.
- **CULTIVATION** Grow in any well-drained soil in full sun.

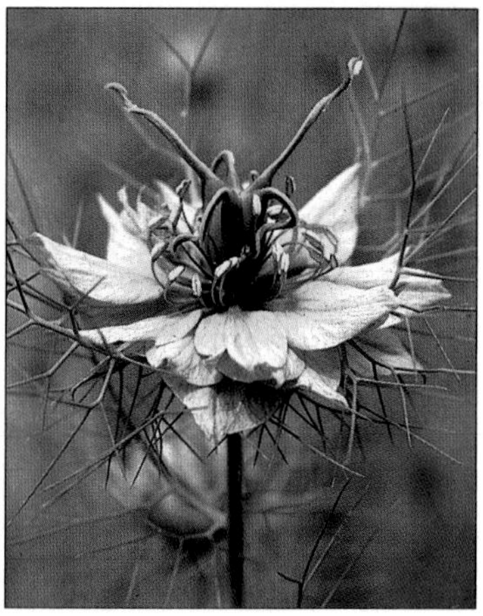

Nigella damascena 'Miss Jekyll'

- **PROPAGATION** Sow seed *in situ* in mid-spring or autumn. Provide cloche protection in winter for autumn-sown plants.
- **PESTS AND DISEASES** Trouble free.

N. damascena (Devil-in-a-bush, Love-in-a-mist). Single-stemmed or branching annual with ovate, finely divided, 2- or 3-pinnatisect, bright green leaves, 12cm (5in) long. In summer, bears terminal, saucer-shaped, pale blue flowers, to 4.5cm (1¾in) across, becoming sky-blue with age, surrounded by a "ruff" of foliage, finely divided at the tips. ↕ to 50cm (20in), ↔ to 23cm (9in). S. Europe, N. Africa. ✻✻✻. **'Blue Midget'** is dwarf; ↕ 25cm (10in). **'Dwarf Moody Blue'** is dwarf, with flowers opening violet, fading to sky-blue; ↕ 20cm (8in). **'Miss Jekyll'** ■ ♀ is tall, with sky-blue flowers; ↕ to 45cm (18in). **'Mulberry Rose'** has large flowers opening creamy pink and deepening to rose-pink; ↕ to 45cm (18in). **Persian Jewel Series** ■ cultivars have sky-blue, deep violet-blue, rose-pink, deep pink, or white flowers; ↕ to 40cm (16in).
***N. hispanica* 'Curiosity'.** Bushy annual bearing broadly ovate, finely divided, 2- or 3-pinnatisect, dark green leaves, to 14cm (5½in) long. Terminal, scented, saucer-shaped, bright blue flowers, to 6cm (2½in) across, with dark eyes and deep maroon-red stamens, are solitary or produced in pairs, in summer. ↕ 60–75cm (24–30in), ↔ to 45cm (18in). ✻✻✻
***N. orientalis* 'Transformer'.** Bushy annual with finely divided, 2- or 3-pinnatisect, broadly ovate, bluish green

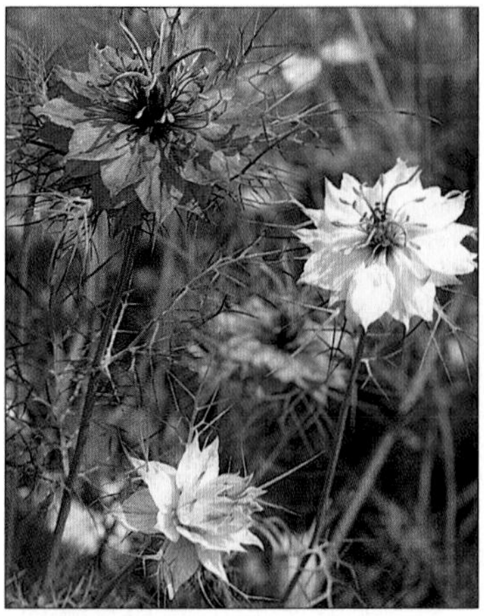

Nigella damascena Persian Jewel Series

N

leaves, to 14cm (5½in) long. In late spring and early summer, bears terminal, solitary yellow flowers, to 4.5cm (1¾in) across. The strongly ribbed seed pods resemble umbrellas when turned inside out, making an unusual addition to dried flower arrangements. ↕ to 45cm (18in), ↔ 22–30cm (9–12in). ❄❄❄

▷**Nightshade, Stinking** see *Hyoscyamus niger*
▷**Ninebark** see *Physocarpus opulifolius*

NIPPONANTHEMUM

ASTERACEAE/COMPOSITAE

Genus of one species of herbaceous or subshrubby perennial from sandy, coastal regions of Japan. It has erect or spreading stems bearing alternate, aromatic leaves crowded together at the ends of the branches. Solitary, daisy-like white flowerheads are produced in summer. Grow *N. nipponicum* in a mixed or herbaceous border, or at the base of a warm, sunny wall.
• **HARDINESS** Frost hardy; may survive temperatures down to -10°C (14°F).
• **CULTIVATION** Grow in very well-drained, moderately fertile soil in full sun. In frost-prone areas, provide a winter mulch over the roots, and protect the leaves with evergreen branches.
• **PROPAGATION** Sow seed at 13°C (55°F) in spring. Divide in early summer.
• **PESTS AND DISEASES** Slugs and aphids may be troublesome.

N. nipponicum. Almost subshrubby perennial with erect or spreading, sparsely branched stems and stalkless, narrowly spoon-shaped, irregularly toothed, aromatic, mid- to dark green leaves, to 9cm (3½in) long. From late summer to late autumn, bears daisy-like white flowerheads, to 6cm (2½in) across, with green disc-florets maturing yellow. ↕↔ 60cm (24in). Japan. ❄❄

▷**Nirre** see *Nothofagus antarctica*
▷**Nodding catchfly** see *Silene pendula*
▷**Nodding ladies' tresses** see *Spiranthes cernua*

NOLANA

SOLANACEAE

Genus of 18 species of often glandular-hairy, erect to spreading annuals, perennials, and subshrubs, usually grown as annuals, found in semi-desert and coastal areas in Peru and Chile. They have simple, alternate or whorled, sometimes succulent leaves. The broadly trumpet-shaped, 5-petalled, blue, pink, or white flowers are borne singly or in clusters in the leaf axils. Grow in a border, or as short-lived container plants in a cool greenhouse. In warm climates, grow perennials in a rock garden.
• **HARDINESS** Half hardy.
• **CULTIVATION** Outdoors, grow in any moderately fertile soil in full sun. Under glass, grow in loam-based potting compost (JI No.2) in full light. Water moderately during the growing season.
• **PROPAGATION** Sow seed at 13–15°C (55–59°F) in early spring, *in situ* in late spring, or in autumn for spring-flowering container plants.
• **PESTS AND DISEASES** Aphids can be a problem.

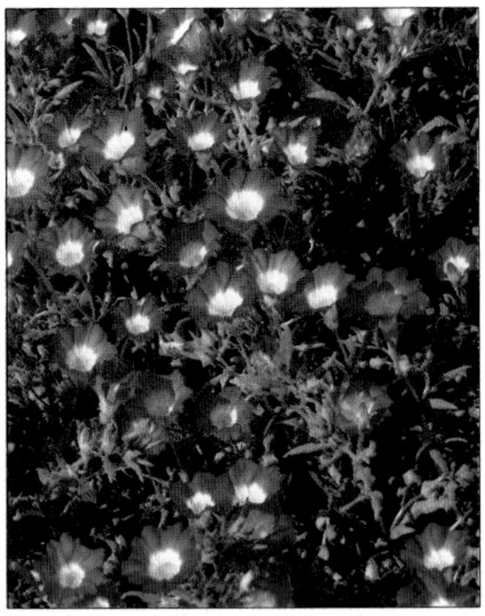
Nolana paradoxa

***N. humifusa* 'Little Bells'.** Spreading, sticky, glandular-hairy annual, perennial, or subshrub with a basal rosette of stalkless, inversely lance-shaped leaves, to 2.5cm (1in) long, and elliptic stem leaves. Lilac-blue flowers, to 2.5cm (1in) across, with broad white throats, streaked lilac-blue, are produced in summer. ↕ to 15cm (6in), ↔ to 45cm (18in). ❄
N. paradoxa ▣ Spreading, fleshy, glandular-hairy annual or perennial with a basal rosette of stalkless, inversely lance-shaped leaves, 5cm (2in) long, and ovate to elliptic stem leaves. In summer, bears dark blue, sometimes purple or purple-blue flowers, to 5cm (2in) across, with yellow throats and white eyes, only opening in full sun. ↕ 20–25cm (8–10in), ↔ to 60cm (24in). ❄

▷***Nolina recurvata*** see *Beaucarnea recurvata*
▷***Nolina tuberculata*** see *Beaucarnea recurvata*

NOMOCHARIS

LILIACEAE

Genus of about 7 species of bulbous perennials from seasonally moist meadows, rocks, and woodland in mountainous areas of W. China, S.E. Tibet, Burma, and N. India. They have linear to lance-shaped or oblong-ovate leaves borne in whorls on the upper halves of the stems, or scattered along them in pairs or threes. In summer, they bear loose racemes of often boldly spotted, saucer-shaped to flat, 6-tepalled flowers, 5–7cm (2–3in) across. They are ideal for a cool woodland garden and effective grown with rhododendrons.

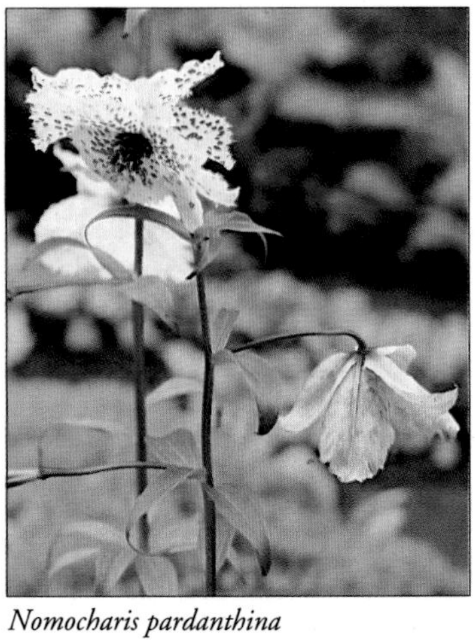
Nomocharis pardanthina

• **HARDINESS** Fully hardy.
• **CULTIVATION** Plant 15cm (6in) deep in winter or spring, in humus-rich, acid soil in partial shade; in cool areas, they may be grown in full sun. They dislike hot, dry conditions; ensure soil is moist in summer but never waterlogged.
• **PROPAGATION** Sow seed at 7–10°C (45–50°F) in autumn or spring. Flowers appear about 4 years after germination.
• **PESTS AND DISEASES** Prone to slug damage.

N. aperta. Bulbous perennial with lance-shaped leaves, 6–10cm (2½–4in) long, in pairs along the stem. In early summer, produces racemes of 5 or 6 nodding, flattish, pale pink flowers, 5–10cm (2–4in) across, spotted deep purple. ↕ 30–80cm (12–32in), ↔ 10cm (4in). W. China. ❄❄❄
N. farreri. Bulbous perennial with linear to lance-shaped leaves, 3.5cm (1½in) long, in whorls up the stem. In early summer, bears racemes of up to 20 nodding, saucer-shaped, white or pale pink flowers, 5–11cm (2–4½in) across, with heavy reddish purple spotting and dark centres. Similar to *N. pardanthina*, but the petals have smooth margins and the leaves are narrower. ↕ 90cm (36in), ↔ 10cm (4in). N.E. Burma. ❄❄❄
N. mairei see *N. pardanthina.*
N. nana see *Lilium nanum.*
N. oxypetala see *Lilium oxypetalum.*
N. pardanthina ▣ syn. *N. mairei.* Bulbous perennial with elliptic to lance-shaped leaves, 2.5–11cm (1–4½in) long, in whorls up the stem. In early summer, bears racemes of 2–20 nodding, saucer-shaped then flat, white or pale pink flowers, 5–9cm (2–3½in) across; they are heavily spotted reddish purple, and have dark centres and fringed petal margins. ↕ 90cm (36in), ↔ 10cm (4in). W. China. ❄❄❄
N. saluenensis. Bulbous perennial with elliptic leaves, 2–4cm (¾–1½in) long, scattered up the stem. In early summer, bears racemes of 1–6 nodding, saucer-shaped flowers, 6–9cm (2½–3½in) across, that vary from pale to mid-pink or white, with light maroon spotting towards the dark purple centres. ↕ 90cm (36in), ↔ 10cm (4in). W. China, N.E. Burma. ❄❄❄

▷***Nopalea cochenillifera*** see *Opuntia cochenillifera*

NOPALXOCHIA

CACTACEAE

Genus of 4 species of freely branching, epiphytic, perennial cacti, very closely related to *Epiphyllum*, from forest in S. Mexico and Central America. They have strap-shaped, jointed, spineless stems, often cylindrical at the bases, with notched margins. In late spring and early summer, funnel- to bell- or cup-shaped, diurnal flowers are borne on slender tubes from the marginal areoles. The flowers last for 3–4 days and are followed in the species by ovoid red fruits, containing seeds encased in jelly-like pulp. Below 10°C (50°F), grow in a temperate or warm greenhouse, or as houseplants. In warmer climates, grow in a courtyard or in a shady border.
• **HARDINESS** Frost tender.
• **CULTIVATION** Under glass, grow in slightly acid, epiphytic cactus compost in bright filtered light, with moderate humidity, away from draughts. During growth, water freely and apply a dilute balanced liquid fertilizer monthly. Keep barely moist when dormant. Outdoors, grow in moist but sharply drained, leafy, gritty soil in a sheltered site in partial shade. See also pp.48–49.
• **PROPAGATION** Sow seed at 19–24°C (66–75°F) in spring. Take cuttings of stem sections after flowering.
• **PESTS AND DISEASES** Vulnerable to mealybugs, especially in early spring.

***N.* 'Achievement'.** Semi-erect, perennial cactus producing strap-shaped stems with rounded margins. Bears yellow flowers, 14cm (5½in) across, with frilled petals. ↕ 45cm (18in) or more, ↔ 40cm (16in). ❀ (min. 10°C/50°F)
N. ackermannii ▣ syn. *Epiphyllum ackermannii.* Erect, perennial cactus with flat, thin, slightly scalloped, fleshy stems, rarely 3-ribbed. The crimson or orange-red flowers have pale yellow-green tubes, 12cm (5in) long, with short pink styles and white stigma lobes. ↕ 45cm (18in) or more, ↔ 40cm (16in). S. Mexico. ❀ (min. 10°C/50°F)
***N.* 'Alba Superba'.** Erect, perennial cactus producing strap-shaped stems with rounded margins. Bears flowers 15–20cm (6–8in) across, with pure white inner petals and pinkish white outer segments. ↕↔ to 50cm (20in). ❀ (min. 10°C/50°F)
***N.* 'Calypso'.** Semi-erect, perennial cactus producing strap-shaped stems with rounded margins and lilac-pink flowers, 12cm (5in) or more across. ↕↔ to 30cm (12in). ❀ (min. 10°C/50°F)
***N.* 'Celestine'.** Erect, perennial cactus producing strap-shaped stems with rounded margins. Bears ruffled, pale reddish pink flowers, 12cm (5in) across. ↕↔ 35cm (14in). ❀ (min. 10°C/50°F)
***N.* 'Chauncey'.** Erect, perennial cactus producing strap-shaped stems with rounded margins. Flowers, 15cm (6in) across, have purple inner petals, each with a red mid-line, and dark red outer segments. ↕ to 60cm (24in), ↔ 45cm (18in). ❀ (min. 10°C/50°F)
***N.* 'Dreamland'.** Erect, perennial cactus producing strap-shaped stems with rounded margins. Flowers, 12cm (5in) across, have pinkish orange petals, each with a deeper, almost red mid-line, and rose-red throats. ↕↔ 50cm (20in). ❀ (min. 10°C/50°F)

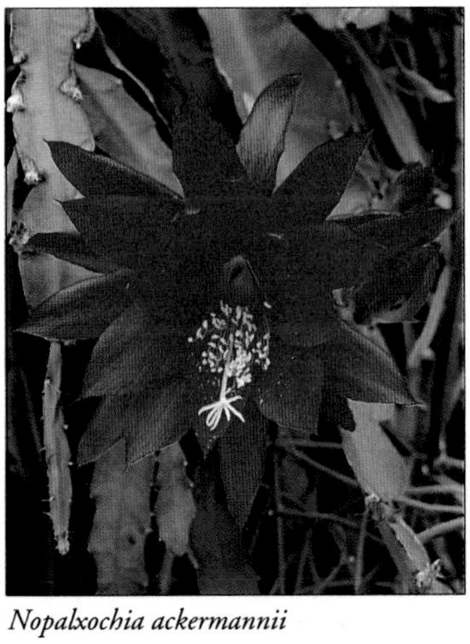
Nopalxochia ackermannii

N

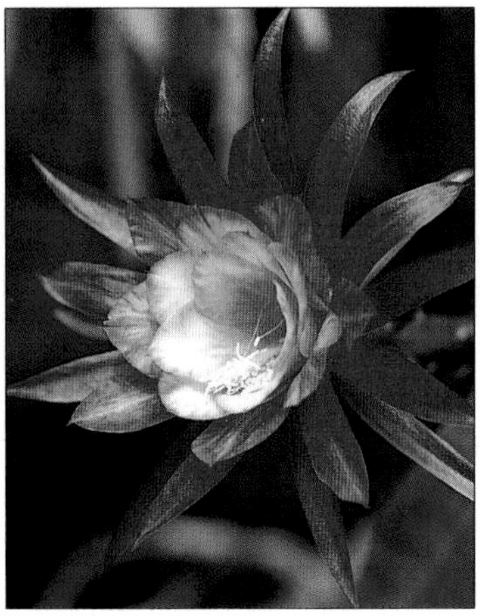

Nopalxochia 'Gloria'

***N.* 'Gloria'** ■ Erect then pendent, perennial cactus bearing slender, strap-shaped stems with minutely notched margins. Produces deep, rich reddish pink flowers, paler in the throats, 10cm (4in) across. ↕ 30cm (12in), ↔ 45cm (18in). ❀ (min. 10°C/50°F)
***N.* 'Helena'.** Erect, perennial cactus with 3-angled, notched stems and minutely spiny areoles. Bears red to violet flowers, 12cm (5in) across, with frilled petals. ↕↔ 45cm (18in). ❀ (min. 10°C/50°F)
***N.* 'Jennifer Ann'** ■ Erect then pendent, perennial cactus with strap-shaped, strongly notched stems. Bears yellow flowers, paler in the throats, to 15cm (6in) across. ↕ 30cm (12in), ↔ 50cm (20in). ❀ (min. 10°C/50°F)

N

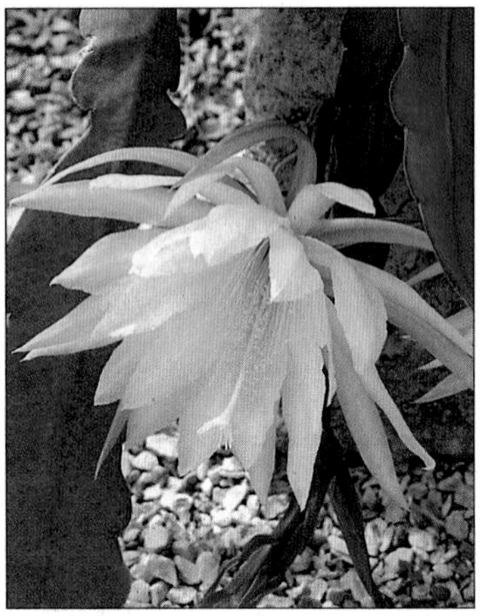

Nopalxochia 'Jennifer Ann'

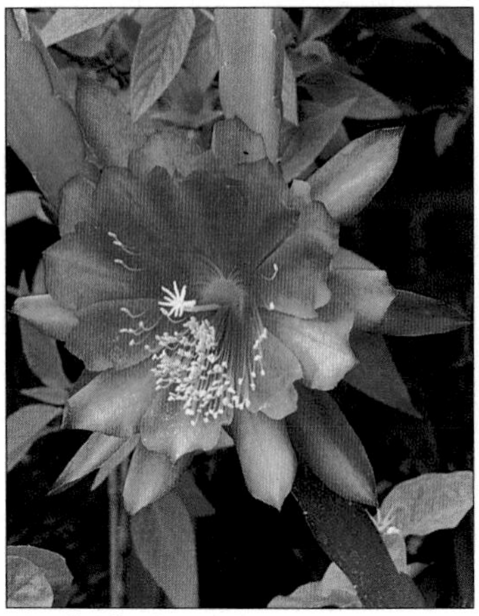

Nopalxochia 'Kismet'

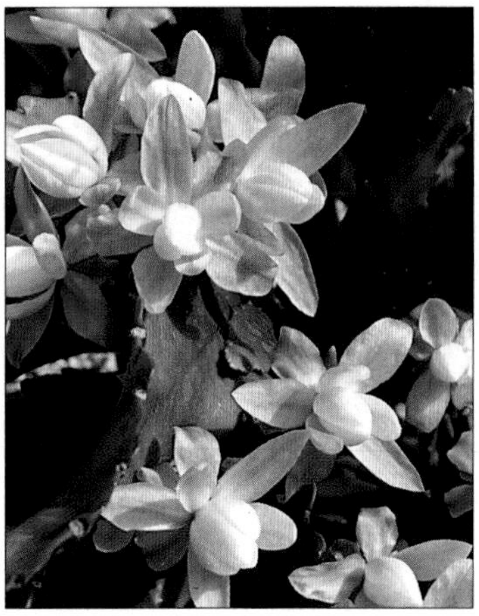

Nopalxochia phyllanthoides 'Deutsche Kaiserin'

***N.* 'King Midas'.** Erect, perennial cactus with strap-shaped or angular stems. Bears bright yellow flowers, to 20cm (8in) across, each with a deep golden mid-stripe and yellowish orange sepals. ↕ to 1m (3ft), ↔ 50cm (20in). ❀ (min. 10°C/50°F)
***N.* 'Kismet'** ■ Perennial cactus producing wide, strap-shaped stems with rounded margins. Bears widely cup-shaped flowers, 16cm (6in) across, in shades of pale purple in the throats and deepening to dark, rich scarlet in the outer segments. ↕↔ to 40cm (16in). ❀ (min. 10°C/50°F)
***N. macdougallii*,** syn. *Epiphyllum macdougallii, Lobeira macdougallii.* Semi-erect, perennial cactus producing flat, 2-winged, scalloped, fleshy stems with inset, marginal areoles. Narrowly trumpet-shaped, lilac-rose flowers, to 8cm (3in) across, have brown-green tubes. ↕ 30cm (12in), ↔ 45cm (18in). S.E. Mexico. ❀ (min. 10°C/50°F)
***N.* 'M.A. Jeans'.** Erect then slightly pendent, perennial cactus producing strap-shaped stems with minutely notched margins. Bears deep pink flowers, 8cm (3in) across. ↕ 30cm (12in), ↔ 50cm (20in). ❀ (min. 10°C/50°F)
***N.* 'Moonlight Sonata'.** Erect, perennial cactus producing strap-shaped stems with rounded margins. Bears flowers, 18cm (7in) across, with white bases, purple-pink petals, and dark violet sepals. ↕ 45cm (18in), ↔ 30cm (12in). ❀ (min. 10°C/50°F)
***N. phyllanthoides* 'Deutsche Kaiserin'** ■ Semi-erect, perennial cactus with strap-shaped, scalloped, fleshy, deep green stems, tapering towards the ends. Bears pink flowers, 7–9cm (3–3½in) across, with white centres. ↕ to 45cm (18in), ↔ 24cm (10in). ❀ (min. 10°C/50°F)
***N.* 'Queen Anne'.** Semi-pendent, perennial cactus producing strap-shaped stems with rounded margins. Bears yellow flowers, 10cm (4in) across. ↕ 24cm (10in), ↔ 40cm (16in). ❀ (min. 10°C/50°F)
***N.* 'Soraya'.** Erect, perennial cactus producing strap-shaped stems with rounded margins. Bears brilliant deep scarlet flowers, 11cm (4½in) across, with broad, almost oval petals. ↕ 24cm (10in), ↔ 20cm (8in). ❀ (min. 10°C/50°F)
***N.* 'Tyke'.** Erect, untidy, perennial cactus producing strap-shaped stems with rounded margins. Reddish orange flowers, 12cm (5in) across, have wide-spreading, twisted petals. ↕ to 50cm (20in), ↔ 45cm (18in). ❀ (min. 10°C/50°F)
***N.* 'Zoe'** ■ Semi-prostrate, perennial cactus producing strap-shaped stems with rounded margins. Bears peach-orange flowers, to 12cm (5in) across, each with 3 rows of petals. ↕↔ 40–50cm (16–20in). ❀ (min. 10°C/50°F)

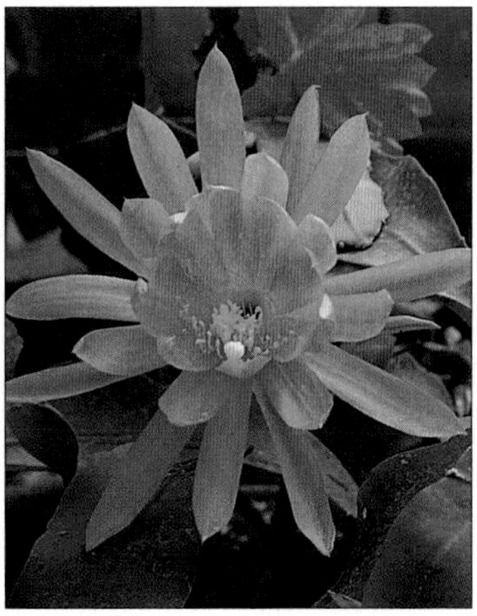

Nopalxochia 'Zoe'

▷**Nordmann fir** see *Abies nordmanniana*
▷**Norway spruce** see *Picea abies*

NOTHOFAGUS

Southern beech

FAGACEAE

Genus of 20 or more species of evergreen or deciduous trees and shrubs from the S. hemisphere (New Guinea and New Caledonia to Australia, New Zealand, and South America), where they occur as forest trees from sea level to the mountains. Leaves are alternate, simple, entire or toothed, sometimes with wavy margins. Flowers and fruits are inconspicuous. They are grown for their habit and foliage, and, in the case of deciduous species, for their attractive autumn colour. Grow as specimen trees in a large garden or woodland garden. In the wild, they often attain much greater heights than in cultivation.

- **HARDINESS** Fully hardy to frost hardy.
- **CULTIVATION** Grow in fertile, moist but well-drained, lime-free soil in full sun. Shelter evergreen species from strong cold winds, at least when young. Pruning group 1.
- **PROPAGATION** Sow seed in a seedbed in autumn. Seed from garden sources may give rise to hybrids.
- **PESTS AND DISEASES** Root rot may be a problem.

***N. alpina* of gardens** see *N. procera.*
N. antarctica ■ ♤ (Antarctic beech, Nirre). Broadly conical, often many-stemmed, deciduous tree or shrub bearing ovate to broadly ovate, glossy, dark green leaves, to 3cm (1¼in) long. Leaves are finely toothed and crinkle-margined, and turn yellow in autumn. ↕ 15m (50ft), ↔ 10m (30ft). S. Chile, S. Argentina. ❄❄❄
N. betuloides ■ ♤ Dense, broadly columnar, evergreen tree with ovate to broadly ovate, blunt-toothed, dark blackish green leaves, to 2.5cm (1in) long, often unequal at the bases, borne on sticky red shoots. ↕ 15m (50ft), ↔ 6m (20ft). Chile, Argentina. ❄❄

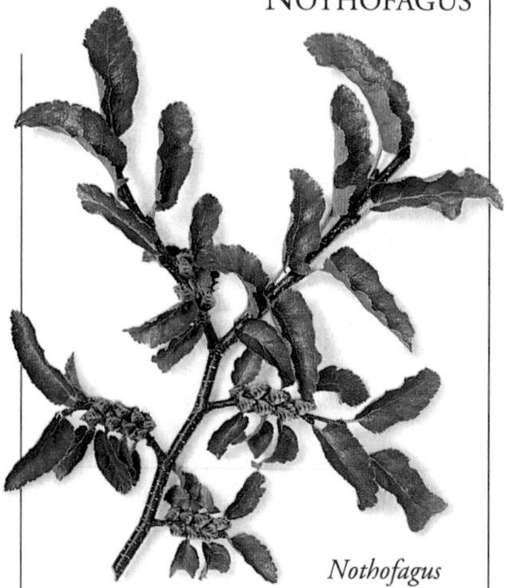

Nothofagus antarctica

N. cunninghamii ♢ (Myrtle beech). Conical, evergreen tree with slender, downy shoots and ovate to triangular-ovate, blunt-toothed, glossy leaves, to 2cm (¾in) long, bronze-red in summer when young. ↕ 12m (40ft), ↔ 8m (25ft). Australia (Victoria, Tasmania). ❄❄
N. dombeyi ■ ♤–♤ Broadly columnar to conical, evergreen tree. Shoots, which are pendulous at the tips, bear narrowly ovate-lance-shaped, finely toothed, dark green leaves, 2–4cm (¾–1½in) long, often unequal at the bases. ↕ 20m (70ft), ↔ 10m (30ft). Chile, Argentina. ❄❄
N. menziesii ♤ (Silver beech). Dense, conical, evergreen tree with silvery white bark when young. Bears broadly ovate to rounded, leathery, dark green leaves, to 2cm (¾in) long, toothed at the margins, pale green when young. ↕ 15m (50ft), ↔ 8m (25ft). New Zealand. ❄❄

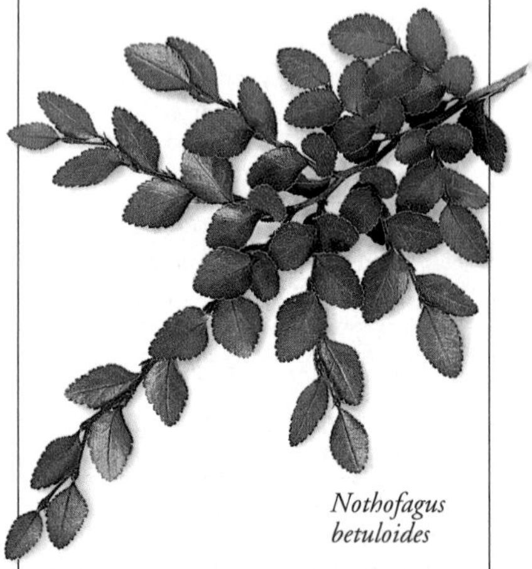

Nothofagus betuloides

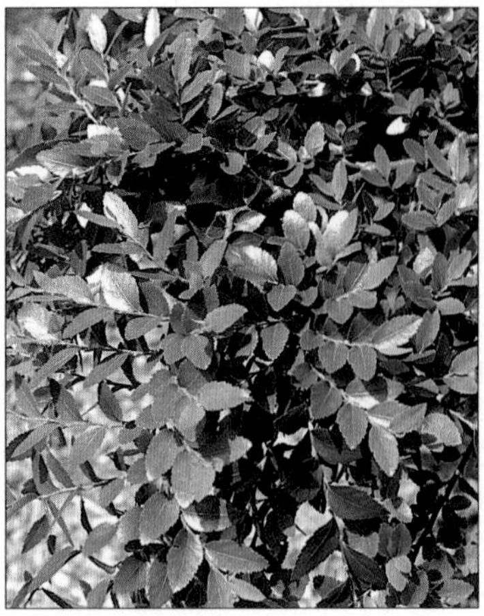

Nothofagus dombeyi

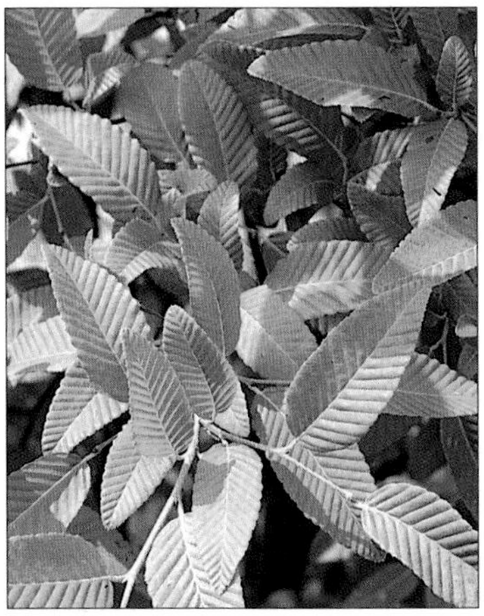

Nothofagus procera

N. obliqua ♢ (Roblé). Fast-growing, narrowly to broadly conical, deciduous tree with arching shoots. Oblong or oblong-lance-shaped, dark green leaves, to 7cm (3in) long, blue-green beneath, with usually 8–10 pairs of veins and doubly toothed margins, turn yellow to orange or red in autumn. ↕20m (70ft), ↔ 15m (50ft). Chile, Argentina. ***

N. procera ■ ♢ syn. *N. alpina* of gardens (Rauli). Fast-growing, broadly conical, deciduous tree. Bears oblong-lance-shaped to elliptic-lance-shaped, matt, slightly scalloped, deep green leaves, to 10cm (4in) or more long, conspicuously marked with 15–18 pairs of veins. Leaves are bronze when young, turning yellow to orange or red in autumn. ↕25m (80ft), ↔ 15m (50ft). Chile, Argentina (Andes). ***

N. pumilio ■ ♢–♢ Columnar, sometimes shrubby, often several-stemmed, deciduous tree bearing oblong to obovate, dark green leaves, to 4cm (1½in) long; each has 5–7 pairs of veins with 2 rounded teeth between each vein. ↕15m (50ft), ↔ 10m (30ft). Chile, Argentina (Andes). ***

N. solandri ♢ (Black beech). Broadly conical, evergreen tree with ovate-elliptic to elliptic-oblong, entire, dark blackish green leaves, to 1.5cm (½in) long, grey-hairy beneath, ending in a short point. ↕15m (50ft), ↔ 10m (30ft). New Zealand. **. **var. *cliffortioides*** (Mountain beech) has ovate, twisted, more sharply pointed leaves.

NOTHOLIRION

LILIACEAE

Genus of 6 species of bulbous perennials, related to *Fritillaria* and *Lilium*, found in open woodland, scrub, and rocky mountains from Afghanistan to W. China. They produce basal tufts of narrowly lance-shaped leaves in winter, followed by racemes of nodding, trumpet- or funnel-shaped flowers in summer. In frost-prone areas, grow in a cool, protected site outdoors, or in a cool greenhouse. They grow best in areas with cool summers.

- **HARDINESS** Frost hardy, but leaves are susceptible to frost damage.
- **CULTIVATION** Plant 10–15cm (4–6in) deep in autumn. Outdoors, plant in deep, humus-rich, well-drained soil in partial shade. Provide protection during periods of prolonged frost. Under glass, plant in large containers in loamless potting compost with added leaf mould and sharp sand, in bright filtered light. Water freely during growth. Keep barely moist when dormant. Bulbs are monocarpic and die after flowering, leaving offsets or a cluster of bulblets that take some time to reach flowering size.
- **PROPAGATION** Sow seed or grow on bulblets in late summer in containers in a cold frame. Remove offsets in autumn.
- **PESTS AND DISEASES** Trouble free.

N. bulbuliferum. Bulbous perennial with narrow, lance-shaped, basal leaves, to 45cm (18in) long. In summer, bears racemes of 10–30 trumpet-shaped, pale lilac flowers, to 4cm (1½in) long, with green tips. ↕ to 1.5m (5ft). ↔ 15cm (6in). Nepal to W. China. **

N. campanulatum. Bulbous perennial with narrow, lance-shaped, basal leaves, to 30cm (12in) long. In summer, bears racemes of up to 20 pendent, deep crimson-purple, green-tipped flowers, to 5cm (2in) long. ↕80cm (32in), ↔ 15cm (6in). N. Burma, W. China. **

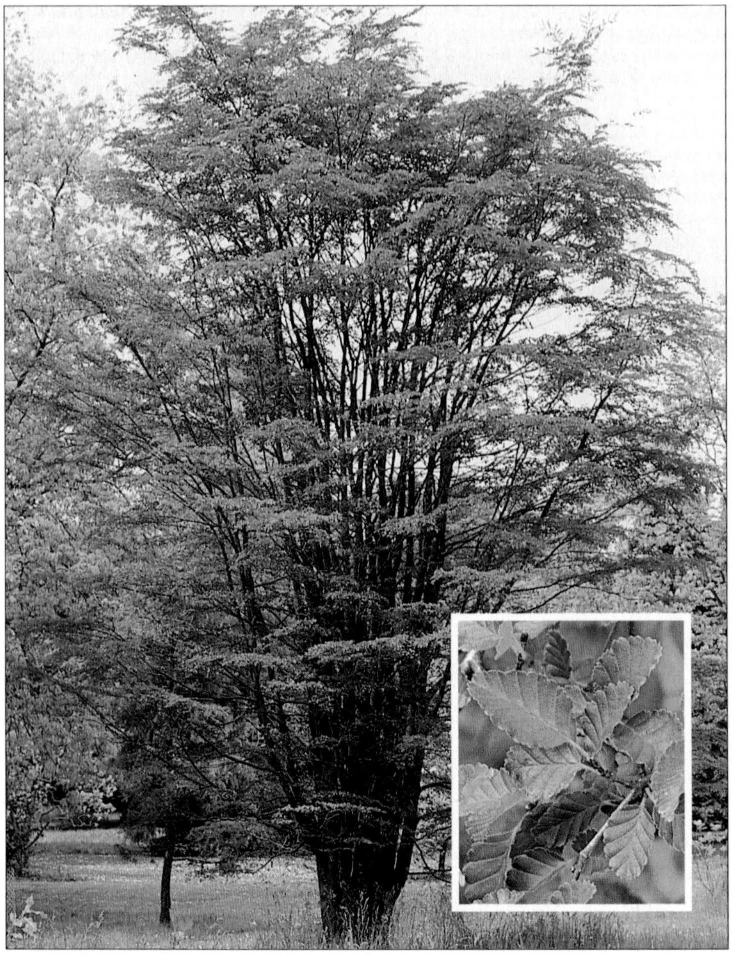

Nothofagus pumilio (inset: leaf detail)

NOTHOSCORDUM

False garlic

ALLIACEAE/LILIACEAE

Genus of about 20 species of bulbous perennials from rocky hillsides and disturbed ground in North and South America. They have linear, basal leaves and, from spring to summer, bear loose umbels of 6-tepalled, funnel-, bell-, or almost star-shaped flowers, borne on erect, leafless stems. They resemble *Allium* but without its characteristic smell. Grow in a rock garden or raised bed. *N. gracile* is best in a wild garden as it increases freely; may become invasive.

- **HARDINESS** Hardy to -10°C (14°F).
- **CULTIVATION** Plant 7cm (3in) deep in any soil in full sun or partial shade in autumn.
- **PROPAGATION** Sow seed as soon as ripe in containers in a cold frame. Remove offsets in autumn.
- **PESTS AND DISEASES** Trouble free.

N. fragrans see *N. gracile.*

N. gracile, syn. *N. fragrans*, *N. inodorum* of gardens. Very vigorous, bulbous perennial with narrow, linear, basal leaves, 20–40cm (8–16in) long. Fragrant umbels of 8–15 small, funnel-shaped, brown- or pink-striped, white or occasionally lilac flowers, 0.9–1.5cm (⅜–½in) long, are borne from spring to summer. ↕25–70cm (10–28in), ↔ 5cm (2in). Mexico, South America. **

***N. inodorum* of gardens** see *N. gracile.*

N. neriniflorum see *Caloscordum neriniflorum.*

▷ ***Notocactus*** see *Parodia*

N. apricus see *P. concinna*
N. brevihamatus see *P. brevihamata*
N. claviceps see *P. claviceps*
N. concinnus see *P. concinna*
N. graessneri see *P. graessneri*
N. haselbergii see *P. haselbergii*
N. magnifica see *P. magnifica*
N. mammulosus see *P. mammulosa*
N. mutabilis see *P. mutabilis*
N. ottonis see *P. ottonis*
N. penicillata see *P. penicillata*
N. rutilans see *P. rutilans*
N. scopa see *P. scopa*
N. submammulosus see *P. mammulosa*

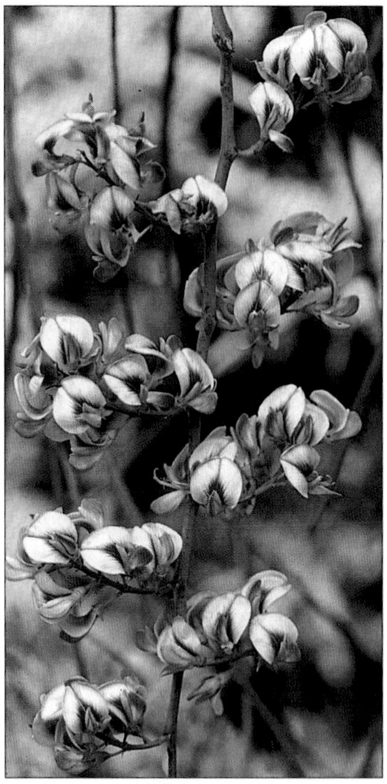

Notospartium glabrescens

NOTOSPARTIUM

LEGUMINOSAE/PAPILIONACEAE

Genus of 3 species of leafless shrubs or trees found on valley sides and river terraces in South Island, New Zealand. They are grown for their elegant habit, green, leafless branches, and pendulous racemes of colourful, pea-like flowers, borne in summer. Grow in a shrub border or at the base of a sunny wall.

- **HARDINESS** Frost hardy.
- **CULTIVATION** Grow in moist but well-drained soil in full sun; shelter from strong winds. Pruning group 9.
- **PROPAGATION** Sow seed in containers in a cold frame in autumn or spring. Take semi-ripe cuttings in summer, with bottom heat.
- **PESTS AND DISEASES** Trouble free.

N. carmichaeliae (Pink broom). Weeping shrub with slender, pendulous, leafless green shoots. Pea-like, purple-veined pink flowers, 8mm (⅜in) long, with broad, standard petals, are borne in dense, slender racemes, to 5cm (2in) long. ↕2–4m (6–12ft), ↔ 1.5m (5ft). New Zealand (South Island). **

N. glabrescens ■ ♀ Upright shrub or small tree with pendulous lower branches and slightly flattened, slender, dark blue-green shoots. Pea-like pink flowers, to 1cm (½in) long, flushed and veined purple, are produced in open racemes, to 5cm (2in) long. ↕3m (10ft), ↔ 2m (6ft) or more. New Zealand (South Island). **

NUPHAR

Spatterdock, Yellow pond lily

NYMPHAEACEAE

Genus of 25 species of deciduous, submerged, aquatic perennials, mainly from temperate regions of the N. hemisphere. They have stout, creeping rhizomes, and both leathery floating leaves and membranous submerged leaves. In summer, they bear solitary, almost spherical flowers, which are held above the water surface. The flowers are followed by berry-like, ovoid to flask-shaped fruits. Generally more vigorous than water lilies (*Nymphaea*), they thrive in deeper, cooler water, forming robust groups of foliage on large natural lakes, where they may cover the water surface completely.

- **HARDINESS** Fully hardy to frost hardy.
- **CULTIVATION** Outdoors, grow vigorous species in water 2m (6ft) deep, anchoring the thick rhizomes in the mud at the bottom. Grow less vigorous species in acid water about 30cm (12in) deep, providing a free root-run. Grow in full sun, and divide frequently for optimum flower production.
- **PROPAGATION** Separate pieces of rhizome that have a growing point attached, and transplant.
- **PESTS AND DISEASES** Trouble free.

N. advena (American spatterdock). Aquatic perennial with floating or upright, thick, tough, leathery, broadly ovate to oblong leaves, to 30cm (12in) long. In summer, bears red-tinged yellow flowers, 4cm (1½in) across, with coppery-red stamens. ↔ indefinite. C. and E. USA. ❄❄❄

N. japonica ■ (Japanese pond lily). Aquatic perennial with narrowly ovate to oblong floating leaves, to 40cm (16in) long, arrow-shaped at the bases, and distinctive, narrow, arrow-shaped, wavy submerged leaves, to 30cm (12in) long. Produces yellow, red-tinted flowers, 5cm (2in) across, in summer. ↔ 1m (3ft). Japan. ❄❄

N. kalmiana. Aquatic perennial with broadly rounded floating leaves, 10cm (4in) long, softly hairy beneath, and distinctive, thin, rounded submerged leaves. In summer, bears orange flowers, 2cm (¾in) across, with yellow margins. ↔ 60–90cm (24–36in). E. USA. ❄❄

N. lutea ■ syn. *N. luteum* (Yellow pond lily). Aquatic perennial with ovate-oblong to rounded, thick, mid- to deep green floating leaves, 40cm (16in) long, and broadly ovate to rounded, wavy-margined, translucent, pale green submerged leaves, each with a deep sinus. In summer, bears yellow flowers, 6cm (2½in) across, with a distinctive, unpleasant smell. ↔ 2m (6ft). Eurasia, N. Africa, E. USA, West Indies. ❄❄❄

N. luteum see *N. lutea.*

N. pumila. Aquatic perennial with broadly ovate floating leaves, 14cm (5½in) long, and broadly ovate to rounded, wavy-margined, translucent, pale green submerged leaves. In summer, bears yellow flowers, to 3cm (1¼in) across. Suitable for a small pool. ↔ 1.4m (4½ft). Europe, Russia (W. Siberia), Japan. ❄❄❄

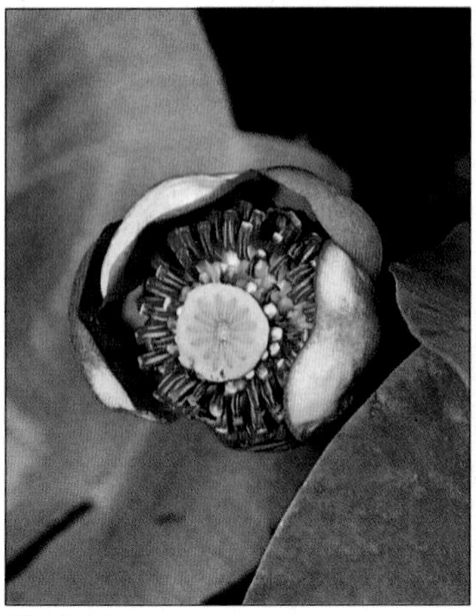

Nuphar japonica

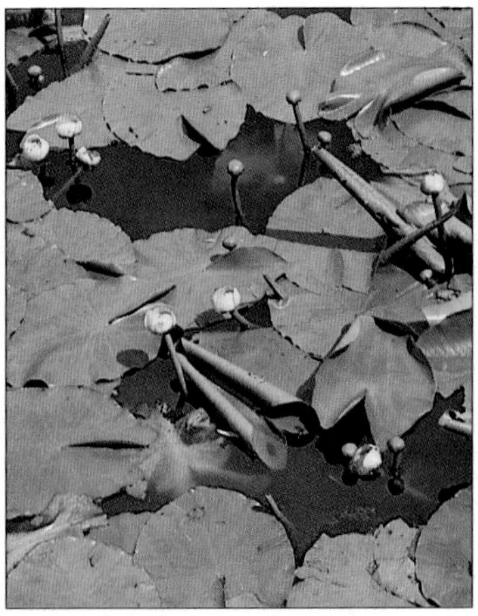

Nuphar lutea

▷**Nutmeg tree, California** see *Torreya californica*
▷**Nutmeg yew** see *Torreya*
▷***Nuttallia*** see *Oemleria*
N. cerasiformis see *O. cerasiformis*
▷***Nyctocereus serpentinus*** see *Peniocereus serpentinus*

NYMANIA

ALTONIACEAE/MELIACEAE

Genus of one species of evergreen shrub from hot, dry areas of South Africa. It is grown for its small, 4-petalled flowers, with 8 long stamens, produced singly from the leaf axils, and its colourful, bladder-like seed pods. The leaves are very narrow and arranged alternately. In frost-prone areas, grow *N. capensis* in a cool greenhouse or conservatory. In warm, dry climates, grow in a border or as a specimen plant.

- **HARDINESS** Frost tender, but may survive short periods at 0°C (32°F).
- **CULTIVATION** Under glass, grow in loam-based potting compost (JI No.2) in full light. In spring and summer, water moderately and apply a balanced liquid fertilizer every month. Water sparingly in winter. Outdoors, grow in fertile, well-drained soil in full sun. Pruning group 8; may need restrictive pruning under glass after fruiting.
- **PROPAGATION** Sow seed at 16°C (61°F) in spring. Root semi-ripe cuttings in summer, with bottom heat.
- **PESTS AND DISEASES** Usually trouble free, although scale insects may be a problem under glass.

N. capensis 🏆 (Chinese lanterns, Klapperbos). Erect to ascending, large shrub or sometimes small tree, usually very open, with rigid branches. The stems are crowded with linear to narrowly oblong leaves, to 5cm (2in) long. Bears 4-petalled flowers, 1.5cm (½in) long, with erect, carmine-red to rose-pink petals, from late winter to early summer. Inflated seed capsules, 2.5–3cm (1–1¼in) long, are off-white, and heavily mottled and suffused carmine-red. ↕ 2–3m (6–10ft) or more, ↔ 1–2m (3–6ft). South Africa (Eastern Cape). ❀ (min. 5–7°C/41–45°F)

NYMPHAEA

Water lily

NYMPHAEACEAE

Genus of 50 species of herbaceous, submerged aquatic perennials occurring worldwide, cultivated for their showy, sometimes fragrant flowers and floating leaves. Water lilies have horizontal or upright rhizomes or stoloniferous tubers, and broadly ovate to rounded, floating leaves, each cleft into 2 lobes, with a basal sinus and a long leaf-stalk. The mostly white, yellow, pink, red, or, in the non-hardy species, blue flowers, borne in summer, each have 4 sepals and numerous narrow petals and stamens. Berry-like fruits, with many seeds, mature under water.

Hardy water lilies, usually day-blooming and with floating flowers, include 2 subgroups: the robust Marliacea Group hybrids, probably derived from *N. alba, N. odorata, N. tuberosa,* and *N. mexicana,* have rounded leaves, and flowers held just above the water; hybrids in the less vigorous Laydekeri Group, derived from *N. alba* and *N. tetragona,* have flowers held on or just above the water, and rounded, often mottled leaves. Tender, tropical water lilies are either day-blooming or night-blooming, with larger, often toothed leaves, and generally bear their flowers well above the water.

Water lilies are a decorative addition to any pool; the shade of their leaves is useful in reducing algae growth. In frost-prone areas, grow tender water lilies in a conservatory in full sun.

- **HARDINESS** Fully hardy to frost tender.
- **CULTIVATION** Grow in undisturbed water in full sun. In summer, plant hardy water lilies in firm, loamy soil; insert the rhizomes just under the surface and cover with washed pea gravel or chippings. Submerge freshly planted containers so that 15–25cm (6–10in) of water covers the young crowns, either by temporarily lowering the water level or by raising the containers on brick plinths. For small rhizomes, reduce the depth to 8cm (3in); increase to 50cm (20in) for the largest rhizomes. Once plants are established, gradually increase the water depth above the crowns to twice the initial planting depth. Contain vigorous water lilies in an aquatic planting basket, or in a specially constructed, permanent planting station, about 1m (3ft) across and 45cm (18in) deep. During active growth, feed container-grown water lilies with proprietary aquatic fertilizer according to the manufacturer's instructions. Remove yellow leaves and dead-head regularly. Divide established plants, whose leaves thrust vertically above the water surface, to maintain flowering.

In frost-prone areas, grow tropical water lilies year-round in baskets in an indoor pool with a minimum temperature of 10°C (50°F) in winter and 21°C (70°F) in summer. In frost-free areas, plant in an outdoor pool in summer, remove the tubers in autumn, and overwinter in damp sand at a minimum of 10°C (50°F). Restart young plants in spring when dividing overwintered tubers. See also pp.52–53.

- **PROPAGATION** Surface-sow seed as soon as ripe, and cover with 2.5cm (1in) of water; germinate hardy species at 10–13°C (50–55°F), tropical species at 23–27°C (73–81°F). The seed heads sink as seeds ripen; enclose in a muslin bag to avoid losses. Divide rhizomes of older plants, or separate offsets. Remove young plantlets from viviparous water lilies in summer, and pot individually in shallow water until established.
- **PESTS AND DISEASES** Susceptible to brown china-mark moth, false leaf-mining midge, water lily beetle, water lily aphid (which overwinters on *Prunus* species), and brown spot, crown rot, and water lily leaf spot.

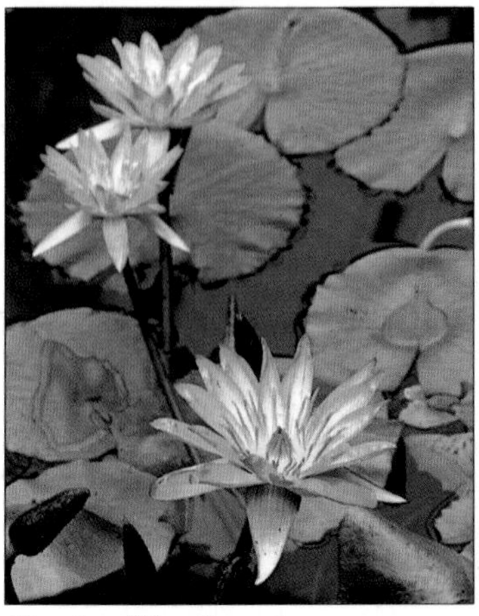

Nymphaea 'Blue Beauty'

N. alba ■ (White water lily). Aquatic perennial with rounded, dark green leaves, often red-green beneath, 30cm (12in) across, with open sinuses. The faintly fragrant white flowers, 20cm (8in) across, with yellow stamens, are cup-shaped, later star-shaped, and day-blooming. ↔ 1.7m (5½ft). Eurasia, N. Africa. ❄❄❄

***N.* 'Albida'** ■ syn. *N.* 'Marliacea Albida'. Aquatic perennial (Marliacea Group) with rounded, dark green leaves, 22cm (9in) across, slightly bronzed when young, with open sinuses. The fragrant, cup-shaped white flowers, 12–15cm (5–6in) across, have yellow stamens. ↔ 0.9–1.2m (3–4ft). ❄❄❄

***N.* 'Amabilis'.** Aquatic perennial with rounded leaves, 24cm (10in) across, with open sinuses, reddish purple when young, maturing to dark green with red-margined, light green undersides. Star-shaped flowers, 15–19cm (6–7in) across, are pink with light pink tips and dark yellow stamens. ↔ 1.5–2.2m (5–7ft). ❄❄❄

***N.* 'American Star'** ■ Aquatic perennial bearing rounded leaves, 25–27cm (10–11in) across, with open sinuses, purple-green when young, with red undersides, maturing to light green. Star-shaped flowers, 15–17cm (6–7in) across, with long, salmon-pink petals tipped paler pink, yellow inner stamens, and pinkish orange outer stamens, are borne well above the water surface. ↔ 1.2–1.5m (4–5ft). ❄❄❄

***N.* 'Attraction'** ■ Aquatic perennial bearing oval, light bronze leaves, to 25–30cm (10–12in) long, with over-lapping lobes, one of which is distinctly raised. Cup-shaped, later star-shaped flowers, to 23cm (9in) across, have dark garnet-red inner petals, lighter towards the margins, and orange-red stamens. ↔ 1.2–1.5m (4–5ft). ❄❄❄

N. 'Aurora' ■ Aquatic perennial with oval, mid-green leaves with maroon mottling, to 16cm (6in) long, with open sinuses. Cup-shaped, later flattened flowers, 10cm (4in) across, with orange stamens, change from yellowish apricot-red through orange-red to a slightly flecked burgundy-red. ↔ 0.9–1.5m (3–5ft). ✻✻✻

N. 'Blue Beauty' ■ Aquatic perennial with oval, toothed, wavy-margined, dark green leaves lightly speckled brown above, to 35cm (14in) across, with partly overlapping lobes. Day-blooming, star-shaped, fragrant, mid-blue flowers, 20–28cm (8–11in) across, have dark yellow stamens. ↔ 1.2–2.2m (4–7ft). ❁ (min. 10°C/50°F)

N. caerulea (Blue lotus). Aquatic perennial with ovate, mid-green leaves, 30–40cm (12–16in) long, purple-spotted beneath, with overlapping lobes. Day-blooming, star-shaped, pale blue flowers, 15cm (6in) across, have paler inner petals and yellow stamens. ↔ 2.5–3m (8–10ft). N. and tropical Africa. ✻

N. capensis ■ (Cape blue water lily). Aquatic perennial with rounded, toothed, wavy-margined, mid-green leaves, 25–40cm (10–16in) across, with slightly overlapping lobes. The young leaves are purple-spotted beneath. Produces day-blooming, star-shaped, fragrant, light blue flowers, 21–25cm (8–10in) across, with dark yellow stamens. ↔ 1.5–2.5m (5–8ft). E. Africa, southern Africa, Madagascar. ❁ (min. 5°C/41°F). **'Rosea'** has leaves tinted red beneath and red-flushed, pale pink flowers.

N. 'Carnea', syn. *N.* 'Marliacea Carnea'. Aquatic perennial (Marliacea Group) with dark green leaves, 19–20cm (7–8in) across, purplish when young, and light pink flowers, 11–12cm (4½–5in) across, with yellow stamens. ↔ 1.2–1.5m (4–5ft). ✻✻✻

***N. caroliniana* 'Nivea'** ■ syn. *N.* 'Caroliniana Nivea'. Aquatic perennial bearing rounded, pale green leaves, 20–25cm (8–10in) across, with slightly open sinuses. Star-shaped, fragrant ivory-white flowers, 12–15cm (5–6in) across, have yellow stamens. ↔ 1.2–1.5m (4–5ft). ✻✻✻

N. 'Caroliniana Nivea' see *N. caroliniana* 'Nivea'.

N. 'Charlene Strawn'. Aquatic perennial with rounded leaves, 20–22cm (8–9in) across, red with purple mottling when young, maturing to mid-green, sometimes marked with purple, and with overlapping lobes. Star-shaped, highly fragrant, yellow flowers, 15–20cm (6–8in) across, have yellow stamens. ↔ 0.9–1.5m (3–5ft). ✻✻✻

N. 'Charles de Meurville'. Aquatic perennial with oval, dark green leaves, 25cm (10in) long, with long, deep sinuses. Star-shaped flowers, 15–17cm (6–7in) across, are dark pinkish red in the centre, fading to pink towards the margins, with orange stamens. ↔ 1.2–1.5m (4–5ft). ✻✻✻

N. 'Chromatella' ■🏆 syn. *N.* 'Marliacea Chromatella'. Aquatic perennial (Marliacea Group) bearing olive-green leaves with bronze markings, 15–20cm (6–8in) across, coppery with purple streaks when young. Canary-yellow flowers, 15cm (6in) across, have broad, incurved petals and golden stamens. ↔ 1.2–1.5m (4–5ft). ✻✻✻

N. x daubenyana (*N. caerulea* x *N. micrantha*). Aquatic, viviparous, hybrid perennial producing ovate, olive- to bronze-green leaves, to 30cm (12in) long, with wavy margins and overlapping lobes, many bearing a plantlet. Day-blooming, cup-shaped, fragrant flowers, 10–18cm (4–7in) across, are light blue with dark margins and yellow stamens. ↔ 0.9–1.2m (3–4ft). Garden origin. ❁ (min. 10°C/50°F)

N. 'Ellisiana'. Aquatic perennial with oval, mid-green leaves, 17–20cm (7–8in) long, with open sinuses; young leaves are dark green, marked purple. Star-shaped, fragrant, bright red flowers, 10–12cm (4–5in) across, have orange-red stamens. ↔ 90cm (36in). ✻✻✻

N. 'Emily Grant Hutchings'. Aquatic perennial bearing rounded, wavy-margined leaves, 25–30cm (10–12in) across, bronze-green above, olive-green beneath, with overlapping nodes. Night-blooming, cup-shaped, dark pink flowers, 15–20cm (6–8in) across, have red stamens. ↔ 1.8–2.2m (6–7ft). ❁ (min. 10°C/50°F)

N. 'Escarboucle' ■🏆 Aquatic perennial with rounded, mid-green leaves, 25–27cm (10–11in) across, brown-tinged when young, with overlapping lobes. Cup-shaped, later star-shaped, vermilion-red flowers, about 15–17cm (6–7in) across, have white-tipped outer petals and dark orange stamens. ↔ 1.2–1.5m (4–5ft). ✻✻✻

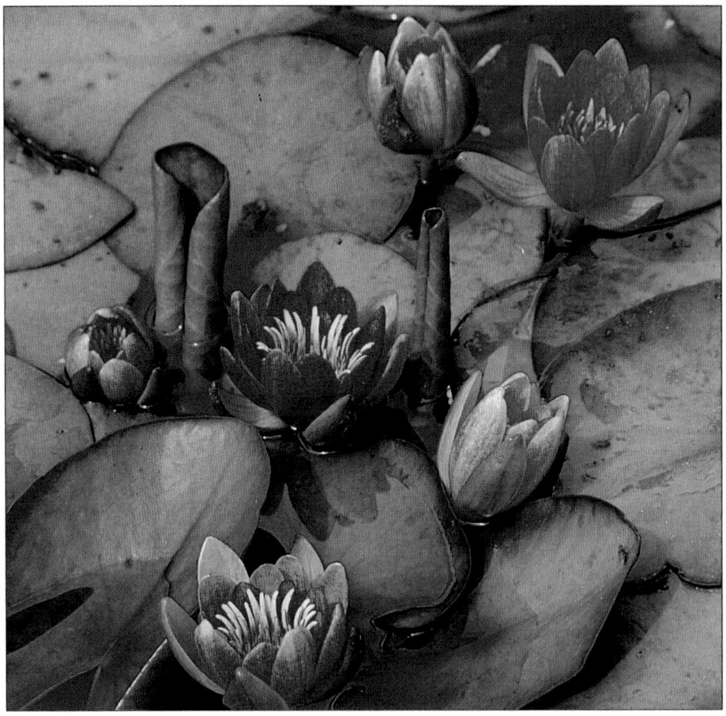

Nymphaea 'Froebelii'

N. 'Firecrest' ■ Aquatic perennial with rounded, mid-green leaves, 22cm (9in) across, dark purple when young, with open sinuses. Star-shaped, deep pink flowers, 15cm (6in) across, with lavender-pink inner petals, have orange inner stamens and pink outer stamens. ↔ 1.2m (4ft). ✻✻✻

N. flava see *N. mexicana.*

N. 'Froebelii' ■ Aquatic perennial with rounded, pale green leaves, 15cm (6in) across, bronzed when young, with open sinuses. Cup-shaped, later star-shaped, burgundy-red flowers, 10–12cm (4–5in) across, have orange-red stamens. ↔ 90cm (36in). ✻✻✻

N. 'Fulgens' ■ syn. *N.* 'Laydekeri Fulgens'. Aquatic perennial (Laydekeri Group) with broadly ovate, dark green leaves, 21cm (8in) long, with overlapping lobes; young leaves are purplish green, marked dark purple. Cup-shaped, burgundy-red flowers, 12–15cm (5–6in) across, have orange-red stamens. ↔ 1.2–1.5m (4–5ft). ✻✻✻

N. 'General Pershing' ■ Aquatic perennial bearing rounded, wavy-margined, olive-green, purple-marked leaves, 23–25cm (9–10in) across, with almost closed sinuses. Day-blooming, cup-shaped, later flat, highly fragrant, lavender-pink flowers, 20–27cm (8–11in) across, have yellow stamens. ↔ 1.5–1.8m (5–6ft). ❁ (min. 10°C/50°F)

N. gigantea (Australian water lily). Aquatic perennial with rounded, toothed, wavy-margined, veined, mid-green leaves, to 60cm (24in) across, tinged pink to purple beneath, with often overlapping lobes. Day-blooming, star-shaped, sky-blue to purplish blue flowers, to 30cm (12in) across, have bright yellow stamens. ↔ 2–3m (6–10ft). N. Papua New Guinea, tropical Australia. ❁ (min. 10°C/50°F)

N. 'Gladstoneana' 🏆 Aquatic perennial with rounded, wavy-margined, dark

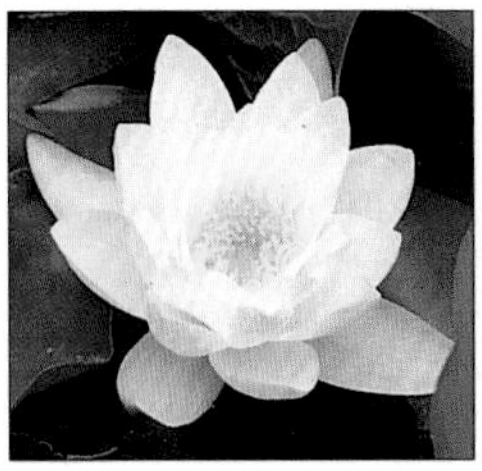

Nymphaea alba

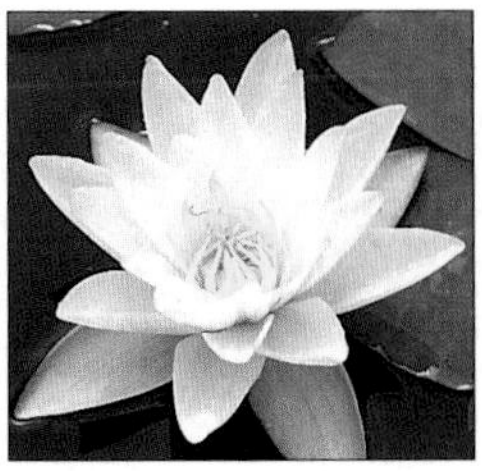

Nymphaea 'Albida'

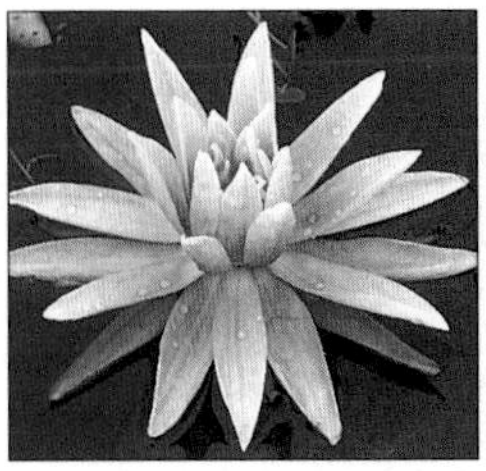

Nymphaea 'American Star'

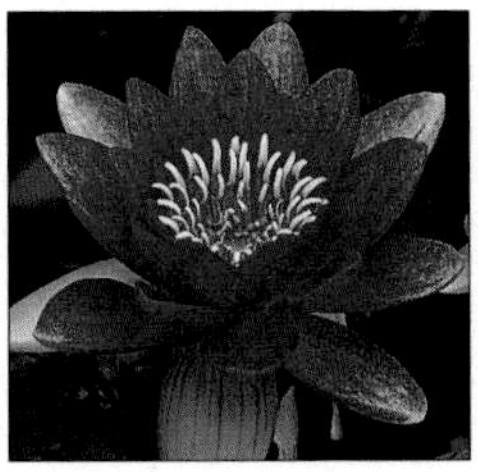

Nymphaea 'Attraction'

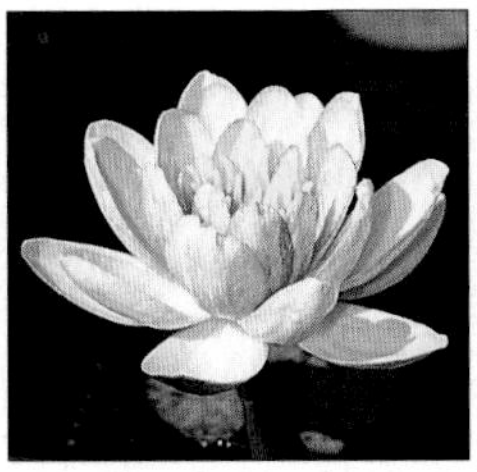

Nymphaea 'Aurora'

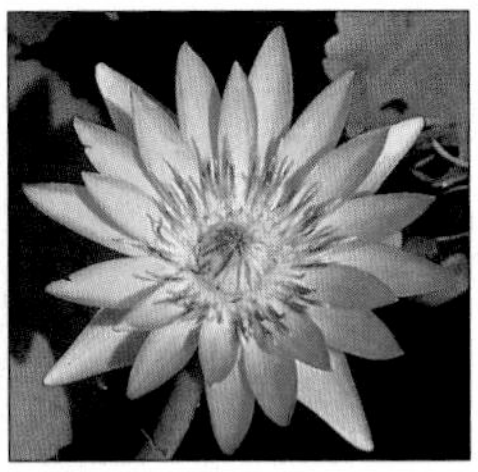

Nymphaea capensis

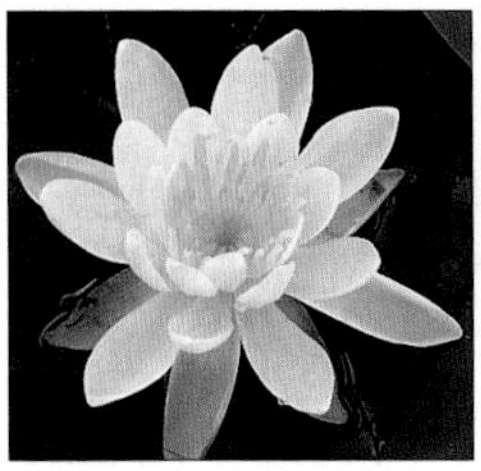

Nymphaea caroliniana 'Nivea'

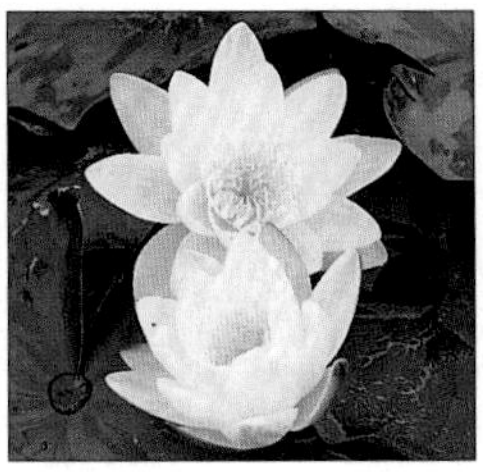

Nymphaea 'Chromatella'

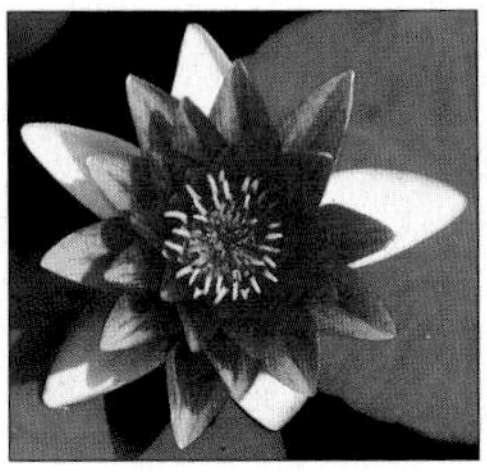

Nymphaea 'Escarboucle'

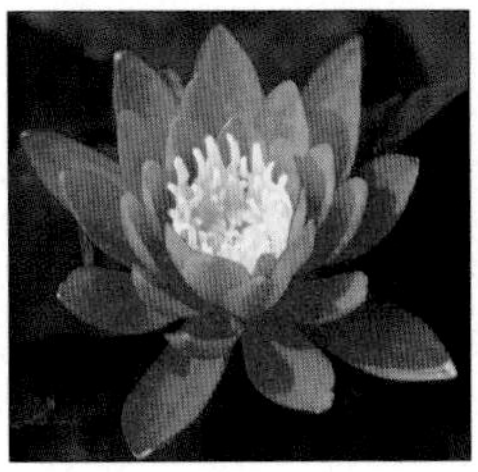

Nymphaea 'Firecrest'

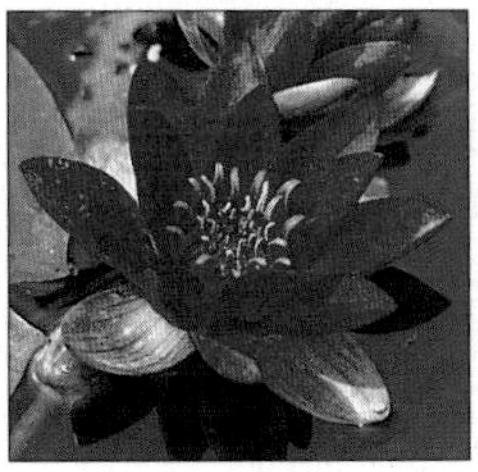

Nymphaea 'Fulgens'

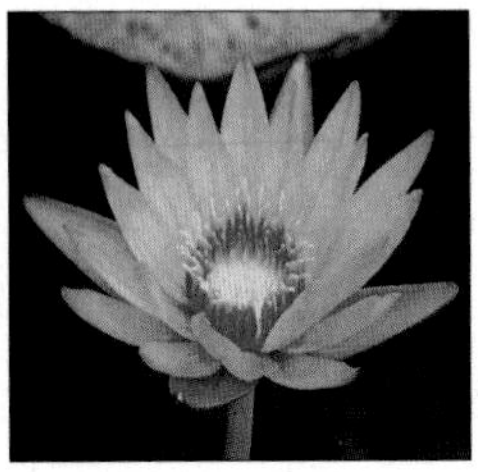

Nymphaea 'General Pershing'

green leaves, 27–30cm (11–12in) across, with toothed margins along the overlapping lobes, and bronzed when young. Star-shaped white flowers, 12–17cm (5–7in) across, have yellow stamens. ↔ 1.5–2.5m (5–8ft). ❄❄❄
N. 'Gloriosa'. Aquatic perennial with broadly ovate, bronze-green leaves, 20–22cm (8–9in) long, with open sinuses; young leaves are light-purple with darker markings and have overlapping lobes. Cup-shaped to star-shaped, bright red flowers, 12cm (5in) across, have orange-red stamens. ↔ 1.5m (5ft). ❄❄❄
N. 'Gonnère' ■ 🏆 Aquatic perennial with rounded, light green leaves, 15–22cm (6–9in) across, with open sinuses; young leaves are bronzed. Globe-shaped, fragrant white flowers, 10–15cm (4–6in) across, have yellow stamens. ↔ 0.9–1.2m (3–4ft). ❄❄❄
N. 'Indiana'. Aquatic perennial with rounded, olive-green leaves, 12cm (5in) long, with open sinuses; young leaves are heavily marked with purplish green. Cup-shaped flowers, gradually flattening to 9–10cm (3½–4in) across, turn from apricot, through apricot-orange, to dark orange-red, and have orange stamens. ↔ 75cm (30in). ❄❄❄
N. 'James Brydon' ■ 🏆 Aquatic perennial with rounded, bronze-green leaves, 17cm (7in) across, with overlapping lobes; young leaves are purplish brown with dark purple markings. Cup-shaped, vivid rose-red flowers, 10–12cm (4–5in) across, have orange-red stamens. ↔ 0.9–1.2m (3–4ft). ❄❄❄
N. 'Laydekeri Fulgens' see *N.* 'Fulgens'.
N. lotus (Egyptian water lily). Aquatic perennial with rounded, toothed, dark green leaves, to 50cm (20in) across, softly hairy beneath, with wavy margins and overlapping nodes. Bears day- or night-blooming, star-shaped, pink-tinged white flowers, to 25cm (10in) across. ↔ 2–3m (6–10ft). Egypt to tropical and S.E. Africa. ❁ (min. 10°C/50°F)
N. 'Louise'. Aquatic perennial with rounded, mid-green leaves, 22–25cm (9–10in) across, with open sinuses; young leaves are slightly bronzed. Cup-shaped, sweetly fragrant red flowers, 15cm (6in) across, have dark yellow stamens. ↔ 1.2–1.5m (4–5ft). ❄❄❄

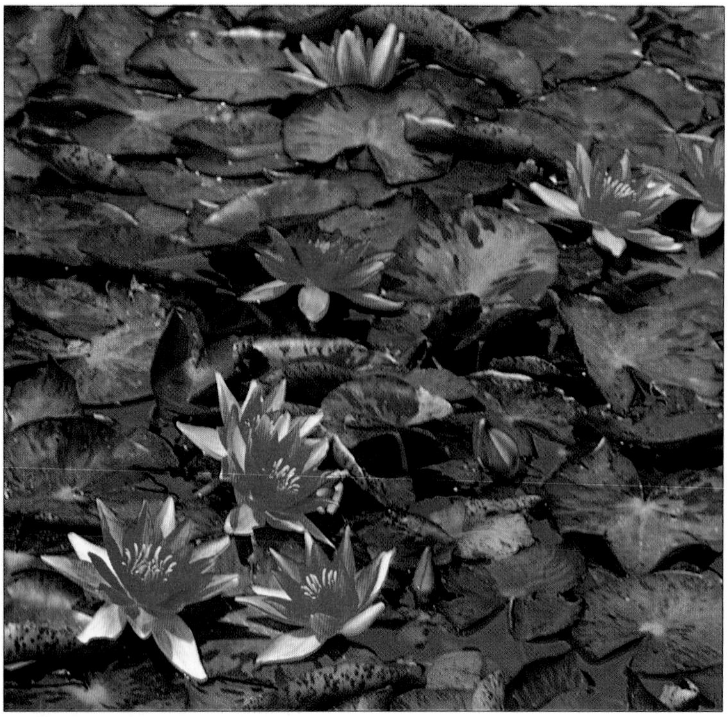
Nymphaea 'Lucida'

N. 'Lucida' ■ Aquatic perennial with broadly ovate, mid-green leaves, to 25cm (10in) long, with large purple markings and open sinuses. Star-shaped flowers, 12–15cm (5–6in) across, have red inner petals, pink-veined, whitish pink outer petals, and yellow stamens. ↔ 1.2–1.5m (4–5ft). ❄❄❄
N. 'Marliacea Albida' see *N.* 'Albida'.
N. 'Marliacea Carnea' see *N.* 'Carnea'.
N. 'Marliacea Chromatella' see *N.* 'Chromatella'.
N. mexicana, syn. *N. flava* (Yellow water lily). Aquatic perennial with ovate to rounded, wavy, toothed, leathery, mid-green leaves, to 18cm (7in) across, with brown marks above, purple beneath, and with open sinuses and overlapping lobes. Bears both floating and aerial, day-blooming, cup-shaped, later star-shaped, slightly fragrant, pale to bright yellow flowers, to 13cm (5in) across. ↔ 2–3m (6–10ft). S. USA, Mexico. ❁ (min. 10°C/50°F)
N. 'Mme Wilfon Gonnère'. Aquatic perennial with rounded leaves, 23–25cm (9–10in) across, with overlapping lobes, slightly bronzed when young, maturing to mid-green; each has a broad yellow stripe in spring that disappears in summer. Peony-like pink flowers, 12cm (5in) across, have light pink outer petals and gold stamens. ↔ 1.2m (4ft). ❄❄❄
N. odorata. Aquatic perennial with ovate to rounded, leathery, glossy, mid-green leaves, 15–30cm (6–12in) across, with open sinuses. Day-blooming, cup-shaped or later star-shaped, fragrant white flowers, 10–22cm (4–9in) across, have yellow stamens. ↔ 1.2–1.8m (4–6ft). N.E. USA. ❄❄❄. **'Sulphurea'** has purple-marked, bronze-green leaves, and fragrant yellow flowers, held slightly above the water. ↔ 0.9–1.2m (3–4ft). **'Sulphurea Grandiflora'** ■ is similar to 'Sulphurea', with marbled, dark green leaves and very large, star-shaped, bright rich yellow flowers. **'Turicensis'** has rounded leaves, 12–15cm (5–6in) across, with rounded lobes and open sinuses, and bears star-shaped, fragrant, soft pink flowers; ↔ 70cm (28in).

N. 'Paul Hariot'. Aquatic perennial with oval leaves, 15–17cm (6–7in) long, with rounded tips to the lobes and open sinuses; leaves are olive-green and purple-speckled when young, maturing to dark green with irregular purple marks. Cup-shaped flowers, 10–12cm (4–5in) across, are creamy apricot, turning light pink, and have orange stamens. ↔ 0.9–1.2m (3–4ft). ❄❄❄
N. 'Pearl of the Pool' ■ Aquatic perennial with rounded, deep green leaves, 25cm (10in) across, with lobes sometimes overlapping and raised, bronzed when young. Star-shaped, fragrant pink flowers, 12–15cm (5–6in) across, have pinkish orange stamens. ↔ 1.2–1.5m (4–5ft). ❄❄❄
N. 'Pink Sensation' ■ Aquatic perennial with rounded, mid-green leaves, to 25cm (10in) across, with narrow sinuses; young leaves are purple-green. Cup-shaped, later star-shaped pink flowers, 12–15cm (5–6in) across, have yellow inner stamens and pink outer stamens. ↔ 1.2m (4ft). ❄❄❄
N. pygmaea see *N. tetragona.*
N. 'Radiant Red'. Aquatic perennial with rounded, mid-green leaves, to 25cm (10in) across, with partly open sinuses. Star-shaped red flowers, 12–15cm (5–6in) across, have long, flecked petals and orange stamens. ↔ 0.9–1.2m (3–4ft). ❄❄❄
N. 'Red Flare'. Aquatic perennial with rounded, heavily toothed, reddish bronze leaves, 25–30cm (10–12in) across, with wavy margins and open sinuses. Night-blooming, flat, dark red flowers, 17–25cm (7–10in) across, have light pink or yellowish stamens and are held well above the water. ↔ 1.5–1.8m (5–6ft). ❁ (min. 10°C/50°F)
N. 'Rembrandt'. Aquatic perennial with rounded, mid-green leaves, 22–25cm (9–10in) across, with open sinuses; young leaves are purplish green. Bears peony-like red flowers, 15–20cm (6–8in) across, with yellow stamens. ↔ 70–120cm (28in–48in). ❄❄❄
N. 'René Gérard' ■ Aquatic perennial with rounded, mid-green leaves, to 25–27cm (10–11in) across, bronzed when young, with partly open sinuses. Star-shaped, rosy-red flowers, 15–22cm (6–9in) across, have strongly flecked, paler outer petals and yellow stamens. ↔ 1.5m (5ft). ❄❄❄

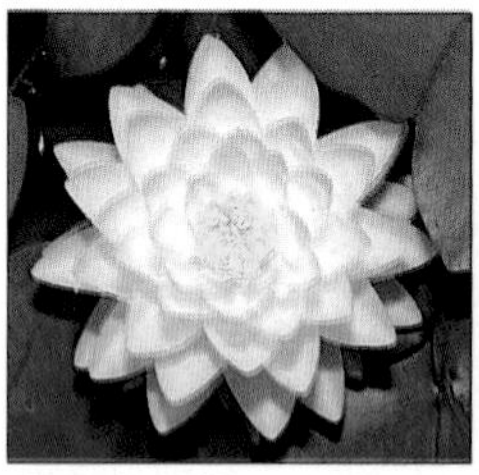
Nymphaea 'Gonnère'

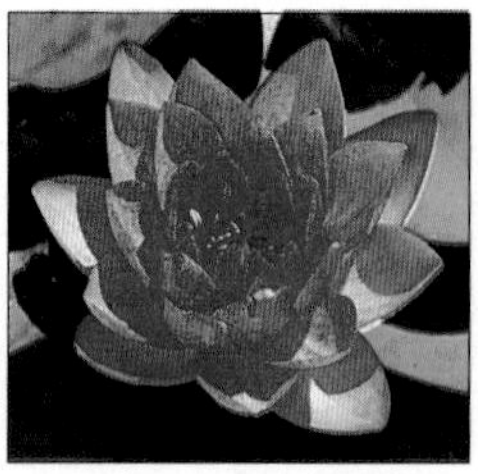
Nymphaea 'James Brydon'

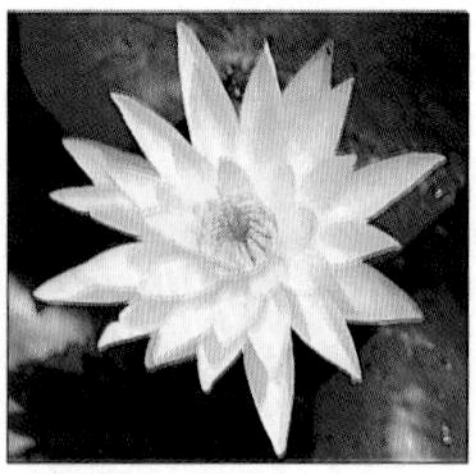
Nymphaea odorata 'Sulphurea Grandiflora'

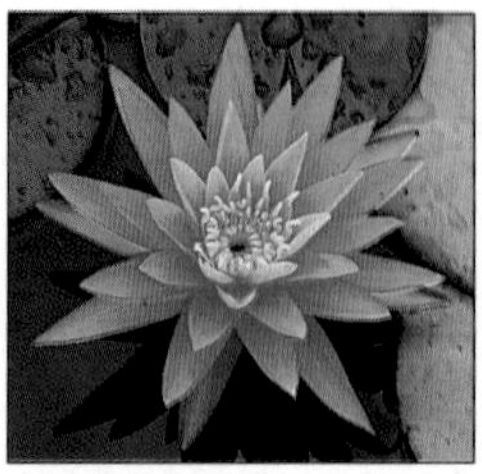
Nymphaea 'Pearl of the Pool'

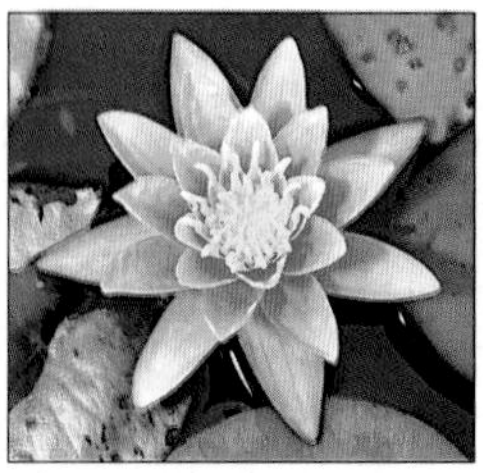
Nymphaea 'Pink Sensation'

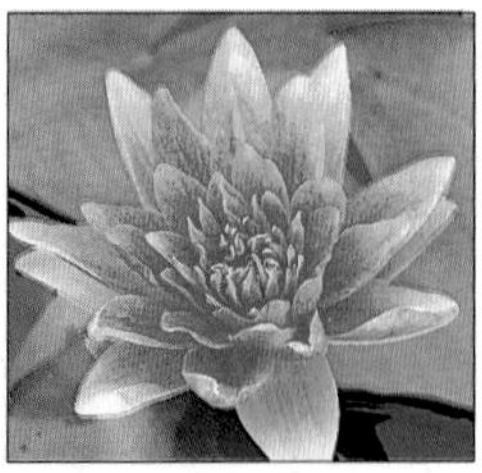
Nymphaea 'René Gérard'

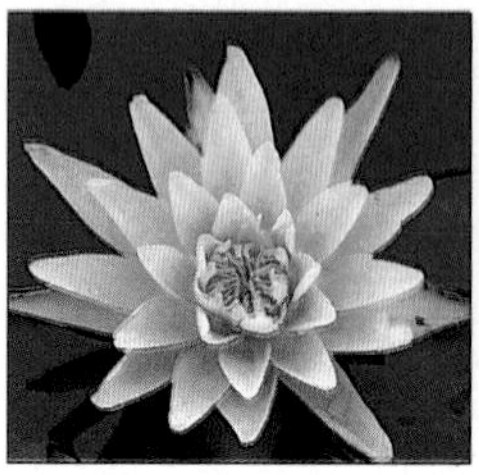
Nymphaea 'Rose Arey'

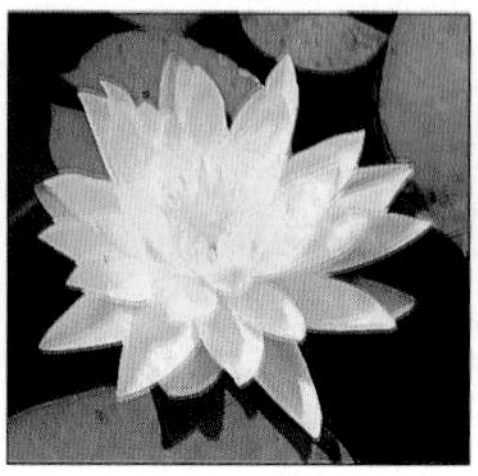
Nymphaea 'Sunrise'

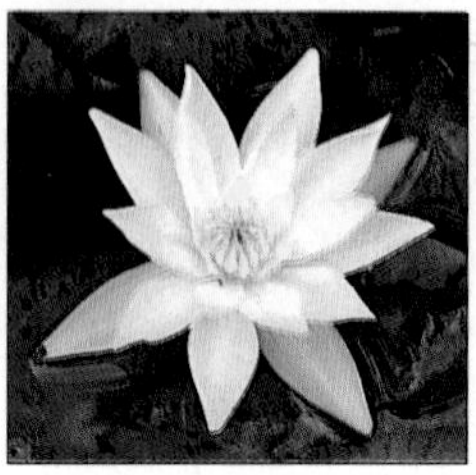
Nymphaea tetragona

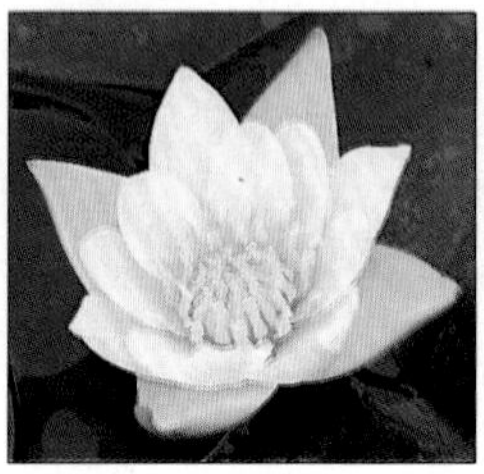
Nymphaea tetragona 'Helvola'

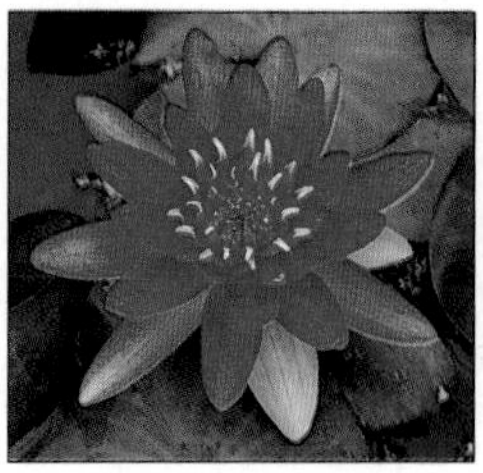
Nymphaea 'Vésuve'

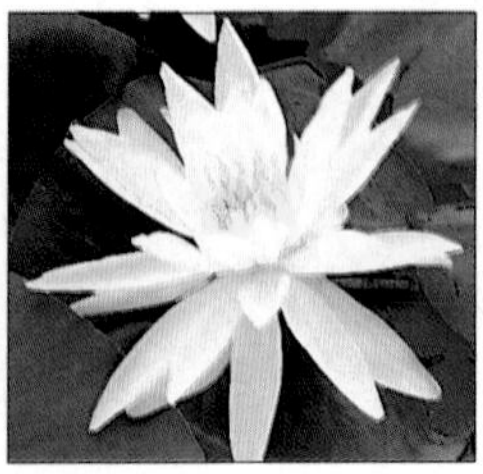
Nymphaea 'Virginalis'

***N.* 'Rose Arey'** ■ Aquatic perennial with rounded, bronze-green leaves, 22cm (9in) across, purple when young, with narrow sinuses. Bears star-shaped, fragrant, deep rose-pink flowers, 17–20cm (7–8in) across, orange-pink toward the margins, with golden stamens. ↔ 1.2–1.5m (4–5ft). ❄❄❄
***N.* 'St. Louis'.** Aquatic perennial with broadly ovate, light green leaves, to 50cm (20in) long, sometimes with wavy margins, purple-marked when young, with open sinuses. Day-blooming, star-shaped, fragrant, lemon-yellow flowers, 20–27cm (8–11in) across, have golden yellow stamens. ↔ 2.5–3m (8–10ft). ❀ (min. 10°C/50°F)
***N.* 'Sunrise'** ■ Aquatic perennial with broadly ovate, dark green leaves, 27cm (11in) long, with open sinuses; young leaves have purple mottling. Bears star-shaped, bright yellow flowers, 17–23cm (7–9in) across, with long, narrow petals and yellow stamens. ↔ 1.2–1.5m (4–5ft). ❄❄
N. tetragona ■ syn. *N. pygmaea.* Aquatic perennial with ovate, dark green, purple-blotched leaves, to 8cm (3in) across, with open sinuses. Day-blooming, cup-shaped, slightly fragrant flowers, 2.5–5cm (1–2in) across, are white with yellow stamens. ↔ 25–40cm (10–16in). N.E. Europe, N. Asia to Japan, N. America. ❄❄. **'Helvola'** ■ has heavily mottled, purple-marked leaves, 12cm (5in) long. Slightly fragrant, vivid yellow flowers, 5–7cm (2–3in) across, have orange-yellow stamens and become star-shaped.
N. tuberosa. Aquatic perennial with rounded, bright green leaves, 10–40cm (4–16in) across, with open sinuses. Day-blooming, cup-shaped, slightly scented white flowers, 10–22cm (4–9in) across, with yellow stamens, are sometimes held 5–8cm (2–3in) above the water. N.E. USA. ↔ to 2.2m (7ft). ❄❄. **'Richardsonii'** has mid-green leaves, 40cm (16in) across, with overlapping lobes. Peony-like white flowers have yellow stamens. ❄❄❄
***N.* 'Vésuve'** ■ Aquatic perennial with rounded, mid-green leaves, 22–25cm (9–10in) across, with open sinuses. Star-shaped, fragrant red flowers, 17cm (7in) across, darkening with age, have inward-curving petals and orange-red stamens. ↔ 1.2m (4ft). ❄❄❄
***N.* 'Virginalis'** ■ Aquatic perennial with rounded, pale green leaves, 22cm (9in) across, purple or bronze when young, with overlapping lobes. Star-shaped, fragrant white flowers, 11–14cm (4½–5½in) across, have yellow stamens. ↔ 0.9–1.2m (3–4ft). ❄❄❄
***N.* 'Virginia'.** Aquatic perennial with ovate, mid-green leaves, 25cm (10in) long, heavily marked with purple, mainly at the margins of older leaves, with open sinuses. Star-shaped, fragrant flowers, 17–20cm (7–8in) across, pale yellow in the centres and off-white towards the outsides, have yellow stamens. ↔ 1.5–1.8m (5–6ft). ❄❄❄
***N.* 'Wood's White Knight'.** Aquatic perennial bearing rounded, mid-green leaves, 30–40cm (12–16in) across, with scalloped, wavy margins and open sinuses. Produces night-blooming, peony-like, fragrant white flowers, 25–30cm (10–12in) across, with yellow stamens. ↔ 2.5–3m (8–10ft). ❀ (min. 10°C/50°F)

NYMPHOIDES

Floating heart

MENYANTHACEAE

Genus of 20 species of rhizomatous, herbaceous, submerged aquatic perennials occurring worldwide. They are often found in shallow, still water in lakes and ponds, where they spread rapidly, the leaves forming a floating carpet. Leaves are rounded with heart-shaped bases, or kidney-shaped, and grow from thin, creeping, branched rhizomes. The yellow or white, fringed flowers, resembling miniature water lilies (*Nymphaea*), are held above the surface of the water. Grow in a wildlife pool with water lilies or *Nuphar* species. In frost-prone areas, grow tender species in a greenhouse pool or aquarium.

- **HARDINESS** Fully hardy to frost tender.
- **CULTIVATION** Outdoors, grow hardy species, and tender species in frost-free areas, in water no deeper than 60cm (2ft). In a small pool, contain within an aquatic planting basket; in a larger pool or lake, growth is limited to the shallow margins. In frost-prone areas, grow tender species in an inert medium in a large aquarium or indoor pool in full light; most are tolerant of a range of water qualities. See also pp.52–53.
- **PROPAGATION** Separate runners during summer.
- **PESTS AND DISEASES** Trouble free.

N. humboldtiana. Rhizomatous, aquatic perennial with spreading runners and kidney-shaped, shiny, pale green leaves, 15cm (6in) across, reddish green beneath, borne on stalks to 1m (3ft) long. In summer, bears funnel-shaped white flowers, to 4cm (1½in) across, with fringed petals. ↔ indefinite. Mexico, West Indies, Central America and tropical South America. ❀ (min. 5°C/41°F)
N. indica (Water snowflake). Rhizomatous, aquatic perennial bearing rounded, glossy, pale green leaves, 5–20cm (2–8in) across, with heart-shaped bases. In summer, bears funnel-shaped white flowers, to 2cm (¾in) across, with yellow centres, and fringed petals covered with hairy white glands. ↔ indefinite. Tropical regions worldwide. ❀ (min. 5°C/41°F)
N. peltata ■ syn. *Limnanthemum nymphoides, L. peltatum, Villarsia nymphoides* (Water fringe, Yellow floating heart). Rhizomatous, aquatic perennial with runners, to 2m (6ft) long, bearing ovate to rounded, mottled, bright mid-green leaves, 5–10cm (2–4in) across. Funnel-shaped, bright golden yellow flowers, 2cm (¾in) across, are produced on long stalks in summer. It is the only species regularly grown outdoors in frost-prone areas. ↔ indefinite. Europe, Asia. ❄❄❄

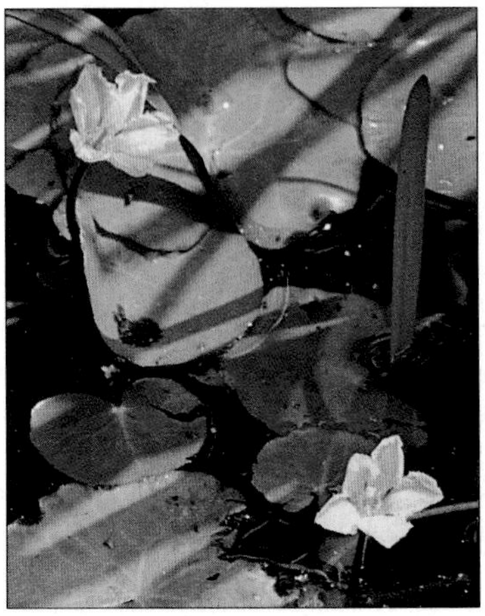

Nymphoides peltata

NYSSA

Tupelo

CORNACEAE/NYSSACEAE

Genus of about 5 species of deciduous trees from woodland and swampland in E. Asia and E. North America. Leaves are simple and alternate. Small, inconspicuous green flowers, borne in clusters in early summer, are followed by small, ovoid blue fruits, about 1cm (½in) long. Grown for their attractive foliage and brilliant autumn colour, they are ideal as specimen trees or in group plantings, and are effective near water.

- **HARDINESS** Fully hardy, but do best in areas with hot summers.
- **CULTIVATION** Grow in fertile, moist but well-drained, neutral to acid soil in sun or partial shade, with shelter from cold, dry winds. Plant as small plants, to 30cm (12in) tall, from containers; it is difficult to transplant them successfully. Pruning group 1; in cool-maritime climates, if it is difficult to maintain a leader, grow as multi-stemmed trees.
- **PROPAGATION** Sow seed in a seedbed in autumn. Take greenwood cuttings in early summer, or semi-ripe cuttings in midsummer.
- **PESTS AND DISEASES** Trouble free.

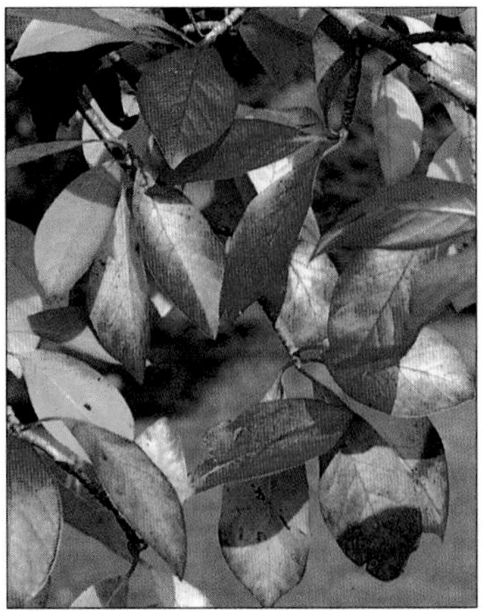

Nyssa sylvatica

N. sinensis ■ ♀ △–▽ (Chinese tupelo). Broadly conical, deciduous tree, sometimes with several stems. Oblong to elliptic, entire, slenderly tapered, dark green leaves, to 20cm (8in) long, are sparsely hairy and bronze-red when young, turning brilliant shades of orange, red, and yellow in autumn, and becoming nearly hairless when mature. ↕↔ 10m (30ft). C. China. ❄❄❄
N. sylvatica ■ △–▽ (Black gum, Sour gum, Tupelo). Broadly conical to columnar, deciduous tree with often drooping lower branches. Bears ovate to obovate, matt or glossy, dark green leaves, to 15cm (6in) long, downy beneath when young, with short, blunt points. Leaves turn vivid orange, yellow, or red in autumn. ↕ 20m (70ft), ↔ 10m (30ft). E. North America. ❄❄❄

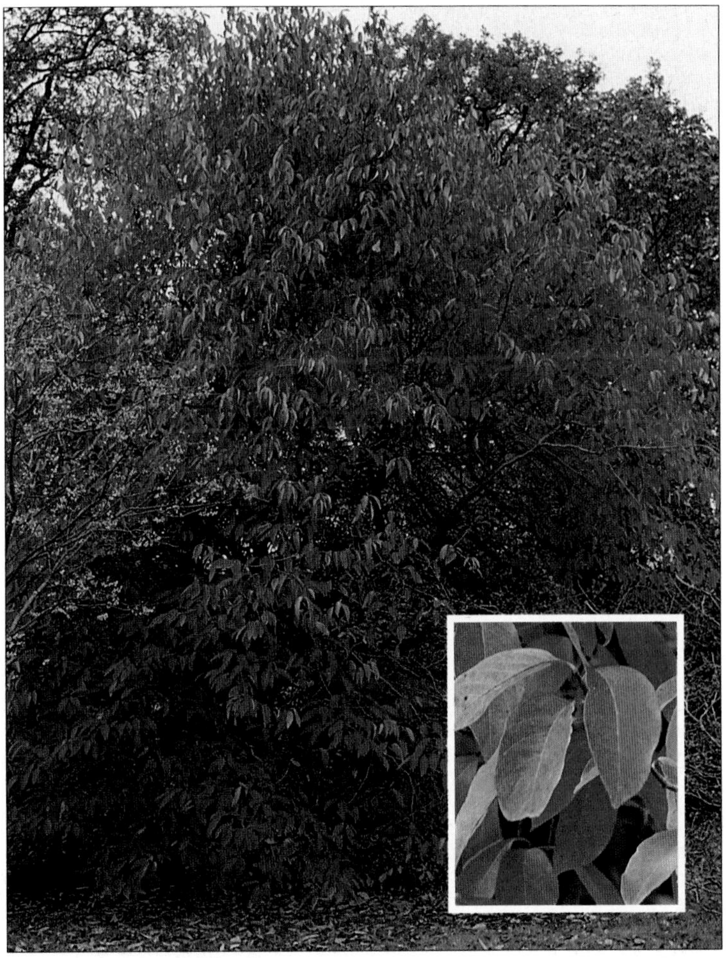

Nyssa sinensis (inset: leaf detail)

N

O

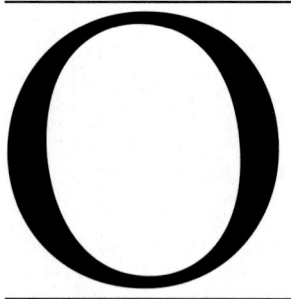

▷**Oak** see *Quercus*
American white see *Quercus alba*
Armenian see *Quercus pontica*
Black see *Quercus velutina*
Black Jack see *Quercus marilandica*
Californian black see *Quercus kelloggii*
Californian live see *Quercus agrifolia*
Canyon see *Quercus chrysolepis*
Chestnut-leaved see *Quercus castaneifolia*
Chinkapin see *Quercus muehlenbergii*
Common see *Quercus robur*
Cork see *Quercus suber*
Daimio see *Quercus dentata*
English see *Quercus robur*
Forest see *Casuarina torulosa*
Holm see *Quercus ilex*
Hungarian see *Quercus frainetto*
Kermes see *Quercus coccifera*
Lebanon see *Quercus libani*
Lucombe see *Quercus* x *hispanica* 'Lucombeana'
Mirbeck's see *Quercus canariensis*
Northern pin see *Quercus ellipsoidalis*
Oregon see *Quercus garryana*
Pedunculate see *Quercus robur*
Pin see *Quercus palustris*
Red see *Quercus rubra*
Scarlet see *Quercus coccinea*
Sessile see *Quercus petraea*
She see *Casuarina*
Shingle see *Quercus imbricaria*
Silky see *Grevillea robusta*
Swamp white see *Quercus bicolor*
Tanbark see *Lithocarpus densiflorus*
Turkey see *Quercus cerris*
Water see *Quercus nigra*
Willow see *Quercus phellos*
▷**Oat grass** see *Arrhenatherum*
Blue see *Helictotrichon sempervivens*
▷**Oats,**
Golden see *Stipa gigantea*
Sea see *Chasmanthium latifolium*
Water see *Zizania*
▷**Obedient plant** see *Physostegia, P. virginiana*

O

OBREGONIA

CACTACEAE

Genus of one species of low-growing, simple, sometimes clustering perennial cactus, closely related to *Ariocarpus*, found on periodically dry, rocky hillsides in N.E. Mexico. Its stems are covered by leaf-like, spirally arranged tubercles. Funnel-shaped flowers are produced from the woolly, depressed centre of each crown during daytime in summer; they are followed by white berries containing pear-shaped, slightly curved seeds. Below 10°C (50°F), grow in a temperate greenhouse; in warm, dry climates, use in a desert garden.
• **HARDINESS** Frost tender.

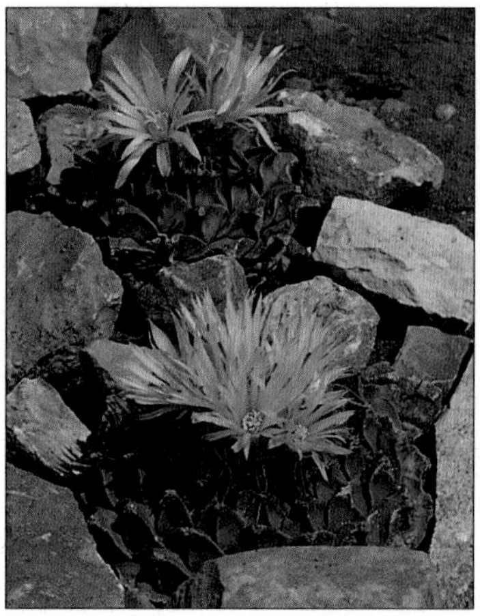

Obregonia denegrii

• **CULTIVATION** Under glass, grow in standard cactus compost in full light with shade from hot sun. From mid-spring to late summer, water moderately and apply a low-nitrogen liquid fertilizer every 4–5 weeks. In autumn, reduce water gradually, then keep completely dry until early spring. Outdoors, grow in sharply drained, neutral to slightly alkaline, gritty, poor, humus-rich soil in full sun. See also pp.48–49.
• **PROPAGATION** Sow seed at 21°C (70°F) in spring or summer.
• **PESTS AND DISEASES** Susceptible to aphids, especially while flowering.

O. denegrii ■ Perennial cactus with a thick, tuberous rootstock and flattened-spherical, greyish green or brownish green stems. Triangular tubercles have woolly hairs in the axils, and areoles at their tips, from which a few bristly spines emerge, but quickly fall. In summer, bears solitary, broadly funnel-shaped, very narrow-petalled, white or pale pink flowers, 2–3.5cm (¾–1½in) across, with yellow centres. ↕ 7–10cm (3–4in), ↔ 12cm (5in). N.E. Mexico. ❄ (min. 7–10°C/45–50°F)

▷**Ocean spray** see *Holodiscus discolor*

OCHAGAVIA

BROMELIACEAE

Genus of 3 species of evergreen, terrestrial perennials (bromeliads) found on exposed, coastal rock faces in Chile. They have almost stemless, spreading rosettes of stiff, spiny-toothed leaves. The spherical inflorescences, produced in summer, sit low in the centres of the rosettes and have conspicuous, narrow bracts and tubular, red or yellow flowers; these are followed by ovoid green berries containing large, spherical brown seeds. Where temperatures regularly drop below 5°C (41°F), grow in a cool greenhouse or as houseplants; in warmer climates, use outdoors in a desert garden.
• **HARDINESS** Frost tender; will sometimes withstand short periods at 0°C (32°F) in a sheltered site.
• **CULTIVATION** Under glass, grow in terrestrial bromeliad compost in full light with low humidity. In growth, water moderately with soft water (avoiding the crown), and apply a half-strength, low-nitrogen liquid fertilizer every 3–4 weeks; keep dry when dormant. Outdoors, grow in moderately

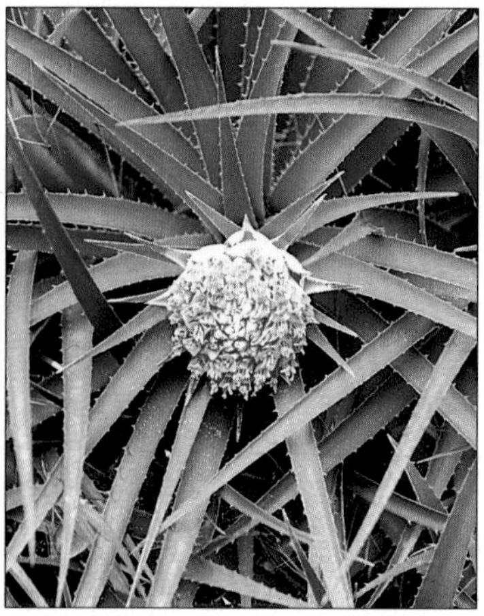

Ochagavia carnea

fertile, humus-rich, gritty, sharply drained soil in full sun. See also p.47.
• **PROPAGATION** Sow seed at 27°C (81°F) as soon as ripe.
• **PESTS AND DISEASES** Susceptible to scale insects.

O. carnea ■ syn. *O. lindleyana*. Terrestrial bromeliad with wide-spreading, dense rosettes of 30–50 stiff, very narrow, linear-lance-shaped, spiny-toothed leaves, 50cm (20in) long, tapering to pointed tips; they are bright dark green above, sometimes with grey-white scales, and densely covered with grey-white scales beneath. In summer, produces many tubular, rose-pink flowers, to 5cm (2in) long, in congested, short-stalked, spherical inflorescences, each with a collar of white and pink bracts. ↕↔ 60cm (24in). C. Chile. ❄ (min. 5°C/41°F)
O. lindleyana see *O. carnea*.

OCHNA

Bird's eye bush

OCHNACEAE

Genus of over 80 species of deciduous or semi-evergreen trees and shrubs from tropical woodland in Africa and Asia, grown for their flowers and fruits. The leathery, often shiny leaves are alternate, simple, and usually minutely toothed. The 5- to 10-petalled, saucer-shaped flowers are solitary, or borne in racemes, panicles, cymes, or umbels. After the petals fall, the calyces and receptacles enlarge and become thick and colourful, contrasting with the shiny, purplish black or black, usually spherical, one-

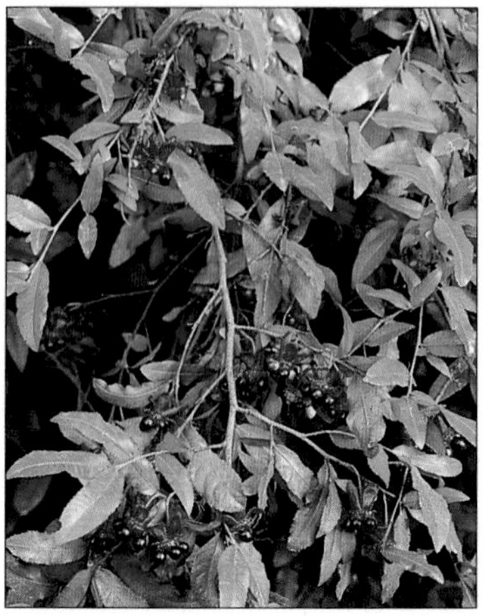

Ochna serrulata

seeded fruits, borne 3–12 on each receptacle. In frost-prone areas, grow in a conservatory or temperate greenhouse; elsewhere, use in a shrub border.
• **HARDINESS** Frost tender.
• **CULTIVATION** Under glass, grow in loam-based potting compost (JI No.3) in full light with shade from hot sun. In growth, water moderately and apply a balanced liquid fertilizer monthly; water sparingly in winter. Outdoors, grow in fertile, moist but well-drained soil in full sun. Pruning group 8; plants under glass need restrictive pruning after flowering.
• **PROPAGATION** Sow seed at 16°C (61°F) in spring. Root semi-ripe cuttings with bottom heat in summer, or air layer in spring.
• **PESTS AND DISEASES** Red spider mites may infest plants under glass.

O. multiflora see *O. serrulata*.
***O. serratifolia* of gardens** see *O. serrulata*.
O. serrulata ■ ◊ syn. *O. multiflora*, *O. serratifolia* of gardens (Mickey Mouse plant). Bushy, semi-evergreen shrub or small tree, with bronze shoots covered with close-set, raised, corky dots. Shiny, bright green leaves, 6cm (2½in) long, are narrowly elliptic and finely toothed. Saucer-shaped flowers, to 2cm (¾in) across, each with 5 or 6 spreading, bright yellow petals, are borne singly or in small cymes, mainly in late spring and summer; after the petals fall, the receptacle and sepals turn glossy red. Produces pendent clusters of 5 or 6 spherical, lustrous black fruit. ↕ 1.5–2.5m (5–8ft), ↔ 1–2m (3–6ft). South Africa. ❄ (min. 7°C/45°F)

OCIMUM

LABIATAE/LAMIACEAE

Genus of 35 species of aromatic annuals and evergreen perennials and shrubs occurring in hot, dry scrub in tropical Africa and Asia. They have erect, usually branching stems, with linear to almost rounded leaves, borne in opposite pairs. The tubular flowers, usually in whorls of 6, are arranged in loose or dense spikes, and have small to large, occasionally brightly coloured bracts. Most species and cultivars have medicinal or culinary uses; *O. basilicum* (basil) and its cultivars are grown as culinary herbs. Grow as annuals in a herb or vegetable garden.
• **HARDINESS** Half hardy to frost tender.
• **CULTIVATION** Grow in light, fertile, well-drained soil in a warm, sheltered site in full sun. Water freely during dry periods in summer. Pinch out flower-heads as soon as they appear, to ensure continued leaf growth.
• **PROPAGATION** Sow seed at 13°C (55°F) in early spring, or sow *in situ* in early summer.
• **PESTS AND DISEASES** May be infested with aphids, and sometimes affected by mildew in hot, dry summers.

O. basilicum (Basil, Sweet basil). Erect, bushy, aromatic annual or short-lived perennial. Narrowly oval to elliptic leaves, to 5cm (2in) long, are entire or toothed, sometimes slightly hairy, and bright green, occasionally flushed deep purple. Produces whorls of 6 tubular, 2- lipped, sometimes pink-purple-tinged, white flowers, to 1cm (½in) long, in lax, slightly hairy spikes in

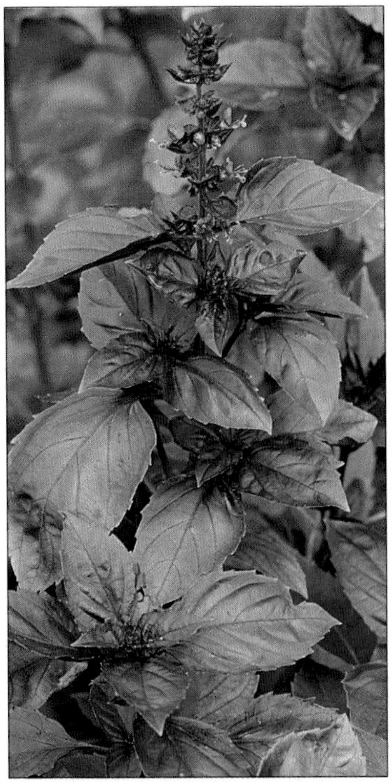

Ocimum basilicum 'Dark Opal'

late summer. ↕30–60cm (12–24in), ↔30cm (12in) if grown as an annual. Tropical and subtropical Asia; widely grown in similar, and Mediterranean climates. ✲. **'Dark Opal'** ■ has red-purple leaves and pink flowers. **var. *minimum*** (Greek bush basil) is compact and rounded, bearing ovate leaves, less than 1cm (½in) long, and flowers 2–3mm (1/16–⅛in) long; ↕↔15–30cm (6–12in). **'Purple Ruffles'** has purple leaves, curled and fringed at the margins.

▷**Oconee bells** see *Shortia galacifolia*
▷**Ocotillo** see *Fouquieria splendens*
▷**Octopus tree** see *Schefflera actinophylla*

x ODONTIODA

ORCHIDACEAE

Hybrid genus of epiphytic, evergreen orchids derived from crosses between *Odontoglossum* and *Cochlioda*; they are vegetatively indistinguishable from *Odontoglossum*. They have ovoid, compressed pseudobulbs, each with 2 linear, mid-green leaves, 20cm (8in) long, at the tip. Erect to arching racemes, 30–45cm (12–18in) tall, of 12 or more rounded to star-shaped flowers, 8cm (3in) across, often with ruffled or crisped margins, arise from the bases of the pseudobulbs at almost any time of the year, most commonly in spring. The flowers range in colour from pastel shades to deep reds, and are often spotted or marked red or yellow.

- **HARDINESS** Frost tender.
- **CULTIVATION** As *Odontoglossum*.
- **PROPAGATION** Divide when the plant fills the pot and "flows" over the sides.
- **PESTS AND DISEASES** Susceptible to red spider mites, aphids, and mealybugs.

x *O.* City of Birmingham (x *O.* Gold Wood x *Odontoglossum harryanum*). Epiphytic orchid with yellow flowers marked purple and bronze. ↕45cm (18in), ↔30cm (12in). ❀ (min. 10°C/50°F; max. 24°C/75°F)
x *O.* Durham Castle 'Lyoth Supreme' (x *O.* Ingmar x x *O.* Trixon). Epiphytic orchid producing brilliantly coloured flowers in rich red and mauve shades. ↕45cm (18in), ↔30cm (12in). ❀ (min. 10°C/50°F; max. 24°C/75°F)
x *O.* Eric Young (x *O.* Golden Rialto x *Odontoglossum* Niamalto). Epiphytic orchid producing light yellow flowers, spotted with deeper yellow. ↕45cm (18in), ↔30cm (12in). ❀ (min. 10°C/50°F; max. 24°C/75°F)
x *O.* Le Nez Point (x *O.* Brocade x x *O.* Trixon). Epiphytic orchid with solid, dark red flowers. ↕45cm (18in), ↔30cm (12in). ❀ (min. 10°C/50°F; max. 24°C/75°F)
x *O.* Mount Bingham ■ (x *O.* Ingera x x *O.* Marzorka). Epiphytic orchid with flowers patterned in red and lilac. ↕45cm (18in), ↔30cm (12in). ❀ (min. 10°C/50°F; max. 24°C/75°F)
x *O.* Petit Port ■ (x *O.* Colwell x x *O.* Margia). Epiphytic orchid bearing rich red flowers with pink-, yellow-, or brown-patterned lips. ↕45cm (18in), ↔30cm (12in). ❀ (min. 10°C/50°F; max. 24°C/75°F)
x *O.* Red Rum (x *O.* Brocade x x *O.* Ingera). Epiphytic orchid with flowers richly patterned in red-mauve and purple. ↕45cm (18in), ↔30cm (12in). ❀ (min. 10°C/50°F; max. 24°C/75°F)

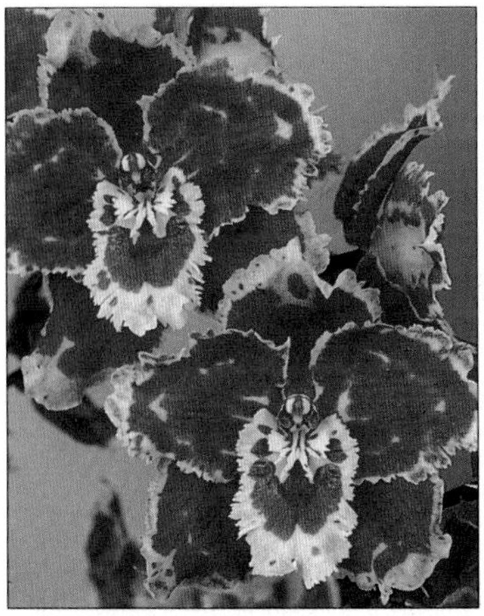

x *Odontioda* Mount Bingham

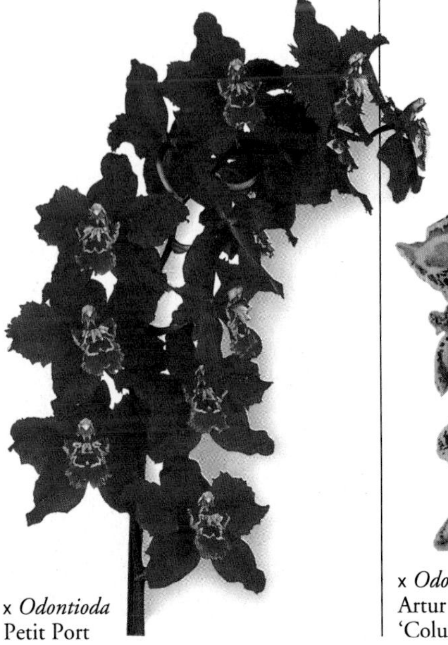

x *Odontioda* Petit Port

x ODONTOCIDIUM

ORCHIDACEAE

Hybrid genus of epiphytic, evergreen orchids derived from crosses between *Odontoglossum* and *Oncidium*; they are vegetatively indistinguishable from *Odontoglossum*. They have rounded or ovoid to conical pseudobulbs (all those described are rounded and compressed), each with 2 linear, mid-green leaves, 23cm (9in) long, at the tip. Tall, arching racemes or panicles of 12 or more flowers, 8cm (3in) across, arise from the base. The predominantly yellow, yellow-brown, or russet-red flowers have large, flared lips.

- **HARDINESS** Frost tender.
- **CULTIVATION** As *Odontoglossum*.
- **PROPAGATION** Divide when the plants overflow their containers.
- **PESTS AND DISEASES** Prone to red spider mites, aphids, and mealybugs.

x *O.* Artur Elle 'Columbien' ■ (*Odontoglossum* Hambühren Gold x *Oncidium tigrinum*). Epiphytic orchid bearing yellow flowers, delicately patterned with chestnut-brown, all year round. ↕45cm (18in), ↔30cm (12in). ❀ (min. 10°C/50°F; max. 24°C/75°F)
x *O.* 'Crowborough' (*Odontoglossum* Golden Guinea x *Oncidium leucochilum*). Epiphytic orchid bearing deep brown and yellow flowers with white lips, mainly in spring. ↕45cm (18in), ↔30cm (12in). ❀ (min. 10°C/50°F; max. 24°C/75°F)
x *O.* 'Purbeck Gold' (*Odontoglossum* Gold Cup x *Oncidium tigrinum*). Epiphytic orchid bearing deep yellow, brown-spotted flowers, with flared yellow lips, mainly in autumn. ↕45cm (18in), ↔30cm (12in). ❀ (min. 10°C/50°F; max. 24°C/75°F)
x *O.* Tiger Hambühren ■ (*Odontoglossum* Goldrausch x *Oncidium tigrinum*). Epiphytic orchid bearing rich yellow flowers, heavily spotted and barred with chestnut-brown, mainly in autumn. ↕45cm (18in), ↔30cm (12in). ❀ (min. 10°C/50°F; max. 24°C/75°F)
x *O.* Tigersun 'Orbec' ■ (*Odontoglossum* Sunmar x *Oncidium tigrinum*). Epiphytic orchid bearing yellow flowers, lightly marked with chestnut-brown, mainly in autumn. ↕45cm (18in), ↔30cm (12in). ❀ (min. 10°C/50°F; max. 24°C/75°F)

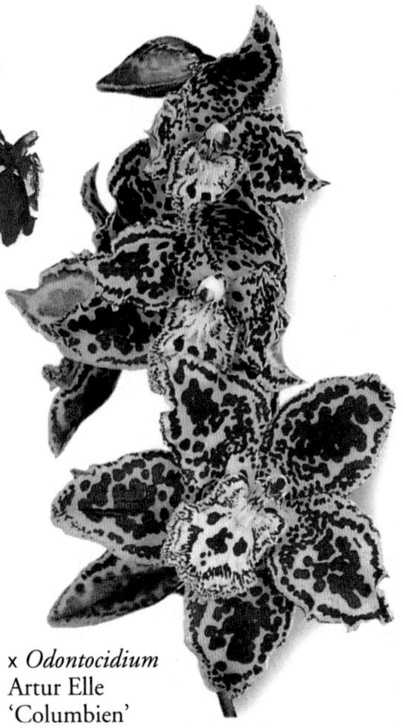

x *Odontocidium* Artur Elle 'Columbien'

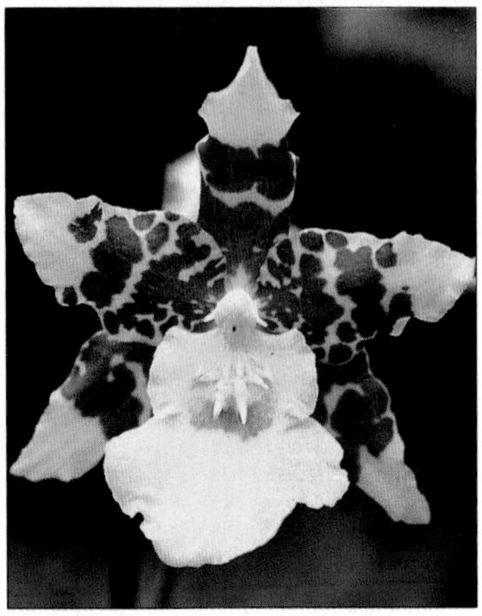

x *Odontocidium* Tiger Hambühren

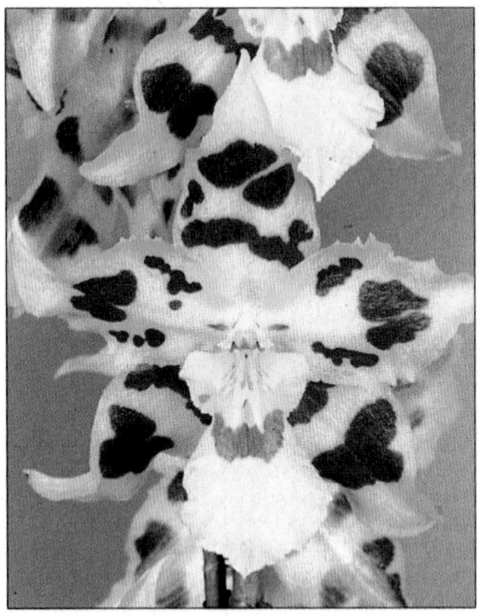

x *Odontocidium* Tigersun 'Orbec'

ODONTOGLOSSUM

ORCHIDACEAE

Genus of about 200 species of evergreen, epiphytic or lithophytic, rhizomatous orchids from mountainous regions, at altitudes of 2,000–3,000m (7,000–10,000ft), in Central and South America. They produce ovoid or oblong-ellipsoid to conical pseudobulbs, each with 1–3 variably shaped, thinly leathery, mid-green leaves at the tip. Flowers are borne in tall or short, erect or arching racemes or panicles arising from the bases of the pseudobulbs, and are highly variable in colour and shape. Many hybrids have been produced that will flower at almost any time of year, with 12 or more flowers in a raceme.

- **HARDINESS** Frost tender.
- **CULTIVATION** Cool-growing orchids. Grow in small pots of epiphytic orchid compost, preferably made with fine-grade bark to suit the fine root system. In summer, provide bright filtered light and high humidity; water and mist freely, and apply fertilizer at every third watering. In winter, provide full light and water sparingly. See also p.46.
- **PROPAGATION** Divide when the plant fills the pot and "flows" over the sides. Hybrids are better retained as one plant; pot on, in late summer or early spring.
- **PESTS AND DISEASES** Prone to red spider mites, aphids, and mealybugs.

O

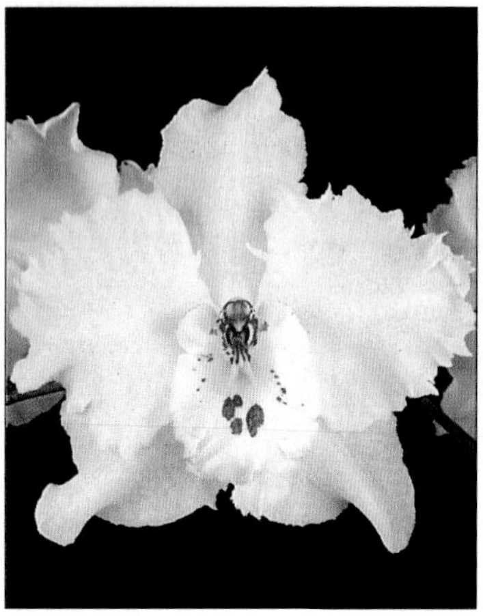

Odontoglossum crispum

O. bictoniense see *Lemboglossum bictoniense.*
O. **Buttercrisp** (*O.* Brimstone Butterfly x *O.* Crispania). Epiphytic orchid with ovoid, compressed pseudobulbs and narrowly oval leaves, 15cm (6in) long. Clear yellow flowers, 6cm (2½in) across, with a few brown spots and brown-spotted, white-margined lips, appear at any time of year. ↕ 30cm (12in), ↔ 25cm (10in). ❄ (min. 10°C/50°F; max. 24°C/75°F)
O. cariniferum. Epiphytic orchid with oblong-ellipsoid, compressed, furrowed pseudobulbs and oblong-elliptic leaves, to 30cm (12in) long. In spring, bears yellow-margined brown flowers, 5cm (2in) across, in erect or arching panicles, 0.6–1.2m (2–4ft) long. ↕ to 1.2m (4ft), ↔ 30cm (12in). Costa Rica, Panama, Colombia, Venezuela. ❄ (min. 10°C/50°F; max. 24°C/75°F)
O. cervantesii see *Lemboglossum cervantesii.*
O. cordatum see *Lemboglossum cordatum.*
O. crispum ■ Epiphytic orchid with ovoid pseudobulbs and linear-elliptic leaves, to 40cm (16in) long. In winter, white flowers, 8cm (3in) across, the lips sometimes yellow and spotted red in the centres, are produced in racemes to 50cm (20in) long. ↕ 50cm (20in), ↔ 25cm (10in). Colombia. ❄ (min. 10°C/50°F; max. 24°C/75°F)
O. grande see *Rossioglossum grande.*
O. harryanum. Epiphytic orchid with slender, ovoid pseudobulbs and elliptic-oblong leaves, to 45cm (18in) long. Flowers, 8cm (3in) across, varying from olive-green to buff or chestnut-brown, with lips lined purplish mauve, appear in racemes to 1–1.2m (3–4ft) long, in winter. ↕ 1–1.2m (3–4ft), ↔ 23cm (9in). Colombia, Peru. ❄ (min. 10°C/50°F; max. 24°C/75°F)
O. odoratum. Epiphytic orchid with ovoid pseudobulbs and narrowly lance-shaped leaves, to 30cm (12in) long. Star-shaped, fragrant flowers, 6cm (2½in) across, pale to deep yellow, dotted and marked dark maroon or red-brown, are produced in panicles to 75cm (30in) long, in spring. ↕ 75cm (30in), ↔ 20cm (8in). Colombia, Venezuela. ❄ (min. 10°C/50°F; max. 24°C/75°F)
O. rossii see *Lemboglossum rossii.*
O. **Royal Occasion** ■ (*O.* Ardentissimum x *O.* Pumistor). Epiphytic orchid with ovoid pseudobulbs and narrowly oval leaves, 30cm (12in) long. White flowers, 6cm (2½in) across, with deep yellow markings in the centres of the lips, are produced in early summer. ↕ 30cm (12in), ↔ 25cm (10in). ❄ (min. 10°C/50°F; max. 24°C/75°F)
O. **Saint Brelade 'Jersey'** (*Lemboglossum rossii* x *O.* Ophyras). Epiphytic orchid with ovoid pseudobulbs and narrowly oval leaves, 15cm (6in) long. Highly decorative, pale mauve flowers, 6cm (2½in) across, with deeper mauve or maroon markings and pale mauve lips marked with white and maroon, are produced in late spring. ↕ 30cm (12in), ↔ 25cm (10in). ❄ (min. 10°C/50°F; max. 24°C/75°F)
O. spectatissimum, syn. *O. triumphans.* Epiphytic orchid producing ovoid pseudobulbs and narrowly elliptic leaves, 40cm (16in) long. In spring, bears erect or arching racemes, to 90cm (36in) long, of golden yellow flowers, heavily barred and spotted chestnut-brown, 10cm (4in) across. ↕ 90cm (36in), ↔ 20cm (8in). Colombia, Venezuela. ❄ (min. 10°C/50°F; max. 24°C/75°F)
O. stellatum see *Lemboglossum stellatum.*
O. triumphans see *O. spectatissimum.*

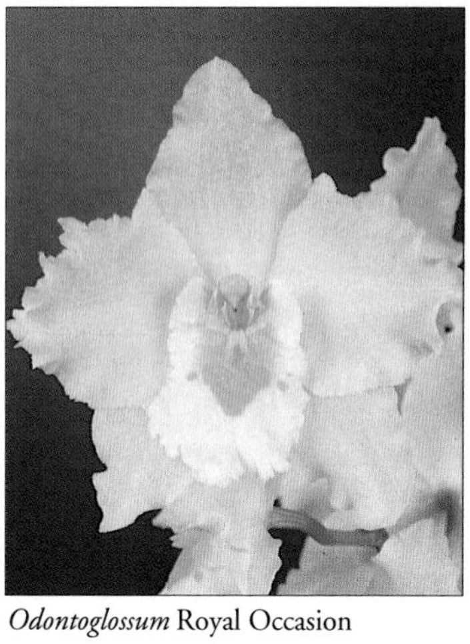

Odontoglossum Royal Occasion

ODONTONEMA

ACANTHACEAE

Genus of 26 species of evergreen perennials and shrubs from woodland in tropical America. They are grown for their terminal racemes or panicles of tubular, brightly coloured flowers, which are 2-lipped or symmetrical. The simple, entire leaves are borne in opposite pairs. Where temperatures fall below 13°C (55°F), grow in a warm greenhouse. In warmer climates, grow in a shrub border.
• **HARDINESS** Frost tender.
• **CULTIVATION** Under glass, grow in loam-based potting compost (JI No.3) in full light with shade from hot sun, and with moderate humidity. During the growing season, water moderately and apply a balanced liquid fertilizer every month; water sparingly in winter. Outdoors, grow in fertile, moist but well-drained soil in full sun. Pruning group 8; plants under glass need restrictive pruning after flowering.
• **PROPAGATION** Sow seed at 16–18°C (61–64°F) in spring. Root greenwood cuttings in early summer, or semi-ripe cuttings with bottom heat in summer.
• **PESTS AND DISEASES** Prone to whiteflies and red spider mites under glass.

O. strictum. Erect shrub, with robust, sparsely branched, rigid stems and oblong, wavy-margined, glossy, deep green leaves, 10–15cm (4–6in) long, with long, sharp points. In winter and spring, bears tubular, 2-lipped, waxy crimson flowers, 2.5cm (1in) long, in slender, erect, compact panicles, to 30cm (12in) long. ↕ 2m (6ft) or more (if unpruned), ↔ 60–100cm (24–39in). Central America. ❄ (min. 13°C/55°F)

x ODONTONIA

ORCHIDACEAE

Hybrid genus of epiphytic, evergreen orchids derived from crosses between *Odontoglossum* and *Miltonia*; they are vegetatively indistinguishable from *Odontoglossum.* They produce ovoid to conical pseudobulbs, each with 2 leaves at the tip. The flowers have large, flat lips and are produced in tall, arching racemes arising from the bases of the pseudobulbs at almost any time of year.
• **HARDINESS** Frost tender.
• **CULTIVATION** As *Odontoglossum.*
• **PROPAGATION** Divide when the plants overflow their containers.
• **PESTS AND DISEASES** Prone to red spider mites, aphids, and mealybugs.

x ***O.*** **Olga** (*Odontoglossum crispum* x x *Odontonia* Thisbe). Epiphytic orchid producing ovoid pseudobulbs and narrowly oval leaves, 30cm (12in) long. White flowers, 8cm (3in) across, with lips marked nut-brown, are borne in tall, arching racemes in winter. ↕ 30cm (12in), ↔ 25cm (10in). ❄ (min. 10°C/50°F; max. 24°C/75°F)

OEMLERIA *syn.* NUTTALLIA, OSMARONIA

ROSACEAE

Genus of one species of deciduous shrub found in forest and canyons in W. North America. It is grown for its simple, alternate, glossy leaves, and its pendent racemes of bell-shaped flowers, both of which appear very early in the year (it is one of the first plants to come into leaf, often in late winter). Male and female flowers are borne on separate plants and both must be grown to bear the small, black, plum-like fruit. Grow in a shrub border or woodland garden.
• **HARDINESS** Fully hardy.
• **CULTIVATION** Grow in fertile, moist but well-drained soil in sun or partial shade. In moist soil, vigorously growing plants may sucker extensively; remove excess suckers to restrict growth. Pruning group 1 or 2.
• **PROPAGATION** Sow seed in a seedbed as soon as ripe. Take greenwood cuttings in early summer. Transplant suckers in autumn.
• **PESTS AND DISEASES** May become chlorotic in shallow, chalky soil.

O. cerasiformis ■ syn. *Nuttallia cerasiformis, Osmaronia cerasiformis* (Indian plum, Oregon plum, Oso berry). Suckering shrub, forming a thicket of upright, eventually arching shoots. These bear narrowly oblong, or lance-shaped to inversely lance-shaped, glossy, dark green leaves, to 9cm (3½in) long, grey-green and softly hairy beneath. Small, bell-shaped, almond-scented

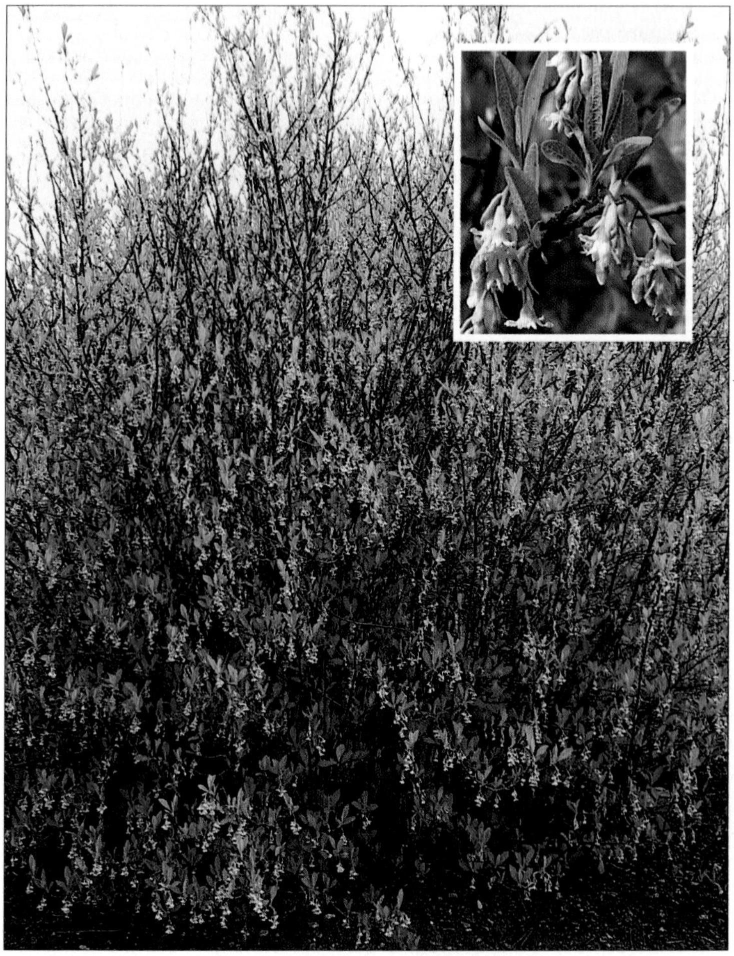

Oemleria cerasiformis (inset: flower detail)

white flowers are produced in pendent racemes, to 10cm (4in) long, in early spring. They are followed on female plants by ovoid, plum-like, purple-black fruit, 2cm (¾in) long. ↕ 2.5m (8ft) or more, ↔ 4m (12ft). W. North America (British Columbia to California). ❄❄❄

OENANTHE

APIACEAE/UMBELLIFERAE

Genus of about 30 species of moisture-loving, hairless perennials from wet meadows, marshland, and shallow water in the N. hemisphere, South Africa, and Australia. Most have alternate, pinnate leaves and bear compound umbels of small, star-shaped white flowers, each with 5 notched petals. They are suitable for damp soil in a bog garden, or for planting as ground cover near a stream or pool. In frost-prone areas, grow tender species in a cool greenhouse. In some species, all parts may cause severe discomfort if ingested; some species are deadly. *O. javanica* is the exception; it is grown as a vegetable in areas where it grows naturally.

• **HARDINESS** Fully hardy to frost tender; *O. javanica* often survives temperatures to -10°C (14°F).

• **CULTIVATION** Grow in any moderately fertile, preferably moist or wet soil, in full sun or partial shade, although quite dry soil is tolerated, especially in partial shade. Shelter from cold, drying winds. In frost-prone areas, provide a dry winter mulch; take cuttings and overwinter in a cold greenhouse to insure against losses.

• **PROPAGATION** Divide in late spring, as growth begins. Take stem-tip cuttings in spring.

• **PESTS AND DISEASES** Susceptible to aphids, and may be damaged by slugs and snails.

O. japonica see *O. javanica*.

O. javanica, syn. *O. japonica*. Spreading perennial with horizontal, rooting stems and celery-like, triangular, pinnate or 2-pinnate leaves, 7–15cm (3–6in) long, with narrowly ovate, toothed, mid-green segments. Compound umbels of star-shaped white flowers, 3mm (⅛in) long, are produced in late summer. ↕ 20–40cm (8–16in), ↔ 90cm (36in). India to Japan, Malaysia, Australia (Queensland). ❄❄. **'Flamingo'** ▣ is grown for its attractive foliage, which is variegated pink, cream, and white.

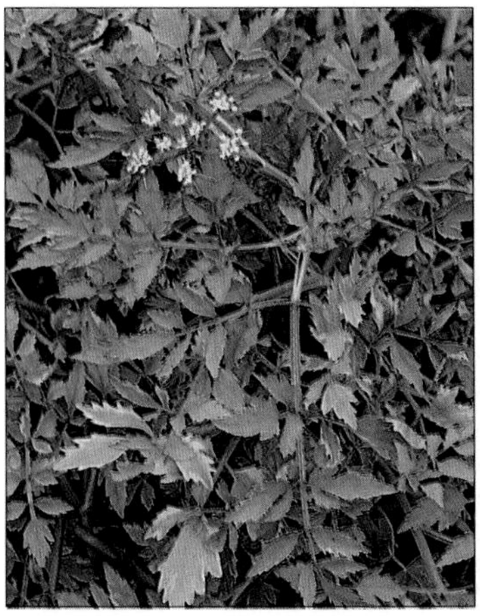

Oenanthe javanica 'Flamingo'

OENOTHERA

Evening primrose, Sundrops

ONAGRACEAE

Genus of about 125 species of annuals, biennials, and perennials, some with tap roots or fibrous roots and a few with rhizomes or runners. Mostly from North America, with a few from South America, they grow in well-drained, sunny sites, such as mountain slopes, although some are from deserts. They have upright or decumbent stems with alternate, more or less lance-shaped, simple or pinnatifid, entire or toothed stem leaves, and occasionally basal rosettes of slightly larger leaves. Evening primroses are grown for their flowers, which are mainly produced over long periods in summer; they are often fragrant, white, yellow, or pink and are large, saucer- to cup-shaped, sometimes trumpet-shaped. Each flower has a long tube and 4 petals, and is either solitary and axillary, or borne in terminal racemes. Individual flowers open at dawn or dusk and fade quickly. Taller species are suitable for a sunny, mixed or herbaceous border; low-growing ones are better for border edging. *O. acaulis*, *O. caespitosa*, and *O. macrocarpa* are excellent for a scree bed or rock garden.

• **HARDINESS** Fully hardy to frost hardy.

• **CULTIVATION** Grow in poor to moderately fertile, well-drained, even stony soil in full sun. *O. fruticosa* prefers slightly more fertile soil. Protect rock garden plants and *O. speciosa* from excessive winter wet.

• **PROPAGATION** Sow seed in containers in a cold frame: annuals and perennials in early spring, biennials in early summer; or sow annuals and biennials *in situ* in autumn. *O. glazioviana* self-seeds prolifically. Divide in early spring, or take softwood cuttings of unflowered shoots of perennials from late spring to midsummer. To avoid damage to tap-rooted species, grow on seedlings and cuttings individually in pots before planting out.

• **PESTS AND DISEASES** Prone to slugs, and sometimes affected by leaf spot and mildew. Root rot may be a problem in wet, heavy soil.

O. acaulis, syn. *O. taraxacifolia*. Clump-forming, short-lived perennial with rosettes of inversely lance-shaped, irregularly pinnatifid, mid-green leaves, 12–20cm (5–8in) long, and a few decumbent stems, to 30cm (12in) or more long. In summer, bears 2–5 trumpet-shaped white flowers, to 8cm (3in) across, from the leaf axils; they open at sunset, and turn pink next day. ↕ 15cm (6in), ↔ to 20cm (8in). Chile. ❄❄❄ (borderline)

O. albicaulis. Spreading annual, biennial, or short-lived perennial, usually grown as a biennial, with basal rosettes of spoon-shaped to ovate, grey-green leaves, to 5cm (2in) long, and white-hairy stems bearing lance-shaped, pinnatifid leaves. In summer, produces solitary, bowl-shaped, scented flowers, to 8cm (3in) across, which open in the evening and are initially white, then cream, and finally pale pink. ↕ 15–30cm (6–12in), ↔ to 30cm (12in). N. America (Rocky Mountains). ❄❄❄

O. berlandieri see *O. speciosa* 'Rosea'.

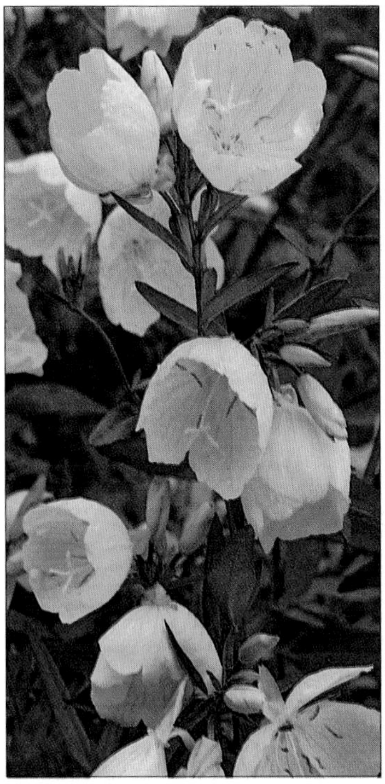

Oenothera fruticosa 'Fyrverkeri'

O. biennis (Evening primrose). Erect, hairy annual or biennial, usually grown as a biennial. Produces large rosettes of oblong to lance-shaped, shallowly toothed, slightly sticky, red-veined, mid-green leaves, 10–30cm (4–12in) long, and lance-shaped stem leaves, to 15cm (6in) long. Bowl-shaped, fragrant flowers, to 5cm (2in) across, initially pale yellow, ageing to dark golden yellow, and opening in the evening, are borne in leafy, spike-like racemes from summer to autumn. Seeds are used to produce evening primrose oil. ↕ 1–1.5m (3–5ft), ↔ to 60cm (24in). E. North America; naturalized in many parts of the world. ❄❄❄

O. caespitosa. Clump-forming biennial or perennial with numerous rosettes of inversely lance-shaped to diamond- or spoon-shaped, entire or irregularly toothed, grey-green leaves, 2–25cm (¾–10in) long. In summer, produces cup-shaped, fragrant white flowers, to 10cm (4in) across, from the rosette leaf axils, several opening at once at sunset; they turn pink with age. ↕↔ to 20cm (8in). W. USA. ❄❄❄

O. deltoides (Desert evening primrose). Erect annual or perennial, branching from the base, with triangularly ovate to lance-shaped, entire to pinnatifid, mid-green leaves, 5–10cm (2–4in) long. Often produces decumbent basal branches in addition to erect stems. In summer, bears solitary, bowl-shaped flowers, 4–8cm (1½–3in) across, initially white then pink, opening in the morning. Needs sharply drained soil. ↕ to 30cm (12in), ↔ to 20cm (8in). USA (Arizona), Mexico (Baja California). ❄❄

O. elata* subsp. *hookeri, syn. *O. hookeri*. Erect perennial or biennial bearing basal rosettes of lance-shaped, slightly toothed, mid-green leaves, 5–12cm (2–5in) long, and hairy, branching stems with smaller leaves. Throughout summer, bears numerous, cup-shaped flowers, 5–7cm (2–3in) across, initially pale yellow becoming orange-red, which open at dusk in terminal spikes. ↕ 90cm (36in), ↔ 30cm (12in). W. North America. ❄❄❄

O. fraseri see *O. fruticosa* subsp. *glauca*.

O. fruticosa, syn. *O. linearis* (Sundrops). Erect perennial or biennial with branched, softly hairy, red-tinged stems bearing lance-shaped to ovate, toothed, mid-green leaves, 2.5–11cm (1–4½in) long, the basal leaves inversely lance-shaped to obovate. From late spring to late summer, produces racemes of 3–10 saucer- to cup-shaped, deep yellow flowers, 2.5–5cm (1–2in) across, opening during the day. ↕ 30–90cm (12–36in), ↔ 30cm (12in). E. North America. ❄❄❄. **'Fireworks'** see 'Fyrverkeri'. **'Fyrverkeri'** ▣ 🏆 syn. 'Fireworks', has purple-brown-flushed leaves, and yellow flowers opening from red buds. **subsp. *glauca*** 🏆 syn. *O. fraseri*, *O. glauca*, *O. tetragona*, has broader, only sparsely hairy, sometimes glaucous leaves, red-tinted when young, and light yellow flowers; E. USA. **'Highlight'** see 'Hoheslicht'. **'Hoheslicht'**, syn. 'Highlight', produces an abundance of bright yellow flowers; ↕ 60cm (24in). **'Yellow River'** has red stems and large, canary-yellow flowers, 4–6cm (1½–2½in) across.

O. glauca see *O. fruticosa* subsp. *glauca*.

O. glazioviana, syn. *O. glazouana*. Erect biennial or short-lived perennial bearing basal rosettes of ovate-lance-shaped, hairy, mid-green leaves, to 20cm (8in) long, with conspicuous white midribs above, red beneath; slightly smaller leaves are borne on the hairy, unbranched, red-spotted stems. In mid- and late summer, produces racemes of bowl-shaped yellow flowers, 5–8cm (2–3in) across, with red-tinged calyces, opening at dusk. ↕ to 1.5m (5ft), ↔ 60cm (24in). N. America. ❄❄❄

O. glazouana see *O. glazioviana*.

O. hookeri see *O. elata* subsp. *hookeri*.

O. linearis see *O. fruticosa*.

O. macrocarpa ▣ 🏆 syn. *O. missouriensis* (Ozark sundrops). Vigorous perennial with trailing, hairy, often red-tinted stems, branching from a central rootstock. Leaves are lance-shaped to ovate, toothed, pale to mid-green, 2–8cm (¾–3in) long, with white midribs. From late spring to early autumn, produces a long succession of solitary, cup-shaped, bright golden yellow flowers, to 12cm (5in) across, with red-flecked calyces, remaining open in daytime. ↕ 15cm (6in), ↔ to 50cm (20in). S. Central USA. ❄❄❄

O. missouriensis see *O. macrocarpa*.

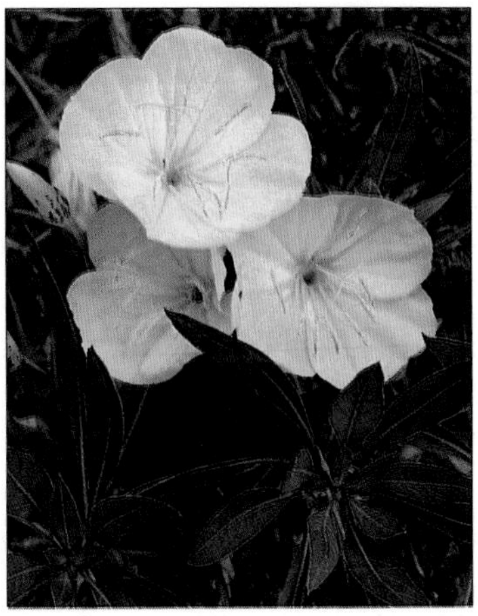

Oenothera macrocarpa

O

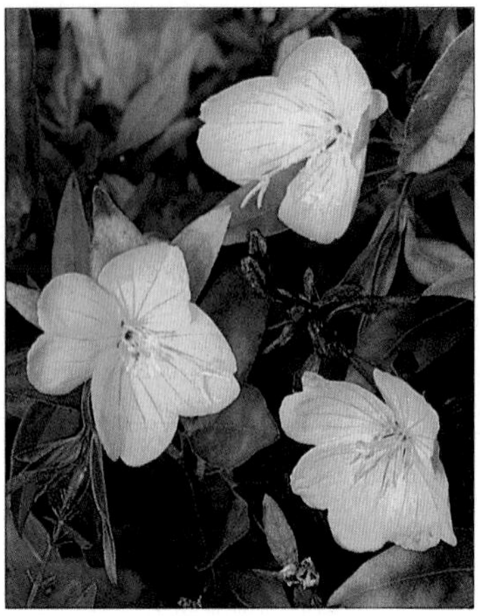

Oenothera perennis

O. perennis ■ syn. *O. pumila* (Sundrops). Clump-forming perennial with rosettes of spoon-shaped to inversely lance-shaped, mid-green leaves, 2.5–5cm (1–2in) long. Loose, leafy, upright, few-flowered racemes of funnel-shaped yellow flowers, to 2cm (¾in) across, open during the day in summer. ↕↔ to 20cm (8in) or more. E. North America. ❄❄❄
O. pumila see *O. perennis.*
O. speciosa. Sometimes invasive perennial, spreading by runners, with basal rosettes of oblong-lance-shaped to lance-shaped, toothed or pinnatifid, mid-green leaves, 2.5–5cm (1–2in) long, and arching stems bearing slightly smaller leaves. Solitary, saucer-shaped to shallowly cup-shaped, very fragrant white flowers, 2.5–6cm (1–2½in) across, sometimes ageing to pink, are produced in long succession from early summer to early autumn, opening during the day. ↕↔ 30cm (12in). S.W. USA to Mexico. ❄❄❄. **'Childsii'** see 'Rosea'. **'Rosea'** ■ syn. *O. berlandieri,* 'Childsii', has smaller white flowers, 4–5cm (1½–2in) across, strongly suffused pink, with deep pink veins and yellow petal bases.

O. taraxacifolia see *O. acaulis.*
O. tetragona see *O. fruticosa* subsp. *glauca.*

▷**Oil palm** see *Elaeis*
African see *E. guineensis*
▷**Oil tree,**
Karum see *Pongamia pinnata*
Macassar see *Cananga odorata*
Poona see *Pongamia pinnata*
▷**Old maid** see *Catharanthus roseus*
▷**Old man** see *Artemisia abrotanum*
▷**Old-man-live-forever** see *Pelargonium cotyledonis*
▷**Old man's beard** see *Clematis*
▷**Old pheasant's eye** see *Narcissus poeticus* var. *recurvus*

OLEA
Olive

OLEACEAE

Genus of about 20 species of evergreen trees and shrubs often found in dry, rocky places in the Mediterranean and Africa to C. Asia and Australasia. They have opposite, leathery leaves, which may be entire or toothed, and produce terminal or axillary panicles of small, 4-lobed, white or off-white flowers; these are followed by edible, ovoid or spherical fruits. Thriving only in areas with a Mediterranean or similar climate, *O. europaea,* the only species cultivated, is of great economic importance for its fruit (olives) and the oil extracted from them. Grow as a specimen tree or in a border; in frost-prone areas, grow in a cool greenhouse or conservatory, or at the base of a sunny, sheltered wall.
• **HARDINESS** Frost hardy.
• **CULTIVATION** Under glass, grow in loam-based potting compost (JI No.3) with additional sharp sand, in full light. During the growing season, water moderately and apply a balanced liquid fertilizer every month; water sparingly in winter. Outdoors, grow in deep, fertile, sharply drained soil in full sun. Pruning group 1; plants under glass need restrictive pruning in spring.

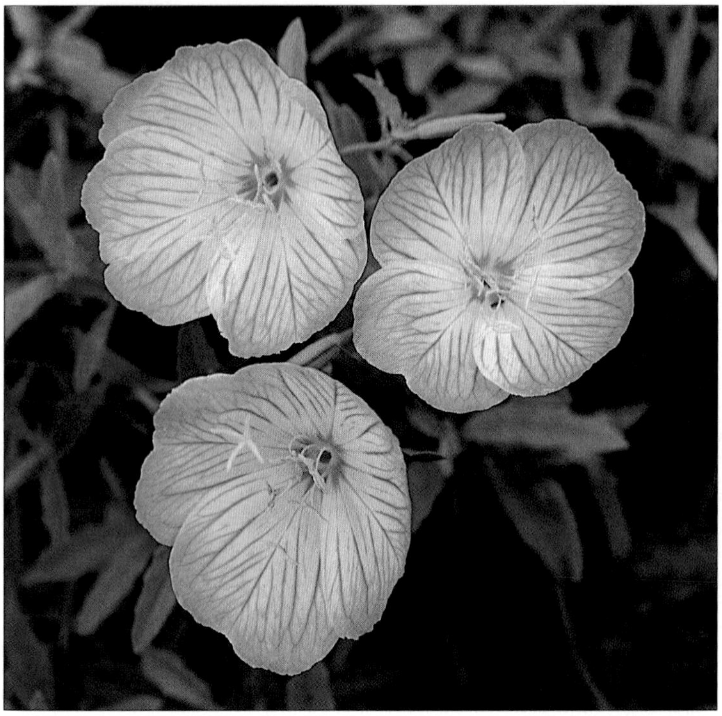

Oenothera speciosa 'Rosea'

• **PROPAGATION** Sow seed at 13–15°C (55–59°F) in spring. Take semi-ripe cuttings in summer.
• **PESTS AND DISEASES** May be infested with scale insects.

O. europaea 🏆 ♀ (Olive). Slow-growing, evergreen tree, developing a rounded head, with opposite, leathery, elliptic to lance-shaped, irregularly toothed leaves, to 8cm (3in) long, grey-green above, silvery grey-green beneath. Tiny, fragrant, creamy white flowers are borne in axillary panicles, to 5cm (2in) long, in summer, followed by edible, spherical to ovoid green fruit (olives), to 4cm (1½in) long, ripening to black. ↕↔ 10m (30ft). Mediterranean. ❄❄

▷**Oleander** see *Nerium*

OLEARIA
Daisy bush

ASTERACEAE/COMPOSITAE

Genus of about 130 species of evergreen shrubs and small trees, and some herbaceous perennials, from a wide variety of habitats, including coastal areas, bogs, forest, riverbanks, and mountain scrub, in Australia. They have generally alternate, occasionally clustered, simple, usually leathery leaves, and are cultivated for their daisy-like flowerheads, often with colourful ray-florets, borne singly, or in corymbs or panicles, in spring or summer. Olearias are suitable for planting in a shrub border, or in a sheltered site if not fully hardy. Some, such as *O.* x *haastii, O. macrodonta,* and *O. traversii,* may be grown as hedges and windbreaks, particularly in coastal areas. In frost-prone climates, grow tender species in a cool or temperate greenhouse.
• **HARDINESS** Fully hardy to frost tender.
• **CULTIVATION** Outdoors, grow in fertile, well-drained soil in full sun, with shelter from cold, drying winds. Under glass, grow in loam-based potting compost (JI No.3) in full light. When in growth, water moderately and apply a balanced liquid fertilizer monthly; water sparingly in winter. Pruning group 8 for early-flowering species, group 9 for late-flowering species; trim lightly to maintain a compact habit. Most species break freely from old wood and tolerate hard pruning.
• **PROPAGATION** Root semi-ripe cuttings in summer, using bottom heat for tender species.
• **PESTS AND DISEASES** Trouble free.

O. albida ♀ (Tanguru). Vigorous, upright shrub or small tree with alternate, oblong to ovate-oblong, wavy-margined leaves, to 10cm (4in) long, dark green above, white-felted beneath. Small, daisy-like white flowerheads, to 7mm (¼in) across, each with 1–5 ray-florets, are borne in panicles, to 5cm (2in) across, in summer. ↕ 5m (15ft), ↔ 3m (10ft). New Zealand (North Island). ❄
***O. albida* of gardens** see *O.* 'Talbot de Malahide'.
O. avicenniifolia ♀ Rounded, bushy shrub or small tree with alternate, elliptic to lance-shaped, dark grey-green leaves, to 10cm (4in) long, pale yellow- or white-felted beneath. Small, daisy-like, fragrant white flowerheads, to 5mm

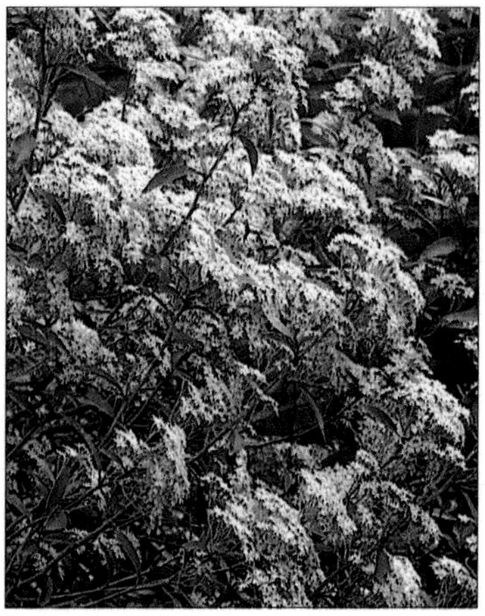

Olearia cheesemanii

(¼in) across, each with usually 1 or 2 ray-florets, are borne in broad corymbs, to 8cm (3in) across, in late summer and early autumn. ↕ 3m (10ft), ↔ 5m (15ft). New Zealand (South Island, Stewart Island). ❄❄❄ (borderline)
O. cheesemanii ■ ♀ syn. *O. rani* of gardens. Upright-branched shrub or small tree with alternate, oblong or elliptic to lance-shaped, slightly toothed, leathery, glossy, dark green leaves, to 9cm (3½in) long, white-felted beneath. Daisy-like white flowerheads, to 9mm (⅜in) across, with yellow centres, are borne in large corymbs, to 20cm (8in) across, in mid- and late spring. ↕ 4m (12ft), ↔ 3m (10ft). New Zealand. ❄❄
O. ciliata. Upright shrub with rough shoots and clustered, rigid, linear, deep green leaves, to 1.5cm (½in) long, the margins strongly rolled back. Solitary, long-stalked, daisy-like flowerheads, 2.5cm (1in) across, blue or white with yellow centres, are produced in spring. ↕ 30cm (12in), ↔ 20cm (8in). Temperate regions of Australia. ❄❄
O. erubescens. Upright shrub with alternate, oblong to lance-shaped, toothed, sometimes lobed, glossy, dark green leaves, to 4cm (1½in) long, sometimes red-tinged when young. In late spring and early summer, daisy-like, yellow-centred white flowerheads, 2.5cm (1in) across, appear singly or in clusters of 2–5, forming leafy panicles, to 45cm (18in) long. ↕ 1.5m (5ft), ↔ 60cm (24in). S.E. Australia. ❄❄
O. frostii. Spreading shrub with alternate, obovate, entire or wavy-toothed, grey-green leaves, to 2.5cm (1in) long, covered with star-like hairs.

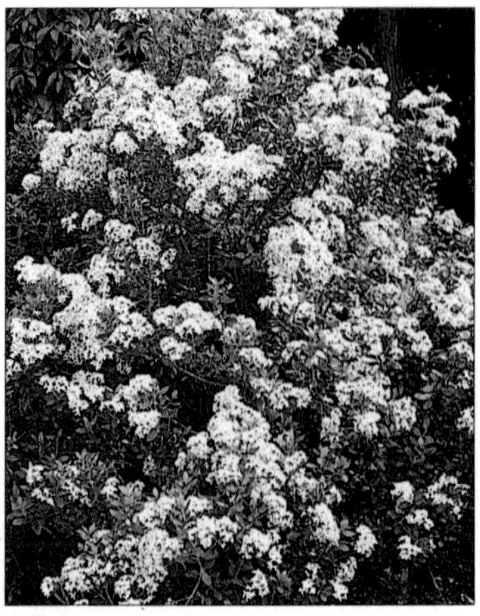

Olearia x *haastii*

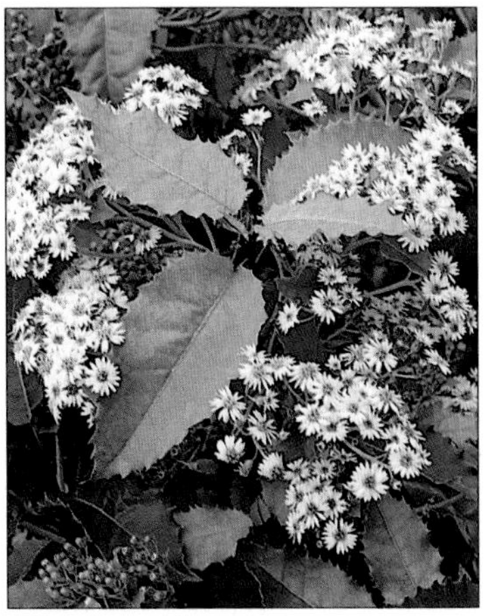
Olearia macrodonta

In midsummer, very showy, yellow-centred mauve flowerheads, resembling Michaelmas daisies, to 4cm (1½in) across, are borne singly or in groups of 2 or 3. ↕60cm (24in), ↔1m (3ft). S.E. Australia (Victoria). ❄

O. gunniana see *O. phlogopappa.*

O.* x *haastii ◼ (*O. avicenniifolia* x *O. moschata*). Dense, bushy shrub with alternate, oval or ovate, glossy, dark green leaves, to 2.5cm (1in) long, white-felted beneath. Dense corymbs, to 8cm (3in) across, of daisy-like, yellow-centred white flowerheads, to 8mm (⅜in) across, appear in mid- and late summer. ↕2m (6ft), ↔3m (10ft) or more. Natural hybrid from New Zealand (South Island). ❄❄❄

***O.* 'Henry Travers'** ♀ syn. *O. semidentata* of gardens. Rounded shrub with slender, white-felted shoots and alternate, lance-shaped, leathery, grey-green leaves, to 8cm (3in) long, white-felted beneath. Solitary, daisy-like flowerheads, 5cm (2in) across, with purple centres and numerous lilac ray-florets, are produced in early and midsummer. ↕2.5m (8ft), ↔2m (6ft). Natural hybrid from New Zealand (Chatham Islands). ❄❄

O. ilicifolia ⚲ (Mountain holly). Dense, spreading, bushy shrub or small tree with alternate, stiff and leathery, narrowly oblong, wavy-margined, sharply toothed, grey-green leaves, to 10cm (4in) long. Daisy-like, fragrant white flowerheads, to 1.5cm (½in) across, with yellow centres, are produced in large corymbs, to 10cm (4in) across, in summer. ↕↔5m (15ft). New Zealand. ❄❄❄ (borderline)

O. insignis see *Pachystegia insignis.*

O. lacunosa. Rounded, strongly branched shrub with densely grey-woolly branchlets. Bears alternate, slender, linear to linear-oblong, sharp-pointed, leathery leaves, 8–17cm (3–7in) long, dark green with yellow midribs above, silver-hairy to pale brown-hairy beneath. Small, daisy-like white flowerheads, 5mm (¼in) across, with yellow centres, are produced in spherical, corymb-like panicles, to 20cm (8in) across, in summer; they are borne more freely in warm, but not dry climates. ↕2–3m (6–10ft), sometimes 4–5m (12–15ft), ↔3m (10ft). New Zealand. ❄❄

O. macrodonta ◼♀⚲ (Arorangi). Vigorous, upright shrub or small tree with alternate, holly-like, ovate-oblong, sharply toothed and pointed, glossy, dark green leaves, to 10cm (4in) long, silver-white-felted beneath. In summer, bears large corymbs, to 15cm (6in) across, of daisy-like, fragrant white flowerheads, to 1cm (½in) across, with reddish brown centres. ↕6m (20ft), ↔5m (15ft). New Zealand. ❄❄❄ (borderline)

***O.* x *mollis* 'Zennorensis'** ♀ syn. *O.* 'Zennorensis'. Dense, rounded shrub with alternate, lance-shaped, sharply toothed leaves, to 10cm (4in) long, glossy, dark olive-green above, densely white-woolly beneath. Daisy-like white flowerheads, 1.5–2cm (½–¾in) across, with yellow centres, are produced in spherical corymbs, 15–20cm (6–8in) across, in late spring. ↕↔2m (6ft). ❄❄❄ (borderline)

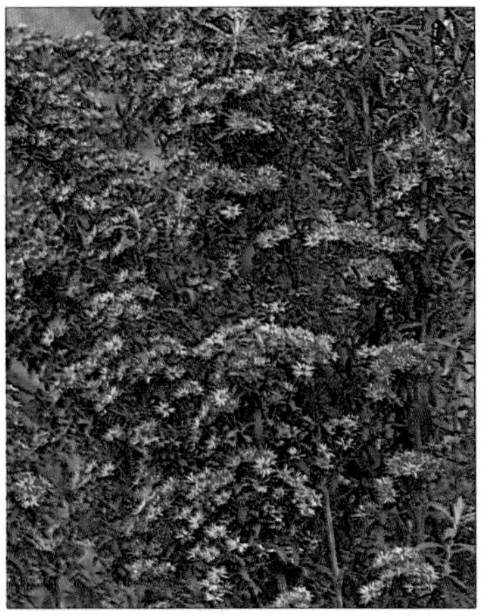
Olearia phlogopappa 'Comber's Pink'

O. moschata (Incense plant). Dense, upright, bushy shrub with alternate, obovate to oblong, leathery, musk-scented, grey-tinged green leaves, to 1.5cm (½in) long, densely white-hairy on both surfaces. Produces dense corymbs of 12–30 daisy-like, yellow-centred white flowerheads, each to 1cm (½in) across, in midsummer. ↕1–2m (3–6ft), ↔1m (3ft). New Zealand (South Island). ❄❄

O. nummulariifolia ◼ Dense, rounded, slow-growing shrub with stout, upright shoots. Bears alternate, small, obovate to rounded, very leathery leaves, to 1cm (½in) long, the margins rolled back, and bright green when young, becoming dark green, and densely white-woolly to buff- or yellow-woolly beneath. Daisy-like, fragrant white flowerheads, 2cm (¾in) across, with cream or pale yellow centres, are produced singly or in clusters of 2 or 3 at the shoot tips in midsummer. ↕↔2m (6ft). New Zealand. ❄❄❄ (borderline)

O. phlogopappa, syn. *O. gunniana, O. stellulata* of gardens. Compact, upright shrub with alternate, oblong to narrowly obovate, wavy-margined, shallowly toothed leaves, to 5cm (2in) long, grey-

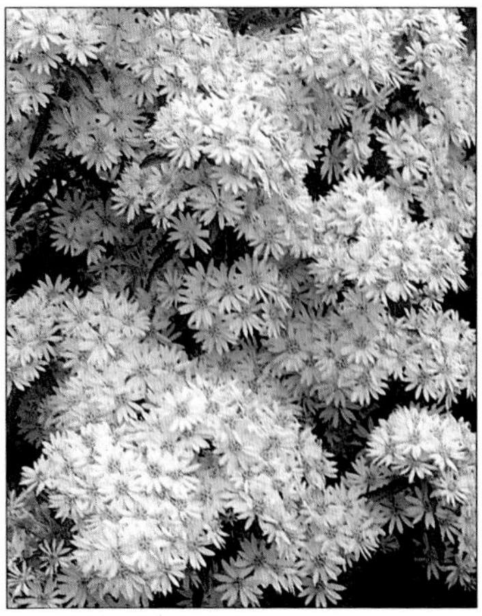
Olearia x *scilloniensis*

green above, densely white-woolly or grey-white-woolly beneath. Daisy-like, usually white, sometimes blue, mauve, or pink flowerheads, 3cm (1¼in) across, with yellow centres, are freely borne in loose, erect corymbs, to 7cm (3in) across, in spring and early summer. ↕↔2m (6ft). S.E. Australia. ❄❄. **'Comber's Blue'** has mid-blue ray-florets. **'Comber's Pink'** ◼ has pink ray-florets.

O. ramulosa ◼ Arching, slender-branched shrub bearing alternate, linear to linear-obovate, dark green leaves, to 1cm (½in) long, the margins rolled back, and densely hairy beneath. Solitary, daisy-like, white, or sometimes blue, mauve, or pink flowerheads, 1.5cm (½in) across, with white centres, are produced in spring, or in late winter under glass. ↕↔1.5m (5ft). Australia. ⚘ (min. 5°C/41°F)

***O. rani* of gardens** see *O. cheesemanii.*

O.* x *scilloniensis ◼ (*O. lirata* x *O. phlogopappa*). Dense, initially upright then rounded shrub, with alternate, elliptic-oblong, wavy-margined, dark green leaves, to 10cm (4in) long, pale green and densely felted beneath. In late spring, daisy-like white flowerheads, to 6cm (2½in) across, with yellow centres, are very profusely borne in corymbs to 7cm (3in) across. ↕↔2m (6ft). Garden origin. ❄❄. **'Master Michael'** has grey-green foliage and blue flowerheads.

***O. semidentata* of gardens** see *O.* 'Henry Travers'.

O. solandri ◼⚲ Dense, upright, bushy shrub or small tree with slender, sticky, yellow-hairy shoots and heather-like, opposite, narrowly spoon-shaped to

O

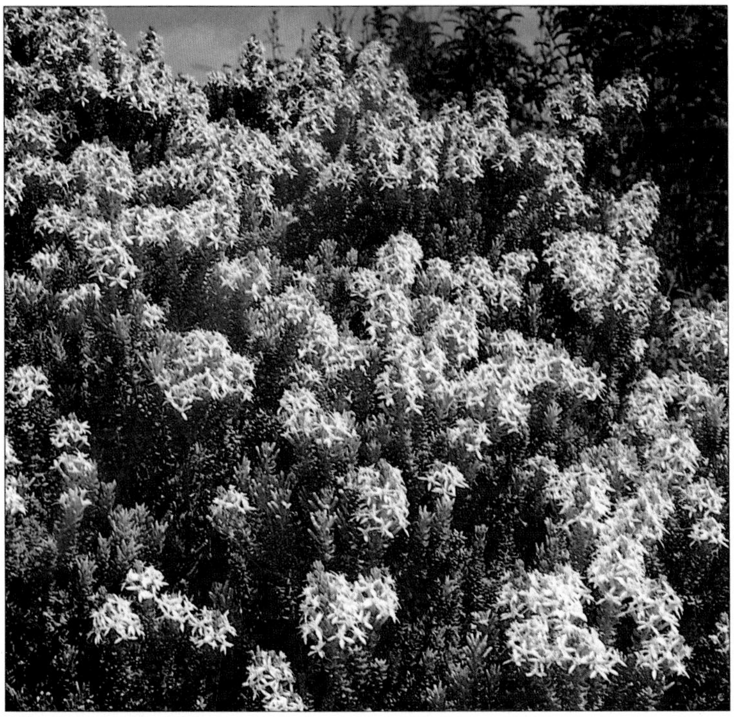
Olearia nummulariifolia

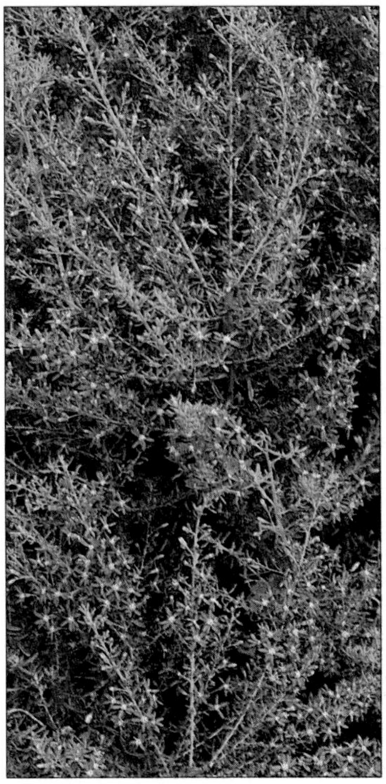
Olearia ramulosa

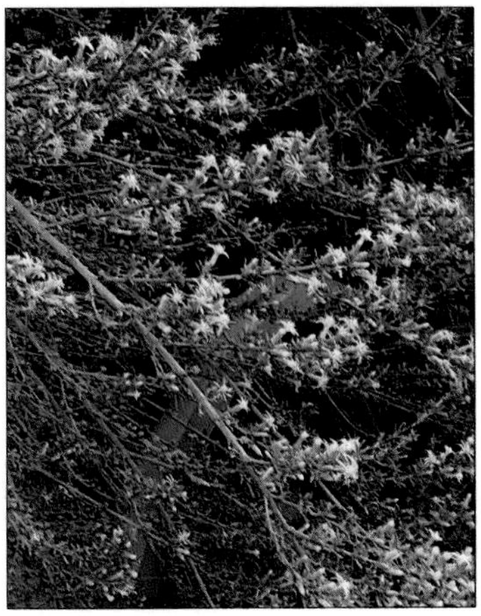
Olearia solandri

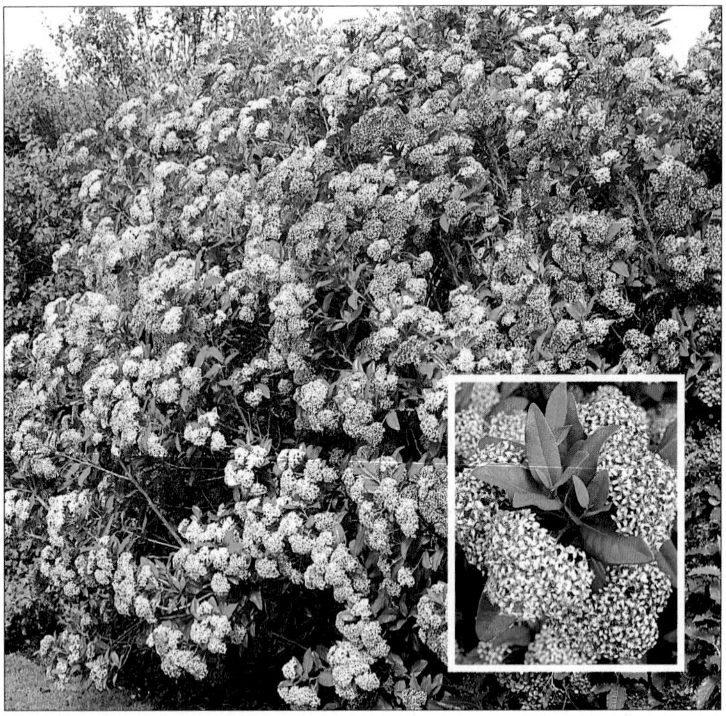

Olearia 'Talbot de Malahide' (inset: flower detail)

narrowly obovate or linear, dark green leaves, to 8mm (3/8in) long, densely white- to yellow-felted beneath. Solitary, daisy-like, very strongly fragrant, pale yellow flowerheads, 8mm (3/8in) across, with about 20 tiny florets, are produced from summer to autumn. ↕↔ 2m (6ft). New Zealand. ❄❄

***O. stellulata* of gardens** see *O. phlogopappa.*

***O.* 'Talbot de Malahide'** ■ syn. *O. albida* of gardens. Dense, upright, bushy shrub with alternate, narrowly ovate, glossy, dark green leaves, to 10cm (4in) long, white- or yellowish-white-felted beneath. Small, daisy-like, fragrant white flowerheads, to 1cm (1/2in) across, each with up to 6 ray-florets and an inconspicuous, brownish yellow centre, are borne in broad corymbs, to 10cm (4in) across, in late summer and early autumn. ↕ 3m (10ft), ↔ 5m (15ft). ❄❄

O. traversii ○ Dense, upright shrub, sometimes a small tree, with stout, angled shoots and opposite, oval to ovate-oblong leaves, to 6cm (2 1/2in) long, glossy, dark green above, white-felted beneath. In early summer, bears relatively inconspicuous, daisy-like, grey-white flowerheads, to 6mm (1/4in) across, without ray-florets, in panicles to 5cm (2in) long. Useful for coastal hedging. ↕ 5–10m (15–30ft), ↔ 3–5m (10–15ft), or more. New Zealand (Chatham Islands). ❄❄❄ (borderline)

O. virgata ■ Arching shrub with smooth, slender, wiry shoots and opposite, narrowly obovate to linear, dark green leaves, to 2cm (3/4in) long, densely white-felted beneath. In summer, small, daisy-like, fragrant, yellowish white flowerheads, 1cm (1/2in) across, each with 3–6 ray-florets and an inconspicuous centre, are profusely borne in opposite clusters, to 4cm (1 1/2in) across, along the branches. ↕↔ 5m (15ft). New Zealand. ❄❄❄ (borderline). **var. *lineata*** has pendulous, softly hairy branchlets with linear leaves, to 4cm (1 1/2in) long, the margins strongly rolled back, and flowerheads with 8–14 ray-florets; ↕ to 2m (6ft); New Zealand (South Island).

***O.* 'Zennorensis'** see *O.* x *mollis* 'Zennorensis'.

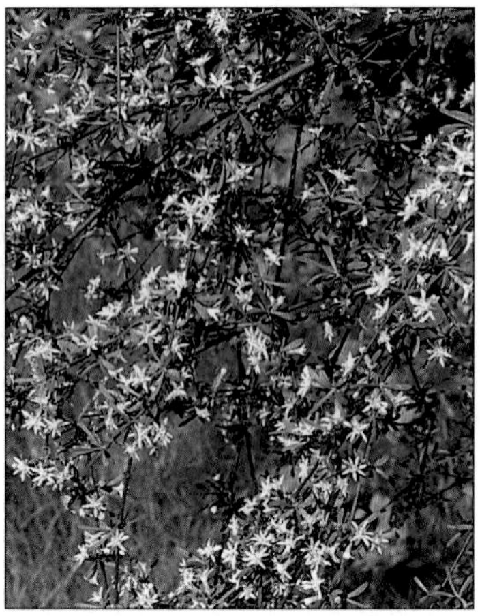

Olearia virgata

▷ **Oleaster** see *Elaeagnus angustifolia*
▷ **Olive** see *Olea, O. europaea*
Fragrant see *Osmanthus fragrans*
▷ ***Oliveranthus elegans*** see *Echeveria harmsii*

OLSYNIUM

IRIDACEAE

Genus of about 12 species of fibrous-rooted, clump-forming perennials, often included in *Sisyrinchium*, found in moist grassland from sea level to subalpine regions in North and South America. They have mostly basal, stem-clasping, linear or lance-shaped leaves, and are grown for their nodding, trumpet-shaped to bell-shaped flowers which are borne in spring. Grow in a shady rock garden, peat bed, or alpine house.

• **HARDINESS** Fully hardy.

• **CULTIVATION** Grow in moist, humus-rich, moderately fertile soil in partial shade. In an alpine house, use a mix of equal parts loam, leaf mould, and grit.

• **PROPAGATION** Sow seed in containers in a cold frame in autumn. Young plants take 2 or 3 years to flower.

• **PESTS AND DISEASES** Trouble free.

O. biflorum, syn. *Phaiophleps biflora, Sisyrinchium odoratissimum.* Slender, clump-forming perennial, with short rhizomes producing upright stems with narrow, rush-like leaves, 4–22cm (1 1/2–9in) long. In late spring or summer, bears cymes of usually 2, occasionally more, trumpet-shaped, fragrant, red-veined, creamy yellow flowers, 2.5cm (1in) long. ↕ 20–35cm (8–14in), ↔ 5cm (2in). Argentina (Patagonia). ❄❄❄

O. douglasii ♀ syn. *Sisyrinchium douglasii, S. grandiflorum* (Grass widow). Clump-forming perennial with upright, slender, rush-like stems sheathed with linear, greyish green leaves, to 10cm (4in) long. In early spring, nodding, bell-shaped, satin-textured, rich purple flowers, to 2cm (3/4in) long, are borne in several terminal spathes, each with 1–4 flowers. ↕ 15–30cm (6–12in), ↔ to 10cm (4in). W. North America. ❄❄❄. **var. *album*** has white flowers.

OMPHALODES

Navelwort

BORAGINACEAE

Genus of about 28 species of annuals, biennials, and perennials, some of which are evergreen or semi-evergreen, from a wide range of habitats in Europe, N. Africa, and Asia. They have clusters of simple leaves either in basal tufts or arranged alternately on stems. In spring and summer, they produce blue or white flowers, similar to forget-me-nots (*Myosotis*), each with a short tube and 5 spreading lobes, usually in terminal racemes or cymes, sometimes singly from the leaf axils. Most are shade-loving, used as ground cover in a border, or rock or woodland garden. Grow *O. luciliae* in a rock garden, scree bed, tufa, or alpine house; use *O. linifolia* in an annual border or for cutting.

• **HARDINESS** Fully hardy.

• **CULTIVATION** Most of the perennials thrive in moist, moderately fertile, humus-rich soil in partial shade. Grow *O. linifolia* in moderately fertile, well-drained soil in sun. Grow *O. luciliae* in tufa, or in very gritty, alkaline soil, in full sun; in an alpine house, use a mix of equal parts loam, leaf mould, and grit, with added limestone chippings.

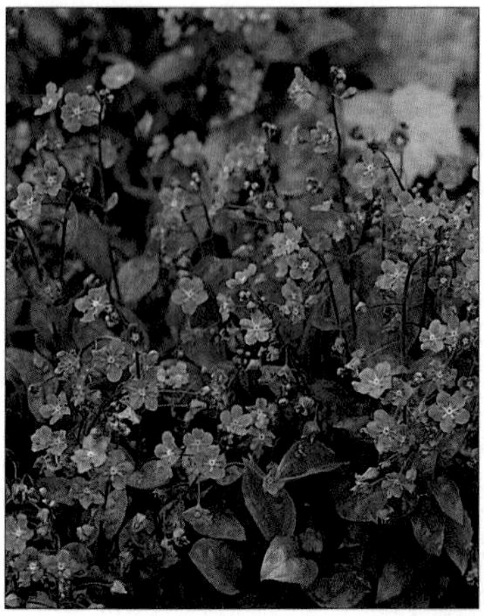

Omphalodes cappadocica

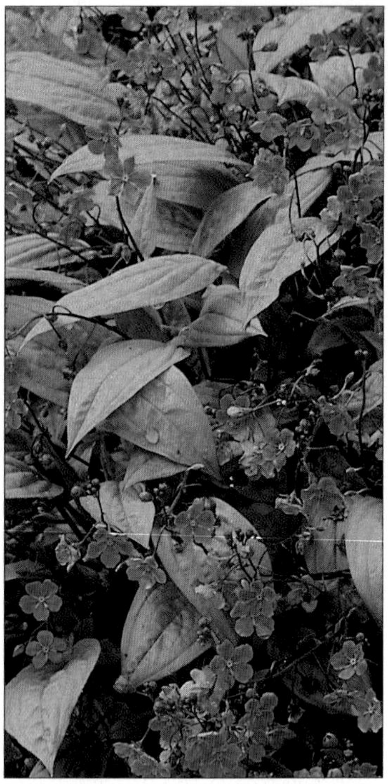

Omphalodes cappadocica 'Cherry Ingram'

• **PROPAGATION** Sow seed in spring: sow annuals *in situ*; sow perennials in containers in a cold frame. Divide perennials in early spring.

• **PESTS AND DISEASES** Very susceptible to damage by slugs and snails.

O. cappadocica ■ ♀ Clump-forming, rhizomatous, evergreen perennial with ovate to heart-shaped, pointed, finely hairy, mid-green, basal leaves, to 10cm (4in) long. Produces loose, terminal racemes, to 25cm (10in) long, of 3–12 white-eyed, azure-blue flowers, each to 5mm (1/4in) across, in early spring. ↕ to 25cm (10in), ↔ to 40cm (16in). Woodland in Turkey. ❄❄❄. **'Cherry Ingram'** ■ is more compact, with larger, deep blue flowers, 7mm (1/4in) across. **'Starry Eyes'** also has larger flowers, to 7mm (1/4in) across, with a central white stripe on each petal.

O. linifolia ■ ♀ (Venus's navelwort). Erect annual, branching from the base, with narrowly lance-shaped to spoon-shaped, sparsely white-hairy, glaucous basal leaves, to 10cm (4in) long, and smaller, very narrow, stalkless stem leaves. From spring to summer, produces loose, terminal racemes of

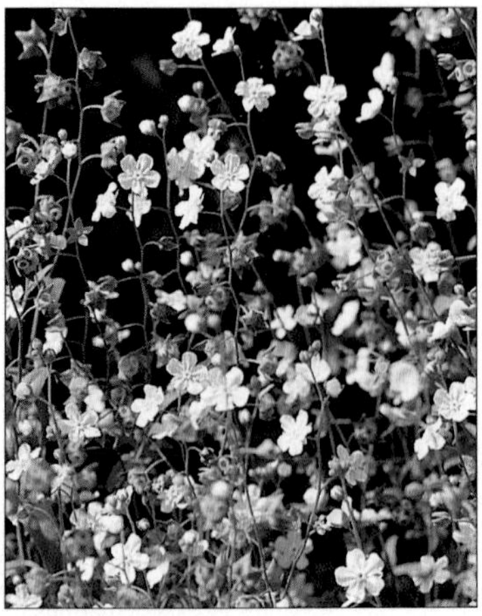

Omphalodes linifolia

O

5–15 tiny, slightly scented, white, or very occasionally pale blue flowers, to 1.5cm (½in) across. Self-seeds readily. ↕30–40cm (12–16in), ↔ to 15cm (6in). Dry, open sites, often in alkaline soil, in S.W. Europe. ❄❄❄

O. luciliae. Clump-forming, semi-evergreen perennial with upright to prostrate stems and ovate to elliptic or oblong, pale grey-blue, basal leaves, to 10cm (4in) long. Produces loose, terminal cymes of 3–15 clear light blue flowers, to 8mm (⅜in) across, often opening pink, over long periods in summer. May be difficult to establish. ↕10cm (4in) or more, ↔ to 15cm (6in). Vertical limestone cliffs, generally in shade, in Greece and Turkey. ❄❄❄

O. verna (Blue-eyed Mary, Creeping forget-me-not). Clump-forming, stoloniferous, semi-evergreen perennial with heart-shaped, ovate to ovate-lance-shaped, pointed, hairy, mid-green, basal leaves, to 20cm (8in) long. Terminal racemes of 5–20 white-eyed, deep bright blue flowers, to 1cm (½in) across, appear in spring. ↕ to 20cm (8in), ↔ 30cm (12in) or more. Moist woodland in S.E. Alps to N. Apennines and to mountains of Romania. ❄❄❄

OMPHALOGRAMMA

PRIMULACEAE

Genus of about 15 species of usually rhizomatous perennials, related to *Primula*, from the Himalayas and the mountains of China. They are grown for their solitary, horizontally borne, salverform flowers, with long tubes and 6–8 spreading lobes, borne in spring or early summer. The lance-shaped to ovate or elliptic, often white-hairy, primula-like, mid- to dark green leaves are borne in rosettes, and arise from a large, dormant winter bud surrounded by scales. They grow best in cool, moist climates; grow in a peat bed, shady rock garden, or in an alpine house.

• **HARDINESS** Fully hardy.

• **CULTIVATION** Grow in cool, moist conditions, in open, moderately fertile, humus-rich, well-drained soil in partial shade. In an alpine house, use a mix of equal parts loam, leaf mould, and grit; move plants to a cool, shady site outdoors during summer.

• **PROPAGATION** Sow seed in containers in an open frame as soon as ripe.

• **PESTS AND DISEASES** Prone to aphids and whiteflies under glass. Young leaves are susceptible to slug and snail damage.

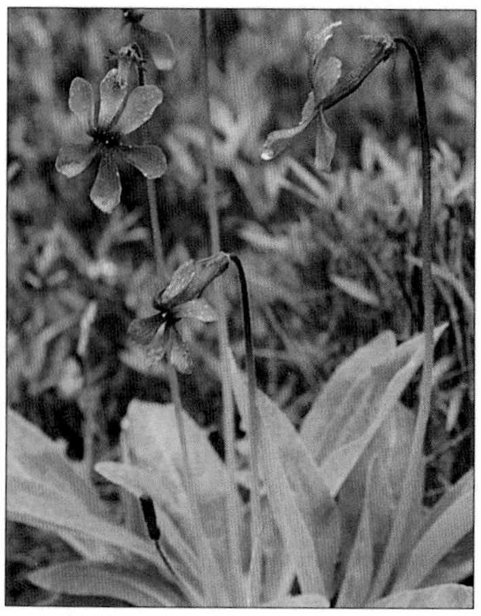

Omphalogramma vinciflorum

O. vinciflorum ■ Rosette-forming perennial, lacking a rhizome but with a large, dormant winter bud. Bears obovate-oblong to oblong, entire to scalloped, hairy, mid-green leaves, to 20cm (8in) long. In spring, produces solitary, salverform flowers, spreading to 5cm (2in) across, with deep violet-purple lobes and darker throats. ↕20cm (8in), ↔ 10cm (4in). China (Yunnan, Sichuan). ❄❄❄

ONCIDIUM

ORCHIDACEAE

Genus of over 450 species of evergreen, terrestrial, epiphytic, or lithophytic orchids found in a variety of habitats, from sea level to altitudes of 3,000m (10,000ft), in Mexico, Central America, South America, and the West Indies. Some oncidiums are compact with fan-like foliage; others have pseudobulbs that bear either 1 large, rigid leaf or 2 smaller, flexible leaves. The flowers are typically yellow, with prominent lips, and are produced in short or tall racemes or panicles from the bases of the plants.

• **HARDINESS** Frost tender.

• **CULTIVATION** Cool- to intermediate-growing orchids. Grow compact species in pots of epiphytic orchid compost; grow those with large, leathery leaves and elongated habit (e.g. *O. flexuosum*) epiphytically on bark or in baskets. In summer, provide high humidity and bright filtered light; those with leathery leaves prefer full light. During the growing season, mist daily and water freely, applying a half-strength fertilizer at every third watering. Provide full light in winter. Keep oncidiums with large pseudobulbs dry in winter; those with small pseudobulbs, or none, require watering all year round. See also p.46.

• **PROPAGATION** Divide when the plants overflow their containers, or remove backbulbs (produced by *O. flexuosum* and *O. tigrinum*) and pot up separately.

• **PESTS AND DISEASES** Prone to aphids, mealybugs, and red spider mites.

O. cavendishianum. Epiphytic orchid with very small pseudobulbs (sometimes none), each with one elliptic to broadly lance-shaped, rigid, leathery leaf, 15–45cm (6–18in) long. In spring, fragrant, waxy, red-spotted yellow flowers, 4cm (1½in) across, with deep yellow lips, are produced in panicles 1.5m (5ft) or more tall. ↕60cm (24in), ↔ 30cm (12in). S. Mexico, Guatemala, Honduras. ⌂ (min. 13°C/55°F; max. 30°C/86°F)

O. crispum. Epiphytic orchid with ovoid pseudobulbs, each with 2 narrowly lance-shaped, leathery leaves, 20cm (8in) long. Chestnut-brown and yellow-spotted flowers, to 8cm (3in) across, are produced in erect to pendent panicles, to 1.1m (3½ft) long, from autumn to spring. ↕60cm (24in), ↔ 30cm (12in). Brazil. ⌂ (min. 13°C/55°F; max. 30°C/86°F)

***O.* Fire Opal** (*O.* Persian Red x *O.* Susan Perreira). Epiphytic orchid with a fan of overlapping, rigid, flattened, linear-oblong leaves, 10cm (4in) long. Highly decorative flowers, 2.5cm (1in) or more across, in shades of rich pink over creamy white, are produced in long racemes several times during the

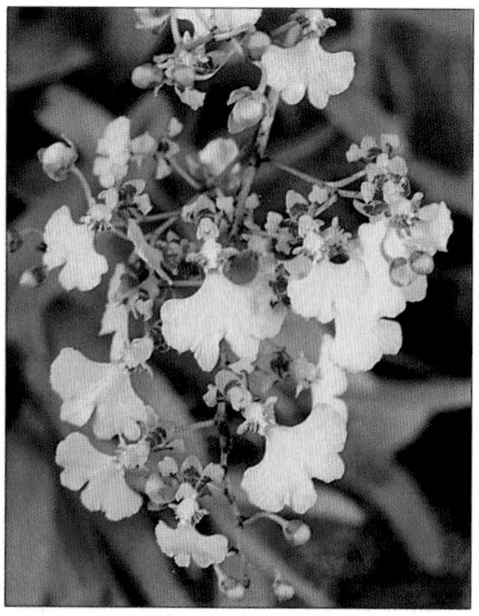

Oncidium flexuosum

year. ↕30cm (12in), ↔ 15cm (6in). ⌂ (min. 13°C/55°F; max. 30°C/86°F)

O. flexuosum ■ ♀ (Dancing doll orchid). Epiphytic orchid with ovoid-oblong pseudobulbs, each with 1 or 2 linear, leathery leaves, to 10–20cm (4–8in) long. From autumn to winter, rich canary-yellow flowers, 2cm (¾in) across, with red-brown markings on the sepals and petals, are clustered towards the tips of panicles to 80cm (32in) long. ↕60cm (24in), ↔ 30cm (12in). S.E. Brazil, Paraguay, Argentina, Uruguay. ⌂ (min. 13°C/55°F; max. 30°C/86°F)

***O.* Gypsy Beauty** (*O.* Phyllis Hetfield x *O.* Thelma Beaumont). Epiphytic orchid with a fan of overlapping, rigid, flattened, linear-oblong leaves, 10cm (4in) long. Highly decorative white and burgundy-red flowers, 2.5cm (1in) or more across, with raspberry lips, are produced in clusters towards the ends of racemes several times during the year. ↕30cm (12in), ↔ 15cm (6in). ⌂ (min. 13°C/55°F; max. 30°C/86°F)

O. longipes. Epiphytic orchid with slender, oblong-ovoid pseudobulbs, each with 2 oblong, soft leaves, to 15cm (6in) long. In spring, produces short racemes of 2–6 yellow flowers, 3.5cm (1½in) across, heavily spotted and streaked red-brown, with yellow lips. ↕12cm (5in), ↔ 15cm (6in). S.E. Brazil. ⌂ (min. 13°C/55°F; max. 30°C/86°F)

O. macranthum, syn. *Cyrtochilum macranthum.* Epiphytic orchid with oblong-conical, fleshy pseudobulbs, each with 2 narrowly inversely lance-shaped to oblong leaves, 25–50cm (10–20in) long. Yellow to brown-gold flowers, 8cm (3in) across, with yellowish white

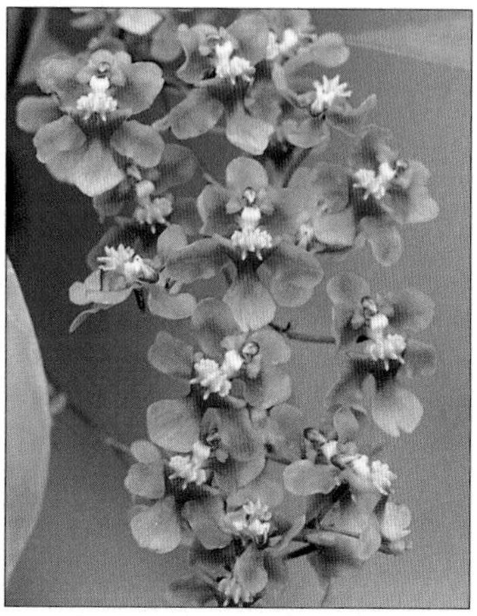

Oncidium ornithorrhynchum

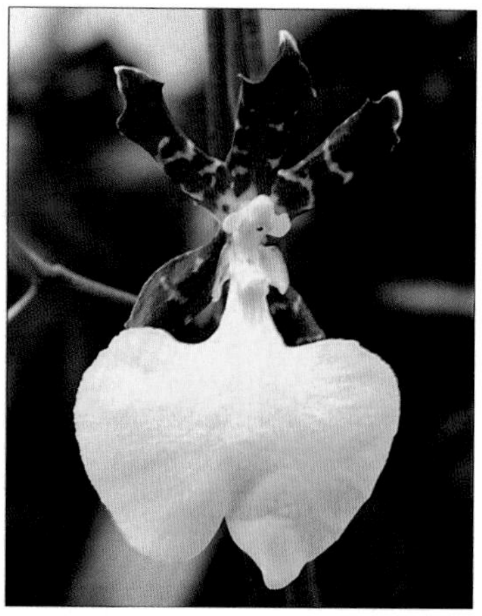

Oncidium tigrinum

lips bordered violet-purple, are borne in lax, spreading panicles, to 3m (10ft) tall, in summer. ↕1m (3ft), ↔ 60cm (24in). Colombia, Ecuador, Peru. ⌂ (min. 13°C/55°F; max. 30°C/86°F)

O. ornithorrhynchum ■ ♀ Epiphytic orchid producing ovoid or ellipsoid pseudobulbs, each with 2 linear-lance-shaped to linear-elliptic, soft leaves, 10–40cm (4–16in) long. In autumn, fragrant, white, pink, or purple-pink flowers, 2–2.5cm (¾–1in) across, with darker pink or lilac-pink lips, are produced in strongly arching panicles, to 50cm (20in) long. ↕15cm (6in), ↔ 23cm (9in). S. Mexico, Guatemala, El Salvador, Costa Rica. ⌂ (min. 13°C/55°F; max. 30°C/86°F)

O. papilio see *Psychopsis papilio.*

O. pusillum, syn. *Psygmorchis pusilla.* Epiphytic orchid with a flattened fan of linear-oblong to oblong-elliptic, fleshy leaves, 6cm (2½in) long. Bears axillary racemes, to 6cm (2½in) long, of 1–4 bright yellow flowers, marked rust-red, to 3cm (1¼in) across, intermittently all year round. ↕↔ 8cm (3in). Central America, South America, West Indies. ⌂ (min. 13°C/55°F; max. 30°C/86°F)

O. sphacelatum. Epiphytic orchid with ribbed, ovoid-ellipsoid pseudobulbs, each with 2 linear-oblong to linear-lance-shaped, semi-leathery leaves, to 1m (3ft) long. In spring, deep yellow flowers, to 3cm (1¼in) across, marked and spotted red-brown, with golden yellow lips, are produced in dense, upright panicles, to 1.5m (5ft) tall. ↕↔ 60cm (24in). Central America, Venezuela. ⌂ (min. 13°C/55°F; max. 30°C/86°F)

O. tigrinum ■ Epiphytic orchid with spherical pseudobulbs, each with 1 or 2 linear-oblong, leathery leaves, 30–50cm (12–20in) long. Fragrant yellow flowers, 5cm (2in) across, with sepals and petals heavily suffused dark red-brown, and with large yellow lips, are produced in long, stout, usually erect panicles, to 1.5m (5ft) tall, in winter. ↕45cm (18in), ↔ 30cm (12in). Mexico. ⌂ (min. 13°C/55°F; max. 30°C/86°F)

▷**Onion** see *Allium*
  False sea see *Ornithogalum longibracteatum*
  Nodding see *Allium cernuum*
  Sea see *Urginea maritima*
  Wild see *Allium cernuum*
▷**Onion couch** see *Arrhenatherum elatius* subsp. *bulbosum* 'Variegatum'

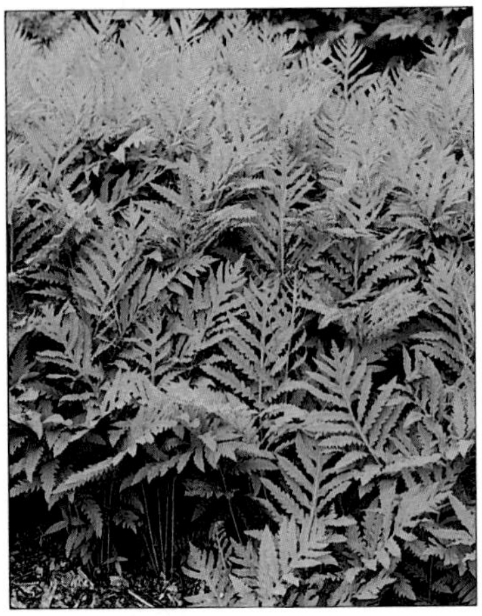

Onoclea sensibilis

ONOCLEA

ATHYRIACEAE/DRYOPTERIDACEAE

Genus of one species of deciduous, terrestrial fern found in damp sites in E. Asia and E. North America. In spring, long-stalked, pinnate or deeply pinnatisect sterile fronds arise singly at short intervals from creeping rhizomes, dying down at the first frost. The fertile fronds are 2-pinnate, with contracted, bead-like black segments curled in to cover the sori, and are borne in late summer, persisting throughout winter. *O. sensibilis* will thrive at the edge of water, or in a damp, shady border.

- **HARDINESS** Fully hardy.
- **CULTIVATION** Grow in a sheltered site, in moist, fertile, humus-rich, preferably acid soil, in light dappled shade (the fronds will burn if exposed to too much sun).
- **PROPAGATION** Sow spores at 15–16°C (59–60°F) as soon as ripe, or divide in spring. See also p.51.
- **PESTS AND DISEASES** Trouble free.

O. sensibilis ■ ♀ (Sensitive fern). Deciduous fern, producing upright then arching, broadly lance-shaped or triangular, pinnate to deeply pinnatisect, pale green sterile fronds, to 1m (3ft) long, in spring; these each have 8–12 pairs of pinnae, which are lobed to wavy-margined or entire. Fertile fronds are borne in late summer, and are stiffly erect, lance-shaped, and 2-pinnate, to 60cm (24in) long; the pinnae are reduced to bead-like black lobes enclosing the sori. The emerging fronds may sometimes be pinkish bronze in spring. ↕ 60cm (24in), ↔ indefinite. E. Asia, E. North America. ✽✽✽

O

ONONIS

Restharrow

LEGUMINOSAE/PAPILIONACEAE

Genus of about 75 species of annuals, perennials, and dwarf shrubs occurring in dry, rocky sites or in grassland, often in alkaline soil, in Europe, the Mediterranean, the Canary Islands, and from N. Africa to Iran. They have alternate, simple or 3-palmate, usually toothed and hairy, clover-like, mostly mid-green leaves, and are grown for their pea-like flowers, borne in panicles, spikes, or racemes in summer. Grow in a rock garden, wall, or sunny bank, or at the front of a mixed or shrub border.

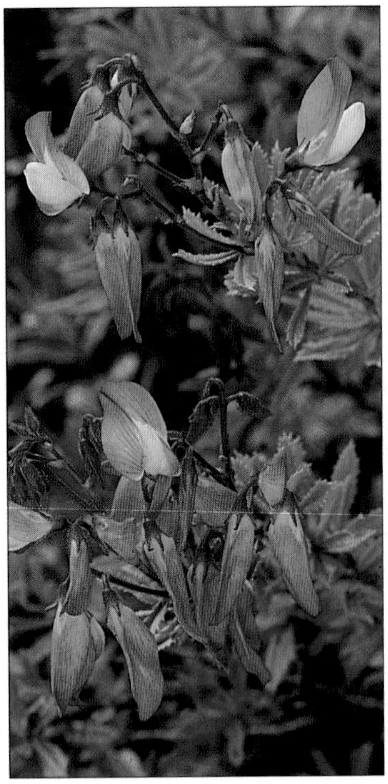

Ononis fruticosa

- **HARDINESS** Fully hardy.
- **CULTIVATION** Grow in a warm, sunny position in moderately fertile, well-drained soil. They may be short-lived, so propagate regularly.
- **PROPAGATION** Sow seed in containers in an open frame in autumn or spring. Take greenwood cuttings of shrubby species in early summer.
- **PESTS AND DISEASES** May be infested with red spider mites under glass.

O. fruticosa ■ (Shrubby restharrow). Short-lived, deciduous shrub with 3-palmate, leathery leaves, 4cm (1½in) long, composed of leaflets that are oblong-lance-shaped and unevenly toothed. Nodding clusters, 5–8cm (2–3in) long, of pea-like pink flowers, each to 2cm (¾in) long, with dark central markings and paler wings, are borne over long periods in summer. ↕↔ to 60cm (24in), occasionally to 1m (3ft). S.E. France, C. Pyrenees, C. and E. Spain. ✽✽✽

O. repens (Common restharrow). Upright or spreading, often stem-rooting, deciduous subshrub, sometimes with soft spines, bearing ovate, simple or 3-palmate leaves, to 2cm (¾in) long, composed of leaflets that are ovate, hairy, and toothed. Open, leafy racemes of pea-like, pink or pink-purple flowers, each to 2cm (¾in) long, are produced throughout summer. ↕ 30–60cm (12–24in), ↔ 50–80cm (20–32in) or more. Europe. ✽✽✽

O. rotundifolia. Upright, deciduous or semi-evergreen, dwarf shrub with 3-palmate leaves, 3cm (1¼in) long, composed of broadly elliptic to rounded, coarsely toothed, hairy leaflets, the terminal leaflet long-stalked. In summer, produces axillary racemes or panicles of pea-like, pale to deep pink or white flowers, to 2cm (¾in) long, striped darker pink. ↕ to 50cm (20in), ↔ to 30cm (12in). S. Europe (S.E. Spain to E. Austria, C. Italy). ✽✽✽

▷ ***Onopordon*** see *Onopordum*

ONOPORDUM

syn. ONOPORDON

Cotton thistle, Scotch thistle

ASTERACEAE/COMPOSITAE

Genus of about 40 erect, rosette-forming biennials from steppes, stony slopes, fallow fields, and disturbed ground in Europe, the Mediterranean, and W. Asia. They have simple to pinnatifid or pinnatisect, spiny-toothed leaves covered in cobweb-like, soft grey hair; the leaves are borne alternately on coarse, usually freely branching, mostly white-woolly stems, the leaf bases often continuing down the stems as very conspicuous wings. Large, round flowerheads, typically thistle-like and without ray-florets, are produced singly or in tight clusters at the stem tips in summer. They may be bright purple, blue-violet, rose-pink, or occasionally white, and are attractive to bees. Cotton thistles readily self-seed and may be grown in a large border, or in a semi-wild or gravel garden.

- **HARDINESS** Fully hardy.
- **CULTIVATION** Grow in fertile, well-drained, neutral to slightly alkaline soil in full sun.
- **PROPAGATION** Sow seed in containers in a cold frame or *in situ* in autumn or spring.
- **PESTS AND DISEASES** Slugs and snails may damage the foliage.

O. acanthium ■ Tap-rooted, rosette-forming biennial with oblong-ovate to lance-shaped or ovate, pinnatifid, spiny-toothed, grey-green leaves, to 35cm (14in) long, sparsely hairy above. In the second year, produces massive, branching, 2- to 4-winged, spiny, hairy, yellow-green stems; in summer, these produce solitary or clustered, round, thistle-like, pale purple or white flower-heads, 4–5cm (1½–2in) across, encased in spine-tipped bracts. ↕ to 3m (10ft), ↔ 1m (3ft). W. Europe to W. and C. Asia. ✽✽✽

O. arabicum see *O. nervosum.*

O. nervosum ♀ syn. *O. arabicum.* Tap-rooted, rosette-forming biennial with oblong-lance-shaped, pinnatisect, spiny toothed, silver-grey leaves, to 50cm (20in) long; they have prominent pale veins and are sparsely hairy beneath. In the second year, produces massive, branching, broad-winged, deeply veined, densely hairy, yellow-tinged stems; in summer, these bear clusters of round, thistle-like, bright purple-red to purple-pink flowerheads, to 3.5cm (1½in) across, encased in spine-tipped bracts. ↕ to 2.5m (9ft), ↔ 1m (3ft). Portugal, Spain. ✽✽✽

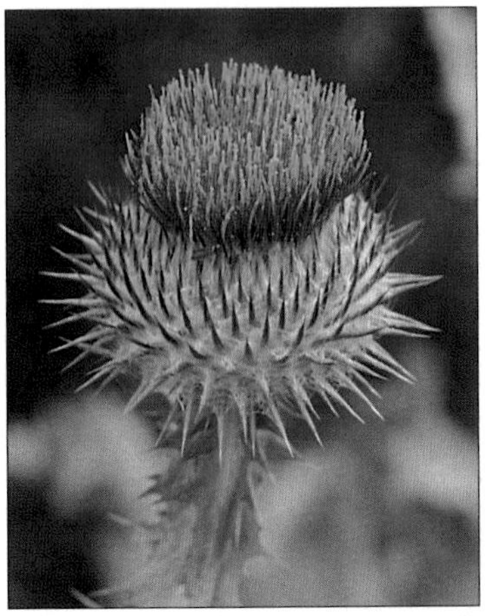

Onopordum acanthium

ONOSMA

BORAGINACEAE

Genus of about 150 species of biennials and often woody-based perennials found in sunny, rocky sites, often rock crevices, from the Mediterranean to Turkey. They are grown for their nodding cymes of narrowly tubular to cylindrical-bell-shaped flowers, mainly yellow, pink, red, or white. The simple, alternate leaves are covered in fine hairs, contact with which may irritate skin. Grow in a scree bed, or in a rock or wall crevice; in wet climates, they grow best in an alpine house or cold greenhouse.

- **HARDINESS** Frost hardy; most will withstand tempertures to -10°C (14°F).
- **CULTIVATION** Outdoors, grow in full sun in a very gritty scree bed, or grow plants on their sides in vertical wall or rock crevices. Protect from excessive rainfall. Under glass, grow in a mix of equal parts loam, leaf mould, and grit; avoid wetting the foliage when watering.
- **PROPAGATION** Sow seed in containers in an open frame in autumn. Take softwood or greenwood cuttings of shrubs in late spring or early summer.
- **PESTS AND DISEASES** May be infested with aphids or whiteflies under glass.

O. alborosea ■ Evergreen, clump-forming perennial with white-hairy, branching stems bearing densely white-bristly-hairy, grey-green leaves, which are spoon- to lance-shaped or obovate to oblong, and to 6cm (2½in) long. In summer, produces congested, terminal cymes of nodding, narrowly tubular-bell-shaped white flowers, to 3cm (1¼in) long; the petal tips quickly darken to pink and sometimes mature to deep purple or violet-blue. ↕↔ 25cm (10in). S.W. Asia. ✽✽

O. frutescens. Upright perennial with unbranched stems covered with tiny, soft hairs. The bristly-hairy, greyish green leaves, to 7cm (3in) long, are lance-shaped to oblong-lance-shaped or linear, with margins rolled back. In summer, bears cymes of cylindrical-bell-shaped, bright yellow flowers, to 2cm (¾in) long, maturing to orange-brown or reddish brown. ↕ 25cm (10in), ↔ to 60cm (24in). Greece, Turkey, Syria. ✽✽

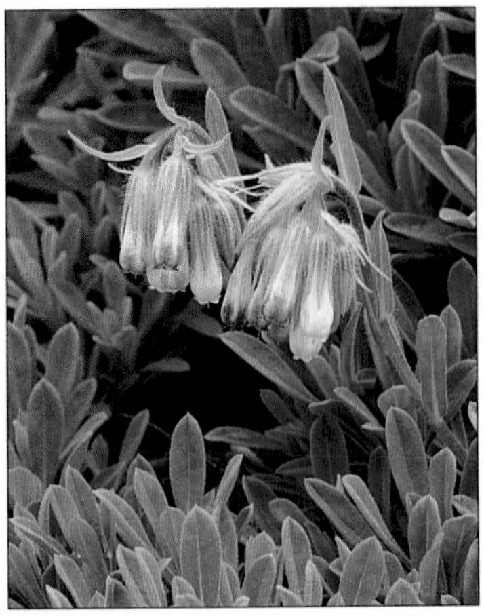

Onosma alborosea

OOPHYTUM

AIZOACEAE

Genus of 2 species of succulent perennials, similar to *Conophytum*, found in dry, hilly areas in Western Cape, South Africa. They have pairs of erect, thick, soft, fleshy leaves, which join to form ovoid, egg-like "bodies" that wither during the dormant period (the name *Oophytum* means "egg plant"). Solitary, daisy-like flowers are produced from a cleft at the top of each body in late summer. In areas where temperatures drop below 7°C (45°F), grow in a temperate greenhouse; in warm, dry climates, grow in a scree bed, raised bed, or desert garden.

- **HARDINESS** Frost tender.
- **CULTIVATION** Under glass, grow in a mix of 2 parts loam to 1 part each sharp sand and leaf mould, in full light with shade from hot sun. Water moderately from late summer to early autumn, and sparingly on warm days from mid-autumn to spring. Keep barely moist when semi-dormant from late spring to midsummer. Outdoors, grow in gritty, poor, humus-rich soil, in full sun with some midday shade. See also pp.48–49.
- **PROPAGATION** Sow seed at 20–25°C (68–77°F), or separate and root complete bodies, in spring or summer.
- **PESTS AND DISEASES** Susceptible to greenflies, especially while flowering.

O. oviforme. Clump-forming, succulent perennial with papillose, glossy, olive-green to bright reddish green leaves, united in pairs to form ovoid bodies, 1cm (½in) across. In late summer, bears daisy-like white flowers, 2cm (¾in) across, with purplish pink tips. ‡ 2cm (¾in), ↔ 10cm (4in). South Africa (Western Cape). ❀ (min. 7°C/45°F)

▷ ***Operculina tuberosa*** see *Merremia tuberosa*

OPHIOPOGON

Lilyturf

CONVALLARIACEAE/LILIACEAE

Genus of about 50 species of evergreen, rhizomatous or tufted perennials, often with swollen, fleshy roots, sometimes also stoloniferous, from shady scrub or woodland in E. Asia, especially China and Japan. They are grown mainly for their dense tufts of somewhat grass-like leaves. Racemes of numerous small, 6-tepalled, semi-spherical to bell-shaped, pinkish white, lilac, or white flowers are produced on leafless stems in summer, followed by spherical to oblong-ellipsoid, glossy, blue or black fruits. Grow as grassy ground cover, for border edging, or in a rock garden or peat bed. In frost-prone areas, grow the less hardy species for seasonal bedding, or in a cool or temperate greenhouse.

- **HARDINESS** Fully hardy to half hardy.
- **CULTIVATION** Outdoors, grow in moist but well-drained, slightly acid, fertile, humus-rich soil in full sun or partial shade. Top-dress annually with leaf mould in autumn. Under glass, grow in loam-based potting compost (JI No.2) in full light or bright indirect light. In growth, water freely and apply a balanced liquid fertilizer monthly; water sparingly in winter.

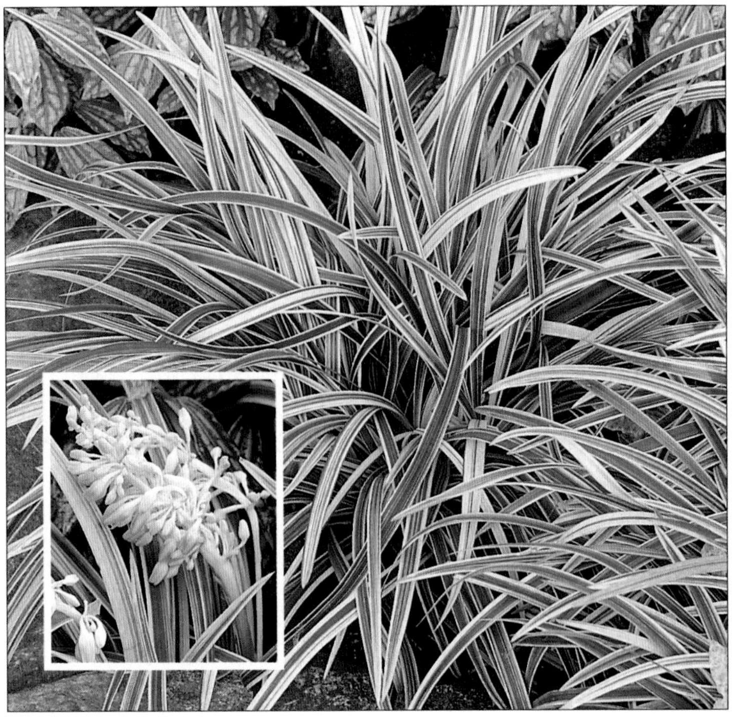

Ophiopogon jaburan 'Vittatus' (inset: flower detail)

- **PROPAGATION** Sow seed in containers in a cold frame as soon as ripe. Divide in spring as growth resumes.
- **PESTS AND DISEASES** Slugs may damage young leaves.

O. jaburan (Jaburan lily, White lilyturf). Tufted, stoloniferous perennial with strap-shaped, leathery, dark green leaves, to 60cm (24in) long. Short bell-shaped, white, sometimes lilac-tinted flowers, 1cm (½in) long, are produced in racemes, to 15cm (6in) long and occasionally curled, in late summer, followed by oblong-ellipsoid, violet-blue fruit, 1cm (½in) long. ‡ to 60cm (24in), ↔ to 30cm (12in). Japan. ❄❄. **'Argenteovittatus'** see 'Vittatus'. **'Javanensis'** see 'Vittatus'. **'Variegatus'** see 'Vittatus'. **'Vittatus'** ■ syn. 'Argenteovittatus', 'Javanensis', 'Variegatus', has pale green leaves that are striped and margined cream, yellow, or white. **'White Dragon'** has leaves boldly striped with white, almost obliterating the green.

O. japonicus. Tuberous-rooted, rhizomatous perennial forming clumps of narrowly linear, curved, rigid, dark green leaves, 20–30cm (8–12in) long. In summer, bears short racemes, 5–8cm (2–3in) long, of small, bell-shaped, white, occasionally lilac-tinged flowers, 5mm (¼in) across, followed by spherical, blue-black berries, 5mm (¼in) across. ‡ 20–30cm (8–12in), ↔ 30cm (12in). Japan. ❄❄❄. **'Kyoto Dwarf'** is compact; ‡↔ 10cm (4in). **'Silver Dragon'** has white-variegated leaves; ‡ to 30cm (12in), ↔ to 15cm (6in).

O. planiscapus. Clump-forming, spreading, rhizomatous perennial with strap-shaped, curving, dark green leaves, 10–35cm (4–14in) long. Short bell-shaped, pale purplish white flowers, to 7mm (¼in) long, are borne in racemes, 4–8cm (1½–3in) long, in summer, followed by spherical, fleshy, dark blue-black fruit, 3–5mm (⅛–¼in) across. ‡ 20cm (8in), ↔ 30cm (12in). ❄❄❄. **'Nigrescens'** ■♀ syn. 'Arabicus', 'Black Dragon', 'Ebony Knight', has almost black leaves.

O. spicatus see *Liriope spicata.*

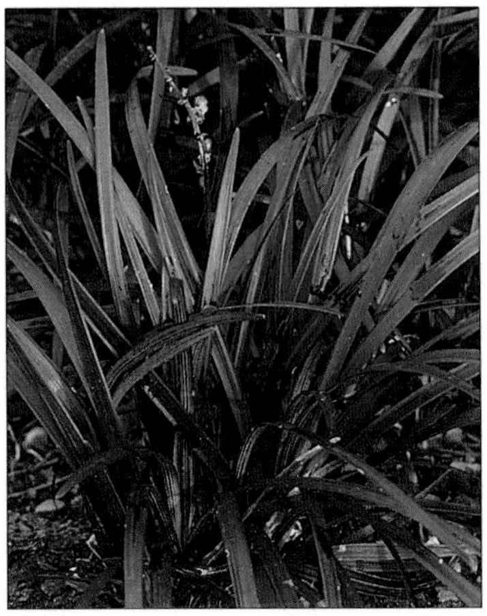

Ophiopogon planiscapus 'Nigrescens'

OPHRYS

ORCHIDACEAE

Genus of about 30 species of deciduous, tuberous, terrestrial orchids from Europe, Mediterranean islands, N. Africa, and W. Asia, occurring in habitats ranging from marshes and grassland to woodland and mountain-sides. They produce rosettes of oblong-ovate, ovate, or lance-shaped, mid-green leaves. From the rosettes arise erect inflorescences with small, bract-like leaves and racemes of 2–12 flowers; each has 3 spreading sepals, 2 petals, and a large lip, often strikingly coloured and resembling the abdomen of a bee or other insect. *Ophrys* species are suitable for a rock garden or for naturalizing in fine turf; in wet, frost-prone climates, they are best grown in an alpine house.

- **HARDINESS** Fully hardy to frost hardy.
- **CULTIVATION** Outdoors, grow in sharply drained, gritty, leafy, humus-rich soil in partial shade. Plant dormant tubers in autumn, at least 5cm (2in) deep. In frost-prone areas, provide a dry winter mulch. In an alpine house, grow in terrestrial orchid compost in bright filtered light. During the growing season, water moderately; keep dry and frost-free when dormant. See also p.46.

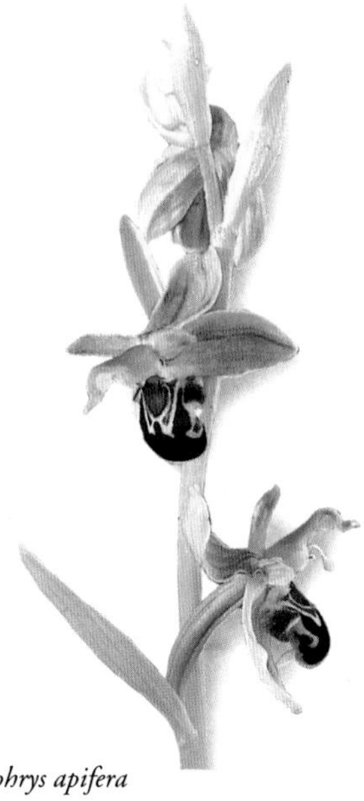

Ophrys apifera

- **PROPAGATION** Separate offsets in autumn.
- **PESTS AND DISEASES** Slugs and snails may cause problems.

O. apifera ■ (Bee orchid). Terrestrial orchid with oblong-ovate leaves, 6cm (2½in) long. Erect racemes, to 30cm (12in) tall, of 2–11 flowers, 2.5cm (1in) across, each with green or purplish pink sepals and petals, and a lip marked red-purple and yellow, are borne in mid-spring and early summer. ‡ 30cm (12in), ↔ 15cm (6in). W., S., and C. Europe, N. Africa, W. Asia. ❄❄❄

O. aranifera see *O. sphegodes.*

O. fuciflora see *O. holoserica.*

O. fusca (Sombre bee orchid). Terrestrial orchid with oblong-ovate or lance-shaped leaves, 6cm (2½in) long. In mid- and late spring, produces erect racemes, to 30cm (12in) tall, of up to 8 variable green or yellow-green flowers, 5cm (2in) across, each with a yellow- or white-margined, bluish, brown, purple, or purplish red lip. ‡ 30cm (12in), ↔ 15cm (6in). Mediterranean, S.W. Romania. ❄❄. **subsp. *iricolor*** ■ has racemes of up to 4 flowers, each with

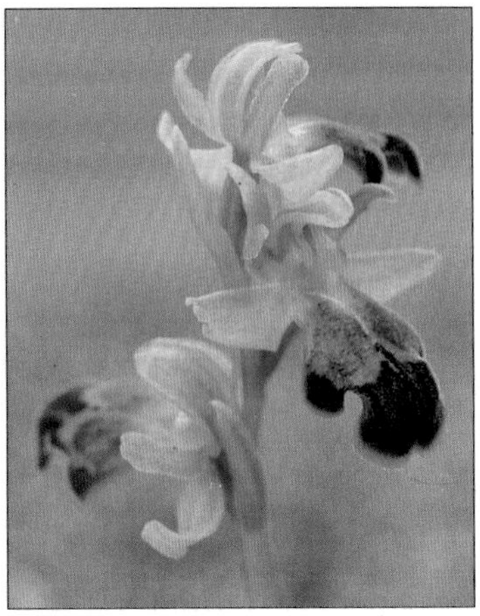

Ophrys fusca subsp. *iricolor*

O

a longer lip that has 2 elongated, iridescent blue patches.

O. holoserica, syn. *O. fuciflora* (Late spider orchid). Terrestrial orchid with ovate-oblong leaves, 6cm (2½in) long. From mid-spring to midsummer, produces short, erect racemes, to 30cm (12in) tall, of 2–6 flowers, 3cm (1¼in) across; each has green, bright pink, or white sepals, pink to purple-pink petals, and a dark brown to dark maroon or ochre lip, sometimes with yellow margins. ↕ 30cm (12in), ↔ 15cm (6in). W., S.W., and C. Europe. ❄❄

O. lutea Terrestrial orchid with ovate leaves, 6cm (2½in) long. Erect racemes, to 30cm (12in) tall, of 2–7 yellow-green flowers, 2.5cm (1in) across, each with a bright yellow lip, dark brown or purplish black in the centre, are borne from mid-spring to early summer. ↕ 30cm (12in), ↔ 15cm (6in). Portugal, Mediterranean. ❄❄

O. speculum see *O. vernixia.*

O. sphegodes, syn. *O. aranifera* (Early spider orchid). Variable, terrestrial orchid with ovate-lance-shaped leaves, 8cm (3in) long. From late spring to midsummer, produces erect racemes, to 45cm (18in) long, of up to 10 flowers, to 2.5cm (1in) across; each has green, occasionally brownish green sepals and petals, and a pale to blackish brown, velvety lip. ↕↔ 15cm (6in). Europe. ❄❄

O. vernixia, syn. *O. speculum* (Mirror orchid). Terrestrial orchid with oblong to lance-shaped leaves, 6cm (2½in) long. In late spring and early summer, produces erect racemes, to 30cm (12in) tall, of up to 15 green flowers, 2.5cm (1in) across, with dark brown stripes; the lip is velvety, black- or brown-margined, with glossy, deep blue, yellow-bordered centres. ↕ 30cm (12in), ↔ 15cm (6in). Portugal, N. Africa, Mediterranean. ❄❄

OPHTHALMOPHYLLUM

AIZOACEAE

Genus, closely related to *Conophytum,* of 19 species of perennial succulents growing wild in dry, hilly areas of Namibia and South Africa. They bear "bodies" of paired, erect, compressed-cylindrical, very fleshy leaves, united for most of their length, with transparent "windows" on the usually flat tops. Solitary, daisy-like flowers are borne from clefts between the paired lobes, during the day in late summer and autumn. In areas where temperatures drop below 10°C (50°F), grow in a temperate greenhouse; in warm, dry climates, grow in a desert garden or in a scree bed or raised bed.

• **HARDINESS** Frost tender.

• **CULTIVATION** Under glass, grow in a mix of 2 parts loam to 1 part each sharp sand and leaf mould, in full light. From late spring to early autumn, water sparingly and apply a dilute, low-nitrogen liquid fertilizer every 4–6 weeks. Reduce water from mid- to late autumn; keep completely dry from winter to mid-spring. Outdoors, grow in gritty, poor, humus-rich soil in full sun. See also pp.48–49.

• **PROPAGATION** Sow seed at 20–25°C (68–77°F), or separate and root complete bodies, in spring or summer.

• **PESTS AND DISEASES** Trouble free.

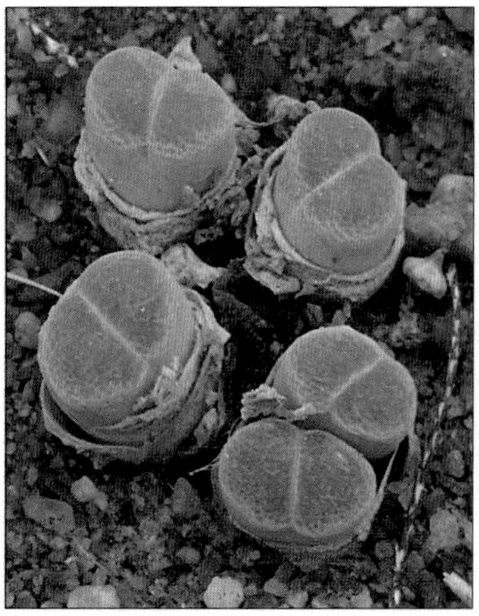

Ophthalmophyllum longum

O. longum ■ syn. *Conophytum longum.* Clump-forming, perennial succulent with grey-green to brown bodies, 2cm (¾in) across, consisting of rounded lobes with translucent dots above and keeled undersides. Daisy-like, white to pale pink flowers, 2cm (¾in) across, are borne in late summer and autumn. ↕ 3cm (1¼in), ↔ indefinite. Namibia, South Africa. ⊛ (min. 5–7°C/41–45°F)

O. maughanii. Clump-forming, perennial succulent producing yellowish green bodies, 2cm (¾in) across, with short, conical lobes. In late summer and autumn, produces daisy-like white flowers, 1.5cm (½in) across. ↕ 4cm (1½in), ↔ indefinite. Namibia, South Africa. ⊛ (min. 5–7°C/41–45°F)

▷**Opium poppy** see *Papaver somniferum*

OPLISMENUS

GRAMINEAE/POACEAE

Genus of 6 species of trailing, annual or perennial grasses from subtropical and tropical forests of Africa, Asia, Polynesia, and Central and South America. They have slender, rooting, leafy stems with flat, lance-shaped to ovate leaves, and bear one-sided racemes of insignificant flowers. Only *O. africanus* 'Variegatus' is of decorative value: in warm areas, it provides excellent ground cover, and is also a useful edging plant; in frost-prone areas, grow as an ornamental plant in a hanging basket in a temperate greenhouse or conservatory.

• **HARDINESS** Frost tender.

• **CULTIVATION** Under glass, grow in loamless or loam-based potting compost (JI No.2) in bright filtered or full light. In growth, water freely and apply a balanced liquid fertilizer every 4 weeks. Water sparingly in winter. Outdoors, grow in any moist but well-drained soil in full sun or partial shade.

• **PROPAGATION** Separate rooted stems in spring; pot up and keep in a propagating case until established.

• **PESTS AND DISEASES** Trouble free.

O. africanus, syn. *O. hirtellus.* Evergreen perennial with wiry stems, spreading and rooting at the nodes, bearing narrowly lance-shaped to ovate, softly hairy, mid-green leaves, to 5cm (2in) long, with long points. Small flowers are produced in one-sided racemes, to 15cm (6in) long, from summer to winter. ↕ 15cm (6in), but may form mounds to 90cm (36in),

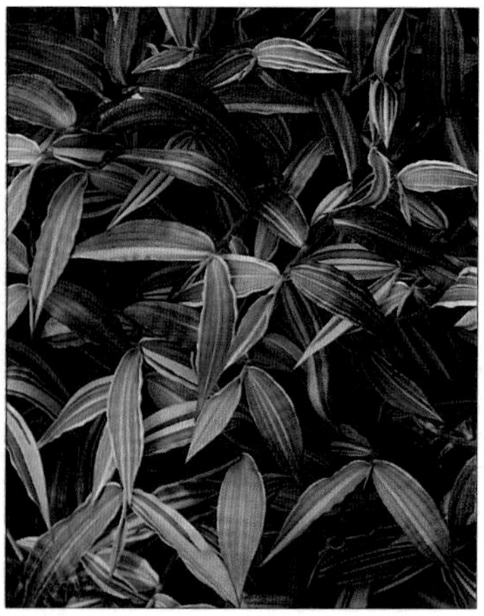

Oplismenus africanus 'Variegatus'

↔ indefinite. Africa, Polynesia, tropical Central and South America. ⊛ (min. 5°C/41°F). **'Variegatus'** ■ 🏆 syn. 'Vittatus', has white-striped leaves, flushed purple-pink.

O. hirtellus see *O. africanus.*

OPUNTIA

CACTACEAE

Genus of about 200 species of perennial cacti, ranging from alpine and ground-cover plants to bushy and tree-like species, from often very arid regions in North, Central, and South America, and the West Indies. They have usually pad-like and flattened, or sometimes cylindrical, club-shaped, or spherical, segmented branches, with areoles producing spines and glochids (barbed spines); a few species have leaf-like scales, which soon fall. On mature plants, funnel- or bowl-shaped flowers are produced singly from the areoles at the tips or sides of the segments; they appear during the day in spring or summer, and are followed by usually spiny, obovoid or spherical fruits (prickly pears). In a few species, these are edible, and contain large, smooth white seeds in pulp.

Where temperatures drop below 10°C (50°F), grow tender species in a cool or temperate greenhouse. In warmer areas, grow opuntias in a desert garden or in a border with other cacti. They are not suitable as houseplants; contact with the bristles causes intense irritation to skin, and they are difficult to remove.

• **HARDINESS** Fully hardy to frost tender.

• **CULTIVATION** Under glass, grow in standard cactus compost in full light or bright filtered light. Large species are best planted directly into a greenhouse border; all dislike root restriction. From early spring to mid-autumn, water freely and apply a balanced liquid fertilizer 3 or 4 times. Keep dry at other times. Outdoors, grow in moderately fertile, sharply drained, gritty, humus-rich soil in full sun. See also pp.48–49.

• **PROPAGATION** Sow pre-soaked seed at 21°C (70°F) in spring. Separate and root stem segments. Handle plants using folded newspaper; dispose of it after use.

• **PESTS AND DISEASES** Vulnerable to scale insects and mealybugs.

O. argentina ■ Tree-like, perennial cactus with thick, bright green stems, cylindrical branches, and flat, oblong segments, 5–12cm (2–5in) long, each with pale brown glochids and usually one spine which is red at first, becoming brown. Wide-spreading, funnel-shaped yellow flowers, 3–4cm (1¼–1½in) across, are produced in summer, followed by edible, ovoid, spineless, purplish red fruit, 5cm (2in) long. ↕ to 15m (50ft), ↔ 3m (10ft). N. Argentina. ⊛ (min. 7–10°C/45–50°F)

O. basilaris. Clump-forming, perennial cactus with velvety, bluish green or pale reddish green stems divided into flat, obovate to nearly rounded segments, 10–20cm (4–8in) long. Brown areoles each have reddish brown glochids and none or 1, rarely up to 5, spines. Bowl-shaped, usually deep purple-red flowers, 6–8cm (2½–3in) across, are borne in summer, followed by spherical to ovoid, dry, velvety, grey-green fruit, 3–4cm (1¼–1½in) long. ↕ 1m (3ft), ↔ to 75cm (30in) or more. S. USA, N. Mexico. ⊛ (min. 7–10°C/45–50°F)

O. bergeriana. Tree-like, perennial cactus with numerous branches divided into flattened, narrowly oblong-oval, pale to fresh green segments, 10–25cm (4–10in) long. Grey areoles each have yellow glochids and 2–5 sheathed, yellow then grey spines. From spring to summer, produces funnel-shaped, bright, deep red flowers, to 6cm (2½in) across, followed by ovoid, spiny red fruit, to 4cm (1½in) long. ↕ to 3.5m (11ft), ↔ 1m (3ft). Origin unknown. ⊛ (min. 7–10°C/45–50°F)

O. chlorotica. Bushy or tree-like, perennial cactus with pale bluish green stems composed of flattened, rounded to obovate segments, to 20cm (8in) long. Grey areoles each bear yellow glochids and 1–6 or more pale yellow or brown spines, which blacken with age. Broadly funnel-shaped yellow flowers, 7cm (3in) across, flushed red outside, are produced from spring to summer; they are followed by ovoid purple fruit, 4cm (1½in) long, with short spines that are lost as the fruit mature. ↕ to 2m (6ft), ↔ 75cm (30in). USA (California, Nevada, New Mexico), N. Mexico. ⊛ (min. 7–10°C/45–50°F)

O. clavarioides. Semi-prostrate, tuberous-rooted, many-branched, perennial cactus with stems divided into cylindrical, inversely conical, flat, or fan-shaped, greyish brown segments, 2cm (¾in) or more long. Whitish grey areoles bear leaf-like, deciduous red scales, to 2mm (1/16in) long, and each areole has 4–10 minute, fine white spines, but no glochids. In late spring

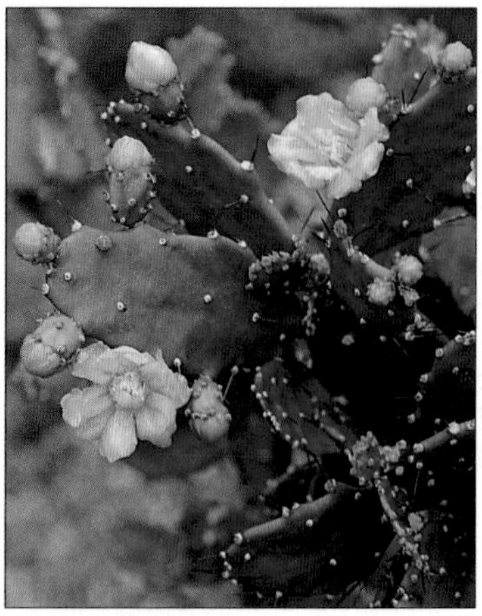

Opuntia argentina

OPUNTIA

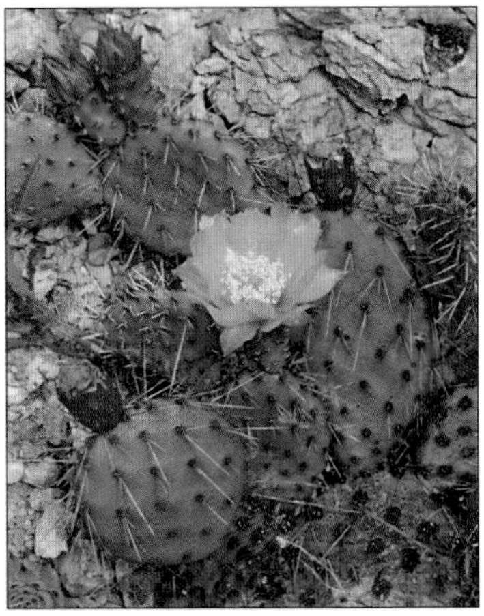

Opuntia erinacea

and summer, produces funnel-shaped, brownish green flowers, 6cm (2½in) across, followed by ellipsoid, spineless, greyish brown fruit, 1.5cm (½in) long. ↕↔ to 10cm (4in). Argentina. ❄ (min. 7–10°C/45–50°F)

O. cochenillifera, syn. *Nopalea cochenillifera.* Shrubby or tree-like, perennial cactus with stems composed of flattened, elliptic to obovate, glossy, dark green segments, 8–25cm (3–10in) long. Mid-green areoles produce yellow glochids, and sometimes 1–3 yellow spines, usually none. Narrowly funnel-shaped, bright red flowers, to 4cm (1½in) across, appear in late spring and summer, followed by ellipsoid, fleshy, spineless red fruit, 2.5–4cm (1–1½in) long. ↕ to 4m (12ft), ↔ 1m (3ft). Mexico. ❄ (min. 7–10°C/45–50°F)

O. compressa, syn. *O. humifusa.* Clump-forming, semi-prostrate, perennial cactus with stems divided into flattened, elliptic to obovate or rounded, greyish green segments, 5–13cm (2–5in) long, often tinged purple, and bearing narrowly wedge-shaped leaves, to 7mm (¼in) long. Brown areoles produce brown glochids, and sometimes 1 or 2 black-tipped white spines. Produces broadly funnel-shaped, bright yellow flowers, 4–6cm (1½–2½in) across, in late spring and summer; they are followed by obovoid, spineless, edible purple or red fruit, 2.5–4cm (1–1½in) long. ↕ 10–30cm (4–12in), ↔ to 1m (3ft) or more. C. and E. USA. ❄ (min. 3–5°C/37–51°F)

O. engelmannii see *O. ficus-indica.*

***O. engelmannii* of gardens** see *O. phaeacantha.*

O. erinacea ■ syn. *O. hystricina.* Clump-forming, perennial cactus producing bluish green stems that are composed of flattened, rounded to broadly obovate segments, 5–10cm (2–4in) long. Brown or white areoles each have yellow glochids and 9 or more thread-like white spines, to 10cm (4in) long. Shallowly bowl-shaped, red, pink, purplish pink, or yellow flowers, 6cm (2½in) across, are produced in summer; they are followed by ovoid, light green, very spiny fruit, to 2cm (¾in) long. ↕ 50cm (20in), ↔ 1.5m (5ft). S.W. USA. ❄ (min. 7–10°C/45–50°F). **var. *ursina*** ■ (Grizzly Bear cactus) bears oblong-elliptic stem segments with numerous very long, thread-like, deflexed spines, to 10cm (4in) long, and produces orange or pink flowers;

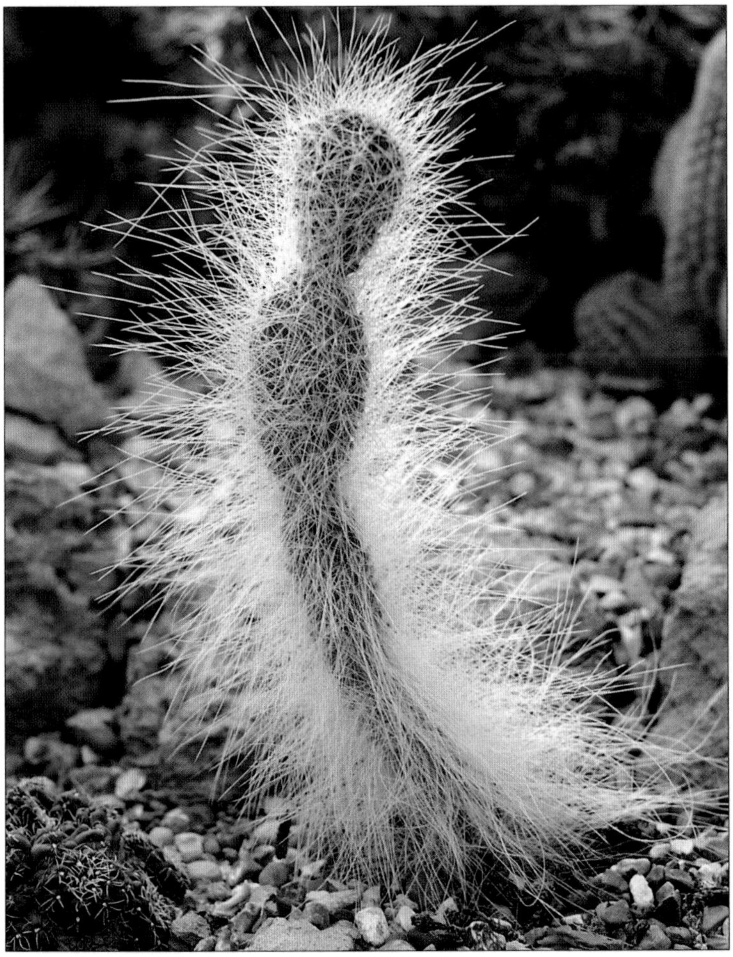

Opuntia erinacea var. *ursina*

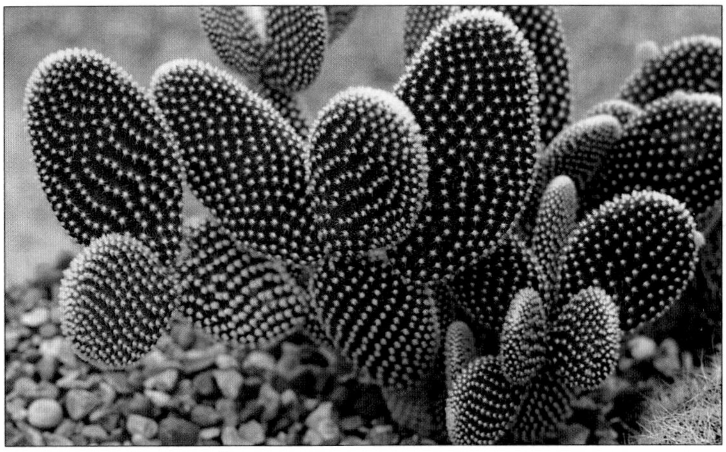

Opuntia microdasys var. *albispina*

↕↔ to 45cm (18in). USA (California, Nevada, Arizona).

O. falcata, syn. *Consolea falcata.* Tree-like, perennial cactus with glossy, dark green stems composed of flattened, oblong to lance-shaped segments, to 35cm (14in) long, marked with small tubercles. White areoles each bear a few brownish white glochids and 2–8 needle-like, rough, pale yellow or yellowish brown spines. Bowl-shaped red flowers, 3–5cm (1¼–2in) across, are borne in late spring and summer, and are followed by ovoid, spineless, dark green fruit, to 4cm (1½in) long. ↕ to 1.5m (5ft), ↔ 75cm (30in). Haiti. ❄ (min. 7–10°C/45–50°F)

O. ficus-indica, syn. *O. engelmannii, O. megacantha* (Indian fig, Prickly pear). Bushy or tree-like, perennial cactus with stems composed of flattened, obovate to oblong, greyish green or mid-green segments, 10–40cm (4–16in) long, with white areoles producing yellow glochids and usually 1 or 2 spines. Bowl-shaped yellow flowers, 10cm (4in) across, are produced in late spring and summer, and are followed by edible, ovoid, spineless purple fruit, to 10cm (4in) long. Some cultivars have yellow, orange, or red fruit. ↕↔ 5m (15ft). Mexico. ❄ (min. 7–10°C/45–50°F)

O. humifusa see *O. compressa.*

O. hystricina see *O. erinacea.*

O. imbricata. Variable, many-branched, perennial cactus with cylindrical, mid-green to bluish green stem segments, 10–40cm (4–16in) long, with very prominent tubercles, and cylindrical leaves, 1.5cm (½in) long. Large yellow areoles each bear yellow glochids and 8–30 brown-sheathed, reddish yellow or white spines. Broadly funnel-shaped, purple or red flowers, usually 4–8cm (1½–3in) across, are produced in late spring and summer, followed by nearly spherical, spineless yellow fruit, 3cm (1¼in) long. ↕ to 3m (10ft), ↔ 1m (3ft). S.W. USA, Mexico. ❄ (min. 7–10°C/45–50°F)

O. megacantha see *O. ficus-indica.*

O. microdasys. Bushy, perennial cactus with stems comprising flattened, oblong, obovate, or almost rounded, velvety, pale to mid-green segments, 6–15cm (2½–6in) long; these are thickly dotted with white areoles bearing minute, yellow, white, or reddish brown glochids and usually no spines. Bowl-shaped, bright yellow flowers, 4–5cm (1½–2in) across, often tinged red on the outside, are produced from spring to summer; they are followed by oblong-ellipsoid, spineless, light purplish red fruit, to 4.5cm (1¾in) long. ↕↔ 40–60cm (16–24in). N. and C. Mexico. ❄ (min. 7–10°C/45–50°F). **var. *albispina*** ■ has dark green stem pads, white glochids, whitish yellow flowers, and darker purple-red fruit. **var. *pallida*** (Bunny ears) has thin, greyish green stem segments, 8–15cm (3–6in) long, with yellow areoles and glochids; ↕↔ 60cm (24in). **var. *rufida***, syn. *O. rufida*, has reddish brown areoles and glochids, no spines, and bowl-shaped, yellow or orange-yellow flowers; ↕↔ 50cm (20in); S. USA, N.W. Mexico.

O. paraguayensis. Semi-erect, perennial cactus with glossy, dark green stems composed of flattened, inversely lance-shaped or narrowly elliptic segments, 18–30cm (7–12in) long, with prominent, yellowish white areoles, tufts of yellow glochids, and usually no spines or one pale yellow spine. Broadly bowl-shaped orange flowers, 8cm (3in) across, are produced in late spring and summer, and are followed by conical, spineless, dark purple fruit, to 7cm (3in) long. ↕ to 2m (6ft), ↔ 1.5m (5ft). Paraguay, Argentina. ❄ (min. 7–10°C/45–50°F)

O. phaeacantha, syn. *O. engelmannii* of gardens. Variable, perennial cactus with stems divided into flattened, obovate or rounded, pale to bluish green, sometimes purple-tinged segments, 10–40cm (4–16in) long. Brown areoles each have a tuft of brown glochids and 1–8 sheathed, brown or red-brown spines. Produces broadly funnel-shaped, sulphur-yellow flowers, 5cm (2in) across, sometimes red-tinged inside, in late spring and summer, followed by ovoid, spineless red fruit, to 4cm (1½in) long. ↕ to 1.5m (5ft), ↔ to 2m (6ft). S.W. USA, N. Mexico. ❄ (min. 7–10°C/45–50°F)

O. pycnantha. Bushy, semi-prostrate, perennial cactus with stems composed of flattened, rounded, slightly softly hairy, dark green segments, 10–18cm (4–7in) long; they are covered with pale brown areoles, each bearing brownish yellow glochids and 3–12 reflexed, yellow or red-brown spines. From spring to summer, produces broadly funnel-shaped, greenish yellow, often red-tinged flowers, 4.5cm (1¾in) across; they are followed by ovoid, very prickly, spiny, dull green fruit, 4cm (1½in) long. ↕↔ 45cm (18in). Mexico (Baja California). ❄ (min. 7–10°C/45–50°F)

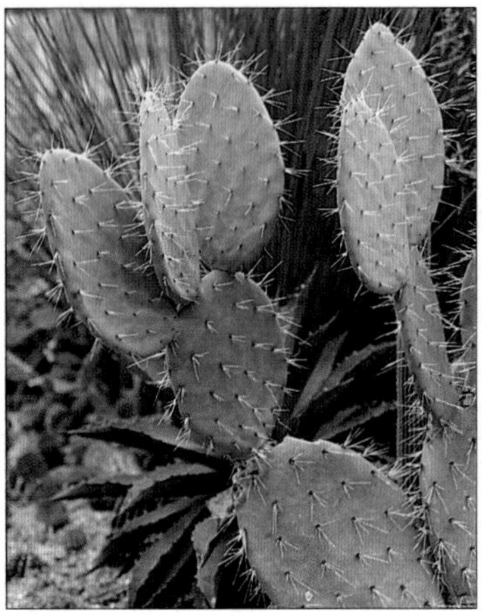

Opuntia robusta

O. robusta ■ Variable, shrubby or tree-like, perennial cactus with stems composed of flat, thick, oval to almost rounded, greyish or bluish green segments, to 40cm (16in) across. Brown areoles bear reddish brown glochids and, in each upper areole, 2–12 sheathed white, pale brown, or yellow spines. Shallowly bowl-shaped yellow flowers, 7cm (3in) across, appear in late spring and summer, followed by spherical to ellipsoid, spineless, deep red fruit, 8cm (3in) long. ↕↔ 2m (6ft) or more. C. Mexico. ❀ (min. 7–10°C/45–50°F)
O. rufida see *O. microdasys* var. *rufida*.
O. subulata. Freely branching, tree-like, perennial cactus, with cylindrical, unsegmented, dark green stems, 5–7cm (2–3in) in diameter; they are covered with oblong tubercles and, on the upper stems, semi-cylindrical, sharp-pointed, more or less evergreen leaves, 5cm (2in) or more long. Yellow areoles each have yellow glochids and 1 or 2 pale yellow spines. Cup-shaped red flowers, 7cm (3in) across, are produced from spring to summer, followed by persistent, oblong-ellipsoid, spineless, dark green fruit, 6–10cm (2½–4in) long. ↕ to 4m (12ft), ↔ to 1.5m (5ft). S. Peru. ❀ (min. 7–10°C/45–50°F)
O. tunicata ■ Densely bushy, freely branching, perennial cactus with whorls of glaucous green stems divided into cylindrical segments, 6–15cm (2½–6in) long. Prominent white areoles have yellow glochids and 6–10 sheathed, off-white or yellow spines. From spring to summer, bears cup-shaped yellow flowers, 3–5cm (1¼–2in) across, followed by spherical to broadly club-

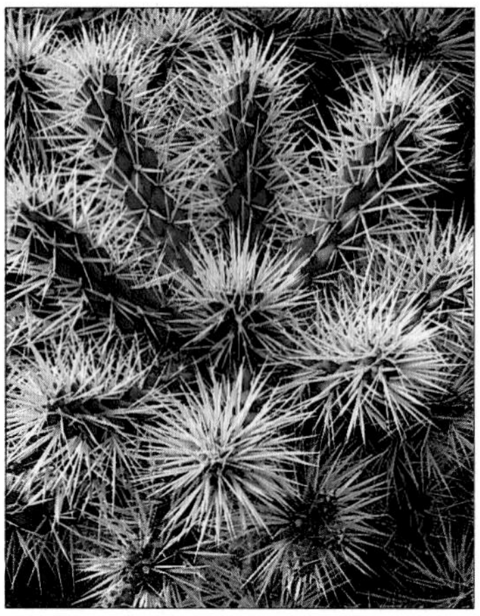

Opuntia tunicata

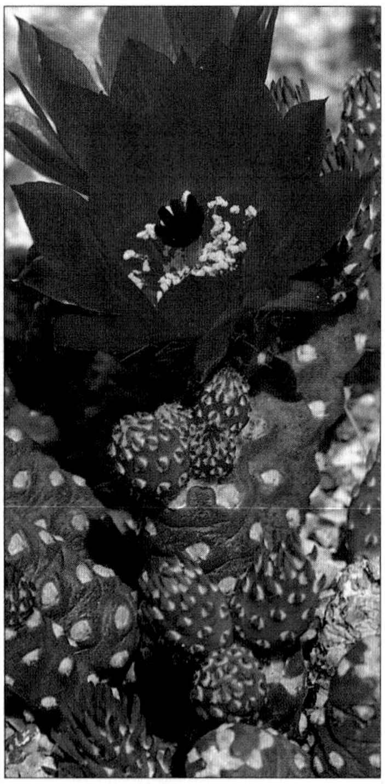

Opuntia verschaffeltii

shaped, spineless, glaucous green fruit, to 3cm (1¼in) long. ↕ 60cm (24in), ↔ 1m (3ft). C. Mexico. ❀ (min. 7–10°C/45–50°F)
O. verschaffeltii ■ Clump-forming, perennial cactus with dull green stems composed of cylindrical segments, 10–20cm (4–8in) or more long, with low tubercles and persistent, cylindrical leaves, to 3cm (1¼in) long. White areoles have yellow glochids and 1–3 or more, hair-like white spines. Cup-shaped, red or orange-red flowers, 4cm (1½in) across, are produced from spring to summer, followed by spherical, spineless red fruit, to 3cm (1¼in) long. ↕ 15cm (6in), ↔ 1m (3ft). Bolivia, N. Argentina. ❀ (min. 7–10°C/45–50°F)
O. vestita (Cotton-pole cactus). Low-growing, perennial cactus with fragile, warty, pale green stems, and cylindrical segments to 20cm (8in) long. Yellow areoles, the upper ones with cylindrical, more or less evergreen leaves, 1cm (½in) long, each produce white glochids and 4–8 white spines intermingled with many fine white hairs, which envelop the stems. Cup-shaped, dark violet-red flowers, 4cm (1½in) across, are borne in late spring and summer, followed by spherical, spineless red fruit, to 2cm (¾in) long. ↕↔ 1m (3ft). Bolivia. ❀ (min. 7–10°C/45–50°F)

▷**Orache, Red** see *Atriplex hortensis*
▷**Orange,**
  Australian mock see *Pittosporum undulatum*
  Japanese bitter see *Poncirus trifoliata*
  Japanese mock see *Pittosporum tobira*
  Mock see *Philadelphus, P. coronarius*
  Osage see *Maclura pomifera*
  Panama see x *Citrofortunella microcarpa*
  Seville see *Citrus aurantium*
  Sweet see *Citrus sinensis* 'Washington'
▷**Orange ball tree** see *Buddleja globosa*
▷**Orange blossom, Mexican** see *Choisya, C. ternata*

ORBEA

ASCLEPIADACEAE

Genus of about 20 species of dwarf, erect to decumbent, mainly clump-forming, leafless, perennial succulents, closely related to *Stapelia*, from semi-arid, hilly, often rocky terrain in E. Africa and South Africa. They have large, warty teeth along the angled stem margins, and produce funnel-shaped, usually 5-lobed, often unpleasantly scented flowers, which attract blue-bottles. The diurnal flowers, borne singly or in few-flowered cymes from summer to autumn, each have a slightly wrinkled, usually flattened corolla, surrounded by a very pronounced, smooth annulus. Below 11°C (52°F), grow in a warm greenhouse; in warm, dry climates, use in a desert garden.
• **HARDINESS** Frost tender.
• **CULTIVATION** Under glass, grow in standard cactus compost, top-dressed with grit. Provide low humidity, with bright filtered light in summer, full light in winter. From spring to early autumn, water moderately, applying a low-nitrogen fertilizer every 3–4 weeks. Keep dry at other times, but water sparingly on warm winter days to prevent shrivelling. Outdoors, grow in gritty, loamy, moderately fertile, humus-rich soil in partial shade. See also pp.48–49.
• **PROPAGATION** Sow seed at 18–21°C (64–70°F) in spring. Take stem-segment cuttings in spring and summer.
• **PESTS AND DISEASES** Susceptible to mealybugs and root mealybugs, and to black rot if overwatered.

O. ciliata, syn. *Diplocyathus ciliata*. Mat-forming succulent with erect, 4-angled, toothed, mid-green stems, the tips tinged red. In summer, bears solitary, bowl-shaped, pale yellow flowers, to 8cm (3in) across, with dark purple-spotted annuli. ↕ 5cm (2in), ↔ to 15cm (6in). South Africa (Northern Cape, Eastern Cape). ❀ (min. 11°C/52°F)
O. variegata ■ syn. *Stapelia variegata* (Starfish cactus, Toad cactus). Variable, clump-forming succulent with erect, obtusely angled, prominently toothed, greyish green stems, often mottled purple. In summer, produces cymes of up to 5 funnel-shaped, flat, densely wrinkled, dark brownish red flowers, 5–9cm (2–3½in) across, patterned white or yellowish white. ↕ 10cm (4in), ↔ to 30cm (12in). South Africa (Eastern Cape). ❀ (min. 11°C/52°F)

ORBEOPSIS

ASCLEPIADACEAE

Genus of about 10 species of leafless, perennial succulents from dry hillsides in Angola, Mozambique, and South Africa. They have angled, freely branching, usually greyish green stems, and bear umbel-like clusters of star-shaped, malodorous flowers during the day in early summer. In areas where temperatures drop below 10°C (50°F), grow in a warm greenhouse; in warm, dry climates, grow in a desert border.
• **HARDINESS** Frost tender.
• **CULTIVATION** Under glass, grow in standard cactus compost and top-dress with grit. Provide low humidity and full light with shade from hot sun. From spring to early autumn, water moderately and apply a low-nitrogen fertilizer every 4 or 5 weeks. Keep dry at other times, but water sparingly on warm winter days to prevent shrivelling. Outdoors, grow in moderately fertile, gritty, loamy, and humus-rich soil, in full sun. See also pp.48–49.
• **PROPAGATION** Sow seed at 18–21°C (64–70°F) in spring. Take stem-segment cuttings in spring and summer.
• **PESTS AND DISEASES** Trouble free.

O. albocastanea, syn. *Caralluma albocastanea*. Semi-erect, succulent perennial that offsets from the base, producing 4-angled, upward-curving, reddish brown stems with pale spots and large, projecting teeth. In early summer,

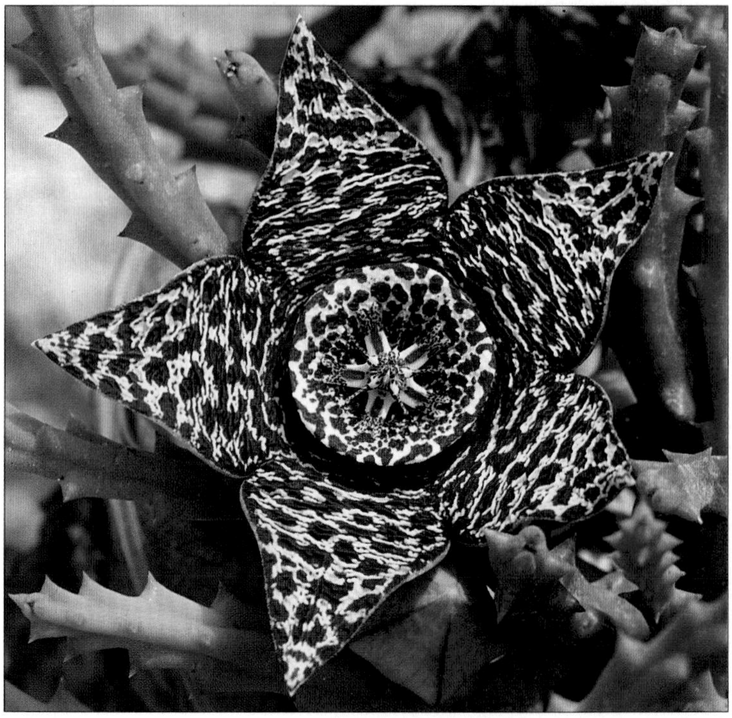

Orbea variegata

star-shaped flowers, 2.5–3cm (1–1¼in) across, are borne in umbel-like clusters of 3–6; they are green outside with red spots, and cream inside with brownish purple spots, the margins having thick, dark red hairs. They have dark brown coronas. ↕ 8cm (3in), ↔ 18cm (7in). Namibia. ❄ (min. 10°C/50°F)
O. lutea, syn. *Caralluma lutea.* Variable, mat-forming, succulent perennial with 4-angled, coarsely toothed, greyish green stems. In early summer, bears dense, umbel-like clusters of 3–26 star-shaped flowers, 4–8cm (1½–3in) across, ranging in colour from reddish brown to maroon or pale lemon-yellow, with yellow-hairy margins and yellow coronas. ↕ 10cm (4in), ↔ 24cm (10in). Southern Africa. ❄ (min. 10°C/50°F)

▷**Orchid,**
Bee see *Ophrys apifera*
Butterfly see *Orchis papilionacea*
Clown see *Rossioglossum grande*
Cradle see *Anguloa*
Dancing doll see *Oncidium flexuosum*
Early purple see *Orchis mascula*
Early spider see *Ophrys sphegodes*
Golden chain see *Dendrochilum*
Green-veined see *Orchis morio*
Heath spotted see *Dactylorhiza maculata*
Jewel see *Goodyera*
Lady's slipper see *Cypripedium, C. calceolus*
Late spider see *Ophrys holoserica*
Marsh see *Dactylorhiza*
Mirror see *Ophrys vernixia*
Moth see *Phalaenopsis*
Pansy see *Miltoniopsis*
Poor man's see *Schizanthus, S. pinnatus*
Robust marsh see *Dactylorhiza elata*
Scorpion see *Arachnis*
Shower see *Congea tomentosa*
Showy lady's slipper see *Cypripedium reginae*
Slipper see *Paphiopedilum*
Sombre bee see *Ophrys fusca*
Spider see *Brassia lawrenceana*
Spotted see *Dactylorhiza*
Swan see *Cycnoches*
Tiger see *Rossioglossum grande*
Tulip see *Anguloa*
▷**Orchids** see p.46
▷**Orchid tree** see *Amherstia nobilis, Bauhinia variegata*

ORCHIS

ORCHIDACEAE

Genus of about 35 species of deciduous, terrestrial orchids from Europe and Asia, mostly occurring in open, grassy places, frequently in poor, dry soil. They have 2 or 3 spherical or ovoid tubers, and rosettes of linear-lance-shaped to oblong-ovate, sometimes purple-spotted, light to dark green leaves. Dense, erect racemes of delicate purple, red, pink, yellow, green, or white flowers, each with a short spur, and sometimes with a pungent odour, are produced from spring to summer. They are suitable for a rock garden or woodland garden, but are usually grown in an alpine house.
• **HARDINESS** Fully hardy to frost hardy.
• **CULTIVATION** In an alpine house, grow in terrestrial orchid compost in bright filtered light. Water moderately in growth; keep dry and frost-free when dormant. Outdoors, grow in fertile,

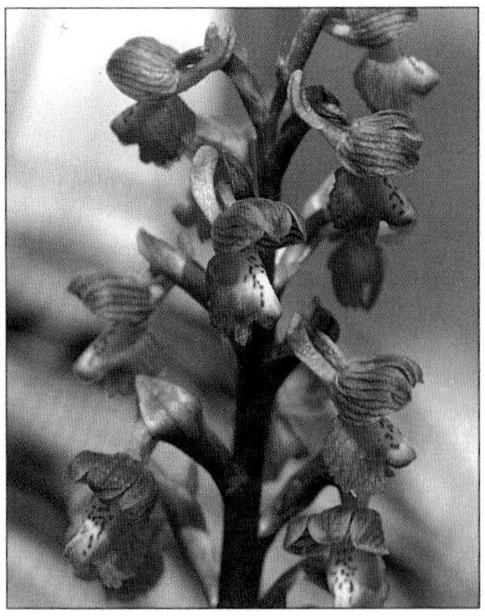

Orchis morio

well-drained, gritty, humus-rich soil in partial shade. *O. morio* and *O. papilionacea* prefer slightly acid to slightly alkaline soil; *O. mascula* prefers moist, neutral to slightly acid soil. Plant dormant tubers in autumn, at least 8cm (3in) deep. In frost-prone areas, provide a dry winter mulch. See also p.46.
• **PROPAGATION** Separate offsets in spring.
• **PESTS AND DISEASES** Slugs and snails may be troublesome.

O. elata see *Dactylorhiza elata.*
O. maderensis see *Dactylorhiza foliosa.*
O. mascula (Early purple orchid). Terrestrial orchid with mid-green, often purple-spotted leaves, 15cm (6in) long. From spring to midsummer, bears light to dark purple flowers, 2cm (¾in) long, in erect racemes, to 30cm (12in) tall. ↕ 30cm (12in), ↔ 15cm (6in). Europe. ✻✻✻
O. morio ■ (Green-veined orchid). Terrestrial orchid with pale to mid-green leaves, 6cm (2½in) long. Pale to deep purple flowers, 2cm (¾in) long, with green veins on the cupped sepals, are borne in erect racemes, to 15cm (6in) tall, from spring to midsummer. ↕ 15–30cm (6–12in), ↔ 8cm (3in). Europe to W. Iran. ✻✻
O. papilionacea (Butterfly orchid). Terrestrial orchid with mid-green leaves, 6cm (2½in) long. In spring and early summer, bears erect racemes, to 15cm (6in) tall, of pale purple to lilac, sometimes reddish brown, darker veined flowers, 2cm (¾in) long, with large, pink-veined lips. ↕ 15–30cm (6–12in), ↔ 8cm (3in). S. Europe to S.W. Asia. ✻✻✻

▷**Oregano** see *Origanum, O. vulgare*

OREOCEREUS

syn. BORZICACTUS

CACTACEAE

Genus of about 6 species of mainly columnar, perennial cacti from mountainous regions in South America. The thick, cylindrical, many-ribbed stems, usually branching from the bases, have tubercles and spiny areoles and, in some species, are covered in long hairs. Solitary, tubular-funnel-shaped flowers are produced during the day in summer, usually near the stem tips. Below 10°C (50°F), grow as houseplants or in a warm greenhouse; in warm, dry climates, grow in a desert garden.

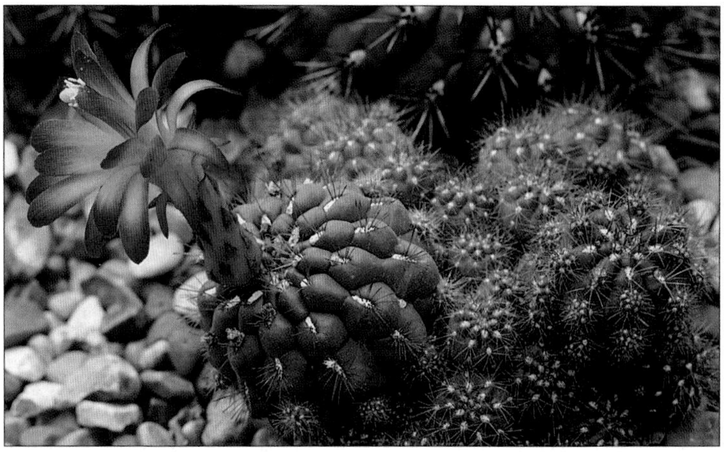

Oreocereus aurantiacus

• **HARDINESS** Frost tender.
• **CULTIVATION** Under glass, grow in a mix of 4 parts standard cactus compost and 1 part limestone chippings, in full light. From spring to summer, water freely; apply a balanced liquid fertilizer monthly. Keep dry at other times. Outdoors, grow in moderately fertile, slightly alkaline, sharply drained, humus-rich soil in full sun. See also pp.48–49.
• **PROPAGATION** Sow seed at 21°C (70°F) in spring or summer.
• **PESTS AND DISEASES** Vulnerable to scale insects.

O. aurantiacus ■ syn. *Borzicactus aurantiacus, Matucana aurantiaca.* Solitary or clustering, perennial cactus with spherical to flattened-spherical or short-cylindrical, warty, dark green stems, each with 11–28 ribs. Elliptic areoles bear 16–22 yellow to reddish brown radial spines, but no centrals. In summer, produces solitary, red-throated, bright orange-red or orange-yellow flowers, to 9cm (3½in) long. ↕↔ 15cm (6in). N. Peru. ❄ (min. 10°C/50°F).
O. celsianus ■ syn. *Borzicactus celsianus.* Slow-growing, clump-forming, perennial cactus with cylindrical, erect stems branching from the bases, each with 10–17 warty ribs. Grey-woolly areoles bear white hairs and yellow to reddish brown spines (7–9 radials and 1–4 much longer centrals). In summer, produces solitary, pale purplish pink flowers, 7–9cm (3–3½in) long, brownish red outside. ↕ 1–3m (3–10ft), ↔ 45cm (18in) or more. Bolivia, N.W. Argentina. ❄ (min. 10°C/50°F)

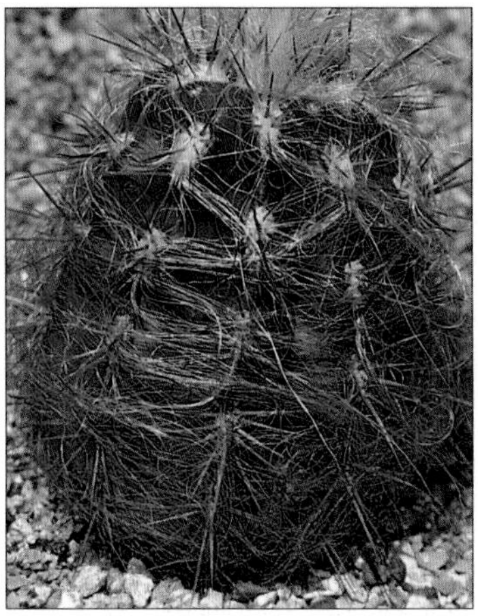

Oreocereus celsianus

O. haynei ■ syn. *Borzicactus haynei, Matucana haynei.* Solitary, occasionally clustering, perennial cactus with spherical to cylindrical, grass-green stems, each with 25–30 ribs and low-set tubercles. Ovoid, thickly set areoles bear yellow wool and spreading, stiff, white to yellowish brown spines (30 or more radials and 3 centrals). Solitary, red and orange to purplish crimson flowers, to 6–7cm (2½–3in) long, are produced in summer. ↕ to 30cm (12in), ↔ 10cm (4in). N. Peru. ❄ (min. 10°C/50°F)
O. hempelianus, syn. *Arequipa hempeliana, Borzicactus leucotrichus.* Solitary, perennial cactus with branching, spherical then short-cylindrical, erect or semi-prostrate, greyish green or glaucous green stems, each with 10–20 warty ribs and yellow wool at the tips. White areoles each bear 11–40 spines (8–30 radials and 3–10 longer centrals). Solitary, bright scarlet to purplish red flowers, to 8cm (3in) long, are produced in summer. ↕ to 40cm (16in), ↔ 10cm (4in). Mountains of S. Peru, N. Chile. ❄ (min. 10°C/50°F)
O. intertexta, syn. *Matucana intertexta.* Clump-forming, perennial cactus with erect, spherical to short-cylindrical, shiny, dark green stems, each with 14–18 warty ribs, often somewhat spiralled. Elliptic areoles each bear yellow spines, reddish brown beneath (16–18 radials and 3–7 longer centrals). In summer, bears solitary, orange-red flowers, 5–7cm (2–3in) across. ↕↔ to 15cm (6in). Peru. ❄ (min. 10°C/50°F)
O. peruviana see *Oroya peruviana.*

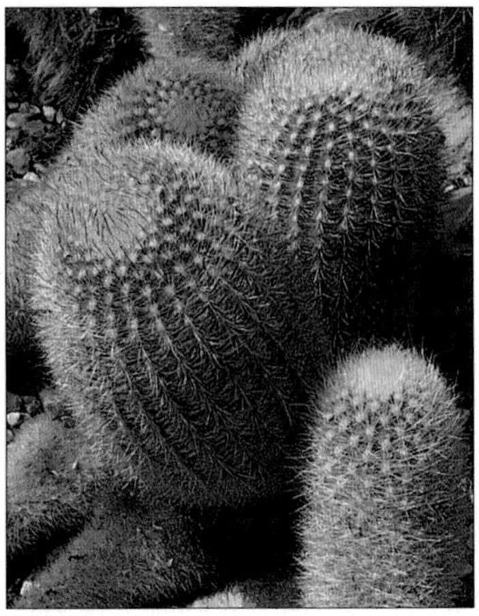

Oreocereus haynei

O

ORIGANUM

Marjoram, Oregano

LABIATAE/LAMIACEAE

Genus of about 20 species of often rhizomatous, summer-flowering, herbaceous perennials and deciduous and evergreen subshrubs from open habitats, often in mountainous areas of the Mediterranean and S.W. Asia. They have spreading to upright stems bearing simple, aromatic leaves in opposite pairs, and inflorescences in spiked whorls, which are sometimes panicle- or corymb-like. The elongated, tubular or funnel-shaped, 2-lipped flowers are borne amid conspicuous, often brightly coloured bracts, which remain attractive for many weeks. Some origanums, *O. dictamnus*, *O. majorana*, *O. onites*, and *O. vulgare* and their cultivars, are used as culinary herbs. Grow smaller species in a rock garden, scree bed, alpine house, or at the front of a border; grow larger ones in a herbaceous border or herb garden. All attract bees and other insects.

• **HARDINESS** Fully hardy to frost hardy.

• **CULTIVATION** Outdoors, grow in full sun in poor to moderately fertile, well-drained, preferably alkaline soil. Grow dwarf perennials and subshrubs in free-draining soil. Some fully hardy species and cultivars resent winter wet, and are best grown in an alpine house; grow in a mix of equal parts loam, leaf mould, and sharp sand. Cut back old, flowered stems in early spring.

• **PROPAGATION** Sow seed in containers in a cold frame in autumn, or at 10–13°C (50–55°F) in spring. Divide in spring, or take basal cuttings in late spring.

• **PESTS AND DISEASES** Susceptible to aphids and red spider mites under glass.

O

O. amanum ■ ♀ Low-spreading, evergreen subshrub with ovate, bright green leaves, to 1.5cm (½in) long, and heart-shaped at the bases. In summer and autumn, curved, funnel-shaped pink flowers, 4cm (1½in) long, with small spreading lobes, are produced in congested, terminal whorls among green bracts, to 2cm (¾in) long, which become flushed purple-pink with age. ↕10–20cm (4–8in), ↔ to 30cm (12in). E. Mediterranean, Turkey. ***

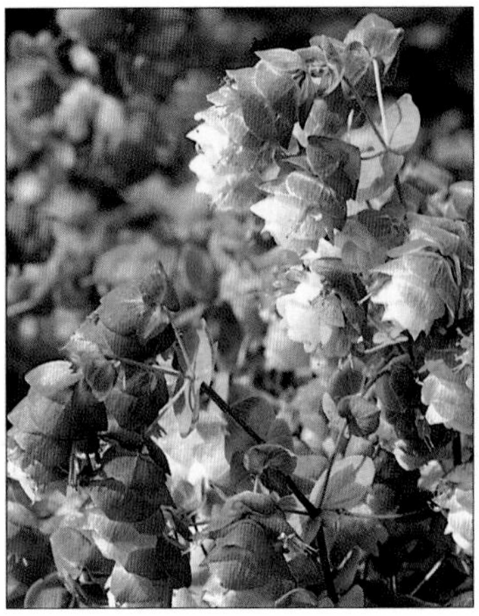

Origanum 'Kent Beauty'

***O.* 'Barbara Tingey'.** Dense, mound-forming, semi-evergreen subshrub, similar to *O. rotundifolium*. Produces rounded, bluish green leaves, purple beneath, 2cm (¾in) long. From summer to autumn, nodding whorls of tubular pink flowers, 1.5cm (½in) long and flared at the mouths, are borne among green bracts, 2cm (¾in) long, which age to deep purple-pink. ↕10cm (4in), ↔ to 20cm (8in). ***

***O.* 'Buckland'.** Upright perennial, with rounded, hairy, grey-green leaves, 1.5cm (½in) long. In summer, whorls of tubular pink flowers, 1.5cm (½in) long, are borne among bracts, 2cm (¾in) long, which are pink from an early age. ↕20cm (8in), ↔ to 15cm (6in). ***

O. dictamnus (Cretan dittany, Hop marjoram). Dome-forming, evergreen subshrub with arching, branching stems bearing rounded-ovate to rounded, densely white-felted, mid-green, sometimes purple-mottled leaves, to 2.5cm (1in) long. In mid- and late summer, bears dense, pendent, panicle-like whorls of small, open funnel-shaped pink flowers, 1cm (½in) long, among hop-like purple bracts, 9–10mm (⅜–½in) long. In wet climates, grow in an alpine house. ↕15cm (6in), ↔ to 20cm (8in). Crete. **

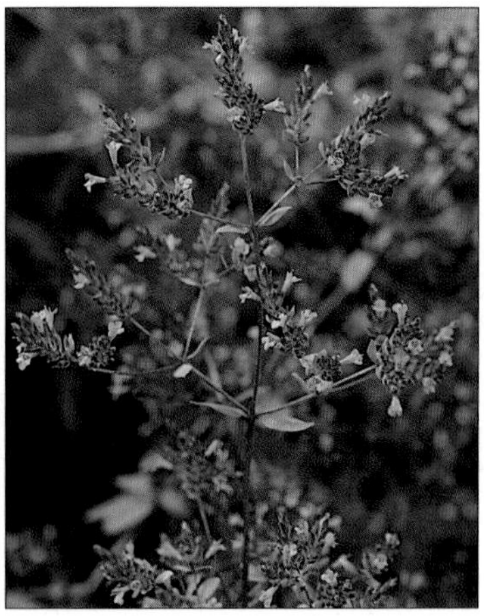

Origanum laevigatum

O. heracleoticum see *O. vulgare* subsp. *hirtum*.

***O.* 'Kent Beauty'** ■ Prostrate, semi-evergreen subshrub with trailing stems clothed in rounded-ovate, bright green leaves, to 2cm (¾in) long. In summer, produces whorls of small, tubular, pale pink to mauve flowers, 1.5cm (½in) long, among deep rose-pink bracts, 2cm (¾in) long. ↕10cm (4in), ↔ to 20cm (8in). ***

O. laevigatum ■ ♀ Woody-based perennial with erect, wiry, red-purple stems and ovate to elliptic, dark green leaves, 1.5–2cm (½–¾in) long, hairy only along the midribs beneath. Loose, panicle-like whorls of numerous tubular, scarcely 2-lipped, purplish pink flowers, 1.5cm (½in) long, are produced from late spring to autumn. The flowers have darker purple calyces, surrounded by red-purple bracts, 1cm (½in) long. ↕to 50–60cm (20–24in), ↔ 45cm (18in). Turkey, Cyprus. ***. **'Herrenhausen'** ■ ♀ has purple-flushed young leaves and winter foliage, and denser whorls of pink flowers; ↕45cm (18in). **'Hopleys'** has large, deep pink flowers, 2cm (¾in) long, and large bracts, 1.5cm (½in) long, borne in narrow whorls; ↕60cm (24in).

O. majorana (Sweet marjoram). Upright, evergreen subshrub, often grown as an annual or biennial, with branching stems bearing ovate or elliptic, softly hairy, grey-green leaves, 0.3–3cm (⅛–1¼in) long. Panicles of tubular, white or pink flowers, 8mm (⅜in) long, with grey-green bracts, to 4mm (⅛in) long, appear from early to late summer. ↕to 80cm (32in), ↔ 45cm (18in). S.W. Europe, Turkey. **

O. microphyllum. Domed, spreading, evergreen subshrub with ovate, downy grey leaves, to 5mm (¼in) long, on slender branches. In summer, bears loose, panicle-like whorls of tubular, pink to purple flowers, 5mm (¼in) long, among purple bracts, to 4mm (⅛in) long. ↕25cm (10in), ↔ to 30cm (12in). Crete. **

O. onites, syn. *Majorana onites* (French marjoram, Pot marjoram). Small, mound-forming, semi-evergreen subshrub with red-hairy stems and ovate to elliptic, bright green leaves, to 2cm (¾in) long, rounded to heart-shaped at the bases. In late summer, produces tubular white flowers, to 6mm (¼in) long, in dense, corymb-like whorls, with green bracts, to 4mm (⅛in) long. Popular herb for Mediterranean dishes. ↕60cm (24in), ↔ 30cm (12in). E. Mediterranean. **

O. rotundifolium ♀ Rhizomatous, woody-based perennial or deciduous, rounded subshrub, with rounded to heart-shaped, blue-grey leaves, to 2.5cm (1in) long. Throughout summer, produces nodding, hop-like whorls of small, tubular, pale pink flowers, to 1.5cm (½in) long, among pale lemon-green bracts, to 2.5cm (1in) long. ↕10–30cm (4–12in), ↔ to 30cm (12in). Turkey, Armenia, Georgia. ***

O. vulgare ■ (Oregano, Wild marjoram). Bushy, rhizomatous, woody-based perennial with upright to spreading stems bearing very aromatic, rounded to ovate, dark green leaves, to 4cm (1½in) long. From midsummer to early autumn, bears loose panicle- or corymb-like whorls of tubular flowers,

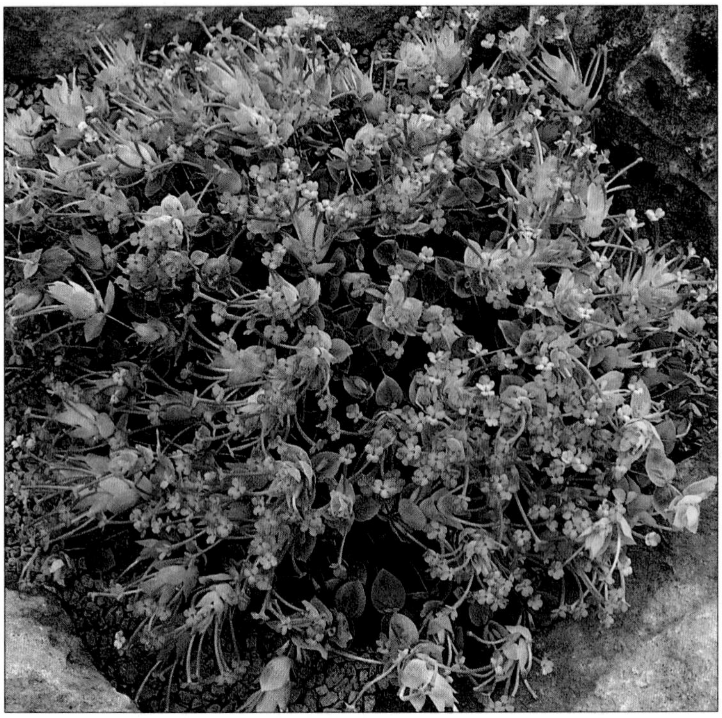

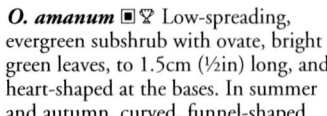

Origanum amanum

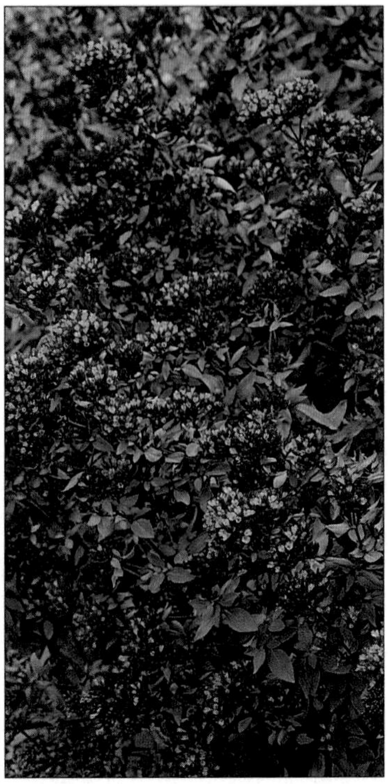

Origanum laevigatum 'Herrenhausen'

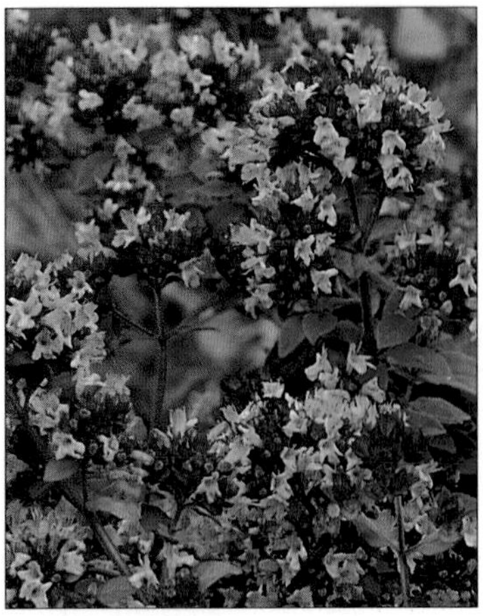

Origanum vulgare

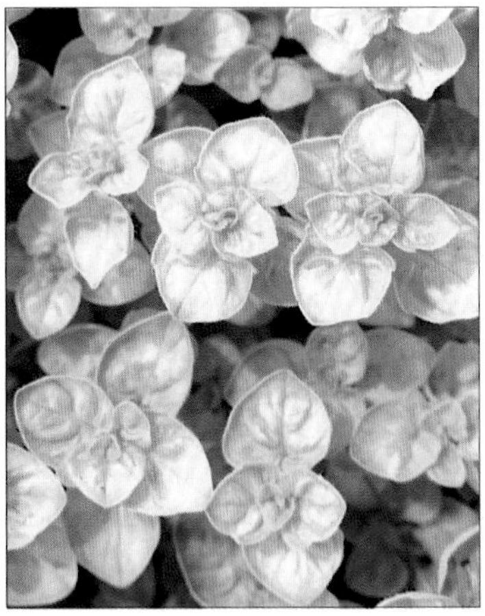

Origanum vulgare 'Aureum'

to 4mm (⅛in) long, varying from deep to pale pink or white, with whorls of leafy, purple-tinted green bracts, to 1cm (½in) long. ↕↔ 30–90cm (12–36in). Europe. ❄❄❄. **'Aureum'** ■ ♀ (Golden wild marjoram) has golden leaves and pink flowers, and spreads less vigorously than the species; ↔ to 30cm (12in). **'Aureum Crispum'**, syn. 'Curly Gold', is more spreading than the species, with curly golden leaves; ↔ 45cm (18in). **'Compactum'** (Compact marjoram) is dense, compact, and dome-forming, with smaller leaves, to 2cm (¾in) long; ↕ to 15cm (6in), ↔ to 30cm (12in). **'Curly Gold'** see 'Aureum Crispum'. **'Gold Tip'**, syn. 'Variegatum', is like 'Aureum Crispum', but the leaves are yellow only at their tips; ↕ 40cm (16in), ↔ 45cm (18in). **'Heiderose'** is upright and bushy in habit, with pink flowers; ↕ to 40cm (16in). **subsp. *hirtum***, syn. *O. heracleoticum*, has a compact habit, with hairy leaves, hairy green bracts, and small heads of white flowers; ↕ 30–70cm (12–28in), ↔ 20–45cm (8–18in); Greece, Turkey. **'Variegatum'** see 'Gold Tip'.

ORIXA

RUTACEAE

Genus of one species of deciduous, spreading, dioecious shrub from woodland and thickets in mountainous regions of China, Korea, and Japan. Cultivated for its elegant, aromatic foliage, it is suitable for a shrub border or woodland garden.

- **HARDINESS** Fully hardy.
- **CULTIVATION** Grow in fertile, well-drained soil in sun or shade. Tolerant of dry soils and exposed positions. Pruning group 1.
- **PROPAGATION** Sow seed in containers in a cold frame in spring. Take semi-ripe cuttings in midsummer.
- **PESTS AND DISEASES** Trouble free.

O. japonica. Spreading, slender-branched, deciduous shrub with simple, alternate, obovate to inversely lance-shaped, aromatic, dark green leaves, to 12cm (5in) long, pale yellow in autumn. Cup-shaped, 4-petalled green flowers, to 5mm (¼in) across, are borne in the leaf axils as the leaves emerge in spring; the males are borne in small panicles, to 3cm (1¼in) long, the females singly. Female plants bear 4-lobed brown fruit, 2cm (¾in) across. ↕ 2.5m (8ft), ↔ 4m (12ft). China, Korea, Japan. ❄❄❄

ORNITHOGALUM

Star-of-Bethlehem

HYACINTHACEAE/LILIACEAE

Genus of 80 species of bulbous perennials found in a variety of habitats, ranging from dry, rocky hillsides to meadows and woodland, in C. and S. Europe, the Mediterranean, former USSR, W. and S.W. Asia, tropical Africa, and South Africa. They are grown for their sometimes corymb-like racemes of often star-, cup-, or funnel-shaped, occasionally scented flowers; usually white, sometimes yellow or orange, they are borne on leafless stems in spring or summer. The leaves are basal, and vary from linear to obovate, sometimes with a silver stripe down the centre. Smaller species are suitable for a rock garden; taller ones for a herbaceous border. In ideal growing conditions, *O. nutans* and *O. umbellatum* may become invasive, but, as with *O. montanum*, are suitable for naturalizing in short turf or beneath shrubs. In frost-prone areas, grow tender species in a cool greenhouse, or grow outdoors and lift in autumn. All parts may cause severe discomfort if ingested, and the sap may irritate skin.

- **HARDINESS** Fully hardy to frost tender.
- **CULTIVATION** Plant bulbs 10cm (4in) deep. Outdoors, plant fully hardy and frost-hardy species in autumn, in moderately fertile, well-drained soil, in a sunny situation. *O. nutans* and *O. umbellatum* tolerate partial shade. Plant half-hardy species in spring for summer flowering; in growth, water freely and lift after flowering; keep frost-free over winter. Under glass, grow tender species in large containers of loam-based potting compost (JI No.2), in full light with shade from hot sun. When in growth, water freely; keep dry when dormant, and repot annually in spring. *O. thyrsoides* may be planted under glass in autumn for spring flowering.
- **PROPAGATION** Sow seed in containers in a cold frame in autumn or spring. Remove offsets when dormant.
- **PESTS AND DISEASES** Trouble free.

O. arabicum. Bulbous perennial with basal rosettes of semi-erect, broadly linear, dark green leaves, to 60cm (24in) long. In early summer, bears corymb-like racemes of 6–25 cup-shaped, scented, white or cream flowers, 3cm (1¼in) across, each with a conspicuous

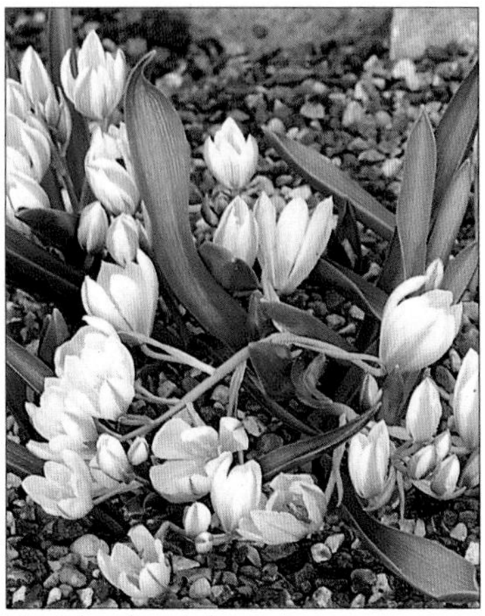

Ornithogalum balansae

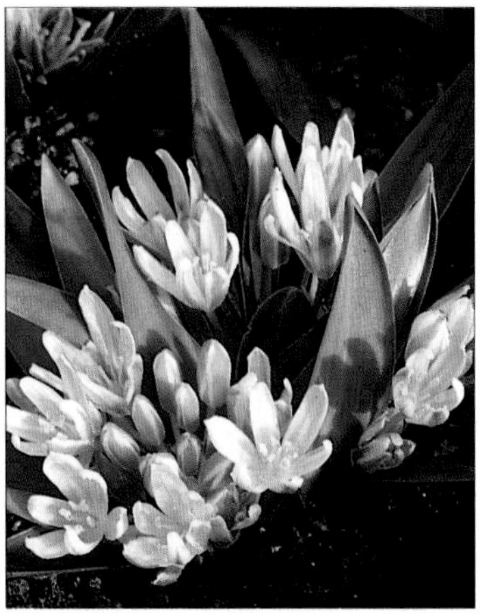

Ornithogalum lanceolatum

black ovary. ↕ 30–80cm (12–32in), ↔ 8cm (3in). Mediterranean. ❄

O. balansae ■ syn. *O. oligophyllum* of gardens. Slender, bulbous perennial with almost prostrate, inversely lance-shaped, glossy, mid-green, basal leaves, to 15cm (6in) long. In early spring, bears corymb-like racemes of 2–5 cup-shaped flowers, 3cm (1¼in) across, glistening white inside, bright green outside. ↕ to 8cm (3in), ↔ 10cm (4in). Balkans, Turkey, Georgia. ❄❄❄

O. caudatum see *O. longibracteatum.*

O. lanceolatum ■ Dwarf, bulbous perennial producing basal rosettes of prostrate, lance-shaped, shiny, mid-green leaves, 10–12cm (4–5in) long. In spring, bears compact, almost stemless racemes of 5–13 star-shaped white flowers, 2–3cm (¾–1¼in) across, striped green on the outsides. ↕ 5–10cm (2–4in), ↔ 10cm (4in). Turkey, Syria, Lebanon. ❄❄❄

O. longibracteatum, syn. *O. caudatum* (False sea onion). Bulbous perennial with lax, strap-shaped, semi-succulent, pale green, basal leaves, to 60cm (24in) long. In summer, bears tall racemes of up to 300 bell-shaped white flowers, to 1.5cm (½in) across, striped green outside, with bracts extending far beyond the flowers. ↕ 1–1.5m (3–5ft), ↔ 15cm (6in). Tropical Africa, South Africa (Northern Cape, Eastern Cape). ❄❄

O. montanum ■ Bulbous perennial producing basal rosettes of prostrate, linear, shiny, pale to greyish green leaves, 10–15cm (4–6in) long. In spring, bears corymb-like racemes of 10–20 star-shaped white flowers, 2cm

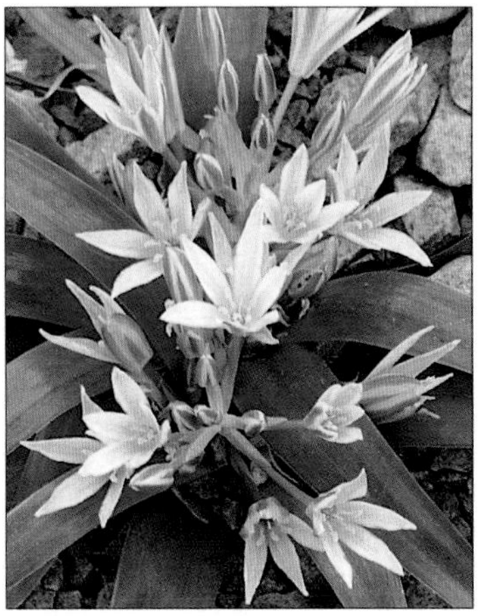

Ornithogalum montanum

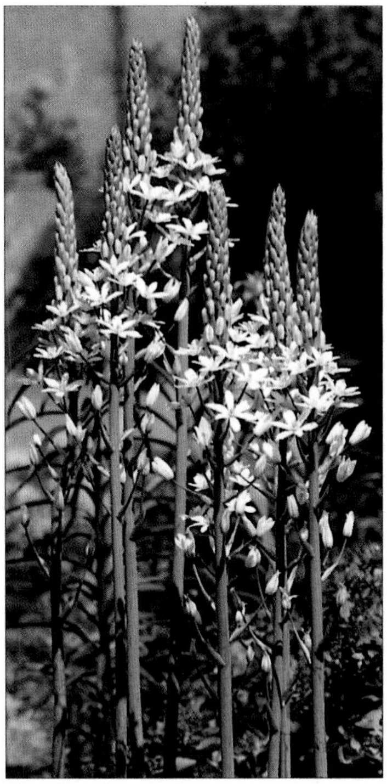

Ornithogalum narbonense

(¾in) across, striped green on the outsides. ↕ 10–25cm (4–10in), ↔ 10cm (4in). S. Europe, Turkey, Lebanon, Israel. ❄❄

O. narbonense ■ Bulbous perennial with semi-erect, linear, grey-green, basal leaves, to 60cm (24in) long. Produces upright, narrowly pyramidal racemes of 25–75 star-shaped white flowers, 2cm (¾in) across, in late spring and early summer. ↕ 30–90cm (12–36in), ↔ 5cm (2in). Mediterranean, Turkey, Caucasus, Iran. ❄❄❄

O. nutans ♀ Bulbous perennial with semi-erect, strap-shaped, bright mid-green, basal leaves, 30–40cm (12–16in) long, each with a central silver stripe above. In spring, bears one-sided racemes of up to 20 semi-pendent, funnel-shaped, silvery white flowers, 3cm (1¼in) across, broadly striped green outside. ↕ 20–60cm (8–24in), ↔ 5cm (2in). Europe, S.W. Asia. ❄❄❄

***O. oligophyllum* of gardens** see *O. balansae.*

O. pyramidale. Bulbous perennial with basal clusters of semi-erect, linear, glossy, mid-green leaves, to 60cm (24in) long, which wither as the flowers open. In late spring and early summer, produces stiff racemes of numerous star-shaped white flowers, 1–2cm (½–¾in) across, striped green on the outsides. ↕ 30–120cm (12–48in), ↔ 7cm (3in). C. Europe, Balkans. ❄❄❄

O. pyrenaicum (Bath asparagus). Bulbous perennial with basal tufts of semi-erect, narrowly linear, grey-green leaves, 20–35cm (8–14in) long, often withering as the flowers open. Long racemes of 25–40 star-shaped, pale yellow flowers, to 1cm (½in) across, broadly or narrowly striped green outside, are produced in early summer. ↕ to 1m (3ft), ↔ 10cm (4in). Europe, Turkey, Caucasus. ❄❄❄

O. saundersiae. Robust, bulbous perennial with erect, strap-shaped, dark green, sometimes greyish green, basal leaves, 60cm (24in) long. In winter or spring, produces dense, corymb-like

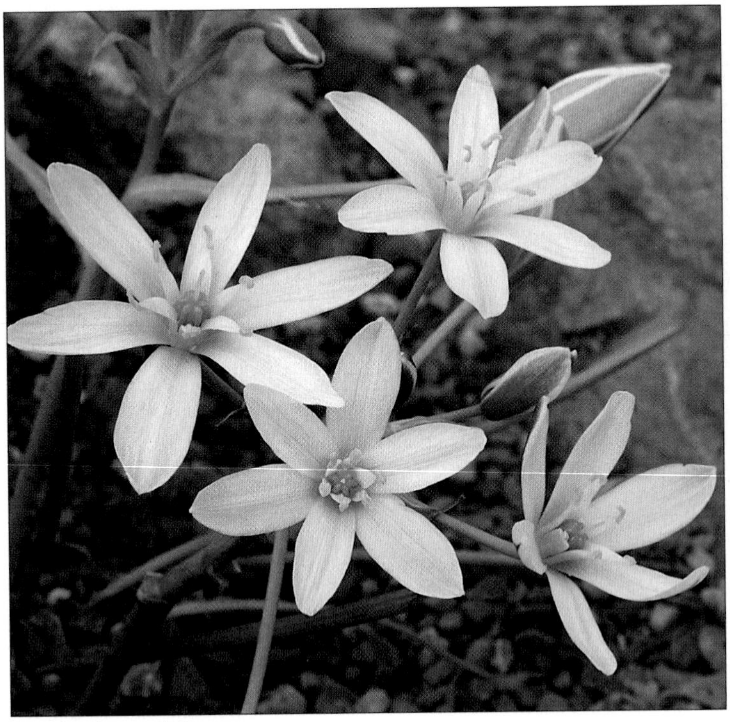

Ornithogalum umbellatum

racemes of cup-shaped, white or creamy white flowers, 2–3cm (¾–1¼in) across, with black or greenish black ovaries. ↕ to 1m (3ft), ↔ 10cm (4in). South Africa (Northern Transvaal, Eastern Transvaal, KwaZulu/Natal), Swaziland. ❄

O. sintenisii. Small, bulbous perennial with basal rosettes of nearly prostrate, linear, recurved and often twisted, mid-green leaves, 20–30cm (8–12in) long. In spring, produces almost stemless racemes of 4–12 open star-shaped white flowers, 2cm (¾in) across, striped green on the outsides. ↕↔ 10cm (4in). Russia, Georgia, Azerbaijan, Iran. ❄❄❄

O. thyrsoides (Chincherinchee). Robust, bulbous perennial with semi-erect, linear to narrowly lance-shaped, mid-green, basal leaves, to 30cm (12in) long, with hairy margins, withering before the flowers open. In spring and early summer, bears dense racemes of many cup-shaped white flowers, 2cm (¾in) across, tinted cream or green at the bases. Excellent for cut flowers. ↕ to 70cm (28in), ↔ 10cm (4in). South Africa (Western Cape). ❄

O. umbellatum ▣ (Star-of-Bethlehem). Bulbous perennial with semi-erect, linear, white-veined, mid-green, basal leaves, to 30cm (12in) long, each with a central silver stripe above; the leaves wither as the flowers open in early summer. Produces corymb-like racemes of 6–20 long-stalked, star-shaped white flowers, 2cm (¾in) across, striped green outside. Increases rapidly. ↕ 10–30cm (4–12in), ↔ 10cm (4in). Europe, Turkey, Syria, Lebanon, Israel, N. Africa. ❄❄❄

ORNITHOPHORA

ORCHIDACEAE

Genus of 1 or possibly 2 species of evergreen, epiphytic orchids from Brazil, occurring in warm, moist, forested areas. They have slender, compressed, ovoid pseudobulbs, each with 2 linear leaves at the tip, and a fine mat of aerial roots. Tiny flowers are borne in slender racemes arising from the bases of the pseudobulbs, and resemble a swarm of insects hovering above the plant.

- **HARDINESS** Frost tender.
- **CULTIVATION** Cool- to intermediate-growing orchids. Grow in epiphytic orchid compost in shallow pots or slatted baskets, or epiphytically on slabs of bark. Provide high humidity and bright filtered light all year. In summer, mist daily, water freely, and apply a quarter-strength fertilizer at every third watering. In winter, water more sparingly, and do not allow to dry out completely. See also p.46.
- **PROPAGATION** Divide when the plant fills the pot and "flows" over the sides.
- **PESTS AND DISEASES** Susceptible to red spider mites, aphids, and mealybugs.

O. radicans, syn. *Sigmatostalix radicans*. Epiphytic orchid with grass-like leaves, 10–18cm (4–7in) long. Intricately patterned, slightly fragrant, white-green or green-yellow flowers, to 8mm (⅜in) across, with cream lips, are borne in racemes 7–15cm (3–6in) long, in autumn. ↕ 10cm (4in), ↔ 30cm (12in). Brazil. ❁ (min. 13°C/55°F; max. 30°C/86°F)

▷ ***Orobus aureus*** see *Lathyrus aureus*
▷ ***Orobus vernus*** see *Lathyrus vernus*

ORONTIUM

Golden club

ARACEAE

Genus of one species of marginal aquatic perennial from E. USA. It has large, thick rhizomes producing oblong to narrowly elliptic, submerged, floating, or aerial leaves, and curious, pencil-like spadices that stand well above the water. Ideal for the margins of an informal pool, it associates well with waterside irises and primulas in early summer.

- **HARDINESS** Fully hardy.
- **CULTIVATION** Grow in deep mud at a pool margin with ample room to spread, or in baskets of loamy soil, in water no

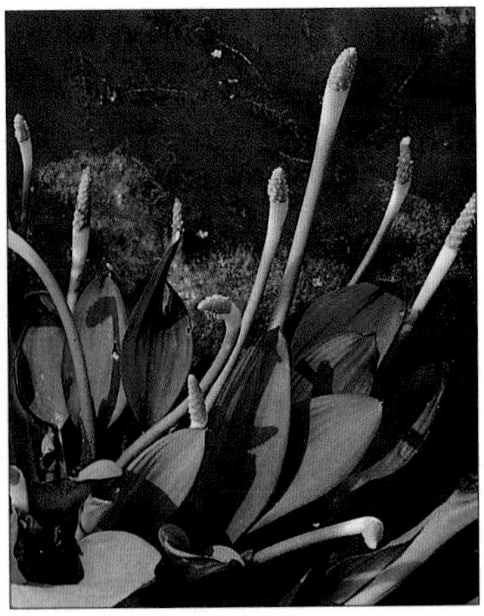

Orontium aquaticum

deeper than 45cm (18in), and in full sun to develop the beauty of the glaucous leaves. Remove the short-lived flower spikes when they fade. See also pp.52–53.

- **PROPAGATION** Sow seed as soon as ripe in a cold frame in trays of loam-based seed compost, and cover with no more than 1–3cm (½–1¼in) of water. Divide the rhizomes in spring.
- **PESTS AND DISEASES** Trouble free.

O. aquaticum ▣ Rhizomatous, marginal aquatic perennial with oblong to narrowly elliptic, submerged, aerial, or floating leaves, to 25cm (10in) long, mid-green and glaucous, often purple-tinted beneath. From late spring to midsummer, bears small, bright yellow flowers near the tops of numerous cylindrical white spadices, 18cm (7in) tall. ↕ 30–45cm (12–18in), ↔ 60–75cm (24–30in). E. USA. ❄❄❄

OROSTACHYS

CRASSULACEAE

Genus of about 10 species of freely offsetting, monocarpic perennials, closely related to *Sedum*, from low to mountainous, rocky areas of Russia, China, North Korea, South Korea, and Japan. They have dense, hemispherical to spherical rosettes of fleshy leaves, and produce erect stems bearing terminal, spike-like racemes or panicles of short-stalked, star-shaped flowers during summer or autumn. The rosettes die after flowering and fruiting. Below 8°C (46°F), grow in a cool greenhouse; in warmer climates, grow in a bed or border with other succulents.

- **HARDINESS** Half hardy to frost tender.
- **CULTIVATION** Under glass, grow in standard cactus compost in full light. From spring to autumn, water freely and apply a half-strength, balanced liquid fertilizer every 4 weeks. Keep almost dry in winter. Outdoors, grow in poor, well-drained soil in full sun. See also pp.48–49.
- **PROPAGATION** Sow seed at 13–18°C (55–64°F), or divide offsets, in spring.
- **PESTS AND DISEASES** Susceptible to mealybugs.

O. chanetii. Clump-forming, perennial succulent with a stoloniferous rootstock and compact, basal rosettes of linear, greyish green leaves, 4cm (1½in) long. Dense, pyramidal, spike-like racemes or panicles, to 20cm (8in) long, of star-shaped white flowers, 1–2cm (½–¾in) across, reddish pink outside, are borne in summer and autumn. ↕ to 20cm (8in) sometimes more, ↔ 10cm (4in). China. ❁ (min. 8°C/46°F)

OROYA

CACTACEAE

Genus of 2 or 3 species of perennial cacti from dry, stony slopes, screes, and cliffs, at altitudes to 4,000m (13,000ft), in Peru. They have flattened-spherical to very short-cylindrical, rarely offsetting stems with numerous warty ribs and spined areoles. Bell- or funnel-shaped flowers are usually borne in a ring around the crown of each stem in summer, followed by obovoid to ovoid red or yellow berries containing black-coated seeds. Where temperatures drop below 13°C (55°F), grow in a warm greenhouse; in warm, dry climates, use in a desert garden.

- **HARDINESS** Frost tender.
- **CULTIVATION** Under glass, grow in standard cactus compost in full light. From spring to autumn, water freely and apply half-strength, balanced liquid fertilizer 3 or 4 times. Keep barely moist in winter. Outdoors, grow in sharply drained, neutral to slightly alkaline, poor, humus-rich soil in full sun. See also pp.48–49.
- **PROPAGATION** Sow seed at 18–21°C (64–70°F) in spring.
- **PESTS AND DISEASES** Susceptible to aphids while flowering.

O. neoperuviana see *O. peruviana*.

O. peruviana ▣ syn. *Oreocereus peruviana, Oroya neoperuviana*. Perennial cactus producing solitary, dull green or bluish green stems, each with up to 35 rounded ribs notched into long tubercles. Linear areoles bear brownish yellow spines (10–30 radials, in comb-like formation, and up to 6 longer centrals). Bell-shaped, pale carmine-red to vermilion, usually yellow-based flowers, 1.5–3cm (½–1¼in) long, are borne in summer. ↕ 15–20cm (6–8in), occasionally more, ↔ to 15cm (6in). Peru. ❁ (min. 13°C/55°F)

▷ ***Orphanidesia*** see *Epigaea*
O. gaultherioides see *E. gaultherioides*
▷ **Orpine** see *Sedum telephium*
Stone see *S. rupestre*
▷ **Orris root** see *Iris germanica* 'Florentina'

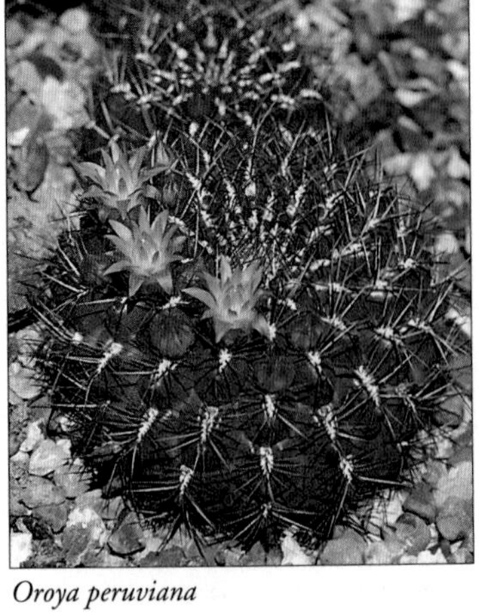

Oroya peruviana

ORTEGOCACTUS

CACTACEAE

Genus of one species of perennial cactus, closely related to *Mammillaria*, from dry areas of S.W. Mexico. It has spherical to short-cylindrical stems, which often offset to form small clusters, with spirally arranged, warty ribs and prominently spined areoles. Solitary, funnel-shaped yellow flowers are produced in summer, followed by orange-yellow or dull red fruit. In areas where temperatures drop below 15°C (59°F), grow in a warm greenhouse; in warm, dry climates, grow in a border with other cacti, or in a raised bed or desert garden.

- **HARDINESS** Frost tender.
- **CULTIVATION** Under glass, grow in standard cactus compost in full light. From spring to early autumn, water freely and apply half-strength, balanced liquid fertilizer every 4–5 weeks. Keep dry at other times. Outdoors, grow in moderately fertile, sharply drained, humus-rich, slightly acid soil in full sun. See also pp.48–49.
- **PROPAGATION** Sow seed at 21°C (70°F) in spring.
- **PESTS AND DISEASES** Vulnerable to mealybugs.

O. macdougallii ▣ syn. *Neobesseya macdougallii*. Clustering, perennial cactus producing spherical to short-cylindrical, pale greyish green stems, 3–4cm (1¼–1½in) thick, covered with large, diamond-shaped tubercles. White-woolly areoles bear black-tipped, white or totally black spines (7 or 8 radials and 1 shorter central spine). Solitary, funnel-shaped yellow flowers, to 3cm (1¼in) long, the outer tepals tinted purple outside, are produced in summer; they are followed by spherical-ellipsoid, orange-yellow or dull red fruit with black-coated seeds. ↕ to 6cm (2½in), ↔ 12cm (5in). S.W. Mexico. ❁ (min. 15°C/59°F)

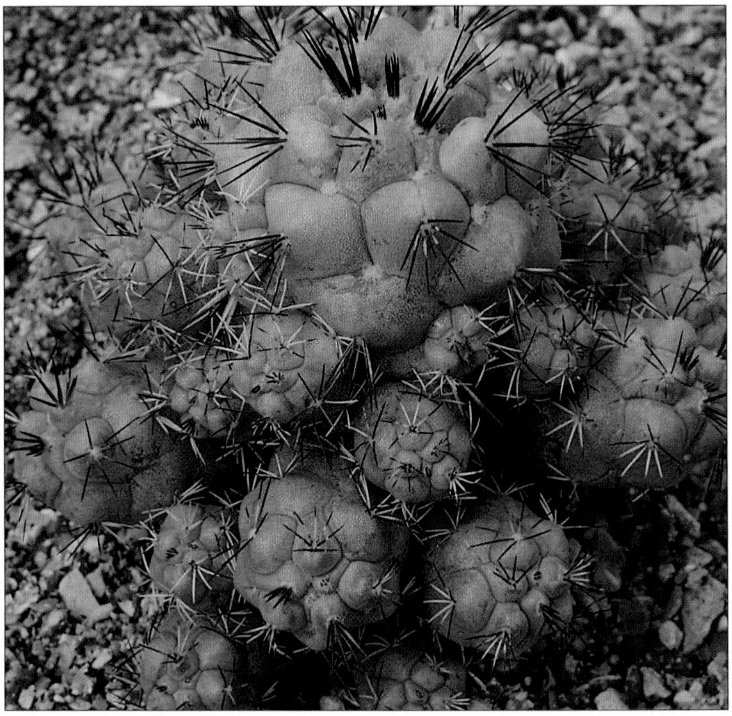

Ortegocactus macdougallii

ORTHOPHYTUM

BROMELIACEAE

Genus of about 18 species of mat-forming, evergreen, semi-succulent, terrestrial perennials (bromeliads) from dry, rocky slopes, to 1,200m (4,000ft) high, in E. Brazil. They spread by stolons to form wide rosettes of usually stemless, softly spiny leaves. In summer, they produce varyingly branched inflorescences with leafy bracts and small, dense clusters of slender, tubular, mainly white flowers. In areas where temperatures drop below 15°C (59°F), grow in a warm greenhouse; in warm, dry climates use in a desert garden.

- **HARDINESS** Frost tender.
- **CULTIVATION** Under glass, grow in terrestrial bromeliad compost in full light. In the growing season, water moderately with soft water, applying half-strength, balanced liquid fertilizer every 3–4 weeks. Keep plants dry in winter. Outdoors, grow in sharply drained, moderately fertile, humus-rich soil in full sun. See also p.47.
- **PROPAGATION** Sow seed at 27°C (81°F) in early spring. Separate offsets in spring.
- **PESTS AND DISEASES** Susceptible to aphids while flowering.

O. navioides, syn. *Cryptanthopsis navioides*. Stemless bromeliad that spreads by stolons to form clustered rosettes of narrowly lance-shaped, finely toothed, sparsely scaly, mid-green leaves, to 30cm (12in) long. In summer, tubular white flowers, to 3cm (1¼in) long, with pale yellowish green sepals and bracts, are produced in few-flowered clusters, sunk in the centre of each rosette. The whole plant often turns bright red or red-purple as the flowers mature. ↕ to 20cm (8in), ↔ to 60cm (24in). E. Brazil. ❁ (min. 15°C/59°F)

O. saxicola. Stemless bromeliad, spreading by stolons to form large clusters of rosettes. Narrowly triangular,

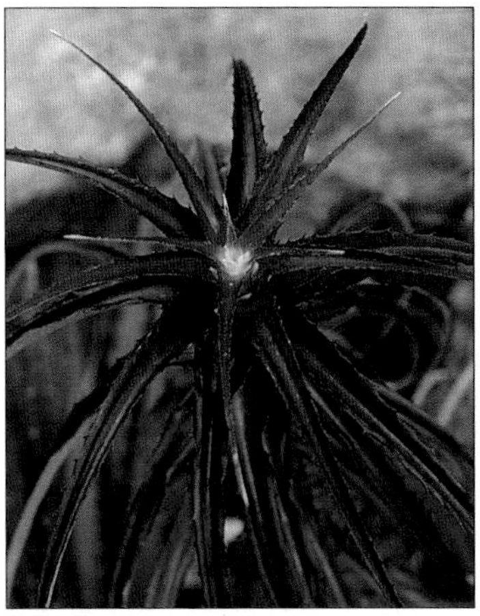

Orthophytum vagans

toothed, pale bright green leaves, 3–6cm (1¼–2½in) long, are usually thick and fleshy. In summer, produces head-like clusters of thick, fleshy bracts and short-stalked, tubular white flowers, to 2cm (¾in) long, with white-margined green sepals, and petals with 2 basal projections. Both the bracts and the flowers are almost hidden in the rosettes. ↕ 8cm (3in), ↔ indefinite. E. Brazil. ❁ (min. 15°C/59°F)

O. vagans ▣ Trailing bromeliad with an elongated, branching caudex, the branches rooting down and forming large, spreading groups. Produces loosely rosetted rows of narrowly triangular, deeply channelled, slightly toothed, bright green leaves, to 10cm (4in) long, scaly beneath, turning red-purple with age. In summer, produces stemless inflorescences of red or orange bracts and 15–30 tubular, apple-green flowers, 2cm (¾in) long, with white-woolly sepals, and stalks 5cm (2in) long. ↕ to 20cm (8in), ↔ indefinite. E. Brazil. ❁ (min. 15°C/59°F)

ORTHROSANTHUS

IRIDACEAE

Genus of 7 species of evergreen perennials occurring in sandy soils in Australia and tropical America. They have narrowly strap-shaped or linear, rigid or arching leaves, arising from short, woody rhizomes. They are grown for their bowl-shaped to open saucer-shaped, 6-tepalled blue flowers, borne in loose, terminal panicles on slender, erect stalks. The flowers are short-lived, but open in succession for 2 weeks or more from late spring to summer. In frost-prone areas grow in a cool greenhouse or conservatory; in warmer areas, grow in a warm, sunny border.

- **HARDINESS** Half hardy to frost tender.
- **CULTIVATION** Under glass, grow in loam-based potting compost (JI No.2), with additional sharp sand and leaf mould, in full light. Water moderately when in growth; keep almost dry when dormant. Repot or top-dress in spring. Outdoors, grow in light, fertile, well-drained, humus-rich soil in full sun.
- **PROPAGATION** Sow seed at 13–18°C (55–64°F), or divide, in spring.
- **PESTS AND DISEASES** Trouble free.

O. chimboracensis. Rhizomatous perennial with stiff, leathery, linear, basal leaves, to 40cm (16in) long, rough to the touch. Loose panicles of shallowly

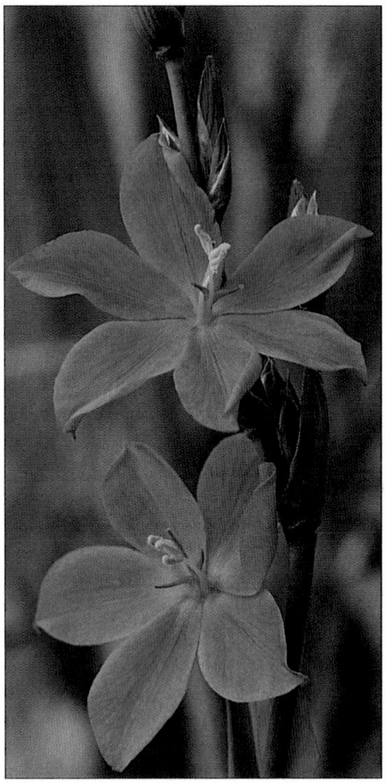

Orthrosanthus multiflorus

bowl-shaped, lavender-blue flowers, 4cm (1½in) across, are produced in summer. ↕ 30–60cm (12–24in), ↔ 30cm (12in). Mexico to Peru. ✻

O. multiflorus ▣ Rhizomatous perennial with rigid, linear, basal leaves, to 45cm (18in) long, with smooth margins. From late spring to summer, bears narrow panicles of open saucer-shaped, pale blue to violet-blue flowers, to 4cm (1½in) across. ↕ 60cm (24in), ↔ 30cm (12in). S.W. Australia. ✻

ORYCHOPHRAGMUS

BRASSICACEAE/CRUCIFERAE

Genus of 2 species of annuals or biennials occurring in fallow fields and on wasteland in C. Asia and China. They have thin, pinnatifid, lower leaves and entire stem-clasping leaves. Cross-shaped flowers, with 4-clawed violet petals, are produced in terminal racemes from late spring to summer. Grow outdoors as a bedding annual or biennial, or, for flowers in late winter and early spring, grow as a short-lived container plant in a cool or temperate greenhouse.

- **HARDINESS** Half hardy.
- **CULTIVATION** Outdoors, grow in fertile, well-drained soil in a warm, sunny site. Under glass, grow in loam-based potting compost (JI No.2) in full light. In growth, water moderately.
- **PROPAGATION** Sow seed *in situ* in spring or early summer or, in frost-free climates, in autumn.
- **PESTS AND DISEASES** Trouble free.

O. violaceus. Annual or biennial with an upright habit, and moderately fast-growing, branching stems bearing thin, pinnatifid, pale green basal leaves, 12–15cm (5–6in) or more long, and smaller, entire, pale green stem-clasping leaves. Produces terminal racemes of 5–25 cross-shaped violet flowers, to 2.5cm (1in) across, in late spring and early summer. ↕ 30–60cm (12–24in), ↔ 30cm (12in). China. ✻

ORYZA

Rice

GRAMINEAE / POACEAE

Genus of about 20 species of annual or perennial, rhizomatous grasses with flat, linear leaves, and panicles of laterally compressed spikelets producing rice-grain seeds when ripe. They are native to tropical and subtropical Africa and Asia, and are widely cultivated in subtropical and tropical regions. *O. sativa* 'Nigrescens' has unusually coloured leaves, and is the only *Oryza* grown for ornamental reasons. Where temperatures fall below 10°C (50°F), grow in a warm greenhouse or conservatory; in warmer areas, grow as a pond marginal or in a bog garden.

- **HARDINESS** Frost tender.
- **CULTIVATION** Under glass, provide full light and use loam-based potting compost (JI No.3) in shallow clay pots, or in fibreglass trays with drainage holes. Keep the soil surface submerged to a depth of about 2.5cm (1in), and refresh water regularly; maintain water temperature at 20–30°C (68–86°F). Drain off as flowerheads form, and keep evenly moist. Algal growth on the soil surface is unsightly but not harmful. Outdoors, grow in very moist, fertile, clay-loam soil, or in pots in shallow water at a pond margin, in full sun.
- **PROPAGATION** Surface-sow seed at 19–24°C (66–75°F) in late winter, in pots standing in containers of water.
- **PESTS AND DISEASES** Trouble free.

***O. sativa* 'Nigrescens'.** Loosely tufted annual, rhizomatous grass with strong, erect stems bearing arching, broadly linear, dark brownish purple leaves, to 1m (3ft) long. Produces spikelets in open, arching panicles, 35cm (14in) long, from midsummer to mid-autumn. ↕75cm (30in), ↔ 30cm (12in). S.E. Asia. ❄ (min. 10°C/50°F)

O

OSBECKIA

MELASTOMATACEAE

Genus of 40–60 species of evergreen perennials, subshrubs, and shrubs from Africa to China, and southwards from Japan to Australia, where they thrive in habitats from grassland to woodland. They are grown for their often showy, 4- or 5-petalled flowers, borne in terminal, leafy panicles or cymes, or sometimes singly, and for their simple, opposite, usually entire, somewhat leathery and bristly-hairy, strongly 3- to 7-veined leaves. Below 13–15°C (55–59°F), grow in a warm greenhouse; in warmer areas, use in a border.

- **HARDINESS** Frost tender.
- **CULTIVATION** Under glass, grow in loam-based potting compost (JI No.3) in bright filtered light or full light, with shade from hot sun. In growth, water freely and apply a balanced liquid fertilizer monthly; water moderately in winter. Outdoors, grow in fertile, moist but well-drained, humus-rich, neutral to acid soil in partial shade or with some midday shade. Pruning group 9; plants under glass need restrictive pruning in early spring.
- **PROPAGATION** Sow seed at 18°C (64°F) in spring. Root semi-ripe cuttings with bottom heat in summer.
- **PESTS AND DISEASES** Prone to scale insects and red spider mites under glass.

O. stellata. Erect shrub, spreading with age, with moderately branched, finely hairy stems and narrowly ovate, hairy-margined, deep green leaves, 6–15cm (2½–6in) long, with long, sharp points; each leaf has 5–7 prominent veins. Bears loose cymes of 4-petalled, saucer-shaped, blue-purple to reddish lilac, pink, or white flowers, 5cm (2in) across, mainly in summer. ↕ 1.2–1.8m (4–6ft), ↔ 1–1.5m (3–5ft). India to China. ❄ (min. 13°C/55°F)

▷ ***Oscularia deltoides*** see *Lampranthus deltoides*

▷ **Osier,**
Common see *Salix viminalis*
Green see *Cornus alternifolia*
Purple see *Salix purpurea*

OSMANTHUS

syn. x OSMAREA

OLEACEAE

Genus of about 15–20 species of evergreen shrubs and small trees from woodland in Asia, the Pacific islands, and S. USA. They are grown for their foliage and flowers: the leaves are lance-shaped to ovate, borne in opposite pairs; the small, tubular, 4-lobed, usually fragrant, white, occasionally yellow or orange flowers are produced in mainly axillary clusters or terminal panicles. The flowers are usually followed by ovoid, blue-black fruits. *Osmanthus* species and cultivars are ideal for a shrub border or woodland garden. *O. delavayi* may be wall-trained; *O.* x *burkwoodii*, *O. delavayi*, and *O. heterophyllus* are very good for hedging and topiary. In frost-prone areas, grow the tender species in a cool or temperate greenhouse.

- **HARDINESS** Fully hardy to frost tender.
- **CULTIVATION** Outdoors, grow in fertile, well-drained soil in sun or partial shade, with shelter from cold, drying winds. Under glass, grow in loam-based potting compost (JI No.3) in full light with shade from hot sun. When in growth, water freely and apply a balanced liquid fertilizer monthly; water sparingly in winter. Pruning group 8 for early-flowering species; group 9 for late-flowering species; all tolerate hard pruning. Trim hedges after flowering, or in spring for *O. heterophyllus*.
- **PROPAGATION** Sow seed in containers in a cold frame as soon as ripe. Root semi-ripe cuttings in summer with bottom heat. Layer in autumn or spring.
- **PESTS AND DISEASES** Trouble free.

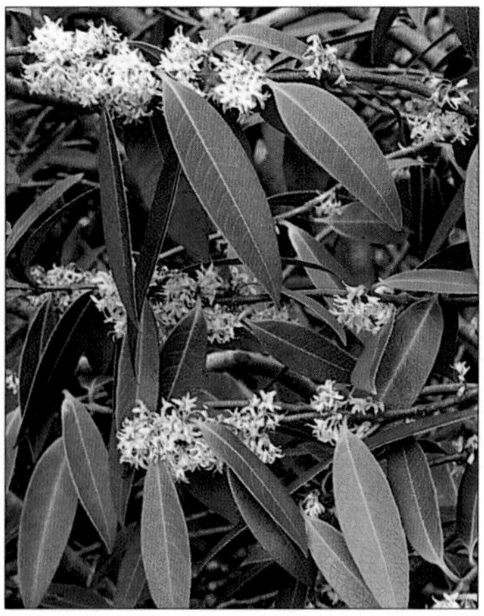

Osmanthus decorus

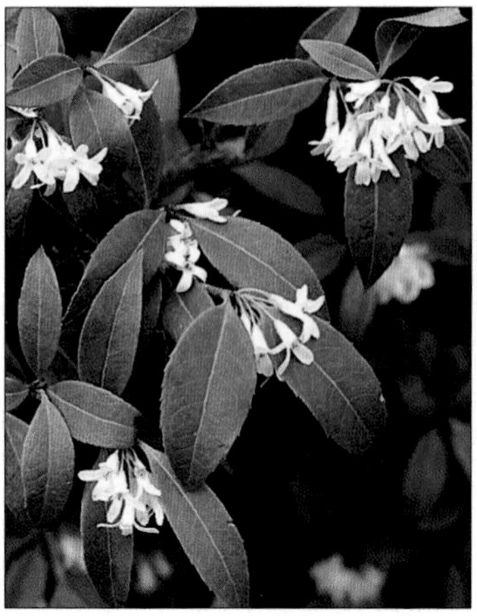

Osmanthus x *burkwoodii*

O. armatus. Dense, rounded shrub with oblong-lance-shaped, sharply spine-toothed, leathery, glossy, dark green leaves, to 15cm (6in) long. Broadly tubular, fragrant, creamy white flowers, with spreading lobes, to 5mm (¼in) across, are borne in axillary clusters in autumn, followed by ovoid, dark violet fruit, to 2cm (¾in) long. ↕ 2.5–5m (8–15ft), ↔ 4m (12ft). W. China. ❄❄

O.* x *burkwoodii ■ ♀ (*O. decorus* x *O. delavayi*), syn. x *Osmarea* x *burkwoodii.* Dense, rounded shrub with oval to ovate, slightly toothed, leathery, glossy, dark green leaves, to 5cm (2in) long. Tubular, very fragrant white flowers, the lobes to 5mm (¼in) across, are profusely borne in small, axillary clusters in mid- and late spring. Seldom produces fruit. ↕↔ 3m (10ft). Garden origin. ❄❄❄

O. decorus ■ syn. *Phillyrea decora.* Dense, rounded, spreading shrub with narrowly oval to oblong, pointed, leathery, glossy, dark green leaves, to 12cm (5in) long, very occasionally with a few teeth. Tubular white flowers, the lobes to 8mm (⅜in) across, are borne in dense, axillary clusters in mid-spring, followed by ellipsoid, blue-black fruit, to 1.5cm (½in) long. ↕ 3m (10ft), ↔ 5m (15ft). Georgia, N.E. Turkey. ❄❄❄

O. delavayi ■ ♀ syn. *Siphonosmanthus delavayi.* Rounded, bushy shrub with arching branches and ovate, finely toothed, leathery, glossy, dark green leaves, to 2.5cm (1in) long. Tubular, very fragrant white flowers, the lobes to 1cm (½in) across, are produced in axillary and terminal clusters in mid- and late spring, followed by ovoid, blue-black fruit, to 1cm (½in) long. ↕ 2–6m (6–20ft), ↔ 4m (12ft) or more. W. China (Sichuan, Yunnan). ❄❄❄

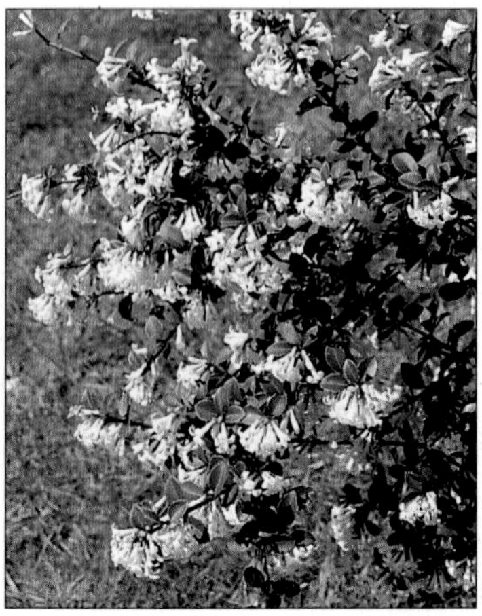

Osmanthus delavayi

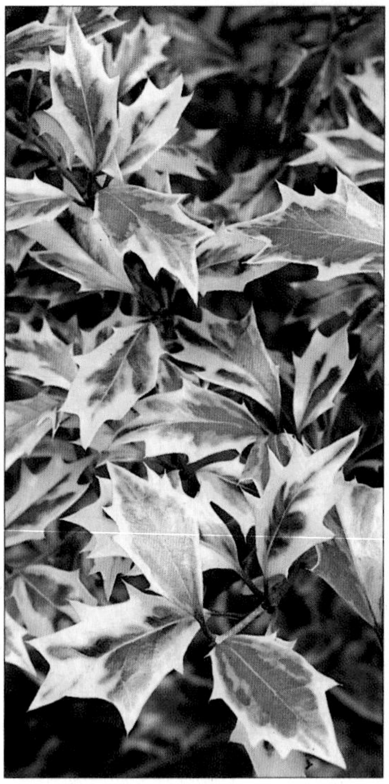

Osmanthus heterophyllus 'Aureomarginatus'

O. forrestii see *O. yunnanensis.*

O.* x *fortunei (*O. fragrans* x *O. heterophyllus*). Upright shrub with holly-like, oval to ovate, leathery, glossy, dark green leaves, to 10cm (4in) long, with spiny margins, but spineless towards the tops of mature plants. Tubular, fragrant white flowers, the lobes to 1cm (½in) across, are produced in axillary clusters from late summer to autumn. Seldom produces fruit. ↕ to 2m (6ft), sometimes to 6m (20ft), ↔ 5m (15ft). Garden origin. ❄❄. **'San José'** has narrower, more spiny leaves.

O. fragrans ◊ (Fragrant olive, Sweet tea). Vigorous, upright shrub or small tree with oblong to oblong-lance-shaped, leathery, entire or finely toothed, glossy, dark green leaves, 10–12cm (4–5in) long. Tubular, very fragrant white flowers, the lobes to 1cm (½in) across, appear singly or in few-flowered, axillary clusters in autumn, and sometimes in spring and summer; they are followed by ovoid, blue-black fruit, to 1cm (½in) long. ↕↔ 6m (20ft). Himalayas, China, Japan. ❄. **f. *aurantiacus*** has orange flowers.

O. heterophyllus. Dense, rounded shrub with holly-like, oval to elliptic-oblong, sharply toothed, leathery, glossy, dark green leaves, to 6cm (2½in) long, often spineless on mature plants. Tubular, fragrant white flowers, the lobes to 5mm (¼in) across, are produced in small, axillary clusters from late summer to autumn, followed by ovoid, blue-black fruit, to 1cm (½in) long. ↕↔ 5m (15ft). Japan, Taiwan. ❄❄. **'Aureomarginatus'** ■ syn. 'Aureus', has yellow-margined leaves. **'Gulftide'** ♀ is compact, with very spiny leaves; ↕ 2.5m (8ft), ↔ 3m (10ft). **'Myrtifolius'** has

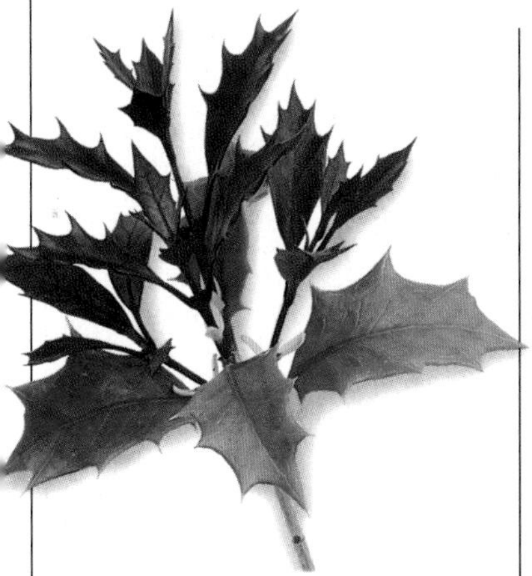

Osmanthus heterophyllus 'Purpureus'

entire, spine-tipped leaves, to 5cm (2in) long; ↕↔ 3m (10ft). **'Purpureus'** ■ has dark blackish purple young leaves. **'Rotundifolius'** has small, spineless leaves, to 4cm (1½in) long, rounded at the tips; ↕↔ 3m (10ft).

O. yunnanensis ♀ syn. *O. forrestii.* Large shrub or small tree, broadly upright at first, later spreading. The oblong to ovate-lance-shaped, spiny-toothed to entire leaves, to 20cm (8in) long, have long, sharp points and are leathery, glossy, dark green, spotted black beneath. Broadly tubular, very fragrant, creamy white flowers, with lobes to 8mm (⅜in) across, are borne in small, axillary clusters in late winter and early spring; they are followed by ovoid, dark purple fruit, to 1.5cm (½in) long, with a white bloom. ↕↔ 10m (30ft) or more. W. China. ✲✲✲ (borderline)

▷**x *Osmarea*** see *Osmanthus*
x *O.* x *burkwoodii* see *O.* x *burkwoodii*
▷***Osmaronia*** see *Oemleria*
O. cerasiformis see *O. cerasiformis*

OSMUNDA

OSMUNDACEAE

Genus of about 12 species of deciduous, terrestrial ferns found in damp places and watersides in all continents except Australasia. Broadly lance-shaped to triangular-ovate or ovate, pinnate, 2-pinnate, or 2-pinnatifid sterile fronds arise from large, erect rhizomes and turn yellow or golden brown in autumn. Distinctive, partially or wholly fertile fronds produce branched clusters of spherical greenish sporangia, which turn rust-brown or blackish on reduced pinnae. Grow in a damp border, or at the margins of a pond or stream.

• **HARDINESS** Fully hardy.

• **CULTIVATION** Grow in moist, fertile, humus-rich, preferably acid soil, in light dappled shade. *O. regalis* prefers a wetter site, but does well in full sun as long as water is plentiful.

• **PROPAGATION** Sow spores at 15–16°C (59–61°F) within 3 days of ripening in summer; they lose viability quickly. Divide clumps from established colonies in autumn or early spring. See also p.51.

• **PESTS AND DISEASES** Trouble free.

O. cinnamomea (Cinnamon fern). Deciduous fern bearing "shuttlecocks" of ovate-lance-shaped, pinnate, pale blue-green sterile fronds, 0.6–1.5m (2–5ft) long, with pinnatifid segments,

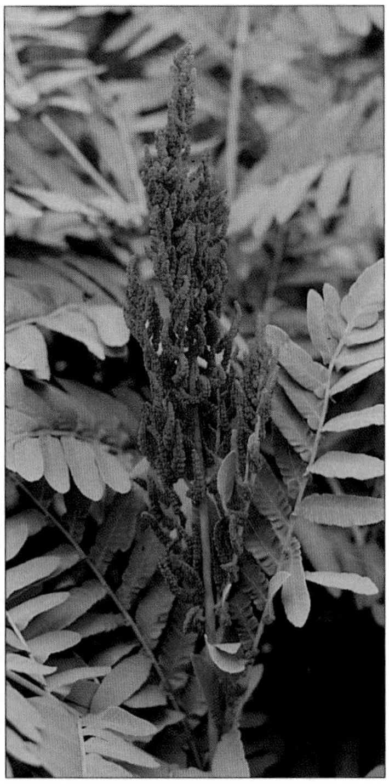

Osmunda regalis

surrounding much narrower, erect fertile fronds, to 1m (3ft) long. The top of each fertile frond is a mass of cinnamon-brown sporangia in summer. ↕ 90cm (36in), ↔ 60cm (24in). E. North America. ✲✲✲

O. claytoniana (Interrupted fern). Deciduous fern bearing "shuttlecocks" of ovate-lance-shaped, pinnate, pale blue-green sterile fronds, to 90cm (36in) long, with pinnatifid segments; they surround taller fertile fronds, similar but with some of the middle pinnae reduced and, in summer, covered in sporangia, which are initially blackish, later yellow-green, then rust-brown. ↕ 90cm (36in), ↔ 60cm (24in). E. North America. ✲✲✲

O. regalis ■𝕐 (Flowering fern, Royal fern). Deciduous fern producing dense clumps of broadly triangular-ovate, 2-pinnate, bright green sterile fronds, 1m (3ft) or more long. In summer, partially fertile fronds, to 2m (6ft) long, have tassel-like tips, with brown or rust-coloured sporangia covering the much smaller pinnae. The fibrous rootstock is the source of osmunda fibre, used as a potting compost for orchids. ↕ 2m (6ft), ↔ 4m (12ft). Temperate and subtropical regions. ✲✲✲. **'Cristata'** has pinnae and segments with crested tips; ↕↔ 1.2m (4ft). **'Purpurascens'** bears attractive red-purple-flushed fronds in spring; ↕↔ 1.2m (4ft). **'Undulata'** bears fronds with wavy segments; ↕↔ 1.2m (4ft).

▷**Oso berry** see *Oemleria cerasiformis*

OSTEOMELES

ROSACEAE

Genus of 3 species of deciduous, semi-evergreen, or evergreen shrubs or small trees from river valleys in China, Japan, Hawaii, and New Zealand. They have alternate, finely pinnate leaves and terminal corymbs of small, cup-shaped, 5-petalled white flowers, followed by spherical to ovoid, red-brown, black, or blue-black fruits, to 8mm (⅜in) across.

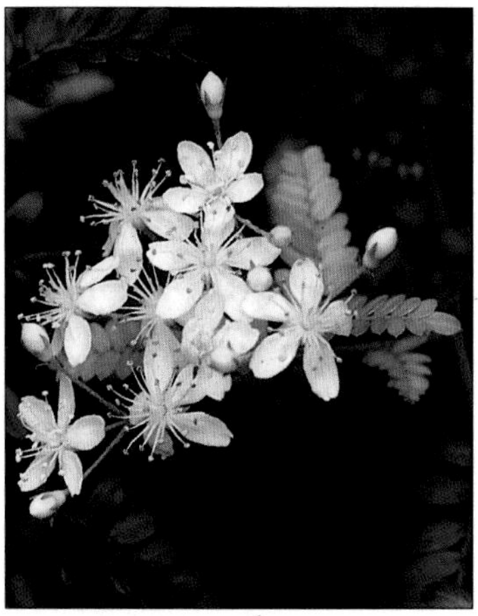

Osteomeles schweriniae

They are best grown in a sheltered shrub border or against a wall. In very cold areas, grow in a cool greenhouse.

• **HARDINESS** Frost hardy to half hardy.

• **CULTIVATION** Outdoors, grow in fertile, well-drained soil in full sun or partial shade, sheltered from strong, cold winds. Under glass, grow in loam-based potting compost (JI No.2) in full light. In growth, water freely and apply a balanced liquid fertilizer monthly; water sparingly in winter. Pruning group 8; may need restrictive pruning under glass.

• **PROPAGATION** Sow seed in containers in a cold frame in autumn. Take semi-ripe cuttings in summer.

• **PESTS AND DISEASES** Trouble free.

O. schweriniae ■ Deciduous or semi-evergreen, arching shrub with long, slender shoots and ovate to oblong-ovate, pinnate leaves, to 7cm (3in) long, consisting of 15–31 ovate-oblong leaflets. In early summer, small, cup-shaped white flowers, to 1.5cm (½in) across, are produced in corymbs, to 8cm (3in) across, at the shoot tips; they are followed by spherical, red-brown, later blue-black fruit. ↕↔ 3m (10ft). S.W. China (Yunnan). ✲✲

OSTEOSPERMUM

ASTERACEAE/COMPOSITAE

Genus of about 70 species of evergreen subshrubs, perennials, and annuals, mostly from southern Africa, but also from the Arabian Peninsula, mainly found in grassland, on rocky mountains, or at forest margins. The alternate leaves are linear to broadly obovate, with entire, toothed, or lobed margins. Osteospermums are grown for their daisy-like, usually white, pink, or yellow flowerheads, sometimes with disc-florets in a contrasting colour, borne singly or in open panicles from late spring to autumn. Numerous cultivars have been selected and named; they have ray-florets varying from deep magenta through deep or pale pink to white or yellow. Grow osteospermums in a border; in frost-prone areas, the half-hardy perennials and subshrubs are best grown as annuals.

• **HARDINESS** Fully hardy to frost tender. Many cultivars will withstand short spells down to -10°C (14°F).

• **CULTIVATION** Grow in light, moderately fertile, well-drained soil in a warm, sheltered site in full sun. Dead-head regularly to prolong flowering. In frost-prone climates, propagate annually and overwinter in frost-free conditions.

• **PROPAGATION** Sow seed at 18°C (64°F) in spring. Root softwood cuttings in late spring or semi-ripe cuttings in late summer.

• **PESTS AND DISEASES** Prone to aphids, downy mildew, and *Verticillium* wilt.

***O. barberae* of gardens** see *O. jucundum.*

***O.* 'Bodegas Pink'.** Semi-upright subshrub with mostly inversely lance-shaped, toothed, mid-green leaves with pale yellow margins. From late spring to autumn, bears solitary, daisy-like flowerheads, 5cm (2in) across, with mauve-pink ray-florets, mauve-purple on the reverse, and dark bluish mauve disc-florets. ↕↔ 45cm (18in). ✲

***O.* 'Buttermilk'** ■𝕐 Upright subshrub with mostly inversely lance-shaped, sparsely toothed, mid-green leaves. Solitary, daisy-like flowerheads, 5cm (2in) across, with white-based, primrose-yellow ray-florets, bronze-yellow on the reverse, and dark bluish mauve disc-florets, are borne from late spring to autumn. ↕↔ 60cm (24in). ✲✲

***O.* 'Cannington Roy'.** Densely spreading subshrub with obovate, sparsely toothed, mid-green leaves. From late spring to autumn, bears solitary, daisy-like flowerheads, 5cm (2in) across, with purple-tipped white ray-florets that age to mauve-pink, mauve-purple on the reverse, and with purple disc-florets. Good ground cover. ↕ 15cm (6in), ↔ 60cm (24in). ✲✲

O. caulescens 𝕐 syn. *O. ecklonis* var. *prostratum* of gardens. Prostrate subshrub with inversely lance-shaped, toothed, mid-green leaves, to 10cm (4in) long. From late spring to autumn, bears solitary, daisy-like flowerheads, 5–6cm (2–2½in) across, with white ray-florets, flushed purple on the reverse, and blue-grey disc-florets. ↕ 10cm (4in), ↔ 60cm (24in). South Africa. ✲✲

O. ecklonis, syn. *Dimorphotheca ecklonis.* Variable, erect to almost prostrate subshrub with inversely lance-shaped, toothed, grey-green leaves, to 10cm (4in) long. From late spring to autumn, bears solitary, daisy-like flowerheads, 5–8cm (2–3in) across, with white ray-florets, indigo-blue on the reverse, and dark blue disc-florets. ↕ 0.6–1.5m (2–5ft), ↔ 0.6–1.2m (24–48in). South Africa (Eastern Cape). ✲✲. **'Blue Streak'** has slate-blue disc-florets and

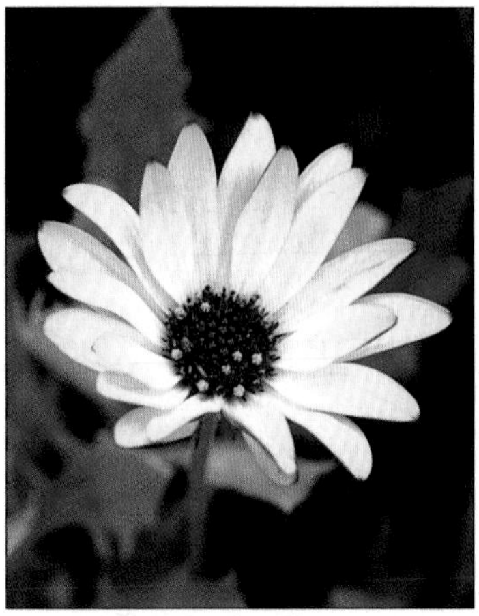

Osteospermum 'Buttermilk'

O

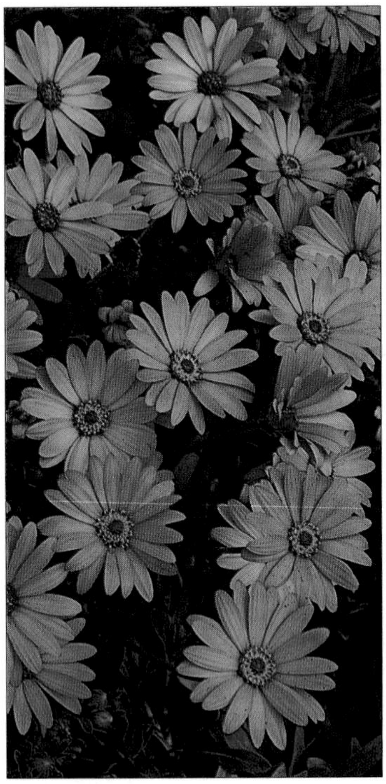

Osteospermum jucundum

white ray-florets, slate-blue on the reverse; ↕↔ 60cm (24in). **var. *prostratum* of gardens** see *O. caulescens*.
O. fruticosum. Woody-based perennial with erect or decumbent stems and obovate to spoon-shaped, slightly fleshy, entire or minutely toothed, mid-green leaves, to 10cm (4in) long, mainly in basal rosettes. Solitary, daisy-like flowerheads, 6–7cm (2½–3in) across, the ray-florets white with purple bases, the disc-florets purplish violet, are borne from late spring to mid-autumn. ↕ to 60cm (24in), ↔ 75cm (30in). South Africa (Western Cape, Eastern Cape, KwaZulu/Natal). ❄❄
O. jucundum ■♀ syn. *Dimorphotheca barberae* of gardens, *O. barberae* of gardens. Neat, clump-forming perennial, spreading by surface rhizomes, with linear to inversely lance-shaped, entire or sparsely toothed, greyish green leaves, 8–10cm (3–4in) long. From late spring to autumn, bears solitary, long-stalked, daisy-like flowerheads, 5cm (2in) across, with mauve-pink to magenta-purple ray-florets, bronze-purple to purple-pink on the reverse, and purple disc-florets that age to gold. ↕ 10–50cm (4–20in), ↔ 50–90cm (20–36in). South Africa

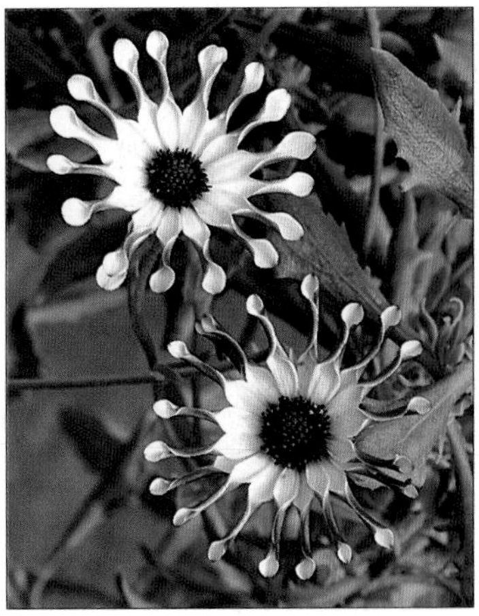

Osteospermum 'Whirligig'

(Northern Transvaal, Orange Free State, KwaZulu/Natal), Swaziland, Lesotho. ❄❄❄. **var. *compactum*** forms neat, compact mats; ↕ 10–20cm (4–8in). **var. *compactum* 'Blackthorn'**, syn. var. *compactum* 'Blackthorn Seedling', has dark purple florets.
***O.* 'Nairobi Purple'** ■ syn. *O.* 'Tresco Purple'. Spreading subshrub with broadly obovate to spoon-shaped, sparsely toothed, bright green leaves, and purplish green stems. From late spring to autumn, bears daisy-like, dark purple flowerheads, 5cm (2in) across, with purple ray-florets, flushed white on the reverse, and black disc-florets. ↕ 15cm (6in), ↔ 90cm (36in). ❄
***O.* 'Tauranga'** see *O.* 'Whirligig'.
***O.* 'Tresco Purple'** see *O.* 'Nairobi Purple'.
***O.* 'Whirligig'** ■♀ syn. *O.* 'Tauranga'. Spreading subshrub with inversely lance-shaped, toothed, grey-green leaves. From late spring to autumn, bears solitary, daisy-like flowerheads, 5–8cm (2–3in) across, with crimped and spoon-shaped white ray-florets, slate-blue or powder-blue on the reverse, and slate-blue disc-florets. ↕↔ 60cm (24in). ❄

OSTROWSKIA

Giant bellflower

CAMPANULACEAE

Genus of one species of tap-rooted perennial from well-drained, stony hillsides in Uzbekistan and Tajikistan. It has thick, unbranched stems which produce whorls of ovate, toothed leaves, and is grown mainly for its racemes of outward-facing, bell-shaped, deep to pale milky-blue flowers. Grow in a sunny, herbaceous or mixed border.

• **HARDINESS** Fully hardy; young growth may be damaged by late frosts.
• **CULTIVATION** Grow in deep, moderately fertile, moist but well-drained soil in full sun. Dies back soon after flowering; when dormant, protect from wet, and provide a dry winter mulch.
• **PROPAGATION** Sow seed singly in containers in a cold frame as soon as ripe; only seed-leaves are produced in the first year. Take care to avoid root damage when potting on and planting out. May produce flowers in the third or fourth year. Take root cuttings in late autumn; they may be slow to become established.
• **PESTS AND DISEASES** Susceptible to slug damage.

O. magnifica ■ Erect, clump-forming perennial with thick, unbranched stems bearing whorls of 4 or 5 ovate, toothed, hairless, somewhat glaucous leaves, 10–15cm (4–6in) long. In early and midsummer, produces few-flowered racemes of outward-facing, open bell-shaped, silver-sheened, pale to deep milky-blue or pale purple flowers, 12–15cm (5–6in) across, veined and suffused lilac. ↕ to 1.5m (5ft), ↔ 45cm (18in). Uzbekistan, Tajikistan. ❄❄❄

OSTRYA

BETULACEAE/CORYLACEAE

Genus of approximately 10 species of monoecious, deciduous trees occurring in woodland in Europe, Asia, North America, and Central America. They have simple, ovate to ovate-oblong or ovate-lance-shaped leaves, arranged alternately. The flowers are produced in catkins, males and females on the same tree, but only the males are conspicuous. Female catkins develop into hop-like fruits in late summer. They are excellent specimen trees for a woodland garden.

• **HARDINESS** Fully hardy.
• **CULTIVATION** Grow in fertile, well-drained soil in sun or partial shade. Pruning group 1.
• **PROPAGATION** Sow seed as soon as ripe in containers in a cold frame, or in a seedbed.
• **PESTS AND DISEASES** Trouble free.

O. carpinifolia ♤–♧ (Hop hornbeam). Broadly conical to rounded tree with hairy shoots and ovate, doubly toothed, lustrous, dark green leaves, to 10cm (4in) long, each with 15–20 pairs of veins; the leaves turn yellow in autumn. Pendulous, yellow male catkins, to 7cm (3in) long, are formed in autumn and open in mid-spring. Hop-like white fruit clusters, 5cm (2in) long, develop in summer and turn brown in autumn. ↕↔ 20m (70ft). S. Europe, Turkey, Syria, Caucasus. ❄❄❄
O. virginiana ■♤ (American hop hornbeam, Ironwood). Conical tree with glandular-hairy shoots and ovate-lance-shaped, sharply, sometimes doubly toothed, dark green leaves, to 12cm (5in) long, each with 11–15 pairs of veins. Pendulous, yellow male catkins, to 5cm (2in) long, are formed in autumn and open in mid-spring; hop-like white fruit clusters, to 5cm (2in) long, develop in summer and turn brown in autumn. ↕ 15m (50ft), ↔ 12m (40ft). E. North America. ❄❄❄

OTHONNA

ASTERACEAE/COMPOSITAE

Genus of about 150 species of evergreen or deciduous, shrubby, succulent perennials and small shrubs, often arising from caudices or thick, tuberous rootstocks. They are found in dry, hilly areas of Tunisia, Algeria, Namibia, and South Africa. They have entire or dissected, fleshy leaves, which are lobed or toothed, and terminal, daisy-like, usually yellow, rarely white or purple flowerheads, produced singly or in corymbs from summer to winter. In areas where temperatures drop below 10°C (50°F), grow tender species as houseplants or in a temperate greenhouse; in warm, dry climates, use in a desert border. Grow *O. cheirifolia* in a raised bed or rock garden, or in a sunny border.

• **HARDINESS** Fully hardy to frost tender.
• **CULTIVATION** Under glass, grow in standard cactus compost in full light. Water moderately during the growing season, more sparingly in winter. Apply a balanced liquid fertilizer 3 or 4 times during summer and autumn. Outdoors, grow in sharply drained, moderately fertile, gritty soil in full sun. See also pp.48–49.
• **PROPAGATION** Sow seed at 18–21°C (64–70°F) in spring. Insert basal or semi-ripe cuttings with bottom heat in late summer. Take basal cuttings of *O. cheirifolia* in early summer.

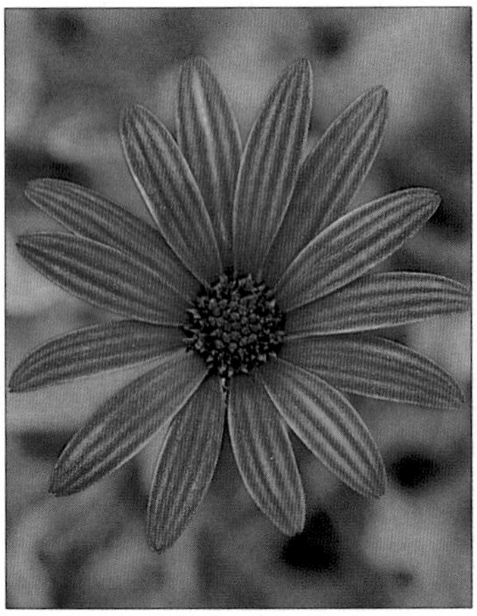

Osteospermum 'Nairobi Purple'

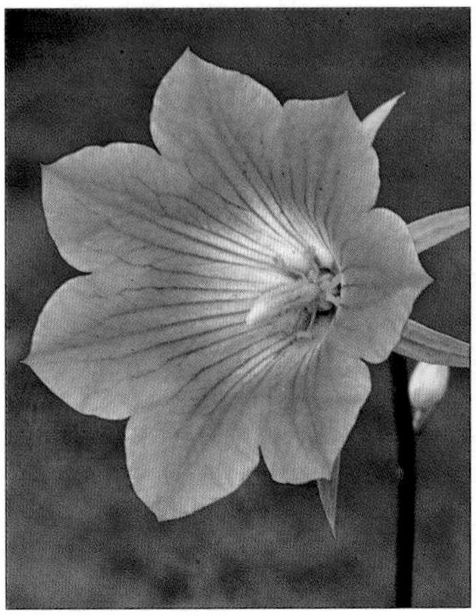

Ostrowskia magnifica

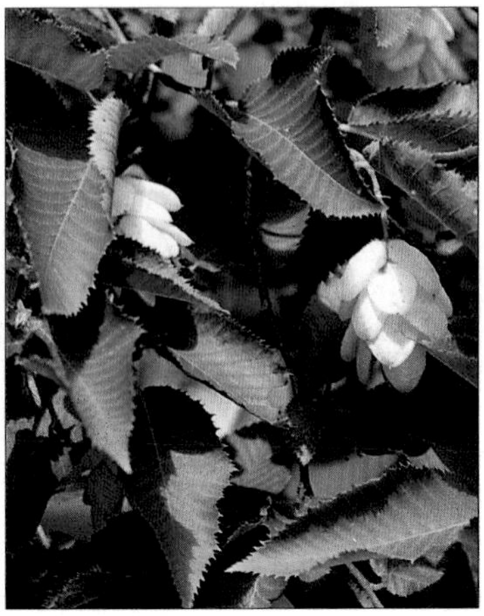

Ostrya virginiana

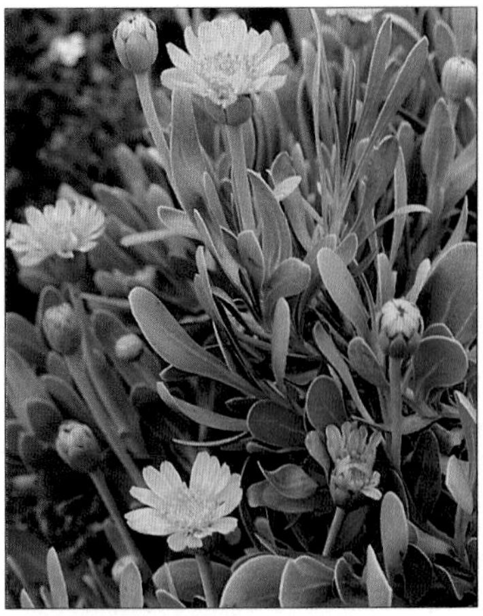

Othonna cheirifolia

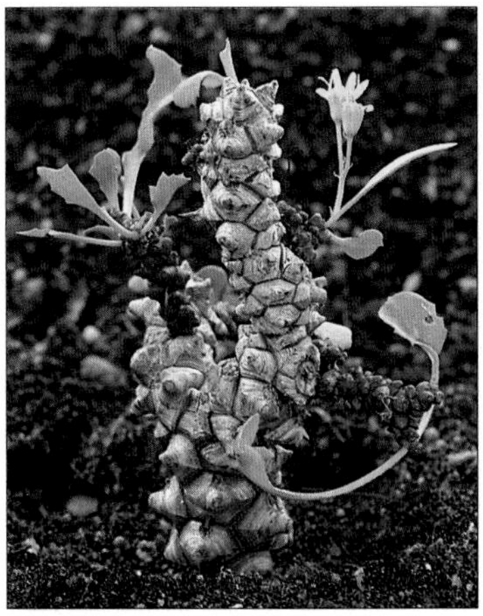

Othonna herrei

• **PESTS AND DISEASES** Prone to red spider mites and aphids.

O. capensis (Little pickles). Evergreen, perennial succulent with cylindrical to cylindrical-obovoid, entire, fleshy, pale green leaves, to 2.5cm (1in) long, often clustered on slender, trailing stems. In summer, bears few-flowered corymbs of daisy-like yellow flowerheads, 1cm (½in) across, which open only in sun. Excellent for a hanging basket. ↕ 20cm (8in), ↔ 1m (3ft). South Africa (Eastern Cape). ❀ (min. 5°C/41°F)
O. cheirifolia ▣ syn. *Othonnopsis cheirifolia*. Spreading, evergreen shrub with branching stems bearing lance- to spoon-shaped, entire, fleshy, pale grey-green leaves, to 8cm (3in) long. In summer, bears solitary, daisy-like yellow flowerheads, about 4cm (1½in) across. ↕ 30cm (12in), ↔ 60cm (24in). N. Africa. ✲✲
O. herrei ▣ Deciduous, perennial succulent with thickened stems and prominent, woody nodules formed from persistent leaf bases. Bears irregularly obovate, wavy-margined, toothed, fleshy, bluish green leaves, 5cm (2in) long, at the tips of short branches. Produces corymbs of daisy-like yellow flowerheads, 2cm (¾in) across, in late autumn and early winter. ↕↔ 10cm (4in). Namibia, South Africa (Northern Cape). ❀ (min. 7–10°C/45–50°F)

▷ ***Othonnopsis cheirifolia*** see *Othonna cheirifolia*

OURISIA

SCROPHULARIACEAE

Genus of approximately 25 species of low-growing, mainly rhizomatous, evergreen or semi-evergreen perennials occurring in alpine regions of Tasmania, New Zealand, South America, and Antarctica. They have mostly radical leaves, which are usually conspicuously veined, but are cultivated for their usually short-tubed flowers, each with 5 spreading lobes, the 3 lower lobes larger than the upper 2. The flowers are produced singly from the leaf axils, or in whorls or racemes on leafless stems. Ourisias grow best in cool, moist climates, and are suitable for a shady rock garden, peat bed, shaded wall, or alpine house.
• **HARDINESS** Fully hardy.
• **CULTIVATION** Grow in reliably moist, fertile, humus-rich soil in partial shade.

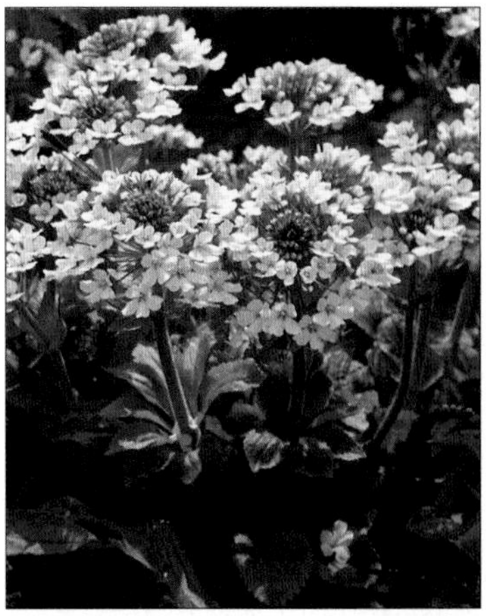

Ourisia macrophylla

Rhizomatous species quickly exhaust soil nutrients, so divide and replant them when they begin to deteriorate. In an alpine house, grow in a mix of 1 part each loam and grit with 2 parts leaf mould, and keep slightly moist in winter; they resent a dry atmosphere.
• **PROPAGATION** Sow seed in containers in a cold frame, as soon as ripe or in early spring. Divide rhizomatous species, or separate rooted sections, in spring. Take stem-tip cuttings of *O. microphylla* in early summer.
• **PESTS AND DISEASES** Often damaged by slugs and snails.

O. caespitosa. Dwarf, mat-forming, evergreen perennial with broadly ovate-spoon-shaped, entire or notched, grey-green leaves, 4–8mm (⅛–⅜in) long. Leafless stems bear up to 5-flowered whorls of tubular, yellow-throated white flowers, to 1.5cm (½in) across, in early summer. ↕ 5cm (2in), ↔ to 20cm (8in). New Zealand. ✲✲✲. **var. *gracilis*** is more compact, with leaves to 6mm (¼in) long, and solitary flowers; ↕ 3cm (1¼in), ↔ 15cm (6in).
O. coccinea. Mat-forming, evergreen perennial with rosettes of broadly elliptic or oblong, toothed, strongly veined, light green leaves, 3–6mm (⅛–¼in) long. Throughout summer, produces loose, terminal racemes of pendent, long-tubed, noticeably 2-lipped scarlet flowers, to 4cm (1½in) long. May spread widely in cool, moist conditions. ↕ 20cm (8in), ↔ 40cm (16in) or more. Chilean Andes. ✲✲✲
O. 'Loch Ewe'. Vigorous, spreading, evergreen perennial, similar to *O. coccinea*, with tight rosettes of broadly oval, leathery, mid-green leaves, 3–6cm (1¼–2½in) long, heart-shaped at the bases. Dense, spike-like racemes of tubular, clear pale pink flowers, 2.5cm (1in) across, are borne in late spring and early summer. ↕ to 20cm (8in), ↔ 30cm (12in). ✲✲✲
O. macrophylla ▣ Mat-forming, evergreen, rhizomatous perennial with ovate to rounded-oblong, coarsely veined, bright green leaves, to 22cm (9in) long. Upright stems produce whorled racemes of many yellow-throated white flowers, to 2cm (¾in) across, in summer. ↕ 30cm (12in) or more, ↔ 40cm (16in) or more. New Zealand. ✲✲✲
O. microphylla ▣ Cushion-forming, semi-evergreen perennial with slender, branching stems clothed in heath-like, pale green leaves, 2mm (¹⁄₁₆in) long, pressed closely to the stems. In late spring and early summer, produces a profusion of solitary, small, tubular, pale pink flowers, 1cm (½in) across, with white centres. ↕ 5cm (2in), ↔ to 15cm (6in). Chile, Argentina. ✲✲✲
O. 'Snowflake' 🏆 Robust, mat-forming, evergreen perennial, similar to *O. caespitosa*, with obovate, spoon-shaped, glossy, dark green leaves, to 1cm (½in) long. Clusters of tubular white flowers, 1–2cm (½–¾in) across, are produced in summer. ↕ 10cm (4in), ↔ to 25cm (10in). ✲✲✲

▷ **Our Lord's candle** see *Yucca whipplei*
▷ **Owl's eyes** see *Huernia zebrina*

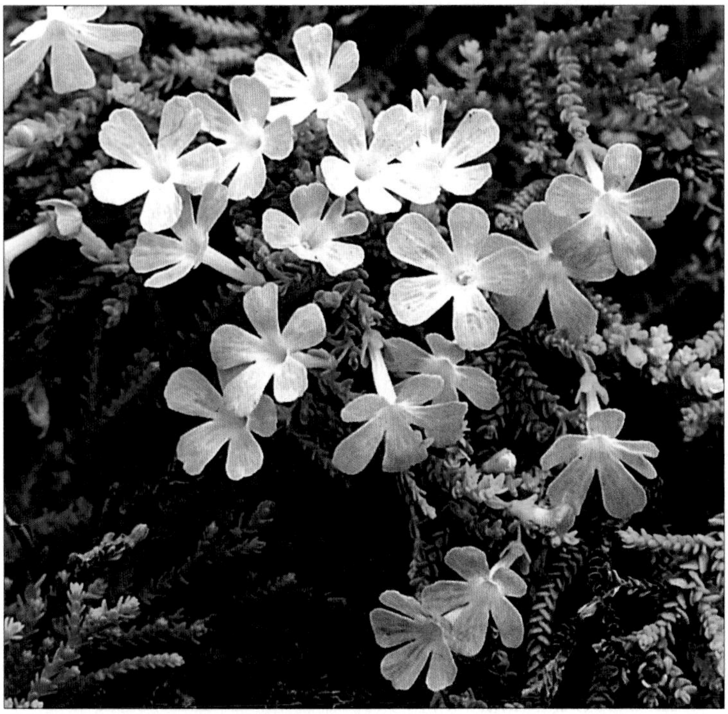

Ourisia microphylla

OXALIS

Shamrock, Sorrel

OXALIDACEAE

Genus of about 500 species of fibrous-rooted, bulbous, rhizomatous, or tuberous annuals and perennials, some of which are very invasive weeds. They occur in open habitats or in woodland, and are widely distributed, with many species from southern Africa and South America. Those grown as ornamentals are valued for their palmate, clover-like foliage (some have leaves that fold at night), and for their funnel- to cup- or bowl-shaped, 5-petalled flowers; these are furled umbrella-like in bud, are borne singly or in cymes, sometimes umbel-like, and usually open only in sunlight, closing in dull weather or at night. Woodland species, such as *O. acetosella* and *O. oregana*, are suitable for naturalizing in a shady site. Many of the hardy species from southern Africa and South America, as well as various cultivars, are suitable for a rock garden, raised bed, trough, or alpine house. In frost-prone areas, grow the less hardy species in a temperate or warm greenhouse.
• **HARDINESS** Fully hardy to frost tender.
• **CULTIVATION** Grow hardy woodland species in moist, fertile, humus-rich soil in full or partial shade. Other hardy species need full sun and well-drained, moderately fertile, humus-rich soil. Under glass, grow in loam-based potting compost (JI No.2) with added grit, in bright filtered light and low humidity. When in growth, water moderately and apply a balanced liquid fertilizer every month. Keep all container-grown plants barely moist when dormant. In an alpine house, grow in a mix of equal parts loam, leaf mould, and grit.
• **PROPAGATION** Sow seed at 13–18°C (55–64°F) in late winter or early spring. Divide in spring; small sections of rhizomatous species root readily with bottom heat.
• **PESTS AND DISEASES** Prone to rust. May be damaged by slugs and snails.

O. acetosella* var. *purpurascens see *O. acetosella* var. *subpurpurascens.*
O. acetosella* var. *rosea see *O. acetosella* var. *subpurpurascens.*
O. acetosella* var. *subpurpurascens ▣ syn. *O. acetosella* var. *purpurascens*, *O. acetosella* var. *rosea*. Creeping, mat-forming, rhizomatous perennial

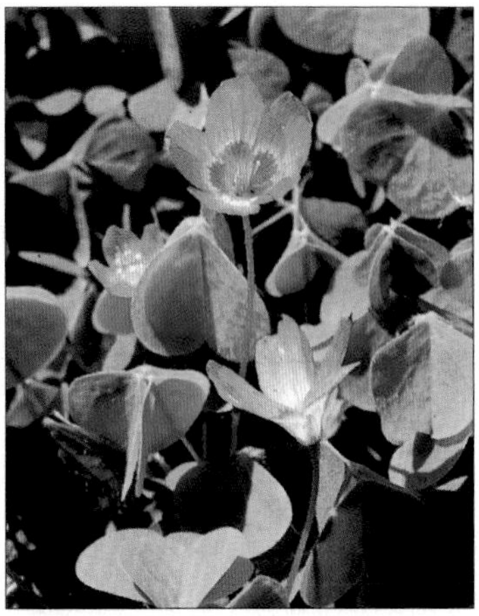

Oxalis acetosella var. *subpurpurascens*

O

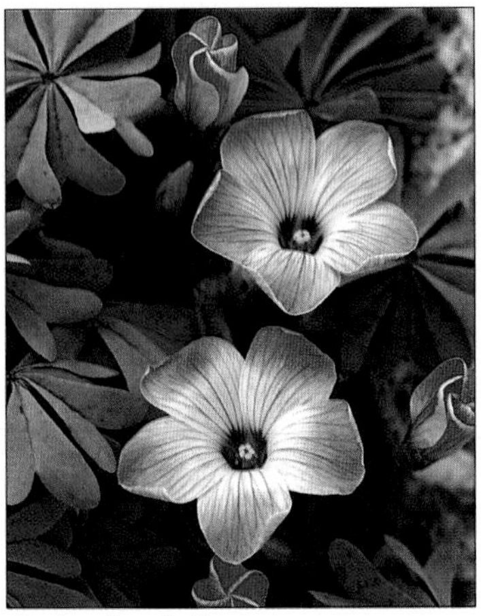
Oxalis adenophylla

with clover-like, pale green leaves, each with 3 inversely heart-shaped, sparsely hairy leaflets, to 2cm (¾in) long. In spring, bears solitary, cup-shaped, dark-veined, rose-pink flowers, 2cm (¾in) across. ↕ 5cm (2in), ↔ indefinite. Woodland in N. hemisphere. ❄❄❄

O. adenophylla ▣ 🏆 Clump-forming perennial with fibre-covered bulbs that produce grey-green leaves, each consisting of 9–22 narrowly and inversely heart-shaped leaflets, to 2cm (¾in) long. In late spring, bears solitary, widely funnel-shaped, purplish pink flowers, about 2.5cm (1in) across, with darker veins and purple throats. ↕ 10cm (4in), ↔ to 15cm (6in). Andes, Chile, Argentina. ❄❄❄

O. bowiei, syn. *O. purpurata* var. *bowiei*. Clump-forming, bulbous perennial with long-stalked, clover-like, leathery leaves, each with 3 rounded to inversely heart-shaped, notched leaflets, 1–2.5cm (½–1in) long, mid-green above, hairy and often purple beneath. Bears loose, umbel-like cymes of 3–12 funnel-shaped, deep purplish pink flowers, to 4cm (1½in) across, with yellow-green tubes, in summer. Very similar to *O. purpurata*, which produces runners and may be invasive. ↕ to 25cm (10in), ↔ to 15cm (6in). South Africa (Western Cape, Eastern Cape, KwaZulu/Natal). ❄❄

O. carnosa see *O. megalorrhiza*.

O. chrysantha. Fibrous-rooted, mat-forming perennial with creeping and rooting, slender stems and white-hairy, light green leaves, each divided into 3 triangular to inversely heart-shaped leaflets, 8mm (⅜in) long. Produces

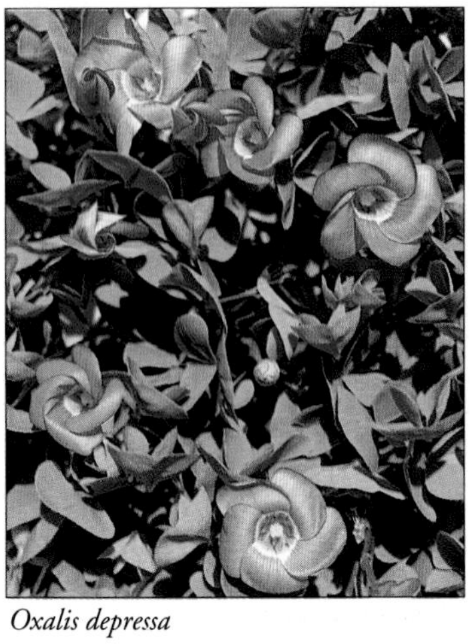
Oxalis depressa

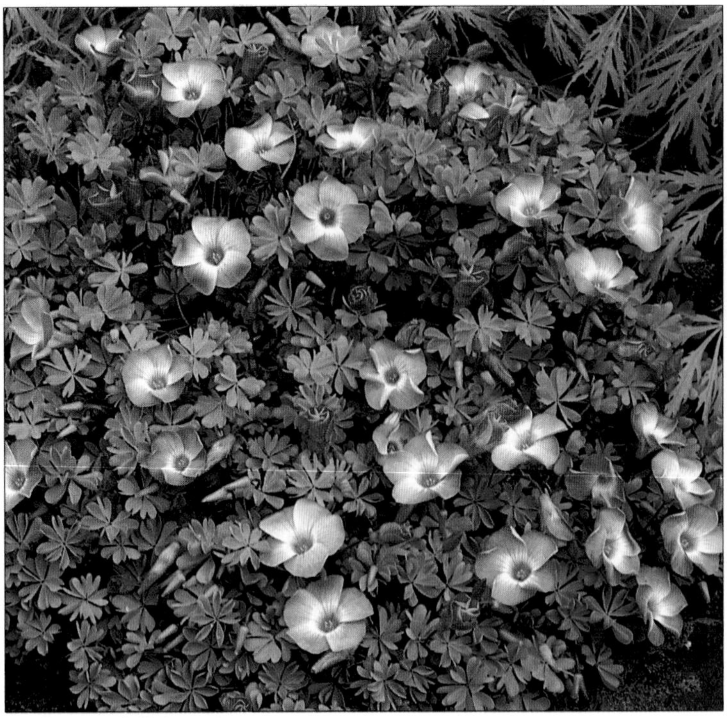
Oxalis enneaphylla 'Rosea'

solitary, funnel-shaped, bright yellow flowers, 1.5–2cm (½–¾in) across, with red markings at the mouths, throughout summer and into autumn. ↕ 5cm (2in), ↔ 30cm (12in) or more. Brazil. ❄❄

O. deppei see *O. tetraphylla.*

O. depressa ▣ syn. *O. inops*. Clump-forming, bulbous perennial with short runners and short-stalked, sometimes sparsely hairy and dark-spotted, grey-green leaves, each divided into 3 triangular-obovate leaflets, to 1cm (½in) long. In summer, bears solitary, widely funnel-shaped, deep rose-pink to purple-pink flowers, to 2cm (¾in) across, with yellow tubes. ↕ 5cm (2in), ↔ to 20cm (8in) or more. Southern Africa. ❄❄❄ (borderline)

O. enneaphylla 🏆 Clump-forming perennial with scaly, branching rhizomes, producing tufts of umbrella-like, somewhat fleshy, hairy, blue-grey leaves, each consisting of 9–20 narrowly oblong, pleated leaflets, to 2cm (¾in) long. Solitary, widely funnel-shaped, fragrant, white to deep red-pink flowers, 2–2.5cm (¾–1in) across, are produced in late spring and early summer. ↕ 8cm (3in), ↔ to 15cm (6in). Patagonia, Falkland Islands. ❄❄❄. **'Minutifolia'** has a more compact habit, with much smaller leaflets, to 1cm (½in) long, and white flowers; ↕ 5cm (2in), ↔ 10cm (4in). **'Rosea'** ▣ has light purple-pink flowers.

O. hedysaroides. Semi-evergreen subshrub with upright, branching, leafy stems, bearing light green leaves, glaucous beneath, each with 3 broadly ovate leaflets, to 2.5cm (1in) long. Produces axillary cymes of 3–6 widely funnel-shaped yellow flowers, to 1.5cm (½in) across, in summer. Suitable for a cool greenhouse. ↕ to 1m (3ft), ↔ to 45cm (18in). Central America. ❄

O. herrerae, syn. *O. succulenta*. Erect, succulent perennial with short-branched, scaly stems. Bears clusters of broad, hairless, mid-green leaves, each with 3 inversely heart-shaped, fleshy leaflets, to 1cm (½in) long, often slightly hairy beneath, on stalks 2–5cm (¾–2in) long. Short-branched cymes of 5–7 bowl-shaped, red-veined yellow flowers, to 1.5cm (½in) across, appear in summer. ↕ to 30cm (12in), ↔ 21cm (8in). Peru, Chile. ⌂ (min. 10°C/50°F)

O. hirta. Variable, bulbous perennial with upright or decumbent, leafy stems bearing almost stalkless, hairy, pale green leaves, each with 3 linear to oblong or obovate leaflets, to 1.5cm (½in) long. In autumn and winter, bears solitary, open funnel-shaped, white, red-pink, or purple flowers, 2cm (¾in) across, with yellow throats. Best in a cool greenhouse in frost-prone climates. ↕ 30cm (12in), ↔ 10cm (4in). South Africa (Western Cape). ❄❄

O. inops see *O. depressa.*

***O.* 'Ione Hecker'** 🏆 Clump-forming, rhizomatous perennial, similar to *O. enneaphylla*, with grey-green leaves, each consisting of 9–15 narrowly oblong leaflets, to 1.5cm (½in) long. In summer, produces solitary, widely funnel-shaped, blue-violet flowers, to 3cm (1¼in) across, conspicuously veined dark purple, and with dark purple throats. ↕ 8cm (3in), ↔ 10cm (4in). ❄❄❄

O. laciniata, syn. *O. squamosoradicosa*. Tuft-forming, rhizomatous perennial, with tiny bulbils, producing tufts of blue-grey, often purple-margined leaves, each with 8–12 inversely heart-shaped, folded, crinkly-margined leaflets, to 1.5cm (½in) long. Solitary, widely funnel-shaped, scented, violet-blue, lilac-blue, red, pink, or white flowers, with light green throats, and to 2.5cm (1in) across, are produced in late spring and summer. Prefers cool conditions. ↕ 5–10cm (2–4in), ↔ 10cm (4in). Patagonia. ❄❄❄

O. lobata ▣ syn. *O. perdicaria*. Clump-forming, bulbous perennial with tuberous roots, producing compact clusters of bright green leaves, each with 3 inversely heart-shaped leaflets, 7mm (¼in) long. The leaves, which appear in spring, die down quickly and reappear

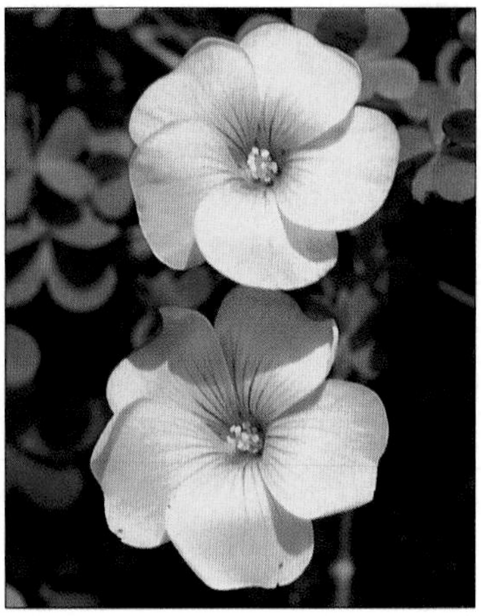
Oxalis lobata

in late summer and autumn at the same time as the solitary, funnel-shaped, bright yellow flowers, often dotted and veined red, 1–2cm (½–¾in) across. ↕↔ to 10cm (4in). Chile. ❄❄

O. megalorrhiza, syn. *O. carnosa*. Slow-growing, succulent perennial with fleshy rhizomes and few-branched, fleshy stems, later becoming woody. These produce terminal clusters of fleshy, glossy, mid-green leaves, each with 3 inversely heart-shaped leaflets, 1–2cm (½–¾in) long. Umbel-like cymes of 2–5 bowl-shaped yellow flowers, to 2cm (¾in) across, are borne in summer and autumn. ↕ 15cm (6in), to 40cm (16in) with age, ↔ to 20cm (8in). Coastal regions of Galapagos Islands, and Peru, Chile, Bolivia. ⌂ (min. 10°C/50°F)

O. obtusa ▣ Slowly spreading, mat-forming, bulbous perennial with runners producing bulbils. It is similar to *O. depressa*, but with shorter-stemmed, hairy, grey-green leaves, each with 3 rounded to triangular-obovate leaflets, 0.5–2.5cm (¼–1in) long. Solitary, widely funnel-shaped, rose-pink, brick-red, or yellow flowers, to 2cm (¾in) across, appear in summer. ↕ 5cm (2in), ↔ 20cm (8in). Namibia, South Africa (Eastern Cape, Southern Cape). ❄❄

O. oregana. Creeping, rhizomatous perennial with hairy, mid-green leaves, each divided into 3 inversely heart-shaped leaflets, 1–3cm (½–1¼in) long. Solitary, cup-shaped, rose-pink, lilac, occasionally white flowers, 2.5cm (1in) across, are produced on slender stems from spring to autumn. ↕ to 20cm (8in), ↔ indefinite. Woodland in W. North America. ❄❄❄

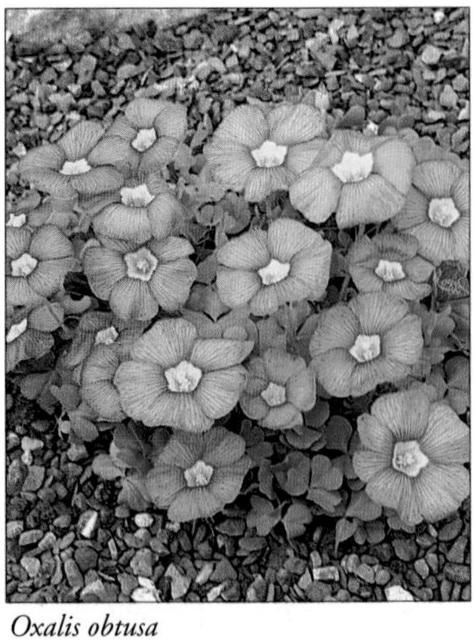
Oxalis obtusa

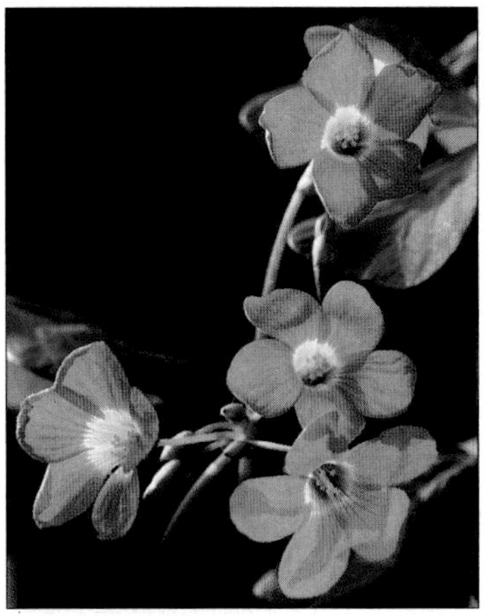

Oxalis tetraphylla

O. perdicaria see *O. lobata.*
O. purpurata* var. *bowiei see *O. bowiei.*
O. purpurea. Variable, bulbous perennial with clusters of silky, white-hairy, dark green leaves, each with 3 diamond-shaped to rounded or broadly obovate leaflets; these are often deep purple beneath, 2cm (¾in) long, and hairy at the margins and on the surfaces. Solitary, widely funnel-shaped, cream, white, pink, or purple flowers, 3–5cm (1¼–2in) across, are produced in autumn and winter. ↕ 10cm (4in), ↔ 15cm (6in). South Africa (Northern Transvaal, Eastern Transvaal, Eastern Cape), Swaziland. ❄❄. **'Ken Aslet'** has bright, deep yellow flowers.
O. squamosoradicosa see *O. laciniata.*
O. succulenta see *O. herrerae.*
O. tetraphylla ■ syn. *O. deppei* (Good luck plant, Lucky clover). Clump-forming, bulbous perennial with mid-green leaves, each consisting of 4 strap-shaped to inversely triangular, entire or notched leaflets, 2–7cm (¾–3in) long, usually banded purple at the bases. In summer, produces loose, umbel-like cymes of 4–12 widely funnel-shaped, reddish purple flowers, with greenish yellow throats, 2–3cm (¾–1¼in) across. ↕↔ to 15cm (6in). Mexico. ❄❄. **'Iron Cross'** ■ has leaflets that each have a V-shaped, dark purple band at the base, combining to form a distinctive cross over the 4 leaflets.
O. versicolor. Clump-forming, bulbous perennial with mid-green leaves, each divided into 3 wedge-shaped-linear to linear, almost hairless leaflets, 1–2cm (½–¾in) long. A profusion of solitary, funnel-shaped white flowers, 2–3cm (¾–1¼in) across, crimson-margined on the reverse and crimson-striped in bud, are produced from late summer to winter. Suitable for an alpine house. ↕ 8cm (3in), ↔ 20cm (8in) or more. Southern Africa. ❄

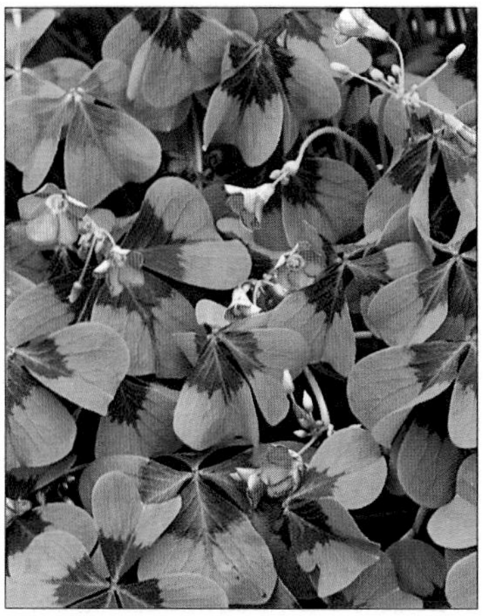

Oxalis tetraphylla 'Iron Cross'

▷ **Ox eye** see *Heliopsis*
▷ **Oxlip** see *Primula elatior*

OXYDENDRUM

ERICACEAE

Genus of one species of deciduous, large shrub or small tree from woodland and streamsides in E. North America. It has rusty-red to grey bark, simple, alternate leaves, which turn vivid red in autumn, and cylindrical to urn-shaped white flowers borne in large, terminal panicles. Cultivated for the autumn colour of its foliage and for its flowers, it is best grown in an open glade in a woodland garden.
• **HARDINESS** Fully hardy.
• **CULTIVATION** Grow in fertile, moist but well-drained, acid soil, preferably avoiding exposed situations. Pruning group 1.
• **PROPAGATION** Sow seed in containers in a cold frame in autumn. Take semi-ripe cuttings in summer.
• **PESTS AND DISEASES** Trouble free.

O. arboreum ■ ◊ (Sorrel tree, Sourwood). Conical to columnar shrub or tree with elliptic to oblong-lance-shaped, toothed, glossy, dark green leaves, to 20cm (8in) long, turning brilliant shades of red, yellow, and purple in autumn. Cylindrical to urn-shaped white flowers, to 6mm (¼in) long, are produced in large panicles, to 25cm (10in) long, in late summer and early autumn. ↕ 10–15m (30–50ft), ↔ 8m (25ft). E. North America. ❄❄❄

▷ ***Oxypetalum*** see *Tweedia*
O. caeruleum see *T. caerulea*
▷ **Oyster plant** see *Mertensia maritima*

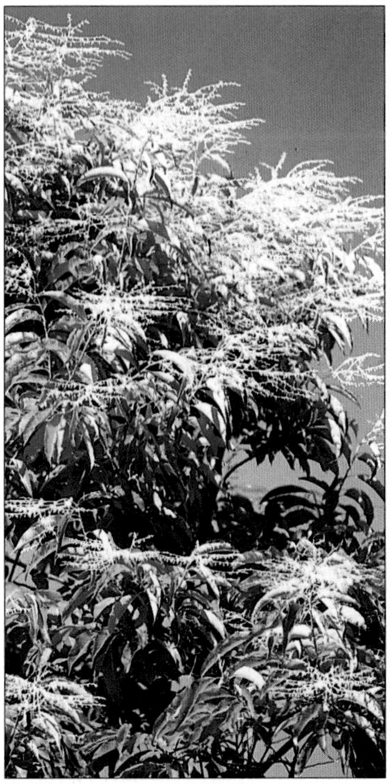

Oxydendrum arboreum

OZOTHAMNUS

ASTERACEAE/COMPOSITAE

Genus of about 50 species of evergreen shrubs and woody-based perennials, closely related to *Helichrysum*, from Australia and New Zealand, where they grow in rocky places and on heathland, from the coast to the mountains. They are cultivated for their often aromatic, usually small, heath-like, alternate leaves, and for their solitary or corymb-like flowerheads, displaying white disc-florets. Grow larger species in a shrub border; smaller species are good in a trough, rock garden, or alpine house.
• **HARDINESS** Fully hardy to half hardy.
• **CULTIVATION** Grow in moderately fertile, well-drained soil in a sheltered site in full sun. *O. coralloides* and *O. selago* need gritty, sharply drained soil; protect from excessive winter wet. In an alpine house, use a mix of equal parts loam, leaf mould, and grit. Pruning group 8.
• **PROPAGATION** Sow seed in containers in an open frame as soon as ripe. Take semi-ripe cuttings in summer.
• **PESTS AND DISEASES** Trouble free.

O. coralloides ■ syn. *Helichrysum coralloides.* Compact, rounded shrub with diamond-shaped, scale-like, leathery leaves, 5mm (¼in) long, white-woolly beneath, and pressed flat to the cylindrical branches. Solitary, terminal, yellowish white, cylindrical flowerheads, 6mm (¼in) across, appear in summer. ↕↔ 60cm (24in). New Zealand. ❄❄
O. ledifolius ■ ♀ syn. *Helichrysum ledifolium* (Kerosene bush). Compact, rounded shrub with yellowish green shoots densely covered with oblong-linear, aromatic, dark green leaves, to 1cm (½in) long, yellow-downy beneath, the margins strongly curved under. In early summer, bears white flowerheads, 5mm (¼in) across, in dense, terminal corymbs, 3–5cm (1¼–2in) across. ↕↔ 1m (3ft). Australia (Tasmania). ❄❄
O. rosmarinifolius ■ syn. *Helichrysum rosmarinifolium.* Compact, upright shrub with rosemary-like, linear, dark green leaves, to 4cm (1½in) long, woolly beneath, the margins curved under. Fragrant white flowerheads, 4mm (⅛in) across, red in bud, are borne in dense, terminal corymbs, 4cm (1½in) across, in early summer. ↕ 2–3m (6–10ft), ↔ 1.5m (5ft). S.E. Australia. ❄❄. **'Silver Jubilee'** ♀ has silvery grey leaves.

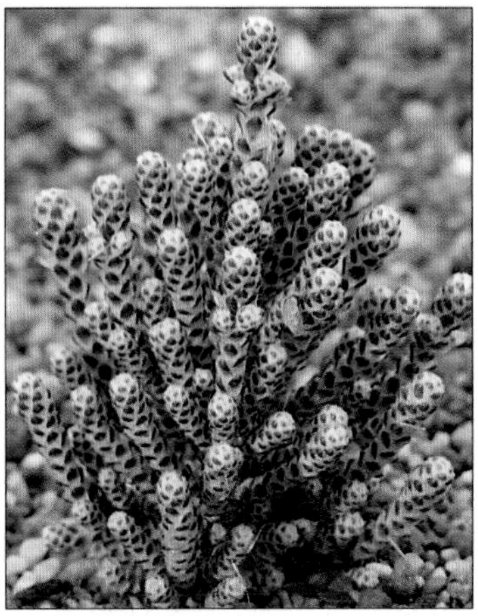

Ozothamnus coralloides

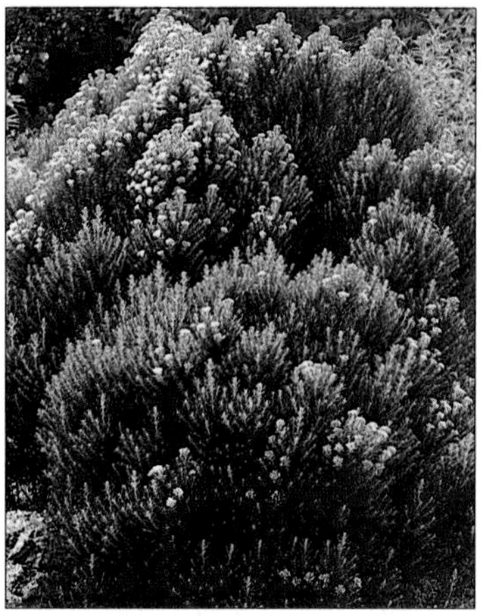

Ozothamnus ledifolius

O. selago ■ syn. *Helichrysum selago.* Dense, upright shrub with rigid shoots densely covered in tiny, ovate to triangular, aromatic leaves, 3mm (⅛in) long, pressed flat to the shoots. Terminal, solitary cream flowerheads, 7mm (¼in) across, are produced in summer. ↕ to 40cm (16in), ↔ 25cm (10in). New Zealand (South Island). ❄❄❄
O. thyrsoideus, syn. *Helichrysum thyrsoideum* (Snow in summer). Upright shrub with linear, aromatic, dark green leaves, to 5cm (2in) long, pressed flat to the shoots. Over a long period in summer, pure white flowerheads, about 4mm (⅛in) across, are produced in dense, rounded corymbs, 2cm (¾in) across, at the shoot tips. ↕ to 3m (10ft), ↔ 2m (6ft). S.E. Australia. ❄❄

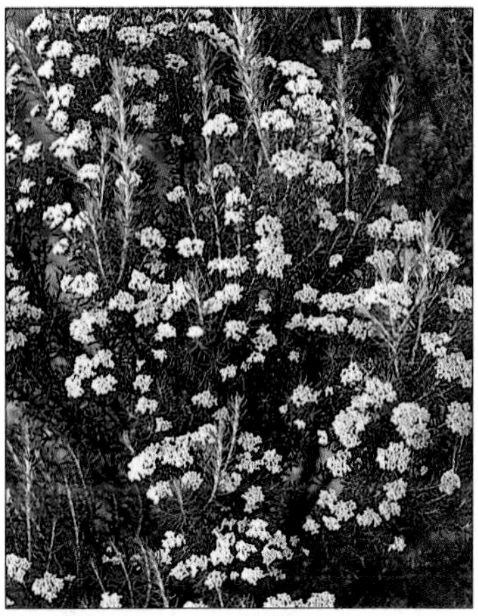

Ozothamnus rosmarinifolius

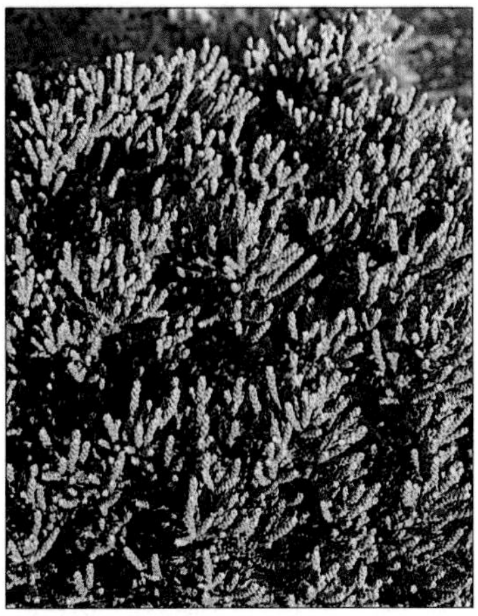

Ozothamnus selago

P

PACHYCEREUS
syn. LOPHOCEREUS

CACTACEAE

Genus of possibly 9 species of columnar, often tree-like, ribbed, perennial cacti from semi-desert areas of the USA and Mexico. These often massive cacti branch from the bases of the main stems, and have large, spiny, usually scaly areoles, sometimes woolly or bristly in the axils. The nocturnal or diurnal, funnel- or bell-shaped, or short, tubular flowers are produced only on mature plants. The bristly, spherical, fleshy fruits contain large, black-coated seeds. Where temperatures drop below 10°C (50°F), grow in a temperate or warm greenhouse. In warmer climates, use in a desert garden.

- **HARDINESS** Frost tender.
- **CULTIVATION** Under glass, grow in standard cactus compost in full light. From spring to summer, water moderately and apply a low-nitrogen liquid fertilizer every 4–5 weeks. Keep dry at other times. Outdoors, grow in moderately fertile, sharply drained soil in full sun. See also pp.48–49.
- **PROPAGATION** Sow seed at 19–24°C (66–75°F) in spring. Take stem-tip cuttings in summer.
- **PESTS AND DISEASES** Vulnerable to scale insects and occasionally mealybugs.

P

P. marginatus. Erect cactus with sometimes sparsely branched, 4- to 7-ribbed, dark green stems, 8–15cm

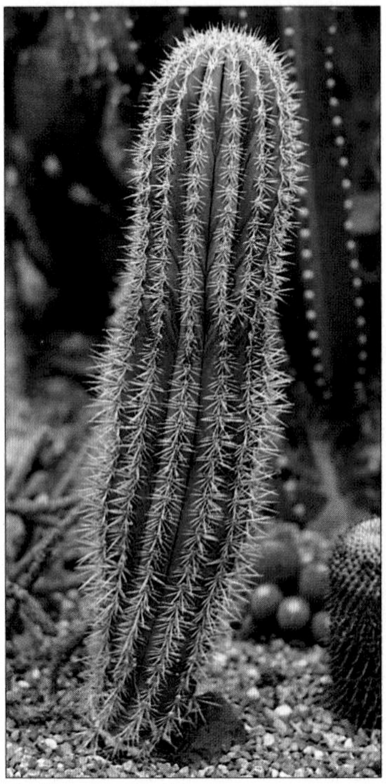

Pachycereus pringlei

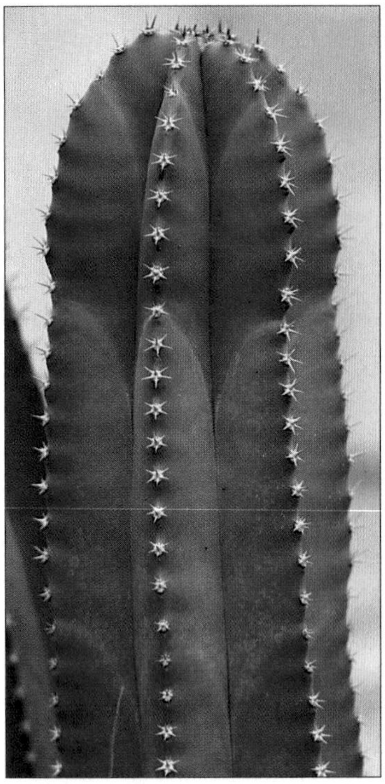

Pachycereus schottii

(3–6in) across, with grey-white areoles bearing brown to grey spines (5–8 radials, 1 or 2 longer centrals). Produces nocturnal and diurnal, tubular, greenish white or pink flowers, 3–5cm (1¼–2in) across, in summer. ↕ to 3–7m (10–22ft), ↔ 1m (3ft). C. and S. Mexico. ❀ (min. 10°C/50°F)

P. pecten-aboriginum. Erect, tree-like cactus with branched, dark bluish green stems, 30cm (12in) thick, each with 10 or 11 acute ribs and grey-white areoles bearing stiff brown spines, fading to grey (8 or 9 radials, 1 or 2 longer centrals). In summer, bears nocturnal and diurnal, funnel-shaped white flowers, 6–8cm (2½–3in) across, with greenish red outer petals. ↕ to 8m (25ft), ↔ 3m (10ft). W. Mexico. ❀ (min. 10°C/50°F)

P. pringlei ■ Tree-like cactus with dark blue-green stems, 1m (3ft) or more thick, and erect branches, each with 10–17 rounded ribs. Grey areoles have reddish to dark brown spines, fading to grey (about 20 radials, 1–3 slightly longer centrals). In summer, bears nocturnal, bell- to funnel-shaped white flowers, 8cm (3in) across, with greenish red outer petals. ↕ to 12–15m (40–50ft), ↔ 3m (10ft). N.W. Mexico. ❀ (min. 10°C/50°F)

P. schottii ■ syn. *Lophocereus schottii.* Erect, columnar cactus with dull dark green stems, to 10–15cm (4–6in) thick, each with 4–9 ribs. Grey-woolly areoles produce almost black spines, fading to grey (4–7 radials, often 1 central). As the plant matures, a spiny, hairy pseudocephalium forms; in summer, it produces nocturnal, slender, funnel-shaped, red, pink, or white flowers, 3–4cm (1¼–1½in) across, green outside, with an unpleasant smell. ↕ 7m (22ft), ↔ 3m (10ft). USA (S. Arizona), N.W. Mexico. ❀ (min. 10°C/50°F). **'Monstrosus'** has misshapen stems, irregular ribs, and spineless areoles; ↕ to 3m (10ft), ↔ 1m (3ft).

P. weberi. Tree-like cactus producing glaucous, blue-green stems, 20cm (8in) or more thick, and erect, 8- to 10-ribbed branches. White-woolly areoles each produce up to 13 spines (6–12 yellowish white, later reddish brown or black radials, 1 longer grey central). In mid-summer, bears nocturnal, funnel-shaped white flowers, yellowish white outside, to 10cm (4in) long. ↕ 10m (30ft), ↔ 3m (10ft) or more. S. Mexico. ❀ (min. 10°C/50°F)

PACHYCORMUS

ANACARDIACEAE

Genus of one species of very variable, slow-growing, deciduous, perennial succulent from desert or semi-desert areas of Mexico. Grey- or silver-barked branches bear pinnate, feathery leaves. Dense, terminal racemes of tiny, cup-shaped flowers are produced by day in summer. Where temperatures drop below 15°C (59°F), grow in a warm greenhouse. In warmer climates, use in a desert garden.

- **HARDINESS** Frost tender.
- **CULTIVATION** Under glass, grow in loam-based potting compost (JI No.2), with added grit, in full light. From mid-spring until the leaves fall, water freely and apply a balanced liquid fertilizer every 6–8 weeks. Keep just moist at other times. Outdoors, grow in sharply drained, moderately fertile soil in full sun. See also pp.48–49.
- **PROPAGATION** Sow seed at 19–24°C (66–75°F) in spring.
- **PESTS AND DISEASES** Young growth is vulnerable to red spider mites.

P. discolor ■ (Elephant tree). Free-branching succulent. The trunk and branches are very swollen, and both contain sponge-like wood and white latex. Pinnate, mid-green leaves, to 8cm (3in) long, consist of 6–8 oval, slightly toothed or lobed leaflets, hairy towards the tips. In summer, bears lax, dense racemes of cup-shaped, white to yellow or red flowers, to 6mm (¼in) long. ↕ 4m (12ft), ↔ 45cm (18in) or more. N.W. Mexico. ❀ (min. 15°C/59°F)

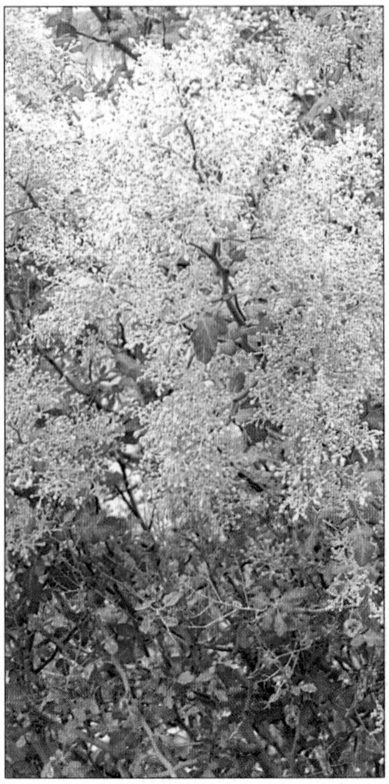

Pachycormus discolor

PACHYCYMBIUM

ASCLEPIADACEAE

Genus of about 30 species of leafless, perennial succulents, formerly classified under *Caralluma*, from mostly hilly terrain in the Arabian Peninsula, E. Africa, Zimbabwe, and South Africa. They have erect or prostrate, 4-angled or rounded, prominently toothed stems, and produce compact cymes of diurnal, bell- or cup-shaped flowers, usually near the stem tips, in summer. Where temperatures drop below 10°C (50°F), grow in a warm greenhouse. In warmer climates, use in a desert garden.

- **HARDINESS** Frost tender.
- **CULTIVATION** Under glass, grow in loam-based potting compost (JI No.2), with added grit or sharp sand, in full light. From mid-spring to early autumn, water moderately and apply a low-nitrogen liquid fertilizer every 6–8 weeks. Keep just moist at other times. Outdoors, grow in moderately fertile, sharply drained soil in full sun. See also pp.48–49.
- **PROPAGATION** Sow seed at 19–24°C (66–75°F) in spring. Take stem-tip cuttings in spring or early summer.
- **PESTS AND DISEASES** Prone to ant damage while flowering.

P. dummeri, syn. *Caralluma dummeri.* Erect, spreading succulent with 4-angled or slightly rounded, greyish green stems, 1.5cm (½in) thick, with dark red stripes. In summer, produces cymes of 1–4, sometimes up to 6, bell-shaped, olive-green to dark green flowers, 4cm (1½in) across, with tapering, spreading lobes, hairy inside, smooth outside. ↕ 10cm (4in), ↔ to 15cm (6in). Uganda, Kenya, Tanzania. ❀ (min. 10°C/50°F)

PACHYPHRAGMA

BRASSICACEAE/CRUCIFERAE

Genus of one species of semi-evergreen, rhizomatous perennial found in moist beech woods in N.E. Turkey and the Caucasus. It produces long-stalked, basal leaves, glossy, dark green at first, becoming duller. Broad, terminal corymbs of 4-petalled white flowers appear just as the leaves develop; the stems later elongate so that the flattened fruit are held above the foliage. A slow-growing, ground-cover plant, *P. macrophyllum* is suitable for planting beneath trees and deciduous shrubs.

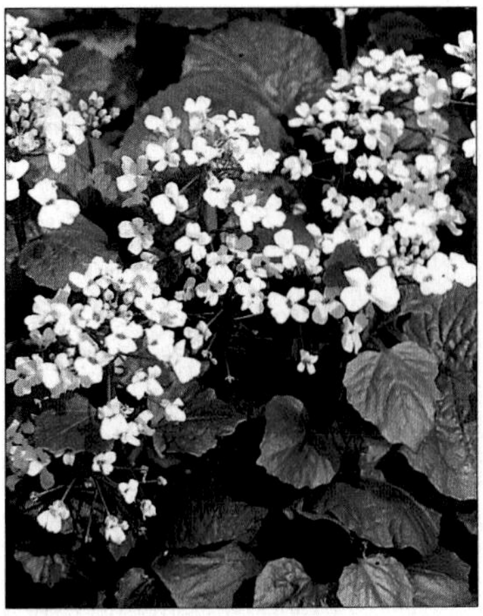

Pachyphragma macrophyllum

• **HARDINESS** Fully hardy.
• **CULTIVATION** Grow in moderately fertile, moist, leafy soil, preferably in partial shade.
• **PROPAGATION** Sow seed in containers in a cold frame in autumn. Divide in spring. Take basal stem cuttings in late spring.
• **PESTS AND DISEASES** Slugs may be a problem.

P. macrophyllum ■ syn. *Thlaspi macrophyllum.* Semi-evergreen perennial with ovate to rounded, scalloped leaves, 2.5–10cm (1–4in) long, produced in basal clusters that partially persist over winter. Flat corymbs of cross-shaped, 4-petalled, unpleasantly scented white flowers, 2cm (¾in) across, with pale green veins, are borne in early spring, followed by distinctive, flat, inversely heart-shaped fruit. ↕ 20–40cm (8–16in), ↔ 60–90cm (24–36in). Caucasus, N.E. Turkey. ❄❄❄

PACHYPHYTUM

CRASSULACEAE

Genus of 12 or more species of rosette-forming, perennial succulents from arid areas of Mexico, closely resembling *Echeveria*, with which it hybridizes. The semi-erect, usually branching, spreading stems become decumbent with age, and bear variably shaped, swollen, fleshy, mid- to dark or grey-green, frequently white-frosted leaves. Racemes of diurnal, bell-shaped flowers are borne on fleshy, sometimes sparsely branched stems, mainly in spring. Where temperatures drop below 7°C (45°F), grow in a temperate greenhouse. In warmer climates, use in a desert garden.
• **HARDINESS** Frost tender.
• **CULTIVATION** Under glass, grow in standard cactus compost in full light, with shade from hot sun. In the growing season, water moderately and apply a low-nitrogen liquid fertilizer every 6–8 weeks. Keep almost dry at other times. Outdoors, grow in moderately fertile, sharply drained soil in full sun, with some midday shade. See also pp.48–49.
• **PROPAGATION** Sow seed at 19–24°C (66–75°F) in spring. Take leaf or stem-tip cuttings in spring or summer.
• **PESTS AND DISEASES** Trouble free.

P. compactum ■ Compact succulent with short-stemmed rosettes of oblong to lance-shaped, white-frosted, dark green leaves, 2–3cm (¾–1¼in) long,

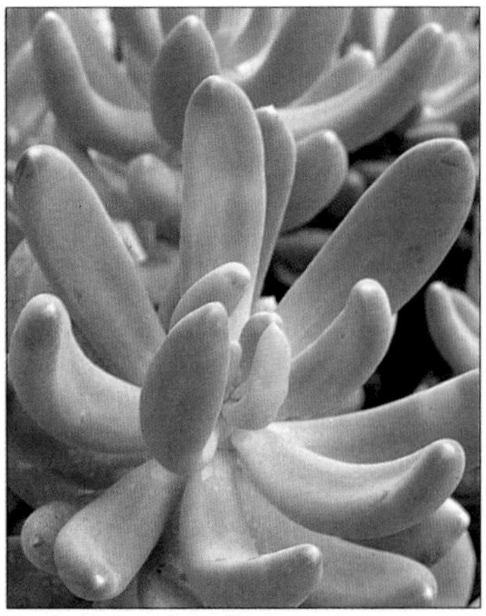
Pachyphytum longifolium

sometimes tinged red-purple, with rounded, angular margins. Racemes of 3–10 pendent, blue-tipped, orange-red flowers, 1cm (½in) long, with pink or green calyces, develop in spring. ↕ 10–15cm (4–6in), ↔ 30cm (12in) or more. Mexico. ❀ (min. 7°C/45°F)

P. hookeri. Clump-forming, long-stemmed succulent with scattered, almost cylindrical, pointed, mid-green leaves, to 5cm (2in) long, with a blue-grey to white bloom; they are slightly flattened on the upper surfaces, with blunt to rounded margins. Racemes of 5–18 yellowish pink flowers, to 1.5cm (½in) long, flushed pale purple-red, with green-tipped pink sepals, are borne in spring. ↕ 60cm (24in), ↔ indefinite. Mexico. ❀ (min. 7°C/45°F)

P. longifolium ■ Rosette-forming succulent with inversely lance-shaped, grey-green leaves, 6–11cm (2½–4½in) long, with a blue-glaucous bloom, blunt or pointed at the tips, and grooved beneath. Racemes of 10–50 white flowers, 1cm (½in) long, strongly suffused red, develop mainly in spring, but also irregularly throughout the year. ↕ 15cm (6in) or more, ↔ 20cm (8in) or more. Mexico. ❀ (min. 7°C/45°F)

P. oviferum ■ (Sugar-almond plant). Clump-forming succulent producing short-stemmed rosettes of obovoid, white-frosted, light green leaves, 2–5cm (¾–2in) long, flushed lavender-blue. Racemes of 10–15 vivid orange-red or greenish red flowers, 1.5cm (½in) long, with pale blue-white calyces, are borne from winter to spring. ↕ 10–12cm (4–5in), ↔ 30cm (12in) or more. Mexico. ❀ (min. 7°C/45°F)

PACHYPODIUM

APOCYNACEAE

Genus of 13 species of shrubby or tree-like, perennial succulents from mostly arid regions of Namibia, South Africa, and Madagascar. Many have swollen, irregularly shaped caudices and very thick, thorny stems. Leaves are simple, entire, and variably shaped; they are usually deciduous but may persist in cultivation. Diurnal, salverform to funnel- or bell-shaped flowers are borne usually in terminal clusters, in summer. Where temperatures drop below 15°C (59°F), grow in a warm greenhouse. In warmer climates, use in a desert garden or as focal points on a lawn.
• **HARDINESS** Frost tender.
• **CULTIVATION** Under glass, grow in standard cactus compost in full light. From late spring to early autumn, water moderately and apply a low-nitrogen liquid fertilizer every 4–5 weeks. Keep dry at other times. Outdoors, grow in moderately fertile, sharply drained soil in full sun. See also pp.48–49.
• **PROPAGATION** Sow seed at 19–24°C (66–75°F), or take stem-tip cuttings, in late spring.
• **PESTS AND DISEASES** Susceptible to aphids while flowering.

P. baronii. Tree-like succulent with a massive, stout, thorny caudex and thick, thorny stems bearing obovate to elliptic, tapering, greyish green leaves, to 15cm (6in) long. Salverform, bright red flowers, to 6cm (2½in) across, develop in summer. ↕ 3m (10ft), ↔ to 1m (3ft). N. Madagascar. ❀ (min. 15°C/59°F)

P. bispinosum. Shrubby succulent with a rugged, partly underground caudex and thin, thorny, fleshy branches bearing lance-shaped to narrowly lance-shaped, roughly hairy, mid-green leaves, 4–8cm (1½–3in) long. Broadly bell-shaped, pink to purple flowers, 3cm (1¼in) across, with recurving white lobes, are produced in summer. ↕ 45cm (18in), ↔ 18cm (7in). South Africa (Eastern Cape). ❀ (min. 15°C/59°F)

P. densiflorum. Shrubby, slow-growing succulent with a thorny caudex, short stem, and short, thick, thorny branches. The obovate to oblong-ovate leaves, to 10cm (4in) long, are mid- to dark green, grey-felted beneath. In summer, bears salverform, bright yellow flowers, to 3cm (1¼in) across, each with prominent yellow anthers forming a cone. ↕ to 45cm (18in), ↔ 12cm (5in) or more. Madagascar. ❀ (min. 15°C/59°F)

P. geayi. Tree-like succulent with a thorny caudex, branching near the top with age. Thorny branches bear linear, greyish green leaves, to 40cm (16in) long, silver-grey-hairy beneath. Salverform, pure white flowers, 8cm (3in) across, are produced in summer. ↕ to 8m (25ft), ↔ to 2m (6ft). S.W. Madagascar. ❀ (min. 15°C/59°F)

P. lamerei ■ Tree-like succulent with a thick caudex branching near the top, with thorns generally in groups of 3. Bears terminal clusters of linear to lance-shaped, shining, dark green leaves, 25–40cm (10–16in) long. Salverform, yellow-throated, creamy white flowers, to 11cm (4½in) across, are borne in summer. ↕ to 6m (20ft), ↔ 2m (6ft). S. and S.W. Madagascar. ❀ (min. 15°C/59°F)

P. namaquanum. Tree-like succulent with a thick, fleshy, thorny, caudex-like trunk, rarely branching, with spirally arranged tubercles, and thorns in groups of 3. Produces terminal rosettes of lance-shaped, slightly hairy, pale green leaves, 12cm (5in) long, with wavy, crisped

P

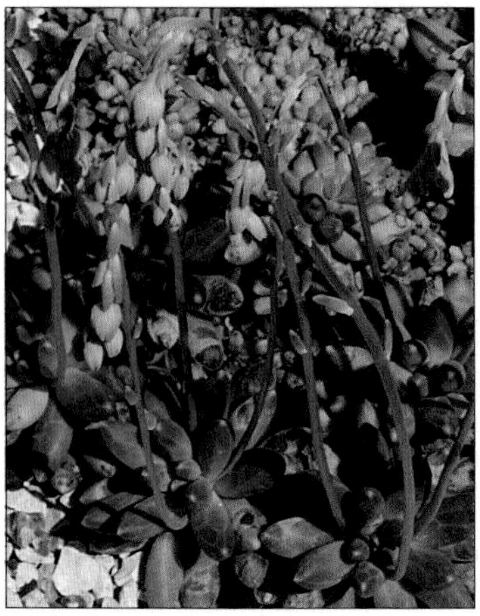
Pachyphytum compactum

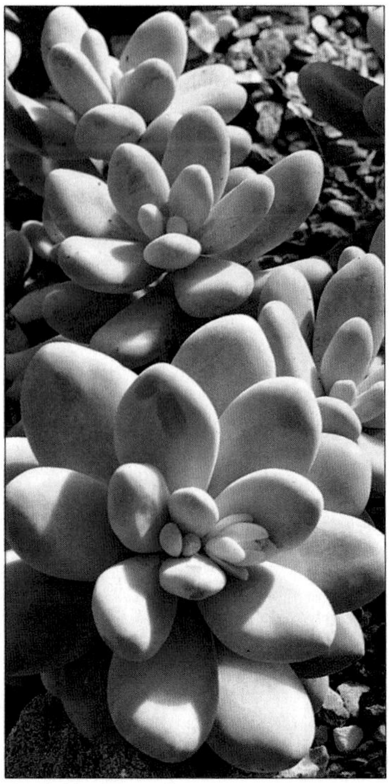
Pachyphytum oviferum

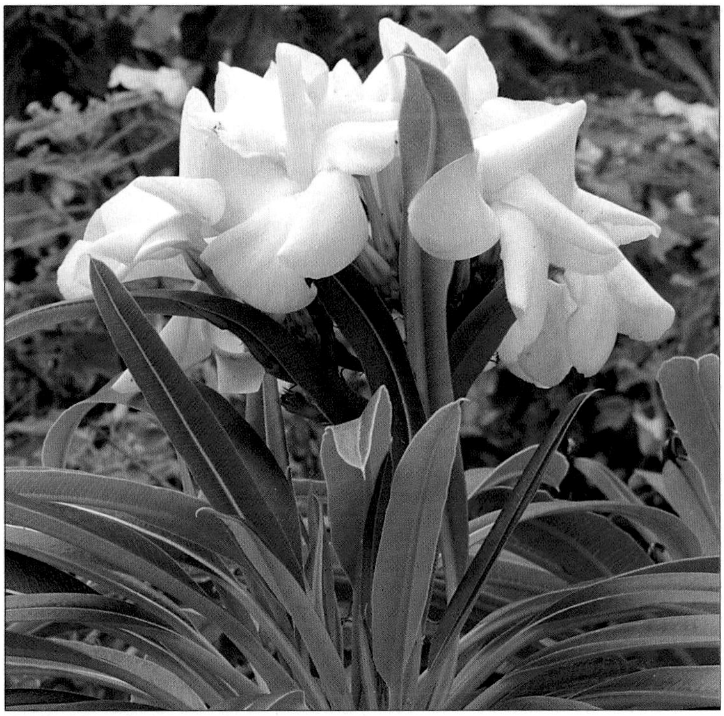
Pachypodium lamerei

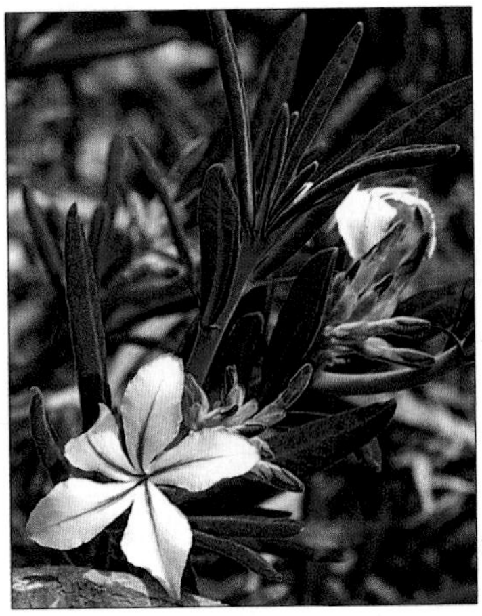
Pachypodium succulentum

margins. In summer, bears tubular, yellow-green and purple-red flowers, striped yellow inside, to 2cm (¾in) long. ↕ to 2.5m (8ft), ↔ 1.5m (5ft). S. Namibia, South Africa (Northern Cape). ❁ (min. 15°C/59°F)
P. rosulatum. Variable, shrubby succulent with a spherical or irregularly shaped, thorny caudex, branching stems, and elliptic, mid- to dark green leaves, to 8cm (3in) long, slightly hairy above. Salverform yellow flowers, to 1.5cm (½in) across, with rounded, flat lobes, are produced in summer. ↕ to 1.5m (5ft), ↔ 1m (3ft) or more. Madagascar. ❁ (min. 15°C/59°F). **var. *borombense*** has inflated, bell-shaped flowers.
P. succulentum ■ Shrubby succulent with a mainly underground caudex. Strong, sturdy branches bear paired thorns and narrowly lance-shaped, minutely hairy, mid- to dark green leaves, to 6cm (2½in) long. Salverform, pink, white, sometimes red-striped, or red flowers, 4cm (1½in) across, with narrow, spreading lobes, develop in summer. ↕↔ 60–90cm (24–36in). South Africa (Orange Free State to Western Cape and Eastern Cape). ❁ (min. 15°C/59°F)

PACHYSANDRA

BUXACEAE

Genus of 4 species of evergreen or semi-evergreen perennials and subshrubs occurring in woodland in China and Japan. They have often rhizome-like, fleshy green stems and upright branches with alternate, broadly ovate to obovate, entire or coarsely toothed, grey- to dark green leaves clustered at their tips. Terminal or axillary spikes of small, unisexual, petalless flowers (the females greenish white, the males with white stamens) are produced in spring or early summer. Cultivated for their foliage, they are useful as ground cover in a shrub border or woodland garden. They spread freely, especially in moist, humus-rich soil.
• **HARDINESS** Fully hardy.
• **CULTIVATION** Grow in any but very dry soil in full or partial shade.
• **PROPAGATION** Divide in spring. Root softwood cuttings in early summer.
• **PESTS AND DISEASES** May be damaged by slugs and snails.

P. terminalis ■🏆 Spreading, evergreen perennial with obovate, coarsely toothed, glossy, dark green leaves, to 10cm (4in)

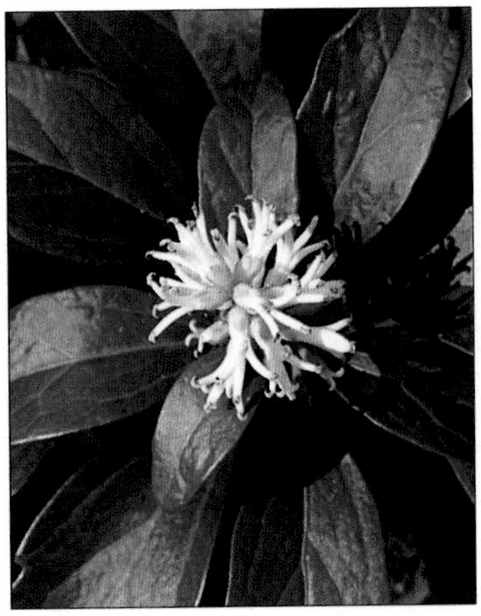
Pachysandra terminalis

long, clustered at the ends of short, smooth stems. Produces tiny white male flowers in spikes, 2–3cm (¾–1¼in) long, in early summer. ↕ 20cm (8in), ↔ indefinite. N. China, Japan. ❄❄❄. **'Green Carpet'** is more compact, with smaller, finely toothed leaves, to 7cm (3in) long; ↕ 15cm (6in), ↔ to 60cm (24in). **'Variegata'** 🏆 is slower-growing, and produces attractive white-margined leaves; ↕ 25cm (10in), ↔ to 60cm (24in).

PACHYSTACHYS

ACANTHACEAE

Genus of 12 species of evergreen perennials and shrubs, closely allied to *Justicia*, from woodland or rainforest in the West Indies and tropical Central and South America. They are cultivated for their tubular, 2-lipped flowers, borne in erect, terminal spikes with large, overlapping, usually brightly coloured bracts. Leaves are opposite and simple, ovate to lance-shaped, and mid- to dark green. Where temperatures drop below 10–15°C (50–59°F), grow in a warm or temperate greenhouse, or as houseplants. In warmer areas, use in a border.
• **HARDINESS** Frost tender.
• **CULTIVATION** Under glass, grow in loam-based potting compost (JI No.2) in full light, with high humidity. During the growing season, water freely and apply a balanced liquid fertilizer monthly. Water moderately in winter. Outdoors, grow in fertile, moist but well-drained soil in full sun. Pruning group 8; may need restrictive pruning under glass.

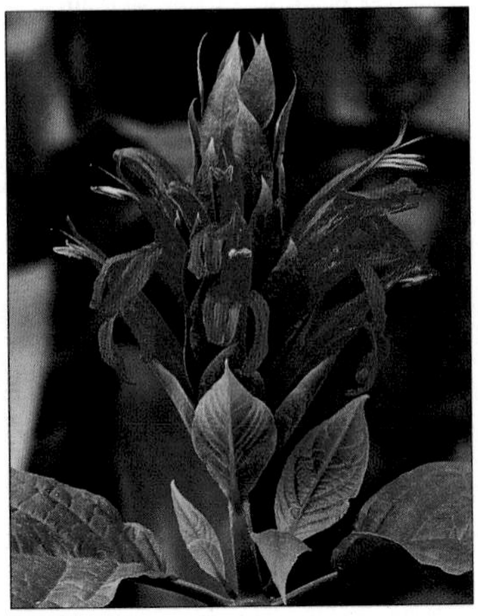
Pachystachys coccinea

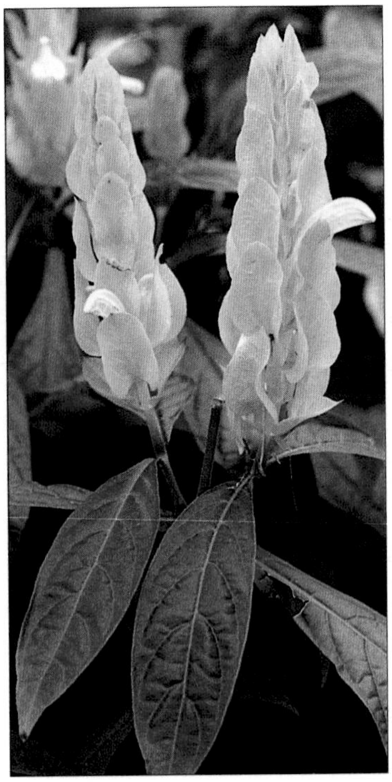
Pachystachys lutea

• **PROPAGATION** Root softwood cuttings with bottom heat in summer.
• **PESTS AND DISEASES** Whiteflies and red spider mites may be troublesome under glass.

P. cardinalis see *P. coccinea*.
P. coccinea ■ syn. *Jacobinia coccinea*, *Justicia coccinea*, *P. cardinalis* (Cardinal's guard). Erect shrub producing robust, simple or sparsely branched stems and ovate-elliptic, strongly veined, lightly wrinkled, dark green leaves, 15–20cm (6–8in) long. In winter, tubular, strongly 2-lipped scarlet flowers, 5cm (2in) long, are borne in terminal spikes, 15cm (6in) long, with 4-ranked, pale green bracts. ↕ to 2m (6ft) or more, ↔ 60–90cm (24–36in). West Indies, N. South America. ❁ (min. 13°C/55°F)
P. lutea ■🏆 (Lollipop plant). Erect shrub with moderately to sparsely branched stems and narrowly ovate, elliptic, or lance-shaped, slender-pointed, strongly veined, mid- to deep green leaves, 8–15cm (3–6in) long. In spring and summer, produces tubular, strongly 2-lipped white flowers, 4–5cm (1½–2in) long, borne in terminal spikes, 10cm (4in) long, with 4-ranked, bright golden yellow bracts. ↕ to 1m (3ft), ↔ 45–75cm (18–30in). Peru. ❁ (min. 13°C/55°F)

PACHYSTEGIA

ASTERACEAE/COMPOSITAE

Genus of one species of evergreen shrub, related to *Olearia*, occurring on cliffs and riverbanks and in rocky places from sea level to mountains in New Zealand. It has alternate, simple leaves, and bears terminal or axillary, solitary flowerheads, to 6cm (2½in) across, with white ray-florets and yellow disc-florets. Grown for its foliage and showy flowers, it is suitable for a rock garden.
• **HARDINESS** Frost hardy.
• **CULTIVATION** Grow in fertile, well-drained soil in full sun; shelter from cold, drying winds. Pruning group 1.
• **PROPAGATION** Sow seed in containers in a cold frame in autumn. Take semi-ripe cuttings in summer.
• **PESTS AND DISEASES** Trouble free.

P. insignis, syn. *Olearia insignis* (Marlborough rock daisy). Spreading shrub with stout, white- or brown-felted shoots and oval to obovate, glossy, dark green leaves, to 15cm (6in) long, grey-green when young, and clustered at the tips of the shoots. In summer, bears long-stalked, daisy-like, solitary white flowerheads, to 6cm (2½in) across, with yellow centres. ↕ 90cm (36in), ↔ 1.2m (4ft). New Zealand (South Island). ❄❄

▷ ***Pachystima*** see *Paxistima*

x PACHYVERIA

CRASSULACEAE

Hybrid genus of mainly rosetted, sometimes clump-forming, perennial succulents, the result of crosses between *Pachyphytum* and *Echeveria*. They have alternate, fleshy, light to mid- or grey-green leaves in very variable shapes, sometimes forming rosettes. Diurnal, bell- or star-shaped flowers are borne in one-sided cymes, in spring or summer. Where temperatures drop below 7°C (45°F), grow in a temperate greenhouse. In warmer areas, use in a desert garden.
• **HARDINESS** Frost tender.
• **CULTIVATION** Under glass, grow in standard cactus compost in full light, with shade from hot sun. From mid-spring to late summer, water moderately and apply a low-nitrogen liquid fertilizer every 6–8 weeks. Keep almost dry at other times. Outdoors, grow in moderately fertile, sharply drained soil in full sun, with some midday shade. See also pp.48–49.
• **PROPAGATION** Take leaf or stem-tip cuttings in spring or summer.
• **PESTS AND DISEASES** Susceptible to mealybugs, especially while flowering.

x *P. glauca* ■ syn. *Echeveria* x *fruticosa*. Rosetted, offsetting succulent with semi-cylindrical, red-tipped, blue-green, white-frosted leaves, to 6cm (2½in) long, with darker markings. Pendent, star-shaped yellow flowers, 1.5cm (½in) long, with recurving red tips, open in terminal, one-sided cymes in spring. ↕ 30cm (12in), ↔ indefinite. ❁ (min. 7°C/45°F)

▷ **Pacific grindelia** see *Grindelia stricta*

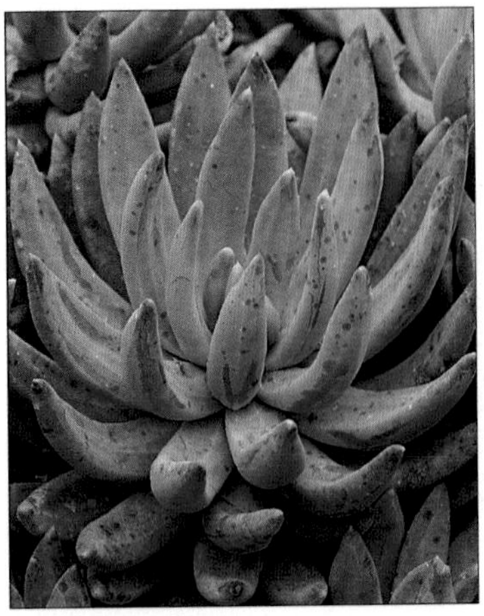
x *Pachyveria glauca*

PAEONIA

Peony

PAEONIACEAE

Genus of 30 or more species of clump-forming herbaceous perennials and deciduous, sometimes suckering shrubs or subshrubs ("tree peonies") found in meadows, scrub, and rocky places from Europe to E. Asia, and in W. North America. They are grown for their large, brightly coloured, sometimes fragrant, showy flowers and bold, dissected leaves. Some bear pod-like fruits, each with 2–5 lobes and large, red or black seeds. Herbaceous peonies, with tuberous rootstocks, comprise the majority of species and cultivars; most cultivars are derived from *P. lactiflora.* Tree peonies have woody stems, often with lax branches.

Peonies have mid- to dark green, sometimes silver-, bluish, or grey-green leaves; these are 2-ternate or occasionally pinnate, with few to many, usually oval to obovate, sometimes linear, entire or lobed leaflets, occasionally softly hairy, especially on the veins beneath.

Peony flowers are usually erect and solitary, or sometimes borne several to a stem. They are saucer-, cup-, or bowl-shaped, sometimes spherical when first open, and each single flower has 5 green sepals and 5–10 brightly coloured petals. Most have a crowded central boss of usually cream or yellow stamens; those with double flowers have either no stamens or a few hidden among the petals. The flowers can be divided into 4 major groups: single, semi-double, double, and anemone-form (see panel). In the descriptions below, flower sizes of herbaceous cultivars are defined as: "small", 5–10cm (2–4in) across; "medium-sized", 10–15cm (4–6in) across; "large", 15–20cm (6–8in) across; or "very large", over 20cm (8in) across. Tree peonies have single to double flowers, 5–30cm (2–12in) across.

Peonies are long-lived plants but they often resent disturbance. Most flower in early summer (only exceptions to this are indicated in the descriptions below). They are ideal for a mixed, herbaceous, or shrub border. If ingested, all parts can cause mild stomach upset.

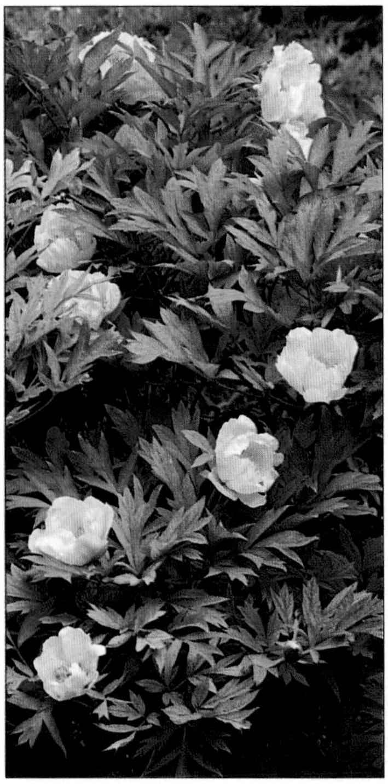

Paeonia 'Argosy'

• **HARDINESS** Fully hardy to frost hardy; young foliage and flower buds may be damaged by late spring frosts.

• **CULTIVATION** Grow in deep, fertile, humus-rich, moist but well-drained soil in full sun or partial shade. Shelter tree peonies from cold, drying winds. Large-flowered cultivars may need support. Pruning group 1 for tree peonies.

• **PROPAGATION** Sow seed in containers outdoors in autumn or early winter (may take 2 or 3 years to germinate). Divide herbaceous peonies in autumn or early spring, or take root cuttings in winter. Take semi-ripe cuttings of tree peonies in summer, or graft in winter.

• **PESTS AND DISEASES** Susceptible to viruses, eelworms, and swift moth larvae. Honey fungus may cause rapid death. Peony grey mould blight (peony wilt) may destroy shoots and buds.

***P.* 'Albert Crousse'.** Herbaceous perennial with deep green leaves and large, double, frilly, rose-pink flowers, flecked with carmine-red in the centres; the outer petals are spreading, the inner ones crowded and ruffled. ‡↔ 85–90cm (34–36in). ❄❄❄

P. albiflora see *P. lactiflora.*

***P.* 'Alice Harding'.** Herbaceous perennial with mid-green leaves and large, double, fragrant, creamy white, amber-tinted flowers with slightly frilled petals, the inner ones incurved. ‡↔ 80–100cm (32–39in). ❄❄❄

***P.* 'America'.** Herbaceous perennial with mid-green leaves and large, single, bowl-shaped, deep crimson flowers, with broad, slightly frilled petals. ‡↔ 0.9–1.1m (3–3½ft). ❄❄❄

P. anomala. Herbaceous perennial with dark green leaves, grey-green beneath, each with 9 narrow-oblong, pinnatifid leaflets, with bristly veins above. Bears single, cup-shaped, bright reddish purple flowers, 7–10cm (3–4in) across, with rounded, wavy petals and golden yellow stamens. ‡↔ 50–60cm (20–24in). Kyrgyzstan, China (E. Tien Shan Mountains). ❄❄❄

***P.* 'Argosy'** ■ syn. *P.* x *lemoinei* 'Argosy'. Compact, deciduous shrub (tree peony) with mid-green leaves deeply divided into pointed lobes. Bears single, cup-shaped, lemon-yellow flowers, marked crimson-purple at the bases, 18cm (7in) across. Difficult to propagate. ‡↔ 2m (6ft). ❄❄❄

P. arietina see *P. mascula* subsp. *arietina.*

***P.* 'Artemis'.** Upright, sparsely branched, deciduous shrub (tree peony) with red-tinged shoots and dark green, red-stalked leaves, blue-green beneath, deeply cut into pointed lobes. Single, cup-shaped, silky yellow flowers, 15cm (6in) across, are borne in late spring. ‡ 2m (6ft), ↔ 1.5m (5ft). ❄❄❄

***P.* 'Auguste Dessert'** ■ Herbaceous perennial with deep green leaves, turning crimson in autumn, and large, semi-double to double, carmine-red flowers, flushed salmon-pink, the silver margins slightly ruffled and uneven. ‡↔ 70–80cm (28–32in). ❄❄❄

***P.* 'Avant Garde'** ■ Herbaceous perennial with abundant mid-green leaves and large, single, bowl-shaped, rose-pink, darker-veined flowers, with yellow stamens. Good for cutting. ‡↔ 90–100cm (36–39in). ❄❄❄

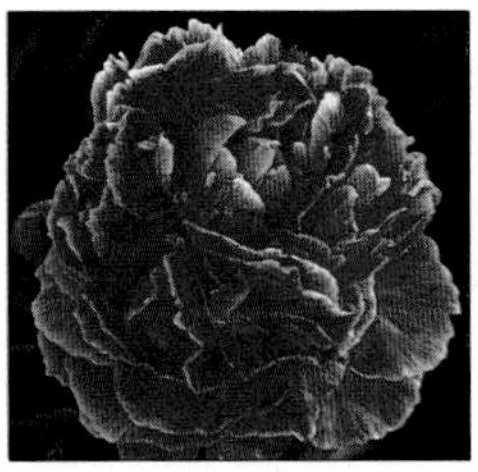

Paeonia 'Auguste Dessert'

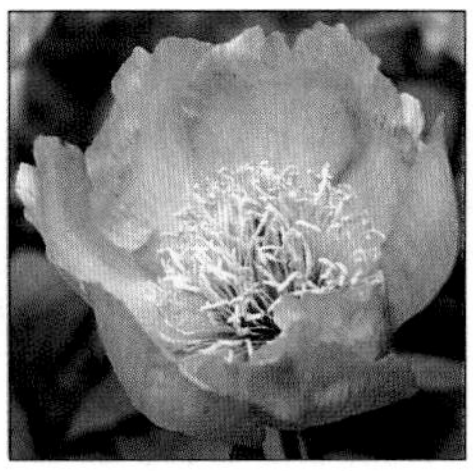

Paeonia 'Avant Garde'

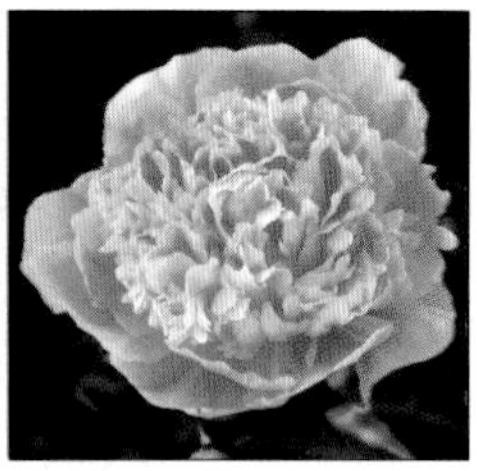

Paeonia 'Ballerina'

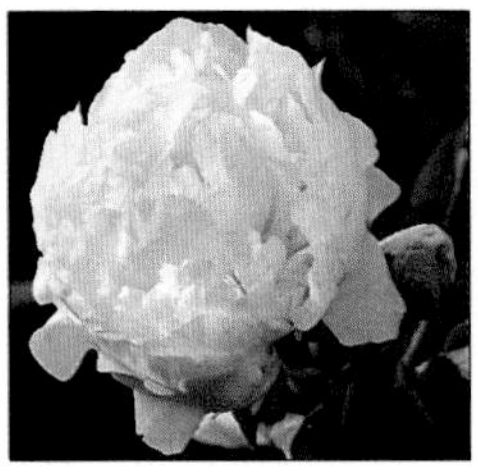

Paeonia 'Baroness Schröder'

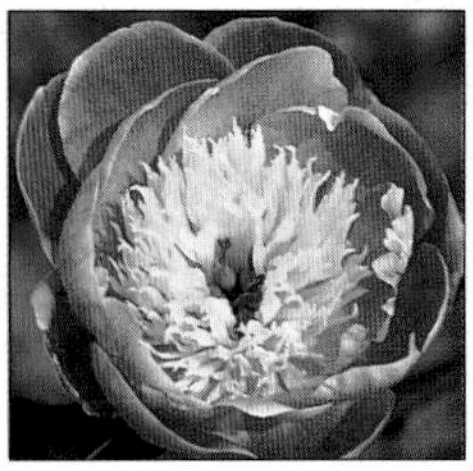

Paeonia 'Bowl of Beauty'

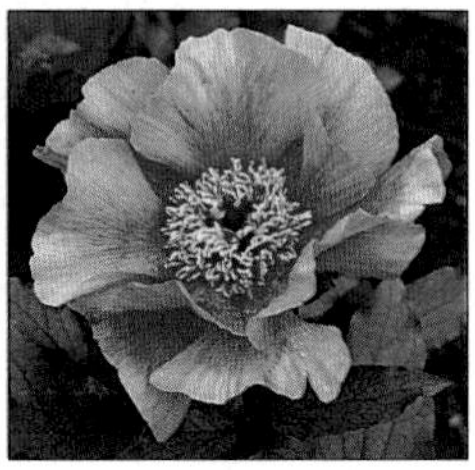

Paeonia cambessedesii

***P.* 'Ballerina'** ■ Herbaceous perennial with deep green leaves, turning red in autumn, and large, double, pink, lilac-flushed flowers, fading almost to white; the outer petals are broad and incurved, the inner ones narrower, curved, and ruffled at the tips. ‡↔ 90–100cm (36–39in). ❄❄❄

***P.* 'Baroness Schröder'** ■ Free-flowering herbaceous perennial with deep green leaves, and large, double, pale pink flowers that fade to white; the outer petals are broad and spreading, the inner ones crowded and incurved, with ruffled margins. ‡↔ 90–100cm (36–39in). ❄❄❄

***P.* 'Barrymore'.** Herbaceous perennial with mid-green leaves and large, anemone-form flowers with pale pink outer petals, fading to pure white as the buds open, and golden yellow petaloids. ‡↔ 80–90cm (32–36cm). ❄❄❄

***P.* 'Bowl of Beauty'** ■ 🏆 Herbaceous perennial with mid-green leaves. Produces very large, anemone-form, carmine-red, pink-tinted flowers with dense, creamy white centres consisting of many crowded, narrow petaloids. ‡↔ 80–100cm (32–39in). ❄❄❄

P. broteroi. Herbaceous perennial with semi-glossy, mid-green leaves, glaucous beneath, each with 9 leaflets, the lower leaves cut into 2 or 3 narrow, pointed lobes, the upper leaves unlobed. In late spring and early summer, bears single, cup-shaped, pink flowers, 10–13cm (4–5in) across, with oval petals and yellow stamens. ‡↔ 40–50cm (16–20in). Portugal, W. and S. Spain. ❄❄

***P.* 'Bunker Hill'.** Herbaceous perennial with deep green leaves and large, double, bright red flowers with ruffled petals. ‡↔ 70–75cm (28–30in). ❄❄❄

P. cambessedesii ■ 🏆 (Majorcan peony). Herbaceous perennial, usually flushed overall with red or purple, especially when young. Purple-veined leaves, dark green above, reddish purple beneath, are each divided into 9 pointed, lance-shaped, elliptic, or ovate leaflets. Produces single, bowl-shaped, deep pink flowers, 6–10cm (2½–4in) across, with wavy-margined petals and yellow stamens with red filaments, in mid- and late spring. ‡↔ 45–55cm (18–22in). Balearic Islands (Majorca). ❄❄

***P.* 'Captivation'.** Herbaceous perennial with deep green leaves. Produces very

PEONY FLOWER FORMS

Peony flowers may be saucer-, cup-, or bowl-shaped, in one of the following forms: **single** – with a whorl of 5–10 broad, overlapping, often slightly incurved petals, and a large, central boss of stamens; **semi-double** – like single peonies, but with 2 or 3 whorls of similar petals; **double** – large, spherical flowers, with narrower, overlapping, often crowded, ruffled petals filling the centres, and stamens inconspicuous or absent; or **anemone-form** (also known as imperial or Japanese) – single or semi-double flowers, with the stamens replaced by narrow, crowded, petal-like structures, known as petaloids (or staminodes).

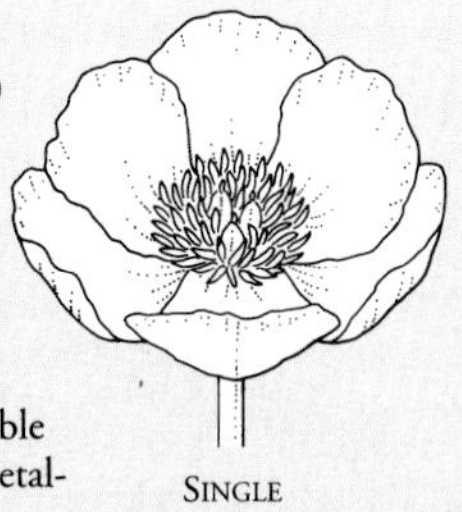

SINGLE

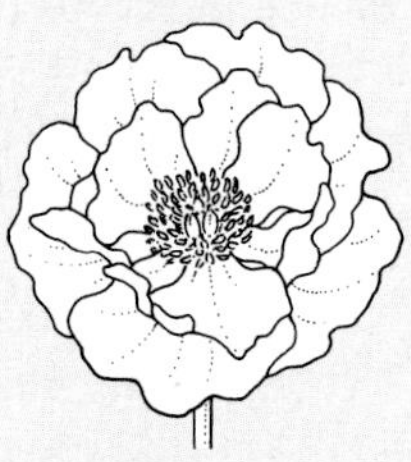

SEMI-DOUBLE

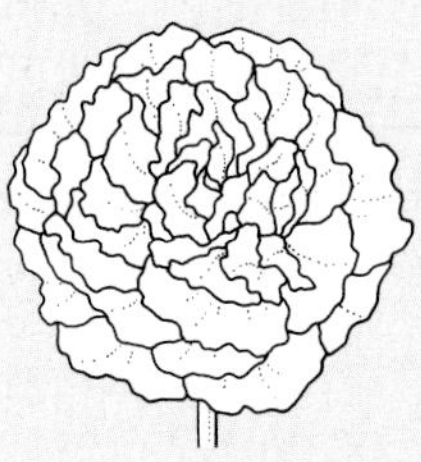

DOUBLE

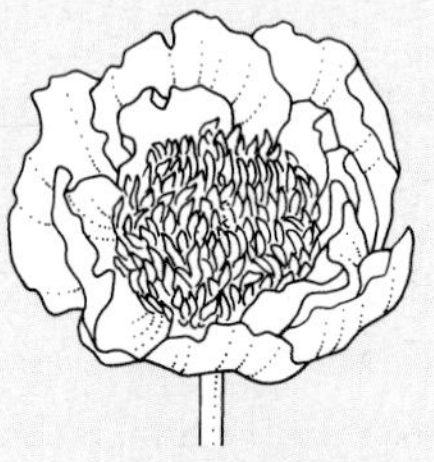

ANEMONE-FORM

P

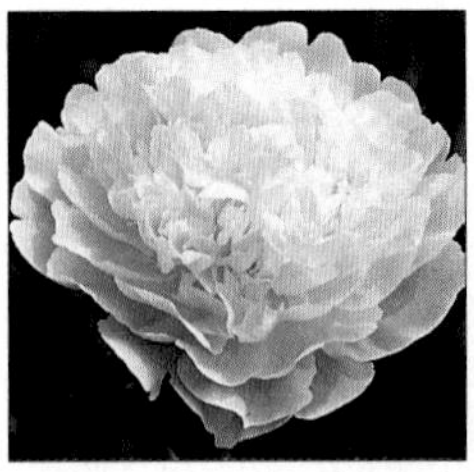
Paeonia 'Cornelia Shaylor'

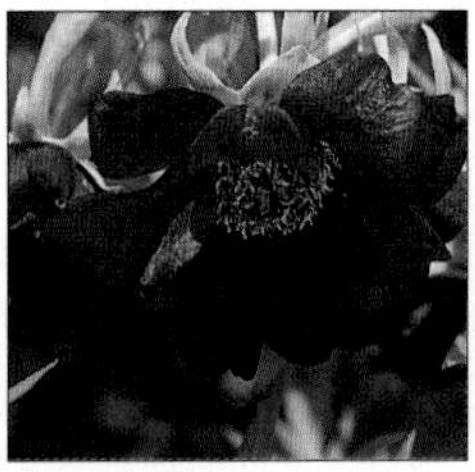
Paeonia delavayi

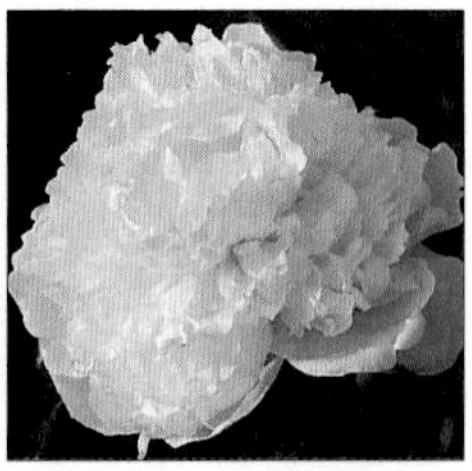
Paeonia 'Duchesse de Nemours'

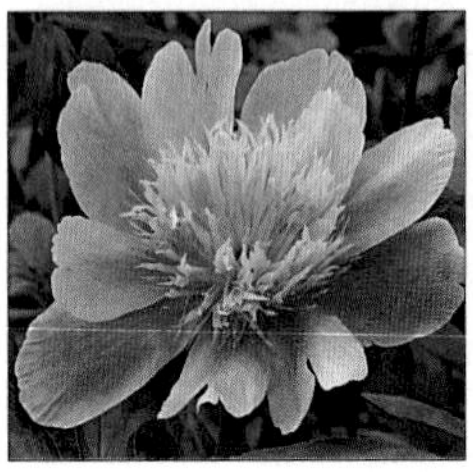
Paeonia 'Evening World'

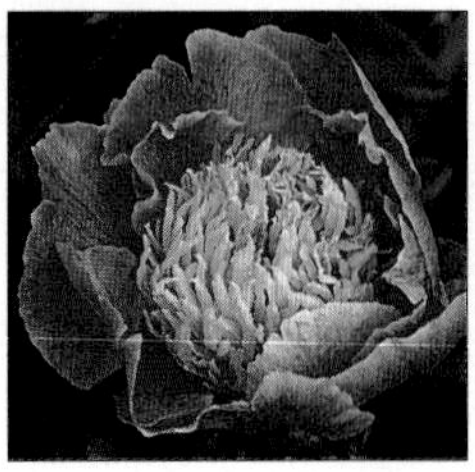
Paeonia 'Globe of Light'

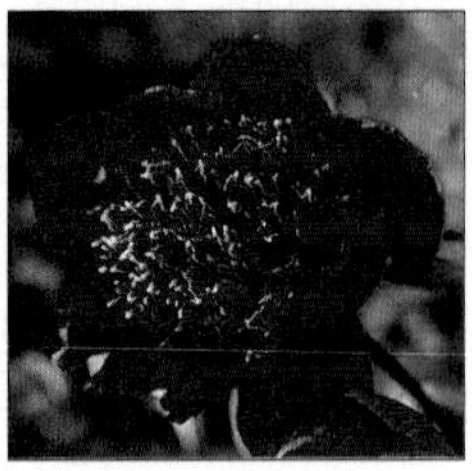
Paeonia 'Instituteur Doriat'

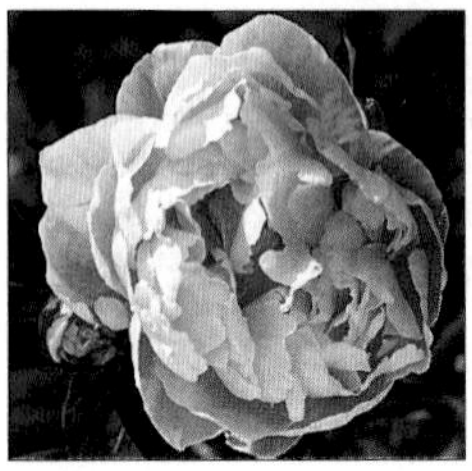
Paeonia 'Kelway's Supreme'

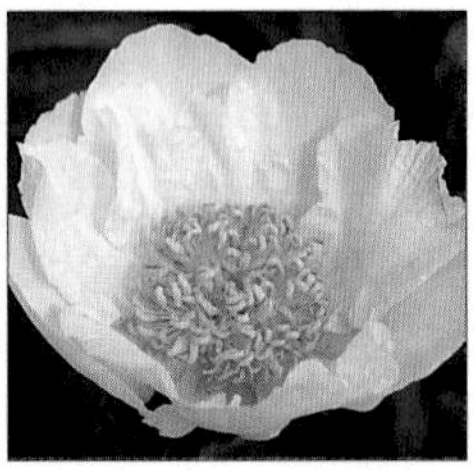
Paeonia 'Krinkled White'

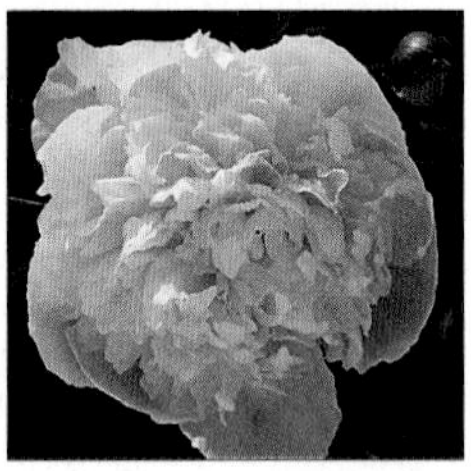
Paeonia 'Laura Dessert'

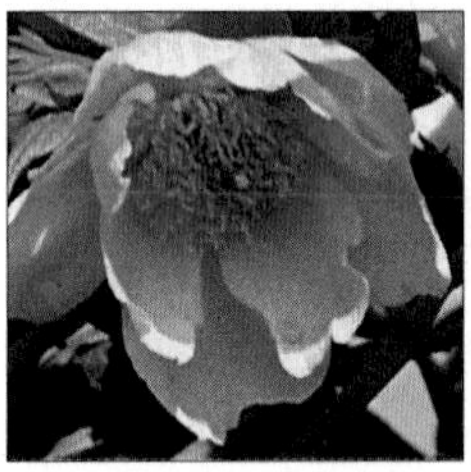
Paeonia lutea var. *ludlowii*

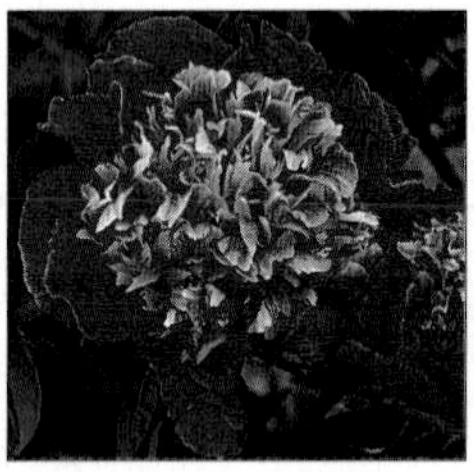
Paeonia 'Magic Orb'

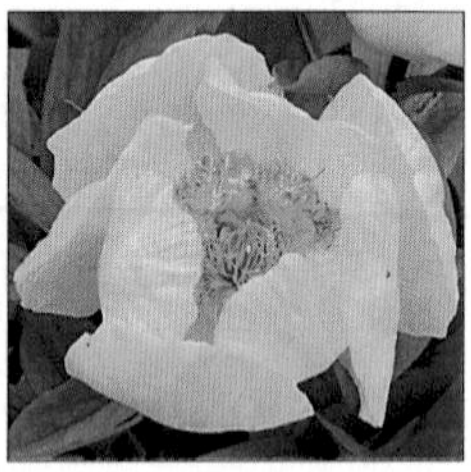
Paeonia mlokosewitschii

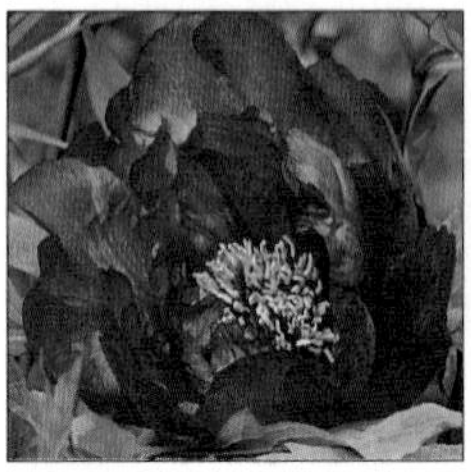
Paeonia 'Mme Louis Henri'

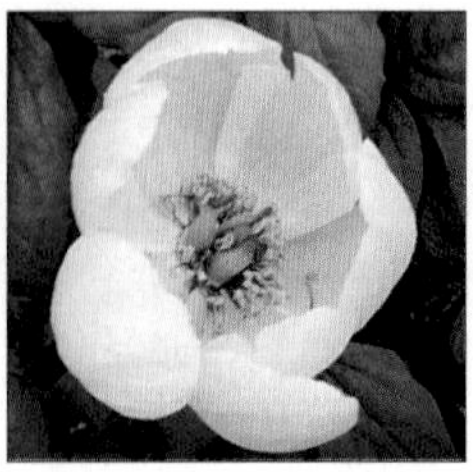
Paeonia obovata var. *alba*

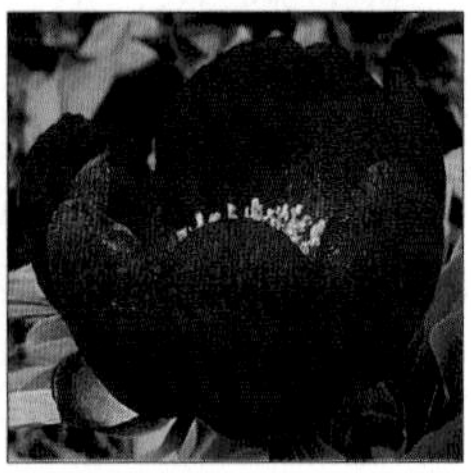
Paeonia officinalis 'Crimson Globe'

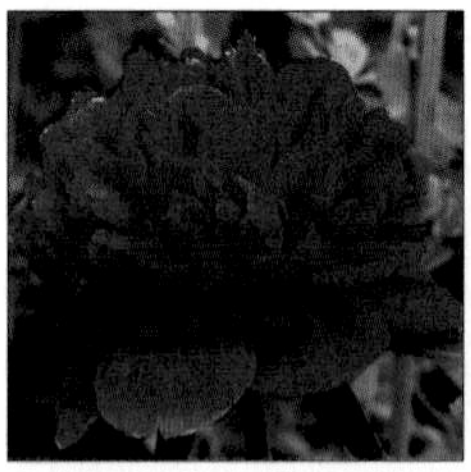
Paeonia officinalis 'Rubra Plena'

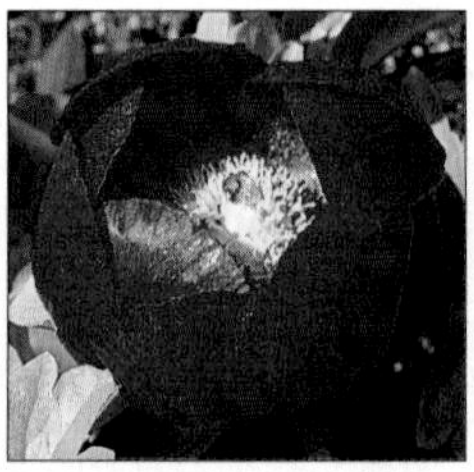
Paeonia peregrina

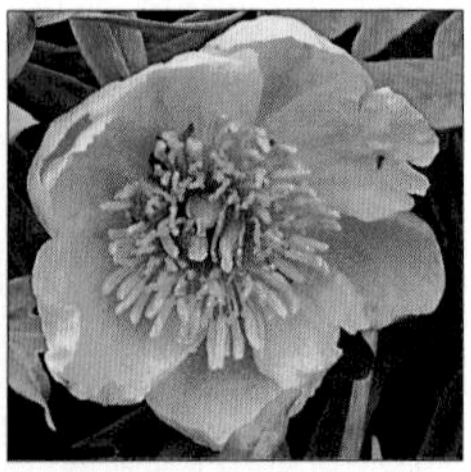
Paeonia potaninii var. *trollioides*

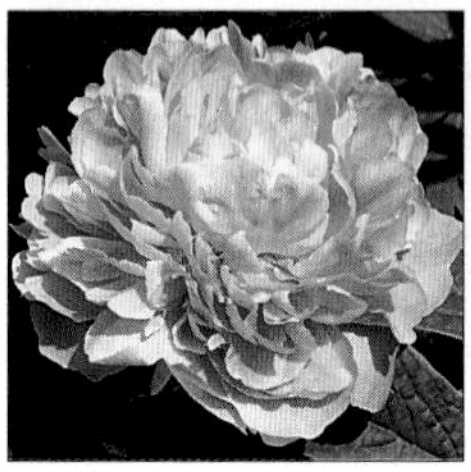
Paeonia 'Sarah Bernhardt'

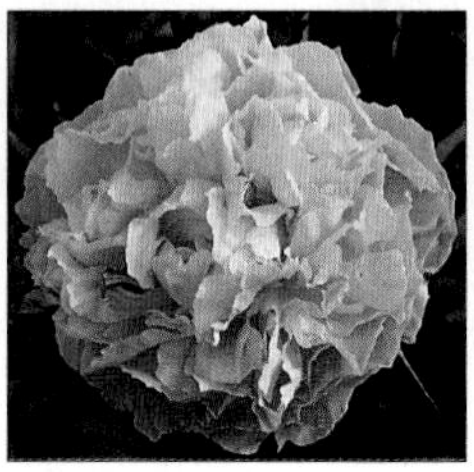
Paeonia 'Shirley Temple'

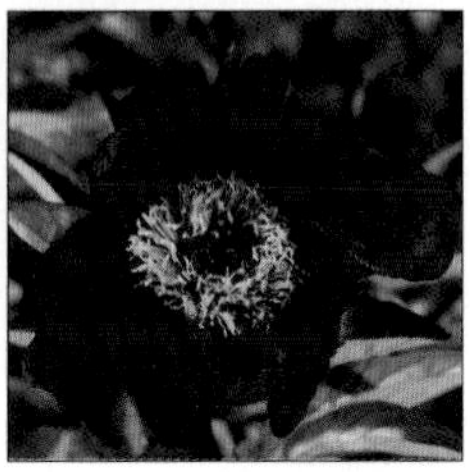
Paeonia 'Sir Edward Elgar'

large, single, bowl-shaped, cherry-red flowers with a silver sheen. ‡↔ 0.9–1.1m (3–3½ft). ❄❄❄

***P.* 'Carnival'.** Herbaceous perennial with deep green leaves. Produces large, double, carmine-red flowers, each with a central mass of dissected, ruffled, cream and rose-pink petals. ‡↔ 80–90cm (32–36in). ❄❄❄

***P.* 'Cheddar Cheese'.** Herbaceous perennial with mid-green leaves. Bears large, double flowers with incurving, ivory-white inner petals and shorter, slightly ruffled yellow outer petals. ‡↔ 90–100cm (36–39in). ❄❄❄

***P.* 'Chocolate Soldier'.** Herbaceous perennial with deep green leaves, flushed bronze when young. Bears large, satiny, deeply cupped, semi-double, deep purple-red flowers with golden stamens. ‡↔ 90–100cm (36–39in). ❄❄❄

P. corallina see *P. mascula*.

***P.* 'Cornelia Shaylor'** ■ Herbaceous perennial with deep green foliage. Bears large, fragrant, double flowers, opening rose-pink but soon fading to bluish white, with dense, ruffled central petals. ‡↔ 80–90cm (32–36in). ❄❄❄

***P.* 'Dayspring'.** Herbaceous perennial with mid-green leaves and medium-sized, single, cup-shaped, fragrant, pale pink flowers, borne several to a stem. ‡↔ 60–70cm (24–28in). ❄❄❄

P. decora see *P. peregrina*.

***P.* 'Defender'** 🏆 Herbaceous perennial with glossy, deep green leaves and medium-sized, single, cup-shaped, deep crimson flowers, with golden yellow stamens. ‡↔ 90–100cm (36–39in). ❄❄❄

P. delavayi ■ 🏆 Upright, sparsely branched, deciduous shrub (tree peony) with 2-pinnate, dark green leaves, blue-green beneath, the leaflets deeply cut into pointed lobes. Bears horizontal to nodding, single, cup-shaped, rich dark red flowers, 10cm (4in) across. ‡ 2m (6ft), ↔ 1.2m (4ft). China. ❄❄❄. **var. *ludlowii*** see *P. lutea* var. *ludlowii*.

***P.* 'Double Cherry'** see *P. suffruticosa* 'Yae-zakura'.

***P.* 'Dresden'.** Vigorous herbaceous perennial with stout stems and deep green leaves that turn red in autumn. Produces large, single, bowl-shaped, ivory-white flowers, flushed rose-pink. ‡↔ 80–85cm (32–34in). ❄❄❄

***P.* 'Duchesse de Nemours'** ■ 🏆 syn. *P.* 'Mrs. Gwyn Lewis'. Robust herbaceous perennial with deep green leaves. Bears large, fragrant, double, pure white flowers, flushed green in bud, with spreading outer petals and dense, unevenly ruffled, yellow-based inner petals. ‡↔ 70–80cm (28–32in). ❄❄❄

P. emodi ■ (Himalayan peony). Herbaceous perennial with erect to arching stems and dark green leaves, each divided into 9 narrow, sometimes 2- or 3-lobed, elliptic leaflets. Semi-pendent, single, cup-shaped, pure white flowers, 10–17cm (4–7in) across, with golden yellow stamens, are borne several to a stem in late spring. ‡↔ 60–80cm (24–32in). W. Himalayas. ❄❄❄

***P.* 'Emperor of India'.** Herbaceous perennial with deep green foliage and large, anemone-form, rich dark red flowers with golden yellow petaloids. ‡↔ 85–90cm (34–36in). ❄❄❄

***P.* 'Evening World'** ■ Herbaceous perennial with mid-green leaves. Bears large, anemone-form flowers with spreading, soft pink outer petals and narrow, paler flesh-pink petaloids. ‡↔ 90–100cm (36–39in). ❄❄❄

***P.* 'Félix Crousse'** 🏆 syn. *P.* 'Victor Hugo'. Herbaceous perennial with deep green leaves and large, fragrant, double, deep crimson-pink flowers, with darker centres and ruffled, silver-margined petals. ‡↔ 70–75cm (28–30in). ❄❄❄

***P.* 'Festiva Maxima'** 🏆 Herbaceous perennial with strong, erect stems and abundant mid-green foliage. Bears very large, fragrant, double white flowers, with loosely arranged, irregularly margined petals, the inner petals with crimson marks at their bases. ‡↔ 90–100cm (36–39in). ❄❄❄

***P.* 'Flamingo'.** Herbaceous perennial with deep green leaves, turning red in autumn. Bears large, double, clear salmon-pink flowers. ‡↔ 75–85cm (30–34in). ❄❄❄

***P.* 'Flight of Cranes'** see *P. suffruticosa* 'Renkaku'.

***P.* 'Floral Rivalry'** see *P. suffruticosa* 'Hana-kisoi'.

***P.* 'Gay Ladye'.** Herbaceous perennial with deep green leaves. Bears medium-sized, single, cup-shaped, vivid deep rose-red flowers with wide-spreading petals. ‡↔ 80–90cm (32–36in). ❄❄❄

***P.* 'Globe of Light'** ■ Herbaceous perennial with mid-green leaves. Bears large, fragrant, anemone-form, rose-pink flowers with golden yellow petaloids. ‡↔ 90–100cm (36–39in). ❄❄❄

P. humilis, syn. *P. officinalis* subsp. *humilis*, *P. officinalis* subsp. *microcarpa*. Herbaceous perennial with hairy stems and leaf-stalks, and mid-green leaves, pale green and densely hairy beneath, each with 9 leaflets deeply cut into narrowly elliptic to oblong lobes. Bears single, bowl- or cup-shaped, purple-red flowers, 10–13cm (4–5in) across, with yellow stamens. ‡↔ 70–80cm (28–32in). S.W. Europe. ❄❄❄

***P.* 'Instituteur Doriat'** ■ Herbaceous perennial with deep green foliage, turning red in autumn. Produces large, anemone-form, velvety, crimson-red flowers with broad, ruffled, silver-margined pink petaloids. ‡↔ 90–100cm (36–39in). ❄❄❄

***P. japonica* of gardens** see *P. lactiflora*.

***P.* 'Kamada Brocade'** see *P. suffruticosa* 'Kamada-nishiki'.

***P.* 'Karl Rosenfield'.** Herbaceous perennial with hairy stems and leaf-stalks, and mid-green leaves with leaflets deeply cut into narrowly elliptic to oblong lobes. Bears large, double, bright deep red flowers, 10–13cm (4–5in) across. ‡↔ 70–80cm (28–32in). ❄❄❄

***P.* 'Kelway's Majestic'.** Herbaceous perennial with deep green leaves. Bears large, anemone-form, fragrant, bright crimson-pink flowers, with slightly ruffled, silver- or gold-flecked, lilac-pink petaloids. ‡↔ 90–100cm (36–39cm). ❄❄❄

***P.* 'Kelway's Supreme'** ■ Robust herbaceous perennial with mid-green foliage. Bears large, fragrant, double or semi-double, pale pink flowers, fading to white, with broad, overlapping petals, often borne in clusters over a long period. ‡↔ 90–100cm (36–39in). ❄❄❄

***P.* 'Knighthood'.** Herbaceous perennial with deep green leaves. Produces large, double, intense wine-red flowers with narrow, crowded, slightly ruffled petals. ‡↔ 70–80cm (28–32in). ❄❄❄

P

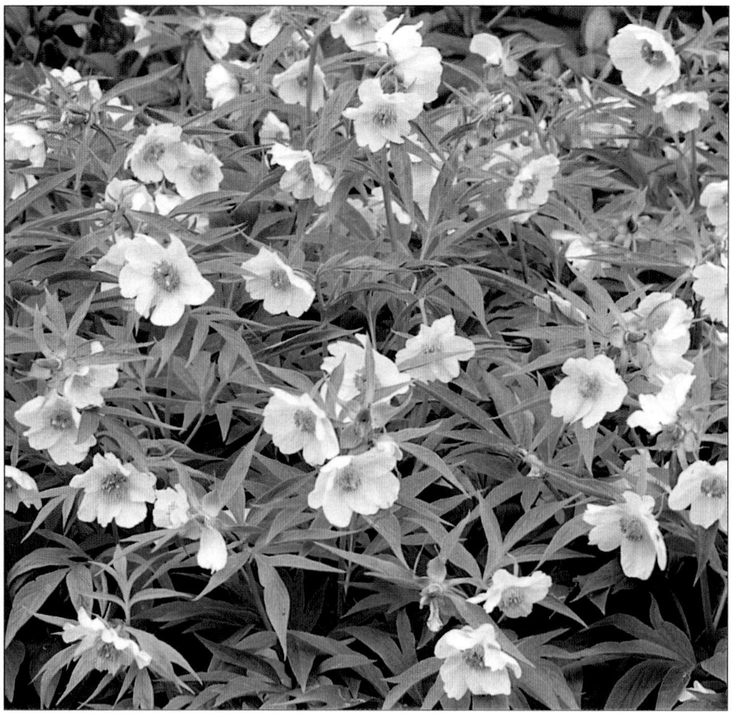

Paeonia emodi

***P.* 'Krinkled White'** ■ Herbaceous perennial with mid-green leaves and strong stems bearing large, single, cup-shaped white, occasionally pink-flushed flowers, with slightly ruffled petals and golden yellow stamens. ↕↔ 75–80cm (30–32in). ✻✻✻
***P.* 'Kronos'.** Upright, sparsely branched, deciduous shrub (tree peony) with red-tinged shoots and red-stalked, dark green leaves, blue-green beneath, deeply cut into pointed lobes. Semi-double, dark red, blue-tinged flowers, 15cm (6in) across, are borne in late spring. ↕ 2m (6ft), ↔ 1.5m (5ft). ✻✻✻
P. lactiflora, syn. *P. albiflora*, *P. japonica* of gardens. Herbaceous perennial with erect, red-mottled stems and dark green leaves, each with 9 elliptic or lance-shaped, rough-margined leaflets, paler and slightly hairy beneath. In early and midsummer, bears usually solitary, single, cup- or bowl-shaped, fragrant, white to pale pink flowers, 7–10cm (3–4in) across, with pale yellow stamens. ↕↔ 50–70cm (20–28in). Russia (E. Siberia), Mongolia, N. and W. China, Tibet. ✻✻✻
***P.* 'Laura Dessert'** ■ 🏆 Herbaceous perennial with pale to mid-green leaves. Bears large, fragrant, double flowers with spreading, pink-flushed, creamy white outer petals and pale canary-yellow, incurving inner petals. ↕↔ 70–75cm (28–30in). ✻✻✻
P.* x *lemoinei (*P. lutea* x *P. suffruticosa*). Upright to spreading, sparsely branched, deciduous shrub (tree peony) with dark green leaves, deeply divided into pointed lobes. Single to double, cup-shaped flowers, 15–20cm (6–8in) across, are white to yellow, often with orange, red, or pink marks. ↕↔ 1.5m (5ft). Garden origin. ✻✻✻. **'Argosy'** see *P.* 'Argosy'. **'L'Espérance'** see *P.* 'L'Espérance'. **'Mme Louis Henri'** see *P.* 'Mme Louis Henri'. **'Souvenir de Maxime Cornu'** see *P.* 'Souvenir de Maxime Cornu'.
***P.* 'L'Espérance'**, syn. *P.* x *lemoinei* 'L'Espérance'. Upright, deciduous shrub (tree peony) with mid-green leaves, each with several deep, pointed lobes. Bears single, cup-shaped, primrose-yellow flowers, 20cm (8in) across, carmine-red at the bases, with red filaments and golden yellow anthers. ↕ 2m (6ft), ↔ 1.5m (5ft). ✻✻✻
P. lobata see *P. peregrina*.
P. lutea. Upright, sparsely branched, deciduous shrub (tree peony) with dark green leaves, blue-green beneath, each with 9 leaflets, deeply cut into pointed lobes. Bears horizontal to nodding, single, cup-shaped, vivid yellow flowers, 6cm (2½in) across. ↕↔ 1.5m (5ft). S.W. China. ✻✻✻. **var. *ludlowii*** ■ 🏆 syn. *P. delavayi* var. *ludlowii*, is more widely grown and more vigorous than the species, with bright green foliage and larger flowers, to 12cm (5in) across, borne in late spring; ↕↔ 2.5m (8ft); S.E. Tibet. **'Superba'** has bronze young foliage, and pink-flushed yellow flowers with red filaments and orange anthers.
***P.* 'Magic Orb'** ■ Herbaceous perennial producing deep green leaves, turning red in autumn. Bears large, fragrant, double flowers with broad, vivid rose-pink outer petals and narrower, more ruffled, incurved, pink-suffused, creamy white inner petals. ↕↔ 90–100cm (36–39in). ✻✻✻
***P.* 'Magnificent Flower'** see *P. suffruticosa* 'Hana-daigin'.
P. mascula ■ syn. *P. corallina*. Erect herbaceous perennial with leaves divided into 9 broadly ovate, obovate, or elliptic leaflets, bluish green above, paler green beneath. Cup- to bowl-shaped flowers are single, deep purplish red, sometimes rose-pink, 7–13cm (3–5in) across, with deep yellow stamens. ↕↔ 60–100cm (24–39in). S. Europe. ✻✻✻. **subsp. *arietina***, syn. *P. arietina*, has narrower, often lobed leaflets, hairy beneath, and reddish pink flowers; ↕↔ 50–75cm (20–30in). E. Europe, Turkey. **subsp. *arietina* 'Northern Glory'** has grey-green leaves and deep pink-purple flowers; ↕↔ 60–70cm (24–28in).
P. mlokosewitschii ■ 🏆 (Caucasian peony). Erect herbaceous perennial with bluish green leaves, each divided into 9 broadly elliptic, ovate, or obovate, blunt, sometimes red-margined leaflets, paler and slightly hairy beneath. In late spring and early summer, bears single, bowl-shaped, lemon-yellow flowers, 10–12cm (4–5in) across, with broad, oval petals and pale yellow stamens. ↕↔ 65–90cm (26–36in). Caucasus. ✻✻✻
***P.* 'Mme Louis Henri'** ■ syn. *P.* x *lemoinei* 'Mme Louis Henri'. Upright, deciduous shrub (tree peony) with mid-green leaves divided into pointed lobes. Bears semi-double, warm orange-yellow flowers, to 17cm (7in) across, heavily flushed orange-red. ↕ 2m (6ft), ↔ 1.5m (5ft). ✻✻✻
***P.* 'Monsieur Jules Elie'** 🏆 Herbaceous perennial with deep green leaves and very large, rounded, double, deep rose-red flowers with a silver sheen. ↕↔ 90–100cm (36–39in). ✻✻✻
***P.* 'Mother of Pearl'.** Herbaceous perennial with attractive, pale bluish green, often red-margined leaves and large, single, cup-shaped, pink-flushed, pale yellow flowers. ↕↔ 70–75cm (28–30in). ✻✻✻
***P.* 'Mrs. Gwyn Lewis'** see *P.* 'Duchesse de Nemours'.
P. obovata 🏆 Herbaceous perennial with erect stems and large, deep green leaves, each with 9 uneven, broadly elliptic leaflets, pale grey-green and slightly hairy beneath. Bears single, cup-shaped, white to purplish red flowers, 7–10cm (3–4in) across, with yellow anthers and green-white or purple filaments. ↕↔ 60–70cm (24–28in). China. ✻✻✻. **var. *alba*** ■ produces white flowers with purple filaments; ↕↔ 70–90cm (28–36in).
P. officinalis (Common peony). Herbaceous perennial with erect stems, slightly hairy at first, and deep green leaves, each divided into 9 leaflets with elliptic to oblong lobes, paler and sometimes hairy beneath. Single, cup-shaped, shiny, deep red or rose-pink flowers, 10–13cm (4–5in) across, with yellow stamens, are borne in early and midsummer. ↕↔ 60–70cm (24–28in). Europe. ✻✻✻. **'Alba Plena'** has large, double white flowers, sometimes flushed pink, the slightly ruffled petals spreading to reveal the carpels at the centre of each flower; ↕↔ 70–75cm (28–30in). **'China Rose'** has dark green leaves and single, deeply cup-shaped, deep salmon-pink flowers with golden yellow stamens; ↕↔ 45–50cm (18–20in). **'Crimson Globe'** ■ produces single, garnet-red flowers with golden yellow stamens; ↕↔ 70–85cm (28–34in). **subsp. *humilis*** see *P. humilis*. **'James Crawford Weguelin'** has bowl-shaped, garnet-red flowers with yellow stamens. **subsp. *microcarpa*** see *P. humilis*. **'Rosea Superba Plena'** has large, double, deep rose-pink flowers with slightly ruffled petals. **'Rubra Plena'** ■ 🏆 has leaves with deep green leaflets, divided into broad, oval segments, and large, double, vivid crimson flowers with satiny, ruffled petals; ↕↔ 70–75cm (28–30in).

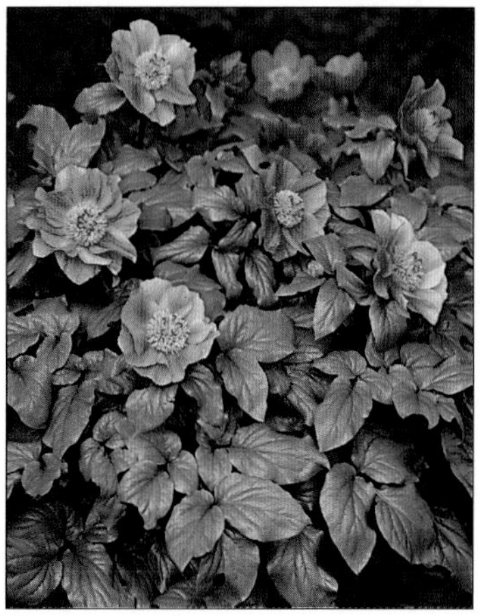

Paeonia mascula

P. peregrina ■ syn. *P. decora*, *P. lobata*. Herbaceous perennial with erect stems and stiff, lustrous, deep green leaves, each with 9 notched or deeply lobed leaflets, bristly on the veins above, usually hairless beneath. Single, bowl-shaped, glistening, deep red flowers, 10–13cm (4–5in) across, with yellow stamens, are borne in late spring and early summer. ↕↔ 50–60cm (20–24in). S. Europe. ✻✻✻. **'Otto Froebel'** 🏆 syn. 'Sunshine', produces deep vermilion flowers with deep yellow stamens. **'Sunshine'** see 'Otto Froebel'.
P. potaninii. Low-growing, deciduous subshrub (tree peony), spreading by suckers, bearing 2-pinnate, dark green leaves with slender lobes. Produces nodding, single, cup- or bowl-shaped, deep maroon-red flowers, 5cm (2in) across, with red filaments. ↕ 60cm (24in), ↔ 1.5m (5ft) or more. W. China. ✻✻✻. **f. *alba*** has white flowers with green filaments. **var. *trollioides*** ■ produces deeply cup-shaped yellow flowers in late spring.
***P.* 'Président Poincaré'.** Herbaceous perennial with deep green leaves, turning red in autumn. Bears large, fragrant, double, deep crimson flowers with ruffled petals in the centres. ↕↔ 90–100cm (36–39in). ✻✻✻
P. rockii see *P. suffruticosa* subsp. *rockii*.
***P.* 'Sarah Bernhardt'** ■ 🏆 Robust herbaceous perennial with erect stems, mid-green leaves, and very large, double, fragrant, rose-pink flowers, the inner petals with ruffled and silvered margins. ↕↔ 90–100cm (36–39in). ✻✻✻
***P.* 'Savage Splendour'.** Upright, sparsely branched, deciduous shrub (tree peony) with mid-green leaves, bluish green beneath, deeply cut into pointed lobes. In late spring or early summer, bears large, solitary, single, cup-shaped white flowers, flushed rose- or lavender-pink. ↕ 2m (6ft), ↔ 1.5m (5ft). ✻✻✻
***P.* 'Shirley Temple'** ■ Herbaceous perennial with deep green leaves. Bears large, double, rose-pink flowers, fading to buff-white, with whorled petals, the innermost paler, narrower, and loosely arranged. ↕↔ 80–85cm (32–34in). ✻✻✻
***P.* 'Silver Flare'.** Herbaceous perennial with deep green leaves and large, single, deeply cup-shaped, fragrant, carmine-red flowers, with silver-margined petals and golden yellow stamens. ↕↔ 90–100cm (36–39in). ✻✻✻
***P.* 'Sir Edward Elgar'** ■ Herbaceous perennial with glossy, dark green leaves, turning red in autumn. Bears abundant large, single, cup-shaped, dark brownish crimson flowers with lemon-yellow stamens. ↕↔ 70–80cm (28–32in). ✻✻✻
P.* x *smouthii (*P. lactiflora* x *P. tenuifolia*). Erect herbaceous perennial with bright green leaves, each divided into 9 leaflets with many, very narrow

P

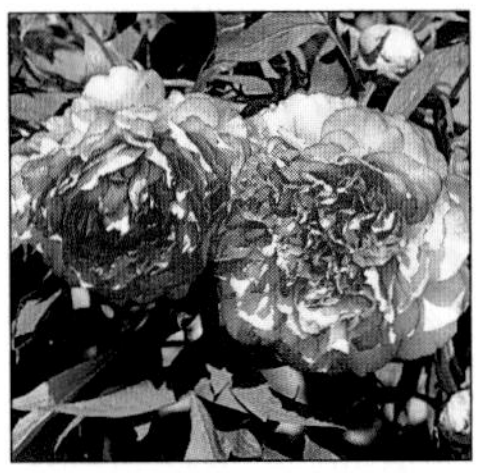
Paeonia 'Souvenir de Maxime Cornu'

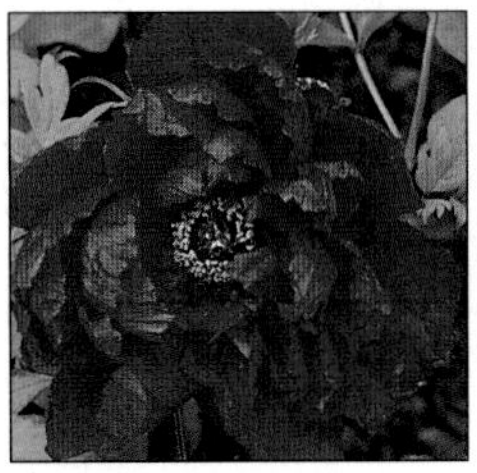
Paeonia suffruticosa 'Cardinal Vaughan'

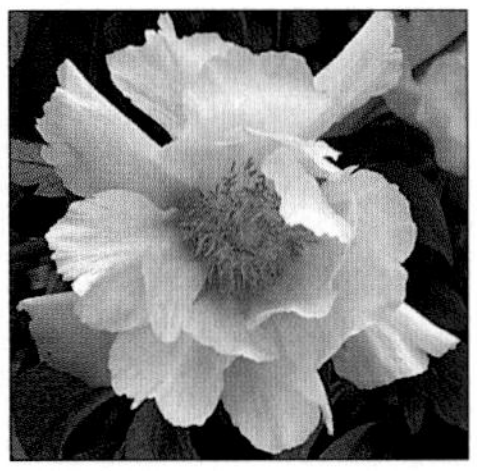
Paeonia suffruticosa 'Godaishu'

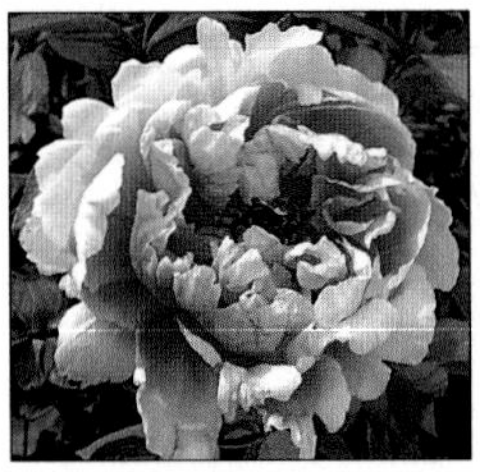
Paeonia suffruticosa 'Reine Elisabeth'

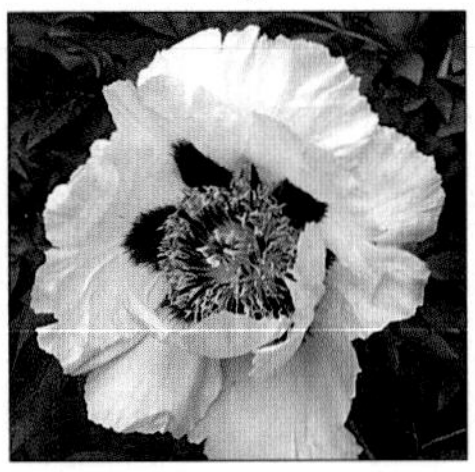
Paeonia suffruticosa subsp. *rockii*

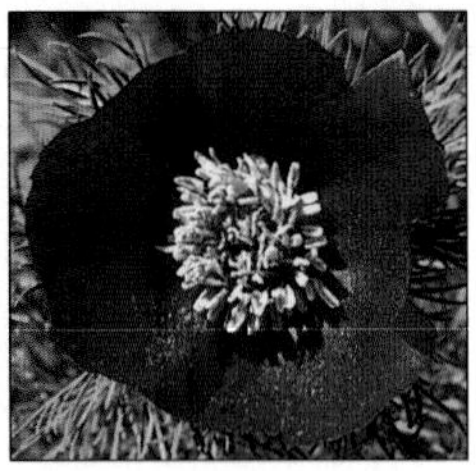
Paeonia tenuifolia

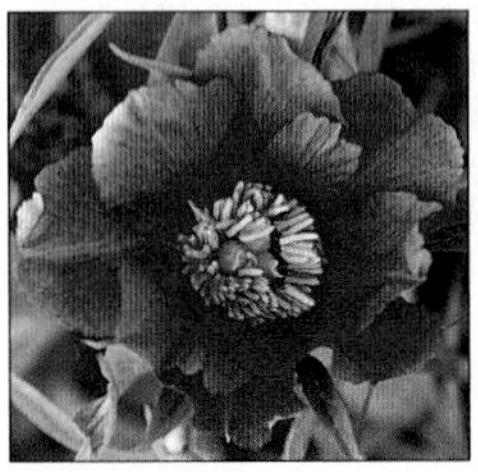
Paeonia veitchii

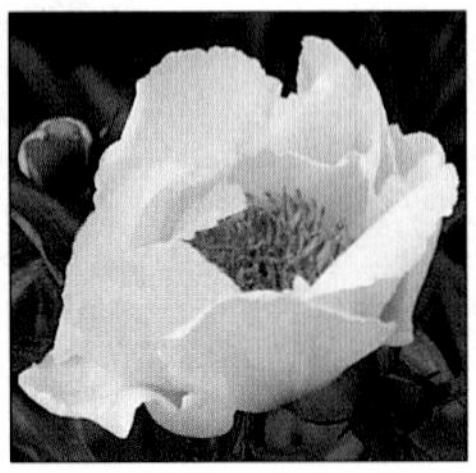
Paeonia 'White Wings'

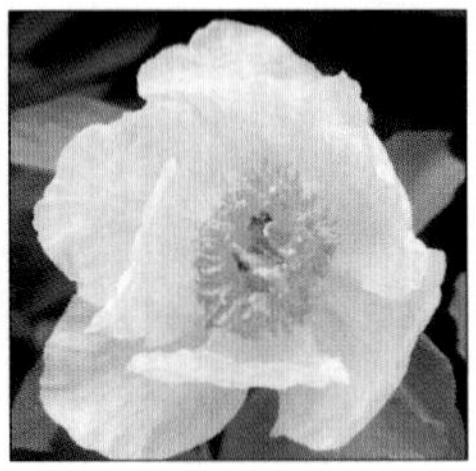
Paeonia wittmanniana

segments. In late spring, bears single, cup-shaped, fragrant, bright red flowers, 7–10cm (3–4in) across, with yellow stamens. A sterile hybrid. ↕↔ 60–80cm (24–32in). Garden origin. ✻✻✻
***P.* 'Souvenir de Maxime Cornu'** ▣ syn. *P.* x *lemoinei* 'Souvenir de Maxime Cornu'. Upright, deciduous shrub (tree peony) with mid-green leaves divided into pointed lobes. Bears double, very fragrant, golden yellow flowers, 20cm (8in) across, the ruffled petal margins strongly suffused dull reddish orange. ↕ 2m (6ft), ↔ 1.5m (5ft). ✻✻✻
P. suffruticosa (Moutan). Upright, sparsely branched, deciduous shrub (tree peony) with dark green leaves, blue-green beneath, each with 9 elliptic or ovate leaflets, deeply cut into pointed lobes. In late spring and early summer, bears single, cup- to bowl-shaped, sometimes scented, white, pink, red, or purple flowers, 15–30cm (6–12in) across, some with maroon marks at the bases. ↕↔ to 2.2m (7ft). China. ✻✻✻. **'Banksii'** has double, purple-red flowers with white tips. **'Cardinal Vaughan'** ▣ has semi-double, ruby-purple flowers. **'Five Continents'** see 'Godaishu'. **'Godaishu'** ▣ syn. 'Five Continents', has semi-double white flowers. **'Hana-daigin'**, syn. *P.* 'Magnificent Flower', has double, violet-purple flowers. **'Hana-kisoi'**, syn. *P.* 'Floral Rivalry', has semi-double, shell-pink flowers. **'Joseph Rock'** see subsp. *rockii*. **'Kamada-nishiki'**, syn. *P.* 'Kamada Brocade', has double, reddish mauve flowers. **'Mrs. William Kelway'** produces double white flowers. **'Reine Elisabeth'** ▣ has semi-double to double, salmon-pink flowers tinged red, with ruffled margins. **'Renkaku'**, syn. *P.* 'Flight of Cranes', has dense, double white flowers with deep yellow stamens. **subsp. *rockii*** ▣ syn. 'Joseph Rock', 'Rock's Variety', *P. rockii*, has semi-double white flowers, marked deep maroon at the bases. **'Rock's Variety'** see subsp. *rockii*. **'Yae-zakura'**, syn. *P.* 'Double Cherry', has double, soft pink flowers.
P. tenuifolia ▣ Herbaceous perennial with deep green leaves, pale and grey-green beneath, with many pointed, linear segments. In late spring and early summer, bears single, cup-shaped, deep red flowers, 7–9cm (3–3½in) across, with yellow stamens. ↕↔ 50–70cm (20–28in). S.E. Europe to S. Russia. ✻✻✻. **'Plena'** has long-lasting, double, rich red flowers.
P. veitchii ▣ Herbaceous perennial with hairless stems and deep green leaves, each divided into 9 lance-shaped, pointed leaflets, hairy along the veins above, pale grey-green and hairless beneath. Usually solitary, semi-pendent, single, cup-shaped, white or pink to pale magenta-pink flowers, 7–9cm (3–3½in) across, with pale lemon stamens, open widely in late spring and early summer. ↕↔ 50–60cm (20–24in). W. China. ✻✻✻. **f. *alba*** has white flowers with yellow stamens; ↕↔ 70–75cm (28–30in). **var. *woodwardii*** is shorter, with hairy stems and leaves hairy beneath, and bears rose-pink flowers; ↕↔ 30–40cm (12–16in).
***P.* 'Victor Hugo'** see *P.* 'Félix Crousse'.
***P.* 'White Wings'** ▣ Herbaceous perennial with glossy, deep green leaves, red in autumn. Large, single, deeply cup-shaped, fragrant, yellowish white flowers have broad, slightly ruffled petals. ↕↔ 75–85cm (30–34in). ✻✻✻
***P.* 'Whitleyi Major'** 🏆 Herbaceous perennial with deep green leaves flushed reddish brown. Bears large, single, cup-shaped, ivory-white flowers with broad, wide-spreading petals and yellow stamens. ↕↔ 80–85cm (32–34in). ✻✻✻
P. wittmanniana ▣ Herbaceous perennial with stiff, hairless stems and shiny, dark green leaves with broadly ovate to broadly elliptic leaflets, paler and downy beneath. In late spring and early summer, bears deeply cup-shaped to almost hemispherical, single, primrose-yellow flowers, 10–13cm (4–5in) across, with yellow anthers and red filaments. ↕↔ 80–110cm (32–42in). N.W. Caucasus. ✻✻✻

▷ **Pagoda flower** see *Clerodendrum paniculatum*
▷ **Pagoda tree** see *Plumeria*
Japanese see *Sophora japonica*
▷ **Paint brush, White** see *Haemanthus albiflos*
▷ **Painted drop-tongue** see *Aglaonema crispum*
▷ **Painted leaf** see *Euphorbia cyathophora*
▷ **Painted net leaf** see *Fittonia*
▷ **Palas** see *Butea monosperma*

PALIURUS

RHAMNACEAE

Genus of about 8 species of spiny, deciduous or evergreen shrubs and trees occurring in dry and rocky places in woodland and at stream margins from S. Europe to E. Asia. The glossy, mid- to dark green leaves are alternate, ovate to broadly ovate, entire or toothed, often with heart-shaped bases. Star-shaped, 5-petalled, yellowish green flowers are produced in small, axillary cymes. The fruits are large, flat, winged discs. Reputed to have been used for Christ's "crown of thorns", *P. spina-christi* is cultivated for its foliage, small flowers, and unusual fruit. Grow in a shrub border or against a wall; can be used for hedging in regions with hot summers.
• **HARDINESS** Frost hardy, but may be hardier in areas with very hot summers.
• **CULTIVATION** Grow in full sun in any well-drained soil. Pruning group 1.
• **PROPAGATION** Sow seed in containers in a cold frame in autumn. Take softwood cuttings in summer.
• **PESTS AND DISEASES** Trouble free.

P. spina-christi ▣ (Christ's thorn, Jerusalem thorn). Bushy, deciduous shrub with slender, thorny shoots and ovate, 3-veined, glossy, bright dark green leaves, to 4cm (1½in) long. Small cymes of tiny, star-shaped yellow flowers are produced in summer, followed by woody fruit, to 2.5cm (1in) across, each with a rounded green wing, turning brown. ↕ 4m (12ft), ↔ 3m (10ft). S. Europe to N. China. ✻✻

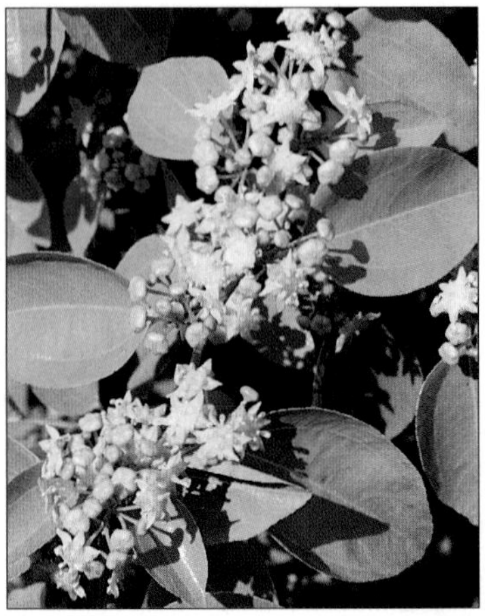
Paliurus spina-christi

▷ **Palm,**
African oil see *Elaeis guineensis*
Alexander see *Archontophoenix alexandrae, Ptychosperma elegans*
Areca see *Chrysalidocarpus lutescens*
Australian fan see *Livistona australis*
Australian ivy see *Schefflera actinophylla*
Bangalow see *Archontophoenix cunninghamiana*
Barbel see *Acanthophoenix*
Betel nut see *Areca catechu*
Blue fan see *Brahea armata*
Blue hesper see *Brahea armata*
Bottle see *Beaucarnea recurvata, Hyophorbe, H. lagenicaulis*
Broom see *Thrinax parviflora*
Burmese fish-tail see *Caryota mitis*
Butterfly see *Chrysalidocarpus lutescens*
Cabbage see *Cordyline, Livistona australis*
Canary Island date see *Phoenix canariensis*
Cardboard see *Zamia furfuracea*
Chilean wine see *Jubaea*
Chinese fan see *Livistona chinensis*
Christmas see *Veitchia merrillii*
Chusan see *Trachycarpus fortunei*
Clustered fish-tail see *Caryota mitis*
Coquito see *Jubaea chilensis*
Date see *Phoenix dactylifera*
Desert fan see *Washingtonia filifera*
Doum see *Hyphaene, H. coriacea*
Dwarf fan see *Chamaerops*
Everglades see *Acoelorraphe wrightii*
Fern see *Cycas, C. circinalis*
Fiji fan see *Pritchardia pacifica*
Fish-tail see *Caryota*
Florida silver see *Coccothrinax argentata*
Gingerbread see *Hyphaene thebaica*
Golden feather see *Chrysalidocarpus lutescens*
Grey goddess see *Brahea armata*
Hesper see *Brahea*
Honey see *Jubaea chilensis*
Illawarra see *Archontophoenix cunninghamiana*
Jaggery see *Caryota urens*
Japanese sago see *Cycas revoluta*
Jelly see *Butia capitata*
Kentia see *Howea forsteriana*
Key see *Thrinax morrisii*
King see *Archontophoenix*
Lady see *Rhapis*
Latan see *Latania*
Lipstick see *Cyrtostachys lakka*
Macaw fat see *Elaeis guineensis*
Manila see *Veitchia merrillii*
Mexican fern see *Dioon edule*
Miniature date see *Phoenix roebelenii*
Miniature fan see *Rhapis excelsa*
Miniature fish-tail see *Chamaedorea metallica*
Needle see *Rhapidophyllum*
New Zealand cabbage see *Cordyline australis*
Northern bangalow see *Archontophoenix alexandrae*
Oil see *Elaeis*
Palmyra see *Borassus flabellifer*
Panama hat see *Carludovica palmata*
Parlour see *Chamaedorea elegans*
Peach see *Bactris gasipaes*
Petticoat see *Copernicia macroglossa*
Piccabeen see *Archontophoenix cunninghamiana*
Porcupine see *Rhapidophyllum hystrix*

P

PAMIANTHE

AMARYLLIDACEAE

Genus of 2 or 3 species of evergreen or deciduous, bulbous perennials from moist, sandy but rocky areas at altitudes of 1,000–2,000m (3,250–7,000ft) in South America. They have false stems formed from the bases of the strap-shaped, keeled leaves, and are grown for their umbels of large, fragrant white spring flowers, resembling daffodils (*Narcissus*), each with 6 spreading outer tepals and an inner "cup". In frost-prone areas, grow in a temperate or warm greenhouse. In warmer regions, grow among small shrubs or in a border.

• **HARDINESS** Frost tender.

• **CULTIVATION** Plant in late summer or early autumn, with the neck of each bulb just above soil level. Under glass, grow in loam-based potting compost (JI No.2), with added grit and well-rotted organic matter, in full light. When in growth, water moderately and apply a balanced liquid fertilizer every month. Water sparingly at other times. Outdoors, grow in moderately fertile, moist but sharply drained soil in full sun.

• **PROPAGATION** Sow seed at 16–21°C (61–70°F) when ripe. Remove offsets in autumn.

• **PESTS AND DISEASES** Trouble free.

P. peruviana ▣ Deciduous, bulbous perennial with a false stem formed by the bases of the semi-erect, strap-shaped, mid-green leaves, 50cm (20in) long, with rounded keels. In spring, produces terminal umbels of 2–4 large, strongly fragrant flowers, 12cm (5in) across, with spreading, creamy white outer petals and bell-shaped, split white "cups" with green central stripes. ↕ to 1.2m (4ft), ↔ 30cm (12in). Peruvian Andes. ❄ (min. 15°C/59°F)

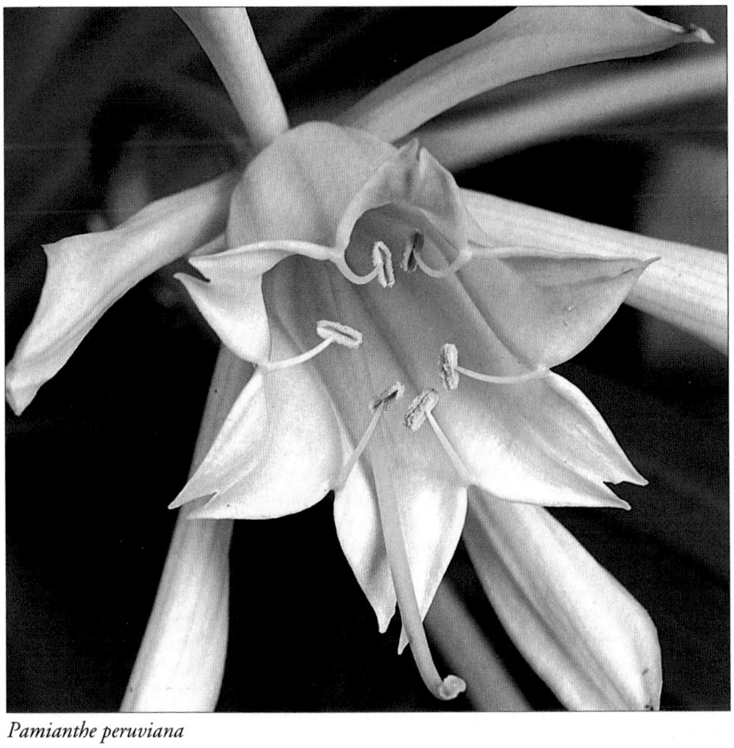

Pamianthe peruviana

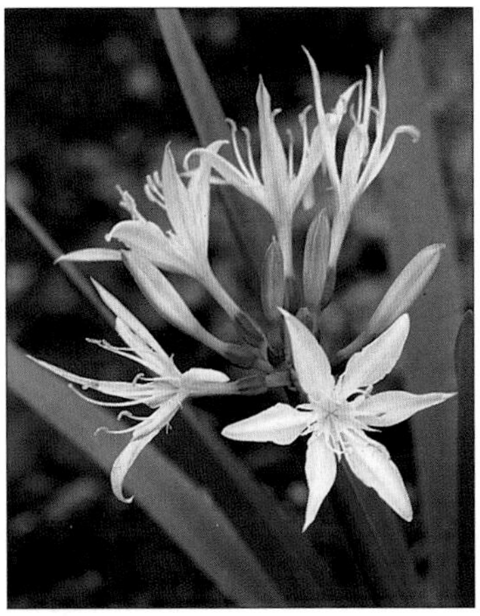

Pancratium illyricum

PANCRATIUM

Sea lily

AMARYLLIDACEAE

Genus of about 16 species of bulbous perennials found in sandy or rocky sites from the Canary Islands, W. Africa to Namibia, and the Mediterranean to tropical Asia. They have 2-ranked, linear to strap-shaped, basal leaves, and produce terminal umbels of showy, fragrant flowers, each with 6 spreading outer petals and a central "cup". Grow against a warm, sunny wall or, in frost-prone areas, in a cool greenhouse.

• **HARDINESS** Half hardy to frost tender. Half-hardy species may withstand occasional temperatures to -5°C (23°F).

• **CULTIVATION** Plant bulbs 15–20cm (6–8in) deep when dormant. Under glass, grow in loam-based potting compost (JI No.2) with added grit, in deep containers or in a greenhouse border, in full light. When in growth, water freely and apply a balanced liquid fertilizer monthly. Keep dry in summer when dormant. Water sparingly in autumn and winter. Outdoors, grow in any sharply drained soil in full sun.

• **PROPAGATION** Sow seed at 13–18°C (55–64°F) when ripe, or remove offsets when dormant.

• **PESTS AND DISEASES** Trouble free.

P. illyricum ▣ Bulbous perennial with semi-erect, broad, strap-shaped, mid-green, glaucous, basal leaves, to 50cm (20in) long. Bears umbels of 10–15 white flowers, 8cm (3in) across, in late spring and early summer. ↕ 40cm (16in), ↔ 15cm (6in). Corsica, Sardinia. ✲

P. maritimum (Sea daffodil). Bulbous perennial with long-necked bulbs and semi-erect, narrow, strap-shaped, grey-green, basal leaves, to 50cm (20in) long. Bears umbels of up to 6 fragrant white flowers, to 10cm (4in) across, in late summer. ↕↔ 30cm (12in). Coastal S.W. Europe, Mediterranean. ✲

PANDANUS

Screw pine

PANDANACEAE

Genus of 250 or more species of dioecious, evergreen shrubs and trees occurring in dry and moist sites throughout tropical regions of Africa, India, Asia, Australasia, and the Pacific islands. The sparsely branched stems of mature plants are often supported by stilt roots. Screw pines are grown for their attractive foliage: the linear, light to dark green leaves are tough and usually spiny-toothed, and borne in 3 spiralling ranks forming terminal rosettes. The small and petalless male and female flowers are produced on separate plants, males in slender, often branched spikes, and females in short, dense, cone-like heads, which develop into small, fruits resembling pineapples when fertilized. Where temperatures fall below 13°C (55°F), grow young plants in a warm greenhouse or as houseplants. In warmer regions, use as specimen plants.

• **HARDINESS** Frost tender.

• **CULTIVATION** Under glass, grow in loam-based potting compost (JI No.2), with added leaf mould and charcoal, in full light, with moderate to high humidity. From spring to summer, water moderately and apply a balanced liquid fertilizer every month. Water sparingly in winter. Outdoors, grow in fertile, moist but well-drained soil in full sun. Pruning group 1.

• **PROPAGATION** Sow seed at 18°C (64°F) as soon as ripe or in spring, first soaking them for 24 hours. Remove suckers or offsets in spring.

• **PESTS AND DISEASES** Scale insects and red spider mites may cause problems under glass.

P. odoratissimus see *P. tectorius.*

P. sanderi. Slow-growing, suckering shrub that seldom branches and rarely flowers. Bears rosettes of arching, linear, minutely spiny yellow leaves, 45–75cm (18–30in) long, becoming green with pale yellow stripes when mature. ↕ 1m (3ft), ↔ 0.75–1.5m (30–60in). Malaysia, possibly Indonesia (Timor). ❄ (min. 13°C/55°F). **'Roehrsianus'** is more robust, and produces leaves to 1m (3ft) long.

P. tectorius ▣ ✾ syn. *P. odoratissimus.* Many-branched, upright tree with thick stilt roots. Whorls of robust branches bear rosettes of linear, long-pointed,

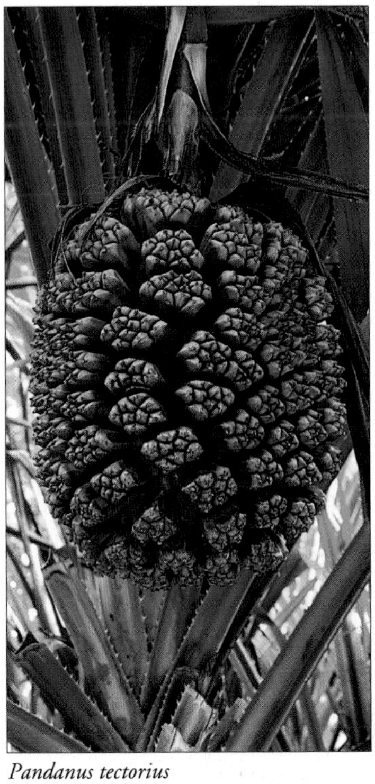

Pandanus tectorius

P

stiffly leathery, bluish green leaves, 1–1.5m (3–5ft) long, with spines along the margins and midribs beneath. Each male flower spike, 20–30cm (8–12in) long, is branched and sheathed in a fragrant white spathe; female flower-heads are small and solitary, about 5cm (2in) across. Flowers are borne mainly in summer, followed by spherical to broadly ovoid fruit, 15–25cm (6–10in) long; they may be yellow or light green flushed red. ↕ 3–6m (10–20ft), ↔ 2–4m (6–12ft). S.E. Asia, Pacific islands. ❀ (min. 13°C/55°F). **var. *bulbosus*** is larger, with fleshier fruit; widely grown in the Pacific; ↕ 4–6m (12–20ft). **var. *laevis*** 🏆 has spineless leaves.

▷ **Panda plant** see *Philodendron bipennifolium*

PANDOREA

BIGNONIACEAE

Genus of 6 species of woody-stemmed, evergreen, twining climbers, rarely shrubs, related to *Tecomaria* and *Tecoma*. They are found in rainforest from sea level to 3,000m (10,000ft) in Malaysia, Papua New Guinea, Australia, and New Caledonia, and are grown for their attractive flowers and foliage. Leaves are opposite or whorled, pinnate, and mid- or dark green, each with up to 7 pairs of leaflets. The fragrant, tubular flowers, each with 5 broad, spreading, petal lobes, the upper 2 smaller than the lower 3, are borne usually in terminal, cyme-like panicles or racemes. In mild climates, they are suitable for a pergola or arch, and look especially effective cascading from a tree. In frost-prone areas, grow in a cool greenhouse.

• **HARDINESS** Frost tender; but *P. jasminoides* and *P. pandorana* may survive temperatures around 0°C (32°F) for short periods, if the wood has been well-ripened in summer.

• **CULTIVATION** Under glass, grow in loam-based potting compost (JI No.3) in full light. When in growth, water moderately and apply a balanced liquid fertilizer monthly. Water sparingly in winter. Outdoors, grow in fertile, moist but well-drained soil in full sun. Provide support for climbing stems. Pruning group 11, after flowering.

• **PROPAGATION** Sow seed at 13–18°C (55–64°F) in spring. Root greenwood cuttings with bottom heat in summer. Layer in spring.

• **PESTS AND DISEASES** Susceptible to red spider mites and aphids under glass.

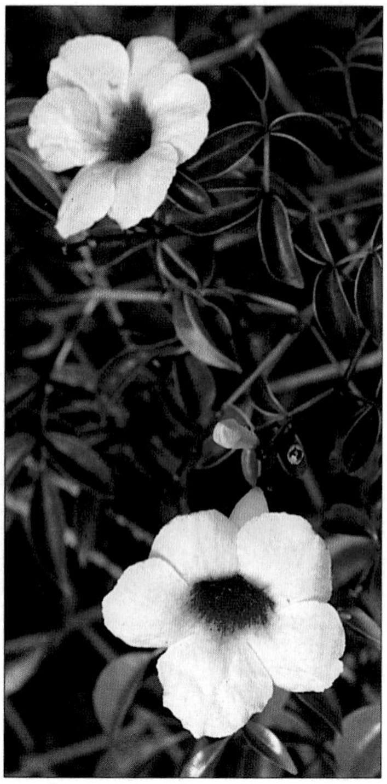

Pandorea jasminoides

P. jasminoides ■ syn. *Bignonia jasminoides* (Bower plant). Vigorous, twining climber with wiry, branching stems, and pinnate leaves composed of 5–9 ovate to lance-shaped, glossy, bright green leaflets, 2.5–5cm (1–2in) long. Tubular flowers with spreading lobes, 4–5cm (1½–2in) across, are white, flushed crimson-pink in the throats, and freely produced in small, cyme-like panicles from spring to summer. ↕ 5m (15ft) or more. Australia (Queensland, New South Wales). ❀ (min. 5°C/41°F). **'Alba'** has pure white flowers. **'Lady Di'** has white flowers with creamy yellow, sometimes orange-yellow throats. **'Rosea'** has pink flowers with deeper pink throats. **'Rosea Superba'** 🏆 produces large pink flowers, to 6cm (2½in) long, with purple-spotted, deep pink throats.

P. lindleyana see *Clytostoma callistegioides.*

P. pandorana, syn. *Bignonia pandorana, Tecoma australis* (Wonga wonga vine). Strong-growing, twining climber with slender, branching stems. Pinnate leaves have usually 6 pairs of ovate to broadly lance-shaped, mid-green leaflets, 3–10cm (1¼–4in) long, deeply and narrowly lobed when young, entire or sometimes scalloped when mature. Tubular, creamy yellow flowers spotted and streaked reddish purple, 1.5–3cm (½–1¼in) across, with spreading lobes, are borne in terminal and axillary cyme-like racemes in winter and spring. ↕ 6m (20ft) or more. E. Australia (including Tasmania), Papua New Guinea, Pacific islands. ❀ (min. 5°C/41°F)

P. ricasoliana see *Podranea ricasoliana.*

PANICUM

Crab grass

GRAMINEAE/POACEAE

Genus of about 470 annual or perennial, deciduous or evergreen grasses occurring in open grassland or wooded areas, often in rocky, moist limestone soil, in tropical regions worldwide, in Europe, and in temperate North America. The leaves are thread-like in bud, usually becoming flat and linear-ovate, and may be light to mid-green, grey-green, or purple. In late summer and autumn, they produce finely branching panicles or racemes of 2-flowered spikelets. Ornamental species are valued mainly for their light, airy flowerheads, suitable for cutting and drying; a number of species, such as millet (*P. miliaceum*), are also valuable fodder crops. Grow in a sunny mixed or herbaceous border.

• **HARDINESS** Fully hardy to half hardy.

• **CULTIVATION** Grow in moderately fertile, well-drained soil in full sun.

• **PROPAGATION** Sow seed at 13–18°C (55–64°F) in spring. Divide perennials between mid-spring and early summer.

• **PESTS AND DISEASES** Trouble free.

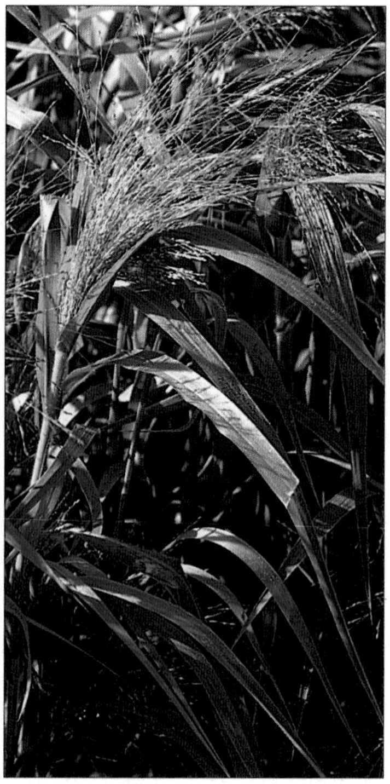

Panicum capillare

P. capillare ■ (Witch grass). Lax, loosely tufted annual with clumps of flat, linear to narrowly lance-shaped, mid-green leaves, to 30cm (12in) long. In late summer and autumn, produces dense panicles, to 45cm (18in) long, of tiny, greenish brown spikelets on hair-fine branchlets. ↕ 60–100cm (24–39in), ↔ 60cm (24in). North America. ❄

P. miliaceum (Millet). Erect, clump-forming annual with flat, narrow, lance-shaped, mid-green, sometimes purple-flushed leaves, to 40cm (16in) long. Produces rigid, intricately branched panicles, to 30cm (12in) long, of slightly pendent, purple-tinged green flowers, borne in small spikelets, to 6mm (¼in) long, in late summer. ↕ to 90cm (36in), ↔ to 23cm (9in). C., S., and E. Europe. ❄❄❄. **'Violaceum'**, syn. *P. violaceum*, has purple-violet leaves and spikelets.

P. violaceum see *P. miliaceum* 'Violaceum'.

P. virgatum (Switch grass). Narrowly upright, rhizomatous, deciduous, perennial grass forming clumps of purple to glaucous, mid-green stems that bear upright, flat, linear, mid-green leaves, to 60cm (24in) long. Leaves turn yellow in autumn and light brown in winter. Produces broad, diffuse, weeping panicles, to 50cm (20in) long, of tiny, purple-green spikelets in early autumn. ↕ 1m (3ft), ↔ 75cm (30in). S. Canada, USA to Central America. ❄❄❄. **'Hänse Herms'**, syn. 'Haense Herms', has a fountain-like habit, and rich reddish purple autumn foliage. **'Heavy Metal'** has stiffer, more erect, metallic blue-grey leaves, turning yellow in autumn. **'Strictum'** is narrowly upright, with leaves that turn bright yellow in autumn; ↕ 1.2m (4ft), ↔ 60cm (24in).

▷ **Pansy** see *Viola, V.* x *wittrockiana*
Mountain see *V. lutea*
Wild see *V. tricolor*

PAPAVER

Poppy

PAPAVERACEAE

Genus of 70 species of annuals, biennials, and perennials occurring in a wide range of habitats from lowlands to high mountains; most are from C. and S. Europe and temperate Asia, a few from South Africa, Australia, W. North America, and subarctic regions. Some annuals are common weeds of arable fields. The usually unbranched, wiry, sometimes hairy stems, which exude latex if damaged, produce a few alternate, mostly radical leaves, which may be simple and toothed, or pinnate to 3-pinnate, pinnatifid or pinnatisect, bristly or smooth, and grey-green or light to dark green. The short-lived flowers are wide-spreading, bowl-, cup-, or saucer-shaped, usually 4-petalled, and brightly coloured, sometimes with basal marks or spots. They are borne singly or in panicles or racemes, the buds often pendent, and are followed by distinctive "pepper-pot" seed pods. Most larger species are spectacular plants for a mixed or herbaceous border; several of the smaller poppies are suitable for a rock garden or an annual border.

• **HARDINESS** Fully hardy to frost hardy.

• **CULTIVATION** Grow in deep, fertile, well-drained soil in full sun, except *P. alpinum* and its cultivars, which require very sharply drained soil.

• **PROPAGATION** Sow seed in spring: for annuals and biennials, sow seed *in situ*; for perennials, sow seed in containers in a cold frame. Divide perennials in spring, or take root cuttings from them in late autumn or early winter.

• **PESTS AND DISEASES** Prone to aphids, pedicel necrosis and fungal wilts, and, in damp conditions, downy mildew.

P. alpinum ■ (Alpine poppy). Tuft-forming, short-lived perennial with variable, 2- or 3-pinnate, sometimes pinnatisect, hairy, grey-green leaves, to

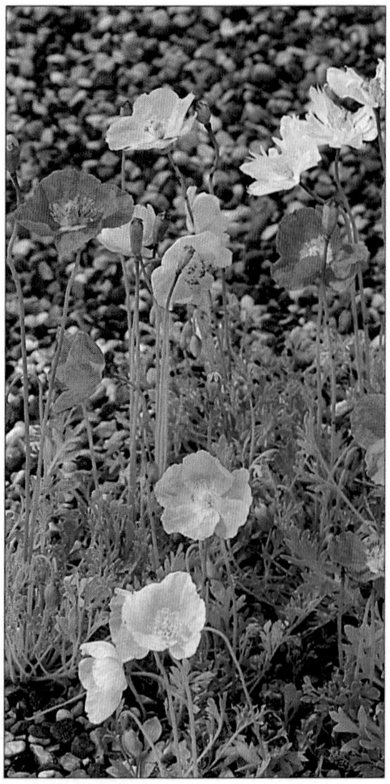

Papaver alpinum

P

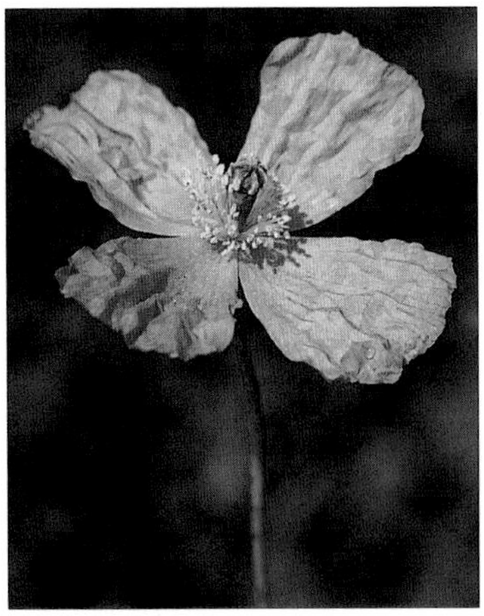

Papaver atlanticum

20cm (8in) long, with linear segments. Solitary, cup- to saucer-shaped, white, yellow, orange, or red flowers, to 4cm (1½in) across, are produced in summer. The name *P. alpinum* is often used to include a range of plants that are now considered distinct species. ↕ 15–20cm (6–8in), ↔ 10cm (4in). Europe (Pyrenees, Alps, Carpathian Mountains). ✻✻✻. **subsp. *burseri*** see *P. burseri.* **subsp. *rhaeticum*** see *P. rhaeticum.*
P. atlanticum ▣ Erect, clump-forming, short-lived perennial with oblong to lance-shaped, coarsely toothed, mid-green leaves, to 15cm (6in) long, very hairy, particularly beneath. In summer, bears solitary, saucer-shaped, soft orange flowers, to 5cm (2in) across, with very hairy sepals. ↕ 30cm (12in), ↔ 15cm (6in). Morocco. ✻✻✻
P. bracteatum ♀ Upright, clump-forming, bristly perennial producing pinnatisect, mid-green leaves, 25–45cm (10–18in) long, with lance-shaped, toothed segments. In early summer, bears solitary, bowl-shaped, blood-red flowers, 10–18cm (4–7in) across, with 4–6 petals, each with a large, elongated black spot at the base. Similar to *P. orientale* but with taller, stiffer stems,

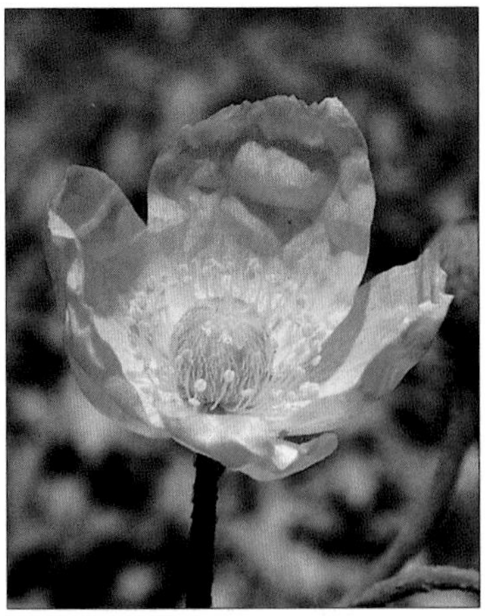

Papaver fauriei

sepal-like bracts below the flowers, and longer spots on the petals. ↕ to 1.2m (4ft), ↔ 90cm (36in). N. Iran. ✻✻✻
P. burseri, syn. *P. alpinum* subsp. *burseri.* Tuft-forming, almost hairless, semi-evergreen, short-lived perennial with 2- or 3-pinnate, grey-green leaves, to 20cm (8in) long, consisting of linear to lance-shaped segments. In summer, produces solitary, saucer-shaped white flowers, to 4cm (1½in) across, with yellow stamens. ↕ 15cm (6in), ↔ 10cm (4in). Europe (Alps, Carpathian Mountains). ✻✻✻
P. commutatum ♀ Erect, branching annual with oval to oblong, pinnatisect, downy, mid-green leaves, to 15cm (6in) long, with lance-shaped segments. Solitary, bowl-shaped, brilliant red flowers, to 8cm (3in) across, spotted black at the petal bases, are borne on softly grey-hairy stems in summer. ↕ to 45cm (18in), ↔ 15cm (6in). Greece (Crete), Turkey, Caucasus, N. Iran. ✻✻✻
P. croceum, syn. *P. nudicaule* of gardens (Arctic poppy, Icelandic poppy). Erect, tuft-forming, hairy perennial, usually grown as a biennial, producing oval, pinnatifid to pinnatisect, densely hairy,

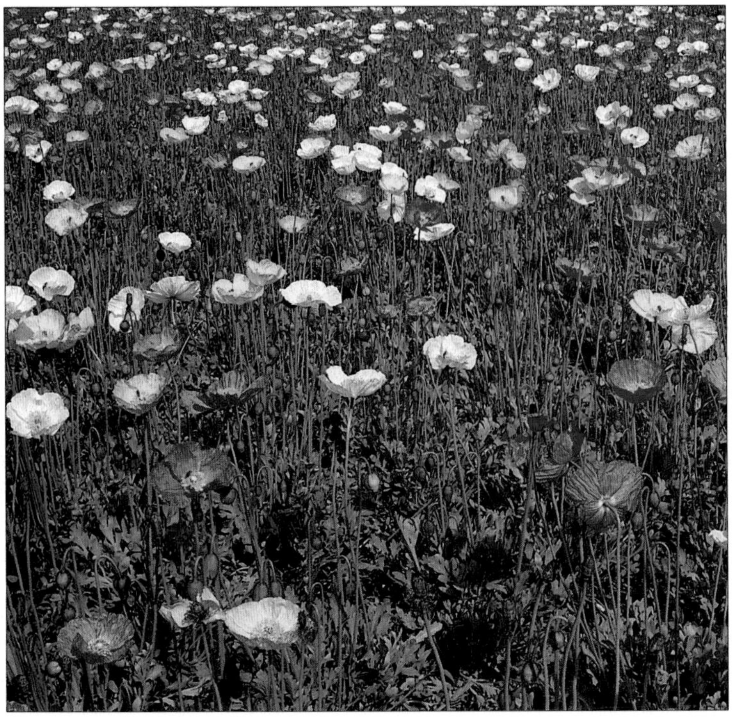

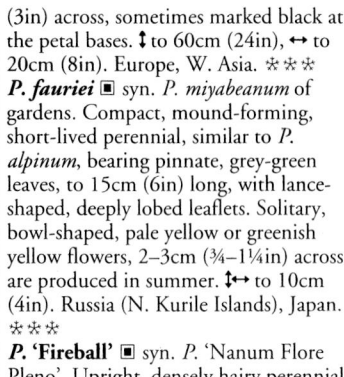

Papaver croceum 'Summer Breeze'

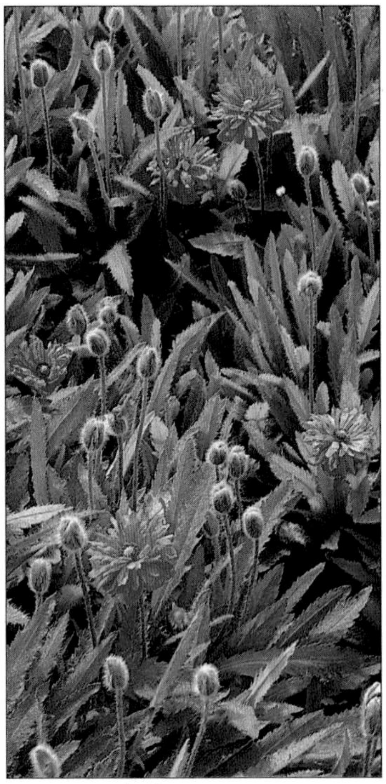

Papaver 'Fireball'

blue-green leaves, 3–15cm (1¼–6in) long, with oblong segments. Solitary, bowl-shaped, occasionally double, fragrant, yellow or white, sometimes orange or pale red flowers, to 8cm (3in) across, are borne on short, hairy stalks in summer. ↕ to 30cm (12in), ↔ to 15cm (6in). Subarctic regions. ✻✻✻. **'Champagne Bubbles'** has large flowers, to 12cm (5in) across, in a range of mostly pastel shades, including red, bronze-yellow, apricot-yellow, pink, and yellow; ↕ to 45cm (18in). **'Garden Gnome'** is dwarf, with flowers mainly in bright shades, including orange-red, yellow, pink, salmon-pink, and white. **'Summer Breeze'** ▣ bears orange, golden yellow, yellow, or white flowers over a very long flowering period; ↕ 30–35cm (12–14in). **'Wonderland'** is dwarf, with large, short-stalked, white, orange, yellow, or red flowers, and is ideal in containers; ↕ to 25cm (10in).
P. dubium (Long-headed poppy). Upright, slender-stemmed, hairy annual with pinnatisect, blue-green leaves, 10–15cm (4–6in) long, with ovate segments. Throughout summer, produces solitary, saucer-shaped, pale scarlet or pinkish red flowers, to 7cm (3in) across, sometimes marked black at the petal bases. ↕ to 60cm (24in), ↔ to 20cm (8in). Europe, W. Asia. ✻✻✻
P. fauriei ▣ syn. *P. miyabeanum* of gardens. Compact, mound-forming, short-lived perennial, similar to *P. alpinum*, bearing pinnate, grey-green leaves, to 15cm (6in) long, with lance-shaped, deeply lobed leaflets. Solitary, bowl-shaped, pale yellow or greenish yellow flowers, 2–3cm (¾–1¼in) across, are produced in summer. ↕↔ to 10cm (4in). Russia (N. Kurile Islands), Japan. ✻✻✻
***P.* 'Fireball'** ▣ syn. *P.* 'Nanum Flore Pleno'. Upright, densely hairy perennial, spreading freely by runners, bearing lance-shaped, conspicuously toothed, bristly, mid-green leaves, to 20cm (8in) long. Solitary, hemispherical, semi-double to double, orange-scarlet flowers, 3–4cm (1¼–1½in) across, with narrow petals, are produced from late spring to midsummer. ↕↔ 30cm (12in). ✻✻✻
P. lateritium. Clump-forming, upright perennial with very hairy, oblong, deeply toothed, mid-green leaves, to 20cm (8in) long. Branching stems produce bowl-shaped, deep orange flowers, to 5cm (2in) across, usually solitary but occasionally in pairs, in mid- and late summer. ↕ 40cm (16in), ↔ 30cm (12in). Turkey. ✻✻✻
***P. miyabeanum* of gardens** see *P. fauriei.*
***P.* 'Nanum Flore Pleno'** see *P.* 'Fireball'.
***P. nudicaule* of gardens** see *P. croceum.*
P. orientale (Oriental poppy). Clump-forming perennial, spreading by runners, with erect, white-bristly stems and pinnatisect, mid-green leaves, to 30cm (12in) long, with lance-shaped, toothed segments. From late spring to midsummer, bears solitary, cup-shaped, orange-scarlet flowers, 10–16cm (4–6in) across, with no bracts; the 4–6 petals have large, bluish black or white basal spots, broader than they are long. ↕ 45–90cm (18–36in), ↔ 60–90cm (24–36in). Caucasus, N.E. Turkey, N. Iran. ✻✻✻. Most plants grown in gardens as cultivars of *P. orientale* are hybrids with *P. bracteatum* and the closely related *P. pseudoorientale;* they are listed here for easy reference.
'Allegro' ▣ has bright orange-scarlet flowers with bold, black basal marks.
'Beauty of Livermere' ▣ ♀ has large, crimson-scarlet flowers, to 20cm (8in) across, with a black mark at the base of each petal; ↕ 0.9–1.2m (3–4ft), ↔ 90cm

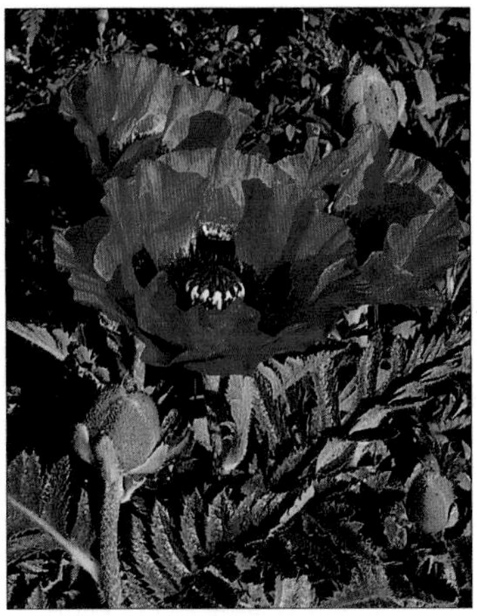

Papaver orientale 'Allegro'

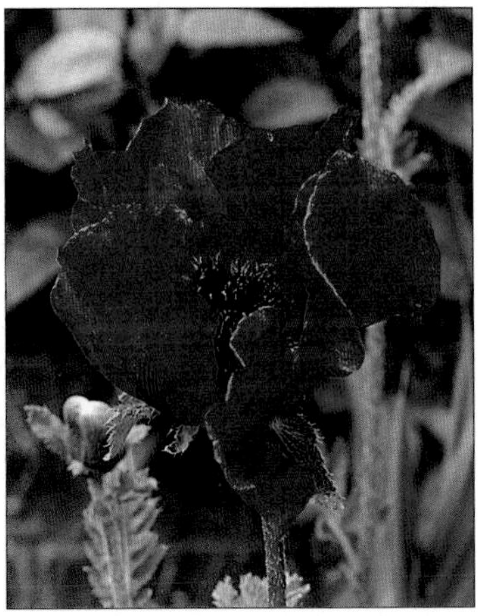

Papaver orientale 'Beauty of Livermere'

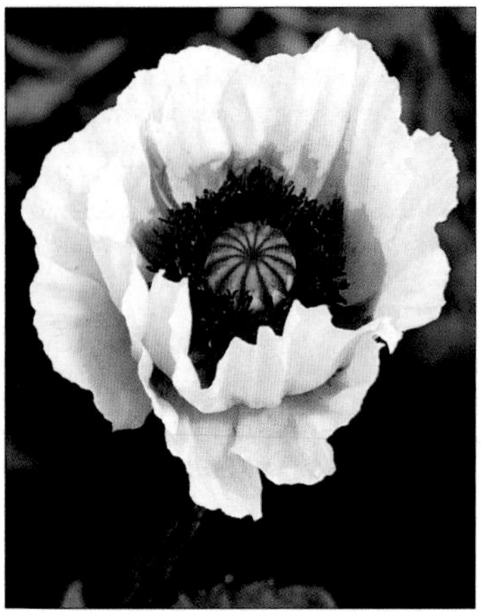

Papaver orientale 'Black and White'

(36in). **'Black and White'** ■♀ produces white flowers with a crimson-black mark at the base of each petal. **'Cedric Morris'** ■♀ has grey-hairy leaves and very large, soft pink flowers, to 16cm (6in) across, the frilled petals each with a black basal mark. **'Indian Chief'** produces deep mahogany-red flowers without spots. **'May Queen'** bears double, orange-red flowers with slightly quilled, unmarked petals. **'Mrs. Perry'** ♀ has pale salmon-pink flowers with black basal marks. **'Perry's White'** has white flowers with maroon-purple centres. **'Picotée'** produces pure white flowers with creased petals that have broad, frilled, orange-pink margins.

P. rhaeticum, syn. *P. alpinum* subsp. *rhaeticum*. Tufted perennial, similar to *P. alpinum*, bearing pinnate, finely hairy, grey-green leaves, to 8cm (3in) long, composed of ovate to lance-shaped segments. Solitary, bowl-shaped, golden yellow or orange flowers, to 5cm (2in) across, are produced in summer. ↕ 15cm (6in), ↔ 10cm (4in). Pyrenees. ❄❄❄

P. rhoeas (Corn poppy, Field poppy, Flanders poppy). Erect, branching, sparsely hairy annual with oblong, pinnatifid to pinnatisect, downy, light green leaves, to 15cm (6in) long, with lance-shaped segments. Solitary, bowl-shaped, brilliant red flowers, to 8cm (3in) across, sometimes marked black at the petal bases, are borne on short, downy stalks in summer. ↕ to 90cm (36in), ↔ to 30cm (12in). Eurasia, N. Africa; also widely naturalized. ❄❄❄. **'Fairy Wings'** see 'Mother of Pearl'. **'Mother of Pearl'** ■ syn. 'Fairy Wings', produces dove-grey, soft pink, or lilac-

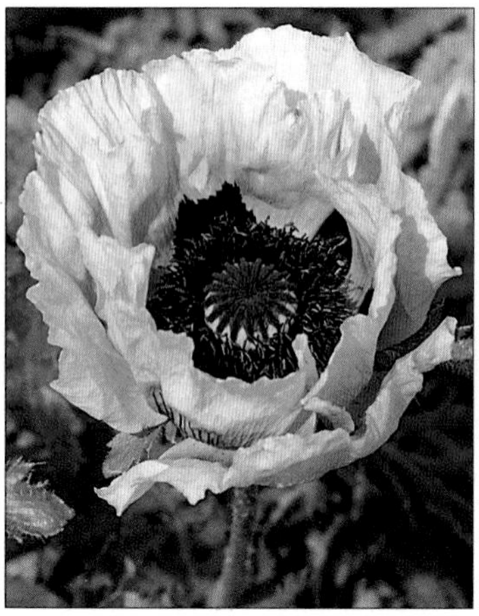

Papaver orientale 'Cedric Morris'

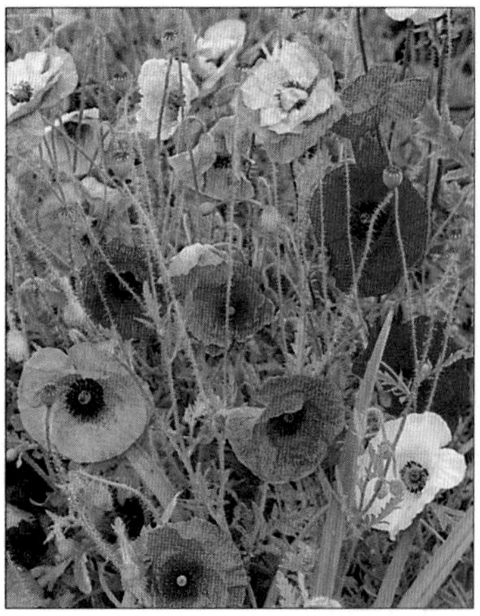

Papaver rhoeas 'Mother of Pearl'

blue flowers, with some paler zoning. **Shirley Series** ■ cultivars have single, semi-double, or double flowers in yellow, pink, orange, or sometimes red, always unmarked at the bases; they need careful selection to maintain the true stock. **Shirley Series 'Reverend Wilks'** has single and semi-double flowers in red, pink, or white, with some picotees and bicolours.

P. rupifragum. Erect, clump-forming perennial with obovate, toothed or lobed, mid-green leaves, to 15cm (6in) long. In summer, produces solitary, bowl-shaped, pale brick-red flowers, to 8cm (3in) across. Similar to *P. atlanticum* except that leaves are hairy only on margins and veins beneath, and sepals are hairless. May self-seed freely. ↕ 45cm (18in), ↔ 20cm (8in). Spain. ❄❄❄

P. somniferum ♀ (Opium poppy). Erect annual with oblong, deeply lobed, glaucous, blue-green leaves, to 12cm (5in) or more long. In summer, leafy stems bear solitary, bowl-shaped, pink, mauve-purple, red, or white flowers, to 10cm (4in) across, sometimes with dark spots at the petal bases. They are followed by large, blue-green seed pods that are good for dried arrangements. All parts may cause mild stomach upset if ingested. ↕ to 1.2m (4ft), ↔ to 30cm (12in). Origin unknown; very widely cultivated and naturalized. ❄❄❄. **'Hen and Chickens'** is grown primarily for its seed heads, with very large pods surrounded by clusters of much smaller capsules. **'Paeony Flowered'** ■ has large, double, frilly flowers in red, purple, pink, salmon-pink, maroon-red,

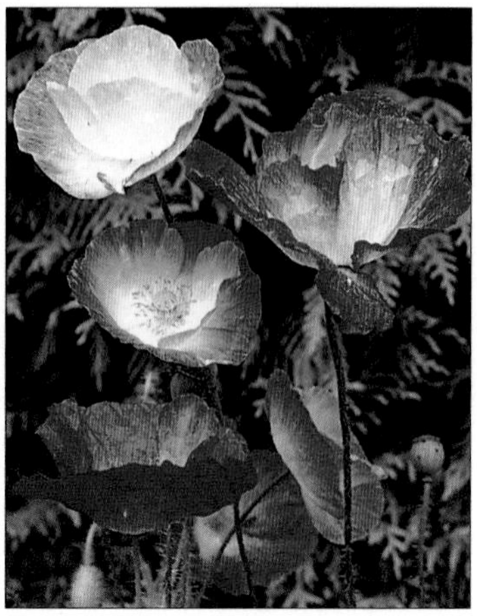

Papaver rhoeas Shirley Series

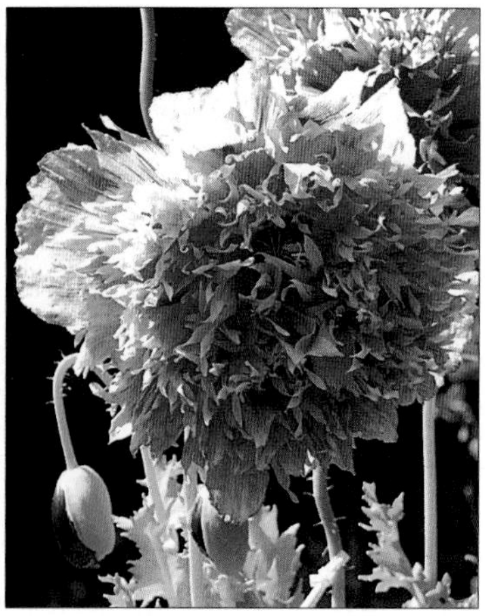

Papaver somniferum 'Paeony Flowered'

or white. **'White Cloud'** produces double white flowers.

P. triniifolium. Erect, branching, hairless or sparsely hairy biennial. In the first year, forms a basal rosette of 3 or 4 ovate to oblong, pinnatisect, glaucous, blue-green leaves, to 7cm (3in) long, with linear segments covered in short yellow hairs. In the summer of the second year, many-branched, leafy stems produce solitary, cup-shaped, orange-pink flowers, to 5cm (2in) across. ↕ to 30cm (12in), ↔ 15cm (6in). E. and S. Turkey. ❄❄❄

▷ **Paperbark** see *Melaleuca*
▷ **Paper bush** see *Edgeworthia*
▷ **Paper mulberry** see *Broussonetia papyrifera*
▷ **Paper rush, Egyptian** see *Cyperus papyrus*

PAPHIOPEDILUM

Slipper orchid

ORCHIDACEAE

Genus of about 60 species of evergreen, mainly terrestrial orchids, some epiphytic or lithophytic, occurring at sea level to over 2,000m (7,000ft), from India to China, S.E. Asia, and Papua New Guinea. They are sympodial, lack pseudobulbs, and produce short stems bearing strap-shaped, lance-shaped, or elliptic to ovate, leathery, sometimes mottled, grey to pale, mid-, or dark green leaves. Each shoot ends in a distinctive solitary flower, or a raceme of 2–8 flowers, each with an upright upper sepal, 2 spreading petals, and 2 lateral sepals united under a variably shaped lip or "pouch". Many hybrids have been developed. Contact with foliage may aggravate skin allergies.

- **HARDINESS** Frost tender.
- **CULTIVATION** Cool- to intermediate-growing orchids. Grow in terrestrial orchid compost, with added crushed bark and dolomitic limestone chips, in pots that constrict the roots. In summer, provide high humidity and bright filtered light, water freely, and apply fertilizer at every third watering. Do not mist. In winter, provide full light and water sparingly; do not allow the compost to dry out completely between waterings. See also p.46.
- **PROPAGATION** Not suitable for division, although cuttings or offshoots may be rooted successfully.
- **PESTS AND DISEASES** Prone to red spider mites, aphids, and mealybugs.

P. appletonianum ■ Terrestrial orchid with elliptic, mottled, mid-green and purple leaves, to 20cm (8in) long. Solitary flowers, 12cm (5in) across, with slender green and rose-pink petals, pale green, darker veined upper sepals, and light brown pouches, appear in winter and spring. ↕ 30cm (12in), ↔ 15cm (6in). Laos, Thailand, Cambodia. ❀ (min. 13°C/55°F; max. 30°C/86°F)

P. argus. Terrestrial orchid with oblong-lance-shaped, pale green leaves with darker mottling, 12–20cm (5–8in) long. In spring, bears solitary flowers, 10cm (4in) across, with dark purple-spotted, off-white petals, pink at the tips; upper sepals have dark green or purple veining; dark green-veined pouches are red above the lips, yellow beneath. ↕ 30cm (12in), ↔ 15cm (6in). Philippines. ❀ (min. 13°C/55°F; max. 30°C/86°F)

P. bellatulum ■ Terrestrial orchid with rigid, leathery, elliptic to strap-shaped leaves, mottled green and grey, to 20cm (8in) long. Solitary, almost stemless, rounded, white or pale yellow flowers, 9cm (3½in) across, with large, dark red spots, are produced in spring. ↕ 12cm (5in), ↔ 15cm (6in). Burma, Thailand. ❀ (min. 13°C/55°F; max. 30°C/86°F)

***P.* Buckhurst 'Mont Millais'** ■ (*P.* Greenville x *P.* Spring Vigil). Terrestrial orchid with strap-shaped to ovate, mid-green leaves, 15cm (6in) long. Solitary yellow flowers, 12cm (5in) across, with white upper sepals, are usually produced in winter. ↕ 30cm (12in), ↔ 20cm (8in). ❀ (min. 13°C/55°F; max. 30°C/86°F)

P. callosum ■ Terrestrial orchid with strap-shaped to elliptic, greyish green leaves, to 25cm (10in) long, with dark green mottling. In spring, bears solitary, maroon and green flowers, 7–9cm (3–3½in) across, with white-striped maroon upper sepals and maroon lips. ↕ 30cm (12in), ↔ 15cm (6in). Thailand, Cambodia, S. Vietnam. ❀ (min. 13°C/55°F; max. 30°C/86°F)

P. delenatii ♀ Terrestrial orchid with rigid, leathery, elliptic to strap-shaped leaves, 10–15cm (4–6in) long, mottled green and grey above, deep purple beneath. In spring, bears almost stalkless white flowers, 8cm (3in) across, with pink lips, singly or in pairs. ↕ 20cm (8in), ↔ 15cm (6in). C. Vietnam. ❀ (min. 13°C/55°F; max. 30°C/86°F)

***P.* Delrosi** (*P. delenatii* x *P. rothschildianum*). Terrestrial orchid with semi-rigid, strap-shaped, linear, purplish green leaves, 15cm (6in) long, lightly mottled greyish green and mid-green. In spring, bears richly coloured pink flowers, 10cm (4in) across, singly or in racemes. ↕↔ 30cm (12in). ❀ (min. 13°C/55°F; max. 30°C/86°F)

P. fairrieanum ■ Terrestrial orchid with strap-shaped, dark green leaves, 9–15cm (3½–6in) long. In autumn, bears solitary, purple-veined, pale green-white flowers, 6–8cm (2½–3in) across, with greenish yellow lips suffused purple brown. ↕↔ 15cm (6in). Himalayas, N.E. India (Sikkim), Bhutan. ❀ (min. 10°C/50°F; max. 30°C/86°F)

***P.* Freckles** ■ (*P.* Burleigh Mohur x *P.* F.C. Puddle). Terrestrial orchid with strap-shaped, mid-green leaves, 15cm (6in) long. In early winter, bears solitary cream flowers, 12cm (5in) across, spotted purple-brown, with pink-flushed lips. ↕ 30cm (12in), ↔ 20cm (8in). ❀ (min. 13°C/55°F; max. 30°C/86°F)

P

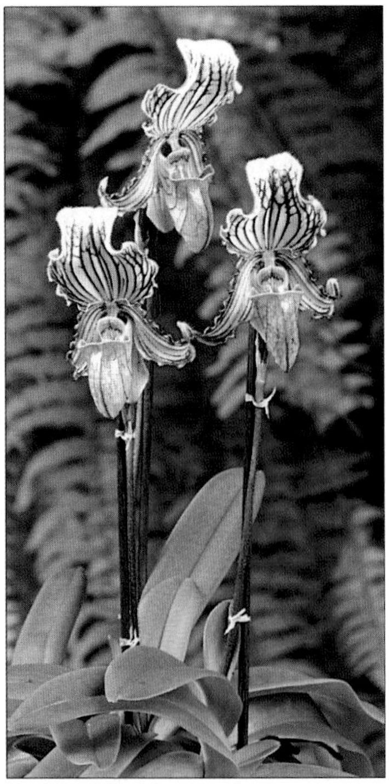
Paphiopedilum fairrieanum

***P.* Goultenianum 'Album'** ■ (*P. callosum* x *P. curtisii*). Terrestrial orchid with broadly ovate, mottled, grey-green and dark green leaves, 10cm (4in) long. Solitary, lime-green and white flowers, 10cm (4in) across, with striped upper sepals, are usually borne in spring. ↕ 30cm (12in), ↔ 20cm (8in). ❄ (min. 13°C/55°F; max. 30°C/86°F)
P. haynaldianum ■ Terrestrial or lithophytic orchid with strap-shaped, light green leaves, to 40cm (16in) long. Racemes of up to 6 slender flowers, to 13cm (5in) across, with green petals tipped and spotted rose-pink, and with spotted upper sepals and greenish brown pouches, are borne in spring. ↕ 45cm (18in), ↔ 30cm (12in). Philippines. ❄ (min. 13°C/55°F; max. 30°C/86°F)
P. hirsutissimum. Terrestrial orchid with linear to strap-shaped, mid-green leaves, to 45cm (18in) long. Solitary flowers, to 14cm (5½in) across, with green and rose-mauve petals, green upper sepals, shaded brown, and greenish brown pouches, are borne in spring. ↕ 15cm (6in), ↔ 20cm (8in). N.E. India, S. China, Thailand. ❄ (min. 10°C/50°F; max. 30°C/86°F)
P. insigne 🏆 Terrestrial orchid with linear to lance-shaped, yellowish green leaves, 20–30cm (8–12in) long. Solitary flowers, 7–10cm (3–3½in) across, with yellow-bronze petals and pouches, and pale green-yellow, spotted upper sepals, appear from autumn to spring. ↕ 15cm (6in), ↔ 25cm (10in). E. Himalayas. ❄ (min. 10°C/50°F; max. 30°C/86°F)
***P.* Joanne's Wine** ■ (*P.* Maudiae x *P.* Vintner's Treasure). Terrestrial orchid with broadly ovate, greyish green leaves, 10cm (4in) long, with dark mottling. In spring, bears solitary flowers, 10cm (4in) across, mostly dark purple and light green. ↕ 23cm (9in), ↔ 20cm (8in). ❄ (min. 13°C/55°F; max. 30°C/86°F)
***P.* Lyric 'Glendora'** ■ (*P.* Lucid x *P.* Paeony). Terrestrial orchid with strap-shaped to ovate, mid-green leaves, 15cm (6in) long. Solitary, rounded flowers, 12cm (5in) across, with deep red and green petals, and white upper sepals with dark red centres, are usually produced in winter. ↕ 30cm (12in), ↔ 20cm (8in). ❄ (min. 13°C/55°F; max. 30°C/86°F)
***P.* Maudiae** 🏆 (*P. callosum* x *P. lawrenceanum*). Terrestrial orchid with attractive, ovate leaves, mottled light and dark green, 12cm (5in) long. Solitary, green-and-white-striped flowers, 10cm (4in) across, are borne in spring or summer. ↕ 30cm (12in), ↔ 15cm (6in). ❄ (min. 13°C/55°F; max. 30°C/86°F). **'Coloratum'** ■ has wine-red flowers with striped upper sepals and greenish white centres.
***P.* Miller's Daughter** ■ (*P.* Chantal x *P.* Dusty Miller). Terrestrial orchid with strap-shaped to ovate, mid-green leaves, 15cm (6in) long. Solitary white flowers, 10cm (4in) across, with pink veins and spots, are usually produced in spring. ↕ 23cm (9in), ↔ 20cm (8in). ❄ (min. 13°C/55°F; max. 30°C/86°F)
P. niveum ■ Terrestrial orchid with rigid, leathery, elliptic to strap-shaped leaves, 10–15cm (4–6in) long, mottled green and grey. Solitary, powder-white flowers, 8cm (3in) across, with small red spots, are borne in summer. ↕↔ 15cm (6in). S. Thailand, N. Malaysia. ❄ (min. 13°C/55°F; max. 30°C/86°F)
P. rothschildianum. Terrestrial orchid with semi-rigid, elliptic to strap-shaped, shiny, mid-green leaves, to 50cm (20in) long. In spring and summer, produces racemes of 2–6 flowers, to 20cm (8in) across, with thin, purple-spotted cream petals, white upper sepals, spotted and striped dark purple, and purplish brown, yellow-rimmed pouches. ↕ 60cm (24in), ↔ 45cm (18in). N. Borneo. ❄ (min. 13°C/55°F; max. 30°C/86°F)
***P.* Silvara 'Jancis'** ■ (*P.* F.C. Puddle x *P.* Sungrove). Terrestrial orchid with narrowly ovate, mid-green leaves, 15cm (6in) long. Solitary white flowers, 10cm (4in) across, with upper sepals peppered orange-brown, are usually borne in spring. ↕ 23cm (9in), ↔ 20cm (8in). ❄ (min. 13°C/55°F; max. 30°C/86°F)
P. sukhakulii ■ 🏆 Terrestrial orchid with narrowly elliptic, mottled, dark grey and mid- and dark green leaves, to 15cm (6in) long. In autumn, bears solitary flowers, 10–12cm (4–5in) across. They have green petals, heavily spotted purplish black, green-striped white upper sepals, and reddish brown pouches. ↕↔ 15cm (6in). Thailand. ❄ (min. 13°C/55°F; max. 30°C/86°F)
***P.* Vanda M. Pearman** ■ (*P. bellatum* x *P. delenatii*). Terrestrial orchid with elliptic to strap-shaped leaves, to 25cm (10in) long, mottled grey and dark green above, purple beneath. From spring to summer, white flowers, 9cm (3½in) across, with pink-flushed pouches, are borne singly or in pairs. ↕ 20cm (8in), ↔ 18cm (7in). ❄ (min. 13°C/55°F; max. 30°C/86°F)
P. venustum ■ Terrestrial orchid with ovate-lance-shaped leaves, to 25cm (10in) long, mottled grey-green and purple. From winter to spring, bears solitary flowers, 8cm (3in) across, with green and rose-red, maroon-spotted petals, green-striped white upper sepals, and yellowish green to reddish brown, prominently veined pouches. ↕↔ 15cm (6in). Himalayas. ❄ (min. 10°C/50°F; max. 30°C/86°F)
P. villosum ■ Terrestrial orchid with strap-shaped, dull mid-green leaves, 25–40cm (10–16in) long. Solitary, glossy, red-brown flowers, 8cm (3in) across, with green and brown upper sepals and light yellow-bronze to green pouches, appear from winter to spring. ↕↔ 15cm (6in). N.E. India, Burma, Thailand, Laos. ❄ (min. 13°C/55°F; max. 30°C/86°F)
***P.* Vintage Harvest 'Applemint'** ■ (*P.* Chianti x *P.* Golden Acres). Terrestrial orchid with strap-shaped, dark green leaves, 15cm (6in) long. In winter, bears solitary, green-yellow flowers, 12cm (5in) across, with cream margins on the upper sepals, turning gold. ↕ 30cm (12in), ↔ 20cm (8in). ❄ (min. 13°C/55°F; max. 30°C/86°F)

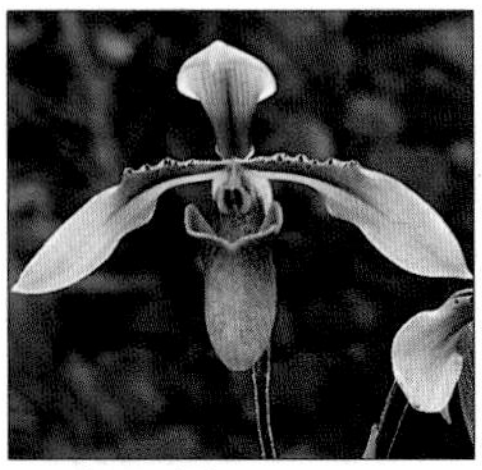
Paphiopedilum appletonianum

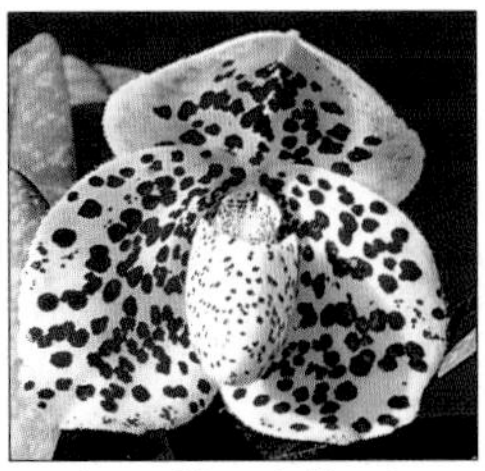
Paphiopedilum bellatulum

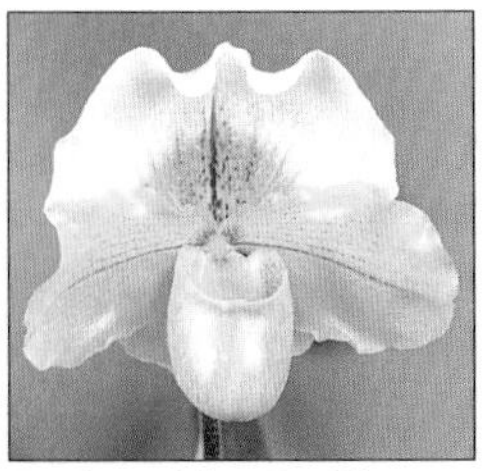
Paphiopedilum Buckhurst 'Mont Millais'

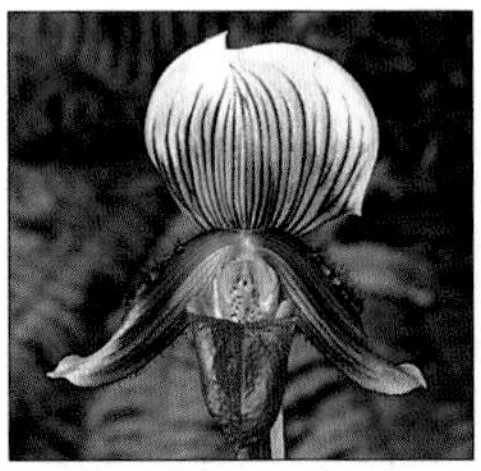
Paphiopedilum callosum

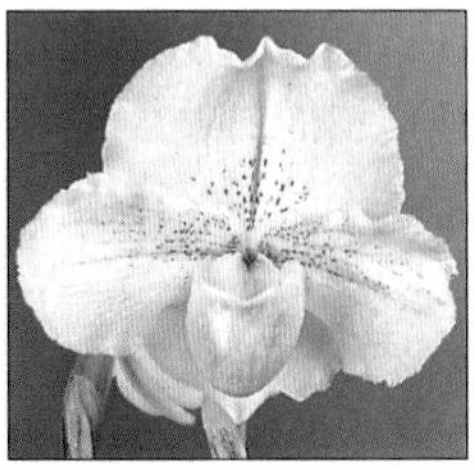
Paphiopedilum Freckles

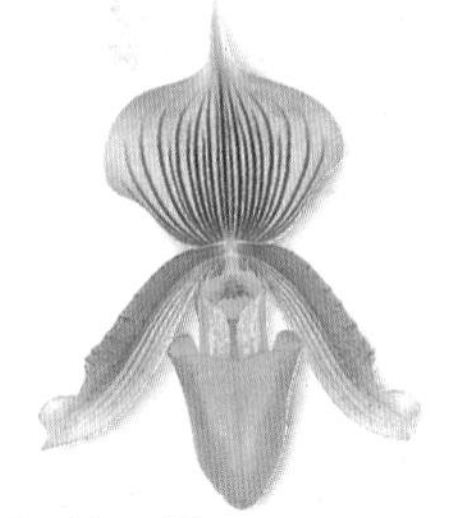
Paphiopedilum Goultenianum 'Album'

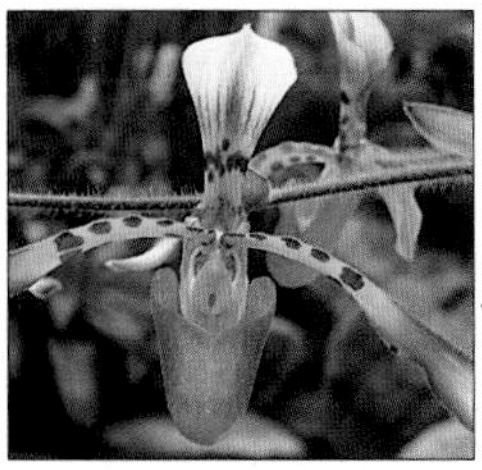
Paphiopedilum haynaldianum

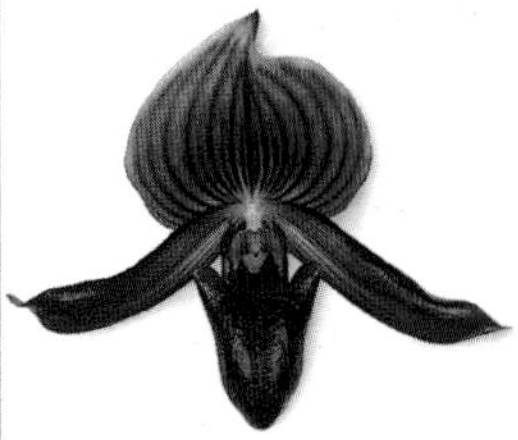
Paphiopedilum Joanne's Wine

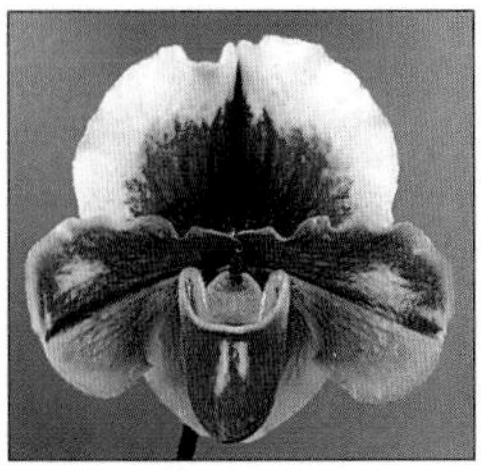
Paphiopedilum Lyric 'Glendora'

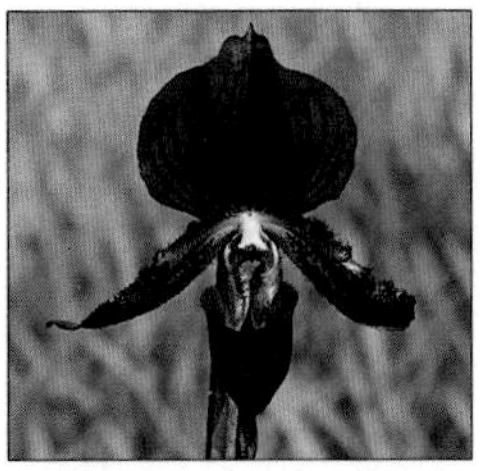
Paphiopedilum Maudiae 'Coloratum'

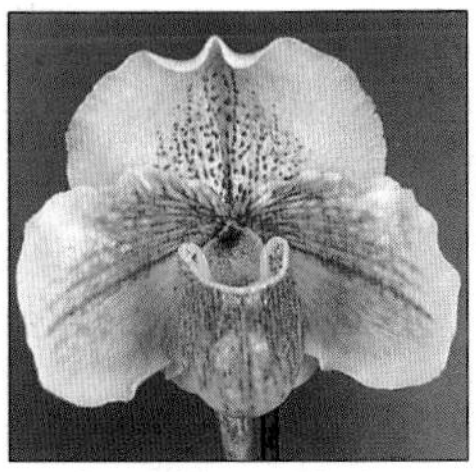
Paphiopedilum Miller's Daughter

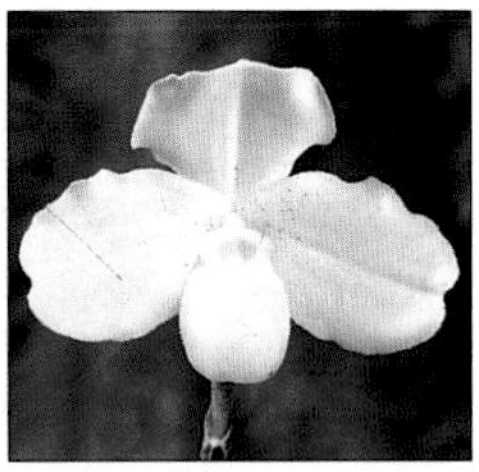
Paphiopedilum niveum

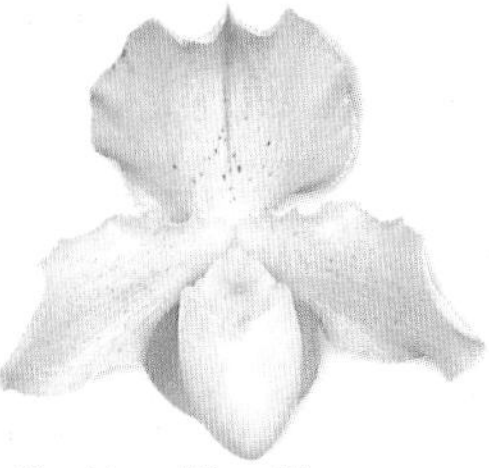
Paphiopedilum Silvara 'Jancis'

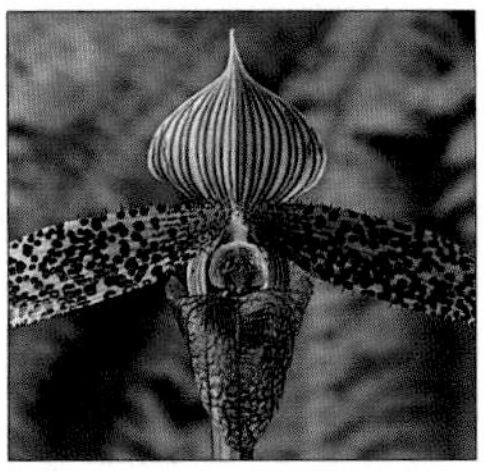
Paphiopedilum sukhakulii

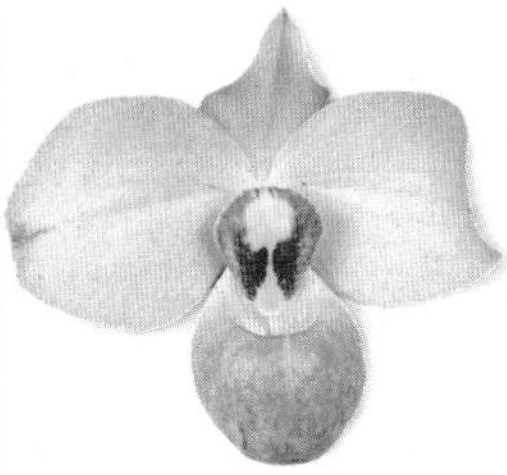
Paphiopedilum Vanda M. Pearman

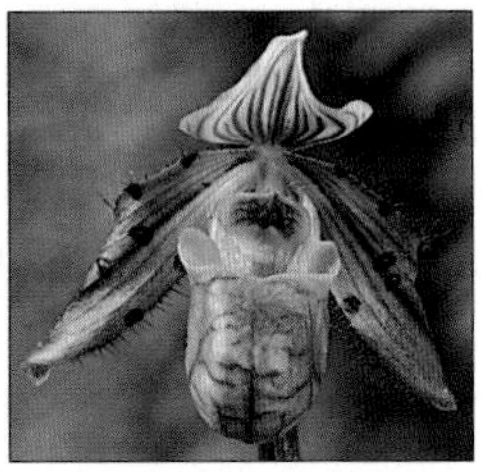
Paphiopedilum venustum

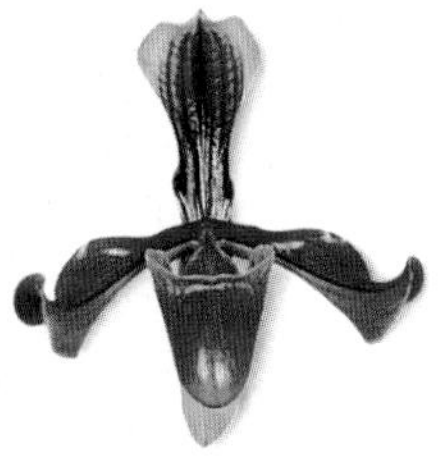
Paphiopedilum villosum

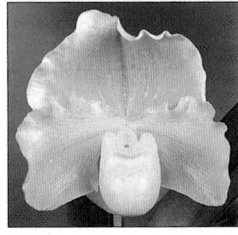

Paphiopedilum Vintage Harvest 'Applemint'

P

▷ **Paprika** see *Capsicum annuum*
▷ **Papyrus** see *Cyperus papyrus*
▷ **Parachute plant** see *Ceropegia sandersonii*

PARADISEA

Paradise lily, St. Bruno's lily

ASPHODELACEAE/LILIACEAE

Genus of 2 species of clump-forming perennials occurring in subalpine or damp meadows and woodland in S. Europe. They have short rhizomes with clustered, fleshy roots and linear, hairless, greyish green, basal leaves. They are cultivated for their loose racemes, borne on slender stems, of trumpet-shaped, 6-tepalled, fragrant flowers, which are excellent for cutting. Grow in a mixed or herbaceous border.

- **HARDINESS** Fully hardy.
- **CULTIVATION** Grow in humus-rich, fertile, moist but well-drained soil in full sun or dappled shade.
- **PROPAGATION** Sow seed in containers in a cold frame as soon as ripe or in spring. Divide after flowering, or in early spring.
- **PESTS AND DISEASES** Slugs may be a problem.

P. liliastrum. Clump-forming perennial producing short rhizomes and grass-like leaves, 12–25cm (5–10in) long. One-sided racemes of white flowers, 3–6cm (1¼–2½in) long, with conspicuous yellow anthers, are borne in late spring or early summer. ↕30–60cm (12–24in), ↔30cm (12in). Mountains of S. Europe. ❄❄❄. **'Major'** ▣ has larger flowers, 5–6cm (2–2½in) long.
P. lusitanicum. Upright, clump-forming perennial with basal rosettes of linear leaves, 30–40cm (12–16in) long. Racemes of 20–25 white flowers, 2cm (¾in) long, are borne in summer. ↕80–120cm (32–48in), ↔30–40cm (12–16in). Portugal, Spain. ❄❄❄

▷ **Paradise flower** see *Solanum wendlandii*

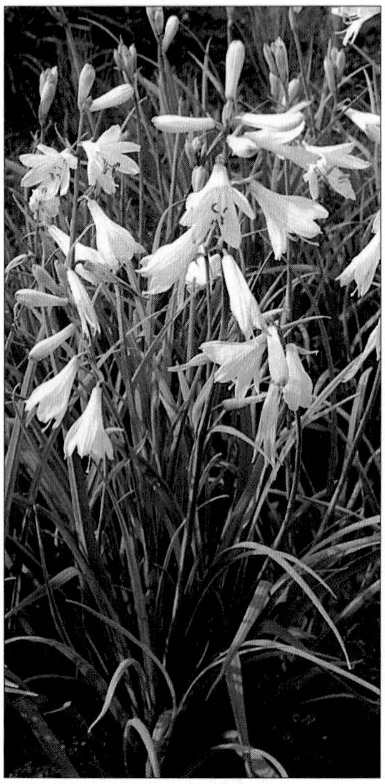

Paradisea liliastrum 'Major'

PARAHEBE syn. DERWENTIA

SCROPHULARIACEAE

Genus of about 30 species of evergreen or semi-evergreen subshrubs and perennials, often classified under *Hebe* or *Veronica*. Most are from Australia and New Zealand, with a few from Papua New Guinea, occurring mainly in sunny and dry, stony habitats or scree. They have woody-based stems, and produce opposite, usually more or less ovate, toothed, mid- to dark green or blue-green leaves, stalkless or with very short stalks. They are cultivated for their erect, axillary racemes of small, saucer-shaped, usually white, pink, lilac, or blue flowers, frequently with contrasting markings; each flower has 4, rarely 5, often pointed, unequal petals. Often mat-forming or decumbent, they are effective tumbling over walls or large rocks, or growing through shrubs, and are also suitable for a gravel bed.

- **HARDINESS** Fully hardy to frost hardy.
- **CULTIVATION** Grow in well-drained, poor to moderately fertile soil in full sun. In frost-prone climates, shelter from cold, drying winds.
- **PROPAGATION** Sow seed in containers in a cold frame as soon as ripe or in spring. Take semi-ripe cuttings in early or midsummer.
- **PESTS AND DISEASES** Slugs may eat young growth.

***P. x bidwillii* 'Kea'.** Prostrate, mat-forming, evergreen subshrub with oblong to obovate, leathery, dark green leaves, to 6mm (¼in) long. Produces short, slender racemes of saucer-shaped, crimson-veined white flowers, to 8mm (⅜in) across, in summer. ↕10cm (4in), ↔15cm (6in). ❄❄❄
P. catarractae ▣🏆 Decumbent or upright, evergreen subshrub with ovate to elliptic or lance-shaped, shallowly to sharply toothed, dark green leaves, to 4cm (1½in) long, tinged purple when young. In summer, produces racemes

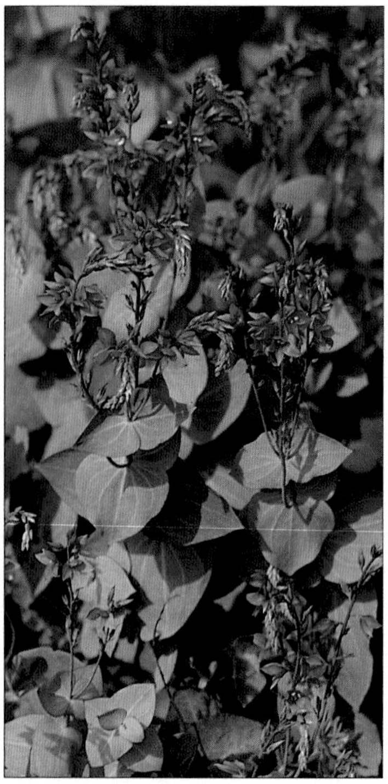

Parahebe perfoliata

of saucer-shaped, purple-veined white flowers, 1cm (½in) across, with red eyes. ↕↔ to 30cm (12in). New Zealand. ❄❄❄
P. hookeriana. Mat-forming, evergreen subshrub with crowded, overlapping, broadly ovate to oblong or oval, deeply toothed, leathery, sparsely hairy, mid-green leaves, to 1.5cm (½in) long. Saucer-shaped, white to lavender-blue flowers, to 1cm (½in) across, each usually with a crimson eye, are borne in racemes in summer. ↕15cm (6in), ↔50cm (20in). New Zealand (North Island). ❄❄❄
P. lyallii. Variable, prostrate, stem-rooting, semi-evergreen shrub with rounded to ovate, leathery, toothed to scalloped, dark green leaves, to 1cm (½in) long. In early summer, bears dense racemes of saucer-shaped, usually purple-veined, white to pink flowers, 1cm (½in) across, with red eyes. ↕25cm (10in), ↔50cm (20in). New Zealand. ❄❄❄
P. perfoliata ▣🏆 syn. *Veronica perfoliata* (Digger's speedwell). Woody-based, evergreen perennial with arching, spreading stems. Bears pairs of broadly ovate, toothed, slightly leathery, glaucous, blue- or grey-green leaves, 5cm (2in) long, overlapping at the bases, each pair arranged at right-angles to the next pair. In late summer, produces racemes of saucer-shaped blue flowers, 6–10mm (¼–½in) across. ↕60–75cm (24–30in), ↔45cm (18in). S.E. Australia. ❄❄

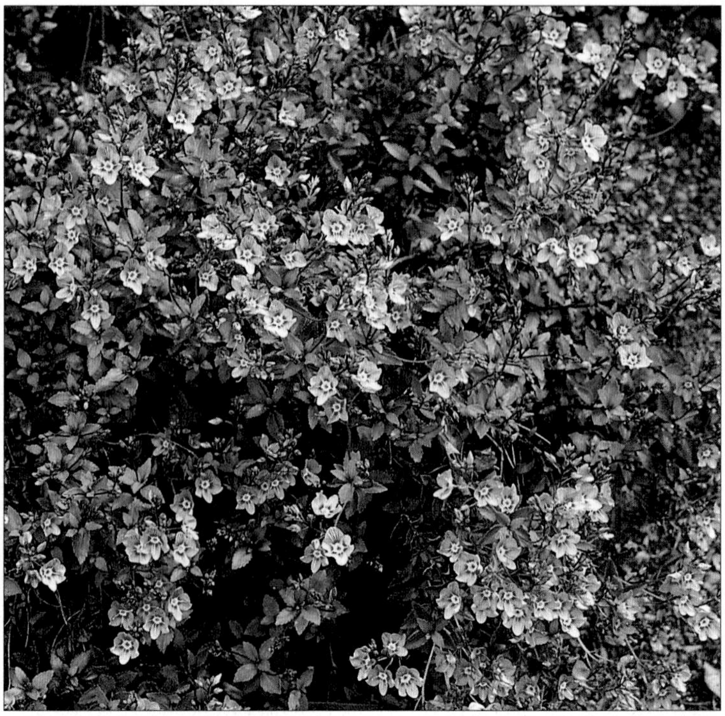

Parahebe catarractae

▷ **Parapara** see *Pisonia umbellifera*

PARAQUILEGIA

RANUNCULACEAE

Genus of 4–6 species of tufted perennials occurring in rock crevices and scree in the Himalayas and mountains of C. Asia and China. They are grown for their solitary, short-stalked, cup-shaped flowers, produced in spring, and for their fern-like, ternate to 3-ternate, often grey or blue-green leaves, arranged alternately. These attractive alpines are suitable for a scree bed, trough, or alpine house, but may be difficult to establish; they grow best in climates with cool summers and cold, dry winters.

- **HARDINESS** Fully hardy.
- **CULTIVATION** Outdoors, grow in poor, sharply drained, alkaline soil in full sun. Protect from winter wet. In an alpine house, grow in a mix of equal parts loam, leaf mould, and grit.
- **PROPAGATION** Sow seed in containers in an open frame as soon as ripe.
- **PESTS AND DISEASES** Susceptible to aphids and red spider mites under glass, and prone to damage by slugs and snails.

P. anemonoides ▣ syn. *P. grandiflora.* Tufted perennial producing long-stalked, 2- or 3-ternate, blue-green leaves, 3cm (1¼in) long, with many, deeply lobed segments. In late spring, produces violet-blue, purple-blue, or pale lilac, occasionally white flowers, 2.5cm (1in) across, with golden nectaries and yellow anthers. ↕↔ to 10cm (4in). C. Asia, Himalayas, W. China. ❄❄❄
P. grandiflora see *P. anemonoides.*

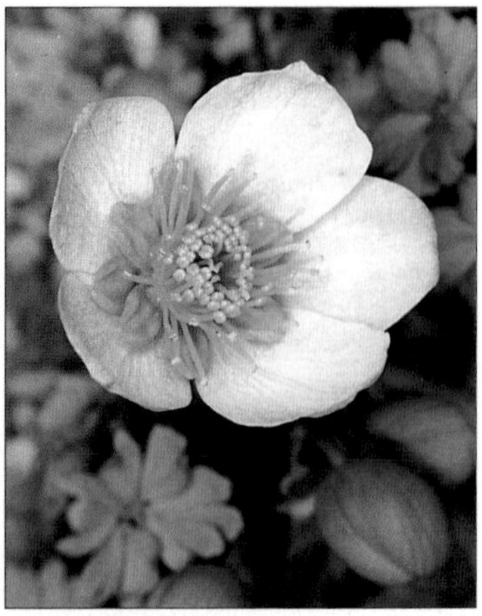

Paraquilegia anemonoides

▷ ***Paraserianthes*** see *Albizia*
P. lophantha see *A. lophantha*
▷ **Parasol tree, Chinese** see *Firmiana simplex*
▷ **Parilla, Yellow** see *Menispermum canadense*

PARIS *syn.* DAISWA

TRILLIACEAE

Genus of about 20 species of rhizomatous perennials occurring in woodland from Europe to the Caucasus, and from the Himalayas to E. Asia. Erect stems each bear a whorl of 4 or more very variable, lance-shaped to ovate, mid- or dark green leaves, just below a solitary, terminal, wheel-shaped, spider-like, or star-shaped flower, with protruding stamens. The flowers are followed by fleshy, capsular fruits with shiny, black or red seeds; these may cause mild stomach upset if ingested. Suitable for a woodland or peat garden.
• **HARDINESS** Fully hardy.
• **CULTIVATION** Grow in moist, fertile, leafy soil in full or partial shade. Leave plants undisturbed to increase year by year.
• **PROPAGATION** Sow seed in containers outdoors in autumn. Divide after the foliage has died down.
• **PESTS AND DISEASES** Slugs may attack rhizomes and young growth.

P. polyphylla, syn. *Daiswa polyphylla.* Slowly spreading perennial with short rhizomes and erect, smooth stems, each producing a whorl of 6–12 oblong to inversely lance-shaped, mid-green leaves, 8–18cm (3–7in) long, rounded at the bases. Solitary, spider-like flowers, each consisting of 4–8 narrow green outer tepals, 2.5–10cm (1–4in) long, and thread-like, yellowish green inner tepals, to 10cm (4in) long, with numerous stamens, are borne in summer. Angled, almost spherical green capsules, to 2cm (¾in) across, split to reveal shiny red seeds when ripe. ↕ 60–90cm (24–36in), ↔ 30cm (12in). Himalayas to Burma, Thailand, W. China. ❄❄❄
P. quadrifolia. Upright perennial with creeping rhizomes and erect stems, each with a whorl of usually 4, sometimes 5 or 6, ovate, mid-green leaves, 5–15cm (2–6in) long. In late spring, bears solitary, star-shaped flowers, 4–7cm (1½–3in) across, with mid-green outer tepals, white inner tepals, and twice as many stamens as inner tepals. Bears blue-black, spherical, berry-like capsules, 1cm (½in) across. ↕ 15–40cm (6–16in), ↔ 30cm (12in). Eurasia. ❄❄❄

PARKINSONIA

CAESALPINIACEAE/LEGUMINOSAE

Genus of more than 12 species of deciduous or evergreen shrubs and trees from dry savannah or scrubland in the drier regions of Africa, S. North America, and Central America. They are grown for their attractive flowers and delicate foliage. The branches have pairs of spines at each node, and bear alternate, 2- or 3-pinnate leaves with very small, light to mid- or yellow-green leaflets. The mostly yellow, red-spotted flowers, with spreading, clawed petals, are borne in short, usually axillary racemes from the upper leaf nodes, followed by leathery or woody, pea-like pods. Grow as specimen trees. In frost-prone areas, grow in a cool or temperate greenhouse.

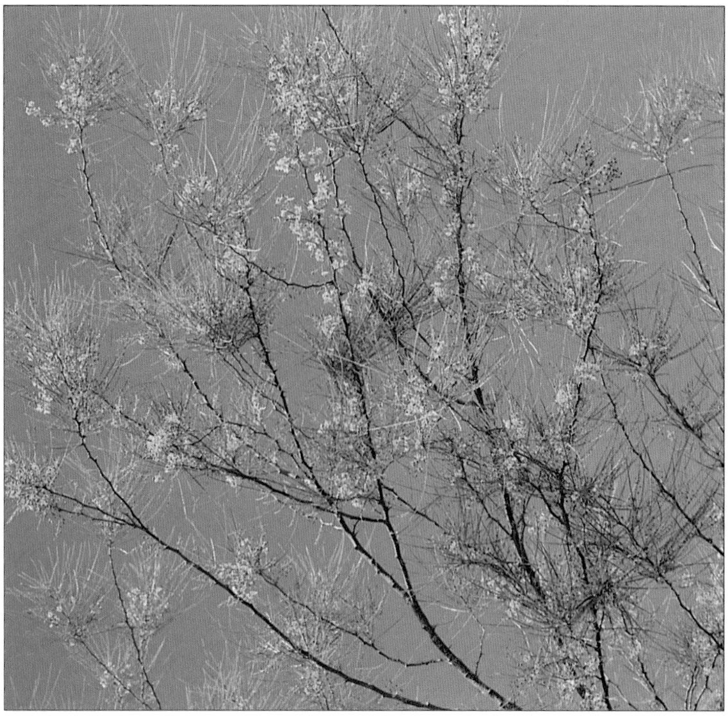

Parkinsonia aculeata

• **HARDINESS** Frost tender.
• **CULTIVATION** Under glass, grow in loam-based potting compost (JI No.3) in full light, with low humidity. From spring to summer, water moderately and apply a balanced liquid fertilizer every month. Water sparingly in winter. Outdoors, grow in fertile, well-drained soil in full sun. Pruning group 1; may need restrictive pruning under glass, after flowering.
• **PROPAGATION** Sow seed at 18–21°C (64–70°F) in spring.
• **PESTS AND DISEASES** Red spider mites may be a problem under glass.

P. aculeata ■ ♀ (Jerusalem thorn). Small, spreading, often weeping, deciduous tree, or occasionally large shrub, bearing spiny green stems and branchlets. Slender, 2-pinnate, stalkless, mid-green leaves, to 30cm (12in) long, have distinctive flat midribs and many tiny, ovate to oblong leaflets, 2–5mm (1/16–¼in) long, often quickly deciduous; they fold up at night. In spring, bears racemes of 2–15 cup-shaped, bright yellow flowers, to 2cm (¾in) across, with orange-spotted standard petals and orange-red stamens. ↕ to 10m (30ft), ↔ 5–8m (15–25ft). S. USA, Mexico; widely naturalized in tropical and subtropical regions. ⊛ (min. 5°C/41°F)

PARNASSIA

Bog star, Grass of Parnassus

PARNASSIACEAE/SAXIFRAGACEAE

Genus of 15 species of herbaceous perennials found in bogs in temperate regions in the N. hemisphere. They produce basal rosettes of broadly ovate, heart-, or kidney-shaped, mid- to dark green leaves. They are grown for their large, solitary, bowl- or saucer-shaped, white to pale yellow flowers, with yellow, nectar-bearing staminodes, borne on upright stems in spring, summer, or early autumn. Grow in wet soil in a rock garden or bog garden.
• **HARDINESS** Fully hardy.
• **CULTIVATION** Grow in humus-rich, poor to moderately fertile, wet but not stagnant soil in full sun.
• **PROPAGATION** Sow seed in containers in a cold frame in autumn; keep moist. Divide in autumn or spring.
• **PESTS AND DISEASES** Susceptible to slug and snail damage.

P. fimbriata. Rosette-forming perennial with kidney-shaped, mid-green basal leaves, 2–5cm (¾–2in) long, and long-stalked, broadly ovate stem leaves, 2cm (¾in) long. Solitary, bowl-shaped white flowers, 3–4cm (1¼–1½in) across, are borne in late summer and early autumn. ↕↔ 20–60cm (8–24in). North America (Alaska to California). ❄❄❄
P. palustris ■ (Grass of Parnassus). Rosette-forming perennial with ovate, heart-shaped, pale green leaves, to 3cm (1¼in) long. Slender stems bear solitary, green-veined white flowers, 2.5cm (1in) across, with yellow nectar glands, in late spring and early summer. ↕ 20cm (8in), ↔ 10cm (4in). N. temperate regions. ❄❄❄

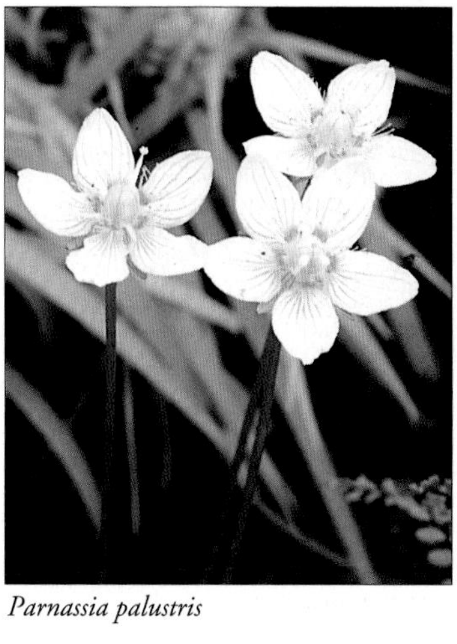

Parnassia palustris

PAROCHETUS

LEGUMINOSAE/PAPILIONACEAE

Genus of 2 species (often confused in cultivation) of trailing, deciduous or evergreen perennials found in montane habitats in E. Africa, the Himalayas to Sri Lanka, S.W. China, and S.E. Asia. They are grown for their clover-like leaves and bright blue, occasionally white, pea-like flowers. Grow in a rock garden or alpine house. *P. africana* is ideal in a hanging basket.
• **HARDINESS** Fully hardy to half hardy.
• **CULTIVATION** Grow in any moist but well-drained soil in partial shade, but protect from winter wet. Plants may be short-lived, so propagate regularly and overwinter young plants under glass. In an alpine house, grow in a mix of equal parts loam-based potting compost (JI No.2), leaf mould, and grit.
• **PROPAGATION** Divide in spring, or separate rooted runners when in growth.
• **PESTS AND DISEASES** May be damaged by slugs and snails.

P. africana ■ (Shamrock pea). Prostrate, mat-forming, non-tuberous, evergreen perennial with freely rooting stems. Each leaf has 3 inversely heart-shaped, rich dark green leaflets, to 3cm (1¼in) long, with bold, dark brown horseshoe markings. Solitary or paired, bright blue flowers, 2.5cm (1in) across, are borne mainly from late autumn to late spring. ↕ 10cm (4in), ↔ 60–100cm (24–39in). Mountains of E. Africa. ❄
P. communis ♀ Prostrate, tuberous-rooted, deciduous perennial with trailing stems. Leaves are divided into 3 inversely heart-shaped, mid-green leaflets, to 2cm (¾in) long, with irregular bronze-brown horseshoe markings. Produces a succession of solitary or paired, bright blue flowers, 2.5cm (1in) across, in late summer and autumn. ↕ 10cm (4in), ↔ 30cm (12in) or more. Himalayas to Sri Lanka, S.W. China, S.E. Asia. ❄❄❄

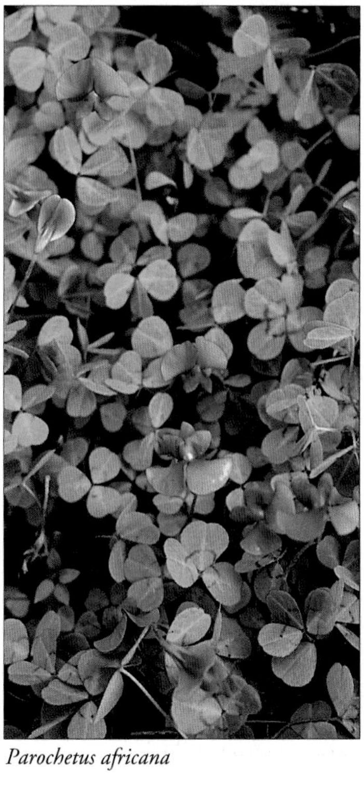

Parochetus africana

PARODIA syn. ERIOCACTUS, NOTOCACTUS, WIGGINSIA

CACTACEAE

Genus of 35–50 species of simple or clustering, mainly spherical, many-ribbed, spiny, perennial cacti, sometimes becoming columnar and sometimes offsetting from the bases. The genus includes many species transferred from *Eriocactus*, *Notocactus*, and *Wigginsia*. They occur mainly in the highlands of Colombia, Brazil, Bolivia, Paraguay, Argentina, and Uruguay. Solitary, diurnal, bell- to funnel-shaped flowers develop near or at the crowns. Where temperatures drop below 10°C (50°F), grow in a warm greenhouse. In warmer climates, use in a desert garden.

- **HARDINESS** Frost tender.
- **CULTIVATION** Under glass, grow in standard cactus compost in full or bright filtered light. From mid-spring to late summer, water moderately and apply a low-nitrogen liquid fertilizer every 6–8 weeks. Keep barely moist at other times. Outdoors, grow in sharply drained, moderately fertile soil in full sun, with some midday shade. See also pp.48–49.
- **PROPAGATION** Sow seed at 19–24°C (66–75°F) in spring or summer.
- **PESTS AND DISEASES** Vulnerable to mealybugs and, while flowering, aphids.

P. brevihamata ■ syn. *Notocactus brevihamatus*. Simple or clustering cactus producing spherical, olive-green stems, each with 20–26 closely set ribs, rounded tubercles, white to yellow areoles, and yellow, later brownish

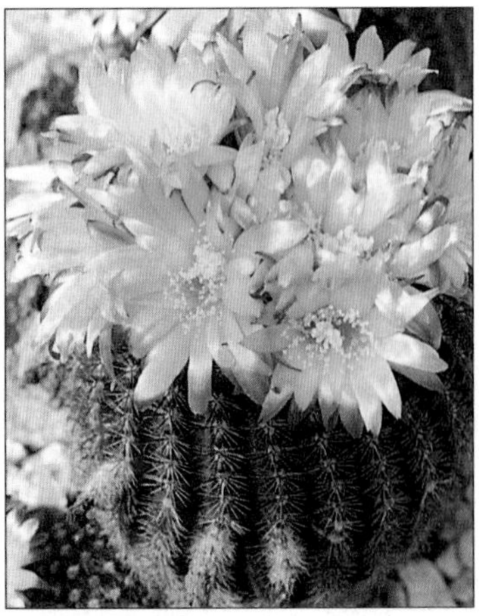

Parodia brevihamata

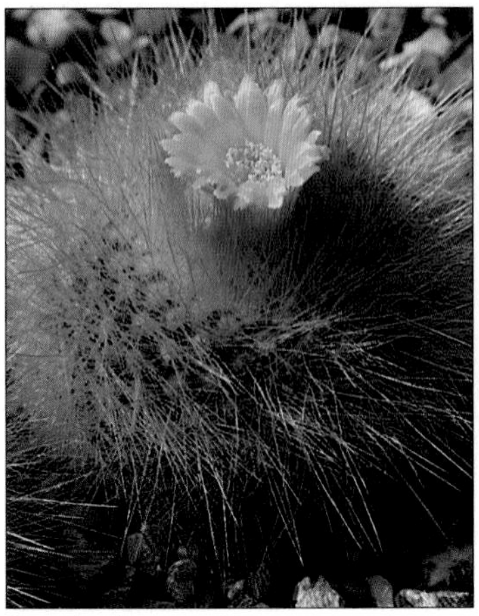

Parodia chrysacanthion

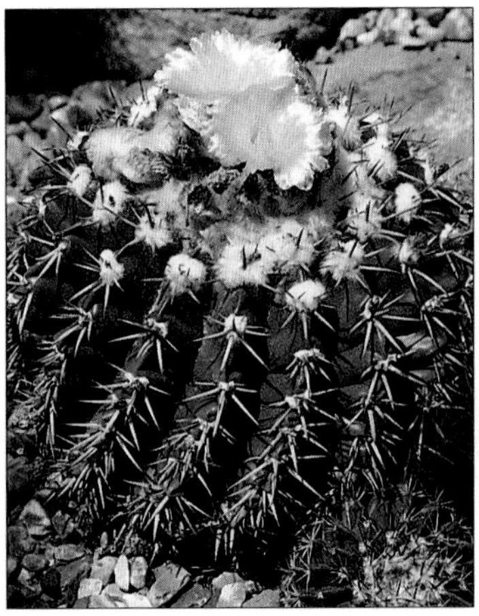

Parodia erinacea

yellow spines (about 16 radials, 1–4 slightly longer centrals). Funnel-shaped, lemon-yellow, sometimes red-tinted flowers, 4cm (1½in) across, are borne in spring. ↕↔ to 6cm (2½in). S. Brazil. ❄ (min. 10°C/50°F)

P. chrysacanthion ■ Simple cactus producing a spherical to depressed-spherical, pale green stem with about 24 spirally arranged, warty ribs, and the crown covered with thick yellow wool. Yellowish white areoles bear yellow spines (30–40 fine radials, 1 or more centrals). Funnel-shaped yellow flowers, 2cm (¾in) across, develop in spring. ↕ 8–12cm (3–5in), ↔ 10cm (4in). N. Argentina. ❄ (min. 10°C/50°F)

P. claviceps, syn. *Notocactus claviceps*. Simple or clustering cactus producing spherical to short-cylindrical, dark green stems, each with 23–30 ribs. White areoles bear wide-spreading, semi-pendent, yellow spines (5–8 radials, 1–3 centrals). Funnel-shaped, sulphur-yellow flowers, 5cm (2in) across, appear in summer. ↕ 10–50cm (4–20in), ↔ 12cm (5in). S. Brazil. ❄ (min. 10°C/50°F)

P. concinna, syn. *Eriocactus apricus*, *Notocactus apricus*, *N. concinnus*. Simple cactus producing a flattened-spherical, 15- to 32-ribbed, dark green stem with a woolly crown, white areoles, and white, pale yellow, brown, or red-brown spines (10–12 radials, 4–6 or more, longer, slightly darker centrals). Funnel-shaped, red-tipped, deep lemon-yellow flowers, 5–8cm (2–3in) across, are produced in spring. ↕ to 6cm (2½in), ↔ 10cm (4in). S. Brazil, Uruguay. ❄ (min. 10°C/50°F)

P. erinacea ■ syn. *Wigginsia erinacea*, *W. vorwerkiana*. Freely offsetting cactus

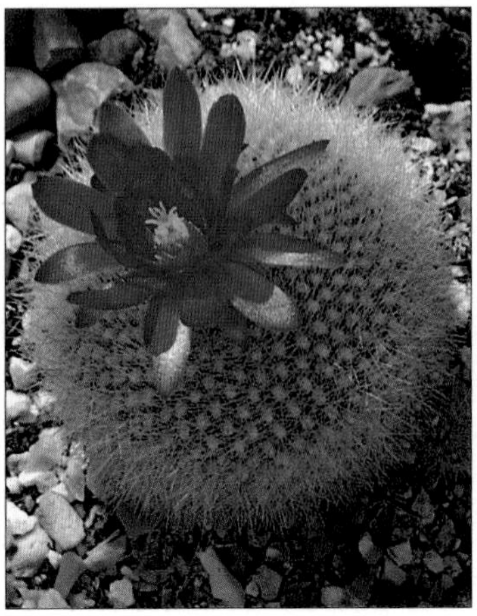

Parodia haselbergii

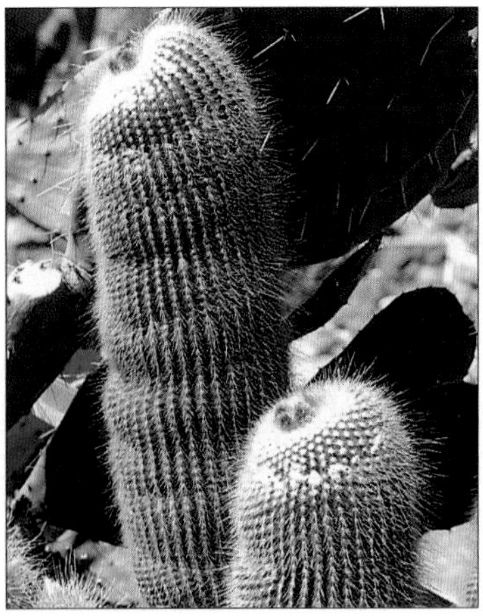

Parodia leninghausii

with spherical to short-cylindrical, light to dark green stems, 6–30cm (2½–12in) thick, each with 15–30 spiralling ribs, grey areoles, and off-white, grey, or brown spines (2–12 radials, 1 longer central). In summer, bears funnel-shaped, glossy yellow flowers, 4cm (1½in) across. ↕ 15cm (6in) or more, ↔ 25cm (10in). S. Brazil, Uruguay, N.E. Argentina. ❄ (min. 10°C/50°F)

P. graessneri, syn. *Notocactus graessneri*. Simple cactus producing a spherical, dark green stem with an angled, spiny crown and 50–60 heavily warty ribs. White areoles bear both pale to golden yellow and pale brown to white spines (about 55 radials, 5 or 6 centrals). In spring, bears funnel-shaped, pale yellow-green flowers, 2cm (¾in) across. ↕ 10–15cm (4–6in), ↔ 10cm (4in). S. Brazil. ❄ (min. 10°C/50°F)

P. haselbergii ■ syn. *Notocactus haselbergii* (Scarlet ball cactus). Simple cactus, rarely offsetting from the base, with a spherical, greyish green stem, to 15cm (6in) thick, with a woolly crown set at an angle, and with 30–60 or more ribs. White-woolly areoles produce yellowish white to yellow spines (25–60 radials, 3–5 slightly longer centrals). Funnel-shaped, bright orange-red or orange-yellow flowers, 1.5cm (½in) across, appear from winter to spring. ↕ 4–15cm (1½–6in), ↔ 18cm (7in) in clusters. S. Brazil. ❄ (min. 10°C/50°F)

P. leninghausii ■ syn. *Eriocactus leninghausii*. Simple or clustering cactus with spherical, later columnar, mid-green stems, each to 10cm (4in) thick, with a woolly crown set at an angle, and with 30–35 ribs. White-woolly areoles bear pale yellow, deeper yellow, or pale brown spines (15–20 or more radials, 3 or 4 centrals). Funnel-shaped, bright yellow or lemon flowers, 4–5cm (1½–2in) across, are borne in summer. ↕ to 60cm (24in), ↔ 20cm (8in) in clusters. S. Brazil. ❄ (min. 10°C/50°F)

P. liliputana see *Blossfeldia liliputana*.

P. magnifica, syn. *Notocactus magnifica*. Simple, sometimes clustering cactus with spherical, later columnar, 11- to 15-ribbed, bluish green stems, to 15cm (6in) thick. Grey-felted areoles bear yellow or brown spines (12–15 or more radials, up to 12 longer centrals). Funnel-shaped, sulphur-yellow flowers, 5cm (2in) across, develop in summer. ↕ 7–15cm (3–6in), ↔ to 45cm (18in). S. Brazil. ❄ (min. 10°C/50°F)

P. mammulosa ■ syn. *Notocactus mammulosus*, *N. submammulosus*. Simple cactus producing a spherical, dark green stem with a woolly crown and 13–21 heavily warty ribs. White areoles bear white, off-white, grey, or pale brown spines (6–25 radials, 2–4 longer centrals). Funnel-shaped, pale to golden yellow flowers, 3.5–5cm (1½–2in) across, with bold red stigmas, develop in summer. ↕ 10–13cm (4–5in), ↔ 6cm (2½in). S. Brazil, Uruguay, N.E. Argentina. ❄ (min. 10°C/50°F)

P. microsperma, syn. *P. mutabilis* var. *sanguiniflora*, *P. sanguiniflora*. Simple cactus producing a depressed-spherical to spherical, sometimes cylindrical, mid-green stem with 15–21 warty ribs. White areoles bear white and red to brown spines (10–25 radials, 3 or 4 longer centrals). Funnel-shaped, yellow

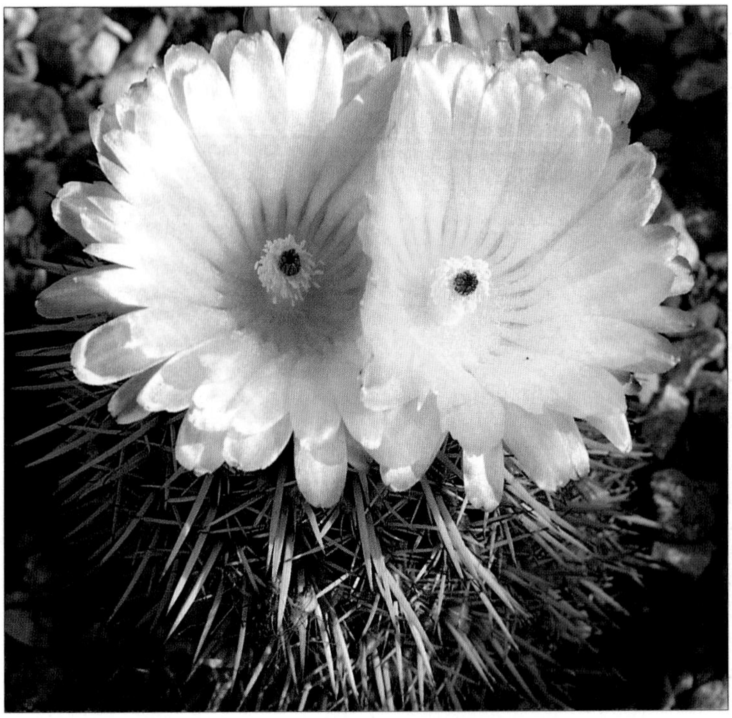

Parodia mammulosa

or red flowers, 3.5cm (1½in) across, are borne from spring to summer. ↕ 20cm (8in), ↔ 10cm (4in). N. Argentina. ❀ (min. 10°C/50°F)
P. mutabilis, syn. *Notocactus mutabilis.* Simple cactus producing a spherical, glaucous, mid-green stem with a white-woolly, brown-spiny crown and 25 or more, spirally arranged, warty ribs. White-woolly areoles bear white and yellow, reddish brown, or orange-brown spines (20–50 fine, almost hair-like, radials, 4–10 strong, sometimes hooked centrals). Funnel-shaped, golden yellow flowers, 3–5cm (1¼–2in) across, are produced from spring to summer. ↕↔ 8cm (3in). N. Argentina. ❀ (min. 10°C/50°F). **var. *sanguiniflora*** see *P. microsperma.*
P. nivosa ■ Simple cactus producing a spherical to short-cylindrical, dull green stem with a white-woolly crown and 16–20 spirally arranged, warty ribs. White-felted areoles have white spines (15–20 radials, 3–5 longer centrals). Funnel-shaped, brilliant red flowers, 3cm (1¼in) across, develop in spring. ↕ 15cm (6in), ↔ 6cm (2½in). N. Argentina. ❀ (min. 10°C/50°F)
P. ocampoi. Clustering cactus with spherical to short-cylindrical, 13- to 20-ribbed, dark green stems, 6cm (2½in) thick, with grey areoles and pale reddish brown spines (8 or 9 radials, 1 smaller central). Funnel-shaped, golden yellow flowers, 3cm (1¼in) across, are borne from spring to summer. ↕ 7–20cm (3–8in), ↔ 15cm (6in). C. Bolivia. ❀ (min. 10°C/50°F)
P. ottonis, syn. *Notocactus ottonis.* Variable, simple, later clustering cactus with spherical or cylindrical, 6- to 15-ribbed, light or dark green or bluish or purplish green stems, 5–15cm (2–6in) thick, each with a white-woolly crown. Pale brown-woolly areoles produce off-white to yellow and brown spines (10–18 radials, 3–6 centrals). Funnel-shaped, deep yellow, rarely orange-red flowers, 4–6cm (1½–2½in) across, are borne in summer. ↕ 3–15cm (1¼–6in), ↔ 18cm (7in). S. Brazil, S. Paraguay, N.E. Argentina, Uruguay. ❀ (min. 10°C/50°F)
P. penicillata ♀ syn. *Notocactus penicillata.* Simple, spherical, later cylindrical cactus producing a mid-green stem with about 17–20 spiralling ribs and close-set tubercles. Brown-woolly areoles bear white, off-white, pale yellow, or pale brown spines (about 40 radials, 10–20 centrals). In summer,

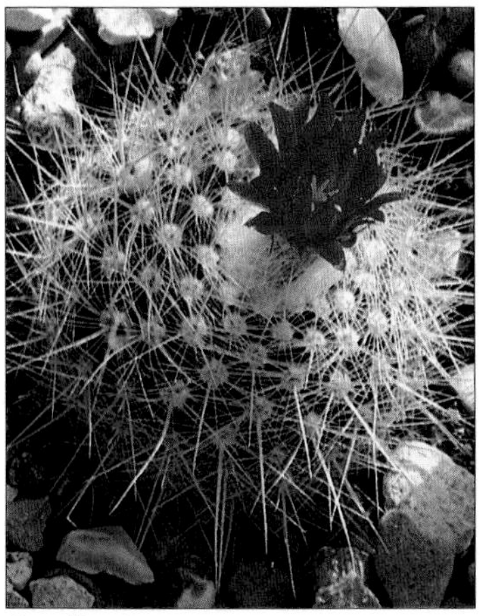

Parodia nivosa

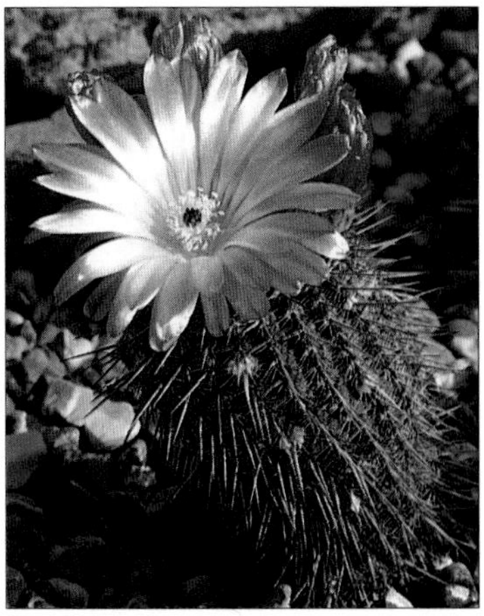

Parodia rutilans

bears funnel-shaped, orange-yellow or vermilion-red flowers, 5cm (2in) across. ↕ 30cm (12in), ↔ 12cm (5in). N. Argentina. ❀ (min. 10°C/50°F)
P. rutilans ■ syn. *Notocactus rutilans.* Simple cactus producing a spherical to cylindrical, bluish dark green stem with a slightly sunken, white-woolly crown and 18–24 spirally arranged ribs. White-woolly areoles produce reddish brown and brown-tipped white spines (14–16 radials, 2 slightly longer centrals). In summer, bears funnel-shaped flowers, 3–4cm (1¼–1½in) across, with pink-tipped petals and yellowish white throats. ↕↔ 5cm (2in). N. Uruguay. ❀ (min. 10°C/50°F)
P. sanguiniflora see *P. microsperma.*
P. schumanniana. Usually simple cactus producing a spherical to cylindrical, mid-green stem with 21–48 straight, acute ribs. White-woolly areoles bear golden yellow, brown, or reddish brown, later grey spines (about 4 radials, 3 or 4 shorter centrals). Produces funnel-shaped, lemon to golden yellow flowers, 4.5–7cm (1¾–3in) across, in summer. ↕ to 1.8m (6ft), ↔ 30cm (12in). S. Paraguay, N.E. Argentina. ❀ (min. 10°C/50°F)
P. scopa, syn. *Notocactus scopa* (Silver ball cactus). Simple or clustering cactus with spherical to cylindrical, 25- to 40-ribbed, dark green stems with spiny, woolly crowns. Grey areoles bear white, pale yellow, red, or brown spines (35–40 or more radials, 3 or 4 longer centrals). Funnel-shaped, bright yellow flowers, 4cm (1½in) across, appear in summer. ↕ 5–50cm (2–20in), ↔ 10cm (4in). S. Brazil, Uruguay. ❀ (min. 10°C/50°F)

PARONYCHIA

Whitlow-wort

CARYOPHYLLACEAE/ILLECEBRACEAE

Genus of about 50 species of annuals and evergreen, mat-forming perennials found mainly in hot, dry habitats around the Mediterranean and in N. Africa, with some in North America. They have linear to lance-shaped, silvery green leaves and dense, axillary cymes of very small, cup-shaped flowers surrounded by conspicuous, translucent silver bracts. Cultivated for their flowers and foliage, they are good carpeting plants for a rock garden.
• **HARDINESS** Fully hardy to half hardy.
• **CULTIVATION** Grow in sharply drained, poor to moderately fertile soil in full sun.
• **PROPAGATION** Divide in spring. Take stem-tip cuttings in early summer.
• **PESTS AND DISEASES** Trouble free.

P. capitata, syn. *P. nivea.* Vigorous, mat-forming perennial with linear-lance-shaped to oblong, silvery grey-green leaves, to 6mm (¼in) long. In summer, bears tiny green flowers in cymes to 1cm (½in) across, enclosed by ornamental, ovate, silvery, papery bracts. ↕ 5cm (2in), ↔ to 30cm (12in). Mediterranean. ✻✻✻
P. kapela* subsp. *serpyllifolia. Very compact, mat-forming perennial with ovate to lance-shaped or elliptic, silvery bluish green leaves, to 4mm (⅛in) long. In summer, bears tiny, greenish white flowers in cymes to 2cm (¾in) across, enclosed by silvery white, papery bracts. ↕ to 5cm (2in), ↔ to 20cm (8in). Mediterranean. ✻✻✻
P. nivea see *P. capitata.*

▷**Parrot feather** see *Myriophyllum aquaticum*

PARROTIA

HAMAMELIDACEAE

Genus of one species of deciduous tree occurring in forests in the Caucasus and N. Iran. *P. persica* is cultivated for its simple, alternate, rich green foliage, attractively coloured in autumn, for its peeling bark, and for its petalless flowers with bright red stamens, borne in dense clusters along the branches in late winter or early spring. Grow as a specimen tree, or in an open site in woodland.
• **HARDINESS** Fully hardy, but flower buds may be damaged by harsh frosts.
• **CULTIVATION** Grow in deep, fertile, moist but well-drained soil in full sun or partial shade. Grow in acid soil for best autumn colour. Pruning group 1.
• **PROPAGATION** Sow seed in containers in a cold frame in autumn. Take greenwood cuttings in early summer, or semi-ripe cuttings in mid- and late summer.
• **PESTS AND DISEASES** Trouble free.

P. persica ■ ♀ ♀ (Persian ironwood). Dense, spreading, short-trunked tree with peeling, grey and fawn bark when mature. Obovate, glossy, rich green leaves, to 12cm (5in) long, turn yellow, orange, and red-purple in autumn. Tiny, spider-like red flowers are borne in spherical clusters, 1cm (½in) across, in late winter or early spring, before the leaves. ↕ 8m (25ft), ↔ 10m (30ft). Caucasus, N. Iran. ✻✻✻. **'Pendula'** ♀ is very compact and weeping. ↕ 1.5m (5ft), ↔ 3m (10ft).

PARROTIOPSIS

HAMAMELIDACEAE

Genus of one species of deciduous shrub found in forests in the W. Himalayas. It is cultivated for its showy flowerheads of petalless flowers, each with 20 or more yellow stamens surrounded by large bracts. Leaves are simple and arranged alternately. Grow as a specimen shrub.
• **HARDINESS** Fully hardy; but late frosts may damage flowerheads.
• **CULTIVATION** Grow in deep, fertile, preferably lime-free, moist but well-drained soil in full sun or partial shade. Pruning group 1.
• **PROPAGATION** Sow seed in containers in a cold frame in autumn. Take greenwood cuttings in early summer, or semi-ripe cuttings in late summer.
• **PESTS AND DISEASES** Trouble free.

P. jacquemontiana ♀ Upright shrub, or sometimes small tree, with very broadly ovate to ovate, mid-green leaves, to 10cm (4in) long. From mid-spring to early summer, bears spider-like flowerheads, to 5cm (2in) across, consisting of yellow-anthered stamens surrounded by conspicuous white bracts. ↕ 6m (20ft), ↔ 4m (12ft). W. Himalayas. ✻✻✻

▷**Parrot leaf** see *Alternanthera ficoidea*
▷**Parrot's beak** see *Lotus berthelotii*
▷**Parrot's bill** see *Clianthus puniceus*
▷**Parrot's flower** see *Heliconia psittacorum*

P

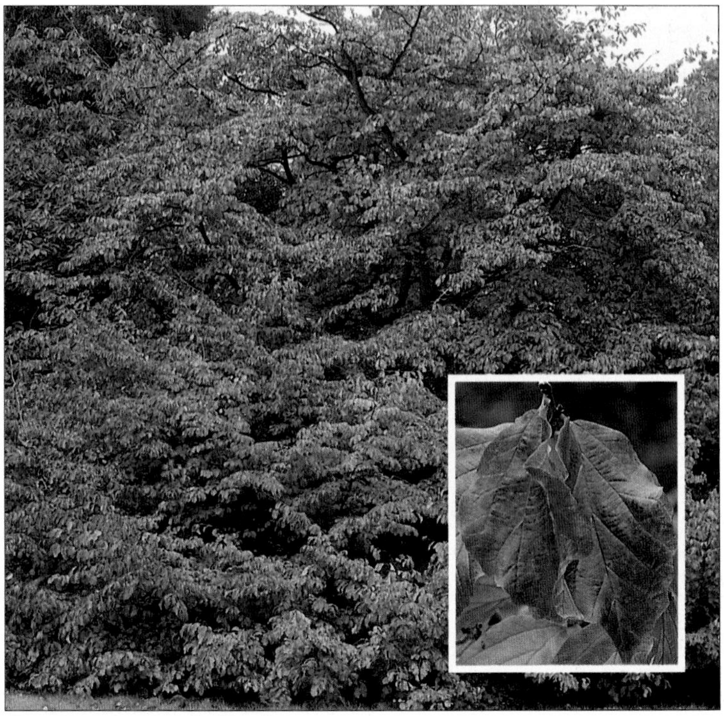

Parrotia persica (inset: leaf detail)

▷**Parsley** see *Petroselinum, P. crispum*
Cow see *Anthriscus sylvestris*
French see *Petroselinum crispum* var. *neapolitanum*
Hamburg see *Petroselinum crispum* var. *tuberosum*
Italian see *Petroselinum crispum* var. *neapolitanum*

PARTHENOCISSUS

Virginia creeper

VITACEAE

Genus of about 10 species of deciduous tendril climbers found in forests in the Himalayas, E. Asia, and North America. Some species are twining, but more commonly they cling by disc-like suckers on the tips of tendrils. They are grown for their lobed or fully divided, palmate leaves, usually brightly coloured in autumn. Clusters of inconspicuous flowers, with 5, sometimes 4, short, thick green petals, are produced in summer, and may be followed by dark blue or black berries, to 8mm (⅜in) across. Grow through a large tree or use to cover a wall or fence. The foliage of wall-grown plants often harbours a variety of wildlife. The berries may cause mild stomach upset if ingested.

• **HARDINESS** Fully hardy; *P. henryana* is frost hardy if not grown against a wall.

• **CULTIVATION** Grow in any fertile, well-drained soil in shade or sun; *P. henryana* usually colours best in partial shade. Young plants may need support initially. Pruning group 11, in early winter and, if necessary, also in summer.

• **PROPAGATION** Sow seed in containers in a cold frame in autumn. Take softwood cuttings in early summer, greenwood cuttings in midsummer, or hardwood cuttings in winter.

• **PESTS AND DISEASES** Trouble free.

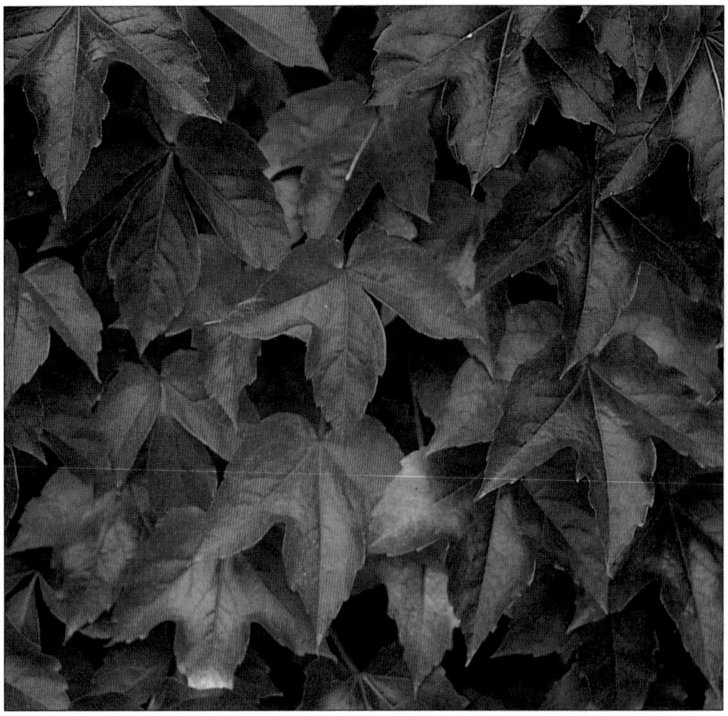

Parthenocissus tricuspidata

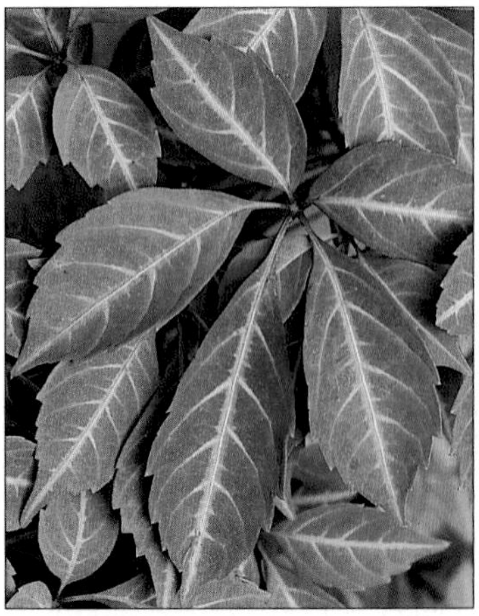

Parthenocissus henryana

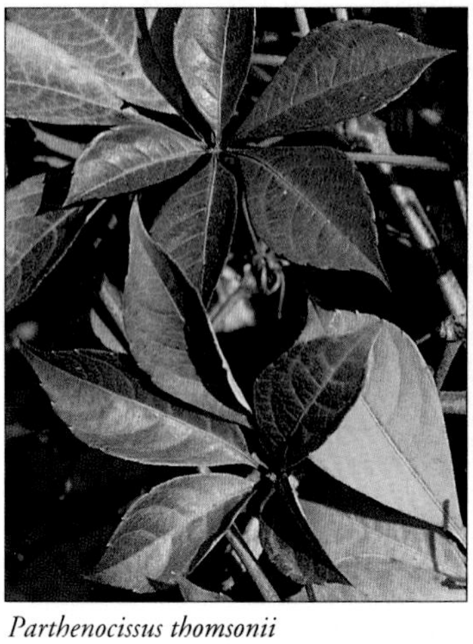

Parthenocissus thomsonii

P. henryana ■ 🏆 syn. *Vitis henryana* (Chinese Virginia creeper). Woody climber with palmate, dark green leaves composed of 3–5 oval, toothed leaflets, to 12cm (5in) long, conspicuously veined white, and sometimes pink in the centres, turning bright red in autumn. ↕10m (30ft). China. ✻✻✻ (borderline)

P. quinquefolia 🏆 syn. *Vitis quinquefolia* (Virginia creeper). Vigorous, woody climber with palmate, dull, mid-green leaves composed of usually 5 oval, sharply toothed leaflets, to 10cm (4in) long, turning brilliant red in autumn. ↕15m (50ft) or more. E. North America. ✻✻✻

P. striata see *Cissus striata.*

P. thomsonii ■ syn. *Cayratia thomsonii, Vitis thomsonii.* Woody climber with palmate, dark green leaves consisting of usually 5 oval, sharply toothed leaflets, to 10cm (4in) long, reddish purple when young, turning purple-green in summer and bright red in autumn. ↕10m (30ft). China, Himalayas. ✻✻✻

P. tricuspidata ■ 🏆 (Boston ivy). Vigorous, woody climber with variable, broadly ovate, deeply toothed, bright green leaves, to 20cm (8in) long, either 3-lobed or with 3 ovate leaflets, turning brilliant red to purple in autumn. ↕20m (70ft). China, Korea, Japan. ✻✻✻. **'Beverley Brook'** has purple-tinged summer foliage, turning brilliant red in autumn. **'Lowii'** ■ has small, deeply 3- to 7-lobed leaves, 10cm (4in) long. **'Veitchii'** ■ syn. *Ampelopsis veitchii*, has dark red-purple foliage in autumn.

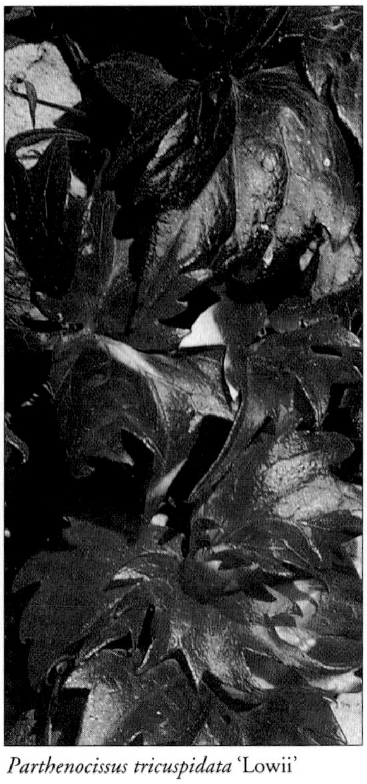

Parthenocissus tricuspidata 'Lowii'

▷**Partridge berry** see *Mitchella, M. repens*

▷**Pasque flower** see *Pulsatilla vulgaris*
Alpine see *P. alpina*
Eastern see *P. patens*

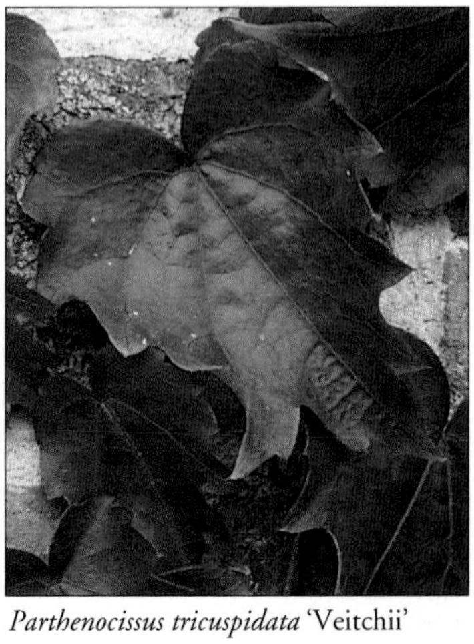

Parthenocissus tricuspidata 'Veitchii'

PASSIFLORA

Granadilla, Passion flower

PASSIFLORACEAE

Genus of more than 400 species of mostly evergreen tendril climbers, and a few annuals, perennials, shrubs, and trees. They occur usually in tropical woodland, on rocks, and in grassland, mainly in tropical North, Central, and South America, and also in tropical Asia, Australia, New Zealand, and the Pacific islands. The leaves are usually alternate, simple or 2- to 9-lobed (mainly 3- or 5-lobed), elliptic to rounded or broadly ovate, and often with prominent nectar glands on the margins or stalks. The exotic flowers are mostly produced singly, sometimes in racemes, from the upper leaf axils. Each has a wide, tubular base and 10, sometimes 5 tepals, that spread out flat, reflex, or form a saucer or bowl shape. A stalk in the centre of each flower bears the ovary and stamens, and is surrounded by one or several rings of fleshy filaments (the corona). The ovoid to spherical, edible, usually yellow fruits are very variable in size. Hardy species are ideal for clothing a wall or trellis. In frost-prone areas, grow tender species in a cool to warm greenhouse. In warmer climates, train over a pergola or arch, or through a tree.

• **HARDINESS** Fully hardy to frost tender. *P.* 'Amethyst', *P. manicata*, and *P.* 'Star of Bristol' may survive temperatures down to 0°C (32°F) if the wood has been well-ripened in summer.

• **CULTIVATION** Under glass, plant in a greenhouse border or in large tubs of loam-based potting compost (JI No.3) in full light, with shade from hot sun. Water freely when in growth, sparingly in winter. Top-dress annually in spring. Outdoors, grow in moderately fertile, moist but well-drained soil in full sun or partial shade, with shelter from cold, drying winds. Pruning group 11 or 12, if necessary, in early spring.

• **PROPAGATION** Sow seed at 13–18°C (55–64°F) in spring. Take semi-ripe cuttings in summer. Layer in spring or autumn.

• **PESTS AND DISEASES** Prone to viruses, especially cucumber mosaic virus, and to red spider mites, whiteflies, mealybugs, and scale insects under glass.

P. alata 🏆 (Maracuja de refresco, Winged-stem passion flower). Robust climber with sparsely branched, 4-

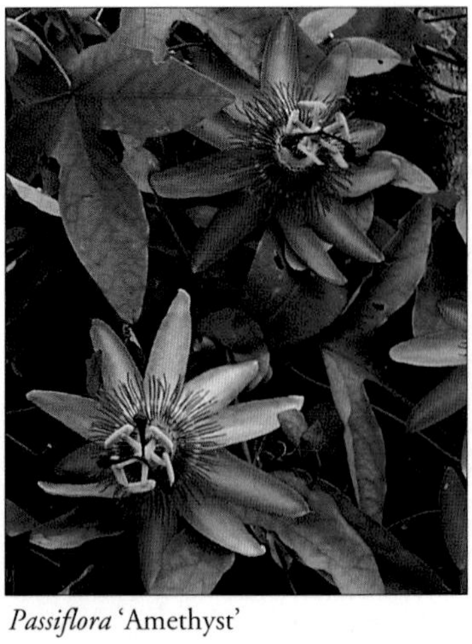

Passiflora 'Amethyst'

P

winged stems and broadly ovate or oblong-ovate, sometimes finely toothed, rich to light green leaves, 8–15cm (3–6in) long. From spring to late summer, bears nodding, fragrant, bowl-shaped, bright carmine-red flowers, 10–12cm (4–5in) across, with curved outer tepals, opening from light crimson buds; coronas have purple, red, and white zones. Bears ovoid to pear-shaped, yellow fruit, 10–15cm (4–6in) long. ↕ to 6m (20ft) or more. Peru to E. Brazil. ❁ (min. 5–7°C/41–45°F)

P.* x *alatocaerulea (*P. alata* x *P. caerulea*) syn. *P.* x *belotii*, *P.* 'Empress Eugenie'. Vigorous climber with slender, 4- or 5-winged, often red-tinted stems. Mid-green leaves, 14cm (5½in) long, each have 3 deep, ovate lobes, the central one largest. From summer to autumn, bears fragrant, bowl-shaped white flowers, 11–13cm (4½–5in) across, the longer inner tepals tinted or dotted purple or red; coronas have blue, purple, and white zones. ↕ 5m (15ft) or more. Garden origin. ❁ (min. 5°C/41°F)

P.* x *allardii (*P. caerulea* 'Constance Elliott' x *P. quadrangularis*). Vigorous, woody tendril climber with 3-lobed, dark green leaves, to 15cm (6in) long. Bowl-shaped, pink-flushed white flowers, to 10cm (4in) or more across, with coronas banded purple, red, and white, are produced from summer to autumn. Bears ovoid, bright orange fruit, to 6cm (2½in) long, without seeds. ↕ 10m (30ft). Garden origin. ❄

***P.* 'Amethyst'** ▣ ♀ syn. *P. amethystina* of gardens, *P.* 'Lavender Lady', *P. violacea* of gardens. Vigorous climber with smooth, slender stems and deeply 3-lobed, membranous, rich green leaves, 6–8cm (2½–3in) long. In late summer and autumn, bears bowl-shaped, purple to purple-blue flowers, to 11cm (4½in) across, with green anthers, tepals that reflex as the flower fades, and darker corona filaments. Bears ellipsoid orange fruit, to 6cm (2½in) long. ↕ 4m (12ft) or more. Garden origin. ❁ (min. 5°C/41°F)

***P. amethystina* of gardens** see *P.* 'Amethyst'.

P. antioquiensis ▣ ♀ syn. *Tacsonia van-volxemii* (Red banana passion flower). Vigorous climber with slender, branched stems and finely toothed, deeply 3-lobed, mid- to deep green leaves, 10–15cm (4–6in) long, downy beneath, each lobe with a slender point; occasionally produces simple, ovate to lance-shaped leaves. Bears long-tubed, bright rose-red, rarely pink flowers, to 14cm (5½in) across, with small violet coronas, mainly in summer. Ellipsoid yellow fruit, to 10cm (4in) long, have a delicate flavour. ↕ 5m (15ft) or more. Colombia. ❁ (min. 5–7°C/41–45°F)

P.* x *belotii see *P.* x *alatocaerulea.*

P. caerulea ▣ ♀ (Blue passion flower). Fast-growing climber with moderately branching, slender, 4-angled, grooved stems bearing rich green leaves, to 10cm (4in) long, divided almost to the base into 3–9, usually 5, oblong lobes. From summer to autumn, bears bowl-shaped, white, sometimes pink-tinged flowers, 7–10cm (3–4in) across, with purple-, blue-, and white-zoned coronas. Ovoid, orange-yellow fruit, to 6cm (2½in) long, are edible but not flavoursome. ↕ 10m (30ft) or more. C. and W. South America. ❄❄. **'Constance Elliott'** ▣ ♀ has fragrant white flowers with pale blue or white filaments. **'Grandiflora'** has flowers to 15cm (6in) across.

P.* x *caeruleoracemosa ▣ ♀ (*P. caerulea* x *P. racemosa*). Variable, vigorous climber with branching, slender, smooth stems and deeply 3- to 5-lobed, rich green leaves, 12–15cm (5–6in) long. From summer to autumn, bears bowl-shaped, red-purple flowers, 10–13cm (4–5in) wide, with spreading corona filaments, deep purple to black at the bases and white above. Produces ovoid green fruit, to 6cm (2½in) long. ↕ 6m (20ft) or more. Garden origin. ❁ (min. 5°C/41°F). **'Eynsford Gem'** is shrubby, with pink-mauve flowers and white filaments.

P. coccinea ▣ syn. *P. fulgens*, *P. velutina* (Red granadilla). Vigorous climber with very slender, smooth, red to purple stems, and oblong-ovate, mid-green leaves, 6–14cm (2½–5½in) long, with soft, red-brown hairs and large, lobe-like teeth. From midsummer to autumn, produces saucer-shaped scarlet flowers, 8–10cm (3–4in) across; coronas have purple, pale pink, and white zones. Spherical to ovoid, finely white-woolly fruit, 5cm (2in) long, ripen orange or yellow with darker stripes. ↕ 4m (12ft) or more. N.W. South America. ❁ (min. 10–13°C/50–55°F)

P. edulis (Passion fruit, Purple granadilla). Vigorous, woody climber with 3-lobed, toothed, glossy, mid-green leaves, to 20cm (8in) long. In summer, bears bowl-shaped white flowers, 7cm (3in) across, green beneath, with wavy, purple-zoned white coronas and ovoid, yellow to purple fruit, 5cm (2in) long. ↕ 5m (15ft). Brazil. ❁ (min. 16°C/61°F)

***P.* 'Empress Eugenie'** see *P.* x *alatocaerulea.*

P.* x *exoniensis ♀ (*P. antioquiensis* x *P. mollissima*) syn. *Tacsonia* x *exoniensis.* Robust climber with branching, slender stems. Downy, rich green leaves, 10cm (4in) long, each have 3 wide-spreading, narrowly lance-shaped, toothed lobes. In summer, produces semi-pendent, long-tubed flowers, 10–13cm (4–5in) wide, dark pink in bud, opening to rose-pink, with short white coronas. Bears banana-shaped fruit, to 9cm (3½in) long, yellow when ripe. ↕ 6m (20ft) or more. Garden origin. ❁ (min. 5°C/41°F)

P. fulgens see *P. coccinea.*

P. incarnata (Maypops). Tendril climber with deeply 3- to 5-lobed, finely toothed, dark green leaves, to 15cm (6in) long. Bowl-shaped, scented, pale purple to nearly white flowers, 8cm (3in) across, with purple and white coronas, are produced in summer, followed by ovoid yellow fruit, to 6cm (2½in) long. ↕ 2m (6ft). E. USA. ❄❄❄

***P.* 'Lavender Lady'** see *P.* 'Amethyst'.

P. manicata ▣ Robust climber with branching, angular stems bearing glossy,

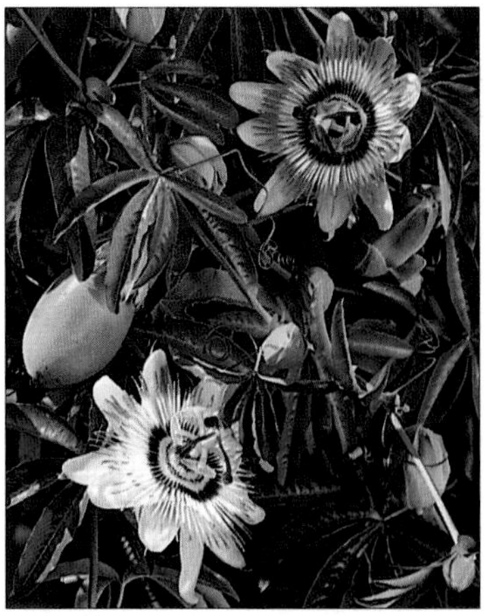

Passiflora caerulea

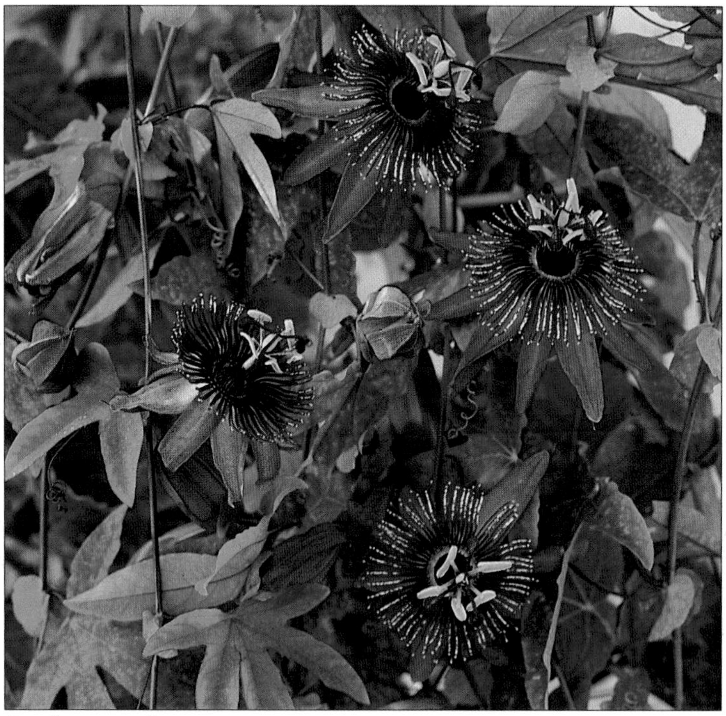

Passiflora x *caeruleoracemosa*

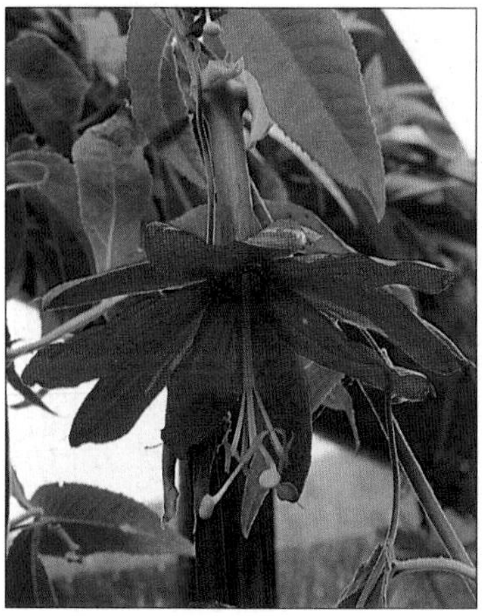

Passiflora antioquiensis

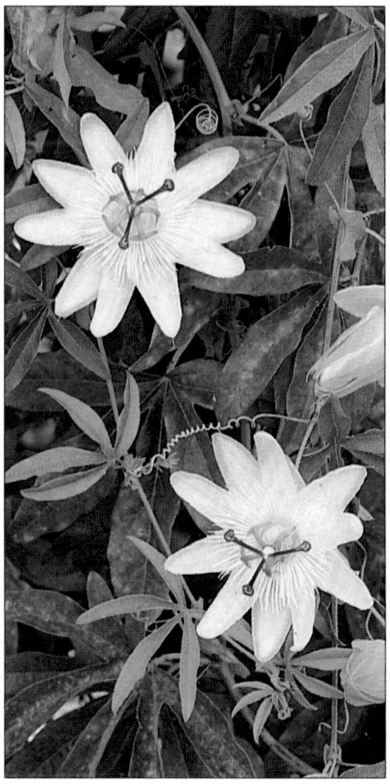

Passiflora caerulea 'Constance Elliott'

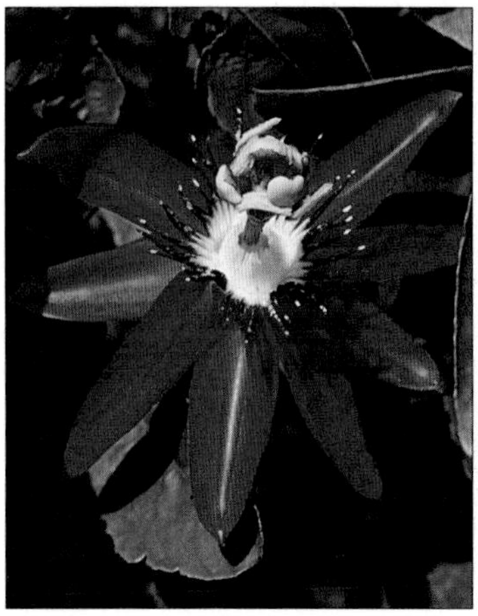

Passiflora coccinea

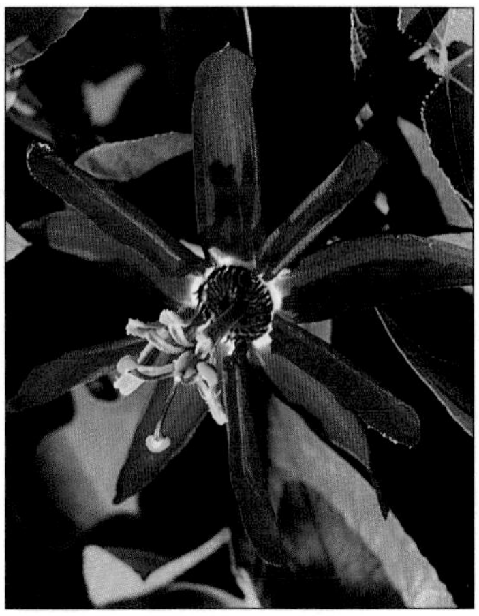

Passiflora manicata

P

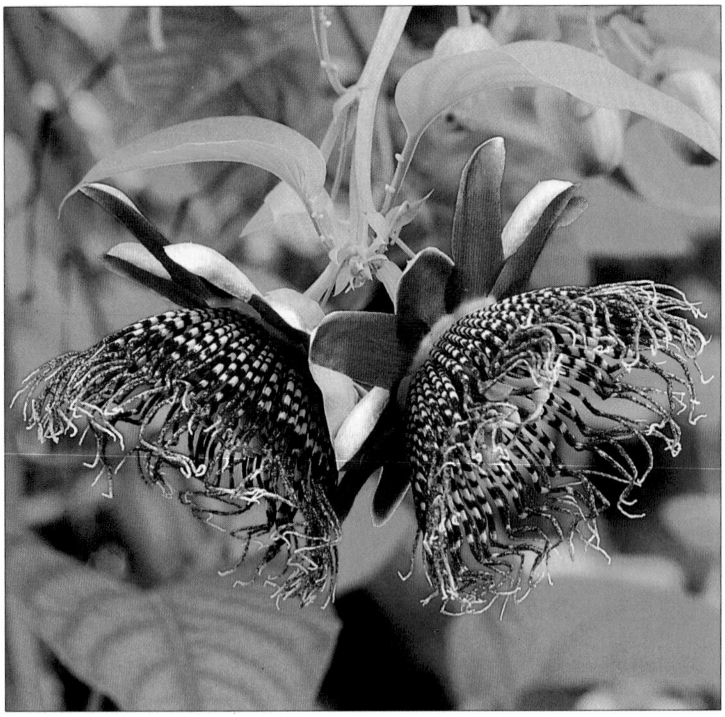

Passiflora quadrangularis

rich green leaves, to 10cm (4in) long, with 3 broad, ovate, sharply toothed lobes, densely woolly beneath. From spring to autumn, produces saucer-shaped, bright red flowers, 10cm (4in) across, white at the bases, with short, purple-blue and white coronas. Bears ovoid, glossy, deep green fruit, to 5cm (2in) long. ↕ 3m (10ft). N. South America. ❄ (min. 5–7°C/41–45°F)

P. mollissima 🏆 syn. *Tacsonia mollissima* (Banana passion flower). Fast-growing climber with moderately branching, slender, downy stems. Softly white-downy, ovate-oblong, mid-green leaves, 10cm (4in) long, have heart-shaped bases and 3 broad, toothed lobes. From midsummer to late autumn, bears pendent, long-tubed, bowl-shaped, pink to coral-pink flowers, 6–9cm (2½–3½in) across; the inner 5 tepals are shorter and darker-tinted than the outer 5, and the corona is reduced to a purple, warty ring. Produces oblong-ovoid, flavoursome yellow fruit, to 8cm (3in) long. ↕ 5m (15ft) or more. N. South America. ❄ (min. 7°C/45°F)

P. organensis. Woody climber with variable, 2-lobed, rarely 3-lobed, usually broadly wedge-shaped, mid-green leaves,

P

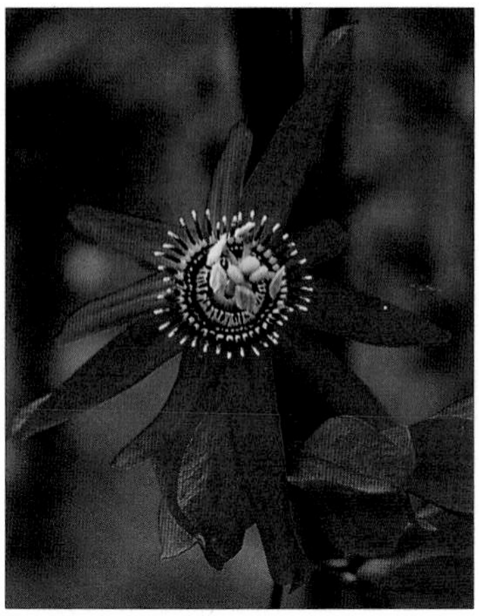

Passiflora racemosa

2–4cm (¾–1½in) long, flecked cream and pink above, purple beneath. In summer, bears bowl-shaped, cream to dark purple flowers, 5cm (2in) across, with similarly coloured coronas. Produces spherical, yellow-green fruit, to 1.5cm (½in) across. ↕ 2.5m (8ft). Brazil. ❄ (min. 16°C/61°F)

P. quadrangularis ▣ 🏆 (Giant granadilla). Strong-growing, tuberous-rooted climber with sparsely branched, 4-angled, winged stems and broadly ovate, rich green leaves, 10–25cm (4–10in) long, with abrupt, slender points. From midsummer to autumn, bears nodding, fragrant, bowl-shaped, pale to deep red flowers, to 12cm (5in) across; they have massive coronas of wavy filaments, 6cm (2½in) long, banded red-purple and white with pink, red, or violet mottling. Greenish yellow to orange, oblong-ovoid fruit, 20–30cm (8–12in) long, have sweetly acid pulp. ↕ 15m (50ft) or more. Central and South America, West Indies. ❄ (min. 13°C/55°F)

P. racemosa ▣ 🏆 (Red passion flower). Vigorous, woody climber with slender, angled stems. The leathery, glossy, mid-green leaves, to 10cm (4in) long, are ovate and simple, or with 3 oblong lobes. Bowl-shaped, bright red flowers, 12cm (5in) across, with purple and white coronas, are borne in pendent racemes, to 30cm (12in) long, in summer and autumn. Produces oblong, deep green fruit, to 8cm (3in) long, becoming paler as they ripen. ↕ 5m (15ft). Brazil. ❄ (min. 16°C/61°F)

P. sanguinea see *P. vitifolia.*

***P.* 'Star of Bristol'** 🏆 Vigorous climber with sparsely branched, slender stems, and rounded, 3- to 5-lobed, dark green leaves, 8–10cm (3–4in) long, the central lobe longest. From summer to autumn, bears saucer- or star-shaped, rich mauve flowers, 10–11cm (4–4½in) across, with darker, spreading coronas. Bears ovoid, bright orange fruit, 5cm (2in) long. ↕ to 4m (12ft). ❄ (min. 5–7°C/41–45°F)

P. velutina see *P. coccinea.*

***P. violacea* of gardens** see *P.* 'Amethyst'.

P. vitifolia, syn. *P. sanguinea.* Vigorous climber with moderately branching, slender, downy, reddish brown stems. Glossy, dark green leaves, 7–14cm (3–5½in) long, have 3 ovate, toothed or scalloped lobes, minutely hairy on the veins. From early summer to autumn, bears bowl-shaped, glowing, bright red flowers, 12–19cm (5–7in) across, with coronas of short, pale red or white filaments and longer, dark red or yellow ones. Produces ovoid, downy, yellow-green fruit, 6cm (2½in) long, with white mottling. ↕ 5m (15ft) or more. Nicaragua to Peru. ❄ (min. 13°C/55°F)

▷ **Passion flower** see *Passiflora*
Banana see *P. mollissima*
Blue see *P. caerulea*
Red see *P. racemosa*
Red banana see *P. antioquiensis*
Winged-stem see *P. alata*

▷ **Passion fruit** see *Passiflora edulis*

PATERSONIA

IRIDACEAE

Genus of 13–18 species of tufted, evergreen, rhizomatous perennials occurring in dry grassland or scrub in Borneo, New Guinea, and Australia. They are cultivated for their short-lived, iris-like, blue or purple, occasionally yellow or white flowers, with 3 broad, spreading outer tepals and 3 smaller, erect inner tepals, the inner ones sometimes absent. They are produced few to many in each inflorescence, on erect to spreading stems in spring or summer. Fans of linear, mid- to grey-green leaves arise from the bases of the stems. In frost-prone areas, grow in a cool greenhouse or conservatory. In warmer areas, grow in a border.

- **HARDINESS** Frost tender.
- **CULTIVATION** Under glass, grow in loam-based potting compost (JI No.2), with added grit, in full light. During the growing season, water freely and apply a balanced liquid fertilizer monthly. Water sparingly in winter. Outdoors, grow in light, fertile, well-drained soil in full sun.
- **PROPAGATION** Sow seed at 13–18°C (55–64°F), or divide, in autumn.
- **PESTS AND DISEASES** Trouble free.

P. glabrata. Rhizomatous perennial with very narrow, mid-green leaves, to 30cm (12in) long. Purple flowers, to 3.5cm (1½in) long, are produced in summer on stems 15cm (6in) long. ↕ to 30cm (12in), ↔ 23cm (9in). Australia (Victoria, New South Wales, Queensland). ❄ (min. 5°C/41°F)

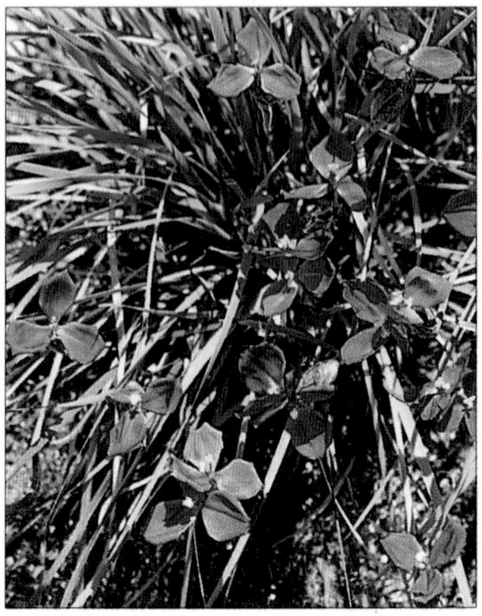

Patersonia sericea

P. occidentalis. Tuft-forming, rhizomatous perennial with few or many mid-green leaves, to 40cm (16in) long. In spring and summer, purple or deep blue flowers, 3.5cm (1½in) long, are borne on stems to 50cm (20in) long. ↕ to 50cm (20in), ↔ 30cm (12in). Australia (Western Australia). ❄ (min. 5°C/41°F)

P. sericea ▣ Rhizomatous perennial with very rigid, erect, mid-green leaves, 55cm (22in) long. Deep purple-blue flowers, 3.5cm (1½in) long, are produced on woolly stems, to 50cm (20in) long, in summer. ↕ 30cm (12in), ↔ 23cm (9in). Australia (Victoria, New South Wales, Queensland). ❄ (min. 5°C/41°F)

P. umbrosa. Rhizomatous perennial with rigid, mid-green leaves, 60–100cm (24–39in) long. In summer, produces blue flowers, 3–4cm (1¼–1½in) long, on stems 80cm (32in) long. ↕ to 1m (3ft), ↔ 30cm (12in). Australia (Western Australia). ❄ (min. 5°C/41°F).

f. *xanthina* has yellow flowers.

PATRINIA

VALERIANACEAE

Genus of about 15 species of clump-forming herbaceous perennials occurring in grassy mountain habitats in Siberia and Japan. They are cultivated for their long-stemmed, sometimes corymb-like panicles of small, 5-lobed, cup-shaped, yellow or white flowers, produced in summer. The leaves are mainly basal, ovate to rounded, lobed, palmate, or pinnate, rarely entire, and mid- to dark green. Grow in a woodland garden or rock garden, in a mixed or herbaceous border, or as ground cover.

- **HARDINESS** Fully hardy.
- **CULTIVATION** Grow in fertile, humus-rich, moist soil in partial or deep shade.

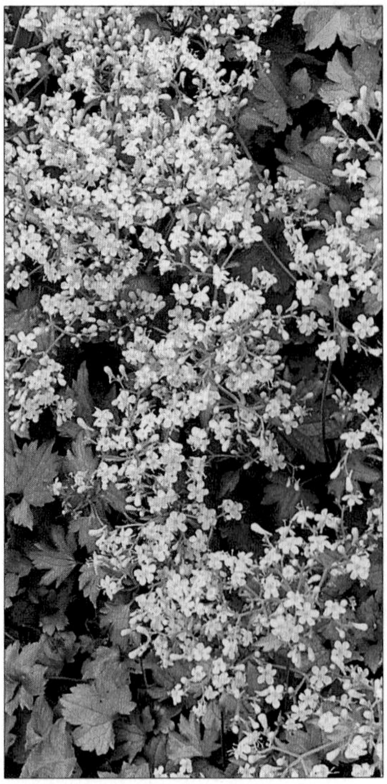

Patrinia triloba var. *palmata*

• **PROPAGATION** Sow seed as soon as ripe in containers in a cold frame. Divide in spring.
• **PESTS AND DISEASES** Young leaves may be damaged by slugs and snails.

P. triloba. Clump-forming, stoloniferous perennial with palmately 3- to 5-lobed, mid-green leaves, 6–10cm (2½–4in) across, turning yellow in autumn. In mid- and late summer, branching, red-tinted stems produce panicles, to 10cm (4in) across, of small, fragrant, cup-shaped yellow flowers, each with a short tube and 5 spreading lobes. ↕ 20–50cm (8–20in), ↔ 15–30cm (6–12in). Japan. ❄❄❄. **var. *palmata*** ▣ has flowers with short spurs.

PAULOWNIA

SCROPHULARIACEAE

Genus of 6 species of deciduous trees occurring in woodland in E. Asia. They produce stout shoots and usually large, hairy, opposite, ovate or 3- to 5-lobed, mid- or yellow-green leaves, often with heart-shaped bases. The flower buds are formed in autumn, and open, before the leaves appear, to bell- to trumpet-shaped, foxglove-like flowers, borne in terminal panicles. Grown for their habit, attractive foliage, and showy flowers, they are fine specimen trees for a lawn. They grow and flower best in climates with long, hot summers. In frost-prone areas, grow as pollards, which will produce very large, ornamental leaves.
• **HARDINESS** Fully hardy; young plants may be damaged by frost.
• **CULTIVATION** Grow in fertile, well-drained soil in full sun. In frost-prone areas, shelter from cold, drying winds. Unripened growth and exposed flower buds may be damaged by late frosts. Pruning group 1, or group 7 if larger leaves are desired.
• **PROPAGATION** Sow seed in containers in a cold frame in autumn or spring. Take root cuttings in winter. Overwinter young plants under glass in their first year.
• **PESTS AND DISEASES** Canker, honey fungus, leaf spot, and powdery mildew may cause problems.

P. fortunei ♀ Broadly columnar tree with stout shoots and ovate, mid-green leaves, to 20cm (8in) long, glossy above and densely hairy beneath. Fragrant flowers, 10cm (4in) long, pale purple outside and creamy white with purple spots inside, are produced in upright panicles in late spring. ↕↔ 8m (25ft). China, Taiwan. ❄❄❄
P. imperialis see *P. tomentosa.*
P. tomentosa ▣Y♀ syn. *P. imperialis* (Empress tree, Foxglove tree, Princess tree). Fast-growing, broadly columnar tree with stout shoots and ovate, sometimes shallowly lobed, bright light green leaves, to 30cm (12in) long, hairy above, densely hairy beneath. Fragrant, pinkish lilac flowers, 5cm (2in) long, with purple and yellow marks inside, are borne in upright panicles in late spring. Very tolerant of atmospheric pollution. ↕ 12m (40ft), ↔ 10m (30ft). China. ❄❄❄

▷ ***Paurotis wrightii*** see *Acoelorraphe wrightii*

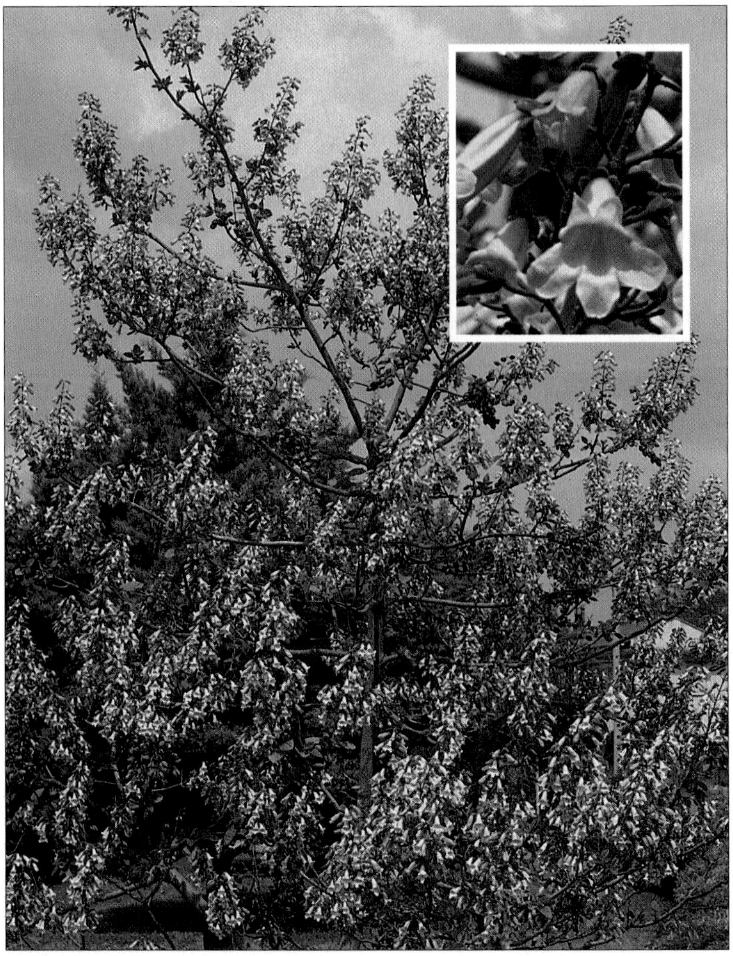

Paulownia tomentosa (inset: flower detail)

PAVETTA

RUBIACEAE

Genus of about 350 species of evergreen shrubs, subshrubs, and trees, related to *Ixora*, found in grassland, thickets, and woodland in tropical and subtropical Africa and Asia. They are grown for their variable, simple leaves, opposite or in whorls of 3, often membranous with tiny black glands, and for their small, tubular flowers with 4 spreading petal lobes (cylindrical to salverform or funnel-shaped), borne in terminal cymes or corymbs. Where temperatures fall below 7°C (45°F), grow in a temperate or warm greenhouse. In warmer regions, grow in a shrub border.
• **HARDINESS** Frost tender.
• **CULTIVATION** Under glass, grow in loam-based potting compost (JI No.3), with added sharp sand, in full light with shade from hot sun, and with high humidity. In spring and summer, water freely and apply a balanced liquid fertilizer monthly. Water sparingly in winter. Outdoors, grow in fertile, moist but well-drained soil in full sun. Pruning group 1; may need restrictive pruning under glass.
• **PROPAGATION** Sow seed at 18–21°C (64–70°F) in spring. Root semi-ripe cuttings in summer, with bottom heat.
• **PESTS AND DISEASES** Trouble free.

P. caffra see *P. capensis.*
P. capensis, syn. *P. caffra*. Bushy, erect then spreading shrub with white-downy stems and obovate, mid-green leaves, to 5cm (2in) long, with pointed tips. Dense, flattened corymbs, 2.5–4cm (1–1½in) across, of white flowers, 2cm (¾in) long, appear in summer, followed by spherical, glossy black fruit, to 1cm (½in) across. ↕↔ 1–2m (3–6ft). South Africa (Western Cape, Eastern Cape). ❀ (min. 7°C/45°F)

PAVONIA

MALVACEAE

Genus of about 150 species of evergreen perennials, subshrubs, and shrubs, often occurring on sandy soils in tropical and subtropical regions of Africa, Asia, the Pacific islands, and North and South America. They are grown for their brightly coloured flowers, solitary, axillary, or borne in terminal, spherical clusters or panicles, mainly in summer. Petals are spreading, or form a tube surrounded by a bell- or cup-shaped calyx, with a whorl of hairy bracts beneath; the stamens and anthers are often protruding. Most have alternate, linear to broadly ovate or oblong, light to dark green leaves, each with a bract-like stipule at the base of the leaf-stalk. In subtropical and tropical gardens, grow among shrubs or in a border. In cooler areas, grow in a warm greenhouse.
• **HARDINESS** Frost tender.
• **CULTIVATION** Under glass, grow in loam-based potting compost (JI No.3) in bright filtered light, with high humidity. When in growth, water freely and apply a balanced liquid fertilizer monthly. Water sparingly in winter. Outdoors, grow in fertile, humus-rich, well-drained soil in full sun or partial shade. Pruning group 1; may need restrictive pruning under glass.
• **PROPAGATION** Sow seed at 19–24°C (66–75°F) in spring. Root semi-ripe cuttings with bottom heat in summer.
• **PESTS AND DISEASES** Red spider mites and whiteflies may be troublesome.

P. x gledhillii (*P. mackoyana* x *P. multiflora*) syn. *P. intermedia* of gardens, *P. multiflora* of gardens. Sparsely branched shrub with pointed, elliptic to lance-shaped, glossy, light green leaves, 10–15cm (4–6in) long, with linear to lance-shaped stipules. In late summer, bears solitary, dark purple flowers, to 3cm (1¼in) long, enclosed in almost cylindrical, hairy calyces with grey-pink teeth, and each with a whorl of red bracts beneath; the stamens have red filaments and chalky, lilac-blue anthers. ↕ to 2m (6ft), ↔ 1m (3ft). Garden origin. ❀ (min. 16–18°C/61–64°F)
***P. intermedia* of gardens** see *P. x gledhillii.*
***P. multiflora* of gardens** see *P. x gledhillii.*

▷ **Pawpaw** see *Asimina triloba*

PAXISTIMA syn. PACHYSTIMA

CELASTRACEAE

Genus of 2 species of low-growing, evergreen shrubs found in rocky sites on mountains and in coniferous woodland in North America. They are grown for their small, opposite, linear to ovate or oblong, sometimes finely toothed, leathery leaves. Tiny, cross-shaped, 4-petalled, greenish white or white flowers, solitary or in axillary clusters, are produced in summer. Grow as ground cover in a rock garden or peat terrace.
• **HARDINESS** Fully hardy.
• **CULTIVATION** Grow in moderately fertile, humus-rich, moist but well-drained soil in full sun or light dappled shade.
• **PROPAGATION** Take semi-ripe cuttings in summer. Remove rooted suckers in spring or autumn.
• **PESTS AND DISEASES** Trouble free.

P. canbyi. Spreading, branching, stem-rooting shrub with stalkless, linear-oblong, sometimes finely toothed, glossy, dark green leaves, to 2cm (¾in) long, with incurved margins. Bears short, pendent clusters of greenish white flowers, 5mm (¼in) across, in summer. ↕ 40cm (16in), ↔ to 1m (3ft). C. North America. ❄❄❄

▷ **Pea,**
Balloon see *Sutherlandia frutescens*
Black coral see *Kennedia nigricans*
Blue see *Clitoria ternatea*
Bush see *Pultenaea procumbens*
Chickling see *Lathyrus sativus*
Coral see *Hardenbergia, Kennedia*
Dusky coral see *Kennedia rubicunda*
Everlasting see *Lathyrus, L. grandiflorus, L. latifolius*
Glory see *Clianthus formosus, C. puniceus*
Heart see *Cardiospermum halicacabum*
Lord Anson's blue see *Lathyrus nervosus*
Perennial see *Lathyrus latifolius, L. sylvestris*
Persian everlasting see *Lathyrus rotundifolius*

P

▷ **Pea cont.**
Purple coral see *Hardenbergia violacea*
Shamrock see *Parochetus africana*
Sturt's desert see *Clianthus formosus*
Swan river see *Brachysema celsianum*
Sweet see *Lathyrus odoratus*
▷ **Peach** see *Prunus persica*
▷ **Peacock flower** see *Tigridia, T. pavonia*
▷ **Peacock plant** see *Calathea makoyana*
▷ **Pear** see *Pyrus*
Common see *Pyrus communis*
Prickly see *Opuntia ficus-indica*
Snow see *Pyrus nivalis*
▷ **Pearl berry** see *Margyricarpus pinnatus*
▷ **Pearl bush** see *Exochorda*
▷ **Pearl everlasting** see *Anaphalis*
▷ **Pearl plant** see *Haworthia pumila*
▷ **Pearlwort** see *Sagina*
▷ **Pea shrub, Russian** see *Caragana frutex*
▷ **Pea tree** see *Caragana arborescens*
▷ **Pecan** see *Carya illinoinensis*
▷ ***Pectinaria pillansii*** see *Stapeliopsis pillansii*

PEDILANTHUS

EUPHORBIACEAE

Genus of about 14 species of variable, bushy, succulent shrubs and small trees occurring mainly in low, rocky terrain in Mexico, Central and South America, the West Indies, and Florida, USA. Many species branch from the roots to form clumps. The fleshy, narrow to broadly ovate, light to mid-green, sometimes white-mottled leaves are usually quickly deciduous. Terminal or axillary cymes of flower-like, tubular bract-cups are produced during the day in summer. Where temperatures drop below 10°C (50°F), grow as houseplants or in a warm greenhouse. In warmer climates, use in a desert garden or shrub border. The stems and leaves contain a milky sap that may cause stomach upset if ingested.

• **HARDINESS** Frost tender.

• **CULTIVATION** Under glass, grow in loam-based potting compost (JI No.2), with added well-rotted organic matter and sharp sand, in bright filtered light. In spring and summer, water moderately and apply a balanced liquid fertilizer every month. Water sparingly in winter. Outdoors, grow in moderately fertile, sharply drained soil in full sun or partial shade. See also pp.48–49.

• **PROPAGATION** Sow seed at 19–24°C (66–75°F) in spring. Take stem-tip cuttings in summer.

• **PESTS AND DISEASES** Trouble free.

P. bracteatus. Bushy, succulent shrub, branching freely from the base, with straight stems. Deciduous, ovate to inversely lance-shaped, white-powdery, mid-green leaves, 10cm (4in) or more long, are keeled beneath, with blunt or pointed tips. In summer, produces green bract-cups, 1.5cm (½in) long, with crimson glands. ↕ 1–3m (3–10ft), ↔ 45cm (18in). N.W. Mexico. ❄ (min. 10°C/50°F)

P. tithymaloides. Upright, bushy, clump-forming, succulent shrub with thin, woody or fleshy, zigzagged stems. Evergreen or deciduous, ovate to elliptic, mid-green leaves, to 8cm (3in) long, are keeled and slightly hairy or powdery beneath. In summer, produces fleshy red bract-cups, to 1.5cm (½in) long, yellow-green at the bases. ↕ 2m (6ft), ↔ to 1m (3ft). USA (Florida) to Venezuela, West Indies. ❄ (min. 10°C/50°F).
'Variegatus' ■ has variably shaped leaves, to 15cm (6in) long, with white or pink variegation; ↔ to 45cm (18in).

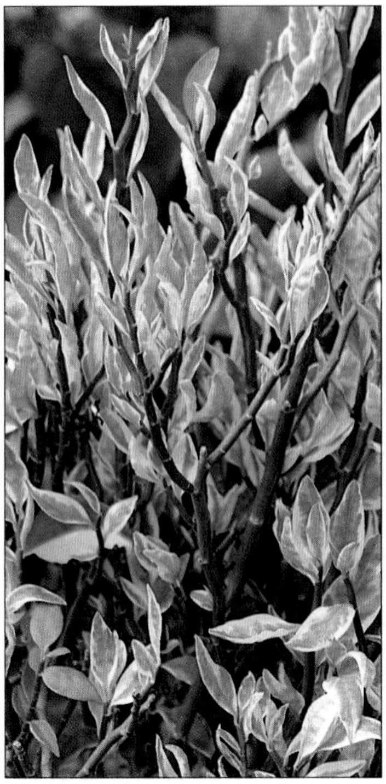

Pedilanthus tithymaloides 'Variegatus'

PEDIOCACTUS

CACTACEAE

Genus of about 6 species of simple or clustering, spherical, perennial cacti occurring in rocky terrain in W. and S. USA. The spiny stems have spiralling, tuberculate ribs. Bell-shaped flowers are produced near or at the stem tips, followed by spherical, pink or greenish yellow fruits. Where temperatures drop below 2°C (36°F), grow as houseplants or in a cool greenhouse. In warmer areas, grow in a raised bed or desert garden.

• **HARDINESS** Frost tender.

• **CULTIVATION** Under glass, grow in standard cactus compost in full light. From spring to summer, water moderately and apply a low-nitrogen fertilizer every 6–8 weeks. Keep dry at other times. Outdoors, grow in moderately fertile, sharply drained soil in full sun. See also pp.48–49.

• **PROPAGATION** Sow seed at 19–24°C (66–75°F) in spring.

• **PESTS AND DISEASES** Susceptible to mealybugs early in the growing season.

P. simpsonii. Simple or clustering cactus with spherical to ovoid, mid-green stems, each with 12 ribs, and white-woolly areoles bearing fine spines (15–25 white radials and 5–10 slightly longer, reddish brown centrals). In spring, white, pink, magenta, yellow, or yellow-green flowers, 1–3cm (½–1¼in) long, are borne singly or in clusters by day. ↕ 12–15cm (5–6in), ↔ to 15cm (6in). W. USA. ❄ (min. 2°C/36°F)

▷ **Peepul** see *Ficus religiosa*

PELARGONIUM

GERANIACEAE

Genus of about 230 species of mainly evergreen perennials, succulents, sub-shrubs, and shrubs, commonly but incorrectly known as geraniums. They occur in a variety of habitats, from mountains to deserts, mostly in South Africa. The many cultivars, derived from about 20 species, are popular garden plants; few species are grown. Leaves are variable, but are usually alternate, palmately lobed or pinnate, sometimes aromatic, often on long stalks. Erect stems bear 5-petalled flowers in terminal, umbel-like clusters (pseudoumbels) referred to in this account as "clusters". The flowers are saucer- or star-shaped, trumpet- or funnel-shaped, or "butterfly"-shaped (the upper 2 petals larger than the lower 3); they are usually borne from spring to summer, although many will flower throughout the year if kept above 7–10°C (45–50°F).

In frost-prone areas, use in containers outside in summer or as bedding plants, and overwinter in a cool greenhouse or conservatory. In frost-free areas, grow in a sunny border. Use scented-leaved cultivars as edging for a border or alongside a path. For winter flowers, grow in a temperate greenhouse or as houseplants. Contact with the foliage may occasionally aggravate skin allergies.

Most cultivars belong to one of the following 6 horticultural groups.

Angel
Very bushy, evergreen perennials and subshrubs, derived mainly from *P. crispum*. They have rounded, sometimes scented, mid-green leaves, 2–3cm (¾–1¼in) long, and clusters of small, single flowers of the regal type (see panel), to 3cm (1¼in) across, in shades of pink, purple, mauve, or white.

Ivy-leaved
Trailing, evergreen perennials with lobed, sometimes pointed, stiff, fleshy, usually mid-green leaves, 2.5–12cm (1–5in) long, very similar to those of ivy (*Hedera helix*). Some cultivars have short-jointed stems. Clusters of single to double flowers, to 4cm (1½in) across, are produced in shades of red, pink, mauve, purple, or white.

Regal
Bushy, evergreen perennials and shrubs, some with short-jointed stems. The leaves are rounded, sometimes lobed or partially toothed, and mid-green, 5–9cm (2–3½in) long. Clusters of single, rarely double flowers, to 4cm (1½in) across, are produced in single or combined shades of red, pink, purple, orange, white, or reddish black.

Scented-leaved
Shrubby, evergreen perennials and shrubs grown mainly for their attractive leaves, which release scent when brushed; each cultivar has a distinct perfume. Leaves are mainly mid-green, sometimes variegated, or gold or silver, and are very variable in shape and size, usually 1.5–12cm (½–5in) long, sometimes toothed, lobed, or deeply incised. They bear clusters of small, single flowers, to 2.5cm (1in) across, in shades of mauve, pink, purple, or white.

Unique
Shrubby, evergreen perennials with rounded or lobed, sometimes incised, mid-green leaves, 5–14cm (2–5½in) across, often with a pungent scent when crushed. They produce clusters of trumpet-shaped, single, white, pink, red, purple, or orange flowers of the regal type (see panel), to 3cm (1¼in) across.

PELARGONIUM GROUPS

Leaves and flower clusters (pseudoumbels) of the 4 main pelargonium groups are shown here. Angel and unique pelargoniums have clusters similar to those of regal pelargoniums.

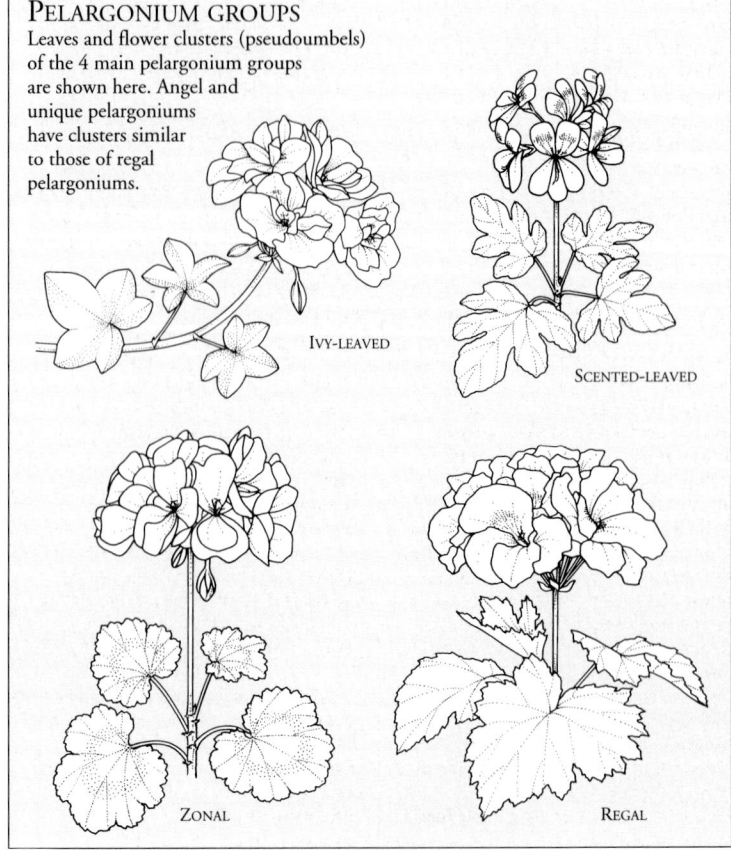

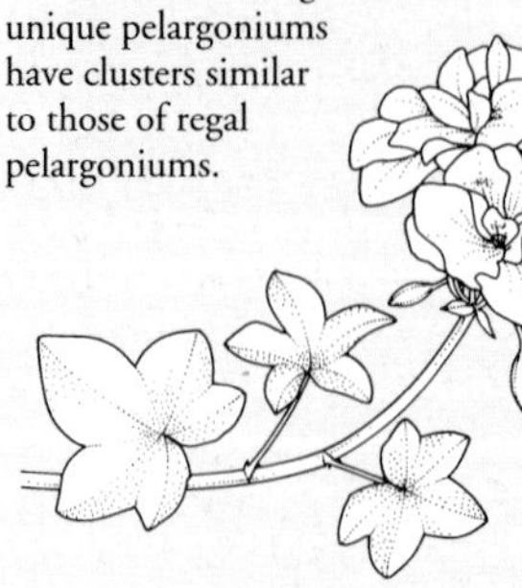

IVY-LEAVED

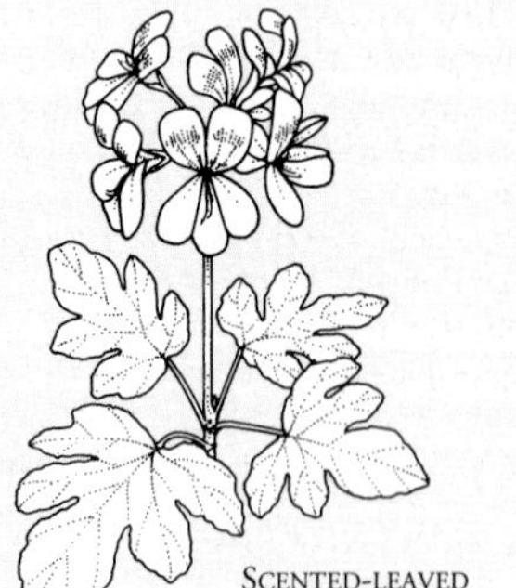

SCENTED-LEAVED

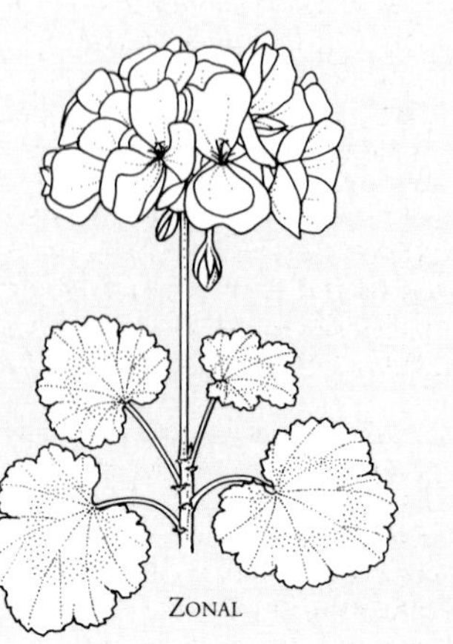

ZONAL

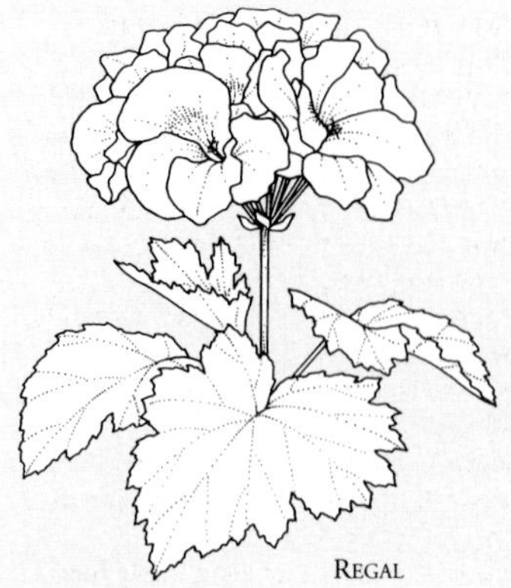

REGAL

P

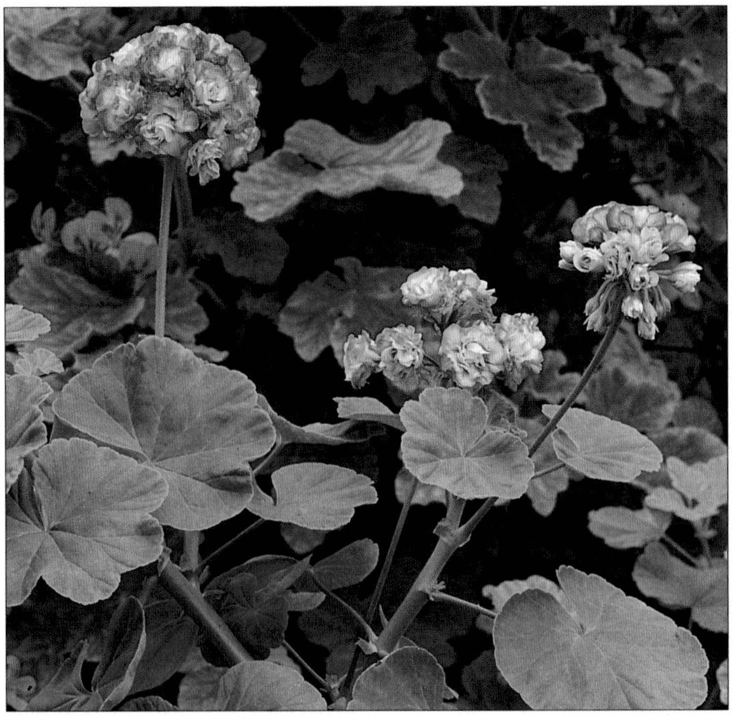

Pelargonium 'Apple Blossom Rosebud'

Zonal
Erect, bushy, succulent-stemmed, evergreen perennials, some with short-jointed stems, derived mainly from *P. inquinans* and *P. zonale.* The leaves are rounded, 4–14cm (1½–5½in) across, light to deep green, often bicoloured or multi-coloured, with zones of dark bronze-green or maroon. Flowers are single, semi-double, or double, to 2.5cm (1in) across, in shades of scarlet, purple, pink, white, orange, or rarely yellow. Rain may damage the blooms of some double-flowered cultivars; these should be grown under glass. As bedding plants, most grow to 60cm (24in) tall; dwarf cultivars are 12–20cm (5–8in) tall, miniature cultivars to 12cm (5in) tall.

There are 2 main groups of zonal pelargoniums: the seed-raised bedding types, mainly comprising the single-flowered F1 hybrids, which flower in the first year and come true to colour and type when raised from seed; and the large-flowered cultivars propagated only from cuttings, which are ideal container plants in a conservatory or as house-plants, or outdoors in frost-free periods.

Zonal pelargoniums can be separated into the following groups:

Cactus-flowered – Flowers, resembling those of cactus dahlias, are single or double, the petals twisted into quills.

Double- and semi-double-flowered – Flowers normally comprise 6 or more open petals.

Fancy-leaved – These are grown mainly for their foliage, which may be silver or gold tricoloured (silver or gold, usually with white and green), bronze and gold, almost black, or butterfly-leaved with a distinct hue in the leaf centre. Flowers are often small and single, rarely double.

Formosum hybrids – Flowers are flat, single or double, with narrow petals. Leaves are deeply incised.

Rosebud – Flowers are double, with rosebud-like centres (the central petals remaining unopened).

Single-flowered – Flowers usually have no more than 5 petals.

Stellar – Flowers are irregularly star-shaped, single or double: the bottom 3 petals are wedge-shaped and broad, the top 2 are much narrower and toothed. The leaves have pointed lobes and, in some cultivars, dark zones, often in the centres.

• **HARDINESS** Mostly frost tender; there are 1 or 2 hardy species from Turkey.
• **CULTIVATION** Under glass, grow in loamless or loam-based potting compost (JI No.2) in full light, with shade from hot sun and good ventilation. Water moderately during growth; apply a balanced liquid fertilizer every 10–14 days in spring and early summer, and a high-potash fertilizer when in flower. Water sparingly in winter. If kept at 7–10°C (45–50°F), plants may flower over winter. Otherwise, cut back by up to two-thirds and keep almost dry. Outdoors, grow in fertile, neutral to alkaline, well-drained soil. Most prefer full sun; regal cultivars prefer partial shade, and zonals tolerate some shade. Lift bedding plants in autumn and over-winter in dry, frost-free conditions; cut back top-growth by one-third and repot in late winter as new growth resumes. Dead-head all pelargoniums regularly.
• **PROPAGATION** Sow seed of species and F1 zonal pelargoniums at 13–18°C (55–64°F) in late winter and early spring. Take softwood cuttings in spring, late summer, or early autumn.
• **PESTS AND DISEASES** Susceptible to vine weevils, leafhoppers, root mealybugs, aphids, caterpillars, western flower thrips, sciarid flies, grey mould (*Botrytis*), and black leg. Zonal pelargoniums are particularly prone to rust, and regal pelargoniums to whiteflies.

***P.* 'Abel Carrière'.** Ivy-leaved pelargonium producing semi-double, light purple flowers, with very dark purple feathering on the upper petals, in clusters 8–9cm (3–3½in) across. ↕45–50cm (18–20in), ↔ 15–20cm (6–8in). ❄ (min. 2°C/36°F)

P. abrotanifolium. Bushy, erect, evergreen, woody-stemmed subshrub. Rounded, finely divided, grey-green leaves, to 1.5cm (½in) long, have linear lobes and smell like southernwood (*Artemisia abrotanum*). Star-shaped, white or pink flowers, 1.5cm (½in) across, are produced in clusters of up to 5, to 5cm (2in) across, from spring to summer. ↕30–40cm (12–16in), ↔ 25–30cm (10–12in). South Africa (Orange Free State, Northern Cape, Western Cape, Eastern Cape). ❄ (min. 2°C/36°F)

P. acetosum ▣ Erect, evergreen perennial with succulent stems bearing obovate, toothed, fleshy, grey-green leaves, 2–6cm (¾–2½in) long, sometimes margined red. From spring to summer, star-shaped, salmon-pink flowers, 2–3.5cm (¾–1½in) across, with long, narrow petals, are borne in sparse clusters, 6–7cm (2½–3in) across. ↕50–60cm (20–24in), ↔ 20–25cm (8–10in). South Africa (Eastern Cape). ❄ (min. 2°C/36°F)

***P.* 'Action'.** Semi-double-flowered zonal pelargonium. Deep pink flowers, with white centres and a small red blaze on each petal, are produced in clusters 9–10cm (3½–4in) across. ↕30–40cm (12–16in), ↔ 15–20cm (6–8in). ❄ (min. 2°C/36°F)

***P.* 'After Glow'.** Single-flowered zonal pelargonium producing pale pink flowers, each with a wide coral-pink ring in the centre, in clusters, 9–10cm (3½–4in) across. ↕30–40cm (12–16in), ↔ 20–25cm (8–10in). ❄ (min. 2°C/36°F)

***P.* 'Alberta'** ▣ Single-flowered zonal pelargonium bearing bicoloured coral-pink and white flowers in clusters 9–10cm (3½–4in) across. ↕40–50cm (16–20in), ↔ 20–25cm (8–10in). ❄ (min. 2°C/36°F)

***P.* 'Alice Crousse'** ▣ 🏆 Short-jointed ivy-leaved pelargonium with double, bright cerise-pink flowers borne in clusters 9cm (3½in) across. ↕25–30cm (10–12in), ↔ 20–25cm (8–10in). ❄ (min. 2°C/36°F)

***P.* 'Amethyst'** ▣ 🏆 Vigorous, short-jointed ivy-leaved pelargonium. Semi-double purple flowers are produced in clusters 9–10cm (3½–4in) across; the upper petals are marked with deep purple and white feathering. ↕25–30cm (10–12in), ↔ 20–25cm (8–10in). ❄ (min. 2°C/36°F)

***P.* 'Ann Hoysted'** ▣ 🏆 Vigorous regal pelargonium bearing clusters, 13–14cm (5–5½in) across, of deep red flowers with almost black upper petals. ↕35–45cm (14–18in), ↔ 20–25cm (8–10in). ❄ (min. 2°C/36°F)

***P.* 'Aphrodite'.** Semi-double-flowered zonal pelargonium producing abundant foliage. Strong stems bear clusters, 10–11cm (4–4½in) across, of pure white flowers. ↕40–45cm (16–18in), ↔ 20–25cm (8–10in). ❄ (min. 2°C/36°F)

***P.* 'Apple Blossom Rosebud'** ▣ 🏆 Rosebud zonal pelargonium bearing bicoloured white and pink flowers in clusters to 8cm (3in) across. ↕30–40cm (12–16in), ↔ 20–25cm (8–10in). ❄ (min. 2°C/36°F)

***P.* 'Aroma'.** Scented-leaved pelargonium with small, rounded, sweet-smelling, grey-green leaves. Bears white flowers in sparse clusters, 2–2.5cm (¾–1in) across. ↕20–25cm (8–10in), ↔ 15–20cm (6–8in). ❄ (min. 2°C/36°F)

***P.* 'Ashfield Serenade'** 🏆 Bushy, single-flowered zonal pelargonium with short, thick stems bearing clusters, 9–10cm (3½in–4in) across, of mauve flowers with white-based, pink upper petals. ↕25–30cm (10–12in), ↔ 20–25cm (8–10in). ❄ (min. 2°C/36°F)

***P.* 'Atomic Snowflake'.** Bushy, scented-leaved pelargonium producing large, 3-lobed, mid-green leaves with yellow variegation and a lemon-rose fragrance. Produces mauve flowers in clusters 2–2.5cm (¾–1in) across. ↕45–50cm (18–20in), ↔ 25–30cm (10–12in). ❄ (min. 2°C/36°F)

***P.* 'Attar of Roses'** 🏆 Scented-leaved pelargonium with 3-lobed, rose-scented leaves. Produces mauve flowers in clusters, 2.5–3cm (1–1¼in) across. ↕50–60cm (20–24in), ↔ 25–30cm (10–12in). ❄ (min. 2°C/36°F)

***P.* 'Attraction'.** Cactus-flowered zonal pelargonium producing double, rose-pink flowers, with red streaks, in clusters, to 7cm (3in) across. ↕20–25cm (8–10in), ↔ 15–20cm (6–8in). ❄ (min. 2°C/36°F)

***P.* 'Autumn Festival'** ▣ Bushy, short-jointed regal pelargonium bearing clusters, 9–10cm (3½–4in) across, of bicoloured salmon-pink and white

P

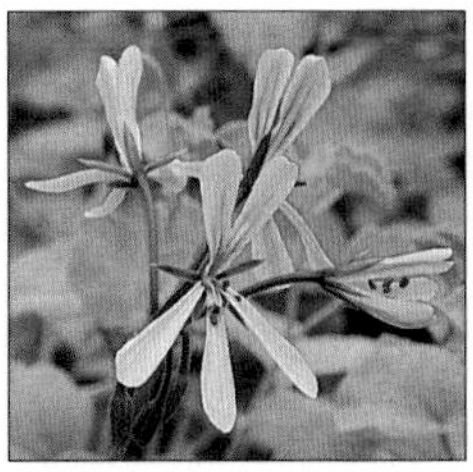

Pelargonium acetosum

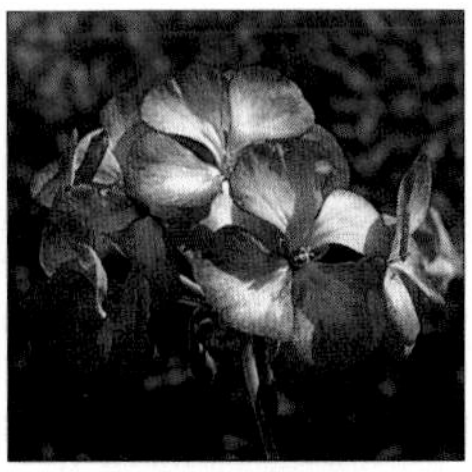

Pelargonium 'Alberta'

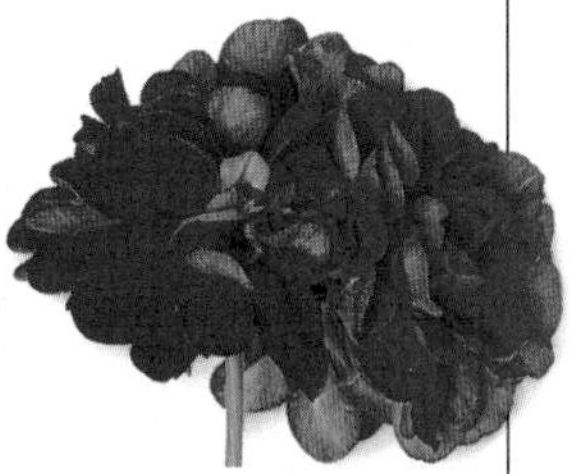

Pelargonium 'Alice Crousse'

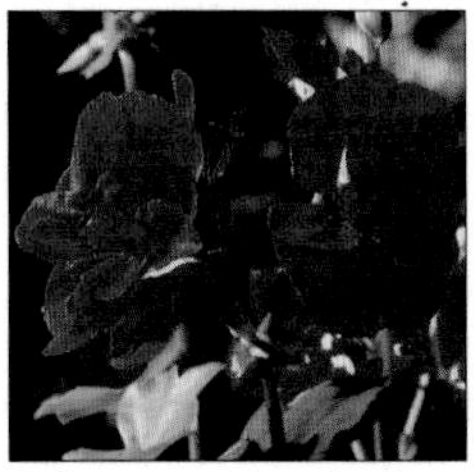

Pelargonium 'Amethyst'

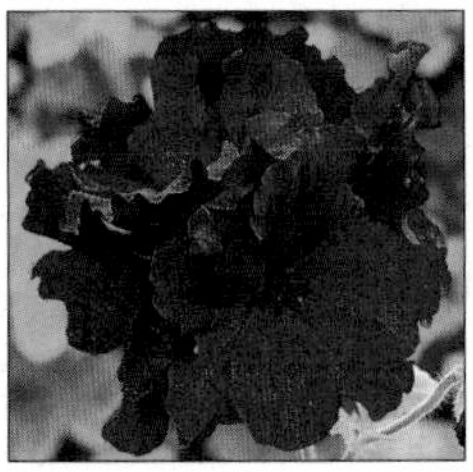

Pelargonium 'Ann Hoysted'

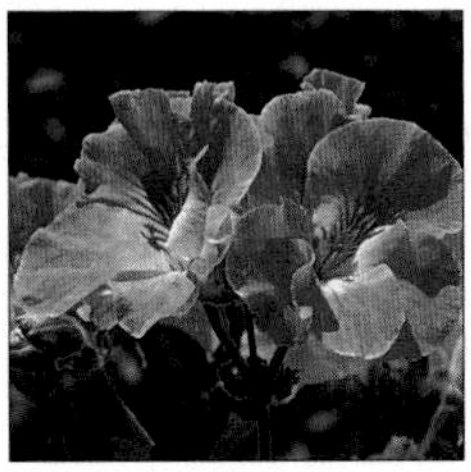

Pelargonium 'Autumn Festival'

flowers with mahogany, feather-like markings in the centres. ↕ 25–30cm (10–12in), ↔ 20–25cm (8–10in). ✿ (min. 2°C/36°F)

***P.* Avanti Series.** Early-flowering, seed-raised, single-flowered zonal pelargoniums with clusters, 10cm (4in) across, of flowers in white or shades of pink, salmon-pink, or red; also available as a mixture. ↕ 35cm (14in), ↔ 25cm (10in). ✿ (min. 2°C/36°F)

***P.* 'Barbe Bleu'.** Ivy-leaved pelargonium with double, purple-black flowers, fading to wine-red in full sun, in clusters 9–10cm (3½–4in) across. ↕ 50–60cm (20–24in), ↔ 20–25cm (8–10in). ✿ (min. 2°C/36°F)

***P.* 'Belinda Adams'** 🏆 Miniature, double-flowered zonal pelargonium bearing clusters, 7cm (3in) across, of white flowers flushed pink. ↕ 10–12cm (4–5in), ↔ 7–10cm (3–4in). ✿ (min. 2°C/36°F)

***P.* 'Ben Franklin'** 🏆 Fancy-leaved zonal pelargonium with rounded silver leaves. Bears clusters, 8–9cm (3–3½in) across, of double, rose-pink flowers. ↕ 30–40cm (12–16in), ↔ 15–20cm (6–8in). ✿ (min. 2°C/36°F)

***P.* 'Bird Dancer'** ■ 🏆 Dwarf, stellar zonal pelargonium with dark-zoned leaves. Bears single flowers, with pale pink lower petals and salmon-pink upper petals, in clusters to 8cm (3in) across. ↕ 15–20cm (6–8in), ↔ 12–15cm (5–6in). ✿ (min. 2°C/36°F)

***P.* 'Blazonry'** ■ Fancy-leaved zonal pelargonium producing rounded, deep cream leaves with rose-pink, mid-green, and purple zones. Single red flowers are borne in clusters 8cm (3in) across. ↕ 25–30cm (10–12in), ↔ 15–20cm (6–8in). ✿ (min. 2°C/36°F)

***P.* 'Bredon'** ■ 🏆 Bushy regal pelargonium bearing clusters, 9–10cm (3½–4in) across, of deep wine-red flowers with a purple-black feathered blaze on each petal. ↕ 40–45cm (16–18in), ↔ 20–25cm (8–10in). ✿ (min. 2°C/36°F)

***P.* 'Brockbury Scarlet'** ■ Cactus-flowered zonal pelargonium. Single scarlet flowers are produced in clusters to 8cm (3in) across. ↕ 25–30cm (10–12in), ↔ 15–20cm (6–8in). ✿ (min. 2°C/36°F)

***P.* 'Brookside Primrose'** ■ Miniature, fancy-leaved zonal pelargonium with dark brown butterfly markings in the centre of each rounded leaf. Double, light pink flowers are borne in clusters 7cm (3in) across. ↕ 10–12cm (4–5in), ↔ 7–10cm (3–4in). ✿ (min. 2°C/36°F)

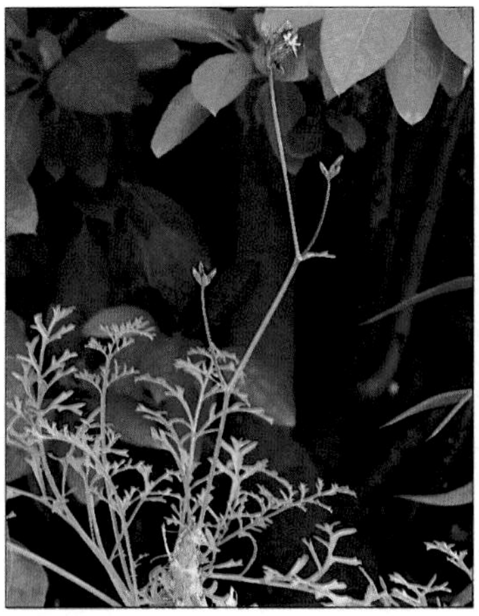

Pelargonium carnosum

***P.* 'Butterfly Lorelei'.** Fancy-leaved zonal pelargonium with yellow butterfly markings in the centre of each rounded leaf. Double, pale salmon-pink flowers are borne in clusters to 8cm (3in) across. ↕ 25–30cm (10–12in), ↔ 15–20cm (6–8in). ✿ (min. 2°C/36°F)

***P.* 'Caligula'** ■ Miniature, double-flowered zonal pelargonium with almost black leaves. Produces clusters, 5–6cm (2–2½in) across, of scarlet flowers. ↕ 10–12cm (4–5in), ↔ 7–10cm (3–4in). ✿ (min. 2°C/36°F)

***P.* 'Capen'.** Bushy, semi-double-flowered zonal pelargonium bearing clusters, 9–10cm (3½in–4in) across, of coral-red flowers. ↕ 40–45cm (16–18in), ↔ 15–20cm (6–8in). ✿ (min. 2°C/36°F)

***P.* 'Carisbrooke'** ■ 🏆 Regal pelargonium with clusters, 9–10cm (3½–4in) across, of pale rose-pink flowers, feathered and blazed wine-red on the upper petals. ↕ 40–45cm (16–18in), ↔ 20–25cm (8–10in). ✿ (min. 2°C/36°F)

P. carnosum ■ Deciduous, perennial succulent with a smooth, swollen stem, 5cm (2in) thick, and fleshy branches, erect and swollen at the joints. Ovate-oblong, pinnate, stalked, slightly hairy, grey-green, very variable leaves, 7–14cm (3–5½in) long, have lobed segments with scalloped margins. Clusters, 4cm (1½in) across, of 2–8 star-shaped, white to pale yellow-green flowers, 1cm (½in) across, are borne in summer. ↕ 40cm (16in), ↔ 25cm (10in). Namibia, South Africa (Northern Cape, Western Cape, Eastern Cape). ✿ (min. 10°C/50°F)

***P.* 'Celebration'.** Vigorous, semi-double-flowered zonal pelargonium producing clusters, 8cm (3in) across, of bicoloured scarlet and white flowers. ↕ 30–40cm (12–16in), ↔ 15–20cm (6–8in). ✿ (min. 2°C/36°F)

***P.* Century Series** 🏆 Compact, seed-raised, single-flowered zonal pelargoniums bearing flowers in shades of red, pink, or white, in clusters to 15cm (6in) across, early in the season. ↕ to 45cm (18in), ↔ 30cm (12in). ✿ (min. 2°C/36°F). **'Century Hot Pink'** ■ has very bright pink flowers.

***P.* Challenge Series.** Compact, seed-raised, single-flowered zonal pelargoniums with clusters to 12cm (5in) across, of flowers in white or shades of red or pink. ↕↔ to 30cm (12in). ✿ (min. 2°C/36°F)

***P.* 'Charlotte Brontë'.** Fancy-leaved zonal pelargonium with rounded, golden yellow, green, and red leaves. Single, salmon-pink flowers are borne in clusters 6–7cm (2½–3in) across. ↕ 25–30cm (10–12in), ↔ 20–25cm (8–10in). ✿ (min. 2°C/36°F)

***P.* Cheerio Series.** Seed-raised, single-flowered zonal pelargoniums bearing flowers in white or shades of pink, salmon-pink, red, or violet, in clusters 10cm (4in) across. ↕↔ 30–40cm (12–16in). ✿ (min. 2°C/36°F)

***P.* 'Chelsworth'.** Miniature, double-flowered zonal pelargonium bearing clusters, 7cm (3in) across, of pinkish orange flowers. ↕ 10–12cm (4–5in), ↔ 7–10cm (3–4in). ✿ (min. 2°C/36°F)

***P.* 'Chew Magna'.** Regal pelargonium with clusters, 9–10cm (3½–4in) across, of pale pink flowers, each petal with a deep red feathered blaze. ↕↔ 30–40cm (12–16in). ✿ (min. 2°C/36°F)

***P.* 'Clorinda'** ■ Vigorous, scented-leaved pelargonium with 3-lobed, cedar-scented leaves. Bears rose-pink flowers in clusters 7cm (3in) across. ↕ 45–50cm (18–20in), ↔ 20–25cm (8–10in). ✿ (min. 2°C/36°F)

***P.* 'Coddenham'** ■ Miniature, double-flowered zonal pelargonium bearing orange-red flowers in clusters 7cm (3in) across. ↕ 10–12cm (4–5in), ↔ 7–10cm (3–4in). ✿ (min. 2°C/36°F)

***P.* 'Contrast'** ■ Fancy-leaved zonal pelargonium with rounded, golden yellow, green, and red leaves. Single scarlet flowers are produced in clusters to 8cm (3in) across. ↕ 25–30cm (10–12in), ↔ 15–20cm (6–8in). ✿ (min. 2°C/36°F)

***P.* 'Copthorne'** 🏆 Vigorous scented-leaved pelargonium with large-lobed leaves exuding an exotic, spicy scent. Bears clusters, 8–9cm (3–3½in) across, of mauve flowers with purple feathering on the upper petals. ↕ 45–50cm (18–20in), ↔ 20–25cm (8–10in). ✿ (min. 2°C/36°F)

P. cotyledonis (Old-man-live-forever). Bushy, deciduous, perennial succulent with short, rough, swollen stems, to 3cm (1¼in) thick. Rounded, rich deep green leaves, 1.5–2cm (½–¾in) long, are heart-shaped at the bases. Clusters, to 6cm (2½in) across, of 5–15 rounded, pure white flowers, to 1.5cm (½in) across, are borne in late spring and early summer. ↕ 30cm (12in), ↔ 15cm (6in). St. Helena. ✿ (min. 10°C/50°F)

***P.* 'Creamery'.** Short-lived, double-flowered zonal pelargonium with pointed leaves. Pale yellow flowers, in clusters 6–7cm (2½–3in) across, colour best when grown in partial shade. ↕ 25–30cm (10–12in), ↔ 10–15cm (4–6in). ✿ (min. 2°C/36°F)

***P. crispum* 'Variegatum'** ■ 🏆 (Variegated lemon-scented pelargonium). Upright scented-leaved pelargonium with cream-margined, mid-green leaves, that release a lemon fragrance when brushed. Pale mauve flowers are produced in clusters, 2–2.5cm (¾–1in) across. ↕ 35–45cm (14–18in), ↔ 12–15cm (5–6in). ✿ (min. 2°C/36°F)

P. cucullatum ■ Shrubby, evergreen perennial with cup-shaped, softly hairy mid-green leaves, to 8cm (3in) long. Bears abundant trumpet-shaped, mauve-purple flowers, to 5cm (2in) across, in clusters 8–9cm (3–3½in) across, from spring to summer. ↕ 60–90cm (24–36in), ↔ 20–25cm (8–10in). South Africa (Western Cape). ✿ (min. 2°C/36°F)

***P.* 'Dale Queen'** ■ Bushy, single-flowered zonal pelargonium producing short-jointed stems. Bears clusters,

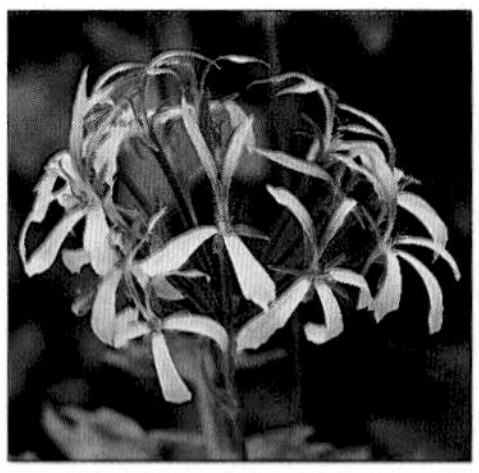

Pelargonium 'Bird Dancer'

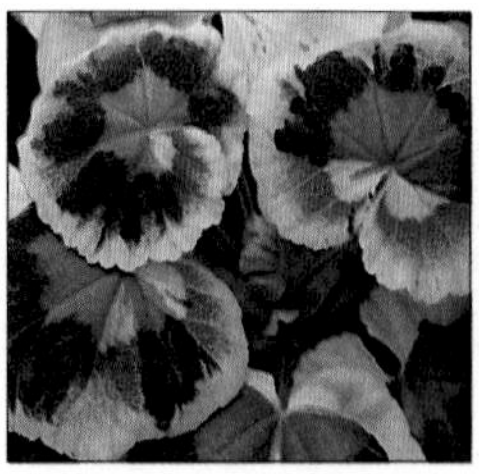

Pelargonium 'Blazonry'

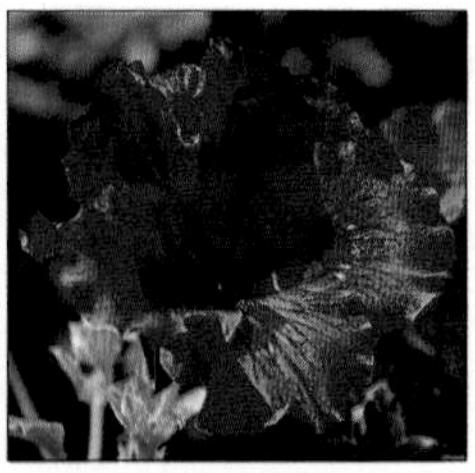

Pelargonium 'Bredon'

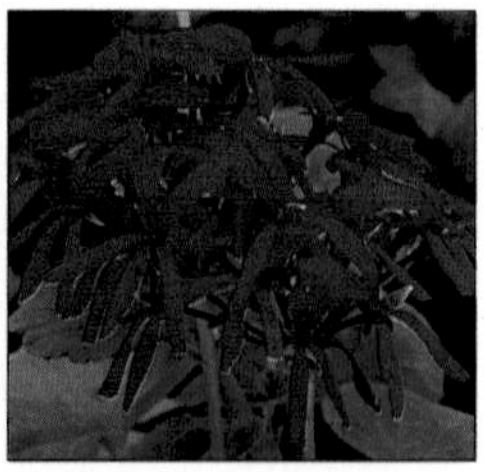

Pelargonium 'Brockbury Scarlet'

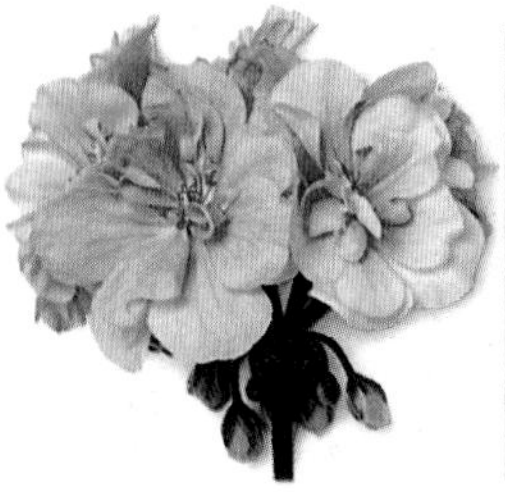

Pelargonium 'Brookside Primrose'

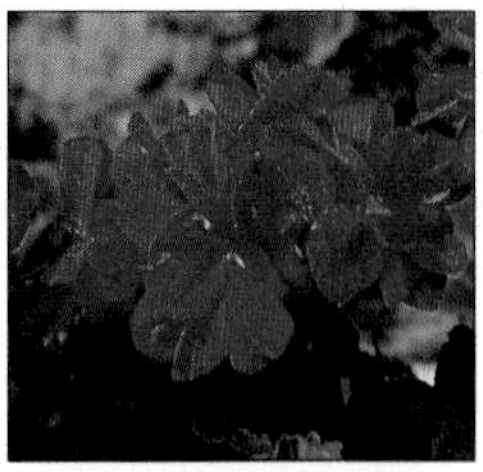

Pelargonium 'Caligula'

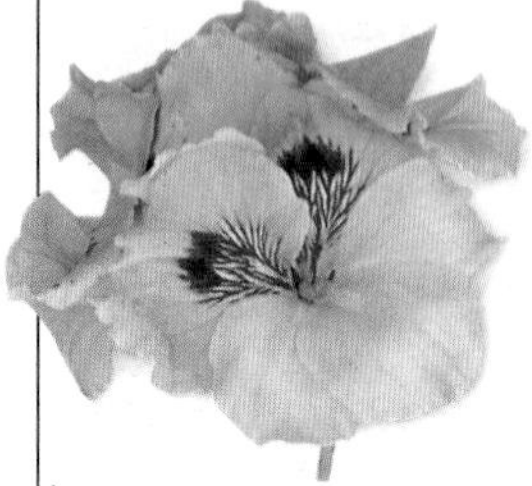

Pelargonium 'Carisbrooke'

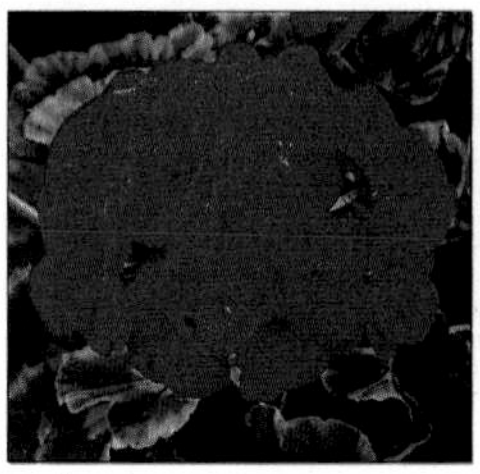

Pelargonium Century Series 'Century Hot Pink'

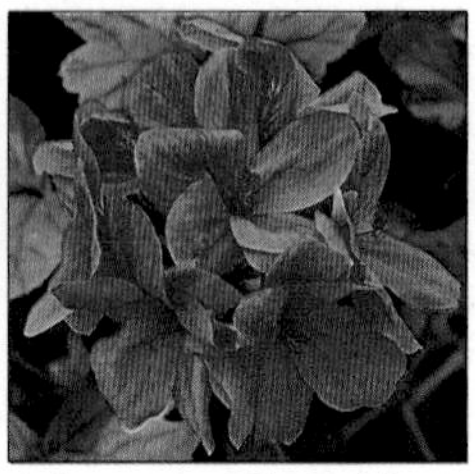

Pelargonium 'Clorinda'

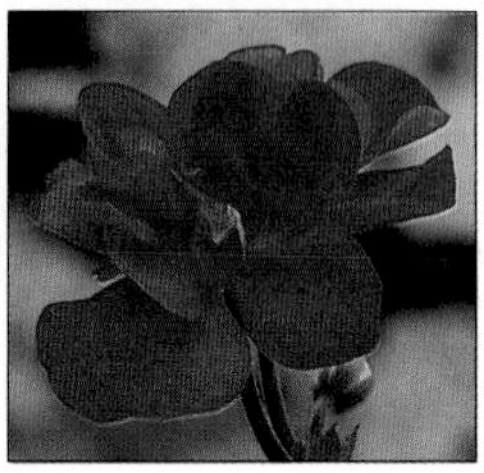

Pelargonium 'Coddenham'

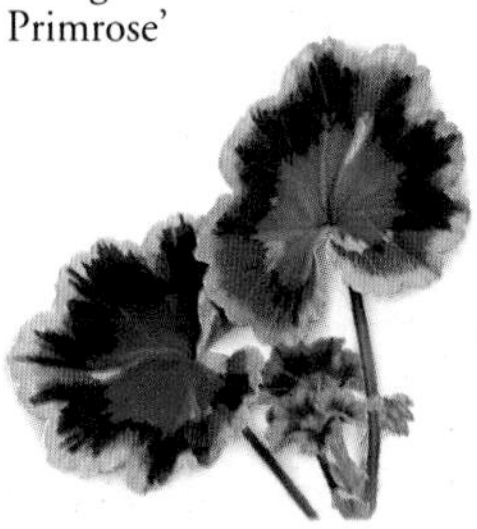

Pelargonium 'Contrast'

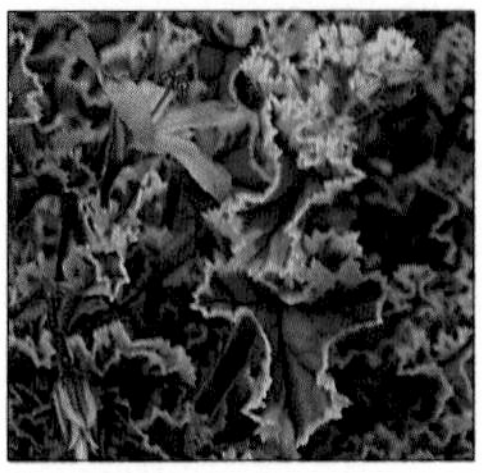

Pelargonium crispum 'Variegatum'

9cm (3½in) across, of pale pink flowers, with darker pink centres. ↕30–40cm (12–16in), ↔15–20cm (6–8in). ❀ (min. 2°C/36°F)

***P.* 'Dame Anna Neagle'** 🏆 Fancy-leaved zonal pelargonium (incorrectly registered as dwarf) producing rounded gold leaves with wide bronze zones. Double, light pink flowers are borne in clusters 6–7cm (2½–3in) across. ↕20–25cm (8–10in), ↔15–20cm (6–8in). ❀ (min. 2°C/36°F)

***P.* 'Davina'.** Miniature, double-flowered zonal pelargonium. Bears clusters, 7cm (3in) across, of salmon-pink flowers, flushed and veined deeper salmon-pink. ↕10–12cm (4–5in), ↔7–10cm (3–4in). ❀ (min. 2°C/36°F)

***P.* 'Dolly Vardon'** ▣🏆 Fancy-leaved zonal pelargonium with rounded, white, red, and green leaves. Bears single scarlet flowers in clusters 7cm (3in) across. ↕25–30cm (10–12in), ↔12–15cm (5–6in). ❀ (min. 2°C/36°F)

***P.* Dynamo Series.** Seed-raised, single-flowered zonal pelargoniums bearing white, deep scarlet, deep rose-pink, or salmon-pink flowers in clusters 12cm (5in) across. ↕40cm (16in), ↔30cm (12in). ❀ (min. 2°C/36°F)

***P.* 'Easter Greeting'** ▣ Low-growing regal pelargonium. Light cerise-pink flowers, with a wine-red blaze on each petal, are borne in clusters 7–9cm (3–3½in) across. ↕25–30cm (10–12in), ↔13–18cm (5–7in). ❀ (min. 2°C/36°F)

P. echinatum. Shrubby, tuberous-rooted, deciduous, perennial succulent with an erect, swollen stem bearing a few grey branches, 1cm (½in) thick, covered with spiny stipules. Heart-shaped, scalloped, grey-green leaves, to 3cm (1¼in) long, with 3–5 shallow lobes, are hairy above, more so beneath. In spring and early summer, produces clusters, to 10cm (4in) across, of 3–8 small, star-shaped, white to pink flowers, 3cm (1¼in) across, with dark red marks on the upper petals. ↕30cm (12in) or more, ↔to 30cm (12in). South Africa (Northern Cape). ❀ (min. 10°C/50°F)

***P.* 'Edmund Lachenal'.** Double-flowered zonal pelargonium with scarlet-based, deep crimson flowers in clusters 10–11cm (4–4½in) across. ↕40–45cm (16–18in), ↔20–25cm (8–10in). ❀ (min. 2°C/36°F)

***P.* Elite Series.** Compact, sturdy, seed-raised, single-flowered zonal pelargoniums, most with attractive leaf zoning, producing clusters, 12cm (5in) across, of flowers in white, salmon-pink, or shades of red or pink. ↕↔25–35cm (10–14in). ❀ (min. 2°C/36°F)

***P.* 'Elizabeth Angus'.** Single-flowered zonal pelargonium bearing clusters, 8–9cm (3–3½in) across, of salmon-pink flowers, each with a small white eye. ↕25–30cm (10–12in), ↔15–20cm (6–8in). ❀ (min. 2°C/36°F)

***P.* 'Emma Hössle'** see *P.* 'Frau Emma Hössle'.

***P.* 'Fair Ellen'** ▣ Scented-leaved pelargonium with deeply lobed leaves that have a strong, spicy perfume. Bears clusters, 5–6cm (2–2½in) across, of purple-pink flowers with toothed petals. ↕30–40cm (12–16in), ↔15–20cm (6–8in). ❀ (min. 2°C/36°F)

***P.* 'Fenton Farm'.** Dwarf, fancy-leaved zonal pelargonium with rounded gold leaves. Tiny, single, white-eyed purple flowers are produced in clusters 4.5–5cm (1¾–2in) across. ↕15–20cm (6–8in), ↔10–12cm (4–5in). ❀ (min. 2°C/36°F)

***P.* 'Filicifolium'.** Scented-leaved pelargonium producing fern-like leaves with a balsam scent. Pale mauve flowers are borne in small clusters, 2–2.5cm (¾–1in) across. ↕25–30cm (10–12in) or more, ↔12–15cm (5–6in). ❀ (min. 2°C/36°F)

***P.* 'Flower of Spring'** ▣🏆 Fancy-leaved zonal pelargonium with rounded silver leaves. Bears single scarlet flowers in clusters 7cm (3in) across. ↕45–60cm (18–24in), ↔20–25cm (8–10in). ❀ (min. 2°C/36°F)

P.* x *fragrans see *P.* 'Fragrans'.

***P.* 'Fragrans'** ▣ syn. *P.* x *fragrans*, *P.* Fragrans Group. Bushy scented-leaved pelargonium with pine-scented, grey-green foliage. Bears clusters, 2.5–3cm (1–1¼in) across, of white flowers. ↕20–25cm (8–10in), ↔15–20cm (6–8in). ❀ (min. 2°C/36°F)

***P.* Fragrans Group** see *P.* 'Fragrans'.

***P.* 'Fragrans Variegatum'.** Bushy scented-leaved pelargonium producing pine-scented, grey-green leaves with cream and white variegation. Bears clusters, 2.5–3cm (1–1¼in) across, of white flowers. ↕20–25cm (8–10in), ↔15–20cm (6–8in). ❀ (min. 2°C/36°F)

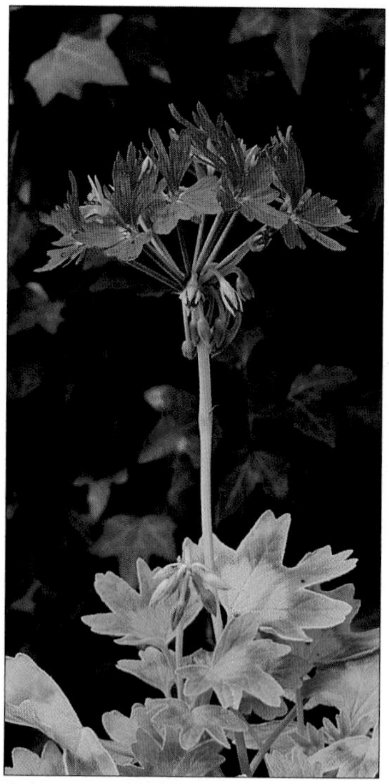

Pelargonium 'Golden Staph'

***P.* 'Fraicher Beauty'** ▣ Double-flowered zonal pelargonium bearing white flowers in clusters, to 13cm (5in) across; the petals have very fine red margins. ↕30–40cm (12–16in), ↔15–20cm (6–8in). ❀ (min. 2°C/36°F)

***P.* 'Francis Parrett'** ▣🏆 Miniature, double-flowered zonal pelargonium producing purple-pink flowers in clusters 7cm (3in) across. ↕10–12cm (4–5in), ↔7–10cm (3–4in). ❀ (min. 2°C/36°F)

***P.* 'Frau Emma Hössle'**, syn. *P.* 'Emma Hössle'. Very bushy, dwarf, double-flowered zonal pelargonium. Mid-pink flowers, with white-based upper petals, are borne in clusters 6–7cm (2½–3in) across. ↕15–20cm (6–8in), ↔10–12cm (4–5in). ❀ (min. 2°C/36°F)

***P.* 'Freckles'** ▣ Seed-raised, single-flowered zonal pelargonium. Produces clusters, 12cm (5in) across, of bright rose-pink flowers, each with a small white eye, and with a darker rose-pink mark at the base of each petal. ↕↔to 30cm (12in). ❀ (min. 2°C/36°F)

***P.* 'Friesdorf'.** Dwarf, fancy-leaved zonal pelargonium with rounded, almost black leaves and narrow-petalled, single crimson flowers in clusters 7cm (3in) across. ↕15–20cm (6–8in), ↔10–12cm (4–5in). ❀ (min. 2°C/36°F)

***P.* 'Frills'.** Miniature, double-flowered zonal pelargonium with pale salmon-pink flowers borne in clusters 4–4.5cm (1½–1¾in) across. ↕10–12cm (4–5in), ↔7–10cm (3–4in). ❀ (min. 2°C/36°F)

***P.* 'Gilbert West'.** Vigorous, single-flowered zonal pelargonium bearing clusters, 9–10cm (3½–4in) across, of magenta flowers; the upper petals have white bases. ↕40–50cm (16–20in), ↔15–20cm (6–8in). ❀ (min. 2°C/36°F)

***P.* 'Golden Brilliantissimum'.** Fancy-leaved zonal pelargonium producing rounded leaves with orange, mid-green, and dark wine-red zones. Double, cherry-red flowers are borne in clusters to 8cm (3in) across. ↕25–30cm (10–12in), ↔12–15cm (5–6in). ❀ (min. 2°C/36°F)

***P.* 'Golden Lilac Mist'.** Bushy, fancy-leaved zonal pelargonium with rounded, bronze-zoned gold leaves. Double, lavender-pink flowers are borne in clusters 7cm (3in) across. ↕25–30cm (10–12in), ↔15–20cm (6–8in). ❀ (min. 2°C/36°F)

***P.* 'Golden Staph'** ▣ Stellar zonal pelargonium with bronze-zoned leaves. Single, orange-red flowers are borne in clusters to 8cm (3in) across. ↕25–30cm (10–12in), ↔12–15cm (5–6in). ❀ (min. 2°C/36°F)

***P.* 'Graveolens' of gardens** ▣ (Rose geranium, Sweet-scented geranium). Vigorous, bushy, erect scented-leaved pelargonium with slightly rough, lobed and cut, mid-green leaves, which have a pungent lemon-rose scent. Sterile mauve flowers are borne in clusters 2.5–3cm (1–1¼in) across. ↕45–60cm (18–24in), ↔20–40cm (8–16in). ❀ (min. 2°C/36°F)

***P.* 'Hans Rigler'.** Vigorous, semi-double-flowered zonal pelargonium producing brilliant scarlet flowers in clusters 10cm (4in) across. ↕30–40cm (12–16in), ↔15–20cm (6–8in). ❀ (min. 2°C/36°F)

***P.* 'Happy Thought'** ▣🏆 Fancy-leaved zonal pelargonium bearing rounded leaves, each with a greenish yellow butterfly marking in the centre. Single,

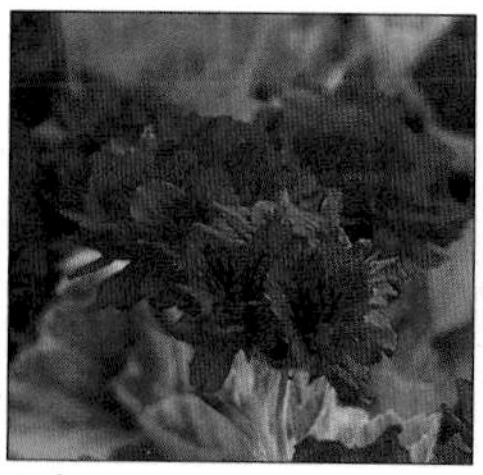

Pelargonium cucullatum

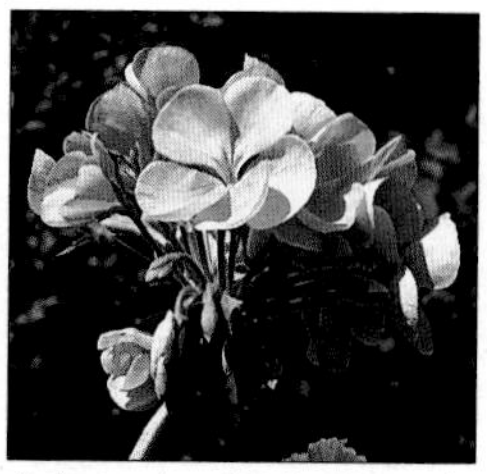

Pelargonium 'Dale Queen'

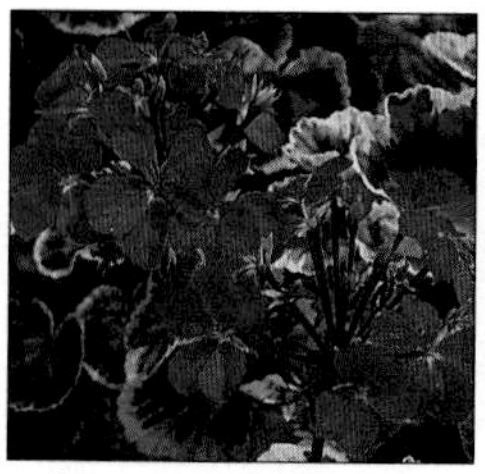

Pelargonium 'Dolly Vardon'

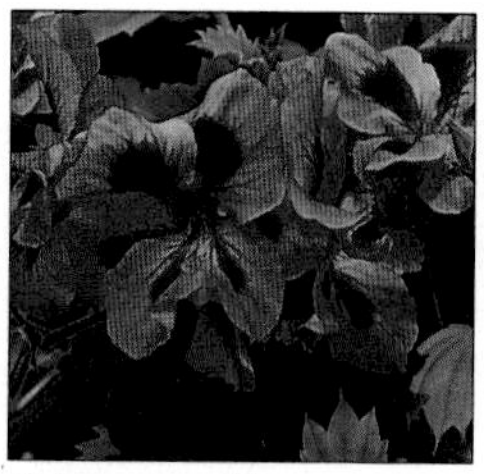

Pelargonium 'Easter Greeting'

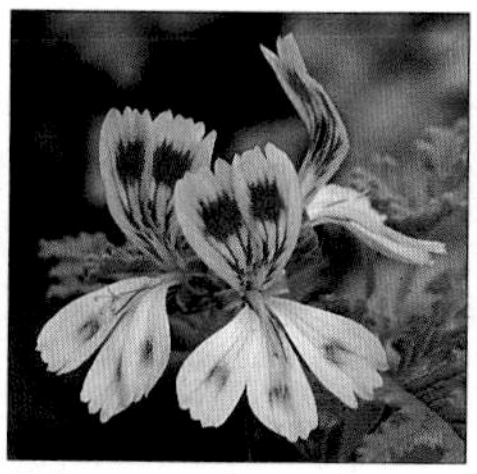

Pelargonium 'Fair Ellen'

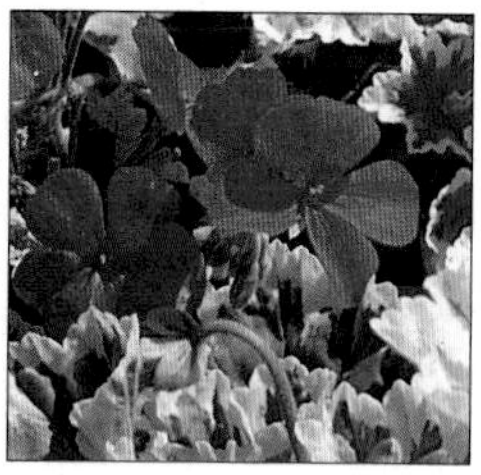

Pelargonium 'Flower of Spring'

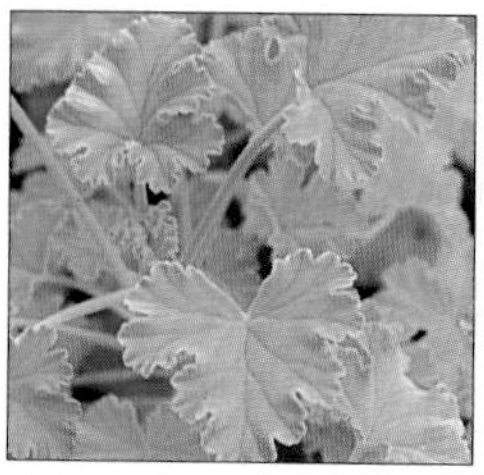

Pelargonium 'Fragrans'

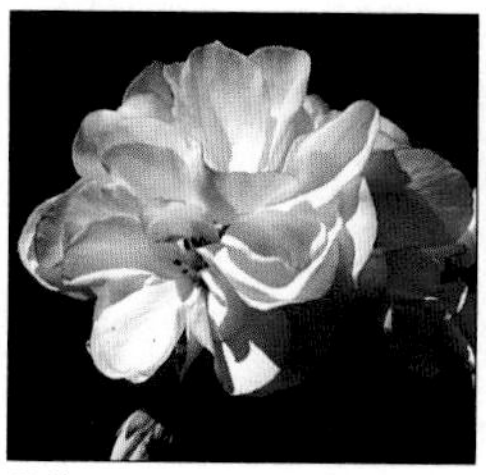

Pelargonium 'Fraicher Beauty'

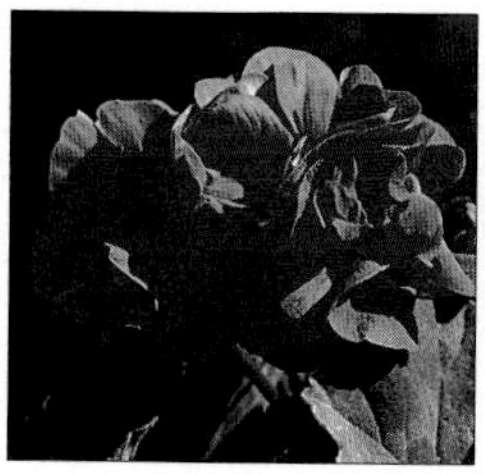

Pelargonium 'Francis Parrett'

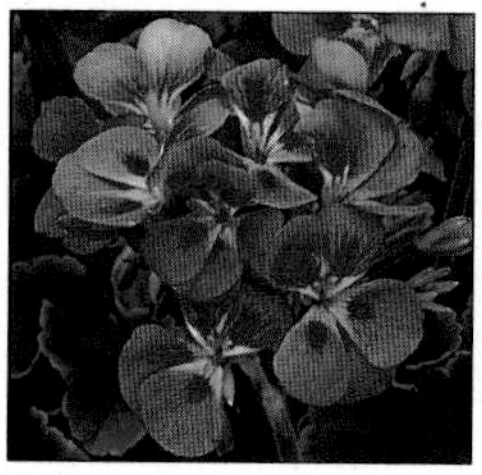

Pelargonium 'Freckles'

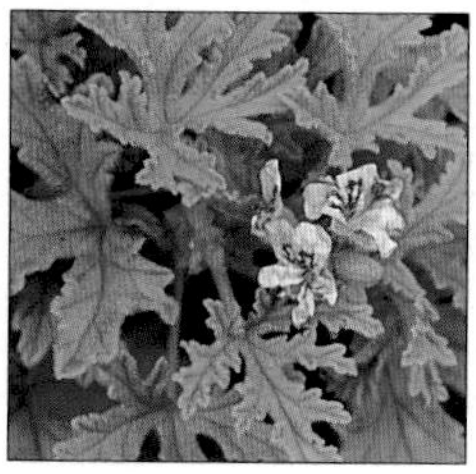

Pelargonium 'Graveolens' of gardens

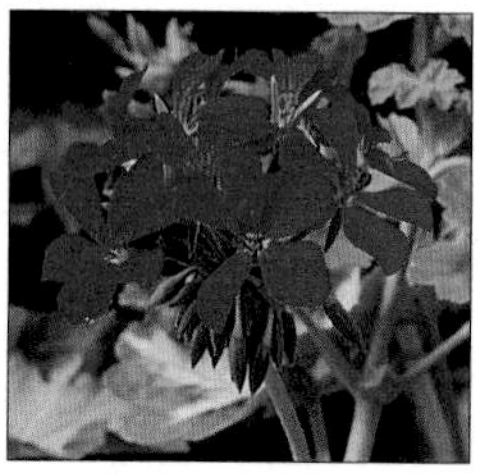

Pelargonium 'Happy Thought'

light crimson flowers are produced in clusters 8–9cm (3–3½in) across. ↕40–45cm (16–18in), ↔20–25cm (8–10in). ❄ (min. 2°C/36°F)

***P.* Horizon Series** ▣ Compact, bushy, seed-raised, single-flowered zonal pelargoniums with strongly zoned foliage. Flowers in white or shades of pink or red are borne in clusters, to 12cm (5in) across, early in the season. Has good wet-weather tolerance. ↕ to 30cm (12in), ↔25cm (10in). ❄ (min. 2°C/36°F). **'Horizon Scarlet'** produces dark, strongly zoned leaves and scarlet flowers.

***P.* 'Icecrystal'.** Semi-double-flowered zonal pelargonium. Bears clusters, to 13cm (5in) across, of white-eyed, lavender-blue flowers with a purple dot on each petal. ↕30–40cm (12–16in), ↔20–25cm (8–10in). ❄ (min. 2°C/36°F)

P. inquinans. Erect, evergreen perennial producing soft, woody stems and rounded, mid-green leaves, 5–6cm (2–2½in) across; they stain fingers red when handled. Saucer-shaped scarlet flowers, 4cm (1½in) across, are borne in clusters, 9cm (3½in) across, from spring to summer. One of the original parents of zonal pelargoniums. ↕60–90cm (24–36in), ↔20–25cm (8–10in). South Africa (Eastern Transvaal, KwaZulu/Natal, Eastern Cape). ❄ (min. 2°C/36°F)

***P.* 'Irene'** ▣🏆 Vigorous, semi-double-flowered zonal pelargonium bearing light cerise-red flowers in clusters 11cm (4½in) across. ↕40–45cm (16–18in), ↔25–30cm (10–12in). ❄ (min. 2°C/36°F)

***P.* 'Isobell'.** Bushy, semi-double-flowered zonal pelargonium producing bright red flowers in clusters 9–10cm (3½–4in) across. ↕25–30cm (10–12in), ↔20–25cm (8–10in). ❄ (min. 2°C/36°F)

***P.* 'Ivalo'** ▣ Bushy, short-jointed, semi-double-flowered zonal pelargonium. Produces clusters, 9–10cm (3½–4in) across, of lavender-pink flowers with purple feathering and marking, and white-based upper petals. ↕25–30cm (10–12in), ↔20–25cm (8–10in). ❄ (min. 2°C/36°F)

***P.* 'Jackie'**, syn. *P.* 'Jackie Gall'. Very bushy, slow-growing, short-jointed ivy-leaved pelargonium with small leaves. Bears clusters, 9cm (3½in) across, of

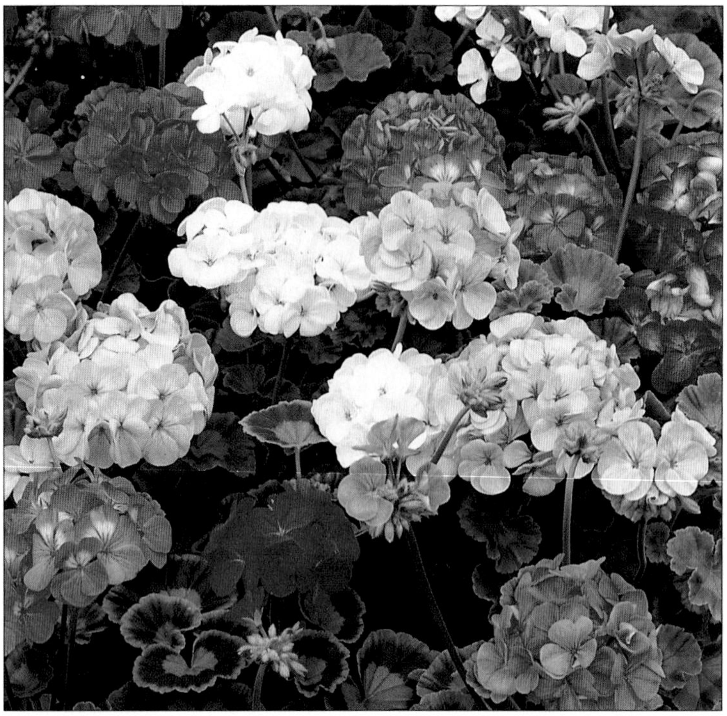

Pelargonium Horizon Series

rosebud-like, double, pale lavender-pink flowers. ↕↔15–20cm (6–8in). ❄ (min. 2°C/36°F)

***P.* 'Jackie Gall'** see *P.* 'Jackie'.

***P.* 'Just William'.** Miniature, double-flowered zonal pelargonium with bright red flowers in clusters 6–7cm (2½–3in) across. ↕10–12cm (4–5in), ↔7–10cm (3–4in). ❄ (min. 2°C/36°F)

***P.* 'Lachsball'** ▣ Vigorous, semi-double-flowered zonal pelargonium bearing clusters, 10cm (4in) across, of deep salmon-pink flowers with tiny white eyes. ↕45–50cm (18–20in), ↔15–20cm (6–8in). ❄ (min. 2°C/36°F)

***P.* 'Lachskönigin'** ▣ Short-jointed ivy-leaved pelargonium with semi-double, rosy salmon-pink flowers borne in clusters 11cm (4½in) across. ↕25–30cm (10–12in), ↔15–20cm (6–8in). ❄ (min. 2°C/36°F)

***P.* 'Lady Plymouth'** ▣🏆 Scented-leaved pelargonium with eucalyptus-scented, silver-margined leaves. Lavender-pink flowers are borne in clusters 3–3.5cm (1¼–1½in) across.

A variant of *P.* 'Graveolens' of gardens. ↕30–40cm (12–16in), ↔15–20cm (6–8in). ❄ (min. 2°C/36°F)

***P.* 'Lavender Grand Slam'** ▣🏆 Bushy regal pelargonium. Produces clusters, 9–10cm (3½–4in) across, of mauve flowers, the upper petals with purple markings and black-purple feathering. ↕30–40cm (12–16in), ↔15–20cm (6–8in). ❄ (min. 2°C/36°F)

***P.* 'Lavender Sensation'.** Bushy regal pelargonium bearing frilly, lavender-pink flowers, with plum markings, in clusters 11–12cm (4½–5in) across. ↕30–40cm (12–16in), ↔15–20cm (6–8in). ❄ (min. 2°C/36°F)

***P.* 'L'Elégante'** ▣🏆 Ivy-leaved pelargonium with silver-green leaves that turn cream-variegated, mid-green, and purple if kept very dry. Single white flowers are borne in clusters to 8cm (3in) across. ↕20–25cm (8–10in), ↔15–20cm (6–8in). ❄ (min. 2°C/36°F)

***P.* 'Lemon Fancy'.** Scented-leaved pelargonium with rough-textured, toothed leaves with a citrus fragrance. Produces mauve flowers in clusters 3–3.5cm (1¼–1½in) across. ↕40–45cm (16–18in), ↔15–20cm (6–8in). ❄ (min. 2°C/36°F)

***P.* 'Leopard'.** Vigorous, bushy ivy-leaved pelargonium producing clusters, 9–10cm (3½–4in) across, of semi-double, purple-pink flowers with wine-red splashes on the upper petals. ↕25–30cm (10–12in), ↔15–20cm (6–8in). ❄ (min. 2°C/36°F)

***P.* 'Leslie Judd'** ▣ Regal pelargonium with pale salmon-pink flowers, feathered wine-red on each petal, borne in clusters 9–10cm (3½–4in) across. ↕40–45cm (16–18in), ↔15–20cm (6–8in). ❄ (min. 2°C/36°F)

***P.* 'Lila Mini Cascade'.** Thin-stemmed ivy-leaved pelargonium with single, lilac-pink flowers borne in clusters 8–9cm (3–3½in) across. ↕45–50cm (18–20in), ↔15–20cm (6–8in). ❄ (min. 2°C/36°F)

***P.* 'Lilian Pottinger'.** Scented-leaved pelargonium with irregular, 3-lobed, toothed, grey-green leaves exuding a camphor-pine fragance. White flowers are produced in clusters 2.5–3cm (1–1¼in) across. ↕20–25cm (8–10in), ↔12–15cm (5–6in). ❄ (min. 2°C/36°F)

***P.* 'Lord Bute'.** Regal pelargonium producing dark reddish black flowers, the petals with dark red margins, in clusters to 10cm (4in) across. ↕45cm (18in), ↔30cm (12in). ❄ (min. 2°C/36°F)

***P.* 'Loverly'.** Bushy, single-flowered zonal pelargonium. Produces clusters, to 8cm (3in) across, of two-toned, salmon-pink flowers. ↕20–25cm (8–10in), ↔12–15cm (5–6in). ❄ (min. 2°C/36°F)

***P.* 'Mabel Grey'** ▣🏆 Scented-leaved pelargonium with deeply cut, rough-textured leaves with a very strong lemon scent. Produces purple flowers in clusters 5cm (2in) across. ↕30–35cm (12–14in), ↔12–15cm (5–6in). ❄ (min. 2°C/36°F)

***P.* 'Magda'.** Double-flowered zonal pelargonium producing clusters, 8cm (3in) across, of pale pink flowers, spotted and streaked scarlet. ↕25–30cm (10–12in), ↔12–15cm (5–6in). ❄ (min. 2°C/36°F)

***P.* 'Mauritania'** ▣ Single-flowered zonal pelargonium. White flowers, tinged rose-pink in the centres, are produced in clusters 9cm (3½in) across.

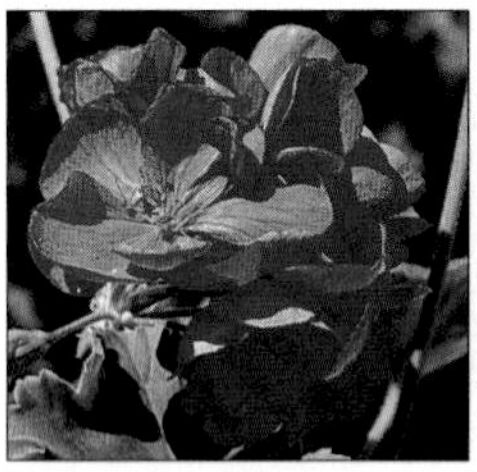

Pelargonium 'Irene'

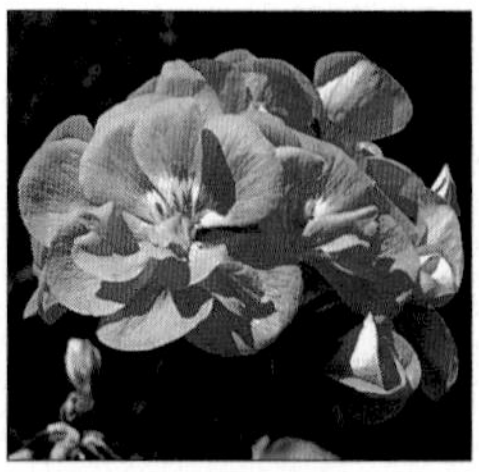

Pelargonium 'Ivalo'

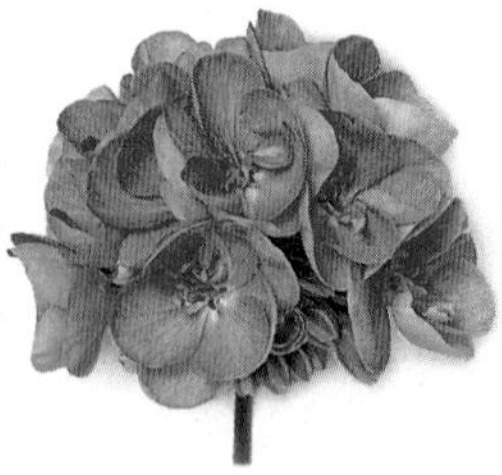

Pelargonium 'Lachsball'

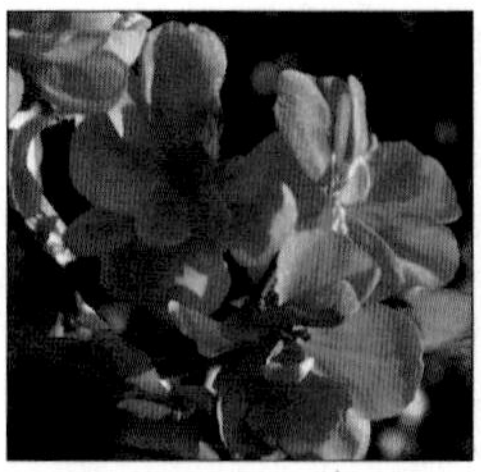

Pelargonium 'Lachskönigin'

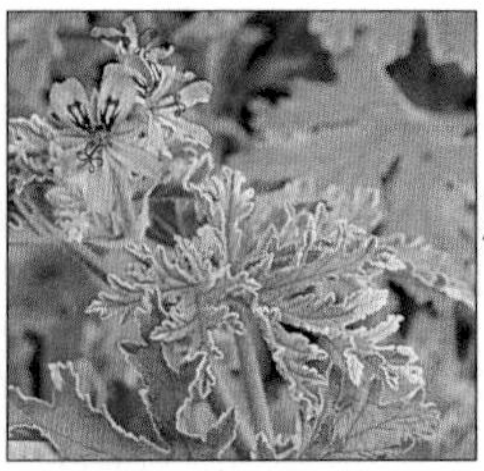

Pelargonium 'Lady Plymouth'

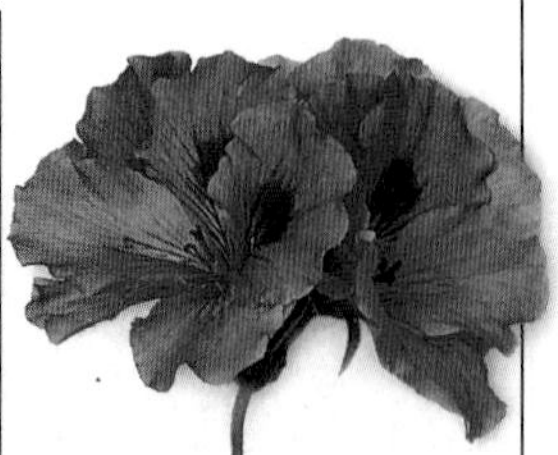

Pelargonium 'Lavender Grand Slam'

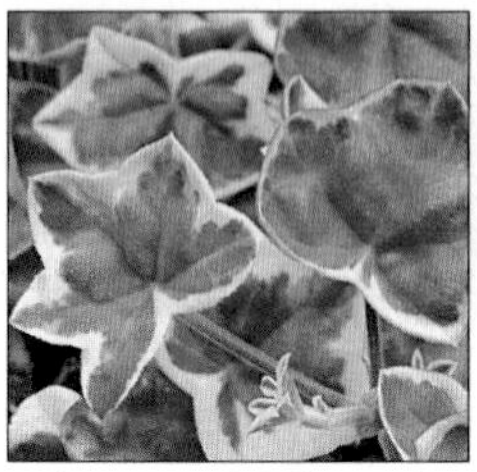

Pelargonium 'L'Elégante'

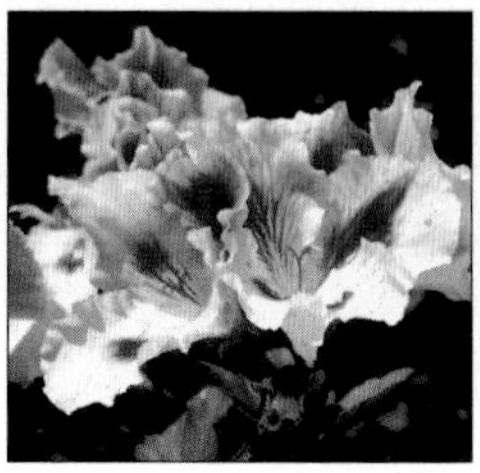

Pelargonium 'Leslie Judd'

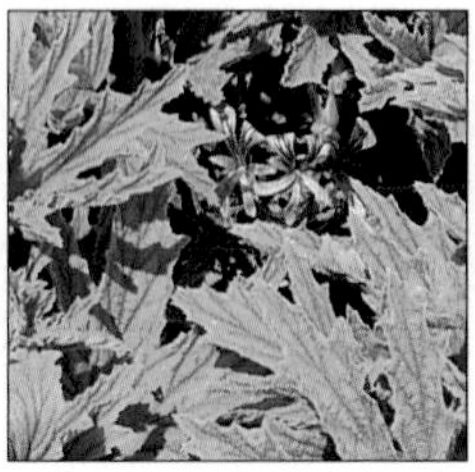

Pelargonium 'Mabel Grey'

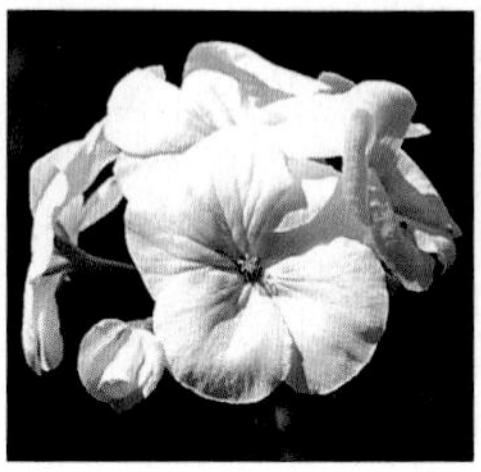

Pelargonium 'Mauritania'

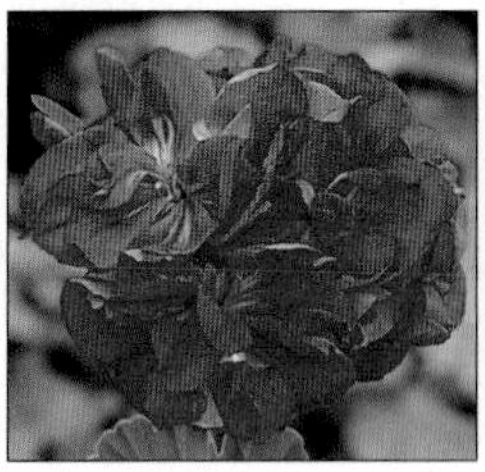

Pelargonium 'Mr. Everaarts'

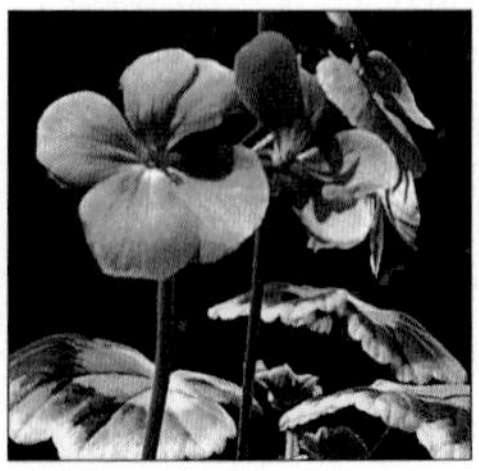

Pelargonium 'Mr. Henry Cox'

↕ 25–30cm (10–12in), ↔ 12–15cm (5–6in). ❄ (min. 2°C/36°F)
***P.* 'Mauve Beauty'.** Slow-growing, short-jointed ivy-leaved pelargonium with double, mauve-pink flowers borne in clusters to 8cm (3in) across. ↕ 20–25cm (8–10in), ↔ 12–15cm (5–6in). ❄ (min. 2°C/36°F)
***P.* 'Mauve Salter Bevis'.** Cactus-flowered zonal pelargonium bearing single, lavender-pink flowers in clusters to 8cm (3in) across. ↕ 25–30cm (10–12in), ↔ 12–15cm (5–6in). ❄ (min. 2°C/36°F)
***P.* 'Miss Wackles'.** Miniature, double-flowered zonal pelargonium producing mid-green leaves with dark brown zones. Produces cerise-red flowers in clusters 4.5–5cm (1¾–2in) across. ↕ 10–12cm (4–5in), ↔ 7–10cm (3–4in). ❄ (min. 2°C/36°F)
***P.* 'Mme Crousse'** 🏆 Very long-jointed ivy-leaved pelargonium with semi-double, pale pink flowers borne in clusters to 7cm (3in) across. ↕ 50–60cm (20–24in), ↔ 15–20cm (6–8in). ❄ (min. 2°C/36°F)
***P.* 'Mme Fournier'** ▣ Miniature, single-flowered zonal pelargonium with purple-black leaves and stems. Scarlet flowers are borne in clusters 4.5–5cm (1¾–2in) across. ↕ 10–12cm (4–5in), ↔ 7–10cm (3–4in). ❄ (min. 2°C/36°F)
***P.* 'Mr. Everaarts'** ▣ Bushy, dwarf, double-flowered pelargonium with bright red-pink flowers borne in clusters 5–6cm (2–2½in) across. ↕ 15–20cm (6–8in), ↔ 10–12cm (4–5in). ❄ (min. 2°C/36°F)
***P.* 'Mr. Henry Cox'** ▣🏆 syn. *P.* 'Mrs. Henry Cox'. Fancy-leaved zonal pelargonium with rounded, golden yellow leaves marked with mid-green, dark purple, and red. Single pink flowers, with small white eyes, are borne in clusters 7cm (3in) across. ↕ 25–30cm (10–12in), ↔ 10–12cm (4–5in). ❄ (min. 2°C/36°F)
***P.* 'Mrs. Henry Cox'** see *P.* 'Mr. Henry Cox'.
***P.* 'Mrs. Pollock'** ▣ Fancy-leaved zonal pelargonium with rounded, golden yellow leaves marked with brownish purple, pink, and mid-green. Single, pinkish orange flowers are borne in clusters 7cm (3in) across. ↕ 25–30cm (10–12in), ↔ 12–15cm (5–6in). ❄ (min. 2°C/36°F)
***P.* 'Mrs. Quilter'** ▣ Fancy-leaved zonal pelargonium bearing rounded gold leaves with wide bronze zones. Single, pale pink flowers are borne in clusters 7cm (3in) across. Leaf colour deepens in full sun. ↕ 30–40cm (12–16in), ↔ 12–15cm (5–6in). ❄ (min. 2°C/36°F)
***P.* 'Mr. Wren'.** Bushy, single-flowered zonal pelargonium with white flowers, overlaid orange, borne in clusters 7cm (3in) across. ↕ 40–45cm (16–18in), ↔ 15–20cm (6–8in). ❄ (min. 2°C/36°F)
***P.* Multibloom Series** ▣🏆 Seed-raised, single-flowered zonal pelargoniums with abundant flowers in white or shades of pink or red, some with white eyes, borne in clusters 8–12cm (3–5in) across. Early flowering over a long period; good wet-weather tolerance. ↕ 25–30cm (10–12in), ↔ 30cm (12in). ❄ (min. 2°C/36°F)
P. odoratissimum. Bushy, spreading, evergreen perennial with rounded, light green leaves, 4–5cm (1½–2in) across, with a scent reminiscent of stored apples. Produces clusters, 2.5–3cm (1–1¼in) across, of 3–10 star-shaped white flowers, to 1.5cm (½in) across, from spring to summer. ↕ 20–25cm (8–10in), ↔ 45–60cm (18–24in). South Africa (KwaZulu/Natal, Northern Transvaal, Eastern Cape, Western Cape). ❄ (min. 2°C/36°F)
***P.* 'Old Spice'** ▣ Bushy, erect scented-leaved pelargonium with rounded, spicy-scented leaves. Bears white flowers in clusters 3–3.5cm (1¼–1½in) across. ↕ 25–30cm (10–12in), ↔ 12–15cm (5–6in). ❄ (min. 2°C/36°F)
***P.* 'Orange Appeal'** ▣ Seed-raised, single flowered zonal pelargonium with clear, bright orange flowers borne in clusters to 7cm (3in) across. ↕ 30–40cm (12–16in), ↔ 30cm (12in). ❄ (min. 2°C/36°F)
***P.* 'Orange Ricard'.** Vigorous, semi-double-flowered zonal pelargonium bearing orange flowers in clusters, 10cm (4in) across. ↕ 40–45cm (16–18in), ↔ 20–25cm (8–10in). ❄ (min. 2°C/36°F)
***P.* Orbit Series.** Very early flowering, seed-raised, single-flowered zonal pelargoniums that branch from the base and have fine leaf zoning. Produces large clusters 12–14cm (5–5½in) across, of flowers in white or shades of pink, orange, or red. ↕ to 35cm (14in), ↔ 25cm (10in). ❄ (min. 2°C/36°F).

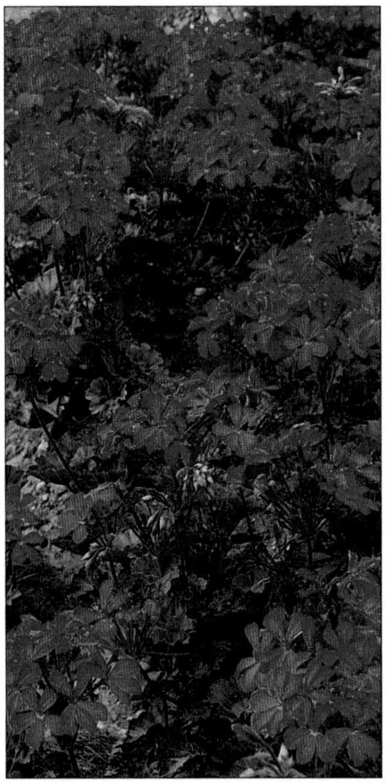

Pelargonium 'Mme Fournier'

'Cherry Orbit' is upright, with purple-zoned leaves and cherry-red flowers.
***P.* 'Palais'.** Vigorous, semi-double-flowered zonal pelargonium bearing pale salmon-pink flowers in clusters 11cm (4½in) across. ↕ 40–45cm (16–18in), ↔ 20–25cm (8–10in). ❄ (min. 2°C/36°F)
***P.* 'Paton's Unique'** ▣🏆 Vigorous unique pelargonium bearing coral-red and pale pink flowers, with small white eyes, in clusters 4–4.5cm (1½–1¾in) across. The leaves release a pungent scent when bruised. ↕ 40–45cm (16–18in), ↔ 15–20cm (6–8in). ❄ (min. 2°C/36°F)
***P.* 'Paul Humphries'** ▣ Bushy, double-flowered zonal pelargonium bearing clusters, 7cm (3in) across, of dark cerise-red flowers, the lower petals tinged purple. ↕ 25–30cm (10–12in), ↔ 15–20cm (6–8in). ❄ (min. 2°C/36°F)
***P.* 'Penve'.** Semi-double-flowered zonal pelargonium with bright magenta-purple flowers with white centres, borne in clusters 10–11cm (4–4½in) across. ↕ 30–40cm (12–16in), ↔ 20–25cm (8–10in). ❄ (min. 2°C/36°F)
***P.* Pinto Series** see *P.* Pulsar Series.
***P.* 'Pixie Rose'** ▣ Stellar zonal pelargonium producing single, rose-red flowers, with small white eyes, in clusters 8–9cm (3–3½in) across. ↕ 25–30cm (10–12in), ↔ 15–20cm (6–8in). ❄ (min. 2°C/36°F)
***P.* 'Polka'** ▣ Vigorous unique pelargonium with clusters, 10cm (4in) across, of orange-red flowers, marked and feathered deep purple on the upper petals; lower petals are pinkish orange. ↕ 45–50cm (18–20in), ↔ 20–25cm (8–10in). ❄ (min. 2°C/36°F)
***P.* 'Prince of Orange'.** Erect, thin-stemmed scented-leaved pelargonium with small, rounded, orange-scented leaves. Bears mauve flowers in clusters 2.5–3cm (1–1¼in) across. ↕ 25–30cm (10–12in), ↔ 15–20cm (6–8in). ❄ (min. 2°C/36°F)
***P.* Pulsar Series**, syn. *P.* Pinto Series. Seed-raised, single-flowered zonal pelargoniums with strongly zoned foliage. Flowers, in white or shades of pink or red, including bicolours, are borne in clusters 12–14cm (5–5½in) across. ↕ 30–35cm (12–14in), ↔ 30cm (12in). ❄ (min. 2°C/36°F). **'Pulsar Scarlet'** ▣ has deep red flowers.
***P.* 'Purple Emperor'** ▣ Regal pelargonium with clusters, 9–10cm (3½–4in) across, of light purple-pink flowers, heavily blazed and feathered deep wine-red on each petal. ↕ 30–40cm (12–16in), ↔ 15–20cm (6–8in). ❄ (min. 2°C/36°F)
***P.* 'Purple Wonder'** ▣ Vigorous, semi-double-flowered zonal pelargonium with cerise-purple flowers borne in clusters 9cm (3½in) across. ↕ 40–45cm (16–18in), ↔ 20–25cm (8–10in). ❄ (min. 2°C/36°F)
P. radens. Vigorous, upright, bushy, evergreen subshrub with triangular, deeply 2-pinnatifid, rough, strongly aromatic, grey-green leaves, 6cm (2½in) long, consisting of oblong segments with margins rolled under. Produces star-shaped, pale to purple-pink flowers, 1.5cm (½in) across, in 2- to 6-flowered clusters, to 6cm (2½in) across, in late spring and summer. ↕ 30–45cm (12–18in), ↔ 20–30cm (8–12in). South Africa (Western Cape, Eastern Cape). ❄ (min. 2°C/36°F)

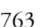

P

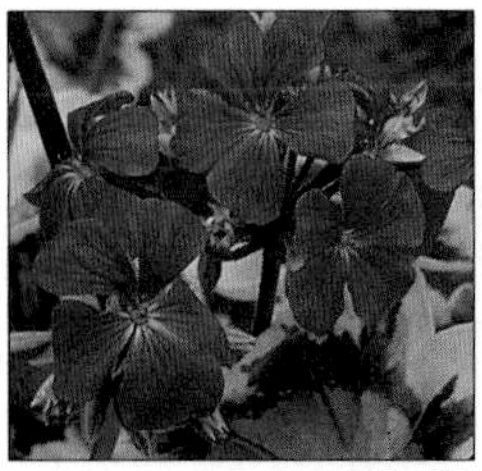

Pelargonium 'Mrs. Pollock'

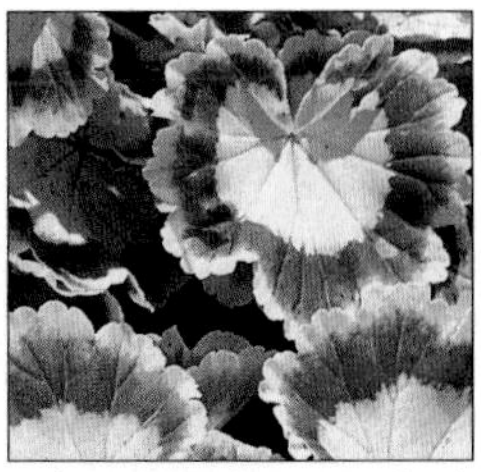

Pelargonium 'Mrs. Quilter'

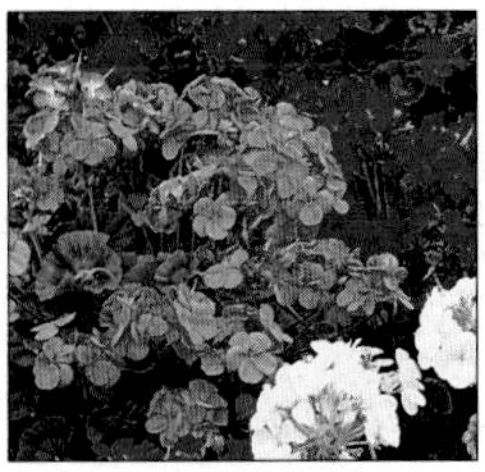

Pelargonium Multibloom Series

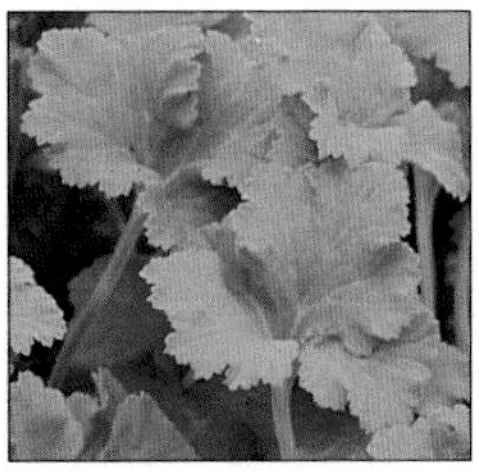

Pelargonium 'Old Spice'

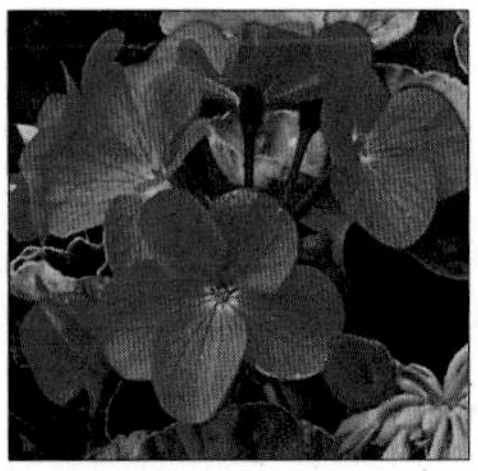

Pelargonium 'Orange Appeal'

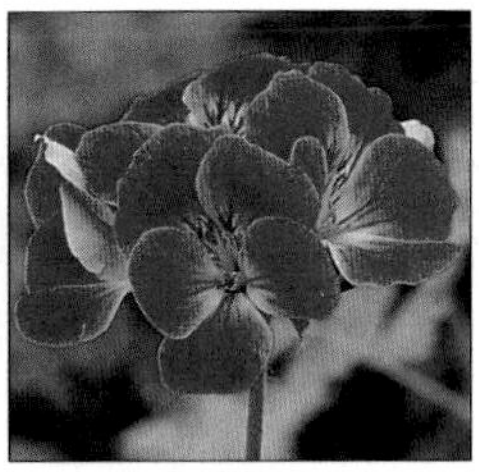

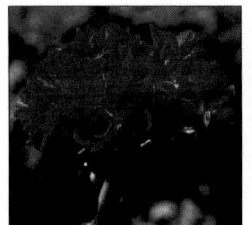

Pelargonium 'Paton's Unique'

Pelargonium 'Paul Humphries'

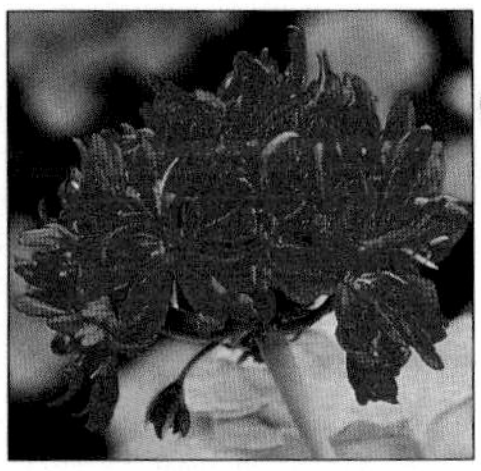

Pelargonium 'Pixie Rose'

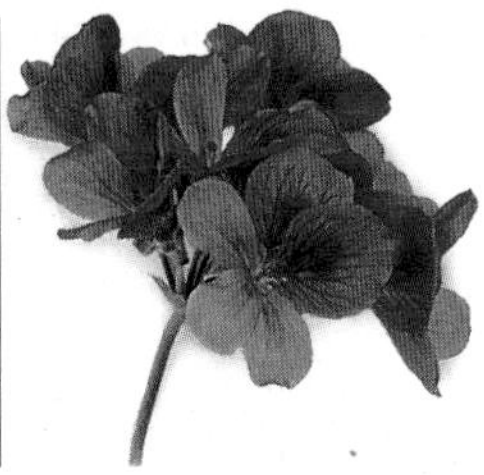

Pelargonium 'Polka'

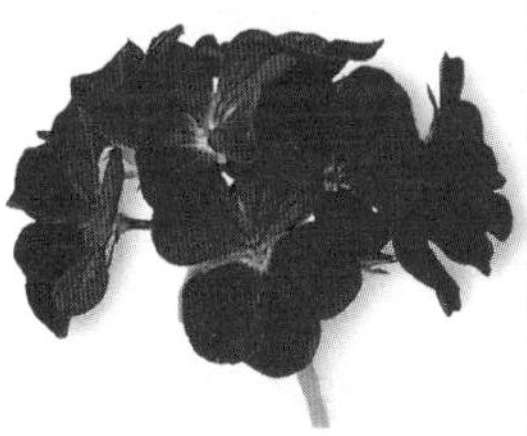

Pelargonium Pulsar Series 'Pulsar Scarlet'

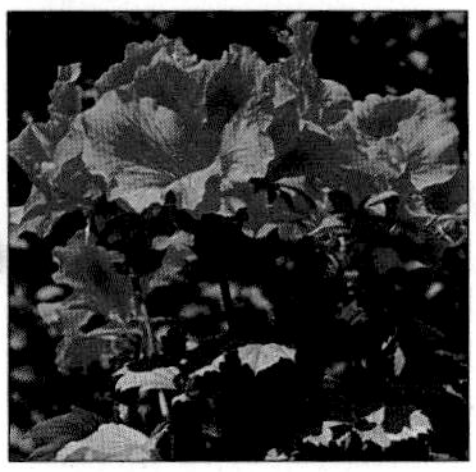

Pelargonium 'Purple Emperor'

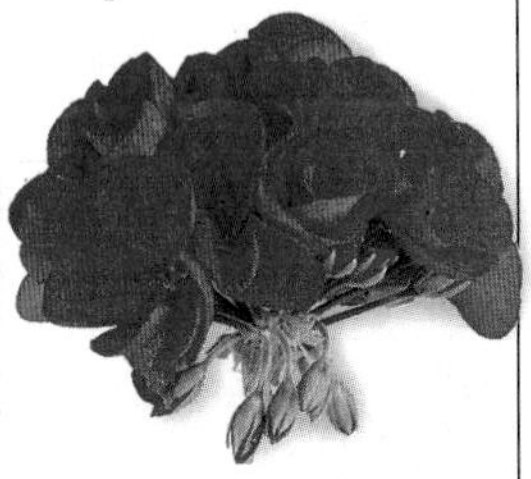

Pelargonium 'Purple Wonder'

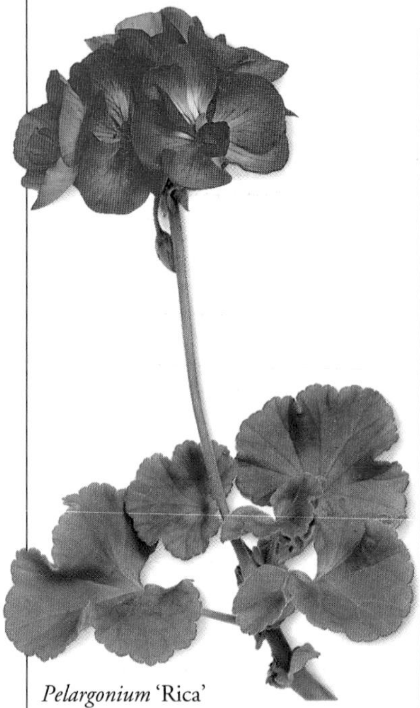

Pelargonium 'Rica'

***P.* 'Rica'** ■ Bushy, semi-double-flowered zonal pelargonium bearing clusters, 10–11cm (4–4½in) across, of deep rose-pink flowers with large white eyes. ↕30–40cm (12–16in), ↔ 15–20cm (6–8in). ❄ (min. 2°C/36°F)
***P.* Ringo 2000 Series.** Seed-raised, single-flowered zonal pelargoniums with very dark zoning on the leaves. Flowers, in white, shades of pink or red, or mixtures, are produced in clusters, 12–14cm (5–5½in) across. ↕30–40cm (12–16in), ↔ 25–35cm (10–14in). ❄ (min. 2°C/36°F)
***P.* 'Rio'.** Single-flowered zonal pelargonium with clusters, to 12cm (5in) across, of rose-pink flowers with a large crimson dot on each petal. ↕30–35cm (12–14in), ↔ 12–15cm (5–6in). ❄ (min. 2°C/36°F)
***P.* 'Robe'** ■ Vigorous, semi-double-flowered zonal pelargonium bearing cerise-crimson flowers in clusters to 8cm (3in) across. ↕40–45cm (16–18in), ↔ 15–20cm (6–8in). ❄ (min. 2°C/36°F)
***P.* 'Rober's Lemon Rose'.** Vigorous, scented-leaved pelargonium with pinnatifid, grey-green leaves, rose-scented with lemon undertones. Produces mauve flowers in clusters 4–4.5cm (1½–1¾in) across. ↕45–50cm (18–20in), ↔ 20–25cm (8–10in). ❄ (min. 2°C/36°F)
***P.* 'Rollisson's Unique'** ■ Unique pelargonium with clusters, 7cm (3in) across, of red-purple flowers with deep purple and white feathering on the upper petals. ↕40–45cm (16–18in), ↔ 15–20cm (6–8in). ❄ (min. 2°C/36°F)
***P.* 'Rouletta'** ■ Vigorous, ivy-leaved pelargonium with semi-double, bicoloured light crimson and white flowers borne in clusters 9cm (3½in) across. May temporarily revert to plain crimson in hot weather. ↕50–60cm (20–24in), ↔ 15–20cm (6–8in). ❄ (min. 2°C/36°F)
***P.* 'Royal Oak'.** Scented-leaved pelargonium with dark green leaves, shaped like oak leaves, with dark central marks, and exuding an exotic, spicy scent. Bears mauve flowers in clusters 2.5–3cm (1–1¼in) across. ↕30–40cm (12–16in), ↔ 25–30cm (10–12in). ❄ (min. 2°C/36°F)
***P.* 'Royal Sovereign'.** Bushy, fancy-leaved zonal pelargonium with rounded bronze and gold leaves. Double red flowers are produced in clusters 7cm (3in) across. ↕25–30cm (10–12in), ↔ 15–20cm (6–8in). ❄ (min. 2°C/36°F)
***P.* 'Samantha Stamps'.** Dwarf, fancy-leaved zonal pelargonium with rounded, bronze-zoned gold leaves. Bears double, pink-flushed white flowers in clusters 8cm (3in) across. ↕20cm (8in), ↔ 15cm (6in). ❄ (min. 2°C/36°F)
***P.* 'Sandra Haynes'.** Bushy, free-flowering regal pelargonium bearing light crimson flowers in clusters 10cm (4in) across. ↕30–40cm (12–16in), ↔ 15–20cm (6–8in). ❄ (min. 2°C/36°F)
***P.* 'Saxifragoides'.** Slow-growing, trailing, possibly ivy-leaved pelargonium with small, succulent leaves. Produces tiny, double, mauve and white flowers in clusters 2.5–3cm (1–1¼in) across. ↕15–20cm (6–8in), ↔ 12–15cm (5–6in). ❄ (min. 2°C/36°F)
***P.* 'Schöne Helena'** ■ Semi-double-flowered zonal pelargonium with clusters, 10–11cm (4–4½in) across, of pale salmon-pink flowers, creamy white towards the petal margins. ↕30–40cm (12–16in), ↔ 20–25cm (8–10in). ❄ (min. 2°C/36°F)
***P.* 'Sefton'** ■ 🏆 Regal pelargonium with clusters, 10cm (4in) across, of cerise-red flowers, each petal with a deep red blaze and feathering. ↕30–40cm (12–16in), ↔ 15–20cm (6–8in). ❄ (min. 2°C/36°F)
***P.* Sensation Series.** Seed-raised, single-flowered zonal pelargoniums, flowering very early and over a long season, with good wet-weather tolerance. Produce clusters, 10–12cm (4–5in) across, of flowers in shades of pink, orange, or red, some with white eyes, including mixtures. ↕to 30cm (12in), ↔ 25cm (10in). ❄ (min. 2°C/36°F). **'Sensation Rose'** has rose-pink flowers.
P. sibthorpiifolium. Stemless perennial arising from a caudex-like base. Stalked, heart-shaped, scalloped, dark green leaves, to 2cm (¾in) long, have minute, soft hairs. Clusters, to 4cm (1½in) across, of 2–6 rounded white flowers, 1.5cm (½in) across, marked and lined red, are borne in early summer. ↕↔ to 15cm (6in). Namibia, South Africa (Northern Cape). ❄ (min. 10°C/50°F)
***P.* 'Snowdrift'.** Short-jointed ivy-leaved pelargonium with double white flowers borne in clusters 7cm (3in) across. ↕25–30cm (10–12in), ↔ 15–20cm (6–8in). ❄ (min. 2°C/36°F)
***P.* 'Sophie Koniger'.** Semi-double-flowered zonal pelargonium with coral-pink flowers borne in clusters 9cm (3½in) across. ↕30–40cm (12–16in), ↔ 20–25cm (8–10in). ❄ (min. 2°C/36°F)
***P.* 'Spellbound'.** Vigorous regal pelargonium with clusters, 10–11cm (4–4½in) across, of pink flowers, overlaid wine-red on the upper petals. ↕30–40cm (12–16in), ↔ 15–20cm (6–8in). ❄ (min. 2°C/36°F)
***P.* 'Spitfire'.** Cactus-flowered zonal pelargonium with silver leaves. Single scarlet flowers are borne in clusters 5–6cm (2–2½in) across. ↕25–30cm (10–12in), ↔ 12–15cm (5–6in). ❄ (min. 2°C/36°F)
***P.* 'Splendide'** ■ Slow-growing, short-branching pelargonium. Butterfly-shaped flowers, 2–3cm (¾–1¼in) across, are borne singly or in clusters, 10–12cm (4–5in) across. Dark red upper petals each have a black spot at the base; lower petals are white, sometimes stained red. ↕25–30cm (10–12in), ↔ 15–20cm (6–8in). ❄ (min. 2°C/36°F)
***P.* 'Standout'.** Vigorous, single-flowered zonal pelargonium producing white-

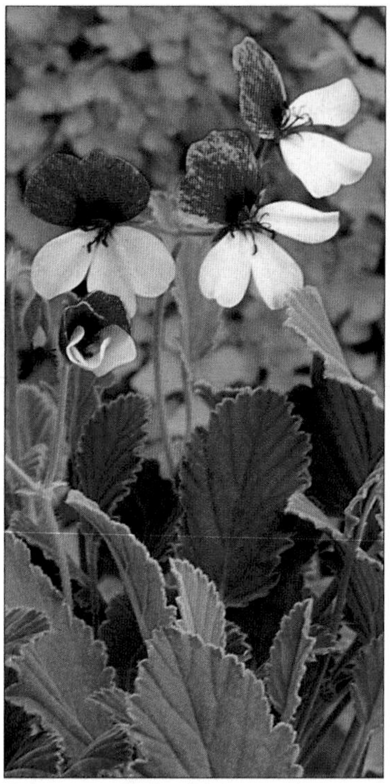

Pelargonium 'Splendide'

centred, coral-pink flowers in clusters 9–10cm (3½–4in) across. ↕45–50cm (18–20in), ↔ 20–25cm (8–10in). ❄ (min. 2°C/36°F)
***P.* 'Summer Showers'.** Ivy-leaved pelargonium bearing single flowers in rose-pink, plum-pink, lavender-blue, or white, in clusters to 12cm (5in) across. ↕to 60cm (24in), ↔ trailing to 90cm (36in). ❄ (min. 2°C/36°F)
***P.* 'Super Nova'.** Stellar zonal pelargonium with double, lilac-pink flowers in clusters 7cm (3in) across. ↕30–40cm (12–16in), ↔ 20–25cm (8–10in). ❄ (min. 2°C/36°F)
***P.* 'Sweet Mimosa'.** Vigorous, scented-leaved pelargonium with deeply lobed, sweet-scented leaves and clusters, 7cm (3in) across, of pink flowers. ↕45–50cm (18–20in), ↔ 20–25cm (8–10in). ❄ (min. 2°C/36°F)
***P.* 'Tavira'** ■ Slow-growing, short-jointed ivy-leaved pelargonium. Semi-double, light cerise-red flowers, feathered wine-red, are produced in clusters to 8cm (3in) across. ↕30–40cm

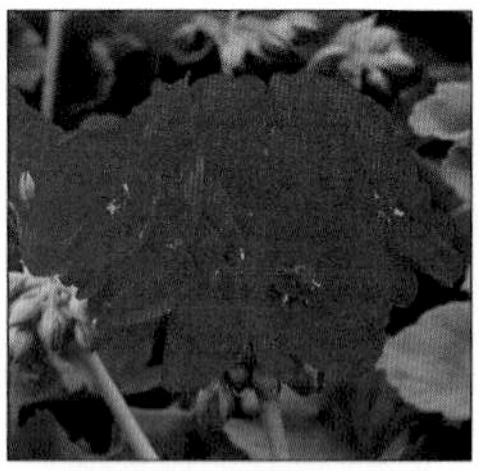

Pelargonium 'Robe'

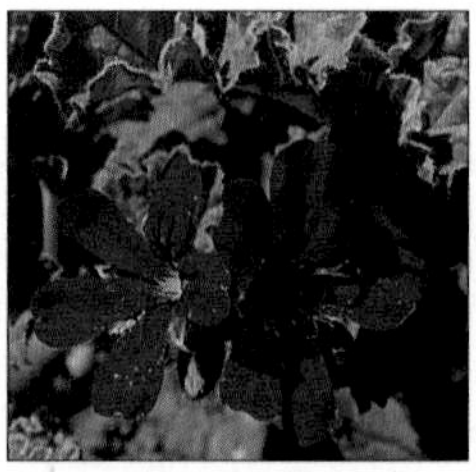

Pelargonium 'Rollisson's Unique'

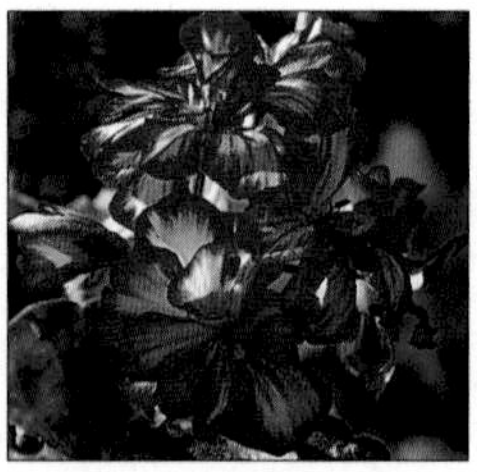

Pelargonium 'Rouletta'

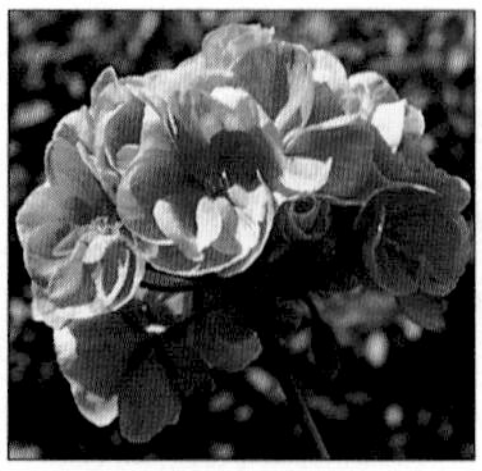

Pelargonium 'Schöne Helena'

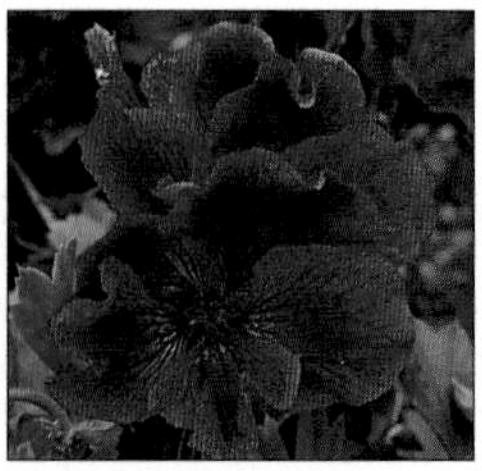

Pelargonium 'Sefton'

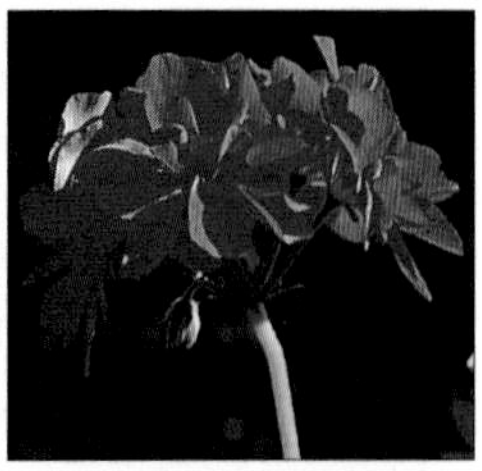

Pelargonium 'Tavira'

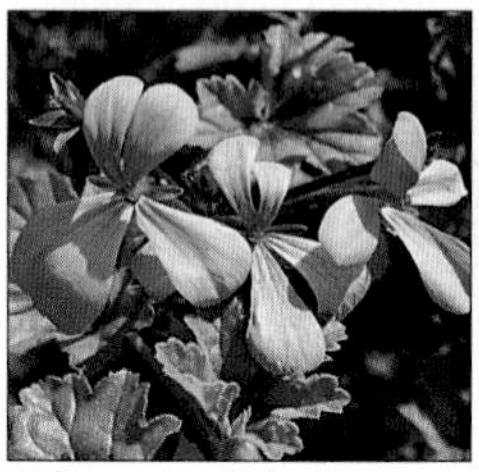

Pelargonium 'The Boar'

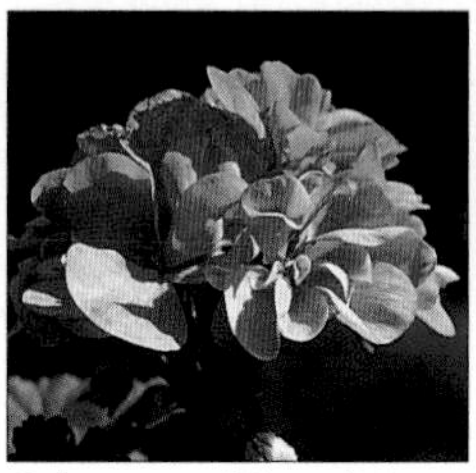

Pelargonium 'Timothy Clifford'

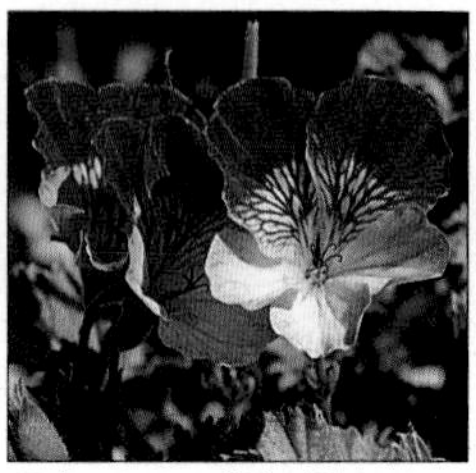

Pelargonium 'Tip Top Duet'

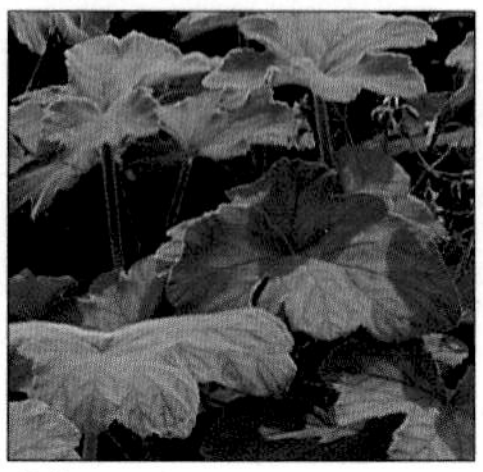

Pelargonium tomentosum

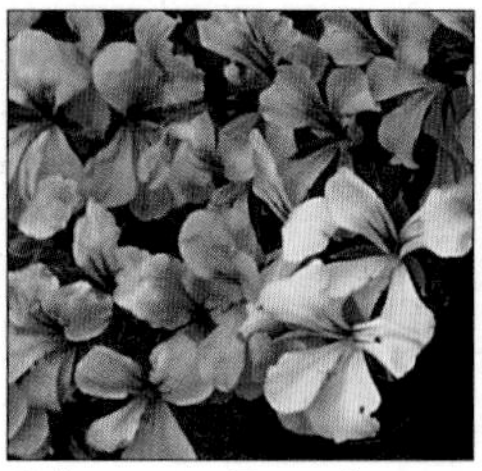

Pelargonium Tornado Series

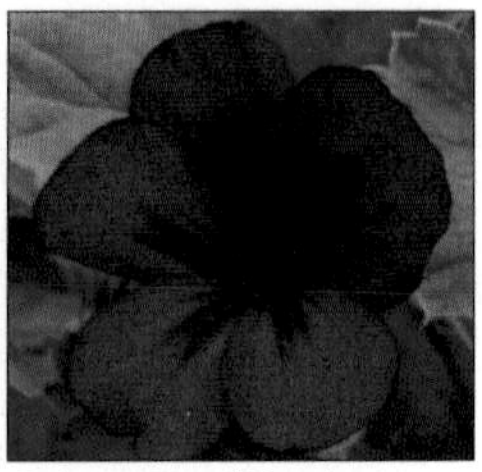

Pelargonium 'Voodoo'

P

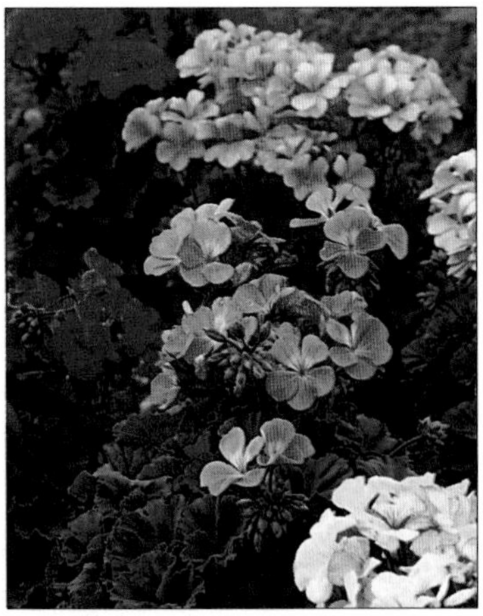

Pelargonium Video Series

(12–16in), ↔ 20–25cm (8–10in). ❀ (min. 2°C/36°F)
P. tetragonum. Shrubby, deciduous, perennial succulent with 3- or 4-angled, erect, smooth, fleshy, pale green stems and broadly heart-shaped, 5-lobed, scalloped, mid-green leaves, 5cm (2in) long. In summer, butterfly-shaped, cream to pale pink flowers, 6cm (2½in) long, with purple-red veins, are borne usually in pairs. ↕ 70cm (28in), ↔ 50cm (20in). South Africa (Eastern Cape, Western Cape). ❀ (min. 10°C/50°F)
***P.* 'The Boar'** ▣ 🏆 Lax, trailing, evergreen perennial producing rounded, mid-green leaves, 6cm (2½in) long, with dark purple-black centres. From spring to summer, bears masses of single, salmon-pink flowers in long-stalked, loose clusters, 7–9cm (3–3½in) across. ↕ 50–60cm (20–24in), ↔ 20–25cm (8–10in). ❀ (min. 2°C/36°F)
***P.* 'Timothy Clifford'** ▣ Miniature zonal pelargonium with very dark green, almost black foliage. Bears double, salmon-pink flowers in clusters 4.5–5cm (1¾–2in) across. ↕ 10–12cm (4–5in), ↔ 7–10cm (3–4in). ❀ (min. 2°C/36°F)
***P.* 'Tip Top Duet'** ▣ 🏆 Angel pelargonium bearing clusters, 4.5–5cm (1¾–2in) across, of very pale pink flowers, the lower petals veined and margined mauve, the upper petals feathered and blazed red-purple. ↕ 30–40cm (12–16in), ↔ 15–20cm (6–8in). ❀ (min. 2°C/36°F)
P. tomentosum ▣ 🏆 (Peppermint-scented geranium). Vigorous, evergreen perennial with heart-shaped, lobed, velvety, peppermint-scented, mid-green leaves, 4–6cm (1½–2½in) long, on scrambling stems. Clusters, 4.5–5cm (1¾–2in) across, of 4–15 butterfly-shaped white flowers, 1.5cm (½in) across, are produced from spring to summer. ↕ 75–90cm (30–36in), ↔ 60–75cm (24–30in). South Africa (Western Cape). ❀ (min. 2°C/36°F)
***P.* Tornado Series** ▣ Neat, compact, early-flowering, seed-raised ivy-leaved pelargoniums. Single lilac or white flowers, in clusters 10–12cm (4–5in) across, are borne on trailing stems. ↕ to 25cm (10in), ↔ 20cm (8in). ❀ (min. 2°C/36°F)
P. triste. Tuberous-rooted herbaceous perennial producing finely pinnate, trailing, mid-green leaves, 18cm (7in) long. From spring to summer, bears clusters, 3–3.5cm (1¼–1½in) across, of 6–20 star-shaped, freesia-scented, nocturnal flowers, 2–3cm (¾–1¼in) across, in yellow, green, or pink, either in combination or with reddish black. ↕ 15–20cm (6–8in), ↔ 45–50cm (18–20in). South Africa (Western Cape, Northern Cape). ❀ (min. 2°C/36°F)
***P.* 'Vancouver Centennial'** 🏆 Stellar zonal pelargonium with bronze and brown leaves. Single orange-red flowers are borne in clusters 7cm (3in) across. ↕ 25–30cm (10–12in), ↔ 15–20cm (6–8in). ❀ (min. 2°C/36°F)
***P.* Video Series** ▣ 🏆 Very dwarf and compact, seed-raised, single-flowered zonal pelargoniums with dark green, strongly zoned foliage. Bear clusters, 8–10cm (3–4in) across, of flowers in shades of pink, or red, salmon-pink, or mixtures. ↕ 20cm (8in), ↔ 18cm (7in). ❀ (min. 2°C/36°F)
***P.* 'Voodoo'** ▣ Unique pelargonium bearing clusters, 7cm (3in) across, of light wine-red flowers, blazed purple-black on each petal. ↕ 50–60cm (20–24in), ↔ 20–25cm (8–10in). ❀ (min. 2°C/36°F)
***P.* 'Wood's Surprise'.** Compact, slow-growing ivy-leaved pelargonium with marbled, cream and mid-green leaves. Bears semi-double, lilac-pink flowers, with white centres, in clusters 5–6cm (2–2½in) across. ↕ 20–25cm (8–10in), ↔ 15–20cm (6–8in). ❀ (min. 2°C/36°F)
***P.* 'Yale'.** Long-jointed, trailing ivy-leaved pelargonium producing semi-double red flowers in clusters to 10cm (4in) across. ↕ 20–25cm (8–10in), ↔ 15–20cm (6–8in). ❀ (min. 2°C/36°F)

▷ **Pelargonium, Variegated lemon-scented** see *Pelargonium crispum* 'Variegatum'
▷ **Pelican's beak** see *Lotus berthelotii*

PELLAEA

ADIANTACEAE

Genus of about 80 species of deciduous or evergreen, terrestrial ferns occurring usually in sheltered sites in semi-desert regions, mainly in South Africa and South America, but also in Canada, the USA, and Australasia. Pinnate or 2-pinnate fronds arise from an erect rhizome in spring. Sori are produced around the segment margins. Grow in a terrace or rock garden. In cool climates, grow tender species in a cool to warm greenhouse.

- **HARDINESS** Frost hardy to frost tender.
- **CULTIVATION** Grow in moderately fertile, moist but well-drained soil in full sun, with some midday shade. In frost-prone areas, grow beneath an over-hanging rock and protect with a dry winter mulch.
- **PROPAGATION** Sow spores at 13–18°C (55–64°F) when ripe. See also p.51.
- **PESTS AND DISEASES** Trouble free.

P. rotundifolia 🏆 (Button fern). Evergreen fern producing a tuft of narrowly oblong, pinnate, leathery, dull dark green fronds, 15–30cm (6–12in) long, with red-flushed midribs, and narrowly oblong to rounded pinnae with finely scalloped margins. Prefers moist, acid soil. ↕ to 30cm (12in), ↔ 40cm (16in). Australia, New Zealand. * *

▷ ***Pellionia*** see *Elatostema*
P. daveauana see *E. repens*
P. pulchra see *E. pulchra*
P. repens see *E. repens*

PELTANDRA

Arrow arum

ARACEAE

Genus of 4 species of rhizomatous, monoecious, marginal aquatic perennials from marshland in E. North America. They have decorative, arrow-shaped or spear-shaped, glossy, mid- or dark green leaves. Tiny male and female flowers are produced on spadices, each surrounded by a longer, sometimes wavy-margined, green or white spathe; they are followed by clusters of green or red berries. Grow these creeping plants on the muddy banks of a wildlife pool or a bog garden; their horizontal surface rhizomes help to stabilize the soil. May become invasive.

- **HARDINESS** Fully hardy.
- **CULTIVATION** Grow in full sun, in the margins of a pond or in baskets of loamy soil in water to 20cm (8in) deep.
- **PROPAGATION** Divide in spring.
- **PESTS AND DISEASES** Trouble free.

P. alba see *P. sagittifolia.*
P. sagittifolia, syn. *P. alba* (White arrow arum). Aquatic perennial producing arrow-shaped, bright green leaves, to 15cm (6in) long, on stalks to 50cm (20in) long. White spathes, 7–10cm (3–4in) long, which open widely, are borne in early summer, followed by red berries. ↕ 45cm (18in), ↔ 60cm (24in). S.E. USA. * * *
P. undulata see *P. virginica.*
P. virginica ▣ syn. *P. undulata* (Green arrow arum). Aquatic perennial with narrowly arrow-shaped, strongly veined, mid-green leaves, 30cm (12in) long, borne on stalks to 45cm (18in) long. Green spathes, 20cm (8in) long, which open only slightly, have wavy, yellow or white margins; they are produced in early summer, and are followed by green berries. ↕ 90cm (36in), ↔ 60cm (24in). E. and S.E. USA. * * *

▷ ***Peltiphyllum*** see *Darmera*
P. peltatum see *D. peltata*

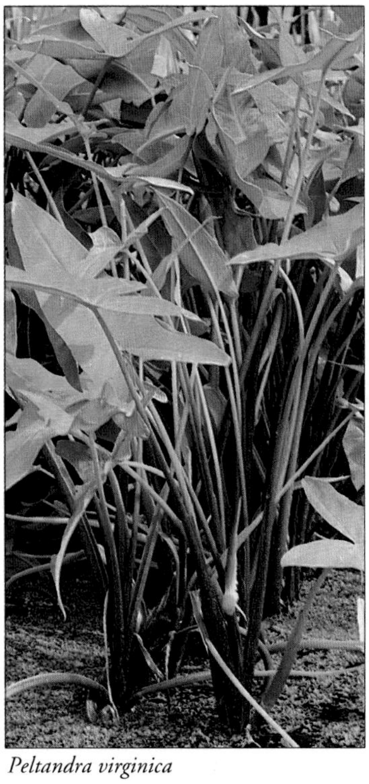

Peltandra virginica

PELTOBOYKINIA

SAXIFRAGACEAE

Genus of 2 species of rhizomatous perennials from mountain woodland in S. Japan. They have peltate, lobed or deeply cut, toothed, glossy, olive- to mid-green leaves: the basal leaves have long leaf-stalks; the stem leaves become progressively smaller and almost stalkless up the stem. Short-lived, small, open bell-shaped, pale greenish yellow flowers are borne in terminal cymes in summer. Grow as ground cover or as foliage plants in a moist, shady position.

- **HARDINESS** Fully hardy.
- **CULTIVATION** Grow in moist, moderately fertile, humus-rich soil in partial shade.
- **PROPAGATION** Sow seed in containers in a cold frame in spring. Divide in autumn or spring.
- **PESTS AND DISEASES** Trouble free.

P. tellimoides, syn. *Boykinia tellimoides.* Clump-forming perennial with rounded to heart-shaped, shallowly lobed, finely toothed, olive- to mid-green leaves, to 30cm (12in) long. Bears pale greenish yellow flowers, 6–10mm (¼–½in) across, in early summer. ↕ to 90cm (36in), ↔ 75cm (30in). Japan. * * *

PELTOPHORUM

CAESALPINIACEAE/LEGUMINOSAE

Genus of 9 species of evergreen trees, related to *Caesalpinia*, occurring in open savannah and dense woodland in tropical regions worldwide. Cultivated mainly as foliage plants, they have often large, alternate, 2-pinnate leaves. Yellow flowers, each with 5 frilled, spreading petals, are produced in racemes or panicles from the uppermost leaf axils. Where temperatures drop below 7°C (45°F), grow in a temperate greenhouse. In warmer climates, grow as specimen or shade trees.

- **HARDINESS** Frost tender.
- **CULTIVATION** Under glass, grow in loam-based potting compost (JI No.3), with added sharp sand, in full light. During growth, water moderately and apply a balanced liquid fertilizer monthly. Water sparingly in winter. Outdoors, grow in fertile, moist but well-drained soil in full sun. Pruning group 1; needs restrictive pruning under glass.
- **PROPAGATION** Sow pre-soaked or scarified seed at 18–21°C (64–70°F) in spring.
- **PESTS AND DISEASES** Prone to red spider mites and whiteflies under glass.

P. pterocarpum ♀ (Flame tree, Yellow flamboyant tree). Fast-growing tree, wide-spreading and freely branching, with rust-red-downy stems. Large, 2-pinnate, deep green leaves are composed of 8–20 pairs of elliptic-oblong leaflets, 2cm (¾in) long. In summer, produces ascending racemes, to 45cm (18in) long, of fragrant, bright yellow flowers, 4cm (1½in) across, with obovate, crinkly petals, each with a central brownish red mark. Elliptic to oblong, winged, purple-brown seed pods are 8–10cm (3–4in) long. ↕ 15m (50ft), ↔ 8–10m (25–30ft). Sri Lanka to Malaysia and N. Australia (coast). ❀ (min. 7°C/45°F)

PENIOCEREUS

CACTACEAE

Genus (now incorporating the genus *Nyctocereus*) of 20 species of thin-stemmed, climbing or prostrate, perennial cacti, sometimes with thick, tuberous roots. They are found in semi-arid areas of S.W. USA, Mexico, and Central America. The branching, ribbed stems usually have only a few spines, and bear axillary, sometimes terminal, solitary, trumpet-shaped flowers, with wide-spreading petals, which open at night in summer. Where temperatures drop below 13°C (55°F), grow in a warm greenhouse. In warmer climates, grow in a desert garden or against a wall.

• **HARDINESS** Frost tender.

• **CULTIVATION** Under glass, grow in a mix of 4 parts standard cactus compost and 1 part well-rotted organic matter in full light, with shade from hot sun. From spring to summer, water freely and apply a low-nitrogen fertilizer every 6–8 weeks. Keep barely moist at other times. Outdoors, grow in sharply drained, moderately fertile soil in full sun, with some midday shade. Stake tall species. See also pp.48–49.

• **PROPAGATION** Sow seed at 19–24°C (66–75°F) in early spring.

• **PESTS AND DISEASES** Vulnerable to mealybugs and aphids, especially while flowering.

P. serpentinus, syn. *Nyctocereus serpentinus*. Climbing or slightly pendent cactus, sometimes branching from the base. Mid-green stems, 5cm (2in) thick, have 10–17 rounded ribs, with areoles bearing about 12 white or brown spines. White flowers, red outside, 15–20cm (6–8in) long, are borne in summer. ↕ 2–3m (6–10ft), ↔ 1m (3ft) or more. Mexico. ❀ (min. 13°C/55°F)

P

PENNISETUM

GRAMINEAE/POACEAE

Genus of approximately 120 species of rhizomatous or stoloniferous, clump-forming, annual and perennial grasses found in woodland and savannah in tropical, subtropical, and warm-temperate zones worldwide. They have linear leaves, and are grown for their feathery, spike-like panicles of clustered, oblong to lance-shaped spikelets, borne in summer and autumn, which are useful for both fresh and dried arrangements. Grow in a mixed border.

• **HARDINESS** Most are hardy to -10°C (14°F). *P. setaceum* is frost hardy. Some are frost tender.

• **CULTIVATION** Grow in preferably light, moderately fertile, well-drained soil in full sun. Cut back dead top-growth by early spring. In frost-prone areas, protect with a dry winter mulch.

• **PROPAGATION** Sow seed at 13–18°C (55–64°F) in early spring. Divide in late spring or early summer.

• **PESTS AND DISEASES** Trouble free.

P. alopecuroides, syn. *P. compressum* (Fountain grass). Clump-forming, densely tufted, evergreen perennial grass with flat, linear, pointed, mid- to dark green leaves, 30–60cm (12–24in) long. In summer and autumn, bears bristly, yellow-green to dark purple spikelets in cylindrical to narrowly oblong panicles, to 20cm (8in) long. ↕ 0.6–1.5m (2–5ft), ↔ 0.6–1.2m (2–4ft). E. Asia to W. Australia. ❄❄. **'Hameln'** ■ is compact and early flowering, with greenish white spikelets, grey-brown when mature, in panicles to 12cm (5in) long. Dark green leaves, to 15cm (6in) long, turn golden yellow in autumn.

P. compressum see *P. alopecuroides*.

P. longistylum see *P. villosum*.

P. macrourum. Densely tufted, clump-forming, evergreen perennial grass with flat or rolled, linear, mid-green leaves, to 60cm (24in) long. In late summer and early autumn, bears pale green, long-bristled spikelets, turning pale brown to purple when mature, in cylindrical, erect or inclined, dense panicles, to 30cm (12in) long. ↕ to 1.8m (6ft), ↔ 1.2m (4ft). Southern Africa. ❄❄

P. orientale ♀ Mound-forming, densely tufted, deciduous perennial grass with upright or arching, narrowly linear, dark green leaves, to 10cm (4in) long. In mid- and late summer, bears softly long-bristled, pink spikelets in long, narrow panicles, to 14cm (5½in) long, resembling bottle brushes. ↕ 60cm (24in), ↔ 75cm (30in). C. and S.W. Asia to N. India. ❄❄

P. rueppellii see *P. setaceum*.

P. setaceum, syn. *P. rueppellii* (Fountain grass). Mound-forming, densely tufted, deciduous perennial grass, often grown as an annual, with upright, narrowly linear, flat or rolled, rough-textured, mid-green leaves, to 30cm (12in) long. From mid-summer to early autumn, bears pink to purplish pink spikelets in plumed, long-bristled, upright to nodding, narrow panicles, to 30cm (12in) long. ↕ 1m (3ft), ↔ 45cm (18in). Tropical Africa, S.W. Asia, Arabian Peninsula. ❄❄. **'Atropurpureum'** see 'Purpureum'. **'Burgundy Giant'** is larger, and is suffused deep burgundy-purple throughout; produces pendulous panicles more than 30cm (12in) long; ↕ 1.5m (5ft), ↔ 60cm (24in). **'Purpureum'**, syn. 'Atropurpureum', has dark purple leaves and deep crimson flowers.

P. villosum ■ syn. *P. longistylum* (Feathertop). Loosely tufted, deciduous perennial grass, often grown as an annual, with upright or arching stems bearing flat or folded, narrowly linear, mid-green leaves, to 15cm (6in) long, and with long hairs just below the flowerheads. In late summer and early autumn, produces cylindrical to almost spherical, plume-like panicles, to 11cm (4½in) long, with soft, feathery pale green or white bristles, becoming purple when mature. ↕↔ 60cm (24in). Mountains of N.E. tropical Africa. ❄❄

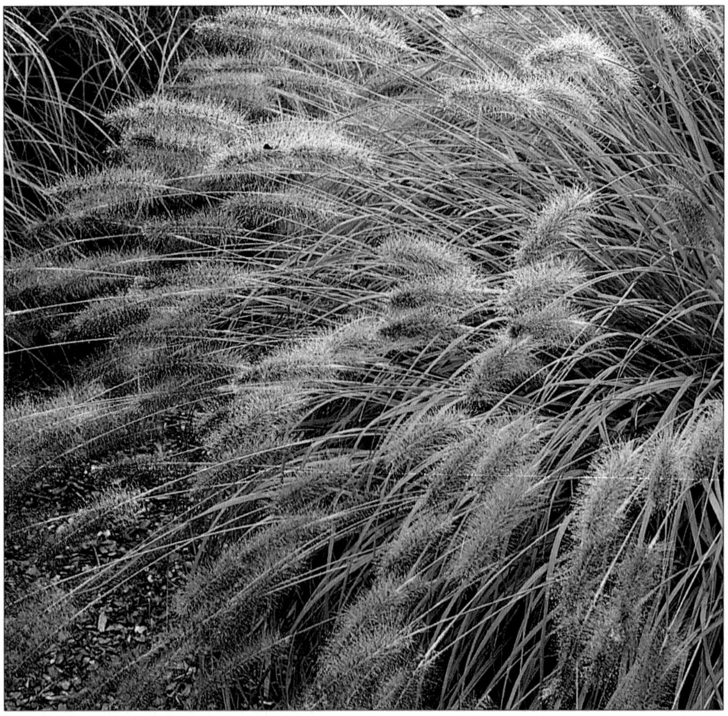

Pennisetum alopecuroides 'Hameln'

▷ **Pennyroyal** see *Mentha pulegium*
▷ **Pennywort** see *Hydrocotyle*

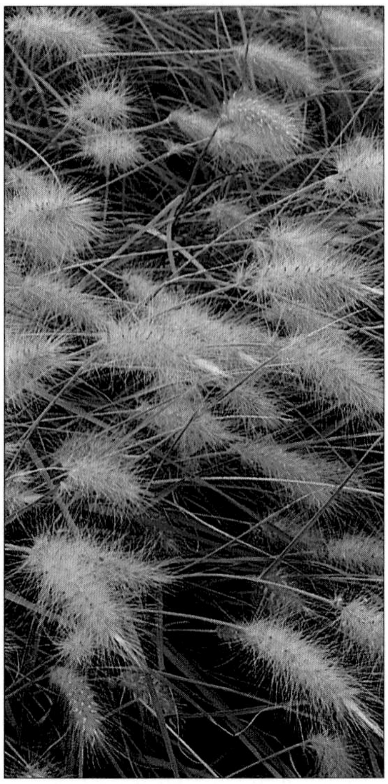

Pennisetum villosum

PENSTEMON

SCROPHULARIACEAE

Genus of approximately 250 species of deciduous, semi-evergreen, or evergreen perennials and subshrubs occurring in a variety of habitats, from open plains to subalpine and alpine areas, in North and Central America. Leaves are stalked or stalkless, usually linear to lance-shaped, and borne in opposite pairs or whorls, or sometimes alternately on the upper parts of the shoots. They are grown for their racemes or panicles of tubular, tubular-bell-shaped, or tubular-funnel-shaped, 2-lipped flowers; the upper lip is usually 2-lobed, the lower lip 3-lobed.

Numerous, bushy, free-flowering cultivars have been developed; most are semi-evergreen with persistent basal growth, and produce racemes or panicles of foxglove-like flowers from early summer to mid-autumn. Other leaf and flower characteristics are very variable: in the descriptions below, leaves are defined simply as narrow or large, and flowers as small or large. Narrow leaves are linear-lance-shaped to lance-shaped, to 7cm (3in) long; large leaves are elliptic to narrowly ovate, usually 12cm (5in) or more long. Small flowers are 2.5–3cm (1–1¼in) long; large flowers are 5–7cm (2–3in) long.

Grow larger species and cultivars in a border or as bedding and smaller ones in a rock garden or at the front of a border.

• **HARDINESS** Fully hardy to half hardy.

• **CULTIVATION** Grow border perennials in fertile, well-drained soil in full sun or partial shade; grow shrubby and dwarf species in poor to moderately fertile, very gritty, sharply drained soil in full sun. In frost-prone areas, protect border perennials with a dry winter mulch. Unless seed is needed, dead-head after flowering to maintain vigour.

• **PROPAGATION** Sow seed in late winter or spring: sow seed of rock garden plants in containers in a cold frame; sow seed of border perennials at 13–18°C (55–64°F). Take softwood cuttings in early summer or semi-ripe cuttings in midsummer. Divide in spring.

• **PESTS AND DISEASES** May be damaged by slugs and snails, and infested with chrysanthemum eelworm. Powdery mildew may be a problem.

***P.* 'Alice Hindley'** ■ ♀ Large-leaved perennial bearing large, tubular-bell-shaped, pale lilac-blue flowers, white

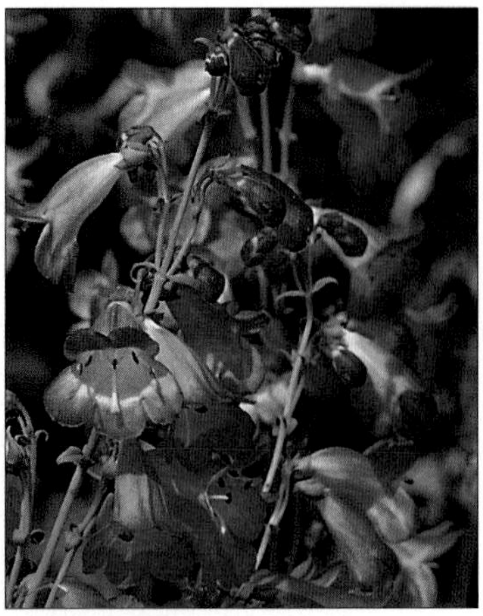

Penstemon 'Alice Hindley'

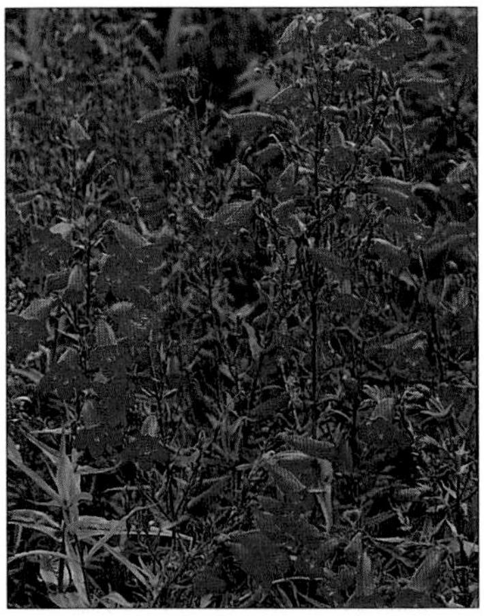

Penstemon 'Andenken an Friedrich Hahn'

inside, tinged mauve-pink outside, from midsummer to early or mid-autumn. ↕90cm (36in), ↔45cm (18in). ✻✻

***P.* 'Andenken an Friedrich Hahn'** ▣ 🏆 syn. *P.* 'Garnet'. Vigorous, bushy, narrow-leaved perennial bearing small, tubular-bell-shaped, deep wine-red flowers from midsummer to early or mid-autumn. ↕75cm (30in), ↔60cm (24in). ✻✻✻ (borderline)

***P.* 'Apple Blossom'** ▣ 🏆 Narrow-leaved perennial bearing small, tubular-bell-shaped, pale pink flowers, with white throats, from midsummer to early or mid-autumn. ↕↔45–60cm (18–24in). ✻✻✻ (borderline)

***P.* 'Barbara Barker'** see *P.* 'Beech Park'.

P. barbatus ▣ syn. *Chelone barbata* (Beardlip penstemon). Erect perennial with semi-evergreen basal rosettes and deciduous stems bearing lance-shaped to linear, entire, sometimes glaucous, mid-green leaves, to 20cm (8in) long. From early summer to early autumn, bears long panicles of pendent, tubular red flowers, tinged pink to carmine-red, 3–4cm (1¼–1½in) long, the reflexed lower lips with yellow beards, the upper ones projecting over them. ↕1.8m (6ft) or more, ↔30–50cm (12–20in). W. USA to Mexico. ✻✻✻

P. barrettiae. Bushy, clump-forming, semi-evergreen perennial with deciduous stems. Ovate to elliptic-ovate, toothed, glaucous, pale green leaves, 4–6cm (1½–2½in) long, are tinged red. In early summer, bears dense racemes of tubular-bell-shaped, lilac-purple flowers, 3.5cm (1½in) long. ↕20–40cm (8–16in), ↔25cm (10in). N.W. USA. ✻✻✻

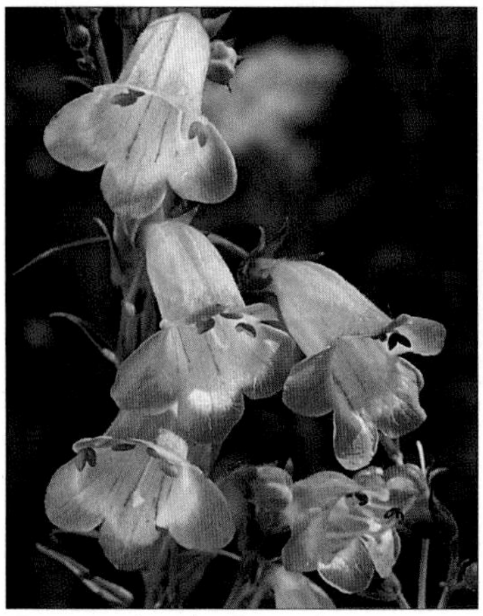

Penstemon 'Apple Blossom'

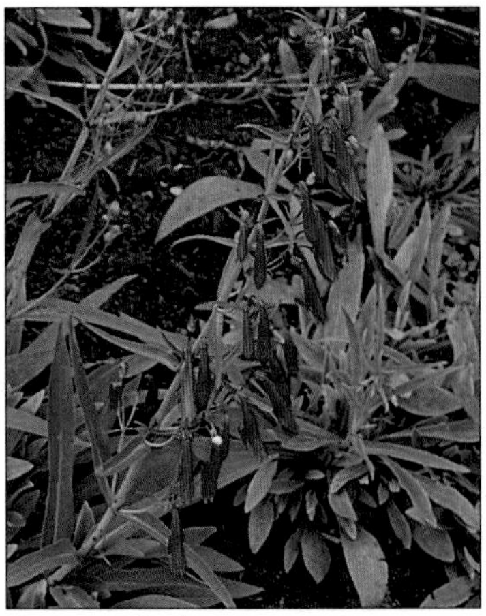

Penstemon barbatus

***P.* 'Beech Park'** 🏆 syn. *P.* 'Barbara Barker'. Large-leaved perennial with large, tubular-bell-shaped, pink and white flowers borne from midsummer to early or mid-autumn. ↕75cm (30in), ↔45cm (18in). ✻✻

***P.* 'Burford Seedling'** see *P.* 'Burgundy'.

***P.* 'Burgundy'** ▣ syn. *P.* 'Burford Seedling'. Large-leaved perennial bearing large, tubular-bell-shaped, wine-red flowers, with white styles and stigmas and white-marked, lighter red throats, from midsummer to early or mid-autumn. ↕90cm (36in), ↔45cm (18in). ✻✻

P. campanulatus, syn. *P. pulchellus.* Upright, semi-evergreen perennial with wiry stems bearing narrowly linear to lance-shaped, toothed, dark green leaves, to 10cm (4in) long. Loose racemes of tubular-bell-shaped, pinkish purple or violet flowers, to 3cm (1¼in) long, are borne in early summer. It is a parent of many hybrids. ↕30–60cm (12–24in), ↔45cm (18in). Mexico, Guatemala. ✻✻

P. cardwellii ▣ Spreading, sometimes stem-rooting, evergreen subshrub with elliptic, finely toothed, mid-green leaves, to 4cm (1½in) long. In early summer, bears few-flowered, raceme-like panicles of slender, tubular-funnel-shaped, deep purple flowers, to 2.5cm (1in) long. ↕10–20cm (4–8in), ↔30cm (12in). USA (Washington, Oregon). ✻✻✻ (borderline)

***P.* 'Charles Rudd'.** Narrow-leaved perennial with purple stems and small, tubular-bell-shaped, magenta-purple

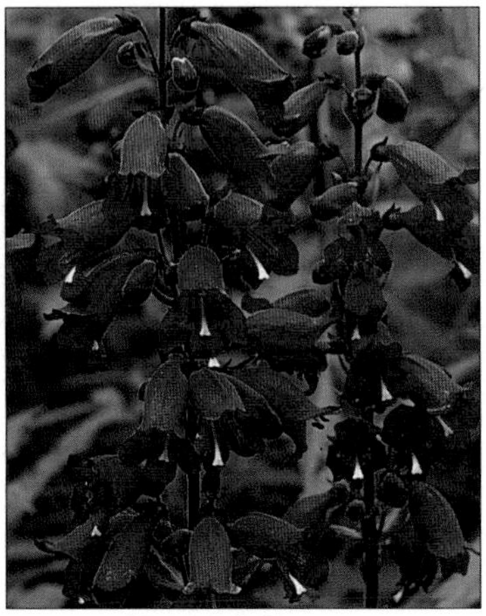

Penstemon 'Burgundy'

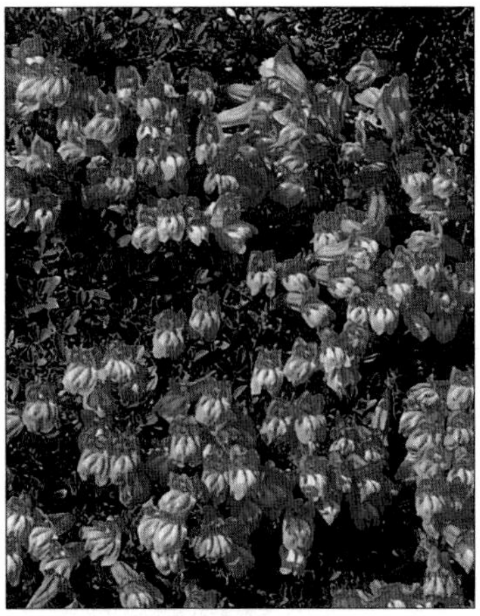

Penstemon cardwellii

flowers, with white throats, borne from midsummer to early or mid-autumn. ↕60cm (24in), ↔45cm (18in). ✻✻✻

***P.* 'Chester Scarlet'** ▣ 🏆 Large-leaved perennial bearing large, tubular-bell-shaped scarlet flowers from midsummer to mid-autumn. ↕60cm (24in), ↔45cm (18in). ✻

P. davidsonii. Prostrate, evergreen subshrub with rounded-elliptic, leathery, entire, mid-green leaves, to 1.5cm (½in) long. In late spring and early summer, bears raceme-like panicles of tubular-funnel-shaped, deep pink to purple flowers, to 4cm (1½in) long. ↕20cm (8in), ↔40cm (16in). Coastal W. USA. ✻✻✻ (borderline). **var. *menziesii*** see *P. menziesii.*

P. diffusus see *P. serrulatus.*

P. digitalis. Vigorous perennial producing semi-evergreen basal rosettes and decidous or semi-evergreen stems often marked reddish purple. Leaves are inversely lance-shaped, entire or sparsely toothed, mid-green, and 10–15cm (4–6in) long. Panicles of tubular-bell-shaped white flowers, 2.5cm (1in) long, sometimes flushed very pale violet, with purple lines inside, are borne from early

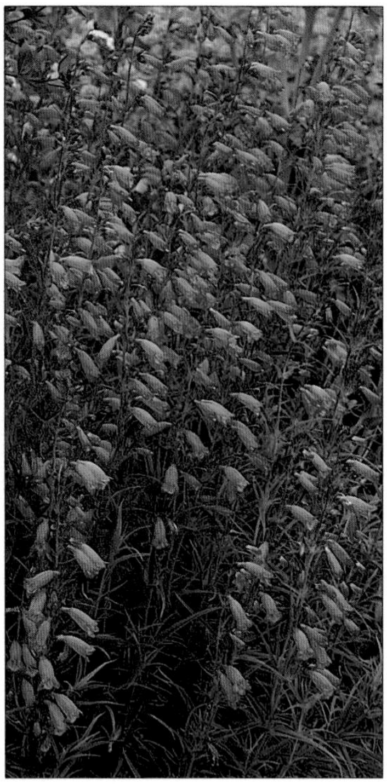

Penstemon 'Evelyn'

to late summer. ↕to 1m (3ft), ↔45cm (18in). E. and S.E. USA. ✻✻✻. **'Husker's Red'** has maroon-red young leaves and pink-tinted white flowers; ↕50–75cm (20–30in), ↔30cm (12in). **'Woodville White'** has white flowers.

P. eatonii (Eaton's firecracker). Upright, woody-based, evergreen or semi-evergreen perennial with lance-shaped-oblong, leathery, mid-green or blue-green leaves, the basal leaves to 15cm (6in) long, the stem leaves shorter. In late summer, bears erect, one-sided panicles of tubular, bright scarlet flowers, 2.5cm (1in) long. ↕30–100cm (12–39in), ↔30–35cm (12–14in). USA (California to Nevada and Utah). ✻✻

***P.* 'Evelyn'** ▣ 🏆 Bushy, narrow-leaved perennial. Small, tubular, rose-pink

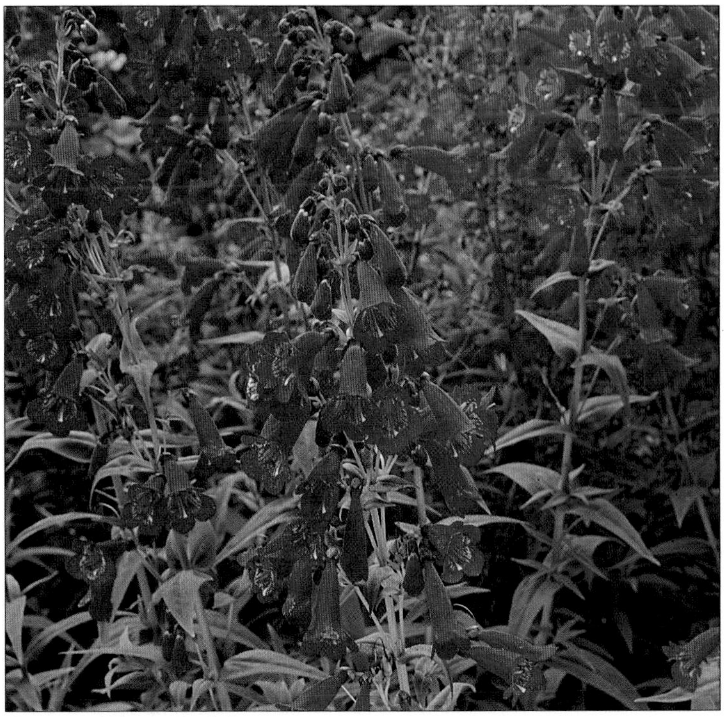

Penstemon 'Chester Scarlet'

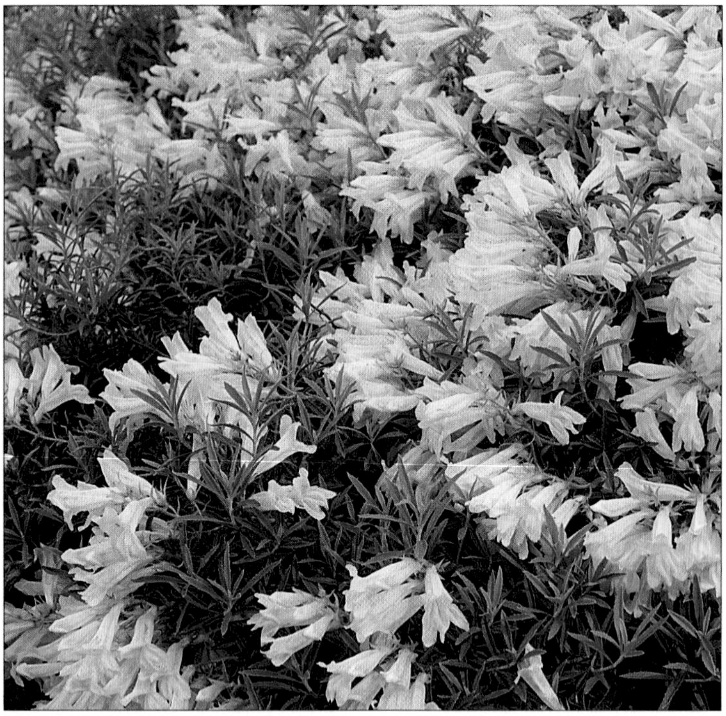
Penstemon fruticosus subsp. *scouleri* f. *albus*

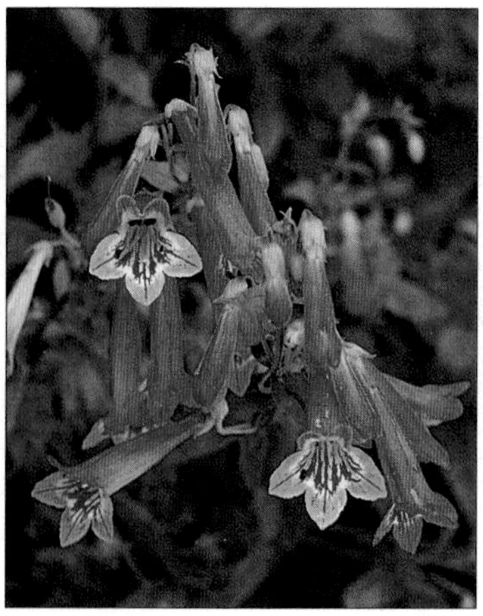
Penstemon isophyllus

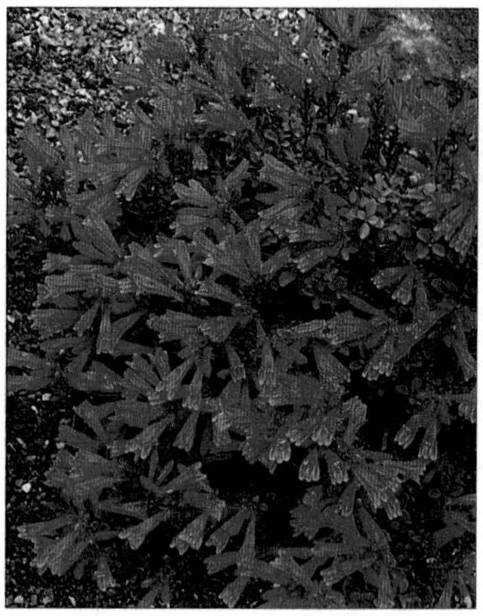
Penstemon newberryi

flowers, paler inside and marked with darker pink lines, are borne from midsummer to early or mid-autumn. ↕45–60cm (18–24in), ↔ 30cm (12in). ✻✻✻
P. 'Firebird' see *P.* 'Schoenholzeri'.
P. fruticosus (Shrubby penstemon). Evergreen, spreading, semi-upright subshrub with lance-shaped to elliptic, toothed, glossy, mid-green leaves, to 5cm (2in) long. Dense racemes of tubular-funnel-shaped, purplish blue flowers, 2.5–3.5cm (1–1½in) long, are borne in late spring and early summer. ↕↔ to 40cm (16in). N. USA. ✻✻✻ (borderline). **subsp. *scouleri*** ♀ syn. *P. scouleri*, has pale to deep purple flowers, to 5cm (2in) long, in summer; W. Canada, N.W. USA. **subsp. *scouleri* f. *albus*** ▣ ♀ bears white flowers; ↕↔ to 30cm (12in).
P. 'Garnet' see *P.* 'Andenken an Friedrich Hahn'.
P. 'George Home' ♀ Narrow-leaved perennial with small, tubular-bell-shaped, wine-red flowers, with white throats, the white extending over the lips, borne from midsummer to early or mid-autumn. ↕75cm (30in), ↔ 45cm (18in). ✻✻✻ (borderline)

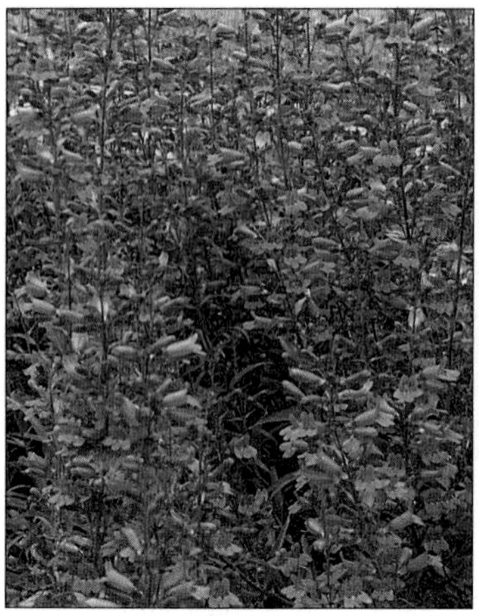
Penstemon heterophyllus

P. heterophyllus ▣ (Foothill penstemon). Evergreen subshrub with linear to lance-shaped, entire, mid-green or bluish green leaves, 2–5cm (¾–2in) long, narrowing at the bases. In summer, produces racemes of tubular-funnel-shaped, pinkish blue flowers, 2.5–3.5cm (1–1½in) long, with blue or lilac lobes. ↕↔ 30–50cm (12–20in). USA (California). ✻✻✻ (borderline). **'Heavenly Blue'** has blue flowers. **subsp. *purdyi*** is compact, with loose racemes of sky-blue flowers; ↕↔ to 20cm (8in). **'True Blue'** is more lax, with racemes of pure bright blue flowers; ↕↔ to 40cm (16in).
P. 'Hidcote Pink' ♀ Narrow-leaved perennial bearing small, tubular, pale pink flowers, with spreading lobes marked with crimson lines inside, from midsummer to early or mid-autumn. ↕60–75cm (24–30in), ↔ 45cm (18in). ✻✻✻ (borderline)
P. hirsutus. Spreading to upright, evergreen subshrub with lance-shaped, toothed, dark green leaves, to 10cm (4in) long. In summer, produces loose racemes of tubular-funnel-shaped, pale violet flowers, 2–5cm (¾–2in) long, with white throats. ↕40–80cm (16–32in), ↔ 30–60cm (12–24in). N.E. North America. ✻✻✻. **'Purpureus'** produces bright clear purple flowers. **var. *pygmaeus*** ▣ is compact and mat-forming, with purple-tinted leaves, 8cm (3in) long; ↕↔ 10cm (4in).

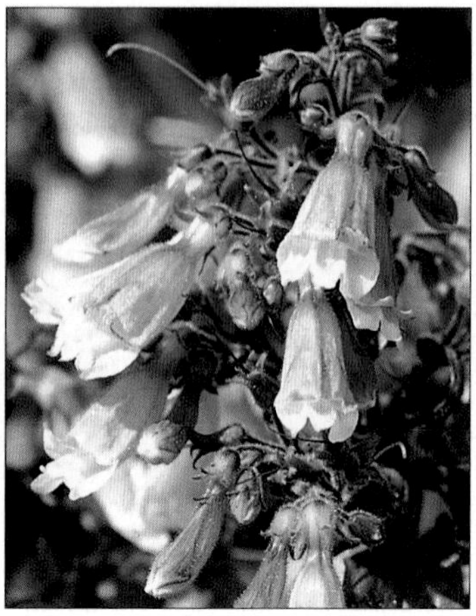
Penstemon hirsutus var. *pygmaeus*

P. 'Hopley's Variegated'. Large-leaved perennial producing mid-green leaves with creamy yellow margins. Bears large, tubular-bell-shaped, lilac-blue flowers with white throats, from midsummer to early or mid-autumn. A variegated version of *P.* 'Alice Hindley'. ↕60cm (24in), ↔ 45cm (18in). ✻✻
P. isophyllus ▣ ♀ Erect, sometimes spreading, evergreen subshrub with lance-shaped, purple-tinged, mid-green leaves, 3–5cm (1¼–2in) long. From early to late summer, produces tubular-bell-shaped, red to deep pink flowers, 4cm (1½in) long, slightly suffused white, in one-sided racemes, to 30cm (12in) long. ↕ to 70cm (28in), ↔ 45cm (18in). Mexico. ✻
P. 'King George V'. Narrow-leaved perennial bearing small, tubular-bell-shaped, bright red flowers, with red-marked white throats, from midsummer to early or mid-autumn. ↕60cm (24in), ↔ 45cm (18in). ✻✻
P. linarioides. Spreading, semi-evergreen subshrub with many slender, upright shoots bearing linear, mid-green leaves, to 2.5cm (1in) long. In summer, produces narrow, spike-like racemes of narrowly tubular-funnel-shaped, pale to deep purple flowers, 1.5–2cm (½–¾in) long, with darker streaks in the throats. ↕50cm (20in), ↔ 25cm (10in). USA (New Mexico, Arizona). ✻✻✻ (borderline)

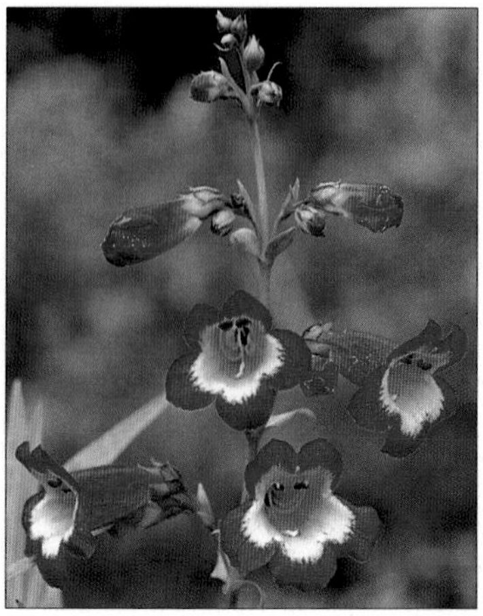
Penstemon 'Maurice Gibbs'

P. 'Maurice Gibbs' ▣ ♀ Large-leaved perennial bearing large, tubular-bell-shaped, cerise-red flowers, with white throats, from midsummer to early or mid-autumn. ↕75cm (30in), ↔ 45cm (18in). ✻✻
P. menziesii, syn. *P. davidsonii* var. *menziesii*. Creeping, mat-forming, semi-evergreen subshrub with elliptic to rounded, minutely toothed, mid-green leaves, to 1.5cm (½in) long. Bears few-flowered racemes of tubular-funnel-shaped, violet-purple flowers, to 3.5cm (1½in) long, in summer. ↕15cm (6in), ↔ 20cm (8in). W. Canada, N.W. USA. ✻✻✻ (borderline)
P. 'Midnight'. Large-leaved perennial bearing large, tubular-bell-shaped, dark indigo-blue flowers from midsummer to early or mid-autumn. ↕90cm (36in), ↔ 45cm (18in). ✻✻
P. 'Mother of Pearl'. Narrow-leaved perennial. From midsummer to early or mid-autumn, produces small, tubular-bell-shaped, pearl-mauve flowers, tinted pink and white, with white throats and red lines. ↕ to 75cm (30in), ↔ 45cm (18in). ✻✻✻ (borderline)
P. 'Myddelton Gem'. Large-leaved perennial with pale green leaves. From

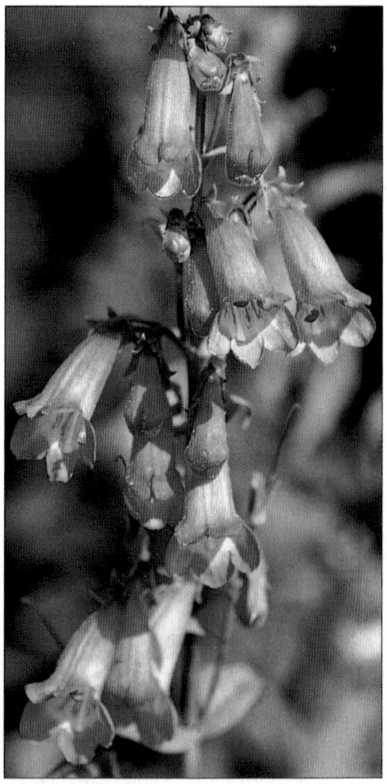
Penstemon 'Pennington Gem'

P

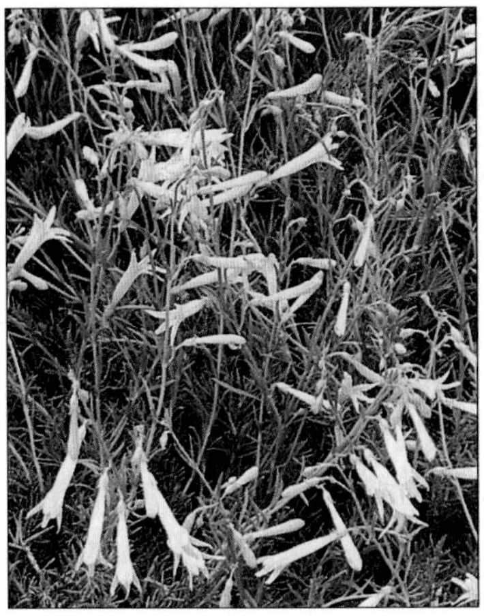

Penstemon pinifolius 'Mersea Yellow'

midsummer to early or mid-autumn, produces large, tubular-bell-shaped, pinkish purple flowers, with white throats. ↕ 75cm (30in), ↔ 45cm (18in). ✻✻

P. newberryi ■ 🏆 Evergreen, mat-forming subshrub with elliptic to ovate, minutely toothed, leathery, dark green leaves, 1.5–4cm (½–1½in) long. In early summer, produces dense racemes of tubular-funnel-shaped, deep red-pink flowers, to 3cm (1¼in) long. ↕ 25cm (10in), ↔ 30cm (12in). USA (Nevada, California). ✻✻✻. **f. *humilior*** is more compact than the species; ↕ 15cm (6in), ↔ 20cm (8in).

***P.* 'Pennington Gem'** ■ 🏆 Narrow-leaved perennial. Large, tubular-bell-shaped, mid-pink flowers, with white throats and purple anthers, are borne from midsummer to early or mid-autumn. ↕ to 75cm (30in), ↔ 45cm (18in). ✻✻

P. pinifolius 🏆 Spreading, evergreen subshrub with crowded, needle-like, pale to mid-green leaves, 1–2.5cm (½–1in) long. In summer, produces loose, terminal, spike-like racemes of narrowly tubular, bright scarlet flowers, each 2.5cm (1in) long. ↕ 40cm (16in), ↔ 25cm (10in). S. USA, Mexico. ✻✻✻ (borderline). **'Mersea Yellow'** ■ has bright deep yellow flowers.

***P.* 'Pink Endurance'.** Upright, woody-based, large-leaved perennial with long, spike-like racemes of small, tubular-funnel-shaped, white-throated, rose-pink flowers, produced in summer. ↕ 40cm (16in), ↔ 30cm (12in). ✻✻✻ (borderline)

P. pulchellus see *P. campanulatus.*

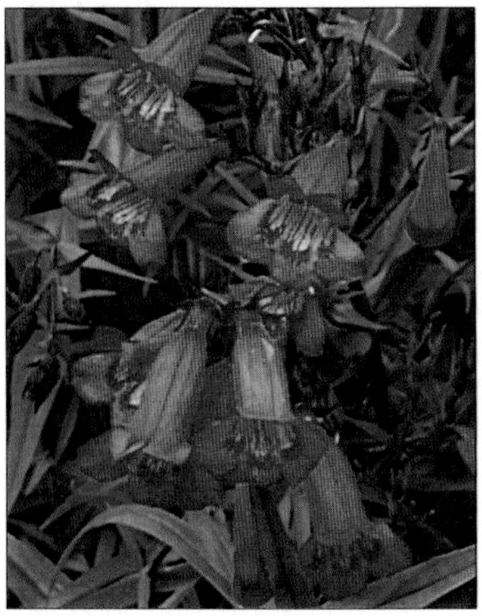

Penstemon 'Schoenholzeri'

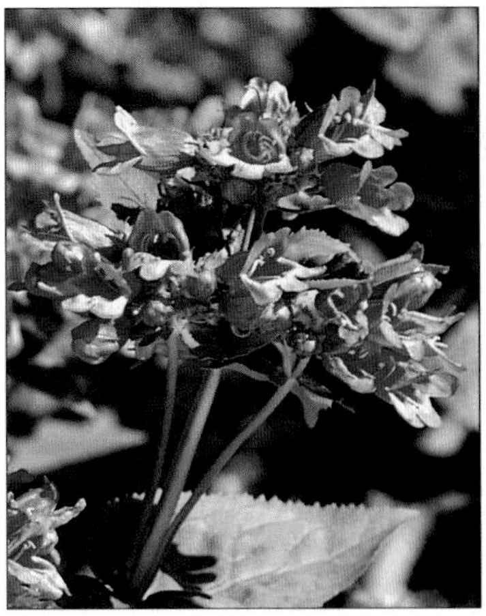

Penstemon serrulatus

P. rupicola 🏆 (Rock penstemon). Prostrate, evergreen subshrub producing elliptic to rounded, leathery, toothed, thick, blue-green leaves, to 2cm (¾in) long. Tubular-funnel-shaped, deep reddish pink flowers, 2.5–3.5cm (1–1½in) long, are borne in late spring or early summer. ↕ to 10cm (4in), ↔ 45cm (18in). Coastal W. USA. ✻✻✻ (borderline). **'Diamond Lake'** is more robust, with pink flowers, 3.5cm (1½in) long. **'Pink Dragon'** is more compact, with pale salmon-pink flowers; ↕ 20cm (8in), ↔ 30cm (12in).

***P.* 'Schoenholzeri'** ■ 🏆 syn. *P.* 'Firebird'. Narrow-leaved perennial bearing large, tubular-bell-shaped scarlet flowers, 7cm (3in) long, from midsummer to early or mid-autumn. ↕ 75cm (30in), ↔ 60cm (24in). ✻✻

P. scouleri see *P. fruticosus* subsp. *scouleri.*

P. serrulatus ■ syn. *P. diffusus* (Cascade penstemon). Spreading, semi-evergreen subshrub with ovate to lance-shaped or elliptic, toothed, glossy, dark green leaves, 2–9cm (¾–3½in) long. Broad, dense, one-sided panicles of narrowly tubular-bell-shaped, pinkish purple flowers, to 2.5cm (1in) long, are borne in late summer. ↕ 50cm (20in), ↔ 30cm (12in). USA (Alaska to Oregon). ✻✻✻

***P.* 'Six Hills'.** Prostrate, evergreen subshrub with rounded, fleshy, grey-green leaves, to 2.5cm (1in) long. In late spring and early summer, produces small, tubular-funnel-shaped, lavender-blue flowers. ↕ 15cm (6in), ↔ 20cm (8in). ✻✻✻

***P.* 'Snow Storm'** see *P.* 'White Bedder'.

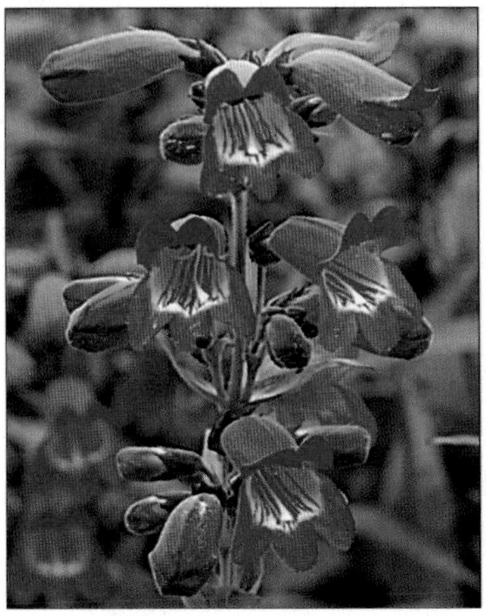

Penstemon 'Sour Grapes'

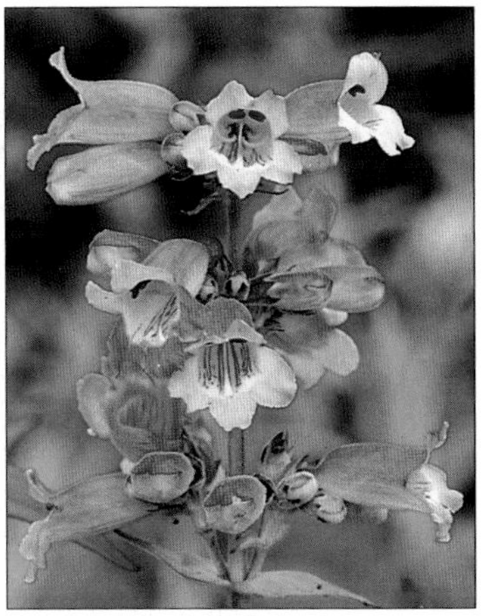

Penstemon 'Stapleford Gem'

***P.* 'Sour Grapes'** ■ Large-leaved perennial. Large, tubular-bell-shaped, greyish blue flowers, suffused rich purple and tinged green, are borne from midsummer to early or mid-autumn. ↕ 60cm (24in), ↔ 45cm (18in). ✻✻

***P.* 'Stapleford Gem'** ■ 🏆 Large-leaved perennial. Large, tubular-bell-shaped, lilac-purple flowers are borne from midsummer to early or mid-autumn; upper lips are pale pink-lilac; lower lips and throats are white with purple lines. ↕ to 60cm (24in), ↔ 45cm (18in). ✻✻✻

P. venustus (Lovely penstemon). Evergreen subshrub with almost stalkless, lance-shaped to oblong, minutely toothed, bluish green leaves, to 8cm (3in) long. Spike-like panicles of tubular-funnel-shaped, pale to deep violet flowers, 2cm (¾in) long, are borne in early summer. ↕ 40–100cm (16–39in), ↔ 30cm (12in). N.W. USA. ✻✻✻ (borderline)

***P.* 'White Bedder'** ■ 🏆 syn. *P.* 'Snow Storm'. Large-leaved perennial bearing large, tubular-funnel-shaped white flowers, becoming pink-tinged, with brown anthers, from midsummer to early or mid-autumn. ↕ 60cm (24in), ↔ 45cm (18in). ✻✻

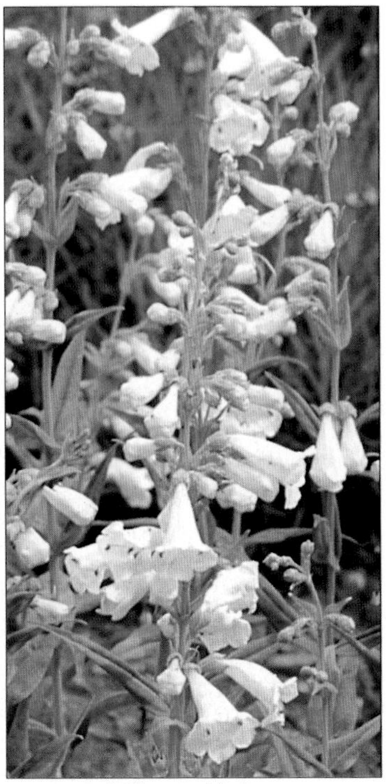

Penstemon 'White Bedder'

▷ **Penstemon,**
Beardlip see *Penstemon barbatus*
Cascade see *Penstemon serrulatus*
Foothill see *Penstemon heterophyllus*
Lovely see *Penstemon venustus*
Rock see *Penstemon rupicola*
Shrubby see *Penstemon fruticosus*

PENTACHONDRA

EPACRIDACEAE

Genus of 3 species of prostrate, evergreen shrubs occurring in boggy meadows in Australia, Tasmania, and New Zealand. They are grown for their heath-like, linear to ovate or elliptic, mid- or dark green leaves, and for their solitary, axillary, small, tubular flowers; the colourful, berry-like fruits are seldom produced in cultivation. They are suitable for a rock garden or peat bank, but grow best in cool climates with mild winters; they are difficult to cultivate in hot, dry conditions.

- **HARDINESS** Frost hardy.
- **CULTIVATION** Grow in moderately fertile, humus-rich, moist but well-drained soil in full sun.
- **PROPAGATION** Sow seed at 13–18°C (55–64°F) as soon as ripe. Take semi-ripe cuttings in summer.
- **PESTS AND DISEASES** Trouble free.

P. pumila. Procumbent shrub with crowded, obovate, hairy, purplish green leaves, to 5mm (¼in) long. In early summer, produces white flowers, to 6mm (¼in) long, with recurving lobes, occasionally followed by orange-red fruit. ↕ 8cm (3in), ↔ 30cm (12in). Australia, New Zealand. ✻✻

PENTAGLOTTIS

Green alkanet

BORAGINACEAE

Genus of one species of evergreen perennial, related to *Anchusa*, occurring in damp, shady habitats, and in hedgerows and woodland margins, in S.W. Europe; it is naturalized in the UK and Belgium. It is valued for its flowers, which resemble forget-me-nots, borne in spring and early summer. The simple leaves are long-stalked in basal rosettes, and stalkless along the branching, erect or ascending stems. Grow in a wild or woodland garden, or in a wildflower border; may self-seed freely.

- **HARDINESS** Fully hardy.
- **CULTIVATION** Grow in humus-rich, damp soil in partial or deep shade. Dead-head after flowering to prevent self-seeding.
- **PROPAGATION** Sow seed in containers in a cold frame when ripe or in early spring. Divide in early spring; the roots are brittle and any pieces left in the soil will sprout freely.
- **PESTS AND DISEASES** Trouble free.

P. sempervirens, syn. *Anchusa sempervirens* (Green alkanet). Bristly, tap-rooted perennial with erect to ascending stems arising from a basal rosette of pointed, ovate to ovate-oblong, mid-green leaves, 10–40cm (4–16in) long; stem leaves are smaller. From spring to early summer, bears leafy cymes of bright blue flowers, to 1cm (½in) across, each with a short tube and 5 spreading lobes. ↕↔ 70–100cm (28–39in). S.W. Europe. ✻✻✻

PENTAS

RUBIACEAE

Genus of up to 40 species of mainly evergreen perennials, biennials, and shrubs from forest margins and scrub in the Arabian Peninsula, tropical Africa, and Madagascar. They are grown for their flat or domed corymbs of salverform flowers, each with 5 spreading petals, which last well as cut flowers. Leaves are ovate to elliptic or lance-shaped, mostly mid-green, and opposite or whorled, on prostrate or erect stems, to 2m (6ft) long. In frost-prone climates, grow in a temperate greenhouse, or in containers outdoors in summer. In warmer areas, grow in a bed or border, or in containers on a patio.

- **HARDINESS** Frost tender.
- **CULTIVATION** Under glass, grow in loam-based potting compost (JI No.2), with added leaf mould and sharp sand, in bright filtered light. During growth, water freely and apply a balanced liquid fertilizer every month. Water sparingly in winter. Outdoors, grow in fertile, well-drained soil in full sun. Pruning group 9, in late winter; plants under glass need restrictive pruning.
- **PROPAGATION** Sow seed at 16–18°C (61–64°F) in spring. Take softwood cuttings at any time of year.
- **PESTS AND DISEASES** Aphids and red spider mites may be troublesome.

***P.* 'California Lavender'.** Dwarf, shrubby perennial with ovate to elliptic or lance-shaped leaves, to 15cm (6in) long. Large, flat corymbs of pale lavender flowers, to 2cm (¾in) across, are borne in summer. ↕35cm (14in), ↔45cm (18in). ❄ (min. 7°C/45°F)
***P.* 'California Pink'.** Compact herbaceous perennial with elliptic to lance-shaped leaves, 8–15cm (3–6in) long. In summer, bears flat corymbs of pink flowers, to 2cm (¾in) across. ↕↔40cm (16in). ❄ (min. 7°C/45°F)
P. carnea see *P. lanceolata*.
P. lanceolata ■ syn. *P. carnea* (Egyptian star cluster, Star cluster). Erect or prostrate, woody-based evergreen perennial or subshrub with ovate to elliptic or lance-shaped, hairy leaves, to 15cm (6in) long. From spring to autumn, bears flat or domed corymbs of long-tubed, pink, magenta, blue, lilac, or white flowers, to 1.5cm (½in) across. ↕2m (6ft), ↔1m (3ft). Yemen to tropical E. Africa. ❄ (min. 7°C/45°F).

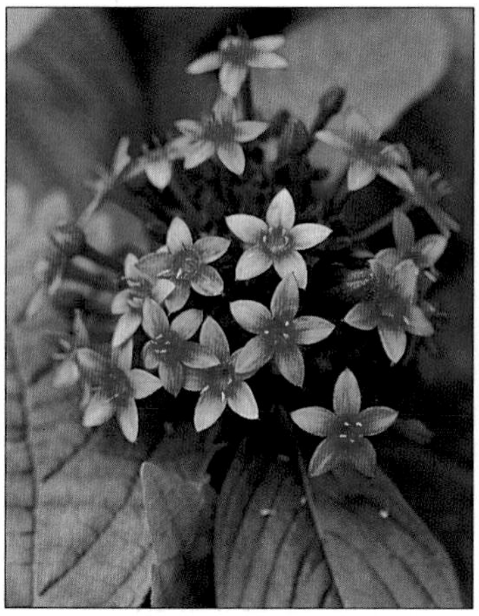

Pentas lanceolata

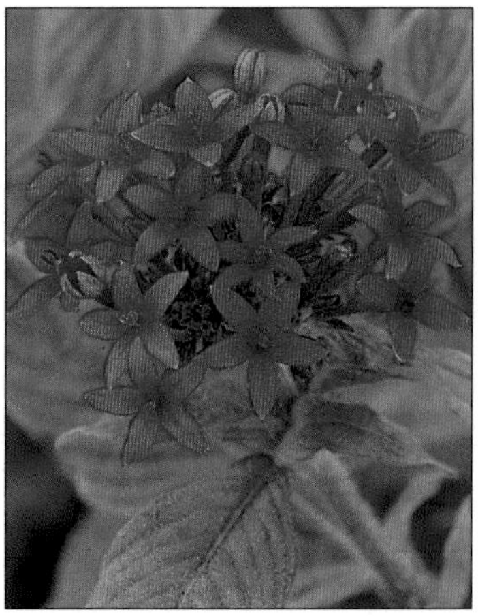

Pentas lanceolata 'Kermesina'

'Avalanche' has white-variegated leaves and white flowers. **'Kermesina'** ■ has red-throated, deep pink flowers. **'New Look'** ■ has dark green leaves and light pink flowers. **subsp. *quartiniana*** has short-tubed, pink to red flowers.
***P.* 'Orchid Star'.** Erect, shrubby perennial with elliptic or lance-shaped, light green leaves, 8–15cm (3–6in) long. Bears domed corymbs of lilac flowers, to 2cm (¾in) across, in summer. ↕45cm (18in), ↔50cm (20in). ❄ (min. 7°C/45°F)
***P.* 'Tu-tone'.** Compact, subshrubby perennial with elliptic or lance-shaped leaves, 8–15cm (3–6in) long. Large, domed corymbs of pink, red-centred flowers, 1–2cm (½–¾in) across, are borne in summer. ↕1m (3ft), ↔60cm (24in). ❄ (min. 7°C/45°F)

▷**Peony** see *Paeonia*
Caucasian see *P. mlokosewitschii*
Common see *P. officinalis*
Himalayan see *P. emodi*
Majorcan see *P. cambessedesii*

PEPEROMIA

PIPERACEAE

Genus of 1,000 or more species of evergreen, sometimes succulent, rosette-forming or erect perennials, some with trailing stems. They occur in tropical and subtropical regions worldwide, in habitats varying from high-altitude cloud forest to near-desert conditions. All have small, short-lived root systems, but absorb water from the atmosphere and store it in their leaf cells. They are grown mainly for their fleshy, often long-stalked, elliptic to ovate or heart-shaped, usually alternate leaves, sometimes in whorls or panicles. Small, white or greenish white flowers are produced in upright, sometimes branched and panicle-like spikes. Flowering is erratic but mainly in late summer. In frost-prone areas, grow in a warm greenhouse or as houseplants; grow trailing species in a hanging basket, and small species in a bottle garden. In tropical areas, grow as ground cover or in a border.

- **HARDINESS** Frost tender.
- **CULTIVATION** Under glass, grow in loamless or loam-based potting compost (JI No.1) in bright indirect light when in active growth, and in full light in winter. Water moderately in summer, sparingly in winter, preferably with tepid, soft water. From spring to summer, maintain moderate to high humidity, mist twice daily, and apply a balanced liquid fertilizer monthly. Outdoors, grow in humus-rich, moist but well-drained soil in partial shade. Most species tolerate poor light, and many of the thicker-leaved species will survive in dry conditions for some time.
- **PROPAGATION** Sow seed at 19–24°C (66–75°F) when ripe. During growth, take softwood, leaf, or leaf bud cuttings, or remove offsets of rosetted variants.
- **PESTS AND DISEASES** Trouble free.

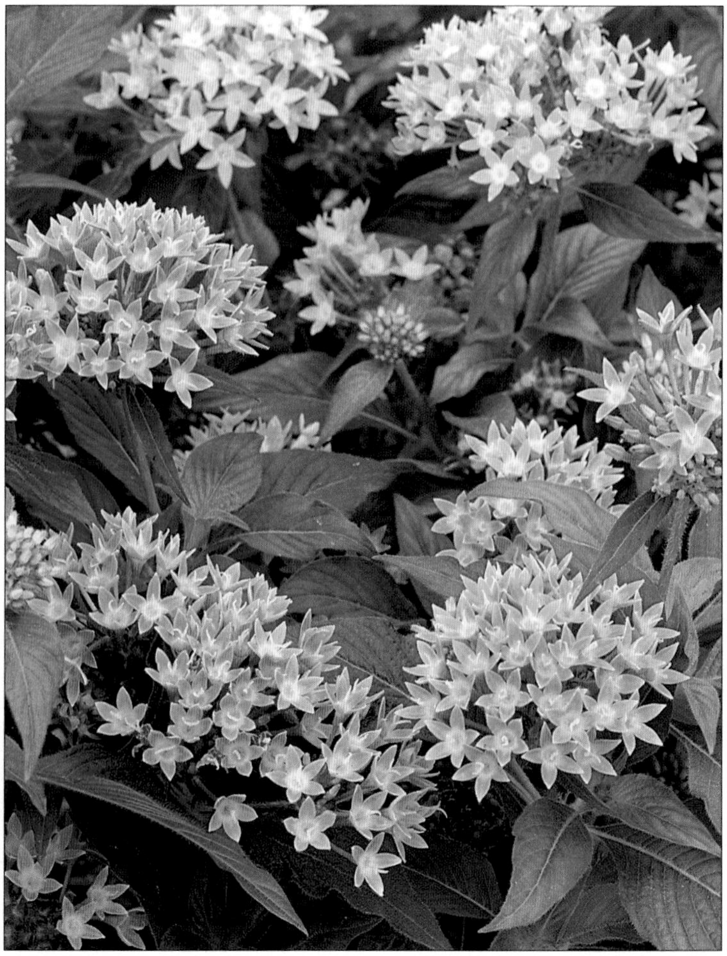

Pentas lanceolata 'New Look'

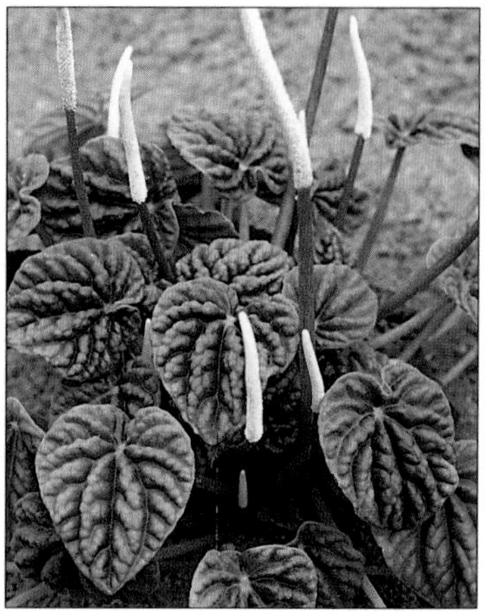

Peperomia caperata

P. argyreia ♕ syn. *P. sandersii* (Watermelon peperomia). Upright, rosette-forming perennial with heart-shaped, leathery, deep green, silver-striped leaves, 5–9cm (2–3½in) long, with long red stems. Bears small green flowers in spikes 5–8cm (2–3in) long. ↕20cm (8in), ↔15cm (6in). N. South America. ❄ (min. 15°C/59°F)
P. caperata ■ Mound-forming perennial with rosettes of long-stemmed, deeply corrugated, heart-shaped, dark green leaves, 2.5–4cm (1–1½in) long. Tiny white flowers are borne in spikes 5–8cm (2–3in) long. ↕↔20cm (8in). Brazil. ❄ (min. 15°C/59°F). **'Emerald Ripple'** ♕ has deep green leaves with

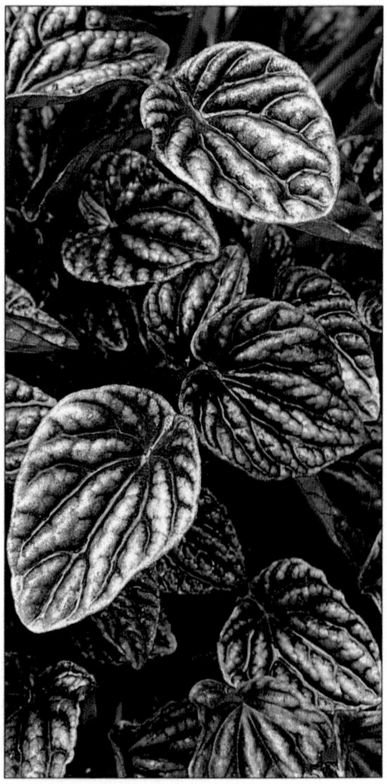

Peperomia caperata 'Luna Red'

P

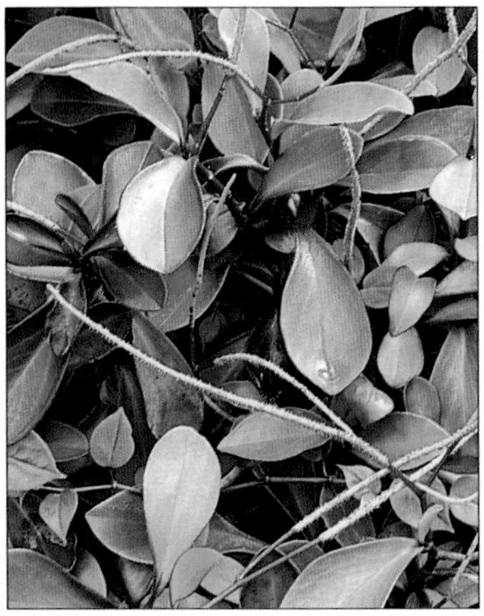

Peperomia clusiifolia

darker stripes along the veins. **'Little Fantasy'** 🏆 is dwarf, with dark green leaves; ↕↔ 8cm (3in). **'Luna Red'** ▣ has dark crimson leaves and stems. **'Tricolor'** is slow-growing, and has pale green leaves with wide cream margins and central pink markings.

P. clusiifolia ▣ Stiff, erect perennial with obovate, slightly concave, mid-green leaves, 4–11cm (1½–4½in) long, often purple-tinged when young. Pale green flowers are borne in spikes 12–19cm (5–7in) long. ↕ 25cm (10in), ↔ 15cm (6in). Brazil. ❄ (min. 15°C/59°F). **'Variegata'** has red-margined, cream-variegated, mid-green leaves.

P. dolabriformis (Prayer peperomia). Robust, erect perennial, becoming woody with age, with succulent, purse-shaped, bright green leaves, 4–5cm (1½–2in) long; the 2 halves of each leaf are folded upwards and fused along the dark green margins. Leafy stems produce panicle-like spikes, 3–7cm (1¼–3in) long, of white flowers. ↕ to 25cm (10in), ↔ 20cm (8in). Peru. ❄ (min. 15°C/59°F)

P. fraseri, syn. *P. resediflora* (Flowering peperomia). Upright, rosette-forming perennial with stiff, heart-shaped, shiny, dark green leaves, 2.5–4.5cm (1–1¾in) long, pale green beneath with red veins. Leafy stems bear panicle-like spikes, to 40cm (16in) long, of white flowers. The only species grown also for its flowers. ↕ 40cm (16in), ↔ 20cm (8in). Ecuador, Colombia. ❄ (min. 15°C/59°F)

P. glabella ▣ (Wax privet peperomia). Spreading perennial with trailing stems and broadly elliptic to slightly obovate, mid-green leaves, 4–6cm (1½–2½in) long, dotted with black glands. Green flowers are borne in spikes 8–12cm (3–5in) long. ↕ 15cm (6in), ↔ 30cm (12in). West Indies, Central and South America. ❄ (min. 15°C/59°F). **'Variegata'** has leaves with creamy yellow margins.

P. griseoargentea, syn. *P. hederifolia* (Ivy-leaf peperomia). Rosette-forming perennial with heart-shaped, silvery grey leaves, 3–6cm (1¼–2½in) long, tinged copper along the veins. Green flowers are borne in spikes 5–9cm (2–3½in) long. ↕ 20cm (8in), ↔ 15cm (6in). Brazil. ❄ (min. 15°C/59°F)

P. hederifolia see *P. griseoargentea.*

P. incana (Felted peperomia). Stiff, semi-erect perennial, later spreading, with succulent, broadly ovate, grey-green leaves, 3–6cm (1¼–2½in) long, covered in white-woolly hairs. Produces green flowers with purple anthers, in spikes 15–20cm (6–8in) long. ↕↔ 30cm (12in). S.E. Brazil. ❄ (min. 15°C/59°F)

P. maculosa (Radiator plant). Robust, erect perennial, becoming untidy as it grows larger, with ovate, shiny, dark green leaves, 12–15cm (5–6in) long, on long stems. Bears spikes, 20cm (8in) or more long, of dark purple flowers. ↕↔ to 20cm (8in). West Indies, Panama, N. South America. ❄ (min. 15°C/59°F)

P. magnoliifolia see *P. obtusifolia.*

P. marmorata ▣ syn. *P. verschaffeltii* (Sweetheart peperomia). Rosette-forming perennial with heart-shaped, dull, mid- or bluish green leaves, 7–12cm (3–5in) long, striped silver-grey, with indented veins. Bears green flowers in spikes to 9cm (3½in) long. ↕↔ to 25cm (10in). S. Brazil. ❄ (min. 15°C/59°F). **'Silver Heart'** has pale green leaves with broad silver stripes.

P. metallica (Red tree). Erect, bushy perennial with elliptic, dark red leaves, 2–3cm (¾–1¼in) long, each with a broad silver band down the centre. Bears red flowers in spikes 3–4cm (1¼–1½in) long. ↕ to 20cm (8in), ↔ 15cm (6in). Peru. ❄ (min. 15°C/59°F)

P. nivalis. Variable, creeping or erect, succulent perennial with fleshy stems containing aniseed-scented sap. Boat-shaped, keeled, fleshy, bright green leaves, 1.5cm (½in) long, white or white flushed pink beneath, are densely crowded at the tips of the stems. Tiny, dull yellow flowers develop in very compressed spikes, to 1.5cm (½in) long. ↕ 10–15cm (4–6in), ↔ indefinite. Peru. ❄ (min. 8°C/46°F)

P. nummulariifolia see *P. rotundifolia.*

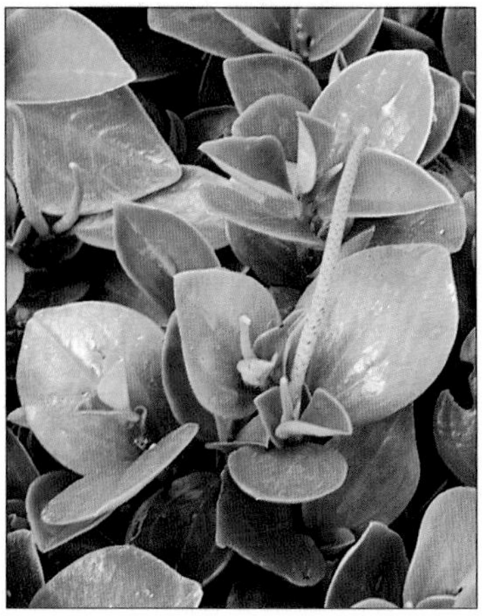

Peperomia glabella

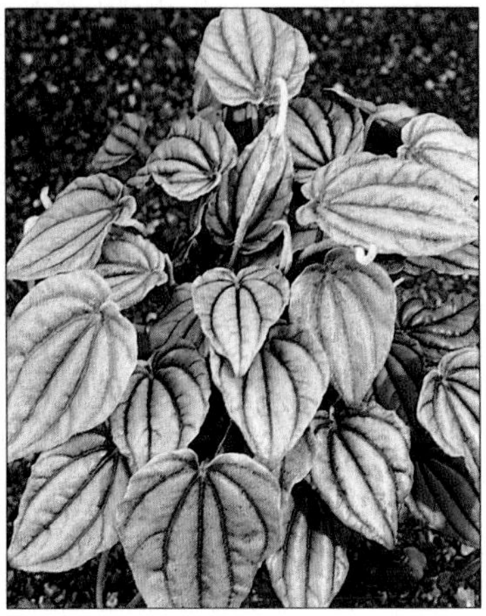

Peperomia marmorata

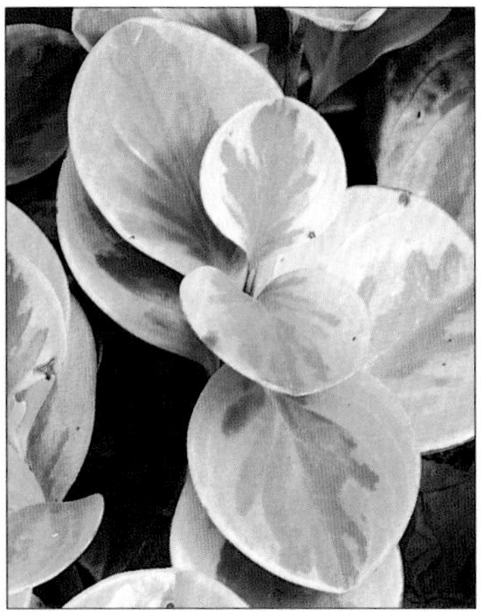

Peperomia obtusifolia 'Variegata'

P. obtusifolia 🏆 syn. *P. magnoliifolia* (Pepper face). Stiff, upright perennial with elliptic, leathery, dull green leaves, 5–15cm (2–6in) long. White flowers are borne in spikes 9–12cm (3½–5in) long. ↕↔ 25cm (10in). ❄ (min. 15°C/59°F). **'Green and Gold'** has leaves with golden yellow margins. **'Variegata'** ▣ has leaves with wide, white or yellow margins.

P. orba, syn. *P.* 'Princess Astrid'. Erect, bushy perennial with ovate, succulent, softly hairy, grey-green leaves, 4–5cm (1½–2in) long, each with a broad silver stripe down the centre. Bears green flowers in spikes 8–12cm (3–5in) long. ↕ to 15cm (6in), ↔ 20cm (8in). Origin unknown. ❄ (min. 15°C/59°F). **'Pixie'**, syn. 'Teardrop', is a dwarf cultivar, with leaves 2–3cm (¾–1¼in) long. Propagate from the smaller shoots. It may revert, producing larger leaves; shoots bearing these should be cut out as they appear. ↕ 8cm (3in), ↔ 10cm (4in). **'Teardrop'** see 'Pixie'.

P. 'Princess Astrid' see *P. orba.*

P. resediflora see *P. fraseri.*

P. rotundifolia, syn. *P. nummulariifolia* (Creeping buttons). Creeping, usually epiphytic, succulent perennial with slender, fleshy stems, often covered with minute, fine hairs or bristles, and bearing rounded to broadly elliptic, fleshy, bright green leaves, 1cm (½in) long. Produces short spikes, 1cm (½in) long, of yellowish white flowers. ↕ 3cm (1¼in), ↔ to 25cm (10in). South Africa, West Indies, Central and South America. ❄ (min. 10°C/50°F)

P. rubella. Erect, branching perennial, becoming untidy with age, with whorls of 4 or 5 elliptic, pale-veined, pale to deep green leaves, to 1.5cm (½in) long, red beneath, giving a copper tinge to the foliage. Green flowers are borne in spikes 2–5cm (¾–2in) long. ↕ to 20cm (8in), ↔ 25cm (10in). West Indies. ❄ (min. 15°C/59°F)

P. sandersii see *P. argyreia.*

P. scandens 🏆 (False philodendron). Trailing perennial with heart-shaped, pale green leaves, 5–7cm (2–3in) long. Produces green flowers in spikes 12–14cm (5–5½in) long. ↕ to 20cm (8in), ↔ 50cm (20in). Mexico to South America. ❄ (min. 15°C/59°F). **'Variegata'** produces leaves with broad yellow margins, but tends to revert to plain green.

P. velutina. Upright, bushy perennial with broadly elliptic, fleshy, velvety, dark green leaves, 2–4.5cm (¾–1¾in) long, with pale veins, and red beneath. Green flowers are produced in spikes 9–10cm (3½–4in) long. ↕ to 30cm (12in), ↔ 20cm (8in). Ecuador. ❄ (min. 15°C/59°F)

P. verschaffeltii see *P. marmorata.*

P. verticillata. Erect, fleshy perennial with rounded to obovate leaves (variable on the same plant), pale green above, red-pink beneath, 0.8–3cm (⅜–1¼in) long, and borne in whorls of 5 at the nodes. Leaves and the lower parts of stems are softly white-hairy. Green flowers are borne in spikes, 2–2.5cm (¾–1in) long. ↕ to 50cm (20in), ↔ to 45cm (18in). W. Indies. ❄ (min. 10°C/50°F)

▷ **Peperomia,**
  Felted see *Peperomia incana*
  Flowering see *Peperomia fraseri*
  Ivy-leaf see *Peperomia griseoargentea*
  Prayer see *Peperomia dolabriformis*
  Sweetheart see *Peperomia marmorata*
  Watermelon see *Peperomia argyreia*
  Wax privet see *Peperomia glabella*

▷ **Pepper** see *Capsicum, Piper*
  Bell see *Capsicum annuum* Grossum Group
  Black see *Piper nigrum*
  Cayenne see *Capsicum annuum* Longum Group
  Cherry see *Capsicum annuum* Cerasiforme Group
  Chilli see *Capsicum, C. annuum, C. annuum* Longum Group
  Cone see *Capsicum annuum* Conioides Group
  Japan see *Zanthoxylum piperitum*
  Mountain see *Drimys lanceolata*
  Red cone see *Capsicum annuum* Fasciculatum Group
  White see *Piper nigrum*

▷ **Pepper bush, Sweet** see *Clethra, C. alnifolia*

▷ **Pepper face** see *Peperomia obtusifolia*

▷ **Peppermint,**
  Mount Wellington see *Eucalyptus coccifera*
  Narrow-leaved black see *Eucalyptus nicholii*
  Sydney see *Eucalyptus piperita*

▷ **Pepper tree** see *Schinus molle*
  Brazilian see *S. terebinthifolius*

▷ **Pepperwort** see *Marsilea*

▷ **Perennials** see pp.38–39

PERESKIA

CACTACEAE

Genus of 16 species of tree-like, scandent, or shrubby, perennial cacti occurring in wooded, often hilly regions of the USA (Florida), Mexico, Central America, tropical South America to N. Argentina, and the West Indies. They have spiny, slightly fleshy branches; some become woody with age. Some have tuberous roots. The fleshy, lance-shaped to rounded or oblong leaves are usually evergreen (deciduous in species with a dormant period). Bowl-shaped flowers, solitary or borne in axillary or terminal corymbs or panicles, open by day from spring to autumn. Where temperatures drop below 10–15°C (50–59°F), grow in a temperate or warm greenhouse. In warm, dry climates, use in a desert garden or courtyard garden.

• **HARDINESS** Frost tender.

• **CULTIVATION** Under glass, grow in standard cactus compost in full light,

P

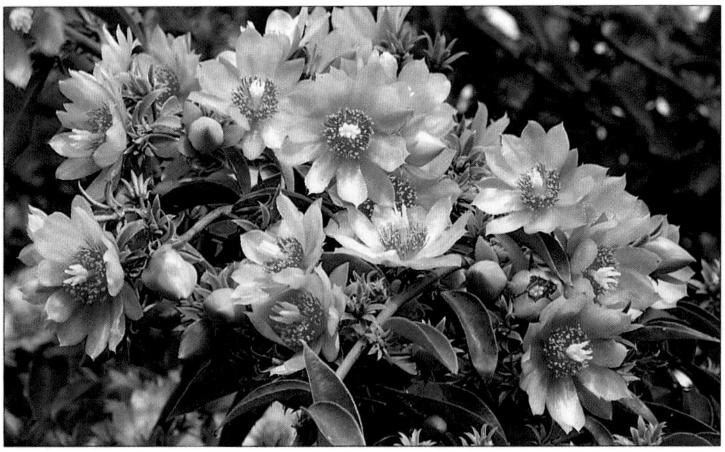

Pereskia aculeata

with shade from the hottest sun. From mid-spring to late summer, water moderately and apply a low-nitrogen fertilizer every 5–6 weeks. Water sparingly in winter. Provide support for stems of climbing species. Outdoors, grow in moderately fertile, sharply drained soil in light dappled shade. See also pp.48–49.
• **PROPAGATION** Sow seed at 19–24°C (66–75°F) in spring. From late spring to summer, take cuttings of stem sections.
• **PESTS AND DISEASES** Susceptible to mealybugs and, while flowering, aphids.

P. aculeata ▣ (Barbados gooseberry). Vigorous, scandent, deciduous cactus producing spiny, fleshy stems and lance-shaped or elliptic to ovate, soft, dark green leaves, to 11cm (4½in) long. Brown areoles bear 1–3 yellowish brown spines. In autumn, produces panicles of long-lasting, scented, creamy white flowers, to 5cm (2in) across, with orange-red stamens. ↕ 8–10m (25–30ft), ↔ indefinite. USA (Florida), West Indies, Paraguay to S. Brazil. ❀ (min. 15°C/59°F). **'Godseffiana'**, syn. var. *godseffiana*, has glossy, peach-coloured leaves when young, often purplish red beneath; ↕ 2–3m (6–10ft), ↔ 1m (3ft).
P. amapola see *P. nemorosa.*
P. argentina see *P. nemorosa.*
P. grandiflorus see *P. grandifolia.*
P. grandifolia ▣ syn. *P. grandiflorus, Rhodocactus grandifolius.* Shrubby, erect, evergreen cactus with thick, spiny stems and narrowly elliptic, ovate, or obovate to lance-shaped leaves, 9–23cm (3½–9in) long. Brown areoles bear up to 8 almost black spines. Corymbs of bright pink to purple-pink flowers, 3–5cm (1¼–2in) across, with white-based petals, are produced from spring to autumn. ↕ to 5m (15ft), ↔ 1m (3ft). Brazil. ❀ (min. 15°C/59°F)

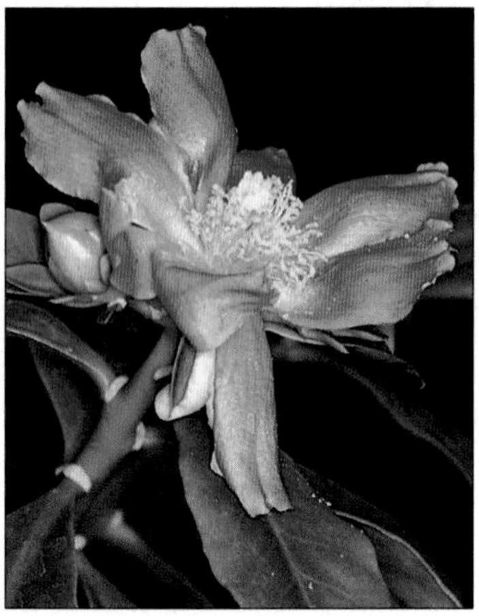

Pereskia grandifolia

P. nemorosa, syn. *P. amapola, P. argentina, P. sacharosa* of gardens. Shrubby, often tree-like, erect, evergreen cactus with smooth green branches and lance-shaped leaves, to 12cm (5in) long. Greyish white areoles bear 3 or more red spines. From spring to summer, bears corymbs of white or pink flowers, 8cm (3in) across. Often confused with *P. sacharosa.* ↕ 6–8m (20–25ft), ↔ 1m (3ft). S. Brazil, Paraguay, Argentina, Uruguay. ❀ (min. 15°C/59°F)
***P. sacharosa* of gardens** see *P. nemorosa.*

PEREZIA

ASTERACEAE/COMPOSITAE

Genus of about 35 species of upright, tufted, sometimes rhizomatous perennials, and occasionally shrubs and annuals, found in open scree in the mountains of South America. The alternate leaves are entire, toothed, or pinnatifid or pinnatisect with toothed and often spiny margined lobes. Daisy- or thistle-like flowerheads are borne singly or in terminal cymes or panicles. Grow in a scree bed or an alpine house; they are intolerant of winter wet.
• **HARDINESS** Fully hardy.
• **CULTIVATION** Grow in fertile, humus-rich, gritty, sharply drained soil in full sun. Protect from winter wet. In an alpine house, grow in a mix of equal parts loam-based potting compost (JI No.1) and grit.
• **PROPAGATION** Sow seed in containers in a cold frame as soon as ripe. Take semi-ripe cuttings in early summer.
• **PESTS AND DISEASES** Aphids, white-flies, and red spider mites may be a problem under glass.

P. linearis. Tufted, hairy-stemmed perennial with dark green leaves, to 3cm (1¼in) long, fringed with fine hairs; basal leaves are narrowly lance-shaped to spoon-shaped, stem leaves are lance-shaped. Bears solitary, short-stemmed, deep blue flowerheads, 2.5cm (1in) or more across, in winter or early spring. ↕ 10cm (4in), ↔ 15cm (6in). S. Andes. ***

▷ **Perfoliate Alexanders** see *Smyrnium perfoliatum*

PERICALLIS

ASTERACEAE/COMPOSITAE

Genus of 15 species of perennials and subshrubs, sometimes grown as annuals, occurring in forests and on slopes and rocky outcrops in the Canary Islands, Madeira, and the Azores. They are grown for their daisy-like flowerheads, solitary or borne in corymbs, appearing from winter to early autumn. Stems are upright to spreading, simple or branching. Leaves are simple, rounded to broadly lance-shaped or arrow-shaped, arranged alternately or in basal rosettes. In frost-prone areas, grow in a cool greenhouse or as houseplants. In warmer climates, grow in a shrub border or use as summer bedding.
• **HARDINESS** Frost tender.
• **CULTIVATION** Under glass, grow in loam-based potting compost (JI No.2) in full light, with shade from hot sun. During growth, water moderately and apply a balanced liquid fertilizer every 2 weeks. Outdoors, grow in fertile, well-drained soil, in full sun with midday shade, or in partial shade. Remove spent blooms to prolong flowering; discard plants when flowering has ceased.
• **PROPAGATION** Sow seed at 13–18°C (55–64°F) from spring to midsummer. Root semi-ripe cuttings in summer.
• **PESTS AND DISEASES** Suceptible to aphids, red spider mites, thrips, white-flies, and chrysanthemum leaf miner.

P. x hybrida, syn. *Cineraria cruentus* of gardens, *C.* x *hybrida, Senecio cruentus, S.* x *hybridus* (Florists' cineraria). Cushion-forming or loosely branched perennial, often grown as an annual, with alternate, ovate, triangular-heart-shaped, mid- to deep green leaves, 25–30cm (10–12in) long. From winter to spring, bears loose, terminal and axillary corymbs, 2.5–8cm (1–3in) across, of flowerheads in single colours and bicolours, in pink, red, blue, white, magenta, lavender-blue, and copper. ↕ 45–60cm (18–24in), ↔ 25–60cm (10–24in). Garden origin. ❀ (min. 7°C/45°F). **'Brilliant'** has large flower-heads, 5cm (2in) across, in a mixture of white, blue, deep red, copper, and rose-pink, and bicolours. **'Chloe'** is an early-flowering mixture, with flowerheads in shades of blue, carmine-red, and pink, and bicolours. **Cindy Series** cultivars are compact; flowerheads are in single colours, as well as in a mixture of blue, carmine-red, copper, and pink; ↕ 20cm (8in), ↔ 30cm (12in). **'Royalty'** is late-flowering, with flowerheads in sky-blue, cherry-red, lilac with a white eye, and bicolours. **'Spring Glory'** ▣ is compact and early-flowering, with abundant flowerheads in blue, copper, carmine-red, and pink, as well as bicolours; ↕ 20cm (8in), ↔ 25cm (10in). **'Star Wars'** is compact, with flowerheads in a mixture of white, blue, rose-pink, carmine-red, and purple; ideal for small containers; ↕ 15cm (6in), ↔ 20cm (8in).

PERILLA

LABIATAE/LAMIACEAE

Genus of 6 species of erect, bushy, aromatic annuals, with 4-angled stems, found in variable habitats, usually in woodland, from India to Japan. They are cultivated for their opposite, simple, usually ovate, mid- or dark green leaves, often flushed or variegated red or bronze. Whorls of insignificant, 2-lipped, 5-lobed, bell-shaped flowers, each encased in a prominent, 2-lipped calyx, are borne in upright spikes in late summer and autumn. *P. frutescens* and its cultivars are the most commonly grown; their decorative, often purple and frilly foliage contrasts well with the flowers of summer bedding plants.
• **HARDINESS** Frost hardy.
• **CULTIVATION** Grow in fertile, moist but well-drained soil in full sun or partial shade.
• **PROPAGATION** Sow seed at 13–18°C (55–64°F) in spring.
• **PESTS AND DISEASES** Trouble free.

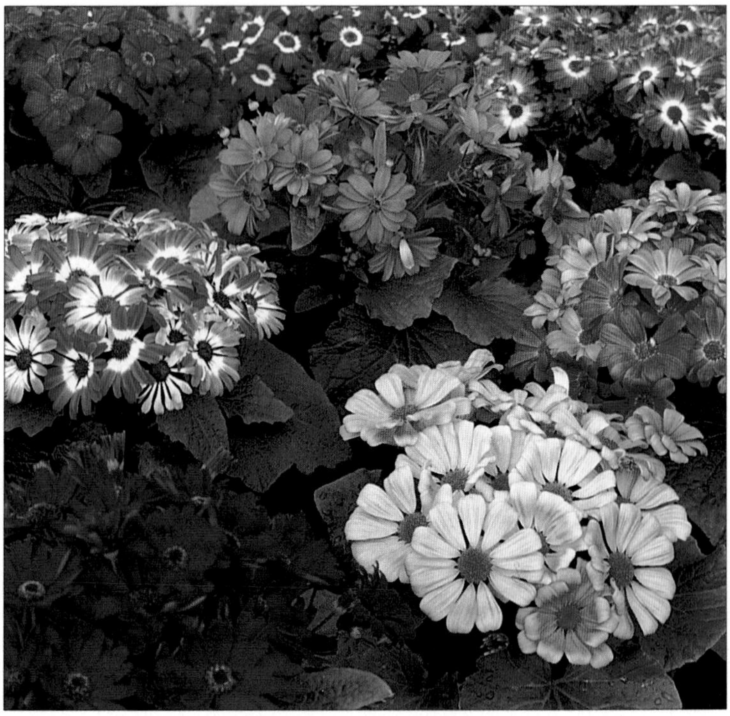

Pericallis x *hybrida* 'Spring Glory'

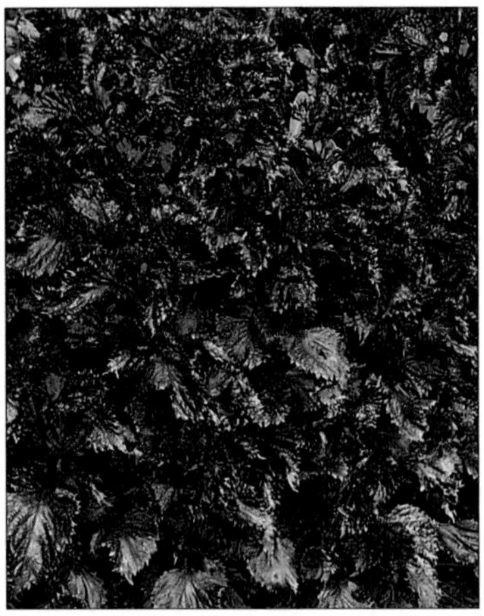

Perilla frutescens var. *crispa*

P. frutescens. Vigorous, hairy annual with broadly ovate, pointed, deeply toothed, long-stalked, mid-green, sometimes purple-flecked leaves, to 12cm (5in) long. Whorls of tiny white flowers are borne in spikes, to 10cm (4in) long, in summer. ↕ to 1m (3ft), ↔ to 30cm (12in). Himalayas to E. Asia. ❄❄. **var. *crispa*** ▣ 𝕐 syn. var. *nankinensis*, has attractive, dark purple or dark bronze, sometimes dark green leaves with frilly margins. **var. *nankinensis*** see var. *crispa*.

PERIPLOCA

ASCLEPIADACEAE

Genus of 11 species of deciduous or evergreen shrubs and climbers found in woodland, in thickets, and on riverbanks in the Mediterranean, tropical Africa, and E. Asia. They are grown for their attractive, lance-shaped to broadly ovate leaves, borne in opposite pairs. Small, star-shaped flowers are produced in terminal or axillary corymbs or cymes. Train *P. graeca*, the most commonly grown species, on wires against a wall, or grow over a pergola, trellis, or similar support. The fruits and sap may cause stomach upset if ingested.

- **HARDINESS** Frost hardy.
- **CULTIVATION** Grow in any well-drained soil in a warm, sheltered site in full sun. Support climbing stems. Pruning group 11, in early spring.
- **PROPAGATION** Sow seed at 13–16°C (55–61°F) in spring. Take semi-ripe cuttings in summer.
- **PESTS AND DISEASES** Trouble free.

P. graeca (Silk vine). Twining, deciduous climber with ovate, glossy, dark green leaves, to 10cm (4in) long. Star-shaped, unpleasantly scented, 5-lobed flowers, 2.5cm (1in) across, greenish yellow outside and purple-brown inside, are borne in long-stalked corymbs of up to 12, in mid- and late summer. They are followed by slender seed pods, to 12cm (5in) long, which open to release silky-tufted seeds. ↕ 9m (28ft). S.E. Europe, S.W. Asia. ❄❄

▷ **Periwinkle** see *Vinca*
Greater see *Vinca major*
Lesser see *Vinca minor*
Madagascar see *Catharanthus, C. roseus*

▷ ***Pernettya*** see *Gaultheria*
P. mucronata see *G. mucronata*
P. prostrata see *G. myrsinoides*
P. tasmanica see *G. tasmanica*

PEROVSKIA

LABIATAE/LAMIACEAE

Genus of 7 species of deciduous subshrubs occurring in rocky sites from C. Asia to the Himalayas, grown for their foliage and flowers. They have opposite, often finely cut and deeply divided, lance-shaped to ovate or oblong, aromatic, grey-green leaves. Terminal panicles of small, tubular, 2-lipped blue flowers are produced in late summer and early autumn. Grow in a mixed or herbaceous border.

- **HARDINESS** Fully hardy.
- **CULTIVATION** Grow in well-drained, poor to moderately fertile soil in full sun. They tolerate dry, chalky soil and coastal conditions. Pruning group 6.
- **PROPAGATION** Root softwood cuttings in late spring, or semi-ripe cuttings in summer.
- **PESTS AND DISEASES** Trouble free.

P. atriplicifolia. Upright subshrub with grey-white shoots and ovate, deeply cut and lobed, grey-green leaves, to 5cm (2in) long. Small, tubular, violet-blue flowers are borne in tall panicles, to 30cm (12in) long, in late summer and early autumn. ↕ 1.2m (4ft), ↔ 1m (3ft). Afghanistan. ❄❄❄

***P.* 'Blue Spire'** ▣ 𝕐 Upright subshrub with grey-white stems bearing ovate, very deeply divided, silver-grey leaves, to 5cm (2in) long. Tubular, violet-blue flowers, in panicles to 30cm (12in) long, are very profusely borne in late summer and early autumn. ↕ 1.2m (4ft), ↔ 1m (3ft). ❄❄❄

***P.* 'Hybrida'.** Upright subshrub with grey-white shoots and ovate, deeply cut, grey-green leaves, to 5cm (2in) long. In late summer and early autumn, bears tubular, dark lavender-blue flowers in tall panicles, to 40cm (16in) long. ↕ 1m (3ft), ↔ 75cm (30in). ❄❄❄

▷ **Persian shield** see *Strobilanthes dyerianus*

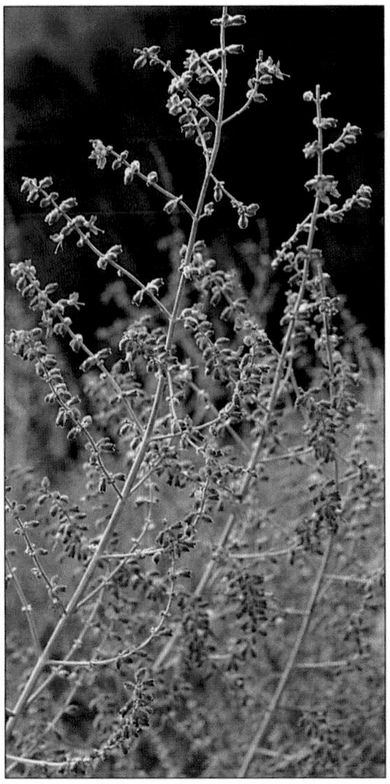

Perovskia 'Blue Spire'

PERSICARIA

syn. ACONOGONON, BISTORTA, TOVARA

POLYGONACEAE

Genus of 50–80 species of annuals, often rhizomatous or stoloniferous perennials, and rarely subshrubs. They may be evergreen, semi-evergreen, or deciduous; some have attractive autumn leaf colour. They are found in a variety of habitats worldwide. Often spreading and sometimes invasive, they have usually fleshy stems and simple, entire, variably shaped, often conspicuously veined leaves comprising long-stalked basal leaves and fewer, smaller, alternate, stalkless leaves on the stems. Spikes or panicles of small, usually long-lasting, funnel-, bell-, or cup-shaped, white, pink, or red flowers are followed by distinctive, usually brownish red, 3-angled or ovoid fruits. Some of the larger perennials are undemanding plants for a border, or as ground cover, and are suitable for naturalizing in a meadow or woodland garden. Grow smaller species in a large rock garden, or at the front of a border. Contact with all parts may irritate skin; the sap may cause mild stomach upset if ingested.

- **HARDINESS** Fully hardy to frost hardy.
- **CULTIVATION** Grow in any moist soil in full sun or partial shade. *P. bistorta* tolerates dry soil.
- **PROPAGATION** Sow seed in containers in a cold frame in spring. Divide perennials in spring or autumn.
- **PESTS AND DISEASES** *P. campanulata* may attract blackfly; *P. virginiana* 'Painter's Palette' may suffer slug or snail damage.

P. affinis, syn. *Polygonum affine*. Mat-forming, evergreen perennial with elliptic-lance-shaped, dark green leaves, 5–15cm (2–6in) long, turning red-bronze in autumn. From midsummer to mid-autumn, bears spikes, 5–8cm (2–3in) long, of cup-shaped, bright

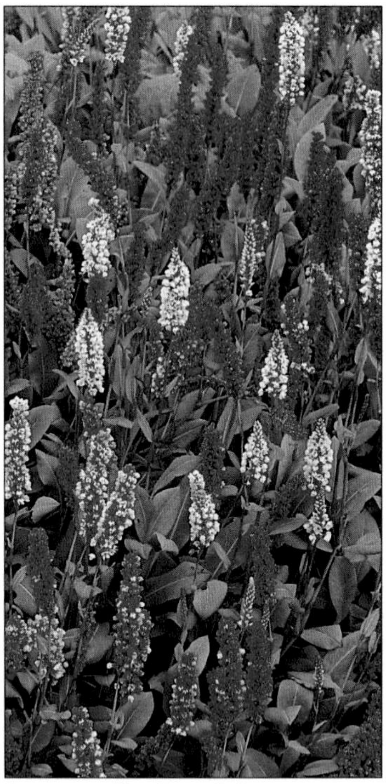

Persicaria affinis 'Superba'

rose-red flowers, to 5mm (¼in) long, fading to pale pink; flowers turn brown with age, providing colour during winter. ↕ to 25cm (10in), ↔ 60cm (24in) or more. Himalayas. ❄❄❄. **'Darjeeling Red'** 𝕐 has large leaves, to 15cm (6in) long, and flowers that open pink and turn red when mature; ↔ 50cm (20in). **'Dimity'** has dense spikes of light pink flowers; leaves turn red in autumn; ↕ 10cm (4in), ↔ 45cm (18in). **'Donald Lowndes'** ▣ 𝕐 has pointed leaves, and produces dense spikes of pale pink flowers, becoming darker when mature; ↕ to 20cm (8in), ↔ 30cm (12in). **'Superba'** ▣ 𝕐 is vigorous, and has pale pink flowers, becoming deep pinkish red, with red calyces; leaves turn rich brown in autumn.

P

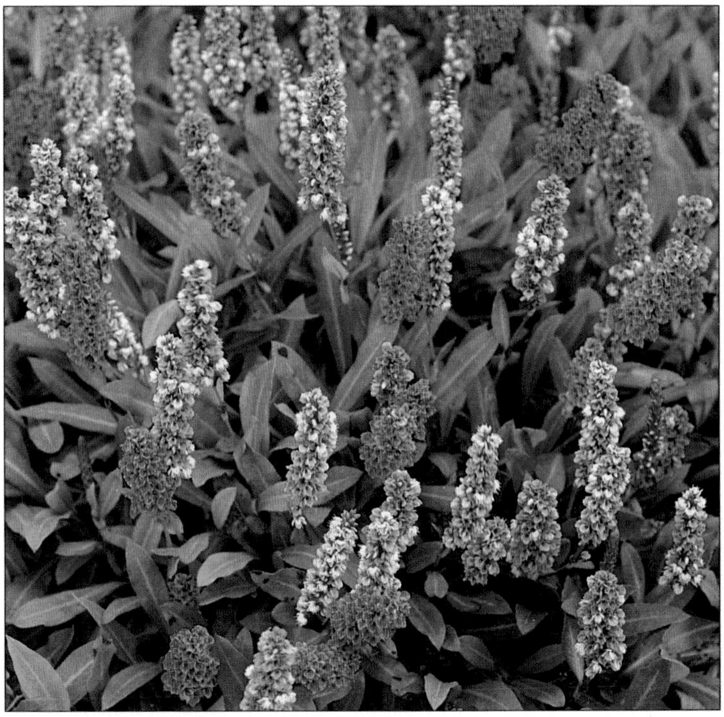

Persicaria affinis 'Donald Lowndes'

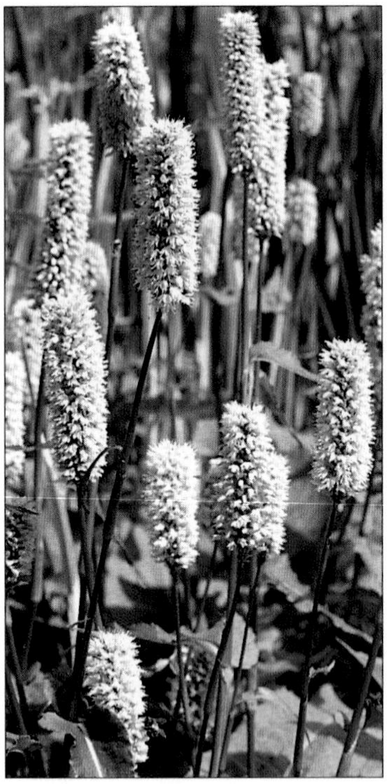
Persicaria bistorta 'Superba'

P. amplexicaulis, syn. *Bistorta amplexicaulis, Polygonum amplexicaule* (Bistort). Robust, clump-forming, semi-evergreen perennial with ovate-lance-shaped, pointed, mid-green leaves, to 25cm (10in) long; they are slightly puckered and prominently veined above, downy beneath. Long-stalked, narrow spikes, to 10cm (4in) long, of narrowly bell-shaped, bright red to purple or white flowers, 5mm (¼in) long, are borne from midsummer to early autumn. ↕↔ to 1.2m (4ft). Himalayas. ❄❄❄. **'Arun Gem'** is low-growing, and produces pendent spikes of dark pink flowers with bronze tips; ↕30cm (12in), ↔ 90cm (36in). **'Firetail'** 🏆 has bright red flowers. **'Inverleith'** forms mounds of dark green leaves, and produces short spikes of dark red flowers; ↕↔ to 45cm (18in).
P. bistorta, syn. *Polygonum bistorta* (Bistort). Vigorous, clump-forming, leafy, hairless, semi-evergreen perennial with broadly ovate, pointed, boldly veined, mid-green leaves, 10–30cm (4–12in) long. Narrowly bell-shaped, pale pink or white flowers, 5mm (¼in) long, are borne in short, dense, cylindrical spikes, 5–7cm (2–3in) long,

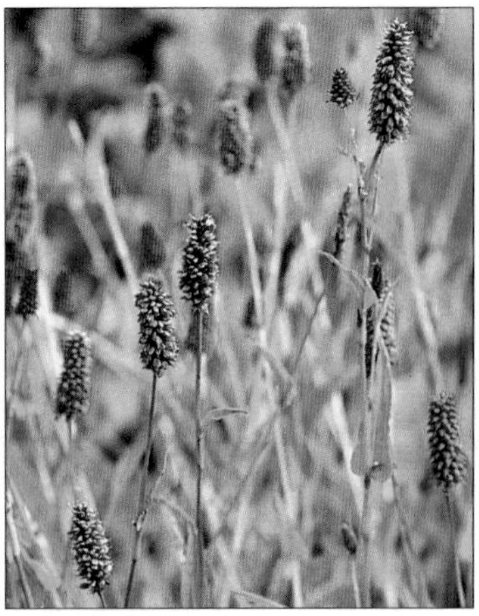
Persicaria macrophylla

from early summer to mid-autumn. ↕75cm (30in), ↔ 90cm (36in). Europe, N. and W. Asia. ❄❄❄. **subsp. *carnea***, syn. *Polygonum carneum*, has deeper pink flowers borne in more spherical spikes; ↕45–70cm (18–28in), ↔ 45cm (18in); Caucasus, N. and E. Turkey. **'Superba'** ■🏆 has dense, spherical spikes of soft pink flowers, freely borne over a long period; ↕ to 90cm (36in).
P. campanulata ■ syn. *Polygonum campanulatum*. Clump-forming, stoloniferous, deciduous or semi-evergreen perennial with sparse, lance-shaped to elliptic-ovate basal leaves, to 15cm (6in) long, and numerous stem leaves; all are hairy, with conspicuous veins, and mid-green above, white or light brown beneath. From midsummer to early autumn, slender stems bear loose, short-stalked panicles, 15cm (6in) long, of bell-shaped, fragrant, pink or white flowers, 5mm (¼in) long. ↕↔ 90cm (36in). N. India, N. Burma, S.W. China. ❄❄❄. **'Southcombe White'** has white flowers.
P. capitata, syn. *Polygonum capitatum*. Branching, stem-rooting, evergreen to deciduous perennial with ovate to elliptic, dark green leaves, to 5cm (2in) long, each with a purple V-shaped band. Bears bell-shaped pink flowers, 2–3mm ($\frac{1}{16}$–⅛in) long, in dense, rounded, short-stemmed panicles, to 1.5cm (½in) across, in summer. Good ground cover; may be invasive. ↕ 8cm (3in), ↔ 50cm (20in) or more. Himalayas. ❄❄
P. macrophylla ■ syn. *Polygonum macrophyllum, P. sphaerostachyum*. Rosette-forming, semi-evergreen perennial with woody crowns and lance-

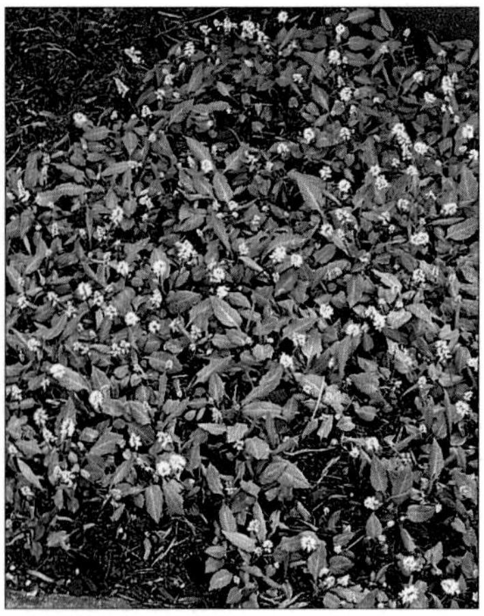
Persicaria tenuicaulis

shaped, boldly veined, mid-green leaves, to 20cm (8in) long. Dense, cylindrical spikes, 1cm (½in) long, of bell-shaped, pink to red flowers, 5mm (¼in) long, are borne from early summer to early autumn. ↕↔ 30cm (12in). Himalayas to S.W. China. ❄❄❄
P. milletii ■ syn. *Polygonum milletii*. Clump-forming, erect, semi-evergreen perennial with linear-lance-shaped, pointed, dark green leaves, to 30cm (12in) long, with prominent midribs and long sheaths. From early summer to late autumn, bears dense, cylindrical spikes, to 4cm (1½in) long, of bell-shaped crimson flowers, 6mm (¼in) long. Similar to *P. macrophylla*, but longer-flowering. ↕↔ to 60cm (24in). Himalayas to S.W. China. ❄❄❄
P. orientale, syn. *Polygonum orientale* (Kiss-me-over-the-garden-gate, Prince's feather, Princess feather). Erect, stout-stemmed, branching, hairy annual with broadly ovate, pointed, mid-green leaves, 10–20cm (4–8in) long, heart-shaped at the bases. Bell-shaped, pink to rose-red or white flowers, to 4mm (⅛in) long, are borne in dense, branching, pendent spikes, 2–8cm (¾–3in) long, in late summer and autumn. ↕ to 1.2m (4ft), ↔ to 60cm (24in). E. and S.E. Asia, Australia. ❄❄❄
P. tenuicaulis ■ syn. *Polygonum tenuicaule*. Slow-growing, mat-forming, deciduous or semi-evergreen perennial with ovate-elliptic, dark green leaves, 3–8cm (1¼–3in) long. Bears short, dense spikes, about 3.5cm (1½in) long, of bell-shaped, fragrant white flowers, 3mm (⅛in) long, in late spring. ↕ 5cm (2in), ↔ 15cm (6in). Japan. ❄❄❄

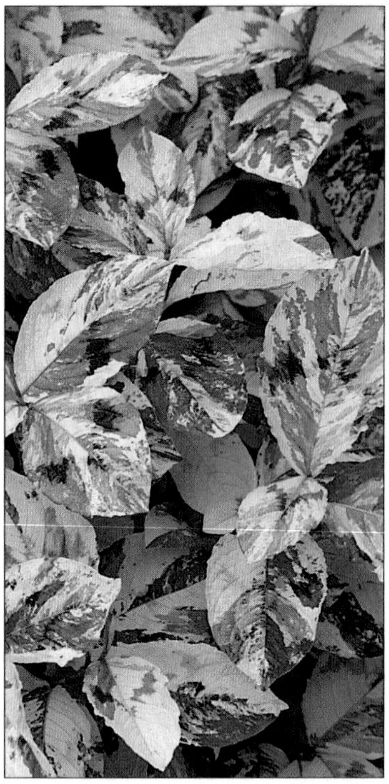
Persicaria virginiana 'Painter's Palette'

P. vacciniifolia ■🏆 syn. *Polygonum vacciniifolium*. Creeping, semi-evergreen perennial with branching, red-tinted stems bearing ovate-elliptic, glossy, mid-green leaves, to 2.5cm (1in) long, turning red in autumn. Bell-shaped, deep pink flowers, 4–6mm (⅛–¼in) long, are produced in narrow, upright spikes, to 8cm (3in) long, in late summer and autumn. ↕ 20cm (8in), ↔ 50cm (20in) or more. Himalayas. ❄❄❄
P. virginiana, syn. *Polygonum virginianum, Tovara virginiana*. Upright herbaceous perennial with ovate to elliptic, mid-green leaves with dark green markings, 8–25cm (3–10in) long. In late summer and early autumn, produces slender, very loose, terminal and axillary spikes, 10–30cm (4–12in) long, of cup-shaped green flowers, 2–3mm ($\frac{1}{16}$–⅛in) across, turning red. ↕ 40–120cm (16–48in), ↔ 60–140cm (24–56in). Himalayas, Japan, E. North America. ❄❄❄. **'Painter's Palette'** ■ produces variegated leaves with central V-shaped brown marks, yellow patches, deep pinkish red tints, and red midribs and stalks.

▷ **Persimmon,**
Chinese see *Diospyros kaki*
Japanese see *Diospyros kaki*

PETASITES

Butterbur, Sweet coltsfoot

ASTERACEAE/COMPOSITAE

Genus of about 15 species of dioecious, rhizomatous perennials from Europe, Asia, and North America, some found in mountainous regions, others in swampy sites, by streams, and in moist woodland. They have long-stalked, heart- to kidney-shaped basal leaves and smaller, short-stalked or stalkless, scale-like stem leaves. Thick stems bear purple, white, or yellow flowerheads, which usually consist of a mixture of disc-florets, ray-florets, and thread-like florets (some fertile, some sterile); they

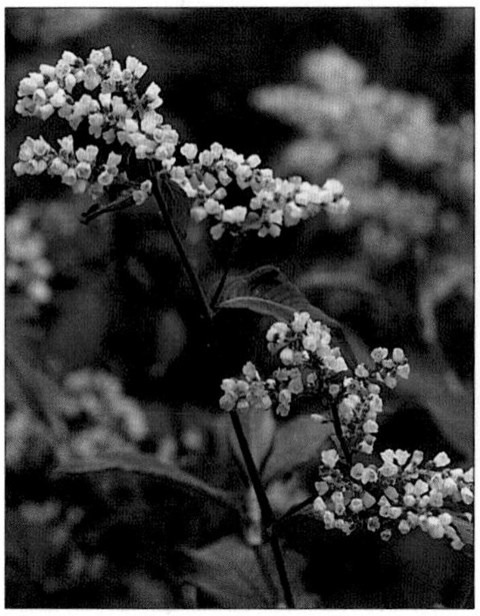
Persicaria campanulata

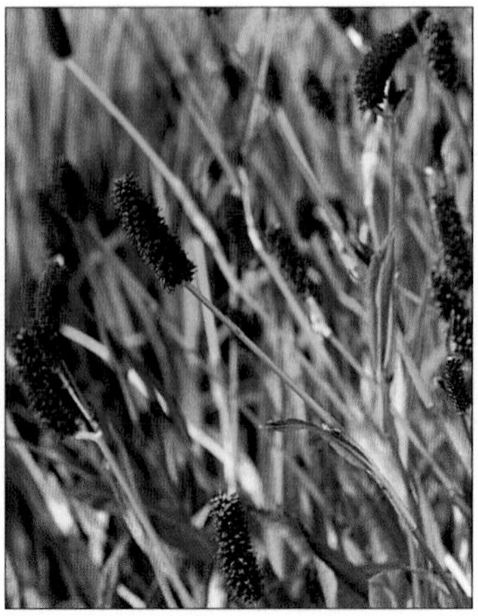
Persicaria milletii

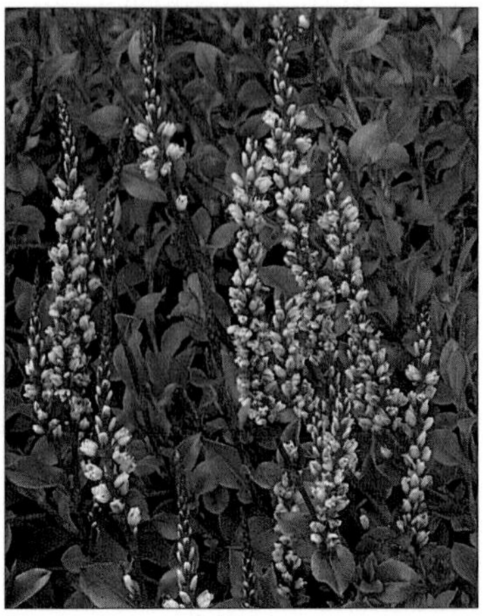
Persicaria vacciniifolia

P

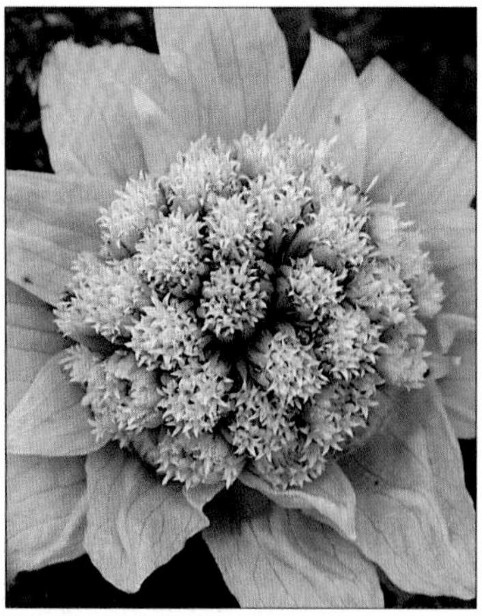

Petasites japonicus

are borne singly or in dense corymbs, racemes, or panicles. Individual plants are either male or female. Grown for their large leaves, they provide good ground cover beside a stream or pool, or in a wild garden, although they may become invasive. The flowers provide early nectar for bees.

- **HARDINESS** Fully hardy to frost hardy. Below -10°C (14°F), new growth of *P. fragrans* may die above ground, but the rhizomes will usually survive.
- **CULTIVATION** Grow in deep, humus-rich, fertile soil that is permanently moist but not stagnant, in partial or full shade. *P. fragrans* tolerates drier soil.
- **PROPAGATION** Divide in spring or autumn.
- **PESTS AND DISEASES** Trouble free.

P. fragrans (Winter heliotrope). Spreading perennial with fleshy rhizomes and kidney-shaped, toothed, basal leaves, to 12cm (5in) across, hairy beneath, borne on stalks to 30cm (12in) long. Short, lax panicles of about 10 strongly vanilla-scented, pale lilac to purple flowerheads, 1cm (½in) across, appear with the leaves from midwinter to early spring. ↕ to 30cm (12in), ↔ 1.5m (5ft). C. Mediterranean. ❄❄

P. japonicus ■ Rhizomatous perennial with kidney-shaped, irregularly toothed, basal leaves, to 80cm (32in) across, hairy beneath, borne on stalks 1m (3ft) long. Densely clustered corymbs of yellowish white flowerheads, to 1.5cm (½in) across, with oblong bracts below, are borne before the leaves in late winter and early spring. May become invasive. ↕ 1.1m (3½ft) ↔ 1.5m (5ft). China, Korea, Japan. ❄❄❄

PETREA

VERBENACEAE

Genus of 30 species of deciduous or semi-evergreen climbers, shrubs, and small trees found in woodland from Mexico to tropical South America. They are grown for their salverform flowers, each with 5 petal lobes, produced in terminal racemes or from the uppermost leaf axils, sometimes forming panicles. Simple, elliptic leaves, with prominent veins, are borne in whorls or opposite pairs. Where temperatures fall below 10–13°C (50–55°F), grow in a warm or temperate greenhouse. In warmer areas, grow in open beds, in borders, or as specimen plants; climbing species look spectacular cascading from a tree.

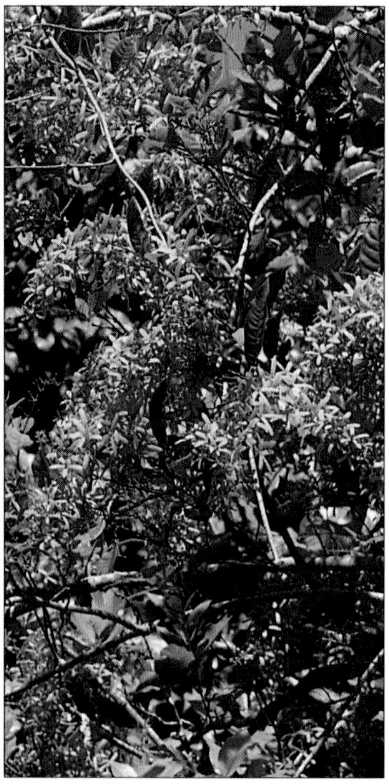

Petrea volubilis

- **HARDINESS** Frost tender.
- **CULTIVATION** Under glass, grow in loam-based potting compost (JI No.3) in full light. When in growth, water moderately and apply a balanced liquid fertilizer every month. Water sparingly in winter. Outdoors, grow in fertile, moist but well-drained soil in full sun. Support climbing stems. Pruning group 11, in late winter or early spring.
- **PROPAGATION** Root semi-ripe cuttings with bottom heat in summer. Layer or air layer in late winter.
- **PESTS AND DISEASES** Scale insects, mealybugs, and red spider mites may be a problem under glass.

P. kohautiana. Woody-stemmed, semi-evergreen climber producing branching, twining stems and stalkless, oblong-elliptic, dark green leaves, 5–20cm (2–8in) long, with heart-shaped bases. Bears erect to nodding panicles, to 60cm (24in) long, of small, salverform, violet to white flowers, from late winter to summer. ↕ to 10m (30ft). West Indies. ❀ (min. 10°C/50°F).

P. volubilis ■ (Purple wreath, Queen's wreath). Woody-stemmed, semi-evergreen climber with branching, twining stems and short-stalked, oblong-elliptic leaves, 10–20cm (4–8in) long, deep green above, paler beneath. Bears erect to arching panicles, 20–35cm (8–14in) long, of small, salverform, amethyst to deep violet flowers, with lilac calyx lobes, from late winter to summer. ↕ to 12m (40ft). Mexico, Central America, Lesser Antilles. ❀ (min. 10°C/50°F). **'Albiflora'** has white flowers.

PETROCALLIS

BRASSICACEAE/CRUCIFERAE

Genus of 2 species of cushion-forming perennials occurring at high altitudes in limestone screes and rocks in the Alps, Pyrenees, and Carpathian mountains. They have palmately 3- to 5-lobed leaves, produced in compact rosettes. Corymbs of 4-petalled flowers are borne on short leafless stems in spring. Grow in an alpine house, scree bed, or trough; they are intolerant of winter wet.

- **HARDINESS** Fully hardy.
- **CULTIVATION** In an alpine house, grow in a mix of 1 part each loam and leaf mould to 2 parts grit. Outdoors, grow in sharply drained, very gritty, poor soil in full sun. Provide protection from winter wet.
- **PROPAGATION** Sow seed in containers in an open frame in autumn. Root rosettes as cuttings in early summer.
- **PESTS AND DISEASES** Aphids, whiteflies, and red spider mites may be troublesome under glass.

P. pyrenaica. Cushion-forming evergreen perennial with dense rosettes of 3-lobed, grey-green leaves, to 6mm (¼in) long. Short-stemmed corymbs of cross-shaped, vanilla-scented, pink-purple, rarely white flowers, to 1cm (½in) across, are borne in spring. ↕ 5cm (2in), ↔ 10cm (4in). Europe (Alps, Pyrenees, Carpathian Mountains). ❄❄❄

PETROCOSMEA

GESNERIACEAE

Genus of about 30 species of evergreen perennials occurring on shady rocks in the mountains of Asia. They produce rosettes of variably shaped, usually lance-shaped to nearly rounded, felted leaves, and are grown for their 5-lobed, tubular to bell-shaped flowers produced in few-flowered, umbel-like clusters in spring. In frost-prone areas, grow in an alpine house or cold greenhouse. In frost-free climates, grow on a shady wall or in a rock crevice.

- **HARDINESS** Half hardy; may be hardy to -2°C (28°F) in a cold greenhouse.
- **CULTIVATION** Under glass, grow in loam-based potting compost (JI No.2), with added grit and leaf mould, in bright indirect light. When in growth, water moderately and apply a balanced liquid fertilizer monthly. Water sparingly in winter. Outdoors, grow in gritty, moderately fertile, humus-rich soil in partial shade.
- **PROPAGATION** Sow seed at 13–18°C (55–64°F) as soon as ripe. Take leaf cuttings in summer.
- **PESTS AND DISEASES** Susceptible to slugs and snails, aphids, and whiteflies.

P. kerrii ■ Rosette-forming perennial with downy, ovate-lance-shaped to oblong, rich green leaves, to 10cm (4in)

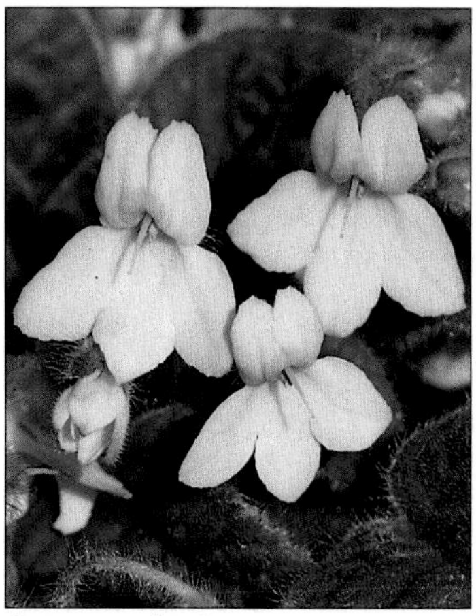

Petrocosmea kerrii

long. In summer, produces short-stemmed, umbel-like clusters of 1–3 short-tubed white flowers, to 1cm (½in) across, with 2-lobed upper lips and 3-lobed lower lips, and yellow throats. ↕ 8cm (3in), ↔ 15cm (6in). Thailand. ❄

PETROPHILE

PROTEACEAE

Genus of about 40 species of evergreen shrubs, allied to *Isopogon*, occurring on heathland, in woodland, and on cliffs, in rocky or sandy soil in Australia. The alternate leaves are linear to broadly triangular, simple, lobed, or pinnate or 2-pinnate, and rigidly leathery. They are cultivated for their unusual flowers, borne in dense spikes or cone-like clusters, surrounded by small bracts, from winter to spring. Each flower is tubular in bud, then splits open to the base into 4 rolled sepals, each with a stamen attached. When the flowers fade, the bracts enlarge and become woody, enclosing the seed pods. In frost-prone areas, grow in a well-ventilated cool greenhouse. In warmer climates, use in a shrub border.

- **HARDINESS** Frost tender, although may survive short spells at 0°C (32°F).
- **CULTIVATION** Under glass, grow in a mix of equal parts loam-based potting compost (JI No.1), grit or perlite, and peat or coir, in full light. When in growth, water moderately and apply a phosphate-free liquid fertilizer every month. Water sparingly in winter. Outdoors, grow in poor, neutral to acid, well-drained, sandy or gritty soil that is low in phosphates and nitrates. Pruning group 1; may need restrictive pruning under glass.
- **PROPAGATION** Sow seed at 18°C (64°F) in spring. Take semi-ripe cuttings with bottom heat in summer.
- **PESTS AND DISEASES** Prone to *Phytophthora* root rot when grown in moist soil and high humidity.

P. linearis. Moderately bushy shrub with wiry stems bearing sickle-shaped, flat, thick, grey-green leaves, 3–8cm (1¼–3in) long, with rounded margins. In spring, produces terminal, ovoid heads, to 5cm (2in) long, of pink flowers, 2.5cm (1in) long; the flowers open to reveal swollen yellow stigmas that turn orange when mature. ↕ to 1m (3ft), ↔ to 80cm (32in). Australia (Western Australia). ❀ (min. 5–7°C/41–45°F)

▷ ***Petrophyton*** see *Petrophytum*

PETROPHYTUM

syn. PETROPHYTON

Rock spiraea

ROSACEAE

Genus of 3 species of evergreen subshrubs, related to *Spiraea*, occurring in screes or rock crevices in the mountains of W. North America. They are grown for their short, dense, spike-like racemes of tiny, fluffy, cup-shaped flowers, each with 5 overlapping petals, produced in summer, and for their neat, compact habit. They form dense mats or mounds of short, prostrate, branching shoots with densely packed, entire, inversely lance-shaped to spoon-shaped, leathery, hairy leaves. Grow in crevices in a rock

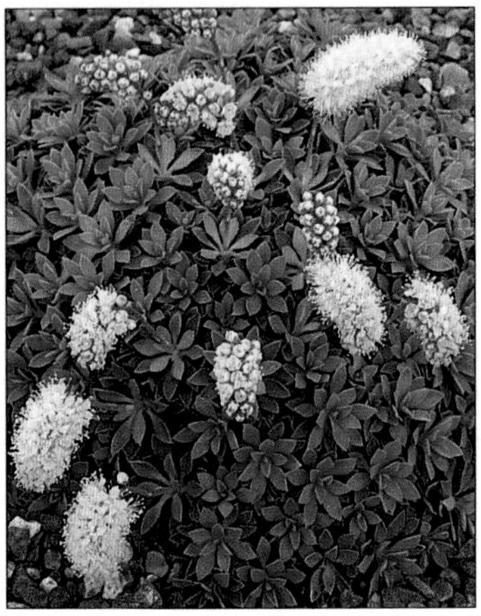

Petrophytum hendersonii

garden, or in tufa, in a trough, or in an alpine house.

- **HARDINESS** Fully hardy in very well-drained soil.
- **CULTIVATION** Grow in poor to moderately fertile, sharply drained, preferably slightly alkaline soil in full sun. In an alpine house, grow in a mix of 1 part each loam and leaf mould and 2 parts grit.
- **PROPAGATION** Sow seed in containers in an open frame in autumn. Take semi-ripe cuttings in early summer. Remove offsets in spring,
- **PESTS AND DISEASES** Aphids and red spider mites may be troublesome under glass.

P. caespitosum. Mat-forming subshrub with dense tufts of spoon-shaped, silky-hairy, bluish green leaves, to 1cm (½in) long. Tiny, cup-shaped, creamy white flowers, with prominent stamens, are produced in conical, spike-like racemes, to 10cm (4in) long, in summer. ↕ 5cm (2in), ↔ 30cm (12in). USA (Rocky Mountains). ❄❄❄

P. hendersonii ■ Dome-forming subshrub with branched stems bearing hairy, spoon-shaped, blue-green leaves, to 2cm (¾in) long. In summer, bears tiny, cup-shaped, white to creamy white flowers in dense, conical, spike-like racemes, to 8cm (3in) long. ↕ 10cm (4in), ↔ 20cm (8in). N.W. USA. ❄❄❄

PETRORHAGIA

CARYOPHYLLACEAE

Genus of about 30 species of annuals and perennials, allied to *Gypsophila* and *Dianthus*, occurring in rocky and sandy habitats in S. and C. Europe. They produce wiry stems, swollen at the nodes, and bear linear to lance-shaped or oblong, sometimes keeled leaves. They are cultivated for their terminal panicles or cymes of 5-petalled, salverform, white, sometimes pink or yellow flowers, borne in summer. Grow in a sunny position on a bank, in a rock garden, or against a wall.

- **HARDINESS** Fully hardy in well-drained soil.
- **CULTIVATION** Grow in any poor to moderately fertile, well-drained soil in full sun.
- **PROPAGATION** Sow seed in containers in a cold frame in autumn. Take stem-tip cuttings in early summer.
- **PESTS AND DISEASES** May be damaged by slugs and snails.

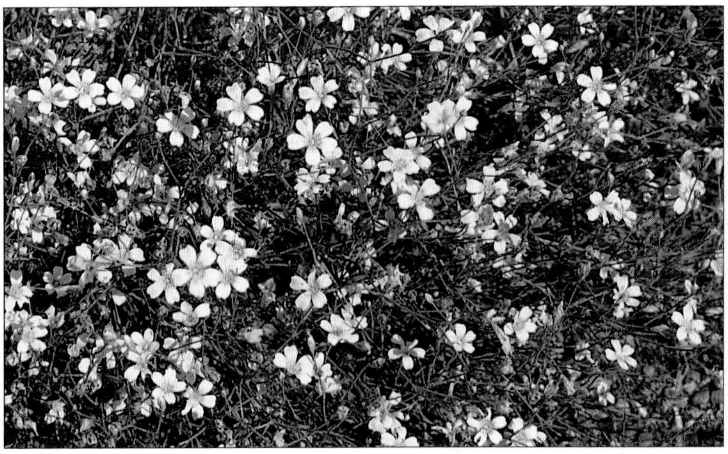

Petrorhagia saxifraga

P. saxifraga ■🏆 syn. *Tunica saxifraga* (Tunic flower). Mat-forming perennial with linear, pointed, grass-like, rich green leaves, about 1cm (½in) long. Delicate cymes of small, salverform, white or pink flowers, 1cm (½in) across, with darker veining, are borne over long periods in summer. C. and S. Europe. ↕ 10cm (4in), ↔ 20cm (8in). ❄❄❄. **'Rosette'** is more compact, with double pink flowers; ↕ 8cm (3in), ↔ 15cm (6in)

PETROSELINUM

Parsley

APIACEAE/UMBELLIFERAE

Genus of 3 species of biennials, with thick rootstocks, occurring in fallow fields and on rocky slopes and waste ground in Mediterranean Europe. The solid, ridged stems bear triangular, pinnate to 3-pinnate, mid-green leaves with toothed leaflets. Terminal, compound umbels of tiny, star-shaped, white or greenish yellow flowers, sometimes tinged red, are produced in the second year, followed by small, ovoid fruits. *P. crispum* (parsley) is grown as a culinary flavouring or garnish, and is widely naturalized in temperate regions; many cultivars are available. Parsley is usually grown as an annual, as the leaves become coarser in the second year. The tuberous-rooted Hamburg parsley (*P. crispum* var. *tuberosum*) is used as a root vegetable. Grow in a herb garden.

- **HARDINESS** Fully hardy.
- **CULTIVATION** Grow in fertile, moist but well-drained soil in full sun or partial shade. For best culinary yield, in winter in frost-prone areas, overwinter in a cold greenhouse or provide cloche protection.
- **PROPAGATION** Sow seed *in situ* from spring to late summer, and keep well watered until germinated. In frost-prone areas, protect late sowings with cloches.
- **PESTS AND DISEASES** Carrot fly larvae may damage roots, and celery fly larvae may tunnel into leaves. The foliage may be affected by leaf spots and by viruses, some transmitted by aphids.

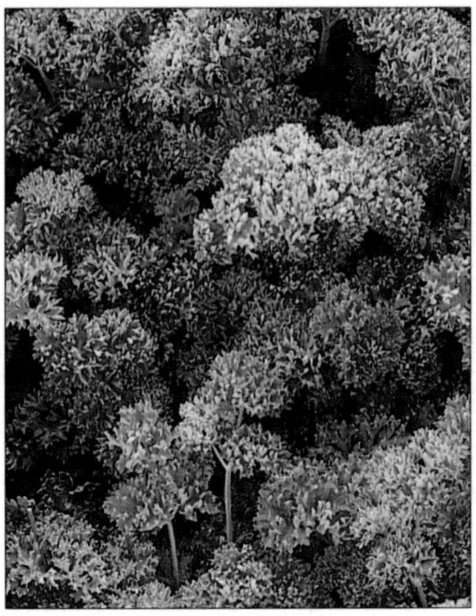

Petroselinum crispum 'Afro'

P. crispum (Parsley). Hairless, clump-forming biennial producing triangular, 3-pinnate, shiny, bright green leaves, divided into ovate, toothed segments, each to 3cm (1¼in) long. In summer of the second year, bears tiny, star-shaped, yellow-green flowers in flat-topped, terminal umbels, 1.5–4cm (½–1½in) across. ↕ 80cm (32in), ↔ 60cm (24in). S. Europe. ❄❄❄. **'Afro'** ■ is upright, with tightly curled, dark green leaves. **'Clivi'** is a compact, dwarf cultivar with dark green leaves; ↕ 20cm (8in), ↔ 30cm (12in). **var. *neapolitanum*** (French parsley, Italian parsley) has leaves with flat segments, and a stronger flavour. **var. *tuberosum*** (Hamburg parsley) produces enlarged, edible roots; ↕ to 35cm (14in), ↔ 30cm (12in).

PETTERIA

LEGUMINOSAE/PAPILIONACEAE

Genus of one species of deciduous shrub, related to *Laburnum*, occurring in mountain scrub in the Balkans, grown for its dense, erect, terminal racemes of fragrant, yellow, pea-like flowers, produced in late spring and summer. It has long-stalked, 3-palmate leaves arranged alternately. Grow in a mixed or shrub border. The seeds may cause stomach upset if ingested.

- **HARDINESS** Fully hardy.
- **CULTIVATION** Grow in well-drained, fertile soil in full sun. Pruning group 1.
- **PROPAGATION** Sow seed in containers outdoors in autumn. Take greenwood cuttings in early summer.
- **PESTS AND DISEASES** Trouble free.

P. ramentacea (Dalmatian laburnum). Upright shrub with 3-palmate, dark green leaves, to 9cm (3½in) long, lighter beneath, comprising elliptic to rounded leaflets. Fragrant yellow flowers, to 2cm (¾in) long, are produced in dense, upright racemes, to 8cm (3in) long, in late spring and early summer. ↕ 2m (6ft), ↔ 1m (3ft). Balkans. ❄❄❄

PETUNIA

SOLANACEAE

Genus of about 40 species of spreading to erect, branching, sticky-hairy annuals and perennials from stony slopes, steppes, and disturbed ground in South America. Simple, ovate to lance-shaped, mid- to dark green leaves are mostly alternate; upper leaves may be opposite. Showy, solitary, 5-lobed, fluted, single or double, saucer- or trumpet-shaped flowers are borne in the upper leaf axils.

Many cultivars have been produced, derived primarily from *P. axillaris*, *P. integrifolia*, and *P. violacea*. Although perennials, they are grown as annuals, and are particularly useful in coastal gardens or in poor soil. The flowers, 3–10cm (1¼–4in) across, are borne from late spring to late autumn, in a variety of colours, mainly pink, red, pale yellow, violet-blue, or white. Some have dark veining, central white "stars", "halos" (throats in contrasting colours), or picotee margins. Leaves are usually 5–12cm (2–5in) long.

The cultivars are divided into two groups. **Grandiflora** petunias have very large flowers, generally to 10cm (4in) across. Many are susceptible to rain damage, and are best grown in sheltered hanging baskets and containers. **Multiflora** petunias are bushier than Grandiflora petunias, with smaller flowers, to 5cm (2in) across, produced in greater quantity. They are usually more tolerant of wet weather, and are ideal for summer bedding or in a mixed border; individual plants may carpet an area up to 1m (3ft) across.

- **HARDINESS** Half hardy.
- **CULTIVATION** Under glass, grow in loam-based potting compost (JI No.1) in full light. When in growth, water freely and apply a high-potassium fertilizer every 2 weeks. Outdoors, grow in light, well-drained soil in full sun, with shelter from wind. Dead-head to prolong flowering.

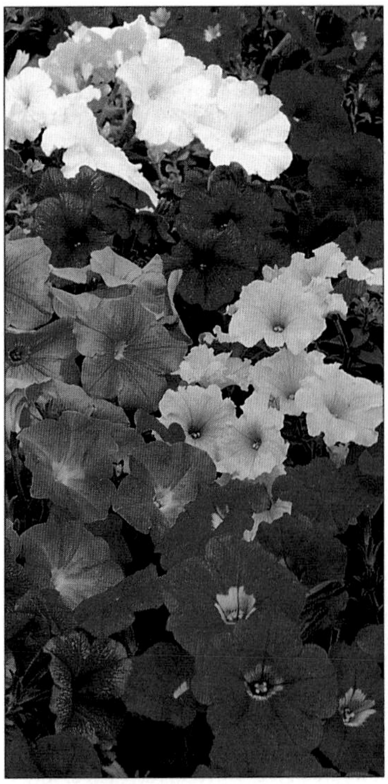

Petunia Carpet Series

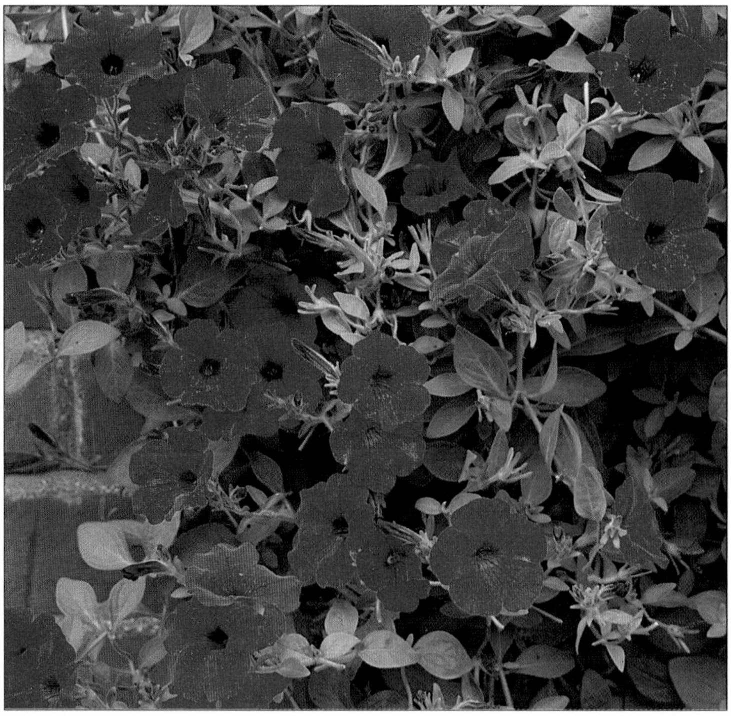

Petunia 'Purple Wave'

• **PROPAGATION** Sow seed at 13–18°C (55–64°F) in autumn or mid-spring. Take softwood cuttings in summer; in frost-prone areas, overwinter young plants under glass.
• **PESTS AND DISEASES** Aphids and slugs may be troublesome. May be affected by fungal foot rot, and by a very wide range of viruses, including alfalfa mosaic virus, tomato spotted wilt virus, tobacco mosaic virus, and potato viruses.

***P.* Aladdin Series** ▣ Grandiflora petunias producing flowers in a range of colours, including strong shades of red and salmon-pink. ↕ to 30cm (12in), ↔ 30–90cm (12–36in). ✲
***P.* Carpet Series** ▣🏆 Multiflora petunias, very compact and spreading, producing flowers in a colour range that includes strong reds and oranges. Ideal for ground cover. ↕ 20–25cm (8–10in), ↔ 30–90cm (12–36in). ✲
***P.* Celebrity Series.** Compact, early-flowering Grandiflora petunias with blooms in a large range of colours, including shades of blue, pink, or red, or pale tones of pink, yellow, or white, some with attractive dark veining. ↕ 23–30cm (9–12in), ↔ 30–90cm (12–36in). ✲. **'Pink Morn'** has pink flowers with pale creamy yellow throats.
***P.* Daddy Series.** Early-flowering Grandiflora petunias bearing large, heavily veined flowers in pastel to deep pink, salmon-pink, purple, or lavender-blue. ↕ to 35cm (14in), ↔ 30–90cm (12–36in). ✲. **'Sugar Daddy'** ▣ has purple flowers with dark veins.
***P.* Dream Series.** Grandiflora petunias bearing white, pink, salmon-pink, magenta, or red flowers. Good wet-weather tolerance for Grandiflora cultivars. ↕ 30–40cm (12–16in), ↔ 30–90cm (12–36in). ✲. **'Salmon Dream'** has salmon-pink flowers.
***P.* Duo Series.** Multiflora petunias with double flowers in a colour range that includes pink, lavender-pink, red, and burgundy, some with dark veining and some bicolours. Tolerant of wet weather, but best in containers or under glass. ↕ to 30cm (12in), ↔ 30–90cm (12–36in). ✲. **'Peppermint'** ▣ has pink flowers with darker rose-pink veining.
***P.* Flash Series.** Compact, early-flowering Grandiflora petunias in a range of colours, including rose-pink, salmon-pink, coral-pink, scarlet, red, sky-blue, blue, and white, all with creamy yellow throats; bicolours are also available. ↕ 23–40cm (9–16in), ↔ 30–90cm (12–36in). ✲
***P.* Horizon Series.** Multiflora petunias with flowers in a colour range, including white, blue, salmon-pink, and red, as well as "halo" cultivars, which have throats in white or shades of red or pink. ↕ 25–35cm (10–14in), ↔ 30–90cm (12–36in). ✲. **'Horizon Red Halo'** ▣ has red flowers with white throats.
***P.* Hula Hoop Series.** Early-flowering Grandiflora petunias with blooms in blue, purple, red, or rose-pink, all with broad, ruffled white margins; also available as a mixture. ↕ 30cm (12in), ↔ 35cm (14in). ✲
***P.* Merlin Series.** Multiflora petunias, very compact and remaining dwarf throughout the season, with flowers mainly in red, rose-pink, or blue, with some picotees. ↕ 20–25cm (8–10in), ↔ 30–90cm (12–36in). ✲
***P.* Mirage Series** 🏆 Multiflora petunias producing large flowers, to 7cm (3in) across, in white or shades of blue, pink, red, or purple, some with darker veining or with central stars. Good wet-weather tolerance. ↕ to 30cm (12in), ↔ 30–90cm (12–36in). ✲. **'Mirage Lavender'** ▣ has deep lavender-blue flowers.
***P.* Picotee Series.** Grandiflora petunias bearing flowers in rich blue, purple, red, or rose-pink, all with broad, ruffled white margins. ↕ 23–40cm (9–16in), ↔ 30–90cm (12–36in). ✲. **'Picotee Rose'** ▣ is compact, with deep rose-pink, white-margined flowers; ↕ to 20cm (8in), ↔ 45cm (18in).
***P.* Polo Series.** Compact Multiflora petunias with flowers in a range of plain, strong colours, some with veining and some bicolours. Extremely tolerant of wet weather. ↕ to 25cm (10in), ↔ 30–90cm (12–36in). ✲
***P.* Primetime Series** ▣ Multiflora petunias with flowers in a range of 24 colours and 5 mixtures (one of the broadest ranges for a Multiflora series); colours include white or shades of blue, pink, salmon-pink, or red, some with dark veins or central stars, or picotee margins. ↕ to 35cm (14in), ↔ 30–90cm (12–36in). ✲. **'Red Veined'** has rose-pink flowers with red veining.
***P.* 'Purple Wave'** ▣ Multiflora petunia with a spreading habit and vibrant magenta flowers. Use as ground cover or in hanging baskets. ↕ 45cm (18in), ↔ 30–90cm (12–36in). ✲
***P.* Supercascade Series.** Grandiflora petunias, very free-flowering over a long period, producing huge flowers, to 12cm (5in) across, in white and blue, lilac-pink, rose-pink, salmon-pink, or deep red. ↕ to 30cm (12in), ↔ 30–90cm (12–36in). ✲
***P.* Surfinia Series.** Grandiflora petunias, more vigorous and branching than other cultivars, with flowers in white and shades of pink, magenta, red, lavender-blue, and blue. They are very free-flowering, with good wet-weather tolerance, and have a trailing habit ideal for hanging baskets. Available only as young plants, propagated from soft-wood cuttings. ↕ 23–40cm (9–16in), ↔ 30–90cm (12–36in). ✲. **'Surfinia Purple'** ▣ has magenta flowers with purple veining.
***P.* Ultra Series.** Early-flowering Grandiflora petunias, compact but spreading, with good wet-weather tolerance. They produce large flowers in a range of 17 colours, including white and shades of blue, pink, and red, or a mixture, some with central stars. ↕ 25–30cm (10–12in), ↔ 30–90cm (12–36in). ✲. **'Rose Star'** ▣ has rose-pink flowers, each with a broad, white central star, creating a striped effect.

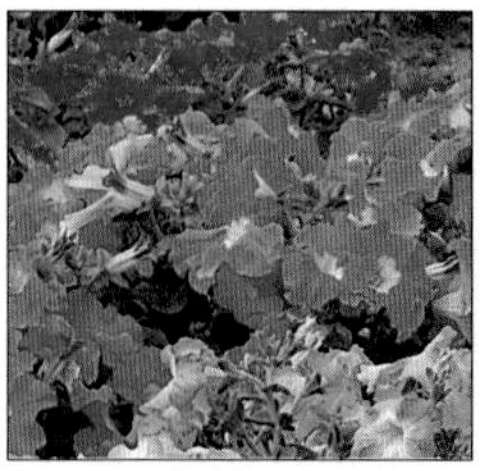

Petunia Aladdin Series

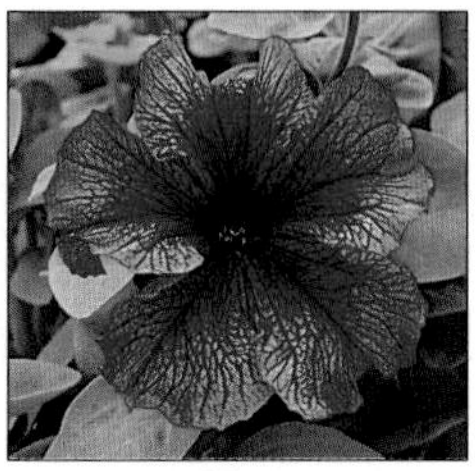

Petunia Daddy Series 'Sugar Daddy'

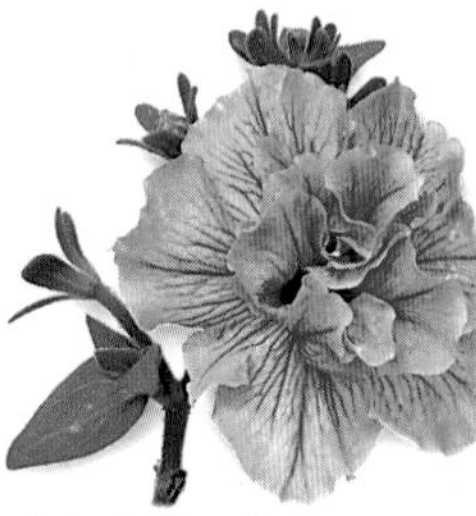

Petunia Duo Series 'Peppermint'

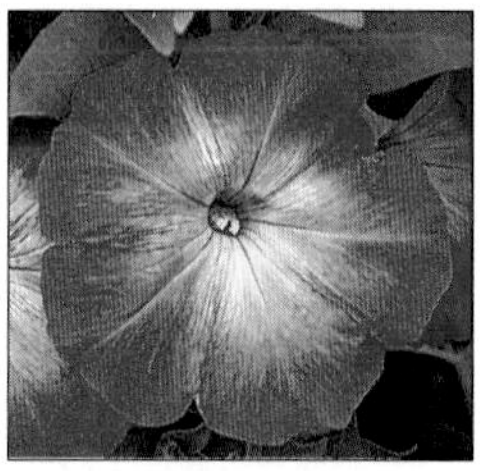

Petunia Horizon Series 'Horizon Red Halo'

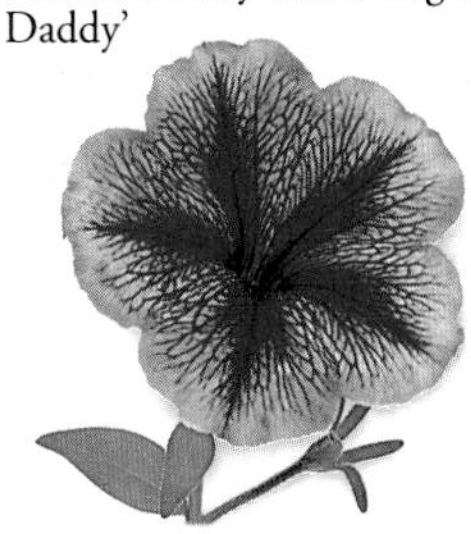

Petunia Mirage Series 'Mirage Lavender'

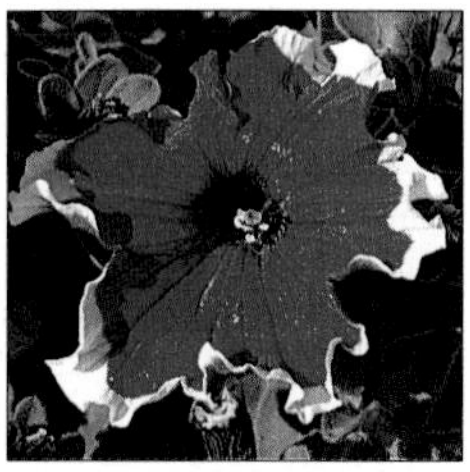

Petunia Picotee Series 'Picotee Rose'

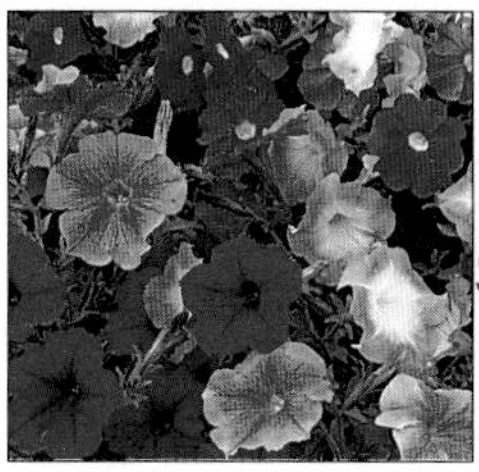

Petunia Primetime Series

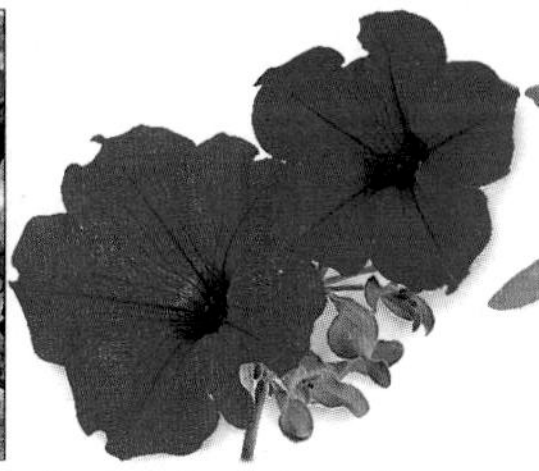

Petunia Surfinia Series 'Surfinia Purple'

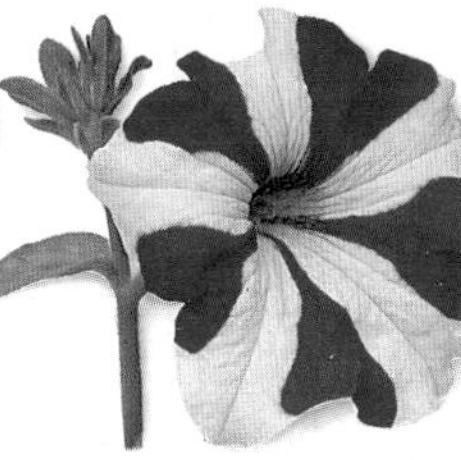

Petunia Ultra Series 'Rose Star'

▷ ***Peucedanum graveolens*** see *Anethum graveolens*

PHACELIA

Scorpion weed

HYDROPHYLLACEAE

Genus of about 150 species of usually erect annuals, biennials, and perennials from variable habitats, including stony slopes, scrub, and woodland, in North and South America. The usually pinnate, sometimes simple leaves are broadly ovate to elliptic or linear, and mostly alternate, the lower ones sometimes opposite. They produce terminal cymes, racemes, or panicles of tubular, bell-shaped, or bowl-shaped, blue, violet, white, or yellow flowers, each with 5 narrow, spreading lobes, and with prominent styles and stamens. The annual species are suitable for a border or a wildlife garden; their nectar-rich flowers attract bees and other insects. Grow *P. sericea* in an alpine house or scree bed; it resents winter wet. Contact with foliage may aggravate skin allergies.
• **HARDINESS** Fully hardy.
• **CULTIVATION** Grow annuals in any fertile, well-drained soil in full sun. Outdoors, grow *P. sericea* in gritty, sharply drained soil in full sun. Protect it from winter wet; in an alpine house, grow in a mix of equal parts loam, leaf mould, and grit.
• **PROPAGATION** Sow seed of annuals *in situ* in spring or early autumn. Sow seed of *P. sericea* in containers in a cold frame in autumn.
• **PESTS AND DISEASES** *P. sericea* is susceptible to aphids and red spider mites under glass.

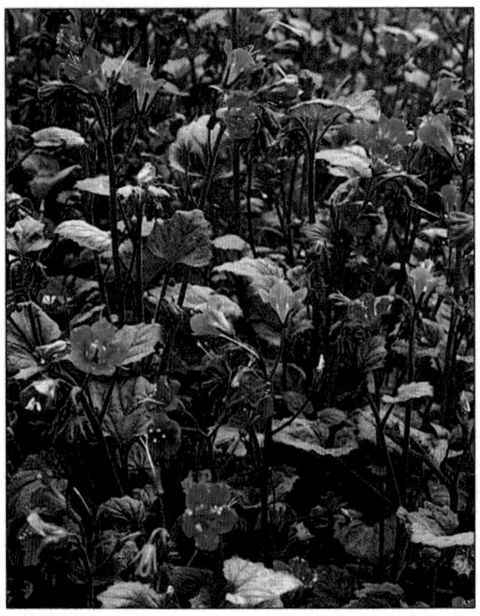

Phacelia campanularia

P. campanularia ■ (Californian bluebell). Erect, compact, intricately branched, glandular-hairy, aromatic annual with simple, ovate to elliptic, coarsely toothed, dark green leaves, to 5cm (2in) long. Lax cymes of upturned, spreading, bell-shaped, dark blue, occasionally white flowers, to 2.5cm (1in) across, are borne in late spring and summer. ↕ 15–30cm (6–12in), ↔ 15cm (6in). USA (S. California). ❄❄❄

P. grandiflora. Vigorous, erect, glandular-hairy annual with simple, broadly ovate to elliptic, irregularly toothed, mid-green leaves, to 20cm (8in) long. Produces erect, densely flowered cymes of upturned, spreading, bell-shaped, lilac-blue or white flowers, to 2cm (¾in) across, in summer. ↕ to 90cm (36in), ↔ to 30cm (12in). USA (S. California). ❄❄❄

P. sericea. Rosette-forming biennial or short-lived perennial with silvery, silky-hairy, deeply pinnatifid leaves, to 10cm (4in) long, with oblong-lance-shaped lobes. Short, dense, panicle-like cymes of bell-shaped, indigo-blue flowers, 6–8mm (¼–⅜in) across, with pale blue anthers and protruding stamens, are produced in summer. ↕ to 55cm (22in), ↔ 10cm (4in). USA (Rocky Mountains). ❄❄❄

P. tanacetifolia. Erect, hairy annual, with pinnatifid to 2-pinnatifid or pinnate, mid-green leaves, to 25cm (10in) long, composed of lance-shaped lobes or pinnae. Dense, curved racemes of spreading, bell-shaped, blue or lavender-blue flowers, to 1.5cm (½in) across, are produced in summer. ↕ to 1.2m (4ft), ↔ to 45cm (18in). USA (California) to Mexico. ❄❄❄

PHAEDRANASSA

Queen lily

AMARYLLIDACEAE

Genus of about 6 species of bulbous perennials from meadows and rocky slopes at high altitudes in South America. They are grown for their colourful, tubular or narrowly funnel-shaped, pendent flowers, borne in terminal umbels of 3–11, from spring to summer. The leaves are basal, lance-shaped to elliptic, and up to 40cm (16in) long, developing with or after the flowers. In frost-prone areas, grow in a cool or temperate greenhouse. In warmer climates, grow in a warm, sunny position in a border.

• **HARDINESS** Frost tender, but will occasionally withstand temperatures to 0°C (32°F) for short periods.

• **CULTIVATION** Under glass, grow in loam-based potting compost (JI No.2) with added sharp sand and leaf mould, in full light. When in growth, water moderately and apply a balanced liquid fertilizer every month. Keep just moist when dormant in autumn and winter. Outdoors, grow in moderately fertile, well-drained soil that does not dry out in summer.

• **PROPAGATION** Sow seed at 13–18°C (55–64°F) when ripe. Remove offsets in autumn.

• **PESTS AND DISEASES** Trouble free.

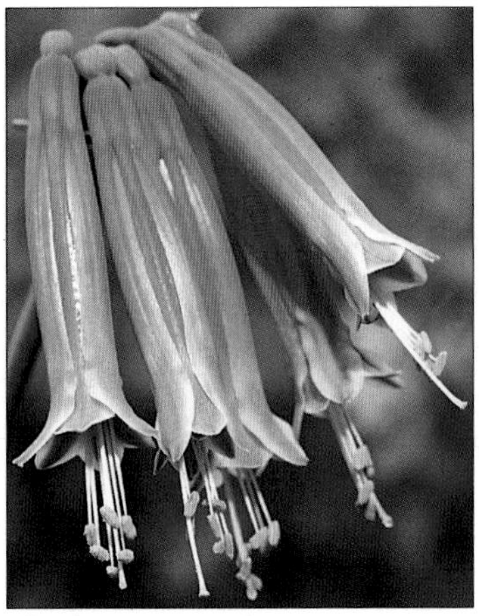

Phaedranassa carmioli

P. carmioli ■ Bulbous perennial producing erect, lance-shaped, mid-green, basal leaves, to 40cm (16in) long, developing with the flowers. From spring to summer, bears umbels of 4–10 pendent, tubular, shiny crimson flowers, 3.5–4.5cm (1½–1¾in) long, with green and yellow tips, and with conspicuous, protruding white anthers. ↕ 50–70cm (20–28in), ↔ 8cm (3in). South America. ❀ (min. 7°C/45°F)

P. dubia. Bulbous perennial producing erect, elliptic, mid-green, basal leaves, to 50cm (20in) long, with the flowers. In summer, produces umbels of 7–9 pendent, tubular, green-tipped, purple-pink flowers, 4.5–5cm (1¾–2in) long, with protruding stamens. ↕ 50–70cm (20–28in), ↔ 8cm (3in). Peru. ❀ (min. 7°C/45°F)

P. tunguraguae. Bulbous perennial with ovoid bulbs and erect, lance-shaped or inversely lance-shaped, glossy, dark green, basal leaves, 30–40cm (12–16in) long, developing after the flowers. Bears umbels of 6–8 pendent, tubular, green-tipped, coral-red flowers, to 3cm (1¼in) long, in summer. ↕ 50–70cm (20–28in), ↔ 8cm (3in). Ecuador. ❀ (min. 7°C/45°F)

P. viridiflora. Bulbous perennial with erect, narrow, bright green, basal leaves, to 40cm (16in) long, appearing with the flowers. Umbels of 3–5 pendent, tubular, yellow and green flowers, 2.5cm (1in) long, are borne in summer. ↕ 60cm (24in), ↔ 8cm (3in). Ecuador, possibly Peru. ❀ (min. 7°C/45°F)

▷ ***Phaedranthus buccinatorius*** see *Distictis buccinatoria*
▷ ***Phaiophleps biflora*** see *Olsynium biflorum*
▷ ***Phaiophleps nigricans*** see *Sisyrinchium striatum*

PHAIUS

ORCHIDACEAE

Genus of about 30 species of deciduous to evergreen, terrestrial and epiphytic orchids from lowland and montane forests in Africa, Madagascar, Asia, Indonesia, N. Australia, and the Pacific islands. They have spherical to ovoid, sometimes stem-like pseudobulbs, each with 3–10 large, folded, lance-shaped to elliptic, mid-green leaves, arranged alternately. Colourful, often spectacular flowers, with entire or lobed lips and spreading petals, are produced in tall, upright, axillary, many-flowered racemes from near the bases of the plants.

• **HARDINESS** Frost tender.

• **CULTIVATION** Intermediate-growing orchids. Grow in terrestrial orchid compost in deep containers that allow room for the copious root system. In summer, provide high humidity and bright filtered light, and water freely, applying fertilizer at every third watering. Once the leaves are fully developed, mist twice daily. In winter, water sparingly and provide full light. See also p.46.

• **PROPAGATION** Divide when the plants "overflow" their containers (take care when dividing to avoid damaging the clustered pseudobulbs).

• **PESTS AND DISEASES** Scale insects, red spider mites, aphids, and mealybugs may be troublesome.

P. flavus, syn. *P. maculatus.* Semi-evergreen orchid with conical pseudobulbs and lance-shaped, mid-green leaves, to 60cm (24in) long, with yellow and white spots. Racemes of fragrant yellow flowers, 8cm (3in) across, with red-brown markings on the lips, are produced in spring. ↕ 1m (3ft), ↔ 60cm (24in). India, Thailand, Malaysia, Indonesia (Java). ❀ (min. 15°C/59°F; max. 30°C/86°F)

P. maculatus see *P. flavus.*

P. tankervilleae ■ Semi-evergreen orchid with ovoid pseudobulbs and several elliptic to lance-shaped, pointed, mid-green leaves, to 1m (3ft) long. In summer, produces racemes of nodding, fragrant, red-brown flowers, 8cm (3in) across, with pink to purplish red lips; throats are yellow and purplish red inside, silvery outside. ↕↔ 1m (3ft). C. China, N. India, Sri Lanka through S.E. Asia to Australia. ❀ (min. 15°C/59°F; max. 30°C/86°F)

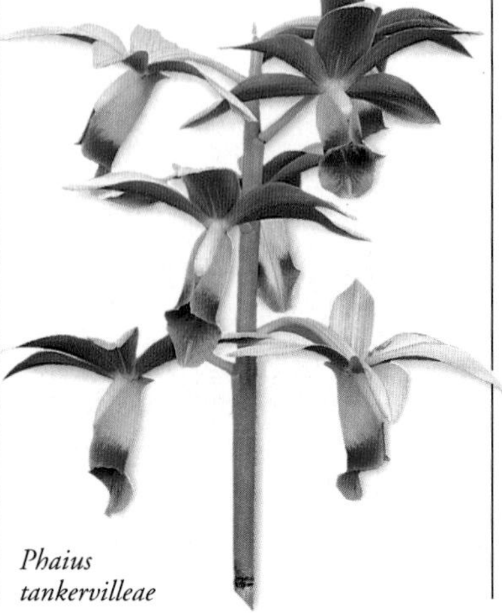

Phaius tankervilleae

PHALAENOPSIS

Moth orchid

ORCHIDACEAE

Genus of approximately 50 species of mostly evergreen, mainly epiphytic, monopodial orchids occurring from sea level to lowland forests in the Himalayas, S.E. Asia, and N. Australia. They each have a short, upward-growing, stem-like rhizome, lacking pseudobulbs and producing 3–6 broadly obovate or oval, upright or semi-pendent, fleshy, mid- to dark green, sometimes mottled leaves. Flowers, in simple or branched racemes, are produced from the bases of the leaves, often throughout the year, remaining in bloom for many months. Many hybrids have been produced.

• **HARDINESS** Frost tender.

• **CULTIVATION** Warm-growing orchids. Grow epiphytically on slabs of bark, or in epiphytic orchid compost in a slatted basket to allow the aerial roots to hang outside. Provide high humidity and bright filtered light all year. From spring to autumn, water freely, mist daily, and apply a balanced fertilizer monthly. In winter, water sparingly, keeping the foliage dry. Support the racemes of flowers to prevent kinking, and cut back flowered stems to a lower node to encourage production of further flowers. See also p.46.

• **PROPAGATION** Not suitable for division, although cuttings or offshoots may be rooted successfully.

• **PESTS AND DISEASES** Red spider mites, aphids, and mealybugs may be a problem.

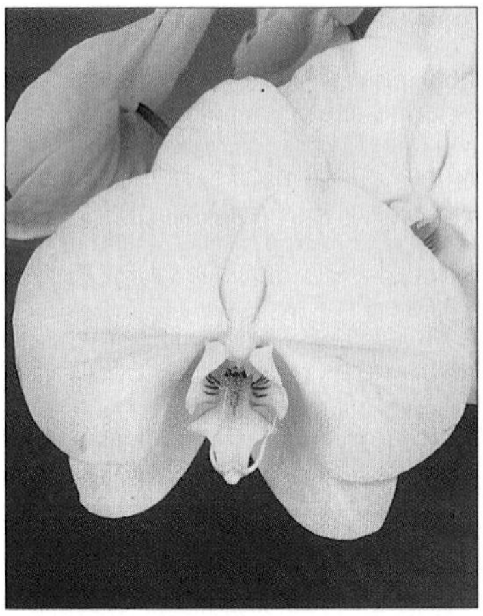

Phalaenopsis Allegria

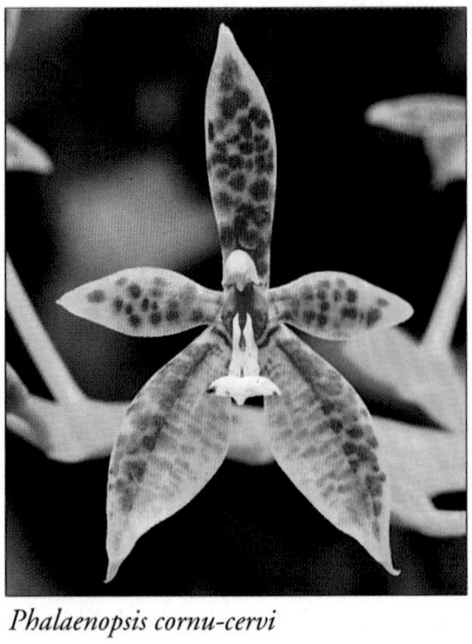

Phalaenopsis cornu-cervi

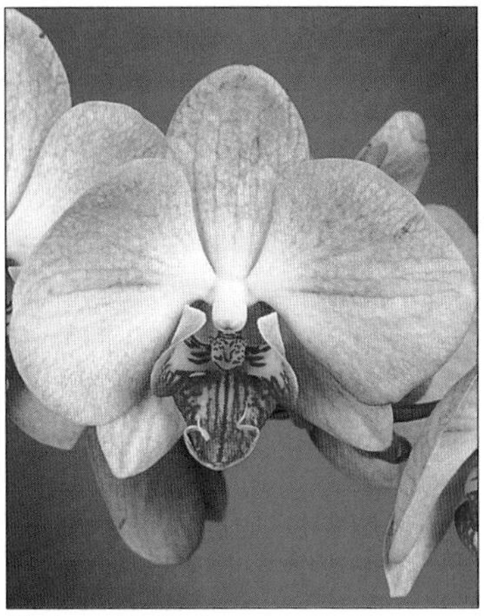

Phalaenopsis Doris

P. Allegria ■ (*P.* Alice Gloria x *P.* Wilma Hughes). Epiphytic orchid with semi-pendent, broadly oval leaves, 30cm (12in) or more long. Numerous large, rounded, heavy, pure white flowers, to 12cm (5in) across, appear in pendent racemes, 1m (3ft) long, throughout the year. ↕ 1m (3ft), ↔ 45cm (18in). ❀ (min. 18°C/64°F; max. 30°C/86°F)
P. amabilis ♀ Epiphytic orchid with semi-pendent, broadly oval leaves, 15–50cm (6–20in) long. Numerous white flowers, 6–10cm (2½–4in) across, with yellow-margined lips and red throat markings, appear in pendent, simple or branched racemes, 1m (3ft) long, from autumn to early spring. ↕↔ 30cm (12in). Philippines, Indonesia to Australia (N.E. Queensland). ❀ (min. 18°C/64°F; max. 30°C/86°F)
P. cornu-cervi ■ Epiphytic orchid with oblong-ovate leaves, to 25cm (10in) long. Star-shaped, fragrant, waxy, yellow-green flowers, 5cm (2in) across, overlaid with red-brown, are borne in succession throughout the year, in short, branched or simple racemes, 15cm (6in) long. ↕ 15cm (6in), ↔ 20cm (8in). Burma, S.E. Asia. ❀ (min. 18°C/64°F; max. 30°C/86°F)
P. Doris ■ (*P.* Elizabethae x *P.* Katherine Siegwart). Epiphytic orchid with semi-pendent, broadly oval, grey-green leaves, 30cm (12in) long. Pink flowers, 8cm (3in) across, with purple-red lips, are borne in arching racemes, 1m (3ft) long, throughout the year. ↕↔ 30cm (12in). ❀ (min. 18°C/64°F; max. 30°C/86°F)
P. equestris ♀ Epiphytic orchid with oblong-ovate leaves, to 20cm (8in) long.

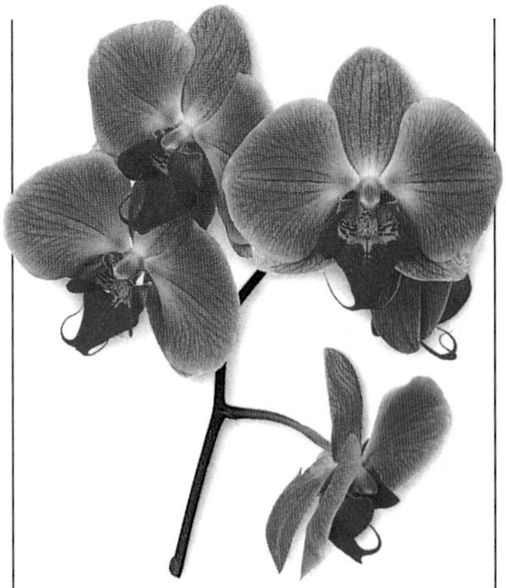

Phalaenopsis Lipperose

From spring to winter, bears simple or branched, erect to arching racemes, 35cm (14in) long, of small, rose-pink flowers, 2cm (¾in) across, with deep pink or purple lips, streaked dark red. ↕↔ 20cm (8in). Philippines, Taiwan. ❀ (min. 18°C/64°F; max. 30°C/86°F)
P. Esmé Hennessy (*P.* Anna Queen x *P.* Pekoe). Vigorous epiphytic orchid with semi-pendent, broadly oval leaves, 30cm (12in) or more long. White flowers, 8cm (3in) across, with faint yellow markings and crimson lips, appear in pendent racemes, 1m (3ft) long, mainly in winter. ↕↔ 30cm (12in). ❀ (min. 18°C/64°F; max. 30°C/86°F)
P. Golden Horizon 'Sunrise' ■ (*P.* Barbara Freed Saltzman x *P.* Golden Buddha). Epiphytic orchid with broadly oval leaves, to 25cm (10in) long. Fleshy, creamy yellow flowers, 6cm (2½in) across, with red-brown stripes and orange-red lips, are borne throughout the year in short racemes, 15cm (6in) long. ↕ 15cm (6in), ↔ 30cm (12in). ❀ (min. 18°C/64°F; max. 30°C/86°F)
P. Henriette Lecoufle 'Boule de Neige' (*P.* Lachésis x *P.* Ramona). Epiphytic orchid with semi-pendent, broadly oval leaves, 30cm (12in) long. Produces large, pure white flowers, 10–12cm (4–5in) across, in pendent racemes, 1m (3ft) long, mainly in winter. ↕ 1m (3ft), ↔ 30cm (12in). ❀ (min. 18°C/64°F; max. 30°C/86°F)
P. Lipperose ■ (*P.* Ruby Wells x *P.* Zada). Epiphytic orchid with semi-pendent, broadly oval leaves, 30cm (12in) long. Pink flowers, 10cm (4in) across, with red lips, appear throughout the year in many-flowered, pendent

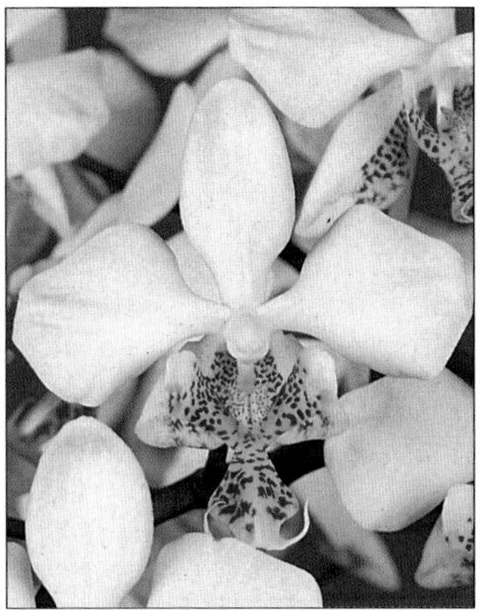

Phalaenopsis stuartiana

racemes, 1m (3ft) long. ↕ 1m (3ft), ↔ 30cm (12in). ❀ (min. 18°C/64°F; max. 30°C/86°F)
P. lueddemanniana. Epiphytic orchid with oblong-ovate leaves, to 30cm (12in) long. In summer, full, rounded, fragrant, waxy white flowers, 5cm (2in) across, with brownish purple bands and pink to purple lips, are borne in succession in short, simple or branched racemes, 15cm (6in) long. ↕ 15cm (6in), ↔ 20cm (8in). Philippines. ❀ (min. 18°C/64°F; max. 30°C/86°F)
P. schilleriana ■ Epiphytic orchid with semi-pendent, broadly elliptic, fleshy leaves, to 45cm (18in) long, dark green spotted with silver-grey above, purple beneath. Numerous rose-pink flowers, 5cm (2in) or more across, with white or yellow lips spotted reddish purple, appear in branching racemes, 1m (3ft) long, in winter and spring. ↕ 60cm (24in), ↔ 30cm (12in). Philippines. ❀ (min. 18°C/64°F; max. 30°C/86°F)
P. stuartiana ■♀ Epiphytic orchid with semi-pendent, broadly oval, mid-green leaves, 35cm (14in) long, mottled grey-green above, purple beneath. In winter, bears branching racemes, 1m (3ft) long, of white flowers, 8cm (3in) across, with yellow marks and brownish red spots on the lower sepals and lips. ↕ 60cm (24in), ↔ 30cm (12in). Philippines. ❀ (min. 18°C/64°F; max. 30°C/86°F)
P. violacea. Epiphytic orchid with broadly oblong leaves, 20–25cm (8–10in) long. In spring and summer, star-shaped, fragrant, waxy, rich violet-purple, yellow, and white flowers, 6cm (2½in) across, with reddish purple lips, are borne in succession in short racemes, 15cm (6in) long. ↕ 15cm (6in), ↔ 30cm (12in). Malaysia, Indonesia (Sumatra), Borneo. ❀ (min. 18°C/64°F; max. 30°C/86°F)
P. Yukimai ■ (*P.* Grace Palm x *P.* Musashino). Epiphytic orchid with broadly oval leaves, 20cm (8in) long. White flowers, 8cm (3in) across, with yellow-tinted, sometimes purple-red lips, appear in racemes 30cm (12in) tall, throughout the year. ↕↔ 30cm (12in). ❀ (min. 18°C/64°F; max. 30°C/86°F)

PHALARIS

GRAMINEAE/POACEAE

Genus of about 15 species of tufted, annual grasses or spreading rhizomatous, perennial grasses found in extremely variable habitats in temperate regions, from dry slopes to moist lake margins. They produce compact panicles of ovate spikelets, each with 1–3 flowers. Leaves are pale to mid-green, usually broadly linear and flat, with short points. *P. arundinacea* and its cultivars need to be controlled if grown in a mixed or herbaceous border, but are good as ground cover, or planted at the side of a pond or stream.

- **HARDINESS** Fully hardy to frost hardy.
- **CULTIVATION** Grow in any soil in full sun or partial shade. Cut back dead foliage in early spring. On variegated cultivars, which may otherwise revert to plain green after midsummer, cut down all but the new young shoots in early summer to encourage fresh growth.
- **PROPAGATION** Divide from mid-spring to midsummer.
- **PESTS AND DISEASES** Trouble free.

P. arundinacea (Reed canary grass, Ribbon grass). Erect, evergreen, rhizomatous, perennial grass with flat, linear, short-pointed, mid-green leaves, to 35cm (14in) long, occasionally striped yellow. In early and midsummer, bears narrow panicles, to 17cm (7in) long, of pale green spikelets, fading to buff with age. ↕ to 1.5m (5ft) in flower, ↔ indefinite. Eurasia, Southern Africa, North America. ✱✱✱. **'Feesey'**, syn. 'Mervyn Feesey', is flushed pink at the stem bases, and has light green leaves with broad white stripes, and panicles with a faint purplish flush; less invasive than the species. **'Mervyn Feesey'** see 'Feesey'. **var. *picta*** ■♀ (Gardeners' garters) has a number of variants with white-striped leaves; ↕ to 1m (3ft).

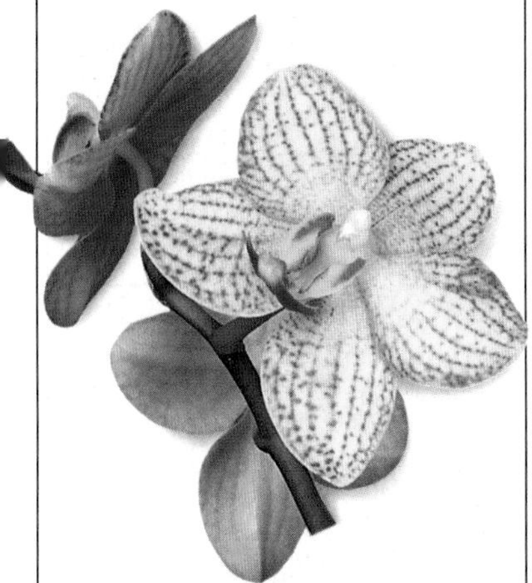

Phalaenopsis Golden Horizon 'Sunrise'

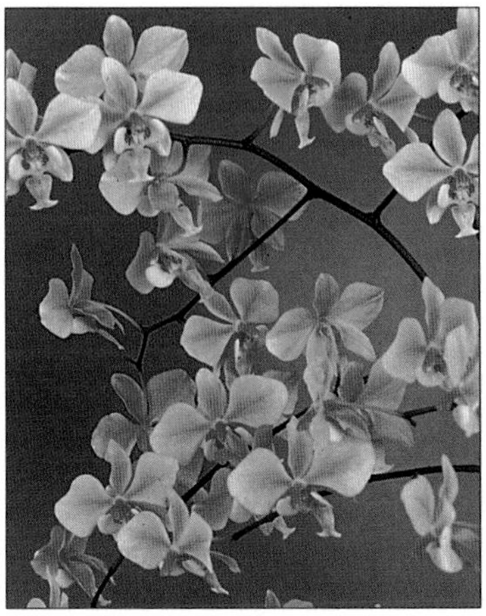

Phalaenopsis schilleriana

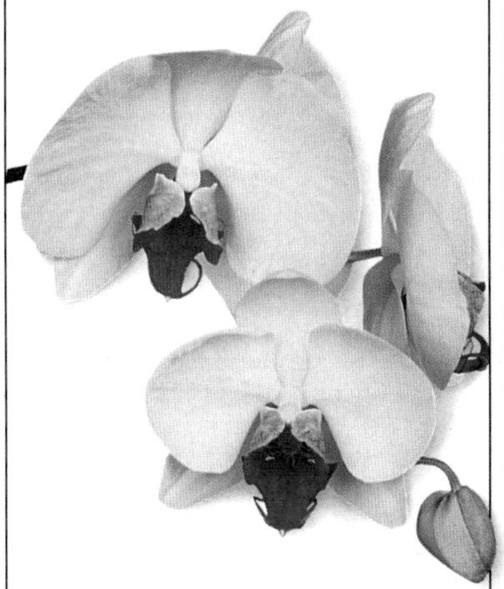

Phalaenopsis Yukimai

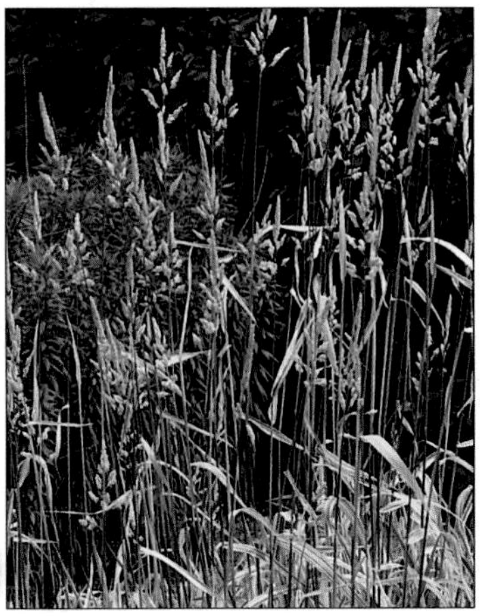

Phalaris arundinacea var. *picta*

▷ **Phanera** see *Bauhinia corymbosa*
▷ ***Phanerophlebia*** see *Cyrtomium*
  P. falcata see *C. falcatum*
  P. fortunei see *C. fortunei*
▷ ***Pharbitis*** see *Ipomoea*
  P. hederacea see *I. hederacea*
  P. purpurea see *I. purpurea*
▷ ***Phaseolus caracalla*** see *Vigna caracalla*
▷ **Pheasant's eye** see *Adonis annua*
  Old see *Narcissus poeticus* var. *recurvus*

PHEBALIUM

RUTACEAE

Genus of 45 species of evergreen trees and shrubs occurring in woodland or open, moist and dry habitats in Australia and New Zealand. They are grown for their foliage and flowers. The simple, alternate, often aromatic, light to dark green leaves are linear to rounded or oblong, sometimes cylindrical. Small, tubular, star- or bell-shaped, 4- or 5-petalled flowers are usually borne singly or in axillary and terminal, umbel-like clusters. Where temperatures regularly fall below 5°C (41°F), grow in a cool greenhouse. In milder climates, grow at the back of a border, or use as a barrier or hedge.
• **HARDINESS** Half hardy to frost tender.
• **CULTIVATION** Under glass, grow in lime-free (ericaceous) potting compost in full light. During growth, water moderately and apply a balanced liquid fertilizer monthly. Water sparingly in winter. Outdoors, grow in neutral to slightly acid, moderately fertile, humus-rich, moist but well-drained soil in full sun. Pruning group 1; may need restrictive pruning under glass after flowering.
• **PROPAGATION** Sow seed at 13–18°C (55–64°F) in spring. Root semi-ripe cuttings with bottom heat in summer.
• **PESTS AND DISEASES** Trouble free.

P

P. squameum ♀ (Bobie-bobie, Satinwood). Large shrub or small tree, erect and lightly to moderately branched if unpruned. Elliptic to oblong-lance-shaped, leathery leaves, 3–10cm (1¼–4in) long, are mid- to deep green above, silver-white scaly with translucent oil glands beneath. In spring or early summer, bears umbel-like clusters of star-shaped white flowers, 8–10mm (⅜–½in) across, with prominent stamens. ↕ 3–6m (10–20ft), ↔ 1.5–3m (5–10ft). Australia (Queensland to Tasmania). ⚘ (min. 5°C/41°F)

PHEGOPTERIS

Beech fern

THELYPTERIDACEAE

Genus of 3 or 4 species of deciduous, terrestrial ferns found on shady banks and rocks in high rainfall areas throughout the N. hemisphere and in S.E. Asia. The pinnate to 2-pinnate or pinnatifid fronds, with pinnatifid or pinnatisect pinnae, arise at random from each erect to creeping rhizome, their fronds turning at right-angles to the light. Round sori, without protective indusia, are produced in 2 rows on the undersides of the frond segments. Beech ferns are ideal for growing in a moist, shady border, or among rocks where the soil does not dry out.

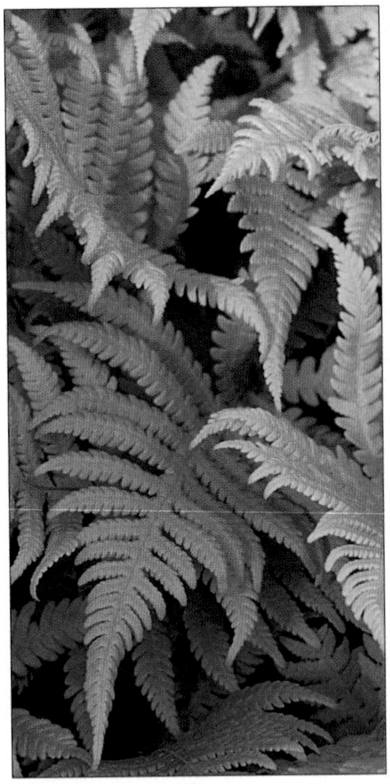

Phegopteris connectilis

• **HARDINESS** Fully hardy.
• **CULTIVATION** Grow in moderately fertile, humus-rich, reliably moist soil, preferably in deep shade.
• **PROPAGATION** Sow spores at 15°C (59°F) as soon as ripe. Divide in spring. See also p.51.
• **PESTS AND DISEASES** Trouble free.

P. connectilis ▣ syn. *Thelypteris phegopteris* (Beech fern). Deciduous fern bearing long-stalked, arrow-shaped to triangular, pinnate, pale green fronds, 30cm (12in) long, with oblong or linear to lance-shaped, deeply pinnatifid pinnae, composed of oblong segments. The lowest pair of pinnae point forwards and downwards. ↕ 30cm (12in), ↔ indeterminate. N. hemisphere. ❄❄❄
P. decursive-pinnata. Deciduous fern producing tufts of narrowly lance-shaped, pinnate or 2-pinnatifid, pale green fronds, to 80cm (32in) long, each tapering gradually to a stalk up to 20cm (8in) long. Pinnae are entire and linear, occasionally pinnatifid. ↕ 80cm (32in), ↔ 40cm (16in). E. Asia. ❄❄❄
P. hexagonoptera, syn. *Thelypteris hexagonoptera* (Broad beech fern). Deciduous fern with long-stalked, triangular, pinnate-pinnatifid fronds, 40cm (16in) long. Similar to *P. connectilis*, but fronds and pinnae are broader, and the lowest pair of pinnae do not point forwards or downwards. ↕ 40cm (16in), ↔ indeterminate. E. North America. ❄❄❄

PHELLODENDRON

RUTACEAE

Genus of 10 species of deciduous, dioecious trees found in moist stream margins in the mountains of E. Asia. They have opposite, pinnate, dull yellowish green to dark green leaves. Small, cup-shaped green male and female flowers are borne in clusters on separate plants in summer, and both must be grown to produce the dark blue-black, spherical fruits, 1cm (½in) across. Grown for their habit and aromatic foliage, usually giving fine autumn colour, they are best used as specimen trees in a garden large enough to accommodate their spreading habit. They thrive in areas with hot summers.
• **HARDINESS** Fully hardy, but young growth may be damaged by late frosts.
• **CULTIVATION** Grow in deep, fertile, well-drained soil in full sun. Pruning group 1.
• **PROPAGATION** Sow seed in containers outdoors in autumn. Root heeled semi-ripe cuttings in midsummer.
• **PESTS AND DISEASES** Trouble free.

P. amurense ♀ (Amur cork tree). Spreading tree with stout shoots, and with thick, corky, pale grey-brown bark when mature. Bears pinnate leaves, to 35cm (14in) long, with up to 13 ovate to lance-shaped, glossy, dark green leaflets, glaucous beneath, turning yellow in autumn. ↕ to 14m (46ft), ↔ 15m (50ft). N.E. Asia. ❄❄❄
P. chinense ▣ ♀ Spreading tree with stout shoots and thin, dark grey-brown bark. Bears pinnate leaves, to 40cm (16in) long, with up to 13 oblong to lance-shaped leaflets, yellow-green above, light green and downy beneath, turning yellow in autumn. ↕ 10m (30ft), ↔ 12m (40ft). C. China. ❄❄❄
P. lavallei ♀ Spreading tree with stout shoots and slightly corky, pale grey-brown bark when mature. Bears pinnate leaves, to 35cm (14in) long, with up to 11 oval to lance-shaped, tapered, matt, mid-green leaflets, downy on the veins beneath, turning yellow in autumn. ↕ 10m (30ft), ↔ 12m (40ft). Japan. ❄❄❄
P. sachalinense ♀ Spreading tree with stout shoots and thin, finely channelled, dark brown bark. Bears pinnate leaves, to 30cm (12in) long, with up to 13 ovate-oblong leaflets, dull green above, smooth and blue-green beneath, turning yellow in autumn. ↕ 10m (30ft), ↔ 12m (40ft). Russia (Sakhalin), Korea, Japan. ❄❄❄

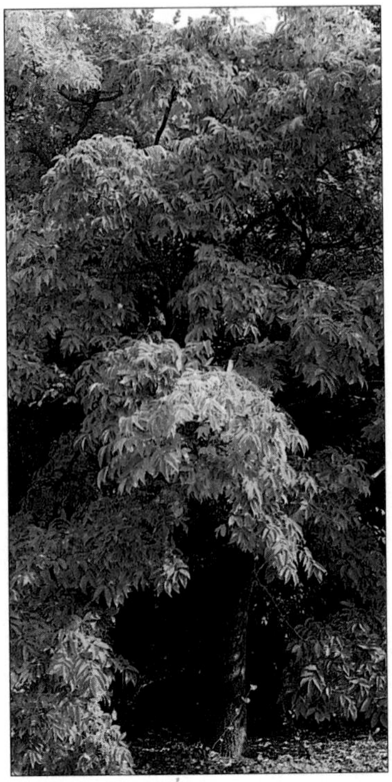

Phellodendron chinense

PHILADELPHUS

Mock orange

HYDRANGEACEAE/PHILADELPHACEAE

Genus of about 40 species of mainly deciduous shrubs found in scrub and on rocky hillsides from E. Europe to the Himalayas, E. Asia, and North and Central America. They are cultivated for their usually fragrant, 4-petalled, cup- or bowl-shaped, sometimes cross-shaped, single, semi-double, or double flowers, produced singly or in racemes, panicles, or cymes. The leaves are simple, mostly ovate, and usually mid-green, arranged in opposite pairs. Grow in a shrub border, or as specimen plants in a woodland garden; larger species and cultivars may be used for screening. Grow *P. mexicanus* against a wall; in frost-prone climates, grow in a cool greenhouse.
• **HARDINESS** Fully hardy to half hardy.
• **CULTIVATION** Grow in any moderately fertile, well-drained soil in full sun or partial shade. *P. microphyllus* needs full sun. Under glass, grow in loam-based potting compost (JI No.3) in full light or bright filtered light. During the growing season, water freely and apply a balanced liquid fertilizer monthly. Keep just moist in winter. Pruning group 2.
• **PROPAGATION** Take softwood cuttings in summer, or hardwood cuttings in autumn or winter.
• **PESTS AND DISEASES** Powdery mildew and aphids may be a problem.

***P.* 'Avalanche'.** Upright, spreading, deciduous shrub with arching branches and elliptic, entire leaves, to 2.5cm (1in) long. Racemes of up to 7 single, cup-shaped, fragrant white flowers, 2.5cm (1in) across, are borne profusely in mid- and late summer. ↕ to 1.5m (5ft), ↔ 3m (10ft). ❄❄❄
***P.* 'Beauclerk'** ▣ 🏆 Slightly arching, deciduous shrub with broadly ovate, toothed leaves, to 6cm (2½in) long. Large, single, cup-shaped white flowers, 5cm (2in) across, with slightly pink-flushed centres, are borne singly or in racemes of 3–5, in early and mid-summer. ↕↔ 2.5m (8ft). ❄❄❄
***P.* 'Belle Etoile'** 🏆 Arching, deciduous shrub with narrowly ovate, tapered, entire leaves, to 9cm (3½in) long. Single, cup-shaped, very fragrant white flowers, 5cm (2in) across, marked pale purple in the centres, are freely borne singly or in 3- to 5-flowered racemes,

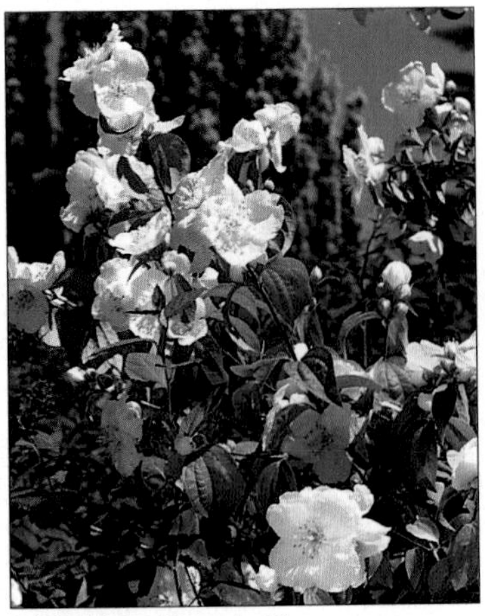

Philadelphus 'Beauclerk'

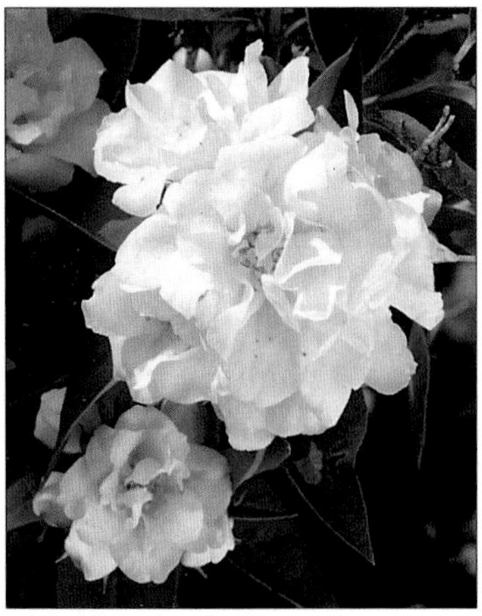

Philadelphus 'Boule d'Argent'

in late spring and early summer. ↕ 1.2m (4ft), ↔ 2.5m (8ft). ❄❄❄

***P.* 'Boule d'Argent'** ■ Arching, compact, bushy, deciduous shrub with broadly ovate, entire, dark green leaves, to 6cm (2½in) long. In early and mid-summer, slightly fragrant, semi-double to double, milk-white flowers, 4.5cm (1¾in) across, are profusely borne in racemes of 5–7. ↕↔ 1.5m (5ft). ❄❄❄

***P.* 'Bouquet Blanc'.** Upright, deciduous shrub with ovate, nearly entire leaves, to 5cm (2in) long. Double to semi-double, fragrant white flowers, 2.5cm (1in) across, are borne singly, in pairs, or in racemes of 3–5, in early or midsummer. ↕ 2m (6ft), ↔ 1.5m (5ft). ❄❄❄

***P.* 'Buckley's Quill'** ■ Upright, deciduous shrub with ovate, entire, dark green leaves, to 8cm (3in) long. Double, fragrant white flowers, 2.5cm (1in) across, each with about 30 quill-like petals, are produced singly or in racemes of 3–5, in early or midsummer. ↕ 2m (6ft), ↔ 1.2m (4ft). ❄❄❄

***P.* 'Burfordensis'** ■ Vigorous, upright, deciduous shrub with ovate, toothed, dark green leaves, to 11cm (4½in) long. Large, single, cup-shaped, slightly fragrant white flowers, to 7cm (3in)

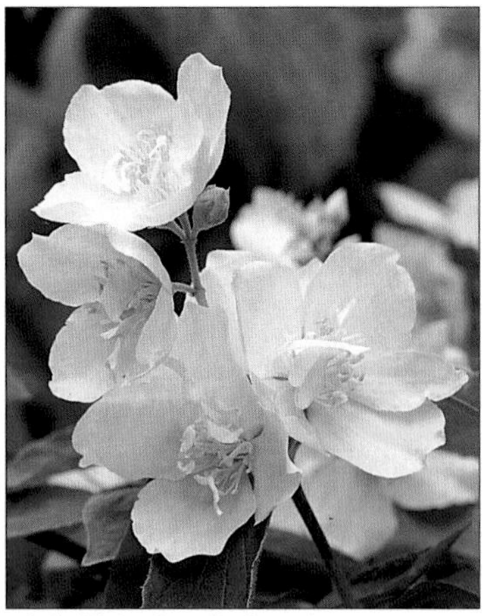

Philadelphus 'Burfordensis'

across, are profusely borne in racemes of 5–9, in early and midsummer. ↕ 3m (10ft), ↔ 2m (6ft). ❄❄❄

P. coronarius (Mock orange). Broadly upright, deciduous shrub with ovate, shallowly toothed leaves, to 10cm (4in) long. Short, terminal racemes of 5–9 cup-shaped, single, very fragrant, creamy white flowers, 2.5cm (1in) across, are produced in early summer. ↕ 3m (10ft), ↔ 2.5m (8ft). S. Europe, Caucasus. ❄❄❄. **'Aureus'** ♀ has golden yellow leaves, turning yellow-green in summer; foliage of flowering shoots may burn in full sun; ↕ 2.5m (8ft), ↔ 1.5m (5ft). **'Variegatus'** ■♀ has leaves with broad white margins, and white flowers; ↕ 2.5m (8ft), ↔ 2m (6ft)

***P.* 'Dame Blanche'** ■ Compact, arching, bushy, deciduous shrub with peeling, dark blackish brown bark and ovate, entire, dark green leaves, to 2cm (¾in) long. Semi-double to nearly double, fragrant, pure white flowers, to 2cm (¾in) across, are freely borne, usually in pairs or in 3- to 5-flowered racemes, in early or midsummer. ↕↔ 2m (6ft). ❄❄❄

P. delavayi. Upright, deciduous shrub with arching branches and ovate,

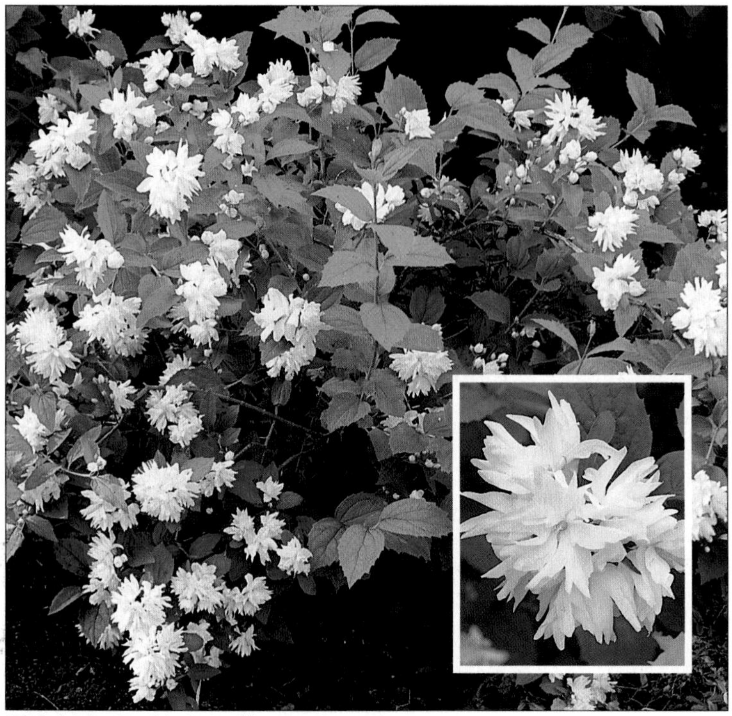

Philadelphus 'Buckley's Quill' (inset: flower detail)

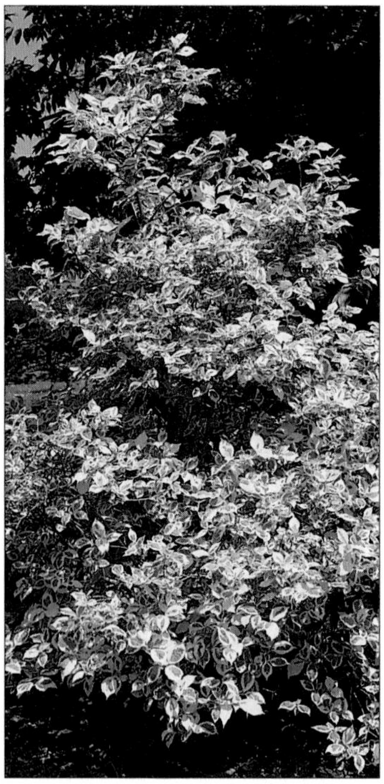

Philadelphus coronarius 'Variegatus'

tapered, sometimes toothed, dark green leaves, to 10cm (4in) or more long. In early or midsummer, bears racemes of 5–9 single, cup-shaped, very fragrant, pure white flowers, 4cm (1½in) across, often purple-flushed on the backs of the sepals. ↕ 3m (10ft), ↔ 2.5m (8ft). W. China, S.E. Tibet, N. Burma. ❄❄. **f. *melanocalyx*** ■ syn. *P. purpurascens*, has white flowers with dark purple sepals.

***P.* 'Girandole'.** Upright, deciduous shrub with ovate leaves, to 5cm (2in) long, nearly entire or each with 1–6 teeth on both margins. Dense, double, fragrant, creamy white flowers, to 4cm (1½in) across, are borne in racemes of up to 7, in early and midsummer. ↕↔ 1.5m (5ft). ❄❄❄

***P.* 'Glacier'.** Upright, deciduous shrub with small, ovate, toothed leaves, to 4cm (1½in) long. Dense racemes of up to 9 double, fragrant white flowers, 2.5cm (1in) across, are borne in midsummer. ↕↔ 1.5m (5ft). ❄❄❄

***P.* 'Innocence'.** Upright, deciduous shrub with arching branches and ovate, entire leaves, to 5cm (2in) long, strongly mottled yellow. Single, or sometimes semi-double, cup-shaped, very fragrant white flowers, 3–3.5cm (1¼–1½in)

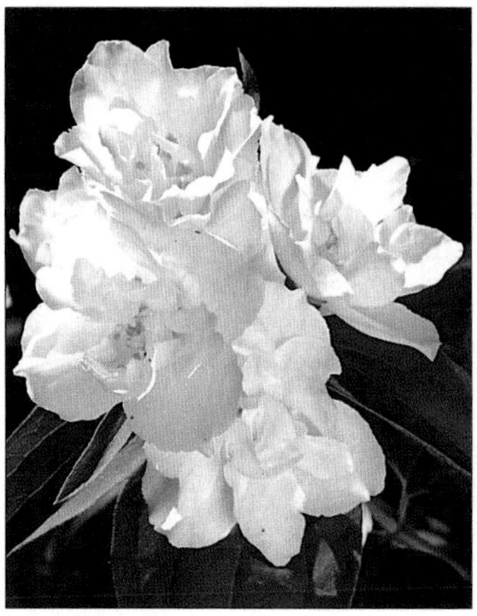

Philadelphus 'Dame Blanche'

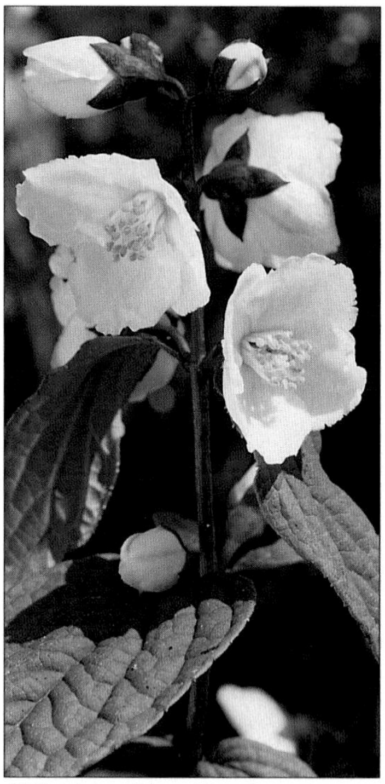

Philadelphus delavayi f. *melanocalyx*

across, usually in 3-flowered racemes, are produced in early or midsummer. ↕ 3m (10ft), ↔ 2m (6ft). ❄❄❄

***P.* 'Lemoinei'** ■ Upright, deciduous shrub with arching branches and ovate, tapered leaves, to 5cm (2in) long, each with 2 or 3 teeth on both margins. Small, single, cup-shaped, extremely fragrant, pure white flowers, 2.5cm (1in) across, are profusely borne in racemes of 3–5, in early or midsummer. ↕↔ 1.5m (5ft). ❄❄❄

P. lewisii. Spreading, deciduous shrub with arching branches and ovate, sometimes finely toothed, bright green leaves, to 10cm (4in) long. Racemes of 5–11 unscented or slightly fragrant, single, cup-shaped, pure white flowers, 4cm (1½in) across, are profusely borne in early or midsummer. ↕↔ 3m (10ft). W. North America (British Columbia to California). ❄❄❄

P. magdalenae. Spreading, bushy, deciduous shrub with ovate, short-pointed, entire leaves, to 6cm (2½in) long. Single, cup-shaped, slightly fragrant, pure white flowers, 2.5cm (1in) across, are borne in racemes of up to 11, in late spring and early summer. ↕↔ 4m (12ft). W. China. ❄❄❄

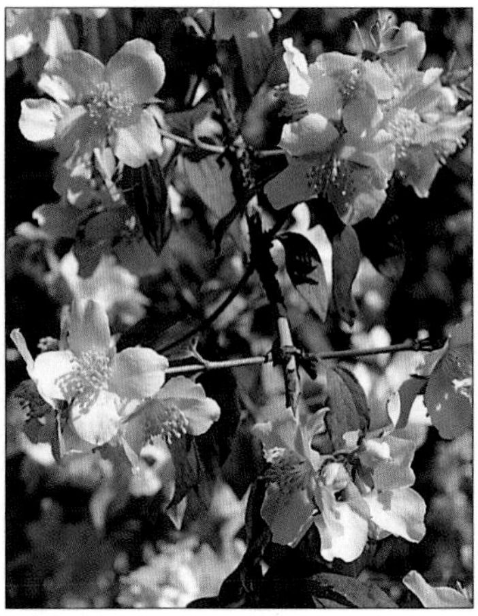

Philadelphus 'Lemoinei'

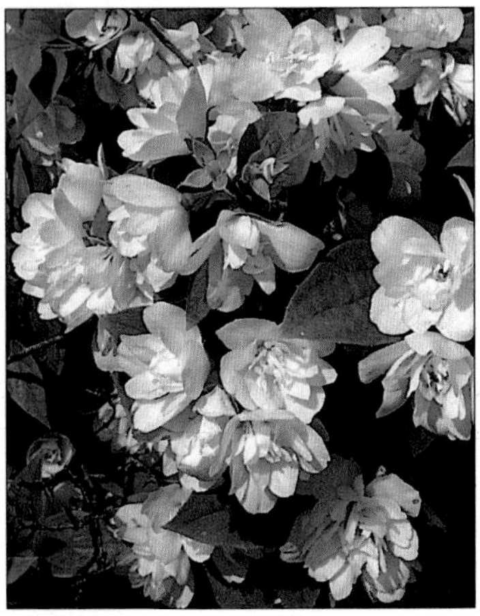

Philadelphus 'Manteau d'Hermine'

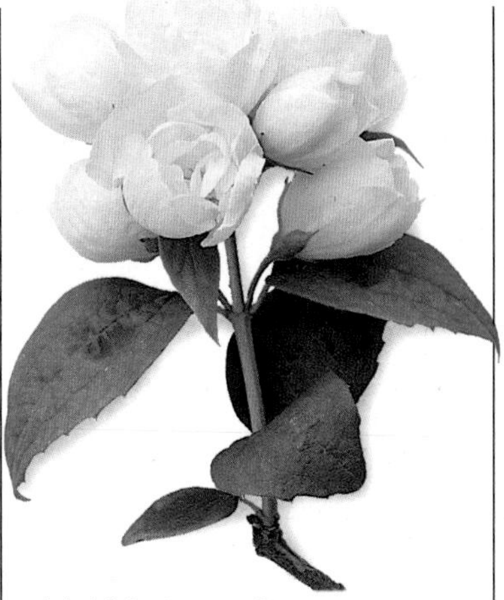

Philadelphus 'Virginal'

P. 'Manteau d'Hermine' ■ 🏆 Bushy, compact, deciduous shrub with arching shoots and elliptic, pointed, entire, pale to mid-green leaves, to 2.5cm (1in) long. Produces double, very fragrant, creamy white flowers, 4cm (1½in) across, usually in racemes of 3, in early and midsummer. ↕75cm (30in), ↔ 1.5m (5ft). ❄❄❄

P. mexicanus. Spreading, evergreen shrub with pendent, bristly shoots and ovate, sometimes sparsely toothed leaves, to 11cm (4½in) long. Single, cup-shaped, strongly rose-scented, creamy white flowers, to 4cm (1½in) across, are borne singly or in racemes of 3, in summer. ↕↔ 2m (6ft) or more. Mexico, Guatemala. ❄. **'Rose Syringa'** has flowers with conspicuous purple-pink markings in the centres.

P. microphyllus ■ Compact, upright, deciduous shrub with peeling, dark chestnut-brown bark and small, elliptic, entire, glossy, mid-green leaves, to 2cm (¾in) long. Solitary or paired, single, cross-shaped, very fragrant, pure white flowers, 2.5cm (1in) across, are borne in early and midsummer. ↕↔ 1m (3ft). S.W. USA. ❄❄❄

P. 'Mont Blanc'. Upright, deciduous shrub with ovate, sparsely toothed leaves, to 3cm (1¼in) long. Single, cross-shaped, fragrant, pure white flowers, to 2.5cm (1in) across, are profusely borne singly or in racemes of up to 5, in early summer. ↕↔ 1m (3ft). ❄❄❄

P. purpurascens see *P. delavayi* f. *melanocalyx.*

P. 'Silberregen', syn. *P.* 'Silver Showers'. Rounded, deciduous shrub with upright, arching shoots and ovate, entire leaves, to 4cm (1½in) long. Solitary, single, cup-shaped, strawberry-scented, pure white flowers, 4cm (1½in) across, are profusely borne in early summer. ↕ 1.2m (4ft), ↔ 1.5m (5ft). ❄❄❄

P. 'Silver Showers' see *P.* 'Silberregen'.

P. subcanus. Erect, deciduous shrub with smooth, grey-brown bark, later peeling, and ovate or ovate-lance-shaped, finely toothed leaves, 4–14cm (1½–5½in) long. In early summer, bears racemes of 5–20 or more shallowly cup-shaped, slightly fragrant white flowers, 2.5–3cm (1–1¼in) across. ↕ 6m (20ft), ↔ 2–3m (6–10ft). S.W. China. ❄

P. 'Sybille' 🏆 Arching, deciduous shrub with broadly ovate, entire leaves, to 5cm (2in) long. In early or midsummer, single, cup-shaped, very fragrant white flowers, to 5cm (2in) across, with conspicuous purple marks in the centres, are profusely borne singly or in racemes of 3–5. ↕ 1.2m (4ft), ↔ 2m (6ft). ❄❄❄

P. 'Virginal' ■ 🏆 Vigorous, upright, deciduous shrub with ovate, entire, dark green leaves, to 8cm (3in) or more long. Double, very fragrant, pure white flowers, 5cm (2in) across, are produced in loose racemes of 5–9, in early or midsummer. ↕ 3m (10ft) or more, ↔ 2.5m (8ft). ❄❄❄

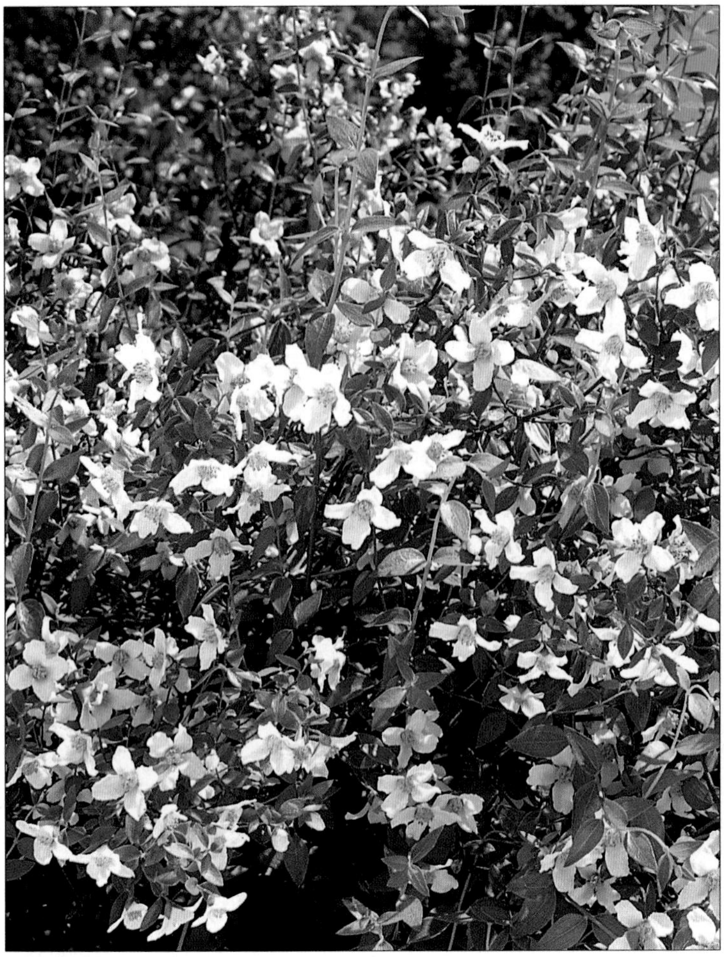

Philadelphus microphyllus

x PHILAGERIA

LILIACEAE/PHILESIACEAE

Hybrid genus of one evergreen shrub, derived from crosses between *Philesia* and *Lapageria.* It is cultivated for its pendent, tubular flowers, produced in summer, and has entire, leathery leaves, arranged alternately. In frost-prone climates, grow in a cool greenhouse. In warmer areas, grow on a moist, shady bank or against a shaded wall.

- **HARDINESS** Frost tender.
- **CULTIVATION** Under glass, grow in lime-free (ericaceous) compost with added sharp sand, in bright indirect light. When in growth, water freely and apply a balanced liquid fertilizer every month. Water sparingly in winter. Outdoors, grow in moderately fertile, humus-rich, reliably moist, acid soil in partial shade. Support climbing stems. Pruning group 12, in spring.
- **PROPAGATION** Layer in autumn.
- **PESTS AND DISEASES** Trouble free.

x P. veitchii (*Lapageria rosea* x *Philesia magellanica*). Twining or scrambling, evergreen shrub producing oblong, 3-veined, glossy, dark green leaves, to 4cm (1½in) long. Pendent, tubular, bright rose-pink flowers, 5cm (2in) long, are borne singly from the leaf axils in summer. ↕ 3–4m (10–12ft). ❀ (min. 2°C/36°F).

PHILESIA

PHILESIACEAE

Genus of one species of evergreen shrub occurring in moist forest in Chile. The alternate leaves are leathery and scale-like. Grown for its showy, trumpet-shaped flowers, produced from the leaf axils in summer and autumn, it is suitable for a moist, shady position.

- **HARDINESS** Frost hardy.
- **CULTIVATION** Grow in moderately fertile, humus-rich, moist but well-drained, acid soil in partial shade. Does not tolerate hot, dry conditions. Pruning group 9.
- **PROPAGATION** Take semi-ripe cuttings in summer, or remove suckers in spring.
- **PESTS AND DISEASES** Trouble free.

P. magellanica. Erect, suckering shrub or, in mild, moist areas, root climber, with oblong, rigid, dark green leaves, to 4cm (1½in) long, blue-white beneath. Trumpet-shaped, waxy, crimson-pink flowers, to 6cm (2½in) long, are borne singly in the leaf axils from midsummer to autumn. ↕ 1m (3ft), ↔ 2m (6ft). Chile. ❄❄

PHILLYREA

OLEACEAE

Genus of 4 species of evergreen shrubs and trees occurring in woodland and rocky places from the Mediterranean to S.W. Asia. Grown for their habit and foliage, they have opposite, linear to ovate-elliptic, yellow-green to dark green leaves. The 4-lobed, salverform white flowers are borne in axillary cymes, followed by spherical or ovoid, blue-black fruits. Grow in a shrub border or woodland garden, or as specimen plants. In frost-prone areas, grow against a sheltered wall.

- **HARDINESS** Fully hardy to frost hardy.
- **CULTIVATION** Grow in fertile, well-drained soil, ideally in full sun, with shelter from cold, dry winds. Tolerates partial shade. Pruning group 1 or 8.
- **PROPAGATION** Root semi-ripe cuttings with bottom heat in summer.
- **PESTS AND DISEASES** Whiteflies may be troublesome.

P. angustifolia. Dense, bushy shrub with narrowly linear, dark green leaves, to 6cm (2½in) long. Inconspicuous, fragrant, greenish white flowers are produced in cymes, 1cm (½in) across, in late spring and early summer, followed by spherical, blue-black fruit, 5mm (¼in) across. ↕↔ 3m (10ft). Mediterranean. ❄❄❄

P. decora see *Osmanthus decorus.*

P. latifolia ■ ◌ Dense, rounded shrub or small tree with oval, glossy, dark green leaves, to 6cm (2½in) long. Inconspicuous, fragrant, greenish white flowers are borne in cymes, 1cm (½in) across, in late spring and early summer, followed by spherical, blue-black fruit, 5mm (¼in) across. ↕↔ to 9m (28ft). Mediterranean, S.W. Asia. ❄❄❄

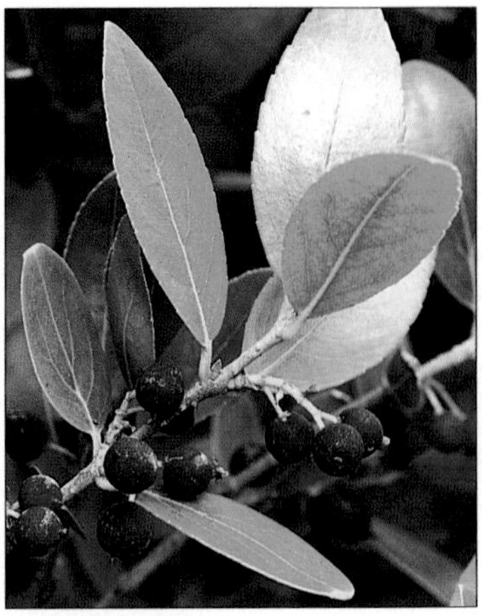

Phillyrea latifolia

PHILODENDRON

ARACEAE

Genus of up to 500 species of often epiphytic, evergreen shrubs, root climbers, or small trees from variable habitats, usually rainforest, in the USA (Florida), Mexico, the West Indies, and Central and tropical South America. They are grown for their leathery, glossy leaves, which may be simple, pinnatifid, or pinnatisect, ovate to oblong, heart-, arrow-, or broadly spear-shaped, and toothed or entire; they are borne alternately, or in tufts or rosettes. Seed-raised species often have a distinct juvenile stage, with leaves quite unlike those of mature plants. Inflorescences, comprising tiny, petalless flowers borne on spadices and enclosed by spathes, are produced intermittently. Where temperatures fall below 15°C (59°F), grow in a warm greenhouse or as houseplants. In warmer areas, train climbing species through a palm tree or against a wall, and grow large shrubs as specimen plants. Small epiphytes are suitable for a large hanging basket. All parts may cause severe discomfort if ingested; contact with sap may irritate skin.

- **HARDINESS** Frost tender.
- **CULTIVATION** Under glass, grow in loamless potting compost in bright filtered or indirect light. During the growing season, water freely and apply a balanced liquid fertilizer every month. In summer, mist twice daily. Water sparingly in winter. Support climbing stems with a moss pole. Outdoors, grow in fertile, humus-rich, moist but well-drained soil in dappled or partial shade. Pruning group 1 for shrubs; group 11 for climbers, in spring; plants under glass may need restrictive pruning.
- **PROPAGATION** Surface-sow seed at 19–24°C (66–75°F) in spring. Take stem-tip or leaf bud cuttings in summer. Layer or air layer in spring.
- **PESTS AND DISEASES** Prone to scale insects and red spider mites under glass.

P. andreanum see *P. melanochrysum.*
P. angustisectum ♀ syn. *P. elegans.* Sparsely branched climber with ovate, pinnatisect, reflexed leaves, 30–60cm (12–24in) long, each with 16–32 slender, finger-like lobes, glossy, deep green above, paler beneath. Green spathes, 15cm (6in) long, are yellow inside, with pink-flushed margins. ↕ 5m (15ft). Colombia. ❄ (min.15°C/59°F)

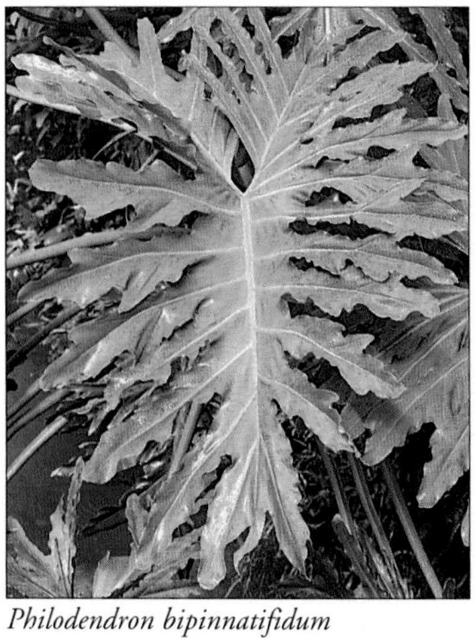
Philodendron bipinnatifidum

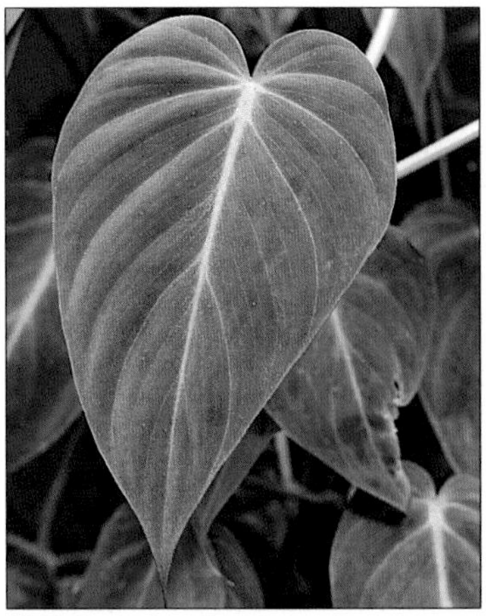
Philodendron melanochrysum

***P. auritum* of gardens** see *Syngonium auritum.*
P. bipennifolium, syn. *P. panduriforme* (Fiddleleaf, Panda plant). Sparsely branched climber with ovate to arrow-shaped, reflexed, lustrous, deep green leaves, 30–45cm (12–18in) long, each with 5 broad lobes, the terminal one longest. Bears greenish cream spathes, to 11cm (4½in) long. ↕ to 5m (15ft) or more. S.E. Brazil. ❄ (min. 15°C/59°F)
P. bipinnatifidum ■ ♀ syn. *P. selloum* (Tree philodendron). Tree-like shrub, usually with a single, robust, erect stem, reclining with age. Very long-stalked, reflexed leaves, to 1m (3ft) long, are broadly ovate, heart-shaped at the bases, and deeply pinnatisect, with many narrow, wavy-margined, semi-glossy, rich green lobes. Green to red-purple spathes, 30cm (12in) long, are cream with red margins inside. ↕↔ to 5m (15ft). S.E. Brazil. ❄ (min. 15°C/59°F). **'German Selloum'** has narrower leaf lobes. **'Variegatum'** has leaves splashed yellow to light green.
P. cordatum (Heart leaf). Fast-growing, moderately to sparsely branched, slender-stemmed climber with glossy, deep green leaves, 30–45cm (12–18in)

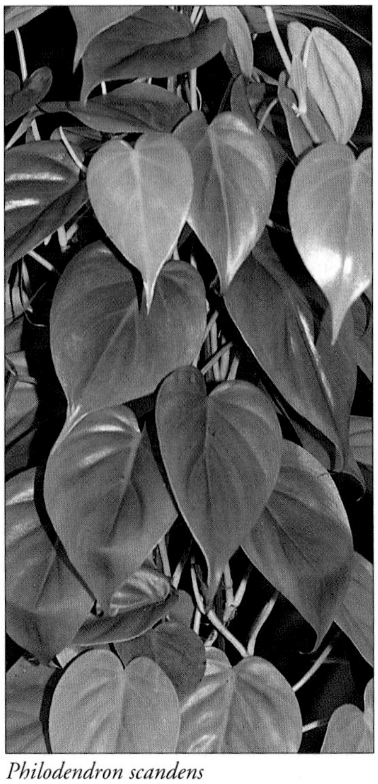
Philodendron scandens

long, ovate-triangular, reflexed, and heart-shaped at the bases, the lower lobes touching or overlapping. Produces green spathes, 10–15cm (4–6in) long. ↕ 3–6m (10–20ft). S.E. Brazil. ❄ (min. 15°C/59°F)
P. domesticum, syn. *P. hastatum* of gardens (Elephant's ear). Usually sparsely branched climber with narrowly triangular to arrow-shaped, reflexed, bright green leaves, 45–60cm (18–24in) long, with wavy margins. Spathes are 12–18cm (5–7in) long, green on the outside, cherry-red inside. ↕ 3–6m (10–20ft). Origin unknown. ❄ (min. 15°C/59°F)
P. elegans see *P. angustisectum.*
P. erubescens ♀ (Blushing philodendron, Red-leaf philodendron). Sturdy-stemmed climber with red-purple stems when young. Ovate-triangular, glossy, dark green leaves, 25–40cm (10–16in) long, heart-shaped at the bases, are coppery red-purple beneath, with purple-tinged stalks. Bears red-purple spathes, 15cm (6in) long, crimson inside, with an unusual aroma. ↕ 3–6m (10–20ft). Colombia. ❄ (min. 15°C/59°F). **'Burgundy'** ♀ is slower-growing, with smaller, red-flushed leaves, to 30cm (12in) long.
***P. hastatum* of gardens** see *P. domesticum.*
P. imbe, syn. *P. sellowianum.* Robust climber with long aerial roots and red-purple stems bearing ovate-oblong to arrow-shaped, reflexed leaves, to 35cm (14in) long; they have a parchment-like texture and are glossy, mid- to dark green above, often flushed or tinted red beneath. Spathes, 15cm (6in) long, are cream and green. ↕ 3–5m (10–15ft). S.E. Brazil. ❄ (min. 15°C/59°F)
P. laciniatum see *P. pedatum.*
P. melanochrysum ■ syn. *P. andreanum* (Black gold philodendron, Velour philodendron). Sparsely branched climber. Bears narrowly ovate to oblong-lance-shaped, reflexed to pendent, velvety blackish green leaves, to 1m (3ft) long, with pale green veins; they have short, slender points and heart-shaped bases (the lobes touch or just overlap). Juvenile plants have much smaller, broader, coppery red leaves. Produces green and white spathes, to 20cm (8in) long. ↕ 3–6m (10–20ft). Colombia. ❄ (min. 15°C/59°F)
P. micans see *P. scandens* f. *micans.*
P. oxycardium see *P. scandens* subsp. *oxycardium.*
P. panduriforme see *P. bipennifolium.*
P. pedatum, syn. *P. laciniatum.* Robust, moderately branching climber. Reflexed, pinnatifid, glossy, deep green leaves, to 45cm (18in) long, are ovate to arrow-shaped, with 5–7 narrowly triangular lobes, the 2 basal lobes sometimes lobed and pointing backwards. Bears green and white spathes, red-flushed at the bases and cream inside, 10–13cm (4–5in) long. ↕ 3–5m (10–15ft). Venezuela to Brazil. ❄ (min. 15°C/59°F)
P. scandens ■ ♀ (Heart leaf, Sweetheart plant). Fast-growing climber producing sparsely to moderately branching, slender stems. Glossy, deep green leaves, sometimes red-purple beneath, are up to 30cm (12in) long on mature plants, 10–15cm (4–6in) long on juveniles; they are rounded, heart-shaped at the bases, and reflexed, with abruptly tapered, slender-pointed tips. Bears green spathes, 15–20cm (6–8in) long, white inside, sometimes red-tinted at the bases. Good as a houseplant. ↕ 3–6m (10–20ft). Mexico, West Indies, S.E. Brazil. ❄ (min. 15°C/ 59°F). **f. *micans***, syn. *P. micans*, has bronze leaves, red-tinted beneath, with larger, overlapping basal leaf lobes. **subsp. *oxycardium***, syn. *P. oxycardium*, has young leaves flushed bronze-brown; E. Mexico.
P. selloum see *P. bipinnatifidum.*
P. sellowianum see *P. imbe.*
P. trifoliatum see *Syngonium auritum.*

▷ **Philodendron,**
Black gold see *Philodendron melanochrysum*
Blushing see *Philodendron erubescens*
False see *Peperomia scandens*
Red-leaf see *Philodendron erubescens*
Tree see *Philodendron bipinnatifidum*
Velour see *Philodendron melanochrysum*

PHLEBODIUM

POLYPODIACEAE

Genus of 10 species of semi-evergreen ferns occurring on trees and rocks in the USA (Florida), Mexico, West Indies, and Central and tropical South America. They have thick, creeping rhizomes, densely covered with golden brown scales, and large, pinnate or pinnatifid, sometimes glaucous fronds. Spores are formed in groups, in one or more rows parallel to the midribs. In frost-prone climates, grow in a warm greenhouse or as houseplants; they are very effective in hanging baskets. In warmer regions, grow in a warm, sheltered border.

- **HARDINESS** Frost tender.
- **CULTIVATION** Under glass, grow in 1 part each loam, medium-grade bark, and charcoal, 2 parts sharp sand, and 3 parts coarse leaf mould. Provide full light or bright filtered light. During growth, water moderately and apply a balanced liquid fertilizer every month. Water sparingly in winter. Outdoors, grow in fertile, well-drained soil in full sun or light dappled shade.
- **PROPAGATION** Sow spores at 19–24°C (66–75°F) as soon as ripe. Divide rhizomes in spring. See also p.51.
- **PESTS AND DISEASES** Scale insects may be a problem.

P. aureum ■ ♀ syn. *Polypodium aureum* (Golden polypody, Hare's foot fern, Rabbit's foot fern). Large, creeping

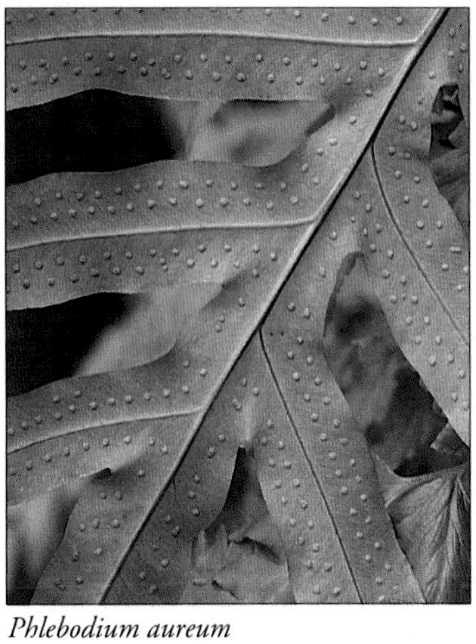
Phlebodium aureum

P

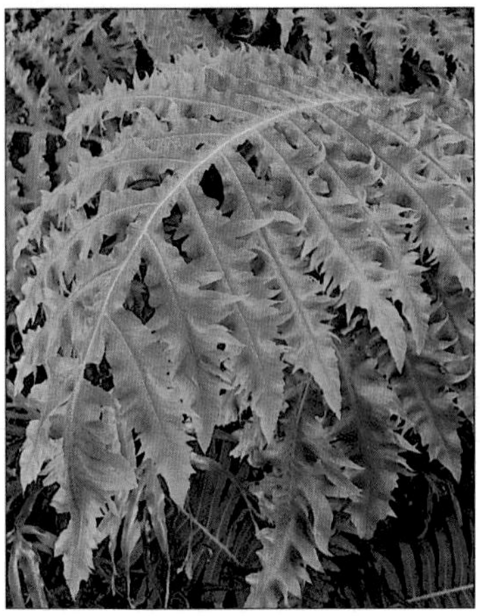

Phlebodium aureum 'Mandaianum'

fern with arching, ovate to oblong or triangular, deeply pinnatifid, glaucous, grey-green fronds, to 1.5m (5ft) long, each with up to 35 narrowly linear to lance-shaped, oblong, or strap-shaped, wavy-margined segments. ↕75cm (30in), ↔ to 1.5m (5ft). USA (Florida), Mexico, West Indies, Central and tropical South America. ❁ (min. 10°C/50°F). **var. *areolatum***, syn. 'Glaucum', has leathery fronds, 60cm (24in) long, with a more pronounced glaucous bloom. **'Glaucum'** see var. *areolatum*. **'Mandaianum'** ■ (Blue fern) has slightly lobed fronds with wavy margins.

PHLOMIS

LABIATAE/LAMIACEAE

Genus of about 100 species of sage-like herbaceous perennials and evergreen shrubs or subshrubs found in rocky sites in Europe, North Africa, and Asia. Leaves are opposite, lance-shaped to ovate, light to grey-green, often with star-shaped hairs. They are grown for their foliage and showy, tubular, dead nettle-like, often hooded, white, yellow, or lilac flowers, borne in dense, axillary whorls on tall, erect stems; they are effective massed in a border. In frost-prone areas, grow against a wall. *P. lanata* is suitable for a rock garden. In winter, seed heads of herbaceous species may be left for their ornamental effect.

- **HARDINESS** Fully hardy to frost hardy.
- **CULTIVATION** Grow in any fertile, well-drained soil in full sun; *P. russeliana* and *P. samia* tolerate some shade. Pruning group 8 or 9.
- **PROPAGATION** Sow seed at 13–18°C (55–64°F) in spring. Divide perennials in spring (preferably) or in autumn. Take softwood cuttings of shrubs in summer.
- **PESTS AND DISEASES** Leafhoppers may be troublesome.

P. bovei* subsp. *maroccana, syn. *P. samia* subsp. *maroccana*. Erect, sticky-hairy perennial with elliptic to oblong, scalloped, grey-green basal leaves, 6–8cm (2½–3in) long, heart-shaped at the bases, and smaller stem leaves. Purple-pink flowers, 4–4.5cm (1½–1¾in) long, with purple spots inside, white-woolly outside, are borne in summer. Similar to *P. samia* but more robust. ↕ to 1.5m (5ft), ↔ 1m (3ft). Mountains in Morocco. ❄❄

P. cashmeriana ■ Erect, densely woolly perennial with ovate to lance-shaped basal leaves, 10–25cm (4–10in) long, yellow-grey above, paler beneath, and smaller stem leaves. In midsummer, hooded, lilac-purple flowers, 2.5cm (1in) long, are borne from the upper leaf axils. ↕ to 90cm (36in), ↔ 60cm (24in). India (Kashmir), W. Himalayas. ❄❄❄

P. chrysophylla 🏆 Rounded, evergreen shrub with stout, spreading branches and elliptic to broadly ovate, grey-green leaves, to 6cm (2½in) long, turning golden green in late summer. Golden yellow flowers, 3cm (1¼in) long, are produced in early summer. ↕ 1m (3ft), ↔ 1.2m (4ft). S.W. Asia. ❄❄

***P.* 'Edward Bowles'.** Upright, evergreen subshrub with large, heart-shaped, wrinkled, grey-green leaves, 15cm (6in) long, woolly beneath. Bears sulphur-yellow flowers, 3cm (1¼in) long, paler on the hoods, in early and midsummer. ↕ 1m (3ft), ↔ 1.5m (5ft). ❄❄

P. fruticosa ■🏆 (Jerusalem sage). Mound-forming, evergreen shrub with upright shoots and sage-like, ovate-lance-shaped, wrinkled, grey-green leaves, to 10cm (4in) long, woolly beneath. In early and midsummer, bears dark golden yellow flowers, 3cm (1¼in) long. ↕ 1m (3ft), ↔ 1.5m (5ft). E. Mediterranean. ❄❄❄ (borderline)

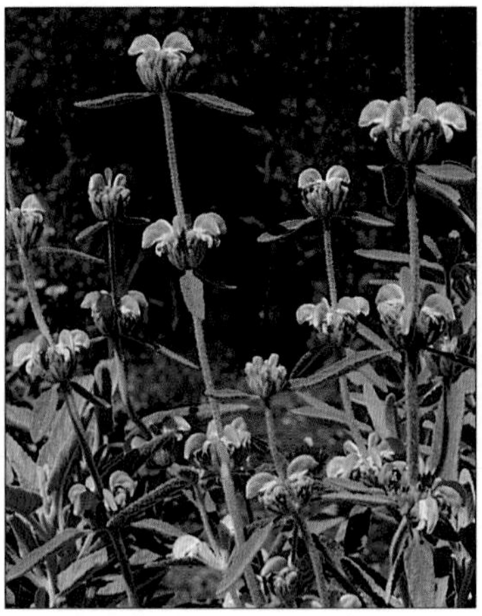

Phlomis italica

P. italica ■ Upright, evergreen shrub bearing oblong-lance-shaped, grey-woolly leaves, to 5cm (2in) long. Lilac-pink flowers, 2cm (¾in) long, are borne in midsummer. ↕ 30cm (12in), ↔ 60cm (24in). Balearic Islands. ❄❄

***P. lanata*.** Compact, mound-forming, evergreen shrub bearing oblong to rounded, deeply veined, scaly, sage-green leaves, to 2.5cm (1in) long. Golden yellow flowers, 2cm (¾in) long, covered with brown hairs, are produced in summer. ↕ 50cm (20in), ↔ 75cm (30in). Greece (Crete). ❄❄

P. longifolia*.** Spreading, evergreen shrub with white-woolly young shoots and lance-shaped, deeply veined, bright green leaves, to 7cm (3in) long, grey-woolly beneath. Dark yellow flowers, to 4cm (1½in) long, with calyx teeth to 3mm (⅛in) long, are produced in summer. ↕ 1.2m (4ft), ↔ 2m (6ft). S.W. Asia. ❄❄. **var. *bailanica has ovate leaves, and flowers with longer calyx teeth, 3–6mm (⅛–¼in) long.

P. purpurea ■ Upright, evergreen shrub with woolly shoots and lance-shaped, leathery, grey-green leaves, to 10cm (4in) long, with star-shaped hairs above, woolly beneath. Purple to pink, occasionally white flowers, 2.5cm (1in) long, are produced in summer. ↕↔ to 60cm (24in). Spain, Portugal. ❄❄

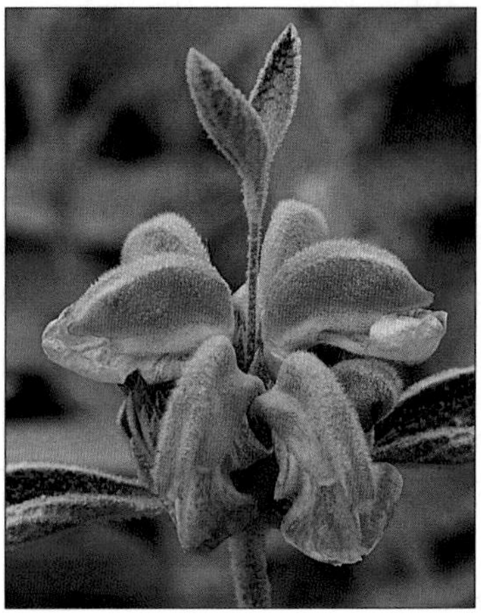

Phlomis purpurea

P. russeliana ■🏆 syn. *P. samia* of gardens, *P. viscosa* of gardens. Erect, hairy perennial, less woolly than *P. cashmeriana* (so appears greener), with mid-green leaves: basal leaves are ovate, 6–20cm (2½–8in) long, heart-shaped at the bases; stem leaves are smaller and scalloped. Hooded, pale yellow flowers, 2.5–3.5cm (1–1½in) long, are borne from late spring to early autumn, mainly in early summer. Often confused with *P. samia*. ↕ to 90cm (36in), ↔ 75cm (30in). Turkey, Syria. ❄❄❄

P. samia*.** Erect perennial producing ovate, scalloped, woolly basal leaves, 10–20cm (4–8in) long, heart-shaped at the bases, and mid-green above, grey beneath, and with smaller stem leaves. Hooded lilac flowers, 3–3.5cm (1¼–1½in) long, tinged rose-pink, especially on the lips, are borne from early to late summer. ↕ to 1m (3ft), ↔ 80cm (32in). S.E. Europe, Turkey. ❄❄❄. **subsp. *maroccana see *P. bovei* subsp. *maroccana*.

***P. samia* of gardens** see *P. russeliana*.

***P. viscosa* of gardens** see *P. russeliana*.

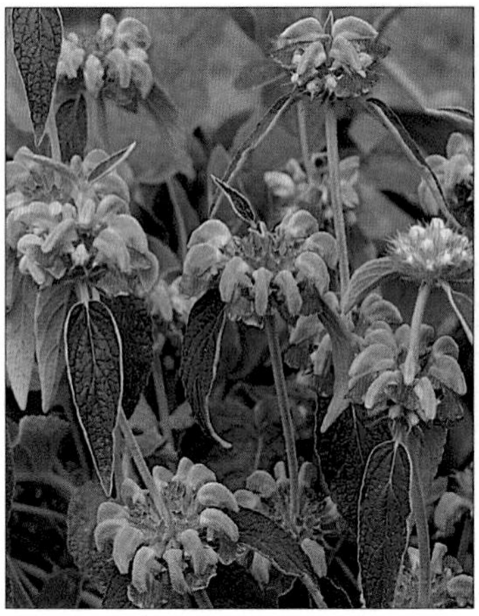

Phlomis cashmeriana

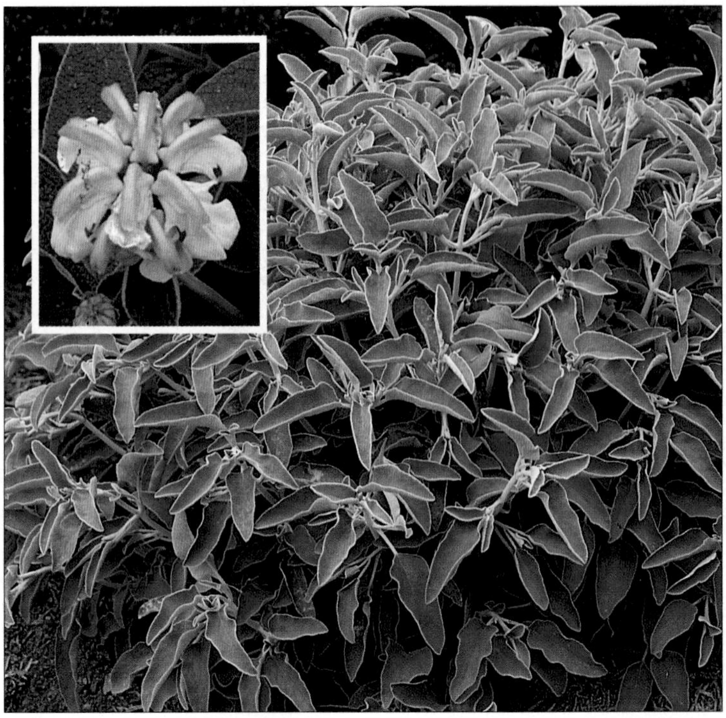

Phlomis fruticosa (inset: flower detail)

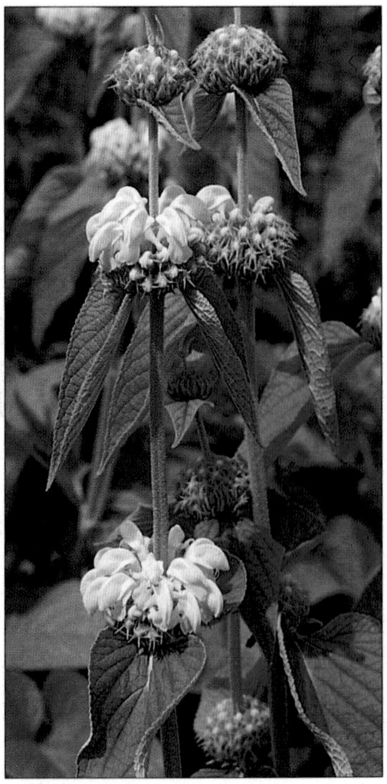

Phlomis russeliana

P

PHLOX

POLEMONIACEAE

Genus of 67 species of evergreen or herbaceous, low-growing or cushion-forming to erect perennials, as well as a few annuals and shrubs, found mostly in North America (one from Siberia, Russia). They are grown for their showy flowers, borne mainly in terminal corymbs or panicle-like cymes, sometimes singly. The flowers are salverform, occasionally funnel-shaped, each with a narrow, tubular base opening to 5 flat, ovate petal lobes, sometimes in a star-shaped arrangement. Leaves are simple, entire, linear to ovate, light to dark green, and often in opposite pairs, the upper leaves sometimes alternate. Mat- and cushion-forming species, from dry, rocky habitats, flower in spring or early summer; grow in a rock garden or alpine house, in a dry wall, or as edging. Woodland species are mainly trailing, and usually flower in early summer; grow in shady sites. The taller "border" phlox are mostly from moist riverside habitats, and produce large corymbs of flowers, usually in midsummer, which are good for cutting. Annuals, from dry rocky slopes and coastal sands, flower from late spring to autumn, and are useful for bedding.

• **HARDINESS** Fully hardy to half hardy.

• **CULTIVATION** Grow annuals in any fertile, well-drained soil in full sun. Perennials and shrubs have varying needs, which may be grouped as set out below. Cut back all tall herbaceous species to the ground in autumn. Dead-head *P. maculata* and *P. paniculata* to prolong flowering. Stake tall cultivars.

1. Grow in fertile, moist soil in full sun or partial shade.

2. Grow in humus-rich, fertile, moist but well-drained soil in partial shade.

3. Grow in well-drained, fertile soil in full sun, or in dappled shade in low rainfall areas.

4. Grow in gritty, sharply drained, poor to moderately fertile soil in full sun. In an alpine house, grow in a mix of equal parts loam, leaf mould, and sharp sand.

• **PROPAGATION** Sow seed of annuals at 13–18°C (55–64°F) in early spring; sow seed of perennials in containers in a cold frame when ripe or in spring. Divide *P. carolina*, *P. maculata*, and *P. paniculata*, and their cultivars, in autumn or spring. Insert basal cuttings in spring, or take root cuttings in early autumn or winter. Take softwood cuttings of non-flowering stems of cushion-forming perennials in spring. Detach rooted pieces of stem from trailing perennials in spring or early autumn.

• **PESTS AND DISEASES** Susceptible to leafy gall, stem eelworms, powdery mildew, and leaf spot.

P. adsurgens ♀ Creeping, stem-rooting, semi-evergreen perennial with prostrate to ascending stems bearing stalkless, rounded to narrowly ovate, light to mid-green leaves, to 2.5cm (1in) long. In late spring and early summer, bears open cymes of salverform, broad-petalled, salmon-pink flowers, to 2.5cm (1in) across, with paler centres. Cultivation group 2. ↕↔ 30cm (12in). N.W. USA. ❄❄❄. **'Red Buttes'** has deep pink flowers with large, overlapping petal lobes. **'Wagon Wheel'** ■ has salmon-pink flowers with very narrow petal lobes, resembling the spokes of a wheel.

***P. amoena* 'Variegata'** see *P.* x *procumbens* 'Variegata'.

P. bifida ■ (Sand phlox). Mound-forming, evergreen perennial with hairy, needle-like, linear leaves, to 6cm (2½in) long. In spring and early summer, bears abundant cymes of salverform, fragrant, deep lavender-blue to white flowers, 2cm (¾in) across, with star-shaped, very deeply cleft petal lobes. Cultivation group 3 or 4. ↕ to 20cm (8in), ↔ 15cm (6in). C. USA. ❄❄❄. **'Colvin's White'** has pure white flowers.

P. bryoides. Cushion-forming, evergreen perennial with hairy, overlapping, lance-shaped leaves, to 5mm (¼in) long. In late spring and early summer, bears solitary, stalkless, salverform, pure white flowers, 1cm (½in) across, towards the shoot tips. May become lax and fail to flower freely in cultivation. Cultivation group 4. ↕ 2–5cm (¾–2in), ↔ 15cm (6in). High altitudes in USA (Oregon, W. Montana to Nevada, W. Nebraska). ❄❄❄

P. carolina (Thick-leaf phlox). Upright and spreading herbaceous perennial bearing thick, lance-shaped to ovate-oblong leaves, 13cm (5in) long. In summer, produces cymes of salverform,

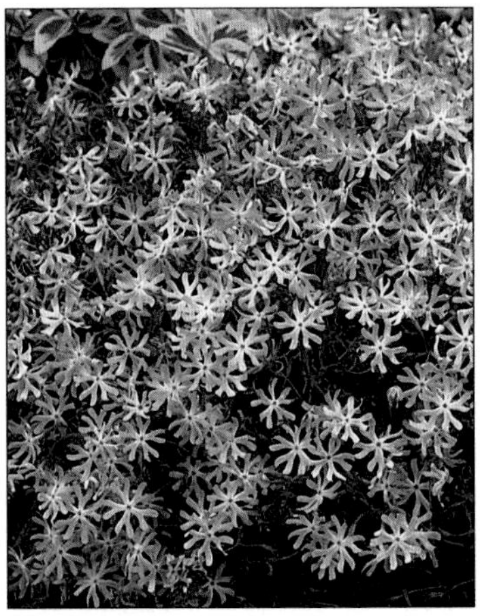

Phlox bifida

purple to pink, rarely white flowers, to 2cm (¾in) across. Cultivation group 1. ↕ 1.2m (4ft), ↔ 45cm (18in). C. and E. USA. ❄❄❄. **'Bill Baker'** ■ produces bright green leaves, to 15cm (6in) long, and bears pink flowers, to 2.5cm (1in) across, in early summer; ↕ 45cm (18in), ↔ 30cm (12in).

***P.* 'Chattahoochee'** ■♀ Short-lived, prostrate, branching, semi-evergreen perennial with purple-tinted stems and lance-shaped leaves, 2–5cm (¾–2in) long, purple-flushed when young. Bears cymes of salverform, lavender-blue flowers, 2–2.5cm (¾–1in) across, with conspicuous red-purple eyes, over long periods in summer and early autumn. Cultivation group 2. ↕ 15cm (6in), ↔ 30cm (12in). ❄❄❄

P. divaricata ♀ (Blue phlox, Wild sweet William). Spreading, stem-rooting, semi-evergreen perennial with ovate, hairy leaves, to 5cm (2in) long, narrower on the flowering stems. In early summer, produces open cymes of salverform, lavender-blue to pale violet and white flowers, 2–3cm (¾–1¼in) across, with notched or unnotched petal lobes. Cultivation group 2. ↕ to 35cm (14in), ↔ 50cm (20in). Woodland in Canada, E. USA. ❄❄❄. **'Dirigo Ice'** ■ has clear, pale blue flowers. **subsp. *laphamii*** ■ has pale to deep lilac-blue flowers with narrow petal lobes.

P. douglasii. Mound-forming, evergreen perennial densely covered with stiff, narrowly lance-shaped, dark green leaves, to 1cm (½in) long. In late spring or early summer, produces salverform, white, lavender-blue, or pink flowers, 1.5cm (½in) across, singly or in twos or threes. Cultivation group 3. ↕ to 20cm (8in), ↔ 30cm (12in). USA (S. Washington to California). ❄❄❄. **'Boothman's Variety'** ■♀ produces violet-pink flowers with dark eyes. **'Crackerjack'** ■♀ is more compact, with reddish magenta flowers; ↕ to 12cm (5in), ↔ to 20cm (8in). **'Iceberg'** ♀ has white flowers, sometimes faintly tinged blue. **'Red Admiral'** ■♀ bears deep crimson flowers. **'Violet Queen'** is compact, with deep violet-purple flowers; ↕ to 10cm (4in), ↔ to 15cm (6in). **'Waterloo'** has crimson flowers.

P. drummondii (Annual phlox). Erect to spreading, bushy, hairy annual with very variable, narrowly inversely lance-shaped to nearly ovate, almost stalkless, stem-clasping leaves, 2.5–8cm (1–3in) long. In late spring, produces cymes of salverform, hairy, purple, pink, red, lavender-blue, or white flowers, to 2.5cm (1in) across, often pale inside, with contrasting marks at the bases of the petal lobes. ↕ 10–45cm (4–18in), ↔ to 25cm (10in) or more. USA (E. Texas). ❄❄. **'African Sunset'** ■ has dusky to deep red flowers. **'Chanal'** ■ is spreading, but still compact, and bears double, almost rose-like pink flowers. **'Dwarf Beauty'** is early flowering, with abundant, very large blooms, to 3cm (1¼in) or more across, in colours including rose-pink, crimson-red, yellow, violet-blue, and white; ↔ 40cm (16in) or more. **'Petticoat'** is dwarf, with very small flowers, to 1.5cm (½in) across, available as a mixture of cream, rose-pink, salmon-pink, and carmine-pink, including bicolours; flowers late, but over a long season; ↕ to 10cm (4in). Cultivars in **Ethnie Pastel Shades Series** are ground-hugging, compact, and very uniform, with flowers in a range of pink and white shades. **Palona Series** cultivars are dwarf and bushy, forming spherical plants, with flowers in white, light blue, violet, salmon-pink, rose-pink, carmine-red, or crimson, some with contrasting eyes. **Palona Series 'Light Salmon'** ■ has pale salmon-pink flowers. **'Promise Pink'** has semi-double, deep salmon-pink flowers. **'Sternenzauber'** ■ syn. 'Twinkle', has

P

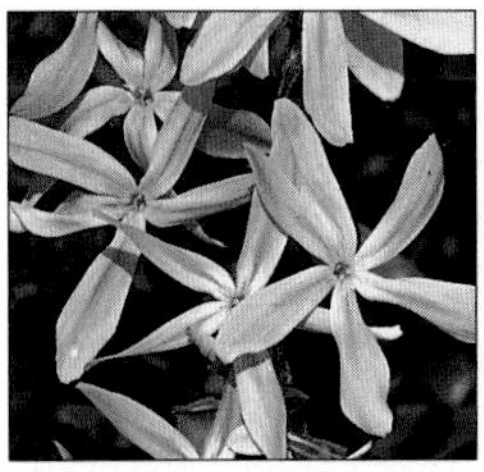

Phlox adsurgens 'Wagon Wheel'

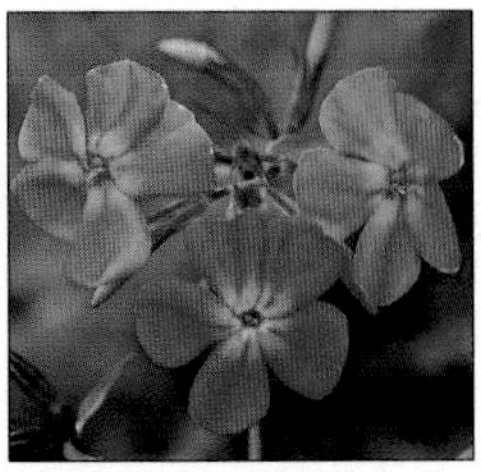

Phlox carolina 'Bill Baker'

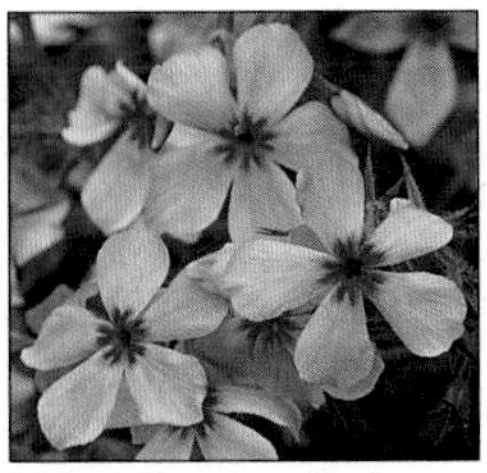

Phlox 'Chatahoochee'

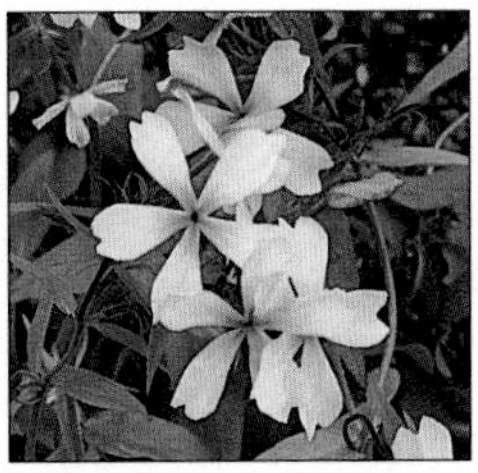

Phlox divaricata 'Dirigo Ice'

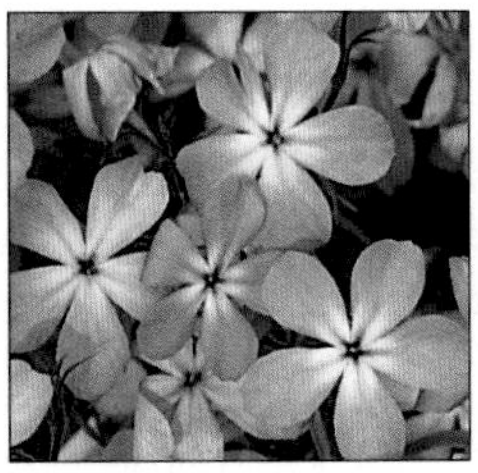

Phlox divaricata subsp. *laphamii*

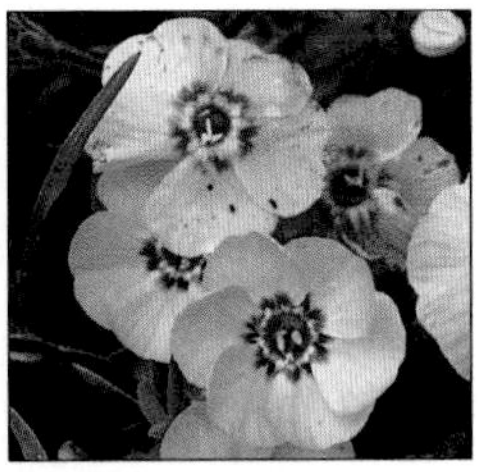

Phlox douglasii 'Boothman's Variety'

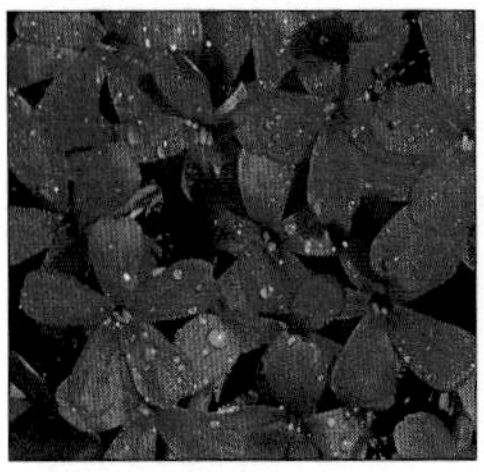

Phlox douglasii 'Crackerjack'

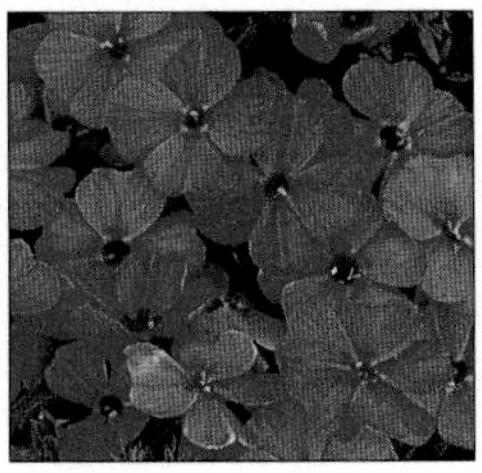

Phlox douglasii 'Red Admiral'

Phlox drummondii 'African Sunset'

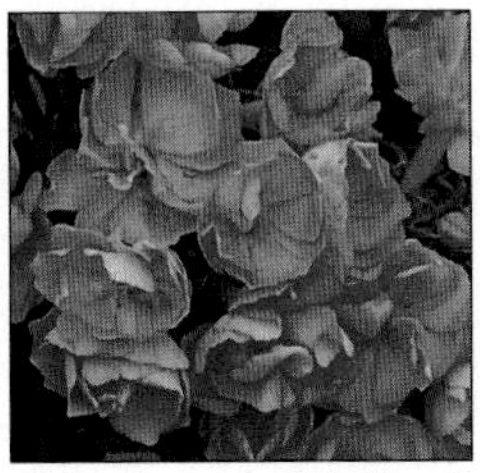

Phlox drummondii 'Chanal'

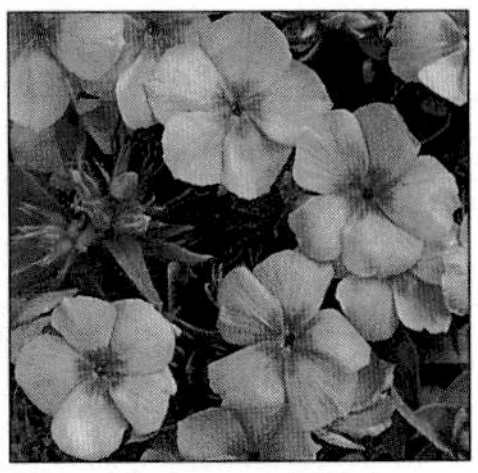

Phlox drummondii Palona Series 'Light Salmon'

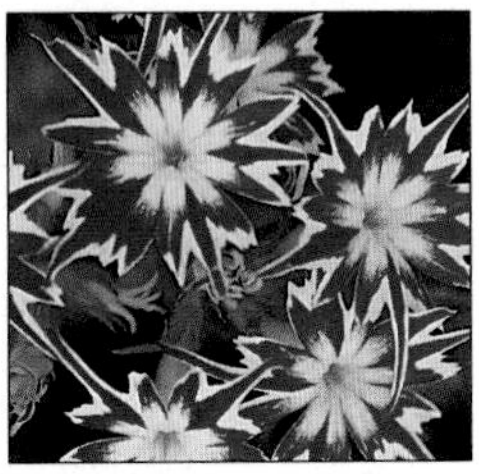

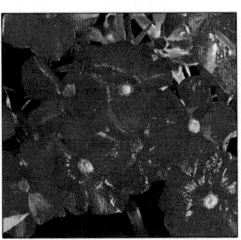

Phlox drummondii 'Sternenzauber'

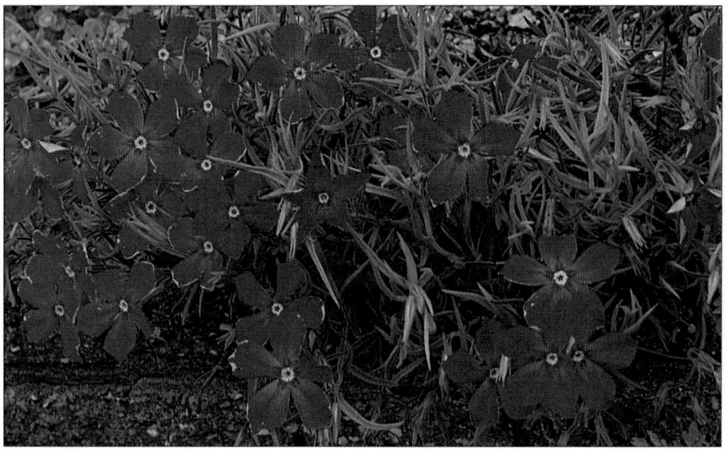
Phlox nana 'Arroya'

tiny flowers, to 2cm (¾in) across, in shades including salmon-pink, rose-pink, and carmine-pink, as well as picotees; petal lobes are often fringed and pointed, appearing star-like. **'Twinkle'** see 'Sternenzauber'.
***P.* 'Emerald Cushion'.** Compact, mound-forming, evergreen perennial, similar to *P. subulata*, with linear to elliptic, light green leaves, to 2cm (¾in) long. In late spring and early summer, bears cymes of salverform, pale violet flowers, 2–2.5cm (¾–1in) across, with narrow, notched petal lobes. Cultivation group 3. ↕ 8cm (3in), ↔ 20cm (8in). ❄❄❄
***P.* 'Fuller's White'.** Clump-forming, semi-evergreen perennial, similar to, but more compact than *P. divaricata*, with ovate leaves, to 5cm (2in) long. In early summer, upright stems bear cymes of salverform, pure white flowers, 2–2.5cm (¾–1in) across, with notched petal lobes. Cultivation group 2. ↕↔ to 20cm (8in). ❄❄❄
P. hoodii. Dwarf, tuft-forming, evergreen perennial with hairy, lance-shaped leaves, to 1cm (½in) long. Bears solitary, salverform, white to pale violet flowers, 1cm (½in) across, in late spring and early summer. Cultivation group 4. ↕ 5cm (2in), ↔ 10cm (4in). USA (Rocky Mountains). ❄❄❄
***P.* 'Kelly's Eye'** ■♀ Vigorous, mound-forming, evergreen perennial, similar to *P. douglasii*, with narrowly lance-shaped, dark green leaves, to 1.5cm (½in) long. In late spring and early summer, bears cymes of salverform, very pale pink flowers, 1.5cm (½in) across, with red-purple eyes. Cultivation group 3. ↕ 10cm (4in), ↔ 30cm (12in) or more. ❄❄❄
P. maculata (Meadow phlox). Erect herbaceous perennial with hairy stems, often red-spotted, and linear to ovate, smooth leaves, 6–13cm (2½–5in) long. In early and midsummer, bears narrowly conical, panicle-like cymes of salverform, fragrant, violet, pink, or white flowers, 2–2.5cm (¾–1in) across. Cultivation group 1. ↕ to 90cm (36in), ↔ 45cm (18in). E. USA. ❄❄❄. **'Alpha'** ♀ produces lilac-pink flowers. **'Omega'** ■♀ has white flowers with lilac-red eyes.
P. mesoleuca see *P. nana* subsp. *ensifolia*.
***P.* 'Millstream'** see *P.* x *procumbens* 'Millstream'.
P. nana (Santa Fe phlox). Deciduous or semi-evergreen perennial, spreading by runners, with trailing or upright shoots, to 20cm (8in) long, sparsely covered with linear to lance-shaped, downy, grey-green leaves, to 4cm (1½in) long. Produces abundant solitary, salverform, bright pink, purple, or white, rarely pale yellow flowers, to 2.5cm (1in) across, from summer to autumn. Cultivation group 4. ↕ to 20cm (8in), ↔ to 30cm (12in). S.W. USA, Mexico. ❄❄❄. **'Arroya'** ■ bears brilliant magenta flowers, with small white eyes, over long periods in summer. **subsp. *ensifolia*,** syn. *P. mesoleuca*, produces white-eyed, soft pink, purple, soft yellow, or white flowers; slower-growing than the species, with shorter shoots, and more difficult to grow. **'Mary Maslin'** ■ has vivid scarlet flowers with yellow eyes. **'Paul Maslin'** has pale yellow flowers with deep purple eyes. **'Tangelo'** has brilliant orange-red flowers with yellow eyes.
P. nivalis ■ (Trailing phlox). Decumbent, evergreen perennial with trailing shoots, to 30cm (12in) long, and hairy, lance-shaped leaves, 2.5cm (1in) long. Bears cymes of salverform, purple, pink, or white flowers, to 1.5cm (½in) across, in summer. Cultivation group 3. ↕ 20cm (8in), ↔ 30cm (12in). C. USA. ❄❄❄. **'Camla'** has very pale pink, almost white flowers.
P. paniculata (Perennial phlox). Erect herbaceous perennial with ovate or lance-shaped to elliptic, toothed, thin leaves, 5–13cm (2–5in) long. Panicle-like cymes of salverform, fragrant, white or pale to dark lilac flowers, 1.5–2.5cm (½–1in) across, are borne from summer to early or mid-autumn. Cultivation group 1. ↕ 1.2m (4ft), ↔ 60–100cm (24–39in). E. USA. ❄❄❄. **'Aida'** has crimson flowers with purple eyes. **'Amethyst'** ♀ produces violet flowers. **'Balmoral'** ■ is vigorous, with large trusses of pink flowers; ↕ 90cm (36in). **'Blue Boy'** is strong-growing, and bears mauve-blue flowers with white eyes; ↕ 90cm (36in). **'Brigadier'** ■♀ has orange-tinged, pinkish red flowers, and deep green leaves. **'Bright Eyes'** ♀ has clear pale pink flowers with red eyes. **'Eva Cullum'** ■ is very free-blooming, producing bright deep pink flowers with darker pink centres. **'Eventide'** ■♀ has lavender-blue flowers; ↕ 90cm (36in). **'Fujiyama'** ■♀ has white flowers; ↕ to 75cm (30in). **'Graf Zeppelin'** ■ has white flowers with red centres. **'Hampton Court'** ■ has dark green foliage and mauve-blue flowers. **'Harlequin'** ■ has leaves with broad, ivory-white margins, and produces reddish purple flowers. **'Le Mahdi'** ♀ produces deep bluish purple flowers with darker eyes; ↕ 1.1m (3½ft). **'Mia Ruys'** ■ bears large white flowers, to 3cm (1¼in) across; ↕ 60cm (24in). **'Mother of Pearl'** ■♀ has pink-tinted white flowers; ↕ 75cm (30in). **'Norah Leigh'** ■ has extensively white-variegated leaves and small, pale lilac flowers, 1.5cm (½in) across, with deeper lilac-pink centres; ↕ 90cm (36in). **'Orange Perfection'** bears deep orange flowers. **'Prince of Orange'** ♀ has orange-red flowers; ↕ to 80cm (32in). **'Prospero'** ♀ has pale lilac flowers with almost white petal margins; ↕ to 90cm (36in). **'Sandringham'** has pale pink flowers with deeper pink centres and widely spaced petal lobes. **'Sir John Falstaff'** has deep salmon-pink flowers with wine-red eyes. **'Starfire'** has dark green leaves and deep crimson-red flowers; ↕ 90cm (36in). **'White Admiral'** ♀ bears white flowers; ↕ 90cm (36in). **'Windsor'** ■♀ has reddish pink flowers with purple-pink eyes.
P.* x *procumbens (*P. stolonifera* x *P. subulata*). Decumbent, mat-forming, semi-evergreen perennial with inversely lance-shaped to elliptic, glossy leaves, 2.5cm (1in) long. Bears open, flat cymes of salverform, bright purple flowers, 2cm (¾in) across, in early summer. Cultivation group 2 or 3. ↕ 10cm (4in), ↔ 30cm (12in). Garden origin. ❄❄❄. **'Millstream'** ♀ syn. *P.* 'Millstream', bears a profusion of deep lavender-pink flowers. **'Variegata'**, syn. *P. amoena* 'Variegata', has leaves with cream margins, and bears deep pink flowers.
P. stolonifera (Creeping phlox). Stoloniferous, spreading herbaceous perennial with obovate, dark green leaves, to 5cm (2in) long. In early summer, upright stems produce open cymes of salverform, pale to deep purple flowers, to 3cm (1¼in) across. Cultivation group 2. ↕ 10–15cm (4–6in), ↔ 30cm (12in) or more. Woodland in C. USA. ❄❄❄. **'Ariane'** ■ has pale green leaves, and white flowers, 3cm (1¼in) or more across, with star-shaped petal lobes and small yellow eyes. **'Blue Ridge'** ♀ bears clear pale blue flowers. **'Mary Belle Frey'** has pink flowers.
P. subulata (Moss phlox). Dense, evergreen perennial forming cushions or mats of hairy, linear to elliptic, bright green leaves, 0.6–2cm (¼–¾in) long. Salverform, purple or red, sometimes violet-purple, lilac, pink, or white flowers, 1.5–2.5cm (½–1in) across, often with star-shaped petal lobes, are produced in few-flowered cymes, rarely singly, in late spring and early summer. Cultivation group 3. ↕ 5–15cm (2–6in),

P

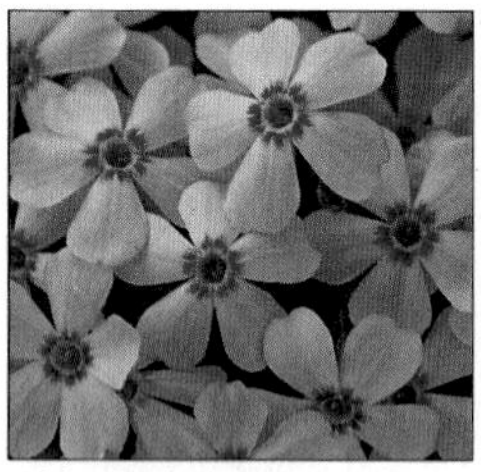
Phlox 'Kelly's Eye'

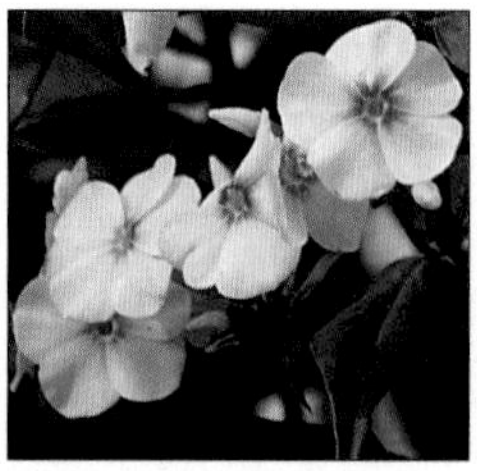
Phlox maculata 'Omega'

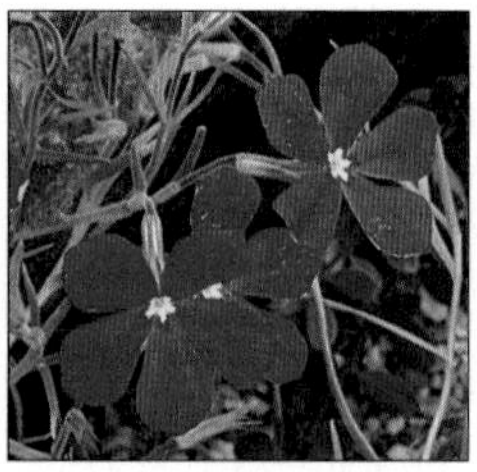
Phlox nana 'Mary Maslin'

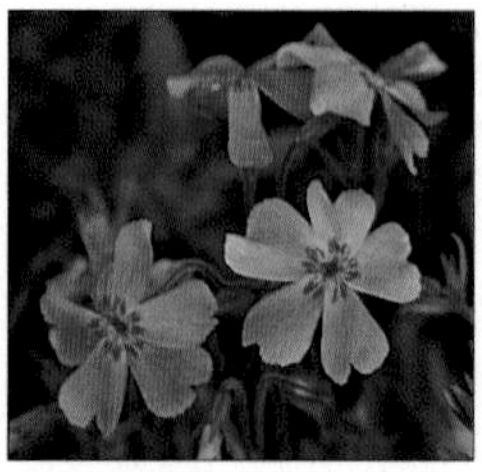
Phlox nivalis

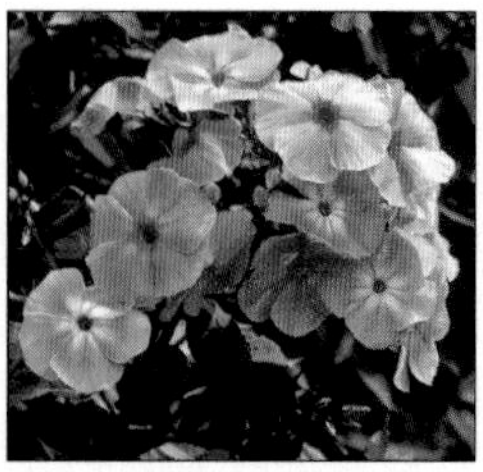
Phlox paniculata 'Balmoral'

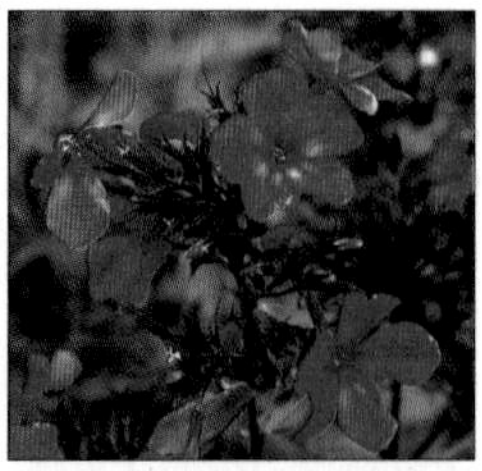
Phlox paniculata 'Brigadier'

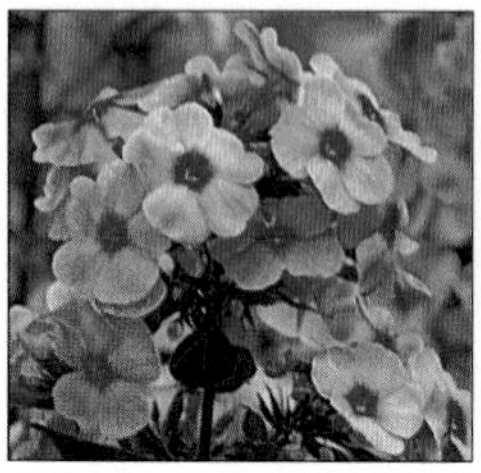
Phlox paniculata 'Eva Cullum'

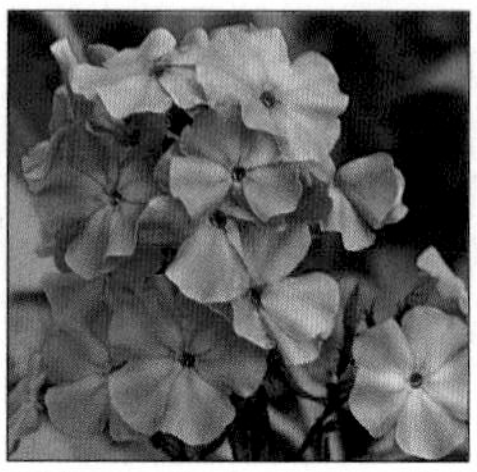
Phlox paniculata 'Eventide'

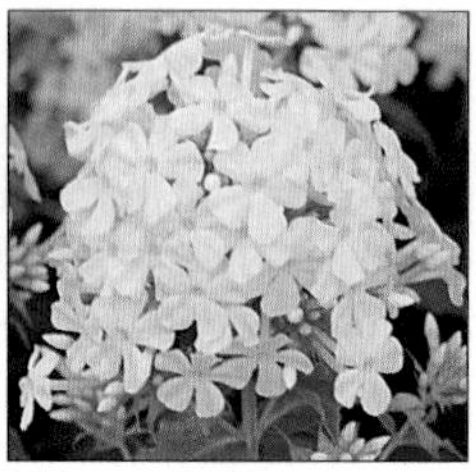
Phlox paniculata 'Fujiyama'

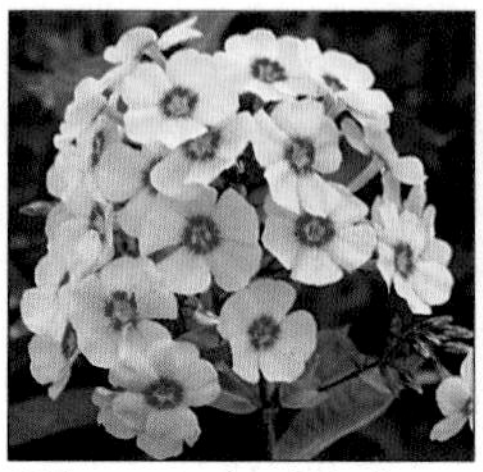
Phlox paniculata 'Graf Zeppelin'

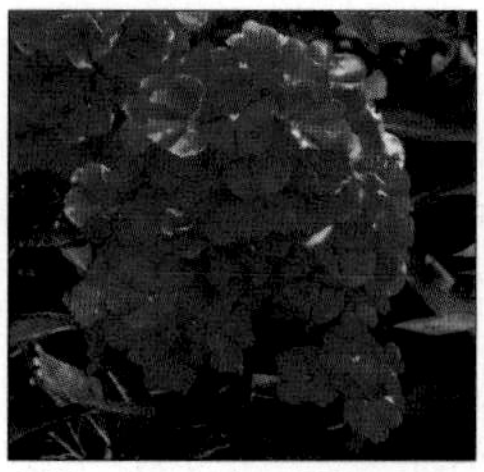
Phlox paniculata 'Hampton Court'

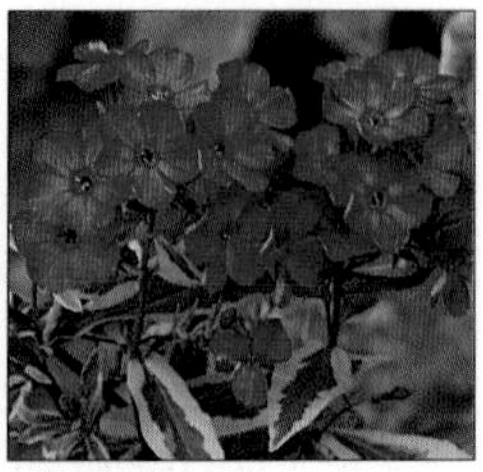
Phlox paniculata 'Harlequin'

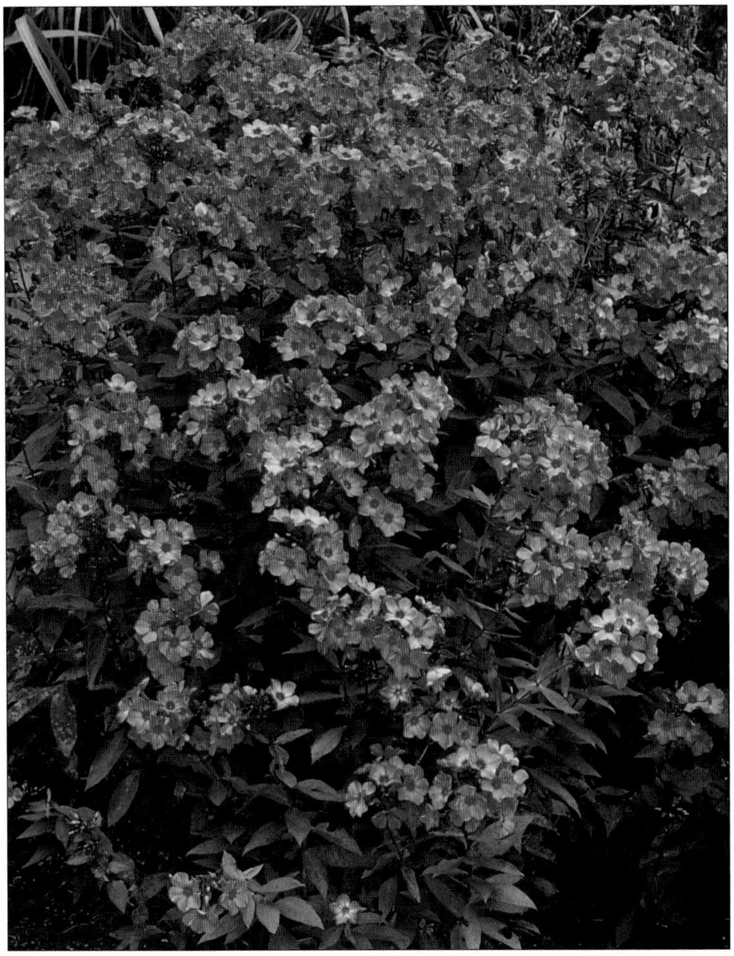

Phlox paniculata 'Windsor'

↔ 50cm (20in) or more. E. to C. USA. ❋❋❋. **'Amazing Grace'** has a lax habit, and bears pale pink flowers with deep pinkish purple eyes. **'G.F. Wilson'** ▣ is vigorous and cushion-forming, and produces deep lavender-blue flowers. **'Marjorie'** ▣ is mat-forming, and bears very large, narrow-petalled, deep pink flowers, 3cm (1¼in) across, each with a darker pink band around a yellow eye. **'McDaniel's Cushion'** 🏆 is vigorous, cushion-forming, and very free-flowering, with very large, very deep pink flowers, to 3.5cm (1½in) across. **'Scarlet Flame'** is vigorous and mat-forming, with deep scarlet flowers. **'Temiskaming'** is slow-growing and cushion-forming, with small, deep magenta flowers, 1.5cm (½in) across.

▷ **Phlox**
Annual see *Phlox drummondii*
Blue see *Phlox divaricata*
Creeping see *Phlox stolonifera*
Meadow see *Phlox maculata*
Moss see *Phlox subulata*
Mountain see *Linanthus grandiflorus*
Perennial see *Phlox paniculata*
Sand see *Phlox bifida*
Santa Fe see *Phlox nana*
Thick-leaf see *Phlox carolina*
Trailing see *Phlox nivalis*

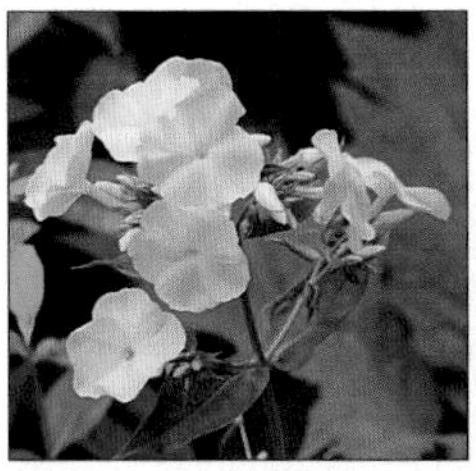

Phlox paniculata 'Mia Ruys'

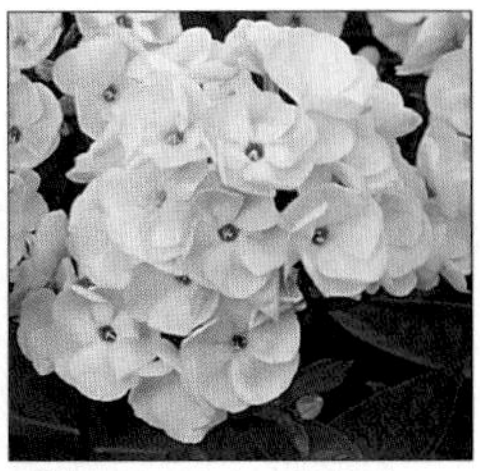

Phlox paniculata 'Mother of Pearl'

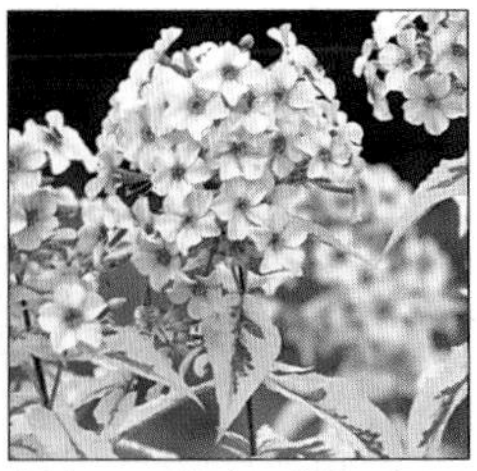

Phlox paniculata 'Norah Leigh'

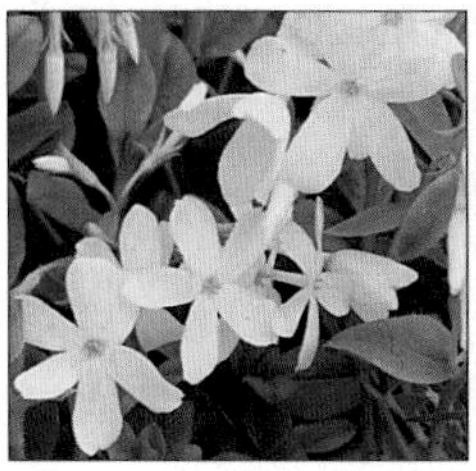

Phlox stolonifera 'Ariane'

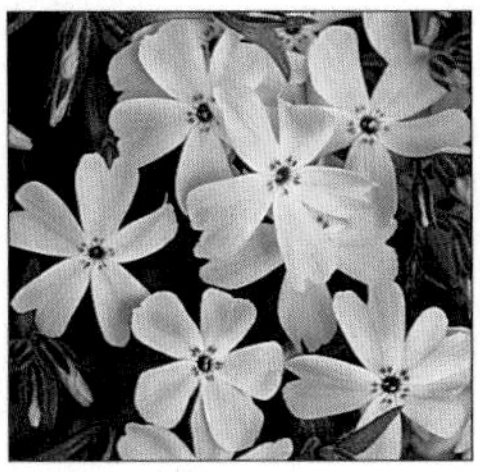

Phlox subulata 'G. F. Wilson'

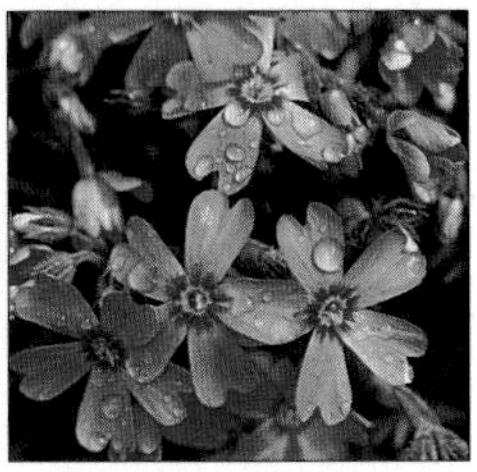

Phlox subulata 'Marjorie'

PHOENIX

ARECACEAE/PALMAE

Genus of 17 species of single- and cluster-stemmed palms occurring in tropical and subtropical forest or low scrub thickets in the Canary Islands, Africa, Crete (Greece), and W. and S. Asia to the Philippines. They have linear to ovate or oblong, pinnate leaves, usually borne in dense, terminal clusters. The bowl-shaped, 3-petalled, cream to yellow flowers are produced in panicles from the lower axils, followed by yellow, orange, red, brown, or black fruits. In frost-prone climates, grow in a warm greenhouse or as houseplants. In warmer areas, use as specimen plants on a lawn.

- **HARDINESS** Frost tender.
- **CULTIVATION** Under glass, grow in loam-based potting compost (JI No.2) in full light, with shade from hot sun. Pot on or top-dress in spring. When in growth, water freely and apply a balanced liquid fertilizer monthly. Water sparingly in winter. Outdoors, grow in fertile, moist but well-drained soil in full sun, with some midday shade.
- **PROPAGATION** Sow seed at 19–24°C (66–75°F) in spring.
- **PESTS AND DISEASES** Prone to scale insects and red spider mites under glass.

P. canariensis 🏆 🌴 (Canary Island date palm). Medium-sized palm with a stout, columnar trunk marked with oblong leaf scars wider than they are long. Spreading to broadly arching leaves, 4–6m (12–20ft) long, consist of many linear, bright mid- to deep green leaflets, set in a single plane. Bowl-shaped, cream to yellow flowers are borne in pendent panicles, 1–1.2m (3–4ft) long, in summer. Fruit are cylindrical to ellipsoid, and yellow flushed red, 2cm (¾in) long, with edible, sweet, but almost dry flesh. ↕ to 15m (50ft), ↔ 12m (40ft). Canary Islands. ⊛ (min. 10–16°C/50–61°F)
P. dactylifera 🌴 (Date palm). Tall, sometimes suckering palm producing a columnar trunk usually clad with old leaf bases, at least towards the top. Leaves, 4–6m (12–20ft) long, are composed of many linear, greyish green leaflets, the lowest ones reduced to spines, arranged in various planes giving a 3-dimensional effect. Bowl-shaped cream flowers appear in long-stalked panicles, 1.5–2m (5–6ft) long, in spring or summer. Ellipsoid to cylindrical, edible, sweet, fleshy, yellow to reddish brown fruit, 2.5–7cm (1–3in) long, are very variable both in texture and flavour. ↕ to 30m (100ft), ↔ 6–12m (20–40ft). Probably N. Africa and W. Asia. ⊛ (min. 10–16°C/50–61°F)
P. humilis see *P. loureirii.*
P. loureirii ❋ syn. *P. humilis.* Small palm, often with clustered stems, bearing leaves to 2m (6ft) long or more, composed of linear, glaucous, bright mid-green leaflets, clustered along the midribs. Bowl-shaped cream flowers appear in panicles, to 1m (3ft) long, usually in summer, followed by ovoid, dry-fleshed, red to black fruit, 1.5–2cm (½–¾in) across. ↕ 2–5m (6–15ft), ↔ 2–4m (6–12ft). Sri Lanka, India to S. China. ⊛ (min. 10–16°C/50–61°F)
P. reclinata ▣ ❋ Small, clustering palm with ascending or leaning, slender

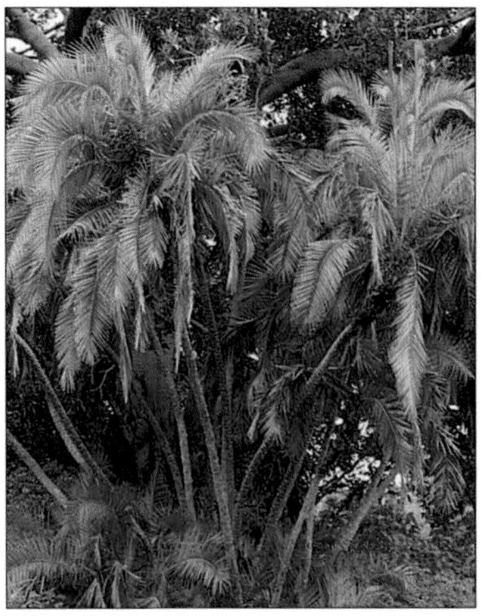

Phoenix reclinata

stems clad with fibrous, red-brown leaf remains. Leaves, to 2.5m (8ft) long, are composed of many linear, mid- to deep green leaflets, usually arranged in several planes. Bowl-shaped cream flowers are produced in panicles, to 1.5m (5ft) long, usually in summer, followed by cylindrical-ellipsoid, edible but dry, orange-red to black fruit, to 2cm (¾in) across. ↕↔ to 10m (30ft). Tropical Africa. ⊛ (min. 10–16°C/50–61°F)
P. roebelenii 🏆 🌴 (Miniature date palm, Pygmy date palm). Small, sometimes clustering palm, often with a narrow skirt of dead leaves. Living leaves, 1–1.2m (3–4ft) long, have many linear, bright deep green leaflets, sometimes with flattened, scale-like hairs beneath. Bowl-shaped cream flowers appear in panicles, to 45cm (18in) long, usually in summer, followed by ellipsoid, edible black fruit, to 1cm (½in) long. ↕ 2m (6ft) or more, ↔ to 2.5m (8ft). Laos. ⊛ (min. 10–16°C/50–61°F)

PHORMIUM

AGAVACEAE/PHORMIACEAE

Genus of 2 species of evergreen perennials found in scrub and swamps, and on hillsides and riverbanks, in areas ranging from coasts to mountains in New Zealand. They form clumps of large, linear, keeled leaves, each folded into a V-shape at the base, and ranging in colour from yellow-green to dark green, with many fine stripes. Cultivars often have attractive, coloured or variegated foliage. Abundant small, tubular, 6-tepalled flowers are produced in erect panicles on leafless stems in summer. They provide a focal point in a border, by a building, or at the edge of a lawn, and are ideal for a coastal garden.

- **HARDINESS** Frost hardy to half hardy; may tolerate temperatures to -12°C (10°F) if given a deep, dry winter mulch.
- **CULTIVATION** Grow in fertile, moist but well-drained soil in full sun. In frost-prone areas, provide a deep, dry mulch in winter.
- **PROPAGATION** Sow seed at 13–18°C (55–64°F) in spring. Divide in spring.
- **PESTS AND DISEASES** Mealybugs may be a problem.

P. colensoi see *P. cookianum.*
P. cookianum 🏆 syn. *P. colensoi* (Mountain flax). Clump-forming perennial with broad, arching, linear, light to yellowish green leaves, to 1.5m (5ft) long. Tubular, yellow-green

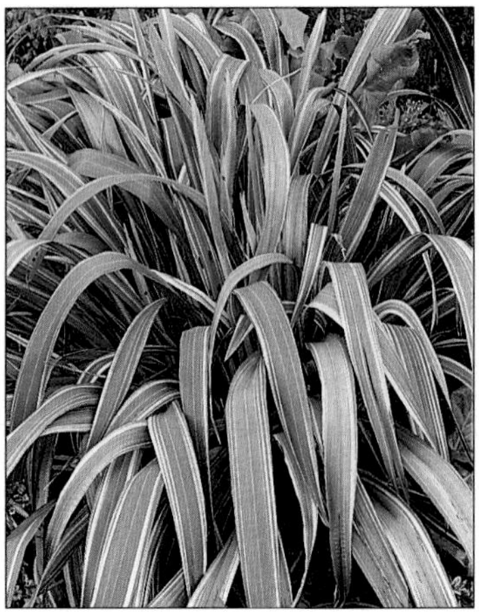
Phormium cookianum subsp. *hookeri* 'Tricolor'

flowers, to 4cm (1½in) long, are borne in upright panicles, 2m (6ft) long, in summer. ↕ to 2m (6ft), ↔ 3m (10ft). New Zealand. ❄❄. **subsp. *hookeri* 'Cream Delight'** 🏆 has leaves with broad bands of creamy yellow in the centres and narrower bands towards the margins. **subsp. *hookeri* 'Tricolor'** ▣ 🏆 has leaves conspicuously margined creamy yellow and red. **'Maori Chief'**, a hybrid of *P. cookianum*, has pink- and red-striped bronze leaves. **'Maori Sunrise**, a hybrid of *P. cookianum*, produces slender, apricot-and-pink-striped leaves with bronze margins. **'Variegatum'** has light green leaves with cream to lime-green stripes and margins.
***P.* 'Sundowner'** ▣ 🏆 Clump-forming perennial with broad, upright, bronze-green leaves, to 1.5m (5ft) long, with dark rose-pink margins. Tubular, yellow-green flowers, to 4cm (1½in) long, are borne in upright panicles, 2m (6ft) long, in summer. ↕↔ to 2m (6ft). ❄❄
P. tenax ▣ 🏆 (New Zealand flax). Clump-forming perennial with rigid, upright, linear leaves, to 3m (10ft) long, dark green above, blue-green beneath. Stout, red-purple panicles, to 4m (12ft)

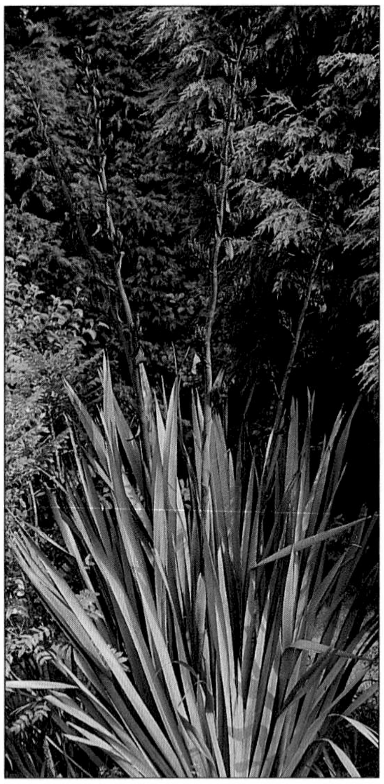
Phormium tenax

long, of tubular, dull red flowers, 5cm (2in) long, are borne in summer. ↕ 4m (12ft), ↔ 2m (6ft). New Zealand. ❄❄. **'Aurora'**, a hybrid of *P. tenax*, has arching bronze leaves striped red, salmon-pink, and yellow; ↕↔ 1.2m (4ft). **'Bronze Baby'**, a dwarf hybrid of *P. tenax*, produces bronze leaves, pendent at the tips; ↕↔ 60–80cm (24–32in). **'Dazzler'** ▣ a hybrid of *P. tenax*, has arching bronze leaves with red, orange, and pink stripes; ↕ 1m (3ft), ↔ 1.2m (4ft). **'Variegatum'** 🏆 produces leaves with creamy yellow stripes at the margins. **'Veitchianum'** has leaves with broad, creamy white stripes.
***P.* 'Yellow Wave'** 🏆 Clump-forming perennial producing broad, arching, yellow-green leaves, to 1m (3ft) long,

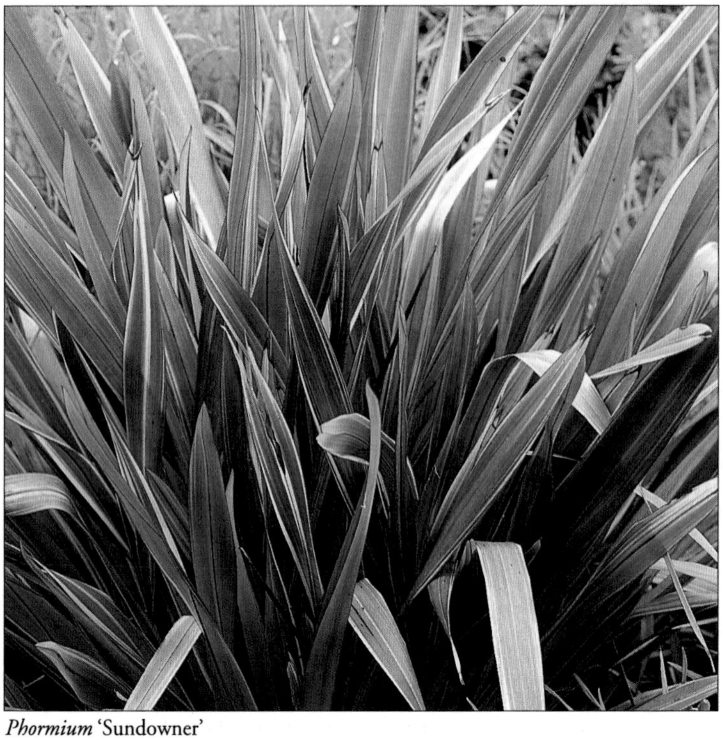
Phormium 'Sundowner'

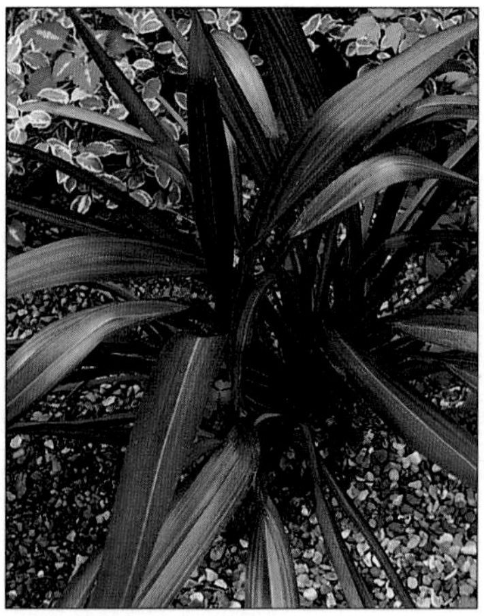
Phormium tenax 'Dazzler'

longitudinally striped mid-green. Tubular, dull red flowers, 5cm (2in) long, in stout, red-purple panicles, to 4m (12ft) long, are borne in summer. ↕ 4m (12ft), ↔ 2m (6ft). ❄❄

PHOTINIA

syn. HETEROMELES, STRANVAESIA

ROSACEAE

Genus of about 60 species of deciduous or evergreen shrubs and trees found in woodland and thickets from the Himalayas to E. and S.E. Asia. Leaves are alternate, lance-shaped to broadly ovate, and mid- or dark green; evergreen leaves are attractive and glossy, often brightly coloured in shades of red when young; deciduous leaves often colour well in autumn. The small, 5-petalled flowers are saucer- to cup-shaped, and are borne in dense, terminal and axillary, corymb-like panicles, followed by spherical or ovoid, usually red fruits, 0.5–1cm (¼–½in) across. Grow deciduous species in a woodland garden, or as specimens on a lawn; grow evergreens in a shrub border or among other trees and shrubs. Use *P.* x *fraseri* cultivars for hedging. In frost-prone areas, grow evergreen shrubs against a wall or in the shelter of trees.

• **HARDINESS** Fully hardy to frost hardy. The early growth of *P. serratifolia* may be damaged by late frosts.

• **CULTIVATION** Grow in fertile, moist but well-drained soil in full sun or partial shade. *P. beauverdiana* and *P. villosa* need acid to neutral soil. Protect frost-hardy species from cold, drying winds. Pruning group 1.

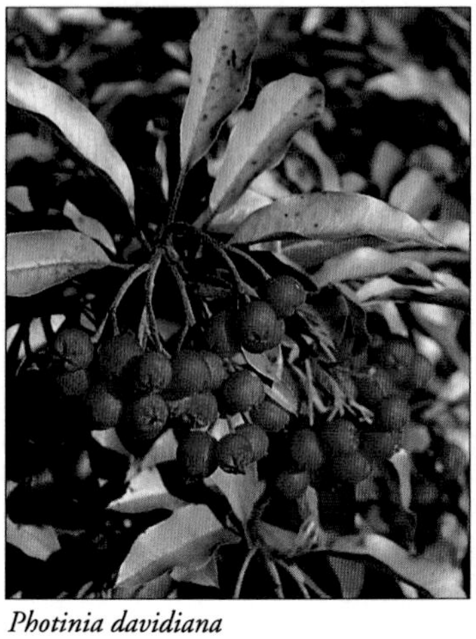
Photinia davidiana

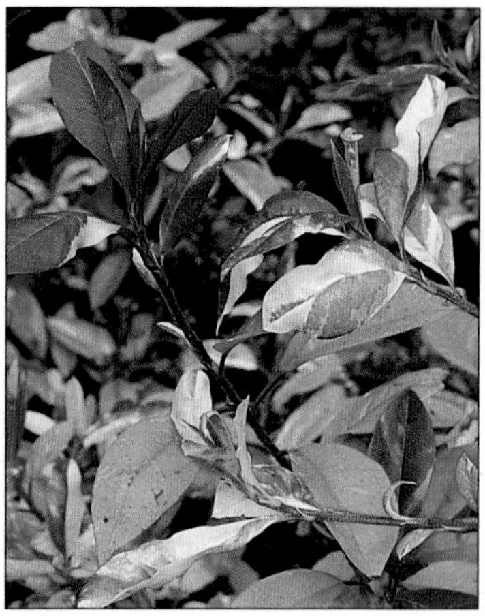
Photinia davidiana 'Palette'

• **PROPAGATION** Sow seed in containers in a cold frame in autumn. Root semi-ripe cuttings with bottom heat in summer.

• **PESTS AND DISEASES** May be affected by fireblight. Susceptible to leaf spot and powdery mildew.

P. beauverdiana 🏆 Ϙ Spreading, deciduous tree with elliptic to obovate, dark green leaves, to 12cm (5in) long, turning red in autumn. In late spring, bears small white flowers in corymb-like panicles, to 5cm (2in) across, followed by ovoid red fruit. ↕ to 10m (30ft), ↔ 6m (20ft). W. China. ❄❄❄
P. davidiana ▣ Ϙ syn. *Stranvaesia davidiana*. Upright, evergreen tree or shrub with elliptic to inversely lance-shaped, tapered, dark green leaves, to 12cm (5in) long; older leaves turn red in autumn. In midsummer, small white flowers are produced in corymb-like panicles, 7cm (3in) across, followed by spherical, bright red fruit. ↕ 8m (25ft), ↔ 6m (20ft). China, Vietnam. ❄❄❄. **'Palette'** ▣ is slow-growing and shrubby, with leaves boldly marked creamy white; ↕ 5m (15ft), ↔ 3m (10ft). **var. *undulata* 'Fructu Luteo'** has yellow fruit.
P.* x *fraseri Ϙ (*P. glabra* x *P. serratifolia*). Upright, evergreen shrub or small tree with inversely lance-shaped to elliptic, leathery, dark green leaves, 10–20cm (4–8in) long, bronze to bright red when young. In mid- and late spring, produces small white flowers in corymb-like panicles, to 15cm (6in) across. ↕↔ 5m (15ft). Garden origin. ❄❄. **'Birmingham'** Ϙ is bushy-headed,

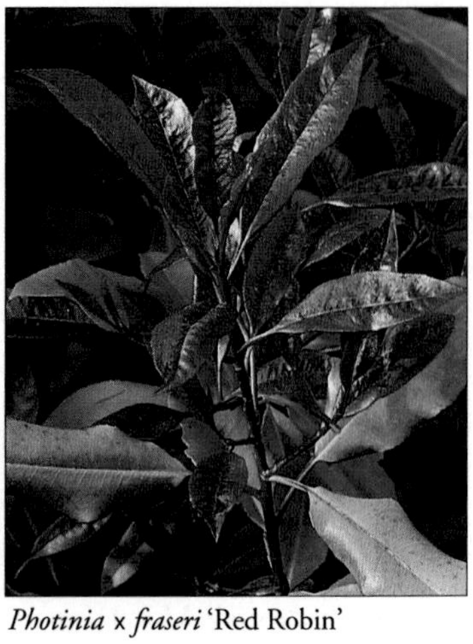
Photinia x *fraseri* 'Red Robin'

P

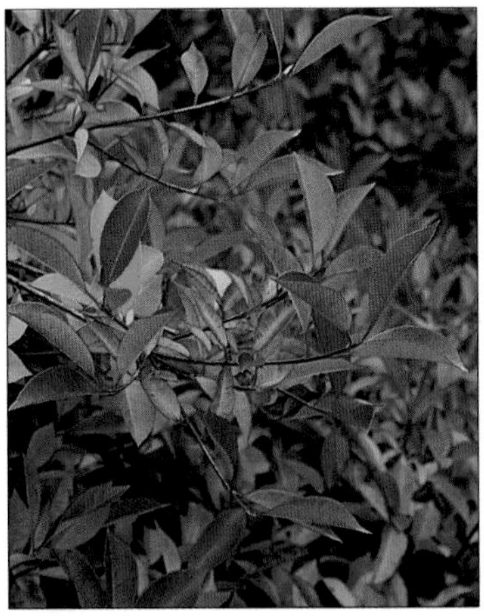

Photinia glabra 'Rubens'

spreading, and often many-stemmed, with oblong to obovate leaves, bright purple-red when young; sometimes bears spherical red fruit. **'Red Robin'** ■♀ is compact, with bright red young foliage.
P. glabra. Dense, rounded, evergreen shrub with elliptic to obovate, dark green leaves, to 9cm (3½in) long, red when young. In early summer, bears flattened, corymb-like panicles, 10cm (4in) across, of small white flowers, followed by spherical red fruit, turning black. ↕↔ 3m (10ft). Japan. ✻✻.
'Rubens' ■ has bright red young foliage.
P. nussia ⚲ syn. *Stranvaesia nussia.* Spreading, often rather spiny, evergreen tree with oblong to obovate, leathery, glossy, dark green leaves, to 10cm (4in) long, paler beneath. In midsummer, bears small white flowers in flattened, corymb-like panicles, to 10cm (4in) across, followed by spherical, downy, orange-red fruit. ↕↔ 6m (20ft). Himalayas to S.E. Asia. ✻✻
***P.* 'Redstart'** ♀⚲ Upright, evergreen shrub or small tree bearing oblong to elliptic, dark green leaves, to 11cm (4½in) long, bronze-red when young, on red shoots. Small white flowers, in dense, corymb-like panicles, 10cm (4in) across, appear in early summer before spherical, yellow-flushed, orange-red fruit. ↕ 5m (15ft), ↔ 3m (10ft). ✻✻✻
P. serratifolia ⚲ syn. *P. serrulata.* Spreading, evergreen tree with peeling, grey and red-brown bark when mature. Oblong to inversely lance-shaped, glossy, shallowly but sharply toothed, dark green leaves, to 20cm (8in) long, are red when young. Bears small white flowers, in flattened, corymb-like panicles, 10–18cm (4–7in) across, in late spring and early summer, followed by spherical red fruit. ↕ 10–12m (30–40ft), ↔ 8m (25ft). China. ✻✻
P. serrulata see *P. serratifolia.*
P. villosa ■♀⚲ Spreading, deciduous tree, sometimes shrubby, with elliptic to obovate, dark green leaves, to 7cm (3in) long, bronze when young, turning orange and red in autumn. Small white flowers in flattened, corymb-like panicles, 4cm (1½in) across, appear in late spring, before ovoid red fruit. ↕↔ 5m (15ft). China, Korea, Japan. ✻✻✻

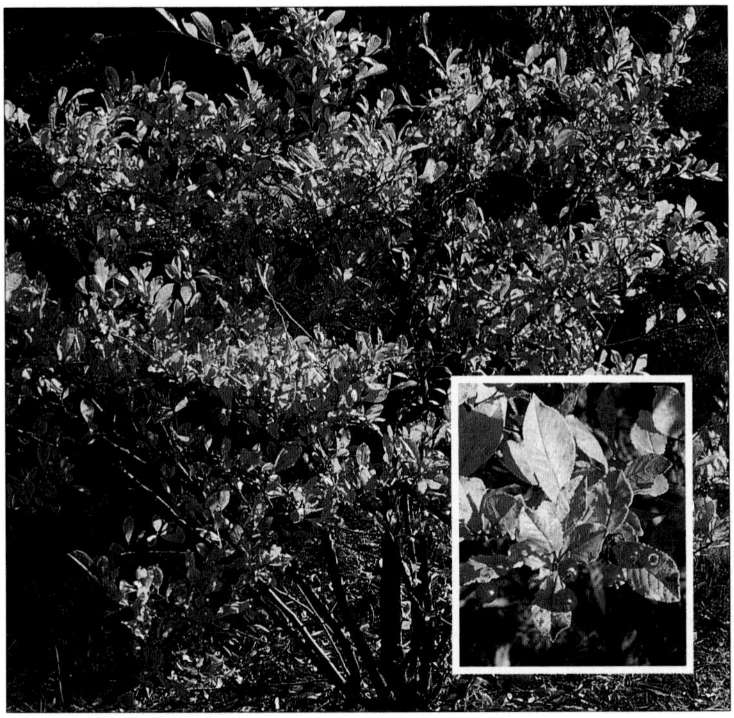

Photinia villosa (inset: leaf detail)

PHRAGMIPEDIUM

ORCHIDACEAE

Genus of 15–20 species of large, evergreen, mainly terrestrial, occasionally lithophytic or epiphytic orchids from Mexico and Central and South America, often found in between rocks or near rivers at low altitudes. They have robust, fleshy, clustered shoots with fibrous roots, but lack pseudobulbs. Leaves are leathery, strap-shaped, often mid-green, and arranged in 2 ranks. Upright stems, arising from the centre of each shoot, bear one or several often brightly coloured flowers in terminal racemes or panicles; some have very long petals, and each has a significant, slipper-shaped lip.
- **HARDINESS** Frost tender.
- **CULTIVATION** Cool-growing orchids. Grow in epiphytic orchid compost in containers that restrict the roots. In summer, provide bright filtered light and high humidity, and apply fertilizer

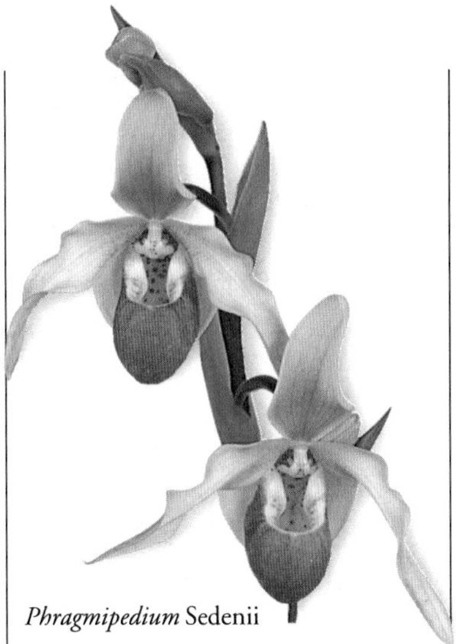

Phragmipedium Sedenii

at every third watering. In winter, provide full light, with some midday shade, water sparingly, and apply fertilizer every 6–8 weeks. See also p.46.
- **PROPAGATION** Divide clustered shoots by separating offshoots before growth begins in late winter or early spring.
- **PESTS AND DISEASES** Prone to red spider mites, aphids, and mealybugs.

P. besseae. Terrestrial or lithophytic orchid with 6–10 strap-shaped, leathery leaves, to 20cm (8in) long. Bright scarlet flowers, 6cm (2½in) across, are borne singly or in short, upright racemes in spring. ↕↔ 15cm (6in). Ecuador, Peru. ❀ (min. 14°C/57°F; max. 30°C/86°F)
P. caudatum. Epiphytic or lithophytic orchid with usually 6–9 strap-shaped, blunt-tipped, leathery, light green leaves, to 60cm (24in) long. In summer, bears upright racemes of very large flowers, 10–15cm (4–6in) across, with very narrow, ribbon-like, dark reddish to greenish brown, pendent petals, 60cm (24in) long, off-white to yellow-green sepals veined darker green or orange, and deep pinkish white lips with pink or brown veins and yellow rims. ↕↔ 60cm (24in). Mexico to Peru. ❀ (min. 14°C/57°F; max. 30°C/86°F)
P. longifolium. Terrestrial orchid with about 6 strap-shaped, leathery leaves, to 1m (3ft) long, with sharp-pointed tips. In autumn, bears racemes of pale yellow-green flowers, 15cm (6in) across, with wavy, purple-margined petals, dark green-veined sepals, and purple-flushed lips. ↕↔ 60cm (24in). Costa Rica, Panama, Colombia, Ecuador. ❀ (min. 14°C/57°F; max. 30°C/86°F)
***P.* Sedenii** ■ (*P. longifolium* x *P. schlimii*). Terrestrial orchid with strap-shaped leaves, to 30cm (12in) long. Erect racemes of rounded, ivory-white flowers, 6cm (2½in) across, flushed and margined rose-pink, with twisted petals and rose-pink lips, appear sporadically throughout the year. ↕↔ 60cm (24in). ❀ (min. 14°C/57°F; max. 30°C/86°F)

PHRAGMITES

Reed

GRAMINEAE/POACEAE

Genus of approximately 4 species of rhizomatous, perennial reed grasses widely distributed in fen, marsh, and riverside habitats in temperate and tropical zones worldwide. They have robust stems bearing deciduous, flat, linear, mid- or slightly grey-green leaves.

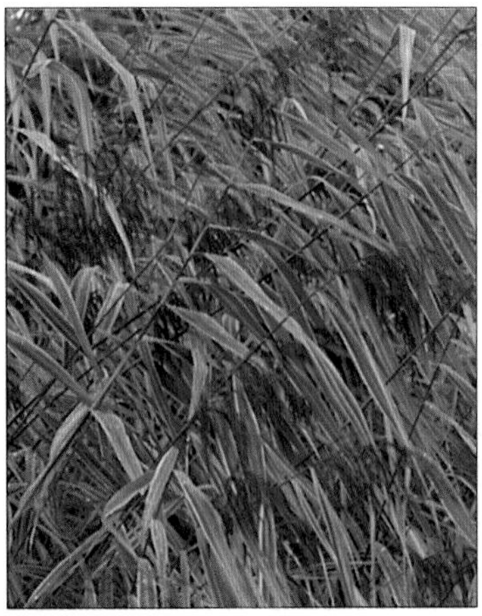

Phragmites australis 'Variegatus'

From late summer to mid- or late autumn, they produce large, plumed, silky-hairy panicles of 3- to 11-flowered spikelets, which are useful for dried arrangements. *P. australis,* the only species commonly grown, is vigorous and invasive, especially at the water's edge. Grow in naturalistic lakeside plantings with ample space. Where space is limited, grow in large containers sunk in water to restrict growth.
- **HARDINESS** Fully hardy.
- **CULTIVATION** Grow in moderately fertile, reliably moist, deep soil in full sun. Cut back dead stems by late winter.
- **PROPAGATION** Divide from early spring to early summer.
- **PESTS AND DISEASES** Trouble free.

P. australis, syn. *P. communis* (Common reed, Norfolk reed). Vigorous, rhizomatous reed grass with robust stems bearing flat, linear, long-pointed, greyish green leaves, to 60cm (24in) long, turning golden russet in autumn. From late summer to mid-autumn, bears spikelets in plume-like, silky-hairy, glistening, dark brownish purple panicles, to 45cm (18in) long. ↕ to 3m (10ft) in flower, ↔ indefinite. Tropical and temperate regions worldwide. ✻✻✻. **'Variegatus'** ■ is less invasive, and has leaves striped golden yellow, fading almost to white.
P. communis see *P. australis.*

PHUOPSIS syn. CRUCIANELLA

RUBIACEAE

Genus of one species of mat-forming, stem-rooting perennial found in open sites on hillsides in the Caucasus Mountains and N.E. Iran. It produces whorls of narrowly elliptic leaves, and is cultivated for its abundant clusters of small, tubular-funnel-shaped, scented flowers, each with 5 spreading petal lobes, borne at the tips of the stems in summer. Grow as ground cover on a bank, in a rock garden, or at the front of a border.
- **HARDINESS** Fully hardy.
- **CULTIVATION** Grow in moderately fertile, gritty, moist but well-drained soil in full sun or partial shade. Cut back after flowering to maintain a compact shape.
- **PROPAGATION** Sow seed in containers in an open frame in autumn. Divide or take stem-tip cuttings from spring to early summer.
- **PESTS AND DISEASES** Trouble free.

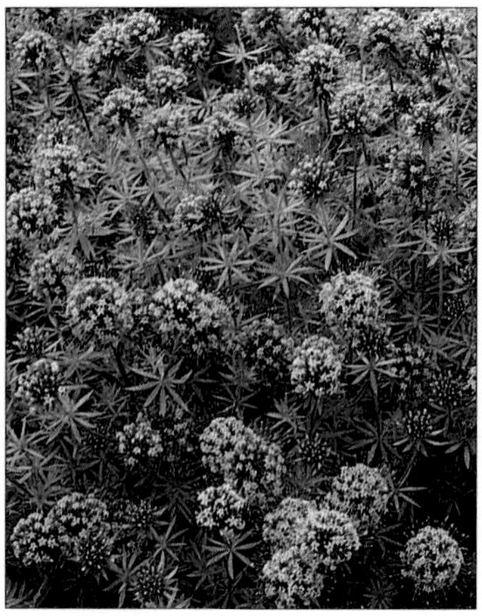

Phuopsis stylosa

P. stylosa ■ syn. *Crucianella stylosa.* Mat-forming perennial with slender, branching stems bearing whorls of 6–8 pointed, narrowly elliptic, musk-scented, pale green leaves, 1.5–2.5cm (½–1in) long. Produces rounded heads of many tiny, tubular-funnel-shaped pink flowers, 1.5–2cm (½–¾in) long, over long periods in summer. ↕ 15cm (6in), ↔ 50cm (20in) or more. Caucasus, N.E. Iran. ❄❄❄

PHYGELIUS

SCROPHULARIACEAE

Genus of 2 species of evergreen shrubs or subshrubs found on wet slopes and streambanks in South Africa. They are cultivated for their panicles of showy, tubular flowers, each with 5 recurved lobes, borne over a long period in summer and often into autumn. The ovate to lance-shaped, dark green leaves are mostly in opposite pairs, the upper leaves sometimes alternate. Grow in a shrub border or herbaceous border, or against a wall. Where temperatures regularly drop below 0°C (32°F), treat as herbaceous perennials. They may spread extensively by suckers, given ideal conditions.

• **HARDINESS** Frost hardy. *P. capensis* is hardy to -10°C (14°F).

• **CULTIVATION** Grow in fertile, moist but well-drained soil in full sun. Dead-head to encourage further flowering. In frost-prone areas, shelter from cold, drying winds, and provide a dry winter mulch. If grown as herbaceous perennials, cut back to the bases in spring; otherwise, pruning group 9.

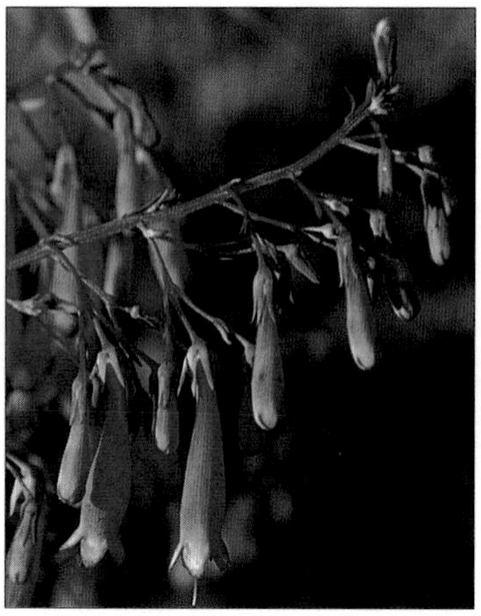

Phygelius aequalis

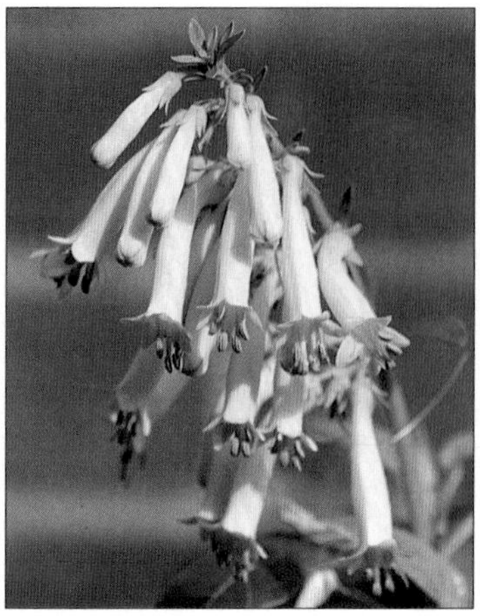

Phygelius aequalis 'Yellow Trumpet'

• **PROPAGATION** Sow seed in containers in a cold frame in spring. Take softwood cuttings in late spring. Remove rooted suckers in spring. Overwinter young plants under glass in frost-prone areas.

• **PESTS AND DISEASES** Figwort weevils and capsid bugs may be a problem.

P. aequalis ■ Upright, suckering shrub with ovate, dark green leaves, to 11cm (4½in) long. In summer, produces upright panicles, to 25cm (10in) long, of nodding, dusky pink flowers, to 6cm (2½in) long, with crimson lobes and yellow throats. ↕↔ 1m (3ft). South Africa. ❄❄. **'Yellow Trumpet'** ■ has pale green leaves, and bears pale creamy yellow flowers.

P. capensis ♀ (Cape figwort). Upright, suckering shrub with ovate, dark green leaves, to 9cm (3½in) long. In summer, bears upright panicles, to 60cm (24in) long, of yellow-throated orange flowers, to 5cm (2½in) long, with orange-red lobes; the flowers turn back towards the stems. ↕ 1.2m (4ft), ↔ 1.5m (5ft). South Africa. ❄❄. **'Coccineus'** has scarlet flowers.

P. x rectus (*P. aequalis* x *P. capensis*). Upright, suckering shrub with ovate,

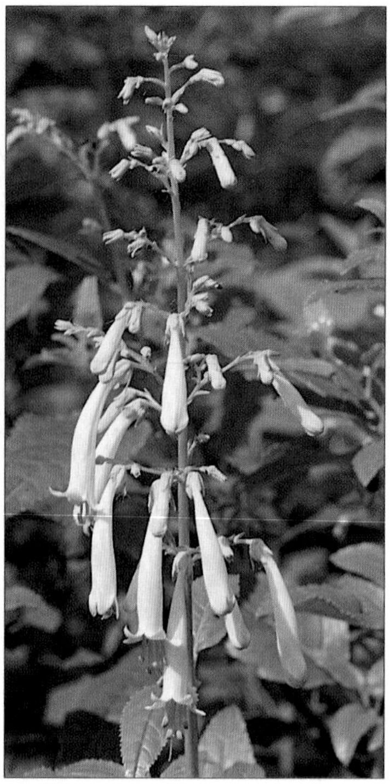

Phygelius x *rectus* 'Moonraker'

dark green leaves, to 10cm (4in) long. In summer, bears pale red flowers, to 6cm (2½in) long, in panicles 15–30cm (6–12in) long. ↕↔ to 1.5m (5ft). Garden origin. ❄❄. **'African Queen'** ■ bears pendent, pale red flowers, with orange-red lobes and yellow mouths, in upright panicles, 30cm (12in) or more long; ↕ 1m (3ft), ↔ 1.2m (4ft). **'Devil's Tears'** has pendent, deep red-pink flowers, turning back towards the stems, with orange-red lobes and yellow throats. **'Moonraker'** ■ has slightly downward-curved, pale creamy yellow flowers. **'Pink Elf'** produces slender, pale pink flowers, with spreading, dark crimson lobes, in panicles to 15cm (6in) long; ↕ 75cm (30in), ↔ 90cm (36in). **'Salmon Leap'** ■ has deeply lobed orange

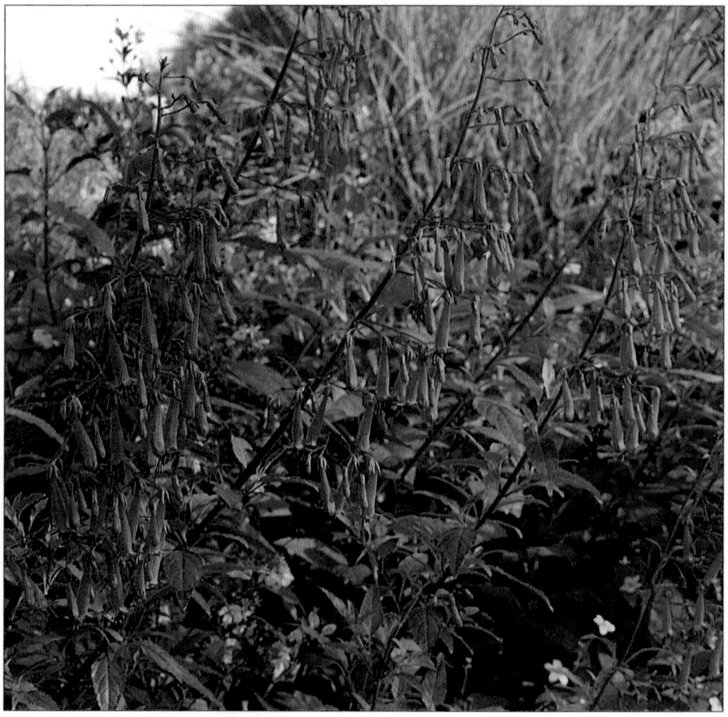

Phygelius x *rectus* 'African Queen'

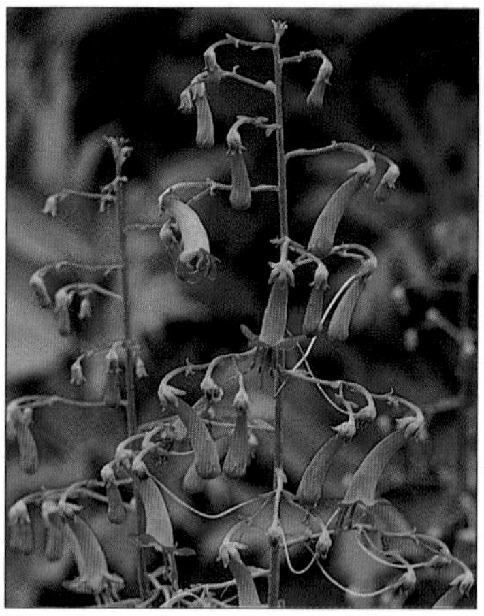

Phygelius x *rectus* 'Salmon Leap'

flowers, turning slightly back towards the stems, in panicles to 45cm (18in) long; ↕ 1.2m (4ft), ↔ 1.5m (5ft). **'Winchester Fanfare'** has pendent, dusky, red-pink flowers.

PHYLICA

Cape myrtle

RHAMNACEAE

Genus of about 150 species of heath-like, evergreen shrubs occurring in a range of habitats from seashores to rocky mountain slopes, mainly in South Africa but also in Madagascar and Tristan da Cunha. Leaves are small, alternate, often densely borne, usually narrow, simple, and entire, often with rolled margins. Each tiny flower either has 5 sometimes petal-like sepals and no petals, or has modified petals forming bristles or filaments. Where temperatures fall below 5°C (41°F), grow in a cool greenhouse. In warmer areas, use in a shrub border, or as a hedge or low windbreak.

• **HARDINESS** Frost tender, but may survive temperatures near 0°C (32°F) in a sheltered site, if the wood has been well ripened in summer.

• **CULTIVATION** Under glass, grow in lime-free (ericaceous) potting compost in full light; ventilate well. When in growth, water moderately and apply a balanced liquid fertilizer monthly. Keep just moist in winter. Outdoors, grow in moderately fertile, humus-rich, moist but well-drained, ideally neutral to acid soil in full sun. Pruning group 10, after flowering; clip hedges after flowering or in midsummer.

• **PROPAGATION** Sow seed at 13–18°C (55–64°F) in spring. Take greenwood cuttings in early summer.

• **PESTS AND DISEASES** Trouble free.

P. plumosa, syn. *P. pubescens.* Moderately bushy, downy shrub with wiry stems. Linear to lance-shaped, mid-green leaves, 1–3cm (½–1¼in) long, have rolled margins, and are dotted with glands above, long-hairy beneath. In spring, bears plume-like inflorescences of tiny, cup-shaped, dark brown flowers, surrounded by leaf-like bracts, 2–3cm (¾–1¼in) long, densely clothed in long, brownish white hairs. ↕ 1–2m (3–6ft), ↔ 0.75–1.5m (1½–5ft). South Africa. ❀ (min. 5°C/41°F)

P. pubescens see *P. plumosa.*

▷ ***Phyllanthus nivosus*** see *Breynia disticha*

P

x PHYLLIOPSIS

ERICACEAE

Hybrid genus of dwarf, evergreen shrubs, derived from crosses between *Phyllodoce* and *Kalmiopsis*. They are grown for their bell-shaped flowers, borne in spring. The stems are upright, bearing simple, alternate, glossy leaves. Grow in a peat bed, or in a shady site in a rock garden.
- **HARDINESS** Fully hardy.
- **CULTIVATION** Grow in moderately fertile, humus-rich, acid, reliably moist soil in deep or partial shade. Pruning group 10, after flowering.
- **PROPAGATION** Take semi-ripe cuttings in summer.
- **PESTS AND DISEASES** Trouble free.

x ***P. hillieri* 'Pinocchio'.** Upright shrub with branching, hairy shoots. Oblong-obovate, glossy, dark green leaves, 2cm (¾in) long, have margins slightly rolled under. Bears erect, terminal racemes of 5-lobed, widely bell-shaped, red-purple flowers, 1cm (½in) across, in late spring. ↕ 20cm (8in), ↔ to 30cm (12in). ❄❄❄

▷ ***Phyllitis*** see *Asplenium*
P. scolopendrium see *A. scolopendrium*
▷ ***Phyllocactus biformis*** see *Disocactus biformis*
▷ ***Phyllocactus eichlamii*** see *Disocactus eichlamii*

PHYLLOCLADUS

Celery pine

PHYLLOCLADACEAE/PODOCARPACEAE

Genus of 5 species of monoecious or dioecious, evergreen, coniferous trees and shrubs found in forests in Indonesia, Malaysia, the Philippines, Tasmania (Australia), and New Zealand. They have 2 kinds of shoots: normal shoots that produce radial, reduced, scale-like, non-functioning leaves, and flattened, modified shoots that form leaf-like, photosynthesizing elements called "phylloclades", which resemble the leaves of celery. Female cones each bear one to several seeds within fleshy, cup-like arils, usually on the edges of the phylloclades. Male cones are catkin-like, borne in terminal groups. Celery pines are unusual specimen plants, and are attractive in spring with their colourful male cones. In frost-prone areas, grow half-hardy species in a cool greenhouse.
- **HARDINESS** Frost hardy to half hardy.
- **CULTIVATION** Under glass, grow in loam-based potting compost (JI No.3), with added leaf mould, in full light. When in growth, water freely and apply a balanced liquid fertilizer every month. Water sparingly in winter. Outdoors, grow in any well-drained soil in full sun.
- **PROPAGATION** Sow seed at 6–12°C (43–54°F) in spring. Take semi-ripe cuttings in summer.
- **PESTS AND DISEASES** Trouble free.

P. trichomanoides ▣ ◊ (Tanekaha). Pyramidal tree with smooth, grey-black bark and whorled branches. Pinnate phylloclades, to 30cm (12in) long, each with 7–15 diamond-shaped segments, are reddish brown when young, then mid-green. In spring, produces spherical, dark blue or black female cones, 2cm (1in) long, and catkin-like,

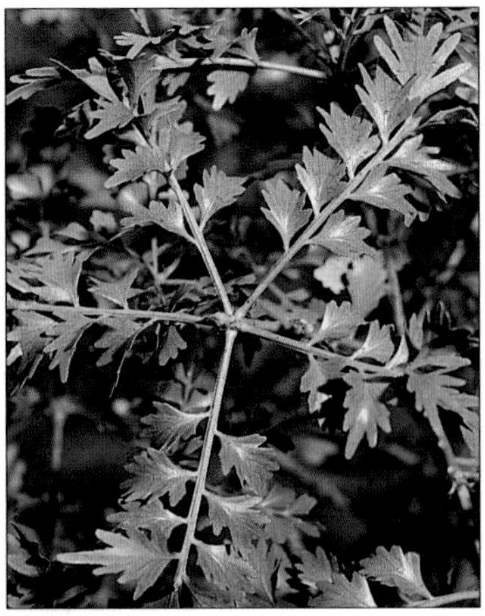

Phyllocladus trichomanoides

cylindrical purple male cones, 1cm (½in) long, ripening red then yellow, borne in clusters of 5–10. ↕ to 12m (40ft) or more, ↔ to 6m (20ft) or more. New Zealand. ❄

PHYLLODOCE

ERICACEAE

Genus of 8 species of spreading or erect, evergreen shrubs and subshrubs from alpine and arctic habitats in the N. hemisphere. Leaves are alternate, linear, leathery, downy beneath, with rolled, toothed margins. Bell-, urn-, or pitcher-shaped, nodding or horizontally held flowers are borne in terminal racemes or umbel-like clusters, sometimes solitary. Grow in a peat bed or rock garden.
- **HARDINESS** Fully hardy.
- **CULTIVATION** Grow in moderately fertile, humus-rich, moist but well-drained, acid soil in partial shade. Pruning group 10, after flowering.
- **PROPAGATION** Sow seed at 6–12°C (43–54°F) in early spring. Take semi-ripe cuttings in summer. Layer in spring.
- **PESTS AND DISEASES** Red spider mites may be a problem under glass.

P. aleutica. Decumbent or scrambling, mat-forming shrub with linear, minutely toothed, bright dark green leaves, 1.5cm (½in) long, softly yellow-downy and with a central white line beneath. In late spring and early summer, bears pendent, umbel-like clusters of urn-shaped, pale yellow-green flowers, to 8mm (⅜in) long. ↕ to 20cm (8in), ↔ 25cm (10in). Japan, Russia (Sakhalin, Kurile Islands, Kamchatka), USA (Alaska). ❄❄❄

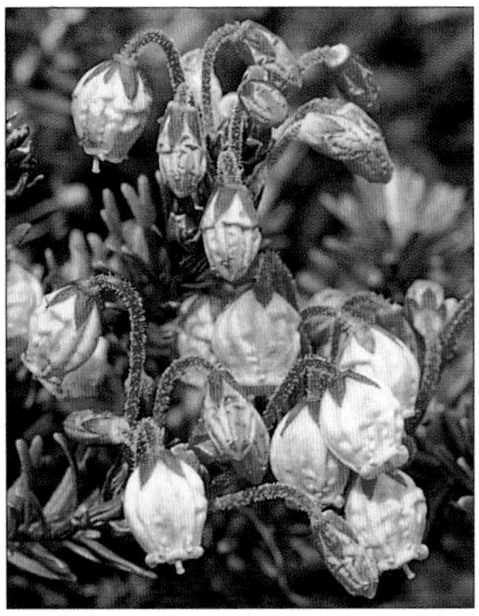

Phyllodoce x *intermedia* 'Drummondii'

P. caerulea 🏆 syn. *P. taxifolia.* Upright shrub with linear, fine-toothed, glossy, dark green leaves, to 1cm (½in) long, downy beneath. Pitcher-shaped, purplish pink flowers, 1cm (½in) long, are produced singly or in umbel-like clusters, in late spring and summer. ↕ 15–22cm (6–9in), ↔ 30cm (12in). Europe, Asia, USA. ❄❄❄

P. empetriformis ▣ Loose, mat-forming shrub with linear, glossy, bright green leaves, 1.5cm (½in) long, with glandular-toothed margins, downy beneath. Bears umbel-like clusters of long-stalked, bell-shaped, purple-pink to rose-red flowers, 9mm (½in) long, in late spring and early summer. ↕ 30cm (12in), ↔ to 40cm (16in). W. North America. ❄❄❄

P. x intermedia (*P. aleutica* var. *glanduliflora* x *P. empetriformis*). Bushy, low-spreading subshrub with linear, glossy, fine-toothed, dark green leaves, 1.5cm (½in) long, downy beneath. In mid-spring, bears umbel-like clusters of pendent, urn-shaped to narrowly bell-shaped, reddish purple to pink flowers, to 6mm (¼in) long, on slender red stalks. ↕ 15–23cm (6–9in), ↔ 35cm (14in). ❄❄❄. **'Drummondii'** ▣ has deep red-purple flowers.

P. nipponica 🏆 Erect subshrub with linear, dark green leaves, to 1cm (½in) long, with white-downy midribs beneath, and minutely glandular-toothed, rolled margins. Loose, umbel-like clusters of pendent, bell-shaped, white, sometimes pink-tinged flowers, 7mm (¼in) long, are borne on upright, red-tinted stalks in late spring and early summer. ↕↔ to 20cm (8in). Japan. ❄❄❄

P. taxifolia see *P. caerulea.*

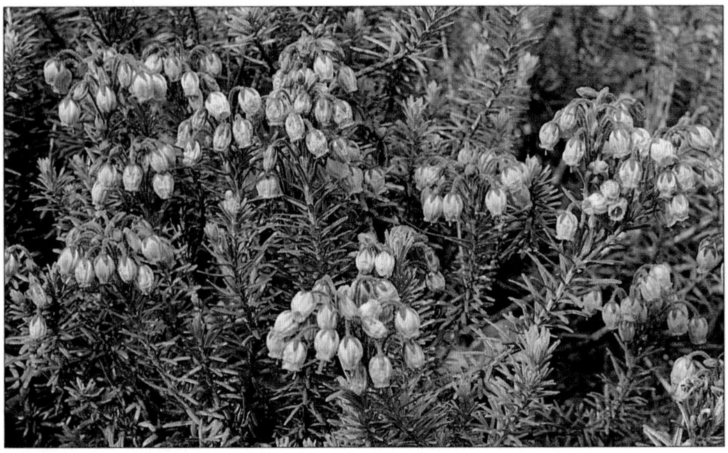

Phyllodoce empetriformis

PHYLLOSTACHYS

GRAMINEAE/POACEAE

Genus of about 80 species of medium-sized to large, evergreen bamboos occurring in deciduous woodland and groves in E. Asia and the Himalayas. They have a branching habit and spreading rhizomes, although in cool-temperate climates they usually form compact clumps. The canes are hollow and grooved, and often zigzag from node to node on young plants. Leaves are yellow-green or light to dark green, narrowly lance-shaped, and tessellated. Valued for their elegant form and foliage, some also for their subtly coloured canes, they are suitable for growing in containers outdoors, as specimen plants, or in groups among shorter shrubs in a border. They thrive in a woodland garden, and may also be used to create a screen.
- **HARDINESS** Fully hardy.
- **CULTIVATION** Grow in fertile, humus-rich, moist but well-drained soil in full sun or dappled shade. In containers, use loam-based potting compost (JI No.3), and apply a balanced liquid fertilizer monthly. In frost-prone climates, shelter from cold, drying winds.
- **PROPAGATION** Divide in spring.
- **PESTS AND DISEASES** Emerging young shoots may be damaged by slugs.

P. aurea 🏆 (Fishpole bamboo, Golden bamboo). Clump-forming, stiffly upright bamboo with grooved canes, bright mid-green at first, becoming brown-yellow when mature; there are cup-shaped swellings beneath each node, and the lower nodes are asymmetrical, distorted, and often densely crowded. Bears narrowly lance-shaped, yellowish to golden green leaves, to 15cm (6in) long. ↕ 2–10m (6–30ft), ↔ indefinite. S.E. China. ❄❄❄. **'Violascens'** see *P. violascens.*

P. aureosulcata (Yellow-groove bamboo). Clump-forming bamboo producing rough, brownish green canes, often zigzagged at the bases, with yellow grooves and striped sheaths. Leaves are narrowly lance-shaped and mid-green, to 17cm (7in) long. ↕ 3–6m (10–20ft), ↔ indefinite. N.E. China. ❄❄❄.

var. *aureocaulis* ▣ has sulphur-yellow canes, occasionally with green stripes near the bases; C. China. **'Spectabilis'** has thick yellow canes with green grooves.

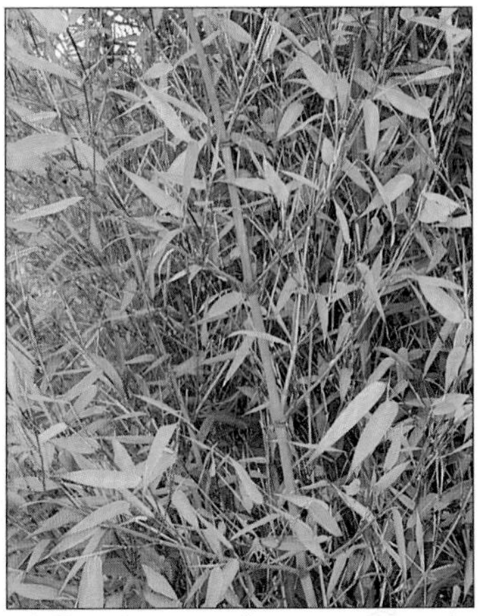

Phyllostachys aureosulcata var. *aureocaulis*

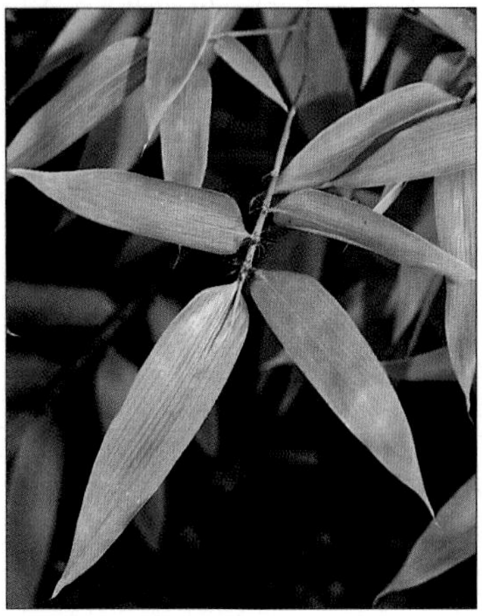

Phyllostachys bambusoides

P. bambusoides ■ (Giant timber bamboo). Clump-forming bamboo with thick, shiny, deep green canes and large, thick leaf sheaths with kinked bristles. Bears broadly lance-shaped, glossy, dark green leaves, to 20cm (8in) long. ↕ 3–8m (10–25ft), ↔ indefinite. China, possibly also Japan. ❄❄❄. **'Allgold'** ■ syn. 'Holochrysa', 'Sulphurea' of gardens, produces rich golden yellow canes, sometimes striped green; occasionally has yellow-striped leaves. **'Holochrysa'** see 'Allgold'. **'Sulphurea' of gardens** see 'Allgold'. **'Violascens'** see *P. violascens.*
P. flexuosa ■ (Zigzag bamboo). Clump-forming bamboo with slightly ribbed, slender, arching canes, often zigzagged between the nodes, bright green at first, turning yellow-brown to almost black with age, and with a waxy white bloom below the nodes. Bears narrowly lance-shaped, fresh green leaves, to 15cm (6in) long, which retain their colour throughout winter. ↕ 2–10m (6–30ft), ↔ indefinite. China. ❄❄❄
P. glauca see *P. violascens.*
***P.* 'Henonis'** see *P. nigra* var. *henonis.*
P. nigra ■🏆 (Black bamboo). Clump-forming bamboo with arching, slender green canes that turn lustrous black in

P

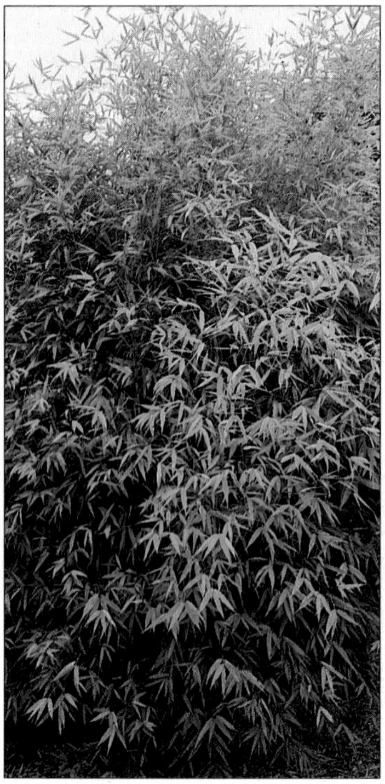

Phyllostachys bambusoides 'Allgold'

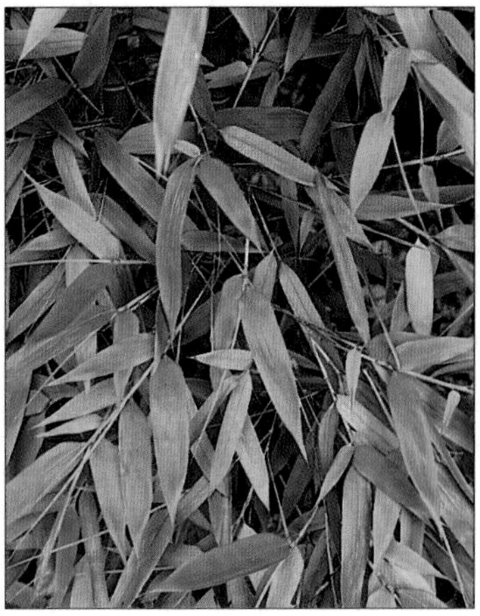

Phyllostachys flexuosa

their second or third year. Produces abundant lance-shaped, dark green leaves, 4–13cm (1½–5in) long. ↕ 3–5m (10–15ft), ↔ 2–3m (6–10ft). E. and C. China. ❄❄❄. **'Boryana'** has green to yellowish green canes with purple-brown marks. **var. *henonis*** ■🏆 syn. *P.* 'Henonis', has bright green canes, turning yellow-green when mature, and glossy leaves, downy and rough when young.
P. violascens, syn. *P. aurea* 'Violascens', *P. bambusoides* 'Violascens', *P. glauca.* Clump-forming then spreading bamboo with swollen green canes, finely striped purple, becoming violet. Bears narrowly lance-shaped, glossy, dark green leaves, to 12cm (5in) long, glaucous beneath. ↕ to 5m (16ft) or more, ↔ 2m (6ft) or more. China. ❄❄❄

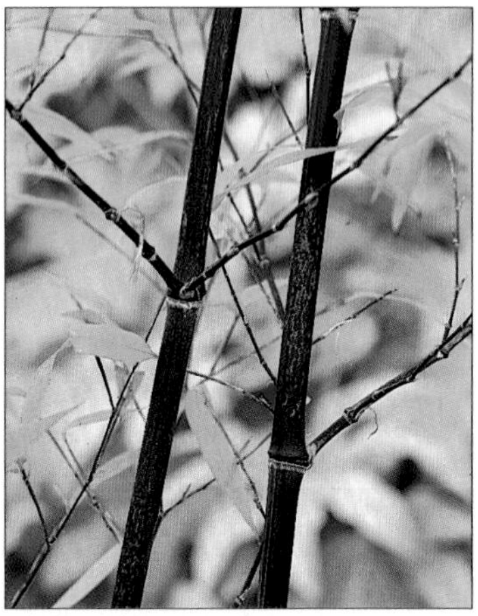

Phyllostachys nigra

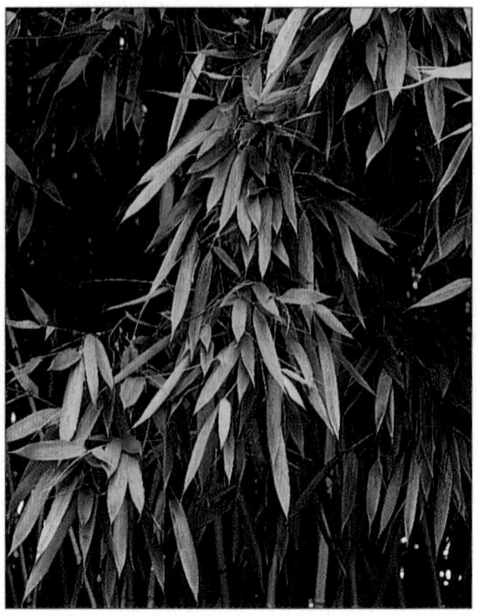

Phyllostachys nigra var. *henonis*

x PHYLLOTHAMNUS

ERICACEAE

Hybrid genus of one upright, evergreen shrub, derived from crosses between *Phyllodoce* and *Rhodothamnus*, grown for its heath-like, alternate, linear leaves and its funnel-shaped flowers, borne in late spring and early summer. Grow in a peat garden or shady rock garden.
• **HARDINESS** Fully hardy.
• **CULTIVATION** Grow in acid, humus-rich, moderately fertile, moist but well-drained soil in partial shade. Shelter from cold, drying winds. Pruning group 10, after flowering.
• **PROPAGATION** Root semi-ripe cuttings in summer.
• **PESTS AND DISEASES** Red spider mites may be troublesome under glass.

x *P. erectus* (*Phyllodoce empetriformis* x *Rhodothamnus chamaecistus*). Evergreen shrub with linear, glossy, dark green leaves, to 1.5cm (½in) long. Produces terminal clusters of 2–10 widely funnel-shaped, deep rose-pink flowers, 1cm (½in) across, in late spring and early summer. ↕ 25cm (10in), ↔ to 30cm (12in). Garden origin. ❄❄❄

▷ ***Phyodina*** see *Callisia*

PHYSALIS

Ground cherry

SOLANACEAE

Genus of about 80 species of upright, bushy, sometimes rhizomatous annuals and perennials found in sunny or lightly shaded, well-drained habitats worldwide, although mostly in the Americas. They have alternate or whorled, entire or pinnatifid, mid-green leaves. Tiny, inconspicuous, bell-shaped flowers, with star-shaped mouths, are produced singly (rarely in small clusters) from the leaf axils; they are followed by spherical, bright red, yellow, or purple, sometimes edible berries, enclosed in decorative, papery, orange to scarlet calyces. In some species, the calyces skeletonize, and persist throughout winter with the berries inside, remaining attractive; they can be used in dried arrangements. They are suitable for a border, although they may become invasive. All parts of *P. alkekengi*, except the fully ripe fruit, may cause mild stomach upset if ingested; contact with foliage may irritate skin.
• **HARDINESS** Fully hardy to frost hardy.
• **CULTIVATION** Grow in any well-drained soil in full sun or partial shade. Cut stems for drying as the calyces begin to colour.
• **PROPAGATION** Sow seed of perennials in containers in a cold frame in spring; sow seed of annuals *in situ* in mid-spring. Divide in spring.
• **PESTS AND DISEASES** Caterpillars may be a problem.

P. alkekengi ■🏆 (Chinese lantern, Japanese lantern). Vigorous, spreading, rhizomatous perennial with triangular-ovate to diamond-shaped leaves, to 12cm (5in) long. Nodding, bell-shaped cream flowers, 2cm (¾in) long, with star-shaped mouths, are produced from the leaf axils in midsummer, followed by large, bright orange-scarlet berries enclosed in papery red calyces, to 5cm

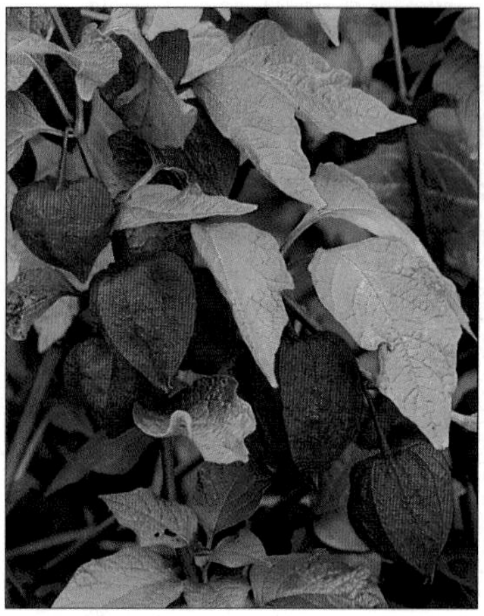

Physalis alkekengi

(2in) across. ↕ 60–75cm (24–30in), ↔ 90cm (36in) or more. C. and S. Europe, W. Asia to Japan. ❄❄❄. **var. *franchetii*** has broadly ovate leaves, and tiny, solitary, creamy white flowers, to 6mm (¼in) long.

PHYSARIA

Bladderpod

BRASSICACEAE/CRUCIFERAE

Genus of 14 species of rosette-forming, often short-lived perennials occurring mainly in the mountains of W. North America, usually in rocky sites and open screes. They are cultivated for their unusual, bladder-like seed pods and their attractive symmetrical rosettes of obovate to lance-shaped, mid-green, often silver-hairy leaves. Raceme-like clusters of 4-petalled, cross-shaped yellow flowers are borne in summer, followed by the inflated seed pods. Grow in a scree bed or alpine house; they are intolerant of excessive winter wet.
• **HARDINESS** Fully hardy.
• **CULTIVATION** Grow in moderately fertile, gritty, sharply drained soil in full sun. Protect from winter wet. In an alpine house, grow in a mix of equal parts loam, leaf mould, and grit.
• **PROPAGATION** Sow seed in containers in an open frame as soon as ripe.
• **PESTS AND DISEASES** Prone to damage by slugs and snails. May be infested with aphids and red spider mites under glass.

P. didymocarpa. Rosette-forming perennial with obovate, silver-grey leaves, 1.5–4cm (½–1½in) long, with a suede-like texture. In summer, bears open clusters of cross-shaped, bright yellow flowers, 2cm (¾in) across, followed by large, inflated, grey-hairy seed pods, 1cm (½in) long. ↕ 8–10cm (3–4in), ↔ to 15cm (6in). W. North America. ❄❄❄

PHYSOCARPUS

ROSACEAE

Genus of about 10 species of deciduous shrubs occurring in thickets and on rocky slopes in E. Asia and North America. They have peeling bark and alternate, ovate to rounded or kidney-shaped, palmately lobed, mid- or dark green leaves. They are cultivated for their foliage and dense, terminal corymbs of small, cup-shaped white flowers, borne in early summer. Grow in a shrub border.

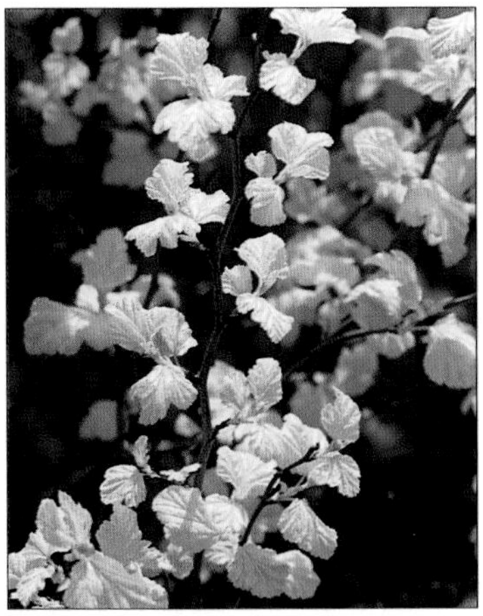

Physocarpus opulifolius 'Dart's Gold'

• **HARDINESS** Fully hardy.
• **CULTIVATION** Grow in preferably acid, fertile, moist but well-drained soil in full sun or partial shade. May become chlorotic if grown in shallow chalk soil. Pruning group 1 or 2.
• **PROPAGATION** Sow seed in containers outdoors in spring or autumn. Take greenwood cuttings in summer. Remove rooted suckers in autumn or spring.
• **PESTS AND DISEASES** Trouble free.

P. opulifolius, syn. *Spiraea opulifolius* (Ninebark). Compact, thicket-forming shrub, spreading by suckers, with arching branches and broadly ovate, 3-lobed, doubly toothed, mid-green leaves, to 8cm (3in) long. Small, cup-shaped, pink-tinged white flowers are produced in dense corymbs, 5cm (2in) across, in early summer, followed by clusters of bladder-like, green-flushed red fruit, 6mm (¼in) long. ↕3m (10ft), ↔5m (15ft). E. North America. ✲✲✲. **'Dart's Gold'** ■ ♀ has bright yellow young foliage; ↕2m (6ft), ↔2.5m (8ft).

PHYSOPLEXIS

CAMPANULACEAE

Genus of one species of tuft-forming, deciduous perennial found in rock crevices in the Alps. Clusters of unusual, bottle-shaped flowers arise from basal tufts of ovate to heart-shaped, toothed leaves. Grow in an alpine house, rock crevice, or scree bed; they are intolerant of winter wet.
• **HARDINESS** Fully hardy.
• **CULTIVATION** Grow in gritty, poor to moderately fertile, sharply drained, preferably alkaline soil in full sun, with some midday shade. Protect from winter wet. In an alpine house, grow in a mix of equal parts loam, leaf mould, and grit.
• **PROPAGATION** Sow seed in containers in an open frame in autumn.
• **PESTS AND DISEASES** Very susceptible to damage by slugs and snails.

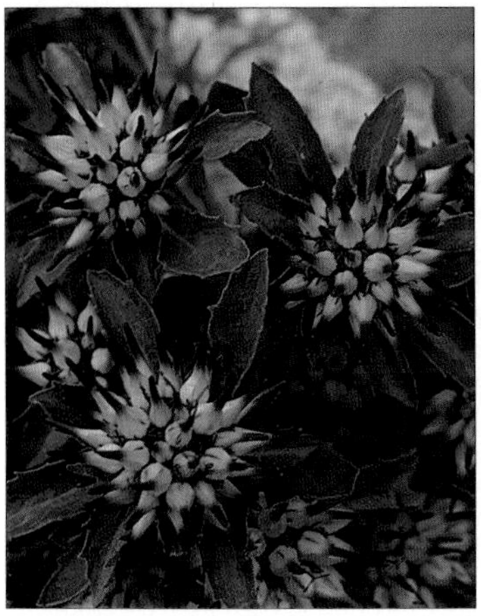

Physoplexis comosa

P. comosa ■ ♀ syn. *Phyteuma comosum*. Tufted, deciduous perennial with ovate to heart-shaped, deeply toothed, mid- to dark green leaves, 2–5cm (¾–2in) long. In late summer, bears terminal clusters of 10–20 bottle-shaped, pale violet flowers, to 2cm (¾in) across, with inflated bases and narrow "necks", and with tapered, deep violet tips. ↕8cm (3in), ↔ to 10cm (4in). Europe (Alps). ✲✲✲

PHYSOSTEGIA

Obedient plant

LABIATAE/LAMIACEAE

Genus of about 12 species of erect, hairless, deciduous, rhizomatous perennials occurring in moist, sunny sites in E. North America. They have square stems and alternate pairs of variable, often toothed leaves. Almost stalkless, tubular, 2-lipped, purple, pink, or white flowers, with flattish upper lips, 3-lobed lower lips, and tubular calyces, are borne in sometimes branched racemes, mainly in summer. The flowers will remain in a new position if they are moved on the stalks, hence the common name. Grow in a border; good for cut flowers.
• **HARDINESS** Fully hardy to frost hardy.
• **CULTIVATION** Grow in fertile, reliably moist soil in full sun or partial shade.
• **PROPAGATION** Sow seed in containers in a cold frame in autumn. Divide in winter or early spring before new growth.
• **PESTS AND DISEASES** Slugs may cause damage. Fungal and bacterial rots may affect damaged rhizomes.

P. speciosa see *P. virginiana*.
P. virginiana, syn. *P. speciosa* (False dragonhead, Obedient plant). Spreading perennial with lance-shaped, elliptic, or spoon-shaped, sharply toothed, mid-green leaves, to 13cm (5in) long. Bears racemes of deep purple or bright lilac-pink, sometimes white flowers, 2–3cm (¾–1¼in) long, with inflated mouths, from midsummer to early autumn. ↕to 1.2m (4ft), ↔60cm (24in) or more. E. North America. ✲✲✲. **'Bouquet Rose'** has pale, lilac-pink flowers. **'Galadriel'** is dwarf, with pale pink-purple flowers; ↕↔ to 45cm (18in). **subsp. *speciosa* 'Variegata'** see 'Variegata'. **'Summer Snow'** ♀ produces white flowers with green calyces; ↕↔ to 60cm (24in). **'Variegata'** ■ syn. subsp. *speciosa* 'Variegata', produces greyish green leaves with white margins, and magenta-pink flowers. **'Vivid'** ■ ♀ forms dense clumps, and bears bright purple-pink flowers; ↕30–60cm (12–24in), ↔30cm (12in).

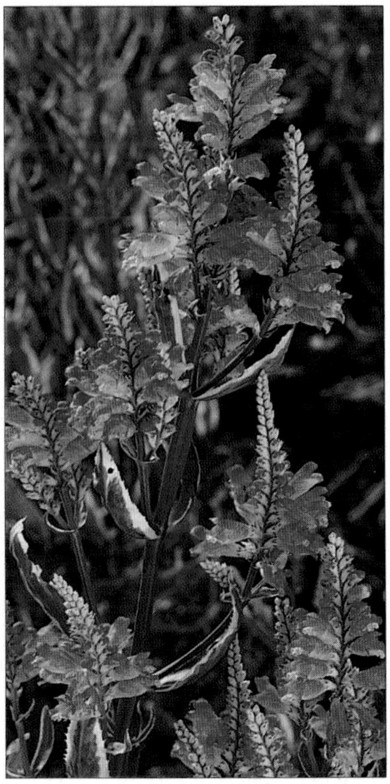

Physostegia virginiana 'Variegata'

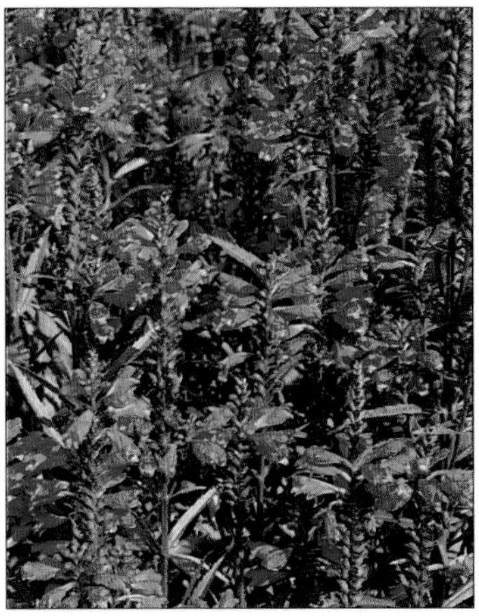

Physostegia virginiana 'Vivid'

PHYTEUMA

Horned rampion

CAMPANULACEAE

Genus of about 40 species of tuft- or clump-forming perennials from open mountain habitats, meadows, and light woodland in Europe and Asia. They have simple, often toothed basal leaves and erect stems with smaller leaves. They are cultivated for their terminal spikes or rounded clusters of stalkless, tubular, narrowly 5-lobed flowers, borne in summer, each flowerhead with a collar of leafy bracts. Grow in a sunny site in a rock garden or at the front of a border.
• **HARDINESS** Fully hardy.
• **CULTIVATION** Grow in moderately fertile, well-drained soil in full sun.
• **PROPAGATION** Sow seed in containers in a cold frame in autumn.
• **PESTS AND DISEASES** Prone to damage by slugs and snails.

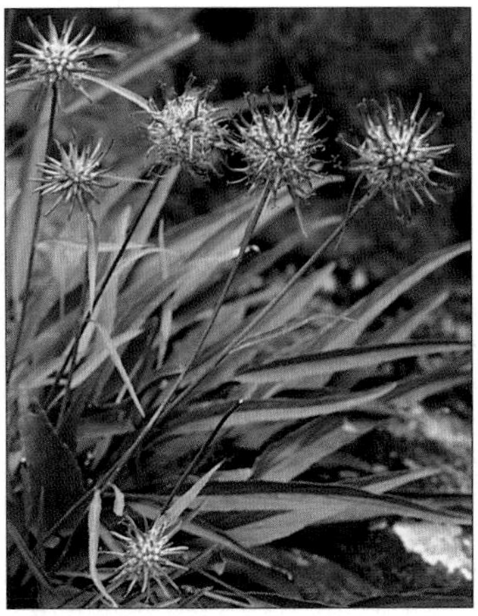

Phyteuma scheuchzeri

P. comosum see *Physoplexis comosa*.
P. humile. Compact, tuft-forming perennial with linear-lance-shaped, sparsely toothed basal leaves, 5–10cm (2–4in) long, and a few shorter stem leaves. In summer, bears violet-blue flowers in rounded clusters, to 2.5cm (1in) across, with linear bracts. ↕15cm (6in), ↔20cm (8in). Europe (C. and S.W. Alps). ✲✲✲
P. scheuchzeri ■ Tuft-forming perennial with linear-lance-shaped, sparsely toothed basal leaves, 5–15cm (2–6in) long, and shorter stem leaves. In summer, bears rounded clusters, 2.5cm (1in) across, of violet-blue flowers with linear bracts. ↕40cm (16in), ↔30cm (12in). Europe (Alps, Apennines). ✲✲✲

PHYTOLACCA

Pokeweed

PHYTOLACCACEAE

Genus of about 25 species of perennials, shrubs, and trees found in open fields or woodland in tropical and subtropical areas of Africa, Asia, and North to South America. They are grown for their attractive autumn foliage colour and their decorative fruits. Leaves are alternate, ovate to elliptic, and entire, and most of the perennial species have coloured stems. Racemes or panicles of small, shallowly cup-shaped, petalless flowers are followed by spherical, dark red to blackish purple berries. Grow in a large border, light woodland, or a waterside planting. All parts may cause severe discomfort if ingested; the fruit of *P. americana* may be lethal if eaten. Contact with the sap may irritate skin.
• **HARDINESS** Fully hardy to half hardy.
• **CULTIVATION** Grow in any fertile, moist soil in full sun or partial shade.
• **PROPAGATION** Sow seed at 13–18°C (55–64°F) in early spring.
• **PESTS AND DISEASES** *P. americana* may be a carrier of several viruses, such as yellows, mosaic, and ringspot.

P. americana ■ syn. *P. decandra* (Pokeweed, Red ink plant). Erect, unpleasant-smelling perennial with branching, red-marked stems and fleshy roots. Ovate to lance-shaped, mid-green

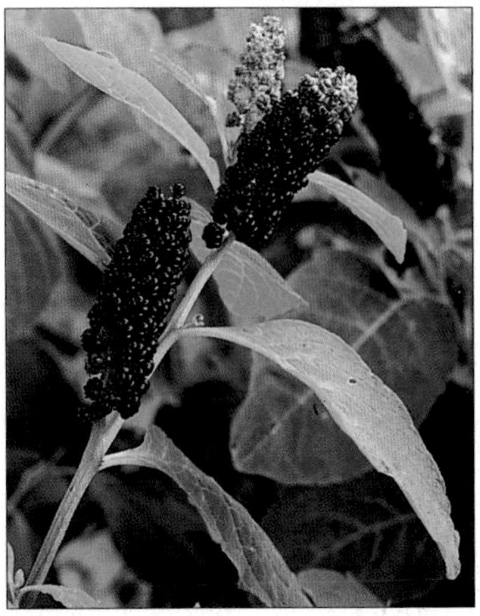

Phytolacca americana

leaves, 15–30cm (6–12in) long, are purple-tinged in autumn. From mid-summer to early autumn, bears white to pink flowers, 8mm (3/8in) across, in racemes 20cm (8in) long; these elongate to 30cm (12in), and are sometimes pendent when bearing the blackish maroon berries (highly toxic if ingested). ↕ to 4m (12ft), ↔ 1m (3ft). E. North America to Mexico. ✻✻✻

P. clavigera see *P. polyandra.*

P. decandra see *P. americana.*

P. polyandra, syn. *P. clavigera.* Erect, shrubby perennial with stems becoming vivid crimson. Ovate to elliptic, mid-green leaves, to 30cm (12in) long, turn yellow in autumn. In late summer, purplish pink flowers, 8mm (3/8in) across, are produced in erect, compact racemes, to 18cm (7in) long, elongating to 30cm (12in) long when bearing the dense masses of black berries. ↕ 2m (6ft), ↔ 60cm (24in). China. ✻✻✻

PICEA
Spruce

PINACEAE

Genus of 30–40 species of monoecious, evergreen, coniferous trees occurring in forest in cool-temperate regions of the N. hemisphere. They have whorled branches and needle-like leaves set singly around the shoots. The woody, oval to oblong-cylindrical female cones, terminal on main shoots and sideshoots, are erect at flowering, later pendent; they ripen in a season from green or red when young, to purple or brown when mature. Ovoid, yellow to red-purple male cones, 2–3cm (3/4–1 1/4in) long, are borne in spring on the previous year's shoots. Spruces are useful for shelter planting or as specimen trees; several cultivars are dwarf or slow-growing.

• **HARDINESS** Fully hardy to frost hardy.

• **CULTIVATION** Grow in any deep, moist but well-drained, ideally neutral to acid soil in full sun. *P. omorika* tolerates alkaline soils; *P. morrisonicola* needs shelter from cold, drying winds.

• **PROPAGATION** Sow seed in containers in a cold frame in spring. Graft cultivars in winter. Take ripewood cuttings of dwarf cultivars in late summer.

• **PESTS AND DISEASES** Adelgids may cause galls, and aphids may cause needle loss. Red spider mites may be trouble-some. Susceptible to honey fungus.

P. abies ▣ ♀ ◊–△ (Christmas tree, Norway spruce). Conical tree when young, columnar when mature, with red-brown bark and orange-brown shoots. Produces blunt, 4-sided, dark green leaves, to 2.5cm (1in) long, pointing forwards and upwards on the shoots, and cylindrical, deep green, later brown female cones, 10–20cm (4–8in) long. The most commonly cultivated spruce. ↕ 20–40m (70–130ft), ↔ 6m (20ft). S. Scandinavia to C. and S. Europe. ✻✻✻. **'Acrocona'** ◊ is small, with pendent branches, and produces abundant cones even on young plants; ↕ 1–3m (3–10ft), ↔ 3–4m (10–12ft). **'Gregoryana'** is a bushy, dwarf shrub, with a tight, rounded habit; ↕↔ 80cm (32in). **'Nidiformis'** ♀ is a spreading, slow-growing, bushy shrub with a hollow "nest" in the centre; ↕ to 1.5m (5ft), ↔ 3–4m (10–12ft). **'Ohlendorffii'** ▣ is a very slow-growing, rounded, bushy shrub, becoming more conical, with short leaves, to 8mm (3/8in) long; ↕ 3m (10ft), ↔ 2–5m (6–15ft). **'Reflexa'** ▣ is prostrate, unless trained on a stem, when it becomes pendent and weeping; ↕ to 15cm (6in), ↔ indefinite.

P. asperata ▣ ♀ △–△ (Dragon spruce). Conical or columnar tree with scaly, purplish grey bark and thick, ridged, yellow-brown shoots, turning ash-grey. Stout, curved, 4-sided, glaucous, blue-green to dark green leaves, 1–2.5cm (1/2–1in) long, point upwards on the shoots. Cylindrical, green, later light brown female cones are 5–15cm (2–6in) long. ↕ 25m (80ft), ↔ 6m (20ft). W. China. ✻✻✻

P. brachytyla △ (Sargent spruce). Conical tree, becoming domed in old age, with cracked grey bark and slender, white or pale brown shoots. Pendent branchlets bear flattened, glossy, mid-green leaves, white beneath, 1–2.5cm (1/2–1in) long, spreading at the sides of the shoots. Bears cylindrical, green, later dark brown female cones, 6–15cm (2 1/2–6in) long. ↕ 25m (80ft), ↔ 6–8m (20–25ft). C. to W. China. ✻✻✻

P. breweriana ▣ ♀ △ (Brewer spruce). Slow-growing, columnar tree with level branches, grey bark, becoming scaly, and pendent side branchlets. Stout, blunt, flattened leaves, glossy, deep green above, whitish green beneath, 2.5–3.5cm (1–1 1/2in) long, are arranged radially on the shoots. Cylindrical, red-brown female cones are 7–14cm (3–5 1/2in) long. ↕ 10–15m (30–50ft), ↔ 3–4m (10–12ft). USA (N. California, S. Oregon). ✻✻✻

P. engelmannii △ (Engelmann spruce). Conical tree with short branches, scaly, red-brown bark, and pale brown shoots. Flexible, slender, 4-sided, bluish green to steel-blue leaves, 1.5–3cm (1/2–1 1/4in) long, are arranged radially, pointing slightly forwards along the shoots. Ovoid to cylindrical, stalkless, light brown female cones, 2.5–7cm (1–3in) long, have flexible scales. ↕ 20–40m (70–130ft), ↔ to 5m (15ft). North America (Rocky Mountains). ✻✻✻

P. glauca ◊–△ (White spruce). Narrowly or broadly conical tree with ash-grey bark, becoming scaly, and buff-white shoots. Four-sided, blue-green leaves, 1–2cm (1/2–3/4in) long, are spreading at the sides of the shoots, overlapping above. Ovoid, green, later light brown female cones are 4–6cm (1 1/2–2 1/2in) long. ↕ to 50m (160ft), ↔ 3–6m (10–20ft). Canada, N. USA. ✻✻✻. **var. *albertiana* 'Conica'** ▣ ♀ syn. 'Albertiana Conica', is a neat, cone-shaped, dwarf, bushy shrub; ↕ 2–6m (6–20ft), ↔ 1–2.5m (3–8ft).

P. jezoensis* subsp. *hondoensis △ (Hondo spruce). Conical tree, becoming gaunt in old age, with large, spreading branches, fissured grey bark, and dense,

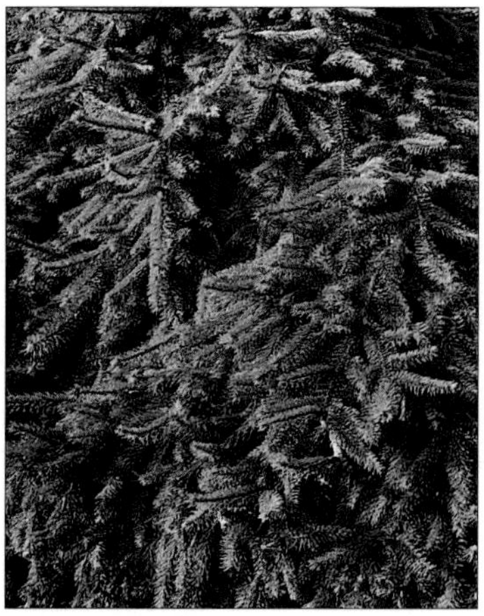
Picea abies 'Reflexa'

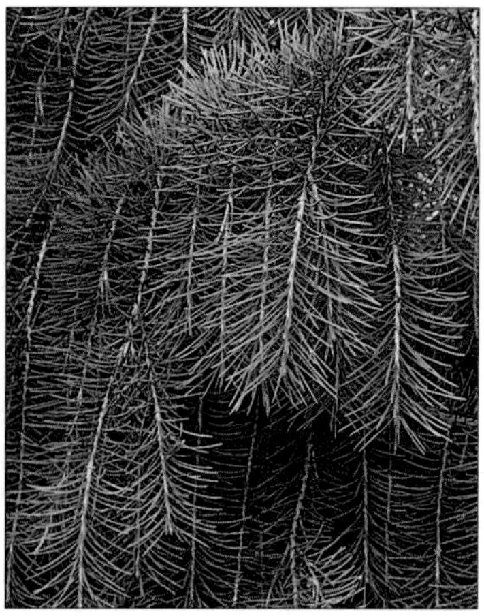
Picea breweriana

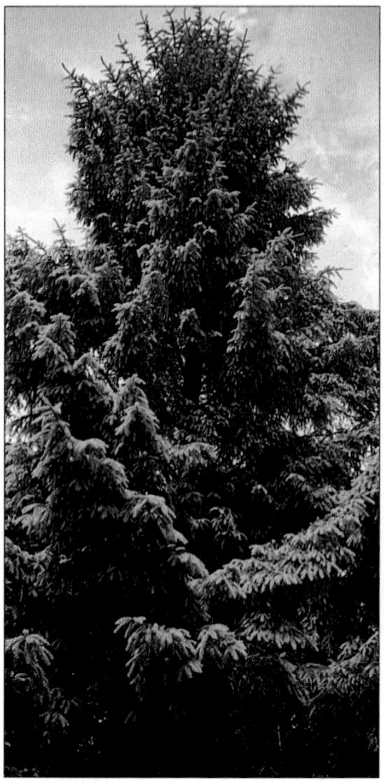
Picea abies

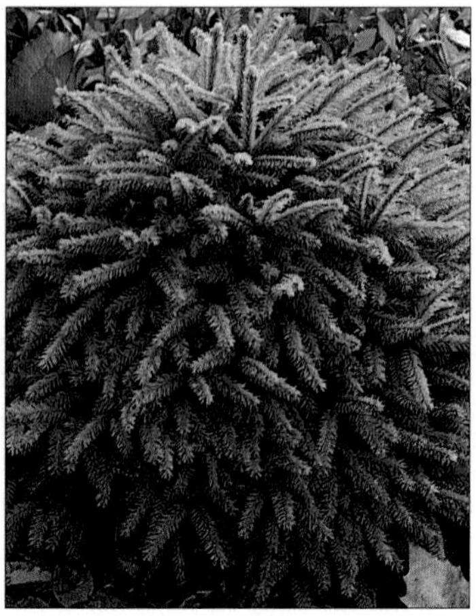
Picea abies 'Ohlendorffii'

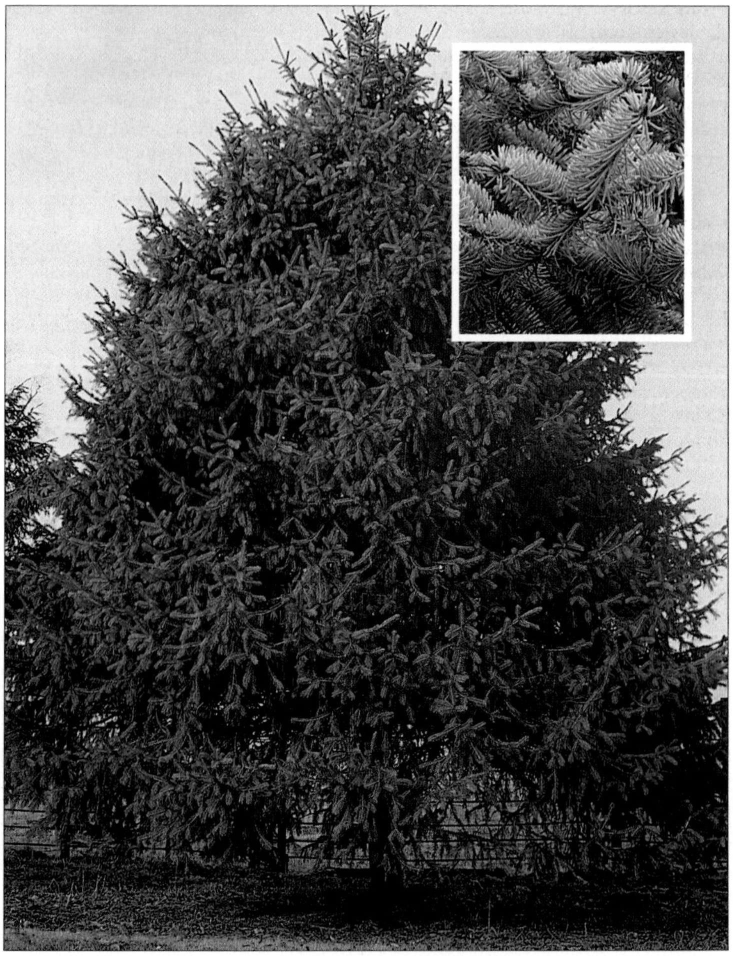
Picea asperata (inset: leaf detail)

P

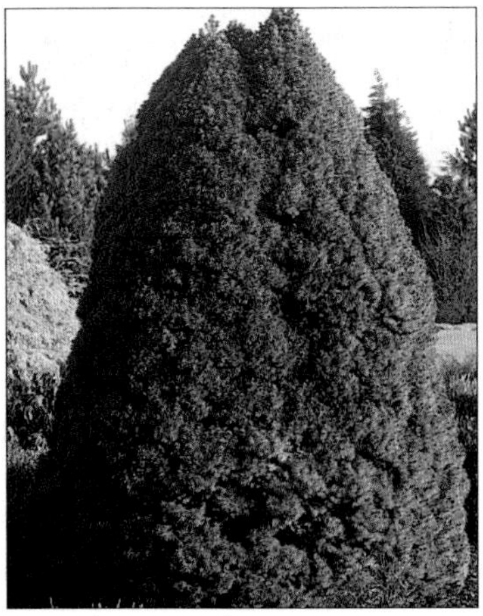

Picea glauca var. *albertiana* 'Conica'

pendent, white or pale brown shoots. Bears flattened, overlapping, glossy, dark green leaves, 1–2cm (½–¾in) long, bright silver beneath. Cylindrical, green, later pale reddish brown female cones, 4–6cm (1½–2½in) long, have thin, stiff scales. ↕ 30m (100ft), ↔ to 8m (25ft). Japan (Honshu). ❄❄❄

P. likiangensis △ (Lijiang spruce). Broadly conical tree with fissured or scaly grey bark and stout, pale brown shoots. Flattened, bluish green leaves, to 1.5cm (½in) long, overlap above the shoots, and spread below. Cylindrical, bright reddish purple, later brown female cones are 7–15cm (3–6in) long. Early-flowering if planted in poor, sandy soil. ↕ 30m (100ft), ↔ 6–9m (20–28ft). S. and W. China, S.E. Tibet. ❄❄❄

P. mariana △ (Black spruce). Conical tree with scaly, grey-brown bark and brown shoots with reddish brown hairs, the lower shoots often layering to form a skirt. Blunt, 4-sided, bluish green leaves are 0.5–2cm (¼–¾in) long. Ovoid, green, later grey-brown female cones, 2–3.5cm (¾–1½in) long, persist on the tree for 2–3 years. ↕ 10–20m (30–70ft), ↔ 2–3m (6–10ft). Canada, N.E. USA. ❄❄❄. **'Nana'** ▣ 🏆 is a rounded, bushy, dwarf shrub with bluish grey foliage; ↕↔ to 50cm (20in).

P. morrisonicola ▣ ◊ (Taiwan spruce). Conical tree with pink-brown or grey-brown bark and very slender, ash-grey shoots. Slender, 4-sided, grass-green leaves, to 1.5cm (½in) long, lie flat on top of the shoots and are spreading below. Oblong-cylindrical purple female cones are 5–7cm (2–3in) long. ↕ to 20m (70ft), ↔ to 5m (15ft). Taiwan. ❄❄

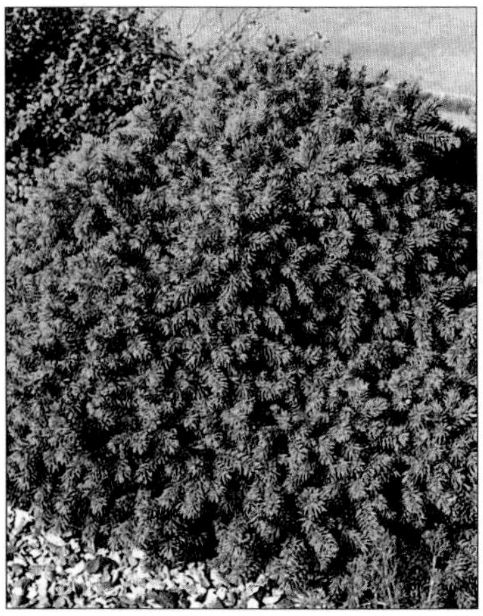

Picea mariana 'Nana'

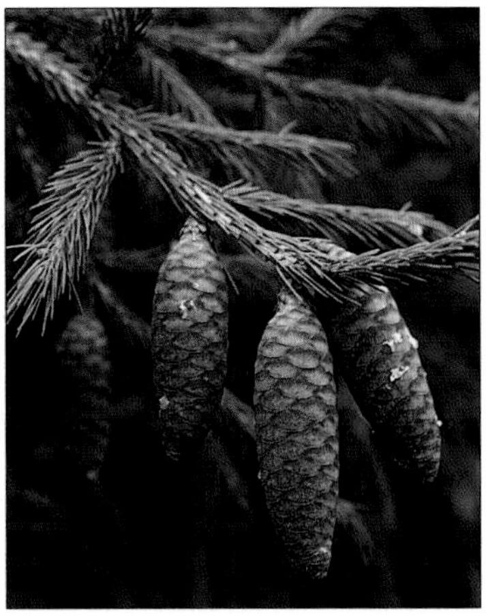

Picea morrisonicola

P. omorika ▣ 🏆 ◊ (Serbian spruce). Narrow, spire-like tree with pendent branches ascending at the tips, brown bark cracking into square plates, and orange-brown shoots with black hairs. Flattened, dark to blue-green leaves, 1–2cm (½–¾in) long, white beneath, lie flat at the sides of the shoots and are spreading below. Bears ovate-oblong, red-brown, later brown female cones, 3–7cm (1¼–3in) long. ↕ 20m (70ft), ↔ 2–3m (6–10ft). Bosnia, Serbia (Drina River valley). ❄❄❄. **'Gnom'** is a dense, broadly conical, dwarf shrub; ↕ to 1.5m (5ft), ↔ 1m (3ft).

P. orientalis 🏆 ◊–▯ (Caucasian spruce, Oriental spruce). Broadly columnar tree, conical when young, with smooth, pink-grey bark, becoming cracked with age, and hairy, grey-brown shoots. Very

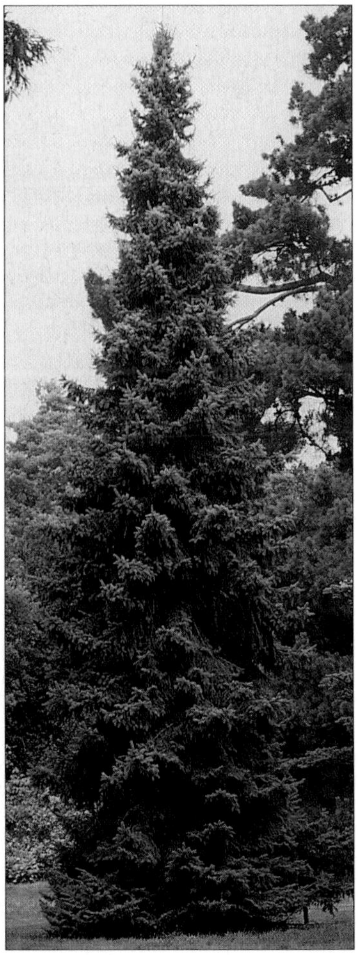

Picea omorika

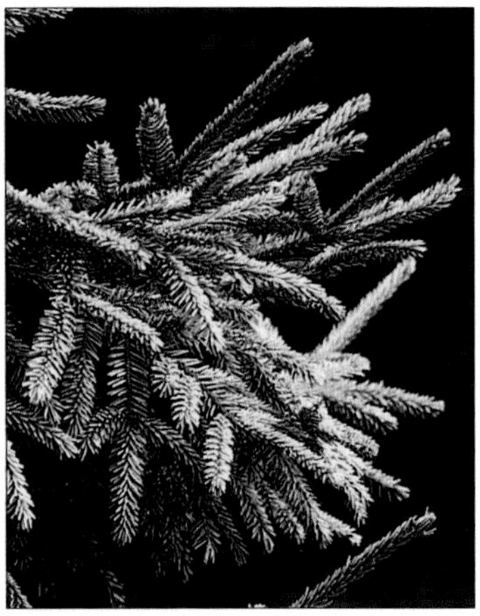

Picea orientalis 'Skylands'

short, blunt, 4-sided, dark green leaves, 6–8mm (¼–⅜in) long, are arranged radially on the shoots. Male cones are deep red. Ovoid-conical, dark purple, later brown female cones are 6–10cm (2½–4in) long. ↕ 30m (100ft), ↔ 6–8m (20–25ft). Caucasus, N.E. Turkey. ❄❄❄. **'Aurea'** 🏆 has bright creamy gold young foliage for 6 weeks in spring. **'Skylands'** ▣ is similar to 'Aurea', but the creamy gold colour lasts all year.

P. pungens ◊–▯ (Colorado spruce). Conical to columnar tree with scaly, purplish grey bark and stout, orange-brown shoots. Stiff, stout, sharp-pointed, 4-sided, bluish grey-green leaves, 1.5–3cm (½–1¼in) long, arranged radially on the shoots, curve upwards, and are covered in glaucous wax. Cylindrical, green, later pale brown female cones are 7–12cm (3–5in) long, with flexible scales. ↕ 15m (50ft), ↔ to 5m (15ft). USA (S. Rocky Mountains from Wyoming to Colorado). ❄❄❄. **'Hoopsii'** 🏆 has glaucous, blue-white foliage. **'Koster'** ▣ 🏆 has glaucous, silvery blue foliage. **'Montgomery'** is a slow-growing, dwarf shrub, with grey-blue leaves and a broad, conical habit; ↕ to 1.5m (5ft), ↔ 1m (3ft). **'Mrs. Cesarini'** is dwarf, with blue-green leaves; ↕ to 2m (6ft), ↔ 1.5m (5ft).

P. purpurea 🏆 ◊–△ (Purple-cone spruce). Columnar or conical tree with flaky, orange-brown bark and slender, densely hairy, buff-white shoots. Slightly flattened, glossy, mid-green leaves, grey-white beneath, 7–12mm (¼–½in) long, lie flat on top of the shoots and are spreading below. Ovoid, purple, later purple-brown female cones are 2.5–4cm

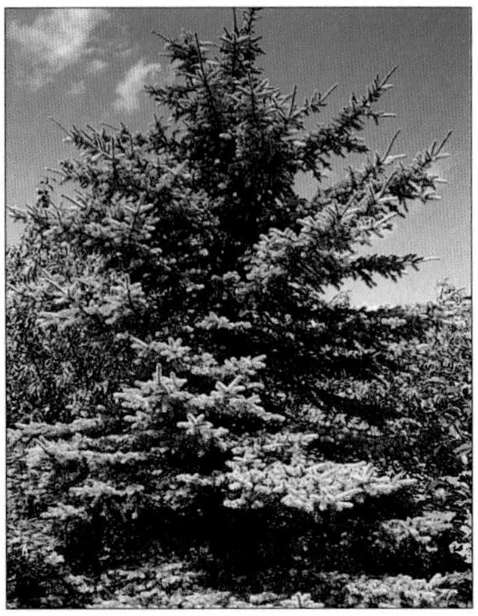

Picea pungens 'Koster'

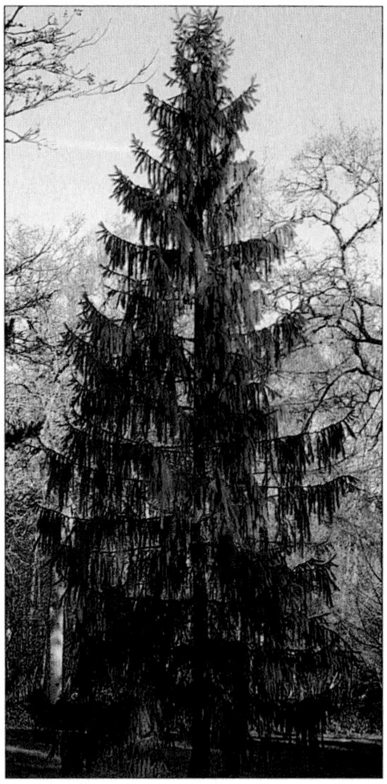

Picea smithiana

(1–1½in) long. ↕ to 20m (70ft), ↔ to 5m (15ft). N.W. China. ❄❄❄

P. sitchensis ◊ (Sitka spruce). Narrowly conical tree with wide-spreading branches when old, purple-brown bark becoming grey, and white shoots. Sharp-pointed, flattened, dark green leaves, white beneath, 2–2.5cm (¾–1in) long, overlap above the shoots, and spread below. Cylindrical, green, later pale brown female cones are 5–10cm (2–4in) long. ↕ 25–50m (80–160ft), ↔ 6–12m (20–40ft). Coastal W. North America (Alaska to California). ❄❄❄

P. smithiana ▣ 🏆 ◊–▯ (Morinda spruce). Conical then columnar tree with spreading branches, pendent branchlets, scaly grey bark, and pale brown shoots. Sparse, incurved, 4-sided, dark green leaves, to 4cm (1½in) long, are arranged radially. Cylindrical, green, later bright brown female cones are 10–20cm (4–8in) long. ↕ 20–30m (70–100ft), ↔ 6–9m (20–28ft). E. Afghanistan to W. Nepal. ❄❄❄

▷ **Pick-a-back plant** see *Tolmiea*
▷ **Pickerel weed** see *Pontederia*, *P. cordata*
▷ **Pickles, Little** see *Othonna capensis*

PICRASMA

SIMAROUBACEAE

Genus of 8 species of deciduous trees occurring in forest in E. and S.E. Asia, the West Indies, Central America, and tropical South America. They have alternate, pinnate leaves, each with a terminal leaflet, and produce axillary, umbel-like panicles of bowl-shaped flowers. *P. quassioides*, the most commonly grown species, is valued for its autumn foliage colour; grow in an open position in a woodland garden, or at a woodland margin.

• **HARDINESS** Fully hardy.

• **CULTIVATION** Grow in fertile, well-drained soil in full sun or partial shade. In frost-prone climates, shelter from cold, drying winds. Pruning group 1.

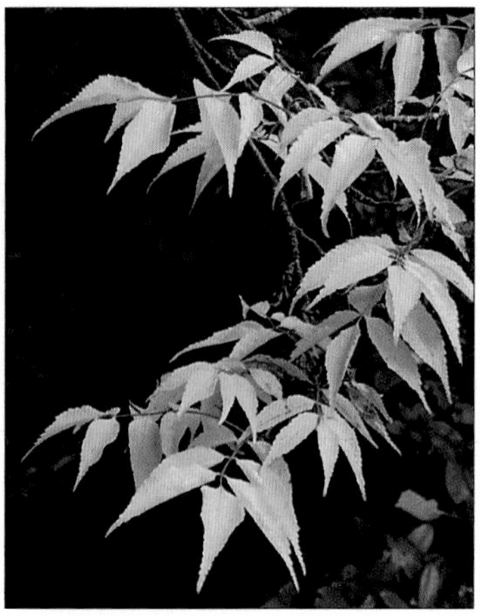
Picrasma quassioides

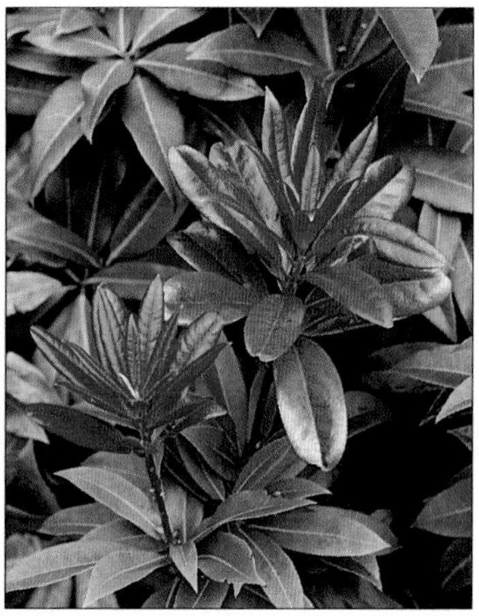
Pieris formosa var. *forrestii* 'Wakehurst'

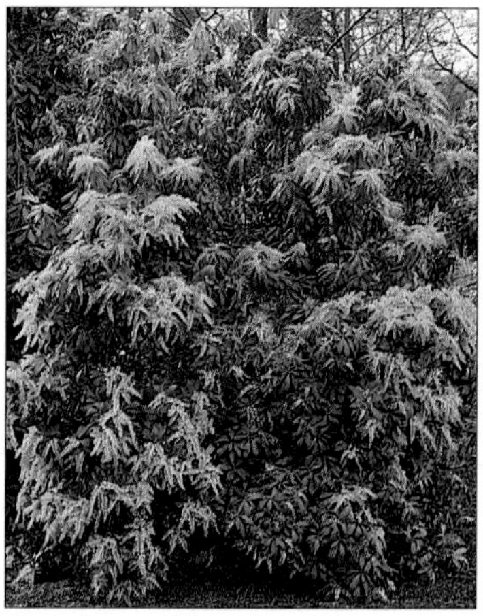
Pieris formosa 'Henry Price'

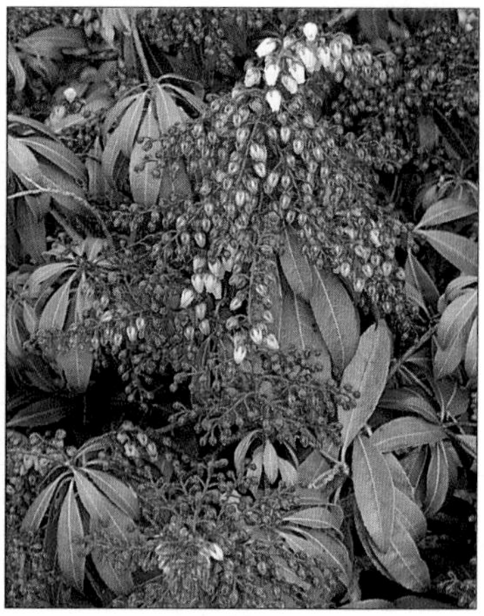
Pieris japonica 'Blush'

• **PROPAGATION** Sow seed in containers in a cold frame in autumn.
• **PESTS AND DISEASES** Trouble free.

P. ailanthoides see *P. quassioides.*
P. quassioides ■ ♀ syn. *P. ailanthoides* (Quassia). Upright tree with pinnate leaves, to 35cm (14in) long, composed of 9–15 ovate, sharply toothed, glossy, mid-green leaflets, turning yellow, orange, and red in autumn. Tiny, bowl-shaped green flowers are produced in umbel-like panicles, to 15cm (6in) long, in early summer. ↕↔ 8m (25ft). N. India, Nepal, Bhutan, China, Korea, Japan. ❄❄❄

PIERIS

ERICACEAE

Genus of 7 species of evergreen shrubs occurring in forest and on hillsides in the Himalayas, E. Asia, North America, and the West Indies. They are grown for their alternate or whorled, oblong or lance-shaped to obovate, glossy, mid- to dark green leaves, often attractively coloured when young, and their terminal panicles of small, urn-shaped flowers, 5–9mm (¼–⅜in) long, usually borne in spring. Grow in a shrub border, or in a peat or woodland garden. Leaves may cause severe discomfort if ingested.
• **HARDINESS** Fully hardy to frost hardy; young growth may be damaged by late frosts.
• **CULTIVATION** Grow in moderately fertile, humus-rich, moist but well-drained, acid soil in full sun or light shade. In frost-prone areas, shelter from cold, drying winds. Pruning group 8.
• **PROPAGATION** Sow seed in containers in a cold frame in spring or autumn. Take greenwood cuttings in early summer, or semi-ripe cuttings in mid- to late summer, with bottom heat.
• **PESTS AND DISEASES** Leaf spot and *Phytophthora* root rot may be a problem.

***P.* 'Bert Chandler'.** Conical shrub with lance-shaped, finely toothed leaves, to 10cm (4in) long, bright pink when young, turning creamy yellow and white, then dark green. Small white flowers are produced only rarely, in pendent panicles to 10cm (4in) long, in spring. ↕ 2m (6ft), ↔ 1.5m (5ft). ❄❄❄
***P.* 'Brouwer's Beauty'.** Dense, erect shrub with obovate to oblong-lance-shaped, lightly toothed, glossy, dark green leaves, 3–8cm (1¼–3in) long. In spring, bears white flowers in semi-erect or pendent, terminal panicles, 5–12cm (2–5in) long. ↕ to 3m (10ft), ↔ to 2m (6ft). ❄❄❄
P. floribunda ■ Compact, rounded shrub with elliptic-ovate, toothed, glossy, dark green leaves, to 8cm (3in) long. White flowers, opening from greenish white buds, are borne in erect, terminal panicles, to 12cm (5in) long, at the shoot-tips, in early and mid-spring. ↕ 2m (6ft), ↔ 3m (10ft). S.E. USA. ❄❄❄
***P.* 'Forest Flame'** 🏆 Compact, upright shrub with slender, inversely lance-shaped, finely toothed, glossy, dark green leaves, to 12cm (5in) long, bright red when young, turning pink, then creamy white, and finally green. White flowers, in erect then pendent, terminal panicles, to 15cm (6in) long, are borne in mid- and late spring. ↕ 4m (12ft), ↔ 2m (6ft). ❄❄
***P. formosa*.** Upright, often suckering, large shrub with oblong, finely toothed, glossy, dark green leaves, to 10cm (4in) long, bronze when young. White flowers are produced in large, semi-erect to pendent, terminal panicles, to 15cm (6in) long, in mid- and late spring. ↕ 5m (15ft), ↔ 4m (12ft). China, Himalayas. ❄❄. **var. *forrestii* 'Charles Michael'** has red young growth, and produces large flowers, 9–11mm (⅜–½in) long, in large panicles, to 18cm (7in) long. **var. *forrestii* 'Jermyns'** 🏆 is spreading, with arching branches and dark red young foliage; produces pendent panicles of white flowers opening from dark red buds; ↕↔ 2.5m (8ft). **var. *forrestii* 'Wakehurst'** ■ 🏆 has brilliant red young foliage. **'Henry Price'** ■ has deeply veined, very dark green leaves, dark bronze-red when young.
P. japonica ■ Compact, rounded shrub with narrowly obovate to elliptic, toothed, glossy, mid-green leaves, to 9cm (3½in) long. White flowers are produced in pendent or semi-erect, terminal panicles, to 15cm (6in) long, clustered at the tips of the shoots, in late winter and spring. ↕ 4m (12ft), ↔ 3m (10ft). E. China, Taiwan, Japan. ❄❄❄. **'Blush'** ■ 🏆 has very dark green leaves and pink-flushed white, later all-white flowers, opening from dark pink buds. **'Christmas Cheer'** has pink-stalked, crimped white flowers, with deep rose-red tips. **'Daisen'** has red flowers, opening from dark pink buds, and

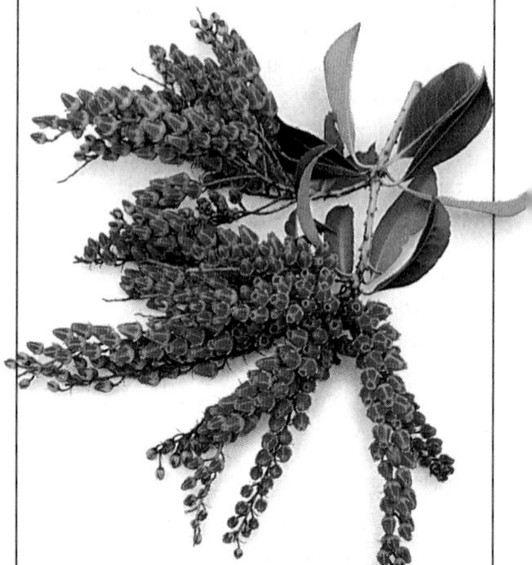
Pieris japonica 'Flamingo'

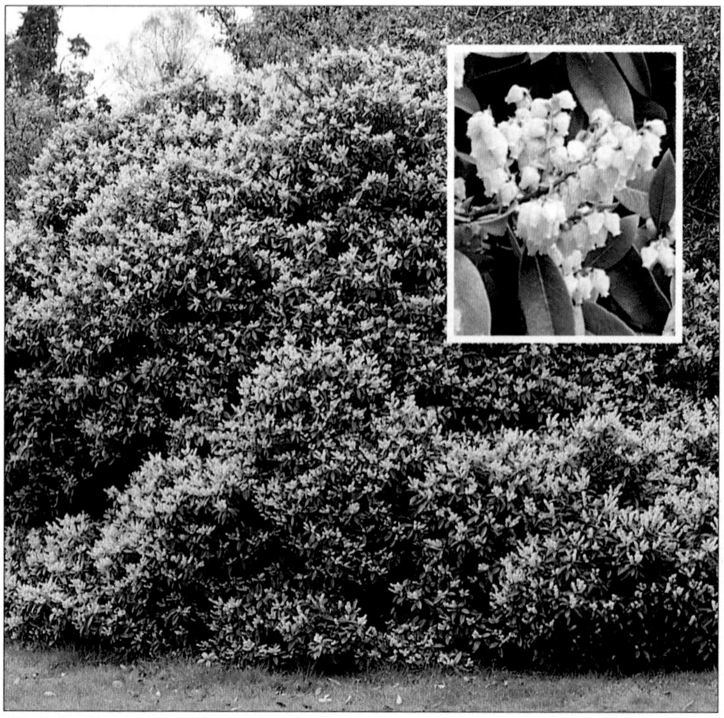
Pieris floribunda (inset: flower detail)

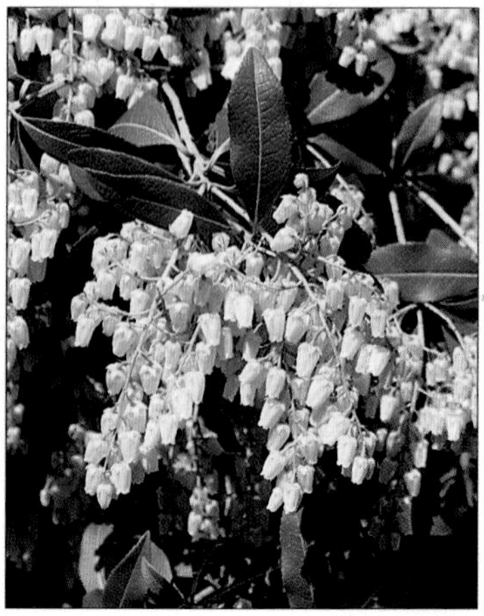
Pieris japonica

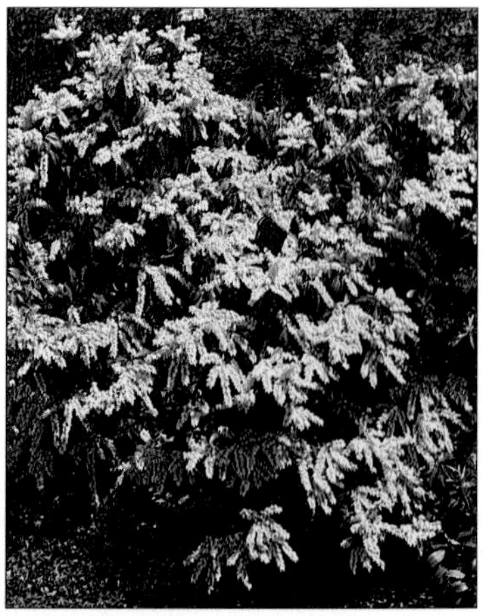
Pieris japonica 'Scarlett O'Hara'

P

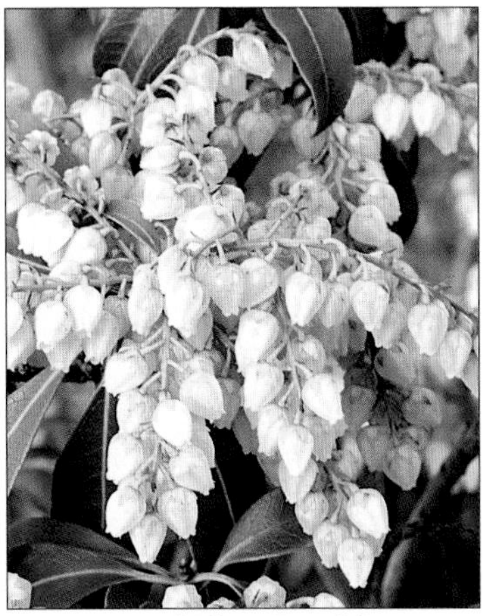

Pieris japonica 'White Cascade'

fading to pink. **'Debutante'** is compact and low-growing, with white flowers in dense, erect panicles, to 12cm (5in) long; ↕↔ 1m (3ft). **'Dorothy Wyckoff'** produces deeply veined, very dark green leaves, turning bronze in cold weather, and purple-red buds, opening pale pink, later turning white. **'Firecrest'** ♀ has deeply veined, dark green leaves, 10cm (4in) long, bright red when young; ↔ 2m (6ft); ❄❄. **'Flamingo'** ▣ has dark red buds, opening dark pink. **'Grayswood'** has brownish red new growth, narrow, dark green leaves, and white flowers borne in long, dense panicles, to 18cm (7in) or more. **'Little Heath'** ♀ is dwarf and compact, with leaves to 3cm (1¼in) long, pink-flushed when young, and with silvery white margins; ↕↔ 60cm (24in). **'Mountain Fire'** ♀ has red young leaves, turning glossy chestnut-brown. **'Purity'** ♀ is compact, and produces white flowers in upright panicles, and pale green leaves when young; ↕↔ 1m (3ft). **'Scarlett O'Hara'** ▣ has white flowers borne in dense panicles. **'Valley Valentine'** ♀ has large panicles of dark dusky red flowers. **'White Cascade'** ▣ has white flowers in long panicles, 18cm (7in) or more long, borne over a long period.
P. nana, syn. *Arcterica nana.* Wiry-stemmed, slow-spreading, cushion-forming, dwarf shrub with ovate-elliptic, leathery, toothed, dark green leaves, to 1cm (½in) long, in pairs or whorls of 3, tinted red-bronze in winter. In late spring and early summer, produces fragrant white flowers in pendent, terminal panicles, to 6cm (2½in) long. ↕ 8cm (3in), ↔ to 30cm (12in). Russia (Kamtchatka), Japan. ❄❄❄

▷**Pigeon berry** see *Duranta erecta*
▷**Pignut** see *Carya glabra*
▷**Pikake** see *Jasminum sambac*

PILEA

URTICACEAE

Genus of about 600 erect or creeping, semi-succulent annuals and evergreen perennials, sometimes woody at the bases, found in rainforest throughout tropical regions worldwide, except Australia. Stems may be branched or unbranched. They are cultivated for their textured, occasionally fleshy, attractively marked, opposite leaves, which are very variable in shape and colour. They also produce wispy, usually insignificant, unisexual, 3- or 4-tepalled

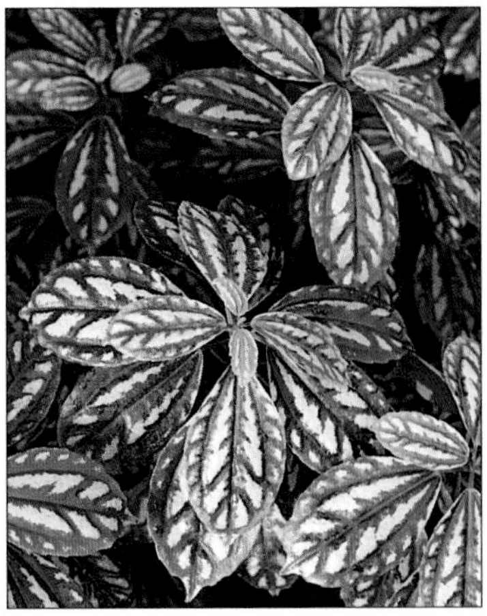

Pilea cadierei

flowers in cymes or panicles, or sometimes singly, from the leaf axils. In frost-prone areas, grow in a warm greenhouse or as houseplants; use trailing species in a hanging basket. In warmer climates, grow as ground cover in a damp, shady border.
• **HARDINESS** Frost tender.
• **CULTIVATION** Under glass, grow in shallow pans of loamless potting compost in bright indirect light, with high humidity. During the growing season, water moderately, allowing the surface to dry out between waterings, and apply a balanced liquid fertilizer every month. Water sparingly in winter. Outdoors, grow in any reliably moist soil in partial or deep shade.
• **PROPAGATION** Sow seed at 19–24°C (66–75°F) in spring. Divide or detach rosettes in spring. Root stem-tip cuttings with bottom heat in spring.
• **PESTS AND DISEASES** May be affected by powdery mildew.

P. cadierei ▣♀ (Aluminium plant). Erect perennial with branches becoming woody at the bases. The obovate to oblong-inversely-lance-shaped, toothed, dark green leaves, 8cm (3in) long, each

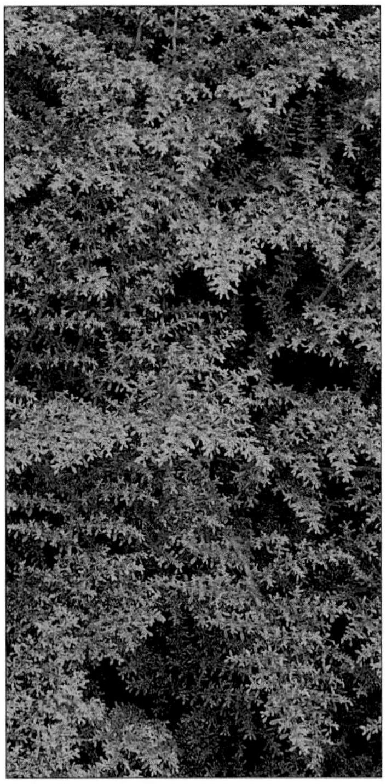

Pilea microphylla

have 4 rows of raised silver patches on the upper surface. ↕ 30cm (12in), ↔ 16–21cm (6–8in). Vietnam. ⊛ (min. 15°C/59°F). **'Minima'** ♀ is compact; ↕ 15cm (6in).
P. grandifolia. Rounded to upright, shrubby perennial producing ovate, coarsely toothed, glossy, dark or bronze-green leaves, 10–20cm (4–8in) long, with pointed tips, sometimes puckered between the veins. ↕ to 1.5m (5ft), ↔ to 80cm (32in). Jamaica. ⊛ (min. 10°C/50°F)
P. involucrata ▣ syn. *P. mollis* (Friendship plant, Panamiga). Trailing or creeping perennial producing tight rosettes of virtually stalkless, ovate to obovate, toothed, dark green leaves, 6cm (2½in) long, with bronze-flushed,

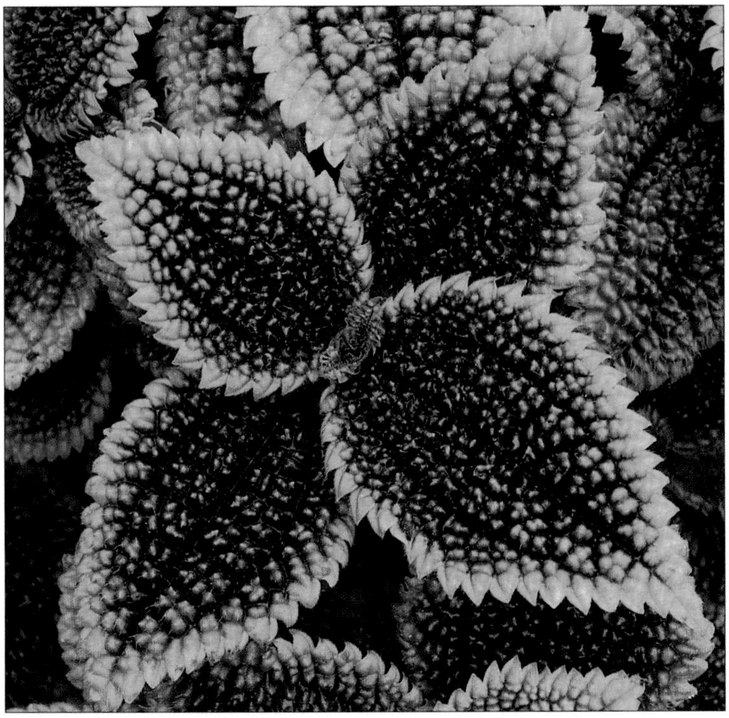

Pilea involucrata

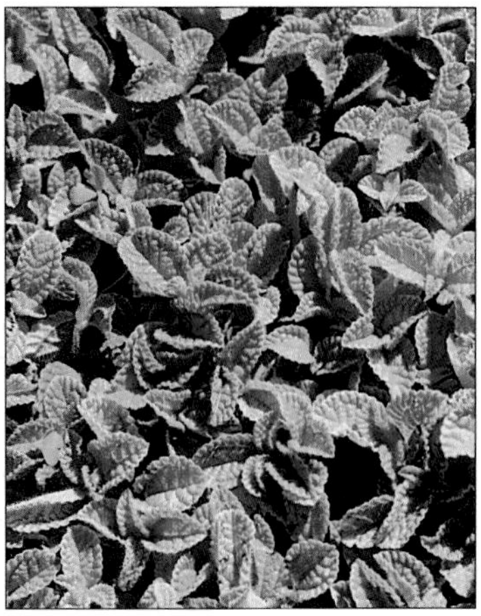

Pilea nummulariifolia

quilted surfaces, sometimes with paler margins. ↕ 3cm (1¼in), ↔ to 30cm (12in). Central and South America. ⊛ (min. 15°C/59°F). **'Moon Valley'** ♀ is more upright and open in habit, and produces ovate, toothed, fresh green leaves, to 10cm (4in) long, with deep purple sunken veins; ↕↔ 30cm (12in).
P. microphylla ▣ (Artillery plant). Densely branching, succulent annual or short-lived perennial with thick, almost erect, fleshy, hairless stems; these bear unequal pairs of obovate to rounded, semi-succulent, bright green leaves, to 1cm (½in) long, with blunt or pointed tips, or rounded leaves, to 3mm (⅛in) long. ↕↔ 30cm (12in). USA (Florida), Mexico, West Indies, South America. ⊛ (min. 15°C/59°F)
P. mollis see *P. involucrata.*
P. nummulariifolia ▣ (Creeping Charlie). Trailing or creeping perennial with frequently branching stems, rooting at the nodes. Rounded, deeply quilted, light green leaves, 2cm (¾in) long, fold inwards slightly at the midribs. ↕ 15cm (6in), ↔ 60cm (24in). West Indies, tropical South America. ⊛ (min. 15°C/59°F)
P. peperomioides ♀ Open-bushy, erect, perennial succulent with thick, fleshy stems covered with persistent stipules. Produces spirally arranged, long-stalked, elliptic to almost rounded, succulent, pale green leaves, 9cm (3½in) long. ↕↔ 30cm (12in) or more. China (Yunnan). ⊛ (min. 10°C/50°F)

PILEOSTEGIA

HYDRANGEACEAE

Genus of 4 species of woody, evergreen root climbers, related to *Hydrangea* and *Schizophragma*, occurring on forest trees and cliffs in India and E. Asia. They have opposite, obovate to oblong, mid-green leaves, and produce dense, terminal, corymb-like panicles of small, cup- or star-shaped, 4- or 5-petalled, creamy white flowers, in late summer and autumn. *P. viburnoides*, the most commonly cultivated species, is valued for its foliage and flowers. Grow on a large tree trunk or a wall.
• **HARDINESS** Hardy to at least -10°C (14°F).
• **CULTIVATION** Grow in fertile, well-drained soil in sun or shade. Pruning group 11, in early spring.
• **PROPAGATION** Root semi-ripe cuttings in summer. Layer in spring.
• **PESTS AND DISEASES** Trouble free.

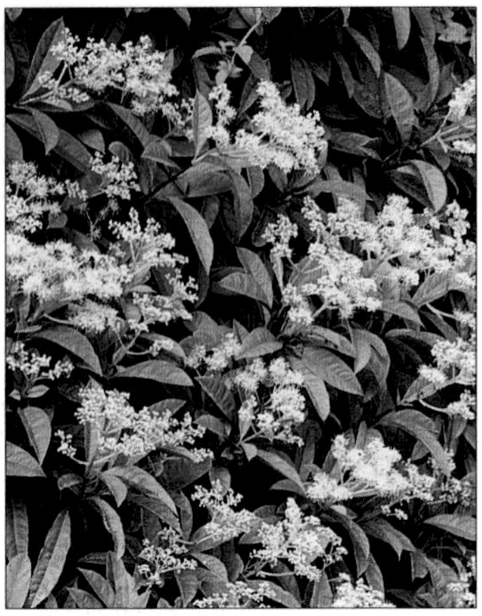

Pileostegia viburnoides

P. viburnoides ■ ♀ syn. *Schizophragma viburnoides*. Evergreen climber with oblong, leathery, dark green leaves, to 15cm (6in) long. Small, star-shaped, creamy white flowers, with prominent stamens, are borne in dense panicles, to 15cm (6in) across, in late summer and autumn. ↕6m (20ft). India, China, Taiwan. ❄❄

▷**Pilewort** see *Ranunculus ficaria*
▷***Pilgerodendron uviferum*** see *Libocedrus uvifera*
▷***Pilocereus senilis*** see *Cephalocereus senilis*

PILOSELLA

ASTERACEAE/COMPOSITAE

Genus of about 20 hairy, rhizomatous or stoloniferous herbaceous perennials from a variety of habitats in Eurasia and North Africa, including grassland, sand dunes, dry slopes, and open woodland. The ovate to narrowly lance-shaped or spoon-shaped, entire or toothed leaves are usually in basal rosettes, sometimes with smaller stem leaves. Greenish yellow or yellow to orange-red, rarely white or red, dandelion-like flowerheads are borne singly or in terminal clusters on usually leafless stems in summer. Grow in a wild garden or meadow, or on dry walls and banks.
• **HARDINESS** Fully hardy.
• **CULTIVATION** Grow in poor to moderately fertile, well-drained or dry soil in full sun or partial shade.
• **PROPAGATION** Sow seed in containers outdoors. Divide in autumn or spring.
• **PESTS AND DISEASES** Trouble free.

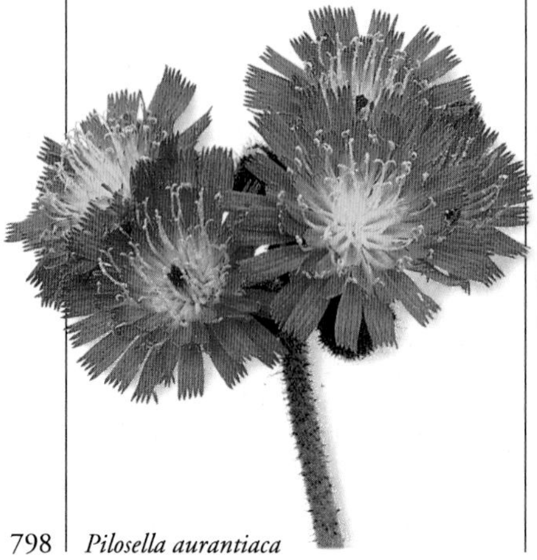

Pilosella aurantiaca

P. aurantiaca ■ syn. *Hieracium aurantiacum, H. brunneocroceum* (Fox and cubs, Orange hawkweed). Stoloniferous perennial with basal rosettes of elliptic to lance-shaped, bluish green leaves, to 20cm (8in) long. In summer, black-hairy stems bear dense clusters of 8–10 orange-red or orange-brown flowerheads, 1.5cm (½in) across. ↕to 20cm (8in), ↔ 90cm (36in). Grassy places in Europe. ❄❄❄

PILOSOCEREUS

CACTACEAE

Genus of 60 species of tree-like or bushy, perennial cacti, branching from the stems or the bases, found in warm, humid, moist areas of Mexico, Central and South America, and the West Indies. The many ribs have spiny, generally densely woolly, hairy areoles, sometimes as long as 5cm (2in), the wool forming skeins covering the ribs. In summer, nocturnal, tubular to bell-shaped flowers are borne from pseudocephaliums, from prominent areoles, or at the crowns, followed by fleshy, fig-like fruits. Below 15°C (59°F), grow in a warm greenhouse. In warmer areas, use as a focal point on a lawn or in a courtyard.
• **HARDINESS** Frost tender.
• **CULTIVATION** Under glass, grow in standard cactus compost in full light. From spring to summer, water freely and apply a balanced liquid fertilizer every 6–8 weeks. Keep just moist at other times. Outdoors, grow in gritty, moderately fertile, sharply drained soil in full sun. See also pp.48–49.
• **PROPAGATION** Sow seed at 19–24°C (66–75°F) in spring.
• **PESTS AND DISEASES** Vulnerable to mealybugs, and to ants if planted out.

P. leucocephalus see *P. palmeri*.
P. palmeri ■ syn. *P. leucocephalus*. Tree-like cactus with a blue-green stem, 5–10cm (2–4in) thick, with 7–9 rounded ribs. The areoles bear dark brown or greyish black spines (8–12 radials, 1 or 2 longer centrals), pale brown or yellow at first. Some areoles become covered with woolly grey hairs, borne more densely at the crown, forming a pseudocephalium. Pinkish purple flowers, 8cm (3in) long, purple-brown outside, are borne in summer. ↕to 6m (20ft), ↔ 1m (3ft). E. Mexico, Central America. ❀ (min. 15°C/59°F)

▷**Pilot plant** see *Silphium laciniatum*

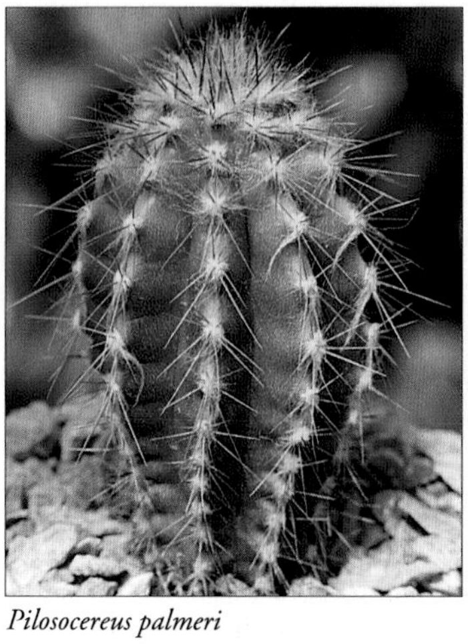

Pilosocereus palmeri

PIMELEA

THYMELAEACEAE

Genus of about 80 species of evergreen shrubs and subshrubs found in scrub, rocky places, and grassland from coastal areas to mountains in Australasia. Those commonly cultivated usually have opposite pairs of ovate to oblong leaves. Tubular, sometimes fragrant flowers, each with 4 spreading lobes, are borne in flat to almost spherical, terminal heads, surrounded by often colourful bracts. They are followed in some species by white, red, green, or black fruits (one-seeded drupes or nuts). In frost-prone areas, grow in containers outdoors and bring under cover in winter, or grow in a cool greenhouse. In warmer climates, grow in a border or a rock garden.
• **HARDINESS** Frost hardy to frost tender.
• **CULTIVATION** Under glass, grow in lime-free (ericaceous) potting compost with added sharp sand, in full light. During growth, water moderately and apply a balanced liquid fertilizer every month. Water sparingly in winter. Outdoors, grow in fertile, well-drained, neutral to acid soil in full sun. Pruning group 8.
• **PROPAGATION** Sow seed in containers in a cold frame in spring. Root semi-ripe cuttings with bottom heat in summer.
• **PESTS AND DISEASES** Red spider mites may be a problem in dry conditions under glass.

P. ferruginea ■ Bushy, domed shrub, at least when young. Densely borne, glossy, mid-green leaves, to 1cm (½in) long, are ovate to oblong, with rolled margins. In late spring and early summer, bears almost spherical heads, to 4cm (1½in) across, of slender-tubed, white-hairy, rose-pink flowers, 8mm (⅜in) across, surrounded by pink to red bracts. ↕ 1–2m (3–6ft), ↔ 1–1.5m (3–5ft). Australia (Western Australia). ❄
P. prostrata ■ Compact, spreading shrub with dark shoots and densely clustered, ovate, grey-green, often red-margined, leathery leaves, to 6mm (¼in) long. In summer, bears flat heads, to 2cm (¾in) across, of tubular, fragrant white flowers, to 6mm (¼in) across, followed by tiny, fleshy, white or red fruit. ↕ 20cm (8in), ↔ 50cm (20in). New Zealand. ❄❄
P. traversii. Upright shrub with densely overlapping, oblong, leathery, grey-

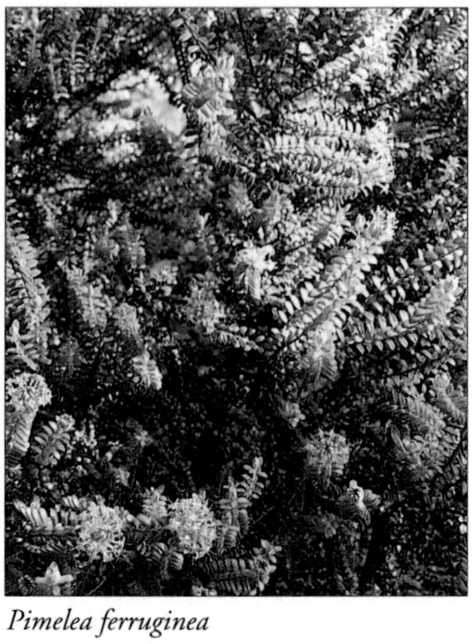

Pimelea ferruginea

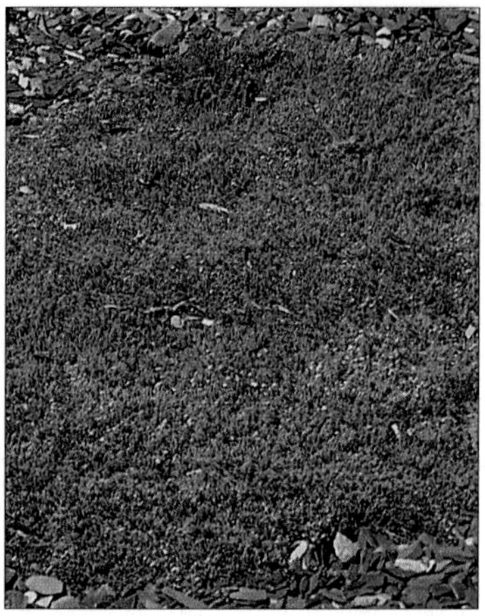

Pimelea prostrata

green, often red-margined leaves, to 1cm (½in) long. Flat heads, 2cm (¾in) across, of up to 20 silky-hairy, tubular, white or pink flowers, 6–8mm (¼–⅜in) across, are borne in summer. ↕↔ 50cm (20in). New Zealand. ❄❄

▷**Pimpernel** see *Anagallis*
Blue see *A. monellii*

PIMPINELLA

APIACEAE/UMBELLIFERAE

Genus of about 150 species of annuals, biennials, and perennials occurring in rough grassland, hedgerows, and woodland in Europe, N. Africa, Asia, and South America. Most have hairy stems, with simple or pinnate leaves, and bear compound umbels of tiny, star-shaped, usually white or yellow, sometimes pink or purple flowers, followed by ovoid-oblong to nearly spherical fruits. Most are suitable for naturalizing in a wild garden; *P. major* 'Rosea' is also effective in a border.
• **HARDINESS** Fully hardy.
• **CULTIVATION** Grow in any, but preferably fertile, moist soil in full sun or partial shade.

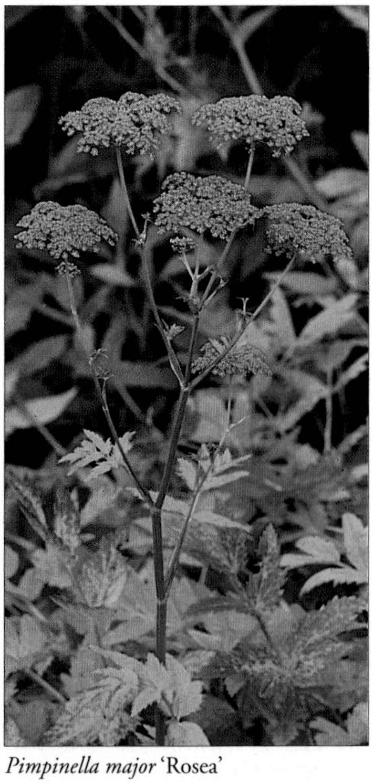

Pimpinella major 'Rosea'

• **PROPAGATION** Sow seed in containers in a cold frame as soon as ripe. Prick out into deep containers, to avoid damage to the tap roots when transplanting later.
• **PESTS AND DISEASES** Susceptible to aphids, slugs, and snails, and to powdery mildew in dry conditions.

P. major. Erect perennial producing triangular to rounded, pinnate, mid-green basal leaves, to 18cm (7in) long, each with 7–13 ovate to lance-shaped, lobed or toothed leaflets, 2–8cm (¾–3in) long, and smaller stem leaves. In mid- and late spring, ridged stems bear tiny, white, greenish white, or pink flowers in compound umbels, 6cm (2½cm) across. ↕ to 1.2m (4ft), ↔ 60cm (24in). Europe to Caucasus. ✻✻✻.
'Rosea' ▣ has both deep pink and pale pink flowers, in early and midsummer.

▷**Pinang** see *Areca catechu*

PINANGA

ARECACEAE/PALMAE

Genus of about 120 species of single- or cluster-stemmed palms occurring in undergrowth in dense, tropical rainforest at low to medium altitudes from the Himalayas to S. China, S.E. Asia, and Papua New Guinea. Simple or pinnate, variably shaped, light to dark green leaves are borne in terminal tufts above distinct crownshafts. Bowl-shaped, 3-petalled flowers are produced in spikes or panicles (erect at first, then becoming pendent) arising from the bases of the crownshafts. In frost-prone areas, grow in a warm greenhouse. In lowland, tropical areas, plant in a shady site near other trees or in a courtyard.
• **HARDINESS** Frost tender.
• **CULTIVATION** Under glass, grow in loam-based potting compost (JI No.3), with added peat and sharp sand, in bright filtered to low light. Pot on or top-dress in spring. During growth, water freely and apply a balanced liquid fertilizer monthly. Water moderately in winter. Outdoors, grow in fertile, moist but well-drained soil in dappled to deep shade.
• **PROPAGATION** Sow seed at 24°C (75°F) in spring.
• **PESTS AND DISEASES** Red spider mites may be troublesome under glass.

P. patula ▣ ✻ Small, cluster-stemmed palm with erect, smooth, cane-like stems with swollen bases. Irregularly pinnate leaves, to 1.5m (5ft) long, each have 16–36 lance-shaped, bright green leaflets. Bowl-shaped green flowers, turning red with age, are borne in recurved panicles, to 1cm (½in) across, usually in summer. ↕↔ to 2.5m (8ft). Indonesia (Sumatra), Borneo. ❀ (min. 16–18°C/61–64°F)

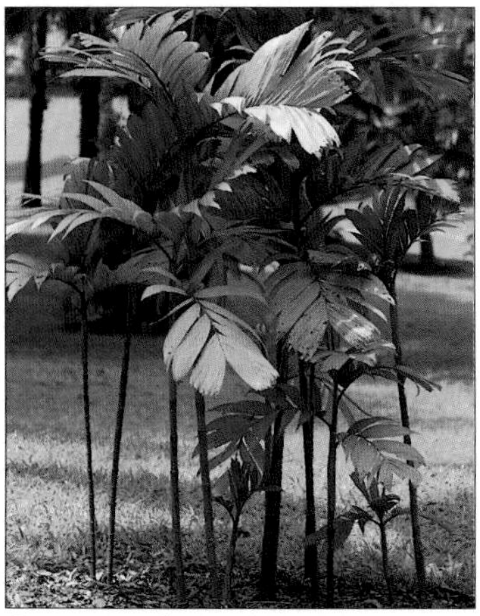

Pinanga patula

▷**Pincushion** see *Leucospermum*
Catherine's see *L. catherinae*
▷**Pincushion flower** see *Isopogon dubius, Scabiosa, S. atropurpurea*
▷**Pine** see *Pinus*
Aleppo see *Pinus halepensis*
Ancient see *Pinus longaeva*
Armand see *Pinus armandii*
Arolla see *Pinus cembra*
Australian see *Casuarina*
Austrian see *Pinus nigra*
Beach see *Pinus contorta*
Bhutan see *Pinus wallichiana*
Big-cone see *Pinus coulteri*
Bishop see *Pinus muricata*
Blue see *Pinus wallichiana*
Bosnian see *Pinus leucodermis*
Bristle cone see *Pinus aristata*
Canary Islands see *Pinus canariensis*
Celery see *Phyllocladus*
Chilean see *Araucaria araucana*
Chinese red see *Pinus tabuliformis*
Cook see *Araucaria columnaris*
Corsican see *Pinus nigra* subsp. *laricio*
Coulter see *Pinus coulteri*
Cowtail see *Cephalotaxus harringtoniana*
Cypress see *Callitris*
Digger see *Pinus sabiniana*
Dwarf mountain see *Pinus mugo*
Dwarf Siberian see *Pinus pumila*
Eastern white see *Pinus strobus*
European black see *Pinus nigra*
Foxtail see *Pinus balfouriana*
Holford see *Pinus* x *holfordiana*
Hoop see *Araucaria cunninghamii*
Jack see *Pinus banksiana*
Japanese black see *Pinus thunbergii*
Japanese red see *Pinus densiflora*
Japanese umbrella see *Sciadopitys verticillata*
Japanese white see *Pinus parviflora*
Jeffrey see *Pinus jeffreyi*
Kauri see *Agathis, A. australis*
King William see *Athrotaxis selaginoides*
Knobcone see *Pinus attenuata*
Korean see *Pinus koraiensis*
Lacebark see *Pinus bungeana*
Limber see *Pinus flexilis*
Lodgepole see *Pinus contorta, P. contorta* var. *latifolia*
Macedonian see *Pinus peuce*
Maritime see *Pinus pinaster*
Mexican weeping see *Pinus patula*
Mexican white see *Pinus ayacahuite*
Monterey see *Pinus radiata*
Montezuma see *Pinus montezumae*
Moreton Bay see *Araucaria cunninghamii*
Mountain see *Pinus uncinata*
New Caledonian see *Araucaria columnaris*
Norfolk Island see *Araucaria heterophylla*
Oyster bay cypress see *Callitris rhomboidea*
Pitch see *Pinus rigida*
Ponderosa see *Pinus ponderosa*
Prince's see *Chimaphila*
Radiata see *Pinus radiata*
Red see *Pinus resinosa*
▷**Pine cont.**
Scots see *Pinus sylvestris*
Screw see *Pandanus*
Shore see *Pinus contorta*
Stone see *Pinus pinea*
Swiss stone see *Pinus cembra*
Tasman celery see *Phyllocladus aspleniifolius*
Tasmanian cypress see *Callitris oblonga*
Umbrella see *Pinus pinea*
Western white see *Pinus monticola*
Western yellow see *Pinus ponderosa*
Weymouth see *Pinus strobus*
▷**Pineapple** see *Ananas*
Red see *A. bracteatus*
Wild see *A. bracteatus*
▷**Pineapple flower** see *Eucomis*
Giant see *E. pallidiflora*
▷**Pineapple guava** see *Acca sellowiana*

PINELLIA

ARACEAE

Genus of about 6 species of tuberous perennials found in deciduous forest, in cultivated fields, and at roadsides in China, Korea, and Japan. The simple, 3-palmate or pedate, basal leaves are rounded to ovate-lance-shaped or heart-shaped. Usually long, fine, black, green, or dark purple spadices, protruding from cylindrical spathes, are produced in summer. Grow in a peat bed or rock garden.
• **HARDINESS** Frost hardy.
• **CULTIVATION** Plant tubers 10–15cm (4–6in) deep in spring. Grow in fertile, humus-rich, well-drained soil in full sun or partial shade.
• **PROPAGATION** Sow seed in containers in a cold frame as soon as ripe. Remove offsets in autumn or early spring, or detach bulbils in late summer.
• **PESTS AND DISEASES** Trouble free.

P. pedatisecta. Tuberous perennial bearing pedate, mid-green leaves, each with 7–11 ovate to lance-shaped segments, 18cm (7in) long. Yellow-green spathes, 10–18cm (4–7in) long, each concealing a yellow-green spadix, rise above the leaves in summer. ↕ 18cm (7in), ↔ 8cm (3in). N. and W. China, Japan. ✻✻
P. ternata. Tuberous perennial with 3-palmate, mid-green leaves, composed of ovate-elliptic to oblong segments, 3–12cm (1¼–5in) long. Produces slightly hooded green spathes, to 7cm (3in) long, each with a protruding, slender green spadix, in summer. ↕ to 20cm (8in), ↔ 5cm (2in). China, Korea, Japan. ✻✻

PINGUICULA

Butterwort

LENTIBULARIACEAE

Genus of about 45 species of spring- or summer-flowering, insectivorous perennials from boggy habitats widely distributed in the N. hemisphere and in South America. They have rosettes of mucilage-secreting, lance-shaped to almost rounded leaves, and leafless stems bearing solitary, spurred, 2-lipped, trumpet-shaped flowers, the upper lip 2-lobed, the lower with 3 widely spreading lobes. Some species die back to resting buds in winter. The sticky leaves trap insects, which are then digested; under

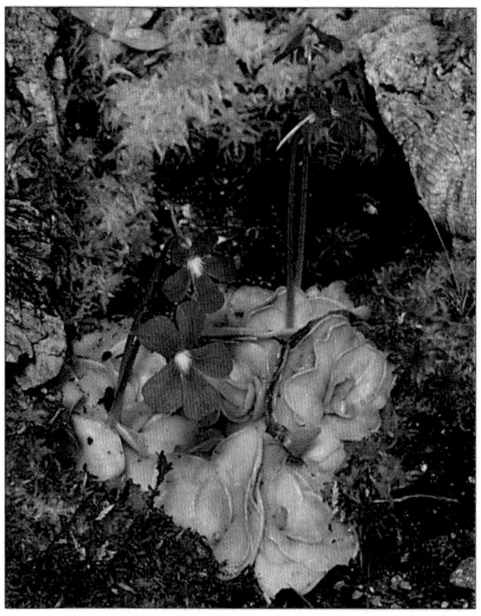

Pinguicula moranensis

glass, butterworts may be used to assist in controlling aphids and whiteflies. In frost-prone areas, grow tender species as houseplants or in a temperate greenhouse. Hardy species are suitable for an alpine house or as bog plants.
• **HARDINESS** Fully hardy to frost tender.
• **CULTIVATION** Under glass, grow in a mixture of equal parts chopped peat and sphagnum moss, with added broken clay pots, in bright filtered light. During growth, water freely and apply a balanced liquid fertilizer every month. Water sparingly in winter. Outdoors, grow in poor, peaty, permanently moist soil in full sun or partial shade.
• **PROPAGATION** Surface-sow seed on damp sphagnum moss at 13–18°C (55–64°F), as soon as ripe. Divide in late winter.
• **PESTS AND DISEASES** Slugs and snails may be troublesome.

P. grandiflora. Rosette-forming perennial with resting buds in winter. Obovate-oblong, sticky, pale green leaves are 3–4.5cm (1¼–1¾in) long. During summer, trumpet-shaped, spurred, dark blue flowers, 2.5cm (1in) across, with widely spreading lobes and white throats, are borne on slender stems. ↕ 15cm (6in), ↔ 10cm (4in). W. Europe. ✻✻✻
P. moranensis ▣ Rosette-forming perennial with ovate, sticky, dull pale green leaves, 6–10cm (2½–4in) long, with inrolled, purple-green margins. Trumpet-shaped, deep carmine-red flowers, to 3cm (1¼in) across, are borne on slender stems in summer. ↕ 15cm (6in), ↔ 10cm (4in). Mexico. ❀ (min. 7°C/45°F)

▷**Pink** see *Dianthus*
Alpine see *Dianthus alpinus*
Carthusian see *Dianthus carthusianorum*
Cheddar see *Dianthus gratianopolitanus*
Chinese see *Dianthus chinensis*
Deptford see *Dianthus armeria*
Fringed see *Dianthus monspessulanus*
Ground see *Linanthus dianthiflorus*
Indian see *Dianthus chinensis*
Maiden see *Dianthus deltoides*
Sea see *Armeria*
Swamp see *Helonias bullata*
▷**Pink shower** see *Cassia javanica*
▷**Piñon,**
Mexican see *Pinus cembroides*
Rocky mountain see *Pinus edulis*
Single-leaf see *Pinus monophylla*

P

PINUS

Pine

PINACEAE

Genus of approximately 120 species of monoecious, evergreen, coniferous trees or shrubs, widely distributed in forests of the N. hemisphere from the Arctic Circle to Central America, Europe, N. Africa, and S.E. Asia. The bark is often fissured, and in some species is divided into irregular, plate-like sections. Pines have small bundles of 2–5, rarely 1 or 6–8, needle-like, light to dark green or yellow-green to bluish or grey-green leaves, which usually persist for 2–4 years, sometimes for longer. The winter buds are usually cylindrical or ovoid, and often resinous. Female cones take 2, or occasionally 3 years to ripen; the seeds are winged in most species. Male cones are yellow and catkin-like, clustered at the shoot bases. Pines are useful as specimen trees, and for shelter and windbreaks; some cultivars and slow-growing species are suitable for a rock garden.

• **HARDINESS** Fully hardy to frost hardy.
• **CULTIVATION** Grow in any well-drained soil in full sun. The 5-needled species may be short-lived in shallow, chalk soil.
• **PROPAGATION** Sow seed of species in containers in a cold frame in spring. Graft cultivars in late winter.
• **PESTS AND DISEASES** Prone to adelgids, aphids, sawfly larvae, honey fungus, pine shoot moth, and various needle cast diseases. Some 5-needled pines are susceptible to white pine blister rust.

P. aristata ▣△ (Bristle cone pine). Dense, conical tree with upturned branch tips, smooth, dark grey bark, and red-brown shoots with pale hairs and ovoid buds. Bright green leaves, 2–4cm (¾–1½in) long, have flecks of white resin and are borne in fives; young needles have blue-white inner sides. Leaves are retained for up to 20 years. Long-ovoid brown female cones, 4–10cm (1½–4in) long, have a bristle-like prickle on each scale. ↕ to 10m (30ft), ↔ to 6m (20ft). USA (Arizona, New Mexico, Colorado). ❄❄❄. **var. *longaeva*** see *P. longaeva.*
P. armandii △ (Armand pine). Broadly conical tree with an open, whorled habit, smooth bark, becoming cracked with age, and olive-green shoots with cylindrical-ovoid buds. Forward-pointing, pendent, shiny, deep green leaves, 10–20cm (4–8in) long, with white inner sides and curved at the bases, are borne in fives. Cylindrical-conical female cones, 12–20cm (5–8in) long, have wingless seeds. ↕ 15–20m (50–70ft), ↔ 6–8m (20–25ft). Tibet, N. Burma, China, Taiwan. ❄❄❄
P. attenuata △ (Knobcone pine). Conical tree with ascending branches, smooth grey bark, becoming fissured and scaly with age, and green-brown shoots with resinous, narrow, spindle-shaped buds. Stiff, slender, grey-green leaves, 8–18cm (3–7in) long, are borne in threes. Ovoid-conical, yellow-brown female cones, swollen on the outer sides, are 9–20cm (3½–8in) long, and may persist for over 20 years. ↕ to 25m (80ft), ↔ to 6–8m (20–25ft). North America (Oregon to Baja California). ❄❄❄
P. ayacahuite ▣△ (Mexican white pine). Conical to broadly conical tree with smooth grey bark, becoming domed and scaly with age, and finely hairy, pale yellow-brown shoots with resinous, conical buds. Forward-pointing, pendent, shiny green leaves, 10–20cm (4–8in) long, with white bands on the inner sides, appear in fives. Very resinous, cylindrical female cones, 20–45cm (8–18in) long, have conical apexes and reflexed scales. ↕ to 30m (100ft), ↔ 6–8m (20–25ft). S. Mexico, Guatemala, Honduras. ❄❄❄
P. balfouriana △ (Foxtail pine). Broad, conical tree with ridged grey bark and hairy, orange-brown shoots with ovoid buds. Dark green leaves, 2–3cm (¾–1¼in) long, with faint white bands on the inner sides, are borne in fives, and retained for 10–20 years. Oblong-cylindrical, purple-brown female cones, 8–14cm (3–5½in) long, have a short prickle on each scale. Similar to *P. aristata,* but does not have flecks of resin on its leaves. ↕ 15m (50ft), ↔ 6–8m (20–25ft). USA (California). ❄❄❄
P. banksiana ◊ (Jack pine). Narrow, conical tree when young, becoming irregular and scruffy with age. It has fissured, red-brown or grey bark, thin, flexible brown shoots, and very resinous, cylindrical buds. Stout, twisted, divergent, yellow-green leaves, 2–4cm (¾–1½in) long, are borne in pairs. Forward-pointing, ovoid-conical, strongly curved, yellow-buff to grey female cones, 4–6cm (1½–2½in) long, are persistent. ↕ 10–20m (30–70ft), ↔ 3–5m (10–15ft). North America (Yukon Territory to Atlantic), south into N.E. USA. ❄❄❄
P. bungeana ▣◊–♤ (Lacebark pine). Columnar or bushy-crowned, slow-growing tree with smooth bark, which flakes in small, round scales to reveal creamy patches that darken through purple to grey-green. Shoots are olive-green with ovoid to ellipsoid buds, and bear hard, shiny, yellow-green leaves, 5–10cm (2–4in) long, in threes. Ovoid female cones, 4–7cm (1½–3in) long, bear seeds with short, brittle wings. ↕ 10–15m (30–50ft), ↔ 5–6m (15–20ft). N. and C. China. ❄❄❄
P. canariensis ▣♀△ (Canary Islands pine). Conical to broadly conical tree, becoming domed with age, with fissured, red-brown bark, yellow shoots, and large, ovate buds. Spreading, grass-green adult leaves, 15–30cm (6–12in) long, are borne in threes. Glaucous blue juvenile leaves are borne singly and are retained for several years. Ellipsoid-ovoid female cones, 9–20cm (3½–8in) long, are borne on long stalks, 2cm (¾in) long. ↕ to 25m (80ft), ↔ 6–9m (20–28ft). Canary Islands. ❄❄
P. cembra ♀◊–♤ (Arolla pine, Swiss stone pine). Narrow, columnar tree with smooth, dark grey bark, becoming fissured with age, and densely brown-hairy shoots with ovate, resinous buds. Dark green leaves, bluish white on the inner sides, 7–9cm (3–3½in) long, are borne in fives. Broad, oblong-conical, bluish green female cones, 6–8cm (2½in–3in) long, are resinous, and bear edible, wingless seeds. ↕ 15–20m (50–70ft), ↔ 6–8m (20–25ft). C. Europe. ❄❄❄
P. cembroides ♤ (Mexican piñon). Domed, rounded tree with scaly, silver-grey bark, fissured red-brown, and orange-brown shoots with ellipsoid buds, which have tapered, reflexed scales. Radially arranged, dark green leaves, 3–6cm (1¼–2½in) long, with glaucous inner sides, are borne in threes, occasionally in pairs. Spherical green female cones, 2.5–4cm (1–1½in) across, ripen to brown, and have wingless seeds. ↕ 10–18m (30–60ft), ↔ 6–8m (20–25ft). S.W. USA, N. Mexico. ❄❄
P. chylla see *P. wallichiana.*
P. contorta ♤ (Beach pine, Lodgepole pine, Shore pine). Broadly conical tree when young, becoming domed with age, with scaly, red-brown bark, shiny, greenish brown shoots, and very resinous, cylindrical buds. Dense, forward-pointing, deep green leaves,

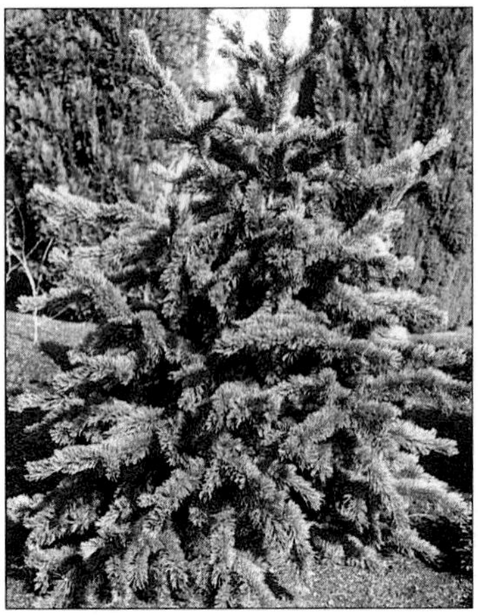
Pinus aristata

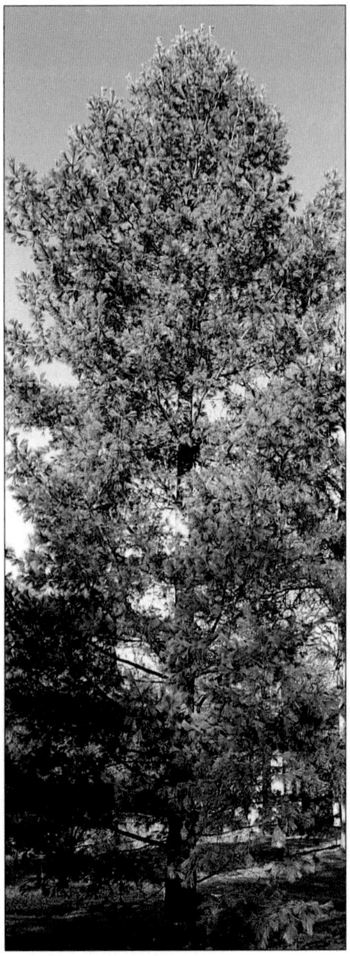
Pinus ayacahuite

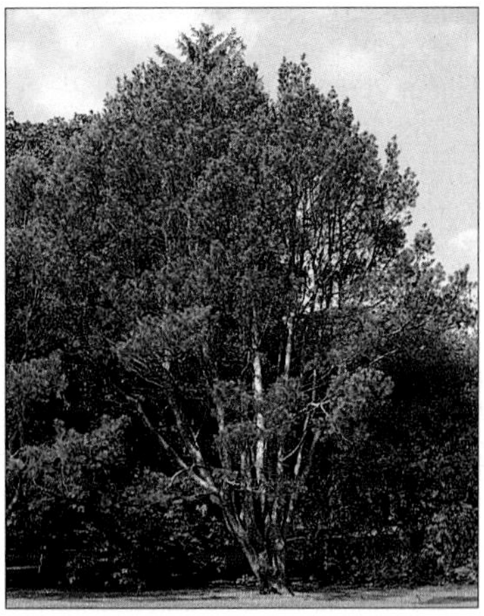
Pinus bungeana

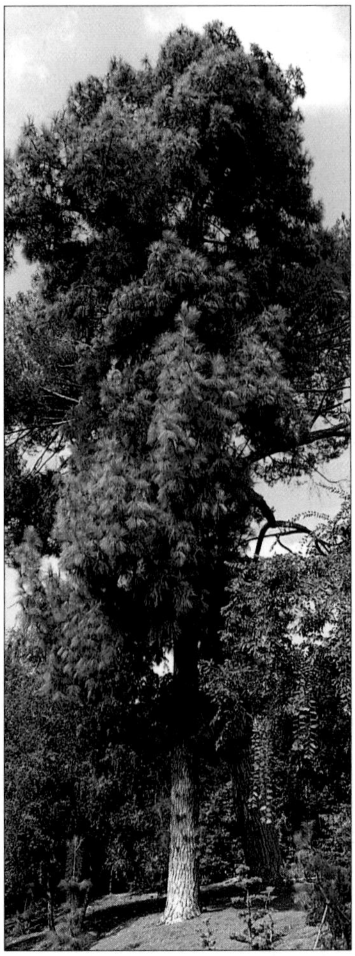
Pinus canariensis

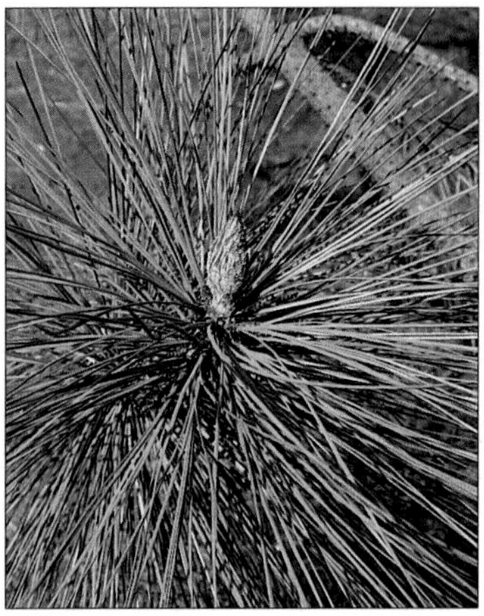
Pinus coulteri

P

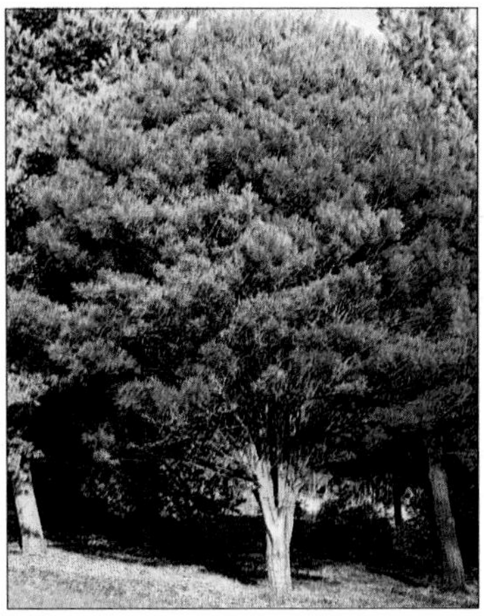

Pinus densiflora 'Umbraculifera'

4–5cm (1½–2in) long, are borne in pairs. Long-conical, yellow-brown to brown female cones, 2.5–7cm (1–3in) long, have reflexed scales, and are persistent. ↕ to 25m (80ft), ↔ to 8m (25ft). Coastal N.W. North America. ❄❄❄. **var. *latifolia*** △ (Lodgepole pine) has a conical habit, flakier bark, and brighter green, spreading leaves, 6–9cm (2½–3½in) long, with ovoid cones, 4cm (1½in) long; Rocky Mountains. **'Spaan's Dwarf'** is dwarf, with a sloping trunk and an open habit, with erect branches; leaves are 1.5cm (½in) long; ↕↔ 75cm (30in).

P. coulteri ▣ Y ○ (Big-cone pine, Coulter pine). Domed tree with grey bark, becoming black-grey and fissured, and brown, glaucous shoots with long, cylindrical to ovoid buds. Radially arranged, stiff, grey-green or bluish green leaves, 20–30cm (8–12in) long, are borne in threes. Massive, ovoid, yellow-brown female cones, 20–35cm (8–14in) long, have stout, forward-pointing spines and large, wingless seeds. ↕ to 25m (80ft), ↔ 8–10m (25–30ft). USA (California), Mexico (Baja California). ❄❄❄

P. densiflora △ (Japanese red pine). Broadly conical to rounded tree, becoming flat-topped, with reddish brown bark, flaky in the upper crown, grey and fissured at the base. The whitish pink shoots have slightly resinous, ovoid buds. Slender, bright green leaves, 8–12cm (3–5in) long, are borne in pairs. Bears long-ovoid, yellow-brown female cones, 3–6cm (1¼–2½in) long. ↕ 15–25m (50–80ft), ↔ 5–7m (15–22ft). N.E. Asia, Japan. ❄❄❄.

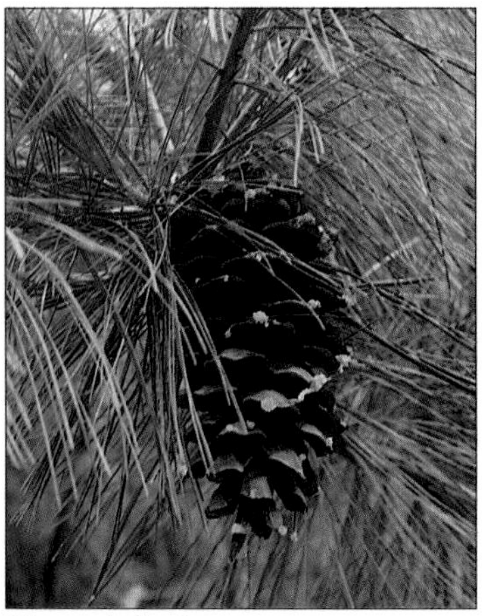

Pinus x *holfordiana*

'Alice Verkade' is a globe-shaped, dwarf selection with bright green leaves; it grows only about 7cm (3in) per year; ↕ 50cm (20in) or more, ↔ 1m (3ft) (when mature). **'Ja-nome'** see 'Oculus Draconis'. **'Oculus Draconis'**, syn. 'Ja-nome', is a large shrub or small tree with two distinctive yellow bands ("dragon's eyes") on each leaf. Bears blue-green female cones. **'Tagyosho'** see 'Umbraculifera'. **'Umbraculifera'** ▣ ○ syn. 'Tagyosho', is a slow-growing, rounded to broadly spreading tree with a domed or umbrella-shaped crown; ↕ 4m (12ft), ↔ 6m (20ft).

P. edulis ○ (Rocky Mountain piñon). Compact, irregular, domed tree with silvery grey bark, orange, bloomed shoots, and ovoid buds. The dark green leaves, 3–6cm (1¼–2½in) long, glaucous on the inner sides, are borne mainly in pairs, and persist for 3–9 years. Spherical, pale brown or green-brown female cones are 3cm (1¼in) long, with wingless seeds. The piñon seeds, or pine kernels, of commerce come mainly from this species. ↕ 6–15m (20–50ft), ↔ 6–8m (20–25ft). S.W. USA. ❄❄

P. excelsa see *P. wallichiana.*

P. flexilis △ (Limber pine). Broadly conical tree, later domed at the top, with smooth grey bark, later fissured; very pliant, hairy green shoots have broadly cylindrical to ovoid buds. Dark green leaves, 4–9cm (1½–3½in) long, are produced in tight bundles of five, and persist for 5–6 years. Long-ovoid, yellow-ochre female cones are 7–15cm (3–6in) long, with wingless seeds. Male cones are red. ↕ 15–20m (50–70ft), ↔ 6–9m (20–28ft). Rocky Mountains from Alberta to Arizona. ❄❄❄

P. griffithii see *P. wallichiana.*

P. halepensis △–○ (Aleppo pine). Conical tree, becoming rounded with age, with scaly, red-brown bark, glaucous grey shoots, and ovate buds with reflexed scales. Slender, sparse, bright green leaves, 6–11cm (2½–4½in) long, are borne in pairs. Long-ovoid, red-brown female cones are 5–12cm (2–5in) long. ↕ to 20m (70ft), ↔ to 6m (20ft). Mediterranean. ❄❄

P. heldreichii* var. *leucodermis see *P. leucodermis.*

P.* x *holfordiana ▣ △ (*P. ayacahuite* x *P. wallichiana*) (Holford pine). Broadly conical tree with grey-brown bark, becoming fissured, and with hairy shoots and cylindrical-conical buds. Blue-green leaves, to 10–20cm (4–8in) long, are borne in fives. Ellipsoid green female cones, 25–30cm (10–12in) long, ripen to buff or yellow-brown. Differs from *P. ayacahuite* in having less reflexed cone scales and smaller seeds, and from *P. wallichiana* in having hairy shoots and wider cones. ↕ to 30m (100ft), ↔ 6–8m (20–25ft). Garden origin. ❄❄❄

P. insignis see *P. radiata.*

P. jeffreyi ▣ Y △ (Jeffrey pine). Broadly conical tree with smooth, deeply fissured black bark and stout, glaucous, grey-green shoots with long, oblong-conical buds. Grey-green or bluish green leaves, 12–26cm (5–10in) long, are borne in threes. Long-ovoid, yellow-grey female cones, 13–30cm (5–12in) long, have rounded bases. ↕ 25–35m (80–120ft), ↔ 6–8m (20–25ft). North America (Oregon to Baja California). ❄❄❄

P. koraiensis △ (Korean pine). Broadly conical tree with smooth, dark grey bark, becoming scaly with age, and green shoots with dense, orange-brown hairs and ovoid to cylindrical buds. Shiny, deep green leaves with silvery white bands on the inner sides, are borne in fives, and are 6–12cm (2½–5in) long. Long-conical, bright green female cones, 9–16cm (3½–6in) long, have large, free-tipped scales and large, wingless seeds. ↕ to 20m (70ft), ↔ to 8m (25ft). Pacific Russia, Korea, N.E. China. ❄❄❄

P. leucodermis Y ◊ syn. *P. heldreichii* var. *leucodermis* (Bosnian pine). Narrow, long-conical tree with scaly, ash-grey bark, glaucous shoots becoming white, and broad, non-resinous, ovoid buds. Dense, forward-pointing, very rigid, dark green leaves, 7–9cm (3–3½in) long, are borne in pairs. Long-conical female cones, 5–10cm (2–4in) long, are cobalt-blue in early summer, ripening to brown. ↕ 15–20m (50–70ft), ↔ 5–6m (15–20ft). Balkans. ❄❄❄. **'Compact Gem'** is dense, with dark green-black leaves growing 2.5cm (1in) per year.

P. longaeva △ syn. *P. aristata* var. *longaeva* (Ancient pine). Small, conical, dense-crowned tree, becoming gnarled in old age, with scaly, dark brown bark, hairy, red-brown shoots, and ovoid-conical buds. Shiny, grey-green leaves, 2.5–3cm (1–1¼in) long, with white inner sides, are borne mainly in fives (some in threes or fours). A few older leaves bear flecks of resin. Ovoid, rust-red female cones, 6–10cm (2½–4in) long, have a small, fragile prickle on each scale. Formerly confused with *P.*

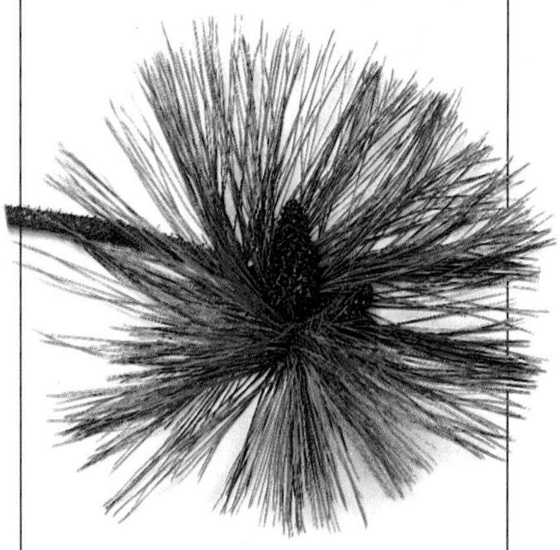

Pinus montezumae

aristata; both have living specimens over 4,700 years old. ↕ to 10m (30ft), ↔ to 6m (20ft). USA (White Mountains of California). ❄❄❄

P. monophylla ○ (Single-leaf piñon). Slow-growing shrub or small tree with a domed crown, smooth, brown or grey bark, becoming fissured with age, and orange shoots with cylindrical-conical buds. Long-persistent, grey-green leaves, 2–5cm (¾–2in) long, are mainly produced singly, and are round in section (occasionally set in pairs and then half-moon-shaped in section). Ovoid, yellow-buff female cones, 8cm (3in) long, have large, wingless seeds. ↕ 5–10m (15–30ft), ↔ to 6m (20ft). S.W. USA. ❄❄

P. montezumae ▣ △ (Montezuma pine). Broadly conical tree, becoming

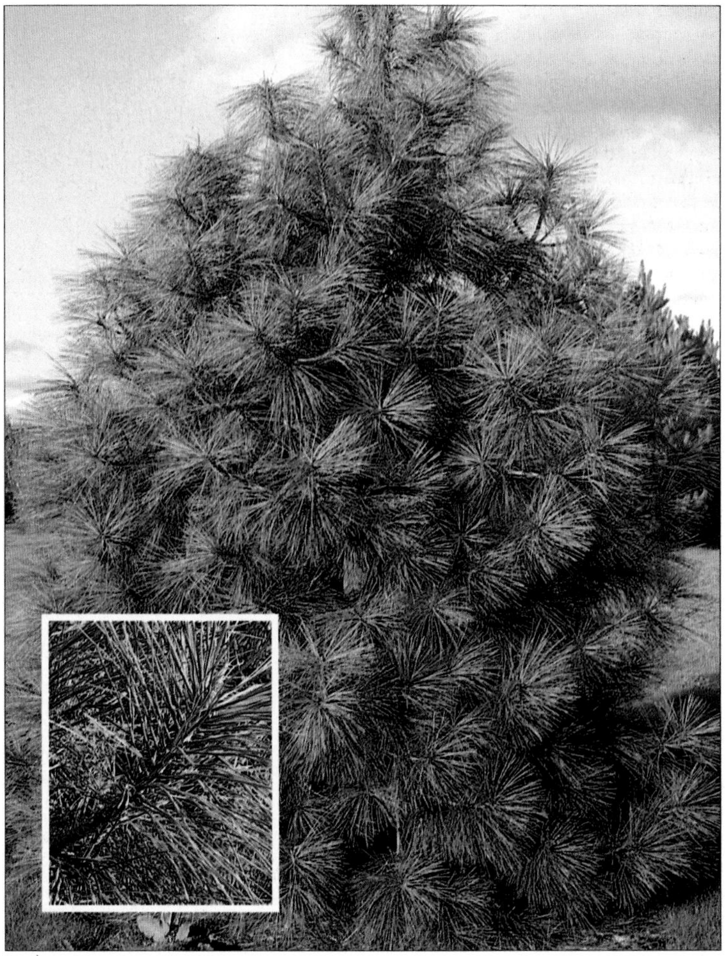

Pinus jeffreyi (inset: leaf detail)

P

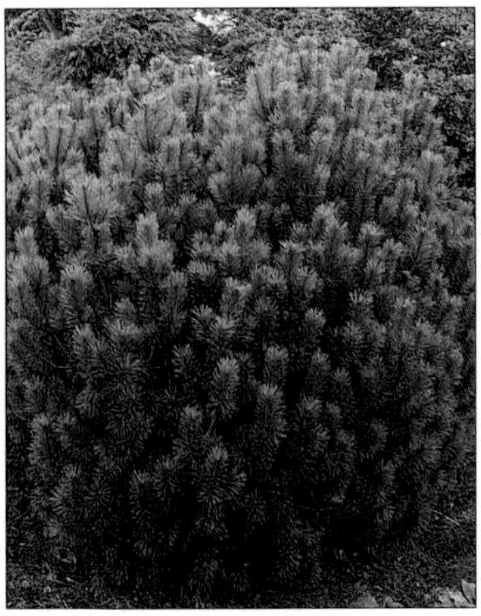

Pinus mugo 'Mops'

domed when old; it has fissured, grey-brown bark, very stout, rough brown shoots, and ovoid-acute buds. Fresh green, pendent leaves, 15–30cm (6–12cm) long, are produced in fives, rarely in sixes or sevens. Bears ovoid to ovoid-conical, yellow to rust-brown female cones, 13–20cm (5–8in) long. ↕15–30m (50–100ft), ↔ 6–9m (20–28ft). C. and S. Mexico to Guatemala. ❄❄ (borderline)

P. monticola ◊ (Western white pine). Narrowly conical tree when young, becoming columnar with age. It has smooth, dark grey bark, becoming plate-like, and brownish green shoots with rust-brown hairs and cylindrical to globose buds. Pale green leaves, 7–10cm (3–4in) long, with bluish green inner sides, are borne in fives. Narrowly conical female cones, 15–30cm (6–12in) long, are green to purple-green when young, yellow-brown when mature. ↕25–40m (80–130ft), ↔ 6–8m (20–25ft). North America (British Columbia to California). ❄❄❄

P. mugo ◊ (Dwarf mountain pine). Shrub or rounded to broadly spreading tree with thick, ascending or spreading branches, scaly grey bark, green shoots, becoming brown, and very resinous, ovoid-oblong buds. Well-spaced, dark to bright green leaves, 3–8cm (1¼–3in) long, are borne in pairs. Ovoid to long-conical, dark brown female cones are 2–6cm (¾–2½in) long and symmetrical at maturity. ↕ to 3.5m (11ft), ↔ to 5m (15ft). C. Europe. ❄❄❄. **'Gnom'** is a squat shrub when young, becoming more rounded. **'Mops'** ▣ ♀ is almost spherical, with green leaves; it grows

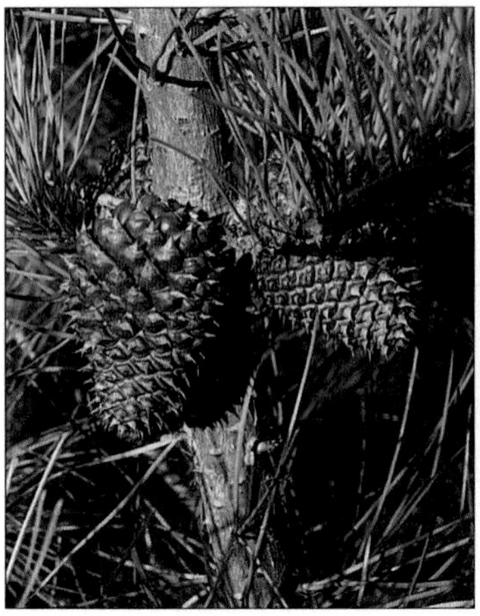

Pinus muricata

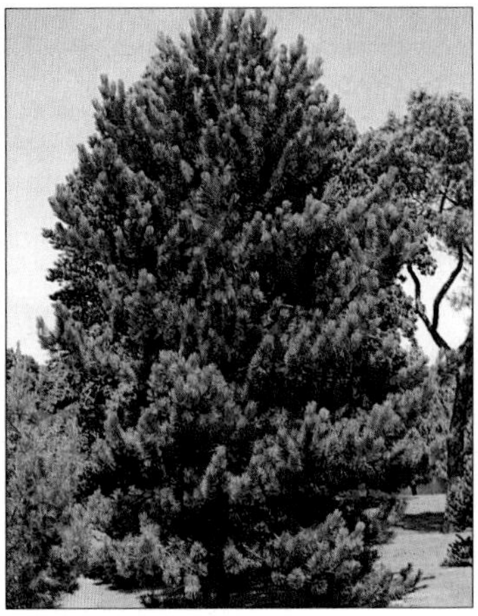

Pinus nigra

approximately 6cm (2½in) per year. **subsp. *uncinata*** see *P. uncinata.*

P. muricata ▣ ♀ ◊–◊ (Bishop pine). Conical tree, becoming broadly domed or columnar with age, with fissured, dark grey bark, orange-brown shoots, and conical to cylindrical buds. Stiff, grey-green or blue-green leaves, 10–15cm (4–6in) long, are borne in pairs, occasionally threes. Oblique, ovoid-conical, nut-brown female cones, 7–9cm (3–3½in) long, have stout spines on the outer scales and persist for 20–30 years. Northern populations in California have blue-green foliage and are faster-growing in cultivation. ↕ to 20m (70ft) ↔ 6–9m (20–28ft). USA (California). ❄❄❄

P. nigra ▣ ♀ ◊–◊ (Austrian pine, European black pine). Domed tree with dense, spreading branches, fissured dark brown or black bark, brown shoots, and broadly ovoid, abruptly sharp-pointed buds with papery scales. Dense, straight, rigid, dark green leaves, 8–16cm (3–6in) long, are borne in pairs. Long-ovoid, yellow-brown female cones are 6–8cm (2½–3in) long. ↕ to 30m (100ft), ↔ 6–8m (20–25ft). Austria, N. Italy to the Balkans. ❄❄❄. **subsp. *laricio*** ♀ syn. var. *maritima* (Corsican pine), is a narrowly conical tree, becoming columnar with age, with dark grey bark, yellow-brown shoots, and narrowly conical, tapered buds. Flexible, well-spaced, grey-green or green leaves are 11–18cm (4½–7in) long; ↕ to 40m (130ft), ↔ to 10m (30ft). France (Corsica), S. Italy (including Sicily). **var. *maritima*** see subsp. *laricio.*

P. parviflora ▣ ♀ ◊ (Japanese white pine). Conical or columnar tree, often with a spreading crown, with scaly, purplish brown bark, greyish brown shoots, and ovoid buds. Deep green leaves, 2–6cm (¾–2½in) long, with whitish blue inner sides, are borne in fives. Ovoid-oblong, red-brown female cones, 5–7cm (2–3in) long, have short-winged seeds. ↕ 10–20m (30–70ft), ↔ 6–8m (20–25ft). Japan. ❄❄❄. **'Adcock's Dwarf'** ♀ is dense and slow-growing, with short, grey-green leaves, 1.5–2.5cm (½–1in) long. **f. *glauca***, syn. 'Glauca', is the most common variant in cultivation; it is small and spreading, with twisted, glaucous foliage.

P. patula ▣ ♀ ◊ (Mexican weeping pine). Rounded to broadly spreading tree with scaly, reddish brown bark, pale green-brown, glaucous shoots, and

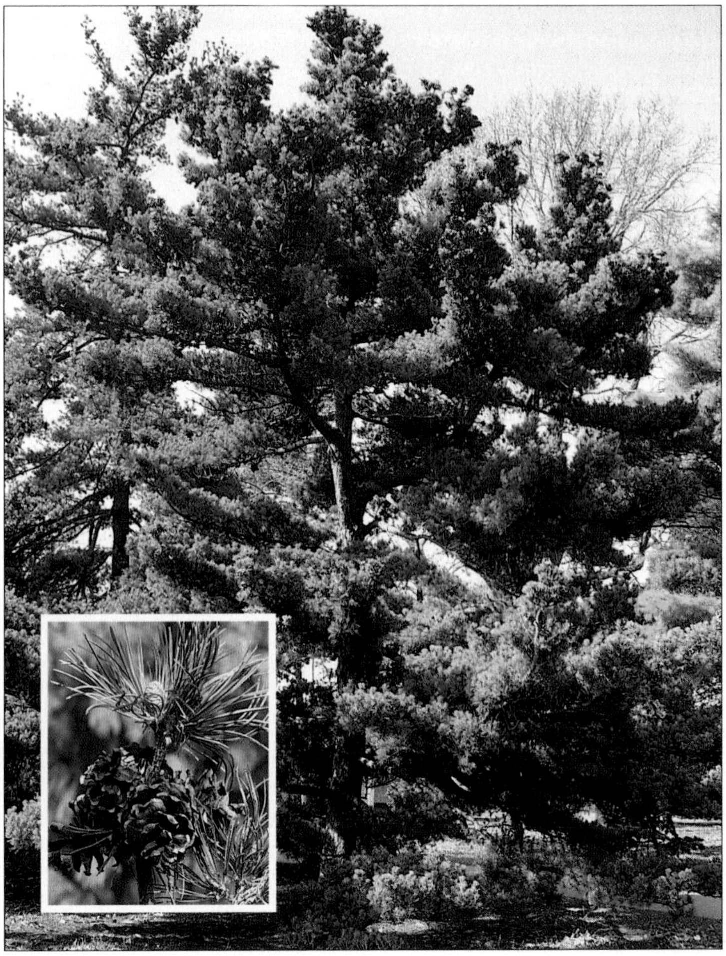

Pinus parviflora (inset: cone detail)

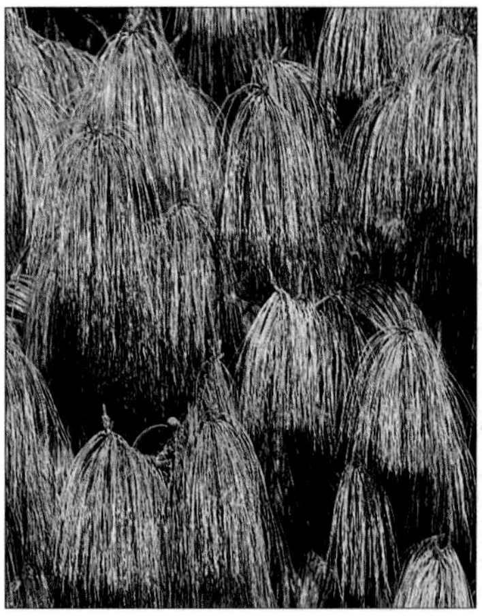

Pinus patula

cylindrical buds. Slender, pendent, shiny, light green leaves, 15–30cm (6–12in) long, are borne in threes, rarely fours or fives. Stalkless, long-conical, yellow to chestnut-brown female cones are 6–10cm (2½–4in) long. Frost tender when young. ↕15–20m (50–70ft), ↔ 6–10m (20–30ft). C. Mexico. ❄❄

P. peuce ▣ ◊ (Macedonian pine). Conical or columnar tree with smooth, grey-green bark, becoming fissured with age, and green, slightly glaucous shoots with ovoid-conical buds. Stiff, grey-green leaves, 7–9cm (3–3½in) long, are borne in fives. Cylindrical-conical green female cones, ripening brown, are 7–16cm (3–6in) long. Tolerates a wide variety of conditions, including very poor soils and harsh climates. ↕25m (80ft), ↔ to 6–8m (20–25ft). S. Balkans to N. Greece. ❄❄❄

P. pinaster ♀ ◊ (Maritime pine). Conical tree, becoming domed, with deeply fissured, orange-brown to purple bark, brown shoots, and spindle-shaped buds that have reflexed scales. Paired, well-spaced, stout, stiff, grey-green leaves are 10–25cm (4–10in) long. Long-ovoid green female cones, 8–22cm (3–9in) long, ripen to chestnut-brown. ↕ to 20m (70ft), ↔ 6–8m (20–25ft). S.W. Europe, Mediterranean. ❄❄❄

P. pinea ▣ ♀ ◊ (Stone pine, Umbrella pine). Conical tree when young, becoming domed, with stout, radiating branches, plate-like, orange-brown bark, orange-brown shoots, and ovate buds. Well-spaced, twisted, glossy green adult leaves, 12–15cm (5–6in) long, are borne in pairs. Solitary, glaucous blue juvenile leaves are retained for several years. Ovoid, shining brown female cones, 12cm (5in) long, ripen in the third year and have wingless seeds. ↕15–20m (50–70ft), ↔ 6–12m (20–40ft). Mediterranean. ❄❄❄

P. ponderosa ♀ ◊–◊ (Ponderosa pine, Western yellow pine). Conical tree, becoming columnar, with deeply fissured bark with smooth, broad plates, and stout, green-brown shoots with oblong-cylindrical buds. Dense, rigid, grey-green leaves, 10–25cm (4–10in) long, are borne in threes, rarely pairs or fives. Ovoid or long-ovoid purple female cones, 6–16cm (2½–6in) long, age to brown. ↕25–35m (80–120ft), ↔ 6–8m (20–25ft). Rocky Mountains from British Columbia to California. ❄❄❄

P. pumila (Dwarf Siberian pine). Spreading, low shrub with branches that are flexible and bend down in cold

P

PINUS

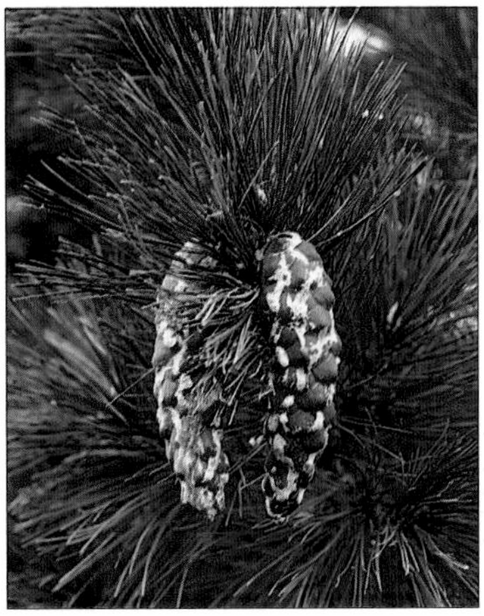

Pinus peuce

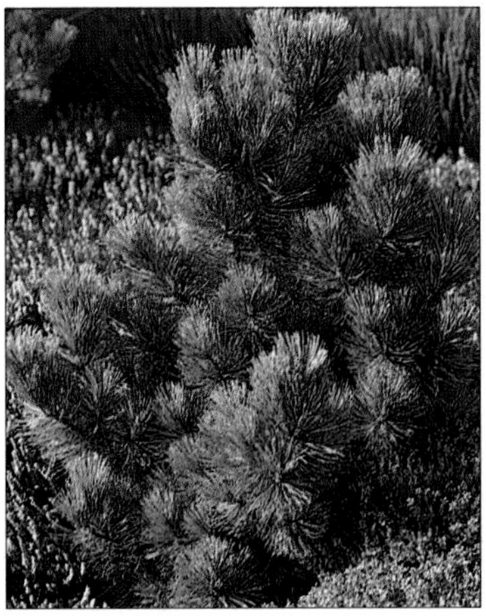

Pinus pumila 'Compacta'

weather, and hairy, green-brown shoots with cylindrical-conical buds. Dark green leaves, 4–6cm (1½–2½in) long, with bright blue inner sides, are borne in fives. Ovoid female cones, violet-purple when young, becoming red- or yellow-brown, are 3–6cm (1¼–2½in) long, with wingless seeds. Male cones are bright red in spring. ↕↔ 2–6m (6–20ft). Russia (Siberia) to Japan, N.E. China. ✻✻✻. **'Compacta'** ▣ is a rounded bush with very dense, grey-green leaves, 5–8cm (2–3in) long, grey-white beneath; ↕↔ 2–3m (10ft).

P. radiata 🏆 ▯–○ syn. *P. insignis* (Monterey pine, Radiata pine). Narrow, conical tree, becoming broadly domed, with heavily ridged black bark, grey-green shoots, and cylindrical buds. Slender, shining, bright green leaves, 10–15cm (4–6in) long, are borne in threes. Very oblique, ovoid, glossy, yellow-brown female cones, 8–15cm (3–6in) long, with 20 swollen outer scales, persist for 20–30 years. Widely planted in forestry throughout the world. ↕ 25–40m (80–130ft), ↔ 8–12m (25–40ft). USA (California). ✻✻✻

P. resinosa △ (Red pine). Conical tree with upswept branches, flaky red bark in the upper crown, scaly, pink-grey bark at the base, and stout, orange to red-brown shoots with ovoid to narrowly conical buds. Yellow-green leaves, 10–15cm (4–6in) long, are produced in pairs and persist for 4–5 years; they snap if bent. Long-ovoid female cones, 4–6cm (1½–2½in) long, are chestnut-brown. Male cones are purple. ↕ 15–25m (50–80ft), ↔ 6–8m (20–25ft). North America (Nova Scotia to West Virginia). ✻✻✻

P. rigida △ (Pitch pine). Conical or ovoid tree, becoming irregular, with fissured, dark grey bark, grey-brown shoots, and cylindrical to ovoid-oblong buds. Thick, stiff, grey-green leaves, 7–14cm (3–5½in) long, are borne in threes. Ovoid-conical, yellow-brown female cones, 3–9cm (1¼–3½in) long, often persist for several years. ↕ to 20m (70ft), ↔ 5–7m (15–22ft). North America (Maine and Ontario south to Georgia). ✻✻✻

P. sabiniana △–○ (Digger pine). Conical or domed tree with fissured grey bark, grey-bloomed shoots, and narrow, cylindrical buds. Flexible, sparse, blue-green or grey-green leaves, 15–30cm (6–12in) long, are borne in threes. Ovoid, dark brown female cones, 10–25cm (4–10in) long, each have a hooked spine and wingless seeds. ↕ to 20m (70ft), ↔ 5–6m (15–20ft). USA (California). ✻✻✻

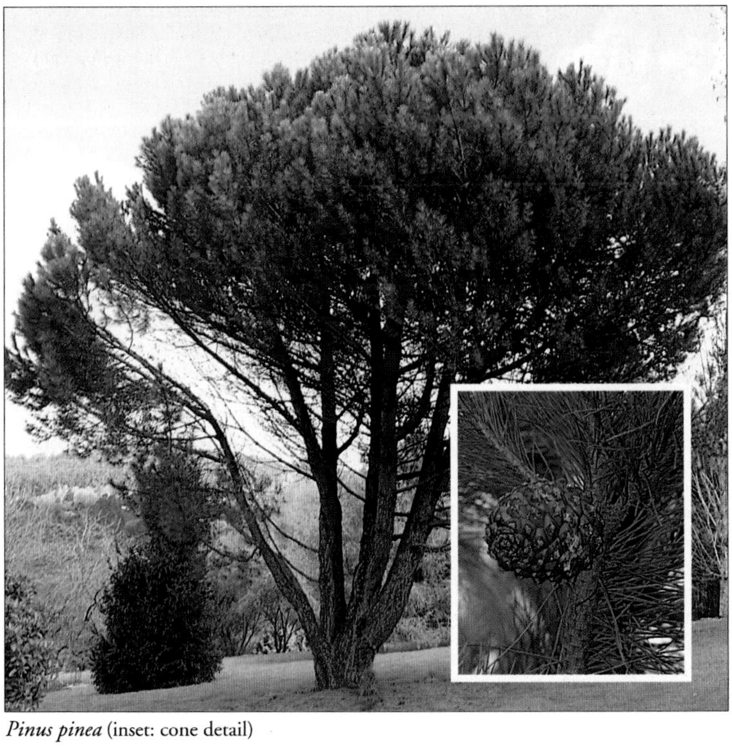

Pinus pinea (inset: cone detail)

P. strobus △–○ (Eastern white pine, Weymouth pine). Slender, conical tree with upswept branches when young, becoming more columnar. It has smooth grey bark, which becomes black and cracked, and slender, olive-brown shoots with ovoid-oblong buds. Slender, grey-green leaves, 8–14cm (3–5½in) long, are borne in fives. Cylindrical, tapered green female cones, ripening to brown, are 8–15cm (3–6in) long. ↕ to 35m (120ft), ↔ 6–8m (20–25ft). North America (Newfoundland to Georgia). ✻✻✻ **'Fastigiata'** ▯ has a narrow, columnar crown of ascending branches.

P. sylvestris ▣ 🏆 △–○ (Scots pine). Conical to columnar-conical tree, becoming domed, with flaky, red-brown or orange bark in the upper crown, ridged, purple-grey bark at the base, and green-brown shoots with oblong-ovate buds. Twisted, blue-green or yellow-green leaves, 5–7cm (2–3in) long, are borne in pairs. Ovoid-conical green female cones, 3–7cm (1¼–3in) long, ripen to grey or red-brown. ↕ 15–30m (50–100ft), ↔ 6–9m (20–28ft). Europe (excluding the far north), temperate Asia. ✻✻✻. **'Argentea'** see 'Edwin Hillier'. **'Aurea'** 🏆 has bright golden yellow foliage in winter, resuming normal colour in spring; ↕ 10–15m (30–50ft). **'Beuvronensis'** 🏆 is a dwarf, rounded bush, to 1m (3ft) high. **'Edwin Hillier'**, syn. 'Argentea', bears bright, silvery blue leaves. **'Fastigiata'** ▯ is narrow and has an upright habit, with ascending branches; ↕ to 8m (25ft), ↔ 1–3m (3–10ft). **'Gold Coin'** ▣ is a slow-growing shrub with intense golden foliage; ↕↔ to 2m (6ft). **'Nana'** see 'Watereri'. **'Watereri'**, syn. 'Nana', is a slow-growing, small tree with an upright habit; ↕ 4m (12ft), ↔ 7m (22ft).

P. tabuliformis △–○ (Chinese red pine). Conical tree when young, becoming flat-topped when old. It has scaly, red-brown bark in the upper crown, fissured grey bark at the base, and yellow-brown shoots with ovoid-conical buds. The leaves, 9–15cm (3½–6in) long, are produced in pairs. Broadly ovoid-conical, dark brown female cones are 4–9cm (1½–3½in) long. ↕ to 15–20m (50–70ft), ↔ 6–10m (20–30ft). N. China. ✻✻✻

P. thunbergiana see *P. thunbergii*.

P. thunbergii △ syn. *P. thunbergiana* (Japanese black pine). Conical tree, becoming rounded, with dark purplish grey bark, yellow-brown shoots, and cylindrical-ovoid buds covered with silky white scales. Thick, dark grey-green leaves, 7–15cm (3–6in) long, are borne in pairs. Long-ovoid, green-brown female cones are 4–7cm (1½–3in) long. Tolerates salt spray. ↕ 15–25m (50–80ft), ↔ 6–8m (20–25ft). N.E. China, Japan, Korea. ✻✻✻

P. uncinata △ syn. *P. mugo* subsp. *uncinata* (Mountain pine). Conical, upright tree, becoming domed with age; it produces scaly, grey-pink bark, orange-brown shoots, and very resinous, small, ovoid buds. Stiff, dark green leaves, 6cm (2½in) long, are produced in pairs. Ovoid, strongly oblique, pale brown female cones are 4–6cm (1½–2½in) long. ↕ 15–20m (50–70ft), ↔ 6–8m (20–25ft). Alps to Spain. ✻✻✻

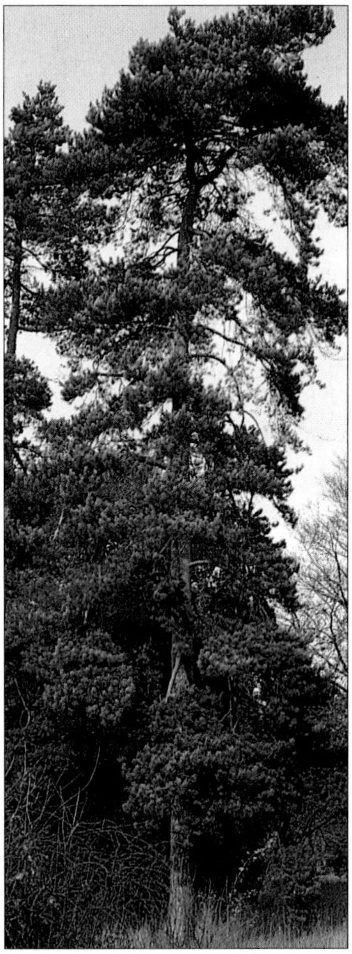

Pinus sylvestris

P. wallichiana 🏆 △–○ syn. *P. chylla*, *P. excelsa*, *P. griffithii* (Bhutan pine, Blue pine). Conical tree when young, developing a broad, domed crown. It has smooth grey bark, becoming scaly and dark brown, and stout, olive-green shoots with cylindrical-conical buds. Arching to pendent, grey-green to glaucous blue leaves are 11–20cm (4½–8in) long, and produced in fives. Ellipsoid green female cones, 10–30cm (4–12in) long, ripening to brown, have forward-pointing scales. ↕ 20–35m (70–120ft), ↔ 6–12m (20–40ft). Himalayas from Afghanistan to N.E. India. ✻✻✻

P

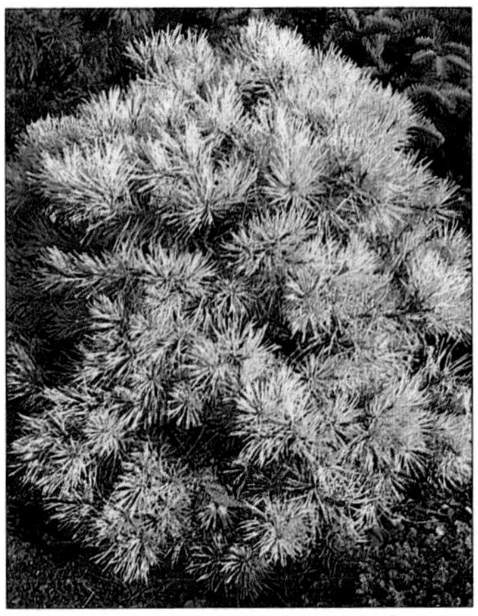

Pinus sylvestris 'Gold Coin'

PIPER

Pepper

PIPERACEAE

Genus of more than 1,000 species of shrubs, climbers, and small trees from very variable habitats throughout tropical regions of the world. Many have a pungent aroma, and some, including *P. nigrum*, are grown as spice crops in tropical regions. They bear alternate, asymmetric, very variable, but often narrowly to broadly ovate to rounded green leaves, heart-shaped at the bases, on stems that are swollen at the nodes. Cylindrical spikes of small (often unisexual) flowers without petals or sepals are followed by single-seeded fruit. In warm, humid, tropical areas with heavy, well-distributed rainfall, peppers are grown in fertile soils, with the shade and support of trees. Fruits are harvested at different stages of ripeness for different uses: dried, green mature fruit for black pepper; ripening green fruit for pickled pink peppercorns; ripened, red or yellow fruit (soaked to remove the outer layer of skin) for white pepper. In temperate zones, *P. nigrum* is grown in a conservatory or warm greenhouse; it may bear fruit under glass. Grow outdoors only in tropical areas.

- **HARDINESS** Frost tender.
- **CULTIVATION** Under glass, grow in loam-based potting compost (JI No.3) with added sharp sand, in bright filtered light and with high humidity. In the growing season, water moderately and apply a balanced liquid fertilizer every month; water sparingly in winter. Outdoors, grow in fertile, well-drained soil in dappled shade. Support climbing stems. Pruning group 11, in late winter.
- **PROPAGATION** Sow seed at 20–24°F (66–75°C) in early spring, or take semi-ripe cuttings in summer.
- **PESTS AND DISEASES** Susceptible to fungal root rot, pepper weevil, and pepper flea beetle.

P. nigrum ■ (Black pepper, White pepper). Evergreen, woody-stemmed, perennial climber with ovate, heart-shaped, leathery, deeply veined, dark green leaves, to 13cm (5in) long. In summer, bears small white flowers in spikes to 11cm (4½in) long, on the side of the swollen stem joint opposite the leaf, followed by spherical fruit that are red when ripe. ↕↔ 4m (12ft) or more. India, Sri Lanka. ❀ (min. 16°C/61°F)

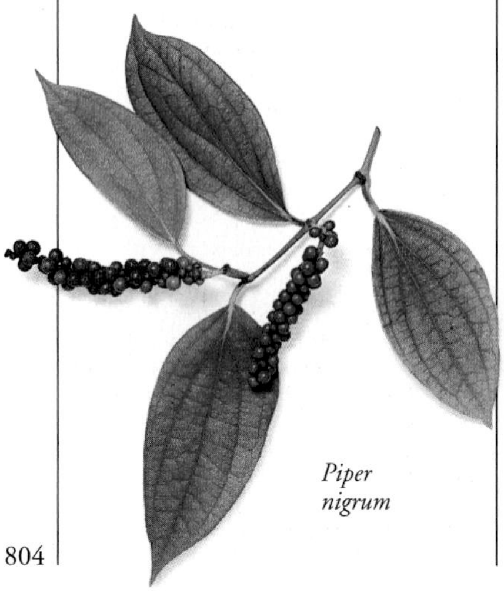

Piper nigrum

PIPTANTHUS

LEGUMINOSAE/PAPILIONACEAE

Genus of 2 species of deciduous or semi-evergreen shrubs occurring in scrub and woodland in the mountains of China and the Himalayas. They have alternate, 3-palmate, mid- to dark green, sometimes grey- or blue-green leaves, occasionally with white hairs and a grey-green surface. Grown for their foliage and pea-like flowers, they are suitable for a shrub border, or for growing against, or training on, a wall.

- **HARDINESS** Frost hardy.
- **CULTIVATION** Grow in fertile, well-drained soil in sun or partial shade. In frost-prone areas, shelter from cold, drying winds. Pruning group 1, or group 13 if wall-trained.
- **PROPAGATION** Sow seed in containers in a cold frame in spring or autumn. Take heeled, semi-ripe basal cuttings in summer.
- **PESTS AND DISEASES** Trouble free.

P. laburnifolius see *P. nepalensis.*
P. nepalensis ■ syn. *P. laburnifolius* (Evergreen laburnum). Open, upright, deciduous or semi-evergreen shrub with 3-palmate leaves composed of lance-shaped, dark blue-green leaflets, to 15cm (6in) long, blue-white beneath. Pea-like, bright yellow flowers, 4cm (1½in) long, are produced in upright, terminal racemes in late spring and early summer, followed by pendent green seed pods, to 22cm (9in) long. ↕ 2.5m (8ft), ↔ 2m (6ft). Himalayas, S.W. China. ❄❄

P. tomentosus. Open, upright, deciduous or semi-evergreen shrub bearing 3-palmate leaves composed of ovate, grey-green leaflets, to 15cm (6in) long, densely silky-hairy beneath. In late spring and early summer, bears pea-like, lemon-yellow flowers, 3cm (1¼in) long, in upright racemes, followed by pendent, woolly seed pods, to 8cm (3in) long. ↕ 2.5m (8ft), ↔ 2m (6ft). S.W. China. ❄❄

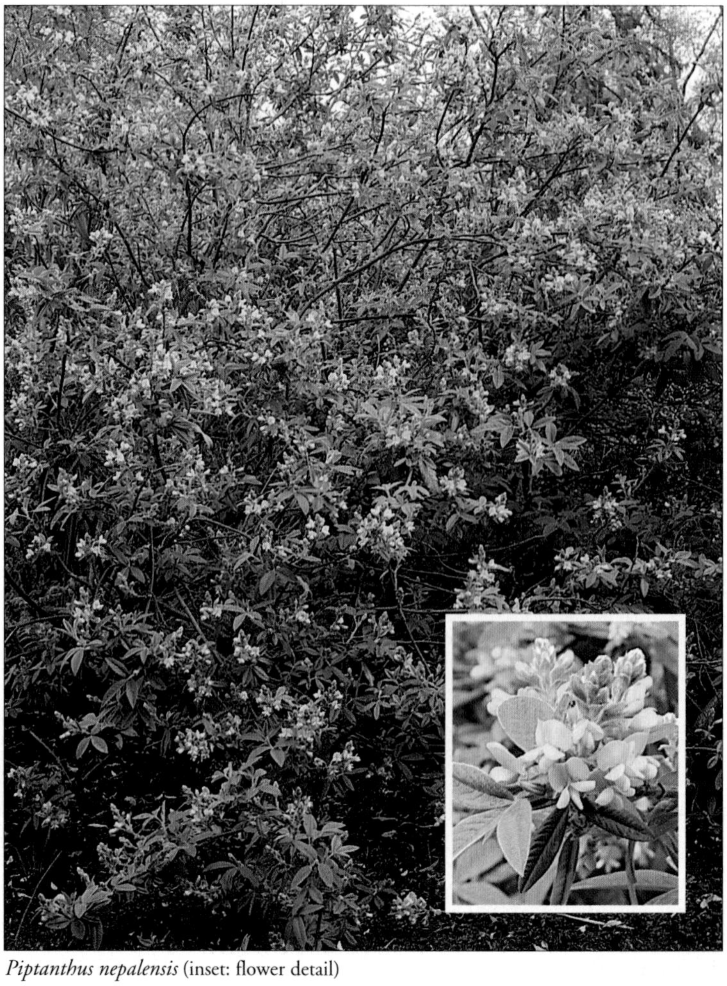

Piptanthus nepalensis (inset: flower detail)

PISONIA

syn. HEIMERLIODENDRON

NYCTAGINACEAE

Genus of 50 species of evergreen trees, shrubs, and climbers from chiefly maritime habitats in tropical regions worldwide, but mainly in North and South America. Cultivated for their attractive leaves, which are simple and entire, and borne alternately, in opposite pairs, or in whorls of 3, they also produce small, funnel-shaped, petalless flowers: the males with tufts of stamens, the females with solitary ovaries that develop into nutlets (achenes). In areas where temperatures fall below 10–13°C (50–55°F), grow in a temperate or warm greenhouse, or as houseplants. In warmer climates, grow as specimen trees, as windbreaks, or as a hedge.

- **HARDINESS** Frost tender.
- **CULTIVATION** Under glass, grow in loam-based potting compost (JI No.3) in full light or bright indirect light. When in growth, water freely and apply a balanced liquid fertilizer every month; water sparingly in winter. Outdoors, grow in fertile, humus-rich, well-drained soil in full sun or partial shade. Pruning group 1; may need restrictive pruning under glass.
- **PROPAGATION** Sow seed at 15–18°C (59–64°F) in spring. Take greenwood cuttings in early summer, or semi-ripe cuttings in mid- to late summer. Air layer in spring.
- **PESTS AND DISEASES** Red spider mites and scale insects may infest greenhouse specimens.

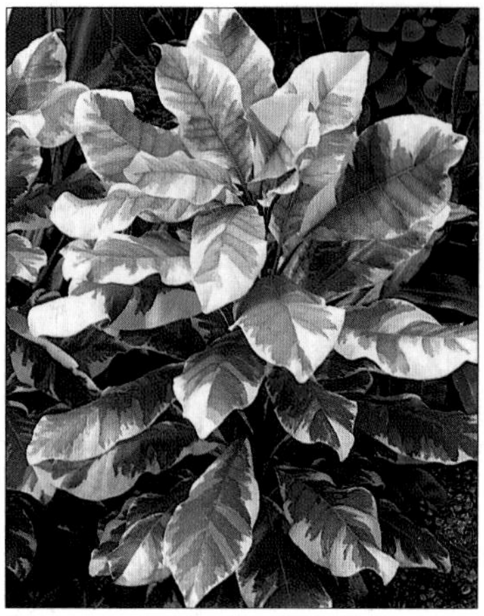

Pisonia umbellifera 'Variegata'

P. brunoniana see *P. umbellifera.*
P. umbellifera ♀ syn. *Heimerliodendron brunonianum, P. brunoniana* (Bird-catcher tree, Parapara). Small tree or large shrub, erect at first, then spreading, and usually freely branching. Densely borne, opposite or whorled, elliptic to lance-shaped leaves, 10–40cm (4–16in) long, are thinly leathery, glossy, and rich green. Bears insignificant, funnel-shaped, pink or yellow flowers, about 4–7mm (⅛–¼in) long, in leafy panicles, intermittently throughout the year. Female sepals are sticky-glandular and elongate, enclosing the nutlets. ↕ 5–20m (15–70ft) sometimes more, ↔ 3–5m (10–15ft). Mauritius to Australia, New Zealand, and Japan (Ogasawara-Shoto). ❀ (min. 10°C/50°F). **'Variegata'** ■ has leaves irregularly splashed and margined creamy white, and pink-tinged stalks.

▷**Pistachio** see *Pistacia*

PISTACIA

Pistachio

ANACARDIACEAE

Genus of 11 species of rounded to upright, dioecious, deciduous and evergreen trees and shrubs from dry habitats in the Mediterranean, C. Asia to Japan, Malaysia, Mexico, and S. USA. They are grown for their foliage, flowers, and fruit (although *P. vera*, which produces the edible pistachio nut, is not grown ornamentally). The alternate leaves are usually pinnate, occasionally ternate or simple; the small, petalless, mostly mid-green flowers appear in usually axillary racemes or panicles, followed by the peppercorn-like fruits. Grow as specimen trees; they thrive in coastal conditions. In frost-prone areas, grow half-hardy species in a cool or warm greenhouse.

- **HARDINESS** Frost hardy to half hardy.
- **CULTIVATION** Under glass, grow in loam-based potting compost (JI No.3)

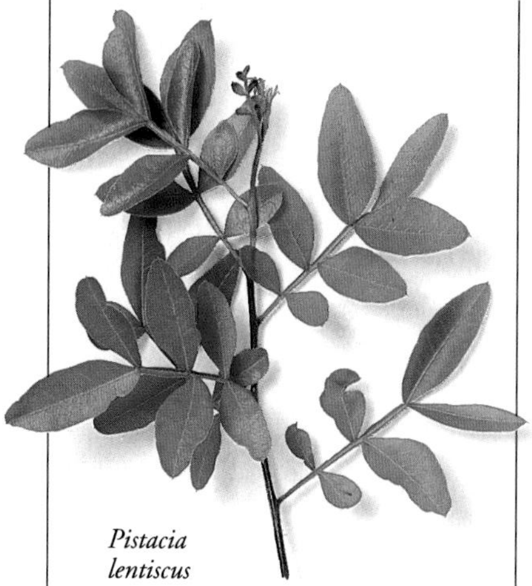

Pistacia lentiscus

with added sharp sand, in full light. During growth, water freely and apply a balanced liquid fertilizer monthly; water sparingly in winter. Outdoors, grow in moderately fertile, sharply drained soil in full sun. Pruning group 1; may need restrictive pruning under glass.

• **PROPAGATION** Sow seed at 25°C (77°F) in early spring. Take greenwood cuttings in late spring or early summer, or semi-ripe cuttings in summer.

• **PESTS AND DISEASES** Prone to fungal root rot; coral spot affects *P. chinensis.*

P. chinensis Q (Chinese mastic). Deciduous tree, erect at first, then spreading. Pinnate leaves, to 25cm (10in) long, each with 10–12 oblong-elliptic, toothed, leathery, glossy, dark green leaflets, with no terminal leaflet, colour well in autumn. Aromatic red flowers are produced with the young leaves in mid- and late spring; the males are in crowded panicles, to 10cm (4in) long, the females in looser panicles, 15–25cm (6–10in) long. The flowers are followed by spherical red fruit, about 3mm (1/8in) across, maturing blue. ↕ 15–25m (50–80ft), ↔ 7–10m (22–30ft). C. and W. China. ✲✲

P. lentiscus ▣ Q (Lentisc, Mastic tree). Evergreen, resinous, aromatic shrub or sometimes small, bushy tree. Pinnate leaves, 10cm (4in) long, with winged stalks and midribs, each have 2–7 pairs of narrowly oblong to ovate, ovate, oblong-lance-shaped, or elliptic, leathery, glossy, dark green leaflets, with no terminal leaflet. In spring or early summer, bears dense panicles, to 3cm (1¼in) long, of male flowers with red stamens, and looser panicles, 6cm (2½in) long, of brownish green female flowers. The flowers are followed by spherical red fruit, 5mm (¼in) across, ripening black. The sap yields mastic, the fragrant gum used in medicine, dentistry, and varnish. ↕↔ 1–3m (3–10ft). Morocco, Canary Islands, Portugal, S. Europe to Greece. ✲

P. terebinthus Q (Terebinth, Turpentine tree). Deciduous, freely branching tree, or sometimes large shrub, with pinnate leaves, 10–20cm (4–8in) long; these each consist of 3–6 pairs of oval, semi-glossy, mid- to rich green leaflets, with a terminal leaflet. In spring or early summer, produces greenish red flowers; the males are in compact panicles, 6–10cm (2½–4in) long, the female in looser panicles, 5–15cm (2–6in) long. The flowers are surrounded by brown bracts, and are followed by obovoid, edible red to purple-brown fruit, to 7mm (¼in) long. The sap yields a fragrant gum, used in cancer treatments. ↕ 6m (20ft) or more, ↔ 2–6m (6–20ft). Portugal to Turkey, Canary Islands, Morocco to Egypt. ✲

PISTIA

Shell flower, Water lettuce

ARACEAE

Genus of one species of evergreen, floating aquatic perennial distributed worldwide in the tropics and subtropics. It is grown for its rosettes of attractive, wedge-shaped leaves, and for the exquisite colouring of its fine, feathery roots (which turn from white to purple, and finally black). Although regarded as a weed in some tropical areas, where its radiating stolons cover the surface of the water, it is an excellent ornamental plant for a sunny, temperate pool, for a greenhouse pool, or for a large aquarium.

• **HARDINESS** Frost tender.

• **CULTIVATION** Grow as a floating aquatic in full sun with some midday shade. In frost-prone areas, lift before the first frosts and overwinter at a minimum of 10°C (50°F); alternatively grow under glass on the surface of an indoor pool (or in baskets at the pool margins), in full light, with shade from hot sun, maintaining a water temperature of 15–22°C (59–72°F). Growth is more rapid the higher the water temperature. See also pp.52–53.

• **PROPAGATION** Separate plantlets in summer.

• **PESTS AND DISEASES** Trouble free.

P. stratiotes ▣ (Shell flower, Water lettuce). Evergreen, floating aquatic perennial with spreading or semi-upright, wedge-shaped, glaucous leaves, to 20cm (8in) long, fluted above and ribbed beneath, borne in floating rosettes. Inconspicuous, tubular flowers are borne in leaf-like spathes in the leaf axils, irregularly throughout the year. ↕ 10cm (4in), ↔ indefinite. Tropics and subtropics worldwide. ❀ (min. 10°C/50°F)

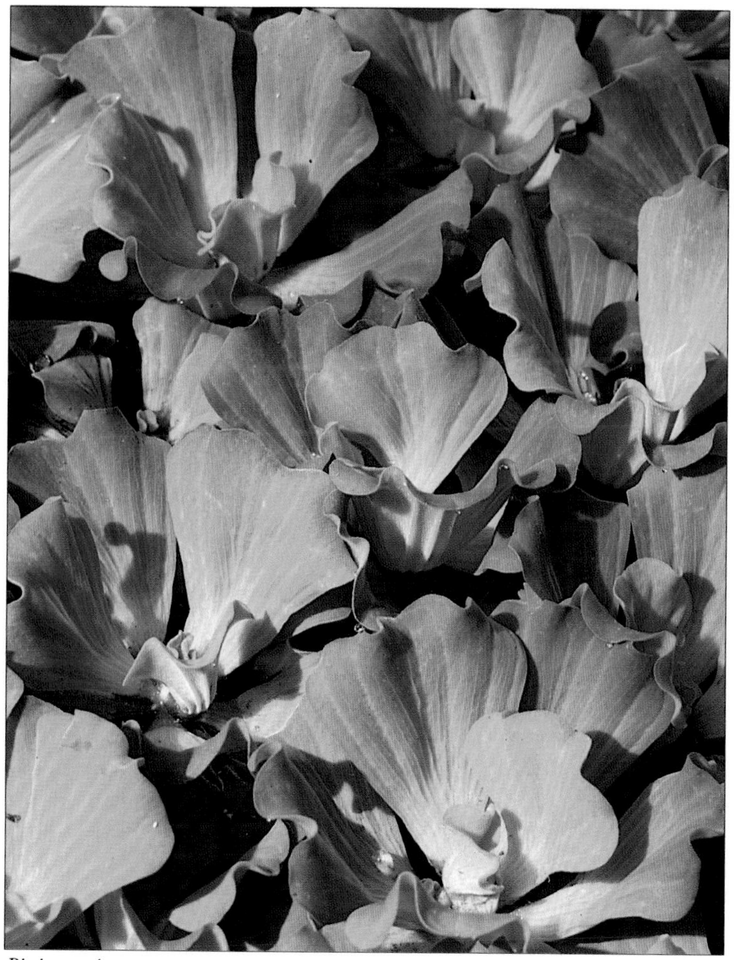

Pistia stratiotes

PITCAIRNIA

BROMELIACEAE

Genus of over 260 species of very variable, rosette-forming, usually evergreen perennials (bromeliads), mostly terrestrial, a few epiphytic. All but one species occur in rocky, generally dry areas of Mexico, Central America, South America, and many West Indian islands. They are cultivated for their linear, lance-shaped, or strap-shaped leaves, which have smooth or spiny margins, and for their bell-shaped, white, yellow, orange, green, or red flowers, which are produced in spikes, racemes, or panicles on branched or unbranched stems. In areas where temperatures drop below 10°C (50°F), grow in a warm greenhouse; in warmer climates, pitcairnias are suitable for a desert garden or moist shrub border.

• **HARDINESS** Frost tender.

• **CULTIVATION** Under glass, grow in standard bromeliad compost in full or bright filtered light. From mid-spring to late autumn, water moderately and apply a nitrogen-based fertilizer every 6–8 weeks. Evergreen species require moderate to high humidity, deciduous species require low humidity. When dormant, protect from cold draughts, keeping deciduous species dry, and evergreen species just moist. Outdoors, grow in moderately fertile, sharply drained soil in sun or partial shade. See also p.47.

• **PROPAGATION** Sow seed at 19–24°C (66–75°F) in spring. Remove offsets in late spring or early summer.

• **PESTS AND DISEASES** Susceptible to scale insects and mealybugs, especially early in the growing season.

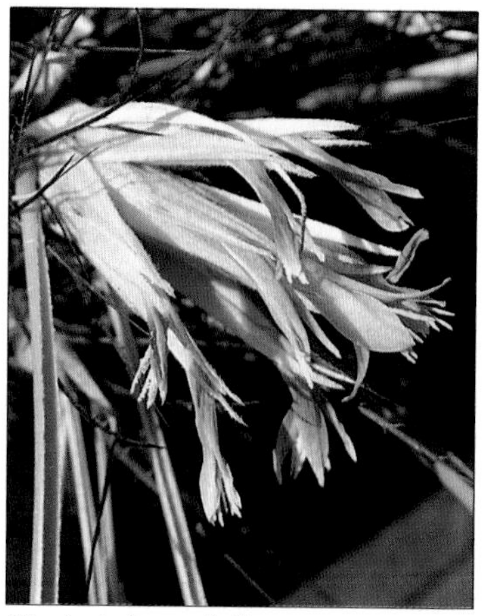

Pitcairnia heterophylla

P. atrorubens. Rosette-forming, epiphytic or terrestrial, evergreen bromeliad with variable leaves: the outer ones are much reduced, smooth-margined, ovate, and very pointed; the lance-shaped inner ones, 60–90cm (24–36in) long, have smooth margins and spiny black stalks. In summer, up to 20 bell-shaped, pale yellow flowers, surrounded by red-purple floral bracts, are produced in spikes, to 30cm (12in) long, on stems with pointed, brownish-purple scape-bracts. ↕ to 90cm (36in), ↔ to 60cm (24in). Mexico, Central America, N.W. South America. ❀ (min. 10°C/50°F)

P. bifrons. Rosette-forming, terrestrial, evergreen bromeliad with strap-shaped, smooth-margined leaves, to 70cm (28in) or more long. During summer, 20–30 bell-shaped, red, red-orange, or yellow flowers, with red or yellow floral bracts, are produced in racemes, 18–27cm (7–11in) long, on white-scaly scapes. ↕↔ 70cm (28in). West Indies (Leeward and Westward Islands, St. Kitts, Guadeloupe). ❀ (min. 10°C/50°F)

P. heterophylla ▣ Epiphytic or terrestrial bromeliad, evergreen for most of the year, but deciduous for a brief period, with a bulbous-based rosette of linear, viciously barbed, spiny outer leaves, to 20cm (28in) long, sometimes reduced to brown spines. Inner leaves, to 70cm (8in) long, are smooth-margined, linear, and white-woolly beneath. During summer, 3–12 bell-shaped, red-pink or white flowers are produced in spikes, to 15cm (6in) long, among red floral bracts, on very short scapes. ↕ 12cm (5in) or more, ↔ to 30cm (12in). Mexico to Venezuela and Peru. ❀ (min. 10°C/50°F)

▷ **Pitcher plant** see *Sarracenia*
Tropical see *Nepenthes*

P

PITTOSPORUM

PITTOSPORACEAE

Genus of approximately 200 species of usually evergreen shrubs and trees, a few epiphytic, found in habitats ranging from sandy savannah to rain-forest, mainly in Australasia, but also in southern Africa, S. and E. Asia, and the Pacific islands. They are grown for their attractive, glossy, often leathery leaves, which are simple, usually entire, and borne alternately or in whorls. The often fragrant, 5-petalled flowers are borne mostly singly in the leaf axils, or in axillary or terminal corymbs, umbels, panicles, or clusters; they are followed by nearly spherical, woody fruits (capsules) that contain usually black seeds embedded in a sticky, brownish yellow mucilage. Where temperatures fall below 0°C (32°F), grow in a cool greenhouse, moving the plants outdoors for the summer. In warmer climates, the trees are fine specimens for a lawn; the shrubs are suitable for a border, and make a good hedge or windbreak, especially in coastal regions.

• **HARDINESS** Frost hardy to frost tender. Half-hardy species may survive short spells at several degrees below 0°C (32°F), provided wood has been well ripened in summer.

• **CULTIVATION** Under glass, grow in loam-based potting compost (JI No.3) in full light. When in growth, water moderately and apply a balanced liquid fertilizer monthly; water sparingly in winter. Outdoors, grow in fertile, moist but well-drained soil in full sun or partial shade, although those with variegated or purple leaves produce the best leaf effect in full sun. In frost-prone climates, shelter from cold, drying winds. Pruning group 1; may need restrictive pruning under glass. Trim hedges in spring and midsummer.

• **PROPAGATION** Sow seed ideally as soon as ripe, or in spring in containers in a cold frame. Take semi-ripe cuttings in summer, or layer or air layer in spring.

• **PESTS AND DISEASES** Red spider mites and scale insects may infest greenhouse specimens. Leaf spot and powdery mildew may cause problems.

P. bicolor ⚲ Large shrub or small tree, erect and bushy, with downy young stems. Alternate, oblong, leathery leaves, 2.5–6cm (1–2½in) long, have rolled margins, and are deep green above, white- to brown-felted beneath. Bears nodding, bell-shaped, fragrant, maroon-crimson flowers, about 1cm (½in) long, singly or in small, axillary clusters, mainly in spring; these are followed by dark red capsules, 1cm (½in) or more across. ↕ 4–5m (12–15ft), occasionally more, ↔ 2–5m (6–15ft). Australia (New South Wales, Victoria, Tasmania). ✲

P. colensoi see *P. tenuifolium* subsp. *colensoi.*

P. crassifolium ⚲ (Karo). Large, monoecious shrub or small tree, usually bushy and erect. It has erect to ascending stems, white- to buff-felted when young, and alternate, leathery leaves, 5–7cm (2–3in) or more long, which are obovate to elliptic, and dark green above, white- or buff-felted beneath. Tubular-bell-shaped, dark red to purple flowers, to 1cm (½in) across, are borne in terminal clusters in early summer: the males in clusters of up to 10, the females in clusters of 5. The flowers are followed by almost spherical brown capsules, to 1.5cm (½in) across. ↕ 5–10m (15–30ft), ↔ 2–5m (6–15ft). New Zealand (North Island). ✲. **'Compactum'** is smaller, denser, and has grey-green leaves, 3–5cm (1¼–2in) long, in tight whorls; ↕ 1.5m (5ft), ↔ 1m (3ft). **'Variegatum'** ▣ has grey-green leaves with broad, irregular, creamy white margins; ↕ 2.5m (8ft).

P. dallii ⚲ Small, broadly upright tree or sometimes large, rounded shrub, opening out with age, with reddish purple stems. Very deep green leaves, alternate, or whorled at the stem tips, are 6–11cm (2½–4½in) long, elliptic to elliptic-oblong, either coarsely and sharply toothed or virtually entire. In summer, produces small, shallowly cup-shaped, fragrant, yellow-green or white flowers, to 0.6–2cm (¼–¾in) across, in dense, terminal, compound umbels; they are followed by ovoid brown capsules, 1cm (½in) long. ↕ to 6m (20ft), ↔ 2–4m (6–12ft). New Zealand (South Island). ✲✲

P. eugenioides 🏆 ⚲ (Lemonwood, Tarata). Small tree, erect and conical when young, becoming rounded with age. Alternate, elliptic to narrowly ovate, wavy-margined leaves, to 13cm (5in) long, are thinly leathery, glossy, light green, and lemon-scented when crushed. Produces star-shaped, fragrant, light greenish yellow flowers, 3mm (⅛in) across, in dense, terminal, compound umbels in summer, followed by ovoid brown capsules, 7mm (¼in) long. ↕ 5–12m (15–40ft), ↔ 2–5m (6–15ft). New Zealand. ✲. **'Variegatum'** ▣ ⚲ produces leaves with bold, irregular, cream to creamy yellow margins. **'Zita Robinson'** ⚲ is similar to the species, but is dense and columnar, with wavy leaf margins.

***P.* 'Garnettii'** ▣ 🏆 Large, bushy shrub, erect at first, then spreading, with alternate, oblong to elliptic leaves, 4–6cm (1½–2½in) long, sparingly hairy below, almost hairless above, greyish green and pink-spotted, with slightly wavy, creamy white margins. In late spring and early summer, bell-shaped, dark purple flowers, about 1cm (½in) long, are borne singly from the leaf axils, followed by almost spherical brown capsules, 1cm (½in) long. ↕ 3–5m (10–15ft), ↔ 2–4m (6–12ft). ✲

P. phillyreoides ⚲ (Desert willow, Weeping pittosporum). Large shrub or small tree of spreading, weeping habit, with softly hairy young stems and alternate, linear-oblong to narrowly lance-shaped, thick leaves, 5–10cm (2–4in) long, mid- to deep green above, paler beneath. In summer, bears bell-shaped, cream to yellow flowers, 1.5cm (½in) long, occasionally singly or more often in axillary, corymb-like clusters. They are followed by almost spherical yellow capsules, 1.5cm (½in) long, which split to disclose sticky, orange-red seeds. ↕ 6–10m (20–30ft), ↔ 3–5m (10–15ft). Dry areas of Australia. ✲

P. ralphii ▣ ⚲ Fast-growing, large shrub or small tree, erect then spreading, with white- to buff-downy young stems, and alternate, elliptic, sometimes wavy-margined leaves, 7–13cm (3–5in) long, semi-lustrous, deep green above, white to buff-felted beneath. In late spring and early summer, bears tubular-bell-shaped, very dark red flowers, to 1cm (½in) long, in loose, terminal, umbel-like clusters, followed by ovoid, hairy, brown capsules, 1.5cm (½in) long. ↕ 3–4m (10–12ft), ↔ 1.5–2.5m (5–8ft). New Zealand (North Island). ✲✲. **'Variegatum'** has greyish green leaves with irregular, fairly wide, creamy white margins. **'Wheeler's Dwarf'** is smaller, very dense, and slow-growing; ↕ 1m (3ft), ↔ 60cm (24in).

P. revolutum. Large, bushy shrub with brown-downy young stems and alternate, ovate to lance-shaped, semi-lustrous, mid- to deep green leaves, 3–11cm (1¼–4½in) long, pale brown and densely woolly beneath, especially on the midribs. In late spring and early summer, produces bell-shaped yellow flowers, 8–10mm (⅜–½in) long, in small, compact, terminal, few-flowered umbels; they are sometimes followed by almost spherical orange capsules, 1cm (½in) or more long, which split to reveal sticky red seeds. ↕ 2–4m (6–12ft), much taller in a warm climate with high rainfall, ↔ 1.5–2.5m (5–8ft). Australia (Queensland, New South Wales). ✲

P. rhombifolium ⚲ (Diamond-leaved laurel). Conical tree, moderately bushy when young, with long-stalked, broadly lance-shaped to diamond-shaped or narrowly oval, lustrous, mid- to deep green leaves, arranged alternately. In summer, produces bell-shaped white flowers, 8–10mm (⅜–½in) long, in axillary or terminal, many-flowered clusters; they are sometimes followed by spherical, bright orange capsules, 1cm (½in) long, which split to reveal the red capsule interior and sticky, glossy black seeds. ↕ 10–20m (30–70ft), ↔ 3–6m (10–20ft). Australia (moist coastal forest in Queensland). ✲

P. tenuifolium ▣ 🏆 ⚲–⚲ (Kohuhu). Large, bushy shrub to small tree, erect and fast-growing when young, broader and slower-growing with age. Produces dark grey to black young stems and alternate, oblong-ovate to elliptic-obovate, usually wavy-margined, thinly leathery, glossy, mid-green leaves, 2.5–6cm (1–2½in) long. In late spring and early summer, bears bell-shaped honey-scented, black-red flowers, 8–10mm (⅜–½in) across, singly or sometimes in small, few-flowered axillary clusters; they are followed by

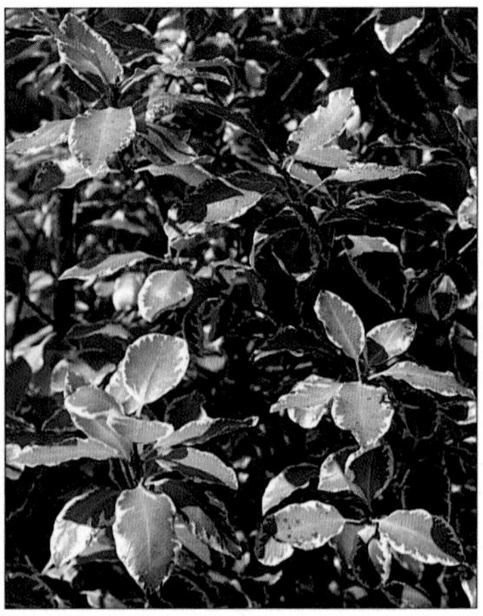

Pittosporum 'Garnettii'

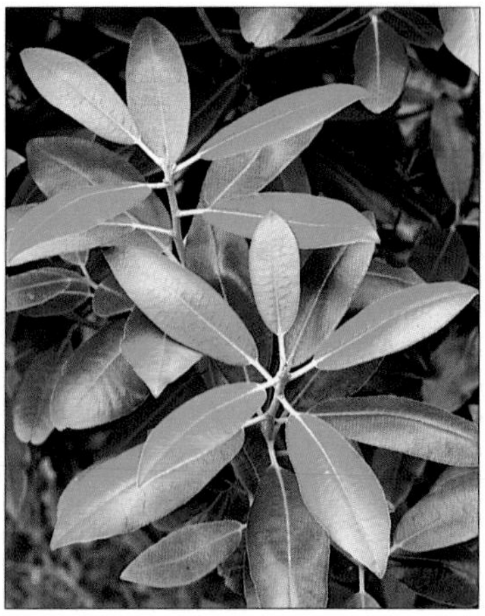

Pittosporum ralphii

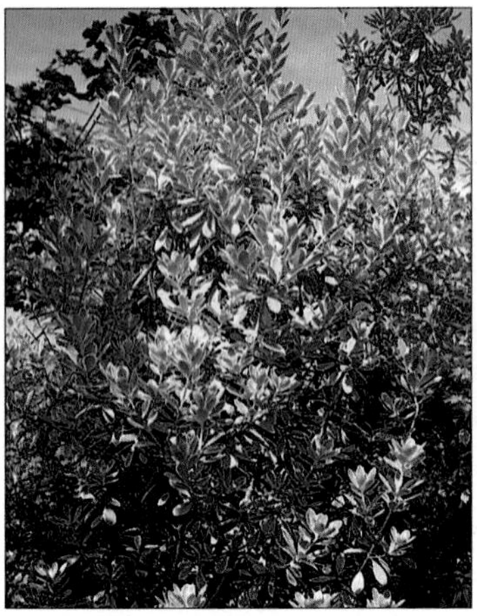

Pittosporum crassifolium 'Variegatum'

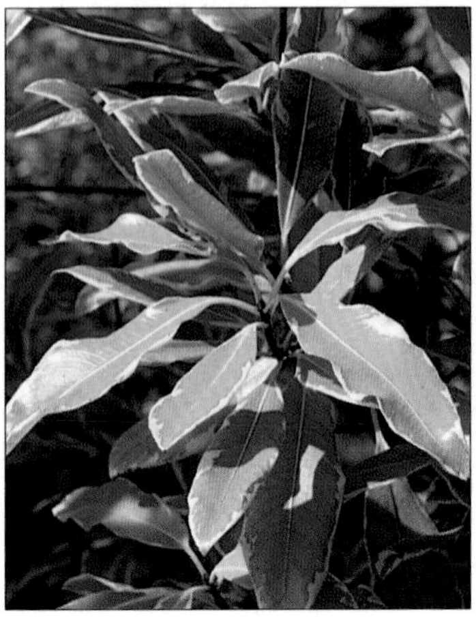

Pittosporum eugenioides 'Variegatum'

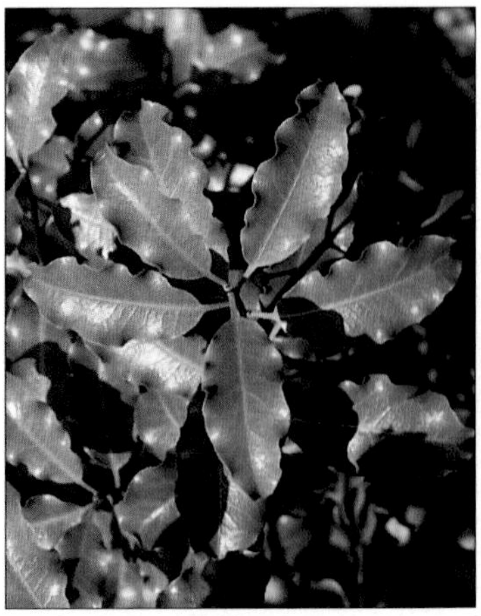

Pittosporum tenuifolium

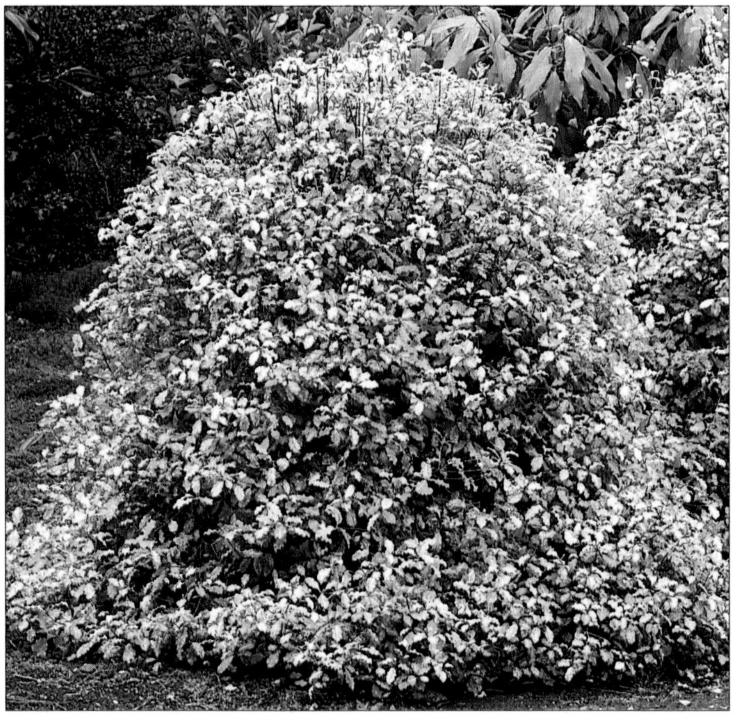

Pittosporum tenuifolium 'Irene Paterson'

grey-black capsules, 1.5cm (½in) long. ↕4–10m (12–30ft), ↔ 2–5m (6–15ft). New Zealand. ✻✻. **'Abbotsbury Gold'** has yellow leaves with irregular green margins; ↕3m (10ft), ↔ 1.5m (5ft). **subsp. *colensoi***, syn. *P. colensoi*, produces softly hairy young stems and broader, thicker leaves, 5–10cm (2–4in) long; ↕8m (25ft), ↔ 1–4m (3–12ft). **'Deborah'** bears small leaves, 2.5cm (1in) long, with cream and green variegation; ↕2m (6ft), ↔ 1m (3ft). **'Golden King'** is erect, with light golden green leaves; ↕ to 3m (10ft), ↔ 1m (3ft). **'Irene Paterson'** ▣ ♀ grows slowly, and bears white leaves speckled and mottled between the veins; ↕ to 1.2m (4ft), ↔ to 60cm (24in). **'Limelight'** bears elliptic, lime-green leaves with dark green, only slightly wavy margins. **'Margaret Turnbull'** is compact, bearing dark green leaves centrally splashed golden yellow; ↕ to 1.8m (6ft), ↔ 1m (3ft). **'Nigricans'** produces black twigs and deep bronze-purple mature leaves. **'Purpureum'** is similar to 'Nigricans' but more open in habit, with purple foliage; ↕3m (10ft), ↔ 1.5m (5ft). **'Silver Queen'** ♀ is compact in growth, and has grey-green

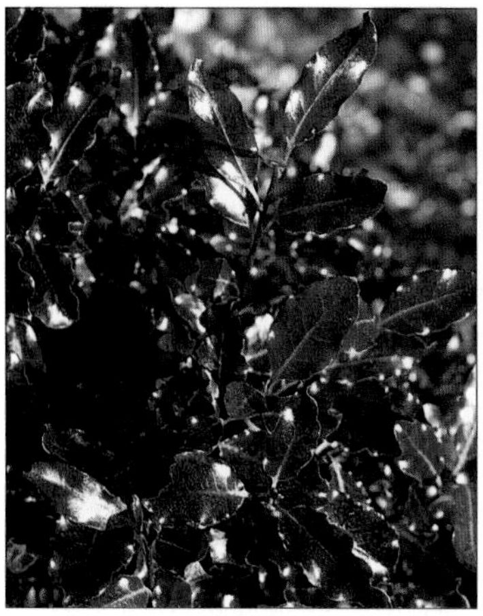

Pittosporum tenuifolium 'Tom Thumb'

leaves with irregular white margins; ↕1–4m (3–12ft), ↔ 2m (6ft). **'Tom Thumb'** ▣ ♀ forms a low bush, and bears foliage flushed bronze-purple; ↕ to 1m (3ft), ↔ 60cm (24in). **'Warnham Gold'** ♀ has golden green leaves that mature golden yellow. **'Wendle Channon'** has light green leaves with cream-coloured margins.

P. tobira ▣ ♀ ☊ (Japanese mock orange). Large shrub or small tree, usually rounded and dense, with erect, sturdy stems and alternate, obovate, leathery leaves, 3–10cm (1¼–4in) long, lustrous and deep green above, paler beneath, and with recurved margins. In late spring and early summer, bears large, handsome, terminal, umbel-like clusters of bell-shaped, very sweetly scented, creamy white flowers, to 2.5cm (1in) across, ageing yellow; they are followed by spherical, yellow-brown capsules with red seeds, 1.5cm (½in) long. ↕2–10m (6–30ft), ↔ 1.5–3m (5–10ft). China, Korea, Japan. ✻. **'Variegatum'** ♀ has congested stems and smaller leaves, 3cm (1¼in) long, with irregular white margins.

P. undulatum ☊ (Australian mock orange, Cheesewood). Dense, rounded

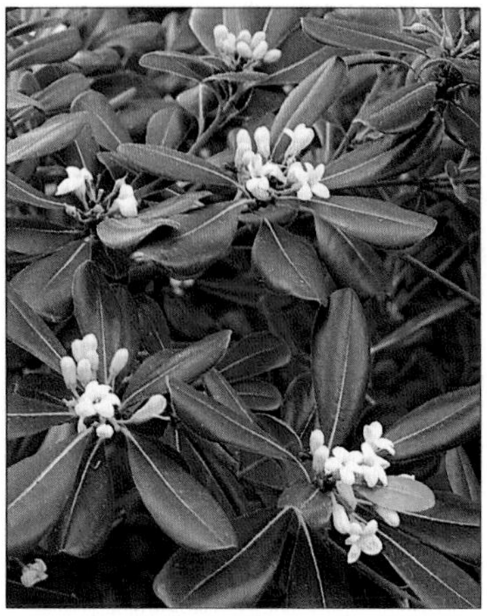

Pittosporum tobira

tree with alternate, oblong-lance-shaped to narrowly oblong-ovate, wavy-margined leaves, 7–15cm (3–6in) long, glossy, deep green above, paler beneath. From late spring to midsummer, bears bell-shaped, fragrant, creamy white flowers, 1.5cm (½in) across, in terminal, umbel-like clusters; they are sometimes followed by spherical, orange to brown capsules, to 1cm (½in) across, which split to reveal sticky, ruby-red seeds. ↕8–15m (25–50ft), sometimes to 24m (80ft), ↔ 3–7m (10–22ft). Australia (Queensland to Tasmania). ✻. **'Variegatum'** has leaves with irregular white margins.

P. viridiflorum Usually free-branching, large shrub or small tree, bearing hairy young stems and alternate, obovate, leathery leaves, 3–10cm (1¼–4in) long; the leaves are lustrous, deep green above, paler beneath, sometimes with margins rolled under. From late spring to midsummer, produces terminal, corymb-like panicles of small, jasmine-scented, yellow-green flowers, to 6mm (¼in) across; they are short-tubed and open trumpet-shaped, with 5 spreading lobes, and are followed by almost spherical brown capsules, 1.5cm (½in) long. ↕3m (10ft), sometimes to 6m (20ft), ↔ 2–3m (6–10ft). South Africa. ❀ (min. 5°C/41°F)

▷ **Pittosporum, Weeping** see *Pittosporum phillyreoides*

PITYROGRAMMA

ADIANTACEAE/PTERIDACEAE

Genus of about 14 species of evergreen, terrestrial ferns, native to woodland and shady rocks in W. North America and tropical areas of Africa, Central America, and South America. They have creeping rhizomes that produce tufts of attractive, triangular, pinnate to 3-pinnate fronds, with a silvery white, yellow, or rarely pink, mealy powder on the undersides. Elongated sori are produced along the veins, without protective indusia. In frost-prone climates, grow in a warm greenhouse or as houseplants. In warmer regions, grow in a sheltered, shady border.

- **HARDINESS** Frost tender.
- **CULTIVATION** Under glass, grow in 1 part each of loam, medium-grade bark, and charcoal, 2 parts sharp sand, and 3 parts coarse leaf mould, in bright filtered light. In the growing season, water moderately, avoiding wetting the foliage, and apply a balanced liquid fertilizer every month. Water sparingly in winter. Outdoors, grow in humus-rich, moist but well-drained soil in partial shade.
- **PROPAGATION** Sow spores at 19–24°C (66–75°F) when ripe. Divide in spring. See also p.51.
- **PESTS AND DISEASES** Trouble free.

P. argentea ▣ Tufted fern bearing long-stalked, arching, broadly triangular, 2- or 3-pinnate fronds, to 60cm (24in) long, with a silvery white or golden yellow bloom beneath. Pinnae are narrowly triangular-ovate, composed of wedge-shaped to broadly oblong-ovate and deeply pinnatifid secondary segments. ↕ to 60cm (24in), ↔ 1m (3ft). Africa, Madagascar, Mascarene Islands. ❀ (min. 10°C/50°F)

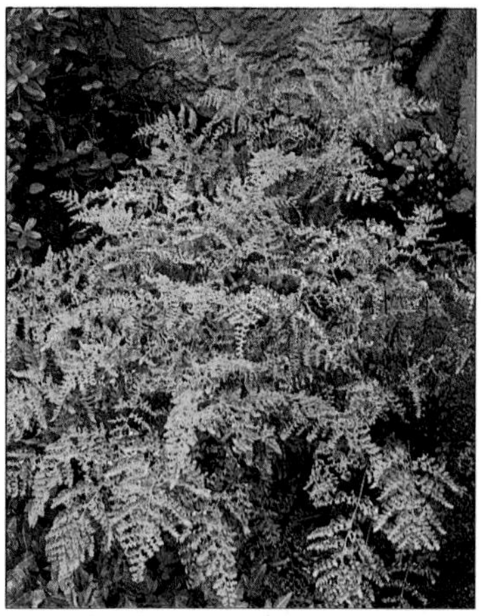

Pityrogramma argentea

P. calomelanos. Neat, tufted fern bearing triangular-ovate, very regularly 2-pinnate, mid-green fronds, to 80cm (32in) long, usually silvery white, rarely pink mealy, on the undersides, with narrowly diamond-shaped segments. ↕ to 30–90cm (12–36in), ↔ to 1m (3ft). Tropical Central America and South America. ❀ (min. 10°C/50°F). **var. *austroamericana*** has a yellow or orange bloom on the undersides of the fronds.

P. chrysophylla. Tufted fern producing very long-stalked, ovate or triangular-ovate, 2- or 3-pinnate, mid-green fronds, 20–60cm (8–24in) tall. Similar to *P. calomelanos*, but the frond undersides are covered with a bright yellow, waxy powder, and the segments are ovate to narrowly diamond-shaped. ↕↔ 10–40cm (4–16in). West Indies, South America. ❀ (min. 10°C/50°F)

P. triangularis, syn. *Gymnogramma triangularis* (Goldback fern). Tufted fern bearing triangular, 2-pinnate, mid- to yellow-green fronds, to 20cm (8in) long, rarely more, the undersides covered with a gold or silver, waxy powder. Pinnae are divided into narrow, triangular or oblong segments. ↕↔ 10–20cm (4–8in). S.W. USA, N.W. Mexico. ❀ (min. 10°C/50°F)

▷ ***Plagianthus lyallii*** see *Hoheria lyallii*
▷ ***Plagiorhegma*** see *Jeffersonia*
P. dubia see *J. dubia*
▷ **Plane** see *Platanus*
London see *P.* x *hispanica*
Oriental see *P. orientalis*

PLANTAGO

Plantain

PLANTAGINACEAE

Genus of some 200 species of mostly rosette-forming annuals, biennials, evergreen perennials and shrubs, many of which are invasive, from very variable habitats worldwide. Grown mainly for their attractive basal rosettes of linear to almost rounded leaves, they also bear tiny, tubular flowers with 4 small petal lobes, in long-stemmed, spherical to oblong spikes, in summer. Grow larger species in a herbaceous border; smaller, alpine species in a rock garden or alpine house. In frost-prone areas, grow tender species in a cool greenhouse.

- **HARDINESS** Fully hardy to frost tender.
- **CULTIVATION** Under glass, grow in 4 parts peat or leaf mould to 1 part grit or sharp sand. Outdoors, grow in preferably neutral to acid, moderately

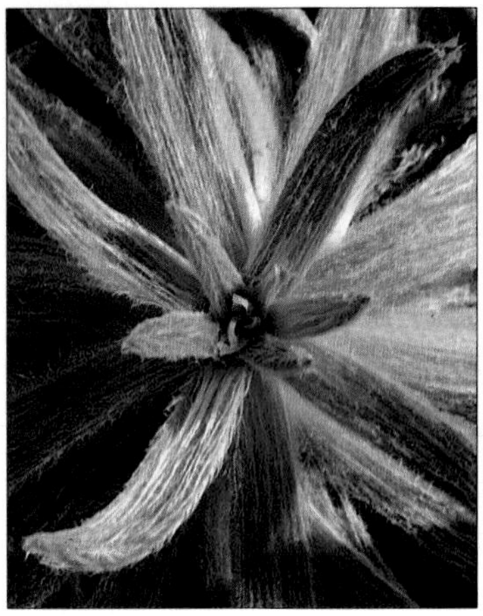

Plantago nivalis

fertile, sharply drained soil in full sun. Protect from winter wet.
• **PROPAGATION** Sow seed in containers in a cold frame in autumn, or divide in spring.
• **PESTS AND DISEASES** Prone to aphids and red spider mites under glass.

P. nivalis ■ Compact perennial with neat rosettes of lance-shaped, very silky-hairy, silver-green leaves, to 1cm (½in) long. In summer, leafless stems, 10cm (4in) long, bear spikes, to 1cm (½in) across, of tiny, tubular, grey-brown flowers. ↕ 2.5cm (1in), ↔ 8cm (3in). Mountains in S. Spain. ❄❄❄

▷**Plantain** see *Musa, Plantago*
French see *Musa acuminata* 'Dwarf Cavendish'
Parrot's see *Heliconia psittacorum*
Water see *Alisma*

PLATANUS

Plane

PLATANACEAE

Genus of about 6 species of deciduous trees found in valley bottoms and watercourses in North America and Mexico, with one species in S.E. Europe and one in S.E. Asia. Planes are grown for their imposing stature and open habit, their large, alternate, palmately lobed leaves, which turn golden brown in autumn, and their flaking bark. The flowers are inconspicuous, but spherical clusters of fruits hang from the shoots throughout winter. They are best as street trees or for large gardens or parks. Planes thrive in urban conditions, but if planted close to buildings their vigorous roots may damage drains. Contact with the basal tufts of hair on the fruits may irritate the skin and respiratory system.
• **HARDINESS** Fully hardy to half hardy, but all grow better in climates with hot summers where the current year's shoots are well-ripened.
• **CULTIVATION** Grow in fertile, well-drained soil in full sun. Pruning group 1.
• **PROPAGATION** Sow seed (of species only) in autumn. Take hardwood cuttings in winter.
• **PESTS AND DISEASES** All except *P. orientalis* are prone to plane anthracnose. The foliage is prone to lacebugs.

P. x acerifolia see *P.* x *hispanica.*
P. x hispanica ■ ♀ ○ (*P. occidentalis* x *P. orientalis*) syn. *P.* x *acerifolia* (London plane). Vigorous, broadly

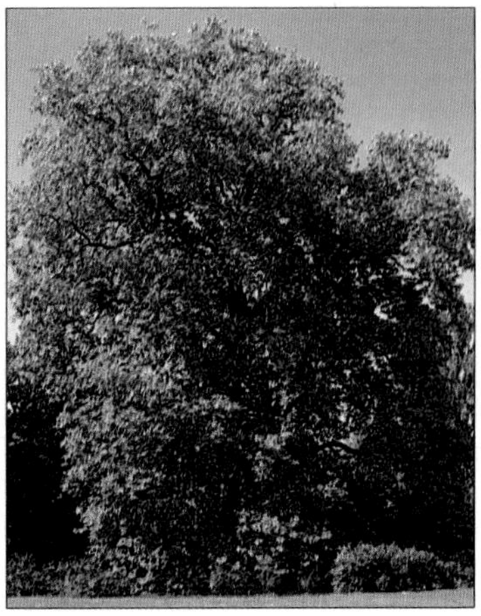

Platanus x *hispanica*

columnar, deciduous tree with flaking brown, grey, and cream bark and very variable but usually sharply 3- to 5-lobed, bright green leaves, to 35cm (14in) long. Green, later brown fruit clusters, 2.5cm (1in) across, are borne in groups of up to 4, and persist during autumn and winter. ↕ 30m (100ft), ↔ 20m (70ft). Garden origin. ❄❄❄. **'Bloodgood'** is fast-growing, drought-tolerant, and relatively resistant to anthracnose. **'Suttneri'** has leaves marked creamy white; ↕ 20m (70ft), ↔ 15m (50ft).
P. occidentalis ○ (American sycamore, Buttonwood). Vigorous, broadly columnar, deciduous tree with flaking brown, grey, and cream bark and usually 3-lobed, bright green leaves, to 20cm (8in) long. Green, later brown fruit clusters, 2.5cm (1in) across, are produced usually singly, rarely in pairs, and persist during autumn and winter. ↕ 25m (80ft), ↔ 20m (70ft) or more. E. and S. North America. ❄❄
P. orientalis ■ ♀ ○ (Oriental plane). Vigorous, spreading, deciduous tree with flaking grey, brown, and cream bark and deeply 5-lobed, glossy green leaves, to 25cm (10in) long. Green, later brown fruit clusters, to 2.5cm (1in) across, are borne in groups of up to 6, and persist during autumn and winter. ↕↔ 30m (100ft) or more. S.E. Europe (widely planted in W. Asia). ❄❄❄
P. racemosa △ (California sycamore). Vigorous, broadly columnar tree with flaking grey bark and deeply 5-lobed, occasionally 3-lobed, dark green leaves, to 15–30cm (6–12in) long, velvety when young. Green, later brown fruit clusters, 2.5cm (1in) across, are produced in groups of 2–7, and persist during autumn and winter. ↕ 25m (80ft), ↔ 20m (70ft) or more. USA (S. California), Mexico. ❄

PLATYCARYA

JUGLANDACEAE

Genus of one species of deciduous, large shrub or small tree from forest in E. Asia. It is cultivated for its long, pinnate leaves that colour yellow in autumn, for its upright catkins, and for its long-lasting, cone-like racemes of fruit. The bark is often used for making a black dye. Best grown as a specimen tree in woodland.
• **HARDINESS** Fully hardy, but young plants may be damaged by frost.
• **CULTIVATION** Grow in fertile, moist but well-drained soil in full sun. Pruning group 1.
• **PROPAGATION** Sow seed in containers in autumn.
• **PESTS AND DISEASES** Trouble free.

P. strobilacea ○ Rounded tree with alternate, pinnate, mid-green leaves, to 30cm (12in) long, composed of 7 to 15 ovate to oblong-lance-shaped, toothed leaflets. In mid- and late summer, tiny flowers are borne in erect, yellow-green catkins: several males, to 10cm (4in) long, surround a single female. Small-winged, green, later brown, fruit are borne in cone-like racemes to 4cm (1½in) long, in autumn, and survive until the following year. ↕↔ 15m (50ft). China, Taiwan, Korea, Japan. ❄❄❄

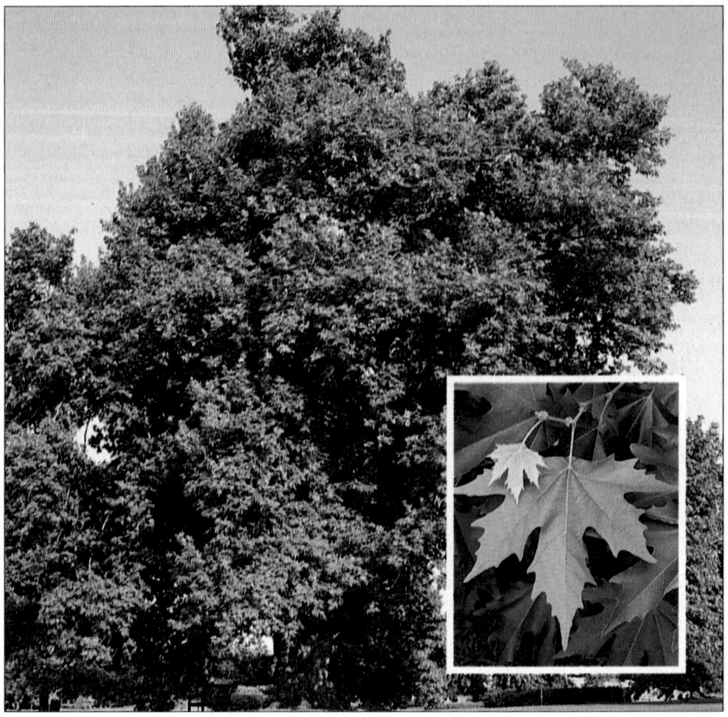

Platanus orientalis (inset: leaf detail)

PLATYCERIUM

Staghorn fern

POLYPODIACEAE

Genus of 15 or more species of evergreen, epiphytic ferns, with short-creeping rhizomes; most are found in temperate and tropical rainforest in Africa, Asia, and Australia, a few in South America. They are grown mainly for their attractive, often elegant foliage, each plant bearing both sterile and fertile fronds. The mid- to deep green sterile fronds are stalkless, rounded to oblong, and entire to irregularly lobed at the upper margins; they become brown and papery, and usually form a persistent "nest" or basket at the base of the plant. The fertile fronds are spreading or pendent to erect, wedge-shaped at the bases, usually grey-green and leathery, and often repeatedly forked; they are shed naturally when old. All fronds are covered on both sides with small, star-shaped hairs. Spores are formed in large patches on the undersides of fertile fronds; in some species, new plants develop from runners on the sides of established nests. In frost-prone climates, grow in a conservatory or cool or temperate greenhouse, or as houseplants, preferably in hanging baskets. In warmer regions, grow epiphytically in a tree.
• **HARDINESS** Frost tender.
• **CULTIVATION** Under glass, grow epiphytically in equal parts coarse leaf mould (or peat), roughly chopped spagnum moss, loam, and charcoal, in bright filtered light. When in growth, water freely, mist daily, and apply a balanced liquid fertilizer every month; water sparingly in winter. Outdoors, grow epiphytically on a tree in partial shade.
• **PROPAGATION** Sow spores at 21°C (70°F) when ripe. Detach plantlets produced from root tips or runners as soon as nests have formed. See also p.51.
• **PESTS AND DISEASES** Scale insects can be a problem.

P. alcicorne (South American staghorn). Epiphytic fern with rounded to kidney-shaped, entire or partially lobed sterile fronds, 15–40cm (6–16in) long, which lie flat, and are mid- to deep green then brown. Leathery, grey-green fertile fronds, 60cm (24in) long, are erect, and divided 2 or 3 times. Spores are formed on frond forks. ↕↔ to 85cm (34in). E. Africa, Madagascar, Seychelles, Mauritius. ❁ (min. 5°C/41°F)
***P. alcicorne* of gardens** see *P. bifurcatum.*
P. bifurcatum ■ ♀ syn. *P. alcicorne* of gardens (Common staghorn fern). Very variable, epiphytic fern with erect or horizontal, rounded to heart- or kidney-shaped sterile fronds, 12–45cm (5–18in) long, which are mid- to deep green then brown, and are entire, wavy, or lobed at the upper margins. Grey-green fertile fronds, to 90cm (36in), are erect, spreading, or pendent, forked 2 or 3 times into strap-shaped, densely hairy segments. Very similar to *P. alcicorne.* A very popular plant, from which many cultivars have been derived. ↕ to 90cm (36in), ↔ 80cm (32in). Java to E. Australia. ❁ (min. 5°C/41°F)

P

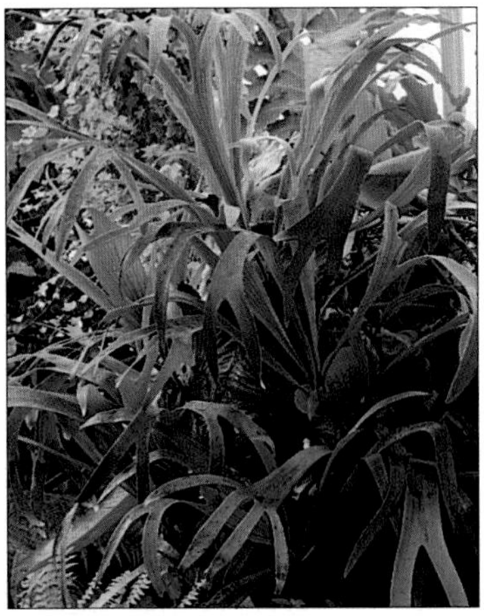

Platycerium bifurcatum

P. elephantotis (Cabbage fern, Elephant's ear fern). Epiphytic fern with erect, rounded to oblong, papery, mid- to deep green then brown sterile fronds, to 90cm (36in) long. Fertile fronds are pendent, wedge-shaped, light grey-green, to 75cm (30in) long. Spores form along frond margins. ↕ to 90cm (36in), ↔ 80cm (32in). Tropical Africa. ❄ (min. 15°C/°59F)
P. grande ♀ Magnificent epiphytic fern bearing bronze to green sterile fronds, to 1m (3ft) tall, rounded to heart- or kidney-shaped, with deeply lobed upper margins; they are papery, may be spreading or lying flat to the branches, and form an impressive crown. Grey-green fertile fronds, to 1.8m (6ft) tall, are pendent, wedge-shaped, leathery, and forked into strap-shaped segments. Spores form in 2 large semicircular patches on the second forks of fertile fronds. ↕ to 1.8m (6ft), ↔ 1.2m (4ft). Philippines, Malaysia, Australia. ❄ (min. 15°C/59°F)
***P. grande* of gardens** see *P. superbum.*
P. hillii ■ Epiphytic fern with rounded, dark green sterile fronds, to 40cm (16in) long, shallowly lobed at the upper margins, and lying flat to the branches. Leathery, light grey-green fertile fronds are erect or arching, broadly wedge-shaped, irregularly forked or palmately lobed above, and 75cm (30in) or more tall. Sometimes considered a variety of *P. bifurcatum.* ↕ 70cm (28in) or more, ↔ 60cm (24in). N.W. Australia, New Guinea. ❄ (min. 10°C/50°F)
P. superbum, syn. *P. grande* of gardens. Very large, epiphytic fern producing a crown of grey to grey-green sterile fronds, to 1.6m (5½ft) tall, deeply lobed at the spreading upper margins, and lying flat on the branches. Greyish green fertile fronds, to 2m (6ft) long, are spreading to pendent, and forked up to 5 times with often twisted segments. Similar to *P. grande* but has only a single spore patch in the first fork of fertile fronds. ↕ to 2m (6ft), ↔ 1.5m (5ft). Australia (Western Australia). ❄ (min. 15°C/59°F)

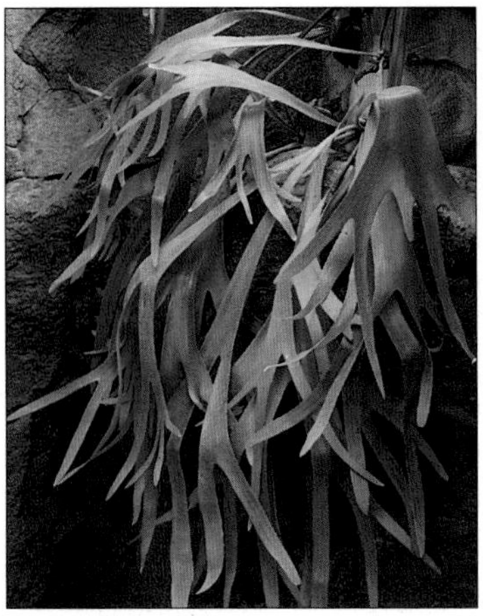

Platycerium hillii

▷ ***Platycladus*** see *Thuja*
P. orientalis see *T. orientalis*

PLATYCODON
Balloon flower
CAMPANULACEAE

Genus of one species of perennial, variable in habit and form, from grassy slopes and mountain meadows in E. Asia. Late emerging, it forms a neat clump of hairless stems with simple, ovate to ovate-lance-shaped, toothed, bluish green leaves. It is cultivated mainly for its clusters of bell-shaped, 5-petalled, mid-blue, dark blue, or lilac-purple flowers, which open from large, balloon-like buds. Suitable for a rock garden or the front of a herbaceous border. It is also good for cutting. Established plants resent disturbance.
- **HARDINESS** Fully hardy.
- **CULTIVATION** Grow in deep, light, fertile, loamy, reliably moist but well-drained soil in full sun or partial shade. Stems may require support.
- **PROPAGATION** Sow seed *in situ* or in containers, in spring. Divide in summer, or detach rooted basal shoots in early summer.
- **PESTS AND DISEASES** Slugs and snails attack young shoots.

P. grandiflorus ■ ♀ Compact, clump-forming perennial with ovate to ovate-lance-shaped, toothed, bluish green leaves, to 5cm (2in) long, borne in whorls on the lower stem, alternately higher up. In late summer, clusters of large, balloon-like buds open to shallow, bell-shaped, 5-petalled, purple-blue flowers, to 5cm (2in) across, with darker blue veins and pointed tips to the petals. ↕ to 60cm (24in), ↔ 30cm (12in). Russia (E. Siberia), N. China (including Manchuria), Korea, Japan. ✲✲✲. **f. *albus*** has white flowers with blue veins. **f. *apoyama*** ♀ has deep violet flowers; ↕ 20cm (8in). **'Mother of Pearl'** see 'Perlmutterschale'. **'Park's Double Blue'** produces double, violet-blue flowers. **'Perlmutterschale'**, syn. 'Mother of Pearl', produces pale pink flowers.

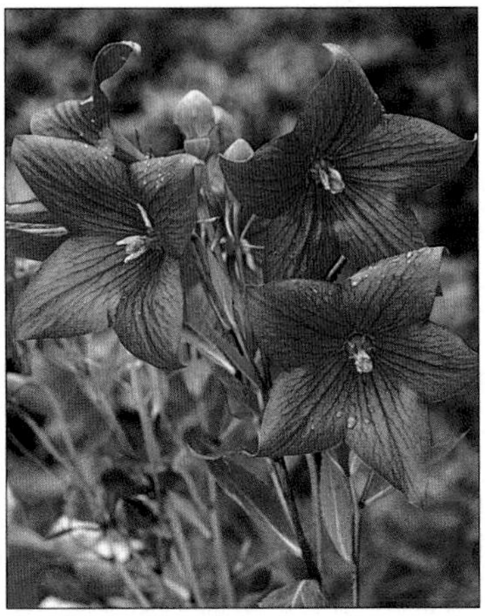

Platycodon grandiflorus

PLATYSTEMON
Californian poppy, Creamcups
PAPAVERACEAE

Genus of one very variable species of erect to spreading, basally branching, hairy annual from grassland, desert margins, and chaparral in W. USA. It has almost stalkless, stem-clasping, entire leaves, sometimes borne in small whorls. It is grown for its short-lived, poppy-like flowers, each with a central boss of flattened stamen filaments, borne in profusion where the climate is neither too hot nor too humid. Suitable for an annual border and rock gardens.
- **HARDINESS** Fully hardy.
- **CULTIVATION** Grow in very light, well-drained soil in full sun.
- **PROPAGATION** Sow seed *in situ* in spring.
- **PESTS AND DISEASES** Trouble free.

P. californicus (Californian poppy, Creamcups). Many-branched, spreading annual bearing linear-oblong to lance-shaped, densely hairy, strongly parallel-veined, grey-green leaves, to 8cm (3in) long. In spring, produces single, slender-stemmed, 6-petalled, creamy yellow flowers, to 2.5cm (1in) across. ↕ 10–30cm (4–12in), ↔ to 23cm (9in). USA (California to Arizona, Utah). ✲✲✲

PLECTRANTHUS
LABIATAE/LAMIACEAE

Genus of 350 species of annuals, evergreen perennials, semi-succulents, and shrubs from Africa, Madagascar, Asia, Australasia, and Pacific islands. Cultivated for their foliage and flowers, they are often upright at first but become trailing or spreading with growth. The heart-shaped to ovate or rounded leaves have usually scalloped, sometimes toothed or wavy margins; they are mostly soft, often slightly furry, and aromatic. The small, tubular, 2-lipped, whorled flowers are borne in terminal panicles, racemes, or spikes. In frost-prone climates, grow in a cool or temperate greenhouse or conservatory, or as houseplants; grow trailing species in hanging baskets, which may be placed outside in summer and autumn. In warmer areas, grow in a sunny border.
- **HARDINESS** Frost tender.
- **CULTIVATION** Under glass, grow in loam-based potting compost (JI No.2) in full light, with shade from hot sun. During the growing season, water freely and apply a balanced liquid fertilizer every month; water moderately during winter. Outdoors, grow in moderately fertile, well-drained soil in dappled shade.
- **PROPAGATION** Sow seed at 19–24°C (66–75°F) when ripe. Divide in mid- or late spring. Take stem-tip cuttings at any time of year.
- **PESTS AND DISEASES** Trouble free.

P. amboinicus. Spreading, often decumbent, evergreen perennial with hairy, ovate, aromatic, mid-green leaves, to 4.5cm (1¾in) long, dotted with glands, and with finely scalloped margins. In summer, bears whorled, tubular, 2-lipped, lilac-pink, mauve, or white flowers, 7–9cm (3–3½in) across, in terminal racemes, to 15cm (6in) long. ↕ 30cm (12in), ↔ 1m (3ft). Tropical to Southern Africa. ❄ (min. 10°C/50°F)
P. argentatus. Erect to spreading, evergreen shrub with silver-hairy stems and densely pubescent, ovate, light grey-green leaves, 5–11cm (2–4½in) long, with scalloped margins. In summer, produces terminal racemes, to 30cm (12in) long, of whorled, tubular, pale bluish white flowers, 9–10mm (⅜–½in) across. ↕↔ 1m (3ft). Australia. ❄ (min. 10°C/50°F)
P. australis (Swedish ivy). Upright then trailing, evergreen perennial producing rounded, glossy, dark green leaves, 2.5–4cm (1–1½in) long, with scalloped margins. Intermittently bears terminal racemes, 20cm (8in) long, of whorled, tubular, white or pale mauve flowers. ↕ 60–90cm (24–36in), ↔ to 1m (3ft). Australia. ❄ (min. 10°C/50°F)
***P. coleoides* of gardens** see *P. forsteri.*
***P. coleoides* 'Variegatus' of gardens** see *P. madagascariensis* 'Variegated Mintleaf'.
P. forsteri, syn. *P. coleoides* of gardens. Upright then trailing, evergreen perennial producing ovate to broadly ovate, hairy, light green leaves, 6–10cm (2½–4in) long, with scalloped margins. Intermittently bears terminal racemes, 15–20cm (6–8in) long, of whorled, tubular, pale mauve or white flowers, 3cm (1¼in) across. ↕ 25cm (10in), ↔ to 1m (3ft). E. Australia, Fiji, New Caledonia. ❄ (min. 10°C/50°F). **'Marginatus'** ■ has leaves with broad, creamy white margins.
P. madagascariensis (Mintleaf). Creeping, shrubby, semi-succulent perennial with square brown stems and rounded, scalloped, firm, fleshy leaves, 3–4cm (1¼–1½in) long, sometimes wrinkled, and coated with white bristles; the leaves smell of mint when crushed. Terminal spikes, 10–15cm (4–6in) long, of whorled, tubular, 2-lipped, pale lavender-blue or white flowers, to 1½cm (½in) across, often dotted with red glands, are borne in early summer. ↕ to 30cm (12in), ↔ indefinite. S.E. Africa, Madagascar. ❄ (min.15°C/59°F). **'Variegated Mintleaf'**, syn. *P. coleoides* 'Variegatus' of gardens, has variegated white leaves.

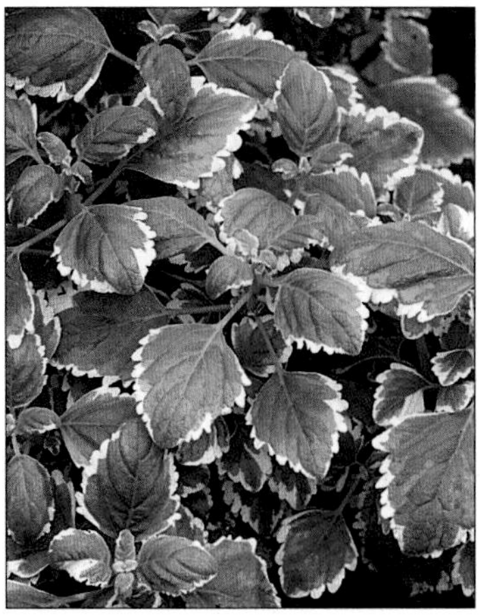

Plectranthus forsteri 'Marginatus'

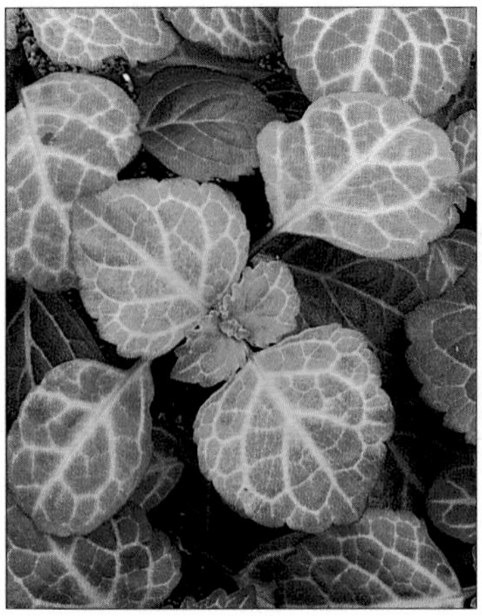
Plectranthus oertendahlii

P. oertendahlii ■ ♀ (Candle plant). Trailing perennial with freely branching, reddish purple stems bearing ovate to almost rounded, scalloped, bronze-green leaves, 3–4cm (1¼–1½in) long, with pale veins above, and undersides with soft purple felting. Loose, terminal racemes, 20cm (8in) long, of whorled, white or light blue flowers, 5mm (¼in) long, are produced at intervals all year round. ↕ 20cm (8in), ↔ trailing to 1m (3ft) or more. South Africa (KwaZulu/Natal). ❀ (min. 10°C/50°F)
P. thyrsoideus, syn. *Coleus thyrsoideus.* Bushy, branching perennial or subshrub, often grown as an annual or a winter-flowering container plant, with hairy stems and heart-shaped, toothed, hairy, mid-green leaves, to 15cm (6in) long. Bright blue flowers, to 1cm (½in) long, are produced in terminal spikes, to 9cm (3½in) long, at various times of the year. ↕ to 90cm (36in), ↔ to 60cm (24in). C. Africa. ❀ (min. 4°C/39°F)
P. verticillatus. Mat-forming, semi-succulent perennial with creeping stems rooting at the nodes. Ovate to rounded, coarsely toothed, soft, fleshy leaves, 1.5–4cm (½–1½in) long, have purplish green undersides. Terminal spikes, 16cm (6in) long, of whorled, tubular, 2-lipped, purple-speckled, white or pale mauve flowers, 1.5–2.5cm (½–1in) across, are produced in summer. ↕ 6–8cm (2½–3in), ↔ indefinite. South Africa (Northern Transvaal, Eastern Transvaal, Eastern Cape), Swaziland, Mozambique. ❀ (min. 10°C/50°F)

P

PLEIOBLASTUS

GRAMINEAE/POACEAE

Genus of about 20 upright, evergreen, woody bamboos usually found in woodland and woodland margins in China and Japan. They are cultivated for their leaves, which are linear to lance-shaped, 5–35cm (2–14in) long, often tessellated, sometimes variegated, and usually white-bristled on the margins. They have generally vigorously spreading rhizomes, and produce thickets of erect woody canes, round in section, and either hollow or almost solid; on the lower part of each cane there are 1–7 branches per node. Spikes or racemes of spikelets, each containing 5–13 florets, are sometimes produced, but flowering occurs only rarely. They are suitable for growing in open glades in a woodland garden.
• **HARDINESS** Fully hardy.

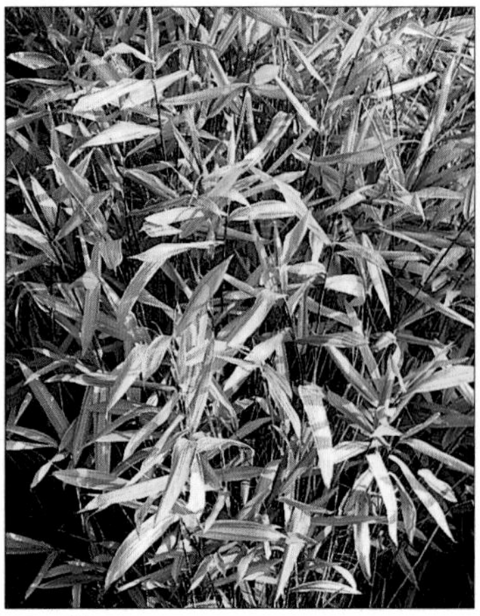
Pleioblastus auricomus

• **CULTIVATION** Grow in fertile, humus-rich, moist but well-drained soil in full sun, or in partial shade if not variegated. Provide shelter from cold, dry winds. Some are vigorous, requiring restraint.
• **PROPAGATION** Separate rhizomes in spring; keep divisions moist until established.
• **PESTS AND DISEASES** Trouble free.

P. auricomus ■ ♀ syn. *Arundinaria auricoma, A. viridistriata, P. viridistriatus.* Upright bamboo with short-running rhizomes and hollow, purple-green canes with hairy nodes. The leaves, to 18cm (7in) long, are linear, brilliant yellow with green stripes, and margined with fine bristles. ↕ to 1.5m (5ft), ↔ 1.5m (5ft). Japan. ❄❄❄
P. humilis, syn. *Arundinaria humilis, Sasa humilis.* Upright bamboo with hollow, dark green canes, 1–3 branches per node, and linear, mid-green leaves, to 20cm (8in) long, sometimes downy beneath. Can be very invasive. ↕ 1.5m (5ft), ↔ 2m (6ft) or more. Japan. ❄❄❄
P. pygmaeus, syn. *Arundinaria pygmaea* (Pygmy bamboo). Upright, woody bamboo with usually solid, mid-green

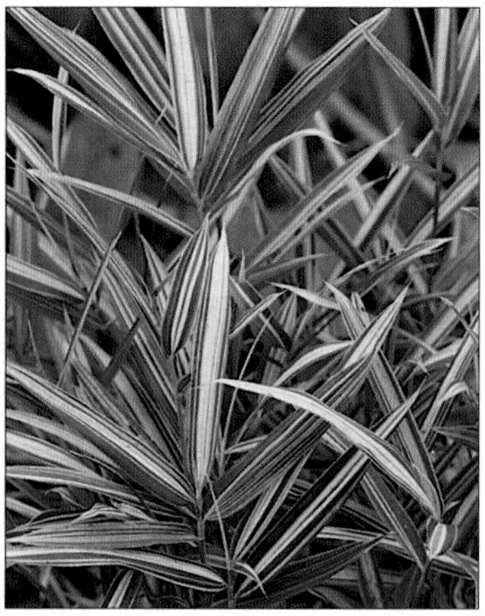
Pleioblastus variegatus

canes, flattened above; they are purplish-green at the tips, with 1 or 2 branches at each node. The leavers are linear, tessellated, downy, mid-green, and 8cm (3in) long. ↕ 40cm (16in), ↔ 1m (3ft). Japan. ❄❄❄. **var. *distichus*** ■ syn. *Arundinaria disticha, A. pygmaea* var. *disticha*, has hollow canes and hairless leaves; ↕ 1m (3ft), ↔ 1.5m (5ft).
***P. simonii* 'Variegatus'**, syn. *Arundinaria simonii* 'Variegata', *P. simonii* f. *variegatus.* Upright, woody bamboo with hollow canes, which have a waxy bloom and 3 branches at each white node. Mid-green, linear to lance-shaped leaves, to 20cm (8in) long, are sometimes striped white, and are finely downy beneath. ↕ 3m (10ft), ↔ 2m (6ft) or more. Japan. ❄❄❄.
f. *variegatus* see *P. simonii* 'Variegatus'.
P. variegatus ■ syn. *Arundinaria fortunei, A. variegata.* Upright, woody bamboo with hollow, pale green canes; the nodes have a white, waxy bloom beneath and each bears 1 or 2 branches. Linear leaves, 14cm (5½in) long, are dark green with cream stripes, and have fine white hairs on both sides. ↕ 75cm (30in), ↔ 1.2m (4ft). Japan. ❄❄❄
P. viridistriatus see *P. auricomus.*

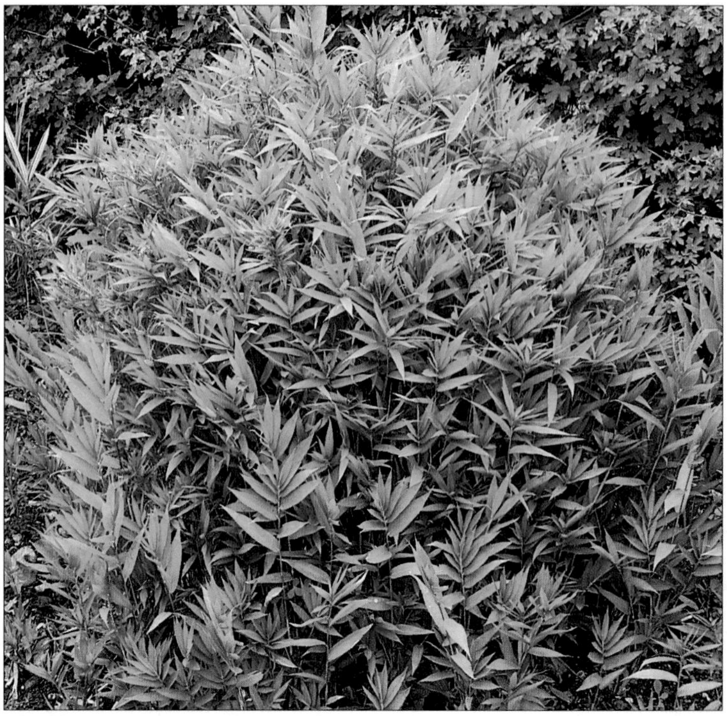
Pleioblastus pygmaeus var. *distichus*

PLEIONE

ORCHIDACEAE

Genus of about 16–20 species of small, deciduous, epiphytic, terrestrial, or lithophytic orchids mainly from wet forest or woodland, at altitudes of 1,000–4,000m (3,250–13,000ft) or higher, from N. India to S. China and Taiwan. They produce short-lived, variably shaped pseudobulbs with 1 or 2 folded, lance-shaped to elliptic, mid-green leaves, 15cm (6in) long, which usually fall before flowering. The often solitary flowers, 8cm (3in) across, are borne on short stems, 5–10cm (2–4in) long, from new growth, at various times of the year. Grow most species in a cool or temperate greenhouse or alpine house, or as houseplants. In areas where temperatures seldom fall below -5°C (23°F), *P. formosana* may be grown in a sheltered rock garden.
• **HARDINESS** Half hardy; some are frost hardy in areas where winter frost is not continuous.
• **CULTIVATION** Cool-growing orchids. Grow in shallow pans of terrestrial or epiphytic orchid compost. Repot annually before flowering. Water freely in spring and summer until the leaves begin to die down, then keep just moist and admit full light. In summer, provide bright filtered light and moderate humidity, mist twice daily, and feed at every third watering. In winter, allow a period of rest, reducing the temperature to 0–2°C (32–35°F). Outdoors, grow *P. formosana* in sharply drained, moderately fertile, leafy, humus-rich soil in a sheltered site in partial shade. Plant in mid-spring. In cold areas, protect from severe weather and excessive wet with an open cloche, from early autumn to spring. See also p.46.
• **PROPAGATION** Divide annually when repotting, discarding old pseudobulbs.
• **PESTS AND DISEASES** Prone to aphids, red spider mites, slugs, and mealybugs.

P. bulbocodioides ■ Terrestrial or lithophytic orchid with almost spherical pseudobulbs, each bearing one folded, lance-shaped to elliptic leaf, to 14cm (5½in) long. In spring, bears solitary, rose-lilac flowers, with white to pink lips spotted with pale brown or purplish pink. ↕ 15cm (6in), ↔ 30cm (12in). Burma, China, Taiwan. ❄ (borderline)
***P.* Eiger** ■ (*P. formosana* x *P. humilis*). Terrestrial or lithophytic orchid with large, pear-shaped pseudobulbs, each bearing one elliptic leaf, to 18cm (7in) long. In mid- and late winter, produces white flowers, shaded pink, 1 or 2 per stem, with white lips marked red, or red and yellow. ↕ 12cm (5in), ↔ 5cm (2in). ❄ (borderline)
P. formosana ■ ♀ Terrestrial or lithophytic orchid with almost spherical pseudobulbs, each bearing one folded, lance-shaped to elliptic leaf, to 14cm (5½in) long. In spring, bears solitary, pale rose-lilac flowers with white lips that have brownish markings, pink margins, and brown or purplish pink spots. ↕ 15cm (6in), ↔ 30cm (12in). E. China, Taiwan. ❄ (borderline)
P. forrestii. Terrestrial or lithophytic orchid with conical pseudobulbs, each bearing one folded, lance-shaped leaf, 10–15cm (4–6in) long. In winter and

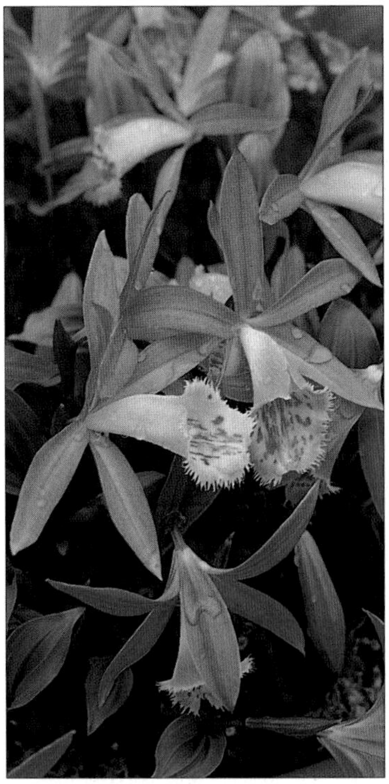

Pleione bulbocodioides

spring, produces solitary yellow flowers with red-dotted lips. ↕ 15cm (6in), ↔ 30cm (12in). China. ✻ (borderline)

P. hookeriana. Epiphytic or lithophytic orchid with conical to ovoid pseudobulbs, each bearing one folded, lance-shaped to elliptic leaf, 5–21cm (2–8in) long. In summer, produces very pale pink to pale purple flowers, 5cm (2in) across, with solitary, white to pale pink lips. ↕ 10cm (4in), ↔ 15cm (6in). Tibet, Nepal, N.E. India, Bhutan, Burma, Laos, N. Thailand, China. ✻ (borderline)

P. humilis. Epiphytic or lithophytic orchid with conical pseudobulbs, each bearing one folded, lance-shaped leaf, 20–30cm (8–12in) long. From winter to spring, produces solitary white flowers with red-streaked lips. ↕ 15cm (6in), ↔ 30cm (12in). Nepal, N.E. India, Burma. ✻ (borderline)

P.* x *lagenaria (*P. maculata* x *P. praecox*). Epiphytic or lithophytic orchid with inverted, cone-shaped pseudobulbs, each bearing 2 folded, lance-shaped leaves, to 30cm (12in) long. Fragrant, pink to rose-lilac to purple flowers, with a yellow central area and purple marks around the margins, are borne 1 or 2 per

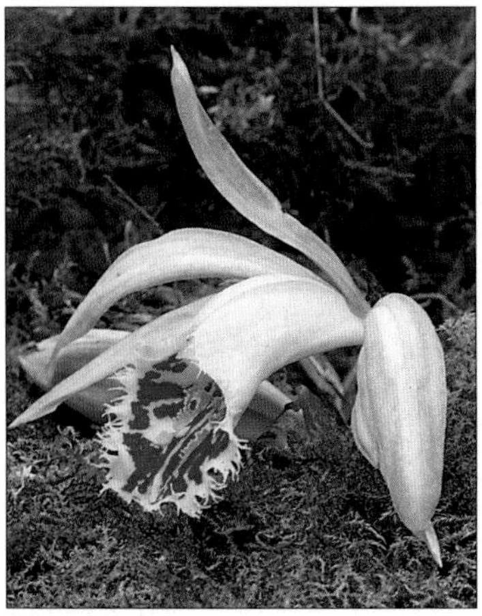

Pleione Eiger

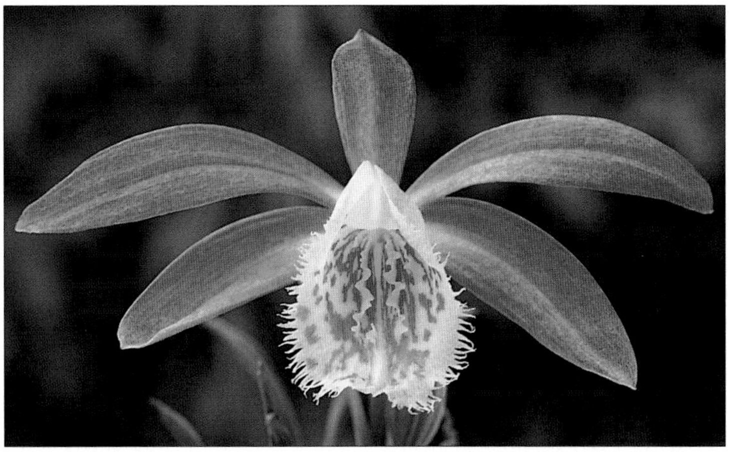

Pleione formosana

pseudobulb, in autumn. ↕ 15cm (6in), ↔ 30cm (12in). India (Assam), possibly S. China. ✻ (borderline)

P. limprichtii. Epiphytic or lithophytic orchid with conical, ovoid or pear-shaped pseudobulbs, each bearing one folded, conical to ovoid leaf, to 14cm (5½in) long. In spring, deep pink to pink-magenta flowers, with rose-red spotted lips, are borne 1 or rarely 2 per pseudobulb. ↕ 15cm (6in), ↔ 30cm (12in). S.W. China, possibly N. Burma. ✻ (borderline)

P. maculata. Epiphytic or lithophytic orchid with barrel-shaped pseudobulbs, each bearing 2 folded, lance-shaped to elliptic leaves, 15–30cm (6–12in) long. In autumn, produces solitary, white or pale cream flowers, sometimes streaked with pink, the lips white with purple markings and a central yellow patch. ↕ 15cm (6in), ↔ 30cm (12in). N. India, Bhutan, Burma, S.W. China, N. Thailand. ✻ (borderline)

P. praecox. Epiphytic or lithophytic orchid with bottle-shaped pseudobulbs, each bearing 2 folded, lance-shaped to narrowly elliptic leaves, to 20cm (8in) long. Solitary, bright rose-purple flowers are produced in autumn. ↕ 15cm (6in), ↔ 30cm (12in). Nepal, N. India (Sikkim), Bhutan, Burma, S.W. China, Thailand. ✻ (borderline)

***P.* Stromboli 'Fireball'** (*P. bulbocodioides* x *P. speciosa*). Epiphytic orchid with conical pseudobulbs, each bearing one folded, lance-shaped to narrowly elliptic leaf, to 25cm (10in) long. In spring, produces solitary, rose-lilac flowers with lips that have reddish pink markings. ↕ 15cm (6in), ↔ 30cm (12in). ✻ (borderline)

PLEIOSPILOS

Living granite

AIZOACEAE

Genus of about 35 species of solitary or clump-forming, stemless, perennial succulents from arid areas of South Africa. They are grown for their unusual form and attractive flowers. Most have 1 or 2, occasionally 3 pairs of often unequal, erect, very fleshy, greyish or yellowish green or brown to red leaves, often with variably coloured dots; they are usually flattened on the upper surfaces, keeled, rounded, or rounded and partly keeled beneath, and united at the bases. The daisy-like, diurnal, yellow or orange flowers, which sometimes have a coconut-like fragrance, open in late summer and early autumn. In areas where temperatures drop below 7°C (45°F), grow as houseplants or in a temperate greenhouse. In warm, dry climates, grow in a raised bed or succulent border.

- **HARDINESS** Frost tender.
- **CULTIVATION** Under glass, grow in standard cactus compost in full light. From early summer to late autumn, water sparingly but regularly and apply a low-nitrogen liquid fertilizer every 4–6 weeks. Keep dry at all other times. Outdoors, grow in low-fertility, sharply drained soil in full sun. See also pp.48–49.
- **PROPAGATION** Sow seed at 19–24°C (66–75°F), or detach offsets, from late spring to summer.
- **PESTS AND DISEASES** Vulnerable to aphids while flowering.

P. bolusii ▣ 🏆 Usually solitary, perennial succulent with one pair of ovoid, grey-green leaves, 4–7cm (1½–3in) long, sometimes tinged red and with dark green dots; they are generally broader than long, with the undersides more rounded and partly keeled. Daisy-like, golden yellow flowers, 6–8cm (2½–3in) across, are solitary or produced in cymes of 2–4 in late summer and early autumn. ↕ 8cm (3in), ↔ 15cm (6in). South Africa (Eastern Cape). ❁ (min. 7°C/45°F)

P. nelii. Solitary, perennial succulent with up to 3 pairs of unequal, almost hemispherical, densely dotted, greyish green leaves, 4–8cm (1½–3in) long, with the tips of the very rounded undersides drawn over the flat upper

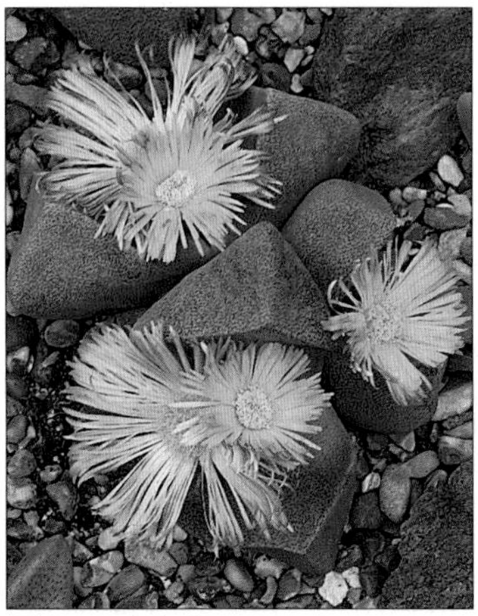

Pleiospilos bolusii

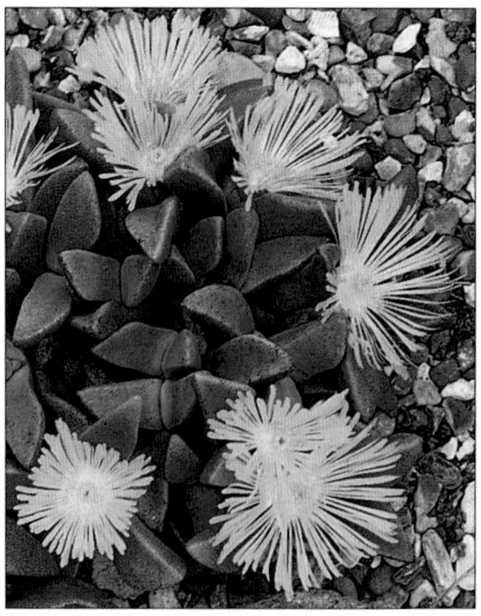

Pleiospilos simulans

surfaces. In late summer and early autumn, produces solitary, daisy-like, orange-pink flowers, 7cm (3in) across. ↕ 7cm (3in), ↔ 12cm (5in). South Africa (Western Cape, Eastern Cape). ❁ (min. 7°C/45°F)

P. simulans ▣ Clump-forming, perennial succulent bearing one pair of slightly unequal, ovate to 3-angled, spreading, densely dotted, reddish, yellowish, or brownish green leaves, 5–8cm (2–3in) long, the keeled undersides thickening towards the tips. Daisy-like, scented, yellow or orange flowers, 6cm (2½in) across, are solitary or produced in cymes of 1–3 in late summer and early autumn. ↕ 10cm (4in), ↔ to 30cm (12in). South Africa (Eastern Cape). ❁ (min. 7°C/45°F)

▷ ***Pleroma macrantha*** see *Tibouchina urvilleana*

PLEUROTHALLIS

ORCHIDACEAE

Genus of about 900 species of mainly small, evergreen, epiphytic or rarely lithophytic orchids found in tropical North, Central, and South America, from Mexico to Peru and Brazil; they occur in forest from low altitudes to over 2,500m (8,000ft). Although extremely variable in form and habit, they typically produce slender stems on creeping rhizomes, with a solitary, lance-shaped to almost rounded, leathery, mid-green leaf at the apex of each stem. One or many flowers, 1.5–3cm (½–1¼in) across, may be produced singly or in racemes from the base of each leaf.

- **HARDINESS** Frost tender.
- **CULTIVATION** Cool- to intermediate-growing orchids. Grow epiphytically on bark, or pot tightly into small containers of epiphytic orchid compost made with fine-grade bark. In summer, provide bright filtered light and high humidity; water freely, mist twice daily, and apply a balanced liquid fertilizer at every third watering. In winter, admit full light and water more sparingly. See also p.46.
- **PROPAGATION** Divide when the plant fills the pot and "flows" over the sides.
- **PESTS AND DISEASES** May be infested by red spider mites, aphids, and mealybugs.

P. grobyi. Small, epiphytic orchid bearing fleshy, lance-shaped to narrowly ovate leaves, 7cm (3in) long, with blunt or rounded tips. Loose racemes of translucent, pale yellow to green flowers, 1cm (½in) long, with scattered purple veins, streaked with brown, are borne above the foliage in summer. ↕ 8cm (3in), ↔ 10cm (4in). Mexico, West Indies, Central and South America. ❄ (min. 10°C/50°F; max. 24°C/75°F)

▷ **Plum,**
Cherry see *Prunus cerasifera*
Date see *Diospyros lotus*
Indian see *Oemleria cerasiformis*
Natal see *Carissa macrocarpa*
Oregon see *Oemleria cerasiformis*

PLUMBAGO

Leadwort

PLUMBAGINACEAE

Genus of 10–15 species of annuals, perennials, and evergreen shrubs and scandent climbers from tropical woodland and scrub in warm-temperate to tropical regions worldwide. They have alternate, simple, entire leaves, and are grown for their terminal, sometimes corymb-like racemes of attractive, white, red, or blue, salverform flowers, each with 5 spreading petal lobes. Where temperatures fall below 7°C (45°F), grow in a cool or temperate greenhouse or conservatory; plants grown in containers can be moved outdoors in summer. In warmer climates, use shrub and perennial species in a mixed or shrub border; train climbers over a pergola or arch.

• **HARDINESS** Half hardy to frost tender.
• **CULTIVATION** Under glass, grow in loam-based potting compost (JI No.3) in full light. Top-dress or pot on in spring. During the growing season, water freely and apply a balanced liquid fertilizer every month; water sparingly in winter. Outdoors, grow in fertile, well-drained soil in full sun. Tie stems to supports. Pruning group 12 for climbers, in early spring; group 8 for shrubs. May need restrictive pruning under glass.
• **PROPAGATION** Sow seed at 13–18°C (55–64°F) in spring, or root semi-ripe cuttings in midsummer with bottom heat. Take softwood cuttings from *P. indica* in late spring or early summer, or insert root cuttings in late winter.
• **PESTS AND DISEASES** Red spider mites, whiteflies, and mealybugs may be a problem under glass.

P. auriculata ▣ 🏆 syn. *P. capensis* (Cape leadwort). Scandent, evergreen shrub, grown as a climber, with slender, whippy, moderately branching stems. Oblong to oblong-spoon-shaped leaves, 4–7cm (1½–3in) long, are mid- to bright matt green, sometimes with a blue-grey tone. Bears long-tubed, sky-blue flowers, 4cm (1½in) long, in dense, terminal, corymb-like racemes, 15cm (6in) across, from summer to late autumn. ↕ 3–6m (10–20ft), ↔ 1–3m (3–10ft). South Africa. ✻. **var. *alba*** bears pure white flowers.
P. capensis see *P. auriculata.*
P. indica, syn. *P. rosea* (Scarlet leadwort). Small, evergreen shrub becoming spreading or semi-scandent if not pruned annually. Ovate-elliptic leaves, 5–11cm (2–4½in) long, are mid- to deep green. Long-tubed, red to deep rose-pink flowers, 2.5cm (1in) long, are

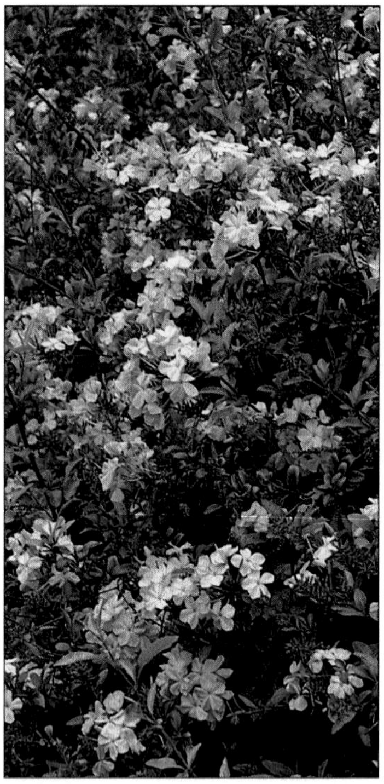

Plumbago auriculata

borne in terminal racemes, 10–30cm (4–12in) long, in winter (earlier if unpruned). ↕ to 2m (6ft), ↔ to 1m (3ft). S.E. Asia. ❄ (min. 7°C/45°F)
P. larpentiae see *Ceratostigma plumbaginoides.*
P. rosea see *P. indica.*

▷ **Plume,**
Brazilian see *Justicia carnea*
Scarlet see *Euphorbia fulgens*
▷ **Plume plant** see *Calomeria amaranthoides*

PLUMERIA

Frangipani, Pagoda tree, West Indian jasmine

APOCYNACEAE

Genus of 7 or 8 species of deciduous or semi-evergreen shrubs and small trees, with succulent stems and very thick, fleshy branches, from tropical and subtropical America. The simple, entire leaves, clustered towards the stem tips, are alternately or spirally arranged. The fragrant, salverform flowers, each with 5 broad petal lobes, are borne in showy, terminal clusters or panicles, often on bare stems or with the young leaves. Below 10°C (50°F), grow in a temperate or warm greenhouse, or as houseplants. In warmer climates, use as specimen plants. The milky sap may cause mild stomach upset if ingested.

• **HARDINESS** Frost tender.
• **CULTIVATION** Under glass, grow in loam-based potting compost (JI No.2) with added sharp sand, in full light. In growth, water moderately and apply a balanced liquid fertilizer monthly; keep almost dry in winter. Outdoors, grow in moderately fertile, well-drained soil in full sun. Pruning group 1; need restrictive pruning under glass.
• **PROPAGATION** Sow seed at 18°C (64°F) in spring. Take ripe cuttings of leafless stem tips in early spring; allow these to dry at the bases before inserting.
• **PESTS AND DISEASES** Red spider mites may be troublesome under glass.

P. acuminata see *P. rubra* var. *acutifolia.*
P. acutifolia see *P. rubra* var. *acutifolia.*
P. alba ▣ ♀ (West Indian jasmine). Large, deciduous shrub or small, spreading tree with robust, sparsely branched, very thick stems. Spirally arranged, lance-shaped, slightly wrinkled, rich green leaves, to 30cm (12in) long, are usually finely hairy beneath. Salverform, yellow-eyed white flowers, 6cm (2½in) across, are produced in terminal panicles from summer to autumn. ↕ to 6m (20ft), ↔ to 4m (12ft). Puerto Rico, Lesser Antilles. ❄ (min. 10–13°C/50–55°F)
P. rubra ▣ ♀ (Common frangipani). Large, deciduous shrub or small, sparsely branched tree, upright in habit, with very thick stems bearing alternately arranged, broadly elliptic to oblong or inversely lance-shaped, mid-green leaves, 20–40cm (8–16in) long, with paler midribs. Salverform, yellow-eyed flowers, 7–10cm (3–4in) across, usually rose-pink but sometimes yellow or red to bronze, are produced in terminal panicles from summer to autumn. ↕ to 7m (22ft), ↔ to 5m (15ft). Mexico to Panama. ❄ (min. 10–13°C/50–55°F). **var. *acutifolia***, syn. *P. acuminata, P. acutifolia*, produces oblong-elliptic, pointed, dark green leaves, to 10cm (4in) long, on long stalks. Terminal panicles of salverform, very fragrant, yellow-centred white flowers, 8–9cm (3–3½in) across, with widely spreading petals, are produced from late summer to autumn. ↕ 4m (12ft), ↔ to 2m (6ft). Mexico to Panama, N. South America, West

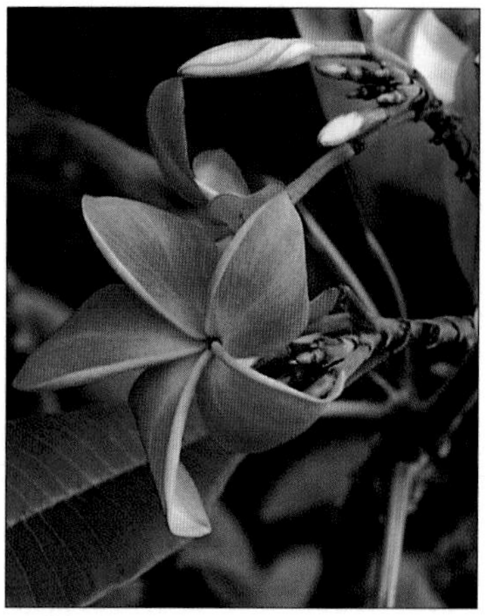

Plumeria rubra

Indies. **f. *tricolor*** bears pink-margined white flowers with yellow eyes.

▷ **Plum yew** see *Cephalotaxus, C. harringtoniana, Prumnopitys andina*
Fortune see *Cephalotaxus fortunei*
▷ **Plush plant** see *Echeveria pulvinata*

POA

Meadow grass, Spear grass

GRAMINEAE/POACEAE

Genus of about 500 species of mainly perennial grasses (some are annuals) found in cool-temperate regions in a wide range of habitats from seashores to alpine zones. They include a number of important fodder, lawn, and pasture grasses. Of variable habit, they are

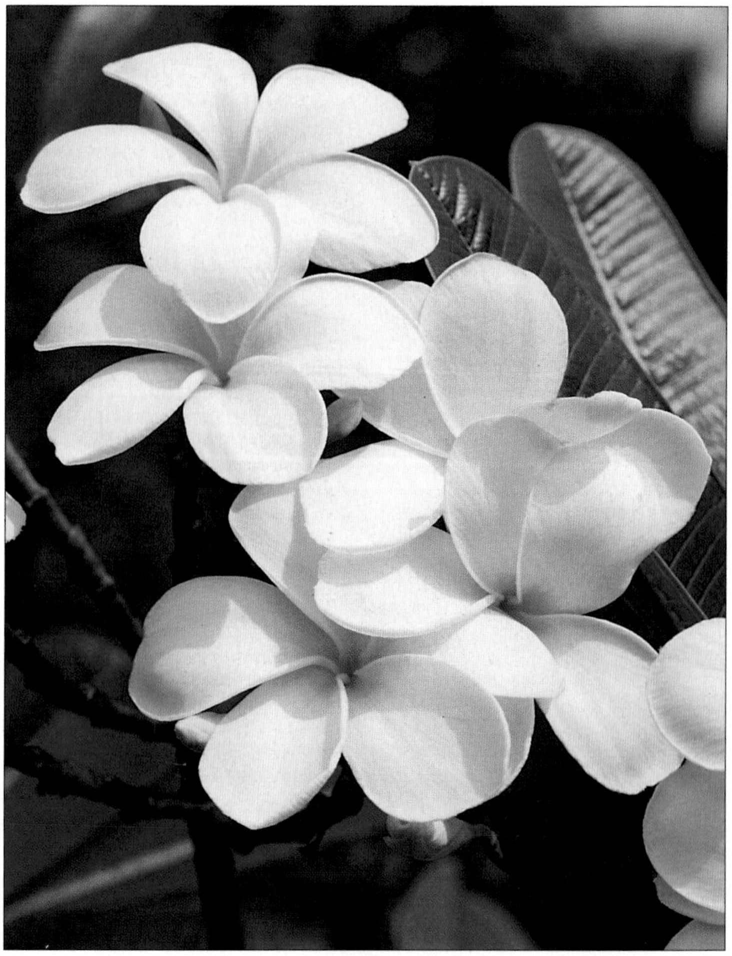

Plumeria alba

P

grown for their narrowly linear, flat to folded leaves and open or compact, summer-flowering panicles. Most cultivated species are grown as turf grasses or for agricultural purposes. *P. alpina* var. *vivipara* is grown as a curiosity, either in a rock garden or at the front of a border. *P. chaixii* and other ornamental species are suitable for a border, and for naturalizing in woodland and other shady situations.

- **HARDINESS** Fully hardy.
- **CULTIVATION** Grow in moderately fertile, medium to light, well-drained soil in full sun or partial shade. Remove flowering stems in autumn to prevent self-seeding; cut back dead foliage in early spring.
- **PROPAGATION** Sow seed in containers in a cold frame in spring or autumn, or divide between mid-spring and early summer. Peg down mature flowerheads of *P. alpina* var. *vivipara* to allow plantlets to root.
- **PESTS AND DISEASES** Trouble free.

P. alpina (Alpine meadow grass). Densely tufted perennial with neat mounds of thick, flat, linear, short-pointed, mid-green leaves, 4–10cm (1½–4in) long. From early to late summer, produces dense, ovoid-pyramidal, short-branched, purplish green flowering panicles, to 7cm (3in) long. ↕30cm (12in), ↔20cm (8in). W. Europe to C. Asia. ❄❄❄. **var. *vivipara*** has panicles in which flower spikelets have been replaced by tiny plantlets.
P. chaixii. Densely tufted perennial bearing flat or folded, unusually broad, linear, glossy, bright green leaves, to 45cm (18in) long and 1cm (½in) wide, each abruptly contracted at the tip to form a "hood". In late spring and early summer, bears open, slightly nodding, straight-branched, ovate to ovate-oblong, pale green, often purple-tinted flowering panicles, to 25cm (10in) long, on strong, erect stems held well above the foliage. ↕1m (3ft), ↔45cm (18in). Europe, S.W. Asia, North America. ❄❄❄

▷**Poached egg plant** see *Limnanthes, L. douglasii*

PODALYRIA

LEGUMINOSAE/PAPILIONACEAE

Genus of about 25 species of evergreen shrubs from woodland, forest margins, and streamsides in southern Africa. They have simple, usually densely hairy leaves with rolled margins, and are grown for their fragrant, pea-like flowers, borne singly or in pairs from the leaf axils. Where temperatures fall below 7°C (45°F), grow in a cool greenhouse. In warmer areas, grow in a shrub border or at the base of a house wall.

- **HARDINESS** Frost tender.
- **CULTIVATION** Under glass, grow in loam-based potting compost (JI No.3) in full light. When in growth, water moderately and apply a balanced liquid fertilizer every month; water sparingly in winter. Outdoors, grow in moderately fertile, moist but well-drained soil in full sun. Pruning group 8; may need restrictive pruning under glass.
- **PROPAGATION** Sow seed at 13–18°C (55–64°F) in spring. Root semi-ripe cuttings with bottom heat in summer.
- **PESTS AND DISEASES** Red spider mites may be troublesome under glass.

P. sericea. Spreading, densely leafy shrub with obovate leaves, 2cm (¾in) long, thickly covered with silver-silky hairs that age to gold. From autumn to spring, produces solitary, upright, pea-like, fragrant, lavender-blue to lavender-pink flowers, 1cm (½in) across, with a purple mark at each petal base. ↕45–90cm (18–36in), ↔45–100cm (18–39in). South Africa (Northern Cape, Western Cape, Eastern Cape). ❀ (min. 7°C/45°F)

▷**Podocarp,**
Tasmanian see *Podocarpus alpinus*
Willowleaf see *Podocarpus salignus*

PODOCARPUS

PODOCARPACEAE

Genus of about 100 species of dioecious, occasionally monoecious, evergreen, coniferous trees and shrubs from forest habitats, mainly in warm-temperate to tropical zones. They are grown for their spirally arranged leaves, which are variable in shape and are mainly borne in 2 ranks. Male and female flowers are usually borne on separate trees: the males are yellow or red, solitary or in axillary clusters of up to 5, or, in some species, borne in narrow, catkin-like cones; the females are green and produced in cone-like structures. Male and female plants are both needed to produce the plum-shaped, rounded to oblong, usually single-seeded fruits, which have fleshy, often red arils at the bases.

Grow as specimens or in a woodland garden; *P. alpinus* and *P. nivalis* are also suitable for a shrub border or large rock garden. *P. macrophyllus* needs long, hot, humid summers to achieve tree stature, remaining shrub-like in cooler areas; it is sometimes used for hedging. The frost-tender species are attractive specimens in warm climates, but need temperate or warm greenhouse protection in frost-prone areas.

- **HARDINESS** Fully hardy to frost tender.
- **CULTIVATION** Tolerant of a range of soils but best in fertile, moist but well-drained, humus-rich soil in full sun, with shelter from cold, dry winds. Most species thrive best in humid or high-rainfall climates.
- **PROPAGATION** Sow seed as soon as ripe, or in containers in an open frame in spring; germination may take as long as 12–18 months. Take semi-ripe cuttings from upright leading shoots in late summer.
- **PESTS AND DISEASES** Trouble free.

P. alpinus (Tasmanian podocarp). Spreading, dense, rounded shrub bearing slender green shoots. Linear, dull green leaves, 6–12mm (¼–½in) long, each with 2 grey bands beneath, are parted on either side of the shoots. Male flowers are produced in yellow, catkin-like cones, female flowers in green cone-like structures. Ovoid, bright red fruit, 6mm (¼in) long, are produced in autumn on female plants. ↕↔ to 2m (6ft). Australia (New South Wales, Tasmania). ❄❄❄
P. andinus see *Prumnopitys andina.*

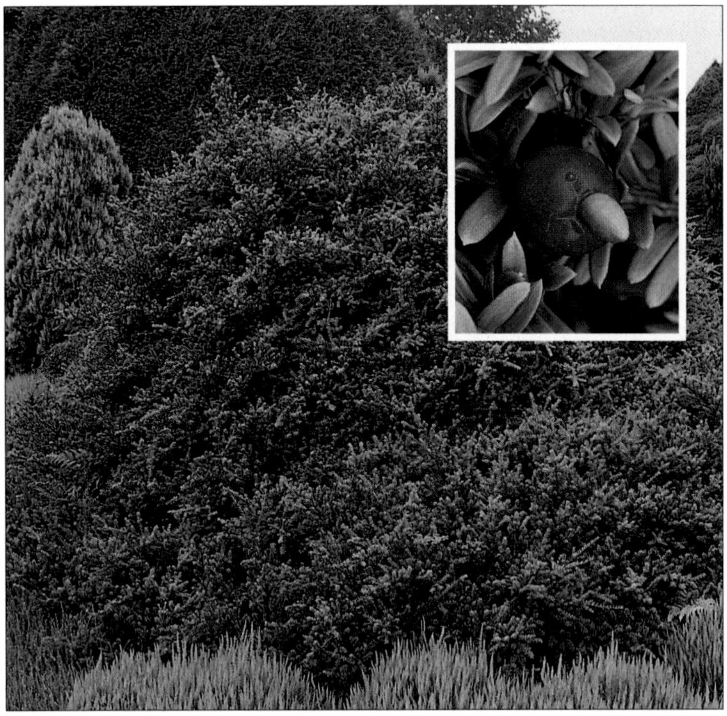

Podocarpus nivalis (inset: fruit detail)

P. macrophyllus ♤ (Kusamaki). Conical tree, becoming domed, with reddish brown bark and erect or spreading, yellowish green shoots. Lance-shaped, firm, leathery leaves, 6–10cm (2½–4in) long, are light green becoming dark green above, each with 2 glaucous bands beneath, and are erect or spreading on the shoots. Male flowers are borne in yellow, catkin-like cones, female flowers in green cone-like structures. Ovoid, reddish purple fruit, about 1cm (½in) long, are borne in autumn on female plants. ↕ to 15m (50ft), ↔6–8m (20–25ft). E. China, Japan. ❄❄
P. nivalis ▣ (Alpine totara). Spreading, dense, rounded shrub, very similar to *P. alpinus*, but with more rigid, linear, green-bronze leaves, 1–2cm (½–¾in) long, set radially around the slender, mid-green shoots, unparted on either side. Male flowers are borne in yellow, catkin-like cones, female flowers in green cone-like structures. Oblong, bright red fruit, 6mm (¼in) long, are produced in autumn on female plants. ↕↔ to 2m (6ft). New Zealand. ❄❄❄
P. salignus ▣ ♀ ♤ (Willowleaf podocarp). Columnar or broadly conical tree with spreading, later pendent branches, fibrous, peeling, red-brown bark, and green shoots that become grey-brown with age. Spreading, linear, often sickle-shaped leaves, 5–11cm (2–4½in) long, are dark bluish green (with a ridge above), and yellow-green beneath; they occur mainly near the shoot tips. The male flowers are borne in yellow, catkin-like cones, female flowers in green cone-like structures. Egg-shaped, green or dark violet fruit, 8mm (⅜in) long, are produced in autumn on female plants. Very graceful as a mature tree. ↕ to 20m (70ft), ↔6–9m (20–28ft). Chile. ❄❄❄

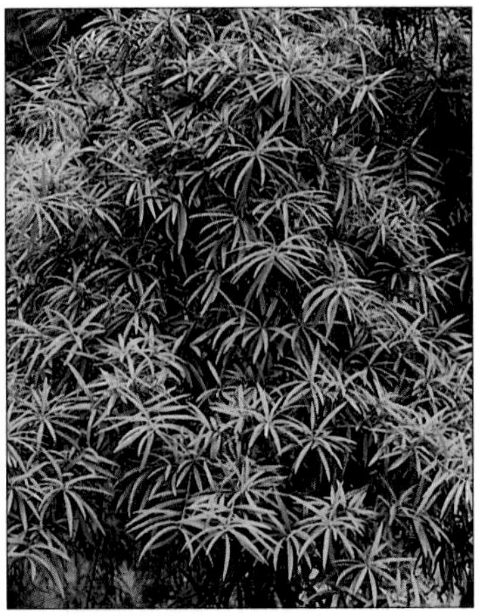

Podocarpus salignus

PODOPHYLLUM

BERBERIDACEAE

Genus of about 9 species of shade-loving, rhizomatous perennials, cultivated for their foliage and flowers, from scrub and forest in North America and from the Himalayas to China and Taiwan. Each plant has 1 or 2 peltate, palmately lobed, radical leaves, sometimes with purplish brown patches between the conspicuous veins; the leaves are pushed up by the lengthening leaf-stalks and emerge looking like tiny, folded umbrellas. Terminal, cup-shaped, pink, white, or red flowers are solitary or produced in small umbels, and are followed by red or yellow fruits, 2.5–5cm (1–2in) long. Podophyllums are suitable for a woodland garden or moist, shady border. All parts of the plants are highly toxic if ingested.

- **HARDINESS** Fully hardy to frost hardy.
- **CULTIVATION** Grow in humus-rich, leafy, moist soil in full or partial shade (*P. peltatum* tolerates drier soil). In cold areas, protect frost-hardy species with a dry winter mulch.
- **PROPAGATION** Sow seed in containers in an open frame as soon as ripe. Divide in spring or late summer.
- **PESTS AND DISEASES** Susceptible to slug damage in spring as the leaves emerge.

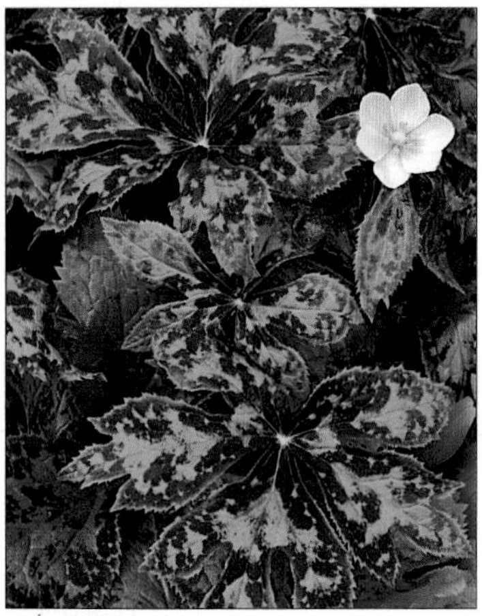

Podophyllum hexandrum

P. emodi see *P. hexandrum*.
P. hexandrum ■ syn. *P. emodi*. Rhizomatous perennial bearing long-stalked, 3- to 5-lobed, deeply toothed, mid-green leaves, to 25cm (10in) long, with purplish brown markings; they unfurl after flowering. Solitary, open cup-shaped, usually 6-petalled, white or pale pink flowers, 2.5–5cm (1–2in) across, with prominent yellow anthers, are borne from late spring to midsummer; they are followed by plum-like, ovoid, fleshy red fruit, to 5cm (2in) long. ↕45cm (18in), ↔ 30cm (12in). N. India (Himalayas) to China. ❄❄❄
P. japonicum see *Ranzania japonica*.
P. peltatum (American mandrake, May apple). Creeping, rhizomatous perennial producing long-stalked, 5- to 9-lobed, toothed, sometimes 2-cleft, glossy leaves, to 30cm (12in) long, well-developed at flowering. Solitary, semi-pendent, shallowly cup-shaped, usually 9-petalled, fragrant, waxy white to pale pink flowers, 5cm (2in) across, are produced beneath the leaves from mid-spring to early summer; they are followed by edible, ovoid, yellowish green fruit, 2.5–5cm (1–2in) long. ↕45cm (18in), ↔ 1.2m (4ft) or more. North America (Ontario and Quebec to Texas and Florida). ❄❄❄
P. pleianthum (Chinese may apple). Rhizomatous perennial with shallowly 6- to 10-lobed, finely toothed, glossy leaves, to 35cm (14in) long. Clusters of 5–8 cup-shaped, deep crimson to purple flowers are borne in the leaf axils in summer, followed by ovoid-spherical, dark red fruit, 2.5cm (1in) long. ↕75cm (30in), ↔ 45cm (18in). C. and S.E. China, Taiwan. ❄❄

PODRANEA

BIGNONIACEAE

Genus of 2 species of woody-stemmed, evergreen climbers from open woodland, one species from Zimbabwe, the other from S. Africa. They have pinnate leaves, borne in opposite pairs, and are cultivated for their 5-lobed, trumpet-shaped, foxglove-like flowers. Where temperatures regularly fall below 0°C (32°F), grow in a cool or temperate greenhouse. In milder climates, they are suitable for a pergola or arch, or cascading from a tree.
• **HARDINESS** Frost tender; may survive short spells near to 0°C (32°F).
• **CULTIVATION** Under glass, grow in loam-based potting compost (JI No.3) in bright filtered light. In growth, water moderately and apply a balanced liquid fertilizer monthly; water sparingly in winter. Outdoors, grow in fertile, moist but well-drained soil in light dappled or partial shade. Pruning group 12, immediately after flowering.
• **PROPAGATION** Sow seed at 13–18°C (55–64°F) in spring, take semi-ripe cuttings in summer, or layer in spring.
• **PESTS AND DISEASES** Prone to red spider mites and mealybugs under glass.

P. ricasoliana, syn. *Pandorea ricasoliana, Tecoma ricasoliana* (Pink trumpet vine). Scandent, twining climber, becoming bushy with age, with pinnate leaves, to 25cm (10in) long, composed of 5–11 lance-shaped to ovate, unevenly toothed, rich green leaflets with slender points. Produces loose, terminal panicles of about 12 trumpet-shaped pink flowers, to 6cm (2½in) long, with red veins, paler tubes, and wavy-margined, round lobes, from winter to summer, depending on temperature. ↕3–5m (10–15ft). South Africa (Eastern Cape, KwaZulu/Natal). ❀ (min. 10°C/50°F)

▷**Pohutakawa** see *Metrosideros*
Common see *M. excelsus*
▷***Poinciana gilliesii*** see *Caesalpinia gilliesii*
▷***Poinciana pulcherrima*** see *Caesalpinia pulcherrima*
▷***Poinciana regia*** see *Delonix regia*
▷**Poinsettia** see *Euphorbia pulcherrima*
Annual see *E. cyathophora*
▷**Poison arrow plant** see *Acokanthera oblongifolia*
▷**Poison bulb** see *Crinum asiaticum*
▷**Poke, Indian** see *Veratrum viride*
▷**Pokeweed** see *Phytolacca, P. americana*
▷**Polar plant** see *Silphium laciniatum*

POLEMONIUM

Jacob's ladder

POLEMONIACEAE

Genus of about 25 species of deciduous, clump-forming or occasionally rhizomatous perennials and annuals, found in stony, arctic or alpine soils, often by streams, or in damp meadows, woodland, or scrub, in Europe, Asia, North America, and Central America. Most have basal clumps of unequally pinnate leaves, usually with numerous leaflets, and erect or decumbent stems bearing smaller leaves. They are grown for their spring and summer flowers,

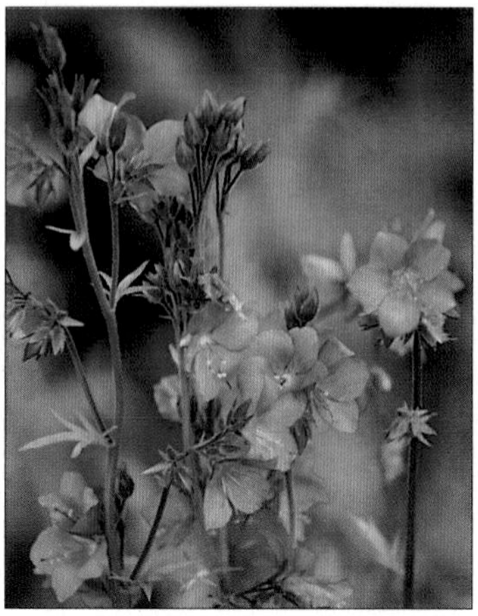

Polemonium caeruleum

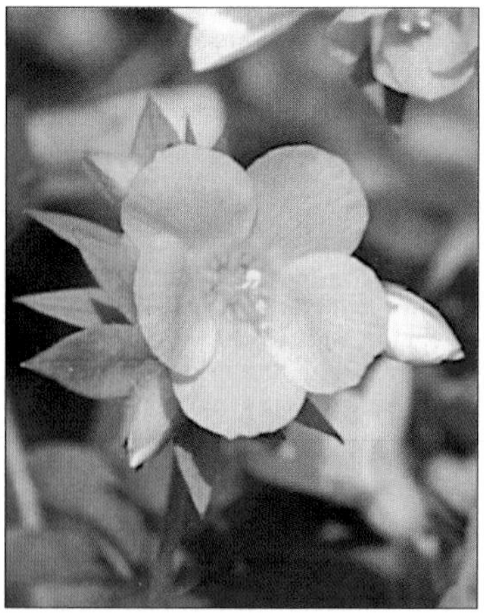

Polemonium carneum

which are bell-shaped, saucer-shaped, narrowly tubular, or funnel-shaped and spreading at the mouths; they are usually white or blue, sometimes purple, pink, or yellow, and either solitary or in terminal or axillary cymes. Grow taller species in a border or wild garden, the smaller, alpine species in a rock garden, scree bed, or alpine house. *P. caeruleum* grows well in grass. *P. brandegeei* and *P. pauciflorum* are usually short-lived.
• **HARDINESS** Fully hardy.
• **CULTIVATION** Grow tall species in any fertile, well-drained but moist soil, preferably in full sun or partial shade. Grow small species in gritty, sharply drained soil in full sun with some midday shade. Dead-head regularly.
• **PROPAGATION** Sow seed in containers in a cold frame in autumn or spring, or divide in spring.
• **PESTS AND DISEASES** Powdery mildew may be a problem.

P. brandegeei. Clump-forming, perennial bearing mainly basal, sticky, pinnate leaves, to 10cm (4in) long, with many lance-shaped leaflets, each to 1.5cm (½in) long. In early summer, upright stems bear short, terminal cymes of long-tubed, funnel-shaped, pale to deep golden yellow, rarely white flowers, to 2.5cm (1in) long. ❄❄❄. **subsp. *mellitum***, syn. *P. mellitum*, bears looser cymes of white or pale cream flowers in summer. ↕20cm (8in), ↔ 15cm (6in). USA (Rocky Mountains).
P. caeruleum ■ (Greek valerian, Jacob's ladder). Clump-forming perennial, mainly hairless but softly hairy near the inflorescences. Bears 2-pinnate leaves, to 40cm (16in) long, each composed of 19–27 oblong-lance-shaped leaflets, 1.5–4cm (½–1½in) long. Lax, terminal or axillary cymes of open bell-shaped, lavender-blue, rarely white flowers, 1–2.5cm (½–1in) across, are produced on erect, branched stems in early summer. ↕30–90cm (12–36in), ↔ 30cm (12in). N. and C. Europe, N. Asia, W. North America. ❄❄❄. **var. *lacteum***, syn. var. *album*, has white flowers.
P. carneum ■ Hairless, clump-forming perennial bearing coarsely divided, pinnate leaves, to 20cm (8in) long, with 13–21 elliptic to ovate leaflets, each 0.7–2cm (¼–¾in) long. Lax, terminal cymes of shallowly bell-shaped, pale pink or yellow, sometimes dark purple or lavender flowers, 1–2.5cm (½–1in) across, with yellow centres, are borne on erect, branched stems in early summer. ↕10–40cm (4–16in), ↔ 20cm (8in). USA (Washington to California). ❄❄❄
P. confertum see *P. viscosum*.
P. eximium, syn. *P. viscosum* var. *eximium*. Compact, clump-forming, perennial bearing crowded tufts of pinnate, glandular-sticky leaves, to 10cm (4in) long, with numerous leaflets, each 6–8mm (¼–⅜in) long, deeply cut into 3 or 5 segments. Erect, branched stems bear dense, terminal cymes of narrowly funnel-shaped to cylindrical, clear blue flowers, 1.5cm (½in) long, in summer. ↕10–30cm (4–12in), ↔ 15cm (6in). High altitudes in W. USA (California, Sierra Nevada). ❄❄❄
P. foliosissimum. Leafy, clump-forming perennial producing a few erect, softly

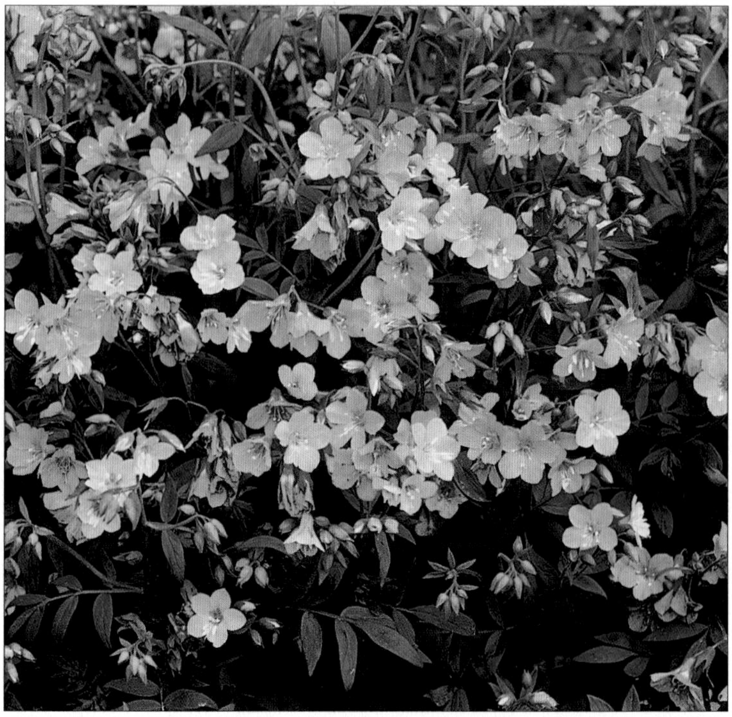

Polemonium 'Lambrook Mauve'

P

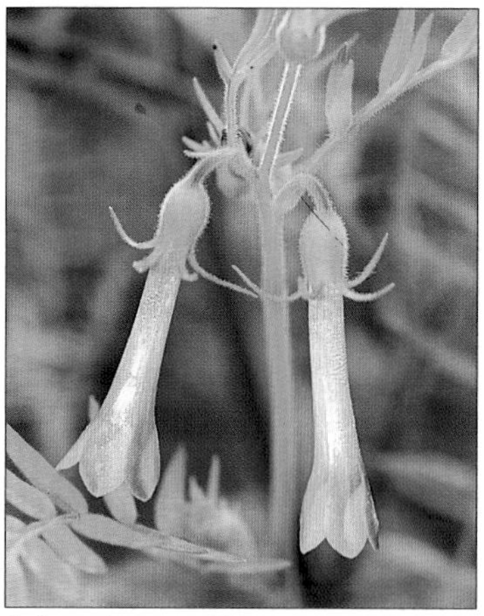

Polemonium pauciflorum

hairy stems. Pinnate leaves, to 15cm (6in) long, each have 11–25 elliptic-lance-shaped leaflets, 1–5cm (½–2in) long. Dense, axillary and terminal cymes of bell-shaped, blue-violet, cream, or white flowers, to 1.5cm (½in) across, are produced in midsummer. ↕75–80cm (30–32in), ↔ 60cm (24in). Central W. USA. ❄❄❄. **var. *flavum*** bears yellow flowers that are shaded orange-red outside; ↕40–70cm (16–28in). USA (S. Arizona, New Mexico).

***P.* 'Lambrook Mauve'** ■🏆 syn. *P. reptans* 'Lambrook Manor', *P. reptans* 'Lambrook Mauve'. Clump-forming perennial forming rounded mounds of neat, pinnate leaves, to 25cm (10in) long, each composed of 7–19 ovate or oblong leaflets, 3–5cm (1¼–2in) long. Erect, branched stems very freely bear lax, terminal cymes of bell-shaped, lilac-blue flowers, 1.5–2cm (½–¾in) across, in late spring and early summer. ↕↔ to 45cm (18in). ❄❄❄

P. mellitum see *P. brandegeei* subsp. *mellitum.*

P. pauciflorum ■ Short-lived, clump-forming perennial with spreading to erect, branched, softly hairy stems and mainly pinnate leaves, to 15cm (6in)

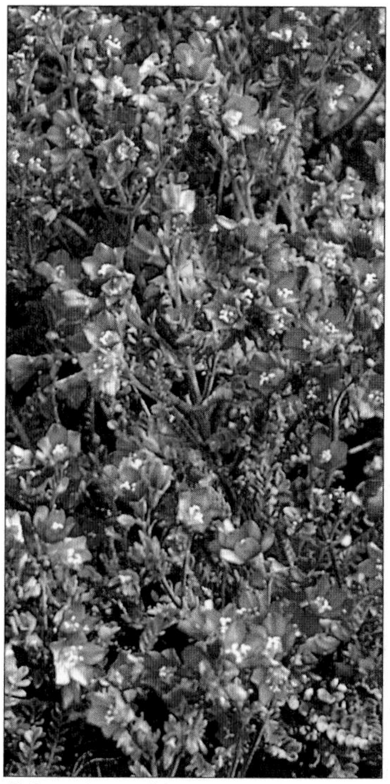

Polemonium pulcherrimum

long, each composed of 11–25 elliptic-lance-shaped leaflets, to 2.5cm (1in) long. From early to late summer, bears horizontal to semi-pendent, narrowly tubular, red-tinted, pale yellow flowers, 4cm (1½in) across, with spreading mouths, either singly or in loose, few-flowered, terminal or axillary cymes. ↕↔ to 50cm (20in). USA (S.E. Arizona, New Mexico). ❄❄❄

P. pulcherrimum ■ Clump-forming perennial with pinnate leaves, to 14cm (5½in) long, each composed of 11–25 ovate leaflets, to 3.5cm (1½in) long. Dense, terminal and axillary cymes of bell-shaped, light blue to purple-blue or white flowers, to 1cm (½in) across, with short tubes, yellow within, are borne on erect, branched stems in early summer. ↕↔ 30cm (12in). North America (Alaska to California). ❄❄❄

***P. reptans* 'Lambrook Manor'** see *P.* 'Lambrook Mauve'.

***P. reptans* 'Lambrook Mauve'** see *P.* 'Lambrook Mauve'.

P. viscosum, syn. *P. confertum.* Clump-forming perennial bearing mainly basal, pinnate leaves, to 20cm (8in) long, with whorls of many palmately 3- or 5-lobed leaflets, each to 1.5cm (½in) long. In summer, produces large, terminal cymes of funnel-shaped, deep blue flowers, to 2–3cm (¾–1¼in) across, on upright, branched stems. ↕5–50cm (2–20in), ↔ 5–20cm (2–8in). North America (mountains from Canada to New Mexico). ❄❄❄. **var. *eximium*** see *P. eximium.*

POLIANTHES

AGAVACEAE

Genus of 13 species of tuberous perennials found in open woodland and at roadsides in sandy areas in Mexico and Texas. They are grown for their showy, loose racemes or spikes of tubular flowers, borne in summer. The mostly basal leaves are lance-shaped or linear. In frost-prone climates, grow in a warm greenhouse or summer border; elsewhere, grow in a sheltered border.

- **HARDINESS** Frost tender.
- **CULTIVATION** Under glass, grow in loam-based potting compost (JI No.2) in full light. During the growing season, water moderately, and apply a balanced liquid fertilizer every 2 weeks. Reduce watering as the leaves die down, and keep dry when dormant. Outdoors, grow in moderately fertile, well-drained soil in full sun. Lift before first frosts and store tubers in sand in frost-free conditions.
- **PROPAGATION** Sow seed at 19–24°C (66–75°F) as soon as ripe. Remove offsets when the plants are dormant.
- **PESTS AND DISEASES** Prone to viruses.

P. geminiflora, syn. *Bravoa geminiflora.* Tuberous perennial with semi-erect, narrow, linear, basal leaves, 30–40cm (12–16in). In summer, produces lax racemes of paired, pendent, tubular, bright orange-red flowers, 2.5cm (1in) long. ↕ to 70cm (28in), ↔ 8cm (3in). Mexico. ❁ (min. 15°C/59°F)

P. tuberosa ■🏆 (Tuberose). Tuberous perennial with semi-erect, thin, linear-lance-shaped leaves, to 45cm (18in) long, in a basal rosette. Spikes of tubular, intensely fragrant, waxy white flowers, 3–6cm (1¼–2½in) long, are

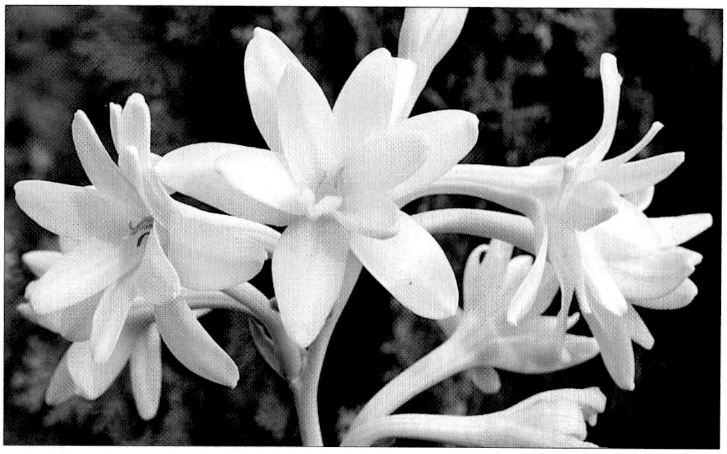

Polianthes tuberosa

produced in summer. ↕ to 1.2m (4ft), ↔ 15cm (6in). Mexico. ❁ (min. 15°C/59°F). **'The Pearl'** bears semi-double flowers.

▷**Policeman's helmet** see *Impatiens glandulifera*

POLIOTHYRSIS

FLACOURTIACEAE

Genus of one species of deciduous tree from mountain woodland in C. China. It is grown for its glossy, dark green leaves and fragrant, papery, greenish white then yellow summer flowers. Grow as a specimen or among trees.

- **HARDINESS** Fully hardy.
- **CULTIVATION** Grow in fertile, well-drained soil in full sun or partial shade, with shelter from cold, drying winds. Pruning group 1.
- **PROPAGATION** Sow seed in containers in an open frame in autumn, or take greenwood cuttings in summer.
- **PESTS AND DISEASES** Trouble free.

P. sinensis ■⚲ Spreading, deciduous tree with grey bark, which is deeply furrowed in mature trees. Ovate, slender-pointed, glossy, dark green leaves, to 15cm (6in) long, red-tinged when young, are arranged alternately, and are borne on red stalks. In mid- and late summer, white buds open to tiny, cup-shaped, fragrant, papery, greenish white then yellow flowers, produced in conical panicles, to 25cm (10in) long. ↕10m (30ft) or more, ↔ 6m (20ft). C. China. ❄❄❄

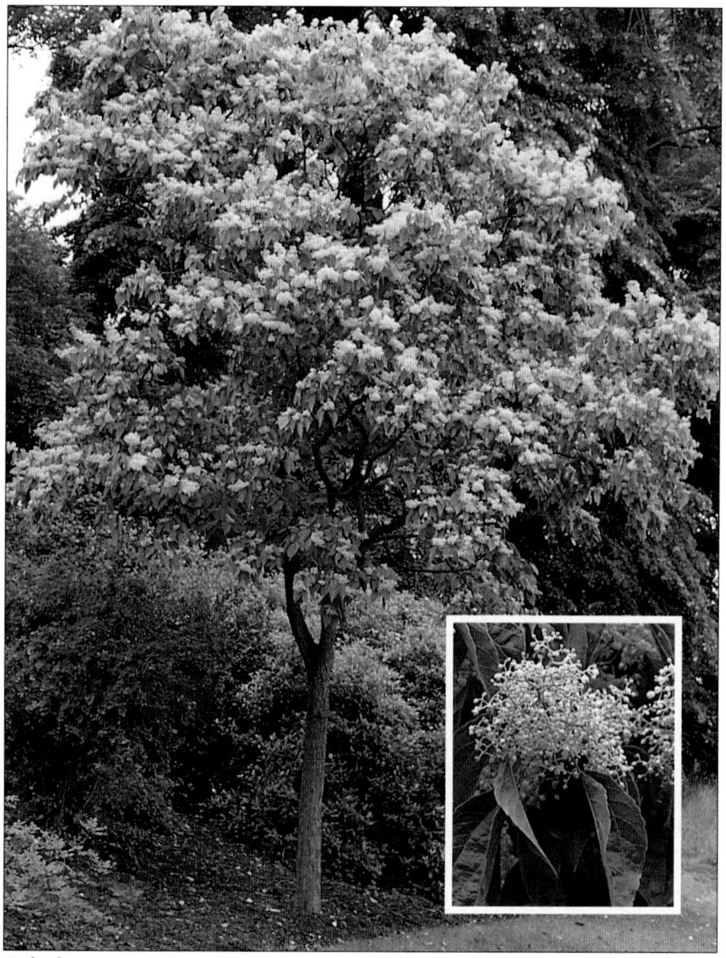

Poliothyrsis sinensis (inset: flower detail)

P

▷ **Polka dot plant** see *Hypoestes, H. phyllostachya*
▷ **Polvillo, Guayacan** see *Tabebuia serratifolia*
▷ **Polyanthus** see *Primula* Polyanthus Group

POLYGALA

Milkwort, Seneca, Snakeroot

POLYGALACEAE

Genus of about 500 species of annuals and evergreen perennials and shrubs distributed in a wide range of habitats worldwide, except in New Zealand, Polynesia, and arctic regions. They are grown for their terminal or axillary racemes of colourful, pea-like flowers, produced in late spring and summer, or in some species in autumn; each flower has 5 sepals, the inner two forming broad, petal-like "wings", and 5 petals, the lowest forming a keel with a fringed apex. The leaves are alternate, opposite, or whorled, linear to rounded, and usually leathery. Grow hardy species in a woodland or rock garden, or in an alpine house. In frost-prone areas, grow tender species in a cool greenhouse or conservatory; in warmer climates, use in a shrub border.

• **HARDINESS** Fully hardy to frost tender.
• **CULTIVATION** Under glass, grow in loamless potting compost in full light, with shade from hot sun. In growth, keep well-ventilated, water freely, and apply a balanced liquid fertilizer monthly; water sparingly in winter. Outdoors, grow in moderately fertile, humus-rich, sharply drained soil in full sun or partial shade. Pruning group 9 for *P.* x *dalmaisiana* and *P. myrtifolia.*
• **PROPAGATION** Sow seed of hardy species in containers in an open frame in autumn; sow seed of tender species at not less than 15°C (59°F) in spring. Take softwood cuttings in early summer, or semi-ripe cuttings in mid- to late summer.
• **PESTS AND DISEASES** Aphids and whiteflies may be a problem under glass.

P

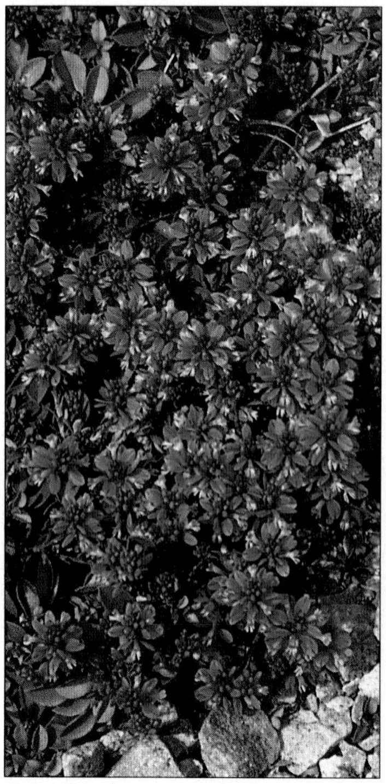

Polygala calcarea

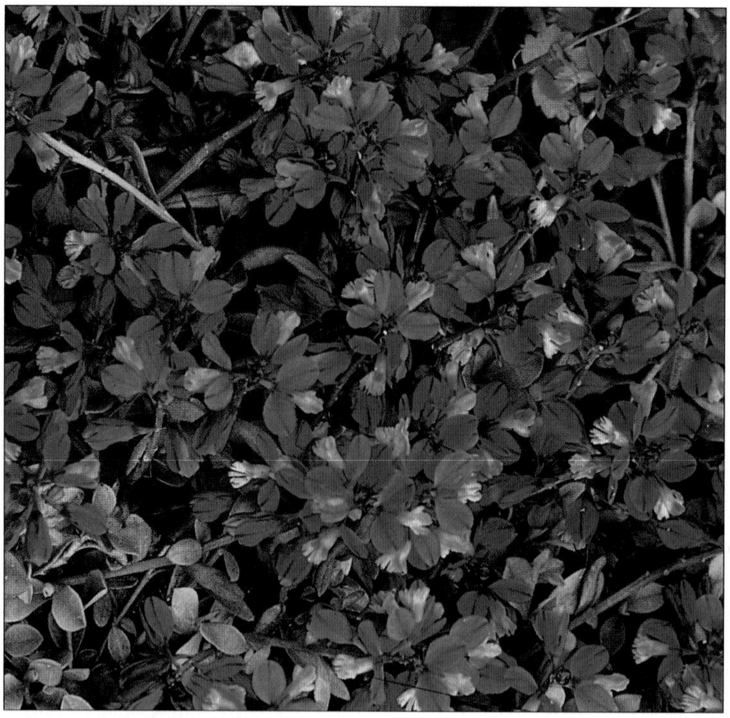

Polygala calcarea 'Bulley's Form'

P. calcarea ■ (Milkwort). Prostrate, creeping, mat-forming, evergreen perennial with basal rosettes of obovate, leathery, mid-green leaves, 1–3.5cm (½–1½in) long. In late spring and early summer, trailing stems bear deep blue flowers, to 7mm (¼in) long, with white-fringed lips, in terminal racemes, to 3cm (1¼in) long. ‡ 5cm (2in), ↔ to 20cm (8in). W. Europe. ❄❄❄. The following cultivars are more robust and free-flowering. **'Bulley's Form'** ■ has larger flowers in a deeper blue. **'Lillet'** ♀ has a compact habit, and produces brighter blue flowers over a long period.
P. chamaebuxus ♀ Small, spreading, evergreen shrub with lance-shaped, leathery, dark green leaves, 1.5–3cm (½–1¼in) long. The flowers, 1.5cm (½in) long, have bright yellow lips, white or pale yellow wings, and a bright yellow keel that ages to purple or brownish crimson; the flowers may be solitary or in pairs, and are produced in the upper leaf axils, mainly in late spring and early summer. ‡ 5–15cm (2–6in), ↔ to 30cm (12in). W. central Europe. ❄❄❄. **var. *grandiflora*** ■ ♀ syn. var. *purpurea*, var. *rhodoptera*, produces flowers with deep purplish pink wings and yellow lips. Alps, Carpathians. **var. *purpurea*** see var. *grandiflora.* **var. *rhodoptera*** see var. *grandiflora.*
P.* x *dalmaisiana ■ ♀ (*P. myrtifolia* x *P. oppositifolia*) syn. *P. myrtifolia* var. *grandiflora* of gardens. Erect, rounded, evergreen shrub, tending to spread with age. Elliptic, ovate, or lance-shaped, glaucous, mid- to deep green leaves, to 2.5cm (1in) long, can be alternate or opposite on the same plant. Leafy, terminal racemes of purple or rose-magenta flowers, 2.5cm (1in) long, with the bases of the keels white, are borne from midsummer to late autumn. ‡↔ 1–2.5m (3–8ft). Garden origin. ❀ (min. 5–7°C/41–45°F)
P. myrtifolia. Erect, bushy, evergreen shrub, spreading with age, with elliptic-oblong or obovate, leathery, mid- to deep green leaves, 2.5–5cm (1–2in) long. Short, leafy, terminal racemes of purple-veined, greenish white flowers, to 2cm (¾in) long, with crested keel petals, are borne from spring to autumn. ‡ 1–2.5m (3–8ft), ↔ 1–2m (3–6ft). South Africa. ❀ (min. 5–7°C/41–45°F). **var. *grandiflora* of gardens** see *P.* x *dalmaisiana.*

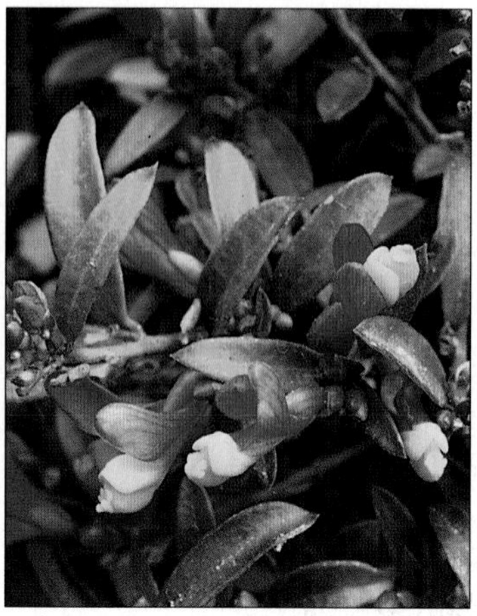

Polygala chamaebuxus var. *grandiflora*

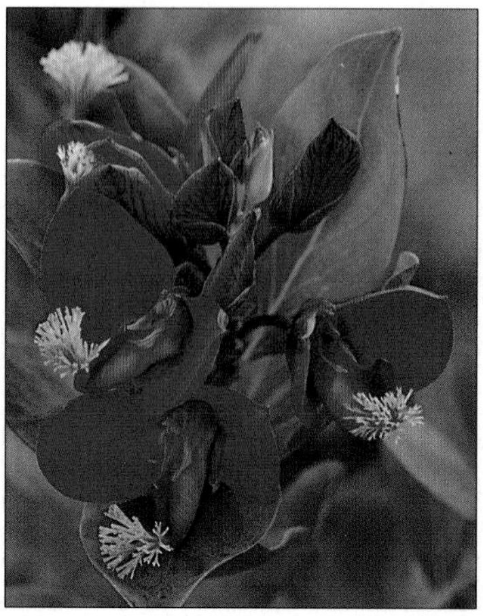

Polygala x *dalmaisiana*

POLYGONATUM

Solomon's seal

CONVALLARIACEAE/LILIACEAE

Genus of about 50 species of rhizomatous perennials from woodland in temperate regions of Eurasia and N. America. Cultivated for their foliage and flowers, they have usually arching stems and alternate, opposite, or whorled, linear to broadly elliptic or ovate, parallel-veined leaves that turn yellow in autumn. Mostly pendent, sometimes erect, tubular to bell-shaped, mainly white or cream, occasionally purple-pink flowers, with green markings, are either solitary or produced in small clusters, often along the lower sides of the stems. The flowers are usually followed by berry-like, spherical, red or black fruits. Solomon's seals are suitable for a shady border, or for a woodland or rock garden. All parts may cause mild stomach upset if ingested.

• **HARDINESS** Fully hardy to frost hardy.
• **CULTIVATION** Grow in fertile, humus-rich, moist but well-drained soil in full or partial shade.
• **PROPAGATION** Sow seed in containers in a cold frame in autumn. Divide rhizomes when growth begins in spring, taking care to avoid damaging young, brittle shoots.
• **PESTS AND DISEASES** Susceptible to slugs and sawfly larvae.

P. biflorum, syn. *P. canaliculatum, P. commutatum, P. giganteum.* Rhizomatous perennial with arching, hairless stems with alternate, narrowly lance-shaped to broadly elliptic leaves, to 18cm (7in) long, with hairless or minutely hairy undersides that are glaucous along the veins. From late spring to midsummer, usually solitary or 2–4 pendent, tubular, greenish white flowers, 1–2.5cm (½–1in) long, are produced in the leaf axils; they are followed by spherical black fruit, 9mm (⅜in) across. ‡ to 0.4–2m (16–72in), ↔ 60cm (24in). S. central Canada, E. North America. ❄❄❄
P. canaliculatum see *P. biflorum.*
P. commutatum see *P. biflorum.*
***P. cyrtonema* of gardens** see *Disporopsis pernyi.*
P. giganteum see *P. biflorum.*
P. hirtum ■ syn. *P. latifolium.* Rhizomatous perennial producing erect stems with alternate, lance-shaped to ovate leaves, 8–15cm (3–6in) long,

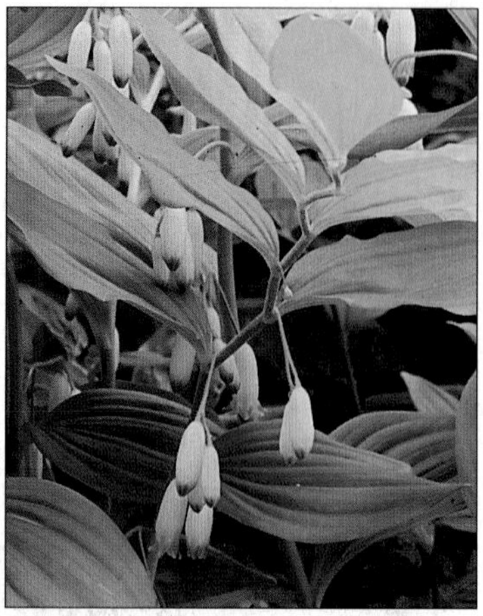

Polygonatum hirtum

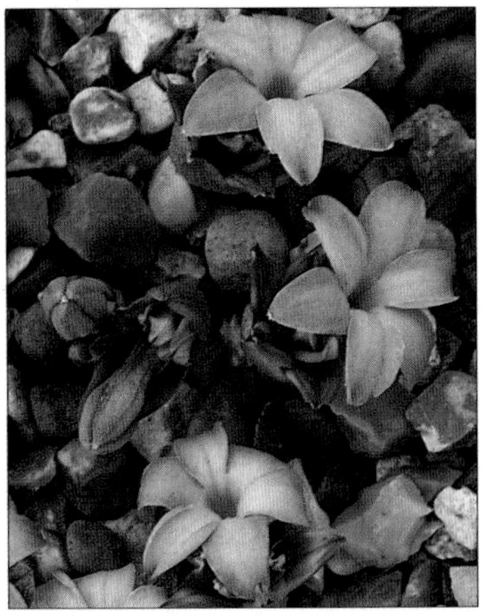

Polygonatum hookeri

slightly hairy beneath. From late spring to midsummer, produces 1–5 pendent, tubular, green-tipped white flowers, 2cm (¾in) long, in the leaf axils; they are followed by spherical black fruit, 6mm (¼in) across. ↕ to 1.2m (4ft), ↔ 60cm (24in). C. and S.E. Europe, Turkey, W. Russia, Caucasus. ***

P. hookeri ▣ Creeping, slowly spreading perennial with upright stems bearing alternate, linear to narrowly elliptic leaves, to 4cm (1½in) long, hairless beneath. In late spring and early summer, produces solitary, erect, pale to deep pink, short-tubed flowers, 2cm (¾in) across, with wide-spreading tepals, in the upper leaf axils; they are followed by spherical black fruit, 3mm (⅛in) across. Suitable for a peat bed. ↕ to 10cm (4in), ↔ to 30cm (12in) or more. E. Himalayas, China. ***

P. humile. Rhizomatous perennial with upright stems bearing lance-shaped to ovate leaves, 4–7cm (1½–3in) long, arranged alternately, and finely hairy on the lower veins. In late spring, produces solitary or paired, pendent, tubular white flowers, to 2cm (¾in) long, in the upper leaf axils; they are followed by spherical, blue-black fruit, to 6mm

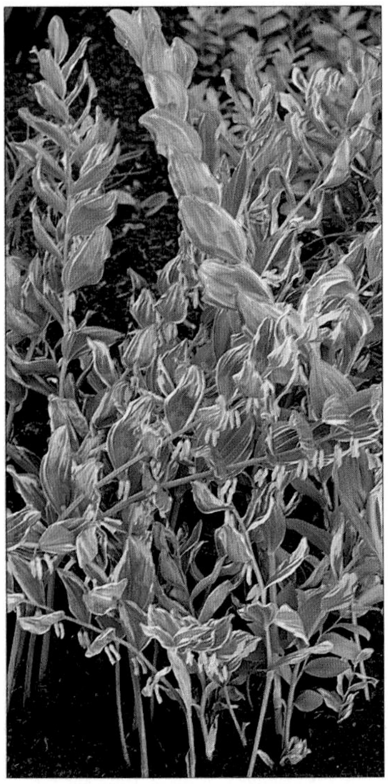

Polygonatum multiflorum 'Striatum'

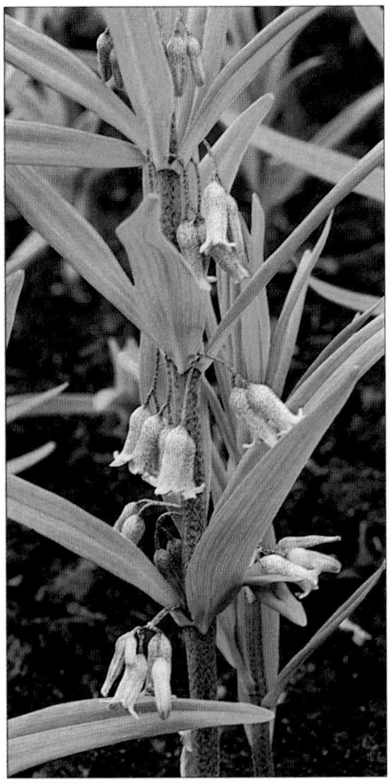

Polygonatum stewartianum

(¼in) across. ↕ 20cm (8in), ↔ 50cm (20in) or more. E. Europe, W. Asia. ***

P. x hybridum 🏆 (*P. multiflorum* x *P. odoratum*) syn. *P. multiflorum* of gardens (Common Solomon's seal). Rhizomatous perennial with scarcely arching, hairless stems bearing alternate, ovate-lance-shaped leaves, to 20cm (8in) long, held horizontally. Pendent, tubular, green-tipped, creamy white flowers, 2cm (¾in) long, slightly constricted around the middle, are produced in late spring, usually 4 per axil; they are followed by spherical, blue-black fruit, to 8mm (⅜in) across. ↕ to 1.5m (5ft), ↔ 30cm (12in). Garden origin. ***

P. latifolium see *P. hirtum.*

P. multiflorum. Rhizomatous perennial with arching, hairless stems bearing ovate-lance-shaped leaves, to 5–15cm (2–6in) long, arranged alternately. In late spring, each lower leaf axil produces 2–6 pendent, tubular, green-tipped white flowers, 1cm (½in) long; they are followed by spherical black fruit, 4–6mm (⅛–¼in) across. ↕ to 90cm (36in), ↔ 25cm (10in). Europe, temperate Asia. ***. **'Striatum'** ▣ syn. 'Variegatum', has leaves striped creamy white.

***P. multiflorum* of gardens** see *P.* x *hybridum.*

P. odoratum, syn. *P. officinale.* Creeping, rhizomatous perennial with arching, angular stems bearing alternate, lance-shaped to ovate, hairless leaves, 5–15cm (2–6in) long, usually in 2 rows. In late spring and early summer, bears 1 or 2 pendent, tubular, fragrant, green-tipped white flowers, to 3cm (1¼in) long, in the upper leaf axils, followed by spherical black fruit, 6mm (¼in) across. ↕ to 85cm (34in), ↔ 30cm (12in). Europe, Caucasus, Russia (Siberia) to Japan. ***. **'Flore Pleno'** 🏆 has double flowers with more extensive green markings. **'Gilt Edge'** has leaves with narrow yellow margins.

P. officinale see *P. odoratum.*

P. stewartianum ▣ Rhizomatous perennial with short, erect, slightly angular, hairless stems bearing whorled, linear-lance-shaped leaves, to 10cm (4in) long. From late spring to mid-summer, produces small clusters of 1–3 pendent, tubular, purple-pink flowers, to 1.5cm (½in) long, in the leaf axils. The spherical red fruit, to 6mm (¼in) across, are spotted purplish white. ↕ 20–90cm (8–36in), ↔ 25cm (10in). Europe, temperate Asia. ***

P. verticillatum (Whorled Solomon's seal). Rhizomatous perennial with erect, slightly angular, hairless stems bearing stalkless, mainly whorled, sometimes opposite, lance-shaped leaves, 6–15cm (2½–6in) long. From late spring to midsummer, produces 1–4 pendent, tubular, greenish white flowers, to 1.5cm (½in) long, in the upper leaf axils; they are followed by spherical red fruit, 5mm (¼in) across. ↕ 20–90cm (8–36in), ↔ 25cm (10in). Europe, Caucasus, Afghanistan. ***

▷ ***Polygonum affine*** see *Persicaria affinis*
▷ ***Polygonum amplexicaule*** see *Persicaria amplexicaulis*
▷ ***Polygonum aubertii*** see *Fallopia aubertii*
▷ ***Polygonum baldschuanicum*** see *Fallopia baldschuanica*
▷ ***Polygonum bistorta*** see *Persicaria bistorta*
▷ ***Polygonum campanulatum*** see *Persicaria campanulata*
▷ ***Polygonum capitatum*** see *Persicaria capitata*
▷ ***Polygonum carneum*** see *Persicaria bistorta* subsp. *carnea*
▷ ***Polygonum macrophyllum*** see *Persicaria macrophylla*
▷ ***Polygonum milletii*** see *Persicaria milletii*
▷ ***Polygonum orientale*** see *Persicaria orientale*
▷ ***Polygonum sphaerostachyum*** see *Persicaria macrophylla*
▷ ***Polygonum tenuicaule*** see *Persicaria tenuicaulis*
▷ ***Polygonum vacciniifolium*** see *Persicaria vacciniifolia*
▷ ***Polygonum virginianum*** see *Persicaria virginiana*

POLYPODIUM

POLYPODIACEAE

Genus of about 75 species of mostly evergreen, usually epiphytic, sometimes terrestrial ferns, mainly from tropical regions of the USA, Central America, and South America, but also from temperate and other tropical regions. They are often found growing on trees, rocks, walls, or well-drained banks and sand dunes. They are cultivated for their sculptural fronds, which are usually lance-shaped, simple to pinnatifid or pinnate, occasionally more divided, and borne at random in 2 rows along creeping, often surface rhizomes. Sori, without indusia, are arranged in rows on each side of the midrib of each frond or pinna. The hardy species are good for a rock garden, mixed border, or bank, especially where winter green and ground cover are required. In frost-prone climates, grow tender species in a warm greenhouse. Elsewhere, the tropical species, which are mostly epiphytic, are suitable for growing in trees.

- **HARDINESS** Fully hardy to frost tender.
- **CULTIVATION** Under glass, grow in equal parts fine-grade bark, perlite, and charcoal. May be grown epiphytically in bright filtered light; wrap the rhizomes in moss and tie to a suitable rooting medium, such as osmunda fibre, and keep moist until established. Water moderately during the growing season; sparingly in winter. Outdoors, grow in moderately fertile, humus-rich, gritty or stony, well-drained soil (*P. cambricum* requires neutral to alkaline soil) in full sun or dappled shade, with shelter from cold, dry winds.
- **PROPAGATION** Sow spores at 15–16°C (59–61°F) when ripe. Divide in spring or early summer. See also p.51.
- **PESTS AND DISEASES** Trouble free.

P. aureum see *Phlebodium aureum.*

P. australe see *P. cambricum.*

P. cambricum, syn. *P. australe*, *P. vulgare* subsp. *serratum* (Southern polypody). Terrestrial, deciduous fern producing broadly lance-shaped to broadly triangular-ovate, pinnate, mid-green fronds, to 60cm (24in) long, with linear or oblong pinnae, the longest usually being the second pair from the base; the pinnae often have toothed margins. New fronds appear in late summer and die back in spring. Sori are conspicuously yellow in winter. ↕ 15–60cm (6–24in), ↔ indefinite. S. and W. Europe. ***. Sterile variants, producing yellow-green fronds with deeply cut margins, are often listed or grown as *P. cambricum.* **'Cristatum'** bears crested frond tips and pinnae. **'Grandiceps'** has much larger crests than 'Cristatum', with the crests at the tips usually wider than the rest of the fronds. **'Omnilacerum Oxford'** has tall, erect, oblong-lance-shaped fronds, to 60cm (24in) long, with lance-shaped pinnae cut irregularly almost to the midribs. **'Willharris'** produces thick-textured, lance-shaped fronds, to 45cm (18in) long, with pinnae deeply divided into long segments.

P. formosanum. Epiphytic, evergreen fern with arching to pendent, ovate to oblong, pinnate, glaucous, pale green fronds, to 50cm (20in) long, composed of spreading, lance-shaped to linear pinnae. The rhizome is conspicuously glaucous, and is very sparsely covered with small scales. ↕↔ to 45cm (18in). China, Taiwan, Japan. *

P. glycyrrhiza ▣ (Licorice fern). Terrestrial, evergreen fern producing

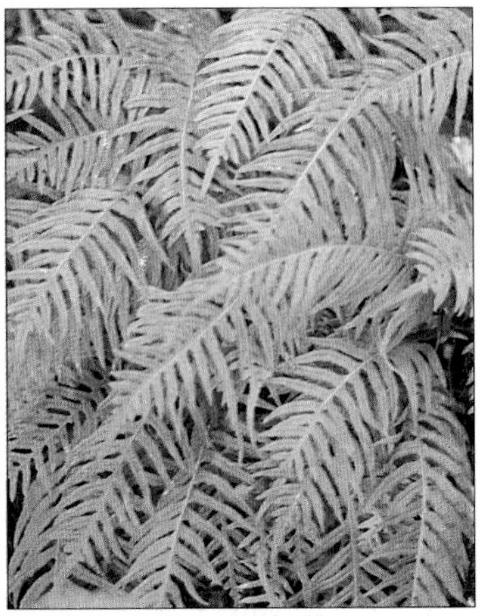

Polypodium glycyrrhiza

P

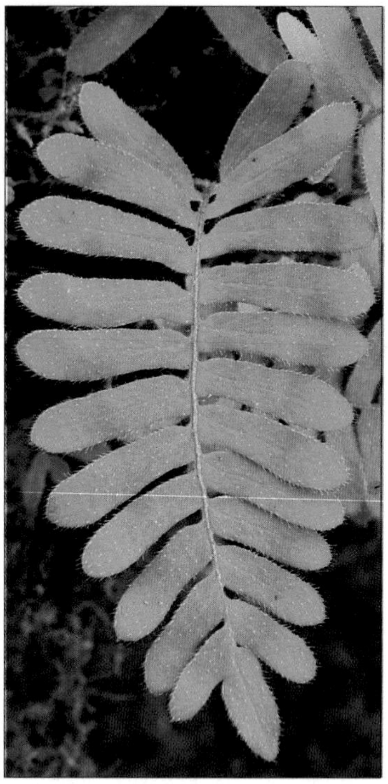

Polypodium polypodioides

lance-shaped, pinnate or very deeply pinnatifid, mid- to dark green fronds, to 35cm (14in) long, comprising sickle-shaped, linear pinnae. Similar to *P. vulgare*, except fronds are darker green, pinnae tips more pointed, and sori smaller. If chewed, the rhizome has a very sweet, licorice taste. ↕ 30cm (12in), ↔ indefinite. North America (Alaska to California). ❄❄❄. **'Longicaudatum'**, syn. *P. vulgare* 'Longicaudatum', has fronds with very long, pointed tips. **Malahatense Group** consists of fertile variants with deeply cut pinnae; they come true from spores.

P. polypodioides ■ (Resurrection fern). Small, semi-evergreen, terrestrial or epiphytic fern with narrowly triangular or oblong, pinnate, fairly leathery, mid-green fronds, to 30cm (12in) tall, covered with scales, and composed of well-spaced, linear or oblong pinnae. Frond margins temporarily roll inwards during dry weather. ↕ to 30cm (12in), ↔ indefinite. Southern Africa, tropical regions of America. ❄

P. scouleri ■ (Leathery polypody). Terrestrial, evergreen fern bearing broadly ovate to triangular, pinnate or very deeply pinnatifid, leathery, thick,

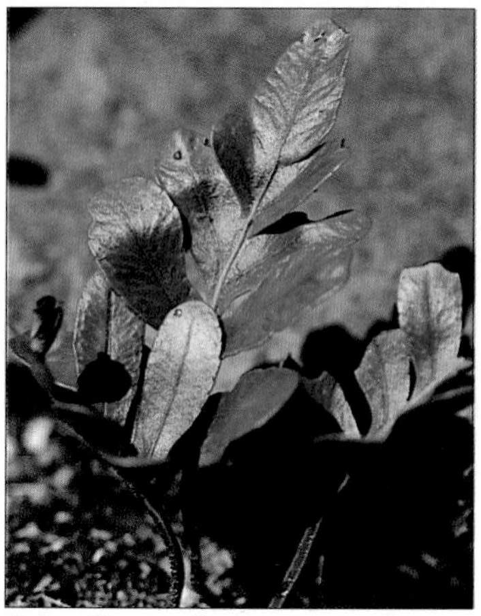

Polypodium scouleri

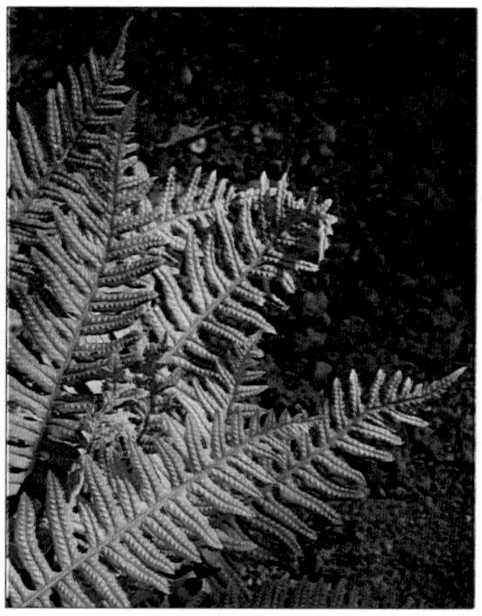

Polypodium vulgare

rigid, glossy, deep green fronds, 30cm (12in) long. Pinnae are spreading, and narrowly oblong. Needs a sheltered site in frost-prone gardens. ↕ 30cm (12in), ↔ indefinite. N.W. North America (coastal belt). ❄❄

P. virginianum (Rockcap fern, Virginian polypody). Terrestrial or epiphytic, evergreen fern, very similar to *P. vulgare*, with arching or pendent, narrowly lance-shaped or triangular to oblong, pinnate or very deeply pinnatifid, leathery to thin, dark green fronds, 25cm (10in) long, composed of lance-shaped to linear or oblong pinnae. ↕ 25cm (10in), ↔ indefinite. E. Asia, North America. ❄❄❄

P. vulgare ■ (Common polypody). Terrestrial or epiphytic, evergreen fern with lance-shaped to oblong, pinnate or very deeply pinnatifid, thin to leathery, dark green fronds, 40cm (16in) long, composed of close, spreading, oblong to linear pinnae. Replaced in warmer sites in Europe by the very similar species, *P. interjectum*, which has ovate-triangular, thin-textured fronds. ↕ 30cm (12in), ↔ indefinite. Mostly in northern regions or on higher ground in Europe, Africa, E. Asia. ❄❄❄. **'Bifidograndiceps'** has large, flat crests; ↕ 30–50cm (12–20in). **'Cornubiense'** ■ is very vigorous, bears both pinnatifid and 3- or 4-pinnatifid fronds, and is excellent as ground cover; ↕ 30–40cm (12–16in). **'Cornubiense Grandiceps'** has 3-pinnate fronds, to 40cm (16in) long, with large, branched, terminal crests. **'Jean Taylor'** is crested, with pinnatifid and 4-pinnatifid fronds, moss-like in appearance; ↕ 20cm (8in). **'Longicaudatum'** see *P. glycyrrhiza* 'Longicaudatum'. **subsp. *serratum*** see *P. cambricum*. **'Trichomanoides Backhouse'** bears pinnatifid and 4-pinnatifid fronds; ↕ 20cm (8in).

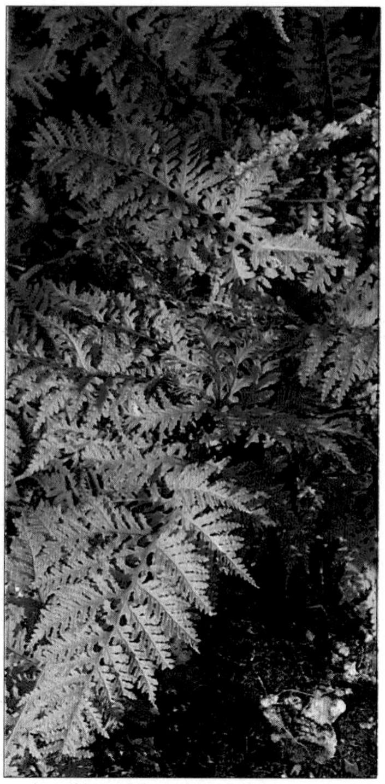

Polypodium vulgare 'Cornubiense'

▷ **Polypody,**
 Common see *Polypodium vulgare*
 Golden see *Phlebodium aureum*
 Leathery see *Polypodium scouleri*
 Limestone see *Gymnocarpium robertianum*
 Southern see *Polypodium cambricum*
 Virginian see *Polypodium virginianum*

POLYSCIAS

ARALIACEAE

Genus of about 100 species of rounded or upright, evergreen shrubs and small trees from tropical regions of Africa, Asia, and the Pacific. They are cultivated for their alternate or spiralling leaves, which may be simple, 3-palmate, or pinnate to 3-pinnate, and tend to be grouped towards the stem tips. The small, usually whitish green flowers have 4–15 tepals, and are most often produced in panicles composed of small umbels, or in terminal clusters; they are followed by small, usually purple to black berries. Below 16°C (61°F), grow in a warm greenhouse or as houseplants. In warmer climates, grow in a shrub border; strong-growing species are also effective for hedging.

• **HARDINESS** Frost tender.

• **CULTIVATION** Under glass, grow in loam-based potting compost (JI No.3) in full light or bright filtered light. In growth, water freely, mist daily, and apply a balanced liquid fertilizer every month. Water sparingly in winter. Outdoors, grow in fertile, humus-rich, moist but well-drained soil in full sun or partial shade. Pruning group 1; trim hedges in late summer and, if necessary, in late winter or early spring; may need restrictive pruning under glass.

• **PROPAGATION** Sow seed at 19–24°C (66–75°F) in spring. Take greenwood cuttings in early summer, or root semi-ripe or ripe, leafless stem sections with bottom heat in summer.

• **PESTS AND DISEASES** Red spider mites, mealybugs, and root-knot eelworms may be troublesome under glass.

P. filicifolia ■ (Chotito, Fern-leaf aralia). Erect, evergreen shrub, sparingly branched (at least when young) unless regularly tip-pruned. Young plants bear arching to semi-pendent, pinnate to 3-pinnate leaves, to 10cm (4in) long, composed of 9–17 narrowly elliptic, bright green leaflets, with purple-tinted midribs. Mature plants produce leaves to 90cm (36in) long, composed of leaflets with entire or finely toothed margins. Star-shaped, whitish green flowers are borne in terminal, umbel-like panicles, in summer, followed by

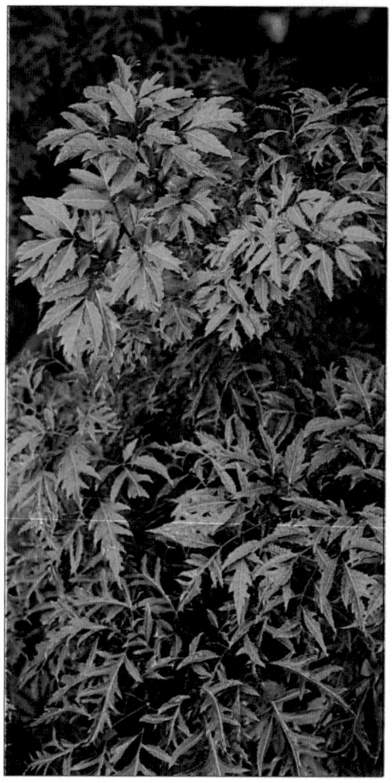

Polyscias filicifolia

black fruit. Flowers and fruit are seldom produced. Probably a hybrid. ↕ to 2–2.5m (6–8ft) or more, ↔ to 1m (3ft) or more. S. Malaysia, Pacific. ❁ (min. 16°C/61°F). **'Marginata'** has leaves with white margins.

P. guilfoylei ♀ (Coffee tree, Geranium aralia). Large, erect, evergreen shrub or small tree, generally sparsely branched, with foliage confined to the stem tips. Pinnate leaves, 30–45cm (12–18in) long, are each composed of 5–9 broadly ovate to oblong-elliptic, shallowly lobed, irregularly spiny-toothed, white- to cream-margined, mid-green leaflets. In summer, mature plants produce brown-budded, 5-petalled, star-shaped, yellow-green flowers in large, loose, terminal, umbel-like panicles, to 50cm (20in) long, followed by spherical, black-purple fruit, 5mm (¼in). ↕ 4–6m (12–20ft), ↔ 1–2.5m (3–8ft). E. Malaysia, W. Pacific. ❁ (min. 16°C/61°F). **'Laciniata'** has pendent, 2-pinnate leaves composed of lance-shaped leaflets with white margins. **'Victoriae'** ■ (Lace aralia) is compact, with much-dissected, fern-like leaves; each leaflet irregularly toothed and white-margined; ↕ 1.5m (5ft), ↔ 80cm (32in).

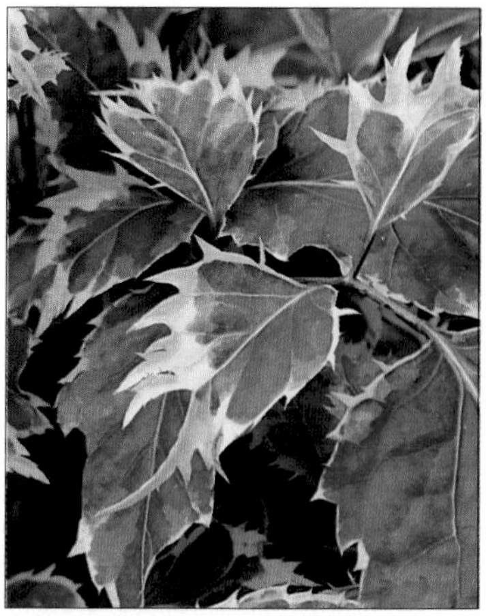

Polyscias guilfoylei 'Victoriae'

POLYSTICHUM

Holly fern, Shield fern

DRYOPTERIDACEAE

Genus of nearly 200 species of usually evergreen, terrestrial ferns found in a range of habitats from alpine cliffs to tropical forests worldwide. They are cultivated for their often lance-shaped, pinnate to 3-pinnate fronds, which arise from erect or short-creeping rhizomes, usually in shapely, "shuttlecock" crowns. The pinnae are holly-like, and sometimes lobed, each lobe ending in a sharp point or bristle. Sori are borne on the undersides of the fronds, each usually protected by a rounded indusium. Grow shield ferns in a rock garden, fernery, or well-drained border. In frost-prone areas, grow tender species in a cool, temperate, or warm greenhouse.

- **HARDINESS** Fully hardy to frost tender.
- **CULTIVATION** Grow in fertile, humus-rich, well-drained soil in deep or partial shade. Remove dead fronds before new ones unfurl. Protect the crowns from excessive winter wet.
- **PROPAGATION** Sow spores at 15–16°C (59–61°F) when ripe. Divide rhizomes in spring. Detach fronds bearing bulbils in autumn. See also p.51.
- **PESTS AND DISEASES** Susceptible to the fungal disease *Taphrina wettsteiniana.*

P. acrostichoides. Terrestrial, evergreen fern producing a shuttlecock of narrowly lance-shaped, pinnate, dark green fronds, 60cm (24in) long, with small, holly-like pinnae. Fertile fronds narrow abruptly towards tips where sori occur. ↕45cm (18in), ↔ 90cm (36in). N.E. North America. ❄❄❄
P. aculeatum 🏆 (Hard shield fern, Prickly shield fern). Terrestrial, evergreen fern bearing narrowly lance-shaped, pinnate or 2-pinnate, often glossy, dark green fronds, 60cm (24in) long or more, forming shuttlecocks. Pinnae are oblong and pinnate or pinnatifid, with spiny-toothed lobes that are unstalked and acutely angled at the point of attachment to the midribs. Reliably evergreen. ↕60cm (24in), ↔ 90cm (36in). N.W. and C. Europe. ❄❄❄. **'Pulcherrimum'** see *P. setiferum* 'Plumosum Bevis'.
P. munitum ▣ (Sword fern). Terrestrial, evergreen fern that bears narrowly lance-shaped, leathery, pinnate, dark green fronds, 90cm (36in) long or more, forming shuttlecocks. Pinnae are linear and spiny-toothed. Larger than *P. acrostichoides,* its fertile fronds do not narrow at the tips. ↕90cm (36in), rarely to 1.5m (5ft), ↔ 1.2m (4ft). N.W. North America. ❄❄❄
P. polyblepharum (Japanese tassel fern). Terrestrial, evergreen fern bearing shuttlecocks of spreading, lance-shaped, 2-pinnate, shiny, dark green fronds, 30–80cm (12–32in) long, covered with golden hairs when they unfurl. Pinnae lobes are oblong-ovate and have spiny-toothed margins. ↕60–80cm (24–32in), ↔ 90cm (36in). South Korea, Japan. ❄❄❄
P. rigens. Terrestrial, evergreen fern producing shuttlecocks of narrowly ovate-oblong, 2-pinnate, leathery, harsh-textured, dull green fronds, 30–45cm (12–18in) long. Broad, lance-shaped pinnae are divided into ovate, spiny-

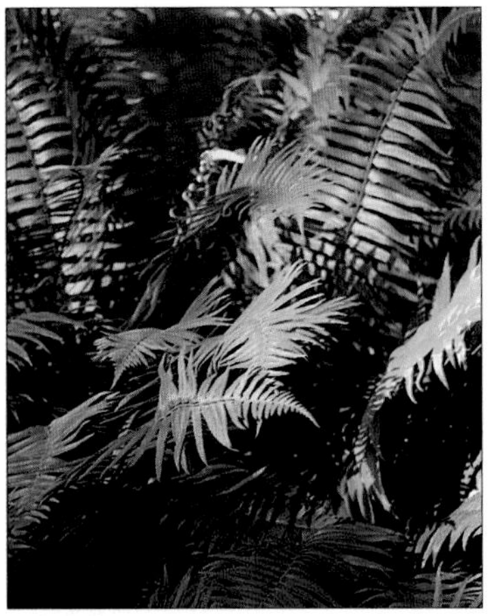

Polystichum munitum

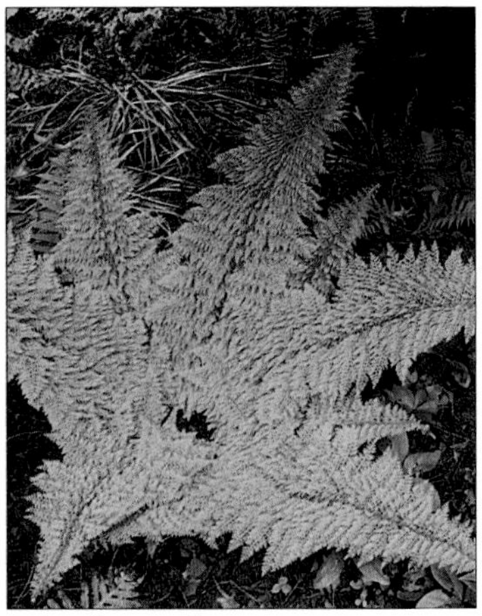

Polystichum setiferum Plumosodivisilobum Group

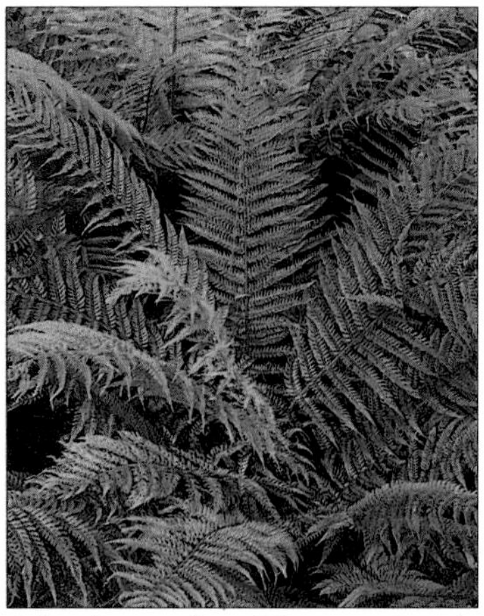

Polystichum setiferum 'Plumosum Bevis'

toothed lobes. In spring, fronds are yellowish green. ↕40cm (16in), ↔ 60cm (24in). Japan. ❄❄❄
P. setiferum 🏆 (Soft shield fern). Terrestrial, evergreen fern with soft, lance-shaped, 2-pinnate, dark green fronds, 30–120cm (12–48in) long, arranged in shuttlecocks. Pinnae lobes are ovate, bristle-toothed, stalked, and obtusely angled at the point of attachment to the midribs. ↕1.2m (4ft), ↔ 90cm (36in). Europe. ❄❄❄. Ferns of **Divisilobum Group** ▣ produce usually spreading, 3-pinnate fronds, comprising narrowed and leathery segments; bulbils often form along the frond midribs. ↕↔ 50–70cm (20–28in) or more. **'Dahlem'** bears almost erect fronds; ↕75cm (30in), ↔ 45cm (18in). **'Herrenhausen'** has broader, spreading fronds; ↕50cm (20in). **'Iveryanum'** has fronds crested at the tips; ↕50cm (20in), ↔ 60cm (24in). **Multilobum Group** ferns produce 3-pinnate fronds similar to those of the Divisilobum Group, but the frond segments are not narrowed or leathery; ↕↔ 60–80cm (24–32in). **Plumosodivisilobum Group** ▣ ferns bear fronds, 4-pinnate at the base, with segments narrowed towards the frond tips; lower pinnae often overlap. **'Plumosomultilobum'** has overlapping, very leafy pinnae, which give it a moss-like appearance; similar to the Plumosodivisilobum Group, but the segments are not narrowed. **'Plumosum Bevis'** ▣ syn. 'Pulcherrimum Bevis', *P. aculeatum* 'Pulcherrimum', has elongated pinnae and segments that sweep gracefully towards the tips. Only very rarely fertile; ↕↔ 60–80cm (24–32in). **'Pulcherrimum Bevis'** see 'Plumosum Bevis'.
P. tsussimense (Korean rock fern). Terrestrial, evergreen fern producing shuttlecocks of broadly lance-shaped, 2-pinnate, dark green fronds, 20–40cm (8–16in) long. The narrow, ovate to oblong-ovate, spiny-toothed pinnae are sharply and abruptly pointed. ↕↔ 40cm (16in). East Asia. ❄❄❄

▷**Pomegranate** see *Punica, P. granatum*
Wild see *Burchellia bubalina*

PONCIRUS *syn.* AEGLE

RUTACEAE

Genus of one species of spiny, deciduous shrub or small tree from woodland in China and Korea. It produces alternate, 3-palmate, dark green leaves, and is cultivated for its 5-petalled, fragrant white flowers and orange-like fruit. Grow in a shrub border or against a sunny wall, or as a very thick, thorny hedge. It is sometimes used as a rootstock for *Citrus* cultivars.

- **HARDINESS** Fully hardy.
- **CULTIVATION** Grow in fertile, well-drained soil in full sun, with shelter from cold, dry winds. Pruning group 1; trim hedges after flowering or fruiting.
- **PROPAGATION** Sow seed in containers in a cold frame in autumn. Take semi-ripe cuttings with bottom heat in summer.
- **PESTS AND DISEASES** Trouble free.

P. trifoliata ♧ (Japanese bitter orange). Rounded, bushy, deciduous shrub or tree with rigid green shoots armed with very sharp spines. Alternate, 3-palmate leaves, 2.5–6cm (1–2½in) long, comprise 3 obovate, dark green leaflets, to 5cm (2in) long, turning yellow in autumn. Solitary, cup-shaped then saucer-shaped, fragrant white flowers, 5cm (2in) across, are borne in late spring and early summer, often again in autumn, followed by orange-like, inedible, green then orange fruit, 4cm (1½in) across. ↕↔ 5m (15ft). N. China, Korea. ❄❄❄

▷**Pondweed** see *Elodea*
Canadian see *Elodea canadensis*
Cape see *Aponogeton distachyos*
Curled see *Potamogeton crispus*

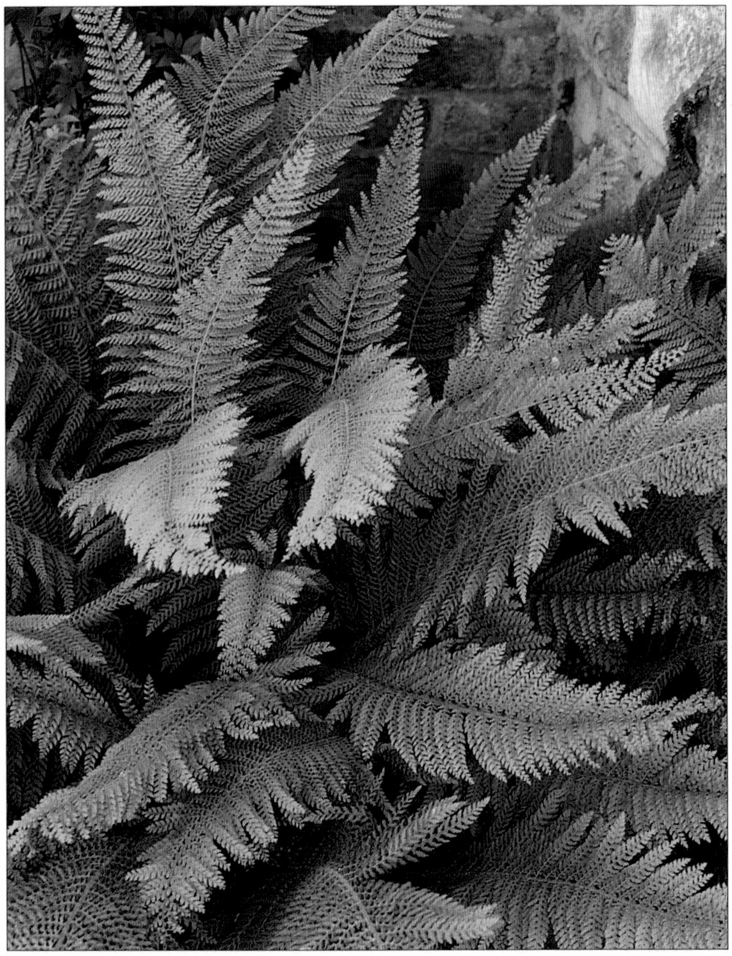

Polystichum setiferum Divisilobum Group

P

PONGAMIA

LEGUMINOSAE/PAPILIONACEAE

Genus of one species of wide-spreading, deciduous or semi-evergreen tree from seashores and riverbanks in Malaysia, Indonesia, N. Australia, and Pacific islands. It has pinnate leaves and axillary racemes of pea-like flowers. In frost-prone climates, grow in a warm greenhouse for its foliage. In tropical areas, it is a fine shade tree, suitable for coasts.

• **HARDINESS** Frost tender.

• **CULTIVATION** Under glass, grow in loam-based potting compost (JI No.3) with added sharp sand, in full light. In growth, water moderately and apply a balanced liquid fertilizer monthly; water sparingly in winter. Outdoors, grow in fertile, well-drained soil in full sun. Pruning group 1; may need restrictive pruning under glass.

• **PROPAGATION** Sow seed at 18–24°C (64–75°F) in spring. Root semi-ripe cuttings in summer with bottom heat.

• **PESTS AND DISEASES** Whiteflies may be a problem under glass.

P. pinnata ◯ (Karum oil tree, Poona oil tree). Many-branched, spreading, deciduous or semi-evergreen tree with a domed head and a usually short trunk. The pinnate, glossy, bright green leaves, 15–30cm (6–12in) long, comprise 5–9 ovate to elliptic leaflets, emerging pink-bronze. In summer and autumn, produces racemes, 13cm (5in) long, of pea-like, mauve-pink or cream flowers, strongly scented when crushed; they have rounded, standard petals, to 1.5cm (½in) across, often incurled. ↕20–25m (70–80ft), ↔15–25m (50–80ft). Malaysia, Indonesia, N. Australia, Pacific islands. ❀ (min. 16°C/61°F)

PONTEDERIA

Pickerel weed

PONTEDERIACEAE

Genus of 5 species of marginal aquatic perennials from freshwater marshes and swamp ditches in North, Central, and South America. They are grown for their neat habit, distinctive foliage, and highly coloured flowers. The thick rootstock produces clumps of often linear or lance-shaped leaves. Terminal spikes of tubular, 2-lipped, usually blue flowers are borne in summer and early autumn. Grow at the margins of a pond or in a large, water-filled tub on a sunny, sheltered patio. Flower spikes may not open fully in cool, wet summers.

• **HARDINESS** Fully hardy to frost hardy.

• **CULTIVATION** Grow in aquatic planting baskets of fertile, loamy soil at the margins of a pool; grow in no more than 10–12cm (4–5in) of water, in full sun. See also pp.52–53.

• **PROPAGATION** Sow seed in containers outdoors as soon as ripe. Divide in late spring when growth starts.

• **PESTS AND DISEASES** Trouble free.

P. cordata ■🏆 (Pickerel weed). Marginal aquatic perennial with erect, lance-shaped, triangular to ovate, glossy, emergent, floating, or submerged leaves, 20cm (8in) wide, with heart-shaped bases, borne on stalks to 25cm (10in) long. In late summer, produces tubular blue flowers in closely packed spikes, 2–16cm (¾–6in) long, on flower-stalks to 35cm (14in) tall. ↕0.9–1.3m (3–4½ft), ↔60–75cm (24–30in). E. North America to Caribbean. ❄❄❄. **var. *lancifolia***, syn. *P. lanceolata*, has narrower leaves, to 12–20cm (5–8in) long, on stalks 60–70cm (24–28in) long. ↕1.2–1.5m (4–5ft), ↔1m (3ft). E. and S. USA, South America. ❄❄ (borderline)

P. lanceolata see *P. cordata* var. *lancifolia.*

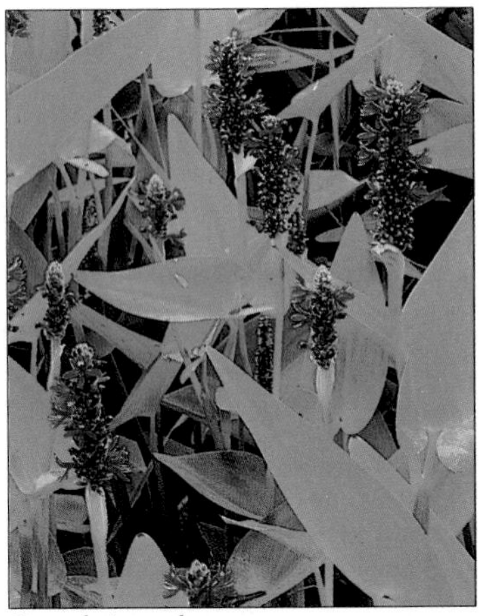

Pontederia cordata

▷**Ponytail** see *Beaucarnea recurvata*
▷**Poplar** see *Populus*
Balsam see *P. balsamifera*
Berlin see *P.* x *berolinensis*
Black see *P. nigra*
Canadian see *P.* x *canadensis*
Chinese necklace see *P. lasiocarpa*
Grey see *P.* x *canescens*
Lombardy see *P. nigra* var. *italica*
Necklace see *P. deltoides*
Western balsam see *P. trichocarpa*
White see *P. alba*
▷**Poppy** see *Papaver*
Alpine see *Papaver alpinum*
Arctic see *Papaver croceum*
California see *Eschscholzia, E. californica*
Californian see *Platystemon, P. californicus*
Celandine see *Stylophorum diphyllum*
Corn see *Papaver rhoeas*
Field see *Papaver rhoeas*
Flanders see *Papaver rhoeas*
Harebell see *Meconopsis quintuplinervia*
Himalayan blue see *Meconopsis betonicifolia, M. grandis*
Horned see *Glaucium*
Icelandic see *Papaver croceum*
Long-headed see *Papaver dubium*
Matilija see *Romneya*
Mexican tulip see *Hunnemannia fumariifolia*
Opium see *Papaver somniferum*
Oriental see *Papaver orientale*
Plume see *Macleaya, M. cordata*
Prickly see *Argemone, A. mexicana*
Red horned see *Glaucium corniculatum*
Snow see *Eomecon*
Tibetan blue see *Meconopsis betonicifolia*
Tree see *Dendromecon, Romneya*
Water see *Hydrocleys nymphoides*
Welsh see *Meconopsis cambrica*
Yellow horned see *Glaucium flavum*
▷**Poppy mallow** see *Callirhoe*
Prairie see *C. involucrata*

POPULUS

Aspen, Cottonwood, Poplar

SALICACEAE

Genus of about 35 species of usually dioecious, mainly deciduous trees found in woodland, valley bottoms, riverbanks, and swampland in N. temperate regions. They are cultivated for their very rapid growth as specimen trees, and for their alternate, ovate, triangular-ovate or diamond-shaped leaves, often aromatic in bud and when unfolding. They have tiny flowers borne in catkins, generally 5–15cm (2–6in) long, mostly in late winter or spring, before the leaves. Male and female flowers are usually borne on separate trees, the females producing copious fluffy white seeds. Most poplars are useful as windbreaks; *P. alba* and *P.* x *canescens* will thrive in coastal sites. The vigorous root systems may damage drains and foundations, particularly on clay soil, so avoid growing poplars within 40m (130ft) of a building.

• **HARDINESS** Fully hardy.

• **CULTIVATION** Tolerant of any, except constantly waterlogged soil, although best in deep, fertile, moist but well-drained soil in full sun. *P. alba* and *P.* x *canescens* tolerate dry conditions; Pruning group 1.

• **PROPAGATION** Take hardwood cuttings in winter. Remove suckers in autumn or late winter.

• **PESTS AND DISEASES** Susceptible to bacterial canker, various fungal diseases (such as honey fungus, rust, and silver leaf), and a variety of insects (such as beetles) and caterpillars, which may eat the foliage or bore into the bark.

P. alba ■◯ (Abele, White poplar). Spreading, deciduous tree with white-hairy young shoots and broadly ovate to almost rounded, wavy-margined to maple-like, deeply 5-lobed leaves, to 10cm (4in) long, dark green above, thickly white-hairy beneath, and turning yellow in autumn. In early spring, bears pendent red male catkins, 7cm (3in) long, or green females, 5cm (2in) long. ↕20–40m (70–130ft), ↔15m (50ft). N. Africa, Turkey, C. and S. former USSR (including S.W. Siberia). ❄❄❄. **f. *pyramidalis*** ■⬮ is pyramidal in shape; ↔5m (15ft). **'Raket'** ■⬮ syn. 'Rocket', is narrowly conical; ↔8m (25ft). **'Richardii'** has leaves that are golden yellow above; ↕15m (50ft), ↔12m (40ft). **'Rocket'** see 'Raket'.

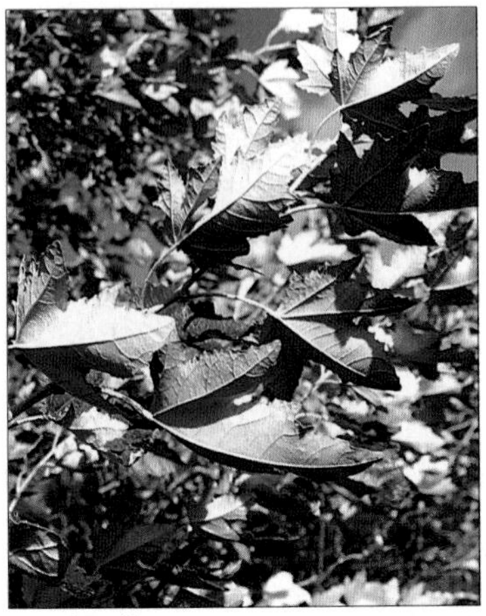

Populus alba

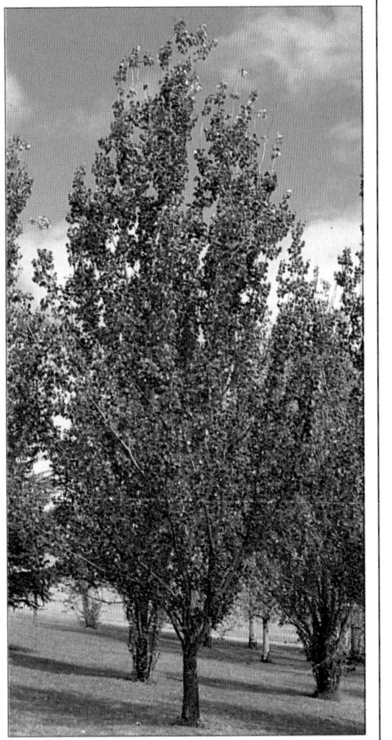

Populus alba f. *pyramidalis*

P. balsamifera ⬮ (Balsam poplar, Tacamahac). Fast-growing, columnar, deciduous tree producing smooth, hairless shoots, balsam-scented buds, and ovate, glossy leaves, to 12cm (5in) long, dark green above, whitish green beneath. Pendent green catkins, the males to 5cm (2in) long, the females to 7cm (3in) long, are produced in early spring. ↕30m (100ft), ↔8m (25ft). North America. ❄❄❄. **var. *michauxii*** produces downy shoots; N. USA.

***P.* 'Balsam Spire'** 🏆⬮ syn. *P.* 'TT 32'. Very fast-growing, narrowly columnar, deciduous tree bearing ovate leaves, 5–12cm (2–5in) long, which are obtuse at the rounded bases and hairy beneath. Cylindrical green female catkins,

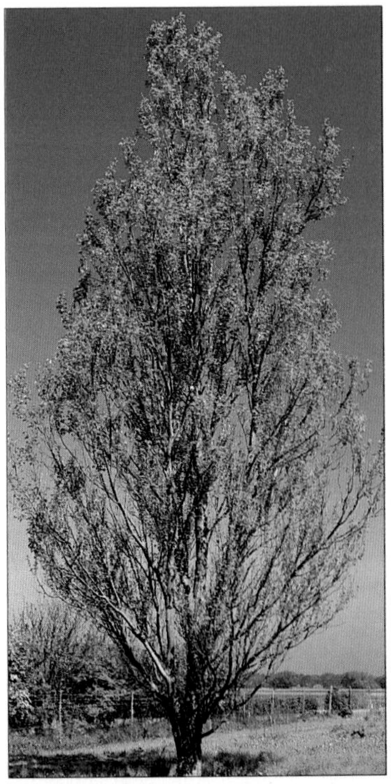

Populus alba 'Raket'

P

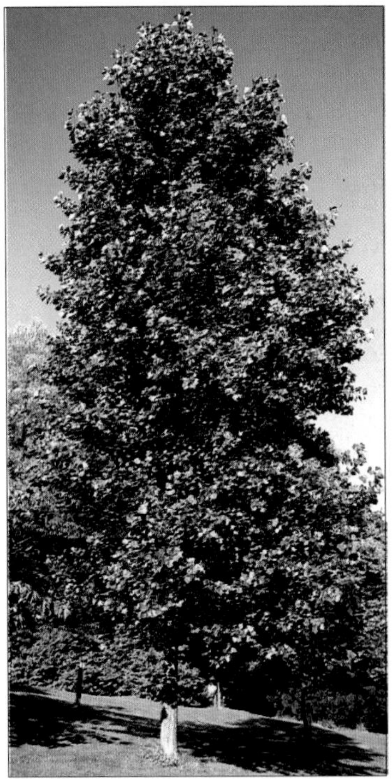
Populus x *canadensis* 'Robusta'

10–14cm (4–5½in) long, are produced from pleasantly aromatic buds in late winter or spring. ↕ 30m (100ft), ↔ 10m (30ft). ✻✻✻

P.* x *berolinensis (*P. laurifolia* x *P. nigra* var. *italica*) (Berlin poplar). • Columnar to broadly columnar, deciduous tree bearing upright branches and ovate, tapered leaves, to 12cm (5in) long, bright green above, whitish green beneath. Red male catkins, 7cm (3in) long, are borne in early spring. ↕ 30m (100ft), ↔ 8m (25ft). Garden origin. ✻✻✻

P.* x *canadensis (*P. deltoides* x *P. nigra*) (Canadian poplar). Fast-growing, conical to columnar, deciduous tree bearing triangular to ovate, scalloped, tapered, glossy, bright green leaves, to 10cm (4in) long, turning yellow in autumn. Red male or green female catkins, each to 10cm (4in) long, are produced in early spring. ↕ 30m (100ft), ↔ 12m (40ft). Garden origin. ✻✻✻. **'Aurea'** syn. 'Serotina Aurea', is columnar and male, producing bronze young leaves in late spring, later turning golden yellow; ↕ 25m (80ft), ↔ 10m (30ft). **'Robusta'** is narrowly conical and male, producing bronze-red young leaves in mid-spring. **'Serotina'** is similar to 'Aurea', but is broadly domed, with spreading branches, and produces grey-green foliage in summer. **'Serotina Aurea'** see 'Aurea'. **'Serotina de Selys'** syn. 'Serotina Erecta', has an upright habit, and produces pale green young leaves and red male catkins.

P.* x *candicans (*P. balsamifera* x *P. deltoides*), syn. *P. gileadensis*, *P.* x *jackii* (Balm of Gilead). Broadly columnar, deciduous tree bearing broadly ovate leaves, to 15cm (6in) long, heart-shaped at the bases, dark green above, whitish green beneath. Green female catkins, to 16cm (6in) long, are produced in early spring. ↕ 25m (80ft), ↔ 15m (50ft). Garden origin. ✻✻✻. **'Aurora'** has leaves conspicuously marked white, cream, and pink; ↕ 15m (50ft), ↔ 6m (20ft).

P.* x *canescens (*P. alba* x *P. tremula*) (Grey poplar). Broadly columnar to spreading, deciduous tree bearing glossy, dark green leaves; these may be broadly ovate, grey-woolly beneath, and to 8cm (3in) long, or rounded, almost hairless, and to 6cm (2½in) long. Red male catkins, to 10cm (4in) long, are borne in early spring. Green catkins, 2–10cm (¾–4in) long, are borne on female trees, which are rarely seen. ↕ to 30m (100ft), rarely to 50m (160ft), ↔ 15m (50ft). Europe. ✻✻✻

P. deltoides (Eastern cottonwood, Necklace poplar). Fast-growing, spreading, deciduous tree bearing oval to triangular, glossy, bright green leaves, to 12cm (5in) long, strongly balsam-scented when young. Red male or green female catkins, each to 10cm (4in) long, are produced in early spring. ↕ 30m (100ft), ↔ 20m (70ft). E. North America. ✻✻✻. **'Siouxland'** is rust-resistant and male.

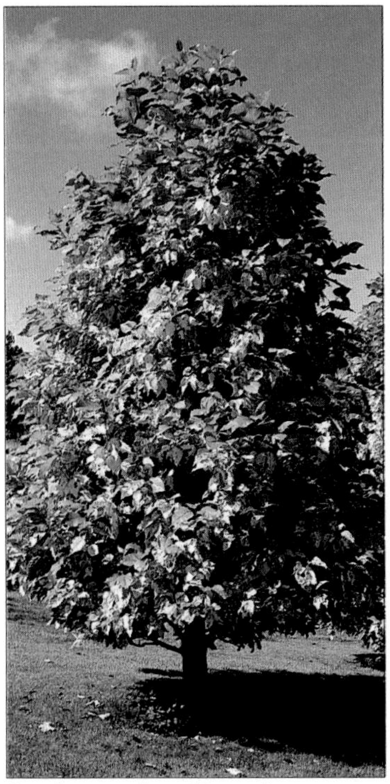
Populus x *candicans* 'Aurora'

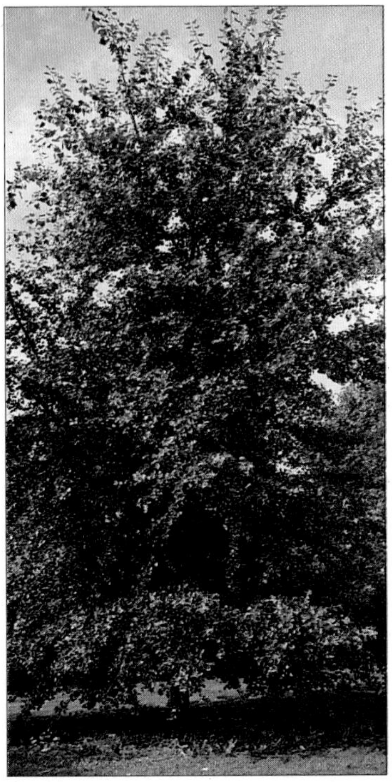
Populus x *canescens*

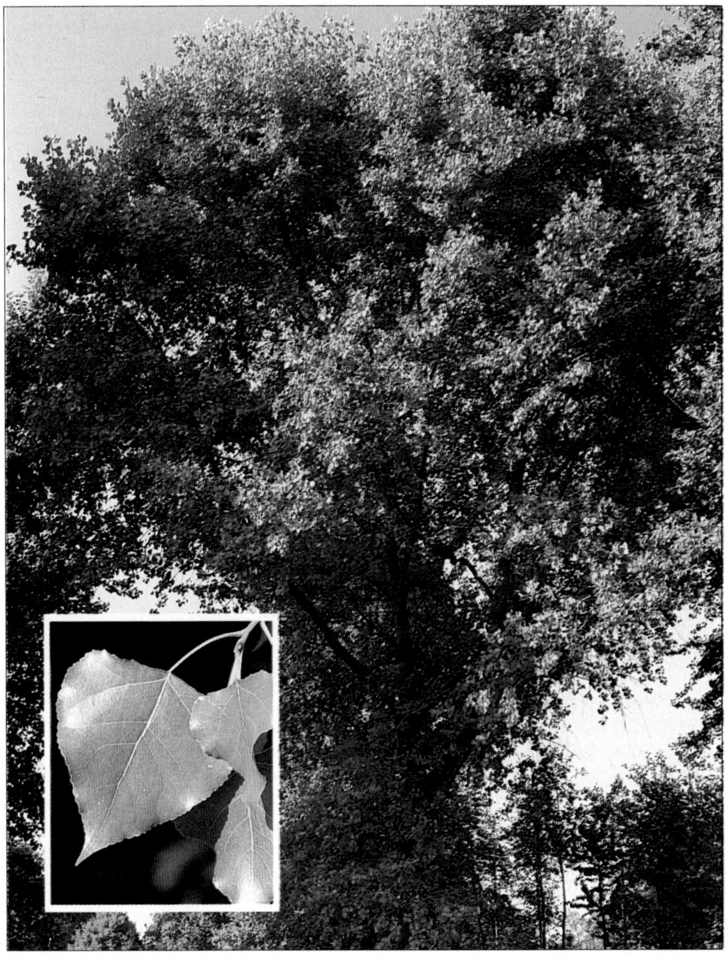
Populus deltoides (inset: leaf detail)

P. fremontii Fast-growing, round-headed, deciduous tree with spreading branches and glossy, yellow-green, broadly triangular leaves, to 8cm (3in) long, which turn yellow in autumn. Pendent red male or green female catkins, both to 10cm (4in) long, open in early spring. ↕ 25m (80ft), ↔ 15m (50ft). W. USA. ✻✻✻

P. gileadensis see *P.* x *candicans.*

P. glauca see *P. jacquemontii* var. *glauca.*

P. grandidentata (Bigtooth aspen). Spreading, deciduous tree with grey-hairy young shoots and ovate leaves, to 12cm (5in) long, grey-woolly at first, dark green above and pale green beneath. Red male catkins, to 6cm (2½in) long, or green females, to 10cm (4in) long, are produced in early spring. ↕ 20m (70ft), ↔ 12m (40ft). E. North America. ✻✻✻

P.* x *jackii see *P.* x *candicans.*

P. jacquemontii* var. *glauca syn. *P. glauca.* Fast-growing, broadly conical, deciduous tree bearing broadly ovate, blue-green leaves, to 17cm (7in) long, on red leaf-stalks marked with darker red veins. The leaves emerge bronze in early spring, and turn yellow in autumn. Pendent catkins are produced in late spring, the red males to 12cm (5in), the green females to 15cm (6in) long. ↕ 20m (70ft), ↔ 10m (30ft). E. Himalayas. ✻✻✻

P. lasiocarpa (Chinese necklace poplar). Broadly conical, later round-headed, deciduous tree bearing stout shoots, hairy when young, and large, heart-shaped, tapered, dark green leaves, to 30cm (12in) long, produced on red stalks. Yellow-green catkins, to 10cm (4in) long, usually containing both male and female flowers, are produced in mid-spring. ↕ 20m (70ft), ↔ 12m (40ft). C. China. ✻✻✻

P. maximowiczii Fast-growing, conical, deciduous tree with hairy young shoots and ovate-elliptic leaves, to 12cm (5in) long, bright green above, whitish green beneath, with green veins. Red male catkins, to 10cm (4in) long, or green females, to 15cm (6in), are borne in early spring. ↕ to 30m (100ft) or more, ↔ 10m (30ft). N.E. Asia. ✻✻✻

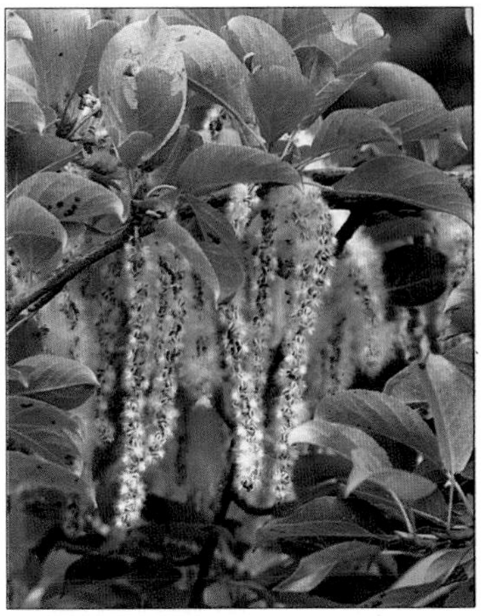
Populus maximowiczii

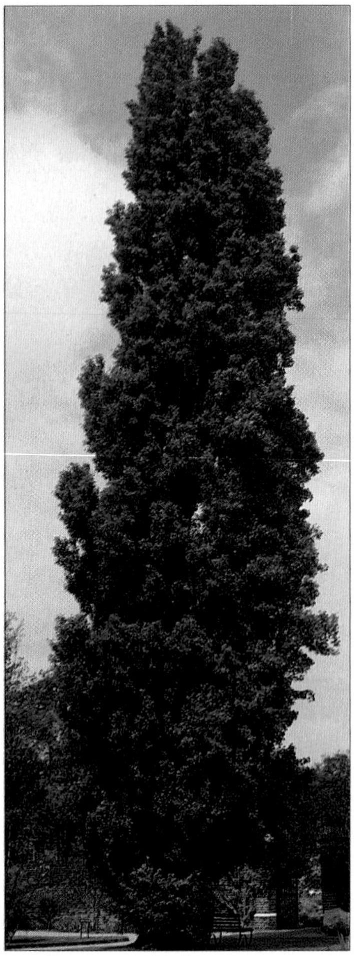
Populus nigra var. *italica*

P. nigra (Black poplar). Fast-growing, spreading, deciduous tree with dark bark and triangular to ovate, tapered, glossy, dark green leaves, to 10cm (4in) long, bronze when young, turning yellow in autumn. Red male or green female catkins, both 5cm (2in) long, are produced in early and mid-spring. ↕35m (120ft), ↔20m (70ft). Europe, N. Africa, C. Asia (including Kazakhstan), Russia (Siberia). ❄❄❄. **'Afghanica'** see 'Thevestina'. **var. *italica*** ■ (Lombardy poplar) is male and narrowly columnar; ↕30m (100ft), ↔5m (15ft). **'Thevestina'** syn. 'Afghanica', is narrowly columnar and female, with striking white bark; ↕30m (100ft), ↔5m (15ft).
P. simonii Columnar, deciduous tree with diamond-shaped-ovate to elliptic,

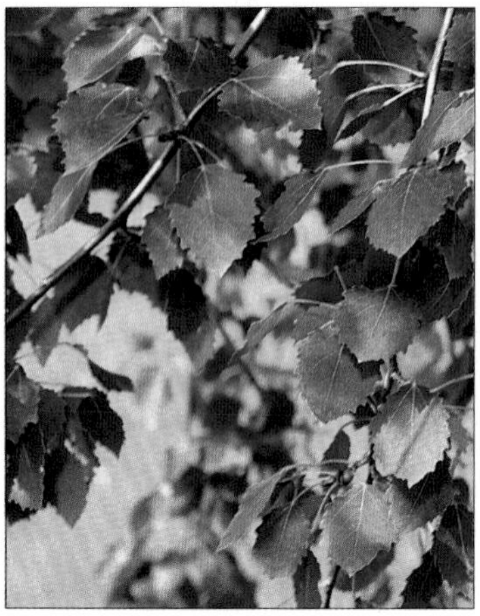
Populus tremula 'Pendula'

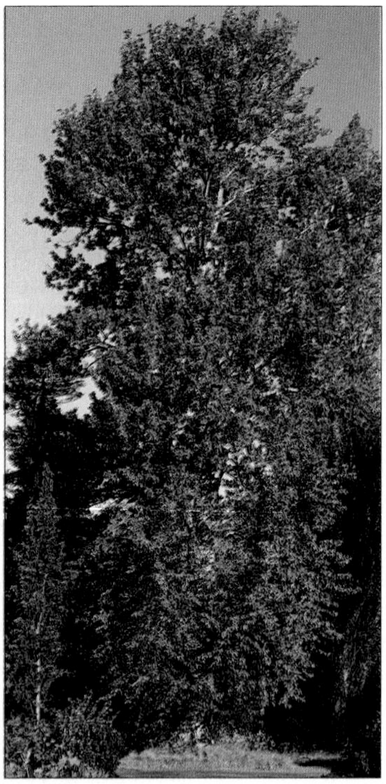
Populus trichocarpa

tapered, dark green leaves, to 12cm (5in) long, emerging yellow-green and balsam-scented very early in spring. Red male or green female catkins, both to 3cm (1¼in) long, are produced in early spring. Susceptible to damage by late frosts. ↕12m (40ft), ↔6m (20ft). N. and W. China. ❄❄❄. **'Fastigiata'** is narrowly upright; ↔3m (10ft).
P. szechuanica Broadly columnar, deciduous tree with ovate-oblong to broadly lance-shaped, smooth, dark green leaves, to 30cm (12in) long, whitish green beneath, bronze when young. Red male catkins, to 10cm (4in) long, or green females, to 15cm (6in), are borne in mid-spring. ↕to 40m (130ft), ↔10m (30ft). W. China. ❄❄❄. **var. *tibetica*** has leaves that are downy beneath, with dark red veins and leaf-stalks.
P. tremula (Common aspen). Vigorous, spreading, deciduous tree or shrub with flat-stalked, rounded to ovate, coarsely toothed, dark green leaves, to 8cm (3in) long, bronze when young, turning yellow in autumn; they tremble and rattle in the breeze. Grey-red male or green female catkins, both to 7cm (3in) long, are produced in early spring. ↕20m (70ft), ↔10m (30ft). Temperate Europe and Asia to China and Japan. ❄❄❄. **'Pendula'** ■ (Weeping aspen) has long, pendent branches; ↕6m (20ft), ↔8m (25ft).
P. tremuloides (American aspen, Quaking aspen). Vigorous, spreading, deciduous tree with flat-stalked, rounded to ovate, finely toothed, glossy, dark green leaves, to 6cm (2½in) long, bronze when young, turning yellow in autumn; light winds cause quivering and rattling of the leaves. Grey-red male or green female catkins, both to 6cm (2½in) long, are produced in early spring. ↕15m (50ft), ↔10m (30ft). W. North America. ❄❄❄
P. trichocarpa ■ (Black cottonwood, Western balsam poplar). Fast-growing, conical, deciduous tree with ovate, glossy leaves, to 20cm (8in) long, dark green above, white beneath, turning yellow in autumn, and strongly balsam-scented when young. Red male catkins, 7cm (3in) long, or green females, to 15cm (6in) long, are borne in mid-spring. ↕30m (100ft) or more, ↔10m (30ft). W. North America. ❄❄❄
***P.* 'TT 32'** see *P.* 'Balsam Spire'.

PORANA

CONVOLVULACEAE

Genus of about 20 species of evergreen, twining climbers or shrubs, closely related to *Ipomoea*, from open or dense woodland in tropical Africa, Asia, and Australia. They have alternate, usually heart-shaped leaves, and are grown for their small, bell- to funnel-shaped, white, blue, or purple flowers, borne singly or in terminal panicles or cymes. Where temperatures drop below 7°C (45°F), grow in a cool or temperate greenhouse. In warmer regions, they are suitable for training over a pergola or arch, or through a shrub.
• **HARDINESS** Frost tender.
• **CULTIVATION** Under glass, grow in loam-based potting compost (JI No.2) in full light. During the growing season, water moderately and apply a balanced liquid fertilizer every 4 weeks; water sparingly in winter, after flowering. Outdoors, grow in fertile, moist but well-drained soil in full sun. Support the climbing stems. Pruning group 11, in early spring.
• **PROPAGATION** Soak seed and sow at 18°C (64°F) in spring. Root greenwood cuttings in early summer, or semi-ripe cuttings with bottom heat in late summer.
• **PESTS AND DISEASES** Prone to red spider mites and whiteflies under glass.

P. paniculata (Bridal bouquet, Snow in the jungle, White corallita). Strong-growing, twining climber bearing slender-pointed, heart-shaped, mid-green leaves, 8–15cm (3–6in) long, smooth above, white-powdery beneath when young. Produces large, terminal panicles, to 30cm (12in) long, of many funnel-shaped, elder-scented white flowers, 8mm (⅜in) across, from summer to early winter. ↕to 9m (28ft). N. India, N. Burma. ⊛ (min. 7°C/45°F)

PORTEA

BROMELIACEAE

Genus of about 7 species of rosette-forming, evergreen, terrestrial perennials (bromeliads) from Brazil, where they usually grow in coastal shrubland and shaded forest, to 600m (2,000ft) high. They are cultivated for their foliage and flowers: the strap-shaped, spiny-margined, fairly stiff leaves are mostly scaly, especially beneath; the tubular, blue or violet flowers are borne in cylindrical heads on long, slender flower-stalks. Where temperatures fall below 15°C (59°F), grow in an indoor garden; in warmer climates, they are suitable for growing outdoors in a desert garden.
• **HARDINESS** Frost tender.
• **CULTIVATION** Under glass, grow in terrestrial bromeliad compost in full light, with shade from hot sun. Water moderately at all times; overwatering often causes root rot. During the

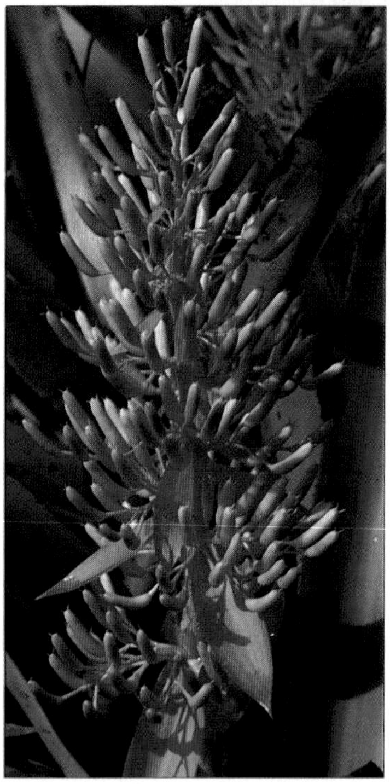
Portea petropolitana

growing season, apply a low-nitrogen fertilizer every 6–8 weeks. Outdoors, grow in humus-rich, leafy, loamy soil in full sun, with some midday shade. See also p.47.
• **PROPAGATION** Sow seed at 19–24°C (66–75°F) in spring or summer. Remove offsets in late spring.
• **PESTS AND DISEASES** Susceptible to beetles when grown outdoors. Scale insects sometimes attack new growth.

P. petropolitana ■ Terrestrial perennial bearing a rosette of strap-shaped, minutely scaly, mid- to dark green leaves, to 80cm (32in) long, with black marginal spines. Large-toothed leaf sheaths have dark brown scales. In summer, the stout, reddish brown scapes produce branched, pendent, compound, cylindrical inflorescences, to 40cm (16in) long, with rose-red bracts. The tubular flowers, to 3cm (1¼in) long, have blue-violet petals and red ovaries. ↕to 1m (3ft), ↔40cm (16in). E. Brazil. ⊛ (min. 15°C/59°F). **var. *extensa*** has more open inflorescences with lilac-blue flowers and purple-tipped green ovaries, borne on arching, coral-red scapes.

▷**Portia tree** see *Thespesia populnea*

PORTULACA

Purslane, Rose moss

PORTULACACEAE

Genus of 100 semi-succulent, mainly erect to trailing annuals, with a few perennials, found in dry, sandy soils in warm-temperate and tropical regions. They have small, fleshy, alternate to sometimes opposite, flat to cylindrical, almost moss-like leaves, which are very variable in colour, often white, green, or red. They are grown for their showy, cup-shaped, rose-like, 4- to 7-petalled, scarlet, carmine, purple, yellow, pink, apricot, or white flowers, which usually have a leafy rosette of foliage below each flowerhead; flowering is best in dry summers. Grow as annuals in a sunny,

P

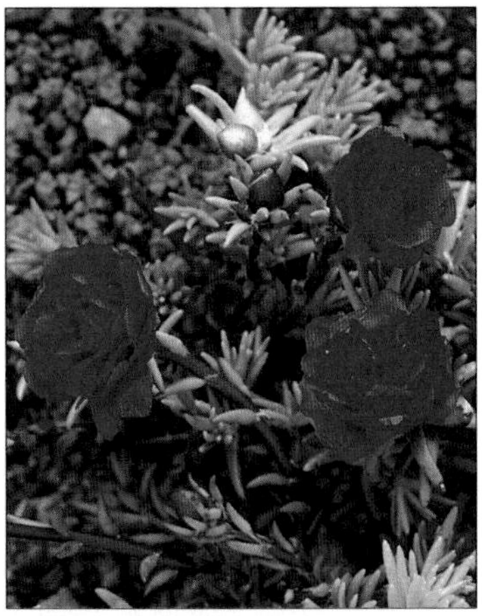

Portulaca grandiflora Sundance Hybrids

dry border or bank, or in a window-box or other container.
• **HARDINESS** Half hardy to frost tender.
• **CULTIVATION** Outdoors, grow in poor, sandy, well-drained soil in full sun.
• **PROPAGATION** Sow seed at 13–18°C (55–64°F) in mid-spring.
• **PESTS AND DISEASES** Prone to aphids. Seedlings are susceptible to damping-off.

P. grandiflora (Rose moss, Sun plant). Spreading, red-stemmed annual with clusters of cylindrical, fleshy, bright green leaves, to 2.5cm (1in) long. In summer, produces single or double, mid- to dark green, satin-textured, rose-pink, red, yellow, or white flowers, to 2.5cm (1in) or more across, sometimes striped and flecked in a contrasting colour. ↕ 10–20cm (4–8in), ↔ 15cm (6in). Brazil, Argentina, Uruguay. ✲. **Minilaca Hybrids** have a neat and compact habit, with large, double flowers, to 5cm (2in) across, in scarlet-red, rose-pink, apricot-pink, creamy yellow, and golden yellow; they are good container plants; ↕ 10–15cm (4–6in). **Sundance Hybrids** ■ are semi-trailing, with large, semi-double or double flowers, to 5cm (2in) across, in a broad range of bright colours; ↕ to 15cm (6in). **Sundial Series** cultivars were bred for longer flowering in poor conditions and cooler climates; they have double flowers in a broad colour range, including an unusual bicolour: white, striped and flecked with lavender-blue.

PORTULACARIA

PORTULACACEAE

Genus of 1–3 species (often considered one variable species) of bushy, perennial, succulent shrubs from semi-arid, hilly lowland in Namibia, South Africa, Swaziland, and Mozambique. Grown mainly for their foliage, they have fleshy stems, leaves, and branches, and inconspicuous, cup- or saucer-shaped flowers in cymes or short racemes. In areas where temperatures fall below 10°C (50°F), grow in a warm greenhouse; in warm, dry climates, use in a shrub border or desert garden.
• **HARDINESS** Frost tender.
• **CULTIVATION** Under glass, grow in loam-based potting compost (JI No.2) with added grit, in full light or bright filtered light. From early spring to early autumn, water freely and apply a low-nitrogen liquid fertilizer every 6–8 weeks; keep almost completely dry at

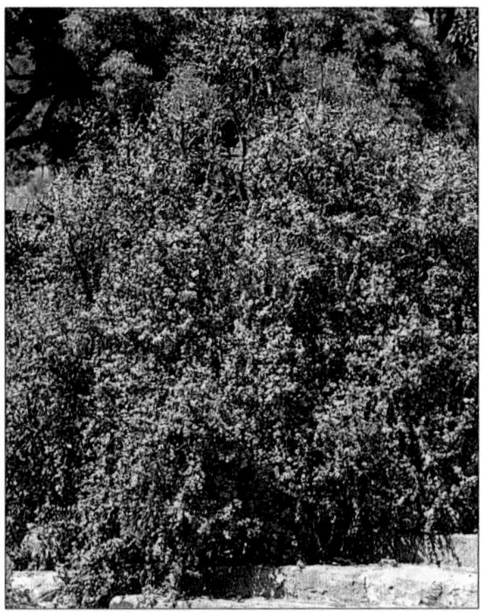

Portulacaria afra 'Foliisvariegatus'

other times. Outdoors, grow in moderately fertile, sharply drained soil in full sun or partial shade. Pruning group 1. See also pp.48–49.
• **PROPAGATION** Root cuttings of stem sections in spring with bottom heat.
• **PESTS AND DISEASES** Susceptible to scale insects.

P. afra. Bushy, succulent shrub with thick, grey-barked stems and jointed, short, twig-like, projecting branches. The obovate, sometimes pointed, opposite, glossy green leaves, to 2cm (¾in) long, are flat above, convex below. Inconspicuous, saucer-shaped, pale pink flowers, 2mm (1/16in) across, are produced in summer. ↕ 2–3m (6–10ft), ↔ 1.5m (5ft). Namibia, South Africa (Northern Cape, Eastern Cape, Northern Transvaal, Eastern Transvaal), Swaziland, Mozambique. ❀ (min. 10°C/50°F). **'Foliisvariegatus'** ■ has yellow-mottled leaves.

POSOQUERIA

RUBIACEAE

Genus of 12–16 species of upright to rounded, evergreen shrubs and trees occurring in habitats from forest to moist ravines in tropical regions of America. They are cultivated for their simple, leathery leaves, produced in opposite pairs, and corymbs of tubular, pendent, salverform, fragrant, white, pink, or red flowers. The flowers each have 5 spreading petal lobes, and are borne in terminal corymbs; they are followed by yellow berries. In areas where temperatures fall below 5–7°C (41–45°F), grow in a cool or temperate greenhouse; elsewhere they are suitable for a shrub border, or as specimens.
• **HARDINESS** Frost tender.
• **CULTIVATION** Under glass, grow in a loam-based potting compost (JI No.2) with added grit, in full light or bright filtered light. From early spring to early autumn, water freely and apply a balanced liquid fertilizer every 6–8 weeks; keep just moist at other times. Outdoors, grow in moderately fertile, sharply drained soil in full sun or partial shade. Pruning group 8; plants under glass need restrictive pruning.
• **PROPAGATION** Take greenwood cuttings in early summer, or semi-ripe cuttings in mid- or late summer.
• **PESTS AND DISEASES** Susceptible to red spider mites, whiteflies, and mealybugs under glass.

P. latifolia ♀ Moderately bushy shrub, or sometimes small, broadly upright tree if unpruned, bearing ovate or oblong to elliptic, prominently veined, rich green leaves, 15–25cm (6–10in) long. In spring, produces dense corymbs of few to many slender-tubed, fragrant white flowers, with long, slender tubes to 15cm (6in) long, 6cm (2½in) across; they are followed by yellow berries, 4–8cm (1½–3in) across. ↕ 2–14m (6–45ft), ↔ 2–6m (6–20ft). Mexico to Brazil, West Indies. ❀ (min. 7°C/45°F)

▷ **Possum haw** see *Ilex decidua, Viburnum acerifolium*

POTAMOGETON

POTAMOGETONACEAE

Genus of 80–100 species of marginal to deep-water aquatic perennials, distributed almost throughout the world, flourishing in freshwater ditches, ponds, canals, and waterways. They are cultivated as oxygenators in water gardens and for their decorative effect in aquariums. The branched, creeping rhizomes spread rapidly in muddy pool bottoms, where they support an interwoven, mat-like network of translucent, linear to lance-shaped submerged leaves, and leathery, opaque, lance-shaped to rounded floating leaves. Inconspicuous flowers are borne in fleshy spikes just above the water.

Grow the hardy species as oxygenators in outdoor pools; *P. crispus* tolerates polluted water better than any other oxygenator, and can also be used in cold-water aquariums. In frost-prone climates, grow tender species in cool-water aquariums; in warmer climates, they are suitable for outdoor pools.
• **HARDINESS** Fully hardy to frost tender.
• **CULTIVATION** In an aquarium, grow in pots of an inert medium in full light. Feed with sachets of proprietary aquarium plant fertilizer. In an outdoor pool, grow in baskets of sandy loam, or root in a muddy pond bottom at a depth of 15–60cm (6–24in), ideally in full sun, or in partial shade. Cut back frequently and thin to keep in check. Submerged leaves may become encrusted with deposits of lime. See also pp.52–53.
• **PROPAGATION** Take cuttings of stem sections in late spring or early summer; the foliage becomes brittle from midsummer onwards.
• **PESTS AND DISEASES** Trouble free.

P. crispus (Curled pondweed). Marginal to deep-water aquatic perennial with cylindrical, branching stems, to 4m (12ft) long, bearing narrowly oblong, almost translucent submerged leaves, about 4cm (1½in) long, wavy-margined when mature, and stalked, pointed, leathery floating leaves. Spikes of inconspicuous, crimson and creamy white flowers, 0.5–1.5cm (¼–½in) across, are produced just above the water surface in summer. ↔ indefinite. Europe, Asia to Australasia. ✲✲✲

▷ **Potato bush, Blue** see *Solanum rantonnetii*
▷ **Potato tree, Chilean** see *Solanum crispum*
▷ **Potato vine** see *Solanum jasminoides, S. wendlandii*

POTENTILLA *syn.* COMARUM

Cinquefoil

ROSACEAE

Genus of about 500 species of shrubs, herbaceous perennials, and a few annuals and biennials, found throughout the N. hemisphere, in habitats ranging from meadows to mountain screes. They are cultivated for their attractive, usually 5-petalled, saucer- to cup-shaped, occasionally star-shaped, white, yellow, orange, pink, or red flowers; they are produced over long periods from spring to autumn, either singly or, more often, in cymes or terminal panicles. The alternate leaves may be pinnate or 3- to 7-palmate, and are often strongly veined and wrinkled. The shrubby potentillas, mainly derived from *P. fruticosa*, are excellent, long-flowering plants for a mixed or shrub border and for low hedges. Many species are also suitable for rock gardens, raised beds, or mixed borders. Most clump-forming hybrids, derived mainly from *P. atrosanguinea* and *P. nepalensis*, are valued for their single, semi-double, or double, mainly red or yellow flowers providing summer and autumn colour in herbaceous borders: they have strawberry-like, 5-palmate, mid- to dark green leaves, 5–10cm (2–4in) long, conspicuously veined and toothed.
• **HARDINESS** Fully hardy.
• **CULTIVATION** Grow in poor to moderately fertile, well-drained soil in full sun. Rock-garden species prefer poor, gritty, sharply drained soil. Pruning group 10 for shrubs, in early or mid-spring.
• **PROPAGATION** Sow seed in containers in a cold frame in autumn or spring. Divide perennials in autumn or spring. Take greenwood cuttings of shrubs in early summer.
• **PESTS AND DISEASES** Trouble free.

P. alba ■ Clump-forming perennial with spreading stems, bearing 5-palmate

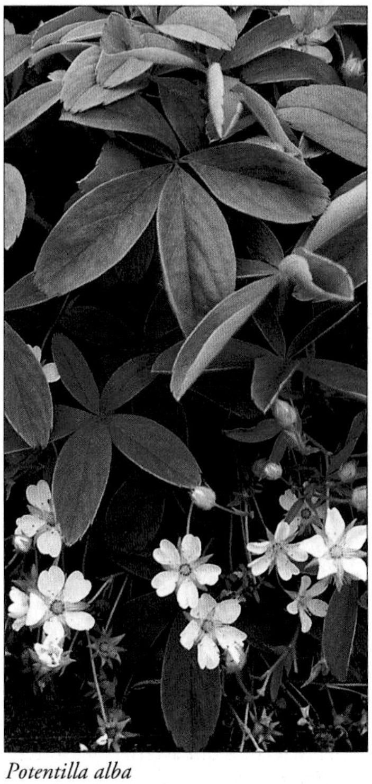

Potentilla alba

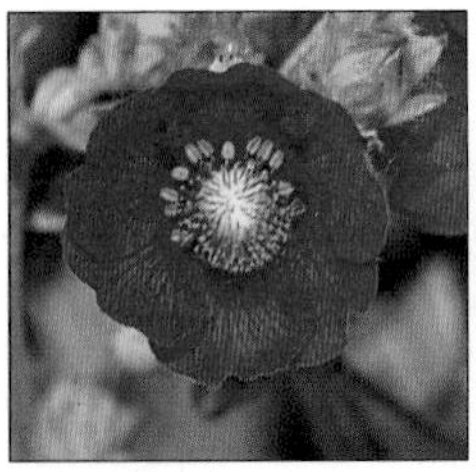
Potentilla atrosanguinea

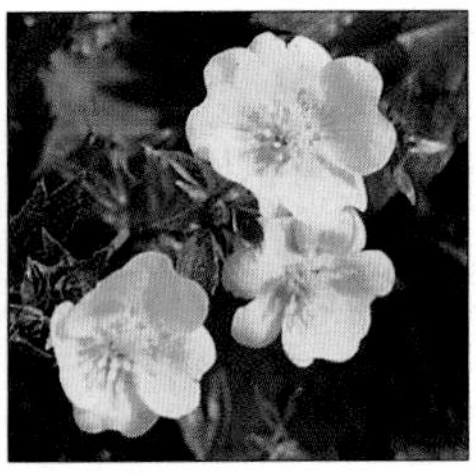
Potentilla aurea

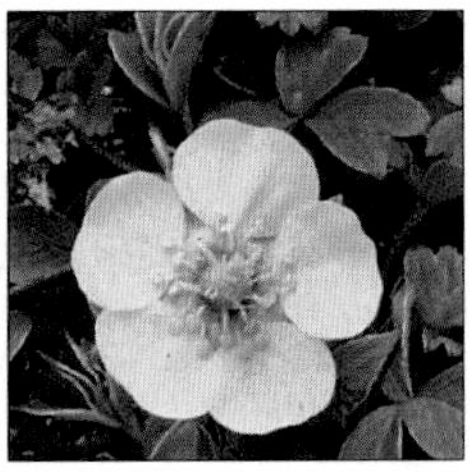
Potentilla eriocarpa

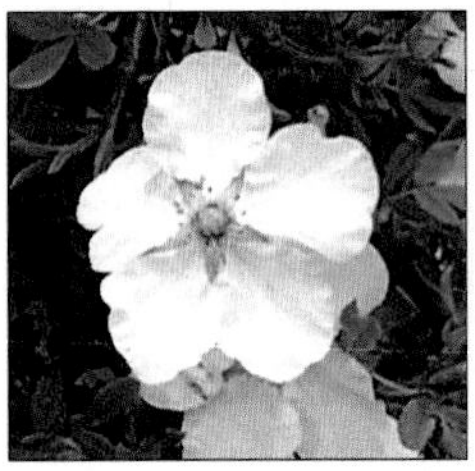
Potentilla fruticosa 'Abbotswood'

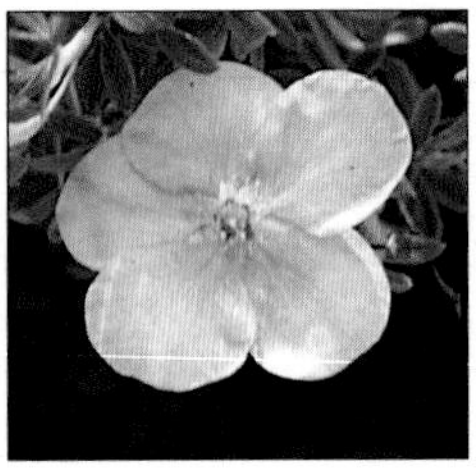
Potentilla fruticosa 'Daydawn'

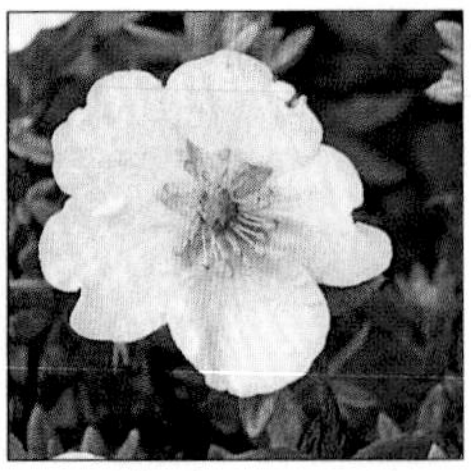
Potentilla fruticosa 'Elizabeth'

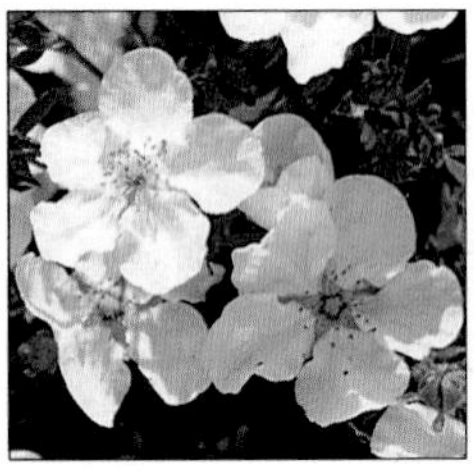
Potentilla fruticosa 'Farrer's White'

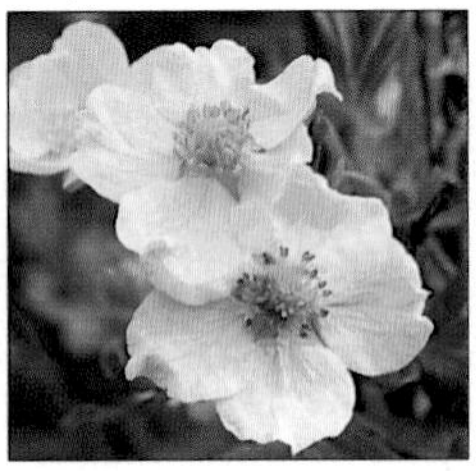
Potentilla fruticosa 'Friedrichsenii'

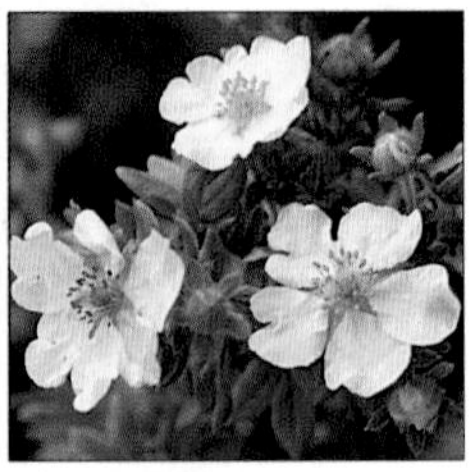
Potentilla fruticosa 'Manchu'

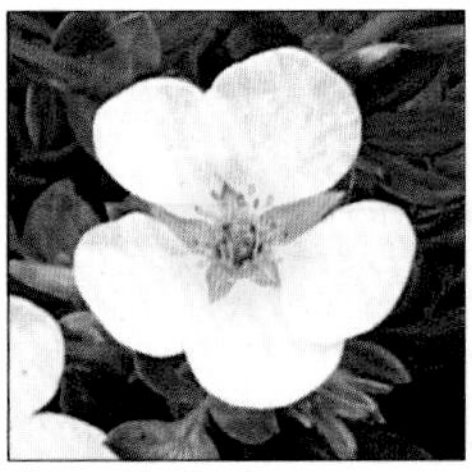
Potentilla fruticosa 'Primrose Beauty'

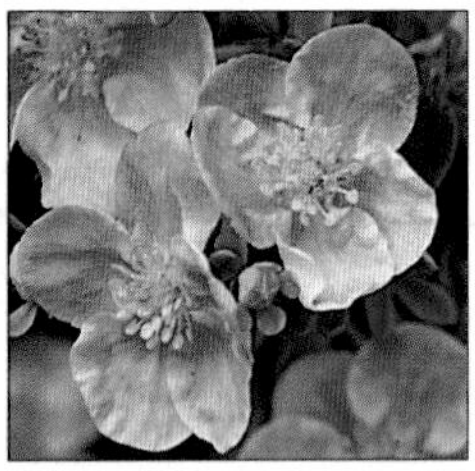
Potentilla fruticosa 'Princess'

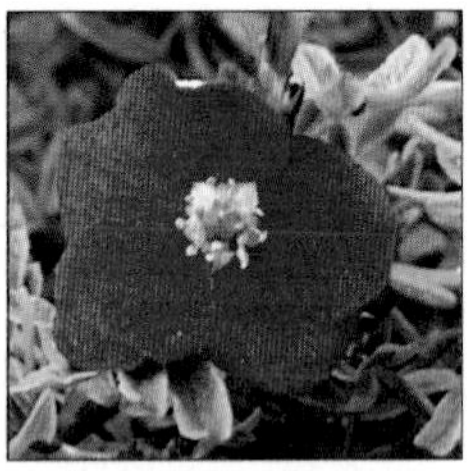
Potentilla fruticosa 'Red Ace'

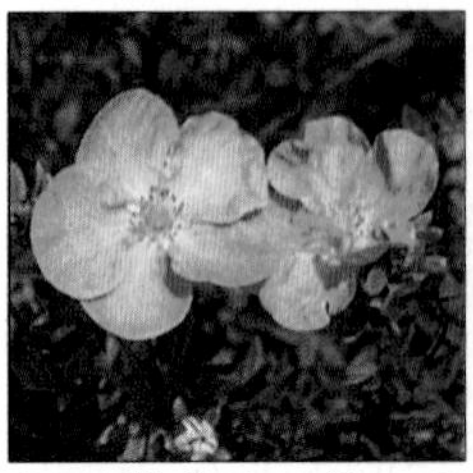
Potentilla fruticosa 'Sunset'

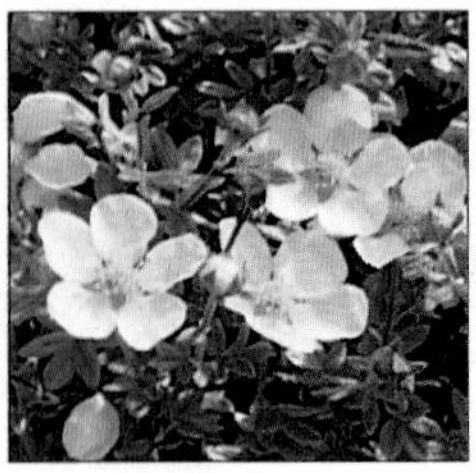
Potentilla fruticosa 'Vilmoriniana'

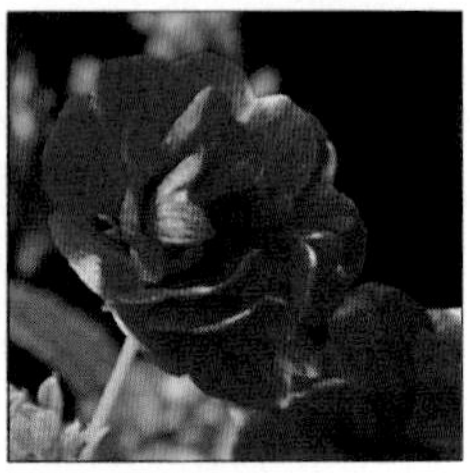
Potentilla 'Gloire de Nancy'

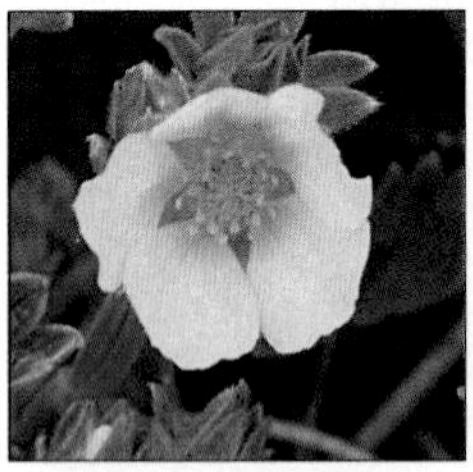
Potentilla megalantha

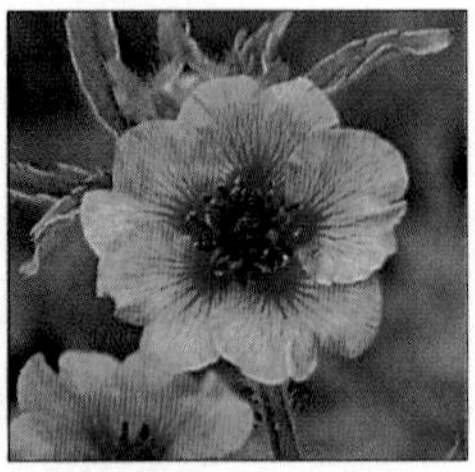
Potentilla nepalensis 'Miss Willmott'

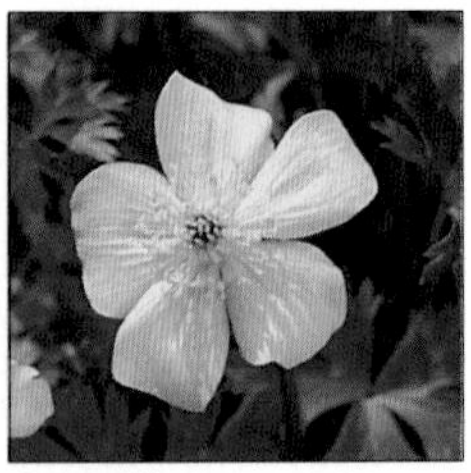
Potentilla neumanniana 'Goldrausch'

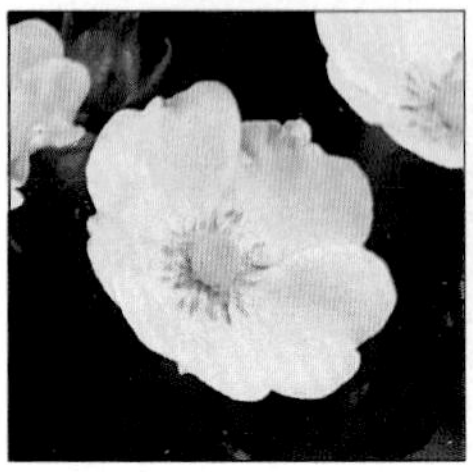
Potentilla recta 'Warrenii'

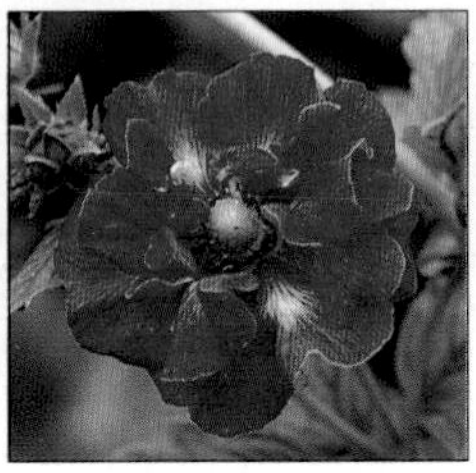
Potentilla 'William Rollison'

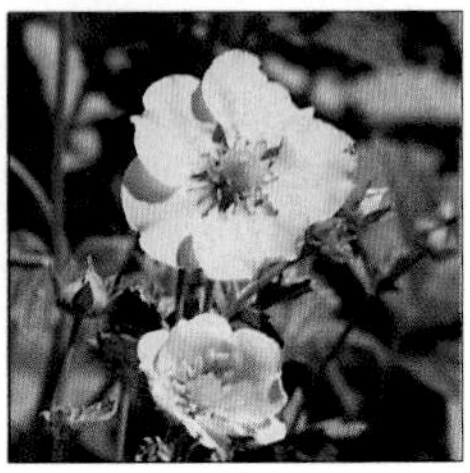
Potentilla 'Yellow Queen'

P

leaves, with oblong to obovate-lance-shaped leaflets, 2–4cm (¾–1½in) long, light green above, silver-silky-hairy beneath. In late spring and early summer, bears loose cymes of flat, saucer-shaped white flowers, 2.5cm (1in) across. ↕ 8cm (3in), ↔ to 30cm (12in). C. and S. Europe. ❄❄❄

P. arbuscula see *P. fruticosa* var. *arbuscula*.

P. atrosanguinea ■ (Himalayan cinquefoil). Clump-forming, hairy perennial bearing 3-palmate, dark green leaves, 5–8cm (2–3in) long, with ovate to elliptic or obovate, toothed leaflets, grey-silky-hairy to densely white-hairy. From summer to autumn, panicle-like cymes of saucer-shaped, yellow, orange, or pale to deep red flowers, 3cm (1¼in) across, are borne on erect, branching, wiry stems. ↕ 45–90cm (18–36in), ↔ 60cm (24in). Himalayas. ❄❄❄. **var. *argyrophylla*** has leaves composed of 3–5 leaflets, and yellow or yellow-orange flowers.

P. aurea ■ Mat-forming perennial with 3- or 5-palmate, glossy, mid-green leaves, to 3cm (1¼in) long, composed of oblong leaflets with sharply toothed, silver-hairy margins. Produces cymes of flat, saucer-shaped, deep golden yellow flowers, 2cm (¾in) across, with overlapping petals, from late spring to summer. ↕ 10cm (4in), ↔ 20cm (8in). Pyrenees, Alps. ❄❄❄

***P. davurica* var. *mandschurica* of gardens** see *P. fruticosa* 'Manchu'.

***P. davurica* 'Veitchii'** see *P. fruticosa* var. *veitchii*.

P. erecta, syn. *P. tormentilla* (Tormentil). Low-growing perennial with trailing, non-rooting stems and usually 3-palmate, rarely 4- or 5-palmate leaves consisting of wedge- to lance-shaped, toothed leaflets, to 2cm (¾in) long, dark green above, silver-silky-hairy beneath. Loose, terminal cymes of slender-stemmed, 4-petalled, saucer-shaped yellow flowers, to 1cm (½in) across, are borne from late spring to summer. Suitable for a wildflower garden. ↕ 10–30cm (4–12in), ↔ to 60cm (24in). Europe, Asia. ❄❄❄

P. eriocarpa ■ Carpet-forming perennial with 3-palmate, bright green leaves, to 3cm (1¼in) long, composed of wedge-shaped, toothed leaflets. Solitary or clustered, short-stalked, cup-shaped, deep yellow flowers, to 4cm (1½in) across, are produced in early summer. ↕ 8cm (3in), ↔ 30cm (12in). Pakistan to China, Himalayas. ❄❄❄

***P.* 'Etna'.** Clump-forming perennial with silver-tinted, deep green leaves, and panicles of semi-double, deep velvety red flowers, 2.5–3cm (1–1¼in) across, with yellow margins, borne in midsummer. ↕ to 45cm (18in), ↔ 60cm (24in). ❄❄❄

***P.* 'Flamenco'.** Clump-forming perennial with deep green leaves, and panicles of single, bright scarlet flowers, 2.5–3cm (1–1¼in) across, borne from late spring to midsummer. ↕ to 45cm (18in), ↔ 60cm (24in). ❄❄❄

P. fragiformis see *P. megalantha*.

P. fruticosa*.** Compact, bushy, deciduous shrub with pinnate leaves, to 4cm (1½in) long, composed of usually 5 or 7 narrowly oblong, dark green leaflets. Saucer-shaped yellow flowers, to 4cm (1½in) across, are borne singly or in cymes of 3 over a long period from late spring to mid-autumn. ↕ 1m (3ft), ↔ 1.5m (5ft). Europe, N. Asia, North America. ❄❄❄. **'Abbotswood'** ■ ♀ has white flowers and dark blue-green leaves; ↕ 75cm (30in), ↔ 1.2m (4ft). **var. *arbuscula, syn. *P. arbuscula*, has grey-green to silvery grey foliage and golden yellow flowers, 4.5cm (1¾in) across; ↔ 1.2m (4ft); Himalayas, China. **'Beesii'** ♀ syn. 'Nana Argentea', is slow-growing and compact, with silver-silky-hairy leaves and golden yellow flowers, 2cm (¾in) across; ↕ 60cm (24in), ↔ 1.2m (4ft). **'Blink'** see 'Princess'. **'Coronation Triumph'** bears profuse bright yellow flowers. **'Daydawn'** ■ ♀ has creamy yellow flowers that are flushed orange-pink; ↔ 1.2m (4ft). **'Elizabeth'** ■ ♀ bears bright yellow flowers, to 4.5cm (1¾in) across. **'Farrer's White'** ■ bears profuse white flowers, 2.5cm (1in) across. **'Friedrichsenii'** ■ is vigorous and upright, with grey-green leaves and pale yellow flowers, 3cm (1¼in) across; ↕ 1.5m (5ft), ↔ 1.2m (4ft). **'Gold Drop'**, syn. 'Goldkugel', *P. parvifolia* 'Gold Drop', is upright, with profuse golden flowers, 2.5cm (1in) across; ↕↔ 1.2m (4ft). **'Goldfinger'** ♀ has large, rich yellow flowers, to 5cm (2in) across. **'Goldkugel'** see 'Gold Drop'. **'Jackman's Variety'** has bright yellow flowers, 3–4cm (1¼–1½in) across. **'Katherine Dykes'** ♀ has profusely borne, canary-yellow flowers. **'Klondike'** ♀ produces bright green leaves and bright yellow flowers. **'Longacre'** ♀ is low-growing and spreading, with bright yellow flowers, to 4cm (1½in) or more across; ↕ 60cm (24in). **'Maanelys'** ♀ syn. 'Moonlight', *P.* 'Manelys', has soft yellow flowers, 3cm (1¼in) across, and grey-green foliage; ↕ 1.2m (4ft), ↔ 2m (6ft). **'Manchu'** ■ syn. *P. davurica* var. *mandschurica* of gardens, is dwarf and mound-forming, with dark pink shoots, silvery grey, silky-hairy leaves, and white flowers, 2.5cm (1in) across; ↕ 30cm (12in), ↔ 75cm (30in). **'Moonlight'** see 'Maanelys'. **'Nana Argentea'** see 'Beesii'. **'Pretty Polly'** has pale pink flowers, 2cm (¾in) across; ↕ 50cm (20in), ↔ 75cm (30in). **'Primrose Beauty'** ■ ♀ has grey-green leaves and pale primrose-yellow flowers, 3.5cm (1½in) across. **'Princess'** ■ syn. 'Blink', is low-growing, with pale pink flowers, 2.5cm (1in) across, fading to white in full sun; ↕ 60cm (24in), ↔ 1m (3ft). **'Red Ace'** ■ has bright vermilion flowers, yellow on the backs of the petals, fading in full sun. **'Royal Flush'** has rich pink flowers with yellow centres, fading to white in full sun; ↕ 45cm (18in), ↔ 75cm (30in). **'Snowbird'** has double white flowers. **'Sunset'** ■ has dark orange flowers, 3cm (1¼in) across, fading in full sun; ↔ 1m (3ft). **'Tangerine'** ♀ has yellow flowers, 3cm (1¼in) across, flushed pale orange-red; ↔ 1m (3ft). **'Tilford Cream'** ♀ is dense and spreading, with creamy white flowers, 3.5cm (1½in) across; ↕ 60cm (24in), ↔ 1m (3ft). **var. *veitchii***, syn. *P. davurica* 'Veitchii', has white flowers, 2.5cm (1in) across. **'Vilmoriniana'** ■ is upright, with silvery grey leaves and creamy white flowers, 4cm (1½in) across; ↕ 1.2m (4ft), ↔ 1m (3ft). **'Yellow Gem'** has a low and spreading habit, producing grey foliage

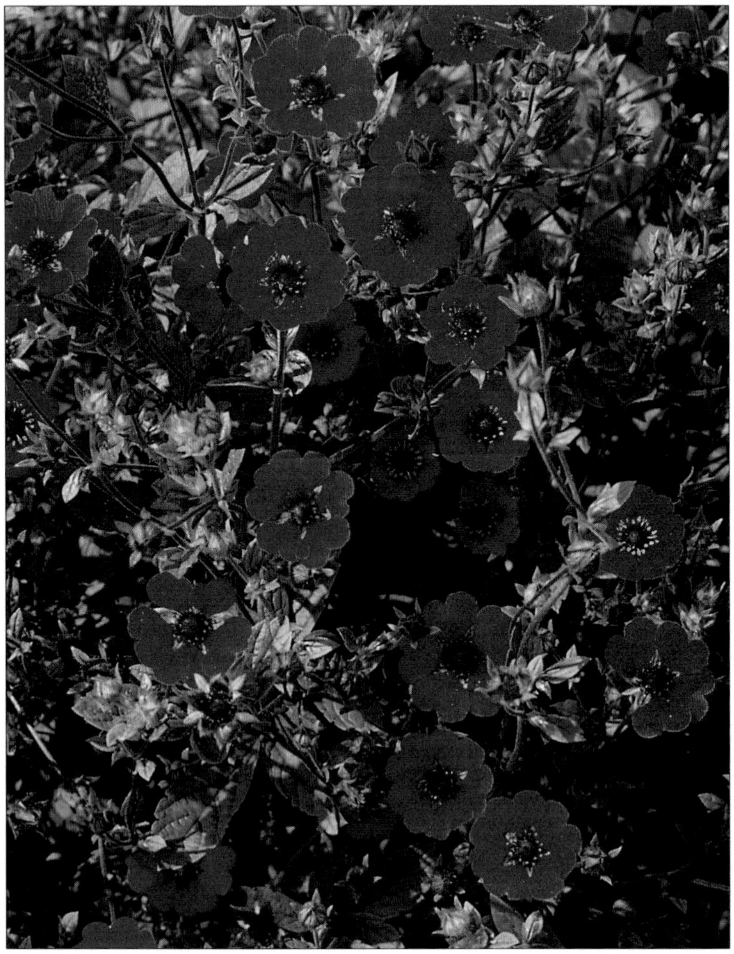

Potentilla 'Gibson's Scarlet'

and ruffled, bright yellow flowers; ↕ 60cm (24in), ↔ 1.2m (4ft).

***P.* 'Gibson's Scarlet'** ■ ♀ Clump-forming perennial with soft green leaves and raceme-like cymes of single, very bright scarlet flowers, 3cm (1¼in) across, from early to late summer. ↕ to 45cm (18in), ↔ 60cm (24in). ***

***P.* 'Gloire de Nancy'** ■ syn. *P.* 'Glory of Nancy'. Clump-forming perennial with dark green leaves, and racemes of double, reddish orange flowers, 2.5–3cm (1–1¼in) across, from early to late summer. ↕ to 45cm (18in), ↔ 60cm (24in). ***

***P.* 'Glory of Nancy'** see *P.* 'Gloire de Nancy'.

***P.* 'Manelys'** see *P. fruticosa* 'Maanelys'.

P. megalantha ■ ♀ syn. *P. fragiformis.* Compact, clump-forming perennial producing 3-palmate leaves, to 8cm (3in) long, with broadly elliptic to obovate, coarsely scalloped leaflets, mid-green and slightly hairy above, grey-green and more hairy beneath. Erect cymes of 3–7 saucer-shaped yellow flowers, 3–4cm (1¼–1½in) across, are produced in mid- and late summer. ↕ 15–30cm (6–12in), ↔ 15cm (6in). E. Asia, Japan. ***

***P.* 'Monsieur Rouillard'.** Clump-forming perennial with mid- to deep green leaves and raceme-like cymes of double, yellow-marked, deep blood-red flowers, 3cm (1¼in) across, borne from early to late summer. ↕ to 45cm (18in), ↔ 60cm (24in). ***

P. nepalensis. Loose, clump-forming perennial with numerous branching, red-tinged, wiry stems bearing 5-palmate, mid-green leaves, 8–10cm (3–4in) long, composed of large, obovate or elliptic, coarsely toothed, hairy leaflets. Throughout summer, bears loose cymes of saucer-shaped, dark crimson flowers, 2.5cm (1in) across, on long leaf-stalks. ↕ 30–90cm (12–36in), ↔ 60cm (24in). W. Himalayas. ***. **'Miss Willmott'** ■ ♀ has cherry-pink flowers suffused yellow, with darker pink centres; ↕ 30–45cm (12–18in). **'Roxana'** has copper-pink flowers with cherry-red centres; ↕ to 45cm (18in).

P. neumanniana, syn. *P. tabernaemontani, P. verna.* Procumbent, mat-forming perennial, similar to *P. eriocarpa*, with 5- or 7-palmate leaves, to 4cm (1½in) long, comprising inversely lance-shaped to obovate, toothed, mid-green leaflets. Bears loose cymes of up to 12 saucer-shaped yellow flowers, to 2.5cm (1in) across, over long periods from spring onwards. ↕ to 10cm (4in), ↔ 30cm (12in). Europe. ***. **'Goldrausch'** ■ produces loose cymes of up to 10 bright golden yellow flowers from spring to early summer; ↕ 10cm (4in), ↔ 20cm (8in). **'Nana'** is more compact; ↕ 8cm (3in), ↔ 15cm (6in).

P. nitida. Densely tufted perennial with palmate, silver-hairy leaves, to 1.5cm (½in) long, comprising 3, rarely 4 or 5, inversely lance-shaped to obovate leaflets. In summer, bears solitary or paired, short-stemmed, saucer-shaped, deep pink, rarely white flowers, 2.5cm (1in) or more across. Attractive alpine for a scree bed; not always free-flowering. ↕ to 10cm (4in), ↔ 15cm (6in). S.W. and S.E. Alps, Apennines. ***

P. palustris, syn. *Comarum palustre* (Marsh cinquefoil). Rhizomatous, woody-based perennial with upright, decumbent stems and pinnate leaves, 3–7cm (1¼–3in) long, composed of 5–7 toothed, oblong, grey-green leaflets, to 6cm (2½in) long. Produces lax cymes of bowl-shaped, purple to maroon flowers, to 3cm (1¼in) across, in early summer. Suitable for the margins of a wildlife pond. ↕ to 50cm (20in), ↔ to 80cm (32in) or more. Europe, W. Asia, North America. ***

***P. parvifolia* 'Gold Drop'** see *P. fruticosa* 'Gold Drop'.

P. recta. Erect, clump-forming, hairy perennial producing 5- or 7-palmate leaves, 10cm (4in) long, with oblong to obovate, toothed, grey-green to mid-green leaflets. Flat cymes of saucer-shaped, pale yellow flowers, to 2.5cm (1in) across, are produced from early to late summer. ↕ 60cm (24in), ↔ 45cm (18in). Europe, Caucasus, Russia (Siberia). ***. **'Citrina'** see var. *pallida.* **'Macrantha'** see 'Warrenii'. **var. *pallida*** ♀ syn. 'Citrina', var. *sulphurea*, produces pale yellow to cream flowers; ↕ 45cm (18in). **var. *sulphurea*** see *var. pallida.* **'Warrenii'** ■ syn. 'Macrantha', produces loose cymes of bright canary-yellow flowers.

P. tabernaemontani see *P. neumanniana.*

P.* x *tonguei ♀ (*P. anglica* x *P. nepalensis*). Clump-forming perennial with long, spreading stems bearing 3- or 5-palmate, dark green leaves, to 5cm (2in) long, composed of obovate leaflets. Over long periods in summer, produces solitary or loose, few-flowered cymes of rather flat, bowl-shaped, apricot-yellow flowers, 1.5cm (½in) across, with deep carmine-red eyes, . ↕ 10cm (4in), ↔ to 30cm (12in). Garden origin. ***

P. tormentilla see *P. erecta.*

P. verna see *P. neumanniana.*

***P.* 'William Rollison'** ■ ♀ Clump-forming perennial with mid-green leaves and raceme-like cymes of semi-double, yellow- or red-orange flowers, 2.5–3cm (1–1¼in) across, with yellow centres and petal backs, from early to late summer. ↕ to 45cm (18in), ↔ 60cm (24in). ***

***P.* 'Yellow Queen'** ■ Clump-forming perennial with mid-green leaves and raceme-like cymes of double or semi-double, pure yellow flowers, 2.5–3cm (1–1¼in) across, from early to late summer. ↕ 30–45cm (12–18in), ↔ 60cm (24in). ***

▷ ***Pothos celatocaulis*** see *Rhaphidophora celatocaulis*

▷ **Pothos, Golden** see *Epipremnum aureum*

x POTINARA

ORCHIDACEAE

Quadrigeneric hybrid genus of evergreen orchids derived from crosses between *Brassavola, Cattleya, Laelia*, and *Sophronitis.* They are vegetatively similar to the 4 parent genera, which are loosely referred to as "cattleyas", and have stout to slender pseudobulbs and 1 or 2 mostly broadly oblong, semi-rigid, leathery leaves. The short racemes of flowers, with usually strong and clear colours, often yellow or red, are borne at the bases of the leaves, with or without sheaths.

- **HARDINESS** Frost tender.

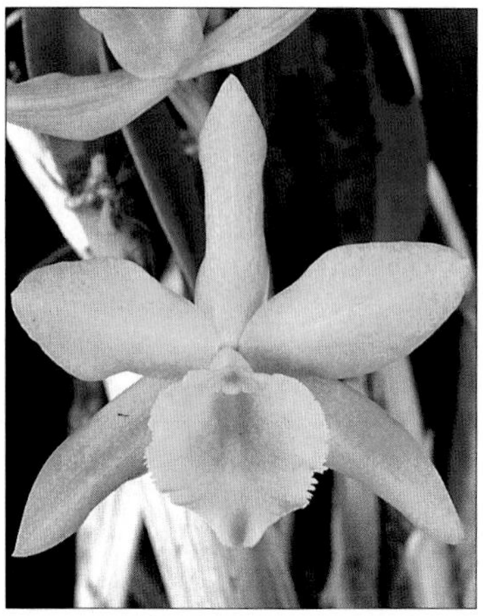

x *Potinara* Cherub 'Spring Daffodil'

- **CULTIVATION** Cool-growing orchids. Grow in pots of epiphytic orchid compost made with coarse bark. When in growth, provide high humidity and bright filtered light, water freely, and feed at every third watering. In winter, admit full light and water sparingly. See also p.46.
- **PROPAGATION** Divide or remove backbulbs in spring.
- **PESTS AND DISEASES** Scale insects, red spider mites, aphids, and mealybugs may be troublesome.

x *P.* Cherub 'Spring Daffodil' ■ (*Cattleya aurantiaca* x *Lowiara* Trinket). Epiphytic orchid with elongated pseudobulbs and semi-rigid, broadly oval leaves, 10cm (4in) long. Clear yellow flowers, 5cm (2in) across, are produced in short racemes in spring. ↕ 15cm (6in), ↔ 20cm (8in). ⌂ (min. 13°C/55°F; max. 30°C/86°F)

▷ **Pouch flower** see *Calceolaria*

▷ **Poui,**
Pink see *Tabebuia rosea*
Yellow see *Tabebuia serratifolia*

▷ **Powder-puff tree** see *Calliandra*

▷ **Prairie cone flower** see *Ratibida*

▷ **Prairie star** see *Lithophragma parviflora*

PRATIA

CAMPANULACEAE

Genus of about 20 species of prostrate, spreading, freely rooting, evergreen perennials, mostly from damp, shady habitats in Africa, Asia, Australia, New Zealand, and South America. They produce alternate, usually stalkless, often toothed, ovate to rounded leaves, and are grown for their mass of solitary, 2-lipped, star-shaped, usually white or blue-purple flowers. Good ground cover in damp soil, they are also suitable for a rock garden or paving crevice, but can be invasive. In areas prone to prolonged or severe frosts, grow frost-hardy species in an alpine house.

- **HARDINESS** Fully hardy to frost hardy.
- **CULTIVATION** Grow in fertile, loamy, reliably moist soil in partial or deep shade; *P. pedunculata* tolerates drier soils. In an alpine house, use a mix of equal parts loam, leaf mould, and grit.
- **PROPAGATION** Divide at any time of year. Keep divisions moist until well-established.
- **PESTS AND DISEASES** Prone to slugs and snails, and to aphids under glass.

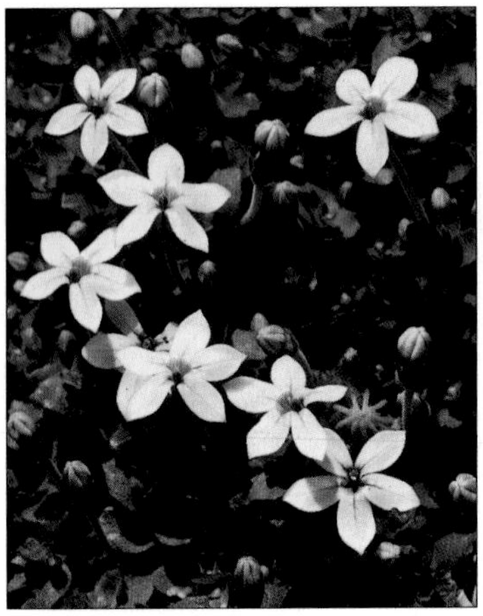

Pratia pedunculata

P. angulata, syn. *Lobelia angulata*. Mat-forming, evergreen perennial with red-tinted stems that spread and root down freely. The broadly ovate to rounded, coarsely toothed leaves are very variable in size, but usually 5–10mm (¼–½in) long. In late spring and early summer, bears short-stalked, axillary, star-shaped, sometimes purple-streaked white flowers, to 1cm (½in) across; they are followed by spherical, red-purple, fleshy fruit, 4mm (⅛in) across. Moderately invasive in moist conditions. ↕ 5cm (2in), ↔ 30–60cm (12–24in). Malaysia, Indonesia, New Zealand. ❄❄❄. **'Treadwellii'**, syn. *P. treadwellii*, is larger in all its parts, and may be very invasive; ↕ 6cm (2½in), ↔ 1m (3ft).
P. pedunculata ◼ syn. *Lobelia pedunculata*. Ground-hugging perennial with ovate to rounded leaves, to 9mm (⅜in) long. Short-stalked, star-shaped, pale blue flowers, to 7mm (¼in) across, are borne over long periods in summer. Invasive, even in dry conditions, but not too rampant. ↕ 1.5cm (½in), ↔ indefinite. Australia. ❄❄❄
P. perpusilla, syn. *Lobelia perpusilla*. Mat-forming perennial bearing tiny, obovate leaves, 3–5mm (⅛–¼in) long, with deeply toothed margins. During summer, bears short-stalked, star-shaped white flowers, 6–10mm (¼–½in) across, with recurving lobes. ↕ to 2cm (¾in), ↔ indefinite. ❄❄. **'Fragrant Carpet'** produces fragrant flowers.
P. treadwellii see *P. angulata* 'Treadwellii'.

▷**Prayer plant** see *Maranta leuconeura*
▷**Prickle ear** see *Acanthostachys*
▷**Prickly Moses** see *Acacia verticillata*
Western see *A. pulchella*
▷**Prickly pear** see *Opuntia ficus-indica*
▷**Pride of Bolivia** see *Tipuana tipu*
▷**Pride of Burma** see *Amherstia nobilis*
▷**Pride of India** see *Koelreuteria paniculata, Lagerstroemia speciosa, Melia azedarach*
▷**Pride of Madeira** see *Echium candicans*
▷**Primavera** see *Cybistax donnell-smithii*
▷**Primrose** see *Primula, P. vulgaris*
Cape see *Streptocarpus*
Desert evening see *Oenothera deltoides*
Evening see *Oenothera, O. biennis*
Fairy see *Primula malacoides*
Japanese see *Primula japonica*

PRIMULA

Primrose

PRIMULACEAE

Genus of about 400 species of mainly herbaceous perennials, some woody-based and evergreen. Occurring in a wide range of habitats from bogs and marshland to alpine areas, they are widely distributed throughout the N. hemisphere, with almost half the species from the Himalayas; a few are also found in the S. hemisphere. They have linear to broadly ovate to obovate, pale to dark green leaves in basal rosettes, and attractive, often salverform, sometimes tubular, bell-shaped or funnel-shaped flowers, with usually spreading petals joined at the bases into tubes. The solitary flowers may be clustered together among the leaves, or borne on slender to stout flower-stalks in umbels, whorls, or racemes. In some primulas, the leaves, flower stems, and calyces may be covered with a white or yellow, waxy meal, or "farina". Primulas can be used for most garden sites, from bog and waterside plantings to borders, rock gardens, and bedding; they can also be grown in an alpine house. A few tender species are grown as cool or temperate greenhouse container plants, or as houseplants.

Primula is a complex genus, divided into many different botanical sections. In gardens, however, only the following 3 major groupings are recognised; they apply to many, but not all primulas.

Auricula primulas
Evergreen primulas, developed from hybrids between *P. auricula* and *P. hirsuta*. They bear umbels of several, usually large, flat-faced, salverform flowers above smooth, leathery, often white-mealy foliage. There are 3 main subgroups: alpine, show, and border.
Alpine Auricula Group – These have the colour of the flower centres in sharp contrast to that of the petals. They may be classed as either light-centred (white or pale in the centres) or gold-centred (yellow or gold in the centres). There is no meal on either leaves or flowers. Grow in an alpine house or rock garden.
Show Auricula Group – These have a distinct circle of white meal, or "paste", in the centre of each flower. They may be described as self-coloured (one colour from the central paste to the petal margins), edged (the paste surrounded by black, feathering out to a green, grey, or white margin), or fancy (the paste surrounded by a colour other than black, with a green, grey, or white margin). Grow in an alpine house.
Border Auricula Group – These are generally robust, garden Auriculas, sometimes white-mealy, and often very fragrant. Grow in a mixed or herbaceous border; excellent for cottage gardens.

Candelabra primulas
Robust herbaceous perennials with several whorls of flowers arranged in tiers up tall, sturdy stems. They are deciduous, dying back to basal buds, or semi-evergreen, dying back to reduced rosettes. Grow in moist shade or woodland; they are seen at their best in groups by streams or in bog gardens.

Primrose-Polyanthus primulas
A very diverse grouping of evergreen, semi-evergreen, or deciduous, winter- to spring-flowering perennial hybrids derived from *P. amoena, P. elatior, P. juliae, P. veris*, and *P. vulgaris*. They have rosettes of broadly ovate to obovate leaves, and mainly large, salverform flowers borne in fascicles (bunched clusters) or umbels, sometimes with both types of inflorescence on the same plant. They occur in a wide range of colours, and are grown as biennials for bedding or containers, as greenhouse container plants, or as perennials for rock gardens, and herbaceous and mixed borders. They are divided into 2 main groups, although interbreeding blurs the distinction between the two.
Primrose Group – Mainly grown as herbaceous perennials, and similar in habit to the 2 main parents, *P. vulgaris* and *P. juliae*. Most produce solitary flowers clustered among the basal rosettes, although a few may have both solitary and umbel-like inflorescences. They are either spring-flowering, if grown without protection, or winter- to spring-flowering, if grown as biennial, greenhouse container plants.
Polyanthus Group – Perennials, usually grown as biennials from summer-sown seed and planted out in autumn to flower through winter and the following spring, or grown under glass as winter- and spring-flowering container plants. A few cultivars are grown as spring-flowering herbaceous perennials; they are propagated by division in autumn, or in spring immediately after flowering. Distinguished from Primrose Group primulas by their long-stalked umbels.

PRIMULA GROUPINGS

The genus *Primula* is classified into many botanical sections. In gardens, however, the 3 informal groupings shown here are the most commonly recognized.

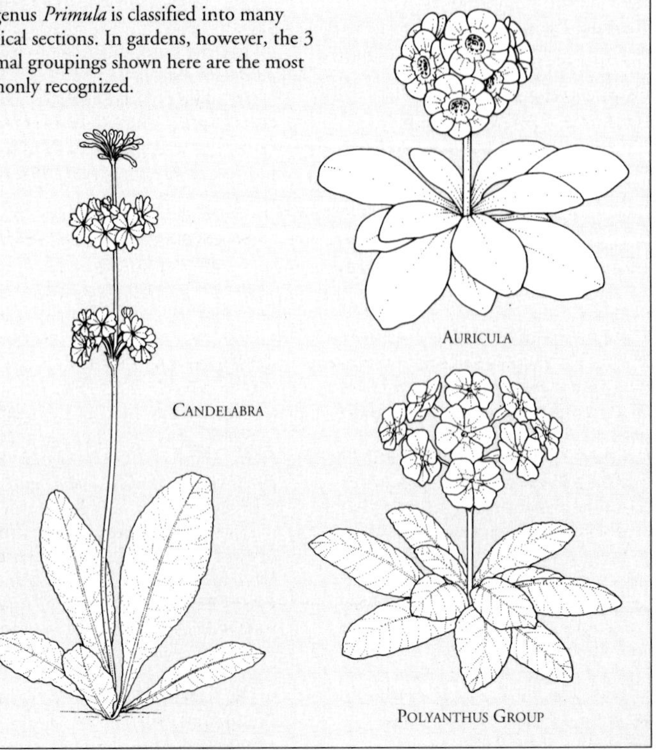

• **HARDINESS** Fully hardy to frost tender.
• **CULTIVATION** For ease of reference, cultivation requirements have been set out in groups, as follows:
1. Full sun or partial shade, in moderately fertile, moist but well-drained, humus-rich soil.
2. Partial shade, in deep, humus-rich, moist, neutral to acid loam soil, or peaty soil. Tolerates full sun if soil remains moist at all times.
3. Deep or partial shade in peaty, gritty, moist but sharply drained acid soil. Protect from excessive winter wet.
4. Under glass in an alpine house or frame. Use a mix of equal parts loam-based potting compost (JI No. 2), leaf mould or peat, and grit. Avoid wetting the foliage of mealy species and hybrids.
5. Full sun with some midday shade, or partial shade, in moist but sharply drained, gritty, humus-rich, slightly alkaline soil.
6. In a cool or temperate greenhouse, or as a houseplant. Use a mix of 4 parts loam-based potting compost (JI No.2) and 1 part each grit and leaf mould (or peat), in bright filtered light. In growth, water freely and apply a half-strength balanced liquid fertilizer every week.
• **PROPAGATION** Surface-sow seed of half-hardy and frost-tender species in early spring. Sow seed of hardy species in containers in an open frame, as soon as ripe or in late winter or early spring. Divide between autumn and early spring. Root basal cuttings or offsets in autumn or early spring. Take root cuttings when dormant in winter.
• **PESTS AND DISEASES** Prone to aphids, red spider mites, leafhoppers, vine weevil, slugs, viruses, primula brown core, and grey mould (*Botrytis*).

P. 'Adrian' ◼ Alpine Auricula primula with oval to rounded, mid-green leaves, to 10cm (4in) long. In spring, produces salverform, light-centred flowers, 3cm (1¼in) across, with purple-blue petals, paler at the margins. Cultivation group 1 or 4. ↕↔ 10cm (4in). ❄❄❄
P. 'Alice Haysom'. Self-coloured show Auricula primula with oval to rounded, mid-green leaves, to 10cm (4in) long. In spring, bears salverform flowers, 3cm

P

(1¼in) across, with cardinal-red petals and golden yellow tubes. Cultivation group 4. ↕↔ 10cm (4in). ❄❄❄

P. allionii ▣ Rosette-forming, evergreen perennial with entire, sometimes scalloped or finely toothed, glandular-hairy, inversely lance-shaped, grey-green leaves, to 5cm (2in) long. In late winter and spring, produces 1- to 5-flowered umbels of salverform flowers, each to 3cm (1¼in) across, varying from white to pink to reddish purple. Each corolla has a flat face and a white eye. Cultivation group 4 (lime-loving). ↕ 7–10cm (3–4in), ↔ to 20cm (8in). Cliffs in S. France and N. Italy. ❄❄❄. There are many named cultivars. **'Snowflake'** is vigorous, with large white flowers, 2.5cm (1in) across, sometimes flushed pink at the margins.

P. alpicola ▣ Rosette-forming, deciduous perennial with elliptic, toothed or scalloped, mid-green leaves, to 10cm (4in) long. In summer, white-mealy stems produce umbels of 6–12 pendent, tubular to funnel-shaped, fragrant, white, yellow, or violet flowers, 1–2.5cm (½–1in) across, with white-mealy eyes. Cultivation group 2. ↕ 50cm (20in), ↔ 30cm (12in). Moist alpine areas in S.E. Tibet. ❄❄❄

P. amoena, syn. *P. elatior* subsp. *meyeri*. Rosette-forming, deciduous perennial with elliptic to spoon-shaped, scalloped or finely toothed leaves, to 17cm (7in) long, bright green above, usually densely hairy beneath. In early spring, hairy stems bear usually one-sided umbels of 6–10 flat to shallowly tubular to funnel-shaped, red-purple, violet-blue, or occasionally white flowers, 2.5cm (1in) across, with yellow eyes. Cultivation group 2 or 4. ↕↔ 15cm (6in). Peaty banks and rocky hillsides in Caucasus and N.E. Turkey. ❄❄❄

P. anisodora, syn. *P. wilsonii* var. *anisodora*. Rosette-forming, semi-evergreen Candelabra primula with obovate, finely toothed, aniseed-scented, mid-green leaves, to 25cm (10in) long. Stout stems produce 3–5 whorls of 8–10 pendent, tubular to bell-shaped, green-eyed, brown-purple flowers, 1.5cm (½in) across, in summer. Cultivation group 2. ↕↔ 60cm (24in). Wet meadows in S.W. China. ❄❄❄

***P.* 'Argus'** ▣ syn. *P.* 'Kingcup'. Very vigorous alpine Auricula primula with oval to rounded, mid-green leaves, to 12cm (5in) long. In spring, produces salverform flowers, to 3cm (1¼in) across, with almost white centres, and

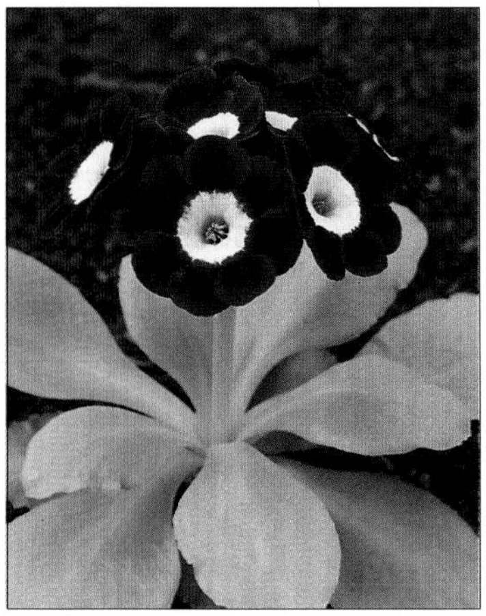

Primula 'Argus'

petals shading from plum-red to beetroot-red. Cultivation group 1 or 4. ↕↔ 10cm (4in). ❄❄❄

P. aurantiaca. Small, rosette-forming, deciduous Candelabra primula with inversely lance-shaped to obovate, finely toothed, dark green leaves, to 20cm (8in) long, with red-purple midribs. In summer, red-tinged stems produce 2–6 whorls of 6–12 salverform, brilliant red-orange flowers, 1.5cm (½in) across. Cultivation group 2. ↕ 30cm (12in), ↔ 40cm (16in). Moist, shaded sites in S.W. China. ❄❄❄

P. aureata ▣ Rosette-forming, evergreen perennial with spoon-shaped to oblong, toothed, white-mealy, mid-green leaves, to 8cm (3in) long. In spring, very short stems, hidden within the foliage, produce umbels of 2–10 salverform, cream to yellow flowers, 3–4cm (1¼–1½in) across, with large, darker yellow eyes. Cultivation group 3 or 4. ↕ 15cm (6in), ↔ 20cm (8in). Moist cliffs and rocky hillsides in Nepal. ❄❄

P. auricula 🏆 Rosette-forming, evergreen, sometimes white-mealy perennial, with usually obovate-spoon-shaped to rounded, entire to toothed, pale green to grey-green leaves, to 12cm (5in) long. Umbels of 2–30 salverform, fragrant, deep yellow flowers, 1.5–2.5cm (½–1in) across, are produced in spring. Cultivation group 1, 4, or 5. ↕ 20cm (8in), ↔ 25cm (10in). Alps, Apennines, Carpathians. ❄❄❄. **var. *albocincta*** ▣ bears grey-green leaves with white margins; Dolomites.

***P.* 'Beatrice Wooster'.** Rosette-forming, evergreen perennial with obovate, scalloped or finely toothed, glandular-hairy, grey-green leaves, to 8cm (3in) long. Large, shallowly cup-shaped, clear pink flowers, to 3cm (1¼in) across, with white eyes, are borne in umbels of 2–10 on short stems in spring. Cultivation group 4 or 5. ↕ 10cm (4in), ↔ 20cm (8in). ❄❄❄

P. beesiana ▣ syn. *P. bulleyana* subsp. *beesiana*. Rosette-forming, deciduous or semi-evergreen Candelabra primula that dies back to basal buds or reduced rosettes. The leaves are inversely lance-shaped to obovate, toothed, mid-green, and to 22cm (9in) long, with red midribs. In summer, stout, white-mealy stems each bear 2–8 whorls of 8–16 salverform, yellow-eyed, reddish pink flowers, 2cm (¾in) across. Cultivation group 2. ↕↔ 60cm (24in). Moist mountain meadows in China. ❄❄❄

P.* x *berninae (*P. hirsuta* x *P. latifolia*). Small, neat, rosette-forming, deciduous perennial with ovate, toothed, mid-green leaves, to 12cm (5in) long. In spring, very short stems produce tubular to cup-shaped purple flowers, 1.5cm (½in) across, singly or in umbels of up to 15. Cultivation group 1 or 4. ↕ 7cm (3in), ↔ 15cm (6in). Garden origin. ❄❄❄. **'Windrush'** produces white-eyed, red-purple flowers, 2cm (¾in) across.

***P.* 'Betty Green'.** Vigorous, rosette-forming, semi-evergreen Primrose Group primula bearing obovate, rich apple-green leaves, to 15cm (6in) long. Tubular to saucer-shaped, vivid crimson flowers, to 4cm (1½in) across, with clear yellow eyes, are produced freely in umbels of 3–25 in spring. Cultivation group 1 or 2. ↕ 10–15cm (4–6in), ↔ 30–40cm (12–16in). ❄❄❄

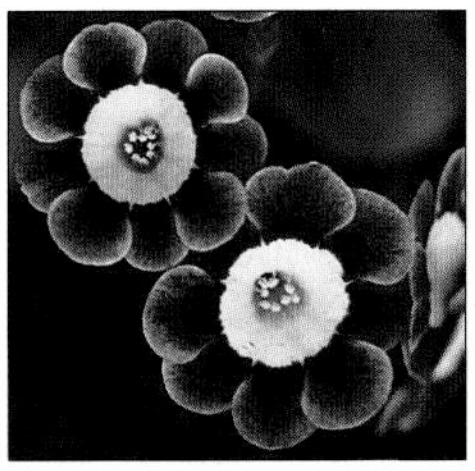

Primula 'Adrian'

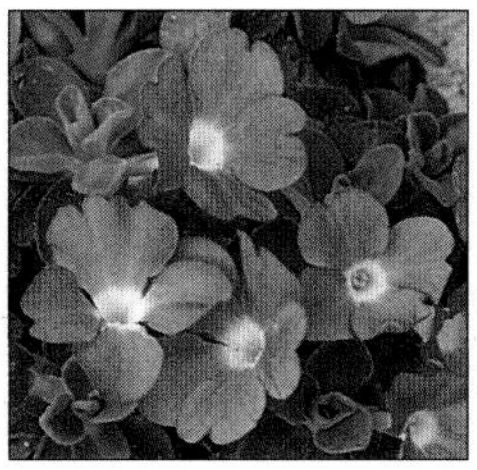

Primula allionii

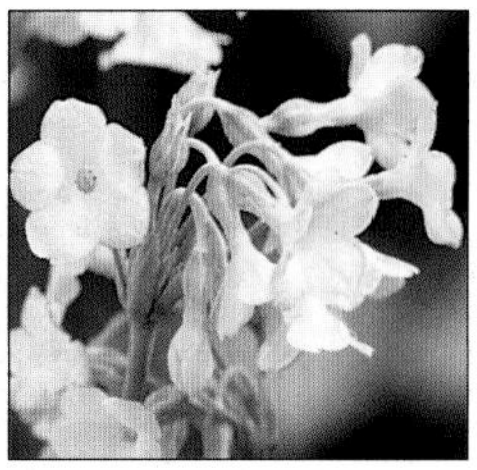

Primula alpicola

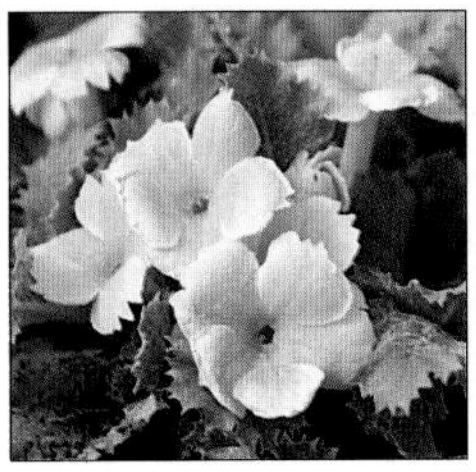

Primula aureata

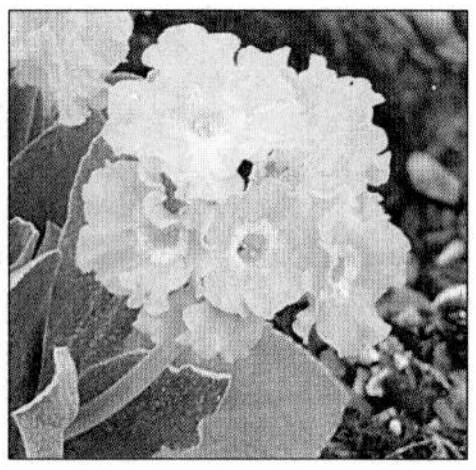

Primula auricula var. *albocincta*

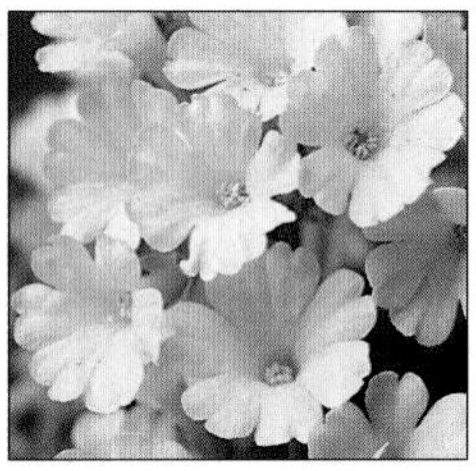

Primula 'Blairside Yellow'

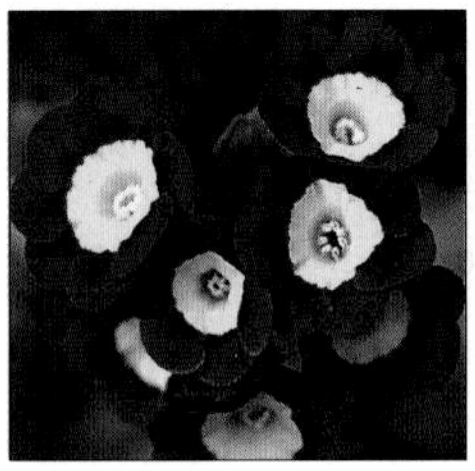

Primula 'Blossom'

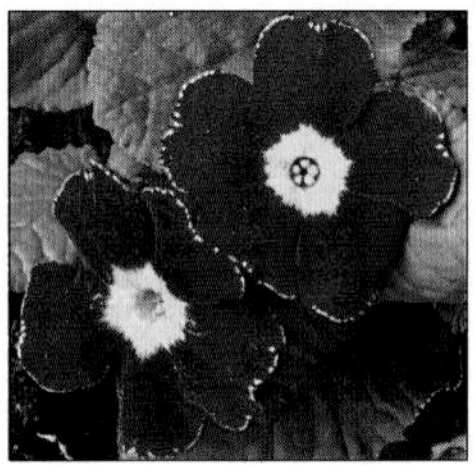

Primula 'Buckland Wine'

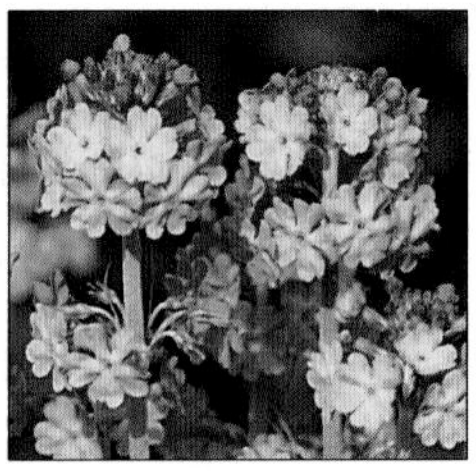

Primula bulleyana

P. bhutanica. Rosette-forming, deciduous perennial, dying back to a large, white-mealy bud in winter. The spoon-shaped, finely toothed, slightly white-mealy, crinkled leaves are mid-green, and to 10cm (4in) long. In late winter and spring, very short stems, hidden within the foliage, each bear umbels of 2–10 salverform, yellow-eyed blue flowers, 2.5cm (1in) across. Cultivation group 3. ↕ 15cm (6in), ↔ 20cm (8in). Mixed forest in Tibet, Bhutan, and India (Assam). ❄❄❄

***P.* 'Blairside Yellow'** ▣ Compact border Auricula primula, with rounded to oval, pale green leaves, to 12cm (5in) long. In early spring, produces open funnel-shaped yellow flowers, to 2.5cm (1in) across. Cultivation group 2 or 5. ↕ 10cm (4in), ↔ 20cm (8in). ❄❄❄

***P.* 'Blossom'** ▣ Vigorous alpine Auricula primula with oval, dark green leaves, 12cm (5in) long. Produces salverform, gold-centred flowers, 2.5cm (1in) across, with shaded crimson petals, in spring. Cultivation group 1 or 4. ↕↔ 10cm (4in). ❄❄❄

P. boothii. Rosette-forming, deciduous perennial with spoon-shaped to elliptic, toothed, dark green leaves, to 15cm (6in) long. Very short stems produce umbels of 2–25 saucer-shaped, yellow-eyed, purple-pink flowers, to 3cm (1¼in) across, in spring. Cultivation group 3 or 4. ↕ 10cm (4in), ↔ 20cm (8in). Moist, peaty areas in E. Himalayas. ❄❄

***P.* 'Broadwell Gold'.** Vigorous border Auricula primula bearing obovate, mid-green leaves, to 15cm (6in) long. In spring, bears salverform, golden yellow flowers, to 4cm (1½in) across, with white-mealy eyes. Cultivation group 1, 2, or 4. ↕↔ 25cm (10in). ❄❄❄

***P.* 'Buckland Wine'** ▣ Compact, rosette-forming, semi-evergreen, Primrose Group primula with oval, bronze-green leaves, to 15cm (6in) long. In spring, produces salverform, wine-red flowers, to 4cm (1½in) across, in umbels of 3–15. Cultivation group 1, 2, or 4. ↕ 10cm (4in), ↔ 25cm (10in). ❄❄❄

P. bulleyana ▣ 🏆 Rosette-forming, semi-evergreen Candelabra primula with ovate to ovate-lance-shaped, toothed, mid-green leaves, to 30cm (12in) long. In summer, stout stems produces 5–7 whorls of 5 to many salverform flowers, 2cm (¾in) across, in crimson fading to orange. Cultivation group 2. ↕↔ 60cm (24in). Hillsides in China. ❄❄❄. **subsp. *beesiana*** see *P. beesiana*.

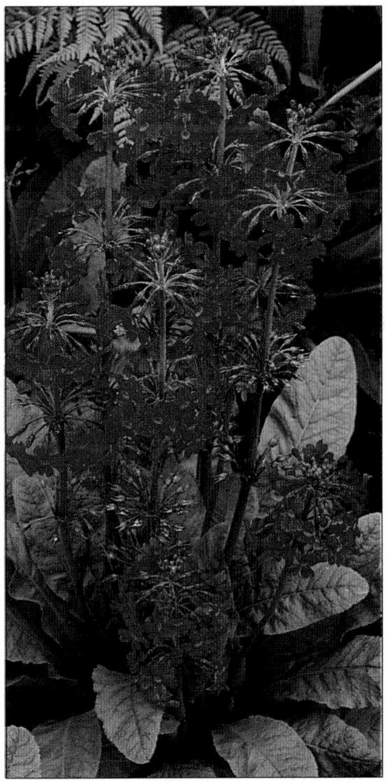

Primula beesiana

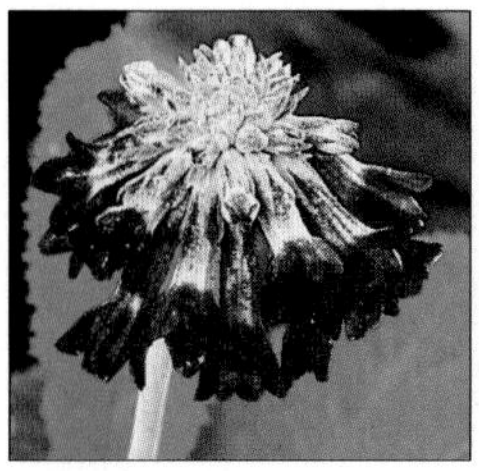
Primula capitata

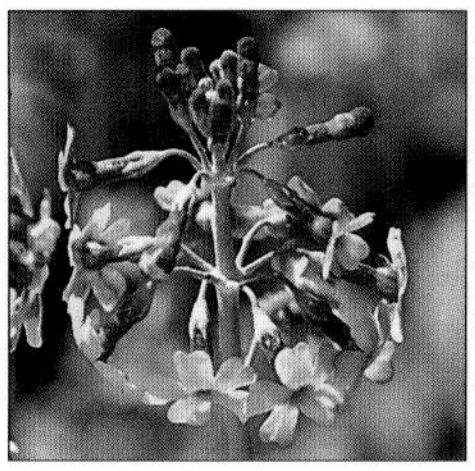
Primula chungensis

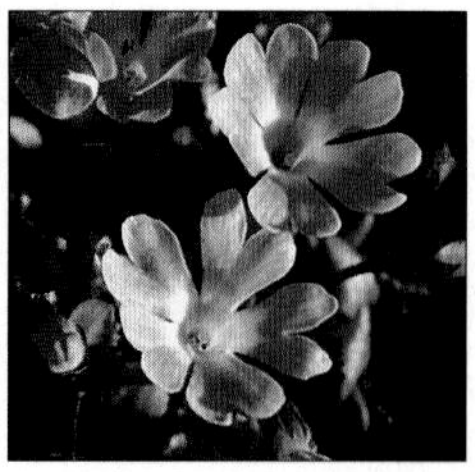
Primula clarkei

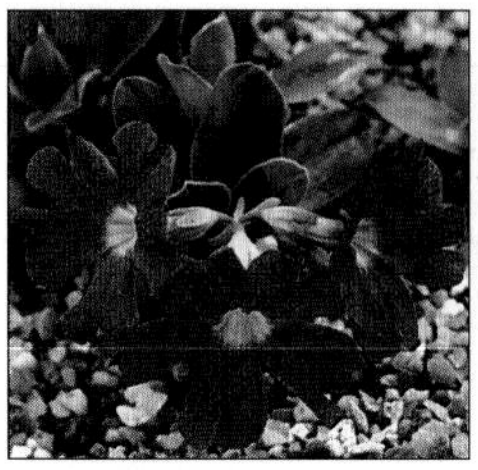
Primula clusiana

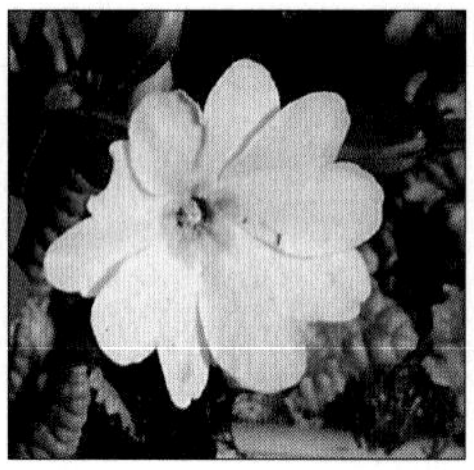
Primula 'Craddock White'

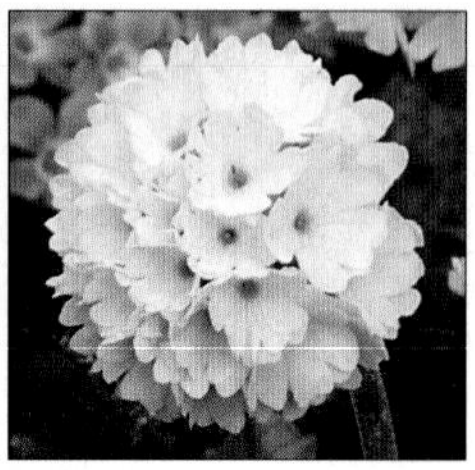
Primula denticulata var. *alba*

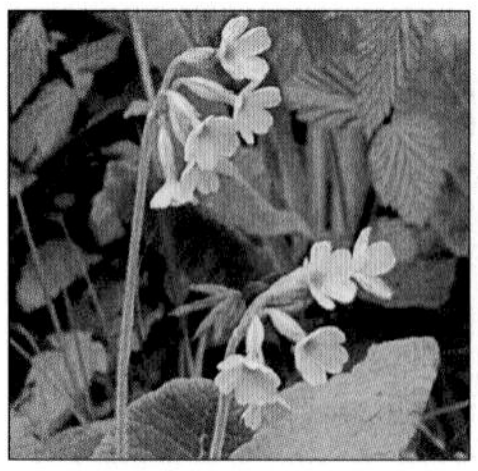
Primula elatior

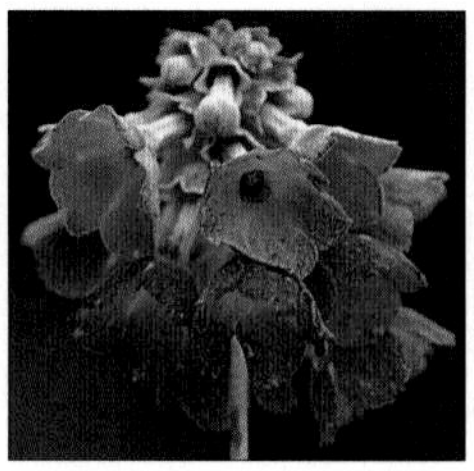
Primula flaccida

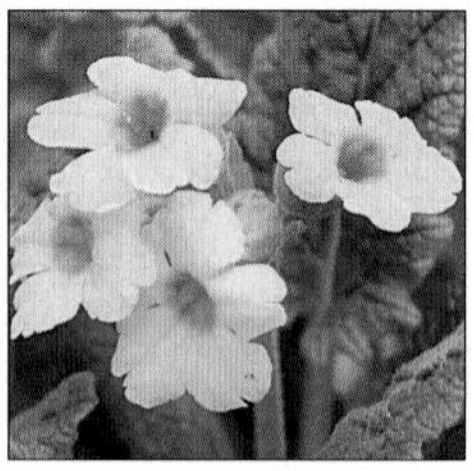
Primula forrestii

P. burmanica. Rosette-forming, deciduous Candelabra primula with inversely lance-shaped, toothed, dull, deep green leaves, to 30cm (12in) long. Stout stems produce up to 6 whorls of 10–18 salverform, yellow-eyed, red-purple flowers, 2cm (¾in) across, in late spring and early summer. Cultivation group 2. ↕↔ 60cm (24in). Meadows and forests in China and Burma. ❄❄❄
P. capitata ■ Rosette-forming, semi-evergreen, short-lived perennial, with inversely lance-shaped or oblong-lance-shaped, finely toothed, usually mealy, pale green leaves, to 15cm (6in) long, white-mealy beneath. Tubular, dark purple flowers, to 1cm (½in) long, with shallowly lobed petals, are borne in flattened, spherical racemes on white-mealy stems, from late spring to early autumn. Cultivation group 2. ↕↔ 40cm (16in). Moist alpine regions in Tibet, Bhutan, and India (Sikkim). ❄❄❄. **subsp. *mooreana*** is vigorous, and larger in all parts; ↕↔ 60cm (24in).
P. chionantha 🏆 Rosette-forming, deciduous perennial with inversely lance-shaped, toothed or almost entire, mid-green leaves, to 25cm (10in) long, covered in yellow or white meal. From late spring to early summer, stout stems produce 1–4 many-flowered whorls of tubular to funnel-shaped, fragrant, milk-white flowers, with or without whitish eyes, to 2.5cm (1in) across. Cultivation group 1 or 2. ↕↔ 60cm (24in). Open, alpine meadows in China. ❄❄❄. **subsp. *melanops*** see *P. melanops.*
***P.* 'Chloe'.** Green-edged show Auricula primula with oval, dark green leaves, to 12cm (5in) long. Salverform, 5- to 7-petalled black flowers, 2.5cm (1in) across, are borne in spring. Cultivation group 4. ↕↔ 10cm (4in). ❄❄❄
P. chungensis ■ Vigorous, rosette-forming, deciduous Candelabra primula with oblong-obovate, toothed and shallowly lobed, mid-green leaves, to 30cm (12in) long. In early summer, stout stems bear 2–5 whorls of up to 12 salverform, fragrant, pale orange flowers, 1.5–2cm (½–¾in) across, with red tubes. Cultivation group 2. ↕ 80cm (32in), ↔ 60cm (24in). Wet, open forest in China and Bhutan. ❄❄❄
P. clarkei ■ Small, rosette-forming, deciduous perennial with rounded to ovate, toothed, pale green leaves, to 5cm (2in) long. In spring, flat, yellow-eyed, rose-pink flowers, to 2cm (¾in) across, are borne in sometimes short-stemmed umbels of 2–6. Cultivation group 2 or 4. ↕ 7cm (3in), ↔ 15cm (6in). Moist hillsides in India (Kashmir). ❄❄❄
P. clusiana ■ Small, rosette-forming, evergreen perennial with oblong to ovate, leathery, dark green leaves, to 8cm (3in) long. In spring, salverform, white-eyed, rose-pink to lilac flowers, to 4cm (1½in) across, are borne singly or in umbels of up to 4. Cultivation group 4 or 5. ↕ 8cm (3in), ↔ 15cm (6in). Austria (N. calcareous Alps). ❄❄❄
P. cockburniana. Rosette-forming, deciduous biennial or short-lived perennial Candelabra primula with oblong to oblong-obovate, mid-green leaves, to 15cm (6in) long, with small, toothed lobes. Slender stems bear 1–3 whorls of 3–8 salverform, red-tinged orange flowers, 1.5cm (½in) across, in summer. Cultivation group 1 or 2. ↕↔ 40cm (16in). Marshy, alpine meadows in China (S.W. Sichuan). ❄❄❄
P. cortusoides. Small, rosette-forming, deciduous perennial with ovate-oblong, softly hairy, toothed, mid-green leaves, to 9cm (3½in) long. Umbels of 2–15 salverform, rose-red, pink to red-violet flowers, to 2cm (¾in) across, are borne in late spring and early summer. Cultivation group 2. ↕↔ 30cm (12in). Woodland in Russia (W. Siberia). ❄❄❄
***P.* 'Craddock White'** ■ Rosette-forming, deciduous or semi-evergreen Primrose Group primula with oval, dark green, bronze-veined leaves, 15cm (6in) long. In spring, salverform, scented white flowers, to 4cm (1½in) across, with yellow eyes, are produced in umbels of 3–8. Cultivation group 2. ↕ 12cm (5in), ↔ 25cm (10in). ❄❄❄
P. cuneifolia. Rosette-forming, deciduous, short-lived perennial with inversely lance-shaped, obovate, or wedge-shaped, coarsely toothed, pale green leaves, to 8cm (3in) long. In summer, salverform, rose-red, yellow-eyed flowers, to 2cm (¾in) across, are borne singly or in umbels of up to 9, on stems ranging from tiny to 30cm (12in) tall. Cultivation group 2 or 4. ↕↔ to 30cm (12in). Russia (Siberia), Japan, North America (E. Alaska to British Columbia, Aleutian Islands). ❄❄❄
P. denticulata 🏆 (Drumstick primula). Robust, rosette-forming, deciduous perennial with oblong-obovate or spoon-shaped, mid-green leaves, to 25cm (10in) long, finely toothed, and white-mealy beneath. Stout stems bear crowded, spherical umbels of tubular to trumpet- or bell-shaped, yellow-eyed, purple flowers, to 2cm (¾in) across, from mid-spring to summer. Cultivation group 1 or 2. ↕↔ 45cm (18in). Moist alpine regions from Afghanistan to S.E. Tibet, Burma, and China. ❄❄❄. **var. *alba*** ■ has white flowers. **'Rubra'** has red-purple flowers.
***P.* 'Dreamer'** ■ Rosette-forming, semi-evergreen or evergreen Primrose Group primula with inversely lance-shaped to obovate, mid-green leaves, 10cm (4in) long. In spring, produces salverform flowers, 4–5cm (1½–2in) across, in cream, apricot, pink, or rose-pink; all bicolours have darker eyes and yellow centres. Cultivation group 6. ↕ 8–10cm (3–4in), ↔ 15–20cm (6–8in). ❄
P. edgeworthii, syn. *P. nana.* Rosette-forming, deciduous perennial with spoon-shaped to triangular-ovate, pale green leaves, to 12cm (5in) long, contracting to a tight rosette or crown in winter. From late winter to spring, very short stems bear umbels of flat, blue, lilac, pink, or white flowers, 3.5cm (1½in) across, with yellow and white eyes. Cultivation group 3 or 4. ↕ 10cm (4in), ↔ 15cm (6in). W. Himalayas. ❄❄❄
P. elatior ■🏆 (Oxlip). Variable, rosette-forming, evergreen or semi-evergreen perennial with ovate to oblong or elliptic, scalloped, mid-green leaves, to 20cm (8in) long, softly hairy beneath. In spring and summer, stiff, upright stems bear one-sided umbels of 2–12 tubular yellow flowers, to 2.5cm (1in) long. Cultivation group 1 or 2. ↕ 30cm (12in), ↔ 25cm (10in). Moist meadows and open woodland in Europe, Turkey to the Altai Mountains, and Russia (Siberia). ❄❄❄. **subsp. *meyeri*** see *P. amoena.*

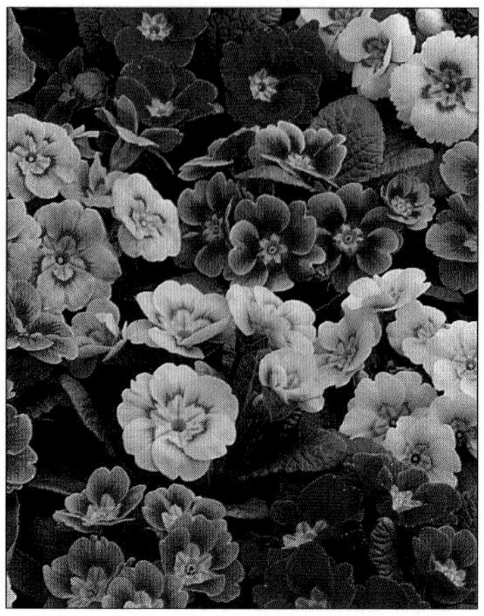
Primula 'Dreamer'

P. ellisiae. Rosette-forming, deciduous perennial with inversely lance-shaped to spoon-shaped, finely toothed, mid-green leaves, to 15cm (6in) long. In summer, sturdy stems produce umbels of 4–8 saucer-shaped, yellow-eyed, pinkish purple flowers, to 2.5cm (1in) across. Cultivation group 1 or 4. ↕↔ 30cm (12in). Moist crevices and ledges in USA (New Mexico). ❄❄❄
***P.* 'E.R. Janes'.** Vigorous, rosette-forming, semi-evergreen Primrose Group primula with broadly oval, toothed, mid-green leaves, to 15cm (6in) long. Masses of salverform, orange-flushed, salmon-pink flowers, 4cm (1½in) across, are borne in fascicles in spring, sometimes again in autumn. Has little foliage at spring flowering. Cultivation group 1 or 2. ↕ 10–15cm (4–6in), ↔ 30–40cm (12–16in). ❄❄❄
P. farinosa. Rosette-forming, deciduous perennial with inversely lance-shaped, sometimes toothed, mid-green leaves, to 10cm (4in) long, and white-mealy beneath. Bears compact umbels of 2–10 tubular, white-mealy, yellow-eyed, lilac-pink flowers, 1.5cm (½in) across, in late spring and early summer. Cultivation group 2 or 4. ↕↔ to 25cm (10in). Moist meadows in Europe, N. Asia, and N. Pacific. ❄❄❄
***P.* 'Finesse'.** Rosette-forming, evergreen or semi-evergreen perennial bearing inversely lance-shaped to obovate, mid-green leaves, 10cm (4in) long. In late winter and early spring, produces salverform flowers, 4.5cm (1¾in) across, in rose-pink, crimson-red, scarlet-red, mauve-blue, purple, light blue, or dark blue; each flower has a thin, "laced" margin in silver or gold. Cultivation group 6. ↕ 8–10cm (3–4in), ↔ 15–20cm (6–8in). ❄
P. flaccida ■🏆 syn. *P. nutans* of gardens. Rosette-forming, deciduous, short-lived perennial with narrowly elliptic or obovate, downy, finely toothed, pale to mid-green leaves, to 20cm (8in) long. In summer, bears conical umbels of 5–15 pendent, broadly tubular to funnel-shaped, white-mealy, lavender-blue to violet flowers, 2.5cm (1in) across. Cultivation group 3 or 4. ↕ 50cm (20in), ↔ 30cm (12in). Open forest and alpine meadows in China. ❄❄❄
P. florindae ■🏆 (Giant cowslip). Rosette-forming, deciduous perennial with ovate, toothed, mid-green leaves, to 45cm (18in) long. Umbels of up to 40 pendent, slender, tubular to funnel-shaped, white-mealy, fragrant, sulphur-yellow flowers, 1–2cm (½–¾in) across, are borne on stout stems in summer. Cultivation group 1 or 2. ↕ to 1.2m (4ft), ↔ 90cm (36in). Marshes and streams in S.E. Tibet. ❄❄❄
P. forrestii ■ Rosette-forming, evergreen, perennial subshrub with ovate-elliptic, scalloped to toothed, dark green leaves, to 20cm (8in) long, wrinkled

P

above, white-mealy beneath. In late spring and summer, stout stems bear umbels of 10–25 salverform, orange-eyed, golden yellow flowers, 1.5–2.5cm (½–1in) across. Cultivation group 4 or 5. ↕ 60cm (24in), ↔ 45cm (18in). Dry, shady crevices in limestone cliffs in China. ✻✻✻

P.* x *forsteri* f. *bileckii (*P. hirsuta* x *P. minima*). Dwarf, rosette-forming, evergreen perennial with wedge-shaped, leathery, toothed, shiny, dark green leaves, 0.5–3cm (½–1¼in) long, with soft, glandular hairs. In late spring, bears umbels of 2 or 3 salverform, red-pink flowers, 1.5–3cm (½–1¼in) across, on very short stems. Cultivation group 2 or 4. ↕ 7cm (3in), ↔ 10cm (4in). Austria (Alps). ✻✻✻

P. frondosa ■ ♀ Rosette-forming, deciduous perennial with spoon-shaped, finely toothed or lobed, mid-green leaves, to 10cm (4in) long, white-mealy beneath. In late spring and early summer, salverform, yellow-eyed, pale pinkish lilac to red-purple flowers, to 1.5cm (½in) across, are borne singly or in loose umbels of up to 30. Cultivation group 2 or 4. ↕ 15cm (6in), ↔ 25cm (10in). Bulgaria (Stara Planina plateau). ✻✻✻

***P.* 'Garryarde Guinevere'** ■ ♀ Vigorous, rosette-forming, evergreen Polyanthus Group primula with oval, toothed, deep bronze leaves, 15cm (6in) long, and salverform, yellow-eyed, purplish-pink flowers, 4cm (1½in) across, borne in umbels of 3–8 in spring. Cultivation group 2. ↕ 12cm (5in), ↔ 25cm (10in). ✻✻✻

P. geraniifolia. Rosette-forming, hairy, deciduous perennial with rounded, 7- to 9-lobed leaves, to 15cm (6in) long, with scalloped margins. Slender stems bear umbels of 2–12 semi-pendent, tubular to bell-shaped, pinkish purple flowers, to 2cm (¾in) across, in late spring and early summer. Cultivation group 2. ↕↔ 30cm (12in). Shady hillsides in India (Sikkim), Nepal, Bhutan, Tibet, and China. ✻✻✻

P. glutinosa. Rosette-forming, evergreen perennial with narrowly inversely lance-shaped to oblong, entire, leathery, sticky, glandular-hairy leaves, to 6cm (2½in) long. In late spring and early summer, cup-shaped, fragrant, blue-violet flowers, to 2cm (¾in) across, are borne singly or in umbels of up to 8. Cultivation group 1 or 4. ↕↔ 10cm (4in). Wet, acid alpine meadows in E. Alps and C. Balkans. ✻✻✻

***P.* Gold Laced Group** ■ Erect, semi-evergreen or evergreen Polyanthus Group primula with oval, sometimes red-tinged, mid-green leaves, 18cm (7in) long. In spring, bears umbels of 3–12 salverform, golden-eyed, very dark mahogany-red or black flowers, to 3cm (1¼in) across, each petal with a narrow gold margin. Cultivation group 2 or 4. ↕ 25cm (10in), ↔ 30cm (12in). ✻✻✻

P. gracilipes ■ Rosette-forming, evergreen or semi-evergreen perennial with oblong to spoon-shaped to elliptic, toothed, mid-green leaves, to 15cm (6in) long. From winter to early summer, umbels of salverform, purple-pink flowers, 1.5–2.5cm (½–1in) across, with white-bordered, orange-yellow eyes, are borne on very short stems hidden within the foliage. Cultivation group 3 or 4. ↕ 10cm (4in), ↔ 20cm (8in). Moist alpine regions in S.E. Tibet and C. Nepal. ✻✻✻

P. griffithii. Rosette-forming, deciduous perennial with ovate to arrow-shaped, toothed, dark bluish green leaves, to 25cm (10in) long, sparsely white-mealy beneath. Bears umbels of 5–12 salverform, yellow-eyed purple flowers, 2.5cm (1in) across, in spring. Cultivation group 3 or 4. ↕ 25cm (10in), ↔ 45cm (18in). Moist hillsides in Tibet and Bhutan. ✻✻✻

P. halleri. Rosette-forming, deciduous perennial with inversely lance-shaped, elliptic to obovate, sometimes finely toothed, white-mealy, mid-green leaves, to 8cm (3in) long. Stout stems bear umbels of up to 20 salverform, yellow-eyed, lilac-pink flowers, to 2cm (¾in) across, in late spring and early summer. Cultivation group 2 or 4. ↕ 30cm (12in), ↔ 25cm (10in). Stony alpine meadows in Alps, Carpathians, Balkans. ✻✻✻

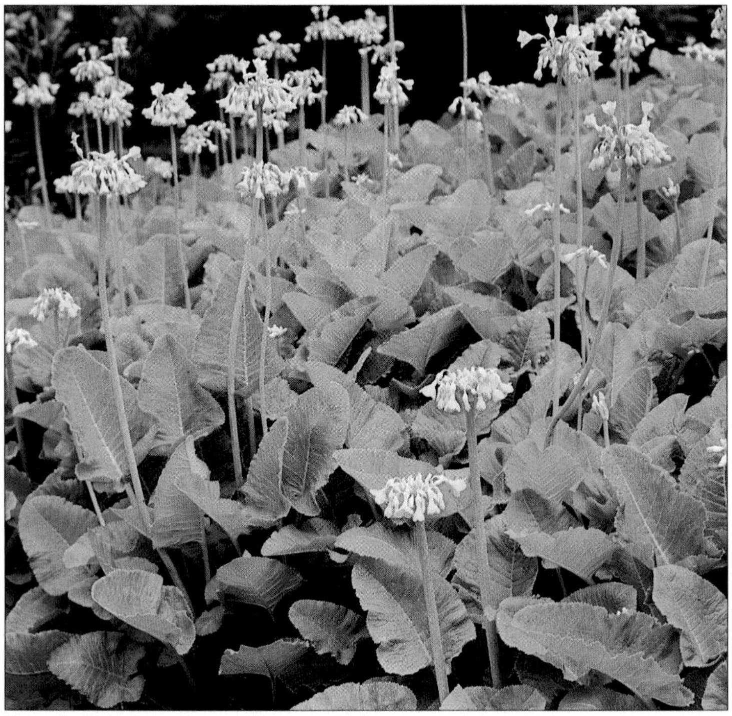
Primula florindae

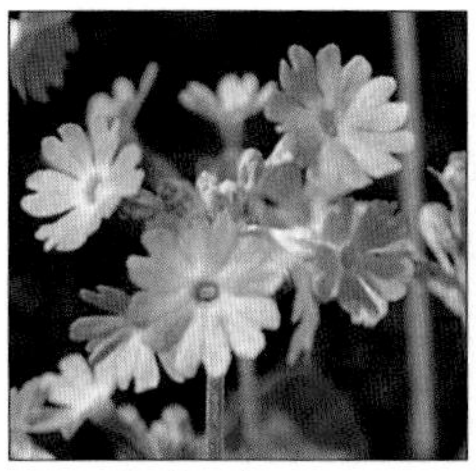
Primula frondosa

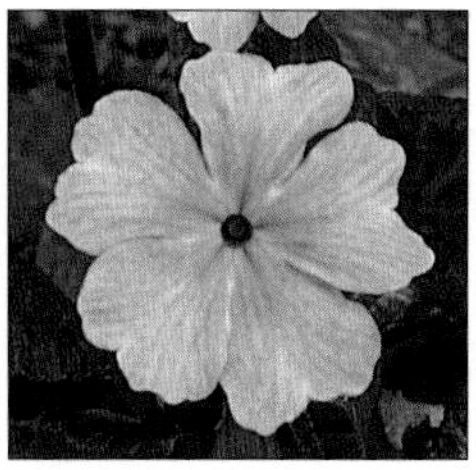
Primula 'Garryarde Guinevere'

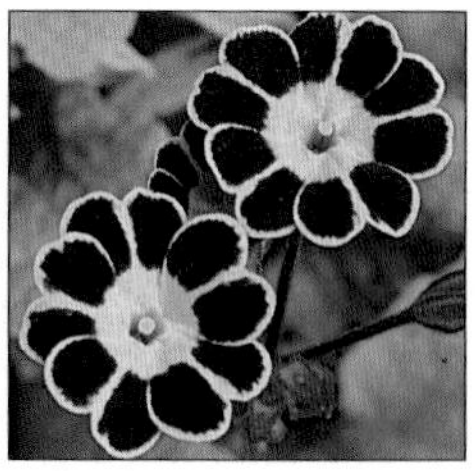
Primula Gold Laced Group

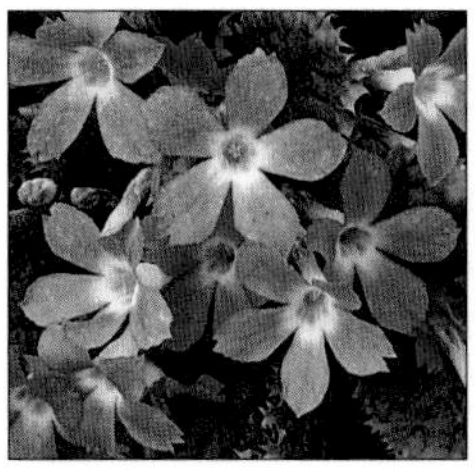
Primula gracilipes

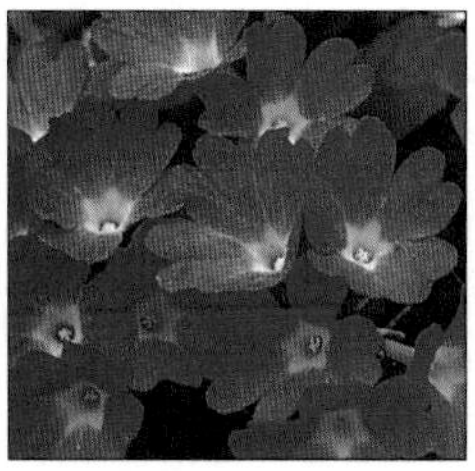
Primula hirsuta

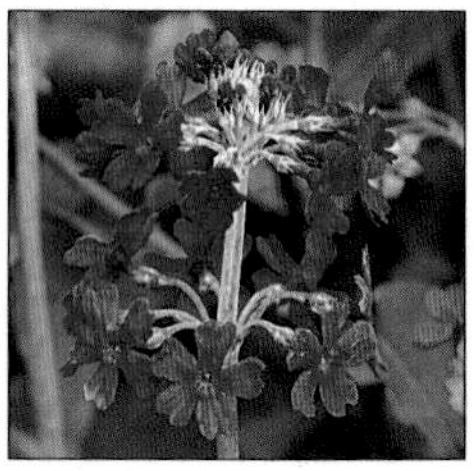
Primula 'Inverewe'

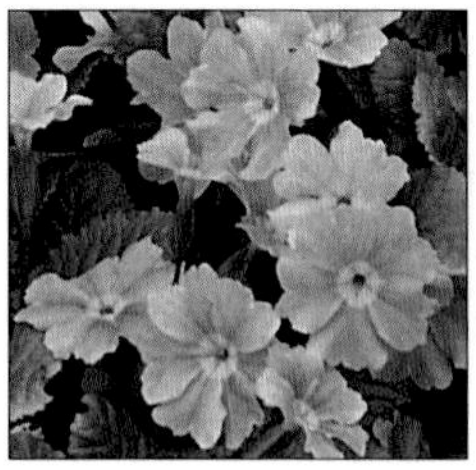
Primula 'Iris Mainwaring'

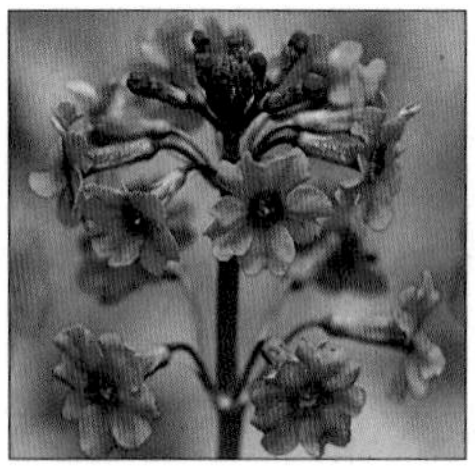
Primula japonica 'Miller's Crimson'

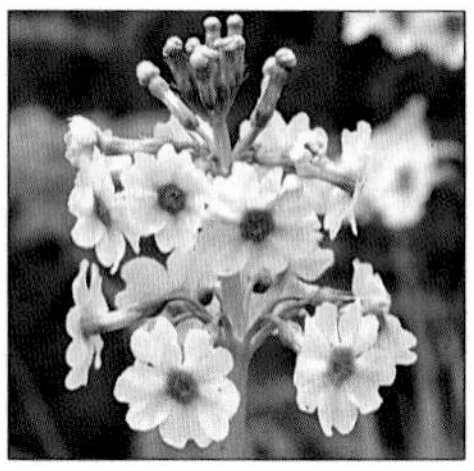
Primula japonica 'Postford White'

P. heucherifolia. Rosette-forming, stoloniferous, hairy, deciduous perennial with long-stalked, rounded leaves, to 15cm (6in) long, with 7–11 triangular lobes. Slender stems bear 3–10 pendent, bell-shaped, mauve-pink to rich purple flowers, 1–2.5cm (½–1in) across, in early summer. Cultivation group 2. ↕↔ 30cm (12in). Shady, rocky hillsides in China (Sichuan). ✻✻✻

P. hirsuta ■ syn. *P. rubra.* Rosette-forming, evergreen perennial with spoon-shaped to obovate, toothed, glandular-hairy, mid-green leaves, to 8cm (3in) long. In late spring and early summer, salverform, usually white-eyed, mauve-pink flowers, 1.5–2.5cm (½–1in) across, are borne singly or in umbels of up to 15, on short stems. Cultivation group 1, 2, or 4. ↕ 10cm (4in), ↔ 25cm (10in). Pyrenees, Alps. ✻✻✻

***P.* 'Hyacinthia'**, syn. *P. marginata* 'Hyacinthia'. Robust, rosette-forming, evergreen perennial with obovate, slightly white-mealy, light green leaves, to 12cm (5in) long. In spring, shallowly tubular to funnel-shaped, 6-lobed, hyacinth-blue flowers, to 3cm (1¼in) across, are borne in umbels of 2–20. Cultivation group 4 or 5. ↕ 15cm (6in), ↔ 20cm (8in). ✻✻✻

***P.* 'Inverewe'** ■ ♀ Vigorous, rosette-forming, semi-evergreen Candelabra primula with oval to lance-shaped, toothed, coarse, mid-green leaves, to 20cm (8in) long. In summer, numerous stems each bear several whorls of 5–15 salverform, brilliant red flowers, to 3cm (1¼in) across. Cultivation group 2. ↕ 75cm (30in), ↔ 60cm (24in). ✻✻✻

P. involucrata. Rosette-forming, deciduous perennial with ovate to oblong, entire or finely toothed, mid-green leaves, to 15cm (6in) long. In late spring and early summer, long, slender stems produce umbels of 2–6 pendent, shallowly tubular to bell-shaped, yellow-eyed white flowers, 1.5–2cm (½–¾in) across. Cultivation group 2. ↕↔ 30cm (12in). Moist alpine meadows from Pakistan to S.W. China. ✻✻✻. **subsp. *yargongensis***, syn. *P. yargongensis*, produces umbels of 3–8 semi-pendent, mauve-pink flowers; S.E. Tibet, China.

P. ioessa. Rosette-forming, deciduous perennial with narrowly oblong or inversely lance-shaped to spoon-shaped, deeply toothed, mid-green leaves, to 20cm (8in) long. Bears umbels of 2–8 pendent, tubular to funnel-shaped, white-mealy, fragrant, mauve-pink to violet or white flowers, 2.5cm (1in) across, in summer. Cultivation group 2, 3, or 4. ↕↔ 30cm (12in). Wet alpine meadows in S.E. Tibet. ✻✻✻

***P.* 'Iris Mainwaring'** ■ Compact, rosette-forming, evergreen or semi-evergreen Primrose Group primula with oval, deep green leaves, to 18cm (7in) long. In spring, delicate, salverform pink flowers, 4cm (1½in) across, with yellow centres, are borne in umbels of 3–8. Cultivation group 1, 2, or 4. ↕ 10–15cm (4–6in), ↔ 30–40cm (12–16in). ✻✻✻

P. japonica ♀ (Japanese primrose). Robust, rosette-forming, deciduous perennial with obovate, oblong, or broadly spoon-shaped, finely scalloped or toothed, pale green leaves, to 25cm (10in) long. Stout stems bearing 1–6 whorls of 5–25 salverform, red-purple to white flowers, 2cm (¾in) across, are borne in late spring and early summer. Cultivation group 2. ↕↔ 45cm (18in). Moist, shady places in Japan. ✻✻✻. **'Miller's Crimson'** ■ has crimson flowers. **'Postford White'** ■ is robust, and has red-eyed, clear white flowers.

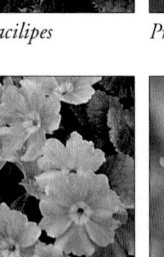

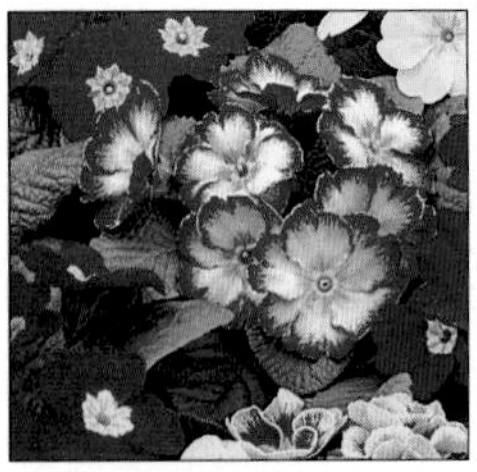
Primula Joker Series

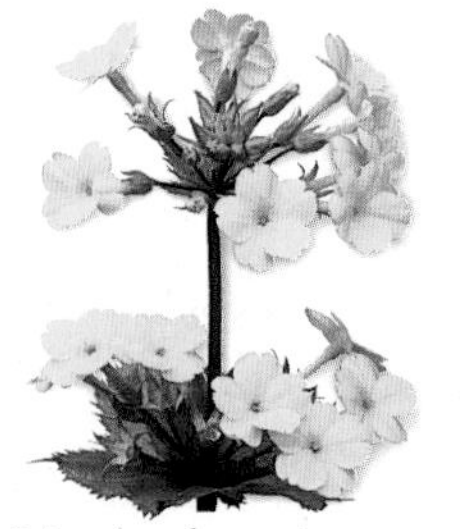
Primula x *kewensis* 'Mountain Spring'

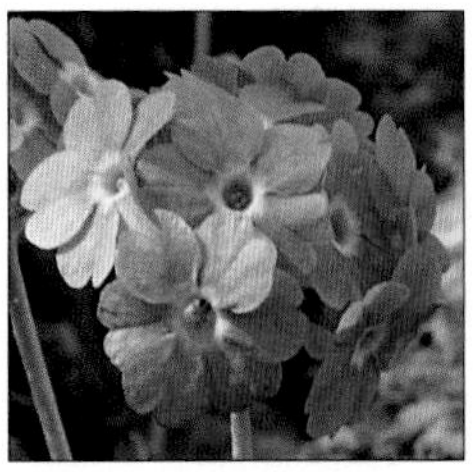
Primula 'Linda Pope'

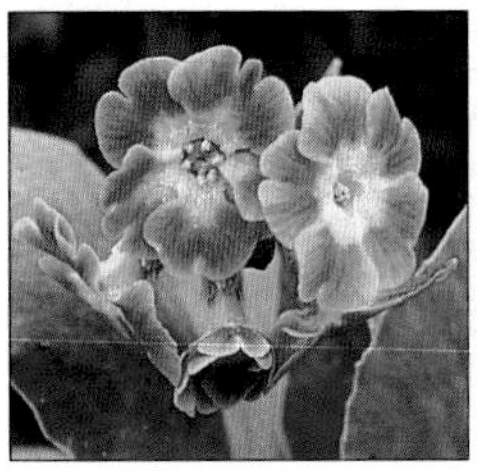
Primula 'Linnet'

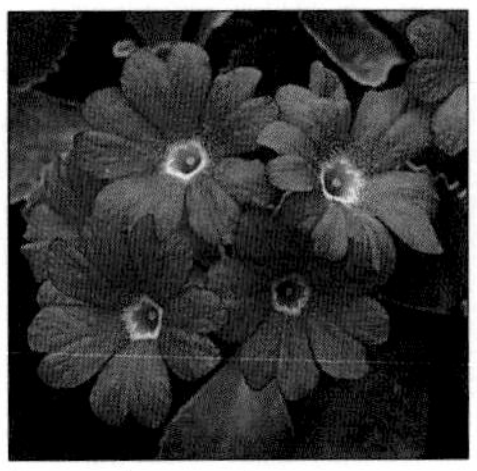
Primula marginata 'Kesselring's Variety'

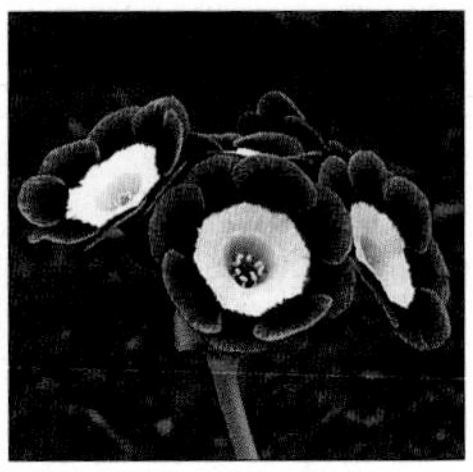
Primula 'Mark'

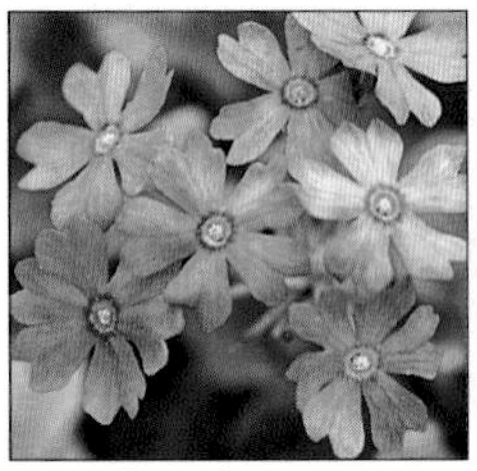
Primula modesta var. faurieae

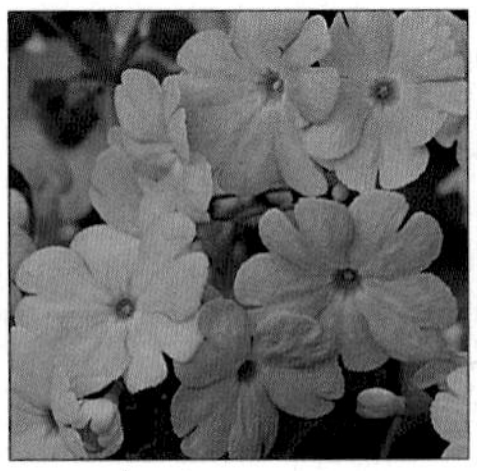
Primula obconica Cantata Series 'Cantata Lavender'

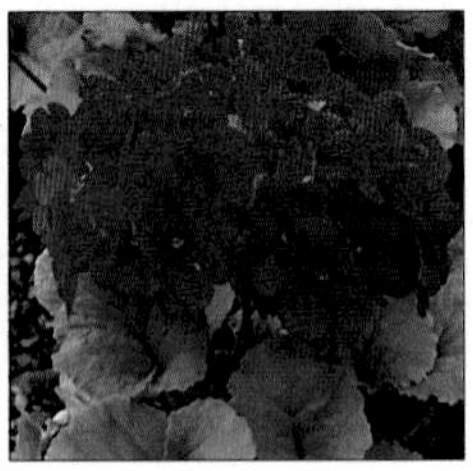
Primula obconica 'Queen of the Market'

P. jesoana. Rosette-forming, hairy, deciduous or semi-evergreen perennial with rounded, deeply 7- to 9-lobed, mid-green leaves, to 30cm (12in) long. Slender stems each bear 1–4 umbels of 2–6 shallowly tubular to bell-shaped, yellow-eyed, pinkish purple or white flowers, 2cm (¾in) across, in late spring and early summer. Cultivation group 2 or 4. ↕↔ 30cm (12in). Mountain areas in C. Japan. **

***P.* 'Johanna'.** Rosette-forming, deciduous perennial bearing inversely lance-shaped, mid-green leaves, to 2cm (¾in) long. In spring, produces few-flowered umbels of salverform, yellow-eyed, clear pink flowers, 1cm (½in) across. Cultivation group 2 or 4. ↕ 10cm (4in), ↔ 15cm (6in). ***

***P.* Joker Series** ■ Compact, rosette-forming, evergreen or semi-evergreen perennials with small, short-stemmed, inversely lance-shaped to obovate, mid-green leaves, 10cm (4in) long. Salverform flowers, 4.5cm (1¾in) across, in a range of colours, including numerous bicolours, with prominent yellow or creamy yellow eyes, are borne in spring. Cultivation group 6. ↕ 8–10cm (3–4in), ↔ 20cm (8in). *

P. juliae. Rosette-forming, semi-evergreen or deciduous perennial with rounded, scalloped, dark green leaves, to 10cm (4in) long, deeply heart-shaped at the bases. In spring and summer, bears solitary, long-stalked, saucer-shaped magenta flowers, to 3cm (1¼in) across, with yellow eyes. Cultivation group 1, 2, or 4. ↕ 7cm (3in), ↔ 25cm (10in). Rocky mountain forest in E. Caucasus. ***

P.* x *kewensis ♀ (*P. floribunda* x *P. sinensis*). Rosette-forming, evergreen perennial with obovate to spoon-shaped, toothed, sparsely white-mealy, mid-green leaves, 15–20cm (6–8in) long. Each stem bears 2–5 whorls of 6–10 long-tubed, salverform, fragrant yellow flowers, to 2cm (¾in) across, in early spring. Cultivation group 6. ↕ to 45cm (18in), ↔ 20cm (8in). Garden origin. *. **'Mountain Spring'** ■ is compact, and bears bright golden yellow flowers; ↕ to 25cm (10in). **'Thurgold'** has clear lemon-yellow flowers.

***P.* 'Kingcup'** see *P.* 'Argus'.

***P.* 'Kinlough Beauty'.** Vigorous, evergreen or semi-evergreen Polyanthus Group primula with oval, dark green green leaves, to 15cm (6in) long. In spring, salverform, salmon-pink flowers, 4cm (1½in) across, with darker pink stripes, are produced in umbels of 3–12. Cultivation group 1, 2, or 4. ↕ 10–15cm (4–6in), ↔ 30–40cm (12–16in). ***

P. kisoana. Rosette-forming, hairy, deciduous perennial with rounded, shallowly lobed, mid-green leaves, to 15cm (6in) long. In spring and early summer, produces umbels of 2–6 tubular to funnel-shaped, pinkish purple flowers, to 3cm (1¼in) across. Cultivation group 2, 3, or 4. ↕ 20cm (8in), ↔ 40cm (16in). Woodland in S.W. Japan. ***

***P.* 'Lady Greer'** ♀ Dainty, evergreen or semi-evergreen Polyanthus Group primula with spoon-shaped, bottle-green leaves, to 12cm (5in) long. In spring, bears salverform, pale yellow flowers, 2cm (¾in) across. Cultivation group 2 or 3. ↕ 10–15cm (4–6in), ↔ 30–40cm (12–16in). ***

P. latifolia. Rosette-forming, deciduous perennial with broadly lance-shaped, glandular-hairy, dull green leaves, to 15cm (6in) long, sometimes toothed at the tips. One-sided umbels of 2–25 salverform, sometimes white-mealy, fragrant, red-purple flowers, 1.5–2cm (½–¾in) across, are produced in late spring and early summer. Cultivation group 1, 2, or 4. ↕ 20cm (8in), ↔ 30cm (12in). Moist, shady, acid cliffs in Pyrenees and Alps. ***

***P.* 'Linda Pope'** ■♀ syn. *P. marginata* 'Linda Pope'. Vigorous, rosette-forming, evergreen or semi-evergreen perennial with oval, toothed, white-mealy, mid-green leaves, 10cm (4in) long. Umbels of 4–16 salverform, mauve-blue flowers, to 3cm (1¼in) across, with white-mealy eyes, are borne in spring. Cultivation group 4 or 5. ↕ 15cm (6in), ↔ 30cm (12in). ***

***P.* 'Lingwood Beauty'.** Rosette-forming, evergreen or semi-evergreen, Primrose Group primula with oval, bright green leaves, to 12cm (5in) long. Umbels of 3–12 salverform crimson flowers, 2.5cm (1in) across, with deep orange eyes, are borne in late spring. Cultivation group 2 or 4. ↕ 10–15cm (4–6in), ↔ 30–40cm (12–16in). ***

***P.* 'Linnet'** ■ Rosette-forming, evergreen perennial bearing obovate, mid-green leaves, to 8cm (3in) long. In spring, bears umbels of salverform, yellow-eyed, orange to rose-pink flowers, 3cm (1¼in) across. Cultivation group 3 or 4. ↕ 10cm (4in), ↔ 20cm (8in). ***

***P.* 'Lismore Yellow'.** Rosette-forming, evergreen perennial with ovate, dark green leaves, to 3cm (1¼in) long. In spring, short stems bear umbels of 2–5 open funnel-shaped, pale yellow flowers, 2.5cm (1in) across. Cultivation group 4 or 5. ↕ 10cm (4in), ↔ 15cm (6in). ***

P. luteola. Rosette-forming, evergreen or semi-evergreen perennial with lance-shaped, sharply double-toothed, mid-green leaves, to 30cm (12in) long. In spring, robust, white-mealy stems bear symmetrical to spherical umbels of 10–25 salverform yellow flowers, 1.5cm (½in) across. Cultivation group 1 or 2. ↕ 35cm (14in), ↔ 45cm (18in). Moist meadows in E. Caucasus. ***

P. macrophylla. Short-lived, rosette-forming, deciduous perennial with lance-shaped to inversely lance-shaped, entire or finely scalloped, mid-green leaves, to 25cm (10in) long, usually white-mealy beneath. In spring, white-mealy stems bear umbels of 5–25 salverform purple flowers, 2cm (¾in) across; the eyes are usually darker or tinged yellow. Cultivation group 2 or 4. ↕ 25cm (10in), ↔ 30cm (12in). Rocky alpine meadows in Himalayas. ***

P. malacoides (Fairy primrose). Erect, rosette-forming, evergreen perennial, usually grown as an annual, with dainty, oval, slightly frilly-margined, softly downy, pale green leaves, to 10cm (4in) long. In winter and spring, flat, single or double, pale lilac-purple, reddish pink, and white flowers, to 1cm (½in) across, are borne in whorls of decreasing size up slender, softly hairy stems. Cultivation group 6. ↕ 30–45cm (12–18in), ↔ 20cm (8in). China. *. **'Benary's Special'** are compact, with blue, yellow, golden orange, scarlet, red-pink, rose-pink, or white flowers; ↕ to 30cm (12in).

P. marginata ♀ Rosette-forming, evergreen or semi-evergreen perennial with obovate to oblong, toothed, leathery, mid-green leaves, to 10cm (4in) long, white-mealy on the margins. In spring, white-mealy stems each bear a symmetrical umbel of 2–20 shallowly tubular to funnel-shaped, faintly fragrant, lavender-blue flowers, to 3cm (1¼in) across, with white-mealy eyes.

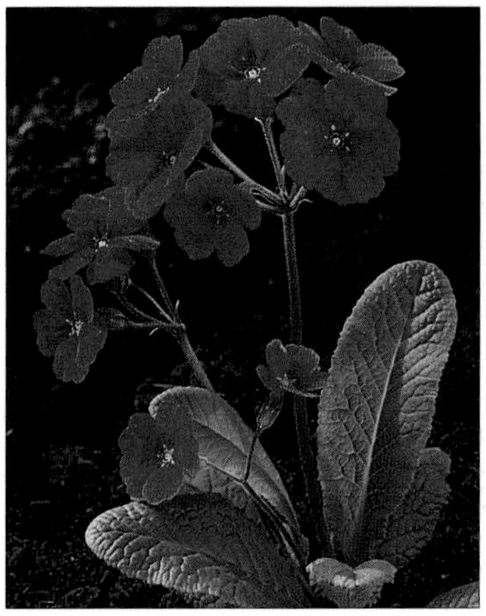
Primula Polyanthus Group Cowichan Series

Cultivation group 4 or 5. ↕ 15cm (6in), ↔ 30cm (12in). Europe (Alps). ***. **'Holden Variety'**, syn. 'Holden Clough', is compact, with small, tubular to funnel-shaped, dark blue flowers, 2cm (¾in) across. **'Hyacinthia'** see *P.* 'Hyacinthia'. **'Ivy Agee'** is vigorous, with heavily white-mealy leaves and lilac-blue flowers with cream eyes. **'Kesselring's Variety'** ■ is moderately vigorous, bearing deep lavender-blue flowers. **'Linda Pope'** see *P.* 'Linda Pope'.

***P.* 'Mark'** ■ Vigorous alpine Auricula primula with oval, vibrant green leaves, to 12cm (5in) long. In spring, bears salverform, light-centred, wine-purple to pink flowers, 2.5cm (1in) across. Cultivation group 4. ↕↔ 10cm (4in). ***

***P.* 'Marven'.** Rosette-forming, evergreen or semi-evergreen perennial with white-mealy, ovate or obovate-oblong, light green leaves, to 10cm (4in) long. In spring, bears umbels of up to 15 tubular to funnel-shaped, deep violet-blue flowers, 3cm (1¼in) across, each with a very dark eye, bordered by a white-mealy zone. Cultivation group 4 or 5. ↕ 10cm (4in), ↔ 25cm (10in). ***

***P.* 'McWatt's Cream'.** Rosette-forming, evergreen or semi-evergreen Polyanthus Group primula with short scapes and spoon-shaped, deep green leaves, 12cm (5in) long. In spring, bears 3- to 12-flowered umbels of salverform cream flowers, 2cm (¾in) across. Cultivation group 1, 2, or 4. ↕ 10–15cm (4–6in), ↔ 30–40cm (12–16in). ***

P. melanops, syn. *P. chionantha* subsp. *melanops*. Rosette-forming, deciduous perennial with lance-shaped, toothed or scalloped, mid-green leaves, to 25cm (10in) long, white-mealy beneath. In late spring, white-mealy stems each bear 1 or 2 umbels of 5–12 narrowly tubular to bell-shaped, fragrant, black-eyed purple flowers, 2cm (¾in) across. Cultivation group 2 or 4. ↕ 35cm (14in), ↔ 50cm (20in). Alpine meadows in China. ***

P. minima. Dwarf, rosette-forming, evergreen perennial with wedge-shaped, leathery, sharply toothed, shiny, dark green leaves, to 3cm (1¼in) long. In late spring, very short stems each bear 1, sometimes 2 salverform, white-eyed, rose-pink, lilac, or white flowers, to 3cm (1¼in) across. Cultivation group 2 or 4. ↕ 7cm (3in), ↔ 20cm (8in). Alpine meadows in E. Alps and Balkans. ***

P

P. modesta. Rosette-forming, deciduous perennial with elliptic to spoon-shaped, wavy-margined or toothed, mid-green leaves, to 8cm (3in) long, white-mealy beneath. In spring and early summer, produces umbels of 2–15 salverform, purple-pink flowers, 1.5cm (½in) across. Cultivation group 1 or 4. ↕↔ 20cm (8in). Moist alpine meadows in Japan. ❄❄❄. **var. *faurieae*** ▣ is smaller, with yellow-eyed, pinkish purple flowers, and broadly ovate, white-mealy leaves with rolled back margins.

P. nana see *P. edgeworthii.*

***P. nutans* of gardens** see *P. flaccida.*

P. obconica. Erect, rosette-forming, evergreen perennial, usually grown as an annual, with fairly coarse, oval to heart-shaped, toothed, mid-green leaves, to 15cm (6in) long. In winter and spring, produces salverform, pink, lilac-blue, red, or white flowers, 2.5–5cm (1–2in) across, sometimes with slightly frilled petal margins, in whorls of decreasing size up stout, hairy stems. Contact with the foliage may irritate skin, and the foliage may cause mild stomach upset if ingested. Cultivation group 6. ↕ 23–40cm (9–16in), ↔ to 25cm (10in). China. ❄❄. **'Appleblossom'**, syn. 'Apricot Brandy', produces large flowers in pale pink, flushing to salmon-pink, then deeper red-pink; ↕ to 20cm (8in). **'Apricot Brandy'** see 'Appleblossom'. **Cantata Series** cultivars are long-blooming, with flowers in carmine-red, pink, rose-pink, apricot-pink, lavender-blue, or white; ↕ 25–30cm (10–12in); **'Cantata Lavender'** ▣ bears lavender-blue flowers. **'Pin Up'** has rose-pink flowers, and is free-flowering. **'Queen of the Market'** ▣ has red-pink flowers; ↕ to 20cm (8in).

***P.* 'Old Yellow Dusty Miller'.** Vigorous border Auricula primula with spoon-shaped, white-mealy, mid-green leaves, to 12cm (5in) long. In spring, produces salverform yellow flowers, 3cm (1¼in) across, with white-mealy eyes. Cultivation group 1. ↕ 15cm (6in), ↔ 25cm (10in). ❄❄❄

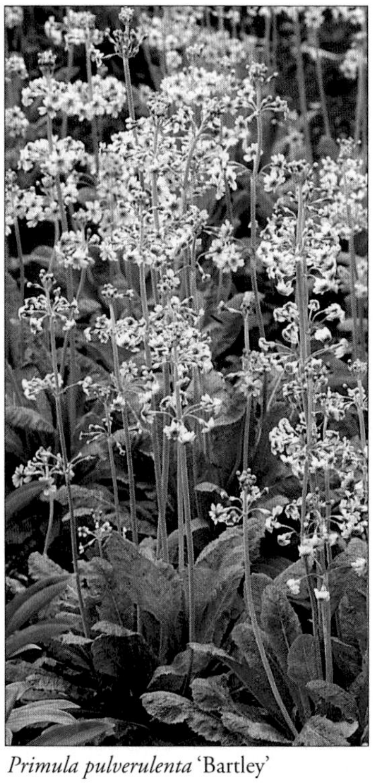

Primula pulverulenta 'Bartley'

***P.* 'Orb'.** Neat show Auricula primula with spoon-shaped or oval, dark green leaves, 12cm (5in) long. In spring, bears salverform, green-margined black flowers, 3cm (1¼in) across. Vigorous and easy to grow. Cultivation group 4. ↕↔ 10cm (4in). ❄❄❄

***P.* 'Our Pat'.** Rosette-forming, evergreen or semi-evergreen Polyanthus Group primula with oval, purple-tinted, bronze-green leaves, to 15cm (6in) long. Umbels of 3–8 rounded, double, dark claret-red flowers, 4cm (1½in) across, are produced very freely in spring. Cultivation group 1, 2, or 4. ↕ 10–15cm (4–6in), ↔ 30–40cm (12–16in). ❄❄❄

P. palinuri ▣ Rosette-forming, evergreen perennial with spoon-shaped to oblong-ovate, sometimes glandular-hairy, more or less toothed, fleshy, mid-green leaves, to 20cm (8in) long. In late winter and early spring, stout stems bear umbels of 3–40 nodding, narrowly funnel-shaped, scented yellow flowers, 1.5cm (½in) across, with white-mealy eyes. Cultivation group 1 or 4; requires full sun. ↕↔ 30cm (12in). Coastal cliffs in S. Italy. ❄❄❄

P. parryi. Rosette-forming, deciduous perennial with obovate to inversely lance-shaped, leathery, entire or finely toothed, mid-green leaves, to 35cm (14in) long, covered in short glands. In spring and summer, stout, erect stems bear one-sided umbels of 3–20 pendent, funnel-shaped, strongly scented, red-purple to magenta flowers, to 3cm (1¼in) across; these are yellow-eyed with dark haloes. Cultivation group 2 or 4. ↕↔ 45cm (18in). Shady mountain areas in W. USA. ❄❄❄

***P.* 'Peter Klein'.** Rosette-forming, semi-evergreen or deciduous perennial with rounded to ovate, bright mid-green leaves, to 6cm (2½in) long. In spring, stout stems produce umbels of 2–5 salverform, bright, deep pink flowers, 2.5cm (1in) across. Cultivation group 2 or 4. ↕↔ 15cm (6in). ❄❄❄

P. petiolaris ▣ Rosette-forming, evergreen perennial with spoon-shaped, finely toothed, mid-green leaves, to 10cm (4in) long. In spring, salverform, magenta-purple flowers, 2cm (¾in) across, yellow-eyed and with thin white borders, are borne singly on short stalks, 2–5cm (¾–2in) long. Cultivation group 3 or 4. ↕ 10cm (4in), ↔ 20cm (8in). Himalayas. ❄❄❄

***P.* Polyanthus Group** (Polyanthus). Rosette-forming, evergreen to semi-evergreen perennials of garden origin, with a complicated parentage believed to include *P. veris, P. elatior, P. vulgaris,* and the red-flowered European primula, *P. juliae.* They form sturdy rosettes of oval, heavily veined, dark green leaves, to 18cm (7in) long, almost corrugated in appearance. Large, salverform, mostly yellow-centred, red, blue, orange, yellow, white, or pink flowers, to 5cm (2in) across, are borne in umbels of 3–15 on thick, hairy stems, to 15cm (6in) long, from late winter to mid-spring. Some seed mixtures are available that produce hardy spring bedding plants. Cultivation group 1, 2, 4, or 6. **Cowichan Series** ▣ cultivars bear bronze-flushed foliage, and flowers in strong, velvety, yellow, blue, red, maroon, or purple, without central yellow eyes. **Crescendo Series** ▣ cultivars are winter-hardy, with large,

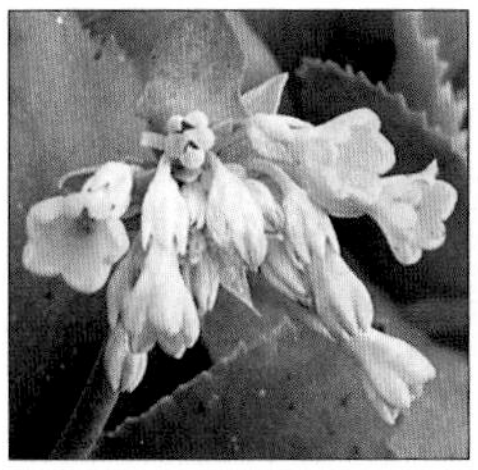

Primula palinuri

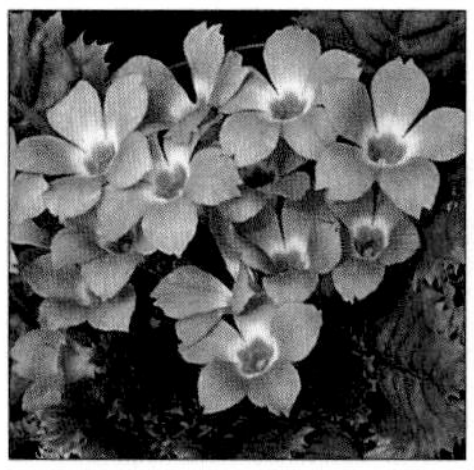

Primula petiolaris

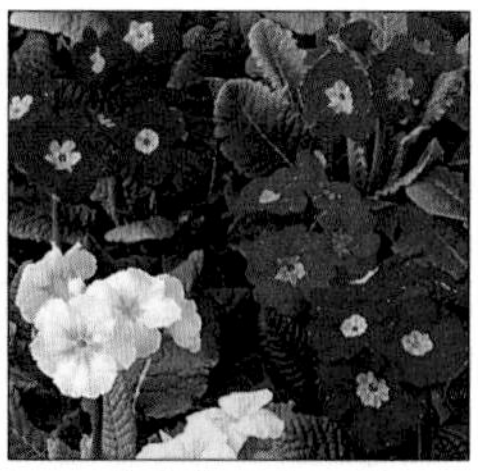

Primula Polyanthus Group Crescendo Series

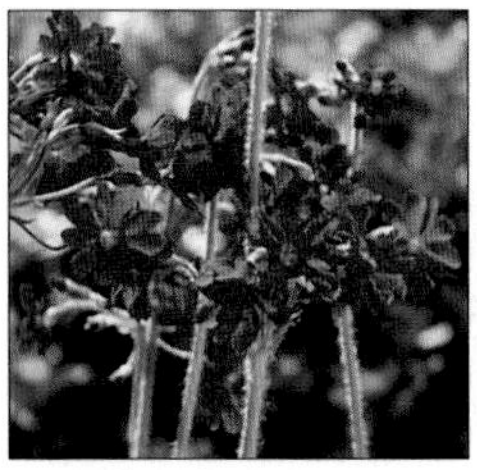

Primula polyneura

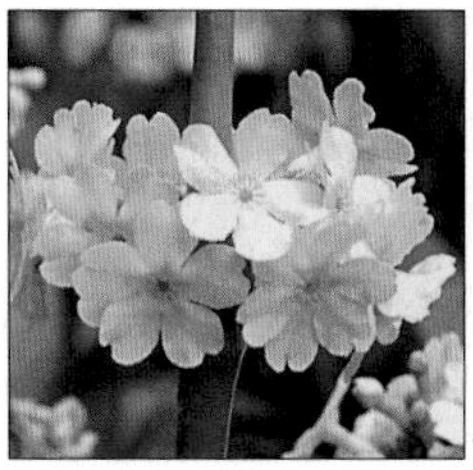

Primula prolifera

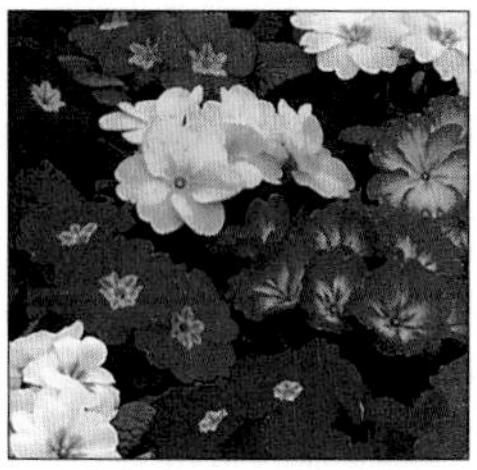

Primula Prominent Series

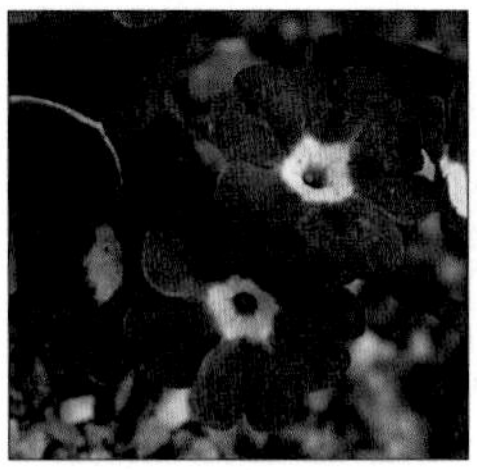

Primula x *pubescens* 'Mrs. J.H. Wilson'

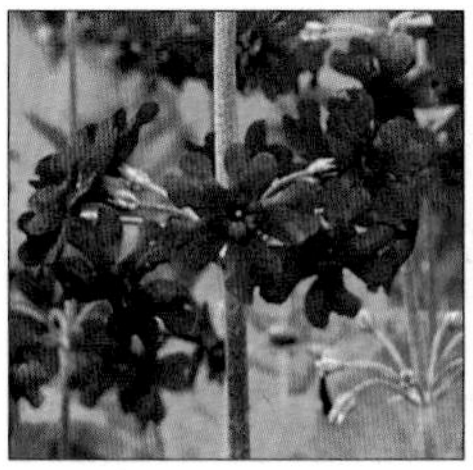

Primula pulverulenta

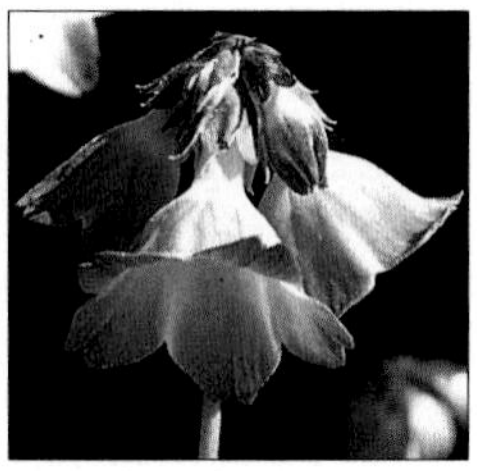

Primula reidii var. *williamsii*

yellow-centred flowers, 5cm (2in) across, available in a number of separate ranges, classified by colour. **Rainbow Series** cultivars are short-stemmed, with yellow-centred flowers in blue, creamy yellow, pink, carmine-red, scarlet-red, white, or yellow, as well as some unusual rusty orange shades.

P. polyneura ▣ Rosette-forming, deciduous perennial with ovate to rounded, 7- to 11-lobed, mid-green leaves, to 30cm (12in) long. Each stem produces 1–3 umbels, each with 2–12 salverform, yellow-eyed, purplish pink flowers, 2.5cm (1in) across, in late spring and summer. Cultivation group 2. ↕↔ 45cm (18in). Woodland in W. China. ❄❄❄

P. prolifera ▣♀ Rosette-forming, evergreen Candelabra primula with spoon- to diamond-shaped, finely toothed, deep green leaves, to 35cm (14in) long. In early summer, stout stems bear 1–7 whorls of 3–12 salverform, fragrant, white-mealy, pale to golden yellow or occasionally dull violet flowers, 2.5cm (1in) across. Cultivation group 2. ↕↔ 60cm (24in). Moist, shady alpine areas from India (Assam) to S.W. China, N. Burma, and Indonesia (Sumatra, Java). ❄❄❄

***P.* Prominent Series** ▣ Dwarf, compact, semi-evergreen or evergreen perennials with inversely lance-shaped to obovate, mid-green leaves, 10cm (4in) long. In mid- and late winter, salverform flowers, 4–5cm (1½–2in) across, are borne in a very wide range of colours, including bicolours. Cultivation group 6. ↕ 8–10cm (3–4in), ↔ 15–20cm (6–8in). ❄

P.* x *pubescens ♀ (*P. auricula* x *P. hirsuta*). Vigorous, rosette-forming, evergreen perennial with obovate to broadly spoon-shaped, sometimes entire, white-mealy, usually mid-green leaves, to 10cm (4in) long. Umbels of few to many salverform flowers, 1.5–2.5cm (½–1in) across, in white, yellow, pink, red, purple, or brown, are borne very freely in spring. Cultivation group 1 or 4. ↕ to 15cm (6in), ↔ 30cm (12in). Garden origin. ❄❄❄. **'Faldonside'** produces dusky red-pink flowers with white eyes; ↕ 7–10cm (3–4in). **'Harlow Car'** has shallowly toothed leaves and large, creamy white flowers, 3cm (1¼in) across; ↕ 7–10cm (3–4in). **'Mrs. J.H. Wilson'** ▣ bears compact rosettes of lance-shaped to obovate, rather thick, grey-green leaves, and fragrant, white-eyed purple flowers; ↕ 7cm (3in). **'Rufus'** has shallowly toothed, pale green leaves, and umbels of up to 16 large, almost brick-red flowers, to 3cm (1¼in) across, with golden yellow eyes; ↕ 8–10cm (3–4in).

P. pulverulenta ▣♀ Rosette-forming, deciduous Candelabra primula with obovate or inversely lance-shaped, finely toothed, mid-green leaves, to 30cm (12in) long. In late spring and early summer, stout, white-mealy stems each bear several whorls of tubular, deep red or red-purple flowers, 2.5cm (1in) across, with darker red or purple eyes. Cultivation group 2. ↕ to 1m (3ft), ↔ 60cm (24in). Wet hillsides in China (Sichuan). ❄❄❄. **'Bartley'** ▣♀ has shell-pink flowers with red eyes.

P. reidii. Robust, rosette-forming, deciduous perennial with oblong to oblong-lance-shaped, scalloped or lobed leaves, to 20cm (8in) long. In summer, bears compact umbels of 3–10 pendent, bell-shaped, fragrant white flowers, 2.5cm (1in) across, often white-mealy on the outsides. Cultivation group 3 or 4. ↕ 5–15cm (2–6in), ↔ 10–15cm (5–6in). N.E. India to C. Nepal (Himalayas). ❄❄❄. **var. *williamsii*** ▣ is more robust, producing flowers that

P

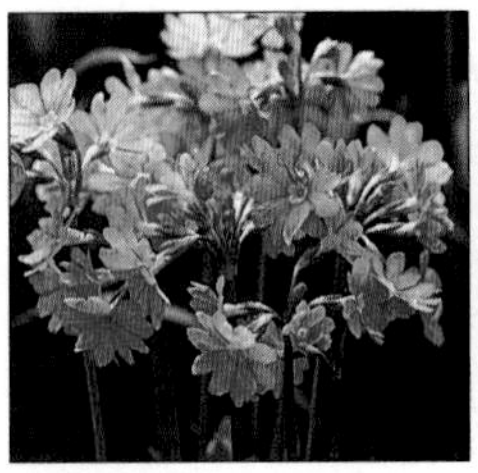
Primula rosea

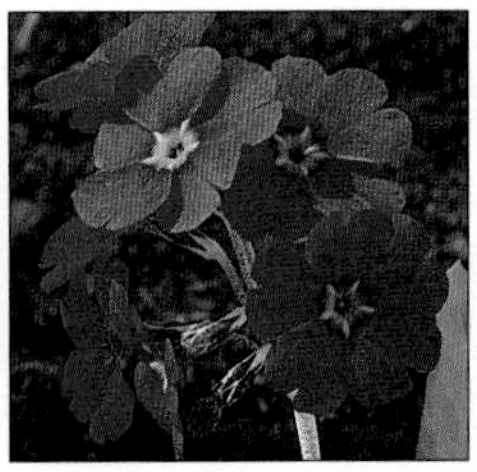
Primula rusbyi

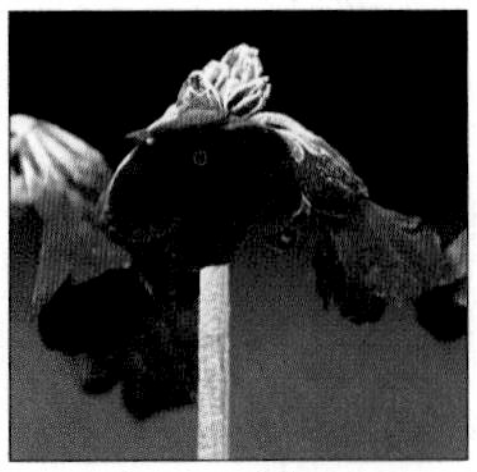
Primula secundiflora

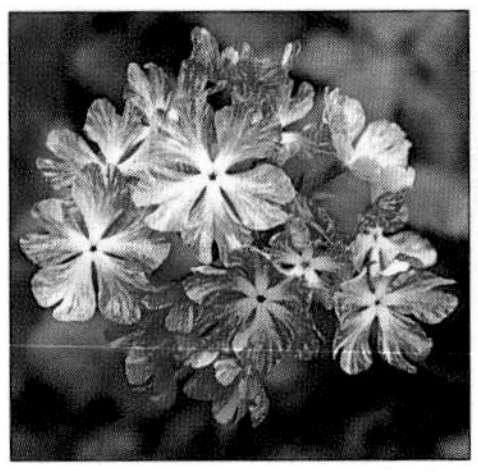
Primula sieboldii 'Wine Lady'

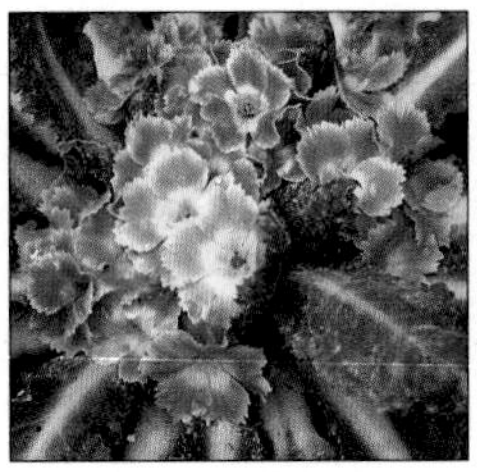
Primula sonchifolia

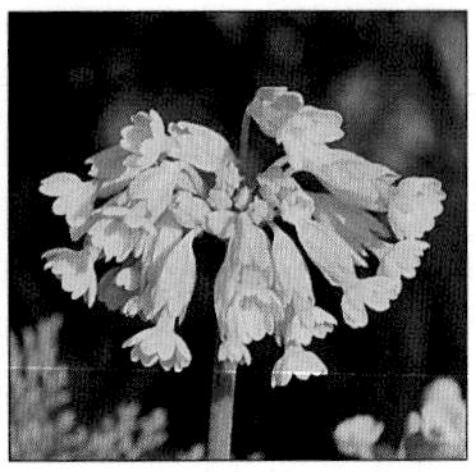
Primula veris

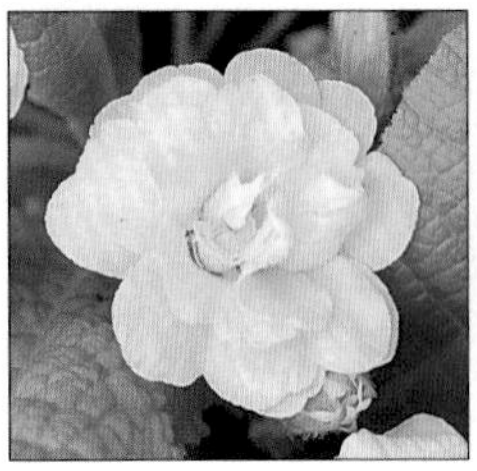
Primula vulgaris 'Double Sulphur'

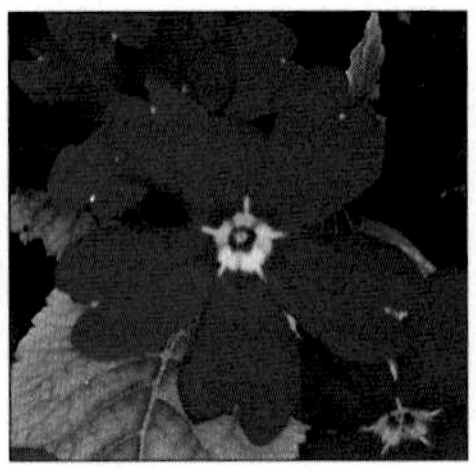
Primula 'Wanda'

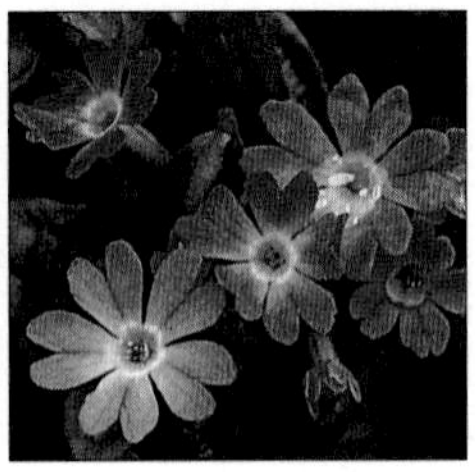
Primula warshenewskiana

are pale blue to white; ↕↔ 15cm (6in); W. and C. Nepal.

P. rosea ■ 🏆 Rosette-forming, deciduous perennial bearing obovate to inversely lance-shaped, scalloped or finely toothed, mid-green, often bronze-flushed leaves, to 20cm (8in) long, tinted red-bronze at first, emerging after the flowers. Umbels of 4–12 salverform, yellow-eyed, red-pink flowers, to 2.5cm (1in) across, are produced in spring. Cultivation group 2. ↕↔ 20cm (8in). Wet meadows from Afghanistan to Nepal. ❄❄❄. **'Grandiflora'** is vigorous, producing larger flowers, to 3cm (1¼in) across; ↕ to 20cm (8in).

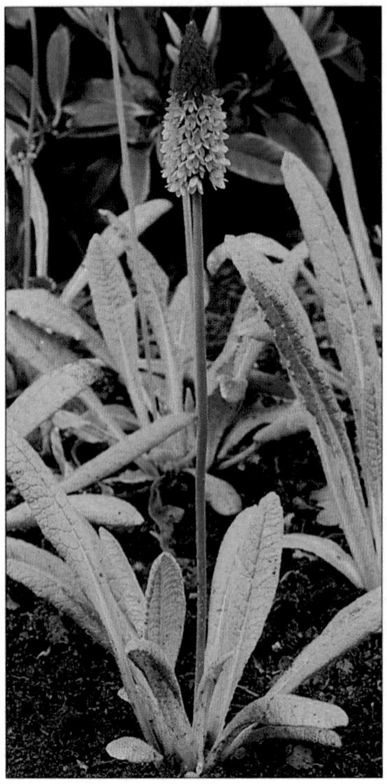
Primula vialii

P. rubra see *P. hirsuta*.

P. rusbyi ■ Rosette-forming, deciduous perennial with elliptic to spoon-shaped, entire or toothed, glandular-hairy, mid-green leaves, 3–10cm (1¼–4in) long. One-sided umbels of 4–12 salverform, rose-red to deep purple flowers, 3cm (1¼in) across, with incurved petals, are produced in spring and summer. Cultivation group 2 or 4. ↕ 20cm (8in), ↔ 35cm (14in). S.E. Arizona, S.W. New Mexico. ❄❄❄

P.* x *scapeosa (*P. bracteosa* x *P. scapigera*). Vigorous, rosette-forming perennial with oblong to spoon-shaped, toothed, mid-green leaves, to 15cm (6in) long. In spring, salverform, pink-purple flowers, 2.5cm (1in) across, are produced singly on short stalks. Cultivation group 3 or 4. ↕ 10cm (4in), ↔ 25cm (10in). Garden origin. ❄❄❄

***P.* 'Schneekissen'**, syn. *P.* 'Snow Cushion'. Very compact, rosette-forming, evergreen Primrose Group primula with rounded, pale green leaves, 10cm (4in) long. Short stems bear umbels of 3–8 salverform, pure white flowers, 2.5cm (1in) across, in spring. Cultivation group 1, 2, or 4. ↕ 8–10cm (3–4in), ↔ 20cm (8in). ❄❄❄

P. secundiflora ■ Rosette-forming, evergreen or semi-evergreen perennial with oblong to obovate or inversely lance-shaped, mid-green leaves, to 30cm (12in) long, with scalloped to toothed margins, and yellow-mealy beneath when young. In summer, stout stems produce one-sided umbels of 5–20 nodding, tubular to bell-shaped, red-purple or deep rose-red flowers, 2.5cm (1in) across. Cultivation group 2. ↕ 60–90cm (24–36in), ↔ 60cm (24in). Wet alpine meadows in S.E. Tibet and W. China. ❄❄❄

P. sieboldii 🏆 Rosette-forming, deciduous perennial with oblong-ovate, lobed, toothed, downy, pale green leaves, to 20cm (8in) long. In late spring and early summer, bears umbels of 2–15 salverform flowers, 2.5cm (1in) across; the flowers are rose-violet to lilac-purple or deep crimson, with white eyes, sometimes pure white. Cultivation group 2. ↕ 30cm (12in), ↔ 45cm (18in). Moist meadows and woodland in Japan. ❄❄❄. **'Musashino'** is vigorous, and bears large, pale rose-pink flowers, 3.5cm (1½in) across, darker beneath. **'Shi-un'** produces fringed flowers that are dark lavender-pink, fading to lavender-blue. **'Snowflake'** is vigorous, producing large white flowers, 3.5cm (1½in) across, with deeply cut petals. **'Sumina'** bears large, wisteria-blue flowers, 3cm (1¼in) across. **'Wine Lady'** ■ produces white flowers, flushed with purple-red.

P. sikkimensis (Himalayan cowslip). Rosette-forming, deciduous perennial with oblong to lance-shaped, elliptic or oblong to inversely lance-shaped, toothed, shining, pale green leaves, to 30cm (12in) long. Produces umbels of numerous pendent, funnel-shaped, white-mealy, yellow or cream flowers, 2.5cm (1in) across, in late spring and early summer. Cultivation group 2. ↕ 60–90cm (24–36in), ↔ 60cm (24in). Wet meadows in Himalayas (W. Nepal to S.W. China). ❄❄❄

P. sinensis. Erect, rosette-forming, evergreen perennial, usually grown as an annual, bearing broadly ovate to rounded, toothed, hairy, bright mid-green leaves, 8–10cm (3–4in) long, often red beneath. In winter and early spring, bears salverform, wavy-margined, purple to pink flowers, to 4cm (1½in) across, in 6- to 10-flowered whorls of decreasing size on thick, hairy stems. ↕↔ 15–20cm (6–8in). Cultivation group 6. Possibly N. China. ❄. **Single Superb Mixed** has flowers in white, pink, red, and lilac-blue; ↕ to 25cm (10in), ↔ to 15cm (6in).

P. sinopurpurea. Rosette-forming, deciduous perennial with oblong-lance-shaped, mid-green leaves, 5–35cm (2–14in) long, yellow-mealy beneath. In late spring and early summer, produces nodding, tubular to funnel-shaped, magenta, purple, and violet flowers, to 3cm (1¼in) across, with pale purple eyes, in umbels of 6–12. Cultivation group 2. ↕ 30–45cm (12–18in), ↔ 30–35cm (12–14in). China. ❄❄❄.

***P.* 'Snow Cushion'** see *P.* 'Schneekissen'.

P. sonchifolia ■ Rosette-forming, deciduous perennial with oblong to obovate, mid-green leaves, to 20cm (8in) long, with small, toothed lobes. In spring, very short stems (elongating in fruit) bear umbels of 3–20 salverform, yellow-eyed, white-margined, lavender-blue flowers, 2.5cm (1in) across. Overwinters as large, white-mealy buds. Cultivation group 3 or 4. ↕ 5cm (2in), ↔ 30cm (12in). Open meadows near the snow line in China, S.E. Tibet, and Burma. ❄❄❄

P. suffrutescens. Mat-forming, evergreen perennial with long rhizomes, and rosettes of wedge-shaped to spoon-shaped, scalloped to toothed, fleshy, dusky green leaves, to 5cm (2in) long. In summer, produces umbels of 2–10 salverform, yellow-eyed, rose-pink to red or purple flowers, 2cm (¾in) across. Cultivation group 1 or 4. ↕ 15cm (6in), ↔ 30cm (12in). USA (California, Sierra Nevada mountains). ❄❄❄

***P.* 'Tawny Port'.** Very dwarf, rosette-forming, evergreen or semi-evergreen Polyanthus Group primula bearing rounded to oval, toothed, maroon-green leaves, 15cm (6in) long. Short stems produce salverform, dark port-wine-coloured flowers, 3.5cm (1½in) across, singly or in umbels of up to 5, over a long period from early to late spring. Cultivation group 1, 2, or 4. ↕ 10–15cm (4–6in), ↔ 15–20cm (6–8in). ❄❄❄

P. veris ■ 🏆 (Cowslip). Very variable, rosette-forming, evergreen or semi-evergreen perennial with oblong-ovate to ovate, sometimes scalloped, mid-green leaves, to 20cm (8in) long. In mid- and late spring, produces umbels of 2–16 salverform, nodding, fragrant, deep yellow flowers, 1.5–2.5cm (½–1in) across. Cultivation group 1 or 2. ↕↔ 25cm (10in). Europe to W. Asia. ❄❄❄

P. vialii ■ 🏆 Rosette-forming, deciduous, often short-lived perennial with broadly lance-shaped to oblong, toothed, softly hairy, mid-green leaves, to 30cm (12in) long. Stiff, stout, white-mealy stems produce dense spikes, to 15cm (6in) long, of many pendent, tubular, blue-violet flowers, 1cm (½in) across, in summer. In bud, the calyces are bright crimson. Cultivation group 2. ↕ 30–60cm (12–24in), ↔ 30cm (12in). Moist mountain areas in China (Sichuan, Yunnan). ❄❄❄

P. villosa. Rosette-forming, evergreen perennial bearing obovate or spoon-shaped to oblong, toothed, fleshy, glandular-hairy leaves, 2–15cm (¾–6in) long. In early summer, red-hairy stems produce umbels of 4–12 salverform, white-eyed, pink to lilac flowers, to 2.5cm (1in) across. Cultivation group 2 or 4. ↕↔ 15cm (6in). Austria (Tyrol). ❄❄❄

P. vulgaris (Primrose). Rosette-forming, evergreen or semi-evergreen perennial with inversely lance-shaped to obovate, toothed to scalloped, deeply veined, bright green leaves, to 25cm (10in) long, softly hairy beneath. From early to late spring, produces clusters of 3–25 salverform, often fragrant, usually pale yellow flowers, 2.5–4cm (1–1½in) across. Cultivation group 2. ↕ 20cm (8in), ↔ 35cm (14in). Open woodland

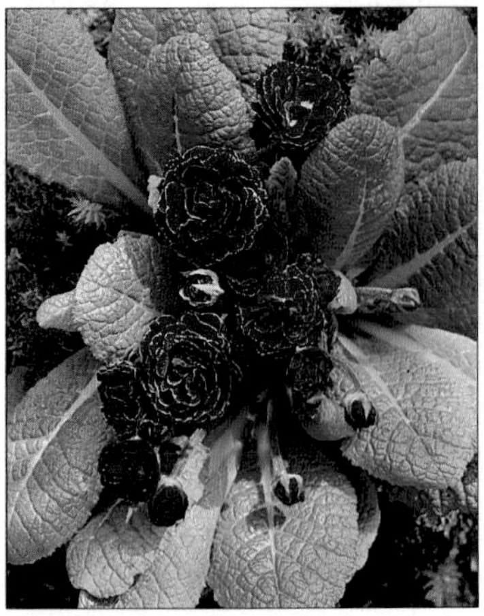
Primula vulgaris 'Miss Indigo'

and shady banks in Europe and W. Turkey. ❄❄❄. Many cultivars have been produced, of which some are hybrids, but with a similar habit to the species, and with double flowers. **'Alba Plena'**, syn. 'Double White', is vigorous and free-flowering, with fully double white flowers on long stalks. **'Double Sulphur'** ■ is vigorous, bearing sage-green leaves and double yellow flowers. **'Double White'** see 'Alba Plena'. **'Jack in the Green'** has single yellow blooms, each backed by a ring of bract-like leaves. **'Ken Dearman'** produces double orange flowers, flushed with shades of yellow and copper. **'Marie Crousse'** is vigorous, with large, scented, double violet flowers, 3cm (1¼in) across, splashed with white. **'Miss Indigo'** ■ is vigorous, and bears double, deep rich purple flowers with creamy white tips. **subsp. *sibthorpii*** ■ 🏆 has wedge-shaped leaves, with usually rose-pink, red, lilac, purple, or white flowers; Balkans, Ukraine (Crimea), Caucasus, Turkey, Armenia.

***P.* 'Wanda'** ■ 🏆 Very vigorous, long-flowering, rosette-forming, evergreen or semi-evergreen perennial with oval, toothed, purplish green leaves, to 12cm (5in) long. Produces clusters of solitary, salverform, dark claret-red flowers, to 3.5cm (1½in) across, in spring. Thrives well in both sun and shade. Cultivation group 1 or 2. ↕10–15cm (4–6in), ↔ 30–40cm (12–16in). ❄❄❄

***P.* Wanda Supreme Series** ■ Evergreen or semi-evergreen perennials bearing small, inversely lance-shaped to obovate, bronze to dark green leaves, 8–10cm (3–4in) long. From winter to mid-spring, bears flowers, 4–5cm (1½–2in) across, in a mixture of different shades of blue, yellow, purple, burgundy, red, rose, and pink bicolours. Cultivation group 1 or 2. ↕8–10cm (3–4in), ↔ 15cm (6in). ❄❄

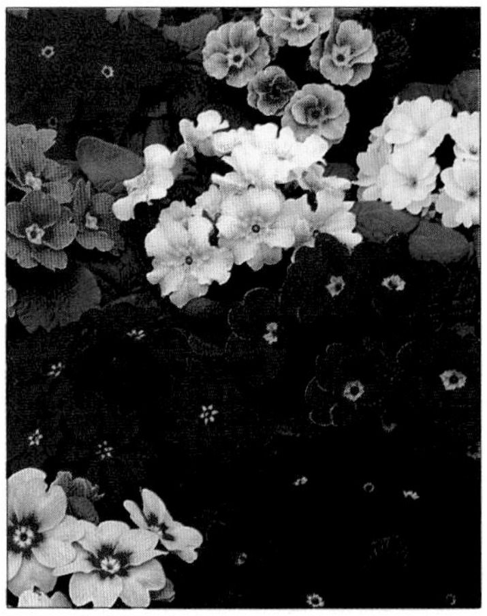

Primula Wanda Supreme Series

P. warshenewskiana ■ Rosette-forming, deciduous perennial with oblong to inversely lance-shaped, finely toothed, dark green leaves, to 7cm (3in) long. Salverform, rose-pink flowers, 1.5cm (½in) across, with white-ringed yellow eyes, are borne singly or in umbels of up to 8, on short stems in late spring to summer. Cultivation group 2 or 4. ↕7cm (3in), ↔ 15cm (6in). Streamsides and wet ground from Tajikistan to Pakistan. ❄❄❄

P. wilsonii* var. *anisodora see *P. anisodora.*

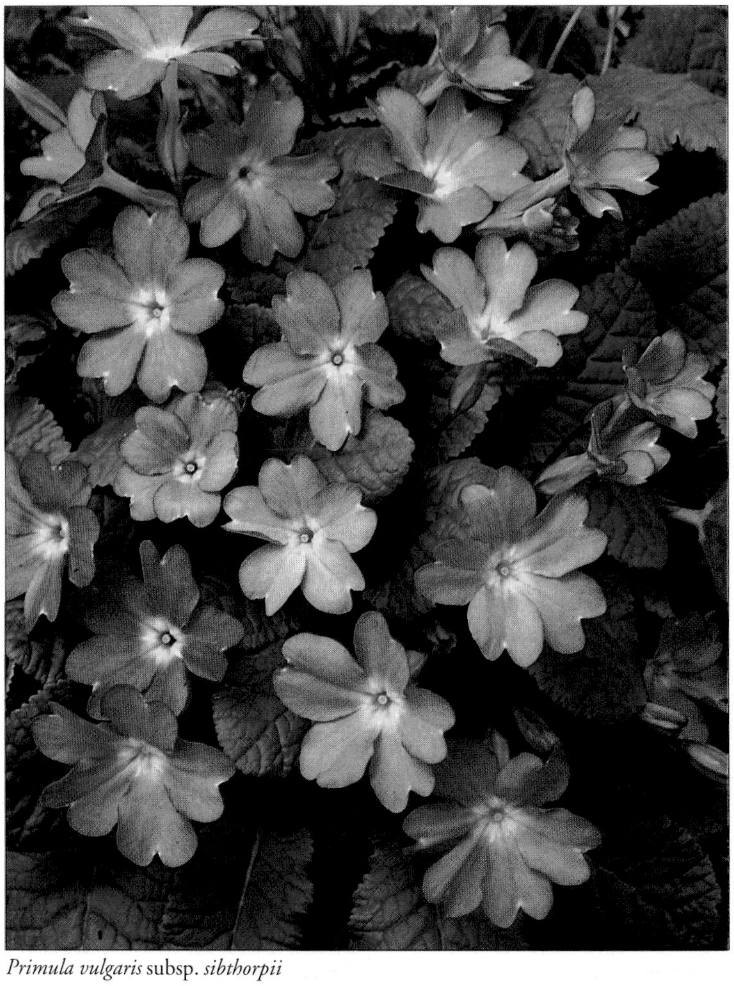

Primula vulgaris subsp. *sibthorpii*

P. wulfeniana. Rosette-forming, evergreen perennial with lance-shaped or elliptic to inversely lance-shaped or obovate, leathery, glandular-hairy, dark green leaves, 1.5–4cm (½–1½in) long. In spring, produces solitary or paired, salverform, rose-red to lilac flowers, to 2.5cm (1in) across, with deeply notched petal lobes. Cultivation group 4 or 5. ↕7cm (3in), ↔ 8cm (3in). Austrian Alps to S. Carpathians. ❄❄❄

P. yargongensis see *P. involucrata* subsp. *yargongensis.*

▷**Primula, Drumstick** see *Primula denticulata*

▷**Prince's feather** see *Amaranthus cruentus, Persicaria orientale*

▷**Princess feather** see *Persicaria orientale*

▷**Princess tree** see *Paulownia tomentosa*

PRINSEPIA

ROSACEAE

Genus of 4 species of arching, spiny, deciduous shrubs found in woodland and thickets in the Himalayas and China. They are cultivated for their linear to elliptic or oblong-lance-shaped leaves, which are rich green on opening, later glossy or dull dark green. They are also valued for their fragrant, cup-shaped, white to yellow flowers, and for their cherry-like, spherical or ovoid, purple or red fruits. Grow in a shrub border, against a wall, or as a hedge; the leaves appear early, and are an excellent foil for other early flowering shrubs.

• **HARDINESS** Fully hardy.

• **CULTIVATION** Grow in fertile, well-drained but not dry soil in full sun, in an open position with room to spread. Pruning group 1; cut out dead wood in summer.

• **PROPAGATION** Sow seed in containers in an open frame in autumn. Take greenwood cuttings in early summer.

• **PESTS AND DISEASES** Trouble free.

P. uniflora ■ Spreading, deciduous shrub with arching shoots bearing sharp spines and alternate, narrowly oblong to linear-oblong, glossy, rich dark green leaves, to 6cm (2½in) long. From early spring to summer, cup-shaped, fragrant white flowers, 1.5cm (½in) across, are produced singly or in clusters of up to 8, along the shoots; they are followed by cherry-like, red or purple fruit, 1cm (½in) across. ↕1.5m (5ft), ↔ 2.5m (8ft). China (N.W. China, Inner Mongolia). ❄❄❄

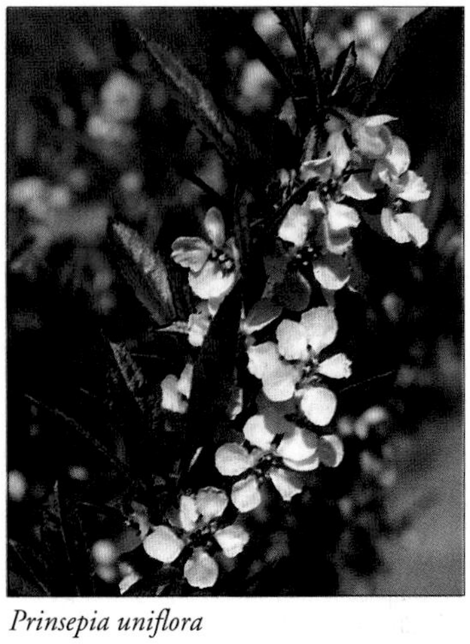

Prinsepia uniflora

PRITCHARDIA

ARECACEAE/PALMAE

Genus of about 37 species of single-stemmed palms from upland areas with high rainfall, on moist hillsides, and in rainforest valleys on volcanic soils in Fiji, Hawaii, and adjacent Pacific islands. They are cultivated for their fan-shaped, rich, mid-green or silvery or greyish green leaves, which are borne in terminal tufts. They produce small, bell-shaped, white, cream, yellow, or orange flowers in spikes or panicles between the leaves. In frost-prone climates, grow in a warm greenhouse. In tropical areas, they are suitable for growing as lawn specimens or in other strategic sites.

• **HARDINESS** Frost tender.

• **CULTIVATION** Under glass, grow in loam-based potting compost (JI No.3) with added sharp sand, in bright filtered light. During the growing season, water freely and apply a liquid feed every month; water sparingly in winter. Outdoors, grow in fertile, moist but well-drained soil in partial shade.

• **PROPAGATION** Sow seed at 24°C (75°F) in spring.

• **PESTS AND DISEASES** Prone to scale insects and red spider mites under glass.

P. gaudichaudii ■ 🌴 Small palm with an erect, columnar trunk and long-stalked, fan-shaped leaves, 1–1.2m (3–4ft) long, deeply cut into many slender lobes, brown-hairy beneath, rich to silvery green above. Bell-shaped yellow flowers are borne in spikes up to 1m (3ft) long, usually in summer. ↕2–5m (6–15ft), ↔ 2.5–3.5m (8–11ft). Hawaii. ❀ (min. 16–18°C/61–64°F)

P. pacifica 🌴 (Fiji fan palm). Small to medium-sized palm with a smooth, slim, columnar trunk. Long-stalked, fan-shaped leaves, 1m (3ft) or more long, are white-downy when young, then smooth, rich green; they are divided for about one-third of their length into slender, pointed lobes. Bell-shaped, white to yellow flowers are borne in stiff panicles, 1m (3ft) long, in summer. ↕to 10m (30ft), ↔ 4–5m (12–15ft). Fiji. ❀ (min. 16–18°C/61–64°F)

▷**Privet** see *Ligustrum*
Amur see *L. amurense*
Chinese see *L. lucidum*
Common see *L. vulgare*
Golden see *L. ovalifolium* 'Aureum'
Japanese see *L. japonicum*

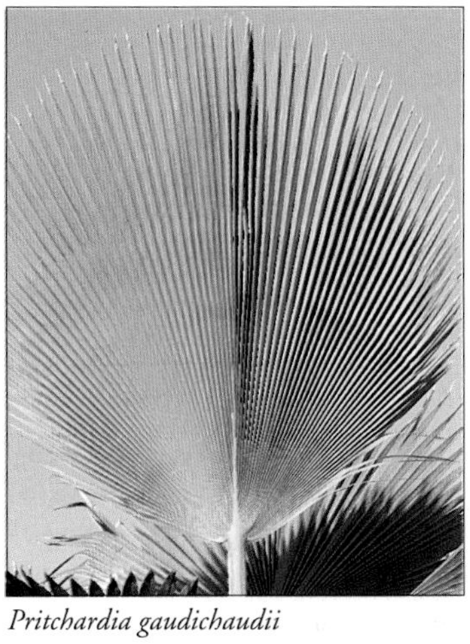

Pritchardia gaudichaudii

P

PROBOSCIDEA

syn. MARTYNIA

Elephant's tusk, Proboscis flower, Unicorn plant

PEDALIACEAE

Genus of about 9 species of erect to spreading, robust, frequently sticky-hairy annuals and perennials found in open plains in tropical North, Central, and South America. They are grown for the tropical effect of their foliage and fruits; the fruits can be dried and used for winter arrangements. The opposite, occasionally alternate, long-stemmed, fairly coarse leaves are rounded to ovate-lance-shaped, entire to palmately or pinnately lobed, and strongly veined. The flowers are borne in racemes, and are funnel- to bell-shaped, 5-lobed, reddish purple, lavender-pink, creamy white, or orange-yellow, with enclosing calyces split to the bases on one side; they are followed by unusually shaped fruits, which each have a pair of strongly upcurved, slender, horn-like beaks or projections at one end, and a fringed crest along the centre of the capsule body. The cultivated species are annuals, and are suitable for a mixed border; they may also be grown as decorative container plants in a cool or temperate greenhouse or conservatory.

• **HARDINESS** Half hardy.

• **CULTIVATION** Under glass, grow in loam-based potting compost (JI No.2) in full light. During the growing season, water freely and apply a balanced liquid fertilizer every 4 weeks. Discard after flowering. Outdoors, grow in fertile, moist but well-drained soil in full sun.

• **PROPAGATION** Sow seed at 21–24°C (70–75°F) in spring.

• **PESTS AND DISEASES** Trouble free.

P. fragrans. Spreading, thick-stemmed, softly hairy annual bearing rounded, broadly ovate to broadly triangular, 5-lobed leaves, to 25cm (10in) long. In summer, produces loose racemes of 8–20 funnel-shaped, fragrant, reddish purple to purple flowers, to 5cm (2in) across; the upper lobes are marked dark purple, each with a strong yellow band extending into the throat. The flowers are followed by narrow, canoe-shaped, crested fruit, to 6cm (2½in) long, with beak-like projections, to 18cm (7in) long, at one end. ↕ to 45cm (18in), ↔ to 90cm (36in). USA (Texas) to Mexico. ✻

P. jussieui see *P. louisianica.*

P. louisianica, syn. *P. jussieui*, *P. proboscidea* (Common devil's claw, Common unicorn plant, Ram's horn). Erect to spreading, thick-stemmed, softly hairy annual with rounded to broadly ovate, unlobed, wavy-margined leaves, 6–20cm (2½–8in) long. In summer, bears open racemes of 8–20 funnel-shaped, creamy white to purple flowers, 3.5–5cm (1½–2in) across, flecked reddish purple and marked yellow within the throats; they are followed by crested, boat-shaped fruit, 10–20cm (4–8in) long, each with a pair of horn-like projections at one end that are longer than the fruit body. ↕ to 45cm (18in), ↔ to 90cm (36in). C. and S.E. USA. ✻

P. proboscidea see *P. louisianica.*

▷**Proboscis flower** see *Proboscidea*

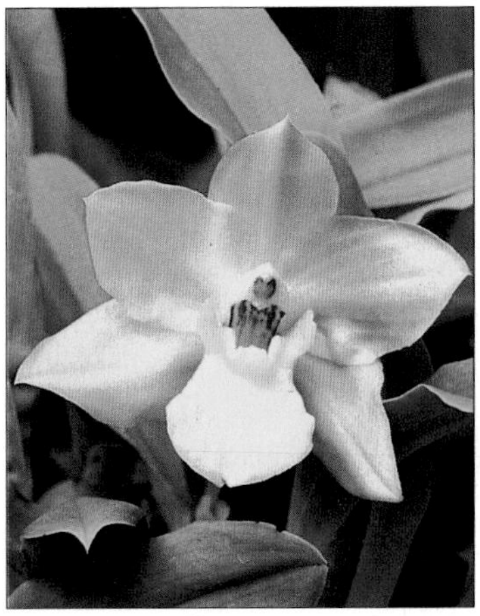

Promenaea xanthina

PROMENAEA

ORCHIDACEAE

Genus of about 15 species of small, evergreen, epiphytic orchids from Brazil, occurring in forest areas at an altitude of around 1,500m (5,000ft). They produce oval pseudobulbs with 1–3 soft-textured, ovate-lance-shaped, light green, apical leaves. Usually yellow or white flowers are borne in ones or twos, rarely more, in short racemes from the bases of the pseudobulbs, mostly in summer and autumn.

• **HARDINESS** Frost tender.

• **CULTIVATION** Cool-growing orchids. Grow in small pots of epiphytic orchid compost made with fine bark, or epiphytically on slabs of bark. During summer, provide high humidity and bright filtered light, water freely (taking care not to overwater), and feed at every third watering. In winter, admit full light and water sparingly. See also p.46.

• **PROPAGATION** Divide when the plant fills the pot and "flows" over the sides, or remove backbulbs.

• **PESTS AND DISEASES** Prone to red spider mites, aphids, and mealybugs.

P. xanthina ■ Epiphytic orchid with clustered, oval pseudobulbs each with 2 broadly oval, soft-textured, light green leaves, 5cm (2in) long. Fragrant, lemon-yellow flowers, 4cm (1½in) across, with red-dotted lips, are borne in summer. ↕ 8cm (3in), ↔ 15cm (6in). Brazil. ❀ (min. 13°C/55°F; max. 30°C/86°F)

▷**Propeller plant** see *Crassula perfoliata* var. *minor*

▷**Prophet flower** see *Arnebia pulchra*

▷***Prosartes*** see *Disporum*

PROSTANTHERA

Mint bush

LABIATAE/LAMIACEAE

Genus of 50 species of bushy, evergreen shrubs and small trees from heathland and dry forest to rainforest and seashore (some species at subalpine and alpine level) in Australia. They are grown for their simple, entire or toothed, aromatic leaves, borne in opposite pairs, and leafy, terminal racemes or panicles of broadly tubular, cup- or bell-shaped, 2-lipped, 5-lobed, white, blue, or purple, occasionally red, yellow, or green flowers. In frost-prone climates, grow all but *P. cuneata* in a cool greenhouse. In

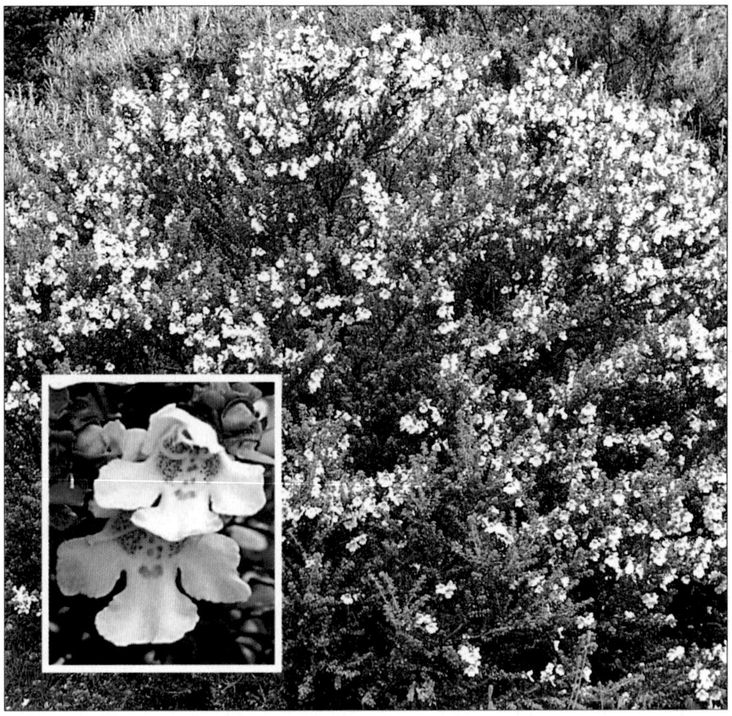

Prostanthera cuneata (inset: flower detail)

warmer areas, grow in a mixed or shrub border, or at the base of a house wall.

• **HARDINESS** Frost hardy to half hardy.

• **CULTIVATION** Under glass, grow in loam-based potting compost (JI No.2) in full light. When in growth, water moderately and apply a balanced liquid fertilizer monthly; water sparingly in winter. Outdoors, grow in moderately fertile, moist but well-drained soil in full sun. Pruning group 8, after flowering; hard pruning may be detrimental.

• **PROPAGATION** Sow seed at 13–18°C (55–64°F) in spring, or take semi-ripe cuttings in summer.

• **PESTS AND DISEASES** Prone to red spider mites and whiteflies under glass.

P. cuneata ■ 🏆 (Alpine mint bush). Bushy, erect to spreading shrub producing woody shoots. Tiny, obovate to rounded, entire leaves, 6mm (¼in) long, with wedge-shaped bases and rolled margins, are glossy, mid- to dark green, and strongly aromatic when crushed. In summer, bears racemes, 20cm (8in) long, of numerous broadly tubular white flowers, 1.5cm (½in) across, with purple and yellow markings within the wide tubes. ↕↔ 30–90cm (12–36in). Australia (subalpine and alpine levels from New South Wales to Tasmania). ✻✻

P. nivea (Snowy mint bush). Moderately bushy shrub, erect at first, then spreading, with slender, square-sectioned stems and entire, narrowly lance-shaped to linear, inrolled, bright green leaves, 2.5–4cm (1–1½in) long. In spring and early summer, bears bell-shaped, pure white, sometimes lavender-blue-tinted flowers, to 2cm (¾in) across, in racemes to 15cm (6in) long. ↕ 2–3m (6–10ft), ↔ 1.5–2m (5–6ft). S.E. Australia. ✻. **var. *induta*** produces lilac flowers and silvery green foliage.

P. ovalifolia ■ (Oval-leaved mint bush). Bushy shrub with erect stems and lance-shaped to inversely lance-shaped, entire, matt, grey-green leaves, to 1.5cm (½in) long. In late spring and early summer, an abundance of cup-shaped purple flowers, 1cm (½in) across, sometimes mauve, or white tinged with lilac, are borne in leafy, terminal racemes, 6–7cm (2½–3in) long. ↕ 2.5–4m (8–12ft), ↔ 1.5–2.5m (5–8ft). E. Australia. ✻

P. rotundifolia ■ 🏆 (Round-leaved mint bush). Bushy, spreading shrub

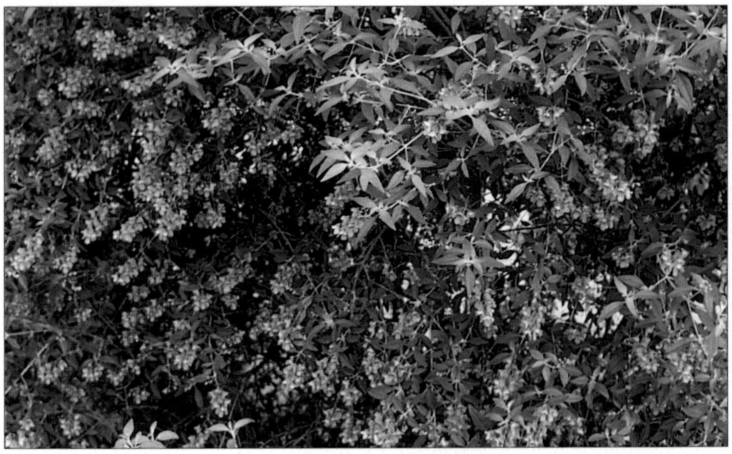

Prostanthera ovalifolia

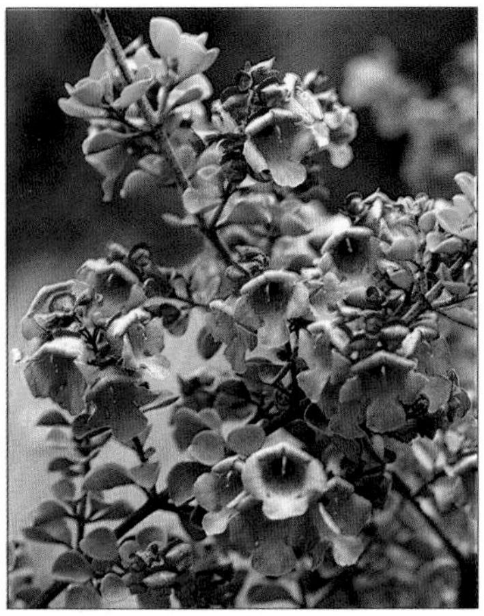

Prostanthera rotundifolia

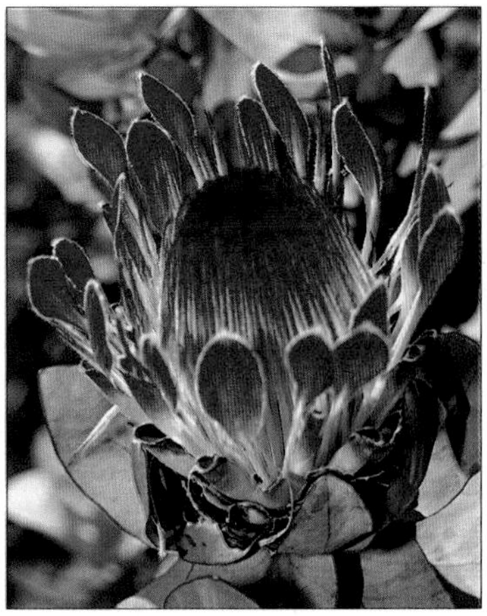

Protea eximia

with slender, hoary stems and rounded to ovate, scarcely toothed leaves, to 1.5cm (½in) long, deep green above, paler beneath. In late spring and early summer, bears bell-shaped, purple to lilac-purple flowers, 1cm (½in) across, in numerous short racemes, to 7cm (3in) long. ↕ 2–4m (6–12ft), ↔ 1–3m (3–10ft). S.E. Australia (including Tasmania). ✻. **var. *rosea***, syn. 'Chelsea Girl', produces grey-green leaves and light rose-pink flowers with mauve anthers.

PROTEA

PROTEACEAE

Genus of 115 species of evergreen shrubs and, rarely, small, usually upright trees found on rocky hillsides and dry scrub from tropical Africa to South Africa. The leaves are alternate to spiralling, simple, entire, and leathery. Proteas are cultivated for their usually solitary and terminal, mainly cone-like clusters or flat heads of small flowers surrounded by petal-like, green, white, pink to purple, or yellow bracts, each cluster resembling a single, large flower. Each floret is tubular, splitting into 4 sepals to reveal the long, straight or curved, usually coloured style. In frost-prone areas, grow in a cool, well-ventilated greenhouse. In warmer areas, use in a mixed or shrub border. Larger species are also fine specimen plants.

- **HARDINESS** Half hardy to frost tender.
- **CULTIVATION** Under glass, grow in a mixture of 1 part loam with added charcoal and 3 parts equal measures of grit (or perlite) and peat, in full light. Water moderately during spring and summer; apply a liquid fertilizer of magnesium sulphate and urea, both at half recommended strength, once in spring and again in early autumn. Water sparingly in winter. Outdoors, grow in poor, neutral to acid, well-drained soil in full sun. Pruning group 1; may need restrictive pruning under glass.
- **PROPAGATION** Sow seed at 13–18°C (55–64°F) as soon as ripe or in spring, or take semi-ripe cuttings in summer.
- **PESTS AND DISEASES** Magnesium deficiency may result in chlorosis of the leaves. Die-back and general failure to thrive usually indicate that the rooting medium is too rich.

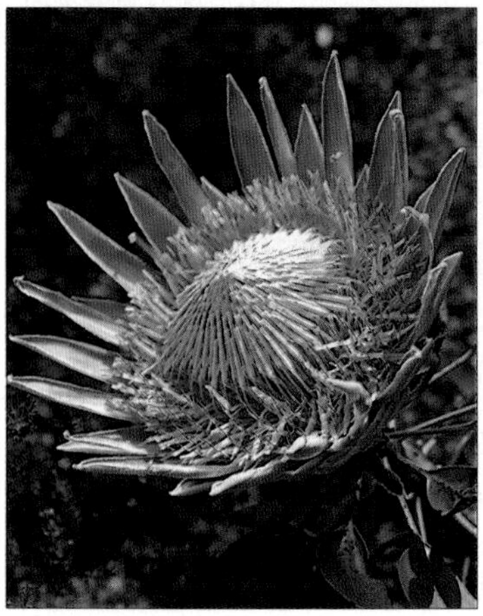

Protea cynaroides

P. barbata see *P. speciosa*.
P. barbigera see *P. magnifica*.
P. compacta. Erect, moderately bushy shrub with oblong to elliptic, stalkless, horny-margined leaves, 5–13cm (2–5in) long. In spring and summer, oblong buds open to obovoid flowerheads, 7–10cm (3–4in) across, with bright pink, rarely white bracts, fringed with white hairs. ↕ 2.5–3.5m (8–11ft), ↔ 1.5–2.5m (5–8ft). South Africa (Western Cape). ✻
P. cynaroides ▣ (King protea). Robust-stemmed, sparsely to moderately branched shrub, often spreading with age. Rounded to elliptic leaves are 8–14cm (3–5½in) long, and are borne on stalks 4–18cm (1½–7in) long. From late spring to summer, produces goblet- or bowl-shaped flowerheads, 12–30cm (5–12in) across, with deep crimson-red to pink or cream bracts. ↕↔ 1–2m (3–6ft). South Africa (Western Cape, Eastern Cape). ✻
P. eximia ▣ ♀ Large shrub or small tree, rounded to broadly columnar, with fairly robust, sparsely branched stems. Ovate leaves are purple-flushed, silvery green, and glaucous, 6–10cm (2½–4in) long, sometimes with red margins, and heart-shaped at the bases. In spring and summer, bears oblong to inversely cone-shaped flowerheads, to 14cm (5½in) across, with red or red-tinted pink bracts, fringed with white hairs. ↕ 3–5m (10–15ft), ↔ 2–3m (6–10ft). South Africa (Western Cape). ✻
P. longifolia, syn. *P. minor*. Erect to spreading shrub with linear, ascending, stalkless, mid- to deep green leaves, 9–20cm (3½–8in) long. During summer, produces oblong to inversely conical flowerheads, 10cm (4in) long, with greenish white to pink bracts, the inner ones fringed with hairs. ↕ 2–3m (6–10ft), ↔ 1.5–2.5m (5–8ft). South Africa (Western Cape). ✻
P. magnifica, syn. *P. barbigera* (Woolly-bearded protea). Erect shrub, often spreading when young, with robust stems and oblong or lance-shaped, wavy-margined, greyish green leaves, 10cm (4in) or more long. From spring to summer, produces densely packed flowerheads, 15cm (6in) across, initially narrowly bell-shaped, opening to cup-shaped, with black-tipped white inner bracts and clear pink outer bracts, fringed with white hairs. ↕↔ 1.5–2.5m (5–8ft). South Africa (Western Cape). ✻
P. mellifera see *P. repens*.
P. minor see *P. longifolia*.
P. repens ▣ ♀ syn. *P. mellifera* (Sugarbush). Erect, moderately bushy shrub or sometimes small tree bearing erect, linear to lance-shaped leaves, to 15cm (6in) long. From spring to summer, produces flowerheads, obovoid in bud, goblet-shaped when open, to 9cm (3½in) across, with hairless bracts, uniformly cream-white or tipped with dark red to pink, and coated with a sticky resin. ↕ 2–4m (6–12ft), ↔ 1.5–3m (5–10ft). South Africa (Western Cape, Eastern Cape). ✻
P. scolymocephala. Rounded shrub with linear to spoon-shaped, tapered, wavy-margined, olive-green leaves, 4–9cm (1½–3½in) long. From late spring to summer, bears bowl-shaped flowerheads, to 5cm (2in) across, with creamy green bracts flushed pink at the tips. ↕ 0.9–1.5m (3–5ft), ↔ 75–120cm (30–48in). South Africa (Western Cape). ✻
P. speciosa, syn. *P. barbata*. Erect, moderately branched shrub with elliptic, leathery, orange-margined, mid-green leaves, 11cm (4½in) long. From summer to autumn, bears oblong-goblet-shaped flowerheads, 8cm (3in) across, with bearded, bright pink to creamy yellow bracts, fringed with tawny brown hairs. ↕ 1m (3ft), ↔ 80cm (32in). South Africa (Western Cape). ✻

▷ **Protea,**
King see *Protea cynaroides*
Woolly-bearded see *Protea magnifica*

PRUMNOPITYS

PODOCARPACEAE

Genus of 10 species of dioecious, occasionally monoecious, evergreen, coniferous trees from forest in Puerto Rico through the Andes to southern Argentina, and from Malaysia to New Zealand. They are upright trees with whorled shoots, grown mainly for their linear or oblong, yew-like foliage. Male and female cones are borne at various times of the year: ovoid or cylindrical male cones are solitary or in groups of 2–20; spherical or ovoid female cones are solitary or borne in groups of up to 8. The fruits are like small, upright plums, but with only a thin, fleshy layer around the seed, and are borne in the leaf axils of short sideshoots. Grow as specimen trees or for hedging. In frost-prone areas, grow tender species in a cool or temperate greenhouse.

- **HARDINESS** Fully hardy to frost tender.
- **CULTIVATION** Grow in moderately fertile, moist but well-drained soil in full sun, with shelter from cold, drying winds. Clip hedges in early summer or midsummer.
- **PROPAGATION** Sow seed in containers outdoors in spring. Take semi-ripe cuttings in late summer.
- **PESTS AND DISEASES** Trouble free.

P. andina △ syn. *Podocarpus andinus* (Plum yew). Dioecious, ovoid tree, conical when young, frequently with several stems, with smooth, grey-brown bark and shoots that are green for 3 years. Linear, soft, dull bluish green leaves, 2–3cm (¾–1¼in) long, parted below the shoot, are more upright above, especially in the sun; each has 2 white bands beneath. Ovoid, white-tinged yellow male cones, 1–2.5cm (½–1in) long, are produced in racemes

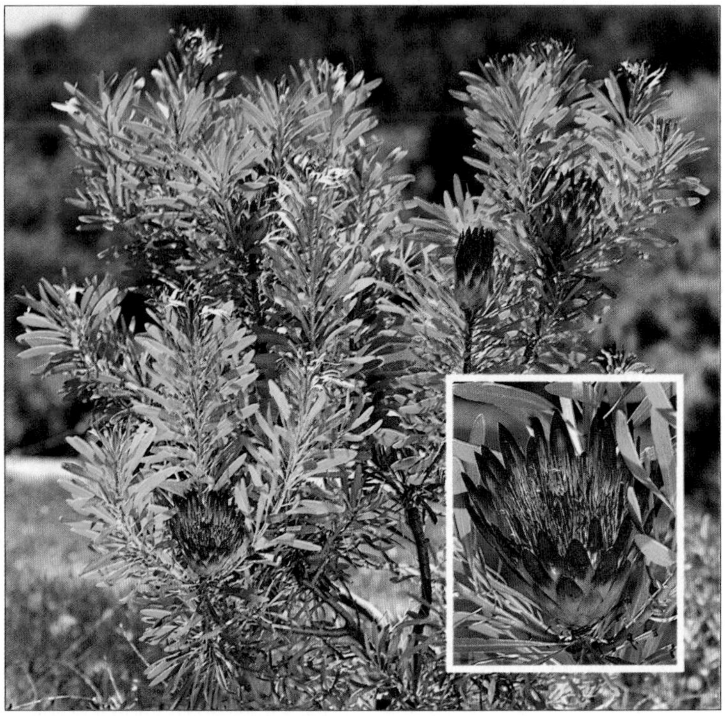

Protea repens (inset: flower detail)

of 5–20 at various times of the year. Plum-shaped, yellowish white fruit, 2cm (¾in) long, have thin, fleshy, edible layers. ↕ 10–20m (30–70ft), ↔ 6–8m (20–25ft). Chile, Argentina. ❄❄❄

PRUNELLA

Self-heal

LABIATAE/LAMIACEAE

Genus of 7 species of spreading, semi-evergreen perennials, rooting freely at the nodes, occurring on dry grassland, on sunny banks, and in open woodland in Europe, Asia, North Africa, and North America. They are grown for their dense, upright spikes or heads of tubular, 2-lipped, white, pink, or violet flowers. The leaves are linear-lance-shaped to broadly ovate, simple or deeply lobed, often rounded at the bases, and either basal or in tufts on the stems. Self-heals are useful ground-covering plants for banks, for the front of a border, or in a wild garden, where they attract bees and other beneficial insects. They are extremely vigorous, and must be sited where they will not swamp other, smaller plants.

- **HARDINESS** Fully hardy.
- **CULTIVATION** Grow in any soil in full sun or partial shade. Dead-head to prevent self-seeding.
- **PROPAGATION** Sow seed at 6–12°C (43–54°F) in spring. Divide in spring or autumn.
- **PESTS AND DISEASES** Susceptible to slugs and snails.

P. grandiflora ■ (Large self-heal). Vigorous, spreading perennial bearing simple, ovate to ovate-lance-shaped, sparsely toothed, deep green leaves, 10cm (4in) long. In summer, leafy stems produce whorls of purple flowers, to 3cm (1¼in) long, with darker lips, in dense, upright spikes. ↕ 15cm (6in), ↔ 1m (3ft) or more. Europe. ❄❄❄. **'Pink Loveliness'** produces clear pink flowers. **'White Loveliness'** produces pure white flowers.

P

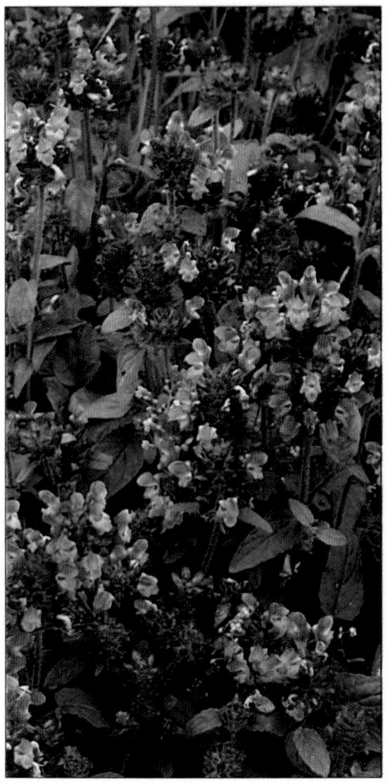

Prunella grandiflora

PRUNUS syn. AMYGDALUS

Ornamental cherry

ROSACEAE

Genus of more than 200 species of deciduous or evergreen, upright, rounded, or occasionally spreading trees or shrubs, widely distributed in N. temperate regions and to the Andes of South America and mountains of S.E. Asia. They occur mainly in woodland, woodland margins, and thickets, but also in a range of other habitats, including coastal sands, rocky places, and cliffs. They have alternate, broadly ovate to lance-shaped, elliptic, oblong, or obovate to almost rounded, usually toothed leaves. Ornamental cherries are cultivated mainly for their white, sometimes pink or red flowers, which are saucer-, bowl-, or cup-shaped, with 5 petals (more in semi-double or double forms); they are usually followed by fleshy, spherical or ovoid fruits. Some, such as *P. maackii* and *P. serrula*, are also grown for their shiny, coloured bark; many, including *P. sargentii*, have good autumn leaf colour. Certain *Prunus* species and cultivars, notably the plum (*P.* x *domestica*), cultivars of the almond (*P. dulcis*), and the peach (*P. persica*), are grown for their edible fruits. Leaves and fruits of most other species may cause severe discomfort if ingested.

They are excellent specimen trees, many being suitable for a small garden. Dense, bushy species, such as *P. laurocerasus* and *P. lusitanica*, are useful for screening and ground cover. *P. cerasifera*, *P.* x *cistena*, *P. incisa*, and *P. spinosa* are suitable for hedging. Grow shrubby species and their cultivars, such as *P. glandulosa* and *P. triloba*, against a wall or in a shrub border.

- **HARDINESS** Fully hardy to frost hardy.
- **CULTIVATION** Grow in any moist but well-drained, moderately fertile soil: deciduous species and cultivars in full sun, evergreens in full sun or partial shade. *P. glandulosa* needs hot sun to ripen its wood. *P. laurocerasus* may become chlorotic on shallow chalk soil. Pruning group 1 for trees and most deciduous shrubs (prune in midsummer in areas where silver leaf is a problem); group 5 for *P. glandulosa* and *P. triloba* (group 13 if wall-trained); group 8 for evergreen shrubs. Trim deciduous hedges after flowering, evergreens in early to mid-spring.
- **PROPAGATION** Sow seed of species in containers outdoors in autumn. Root greenwood cuttings of deciduous species in early summer, and semi-ripe cuttings of evergreens in midsummer, both with bottom heat. Bud cultivars in summer, or graft in early spring.
- **PESTS AND DISEASES** Susceptible to damage from aphids, caterpillars, and bullfinches. Diseases include peach leaf curl (on *P. dulcis* and *P. persica*), silver leaf, honey fungus, blossom wilt, and *Taphrina wiesneri*, which causes witches' brooms (abnormal, crowded shoots).

***P.* 'Accolade'** ■ 🏆 ○ Spreading, deciduous tree with oblong, tapered, dark green leaves, to 10cm (4in) long. Clusters of 3 semi-double, pale pink flowers, 4cm (1½in) across, open from dark pink buds in early spring. ↕↔ 8m (25ft). ❄❄❄

***P.* 'Amanogawa'** 🏆 ◊ Upright, deciduous tree bearing obovate leaves, to 12cm (5in) long, yellowish bronze in spring while still folded, often red, yellow, and green on the same tree, at the same time, in autumn. In late spring, bears dense clusters of saucer-shaped or semi-double, fragrant, pale pink flowers, 4cm (1½in) across, held vertically on stout stalks. ↕ 8m (25ft), ↔ 4m (12ft). ❄❄❄

P.* x *amygdalopersica ○ (*P. dulcis* x *P. persica*) syn. *P.* x *persicoides*. Spreading, deciduous tree bearing lance-shaped, tapered, mid-green leaves, to 12cm (5in) long, with sharply toothed margins. Solitary, saucer-shaped, light pink flowers, 5cm (2in) across, are borne in early and mid-spring, followed by spherical, peach-like, dry-fleshed green fruit, 4cm (1½in) across. ↕↔ 7m (22ft). Garden origin. ❄❄❄. **'Pollardii'** bears large, rich pink flowers in early spring.

P. avium ■ 🏆 ○ (Gean, Wild cherry). Spreading, deciduous tree with red-banded bark and ovate-oblong, dark green leaves, to 15cm (6in) long, bronze when young, turning red and yellow in autumn. Bowl-shaped white flowers, 3cm (1¼in) across, are borne in umbels in mid-spring, followed by heart-shaped to ovoid red fruit, 1cm (½in) across. ↕ 20m (70ft), ↔ 10m (30ft). Europe, N. Africa, S.W. Asia, Russia (W. Siberia). ❄❄❄. **'Plena'** ■ 🏆 has double flowers and red autumn colour; ↕↔ 12m (40ft).

P.* x *blireana 🏆 ○ Spreading, deciduous shrub or small tree bearing ovate, red-purple leaves, to 6cm (2½in) long, turning dark green in summer. Solitary, double pink flowers, 3cm (1¼in) across, are produced before the leaves in early and mid-spring. ↕↔ 4m (12ft). Garden origin. ❄❄❄

P. campanulata ○ (Bell-flowered cherry, Taiwan cherry). Spreading, deciduous tree bearing ovate, tapered mid-green leaves, to 10cm (4in) long. Shallowly bowl-shaped, pink or red flowers, 2cm (¾in) across, in umbels of 2–5, are borne before or with the leaves in early and mid-spring, followed by ovoid, cherry-like red fruit, to 1.5cm (½in) across. ↕↔ 8m (25ft). S. China, Taiwan, S. Japan. ❄❄

P. cerasifera ○ (Cherry plum, Myrobalan). Rounded, deciduous tree with ovate to obovate, dark green leaves, to 6cm (2½in) long. Solitary, bowl-shaped white flowers, 2.5cm (1in) across, are borne along bare shoots in early spring, with the leaves, and are sometimes followed by spherical, plum-like, edible, red or yellow fruit, 3cm (1¼in) across. ↕↔ 10m (30ft). S.E. Europe, S.W. Asia. ❄❄❄. **'Nigra'** ■ 🏆 syn. 'Pissardii Nigra', has dark purple leaves, red when young, and pink flowers. **'Pissardii'**, syn. *P. pissardii*, has dark red-purple leaves, and pale pink flowers that fade to white. **'Pissardii Nigra'** see 'Nigra'. **'Thundercloud'** ■ has pink flowers and dark purple foliage.

***P.* 'Cheal's Weeping'** ■ 🏆 ♈ syn. *P.* 'Kiku-shidare-zakura'. Weeping, deciduous tree bearing lance-shaped, tapered, mid-green leaves, to 10cm (4in) long, bronze when young. Fully double, bright pink flowers, 4cm (1½in) across, are borne in dense clusters, before or with the leaves, in mid- and late spring. ↕↔ 3m (10ft). ❄❄❄

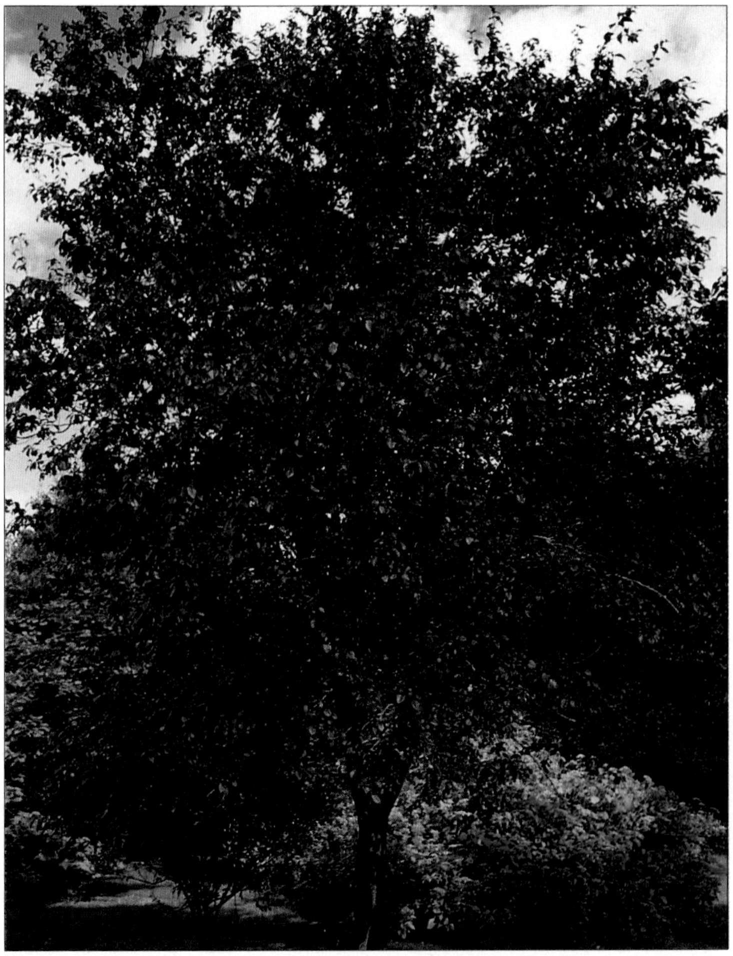

Prunus cerasifera 'Nigra'

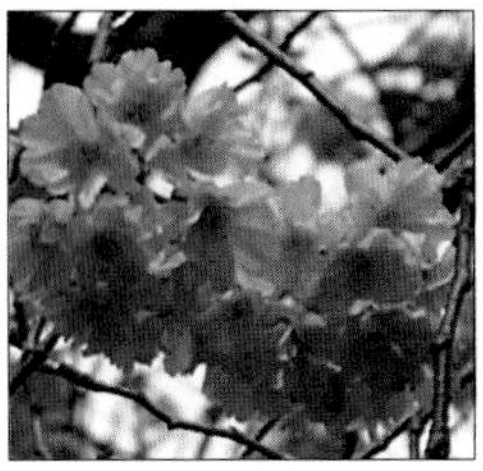
Prunus 'Accolade'

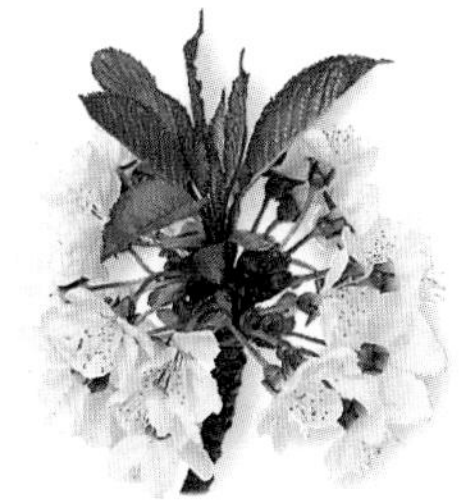
Prunus avium

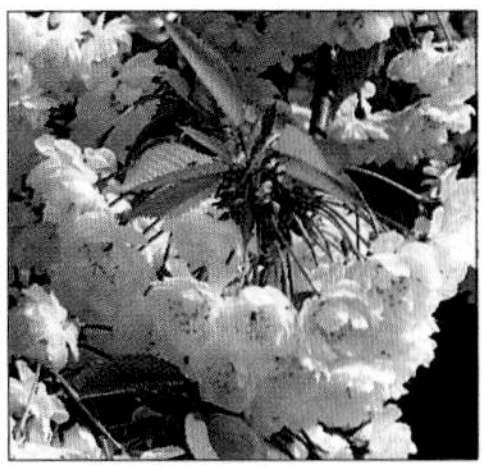
Prunus avium 'Plena'

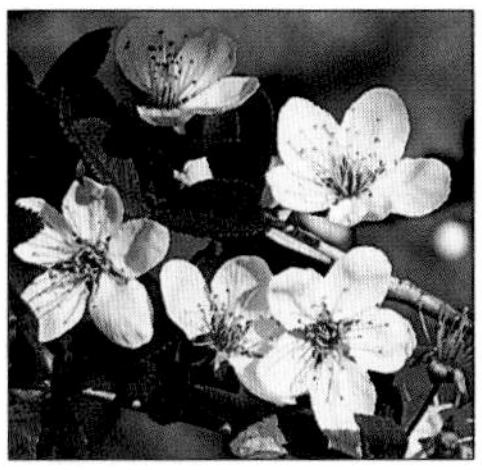
Prunus cerasifera 'Thundercloud'

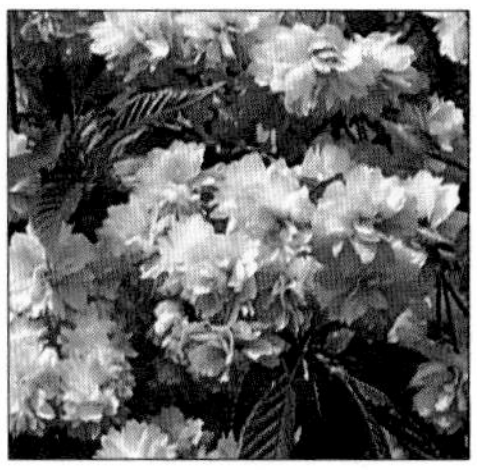
Prunus 'Cheal's Weeping'

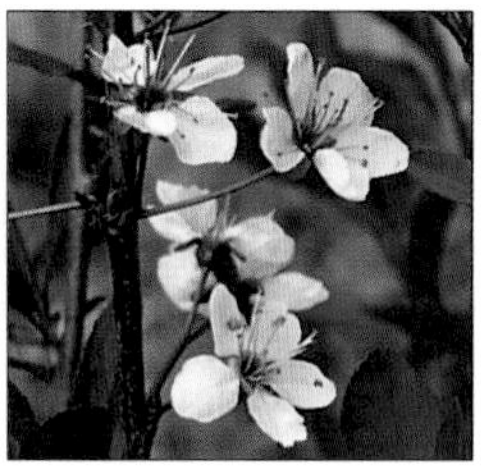
Prunus x *cistena*

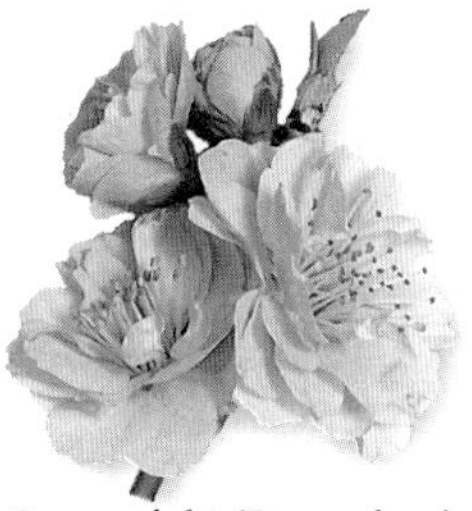
Prunus dulcis 'Roseoplena'

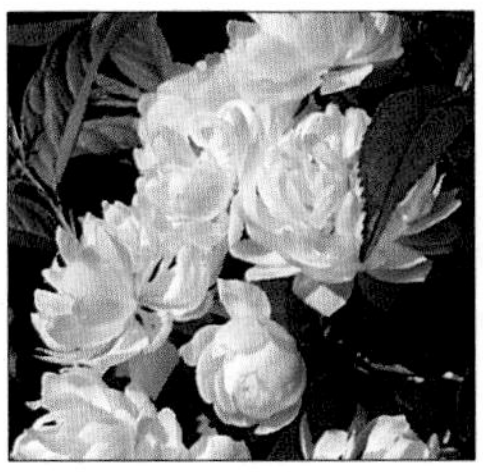
Prunus glandulosa 'Alba Plena'

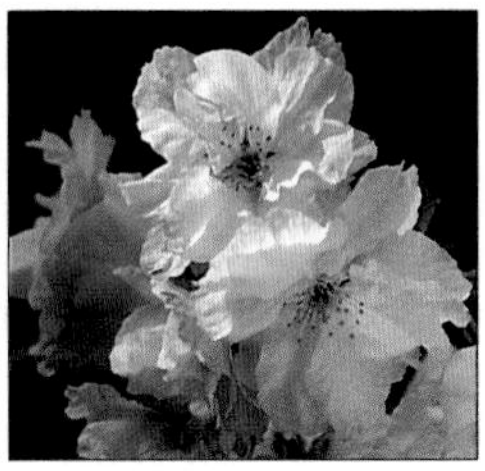
Prunus 'Hokusai'

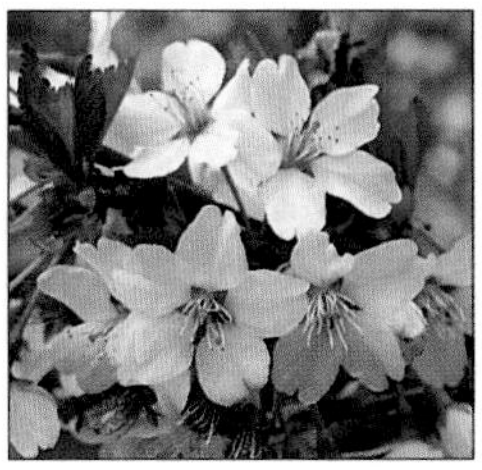
Prunus incisa

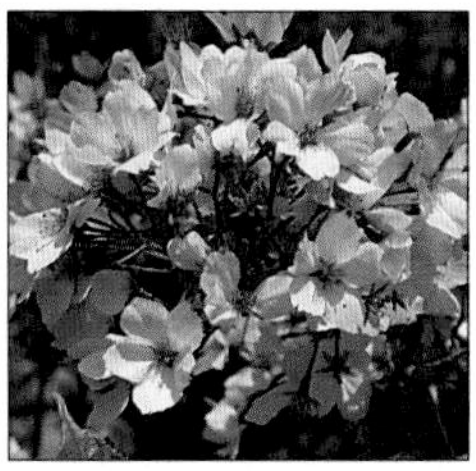
Prunus jamasakura

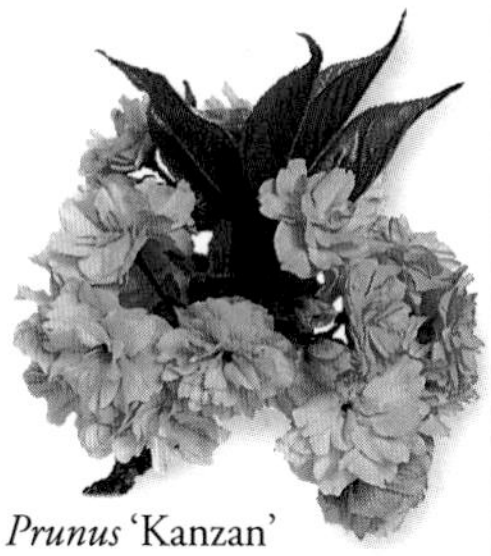
Prunus 'Kanzan'

***P.* 'Chôshû-hizakura'** ♀⚲ Broadly upright, deciduous tree with elliptic, tapered, dark green leaves, to 15cm (6in) long, bronze-red when young. Bowl-shaped or semi-double, mid-pink flowers, 3cm (1¼in) across, are borne in clusters of 2–4 in mid-spring. ↕7m (22ft), ↔ 6m (20ft). ❄❄❄
P.* x *cistena ▣♀ (*P. cerasifera* 'Atropurpurea' x *P. pumila*). Slow-growing, upright, deciduous shrub with oval, red-purple leaves, to 6cm (2½in) long, red when young. Solitary, bowl-shaped white flowers, 1cm (½in) across, are produced in late spring, sometimes followed by spherical, cherry-like, dark purple fruit, 2cm (¾in) across. ↕↔ 1.5m (5ft). Garden origin. ❄❄❄
P. davidiana ⚲ Spreading, deciduous tree with slender, lance-shaped, long-pointed, somewhat glossy, dark green leaves, to 12cm (5in) long. Solitary, saucer-shaped, white or pale pink flowers, 2.5cm (1in) across, stalkless or almost so, are borne before the leaves in early spring, followed by spherical, woolly yellow fruit, to 3cm (1¼in) across. Flowers may be damaged by late frosts. ↕↔ 8m (25ft). China. ❄❄❄
P. dulcis ⚲ (Common almond). Upright, spreading, deciduous tree with lance-shaped, finely toothed, tapered, dark green leaves, to 12cm (5in) long. Solitary or paired, bowl-shaped, pink or white flowers, 5cm (2in) across, are produced on bare shoots in early spring, followed by ovoid, velvety green fruit, to 6cm (2½in) long, each containing an edible nut. ↕↔ 8m (25ft). N. Africa, C. and S.W. Asia. ❄❄❄. **'Roseoplena'** ▣ bears double pink flowers.
***P.* 'Fudan-zakura'** ⚲ syn. *P. serrulata* f. *semperflorens.* Small, spreading, deciduous tree with ovate, mid-green leaves, 6–12cm (2½–5in) long, rough on the upper surfaces. Intermittently from late autumn to mid-spring, soft pink buds open to shallowly cup-shaped, single white flowers, 4cm (1½in) across, in short-stalked clusters. ↕↔ 5m (15ft). ❄❄❄
P. glandulosa. Rounded, deciduous shrub bearing narrowly ovate or elliptic, finely toothed, pale to mid-green leaves, to 10cm (4in) long. In late spring, bowl-shaped, white to pale pink flowers, to 1cm (½in) across, are borne singly or in pairs, densely clustered along the branches; they are followed by spherical, dark red fruit, to 1cm (½in) across. ↕↔ 1.5m (5ft). N. and C. China, Japan. ❄❄❄. **'Alba Plena'** ▣♀ has double, pure white flowers. **'Rosea Plena'** see 'Sinensis'. **'Sinensis'** ♀ syn. 'Rosea Plena', has double pink flowers.
***P.* 'Hally Jolivette'** ▣⚲ Rounded, bushy, deciduous tree or shrub with ovate, dark green leaves, to 5cm (2in) long. Double white flowers, 3cm (1¼in) across, in clusters of up to 5, open from pink buds in mid- and late spring. ↕↔ 5m (15ft). ❄❄❄
***P.* 'Hillieri'** ⚲ Spreading, deciduous tree with elliptic, dark green leaves, to 10cm (4in) long, bronze when young, orange-red in autumn. Many bowl-shaped, soft pink flowers, 4cm (1½in) across, are produced in clusters of up to 4, in mid-spring. ↕↔ 10m (30ft). ❄❄❄
***P.* x *hillieri* 'Spire'** see *P.* 'Spire'.
***P.* 'Hokusai'** ▣⚲ syn. *P.* 'Uzuzakura'. Spreading, deciduous tree with oval, dark green leaves, to 12cm (5in) long, bronze when young, orange and red in autumn. In mid- and late spring, bears double, pale pink flowers, 5cm (2in) across, singly or in dense clusters of up to 6. ↕6m (20ft), ↔ 8m (25ft). ❄❄❄
***P.* 'Hosokawa'** see *P.* 'Mount Fuji'.
***P.* 'Ichiyo'** ♀⚲ Spreading, deciduous tree with elliptic, dark green leaves, to 10cm (4in) long, bronze when young. Wide-open, double, soft pink flowers, 5cm (2in) across, are borne in long, pendent clusters of 3 or 4 in mid- and late spring. ↕↔ 8m (25ft). ❄❄❄
P. ilicifolia ⚲ (Holly-leaved cherry). Compact, spreading, rounded, evergreen shrub or small tree with broadly lance-shaped to ovate, holly-like, sharply toothed, leathery, glossy, dark green leaves, to 5–7cm (2–3in) long. In summer, bowl-shaped white flowers, to 8mm (⅜in) across, are borne in racemes to 7cm (3in) long. Spherical, cherry-like red fruit, to 1.5cm (½in) across, ripen to blue-black. ↕to 9m (28ft), ↔ 6m (20ft). USA (California). ❄❄
P. incisa ▣⚲ (Fuji cherry). Spreading, deciduous, rounded shrub, rarely tree-like, with ovate to obovate, sharply toothed, dark green leaves, to 6cm (2½in) long, bronze-red when young, turning orange-red in autumn. Saucer-shaped, white or pale pink flowers, 2cm (¾in) across, solitary or in clusters of 2 or 3, are borne before the leaves in early and mid-spring; they are followed by ovoid, cherry-like, purple-black fruit, to 8mm (⅜in) long. ↕↔ 8m (25ft). S.W. Japan. ❄❄❄. **'February Pink'** bears pale pink flowers over a long period in winter and early spring. **'Kojo-no-mai'** has oblong to lance-shaped leaves, 0.6–3cm (¼–1¼in) long, yellow-green when young, turning mid-green in summer. Light red buds open to pale red flowers, 1.5cm (½in) across, borne singly or in pairs. ↕↔ 2.5m (8ft). **'Praecox'** ♀ has pink buds that open to white flowers in late winter.
P. jamasakura ▣⚲ syn. *P. serrulata* var. *spontanea* (Hill cherry). Spreading, deciduous tree with oblong, dark green leaves, to 12cm (5in) long, bronze-red when young, turning red and yellow in autumn. In mid- and late spring, bears a profusion of cup-shaped white flowers, 3cm (1¼in) across, in clusters of 3–5, followed by ovoid, cherry-like, magenta-red fruit, to 1cm (½in) long. ↕↔ 12m (40ft). China, Korea, Japan. ❄❄❄
***P.* 'Jo-nioi'** ⚲ Spreading, deciduous tree with elliptic, mid-green leaves, to 10cm (4in) long, pale bronze when young. Bowl-shaped, fragrant white flowers, 4cm (1½in) across, in clusters of 3–5, open from pink buds in mid-spring. ↕↔ 10m (30ft). ❄❄❄
***P.* 'Kanzan'** ▣♀⚲ Upright, deciduous tree, vase-shaped when young, spreading wider with age, with ovate, dark green leaves, to 12cm (5in) long, bronze when young. Double, deep pink flowers, 5cm (2in) across, are profusely borne in clusters of 2–5 in mid- and late spring, before and as the leaves emerge. ↕↔ 10m (30ft). ❄❄❄
***P.* 'Kiku-shidare-zakura'** see *P.* 'Cheal's Weeping'.
***P.* 'Kursar'** ♀⚲ Spreading, deciduous tree with elliptic, dark green leaves, to 12cm (5in) long, bronze when young. Saucer-shaped, dark pink flowers, 2cm (¾in) across, are profusely borne in clusters of 3 or 4 in early spring, before the leaves. ↕↔ 8m (25ft). ❄❄❄

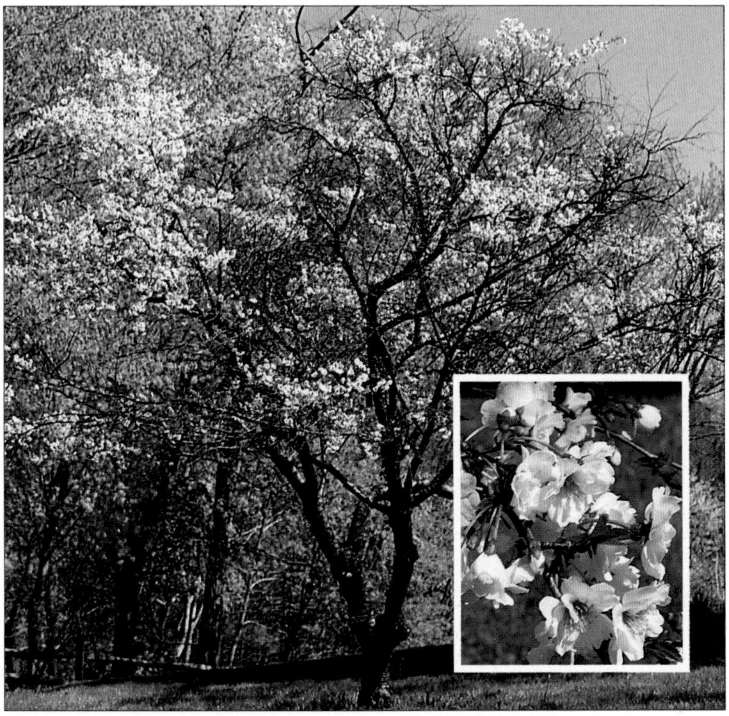
Prunus 'Hally Jolivette' (inset: flower detail)

P

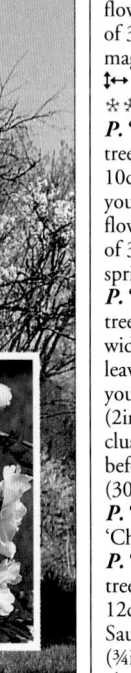

PRUNUS

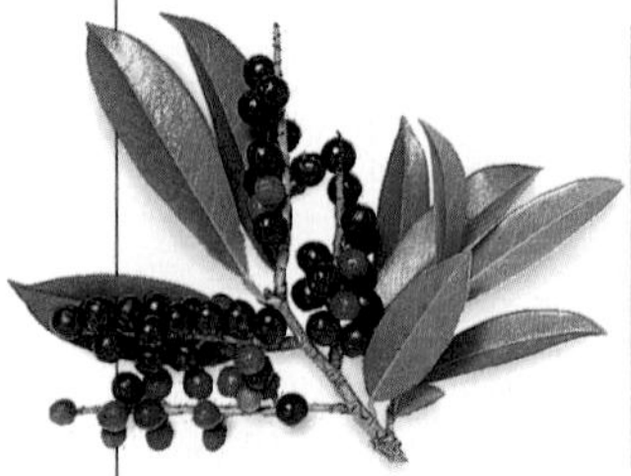
Prunus laurocerasus

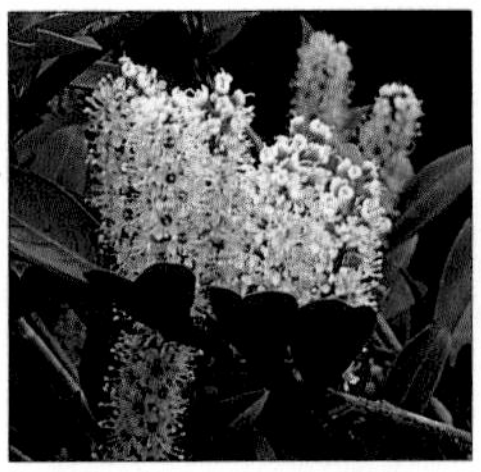
Prunus laurocerasus 'Otto Luyken'

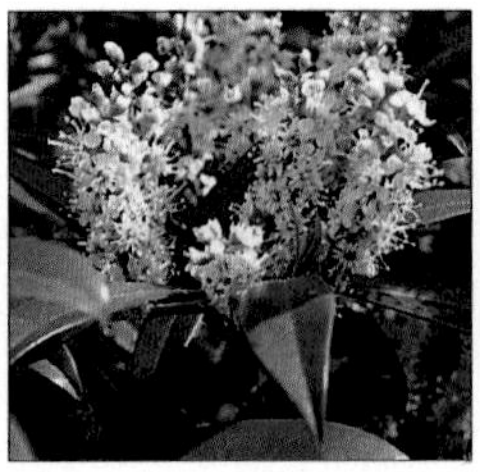
Prunus laurocerasus 'Zabeliana'

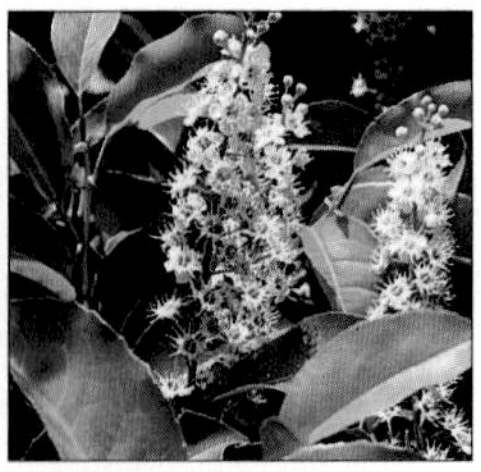
Prunus lusitanica subsp. *azorica*

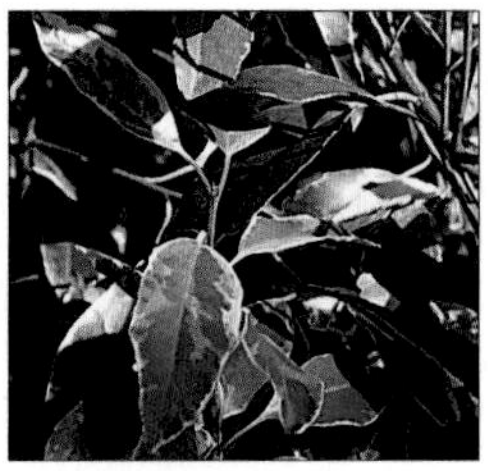
Prunus lusitanica 'Variegata'

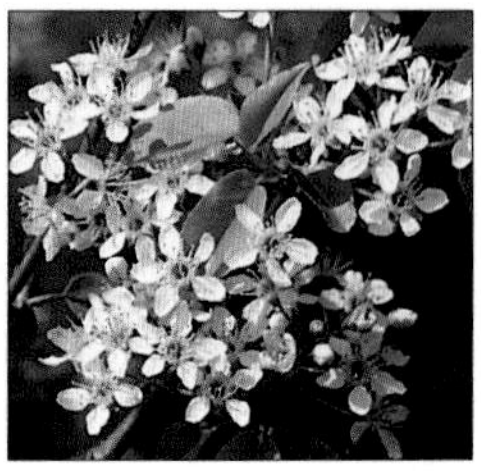
Prunus mahaleb

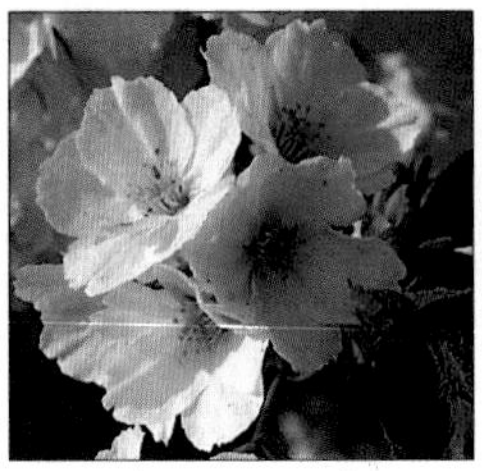
Prunus 'Mount Fuji'

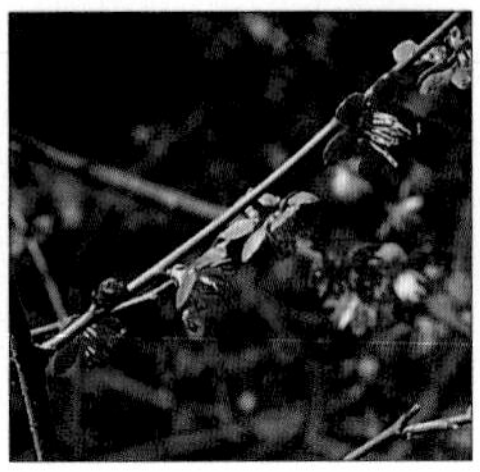
Prunus mume 'Beni-chidori'

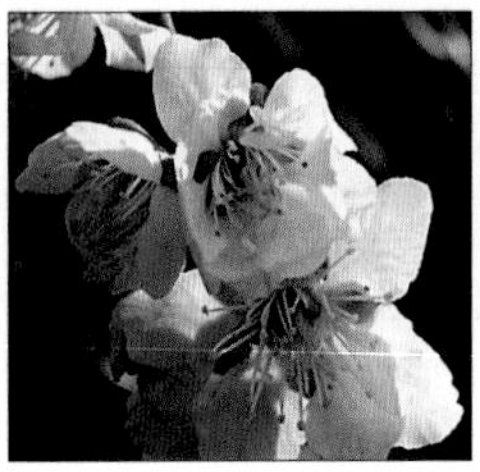
Prunus mume 'Omoi-no-mama'

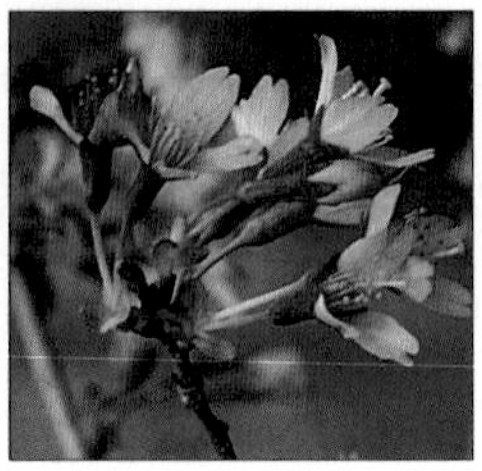
Prunus 'Okame'

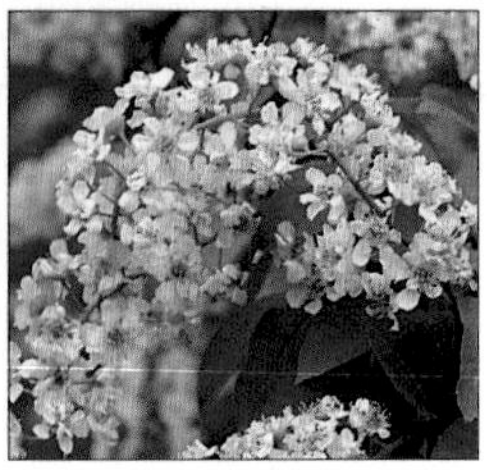
Prunus padus

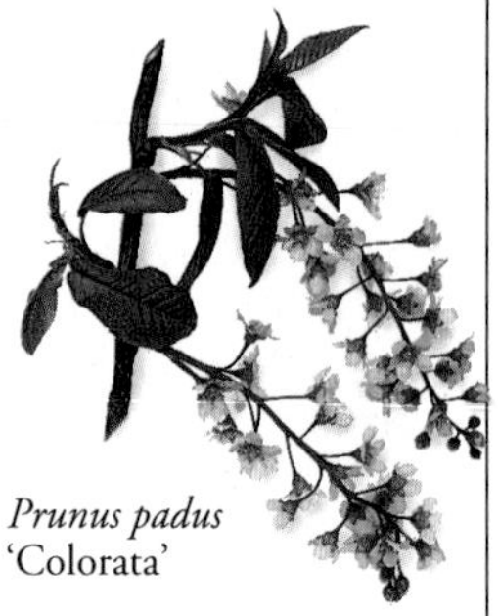
Prunus padus 'Colorata'

P. laurocerasus ▣🏆 (Cherry laurel, Laurel). Dense, bushy, evergreen shrub, becoming spreading and tree-like with age, with oblong, glossy leaves, to 15cm (6in) long, dark green above, pale green beneath. In mid- and late spring, cup-shaped, fragrant white flowers, 8mm (3/8in) across, are produced in upright racemes, 5–12cm (2–5in) long, followed by conical, cherry-like red fruit, 1cm (1/2in) across, ripening to black. ↕8m (25ft), ↔10m (30ft). E. Europe, S.W. Asia. ❄❄❄. **'Camelliifolia'** is upright, with conspicuously twisted leaves; ↔4m (12ft). **'Castlewellan'** see 'Marbled White'. **'Green Carpet'** see 'Grünerteppich'. **'Grünerteppich'**, syn. 'Green Carpet', is low and spreading, with leaves to 12cm (5in) long; ↕1m (3ft), ↔3m (10ft). **'Herbergii'** has a compact habit, with narrow leaves; ↕↔3m (10ft). **'Marbled White'**, syn. 'Castlewellan', has leaves conspicuously marked white; ↕↔5m (15ft). **'Otto Luyken'** ▣🏆 is very compact, with narrow, pointed, dark green leaves, to 11cm (4½in) long; frequently flowers again in autumn; ↕1m (3ft), ↔1.5m (5ft). **'Rotundifolia'** is vigorous and upright, excellent for hedging; ↕5m (15ft), ↔4m (12ft). **'Schipkaensis'** is spreading, and flowers profusely; ↕2m (6ft), ↔3m (10ft). **'Zabeliana'** ▣ has a low and wide-spreading habit, very narrow leaves, and often flowers again in autumn; ↕1m (3ft), ↔2.5m (8ft).

P. lusitanica 🏆△ (Laurel, Portugal laurel). Dense, bushy, evergreen shrub or tree with red-stalked, ovate to elliptic, glossy, dark green leaves, to 12cm (5in) long. Cup-shaped, fragrant white flowers, 1.5cm (1/2in) across, are borne in slender, ascending, spreading, or pendent racemes, to 25cm (10in) long, in early summer, followed by ovoid, cherry-like red fruit, 1cm (1/2in) across, ripening to black. ↕↔ to 20m (70ft). S.W. Europe. ❄❄. **subsp. *azorica*** ▣🏆 has broader leaves, and racemes to 10cm (4in) long; Azores. **'Variegata'** ▣ has leaves narrowly margined with white.

P. maackii ▣△ (Manchurian cherry). Conical, deciduous tree or shrub with peeling, yellow-brown bark and ovate, dark green leaves, to 8cm (3in) long, turning yellow in autumn. In mid-spring, produces dense racemes, 5–8cm (2–3in) long, each with 6–10 bowl-shaped, fragrant white flowers, 1cm (1/2in) across; they are followed by spherical, cherry-like, glossy black fruit, 5mm (1/4in) across. ↕10m (30ft), ↔8m (25ft). N.E. Asia. ❄❄❄

P. mahaleb ▣♧ (Saint Lucie cherry). Spreading, deciduous tree with rounded, glossy, dark green leaves, to 6cm (2½in) long, turning yellow in autumn. In mid- and late spring, bowl-shaped, very fragrant white flowers, 1.5cm (1/2in) across, are produced in racemes to 5cm (2in) long; they are followed by ovoid, glossy red cherries, 6mm (1/4in) long, ripening to black. ↕10m (30ft), ↔8m (25ft). Europe. ❄❄❄

***P.* 'Mount Fuji'** ▣🏆♧ syn. *P.* 'Hosokawa', *P.* 'Shirotae'. Spreading, deciduous tree with slightly arching branches and elliptic, dark green leaves, to 12cm (5in) long, pale green when young, orange and red in autumn. In mid-spring, bears cup-shaped or semi-double, fragrant white flowers, 5cm (2in) across, in pendent clusters of 2 or 3. ↕6m (20ft), ↔8m (25ft). ❄❄❄

P. mume ♧ (Japanese apricot). Spreading, deciduous tree producing green shoots and rounded, tapered, dark green leaves, to 10cm (4in) long. Bowl-shaped, fragrant, white to dark pink flowers, 2.5cm (1in) across, are produced singly or in pairs, on bare shoots, in late winter and early spring; they are followed by spherical, softly hairy, apricot-like, sour to bitter, edible yellow fruit, to 3cm (1¼in) across. ↕↔9m (28ft). China, Korea. ❄❄❄. **'Beni-chidori'** ▣ syn. 'Benishidore', is upright and shrubby, with dark pink flowers; ↕↔2.5m (8ft). **'Dawn'** bears double, ruffled pink flowers. **'Omoi-no-mama'** ▣ syn. 'Omoi-no-wac', is upright and shrubby, with semi-double, pink-flushed white flowers; ↕↔2.5m (8ft). **'Pendula'** ♧ has weeping branches and pink flowers; ↕↔6m (20ft). **'W.B. Clarke'** ♧ is weeping, with double pink flowers; ↕↔6m (20ft).

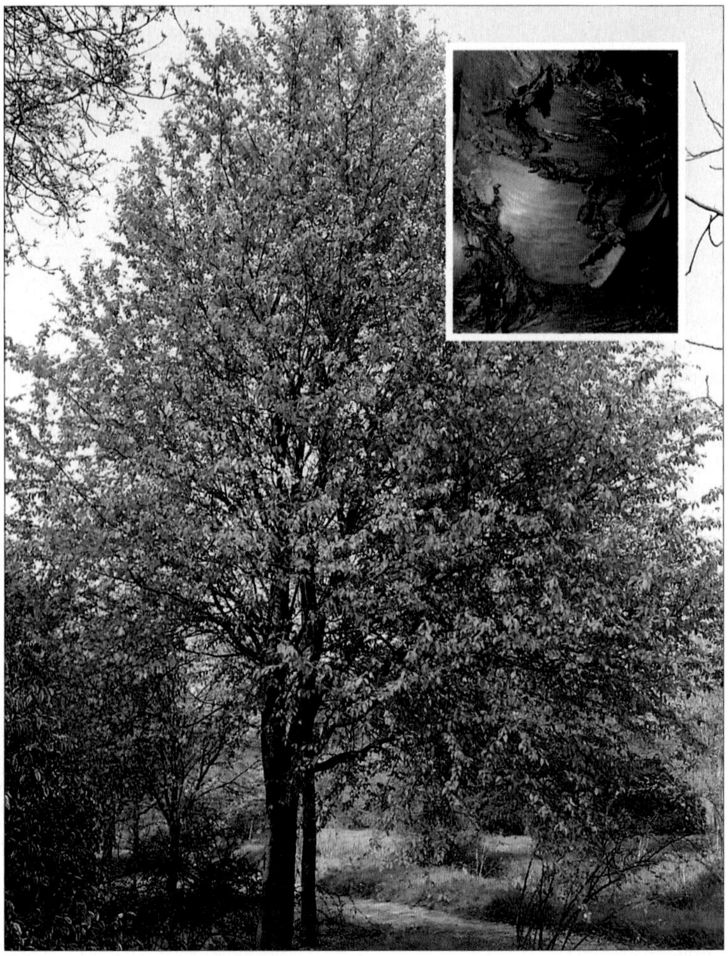
Prunus maackii (inset: bark detail)

***P.* 'Okame'** ▣🏆♧ Bushy, deciduous tree or shrub with narrowly oval, sharply toothed, dark green leaves, to 8cm (3in) long, turning orange and red in autumn. In early spring, profuse, cup-shaped, carmine-pink flowers, 2–2.5cm (3/4–1in) across, are borne in clusters of 2–5. ↕10m (30ft), ↔8m (25ft). ❄❄❄

P. padus ▣♧ (Bird cherry). Spreading, deciduous tree or shrub, conical when young. Elliptic, dark green leaves, to 10cm (4in) long, turn red or yellow in autumn. Pendent racemes, to 15cm (6in) long, of cup-shaped, fragrant white flowers, to 1.5cm (1/2in) across, are produced in late spring, followed by spherical, pea-like, glossy black fruit, 8mm (3/8in) across. ↕15m (50ft), ↔10m (30ft). Europe, N. Asia to C. Japan. ❄❄❄. **'Albertii'** bears abundant flowers in dense racemes. **'Colorata'** ▣🏆 has reddish purple young foliage and pink flowers. **'Plena'** has double flowers. **'Watereri'** ▣🏆 has flowers in slender racemes, to 20cm (8in) long.

***P.* 'Pandora'** ▣🏆♧ Spreading, deciduous tree, upright when young, with oval, dark green leaves, to 7cm (3in) long, bronze when young, turning orange and red in autumn. In early spring, masses of solitary, cup-shaped, pale pink flowers, 3cm (1¼in) across, open before the leaves, from dark pink buds. ↕10m (30ft), ↔8m (25ft). ❄❄❄

***P. pendula* 'Pendula Rosea'** see *P.* x *subhirtella* 'Pendula Rosea'.

***P. pendula* 'Pendula Rubra'** see *P.* x *subhirtella* 'Pendula Rubra'.

P. pensylvanica ♧ (Pin cherry). Spreading, deciduous tree or shrub with peeling, red-banded bark and ovate to

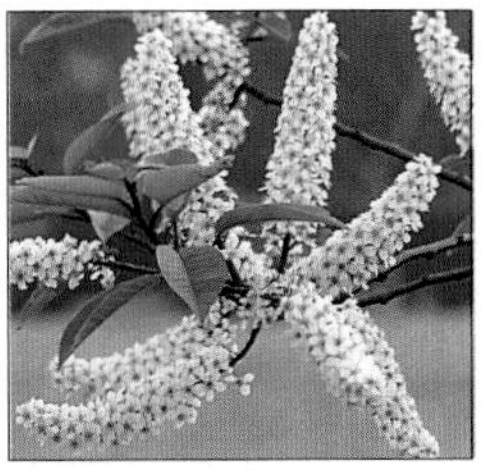
Prunus padus 'Watereri'

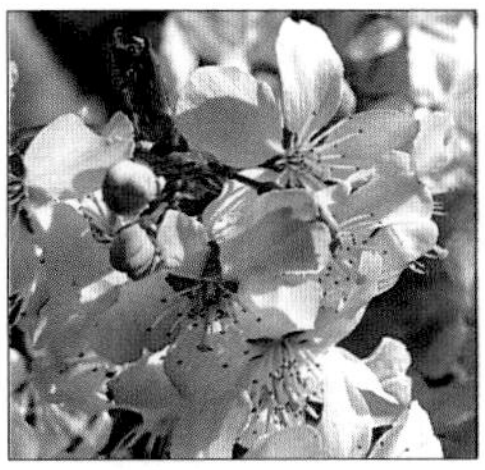
Prunus 'Pandora'

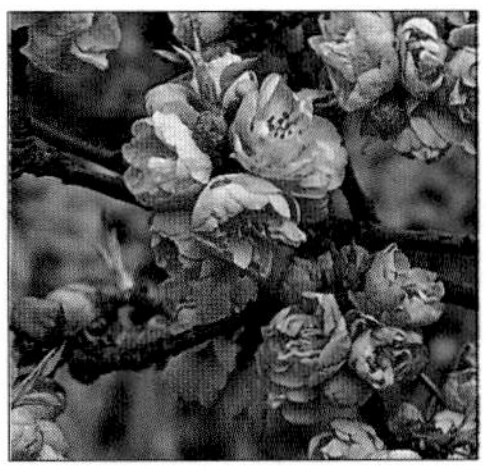
Prunus persica 'Klara Meyer'

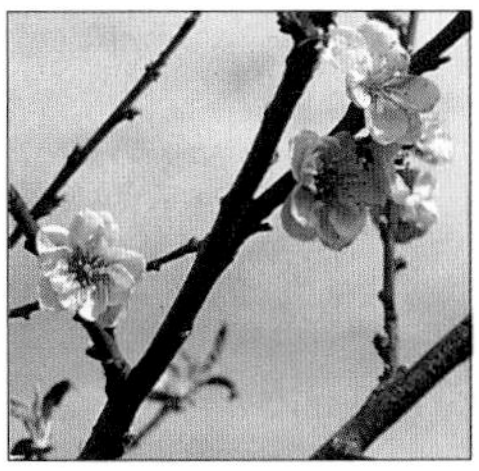
Prunus persica 'Prince Charming'

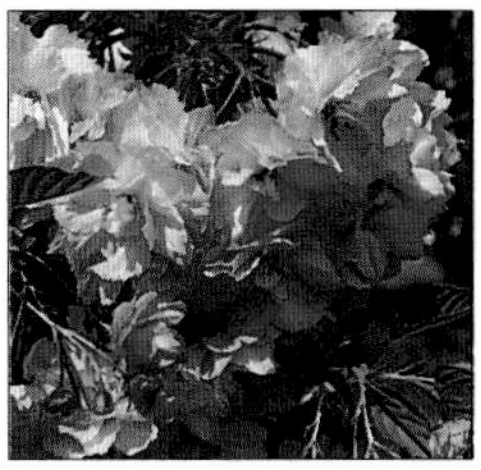
Prunus 'Pink Perfection'

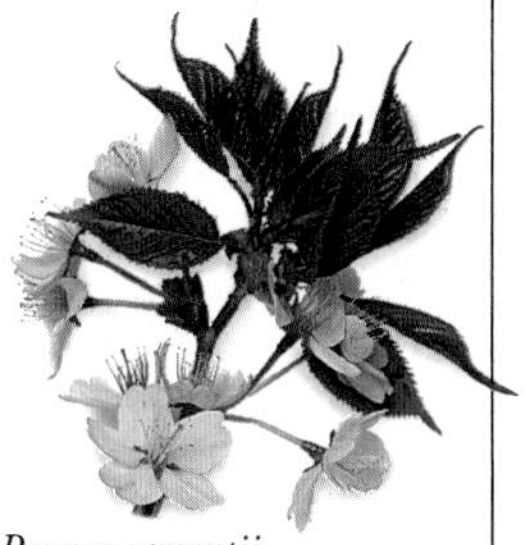
Prunus sargentii

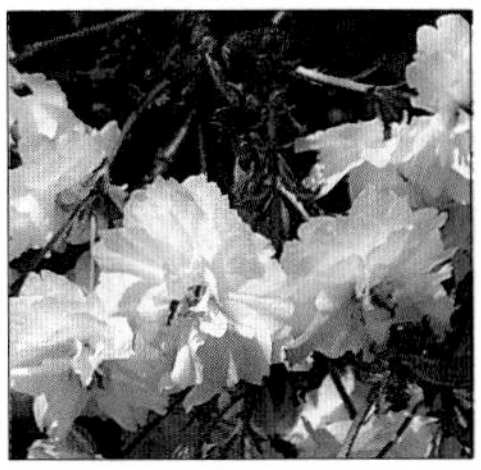
Prunus 'Shirofugen'

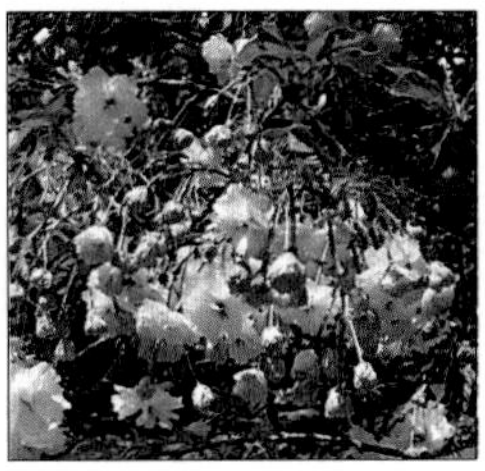
Prunus 'Shôgetsu'

Prunus spinosa 'Purpurea'

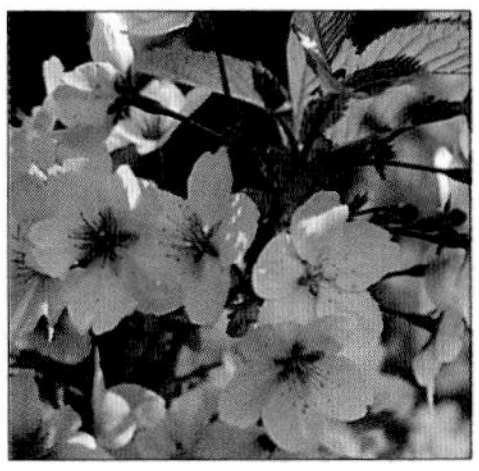
Prunus 'Spire'

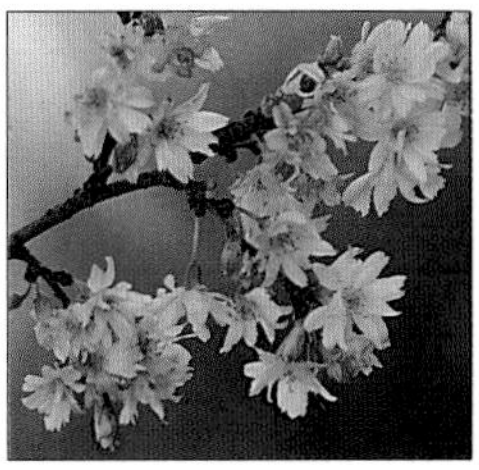
Prunus x *subhirtella* 'Autumnalis Rosea'

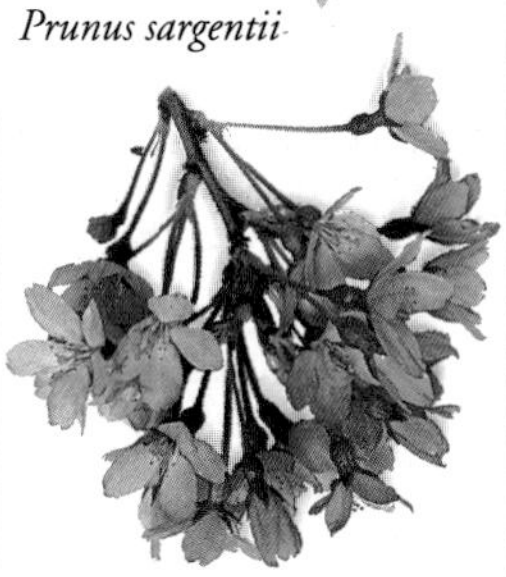
Prunus x *subhirtella* 'Pendula Rosea'

oblong-lance-shaped, bright green leaves, to 11cm (4½in) long, turning yellow and red in autumn. In mid- and late spring, cup-shaped white flowers, 1.5cm (½in) across, are borne before or with the leaves, in stalkless umbels of 3–6, followed by spherical red fruit, 5mm (¼in) across. ↕↔ to 10m (30ft). North America. ✱✱✱. **'Stockton'** has double flowers and red autumn colour.

P. persica ◯ (Peach). Spreading, deciduous tree with narrowly elliptic, slender-pointed, glossy, mid- to dark green leaves, to 15cm (6in) long. Bears solitary, bowl-shaped, pink or red flowers, 4cm (1½in) across, in late spring, before the leaves, followed by spherical, downy, edible, red-blushed yellow fruit, 8cm (3in) across. ↕↔ 8m (25ft). China. ✱✱✱. **'Helen Borchers'** has semi-double, rose-pink flowers, 6cm (2½in) across. **'Klara Meyer'** ▣ has double, bright pink flowers. **'Peppermint Stick'** bears double white flowers with red stripes. **'Prince Charming'** ▣ ◯ is upright, with double, dark pink flowers; ↕ 4m (12ft), ↔ 1.5m (5ft).

P.* x *persicoides see *P.* x *amygdalopersica.*

***P.* 'Pink Perfection'** ▣ ♀ ◯ Spreading, deciduous tree with oblong, dark green leaves, to 12cm (5in) long, bronze when young. Double pink flowers, 5cm (2in) across, open in long, pendent clusters of 3–5 in late spring. ↕↔ 8m (25ft). ✱✱✱

***P.* 'Pink Star'** see *P.* x *subhirtella* 'Stellata'.

P. pissardii see *P. cerasifera* 'Pissardii'.

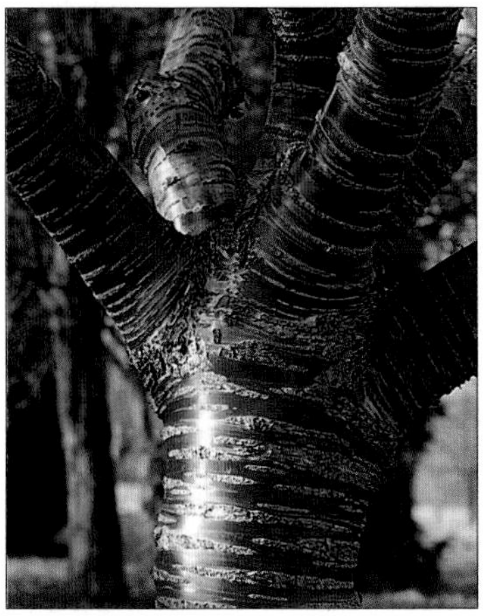
Prunus serrula

P. sargentii ▣ ♀ ◯ (Sargent cherry). Spreading, deciduous tree with elliptic, tapered, dark green leaves, to 12cm (5in) long, red when young, turning brilliant orange-red in early autumn. Bowl-shaped, pale pink flowers, 4cm (1½in) across, are produced in umbels of 2–4 in mid-spring; they are followed by ovoid, cherry-like, glossy crimson fruit, to 1cm (½in) long. ↕ to 20m (70ft), ↔ 15m (50ft). Russia (Sakhalin), Korea, Japan. ✱✱✱. **'Columnare'** ◯ is narrow and upright; ↔ 3m (10ft).

P. serotina ◯ (Black cherry, Wild rum cherry). Broadly columnar, deciduous tree with elliptic, glossy, dark green leaves, to 12cm (5in) long, turning yellow or red in autumn. In late spring and early summer, bowl-shaped, fragrant white flowers, 1.5cm (½in) across, are borne in racemes to 15cm (6in) long; they are followed by spherical, edible red fruit, 1cm (½in) across, ripening to black. ↕ to 35m (120ft). North America. ✱✱✱

P. serrula ▣ ♀ ◯ Rounded, deciduous tree with peeling, glossy, copper-brown bark and lance-shaped, tapered, dark green leaves, to 10cm (4in) long, turning yellow in autumn. Bowl-shaped white flowers, 2cm (¾in) across, solitary or in umbels of 2–4, are borne as the leaves emerge in late spring, followed by ovoid, cherry-like fruit, 1cm (½in) long. ↕↔ 10m (30ft). W. China. ✱✱✱

P. serrulata* f. *semperflorens see *P.* 'Fudan-zakura'.

P. serrulata* var. *spontanea see *P. jamasakura.*

***P.* 'Shirofugen'** ▣ ♀ ◯ Spreading, deciduous tree bearing oblong, dark green leaves, to 12cm (5in) long, bronze-red when young, turning orange-red in autumn. Clusters of 3–5 double, fragrant white flowers, 5cm (2in) across, open from pink buds in late spring; they turn pink before they fall. ↕ 8m (25ft), ↔ 10m (30ft). ✱✱✱

***P.* 'Shirotae'** see *P.* 'Mount Fuji'.

***P.* 'Shôgetsu'** ▣ ♀ ◯ Rounded, deciduous tree bearing oblong, mid-green leaves, to 12cm (5in) long, bronze when young, turning orange and red in autumn. Frilly-margined, double, pink and white flowers, 5cm (2in) across, in pendent clusters of 3–6, open from pink buds in late spring. ↕ 5m (15ft), ↔ 8m (25ft). ✱✱✱

P. spinosa ◯ (Blackthorn, Sloe). Dense, bushy, spiny, deciduous shrub or tree with elliptic to obovate, mid- to deep green leaves, to 5cm (2in) long. Solitary, rarely paired, bowl-shaped white flowers, to 1.5cm (½in) across, are borne before the leaves in early and mid-spring; they are followed by spherical, edible, glaucous black fruit, 1.5cm (½in) across. ↕ 5m (15ft), ↔ 4m (12ft). Europe to Russia (W. Siberia), Mediterranean. ✱✱✱. **'Purpurea'** ▣ has red leaves, later turning dark red-purple, and pale pink flowers.

***P.* 'Spire'** ▣ ♀ ◯ syn. *P.* x *hillieri* 'Spire'. Vase-shaped, deciduous tree, conical when young, with obovate, dark green leaves, to 10cm (4in) long, bronze when young, turning orange and red in autumn. Bowl-shaped, pale pink flowers, 4cm (1½in) across, in clusters of 3–5, are produced as the leaves emerge in mid-spring. ↕ 10m (30ft), ↔ 6m (20ft). ✱✱✱

P.* x *subhirtella ◯ (*P. incisa* x *P. pendula*) (Higan cherry, Rosebud cherry). Spreading, deciduous tree with broadly elliptic or ovate, sometimes 3-lobed, sharply toothed, dark green leaves, to 8cm (3in) long, pale bronze when young, turning yellow in autumn. Bowl-shaped, white or pink flowers, 2cm (¾in) across, are borne in clusters of 2–5, intermittently from autumn to spring, before or with the leaves; they are sometimes followed by ovoid, cherry-like, red, later nearly black fruit, 8mm (⅜in) long. ↕↔ 8m (25ft). Japan. ✱✱✱. **'Autumnalis'** ♀ bears semi-double, pink-tinged white flowers in mild periods between autumn and spring. **'Autumnalis Rosea'** ▣ ♀ is similar to 'Autumnalis' but produces pink flowers. **'Fukubana'** ♀ produces semi-double, dark rose-pink flowers. **'Pendula Rosea'** ▣ ♀ ◯ syn. *P. pendula* 'Pendula Rosea', has weeping branches and rose-pink flowers. **'Pendula Rosea Plena'** ▣ ◯ has weeping branches and semi-double, rose-pink flowers. **'Pendula Rubra'** ◯ syn. *P. pendula* 'Pendula Rubra', has weeping branches

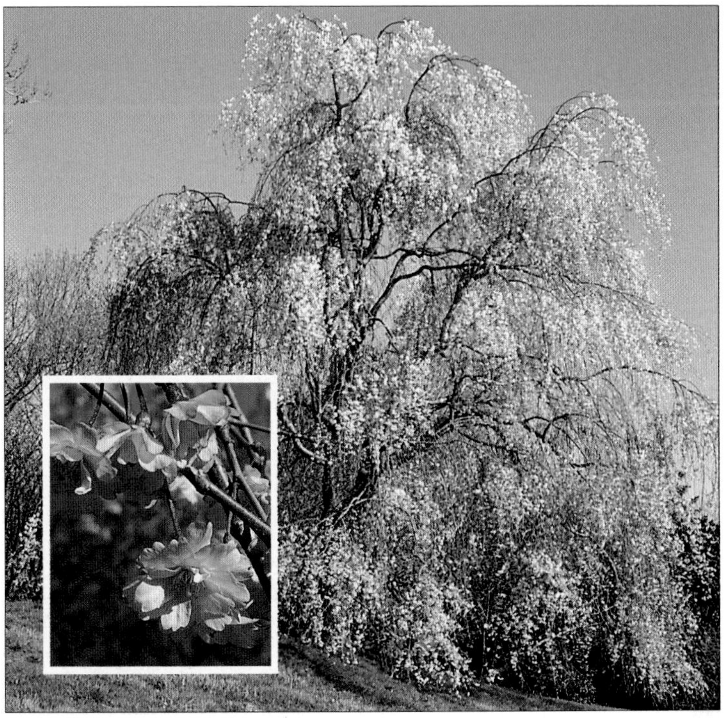
Prunus x *subhirtella* 'Pendula Rosea Plena' (inset: flower detail)

P

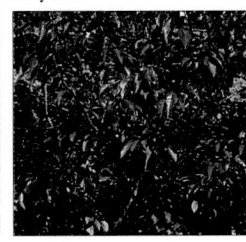

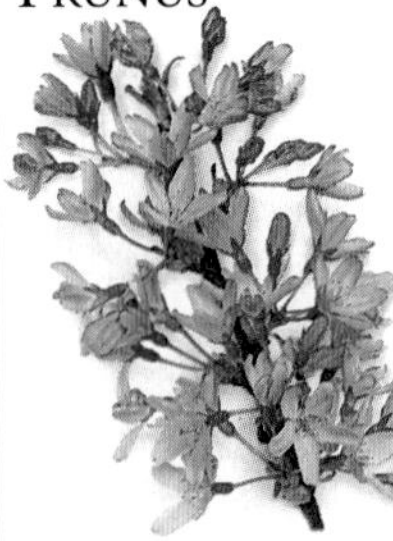
Prunus x *subhirtella* 'Stellata'

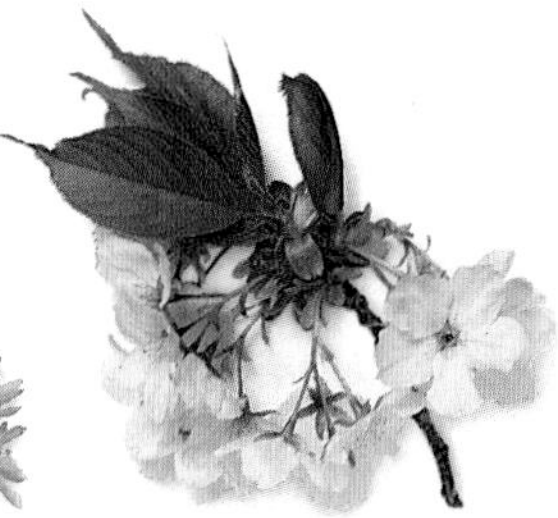
Prunus 'Taihaku'

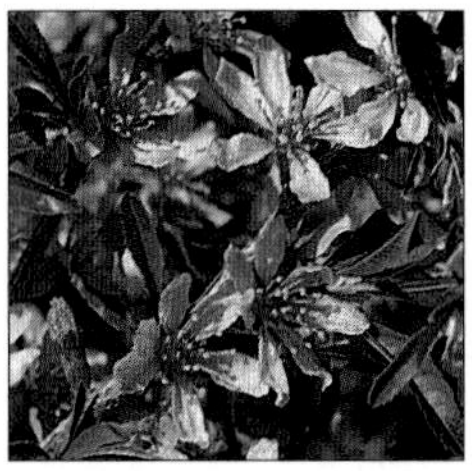
Prunus tenella

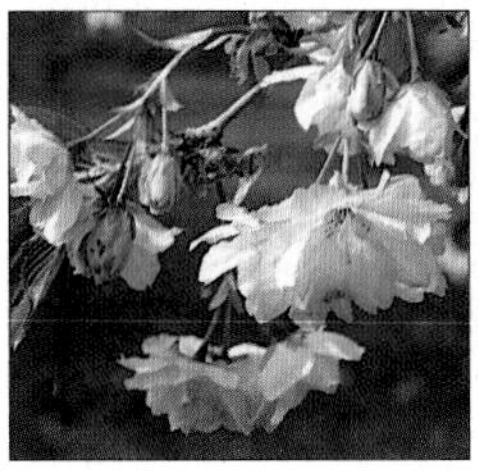
Prunus 'Ukon'

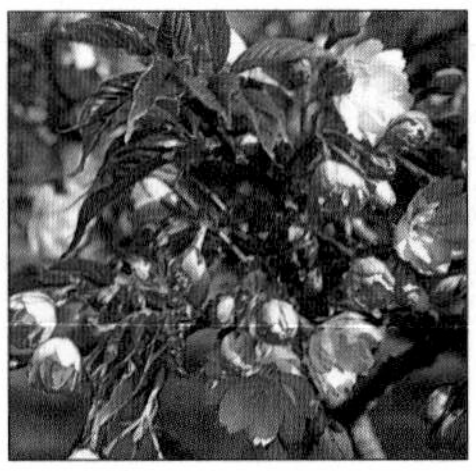
Prunus 'Yae-murasaki'

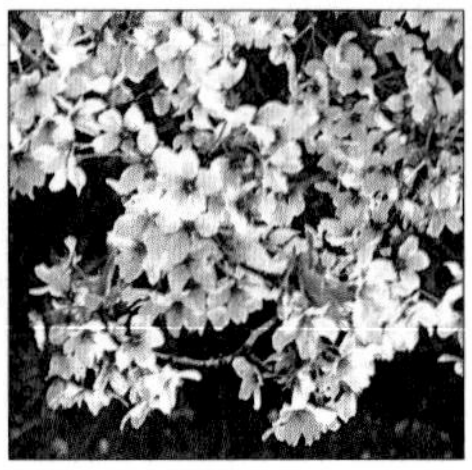
Prunus x *yedoensis*

and dark pink flowers. **'Stellata'** ■ syn. *P.* 'Pink Star', has pale pink flowers, red in bud, with narrow, pointed petals.
***P.* 'Taihaku'** ■🏆⌂ (Great white cherry). Vigorous, spreading, deciduous tree bearing elliptic, dark green leaves, to 20cm (8in) long, bronze when young. Bowl-shaped white flowers, to 6cm (2½in) across, are produced in clusters of up to 4 in mid-spring. ↕8m (25ft), ↔ 10m (30ft). ❄❄❄
P. tenella ■ (Dwarf Russian almond). Bushy, deciduous shrub with upright shoots and obovate to inversely lance-shaped, glossy, dark green leaves, to 8cm (3in) long. Bowl-shaped, bright pink flowers, to 3cm (1¼in) across, solitary or in profuse clusters of 2 or 3, are produced with the young leaves in mid- and late spring; they are followed by ovoid, almond-like, velvety, grey-yellow fruit, to 2.5cm (1in) long. ↕to 1.5m (5ft), ↔ 1.5m (5ft). C. Europe to Russia (Siberia). ❄❄❄. **'Fire Hill'** 🏆 has very dark pink flowers.
***P.* 'Trailblazer'** ⌂ Broadly upright, deciduous tree with oval, red-purple leaves, to 8cm (3in) long. Solitary, bowl-shaped, white or pale pink flowers, 2cm (¾in) across, are borne before the leaves in mid-spring, and are sometimes followed by plum-like, edible red fruit, 6cm (2½in) across. ↕10m (30ft), ↔ 6m (20ft). ❄❄❄

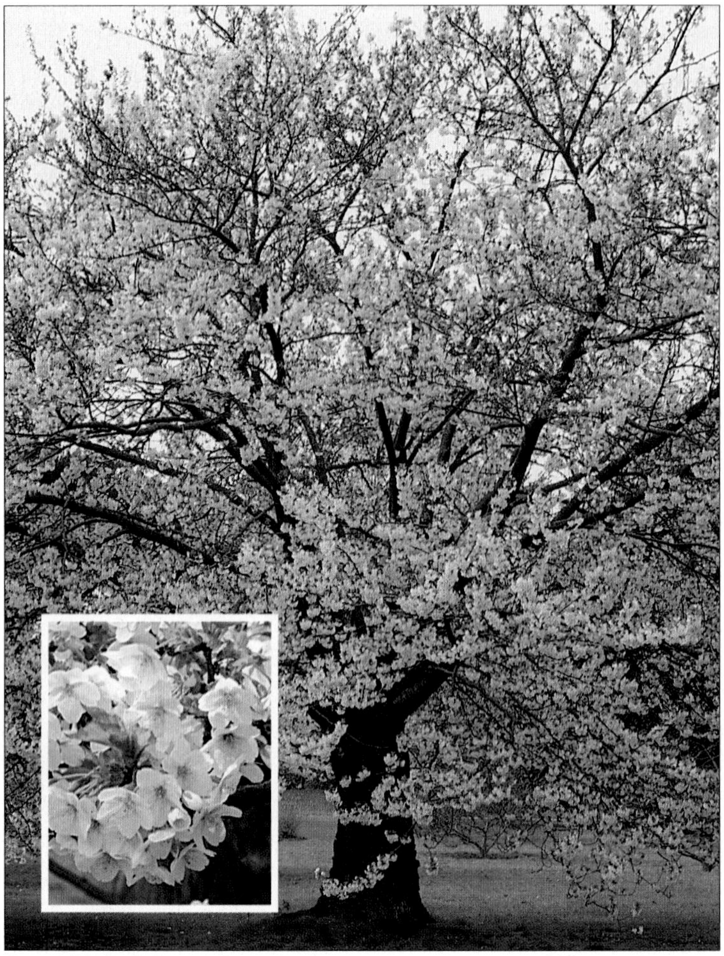
Prunus 'Umineko' (inset: flower detail)

P. triloba ⌂ (Flowering almond). Densely branched, deciduous shrub or small tree bearing broadly elliptic, often 3-lobed leaves, 4–8cm (1½–3in) long, dark green above, mid-green and softly hairy beneath. Solitary or paired, bowl-shaped pink flowers, 2–3.5cm (¾–1½in) across, are produced in early and mid-spring; they are followed by spherical red fruit, 1cm (½in) across. ↕↔ 3m (10ft). China. ❄❄❄.
'Multiplex' 🏆 is spreading, bearing oval leaves, to 6cm (2½in) long. Double pink flowers, 4cm (1½in) across, are produced in mid-spring. ↕↔ 4m (12ft).
***P.* 'Ukon'** ■🏆⌂ Vigorous, spreading, deciduous tree with elliptic, tapered, dark green leaves, to 12cm (5in) long, bronze when young. Clusters of 3–6 double flowers, 4cm (1½in) across, yellowish white on the outsides and slightly pink at the tips, open from pink buds in mid-spring. ↕8m (25ft), ↔ 10m (30ft). ❄❄❄
***P.* 'Umineko'** ■⌂ Upright, deciduous tree with ovate, sharply toothed, dark green leaves, to 7cm (3in) long, pale green when young. Cup-shaped white flowers, 4cm (1½in) across, are borne in clusters of 2 or 3 in mid-spring, with the young leaves. ↕8m (25ft), ↔ 3m (10ft). ❄❄❄
***P.* 'Uzuzakura'** see *P.* 'Hokusai'.
P. virginiana ⌂ (Choke cherry, Virginian bird cherry). Conical, often suckering, deciduous tree or shrub with broadly obovate to broadly elliptic, glossy, mid- to dark green leaves, to 10cm (4in) long. In late spring, bears cup-shaped white flowers, 1cm (½in) across, in dense racemes, to 10cm (4in) long; they are followed by spherical, red to purple fruit, 8mm (⅜in) across. ↕10m (30ft), ↔ 8m (25ft). North America. ❄❄❄. **'Shubert'** produces leaves that turn dark red-purple in summer.
***P.* 'Yae-murasaki'** ■⌂ Spreading, very slow-growing, deciduous tree with elliptic, tapered, mid-green leaves, to 12cm (5in) long, bronze when young, turning orange-red in autumn. In mid-spring, bears semi-double, dark pink flowers, 4cm (1½in) across, in clusters of 2–4. ↕5m (15ft), ↔ 8m (25ft). ❄❄❄
P.* x *yedoensis ■🏆⌂ (*P. speciosa* x *P.* x *subhirtella*) (Yoshino cherry). Spreading, deciduous tree bearing arching branches and elliptic, dark green leaves, to 11cm (4½in) long. In early spring, before the leaves, produces a profusion of racemes of 5 or 6 bowl-shaped, pale pink flowers, 4cm (1½in) across, fading to nearly white. ↕to 15m (50ft), ↔ 10m (30ft). Japan. ❄❄❄.
'Shidare-yoshino' ⌂ syn. 'Pendula', 'Perpendens', has weeping branches arching to the ground.

PSEUDERANTHEMUM

ACANTHACEAE

Genus of about 60 species of evergreen perennials, subshrubs, and shrubs from woodland habitats in tropical regions worldwide. They are grown primarily for their variegated or coloured leaves, which are opposite, simple, and entire or toothed. The long, tubular, 2-lipped, white, blue, purple, or red flowers, sometimes marked with yellow, are produced in spikes, racemes, or cymes. In areas where temperatures fall below

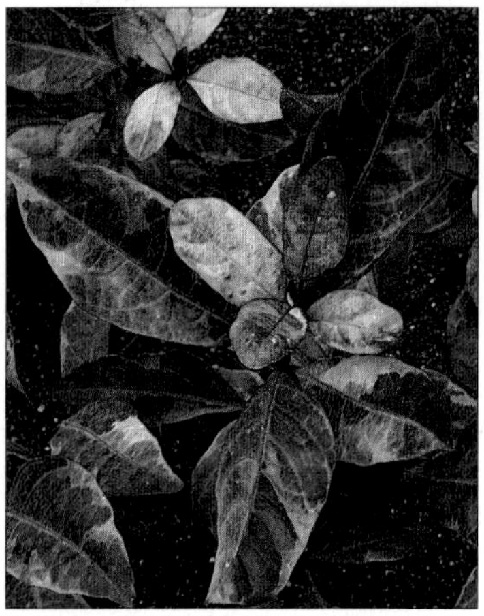
Pseuderanthemum atropurpureum 'Variegatum'

13°C (55°F), grow as foliage plants in a warm greenhouse. In tropical climates, they are suitable for growing in a shrub border.

- **HARDINESS** Frost tender.
- **CULTIVATION** Under glass, grow in loam-based potting compost (JI No.2) in bright filtered light, providing high humidity. During the growing season, water moderately and apply a balanced liquid fertilizer every month; water sparingly in winter. Outdoors, grow in fertile, moist, but well-drained soil in full sun with some midday shade, or in partial shade. Pruning group 9; needs restrictive pruning under glass.
- **PROPAGATION** Root semi-ripe cuttings in midsummer with bottom heat.
- **PESTS AND DISEASES** May be infested by red spider mites and whiteflies under glass.

P. atropurpureum, syn. *Eranthemum atropurpureum.* Erect, open shrub, the stems sparsely branched unless pinched out at intervals when young. Ovate to broadly elliptic leaves, 10–15cm (4–6in) long, are deep purple, sometimes metallic green, spotted yellow, pinkish purple, pink, green, and white. During summer, tubular white flowers, spotted rose-red or purple at the bases, 2.5cm (1in) long, are borne in dense, terminal spikes, to 18cm (7in) long. ↕0.9–1.5m (3–5ft), ↔ 30–75cm (12–30in). Polynesia. ❀ (min. 13°C/55°F).
'Variegatum' ■ syn. 'Tricolor', bears bronze-purple leaves, splashed and suffused creamy yellow and pink, and has pink flowers.

PSEUDOCYDONIA

ROSACEAE

Genus of one species of deciduous or semi-evergreen shrub or tree from temperate woodland in China. It has simple, dark green leaves, but is grown mainly for its peeling bark, cup-shaped pink flowers, and large, edible yellow fruit. It is best cultivated as a specimen tree, but will achieve tree stature only in regions with long, hot summers; in areas with cool summers, it remains shrubby and is best trained against a warm, sunny wall.

- **HARDINESS** Fully hardy in areas with hot summers, but otherwise frost hardy.
- **CULTIVATION** Grow in fertile, well-drained soil in full sun. Provide a warm site, sheltered from severe frost, and, in

P

areas with cool summers, sheltered from cold, drying winds. Pruning group 1, or group 13 if wall-grown.
• **PROPAGATION** Sow seed in containers outdoors in autumn.
• **PESTS AND DISEASES** Trouble free.

P. sinensis ♤ syn. *Cydonia sinensis.* Spreading shrub or small tree bearing peeling grey and white bark, and oval, finely toothed, dark green leaves, to 10cm (4in) long. Solitary, cup-shaped pink flowers, 4cm (1½in) across, are produced in mid- and late spring, followed, after hot summers, by ovoid yellow fruit, 15cm (6in) long. ↕↔ 6m (20ft). China. ✱✱

▷ ***Pseudodrynaria coronans*** see *Aglaomorpha coronans*
▷ ***Pseudofumaria*** see *Corydalis*
P. lutea see *C. lutea*
▷ ***Pseudogynoxys chenopodioides*** see *Senecio confusus*

PSEUDOLARIX

PINACEAE

Genus of one species of monoecious, deciduous, coniferous tree occurring in forest in China, with linear leaves borne in rosettes on short shoots (as in *Larix*). It is grown mainly for the outstanding golden orange colour of its autumn foliage. The female cones have large, triangular green scales and release the seeds by disintegrating; the male cones are catkin-like and clustered on short shoots. It is an excellent specimen tree, but is initially slow-growing, and is best grown in regions with long, hot summers.
• **HARDINESS** Fully hardy.
• **CULTIVATION** Grow in deep, fertile, acid to neutral, well-drained soil in a warm, sheltered site in full sun. Protect from cold, drying winds.
• **PROPAGATION** Sow seed in containers outoors in spring. Take greenwood cuttings in early summer.
• **PESTS AND DISEASES** Trouble free.

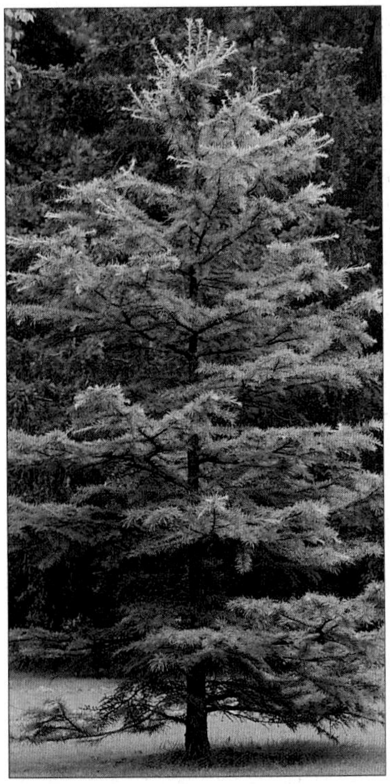
Pseudolarix amabilis

P. amabilis ▣ ♀ ♤ syn. *P. kaempferi* (Golden larch). Broadly conical or flattened, open-crowned tree with spreading branches, grey bark furrowed with raised, plate-like pieces, and purple, later greyish purple shoots with ovoid buds. Linear, soft, fresh green leaves, 2–5cm (¾–2in) long, turning golden orange in autumn, are borne on both long and short shoots. Erect, ovoid, yellow-green female cones, 6–8cm (2½–3in) long, ripening to brown, are spiky due to the free tips of the scales. ↕ to 15–20m (50–70ft), ↔ 6–12m (20–40ft). S. and E. China. ✱✱✱
P. kaempferi see *P. amabilis.*

▷ ***Pseudomuscari azureum*** see *Muscari azureum*

PSEUDOPANAX

ARALIACEAE

Genus of 12–20 species of evergreen trees and shrubs from forest and scrub in Tasmania (Australia), New Zealand, and Chile. Cultivated for their upright habit, foliage, and fruits, they are valuable architectural or specimen plants. The alternate, simple or palmate, entire or variously toothed leaves may vary greatly in shape, depending on the age of the plant. Inconspicuous, 4- or 5-petalled green flowers are borne mainly in winter, in terminal or, less commonly, lateral umbels, clusters, racemes, or mixtures of these. Male and female flowers usually grow on separate plants; both are required to produce the fruits, which are drupe-like, each with 2–5 stones. Grow in a warm, sheltered shrub border. In frost-prone areas, grow tender species in a cool greenhouse or conservatory.
• **HARDINESS** Frost hardy to frost tender.
• **CULTIVATION** Under glass, grow in loam-based potting compost (JI No.3), with added sharp sand, in full light with shade from hot sun, or in bright filtered light. In growth, water moderately and apply a balanced liquid fertilizer every month; water sparingly in winter. Outdoors, grow in fertile, well-drained soil in full sun or partial shade. In frost-prone areas, shelter from cold, drying winds. Pruning group 1; may need restrictive pruning under glass.
• **PROPAGATION** Sow seed in autumn or spring: seed of tender species at 19–24°C (66–75°F); seed of hardy species in containers in a cold frame. Take semi-ripe cuttings, or air layer, in summer.
• **PESTS AND DISEASES** Trouble free.

P. arboreus ♤ syn. *Neopanax arboreum* (Five finger, Whauwhaupaku). Bushy, round-headed, evergreen tree or sometimes large shrub, with long-stalked, 5- or 7-palmate, glossy, deep green leaves, composed of stalked, narrowly oblong to oblong-obovate, toothed leaflets, 10–20cm (4–8in) long. In winter, bears star-shaped, purple-budded cream flowers in compound umbels, to 20cm (8in) across, followed by black-purple fruit, 6mm (¼in) across. ↕ 4–8m (12–25ft), ↔ 2.5–5m (8–15ft). New Zealand. ❀ (min. 2°C/36°F)
P. crassifolius ♤ (Lancewood). Evergreen tree, unbranched for many years, with long, slender seedling leaves, to 60cm (24in) long, and downward-

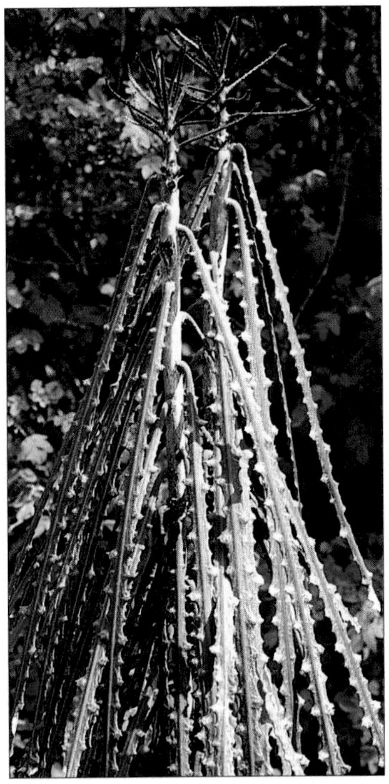
Pseudopanax ferox

pointing, dark green mature leaves, to 1m (3ft) long or more. Seedling leaves are simple, ovate to lance-shaped, membranous, coarsely toothed or lobed; mature leaves are linear, rigid, somewhat variegated, with red midribs and spine-tipped teeth. Mature plants develop a rounded head and narrow, spreading, linear to linear-obovate, 3- or 5-palmate, leathery leaves, with linear or sword-shaped leaflets, 20cm (8in) long. Star-shaped, greenish white flowers are produced in umbels, 7–10cm (3–4in) across, in summer and early autumn; they are followed on female or hermaphrodite flowers by spherical black fruit, 5mm (¼in) across. ↕ to 15m (50ft) ↔ 2m (6ft). New Zealand. ✱✱
P. ferox ▣ ♤ (Toothed lancewood). Upright, dioecious, evergreen tree, later developing a small, rounded head. Young plants produce simple, pendent, narrow, linear, sharply pointed, coarsely and jaggedly toothed, dark bronze-green mature leaves, to 45cm (18in) long, marked white or grey. Mature plants bear spreading, linear, dark green leaves, to 15cm (6in) long. Green flowers are borne in umbel-like panicles, to 10cm (4in) across, in summer and early

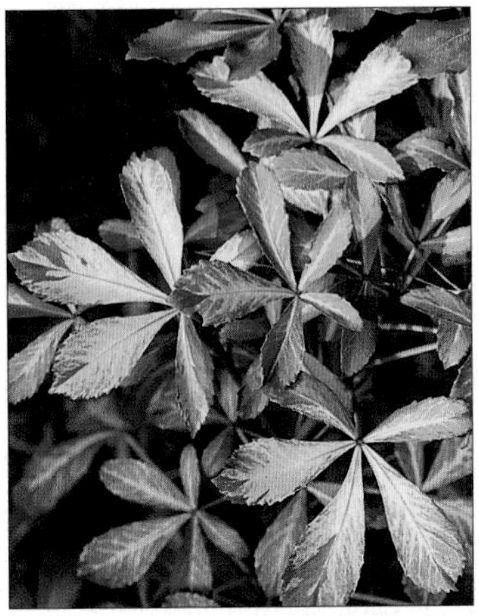
Pseudopanax lessonii 'Gold Splash'

autumn; they are followed on female plants by ovoid black fruit, 8mm (⅜in) across. ↕ 5m (15ft), ↔ 2m (6ft). New Zealand. ✱✱
P. laetus ♤ Rounded, dioecious, evergreen tree or shrub with stout shoots, and 5- or 7-palmate leaves composed of long-stalked, obovate, leathery, dark green leaflets, to 30cm (12in) long. In winter, bears greenish purple flowers in compound umbels, to 20cm (8in) across, followed on female plants by spherical, purple-black fruit, 5mm (¼in) across. ↕ 6m (20ft), ↔ 3m (10ft). New Zealand (North Island). ✱✱
P. lessonii ♤ (Houpara). Erect to spreading, evergreen, large shrub or small tree, with stout branches. The deep green leaves are 3- or 5-palmate: on juvenile plants they have 5 lance-shaped, coarsely and irregularly toothed leaflets, to 12cm (5in) long; on mature plants, they comprise 3 smaller, stalkless, obovate, entire to sparsely toothed leaflets, to 10cm (4in) long. Yellowish green flowers are borne in compound umbels, 10cm (4in) across, in summer; they are followed by oblong, purple-black fruit, 5mm (¼in) long. ↕ 3–6m (10–20ft), ↔ 2–4m (6–12ft). New Zealand (North Island, Three Kings Island). ❀ (min. 2°C/36°F). **'Gold Splash'** ▣ ♀ has yellow-marked leaves. **'Purpureus'** ♀ has bronze-purple foliage.

▷ ***Pseudorhipsalis alata*** see *Disocactus alatus*
▷ ***Pseudorhipsalis macrantha*** see *Disocactus macranthus*

PSEUDOSASA

GRAMINEAE/POACEAE

Genus of 3–6 species of woody, upright, spreading to clump-forming, evergreen, rhizomatous, perennial bamboos, often thicket-forming, found in woodland and along roads or tracks in China, Japan, and Taiwan. They are cultivated for their woody canes, which are erect, cylindrical, simple-branched or sometimes 3-branched at each upper node, and to 6m (20ft) high. The mid- or dark green leaves are lance-shaped or oblong, hairless, and somewhat tessellated. Rarely, spikelets of 2 to 8 flowers are borne in terminal, lax panicles. Grow in a woodland or wild garden, or as screening plants; they can be vigorous and invasive, and need room to spread.
• **HARDINESS** Fully hardy.
• **CULTIVATION** Grow in fertile, moist but well-drained soil in full sun or partial shade. If plants do flower, cut back to the bases, and apply a general-purpose fertilizer and deep organic mulch; this usually restores vigour.
• **PROPAGATION** Divide clumps in spring; keep moist until established.
• **PESTS AND DISEASES** Trouble free.

P. japonica. Upright, eventually thicket-forming, spreading, rhizomatous bamboo. Canes are olive green when young, maturing to pale beige. Lance-shaped or oblong, tessellated, dark green leaves, to 35cm (14in) long, are silver-grey beneath and have yellow midribs. Spikelets of 2–8 green flowers are borne in lax panicles, although flowering is rare. ↕ 6m (20ft), ↔ indeterminate. Japan. ✱✱✱

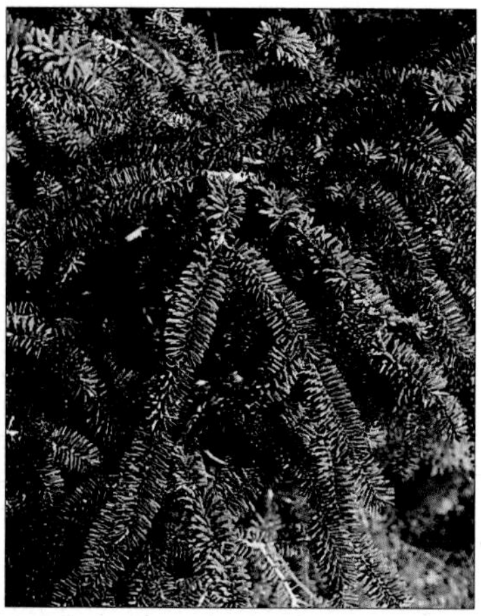

Pseudotsuga menziesii 'Fretsii'

PSEUDOTSUGA

PINACEAE

Genus of 6–8 species of tall, evergreen, coniferous trees from forest in China, Taiwan, Japan, W. North America, and Mexico. The linear leaves, arranged radially on the shoots, develop from pointed, many-scaled buds that are unique to the genus. The female cones have protruding, trident-shaped bract scales; the male cones are cylindrical. They are imposing specimen trees.

• **HARDINESS** Fully hardy.
• **CULTIVATION** Grow in any well-drained, non-chalky soil, in full sun.
• **PROPAGATION** Sow seed in containers outdoors in spring. Graft cultivars in late winter.
• **PESTS AND DISEASES** The foliage is attacked by Douglas fir adelgids.

P. douglasii see *P. menziesii.*
P. menziesii ♀ ⌂–♀ syn. *P. douglasii, P. taxifolia* (Douglas fir). Broadly conical tree when young, becoming columnar with spreading branches. The bark is smooth and grey at first, then thick, corky, deeply ridged, and red-brown. Ovoid, sharp-pointed, red-brown buds open to linear, soft, dark green leaves, 1.5–3cm (½–1¼in) long, loosely parted on the shoots, each with 2 white bands beneath. Ovoid-conical female cones, 7–10cm (3–4in) long, have long, erect bracts. ↕ 25–50m (80–160ft), ↔ 6–10m (20–30ft). W. North America (British Columbia to California). ✲✲✲.
'Fretsii' ■ is slow-growing, forming a small, spreading, conical tree, with dull green leaves, 0.8–1cm (⅜–½in) long; ↕ to 6m (20ft). **var. *glauca*** ■ (Blue Douglas fir) has smaller cones, 4.5–6cm (1¾–2½in) long, with reflexed bracts; the leaves are blue-glaucous, and the grey or black bark is thinner and more scaly. **'Oudemansii'** is slow-growing, with short leaves, 1.5–2cm (½–¾in) long; ↕ 5–10m (15–30ft).
P. taxifolia see *P. menziesii.*

PSEUDOWINTERA

WINTERACEAE

Genus of 3 species of aromatic, evergreen trees and shrubs from mountain forest in New Zealand. They are cultivated mainly for their alternate, broadly elliptic, leathery leaves, which have obvious glands. Cup-shaped, greenish yellow to white flowers are produced in axillary clusters, and are followed by spherical, dark red or black fruits. Pseudowinteras grow best in a sheltered border or woodland situation. In frost-prone areas, grow less hardy species in a cool greenhouse.

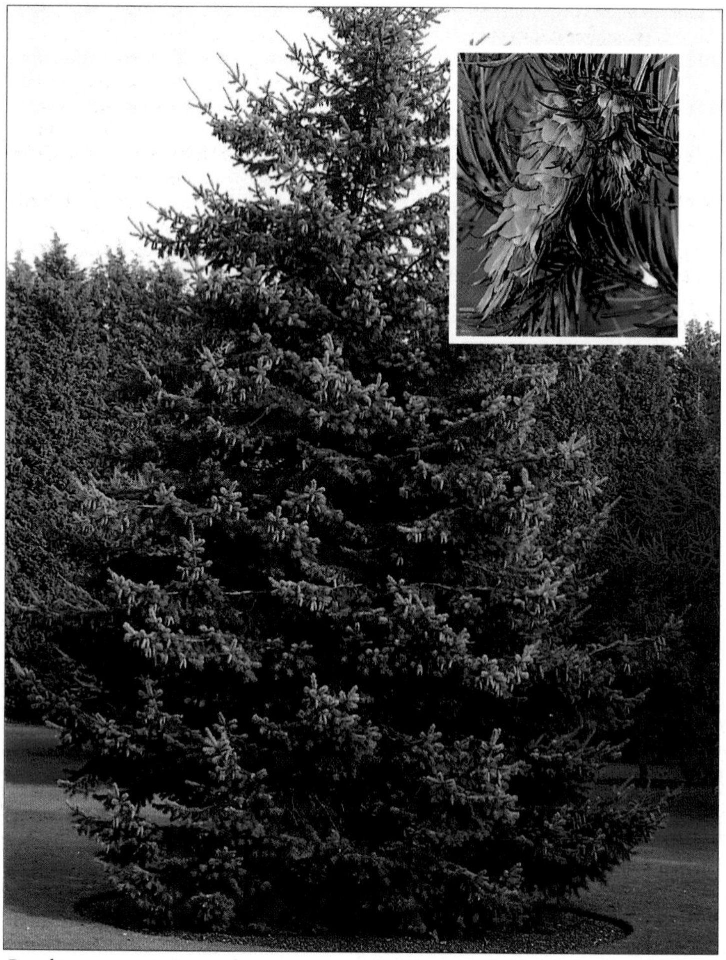

Pseudotsuga menziesii var. *glauca* (inset: cone detail)

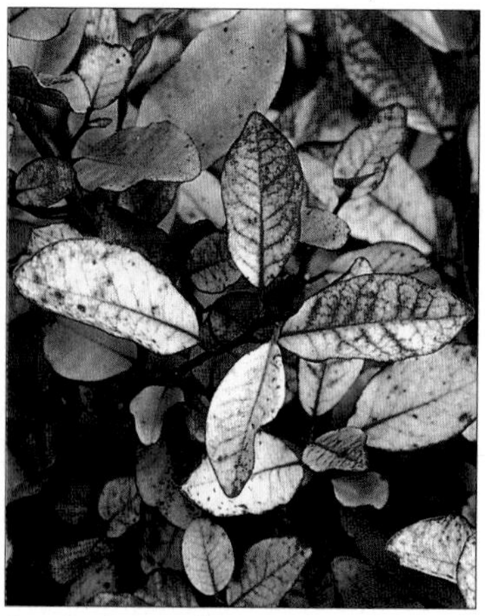

Pseudowintera colorata

• **HARDINESS** Frost hardy to half hardy.
• **CULTIVATION** Under glass, grow in loam-based potting compost (JI No.3) in full light or bright filtered light. During growth, water freely, applying a balanced liquid fertilizer monthly; water sparingly at all other times. Outdoors, grow in humus-rich, preferably neutral to acid, moist but well-drained soil in full sun or partial shade. Pruning group 8; may need restrictive pruning under glass.
• **PROPAGATION** Sow seed at 13–18°C (55–64°F) in autumn or spring. Root semi-ripe cuttings in midsummer with bottom heat.
• **PESTS AND DISEASES** Trouble free.

P. colorata ■ syn. *Drimys colorata.* Spreading, bushy shrub bearing broadly elliptic, leathery, yellow-green leaves, to 8cm (3in) long, marked pink and margined dark red-purple above, glaucous beneath. In mid-spring, bears clusters of 2–5 or more, cup-shaped, greenish yellow flowers, 1cm (½in) across, followed by spherical red, later black berries, 5mm (¼in) across. ↕ 1m (3ft), ↔ 1.5m (5ft). New Zealand. ✲✲

▷ ***Pseudozygocactus epiphylloides*** see *Hatiora epiphylloides*

PSILOTUM

Fork fern

PSILOTACEAE

Genus of 2 species of terrestrial or epiphytic, evergreen, rhizomatous, fern-like perennials from moist tropical and warm-temperate forest or woodland worldwide. They are grown for their upright, spreading, or pendent habit, and for their distinctive, repeatedly forked, triangular or flattened, yellow-green stems, 1–3mm (1⁄16–⅛in) thick, which may die back in winter. The leaves are very small and inconspicuous, and the stems sometimes bear small, spherical, 3-lobed sporangia in the axils of minute bracts. In frost-prone areas, grow in a cool or temperate greenhouse, and leave undisturbed for long periods; in warmer areas, grow beneath shrubs or tree ferns.

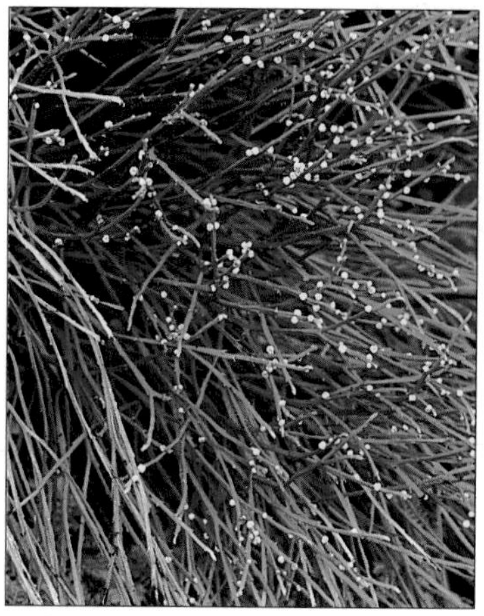

Psilotum nudum

• **HARDINESS** Frost tender.
• **CULTIVATION** Under glass, grow in 1 part each of loam, medium-grade bark, and charcoal, 2 parts sharp sand, and 3 parts coarse leaf mould; or grow epiphytically on tree-fern bark. Provide bright filtered light and high humidity. In growth, water and mist freely, and apply a balanced liquid fertilizer every month; water sparingly in winter. Outdoors, grow in moderately fertile, moist but well-drained soil in light dappled shade.
• **PROPAGATION** Sow spores at 21°C (70°F) when ripe. Divide established plants in spring. See also p.51.
• **PESTS AND DISEASES** Trouble free.

P. nudum ■ Bushy, evergreen, fern-like perennial with upright, spreading, or pendent, branching, yellow-green, triangular stems, to 60cm (24in) long. Dull yellow sporangia, 3mm (⅛in) wide, are produced on the upper parts of the stems. Leaves are sparse and scale-like, 2mm (1⁄16in) long. ↕↔ 60cm (24in). Tropical to warm-temperate areas worldwide. ❀ (min. 5°C/41°F)

PSYCHOPSIS

ORCHIDACEAE

Genus of about 5 species of small, evergreen, epiphytic orchids from lowland to mountainous forest, at altitudes of up to 1,000m (3,250ft), in Central America, South America, and Trinidad. They have compressed, clustered, oval pseudobulbs, and solitary, semi-rigid, oblong-elliptic leaves, which are mottled dark green and dull purple. Butterfly-

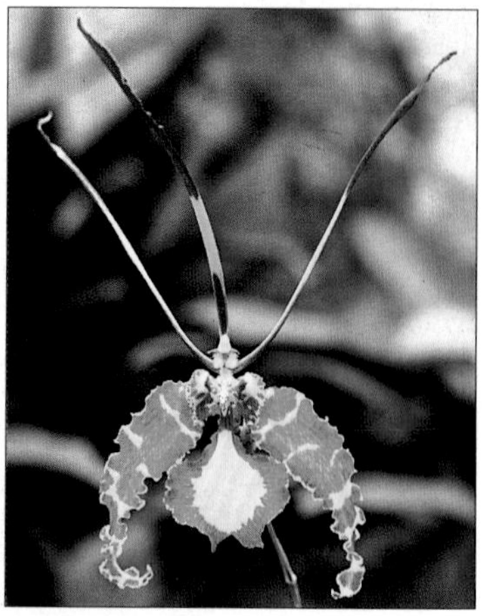

Psychopsis papilio

P

like flowers are borne over a long period in long, slender, few-flowered, jointed racemes, occasionally singly, from the base of each pseudobulb.

- **HARDINESS** Frost tender.
- **CULTIVATION** Intermediate-growing orchids. Grow in epiphytic orchid compost or epiphytically on slabs of bark. Throughout the year, provide full light and high humidity, and water sparingly. During summer, mist rather than water, and feed every week. See also p.46.
- **PROPAGATION** Divide when the plant fills the pot and "flows" over the sides.
- **PESTS AND DISEASES** May be infested by red spider mites, aphids, and mealybugs.

P. papilio ■ syn. *Oncidium papilio.* Epiphytic orchid with spherical pseudobulbs, each producing a single, ovate to elliptic leaf, 12–25cm (5–10in) long. Orange-brown flowers, 15cm (6in) across, slightly mottled greenish yellow, with yellow and brown mottled lips, are borne in few-flowered racemes, to 1.2m (4ft) long, throughout the year. ↕60cm (24in), ↔30cm (12in). Trinidad, Venezuela, Colombia, Ecuador, Peru. ❁ (min. 10°C/50°F; max. 30°C/86°F)

▷ ***Psygmorchis pusilla*** see *Oncidium pusillum*

PSYLLIOSTACHYS

Statice

PLUMBAGINACEAE

Genus of about 6–8 species of erect, usually rosette-forming annuals found in sandy soils on plains and in foothills from Syria to Iran and C. Asia. They have mostly basal, deeply lobed or occasionally simple and entire, oblong or lance-shaped to obovate, light to mid-green leaves. From spring to autumn, they produce branching or simple spikes of tiny, tubular, pink or white flowers, each with 5 spreading lobes. Statices are suitable for the front of an annual border, and are tolerant of coastal conditions. They are also excellent for cutting and drying.

- **HARDINESS** Fully hardy to half hardy.
- **CULTIVATION** Grow in fertile, moist but well-drained soil in a warm, sheltered site in full sun.
- **PROPAGATION** Sow seed at 21°C (70°F) in spring.
- **PESTS AND DISEASES** Prone to grey mould (*Botrytis*) and powdery mildew.

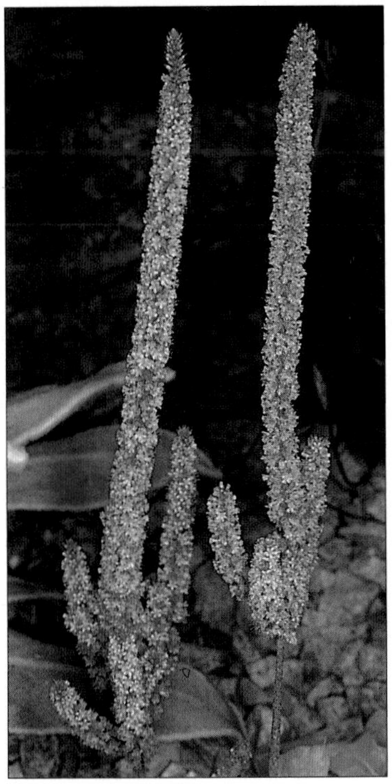

Psylliostachys suworowii

P. spicata, syn. *Limonium spicatum, Statice spicata.* Rosette-forming annual with deeply lobed, inversely lance-shaped leaves, 5–15cm (2–6in) long; the leaf-stalks and midribs are densely clothed in long hairs. Rose-pink flowers are borne in terminal spikes, to 9cm (3½in) long, and shorter, lateral spikes, from summer to early autumn. ↕30–45cm (12–18in), ↔ to 30cm (12in). Ukraine (Crimea), Caucasus, Iran. ✲

P. suworowii ■ syn. *Limonium suworowii, Statice suworowii.* Rosette-forming annual bearing simple, basal, inversely lance-shaped to oblong-obovate, wavy-margined to slightly lobed, light green leaves, to 15cm (6in) long. Rose-pink flowers, are borne in narrow, cylindrical, branching spikes, to 20cm (8in) long, from summer to early autumn. ↕30–45cm (12–18in), ↔ to 30cm (12in). Iran, W. Turkmenistan, N. Afghanistan, C. Asia. ✲

PTELEA

RUTACEAE

Genus of 3 or more species of aromatic, deciduous trees and shrubs found in thickets and on rocky slopes in North America. Cultivated for their 3-palmate, strongly scented leaves, they also bear corymbs of inconspicuous, cup-shaped or star-shaped, sometimes unisexual, greenish white flowers, followed by winged, more or less rounded and flattened fruits. Suitable for growing in a shrub border or as lawn specimens.

- **HARDINESS** Fully hardy to frost hardy.
- **CULTIVATION** Grow in fertile, well-drained soil in full sun or dappled shade. Pruning group 1.
- **PROPAGATION** Sow seed in containers outdoors in autumn or spring. Take greenwood cuttings in early summer.
- **PESTS AND DISEASES** Trouble free.

P. trifoliata ♀ (Hop tree). Upright, deciduous shrub with aromatic bark and alternate, 3-palmate, scented, dark green leaves, to 12cm (5in) long, with ovate to elliptic leaflets. Corymbs of star-shaped, greenish white flowers are borne in summer, followed by winged, rounded and flattened, pale green fruit, to 2.5cm (1in) across. ↕8m (25ft), ↔4m (12ft). North America (Ontario to Connecticut, Michigan, Iowa, Florida, Texas, and N. Mexico). ✲✲✲. **'Aurea'** ■♀ bears bright yellow to yellow-green leaves, turning dark green, then yellow in autumn; ↕5m (15ft).

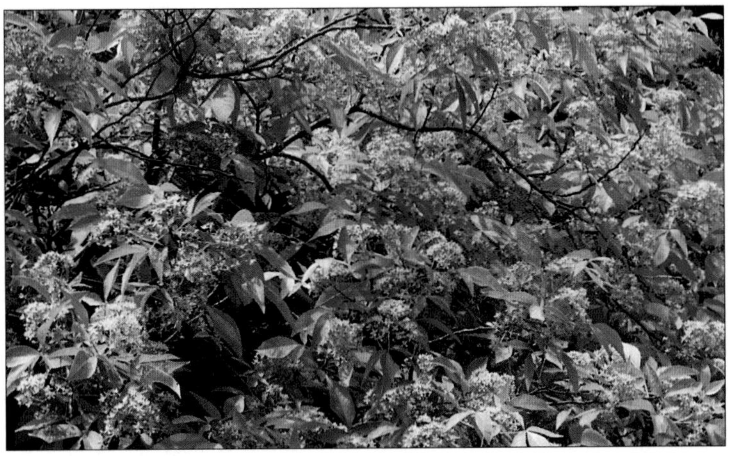

Ptelea trifoliata 'Aurea'

PTERIS

Brake

ADIANTACEAE/PTERIDACEAE

Genus of approximately 280 species of deciduous, semi-evergreen, and evergreen, terrestrial ferns, found mainly in tropical and subtropical forests throughout the world. The rhizomes are stout and erect to slender and short-creeping. Brakes are cultivated for their closely spaced fronds, which are pinnatisect or pinnate to 4-pinnate, and range from less than 30cm (12in) long to 3m (10ft). Spores form at the frond margins, which curl under to protect them. In frost-prone climates, grow the tender species and cultivars in a cool or temperate greenhouse, or as houseplants. In warmer areas, use singly as feature plants, or in mixed foliage plantings.

- **HARDINESS** Frost hardy to frost tender.
- **CULTIVATION** Under glass, grow in 1 part each of sharp sand, coarse leaf mould, and charcoal, and 2 parts loam-based potting compost (JI No.2), in bright filtered light and high humidity; *P. cretica* and *P. vittata* prefer slightly alkaline soil, so add limestone chips. In growth, water freely, applying a high-nitrogen liquid fertilizer monthly; water sparingly in winter. Outdoors, grow in any moist but well-drained soil (except chalky soil), with added leaf mould, in partial or deep shade.
- **PROPAGATION** Sow spores at 21°C (70°F) when ripe. Divide plants with creeping, branched rhizomes in spring. See also p.51.
- **PESTS AND DISEASES** Prone to scale insects and leaf eelworms under glass. In still, humid conditions, sooty mould may occur if water settles on the fronds.

P. argyraea ■ (Silver brake). Evergreen fern with erect rhizomes bearing erect, pinnate or 2-pinnate fronds, 60–100cm (24–39in) long, each with up to 6 pairs

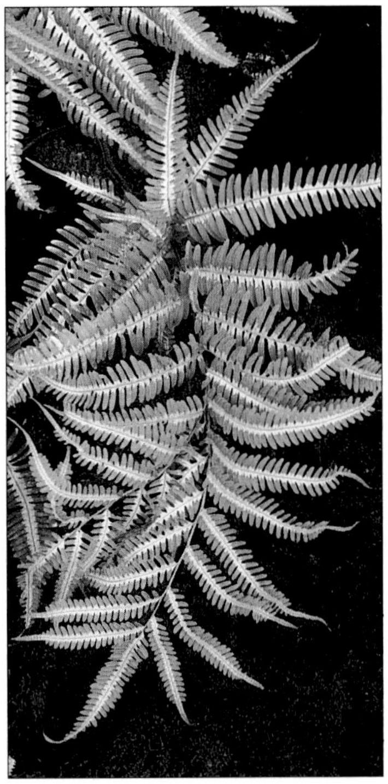

Pteris argyraea

of oblong, dark green pinnae with broad, silvery white stripes down their centres. The pinnatisect pinnae are composed of numerous linear-oblong lobes; the lowest pair are usually forked. Requires shade. ↕↔ to 1m (3ft). Tropics. ❁ (min. 10°C/50°F)

P. biaurita. Evergreen fern with erect rhizomes producing erect, oblong or triangular-oblong, pinnate, light apple-green fronds, to 1.3m (4½ft) long, each with 5–15 pairs of pinnatisect pinnae, the lowest pair usually forked. Similar to *P. argyraea*, but pinnae lack the central white streaks. Thrives in damp shade. ↕0.6–1.5m (24–60in), ↔40–150cm (16–60in). Tropics. ❁ (min. 10°C/50°F)

P. cretica ♀ Evergreen fern with a short-creeping, many-branched rhizome. Produces arching, crowded, ovate or rounded, pinnate, pale green fronds, 30–70cm (12–28in) long, each with 1–5 pairs of narrowly lance-shaped, simple or forked pinnae. Fertile fronds are taller and have narrower pinnae than sterile fronds. Some clones are half hardy. ↕ to 75cm (30in), ↔60cm (24in). Europe, Africa, Asia. ❁ (min. 2°C/36°F). **'Albolineata'** ■♀ has a broad white band along the centre of

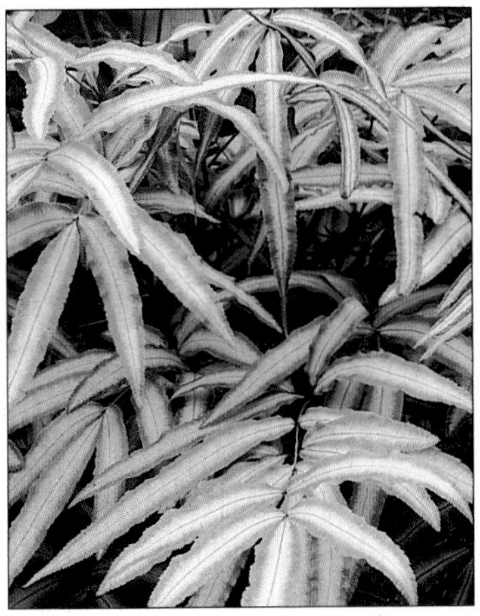

Pteris cretica 'Albolineata'

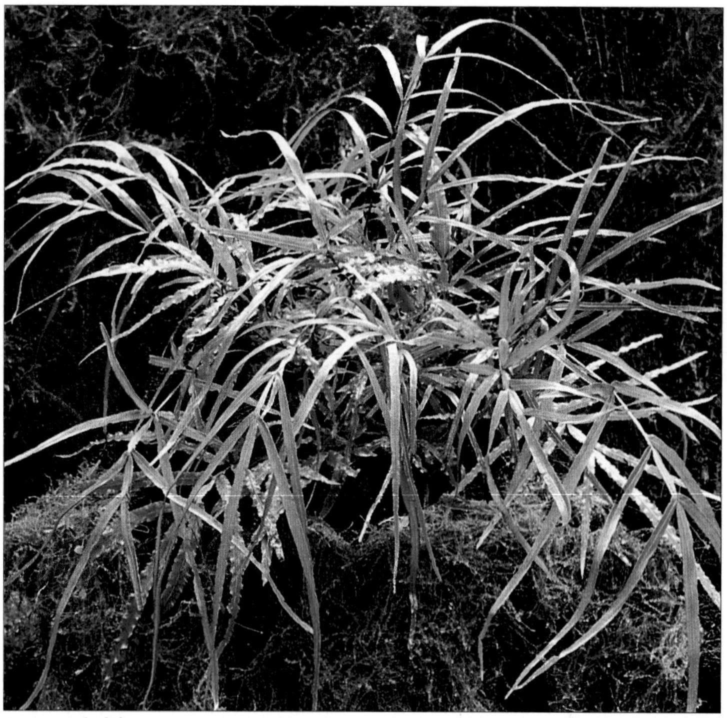

Pteris multifida

each pinna, and is easier to grow than the species; ❄❄ (borderline). **'Childsii'** has broader pinnae than the species, with incised margins and small crested tips. Possibly of hybrid origin; ↕ to 50cm (20in), ↔ 30cm (12in). **'Distinction'** is smaller than the species, and has deeply lobed pinnae with branched tips; ↕↔ 40cm (16in). **'Mayi'** is similar to 'Albolineata', but has crested pinnae tips. **'Parkeri'** is a vigorous cultivar, with broader, mid- to dark green pinnae; ↕ to 90cm (36in), ↔ 60cm (24in). **'Rivertoniana'** is strong-growing, with pinnae margins that are deeply but irregularly cut into narrow lobes. **'Wimsettii'** has a compact habit; the margins of the pinnae are deeply and irregularly lobed, with the tips often crested; ↕↔ 45cm (18in).

P. dentata. Evergreen fern that forms clumps of triangular to ovate, very variably divided, 2- or 3-pinnate, bright green fronds, to 1.5m (5ft) long, arising from short-creeping to erect rhizomes. Sterile fronds have pinnae segments with finely toothed margins, but on fertile fronds the margins are entire. ↕ 0.5–1.8m (20–72in), ↔ 0.6–1.5m (24–60in). Tropical Africa, South Africa, Arabian Peninsula. ❄ (min. 10°C/50°F)

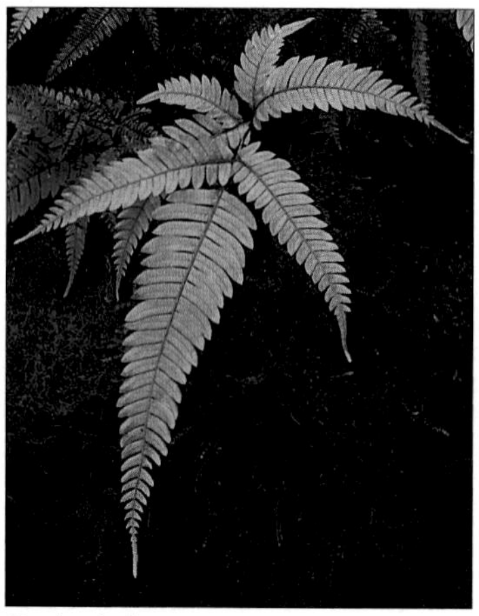

Pteris tricolor

P. ensiformis (Sword brake). Evergreen fern with short-creeping, branched rhizomes producing narrow-triangular, 2-pinnate, dark green fronds, often greyish white around the midribs. Fertile fronds, up to 40cm (16in) long, have 4 or 5 pairs of linear pinnae, each with a few toothed segments at the base. Sterile fronds are shorter, and have narrower pinnae with entire margins. ↕↔ 30cm (12in). Himalayas to Japan, Philippines, Polynesia, tropical Australia. ❄ (min. 10°C/50°F). **'Arguta'** has dark green fronds with strongly contrasting silver-white central midribs. **'Evergemiensis'** has silver markings similar to 'Arguta'. **'Victoriae'** has white bands running either side of the midribs.

P. fauriei. Small, neat, evergreen fern with erect rhizomes producing arching, broadly triangular to ovate, mid-green fronds, 20–60cm (8–24in) long, each with 3–5 pairs of oblong, deeply pinnatisect pinnae. ↕ to 45cm (18in), ↔ 60cm (24in). China, Japan. ❄ (min. 10°C/50°F)

P. multifida ■ (Spider brake). Evergreen fern with short-creeping to erect, many-branched rhizomes producing numerous erect, ovate, light green fronds, 20–50cm (8–20in) long. Each frond is 2-pinnate at the base, pinnatisect above, with 3–5 pairs of pinnae. Pinnae are linear, with long, tapering tips, the upper ones decurrent to the stem. ↕ to 45cm (18in), ↔ 23cm (9in). China, Korea, Japan to Taiwan, Indonesia. ❄ (min. 10°C/50°F). **'Corymbifera'** has crested pinnae tips.

P. tremula (Shaking brake, Tender brake). Evergreen fern with an erect rhizome producing ovate, arching, light green fronds, to 2m (6ft) tall, 3- or 4-pinnate at the base, with overlapping pinnae giving a feathery appearance. Pinnae are narrowly oblong to linear, with finely toothed margins. Fast-growing, and may become invasive. ↕ to

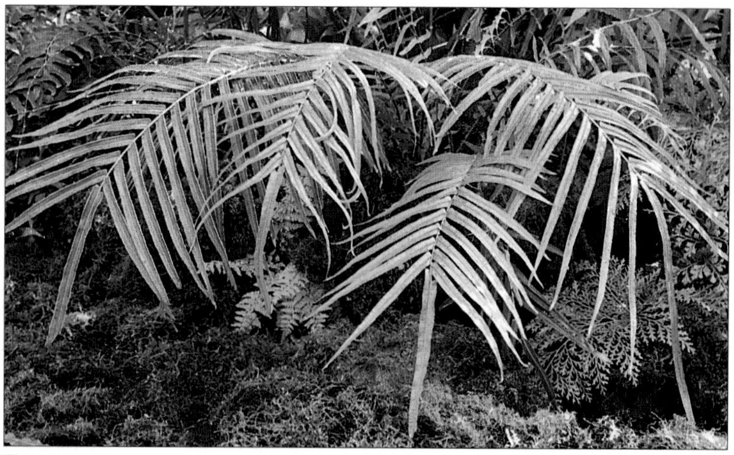

Pteris vittata

1.5m (5ft), ↔ 1m (3ft). New Zealand, Australia, Fiji. ❄ (min. 10°C/ 50°F)

P. tricolor ■ (Painted brake). Evergreen fern with erect, ovate, pinnate fronds, 40–60cm (16–24in) long, arising from creeping, branched rhizomes. Fertile fronds have 2–5 pairs of pinnatisect, oblong pinnae; they are red-purple when young, ageing to mid-green, but stalks and midribs remain purple. ↕ to 60cm (24in), ↔ 60cm (24in). Malacca. ❄ (min. 10°C/50°F)

P. umbrosa (Jungle brake). Evergreen fern with short-creeping, many-branched rhizomes. Triangular-ovate, shining, dark green, erect fronds, to 1m (3ft) tall, are 2-pinnatisect with 3–7 pairs of narrowly lance-shaped lobes, the lower ones divided into 3 or 5 segments. The fronds are similar in appearance to those of *P. cretica*, but are much more robust and luxuriant. ↕ to 1.2m (4ft), ↔ 1m (3ft). Australia. ❄ (min. 10°C/50°F)

P. vittata ■ Evergreen fern with short-creeping rhizomes covered with golden scales. Fronds are erect, oblong, pinnate, to 1m (3ft) tall, with up to 40 pairs of simple, linear, dark green pinnae. Tolerates chalk and some exposure to sun. ↕ to 1m (3ft), ↔ 60cm (24in). Tropical and warm-temperate regions of Europe, Africa, Asia, Australasia. ❄ (min. 2°C/36°F)

PTEROCACTUS

CACTACEAE

Genus of 9 species of dwarf, shrub-like cacti occurring in hilly regions of Argentina. They arise from tuberous rootstocks, and branch from the bases to produce somewhat club-shaped stems. The areoles bear very fine, almost hair-like spines and minute glochids. Small, white or yellow to reddish brown and coppery, diurnal flowers, without tubes, are produced terminally in early summer. In frost-prone climates, grow in a cool greenhouse or in a bowl garden; in warmer regions, they are suitable for growing outdoors in a desert garden.

• **HARDINESS** Frost tender.

• **CULTIVATION** Under glass, grow in standard cactus compost in full light. From spring to summer, water moderately and apply a low-nitrogen liquid fertilizer every 4 or 5 weeks. Keep completely dry at other times. Outdoors, grow in poor, sharply drained soil in full sun. See also pp.48–49.

• **PROPAGATION** Sow seed at 19–24°C (66–75°F) in spring. Take basal cuttings in spring or early summer.

• **PESTS AND DISEASES** Susceptible to mealybugs.

P. fischeri. Short-stemmed, shrub-like cactus producing spherical or ovoid, cylindrical, jointed, brown-green stems, 2cm (¾in) thick. White areoles bear about 16 spines (12 yellow radial spines and 4 longer, brownish yellow centrals). White flowers, 4cm (1½in) or more across, are produced in early summer. ↕ 15cm (6in), ↔ to 20cm (8in). S. Argentina. (Neuquen, Rio Negro). ❄ (min. 2–7°C/36–45°F)

P. kuntzei see *P. tuberosus.*

P. tuberosus ■ syn. *P. kuntzei.* Shrub-like cactus producing cylindrical, brown or green-brown stems, to 0.8–1.5cm (⅜–½in) thick, with a vertical violet line below each areole. The grey areoles bear minute, off-white spines that lie flat on the stems. Pale yellow flowers, 3–5cm (1¼–2in) across, sometimes tinged orange-brown or coppery brown, are produced in early summer. ↕↔ to 40cm (16in). Argentina (Mendoza). ❄ (min. 2–7°C/36–45°F)

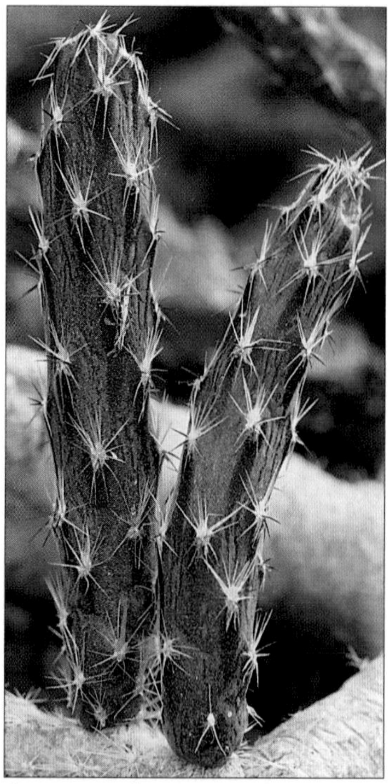

Pterocactus tuberosus

P

PTEROCARYA

Wing nut

JUGLANDACEAE

Genus of about 10 species of fast-growing, deciduous trees found in woodland and on riverbanks, mainly in the mountains of Asia, from the Caucasus to Japan. They are cultivated for their attractive, spreading habit, for their large, alternate, more or less oblong, pinnate leaves, composed of 5–27 leaflets, which colour yellow in autumn, and for their long, pendent spikes of winged fruit, which are produced over a long period in summer. Inconspicuous green male and female flowers are produced in separate catkins in spring as the leaves emerge. Wing nuts grow to a considerable size, so site in a large garden or park.

• **HARDINESS** Fully hardy, but foliage may be damaged by late frosts.
• **CULTIVATION** Grow in deep, fertile, moist but well-drained soil in full sun. Pruning group 1; remove unwanted suckers as they appear.
• **PROPAGATION** Sow seed in containers outdoors in autumn. Remove rooted suckers in autumn.
• **PESTS AND DISEASES** Trouble free.

P. fraxinifolia 🏆 🌳 (Caucasian wing nut). Vigorous, spreading tree bearing pinnate leaves, to 40cm (16in) long, with cylindrical midribs; the leaves are composed of 23 or more, oblong to ovate, glossy, dark green leaflets. Small, winged green fruit are produced in pendent spikes, to 50cm (20in) long, in summer. ↕ 25m (80ft), ↔ 20m (70ft). Caucasus, N. Iran. ❄❄❄

P. x rehderiana 🌳 (*P. fraxinifolia* x *P. stenoptera*). Very vigorous, spreading, strongly suckering tree bearing pinnate leaves, to 20cm (8in) long, with slightly winged midribs; the leaves are composed of up to 21 oblong to ovate, glossy, dark green leaflets. Small, winged green fruit are produced in pendent spikes, to 45cm (18in) long, in summer. ↕ 25m (80ft), ↔ 20m (70ft). Garden origin. ❄❄❄

P. rhoifolia 🌳 (Japanese wing nut). Spreading tree with pinnate leaves, to 40cm (16in) long; the leaves are composed of up to 21 ovate-oblong, tapered, glossy, mid-green leaflets. Small, winged green fruit are produced in pendent spikes, to 30cm (12in) long, in summer. ↕ 30m (100ft), ↔ 25m (80ft). Japan. ❄❄❄

P. stenoptera ▣ 🌳 (Chinese wing nut). Spreading tree with pinnate leaves, to 40cm (16in) long, with winged midribs; the leaves comprise up to 21 oblong, bright green leaflets, the terminal leaflet often absent. Small, winged green fruit are produced in pendent spikes, to 30cm (12in) long, in summer. ↕ 25m (80ft), ↔ 15m (50ft). China. ❄❄❄

PTEROCELTIS

ULMACEAE

Genus of one species of deciduous tree found near streams, in rocky places, and in valleys in the mountains of China. It is cultivated for its habit, peeling bark, bright green foliage, and winged green fruit. Inconspicuous, very small green flowers are produced in spring. Best grown as a specimen tree.

• **HARDINESS** Fully hardy.
• **CULTIVATION** Grow in fertile, moist but well-drained soil in full sun. Pruning group 1.
• **PROPAGATION** Sow seed in containers outdoors in autumn.
• **PESTS AND DISEASES** Trouble free.

P. tatarinowii 🌳 Spreading tree with arching branches, flaking grey bark, and ovate, tapered, 3-veined, bright green leaves, to 10cm (4in) long, with toothed margins. The tiny, green male flowers are produced in stalkless clusters; the very small, green female flowers are solitary. Both male and female flowers are produced in spring, from the leaf axils; they are followed by round, winged green fruit, 2cm (¾in) across, in autumn. ↕↔ 10m (30ft). N. and C. China. ❄❄❄

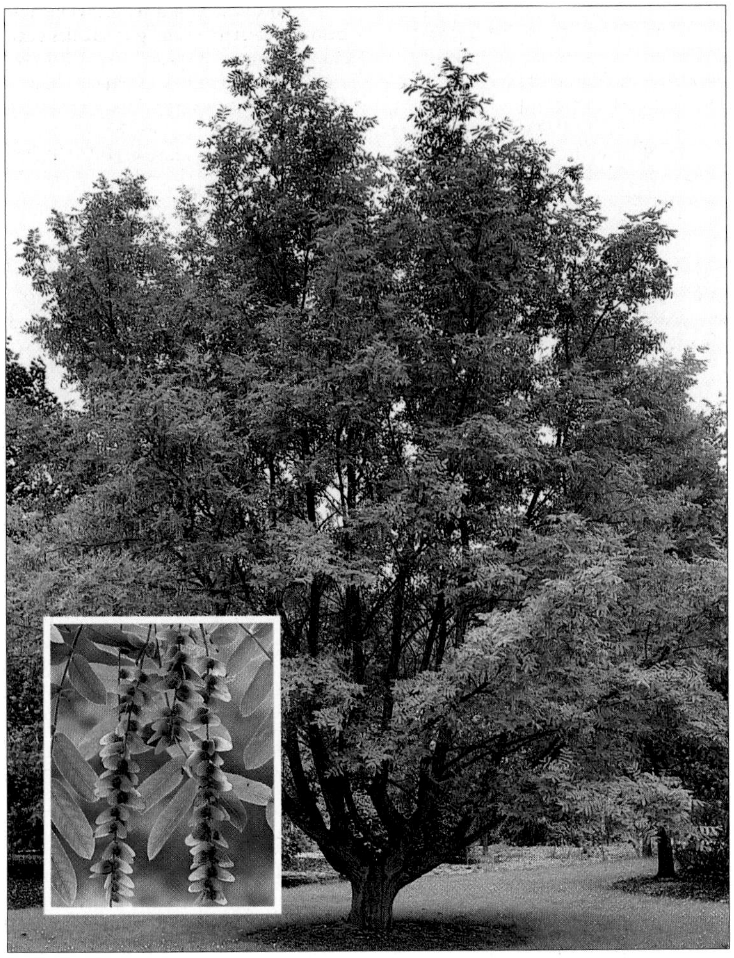

Pterocarya stenoptera (inset: fruit detail)

PTEROCEPHALUS

DIPSACACEAE

Genus of approximately 25 species of annuals, perennials, and evergreen shrubs, occurring on rocky slopes, roadsides, and waste ground from the Mediterranean and tropical Africa to C. Asia, the Himalayas, and W. China. They have opposite, simple, entire or pinnatifid leaves, sometimes with scalloped margins. They are cultivated for their scabious-like, pink or mauve flowerheads, produced on long stems in summer, and the attractive, papery seed heads that follow. *P. perennis*, the only species widely grown, is suitable for a rock garden or the front of a border.

• **HARDINESS** Fully hardy.
• **CULTIVATION** Grow in any well-drained soil in full sun.
• **PROPAGATION** Sow seed in containers in a cold frame in autumn. Take stem-tip cuttings in summer.
• **PESTS AND DISEASES** Trouble free.

P. perennis ▣ syn. *P. parnassi.* Evergreen, mat-forming perennial bearing opposite, ovate to fiddle-shaped, hairy, grey-green leaves, to 4cm (1½in) long, scalloped at the margins. During summer, long stems, to 8cm (3in) long, bear solitary, dense, flattened heads of tubular, pale pinkish purple flowers, to 4cm (1½in) across; they are followed by papery seed heads. ↕ 8cm (3in), ↔ 20cm (8in). Greece. ❄❄❄

P. parnassi see *P. perennis.*

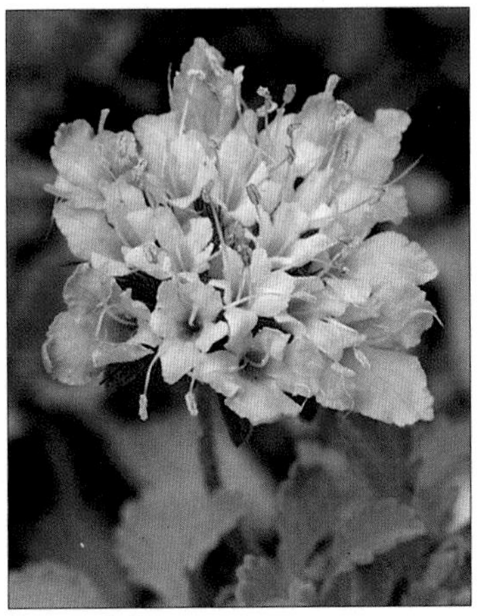

Pterocephalus perennis

PTERODISCUS

PEDALIACEAE

Genus of 18 species of succulent perennials and subshrubs found in semi-desert, rocky regions from tropical E. to S.W. Africa. They have a swollen caudex, tuberous roots, and solitary or branching stems. They are grown for their foliage and flowers: the leaves are very variable, light to dark green, and have entire, toothed, or deeply cut margins; the 5-lobed, funnel- to bell-shaped flowers are slightly 2-lipped, diurnal, usually yellow, orange, red, purple, or white, and are produced singly from the leaf axils in summer. In areas where temperatures fall below 15°C (59°F), grow as houseplants or in a warm greenhouse; in warm, dry climates, grow in a succulent border.

• **HARDINESS** Frost tender.
• **CULTIVATION** Under glass, grow in standard cactus compost in full light. From spring to summer, water sparingly and apply a low-nitrogen liquid fertilizer every 4–6 weeks. Keep dry at other times. Outdoors, grow in moderately fertile, sharply drained soil in full sun. Protect from excessive wet. See also pp.48–49.
• **PROPAGATION** Sow seed in spring at 19–24°C (66–75°F).
• **PESTS AND DISEASES** Trouble free.

P. luridus. Succulent with a conical, fleshy caudex, 8cm (3in) thick towards the base, covered with a smooth grey bark. Spreading, slightly white-frosted stems bear oblong, dark green leaves, 8cm (3in) long, with white or blue undersides and entire margins. Funnel-shaped yellow flowers, 2.5–5cm (1–2in) long, spotted red outside, are produced in summer. ↕ 50cm (20in), ↔ 15cm (6in). S.W. Africa. ❀ (min. 15°C/59°F)

P. speciosus. Succulent with a conical to spherical, fleshy caudex, 6cm (2½in) thick towards the base, and stems bearing linear-oblong, dark green leaves, to 6cm (2½in) long, with irregularly toothed margins. Funnel-shaped, pale reddish purple flowers, 3cm (1¼in) long, are produced in summer. ↕ 15cm (6in), ↔ 10cm (4in). South Africa (Northern Transvaal, Eastern Cape). ❀ (min. 15°C/59°F)

PTEROPOGON

ASTERACEAE/COMPOSITAE

Genus of 10 erect to slightly spreading, slender-stemmed, white-woolly annuals, previously part of the genus *Helipterum*, from semi-arid regions of South Africa and Australia. They bear alternate, narrowly lance-shaped, light to mid-green, white-woolly leaves, but are cultivated for their long-stemmed, leafy clusters of small, rounded, papery, daisy-like, usually yellow flowerheads, borne from summer to early autumn. Suitable for an annual or mixed border. The flowerheads are good for drying, the clustered blooms of *P. humboldtianus* turning an attractive metallic green.

• **HARDINESS** Half hardy.
• **CULTIVATION** Grow in poor, sharply drained soil in full sun.
• **PROPAGATION** Sow seed *in situ* in late spring.
• **PESTS AND DISEASES** Prone to aphids.

P. humboldtianus, syn. *Helipterum humboldtianum*. Erect, single-stemmed or slightly branching annual with narrowly lance-shaped, white-woolly leaves, to 3cm (1¼in) long. Slightly fragrant, straw-textured yellow flowers are produced in flowerheads to 8cm (3in) across, from summer to early autumn. ↕ to 45cm (18in), ↔ to 15cm (6in). S. Australia. ❄

PTEROSTYRAX

STYRACACEAE

Genus of 4 species of spreading, deciduous trees or shrubs, with peeling, aromatic bark, occurring in mountain woodland in China and Japan. They are cultivated for their alternate, oblong to ovate, pale green leaves, pendent panicles of fragrant, 5-lobed white flowers, and unusual, ribbed or winged fruits. Grow as shrubs or as single- or multiple-stemmed specimen trees in a lawn or woodland setting.

- **HARDINESS** Fully hardy.
- **CULTIVATION** Grow in deep, fertile, well-drained, neutral to acid soil in full sun or partial shade. Pruning group 1.
- **PROPAGATION** Sow seed in containers outdoors in autumn. Take semi-ripe cuttings in summer.
- **PESTS AND DISEASES** Trouble free.

P. hispida ♀ ♀ (Epaulette tree). Spreading tree or shrub with peeling, aromatic grey bark and oblong to ovate, pale green leaves, to 20cm (8in) long. Bell-shaped, fragrant white flowers, 1cm (½in) across, each with 5 lobes divided almost to the base, are borne in pendent panicles, to 20cm (8in) long, in early and midsummer, followed by oblong, 5-ribbed fruit, to 1cm (½in) long, covered in yellow-brown bristles. ↕ 15m (50ft), ↔ 12m (40ft). China, Japan. ❄❄❄

▷ ***Ptilotrichum spinosum*** see *Alyssum spinosum*

P

PTILOTUS

AMARANTHACEAE

Genus of about 100 species of annuals, herbaceous perennials, and subshrubs from open scrub in Australia. They are grown for their dense, rounded, ovoid or conical to cylindrical spikes of tiny, 5-tepalled, white, yellow, pink, mauve, purple, or green flowers, often enhanced by long white hairs. The leaves are alternate and usually narrow. In frost-prone areas, grow in a cool greenhouse or in an alpine house, or as annual summer bedding plants; in warmer areas, grow in a border or rock garden.

- **HARDINESS** Frost hardy.
- **CULTIVATION** Under glass, grow in loam-based potting compost (JI No.2) in full light. During the growing season, water moderately and apply a balanced liquid fertilizer monthly; keep almost dry in winter. Outdoors, grow in fertile, sharply drained soil in full sun; avoid wet conditions.
- **PROPAGATION** Sow seed at 13–16°C (55–61°F) in spring. Take root cuttings in early spring.
- **PESTS AND DISEASES** Trouble free.

P. exaltatus (Pink mulla mulla). Robust, bushy perennial with rosettes of oblong-lance-shaped, thick, wavy-margined, bluish green leaves, to 8cm (3in) long, often tinged red. Very small, white to pink or red flowers, with hairy brown bracts, are borne in conical, later cylindrical spikes, to 15cm (6in) long, from winter to summer. ↕ to 30cm (12in) or more, ↔ 60cm (24in). Australia. ❄❄

P. manglesii, syn. *Trichinium manglesii*. Erect or spreading perennial bearing rosettes of narrow to broadly ovate, thick, smooth-margined, white-hairy, mid-green leaves, 2.5–8cm (1–3in) long. The lower leaves are borne on long stalks; the upper leaves are smaller and stalkless. In summer, very small, pink to violet flowers, with dark brown bracts, are produced in round to ovoid, white-hairy spikes, 8–10cm (3–4in) long. ↕↔ 10–40cm (4–16in). Australia. ❄❄

PTYCHOSPERMA

ARECACEAE/PALMAE

Genus of about 30 species of single- or cluster-stemmed palms found in moist forest habitats from coastal lowlands to mountain valleys, from Micronesia to Australia, New Guinea, and the Solomon Islands. Pinnate, oblong-elliptic, glossy leaves are composed of linear leaflets. Greenish white or greenish yellow, 3-petalled flowers are produced in panicles below the leaves, followed by spherical to ovoid, red, orange, or purplish black fruits. In frost-prone climates, grow in a warm greenhouse, or as houseplants. In tropical regions, grow as specimens in a small lawn, or to add height and interest to a shrub border.

- **HARDINESS** Frost tender.
- **CULTIVATION** Under glass, grow in loam-based potting compost (JI No.3) with added well-rotted organic matter and sharp sand, in bright indirect light. Pot on or top-dress in spring; during the growing season, water freely and apply a balanced liquid fertilizer every month. Water sparingly in winter. Outdoors, grow in fertile, moist but well-drained soil in partial shade.
- **PROPAGATION** Sow seed at 24°C (75°F) in spring.
- **PESTS AND DISEASES** Prone to scale insects and red spider mites under glass.

P. alexandrae see *Archontophoenix alexandrae*.

P. elegans ♈ syn. *Seaforthia elegans* (Alexander palm, Solitaire palm). Small to medium-sized palm with a slender, columnar trunk, ringed with old leaf scars. The woolly crownshaft produces pinnate, short-stalked leaves, 1–2.5m (3–8ft) long, composed of many broadly linear, mid-green leaflets with notched or toothed tips. In summer, fragrant, greenish white flowers, each to 8mm (⅜in) across, are produced in nodding panicles, 30–60cm (12–24in) long; they are followed by ovoid, bright red fruit, 2cm (¾in) across. ↕ 8–12m (25–40ft), ↔ 2–4m (6–12ft). N.E. Australia. ❀ (min. 16°C/61°F)

P. macarthurii ▣ ✾ Small, cluster-stemmed palm with slender, ring-scarred trunks. Pinnate, short-stalked leaves, 1.5m (5ft) long, are composed of many linear, bright green leaflets with ragged-toothed tips. Greenish yellow flowers, each to 8mm (⅜in) across, are produced in panicles 30–45cm (12–18in) long, usually in summer; they are followed by ovoid red fruit, 1.5cm (½in) long. ↕ 3–7m (10–22ft), ↔ 2–4m (6–12ft). New Guinea, N.E. Australia (Cape York Peninsula). ❀ (min. 16°C/61°F)

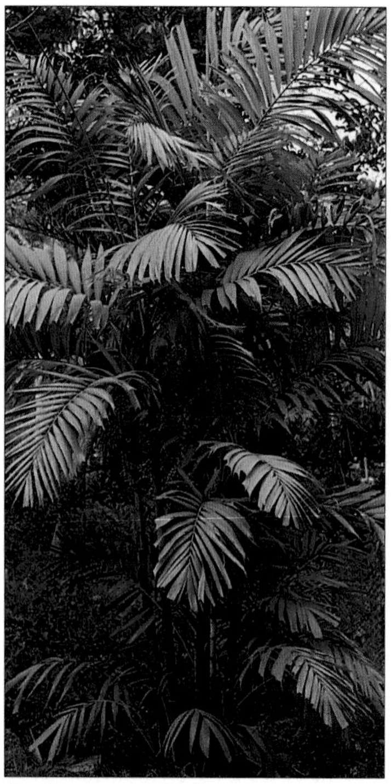

Ptychosperma macarthurii

▷ **Puccoon, Red** see *Sanguinaria*

▷ **Pudding pipe-tree** see *Cassia fistula*

PUERARIA

LEGUMINOSAE/PAPILIONACEAE

Genus of 17 species of mainly woody-stemmed, deciduous or evergreen, twining climbers from thickets and woodland in S.E. Asia and Japan. They are grown for their alternate, 3-palmate or pinnate leaves and for their axillary or terminal racemes of pea-like flowers. *P. lobata*, the only species commonly cultivated, is extremely vigorous and must be sited with care. It is suitable for growing as ground cover, for screening an unsightly building, or for covering a tall tree stump. In frost-prone areas, it may also be grown as an annual.

- **HARDINESS** Frost hardy to frost tender.
- **CULTIVATION** Grow in fertile, moist but well-drained soil in full sun or partial shade. Support twining stems. Pruning group 11, in spring.
- **PROPAGATION** Sow seed at 13–18°C (55–64°F) in spring.
- **PESTS AND DISEASES** Trouble free.

P. hirsuta see *P. lobata*.

P. lobata, syn. *P. hirsuta*, *P. thunbergiana* (Japanese arrowroot, Kudzu vine). Very vigorous, deciduous, twining climber, with a large tuber, sometimes grown as an annual. Bears 3-palmate leaves composed of ovate to diamond-shaped, lobed leaflets, the central one largest, to 18cm (7in) long. In autumn, fragrant, pea-like purple flowers, 2cm (¾in) long, are produced in erect racemes, to 25cm (10in) long. ↕ to 20m (70ft) or more (sometimes reaches half this in one year). China, Japan, Pacific islands. ❄❄

P. thunbergiana see *P. lobata*.

PULMONARIA

Lungwort

BORAGINACEAE

Genus of about 14 species of deciduous or evergreen, low-growing perennials, with slowly spreading rhizomes. They are found in Europe and Asia, on acid to alkaline soils in a wide range of habitats, including mountainous areas, moist, subalpine woodland, and streamsides. They are grown for their early flowers, often among the first perennial blooms, in late winter or spring, and for their simple, ovate to elliptic or oblong, hairy basal leaves, which are often attractively spotted white or silver. The stem leaves are few, smaller, and more or less stalkless. Regular, funnel-shaped flowers, 5–10mm (¼–½in) across, with 5 spreading lobes, are borne in terminal cymes; the flowers may be pink, red, violet, purple, blue, or white, with either long (pin) or short (thrum) styles; blue, purple, or violet flowers may often be pink in bud. After flowering, new "summer" leaves develop, showing the markings at their best. Lungworts are good ground-cover plants for a shady position: grow in woodland, among shrubs, in a wild garden, or at the front of a border. They are attractive to bees.

- **HARDINESS** Fully hardy.
- **CULTIVATION** Grow in humus-rich, fertile, moist but not waterlogged soil, in full or partial shade; *P. officinalis* will tolerate full sun. Remove old leaves after flowering. Divide every 3–5 years.
- **PROPAGATION** Sow seed in containers outdoors as soon as ripe. Lungworts hybridize freely in cultivation, and plants raised from seed of species in gardens often do not come true. Divide after flowering, or in autumn. Take root cuttings in midwinter.
- **PESTS AND DISEASES** Prone to powdery mildew in dry conditions. Slugs and snails may damage new growth.

P. angustifolia ♀ (Blue cowslip). Open clump-forming, rhizomatous, usually deciduous perennial with lance-shaped, unspotted, mid- to dark green leaves, 40cm (16in) long. Funnel-shaped, rich blue flowers are borne profusely on erect then spreading stems, from early to late spring. ↕ 25–30cm (10–12in), ↔ 45cm (18in). C., N.E., and E. Europe. ❄❄❄. **subsp. *azurea*** ▣ syn. *P. azurea*, has brighter blue flowers, tinted red in bud; ↕ to 25cm (10in). **'Beth's Pink'** see *P.*

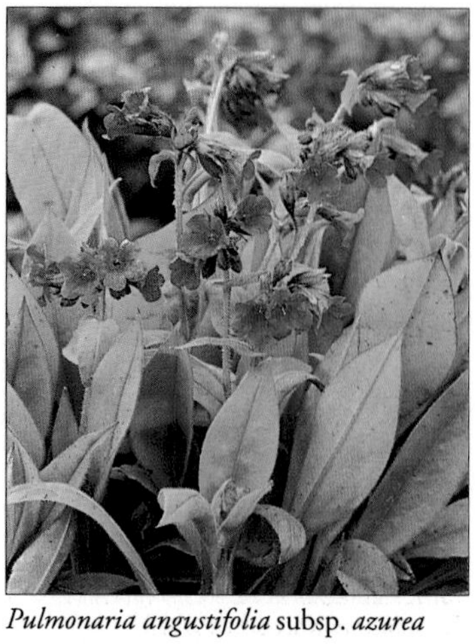

Pulmonaria angustifolia subsp. *azurea*

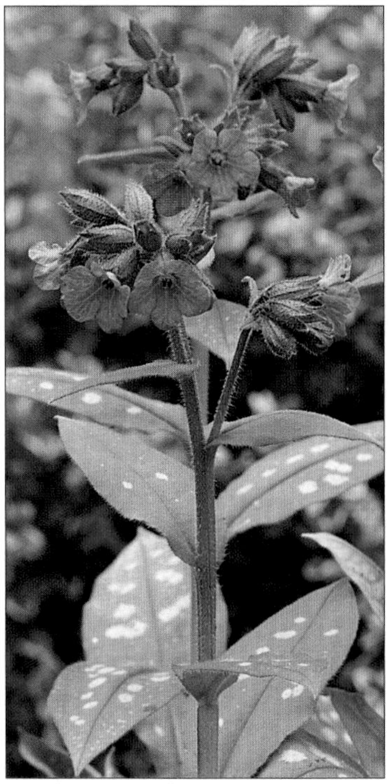

Pulmonaria 'Lewis Palmer'

'Beth's Pink'. **'Blaues Meer'** produces bright blue flowers very freely.
P. azurea see *P. angustifolia* subsp. *azurea.*
***P.* 'Beth's Pink'**, syn. *P. angustifolia* 'Beth's Pink'. Clump-forming, rhizomatous, deciduous perennial with ovate, white-spotted, dark green leaves, to 25cm (10in) long, narrowing abruptly to the leaf-stalks. In mid- and late spring, bears funnel-shaped, deep coral-pink flowers. ↕ to 30cm (12in), ↔ 45cm (18in). ❄❄❄
***P.* 'Blue Ensign'.** Clump-forming, rhizomatous, deciduous perennial with ovate, unspotted, dark green leaves, to 25cm (10in) long, and large, blue-violet flowers, borne in spring. ↕ to 35cm (14in), ↔ to 45cm (18in). ❄❄❄
***P.* 'Lewis Palmer'** ▣🏆 syn. *P. longifolia* 'Lewis Palmer'. Clump-forming, rhizomatous, deciduous perennial with lance-shaped, softly hairy, dark green basal leaves, to 30cm (12in) long, irregularly splashed and spotted greenish white, and ovate-lance-shaped stem leaves. In early spring, bears funnel-shaped flowers that open pink and become bright blue. ↕ 35cm (14in), ↔ 45cm (18in). ❄❄❄

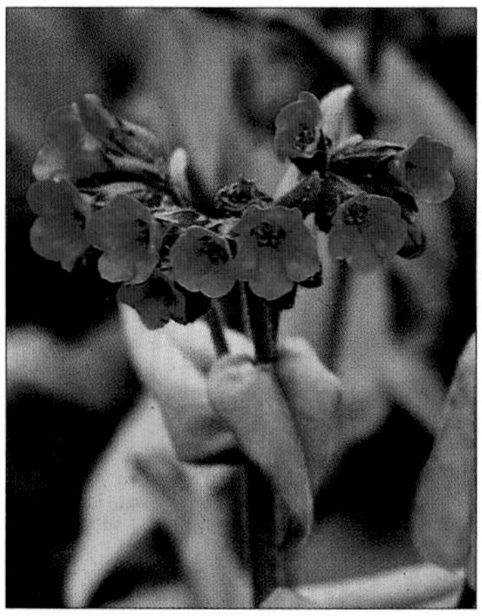

Pulmonaria 'Mawson's Blue'

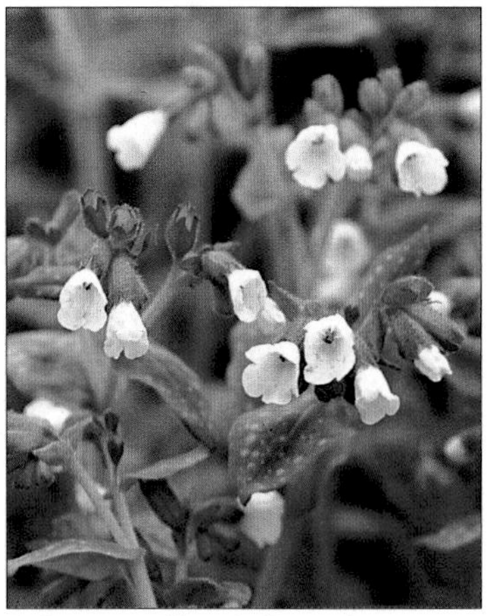

Pulmonaria officinalis 'Sissinghurst White'

P. longifolia. Densely clump-forming, rhizomatous, deciduous perennial with narrowly lance-shaped, dark green leaves, to 45cm (18in) long, spotted silvery white. Dense cymes of long-lasting, funnel-shaped, blue-purple to almost blue flowers are borne from late winter to late spring. ↕ to 30cm (12in), ↔ 45cm (18in). W. Europe, including Sweden and Britain. ❄❄❄. **'Bertram Anderson'** has longer, narrower, more strongly marked leaves, and brighter blue flowers. **'Lewis Palmer'** see *P.* 'Lewis Palmer'.
***P.* 'Mawson's Blue'** ▣ syn. *P.* 'Mawson's Variety'. Erect to spreading, rhizomatous, deciduous perennial bearing ovate to elliptic, softly hairy, unspotted, dark green leaves, to 30cm (12in) long. Produces dark blue flowers in spring. ↕ to 35cm (14in), ↔ to 45cm (18in). ❄❄❄
***P.* 'Mawson's Variety'** see *P.* 'Mawson's Blue'.
P. mollis, syn. *P. montana.* Vigorous, clump-forming, rhizomatous, deciduous perennial bearing elliptic to narrowly ovate, softly hairy, unspotted, mid-green leaves, to 45cm (18in) long. From late winter to mid-spring, produces funnel-shaped, rich blue flowers, sometimes pink-tinged fading to purplish blue. ↕ to 45cm (18in), ↔ 60cm (24in). Belgium, N.W. France, W. Germany, W. Switzerland. ❄❄❄
P. montana see *P. mollis.*
P. officinalis (Jerusalem cowslip, Soldiers and sailors, Spotted dog). Open clump-forming, rhizomatous, evergreen perennial with ovate, bristly, white-

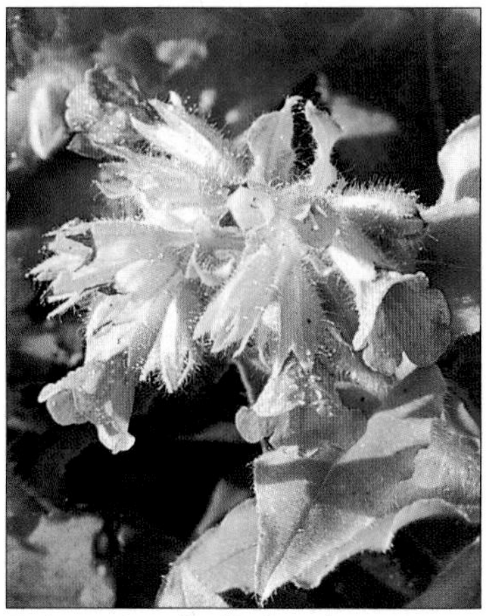

Pulmonaria rubra 'Redstart'

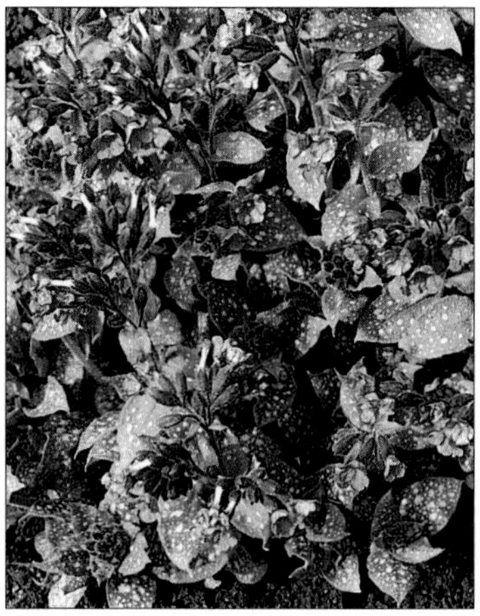

Pulmonaria saccharata

spotted, bright mid-green leaves, 10–13cm (4–5in) long, heart-shaped at the bases. From early to late spring, bears funnel-shaped flowers, opening pink and becoming reddish violet then blue. ↕ 25cm (10in), ↔ 45cm (18in). Europe. ❄❄❄. **'Cambridge Blue'**, syn. 'Cambridge', bears heart-shaped leaves and abundant pale blue flowers, pink-tinted on opening; ↕ to 30cm (12in). **'Sissinghurst White'** ▣🏆 syn. *P. saccharata* 'Sissinghurst White', bears leaves 20–25cm (8–10in) long, with numerous white spots, and pure white flowers opening from pale pink buds; ↕ to 30cm (12in). **'White Wings'** bears pink-eyed white flowers in late spring.
P. rubra 🏆 Loosely clump-forming, rhizomatous, leafy, evergreen perennial with elliptic, almost diamond-shaped, velvety, unspotted, matt, bright green leaves, to 60cm (24in) long. Funnel-shaped, bright brick-red to salmon-red flowers are borne over a long period from late winter to mid-spring. ↕ to 40cm (16in), ↔ 90cm (36in). S.E. Europe. ❄❄❄. **var. *alba*** see var. *albocorollata.* **var. *albocorollata***, syn. var. *alba*, has white flowers; ↕ to 30cm (12in). **'Barfield Pink'** has pink-and-white-striped flowers; ↕ to 30cm (12in). **'Bowles' Red'** has leaves with pale green spots, and coral-red flowers. **'David Ward'** has strongly white-variegated, sage-green leaves, with cream margins, and coral-red flowers; ↕ to 30cm (12in). **'Redstart'** ▣ has coral-red flowers and is often the first pulmonaria to flower, in midwinter.
P. saccharata ▣ (Jerusalem sage). Clump-forming, rhizomatous, evergreen perennial with elliptic, white-spotted, mid-green leaves, to 27cm (11in) long, the stem leaves nearly as large as the basal leaves. From late winter to late spring, bears funnel-shaped, red-violet, violet, or white flowers, with dark green calyces. ↕ 30cm (12in), ↔ 60cm (24in). S.E. France, N. and C. Italy. ❄❄❄. Cultivars in **Argentea Group** 🏆 have almost completely silver leaves, and flowers opening red, ageing to dark violet. **'Frühlingshimmel'** ▣ has many-spotted leaves, and light blue flowers with darker blue-purple eyes and calyces; ↕ 25cm (10in). **'Leopard'** has many-spotted, dark green leaves, and red, pink-tinted flowers. **'Mrs. Moon'** has pink buds opening to bluish lilac flowers. **'Pink Dawn'** bears deep pink flowers ageing to violet. **'Sissinghurst White'** see *P. officinalis* 'Sissinghurst White'.
P. vallarsae. Clump-forming, rhizomatous, deciduous perennial with elliptic-oblong, wavy-margined, densely softly hairy, dark green leaves, 20cm (8in) long, narrowing abruptly to the leaf-stalks; they have bright green or whitish green spots, in rare cases none. Funnel-shaped violet flowers, becoming more purple with age, are borne on glandular-hairy stems from early to late spring. ↕ 15–30cm (6–12in), ↔ 60cm (24in). Italy. ❄❄❄. **'Margery Fish'** 🏆 has bright green leaves, 15cm (6in) long, densely silvered on the upper surfaces, with the midribs and margins spotted. The flowers are coral-pink to red-violet, becoming violet; ↕ 18–28cm (7–11in).

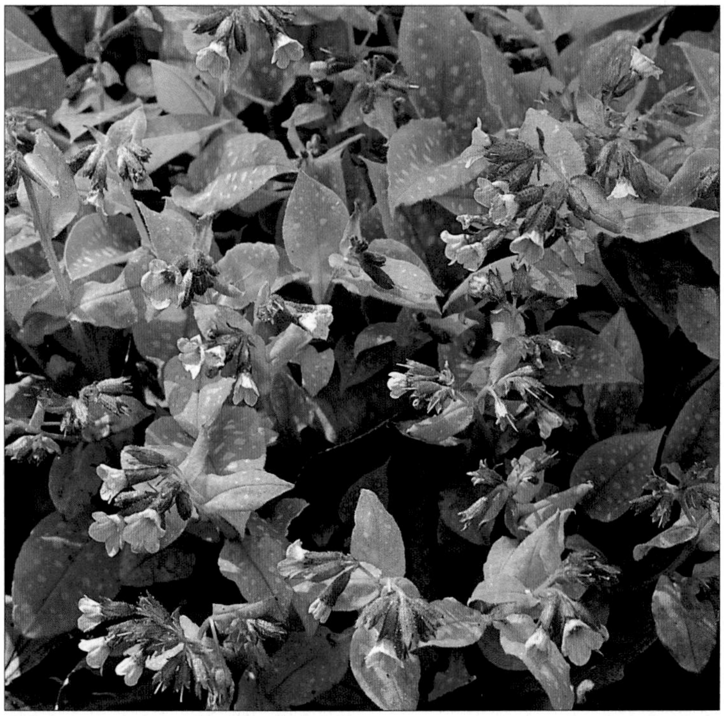

Pulmonaria saccharata 'Frühlingshimmel'

PULSATILLA

RANUNCULACEAE

Genus of about 30 species of clump-forming, deciduous perennials (sometimes with a few overwintering leaves) with a coarsely fibrous rootstock, found mainly in short turf and alpine meadows in Eurasia and N. America. They are cultivated for their finely dissected, fern-like leaves and their solitary, usually silky-hairy, bell- or cup-shaped flowers, produced in spring and early summer. The flowers are followed by spherical seed heads with silver-silky, plume-like styles, borne on stems that often elongate considerably after flowering; heights given below are for plants in flower. Grow in a rock garden, scree bed, or alpine house. All parts of the plant may cause mild stomach upset if ingested, and, in rare instances, contact with the sap may irritate skin.

• **HARDINESS** Fully hardy.

• **CULTIVATION** Grow in fertile, very well-drained soil in full sun; *P. vernalis* needs very gritty, moist but sharply drained soil in a scree bed, and requires protection from excessive winter wet. Pulsatillas resent root disturbance and may be difficult to establish, so plant when small and leave undisturbed. In an alpine house, use a mix of equal parts loam-based potting compost (JI No.1) and grit.

• **PROPAGATION** Sow seed as soon as ripe in containers in an open frame. Take root cuttings in winter.

• **PESTS AND DISEASES** Young growth may be attacked by slugs and snails.

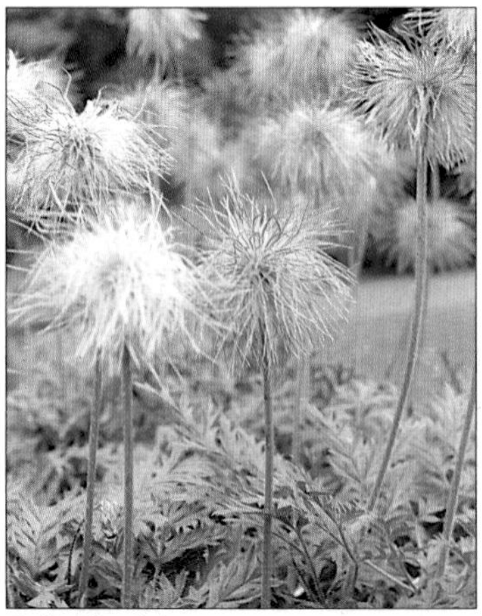

Pulsatilla alpina

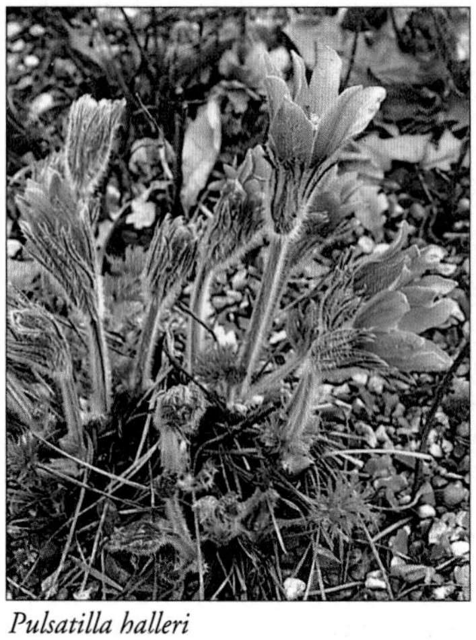

Pulsatilla halleri

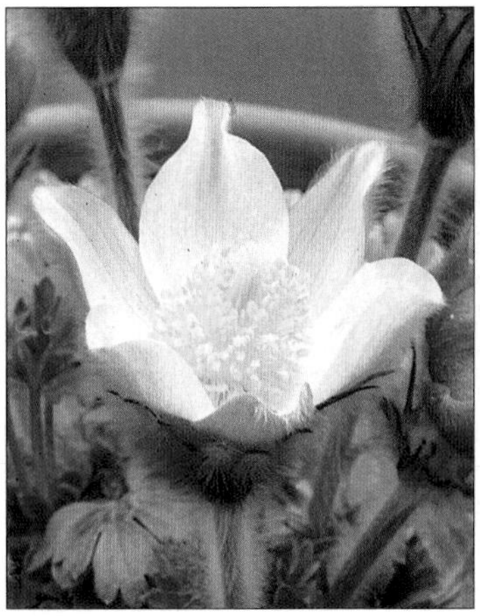

Pulsatilla vernalis

P. alpina ■ (Alpine pasque flower). Clump-forming perennial with finely divided, 2-pinnate, hairy, mid-green leaves, 6–12cm (2½–5in) long, composed of 30–80 toothed leaflets. In spring, bears cup-shaped white flowers, to 6cm (2½in) across, with silky-hairy petals, blue-tinted on the reverse, and yellow stamens, followed by ornamental seed heads (pictured). ↕ 15–30cm (6–12in), ↔ 20cm (8in). Mountains in C. Europe. ❄❄❄. **subsp. *apiifolia*** ♀ syn. subsp. *sulphurea*, has pale yellow flowers, and usually occurs in acid soils. **subsp. *sulphurea*** see subsp. *apiifolia*.
P. halleri ■ ♀ Tufted perennial, densely clothed in long silver hairs, with pinnate, light green leaves, 5–18cm (2–7in) long, comprising 3–5 pinnatifid leaflets with oblong-lance-shaped lobes; the terminal leaflet is long-stalked. Erect, silky-hairy, bell-shaped, violet-purple to lavender-blue flowers, to 9cm (3½in) across, are produced with the leaves in late spring. ↕ 20cm (8in), ↔ 15cm (6in). C. and S.E. Europe, Crimea. ❄❄❄. **subsp. *grandis***, syn. *P. vulgaris* subsp. *grandis*, has silvery golden brown hairs. It bears very finely divided leaves after the shallowly bell-shaped, lavender-blue flowers, which have rounded segments; C. Europe, Ukraine.
P. patens (Eastern pasque flower). Clump-forming perennial with rounded-heart-shaped, roughly hairy, 3- to 7-palmate, mid-green leaves, to 12cm (5in) long; each of the leaflets is divided into 15–80 linear to linear-lance-shaped segments. In late spring, bears erect, broadly cup-shaped, blue-violet, lilac, or occasionally yellowish or

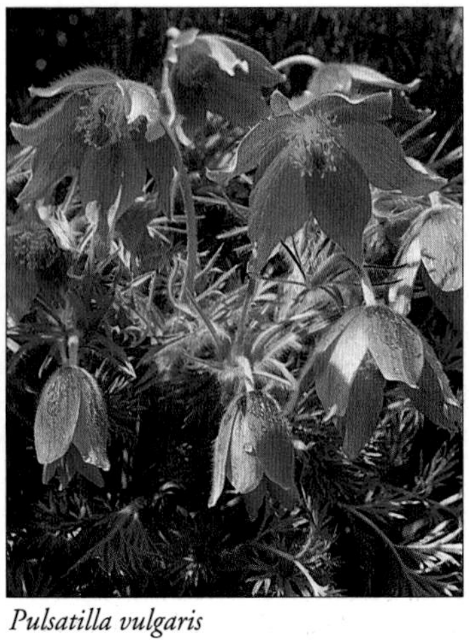

Pulsatilla vulgaris

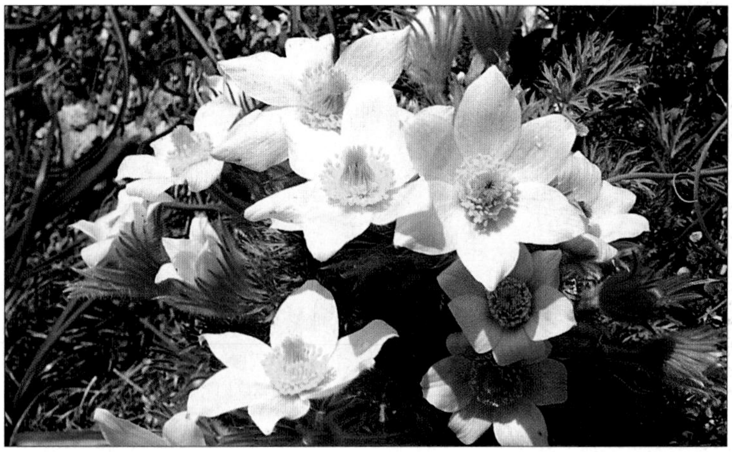

Pulsatilla vulgaris f. *alba*

yellowish white flowers, 5–8cm (2–3in) across. ↕ 15cm (6in), ↔ 10cm (4in). E. Europe, Russia (Siberia), North America. ❄❄❄
P. vernalis ■ ♀ Clump-forming perennial (with basal leaves overwintering) bearing clusters of finely cut, very sparsely hairy, pinnate, light green leaves, 6–12cm (2½–5in) long, comprising 3–5 deeply toothed leaflets. In spring, pendent buds open to erect, bell-shaped white flowers, to 6cm (2½in) across, deeply flushed with bluish violet and silky on the outside. ↕↔ to 10cm (4in). Mountains from Spain to Scandinavia, Bulgaria, and Russia (Siberia). ❄❄❄
P. vulgaris ■ ♀ (Pasque flower). Clump-forming perennial with finely divided, pinnate, light green leaves, 8–20cm (3–8in) long, comprising 7–9 leaflets, each 2- or 3-pinnatisect; the lobes are linear to linear-lance-shaped, very hairy when young. In spring, bears upright or semi-pendent, bell-shaped or narrowly bell-shaped, silky-hairy flowers, 4–9cm (1½–3½in) across, in shades of deep to pale purple, occasionally white. ↕ 10–20cm (4–8in), ↔ 20cm (8in). UK, W. France to Ukraine. ❄❄❄. **f. *alba*** ■ ♀ produces pure white flowers of variable size. **subsp. *grandis*** see *P. halleri* subsp. *grandis*. **'Rode Klokke'** syn. 'Rote Glocke', bears deep red flowers.

PULTENAEA

LEGUMINOSAE/PAPILIONACEAE

Genus of about 120 species of evergreen shrubs from dry forest in Australia. They are cultivated for their usually alternate, occasionally opposite, linear to almost rounded leaves, and for their pea-like flowers. The axillary, usually yellow or pink flowers have notched standard petals, and are produced singly or in clusters, which are often crowded into apparently terminal heads. In frost-prone areas, grow in a cool greenhouse; in warmer areas, grow in a shrub border, or at the base of a wall.

• **HARDINESS** Half hardy to frost tender.

• **CULTIVATION** Under glass, grow in loamless potting compost with added sharp sand, in full light. In growth, water moderately and apply a balanced liquid fertilizer every month; water sparingly in winter. Outdoors, grow in moderately fertile, well-drained soil in full sun. Pruning group 8; may need restrictive pruning under glass.

• **PROPAGATION** Sow seed at 13–18°C (55–64°F) in autumn or spring. Root semi-ripe cuttings with bottom heat in summer.

• **PESTS AND DISEASES** Grey mould may be a problem in damp conditions.

P. procumbens (Bush pea, Eggs and bacon). Low, spreading to mat-forming shrub with alternate, narrowly elliptic, mid- to deep greyish green leaves, 0.8–1cm (⅜–½in) long, with upfolded sides and reflexed points. In spring and early summer, pea-like, orange-red flowers, 1cm (½in) across, shaded orange-yellow, are produced in small, apparently terminal heads. ↕ 15–30cm (6–12in), ↔ 40cm (16in) or more. Australia (New South Wales, Victoria). ❀ (min. 5°C/41°F)

PUNICA

Pomegranate

LYTHRACEAE/PUNICACEAE

Genus of 2 species of rounded, deciduous shrubs or trees found in scrub, one species occurring from S.E. Europe and S.W. Asia to the Himalayas, the other from Socotra (Yemen). They have mostly opposite, narrowly oblong, entire leaves, and are grown for their showy, funnel-shaped, bright red flowers and large, spherical, edible fruits. In frost-prone areas, grow in a cool greenhouse or against a sunny wall, either as free-standing shrubs or fan-trained; in warmer areas, use as specimen trees, in a shrub border, or as hedging.

• **HARDINESS** Frost hardy; they require long, hot summers to produce fruit.

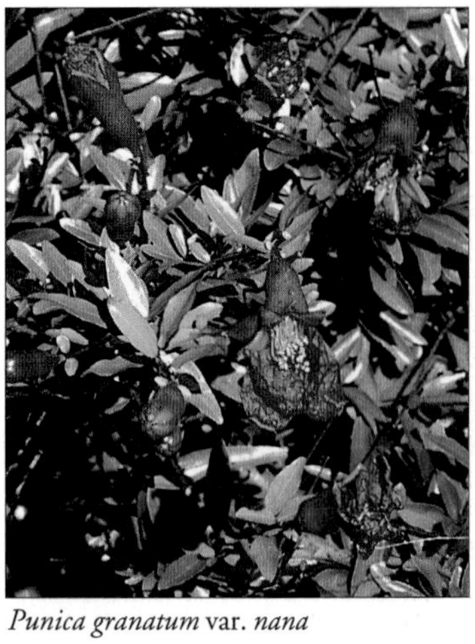

Punica granatum var. *nana*

P

• **CULTIVATION** Under glass, plant directly in a greenhouse border or in large containers of loam-based potting compost (JI No.2) in full light. When in growth, water freely and apply a balanced liquid fertilizer every month; water sparingly in winter. A temperature of 13–16°C (55–61°F) in autumn is required for fruit to ripen. Outdoors, grow in fertile, well-drained soil in full sun. Pruning group 1, from spring to summer; group 13 if wall-trained. Remove wayward shoots in spring.
• **PROPAGATION** Sow seed at 13–18°C (55–64°F) in spring. Root semi-ripe cuttings with bottom heat in summer.
• **PESTS AND DISEASES** Trouble free.

P. granatum ♀ (Pomegranate). Upright, sometimes spiny shrub or small, rounded tree with opposite, narrowly oblong, glossy, bright green leaves, coppery or red-veined when young, to 8cm (3in) long. Over a long period in summer, bears funnel-shaped, 5-petalled, bright orange-red flowers, to 4cm (1½in) across, singly or in clusters of up to 5, followed by spherical, yellow-brown, edible fruit, to 12cm (5in) across. ↕6m (20ft), ↔5m (15ft). S.E. Europe to Himalayas. ❄❄. **var. *nana*** ▣ is a compact, rounded shrub that fruits very freely; ↕↔30–100cm (12–39in). **f. *plena*** ♀ produces double flowers.

▷**Purslane** see *Claytonia, Portulaca*
Rock see *Calandrinia umbellata*
Tree see *Atriplex halimus*
Water see *Ludwigia palustris*

PUSCHKINIA

HYACINTHACEAE/LILIACEAE

Genus of one species of bulbous perennial, related to *Chionodoxa* and *Scilla*, occurring in the Middle East, in damp flushes in grassland where snow has recently melted. It is grown for its small, densely packed racemes of bell-shaped, pale blue flowers with darker blue stripes, borne in spring. The bulbs each have 2 semi-erect, basal leaves. Grow in a rock garden or among shrubs.
• **HARDINESS** Fully hardy.
• **CULTIVATION** Grow in any well-drained soil in full sun or light dappled shade.
• **PROPAGATION** Sow seed in containers in a cold frame in summer or autumn. Remove offsets in summer as the leaves die down.
• **PESTS AND DISEASES** Prone to viruses.

P. libanotica see *P. scilloides* var. *libanotica*.
P. scilloides ▣ Small, bulbous perennial with 2 semi-erect, linear, basal leaves, 15cm (6in) long. In spring, produces compact racemes of 4–10 open bell-shaped, very pale, bluish white flowers, 1cm (½in) across, with a dark blue stripe on each petal. ↕to 20cm (8in), ↔5cm (2in). Caucasus, Turkey, Lebanon, N. Iraq, N. Iran. ❄❄❄. **var. *libanotica*** ▣ syn. *P. libanotica*, has smaller white flowers, 7–8mm (¼–⅜in) across, rarely striped blue, with long, sharply pointed lobes; Turkey, Lebanon.

▷**Pussy ears** see *Cyanotis somaliensis*
▷**Pussy-toes** see *Antennaria*

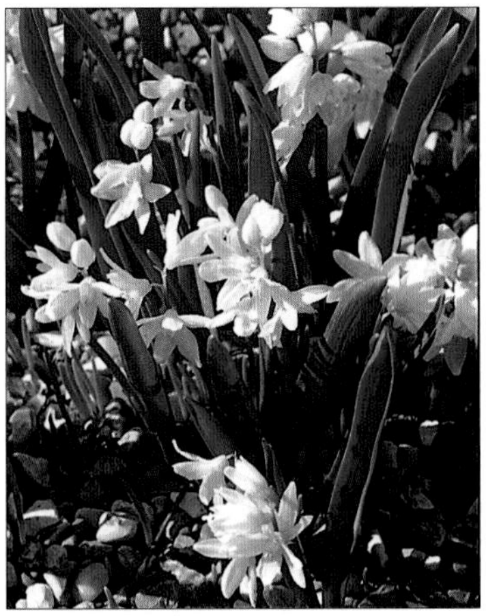

Puschkinia scilloides var. *libanotica*

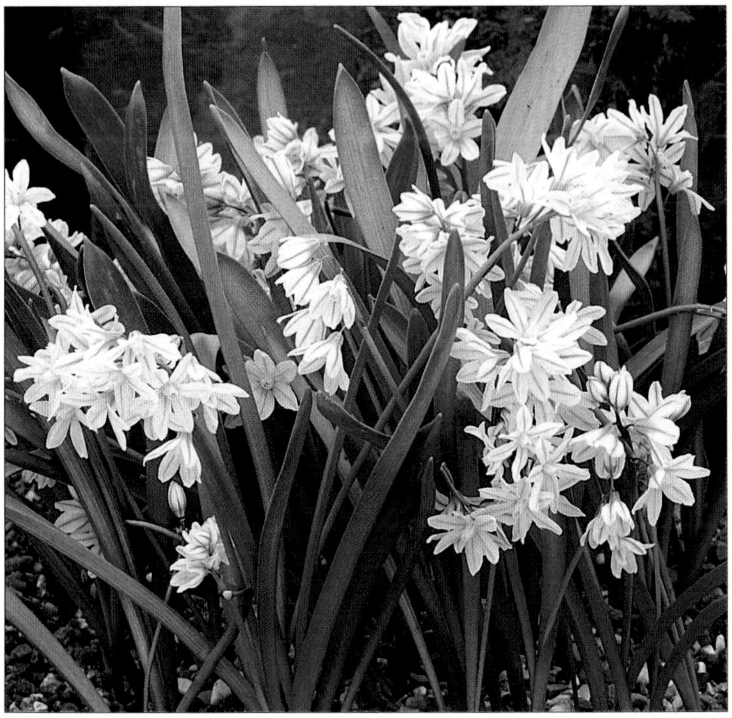

Puschkinia scilloides

PUTORIA

RUBIACEAE

Genus of 3 species of dwarf, evergreen shrubs occurring in sunny, rocky areas around the Mediterranean. They bear opposite, lance-shaped to obovate or oblong, malodorous, leathery, lustrous, rich, mid-green leaves, but they are cultivated for their long-tubed, funnel-shaped, pink to purple flowers, produced singly or in clusters from early to late summer. *P. calabrica*, the only cultivated species, is suitable for growing in a rock garden or at the base of a warm, sunny wall.
• **HARDINESS** Fully hardy.
• **CULTIVATION** Grow in any well-drained soil in full sun.
• **PROPAGATION** Sow seed in containers in a cold frame in spring. Take softwood cuttings in early summer.
• **PESTS AND DISEASES** Trouble free.

P. calabrica (Stinking madder). Slow-growing, spreading shrub with elliptic-lance-shaped, leathery, mid-green leaves, 2cm (¾in) long, foetid if crushed. Produces dense, terminal clusters of funnel-shaped pink flowers, to 1.5cm (½in) long, from early to late summer. ↕8cm (3in), ↔to 30cm (12in). Mediterranean. ❄❄❄

PUYA

BROMELIACEAE

Genus of about 170 species of terrestrial, evergreen perennials (bromeliads) from rocky slopes, to 2,000m (6,500ft) high, in Andean South America, Costa Rica, Colombia, Guyana, N. Brazil, and N. central Argentina. They have erect or widely spreading rosettes of linear leaves with coarse marginal spines; young leaf-blades are upright, mature ones are outspread. The leaf sheaths are prominent, often forming bulbous bases. The flowers are trumpet- or bell-shaped, in colours from white, greenish yellow, and sea-green to ice-blue or violet; they are usually produced in erect panicles, the branches having sterile tips (which act as perches for humming-bird pollinators). Flowers are followed by green fruit capsules containing winged seeds. Puyas tolerate cold more than most bromeliads. In frost-prone areas, grow in a conservatory or cool greenhouse; in warmer climates, use in a raised bed.
• **HARDINESS** Frost hardy (borderline) to frost tender.
• **CULTIVATION** Under glass, grow in terrestrial bromeliad compost in full light. From mid-spring to late summer, water moderately and apply a low-nitrogen liquid fertilizer every 6–8 weeks; water sparingly at other times. Outdoors, grow in any well-drained soil in full sun. Protect from winter wet. See also p.47.
• **PROPAGATION** Sow seed at 19–24°C (66–75°F) as soon as ripe.
• **PESTS AND DISEASES** New growth is susceptible to scale insects.

P. berteroniana ▣ Bromeliad with a caudex-like stem bearing spreading, terminal rosettes of lance-shaped, arching, dark green leaves, 60–100cm (24–39in) long, white-scaly beneath. In early summer, produces loose, pyramidal panicles, over 1m (3ft) long, of funnel-shaped, rich bluish green or deep blue-green flowers, 5cm (2in) long, with bright orange-yellow stamens. Will tolerate brief periods below 0°C (32°F). ↕to 2m (6ft), ↔3m (10ft). C. Chile. ❄❄ (borderline)
P. caerulea see *P. coerulea*.
P. chilensis ▣ Bromeliad with a very woody, caudex-like stem, sometimes branched, bearing spreading, dense, terminal rosettes of lance-shaped, stiff, leathery, mid-green leaves, 1m (3ft) long, with marginal spines. In summer, produces bell- to trumpet-shaped, yellow or green flowers, to 5cm (2in) long, with green sepals, in loosely branched panicles, 1.5m (5ft) long; the

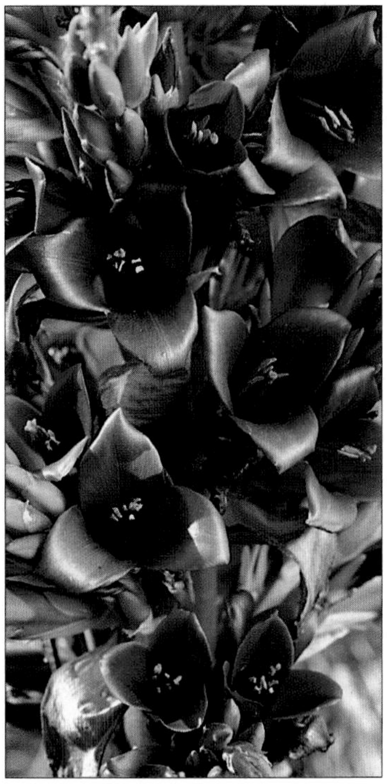

Puya berteroniana

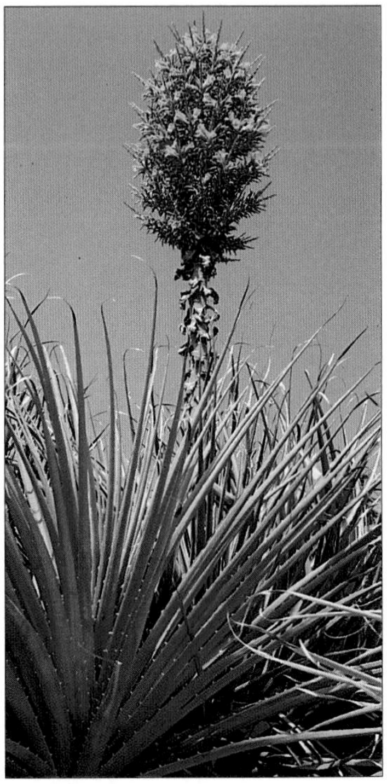

Puya chilensis

P

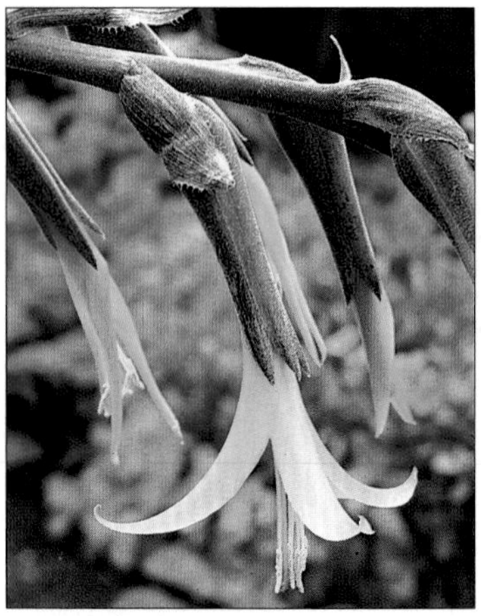

Puya mirabilis

upper parts of the panicle branches are covered with reduced bracts. ↕ 5m (15ft), ↔ 2m (6ft) or more. C. Chile. ❄

P. coerulea, syn. *P. caerulea.* Extremely variable bromeliad producing well-developed, erect, stout stems, each with terminal, spreading rosettes of lance-shaped leaves, to 60cm (24in) long, the leaf-blades ash-white, the margins with hooked, reddish brown spines, to 5mm (¼in) long. In summer, produces tubular, erect, stalked, dark blue flowers, 5cm (2in) or more long, in racemes or panicles, 40cm (16in) or more long. ↕↔ to 2m (6ft). C. Chile. ❄

P. mirabilis ▣ Stemless bromeliad bearing terminal, spreading rosettes of loose, linear-lance-shaped, finely toothed, white to brownish green leaves, to 60cm (24in) long. In summer, bears loose, simple racemes, to 50cm (20in) long, of funnel-shaped, yellowish green flowers, 10cm (4in) long. ↕↔ to 60cm (24in). Bolivia, N. Argentina. ❀ (min. 5°C/41°F)

P. raimondii ▣ Bromeliad with a thick, caudex-like stem, to 50cm (20in) across. Produces broadly lance-shaped, often red-suffused, bright green leaves, to 2m (6ft) long, densely scaly beneath, in a dense, globular, terminal rosette. In summer, tubular, greenish white, rarely purple flowers, 5cm (2in) long, are borne in a cylindrical, compound raceme, to 5m (15ft) long. ↕ to 2m (6ft), ↔ 1m (3ft). Peru, Bolivia. ❀ (min. 5°C/41°F)

P

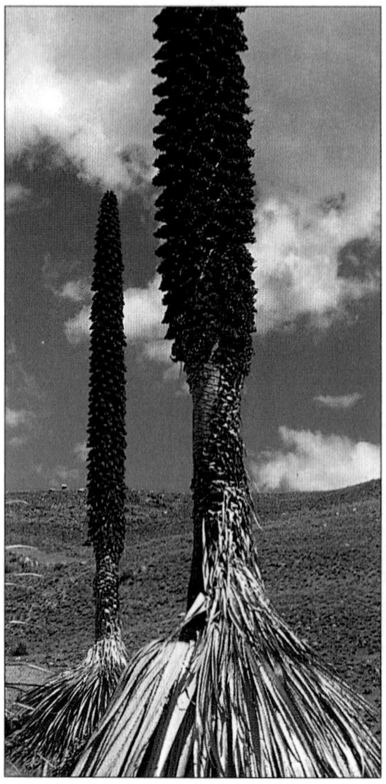

Puya raimondii

PYCNOSTACHYS

LABIATAE/LAMIACEAE

Genus of 40 species of erect, evergreen perennials or soft-stemmed shrubs occurring in forest margins in tropical and southern Africa and Madagascar. They are cultivated for their dense, terminal spikes of 2-lipped, tubular, deep blue flowers. The leaves are opposite or in whorls, linear, lance-shaped, or ovate, and are rather pungent when crushed. In frost-prone areas, grow in a warm greenhouse or conservatory. In warmer areas, they are suitable for growing in a shrub border.

• **HARDINESS** Frost tender.

• **CULTIVATION** Under glass, grow in loam-based potting compost (JI No.2) with added sharp sand, in full light. During the growing season, water freely and apply a balanced liquid fertilizer every month; water sparingly in winter. Outdoors, grow in fertile, well-drained soil in full sun.

• **PROPAGATION** Sow seed at 15–18°C (59–64°F) in spring. Take softwood cuttings at any time.

• **PESTS AND DISEASES** Whiteflies may be troublesome.

P. dawei ▣ Pyramidal, evergreen perennial bearing opposite, linear, mid-green leaves, to 30cm (12in) long, red beneath, with long, sharp points and toothed margins. In summer, produces tubular, cobalt-blue flowers, to 2.5cm (1in) long, in dense, terminal spikes, 15cm (6in) long. ↕ 1.8m (6ft), ↔ 90cm (36in). Tropical Africa. ❀ (min. 12°C/54°F)

P. urticifolia. Erect, soft-stemmed, evergreen shrub, becoming somewhat woody at the base and branching freely, with opposite, narrowly ovate, hairless or softly hairy, mid-green leaves, to 12cm (5in) long, often with toothed margins. In winter, tubular, deep blue flowers, 1–2cm (½–¾in) long, sometimes white with a blue tinge, are produced in dense, terminal spikes, to 10cm (4in) long. ↕ 2.5m (8ft), ↔ 1.2m (4ft). Tropical Africa and Mozambique. ❀ (min. 12°C/54°F)

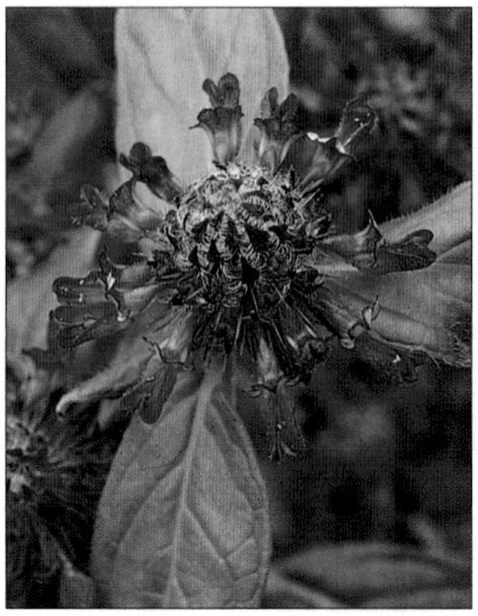

Pycnostachys dawei

PYRACANTHA

Firethorn

ROSACEAE

Genus of 7 species of spiny, evergreen, spreading to erect shrubs, occasionally trees, found in scrub and woodland margins from S. Europe to S.W. Asia, the Himalayas, China, and Taiwan. They are cultivated for their foliage, flowers, and, in particular, fruit: the variably shaped leaves are alternate and often have toothed margins; the 5-petalled white flowers are hawthorn-like and borne in compound corymbs; the showy, spherical berries that follow them in autumn are yellow, orange, or red. Grow firethorns as free-standing shrubs in a shrub border, or against a wall, or for hedging. The seeds may cause mild stomach upset if ingested.

• **HARDINESS** Fully hardy to frost hardy.

• **CULTIVATION** Grow in fertile, well-drained soil in full sun or partial shade. In frost-prone areas, shelter from cold, drying winds. Pruning group 1 for free-standing shrubs. Trim hedging in early to midsummer. On wall-trained plants, tie in any shoots needed to extend the framework, and cut back unwanted shoots to the main stem. After flowering in midsummer, shorten lateral shoots to 2 or 3 leaves from the base to expose the developing berries. In spring, remove old fruit trusses to make way for new growth.

• **PROPAGATION** Sow seed in containers in a cold frame in autumn. Root semi-ripe cuttings with bottom heat in summer.

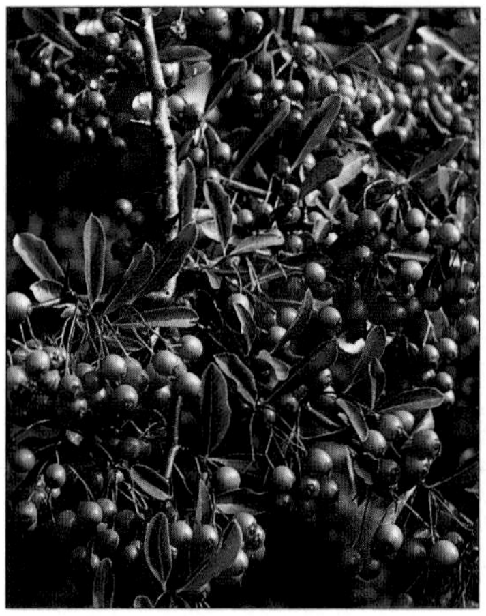

Pyracantha 'Golden Charmer'

• **PESTS AND DISEASES** Susceptible to aphids, caterpillars, scale insects, leaf miners, coral spot, fireblight, and scab.

P. angustifolia. Dense, bushy shrub with narrowly oblong or obovate, dark green leaves, to 5cm (2in) long, grey-felted beneath. Small white flowers are produced in corymbs in midsummer; they are followed by orange-yellow berries, 8mm (⅜in) across. ↕↔ 3m (10ft). W. China. ❄❄

P. atalantioides. Vigorous shrub with upright, arching shoots and oblong-elliptic to lance-shaped, glossy, dark green leaves, to 8cm (3in) long. In spring, small white flowers are borne in corymbs; they are followed by persistent, bright orange-red berries, to 7mm (¼in) across. ↕ to 6m (20ft),

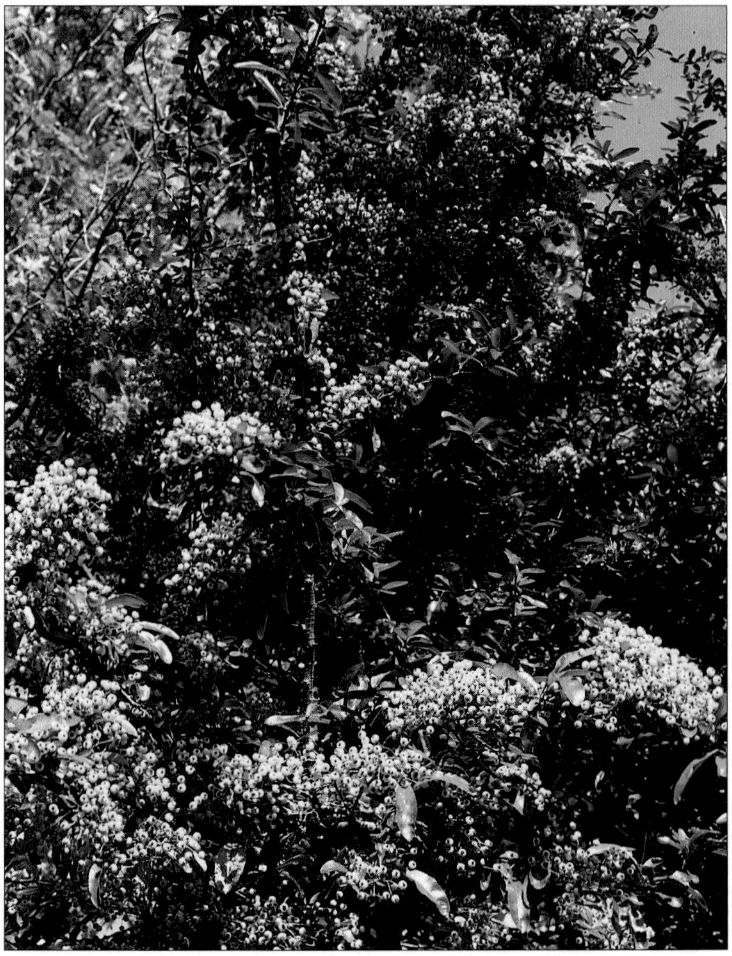

Pyracantha atalantioides 'Aurea'

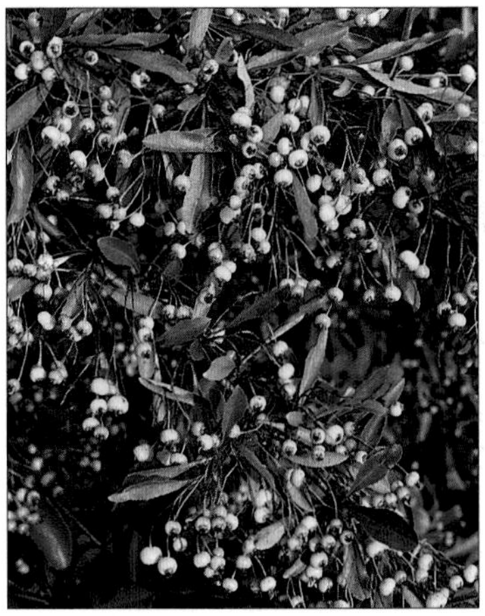

Pyracantha 'Golden Dome'

↔ 4m (12ft). C. China. ✻✻. **'Aurea'** ■ bears yellow berries.
P. coccinea. Dense, bushy shrub with ovate-lance-shaped, dark green leaves, to 2–4cm (¾–1½in) long. Small, creamy white flowers are borne in corymbs in early summer, followed by bright scarlet berries, 5mm (¼in) across. ↕↔ 4m (12ft). S.E. Europe to Caucasus. ✻✻✻. **'Lalandei'** has an upright habit and a profusion of bright orange-red berries, 7–8mm (¼–⅜in) across; ↕ to 6m (20ft).
***P.* 'Golden Charmer'** ■ Vigorous, bushy shrub with arching branches and inversely lance-shaped, glossy, bright green leaves, to 5cm (2in) long. Small white flowers are produced in corymbs in early summer, followed by bright orange-red berries, 9mm (⅜in) across. ↕↔ 3m (10ft). ✻✻✻
***P.* 'Golden Dome'** ■ Spreading shrub, forming a dense mound of arching branches bearing oblong, glossy, dark green leaves, to 6cm (2½in) long. In early summer, small white flowers are produced in corymbs; they are followed by an abundance of golden yellow berries, 5mm (¼in) across. ↕ 2m (6ft), ↔ 3m (10ft). ✻✻✻
***P.* 'Harlequin'**, syn. *P.* 'Variegated'. Spreading shrub with oblong, dark green leaves, 5cm (2in) long, strikingly marked creamy white, flushed pink when young. Small white flowers are produced in corymbs in early summer, followed by red berries, 5mm (¼in) across. Best grown against a wall. ↕ 1.5m (5ft), ↔ 2m (6ft). ✻✻
P. koidzumii. Erect shrub with inversely lance-shaped, glossy, dark green leaves, to 5cm (2in) long. Small

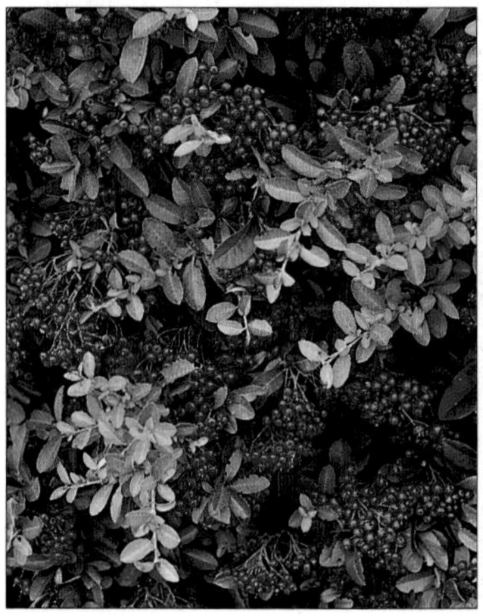

Pyracantha 'Mohave'

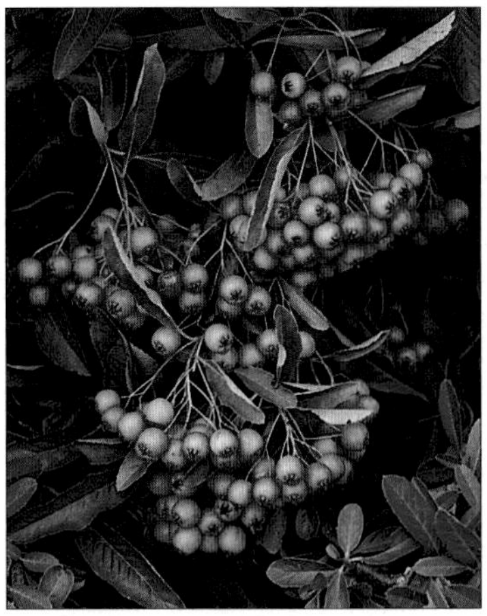

Pyracantha 'Orange Glow'

white flowers are produced in corymbs in early summer, followed by orange-red berries, 7mm (¼in) across. ↕ 3m (10ft), ↔ 4m (12ft). Taiwan. ✻✻. **'Rosedale'** has arching branches and bright red berries, 9mm (⅜in) across.
***P.* 'Mohave'** ■ Vigorous, bushy shrub with oval, dark green leaves, to 6cm (2½in) long. In early summer, small white flowers are produced in corymbs, followed by long-lasting red berries, 9mm (⅜in) across. ↕ 4m (12ft), ↔ 5m (15ft). ✻✻
***P.* 'Orange Charmer'.** Vigorous, bushy shrub with arching branches and elliptic to obovate, glossy, bright green leaves, to 5cm (2in) long. Small white flowers are borne in corymbs in early summer, followed by dark orange berries, 9mm (⅜in) across. ↕↔ 3m (10ft). ✻✻✻
***P.* 'Orange Glow'** ■🏆 Upright, later spreading, loosely branched shrub with broadly elliptic to obovate, glossy, dark green leaves, 2–4cm (¾–1½in) long. Small white flowers are produced in corymbs in late spring, followed by a profusion of persistent, orange-red to dark orange berries, 7–8mm (¼–⅜in) across. ↕↔ 3m (10ft). Probably a cultivar of *P. fortuneana.* ✻✻✻

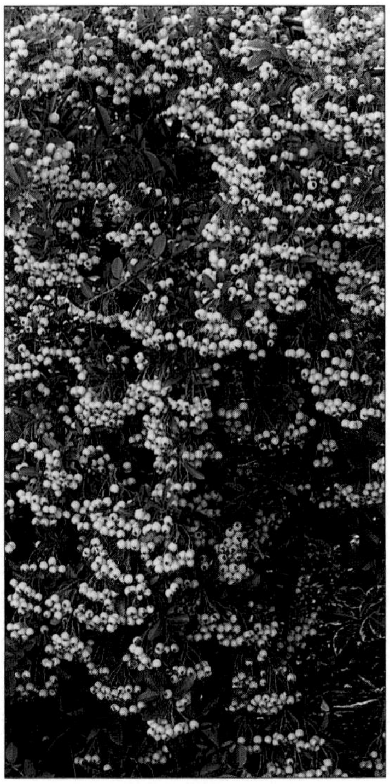

Pyracantha 'Soleil d'Or'

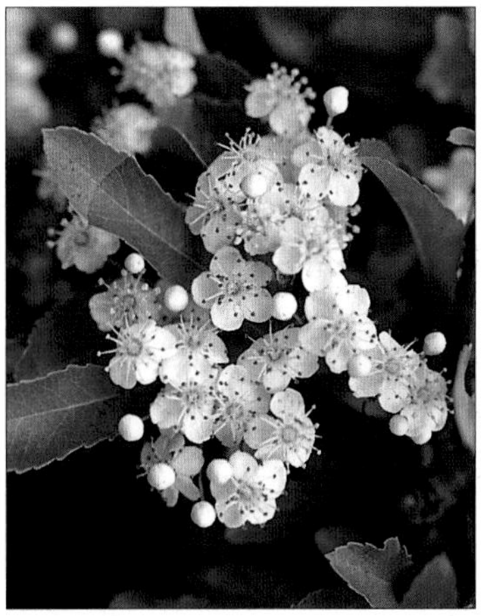

Pyracantha x *watereri*

P. rogersiana 🏆 Spreading shrub with arching branches and inversely lance-shaped to narrowly obovate, glossy, bright green leaves, to 4cm (1½in) long. Small white flowers are produced in corymbs in spring, followed by orange-red berries, 8mm (⅜in) across. ↕↔ 4m (12ft). W. China. ✻✻. **f. *flava*** 🏆 has yellow berries.
***P.* 'Santa Cruz'.** Low, compact, spreading shrub with oblong, dark green leaves, to 8cm (3in) long. Small white flowers are produced in corymbs in early summer, followed by small red berries, 6–8mm (¼–⅜in) across. ↕ 1m (3ft), ↔ 2m (6ft). ✻✻
***P.* 'Shawnee'.** Spreading shrub with narrowly elliptic, glossy, dark green leaves, to 5cm (2in) long. Small white flowers are borne in corymbs in early summer, followed by slightly flattened, orange-yellow berries, 9mm (⅜in) across. ↕ 3m (10ft), ↔ 4m (12ft). ✻✻
***P.* 'Soleil d'Or'** ■ Upright shrub with red-tinged shoots and broadly elliptic, glossy, dark green leaves, 6cm (2½in) long. Small white flowers are produced in corymbs in early summer, followed by a profusion of golden yellow berries, 1cm (½in) across. ↕ 3m (10ft), ↔ 2.5m (8ft). ✻✻✻
***P.* 'Teton'.** Vigorous, upright shrub with oblong, wavy-margined, glossy, bright green leaves, to 5cm (2in) long. Small white flowers are produced in corymbs in early summer, followed by an abundance of yellow-orange berries, 6mm (¼in) across. ↕ 5m (15ft), ↔ 3m (10ft). ✻✻✻
***P.* 'Variegated'** see *P.* 'Harlequin'.
P.* x *watereri ■🏆 (*P. atalantioides* x *P. rogersiana*). Dense, upright shrub with elliptic, dark green leaves, to 6cm (2½in) long. In early summer, small white flowers are produced in corymbs, followed by bright red berries, 8mm (⅜in) across. ↕↔ 2.5m (8ft). Garden origin. ✻✻✻

▷ **Pyramid tree, Queensland** see *Lagunaria patersonia*
▷ ***Pyrethropsis*** see *Rhodanthemum*
P. atlantica see *R. atlanticum*
P. catananche see *R. catananche*
P. gayana see *R. gayanum*
P. hosmariensis see *R. hosmariense*
P. maresii see *R. maresii*
▷ ***Pyrethrum*** see *Tanacetum*
P. coccineum see *Tanacetum coccineum*
P. parthenium see *Tanacetum parthenium*

▷ ***Pyrethrum* cont.**
P. ptarmiciflorum see *Tanacetum ptarmiciflorum*
P. radicans see *Leucanthemopsis pectinata*
P. roseum see *Tanacetum coccineum*
▷ **Pyrethrum** see *Tanacetum coccineum*

PYROLA

Shinleaf, Wintergreen

ERICACEAE/PYROLACEAE

Genus of 35 species of creeping, rhizomatous, evergreen perennials from woodland and moorland in the N. hemisphere. They are grown for their basal clusters of alternate, simple, usually rounded to ovate, long-stalked, mid- to dark green leaves, and their upright racemes of cup- to bowl-shaped, usually white, occasionally pink or red flowers, borne in summer. They can be difficult to establish, possibly needing a mycorrhizal association with specific, soil-dwelling fungi. Grow in a woodland garden, peat bed, or rock garden.
• **HARDINESS** Fully hardy.
• **CULTIVATION** Grow in fertile, acid, leafy, moist but well-drained soil in partial or dappled shade.
• **PROPAGATION** Surface-sow seed in containers of damp sphagnum moss as soon as ripe. Divide with care in spring; roots resent disturbance.
• **PESTS AND DISEASES** Very susceptible to attack by slugs and snails.

P. rotundifolia (Round-leaved winter-green, Wild lily-of-the-valley). Creeping perennial with basal clusters of rounded or broadly oval, mid- to dark green leaves, 2–6cm (¾–2½in) long. In summer, produces upright stems bearing loose racemes of up to 20 cup-shaped, pure white, rarely pink-tinged flowers, 0.8–1.5cm (⅜–½in) across, with incurving petals. ↕ 20cm (8in), ↔ 15cm (6in). Europe, North America. ✻✻✻

PYROSTEGIA

BIGNONIACEAE

Genus of 3 or 4 species of woody-stemmed, evergreen tendril climbers found in tropical woodland in South America. Leaves, produced in opposite pairs, each have 2 or 3 leaflets and some-times a terminal, 3-branched tendril. The tubular or bell-shaped, usually orange or red flowers each have a tapered base and club-like tip, with 5 short petal lobes. Where temperatures fall below 10–13°C (50–55°F), grow in a temperate or warm greenhouse. In warmer areas, grow over a pergola or arch, or allow to cascade from a tree.
• **HARDINESS** Frost tender.
• **CULTIVATION** Under glass, grow in loam-based potting compost (JI No.2) with added leaf mould and sharp sand, in full light. During the growing season, water moderately and apply a balanced liquid fertilizer monthly; water sparingly in winter. Outdoors, grow in fertile, moist but well-drained soil in full sun. Support climbing stems. Pruning group 11 or 12, after flowering.
• **PROPAGATION** Sow seed at 16°C (61°F) in spring. Root semi-ripe cuttings with bottom heat in summer.
• **PESTS AND DISEASES** May be infested with scale insects and red spider mites under glass.

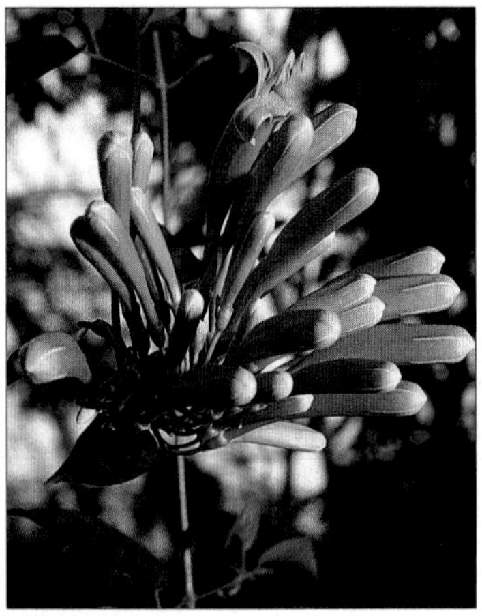

Pyrostegia venusta

P. ignea see *P. venusta.*
P. venusta ■ syn. *P. ignea* (Golden shower). Very vigorous climber with numerous slender stems, and opposite leaves composed of ovate to oblong-lance-shaped, rich green leaflets, to 8cm (3in) long. Bears a profusion of curved, tubular, waxy, golden to reddish orange flowers, 6cm (2½in) long, in terminal clusters, mainly in winter. ↕10m (30ft) or more. Bolivia to Brazil, Paraguay, N. Argentina. ❀ (min. 10–13°C/50–55°F)

▷ ***Pyrrhocactus crispus*** see *Neoporteria crispa*

PYRROSIA
Felt fern

POLYPODIACEAE

Genus of about 100 species of epiphytic and terrestrial, evergreen ferns with long-creeping rhizomes, mainly from tropical forest in North and South America, but also found in temperate areas in E. Asia. They are cultivated for their very small to large, mostly simple, linear to almost rounded, sometimes palmately lobed, thick, leathery fronds, the undersides of which are usually densely covered with matted and felt-like, star-shaped, branched hairs. In frost-prone climates, grow in a container or hanging basket in a temperate greenhouse; elsewhere, grow epiphytically on a tree or on other mossy supports, or in a sheltered, shady border.
• **HARDINESS** Frost hardy to frost tender.
• **CULTIVATION** Under glass, grow in a mix of 1 part each loam, medium-grade bark, and charcoal, 2 parts sharp sand, and 3 parts coarse leaf mould. Provide bright filtered or indirect light, with high humidity. In growth, water freely and apply a balanced liquid fertilizer monthly; water sparingly in winter. Outdoors, grow in moderately fertile, leafy, well-drained soil in partial shade.
• **PROPAGATION** Sow spores at 21°C (70°F) when ripe. Divide in spring. See also p.51.
• **PESTS AND DISEASES** Scale insects may be troublesome.

P. lingua ■ (Japanese felt fern, Tongue fern). Evergreen fern bearing simple, lance-shaped to ovate, leathery, glossy, dark green fronds, to 30cm (12in) long, sparsely hairy above, densely covered with star-shaped hairs beneath. Spores form in patches over a large part of the undersides of the fronds. ↕10–20cm (4–8in), ↔30cm (12in). E. Asia, China, Taiwan, Japan (Ryukyu Islands). ❀ (min. 10°C/50°F). **'Cristata'** has fronds repeatedly forked at the tips.

PYRUS
Pear

ROSACEAE

Genus of about 30 species of upright, mainly deciduous trees and shrubs, found in woodland, in rocky places, and on hillsides in Europe, W. to E. Asia, and N. Africa. They are grown for their habit, flowers, and fruits. The leaves are alternate, entire or very rarely lobed, ovate to oblong, elliptic, or oval, the margins often with forward-pointing teeth; some have good autumn colour. The 5-petalled, saucer- to bowl-shaped flowers, borne in umbel-like racemes, are white, occasionally pink, and usually have red anthers. The fruits are spherical to typically pear-shaped; numerous cultivars have been bred specifically for the production of culinary and dessert pears. Ornamental pears are best grown as specimen trees on a lawn; the smaller ones, such as *P. salicifolia* 'Pendula', and those of narrow habit, such as *P. calleryana* 'Chanticleer', are particularly suitable for growing in a small garden.
• **HARDINESS** Fully hardy.
• **CULTIVATION** Grow in any fertile, well-drained soil in full sun. Pruning group 1.
• **PROPAGATION** Sow seed in an open frame or in a seedbed in autumn. Bud in summer, or graft in winter.
• **PESTS AND DISEASES** Susceptible to aphids, caterpillars, leaf midges, and mites. They are also prone to fireblight, honey fungus, powdery mildew, canker, brown rot, and scab.

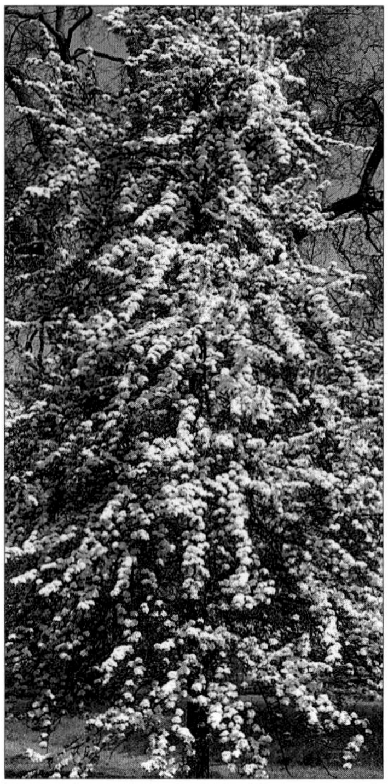

Pyrus communis

P. calleryana △ Broadly conical, often very thorny, deciduous tree with ovate to broadly ovate, finely scalloped or toothed, glossy, dark green leaves, to 8cm (3in) long, turning red in late autumn. White flowers, 2cm (¾in) across, are borne in umbel-like racemes of up to 12, in early and mid-spring, followed in autumn by spherical brown fruit, 1cm (½in) across. ↕↔15m (50ft). China. ❄❄❄. **'Autumn Blaze'** has red-purple autumn colour. **'Bradford'** ⬯ is narrowly conical, becoming broader with age, and thornless; ↔12m (40ft). **'Capital'** ⬯ is narrowly conical, with copper autumn colour; ↕12m (40ft), ↔5m (15ft). **'Chanticleer'** ■🏆⬯ is narrowly conical; ↔6m (20ft).
P. communis ■🏆△ (Common pear). Columnar, occasionally thorny, deciduous tree with ovate to elliptic, glossy, dark green leaves, to 10cm (4in) long, with fine, forward-pointing teeth. White flowers, 4cm (1½in) across, often tinged pink in bud, are borne in umbel-like racemes of 5–9 in mid-spring; they are followed by edible, pear-shaped to spherical, green to yellow fruit, to 10cm (4in) long. Parent of numerous fruit-bearing cultivars. ↕15m (50ft), ↔10m (30ft). S. Europe, S.W. Asia. ❄❄❄. **'Beech Hill'** ⬯ is narrowly conical, with leaves that turn orange and red in autumn; ↕10m (30ft), ↔7m (22ft).
P. japonica see *Chaenomeles speciosa.*
P. nivalis △ (Snow pear). Broadly conical, thornless, deciduous tree with elliptic to obovate, entire or shallowly scalloped, silvery grey leaves, to 8cm (3in) long, white-hairy beneath. In mid-spring, bears white flowers, 3cm (1¼in) across, in umbel-like racemes of 6–9, followed by spherical, yellow-green fruit, 4cm (1½in) across. ↕12m (40ft), ↔8m (25ft). C. and S.E. Europe. ❄❄❄
P. salicifolia ⌓ Spreading, deciduous tree with pendent shoots and lance-shaped to narrowly elliptic, willow-like, grey-felted leaves, to 9cm (3½in) long, becoming hairless with age. Creamy white flowers, 2cm (¾in) across, are borne in dense, umbel-like racemes of 6–8 in spring, followed by pear-shaped green fruit, 3cm (1¼in) long. ↕8m (25ft), ↔6m (20ft). S.E. Europe, Caucasus, Turkey, N.W. Iran. ❄❄❄. **'Pendula'** ■🏆⌓ has stiffly weeping branches; ↕5m (15ft), ↔4m (12ft).
P. ussuriensis △ Broadly conical, deciduous tree with broadly oval, glossy, dark green leaves, to 10cm (4in) long. White flowers, 3cm (1¼in) across, are borne in umbel-like racemes of 6–9 in mid-spring, followed by almost spherical green fruit, 4cm (1½in) across. ↕12m (40ft), ↔8m (25ft). N.E. Asia. ❄❄❄

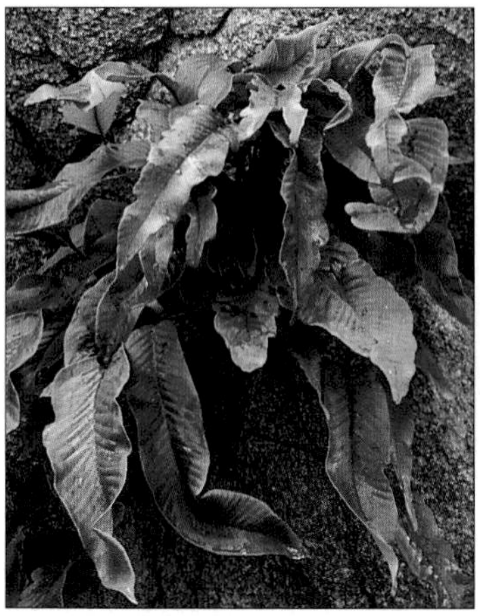

Pyrrosia lingua

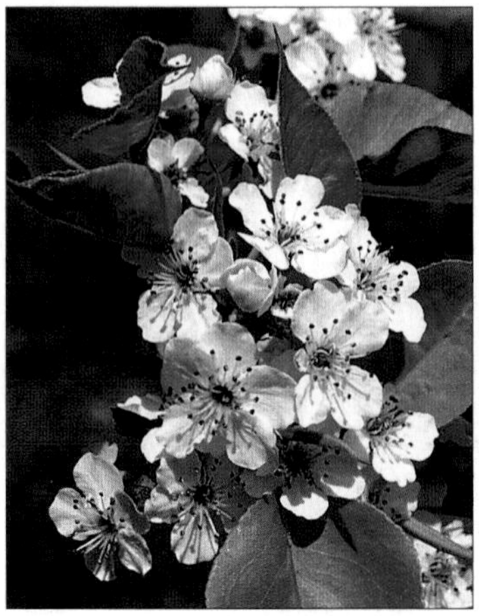

Pyrus calleryana 'Chanticleer'

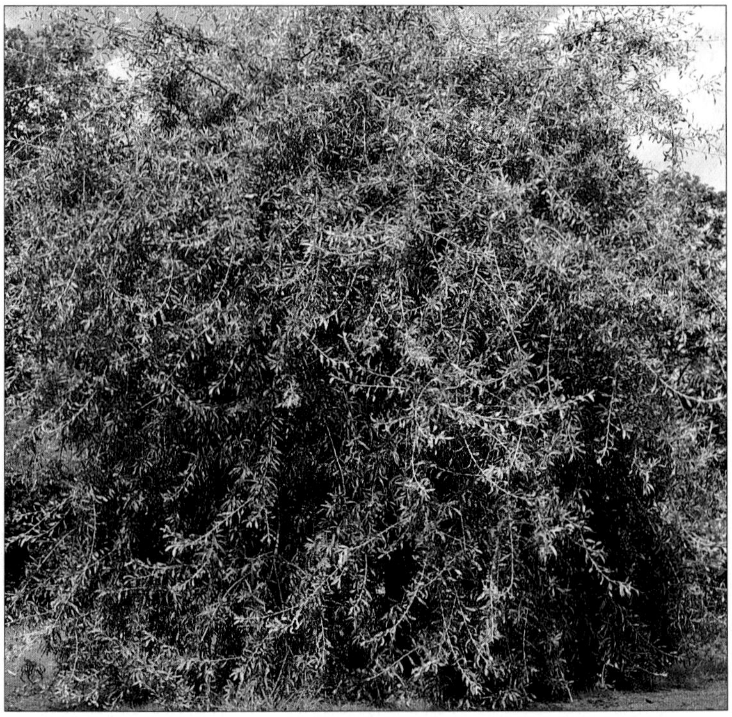

Pyrus salicifolia 'Pendula'

Q

▷ **Quaking grass** see *Briza*
Common see *B. media*
Greater see *B. maxima*
Lesser see *B. minor*
▷ **Quamash** see *Camassia, C. quamash*
▷ ***Quamoclit coccinea*** see *Ipomoea coccinea*
▷ ***Quamoclit lobata*** see *Ipomoea lobata*
▷ ***Quamoclit pennata*** see *Ipomoea quamoclit*

QUAQUA

ASCLEPIADACEAE

Genus of 14 species of perennial succulents, closely related to *Caralluma*, from hilly, often rocky terrain in S. Namibia and South Africa, grown for their prominently to shallowly lobed, bowl-shaped flowers, which are borne singly or in clusters during daytime in early summer. Where temperatures fall below 10°C (50°F), grow in a warm greenhouse; in warm, dry climates, use in a raised bed with other succulents.

- **HARDINESS** Frost tender.
- **CULTIVATION** Under glass, grow in a mix of equal parts loam-based potting compost (JI No.2) and sharp grit, in full light with shade from hot sun. During growth, water freely and apply a dilute balanced fertilizer 2 or 3 times. Keep barely moist in winter. Outdoors, grow in gritty, sharply drained, moderately fertile soil in full sun with some midday shade. See also pp.48–49.
- **PROPAGATION** Sow seed at 18–21°C (64–70°F) in spring. Take stem cuttings in late summer.
- **PESTS AND DISEASES** Prone to aphids.

Q. pillansii, syn. *Caralluma pillansii*. Erect, freely branching succulent with prominently 4-angled, sturdy, dark grey-green stems, to 2.5cm (1in) thick, spotted red, and bearing compressed brown teeth with spine-like tips. Dense clusters of 4–20 bowl-shaped, purple-brown flowers, to 2.5cm (1in) across, with purple- or red-spotted, greyish green lobes, develop from the stem grooves in early summer. ‡↔ to 30cm (12in). S. Namibia, South Africa (Western Cape). ❀ (min. 10°C/50°F)

▷ **Quassia** see *Picrasma quassioides*
▷ **Queen Anne's lace** see *Anthriscus sylvestris*
▷ **Queen Anne's thimbles** see *Gilia capitata*
▷ **Queencup** see *Clintonia uniflora*
▷ **Queen of the meadows** see *Filipendula ulmaria*
▷ **Queen of the night** see *Selenicereus grandiflorus*
▷ **Queen of the prairies** see *Filipendula rubra*
▷ **Queen's tears** see *Billbergia nutans*

QUERCUS

Oak

FAGACEAE

Genus of about 600 species of monoecious, deciduous, semi-evergreen or evergreen trees and shrubs, widely distributed in woodland and scrub in the N. hemisphere, and grown for their habit and foliage. They have usually fissured bark, downy to hairless shoots, and alternate, entire, lobed, or toothed leaves, which in some deciduous species give excellent autumn colour. The tiny male and female flowers are produced separately on the same plant in late spring and early summer; the males are borne in pendent catkins, the females singly, in pairs, or in racemes, followed by usually ovoid brown nuts (acorns) in scaly cups. The acorns are mostly 1–3cm (½–1¼in) long, sometimes more, and solitary or paired, but in some species are borne in racemes. Oak trees are best as specimens in a large garden or a park.

- **HARDINESS** Fully hardy to frost hardy.
- **CULTIVATION** Grow in deep, fertile, well-drained soil in sun or partial shade; evergreen species prefer full sun. Shelter oaks of borderline hardiness from frost and cold winds. They are lime-tolerant unless stated otherwise. Pruning group 1.
- **PROPAGATION** Sow seed in containers in a cold frame or seedbed as soon as ripe. Graft in mid-autumn or late winter.
- **PESTS AND DISEASES** Susceptible to oak wilt, honey fungus, powdery mildew, aphids, gall wasps, and various bracket fungi. Knopper gall can disfigure acorns.

Q. acutissima ♀ syn. *Q. serrata*. Rounded, deciduous tree with fissured, corky, ashen-grey to black bark and long-lasting, sweet-chestnut-like, oblong-lance-shaped to obovate, glossy, mid-green leaves, to 20cm (8in) long, margined with bristle-tipped teeth. Solitary, ovoid acorns are borne in cups covered with slender, long, hairy scales. ‡↔ 15–20m (50–70ft). Himalayas, China, Korea, Japan. ❄❄❄
Q. aegilops see *Q. macrolepis*.
Q. agrifolia ▣ ♀ (Californian live oak). Spreading, evergreen tree or shrub with ridged, grey to reddish brown bark and convex, ovate-elliptic to broadly elliptic, spiny-toothed, glossy, dark green leaves, to 7cm (3in) long. Bears solitary, slender, ovoid, pointed acorns, to 3.5cm (1½in) long. ‡↔ 10m (30ft). USA (California). ❄❄❄
Q. alba ♀ (American white oak). Spreading, deciduous tree with peeling, pale grey to brown bark. The obovate, oblong, or elliptic, deeply lobed, bright green leaves, to 22cm (9in) long, often pink-tinged when young, turn purple-red in autumn. Solitary acorns are ovoid-oblong. Needs lime-free soil. ‡↔ 30m (100ft). E. North America. ❄❄❄
Q. aliena ♀ Spreading, deciduous tree with fissured, grey-brown bark, obovate, prominently toothed and veined, glossy, bright green leaves, to 20cm (8in) long, blue-green beneath, and stalked, ovoid acorns. ↕25m (80ft), ↔ 12m (40ft). China, Korea, Japan. ❄❄❄
Q. bicolor ♀ (Swamp white oak). Spreading, deciduous tree with peeling, fissured, grey-brown bark and oblong-obovate or obovate, shallowly lobed, glossy, dark green leaves, to 16cm (6in) long, white-hairy beneath when young, orange to bright red in autumn. Long-stalked acorns are oblong-ovoid. ↕20m (70ft), ↔ 15m (50ft). S.E. USA. ❄❄❄
Q. borealis see *Q. rubra*.
Q. canariensis ▣ ♀ ♀ (Mirbeck's oak). Deciduous or semi-evergreen tree, narrow when young, broadening with age, with rugged, thick black bark. Obovate-oblong to obovate, shallowly lobed, rich green leaves, to 18cm (7in) long, turn yellow-brown in autumn. Ovoid acorns are borne in clusters of up to 4. ↕30m (100ft), ↔ 15m (50ft). S.W. Europe, N. Africa. ❄❄❄
Q. castaneifolia ▣ ♀ (Chestnut-leaved oak). Fast-growing, spreading, deciduous tree with rough, corky brown bark and sweet-chestnut-like, elliptic-oblong to oblong-lance-shaped, triangular-toothed, glossy, dark green leaves, to 16cm (6in) long, grey beneath. Ovoid acorns, in long-scaled cups, are solitary or in groups of up to 5. ↕25m (80ft), ↔ 20m (70ft). Caucasus, N. Iran. ❄❄❄. **'Green Spire'** ♀ ♀ has upright branches; ↔ 10m (30ft).
Q. cerris ♀ ♀ (Turkey oak). Fast-growing, spreading, deciduous, very variable tree with grey-white bark, splitting into thick plates, and oblong-elliptic to oblong-lance-shaped, deeply lobed or toothed, dark green leaves, to 12cm (5in) long, pale green beneath and yellow-brown in autumn. Ellipsoid acorns, 2.5–4cm (1–1½in) long, in cups densely covered with long, slender scales, are solitary or in groups of 2–4. ↕30m (100ft), ↔ 25m (80ft). C. and S. Europe. ❄❄❄. **'Argenteovariegata'** ▣ syn. 'Variegata', has leaves margined with creamy yellow, later creamy white; ↕15m (50ft), ↔ 12m (40ft).
Q. chrysolepis ♀ (Canyon oak). Spreading, evergreen tree or shrub with scaly, whitish grey or red-tinted bark and oblong-ovate to elliptic, spiny-toothed, leathery, shining, dark green leaves, to 6cm (2½in) long, grey- or yellow-hairy beneath. Ovoid to oblong-ovoid acorns, 2.5–5cm (1–2in) long, are borne in felted cups. ↕20m (70ft), ↔ 10m (30ft). USA (California). ❄❄
Q. coccifera ♀ (Kermes oak). Bushy, compact, evergreen shrub or tree with smooth grey bark, cracking with age, and holly-like, ovate to oblong-lance-shaped, spiny-margined, glossy, dark green leaves, 3–5cm (1¼–2in) long. Bears solitary, spherical or ovoid acorns in very spiny cups. ↕to 10m (30ft), ↔ 4–6m (12–20ft). Mediterranean. ❄❄
Q. coccinea ▣ ♀ (Scarlet oak). Rounded, deciduous tree with pale grey-brown bark in scaly plates. Glossy, dark green leaves, to 15cm (6in) long, are elliptic, with deep lobes ending in bristle-tipped teeth, and tufts of hairs in the vein axils beneath; the leaves turn bright red in autumn. Acorns are ovoid to nearly spherical. Requires lime-free soil. ↕20m (70ft), ↔ 15m (50ft). E. North America. ❄❄❄. **'Splendens'** ♀ is very dark red in autumn.
Q. conferta see *Q. frainetto*.
Q. dentata ▣ ♀ (Daimio oak). Rugged, spreading, stoutly branched, deciduous tree with fissured brown bark, splitting into grey, scaly plates. Produces obovate, shallowly lobed to wavy-margined, dark green leaves, to 30cm (12in) or more long. Bears ovoid to nearly spherical, solitary acorns. Requires acid soil. ↕15m (50ft), ↔ 10m (30ft). E. Asia. ❄❄❄
Q. ellipsoidalis ▣ ♀ (Northern pin oak). Spreading, deciduous tree with

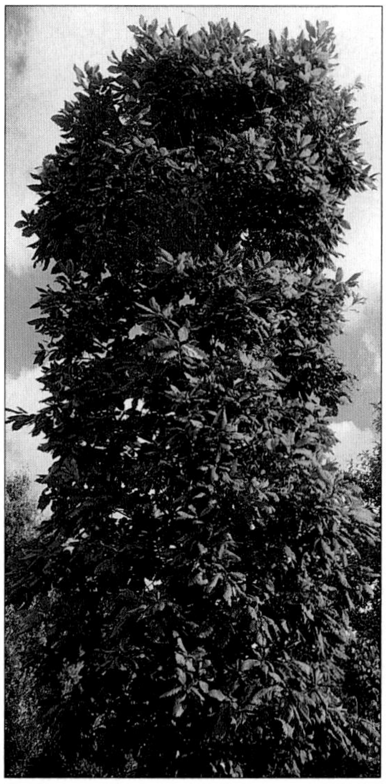

Quercus canariensis

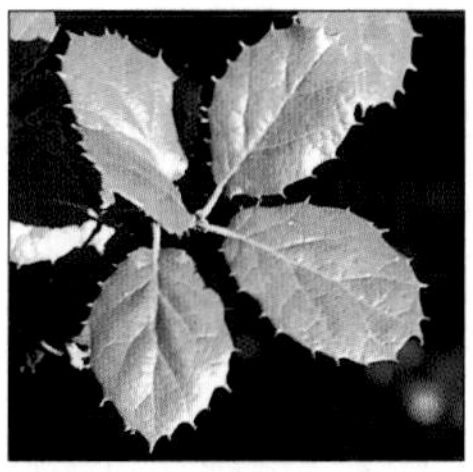

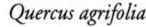

Quercus agrifolia

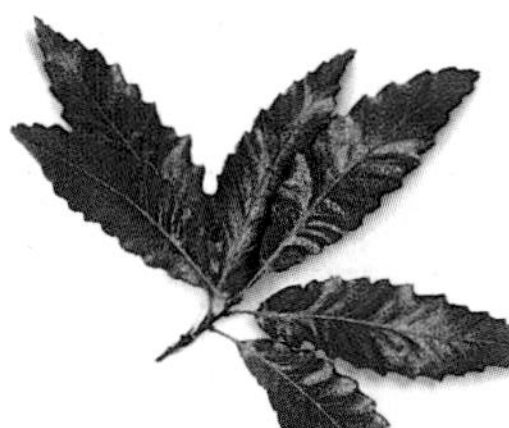

Quercus castaneifolia

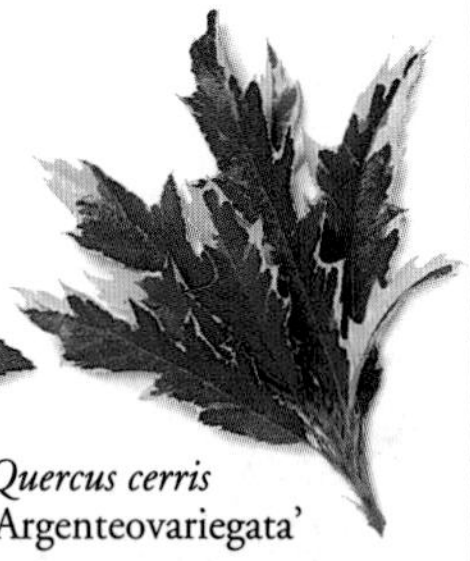

Quercus cerris 'Argenteovariegata'

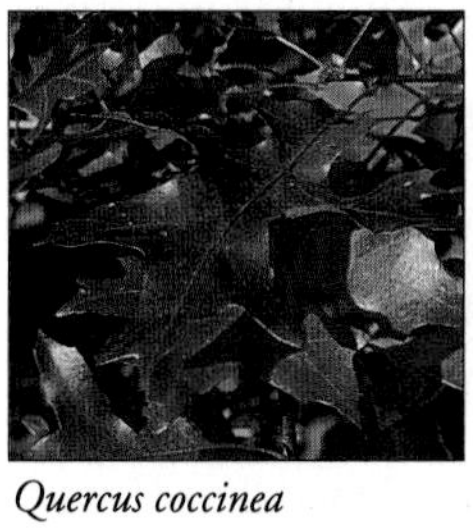

Quercus coccinea

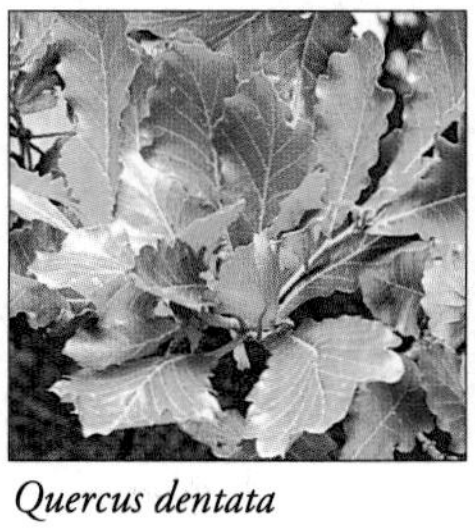

Quercus dentata

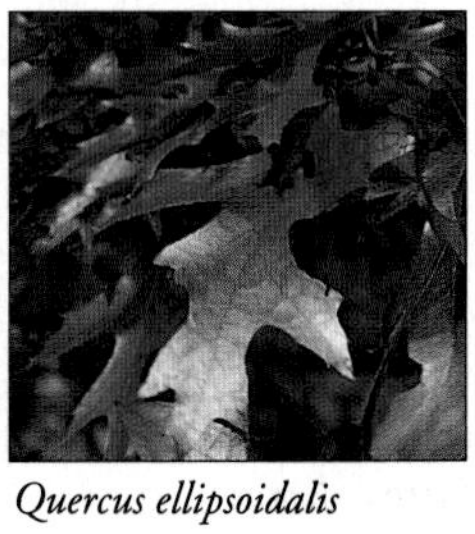

Quercus ellipsoidalis

Q

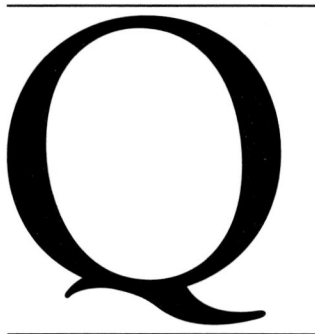

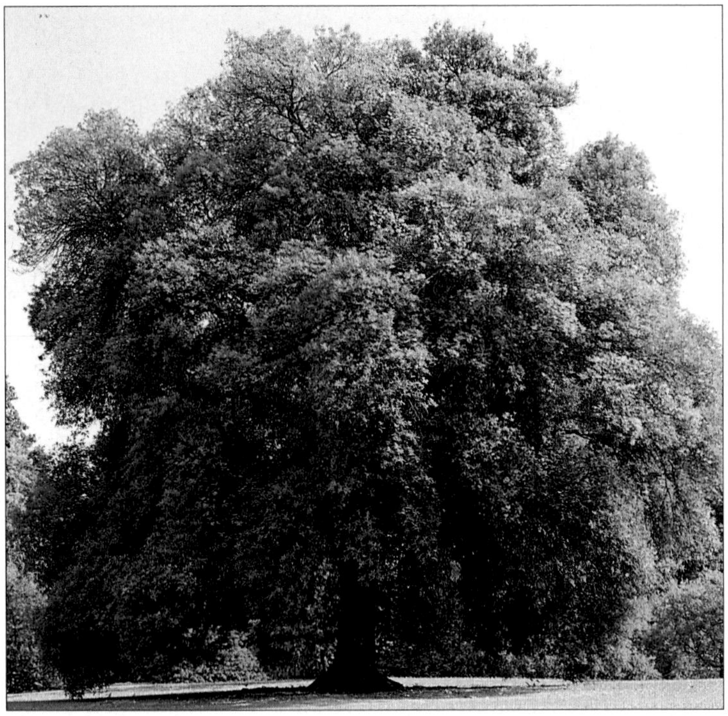

Quercus ilex

smooth grey bark. Glossy, dark green leaves, to 13cm (5in) long, are elliptic with wedge-shaped bases, and deeply cut into bristle-tipped lobes; they turn red-purple in autumn. Acorns are ellipsoid. Needs lime-free soil. ↕20m (70ft), ↔15m (50ft). Central N. USA. ✻✻✻

Q. falcata ♀ Spreading, deciduous tree with fissured, grey-brown bark. Elliptic, dark green leaves, 9–22cm (3½–9in) long, white- or grey-hairy beneath, are deeply cut into bristle-tipped, usually curved lobes, the terminal lobe often long. Bears broadly ellipsoid to spherical acorns. Requires lime-free soil. ↕15m (50ft), ↔12m (40ft). S.E. USA. ✻✻✻

Q. frainetto ♀ syn. *Q. conferta* (Hungarian oak). Fast-growing, spreading, deciduous tree with rugged, dark grey bark and obovate, dark green leaves, to 20cm (8in) long, cut into numerous rounded lobes and turning yellow-brown in autumn. Ellipsoid to ovoid-oblong acorns are borne in clusters of 2–4. ↕30m (100ft), ↔20m (70ft). S.E. Europe. ✻✻✻. **'Hungarian Crown'** 🏆♀ is compact and upright; ↕20m (70ft), ↔10m (30ft).

Q. garryana ▣♀ (Oregon oak). Rounded, deciduous tree with shallowly

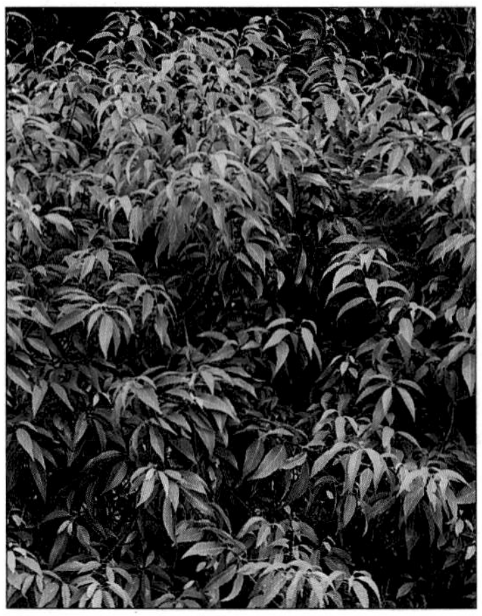

Quercus myrsinifolia

cracked, pale grey bark and orange-red, hairy young shoots. Glossy, oblong-obovate, dark green leaves, to 15cm (6in) long, have up to 5 deep, entire lobes each side. The solitary, ovoid acorns are sweet and edible. ↕↔10m (30ft). W. North America. ✻✻✻

Q.* x *heterophylla ▣♀ (*Q. phellos* x *Q. rubra*). Spreading, deciduous tree with smooth, pale grey bark. Oblong-lance-shaped to obovate, entire to shallowly bristle-toothed, glossy, mid-green leaves, are to 15cm (6in) long, turning orange to red in autumn. Bears ovoid acorns in very shallow cups. Requires lime-free soil. ↕20m (70ft), ↔15m (50ft). E. USA. ✻✻✻

Q.* x *hispanica ♀ (*Q. cerris* x *Q. suber*), syn. *Q.* x *pseudosuber*. Upright, semi-evergreen tree with corky, grey-brown bark and very variable (often fiddle-shaped, lobed, or oblong-elliptic), glossy, dark green leaves, to 5cm (2in) long, white-hairy beneath. Oblong-ovoid acorns are to 4cm (1½in) long. ↕12m (40ft), ↔8m (25ft). Garden origin. ✻✻✻. **'Diversifolia'**, syn. *Q.* x *lucombeana* 'Diversifolia', has unusual leaves: in some, the central portions are reduced to narrow strips; others are fiddle- or spoon-shaped; ↔4–5m (12–15ft). **'Lucombeana'** ▣🏆♀ syn. *Q.* x *lucombeana*, *Q.* x *lucombeana* 'William Lucombe' (Lucombe oak) has ovate to oblong leaves, to 12cm (5in) long; ↕25m (80ft), ↔20m (70ft).

Q. ilex ▣🏆♀ (Holm oak). Rounded, evergreen tree with smooth, dark grey bark and very variable, usually oblong-ovate to lance-shaped, entire or toothed, glossy, dark green leaves, to 8cm (3in) long, grey-hairy beneath, and silvery grey when young. Bears oblong-ovoid to nearly rounded acorns, solitary or in groups of 2 or 3. ↕25m (80ft), ↔20m (70ft). S.W. Europe. ✻✻. **'Fordii'** has narrowly oblong, wavy-margined leaves.

Q. ilicifolia ♀ Spreading, deciduous small tree or shrub with smooth grey bark and obovate to elliptic leaves, to 10cm (4in) long, each with usually 5 bristle-tipped, triangular lobes, dark green above and grey-hairy beneath; they turn red or yellow in autumn. Bears paired, ovoid to nearly spherical acorns. ↕6m (20ft), ↔5m (15ft). E. USA. ✻✻✻

Q. imbricaria ♀ (Shingle oak). Spreading, deciduous tree with smooth, grey-brown bark and oblong to lance-shaped or obovate, entire, glossy, dark green leaves, to 18cm (7in) long, grey-hairy beneath, and turning yellow-brown in autumn. Bears solitary, nearly spherical acorns. ↕20m (70ft), ↔15m (50ft). C. and E. USA. ✻✻✻

Q. kelloggii ♀ (Californian black oak). Rounded, deciduous tree with cracked, dark brown bark and elliptic, deeply lobed, glossy, dark green leaves, 8–22cm (3–9in) long; they each have usually 7 bristle-tipped lobes, and turn yellow-brown in autumn. Produces ovoid-oblong acorns, to 3.5cm (1½in) long. ↕20m (70ft), ↔15m (50ft). USA (Oregon, California). ✻✻✻

Q. laurifolia ▣♀ Rounded, deciduous tree with fissured, grey-black bark and narrowly oblong to obovate, entire to 3-lobed, smooth, glossy, dark green leaves, to 10cm (4in) long, bronze when young, lasting well into winter. Acorns are spherical-ovoid. Requires lime-free soil. ↕↔20m (70ft). S.E. USA. ✻✻✻

***Q.* x *libanerris* 'Rotterdam'** ♀ Fast-growing, spreading, deciduous tree with fissured grey bark and oblong, sharply toothed and lobed, glossy, dark green leaves, to 12cm (5in) long, grey-hairy beneath. Acorns are similar to those of *Q. cerris*. ↕probably 20m (70ft), ↔15m (50ft). Recent garden origin. ✻✻✻

Q. libani ♀ (Lebanon oak). Rounded, deciduous or semi-evergreen tree with smooth, later fissured, grey bark and slender shoots. Chestnut-like, oblong-lance-shaped to oblong, glossy, dark green leaves, to 10cm (4in) long, with numerous bristly marginal teeth, last well into winter. Acorns are ovoid to cylindrical. ↕↔15m (50ft). Turkey, Syria, N. Iraq, N. Iran. ✻✻✻

Q. lobata ♀ Slow-growing, spreading, deciduous tree with deeply furrowed, grey to brown bark. Obovate, dark green leaves, to 8cm (3in) long, are each deeply divided into 11 rounded lobes, and are finely hairy beneath. Bears ovoid, sweet, edible acorns, to 4cm (1½in) long. ↕16m (52ft), ↔15m (50ft). USA (California). ✻✻✻

Q.* x *lucombeana see *Q.* x *hispanica* 'Lucombeana'.

***Q.* x *lucombeana* 'Diversifolia'** see *Q.* x *hispanica* 'Diversifolia'.

***Q.* x *lucombeana* 'William Lucombe'** see *Q.* x *hispanica* 'Lucombeana'.

Q. macranthera ▣♀ Fast-growing, spreading, deciduous tree with fissured, grey-brown bark and stout, hairy shoots. Obovate, mid- to dark green leaves, to 19cm (7in) long, have numerous rounded lobes, cut more deeply towards the bases. Bears solitary, ovoid-ellipsoid acorns. ↕20m (70ft), ↔15m (50ft). Caucasus, N. Iran. ✻✻✻

Q. macrocarpa ▣♀ Slow-growing, spreading, deciduous tree with ridged, dark brown bark and corky, hairy shoots. Glossy, dark green leaves, to 25cm (10in) long, white-hairy beneath, are obovate to oblong-obovate, with deep and irregular lobes. Solitary, ovoid

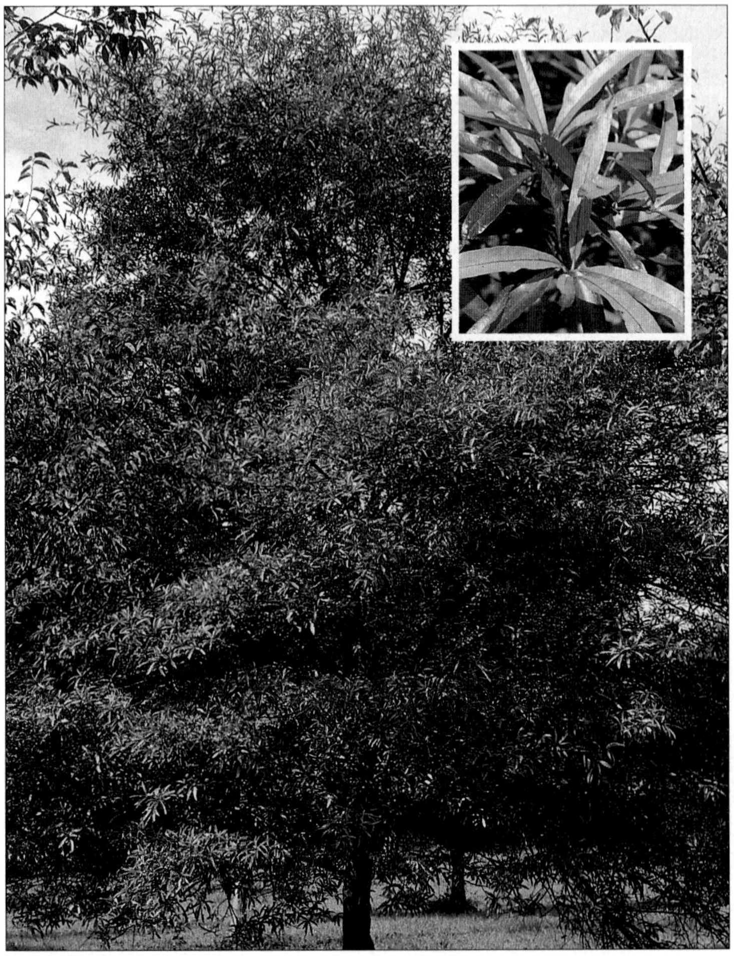

Quercus phellos (inset: autumn leaf colour)

Q

acorns, to 5cm (2in) long, are borne in large, fringed cups. ↕ 15m (50ft), ↔ 10m (30ft). E. North America. ❄❄❄
Q. macrolepis ▣ ♀ syn. *Q. aegilops*. Spreading, deciduous or semi-evergreen, often broad-crowned tree with fissured, dark grey bark. Ovate to oblong, grey-green leaves, to 10cm (4in) long, with angular, bristle-tipped lobes, are densely white-hairy or yellowish white-hairy on both surfaces. Bears acorns, to 4.5cm (1¾in) long, singly or in clusters of 2 or 3, in unusually large, scaly cups, to 6cm (2½in) across. ↕ 15m (50ft), ↔ 12m (40ft). S.E. Europe, Turkey. ❄❄
Q. marilandica ▣ ♀ (Black Jack oak). Spreading, deciduous small tree with very rough, black-brown bark. Broadly obovate, glossy, dark green leaves, 6–17cm (2½–7in) long, each end in 3 bristle-tipped lobes, and turn yellow, red, or brown in autumn. Produces ovoid acorns. Requires lime-free soil. ↕ 12m (40ft), ↔ 15m (50ft). S.E. USA. ❄❄❄
Q. mongolica ♀ Spreading, deciduous tree with rough grey bark and obovate, dark green leaves, to 20cm (8in) or more long, with rounded lobes. Produces ovoid to ellipsoid acorns. ↕ 20m (70ft), ↔ 15m (50ft). E. Asia. ❄❄❄. **var. *grosseserrata*** has leaves with acutely triangular and tooth-like lobes.
Q. muehlenbergii ▣ ♀ (Chinkapin oak). Rounded, deciduous tree with grey, scaly bark and elliptic to obovate, pointed, glossy, dark green or yellow-green leaves, to 15cm (6in) long, whitish green beneath, triangularly lobed and with numerous curved teeth, turning yellow-brown in autumn. Produces

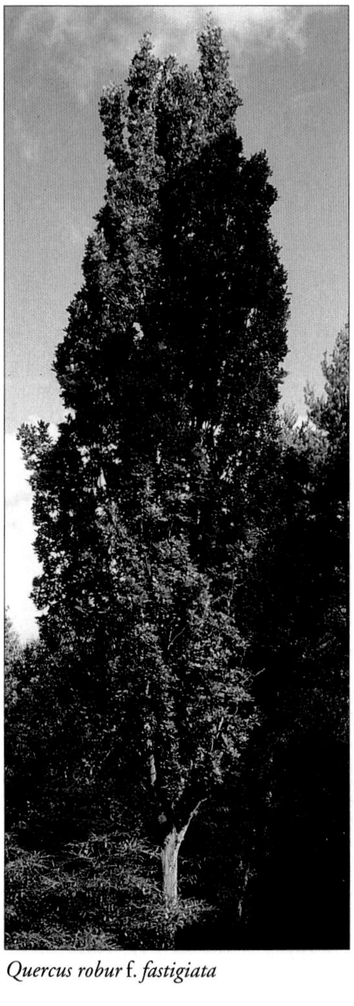
Quercus robur f. *fastigiata*

ovoid acorns. ↕ 15m (50ft), ↔ 12m (40ft). E. USA. ❄❄❄
Q. myrsinifolia ▣ ♀ Rounded, evergreen tree or shrub with smooth, dark grey bark and lance-shaped, tapered, weakly toothed, glossy, dark green leaves, to 12cm (5in) long, bronze-red when young. Solitary, ovoid-oblong acorns are borne in distinctively ringed cups. ↕ 12m (40ft), ↔ 10m (30ft). S. China, Laos, Japan. ❄❄
Q. nigra ▣ ♠ (Water oak). Broadly conical, deciduous tree with smooth, brown then dark grey bark. Variable, dark green leaves, 4–15cm (1½–6in) long, are narrowly obovate or spoon-shaped, rarely elliptic, usually 3-lobed, and retained late on the tree. Acorns are spherical. Needs lime-free soil. ↕ 15m (50ft), ↔ 12m (40ft). S.E. USA. ❄❄❄
Q. palustris ▣ ♀ ♠ (Pin oak). Fast-growing, broadly conical, deciduous tree with pendent lower branches and smooth grey bark. Elliptic, deeply lobed, glossy, mid-green leaves, to 15cm (6in) long, are broadly tapered at the bases; they have large tufts of hairs in the leaf vein axils beneath, and turn scarlet to red-brown in autumn. Acorns are nearly spherical. ↕ 20m (70ft), ↔ 12m (40ft). E. USA. ❄❄❄. **'Sovereign'** has spreading lower branches.
Q. pedunculata see *Q. robur*.
Q. petraea ♀ ♀ syn. *Q. sessiliflora* (Sessile oak). Spreading, deciduous tree with ridged grey bark and yellow-stalked, ovate, obovate, or oblong, dark green leaves, 6–17cm (2½–7in) long, margined with rounded lobes. Stalkless, ovoid to oblong-ovoid acorns are borne singly or in clusters of 2–5. ↕ 30m (100ft), ↔ 25m (80ft). Europe. ❄❄❄. **'Columna'** ◊ is upright and columnar, with oblong, lobed or entire, bluish green leaves; ↕ 20m (70ft), ↔ 6m (20ft).
Q. phellos ▣ ♀ ♀ syn. *Q. pumila* (Willow oak). Spreading, deciduous tree with smooth grey bark and willow-like, entire or slightly wavy-margined, slender, linear to narrowly oblong, bright dark green leaves, to 12cm (5in) long; in autumn, they turn yellow, then brown. Acorns are spherical. ↕ 20m (70ft), ↔ 15m (50ft). E. USA. ❄❄❄
Q. phillyreoides ▣ ♀ Spreading, evergreen tree with smooth, brownish grey to dark grey bark and oblong to ovate-oblong, toothed, dark green leaves, to 6cm (2½in) long, often bronze when young. Ovoid acorns are borne in cone-shaped cups. ↕↔ 10m (30ft). China, S. Japan. ❄❄❄
Q. pontica ♀ (Armenian oak). Shrubby or oval-headed, deciduous, small tree with shallowly fissured, pale grey-brown bark and stout reddish shoots. Obovate or elliptic to broadly elliptic, bright mid-green leaves, to 25cm (10in) long, with numerous parallel veins ending in small, pointed teeth, turn yellow-brown in autumn. Ovoid acorns are borne singly or in stout-stalked clusters of 2–5, at the shoot tips. ↕ 6m (20ft), ↔ 5m (15ft). N.E. Turkey, Caucasus. ❄❄❄
Q. x pseudosuber see *Q.* x *hispanica*.
Q. pubescens ♀ Spreading, deciduous tree with deeply furrowed, grey to black bark and densely hairy shoots. Oblong-ovate, grey-green leaves, to 10cm (4in) long, hairy beneath, have rounded lobes ending in small, pointed teeth. Ovoid acorns are borne singly or in groups of up to 4. ↕ 10–20m (30–70ft), ↔ 15m

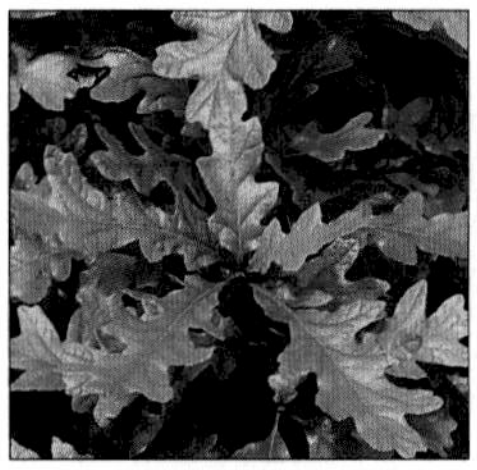
Quercus garryana

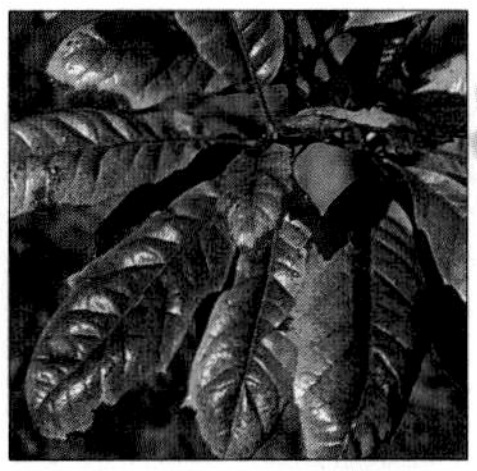
Quercus x *heterophylla*

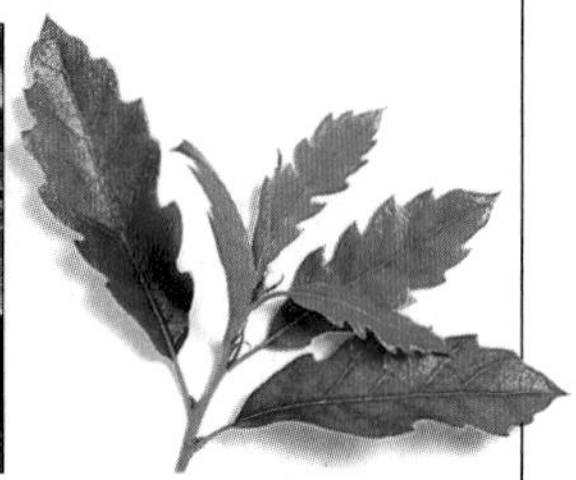
Quercus x *hispanica* 'Lucombeana'

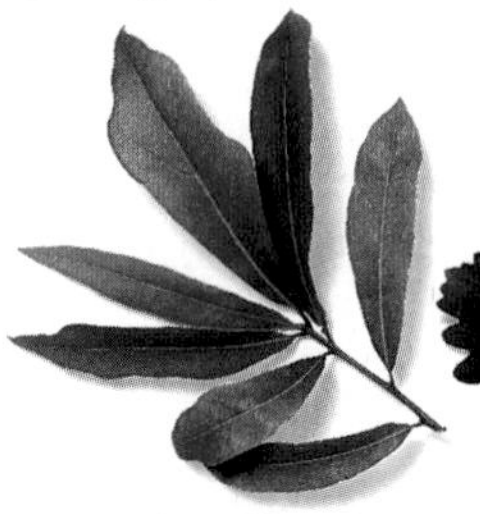
Quercus laurifolia

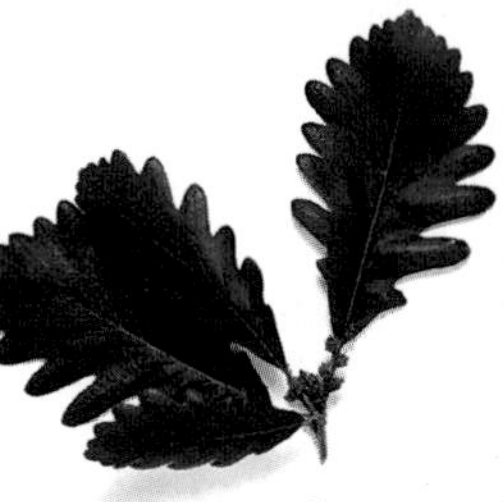
Quercus macranthera

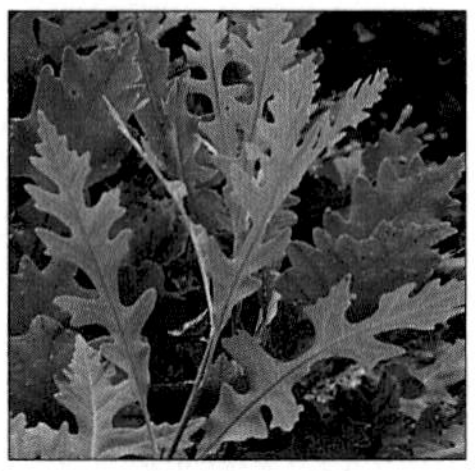
Quercus macrocarpa

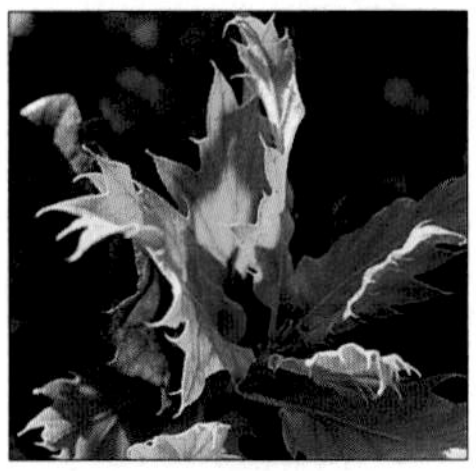
Quercus macrolepis

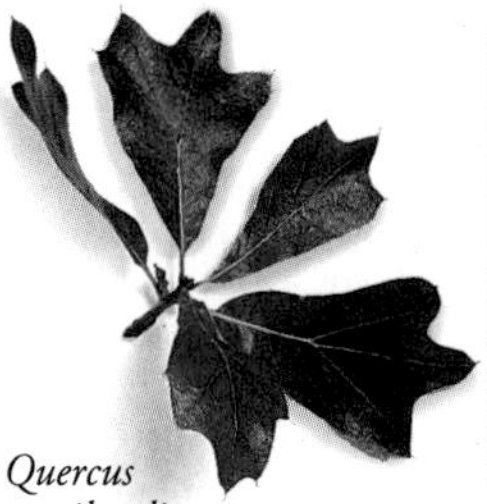
Quercus marilandica

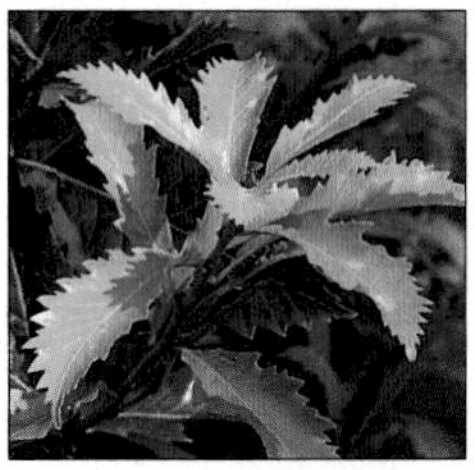
Quercus muehlenbergii

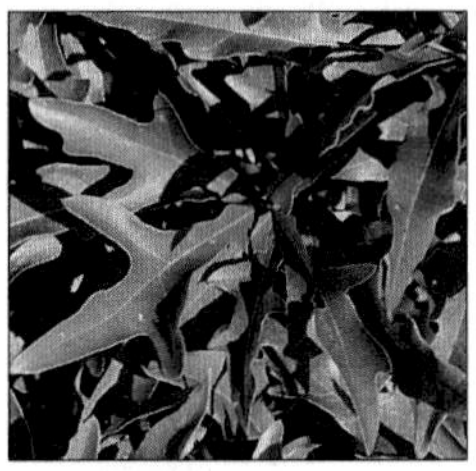
Quercus nigra

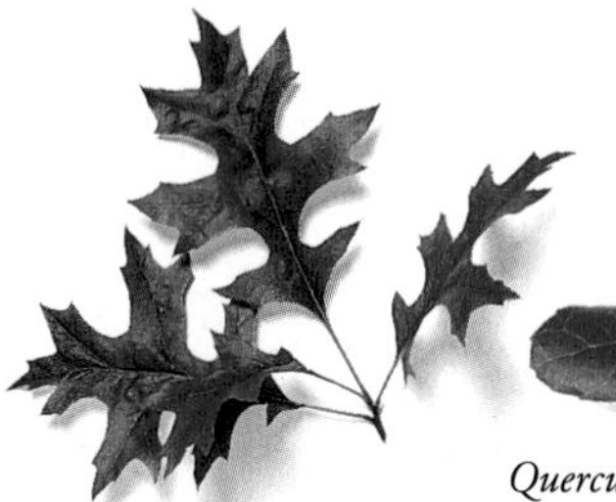
Quercus palustris

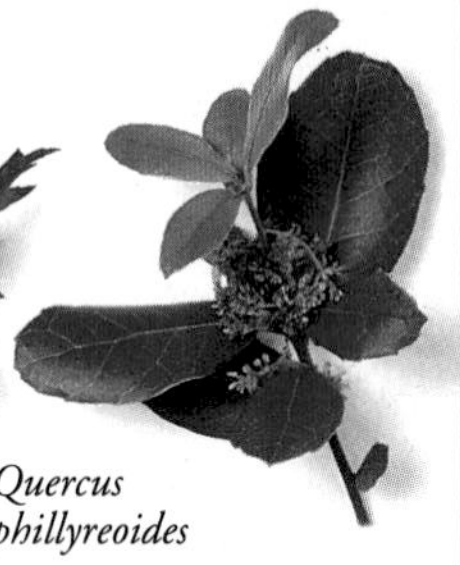
Quercus phillyreoides

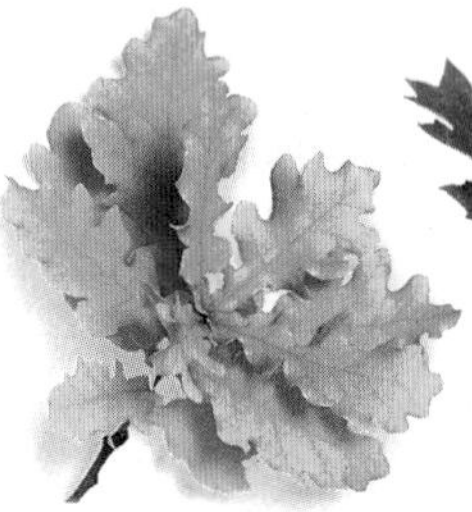
Quercus robur 'Concordia'

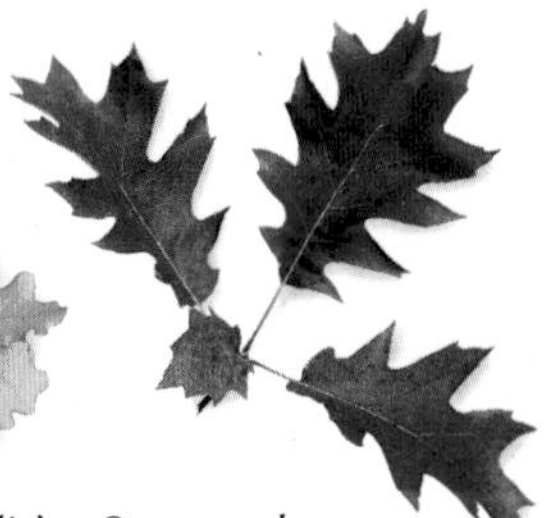
Quercus rubra

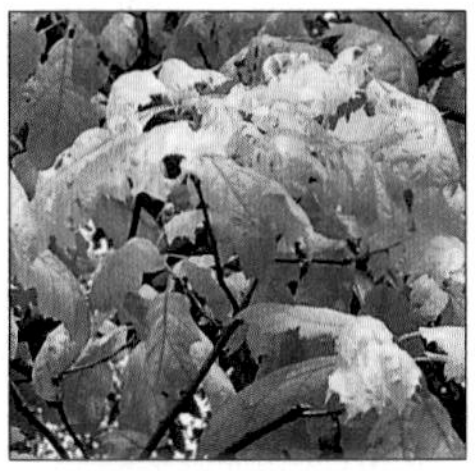
Quercus rubra 'Aurea'

(50ft). C. and S. Europe, Turkey, Ukraine (Crimea). ❄❄❄
Q. pumila see *Q. phellos*.
Q. pyrenaica ♀ Broadly columnar, deciduous tree with furrowed, brown to black bark and often pendent, downy shoots. Obovate, elliptic, or broadly oblong, deeply lobed and toothed, glossy, dark green leaves, to 16cm (6in) long, downy when young, emerge in late spring. The oblong-ovoid acorns are produced in clusters of 2–4. ↕ 20m (70ft), ↔ 12m (40ft). France, Spain, Portugal, Morocco. ❄❄❄
Q. robur ♀ ♀ syn. *Q. pedunculata* (Common oak, English oak, Pedunculate oak). Rugged, spreading, deciduous tree with fissured, grey-brown bark. Dark green, very short-stalked leaves, to 14cm (5½in) long, are ovate-oblong, with rounded lobes, each base with two small, ear-like lobes. Ovoid acorns are borne singly or in clusters of 2 or 3. ↕ 35m (120ft), ↔ 25m (80ft). Europe. ❄❄❄. **'Concordia'** ▣ has bright yellow young foliage, turning green; ↕↔ 10m (30ft). **f. *fastigiata*** ▣ ◊ has upright branches; ↕↔ 15m (50ft). **f. *pendula*** ♀ has weeping shoots.
Q. rubra ▣ ♀ ♀ syn. *Q. borealis* (Red oak). Fast-growing, spreading, deciduous tree with smooth, greyish brown or dark grey bark. Elliptic, matt, dark green leaves, to 20cm (8in) long, cut into bristle-tipped lobes, turn yellow- to red-brown in autumn. Acorns are hemispherical. Requires lime-free soil. ↕ 25m (80ft), ↔ 20m (70ft). E. North America. ❄❄❄. **'Aurea'** ▣ has golden yellow leaves in spring, turning green; ↕ 15m (50ft), ↔ 10m (30ft).
Q. serrata see *Q. acutissima*.
Q. sessiliflora see *Q. petraea*.
Q. shumardii ♀ Broadly columnar, deciduous tree with smooth grey bark. Leaves are glossy, dark green, to 18cm

Q

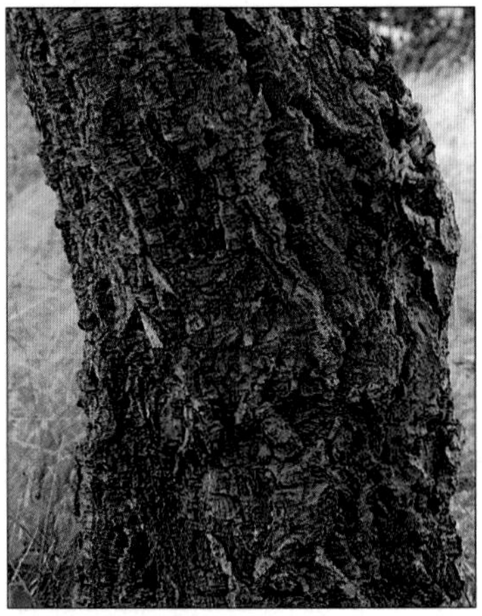

Quercus suber

(7in) long, elliptic to elliptic-obovate, truncate, each with up to 9 lobes ending in bristle-tipped teeth, and turn red to red-brown in autumn. Acorns are ovoid. Requires lime-free soil. ↕ 20m (70ft), ↔ 12m (40ft). S.E. USA. ❄❄❄

Q. suber ▣ ♀ (Cork oak). Rounded, evergreen tree with thick, corky bark (the cork of commerce). Ovate-oblong, toothed, rigid, dark green leaves, to 7cm (3in) long, are grey-hairy beneath. Bears ovoid-oblong acorns. ↕↔ 20m (70ft). W. Mediterranean, N. Africa. ❄❄

Q.* x *turneri ♀ (*Q. ilex* x *Q. robur*). Dense, rounded, semi-evergreen tree with fissured, brownish grey to dark grey bark and obovate, shallowly lobed, dark green leaves, to 12cm (5in) long. Bears ovoid acorns in clusters of 3–7. ↕↔ 20m (70ft). Garden origin. ❄❄❄

Q. velutina ♀ (Black oak). Fast-growing, spreading, deciduous tree with ridged, dark brown, almost black bark. Elliptic, glossy, dark green leaves, to 25cm (10in) long, each with up to 7 pointed, deep lobes, turn red-brown in autumn. Acorns are more or less spherical. Requires lime-free soil. ↕ 30m (100ft), ↔ 25m (80ft). E. North America. ❄❄❄

Q. wislizeni ▣ ♀ Spreading, evergreen tree or shrub with blackish or reddish brown bark and broadly lance-shaped to broadly elliptic, usually spiny-toothed, glossy, dark green leaves, 2.5–4cm (1–1½in) long. Bears solitary, oblong-ellipsoid acorns, to 4cm (1½in) long. ↕ to 20m (70ft), ↔ 12m (40ft). USA (California). ❄❄

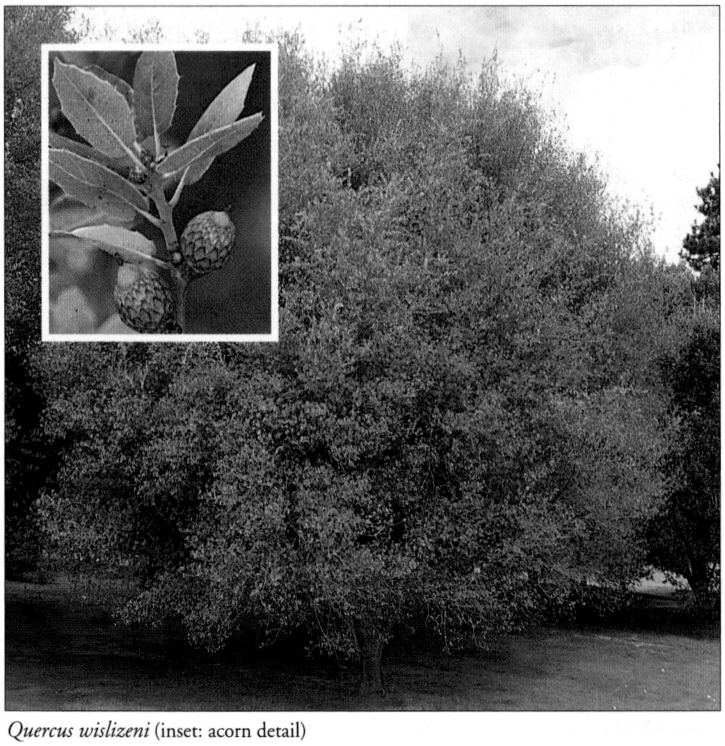

Quercus wislizeni (inset: acorn detail)

QUESNELIA

BROMELIACEAE

Genus of approximately 15 species of almost stemless, evergreen, terrestrial or epiphytic perennials (bromeliads), some rhizomatous, found in scrub, woodland, or rainforest in E. Brazil, to 2,000m (6,500ft). They are cultivated for their rosetted, lance-shaped, spiny-margined, thick, stiff leaves and their upright or pendent, ellipsoid or cylindrical, dense or lax inflorescences of ovoid or tubular flowers, borne among showy bracts from late spring to summer. Below 13°C (55°F), grow as houseplants or in a warm greenhouse; elsewhere, grow in a humid, moist part of the garden.

• **HARDINESS** Frost tender.

• **CULTIVATION** Under glass, grow in epiphytic or terrestrial bromeliad compost in bright filtered light. Water moderately at all times and regularly mist lightly. Apply a nitrogen-based fertilizer monthly during the growing season. Outdoors, grow in open, coarse, humus-rich, moist but well-drained soil in partial shade. See also p.47.

• **PROPAGATION** Sow seed at 27°C (81°F) as soon as ripe. Remove offsets in late spring or summer.

• **PESTS AND DISEASES** Young growth is vulnerable to scale insects.

Q. liboniana ▣ Epiphytic perennial with funnel-shaped rosettes of lance-shaped, stiff, minutely brown-scaly, dark green leaves, 75–80cm (30–32in) long, margined with straight or curved spines. From late spring to summer, bears simple or few-branched inflorescences,

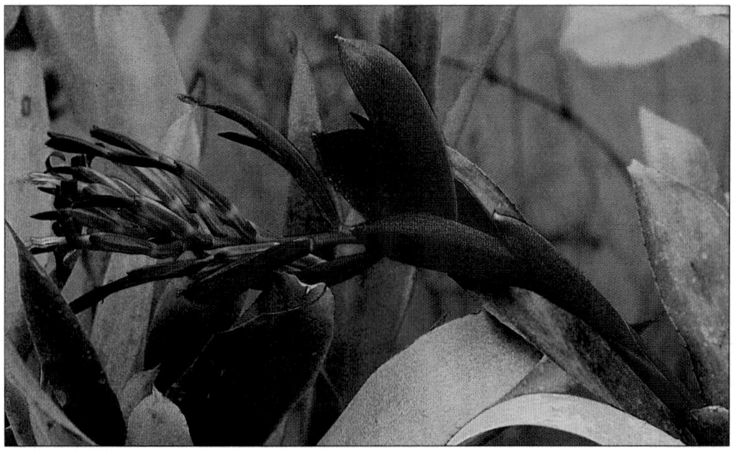

Quesnelia liboniana

10cm (4in) long, comprising orange-red bracts and tubular, deep purple-blue flowers, 5cm (2in) long, with yellow sepals, flushed orange-red. ↕↔ 75cm (30in). E. Brazil. ❁ (min. 13°C/55°F)

Q. marmorata, syn. *Aechmea marmorata*. Epiphytic, rhizomatous perennial with tubular rosettes of thick, 2-ranked, lance-shaped, greyish green leaves, 40–60cm (16–24in) long, marbled and banded lilac and green, with pinkish grey marginal spines. From late spring to summer, bears pyramid-shaped, terminal inflorescences, 20cm (8in) long, consisting of tiny pink floral bracts and ovoid, blue or purple flowers, 3cm (1¼in) long, with blue-purple sepals. ↕ 60cm (24in), ↔ 30cm (12in) or more. E. Brazil. ❁ (min. 13°C/55°F)

Q. quesneliana. Rhizomatous, terrestrial perennial with broad rosettes of 6–10 lance-shaped, brown-spiny, bright green leaves, 70–90cm (28–36in) long, cross-banded with greyish lilac scales beneath. From late spring to summer, bears cylindrical or narrowly ellipsoid inflorescences, 15cm (6in) long; these consist of overlapping pink, later white scales and spirally arranged, wavy-margined, red to rose-pink bracts, which almost hide the oval, blue-margined white flowers, 3.5cm (1½in) long, with red sepals. ↕↔ to 75cm (30in) or more. E. Brazil. ❁ (min. 13°C/55°F)

▷**Quick** see *Crataegus monogyna*
▷**Quickthorn** see *Crataegus monogyna*
▷**Quince** see *Cydonia*
Common see *Cydonia oblonga*
Flowering see *Chaenomeles*
Japanese see *Chaenomeles, C. japonica*
Maule's see *Chaenomeles japonica*

QUISQUALIS

COMBRETACEAE

Genus of about 16 species of woody-stemmed, evergreen climbers or scandent shrubs from tropical forest in Africa, South Africa, Indonesia, and Malaysia. They are cultivated for their small, tubular, 5-lobed flowers, borne in terminal or axillary racemes or panicles. Leaves are simple and usually produced in opposite pairs. Where temperatures fall below 13°C (55°F), grow in a warm greenhouse. In tropical climates, use to clothe an arch or wall.

• **HARDINESS** Frost tender.

• **CULTIVATION** Under glass, grow in loam-based potting compost (JI No.3) in full light with shade from hot sun. In growth, water freely and apply a balanced liquid fertilizer every month. Water sparingly in winter. Outdoors, grow in moderately fertile, moist but well-drained soil in full sun with some midday shade. Pruning group 11, in late winter or early spring.

• **PROPAGATION** Sow seed at 18°C (64°F) in spring. Root softwood cuttings with bottom heat in late spring. Layer in spring.

• **PESTS AND DISEASES** Prone to red spider mites and mealybugs under glass.

Q. indica ▣ (Rangoon creeper). Freely branching, perennial climber, erect and shrub-like when young. Mid- to deep green leaves, 8–18cm (3–7in) long, are elliptic to elliptic-oblong with rounded to heart-shaped bases, long, sharp tips, and prominent veins. In summer and autumn, bears slender-tubed, fragrant flowers, 4–7cm (1½–3in) long, with 5 spreading lobes, in pendent, terminal racemes, 10cm (4in) long; initially white, they change to pink and purplish red then bright red over a 3-day period. ↕ to 20m (70ft) or more. Tropical Africa and S.E. Asia. ❁ (min. 13°C/55°F)

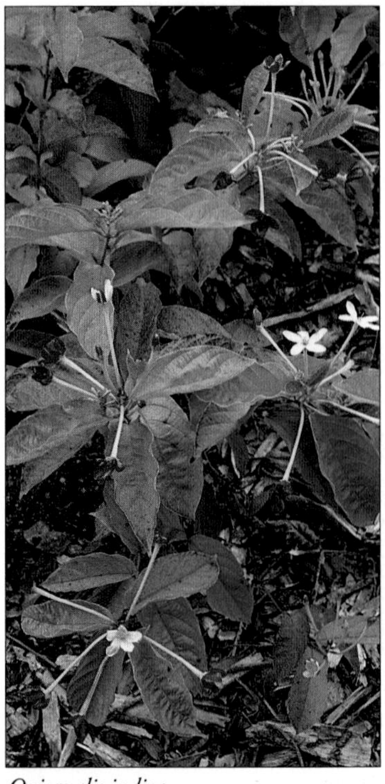

Quisqualis indica

Q

R

- ▷ **Rabbit's foot** see *Maranta leuconeura* 'Kerchoveana'
- ▷ **Rabbit's tracks** see *Maranta leuconeura* 'Kerchoveana'
- ▷ **Radiator plant** see *Peperomia maculosa*
- ▷ **Raffia** see *Raphia*
- ▷ **Ragged robin** see *Lychnis flos-cuculi*
- ▷ **Ragwort, Leopard's bane** see *Senecio doronicum*
- ▷ **Rainbow plant, Marbled** see *Billbergia* Fantasia Group
- ▷ **Rainbow star** see *Cryptanthus bromelioides*
- ▷ **Rain flower** see *Zephyranthes*
- ▷ **Raisin-tree** see *Hovenia dulcis*

RAMONDA

GESNERIACEAE

Genus of 3 species of rosette-forming, evergreen perennials from shady rock crevices and cliff faces in N.E. Spain, the Pyrenees, and Balkan mountains. They are grown for their hairy, crinkled leaves, of variable shape and colour, and their flat or shallowly cup-shaped, colourful flowers. The flowers are often slightly 2-lipped, with 4 or 5, rarely 6 petals, and are borne singly or in cyme-like panicles on slender, leafless stems, in late spring and early summer. Grow in a rock garden, a peat bed, in crevices in a stone wall, or in an alpine house.

• **HARDINESS** Fully hardy, but intolerant of excessive winter wet.

• **CULTIVATION** In an alpine house, grow in equal parts loam, leaf mould, and grit, in bright filtered light with shade from hot sun. Outdoors, grow in moist but well-drained, humus-rich, moderately fertile soil in partial shade. Plants are best grown on their sides to avoid accumulations of moisture in the rosettes, which may cause rotting in winter. Leaves wither in dry conditions, but recover if watered thoroughly.

• **PROPAGATION** Sow seed very thinly in containers in a cold frame as soon as ripe. Seedlings develop slowly, so do not prick out until they have several leaves. Root rosettes in early summer, or root leaf cuttings in early autumn.

• **PESTS AND DISEASES** Very susceptible to slug and snail damage.

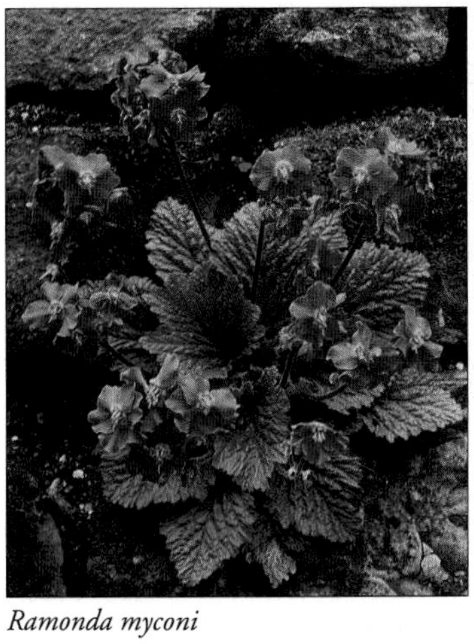

Ramonda myconi

R. myconi ▣ 🏆 syn. *R. pyrenaica*. Rosette-forming, evergreen perennial with elliptic to very broadly ovate, hairy, slightly crinkled, dark green leaves, to 8cm (3in) long. Cyme-like panicles of outward-facing, flat, 5-petalled flowers, 2.5 cm (1in) across, usually deep violet-blue with yellow anthers, are produced in late spring and early summer; pink- and white-flowered variants also occur. ↕10cm (4in), ↔ to 20cm (8in). Pyrenees, N.E. Spain. ❄❄❄

R. nathaliae 🏆 Rosette-forming, evergreen perennial with elliptic to broadly ovate, hairy, slightly crinkled, glossy, pale green leaves, to 5cm (2in) long, entire or with slightly scalloped margins. In late spring and early summer, bears cyme-like panicles of outward-facing, flattish, 4-petalled, deep mauve-blue flowers, to 3.5cm (1½in) across, with orange-yellow eyes and yellow anthers. ↕↔ 10cm (4in). Bosnia & Herzegovina, Macedonia, N. Greece. ❄❄❄

R. pyrenaica see *R. myconi*.

R. serbica. Rosette-forming, evergreen perennial with narrowly obovate, hairy, crinkled, irregularly scalloped, pale green leaves, to 5cm (2in) long. In late spring and early summer, outward-facing, saucer- to cup-shaped, lilac-blue flowers, 3.5cm (1½in) across, each with 5, sometimes 6 petals and violet-blue anthers, open singly or in pairs in cyme-like panicles. ↕10cm (4in), ↔ 15cm (6in). Croatia, Yugoslavia, Albania, W. Greece, N.W. Bulgaria. ❄❄❄

- ▷ **Rampion, Horned** see *Phyteuma*
- ▷ **Ram's horn** see *Proboscidea louisianica*
- ▷ **Rangoon creeper** see *Quisqualis indica*

RANUNCULUS

Buttercup, Crowfoot

RANUNCULACEAE

Genus of about 400 species of annuals, biennials, and mainly deciduous, sometimes evergreen perennials, widely distributed in temperate regions of the world. They are found in a range of habitats, varying from damp woodland to grassland, and from mountain screes and summer-dry sites to bogs or shallow water. They may be rhizomatous, tuberous, fibrous-rooted, or spread by runners. The leaves form basal rosettes or are sometimes stem-clasping; they are very variable in shape, and may be simple and entire, toothed to palmately lobed, or pinnatisect. Buttercups are grown for their bowl-shaped, or cup- to saucer-shaped, usually 5-petalled, mainly yellow, but also white, pink, orange, or red flowers, which are borne singly or in cyme-like panicles in spring, summer, or occasionally in autumn. Buttercups are suitable for a wide range of sites (see cultivation groups below). Contact with the sap may irritate skin.

• **HARDINESS** Most are fully hardy. *R. asiaticus* is half hardy.

• **CULTIVATION** Buttercups have a range of cultivation requirements; for ease of reference, they have been divided into groups as follows:

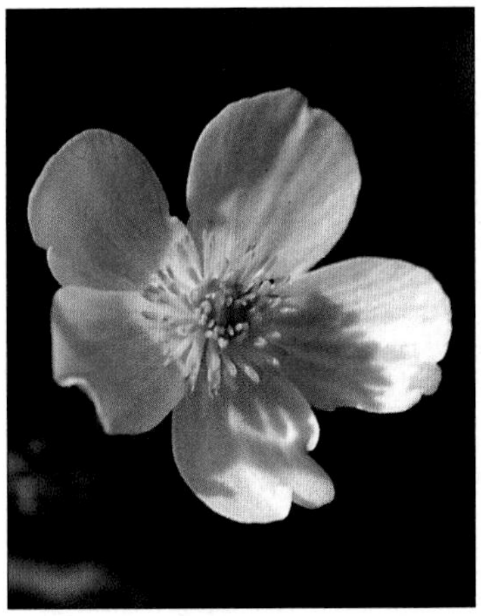

Ranunculus aconitifolius

1. Woodland buttercups, best in partial or full shade in moist, humus-rich soil.
2. Buttercups easily grown in sun or partial shade, in fertile, moist but well-drained soil; grow in a border or rock garden.
3. High alpine buttercups, best grown in gritty, humus-rich, sharply drained soil in a scree bed in full sun, or in an alpine house in a mix of equal parts loam, leaf mould, and grit in full light.
4. Aquatic or bog plants, best grown in mud at a pond margin or streamside. Grow *R. aquatilis* in 15–60cm (6–24in) of still or fast-moving water; grow *R. lingua* and *R. flammula* in 15–22cm (6–9in) of still or slow-moving water.
5. Tuberous buttercups (except *R. ficaria*) that require a dry, dormant period in summer; best in a bulb frame or alpine house in a mix of equal parts loam, leaf mould, and grit in full light.

• **PROPAGATION** Sow seed of most alpine species in pans in an open frame when seed is still slightly green; germination is erratic, and pans should be retained for several years if seeds fail to germinate in the first year. Sow seed of perennials, aquatic perennials, and mat-forming alpines in containers in a cold frame as soon as ripe, or divide in spring or autumn. Divide tuberous species, or detach basal bulbils (where these form), in spring or autumn.

• **PESTS AND DISEASES** Vulnerable to slug and snail damage, aphids, and powdery mildew.

R. aconitifolius ▣ (Bachelor's buttons). Clump-forming, hairy, fibrous-rooted perennial producing palmately 3- to 5-lobed, toothed, glossy, dark green, basal leaves, to 20cm (8in) long. In late spring and early summer, freely branched stems bear numerous red-tinged buds that open to panicles of saucer-shaped white flowers, 1–2cm (½–¾in) across, with red- or purple-backed sepals. Cultivation group 1 or 2. ↕60cm (24in), ↔ 45cm (18in). C. Europe. ❄❄❄. **'Flore Pleno'** ▣ 🏆 (Fair maids of France, Fair maids of Kent, White bachelor's buttons) has long-lasting, double white flowers with numerous small petals.

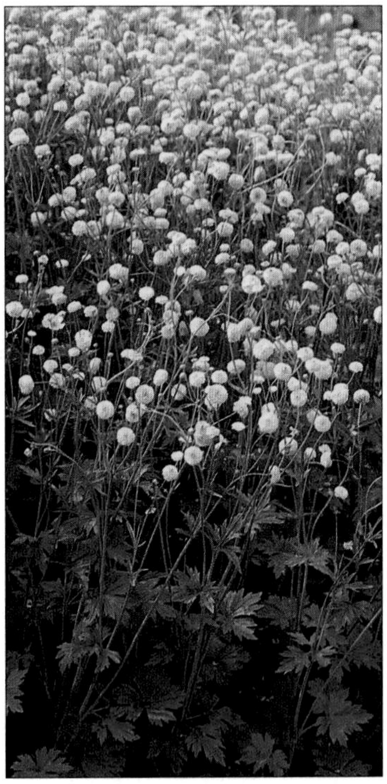

Ranunculus acris 'Flore Pleno'

R. acris (Meadow buttercup). Erect, hairy, fibrous-rooted perennial, sometimes with short rhizomes. The long-stalked, broadly ovate, palmately 3- to 7-lobed, mid-green, basal leaves, 8cm (3in) long, have toothed lobes, which are sometimes further subdivided. Many-branched stems bear panicles of numerous saucer-shaped, glossy, golden yellow flowers, to 2.5cm (1in) across, in early and midsummer. Cultivation group 1 or 2. ↕20–90cm (8–36in), ↔ 22cm (9in). Europe and W. Asia. ❄❄❄. **'Farrer's Yellow'** has pale yellow flowers. **'Flore Pleno'** ▣ bears double, rosetted, many-petalled yellow flowers.

R

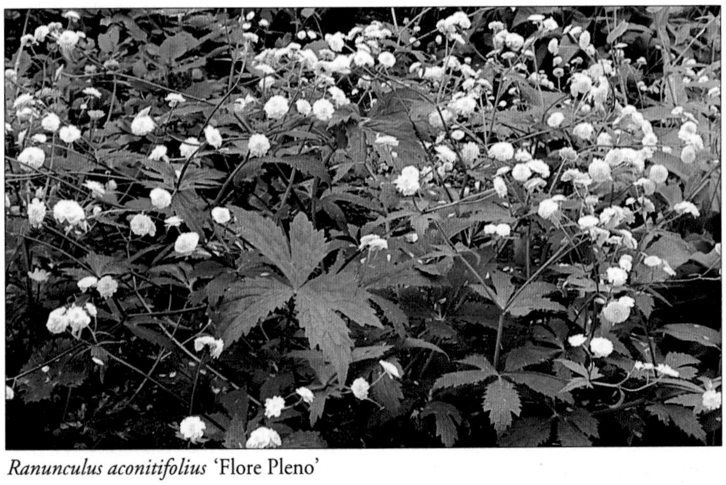

Ranunculus aconitifolius 'Flore Pleno'

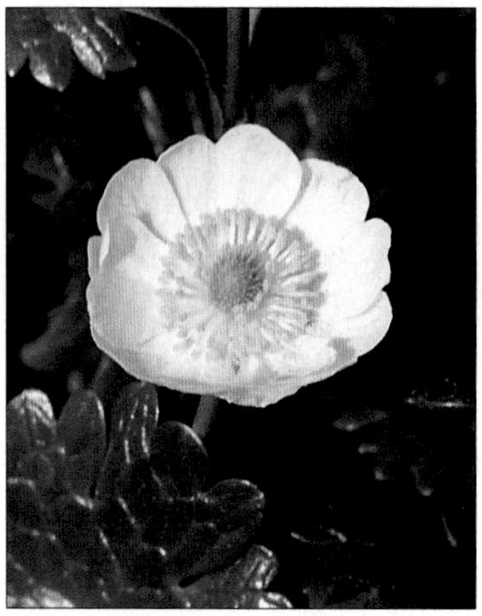

Ranunculus alpestris

R. alpestris ■ Short-lived, tufted, occasionally evergreen perennial with fibrous roots. The kidney-shaped, palmately 3- to 5-lobed, basal leaves, are 3–5cm (1¼–2in) long, round-toothed, glossy and dark green. From late spring to midsummer, bears cup-shaped white flowers, to 2cm (¾in) across, singly or occasionally in clusters of 2 or 3. Cultivation group 3. ↕↔ to 10cm (4in). Mountains of C. and S. Europe. ✽✽✽
R. amplexicaulis. Clump-forming perennial with fibrous roots and ovate-lance-shaped, entire, sometimes sparsely hairy, grey-green basal leaves, to 7cm (3in) long, and smaller leaves clasping the upright, branching stems. In early summer, bears cyme-like panicles of up to 5 cup-shaped white flowers, each 2–2.5cm (¾–1in) across. Cultivation group 2. ↕ to 30cm (12in), ↔ 20cm (8in). Pyrenees, N. and C. Spain. ✽✽✽
R. aquatilis ■ (Water crowfoot). Aquatic annual or usually evergreen perennial with submerged, branched, slender stems and dark green leaves, 3–8cm (1¼–3in) long. The kidney-shaped to rounded, floating leaves are deeply divided into 3–7 lobes; the submerged leaves have many thread-like segments. Solitary, bowl- or saucer-shaped, white-based yellow flowers, 2cm (¾in) across, are borne on the water's surface in midsummer. Cultivation group 4. ↔ indefinite. Europe. ✽✽✽
R. asiaticus ■ (Persian buttercup). Tuberous, fibrous-rooted perennial with long-stalked, broadly ovate to rounded, deeply 3-lobed, hairy, pale to dark green, basal leaves, to 14cm (5½in) long, the lobes further subdivided and

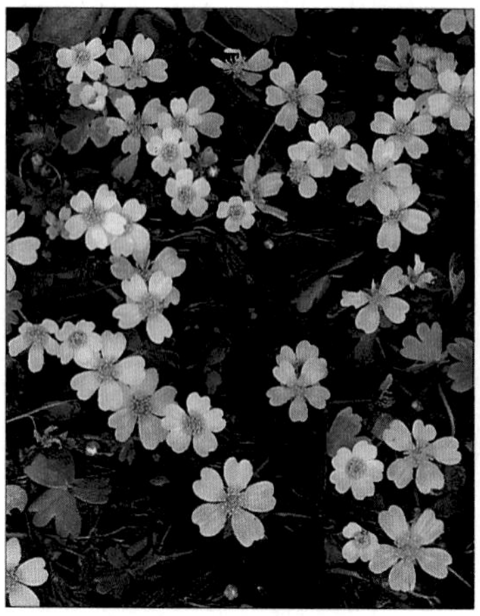

Ranunculus aquatilis

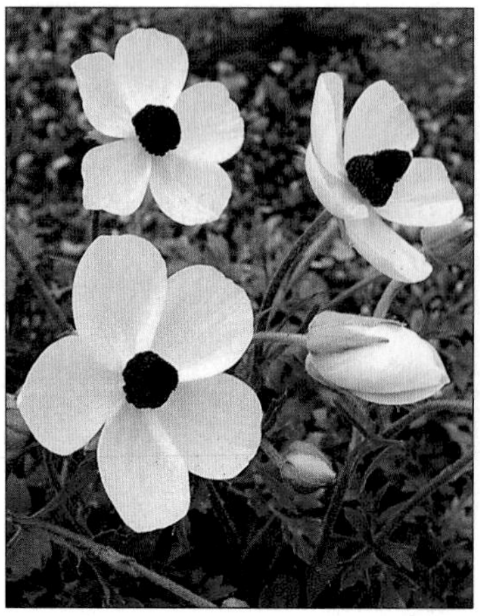

Ranunculus asiaticus

toothed. Branching flowering stems bear 1–4 cup-shaped, red, pink, yellow, or white flowers, 3–5cm (1¼–2in) across, with purple-black centres, in late spring and early summer. Cultivation group 5. ↕ 20–45cm (8–18in), ↔ 20cm (8in). E. Mediterranean, N.E. Africa, S.W. Asia. ✽. **Turban Group** cultivars have double flowers.
R. bulbosus (Bulbous buttercup). Erect, hairy, sometimes semi-evergreen perennial with fibrous roots and a swollen, corm-like stem base. Ovate, 3-lobed, dark green basal and lower stem leaves, to 12cm (5in) long, each have a long-stalked middle segment. In late spring and early summer, bears branched, cyme-like panicles of several saucer-shaped, rich golden yellow flowers, 2–3cm (¾–1¼in) across, with reflexed, paler yellow sepals. Cultivation group 2. ↕ 15–40cm (6–16in), sometimes to 80cm (32in), ↔ 30cm (12in). Europe, N. Africa, Caucasus. ✽✽✽. **var. *farreri*** see 'F.M. Burton'. **'F.M. Burton'**, syn. var. *farreri*, bears glossy, pale creamy yellow flowers. **'Speciosus Plenus' of gardens** see *R. constantinopolitanus* 'Plenus'.
R. bullatus. Tuberous perennial with broadly obovate, puckered, glossy, dark green, basal leaves, to 10cm (4in) long, hairy beneath, and often with 3 shallow lobes or teeth at the tips. In autumn, short, unbranched stems each bear 1 or 2 bowl-shaped, violet-scented, shining yellow flowers, 2.5cm (1in) across. Unusual in being autumn-flowering and scented. Cultivation group 5. ↕↔ to 10cm (4in). W. to E. Mediterranean, (including Spain and Portugal). ✽✽

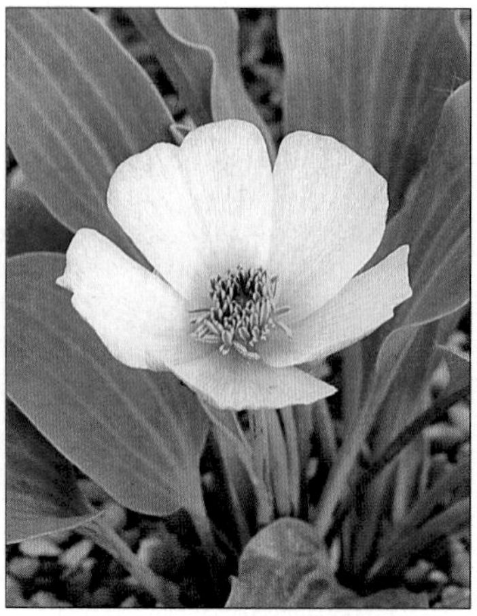

Ranunculus calandrinioides

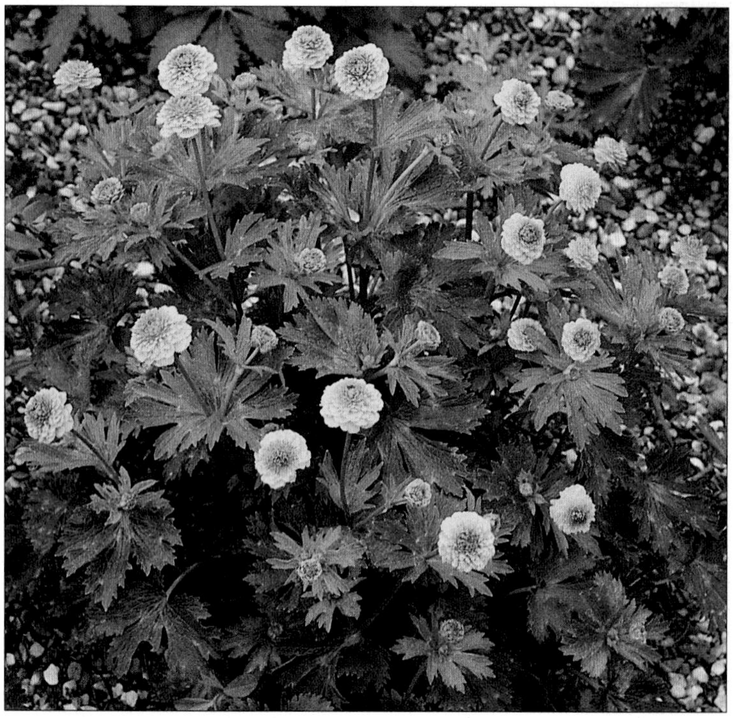

Ranunculus constantinopolitanus 'Plenus'

R. calandrinioides ■ 🏆 Clump-forming perennial with thick, fleshy roots and broadly lance-shaped to ovate-lance-shaped, hairless, blue-green leaves, to 7cm (3in) long, dying down in summer. In late winter and early spring, unbranched stems bear short, cyme-like panicles of up to 3 cup-shaped, usually pink-flushed white flowers, to 5cm (2in) across. Cultivation group 3 or 5. ↕ 20cm (8in), ↔ 15cm (6in). Atlas Mountains. ✽✽✽
R. constantinopolitanus. Clump-forming perennial with short rhizomes and deeply 3-lobed, mid-green basal and lower stem leaves, 3–10cm (1¼–4in) long. From mid-spring to midsummer, branched stems bear cyme-like panicles of 3–8 bowl-shaped, glossy, bright yellow flowers, to 3cm (1¼in) across, with reflexed, pale yellow sepals. Cultivation group 1 or 2. ↕ 30–70cm (12–28in), ↔ 30cm (12in). E. Europe, Balkans, Cyprus, Syria, Iraq, Iran, Caucasus, Ukraine (Crimea). ✽✽✽. **'Plenus'** ■ syn. *R. bulbosus* 'Speciosus Plenus' of gardens, *R. gouanii* 'Plenus', *R. speciosus* 'Flore Pleno', produces double yellow flowers; ↕ 30cm (12in), ↔ 15cm (6in).

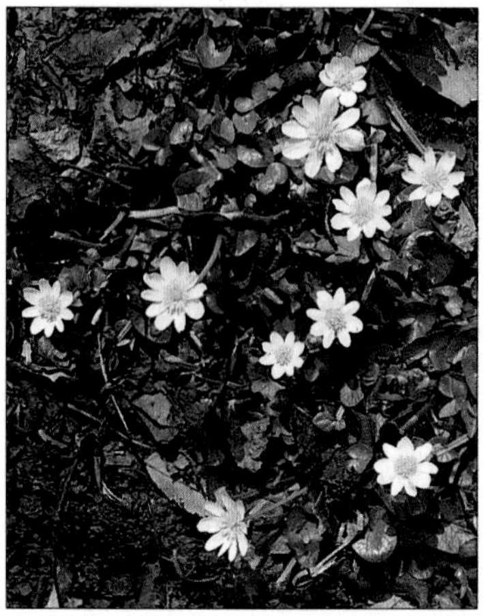

Ranunculus ficaria f. *albus*

R. crenatus. Rosette-forming, semi-evergreen perennial with fibrous roots and rounded, glossy, mid-green leaves, 5–15mm (¼–½in) long, toothed or shallowly 3-lobed at the tips. In summer, flowering stems bear solitary, or occasionally pairs of shallowly cup-shaped white flowers, 2.5cm (1in) across. Cultivation group 3. ↕↔ to 8cm (3in). E. Alps, C. Apennines, mountains of Balkan peninsula, S. and E. Carpathians. ✽✽✽
R. ficaria (Lesser celandine, Pilewort). Very variable, tuberous perennial with long-stalked, broadly heart-shaped, glossy, usually dark green, basal leaves, 2–5cm (¾–2in) long, often with silver or bronze markings and scalloped or toothed margins. In early spring, bears usually solitary, shallowly cup-shaped, brilliant, shining, golden yellow flowers, 2–3cm (¾–1¼in) across, fading to white with age. The leaves die down after flowering. Some variants produce axillary bulbils and are extremely invasive. Cultivation group 1. ↕ 5cm (2in), ↔ to 30cm (12in) or more. Europe, N.W. Africa, S.W. Asia. ✽✽✽. **f. *albus*** ■ has very pale yellow flowers, fading to white, and leaves marked dark bronze. **f. *aurantiacus*** ■ syn. 'Cupreus', has silvery leaves, each with a bronze central mark, and deep coppery orange flowers, darker on the reverse. **'Brazen Hussy'** produces glossy, deep chocolate-brown leaves, and shining, golden yellow flowers with a bronze reverse. Seedlings often have bronze leaves. **'Collarette'** produces leaves with bronze central bands, and double yellow flowers with anemone-form centres. **'Cupreus'** see f. *aurantiacus*. **'Double Bronze'** bears double yellow flowers with a bronze reverse to the petals. **'Double Cream'** see 'Double Mud'. **'Double Mud'**, syn. 'Double Cream', has double cream flowers, with a grey-tinted reverse to the petals. **'Salmon's White'** bears pale green leaves with bronze marks, and cream flowers, tinted blue-purple on the reverse of the petals.

R

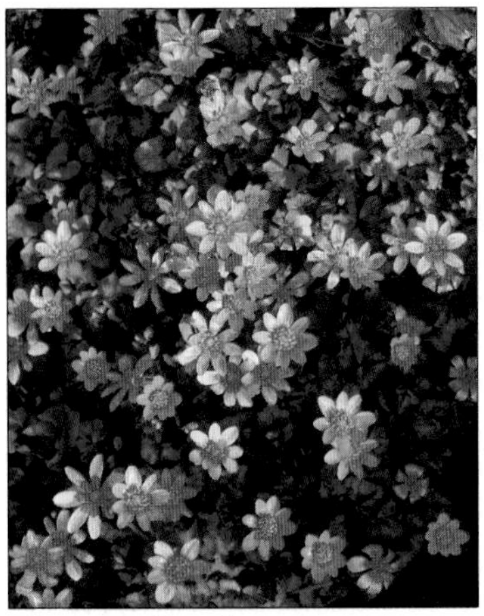

Ranunculus ficaria f. *aurantiacus*

R. flammula (Lesser spearwort). Marginal aquatic perennial with semi-erect, red-tinted green stems bearing broadly ovate to linear-lance-shaped, dark green leaves, 1–2.5cm (½–1in) long. Shallowly cup-shaped, bright yellow flowers, 2cm (¾in) across, are borne in few-flowered, cyme-like panicles, or sometimes singly, in early summer. Cultivation group 4. ↕70cm (28in), ↔ 75cm (30in). Europe, Asia. ❄❄❄
R. glacialis. Hummock-forming perennial with fibrous roots and very broadly ovate, deeply 3-lobed, slightly fleshy, hairless, dark green leaves, 3–8cm (1¼–3in) long. In late spring and early summer, flowering stems bear solitary, occasionally 2 or 3, shallowly cup-shaped, white or pink flowers, 2–3cm (¾–1¼in) across, flushed deep pink after fertilization. Protect from excessive winter wet. Cultivation group 3. ↕5–25cm (2–10in), ↔ 5cm (2in). Spain (Sierra Nevada), Pyrenees, Alps, Greenland. ❄❄❄
***R. gouanii* 'Plenus'** see *R. constantinopolitanus* 'Plenus'.
R. gramineus ■♀ Clump-forming perennial, very variable in size and habit, with basal clusters of grass-like, linear to lance-shaped, very finely hairy, glaucous leaves, to 20cm (8in) long. In late spring and early summer, branched flowering stems bear 1–3 cup-shaped, lemon-yellow flowers, to 2cm (¾in) across. Cultivation group 2. ↕ to 30cm (12in), ↔ to 15cm (6in). S.W. Europe. ❄❄❄
R. insignis. Semi-evergreen, clump-forming perennial, similar to *R. lyallii*,

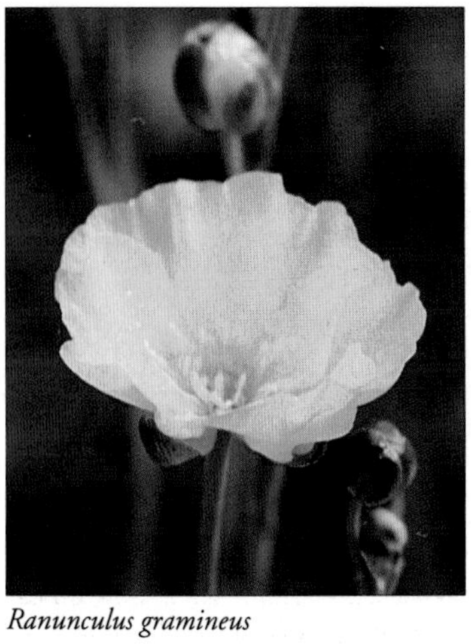

Ranunculus gramineus

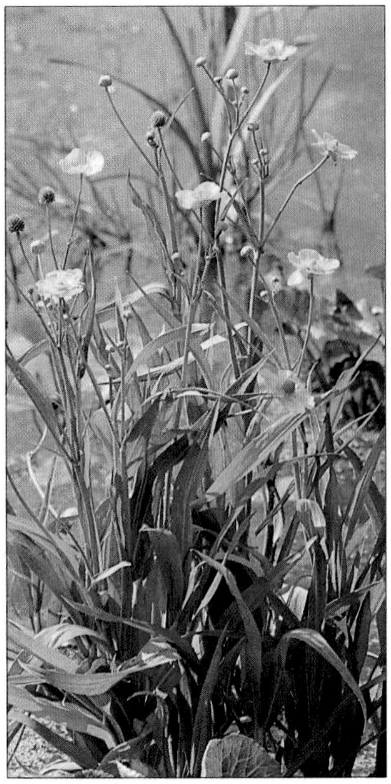

Ranunculus lingua

with ovate-lance-shaped, leathery, dark green, basal leaves, to 15cm (6in) long, brown-hairy beneath. In summer, bears panicles of 5–20 shallowly cup-shaped, deep yellow flowers, 2–5cm (¾–2in) across. Cultivation group 1 or 2. ↕ to 60cm (24in), ↔ to 30cm (12in). New Zealand. ❄❄❄
R. lingua ■ (Greater spearwort). Marginal aquatic perennial with erect, hollow stems. Non-flowering stems bear long-stalked, ovate to ovate-oblong, blue-green leaves, to 20cm (8in) long, with heart-shaped bases. In early summer, branched flowering stems, with short-stalked, linear to lance-shaped leaves, bear cup-shaped, golden yellow flowers, 5cm (2in) across, singly or in few-flowered, cyme-like panicles. Cultivation group 4. ↕1.5m (5ft), ↔ 2m (6ft). Europe to Siberia. ❄❄❄
R. lyallii (Giant buttercup, Mount Cook lily). Semi-evergreen, clump-forming, rhizomatous perennial with peltate, rounded, scalloped, leathery, dark green, basal leaves, to 30cm (12in) long, becoming progressively smaller up the branching stems. Cyme-like panicles of 5–15 cup-shaped white flowers, 5cm (2in) across, are borne in summer.

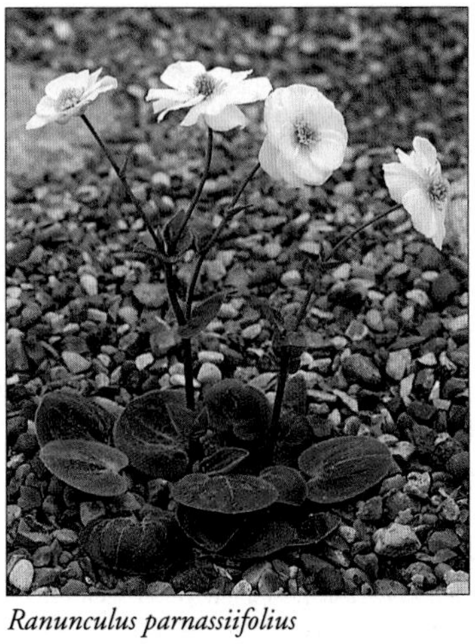

Ranunculus parnassiifolius

Requires cool conditions. Cultivation group 1 or 2. ↕ to 1m (3ft), ↔ to 35cm (14in). Rocky areas in New Zealand. ❄❄❄ (borderline)
***R. montanus* 'Molten Gold'** ♀ Vigorous, mat-forming, rhizomatous perennial producing rounded-obovate, 3- to 5-lobed, glossy, deep green basal leaves, to 4cm (1½in) long, and narrower stem leaves. In early summer, short flowering stems each bear 1–3 shallowly cup-shaped, shining, bright gold-yellow flowers, 2–3cm (¾–1¼in) across. Cultivation group 2. ↕10cm (4in), ↔ 30cm (12in). ❄❄❄
R. parnassiifolius ■ Rosette-forming perennial with fibrous roots and broadly lance-shaped to ovate-heart-shaped, hairy, dark green, basal leaves, to 5cm (2in) long. In early summer, stems bear solitary, occasionally 2 or 3, cup-shaped flowers, 2.5cm (1in) across, opening white but often turning pink with age, usually finely pink- or red-veined. Cultivation group 3. ↕15cm (6in), ↔ 10cm (4in). High screes in the Alps, Pyrenees, N. Spain. ❄❄❄
***R. repens* 'Pleniflorus'**, syn. *R. repens* var. *pleniflorus* (Double creeping buttercup). Erect, fast-spreading, hairy, stoloniferous perennial. Long-stalked, triangular-ovate, mid-green basal and lower stem leaves, 9cm (3½in) long, each have 3 lobes, further cut into 3 toothed segments, the middle lobe long-stalked. Branched stems bear cyme-like panicles of double, glossy, bright yellow flowers, 1.5–2cm (½–¾in) across, with tightly packed petals and pale yellow sepals, from late spring to midsummer. Cultivation group 1 or 2. ↕30–60cm (12–24in), ↔ 2m (6ft). ❄❄❄
R. repens* var. *pleniflorus see *R. repens* 'Pleniflorus'.
***R. speciosus* 'Flore Pleno'** see *R. constantinopolitanus* 'Plenus'.

RANZANIA

BERBERIDACEAE

Genus of one species of herbaceous perennial found in deciduous mountain woodland in S. Japan. It has short rhizomes, and is grown for its attractive foliage and flowers. Smooth stems, with opposite, 3-palmate leaves at their tips, bear pendent, bell-shaped flowers, either singly or in few-flowered cymes, before the leaves have fully developed; the long flower-stalks become upright as berries form. Grow in a woodland garden or shady border.
• **HARDINESS** Hardy to -10°C (14°F), but late frosts may damage new growth.
• **CULTIVATION** Grow in moist, leafy, humus-rich soil in partial or deep shade.
• **PROPAGATION** Sow seed in containers in a cold frame in autumn; seedlings will flower in about 4 years. Divide in early spring.
• **PESTS AND DISEASES** Susceptible to slug damage in spring.

R. japonica, syn. *Podophyllum japonicum.* Rhizomatous perennial with smooth stems, each bearing 2 or 3 opposite, broadly triangular leaves, to 8cm (3in) long, composed of 3 broadly ovate to heart-shaped leaflets, mid-green above, bluish green beneath. In mid- and late spring, long flower-stalks bear pendent, bowl-shaped, pale mauve-blue flowers, 2.5–3cm (1–1¼in) across, each with 6 large, pointed tepals and 6 small petals that recurve with age. The flowers are followed by elliptic white berries, to 1.5cm (½in) long. ↕ to 30cm (12in), ↔ 20cm (8in). S. Japan (N. Hondo). ❄❄

RAOULIA

ASTERACEAE/COMPOSITAE

Genus of about 20 species of evergreen perennials or subshrubs from screes and open rocky places at high and low altitudes in New Zealand. They form mats or cushions of dense, overlapping, linear to diamond- or spoon-shaped, silvery leaves. The usually small, disc-shaped flowerheads are borne singly or in few-flowered, terminal clusters. They thrive in regions with cool summers and mild winters, and are excellent foliage plants for a rock garden, raised bed or scree bed, or for an alpine house.
• **HARDINESS** Hardy to about -10°C (14°F) in well-drained soil.
• **CULTIVATION** Under glass, grow in a mix of equal parts loam, leaf mould, and sharp sand, with a top dressing of grit, in bright filtered light. When in growth, water freely (avoiding the foliage); keep just moist in winter. Outdoors, grow in gritty, humus-rich, moist but sharply drained soil in full sun, or in partial shade in warm, dry areas. Protect from excessive winter wet.
• **PROPAGATION** Divide or separate rooted stems of mat-forming species in spring. Root new rosettes of cushion-forming species as cuttings in early summer in partial shade; water carefully and moderately until rooted.
• **PESTS AND DISEASES** Prone to red spider mites and aphids under glass.

R. australis ■ syn. *R. lutescens.* Prostrate, mat-forming, grey-silver perennial with branching, rooting stems, densely clothed in overlapping, spoon-shaped, silver-hairy leaves, 2mm ($\frac{1}{16}$in) long. In summer, bears sulphur-yellow flowerheads, 5mm (¼in) across. Plants sold under this name are often variants of *R. hookeri.* ↕1cm (½in), ↔ 30cm (12in) or more. New Zealand. ❄❄
R. eximia (Vegetable sheep). Extremely dense, cushion-forming perennial with tightly packed rosettes of overlapping, oblong to ovate, grey-hairy leaves, to 2mm ($\frac{1}{16}$in) long. Yellowish white flowerheads, to 3mm (⅛in) across, are borne in late spring or summer. Resents winter wet; best grown in an alpine

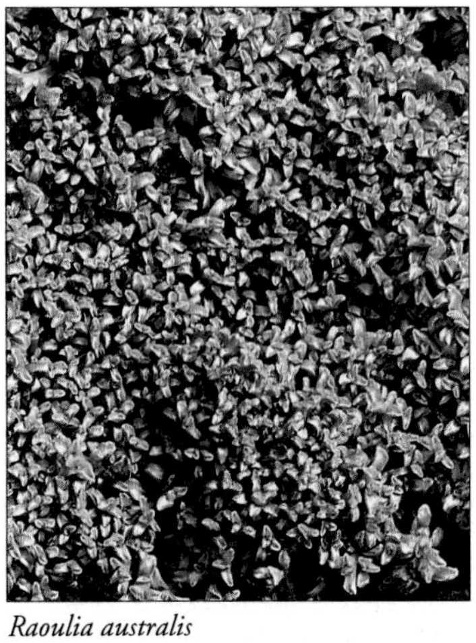

Raoulia australis

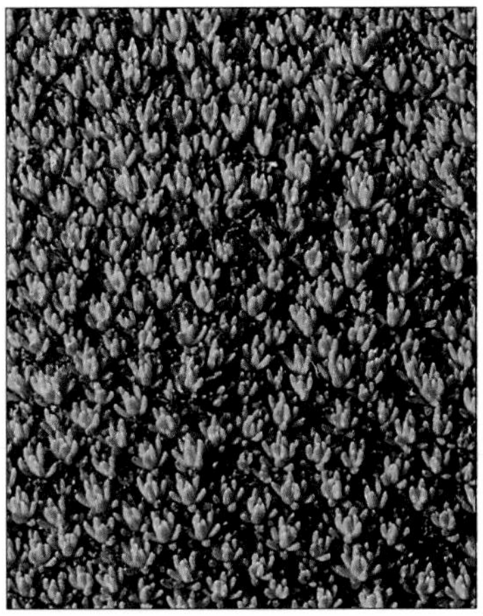

Raoulia haastii

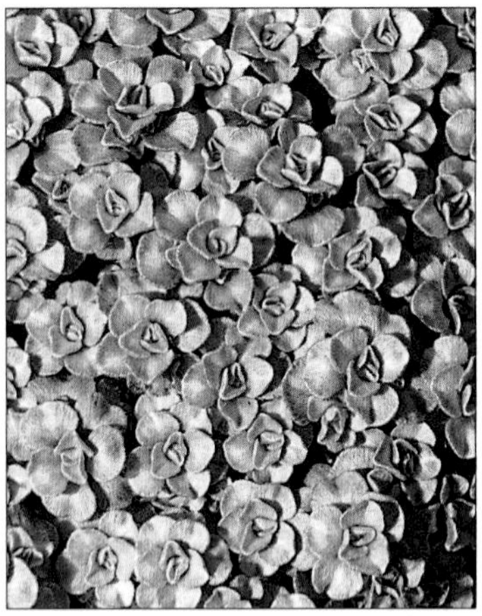

Raoulia hookeri var. *alboserícea*

house. ↕5cm (2in), ↔ to 10cm (4in). New Zealand. ✻✻

R. haastii ▣ Dense, cushion-forming perennial with loosely overlapping, ovate to linear-oblong, silky-hairy leaves, to 5mm (¼in) long; pale green at first, they darken in summer, becoming brown-tinted in winter. In spring, bears yellow flowerheads, to 5mm (¼in) across. ↕1cm (½in), ↔ 30cm (12in) or more. New Zealand. ✻✻

R. hookeri* var. *alboserícea ▣ Mat-forming perennial producing branching, rooting stems clothed in closely overlapping, narrowly obovate-spoon-shaped leaves, 2mm (1⁄16in) long, covered with white-silky hairs. Silky-hairy, pale green or straw-coloured flowerheads, to 7mm (¼in) across, are borne briefly in summer. Similar to, but less tolerant of winter wet than *R. australis.* ↕1cm (½in), ↔ to 20cm (8in). New Zealand (North Island). ✻✻

R. leontopodium see *Leucogenes leontopodium.*

R.* x *loganii see x *Leucoraoulia loganii.*

R. lutescens see *R. australis.*

RAPHIA

Raffia

ARECACEAE/PALMAE

Genus of about 30 species of massive, single- or cluster-stemmed, spreading, monocarpic palms, mainly found in moist, wet, or swampy sites and by streams in Central and South America, Africa, and Madagascar. Some species have short, underground stems (caudices) and appear to be stemless. The pinnate, light to mid-green leaves, with folded linear leaflets, are produced in terminal heads or tufts. Panicles of bowl-shaped, 3-petalled flowers are borne either between the leaves or just beneath the lowest leaf. In frost-prone areas, grow young specimens as house-plants or in a warm greenhouse or conservatory. In tropical areas, use the stemless species in a border, and those with stems as specimens on a lawn.

• **HARDINESS** Frost tender.

• **CULTIVATION** Under glass, grow in loamless potting compost in bright filtered light. In the growing season, water freely and apply a balanced liquid fertilizer monthly; water moderately in winter. Pot on or top-dress in spring. Outdoors, grow in moist, moderately fertile, humus-rich soil in partial shade.

• **PROPAGATION** Sow seed at 27°C (81°F) in spring.

• **PESTS AND DISEASES** Red spider mites may be a problem under glass.

R. farinifera 🌴 Large, spreading palm with a sturdy trunk covered in old leaf bases. Erect to arching leaves, to 20m (70ft) long, each have numerous linear leaflets to 2m (6ft) long; they are waxy, light to mid-green above, and waxy, powdery white beneath. Green flowers, 8–15mm (⅜–½in) across, are borne in panicles to 3m (10ft) long, in summer, followed by ovoid to ellipsoid, scaly orange fruit, 7–10cm (3–4in) long. ↕ to 25m (80ft), ↔ to 20m (70ft) or more. Tropical Africa, Madagascar. ❀ (min. 16°C/61°F)

▷ ***Raphidophora*** see *Rhaphidophora*
▷ **Raripila, Red** see *Mentha* x *smithiana*
▷ **Raspberry, Flowering** see *Rubus odoratus*
▷ **Rasp fern, Common** see *Doodia media*
▷ **Rata** see *Metrosideros, M. robustus*
Northern see *M. robustus*

RATIBIDA

Mexican hat, Prairie cone flower

ASTERACEAE/COMPOSITAE

Genus of 5 or 6 species of biennials and perennials, mainly found on prairies in North America and Mexico. Woody-based crowns produce erect stems, branching above the middle, that bear alternate, pinnate to pinnatifid leaves and solitary, terminal flowerheads. They are cultivated for their daisy-like flowerheads, which have a few long, yellow or yellow-brown ray-florets and prominent, spherical or cone-shaped centres of brown disc-florets. Grow in a sunny border, gravel garden, or wild-flower meadow. The flowerheads are good for cutting.

• **HARDINESS** Fully hardy.

• **CULTIVATION** Grow in dry, well-drained, neutral to slightly alkaline, moderately fertile soil in full sun. Ratibidas are drought-resistant.

• **PROPAGATION** Sow seed in containers in a cold frame in early spring. Divide perennials in spring when young (the roots become woody with age).

• **PESTS AND DISEASES** Trouble free.

R. columnifera ▣ syn. *Lepachys columnifera, Rudbeckia columnifera.* Erect perennial, sometimes grown as a biennial or annual, with pinnate, hairy, greyish green leaves, 3–15cm (1¼–6in) long; the leaflets are usually linear, entire, and often pinnatifid. From early summer to early autumn, long, thin, branching stems bear daisy-like flower-heads, to 8cm (3in) across, with reflexed yellow ray-florets and large, columnar centres of green, then brown disc-florets. ↕ to 80cm (32in), ↔ 30cm (12in). S.W. Canada, W. and C. USA to New Mexico. ✻✻✻. **f. *pulcherrima*** bears flowerheads with purple-brown or reddish brown ray-florets; ↕30cm (12in), ↔ 20cm (8in).

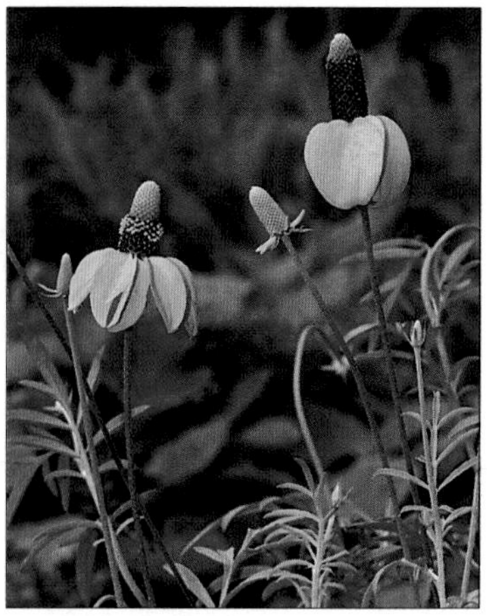

Ratibida columnifera

R. pinnata, syn. *Lepachys pinnata* (Drooping coneflower, Grey-head coneflower). Upright, stout-stemmed, branching perennial, sometimes grown as a biennial or annual. Pinnate, toothed, bluish green leaves, 2–12cm (¾–5in) long, with lance-shaped, sparsely hairy leaflets, are borne mainly on the lower, unbranched portion of the stems. From summer to autumn, bears long-stemmed, daisy-like flowerheads, to 12cm (5in) across, with bright yellow ray-florets and red-brown disc-florets forming prominent, oval, cone-shaped centres. ↕ to 1.2m (4ft), ↔ to 45cm (18in). C. North America. ✻✻✻

▷ **Rattan cane** see *Calamus rotang*
▷ **Rattan vine** see *Berchemia scandens*
▷ **Rattlebox** see *Crotalaria*
▷ **Rattlesnake plant** see *Calathea lancifolia*
▷ **Rauli** see *Nothofagus procera*

RAVENALA

Traveller's tree

STRELITZIACEAE

Genus of one species of small, evergreen tree, occurring in open rainforest or deforested areas in Madagascar, grown for its foliage, spathes, and palm-like habit. The large, alternate, long-stalked, banana-like leaves have expanded leaf bases that accumulate water. Boat-shaped spathes, enclosing cymes of tiny, 3-petalled flowers, are produced from the leaf axils. Where temperatures fall below 16–18°C (61–64°F), grow in a warm greenhouse. In tropical regions, use as a distinctive specimen tree.

• **HARDINESS** Frost tender.

• **CULTIVATION** Under glass, grow in loam-based potting compost (JI No.3) in full light, with high humidity. Water freely in spring and summer, applying a balanced liquid fertilizer monthly; water more sparingly in winter. Outdoors, grow in fertile, moist, but well-drained soil in full sun. Provide shelter from strong winds.

• **PROPAGATION** Sow seed at 20–21°C (68–70°F), or remove rooted suckers, in spring.

• **PESTS AND DISEASES** Red spider mites may be a problem under glass.

R. madagascariensis 🌴 Large, erect tree with an unbranched, palm-like trunk topped by a fan-shaped crown of 2-ranked, paddle-shaped, leathery, lustrous, rich green leaves. The oblong leaf-blades, 2–4m (6–12ft) long, are borne on thick, grooved stalks, of about the same length, closely overlapping at the bases. On mature plants, tiny, narrow white flowers, each with 6 tepals, emerge from pointed, boat-shaped, greenish white spathes, a few at a time, in summer; they are followed by fruit capsules that contain seeds with bright blue arils. ↕10–16m (30–52ft), ↔ 3–6m (10–20ft). Madagascar. ❀ (min. 16–18°C/61–64°F)

REBUTIA

syn. SULCOREBUTIA, WEINGARTIA

CACTACEAE

Genus of about 40 species of mostly dwarf, clump-forming, simple or clustering, perennial cacti found in mountainous terrain, to 4,000m (13,000ft) high, in Bolivia and N. and N.W. Argentina. They are cultivated for their habit and colourful flowers. The spherical to short-cylindrical, ribbed stems are divided into low tubercles in some species. The areoles have mainly short, bristly spines and, in summer, those near the stem bases bear many trumpet-shaped, diurnal flowers. In frost-prone regions, grow in a temperate greenhouse or as houseplants. In warm, dry areas, use in a desert garden or a raised bed.

• **HARDINESS** Frost tender.

• **CULTIVATION** Under glass, grow in standard cactus compost in full light, with low humidity. From spring to summer, water moderately and apply a balanced liquid fertilizer 3 or 4 times; keep completely dry at other times. Outdoors, grow in moderately fertile, gritty, sharply drained soil in full sun. See also pp.48–49.

• **PROPAGATION** Sow seed at 21°C (70°F) in early spring, or remove offsets in spring or summer.

• **PESTS AND DISEASES** Prone to mealy-bugs early in the growing season.

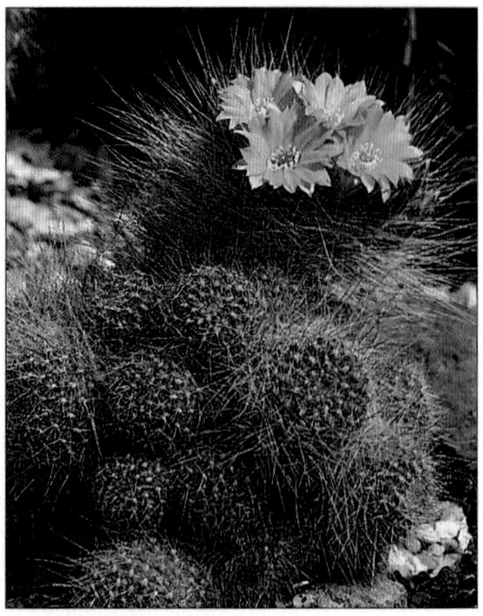

Rebutia aureiflora

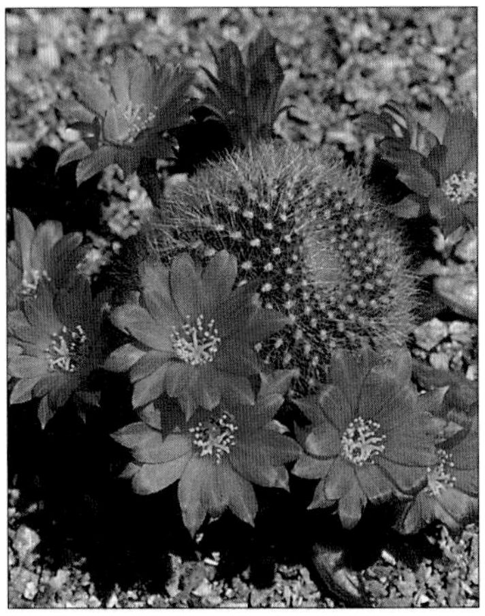
Rebutia fiebrigii

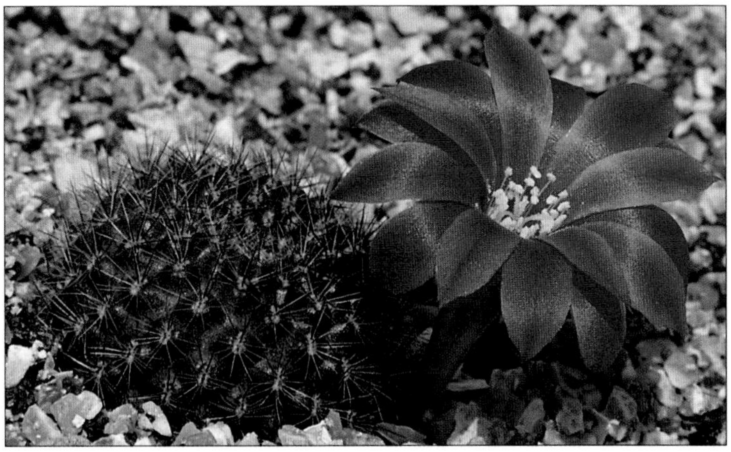
Rebutia minuscula

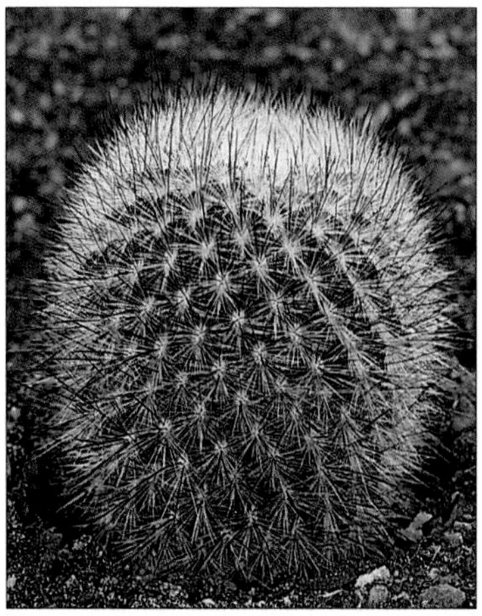
Rebutia tiraquensis

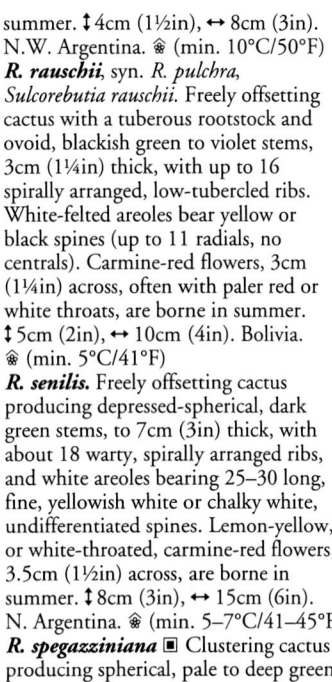

R. aureiflora ■ 🏆 Freely clustering cactus with depressed-spherical to spherical, mid-green to greenish violet, often red-tinged stems, to 3.5cm (1½in) thick. The stems are covered with prominent, spirally arranged tubercles set with white areoles and greyish white spines (10–16 radials and 1–4 longer centrals). White-throated, yellow or yellowish orange, sometimes orange, red, or purple flowers, 4cm (1½in) across, are borne in summer. ↕ 10cm (4in), ↔ to 20cm (8in). N.W. Argentina. ❄ (min. 5°C/41°F)
R. fiebrigii ■ syn. *R. muscula.* Variable, clustering cactus with spherical to ovoid or depressed-spherical, dark green stems, 6cm (2½in) thick, with up to 18 ribs. White areoles bear 30–40 white radial spines and 2–5 longer, brownish white centrals. Bright yellowish brown or bright orange to red flowers, 2–3.5cm (¾–1½in) across, are borne in summer. ↕ 10cm (4in), ↔ to 15cm (6in). Bolivia, N.W. Argentina. ❄ (min. 5°C/41°F)
R. heliosa. Initially simple, later clustering cactus producing depressed-spherical to cone-shaped, greyish green stems, to 2.5cm (1in) thick, with 15–40 low-tubercled, spirally arranged ribs. Brown-felted areoles have 24–26 tiny, comb-like, undifferentiated white spines. In summer, bears orange or deep rose-red flowers, 4cm (1½in) across; the inner petals often have a central lilac stripe. ↕ 10cm (4in), ↔ 15cm (6in). Bolivia. ❄ (min. 5°C/41°F)
R. krainziana ■ Clustering cactus with depressed-spherical, warty, bright to dull green stems, 4cm (1½in) thick. The stems have 20 or more, spirally arranged ribs, and close-set white areoles with 8–12 tiny, undifferentiated white spines. Bright red flowers, to 5cm (2in) across, sometimes with a violet sheen and violet throats, are borne in summer. ↕ 5cm (2in), ↔ 20cm (8in). Probably of garden origin. ❄ (min. 5°C/41°F)
R. minuscula ■ syn. *R. violaciflora.* Freely clustering cactus with slightly flattened, spherical, dull mid- to dark green stems, 5cm (2in) thick, with 16–20 warty, spirally arranged ribs, and brown areoles bearing 25–30 undifferentiated white spines. Bright pinkish purple flowers, 3–4cm (1¼–1½in) across, are produced in summer. ↕ 5cm (2in), ↔ 12cm (5in). N. Argentina. ❄ (min. 5°C/41°F)
R. muscula see *R. fiebrigii.*
R. neocumingii ■ syn. *Weingartia neocumingii.* Simple cactus, of variable form and shape, with hemispherical to spherical, bright dark green stems, 10cm (4in) thick. The stems have 16–18 warty ribs, white areoles, and brown-tipped yellow spines (16–20 radials and 3–10 thicker centrals). Orange or yellow flowers, 2cm (¾in) or more across, are borne in summer. ↕ 20cm (8in), ↔ 10cm (4in). Bolivia. ❄ (min. 5°C/41°F)
R. pulchra see *R. rauschii.*
R. pygmaea. Simple or clustering cactus producing ovoid to short-cylindrical, mid- to dark green stems, 1–2cm (½–¾in) thick, with tubercles arranged in 8–12 spiral rows and white spines, 2–3mm (1/16–⅛in) long (9–11 radials, no centrals). Solitary, pink-purple flowers, 2–2.5cm (¾–1in) across, are borne on the lower parts of the stems in summer. ↕ 4cm (1½in), ↔ 8cm (3in). N.W. Argentina. ❄ (min. 10°C/50°F)
R. rauschii, syn. *R. pulchra, Sulcorebutia rauschii.* Freely offsetting cactus with a tuberous rootstock and ovoid, blackish green to violet stems, 3cm (1¼in) thick, with up to 16 spirally arranged, low-tubercled ribs. White-felted areoles bear yellow or black spines (up to 11 radials, no centrals). Carmine-red flowers, 3cm (1¼in) across, often with paler red or white throats, are borne in summer. ↕ 5cm (2in), ↔ 10cm (4in). Bolivia. ❄ (min. 5°C/41°F)
R. senilis. Freely offsetting cactus producing depressed-spherical, dark green stems, to 7cm (3in) thick, with about 18 warty, spirally arranged ribs, and white areoles bearing 25–30 long, fine, yellowish white or chalky white, undifferentiated spines. Lemon-yellow, or white-throated, carmine-red flowers, 3.5cm (1½in) across, are borne in summer. ↕ 8cm (3in), ↔ 15cm (6in). N. Argentina. ❄ (min. 5–7°C/41–45°F)
R. spegazziniana ■ Clustering cactus producing spherical, pale to deep green stems, 5cm (2in) thick, with about 18 prominently warty ribs, white-felted areoles, and white spines (14 radials and 3–6 shorter centrals). Pale vermilion to dark red flowers, 2.5–3cm (1–1¼in) across, are borne in summer. ↕ to 10cm (4in), ↔ to 20cm (8in). N.W. Argentina. ❄ (min. 5–7°C/41–45°F)
R. spinosissima. Freely offsetting cactus producing spherical, bright green stems, 5–6cm (2–2½in) thick, with 15 or more warty, spirally arranged ribs, white-hairy areoles, and white spines (numerous radials and 5 or 6 thicker, brown-tipped centrals). Pale orange to mid-red flowers, 3–4cm (1¼–1½in) across, are borne in summer. ↕ to 10cm (4in), ↔ 15cm (6in). N. Argentina. ❄ (min. 5–7°C/41–45°F)
R. tiraquensis ■ Upright cactus with mid-green stems, simple at first, but eventually clump-forming, covered in spirally arranged tubercles. Elongated areoles, to 7mm (¼in) long, bear 2–4 reddish brown central spines, 6–7cm (2½–3in) long, and 14–18 glassy white radials. Solitary, funnel-shaped, purple or magenta flowers, 3.5cm (1½in) across, are borne in summer. ↕ 9–10cm (3½–4in), ↔ 10cm (4in). Bolivia. ❄ (min. 7–10°C/45–50°F)
R. violaciflora see *R. minuscula.*

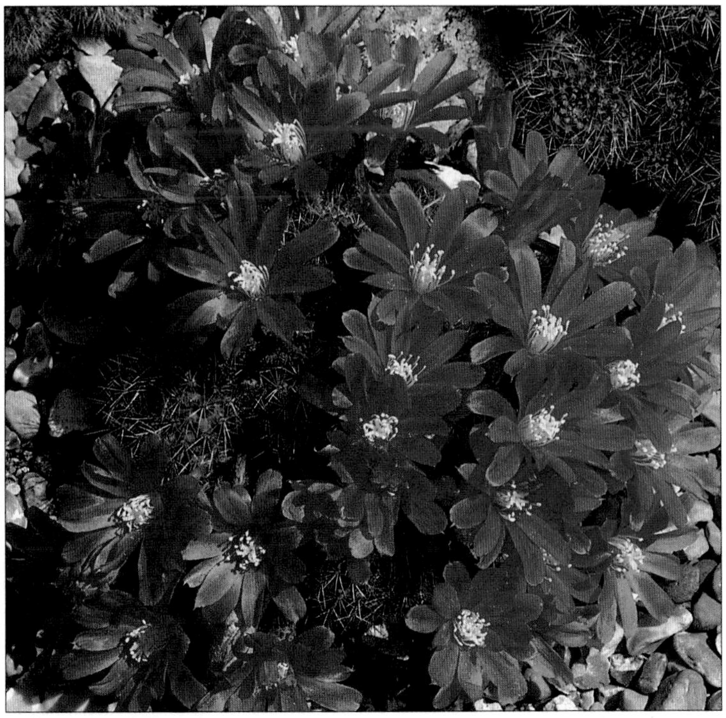
Rebutia spegazziniana

R

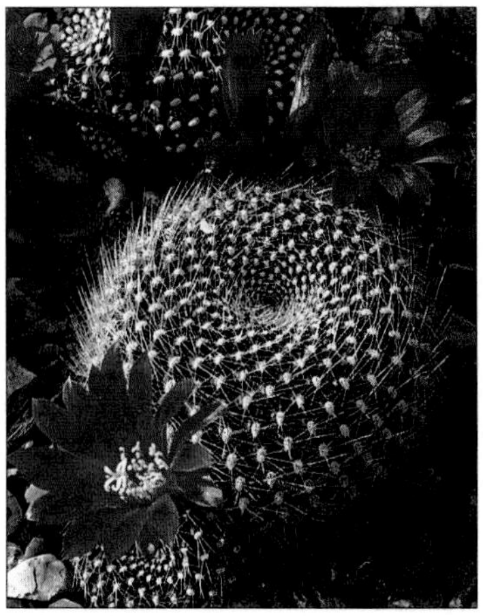
Rebutia krainziana

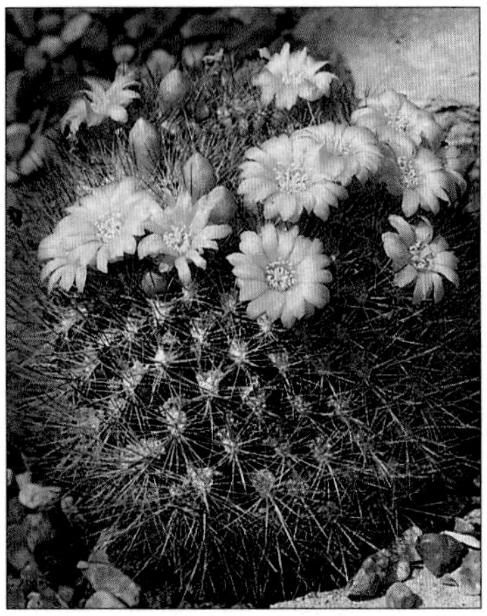
Rebutia neocumingii

▷ ***Rechsteineria leucotricha*** see *Sinningia canescens*
▷ **Redbud,**
California see *Cercis occidentalis*
Chinese see *Cercis chinensis*
Eastern see *Cercis canadensis*
Western see *Cercis occidentalis*
▷ **Red cloak, Brazilian** see *Megaskepasma erythrochlamys*
▷ **Red cole** see *Armoracia rusticana*
▷ **Red hot poker** see *Kniphofia*
▷ **Red ink plant** see *Phytolacca americana*
▷ **Red pine** see *Pinus resinosa*
Chinese see *P. tabuliformis*
Japanese see *P. densiflora*
▷ **Red tree** see *Peperomia metallica*
▷ **Redwood,**
Coastal see *Sequoia sempervirens*
Dawn see *Metasequoia glyptostroboides*
Giant see *Sequoiadendron giganteum*
Sierra see *Sequoiadendron giganteum*
▷ **Reed** see *Phragmites*
Burr see *Sparganium*
Common see *Phragmites australis*
Giant see *Arundo donax*
Norfolk see *Phragmites australis*
▷ **Reedmace** see *Typha*
Narrow-leaved see *T. angustifolia*

REHDERODENDRON

STYRACACEAE

Genus of 9 species of deciduous shrubs and trees from mountain woodland in China and Vietnam. They are valued for their cup-shaped, 5-petalled white flowers, borne in leafless, axillary, cyme-like panicles or racemes, and their oblong or elliptic, ribbed, woody fruits. The leaves are alternate and finely toothed. *R. macrocarpum*, the only species usually cultivated, is ideal for a woodland garden.

• **HARDINESS** Hardy to -10°C (14°F).
• **CULTIVATION** Grow in fertile, moist but well-drained, neutral to acid soil in sun or partial shade, sheltered from cold, dry winds. Pruning group 1.
• **PROPAGATION** Sow seed in containers in a cold frame as soon as ripe. Root semi-ripe cuttings in summer.
• **PESTS AND DISEASES** Trouble free.

R. macrocarpum ♀ Small, broadly upright, deciduous tree with red young shoots and elliptic to oblong, glossy, dark green leaves, to 15cm (6in) long. As the leaves emerge in late spring, bears cyme-like racemes of 6–10 cup-shaped, fragrant, creamy white flowers, 6cm (2½in) across. Flowers are followed by pendent, ellipsoid, green, then red fruit, to 7cm (3in) long. ↕ 10m (30ft), ↔ 7m (22ft). W. China. ✲✲

REHMANNIA

SCROPHULARIACEAE

Genus of 8 or 9 species of perennials, sometimes grown as biennials, from woodland and stony sites in China. They are cultivated for their large, foxglove-like flowers, which are 2-lipped and borne in terminal racemes. The leaves, arranged in basal rosettes, are large, obovate to oblong, shallowly lobed or toothed, conspicuously veined, and hairy. Grow at the front of a sunny border; in regions with mild, damp winters grow permanently, or over-winter, in a cool greenhouse.

• **HARDINESS** Fully hardy to frost hardy.
• **CULTIVATION** Under glass, grow in loam-based potting compost (JI No.2) in bright filtered light. When in growth, water freely and apply a balanced liquid fertilizer monthly; keep just moist in winter. Outdoors, grow in well-drained, moderately fertile, humus-rich soil in a sheltered site in full sun. In regions where winters are mild and damp, lift in autumn, pot up, and overwinter in a cool, dry place, at 7°C (45°F).
• **PROPAGATION** Sow seed at 13–16°C (55–61°F) in late winter; seedlings will flower in 12–14 months. Take root cuttings in late autumn, or softwood cuttings from basal shoots before flowering. Separate and pot up runners in spring.
• **PESTS AND DISEASES** Susceptible to slug and snail damage.

***R. angulata* of gardens** see *R. elata.*
R. elata ■ syn. *R. angulata* of gardens (Chinese foxglove). Rosette-forming perennial with obovate, lobed or toothed, conspicuously veined, hairy, mid-green, basal leaves, 20–25cm (8–10in) long. Branched stems bear leafy racemes of semi-pendent, tubular flowers, 7–10cm (3–4in) long, from summer to autumn. The flowers have bright, pinkish purple lips and paler tubes; they are red-spotted, especially in the throats. ↕ to 1.5m (5ft), ↔ 50cm (20in). China. ✲✲✲
R. glutinosa ♀ Sticky, purple-hairy perennial with slender runners and rosettes of obovate, scalloped, conspicuously veined, basal leaves, to 10cm (4in) long, mid-green above and often red-tinted beneath. From mid-spring to summer, branched, leafy stems bear pendent, tubular flowers, to 5cm (2in) long, in few-flowered, cyme-like racemes, or singly on long flower-stalks, from the leaf axils. The flowers have reddish brown tubes, marked with darker reddish purple veins, and pale yellow-brown lips. ↕ 15–30cm (6–12in), ↔ to 30cm (12in). N. China. ✲✲✲

REINECKEA

CONVALLARIACEAE/LILIACEAE

Genus of one species of rhizomatous, evergreen perennial from deciduous woodland or sandy open areas among shrubs in China and Japan. It is grown for its arching, pale green leaves and spikes of tiny, fragrant pink flowers. *R. carnea* provides attractive, leafy ground cover, but rarely flowers freely or bears its spherical red berries in areas with cool summers.

• **HARDINESS** Fully hardy.
• **CULTIVATION** Grow in moist but well-drained, humus-rich, neutral or acid soil in partial shade.
• **PROPAGATION** Sow seed in containers in a cold frame as soon as ripe. Separate rhizomes from the margins of established clumps in spring.
• **PESTS AND DISEASES** Susceptible to damage from slugs and snails.

R. carnea. Evergreen, rhizomatous perennial with tufts of arching, linear-lance-shaped, glossy, mid- to dark green leaves, 15–35cm (6–14in) long, borne in 2 ranks at the ends of the rhizomes. In late spring, bears dense, terminal spikes of shallowly cup-shaped, pale to deep pink flowers, to 1cm (½in) across, each with 6 segments, the tips reflexing with age. In areas with warm summers, spherical red berries, 8–10mm (⅜–½in) across, are produced in autumn. ↕ 20cm (8in), ↔ 40cm (16in) or more. China, Japan. ✲✲✲

REINWARDTIA

LINACEAE

Genus of 1 or 2 species of evergreen shrubs or subshrubs, related to flaxes (*Linum*), found in mountain woodland from Pakistan to S.W. China and S.E. Asia. The alternate, elliptic- to oblong-obovate leaves may be entire or toothed. They are grown for their funnel-shaped flowers, each with 5 spreading petal

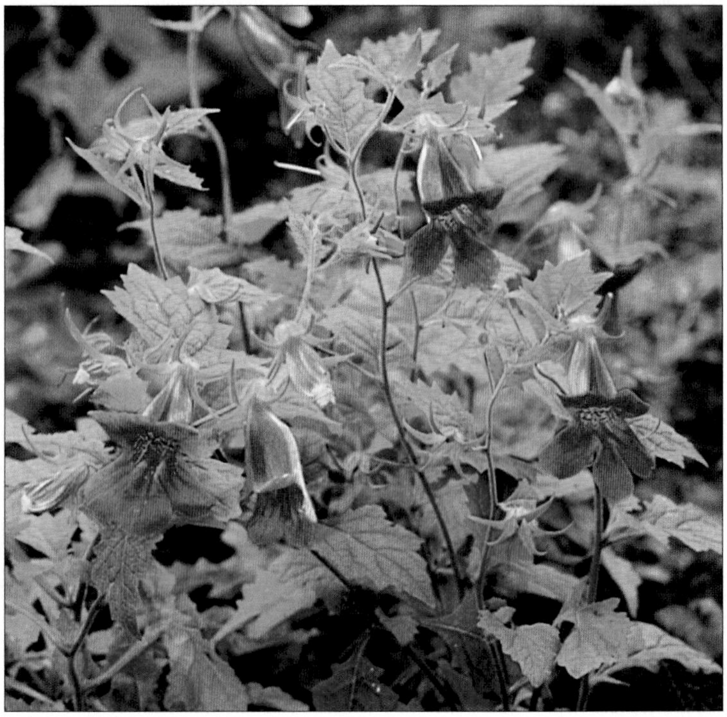

Rehmannia elata

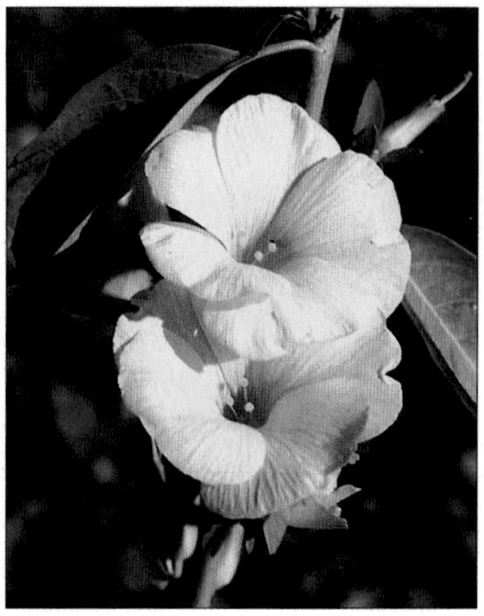

Reinwardtia indica

lobes, borne in terminal or axillary, cyme-like clusters, occasionally singly. Where temperatures fall below 7°C (45°F), grow in a temperate greenhouse. In milder regions, grow at the base of a sunny wall, or in a courtyard garden.

• **HARDINESS** Frost tender.
• **CULTIVATION** Under glass, grow in loamless or loam-based potting compost (JI No.3) in full light, with shade from hot sun and moderate humidity. In growth, mist regularly, water freely, and apply a balanced liquid fertilizer monthly; water moderately at other times. Winter flowers are borne most freely with a minimum temperature of 13°C (55°F). Outdoors, grow in fertile, moist but well-drained, humus-rich soil in full sun. Pruning group 8; tip-prune young plants to encourage branching.
• **PROPAGATION** Sow seed at 16–18°C (61–64°F) in spring. Root softwood cuttings in early summer.
• **PESTS AND DISEASES** Red spider mites may be a problem under glass.

R. indica ■ syn. *R. tetragyna, R. trigyna* (Yellow flax). Open, erect to spreading shrub with elliptic- to oblong-obovate, finely toothed, deep green to greyish green leaves, 3–8cm (1¼–3in) long. From autumn to late spring, produces funnel-shaped, bright golden yellow flowers, 3–5cm (1¼–2in) across, singly or in short, cyme-like clusters from the leaf axils. ↕↔ 60–90cm (24–36in). Pakistan, N. India, Burma, S.W. China, S.E. Asia. ❀ (min. 7°C/45°F)
R. tetragyna see *R. indica.*
R. trigyna see *R. indica.*

RESEDA

Mignonette

RESEDACEAE

Genus of 55–60 species of erect to spreading, branching, and occasionally rosette-forming annuals and perennials from stony hillsides, scrub, or field margins, mainly in the Mediterranean and S.W. Asia, but also in E. Africa and N.W. India. They have alternate, small, variably shaped, entire, toothed, or pinnatifid, prominently veined, mostly mid-green leaves. Star-shaped, greenish white or greenish yellow, sometimes red-tinged flowers, each with 4–10 narrow petals, are borne in long, unbranched or branching, spike-like racemes from spring to autumn. *R. odorata* has been grown for centuries, mainly for its fragrant flowers, which hold their scent

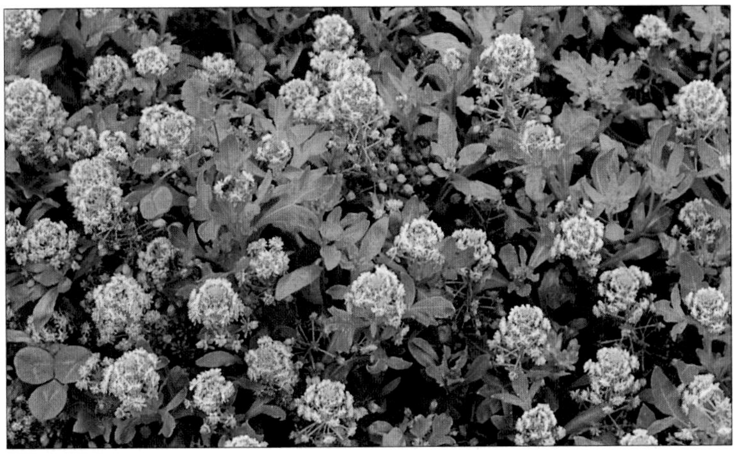

Reseda odorata

for months even when cut and dried; modern cultivars have larger, more strongly coloured flowers, which tend to be less fragrant. All are attractive to bees, and are ideal for a mixed or herbaceous border, or for a wildflower garden.

• **HARDINESS** Fully hardy.

• **CULTIVATION** Grow in well-drained, moderately fertile, preferably alkaline soil in full sun or partial shade. Deadhead to prolong flowering.

• **PROPAGATION** Sow seed at 13°C (55°F) in late winter, or *in situ* in early spring or autumn. Where temperatures fall below -5°C (23°F), provide cloche protection for autumn-sown seedlings.

• **PESTS AND DISEASES** Trouble free.

R. odorata ■ (Common mignonette). Erect to slightly spreading, hairless annual with branching, strongly ribbed stems and entire, elliptic to spoon-shaped, sometimes 3-lobed leaves, to 10cm (4in) long. From summer to early autumn, bears loose, conical, raceme-like heads of tiny, star-shaped, highly fragrant, yellowish green or white to reddish green flowers, to 7mm (¼in) across; each flower has 4–7 petals and a central tuft of orange stamens. ↕ 30–60cm (12–24in), ↔ to 23cm (9in). N. Africa. Widely naturalized. ❄❄❄

▷ **Restharrow** see *Ononis*
  Common see *O. repens*
  Shrubby see *O. fruticosa*

▷ **Resurrection plant** see *Selaginella lepidophylla*

RETAMA *syn.* LYGOS

LEGUMINOSAE/PAPILIONACEAE

Genus, related to *Genista*, of 4 species of deciduous shrubs found on sandy and rocky soils in the Canary Islands, the Mediterranean, and W. Asia. They have willowy, dark green stems with alternate, mid-green leaves that soon fall, and pea-like, yellow or white flowers borne in dense, axillary racemes. *R. monosperma*, the only species usually cultivated, has an elegant, arching habit and fragrant flowers. In frost-prone areas, grow in a cool greenhouse. In warmer areas, grow in a sheltered border or at the base of a warm, sunny wall.

• **HARDINESS** Half hardy.

• **CULTIVATION** Under glass, grow in loam-based potting compost (JI No.2) in full light. When in growth, water moderately; keep just moist in winter. Outdoors, grow in moderately fertile, sharply drained soil in full sun, in a sheltered position. Pruning group 3, although pruning is seldom needed; do not cut back into old wood.

• **PROPAGATION** Sow seed in containers in a cold frame in spring. Root semi-ripe cuttings in summer.

• **PESTS AND DISEASES** Trouble free.

R. monosperma, syn. *Genista monosperma.* Graceful, deciduous shrub with slender, arching, silky grey stems and a few linear leaves, to 2cm (¾in) long, which soon fall. Small, very fragrant, pea-like white flowers are produced in dense, axillary racemes, to 4cm (1½in) long, in early spring. ↕ to 4m (12ft), ↔ 1.5m (5ft). Portugal, Spain, N. Africa, Canary Islands. ❄

▷ **Rewarewa** see *Knightia excelsa*

▷ ***Reynoutria*** see *Fallopia*

RHAMNUS

RHAMNACEAE

Genus of 125 or more species of usually thorny, deciduous or evergreen shrubs and trees, widely distributed in N. temperate regions, with a few in the S. hemisphere. They occur in woodland, heathland, scrub, fens, bogs, or rocky places, often on alkaline soils. They are cultivated primarily for their foliage, which has good autumn colour in some deciduous species, and for their decorative fruits. The leaves are opposite or alternate. Tiny, hermaphrodite or unisexual, cup-shaped flowers, 2–4mm ($\frac{1}{16}$–⅛in) across, with 4 or 5 petals, are borne in axillary racemes or umbel-like clusters; they are often fragrant and usually yellowish white, greenish white, or white. Some flowers, particularly those of *R. frangula*, are very attractive to bees. Grow in a shrub border; *R. cathartica* and *R. frangula* may be used as hedging, or in a wild or woodland garden. All parts may cause severe discomfort if ingested.

• **HARDINESS** Fully hardy to frost hardy.

• **CULTIVATION** Grow in moderately fertile soil in full sun or partial shade. *R. cathartica*, *R. frangula*, and *R. imeretina* prefer moist soils. *R. alaternus* needs well-drained soil in full sun. Pruning group 1; trim hedges in early spring. Cut out reverting shoots on *R. alaternus* 'Argenteovariegata' when seen.

• **PROPAGATION** Sow seed in containers in a cold frame as soon as ripe. Root semi-ripe cuttings of evergreen species in summer. Root greenwood cuttings of deciduous species in early summer, or layer in autumn or spring.

• **PESTS AND DISEASES** Trouble free.

R. alaternus (Italian buckthorn). Erect to spreading, evergreen shrub with ovate to oblong, leathery, glossy, dark green leaves, to 7cm (3in) long. Unisexual and hermaphrodite, yellow-green flowers are borne in axillary clusters in late spring and early summer; they are followed by spherical red fruit, 6mm (¼in) across, ripening to black in late summer. ↕ 5m (15ft), ↔ 4m (12ft). Portugal, Morocco, Mediterranean, Ukraine (Crimea). ❄❄. **'Argenteovariegata'** ■ ♀ syn. 'Variegata', has grey-green leaves with conspicuous white margins.

R. californica (Coffeeberry). Upright, evergreen or semi-evergreen shrub with red shoots and oblong to oval, glossy, mid-green leaves, to 8cm (3in) long. In late spring and early summer, bears axillary clusters of hermaphrodite, yellowish white flowers. Spherical red fruit, 6mm (¼in) across, ripen to purple-black in late summer and autumn. ↕ 4m (12ft), ↔ 3m (10ft). W. USA. ❄❄

R. cathartica (Common buckthorn). Dense, thicket-forming, spiny, deciduous shrub, sometimes a small tree, with oval to ovate or elliptic, glossy, dark green leaves, to 6cm (2½in) long, turning yellow in autumn. Axillary clusters of unisexual, yellowish green flowers are borne in late spring and early summer. In autumn, bears spherical red fruit, to 6mm (¼in) across, ripening to black. ↕ 6m (20ft), ↔ 5m (15ft). Europe, N.W. Africa, Asia. ❄❄❄

R. frangula (Alder buckthorn). Bushy, spreading, deciduous shrub with oval to obovate, glossy, dark green leaves, to 7cm (3in) long, turning red in autumn. In late spring and early summer, bears axillary clusters of hermaphrodite green flowers, followed by fleshy, spherical red fruit, to 1cm (½in) across, ripening to black in autumn. ↕↔ 5m (15ft). Europe, N. Africa, Russia to Altai Mountains. ❄❄❄

R. imeretina. Open, spreading, deciduous shrub with stout shoots and oblong to oval, conspicuously veined, dark green leaves, to 30cm (12in) long, turning bronze-purple in autumn. In early summer, bears unisexual green flowers in axillary clusters, followed in late summer and autumn by spherical red fruit, 5mm (¼in) across, ripening to black. ↕ 3m (10ft), ↔ 5m (15ft). Georgia, E. Turkey, Armenia. ❄❄❄

RHAPHIDOPHORA

syn. RAPHIDOPHORA

ARACEAE

Genus of 60 species of evergreen root climbers and trailers from woodland in tropical S. and S.E. Asia and the Pacific islands. They are cultivated for their attractive leaves, which are short-stalked and entire on young plants, and long-stalked, larger, and pinnatifid or pinnate on mature specimens. In summer, mature plants grown outdoors produce yellow spadices of tiny, petalless flowers, surrounded by boat-shaped, yellow to green spathes. In frost-prone regions, grow as houseplants, or in a warm greenhouse or conservatory. In tropical

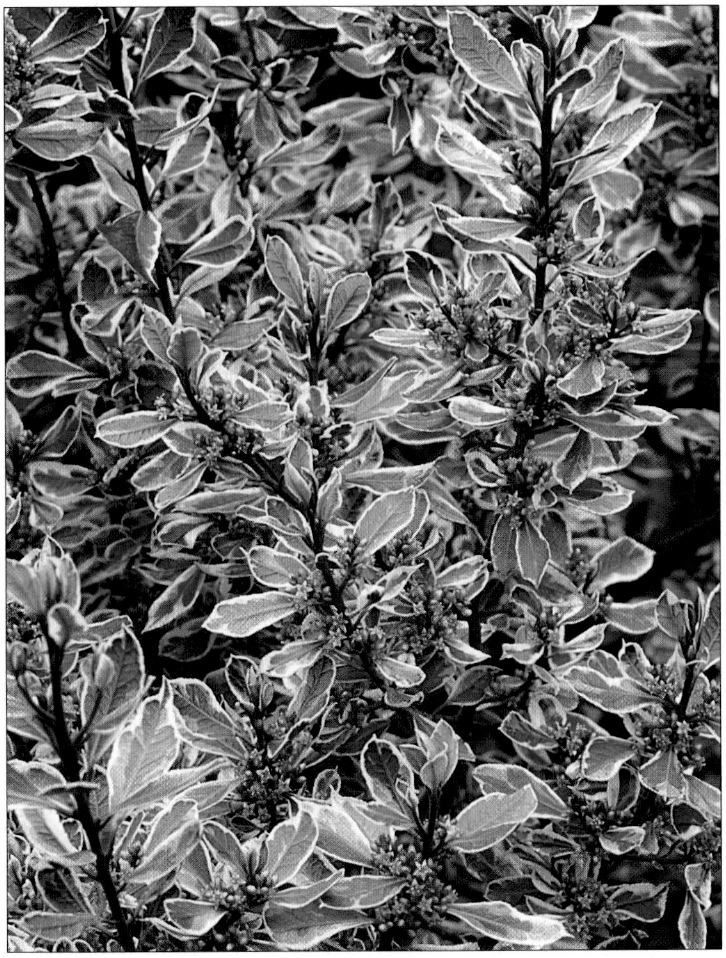

Rhamnus alaternus 'Argenteovariegata'

climates, grow through a tree or on a damp shady wall.
• **HARDINESS** Frost tender.
• **CULTIVATION** Under glass, grow in equal parts loam, leaf mould, bark, and sharp sand in bright filtered light. Provide moderate humidity, draught-free conditions, and the support of a moss pole or similar structure. When in full growth, water moderately, mist regularly, and apply a balanced liquid fertilizer every 2–3 weeks; water sparingly in winter. Outdoors, grow in moist, humus-rich soil in partial shade. Pruning group 11, after flowering; pruning is seldom needed.
• **PROPAGATION** Sow seed at 18–21°C (64–70°F) in spring. Root stem-tip or leaf-bud cuttings, or air layer, in spring or early summer.
• **PESTS AND DISEASES** Prone to scale insects and red spider mites under glass.

R. celatocaulis, syn. *Monstera latevaginata* of gardens, *Pothos celatocaulis, R. pinnata* (Shingle plant). Erect, sparsely branched climber mostly grown in its juvenile phase, when it has short-stalked, elliptic-ovate, entire, blue-green leaves, to 10cm (4in) long, closely overlapping and lying flat along the stems. Mature leaves are entire, pinnatifid, or pinnatisect, and 20–40cm (8–16in) long, with stalks of the same length. In summer, produces yellow spathes, 10–15cm (4–6in) long, singly from the leaf axils on long stems. ↕ 10m (30ft). Borneo. ⊛ (min. 15°C/59°F)
R. decursiva ▣ Erect, robust climber usually cultivated in its adult phase, when it has thick, stiff, sparsely branched, slow-growing stems and oblong, pinnatisect, leathery, lustrous, rich green leaves, 50–90cm (20–36in) long. Juvenile leaves are arranged in 2 ranks and are broadly ovate, entire, and mid-green, to 30cm (12in) long. Fleshy yellow spathes, 14–18cm (5½–7in) long, are produced singly from the leaf axils in summer. ↕ to 10m (30ft). N. Burma, India, Sri Lanka. ⊛ (min. 15°C/59°F)
R. pinnata see *R. celatocaulis*.

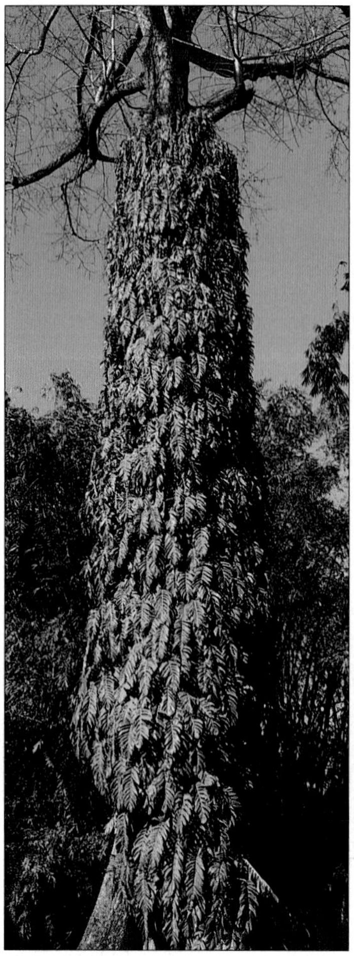
Rhaphidophora decursiva

RHAPHIOLEPIS

ROSACEAE

Genus of about 3–5, possibly up to 15 species of evergreen shrubs and trees from scrub in S.E. and E. Asia. They are grown for their alternate, often toothed leaves, which are glossy, dark green, and leathery, and for their fragrant, apple-blossom-like, star-shaped flowers borne in erect, terminal racemes or panicles in spring or summer. Grow in a sheltered border, or at the base of a warm, sunny wall. In frost-prone areas, grow half-hardy species in a cool greenhouse.
• **HARDINESS** Frost hardy to half hardy.
• **CULTIVATION** Under glass, grow in loam-based potting compost (JI No.3) in full light. In the growing season, water moderately and apply a balanced liquid fertilizer monthly; water sparingly in winter. Outdoors, grow in moist but well-drained, moderately fertile soil in full sun, with shelter from cold, drying winds. Pruning group 8.
• **PROPAGATION** Root semi-ripe cuttings in late summer. Layer in autumn.
• **PESTS AND DISEASES** Trouble free.

R. x delacourii (*R. indica* x *R. umbellata*). Dome-shaped, evergreen shrub with broadly obovate to inversely lance-shaped, shallowly toothed, leathery, dark green leaves, to 7cm (3in) long. Star-shaped pink flowers, to 2cm (¾in) across, are produced in erect, broadly conical panicles, to 10cm (4in) long, in spring or summer. ↕ 2m (6ft), ↔ 2.5m (8ft). Garden origin. ❄❄. **'Coates' Crimson'** bears dark pink flowers. **'Enchantress'** is compact, with rose-pink flowers. **'Indian Princess'** produces bright pink flowers fading to white. **'Spring Song'** bears pale pink flowers over an extended period. **'White Enchantress'** is dwarf and compact, bearing pure white flowers.
R. indica (Indian hawthorn). Bushy, spreading, evergreen shrub producing narrowly elliptic to lance-shaped, deeply toothed, leathery, glossy, dark green leaves, to 7–11cm (3–4½in) long. In spring or early summer, bears white flowers, to 1.5cm (½in) across, with pink-flushed centres, in loose racemes or panicles, to 8cm (3in) long. ↕ 1.5m (5ft), ↔ 2m (6ft). China. ❄
R. japonica see *R. umbellata*.
R. ovata see *R. umbellata*.
R. umbellata ▣ ♀ syn. *R. japonica, R. ovata*. Bushy, evergreen shrub with oval to obovate or inversely lance-shaped, leathery, dark green, shallowly toothed leaves, to 9cm (3½in) long. White flowers, to 2cm (¾in) across, sometimes tinted rose-pink, are borne in conical racemes, to 10cm (4in) long, in early summer. ↕↔ 1.5m (5ft). Korea, Japan. ❄❄

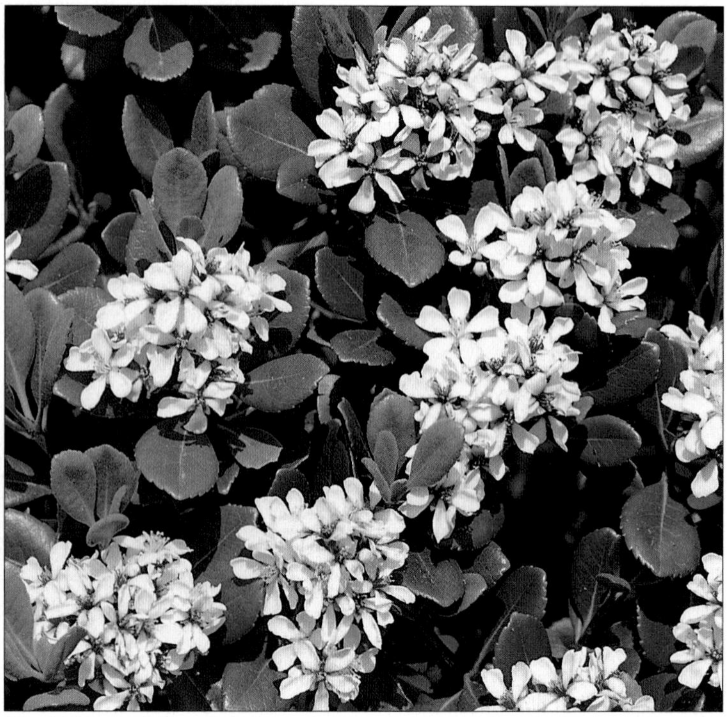
Rhaphiolepis umbellata

RHAPIDOPHYLLUM

Needle palm

ARECACEAE/PALMAE

Genus of one species of almost stemless palm from wooded, swampy areas in coastal S.E. USA. It is grown for its fan-shaped, palmately lobed leaves, cut almost to the midribs. The tiny, bowl-shaped, 3-petalled flowers are borne in small panicles among the leaf sheaths. In frost-prone areas, grow in a cool or temperate greenhouse. In warmer areas, use as a lawn or courtyard specimen.
• **HARDINESS** Frost tender, but will survive short spells around 0°C (32°F), if ripened by warm summers.
• **CULTIVATION** Under glass, grow in loam-based potting compost (JI No.2) in bright filtered light. When in growth, water freely and apply a balanced liquid fertilizer monthly; water more sparingly in winter. Pot on or top-dress in spring. Outdoors, grow in any moderately fertile, moist but well-drained soil in partial shade.
• **PROPAGATION** Sow seed at 16–18°C (61–64°F) in spring. Remove smaller suckers in spring.
• **PESTS AND DISEASES** Red spider mites, mealybugs, and scale insects may be a problem under glass.

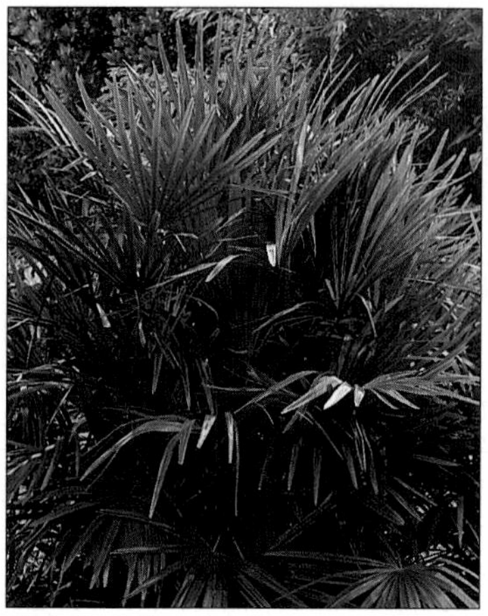
Rhapidophyllum hystrix

R. hystrix ▣ ❄ (Blue palmetto, Porcupine palm). Small, slow-growing, clump-forming palm with a short-branching stem system below or at the soil surface. Sheaths at the bases of the leaf-stalks bear long, erect spines; each smooth, erect leaf-stalk bears a deeply lobed leaf-blade, to 1m (3ft) long, with 5–12 lobes, bright green above, tinted blue-grey beneath. Tiny, bowl-shaped, purplish red flowers, borne in summer, are hidden by the foliage. ↕ 1.5–2m (5–6ft), ↔ 2–4m (6–12ft). USA (S. Carolina to Florida and Mississippi). ⊛ (min. 7–10°C/45–50°F)

RHAPIS

Lady palm

ARECACEAE/PALMAE

Genus of 12 species of small, cluster-stemmed palms found in shady tropical and subtropical forest from S. China to S.E. Asia. The light or mid-green leaves, arranged in spirals or loose tufts at the stem tips, are divided almost to the bases into 2–10 or more lobes. Bowl-shaped, 3-petalled flowers are borne in short panicles between the leaves. In frost-prone areas, grow in a temperate or warm greenhouse, or as houseplants. In frost-free regions, use in a shady border or to add foliage interest to other plantings.
• **HARDINESS** Frost tender.
• **CULTIVATION** Under glass, grow in loamless potting compost in bright filtered light. In the growing season, water freely and apply a balanced liquid fertilizer monthly; water moderately in winter. Pot on or top-dress in spring. Outdoors, grow in any moderately fertile, moist but well-drained soil in dappled shade.
• **PROPAGATION** Sow seed at 27°C (81°F), or divide, in spring.
• **PESTS AND DISEASES** Red spider mites may be a problem under glass.

R

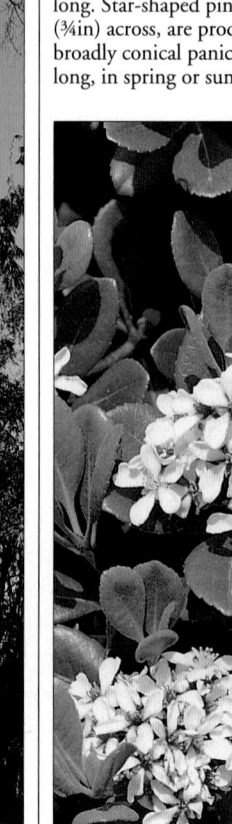

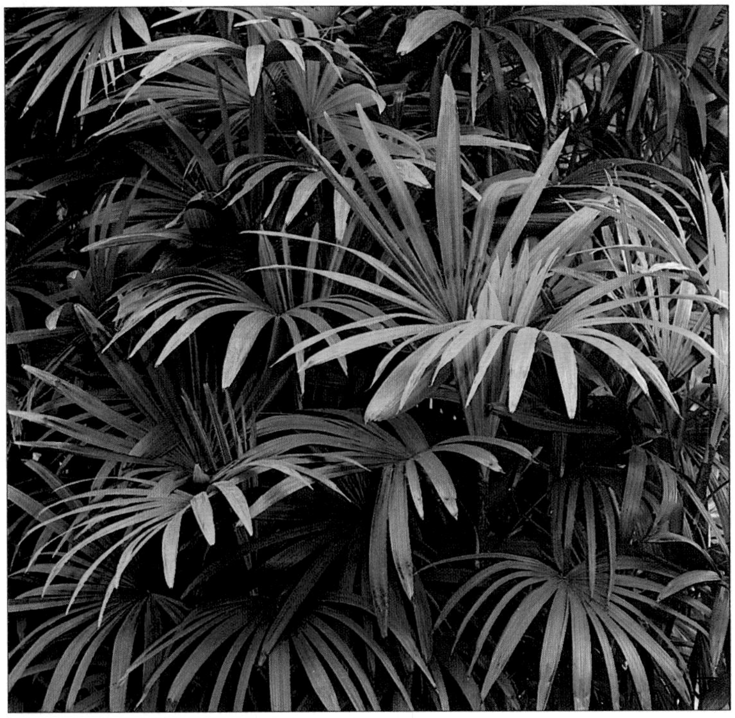

Rhapis excelsa

R. excelsa ▣🏆✱ syn. *R. flabelliformis* (Miniature fan palm). Small, clump-forming palm with slender, erect, bamboo- or reed-like stems. The long-stalked, deeply lobed, lustrous, dark green leaves, 20–30cm (8–12in) long, each have 3–10 broadly to narrowly lance-shaped, puckered lobes. Tiny, bowl-shaped cream flowers are borne in panicles, to 12cm (5in) long, among the leaves, in summer. ↕↔ 1.5–5m (5–15ft). S. China. ❀ (min. 10–13°C/50–55°F). **'Variegata'** has leaves with white-striped lobes. **'Zuikonishiki'** has leaves with yellow-variegated lobes; ↕ to 60cm (24in), rarely more.
R. flabelliformis see *R. excelsa.*

▷ ***Rhazya*** see *Amsonia*
R. orientalis see *A. orientalis*

RHEUM
Rhubarb

POLYGONACEAE

Genus of about 50 species of rhizomatous, often tough or woody perennials found in a range of habitats, from marshy meadows and streamsides to scrub and rocky slopes, in E. Europe and C. Asia to the Himalayas and China. Unlike *R.* x *hybridum,* which is grown for its edible leaf-stalks, the rhubarbs described below are cultivated for their imposing, large, basal leaves and tall flower panicles. A few species from mountainous regions in Asia are dwarf with small flower spikes. The rounded, entire to palmately lobed leaves often emerge from bright red buds; the leaves are sometimes crimson-purple when young, usually with coarse teeth and conspicuous veins and midribs. Large panicles of tiny, petalless, star-shaped flowers are borne on hollow, leafless, flowering stems in summer; they have large, colourful, showy bracts in some species. The flowers are followed by small, triangular, winged, usually brown fruits. Grow rhubarbs near water, or in a moist border or woodland garden. The leaves may cause severe discomfort if ingested.

- **HARDINESS** Fully hardy.
- **CULTIVATION** Grow in deep, moist, humus-rich soil in full sun or partial shade. *R. alexandrae* prefers wet, marshy soil. Mulch annually in early spring with well-rotted organic matter. *R. nobile* may prove difficult to establish.
- **PROPAGATION** Sow seed in containers in a cold frame in autumn. Divide in early spring.
- **PESTS AND DISEASES** Susceptible to damage by slugs, and prone to crown rot and viruses.

***R.* 'Ace of Hearts'** ▣ syn. *R.* 'Ace of Spades'. Rhizomatous perennial with elongated, heart-shaped, entire, dark green leaves, to 35cm (14in) long, red-veined above and purple-red beneath. In mid- and late summer, numerous tiny, star-shaped, very pale pink to white flowers open in panicles to 1.2m (4ft) long. ↕ to 1.2m (4ft), ↔ 90cm (36in). ✻✻✻
***R.* 'Ace of Spades'** see *R.* 'Ace of Hearts'.
R. alexandrae. Rhizomatous perennial with rosetted, oblong-ovate, entire, glossy, dark green leaves, to 20cm (8in) long, with heart-shaped bases and prominent veins. In early summer, bears narrow, arching, then pendent panicles, 60cm (24in) long, of tiny, star-shaped, yellow-green flowers, which are almost hidden by creamy white or greenish cream bracts, to 10cm (4in) or more long. ↕ to 1.5m (5ft), ↔ 60cm (24in). W. China, Tibet. ✻✻✻
R. nobile. Rhizomatous perennial, similar to *R. alexandrae,* with broadly ovate, entire, glossy, dark green leaves, to 30cm (12in) or more long, veined and margined red. In midsummer, bears panicles, 60cm (24in) long, of showy, arching to pendent, overlapping cream bracts, to 15cm (6in) long, which conceal short, erect clusters of tiny, star-shaped green flowers. ↕ to 2m (6ft), ↔ 60cm (24in). Himalayas, Nepal to S.E. Tibet. ✻✻✻
R. palmatum 🏆 (Chinese rhubarb). Rhizomatous perennial with a massive rootstock and thick leaf-stalks that bear broadly ovate to rounded, palmately 3–9 lobed, coarsely toothed, dark green leaves, to 90cm (36in) long, purple-red or red and softly hairy beneath. In early summer, numerous tiny, star-shaped, creamy green to deep red flowers are borne in panicles to 2m (6ft) long. ↕ to 2.5m (8ft), ↔ to 1.8m (6ft). N.W. China, N.E. Tibet. ✻✻✻.
'Atropurpureum' see 'Atrosanguineum'.
'Atrosanguineum' ▣ syn. 'Atropurpureum', has leaves that emerge from almost scarlet buds; the leaves are vivid crimson-purple when young, fading gradually to dark green above. Bears clustered panicles of rich cerise-pink flowers. **'Bowles' Crimson'** has darker red flowers, and leaves that are crimson beneath. **var. *tanguticum*** has leaves with jagged leaflets, emerging reddish green and becoming dark green, often purple-tinted, with age. Massive flowering stems bear erect panicles of numerous white, pink, or crimson flowers; ↕ 2m (6ft).

▷ **Rheumatism root** see *Jeffersonia diphylla*

RHEXIA
Meadow beauty

MELASTOMATACEAE

Genus of about 10 species of bristly perennials, some tuberous, others woody-based, from swamps or moist meadows in E. North America. They have square stems and opposite, oblong to ovate-lance-shaped, almost stalkless leaves with entire, usually hairy to bristly margins. They are cultivated for their shallowly saucer-shaped flowers, each with a short tube, 4 widely parted petals, and 8 prominent stamens, borne singly or in terminal cymes in summer. Grow in a sheltered border, bog garden, or wild garden.

- **HARDINESS** Fully hardy to frost hardy.
- **CULTIVATION** Grow in constantly moist, acid soil in full sun. In frost-prone areas that do not experience snow cover, protect the crown with a deep winter mulch. They dislike disturbance.
- **PROPAGATION** Sow seed at 13–18°C (55–64°F) in spring; before planting out, grow seedlings on, in containers in a cold frame, for up to 2 years to obtain strong plants. Divide in spring.
- **PESTS AND DISEASES** Susceptible to slug damage.

R. virginica (Meadow beauty). Bristly, tuberous perennial with square, slightly winged stems. Almost stalkless, oval to oblong-lance-shaped, mid-green leaves, to 5cm (2in) long, are hairy above, with

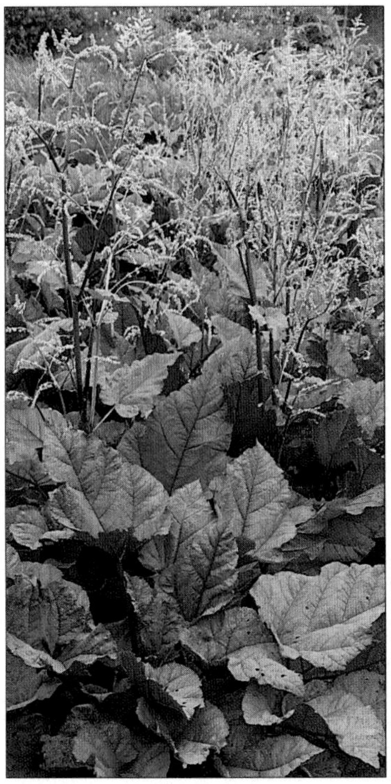

Rheum 'Ace of Hearts'

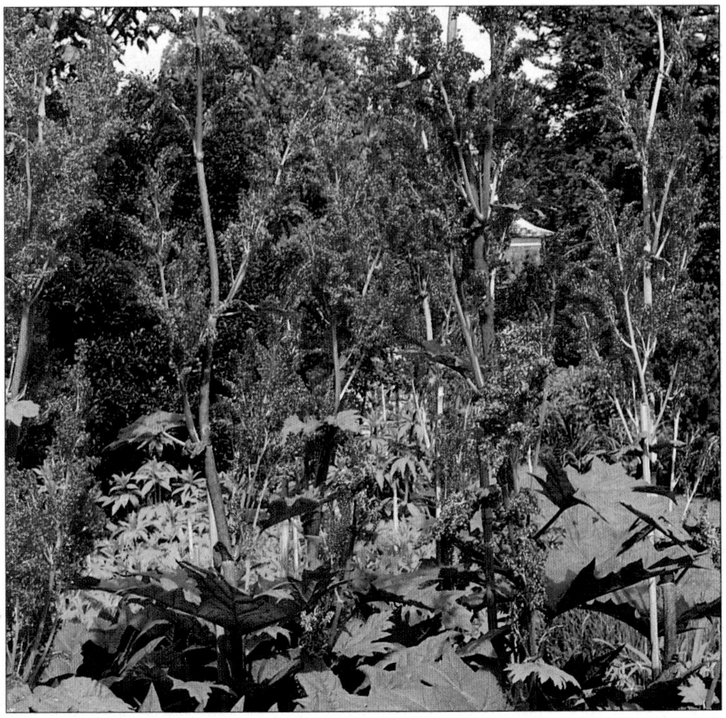

Rheum palmatum 'Atrosanguineum'

3–5 prominent veins and hair-fringed margins. In mid- and late summer, few-flowered cymes of shallowly saucer-shaped, short-tubed purple flowers, 4cm (1½in) across, open from red-bristly buds. ↕22–45cm (9–18in), ↔15cm (6in). E. North America (Nova Scotia to Texas). ❄❄❄

▷ ***Rhipsalidopsis*** see *Hatiora*
R. gaertneri see *H. gaertneri*
R. rosea see *H. rosea*

RHIPSALIS

CACTACEAE

Genus of about 50 species of mostly epiphytic or rock-dwelling perennial cacti from wooded and forested areas of Central and South America and the West Indies, with one species found in tropical Africa, Madagascar, and Sri Lanka. They often have aerial roots and freely branching stems, which vary in shape from cylindrical to winged, or flat and leaf-like, and may be ribbed or angled, some having spines or bristles. Small, funnel-shaped, diurnal flowers are borne singly or in small clusters from the areoles, mainly from spring to summer. These are followed by fleshy, berry-like, usually spherical fruits. In frost-prone areas, grow as houseplants in containers or hanging baskets, or in a temperate or warm greenhouse. In frost-free regions, grow epiphytically on a tree, or in a sheltered, humid border.

• **HARDINESS** Frost tender.
• **CULTIVATION** Under glass, grow in epiphytic cactus compost in bright filtered or indirect light with moderate to high humidity. Mist daily in warm weather. In growth, water freely and apply a balanced liquid fertilizer 3 or 4 times; water sparingly at other times. Outdoors, grow in an open site in fertile, humus-rich, moist but sharply drained soil in partial shade. See also pp.48–49.
• **PROPAGATION** Sow seed at 19–24°C (66–75°F), or root cuttings of stem sections, in spring or summer.
• **PESTS AND DISEASES** Susceptible to mealybugs.

R. baccifera, syn. *R. cassutha* (Mistletoe cactus). Pendent, epiphytic cactus with aerial roots and cylindrical, sparsely branched, mid-green stems, 4–6mm (⅛–¼in) thick. Minute areoles bear clusters of funnel-shaped white flowers, 5–10mm (¼–½in) long, from winter to

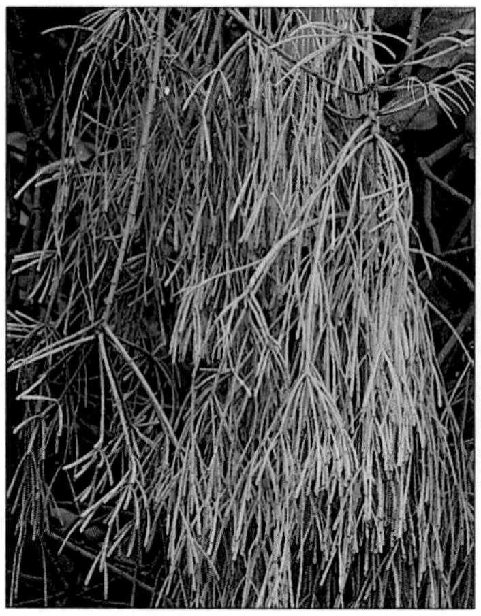
Rhipsalis capilliformis

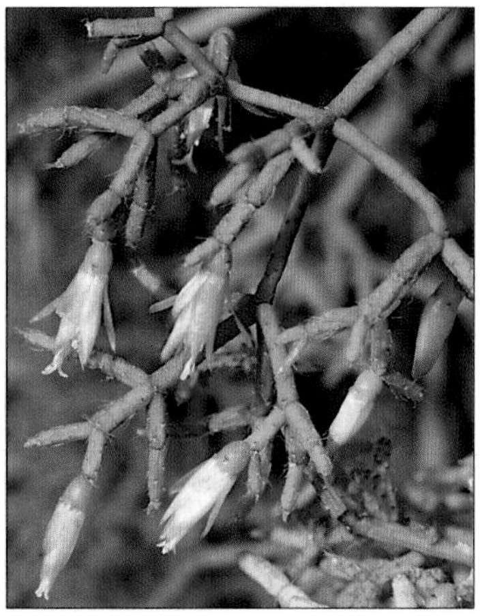
Rhipsalis cereuscula

spring, followed by spherical, pale pink or translucent white fruit, 5–8mm (¼–⅜in) across. ↕to 4m (12ft), ↔60cm (24in). Africa, Madagascar, Sri Lanka, Tropical America. ❁ (min. 7–12°C/45–54°F)
R. capilliformis ■ Pendent, epiphytic cactus producing cylindrical, jointed, pale green stems with bunches of side branches, 2–3mm (1/16–⅛in) thick. The stems have slightly woolly, bristly areoles and, near the tips of the joints, minute, bristleless areoles bearing clusters of funnel-shaped, glossy, greenish white flowers, to 8mm (⅜in) long, in late spring. These are followed by spherical white fruit, 4–5mm (⅛–¼in) across. ↕40cm (16in) or more, ↔30cm (12in). E. Brazil. ❁ (min. 7–12°C/45–54°F)
R. cassutha see *R. baccifera*.
R. cereuscula ■ Erect then pendent, epiphytic cactus producing cylindrical, many-branched, mid-green stems, 4mm (⅛in) thick, with whorls of short, jointed branches. In spring, woolly, few-bristled areoles at the tips of the short branches bear usually solitary, narrowly funnel-shaped white flowers, 1.5cm (½in) long, with pinkish green sepals. These are followed by obovoid white fruit, 5mm (¼in) across. ↕to 60cm (24in), ↔40cm (16in). Brazil, Paraguay, Argentina. ❁ (min. 7–12°C/45–54°F)
R. crispata. Semi-pendent, epiphytic cactus producing branching, flat, leaf-like, light green stems, 2–4cm (¾–1½in) thick, with elliptic, inversely lance-shaped or obovate segments, with sometimes 3-winged, scalloped margins. In early summer, minute, spineless areoles bear solitary, funnel-shaped,

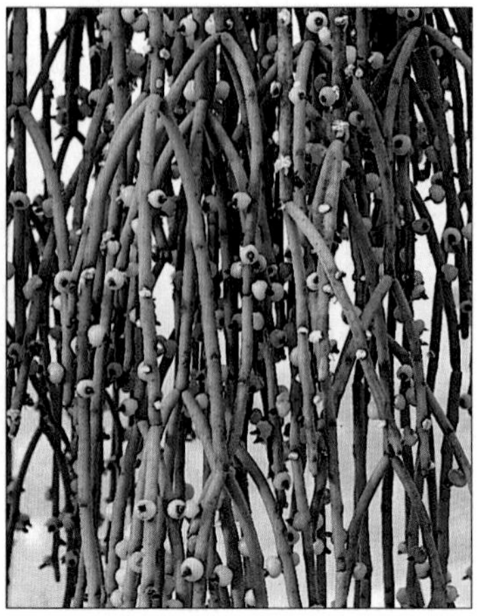
Rhipsalis floccosa

creamy white flowers, 1.5cm (½in) across, followed by spherical white, sometimes red-flushed fruit, 8–10mm (⅜–½in) across. ↕60cm (24in), ↔ indefinite. S.E. Brazil. ❁ (min. 7–12°C/45–54°F)
R. fasciculata. Erect or semi-pendent, epiphytic cactus producing cylindrical, branching, pale bluish green stems, 6mm (¼in) thick, with woolly, few-bristled areoles along the margins. In early summer, the areoles bear funnel-shaped, white or pale greenish white flowers, to 8mm (⅜in) long, singly or in small clusters. They are followed by spherical white fruit, 4–5mm (⅛–¼in) across. ↕to 60cm (24in), ↔to 30cm (12in). Brazil. ❁ (min. 7–12°C/45–54°F)
R. floccosa ■ syn. *R. tucumanensis.* Pendent, epiphytic cactus with aerial roots and cylindrical, branching, mid-green stems, to 1cm (½in) thick. Stem segments are arranged in whorls of 2–6, and have slightly woolly, sunken areoles bearing solitary, funnel-shaped, pink-tipped, white or creamy white flowers, 1.5cm (½in) long, from winter to spring. These are followed by spherical white, sometimes pink-tinged fruit, 5–10mm (¼–½in) across. ↕45cm (18in), ↔24cm (10in). Brazil, Bolivia, N. Paraguay, Argentina. ❁ (min. 7–12°C/45–54°F)
R. paradoxa. Pendent, epiphytic cactus with aerial roots and branching, mid-green stems, 3–5cm (1¼–2in) thick. Stems have long, 3-angled segments, twisted into shorter segments every 2–6cm (¾–2½in), with white wool at the top of each angle. Funnel-shaped white flowers, 2cm (¾in) across, are borne singly from sunken areoles in late spring. They are followed by spherical red fruit, 8mm (⅜in) across. ↕1m (3ft) or more, ↔ indefinite. S.E. Brazil. ❁ (min. 7–12°C/45–54°F)
R. tucumanensis see *R. floccosa*.

RHODANTHE

syn. ACROCLINIUM
Strawflower

ASTERACEAE/COMPOSITAE

Genus of over 40 species of erect, drought-tolerant annuals, perennials, and subshrubs, frequently included in the genera *Acroclinium* and *Helipterum*, occurring in arid areas of Australia. They are cultivated for their solitary or corymb-like clusters of daisy-like, straw-textured, "everlasting", single to double,

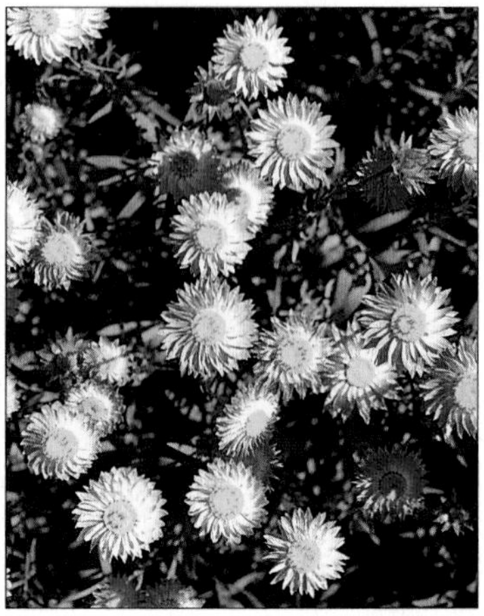
Rhodanthe chlorocephala subsp. *rosea*

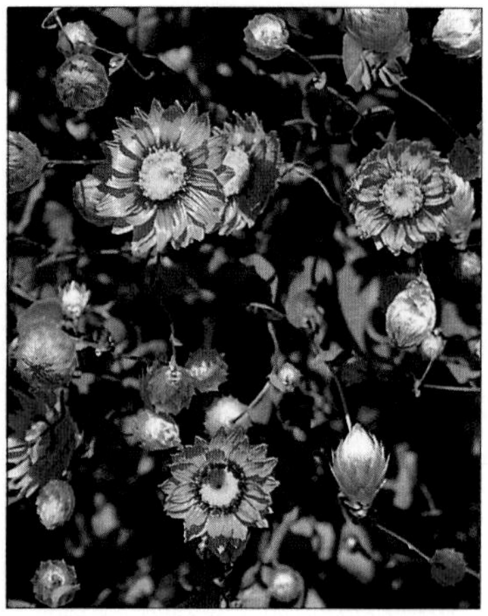
Rhodanthe manglesii

yellow, white, or pink flowerheads, borne mainly in summer. The alternate leaves are entire, linear to oblong or obovate, and mid- to grey-green. Grow in an annual or mixed border; the perennials and subshrubs are usually grown as annuals, even in frost-free areas. The flowerheads are excellent for dried flower arrangements.

• **HARDINESS** Half hardy.
• **CULTIVATION** Grow in light, well-drained, preferably poor soil in full sun. Cut for drying before flowerheads are fully open, and hang upside down in a cool, dry, dark place.
• **PROPAGATION** Sow seed at 16°C (61°F) in early spring and plant out when all danger of frost has passed, or sow *in situ* in mid-spring.
• **PESTS AND DISEASES** Seedlings and young plants are prone to aphids and slug damage.

R. chlorocephala* subsp. *rosea ■ syn. *Acroclinium roseum, Helipterum roseum.* Fast-growing, erect annual producing linear, pointed, stem-clasping, grey-green leaves, to 3.5cm (1½in) long. In summer, bears solitary, daisy-like flowerheads, 2.5–8cm (1–3in) across, with yellow disc-florets surrounded by spreading, papery, white or rose-pink bracts, often with white bases; they close in dull weather. ↕30–60cm (12–24in), ↔15cm (6in). S.W. Australia. ❄
R. manglesii ■ syn. *Helipterum manglesii.* Erect, bushy annual with oblong to ovate, pointed, grey-green leaves, to 10cm (4in) long. From summer to early autumn, bears stiff-stemmed clusters of small, daisy-like flowerheads, to 3cm (1¼in) across, with light yellow disc-florets surrounded by decorative, spreading, papery, red, pink, or white bracts. ↕60cm (24in), ↔15cm (6in). W. Australia. ❄

RHODANTHEMUM

syn. CHRYSANTHEMOPSIS, PYRETHROPSIS

ASTERACEAE/COMPOSITAE

Genus of about 10 species of mat-forming, often rhizomatous perennials and subshrubs, previously included in the genera *Chrysanthemum* or *Leucanthemum*, from exposed rocky areas in N. Africa, with one species from Spain. They are cultivated for their solitary, large, daisy-like flowerheads, surrounded by prominent, usually green bracts, borne on erect, branched or unbranched stems, mainly in spring and

R

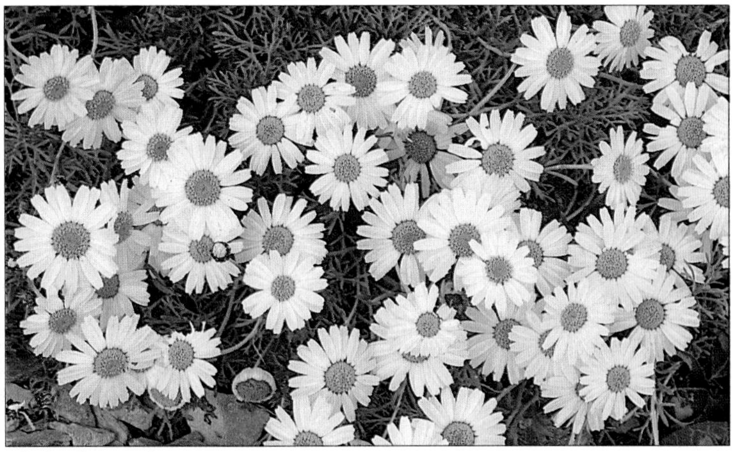
Rhodanthemum hosmariense

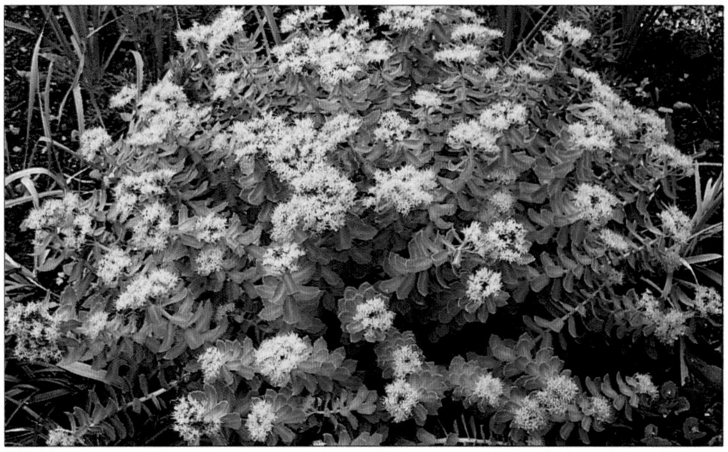
Rhodiola rosea

summer. The deeply or shallowly 3-lobed leaves are hairy and sometimes silvery. Grow in a sunny rock garden, a raised bed, at the base of a warm, sunny wall, or in an alpine house.
• **HARDINESS** Most are hardy to -10°C (14°F) in very well-drained soil, but resent excessive winter wet.
• **CULTIVATION** Under glass, grow in loam-based potting compost (JI No.2) in full light. In the growing season, water freely and apply a balanced liquid fertilizer monthly; water moderately in winter. Outdoors, grow in moderately fertile, very well-drained soil in full sun.
• **PROPAGATION** Sow seed in containers in a cold frame in spring. Root softwood cuttings in early summer.
• **PESTS AND DISEASES** Susceptible to aphids and red spider mites under glass.

R. atlanticum, syn. *Chrysanthemum atlanticum, Pyrethropsis atlantica.* Prostrate, rhizomatous perennial with unbranched stems and 3-lobed, hairy, mid-green leaves, to 4cm (1½in) long, the middle lobe divided into 3, the outer lobes finely divided. In summer, bears solitary, daisy-like flowerheads, 3cm (1¼in) across, with white ray-florets, flushed pink beneath, and yellow disc-florets. ↕ 8cm (3in), ↔ 30cm (12in). Morocco. ❄❄
R. catananche, syn. *Chrysanthemum catananche, Pyrethropsis catananche.* Rhizomatous perennial producing unbranched stems and hairy, silver-grey leaves, to 6cm (2½in) long, irregularly cut into 3 toothed lobes. In summer, bears solitary, daisy-like flowerheads, to 5cm (2in) across, with cream ray-florets, each with a maroon stripe, surrounding a small centre of deep yellow disc-florets. ↕ 15cm (6in), ↔ 30cm (12in). Morocco. ❄❄
R. gayanum, syn. *Chrysanthemum gayanum, Pyrethropsis gayana.* Semi-erect subshrub with branching stems and deeply 3-lobed, softly hairy, grey-green leaves, 2.5cm (1in) long. In summer, freely bears solitary, daisy-like flowerheads, 2.5–4cm (1–1½in) across, with rose-pink or white, pink-backed ray-florets and brown disc-florets. ↕↔ to 30cm (12in). Morocco, Algeria. ❄❄
R. hosmariense ■ 🏆 syn. *Chrysanthemum hosmariense, Leucanthemum hosmariense, Pyrethropsis hosmariensis.* Spreading, bushy subshrub with stalkless, softly hairy, intensely silver, deeply 3-lobed leaves, to 4cm (1½in) long. From early spring to autumn, bears solitary, short-stemmed, daisy-like flowerheads, to 5cm (2in) across, with white ray-florets and wide centres of yellow disc-florets. The flowerheads are surrounded by silvery bracts, the outer ones with distinctive black margins. It is the easiest species to grow in the open garden; in an alpine house it flowers for most of the year, if dead-headed. ↕ 10–30cm (4–12in), ↔ 30cm (12in). Morocco (Atlas Mountains). ❄❄
R. maresii, syn. *Chrysanthemum maresii, Pyrethropsis maresii.* Spreading subshrub, similar to *R. hosmariense*, with deeply 3-lobed, softly hairy, silver-green leaves, to 6cm (2½in) long. In summer, bears solitary, daisy-like flowerheads, 2–4cm (¾–1½in) across, with yellow ray-florets and yellow disc-florets that become increasingly purple-tinged with age. ↕ 10–30cm (4–12in), ↔ 30cm (12in). Algeria. ❄❄

RHODIOLA

CRASSULACEAE

Genus of about 50 species of perennials, some dioecious, widely distributed in the N. hemisphere in sunny, rocky habitats. They have thick, fleshy rhizomes producing scaly brown basal leaves, and stiffly erect, unbranched or occasionally branched stems that bear alternate, triangular-ovate to lance-shaped, often toothed, fleshy, grey-green stem leaves. The small, star-shaped, green, yellow, orange, or red flowers, with 8–10 prominent stamens, are borne in dense, rounded, terminal, corymb- or raceme-like heads, and may be unisexual or bisexual. Rhodiolas are cultivated for their foliage and flowers, and are suitable for a rock garden, or the front of a mixed or herbaceous border.
• **HARDINESS** Fully hardy.
• **CULTIVATION** Grow in moderately fertile soil in full sun.
• **PROPAGATION** Sow seed in containers in a cold frame in spring or autumn. Divide rhizomes in spring or early summer. Root leaf cuttings in summer.
• **PESTS AND DISEASES** Prone to aphids.

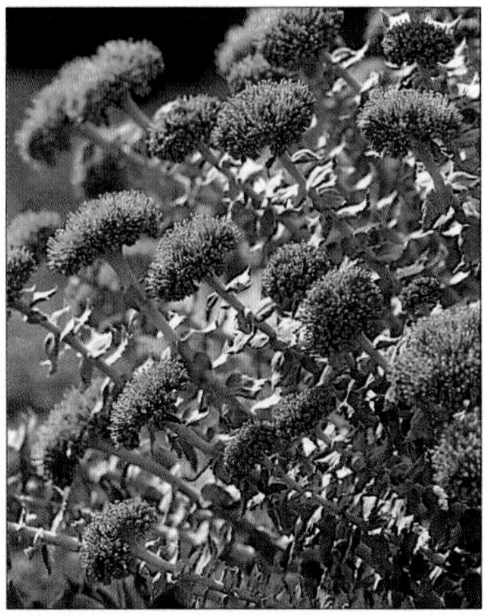
Rhodiola heterodonta

R. heterodonta ■ syn. *Sedum heterodontum, S. rosea* var. *heterodontum.* Erect, hairless, dioecious, rhizomatous perennial with branching stems of ovate, fleshy, greyish green leaves, 2.5–3cm (1–1¼in) long, either entire or with a few coarse teeth. In late spring and early summer, bears dense, terminal cymes of numerous star-shaped yellow flowers, 3mm (⅛in) across, opening from rounded red buds in late spring and early summer. Male flowers have red or purple-red anthers that colour the whole of the flowerheads; females have purple-tipped carpels. ↕↔ to 40cm (16in). Afghanistan, Pamir Mountains, W. Himalayas, Tibet. ❄❄❄
R. rosea ■ syn. *Sedum rosea, S. rhodiola* (Roseroot). Variable, clump-forming, dioecious, rhizomatous perennial with purple stems bearing broadly ovate to narrowly inversely lance-shaped, entire or irregularly toothed, glaucous, fleshy, grey-green leaves, to 4cm (1½in) long, with red-tinted tips. In summer, bears dense, terminal, corymb- or umbel-like heads of numerous male or female, yellow-green flowers, 6mm (¼in) across, opening from slightly pink buds. ↕ 5–30cm (2–12in), ↔ 20cm (8in). Throughout N. hemisphere. ❄❄❄. **subsp. *integrifolia*** has smaller leaves, and red-purple, sometimes green flowers often borne on reddish green stems.
R. wallichiana, syn. *Sedum crassipes, S. wallichianum.* Erect, rhizomatous, hairless perennial with linear-lance-shaped, slightly toothed, mid-green leaves, 1–3cm (½–1¼in) long. In early summer, bears dense but few-flowered, terminal, corymb-like flowerheads with bisexual, star-shaped, pale yellow to greenish white flowers, 5–10mm (¼–½in) across, sometimes tinged pink. ↕ to 35cm (14in), ↔ 30cm (12in). W. Himalayas, W. China, Tibet. ❄❄❄

▷ ***Rhodocactus grandifolius*** see *Pereskia grandifolia*

RHODOCHITON

SCROPHULARIACEAE

Genus of 3 species of deciduous, perennial climbers found in woodland in Mexico. They are cultivated for their flowers, which have pendent, long-tubed corollas, with 5 rounded segments, and inflated calyces. Twining leaf-stalks bear alternate, simple, sparsely toothed leaves. In frost-prone areas, grow as annuals outdoors, or in a cool greenhouse. In frost-free areas, use to cover a pergola or arch.
• **HARDINESS** Frost tender.
• **CULTIVATION** Under glass, grow in loam-based potting compost (JI No.2) in full light with shade from hot sun. When in growth, water freely and apply a balanced liquid fertilizer monthly; keep just moist in winter. Pot on in spring. Outdoors, grow in fertile, humus-rich, moist but well-drained soil in full sun.
• **PROPAGATION** Sow seed at 15–18°C (59–64°F) as soon as ripe or in spring.
• **PESTS AND DISEASES** Prone to red spider mites and whiteflies under glass.

R. atrosanguineus ■ 🏆 syn. *R. volubile.* Slender-stemmed climber producing heart-shaped, rich green leaves, 4–8cm (1½–3in) long. Long, pendent stalks bear solitary, tubular, black to reddish purple flowers, 4.5cm (1¾in) long, with cup-shaped, rose-pink or mauve calyces, from summer to autumn. ↕ to 3m (10ft), sometimes more. Mexico. ❀ (min. 3–5°C/37–41°F)
R. volubile see *R. atrosanguineus.*

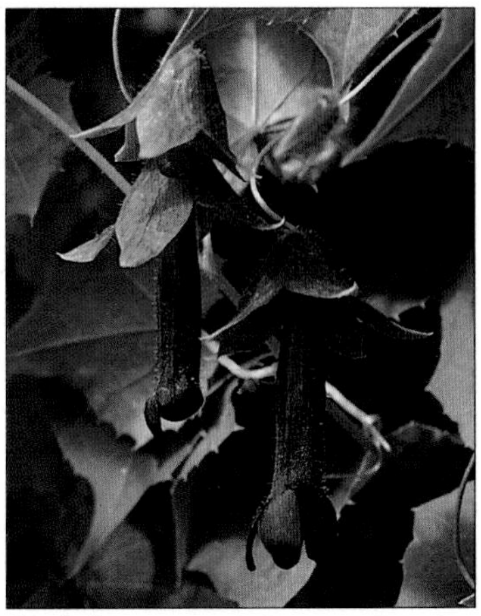
Rhodochiton atrosanguineus

RHODODENDRON

syn. AZALEA

ERICACEAE

Genus of 500–900 species of evergreen and deciduous trees and shrubs, sometimes epiphytic, from Europe, Asia, Australasia, and North America, particularly S.W. China, Tibet, Burma, N. India, and New Guinea. They occur in diverse habitats, from dense forest to alpine tundra, and from sea level to high altitudes. They vary greatly in habit (see panel below), and may reach a height of 25m (80ft) or creep at ground level to form prostrate shrubs.

The leaves are mostly lance-shaped and mid- to dark green, ranging in size from 4mm (⅛in) to 75cm (30in) long. All hybrids described below conform to one of the following leaf length ranges: very large, 45–75cm (18–30in) long; large, 15–45cm (6–18in) long; medium-sized, 5–15cm (2–6in) long; small, 1–5cm (½–2in) long; very small, 4–10mm (⅛–½in) long. Some have leaves and young stems covered with an indumentum (a dense woolly covering of hairs or scales); a few have leaves that are aromatic when crushed.

Rhododendrons are grown mainly for their spectacular, sometimes strongly scented flowers, which are borne singly or in lateral or terminal racemes (known as trusses), from late autumn to late summer. The individual flowers vary greatly in size and shape (see panel below), but are usually 5-lobed, and often marked with flares or spots inside, on the upper or lower lobes or in the throats; some also have conspicuous or brightly coloured, basal nectar pouches inside. There are thousands of hybrids, encompassing nearly every flower colour. Some rhododendrons also have attractive young growth, which ranges in colour from red to bronze-brown or metallic blue-green; a few have decorative, exfoliating bark, which may be any colour from brown-pink or deep maroon to silvery grey. A number of the deciduous rhododendrons are valued for their autumn colour.

Rhododendrons have a wide range of garden uses: dwarf alpine varieties are effective in a rock garden; larger woodland rhododendrons are excellent for brightening shady areas; the "iron clad" (or "hardy hybrid") rhododendrons are tolerant of more exposed sites and also suitable for hedges or informal screens; and many of the modern compact hybrids are ideal for growing on shaded patios, or in containers or tubs. In frost-prone areas, tender rhododendrons, including Vireyas, are best grown in a conservatory or cool greenhouse. The nectar of some rhododendron flowers may cause severe discomfort if ingested.

In horticulture, rhododendrons are often divided into 4 main groups: evergreen rhododendrons, Vireya rhododendrons, azaleas, and azaleodendrons.

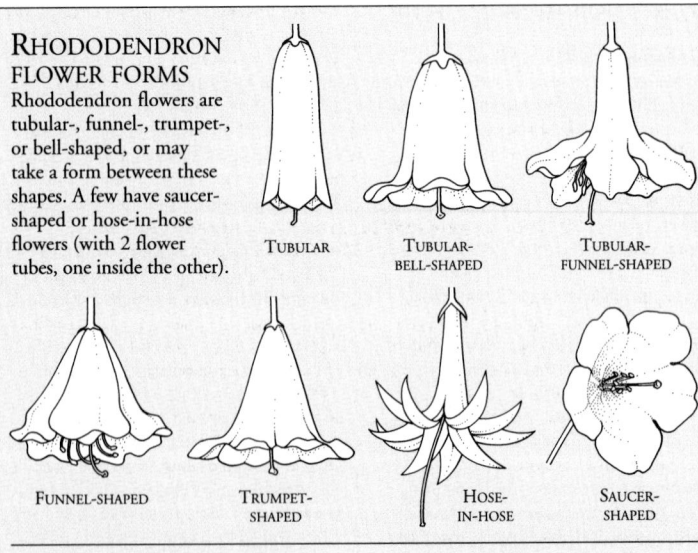

RHODODENDRON FLOWER FORMS

Rhododendron flowers are tubular-, funnel-, trumpet-, or bell-shaped, or may take a form between these shapes. A few have saucer-shaped or hose-in-hose flowers (with 2 flower tubes, one inside the other).

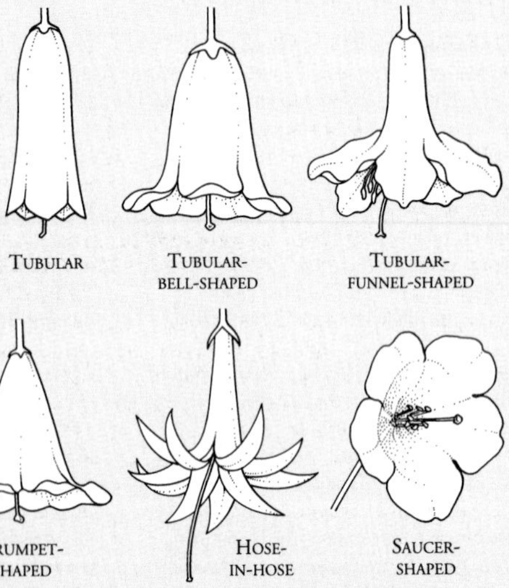

RHODODENDRON HABITS

Evergreen rhododendrons vary in habit from small shrubs to large trees. Azaleas and Vireyas are both shrubby.

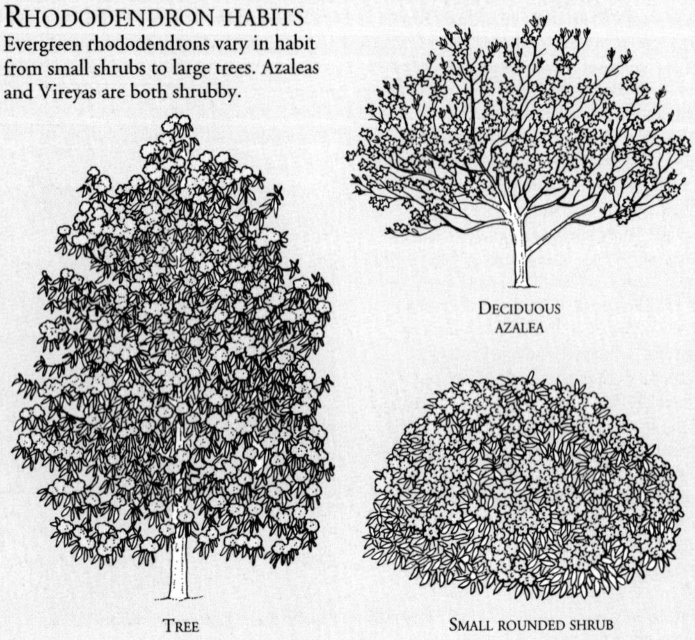

Evergreen rhododendrons

Unless otherwise stated, all evergreen shrubs and trees described on the following pages fall into this group, which includes the "iron clad" rhododendrons (often known as "hardy hybrids"), derived from *R. catawbiense*, *R. ponticum*, and *R. caucasicum* crosses. Evergreen rhododendrons vary in habit from small, cushion-forming shrubs to tree rhododendrons. They have small to large leaves and flowers in a variety of shapes, sizes, and colours.

Vireya rhododendrons

Sometimes known as Malesian rhododendrons, these are evergreen, usually epiphytic shrubs from tropical areas of S.E. Asia, and are frost tender. They have scaly leaves and stems. The flowers are extremely varied in shape, colour, and season; a range of plants will give flowers throughout the year. Grow in a cool greenhouse or conservatory. Containers will restrict the spread of larger plants.

Evergreen and deciduous azaleas

These are small to medium-leaved shrubs belonging to the botanical Section *Azalea* within the genus *Rhododendron*, and commonly known to gardeners as azaleas. They bear a profusion of small to large trusses of usually small flowers in a variety of shapes. Azalea hybrids may be further divided into the following subgroups:

***Deciduous hybrid azaleas* – Ghent (Gandavense) hybrids** are Belgian-raised, fully hardy azaleas, resulting from crosses between American azalea species and *R. luteum*. The funnel-shaped, white, yellow, orange, pink, or red flowers, borne in early summer, are long-tubed, sometimes double, and usually scented. **Knap Hill-Exbury hybrids** are English hybrid azaleas with complex origins (American azalea species x *R. molle*), characterized by large trusses of trumpet-shaped, scented or scentless flowers, in a wide range of bright colours, borne in mid- to late spring. **Mollis hybrids** have Dutch and Belgian origins, and are a result of crossing selections of *R. molle* subsp. *japonicum* and *R. molle*. Funnel-shaped, unscented flowers, in a wide range of colours, including cream, yellow, pink, orange, or red, are borne before the leaves in late spring. **New Zealand Ilam hybrids** are a further selection developed from Knap Hill-Exbury hybrids. **Occidentale hybrids** are English azaleas, raised by crossing Mollis hybrids with *R. occidentale*. Funnel-shaped, usually scented, pink or white flowers are borne in summer, later than those of Ghent hybrids. **Rustica (Rustica Flore Pleno) hybrids** are sweet-scented, double-flowered azaleas, resulting from crosses between double-flowered Ghent hybrids and *R. molle* subsp. *japonicum*. Funnel-shaped, hose-in-hose, yellow, cream, white, pink, or red flowers are borne in late spring and early summer on compact bushes.

***Evergreen hybrid azaleas* – Gable hybrids** are azaleas raised by Joseph B. Gable in Pennsylvania, USA, using mainly *R. kaempferi* and *R. yedoense* var. *poukhanense* with other species and hybrids. The unscented flowers are funnel-shaped, mostly pink, red, or white, and borne in late spring and early summer. **Glenn Dale hybrids** are varied, complex azaleas raised in Glenn Dale, Maryland, USA. The relatively large, scented, funnel-shaped flowers, usually white or pink to red, are borne from spring to early summer. Some are frilled, semi-double, or multicoloured. **Indian (Indica) hybrids** are complex azaleas, mostly of Belgian origin, bred from *R. simsii*, *R. mucronatum*, *R. indicum*, and other species. In winter, they produce large, funnel-shaped, unscented flowers in a wide range of colours, and are popular for growing indoors in containers for winter decoration. **Kaempferi hybrids** are Dutch azaleas raised from *R. kaempferi*, *R.* 'Malvaticum', and *R.* 'Maxwellii'. They are taller, more hardy, and later-flowering than Kurume hybrids (below), which are also derived from *R. kaempferi.* They bear funnel-shaped, unscented, white, pink, or red flowers in spring, on bushes about 1.2m (4ft) tall. **Kurume hybrids** are Japanese-raised dwarf azaleas, originating from crosses between *R. kaempferi*, *R. kiusianum*, and *R.* 'Obtusum'. Numerous, very small, funnel-shaped, unscented flowers are borne in a wide range of colours in spring. They are particularly effective in massed plantings. **Kyushu hybrids** are very hardy Japanese azaleas. They are the result of a complex breeding programme, using *R. kiusianum* with other dwarf species to produce low-growing, compact plants with small, shiny leaves. They are exceptionally hardy, to -30°C (-22°F), and ideal for cold climates. Small, funnel-shaped, unscented flowers, in a wide range of colours, are borne in spring. **Oldhamii hybrids** are dwarf azaleas raised at Exbury, England. The large, funnel-shaped flowers are unscented and borne in a wide range of colours in spring. **Satsuki hybrids** are Japanese-raised azaleas, originally used for bonsai work. They have been bred using mainly *R. indicum* and *R. simsii.* Half hardy with a low, twiggy habit, they bear large, funnel-shaped, unscented flowers in white, pink, red, or purple, in summer. They have a tendency to sport. **Shammarello hybrids** were raised by Shammarello in N. Ohio, USA. They are ideal for growing in very cold climates, and are hardy from -20 to -26°C (-10 to -20°F). Many have been raised by crossing *R.* 'Hino-crimson' with *R. yedoense* var. *poukhanense.* They have small, trumpet-shaped, unscented flowers in a range of colours, borne in late spring. **Vuyk (Vuykiana) hybrids** were bred by Vuyk van Nes Nurseries in Holland, using a complex cross of *R. kaempferi* and *R. mucronulatum*, and probably other species. They bear very showy, medium-sized, funnel-shaped, unscented flowers in a range of colours, in late spring.

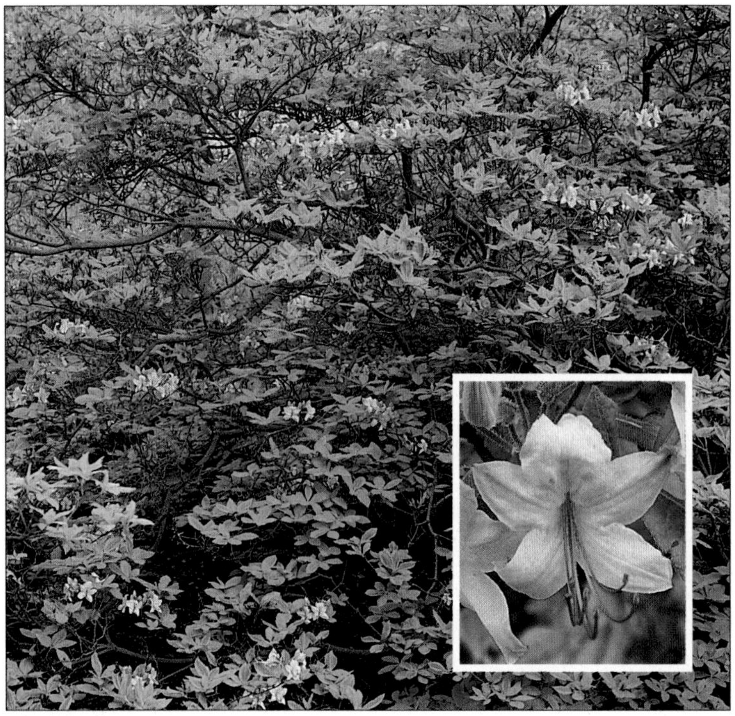

Rhododendron austrinum (inset: flower detail)

Azaleodendrons
This is a group of hybrids between deciduous azaleas and evergreen hybrid rhododendrons. They are generally fully hardy, semi-evergreen shrubs, 1–2.5m (3–8ft) tall, flowering in late spring and early summer. They produce cream, yellow, pink, or mauve flowers, some of which are fragrant.

• **HARDINESS** Fully hardy to frost tender.
• **CULTIVATION** Under glass, grow tender rhododendrons in lime-free (ericaceous) potting compost in bright filtered light with moderate to high humidity. When in growth, water freely with soft water and apply a balanced liquid fertilizer monthly; keep just moist in winter.

For Vireyas, use well-crocked containers and incorporate granulated bark, rotted bracken litter, or conifer needles to keep the compost open. Vireyas will tolerate a maximum day temperature of 32°C (90°F).

Indian hybrids grown as winter-flowering houseplants should be misted daily until the flower buds show colour; provide a maximum temperature of 13–16°C (55–61°F) when in bloom. Remove spent flowers and repot after flowering, then transfer to a cool greenhouse or window-sill in bright, indirect light. For the summer months, plunge pots in a shaded, well-ventilated cold frame and keep cool, moist, and humid; protect from any autumn frosts; bring plants indoors in early winter.

Outdoors, grow rhododendrons in moist but well-drained, leafy, humus-rich, acid soil (ideally pH4.5–5.5). Shallow planting is essential: all rhododendrons are surface-rooting and will not tolerate deep planting. Most large-leaved species and hybrids require dappled shade in sheltered woodland conditions; avoid the deep shade immediately beneath a tree canopy. Most of the other groups, including the "iron clads" and "hardy hybrids", thrive in light dappled shade or part-day shade, but not early morning sun; they will tolerate a more open site if given shelter from cold, dry winds. Most dwarf alpine species will tolerate full sun in cooler climates, provided the soil remains moist. Avoid frost pockets to reduce the risks of waterlogging and bark split. Mulch annually with leaf mould. After flowering, dead-head where practical, to promote vegetative growth rather than seed production. Pruning group 8.

• **PROPAGATION** Surface-sow seed at 13–18°C (55–64°F) in ericaceous (lime-free) propagating compost or fine moss peat, as soon as ripe or in early spring. Sow seed of hardy dwarf species and hybrids in containers in a cold frame as soon as ripe. Rhododendrons hybridize freely and garden-collected seed may not come true; however, seed collected from species in the wild or from hand-pollinated garden plants will generally produce plants that are true to type. Root semi-ripe cuttings in late summer. Layer in autumn. Graft in late winter or late summer.
• **PESTS AND DISEASES** Susceptible to vine weevil, rhododendron and azalea whiteflies, leafhoppers, lacebugs, scale insects, caterpillars, aphids, powdery mildew, bud blast, honey fungus, rust, leafy gall, petal blight, silver leaf, *Phytophthora* root rot, and lime-induced chlorosis (if soil is not sufficiently acid).

***R.* 'A. Bedford'** see *R.* 'Arthur Bedford'.
***R.* 'Addy Wery'** ♀ Evergreen Kurume azalea with small leaves. In mid- and late spring, bears an abundance of funnel-shaped, vermilion-red flowers, 4.5cm (1¾in) long, in small trusses. ↕↔ 1.2m (4ft). ❄❄❄
R. adenogynum ◐ syn. *R. adenophorum.* Evergreen shrub or small tree with elliptic or narrowly elliptic, dark green leaves, 6–11cm (2½–4½in) long; the undersides have a thick, tawny indumentum, yellowish brown at first, becoming olive-brown when mature. Trusses of 4–12 funnel-shaped, pink-tinged white flowers, 3–4.5cm (1¼–1¾in) long, spotted crimson inside, or each with a reddish pink mark, are borne in mid-spring. ↕↔ 2.5m (8ft). S.W. China. ❄❄❄
R. adenophorum see *R. adenogynum.*
R. albrechtii ▣ ♀ Twiggy, deciduous azalea with obovate, finely toothed, dark green leaves, 4–12cm (1½–5in) long, grey-downy beneath. Trusses of 3–5 widely bell-shaped, deep to purplish rose-pink flowers, 4–5cm (1½–2in) across, spotted olive-green inside, are borne in mid-spring. Tolerates full sun. ↕↔ 2.5m (8ft). Japan. ❄❄❄
***R.* 'Alison Johnstone'** ▣ Evergreen shrub producing small, elliptic leaves with a metallic lustre. In spring, bears loose trusses of pendent, tubular-bell-shaped, pale yellow flowers, 4cm (1½in) long, flushed peach-pink inside. Prefers a sunny, sheltered site. ↕↔ 2m (6ft). ❄❄❄
***R.* 'Angelo'.** Tall, evergreen shrub with an open habit and medium-sized to large leaves. Trusses of 9–10 funnel-shaped, fragrant, very pale pink or white flowers, 13cm (5in) long, open in late spring and early summer. ↕↔ 4m (12ft). ❄❄❄
***R.* 'Anna Baldsiefen'** ♀ Dwarf, compact, evergreen shrub of upright habit, with small, oblong-ovate leaves, turning bronze-red in winter. In early spring, bears dense trusses of numerous funnel-shaped, bright pink flowers, 3cm (1¼in) long, with deeper pink margins. ↕↔ 1m (3ft). ❄❄❄
***R.* 'Anna Rose Whitney'** ♀ Evergreen shrub with large leaves. In late spring, bears loose, rounded trusses of widely funnel-shaped, deep rose-pink flowers, 6–10cm (2½–4in) across, spotted brown inside. ↕↔ 4m (12ft). ❄❄❄
R. arboreum ▣ ◐ Evergreen tree producing inversely lance-shaped, dark green leaves, 7–19cm (3–7in) long, with a silvery, fawn, or cinnamon-brown indumentum beneath. Dense trusses of tubular-bell-shaped, red, pink, or white flowers, 3–5cm (1¼–2in) long, with black nectar pouches and black spots inside, are borne in early spring. ↕ 12m (40ft), ↔ 4m (12ft). China to Thailand, N. India, Bhutan, Sri Lanka. ❄❄
***R.* 'Arctic Tern'** see x *Ledodendron* 'Arctic Tern'.
R. argyrophyllum ▣ Evergreen shrub with oblong to lance-shaped, dark green leaves, 3–6cm (1¼–2½in) long, with grey-white hairs beneath. In mid- and late spring, bears lax trusses of funnel- to bell-shaped, mid- to pale pink flowers, 3–6cm (1¼–2½in) long, spotted deep pink inside. ↕ 6m (20ft), ↔ 2.5m (8ft). S.W. China. ❄❄❄
R. arizelum see *R. rex* subsp. *arizelum.*
***R.* 'Arthur Bedford'**, syn. *R.* 'A. Bedford'. Vigorous, evergreen shrub with large leaves. In early summer, bears pyramid-shaped trusses of funnel-shaped, light mauve flowers, 5–9cm (2–3½in) long, each with a deep brown-red flare in the throat. Tolerant of sun. ↕↔ 3m (10ft). ❄❄❄
R. augustinii ▣ ◐ Bushy, evergreen shrub or small tree producing oblong to lance-shaped, mid- to dark green leaves, 4–11cm (1½–4½in) long. Trusses of 2–5 broadly funnel-shaped, pale to deep blue or lavender-blue flowers, to 7cm (3in) across, spotted greenish brown inside, open in mid-spring. Will grow in full sun. ↕↔ 2.2m (7ft). China. ❄❄❄
R. auriculatum ◐ Multi-stemmed, spreading, evergreen shrub or small tree producing oblong to lance-shaped, dark green leaves, 15–30cm (6–12in) long, with ear-like lobes at their bases. In late summer, bears loose trusses of funnel-shaped, 7-lobed, very fragrant white flowers, 8–11cm (3–4½in) long, tinted green inside. ↕ to 10m (30ft), ↔ 5m (15ft). W. China. ❄❄❄
R. austrinum ▣ ♀ syn. *R. prinophyllum.* Deciduous azalea with elliptic-obovate, dark green leaves, 3–9cm (1¼–3½in) long, sparsely hairy above, glaucous, grey-green and more hairy beneath. Trusses of 5–9 tubular-funnel-shaped, pale to deep pink flowers, 3.5cm (1½in) long, are borne in late spring. Will tolerate full sun. ↕↔ 3m (10ft). USA (Florida to Mississippi). ❄❄❄
***R.* 'Azor'.** Vigorous, evergreen shrub of open habit, with medium-sized leaves. In midsummer, bears loose trusses of funnel-shaped, fragrant, salmon-pink flowers, 6–9cm (2½–3½in) long, spotted red-brown inside. ↕↔ 4m (12ft). ❄❄❄
***R.* 'Azuma-kagami'** ▣ ♀ Compact, evergreen Kurume azalea with small leaves. In mid-spring, bears numerous small trusses of hose-in-hose, bright pink flowers, 3cm (1¼in) long. ↕↔ 1.2m (4ft). ❄❄❄
R. bakeri see *R. calendulaceum.*
R. barbatum ◐ Multi-stemmed, tall, evergreen shrub or small tree with bristly

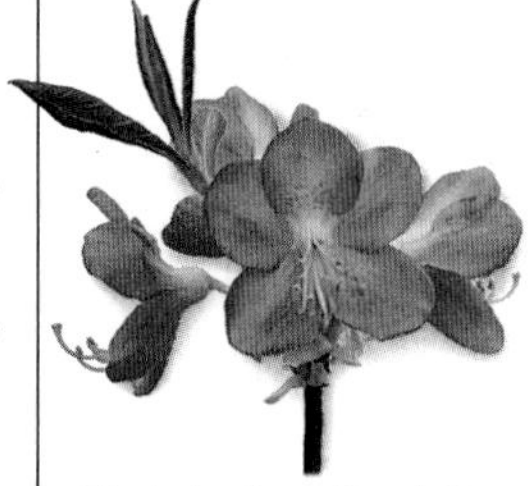

Rhododendron albrechtii

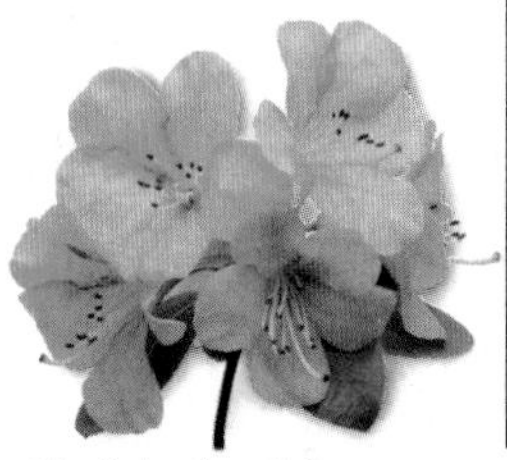

Rhododendron 'Alison Johnstone'

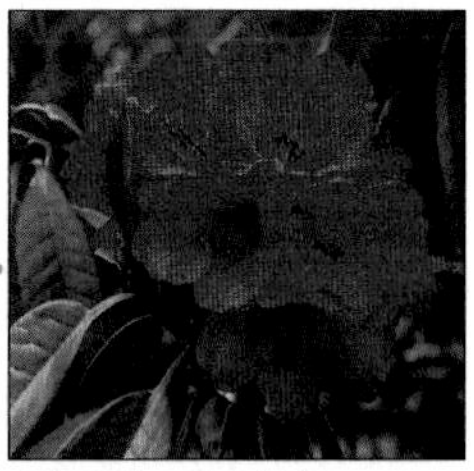

Rhododendron arboreum

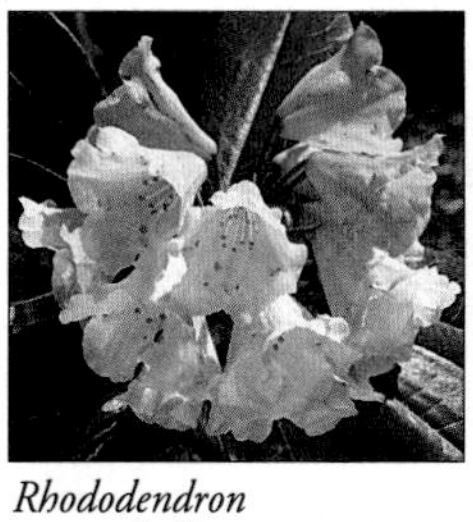

Rhododendron argyrophyllum

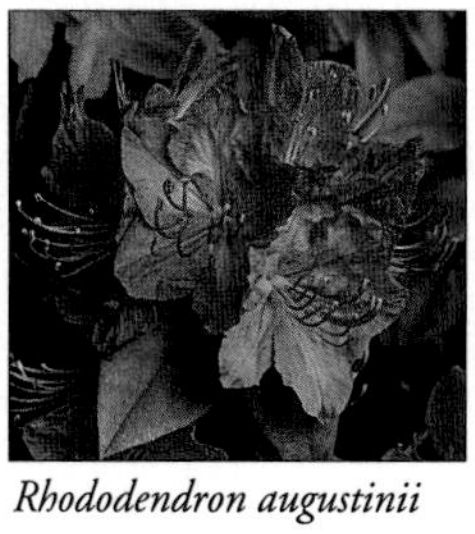

Rhododendron augustinii

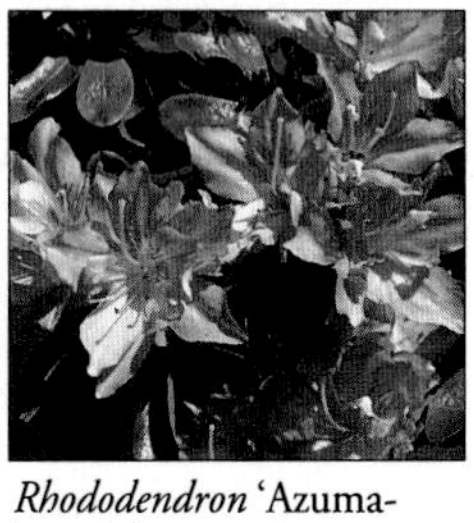

Rhododendron 'Azuma-kagami'

leaf-stalks and young stems, and peeling, reddish purple bark. Produces elliptic to obovate, dark green leaves, 9–19cm (3½–7in) long. Tight trusses of tubular to bell-shaped, bright scarlet flowers, 3.5–5cm (1½–2in) long, with crimson-black nectar pouches inside, are borne in early spring. ↕↔ 6m (20ft). Himalayas. ❄❄❄

***R.* 'Beauty of Littleworth'** ▣ ♡ Vigorous, showy, evergreen shrub with large leaves. In late spring, bears cone-shaped trusses of funnel-shaped, fragrant white flowers, 10–15cm (4–6in) long, spotted crimson inside. Only suitable for dappled shade. ↕↔ 4m (12ft). ❄❄❄

***R.* 'Beethoven'** ▣ ♡ Dwarf, evergreen Vuyk azalea with small leaves. In late spring, bears lax trusses of funnel-shaped, fringe-petalled, magenta-pink flowers, 5cm (2in) long, each with a deeper mauve mark inside. ↕↔ 1.3m (4½ft). ❄❄❄

***R.* 'Berryrose'** ♡ Mound-forming, evergreen shrub with sparse, medium-sized leaves. Compact trusses of tubular-funnel-shaped, bright apricot-orange flowers, 10cm (4in) long, are borne in late spring. ↕↔ 1.5m (5ft). ❄❄❄

***R.* 'Blue Diamond'** ▣ Dwarf, small-leaved, evergreen shrub with a compact, upright habit. In mid- and late spring, bears trusses of up to 5 funnel-shaped, violet-blue flowers, 5cm (2in) long. Prefers full sun. ↕↔ 1.5m (5ft). ❄❄❄

***R.* 'Blue Peter'** ▣ ♡ Large-leaved, evergreen shrub of open habit. In early summer, bears tight, rounded trusses of funnel-shaped, lavender-blue flowers, 7cm (3in) long, with frilled petals and purple marks inside. Tolerates full sun. ↕↔ 3m (10ft). ❄❄❄

***R.* 'Blue Tit'.** Dwarf, compact, evergreen shrub with small leaves that are a distinctive yellowish green when young, mid-green when mature. Trusses of 2 or 3 funnel-shaped, grey-blue flowers, 0.7–2.5cm (¼–1in) long, are borne at the tips of the shoots in early and mid-spring. Suitable for a rock garden in full sun. ↕↔ 1m (3ft). ❄❄❄

***R.* 'Bow Bells'** ♡ Free-flowering, compact, evergreen shrub with small to medium-sized, broadly ovate to rounded leaves, reddish bronze when young, mid-green when mature. In late spring, bears lax trusses of long-stalked, bell-shaped, light pink flowers, 5–6cm (2–2½in) long. ↕↔ 2m (6ft). ❄❄❄

R. brachysiphon see *R. maddenii.*

***R.* 'Britannia'** ♡ Low but relatively broad, evergreen shrub with medium-sized, pale green leaves. Dense trusses of bell-shaped, bright scarlet flowers, 5–7cm (2–3in) long, are borne in early summer. ↕ 1.5m (5ft), ↔ 2.2m (7ft). ❄❄❄

R. bullatum see *R. edgeworthii.*

R. bureaui see *R. bureavii.*

R. bureavii ▣ ♡ syn. *R. bureaui.* Multi-stemmed, evergreen shrub producing ovate to lance-shaped, dark green leaves, 4.5–12cm (1¾–5in) long, initially covered with a light brown indumentum above and a woolly, bright orange-brown indumentum beneath. In mid-spring, bears neat trusses of tubular-bell-shaped, white or soft pink, crimson-spotted flowers, 2.5–4cm (1–1½in) long. ↕↔ 3m (10ft). S.W. China. ❄❄❄

R. calendulaceum, syn. *R. bakeri.* Robust, deciduous azalea with elliptic-oblong, mid-green leaves, 3.5–9cm (1½–3½in) long, softly hairy on both sides. In late spring and early summer, bears lax trusses of funnel-shaped, bright orange to scarlet flowers, to 5cm (2in) long, usually opening with the leaves, or just after they emerge. Prefers full sun. ↕↔ 2.5m (8ft). E. USA. ❄❄❄

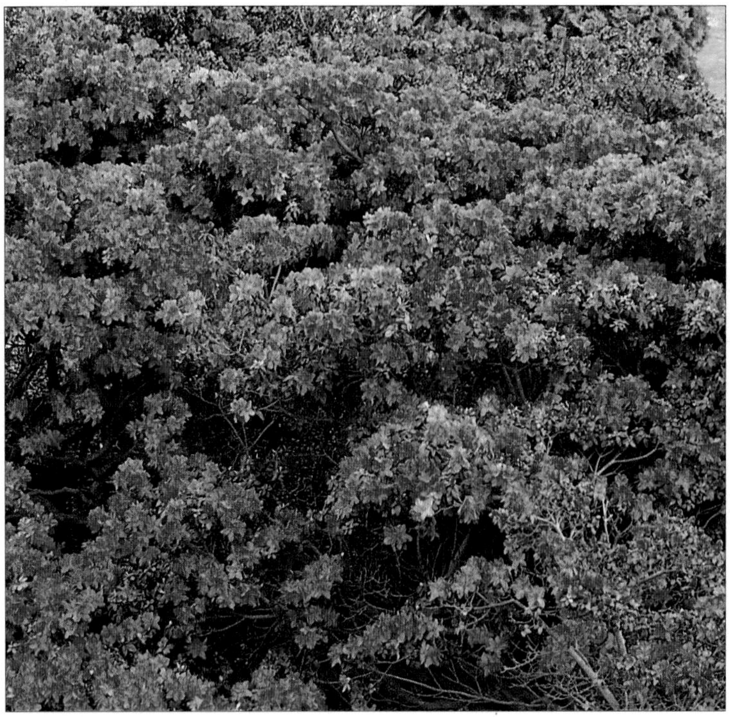

Rhododendron 'Blue Diamond'

R. calophytum ▣ ♡ ◌ Many-stemmed, evergreen shrub or small tree with oblong to inversely lance-shaped, dark green leaves, 14–30cm (5½–12in) long. In early spring, bears large trusses of broadly bell-shaped, 5- to 7-lobed, fragrant, pale pink flowers, to 7cm (3in) across, with basal, carmine-red marks in the throats. ↕ 10m (30ft), ↔ 6m (20ft). S.W. China, Tibet. ❄❄❄

R. calostrotum ▣ Compact, dwarf, evergreen shrub with oblong-ovate to rounded leaves, 1–3cm (½–1¼in) long, scaly and glaucous above, with dense brown scales beneath. In late spring and early summer, freely bears solitary or pairs of saucer-shaped, bright rose-purple flowers, 2–4cm (¾–1½in) across, often with purple spots on the upper lobes. Tolerates full sun if kept moist. ↕ 75cm (30in), ↔ 90cm (36in). N.E. India, Tibet, W. China. ❄❄❄. **subsp. *keleticum*** ♡ syn. *R. keleticum,* is almost prostrate, with glossy, dark green leaves, 2–9mm ($^{1}/_{16}$–⅜in) long, densely brown-scaly beneath. Bears trusses of up to 3 widely funnel-shaped, purplish crimson flowers, crimson-spotted inside; ↕ 30cm (12in), ↔ 90cm (36in). S.E. Tibet, S.W. China, N.E. Burma.

R. campanulatum ▣ ◌ Vigorous, evergreen shrub or small tree producing oblong-elliptic, dark green leaves, 7–14cm (3–5½in) long, with a dense, suede-like brown indumentum beneath. In mid-spring, bears trusses of 8–15 broadly bell-shaped, lilac-blue, sometimes white flowers, 5cm (2in) across, with darker spots inside. ↕↔ 4m (12ft). Himalayas. ❄❄❄

R. campylocarpum ▣ ◌ Robust, evergreen shrub or small tree with neat, elliptic-ovate, dark green leaves, 3–10cm (1¼–4in) long, pale grey-green beneath. Trusses of 3–15 delicate, bell-shaped, pale to mid-yellow flowers, 2.5–4cm (1–1½in) long, are borne in mid-spring. Some variants have deep red basal marks inside. ↕ to 5m (15ft), ↔ 4m (12ft). S.E. Tibet, S.W. China, N.E. Burma. ❄❄❄

R. campylogynum. Dwarf, compact, evergreen shrub with inversely lance-shaped leaves, 1–3.5cm (½–1½in) long, glossy, dark green above, often off-white or silver beneath. In late spring, bears small trusses of long-stemmed, nodding, broadly bell-shaped flowers, 1–2.5cm (½–1in) long, varying in colour from white or pink to purple or purplish black. Suitable for growing in a rock garden in full sun. ↕↔ 75cm (30in). E. India (Arunachal Pradesh), Tibet, W. China, N.E. Burma. ❄❄❄

R. camtschaticum. Deciduous shrub with an unusual, dwarf, procumbent habit and obovate, hairy-margined, mid-green leaves, 2–5cm (¾–2in) long, on hairy shoots. Saucer-shaped, reddish purple or pink flowers, 2.5cm (1in) across, each with a leafy calyx, are borne singly or in pairs in late spring and early summer. ↕ to 30cm (12in), ↔ 90cm (36in). E. Asia, Alaska. ❄❄❄

***R.* 'Carita'** ▣ Neat, evergreen shrub, becoming more open with age, with medium-sized leaves. In mid-spring, bears flat-topped trusses of funnel-shaped flowers, 5cm (2in) long, pale pink to pale lemon yellow, each with a small, cerise-red, basal flash in the throat. ↕↔ 2.5m (8ft). ❄❄❄

***R.* 'Carmen'** ♡ Dwarf, evergreen shrub with small, dark green leaves. Loose trusses of 2–5 tubular-bell-shaped, waxy, dark red flowers, 3–6cm (1¼–2½in) long, are produced in mid-spring. ↕ 1m (3ft), ↔ 1.2m (4ft). ❄❄❄

R. carolinianum see *R. minus.*

R. catawbiense. Evergreen shrub with oblong-ovate, glossy, dark green leaves, 7–15cm (3–6in) long, paler beneath. Large trusses of funnel-bell-shaped, reddish purple flowers, 3–4.5cm (1¼–1¾in) long, are produced in late spring and early summer. Thrives in full sun; very hardy. ↕↔ 3m (10ft). E. North America. ❄❄❄

***R.* 'Catawbiense Album'.** Vigorous, shrubby, evergreen "iron clad" rhododendron with medium-sized leaves. In early summer, pale lilac buds open to conical trusses of bell-shaped white flowers, 6–8cm (2½–3in) long, with green flashes in the throats. Tolerates sun and wind. ↕↔ 3m (10ft). ❄❄❄

***R.* 'Cécile'** ▣ ♡ Vigorous, deciduous Knap Hill-Exbury azalea with medium-sized leaves. In late spring, dark salmon-pink buds open to dense, rounded trusses of tubular-funnel-shaped, clear salmon-pink flowers, 5cm (2in) long, with yellow flares in the throats. ↕↔ 2.2m (7ft). ❄❄❄

***R.* 'Chikor'.** Dwarf, evergreen shrub with a neat habit and small, dark green leaves, bronze-tinted in winter. Trusses of 3–6 saucer-shaped, clear yellow flowers, 3cm (1¼in) across, are borne in mid-spring. ↕↔ 60cm (24in). ❄❄❄

***R.* 'Chionoides'.** Dense, evergreen shrub with medium-sized leaves. In mid- and late spring, bears dense trusses of funnel-shaped, pure white flowers, 5cm (2in) long, each with a conspicuous yellow flare on the inside of the upper lobe. Tolerant of wind, sun, and heat. ↕↔ 2m (6ft). ❄❄❄

***R.* 'Christmas Cheer'** ♡ Dense, compact, evergreen shrub with medium-sized leaves. Numerous trusses of funnel-shaped, whitish pink flowers, 4.5cm (1¾in) long, open in late winter and early spring. ↕↔ 2m (6ft). ❄❄❄

R. ciliatum ♡ Semi-dwarf, compact, evergreen shrub with oblong-elliptic leaves, 4.5–9cm (1¾–3½in) long, dark green above, paler green beneath, and with hairy margins. Small trusses of 2–4 tubular-bell-shaped, pinkish white flowers, 2–3cm (¾–1¼in) long, open in early and mid-spring. Tolerates full sun. ↕↔ 2m (6ft). E. Himalayas. ❄❄

***R.* 'Cilpinense'** ▣ ♡ Showy, compact, small-leaved, evergreen shrub. In early spring, bears profuse trusses of up to 3 funnel-shaped, pale to mid-pink flowers, 4.5–5cm (1¾–2in) long. Flowers are vulnerable to early frosts. ↕↔ 1.1m (3½ft). ❄❄❄

R. cinnabarinum ▣ Vigorous, erect, evergreen shrub producing neat, aromatic, elliptic-obovate, hairless, dark green leaves, 3–9cm (1¼–3½in) long, with a metallic grey-green sheen above, scaly beneath. Loose trusses of pendent, narrowly tubular-bell-shaped, waxy, red, sometimes yellow, orange, apricot-pink, or reddish purple flowers, 2.5–3.5cm (1–1½in) long, are borne from mid-spring to early summer. ↕ 6m (20ft), ↔ 2m (6ft). Himalayas to N. Burma. ❄❄❄. **subsp. *xanthocodon*** ▣ ♡ syn. *R. xanthocodon,* bears trusses of 5–10 rich yellow flowers. E. India, Bhutan, Tibet, China.

***R.* 'Cinnkeys'.** Erect, evergreen shrub with medium-sized, narrowly oblong, glossy leaves. In mid- and late spring, bears multiple trusses of narrowly tubular flowers, 4cm (1½in) long, with clear red tubes and yellow lobes with a light, waxy bloom. ↕↔ 2.2m (7ft). ❄❄❄

***R.* 'Coccineum Speciosum'** ♡ Bushy, deciduous Ghent azalea with small, dark green leaves, turning yellow or orange in autumn. In early summer, bears lax trusses of funnel-shaped, fragrant, rich

R

orange-red flowers, to 5cm (2in) long. ↕↔ 2m (6ft). ❄❄❄

***R.* 'Corneille'** ▣ 🏆 Deciduous, tall-growing Ghent azalea of open habit, with small leaves. Domed trusses of open trumpet-shaped, honeysuckle-like, fragrant cream flowers, 4cm (1½in) long, strongly suffused pink on the outside, are borne in early summer. ↕↔ 1.5–2.5m (5–8ft). ❄❄❄

***R.* 'Cottage Garden's Pride'** see *R.* 'Mrs. G.W. Leak'.

***R.* 'Crest'** ▣ 🏆 syn. *R.* 'Hawk Crest'. Evergreen shrub of open habit, with medium-sized leaves. In mid-spring, orange-yellow buds open to trusses of up to 12 long-lasting, broadly funnel-shaped, primrose-yellow flowers, 10cm (4in) long. ↕↔ 3.5m (11ft). ❄❄❄

R. cubittii ▣ Evergreen shrub with purple-brown young shoots and oblong-elliptic, leathery, sparsely scaly, mid- to dark green leaves, to 10cm (4in) long. In mid- and late spring, bears funnel-shaped, white to pale pink flowers, to 10cm (4in) long, with brownish or orange-yellow markings. ↕ 1.5m (5ft), ↔ to 1m (3ft). N. Burma. ❄

***R.* 'Cunningham's White'.** Compact, evergreen shrub with medium-sized leaves. In late spring, mauve buds open to lax trusses of funnel-shaped white flowers, 5–6cm (2–2½in) long, with yellow to green-brown markings inside. ↕↔ 2.2m (7ft). ❄❄❄

***R.* 'Curlew'** 🏆 Dwarf, spreading, small-leaved, evergreen shrub. In mid-spring, bears numerous trusses of 2 or 3 broadly funnel-shaped, bright yellow flowers, 5cm (2in) across, spotted greenish brown inside. ↕↔ 60cm (24in). ❄❄❄

***R.* 'Cynthia'** ▣ 🏆 syn. *R.* 'Lord Palmerston'. Large, evergreen shrub with large leaves. In late spring, bears pyramidal trusses of funnel-shaped, deep rose-pink to magenta flowers, 8cm (3in) long, with deep crimson markings on the insides of the upper lobes. Grows well in sun. ↕↔ 6m (20ft). ❄❄❄

R. dauricum. Deciduous or semi-evergreen shrub with small, elliptic, leathery, glossy, dark green leaves, 1–3.5cm (½–1½in) long, scaly beneath, turning purple-brown in winter. In mid- and late winter, bears small trusses of funnel-shaped, vivid rose-purple flowers, 1.5–2cm (½–¾in) long. Very hardy; suitable for an open site. ↕↔ 1.5m (5ft). E. Asia. ❄❄❄

R. davidsonianum ▣ 🏆 Vigorous, evergreen shrub producing lance-shaped to oblong-lance-shaped, glossy, dark green leaves, 3–7cm (1¼–3in) long, densely brown-scaly beneath. In mid-spring, bears trusses of 2–6 broadly funnel-shaped, pale pink to purplish pink flowers, to 4.5cm (1¾in) across, sometimes spotted red inside. Grow in full sun or partial shade. ↕ to 4m (12ft), ↔ 3m (10ft). W. China. ❄❄❄

***R.* 'Daviesii'** 🏆 Compact, deciduous Ghent azalea with small leaves. In late spring and early summer, bears lax trusses of tubular to funnel-shaped, fragrant white flowers, to 7cm (3in) long, with yellow flares inside. ↕↔ 1.5m (5ft). ❄❄❄

R. decorum ▣ ○ Large shrub or small tree with rough, fissured bark and oblong-ovate, dark green leaves, 6–20cm (2½–8in) long, glaucous beneath. In late spring and early summer, bears trusses of 7–10 funnel- to bell-shaped, 6- or 7-lobed, strongly scented white flowers, 4.5–11cm (1¾–4½in) long, sometimes faintly tinged pink, often with greenish yellow bases. ↕ 6m (20ft), ↔ 2.5m (8ft). China. ❄❄❄

R. degronianum* subsp. *heptamerum see *R. metternichii.*

R. degronianum* subsp. *yakushimanum see *R. yakushimanum.*

R. dichroanthum. Compact, evergreen shrub producing obovate to inversely lance-shaped, dark green leaves, 4–4.5cm (1½–1¾in) long, with a thin, pale fawn indumentum beneath. In late spring and early summer, bears trusses of 4–8 fleshy, tubular to bell-shaped, yellow to orange or orange-red flowers, 3.5–5cm (1½–2in) long. Grows well in full sun. ↕ to 2m (6ft), ↔ 2.2m (7ft). N.E. Burma, W. China. ❄❄❄

R. discolor see *R. fortunei* subsp. *discolor.*

***R.* 'Doc'** ▣ 🏆 Small, compact, evergreen shrub with medium-sized leaves. In late spring, bears rounded trusses of funnel-shaped, wavy-margined, rose-pink flowers, 4cm (1½in) long, with deeper pink margins and spots, fading to white. ↕↔ 1.2m (4ft). ❄❄❄

***R.* 'Doncaster'.** Evergreen shrub with distinctive, concave, wavy-margined, medium-sized leaves. Full, dense trusses of funnel-shaped, dark red flowers, to 8cm (3in) long, each with a black-spotted flare inside, are borne in mid- and late spring. ↕↔ 2.2m (7ft). ❄❄❄

***R.* 'Dopey'** 🏆 Upright, compact, evergreen shrub with medium-sized leaves. In late spring, bears neat, full trusses of long-lasting, bell-shaped, glossy red flowers, 5–7cm (2–3in) long, with dark brown spots inside, paler towards the margins. ↕↔ 2m (6ft). ❄❄❄

***R.* 'Dora Amateis'** ▣ 🏆 Reliable, semi-dwarf, compact, evergreen shrub with small leaves. In spring, bears lax trusses of 6–8 broadly funnel-shaped white flowers, 2–3cm (¾–1¼in) long, the insides flushed pink with small green flecks. ↕↔ 60cm (24in). ❄❄❄

***R.* 'Dr. Herman Sleumer'.** Evergreen Vireya rhododendron with medium-sized leaves. Intermittently bears trusses of 5 or 6 bell-shaped pink flowers, 4–6cm (1½–2½in) long, with cream throats, from winter to summer. ↕ 1.2m (4ft), ↔ 1m (3ft). ❀ (min. 5°C/41°F)

R. edgeworthii 🏆 syn. *R. bullatum.* Evergreen, epiphytic shrub with elliptic to ovate, wrinkled, dark green leaves, 5–10cm (2–4in) long; the shoots and undersides of the leaves have a thick, tawny indumentum. In mid-spring, bears trusses of 2 or 3 broadly funnel-shaped, strongly scented flowers, 6–15cm (2½–6in) across, white to pale pink or pink, flushed deep red outside. ↕↔ 2.5m (8ft). E. Himalayas. ❄❄

***R.* 'Edmund de Rothschild'.** Vigorous, upright, leggy, evergreen shrub with medium-sized leaves. In early summer, bears dense trusses of 20 or more funnel-shaped, deep red flowers, 9cm (3½in) long, heavily spotted darker red inside. ↕↔ 3m (10ft). ❄❄❄

***R.* 'Elisabeth Hobbie'** 🏆 Dense, compact, semi-dwarf, evergreen shrub with medium-sized, rounded leaves. In early and mid-spring, produces lax trusses of 6–10 narrowly funnel-shaped, scarlet-red flowers, 6cm (2½in) long, faintly spotted darker red inside. ↕↔ 75cm (30in). ❄❄❄

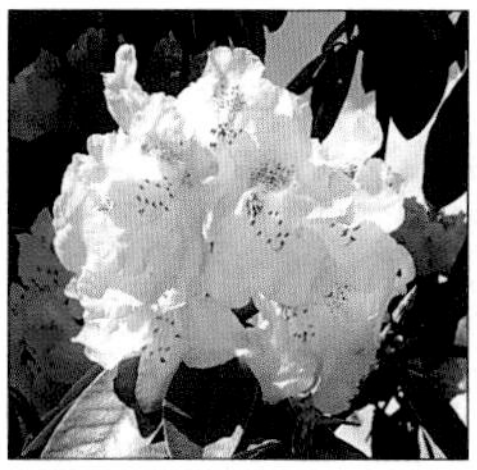

Rhododendron 'Beauty of Littleworth'

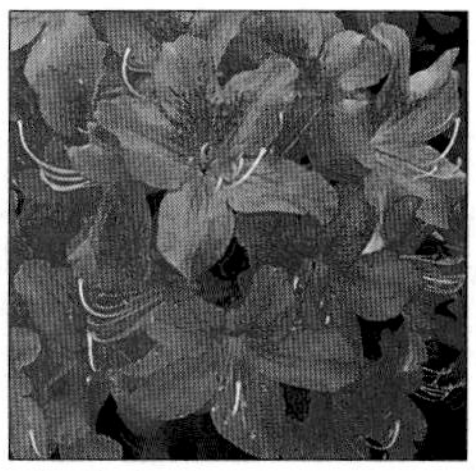

Rhododendron 'Beethoven'

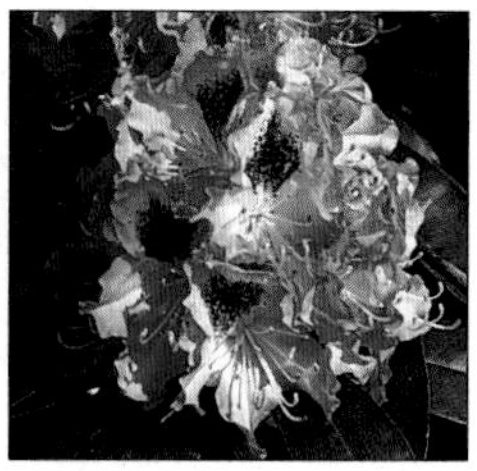

Rhododendron 'Blue Peter'

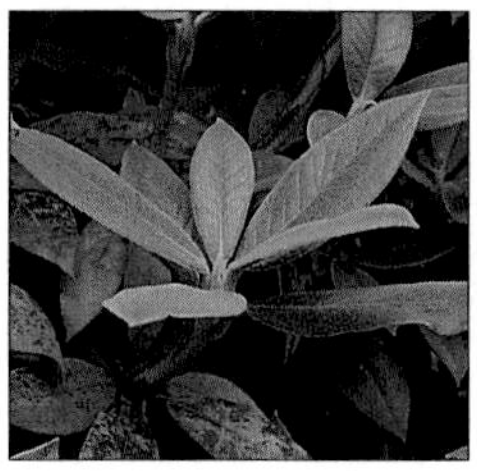

Rhododendron bureavii

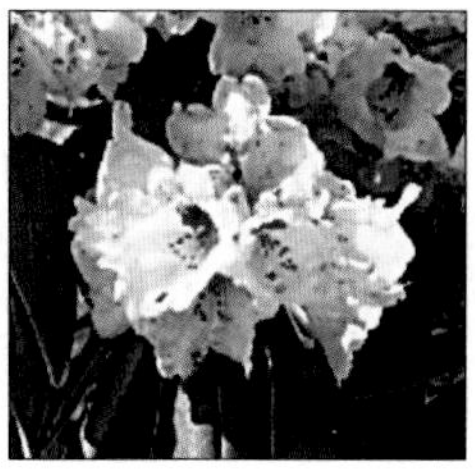

Rhododendron calophytum

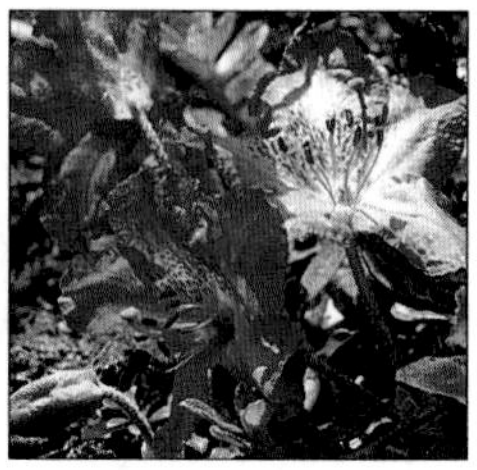

Rhododendron calostrotum

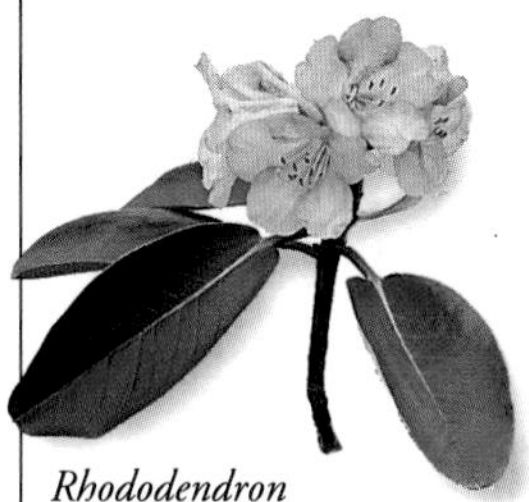

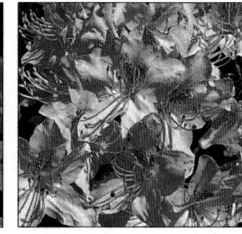

Rhododendron campanulatum

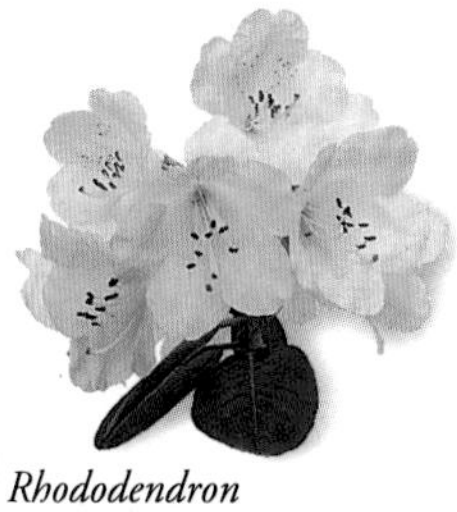

Rhododendron campylocarpum

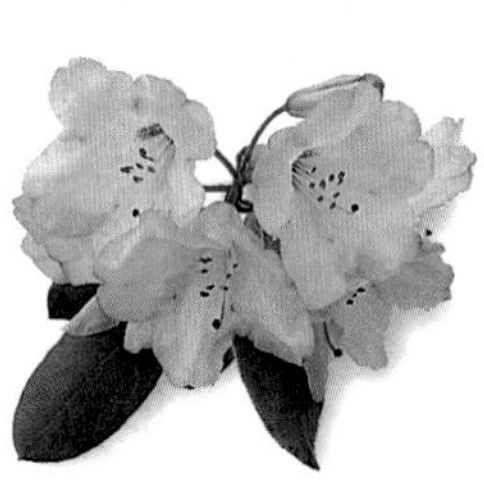

Rhododendron 'Carita'

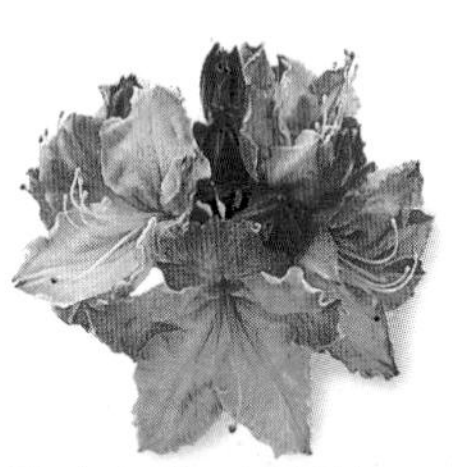

Rhododendron 'Cécile'

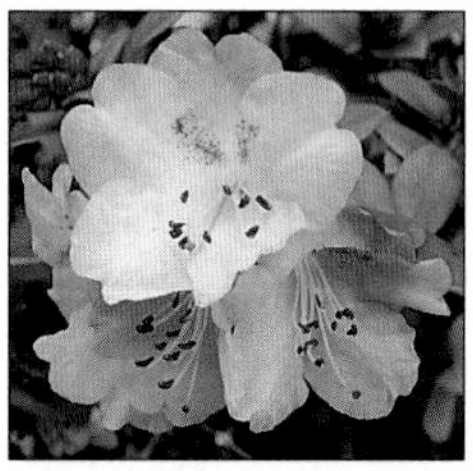

Rhododendron 'Cilpinense'

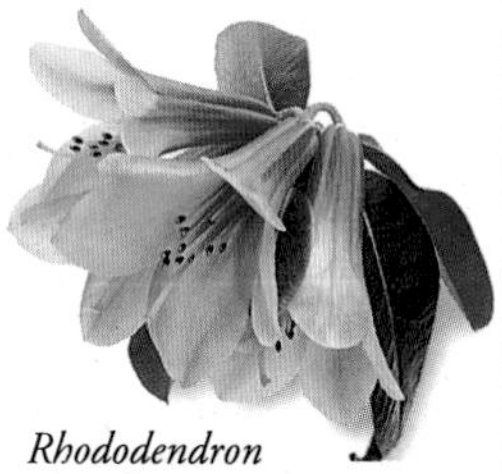

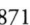

Rhododendron cinnabarinum

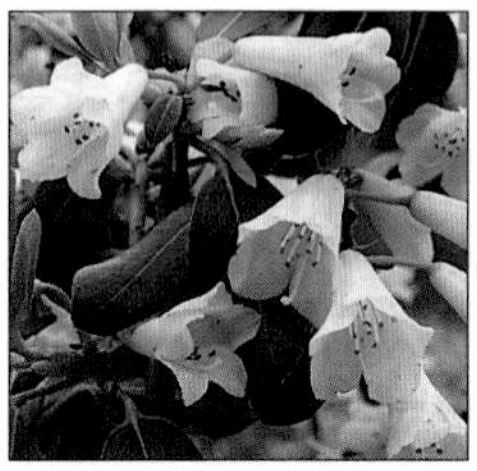

Rhododendron cinnabarinum subsp. *xanthocodon*

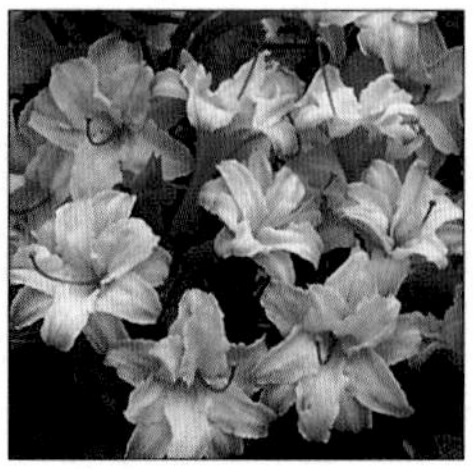

Rhododendron 'Corneille'

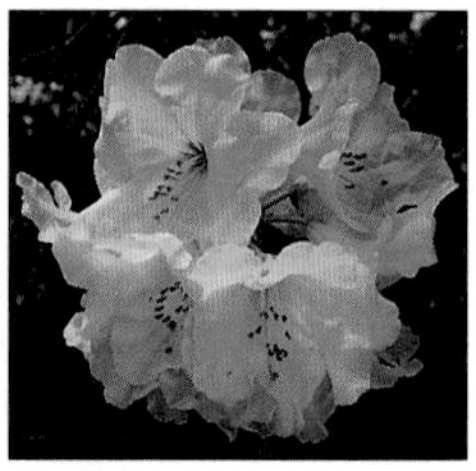

Rhododendron 'Crest'

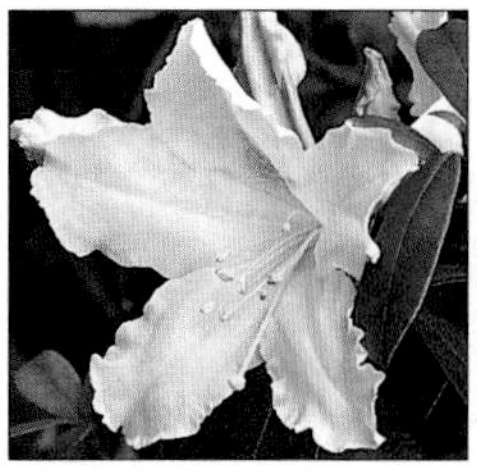

Rhododendron cubittii

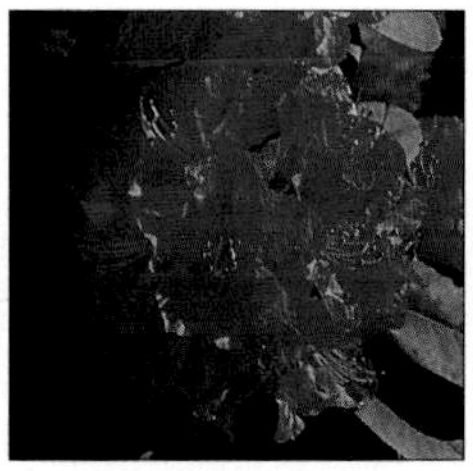

Rhododendron 'Cynthia'

Rhododendron davidsonianum

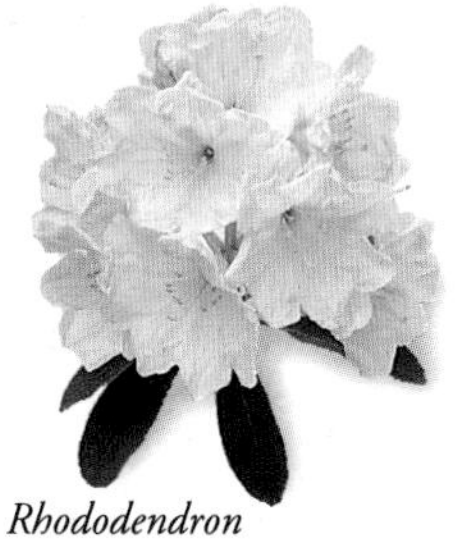

Rhododendron decorum

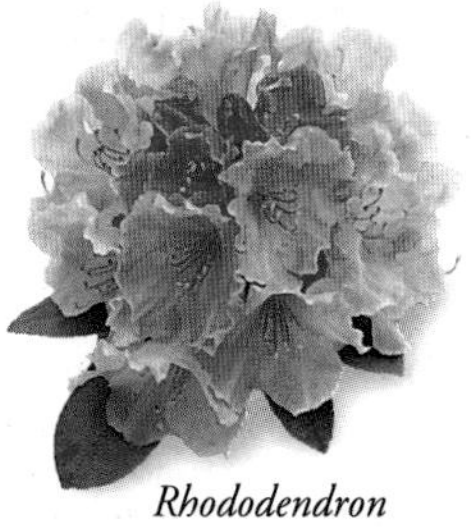

Rhododendron 'Doc'

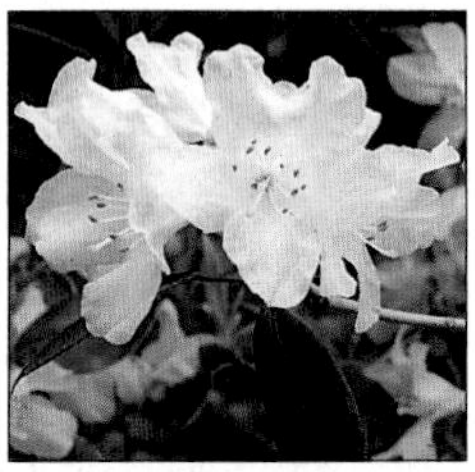

Rhododendron 'Dora Amateis'

R

***R.* 'Elizabeth'** ■ Compact, dwarf, evergreen shrub with small leaves. In spring, bears trusses of up to 5 funnel-shaped, bright red flowers, 6–8cm (2½–3in) long, in such abundance that they may almost hide the foliage. Suitable for sun. ↕↔ 1m (3ft). ❄❄❄

***R.* 'Elizabeth Lockhart'.** Compact, semi-dwarf, evergreen shrub with small, rounded, shiny, deep maroon-purple leaves. In mid-spring, bears loose trusses of bell-shaped, cherry-red flowers, 5cm (2in) long. Remove any growth that reverts to green. ↕↔ 1m (3ft). ❄❄❄

***R.* 'Elsie Lee'.** Dwarf, evergreen Shammarello azalea with small leaves. In late spring, bears numerous small trusses of broadly funnel-shaped, semi-double, light reddish-purple flowers, 5–7cm (2–3in) across. Suitable for full sun and exposed sites. Very hardy. ↕↔ 1m (3ft). ❄❄❄

R. eriogynum see *R. facetum*.

***R.* 'Fabia'** ■ ♀ Evergreen shrub with medium-sized leaves. Loose trusses of long-lasting, funnel-shaped, orange-red flowers, to 7cm (3in) long, marked pale brown inside, are borne in late spring. ↕↔ 2m (6ft). ❄❄

R. facetum ♢ syn. *R. eriogynum*. Evergreen shrub or small tree with a woolly white indumentum on young shoots. Oblong-elliptic to inversely lance-shaped leaves, 10–19cm (4–7in) long, are matt, mid-green above, glossy beneath. In early summer, produces trusses of 8–16 tubular-bell-shaped, bright scarlet flowers, 4–5cm (1½–2in) long, with deep purple nectar pouches. ↕ 10m (30ft), ↔ 2.5m (8ft). Burma, China. ❄❄

R. falconeri ■ ♀ ♢ Multi-stemmed, evergreen tree with flaking, red-brown bark. Broadly elliptic to obovate, dark green leaves, 18–35cm (7–14in) long, have a dense, woolly brown indumentum beneath and on the leaf-stalks. In mid-spring, bears large trusses of 20–25 widely bell-shaped, fleshy, creamy white or yellow flowers, 4–5cm (1½–2in) long, sometimes pink-tinged, often with purple marks inside. ↕ to 12m (40ft), ↔ 5m (15ft). E. Himalayas. ❄❄❄

R. fastigiatum. Compact, dwarf, alpine rhododendron with broadly elliptic to ovate-oblong, glaucous, mid-green leaves, 0.5–1.5cm (¼–½in) long, with tan scales beneath. Abundant trusses of up to 5 funnel-shaped, purplish blue flowers, 1–2cm (½–¾in) long, are borne in mid-spring. Suitable for full sun. ↕↔ 1m (3ft). W. China. ❄❄❄

***R.* 'Fastuosum Flore Pleno'** ■ ♀ Dome-shaped, shrubby, "iron clad" rhododendron with medium-sized leaves. Long-lasting trusses of funnel-shaped, wavy-margined, double mauve flowers, 5–7cm (2–3in) long, with brown-crimson flashes inside, are borne in late spring and early summer. ↕↔ 4m (12ft). ❄❄❄

R. ferrugineum (Alpenrose). Compact, evergreen shrub producing narrowly to broadly elliptic, glossy, dark green leaves, 2–4cm (1–1½in) long, the leaf-stalks and undersides covered in red-brown scales. In early summer, bears trusses of 6–8 tubular, rose-pink to crimson, occasionally white flowers, 1.5cm (½in) long, with spreading lobes. Prefers full sun. ↕ to 1.5m (5ft), ↔ 1.2m (4ft). C. Europe. ❄❄❄

R. fictolacteum see *R. rex* subsp. *fictolacteum*.

***R.* 'Firefly'** see *R.* 'Hexe'.

R. forrestii. Prostrate, creeping, evergreen shrub with neat, broadly obovate to rounded, glossy, dark green leaves, 1–3cm (½–1¼in) long, purple beneath. Tubular to bell-shaped, fleshy scarlet flowers, 3–3.5cm (1¼–1½in) long, with dark carmine-red nectar pouches, are borne singly or in pairs in mid-spring. ↕ 20cm (8in), ↔ 1.5m (5ft). Tibet, China (Yunnan), N.E. Burma. ❄❄❄

R. fortunei ♢ Evergreen shrub or small tree with oblong-elliptic to oblong leaves, 8–18cm (3–7in) long, matt, dark green above, paler green beneath. Trusses of 6–12 broadly funnel-shaped, 7-lobed, fragrant, pink or lilac-pink flowers, 6–8cm (2½–3in) across, are borne in mid- and late spring. ↕ 10m (30ft), ↔ 2.5m (8ft). China. ❄❄❄. **subsp. *discolor*** ■ ♀ syn. *R. discolor*, has a more open habit, and bears trusses of 8–10 funnel- to bell-shaped, white, pink, or rose-pink flowers, in early and midsummer. ↕ 6m (20ft), ↔ 3m (10ft).

***R.* 'Fragrantissimum'** ■ ♀ Lax, evergreen shrub with hairy, medium-sized leaves. In mid-spring, bears trusses of up to 4 broadly funnel-shaped, nutmeg-scented, white, sometimes pink-flushed flowers, 6cm (2½in) long, with yellow throats. ↕↔ 2m (6ft). ❄

***R.* 'Freya'** ■ Deciduous, compact, bushy Rustica azalea with small leaves. Flat-domed trusses of funnel-shaped, hose-in-hose, fragrant, pink-flushed, salmon-orange flowers, 4cm (1½in) long, are borne in late spring and early summer. Suitable for sun. ↕↔ 1.5m (5ft). ❄❄❄

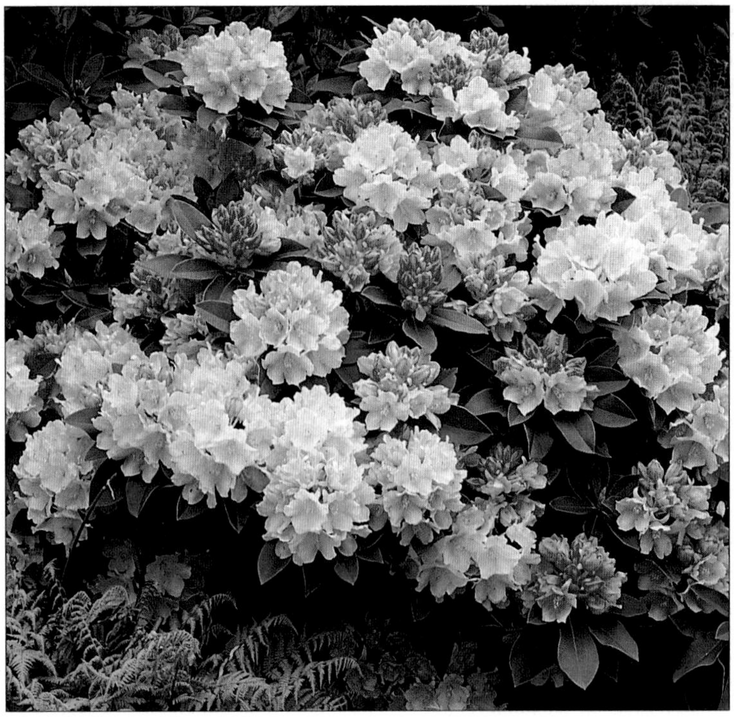

Rhododendron 'Golden Torch'

***R.* 'Frome'** ■ Deciduous Knap Hill-Exbury azalea of open habit, with medium-sized leaves. In late spring, bears frilled, wavy-margined, broadly funnel-shaped, saffron-yellow flowers, 7cm (3in) long, overlaid with red in their throats. Suitable for an open site. ↕↔ 1.5m (5ft). ❄❄❄

R. fulgens. Rounded, evergreen shrub with smooth, peeling, pink-grey to red-brown bark. The broadly ovate to obovate, glossy, dark green leaves, 7–11cm (3–4½in) long, have a dense, reddish brown indumentum beneath. Compact trusses of 10–15 tubular to bell-shaped, crimson-scarlet flowers, 2–3.5cm (¾–1½in) long, with black-red nectar pouches, are borne in early spring. ↕ 4m (12ft), ↔ 3m (10ft). E. Himalayas, Tibet. ❄❄❄

R. fulvum ■ ♀ ♢ Large, evergreen shrub or small tree with inversely lance-shaped to elliptic leaves, 8–22cm (3–9in) long, glossy, dark green above, with a red-brown to fawn indumentum beneath. Compact trusses of up to 20 tubular-bell-shaped white flowers, 2.5–4.5cm (1–1¾in) long, flushed rose-pink to deep rose-pink, sometimes each with a basal crimson mark, open in early and mid-spring. ↕ 5m (15ft), ↔ 3m (10ft). E. Himalayas, China. ❄❄❄

***R.* 'Furnivall's Daughter'** ■ ♀ Upright, rounded, showy, evergreen shrub with medium-sized leaves. In late spring and early summer, bears compact trusses of funnel-shaped, bright pink flowers, 9cm (3½in) long, each with a bold, strawberry-red flare in the throat. ↕↔ 3m (10ft). ❄❄❄

***R.* 'George Budgen'.** Vigorous, evergreen, compact Vireya rhododendron with medium-sized leaves. Trusses of up to 5 tubular-funnel-shaped flowers, 8cm (3in) long, bright orange at the petal tips, shading to rich yellow at the centres, are borne intermittently from winter to summer. ↕ 1.3m (4½ft), ↔ 1–1.2m (3–4ft). ❀ (min. 5°C/41°F)

***R.* 'George Reynolds'** ■ Deciduous, bushy Knap Hill-Exbury azalea with medium-sized leaves. Large trusses of broadly funnel-shaped yellow flowers, 6–8cm (2½–3in) long, flushed pink in bud, are borne with or before the leaves, in mid-spring. Suitable for full sun. ↕↔ 2m (6ft). ❄❄❄

***R.* 'Gibraltar'** ♀ Vigorous, deciduous Knap Hill-Exbury azalea with medium-sized leaves. In spring, crimson-orange buds open to dense trusses of funnel-shaped, brilliant orange flowers, 6–8cm (2½–3in) long, each with a distinct yellow flash and crinkled petals. Suitable for full sun. ↕↔ 1.5m (5ft). ❄❄❄

***R.* 'Ginny Gee'** ♀ Dwarf, evergreen shrub forming dense, cushion-like mats of small, dark green leaves. Multiple trusses of tubular-funnel-shaped, pale purplish pink flowers, 2.5cm (1in) long, fading to white-pink, cover the leaves in mid-spring. Suitable for sun. ↕↔ 60–90cm (24–36in). ❄❄❄

R. glaucophyllum. Compact, semi-dwarf, evergreen shrub with oblong to elliptic-lance-shaped, aromatic leaves, 3.5–6cm (1½–2½in) long, matt, dark green above, white-glaucous and scaly beneath. In mid-spring, bears lax trusses of 4–10 bell-shaped, white, rose-pink, or pinkish purple flowers, 1–3cm (½–1¼in) long. Suitable for full sun. ↕↔ 1.5m (5ft). E. Himalayas. ❄❄❄

***R.* 'Gloria Mundi'** ■ Deciduous, twiggy Ghent azalea with small leaves. In early summer, bears lax trusses of honeysuckle-like, tubular-funnel-shaped, fragrant orange flowers, 4–7cm (1½–3in) long, with yellow flares inside and frilled margins. Suitable for full sun. ↕↔ 2m (6ft). ❄❄❄

***R.* 'Glory of Littleworth'** ■ Semi-evergreen azaleodendron of untidy habit, with medium-sized leaves. Compact trusses of broadly funnel-shaped, creamy white flowers, 5–6cm (2–2½in) long, with bright orange-red flashes on the upper petals, open from mid-spring to early summer. ↕↔ 1.5m (5ft). ❄❄❄

***R.* 'Glowing Embers'** ■ Striking, deciduous Knap Hill-Exbury azalea with medium-sized leaves. Conical trusses of

R

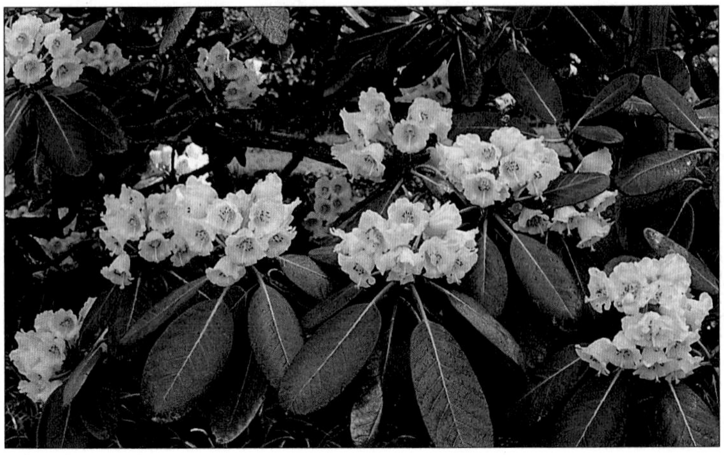

Rhododendron falconeri

broadly funnel-shaped, vivid reddish orange flowers, 7cm (3in) long, each marked orange in the throat, are produced in mid-spring. Suitable for sun. ↕↔ 2m (6ft). ❄❄❄

***R.* 'Goldbukett'**, syn. *R.* 'Golden Bouquet'. Evergreen shrub producing medium-sized leaves. In late spring and early summer, bears loose trusses of 10–14 funnel-shaped, creamy yellow flowers, 5–6cm (2–2½in) long, spotted red-purple inside. Very hardy. ↕↔ 2m (6ft). ❄❄❄

***R.* 'Gold Crown'** see *R.* 'Goldkrone'.

***R.* 'Golden Bouquet'** see *R.* 'Goldbukett'.

***R.* 'Golden Fleece'** see *R.* 'Princess Anne'.

***R.* 'Golden Torch'** ■ 🏆 Compact, upright, evergreen shrub with medium-sized leaves. In late spring and early summer, salmon-pink buds open to rounded trusses of funnel-shaped, soft yellow flowers, 4–5cm (1½–2in) long, fading to pale yellow or cream. ↕↔ 1.5m (5ft). ❄❄❄

***R.* 'Goldkrone'** ■ syn *R.* 'Gold Crown'. Low-growing, compact, evergreen shrub with medium-sized leaves. Trusses of 16–18 funnel- to bell-shaped, bright golden yellow flowers, 5–7cm (2–3in) long, delicately spotted ruby-red inside, are borne in succession in mid-spring. Very hardy. ↕↔ 1.5m (5ft). ❄❄❄

***R.* 'Goldsworth Orange'.** Upright, evergreen shrub, of dense, compact habit, with medium-sized leaves. In early summer, bears full trusses of tubular-funnel-shaped, salmon-pink flowers, 6cm (2½in) long, with subtle orange shading. ↕↔ 2m (6ft). ❄❄❄

***R.* 'Gomer Waterer'** 🏆 Compact, evergreen shrub with medium-sized leaves. In late spring and early summer, lilac-pink buds open to hemispherical trusses of funnel-shaped white flowers, to 8cm (3in) long, flushed mauve-pink at the margins, each with a bold yellow-brown flare in the throat. Very tolerant of sun, heat, and wind. ↕↔ 2m (6ft). ❄❄❄

***R.* 'Grace Seabrook'.** Vigorous, evergreen shrub with medium-sized leaves. In early and mid-spring, bears tight trusses of funnel-shaped, deep blood-red flowers, 8cm (3in) long, paling towards the margins. Very hardy. ↕↔ 2m (6ft). ❄❄❄

***R.* 'Greeting'.** Dwarf, evergreen Glenn Dale azalea with small leaves. In early and mid-spring, bears lax trusses of funnel-shaped, wavy-margined, bright orange-red flowers, 5cm (2in) long. Grow in full sun or partial shade. ↕↔ 1m (3ft). ❄❄❄

R. griersonianum ■ Striking, evergreen shrub with bristly, woolly shoots. Elliptic to oblong-lance-shaped, matt, olive-green leaves, 10–20cm (4–8in) long, have a loose brown indumentum beneath. In late spring and early summer, trusses of 5–12 tubular-bell-shaped scarlet flowers, 6–8cm (2½–3in) long, open from buds with long, tapering scales. ↕↔ 3m (10ft). W. China, N.E Burma. ❄❄❄

R. griffithianum ♀ Evergreen, large shrub or tree with peeling, smooth, red-brown bark. Oblong-elliptic, pale green leaves, 10–30cm (4–12in) long, are slightly glaucous beneath. Trusses of 3–6 open bell-shaped, fragrant, white or pale pink flowers, 4.5–8cm (1¾–3in) long, spotted green inside, open in mid-spring. ↕ 6m (20ft), ↔ 2.5m (8ft). C. and E. Himalayas, Bhutan. ❄❄

***R.* 'Gumpo'**, syn. *R. indicum* var. *eriocarpum* 'Gumpo'. Late-flowering, dwarf, evergreen Satsuki azalea with small leaves. In early summer, bears few-flowered trusses of funnel-shaped, wavy-petalled, white, sometimes pink or pink-flushed white flowers, 6–8cm (2½–3in) long. Heat-tolerant. ↕↔ 1m (3ft). ❄❄❄

R. haematodes. Slow-growing, compact, evergreen shrub producing oblong-obovate, dark green leaves, 4.5–10cm (1¾–4in) long, with a dense, reddish-brown indumentum beneath. In late spring, bears lax trusses of 6–10 tubular-bell-shaped, fleshy crimson flowers, 3.5–4.5cm (1½–1¾in) long. ↕↔ 2m (6ft). China (Yunnan). ❄❄❄

***R.* 'Halfdan Lem'** ■ Very vigorous, lax, evergreen shrub with large leaves. In mid- and late spring, bears tight trusses of broadly funnel-shaped red flowers, 9cm (3½in) long, spotted dark red, fading to pink with age. ↕↔ 2.5m (8ft). ❄❄❄

***R.* 'Hatsugiri'** ■ 🏆 Compact, dwarf, evergreen Kurume azalea with small leaves. In spring, bears trusses of up to 3 broadly funnel-shaped, bright crimson-purple flowers, 0.7–2.5cm (¼–1in) long. Will tolerate sun. ↕↔ 60cm (24in). ❄❄❄

***R.* 'Hawk Crest'** see *R.* 'Crest'.

***R.* 'Hexe'**, syn. *R.* 'Firefly'. Dwarf, evergreen Indian azalea of neat habit, with small leaves. In spring, bears lax trusses of numerous hose-in-hose, glowing crimson flowers, 3–4cm (1¼–1½in) long. ↕↔ 60cm (24in). ❄❄

***R.* 'Hino-crimson'** 🏆 Dwarf, evergreen Kurume azalea of dense habit, with small leaves. In spring, bears abundant funnel-shaped, brilliant red flowers, 0.7–2.5cm (¼–1in) long, in rounded trusses. ↕↔ 60cm (24in). ❄❄❄

***R.* 'Hinode-giri'** ■ 🏆 Compact, dwarf, evergreen Kurume azalea with small leaves. In spring, bears domed trusses of numerous broadly funnel-shaped, bright crimson flowers, 1–2.5cm (½–1in) long. Prefers full sun. ↕↔ 60cm (24in). ❄❄❄

***R.* 'Hino-mayo'** ■ 🏆 Dwarf, small-leaved, evergreen Kurume azalea of dense, compact habit. From mid-spring to early summer, produces lax trusses of broadly funnel-shaped, clear pink flowers, 1–2.5cm (½–1in) long. Will tolerate full sun. ↕↔ 60cm (24in). ❄❄❄

R. hippophaeoides ■ Upright, semi-dwarf, evergreen shrub with narrowly lance-shaped, aromatic, scaly, grey-green leaves, 2–3cm (¾–1¼in) long. In early and mid-spring, bears trusses of 6–8 funnel-shaped, lavender-blue or pale lilac flowers, 0.5–2.5cm (¼–1in) long. Prefers full sun. ↕ 1.5m (5ft), ↔ 75cm (30in). S.W. China. ❄❄❄

R. hodgsonii ♀ Evergreen tree or large shrub with attractive, peeling, red-brown to grey bark and oblong-elliptic leaves, 17–24cm (7–10in) long, glossy, dark green above, with a pale brown indumentum beneath. Compact trusses of 15–20 tubular-bell-shaped, fleshy, crimson, purple, or rose-purple flowers, 3–5cm (1¼–2in) long, each usually with 7 or 8, occasionally up to 10 lobes, open in mid- and late spring. ↕ to 11m (35ft), ↔ 6m (20ft). E. Himalayas. ❄❄❄

***R.* 'Homebush'** ■ 🏆 Compact, bushy, deciduous Knap Hill-Exbury azalea with

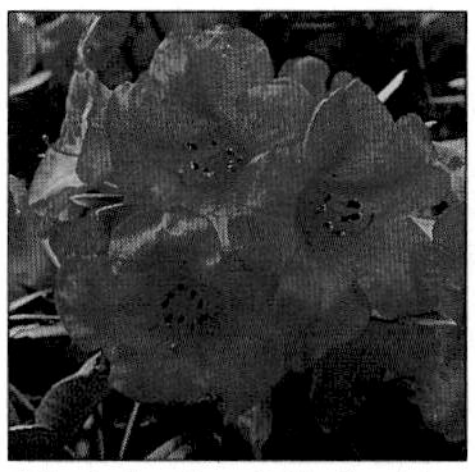
Rhododendron 'Elizabeth'

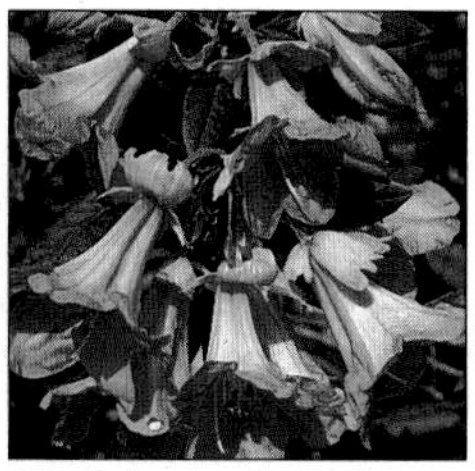
Rhododendron 'Fabia'

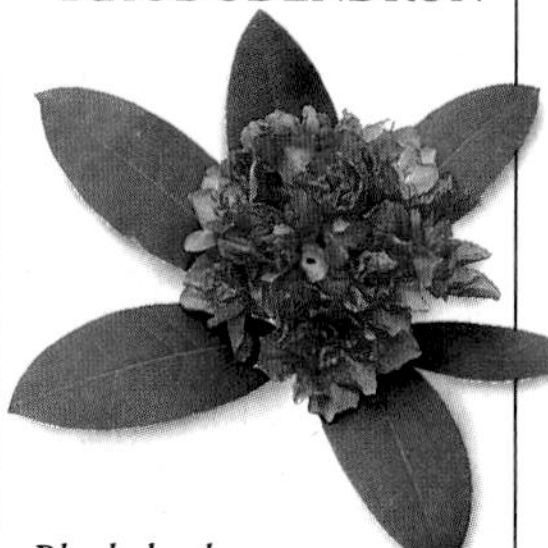
Rhododendron 'Fastuosum Flore Pleno'

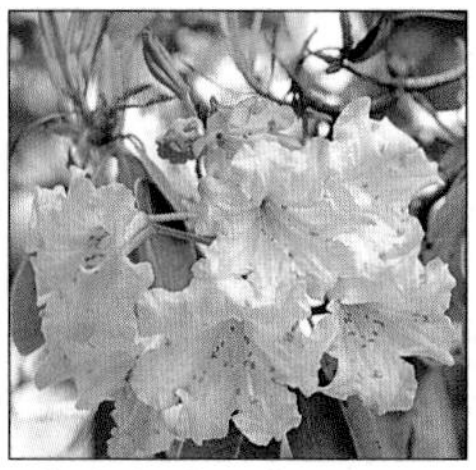
Rhododendron fortunei subsp. *discolor*

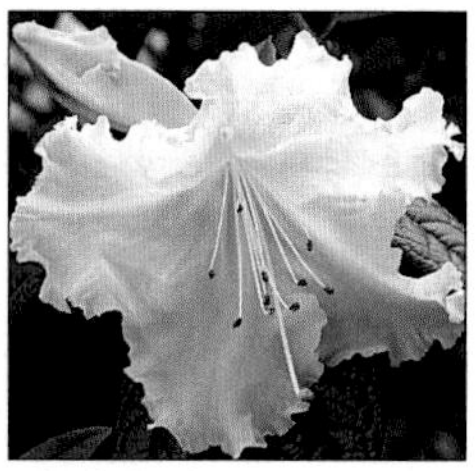
Rhododendron 'Fragrantissimum'

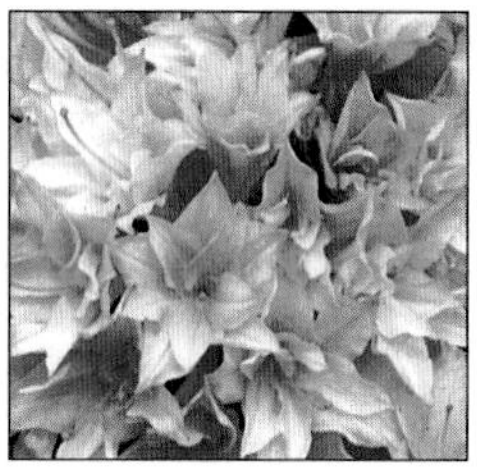
Rhododendron 'Freya'

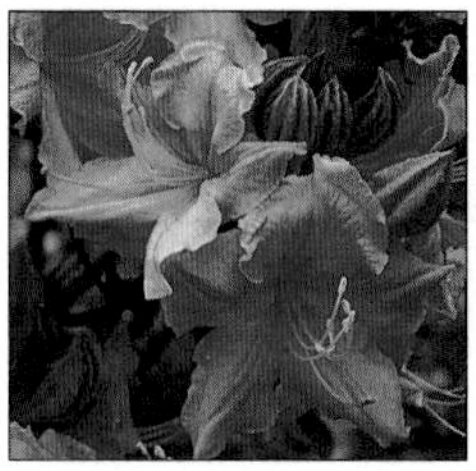
Rhododendron 'Frome'

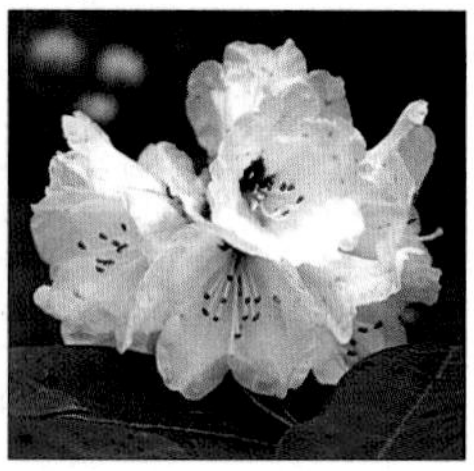
Rhododendron fulvum

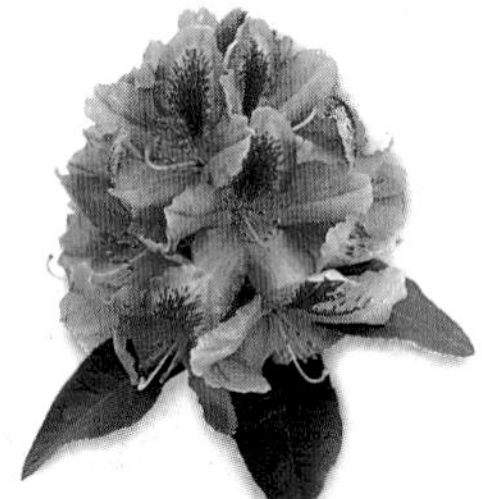
Rhododendron 'Furnivall's Daughter'

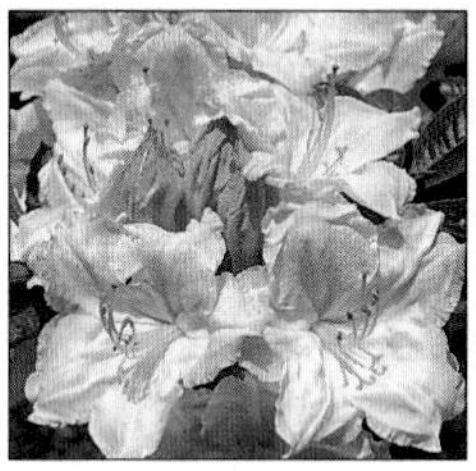
Rhododendron 'George Reynolds'

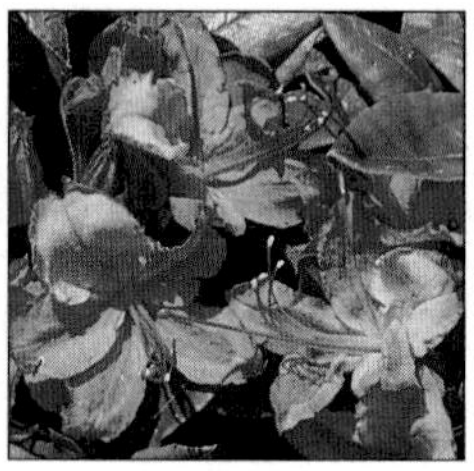
Rhododendron 'Gloria Mundi'

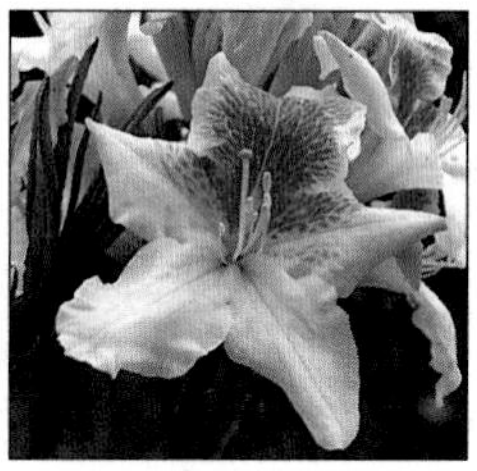
Rhododendron 'Glory of Littleworth'

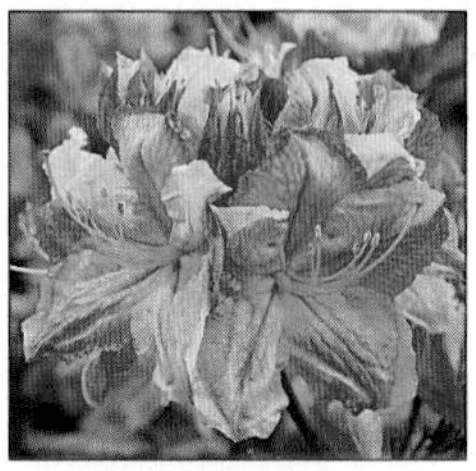
Rhododendron 'Glowing Embers'

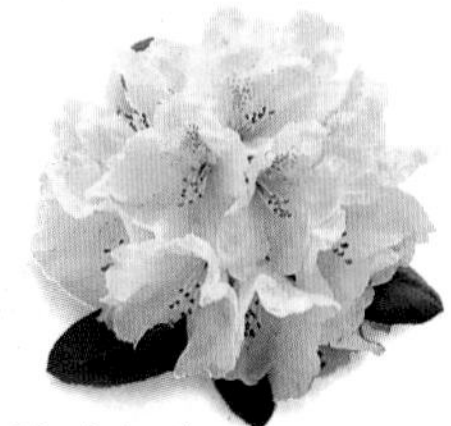
Rhododendron 'Goldkrone'

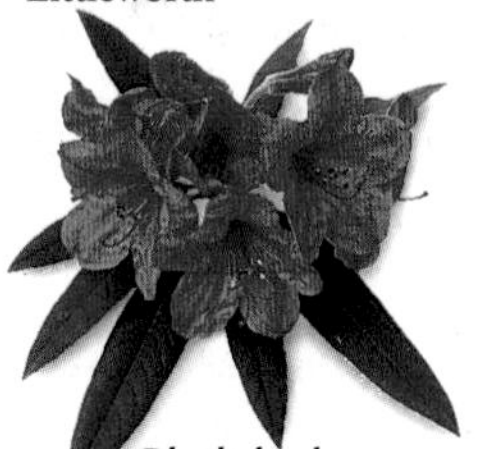
Rhododendron griersonianum

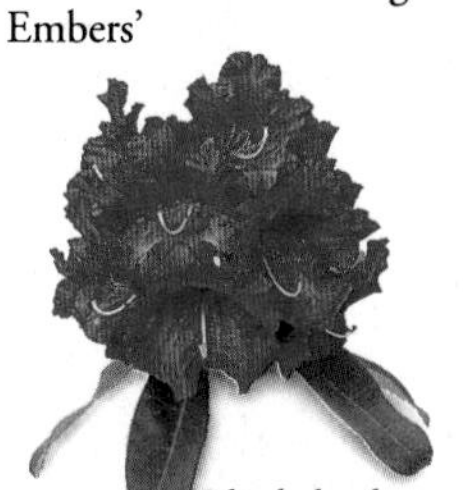
Rhododendron 'Halfdan Lem'

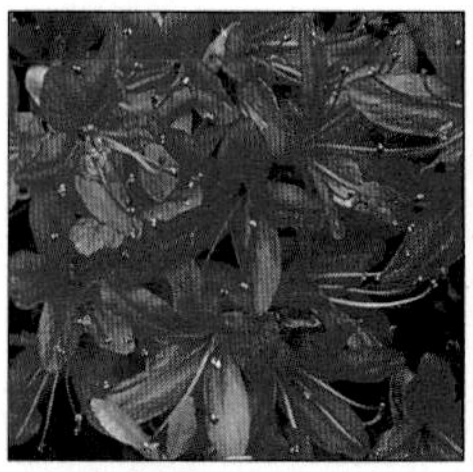
Rhododendron 'Hatsugiri'

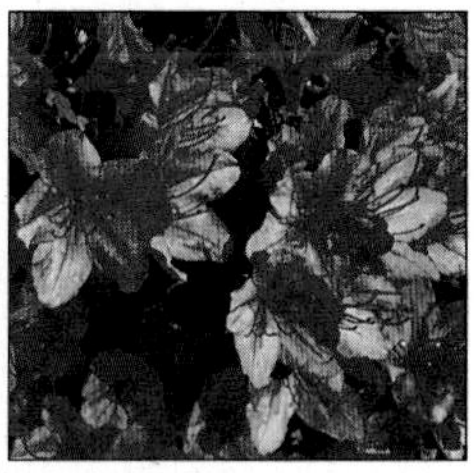
Rhododendron 'Hinode-giri'

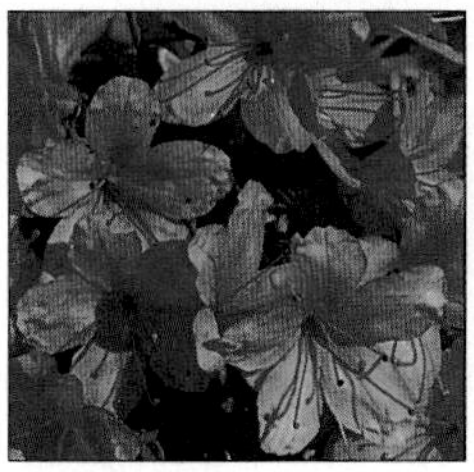
Rhododendron 'Hino-mayo'

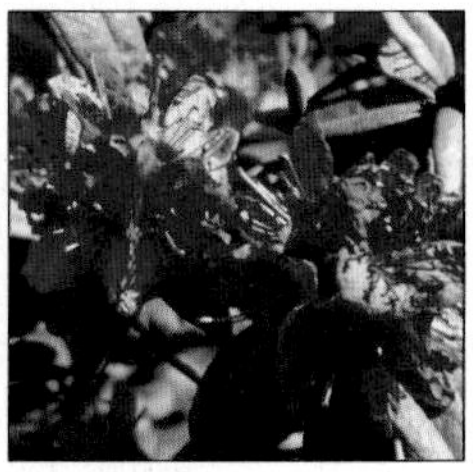
Rhododendron hippophaeoides

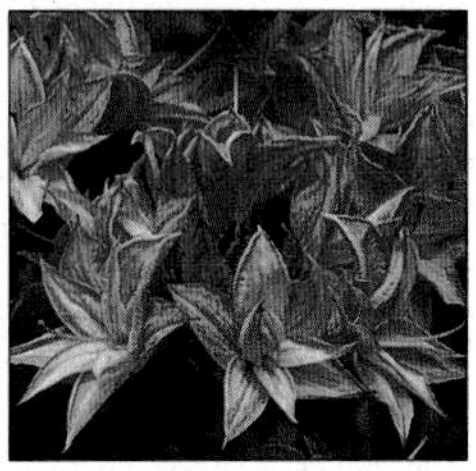
Rhododendron 'Homebush'

R

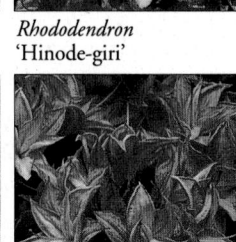

medium-sized leaves. In late spring, bears tight, rounded trusses of trumpet-shaped, semi-double, bright pink flowers, 3cm (1¼in) long, with paler pink shading. ↕↔ 1.5m (5ft). ✲✲✲
***R.* 'Hotei'** 🏆 Dense, evergreen shrub with medium-sized leaves. In mid- and late spring, bears slightly open trusses of funnel-shaped, deep yellow flowers, 5cm (2in) long, each with a prominent calyx. ↕↔ 1.5–2.5m (5–8ft). ✲✲✲
***R.* 'Humming Bird'.** Neat, compact, dome-shaped, evergreen shrub with small, rounded, glossy leaves. In early and mid-spring, bears loose trusses of 4 or more, nodding, widely bell-shaped, cherry-red flowers, 5–6cm (2–2½in) across. ↕↔ 1.5m (5ft). ✲✲✲
***R.* 'Hydon Dawn'** ▣ 🏆 Very compact, low-growing, evergreen shrub with medium-sized leaves. From mid-spring to early summer, bears tight trusses of funnel-shaped, frilled, pale pink flowers, 5cm (2in) long, fading to white. Tolerates full sun. ↕↔ 1.5m (5ft). ✲✲✲
***R.* 'Hydon Hunter'** 🏆 Vigorous, open shrub with medium-sized leaves. In early summer, bears compact trusses of narrowly bell-shaped flowers, 5cm (2in) long, with red rims fading to pink in the centres and spotted orange inside. Grow in sun. ↕↔ 1.5m (5ft). ✲✲✲
***R.* 'Ilam Cream'** ▣ Evergreen shrub producing large leaves. Lax trusses of lilac-pink buds open to funnel-shaped, fragrant, creamy yellow flowers, 6–9cm (2½–3½in) long, in late spring and early summer. ↕↔ 4m (12ft). ✲✲✲
R. impeditum 🏆 Compact, dwarf, evergreen shrub with tiny, elliptic-ovate, aromatic, scaly, grey-green leaves, 4–15mm (⅛–½in) long. In mid- and late spring, bears abundant broadly funnel-shaped, purplish blue flowers, 2–2.5cm (¾–½in) long, singly or in pairs. ↕↔ 60cm (24in). W. China. ✲✲✲
***R.* 'I.M.S.'** see *R.* 'Irene Stead'.
***R. indicum* var. *eriocarpum* 'Gumpo'** see *R.* 'Gumpo'.
R. insigne 🏆 Compact, dome-shaped, evergreen shrub with elliptic to lance-shaped, stiff leaves, 7–13cm (3–5in) long, glossy, dark green above, copper beneath. In late spring and early summer, bears trusses of 8–15 bell-shaped, pinkish white flowers, to 4cm (1½in) long, the insides striped rose-pink with crimson spots. Tolerates full sun. ↕↔ 4m (12ft). W. China. ✲✲✲
***R.* 'Irene Koster'** ▣ 🏆 Deciduous Occidentale azalea with medium-sized leaves. Bold trusses of delicate, funnel-shaped, fragrant, pink-suffused yellow flowers, 6cm (2½in) long, with orange-yellow flashes inside, open in late spring and early summer. ↕↔ 2m (6ft). ✲✲✲
***R.* 'Irene Stead'** ▣ syn. *R.* 'I.M.S.'. Vigorous, evergreen shrub with large leaves and deep purple leaf-stalks. In late spring, flower buds open to very large trusses of funnel-shaped, fragrant, soft pink flowers, 6–9cm (2½–3½in) long. ↕↔ 4m (12ft). ✲✲✲
***R.* 'Irohayama'** ▣ 🏆 Compact, dwarf, small-leaved, evergreen Kurume azalea. Small trusses of abundant funnel-shaped white flowers, 4–5cm (1½–2in) long, margined pale lavender, open in spring. Grow in sun. ↕↔ 60cm (24in). ✲✲✲
R. irroratum 🗨 Evergreen, large shrub or small tree with inversely lance-shaped to elliptic leaves, 7–14cm (3–5½in) long, mid-green above, paler beneath. Trusses of up to 15 tubular-bell-shaped white flowers, 3.5–5cm (1½–2in) long, sometimes suffused pale pink, and variably crimson-spotted within, open in early spring. Grow in sun. ↕ 8m (25ft), ↔ 4m (12ft). China (Yunnan, Sichuan), Vietnam, Indonesia, Laos. ✲✲✲
***R.* 'Jalisco'.** Evergreen shrub of open habit, with medium-sized leaves. In late spring and early summer, bears semi-pendent trusses of funnel-shaped, yellow or apricot-yellow flowers, 6cm (2½in) long, marked and streaked red-brown in the throats. ↕↔ 2.2m (7ft). ✲✲
R. japonicum see *R. molle* subsp. *japonicum.*
R. jasminiflorum. Evergreen Vireya rhododendron with a lax, untidy habit. Elliptic to lance-shaped or oblong, dark green leaves, 2.5–5cm (1–2in) long, arranged in whorls of 3–5, have small but distinct brown scales beneath. Trusses of 5–12 trumpet-shaped, sweet-scented flowers, 3.5–5cm (1½–2in) long, often opening pale pink and fading to white, with red flower-stalks, are borne intermittently from summer to winter. ↕ 1m (3ft), ↔ 1–2m (3–6ft). W. Malaysia, Philippines, Sumatra. ❁ (min. 5°C/41°F)
***R.* 'Jean Mary Montague'** see *R.* 'The Hon. Jean Marie de Montague'.
***R.* 'John Cairns'** ▣ 🏆 Striking, robust, small-leaved, evergreen Kaempferi azalea, of compact, upright habit. Flat-headed trusses of abundant funnel-shaped, orange-red flowers, 4–4.5cm (1½–1¾in) long, are borne in spring. Grow in sun. ↕↔ 1.5m (5ft). ✲✲✲
R. kaempferi ▣ 🏆 Loosely branched, erect, semi-evergreen azalea with glossy, mid-green leaves, 1–5cm (1½–2in) long, ovate to lance-shaped in spring, smaller and elliptic-obovate in summer. In late spring and early summer, bears trusses of 2–4 broadly funnel-shaped flowers, 2–3cm (¾–1¼in) long, in shades of red. Prefers full sun. ↕ 3m (10ft), ↔ 1.5m (5ft). Korea, Japan. ✲✲✲
R. keiskei ▣ Compact, dwarf or semi-dwarf, evergreen shrub with small, oblong-lance-shaped, dark green leaves, 2.5–8cm (1–3in) long, slightly scaly above, densely scaly beneath. Trusses of 2–5 broadly funnel-shaped, pale to lemon-yellow flowers, to 5cm (2in) across, are borne freely in mid- and late spring. ↕ 25–90cm (10–36in), ↔ 1.2m (4ft). S. Japan. ✲✲✲. **'Yaku Fairy'** 🏆 is prostrate; ↕ 15cm (6in).
R. keleticum see *R. calostrotum* subsp. *keleticum.*
***R.* 'Ken Janeck'** see *R. yakushimanum* 'Ken Janeck'.
R. kesangiae 🗨 Vigorous, evergreen shrub or small tree with very large, broadly elliptic to obovate, glossy, dark green leaves, 20–30cm (8–12in) long, with a silver-fawn indumentum beneath. In mid- and late spring, bears compact trusses of 15–25 bell-shaped, rose-pink flowers, 3–5cm (1¼–2in) long, with red nectar pouches. ↕ 12m (40ft), ↔ 8m (25ft). Bhutan. ✲✲✲
***R.* 'Kilimanjaro'** ▣ 🏆 Vigorous, evergreen shrub with medium-sized leaves. From mid-spring to early summer, bears very large trusses of funnel-shaped, bright deep red flowers, 15cm (6in) long, spotted crimson on the lobes. ↕↔ 2.2m (7ft). ✲✲✲
***R.* 'Kirin'** ▣ 🏆 Free-flowering, evergreen, compact, dwarf Kurume azalea with small leaves. In mid-spring, bears small trusses of hose-in-hose, deep pink flowers, 3cm (1¼in) long, shaded a delicate silvery rose-pink. Suitable for sun. ↕↔ 1.5m (5ft). ✲✲✲
R. kiusianum ▣ 🏆 Dwarf, semi-evergreen shrub with variable, broadly elliptic to obovate, short-bristled, mid-green leaves, 0.5–2cm (¼–¾in) long, larger in spring than in summer. Trusses of 2 or 3 funnel-shaped, pink or purple, sometimes white flowers, 1.5–2cm (½–¾in) long, are borne in late spring and early summer. Prefers full sun. ↕↔ 1.2m (4ft). Japan. ✲✲✲
***R.* 'Klondyke'** 🏆 Striking, deciduous Knap Hill-Exbury azalea with medium-sized leaves. In late spring, red-flushed buds open to large trusses of funnel-shaped, glowing orange-gold flowers, 6cm (2½in) long, tinted red on the reverse of the petals. Grow in full sun. ↕↔ 2m (6ft). ✲✲✲
***R.* 'Kluis Sensation'** 🏆 Relatively slow-growing, evergreen shrub with medium-sized leaves. In late spring and early summer, bears tight trusses of funnel-shaped, slightly frilled, dark red-scarlet flowers, 4.5–5cm (1¾–2in) long, spotted crimson inside. Very tolerant of heat and sun. ↕↔ 2.2m (7ft). ✲✲✲
R. konorii. Erect, evergreen Vireya rhododendron producing obovate to broadly elliptic, dull, mid-green leaves, 11–14cm (4½–5½in) long, with small brown scales beneath. From summer to winter, intermittently bears trusses of 4–7 elongated, funnel-shaped, usually 7-lobed, fragrant flowers, 7–9cm (3–3½in) long, pale to deep pink, or pink fading to white, with prominent cream stamens. ↕ 2m (6ft), ↔ 1.5m (5ft). New Guinea. ❁ (min. 5°C/41°F)
***R.* 'Kure-no-yuki'** ▣ 🏆 syn. *R.* 'Snowflake'. Compact, dwarf, evergreen Kurume azalea with small leaves. Freely bears trusses of 2 or 3 hose-in-hose white flowers, 0.5–2.5cm (¼–1in) long, in mid-spring. ↕↔ 1m (3ft). ✲✲✲
R. lacteum. Large, densely branched, evergreen shrub producing oblong-elliptic, dark green leaves, 8–17cm (3–7in) long, with a brown indumentum beneath. Trusses of 20–30 broadly bell-shaped, pale yellow flowers, 5cm (2in) across, sometimes with crimson marks inside, are borne in mid- and late spring. ↕↔ 5m (15ft). China (Sichuan, Yunnan), Burma. ✲✲✲
***R.* 'Lady Alice Fitzwilliam'** 🏆 Open, evergreen shrub with medium-sized leaves. In mid-spring, bears trusses of 2 or 3 funnel-shaped, nutmeg-scented pink flowers, 10cm (4in) long, maturing to white with yellow-marked throats. ↕↔ 2m (6ft). ✲✲
***R.* 'Lady Clementine Mitford'** 🏆 Shrubby, spreading, evergreen "iron clad" rhododendron, with medium-sized leaves. In late spring and early summer, bears compact trusses of funnel-shaped flowers, to 8cm (3in) long, peach-pink at the margins of the petals, shading to white at the centres, with V-shaped markings of red-brown to green spots in the throats. ↕↔ 2.5m (8ft). ✲✲✲
***R.* 'Lady Eleanor Cathcart'** 🏆 🗨 Shrubby, evergreen "iron clad" rhododendron with arching, medium-sized leaves. In late spring, bears rounded trusses of funnel-shaped, pale pink flowers, 5–6cm (2–2½in) long, with dark maroon flares inside. Suitable for sun. ↕↔ 4m (12ft). ✲✲✲
R. laetum ▣ Erect, evergreen Vireya rhododendron with elliptic to broadly elliptic, glossy, dark green leaves, 5–9cm (2–3½in) long, with tiny scales beneath. In spring, bears trusses of 5–12 funnel-shaped, golden yellow flowers, 4.5cm (1¾in) long, later suffused orange-red, on red flower-stalks. ↕↔ 1.5m (5ft). N.W. New Guinea. ❁ (min. 5°C/41°F)
***R.* 'Lavender Girl'** ▣ 🏆 Evergreen, large-leaved shrub with domed trusses of funnel-shaped, fragrant, pink-mauve flowers, to 10cm (4in) long, fading to near white in the centres. Blooms open in late spring and early summer, earlier than most other hybrids with lavender-blue or mauve-pink flowers. Grow in an open site. ↕↔ 2.5m (8ft). ✲✲✲

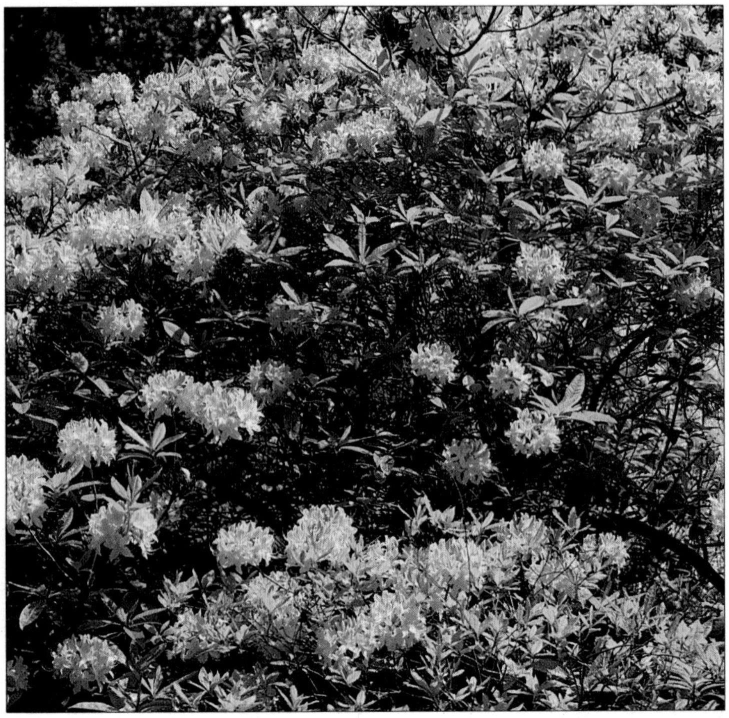

Rhododendron luteum

***R.* 'Ledifolium'** see *R. mucronatum.*
***R.* 'Lem's Cameo'** ■🏆 Evergreen shrub producing medium-sized leaves, brown-bronze when young. In mid-spring, bears large, domed trusses of funnel-shaped, frilled, pale peach flowers, 9cm (3½in) long, fading to apricot-cream or pink, and marked and spotted red in the throats. ↕↔ 2.2m (7ft). ❄❄❄
R. lepidostylum 🏆 Distinctive, dome-shaped, dwarf, evergreen shrub with densely bristly shoots. Small, oblong-oval, obovate, or ovate leaves, 3–3.5cm (1¼–1½in) long, intensely glaucous above, golden scaly beneath, have margins fringed with hairs. Broadly funnel-shaped yellow flowers, 4cm (1½in) across, sparsely bristly outside, are borne singly or in pairs, in late spring and early summer. ↕↔ 1m (3ft). W. China. ❄❄❄
R. leucaspis ■ Densely branched, dwarf, evergreen shrub with bristly calyces and shoots, and broadly elliptic, dark green leaves, 3–4.5cm (1¼–1¾in) long, bristly above, scaly and yellowish green beneath. In early spring, bears trusses of up to 3 saucer-shaped white flowers, 5cm (2in) across, with chocolate-brown anthers. ↕ 1m (3ft), ↔ 1.5m (5ft). S.E. Tibet. ❄❄
R. lindleyi 🏆 Evergreen, epiphytic shrub, of untidy habit, with peeling, reddish brown bark. Lance-shaped to oblong-lance-shaped, olive-green leaves, 9–13cm (3½–5in) long, are glaucous and scaly beneath. In late spring and early summer, bears trusses of up to 6 tubular to funnel-shaped, heavily scented white flowers, 7–10cm (3–4in) long, each with a yellow or orange flare within. ↕ 3m (10ft), ↔ 2m (6ft). E. Himalayas. ❄❄
***R.* 'Lionel's Triumph'.** Tall, large-leaved evergreen shrub with an open habit. Large trusses of funnel-shaped, creamy yellow flowers, 10cm (4in) long, with crimson-spotted throats and pink-flushed margins, open from pink buds in mid-spring. Grow in partial shade. ↕↔ 4m (12ft). ❄❄❄
***R.* 'Loderi King George'** ■🏆 Large, evergreen shrub of open habit, with large leaves. In late spring and early summer, pale pink buds open to huge trusses of funnel-shaped, fragrant, pure white flowers, 9–11cm (3½–4½in) long, with subtle green markings in the throats. ↕↔ 4m (12ft). ❄❄❄
***R.* 'Loderi Venus'** 🏆 Evergreen, large-leaved shrub of open habit. In late spring and early summer, bears large trusses of funnel-shaped, fragrant, mid-pink flowers, 9–11cm (3½–4½in) long, fading to pale pink, the throats slightly green-marked. ↕↔ 4m (12ft). ❄❄❄
***R.* 'Loder's White'** 🏆 Vigorous, evergreen shrub with large leaves. In midsummer, bears large, conical trusses of long-lasting, funnel-shaped, slightly fragrant white flowers, 9–10cm (3½–4in) long, with red flecks inside. Thrives in sun. ↕↔ 3m (10ft). ❄❄❄
***R.* 'Lord Palmerston'** see *R.* 'Cynthia'.
***R.* 'Louise Dowdle'** ■ Compact, evergreen Glenn Dale azalea with medium-sized leaves. In spring, bears compact trusses of funnel-shaped, vivid red-purple flowers, 4cm (1½in) long, the throats with bright rose-red marks. Suitable for full sun. ↕↔ 1m (3ft). ❄❄❄
R. lutescens ■ Graceful, bushy, erect, semi-evergreen shrub with ovate-oblong to lance-shaped, sparsely scaly leaves, 5–9cm (2–3½in) long, bronze when young, maturing to dull green, and paler green with yellow scales beneath. In early spring, bears trusses of 3–6 broadly funnel-shaped, primrose-yellow flowers, 2.5cm (1in) across, spotted green inside. ↕↔ 5m (15ft). S.W. China. ❄❄❄
R. luteum ■🏆 Deciduous azalea of open habit, with oblong to lance-shaped, mid-green leaves, 5–10cm (2–4in) long, sparsely hairy above and beneath. Trusses of 7–12 funnel-shaped, strongly scented, sticky yellow flowers, 3.5cm (1½in) long, open in late spring and early summer. Prefers full sun. ↕↔ 4m (12ft). E. Europe to Caucasus. ❄❄❄
R. macabeanum 🏆Ϙ Evergreen shrub or tree with large, oblong-ovate, dark green leaves, 20–30cm (8–12in) long, with a woolly, pale fawn indumentum beneath. In mid-spring, bears huge trusses of up to 20 broadly bell-shaped, creamy to deep yellow flowers, 5–6cm (2–2½in) across, with purple marks inside, and purple nectar pouches. ↕ 15m (50ft), ↔ 6m (20ft). India (Manipur). ❄❄❄
R. macgregoriae ■ Bushy, evergreen Vireya rhododendron with ovate-lance-shaped to ovate-elliptic, glossy, dark green leaves, 4–9cm (1½–3½in) long, minutely scaly beneath. Trusses of up to 25 short, widely funnel- to bell-shaped, usually yellow or orange, occasionally pink flowers, to 1–3cm (½–1¼in) long, with protruding brown stamens, open in winter. ↕ to 5m (15ft), ↔ 1–2m (3–6ft). New Guinea. ⌂ (min. 5°C/41°F)
R. macrophyllum. Large, free-flowering, evergreen shrub with oblong-obovate to elliptic leaves, 7–17cm (3–7in) long, dark green above, paler green beneath. In late spring and early summer, bears compact trusses of 15–20 funnel-shaped, rose-purple to pink, sometimes white flowers, 3–4cm (1¼–1½in) long, with red-brown spots inside. Suitable for sun. ↕↔ to 5m (15ft). W. North America. ❄❄❄
R. maddenii 🏆 syn. *R. brachysiphon.* Multi-stemmed, evergreen shrub with peeling, grey-brown bark. Leaves, varying from lance-shaped or obovate to elliptic, are 6–18cm (2½–7in) long, dark green above, and densely brown-scaly beneath. In late spring and early summer, bears trusses of 2–4 funnel-shaped, strongly scented white flowers, 6–10cm (2½–4in) long, sometimes flushed rose-pink. ↕↔ 2.5m (8ft). Himalayas, S.W. China, Burma. ❄❄
R. mallotum Ϙ Evergreen, upright shrub or small tree producing obovate, stiff leaves, 10–13cm (4–5in) long, dark green and hairless above, with a woolly, reddish brown indumentum beneath. Trusses of up to 15 tubular-bell-shaped, fleshy scarlet flowers, 4–4.5cm (1½–1¾in) long, are borne in early spring. ↕ 6–7m (20–22ft), ↔ 3m (10ft). W. China, N.E. Burma. ❄❄❄
***R.* 'Martha Isaacson'.** Sturdy, semi-evergreen azaleodendron with medium-sized, maroon-tinted leaves. In late spring and early summer, bears rounded trusses of funnel-shaped, slightly scented white flowers, 4cm (1½in) long, with vivid pink stripes. Prefers full sun. ↕↔ 2.5m (8ft). ❄❄❄
***R.* 'May Day'** ■🏆 Low-growing, spreading, large-leaved evergreen shrub. In mid-spring, freely bears loose trusses

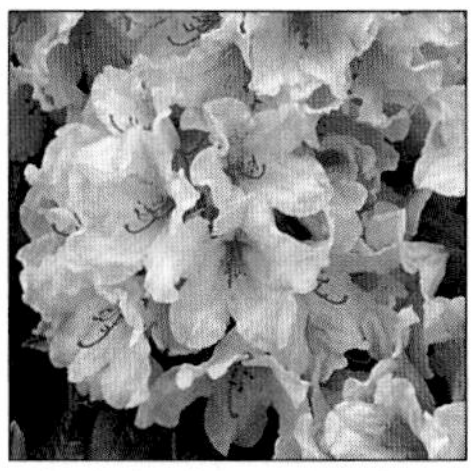
Rhododendron 'Hydon Dawn'

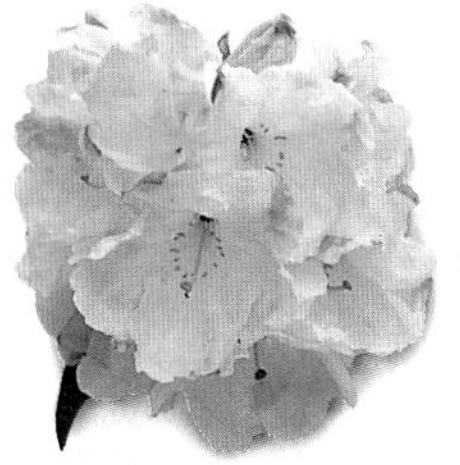
Rhododendron 'Ilam Cream'

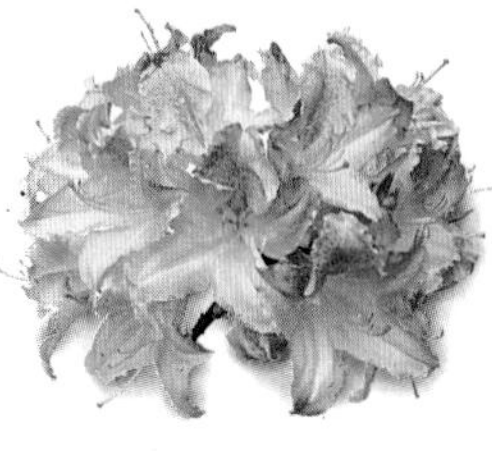
Rhododendron 'Irene Koster'

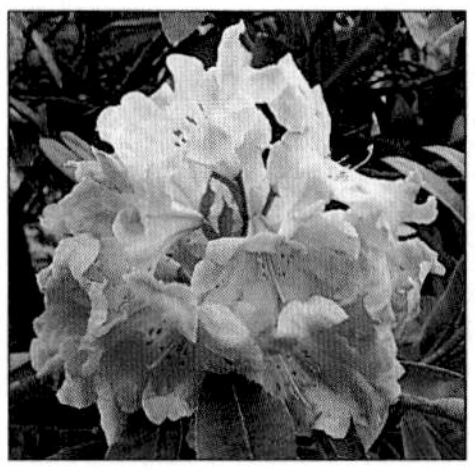
Rhododendron 'Irene Stead'

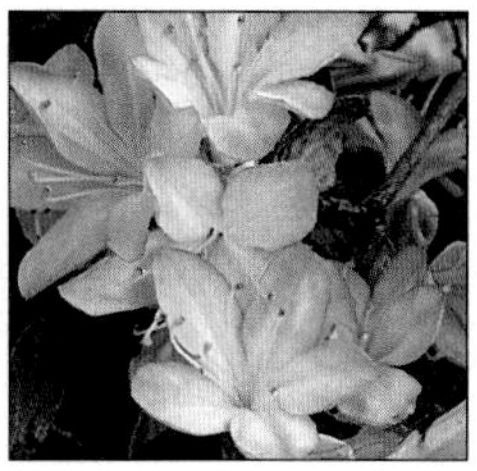
Rhododendron 'Irohayama'

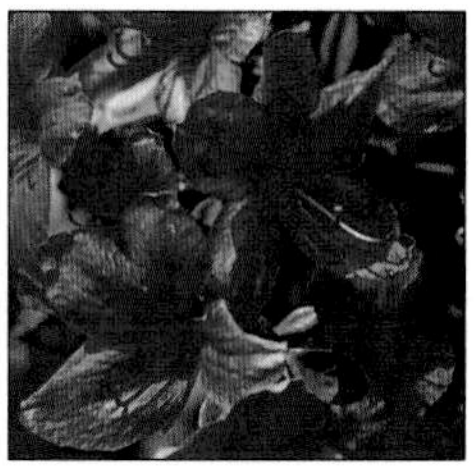
Rhododendron 'John Cairns'

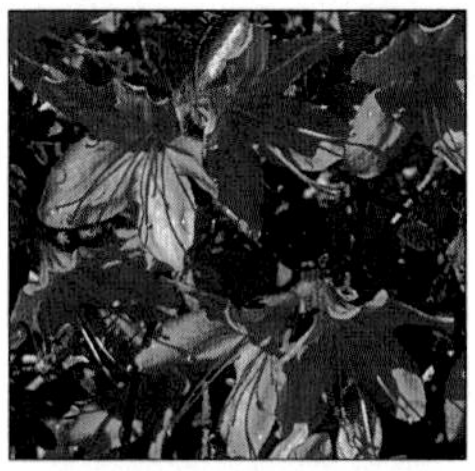
Rhododendron kaempferi

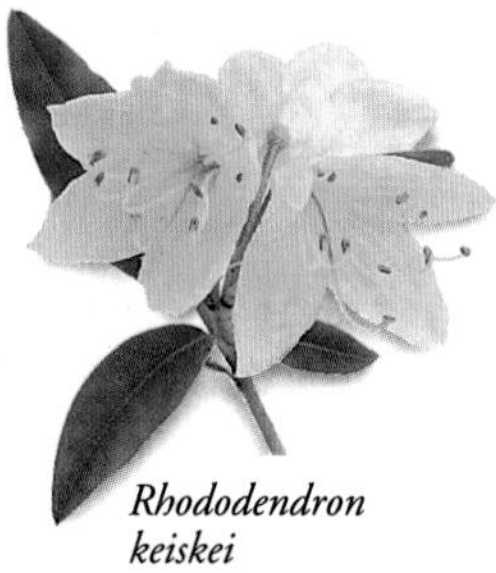
Rhododendron keiskei

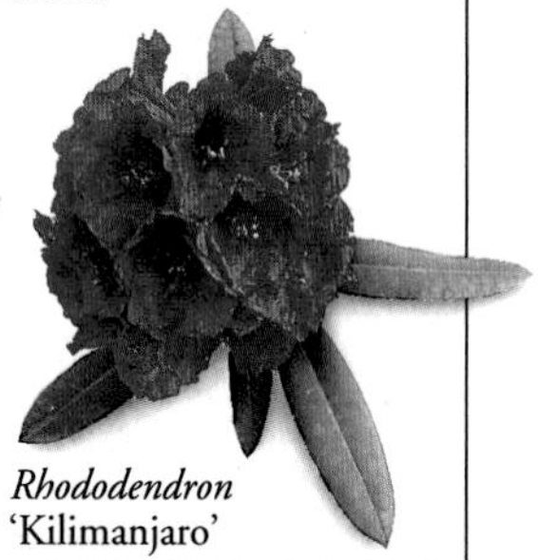
Rhododendron 'Kilimanjaro'

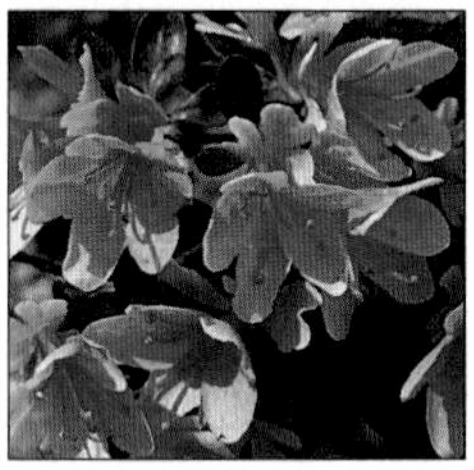
Rhododendron 'Kirin'

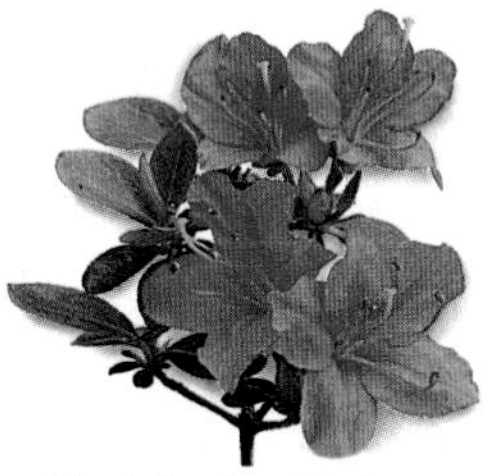
Rhododendron kiusianum

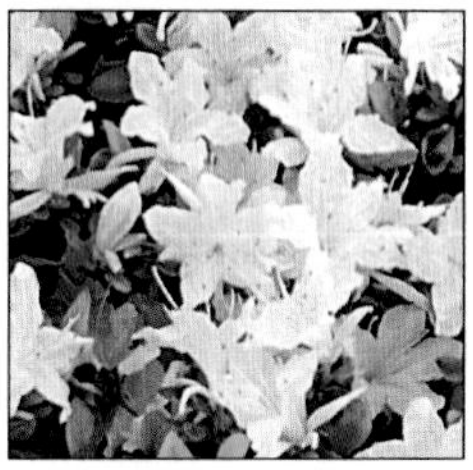
Rhododendron 'Kure-no-yuki'

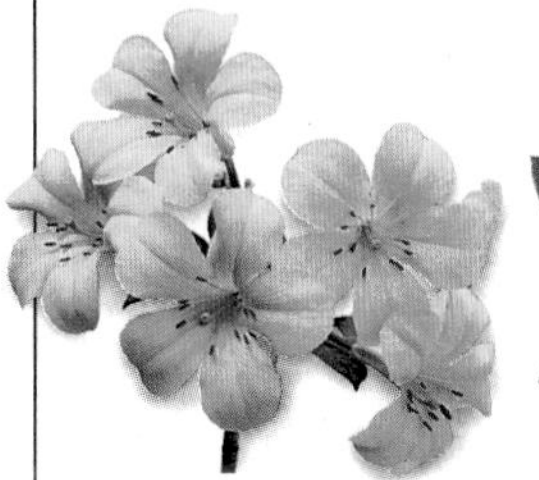
Rhododendron laetum

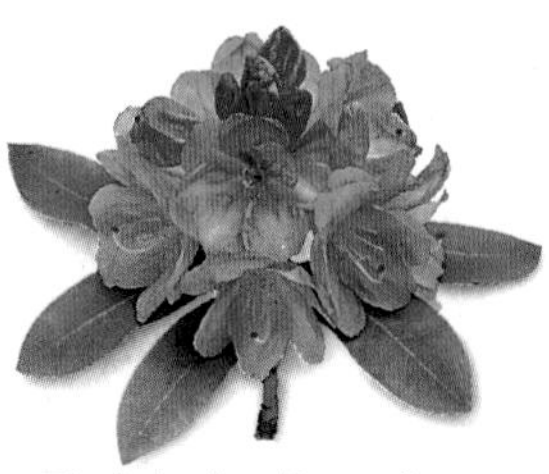
Rhododendron 'Lavender Girl'

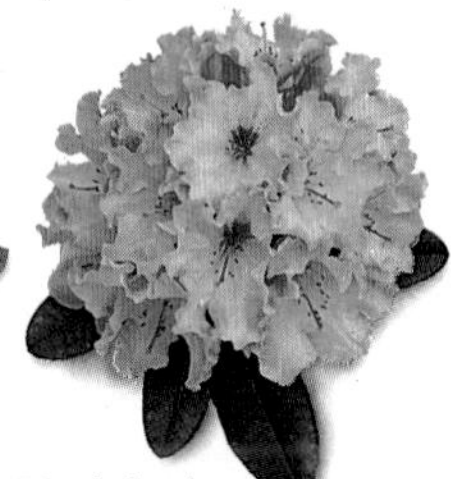
Rhododendron 'Lem's Cameo'

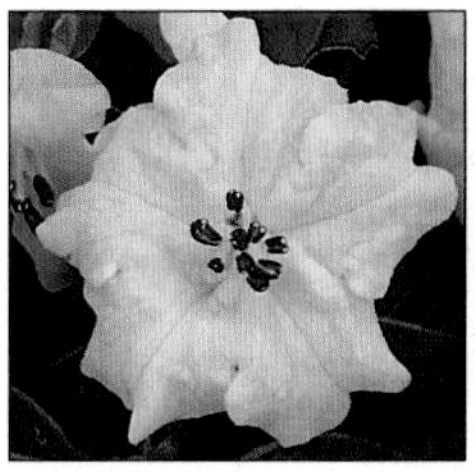
Rhododendron leucaspis

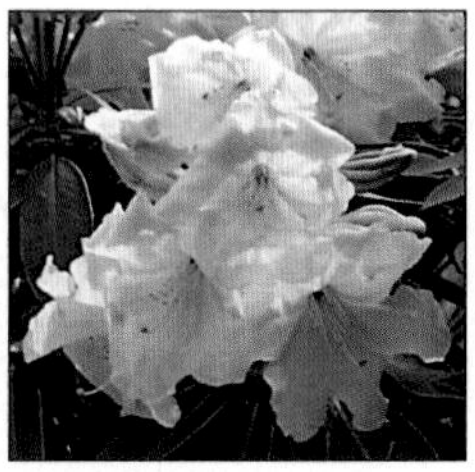
Rhododendron 'Loderi King George'

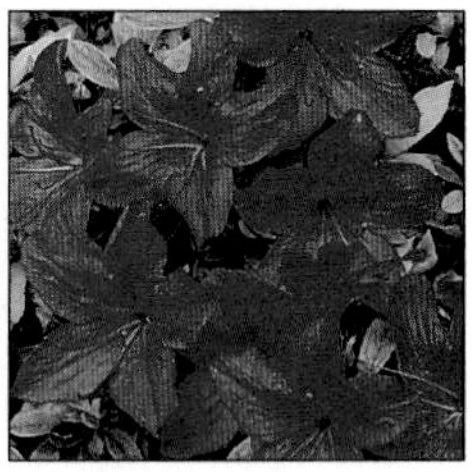
Rhododendron 'Louise Dowdle'

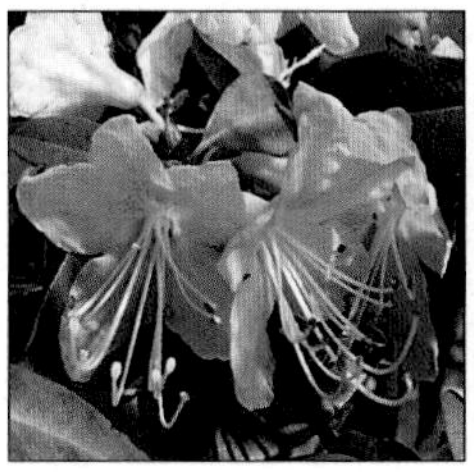
Rhododendron lutescens

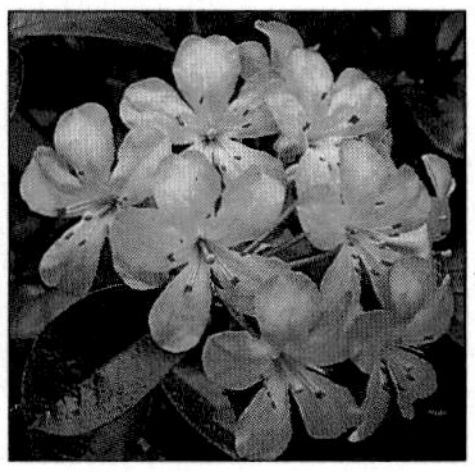
Rhododendron macgregoriae

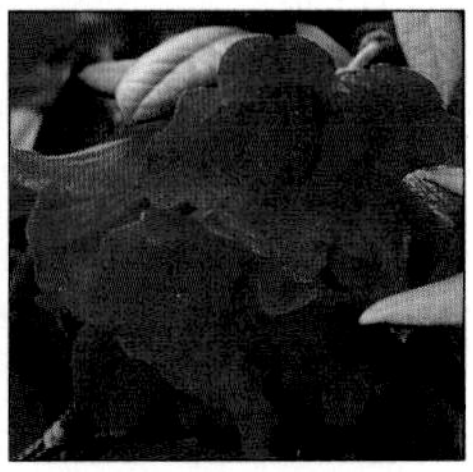
Rhododendron 'May Day'

R

of funnel-shaped scarlet flowers, 7cm (3in) long, with petal-like calyces. Tolerates full sun. ↕↔ 1.5m (5ft). ❄❄❄

***R.* 'Medway'** ▣ Deciduous, bushy Knap Hill-Exbury azalea of open habit, with medium-sized leaves. In late spring, bears trusses of trumpet-shaped, pale pink flowers, 6cm (2½in) long, with darker margins, orange-flashed throats, and frilled petals. ↕↔ 1.5–2.5m (5–8ft). ❄❄❄

***R. mekongense* Viridescens Group**, syn. *R. viridescens*. Distinctive, semi-dwarf, evergreen shrubs with oblong-oval, pale blue-green leaves, 5cm (2in) long, glaucous above, paler and scaly beneath. Trusses of 4 or 5 broadly funnel-shaped, pale yellow flowers, 2cm (¾in) long, with green spots inside, are borne in late spring and early summer. Suitable for full sun. ↕↔ 1.2m (4ft). S.E. Tibet, S.W. China. ❄❄❄

R. metternichii ▣ syn. *R. degronianum* subsp. *heptamerum*. Evergreen shrub with oblong to inversely lance-shaped leaves, 8–14cm (3–5½in) long, often red when young, maturing to glossy, deep green above, with a thick brown indumentum beneath. In mid-spring, bears trusses of up to 12 funnel- to bell-shaped, 5- to 7-lobed, pale to deep pink flowers, 3–4.5cm (1¼–1¾in) long, sometimes lined deeper pink inside. Will tolerate full sun. ↕↔ 2m (6ft). N. Japan. ❄❄❄

R. minus, syn. *R. carolinianum*. Evergreen shrub with ovate-elliptic to elliptic, dark green leaves, 5–11cm (2–4½in) long, brown-scaly beneath. In late spring and early summer, bears trusses of 6–12 funnel- to bell-shaped, pink-purple, pink, or white flowers, 2–3.5cm (¾–1½in) long, with green-brown spots. Very hardy; suitable for an open site. ↕↔ 4m (12ft). E. North America. ❄❄❄

***R.* 'Moerheim'** 🏆 Free-flowering, dwarf, evergreen shrub with small, dark green leaves that turn maroon in winter. Bears small trusses of funnel-shaped, violet-blue flowers, 3cm (1¼in) long, in abundance in mid-spring. Very hardy; prefers full sun. ↕↔ 60cm (24in). ❄❄❄

R. molle* subsp. *japonicum, syn. *R. japonicum*. Vigorous, deciduous azalea of upright habit, with obovate, obovate-oblong, or inversely lance-shaped leaves, 5–10cm (2–4in) long, mid-green above, paler bluish green beneath. Trusses of 2–12 widely funnel-shaped, often scented, orange-red, occasionally yellow flowers, 6–9cm (2½–3½in) long, softly hairy outside, are borne before the leaves, in late spring. Tolerates full sun. ↕↔ 2.2m (7ft). C. and E. Japan. ❄❄❄

***R.* 'Moonshine Crescent'.** Evergreen shrub of open, upright habit, with medium-sized leaves. In mid-spring, dome-shaped trusses of bell-shaped, primrose-yellow flowers, 5–7cm (2–3in) long, open from red winter buds. ↕↔ 2–2.5m (6–8ft). ❄❄❄

R. moupinense 🏆 Compact, dwarf, evergreen shrub with narrowly ovate, elliptic, or obovate, glossy, dark green leaves, 3–5cm (1¼–2in) long, paler green and minutely scaly beneath. Trusses of up to 3 funnel-shaped, white, pink, or deep rose-pink flowers, 3–4cm (1¼–1½in) long, sometimes spotted purple inside, are borne in late winter and early spring. ↕↔ 1.2m (4ft). W. China. ❄❄❄

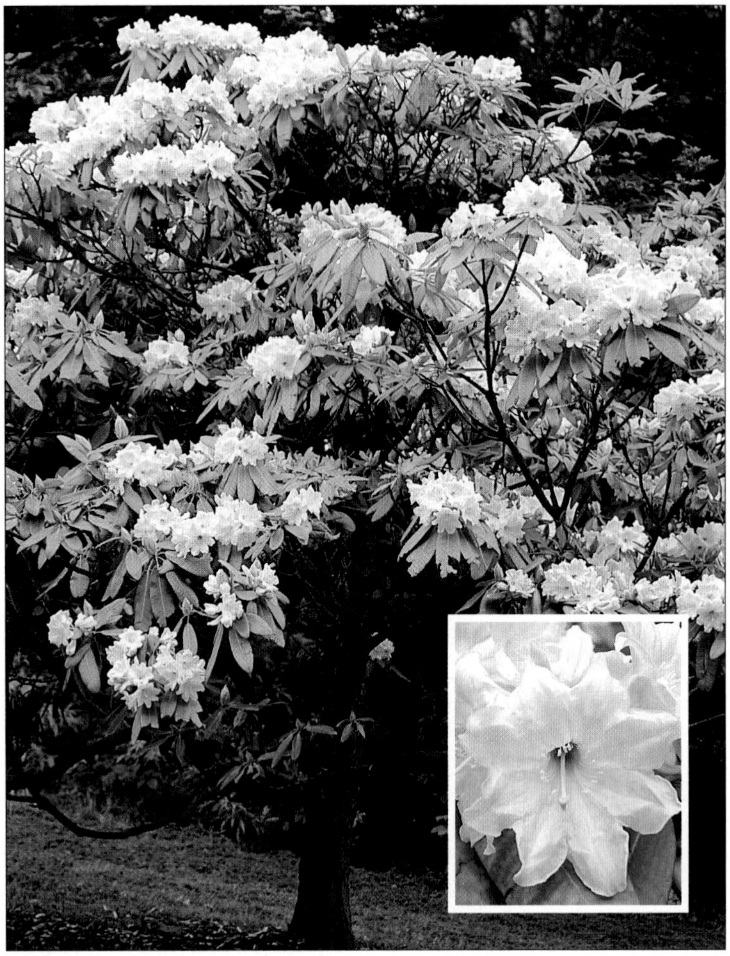

Rhododendron 'Polar Bear' (inset: flower detail)

***R.* 'Mrs. A.T. de la Mare'** 🏆 Upright, compact, evergreen shrub with medium-sized leaves. Domed trusses of funnel-shaped, frilled, slightly fragrant, pale pink flowers, 9cm (3½in) long, fading to white, with green-spotted throats, are borne in late spring. ↕↔ 3m (10ft). ❄❄❄

***R.* 'Mrs. Furnival'** ▣🏆 Compact, evergreen shrub with medium-sized leaves. From an early age, bears neat trusses of funnel-shaped, light rose-pink flowers, to 8cm (3in) long, each with a bold, brownish red flare inside, in late spring. Suitable for partial shade or full sun. ↕↔ 2.2m (7ft). ❄❄❄

***R.* 'Mrs. G.W. Leak'** ▣ syn. *R.* 'Cottage Garden's Pride'. Compact, evergreen shrub with medium-sized leaves. In mid-spring, bears upright trusses of funnel-shaped, light rose-pink flowers, 10–15cm (4–6in) long, each with a deep brown and crimson central flare. ↕↔ 4m (12ft). ❄❄❄

***R.* 'Mrs. T.H. Lowinsky'** ▣🏆 Free-flowering, vigorous, evergreen shrub with medium-sized leaves. Dense trusses of funnel-shaped, pink-flushed white flowers, to 8cm (3in) long, each with a bright orange-brown flare inside and reflexed lobes, open from lavender-pink buds in early summer. Grow in sun. ↕↔ 2.2–3m (7–10ft). ❄❄❄

R. mucronatum ▣ syn. *R.* 'Ledifolium'. Spreading, semi-evergreen shrub with lance-shaped to ovate- or oblong-lance-shaped, hairy, mid-green leaves, 3–6cm (1¼–2½in) long. In mid-spring, freely bears trusses of 2 or 3 widely funnel-shaped, fragrant white, occasionally pink flowers, 6–7cm (2½–3in) across. Grows well in full sun. ↕↔ 1.2–1.5m (4–5ft). Origin uncertain. ❄❄❄

***R. mucronulatum*.** Dwarf to medium-sized, deciduous shrub of erect habit, with lance-shaped, dark green leaves, 4–6cm (1½–2½in) long, scaly beneath. Solitary, funnel-shaped, pinkish purple, pink, or occasionally white flowers, 2–2.5cm (¾–1in) long, are borne from midwinter to early spring. Grow in full sun. ↕ 0.3–2.5m (1–8ft), ↔ 1m (3ft). E. Russia, N. and C. China, Mongolia. ❄❄❄

***R. nakaharae*.** Prostrate, compact, evergreen shrub with small, bristly leaves, 2.5cm (1in) long, shiny, dark green above, paler green beneath. Trusses of up to 3 funnel- to bell-shaped, dark orange-red to rose-red flowers, 1–2cm (½–¾in) long, are borne in early and midsummer. ↕ 30cm (12in), ↔ 2m (6ft). Taiwan. ❄❄❄

***R.* 'Naomi'** ▣♀ Tall, evergreen shrub or small tree with medium-sized leaves. In mid-spring, produces large trusses of widely funnel-shaped, fragrant, pale lavender-pink flowers, 9cm (3½in) across, shading to greenish yellow in the throats and each with a subtle brown stripe. ↕↔ 5m (15ft). ❄❄❄

***R.* 'Narcissiflorum'** ▣🏆 Compact, vigorous, deciduous Ghent azalea with medium-sized leaves. In late spring and early summer, bears compact trusses of hose-in-hose, sweetly scented, pale yellow flowers, 3cm (1¼in) long, darker yellow towards the centres and on the outsides of the petals. ↕↔ 1.5–2.5m (5–8ft). ❄❄❄

***R.* 'Ne Plus Ultra'.** Vigorous, upright, evergreen Vireya rhododendron with medium-sized leaves. Trusses of up to 14 tubular-funnel-shaped, bright red flowers, 5–6cm (2–2½in) long, with purplish pink throats, are produced intermittently from summer to winter. ↕ 1.5m (5ft), ↔ 1m (3ft). ❀ (min. 5°C/41°F)

R. neriiflorum ▣ Evergreen shrub producing elliptic to oblong or inversely lance-shaped, dark green leaves, 4–11cm (1½–4½in) long, glaucous beneath. In mid- and late spring, bears trusses of 5–12 tubular-bell-shaped, fleshy, bright scarlet to crimson flowers, 3.5–4.5cm (1½–1¾in) long. Suitable for full sun. ↕ to 6m (20ft), ↔ 4m (12ft). Tibet, China, Burma. ❄❄❄

R. niveum 🏆♀ Distinctive, evergreen shrub or tree with white-felted shoots and inversely lance-shaped to elliptic leaves, 11–17cm (4½–7in) long, dark green above, with a white-fawn indumentum beneath. In mid-spring, bears compact trusses of 15–30 tubular-bell-shaped, smoky blue to purple-lilac flowers, 3–3.5cm (1¼–1½in) long, with dark purple nectar pouches inside. ↕ to 6m (20ft), ↔ 4m (12ft). India (Sikkim), Bhutan. ❄❄❄

***R.* Nobleanum Group** ▣♀ syn. *R.* x *pulcherrimum*. Robust, evergreen shrubs or small trees producing medium-sized to large leaves. Compact trusses of broadly funnel-shaped flowers, 5cm (2in) across, which may be rose-red, pink, or white (depending on the clone), are borne intermittently in mild weather, from late autumn to early spring. ↕↔ 5m (15ft). ❄❄❄

***R.* 'Nova Zembla'** ▣ Evergreen shrub with medium-sized leaves. Full, rounded trusses of broadly funnel-shaped, deep red flowers, 4–5cm (1½–2in) long, spotted darker red inside, are produced in mid- and late spring. ↕↔ 1.5–3m (5–10ft). ❄❄❄

R. nuttallii 🏆♀ Evergreen shrub or small tree of open habit, with oblong to oblong-ovate leaves, 17–26cm (7–10in) long, strongly puckered, dark green above, densely scaly beneath. Trusses of 3–6 very large, tubular to bell-shaped, strongly scented, yellow or creamy white flowers, 8–13cm (3–5in) long, suffused yellow in the throats, are borne in mid-spring. ↕↔ to 10m (30ft). N.E. India to W. China. ❄

R. occidentale ▣🏆 Deciduous shrub with elliptic to oblong-lance-shaped leaves, 3–9cm (1¼–3½in) long, glossy, mid-green above, glaucous beneath. In early summer, bears trusses of 6–12 broadly funnel-shaped, sweetly scented, usually creamy white or pale pink flowers, 6–8cm (2½–3in) across, each with a yellow or yellow-orange mark inside. Grow in sun. ↕↔ 3m (10ft). W. North America. ❄❄❄

***R.* 'Odee Wright'** ▣🏆 Compact, sometimes low-growing, dense, evergreen shrub with medium-sized leaves. In mid-spring, peach-coloured buds open to trusses of up to 15 broadly funnel-shaped, greenish yellow flowers, to 15cm (6in) long, tinted pink, and spotted carmine-red in the throats. Grow in full sun. ↕↔ 1.5m (5ft). ❄❄❄

***R.* 'Olive'** ▣ Free-flowering, upright, small to medium-sized, evergreen shrub producing small, ovate-elliptic leaves, mid-green above, paler green beneath. Trusses of 2 or 3 funnel-shaped flowers, 4cm (1½in) long, mauve-pink with

R

deeper spots inside, are borne in early spring. ↕ 1.2m (4ft), ↔ 1m (3ft). ❄❄❄
R. orbiculare ○ Evergreen shrub or tree producing distinctive, rounded, matt, mid-green leaves, 7–13cm (3–5in) long, glaucous beneath, with heart- or ear-shaped bases. Loose trusses of 7–12 broadly bell-shaped, rose- to deep pink flowers, 5–7cm (2–3in) long, are borne in mid- and late spring. Grow in sun. ↕↔ 3m (10ft). W. China. ❄❄❄
R. oreodoxa ■ ○ Evergreen shrub or small tree with obovate-elliptic, dark green leaves, 6–9cm (2½–3½in) long, pale bluish green and glaucous beneath. In mid-spring, bears abundant trusses of 10–12 tubular- to broadly bell-shaped, usually 7-lobed pink flowers, 5cm (2in) long, sometimes purple-spotted inside. Tolerates full sun. ↕ 3–5m (10–15ft), ↔ 3m (10ft). W. China. ❄❄❄
R. oreotrephes ■ Evergreen shrub producing oblong-elliptic, mid- or grey-green leaves, 2–8cm (¾–3in) long, usually with purple, red-brown, or grey scales, and glaucous beneath. In mid- and late spring, bears trusses of 3–11 funnel- to bell-shaped, mauve, purple, or rose-pink flowers, 2.5–3.5cm (1–1½in) long, sometimes purple-spotted inside. Thrives in sun. ↕↔ 5m (15ft). Tibet, China, Burma. ❄❄❄
R. pachysanthum ■ ♀ Evergreen, mound-forming shrub. Lance-shaped to oval leaves, 4–10cm (1½–4in) long, have a conspicuous silver-brown indumentum above, and a dense silver indumentum beneath, later becoming rich brown. In mid-spring, bears trusses of 11 or more funnel- to bell-shaped, pale rose-pink flowers, to 4cm (1½in) long, with variable markings inside. Grow in sun. ↕ 1.5–2.5m (5–8ft), ↔ 2.5m (8ft). Taiwan. ❄❄❄
***R.* 'Palestrina'** ■ ♀ Compact, evergreen Vuyk azalea with small leaves. Trusses of 2 or 3 open funnel-shaped, pure white flowers, 6–10cm (2½–4in) long, with faint green markings in the throats, are borne freely in late spring. ↕↔ 1.2m (4ft). ❄❄❄
***R.* 'Patty Bee'** ♀ Free-flowering, dwarf, evergreen shrub, of compact, rounded habit, with small leaves turning purple-bronze in winter. Compact trusses of broadly funnel-shaped, clear pale yellow flowers, 5cm (2in) across, smother the foliage in early and mid-spring. Prefers full sun; very hardy. ↕↔ 75cm (30in). ❄❄❄
R. pemakoense. Dwarf, dense, compact, evergreen shrub with small, elliptic to obovate leaves, 2–3cm (¾–1¼in) long, glossy, dark green above, glaucous beneath. Abundant trusses of up to 3 bell-shaped, pink to rose-purple flowers, 3.5–4.5cm (1½–1¾in) long, open in early and mid-spring. ↕↔ 60cm (24in). N.E. India, S.E. Tibet. ❄❄❄
***R.* 'Penheale Blue'** ♀ Free-flowering, low-growing, compact, evergreen shrub with small leaves. Clustered trusses of funnel-shaped, red-flushed, bright violet-blue flowers, 2.5cm (1in) long, are borne in early and mid-spring. Suitable for full sun. ↕↔ 1–1.2m (3–4ft). ❄❄❄
***R.* 'Percy Wiseman'** ♀ Low-growing, compact, evergreen shrub with medium-sized leaves. In mid- and late spring, bears rounded trusses of funnel-shaped, peach-pink and cream flowers, 5cm (2in) long, fading to creamy white, with green markings in the throats. Suitable for full sun. ↕↔ 2m (6ft). ❄❄❄
***R.* 'Persil'** ■ ♀ Deciduous, bushy Knap Hill-Exbury azalea producing medium-sized leaves. Funnel-shaped, pure white flowers, to 6cm (2½in) long, each with a bold orange-yellow flare inside, open in mid-spring. ↕↔ 2m (6ft). ❄❄❄
***R.* 'Peter John Mezitt'** ♀ syn. *R.* 'P.J. Mezitt'. Dwarf, compact, evergreen shrub with small, ovate, dark green leaves, which turn brownish purple in winter if grown in full sun. Trusses of 4–9 small, frost-resistant, broadly funnel-shaped, bright lavender-pink flowers, 4.5cm (1¾in) long, are borne in very early spring. Very hardy. ↕↔ 1.2m (4ft). ❄❄❄
***R.* 'Pink Pearl'** ■ Vigorous, evergreen shrub of open, erect habit, with large leaves. In mid- and late spring, bears abundant tall trusses of funnel-shaped, soft pink flowers, 10–12cm (4–5in) long, fading to white. Thrives in sun. ↕↔ 4m (12ft). ❄❄❄
***R.* 'P.J. Mezitt'** see *R.* 'Peter John Mezitt'.
***R.* 'Polar Bear'** ■ ♀ ○ Late-flowering, vigorous, multi-stemmed, evergreen shrub or small tree with large leaves. In late summer, bears large trusses of tubular-funnel-shaped, strongly scented white flowers, 4.5–10cm (1¾–4in) long, with light brown-flecked, pale green throats. ↕ 5m (15ft), ↔ 4m (12ft). ❄❄❄
R. ponticum. Vigorous, evergreen shrub with inversely lance-shaped to broadly elliptic leaves, 6–18cm (2½–7in) long, glossy, dark green above, paler beneath. In early summer, bears trusses of 10–15 broadly funnel-shaped, reddish purple, occasionally white flowers, to 5cm (2in) long, often spotted yellowish green inside. ↕ 6–8m (20–25ft), ↔ 6m (20ft). Portugal, Spain, Lebanon, Turkey, Armenia, Caucasus. ❄❄❄
R. x praecox see *R.* 'Praecox'.
***R.* 'Praecox'** ♀ syn. *R.* x *praecox.* Early-flowering, sometimes low-growing, evergreen shrub producing small leaves. In late winter and early spring, trusses of 2 or 3 widely funnel-shaped, rose-purple flowers, 4–4.5cm (1½–1¾in) across, are borne at the shoot tips. Thrives in full sun; suitable as a hedge. ↕↔ 1.3m (4½ft). ❄❄❄
***R.* 'President Roosevelt'** ■ Slow-growing, weakly branched, evergreen shrub with splashes of bright yellow on its medium-sized, glossy, dark green leaves. In early and mid-spring, bears conical trusses of funnel-shaped, bright red flowers, 4–5cm (1½–2in) long, fading to white in the centres. ↕↔ 2m (6ft). ❄❄❄
***R.* 'Princess Anne'** ♀ syn. *R.* 'Golden Fleece'. Compact, rounded, semi-dwarf, evergreen shrub with small, ovate, mid-green leaves, bronze when young and during cold winters. Domed trusses of funnel-shaped, pale yellow, green-tinged flowers, 5cm (2in) long, are borne in abundance in mid-spring. Prefers full sun. ↕↔ 75–120cm (30–48in). ❄❄❄
R. prinophyllum see *R. austrinum.*
R. pseudochrysanthum ♀ Dome-shaped, evergreen shrub producing ovate to elliptic, rigid, thick, dark green leaves, 3–8cm (1¼–3in) long, with a thin grey indumentum above; the undersides are glossy, with midrib indumentum only. In mid-spring, bears trusses of 5–10 bell-shaped, pale pink or white flowers,

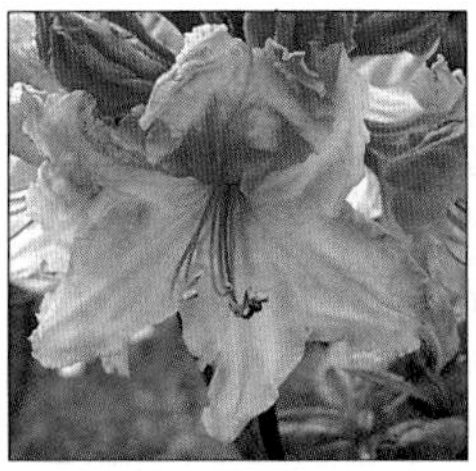
Rhododendron 'Medway'

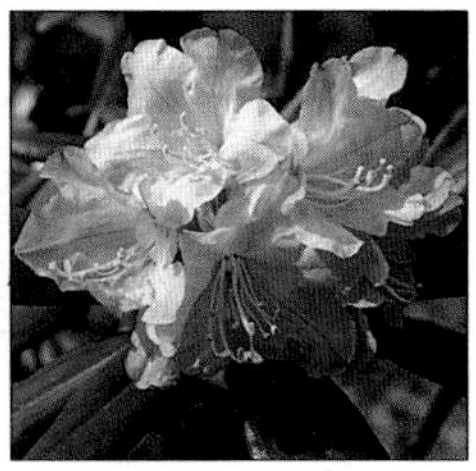
Rhododendron metternichii

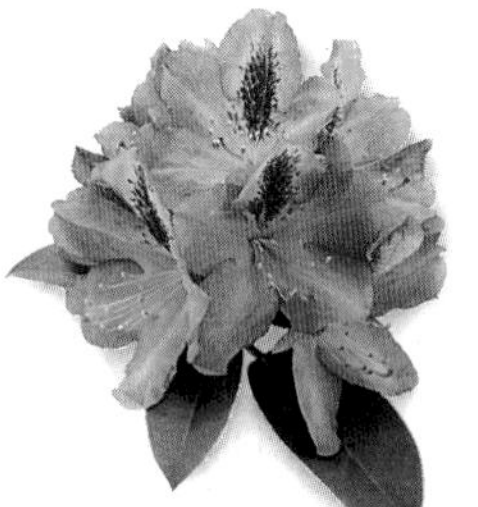
Rhododendron 'Mrs. Furnival'

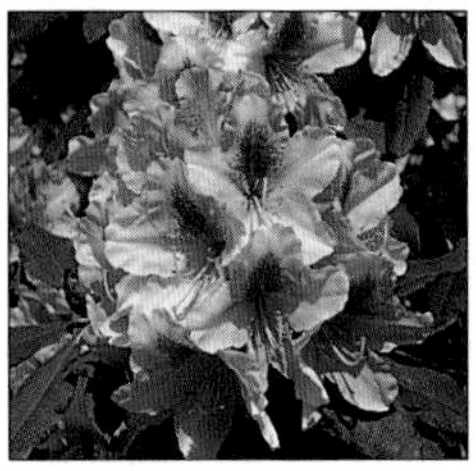
Rhododendron 'Mrs. G.W. Leak'

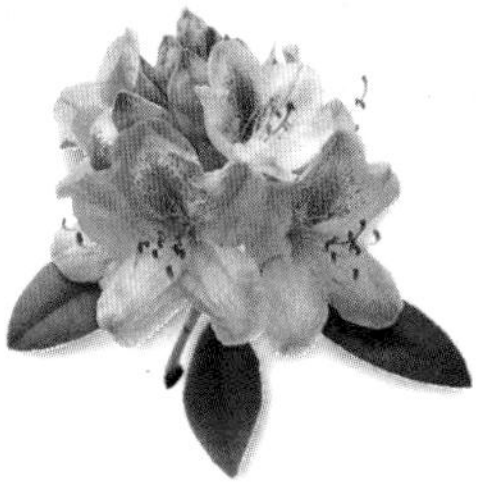
Rhododendron 'Mrs. T.H. Lowinsky'

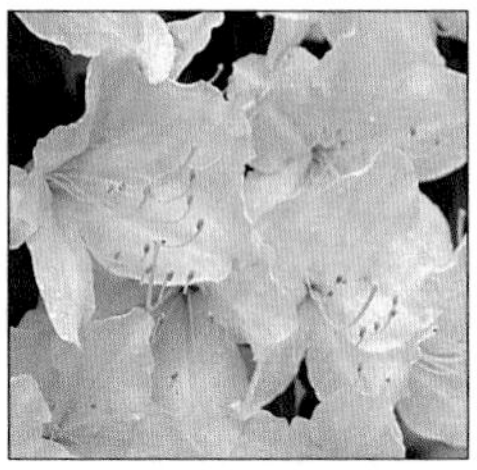
Rhododendron mucronatum

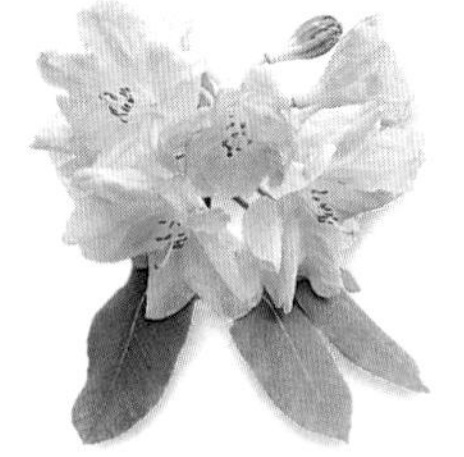
Rhododendron 'Naomi'

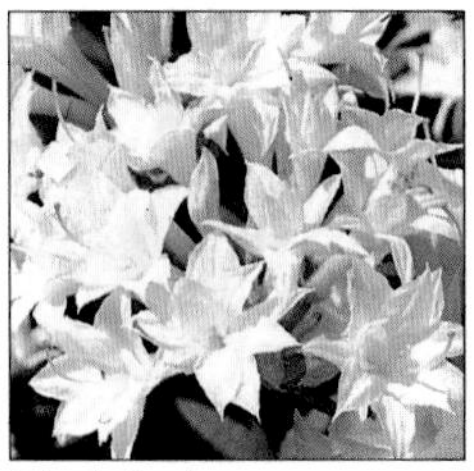
Rhododendron 'Narcissiflorum'

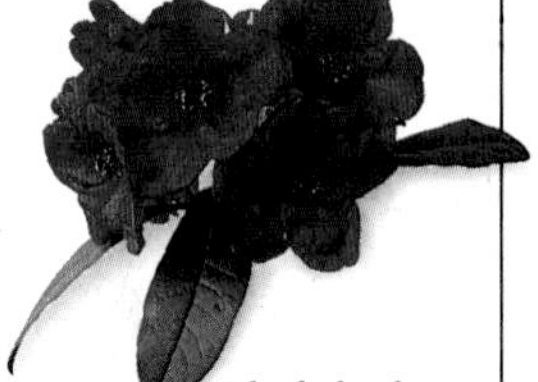
Rhododendron neriiflorum

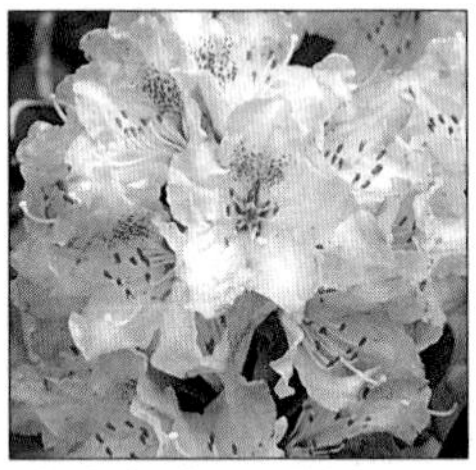
Rhododendron Nobleanum Group

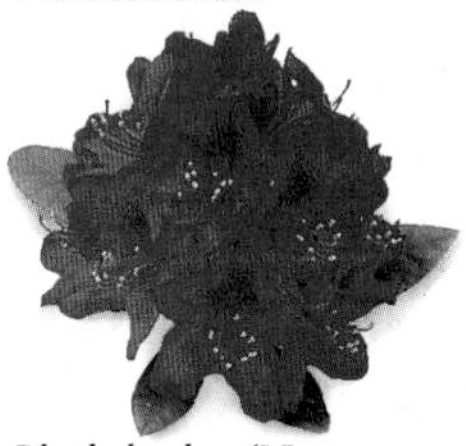
Rhododendron 'Nova Zembla'

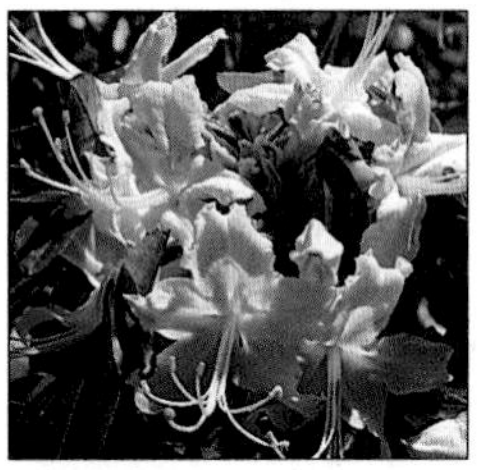
Rhododendron occidentale

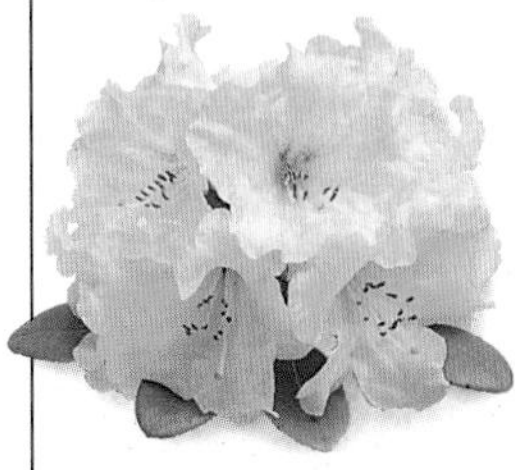
Rhododendron 'Odee Wright'

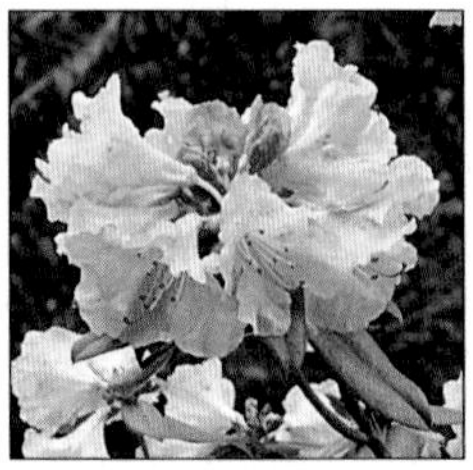
Rhododendron 'Olive'

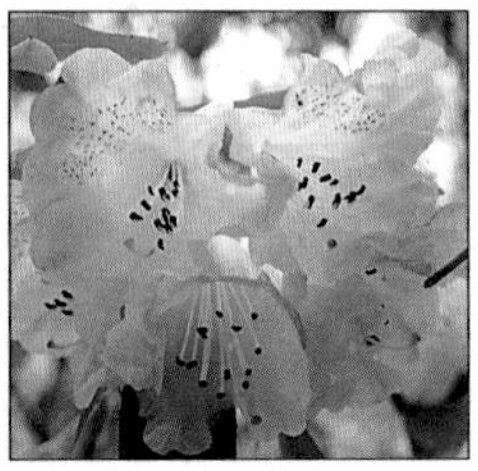
Rhododendron oreodoxa

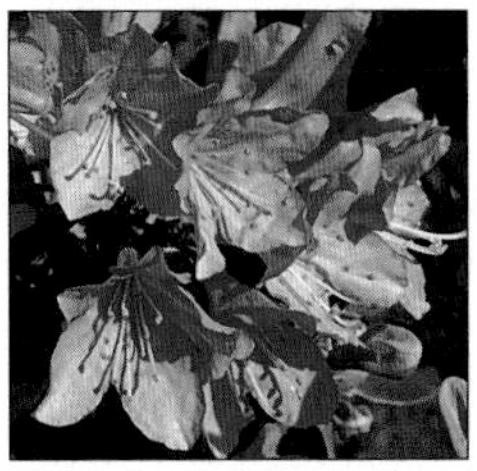
Rhododendron oreotrephes

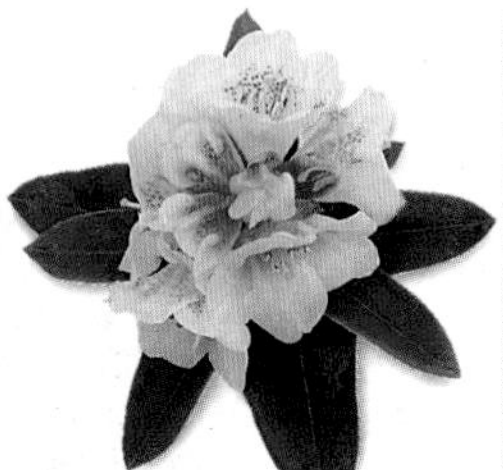
Rhododendron pachysanthum

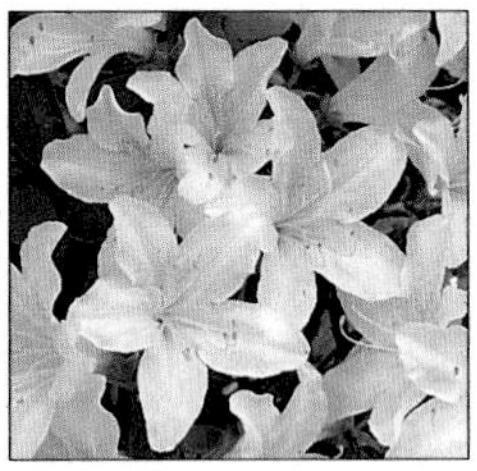
Rhododendron 'Palestrina'

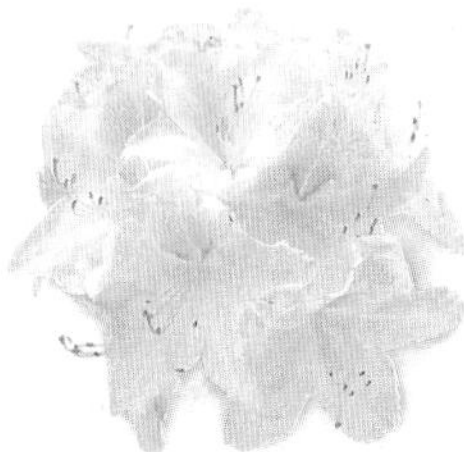
Rhododendron 'Persil'

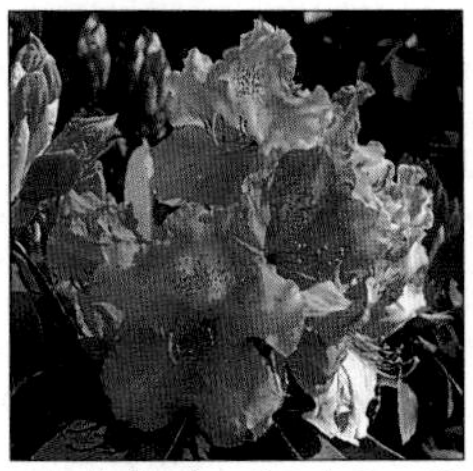
Rhododendron 'Pink Pearl'

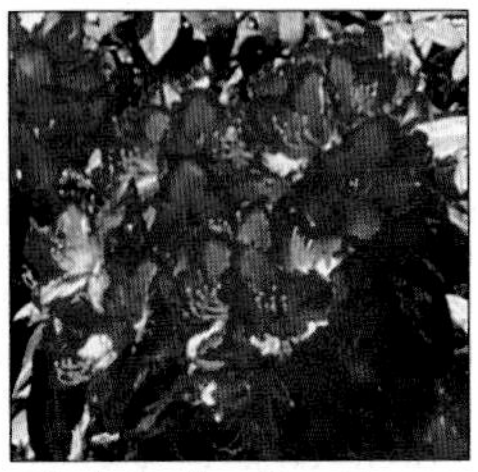
Rhododendron 'President Roosevelt'

R

3–4cm (1¼–1½in) long, deeply lined with dark pink outside and spotted with dark pink inside. Suitable for full sun. ↕↔ to 3m (10ft). Taiwan. ❄❄❄

***R.* 'Ptarmigan'** ■ ♀ Free-flowering, drought-resistant, dwarf, evergreen shrub with a spreading habit and small, dark green leaves. Clustered trusses of funnel-shaped, pure white flowers, 2.5cm (1in) long, virtually smother the foliage in early and mid-spring. ↕↔ 45–90cm (18–36in). ❄❄❄

R.* x *pulcherrimum see *R.* Nobleanum Group.

***R.* 'Purple Splendour'** ■ ♀ Evergreen shrub with medium-sized leaves. In late spring and early summer, bears trusses of about 15 striking, frilled, funnel-shaped, deep purple-blue flowers, to 8cm (3in) long, each with a purple-black basal mark inside. Suitable for full sun. ↕↔ 3m (10ft). ❄❄❄

***R.* 'Queen Elizabeth II'** ■ ♀ Strong-growing, evergreen shrub of open habit, with medium-sized leaves. Full trusses of 10–12 funnel-shaped, very pale, clear greenish yellow flowers, 11–12cm (4½–5in) long, are borne in mid- and late spring. ↕↔ 1.5–3m (5–10ft). ❄❄❄

R. racemosum ■ Stiffly branched, evergreen shrub producing broadly obovate to oblong-elliptic, mid- to dark green leaves, 1.5–5cm (½–2in) long, glaucous beneath. Bears abundant trusses of up to 4 widely funnel-shaped, deep rose-red, pink, or white flowers, to 3cm (1¼in) across, along the stems in early and mid-spring. ↕↔ 2m (6ft). W. China. ❄❄❄

***R.* 'Razorbill'** ♀ Free-flowering, compact, semi-dwarf, evergreen shrub with small, crinkled, dark green leaves. In early and mid-spring, bears conical trusses of distinctive, upward-facing, tubular, light rose-pink flowers, 2cm (¾in) long, flushed deep pink inside. ↕↔ 1.1–1.3m (3½–4½ft). ❄❄❄

R. rex ○ Evergreen, large shrub or small tree producing inversely lance-shaped leaves, 25–45cm (10–18in) long, with a cinnamon-brown indumentum above when young, becoming wrinkled, dark green, with a thick, cinnamon-brown or darker brown indumentum beneath. In mid- and late spring, bears trusses of 12–25 bell-shaped, 7- or 8-lobed, white-tinged pink flowers, 4–5cm (1½–2in) long, each with a crimson basal mark and sometimes heavily spotted crimson. Requires a sheltered site in light woodland. ↕↔ 12m (40ft). China (Sichuan, Yunnan). ❄❄❄. **subsp. *arizelum*** ■ syn. *R. arizelum*, has obovate leaves, 13–22cm (5–9in) long, and usually yellow, sometimes pink, rarely white flowers, with crimson marks in the throats; ↕↔ 8m (25ft), China (W. Yunnan), N.E. Burma. **subsp. *fictolacteum*** ■ syn. *R. fictolacteum*, has oblong-ovate to lance-shaped leaves, 11–30cm (4½–12in) long, and bears trusses of 12–25 white, sometimes pink-tinged flowers with crimson throats and sometimes crimson spotting; S.E. Tibet, China (W. Yunnan), N.E. Burma.

***R.* 'Rose Bud'** ■ ♀ Compact, low-growing, evergreen Kurume azalea with small leaves. In mid-spring, bears an abundance of small trusses of rosebud-like, funnel-shaped, rose-pink flowers, 3cm (1¼in) long. Thrives in sun. ↕↔ 60–90cm (24–36in). ❄❄❄

***R.* 'Roza Harrison'** see *R.* 'Roza Stevenson'.

***R.* 'Roza Stevenson'** ■ ♀ syn. *R.* 'Roza Harrison'. Vigorous, open, erect, evergreen shrub with medium-sized leaves. In mid- and late spring, bears abundant loose trusses of 10–12 saucer-shaped, clear lemon-yellow flowers, 15cm (6in) across. ↕↔ 1.5–4m (5–12ft). ❄❄❄

R. rubiginosum ○ Evergreen shrub or small tree with lance-shaped or oblong to elliptic-lance-shaped, dark green leaves, 5–12cm (2–5in) long, red-brown and scaly beneath. In mid- and late spring, bears trusses of 4–8 funnel- to bell-shaped, rose-pink to lilac-purple flowers, 1.5–3.5cm (½–1½in) long, brown-spotted inside. Thrives in sun. ↕ 10m (30ft) or more, ↔ 6m (20ft). S.E. Tibet, S.W. China, N. Burma. ❄❄❄

R. russatum ■ ♀ Dwarf, compact, evergreen shrub with narrowly to broadly elliptic or oblong, dark green leaves, to 4cm (1½in) long, brown to red-brown and scaly beneath. In mid- and late spring, bears trusses of 4–6 broadly funnel-shaped, reddish purple to indigo-blue, occasionally white flowers, 1–2cm (½–¾in) across. Prefers full sun. ↕ to 1.5m (5ft), ↔ 1.2m (4ft). S.W. China. ❄❄❄

***R.* 'St. Valentine'** ■ syn. *R.* 'Valentine'. Evergreen Vireya rhododendron of spreading habit, with small, elliptic leaves. Trusses of 3–5 pendent, tubular-bell-shaped, bright red flowers, 4cm (1½in) long, are borne in spring. ↕ 1.5m (5ft), ↔ 2m (6ft). ❀ (min. 5°C/41°F)

***R.* 'Sappho'** ■ ♀ Free-flowering, tall, evergreen shrub with medium-sized leaves. Funnel-shaped white flowers, 7–9cm (3–3½in) long, attractively flared purple-black in the throats, are borne in high-domed trusses in early summer. Grow in full sun. ↕↔ 3m (10ft). ❄❄❄

R. sargentianum ♀ Compact, dwarf, evergreen shrub with bristly, scaly shoots and broadly elliptic, aromatic leaves, to 1.5cm (½in) long, glossy mid-green above, densely golden scaly beneath. From mid-spring to early summer, bears flattened trusses of 5–7 tubular, lemon-yellow or cream flowers, to 1cm (½in) long, with spreading lobes. ↕↔ 60cm (24in). W. China. ❄❄❄

***R.* 'Satan'** ♀ Bushy, free-flowering, deciduous Knap Hill-Exbury azalea with medium-sized leaves. In mid-spring, produces bold trusses of funnel-shaped, bright red flowers, 5cm (2in) long. Grow in full sun. ↕↔ 2m (6ft). ❄❄❄

***R.* 'Scarlet Wonder'** ♀ Free-flowering, compact, semi-dwarf, evergreen shrub with small leaves. In mid-spring, bears loose trusses of 4–7 funnel-shaped, slightly frilled, bright cardinal-red flowers, 5cm (2in) long. ↕↔ 1.2–2m (4–6ft). ❄❄❄

R. schlippenbachii ♀ Deciduous, densely branched azalea with obovate or broadly ovate leaves, 2.5–11cm (1–4½in) long, dark green above, paler green beneath, borne in whorls of 5 at the branch tips. In mid- and late spring, produces trusses of 3–6 flat or saucer-shaped, pale pink or rose-pink, sometimes white flowers, 3–5cm (1¼–2in) across, spotted reddish pink on the upper lobes. ↕↔ to 5m (15ft). China (N. Manchuria), Korea. ❄❄❄

***R.* 'Scintillation'.** Evergreen shrub with medium-sized leaves. In early summer, bears dense, rounded trusses of funnel-shaped, pale pink flowers, 6–7cm (2½–3in) long, each with a bronze to pinkish brown flare in the throat. ↕↔ 2.2m (7ft). ❄❄❄

***R.* 'Seta'** ■ ♀ Free-flowering, evergreen shrub of open habit, with small leaves. In early spring, bears upright, clustered trusses of tubular-bell-shaped, light pink flowers, 3.5cm (1½in) long, striped deep pink on the outsides. ↕↔ 1–1.5m (3–5ft). ❄❄❄

***R.* 'Seven Stars'** ■ ♀ Vigorous, upright, evergreen shrub with medium-sized leaves. In mid-spring, bears rounded trusses of funnel-shaped, pale pinkish white flowers, 5cm (2in) across, flushed deep red-purple on the outsides on opening. ↕↔ 4m (12ft). ❄❄

***R.* 'Shamrock'.** Free-flowering, compact, dwarf, spreading, evergreen shrub with small leaves. In early and mid-spring, pale green buds open to trusses of 5–9 funnel-shaped, pale yellow flowers, 0.7–2.5cm (¼–1in) across, tinged green and spotted yellow inside. Very hardy; tolerates sun and drought. ↕↔ 75cm (30in). ❄❄❄

***R.* 'Silver Moon'.** Dwarf, broadly spreading, evergreen Glenn Dale azalea with small leaves. Abundant, funnel-shaped white flowers, 6–8cm (2½–3in) long, marked pale green inside, are borne in rounded trusses in mid-spring. Grow in sun. ↕↔ 1–1.5m (3–5ft). ❄❄❄

***R.* 'Silver Slipper'** ♀ Bushy, deciduous Knap Hill-Exbury azalea producing medium-sized leaves. Domed trusses of funnel-shaped white flowers, 6cm (2½in) across, flushed pink with central orange flares inside, are borne freely in

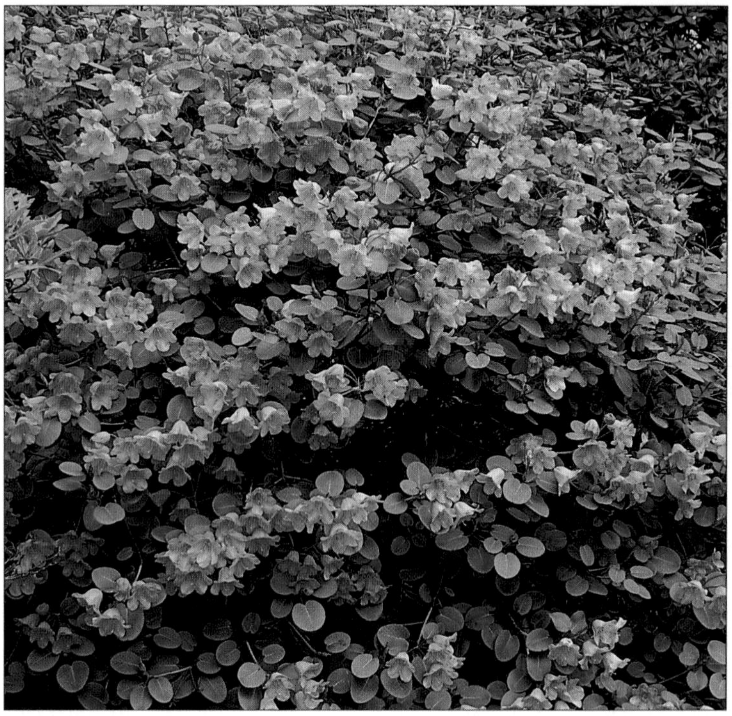

Rhododendron 'Temple Belle'

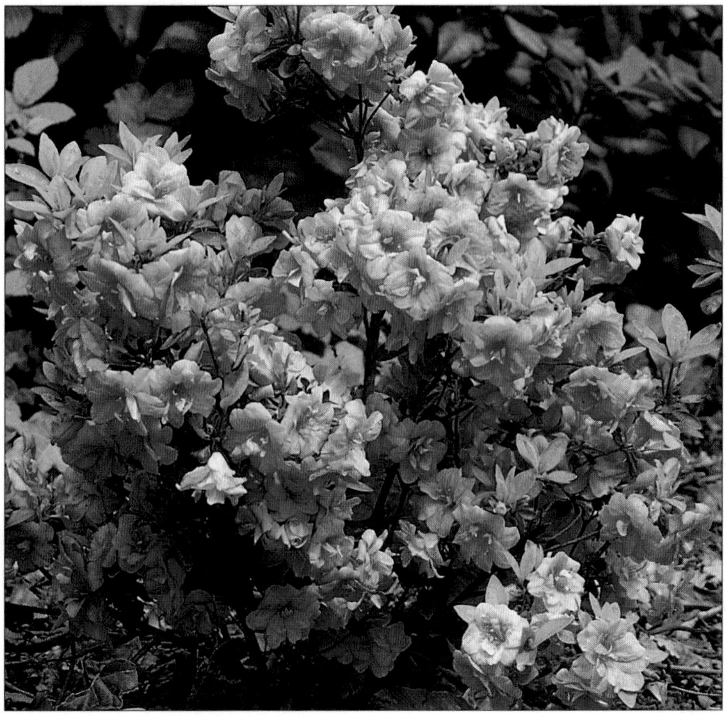

Rhododendron 'Rose Bud'

R

mid-spring. Suitable for sun. ↕↔ 2m (6ft). ***

R. sinogrande ■ ♀ ○ Evergreen shrub or small tree with very large, oblong to lance-shaped, glossy, dark green leaves, to 75cm (30in) long, with a smooth, silver to buff indumentum beneath. In mid- and late spring, bears trusses of 20–30 widely bell-shaped, pale yellow to creamy white flowers, 5cm (2in) long, marked crimson inside. ↕↔ 10m (30ft). Tibet, China, Burma. ***

***R.* 'Sir Charles Lemon'** ♀ Tall, erect, evergreen shrub producing medium-sized, dark green leaves with a cinnamon-brown indumentum beneath. In mid- and late spring, bears abundant dense trusses of funnel-shaped, pure white flowers, 4cm (1½in) across, speckled red inside. Grow in full sun. ↕ 6m (20ft), ↔ 4m (12ft). ***

R. smirnowii. Evergreen shrub producing oblong to lance-shaped, dark green leaves, 7–14cm (3–5½in) long, with a thick, woolly, fawn indumentum beneath. Trusses of 10–12 funnel- to bell-shaped, pale to deep rose-purple flowers, to 4cm (1½in) long, are borne in late spring and early summer. Very hardy. ↕ to 4m (12ft), ↔ 5m (15ft). N.E. Turkey, Georgia, Caucasus. ***

***R.* 'Snowdrift'.** Deciduous, bushy Mollis azalea with medium-sized leaves. Dense trusses of narrowly funnel-shaped white flowers, with yellow-orange marks in the throats, are borne in spring before the leaves. Suitable for full sun. ↕↔ 2.5m (8ft). ***

***R.* 'Snowflake'** see *R.* 'Kure-no-yuki'.

***R.* 'Snow Lady'** ♀ Compact, evergreen, semi-dwarf shrub with medium-sized leaves. In early spring, freely bears lax trusses of 2–5 funnel-shaped, pure white flowers, 2.5–4cm (1–1½in) long. Flowers best in a sunny, but sheltered site. ↕↔ 1m (3ft). ***

***R.* 'Songbird'.** Evergreen, compact, semi-dwarf shrub with small leaves. Neat trusses of small, funnel-shaped, vivid violet-blue flowers are borne in profusion in early spring. Very hardy; suitable for full sun. ↕↔ 1.2m (4ft). ***

R. souliei ■ Evergreen shrub with ovate-rounded leaves, 6–8cm (2½–3in) long, metallic blue-green above when young, becoming mid-green with age, light green and glaucous beneath. In late spring and early summer, bears trusses of 5–8 saucer-shaped, pink or rose-red, occasionally white flowers, 5–8cm (2–3in) long. ↕ to 5m (15ft), ↔ 4m (12ft). W. China. ***

***R.* 'Spek's Brilliant'** ■ ♀ Deciduous Mollis azalea with medium-sized leaves. In late spring and early summer, produces full trusses of funnel-shaped, bright orange-scarlet flowers, 2.5–6cm (1–2½in) across, with deeper orange-scarlet flares inside. Suitable for full sun. ↕↔ 2.5m (8ft). ***

***R.* 'Spek's Orange'** ■ ♀ Deciduous, bushy Mollis azalea with medium-sized leaves. In late spring and early summer, bears dense trusses of broadly funnel-shaped, bright reddish orange flowers, 6cm (2½in) long. Suitable for full sun. ↕↔ 2.5m (8ft). ***

***R.* 'Strawberry Ice'** ■ ♀ Bushy, deciduous Knap Hill-Exbury azalea with medium-sized leaves. Rounded trusses of broadly funnel-shaped, pale flesh pink flowers, 6–7cm (2½–3in) long, heavily veined and mottled deeper pink at the petal margins, with deep yellow-marked throats, are borne in late spring. Thrives in full sun. ↕↔ 2m (6ft). ***

R. strigillosum. Large, dome-shaped, evergreen shrub with densely bristly shoots and recurved, oblong to lance-shaped leaves, 7–14cm (3–5½in) long, bright green above, scaly and brown-hairy beneath. From late winter to mid-spring, bears trusses of 8–12 tubular-bell-shaped, glossy crimson-scarlet flowers, 4–6cm (1½–2½in) long. ↕↔ 6m (20ft). W. China. ***

***R.* 'Susan'** ■ ♀ Vigorous but compact, evergreen shrub with medium-sized leaves. In mid-spring, bears trusses of 12–16 funnel-shaped, cool mauve-blue flowers, 6cm (2½in) long, with darker margins, fading to near white. ↕↔ 3m (10ft). ***

R. sutchuenense ■ ○ Spreading, evergreen shrub or small tree with oblong to lance-shaped leaves, 11–25cm (4½–10in) long, matt, mid-green above, paler green beneath. From late winter to mid-spring, bears trusses of 8–12 broadly bell-shaped, rose-pink or pale lilac flowers, to 8cm (3in) across, often with purple spots inside. ↕↔ 8m (25ft). W. China. ***

***R.* 'Taylorii'.** Erect, evergreen Vireya rhododendron with medium-sized, narrowly elliptic leaves. From winter to spring, intermittently bears rounded trusses of up to 15 funnel-shaped pink flowers, 5–8cm (2–3in) long. ↕ 1.5m (5ft), ↔ 1m (3ft). ❀ (min. 5°C/41°F)

***R.* 'Temple Belle'** ■ ♀ Low-growing, compact, evergreen shrub producing medium-sized, rounded, pale green leaves. Loose trusses of 3–5 bell-shaped, clear pink flowers, 5–6cm (2–2½in) long, are borne freely in early and mid-spring. ↕↔ 2m (6ft). ***

***R.* 'Tessa Roza'** ♀ Early-flowering, low-growing, upright, evergreen shrub with small leaves. In late winter and early spring, produces trusses of 3 funnel-shaped, deep rose-pink flowers, 3–4cm (1¼–1½in) long, spotted deep carmine-red inside. ↕↔ 1.5m (5ft). ***

***R.* 'The Hon. Jean Marie de Montague'**, syn. *R.* 'Jean Mary Montague'. Free-flowering, compact, evergreen shrub with medium-sized leaves. Dense trusses of funnel-shaped, scarlet-crimson flowers, 5–7cm (2–3in) long, are borne in mid-spring. Tolerates heat, sun, and an exposed site. ↕↔ 2.5m (8ft). ***

R. thomsonii ■ ○ Evergreen shrub or small tree with smooth, peeling, purple-brown bark and broadly ovate leaves, 3–11cm (1¼–4½in) long, dark green above, glaucous beneath. Pendent trusses of 6–12 bell-shaped, waxy, fleshy, deep blood-red flowers, 3.5–5cm (1½–2in) long, with large calyces, open in mid- and late spring. ↕↔ 6m (20ft). Himalayas, W. China. ***

***R.* 'Titian Beauty'** ■ ♀ Low-growing, compact, evergreen shrub producing medium-sized, deep green leaves, with a thin brown indumentum beneath. Lax trusses of tubular-bell-shaped, waxy, rich red flowers, 3.5–5cm (1½–2in) long, are borne on long flower-stalks above the foliage, in late spring and early summer. Suitable for full sun. ↕↔ 2m (6ft). ***

R. tsariense. Evergreen shrub producing elliptic-obovate, dark green leaves, 3.5–6cm (1½–2½in) long, with a rich

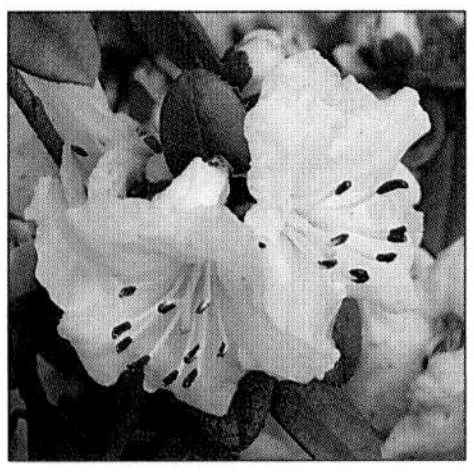

Rhododendron 'Ptarmigan'

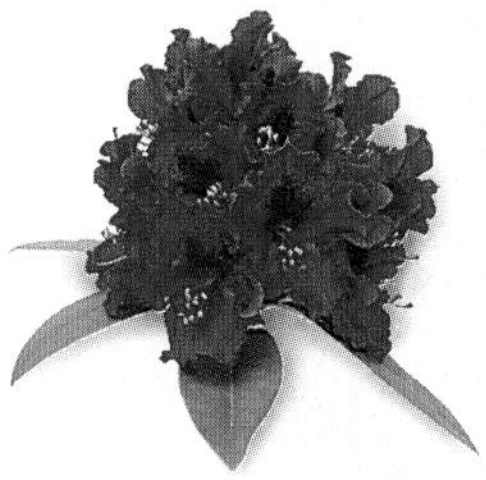

Rhododendron 'Purple Splendour'

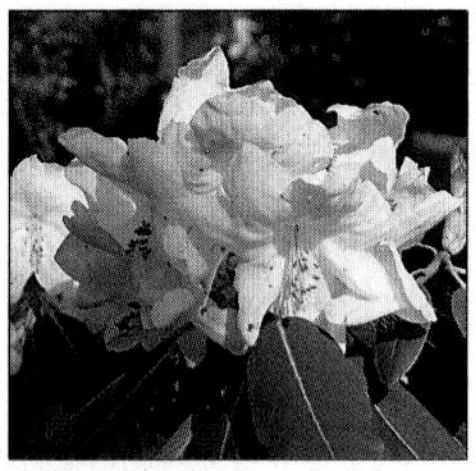

Rhododendron 'Queen Elizabeth II'

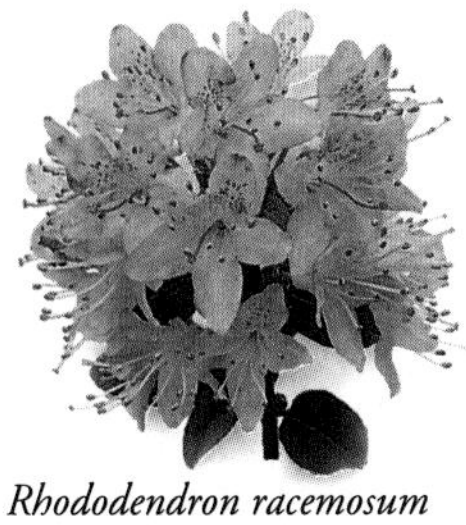

Rhododendron racemosum

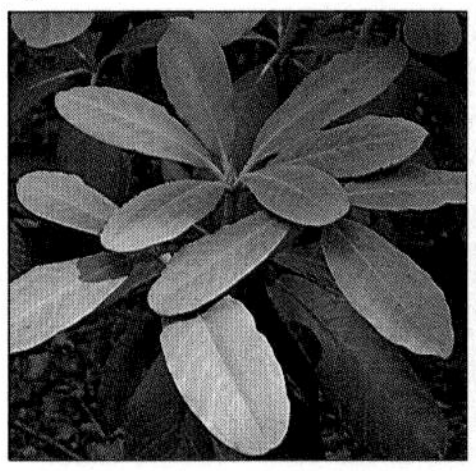

Rhododendron rex subsp. *arizelum*

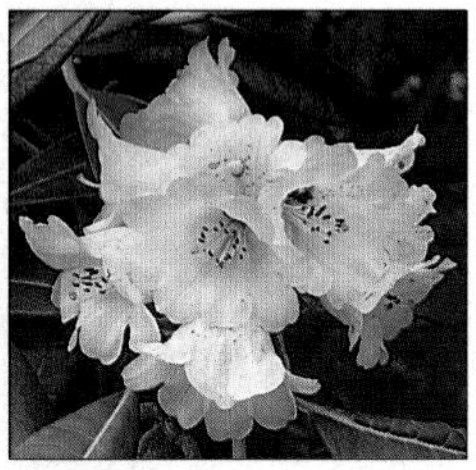

Rhododendron rex subsp. *fictolacteum*

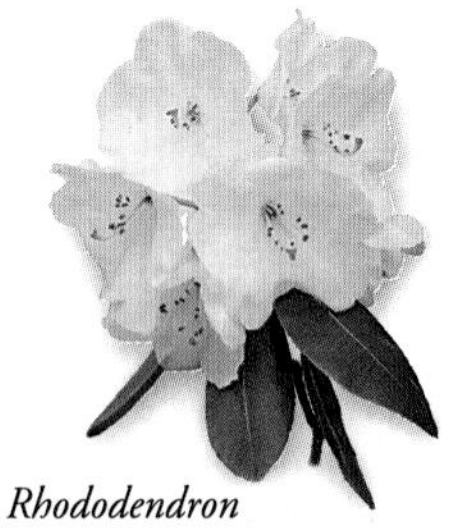

Rhododendron 'Roza Stevenson'

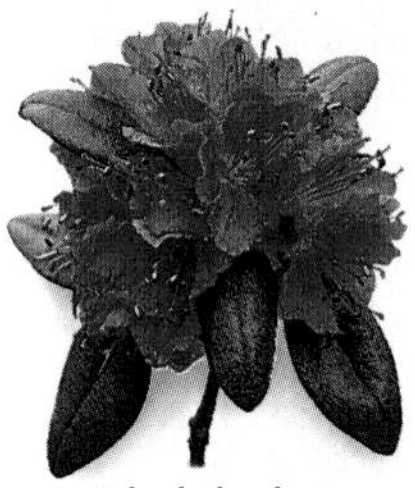

Rhododendron russatum

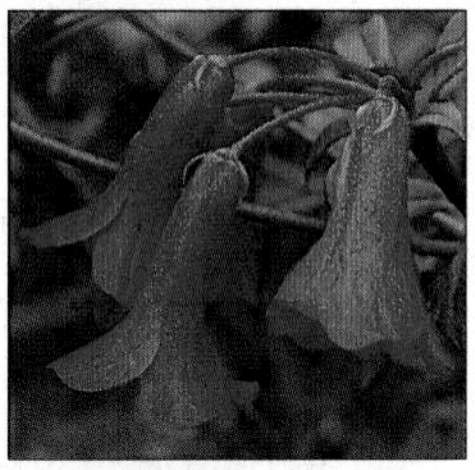

Rhododendron 'St. Valentine'

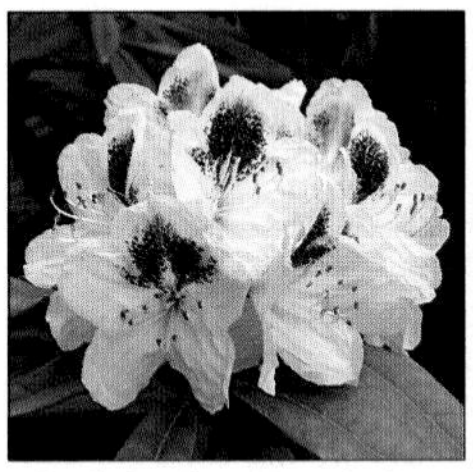

Rhododendron 'Sappho'

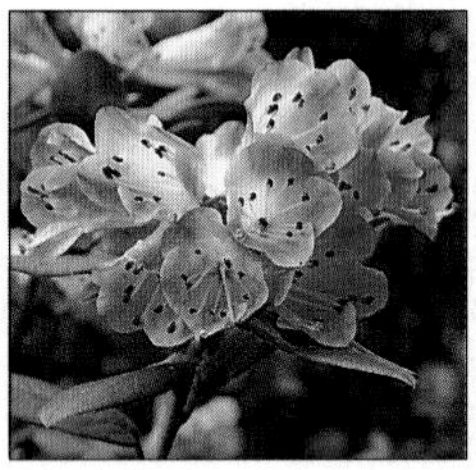

Rhododendron 'Seta'

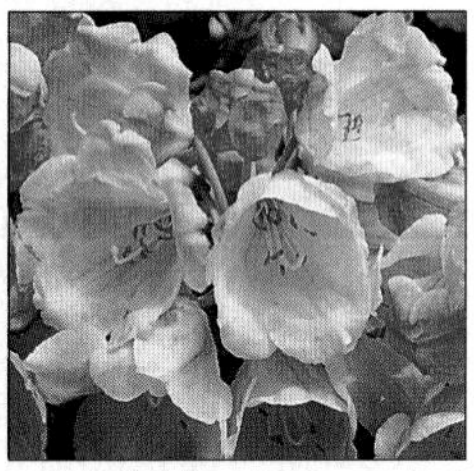

Rhododendron 'Seven Stars'

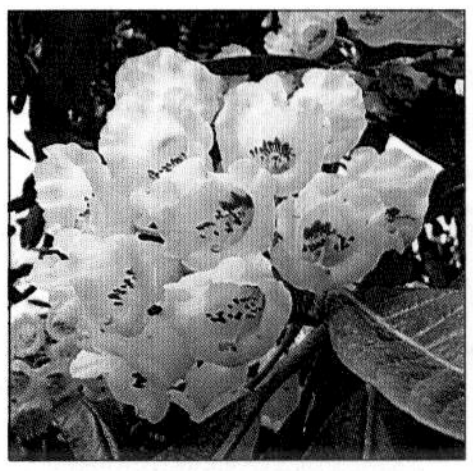

Rhododendron sinogrande

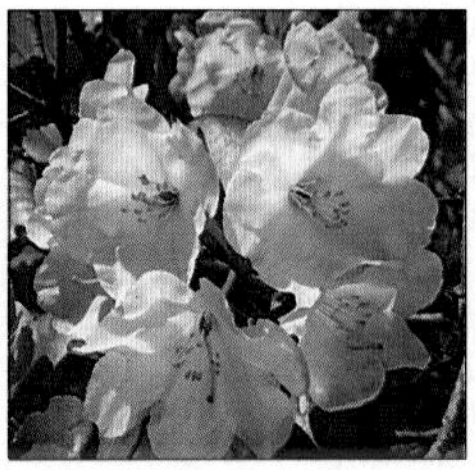

Rhododendron souliei

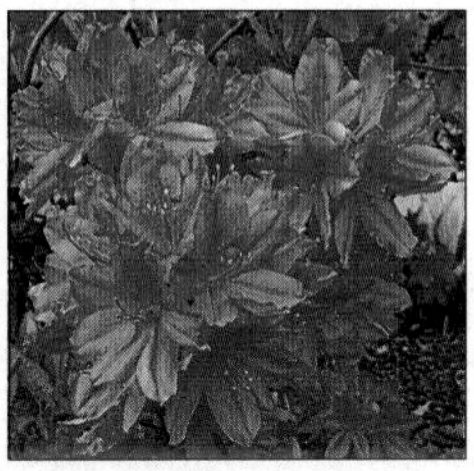

Rhododendron 'Spek's Brilliant'

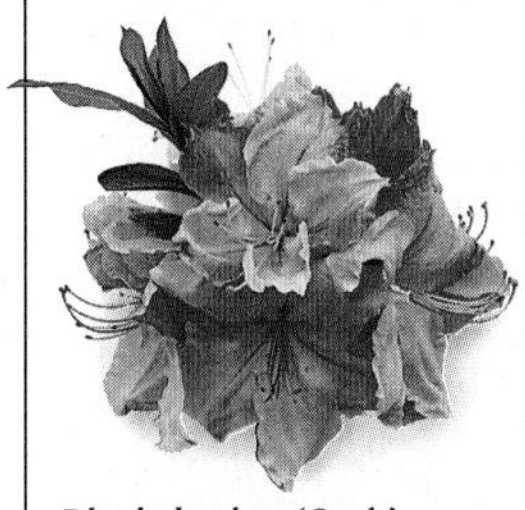

Rhododendron 'Spek's Orange'

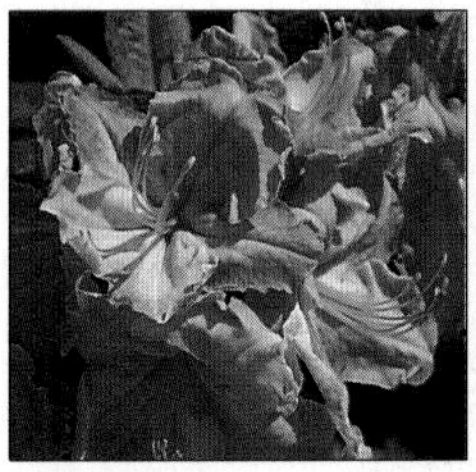

Rhododendron 'Strawberry Ice'

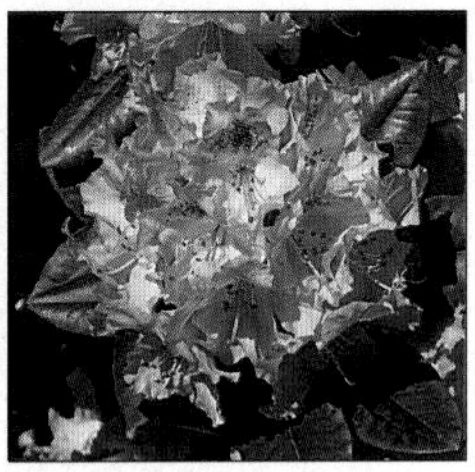

Rhododendron 'Susan'

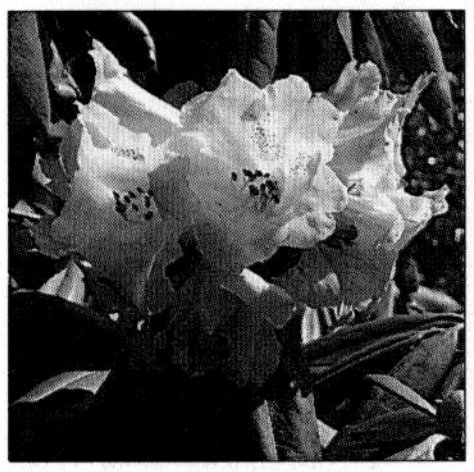

Rhododendron sutchuenense

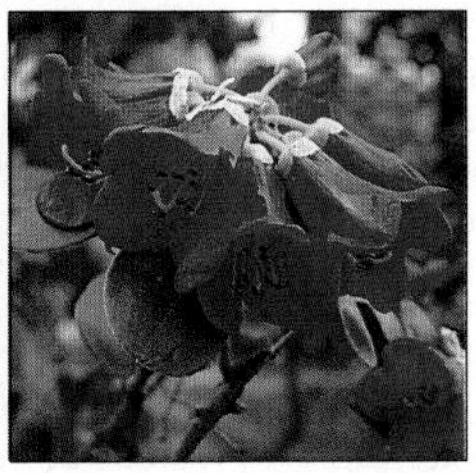

Rhododendron thomsonii

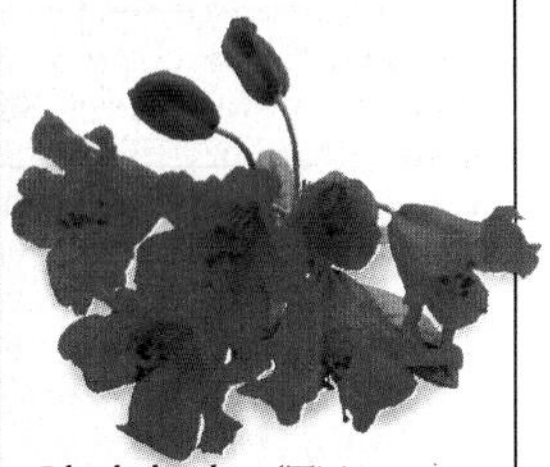

Rhododendron 'Titian Beauty'

R

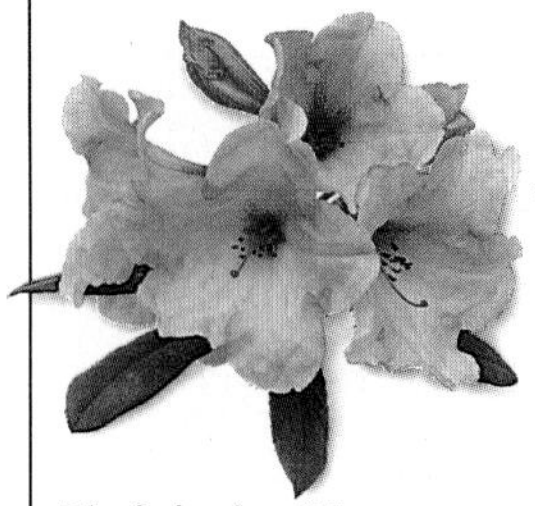
Rhododendron 'Vanessa Pastel'

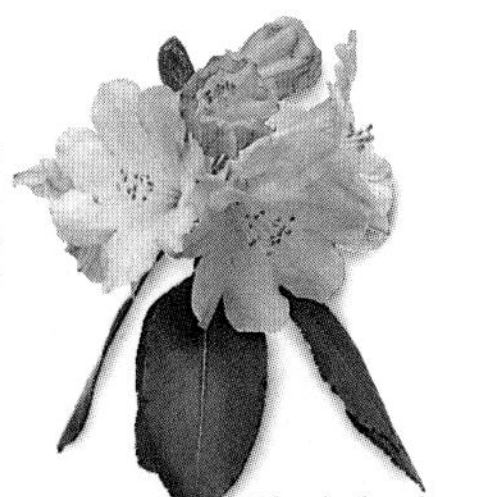
Rhododendron vernicosum

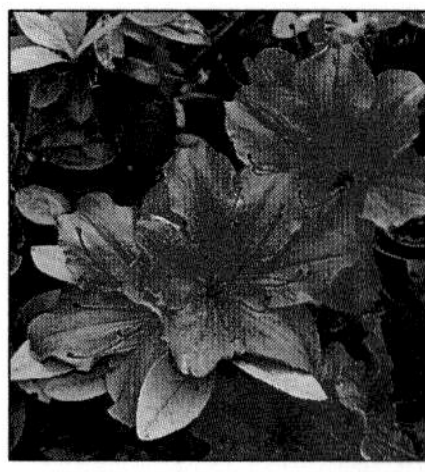
Rhododendron 'Vuyk's Rosyred'

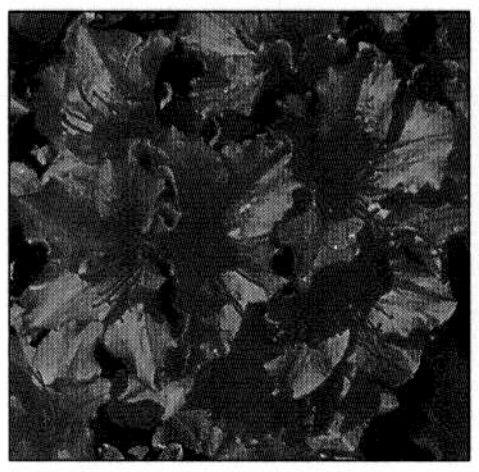
Rhododendron 'Vuyk's Scarlet'

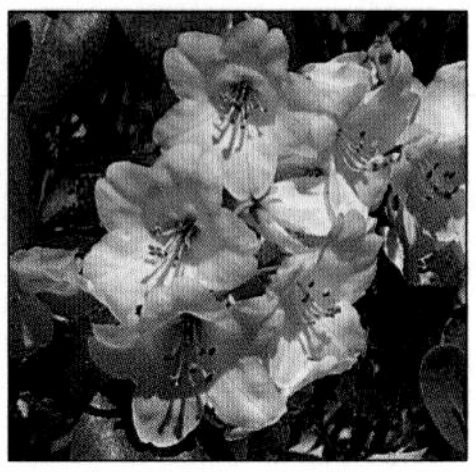
Rhododendron wardii

Rhododendron yakushimanum

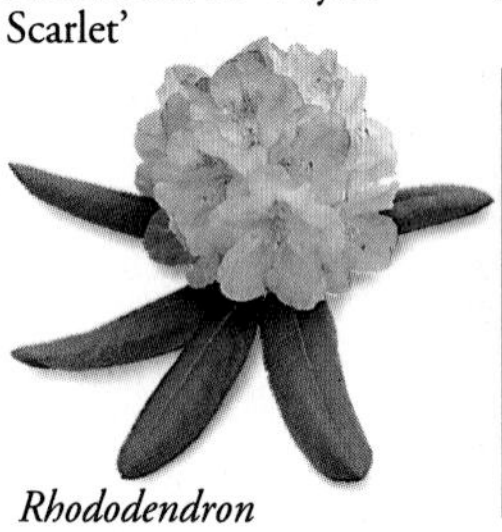
Rhododendron yakushimanum 'Ken Janeck'

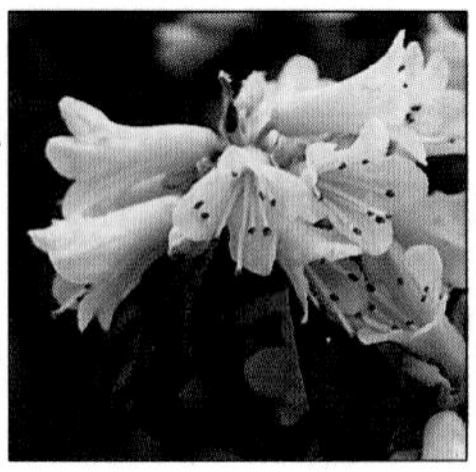
Rhododendron 'Yellow Hammer'

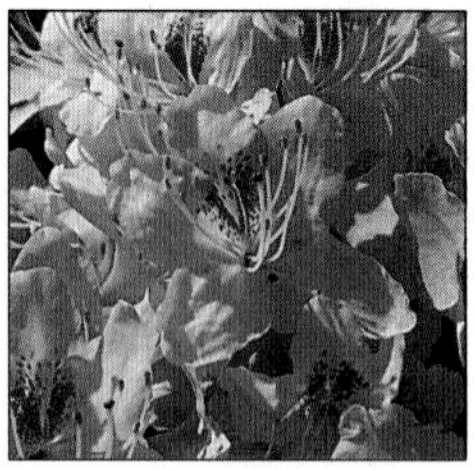
Rhododendron yunnanense

cinnamon-brown indumentum beneath. Trusses of 3 or 4 bell-shaped white flowers, 2.5–3.5cm (1–1½in) long, tinged pink and frequently spotted red inside, are borne from early to late spring. ↕↔ 4m (12ft). E. Himalayas, Tibet, Bhutan. ❄❄❄

***R.* 'Valentine'** see *R.* 'St. Valentine'.

***R.* 'Vanessa Pastel'** ■ ♀ Free-flowering, compact, evergreen shrub producing medium-sized leaves. In early summer, bears lax trusses of funnel-shaped, creamy pink flowers, 6cm (2½in) long, stained red on the outsides and with red-marked throats. ↕↔ 2m (6ft). ❄❄

R. vaseyi ♀ Deciduous azalea with elliptic to elliptic-oblong, hairless, shiny, dark green leaves, 5–12cm (2–5in) long, paler green beneath. In mid- and late spring, trusses of 4–8 broadly funnel-shaped, rose-pink, pale pink, or white flowers, 4cm (1½in) long, spotted red, are borne before the leaves. Suitable for full sun. ↕↔ 5m (15ft). E. North America. ❄❄❄

R

R. vernicosum ■ ◐ Evergreen shrub or small tree of variable habit, with elliptic to ovate-elliptic or obovate-elliptic, dull, mid-green leaves, 5–10cm (2–4in) long, slightly glaucous beneath. In late spring, produces trusses of 6–12 funnel- to bell-shaped, 6- or 7-lobed flowers, 3.5–5cm (1½–2in) long, bright rose-pink, lavender-pink, or white, sometimes marked crimson inside. ↕↔ 6m (20ft). W. China. ❄❄❄

***R.* 'Vida Brown'.** Slow-growing, evergreen Kurume azalea of low, compact habit, with small leaves. Hose-in-hose, rose-pink flowers, 4cm (1½in) long, are borne in small trusses in mid-spring. ↕ 75cm (30in), ↔ 1.2m (4ft). ❄❄❄

R. viridescens see *R. mekongense* Viridescens Group.

R. viscosum ♀ Deciduous azalea with hairy shoots and elliptic-obovate to oblong-obovate, dark green leaves, 1.5–3cm (½–1¼in) long, often glaucous beneath. In early and midsummer, bears trusses of 4–12 narrowly tubular to funnel-shaped, fragrant, pink-suffused white flowers, 2–3cm (¾–1¼in) long. Thrives in damp soil in sun. ↕↔ 2.5m (8ft). E. North America. ❄❄❄

***R.* 'Vuyk's Rosyred'** ■ ♀ Low-growing, dwarf, evergreen Vuyk azalea with small leaves. Bears a profusion of funnel-shaped, satiny, deep rose-pink flowers, 5cm (2in) long, each with a darker pink flare inside, in pairs in mid-spring. Suitable for full sun. ↕ 75cm (30in), ↔ 1.2m (4ft). ❄❄❄

***R.* 'Vuyk's Scarlet'** ■ ♀ Dwarf, evergreen Vuyk azalea with small leaves. In mid-spring, bears abundant solitary or paired, funnel-shaped, crimson-scarlet flowers, 6–7cm (2½–3in) long, with wavy-margined lobes. Tolerates full sun, especially in frost-prone areas. ↕ 75cm (30in), ↔ 1.2m (4ft). ❄❄❄

R. wardii ■ ◐ Evergreen shrub or small tree with oblong-elliptic to broadly obovate, hairless, dark green leaves, 6–11cm (2½–4½in) long, paler green beneath. Trusses of 7–14 broadly funnel-shaped flowers, 4–5cm (1½–2in) long, in various shades of yellow, sometimes with basal crimson marks inside, are borne in late spring and early summer. ↕ 6m (20ft), ↔ 5m (15ft). S.E. Tibet, S.W. China. ❄❄❄

***R.* 'Wigeon'.** Free-flowering, semi-dwarf, evergreen shrub with small leaves. In mid-spring, bears neat trusses of numerous saucer-shaped, rich lavender-pink flowers, 2.5cm (1in) long, with deeper spotting on the upper lobes inside. Very hardy; suitable for full sun. ↕↔ 1.2m (4ft). ❄❄❄

R. williamsianum ♀ Dome-shaped, evergreen shrub with ovate-rounded leaves, 2–4.5cm (¾–1¾in) long, brown when young, bright green above and glaucous beneath when mature. Loose trusses of 2 or 3 bell-shaped flowers, 3–4cm (1¼–1½in) long, in various shades of pink, occasionally white, are borne in abundance in mid- and late spring. Thrives in full sun. ↕ to 1.5m (5ft), ↔ 1.2m (4ft). W. China. ❄❄❄

***R.* 'Winsome'** ■ ♀ Compact, dense, sometimes low-growing, evergreen shrub with medium-sized, mid-green leaves, bronze when young. Loose trusses of funnel-shaped, cherry-pink flowers, 5–6cm (2–2½in) long, open in early and mid-spring. Suitable for sun or partial shade. ↕↔ 1.5m (5ft). ❄❄❄

***R.* 'Wombat'** ■ Prostrate, vigorous, evergreen azalea with small leaves. Lax trusses of funnel-shaped pink flowers,

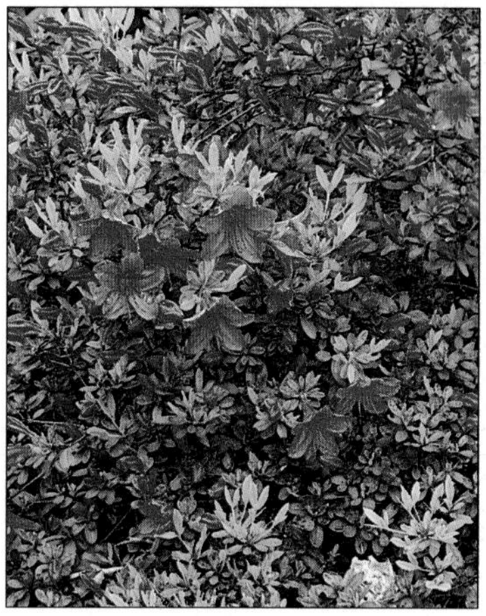
Rhododendron 'Wombat'

1–2cm (½–¾in) long, are produced in abundance in early summer. Provides excellent ground cover in full sun. ↕ 25cm (10in), ↔ 1.2m (4ft). ❄❄❄

R. xanthocodon see *R. cinnabarinum* subsp. *xanthocodon.*

***R.* 'Yaku Princess'.** Dense, compact, low-growing, evergreen shrub producing medium-sized, olive-green leaves, with a buff indumentum beneath. Spherical trusses of funnel-shaped, pinkish white flowers, 5–6cm (2–2½in) long, each with a deeper pink mark and greenish spots inside, are borne in mid- and late spring. Suitable for full sun. ↕↔ 1.5m (5ft). ❄❄❄

R. yakushimanum ■ syn. *R. degronianum* subsp. *yakushimanum.* Tightly dome-shaped, evergreen shrub with recurved, linear to lance-shaped, glossy, dark green leaves, 8–14cm (3–5½in) long, with a thick, reddish brown indumentum beneath. Young foliage has a pale cinnamon-brown indumentum on the upper surfaces, which is lost as the leaves mature. In mid-spring, trusses of 5–10 deep rose-pink buds open to tubular-funnel-shaped flowers, 3–4.5cm (1¼–1¾in) long, fading to pale pink or white. Very hardy; suitable for full sun. ↕↔ to 2m (6ft). Japan (Yakushima Island). ❄❄❄. **'Ken Janeck'** ■ syn. *R.* 'Ken Janeck', is low-growing, bearing full trusses of funnel-shaped white flowers, 4–5cm (1½–2in) long, lined with pinkish purple and spotted with green; ↕ 1.2m (4ft), ↔ 1.3m (4½ft).

***R.* 'Yellow Hammer'** ■ ♀ Erect, free-flowering, evergreen shrub with small leaves. Produces small, tightly packed trusses of 2 or 3 tubular, canary-yellow flowers, 2.5–3cm (1–1¼in) long, in early and mid-spring, and frequently again in autumn. Grow in sun. ↕↔ 2m (6ft). ❄❄❄

R. yunnanense ■ Vigorous, evergreen or semi-evergreen shrub with lance-shaped, narrowly elliptic, or elliptic, scaly leaves, 3–10cm (1¼–4in) long, bright green above, paler green beneath. In late spring, bears trusses of 3–5 broadly funnel-shaped, pink, pale rose-pink, lavender-pink, or white flowers, 2–3cm (¾–1¼in) long, sometimes with crimson marks, or crimson-spotted inside. Thrives in sun. ↕ to 6m (20ft), ↔ 4m (12ft). S.E. Tibet, W. China, Burma. ❄❄❄

▷**Rhododendron, Indian** see *Melastoma malabathricum*

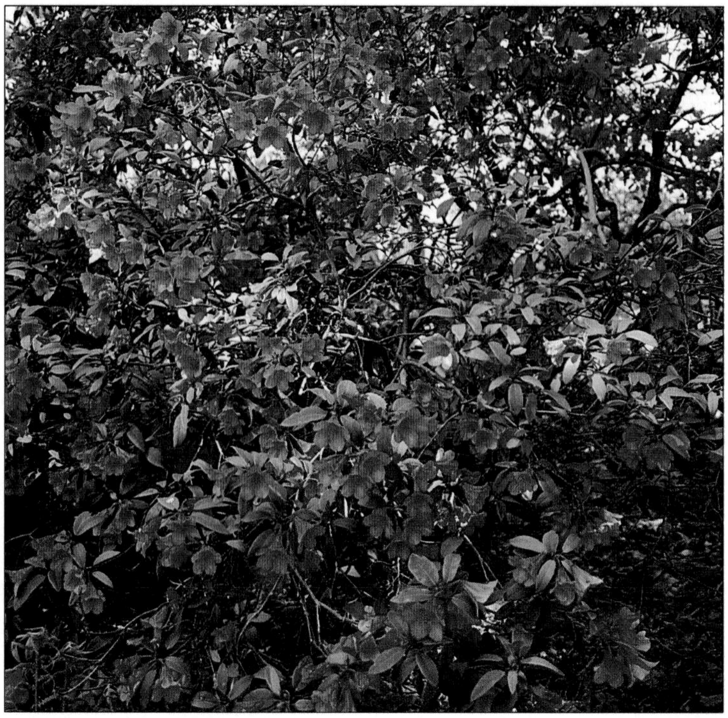
Rhododendron 'Winsome'

RHODOHYPOXIS

HYPOXIDACEAE

Genus of 6 species of small, clump-forming herbaceous perennials, with corm-like rootstocks, from open meadows in areas with heavy summer rainfall in the eastern provinces of South Africa, and Swaziland. The basal leaves are lance-shaped and hairy. Short-stalked, almost flat, white, pink, red, or deep purple flowers are produced over long periods in summer. Each flower has 6 overlapping tepals, arranged in 2 ranks of 3, which are fused at the bases to form a tube; the outer tepals are broader than the inner ones. Grow in a trough, rock garden, or alpine house.

• **HARDINESS** Fully hardy to frost hardy; to survive lower temperatures, plants must be kept almost dry in winter.

• **CULTIVATION** Under glass, grow in a mix of equal parts lime-free (ericaceous) potting compost, leaf mould, and sharp sand, in full light. When in growth, water freely and apply a balanced liquid fertilizer monthly; keep just moist in winter. Outdoors, grow in well-drained, moderately fertile, humus-rich soil in full sun, with protection from excessive winter wet. *R. milloides* thrives in damp conditions, and will tolerate more winter wet.

• **PROPAGATION** Sow seed at 6–12°C (45–54°F) as soon as ripe or in spring. Divide established clumps, or separate offsets, in late autumn.

• **PESTS AND DISEASES** Susceptible to red spider mites and thrips under glass.

R. baurii ♀ Clump-forming perennial with basal clusters of narrowly lance-shaped, keeled, folded leaves, to 10cm (4in) long. The leaves are dull greyish green, and very hairy on both surfaces and at the margins. Solitary, pale to deep reddish pink flowers, to 2cm (¾in) across, are produced on stalks 5–10cm (2–4in) tall, throughout summer. ↕↔ 10cm (4in). South Africa. ✲✲. The

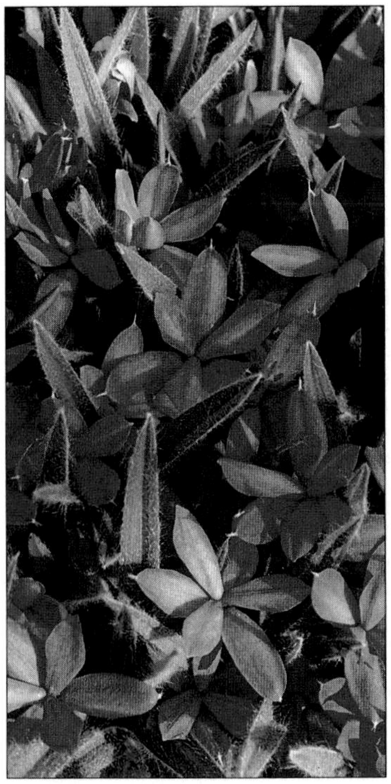

Rhodohypoxis baurii 'Albrighton'

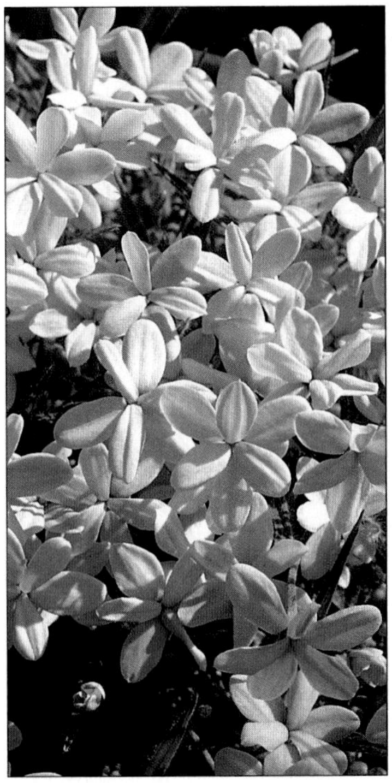

Rhodohypoxis baurii 'Margaret Rose'

following cultivars, derived mainly from *R. baurii* and *R. baurii* var. *platypetala*, are generally large-flowered and vigorous. **'Albrighton'** ■ has deep red-pink flowers. **'Harlequin'** has pink-flushed white flowers, to 1.5cm (½in) across, with distinct pink margins. **'Helen'**, syn. *R.* 'Tetra White', has very large white flowers, 3cm (1¼in) or more across. **'Margaret Rose'** ■ has clear pink flowers. **var. *platypetala*** is more robust than *R. baurii*, with wider, grey-green leaves and white, rarely pink flowers, to 3cm (1¼in) across; ↕ 12cm (5in), ↔ 15cm (6in). **'Tetra Pink'** and **'Tetra Red'** have large flowers, 3cm (1¼in) or more across, in pink and reddish purple, respectively; flowers become smaller after 2–3 years.

R. milloides. Vigorous, clump-forming perennial with runners, and with erect, hairless or sparsely hairy, linear-lance-shaped, keeled, folded, light green, basal leaves, to 17cm (7in) long. Cerise or dark crimson, occasionally deep pink or white flowers, to 3.5cm (1½in) across, are produced on hairy flower-stalks, to 12cm (5in) or more tall, over long periods in summer. ↕ 15cm (6in), ↔ 20cm (8in). South Africa. ✲✲✲

***R.* 'Tetra White'** see *R. baurii* 'Helen'.

RHODOPHIALA

AMARYLLIDACEAE

Genus, closely related to *Hippeastrum*, of about 35 species of bulbous perennials from coastal sands to rocky, dry sites in the mountains of Uruguay, Argentina, and Chile. They are grown for their funnel-shaped flowers, borne in umbels on leafless stems in summer or autumn. The basal leaves are linear and mid-green. Grow in an alpine house; in frost-free areas, however, *R. advena* and *R. pratensis* may be grown outdoors against a warm, sunny wall.

• **HARDINESS** Half hardy to frost tender; *R. advena*, *R. bifida*, and *R. pratensis* may withstand occasional falls to around -5°C (23°F).

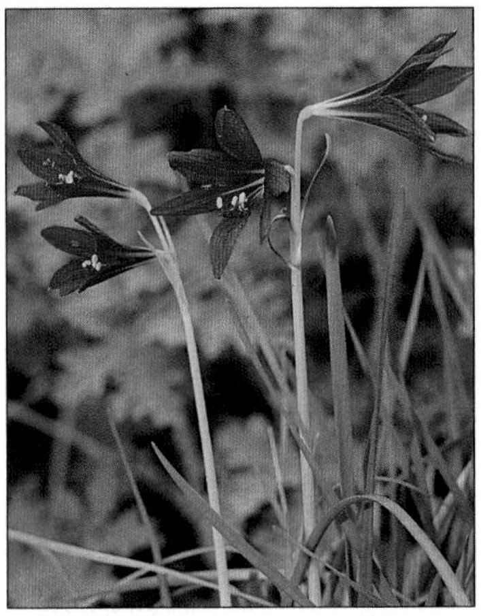

Rhodophiala advena

• **CULTIVATION** Under glass, plant bulbs with the necks and shoulders above soil level, in autumn. Grow in loam-based potting compost (JI No.2) in full light or bright filtered light. Water sparingly until plants are in active growth, then water moderately and apply a half-strength balanced liquid fertilizer every 2–3 weeks. Keep dry when dormant. Avoid root disturbance; pot on only every 3 years. Outdoors, plant bulbs 15–20cm (6–8in) deep in moderately fertile, well-drained soil in full sun. Provide a deep, dry winter mulch in cold areas.

• **PROPAGATION** Sow seed at 16°C (61°F) as soon as ripe. Remove offsets in autumn or winter.

• **PESTS AND DISEASES** Trouble free.

R. advena ■ syn. *Hippeastrum advenum.* Bulbous perennial producing umbels of 2–6 horizontal, open funnel-shaped, red, yellow, or pink flowers, 5cm (2in) across, in late summer and early autumn, just before the semi-erect, linear, basal leaves, 15–30cm (6–12in) long, emerge. ↕ 30–50cm (12–20in), ↔ 10cm (4in). Chile. ✲

R. bifida, syn. *Hippeastrum bifidum.* Bulbous perennial producing umbels of up to 5 erect, narrowly funnel-shaped, bright deep red flowers, 5cm (2in) long, in summer; flowers are borne as, or just before, the semi-erect, linear, basal leaves, to 45cm (18in) long, emerge. ↕ to 30cm (12in), ↔ 10cm (4in). Argentina, Uruguay. ✲

R. pratensis, syn. *Hippeastrum pratense.* Bulbous perennial bearing umbels of 2–8 horizontal, broadly funnel-shaped red flowers, 5–7cm (2–3in) across, in early summer, at the same time as the semi-erect, linear, basal leaves, 30–50cm (12–20in) long. ↕ to 60cm (24in), ↔ 10cm (4in). Chile. ✲

RHODOTHAMNUS

ERICACEAE

Genus of 2 species of dwarf, evergreen shrubs found in pockets of humus-rich soil, often among limestone rocks, in the eastern Alps and Turkey. They have glossy, dark green foliage, and are grown for their solitary, occasionally clustered, cup-shaped pink flowers, produced in profusion from the leaf axils in early summer. Grow in a rock garden, peat bed, or alpine house. They are not easy to establish.

• **HARDINESS** Fully hardy.

• **CULTIVATION** Under glass, grow in loam-based potting compost (JI No.2) with additional leaf mould, in full light. In the growing season, water freely and apply a balanced liquid fertilizer monthly; water more sparingly in winter. Outdoors, grow in moderately fertile, humus-rich, acid or alkaline, moist soil with a cool root run. They prefer full sun, but partial shade is tolerated, especially in drier areas. Avoid root disturbance.

• **PROPAGATION** Sow seed in containers in an open frame in autumn. Root semi-ripe cuttings in summer.

• **PESTS AND DISEASES** Susceptible to aphids and red spider mites under glass.

R. chamaecistus. Semi-prostrate, evergreen shrub with elliptic to inversely lance-shaped, glossy, bright dark green leaves, 6–10mm (¼–½in) long, paler beneath, fringed with bristly white hairs. In late spring and early summer, abundant cup-shaped, 5-petalled, pale clear pink flowers, to 3cm (1¼in) across, with red eyes, are produced singly from the leaf axils or in few-flowered terminal clusters. ↕ 20cm (8in), ↔ 25cm (10in). E. Alps. ✲✲✲

RHODOTYPOS

ROSACEAE

Genus of one species of deciduous shrub occurring in scrub and woodland in China and Japan. It has opposite, ovate, toothed leaves, but is cultivated mainly for its large, papery, 4-petalled white flowers, borne over a long period from spring to summer, and its shiny black berries. Grow in a shrub border or woodland garden.

• **HARDINESS** Fully hardy.

• **CULTIVATION** Grow in moderately fertile, moist but well-drained soil, preferably in sun, although partial shade is tolerated. Pruning group 1 or 2.

• **PROPAGATION** Sow seed in a seedbed, or in containers in a cold frame, in autumn. Root greenwood cuttings in early summer, or semi-ripe cuttings in late summer.

• **PESTS AND DISEASES** Trouble free.

R. kerrioides see *R. scandens.*

R. scandens ■ syn. *R. kerrioides.* Deciduous shrub with arching shoots and ovate, tapered, sharply toothed, deeply veined, mid-green leaves, to 6cm (2½in) long. In late spring and early summer, 4-petalled white flowers, 4cm

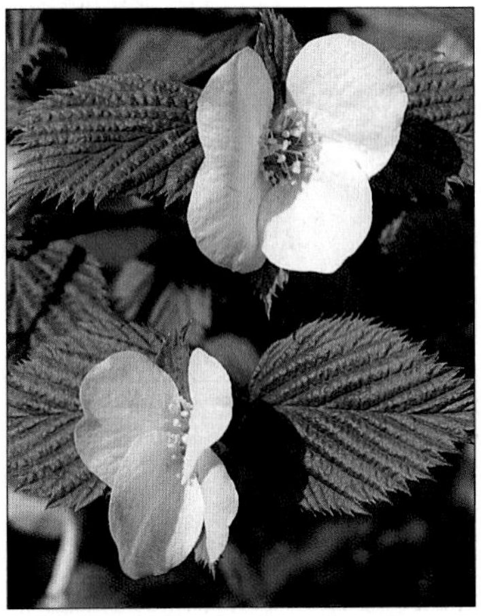

Rhodotypos scandens

(1½in) across, are produced singly from the shoot tips; they are followed by spherical, glossy black berries, to 8mm (⅜in) across. ↕↔ 1.5m (5ft). China, Japan. ❄❄❄

▷ ***Rhoeo discolor*** see *Tradescantia spathacea*

▷ ***Rhoeo spathacea*** see *Tradescantia spathacea*

RHOICISSUS

VITACEAE

Genus of 10–12 species of evergreen trees and woody-stemmed tendril climbers or scramblers from woodland in tropical Africa and South Africa. The leaves are alternate, and simple or 3-, occasionally 5-palmate, with entire or toothed leaflets. Tendrils are produced opposite the leaves. Tiny, yellowish green flowers are borne in small cymes that are almost hidden by the leaves; they are followed by red to purple berries. Where temperatures fall below 7°C (45°F), grow in a cool or temperate greenhouse, or as houseplants; elsewhere, use to clothe a wall, pergola, or arch.

- **HARDINESS** Frost tender.
- **CULTIVATION** Under glass, grow in loam-based potting compost (JI No.2) in full light. In the season, water moderately and apply a balanced liquid fertilizer monthly; water sparingly in winter. Outdoors, grow in fertile, moist but well-drained soil in full sun. Pruning group 11, in early spring.
- **PROPAGATION** Sow seed at 13°C (55°F) in spring. Root semi-ripe cuttings with bottom heat in summer. Layer in spring.
- **PESTS AND DISEASES** Red spider mites and powdery mildew may be a problem.

R. capensis ◼🏆 syn. *Cissus capensis, Vitis capensis* (Cape grape). Robust climber with tuberous roots and very long, forked tendrils. Leathery, lustrous, dark green leaves, 10–20cm (4–8in) long, are rounded to kidney-shaped, and bluntly 5-angled, with broad, wavy teeth. Insignificant, yellowish green flowers are borne in spring, and are followed by grape-like, spherical, blackish red berries. ↕5m (15ft) or more. South Africa. ❀ (min. 7°C/45°F)

R. rhombifolia see *Cissus rhombifolia.*

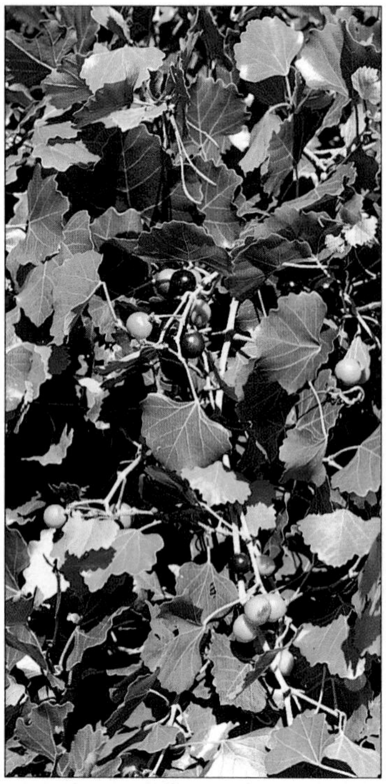

Rhoicissus capensis

RHOMBOPHYLLUM

AIZOACEAE

Genus of 3 species of very fleshy, usually compact, mat-forming, perennial succulents occurring on hillsides and often in the lowlands of South Africa. The crowded, fleshy leaves are linear or semi-cylindrical, expanded towards the middle, and opposite or united at the bases; they are mid- to dark greyish green, with white or translucent spots, and margins that are entire or have 1 or 2 short teeth. Attractive, daisy-like, bright golden yellow flowers, which open during the day, are produced singly or in cymes of 3–7 in summer. In frost-prone regions, grow in a temperate greenhouse. In warm, dry climates, grow outdoors in a raised bed or desert garden.

- **HARDINESS** Frost tender.
- **CULTIVATION** Under glass, grow in standard cactus compost in full light with low humidity. In spring and summer, water moderately and apply a dilute, low-nitrogen fertilizer monthly; keep completely dry at other times. Outdoors, grow in poor to moderately fertile, sharply drained soil in full sun. See also pp.48–49.
- **PROPAGATION** Sow seed at 19–24°C (66–75°F), or divide offsets, in spring or summer.
- **PESTS AND DISEASES** Prone to aphids while flowering.

R. rhomboideum ◼ Clump-forming succulent with 4 or 5 uneven pairs of semi-cylindrical, white-spotted, dark greyish green leaves, 2.5–5cm (1–2in) long; the upper surfaces of the leaves are more or less flat, the undersurfaces are rounded, thickened, and keeled towards the tips, with paler green, occasionally toothed margins. Golden yellow flowers, 3cm (1¼in) across, tinged red on the reverse of the petals, are produced in summer. ↕5cm (2in), ↔15cm (6in). South Africa (Eastern Cape). ❀ (min. 7°C/45°F)

▷ **Rhubarb** see *Rheum*
Chinese see *R. palmatum*

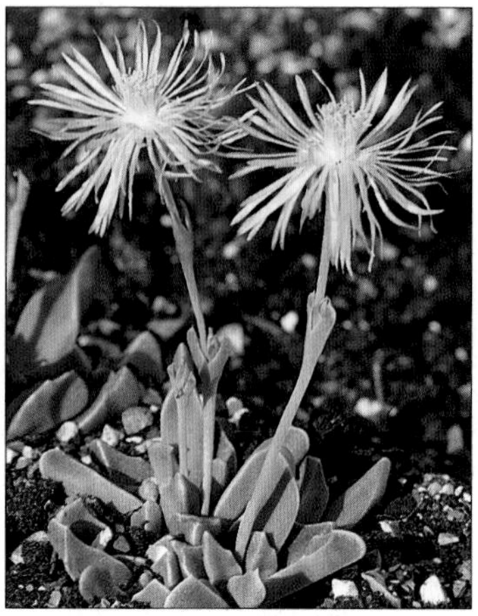

Rhombophyllum rhomboideum

RHUS syn. TOXICODENDRON

Sumach

ANACARDIACEAE

Genus of about 200 species of deciduous or evergreen shrubs, trees, and woody climbers, widely distributed in temperate and subtropical North America, South Africa, E. Asia, and N.E. Australia. They are found in woodland, thickets, dry sites, bogs, and on rocky slopes. Sumachs are grown mainly for their alternate, simple, pinnate, or palmate leaves, which in many species and cultivars turn brilliant shades of yellow, red, or orange in autumn; some also produce showy fruit clusters. The inconspicuous flowers, usually 2mm (1/16in) across, are borne in spring or summer in terminal, normally erect, ovoid, or conical to pyramidal panicles. In autumn, they are followed by spherical, usually red fruits, 4–6mm (⅛–¼in) across. *R. glabra, R.* x *pulvinata,* and *R. typhina* usually produce male and female flowers on separate plants; plants of both sexes must be grown together to obtain fruit. Grow in a shrub border or woodland garden, or as specimen plants. In frost-prone areas, grow tender species in a cool greenhouse. All parts of *R. radicans* and *R. verniciflua* are highly toxic if ingested; contact with their foliage, and that of a number of related species, including *R. succedanea,* may aggravate skin allergies.

- **HARDINESS** Fully hardy to frost tender.
- **CULTIVATION** Grow in moist but well-drained, moderately fertile soil, in full sun to obtain best autumn colour. Suckering species, such as *R. typhina,* may be invasive. Pruning group 1, or group 7 for *R. typhina, R.* x *pulvinata,* and *R. glabra.*
- **PROPAGATION** Sow seed in a seedbed in autumn. Root semi-ripe cuttings in summer, or insert root cuttings in winter. Separate suckers when dormant.
- **PESTS AND DISEASES** Prone to coral spot and *Verticillium* wilt.

R. aromatica (Fragrant sumach). Mound-forming, suckering, deciduous shrub with spreading shoots. The 3-palmate, aromatic leaves, to 10cm (4in) long, are softly hairy or almost hairless, with ovate or obovate, sharply toothed, dark green leaflets, turning orange to red-purple in autumn. Tiny yellow flowers are borne in small, erect, ovoid panicles, 2cm (¾in) long, in mid-spring, followed by spherical red fruit. ↕1–1.5m (3–5ft), ↔1.5m (5ft). E. North America. ❄❄❄

R. chinensis ▢ Upright, deciduous tree with stout, downy shoots bearing pinnate leaves, to 40cm (16in) long, with winged stalks and 7–13 ovate-oblong, mid-green leaflets, turning red in autumn. In late summer, bears yellowish white flowers in erect, conical panicles, to 25cm (10in) long, followed by spherical, orange-red fruit. ↕↔ 6m (20ft). E. Asia. ❄❄❄ (borderline)

R. copallina ▢ (Dwarf sumach, Shining sumach). Upright, deciduous shrub or tree with long, branching, softly hairy, reddish green shoots. Pinnate leaves, to 35cm (14in) long, have winged stalks, and 9–15 oblong-lance-shaped, glossy, dark green leaflets, turning bright red in

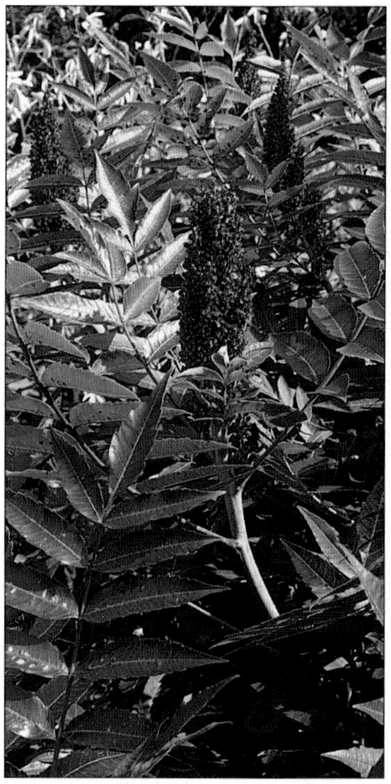

Rhus glabra

autumn. In summer, bears yellow-green flowers in erect, conical panicles, to 15cm (6in) long, followed by spherical red fruit. ↕↔ 1.5m (5ft) or more. E. North America. ❄❄❄

R. cotinoides see *Cotinus obovatus.*

R. cotinus see *Cotinus coggygria.*

R. glabra ◼ (Scarlet sumach, Smooth sumach). Bushy, suckering, deciduous shrub producing smooth, hairless shoots and pinnate leaves, to 45cm (18in) long, with 15–31 oblong-lance-shaped, toothed, glossy, bluish green leaflets, turning rich red in autumn. In summer, bears yellow-green flowers in upright, conical panicles, to 25cm (10in) long; they are followed on female plants by spherical red fruit. ↕↔ 2.5m (8ft) or more. North America, Mexico. ❄❄❄.

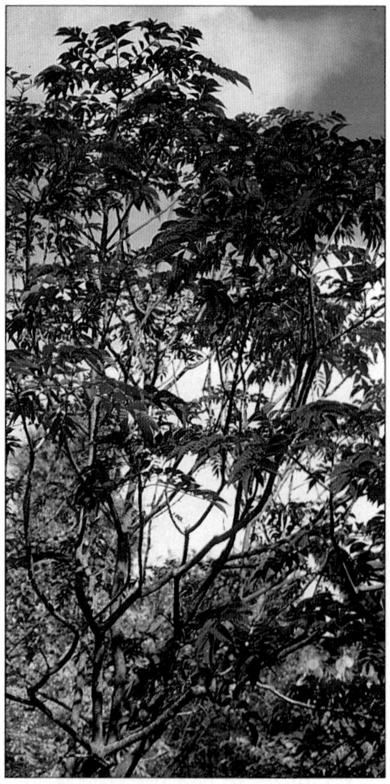

Rhus trichocarpa

R

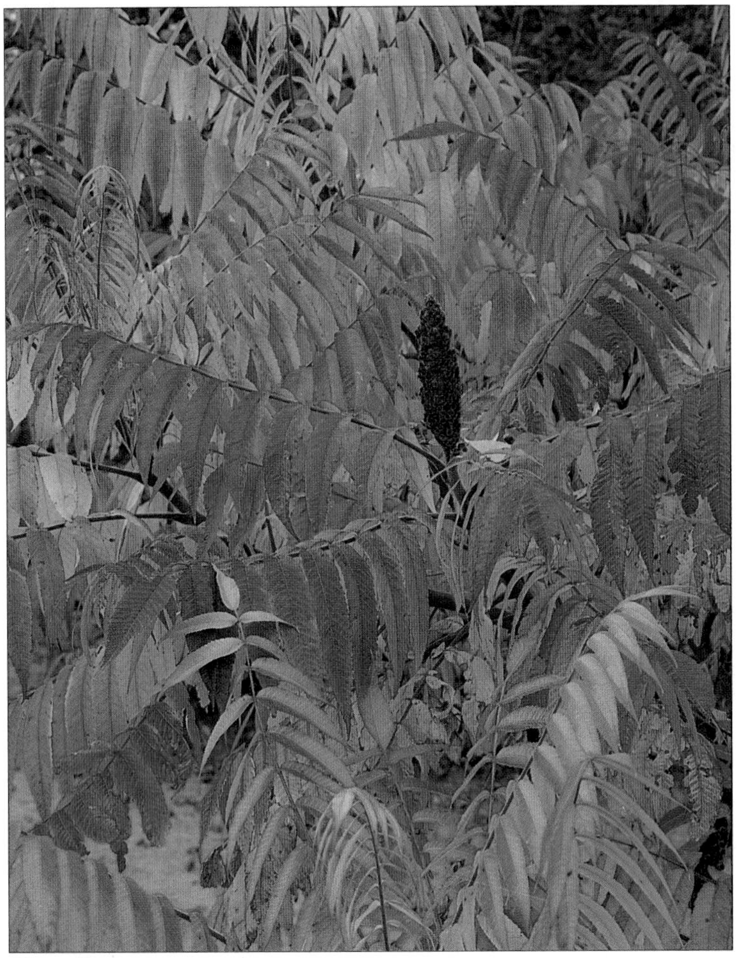

Rhus typhina

'Laciniata' of gardens see *R.* x *pulvinata* 'Red Autumn Lace'.
R. potaninii ◌ Rounded, deciduous tree with hairless or finely hairy shoots and pinnate leaves, to 35cm (14in) long, composed of 7–11 oblong to oblong-lance-shaped, dark green leaflets, turning red in autumn. Creamy white flowers are borne in pendent, pyramidal panicles, 20cm (8in) long, in summer, followed by spherical, hairy red fruit. ↕12m (40ft), ↔8m (25ft). China. ***
***R.* x *pulvinata* 'Red Autumn Lace'** ♀ syn. *R. glabra* 'Laciniata' of gardens. Spreading, suckering, deciduous shrub with smooth shoots and pinnate leaves, to 50cm (20in) or more long, composed of 11–13 oblong-lance-shaped, rich green leaflets, turning orange to red-

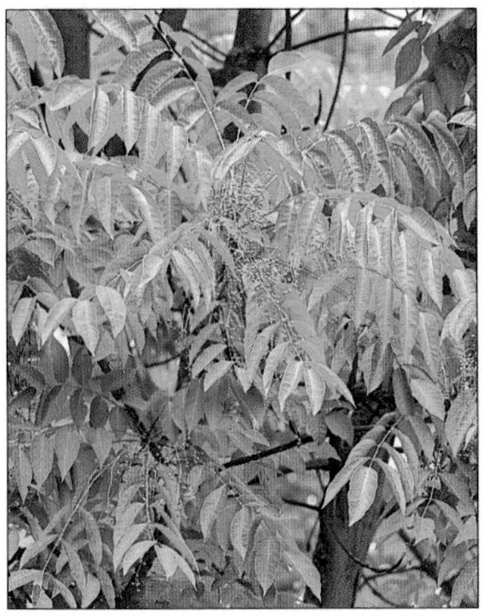

Rhus verniciflua

purple in autumn. Yellow-green flowers are borne in erect, conical panicles, to 20cm (8in) long, in summer, followed by spherical, bristly red fruit. ↕3m (10ft), ↔5m (15ft). ***
R. succedanea ◌ syn. *Toxicodendron succedaneum* (Wax tree). Spreading, deciduous tree with softly hairy young shoots. Pinnate leaves, to 30cm (12in) long, have 9–15 ovate-oblong, glossy, dark green leaflets, turning red in autumn. Yellow-green flowers are borne in dense, erect, conical panicles, to 12cm (5in) long, in summer, followed by spherical, waxy, yellow-brown fruit. ↕↔10m (30ft). E. Asia. **
R. trichocarpa ■ ◌ Spreading, deciduous tree or shrub with softly hairy young shoots, later becoming hairless. Pinnate leaves, to 50cm (20in) long, have 13–17 broadly ovate, usually entire, dark green leaflets, pink-tinged when young, turning red-purple to orange in autumn. In summer, bears yellow flowers in erect, conical panicles, to 10cm (4in) long, followed by spherical, bristly, brownish yellow fruit. ↕↔6m (20ft). C. China, Korea, Japan. ***
R. typhina ■ ♀ ◌ (Stag's horn sumach, Velvet sumach). Upright, suckering, deciduous shrub or tree with densely velvety red shoots, resembling a stag's horns. Pinnate leaves, to 60cm (24in) long, have 11–31 oblong-lance-shaped, dark green leaflets, turning brilliant orange-red in autumn. Yellow-green flowers are produced in erect, conical panicles, to 20cm (8in) long, in summer; they are followed on female plants by dense clusters of spherical, hairy, deep crimson-red fruit. ↕5m (15ft) or more, ↔6m (20ft). E. North America. ***. **'Dissecta'** ♀ syn. 'Laciniata' of gardens, is female and shrubby, with finely cut leaflets; ↕2m (6ft), ↔3m (10ft).
R. verniciflua ■ ◌ syn. *Toxicodendron vernicifluum* (Varnish tree). Spreading, deciduous tree with softly hairy young shoots, later becoming hairless. Pinnate leaves, to 60cm (24in) long, have 7–13 broadly ovate, glossy, bright green leaflets, turning red in autumn. Yellow-green flowers are produced in lax, semi-pendent panicles, to 20cm (8in) long, in summer, followed by spherical, pale yellow fruit. ↕15m (50ft), ↔10m (30ft). E. Asia. ***

▷ ***Rhynchelytrum*** see *Melinis*
R. repens see *M. repens*
R. roseum see *M. repens*

RHYNCHOSTYLIS

ORCHIDACEAE

Genus of about 6 species of evergreen, monopodial, epiphytic orchids from warm, moist forest in India, Malaysia, Indonesia, the Philippines, Thailand, Laos, Burma, and Sri Lanka. They have thick, rigid, aerial roots, and produce 8–10 pairs of semi-rigid, linear to strap-shaped leaves at the apexes of short, stout stems. Many small flowers are borne in dense, upright or pendent racemes that arise laterally from the bases of the leaves from spring to winter.
- **HARDINESS** Frost tender.
- **CULTIVATION** Intermediate-growing orchids. Grow in epiphytic orchid compost in half-pots or (preferably) in slatted baskets. Provide high humidity, full light, and shade from hot sun. In summer, water freely, mist daily, and apply a balanced liquid fertilizer at every third watering; water moderately in winter. Disturb as little as possible. See also p.46.
- **PROPAGATION** Divide when the plant fills the container and "flows" over the sides. Cuttings or offshoots may be rooted successfully.
- **PESTS AND DISEASES** Red spider mites, aphids, and mealybugs may be a problem.

R. gigantea. Epiphytic orchid with linear, mid-green leaves, 25cm (10in) long. Fragrant, waxy, pale purple-spotted, white or deep violet flowers, to 4cm (1½in) across, are borne in pendent racemes, 20–25cm (8–10in) long, from autumn to winter. ↕↔30cm (12in). Burma, Thailand, Laos. ❀ (min. 13–15°C/55–59°F; max. 30°C/86°F)
R. retusa. Epiphytic orchid with linear to oblong, bluish green leaves, 25cm (10in) long. Fragrant, waxy white flowers, to 3cm (1¼in) across, spotted purple or pink, with purple lips, are produced in pendent racemes, to 30cm (12in) long, in summer. ↕15cm (6in), ↔25cm (10in). India, Burma, Sri Lanka to Malaysia, Philippines. ❀ (min. 13–15°C/55–59°F; max. 30°C/86°F)

▷ **Ribbon bush** see *Homalocladium*, *Hypoestes aristata*
▷ **Ribbon grass** see *Phalaris arundinacea*
▷ **Ribbon plant** see *Chlorophytum comosum*, *Dracaena sanderiana*
▷ **Ribbonwood** see *Hoheria sexstylosa*

RIBES

Flowering currant

GROSSULARIACEAE/SAXIFRAGACEAE

Genus of about 150 species of mainly deciduous, occasionally evergreen, sometimes spiny shrubs, widely distributed in woodland, scrub, and rocky places. Most are found in N. temperate regions; some occur in South America. Some species, such as blackcurrant (*R. nigrum*), redcurrant (*R. rubrum*), and gooseberry (*R. uva-crispa*), are grown for their edible fruits; those described below are cultivated primarily for their flowers. The leaves are alternate and often 3- to 5-lobed. Small, tubular, cup- or bell-shaped flowers, each with small petals and 4, rarely 5, larger, spreading sepals, are borne singly or in pendent racemes, mostly in spring or summer. The berry-like fruits are spherical or ovoid, and vary in colour from red or black to green or white. Grow in a shrub border; *R. speciosum* and *R. viburnifolium* are best grown against a wall. *R. sanguineum* may be used as informal hedging.
- **HARDINESS** Fully hardy to frost hardy.
- **CULTIVATION** Grow in moderately fertile, well-drained soil in full sun. *R. laurifolium* will grow well in partial shade; *R. sanguineum* 'Brocklebankii' should be shaded from the hottest sun. Pruning group 2; group 13 if wall-grown, in late summer. Trim hedges after flowering.
- **PROPAGATION** Root hardwood cuttings of deciduous flowering currants in winter. Root semi-ripe cuttings of evergreens in summer.
- **PESTS AND DISEASES** Aphids, leaf spot, powdery mildew, honey fungus, and coral spot may be a problem.

R. alpinum. Compact, mound-forming, much-branched, deciduous shrub with spineless shoots and broadly ovate, 3- to 5-lobed, mid-green leaves, to 5cm (2in) long, often smaller. In spring, bears bell-shaped, greenish yellow flowers (males and females on separate plants) in erect racemes, to 4cm (1½in) long; they are followed on female plants by spherical, dark red fruit, 7mm (¼in) long. ↕60cm (24in), ↔90cm (36in). N. Europe to Russia (Siberia). ***. **'Aureum'** ■ is female, and has bright yellow leaves, becoming paler in summer. R
***R. aureum* of gardens** see *R. odoratum*.
R.* x *gordonianum (*R. petraeum* x *R. sanguineum*). Spreading, spineless,

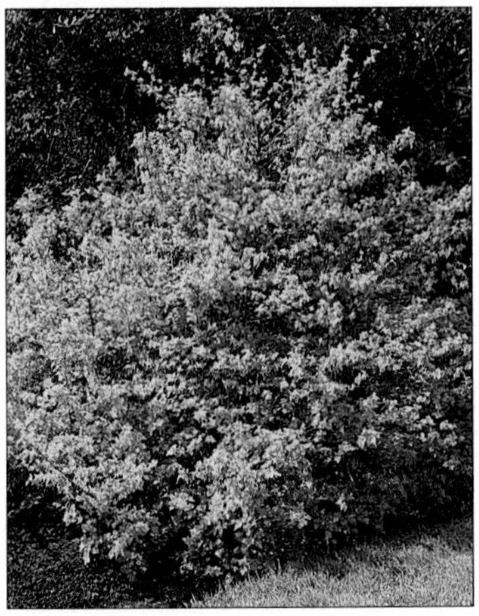

Ribes alpinum 'Aureum'

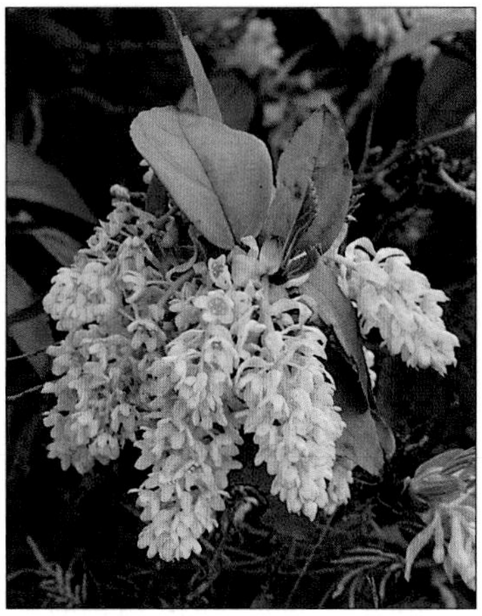

Ribes laurifolium

deciduous shrub with rounded, 3- to 5-lobed, toothed, aromatic, dark green leaves, to 5cm (2in) long. Tubular, 5-lobed flowers, red outside and yellow within, open in dense, pendent racemes, to 7cm (3in) long, in early summer. It is not known to produce fruit and is probably sterile. ↕ 2m (6ft), ↔ 2.5m (8ft). Garden origin. ✻✻✻

R. laurifolium ■ Spreading, spineless, dioecious, evergreen shrub with ovate-oblong, scalloped, leathery, dark green leaves, 5–10cm (2–4in) long. In late winter and early spring, bears cup-shaped, greenish yellow flowers in pendent racemes, the males to 5cm (2in) long, the females to 2.5cm (1in) long. Female flowers are followed by ovoid fruit, to 1cm (½in) long, red at first, ripening to black. ↕ 1m (3ft), ↔ 1.5m (5ft). W. China. ✻✻✻

R. odoratum ■ syn. *R. aureum* of gardens (Buffalo currant). Spineless, erect, deciduous shrub with hairy young shoots (hairless in the true *R. aureum*). Broadly ovate, 3- to 5-lobed, toothed, bright green leaves, to 8cm (3in) long, turn red and purple in autumn. In mid- and late spring, bears tubular, fragrant yellow flowers in pendent racemes, to 5cm (2in) long, followed by spherical black fruit, to 1cm (½in) across. ↕↔ 2m (6ft). C. USA. ✻✻✻

R. sanguineum (Flowering currant). Upright, spineless, deciduous shrub with rounded, 3- to 5-lobed, toothed, aromatic, dark green leaves, 5–10cm (2–4in) long, heart-shaped at the bases, and slightly hairy above, white-hairy beneath. Tubular, deep pinkish red flowers are borne in pendent racemes,

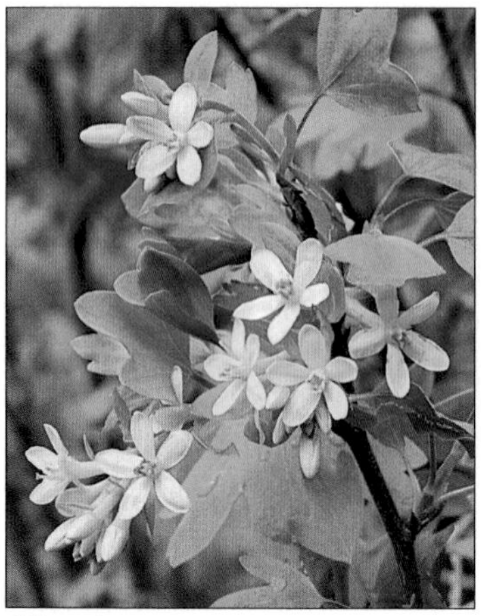

Ribes odoratum

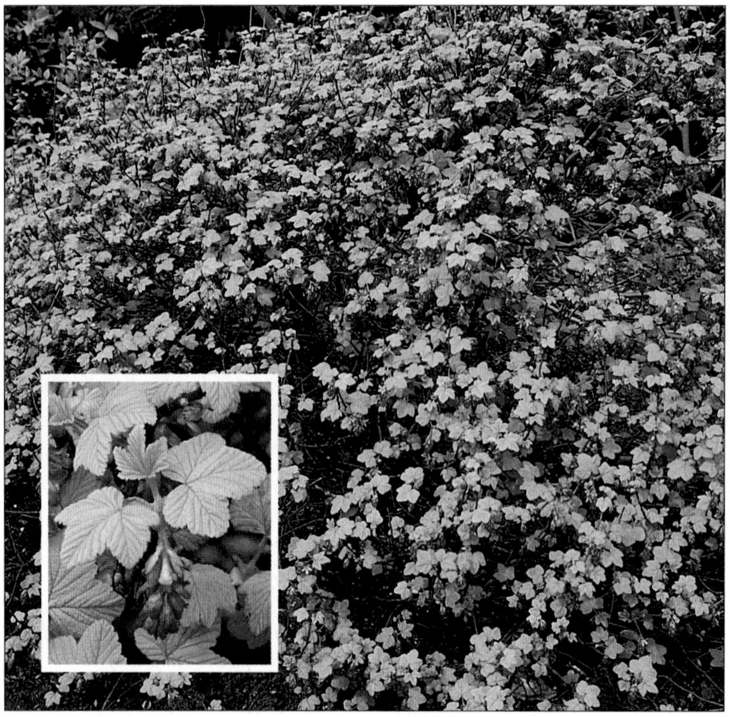

Ribes sanguineum 'Brocklebankii' (inset: leaf and flower detail)

5–10cm (2–4in) long, in spring, followed by spherical, glaucous, blue-black fruit, 5mm (¼in) across. ↕↔ 2m (6ft). W. North America. ✻✻✻. **'Brocklebankii'** ■♀ is slow-growing, with bright yellow leaves, paler in summer, and pale pink flowers; ↕↔ 1.2m (4ft). **'King Edward VII'** is compact and upright, with dark red flowers. **'Pulborough Scarlet'** ■♀ is vigorous, and bears dark red, white-centred flowers; ↕ 3m (10ft), ↔ 2.5m (8ft). **'Tydeman's White'** ♀ has pure white flowers; ↕↔ 2.5m (8ft).

R. speciosum ♀ (Fuchsia-flowered currant). Upright, spiny, deciduous shrub with bristly shoots, red when young, and broadly ovate, 3- to 5-lobed, glossy, mid-green leaves, 1–4cm

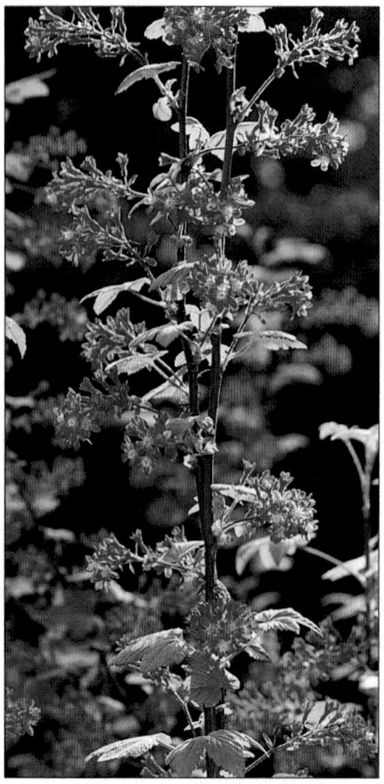

Ribes sanguineum 'Pulborough Scarlet'

(½–1½in) long. In mid- and late spring, bears slender, bell-shaped, dark red flowers, with protruding red stamens, in small, pendent racemes, 2.5cm (1in) long. Flowers are followed by spherical, bristly red fruit, to 1cm (½in) across. ↕ 2m (6ft), sometimes more, ↔ 2m (6ft). USA (California). ✻✻✻ (borderline)

R. viburnifolium. Arching, spineless, evergreen shrub with long, pendent or semi-climbing, spineless shoots and broadly ovate to elliptic, aromatic, glossy, dark green leaves, to 4cm (1½in) long. In mid-spring, bears tiny, bell-shaped pink flowers in small, erect racemes, to 2.5cm (1in) long, followed by ovoid red fruit, to 8mm (⅜in) long. ↕↔ 2.5m (8ft). USA (S. California). ✻✻

▷**Rice** see *Oryza*
Annual wild see *Zizania aquatica*
Canadian wild see *Zizania aquatica*
Water see *Zizania aquatica*
Wild see *Zizania*
▷**Rice-paper plant** see *Tetrapanax papyrifer*

RICHEA

EPACRIDACEAE

Genus of 11 species of evergreen shrubs and small trees found in moist forest in Australia, often at high altitudes. They have crowded branches with spiralling, alternate, narrow leaves, overlapping at the bases. The small, ovoid to conical or bottle-shaped flowers are borne in terminal spikes or panicles; they are open at the bases and almost closed at the tips, quickly losing their petals and leaving the stamens and stigmas exposed. In frost-prone areas, grow half-hardy and tender species in a cool greenhouse or conservatory. In frost-free areas, grow the shrubby species at the base of a warm, sunny wall or in a shrub border; use the trees as specimen plants.

- **HARDINESS** Frost hardy to half hardy.
- **CULTIVATION** Under glass, grow in lime-free (ericaceous) potting compost in full light. When in growth, water

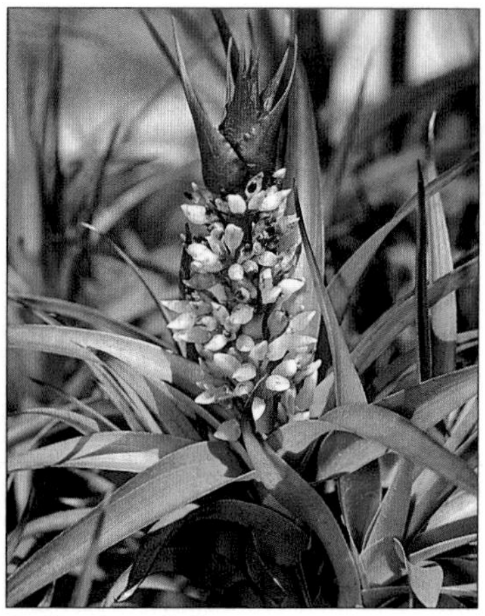

Richea dracophylla

freely and apply a half-strength balanced liquid fertilizer monthly; water sparingly in winter. Outdoors, grow in moist but well-drained, poor to moderately fertile, humus-rich, neutral to acid soil in full sun; shelter from cold, dry winds. Pruning group 9.

- **PROPAGATION** Surface-sow seed in containers outdoors, ideally as soon as ripe or in spring (germination is unreliable). Root semi-ripe cuttings with bottom heat in late summer.
- **PESTS AND DISEASES** Trouble free.

R. dracophylla ■♀ Medium to large shrub or small tree with sparse, erect branches. Spreading, spiralling, flexuous, lance-shaped, dark green leaves, 15–30cm (6–12in) long, with tapering, red-tinged tips, are crowded at the ends of the stems. Small, obovoid white flowers are produced in dense, upright panicles, 15–25cm (6–10in) long, in summer. ↕ 2–5m (6–15ft), ↔ 0.6–1.5m (2–5ft). Australia (Tasmania). ✻

RICINUS

EUPHORBIACEAE

Genus of one species of erect, very fast-growing, mound-forming, suckering, monoecious, evergreen shrub, widely naturalized in wasteland, at roadsides, and on stony slopes, from N.E. Africa to W. Asia. It is grown mainly for its large, glossy, palmately lobed leaves. Spikes of small, cup-shaped flowers are followed by prickly, ovoid capsules. In frost-prone areas, grow as an annual in a cool greenhouse or conservatory, or as a specimen plant for summer bedding. In warmer

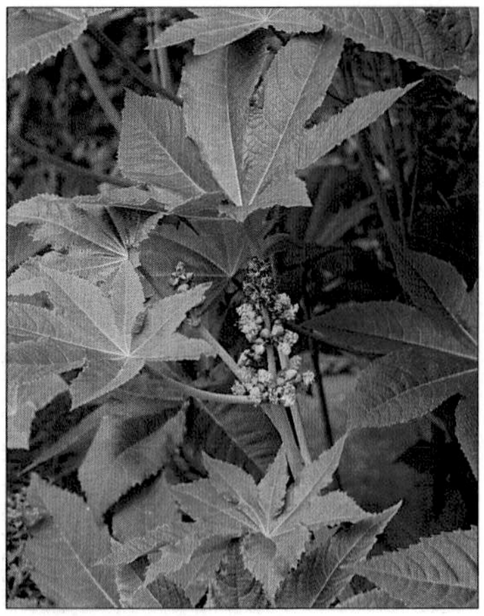

Ricinus communis

R

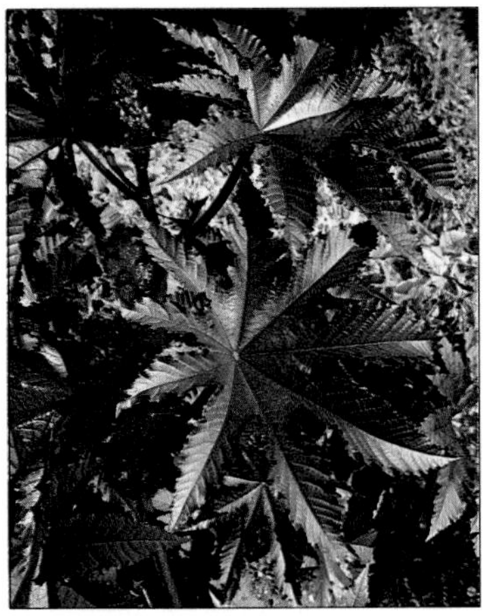

Ricinus communis 'Impala'

climates, grow in a border. All parts of *R. communis*, particularly the seeds, are highly toxic if ingested; contact with the foliage may aggravate skin allergies.
• **HARDINESS** Half hardy.
• **CULTIVATION** Under glass, grow in loam-based potting compost (JI No.2) in full light. In growth, water freely and apply a balanced liquid fertilizer monthly; water sparingly in winter. Outdoors, grow in fertile, humus-rich, well-drained soil in full sun. Stake in exposed sites. Plants grown on poor soils tend to produce flowers at the expense of vegetative growth and bear smaller leaves. Pruning group 9; plants grown under glass may need restrictive pruning.
• **PROPAGATION** Soak seed for 24 hours before sowing in late spring; sow singly into 9cm (3½in) pots, at 21°C (70°F). Grow young plants on at 13°C (55°F); pot on into 13cm (5in) pots before they become pot-bound, to prevent premature flower production. Plant out when all danger of frost has passed.
• **PESTS AND DISEASES** Red spider mites may be a problem under glass.

R. communis ▣ (Castor oil plant). Erect, branching shrub, usually grown as an annual, with alternate, very broadly ovate, deeply 5- to 12-lobed, toothed, glossy, mid-green, reddish purple, or bronze-red leaves, 15–45cm (6–18in) long. Greenish yellow flowers, to 2.5cm (1in) long, are borne in ovoid spikes, to 15cm (6in) long, in summer; the female flowers are borne above the males at the tips of the spikes, and each female has a prominent red stigma. The flowers are followed by spherical, reddish brown capsules, covered with soft brown spines. ↕ to 1.8m (6ft) or more, ↔ to 1m (3ft) as an annual; ↕ to 10m (30ft), ↔ to 4m (12ft) as a shrub. N.E. Africa to W. Asia. ✻. Heights given for cultivars are for annual growth. **'Carmencita'** 🏆 is tall and well-branched, with dark bronze-red foliage and bright red female flowers; ↕ 2–3m (6–10ft). **'Impala'** ▣ is compact, with reddish purple foliage and yellowish green male flowers; young shoots and leaves are carmine-red; ↕ 1.2m (4ft). **'Red Spire'** is tall, with red stems and bronze-flushed leaves; ↕ 2–3m (6–10ft). **'Zanzibarensis'** ▣ is tall, producing large, white-veined, mid-green leaves, 50cm (20in) long; ↕ 2–3m (6–10ft).

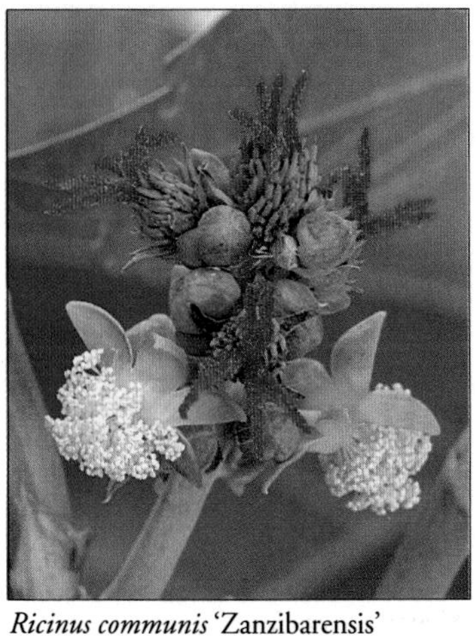

Ricinus communis 'Zanzibarensis'

RIGIDELLA

IRIDACEAE

Genus, closely related to *Tigridia*, of 4 species of bulbous perennials from dry pine to cloud forest in Central America. They are cultivated for their iris-like, brightly coloured flowers, borne in succession in spring or summer. The long, broadly lance-shaped, many-folded leaves are reduced to short, sharp-pointed, leaf-like bracts on the flowering stems. In frost-prone areas, grow in a cool greenhouse. In warmer areas, grow at the base of a sunny wall or in a warm site where the soil dries out in summer.
• **HARDINESS** Half hardy, but may withstand short spells at -5°C (23°F).
• **CULTIVATION** Plant bulbs 10cm (4in) deep in spring. Under glass, grow in deep containers of loam-based potting compost (JI No.2) with added sharp sand, in full light. Water moderately in growth; keep completely dry in winter. Pot on in spring. Outdoors, grow in humus-rich, well-drained soil in full sun; in frost-prone regions, lift for frost-free winter storage.
• **PROPAGATION** Sow seed at 13–18°C (55–64°F) in spring.
• **PESTS AND DISEASES** Trouble free.

R. flammea. Bulbous perennial with lance-shaped basal leaves, to 30cm (12in) long, and shorter, sheathing stem leaves. Short-lived, iris-like, semi-pendent, brilliant scarlet flowers, 10cm (4in) across, with striking purple markings at the bases of the petals, are borne in succession before the leaves in spring or early summer. ↕ 1–1.5m (3–5ft), ↔ 30cm (12in). Mexico. ✻

▷**Rimu** see *Dacrydium cupressinum*

ROBINIA

LEGUMINOSAE/PAPILIONACEAE

Genus of about 20 species (or only 4, according to some authorities) of deciduous, sometimes bristly or thorny trees and shrubs found in woodland and thickets in the USA. They are cultivated for their alternate, pinnate leaves, and pendent racemes of pea-like flowers, borne in late spring and early summer. Grow the trees as specimen plants; shrubby robinias are suitable for a large shrub border. *R. hispida* is effective grown against a sunny wall. All parts may cause severe discomfort if ingested.
• **HARDINESS** Fully hardy.
• **CULTIVATION** Grow in full sun in moderately fertile, moist but well-drained soil; they will tolerate poor, dry soils. Shelter from strong winds, as the branches are brittle. Suckers from *R. pseudoacacia* may be a problem. Pruning group 1; *R. pseudoacacia* 'Frisia' also group 7. Prune in late summer or early autumn to prevent bleeding.
• **PROPAGATION** Sow seed in containers in a cold frame in autumn. Insert root cuttings or graft in winter. Remove suckers in autumn.
• **PESTS AND DISEASES** Trouble free.

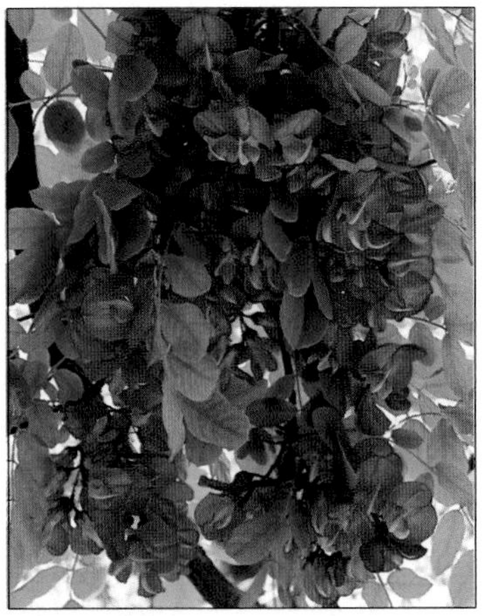

Robinia hispida

***R. x ambigua* 'Decaisneana'** 🌳 Spreading, nearly thornless tree with pinnate, dark green leaves, to 25cm (10in) long, composed of up to 23 ovate leaflets. Pale pink flowers, 2.5cm (1in) long, are borne in pendent racemes, to 15cm (6in) long, in early summer, followed by smooth, dark brown seed pods, 10cm (4in) long. ↕ 15m (50ft), ↔ 10m (30ft). ✻✻✻
R. fertilis see *R. hispida* var. *fertilis.*
R. hispida ▣🏆 (Bristly locust, Rose acacia). Upright, suckering shrub with bristly shoots and pinnate, dark green leaves, to 30cm (12in) long, composed of 9–13 ovate to broadly elliptic leaflets. In late spring and early summer, bears light rose-pink flowers, 3cm (1¼in) long, in pendent racemes, to 12cm (5in) long, followed by bristly brown seed pods, 4–6cm (1½–2½in) long. ↕ 2.5m (8ft), ↔ 3m (10ft). S.E. USA. ✻✻✻. **var. *fertilis***, syn. *R. fertilis*, has dense, spreading bristles on shoots and leaves, and narrow, oblong-ovate to elliptic leaflets; ↕↔ 2m (6ft). **var. *kelseyi***, syn. *R. kelseyi*, is similar to *R. hispida* but has bristles only on the flower-stalks and raceme axes; leaves have oblong to ovate leaflets. It bears bright rose-pink flowers very freely. **'Monument'** is compact and conical, with sparsely bristly shoots and lilac-pink flowers; ↕ 4m (12ft).
***R.* 'Idaho'** ▣🌳 Open, spreading tree with arching branches and pinnate, mid- to dark green leaves, to 25cm (10in) long, with 15 oval leaflets. In late spring and early summer, produces fragrant, dark pink flowers, 2.5cm (1in) long, in pendent racemes, to 20cm (8in) long. It is sterile and does not bear seed pods. ↕ 12m (40ft), ↔ 10m (30ft). ✻✻✻
R. kelseyi see *R. hispida* var. *kelseyi.*
R. luxurians see *R. neomexicana.*
R. x margaretta see *R. x slavinii.*
***R. x margaretta* 'Casque Rouge'** see *R. x slavinii* 'Casque Rouge'.
***R. x margaretta* 'Pink Cascade'** see *R. x slavinii* 'Casque Rouge'.

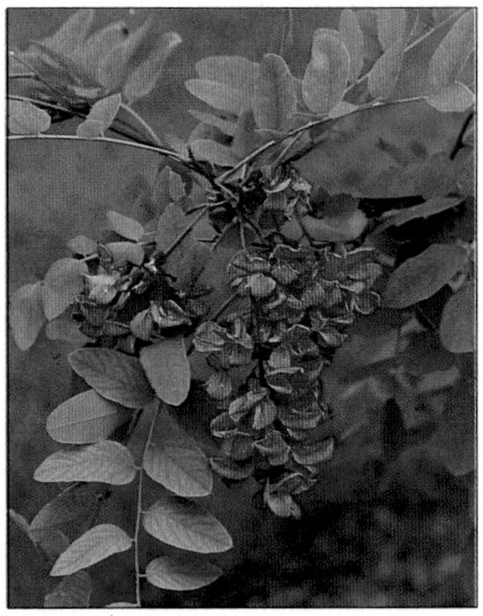

Robinia 'Idaho'

R. neomexicana 🌳 syn. *R. luxurians* (New Mexico locust). Upright, thicket-forming, spiny shrub or small tree with pinnate, hairy, blue-green leaves, to 20cm (8in) long, composed of 13 to 25 lance-shaped, narrowly ovate or oblong leaflets. In early summer, bears pink flowers, 2.5cm (1in) long, in pendent racemes, to 10cm (4in) long, followed by sparsely glandular brown seed pods, to 10cm (4in) long. ↕ 6m (20ft), ↔ 5m (15ft). USA (New Mexico, Arizona). ✻✻✻
R. pseudoacacia 🏆🌳 (Black locust, False acacia, Locust). Fast-growing, suckering, broadly columnar tree with usually spiny shoots. Pinnate, dark green leaves, to 30cm (12in) long, have up to 23 lance-shaped or elliptic to ovate, blunt leaflets. In early and midsummer, bears fragrant white flowers, 2cm (¾in) long, in pendent racemes, to 20cm (8in) long, followed by smooth, dark brown seed pods, 10cm (4in) long. ↕ 25m (80ft), ↔ 15m (50ft). E. USA. ✻✻✻. The following selections do not flower freely. **'Bessoniana'** 🌳 is erect when young, later rounded; ↕ 15m (50ft), ↔ 10m (30ft). **'Fastigiata'** see 'Pyramidalis'. **'Frisia'** ▣🏆🌳 has golden

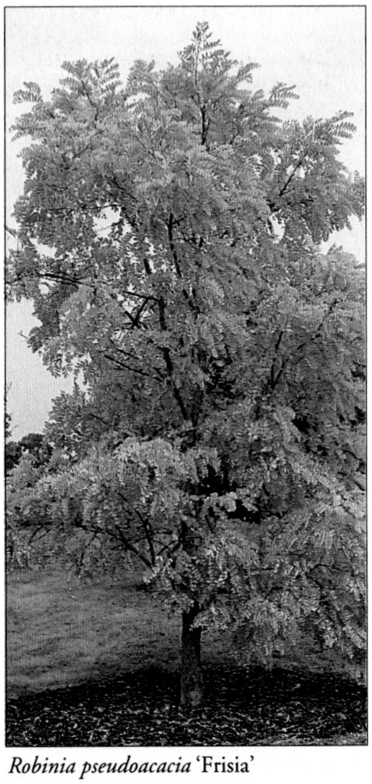

Robinia pseudoacacia 'Frisia'

R

yellow foliage, turning yellow-green in summer, then orange-yellow in autumn; ↕ 15m (50ft), ↔ 8m (25ft). **'Inermis'** see 'Umbraculifera'. **'Pyramidalis'** ◊ syn. 'Fastigiata', is narrowly columnar with upright, spineless shoots; ↕ 15m (50ft), ↔ 3m (10ft). **'Tortuosa'** ♀ is slow-growing with twisted shoots; ↕ 15m (50ft), ↔ 10m (30ft). **'Umbraculifera'** ♀ syn. 'Inermis' (Mop-head acacia), has a rounded crown; ↕↔ 6m (20ft).

R.* x *slavinii 🏆 ♀ (*R. hispida* var. *kelseyi* x *R. pseudoacacia*), syn. *R.* x *margaretta*. Open, rounded, spiny tree or shrub with bristly young branches and pinnate, dark green leaves, to 20cm (8in) long, composed of up to 19 ovate leaflets. Fragrant, lilac-pink to dark pink flowers, 2cm (¾in) long, are borne in pendent racemes, to 15cm (6in) long, in late spring; they are followed by brown, warty seed pods, to 10cm (4in) long. ↕↔ 10m (30ft). Garden origin. ❄❄❄. **'Casque Rouge'** syn. *R.* x *margaretta* 'Casque Rouge', *R.* x *margaretta* 'Pink Cascade', has dark purple-pink flowers.

▷ **Roblé** see *Nothofagus obliqua*
▷ ***Rochea coccinea*** see *Crassula coccinea*
▷ ***Rochea falcata*** see *Crassula perfoliata* var. *minor*
▷ **Rock cress** see *Arabis*
▷ **Rocket, Sweet** see *Hesperis matronalis*
▷ **Rock rose** see *Cistus, Helianthemum*
Montpellier see *Cistus monspeliensis*
Sydney see *Boronia serrulata*

RODGERSIA

SAXIFRAGACEAE

Genus of 6 species of vigorous, clump-forming, rhizomatous perennials occurring in moist woodland and scrub, and at streamsides, in the mountains of Burma, China, Korea, and Japan. They have large, long-stalked, palmate or pinnate, sometimes bronze-tinted, basal leaves, in some species turning shades of red and brown in autumn. In summer, tall stems bear star-shaped, petalless, white or pink flowers, each 7–8mm (¼–⅜in) across, in large, fluffy, pyramidal panicles. These are followed by dark red or brown, capsular fruits. Grow near water, in a bog garden or moist border, or use for naturalizing at woodland margins.

- **HARDINESS** Fully hardy, but young leaves may be damaged by late frosts.
- **CULTIVATION** Grow in humus-rich, moist soil in full sun or partial shade, sheltered from cold, drying winds. They resent drought, but will tolerate drier conditions with more shade.
- **PROPAGATION** Sow seed in containers in a cold frame in spring. Divide in early spring.
- **PESTS AND DISEASES** Slugs may damage young leaves.

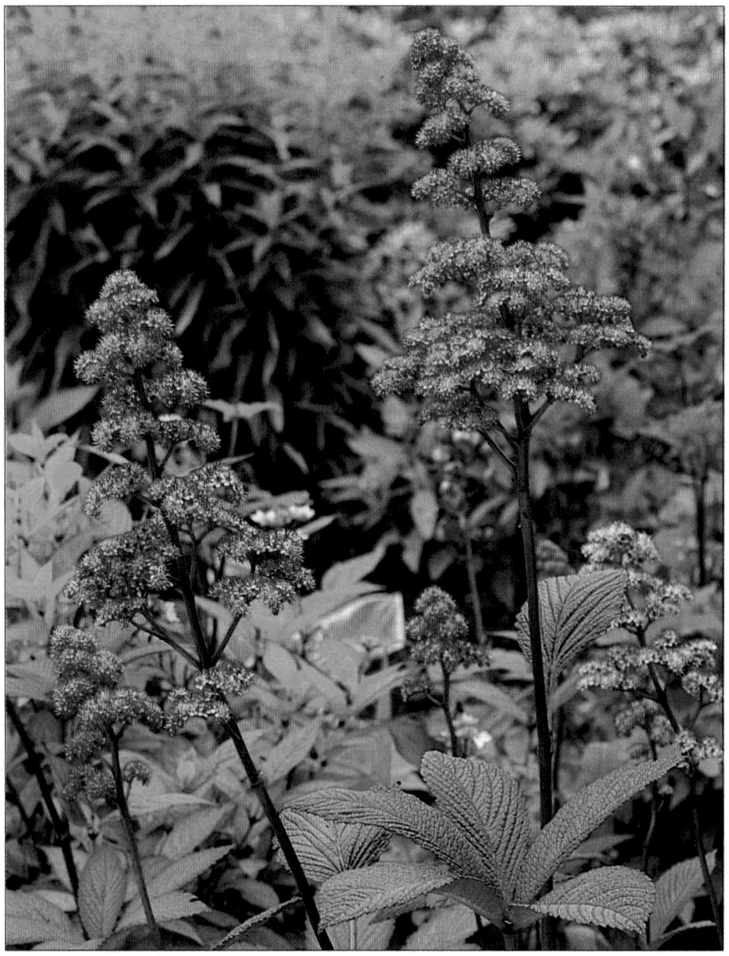
Rodgersia pinnata 'Superba'

R. aesculifolia ▣ 🏆 Clump-forming, rhizomatous perennial producing horse-chestnut-like, palmate, crinkled, mid-green leaves, to 25cm (10in) long. The leaves have densely woolly, red-brown stalks and veins, and usually 7, sometimes 5–9, obovate, toothed leaflets. In midsummer, bears numerous star-shaped, white or pink flowers in large panicles, to 60cm (24in) long. ↕ to 2m (6ft), ↔ 1m (3ft). N. China. ❄❄❄

R. japonica see *R. podophylla*.

R. pinnata. Rhizomatous, clump-forming perennial producing pinnate, or partially pinnate or palmate, crinkled, heavily veined, glossy, dark green leaves, to 90cm (36in) long; leaves have reddish green stalks and 5–9 obovate-inversely-lance-shaped leaflets. In mid- and late summer, reddish green stems bear star-shaped, yellowish white, pink, or red flowers in panicles 30–70cm (12–28in) long. ↕ to 1.2m (4ft), ↔ 75cm (30in). China (Sichuan, Yunnan). ❄❄❄. **'Superba'** ▣ 🏆 has purplish bronze young leaves, sometimes with fewer leaflets than in the species, and bright pink flowers.

R. podophylla ▣ 🏆 syn. *R. japonica*. Clump-forming, rhizomatous perennial with palmate leaves, to 40cm (16in) long, composed of usually 5 large, jagged, obovate, 3- to 5-lobed leaflets, crinkled and bronze when young, becoming smoother, glossy, and mid-green, with brown hairs. The leaves turn bronze-red in autumn. In mid- and late summer, bears star-shaped, creamy green flowers in panicles 30cm (12in) long. ↕ to 1.5m (5ft), ↔ to 1.8m (6ft). Korea, Japan. ❄❄❄

R. sambucifolia ▣ Clump-forming, rhizomatous perennial with elder-like, pinnate, hairy, dark green leaves, to 75cm (30in) long, with usually 7, sometimes 3–11, oblong-lance-shaped, toothed leaflets. In early and mid-summer, bears star-shaped, white or pink flowers in dense panicles, to 45cm (18in) long, arching at the tips. ↕↔ 90cm (36in). W. China. ❄❄❄

R. tabularis see *Astilboides tabularis*.

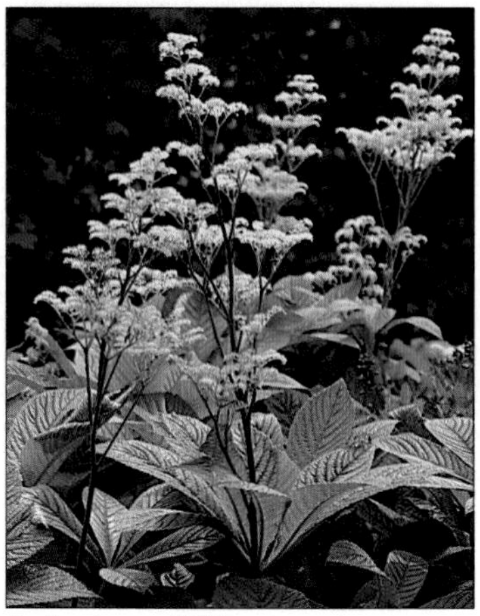
Rodgersia aesculifolia

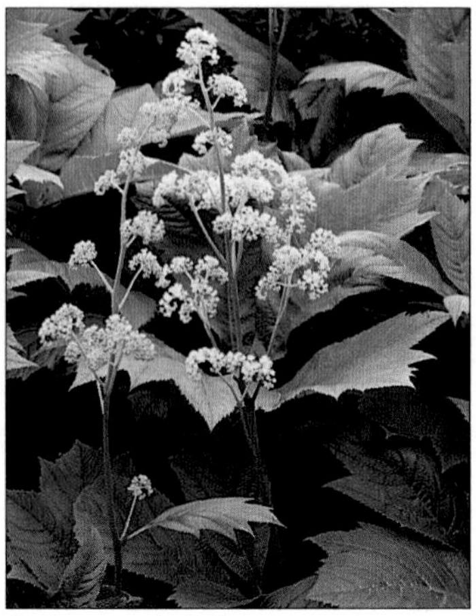
Rodgersia podophylla

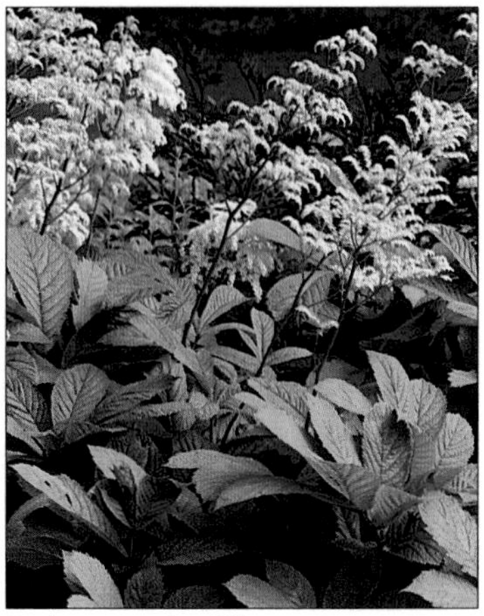
Rodgersia sambucifolia

RODRIGUEZIA

ORCHIDACEAE

Genus of about 30 species of evergreen, rhizomatous, epiphytic orchids from warm, moist, forest areas of Central and South America. They have fine, aerial, sometimes mat-forming roots, ovoid pseudobulbs partially enveloped by overlapping leaf-sheaths, and narrowly strap-shaped to oblong, leathery, mid-green leaves. They are grown mainly for their fragrant flowers, borne in pendent racemes arising from the bases of the pseudobulbs.

- **HARDINESS** Frost tender.
- **CULTIVATION** Intermediate-growing orchids. Grow in small containers of epiphytic orchid compost made with fine-grade bark, or grow epiphytically on bark. Provide full light with shade from hot sun, and high humidity. In summer, water freely, mist daily, and apply a balanced liquid fertilizer at every third watering; water more sparingly in winter. See also p.46.
- **PROPAGATION** Divide when the plant fills the pot and "flows" over the sides.
- **PESTS AND DISEASES** Prone to red spider mites, aphids, and mealybugs.

R. venusta. Epiphytic orchid with compressed, ovoid pseudobulbs, each producing several narrowly oblong, leathery leaves, 15cm (6in) long. Arching racemes of many very fragrant, pure white flowers, 3cm (1¼in) across, with yellow-marked lips, are borne in autumn. ↕↔ 15cm (6in). E. Brazil. ❄ (13°C/55°F; max. 30°C/86°F)

ROHDEA

CONVALLARIACEAE/LILIACEAE

Genus of one species of rhizomatous perennial from woodland in S.W. China and Japan, grown for its basal rosettes of fleshy, dark green leaves, and erect spikes of narrowly bell-shaped flowers, borne in early spring. Grow in a woodland garden or damp, shady border.

- **HARDINESS** Frost hardy; will tolerate occasional falls in temperature to around -10°C (14°F).
- **CULTIVATION** Grow in humus-rich, moist, moderately fertile soil in deep or partial shade.
- **PROPAGATION** Sow seed in containers in a cold frame in autumn. Divide in spring.
- **PESTS AND DISEASES** Prone to damage by slugs, snails, and vine weevil larvae.

R. japonica. Rosetted, rhizomatous perennial with thick, semi-erect, usually inversely lance-shaped, leathery, dark green leaves, 28–45cm (11–18in) long. In early spring, erect stems bear dense spikes, 2.5–5cm (1–2in) long, of narrowly bell-shaped, greenish white flowers, to 5mm (¼in) across, followed by fleshy red berries. ↕ 25cm (10in), ↔ 20cm (8in). S.W. China, Japan. ✻✻

ROMANZOFFIA

HYDROPHYLLACEAE

Genus of 4 species of low-growing, clump-forming perennials, with tuber-like roots, from shaded, rocky, alpine, or woodland habitats in W. North America and the Aleutian Islands. They produce tufts of rounded or kidney-shaped, lobed or deeply scalloped leaves, which die back after flowering and re-emerge in autumn. The bell- or funnel-shaped flowers, each with 5 rounded petal lobes and conspicuous anthers, are borne in raceme-like cymes in early summer. Suitable for a woodland garden, rock garden, peat bed, or for growing in an alpine house.

• **HARDINESS** Fully hardy.
• **CULTIVATION** Grow in moist but well-drained, humus-rich, neutral to acid soil in deep or partial shade.
• **PROPAGATION** Sow seed in containers in an open frame as soon as ripe. Divide in early spring.
• **PESTS AND DISEASES** Susceptible to damage by slugs and snails.

R. sitchensis, syn. *R. suksdorfii.* Tufted perennial with swollen roots and kidney-shaped, deeply lobed, glossy, dark green leaves, 2.5cm (1in) long. In early summer, bears small, funnel-shaped white flowers, 8mm (⅜in) long, with yellow petal bases and deep yellow anthers, in branching, terminal, raceme-like cymes, to 15cm (6in) long. ↕ 30cm (12in), ↔ to 15cm (6in). W. North America (Alaska to Montana). ✻✻✻
R. suksdorfii see *R. sitchensis.*

ROMNEYA

Matilija poppy, Tree poppy

PAPAVERACEAE

Genus of 2 species of suckering, woody-based, subshrubby perennials found in chaparral and sage scrub in S. California, USA, and N. Mexico. They are grown for their glaucous foliage and fragrant, showy white flowers. The leaves are alternate, and pinnatifid to pinnatisect; the poppy-like, solitary, terminal, 6-petalled flowers, with bright yellow stamens, are borne in summer. Grow in a border or, in frost-prone areas, against a warm, sunny wall.

• **HARDINESS** Frost hardy.
• **CULTIVATION** Grow in fertile, well-drained soil in full sun, sheltered from strong, cold winds. Provide a deep, dry winter mulch. Tree poppies are sometimes difficult to establish and resent transplanting, but may eventually spread vigorously by suckers. Usually cut back to the base by frost; in warmer areas, pruning group 6.
• **PROPAGATION** Sow seed at 13–16°C (55–61°F) in spring. Root basal cuttings in spring; insert root cuttings in winter.
• **PESTS AND DISEASES** *Verticillium* wilt and caterpillars may be a problem.

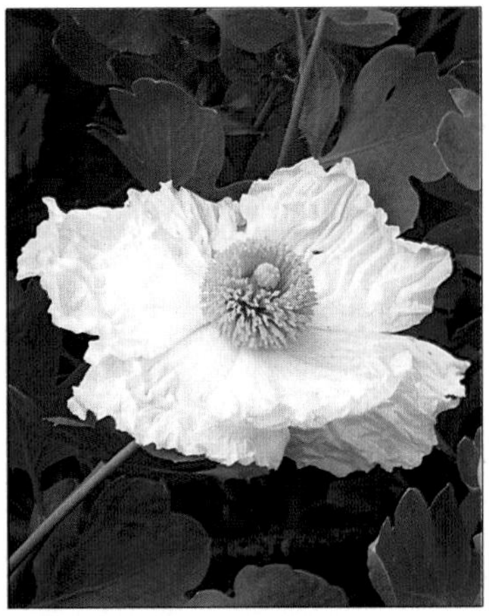

Romneya coulteri 'White Cloud'

R. coulteri ♀ Upright, deciduous subshrub producing ovate to rounded, pinnatifid, intensely glaucous, grey-green leaves, to 12cm (5in) long, with 3–5 lance-shaped to ovate lobes. Solitary, shallowly cup-shaped white flowers, to 12cm (5in) across, with prominent yellow stamens, are borne over a long period in summer. ↕ 1–2.5m (3–8ft), ↔ indefinite. ✻✻. **'White Cloud'** ■ is vigorous and fast-spreading, with very glaucous foliage.

ROMULEA

IRIDACEAE

Genus of about 80 species of small, cormous perennials from a range of habitats including mountainous areas and coastal cliff tops in Europe, the Mediterranean, N. Africa, and South Africa. They are grown for their colourful, crocus-like flowers, produced in spring on very short, slender stems. The flowers often open only at midday, closing in the evening. Each plant produces up to 6 erect, or recurved and arching, thread-like, basal leaves, 5–40cm (2–16in) long. Grow in a sunny rock garden, or in containers in an alpine house. Half-hardy species are best grown in a cool greenhouse.

• **HARDINESS** Frost hardy to half hardy.
• **CULTIVATION** Plant corms 8cm (3in) deep in autumn. Under glass, grow in loam-based potting compost (JI No.2) with additional grit, in full light. In the growing season, water moderately and apply a balanced liquid fertilizer monthly. After flowering, reduce water gradually; keep completely dry when

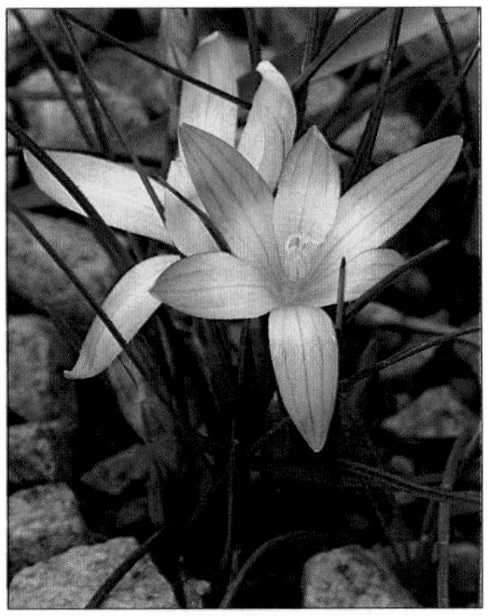

Romulea bulbocodium

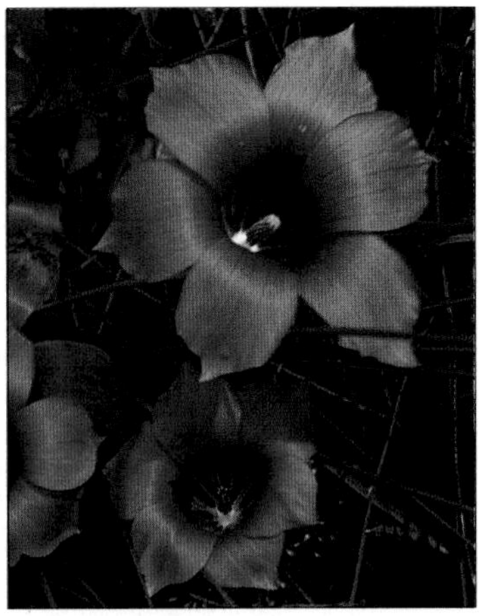

Romulea sabulosa

dormant in summer. Outdoors, grow in moderately fertile, well-drained soil in full sun.
• **PROPAGATION** Sow seed at 6–12°C (45–54°F) in autumn, or remove offsets when dormant.
• **PESTS AND DISEASES** Trouble free.

***R. bulbocodioides* of gardens** see *R. flava.*
R. bulbocodium ■ syn. *R. grandiflora.* Small, cormous perennial with recurved, linear, channelled, mid-green, basal leaves. In spring, stems bear up to 5 upright, funnel-shaped, pale to deep lilac-purple flowers, 2.5cm (1in) long, with white or yellow centres. ↕ 5–10cm (2–4in), ↔ 5cm (2in). Mediterranean, Portugal, N.W. Spain, Bulgaria. ✻✻. **var. *crocea*** has yellow flowers.
R. flava, syn. *R. bulbocodioides* of gardens. Cormous perennial with upright, sheathing, linear, mid-green, basal leaves. In spring, produces up to 4 solitary, funnel-shaped, yellowish green, sometimes white or blue flowers, 3–4cm (1¼–1½in) long, with yellow centres. ↕ 10cm (4in), ↔ 5cm (2in). South Africa (Western Cape, Northern Cape, Eastern Cape). ✻
R. grandiflora see *R. bulbocodium.*
R. longituba see *R. macowanii* var. *alticola.*
R. macowanii* var. *alticola, syn. *R. longituba.* Cormous perennial with erect or recurved, linear, mid-green, basal leaves. In summer, stems bear up to 3 tubular, bright yellow flowers, 3–6cm (1¼–2½in) long, with orange-yellow centres. ↕ 8cm (3in), ↔ 5cm (2in). Lesotho (Drakensberg mountains), South Africa. ✻✻
R. requienii. Cormous perennial with arching to almost prostrate, linear, mid-green, basal leaves. Stems with up to 3 funnel-shaped violet flowers, 5cm (2in) long, sometimes veined darker violet, and with paler violet or white centres, are produced in spring. ↕↔ 12cm (5in), ↔ 5cm (2in). Mediterranean, France (Corsica), Italy (Sardinia). ✻✻
R. sabulosa ■ Showy, cormous perennial with upright or recurved, linear, mid-green, basal leaves. In early spring and summer, stems bear up to 4 funnel-shaped flowers, 5cm (2in) long; the flowers are bright shining scarlet to ruby red, with black centres, sometimes with paler margins, and open wide in the sun. ↕ 10–20cm (4–8in), ↔ 5cm (2in). South Africa (Western Cape, Eastern Cape). ✻

RONDELETIA

RUBIACEAE

Genus of 125–150 species of evergreen shrubs and trees from tropical woodland in Central and South America. The simple, leathery to paper-thin leaves are borne in opposite pairs or whorls of 3. They are grown for their small, tubular to salverform, sometimes fragrant flowers, each with 4–6 spreading petal lobes, which are borne in large, axillary or terminal panicles, cymes, or corymbs. Where temperatures fall below 12°C (54°F), grow in a temperate or warm greenhouse. In warmer areas, grow in a shrub border.

• **HARDINESS** Frost tender.
• **CULTIVATION** Under glass, grow in loam-based potting compost (JI No.3) with added leaf mould, in full light with shade from hot sun. Water freely in growth, and apply a balanced liquid fertilizer monthly; water moderately in winter. Outdoors, grow in fertile, moist but well-drained soil in sun or partial shade. Pruning group 9; plants under glass may need restrictive pruning.
• **PROPAGATION** Root semi-ripe cuttings with bottom heat in summer.
• **PESTS AND DISEASES** Prone to red spider mites, mealybugs, and whiteflies.

R. amoena ■♀ Bushy, rounded shrub or small tree with smooth to downy stems and elliptic or ovate-oblong leaves, 8–15cm (3–6in) long, glossy, mid-green above, brown-hairy or hairless beneath. In summer, bears axillary or terminal cymes or panicles, 5–15cm (2–6in) long, of small, salverform, fragrant, pink or white flowers with bearded yellow throats. ↕ 1.5–5m (5–15ft) or more, ↔ 1.5–4m (5–12ft). Mexico, Guatemala, Panama. ❀ (min. 12°C/54°F)
R. odorata, syn. *R. speciosa.* Bushy shrub, often with downy to felted stems, producing ovate to oblong, puckered, wavy-margined leaves, to 10cm (4in) long, deep green above, paler green beneath. Tubular, fragrant, orange to red, yellow-throated flowers are borne in dense, terminal cymes, corymbs, or panicles, 10cm (4in) long, in autumn. ↕ to 3m (10ft), ↔ to 2.5m (8ft). Cuba, Panama. ❀ (min. 12°C/54°F)
R. speciosa see *R. odorata.*

▷ ***Rooksbya euphorbioides*** see *Neobuxbaumia euphorbioides*
▷ **Rooistompie** see *Mimetes cucullatus*

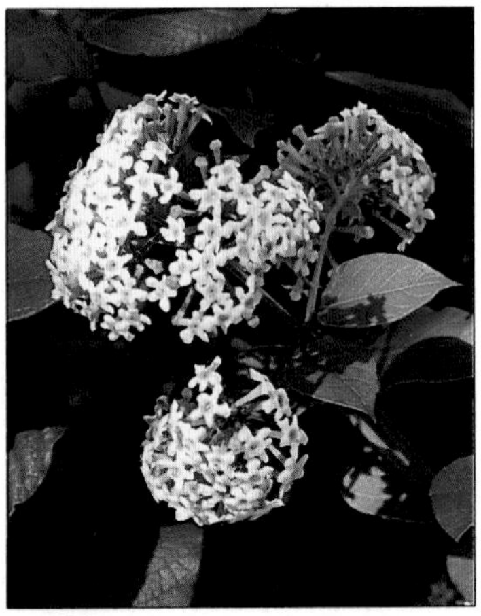

Rondeletia amoena

R

ROSA

Rose

ROSACEAE

Genus of about 150 species of semi-evergreen or deciduous, perennial shrubs and climbers, some of which have been in cultivation for many centuries. They are found in a wide variety of habitats in Asia, Europe, N. Africa, and North America. Roses have erect, arching, scrambling, or sometimes trailing, often thorny or prickly stems. The alternate leaves range from 2.5cm (1in) long in miniature roses to 18cm (7in) or more long in bush, shrub, and climbing roses; each leaf usually has 5 or 7 sometimes toothed, variably shaped leaflets.

Roses are grown for their attractive and often very fragrant flowers, borne mainly in summer and autumn, and sometimes also for their fruits, known as hips. The flowers are solitary or borne in corymbs (referred to in this account as clusters), are sometimes remontant, and vary greatly in colour, size, and form (see panel below). Roses are suitable for a range of garden situations: as specimen plants or standards, for a shrub or mixed border, as hedges, or as climbers to clothe walls, trees, pillars, pergolas, and arbours. Groups of roses are often grown together in a single bed; a well-chosen mix of cultivars will ensure a long summer display. Miniature roses are suitable for a rock garden, raised bed, or containers. The flowers of all roses are popular for cutting.

Many modern rose cultivars are known by their trademark names rather than by their registered cultivar names; where this is the case, the plant is listed below under its trademark name, with the cultivar name given as a synonym. For reasons of space, these cultivar names have not been cross-referenced.

Rose species and cultivars are often regarded as 2 separate groups. Cultivars are further divided into Old Garden and Modern roses, the many subgroups of which are described below.

Species, or wild, roses (including inter-specific hybrids, which share most of the characteristics of their parent species) are either shrubs or climbers, mostly bearing single, 5-petalled, often fragrant flowers in early summer, usually in one flush on short shoots from second-year wood; the flowers are followed by red or black hips.

Cultivars, derived initially from crossing species roses, number many thousands, and are very varied in habit. In the subgroup descriptions below, leaflet lengths are defined as: small, up to 4cm (1½in); medium-sized, 4–7cm (1½–3in); large, over 7cm (3in). The flowers, in a range of shapes, are borne mainly in summer, over a longer period than in species roses; they are often remontant. Flowers are either single (having 8 petals or fewer), semi-double (8–20 petals), double (20 petals or more), or fully double (over 30 petals). "Single to fully double", as used below, means that the flowers may be single, semi-double, double, or fully double.

ROSE FLOWER FORMS

Flat – Open, usually single or semi-double flowers with petals that are almost flat.
Cupped – Open, single to fully double flowers with petals that curve outwards and upwards from the centre.
Rounded – Usually double or fully double flowers with even-sized, overlapping petals forming a bowl shape or more rounded form.
High-centred – Semi-double to fully double flowers with high, tight centres.
Urn-shaped – Semi-double to fully double flowers with inner petals that curve inwards to form an urn-shape, and outer petals that are flatter and more spreading.
Rosette-shaped – Almost flat, double or fully double flowers with slightly overlapping, often uneven petals.
Quartered-rosette – Almost flat, double or fully double flowers with the petals, often of uneven size, arranged so that the flower appears divided into 4 sections.
Pompon – Small, rounded, double or fully double flowers, usually in clusters, with masses of small petals.

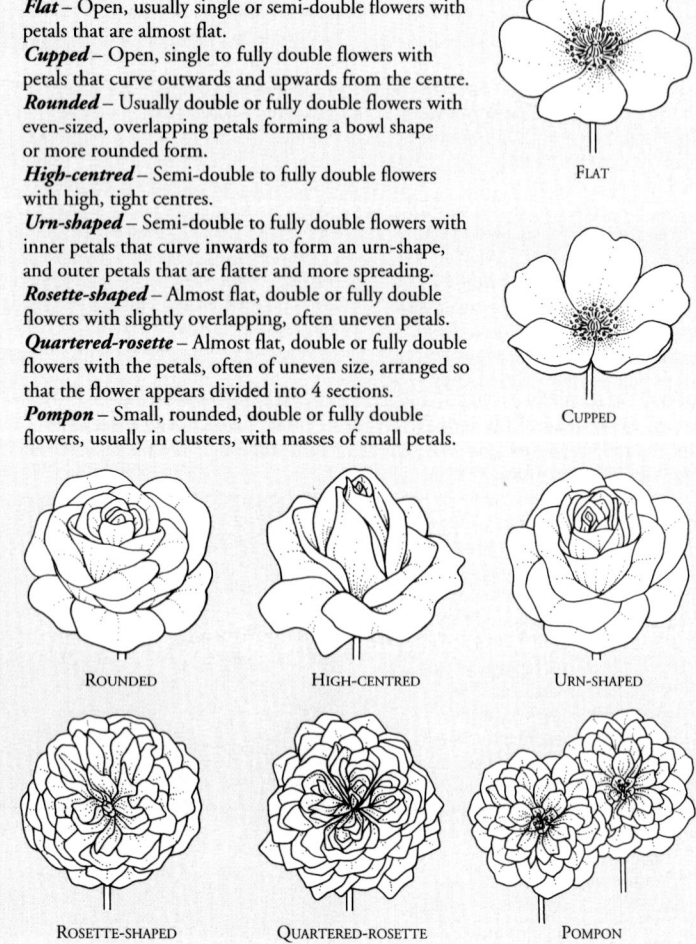

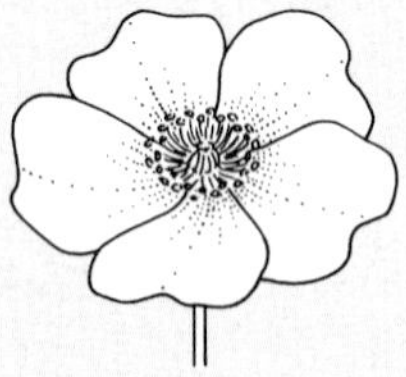
FLAT

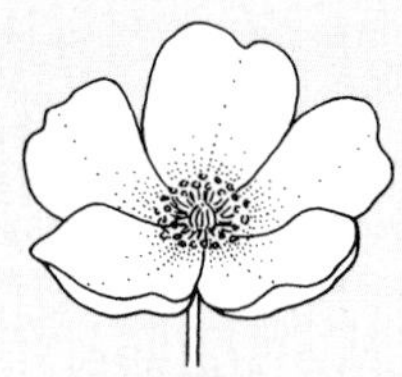
CUPPED

ROUNDED

HIGH-CENTRED

URN-SHAPED

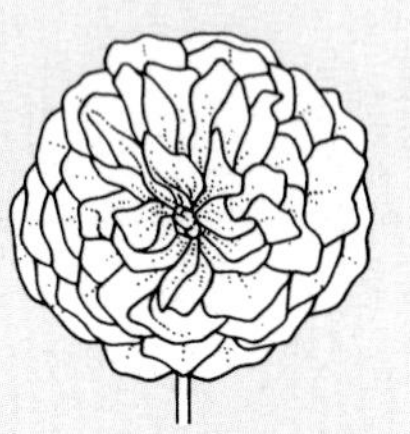
ROSETTE-SHAPED

QUARTERED-ROSETTE

POMPON

Old Garden roses

Alba – Large, free-branching shrub roses, varying greatly in size, with only a few prickles on the stems. They have greyish green leaves with medium to large, oval leaflets, and bear clusters of 5–7 semi- to fully double, scented flowers in midsummer, on shoots from second-year wood. Very hardy. Most are suitable for a border, as hedges, or as specimen plants.

Bourbon – Large, open, remontant shrub roses, often with long, smooth or prickly stems, which may be trained to climb. They have often glossy leaves with medium-sized, oval leaflets, and most bear numerous scented, double or fully double flowers, usually in clusters of 3, in flushes in summer and usually autumn. Flowers are borne on short shoots from second-year wood and on new wood. Ideal for a border, or for training on a fence, wall, or pillar.

Boursault – Climbing roses with long, arching, usually smooth stems, and dark green leaves with medium to large, oval leaflets. They bear semi-double or double, slightly scented flowers, singly or in clusters of 3, in early summer, on short shoots from second-year wood. Grow against a sheltered wall or fence.

Centifolia (Provence) – Lax, thorny shrub roses producing matt, dark green leaves with small to medium-sized, oval leaflets. Double or fully double, often scented flowers, are borne singly or in clusters of 3 in summer, on shoots from second-year wood. Grow in a border.

China – Spindly, remontant shrub roses with mostly smooth stems, bearing only a few reddish brown prickles, and glossy leaves comprised of small to medium-sized, lance-shaped leaflets. They bear single to fully double, sometimes scented flowers, singly or in clusters of 3–13, in flushes from summer to autumn. Flowers are borne on short shoots from second-year wood and on new wood. Use in a border, or grow against a low wall in a sheltered site.

Damask – Open shrub roses with prickly stems and downy leaves with medium to large, oval leaflets. They bear semi- to fully double, often very fragrant flowers, singly or in loose clusters of 5–7, mainly in summer, on shoots from second-year wood; a few also flower on new wood in autumn. Ideal for a border or for training on a support.

Gallica – Shrub roses of dense, free-branching habit, with usually thorny stems, and mostly dull, dark green leaves with medium-sized, oval leaflets. In summer, they bear single to fully double, mostly scented flowers, often in clusters of 3, on shoots from second-year wood. Use in a bed or as hedges.

Hybrid Perpetual – Free-branching, remontant shrub roses with upright, prickly growth and dark green leaves with medium to large, oval leaflets. They bear often scented, fully double flowers, singly or in clusters of 3, in flushes from summer to autumn, on shoots from second-year wood and on new wood. Ideal for a bed or border.

Moss – Often lax shrub roses with moss-like, furry growth on the stems and calyces, and mostly dark green leaves with medium to large, oval leaflets. Semi- to fully double, usually fragrant flowers, often in clusters of 3 or more, are borne on very thorny shoots from second-year wood in summer. Suitable for a bed or border.

Noisette – Remontant climbing roses with smooth stems and usually glossy leaves comprising medium to large, oval or lance-shaped leaflets. They bear large clusters of 3–15 slightly spice-scented, normally double to fully double flowers, in flushes from summer to autumn. Flowers are borne on shoots from second-year wood, occasionally on new wood. Grow against a sheltered wall.

Portland – Upright, compact, remontant shrub roses with thorny stems and usually dark green leaves composed of medium to large, oval leaflets. Semi- to fully double, usually scented flowers are borne, singly or in clusters of 3, in flushes from summer to autumn, mainly on shoots from second-year wood. Grow in a bed or border.

Scots (or ***Scotch***) – Suckering shrub roses, selections or hybrids of *R. pimpinellifolia*, of low, spreading, rarely upright habit, with prickly stems and dark green leaves comprising small to medium-sized, oval leaflets. The single to double, occasionally scented flowers are solitary or borne in clusters of 3 or more, on short stems from second-year wood, usually in early summer. Suitable for a bed or border.

Sempervirens – Vigorous, semi-evergreen climbing or rambler roses with shiny, light green leaves composed of small to medium-sized, lance-shaped leaflets. Arching, thorny stems bear clusters of 3–15 unscented, semi- to fully double flowers in summer, on short stems from second-year wood. Use to clothe a fence or pergola, or in informal, unconfined plantings.

Sweet Briar – Vigorous, free-branching shrub roses with usually thorny stems and sweetly scented, dark green leaves composed of small to medium-sized, oval leaflets. In summer, they bear single to double, usually scented flowers, singly or in clusters of up to 7, on short shoots from second-year wood. Use as hedges, as specimen plants, or in a large border.

Tea – Remontant shrub and climbing roses with smooth to thorny stems, sometimes bearing a few large red prickles, and medium-sized, glossy, light or sometimes dark green leaves with lance-shaped leaflets. Semi- to fully double, spice-scented flowers are borne singly or in clusters of 3, in flushes from summer to autumn, on shoots from second-year wood and on new wood. Grow in a sheltered site in a bed or border, or against a wall.

Modern roses

Climber – Often vigorous climbing roses with thorny, arching, stiff stems and often dense, glossy, mid- to dark green foliage. They bear often scented flowers in a variety of forms, singly or in clusters of 3–7 or more. Some bloom in summer only, on short shoots from second-year wood; many are remontant and also flower on new wood. Train against a wall or fence, or use to cover garden structures.

Cluster-flowered bush (Floribunda) – Remontant, free-branching shrub roses of upright or bushy habit, usually with prickly stems and glossy, dark green leaves composed of medium-sized, oval or lance-shaped leaflets. The single to fully double, sometimes scented flowers are usually in clusters of 3–25, rarely solitary, and borne continuously from summer to autumn on shoots from second-year wood and on new wood. Use in a border or as hedges.

Dwarf cluster-flowered bush (Patio) – Remontant shrub roses with compact growth, sometimes prickly stems, and usually glossy leaves composed of small to medium, oval or lance-shaped leaflets. They bear clusters of 3–11 single to double, usually unscented flowers in flushes from summer to autumn, on shoots from second-year wood and on new wood. Suitable for a bed or border, as low hedges, and for containers.

Ground-cover bush or shrub – Spreading and trailing roses, mostly with prickly stems, producing often glossy leaves with small to medium-sized, lance-shaped leaflets. They bear clusters of numerous single to fully double, sometimes scented flowers; some flower in summer only, on short shoots from second-year wood; some are remontant, and also flower on new wood. Many bear flowers all along the stems. Ideal for a bed, bank, container, or for trailing over walls.

Large-flowered bush (Hybrid Tea) – Remontant, free-branching shrub roses of upright or bushy habit, with usually thorny stems and glossy or matt, mid- to dark green leaves with medium-sized to large, oval or lance-shaped leaflets. Large, usually double, often scented flowers are solitary or borne in clusters of 3 in flushes from summer to autumn, on shoots from second-year wood and on new wood. Use as hedges or in a formal bed, and for cut flowers.

Miniature bush – Remontant shrub roses with very compact, sparsely thorny, short growth, and leaves with very small, usually lance-shaped leaflets. Sprays of 3–11 tiny, single to fully double, rarely scented flowers are borne in flushes from summer to autumn, on very short shoots from second-year wood and on new wood. Ideal for edging paths, or for a raised bed, rock garden, or container.

Miniature climber – Remontant climbing roses with restrained, sparsely thorny growth, and leaves comprised of very small, lance-shaped leaflets. Clusters of 3–9 tiny, single to fully double, rarely scented flowers are borne in flushes from summer to autumn, on shoots from second-year wood and on new wood. Grow against a low wall, fence, or pillar.

Miniature ground-cover bush or shrub – Remontant miniature roses with very compact, spreading, sparsely thorny growth, and leaves with usually very small, lance-shaped leaflets. They bear clusters of 3–11 tiny, single to fully double, rarely scented flowers in flushes from summer to autumn, on short shoots from second-year wood and on new wood. Use for edging a path or driveway, or in a raised bed, rock garden, or container.

Polyantha – Remontant, compact-growing shrub roses with sparsely thorny stems, and glossy leaves with small, lance-shaped leaflets. Sprays of many small, single to double, rarely scented flowers are borne in flushes from summer to autumn, on short shoots from second-year wood and on new wood. Suitable for a bed or border, as hedges, and for containers.

Rambler – A diverse group of vigorous climbing roses with long, arching, thorny, sometimes lax stems and dense foliage. They have usually glossy leaves with small, lance-shaped leaflets, and bear clusters of 3–21 single to fully double, sometimes scented flowers, mainly in summer, on short shoots from second-year wood. Train over a fence or pergola, on walls, or into a tree.

Rugosa – Hardy shrub roses with tough, wrinkled, usually bright green leaves with medium to large, oval or lance-shaped leaflets and prickly stems. Most bear single or semi-double, scented flowers, in clusters of 3–11, throughout summer and autumn, on shoots from second-year wood and on new wood. They are often followed by tomato-like, usually red hips. Use as hedges, for a bed or border, or as specimen plants.

Shrub – A very diverse group, including the hybrid musk roses. They are usually larger than bush roses, with often thorny stems, and produce leaves with medium-sized to large, oval or lance-shaped leaflets. The usually scented, single to fully double flowers are borne in few- to many-flowered clusters, sometimes singly, from summer to autumn; some bloom in summer only from second-year wood; most are remontant and also flower on new wood. Ideal for a border or bed, or as hedges; some are also excellent specimen plants.

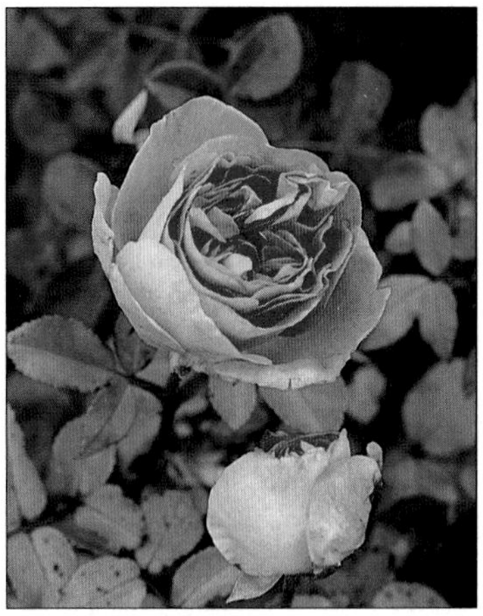

Rosa 'Abraham Darby'

• **HARDINESS** Fully hardy to frost hardy.

• **CULTIVATION** Roses tolerate a wide range of conditions, but usually prefer an open site in full sun. They thrive on moderately fertile, humus-rich, moist but well-drained soil. Soil in which roses have recently been grown is unsuitable for new plantings because of the build-up of harmful soil organisms. In such cases, either exchange the soil, which may be used elsewhere, sterilize the soil with a proprietary remedy, or choose a fresh planting site. The best time for planting is winter or early spring, during a frost-free spell. For best flowering, apply a balanced fertilizer and mulch in late winter or early spring. In spring and summer, apply a balanced liquid fertilizer every 3 weeks. The height and spread measurements in the descriptions below are for pruned plants; unpruned, roses grow much larger.

Most roses sold have been budded on the rootstock of a wild rose to ensure vigorous growth. The rootstock may produce shoots, known as "suckers", which should be removed at their point of origin as soon as seen. To identify a sucker, check that it originates from the rootstock itself, and not from above the point where the plant was budded.

Rain may damage the flowers of some roses, causing the petals to form "balls".

• **PROPAGATION** Root hardwood cuttings in autumn. Bud in summer.

• **PESTS AND DISEASES** Susceptible to aphids, leafhoppers, red spider mites, scale insects, caterpillars, sawfly larvae, and leaf-cutting bees; rabbits and deer may cause damage. Prone to black spot, rust, powdery mildew, die-back, canker, crown gall, honey fungus, soil sickness, viruses, and downy mildew.

***R.* 'Abbeyfield Rose'** 🏆 syn. *R.* 'Cocbrose'. Large-flowered bush rose of compact habit, with masses of glossy, dark green leaves. High-centred, double, deep rose-pink flowers, 10cm (4in) across, are borne freely from summer to autumn. ↕↔ 60cm (24in). ✲✲✲

***R.* 'Abraham Darby'** ▣ syn. *R.* 'Auscot'. Shrub rose with a strong,

PRUNING REQUIREMENTS

On planting, shorten thick roots to 25cm (10in) and remove damaged ones. Reduce top-growth to 3–5 strong shoots, and cut these back to outward-facing buds: to 8–15cm (3–6in) above ground for large- and cluster-flowered bushes and dwarf variants; to 40cm (16in) for ramblers; to 20–30cm (8–12in) for other groups. For climbers and standards, remove only dead, diseased, damaged, weak, or crossing shoots.

When in growth, remove dead, damaged, and diseased wood, suckers, and blind shoots, and prune as below. Dead-head all roses unless hips are wanted. In autumn, trim long shoots back by 15–30cm (6–12in) to reduce wind rock. Avoid pruning in frosty weather when roses are dormant; delay until early spring in areas with severe winters. Prune in the cooler months in warm climates, to simulate dormancy.

The pruning chart below gives specific advice for individual rose groups. For standard roses, prune according to the type of rose that forms the head; leave weeping standards unpruned on planting and for 2 subsequent years, to develop their form.

GROUP	SEASON	FOR MAINTENANCE	FOR RENEWAL
LARGE-FLOWERED BUSH, TEA, HYBRID PERPETUAL	Late winter to early spring	Cut back main stems to 20–25cm (8–10in) above ground in temperate climates; to 45–60cm (18–24in) in warm climates. Reduce sideshoots to 2 or 3 buds or 10–15cm (4–6in). Remove weak, spindly shoots.	Cut back ⅓ of oldest stems almost to the base; repeat for rest of old stems over next 2 or 3 years.
CLUSTER-FLOWERED BUSH (INC. DWARF CULTIVARS), MINIATURE BUSH, POLYANTHA	Late winter to early spring	Cut back main stems to 25–45cm (10–18in) above ground; reduce sideshoots to 2 or 3 buds. Cut back stems and side-shoots of dwarf cultivars and miniature bushes by ⅓–½.	As above.
CLIMBERS (INC. MINIATURE CULTIVARS), BOURSAULT, NOISETTE, AND CLIMBING BOURBON	Late autumn to early spring	In the first 2 years, cut out only dead, diseased, or damaged wood; train stems on to wires or other, preferably horizontal supports. From year 3, prune main shoots to within designated area for growth; reduce sideshoots by ⅔, or to 3 or 4 buds.	Cut back 1 or 2 of oldest stems to 30–45cm (12–18in) above ground. Repeat every 1–3 years.
RAMBLER, SEMPERVIRENS	Summer, after flowering	In the first 2 years, train stems on to support; reduce sideshoots only, by ⅔ or to 2–4 buds. In year 3, reduce sideshoots as before, and begin renewal pruning.	Cut out ¼–⅓ of flowered stems at the base. New shoots arise from base.
GROUND-COVER BUSH (INC. MINIATURE CULTIVARS)	Late winter to early spring	Cut back to outward-facing buds to confine to designated area for growth. Shorten sideshoots if overcrowded.	Cut out ⅕–¼ of oldest flowered stems.
SPECIES, SHRUB, MINIATURE BUSH, RUGOSA	Late summer, after flowering	For non-remontant roses, prune main stems lightly, or cut back by up to ⅓, as necessary; reduce sideshoots by ½–⅔. For remontant roses, see below.	As above.
BOURBON, CHINA, PORTLAND; & remontant roses of group above	Late winter to early spring	As for category above, but during the dormant season.	As above.
ALBA, CENTIFOLIA, DAMASK, MOSS, SCOTS, SWEET BRIAR	Late summer	Immediately after flowering, prune main stems lightly or cut back by ¼–⅓, as necessary; reduce sideshoots by ⅔.	Cut out up to ¼ of oldest stems; cut back rest by ⅓.
GALLICA	Late summer	Cut back overlong shoots by up to ⅓; reduce sideshoots by ⅔.	Cut out 1 or 2 of oldest stems every 1–3 years.

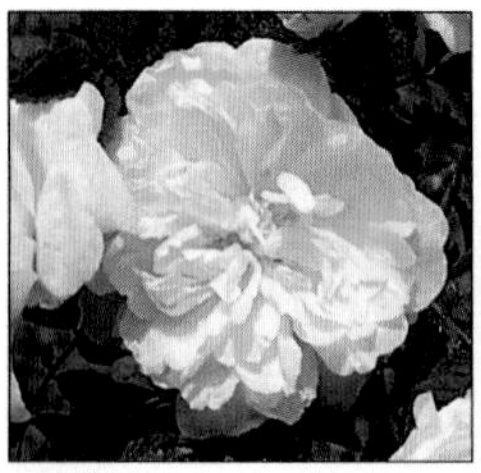
Rosa 'Agnes'

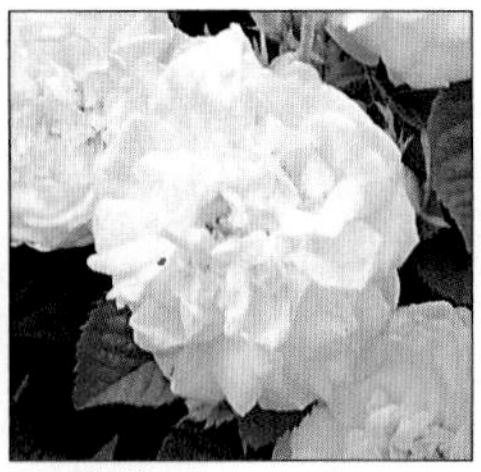
Rosa 'Alba Maxima'

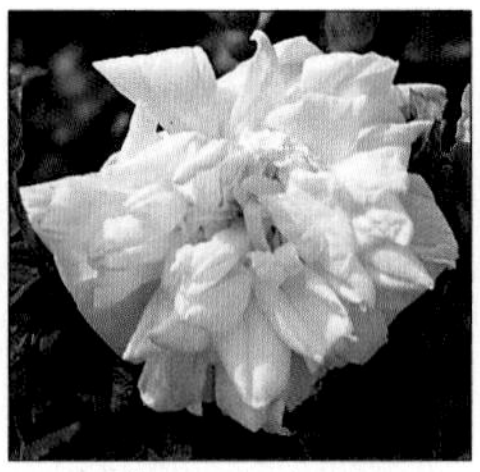
Rosa 'Albéric Barbier'

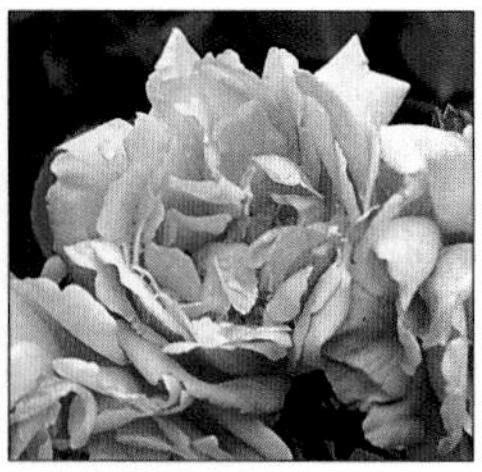
Rosa 'Albertine'

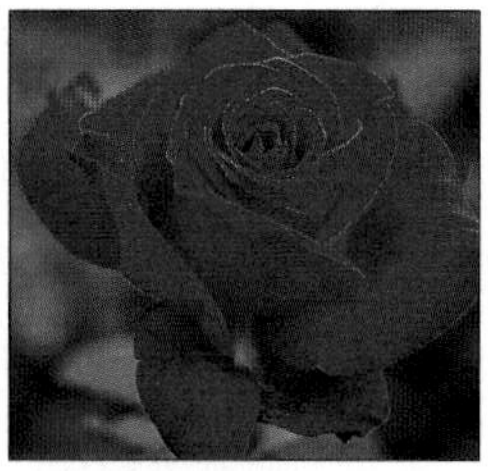
Rosa 'Alec's Red'

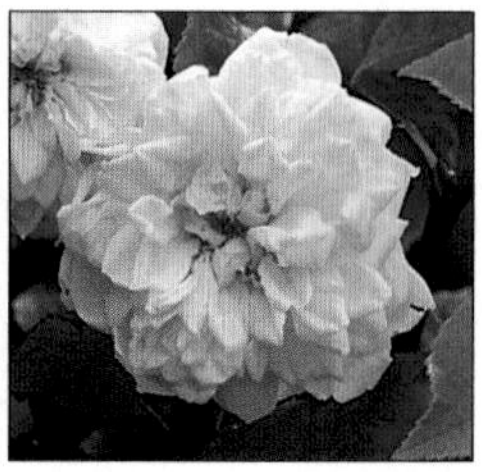
Rosa 'Alister Stella Gray'

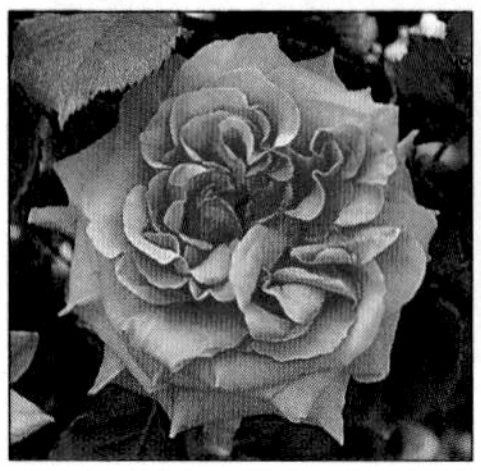
Rosa 'Aloha'

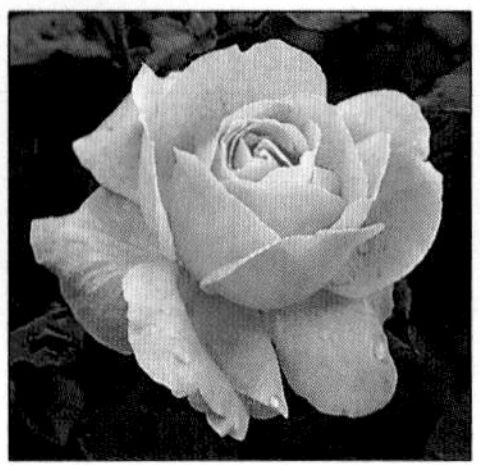
Rosa 'Alpine Sunset'

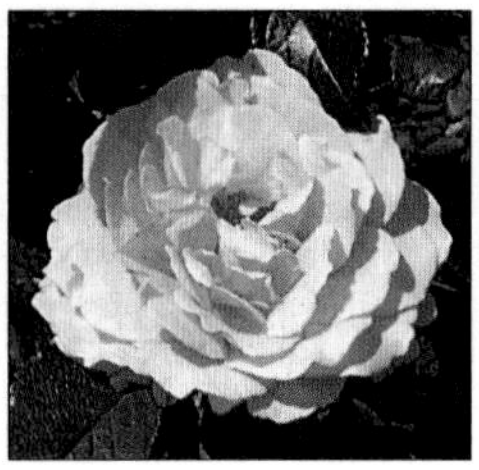
Rosa 'Amber Queen'

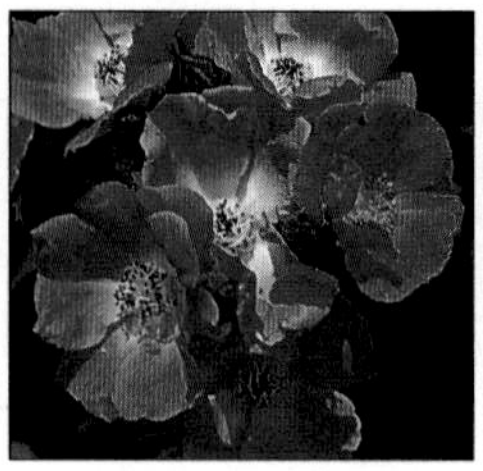
Rosa 'American Pillar'

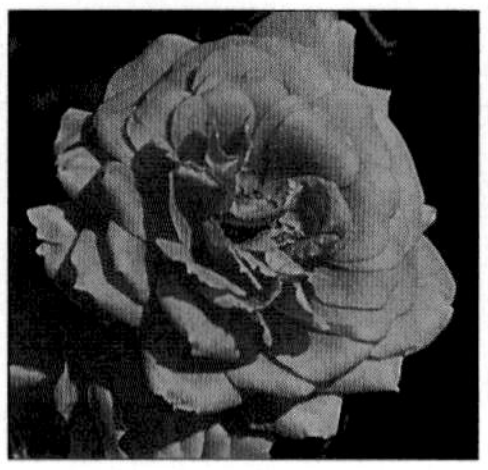
Rosa 'Angela Rippon'

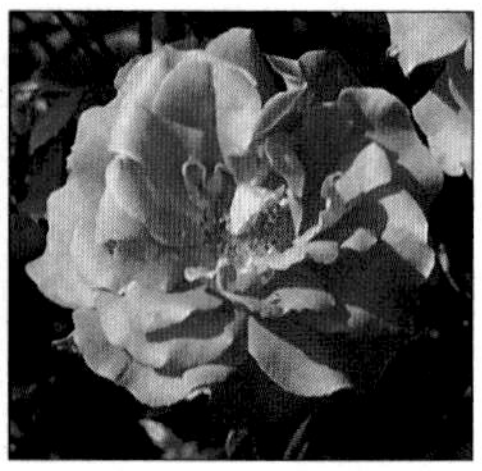
Rosa 'Anisley Dickson'

bushy habit and large, glossy, dark green leaves. Cupped, fully double, fruit-scented, apricot-pink flowers, 11cm (4½in) across, are borne from summer to autumn. ↕↔ 1.5m (5ft). ❄❄❄

***R.* 'Adélaïde d'Orléans'** 🏆 Sempervirens rambler rose producing long, slender stems and matt, light green leaves. Clusters of pendent, cupped, semi-double, lightly scented, light pink flowers, 4cm (1½in) across, are borne in midsummer. ↕ 5m (15ft), ↔ 3m (10ft). ❄❄

***R.* 'Agnes'** ■ Rugosa rose with upright stems, dark green leaves and cupped, double, scented, light yellow flowers, 10cm (4in) across, produced in summer (a few borne later). ↕ 2m (6ft), ↔ 1.2m (4ft). ❄❄❄

***R.* 'Aimée Vibert'**, syn. *R.* 'Bouquet de la Mariée'. Noisette climbing rose with long stems and glossy, dark green leaves. Cupped, fully double, lightly scented white flowers, 8cm (3in) across, are borne in large clusters from summer to autumn. May be grown as a shrub. ↕ 3–5m (10–15ft), ↔ 3m (10ft). ❄❄

***R.* x *alba* 'Maxima'** see *R.* 'Alba Maxima'.

***R.* 'Alba Maxima'** ■🏆 syn. *R.* x *alba* 'Maxima' (Great white rose, Jacobite rose, White rose of York). Alba rose of vigorous, upright habit, with greyish green leaves. Flat, double, sweet-scented, creamy white flowers, 8cm (3in) across, are borne in midsummer. ↕ 2.2m (7ft), ↔ 1.5m (5ft). ❄❄❄

***R.* x *alba* 'Semiplena'** see *R.* 'Alba Semiplena'.

***R.* 'Alba Semiplena'** 🏆 syn. *R.* x *alba* 'Semiplena'. Alba rose of vigorous, bushy habit, with greyish green leaves. In midsummer, produces flat, semi-double, scented white flowers, 8cm (3in) across. ↕ 2.2m (7ft), ↔ 1.5m (5ft). ❄❄❄

***R.* 'Albéric Barbier'** ■🏆 Vigorous, semi-evergreen rambler with pendent growth and glossy, dark green leaves. Clusters of rosette-shaped, fully double, slightly fragrant, creamy white flowers, 8cm (3in) across, aging to pure white, are produced in summer. ↕ to 5m (15ft), ↔ 3m (10ft). ❄❄❄

***R.* 'Albertine'** ■🏆 Vigorous, rampant rambler with arching, prickly, reddish green stems and mid-green leaves. Rounded to cupped, fully double, sweetly scented, light salmon-pink flowers, 8cm (3in) across, are borne freely in midsummer. ↕ to 5m (15ft), ↔ 4m (12ft). ❄❄❄

***R.* 'Alec's Red'** ■ Large-flowered bush rose with mid-green leaves and high-centred, fully double, strongly fragrant red flowers, 15cm (6in) across, borne from summer to autumn. ↕ 1m (3ft), ↔ 60cm (24in). ❄❄❄

***R.* 'Alexander'** ■🏆 Vigorous large-flowered bush rose with shiny, dark green foliage. Urn-shaped, double, bright red flowers, 12cm (5in) across, often with scalloped petals, are borne on long stems from summer to autumn. ↕ to 2m (6ft), ↔ 80cm (32in). ❄❄

***R.* 'Alister Stella Gray'** ■🏆 syn. *R.* 'Golden Rambler'. Noisette climbing rose with long, vigorous, arching stems and mid-green foliage. Quartered-rosette, fully double, musk-scented flowers, 6cm (2½in) across, yolk-yellow fading to white, are borne freely from summer to autumn. ↕ to 5m (15ft), ↔ 3m (10ft). ❄❄

***R.* 'Aloha'** ■ Strong-stemmed climber with leathery, dark green leaves. Bears rounded, fully double, sweetly scented, rose-pink and salmon-pink flowers, 9cm (3½in) across, from summer to autumn. May be maintained as a shrub by pruning. ↕ to 3m (10ft), ↔ 2.5m (8ft). ❄❄❄

***R.* 'Alpine Sunset'** ■ Large-flowered bush rose of neat habit, with glossy, light green leaves. From summer to autumn, bears rounded, fully double, fragrant, light peach-yellow flowers, 18cm (7in) across, edged pink. ↕↔ 60cm (24in). ❄❄❄

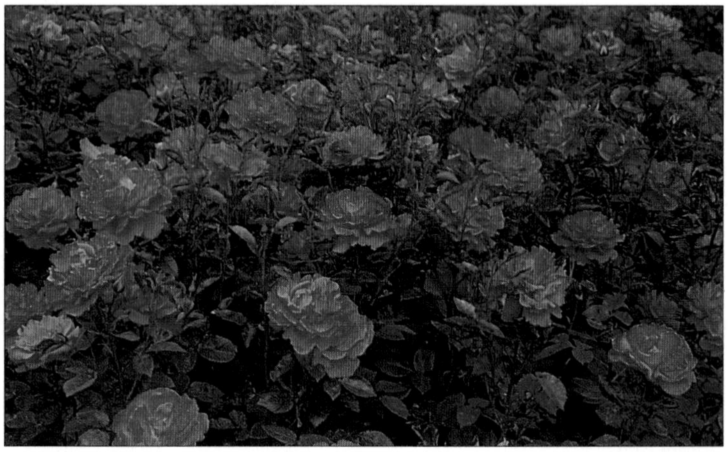
Rosa 'Alexander'

***R.* 'Altissimo'** 🏆 Climber with dark green leaves and cupped, single, bright red flowers, 12cm (5in) across, showing yellow stamens, borne from summer to autumn. ↕ 3m (10ft), ↔ 2.5m (8ft). ❄❄❄

***R.* 'Amanda'** see *R.* 'Red Ace'.

***R.* 'Amberlight'** see *R.* 'Fyvie Castle'.

***R.* 'Amber Queen'** ■🏆 syn. *R.* 'Harroony', *R.* 'Prinz Eugen van Savoyen'. Cluster-flowered bush rose of neat, spreading habit, with leathery, dark green foliage, reddish green when young. Cupped, fully double, fragrant, amber-yellow flowers, 8cm (3in) across, are borne from summer to autumn. ↕ 50cm (20in), ↔ 60cm (24in). ❄❄❄

***R.* 'America'**. Free-branching climber producing mid-green leaves. From summer to autumn, bears cupped, fully double, fragrant, coral- to salmon-pink flowers, 10cm (4in) across. ↕ to 4m (12ft), ↔ 2.5m (8ft). ❄❄❄

***R.* 'American Pillar'** ■ Rampant rambler with long stems and leathery, glossy, mid-green foliage. Large clusters of cupped, single, carmine-red flowers, 5cm (2in) across, with white eyes, are borne freely in midsummer. ↕ to 5m (15ft), ↔ 4m (12ft). ❄❄❄

***R.* 'Andeli'** see *R.* 'Double Delight'.

***R.* x *anemonoides* 'Ramona'** see *R.* 'Ramona'.

***R.* 'Angela Rippon'** ■ syn. *R.* 'Ocarina', *R.* 'Ocaru'. Miniature bush rose of upright habit, with many dark green leaves. Bears urn-shaped, fully double, rose- to salmon-pink flowers, 4cm (1½in) across, from summer to autumn. ↕ 45cm (18in), ↔ 30cm (12in). ❄❄❄

***R.* 'Angel Face'**. Spreading cluster-flowered bush rose with leathery, dark green leaves. From summer to autumn, bears cupped, fully double, scented, deep mauve flowers, 10cm (4in) across. ↕ 1m (3ft), ↔ 60cm (24in). ❄❄❄

***R.* 'Angelita'** see *R.* 'Snowball'.

***R.* 'Anisley Dickson'** ■🏆 syn. *R.* 'Dickimono', *R.* 'Dicky'. Vigorous cluster-flowered bush rose with shiny, dark green leaves and large clusters of high-centred, double, deep reddish salmon-pink flowers, 8cm (3in) across, borne from summer to autumn. ↕ 1m (3ft), ↔ 75cm (30in). ❄❄❄

***R.* 'Anna Ford'** ■🏆 syn. *R.* 'Harpiccolo'. Dwarf cluster-flowered bush rose of compact habit, with dark green leaves. Bears many urn-shaped, semi-double, orange-red flowers, 4cm (1½in) across, opening flat, from summer to autumn. ↕ 45cm (18in), ↔ 40cm (16in). ❄❄❄

***R.* 'Anna Livia'** 🏆 syn. *R.* 'Kormetter', *R.* 'Trier 2000'. Vigorous cluster-flowered bush rose with leathery, mid-green foliage. Large sprays of rounded, double pink flowers, 8cm (3in) across, are borne freely from summer to autumn. ↕ 75cm (30in), ↔ 60cm (24in). ❄❄❄

***R.* 'Anne Harkness'** ■ syn. *R.* 'Harkaramel'. Cluster-flowered bush rose of vigorous, tall habit, with mid-green foliage. Urn-shaped, double, apricot-yellow flowers, 8cm (3in) across, are borne in spectacular, many-flowered sprays from late summer to autumn. ↕ 1.2m (4ft), ↔ 60cm (24in). ❄❄❄

***R.* 'Apricot Nectar'**. Cluster-flowered bush rose with mid-green leaves and rounded, fully double, scented, apricot to apricot-pink flowers, 10cm (4in) across, borne in tight clusters from summer to autumn. ↕ to 80cm (32in), ↔ 65cm (26in). ❄❄❄

***R.* 'Arizona'**, syn. *R.* 'Tocade', *R.* 'Werina'. Large-flowered bush rose with shiny, dark green leaves. Urn-shaped, double, sweet-scented, orange-yellow flowers, 10cm (4in) across, are borne

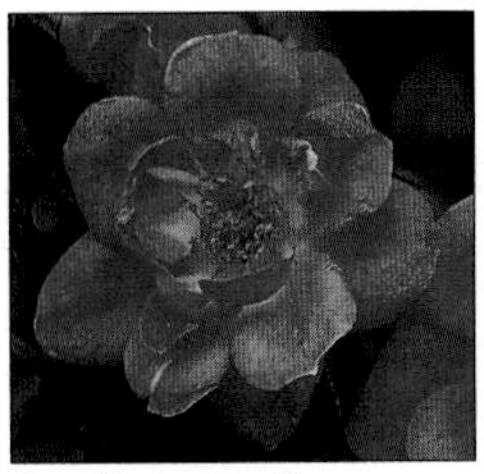
Rosa 'Anna Ford'

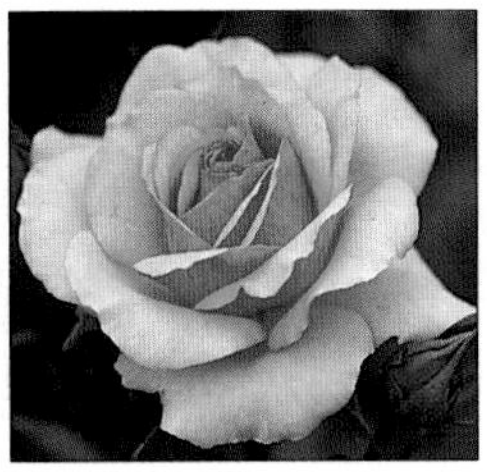
Rosa 'Anne Harkness'

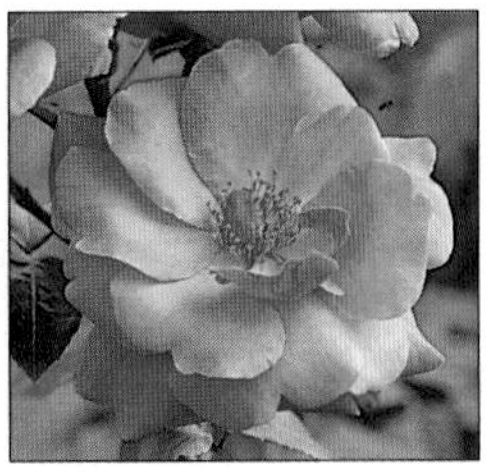
Rosa 'Armada'

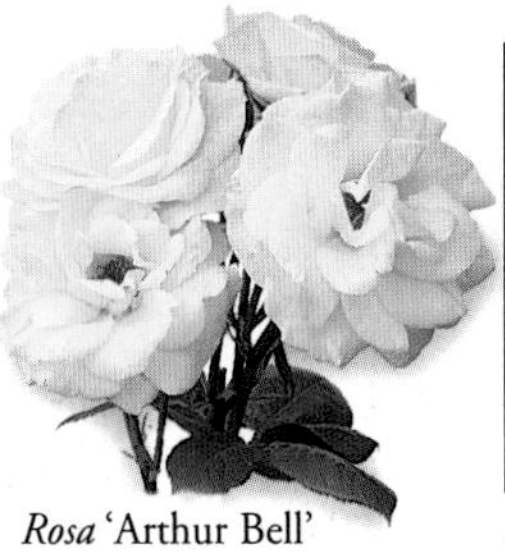
Rosa 'Arthur Bell'

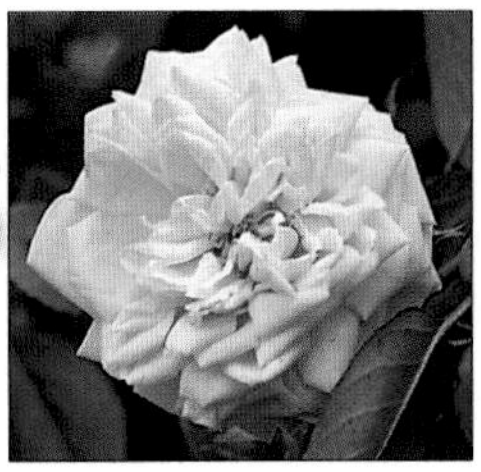
Rosa 'Awakening'

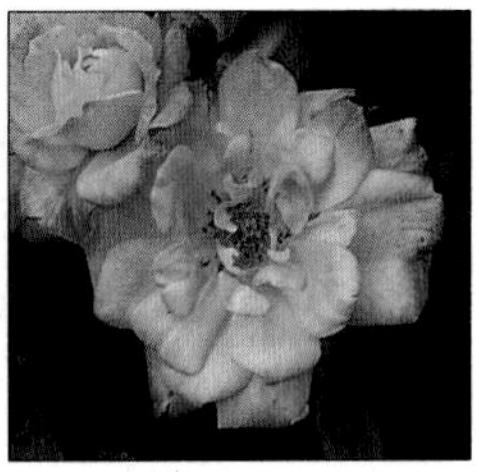
Rosa 'Baby Masquerade'

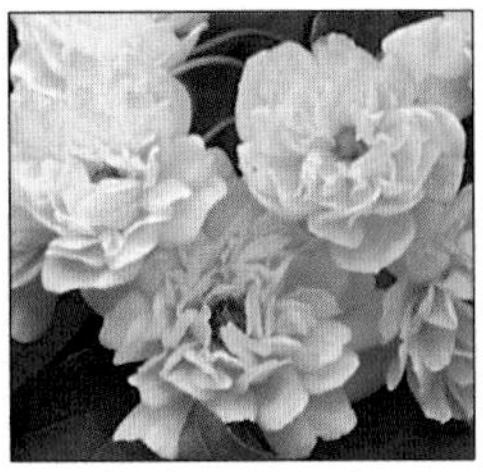
Rosa banksiae 'Lutea'

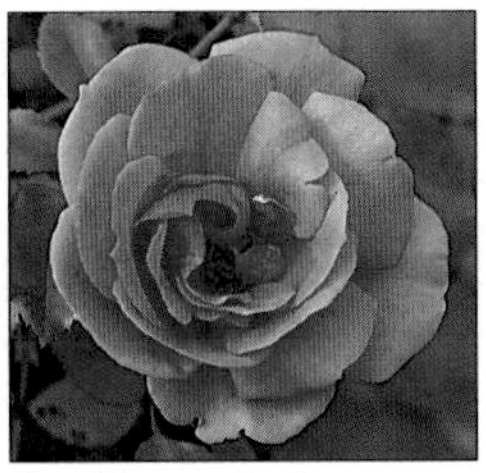
Rosa 'Bantry Bay'

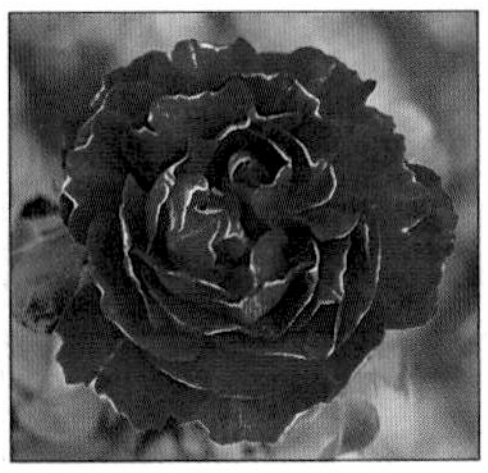
Rosa 'Baron Girod de l'Ain'

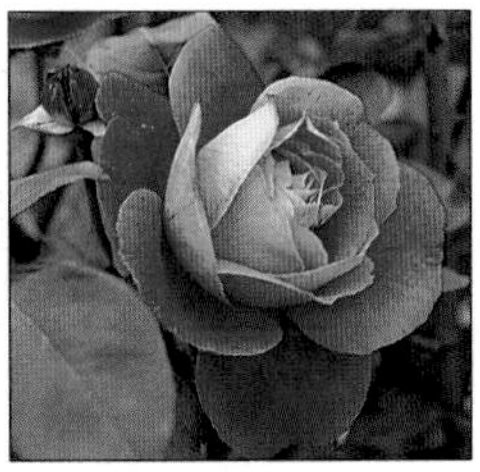
Rosa 'Baronne Edmond de Rothschild'

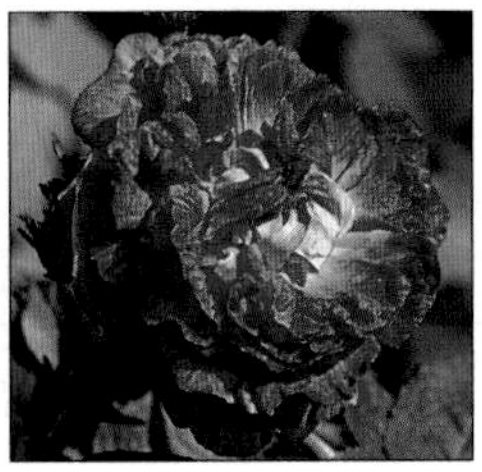
Rosa 'Belle de Crécy'

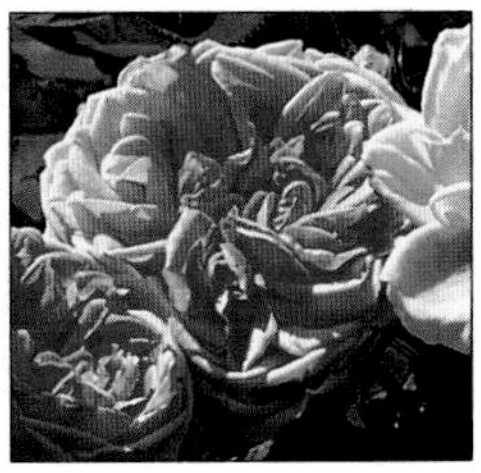
Rosa 'Blairii Number Two'

from summer to autumn. ↕ to 1.5m (5ft), ↔ 75cm (30in). ❄❄❄
***R.* 'Arizona Sunset'.** Miniature bush rose of spreading habit, with mid-green foliage. From summer to autumn, bears cupped, double flowers, 4.5cm (1¾in) across, light yellow, flushed orange-red. ↕↔ 40cm (16in). ❄❄❄
***R.* 'Armada'** ■ syn. *R.* 'Haruseful'. Vigorous, free-branching shrub rose with glossy, dark green leaves. Cupped, semi-double, scented, deep rose-pink flowers, 8cm (3in) across, are borne from summer to autumn. ↕ 1.5m (5ft), ↔ 1.2m (4ft). ❄❄❄
***R.* 'Arthur Bell'** ■🏆 Cluster-flowered bush rose with shiny, bright green leaves. Cupped, double, fragrant, yellow to cream flowers, 8cm (3in) across, are produced from summer to autumn. ↕ 1m (3ft), ↔ 60cm (24in). ❄❄❄
***R.* 'Avon'**, syn. *R.* 'Fairy Lights', *R.* 'Poulmulti', *R.* 'Sunnyside'. Ground-cover rose of compact habit, with dark green leaves. Clusters of flat, semi-double, pale pink to pearl-white flowers, 4.5cm (1¾in) across, are borne along the stems from summer to autumn. ↕ 35cm (14in), ↔ 1m (3ft). ❄❄❄
***R.* 'Awakening'** ■ syn. *R.* 'Probuzini'. Climber with shiny, mid-green leaves. Clusters of cupped, fully double, fragrant, pale pearl-pink flowers, 8cm (3in) across, are borne from summer to autumn. Tolerates a partially shaded site. ↕ 3m (10ft), ↔ 2.5m (8ft). ❄❄❄
***R.* 'Ayrshire Splendens'** see *R.* 'Splendens'.
***R.* 'Baby Carnival'** see *R.* 'Baby Masquerade'.
***R.* 'Baby Love'.** Dwarf cluster-flowered rose of shrubby growth and dense, upright habit. Shallowly cupped, single, bright yellow flowers, 5cm (2in) across, are borne freely close to the mid-green foliage, from summer to autumn. ↕ 1.1m (3½ft), ↔ 75cm (30in). ❄❄❄
***R.* 'Baby Masquerade'** ■ syn. *R.* 'Baby Carnival'. Miniature bush rose of dense, twiggy habit, with dark green leaves and clusters of many rosette-shaped, double, yellow-pink flowers, 2.5cm (1in) across, borne from summer to autumn. ↕↔ 40cm (16in). ❄❄❄
***R.* 'Bad Nauheim'** see *R.* 'National Trust'.
***R.* 'Ballerina'** ■🏆 Polyantha shrub rose of dense, spreading habit, with mid-green leaves. Spectacular in flower, it bears many shallowly cupped, single, white-centred, light pink flowers, 3cm (1¼in) across, in mop-headed clusters, from summer to autumn. ↕ to 1.5m (5ft), ↔ 1.2m (4ft). ❄❄❄
R. banksiae*,** syn. *R. banksiae* var. *alba*, *R. banksiae* 'Alba Plena' (Double white banksian rose). Climbing species rose with long, slender, smooth stems and small, pale green leaves composed of 3–7 oblong-lance-shaped to elliptic-ovate leaflets, 3–6cm (1¼–2½in) long. Clusters of many rosette-shaped, double, violet-scented white flowers, 2.5cm (1in) across, with notched petals, are produced in late spring. Protect from frost for best results. Prune spent wood only. ↕ to 12m (40ft), ↔ to 6m (20ft). W. and C. China. ❄❄. **var. *alba see *R. banksiae*. **'Alba Plena'** see *R. banksiae*. **'Lutea'** ■🏆 syn. var. *lutea* (Yellow banksian rose) bears fully double yellow flowers, 2cm (¾in) across. Requires a sheltered wall; ↕↔ to 6m (20ft). **'Lutescens'**, syn. f. *lutescens*, produces single, strongly scented yellow flowers. **var. *normalis*** (Single white banksian rose) bears single, fragrant white flowers on prickly stems; ↕↔ to 12m (40ft).
***R.* 'Bantry Bay'** ■ Climber of upright, free-branching habit, with dark green leaves. Clusters of cupped, semi-double, lightly scented, deep pink flowers, 9cm (3½in) across, are borne from summer to autumn. ↕ 4m (12ft), ↔ 2.5m (8ft). ❄❄❄
***R.* 'Baron Girod de l'Ain'** ■ Hybrid Perpetual rose of vigorous habit, with moderately prickly stems and leathery, dark green leaves. From summer to autumn, bears cupped, fully double, scented crimson, white-edged flowers, 10cm (4in) across, with wavy-margined petals. ↕ 1.2m (4ft), ↔ 1m (3ft). ❄❄❄
***R.* 'Baronne Edmond de Rothschild'** ■ syn. *R.* 'Meigriso'. Vigorous large-flowered bush rose producing leathery, glossy, mid-green foliage. Rounded, fully double, fragrant, ruby-red flowers, 12cm (5in) across, with a pale pink reverse to the petals, are borne from summer to autumn. ↕ 90cm (36in), ↔ 75cm (30in). ❄❄❄
***R.* 'Baronne Prévost'** 🏆 Erect Hybrid Perpetual rose with prickly stems and dark green leaves. Quartered-rosette, fully double, scented pink flowers, 10cm (4in) across, are borne from summer to autumn. ↕ to 1.5m (5ft), ↔ 1m (3ft). ❄❄❄
***R.* 'Beauty of Glazenwood'** see *R.* x *odorata* 'Pseudindica'.
***R.* 'Belle Amour'.** Alba rose of upright habit, with grey-green foliage. Camellia-like, rounded, semi-double, myrrh-scented, light salmon-pink flowers, 9cm (3½in) across, cupped on opening, are borne in midsummer, followed by spherical red hips. ↕ 2m (6ft), ↔ 1.2m (4ft). ❄❄❄
***R.* 'Belle Courtisane'** see *R.* 'Königin von Dänemark'.
***R.* 'Belle de Crécy'** ■🏆 Gallica rose of lax habit, with bristly stems and greyish green leaves. In summer, bears quartered-rosette, full-petalled, fully double, fragrant, deep pink to purple flowers, 8cm (3in) across, showing green centres as they open. ↕ 1.2m (4ft), ↔ 1m (3ft). ❄❄❄
***R.* 'Belle de Londres'** see *R.* 'Compassion'.
***R.* 'Belle of Portugal'** see *R.* 'Belle Portugaise'.
***R.* 'Belle Portugaise'**, syn. *R.* 'Belle of Portugal'. Very vigorous, climbing Tea rose with glossy, olive green leaves and high-centred, semi-double, fragrant, light salmon-pink flowers, 12cm (5in) across, borne in summer. ↕ to 5m (15ft), ↔ 3m (10ft). ❄❄
***R.* 'Berkeley'** see *R.* 'Tournament of Roses'.
***R.* 'Big Purple'**, syn. *R.* 'Nuit d'Orient', *R.* 'Stebigpu'. Vigorous large-flowered bush rose with dark green leaves. Bears high-centred, fully double, strongly scented, deep beetroot-purple flowers, 12cm (5in) across, from summer to autumn. ↕ 1.1m (3½ft), ↔ 70cm (28in). ❄❄❄
***R.* 'Bizarre Triomphant'** see *R.* 'Charles de Mills'.
***R.* 'Blairii Number Two'** ■🏆 Vigorous, climbing Bourbon rose with mid-green leaves, reddish green when young. In summer, bears clusters of usually 3–5 double, fragrant, light pink flowers, 8cm (3in) across, rounded at

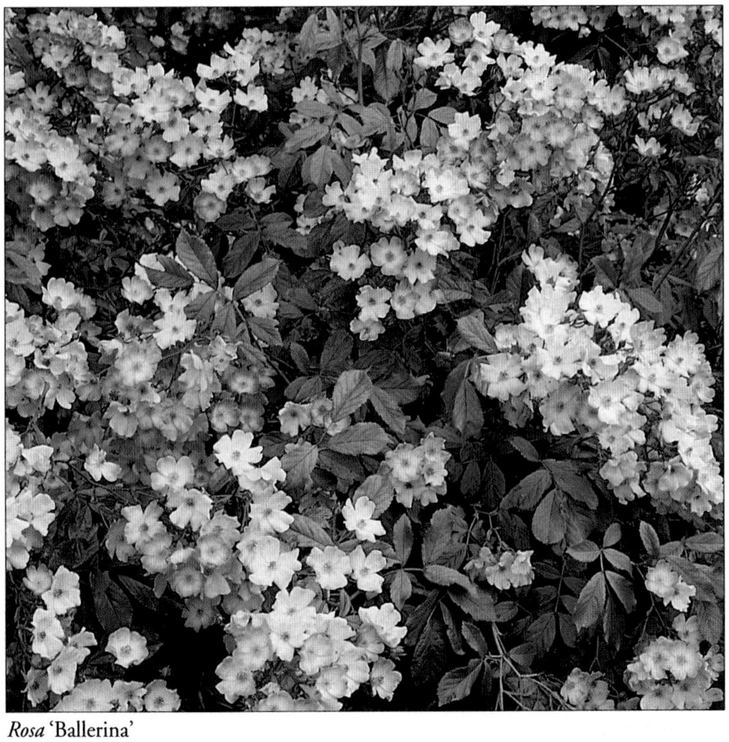
Rosa 'Ballerina'

R

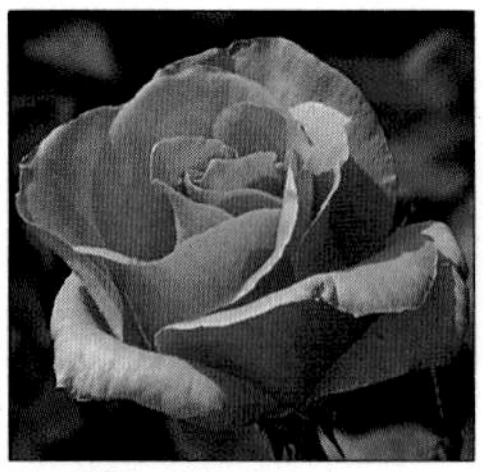
Rosa 'Blessings'

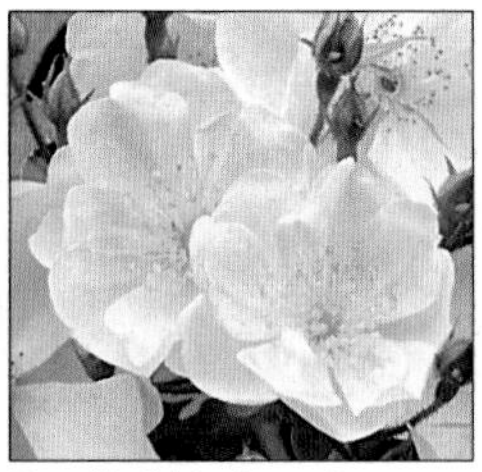
Rosa 'Bobbie James'

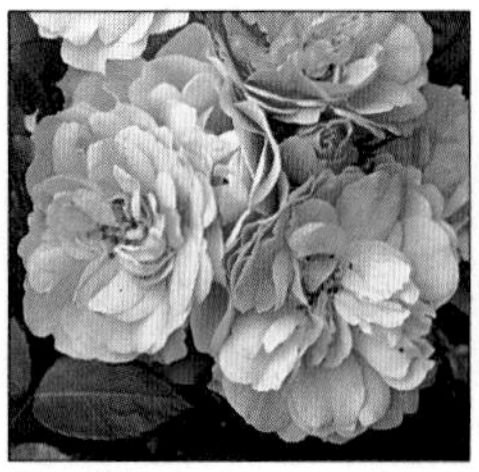
Rosa 'Bonica'

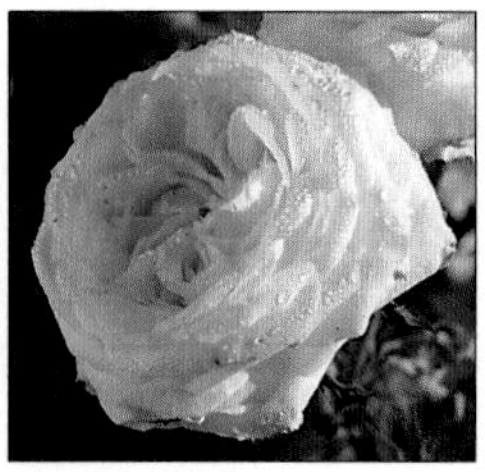
Rosa 'Boule de Neige'

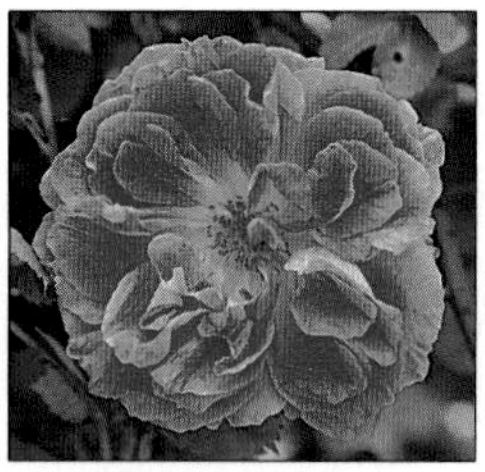
Rosa 'Bourbon Queen'

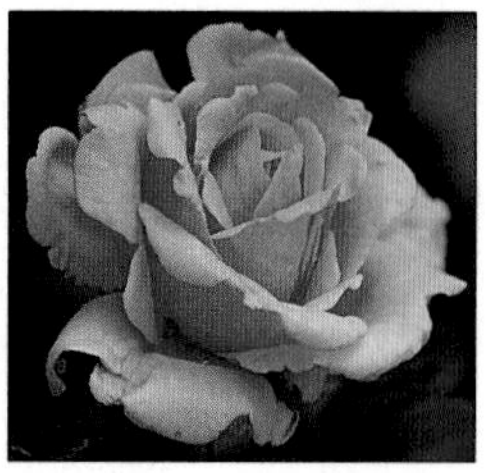
Rosa 'Breath of Life'

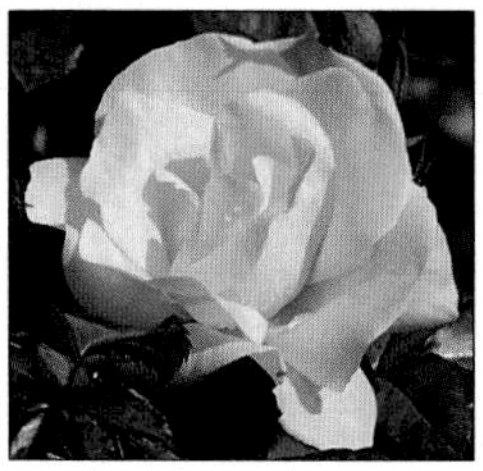
Rosa 'Bright Smile'

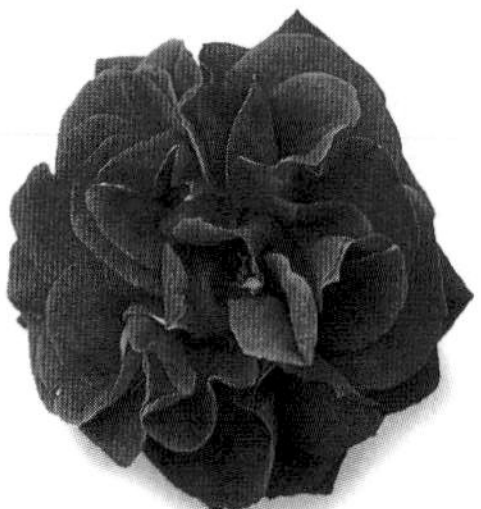
Rosa 'Brown Velvet'

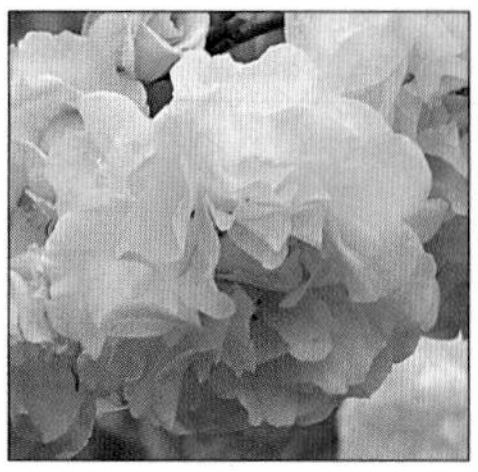
Rosa 'Buff Beauty'

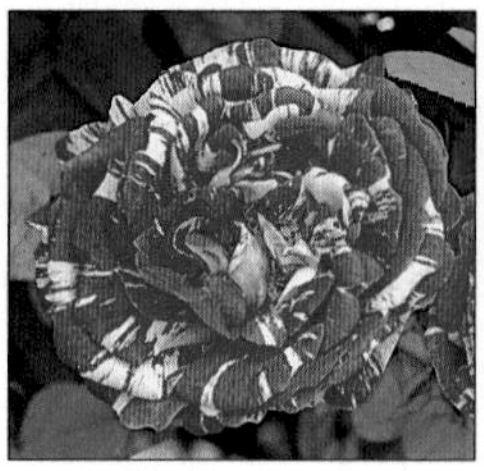
Rosa 'Camaïeux'

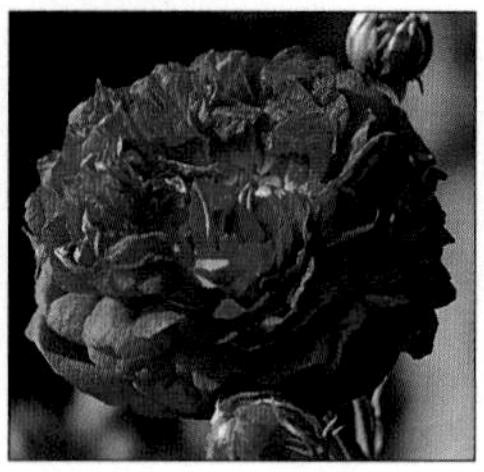
Rosa 'Cardinal de Richelieu'

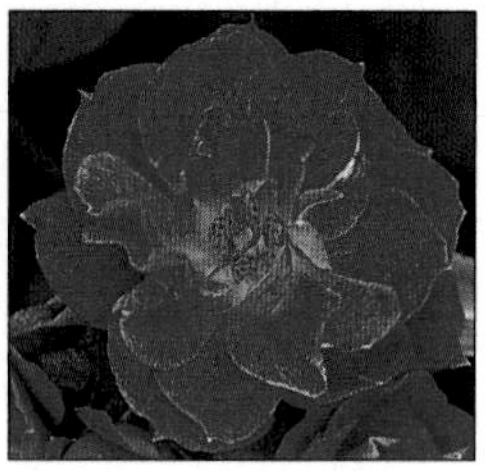
Rosa 'Cardinal Hume'

first, opening flat. Prone to mildew. ↕ to 4m (12ft), ↔ 2m (6ft). ❄❄❄

***R.* 'Blanc Double de Coubert'** 🏆 Rugosa rose of dense, spreading habit, with leathery, mid-green foliage. From summer to autumn, bears loose-petalled, cupped to flat, semi-double, fragrant white flowers, 8cm (3in) across, with yellow stamens, followed in some years by spherical red hips. ↕ 1.5m (5ft), ↔ 1.2m (4ft). ❄❄❄

***R.* 'Blanche Moreau'.** Moss rose of lax growth, with dark green leaves. In summer, bears cupped, fully double, fragrant white flowers, 10cm (4in) across, with brownish green mossing on the stems and calyces. ↕ 1.5m (5ft), ↔ 1.2m (4ft). ❄❄❄

***R.* 'Blaze'.** Branching climber with mid-green leaves and clusters of cupped, semi-double red flowers, 6cm (2½in) across, borne freely from summer to autumn. ↕↔ 2.5m (8ft). ❄❄❄

***R.* 'Blessings'** ■ 🏆 Vigorous large-flowered bush rose with dark green leaves. Bears urn-shaped, fully double, scented, salmon-pink flowers, 10cm (4in) across, from summer to autumn. ↕ 1.1m (3½ft), ↔ 75cm (30in). ❄❄❄

***R.* 'Blue Moon'**, syn. *R.* 'Mainzer Fastnacht', *R.* 'Sissi'. Branching large-flowered bush rose with dark green leaves. Bears high-centred, fully double, fragrant, lilac-mauve flowers, 10cm (4in) across, from summer to autumn. ↕ 1m (3ft), ↔ 70cm (28in). ❄❄❄

***R.* 'Blue Rambler'** see *R.* 'Veilchenblau'.

***R.* 'Blush Noisette'** see *R.* 'Noisette Carnée'.

***R.* 'Blush Rambler'.** Vigorous rambler with long, arching stems and masses of shiny, mid-green leaves. Large, dense clusters of cupped, semi-double, light pink flowers, 4cm (1½in) across, are borne in late summer. ↕ 4m (12ft), ↔ 5m (15ft). ❄❄❄

***R.* 'Bobbie James'** ■ 🏆 Rampant rambler producing glossy leaves, reddish green when young, maturing mid-green. Large clusters of cupped, semi-double, scented, creamy white flowers, 5cm (2in) across, are produced in summer. ↕ to 10m (30ft), ↔ 6m (20ft). ❄❄❄

***R.* 'Bonica'** ■ 🏆 syn. *R.* 'Bonica '82', *R.* 'Meidonomac'. Vigorous shrub rose of low, spreading habit, with dense, glossy, rich green foliage. Large sprays of cupped, fully double, rose-pink flowers, 7cm (3in) across, are borne from summer to autumn. ↕ 85cm (34in), ↔ 1.1m (3½ft). ❄❄❄

***R.* 'Bonica '82'** see *R.* 'Bonica'.

***R.* 'Boule de Neige'** ■ Bourbon rose of vigorous, uneven growth, with glossy, dark green leaves. From summer to autumn, bears cupped to rosette-shaped, fully double, fragrant, pink-touched white flowers, 8cm (3in) across. ↕ 1.5m (5ft), ↔ 1.2m (4ft). ❄❄❄

***R.* 'Bouquet de la Mariée'** see *R.* 'Aimée Vibert'.

***R.* 'Bourbon Queen'** ■ syn. *R.* 'Souvenir de la Princesse de Lamballe'. Vigorous Bourbon rose with long, leafy stems and mid-green foliage. Clusters of numerous cupped, double, scented, magenta to rose-pink flowers, 8cm (3in) across, are borne mainly in summer. ↕ to 2.5m (8ft), ↔ 1.5m (5ft). ❄❄❄

R. bracteata (Chickasaw rose, Macartney rose). Fast-growing, semi-evergreen species rose producing prickly, brownish green stems and glossy, dark green leaves, each with 5–11 obovate to elliptic leaflets, 2–5cm (¾–2in) long. From summer to autumn, bears cupped to flat, single, lightly scented white flowers, 9cm (3½in) across, with gold stamens and curling petals, followed by spherical orange hips. ↕↔ to 6m (20ft). S.E. China, Taiwan. ❄❄

***R.* 'Brandy'.** Large-flowered bush rose producing dark green leaves. Bears high-centred, double, lightly scented apricot flowers, 10cm (4in) across, from summer to autumn. ↕ 1.1m (3½ft), ↔ 75cm (30in). ❄❄

***R.* 'Brass Ring'** see *R.* 'Peek A Boo'.

***R.* 'Breath of Life'** ■ syn. *R.* 'Harquanne'. Upright climber with mid-green leaves and rounded, fully double, scented, apricot to apricot-pink flowers, 10cm (4in) across, borne from summer to autumn. ↕ 2.5m (8ft), ↔ 2.2m (7ft). ❄❄❄

***R.* 'Brigadoon'** syn. *R.* 'Jacpal'. Large-flowered bush rose with dark green leaves. From summer to autumn, bears high-centred, double, lightly scented, strawberry-red flowers, 12cm (5in) across, margined pale pink. ↕ 1m (3ft), ↔ 70cm (28in). ❄❄❄

***R.* 'Bright Smile'** ■ syn. *R.* 'Dicdance'. Low-growing cluster-flowered bush rose with glossy, bright green leaves. Well-spaced clusters of flat, semi-double, scented yellow flowers, 8cm (3in) across, are borne freely from summer to autumn. ↕↔ 45cm (18in). ❄❄❄

***R.* 'Brite Lites'** see *R.* 'Princess Alice'.

***R.* 'Broadway'**, syn. *R.* 'Burway'. Large-flowered bush rose with glossy, dark green foliage. From summer to autumn, bears high-centred, fully double, spice-scented, orange-yellow flowers, 10cm (4in) across, the outer petals flushed with pink. ↕ 1m (3ft), ↔ 60cm (24in). ❄❄❄

***R.* 'Brown Velvet'** ■ syn. *R.* 'Colorbreak', *R.* 'Maccultra'. Cluster-flowered bush rose with glossy, dark green leaves. Bears fully double, brownish orange flowers, 8cm (3in) across, quartered-rosette on opening, from summer to autumn. ↕ 1m (3ft), ↔ 60cm (24in). ❄❄❄

***R.* 'Buffalo Bill'** see *R.* 'Regensberg'.

***R.* 'Buff Beauty'** ■ 🏆 Shrub rose of rounded habit, with dense, dark green leaves. Freely bears large clusters of cupped, fully double, lightly fragrant flowers, 9cm (3½in) across, apricot fading to buff, in summer, a few later. ↕↔ 1.2m (4ft). ❄❄❄

***R.* 'Burgund '81'** see *R.* 'Loving Memory'.

***R.* 'Burning Sky'** see *R.* 'Paradise'.

R. californica. Shrubby species rose with bristly shoots and dull, mid-green leaves, each composed of 5–7 ovate to broadly elliptic leaflets, 1–3cm (½–1¼in) long. Clusters of flat, single, scented, lilac-pink flowers, 4cm (1½in) across, are borne freely in summer, a few later in autumn, before the spherical, orange-red hips. ↕ 1.5–2.5m (5–8ft), ↔ 1.2–2m (4–6ft). USA (S. Oregon to S. California), N.W. Mexico. ❄❄❄.

'Plena' see *R. nutkana* 'Plena'.

***R.* 'Camaïeux'** ■ Gallica rose of dense habit, with mid-green foliage. Cupped, fully double, scented, light pink flowers, 9cm (3½in) across, striped with crimson-purple to lilac-grey, are borne in summer. ↕↔ 80cm (32in). ❄❄❄

***R.* 'Camelot'.** Vigorous, tall cluster-flowered bush rose with leathery, dark green leaves. From summer to autumn, bears cupped, fully double, spice-scented, coral pink flowers, 9cm (3½in) across. ↕ 1.5m (5ft), ↔ 1m (3ft). ❄❄❄

***R.* 'Canary Bird'** see *R. xanthina* 'Canary Bird'.

***R.* 'Capitaine John Ingram'** 🏆 Vigorous, bushy Moss rose with dark green leaves and clusters of peony-like, pompon-shaped, fully double, fragrant, dark crimson to purple flowers, 8cm (3in) across, with a lilac-pink reverse to the petals, borne in summer. ↕ 1.2m (4ft), ↔ 1m (3ft). ❄❄❄

***R.* 'Cardinal de Richelieu'** ■ 🏆 Gallica rose of vigorous, compact, lax habit, with smooth stems and dense, dark green foliage. Rounded, fully double, fragrant, deep burgundy-purple flowers, 8cm (3in) across, are borne in summer. ↕ 1m (3ft), ↔ 1.2m (4ft). ❄❄❄

***R.* 'Cardinal Hume'** ■ syn. *R.* 'Harregale'. Vigorous shrub rose of spreading habit, with dense, dark green leaves. Bears dense clusters of cupped, double, lightly scented, reddish purple flowers, 8cm (3in) across, from summer to autumn. ↕ 80cm (32in), ↔ 1.1m (3½ft). ❄❄❄

***R.* 'Carefree Wonder'**, syn. *R.* 'Meipitac'. Free-branching, leafy shrub rose of rounded, bushy habit, with mid-green leaves. From summer to autumn, freely bears clusters of cupped, double pink flowers, 9cm (3½in) across, with a pale pink reverse to the petals. ↕ 75cm (30in), ↔ 60cm (24in). ❄❄❄

***R.* 'Caribia'** see *R.* 'Harry Wheatcroft'.

***R.* 'Carl Philip'** see *R.* 'The Times'.

***R.* 'Casino'** ■ syn. *R.* 'Gerbe d'Or', *R.* 'Macca'. Climber with sparse, dark green leaves and rounded, fully double, fragrant yellow flowers, 9cm (3½in) across, sometimes opening quartered-rosette, borne from summer to autumn. ↕ 3m (10ft), ↔ 2.2m (7ft). ❄❄❄

***R.* 'Catherine Mermet'.** Vigorous, shrubby Tea rose with shiny, mid-green leaves and high-centred, fully double, scented, beige-pink flowers, 10cm (4in) across, with a mauve tinge, borne from summer to autumn. ↕ 1.2m (4ft), ↔ 1.1m (3½ft). ❄❄

***R.* 'Cécile Brunner'** ■ 🏆 syn. *R.* 'Mignon', *R.* 'Sweetheart Rose'. China rose of upright growth, with sparse, dark green leaves. Perfectly formed, urn-shaped, fully double, light pink flowers, 4cm (1½in) across, are borne from summer to autumn. ↕ 75cm (30in), ↔ 60cm (24in). ❄❄❄

***R.* 'Céleste'** ■ 🏆 syn. *R.* 'Celestial'. Vigorous, spreading Alba rose with greyish green foliage. Clusters of cupped, double, fragrant, light pink flowers, 8cm (3in) across, are produced in midsummer. ↕ 1.5m (5ft), ↔ 1.2m (4ft). ❄❄❄

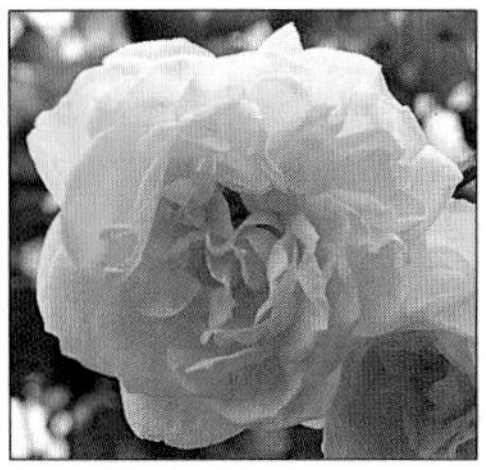
Rosa 'Casino'

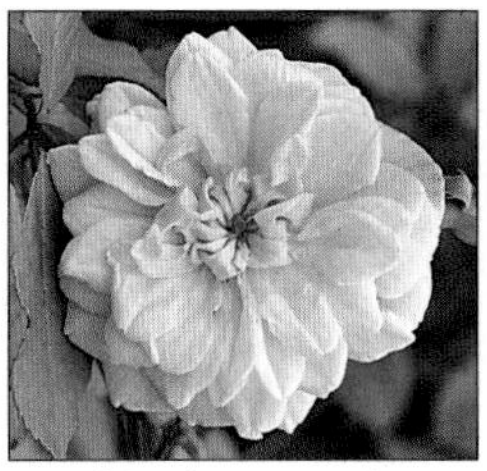
Rosa 'Cécile Brunner'

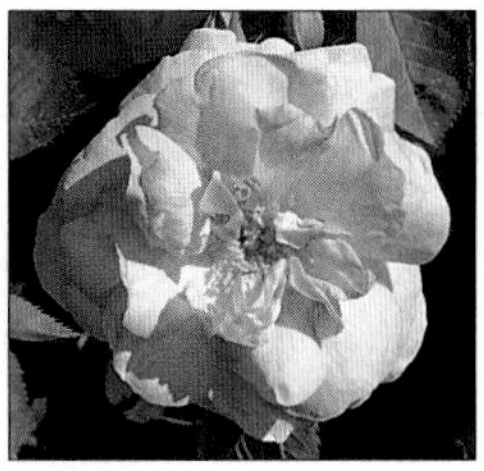
Rosa 'Céleste'

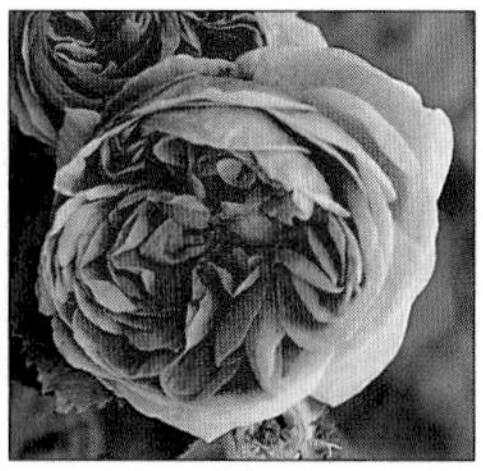
Rosa x *centifolia* 'Muscosa'

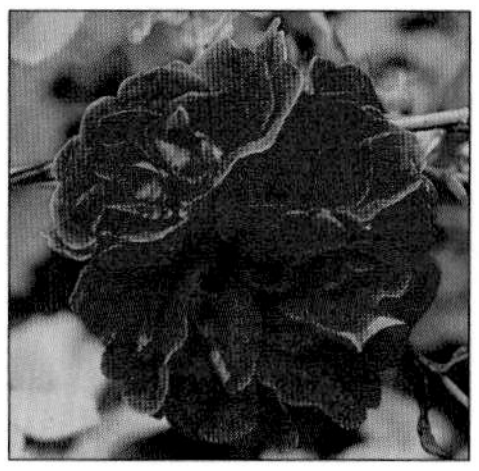
Rosa 'Cerise Bouquet'

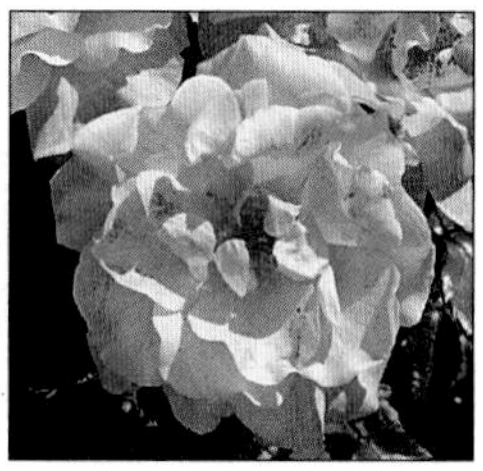
Rosa 'Champagne Cocktail'

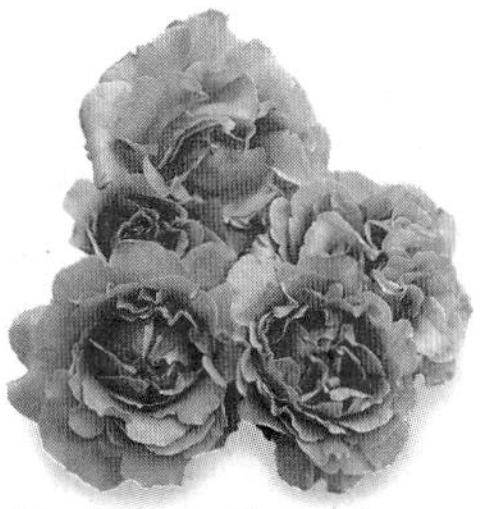
Rosa 'Cherry Brandy'

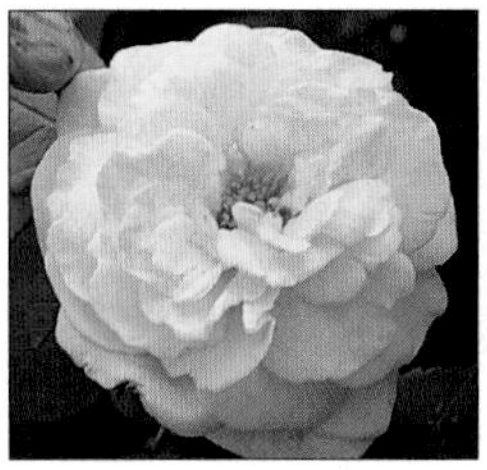
Rosa 'Chinatown'

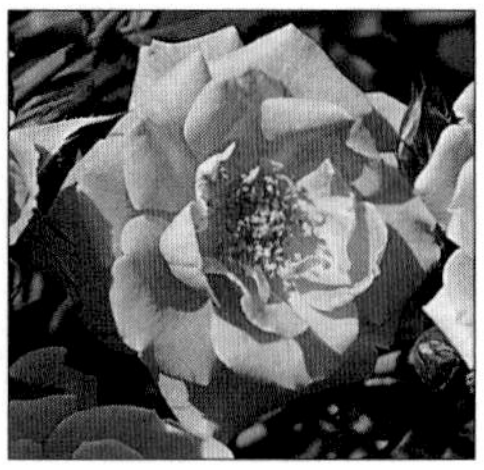
Rosa 'Cider Cup'

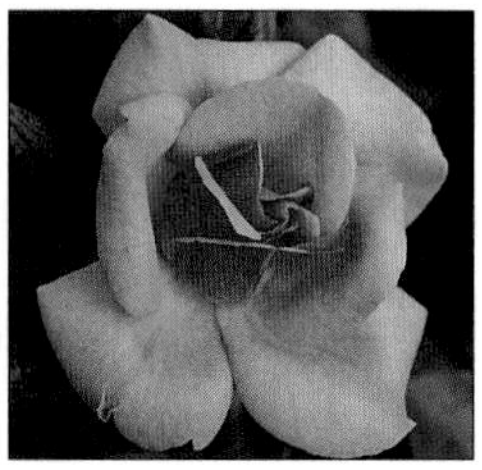
Rosa 'City Girl'

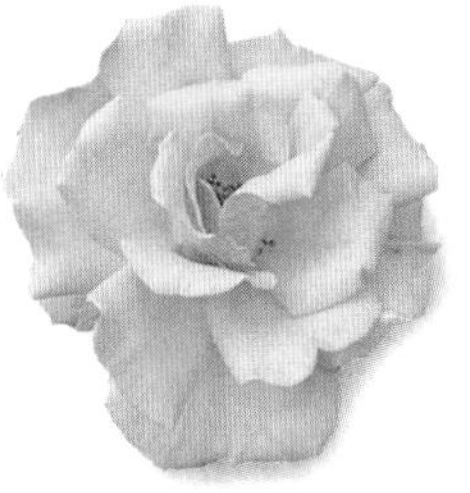
Rosa 'City of London'

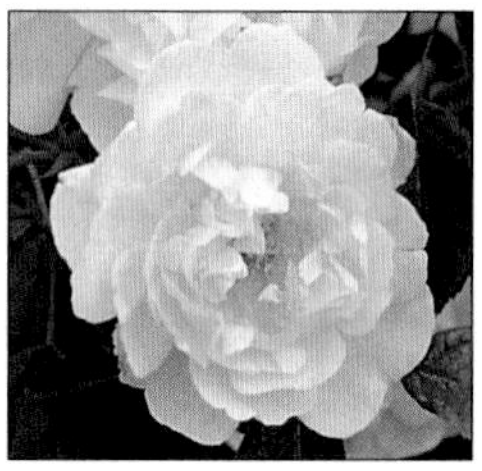
Rosa 'City of York'

***R.* 'Celestial'** see *R.* 'Céleste'.
R.* x *centifolia. Vigorous Centifolia rose of branching habit, with arching, dull, mid-green leaves comprising 5–7 broadly ovate leaflets, to 5cm (2in) long. In summer, bears cupped, fully double, very fragrant, deep rose-pink, sometimes red or white flowers, 9cm (3½in) across. ↕1.5m (5ft), ↔ 1.2m (4ft). Garden origin. ❄❄❄. **'Cristata'** 🏆 syn. *R.* 'Chapeau de Napoléon', *R.* 'Cristata' (Crested moss rose) has a lax, branching habit, and double, rose-pink flowers on bowing stems. It has no true moss, but mossy tufts on the calyces. Best grown on a support. **'Muscosa'** ▣🏆 (Common moss rose) is a vigorous, branching Moss rose with dull, dark green leaves, and dense moss on the stems and calyces. Rounded to cupped pink flowers are 8cm (3in) across. **var. *pomponia*** see *R.* 'De Meaux'.
***R.* 'Cerise Bouquet'** ▣🏆 Very vigorous shrub rose of arching habit, producing small, greyish green leaves. In summer, bears a spectacular display of flat, semi-double, cherry-red flowers, 6cm (2½in) across. ↕↔ to 3.5m (11ft). ❄❄❄
***R.* 'C.F. Meyer'** see *R.* 'Conrad Ferdinand Meyer'.
***R.* 'Champagne Cocktail'** ▣ syn. *R.* 'Horflash'. Cluster-flowered bush rose with dark green leaves. From summer to autumn, bears open clusters of cupped, double, scented, light yellow flowers, 9cm (3½in) across, with pink markings. ↕1m (3ft), ↔ 70cm (28in). ❄❄❄
***R.* 'Champneys' Pink Cluster'.** Vigorous Noisette climbing rose with arching, smooth stems and shiny, light green leaves. From summer to autumn, bears large clusters of cupped, double, fragrant pink flowers, 5cm (2in) across. ↕2.5–4m (8–12ft), ↔ 2.5m (8ft). ❄❄
***R.* 'Chapeau de Napoléon'** see *R.* x *centifolia* 'Cristata'.
***R.* 'Charles de Mills'** ▣🏆 syn. *R.* 'Bizarre Triomphant'. Upright, arching Gallica rose with smooth stems and mid-green foliage. In summer, pink buds open to quartered-rosette, fully double, fragrant, magenta-pink flowers, 10cm (4in) across. ↕↔ 1.2m (4ft) or more. ❄❄❄
***R.* 'Cheerio'** see *R.* 'Playboy'.
***R.* 'Cherish'**, syn. *R.* 'Jacsal'. Cluster-flowered bush rose of compact habit, with dark green leaves. High-centred, double, light pink flowers, 8cm (3in) across, the petals with white bases inside, open from summer to autumn. ↕70cm (28in), ↔ 60cm (24in). ❄❄❄
***R.* 'Cherry Brandy'** ▣ syn. *R.* 'Arocad', *R.* 'Tanryrandy'. Fast-growing, large-flowered bush rose of uneven habit, with dense, glossy, bright green leaves. High-centred to cupped, double orange flowers, 9cm (3½in) across, suffused salmon-pink, are borne singly and in open clusters from summer to autumn. ↕75cm (30in), ↔ 60cm (24in). ❄❄❄
***R.* 'Child's Play'**, syn. *R.* 'Savachild'. Miniature bush rose of upright habit, with dark green leaves. Produces high-centred, double, bicoloured, pink and white flowers, 4cm (1½in) across, from summer to autumn. ↕35cm (14in), ↔ 25cm (10in). ❄❄❄
***R.* 'China Doll'.** Miniature bush rose with leathery, mid-green leaves and cupped, double, china-pink flowers, 4cm (1½in) across, borne from summer to autumn. ↕↔ 45cm (18in). ❄❄❄
***R.* 'Chinatown'** ▣🏆 syn. *R.* 'Ville de Chine'. Vigorous cluster-flowered bush rose with strong, uneven growth and abundant, glossy, dark green leaves. From summer to autumn, produces rounded, double, scented yellow flowers, 10cm (4in) across, flushed pink. ↕1.2m (4ft), ↔ 1m (3ft). ❄❄❄
R. chinensis* var. *minima see *R.* 'Rouletii'.
***R. chinensis* 'Mutabilis'** see *R.* x *odorata* 'Mutabilis'.
***R. chinensis* 'Semperflorens'** see *R.* x *odorata* 'Semperflorens'.
***R. chinensis* 'Viridiflora'** see *R.* x *odorata* 'Viridiflora'.
***R.* 'Christian IV'** see *R.* 'The Times'.
***R.* 'Chrysler Imperial'.** Neat large-flowered bush rose producing dark green leaves. From summer to autumn, bears high-centred, fully double, very fragrant, deep red flowers, 12cm (5in) across. Prefers a sheltered site. ↕1m (3ft), ↔ 60cm (24in). ❄❄❄
***R.* 'Cider Cup'** ▣ syn. *R.* 'Dicladida'. Dwarf cluster-flowered bush rose of neat habit, with dense, glossy, mid-green foliage. From summer to autumn, bears well-spaced clusters of high-centred, double, deep apricot-pink flowers, 4cm (1½in) across. ↕45cm (18in), ↔ 30cm (12in). ❄❄❄
***R.* 'City Girl'** ▣ syn. *R.* 'Harzorba'. Free-branching climber producing glossy, dark green leaves. From summer to autumn, bears clusters of cupped, semi-double, scented, salmon-pink flowers, 11cm (4½in) across. ↕↔ 2.2m (7ft). ❄❄❄
***R.* 'City of Belfast'**, syn. *R.* 'Macci'. Cluster-flowered bush rose of compact habit, with glossy, dark green foliage and cupped, double scarlet flowers, 6cm (2½in) across, borne from summer to autumn. ↕↔ 60cm (24in). ❄❄❄
***R.* 'City of Leeds'.** Vigorous cluster-flowered bush rose producing dark green foliage. Freely bears cupped to flat, semi-double, salmon-pink flowers, 9cm (3½in) across, from summer to autumn. ↕75cm (30in), ↔ 60cm (24in). ❄❄❄
***R.* 'City of London'** ▣🏆 syn. *R.* 'Harukfore'. Cluster-flowered bush rose or climbing rose of spreading, uneven habit, with glossy mid-green leaves. Loosely formed, rounded to flat, semi-double to double, fragrant, light pink flowers, 8cm (3in) across, are produced from summer to autumn. ↕80cm (32in), ↔ 75cm (30in). ❄❄❄
***R.* 'City of York'** ▣ syn. *R.* 'Direktor Benschop'. Climber with glossy, bright green foliage. Clusters of cupped, semi-double, scented, creamy white flowers, 6cm (2½in) across, are borne in early summer. ↕to 4m (12ft), ↔ 3m (10ft). ❄❄❄
***R.* 'Clarissa'**, syn. *R.* 'Harprocrustes'. Cluster-flowered bush rose producing

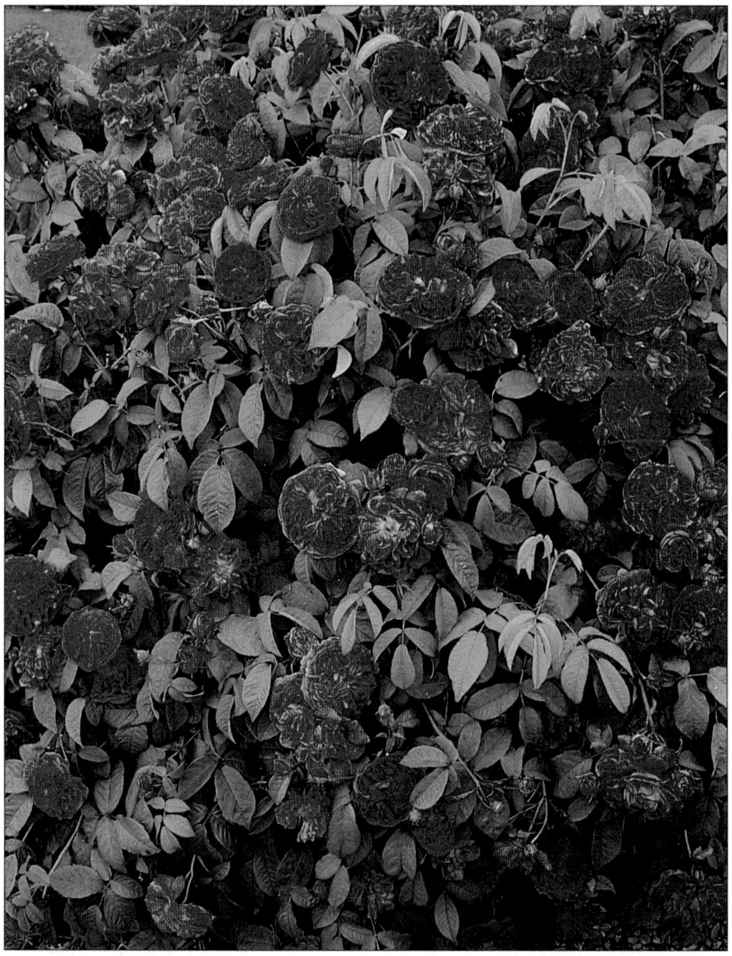
Rosa 'Charles de Mills'

R

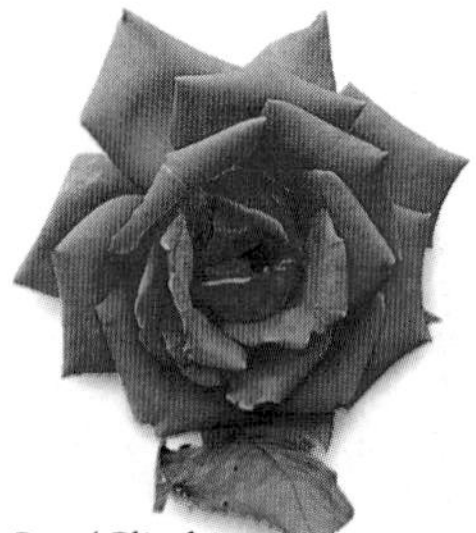
Rosa 'Climbing Mrs. Sam McGredy'

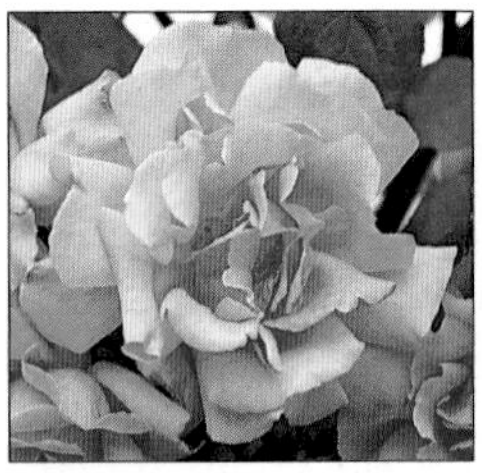
Rosa 'Compassion'

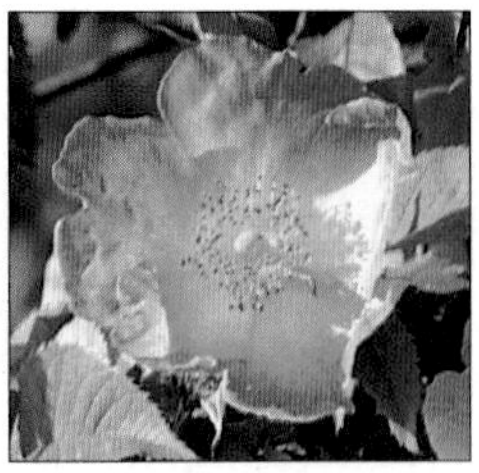
Rosa 'Complicata'

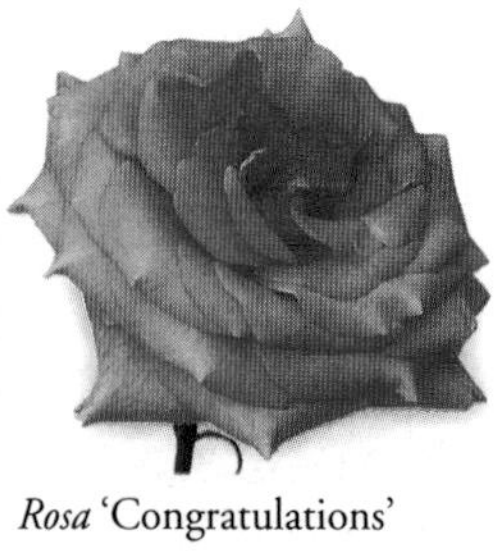
Rosa 'Congratulations'

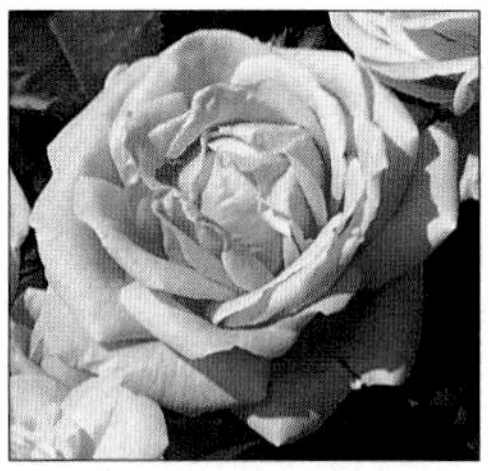
Rosa 'Conrad Ferdinand Meyer'

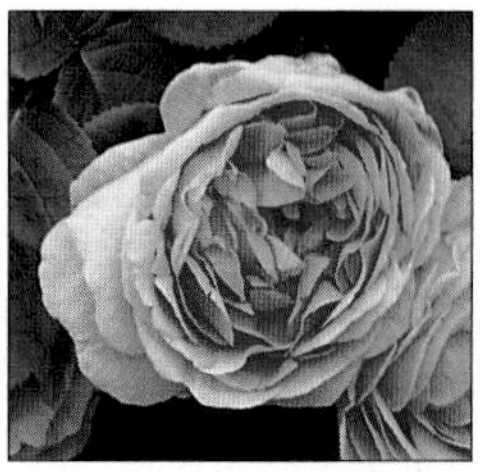
Rosa 'Constance Spry'

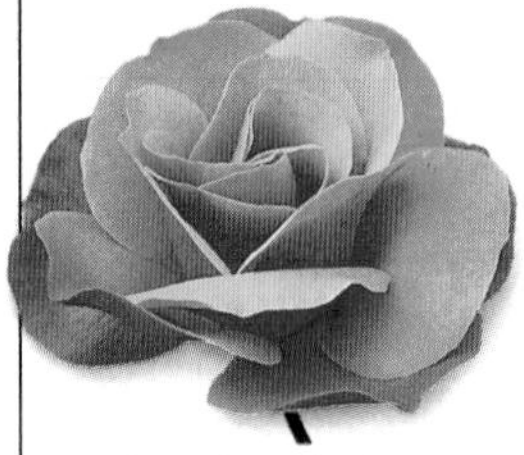
Rosa 'Cordon Bleu'

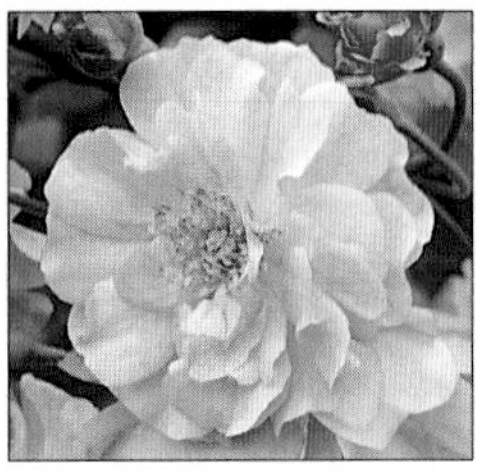
Rosa 'Cornelia'

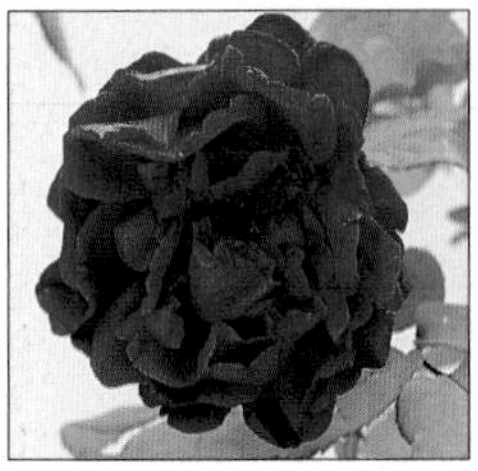
Rosa 'Crimson Glory'

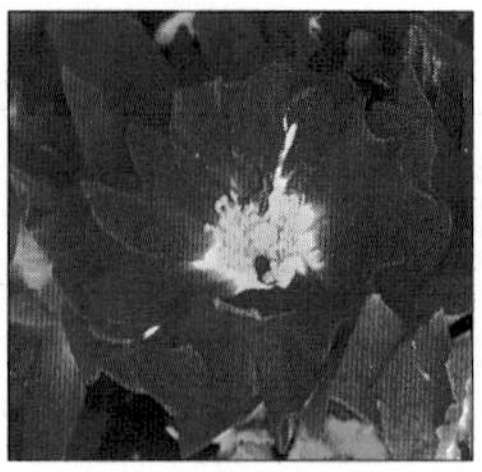
Rosa 'Crimson Shower'

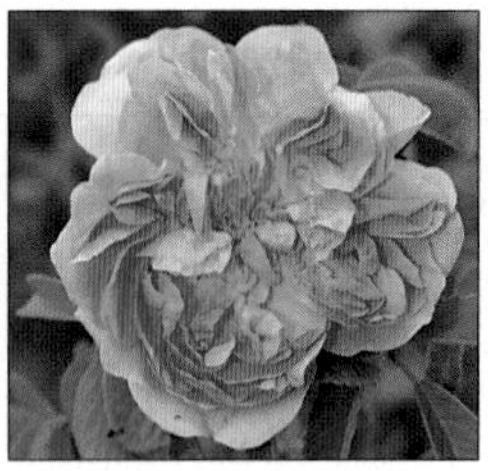
Rosa x *damascena* var. *semperflorens*

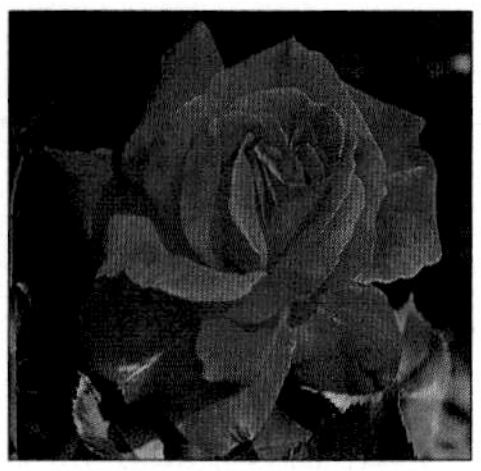
Rosa 'Danse du Feu'

many small, glossy, dark green leaves. Abundant urn-shaped, fully double apricot flowers, 5cm (2in) across, are borne on long stems from summer to autumn. ↕ 80cm (32in), ↔ 45cm (18in). ❄❄❄

***R.* 'Class Act'**, syn. *R.* 'First Class', *R.* 'Jacare', *R.* 'White Magic'. Cluster-flowered bush rose producing dark green leaves and loosely formed, flat, semi-double white flowers, 8cm (3in) across, from summer to autumn. ↕ 1m (3ft), ↔ 75cm (30in). ❄❄❄

***R.* 'Climbing Cécile Brunner'** 🏆 Vigorous climber with strong growth and sparse, dark green leaves composed of lance-shaped leaflets. From summer to autumn, bears exquisitely formed, urn-shaped, double, light pink flowers, 4cm (1½in) across. ↕↔ 4m (12ft). ❄❄❄

***R.* 'Climbing Crimson Glory'.** Climber of branching habit, with fairly sparse, mildew-prone, dark green leaves and prickly stems. Cupped, fully double, intensely fragrant, dark crimson flowers, 11cm (4½in) across, are borne on bowing stems from summer to autumn. ↕ to 5m (15ft), ↔ 2.5m (8ft). ❄❄❄

***R.* 'Climbing Ena Harkness'.** Climber of branching habit, with mid-green foliage and high-centred, fully double, fragrant, bright crimson flowers, 12cm (5in) across, borne from summer to autumn. ↕ 5m (15ft), ↔ 2.5m (8ft). ❄❄❄

***R.* 'Climbing Etoile de Hollande'** 🏆 Climber with rampant, open growth, dark green foliage, and cupped, double, very fragrant, dark crimson flowers, 11cm (4½in) across, borne mainly in summer. ↕ to 6m (20ft), ↔ 5m (15ft). ❄❄❄

***R.* 'Climbing Iceberg'** ▣ 🏆 Climber with strong, well-branched growth and dense, light green foliage. Showy clusters of numerous cupped, double white flowers, 8cm (3in) across, are borne freely from summer to autumn. ↕↔ 3m (10ft). ❄❄❄

***R.* 'Climbing Lady Hillingdon'** 🏆 Climbing Tea rose with stiff, vigorous growth, purplish green wood, and glossy, dark green foliage. From summer to autumn, high-centred to cupped, semi-double to double, fragrant, light apricot-yellow flowers, 9cm (3½in) across, are borne on nodding stems. ↕ to 5m (15ft), ↔ 2.5m (8ft). ❄❄❄

***R.* 'Climbing Little White Pet'** see *R.* 'Félicité Perpétue'.

***R.* 'Climbing Mrs. Sam McGredy'** ▣ 🏆 Vigorous climber with a stiff, branching habit and sparse dark green foliage. Urn-shaped, fully double, copper-red to salmon-pink flowers, 11cm (4½in) across, are borne mainly in summer. ↕↔ 3m (10ft). ❄❄❄

***R.* 'Climbing Orange Meillandina'** see *R.* 'Climbing Orange Sunblaze'.

***R.* 'Climbing Orange Sunblaze'**, syn. *R.* 'Climbing Orange Meillandina', *R.* 'Meijikatarsar'. Miniature climber with upright, branching growth and many dark green leaves. Cupped, fully double, bright orange-red flowers, 4cm (1½in) across, are borne from summer to autumn. ↕ 1.5m (5ft), ↔ 1.2m (4ft). ❄❄❄

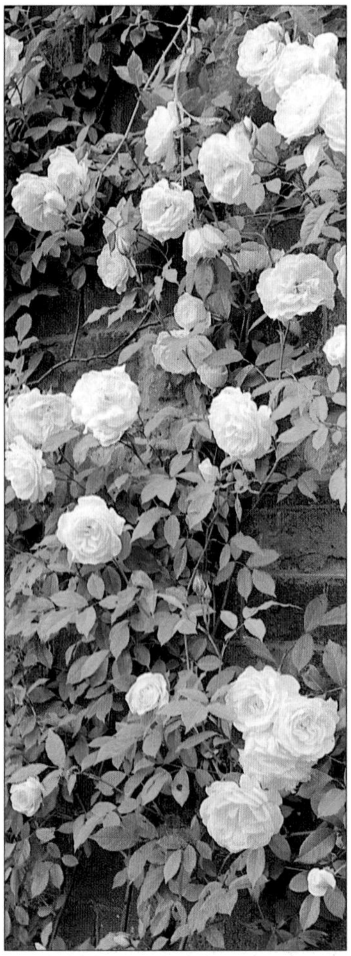
Rosa 'Climbing Iceberg'

***R.* 'Climbing Pompon de Paris'.** Vigorous, miniature China climbing rose with spreading, arching growth and abundant matt, mid-green foliage. Many-flowered clusters of cupped, fully double, rose-red flowers, 2.5cm (1in) across, are borne in early summer. ↕ to 4m (12ft), ↔ 2.5m (8ft). ❄❄❄

***R.* 'Climbing Shot Silk'** 🏆 Branching climber with shiny, deep green foliage. Urn-shaped to cupped, double, sweet-scented flowers, 10cm (4in) across, salmon-pink suffused yellow, are borne mainly in summer. ↕ 3m (10ft), ↔ 2.5m (8ft). ❄❄❄

***R.* 'Colorbreak'** see *R.* 'Brown Velvet'.

***R.* 'Color Magic'.** Large-flowered bush rose of branching habit, producing dark green leaves. Cupped, wide-opening, double flowers, 12cm (5in) across, ivory becoming deep pink, are borne freely from summer to autumn. ↕ 1.1m (3½ft), ↔ 75cm (30in). ❄❄

***R.* 'Commandant Beaurepaire'**, syn. *R.* 'Panachée d'Angers'. Vigorous, bushy, spreading Bourbon rose with wavy, pale green leaves. From summer to autumn, bears cupped, double, fragrant pink flowers, 10cm (4in) across, with purple and white stripes. ↕↔ 1.2m (4ft). ❄❄❄

***R.* 'Compassion'** ▣ 🏆 syn. *R.* 'Belle de Londres'. Climber with upright, free-branching growth and dark green leaves. Rounded, fully double, fragrant flowers, 10cm (4in) across, salmon-pink suffused apricot, are borne from summer to autumn. ↕ 3m (10ft), ↔ 2.5m (8ft). ❄❄❄

***R.* 'Complicata'** ▣ 🏆 Very vigorous Gallica rose with strong, arching, open growth and greyish green leaves. In summer, bears clusters of cupped to flat, single pink flowers, 11cm (4½in) across, with paler centres and folded petals. ↕ 2.2m (7ft), ↔ 2.5m (8ft). ❄❄❄

***R.* 'Comte de Chambord'** see *R.* 'Mme Knorr'.

***R.* 'Comtesse de Labarthe'** see *R.* 'Duchesse de Brabant'.

***R.* 'Comtesse Ouwaroff'** see *R.* 'Duchesse de Brabant'.

***R.* 'Congratulations'** ▣ syn. *R.* 'Korlift', *R.* 'Sylvia'. Tall, vigorous large-flowered bush rose with dark green leaves. Neatly formed, urn-shaped, fully double, rose-pink flowers, 11cm (4½in) across, are borne on long stems from summer to autumn. ↕ 1.5m (5ft), ↔ 1m (3ft). ❄❄❄

***R.* 'Conrad Ferdinand Meyer'** ▣ syn. *R.* 'C.F. Meyer'. Strong, vigorous shrub rose with prickly, arching stems and coarse, greyish green leaves. Bears cupped, fully double, fragrant, silvery pink flowers, 10cm (4in) across, mainly in summer, a few in autumn. Prone to rust. ↕ 2.5m (8ft), ↔ 2m (6ft). ❄❄❄

***R.* 'Conservation'** ▣ syn. *R.* 'Cocdimple'. Vigorous, dwarf cluster-flowered bush rose with glossy, mid-green leaves. From summer to autumn, freely bears dense clusters of cupped, semi-double, apricot-pink flowers, 6cm (2½in) across. ↕↔ 45cm (18in). ❄❄❄

***R.* 'Constance Spry'** ▣ 🏆 Shrub rose of arching habit, which will climb if supported, with dense, greyish green leaves. Rounded, fully double, myrrh-scented pink flowers, 12cm (5in) across, are borne on nodding stems in summer. ↕ 2m (6ft), ↔ 1.5m (5ft) as a shrub; ↕↔ 3m (10ft) as a climber. ❄❄❄

***R.* 'Cordon Bleu'** ▣ *R.* 'Harubasil'. Large-flowered bush rose with dark green foliage and cupped, double, scented, reddish apricot flowers, 10cm (4in) across, borne from summer to autumn. ↕ 1m (3ft), ↔ 60cm (24in). ❄❄❄

***R.* 'Cornelia'** ▣ 🏆 Vigorous shrub rose of arching, spreading habit, producing dense, dark green leaves with lance-shaped leaflets. From summer to autumn, bears large clusters of many rosette-shaped, double, pink-tinged flowers, 5cm (2in) across, copper at the centres. ↕↔ 1.5m (5ft). ❄❄❄

***R.* 'Crimson Glory'** ▣ Large-flowered bush rose of branching habit, with sparse, mildew-prone, dark green leaves and prickly stems. Cupped, fully double, intensely fragrant, dark crimson flowers, 11cm (4½in) across, are borne on bowing stems from summer to autumn. ↕↔ 60cm (24in). ❄❄❄

***R.* 'Crimson Shower'** ▣ 🏆 Rambler with lax stems and many glossy, bright green leaves. Dense clusters of rosette-shaped, double crimson flowers, 3cm (1¼in) across, are produced from late summer to autumn. ↕ to 2.5m (8ft), ↔ 2.2m (7ft). ❄❄❄

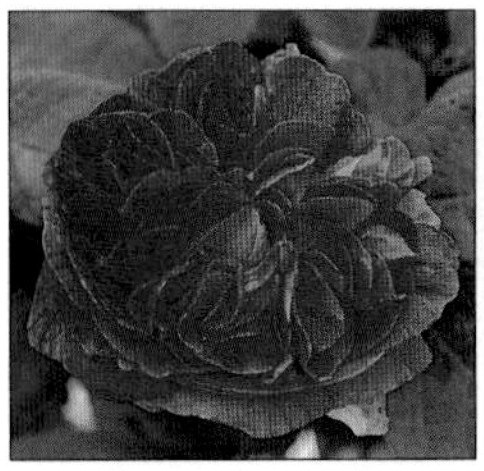
Rosa 'De la Maître d'Ecole'

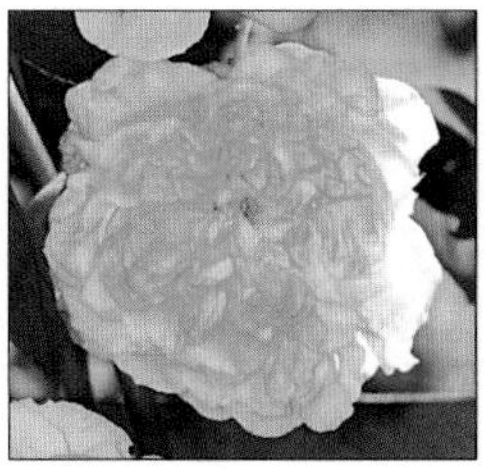
Rosa 'Desprez à Fleur Jaune'

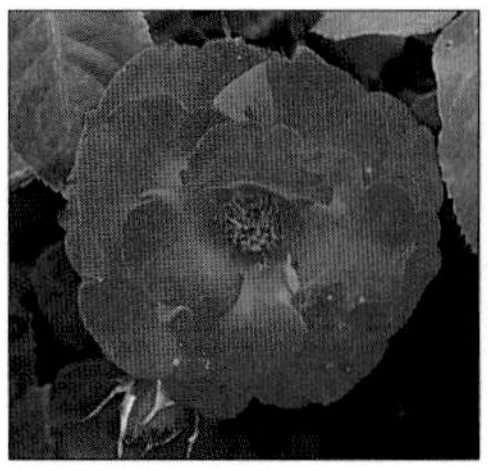
Rosa 'Disco Dancer'

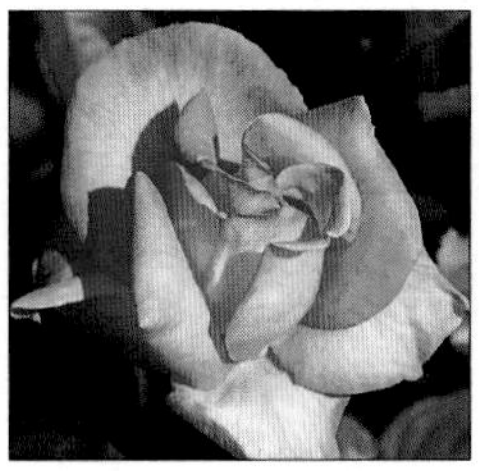
Rosa 'Doris Tysterman'

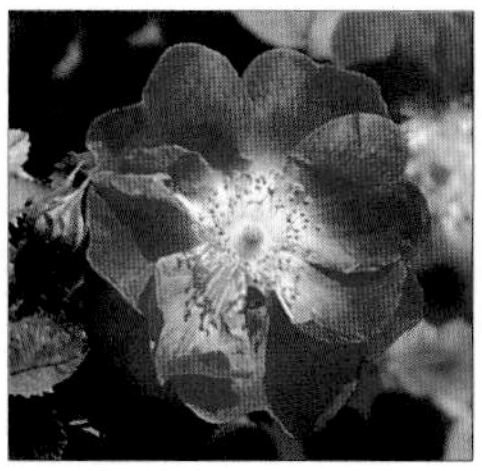
Rosa 'Dortmund'

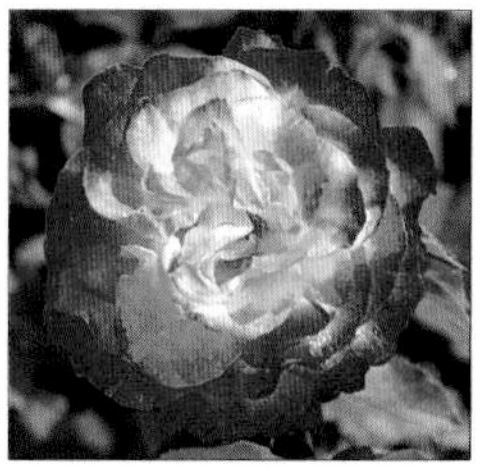
Rosa 'Double Delight'

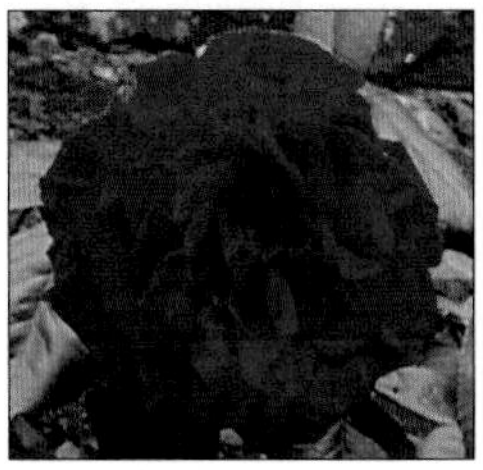
Rosa 'Dublin Bay'

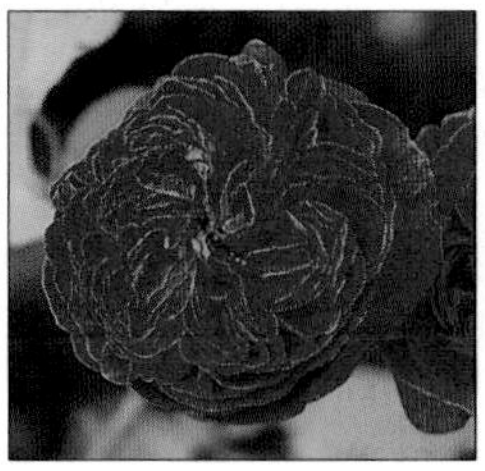
Rosa 'Duc de Guiche'

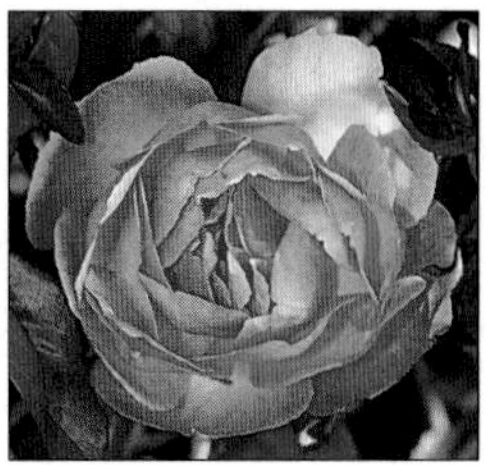
Rosa 'Duchesse de Brabant'

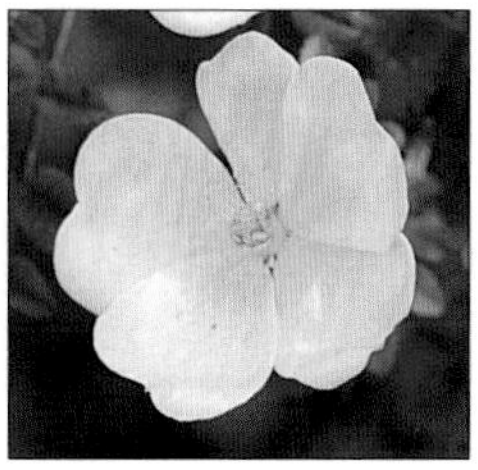
Rosa 'Dunwich Rose'

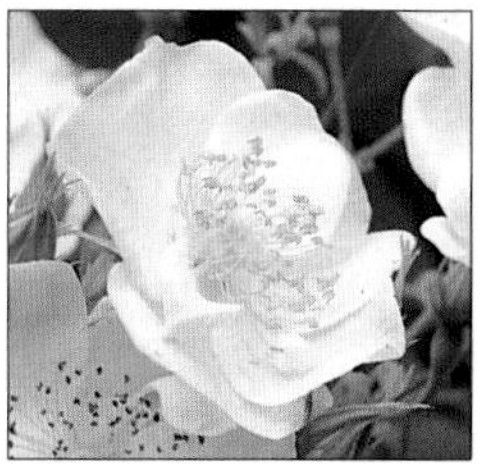
Rosa 'Dupontii'

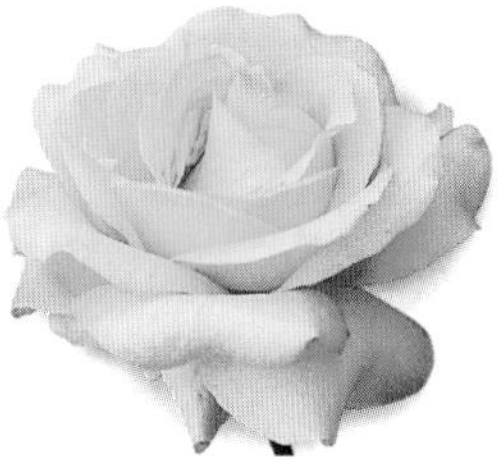
Rosa 'Dutch Gold'

***R.* 'Cristata'** see *R.* x *centifolia* 'Cristata'.
***R.* 'Cuisse de Nymphe'** see *R.* 'Great Maiden's Blush'.
***R.* 'Cupcake'**, syn. *R.* 'Spicup'. Vigorous miniature bush rose of compact, bushy habit, with glossy, mid-green leaves. High-centred, fully double, mid-pink flowers, 4cm (1½in) across, are borne from summer to autumn. ↕35cm (14in), ↔ 30cm (12in). ***
***R.* 'Dainty Bess'.** Branching large-flowered bush rose with leathery, dark green leaves. Flat, single, scented, pale pink flowers, 9cm (3½in) across, with maroon stamens, are borne from summer to autumn. ↕1m (3ft), ↔ 60cm (24in). ***
R.* x *damascena (Damask rose). Vigorous Damask rose with arching, prickly stems and dull, greyish green leaves, each composed of 5, rarely 7, ovate to elliptic leaflets, to 6cm (2½in) long. In summer, bears clusters of 3–11 cupped to flat, semi-double, fragrant, pale pink to white flowers, 8cm (3in) across. Middle East. ↕2m (6ft), ↔ 1.5m (5ft). ***. **var. *bifera*** see var. *semperflorens*. **var. *semperflorens*** ■ syn. var. *bifera*, *R.* 'Quatre Saisons' (Autumn damask rose, Four seasons rose, Rose of Castille) has an open, arching habit and light green leaves. Loosely formed, rose-pink flowers, 9cm (3½in) across, are produced in lax clusters, mainly in summer and sporadically in autumn. Best in a sunny position; ↕1.5m (5ft), ↔ 1.2m (4ft). **'Versicolor'** (York and Lancaster rose) has a twiggy, untidy habit, and bears loosely cupped, double, pink-tinged white flowers, 6cm (2½in) across; ↕1.5m (5ft), ↔ 1.2cm (4ft).

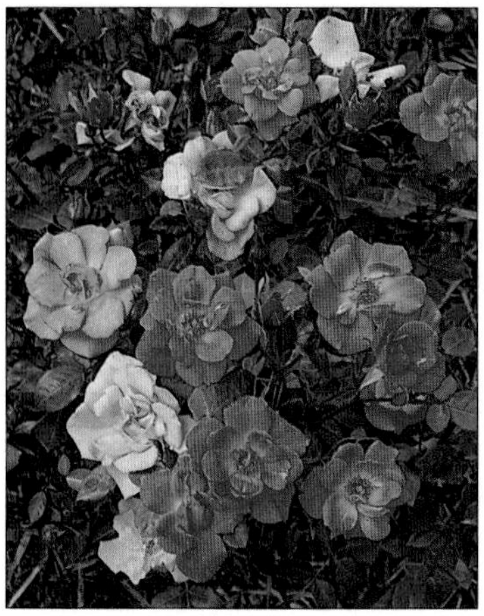
Rosa 'Conservation'

***R.* 'Danse du Feu'** ■ syn. *R.* 'Spectacular'. Stiffly branched climber bearing abundant glossy, mid-green leaves. Rounded, double scarlet flowers, 8cm (3in) across, are produced from summer to autumn. ↕↔ 2.5m (8ft). ***
***R.* 'Darling Flame'**, syn. *R.* 'Meilucca', *R.* 'Minuetto'. Bushy, well-branched miniature bush rose producing glossy, dark green leaves. Urn-shaped, double, orange-red flowers, 4cm (1½in) across, are borne freely from summer to autumn. ↕40cm (16in), ↔ 30cm (12in). ***
***R.* 'Dearest'.** Cluster-flowered bush rose of neat, spreading habit, with dark green leaves. Large clusters of camellia-like, rounded, double, fragrant, light rose-pink flowers, 8cm (3in) across, are borne from summer to autumn. ↕↔ 60cm (24in). ***
***R.* 'Deep Secret'**, syn. *R.* 'Mildred Scheel'. Vigorous large-flowered bush rose with glossy, dark green foliage. Rounded, fully double, scented, deep crimson flowers, 10cm (4in) across, are borne from summer to autumn. ↕1m (3ft), ↔ 75cm (30in). ***
***R.* 'De la Maître d'Ecole'** ■ 🏆 Gallica rose of bushy, spreading habit, with mid-green foliage. Quartered-rosette, fully double, fragrant, carmine-red to light pink flowers, 10cm (4in) across, are borne on bowed stems in summer. ↕1m (3ft), ↔ 1.1m (3½ft). ***
***R.* 'De Meaux'**, syn. *R.* x *centifolia* var. *pomponia*, *R.* 'Rose de Meaux' (Pompon rose). Dwarf Centifolia rose of upright habit, with bright green leaves. Clusters of pompon, fully double, scented, rose-pink flowers, 4cm (1½in) across, are borne in summer. ↕1m (3ft), ↔ 75cm (30in). ***
***R.* 'Desprez à Fleur Jaune'** ■ 🏆 syn. *R.* 'Jaune Desprez'. Vigorous Noisette climbing rose with arching growth and light green leaves. Flat, fully double, scented, pale creamy apricot flowers, 8cm (3in) across, are borne mainly in summer. ↕↔ 5m (15ft). **
***R.* 'Dicky'** see *R.* 'Anisley Dickson'.
***R.* 'Direktor Benschop'** see *R.* 'City of York'.
***R.* 'Disco Dancer'** ■ syn. *R.* 'Dicinfra'. Free-branching, vigorous cluster-flowered bush rose with dense, glossy, mid-green foliage. Showy, cupped, double, bright orange-scarlet flowers, 6cm (2½in) across, are produced from summer to autumn. ↕75cm (30in), ↔ 60cm (24in). ***
***R.* 'Dolly Parton'.** Large-flowered bush rose with dark green foliage and high-centred, fully double, fragrant, vivid orange-red flowers, 11cm (4½in) across, borne from summer to autumn. ↕1.2m (4ft), ↔ 60cm (24in). **
***R.* 'Donatella'** see *R.* 'Granada'.
***R.* 'Doris Tysterman'** ■ Tall large-flowered bush rose producing glossy, dark green foliage. High-centred, double, orange-red flowers, 10cm (4in) across, are borne from summer to autumn. ↕1.2m (4ft), ↔ 75cm (30in). ***
***R.* 'Dorothy Perkins'.** Lax rambler with many glossy, dark green leaves. Bears dense clusters of rosette-shaped, double, rose-pink flowers, 2cm (¾in) across, in late summer. ↕↔ to 3m (10ft). ***
***R.* 'Dortmund'** ■ Upright climber with dense, glossy, dark green leaves. Showy clusters of flat, single red flowers, 10cm (4in) across, each with a white eye, are borne freely from summer to autumn. ↕3m (10ft), ↔ 2m (6ft). ***
***R.* 'Double Delight'** ■ syn. *R.* 'Andeli'. Large-flowered bush rose of uneven, branching habit, with dull, mid-green foliage. From summer to autumn, bears rounded, fully double, sweet-scented flowers, 12cm (5in) across, pale pink, margined and flushed carmine-red. The flowers spoil in rain. ↕1m (3ft), ↔ 60cm (24in). ***
***R.* 'Drummer Boy'**, syn. *R.* 'Harvacity'. Spreading, dwarf cluster-flowered bush rose producing mid-green foliage. Dense sprays of cupped, double, bright crimson flowers, 5cm (2in) across, are borne freely from summer to autumn. ↕↔ 50cm (20in). ***
***R.* 'Dublin Bay'** ■ 🏆 Free-branching climber, which may be pruned to form a shrub. Bears glossy, dark green leaves and clusters of cupped, double, bright crimson flowers, 10cm (4in) across, from summer to autumn. ↕↔ 2.2m (7ft). ***
***R.* 'Duc de Guiche'** ■ 🏆 Gallica rose of spreading habit, with dark green leaves. Fully double, crimson-purple flowers, 10cm (4in) across, opening flat and quartered-rosetted, are produced in summer. ↕↔ 1.2m (4ft). ***
***R.* 'Duchesse de Brabant'** ■ syn. *R.* 'Comtesse de Labarthe', *R.* 'Comtesse Ouwaroff'. Tea rose of spreading, shrubby habit, with mid- to dark green leaves. Cupped, silky-petalled, double, scented, rose-pink flowers, 11cm (4½in) across, are borne from summer to autumn. ↕1.2m (4ft) or more, ↔ 1m (3ft). **
***R.* 'Duchesse d'Istrie'** see *R.* 'William Lobb'.
***R.* 'Duchess of Portland'** see *R.* 'Portlandica'.
***R.* 'Duet'.** Vigorous large-flowered bush rose producing leathery, mid-green leaves. High-centred, double flowers, 10cm (4in) across, in two shades of pink, are borne freely from summer to autumn. Good for cut flowers. ↕1.2m (4ft), ↔ 60cm (24in). ***
***R.* 'Duftzauber '84'** see *R.* 'Royal William'.
***R.* 'Dunwich Rose'** ■ syn *R.* *pimpinellifolia* 'Dunwichensis'. Vigorous, twiggy Scots rose with a low, hummock-forming habit and dark green leaves. In early summer, bears a profusion of short-stemmed, cupped to flat, single, scented, creamy white flowers, 6cm (2½in) across, with prominent gold stamens. ↕65cm (26in), ↔ 1.2m (4ft). ***
***R.* 'Dupontii'** ■ syn. *R.* *moschata* var. *nivea* (Snowbush rose). Shrub rose of upright, shrubby habit, with grey-green foliage. Cupped to flat, single, fragrant, creamy white flowers, 6cm (2½in) across, showing yellow anthers, are borne freely in midsummer. ↕↔ 2.2m (7ft). ***
***R.* 'Dutch Gold'** ■ Vigorous large-flowered bush rose producing large, dark green leaves. Rounded, fully double, scented yellow flowers, 15cm (6in) across, are borne from summer to autumn. ↕1.1m (3½ft), ↔ 75cm (30in). ***
***R.* 'Easlea's Golden Rambler'.** Rambler with leathery, dark green leaves and loosely formed, rounded, fully double, scented flowers, 10cm (4in) across, bright yellow flecked with red, borne in summer. ↕to 6m (20ft), ↔ 5m (15ft). ***

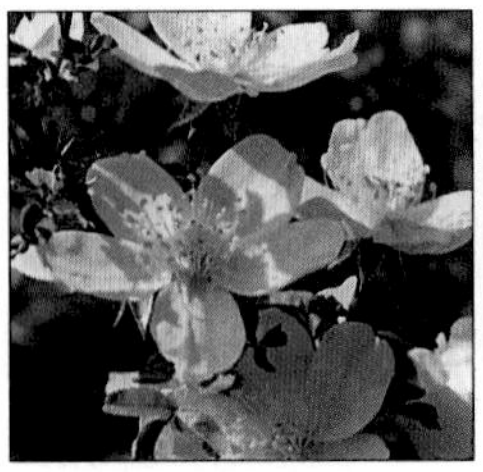
Rosa ecae

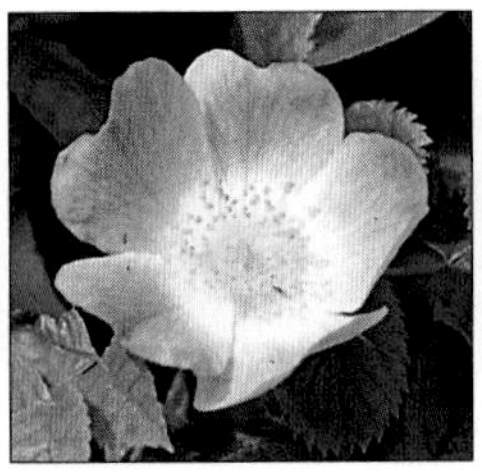
Rosa eglanteria

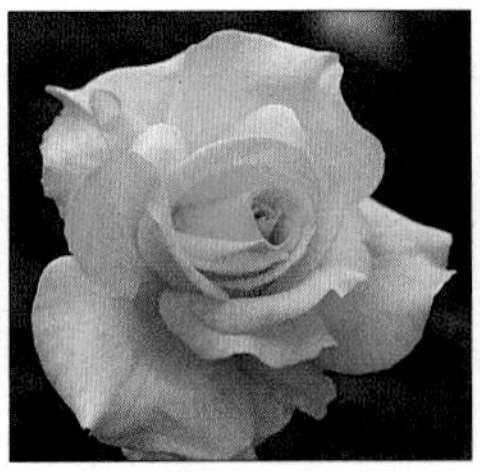
Rosa 'Elina'

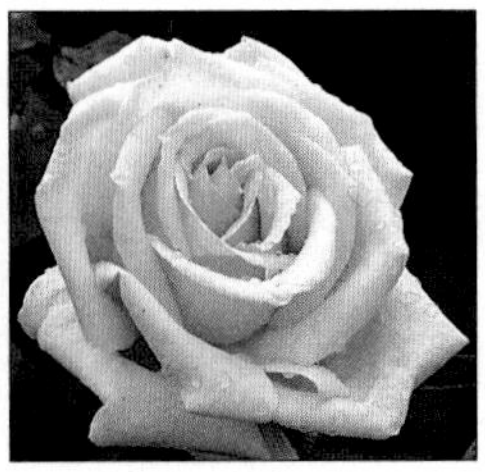
Rosa 'Elizabeth Harkness'

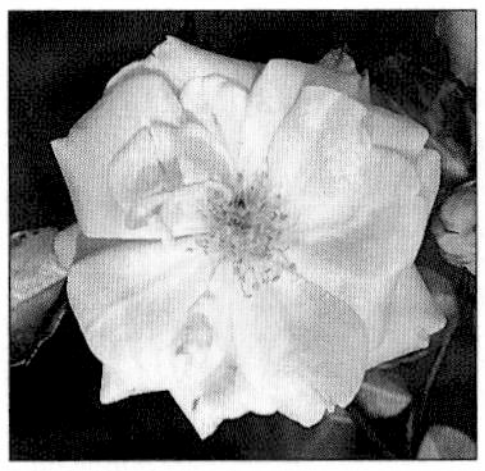
Rosa 'Emily Gray'

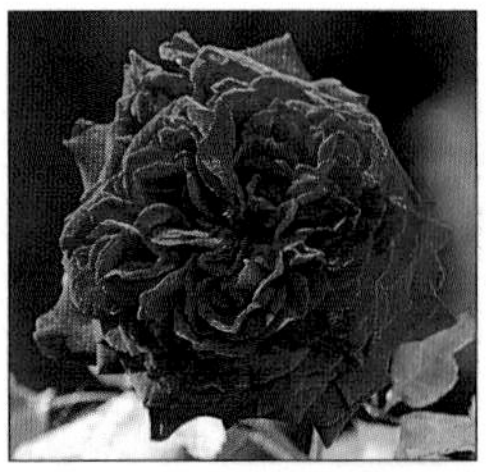
Rosa 'Empereur du Maroc'

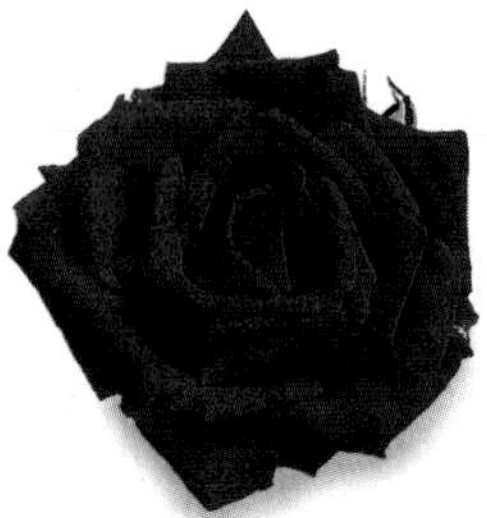
Rosa 'Ena Harkness'

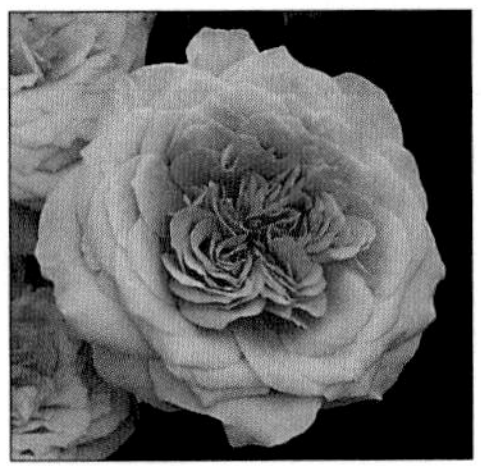
Rosa 'English Garden'

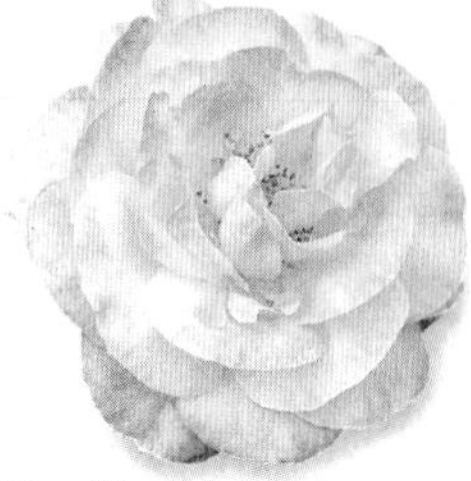
Rosa 'English Miss'

Rosa 'Ernest H. Morse'

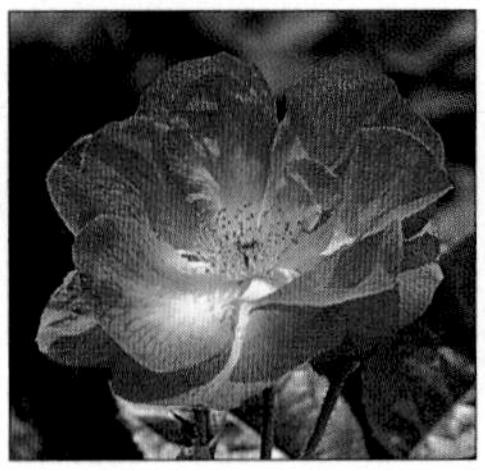
Rosa 'Escapade'

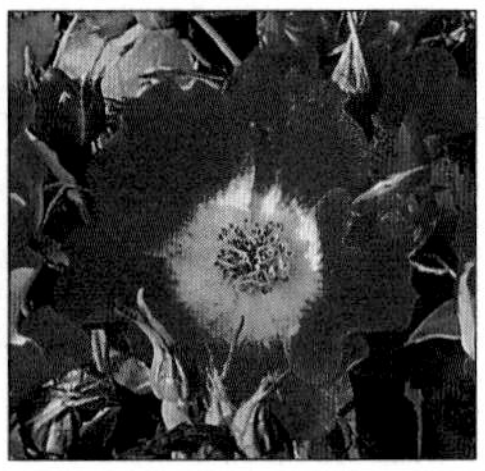
Rosa 'Eye Paint'

R. ecae ■ Erect, wiry, suckering species rose with red stems and small, fern-like, mid-green leaves, each composed of 5–9 broadly elliptic to obovate leaflets, 4–8mm (⅛–⅜in) long. Cupped, single, musk-scented, bright yellow flowers, 2cm (¾in) across, are produced along the stems in late spring. Liable to die-back. ↕1.5m (5ft), ↔1.2m (4ft). Turkmenistan, Uzbekistan, Tajikistan, N.E. Afghanistan, N.W. Pakistan. ❄❄

R. eglanteria ■♀ syn. *R. rubiginosa* (Eglantine rose, Sweet briar). Vigorous, arching, prickly species rose with apple-scented, dark green leaves composed of 5–9 ovate leaflets, 2.5–4cm (1–1½in) long. Cupped, single, rose-pink flowers, 2.5cm (1in) across, are produced in midsummer, followed by ovoid to spherical red hips in autumn. ↕↔ to 2.5m (8ft). Europe, N. Africa to W. Asia. ❄❄❄

***R.* 'E.H. Morse'** see *R.* 'Ernest H. Morse'.

***R.* 'Electron'** see *R.* 'Mullard Jubilee'.

***R. elegantula* 'Persetosa'**, syn. *R. elegantula* f. *persetosa*, *R. farreri* f. *persetosa.* Upright species rose with wiry stems, red-bristled when young, and pale grey-green leaves, each composed of 7–11 narrowly ovate to elliptic, fern-like leaflets, 1.5cm (½in) long, reddening in autumn. Shallowly cupped, single, light pink flowers, 2cm (¾in) across, are produced in summer; they are followed by ovoid, orange-red hips. ↕↔ 2m (6ft). N.W. China. ❄❄❄

R. elegantula* f. *persetosa see *R. elegantula* 'Persetosa'.

***R.* 'Elina'** ■♀ syn. *R.* 'Dicjana', *R.* 'Peaudouce'. Vigorous large-flowered bush rose with abundant dark green foliage. Rounded, fully double, scented, ivory-white flowers, 15cm (6in) across, with lemon-yellow centres, are borne freely from summer to autumn. ↕1.1m (3½ft), ↔75cm (30in). ❄❄❄

***R.* 'Elizabeth Harkness'** ■ Large-flowered bush rose of neat habit, with dark green leaves. High-centred to rounded, fully double, fragrant, creamy pink flowers, 12cm (5in) across, are produced from summer to autumn. ↕80cm (32in), ↔60cm (24in). ❄❄❄

***R.* 'Elizabeth of Glamis'**, syn. *R.* 'Irish Beauty'. Cluster-flowered bush rose producing mid-green foliage. From summer to autumn, bears well-spaced sprays of cupped, double, scented, light orange-pink flowers, 9cm (3½in) across. ↕75cm (30in), ↔60cm (24in). ❄❄❄

***R.* 'Emily Gray'** ■ Semi-evergreen rambler with lax stems covered in lustrous, dark green leaves. In summer, bears small clusters of loosely formed, rounded, double, scented, butter-yellow flowers, 5cm (2in) across. ↕ to 5m (15ft), ↔3m (10ft). ❄❄❄

***R.* 'Empereur du Maroc'** ■ Hybrid Perpetual rose of compact, shrubby habit, with mid-green leaves. Quartered-rosette, fully double, fragrant, maroon-crimson flowers, 8cm (3in) across, are borne freely on bowed stems in summer, sparsely in autumn. ↕1.2m (4ft), ↔1m (3ft). ❄❄❄

***R.* 'Empress Josephine'** see *R.* x *francofurtana.*

***R.* 'Ena Harkness'** ■ Large-flowered bush rose of branching habit, with mid-green leaves. High-centred, double, fragrant, bright crimson flowers, 10cm (4in) across, are borne from summer to autumn. ↕75cm (30in), ↔60cm (24in). ❄❄❄

***R.* 'English Garden'** ■ syn. *R.* 'Ausbuff'. Upright shrub rose with light green leaves and rosette-shaped, double, lightly scented flowers, 10cm (4in) across, buff yellow, paling towards the edges, borne from summer to autumn. ↕1m (3ft), ↔75cm (30in). ❄❄❄

***R.* 'English Miss'** ■ Cluster-flowered bush rose of neat, spreading habit, with leathery, dark green leaves. Wide clusters of camellia-like, cupped, fully double, fragrant, pale pink flowers, 8cm (3in) across, are borne from summer to autumn. ↕75cm (30in), ↔60cm (24in). ❄❄❄

***R.* 'Ernest H. Morse'** ■ syn. *R.* 'E.H. Morse'. Large-flowered bush rose with semi-glossy, dark green foliage. High-centred, double, very fragrant crimson flowers, 12cm (5in) across, are freely produced from summer to autumn. ↕75cm (30in), ↔60cm (24in). ❄❄❄

***R.* 'Escapade'** ■♀ syn. *R.* 'Harpade'. Vigorous cluster-flowered bush rose of dense habit, with abundant light green foliage. Showy, cupped, semi-double, scented, pink-violet flowers, 8cm (3in) across, each with a white eye, are borne freely from summer to autumn. ↕75cm (30in), ↔60cm (24in). ❄❄❄

***R.* 'Esmeralda'** see *R.* 'Keepsake'.

***R.* 'Essex'**, syn. *R.* 'Pink Cover', *R.* 'Poulnoz'. Ground-cover rose of dense habit, with dark green leaves. From summer to autumn, clusters of many small, cupped, single, light reddish pink flowers, 2.5cm (1in) across, with whitish pink centres, are borne freely along the stems. ↕60cm (24in), ↔1.2m (4ft). ❄❄❄

***R.* 'Euphrates'**, syn. *R.* 'Harunique'. Prickly, hummock-forming shrub rose with light green leaves composed of narrow leaflets. In summer, produces clusters of numerous cupped, single, salmon- to rose-pink flowers, 2cm (¾in) across, with scarlet at the petal bases. ↕60cm (24in), ↔75cm (30in). ❄❄❄

***R.* 'Evelyn Fison'**, syn. *R.* 'Irish Wonder'. Cluster-flowered bush rose with sparse, glossy, dark green foliage. Many neatly formed, rounded, double, bright deep red flowers, 6cm (2½in) across, are borne from summer to autumn. ↕70cm (28in), ↔60cm (24in). ❄❄❄

***R.* 'Excelsa'**, syn. *R.* 'Red Dorothy Perkins'. Lax rambler with abundant shiny, mid-green leaves. In summer, bears dense clusters of rosette-shaped, fully double crimson flowers, 2cm (¾in) across. Prone to mildew. ↕4m (12ft), ↔3m (10ft). ❄❄❄

***R.* 'Eye Paint'** ■ syn. *R.* 'Maceye', *R.* 'Tapis Persan'. Vigorous cluster-flowered bush or shrub rose with dense, dark green foliage. Large clusters of cupped to flat, single scarlet flowers, 5cm (2in) across, with white eyes, are borne from summer to autumn. ↕1.1m (3½ft), ↔75cm (30in). ❄❄❄

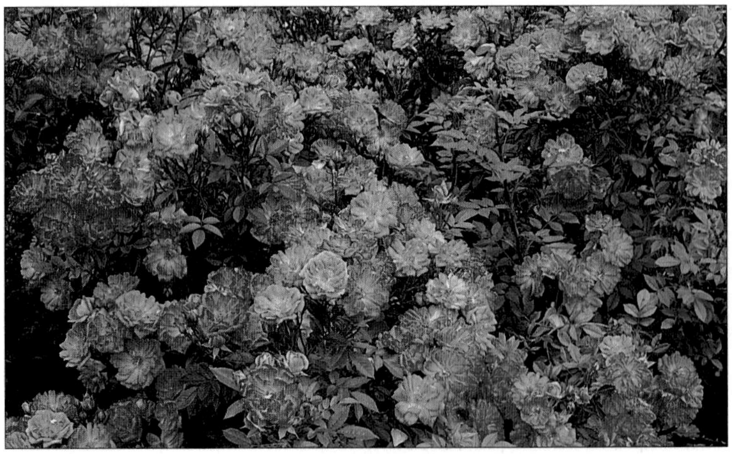
Rosa 'Ferdy'

***R.* 'Fairyland'**, syn. *R.* 'Harlayalong'. Polyantha shrub rose of vigorous, arching, spreading habit, with small, dark green leaves. Large sprays of many rosette-shaped, double, scented, pale pink flowers, 4cm (1½in) across, are borne from summer to autumn. ↕75cm (30in), ↔1.2m (4ft). ❄❄❄

***R.* 'Fairy Lights'** see *R.* 'Avon'.

***R.* 'Fanny Bias'** see *R.* 'Gloire de France'.

***R.* 'Fantin-Latour'** ■♀ Vigorous Centifolia rose of open habit, producing broad, dark green leaves. Cupped to flat, fully double, fragrant, light pink flowers, 10cm (4in) across, each with a green button eye, are borne in summer. ↕1.5m (5ft), ↔1.2m (4ft). ❄❄❄

R. farreri* f. *persetosa see *R. elegantula* 'Persetosa'.

R. fedtschenkoana. Very vigorous, suckering species rose with arching, bristly stems and pale grey-green leaves with 5–9 elliptic to obovate leaflets, 2.5cm (1in) long. Single, flat white flowers, 4.5cm (1¾in) across, with yellow stamens, are borne in clusters of up to 4 blooms, mainly in summer; they are followed by pear-shaped, orange-red hips. ↕↔ 2.2m (7ft). C. Asia. ❄❄❄

***R.* 'Fée des Neiges'** see *R.* 'Iceberg'.

***R.* 'Felicia'** ■♀ Vigorous shrub rose with abundant dark green leaves. Large clusters of cupped, double, scented, light pink flowers, 8cm (3in) across, flushed yellow-apricot, are borne from summer to autumn. ↕1.5m (5ft), ↔2.2m (7ft). ❄❄❄

R

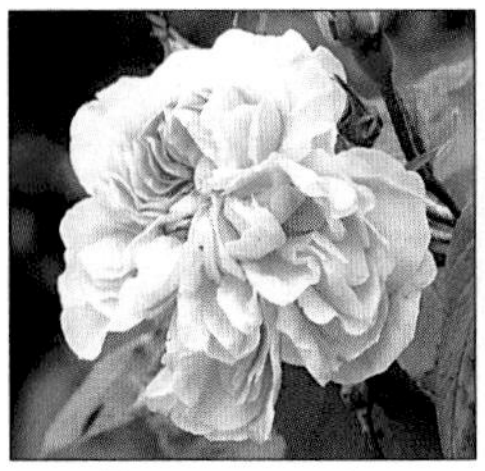
Rosa 'Fantin-Latour'

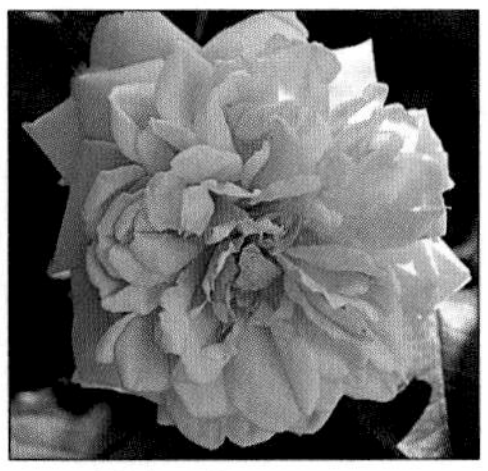
Rosa 'Felicia'

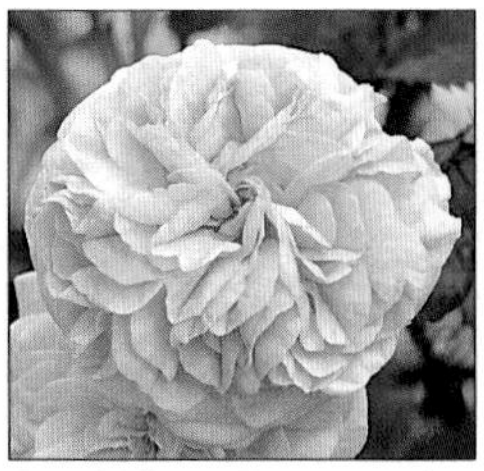
Rosa 'Félicité Parmentier'

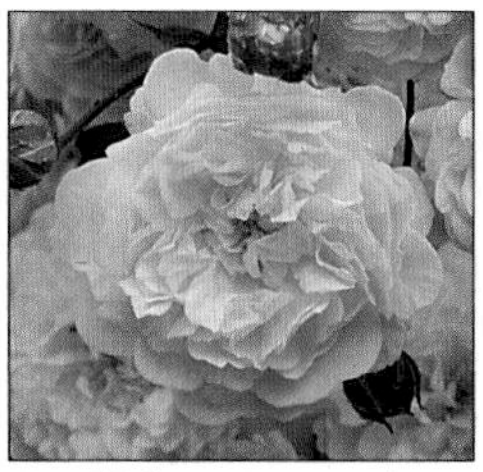
Rosa 'Félicité Perpétue'

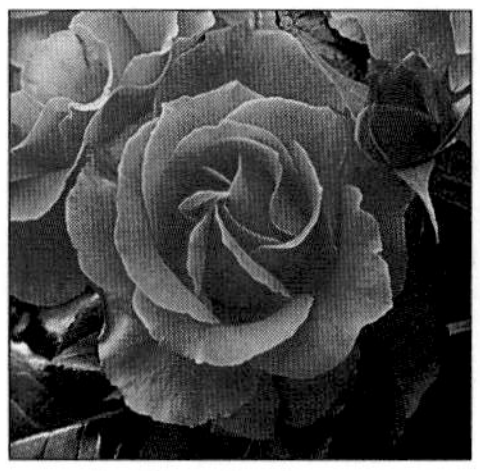
Rosa 'Fellowship'

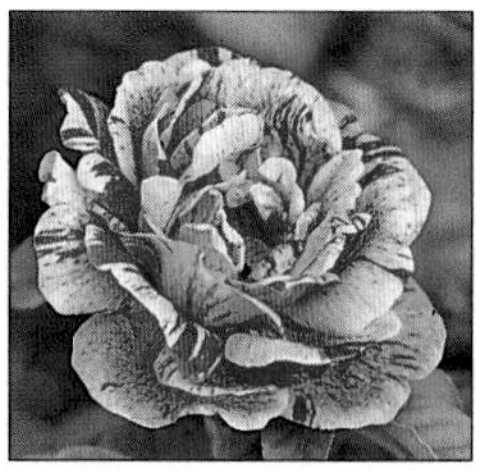
Rosa 'Ferdinand Pichard'

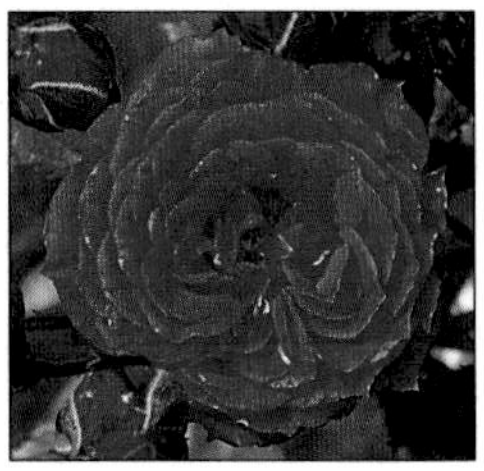
Rosa 'Fire Princess'

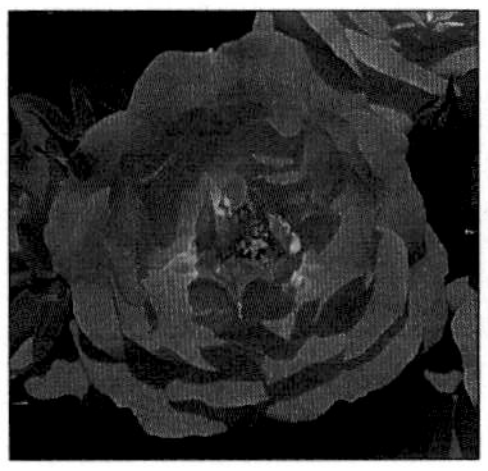
Rosa 'Flower Carpet'

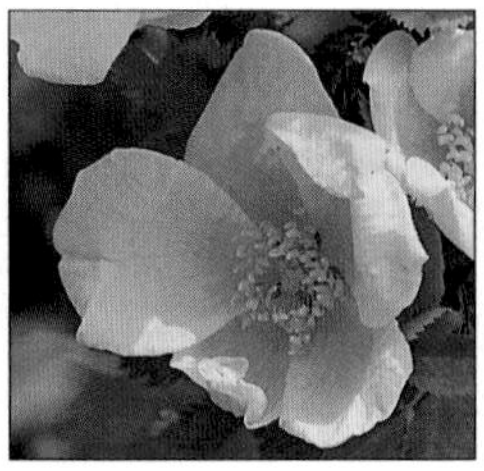
Rosa foetida

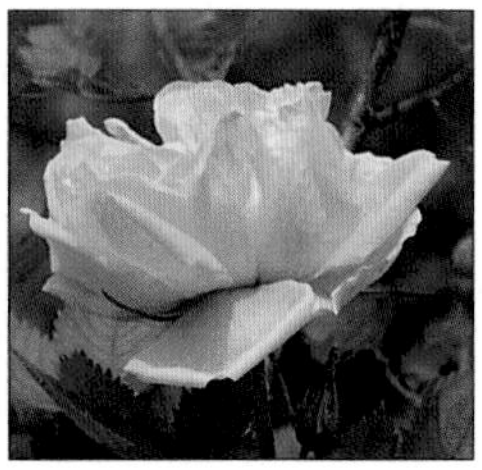
Rosa foetida 'Persiana'

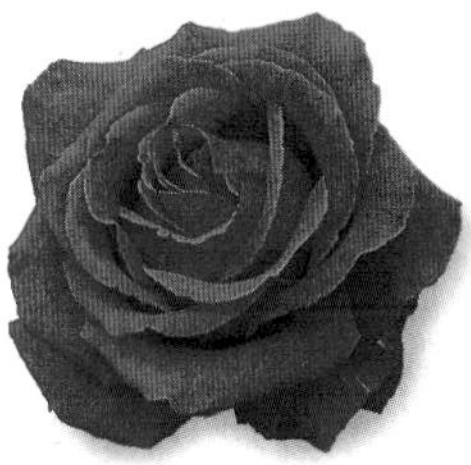
Rosa 'Fragrant Cloud'

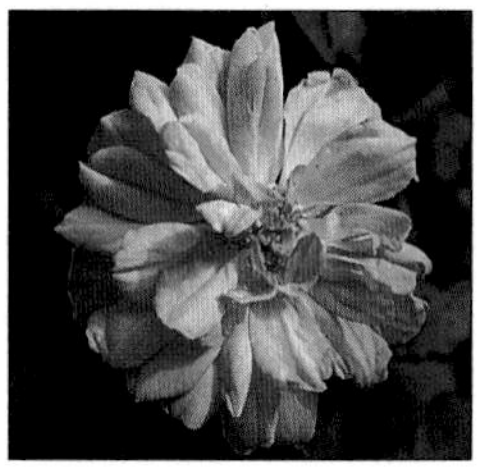
Rosa 'François Juranville'

***R.* 'Félicité et Perpétue'** see *R.* 'Félicité Perpétue'.
***R.* 'Félicité Parmentier'** ■ 🏆 Vigorous Alba rose of upright, compact habit, producing abundant grey-green leaves. In midsummer, bears quartered-rosette, fully double, fragrant, cream to pale pink flowers, 6cm (2½in) across. ↕ 1.3m (4½ft), ↔ 1.2m (4ft). ❄❄❄
***R.* 'Félicité Perpétue'** ■ 🏆 syn. *R.* 'Climbing Little White Pet', *R.* 'Félicité et Perpétue'. Sempervirens rambler rose with long, slender stems clothed in dense, dark green leaves. Rosette-shaped, fully double, pale pink to white flowers, 4cm (1½in) across, are borne freely in summer. ↕ to 5m (15ft), ↔ to 4m (12ft). ❄❄❄
***R.* 'Fellowship'** ■ syn. *R.* 'Harwelcome'. Vigorous cluster-flowered bush rose with even growth and abundant glossy, mid-green foliage. Well-spaced clusters of cupped, double, scented, deep orange flowers, 9cm (3½in) across, are borne freely from summer to autumn. ↕ 75cm (30in), ↔ 60cm (24in). ❄❄❄
***R.* 'Ferdi'** see *R.* 'Ferdy'.
***R.* 'Ferdinand Pichard'** ■ 🏆 Upright, compact Hybrid Perpetual rose with smooth stems and long, light green leaves. Cupped, double, fragrant, pale pink flowers, 8cm (3in) across, with pink and red stripes, are produced from summer to autumn. ↕ 1.5m (5ft), ↔ 1.2m (4ft). ❄❄❄
***R.* 'Ferdy'** ■ syn. *R.* 'Ferdi', *R.* 'Keitoly'. Cluster-flowered shrub rose of uneven, spiky growth, with fine-cut, mid-green leaves. Dense clusters of cupped to flat, double, bright pink flowers, 2.5cm (1in) across, wreathe the stems from summer to autumn. ↕ 80cm (32in), ↔ 1.2m (4ft). ❄❄❄
***R.* 'Festival'**, syn. *R.* 'Kordialo'. Compact, dwarf cluster-flowered bush rose with abundant dark green leaves. From summer to autumn, bears dense clusters of rounded, semi-double, crimson-scarlet flowers, 4.5cm (1¾in) across, with a silvery white reverse to the petals. ↕ 60cm (24in), ↔ 50cm (20in). ❄❄❄
***R. filipes* 'Kiftsgate'** ■ 🏆 syn. *R.* 'Kiftsgate'. Rampant climber producing abundant glossy, light green leaves, each composed of 5–7 narrowly elliptic to narrowly ovate leaflets, 5–8cm (2–3in) long. Large clusters of cupped, single, fragrant, creamy white flowers, 2.5cm (1in) across, are borne in late summer. ↕ to 10m (30ft), ↔ 6m (20ft). ❄❄❄
***R.* 'Fiona'**, syn. *R.* 'Meibeluxen'. Cluster-flowered shrub rose with a wide, spreading habit and shiny dark green leaves. Large clusters of cupped to flat, double red flowers, 6cm (2½in) across, are borne from summer to autumn. ↕ 80cm (32in), ↔ 1.2m (4ft). ❄❄❄
***R.* 'Fire Princess'** ■ Upright miniature bush rose with glossy, mid-green leaves. Rosette-shaped, fully double scarlet flowers, 4cm (1½in) across, are borne from summer to autumn. ↕ 45cm (18in), ↔ 30cm (12in). ❄❄❄
***R.* 'First Class'** see *R.* 'Class Act'.
***R.* 'First Prize'.** Large-flowered bush rose of vigorous, spreading habit, with leathery, dark green foliage. High-centred, double, scented, two-toned pink flowers, 13cm (5in) across, are borne from summer to autumn. ↕ 1.2m (4ft), ↔ 75cm (30in). ❄❄❄
***R.* 'Flower Carpet'** ■ 🏆 syn. *R.* 'Heidetraum', *R.* 'Noatraum'. Vigorous ground-cover rose with abundant, shiny, bright green leaves. Showy clusters of cupped, double, deep rose-pink flowers, 5cm (2in) across, are borne freely along the stems from summer to autumn. ↕ 75cm (30in), ↔ 1.2m (4ft). ❄❄❄
R. foetida ■ (Austrian briar, Austrian yellow rose). Species rose of upright, open habit, with arching, brownish green stems and pale green leaves, each comprised of 5–7 elliptic to obovate leaflets, 2–4cm (¾–1½in) long. Cupped, single, pungent, bright yellow flowers, 5cm (2in) across, are borne in early summer; the flowers are followed by spherical red hips. Susceptible to die-back in hard winters. ↕↔ 1.5m (5ft). W. to C. Asia. ❄❄. **'Bicolor'**, syn. *R.* 'Rose Capucine' (Austrian copper rose), a sport of *R. foetida*, has vivid nasturtium-orange flowers with a yellow reverse to the petals. **'Persiana'** ■ syn. var. *persiana* (Persian yellow rose) has gaunt, arching growth, small, fern-like leaves, and fully double yellow flowers, 6cm (2½in) across; ↔ 1.2m (4ft).
***R.* 'Fontaine'** see *R.* 'Fountain'.
***R.* 'Fountain'**, syn. *R.* 'Fontaine', *R.* 'Red Prince'. Vigorous cluster-flowered shrub rose with strong, upright growth and glossy, dark green leaves. From summer to autumn, bears large clusters of cupped, double, scented, bright crimson flowers, 12cm (5in) across. ↕ 2m (6ft), ↔ 1.2m (4ft). ❄❄❄
***R.* 'Fragrant Cloud'** ■ syn. *R.* 'Tanellis'. Large-flowered bush rose with branching growth and abundant, dark green leaves. Rounded, double, intensely fragrant, dusky scarlet flowers, 11cm (4½in) across, are borne freely from summer to autumn. ↕ 75cm (30in), ↔ 60cm (24in). ❄❄❄
***R.* 'Fragrant Delight'.** Cluster-flowered bush rose of willowy, uneven habit, with abundant reddish green foliage. Freely bears large sprays of urn-shaped, double, scented, salmon-pink flowers, 8cm (3in) across, from summer to autumn. ↕ 1m (3ft), ↔ 75cm (30in). ❄❄❄
***R.* 'Fragrant Dream'**, syn. *R.* 'Dicodour'. Upright, branching large-flowered bush rose producing dark green foliage. High-centred to rounded, double, fragrant, light apricot flowers, 12cm (5in) across, are borne from summer to autumn. ↕ 80cm (32in), ↔ 75cm (30in). ❄❄❄
***R.* 'Fragrant Surprise'** see *R.* 'Samaritan'.
***R.* 'Francine Austin'**, syn. *R.* 'Ausram'. Cluster-flowered shrub rose of arching, open habit, with long, light green leaves. Small sprays of many pompon, double, scented white flowers, 4cm (1½in) across, are borne on bowed stems from summer to autumn. ↕ 1m (3ft), ↔ 1.2m (4ft). ❄❄❄
R.* x *francofurtana 🏆 syn. *R.* 'Empress Josephine'. Bushy, wide-spreading Gallica rose with smooth stems and greyish green leaves composed of 5–7 broadly ovate leaflets, to 5cm (2in) long. Loosely formed, rounded, semi-double flowers, 9cm (3½in) across, with wavy-margined, bright pink petals and deeper pink veining, open in summer, followed by inversely cone-shaped red hips. ↕↔ 1.2m (4ft). Garden origin. ❄❄❄
***R.* 'François Juranville'** ■ 🏆 Rambler with abundant, shiny, dark green leaves and clusters of rosette-shaped, fully double, apple-scented, light salmon-pink flowers, 8cm (3in) across, borne in summer. ↕ 6m (20ft), ↔ 5m (15ft). ❄❄❄
***R.* 'Frau Dagmar Hartopp'** see *R.* 'Fru Dagmar Hastrup'.

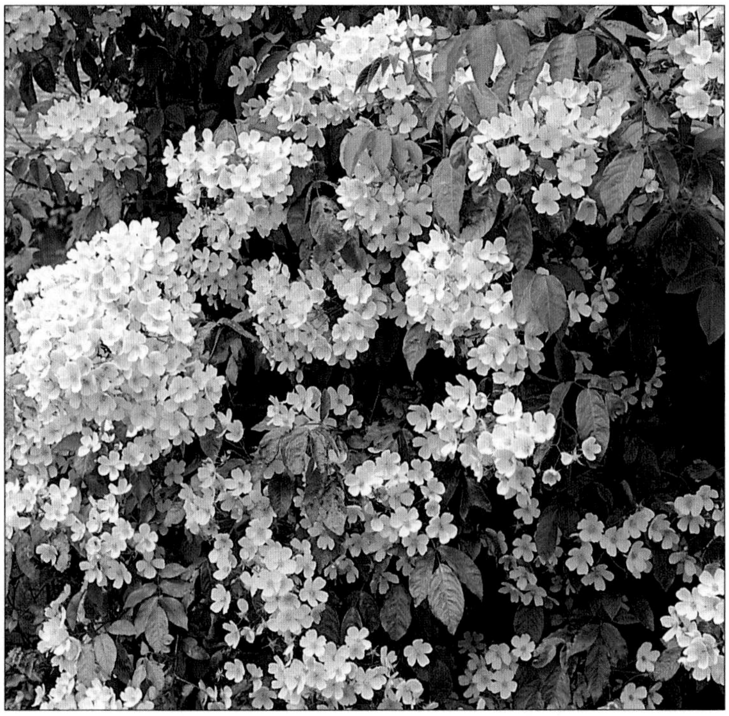
Rosa filipes 'Kiftsgate'

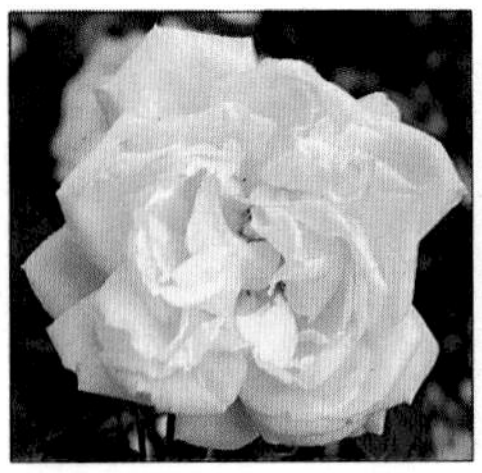
Rosa 'Frau Karl Druschki'

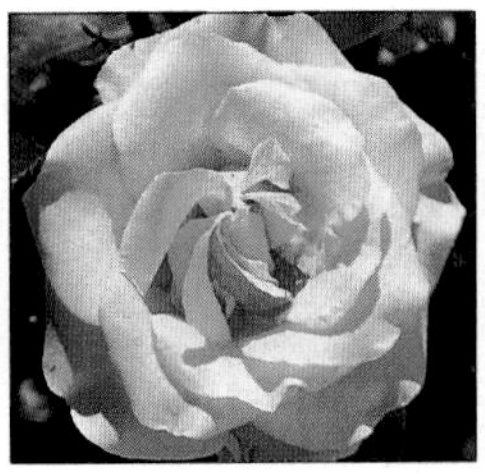
Rosa 'Freedom'

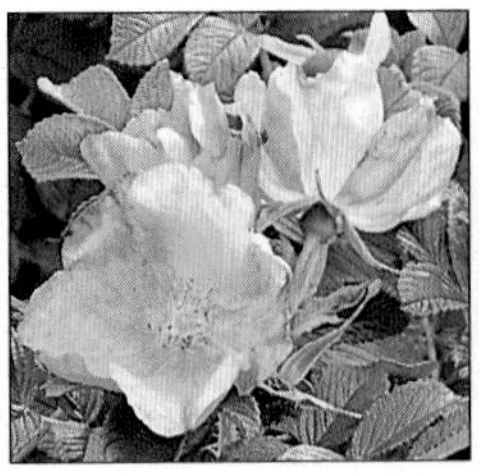
Rosa 'Fru Dagmar Hastrup'

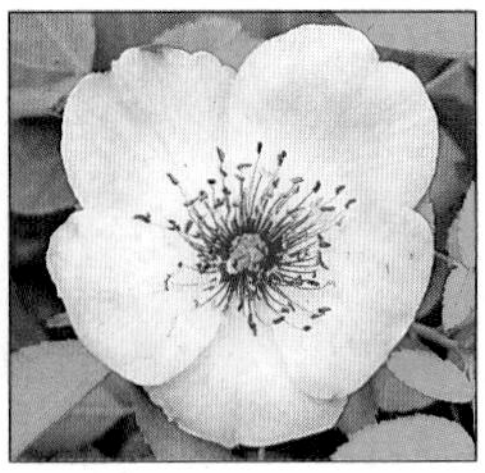
Rosa 'Frühlingsmorgen'

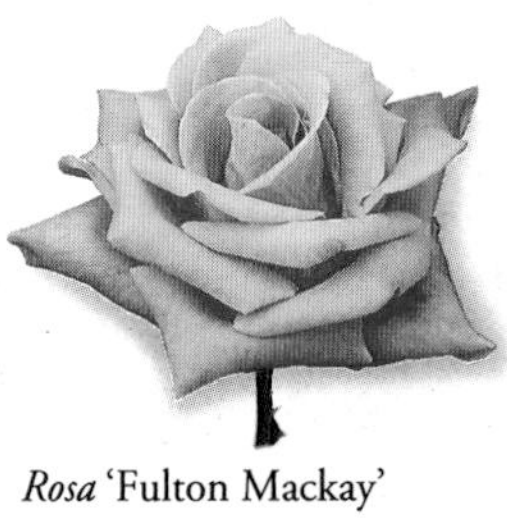
Rosa 'Fulton Mackay'

Rosa gallica var. *officinalis*

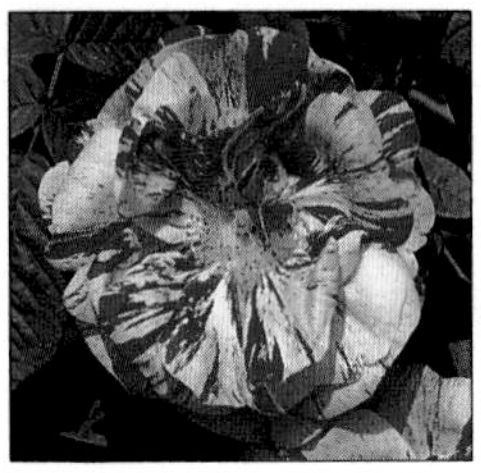
Rosa gallica var. *officinalis* 'Versicolor'

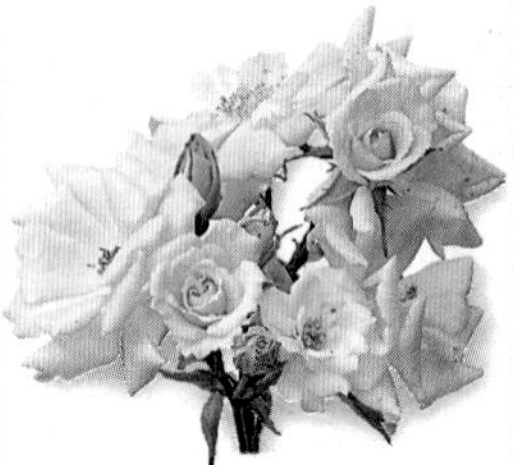

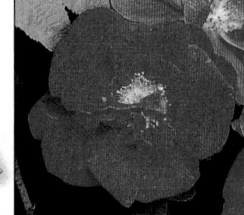
Rosa 'Gentle Touch'

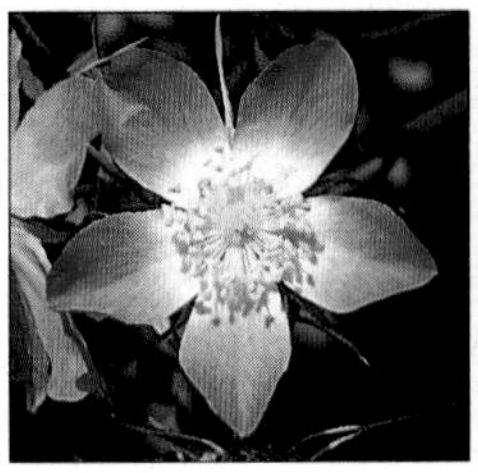
Rosa glauca

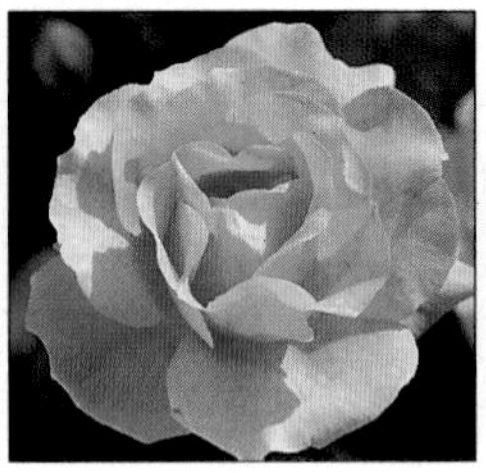
Rosa 'Glenfiddich'

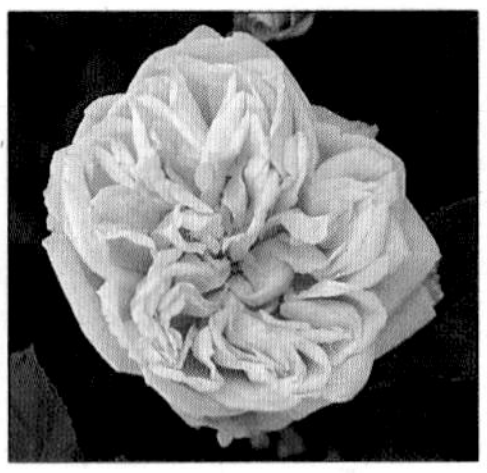
Rosa 'Gloire de Dijon'

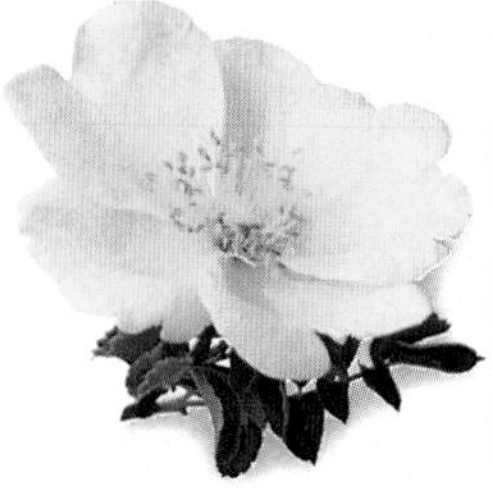
Rosa 'Golden Chersonese'

***R.* 'Frau Karl Druschki'** ■ syn. *R.* 'Reine des Neiges', *R.* 'Snow Queen', *R.* 'White American Beauty'. Vigorous Hybrid Perpetual rose with strong, arching stems, mid-green leaves, and high-centred, fully double, milk-white flowers, 11cm (4½in) across, borne from summer to autumn. ↕ to 1.5m (5ft), ↔ 1.2m (4ft). ❄❄❄
***R.* 'Fred Loads'** ♀ Vigorous cluster-flowered bush rose of gaunt habit, producing dark green leaves. Many showy, cupped to flat, semi-double, vermilion-orange flowers, 9cm (3½in) across, are borne from summer to autumn. ↕ 2m (6ft), ↔ 1m (3ft). ❄❄❄
***R.* 'Freedom'** ■♀ syn. *R.* 'Dicjem'. Large-flowered bush rose of uneven growth, with many shoots and abundant glossy, mid-green foliage. Rounded, double, stiff-petalled, bright yellow flowers, 9cm (3½in) across, are borne freely from summer to autumn. ↕ 75cm (30in), ↔ 60cm (24in). ❄❄❄
***R.* 'French Lace'**, syn. *R.* 'Jaclace'. Upright cluster-flowered bush rose with well-branched growth and mid-green foliage. From summer to autumn, bears high-centred, fully double, scented white flowers, 9cm (3½in) across. ↕ 1m (3ft), ↔ 60cm (24in). ❄❄❄
***R.* 'Friesia'** see *R.* 'Korresia'.
***R.* 'Fru Dagmar Hastrup'** ■♀ syn. *R.* 'Frau Dagmar Hartopp'. Sturdy Rugosa rose of spreading habit, producing leathery mid-green leaves. Shallowly cupped, single, clove-scented, light pink flowers, 9cm (3½in) across, are borne mainly in summer, followed by tomato-shaped, dark red hips in autumn. ↕ 1m (3ft), ↔ 1.2m (4ft). ❄❄❄
***R.* 'Frühlingsgold'** ♀ syn. *R.* 'Spring Gold'. Vigorous shrub rose with strong, arching branches, covered in downy red bristles when young, and with toothed, matt, light green leaves. Cupped, semi-double, scented, pale yellow flowers, 10cm (4in) across, with golden stamens, are borne mainly in early summer. ↕ 2.5m (8ft), ↔ 2.2m (7ft). ❄❄❄
***R.* 'Frühlingsmorgen'** ■ syn. *R.* 'Spring Morning'. Open, free-branching shrub rose with greyish green leaves. Shallowly cupped, single, hay-scented pink flowers, 12cm (5in) across, with primrose-yellow centres and maroon stamens, are produced in early summer. ↕ 2m (6ft), ↔ 1.5m (5ft). ❄❄❄
***R.* 'Fulton Mackay'** ■ syn. *R.* 'Cocdana'. Large-flowered bush rose with handsome, glossy, mid-green foliage. High-centred, double, scented, golden apricot, pink-flushed flowers, 12cm (5in) across, are borne from summer to autumn. ↕ 75cm (30in), ↔ 60cm (24in). ❄❄❄
***R.* 'Fyvie Castle'**, syn. *R.* 'Amberlight', *R.* 'Cocbamber'. Large-flowered bush rose of neat, branching habit, with mid-green foliage. Rounded, fully double, scented flowers, 13cm (5in) across, apricot-pink flushed amber, are borne from summer to autumn. ↕↔ 60cm (24in). ❄❄❄
R. gallica* var. *officinalis ■♀ syn. *R. officinalis* (Apothecary's rose, Crimson damask rose, Provins rose, Red rose of Lancaster). Species rose of neat, rounded habit, producing rough, dark green leaves with 3–5, rarely 7, broadly elliptic to almost rounded leaflets, 2.5–8cm (1–3in) long. Cupped to flat, semi-double, scented, pinkish red flowers, 8cm (3in) across, are borne singly or in clusters of 2–4 in summer, followed by spherical to ellipsoid, orange-red hips. ↕ 80cm (32in), ↔ 1m (3ft). ❄❄❄.
'Versicolor' ■♀ (Rosa mundi rose) is compact, with pale pink flowers, striped reddish pink.
***R.* 'Garden Party'.** Vigorous large-flowered bush rose with mid-green leaves. From summer to autumn, bears high-centred, double, fragrant white flowers, 12cm (5in) across, margined pale pink. ↕ 1.2m (4ft), ↔ 80cm (32in). ❄❄❄
***R.* 'Garnette'**, syn. *R.* 'Garnette Red'. Cluster-flowered bush rose with dark green leaves and tight clusters of cupped to flat, fully double, firm-petalled, garnet-red flowers, 6cm (2½in) across, borne from summer to autumn. ↕ 1m (3ft), ↔ 45cm (18in). ❄❄❄
***R.* 'Garnette Red'** see *R.* 'Garnette'.
***R.* 'Gentle Touch'** ■♀ syn. *R.* 'Diclulu'. Dwarf cluster-flowered bush rose of neat habit, producing dark green leaves. Sprays of urn-shaped, semi-double, pale salmon-pink flowers, 5cm (2in) across, are borne close to the foliage from summer to autumn. ↕ 50cm (20in), ↔ 40cm (16in). ❄❄❄
***R.* 'Gerbe d'Or'** see *R.* 'Casino'.
***R.* 'Gertrude Jekyll'** ♀ syn. *R.* 'Ausbord'. Lanky large-flowered shrub rose with greyish green leaves. Cupped, double, fragrant, deep pink flowers, 10cm (4in) across, with infolded petals, are borne from summer to autumn. ↕ 1.5m (5ft), ↔ 1m (3ft). ❄❄❄
***R.* 'Gingernut'**, syn. *R.* 'Coccrazy'. Dwarf cluster-flowered bush rose of vigorous, short, spreading habit, with glossy, mid-green leaves. From summer to autumn, freely bears cupped, double flowers, 6cm (2½in) across, bronze-orange, with reddish tints on the reverse of the petals. ↕ 40cm (16in), ↔ 45cm (18in). ❄❄❄
***R.* 'Gioia'** see *R.* 'Peace'.
***R.* 'Gipsy Boy'** see *R.* 'Zigeunerknabe'.
R. glauca ■♀ syn. *R. rubrifolia.* Vigorous, arching species rose with reddish green stems and greyish purple leaves, each composed of 5–9 ovate to narrowly elliptic leaflets, 2.5–4cm (1–1½in) long. Flat, single, cerise-pink flowers, 4cm (1½in) across, with paler pink centres and gold stamens, are borne in small clusters in summer; they are followed by many spherical red hips in autumn. ↕ 2m (6ft), ↔ 1.5m (5ft). Mountains of C. and S. Europe. ❄❄❄
***R.* 'Glenfiddich'** ■ Cluster-flowered bush rose with glossy, dark green leaves. Produces clusters of urn-shaped, double, scented, amber to yellow flowers, 10cm (4in) across, from summer to autumn. ↕ 80cm (32in), ↔ 60cm (24in). ❄❄❄
***R.* 'Gloire de Dijon'** ■♀ (Old glory rose). Vigorous, stiffly branching Noisette or climbing Tea rose with glossy, dark green leaves. Quartered-rosette, fully double, scented, creamy buff flowers, 10cm (4in) across, are borne from summer to autumn. ↕ to 5m (15ft), ↔ 4m (12ft). ❄❄❄
***R.* 'Gloire de France'**, syn. *R.* 'Fanny Bias'. Lax Gallica rose with crisp, dark green foliage. Quartered-rosette, fully double, fragrant, lilac-pink flowers, 8cm (3in) across, are borne freely in summer. ↕ 1m (3ft), ↔ 1.2m (4ft). ❄❄❄
***R.* 'Gloria Dei'** see *R.* 'Peace'.
***R.* 'Golden Cherry'** see *R. laevigata.*
***R.* 'Golden Chersonese'** ■ syn. *R.* 'Hilgold'. Vigorous, upright shrub rose

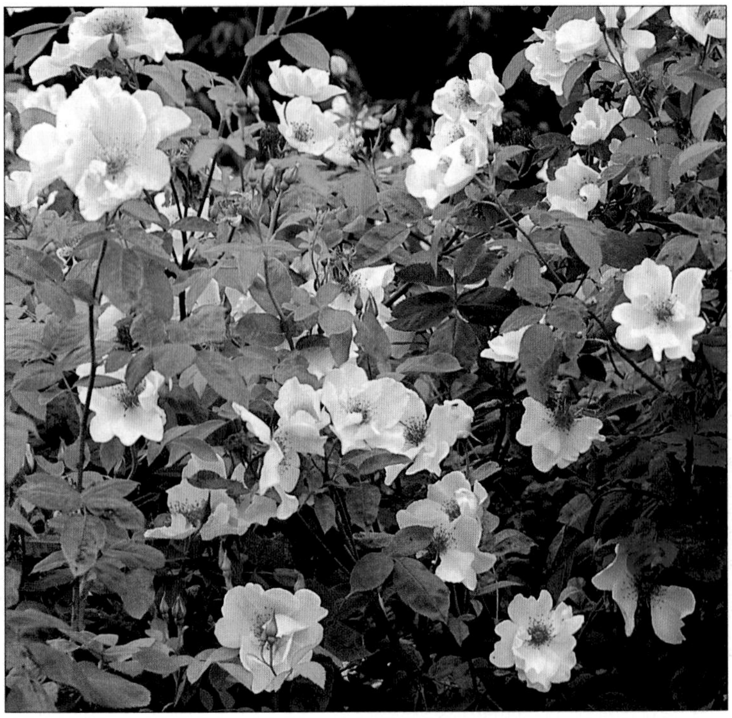
Rosa 'Golden Wings'

R

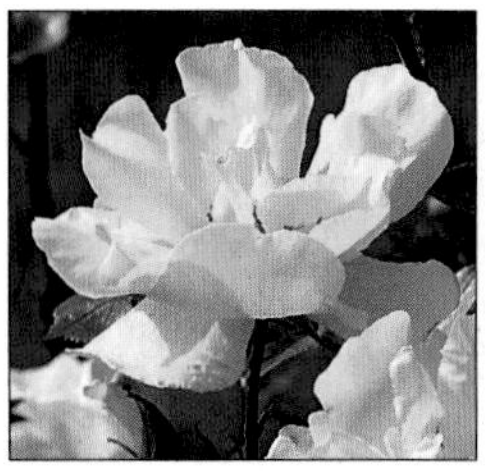
Rosa 'Golden Showers'

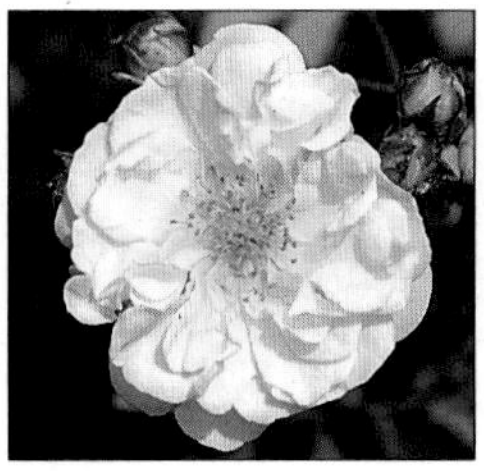
Rosa 'Goldfinch'

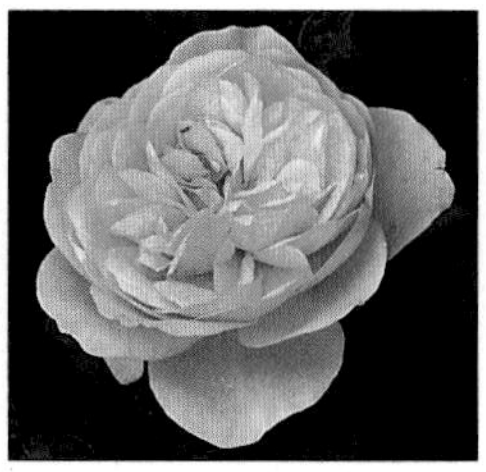
Rosa 'Graham Thomas'

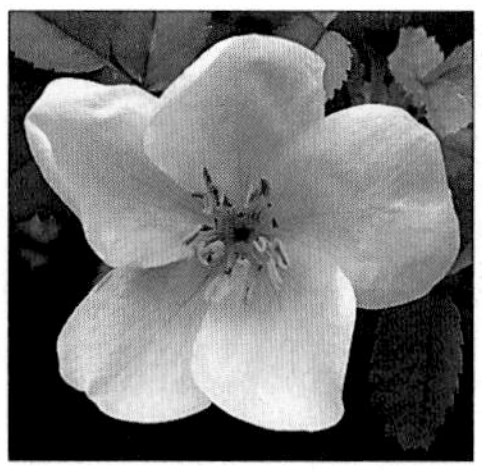
Rosa 'Grandiflora'

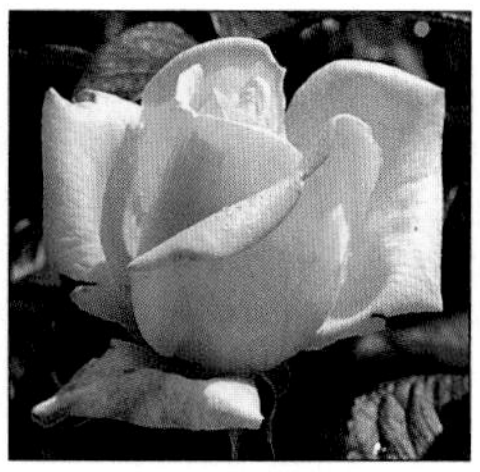
Rosa 'Grandpa Dickson'

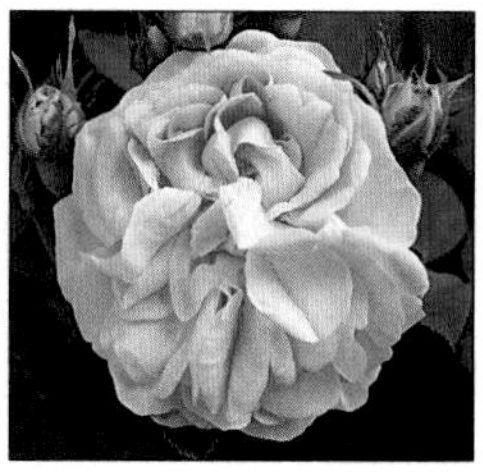
Rosa 'Great Maiden's Blush'

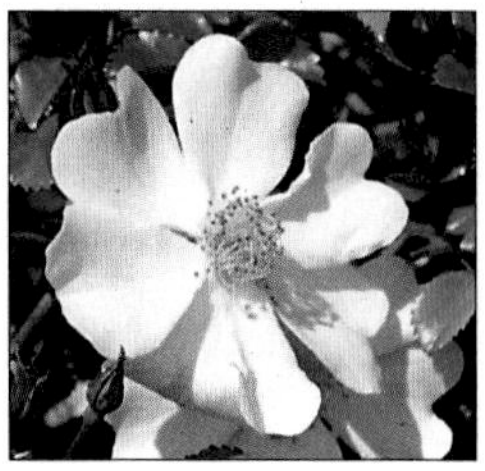
Rosa 'Grouse'

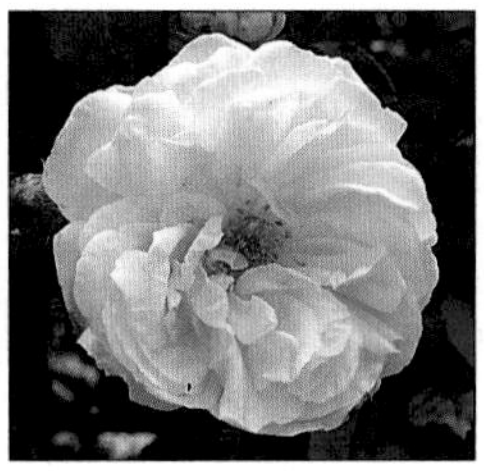
Rosa 'Gruss an Aachen'

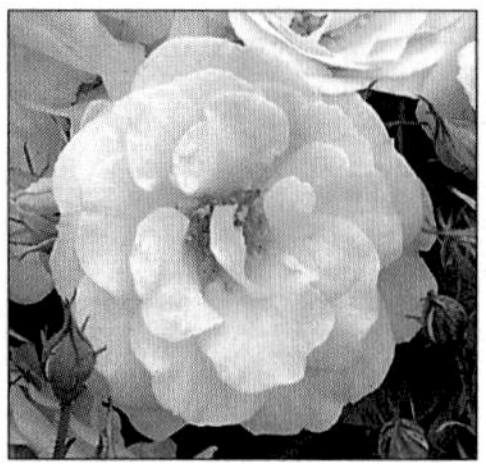
Rosa 'Hakuun'

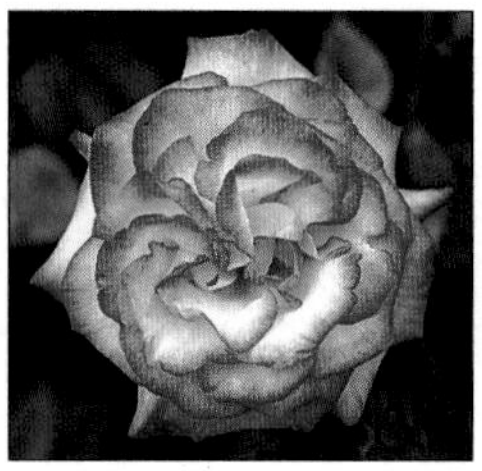
Rosa 'Handel'

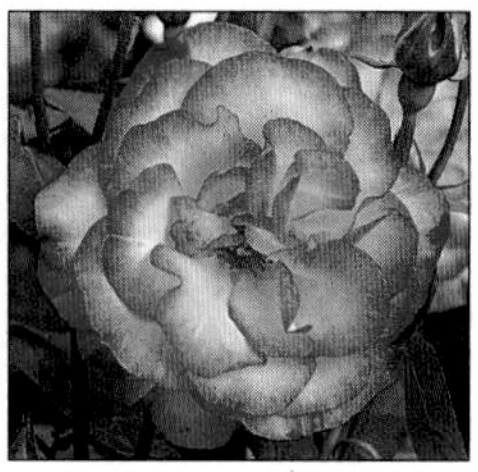
Rosa 'Hannah Gordon'

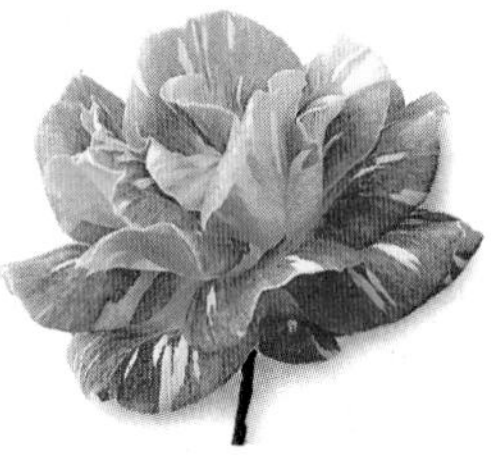
Rosa 'Harry Wheatcroft'

with arching, reddish green stems and fern-like, mid-green leaves. Cupped to flat, single, bright yellow flowers, 4cm (1½in) across, are borne along the branches in early summer. ↕ 2.2m (7ft), ↔ 1.5m (5ft). ❄❄❄

***R.* 'Golden Rambler'** see *R.* 'Alister Stella Gray'.

***R.* 'Golden Showers'** ■ ♀ Stiff, upright climber with glossy, dark green leaves. Numerous cupped, double, fragrant, clear yellow flowers, 10cm (4in) across, are borne from summer to autumn. ↕ to 3m (10ft), ↔ 2m (6ft). ❄❄❄

***R.* 'Golden Sunblaze'** see *R.* 'Rise 'n' Shine'.

***R.* 'Golden Wings'** ■ ♀ Dense, spreading shrub rose with many prickly stems and light green leaves. Shallowly cupped, single, scented, pale yellow flowers, 12cm (5in) across, are borne from summer to autumn. ↕ 1.1m (3½ft), ↔ 1.3m (4½ft). ❄❄❄

***R.* 'Goldfinch'** ■ Vigorous, arching rambler producing abundant light green leaves. Masses of rosette-shaped, double, scented flowers, 4cm (1½in) across, deep yellow fading to creamy white, are borne in summer. ↕ 2.5m (8ft), ↔ 2m (6ft). ❄❄❄

***R.* 'Gold Medal'**, syn. *R.* 'Aroyqueli'. Upright, vigorous large-flowered bush rose with dark green leaves. High-centred, fully double, deep yellow flowers, 9cm (3½in) across, with a light, fruity fragrance, are borne from summer to autumn. ↕ 1.1m (3½ft), ↔ 70cm (28in). ❄❄❄

***R.* 'Gold of Ophir'** see *R.* x *odorata* 'Pseudindica'.

***R.* 'Goldsmith'** see *R.* 'Simba'.

***R.* 'Gourmet Popcorn'**, syn. *R.* 'Weopop'. Vigorous, rounded miniature bush rose with dark green leaves. From summer to autumn, bears clusters of numerous cupped to flat, semi-double, honey-scented white flowers, 2cm (¾in) across. ↕↔ 40cm (16in). ❄❄❄

***R.* 'Graham Thomas'** ■ ♀ syn. *R.* 'Ausmas'. Vigorous shrub rose of lax, arching habit, with bright green leaves. Quartered-rosette to cupped, fully double, scented yellow flowers, 11cm (4½in) across, are borne from summer to autumn. ↕ 1.2m (4ft), ↔ 1.5m (5ft). ❄❄❄

***R.* 'Granada'**, syn. *R.* 'Donatella'. Vigorous large-flowered bush rose with leathery, dark green leaves. High-centred, double, slightly fragrant flowers, 11cm (4½in) across, blended rose-pink, red, and lemon-yellow, are borne from summer to autumn. ↕ 1.2m (4ft), ↔ 75cm (30in). ❄❄

***R.* 'Grandiflora'** ■ syn *R. pimpinellifolia* var. *altaica*. Vigorous Scots rose of upright habit, with twiggy stems and dark green leaves. Cupped to flat, single, scented, creamy white flowers, 6cm (2½in) across, with yellow stamens are borne in early summer. ↕ to 2m (6ft), ↔ 1.2m (4ft). ❄❄❄

***R.* 'Grandpa Dickson'** ■ syn. *R.* 'Irish Gold'. Large-flowered bush rose of neat habit, with glossy, light green leaves. High-centred, fully double, primrose-yellow flowers, 18cm (7in) across, are borne from summer to autumn. ↕ 75cm (30in), ↔ 60cm (24in). ❄❄❄

***R.* 'Great Maiden's Blush'** ■ syn. *R.* 'Cuisse de Nymphe', *R.* 'La Séduisante'. Vigorous Alba rose with strong, arching stems and grey-green leaves. Cupped, fully double, very fragrant, pinkish white flowers, 8cm (3in) across, with infolded petals, are borne freely in midsummer. ↕ 2m (6ft), ↔ 1.3m (4½ft). ❄❄❄

***R.* 'Grouse'** ■ syn. *R.* 'Immensee', *R.* 'Korimro', *R.* 'Lac Rose'. Very vigorous, trailing ground-cover rose with shiny, dark green leaves. Flat, single, scented, light pink to near white flowers, 4cm (1½in) across, are borne close to the stems in summer. ↕ 60cm (24in), ↔ 3m (10ft). ❄❄❄

***R.* 'Gruss an Aachen'** ■ Erect cluster-flowered bush rose with leathery, dark green foliage. Rounded, fully double, scented, pale pink to creamy white flowers, 8cm (3in) across, are borne from summer to autumn. ↕↔ 45cm (18in). ❄❄

***R.* 'Guinée'.** Vigorous, stiffly branched climber producing leathery, dark green leaves. In summer, bears cupped, fully double, fragrant, blackish red flowers, 11cm (4½in) across. ↕ 5m (15ft), ↔ 2.2m (7ft). ❄❄❄

***R.* 'Guletta'** see *R.* 'Rugul'.

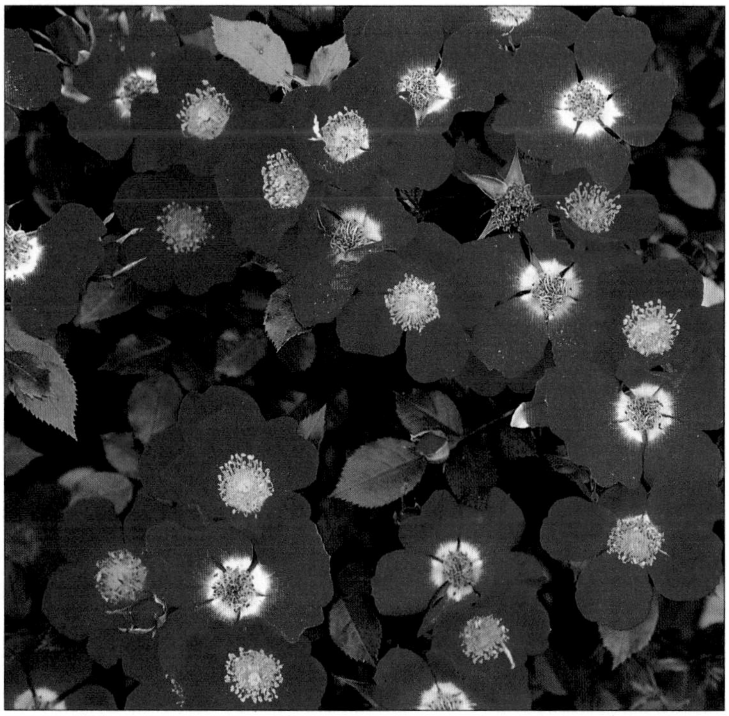
Rosa 'Hampshire'

***R.* 'Hakuun'** ■ Dwarf cluster-flowered bush rose of low, compact habit, with light green foliage. Masses of high-centred to rounded, semi-double, buff to creamy white flowers, 6cm (2½in) across, open from summer to autumn. ↕ 40cm (16in), ↔ 45cm (18in). ❄❄❄

***R.* 'Hampshire'** ■ syn. *R.* 'Korhamp'. Prostrate ground-cover rose producing glossy, mid-green leaves. From summer to autumn, bears clusters of many flat, single scarlet flowers, 5cm (2in) across, with yellow centres fading to white. ↕ 30cm (12in), ↔ 75cm (30in). ❄❄❄

***R.* 'Handel'** ■ ♀ Climber of stiff, erect habit, with glossy, dark green leaves. Open clusters of urn-shaped, double, lightly scented cream flowers, 8cm (3in) across, with pinkish red margins, are borne from summer to autumn. ↕ 3m (10ft), ↔ 2.2m (7ft). ❄❄❄

***R.* 'Hannah Gordon'** ■ syn. *R.* 'Korweiso', *R.* 'Raspberry Ice'. Cluster-flowered bush rose of spreading, open habit, with dark green leaves. From summer to autumn, bears sprays of cupped, double, pale pink flowers, 8cm (3in) across, margined reddish pink. ↕ 80cm (32in), ↔ 65cm (26in). ❄❄❄

***R.* 'Harisonii'** see *R.* x *harisonii* 'Harison's Yellow'.

***R.* x *harisonii* 'Harison's Yellow'** ♀ syn. *R.* 'Harisonii'. Suckering Scots rose of gaunt habit, with prickly, dark brown stems and small, fern-like, mid-green leaves with 5–7 oval leaflets, 2cm (¾in) long. In summer, bears cupped, semi-double, bright deep yellow flowers, 5cm (2in) across, on short stems, followed by spherical-oblong, blackish red hips. ↕ 2m (6ft), ↔ 1.2m (4ft). ❄❄❄. **'Williams' Double Yellow'**, syn. *R.* 'Williams' Double Yellow', has a suckering, branching habit, and bears loosely double, fragrant flowers.

***R.* 'Harpade'** see *R.* 'Escapade'.

***R.* 'Harry Wheatcroft'** ■ syn. *R.* 'Caribia'. Vigorous large-flowered bush rose with glossy, reddish green leaves. Bears high-centred, double, scarlet-red flowers, 12cm (5in) across, with yellow-striped petals, from summer to autumn. ↕ 1m (3ft), ↔ 60cm (24in). ❄❄❄

***R.* 'Harvest Fayre'**, syn. *R.* 'Dicnorth'. Cluster-flowered bush rose with uneven growth and yellowish green leaves. Showy, rounded, double, apricot-orange flowers, 6cm (2½in) across, are borne

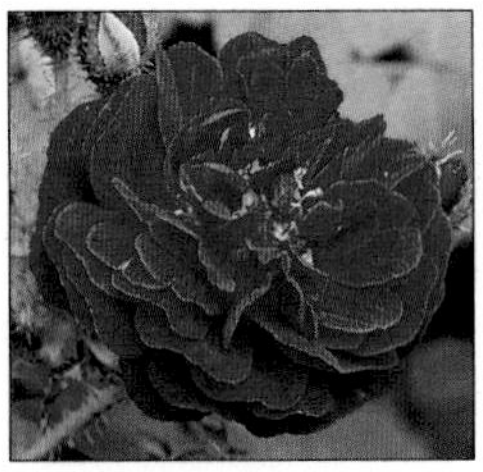
Rosa 'Henri Martin'

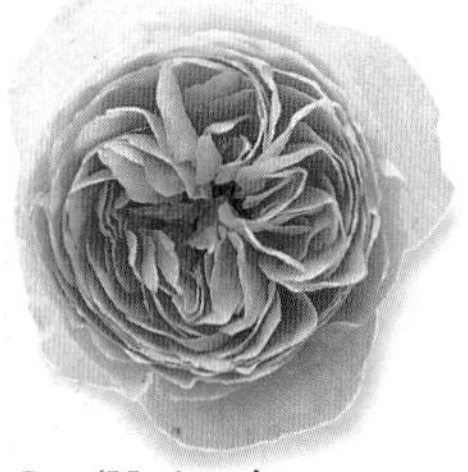
Rosa 'Heritage'

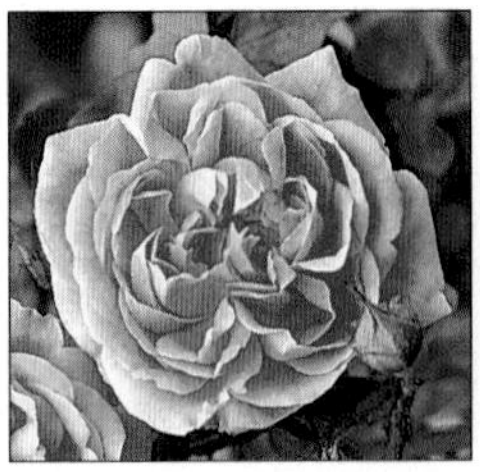
Rosa 'Hermosa'

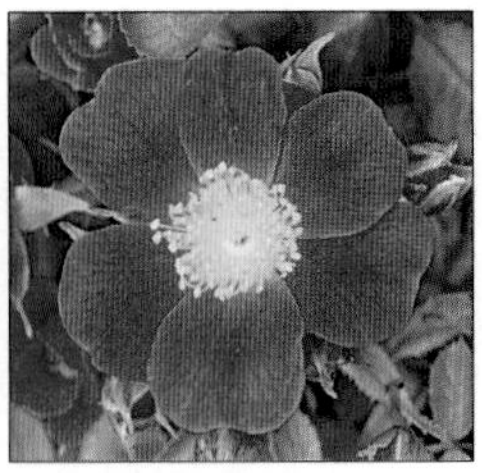
Rosa 'Hertfordshire'

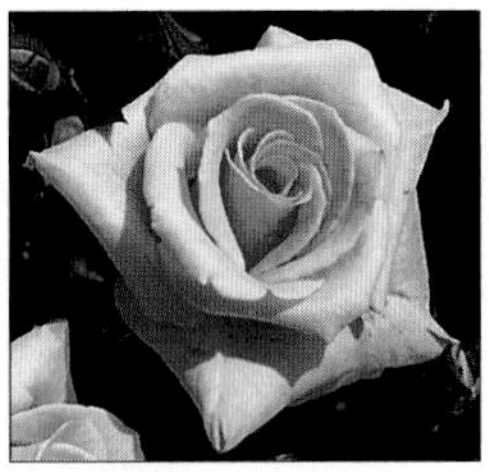
Rosa 'High Hopes'

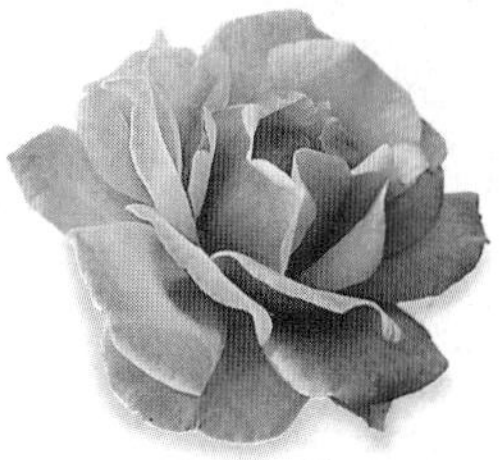
Rosa 'High Sheriff'

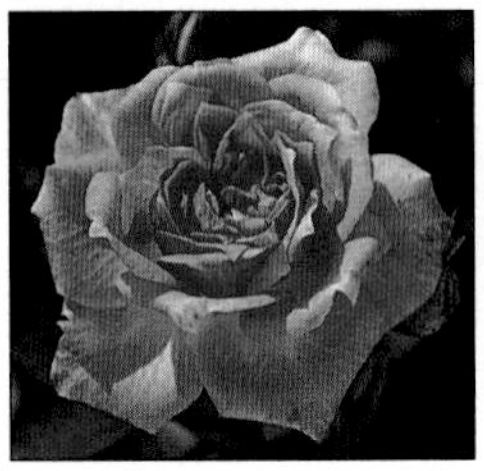
Rosa 'Hula Girl'

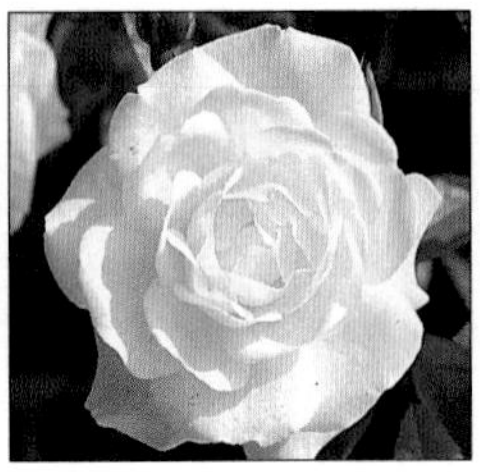
Rosa 'Iceberg'

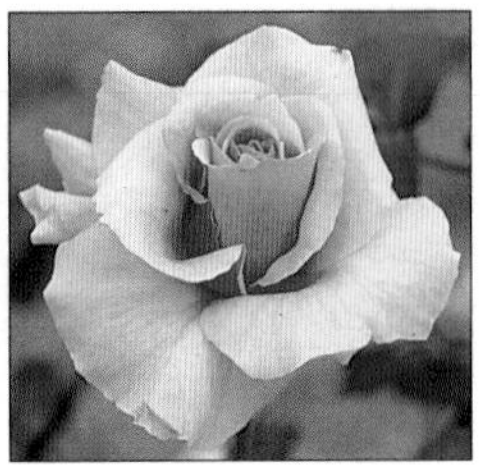
Rosa 'Iced Ginger'

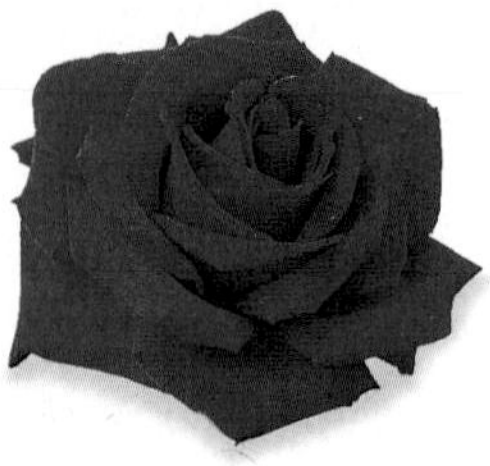
Rosa 'Ingrid Bergman'

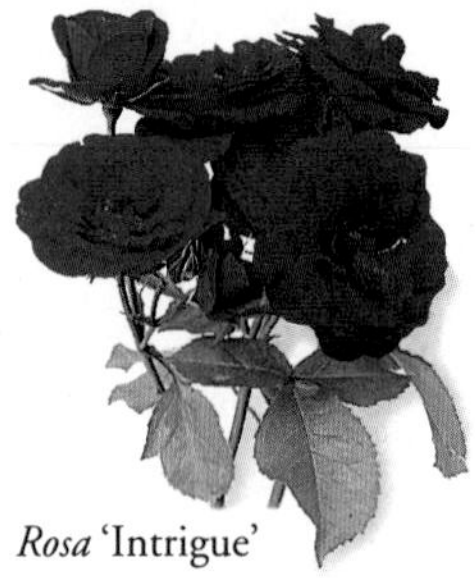
Rosa 'Intrigue'

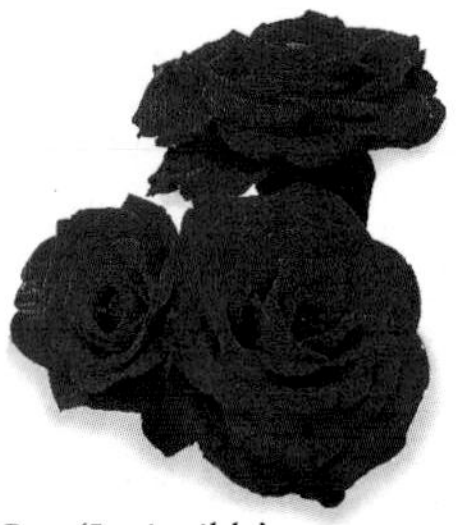
Rosa 'Invincible'

freely from summer to autumn. ↕75cm (30in), ↔ 60cm (24in). ***
***R.* 'Heart Throb'** see *R.* 'Paul Shirville'.
***R.* 'Heckenzauber'** see *R.* 'Sexy Rexy'.
***R.* 'Heidekönigin'** see *R.* 'Pheasant'.
***R.* 'Heideröslein'** see *R.* 'Nozomi'.
***R.* 'Heidetraum'** see *R.* 'Flower Carpet'.
***R.* 'Hello'**, syn. *R.* 'Cochello'. Dwarf cluster-flowered bush rose with dense, mid-green foliage. Numerous cupped to flat, single crimson flowers, 5cm (2in) across, with white eyes, are borne freely from summer to autumn. ↕↔ 45cm (18in). ***
***R.* 'Helmut Schmidt'** see *R.* 'Simba'.
***R.* 'Henri Martin'** ■ 🏆 (Red moss rose). Vigorous Moss rose of arching growth, with rough, dark green leaves. Rounded, double, scented crimson flowers, 8cm (3in) across, with light green moss on the stems and sepals, open in summer. ↕ to 2m (6ft), ↔ 1.2m (4ft). ***
***R.* 'Heritage'** ■ syn. *R.* 'Ausblush'. Vigorous shrub rose with dark green leaves. Open clusters of cupped, fully double, lemon-scented, light pink flowers, 11cm (4½in) across, with infolded petals, are borne from summer to autumn. ↕↔ 1.2m (4ft). ***
***R.* 'Hermosa'** ■ syn. *R.* 'Mélanie Lemaire', *R.* 'Mme Neumann'. Upright, bushy China rose with greyish green leaves, and rounded, double, scented, rose-pink flowers, 7cm (3in) across, borne freely from summer to autumn. ↕1m (3ft), ↔ 60cm (24in). ***
***R.* 'Hertfordshire'** ■ syn. *R.* 'Kortenay'. Ground-cover rose of compact, uneven, spiky habit, with dense, bright green leaves. Flat, single, carmine-pink flowers, 4.5cm (1¾in) across, with paler pink centres, are borne freely in large clusters on short stems, from summer to autumn. ↕45cm (18in), ↔ 1m (3ft). ***
***R.* 'Hiawatha'.** Vigorous, spreading rambler with leathery, semi-glossy, dark green foliage. In summer, bears large clusters of cupped, single crimson flowers, 4cm (1½in) across, with white eyes. ↕5m (15ft), ↔ 4m (12ft). ***
***R.* 'Highdownensis'** 🏆 syn. *R. moyesii* 'Highdownensis'. Vigorous shrub rose with dense growth and mid-green leaves, reddish green when young. Flat, single, deep pink flowers, 5cm (2in) across, with yellow stamens, borne close to the branches in summer, are followed by large, flask-shaped scarlet hips. ↕3m (10ft), ↔ 2m (6ft). ***
***R.* 'High Hopes'** ■ syn. *R.* 'Haryup'. Stiff, vigorous, arching climber with glossy, dark green leaves. Urn-shaped to rounded, double, scented, light rose-pink flowers, 8cm (3in) across, are borne freely from summer to autumn. ↕4m (12ft), ↔ 2.5m (8ft). ***
***R.* 'High Sheriff'** ■ syn. *R.* 'Harwellington'. Tall, free-branching, vigorous large-flowered bush rose with glossy, mid-green foliage. From summer to autumn, bears high-centred, double, peach-orange flowers, 10cm (4in) across, red on the reverse of the petals. ↕1.2m (4ft), ↔ 70cm (28in). ***
***R.* 'Hilgold'** see *R.* 'Golden Chersonese'.
***R.* 'Hotline'**, syn. *R.* 'Aromikeh'. Fast-growing, compact miniature bush rose with light mossing and mid-green leaves. High-centred to cupped, semi-double, mid-red flowers, 4cm (1½in) across, are borne from summer to autumn. ↕45cm (18in), ↔ 35cm (14in). ***
***R.* 'Hugh Dickson'.** Vigorous Hybrid Perpetual rose with lanky, arching, prickly stems and rough, dark green leaves. Rounded, fully double, fragrant crimson flowers, 10cm (4in) across, are borne from summer to autumn. ↕2.5m (8ft), ↔ 1.5m (5ft), trained against a support; ↕1.5m (5ft), ↔ 2.5m (8ft), if pegged down. ***
R. hugonis see *R. xanthina* f. *hugonis.*
***R.* 'Hula Girl'** ■ Miniature bush rose of neat, upright habit, with semi-glossy, mid-green foliage. Urn-shaped, fully double, lightly scented, pale orange-pink flowers, 3cm (1¼in) across, are borne from summer to autumn. ↕50cm (20in), ↔ 30cm (12in). ***
***R.* 'Iceberg'** ■ 🏆 syn. *R.* 'Fée des Neiges', *R.* 'Korbin', *R.* 'Schneewittchen'. Vigorous cluster-flowered bush rose of rounded habit, with abundant light green foliage. Large clusters of many cupped, double, creamy to pure white flowers, 7cm (3in) across, are borne freely from summer to autumn. ↕80cm (32in), ↔ 65cm (26in). ***
***R.* 'Iced Ginger'** ■ Cluster-flowered bush rose of lanky habit, with sparse, light green foliage. High-centred, fully double, buff to copper-pink flowers, 11cm (4½in) across, are borne from summer to autumn. ↕1m (3ft), ↔ 70cm (28in). ***
***R.* 'Immensee'** see *R.* 'Grouse'.
***R.* 'Incarnata'** see *R.* 'Maiden's Blush'.
***R.* 'Indian Summer'**, syn. *R.* 'Peaperfume'. Large-flowered bush rose of compact habit and uneven growth, with dark green foliage. Rounded, fully double, fragrant, creamy orange flowers, 11cm (4½in) across, are borne from summer to autumn. ↕55cm (22in), ↔ 60cm (24in). ***
***R.* 'Ingrid Bergman'** ■ 🏆 syn. *R.* 'Poulman'. Large-flowered bush rose of branching habit, with leathery, dark green leaves. High-centred, fully double, dark red flowers, 11cm (4½in) across, are produced from summer to autumn. ↕80cm (32in), ↔ 65cm (26in). ***
***R.* 'Integrity'** see *R.* 'Savoy Hotel'.
***R.* 'Intrigue'** ■ syn. *R.* 'Lavaglut'. Vigorous, cluster-flowered bush rose of compact habit, with glossy, purplish green leaves. Rounded, double, dark red flowers, 7cm (3in) across, are borne in large clusters from summer to autumn. ↕70cm (28in), ↔ 60cm (24in). **
***R.* 'Invincible'** ■ syn. *R.* 'Runatru'. Cluster-flowered bush rose of neat habit, with glossy, dark green foliage. Cupped, double, bright crimson flowers, 9cm (3½in) across, are borne in open clusters from summer to autumn. ↕70cm (28in), ↔ 50cm (20in). ***
***R.* 'Irish Beauty'** see *R.* 'Elizabeth of Glamis'.
***R.* 'Irish Gold'** see *R.* 'Grandpa Dickson'.
***R.* 'Irish Wonder'** see *R.* 'Evelyn Fison'.
***R.* 'Ispahan'** ■ 🏆 syn. *R.* 'Pompon des Princes', *R.* 'Rose d'Isfahan'. Vigorous Damask rose with abundant grey-green foliage. Cupped, double, fragrant, clear pink flowers, 8cm (3in) across, are borne throughout summer. ↕1.5m (5ft), ↔ 1.2m (4ft). ***
***R.* 'Jack Dayson'** see *R.* 'Perfect Moment'.
***R.* 'Jacqueline du Pré'** ■ 🏆 Vigorous, arching shrub rose with shiny, dark green leaves. Cupped, semi-double, musk-scented ivory flowers, 10cm (4in) across, with scalloped petals and red stamens, are borne from early summer to autumn. ↕1.5m (5ft), ↔ 1.2m (4ft). ***
***R.* 'Jacques Cartier'** see *R.* 'Marchesa Boccella'.
***R.* 'Jaune Desprez'** see *R.* 'Desprez à Fleur Jaune'.
***R.* 'Jeanne Lajoie'.** Miniature climber of bushy habit, producing glossy, dark green leaves and high-centred, fully double, lavender-pink flowers, 4.5cm (1¾in) across, from summer to autumn. ↕ to 2m (6ft) on a support, ↔ 70cm (28in). ***
***R.* 'Jenny Duval'** see *R.* 'Président de Sèze'.
***R.* 'John Cabot'** ■ Vigorous shrub rose producing abundant light green leaves. Clusters of cupped, double, scented magenta flowers, 6cm (2½in) across, are borne from summer to autumn. ↕1.5m (5ft), ↔ 1.2m (4ft). ***
***R.* 'John Waterer'.** Vigorous large-flowered bush rose producing deep green leaves. Bears long-petalled, high-centred, fully double, dark crimson flowers, 10cm (4in) across, from summer to autumn. ↕1.1m (3½ft), ↔ 70cm (28in). ***
***R.* 'Josephine Bruce'.** Large-flowered bush rose with short, splayed growth and dark green foliage. From summer to autumn, bears high-centred, double, fragrant, rich blackish crimson flowers, 12cm (5in) across. Prone to mildew. ↕75cm (30in), ↔ 60cm (24in). ***
***R.* 'Joseph's Coat'.** Vigorous, branching climber or shrub rose with dark green leaves. Showy clusters of urn-shaped to cupped, double yellow flowers, 8cm (3in) across, suffused orange-pink and red, are borne from summer to autumn. ↕↔ 3m (10ft) as a climber; ↕ to 1.2m (4ft), ↔ 1m (3ft) as a shrub. ***
***R.* 'Judy Garland'**, syn. *R.* 'Harking'. Vigorous cluster-flowered bush rose with semi-glossy, mid-green foliage. Cupped, double, lightly scented yellow flowers, 7cm (3in) across, the petals margined orange-red, are borne freely from summer to autumn. ↕75cm (30in), ↔ 65cm (26in). ***
***R.* 'Julia's Rose'** ■ Large-flowered bush rose with spindly, branching growth and sparse reddish green foliage. High-centred, double, brownish pink to buff flowers, 10cm (4in) across, are borne from summer to autumn. ↕75cm (30in), ↔ 45cm (18in). ***
***R.* 'Just Joey'** ■ 🏆 Large-flowered bush rose of open, branching habit, with sparse, dark green foliage. Rounded, fully double, fragrant, copper-pink flowers, 12cm (5in) across, with wavy-margined petals, are borne from summer

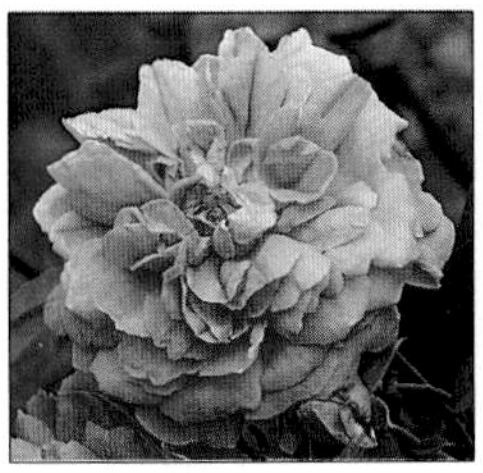
Rosa 'Ispahan'

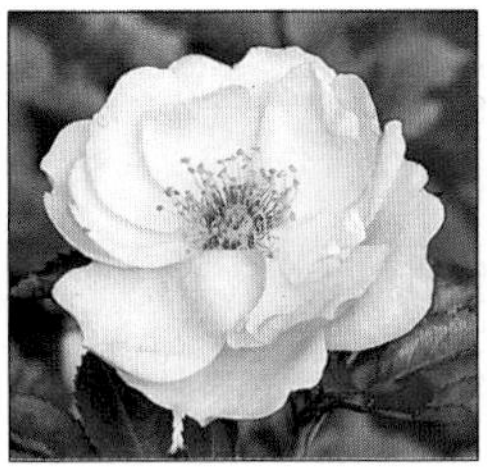
Rosa 'Jacqueline du Pré'

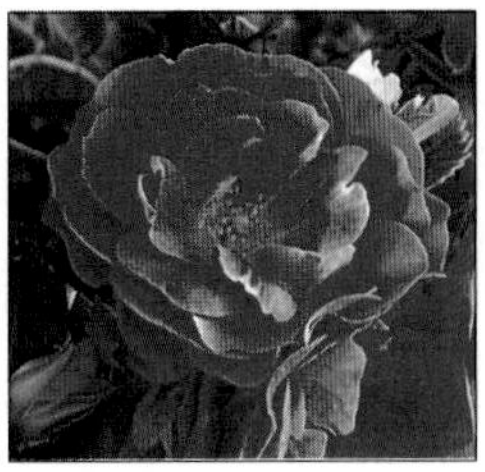
Rosa 'John Cabot'

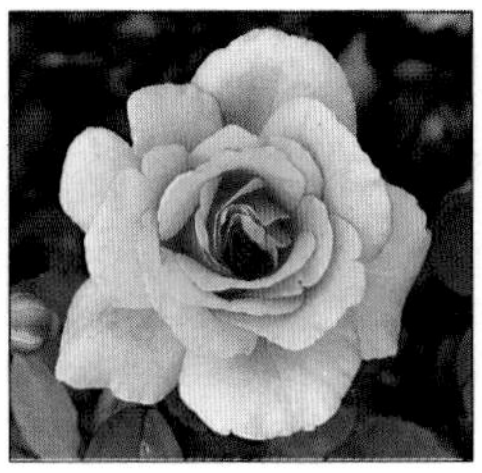
Rosa 'Julia's Rose'

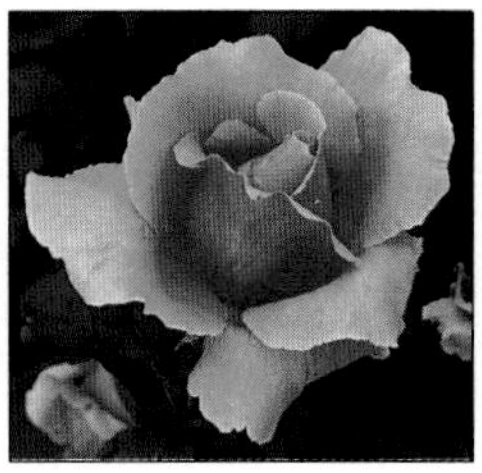
Rosa 'Just Joey'

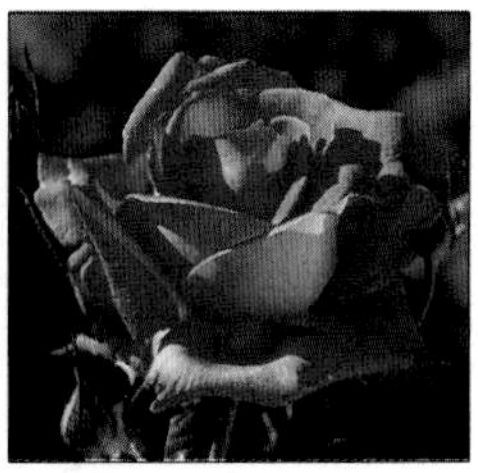
Rosa 'Keepsake'

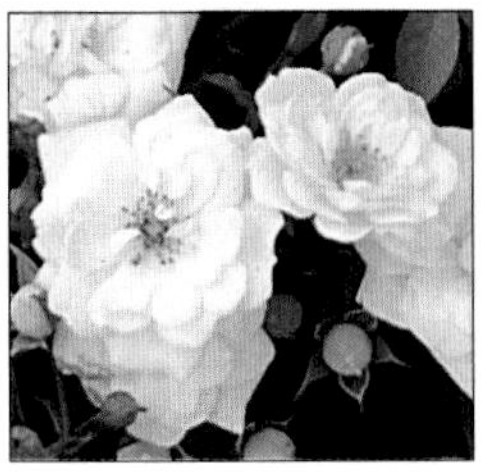
Rosa 'Kent'

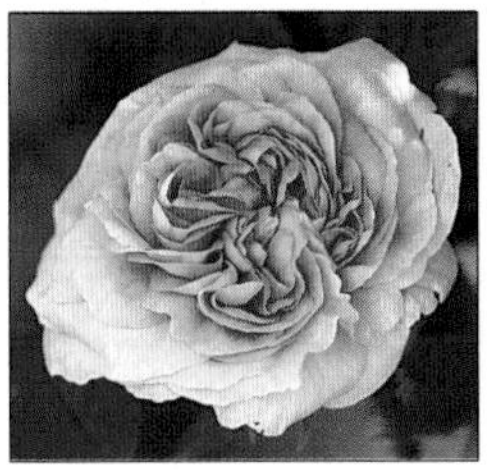
Rosa 'Königin von Dänemark'

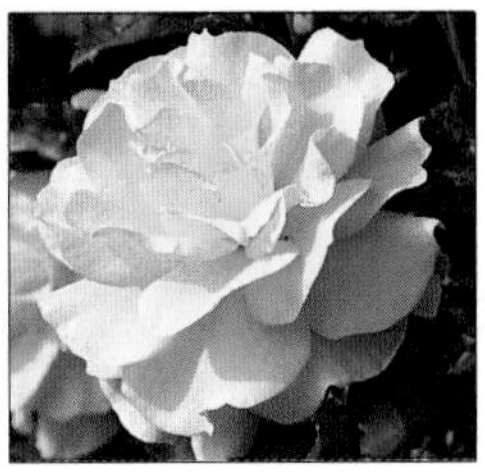
Rosa 'Korresia'

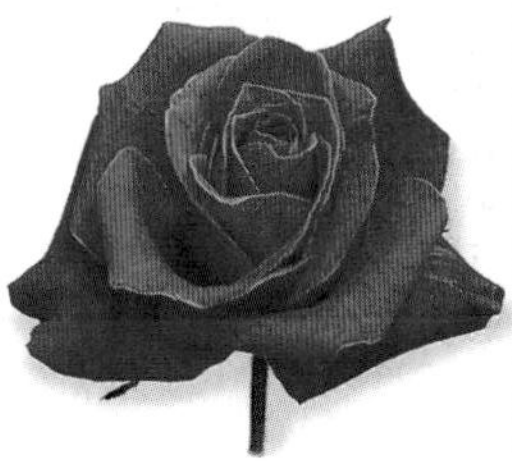
Rosa 'Lady Mitchell'

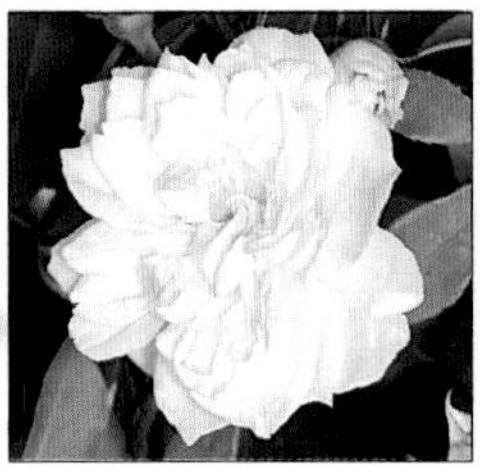
Rosa 'Lamarque'

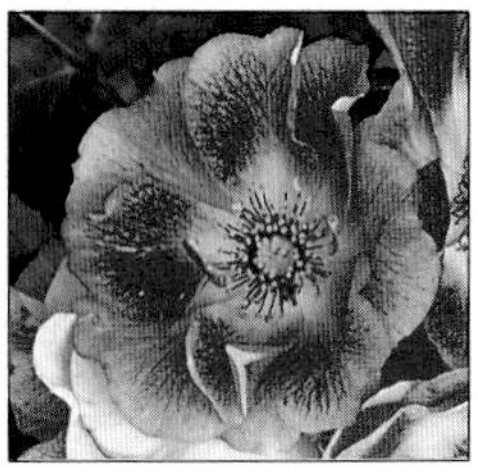
Rosa 'Laughter Lines'

to autumn. ↕75cm (30in), ↔70cm (28in). ❄❄❄

***R.* 'Katharina Zeimet'**, syn. *R.* 'White Baby Rambler'. Vigorous Polyantha bush rose producing abundant dark green leaves. From summer to autumn, bears dense clusters of cupped, double white flowers, 4.5cm (1¾in) across. ↕↔50cm (20in) or more. ❄❄❄

***R.* 'Kathleen Harrop'.** Bourbon rose of arching, lax habit, with dark green leaves. Cupped, double, fragrant, pale pink flowers, 8cm (3in) across, are borne from summer to autumn. Susceptible to mildew. ↕2.5m (8ft), ↔2m (6ft). ❄❄❄

***R.* 'Keepsake'** ■ syn. *R.* 'Esmeralda', *R.* 'Kormalda'. Large-flowered bush rose of uneven habit, with dark green leaves. From summer to autumn, bears well-formed, high-centred, fully double, lightly scented, deep pink flowers, 12cm (5in) across. ↕75cm (30in), ↔60cm (24in). ❄❄❄

***R.* 'Kent'** ■ syn. *R.* 'Poulcov', *R.* 'Pyrenees', *R.* 'White Cover'. Compact, spreading, ground-cover shrub rose with shiny, dark green leaves. Cupped to flat, semi-double white flowers, 4.5cm (1¾in) across, are borne on short stems from summer to autumn. ↕45cm (18in), ↔1m (3ft). ❄❄❄

***R.* 'Kew Rambler'.** Vigorous rambler with stiff but pliable growth and dense, grey-green leaves. Clusters of cupped, single, scented pink flowers, 4cm (1½in) across, each with a white eye and yellow stamens, are borne in summer. ↕5m (15ft), ↔4m (12ft). ❄❄❄

***R.* 'Kiftsgate'** see *R. filipes* 'Kiftsgate'.

***R.* 'King's Ransom'.** Large-flowered bush rose producing leathery, glossy, dark green leaves. Bears urn-shaped to cupped, fully double, lightly scented yellow flowers, 12cm (5in) across, on long stems from summer to autumn. ↕75cm (30in), ↔60cm (24in). ❄❄❄

***R.* 'Königin von Dänemark'** ■♀ syn. *R.* 'Belle Courtisane', *R.* 'Queen of Denmark'. Vigorous, lax Alba rose with dull, bluish green leaves. In midsummer, bears quartered-rosette, fully double, very fragrant, deep to light pink flowers, 9cm (3½in) across, with green button eyes. ↕1.5m (5ft), ↔1.2m (4ft). ❄❄❄

***R.* 'Königliche Hoheit'** see *R.* 'Royal Highness'.

***R.* 'Korbin'** see *R.* 'Iceberg'.

***R.* 'Kordes Robusta'** see *R.* 'Robusta'.

***R.* 'Korp'**, syn. *R.* 'Prominent'. Cluster-flowered bush rose with uneven growth and dark green foliage. Cupped, stiff-petalled, fully double, vivid orange-red flowers, 9cm (3½in) across, are borne on long stems from summer to autumn. ↕1m (3ft), ↔65cm (26in). ❄❄❄

***R.* 'Korresia'** ■ syn. *R.* 'Friesia', *R.* 'Sunsprite'. Compact cluster-flowered bush rose with light green leaves. Sprays of urn-shaped to cupped, double, fragrant, bright yellow flowers, 8cm (3in) across, with wavy-margined petals, are borne from summer to autumn. ↕75cm (30in), ↔60cm (24in). ❄❄❄

***R.* 'La Belle Sultane'** see *R.* 'Violacea'.

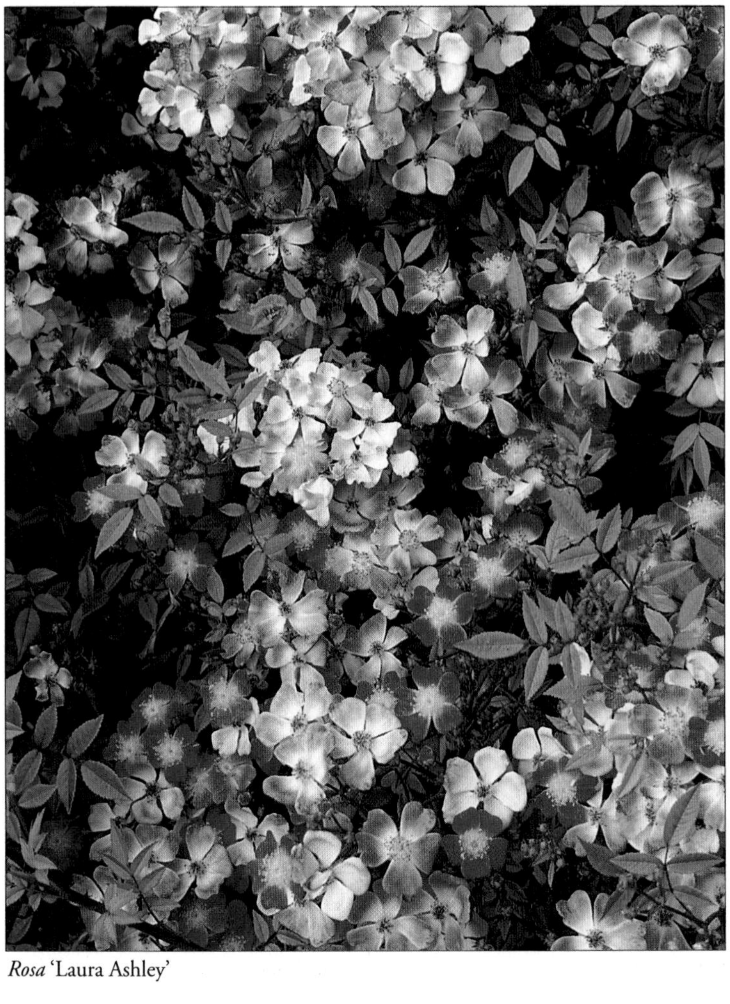
Rosa 'Laura Ashley'

***R.* 'Lac Rose'** see *R.* 'Grouse'.

***R.* 'Lady Mitchell'** ■ syn. *R.* 'Haryearn'. Large-flowered bush rose with dark green leaves and rounded, fully double, scented, deep pink flowers, 13cm (5in) across, borne from summer to autumn. ↕1m (3ft), ↔65cm (26in). ❄❄❄

***R.* 'Lady Penzance'.** Vigorous, twiggy, free-branching Sweet Briar rose with apple-scented, shiny, dark green leaves. Cupped, single, copper-pink and yellow flowers, 4cm (1½in) across, are borne briefly in midsummer, followed by ovoid red hips. ↕↔2m (6ft). ❄❄❄

R. laevigata, syn. *R.* 'Golden Cherry' (Camellia rose, Cherokee rose). Vigorous species rose with large prickles, arching stems, and attractive, glossy, dark green leaves, each with 3, rarely 5, lance-shaped to elliptic or ovate leaflets, 3–6cm (1¼–2½in) long. Solitary, flat, single, scented white flowers, to 10cm (4in) across, with scalloped petals and gold stamens, are borne in summer; they are followed by pear-shaped, bristly, brownish orange-red hips. Evergreen in mild climates. ↕↔2–6m (6–20ft). E. and S. China, Taiwan, S.E. Asia. ❄❄

***R.* 'L'Aimant'**, syn. *R.* 'Harzola'. Vigorous cluster-flowered bush rose with dark green foliage. Cupped, double, fragrant, reddish salmon-pink flowers, 9cm (3½in) across, are borne from summer to autumn. ↕1m (3ft), ↔75cm (30in). ❄❄❄

***R.* 'Lamarque'** ■ Vigorous Noisette climbing rose with smooth stems and limp, shiny, bright green foliage. Flat, quartered-rosette, fully double, fragrant, yellowish white flowers, 9cm (3½in) across, are borne on nodding stems from summer to autumn. ↕to 5m (15ft), ↔2.5m (8ft). ❄❄

***R.* 'Landora'** see *R.* 'Sunblest'.

***R.* 'La Reine Victoria'** see *R.* 'Reine Victoria'.

***R.* 'La Royale'** see *R.* 'Maiden's Blush'.

***R.* 'La Séduisante'** see *R.* 'Great Maiden's Blush'.

***R.* 'Las Vegas'**, syn. *R.* 'Korgane'. Vigorous large-flowered bush rose with glossy, mid-green foliage. From summer to autumn, bears urn-shaped, double, deep orange flowers, 10cm (4in) across, with a yellow reverse to the petals. ↕1m (3ft), ↔65cm (26in). ❄❄❄

***R.* 'Laughter Lines'** ■ syn. *R.* 'Dickerry'. Cluster-flowered bush rose of upright habit, with crisp, dark green foliage. Cupped, semi-double, rose-pink flowers, opening wide to 9cm (3½in) across, with red, gold, and white markings, are borne from summer to autumn. ↕70cm (28in), ↔60cm (24in). ❄❄❄

***R.* 'Laura Ashley'** ■ syn. *R.* 'Chewharla'. Dense, compact ground-cover rose producing abundant mid-green leaves. Large clusters of cupped to flat, single, magenta-pink to lilac flowers, 3cm (1¼in) across, with pale yellow centres, cover the plant from summer to autumn. ↕60cm (24in), ↔1.2m (4ft). ❄❄❄

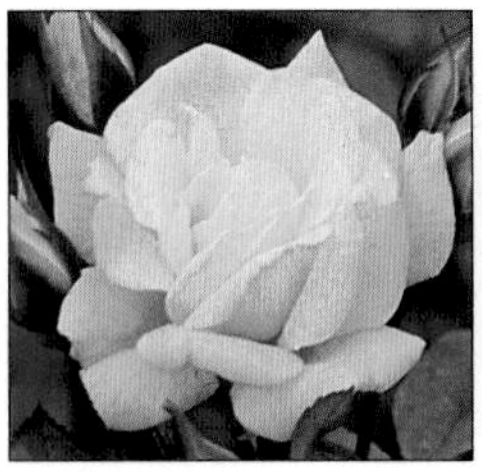

Rosa 'Laura Ford'

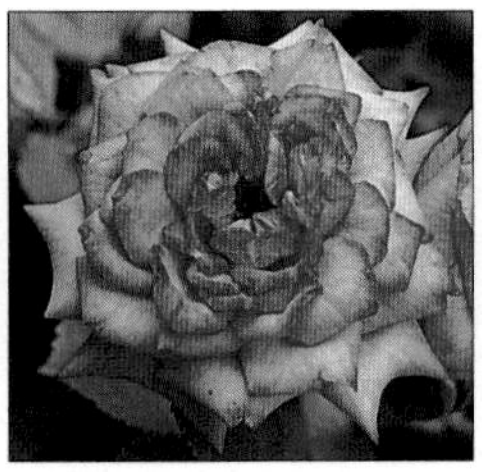

Rosa 'Lavender Jewel'

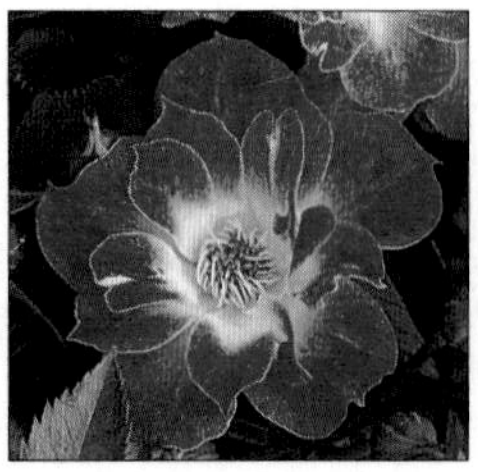

Rosa 'Little Artist'

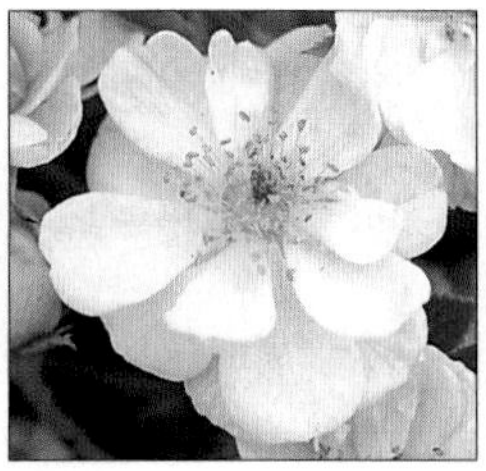

Rosa 'Little Bo-Peep'

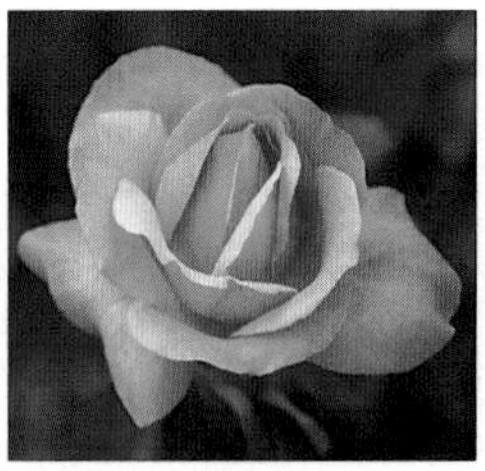

Rosa 'Lovely Lady'

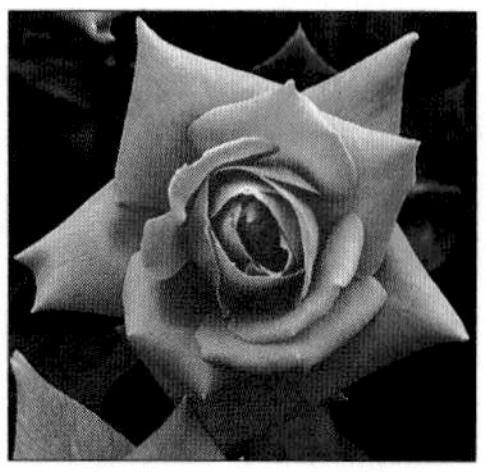

Rosa 'Lovers' Meeting'

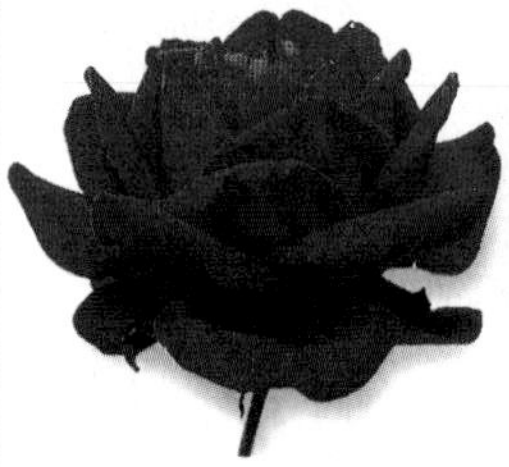

Rosa 'Loving Memory'

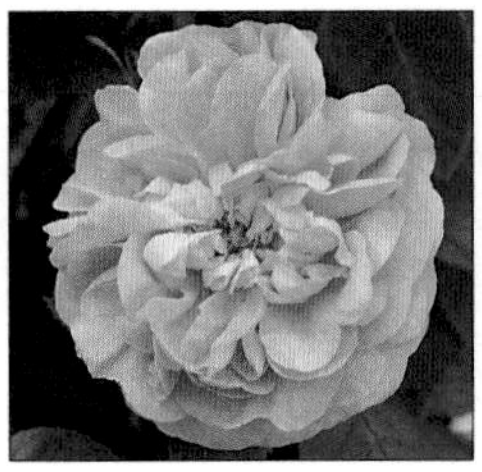

Rosa 'Maiden's Blush'

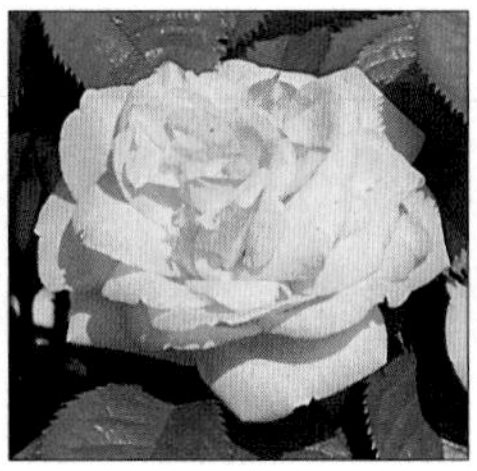

Rosa 'Maigold'

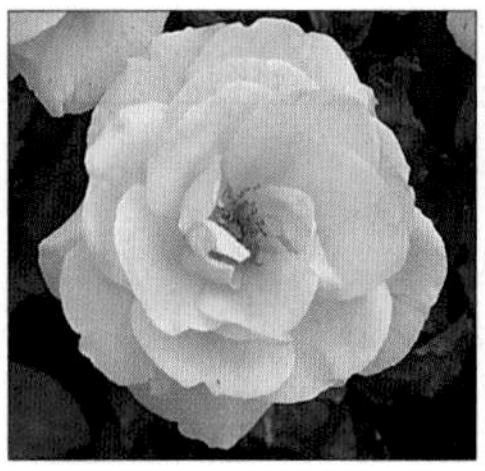

Rosa 'Many Happy Returns'

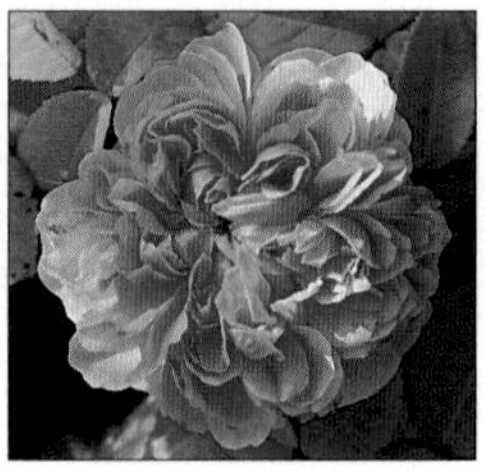

Rosa 'Marchesa Boccella'

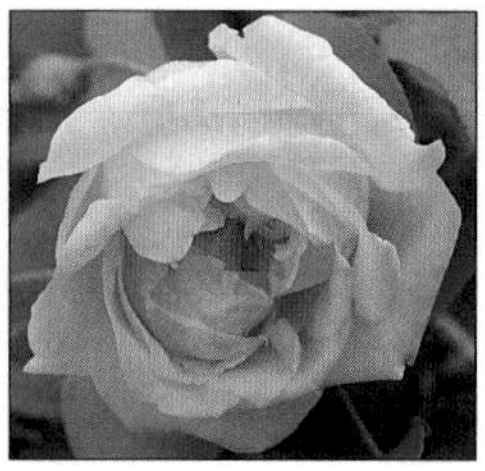

Rosa 'Maréchal Niel'

***R.* 'Laura Ford'** ▣ syn. *R.* 'Chewarvel'. Stiff, upright, miniature climber with abundant shiny, light green leaves. From summer to autumn, bears clusters of urn-shaped to flat, semi-double, lightly scented yellow flowers, 4.5cm (1¾in) across, becoming pink tinged with age. ↕2.2m (7ft), ↔ 1.2m (4ft). ❄❄❄

***R.* 'Lavender Jewel'** ▣ Miniature bush rose of neat, spreading habit, with dark green foliage. Cupped, double, lavender-pink flowers, 4cm (1½in) across, are produced in clusters from summer to autumn. ↕↔ 30cm (12in). ❄❄❄

***R.* 'L.D. Braithwaite'**, syn. *R.* 'Auscrim'. Open shrub rose producing greyish green leaves. Loosely formed, rosette-shaped, fully double, scented, bright crimson flowers, 9cm (3½in) across, with infolded petals, are borne from summer to autumn. ↕ 1m (3ft), ↔ 1.2m (4ft). ❄❄❄

***R.* 'Leda'** (Painted damask rose). Lax Damask rose with prickly stems and grey-green leaves. In summer, bears rosette-shaped, fully double, fragrant, carmine-tipped white flowers, 7cm (3in) across, with button centres, reflexing into a ball. ↕↔ 1m (3ft). ❄❄❄

***R.* 'Legnews'** see *R.* 'News'.

***R.* 'Lemon Pillar'** see *R.* 'Paul's Lemon Pillar'.

***R.* 'Leverkusen'.** Vigorous, arching climber producing toothed, glossy, deep green leaves. Clusters of wide-opening, rosette-shaped, double, lightly scented, pale yellow flowers, 8cm (3in) across, are borne from summer to autumn. May be grown as a shrub. ↕ 3m (10ft), ↔ 2.2m (7ft). ❄❄❄

***R.* 'Little Artist'** ▣ syn. *R.* 'Top Gear'. Neat, upright miniature bush rose with mid-green foliage. Cupped to flat, semi-double red flowers, 4.5cm (1¾in) across, with white markings, are borne on short, stiff stems from summer to autumn. ↕↔ 30cm (12in). ❄❄❄

***R.* 'Little Bo-Peep'** ▣ syn. *R.* 'Poullen'. Dwarf cluster-flowered bush rose of low, spreading habit, with dark green foliage. Dense clusters of many rounded to flat, semi-double, light pink flowers, 4cm (1½in) across, are borne close to the plant from summer to autumn. ↕ 30cm (12in), ↔ 50cm (20in). ❄❄❄

***R.* 'Little White Pet'** ▣🏆 syn. *R.* 'White Pet'. Vigorous, free-branching Polyantha rose with deep green foliage. From summer to autumn, red buds open to dense sprays of rosette-shaped, fully double white flowers, 4cm (1½in) across. ↕ 45cm (18in), ↔ 55cm (22in) with hard pruning. ❄❄❄

***R. longicuspis* of gardens** see *R. mulliganii.*

***R.* 'L'Ouche'** see *R.* 'Louise Odier'.

***R.* 'Louise Odier'**, syn. *R.* 'L'Ouche', *R.* 'Mme de Stella'. Bourbon rose of slender, arching growth, with light grey-green foliage. Camellia-shaped, rosetted, fully double, fragrant pink flowers, 9cm (3½in) across, with lilac tints, are borne from summer to autumn. ↕ 2m (6ft), ↔ 1.2m (4ft). ❄❄❄

***R.* 'Lovely Lady'** ▣🏆 syn. *R.* 'Dicjubell'. Large-flowered bush rose with a vigorous, free-branching habit and abundant glossy, mid-green leaves. Urn-shaped, fully double, scented, salmon-pink flowers, 10cm (4in) across, are borne from summer to autumn. ↕ 75cm (30in), ↔ 60cm (24in). ❄❄❄

***R.* 'Lovers' Meeting'** ▣ Free-branching large-flowered bush rose of vigorous, spreading habit, with bronze-green foliage. High-centred, double, reddish orange flowers, 9cm (3½in) across, are borne singly and in wide sprays from summer to autumn. ↕↔ 75cm (30in). ❄❄❄

***R.* 'Loving Memory'** ▣ syn. *R.* 'Burgund '81', *R.* 'Korgund'. Robust large-flowered bush rose with dull, dark green leaves. High-centred, fully double, lightly scented, dark red flowers, 12cm (5in) across, are borne on strong, stiff stems from summer to autumn. ↕ 1.1m (3½ft), ↔ 75cm (30in). ❄❄❄

R. lucida see *R. virginiana.*

***R.* 'Lü E'** see *R.* x *odorata* 'Viridiflora'.

***R.* 'Macrantha Raubritter'** see *R.* 'Raubritter'.

R. macrophylla. Vigorous species rose producing red stems and mid-green leaves, each composed of 7–11 oval leaflets, to 6cm (2½in) long. Flat, single, scented red flowers, 5–7cm (2–3in) across, are borne singly or in clusters of up to 5 in summer, followed by flask-shaped red hips. ↕ 4m (12ft), ↔ 3m (10ft). Himalayas, from Pakistan to W. China. ❄❄❄

***R.* 'Magenta'.** Shrubby, spreading cluster-flowered bush rose with leathery, dark green leaves. Quartered-rosette, fully double, fragrant, pink-magenta flowers, 9cm (3½in) across, are borne in heavy clusters on bowed stems from summer to autumn. ↕ 1.5m (5ft), ↔ 1.2m (4ft). ❄❄❄

***R.* 'Magic Carrousel'.** Miniature bush rose of neat, bushy habit, with glossy, mid-green leaves. Rosette-shaped, double, pale yellow flowers, 4cm (1½in) across, with crimson edging, are produced from summer to autumn. ↕ 40cm (16in), ↔ 30cm (12in). ❄❄❄

***R.* 'Maiden's Blush'** ▣ syn. *R.* 'Incarnata', *R.* 'La Royale'. Vigorous, upright, arching Alba rose with dull, bluish green foliage. Cupped, fully double, fragrant, very pale pink flowers, 7cm (3in) across, with irregular centres, are borne in midsummer. ↕ 1.2m (4ft), ↔ 90cm (36in). ❄❄❄

***R.* 'Maigold'** ▣🏆 Strong, stiff-growing climber with very prickly, arching stems and leathery, dark green leaves. Cupped, semi-double, scented, bronze-yellow flowers, 10cm (4in) across, are borne freely in early summer and sparsely again in autumn. ↕↔ 2.5m (8ft). ❄❄❄

***R.* 'Mainzer Fastnacht'** see *R.* 'Blue Moon'.

***R.* 'Many Happy Returns'** ▣🏆 syn. *R.* 'Harwanted', *R.* 'Prima'. Cluster-flowered bush rose of shrubby habit, with attractive, shiny, mid-green foliage. Cupped, semi-double, scented, pale pink flowers, 10cm (4in) across, are borne in dense clusters from summer to autumn. ↕↔ 75cm (30in). ❄❄❄

***R.* 'Marchesa Boccella'** ▣🏆 syn. *R.* 'Jacques Cartier'. Portland rose of dense habit, with abundant light green foliage. Quartered-rosette, fully double, scented, rose-pink flowers, 11cm (4½in) across, are borne on short stems from summer to autumn. ↕ 1.2m (4ft), ↔ 1m (3ft). ❄❄❄

***R.* 'Maréchal le Clerc'** see *R.* 'Touch of Class'.

***R.* 'Maréchal Niel'** ▣ Vigorous Noisette or climbing Tea rose with long, shiny, rich green leaves. High-centred, fully double, scented, clear yellow flowers, 10cm (4in) across, are produced on nodding stems from summer to

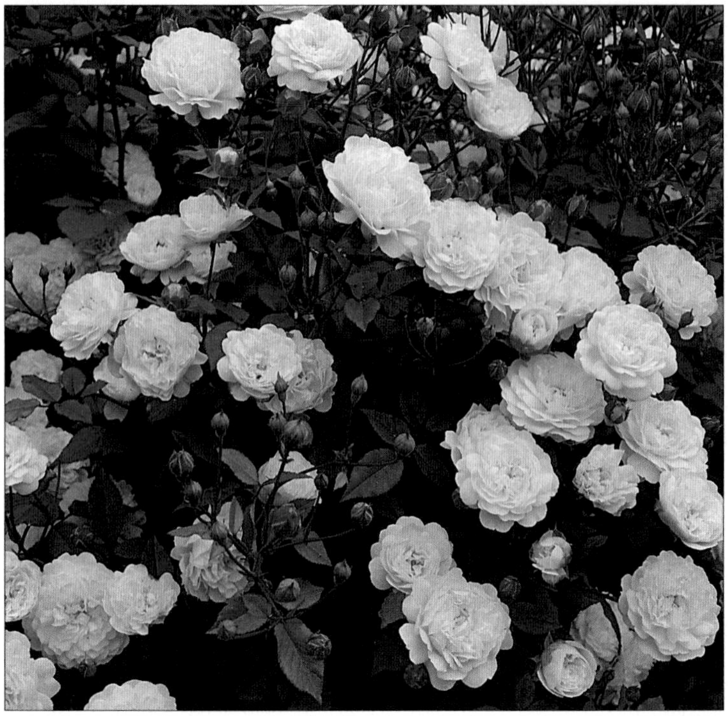

Rosa 'Little White Pet'

R

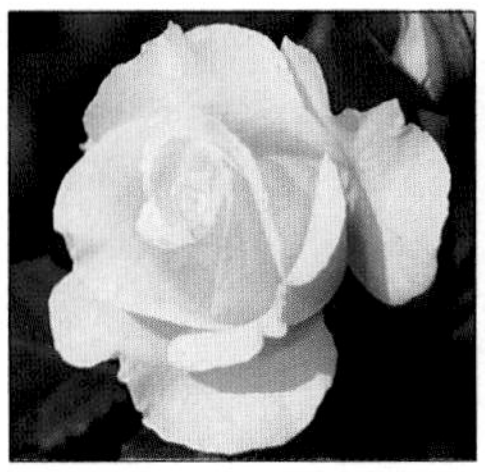
Rosa 'Margaret Merril'

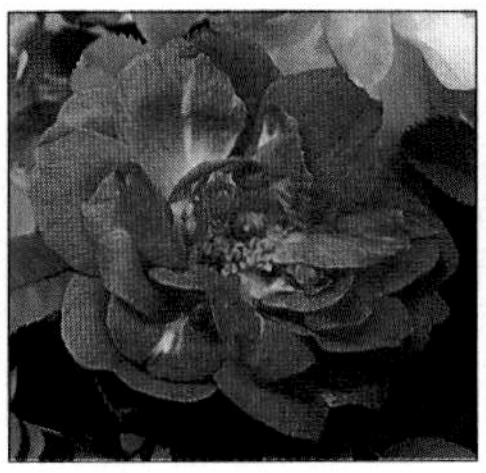
Rosa 'Marguerite Hilling'

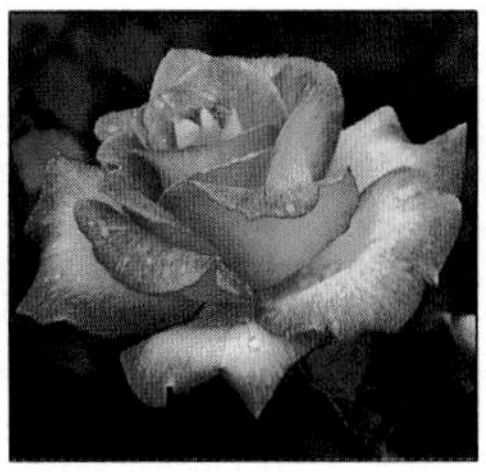
Rosa 'Marion Harkness'

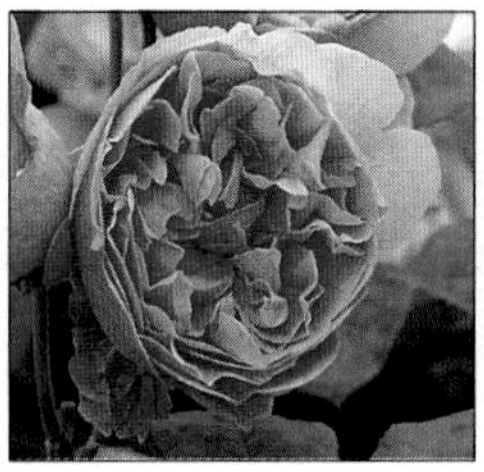
Rosa 'Mary Rose'

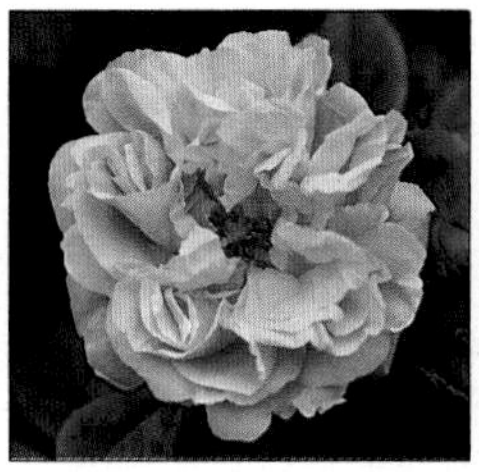
Rosa 'May Queen'

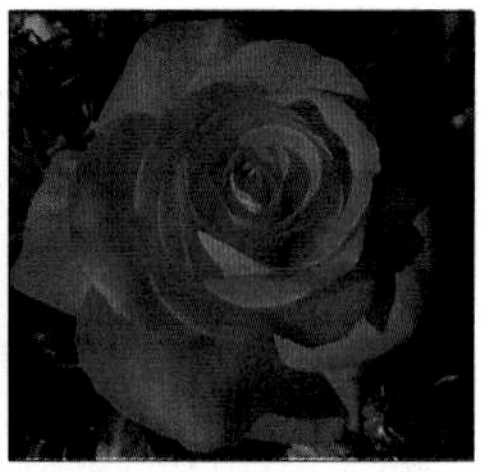
Rosa 'Melody Maker'

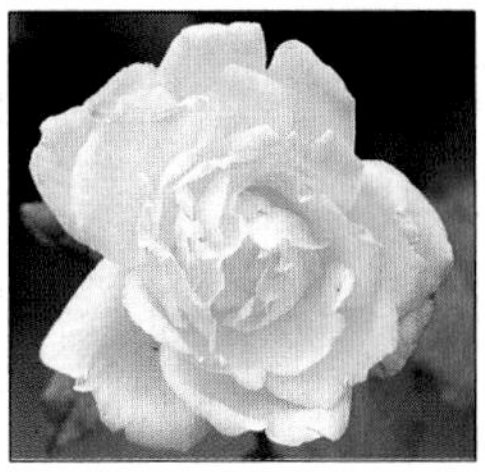
Rosa 'Mme Alfred Carrière'

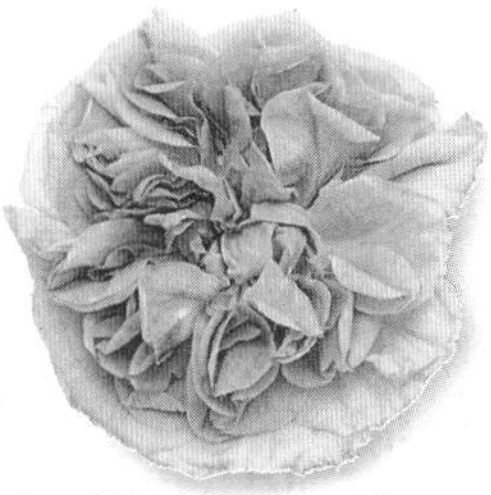
Rosa 'Mme de Sancy de Parabère'

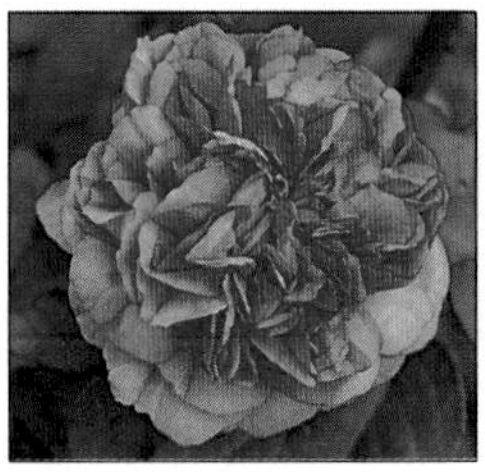
Rosa 'Mme Ernst Calvat'

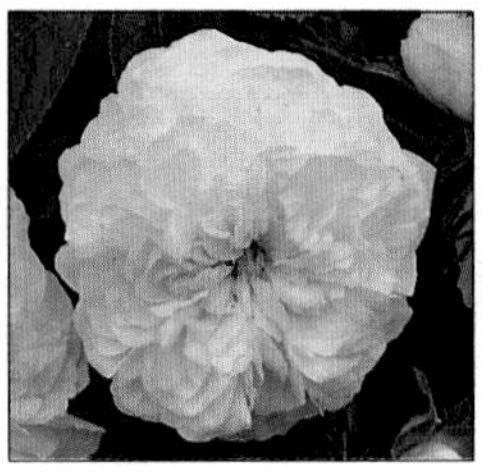
Rosa 'Mme Hardy'

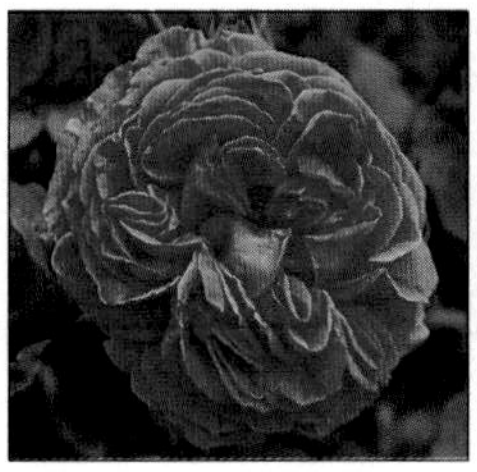
Rosa 'Mme Isaac Pereire'

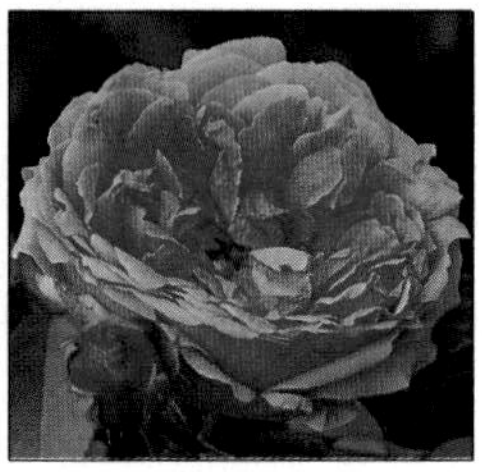
Rosa 'Mme Knorr'

autumn. ↕ to 5m (15ft), ↔ 2.5m (8ft). ❄❄❄ (borderline)

***R.* 'Margaret Merril'** ■ 🏆 syn. *R.* 'Harkuly'. Cluster-flowered bush rose with crisp, dark green leaves. Bears high-centred to cupped, double, fragrant, pale pink to white flowers, 10cm (4in) across, with maroon stamens, singly or in clusters from summer to autumn. ↕ 80cm (32in), ↔ 60cm (24in). ❄❄❄

***R.* 'Marguerite Hilling'** ■ 🏆 syn. *R.* 'Pink Nevada'. Vigorous, arching shrub rose with red stems and dense, light green foliage. Flat, semi-double, scented, rose-pink flowers, 10cm (4in) across, with deeper shading, are borne freely in early summer and sparsely in autumn. ↕↔ 2.2m (7ft). ❄❄❄

***R.* 'Mariandel'** see *R.* 'The Times'.

***R.* 'Marion Harkness'** ■ syn. *R.* 'Harkantabil'. Large-flowered bush rose of well-branched habit, with glossy, dark green leaves. Rounded, double yellow flowers, 9cm (3½in) across, shaded orange-red towards the petal tips, are borne freely from summer to autumn. ↕ 75cm (30in), ↔ 60cm (24in). ❄❄❄

***R.* 'Marjorie Fair'**, syn. *R.* 'Red Ballerina', *R.* 'Red Yesterday'. Dense Polyantha shrub rose with glossy, mid-green leaves. Mop-headed clusters of many cupped, single, wine-red flowers, 4.5cm (1¾in) across, each with a white eye, are borne from summer to autumn. ↕↔ 1.2m (4ft). ❄❄❄

***R.* 'Marlena'.** Cluster-flowered bush rose of compact habit, with dark green leaves. Sprays of cupped, double, bright crimson flowers, 6cm (2½in) across, are borne freely from summer to autumn. ↕↔ 45cm (18in). ❄❄❄

***R.* 'Mary Rose'** ■ syn. *R.* 'Ausmary'. Shrub rose of upright, uneven growth, with matt, mid-green leaves. Cupped, double, scented, deep rose-pink flowers, 9cm (3½in) across, are borne from summer to autumn. ↕ 1.2m (4ft), ↔ 1m (3ft). ❄❄❄

***R.* 'Masquerade'.** Vigorous cluster-flowered bush rose of compact habit, with leathery, dark green leaves. From summer to autumn, bears sprays of cupped to flat, semi-double flowers, to 6cm (2½in) across, changing in colour from yellow to pink and dark red. ↕ 80cm (32in), ↔ 60cm (24in). ❄❄❄

***R.* 'Matangi'** syn. *R.* 'Macman'. Compact cluster-flowered bush rose with abundant glossy, dark green leaves. Showy, open-cupped, double, rich orange-red flowers, 9cm (3½in) across, with white in the centres and on the reverse of the petals, are borne from summer to autumn. ↕ 80cm (32in), ↔ 60cm (24in). ❄❄❄

***R.* 'Matthias Meilland'** syn. *R.* 'Meifolio'. Cluster-flowered bush rose with glossy, dark green foliage. Cupped, double, bright deep scarlet flowers, 8cm (3in) across, are borne from summer to autumn. ↕ 75cm (30in), ↔ 60cm (24in). ❄❄❄

***R.* 'May Queen'** ■ Vigorous, arching rambler with abundant glossy, mid-green foliage. In summer, bears clusters of quartered-rosette, apple-scented, double, clear rose-pink flowers, 8cm (3in) across. ↕ 4m (12ft), ↔ 3m (10ft). ❄❄❄

***R.* 'Meg'.** Stiff, vigorous climber with dark green leaves. Bears open clusters of cupped to flat, semi-double, fragrant, pink-apricot to pink flowers, 12cm (5in) across, with red stamens, from summer to autumn. ↕↔ 4m (12ft). ❄❄❄

***R.* 'Mélanie Lemaire'** see *R.* 'Hermosa'.

***R.* 'Melody Maker'** ■ syn. *R.* 'Dicqueen'. Cluster-flowered bush rose of dense habit, with abundant dark green foliage. Freely bears rounded, fully double, light scarlet flowers, 9cm (3½in) across, from summer to autumn. ↕ 70cm (28in), ↔ 60cm (24in). ❄❄❄

***R.* 'Mermaid'** 🏆 Vigorous, slow-growing climber with stiff, red-brown stems, hooked thorns, and shiny, dark green leaves. From summer to autumn, bears cupped to flat, single, primrose-yellow flowers, 11cm (4½in) across, with sulphur-yellow stamens. ↕↔ to 6m (20ft). ❄❄❄

***R.* 'Mevrouw Nathalie Nypels'** 🏆 Cluster-flowered Polyantha rose of neat habit, with glossy, mid-green leaves. Freely bears cupped, semi-double, rose-pink flowers, 6cm (2½in) across, from summer to autumn. ↕ 75cm (30in), ↔ 60cm (24in). ❄❄❄

***R.* 'Michèle Meilland'.** Large-flowered bush rose of well-branched, leafy habit, with mid-green foliage. Neatly formed, urn-shaped, double, light pink flowers, 9cm (3½in) across, are borne from summer to autumn. Excellent for flower arrangements. ↕ 1m (3ft), ↔ 60cm (24in). ❄❄❄

***R.* 'Mignon'** see *R.* 'Cécile Brunner'.

***R.* 'Mildred Scheel'** see *R.* 'Deep Secret'.

***R.* 'Minuetto'** see *R.* 'Darling Flame'.

***R.* 'Mischief'.** Large-flowered bush rose producing abundant but rust-prone, mid-green leaves. Urn-shaped, double, scented, pink-orange to pink flowers, 10cm (4in) across, are borne from summer to autumn. ↕ 1m (3ft), ↔ 60cm (24in). ❄❄❄

***R.* 'Mme Alfred Carrière'** ■ 🏆 Noisette climbing rose with slender, smooth stems and pale green foliage. Rounded, fully double, fragrant, pale pink to white flowers, 6cm (2½in) across, are borne from summer to autumn. ↕ 5m (15ft), ↔ 3m (10ft). ❄❄❄

***R.* 'Mme A. Meilland'** see *R.* 'Peace'.

***R.* 'Mme Butterfly'.** Large-flowered bush rose with stiff growth and sparse, mid-green foliage. Neatly formed, urn-shaped to cupped, double, fragrant, light pink flowers, 8cm (3in) across, are borne from summer to autumn. ↕ 1m (3ft), ↔ 60cm (24in). ❄❄❄

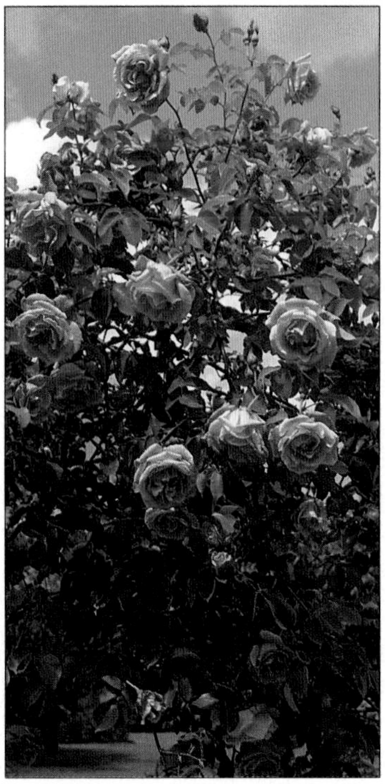
Rosa 'Mme Grégoire Staechelin'

***R.* 'Mme de la Roche-Lambert'** see *R.* 'Mme Delaroche-Lambert'.

***R.* 'Mme Delaroche-Lambert'** 🏆 syn. *R.* 'Mme de la Roche-Lambert'. Upright, arching Moss rose with rough, dull, light to mid-green leaves and brownish green moss. Rounded, fully double, scented, purplish pink flowers, 8cm (3in) across, some with button centres, are borne mainly in summer, sometimes also in autumn. ↕ 1.2m (4ft), ↔ 1m (3ft). ❄❄❄

***R.* 'Mme de Sancy de Parabère'** ■ Vigorous, arching Boursault climbing rose with smooth green wood and dark green leaves. Rosette-shaped, double, clear rose-pink flowers, 12cm (5in) across, are borne in early summer. ↕ 5m (15ft), ↔ 3m (10ft). ❄❄

***R.* 'Mme de Stella'** see *R.* 'Louise Odier'.

***R.* 'Mme Ernst Calvat'** ■ Vigorous, arching Bourbon rose with dark green leaves, purplish green when young. From summer to autumn, produces quartered-rosette, fully double, fragrant, rose-pink flowers, 15cm (6in) across. ↕ 2m (6ft), ↔ 1.2m (4ft). ❄❄❄

***R.* 'Mme Grégoire Staechelin'** ■ 🏆 syn. *R.* 'Spanish Beauty'. Very vigorous, arching climber with masses of large, dark green leaves. Rounded, fully double flowers, 12cm (5in) across, with ruffled, red-flushed, clear pink petals, are borne in early summer. Flowers are followed by large, spherical red hips. ↕ to 6m (20ft), ↔ 4m (12ft). ❄❄❄

***R.* 'Mme Hardy'** ■ 🏆 Vigorous, upright Damask rose with abundant leathery, dark green leaves. Quartered-rosette, fully double, fragrant white flowers, 10cm (4in) across, each with a green button eye, are produced in summer. ↕ 1.5m (5ft), ↔ 1.2m (4ft). ❄❄❄

***R.* 'Mme Hébert'** see *R.* 'Président de Sèze'.

***R.* 'Mme Isaac Pereire'** ■ 🏆 Vigorous, arching Bourbon shrub or climbing rose with large, dark green leaves. From summer to autumn, bears quartered-rosette, fully double, fragrant, deep purplish pink flowers, 15cm (6in) across. ↕ 2.2m (7ft), ↔ 2m (6ft). ❄❄❄

***R.* 'Mme Knorr'** ■ 🏆 syn. *R.* 'Comte de Chambord'. Bushy, leafy, vigorous Portland rose with mid-green foliage. From summer to autumn, bears

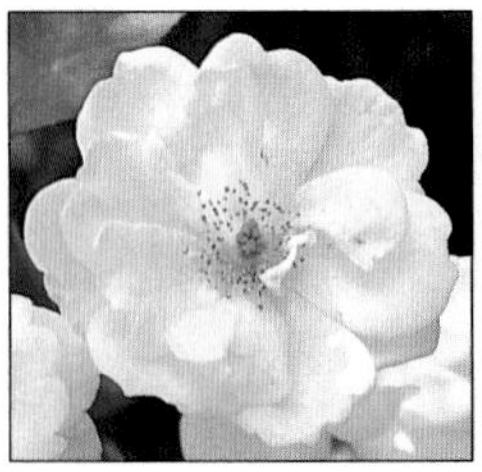
Rosa 'Moonlight'

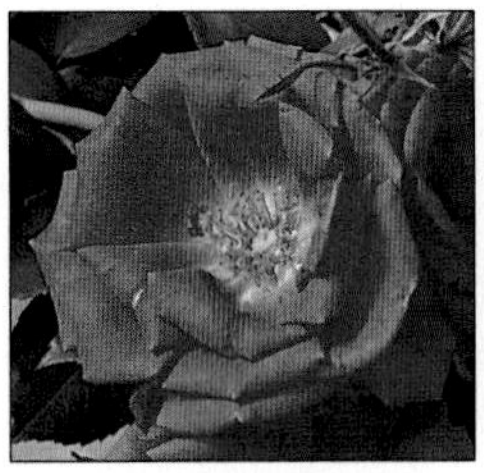
Rosa 'Morning Jewel'

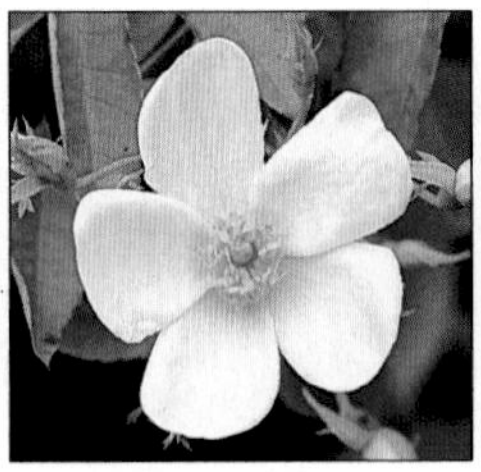
Rosa moschata

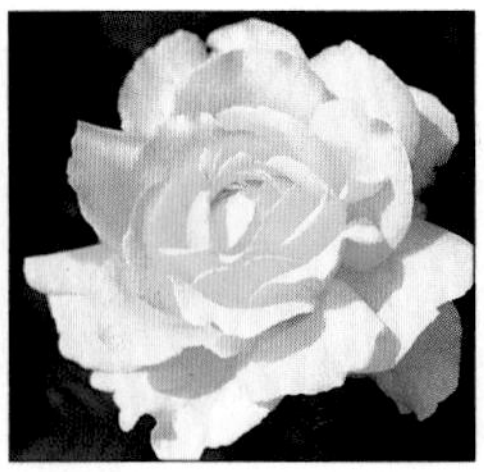
Rosa 'Mountbatten'

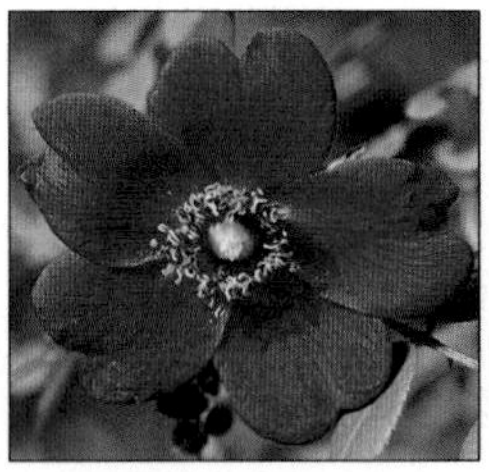
Rosa moyesii 'Geranium'

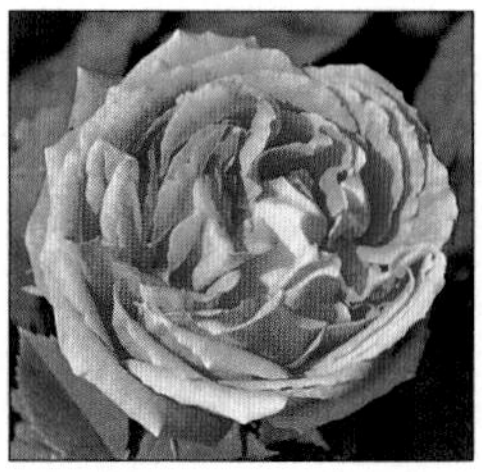
Rosa 'Mrs. John Laing'

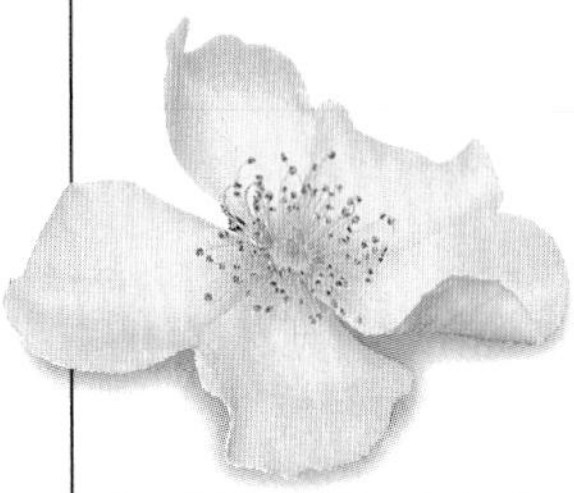
Rosa 'Mrs. Oakley Fisher'

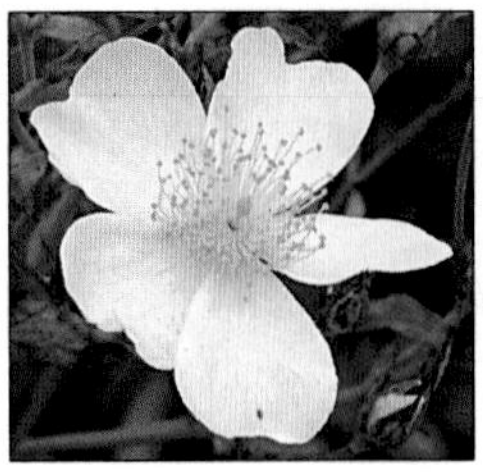
Rosa mulliganii

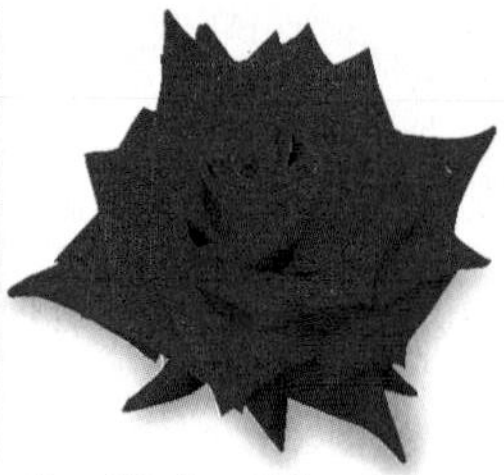
Rosa 'National Trust'

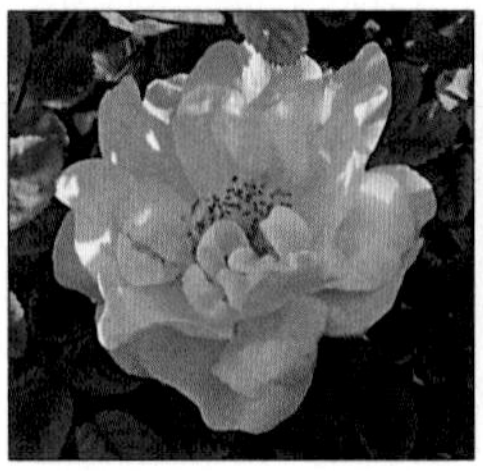
Rosa 'Nevada'

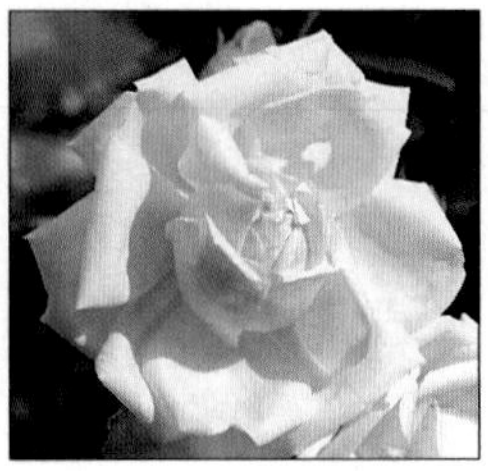
Rosa 'New Dawn'

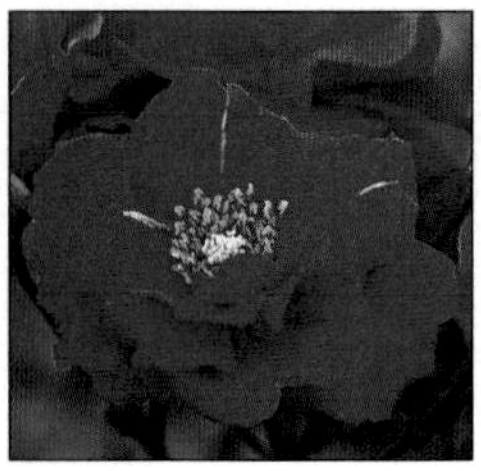
Rosa 'News'

quartered-rosette, fully double, fragrant, lilac-tinted pink flowers, 10cm (4in) across ↕ 1.2m (4ft), ↔ 1m (3ft). ❄❄❄
***R.* 'Mme Legras de St. Germain'.** Upright Alba rose with smooth stems and greyish green leaves. Rosette-shaped, fully double, fragrant, lemon-white flowers, 9cm (3½in) across, are borne in midsummer. May be trained on a support. ↕↔ 2m (6ft) as a shrub; ↕ to 5m (15ft) as a climber. ❄❄❄
***R.* 'Mme Neumann'** see *R.* 'Hermosa'.
***R.* 'Mme Pierre Oger'.** Lax Bourbon rose with slender stems and light green leaves. From summer to autumn, bears cupped, double, scented, creamy pink flowers, 8cm (3in) across, marked with lilac. ↕ 2m (6ft), ↔ 1.2m (4ft). ❄❄❄
***R.* 'Mme Plantier'** ■ Vigorous, arching Alba shrub or Noisette climbing rose with long, smooth, mid-green leaves. In midsummer, bears clusters of cupped, fully double, scented white flowers, 7cm (3in) across, reflexing into a ball. ↕ 2m (6ft), ↔ to 6m (20ft) on a support, ↔ 2.5m (8ft) grown as a shrub. ❄❄❄
***R.* 'Montezuma'.** Tall, strong large-flowered bush rose with stiff stems and leathery leaves. High-centred, fully double, salmon-pink to red flowers, 9cm (3½in) across, are borne singly and in large sprays from summer to autumn. ↕ 1.3m (4½ft), ↔ 70cm (28in). ❄❄❄
***R.* 'Moonlight'** ■ Shrub rose of dense habit, with stems and leaves both reddish green. Clusters of flat, semi-double, scented, lemon-white flowers, 4.5cm (1¾in) across, are borne freely from summer to autumn. ↕↔ 1.2m (4ft). ❄❄❄
***R.* 'Morning Jewel'** ■🏆 Vigorous, free-branching climber producing glossy, mid-green leaves. Clusters of cupped, double, scented, bright pink flowers, 9cm (3½in) across, are borne from summer to autumn. Tolerates partial shade. ↕ 3m (10ft), ↔ 2.5m (8ft). ❄❄❄
R. moschata ■ (Musk rose). Species rose of tall, lax habit, with dark green stems and purplish green leaves, each comprising 5–7 broadly ovate to broadly elliptic leaflets, 1.5–4cm (½–1½in) long. Few-flowered, loose clusters of flat, single to semi-double, musk-scented, milk-white flowers, 5cm (2in) across, are borne from late summer to autumn; they are followed by spherical to ovoid, orange-red hips. ↕↔ to 3m (10ft). W. Asia. ❄❄. **var. *nivea*** see *R.* 'Dupontii'.
***R.* 'Mountbatten'** ■🏆 syn. *R.* 'Harmantelle'. Vigorous cluster-flowered bush rose of shrubby habit, with crisp, leathery, bright green leaves. Rounded, fully double, scented yellow flowers, 10cm (4in) across, are produced from summer to autumn. ↕ 1.2m (4ft), ↔ 75cm (30in). ❄❄❄
R. moyesii. Vigorous, arching species rose producing mid- to dark green leaves, each comprising 7–13 small, broadly elliptic to ovate leaflets, 1–4cm (½–1½in) long. Flat or cupped, single, deep scarlet or pink flowers, 5cm (2in) across, with yellow stamens, are borne singly or in small clusters in summer; they are followed by large, flask-shaped red hips. ↕ 4m (12ft), ↔ 3m (10ft). W. China. ❄❄❄. **var. *fargesii*** is less vigorous, and has pink flowers; ↕ 2.5m (8ft), ↔ 1.5m (5ft). **'Geranium'** ■🏆 has a compact habit, and bears brighter, cherry-red flowers with cream stamens, followed by orange-red hips; ↕ 2.5m (8ft), ↔ 1.5m (5ft). **'Highdownensis'** see *R.* 'Highdownensis'.
***R.* 'Mr. Lincoln'.** Stiff-stemmed, large-flowered bush rose of upright habit, with leathery, dull, dark green foliage. High-centred to cupped, fully double, fragrant, dark velvety red flowers, 12cm (5in) across, are produced from summer to autumn. ↕ 1.1m (3½ft), ↔ 60cm (24in). ❄❄❄

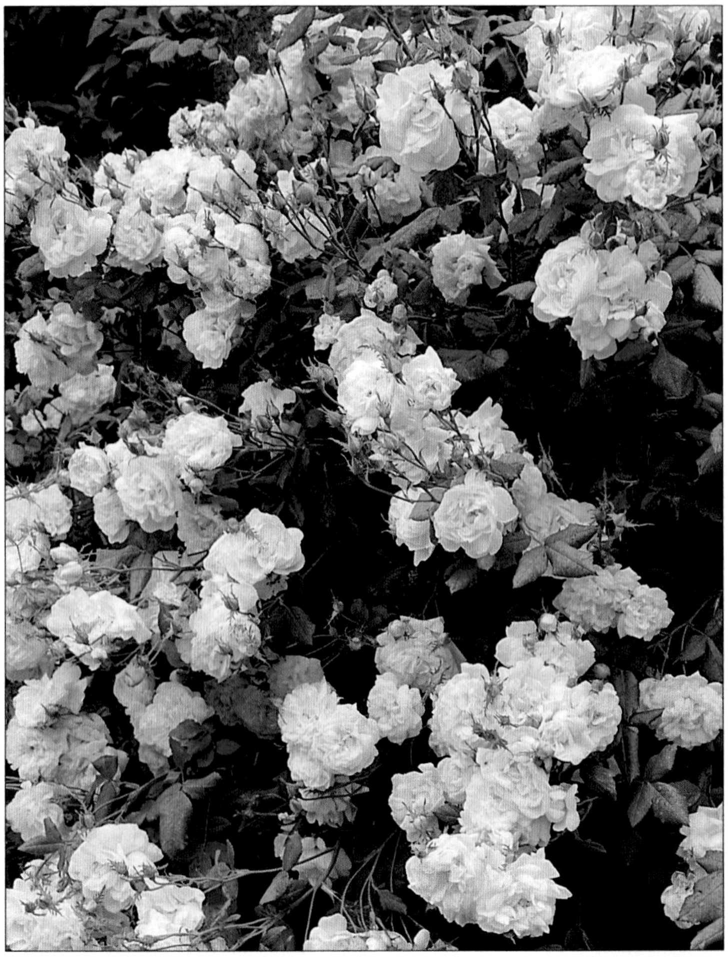
Rosa 'Mme Plantier'

***R.* 'Mrs. John Laing'** ■ Hybrid Perpetual rose with abundant light green foliage. From summer to autumn, bears rounded, fully double, fragrant, silvery pink flowers, 12cm (5in) across. ↕ 1m (3ft), ↔ 75cm (30in). ❄❄❄
***R.* 'Mrs. Oakley Fisher'** ■🏆 Large-flowered bush rose with spindly stems and sparse, bronze-green foliage. From summer to autumn, bears cupped to flat, single, scented apricot flowers, 7cm (3in) across, fading to pale buff with age. ↕↔ to 1m (3ft). ❄❄❄
***R.* 'Mullard Jubilee'**, syn. *R.* 'Electron'. Vigorous large-flowered bush rose producing abundant mid-green leaves. Urn-shaped, fully double, scented, deep rose-pink flowers, 12cm (5in) across, are borne from summer to autumn. ↕ 75cm (30in), ↔ 60cm (24in). ❄❄❄
R. mulliganii ■🏆 syn. *R. longicuspis* of gardens. Rampant species rose with large, shiny, greyish green leaves, each comprising 5–7 elliptic-ovate to oblong-ovate leaflets, to 6cm (2½in) long. Large clusters of many pendent, cupped to flat, single white flowers, to 6cm (2½in) across, are borne on slender flower-stalks in summer. ↕ to 6m (20ft), ↔ 3m (10ft). W. China. ❄❄❄
R. multiflora. Upright, arching, very vigorous species rose producing masses of dull, light to mid-green leaves, each with 7–9, rarely 5–11, obovate or elliptic leaflets, 1.5–5cm (½–2in) long. Large clusters of cupped to flat, single, fruit-scented white flowers, to 3cm (1¼in) across, fading to red, are borne freely but fleetingly in summer, followed by ovoid to spherical red hips, to 7mm (¼in) long. ↕ to 5m (15ft), ↔ 3m (10ft). Japan, Korea. ❄❄❄
***R.* 'Mutabilis'** see *R.* x *odorata* 'Mutabilis'.
***R.* 'National Trust'** ■ syn. *R.* 'Bad Nauheim'. Compact large-flowered bush rose with abundant dark green foliage. Neatly formed, urn-shaped, fully double, scarlet-crimson flowers, 10cm (4in) across, are borne freely from summer to autumn. ↕↔ 60cm (24in). ❄❄❄
***R.* 'Nevada'** ■🏆 Vigorous, arching shrub rose with red stems and dense, light green leaves. Flat, semi-double, scented, creamy white flowers, 10cm (4in) across, are borne freely in early summer and sparsely in autumn. ↕↔ 2.2m (7ft). ❄❄❄

R

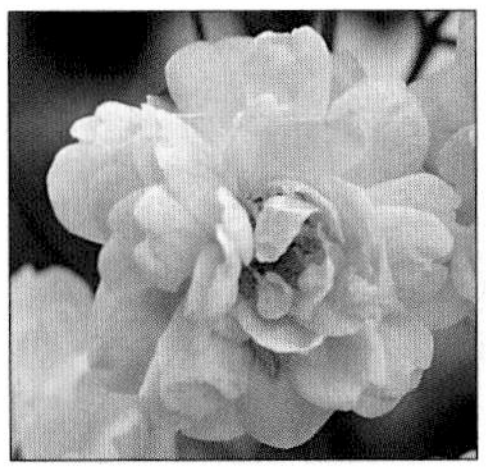
Rosa 'Noisette Carnée'

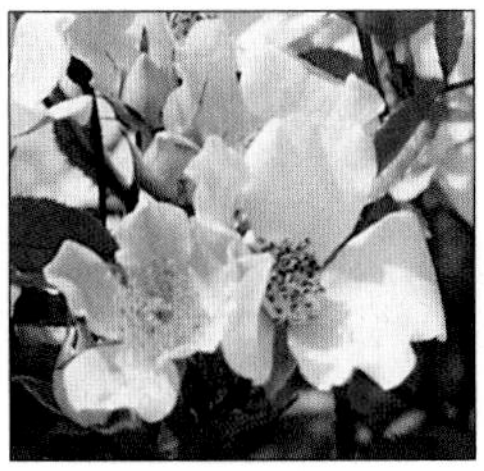
Rosa 'Nozomi'

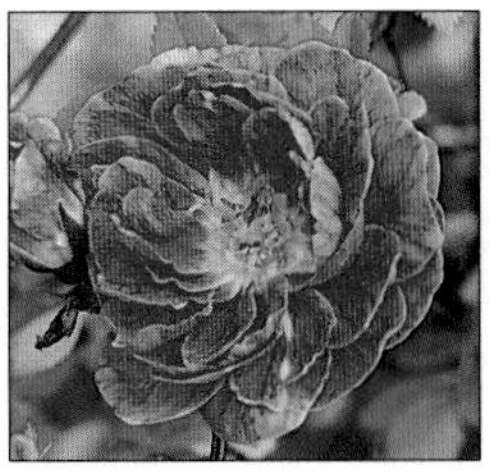
Rosa nutkana 'Plena'

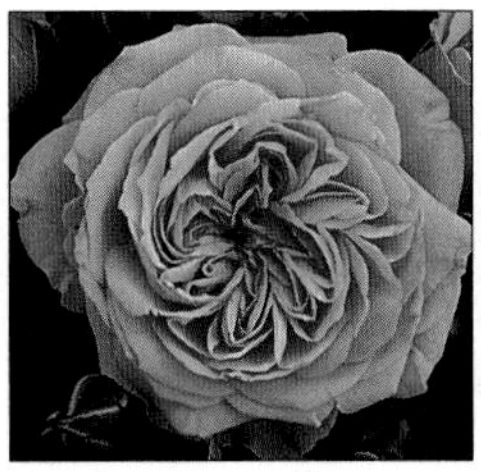
Rosa 'Octavia Hill'

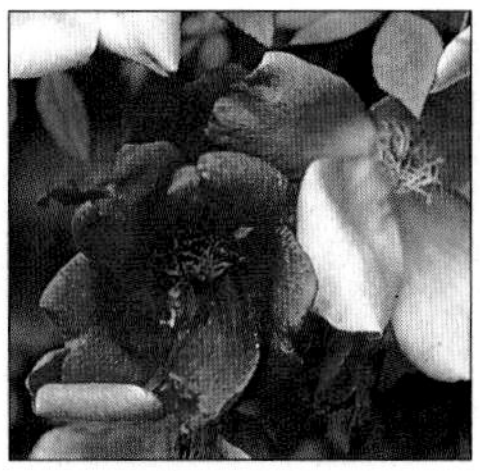
Rosa x *odorata* 'Mutabilis'

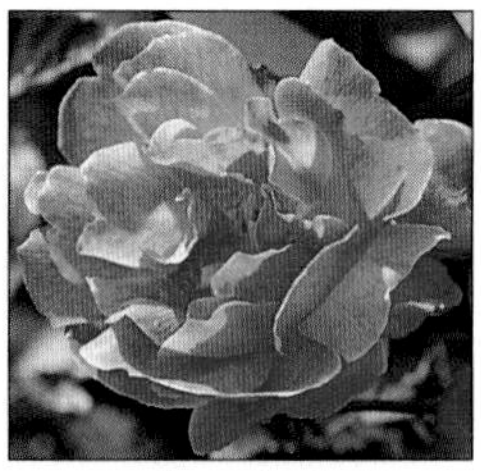
Rosa x *odorata* 'Pallida'

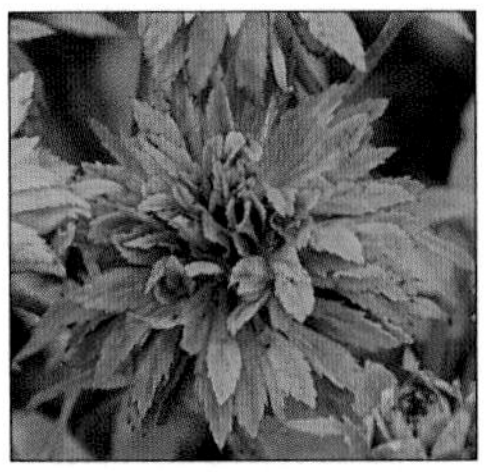
Rosa x *odorata* 'Viridiflora'

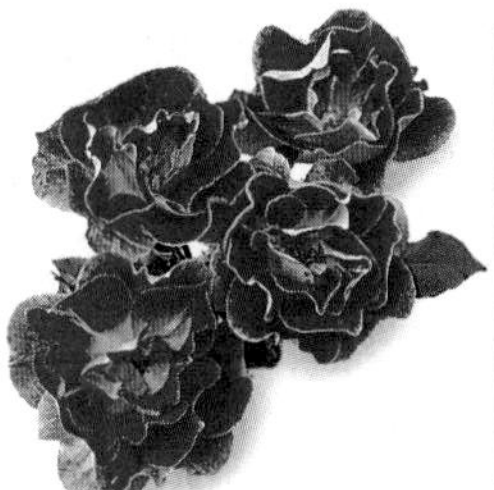
Rosa 'Old Master'

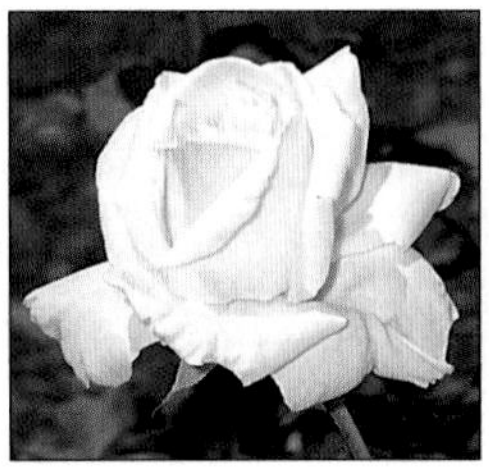
Rosa 'Ophelia'

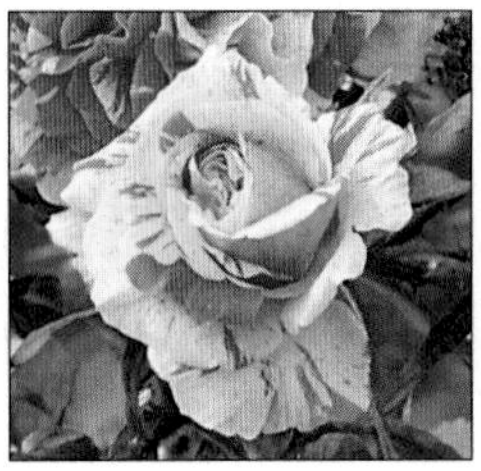
Rosa 'Oranges and Lemons'

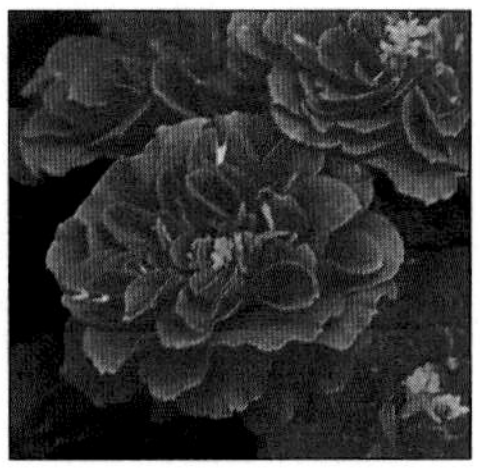
Rosa 'Orange Sunblaze'

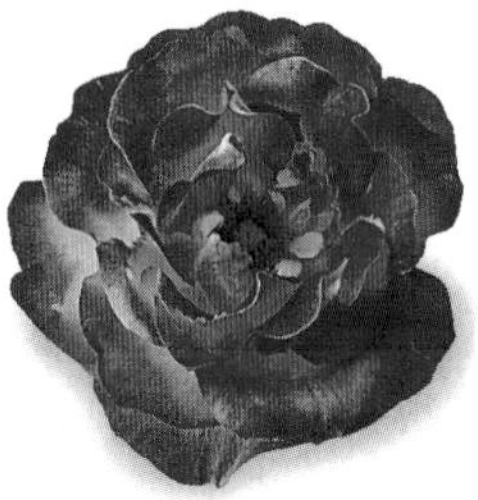
Rosa 'Painted Moon'

***R.* 'New Dawn'** ■ 🏆 syn. *R.* 'The New Dawn'. Climber of vigorous, arching habit, with shiny, mid-green leaves. From summer to autumn, bears clusters of cupped, double, fragrant, pale pearl-pink flowers, 8cm (3in) across. Tolerates a partially shaded site. ↕ 3m (10ft), ↔ 2.5m (8ft). ❄❄❄

***R.* 'News'** ■ syn. *R.* 'Legnews'. Cluster-flowered bush rose with dark green foliage. Cupped, wide-opening, double, scented, bright beetroot-purple flowers, 8cm (3in) across, are borne from summer to autumn. ↕ 60cm (24in), ↔ 50cm (20in). ❄❄❄

***R.* 'Nigel Hawthorne'**, syn. *R.* 'Harquibbler'. Hummock-forming shrub rose with wiry, prickly stems and wrinkled, mid-green leaves. Cupped to flat, single, pale salmon-pink flowers, 5cm (2in) across, each with a deep scarlet eye, are borne in summer. ↕ 60cm (24in), ↔ 75cm (30in). ❄❄❄

***R.* 'Niphetos'.** Branching, climbing Tea rose with lance-shaped, pale green leaves. Pointed buds open to rounded, double, scented, creamy white flowers, 12cm (5in) across, borne on nodding stems, mainly in summer, a few later. ↕ 3m (10ft), ↔ 2.5m (8ft). ❄❄❄

***R.* 'Noisette Carnée'** ■ syn. *R.* 'Blush Noisette'. Branching Noisette climbing rose that can be grown as a shrub, with lax stems and matt, mid-green foliage. Cupped, double, spice-scented, pale pink flowers, 4cm (1½in) across, are produced from summer to autumn. ↕ 2–4m (6–12ft), ↔ 2–2.5m (6–8ft). ❄❄❄

***R.* 'Normandica'** see *R.* 'Petite de Hollande'.

***R.* 'Northamptonshire'** syn. *R.* 'Mattdor'. Spreading ground-cover rose with shiny, dark green foliage. Large sprays of cupped, semi-double, pearl-white flowers, 4.5cm (1¾in) across, are borne freely from summer to autumn. ↕ 45cm (18in), ↔ 1m (3ft). ❄❄❄

***R.* 'Nozomi'** ■ 🏆 syn. *R.* 'Heideröslein'. Trailing ground-cover rose producing shiny, dark green leaves. Clusters of flat, single, pale pink-white flowers, 2.5cm (1in) across, cover the plant in summer. ↕ 45cm (18in) or to 1.5m (5ft) when trained on a pillar, ↔ 1.2m (4ft). ❄❄❄

***R.* 'Nuit d'Orient'** see *R.* 'Big Purple'.

***R.* 'Nuits de Young'** (Old black rose). Erect Moss rose with wiry stems, brownish green mossing, and dark green leaves. In summer, bears flat, double, scented, dark maroon-purple flowers, 5cm (2in) across, showing yellow stamens. ↕ 1.2m (4ft), ↔ 1m (3ft). ❄❄❄

R. nutkana (Nootka rose). Robust species rose with brownish green stems and toothed, mid-green leaves, each with 5–9 ovate to elliptic leaflets, 2–5cm (¾–2in) long. In summer, bears usually solitary, cupped, single, reddish pink flowers, 5–7cm (2–3in) across, followed by spherical, purplish red hips. ↕ to 3m (10ft), ↔ 2m (6ft). North America (Alaska to N. California). **'Plena'** ■ 🏆 syn. *R. californica* 'Plena', has semi-double pink flowers; ↕ 1.5–2.5m (5–8ft), ↔ 1.2–2m (4–6ft). ❄❄❄

***R.* 'Ocarina'** see *R.* 'Angela Rippon'.

***R.* 'Octavia Hill'** ■ Vigorous shrub rose with abundant glossy, dark green leaves. Sprays of several quartered-rosette, double, scented, clear rose-pink flowers, 8cm (3in) across, are borne from summer to autumn. ↕↔ 1.1m (3½ft). ❄❄❄

R.* x *odorata (*R. chinensis* x *R. gigantea*). Shrubby or climbing China rose with lax, prickly stems and light green leaves comprising 3–5 narrowly ovate leaflets, 4–6cm (1½–2½in) long. From summer to autumn, bears rounded, double, white, pale pink, or pale yellow flowers, 5–8cm (2–3in) across. ↕↔ 2m (6ft) as shrub; ↕ 5m (15ft), ↔ 3–4m (10–12ft) as a climber. Garden origin. ❄❄. **'Mutabilis'** ■ 🏆 syn. *R. chinensis* 'Mutabilis', *R.* 'Mutabilis', *R.* 'Tipo Ideale', is shrubby, with reddish purple, sparsely prickly stems that will climb if supported, and glossy dark green leaves, flushed purple. Bears cupped, single flowers, 6cm (2½in) across, which change from light yellow to copper-pink and then to deep pink. ↕ 1.2m (4ft), ↔ 1m (3ft) as a shrub; ↕ to 3m (10ft), ↔ 2m (6ft) as a climber. ❄❄❄ (borderline). **'Pallida'** ■ (Old blush China rose, Parsons' pink China rose) is bushy, with shiny, mid-green leaves. It freely bears cupped, double pink flowers, 6cm (2½in) across. ↕ 1m (3ft), sometimes to 3m (10ft) in mild climates, ↔ 80cm (32in). ❄❄❄. **'Pseudindica'**, syn. *R.* 'Beauty of Glazenwood', *R.* 'Gold of Ophir', *R.* 'San Rafael' (Fortune's double yellow rose) is a lax climber with glossy, light green leaves. It bears high-centred to cupped, semi-double, scented, copper-red to yellow flowers, 5cm (2in) across. ↕ 2.5–5m (8–15ft), ↔ 1.5–3m (5–10ft). ❄❄. **'Semperflorens'**, syn. *R. chinensis* 'Semperflorens' (Slater's crimson China rose) is open-branched, with dark green leaves and semi-double, crimson-red flowers, 6cm (2½in) across. ↕↔ 1m (3ft). ❄❄❄ (borderline). **'Viridiflora'** ■ syn. *R. chinensis* 'Viridiflora', *R.* 'Lü E', *R.* 'Viridiflora' (Green rose) is upright, with shiny, dark green leaves and sprays of rosette-shaped, double flowers, 5cm (2in) across, green ageing to purplish green, with narrow petals that resemble sepals. ↕ 75cm (30in), ↔ 60cm (24in). ❄❄❄

R. officinalis see *R. gallica* var. *officinalis*.

***R.* 'Old Master'** ■ syn. *R.* 'Macesp'. Vigorous cluster-flowered bush rose with glossy, dark green leaves. Cupped, semi-double flowers, 11cm (4½in) across, shaded and marked carmine-red on a white background, are produced from summer to autumn. ↕ 80cm (32in), ↔ 60cm (24in). ❄❄❄

***R.* 'Olympiad'** syn. *R.* 'Macauck'. Large-flowered bush rose with mid-green foliage and high-centred, fully double, velvety, bright red flowers, 10cm (4in) across, borne from summer to autumn. Flowers last well when cut. ↕ 1.2m (4ft), ↔ 65cm (26in). ❄❄❄

R. omeiensis* f. *pteracantha see *R. sericea* subsp. *omeiensis* f. *pteracantha*.

***R.* 'Opa Pötschke'** see *R.* 'Precious Platinum'.

***R.* 'Ophelia'** ■ Large-flowered bush rose with stiff growth and sparse, dark green foliage. Neatly formed, urn-shaped to cupped, double, fragrant, creamy pale pink flowers, 8cm (3in) across, are produced from summer to autumn. ↕ 1m (3ft), ↔ 60cm (24in). ❄❄❄

***R.* 'Oranges and Lemons'** ■ syn. *R.* 'Macoranlem'. Vigorous cluster-flowered bush rose with shiny, dark green foliage, reddish green when young. From summer to autumn, bears rounded, fully double flowers, 10cm (4in) across, with stiff, infolded, orange-yellow petals, striped scarlet, fading to pinkish red. ↕ 80cm (32in), ↔ 60cm (24in). ❄❄❄

***R.* 'Orange Sensation'.** Vigorous, spreading cluster-flowered bush rose producing shiny, light green foliage. Rounded, double, scented, bright orange-red flowers, 8cm (3in) across, are borne from summer to autumn. ↕ 70cm (28in), ↔ 60cm (24in). ❄❄❄

***R.* 'Orange Sunblaze'** ■ syn. *R.* 'Meijikitar', *R.* 'Sunblaze'. Miniature bush rose of compact habit, with dense, dark green leaves. Cupped, fully double, bright orange-red flowers, 4cm (1½in) across, are borne from summer to autumn. ↕↔ 30cm (12in). ❄❄❄

***R.* 'Orange Triumph'.** Stiff, vigorous Polyantha rose with glossy, dark green leaves. Full, showy clusters of cupped, double, dull red flowers, 4cm (1½in) across, are borne from summer to autumn. ↕ 1m (3ft), ↔ 75cm (30in). ❄❄❄

***R.* 'Paestana'** see *R.* 'Portlandica'.

***R.* 'Painted Moon'** ■ syn. *R.* 'Dicpaint'. Leafy, spreading large-flowered bush rose producing mid-green foliage. Wide sprays of cupped, double flowers, 9cm (3½in) across, light yellow, strongly suffused pink and crimson, are borne from summer to autumn. ↕ 75cm (30in), ↔ 60cm (24in). ❄❄❄

***R.* 'Panachée d'Angers'** see *R.* 'Commandant Beaurepaire'.

***R.* 'Papa Meilland'.** Large-flowered bush rose with a lanky habit and olive-green leaves. High-centred, fully double, very fragrant, dark velvet-crimson flowers, 12cm (5in) across, are borne on long stems from summer to autumn. Prone to mildew. ↕ 1m (3ft), ↔ 60cm (24in). ❄❄

***R.* 'Paradise'**, syn. *R.* 'Burning Sky', *R.* 'Wezeip'. Vigorous large-flowered bush rose producing glossy, dark green leaves. From summer to autumn, bears high-centred, double, scented, lavender-pink flowers, 10cm (4in) across, edged ruby-red. ↕ 1.2m (4ft), ↔ 70cm (28in). ❄❄❄

***R.* 'Parkdirektor Riggers'.** Stiff, vigorous climber with glossy, dark green leaves. Large clusters of cupped, semi-double scarlet flowers, 6cm (2½in) across, with wavy-margined petals, are borne from summer to autumn. ↕ 4m (12ft), ↔ 2.5m (8ft). ❄❄❄

***R.* 'Party Girl'.** Bushy, compact miniature bush rose with dark green leaves. Neatly formed, high-centred, double, scented, apricot-yellow flowers, 3cm (1¼in) across, suffused salmon-pink, are borne from summer to autumn. ↕↔ 35cm (14in). ❄❄❄

***R.* 'Pascali'.** Large-flowered bush rose with sparse, dark green foliage. Neatly

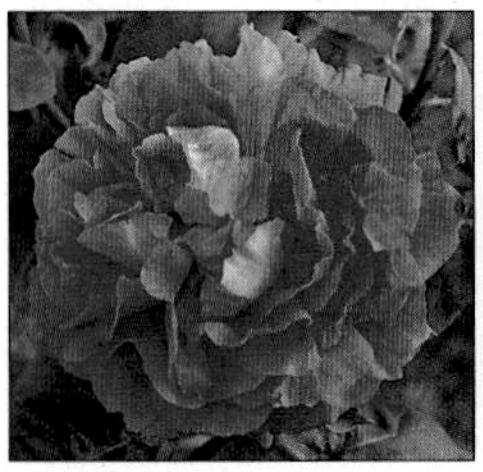
Rosa 'Paul Neyron'

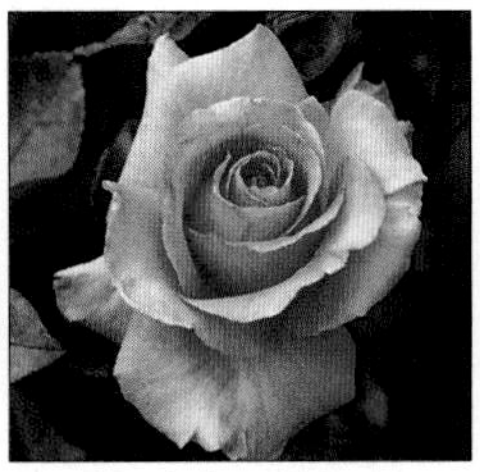
Rosa 'Paul Shirville'

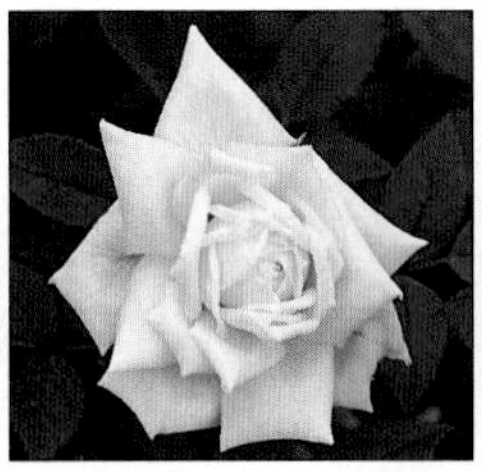
Rosa 'Paul's Lemon Pillar'

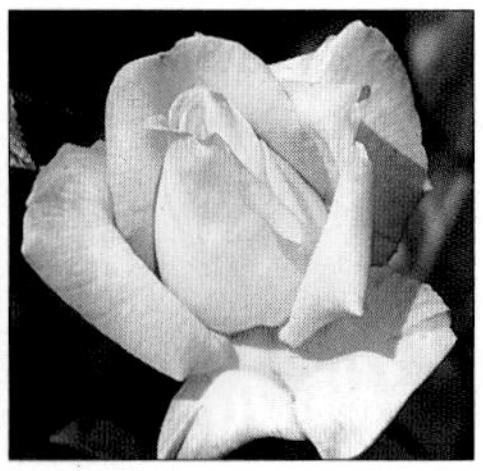
Rosa 'Peace'

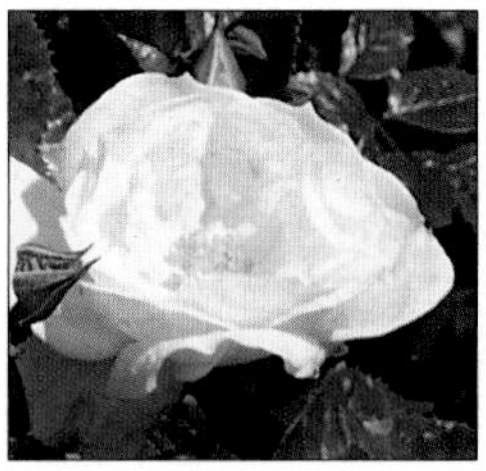
Rosa 'Pearl Drift'

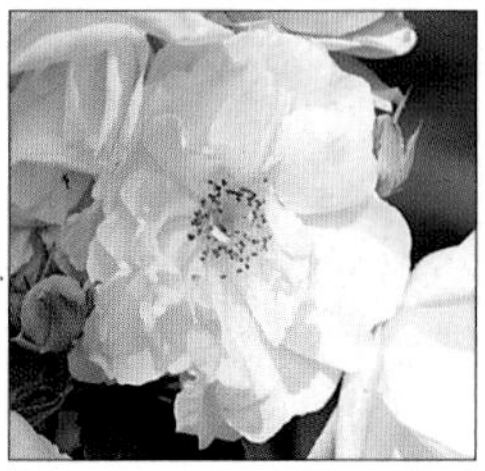
Rosa 'Penelope'

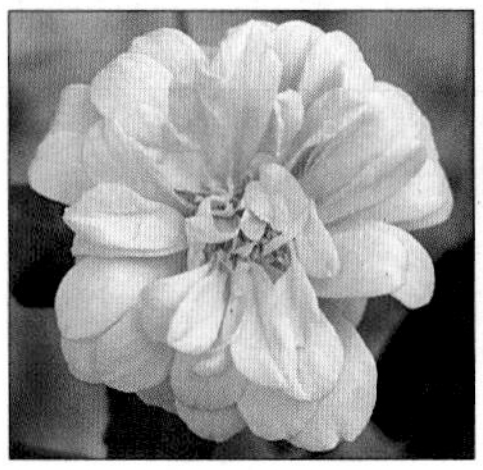
Rosa 'Perle d'Or'

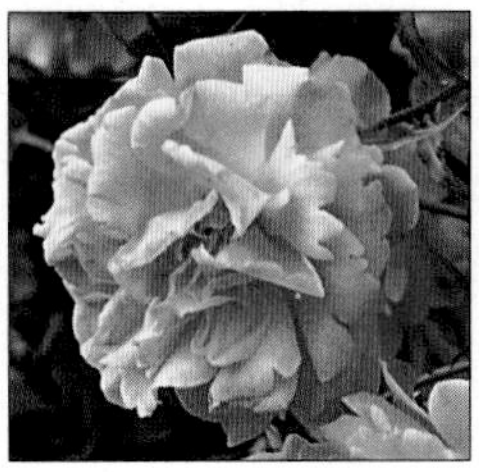
Rosa 'Pheasant'

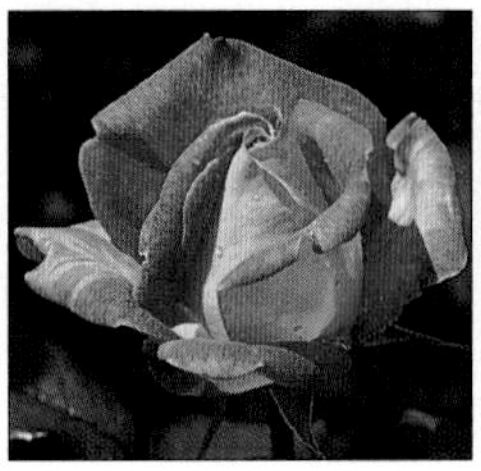
Rosa 'Piccadilly'

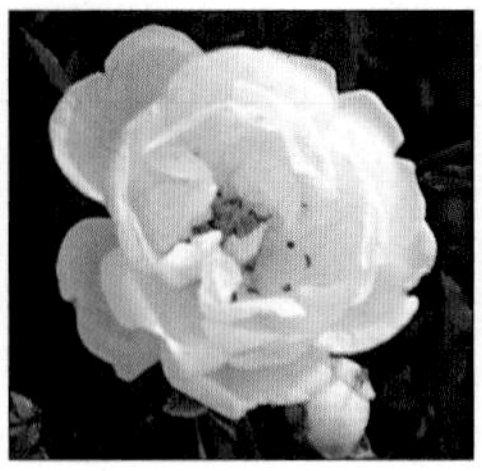
Rosa pimpinellifolia 'Plena'

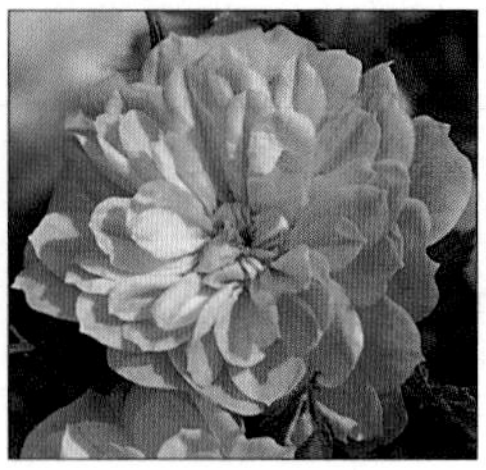
Rosa 'Pink Bells'

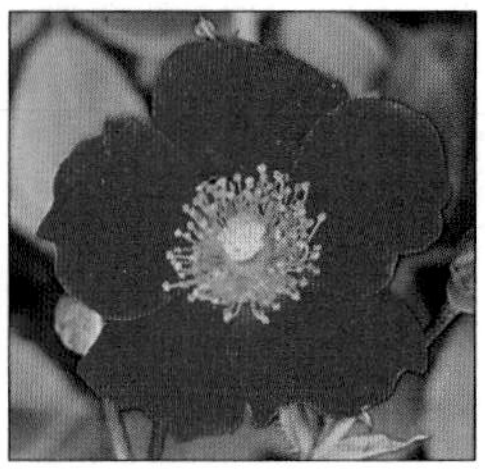
Rosa 'Pink Chimo'

formed, urn-shaped, double white flowers, 9cm (3½in) across, are borne from summer to autumn. ↕75cm (30in), ↔ 50cm (20in). ❄❄❄

***R.* 'Paul Neyron'** ■ Vigorous, upright Hybrid Perpetual rose producing olive-green leaves. Rounded, fully double, scented flowers, to 15cm (6in) across, with ruffled, lilac-tinged, deep pink petals, are borne from summer to autumn. ↕1.5m (5ft), ↔ 1.2m (4ft). ❄❄❄

***R.* 'Paul Ricault'.** Hybrid Perpetual rose of open, lax habit, with arching, prickly stems and mid-green leaves. Rounded buds open to flat, quartered-rosette, fully double, fragrant, deep pink flowers, 8cm (3in) across, from summer to autumn. ↕1.5m (5ft), ↔ 1.2m (4ft). ❄❄

***R.* 'Paul's Himalayan Musk'** 🏆 syn. *R.* 'Paul's Himalayan Rambler'. Rampant climber with trailing shoots and arching, dark green leaves. Large clusters of rosette-shaped, double, pale pink flowers, 4cm (1½in) across, are borne freely in summer. Effective trained on a tree. ↕↔ 10m (30ft). ❄❄❄

***R.* 'Paul's Himalayan Rambler'** see *R.* 'Paul's Himalayan Musk'.

***R.* 'Paul Shirville'** ■🏆 syn. *R.* 'Harqueterwife', *R.* 'Heart Throb'. Large-flowered bush rose of spreading, shrubby habit, with dark reddish green foliage. High-centred, double, fragrant, rose-pink to salmon-pink flowers, 10cm (4in) across, are borne from summer to autumn. ↕1m (3ft), ↔ 75cm (30in). ❄❄❄

***R.* 'Paul's Lemon Pillar'** ■ syn. *R.* 'Lemon Pillar'. Stiff, upright climber with dark green leaves and high-centred to rounded, fully double, lemon-scented white flowers, 12cm (5in) across, borne in summer. ↕4m (12ft), ↔ 3m (10ft). ❄❄❄

***R.* 'Paul's Scarlet Climber'.** Very vigorous, arching climber with dense, semi-glossy, mid-green foliage. Clusters of many cupped, double, bright red flowers, 8cm (3in) across, are borne freely in summer. ↕↔ 3m (10ft). ❄❄❄

***R.* 'Paul Transon'** 🏆 Vigorous, lax rambler producing shiny, dark green foliage. Flat, fully double, scented, copper- to salmon-pink flowers, 8cm (3in) across, with pleated petals, are borne in summer, also later in warm sites. ↕3m (10ft), ↔ 2.5m (8ft). ❄❄❄

***R.* 'Peace'** ■🏆 syn. *R.* 'Gioia', *R.* 'Gloria Dei', *R.* 'Mme A. Meilland'. Vigorous, shrubby large-flowered bush rose with glossy, dark green foliage. High-centred to rounded, fully double, scented, pink-tinged yellow flowers, 15cm (6in) across, are produced from summer to autumn. ↕1.2m (4ft), ↔ 1m (3ft). ❄❄❄

***R.* 'Pearl Drift'** ■ syn. *R.* 'Leggab'. Vigorous shrub rose of spreading habit, with abundant glossy, dark green leaves. From summer to autumn, bears clusters of cupped, semi-double, scented, pale pink flowers, 10cm (4in) across. ↕1m (3ft), ↔ 1.2m (4ft). ❄❄❄

***R.* 'Peaudouce'** see *R.* 'Elina'.

***R.* 'Peek A Boo'**, syn. *R.* 'Brass Ring', *R.* 'Dicgrow'. Dense, cushion-forming, dwarf cluster-flowered bush rose with narrow, dark green leaves. Sprays of many urn-shaped, double, apricot-pink flowers, 4cm (1½in) across, are borne freely from summer to autumn. ↕↔ 45cm (18in). ❄❄❄

***R.* 'Peer Gynt'.** Vigorous large-flowered bush rose with abundant rich green foliage. Rounded, fully double, lightly scented yellow flowers, 11cm (4½in) across, edged reddish pink, are borne from summer to autumn. ↕80cm (32in), ↔ 60cm (24in). ❄❄❄

***R.* 'Penelope'** ■🏆 Bushy, dense shrub rose with dark green leaves. Large clusters of well-spaced, cupped to flat, semi-double, scented, pale creamy pink flowers, 7cm (3in) across, are borne from summer to autumn. ↕↔ 1.1m (3½ft). ❄❄❄

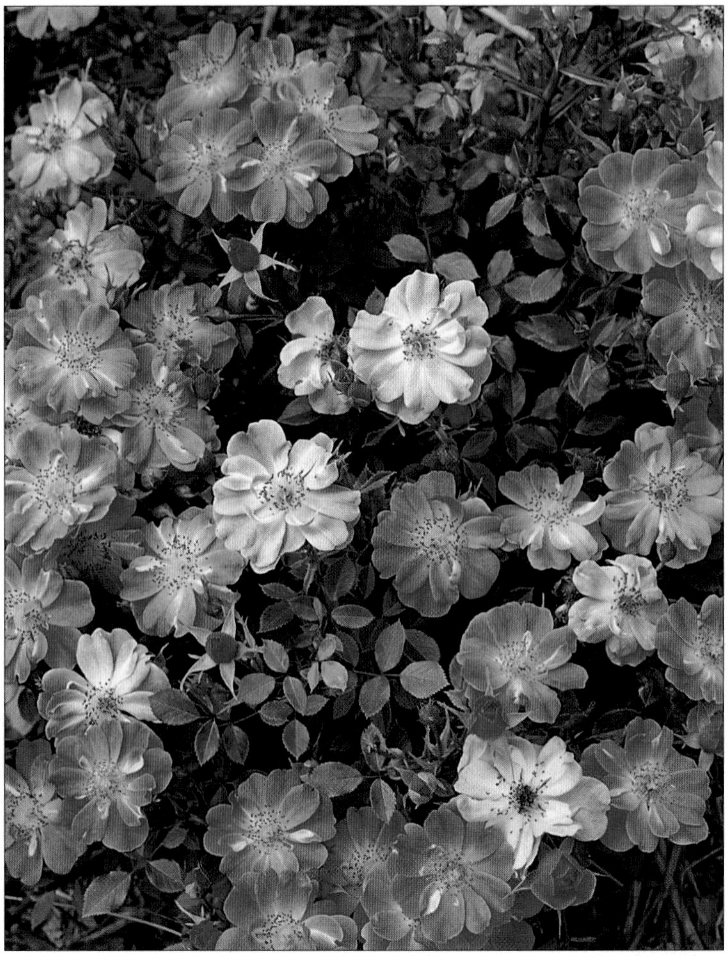
Rosa 'Petit Four'

***R.* 'Perfect Moment'**, syn. *R.* 'Jack Dayson', *R.* 'Korwilma'. Vigorous large-flowered bush rose with glossy, dark green foliage. Rounded, double flowers, 9cm (3½in) across, orange-red shaded with yellow, are borne on stiff stems from summer to autumn. ↕1.1m (3½ft), ↔ 70cm (28in). ❄❄❄

***R.* 'Perle d'Or'** ■🏆 syn. *R.* 'Yellow Cécile Brunner'. China rose forming a leafy, twiggy shrub with glossy, dark green foliage. From summer to autumn, neatly formed, urn-shaped, fully double, pale apricot flowers, 4cm (1½in) across, are borne in clusters on slender stems. ↕to 1.2m (4ft), ↔ 1m (3ft). ❄❄❄

***R.* 'Pernille Poulsen'.** Vigorous cluster-flowered bush rose with light green foliage. Urn-shaped, semi-double, salmon-pink flowers, 9cm (3½in) across, are borne freely from summer to autumn. ↕↔ 65cm (26in). ❄❄

***R.* 'Perpetual White Moss'** see *R.* 'Quatre Saisons Blanche Mousseuse'.

***R.* 'Petite de Hollande'**, syn. *R.* 'Normandica', *R.* 'Petite Junon de Hollande', *R.* 'Pompon des Dames'. Vigorous, compact, bushy Centifolia rose with mid-green leaves. Clusters of rounded, fully double, many-petalled, fragrant, rose-pink flowers, 5cm (2in) across, are borne in summer. ↕↔ 1m (3ft). ❄❄❄

***R.* 'Petite Junon de Hollande'** see *R.* 'Petite de Hollande'.

***R.* 'Petite Lisette'.** Damask rose with toothed, greyish green leaves. Well-spaced clusters of pompon, fully double, scented, rose-pink flowers, 2.5cm (1in) across, with infolded centre petals, are borne in summer. ↕↔ 1m (3ft). ❄❄❄

***R.* 'Petit Four'** ■ syn. *R.* 'Interfour'. Compact, leafy, dwarf cluster-flowered bush rose with mid-green foliage and many flat, semi-double, pink and white flowers, 4cm (1½in) across, borne from summer to autumn. ↕↔ 40cm (16in). ❄❄❄

***R.* 'Pheasant'** ■ syn. *R.* 'Heidekönigin', *R.* 'Kordapt'. Ground-cover rose of creeping habit, producing abundant glossy, mid-green leaves. Cupped, double pink flowers, 5cm (2in) across, showing yellow stamens, are borne in

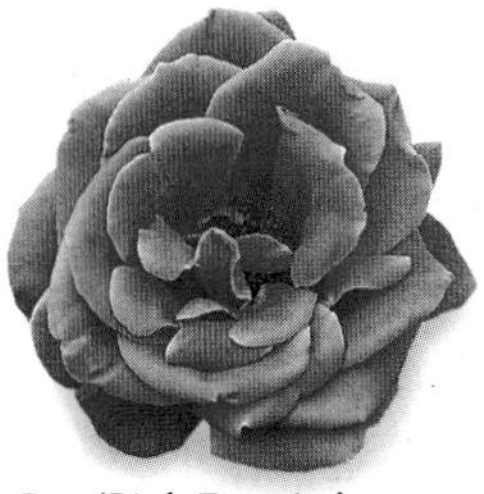
Rosa 'Pink Favorite'

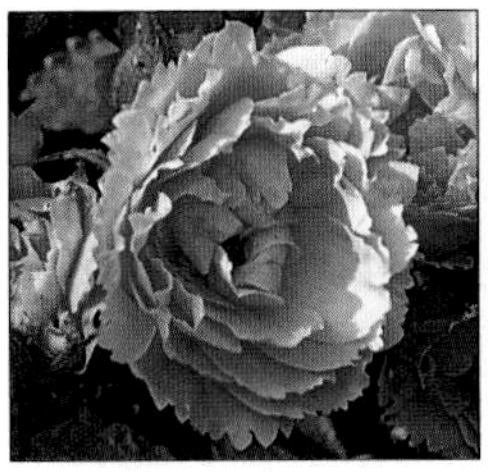
Rosa 'Pink Grootendorst'

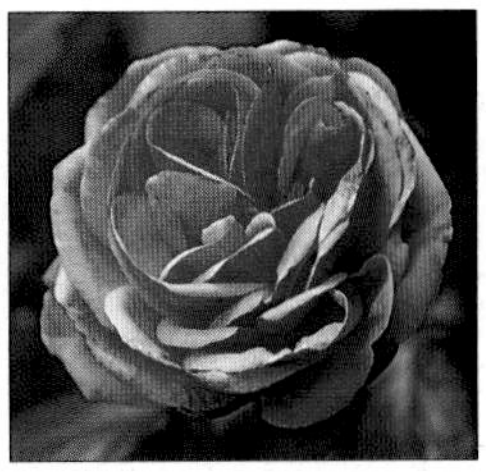
Rosa 'Pink Perpetue'

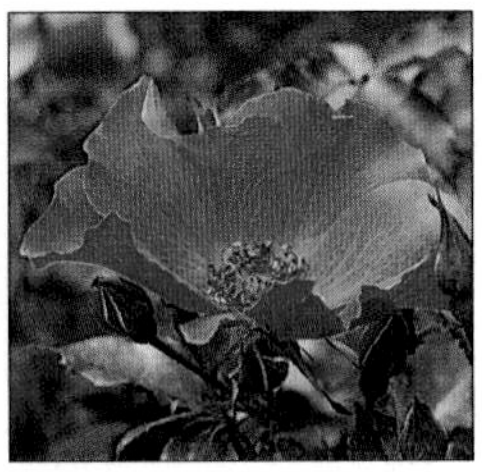
Rosa 'Playgirl'

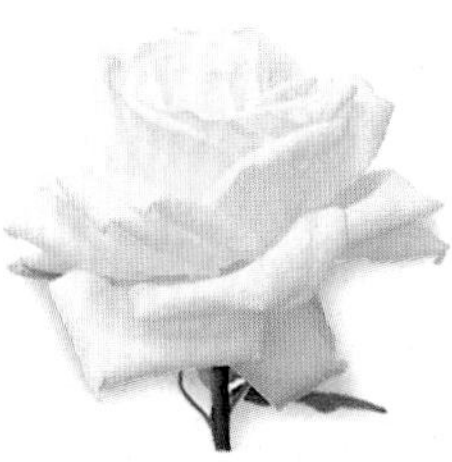
Rosa 'Polar Star'

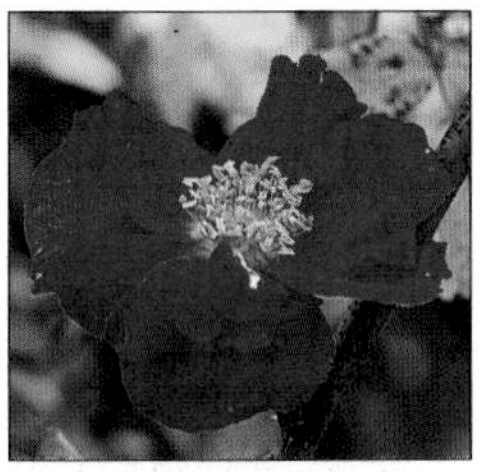
Rosa 'Portlandica'

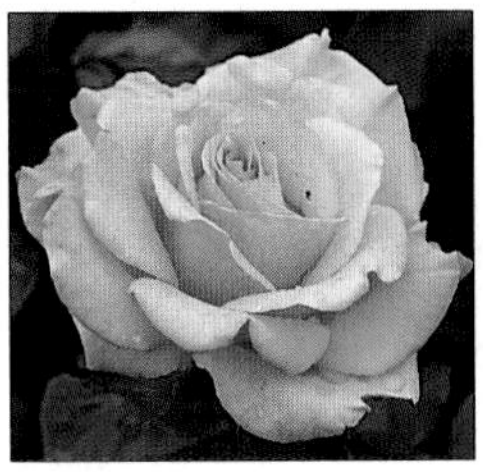
Rosa 'Pot o' Gold'

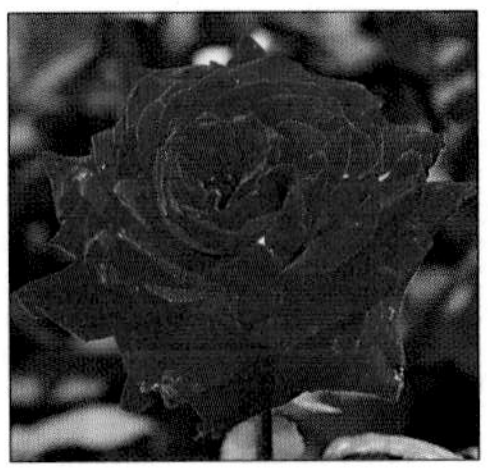
Rosa 'Precious Platinum'

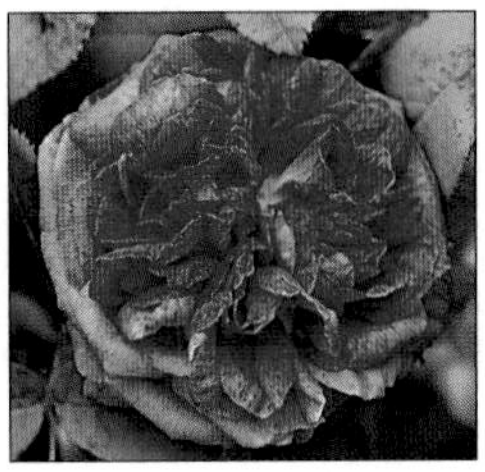
Rosa 'Président de Sèze'

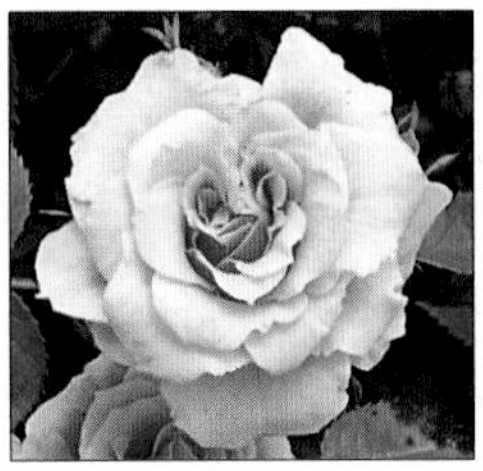
Rosa 'Pretty Polly'

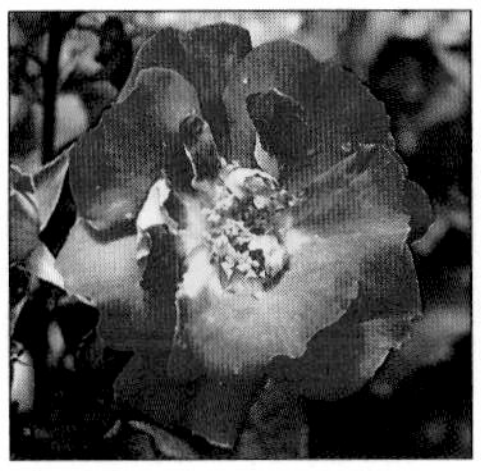
Rosa 'Pride of Maldon'

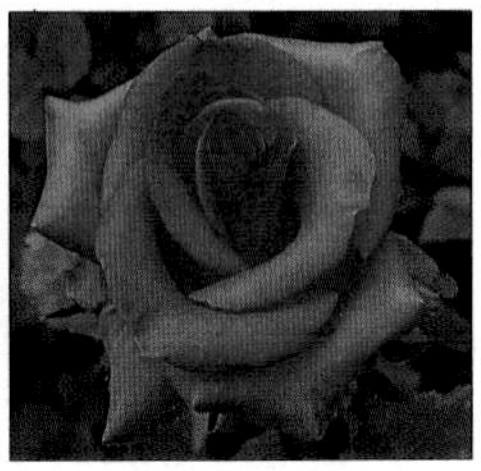
Rosa 'Prima Donna'

clusters along the stems in summer. ↕50cm (20in), ↔3m (10ft). ❄❄❄
***R.* 'Phyllis Bide'** 🏆 Vigorous climber with many lax shoots and shiny, mid-green leaves with narrow leaflets. From summer to autumn, bears wide clusters of rosette-shaped, double flowers, yellow flushed pink, 5cm (2in) across. ↕2.5m (8ft), ↔1.5m (5ft). ❄❄❄
***R.* 'Piccadilly'** ■ Vigorous large-flowered bush rose producing abundant glossy, reddish green foliage. From summer to autumn, bears high-centred, double, bicoloured, red and yellow flowers, 12cm (5in) across. ↕80cm (32in), ↔60cm (24in). ❄❄❄
***R.* 'Piccolo'**, syn. *R.* 'Tanolokip'. Cluster-flowered bush rose with glossy, dark green leaves. Cupped to flat, double, orange-red flowers, 6cm (2½in) across, are borne from summer to autumn. ↕↔50cm (20in). ❄❄❄
R. pimpinellifolia, syn. *R. spinosissima* (Burnet rose, Scotch rose, Scots rose). Dense, spreading, prickly species rose of suckering habit, with small, fern-like, dark green leaves composed of 7–9, rarely 11, broadly elliptic or broadly obovate to almost rounded leaflets, 0.5–2cm (¼–¾in) long. Solitary, cupped, single, creamy white flowers, 4cm (1½in) across, are borne freely in early summer, followed by spherical, purplish black hips. ↕to 1m (3ft), ↔1.2m (4ft). W. and S. Europe, S.W. and C. Asia to China and Korea. ❄❄❄.
var. *altaica* see *R.* 'Grandiflora'.
'Dunwichensis' see *R.* 'Dunwich Rose'.
'Plena' ■ has double white flowers.
***R.* 'Pink Bells'** ■ syn. *R.* 'Poulbells'. Vigorous, spreading ground-cover rose of dense habit, with abundant, mid-green foliage. Pompon, fully double, bright pink flowers, 2.5cm (1in) across, are borne along the stems in summer. ↕75cm (30in), ↔1.5m (5ft). ❄❄❄
***R.* 'Pink Chimo'** ■ syn. *R.* 'Interchimp'. Vigorous ground-cover shrub rose with abundant dark green leaves. Cupped to flat, semi-double, deep pink flowers, 5cm (2in) across, are borne freely along the stems from summer to autumn. ↕60cm (24in), ↔1.5m (5ft). ❄❄❄
***R.* 'Pink Cover'** see *R.* 'Essex'.
***R.* 'Pink Favorite'** ■ Branching large-flowered bush rose with long, shiny dark green leaves. High-centred to cupped, double, bright rose-pink flowers, deeper in bud, 9cm (3½in) across, are borne freely from summer to autumn. ↕75cm (30in), ↔60cm (24in). ❄❄❄
***R.* 'Pink Grootendorst'** ■🏆 Rugosa rose of upright, dense habit, with prickly stems and coarse, leathery, dark green leaves. Crowded clusters of rosette-shaped, double, rose-pink flowers, 4cm (1½in) across, with frilled petals, are borne from summer to autumn. ↕1.3m (4½ft), ↔1.1m (3½ft). ❄❄❄
***R.* 'Pink Nevada'** see *R.* 'Marguerite Hilling'.
***R.* 'Pink Parfait'.** Cluster-flowered bush rose of neat habit, producing mid-green foliage. High-centred to cupped, double flowers, 9cm (3½in) across, in shades of light pink, are borne freely from summer to autumn. ↕70cm (28in), ↔60cm (24in). ❄❄❄
***R.* 'Pink Perpetue'** ■ Stiffly branched climber with leathery, dark green leaves. Rounded to cupped, double, scented pink flowers, 8cm (3in) across, with a deeper pink reverse to the petals, are borne from summer to autumn. ↕to 3m (10ft), ↔2.5m (8ft). ❄❄❄
***R.* 'Pink Symphony'** see *R.* 'Pretty Polly'.
***R.* 'Playboy'** ■ syn. *R.* 'Cheerio'. Cluster-flowered bush rose with dense, glossy, dark green foliage. From summer to autumn, bears cupped, semi-double, orange-yellow flowers, 8cm (3in) across, shaded scarlet, with reflexed petals. ↕75cm (30in), ↔65cm (26in). ❄❄❄
***R.* 'Playgirl'** ■ syn. *R.* 'Morplag'. Cluster-flowered bush rose with dark green foliage and sprays of cupped, single, deep rose-pink flowers, 8cm (3in) across, with golden stamens, borne freely from summer to autumn. ↕75cm (30in), ↔65cm (26in). ❄❄❄
***R.* 'Poesie'** see *R.* 'Tournament of Roses'.
***R.* 'Polar Star'** ■ syn. *R.* 'Polarstern', *R.* 'Tanlarpost'. Vigorous, free-branching large-flowered bush rose with dark green leaves. High-centred, fully double, creamy white flowers, 11cm (4½in) across, are borne on long, stiff stems, from summer to autumn. ↕1m (3ft), ↔70cm (28in). ❄❄❄
***R.* 'Polarstern'** see *R.* 'Polar Star'.
***R.* 'Pompon de Paris'** see *R.* 'Rouletii'.
***R.* 'Pompon des Dames'** see *R.* 'Petite de Hollande'.
***R.* 'Pompon des Princes'** see *R.* 'Ispahan'.
***R.* 'Popcorn'.** Vigorous miniature bush rose of compact habit, producing small, glossy, dark green leaves. Clusters of numerous cupped to flat, semi-double, honey-scented white flowers, 2.5cm (1in) across, showing yellow stamens, cover the plant from summer to autumn. ↕↔30cm (12in). ❄❄❄
***R.* 'Portlandica'** ■ syn. *R.* 'Duchess of Portland', *R.* 'Paestana' (Portland rose). Vigorous Portland rose of shrubby habit, with dark green leaves. Cupped, single to semi-double, cerise-red flowers, 8cm (3in) across, with golden stamens, are borne in summer, and again in autumn if dead-headed. ↕↔1m (3ft). ❄❄❄

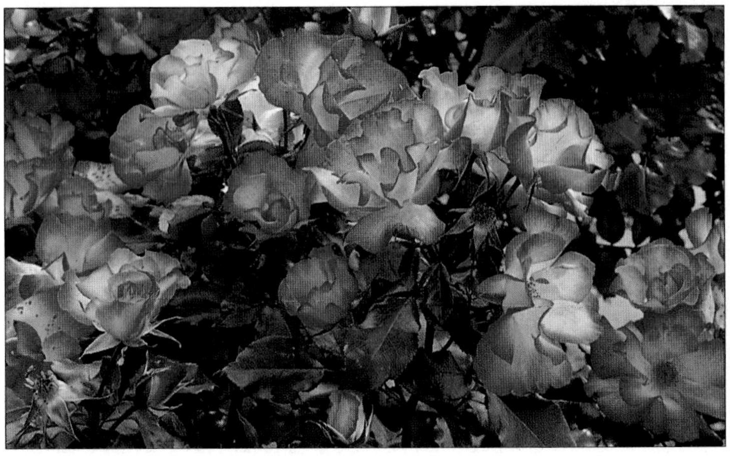
Rosa 'Playboy'

***R.* 'Pot o' Gold'** ■ syn. *R.* 'Dicdivine'. Large-flowered bush rose of neat, spreading habit, with abundant, mid-green foliage. Rounded, fully double, fragrant, golden yellow flowers, 9cm (3½in) across, are borne from summer to autumn. ↕75cm (30in), ↔60cm (24in). ❄❄❄
***R.* 'Precious Platinum'** ■ syn. *R.* 'Opa Pötschke'. Vigorous large-flowered bush rose of uneven growth, producing glossy, dark green leaves. Rounded, fully double, bright crimson-scarlet flowers, 10cm (4in) across, are borne from summer to autumn. ↕1m (3ft), ↔65cm (26in). ❄❄❄
***R.* 'Preference'** see *R.* 'Princesse de Monaco'.
***R.* 'Président de Sèze'** ■🏆 syn. *R.* 'Jenny Duval', *R.* 'Mme Hébert'. Vigorous Gallica rose of open habit, with greyish green foliage. Quartered-rosette, fully double, fragrant, pale lilac-pink flowers, 10cm (4in) across, with deep magenta margins, are borne in summer. ↕↔1.2m (4ft). ❄❄❄
***R.* 'Pretty Polly'** ■ syn. *R.* 'Meitonje', *R.* 'Pink Symphony', *R.* 'Sweet Sunblaze'. Dwarf cluster-flowered bush rose of compact, rounded habit, with abundant dark green leaves. Many cupped, fully double, rose-pink flowers, 4.5cm (1¾in) across, are borne from summer to autumn. ↕40cm (16in), ↔45cm (18in). ❄❄❄
***R.* 'Pride of Maldon'** ■ syn. *R.* 'Harwonder'. Vigorous cluster-flowered bush rose of dense, leafy growth, with lustrous, dark green leaves. From summer to autumn, bears many showy, cupped, semi-double orange flowers, 9cm (3½in) across, with a yellow reverse to the petals. ↕75cm (30in), ↔60cm (24in). ❄❄❄
***R.* 'Prima'** see *R.* 'Many Happy Returns'.
***R.* 'Prima Ballerina'.** Vigorous large-flowered bush rose, often with scaly marks on the stems, producing leathery, mid-green leaves. Urn-shaped, double, fragrant, warm rose-pink flowers, 10cm (4in) across, are borne from summer to autumn. ↕1m (3ft), ↔60cm (24in). ❄❄❄
***R.* 'Prima Donna'** ■ syn. *R.* 'Tobone'. Tall large-flowered bush rose producing mid-green leaves. High-centred, double, deep pink flowers, 10cm (4in) across, are produced on long stems from

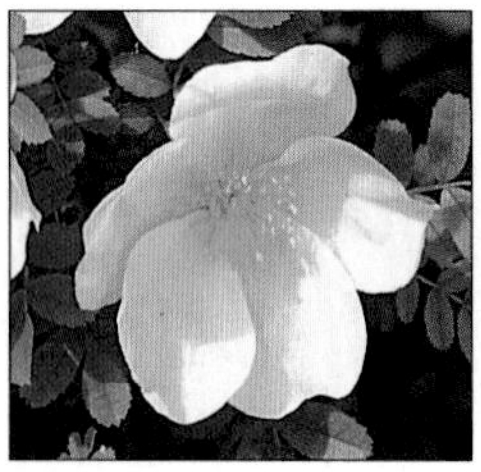
Rosa primula

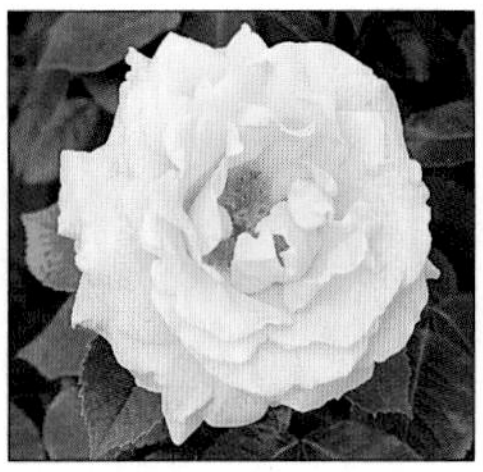
Rosa 'Princess Michael of Kent'

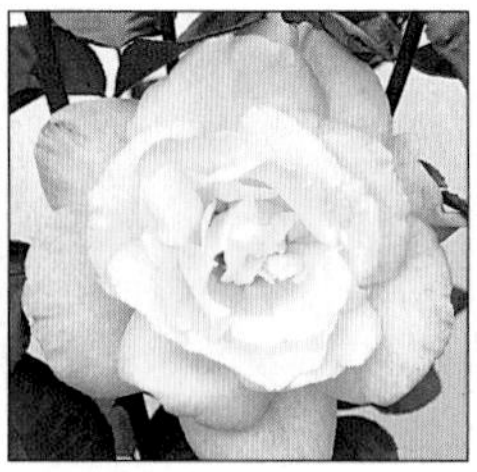
Rosa 'Pristine'

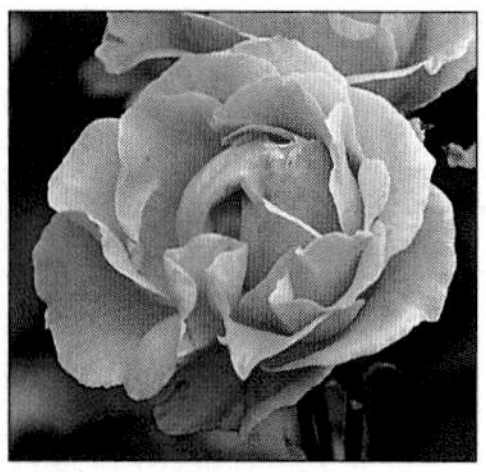
Rosa 'Queen Elizabeth'

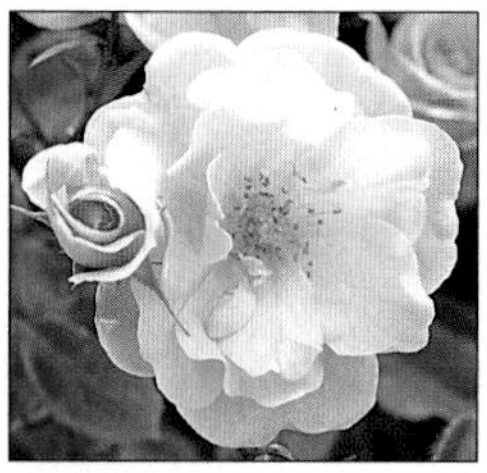
Rosa 'Queen Mother'

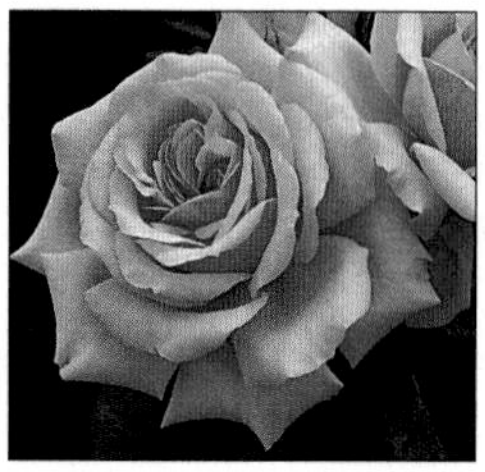
Rosa 'Radox Bouquet'

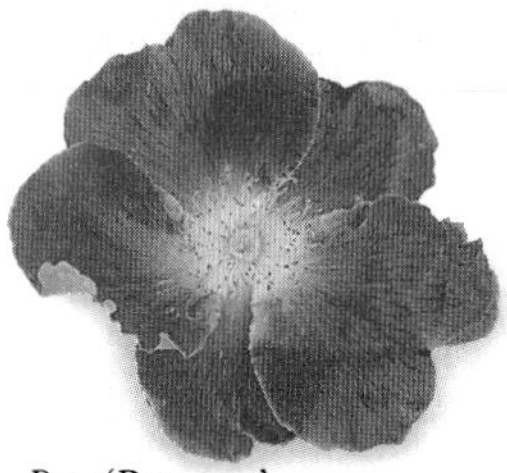

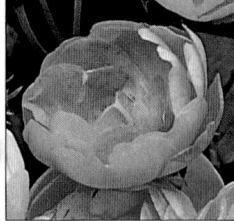
Rosa 'Ramona'

Rosa 'Raubritter'

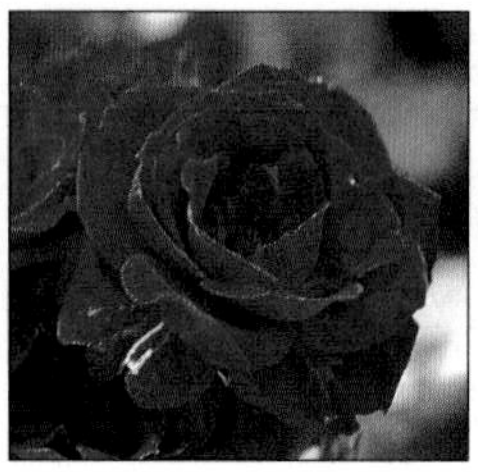
Rosa 'Red Ace'

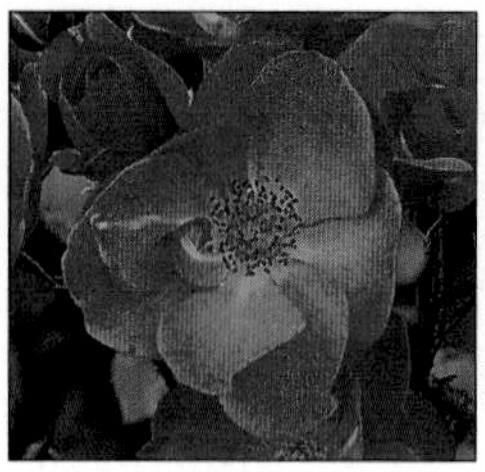
Rosa 'Red Blanket'

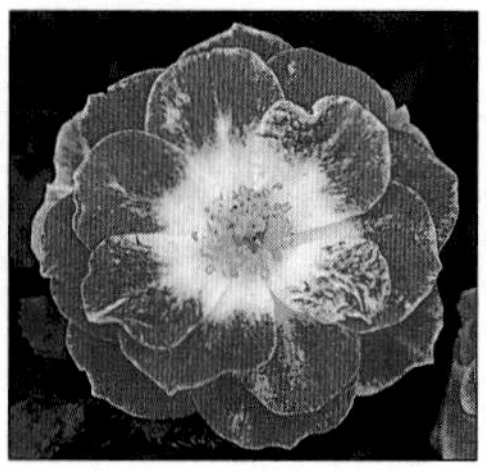
Rosa 'Regensberg'

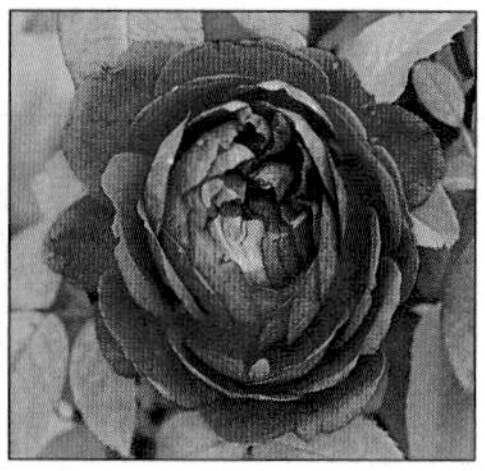
Rosa 'Reine des Violettes'

summer to autumn. ↕ 1.2m (4ft), ↔ 70cm (28in). ❄❄❄

R. primula ▣ 🏆 (Incense rose). Erect to arching species rose with aromatic, dense, fern-like, mid-green leaves comprising 9, rarely 7–13, elliptic to obovate or inversely lance-shaped leaflets, to 2cm (¾in) long, on slender, reddish green stems. Solitary, cupped, single, scented, pale primrose-yellow flowers, to 5cm (2in) across, are borne in late spring; they are followed by spherical to inversely cone-shaped, brownish maroon hips. ↕ to 3m (10ft), ↔ 2m (6ft). Asia (Turkmenistan to N. China). ❄❄❄ (borderline)

***R.* 'Prince Charles'.** Arching, lax Bourbon rose with smooth stems and leathery, dark green leaves. Loosely formed, rounded to cupped, double, fragrant, crimson-purple flowers, 10cm (4in) across, fading to lilac-red, are borne in summer. ↕ to 1.5m (5ft), ↔ 1.3m (4ft). ❄❄❄

***R.* 'Princess Alice'** ▣ syn. *R.* 'Brite Lites', *R.* 'Hartanna, *R.* 'Zonta Rose'. Cluster-flowered bush rose of narrow habit, with mid-green leaves comprising lance-shaped leaflets. Long-stemmed sprays of rounded, double, bright yellow flowers, 6cm (2½in) across, are borne from summer to autumn. ↕ 1.1m (3½ft), ↔ 60cm (24in). ❄❄❄

***R.* 'Princesse de Monaco'**, syn. *R.* 'Meimagarmic', *R.* 'Preference'. Vigorous, branching large-flowered bush rose producing dark green foliage. High-centred, fully double, fragrant white flowers, 11cm (4½in) across, with pink-margined petals, are borne from summer to autumn. ↕ 1m (3ft), ↔ 65cm (26in). ❄❄❄

***R.* 'Princess Michael of Kent'** ▣ syn. *R.* 'Harlightly'. Neat cluster-flowered bush rose with glossy, bright green foliage. Rounded, fully double, scented yellow flowers, 9cm (3½in) across, are borne from summer to autumn. ↕ 60cm (24in), ↔ 50cm (20in). ❄❄❄

***R.* 'Prinz Eugen van Savoyen'** see *R.* 'Amber Queen'.

***R.* 'Pristine'** ▣ syn. *R.* 'Jacpico'. Vigorous large-flowered bush rose producing dark green leaves with very large leaflets. From summer to autumn, bears high-centred, double, scented flowers, 12cm (5in) across, ivory flushed pale pink with long, overlapping petals. ↕ 1.2m (4ft), ↔ 75cm (30in). ❄❄❄

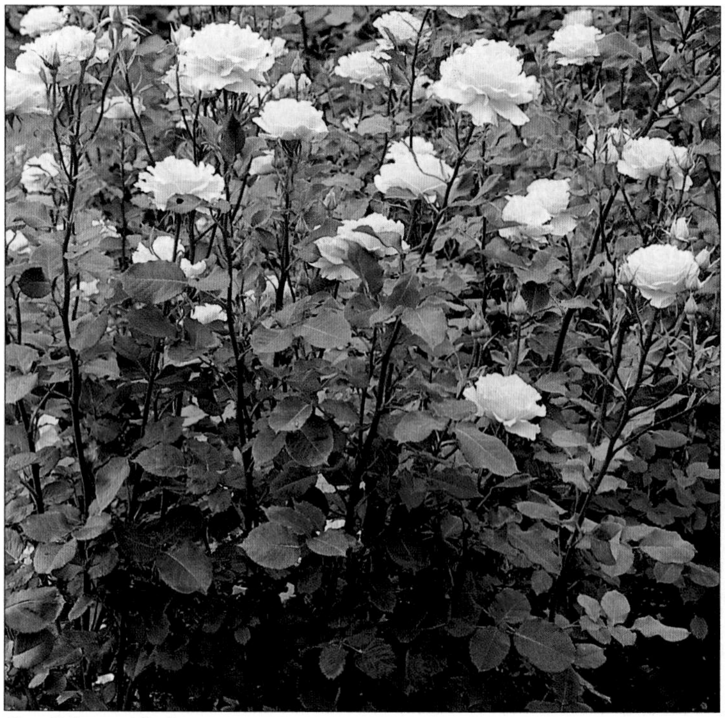
Rosa 'Princess Alice'

***R.* 'Probuzini'** see *R.* 'Awakening'.

***R.* 'Prominent'** see *R.* 'Korp'.

***R.* 'Prosperity'** 🏆 Dense, arching shrub rose with many dark green leaves. From summer to autumn, bears large clusters of rosette-shaped, double, scented, creamy white flowers, 5cm (2in) across, flushed pale pink. ↕ to 2.5m (8ft), ↔ 1.2m (4ft). ❄❄❄

***R.* 'Pyrenees'** see *R.* 'Kent'.

***R.* 'Quatre Saisons'** see *R.* x *damascena* var. *semperflorens.*

***R.* 'Quatre Saisons Blanche Mousseuse'**, syn. *R.* 'Perpetual White Moss', *R.* 'Rosier de Thionville'. Open, arching Moss rose, a sport of *R.* x *damascena* var. *semperflorens*, with light green leaves, and stems and buds covered with stiff, brownish green moss. Loosely formed, cupped to flat, double, fragrant white flowers, 9cm (3½in) across, are borne in summer, and sporadically in autumn. ↕ 1.5m (5ft), ↔ 1.2m (4ft). ❄❄❄

***R.* 'Queen Elizabeth'** ▣ 🏆 syn. *R.* 'The Queen Elizabeth'. Vigorous cluster-flowered bush rose with leathery, dark green leaves. Rounded, fully double pink flowers, 10cm (4in) across, are borne on long, stiff stems from summer to autumn. ↕ to 2.2m (7ft), ↔ 1m (3ft). ❄❄❄

***R.* 'Queen Mother'** ▣ 🏆 syn. *R.* 'Korquemu'. Dwarf cluster-flowered bush rose of spreading habit, with abundant glossy, mid-green foliage. Many cupped to flat, semi-double, clear pink flowers, 6cm (2½in) across, are borne from summer to autumn. ↕ 40cm (16in), ↔ 60cm (24in). ❄❄❄

***R.* 'Queen of Beauty & Fragrance'** see *R.* 'Souvenir de la Malmaison'.

***R.* 'Queen of Denmark'** see *R.* 'Königin von Dänemark'.

***R.* 'Queen of the Violets'** see *R.* 'Reine des Violettes'.

***R.* 'Radox Bouquet'** ▣ syn. *R.* 'Harmusky', *R.* 'Rosika'. Cluster-flowered bush rose producing shiny, mid-green foliage. Rosette-shaped, fully double, fragrant, rose-pink flowers, 9cm (3½in) across, are borne from summer to autumn. ↕ 1m (3ft), ↔ 60cm (24in). ❄❄❄

***R.* 'Rambling Rector'** ▣ 🏆 Rampant rambler with strong, arching stems and abundant grey-green foliage. Clusters of many cupped to flat, semi-double, scented, creamy white flowers, 4cm (1½in) across, showing golden stamens, are borne in summer, followed by spherical red hips in autumn. ↕↔ 6m (20ft). ❄❄❄

***R.* 'Ramona'** ▣ syn. *R.* x *anemonoides* 'Ramona', *R.* 'Red Cherokee'. Stiff, open climber with sparse, dark green leaves. Flat, single, carmine-red flowers, 10cm (4in) across, with a greyish red reverse to the petals and gold stamens, are borne in early summer. ↕ 2.5m (8ft), ↔ 3m (10ft). ❄❄

***R.* 'Raspberry Ice'** see *R.* 'Hannah Gordon'.

***R.* 'Raubritter'** ▣ syn. *R.* 'Macrantha Raubritter'. Shrub rose of lax, spreading habit, with dark greyish green leaves. Clusters of many rounded, semi-double pink flowers, 5cm (2in) across, are borne in summer. ↕ to 1m (3ft), ↔ 2m (6ft). ❄❄❄

***R.* 'Red Ace'** ▣ syn. *R.* 'Amanda', *R.* 'Amruda'. Compact miniature bush rose with mid-green foliage. Clusters of rounded, semi-double, dark crimson flowers, 4cm (1½in) across, are borne from summer to autumn. ↕ 35cm (14in), ↔ 30cm (12in). ❄❄❄

***R.* 'Red Ballerina'** see *R.* 'Marjorie Fair'.

***R.* 'Red Blanket'** ▣ 🏆 syn. *R.* 'Intercell'. Ground-cover shrub rose of spreading habit, with abundant dark green leaves. Semi-double flowers, opening flat, to 7cm (3in) across, are rose-red paling to white at the petal bases, and are borne in wide, showy clusters from summer to autumn. ↕ 75cm (30in), ↔ 1.2m (4ft). ❄❄❄

***R.* 'Red Cascade'**, syn. *R.* 'Moorcap'. Miniature climber of dense, spreading habit, with dark green leaves. Tight clusters of cupped, fully double, dark red flowers, 4cm (1½in) across, are borne from summer to autumn. ↕↔ to 1.5m (5ft). ❄❄❄

***R.* 'Red Cherokee'** see *R.* 'Ramona'.

***R.* 'Red Dorothy Perkins'** see *R.* 'Excelsa'.

***R.* 'Red Prince'** see *R.* 'Fountain'.

***R.* 'Red Yesterday'** see *R.* 'Marjorie Fair'.

***R.* 'Regensberg'** ▣ syn. *R.* 'Buffalo Bill', *R.* 'Macyoumis', *R.* 'Young Mistress'.

R

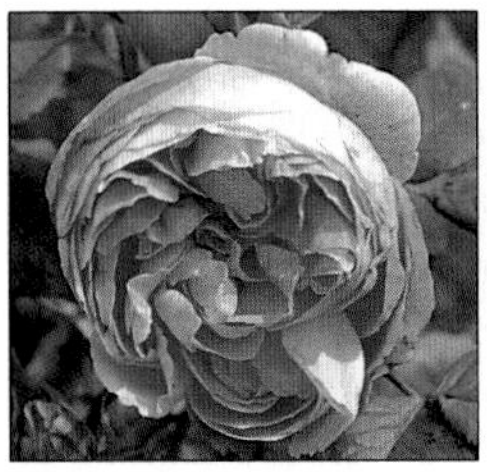
Rosa 'Reine Victoria'

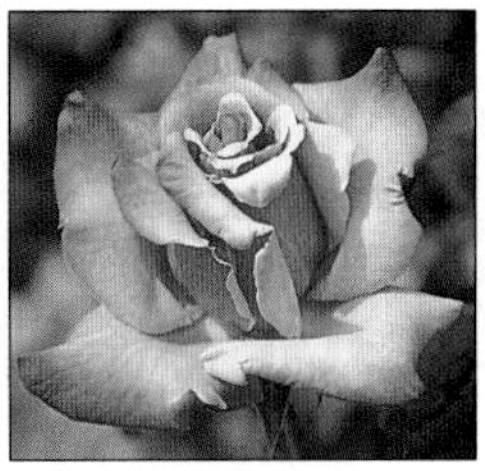
Rosa 'Remember Me'

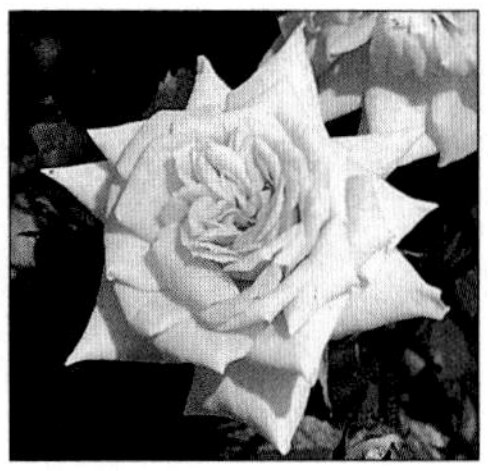
Rosa 'Rise 'n' Shine'

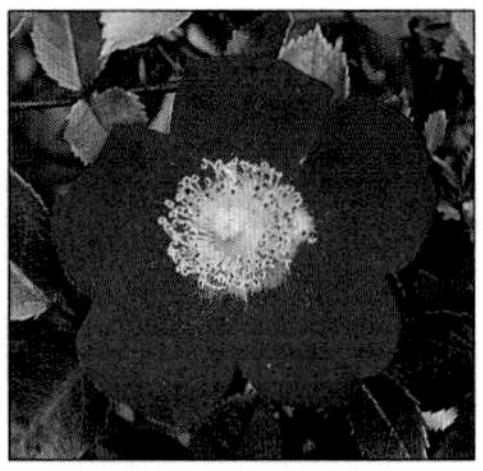
Rosa 'Robin Redbreast'

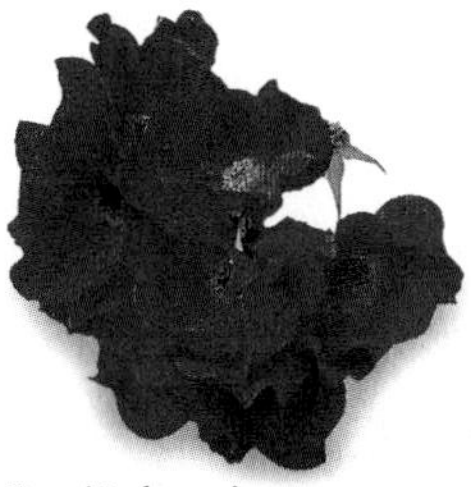
Rosa 'Robusta'

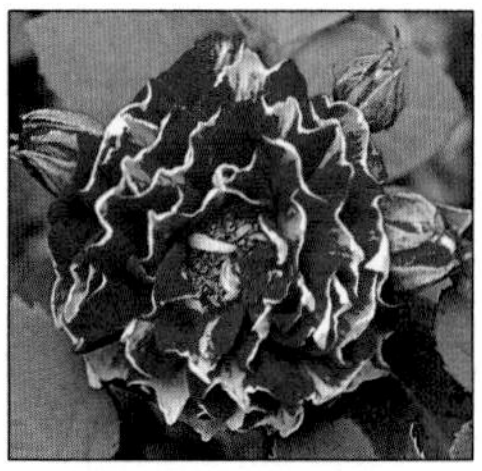
Rosa 'Roger Lambelin'

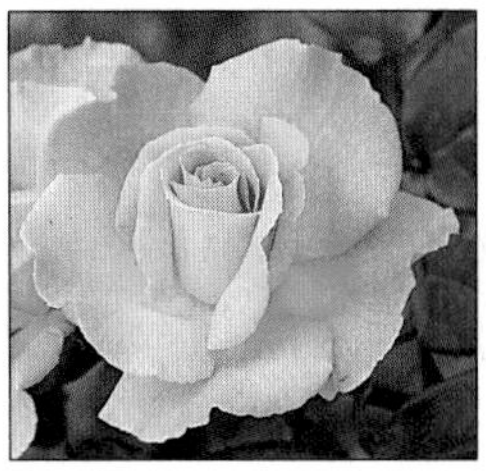
Rosa 'Rosemary Harkness'

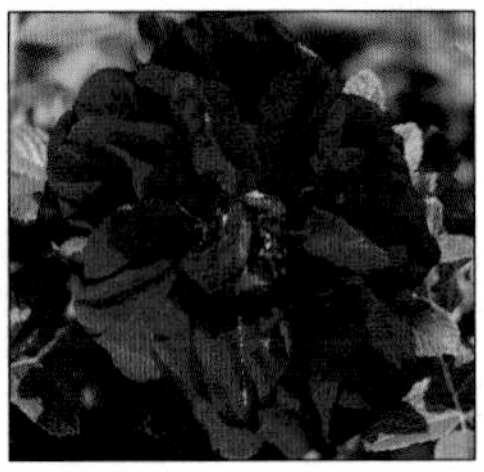
Rosa 'Roseraie de l'Haÿ'

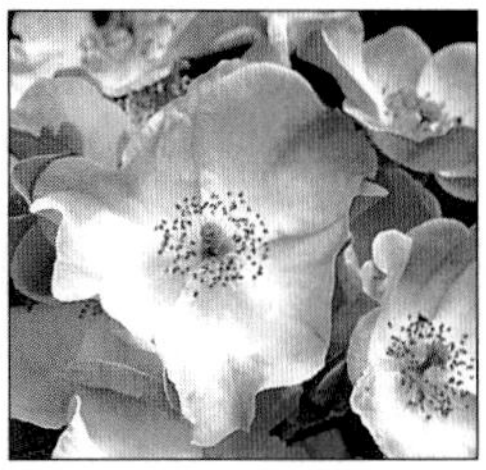
Rosa 'Rosy Cushion'

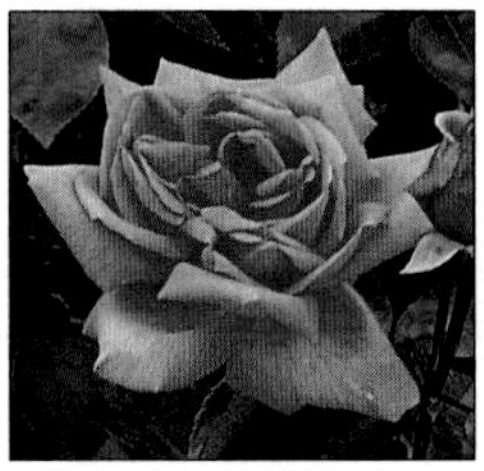
Rosa 'Rosy Mantle'

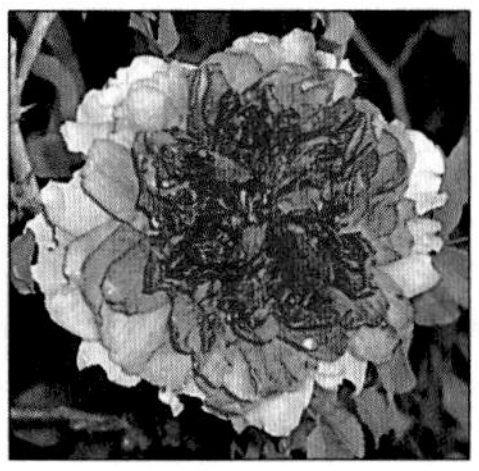
Rosa roxburghii

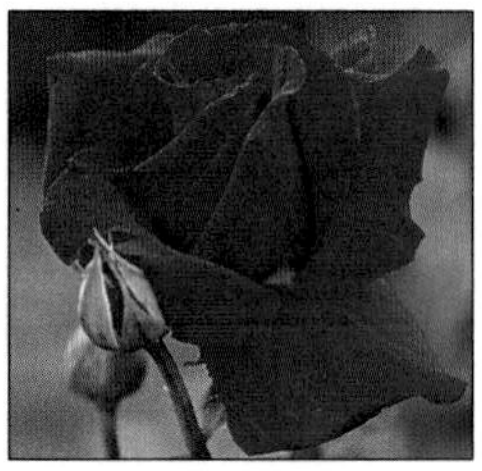
Rosa 'Royal William'

Cluster-flowered bush rose of short, dense habit, with glossy, mid-green leaves. Cupped, double flowers, opening to 11cm (4½in) across, deep pink marked with white, are borne in dense clusters from summer to autumn. ↕40cm (16in), ↔ 50cm (20in). ❄❄❄
***R.* 'Reine des Neiges'** see *R.* 'Frau Karl Druschki'.
***R.* 'Reine des Violettes'** ■ syn. *R.* 'Queen of the Violets'. Arching Hybrid Perpetual rose with smooth stems and greyish green leaves. From summer to autumn, bears quartered-rosette, fully double, fragrant, violet-purple flowers, 8cm (3in) across. ↕1.5m (5ft), ↔ 1.2m (4ft). ❄❄❄
***R.* 'Reine Victoria'** ■ syn. *R.* 'La Reine Victoria'. Lax Bourbon rose with slender stems and light green leaves. Cupped, double, scented, light rose-pink flowers, 8cm (3in) across, are borne from summer to autumn. ↕2m (6ft), ↔ 1.2m (4ft). ❄❄❄
***R.* 'Remember Me'** ■♀ syn. *R.* 'Cocdestin'. Vigorous large-flowered bush rose of stiff habit, with abundant glossy, dark green leaves. High-centred, fully double, copper-orange flowers, 9cm (3½in) across, are borne singly and in wide sprays from summer to autumn. ↕1m (3ft), ↔ 60cm (24in). ❄❄❄
***R.* 'Rise 'n' Shine'** ■ syn. *R.* 'Golden Sunblaze'. Miniature bush rose of upright habit, with dark green leaves. Urn-shaped, fully double yellow flowers, 4cm (1½in) across, are borne from summer to autumn. ↕40cm (16in), ↔ 25cm (10in). ❄❄❄
***R.* 'Robert le Diable'.** Centifolia rose of bushy, lax habit, with narrow, dark green leaves. In summer, bears cupped to flat, semi-double, scented purple flowers, 8cm (3in) across, shaded slate-grey and splashed with cerise-red. ↕↔ 1m (3ft). ❄❄❄
***R.* 'Robin Redbreast'** ■ syn. *R.* 'Interrob'. Dwarf ground-cover rose of dense habit, with many shiny, mid-green leaves. Dense clusters of cupped to flat, single, dark red flowers, 4.5cm (1¾in) across, with pale white centres, are produced from summer to autumn. ↕45cm (18in), ↔ 60cm (24in). ❄❄❄

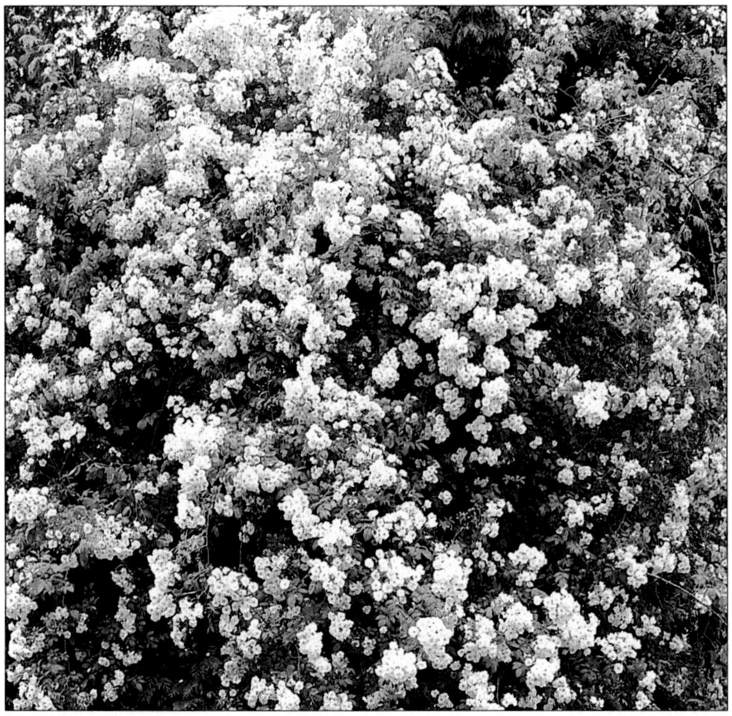
Rosa 'Rambling Rector'

***R.* 'Robusta'** ■ syn. *R.* 'Kordes Robusta'. Vigorous, stiff-growing Rugosa rose with prickly stems and leathery, dark green leaves. Clusters of cupped, single, wine-red flowers, 6cm (2½in) across, with wavy-margined petals, are produced from summer to autumn. ↕1.5m (5ft), ↔ 1m (3ft). ❄❄❄
***R.* 'Rock 'n' Roll'** see *R.* 'Tango'.
***R.* 'Roger Lambelin'** ■ Hybrid Perpetual rose with a shrubby habit, which produces dark green leaves. Loosely formed, rounded, double, fragrant flowers, 7cm (3in) across, with maroon, white-margined petals, are borne mainly in summer. Prone to rust. ↕↔ 1m (3ft). ❄❄❄
***R.* 'Rose Capucine'** see *R. foetida* 'Bicolor'.
***R.* 'Rose de Meaux'** see *R.* 'De Meaux'.
***R.* 'Rose des Maures'** see *R.* 'Sissinghurst Castle'.
***R.* 'Rose d'Isfahan'** see *R.* 'Ispahan'.
***R.* 'Rose Gaujard'.** Strong-growing large-flowered bush rose with abundant glossy, dark green foliage. Urn-shaped, double, cherry-red flowers, 10cm (4in) across, with a pale pink reverse to the petals, are borne from summer to autumn. ↕1m (3ft), ↔ 75cm (30in). ❄❄❄
***R.* 'Rose-Marie Viaud'.** Vigorous rambler with conspicuously veined, light green leaves. Sprays of rosette-shaped, double, lavender-pink to purple flowers, 4cm (1½in) across, fading to greyish mauve, are produced in summer. ↕ to 5m (15ft), ↔ 2.5m (8ft). ❄❄❄
***R.* 'Rosemary Harkness'** ■ syn. *R.* 'Harrowbond'. Vigorous large-flowered bush rose of shrubby habit, with glossy, dark green foliage. Urn-shaped buds open to rounded, double, fragrant, orange to salmon-pink flowers, 10cm (4in) across, from summer to autumn. ↕↔ 80cm (32in). ❄❄❄
***R.* 'Roseraie de l'Haÿ'** ■♀ Vigorous, dense Rugosa rose with leathery, wrinkled, light green leaves. Cupped to flat, double, strongly scented, rich purple-red flowers, 11cm (4½in) across, are borne from summer to autumn. ↕2.2m (7ft), ↔ 2m (6ft). ❄❄❄
***R.* 'Rosette Delizy'.** Vigorous, upright, shrubby Tea rose with glossy, dark green leaves. From summer to autumn, bears high-centred, double, tea-scented, pale yellow flowers, 9cm (3½in) across, flushed apricot-pink. ↕ to 1.2m (4ft), ↔ 1m (3ft). ❄❄
***R.* 'Rosier de Thionville'** see *R.* 'Quatre Saisons Blanche Mousseuse'.
***R.* 'Rosika'** see *R.* 'Radox Bouquet'.
***R.* 'Rosy Cushion'** ■♀ syn. *R.* 'Interall'. Dense, spreading shrub rose with abundant glossy, dark green leaves. From summer to autumn, bears clusters of cupped, semi-double, scented pink flowers, 6cm (2½in) across, with off-white centres. ↕1m (3ft), ↔ 1.2m (4ft). ❄❄❄
***R.* 'Rosy Mantle'** ■ Stiff climber of open habit, with sparse dark green leaves. High-centred, fully double, fragrant, rose- to salmon-pink flowers, 10cm (4in) across, are borne from summer to autumn. ↕2.5m (8ft), ↔ 2m (6ft). ❄❄❄
***R.* 'Rouletii'**, syn. *R. chinensis* var. *minima*, *R.* 'Pompon de Paris'. Compact miniature China rose with thin stems and mid-green leaves comprising many lance-shaped leaflets. Cupped, double, deep pink flowers, 2cm (¾in) across, are borne freely from summer to autumn. ↕↔ 20cm (8in). ❄❄❄
R. roxburghii ■ syn. *R. roxburghii* 'Plena' (Burr rose, Chestnut rose, Chinquapin rose). Vigorous, stiff-growing species rose with flaky bark and light to mid-green leaves, each comprised of 7, rarely 17–19, narrowly ovate to obovate leaflets, 1.5–2.5cm (½–1in) long. Solitary, neatly formed, rounded, double, lilac-pink flowers, 8cm (3in) across, open from prickly buds in summer. ↕↔ 2m (6ft). E. Asia. ❄❄❄.
'Plena' see *R. roxburghii.*
***R.* 'Royal Dane'** see *R.* 'Troika'.
***R.* 'Royal Highness'**, syn. *R.* 'Königliche Hoheit'. Large-flowered bush rose producing strong stems and leathery, dark green leaves. High-centred, fully double, fragrant, pearl-pink flowers, 12cm (5in) across, are borne from summer to autumn. ↕1.1m (3½ft), ↔ 60cm (24in). ❄❄❄
***R.* 'Royal William'** ■♀ syn. *R.* 'Duftzauber '84', *R.* 'Korzaun'. Vigorous, large-flowered bush rose with dark green leaves. High-centred, fully double, fragrant, deep crimson flowers, 12cm (5in) across, are borne from summer to autumn. ↕1m (3ft), ↔ 75cm (30in). ❄❄❄
R. rubiginosa see *R. eglanteria.*

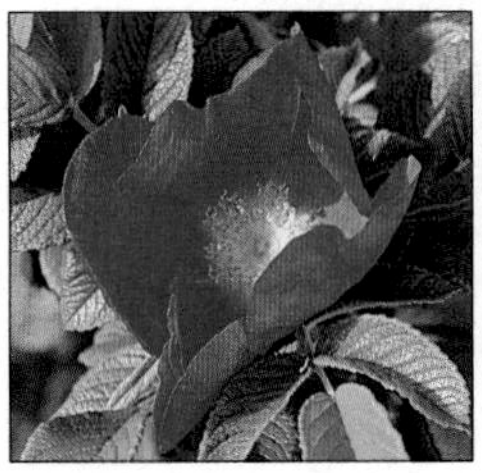
Rosa rugosa

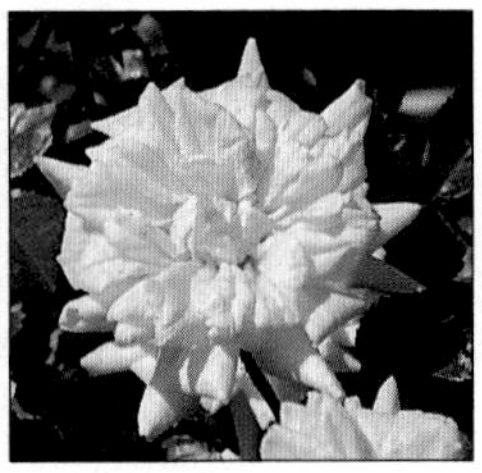
Rosa 'Rugul'

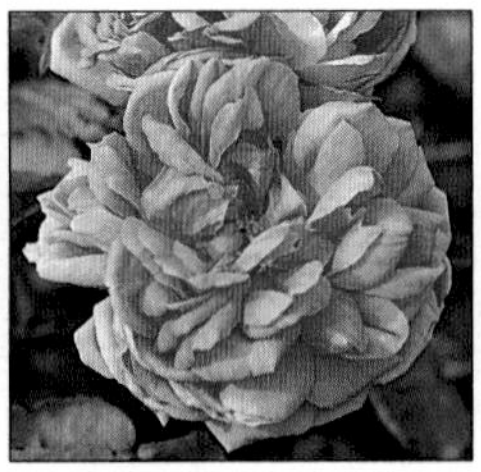
Rosa 'Salet'

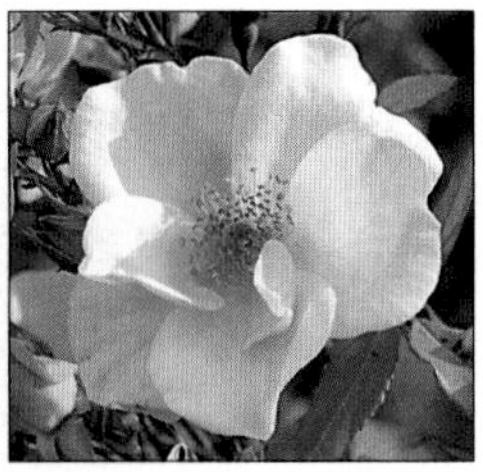
Rosa 'Sally Holmes'

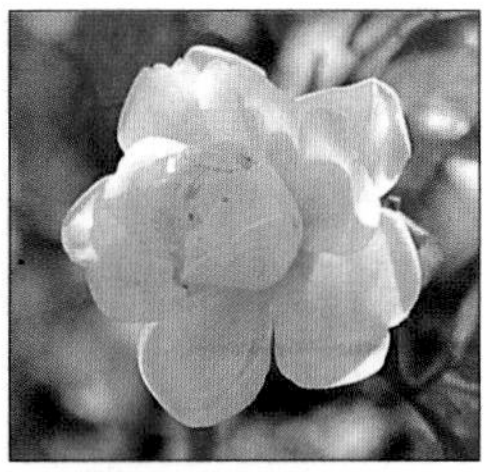
Rosa 'Sanders' White Rambler'

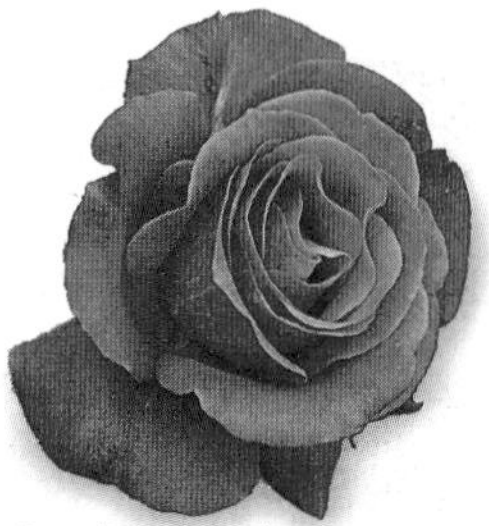
Rosa 'Sandringham Centenary'

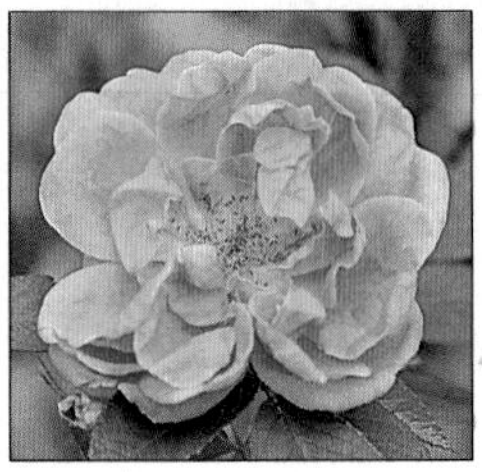
Rosa 'Sarah van Fleet'

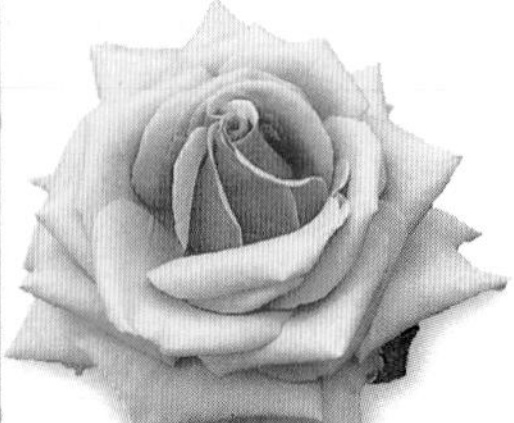
Rosa 'Savoy Hotel'

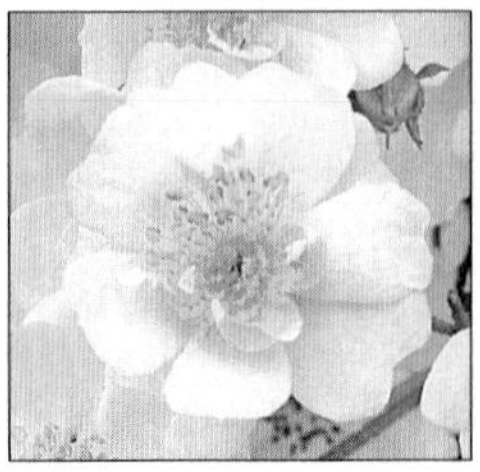
Rosa 'Seagull'

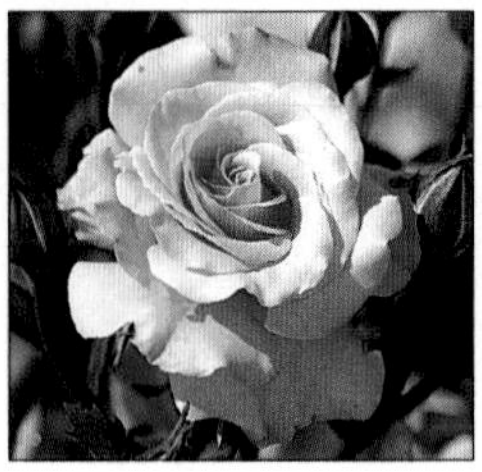
Rosa 'Sexy Rexy'

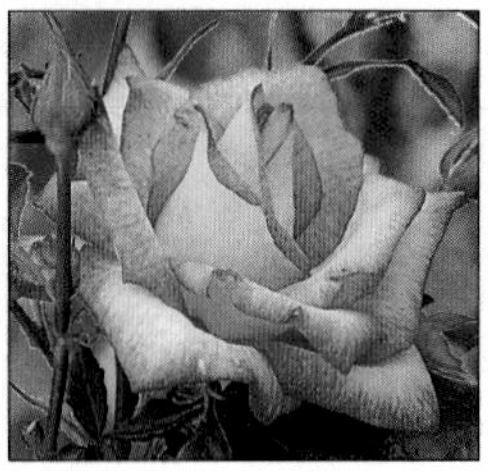
Rosa 'Sheila's Perfume'

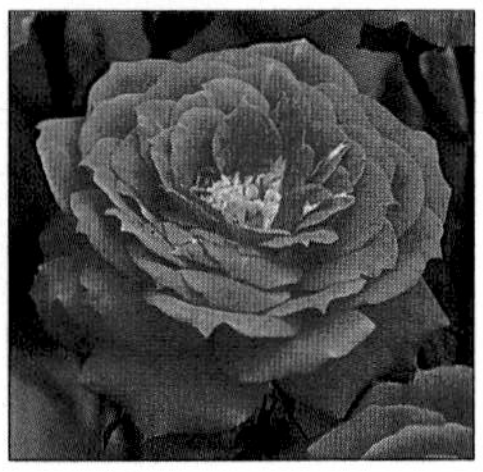
Rosa 'Sheri Anne'

R. rubrifolia see *R. glauca*.
R. rugosa ■ (Hedgehog rose, Japanese rose, Ramanas rose). Vigorous, dense species rose with very prickly stems and wrinkled, leathery, dark green leaves, each composed of 7–9, rarely up to 11, narrowly oblong leaflets, 2.5–5cm (1–2in) long. Cupped, single, fragrant, violet-carmine-red flowers, 8cm (3in) across, showing yellow stamens, are borne singly or in small clusters from summer to autumn, followed by tomato-shaped, red to orange-red hips. Good as a hedge. ↕↔ 1–2.5m (3–8ft). E. Russia, N. China, Korea, Japan. ❄❄❄. **var. *alba*** 🏆 has white flowers, to 9cm (3½in) across, opening from pale pink buds. **var. *rosea*** ■ has rose-pink flowers. **var. *rubra*** 🏆 syn. f. *rubra*, has purplish red flowers. **'Scabrosa'** see *R.* 'Scabrosa'.
***R.* 'Rugul'** ■ syn. *R.* 'Guletta', *R.* 'Tapis Jaune'. Compact, dwarf cluster-flowered bush rose of dense habit, with bright green foliage. Cupped to flat, double yellow flowers, 5cm (2in) across, are produced from summer to autumn. ↕30cm (12in), ↔ 35cm (14in). ❄❄❄
***R.* 'St. Cecilia'**, syn. *R.* 'Ausmit'. Upright shrub rose with mid-green leaves and neatly spaced, cupped, fully double, myrrh-scented, pale apricot-pink to white flowers, 10cm (4in) across, borne on bowed stems from summer to autumn. ↕1m (3ft), ↔ 75cm (30in). ❄❄❄
***R.* 'St. Nicholas'.** Vigorous, erect, prickly Damask rose with abundant downy, dark green foliage. Cupped, semi-double, scented, rose-pink flowers, 12cm (5in) across, with golden stamens, are borne in summer, followed by ellipsoid, orange-red hips. ↕to 2m (6ft), ↔ 1.2m (4ft). ❄❄❄
***R.* 'Salet'** ■ Upright, arching Moss rose with lightly mossed stems and matt, pale green foliage. Bears rounded, double, fragrant, clear rose-pink flowers, 7cm (3in) across, mainly in summer. ↕1.2m (4ft), ↔ 1m (3ft). ❄❄❄
***R.* 'Sally Holmes'** ■🏆 Upright, narrow shrub rose with glossy, dark green leaves. Large clusters of many wide, cupped, single, scented, creamy white flowers, 9cm (3½in) across, are borne on long stems from summer to autumn. ↕2m (6ft), ↔ 1m (3ft). ❄❄❄

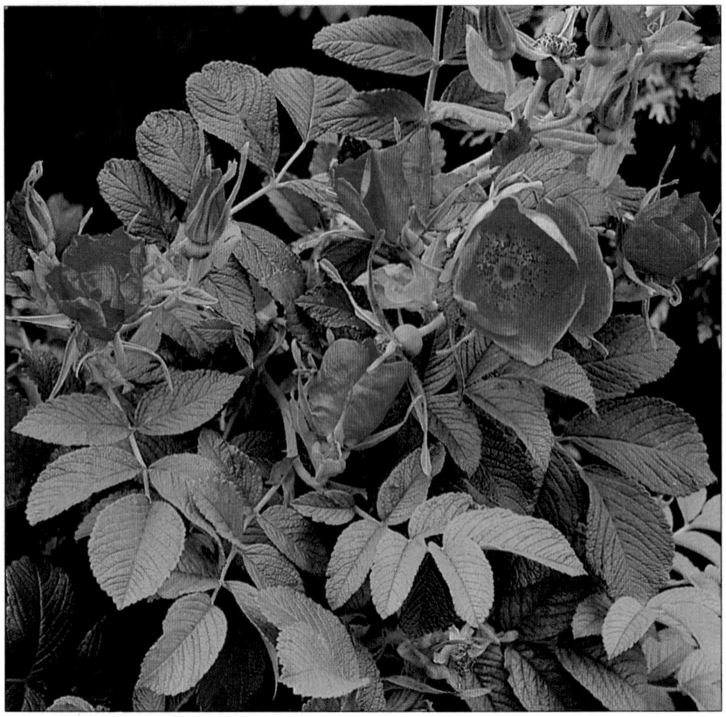
Rosa rugosa var. *rosea*

***R.* 'Samaritan'**, syn. *R.* 'Fragrant Surprise', *R.* 'Harverag'. Large-flowered bush rose with abundant glossy, mid-green foliage. From summer to autumn, wide sprays of pointed buds open to quartered-rosette, fully double, scented flowers, 9cm (3½in) across, which age from apricot-pink to orange-red. ↕70cm (28in), ↔ 60cm (24in). ❄❄❄
***R.* 'Sanders' White Rambler'** ■🏆 Vigorous, arching rambler of lax growth, with abundant glossy, light green leaves. Sprays of many rosette-shaped, fully double, scented white flowers, 5cm (2in) across, cover the plant in late summer. ↕↔ to 4m (12ft). ❄❄❄
***R.* 'Sandringham Centenary'** ■ Vigorous large-flowered bush rose producing dark green leaves. High-centred, double, rose- to salmon-pink flowers, 11cm (4½in) across, are borne from summer to autumn. ↕1.2m (4ft), ↔ 75cm (30in). ❄❄❄
***R.* 'San Rafael'** see *R.* x *odorata* 'Pseudindica'.
***R.* 'Sarah van Fleet'** ■ Vigorous, erect to arching Rugosa rose producing large, wrinkled, bronze-green leaves. Cupped, semi-double, fragrant, clear light pink flowers, 8cm (3in) across, showing yellow stamens, are borne from summer to autumn. ↕2.5m (8ft), ↔ 1.5m (5ft). ❄❄❄
***R.* 'Savoy Hotel'** ■🏆 syn. *R.* 'Harvintage', *R.* 'Integrity'. Vigorous large-flowered bush rose with strong stems and dark green leaves. From summer to autumn, bears high-centred to rounded, fully double, light pink flowers, 11cm (4½in) across, with a deeper pink reverse to the petals. ↕80cm (32in), ↔ 60cm (24in). ❄❄❄
***R.* 'Scabrosa'** 🏆 syn. *R. rugosa* 'Scabrosa'. Vigorous, dense-growing Rugosa rose of rounded habit, with wrinkled, leathery, light green leaves. Cupped, single, fragrant, reddish mauve flowers, 10cm (4in) across, with prominent yellow stamens, are borne from summer to autumn, followed by tomato-shaped red hips. ↕↔ 1.7m (5½ft). ❄❄❄
***R.* 'Scarlet Fire'** see *R.* 'Scharlachglut'.
***R.* 'Scarlet Glow'** see *R.* 'Scharlachglut'.
***R.* 'Scharlachglut'** 🏆 syn. *R.* 'Scarlet Fire', *R.* 'Scarlet Glow'. Very vigorous, arching shrub or climbing rose of open habit, with dark green leaves. Showy, cupped, single, bright crimson-scarlet flowers, 12cm (5in) across, with golden stamens, are borne freely in summer, followed by pear-shaped, bright red hips. ↕to 3m (10ft), ↔ 2m (6ft). ❄❄❄
***R.* 'Schneewittchen'** see *R.* 'Iceberg'.
***R.* 'Schneezwerg'** 🏆 syn. *R.* 'Snow Dwarf'. Rugosa rose of dense, bushy, even habit, with wrinkled, mid-green leaves. From summer to autumn, bears flat, semi-double, scented white flowers, 8cm (3in) across, showing yellow stamens; they are followed by tomato-shaped, orange-red hips. ↕1.2m (4ft), ↔ 1.5m (5ft). ❄❄❄
***R.* 'Schoolgirl'.** Stiff, lanky, large-flowered climber producing sparse deep green leaves. High-centred to rounded, fully double, scented, deep apricot flowers, 10cm (4in) across, are borne from summer to autumn. ↕3m (10ft), ↔ 2.5m (8ft). ❄❄❄
***R.* 'Seagull'** ■🏆 Rampant rambler of arching habit, with greyish green leaves. Large clusters of numerous cupped to flat, single to semi-double white flowers, 2.5cm (1in) across, with golden stamens, cover the plant in summer. ↕to 6m (20ft), ↔ 4m (12ft). ❄❄❄
R. sericea* subsp. *omeiensis* f. *pteracantha, syn. *R. omeiensis* f. *pteracantha* (Winged thorn rose). Stiff, upright, vigorous species rose with large, translucent red prickles, to 3cm (1¼in) or more wide and 2cm (¾in) tall, on young stems. Small, fern-like, light green leaves each have 11–17 elliptic, oblong, or obovate leaflets, 1–3cm (½–1¼in) long. Solitary, flat, usually 4-petalled white flowers, 2.5–6cm (1–2½in) across, are borne briefly along the stems in summer. ↕2.5m (8ft), ↔ 2.2m (7ft). W. China. ❄❄❄
***R.* 'Sexy Rexy'** ■🏆 syn. *R.* 'Heckenzauber', *R.* 'Macrexy'. Cluster-flowered bush rose producing abundant glossy, dark green foliage. Showy, heavy heads of camellia-like, rounded, fully double, rose-pink flowers, 8cm (3in) across, are borne from summer to autumn. ↕70cm (28in), ↔ 60cm (24in). ❄❄❄
***R.* 'Sheila's Perfume'** ■ syn. *R.* 'Harsherry'. Cluster-flowered bush rose with glossy, dark green leaves. Urn-shaped, double, fragrant yellow flowers, 9cm (3½in) across, strongly marked and veined with red, are borne singly or in

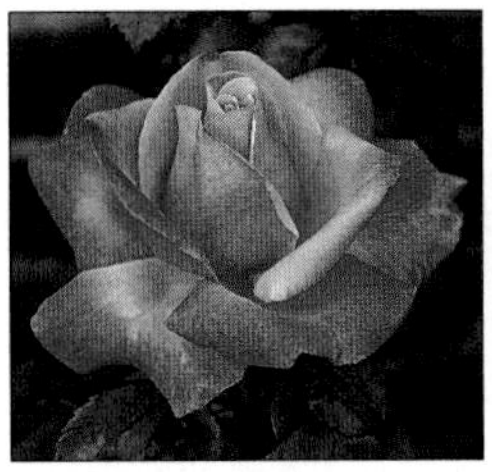
Rosa 'Silver Jubilee'

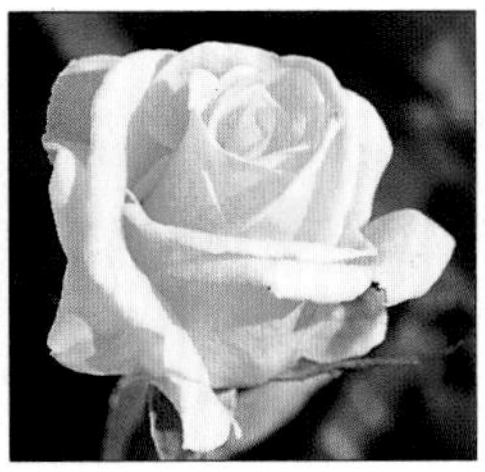
Rosa 'Simba'

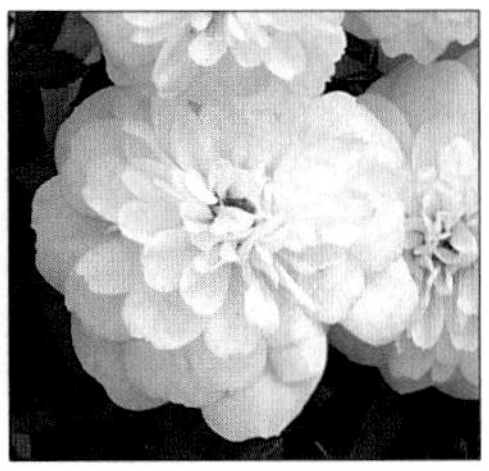
Rosa 'Snowball'

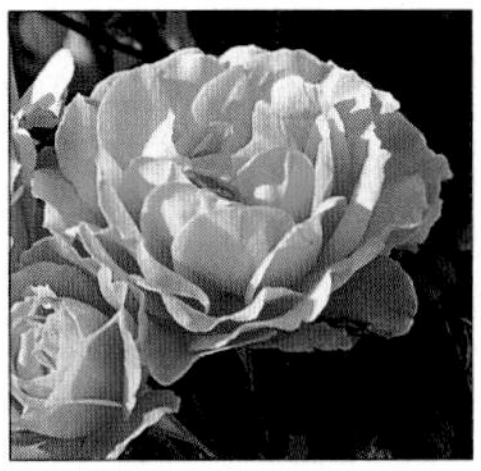
Rosa 'Southampton'

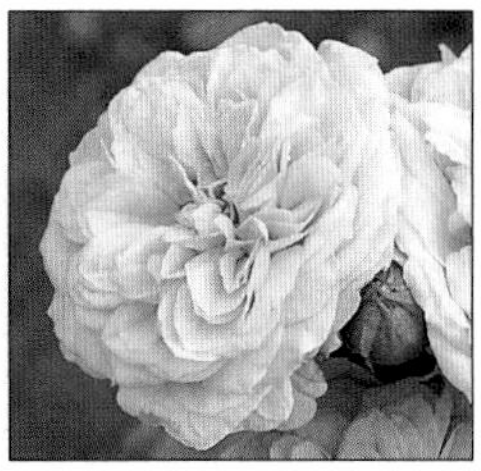
Rosa 'Souvenir de la Malmaison'

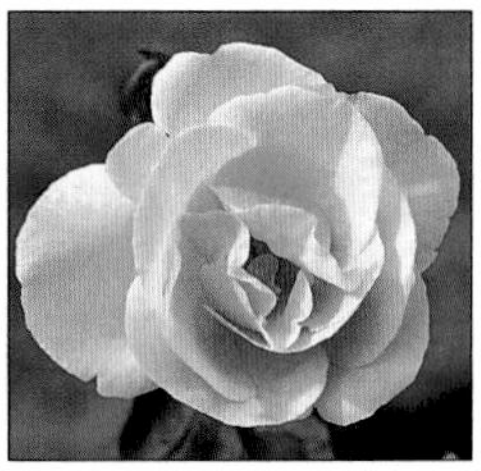
Rosa 'Souvenir de St. Anne's'

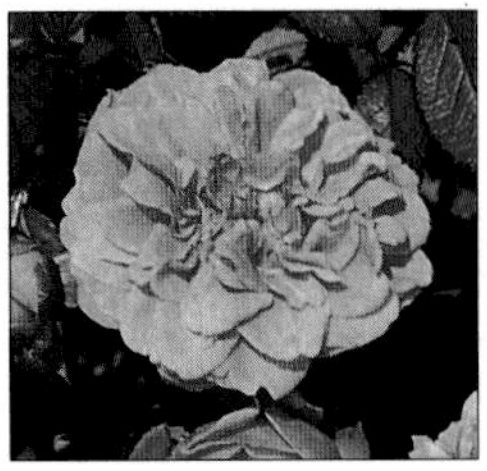
Rosa 'Stacey Sue'

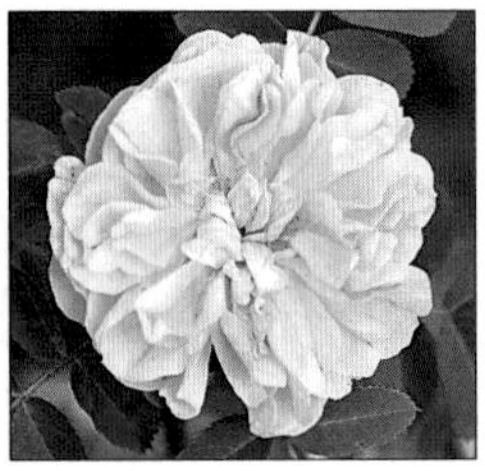
Rosa 'Stanwell Perpetual'

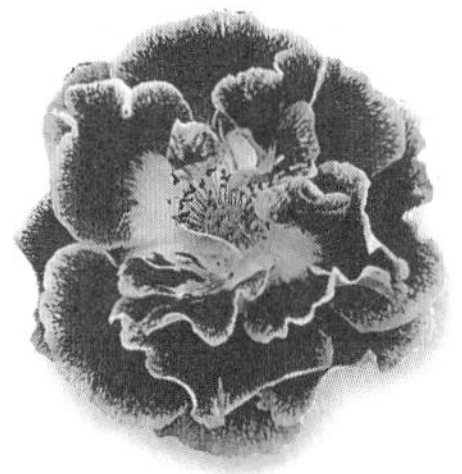
Rosa 'Sue Lawley'

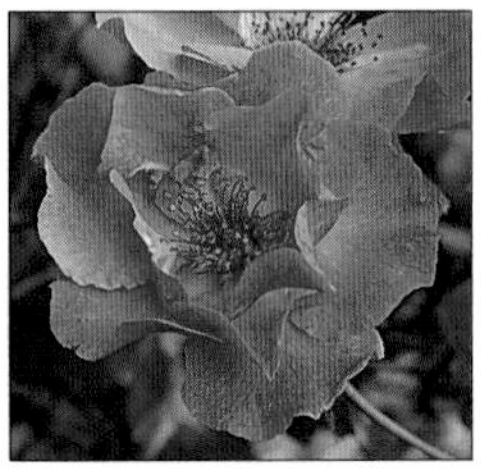
Rosa 'Summer Wine'

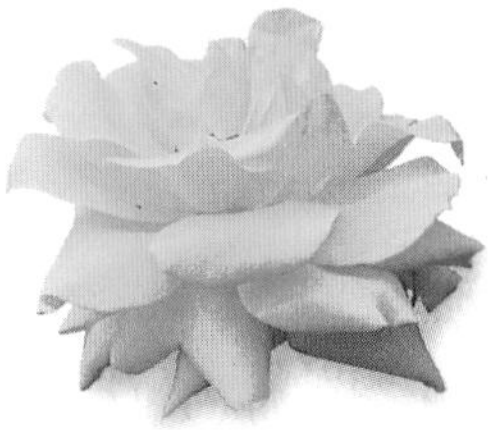
Rosa 'Sunblest'

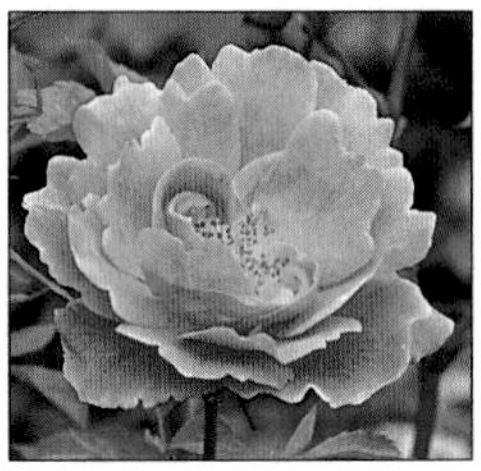
Rosa 'Surrey'

open clusters from summer to autumn. ↕75cm (30in), ↔ 60cm (24in). ✻✻✻

***R.* 'Sheri Anne'** ▣ Miniature bush rose of neat, upright habit, with glossy, mid-green leaves. From summer to autumn, bears clusters of many urn-shaped, double, light orange-red flowers, 2.5cm (1in) across, the petals with yellow bases. ↕35cm (14in), ↔ 30cm (12in). ✻✻✻

***R.* 'Shocking Blue'** syn. *R.* 'Korblue'. Cluster-flowered bush rose with dark green leaves. Urn-shaped buds open to rounded, fully double, fragrant, lilac-purple flowers, 10cm (4in) across, borne singly or in clusters from summer to autumn. ↕75cm (30in), ↔ 60cm (24in). ✻✻✻

***R.* 'Silver Jubilee'** ▣🏆 Large-flowered bush rose of dense, leafy habit, with dark green leaves. High-centred, fully double, rose-pink flowers, to 12cm (5in) across, flushed peach- or salmon-pink, are borne singly or in open clusters on strong stems from summer to autumn. ↕1.1m (3½ft), ↔ 60cm (24in). ✻✻✻

***R.* 'Silver Moon'.** Vigorous, free-branching climber with long, arching stems and glossy, dark green leaves. In summer, freely bears clusters of cupped, semi-double, scented, creamy white flowers, 10cm (4in) across. ↕to 6m (20ft), ↔ 3m (10ft). ✻✻✻

***R.* 'Simba'** ▣ syn. *R.* 'Goldsmith', *R.* 'Helmut Schmidt', *R.* 'Korbelma'. Large-flowered bush rose of neat habit, with mid-green leaves. Urn-shaped buds open to well-formed, rounded, fully double yellow flowers, 9cm (3½in) across, borne from summer to autumn. ↕60cm (24in), ↔ 50cm (20in). ✻✻✻

***R.* 'Sissi'** see *R.* 'Blue Moon'.

***R.* 'Sissinghurst Castle'** syn. *R.* 'Rose des Maures'. Gallica rose of upright, free-suckering habit, with slender, firm stems and dark green leaves. Cupped to flat, semi-double, scented, deep maroon-crimson flowers, 6cm (2½in) across, showing yellow stamens, are borne in summer. ↕↔ 1m (3ft). ✻✻✻

***R.* 'Snowball'** ▣ syn. *R.* 'Angelita', *R.* 'Macangel'. Compact miniature bush rose of spreading habit, with many tiny, bright green leaves. Clusters of pompon, narrow-petalled, fully double white flowers, 2.5cm (1in) across, are borne from summer to autumn. ↕20cm (8in), ↔ 30cm (12in). ✻✻✻

***R.* 'Snow Carpet'** 🏆 syn. *R.* 'Maccarpe'. Prostrate, creeping miniature ground-cover rose with bright green leaves. In summer, bears pompon, fully double, creamy white flowers, 3cm (1¼in) across. ↕15cm (6in), ↔ 45cm (18in). ✻✻✻

***R.* 'Snow Dwarf'** see *R.* 'Schneezwerg'.

***R.* 'Snow Queen'** see *R.* 'Frau Karl Druschki'.

***R.* 'Sommerwind'** see *R.* 'Surrey'.

***R.* 'Southampton'** ▣🏆 syn. *R.* 'Susan Ann'. Cluster-flowered bush rose with shiny, dark green leaves. High-centred, double, scented apricot flowers, 8cm (3in) across, flushed with red, are borne singly or in clusters on firm stems from summer to autumn. ↕1.1m (3½ft), ↔ 70cm (28in). ✻✻✻

***R.* 'Souvenir de la Malmaison'** ▣ syn. *R.* 'Queen of Beauty & Fragrance'. Dense, spreading Bourbon rose with dark green foliage and quartered-rosette, fully double, spice-scented, pale pink to white flowers, 12cm (5in) across, borne from summer to autumn. Rain may spoil flowers. ↕↔ to 1.5m (5ft). ✻✻✻

***R.* 'Souvenir de la Princesse de Lamballe'** see *R.* 'Bourbon Queen'.

***R.* 'Souvenir de St. Anne's'** ▣🏆 Vigorous Bourbon rose producing abundant dark green foliage. Wide-opening, cupped, semi-double, scented, pearl-pink flowers, 9cm (3½in) across, are borne freely from summer to autumn. ↕1.5m (5ft), ↔ 1.2m (4ft). ✻✻✻

***R.* 'Spanish Beauty'** see *R.* 'Mme Grégoire Staechelin'.

***R.* 'Spanish Shawl'** see *R.* 'Sue Lawley'.

***R.* 'Spectacular'** see *R.* 'Danse du Feu'.

R. spinosissima see *R. pimpinellifolia.*

***R.* 'Splendens'**, syn. *R.* 'Ayrshire Splendens' (Myrrh-scented rose). Vigorous climber with dark green leaves. In summer, purple-red buds open to loosely formed, cupped, double, myrrh-scented, pale creamy pink flowers, 4.5cm (1¾in) across, with orange-yellow stamens. ↕to 8m (25ft), ↔ 3m (10ft). ✻✻✻

***R.* 'Spring Gold'** see *R.* 'Frühlingsgold'.

***R.* 'Spring Morning'** see *R.* 'Frühlingsmorgen'.

***R.* 'Stacey Sue'** ▣🏆 Miniature bush rose of neat, spreading habit, with dark green leaves. Rosette-shaped, fully double, rose-pink flowers, 2.5cm (1in) across, are borne in dense sprays from summer to autumn. ↕25cm (10in), ↔ 30cm (12in). ✻✻✻

***R.* 'Stanwell Perpetual'** ▣ Scots rose of spreading, twiggy habit, with prickly stems and fern-like, dark greyish green leaves. Loosely formed, cupped, fully double, scented, pale pink flowers, 8cm (3in) across, are borne singly on thin stems from summer to autumn. ↕1m (3ft), ↔ 1.2m (4ft). ✻✻✻

***R.* 'Starina'**, syn. *R.* 'Meigabi'. Neat miniature bush rose with shiny, dark green leaves. High-centred, fully double, orange-red flowers, 4cm (1½in) across, are borne from summer to autumn. ↕↔ 35cm (14in). ✻✻✻

***R.* 'Stars 'n' Stripes'.** Miniature bush rose of uneven, spreading habit, with small, dark green leaves. From summer to autumn, bears cupped, semi-double flowers, 4.5cm (1¾in) across, pale pink to white, striped strawberry-red. ↕30cm (12in), ↔ to 70cm (28in). ✻✻✻

R. stellata* var. *mirifica (Sacramento rose). Species rose of suckering habit, with springy, wiry, prickly stems and mid-green leaves, each with 3–5 deeply cut, gooseberry-like, wedge-shaped leaflets, 0.7–1cm (¼–½in) long. In summer bears solitary, wide-opening, cupped to flat, single, scented, pink to deep rose-purple flowers, 3.5–6cm (1½–2¼in) across. ↕to 1.1m (3½ft), ↔ 1.2m (4ft). USA (New Mexico). ✻✻✻

***R.* 'Sterling Silver'.** Large-flowered, not very robust bush rose with sparse leathery, mid-green foliage. From summer to autumn, bears high-centred to cupped, double, fragrant, lilac-mauve flowers, 9cm (3½in) across. ↕80cm (32in), ↔ 60cm (24in). ✻✻✻

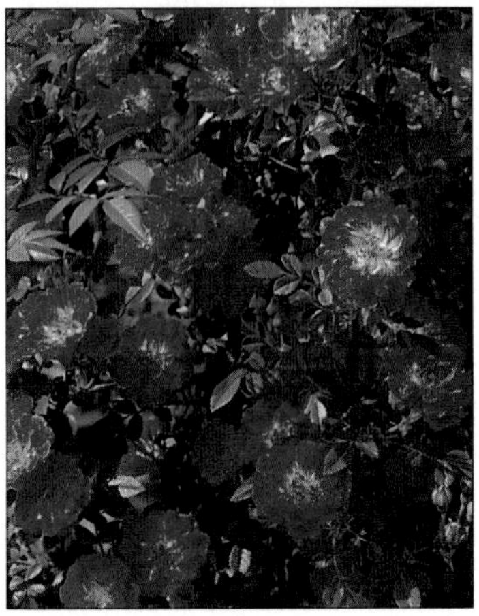
Rosa 'Suma'

***R.* 'Stretch Johnson'** see *R.* 'Tango'.

***R.* 'Sue Lawley'** ▣ syn. *R.* 'Macspash', *R.* 'Spanish Shawl'. Cluster-flowered bush rose with dark green leaves. From summer to autumn, bears sprays of cupped, wide-opening, double, carmine-red flowers, 9cm (3½in) across, with paler pink or white centres and petal margins. ↕↔ 60cm (24in). ✻✻✻

***R.* 'Suma'** ▣🏆 syn. *R.* 'Harsuma'. Prostrate ground-cover shrub rose with shiny, dark green foliage, turning burnished crimson in autumn. Clusters of rosette-shaped, double, ruby-red to deep pink flowers, 3cm (1¼in) across, are borne along the stems from summer to autumn. ↕50cm (20in), ↔ 1.5m (5ft). ✻✻✻

***R.* 'Summer Wine'** ▣🏆 syn. *R.* 'Korizont'. Climber with stiff, branching growth and mid-green leaves. Cupped, single, scented, coral-pink flowers, 10cm (4in) across, shaded yellow at the bases and with folded petals, are produced from summer to autumn. ↕3m (10ft), ↔ 2.2m (7ft). ✻✻✻

***R.* 'Sunblaze'** see *R.* 'Orange Sunblaze'.

***R.* 'Sunblest'** ▣ syn. *R.* 'Landora'. Large-flowered bush rose producing shiny, mid-green leaves. Pointed buds open to cupped, double yellow flowers, 9cm (3½in) across, borne freely from summer to autumn. ↕1m (3ft), ↔ 60cm (24in). ✻✻✻

***R.* 'Sunnyside'** see *R.* 'Avon'.

***R.* 'Sunsprite'** see *R.* 'Korresia'.

***R.* 'Super Star'**, syn. *R.* 'Tanorstar', *R.* 'Tropicana'. Large-flowered bush rose of open, uneven habit, with small, dark green leaves. Rounded, fully double, lightly scented, vermilion to pale scarlet flowers, 11cm (4½in) across, are borne from summer to autumn. ↕1.1m (3½ft), ↔ 1m (3ft). ✻✻✻

***R.* 'Surrey'** ▣🏆 syn. *R.* 'Korlanum', *R.* 'Sommerwind', *R.* 'Vent d'Eté'. Vigorous, mound-forming ground-cover shrub rose with abundant dark green foliage. Clusters of cupped, double, rose-pink flowers, 6cm (2½in) across, are borne along the stems from summer to autumn. ↕80cm (32in), ↔ 1.2m (4ft). ✻✻✻

***R.* 'Susan Ann'** see *R.* 'Southampton'.

***R.* 'Sutter's Gold'.** Spindly large-flowered bush rose with sparse leathery, dark green foliage. High-centred buds

ROSA

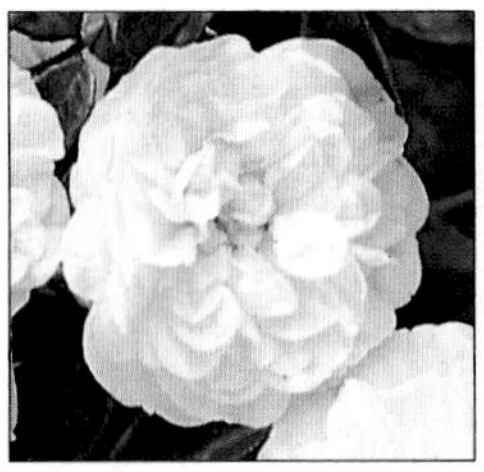
Rosa 'Swany'

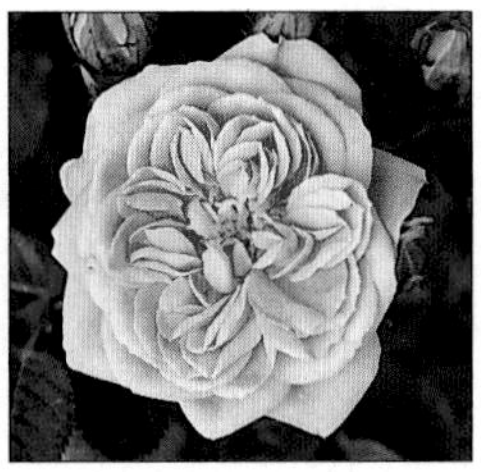
Rosa 'Sweet Dream'

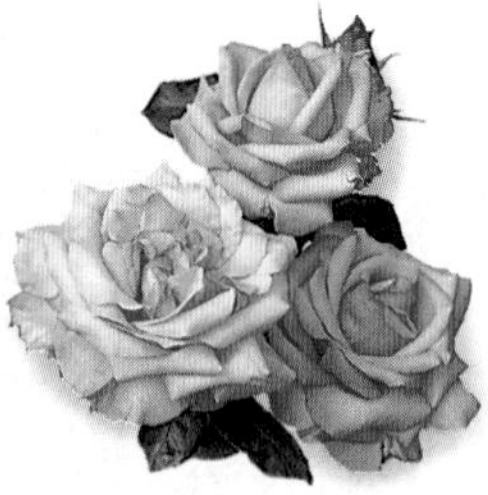
Rosa 'Sweetheart'

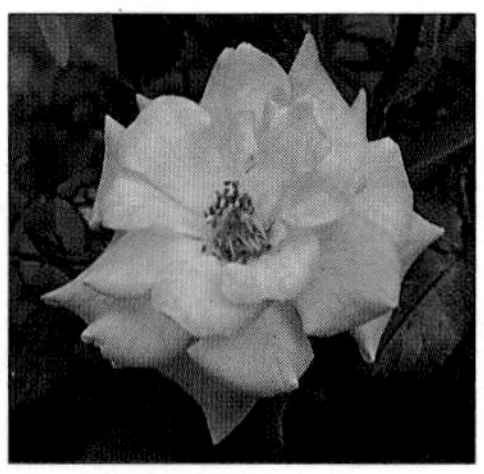
Rosa 'Sweet Magic'

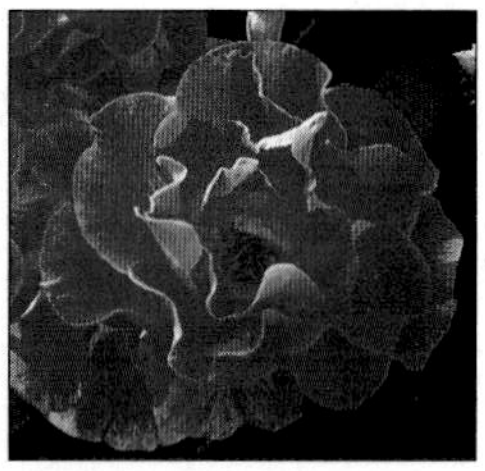
Rosa 'Tango'

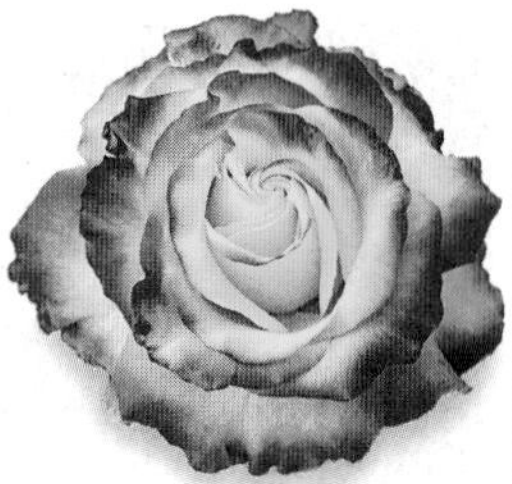
Rosa 'Tequila Sunrise'

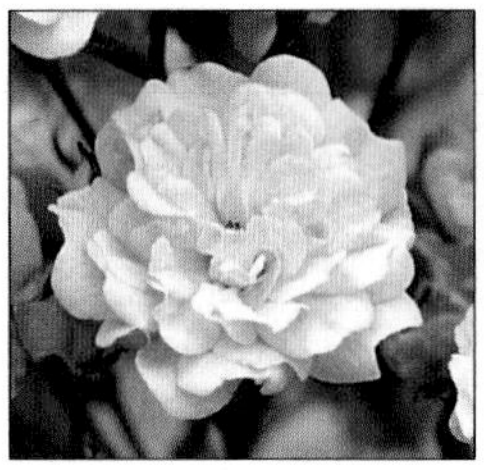
Rosa 'The Fairy'

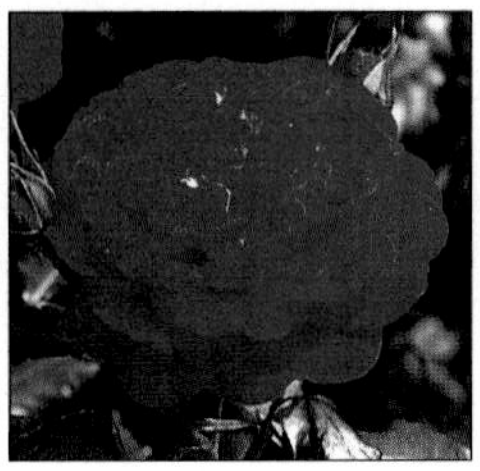
Rosa 'The Times'

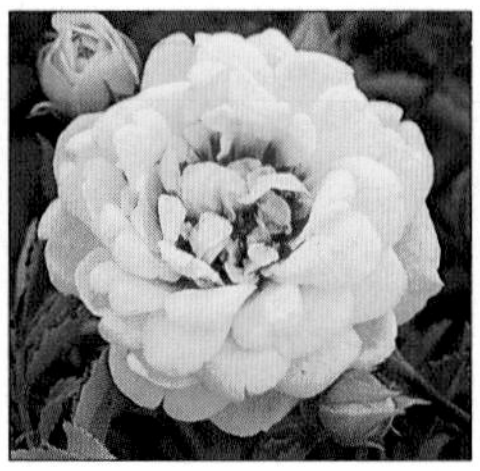
Rosa 'Tigris'

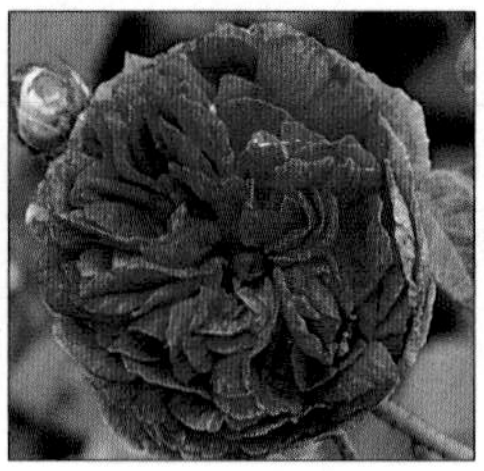
Rosa 'Tour de Malakoff'

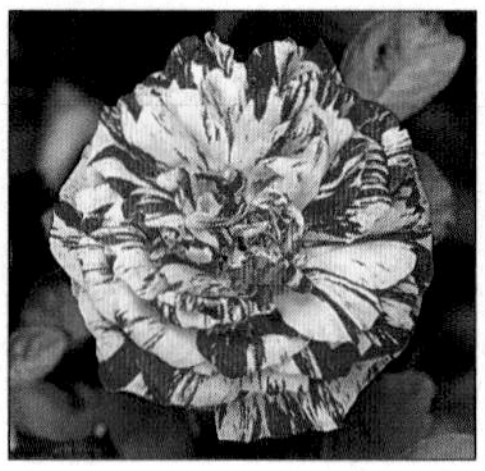
Rosa 'Tricolore de Flandre'

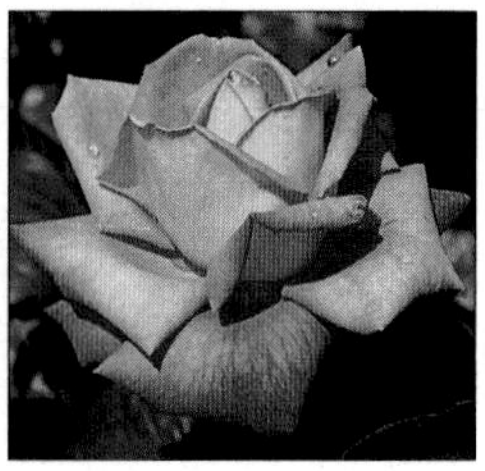
Rosa 'Troika'

open to loosely formed, high-centred, double, fragrant, golden orange flowers, 11cm (4½in) across, overlaid with red, from summer to autumn. ↕1m (3ft), ↔60cm (24in). ***

***R.* 'Swany'** ■ ♀ syn. *R.* 'Meiburenac'. Vigorous, dense ground-cover shrub rose with shiny, dark green leaves. Profuse clusters of numerous flat, fully double white flowers, 5cm (2in) across, are borne from summer to autumn. ↕to 75cm (30in), ↔to 1.7m (5½ft). ***

***R.* 'Sweet Dream'** ■ ♀ syn. *R.* 'Fryminicot'. Dwarf cluster-flowered bush rose of neat, leafy habit, with mid-green foliage. Dense clusters of cupped, fully double, peach-apricot flowers, 6cm (2½in) across, are borne on stiff stems from summer to autumn. ↕40cm (16in), ↔35cm (14in). ***

***R.* 'Sweetheart'** ■ syn. *R.* 'Cocapeer'. Large-flowered bush rose of upright habit, with dense, light green foliage. Rounded, double, fragrant, rose-pink flowers, 11cm (4½in) across, are borne from summer to autumn. ↕90cm (36in), ↔60cm (24in). ***

***R.* 'Sweetheart Rose'** see *R.* 'Cécile Brunner'.

***R.* 'Sweet Juliet'**, syn. *R.* 'Ausleap'. Large-flowered shrub rose of prolific growth, with mid-green leaves. Cupped, fully double, tea-scented, apricot-yellow flowers, 10cm (4in) across, are borne from summer to autumn. ↕1.1m (3½ft), ↔1m (3ft). ***

***R.* 'Sweet Magic'** ■ ♀ syn. *R.* 'Dicmagic'. Neat, dwarf cluster-flowered bush rose with bright green leaves. From summer to autumn, well-spaced clusters of urn-shaped buds open to cupped, double, apricot-orange and yellow flowers, 4cm (1½in) across. ↕↔35cm (14in). ***

***R.* 'Sweet Sunblaze'** see *R.* 'Pretty Polly'.

***R.* 'Sylvia'** see *R.* 'Congratulations'.

***R.* 'Sympathie'** ■ Free-branching, vigorous climber with dense, glossy, dark green foliage. Cupped, fully double, bright deep red flowers, 8cm (3in) across, are borne from summer to autumn, usually in clusters. ↕3m (10ft), ↔2.5m (8ft). ***

***R.* 'Taifun'** see *R.* 'Typhoon'.

***R.* 'Tall Story'** ♀ syn. *R.* 'Dickooky'. Ground-cover shrub rose with abundant glossy, light green leaves. Graceful sprays of cupped, semi-double, scented, light primrose-yellow flowers, 6cm (2½in) across, are borne on bowed stems from summer to autumn. ↕75cm (30in), ↔1.2m (4ft). ***

***R.* 'Tanellis'** see *R.* 'Fragrant Cloud'.

***R.* 'Tango'** ■ ♀ syn. *R.* 'Macfirwal', *R.* 'Rock 'n' Roll', *R.* 'Stretch Johnson'. Cluster-flowered bush rose with mid-green leaves. From summer to autumn, bears cupped, wide-opening, semi-double, orange-red flowers, 6cm (2½in) across, with petals margined yellowish white and yellow on the reverse sides. ↕75cm (30in), ↔60cm (24in). ***

***R.* 'Tanryrandy'** see *R.* 'Cherry Brandy'.

***R.* 'Tapis d'Orient'** see *R.* 'Yesterday'.

***R.* 'Tapis Jaune'** see *R.* 'Rugul'.

***R.* 'Tapis Persan'** see *R.* 'Eye Paint'.

***R.* 'Tequila Sunrise'** ■ ♀ syn. *R.* 'Dicobey'. Large-flowered bush rose of open habit, with glossy, dark green leaves. Wide sprays of rounded, fully double yellow flowers, 10cm (4in) across, with scarlet-margined petals, are borne freely from summer to autumn. ↕75cm (30in), ↔60cm (24in). ***

***R.* 'The Fairy'** ■ ♀ Dwarf Polyantha rose of dense, cushion-forming habit, with abundant shiny, mid-green leaves. Rosette-shaped, double, light pink flowers, 2.5cm (1in) across, are borne freely from late summer to autumn. ↕↔60–90cm (24–36in). ***

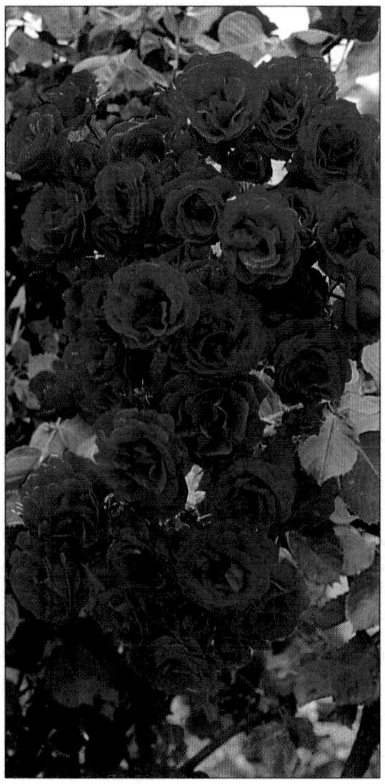
Rosa 'Sympathie'

***R.* 'The New Dawn'** see *R.* 'New Dawn'.

***R.* 'The Queen Elizabeth'** see *R.* 'Queen Elizabeth'.

***R.* 'The Times'** ■ ♀ syn. *R.* 'Carl Philip', *R.* 'Christian IV', *R.* 'Korpeahn', *R.* 'Mariandel'. Cluster-flowered bush rose of spreading habit, with abundant purplish green leaves. Cupped to flat, double, dark crimson flowers, 8cm (3in) across, are borne in wide clusters from summer to autumn. ↕60cm (24in), ↔75cm (30in). ***

***R.* 'Thisbe'.** Leafy, bushy cluster-flowered shrub rose producing mid-green leaves with lance-shaped leaflets. Rosette-shaped, fully double, scented, buff yellow flowers, 4.5cm (1¾in) across, fading to cream and showing amber stamens, are borne from summer to autumn. ↕↔1.2m (4ft). ***

***R.* 'Tigris'** ■ syn. *R.* 'Harprier'. Cushion-forming, spreading shrub rose with wiry, prickly, gooseberry-like stems and pale green leaves. In summer, bears pompon, double, canary-yellow flowers, 3cm (1¼in) across, with dark red eyes. ↕45cm (18in), ↔60cm (24in). ***

***R.* 'Tipo Ideale'** see *R.* x *odorata* 'Mutabilis'.

***R.* 'Tobone'** see *R.* 'Prima Donna'.

***R.* 'Tocade'** see *R.* 'Arizona'.

***R.* 'Top Gear'** see *R.* 'Little Artist'.

***R.* 'Touch of Class'**, syn. *R.* 'Kricarlo', *R.* 'Maréchal le Clerc'. Large-flowered bush rose with dark green leaves. High-centred, double flowers, 12cm (5in) across, pale creamy pink suffused with coral-pink, are borne on long stems from summer to autumn. ↕1.1m (3½ft), ↔70cm (28in). ***

***R.* 'Tour de Malakoff'** ■ Centifolia rose of lax, spreading habit, with dark green leaves. Cupped, double, fragrant flowers, 12cm (5in) across, purplish magenta fading to greyish violet, are borne in summer. ↕2m (6ft), ↔1.5m (5ft). ***

***R.* 'Tournament of Roses'**, syn. *R.* 'Berkeley', *R.* 'Jacient', *R.* 'Poesie'. Strong-growing large-flowered bush rose with glossy, dark green leaves. Rounded, double, light rose- to salmon-pink flowers, 10cm (4in) across, are borne from summer to autumn. ↕1.1m (3½ft), ↔60cm (24in). ***

***R.* 'Tricolore de Flandre'** ■ Vigorous Gallica rose of bushy, upright habit, with dull, dark green leaves. Cupped to flat, fully double, fragrant, pale pink flowers, 6cm (2½in) across, striped with pink and purple, are borne in summer. ↕↔1m (3ft). ***

***R.* 'Trier 2000'** see *R.* 'Anna Livia'.

***R.* 'Troika'** ■ ♀ syn. *R.* 'Royal Dane'. Vigorous, branching large-flowered bush rose with abundant semi-glossy, mid-green leaves. High-centred, double, fragrant, reddish orange flowers, 15cm (6in) across, with pink flushes, are produced from summer to autumn. ↕1m (3ft), ↔75cm (30in). ***

***R.* 'Tropicana'** see *R.* 'Super Star'.

***R.* 'Trumpeter'** ■ ♀ syn. *R.* 'Mactru'. Cluster-flowered bush rose of neat habit, with deep green foliage. Showy, cupped, fully double, vivid orange-red flowers, 6cm (2½in) across, are borne from summer to autumn. ↕60cm (24in), ↔50cm (20in). ***

***R.* 'Tuscany Superb'** ■ ♀ (Double velvet rose). Vigorous, rounded Gallica rose with dark green leaves. In summer, erect stems bear cupped to flat, double, scented, deep crimson-maroon to purple flowers, 5cm (2in) across, showing gold stamens. ↕↔1m (3ft). ***

***R.* 'Typhoon'** ■ syn. *R.* 'Taifun'. Large-flowered bush rose of even, spreading habit, with burnished, dark green leaves. Rounded, fully double, fragrant, salmon- to orange-pink flowers, 10cm (4in) across, are borne from summer to autumn. ↕75cm (30in), ↔65cm (26in). ***

***R.* 'Valencia'** ■ syn. *R.* 'Koreklia'. Large-flowered bush rose of open habit, with leathery, glossy, dark green foliage. From summer to autumn, bears high-centred, fully double, fragrant, amber-yellow flowers, 10cm (4in) across. ↕75cm (30in), ↔65cm (26in). ***

***R.* 'Valentine Heart'** ■ syn. *R.* 'Dicogle'. Cluster-flowered bush rose of open habit, with dark green foliage. From summer to autumn, pale scarlet buds open to cupped, semi-double, scented, pale pink and deeper pink flowers, 7cm (3in) across, with infolded, frilled petals at the centres. ↕60cm (24in), ↔50cm (20in). ***

***R.* 'Variegata di Bologna'.** Willowy, arching, smooth-wooded Bourbon rose

R

ROSA

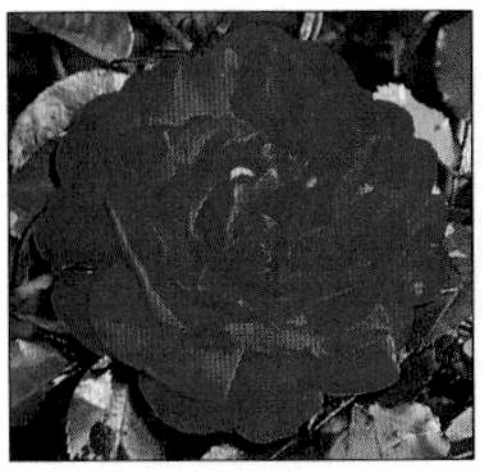
Rosa 'Trumpeter'

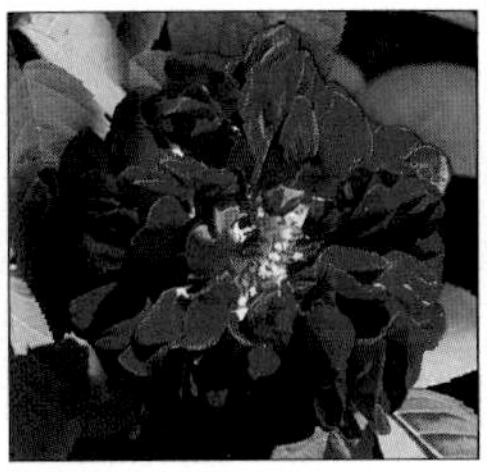
Rosa 'Tuscany Superb'

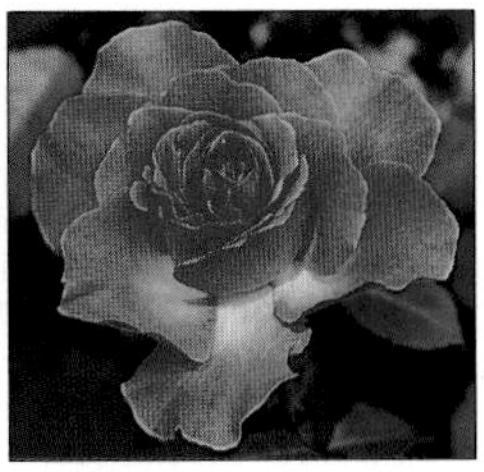
Rosa 'Typhoon'

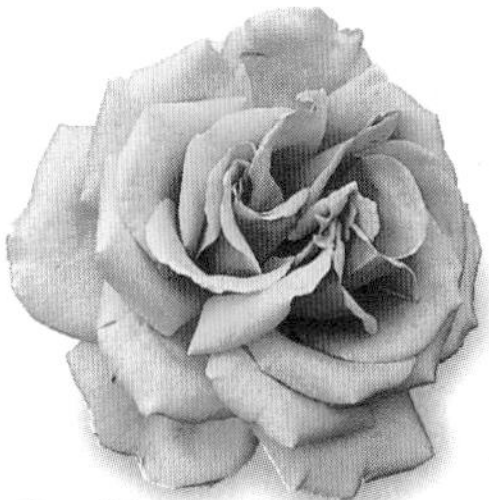
Rosa 'Valencia'

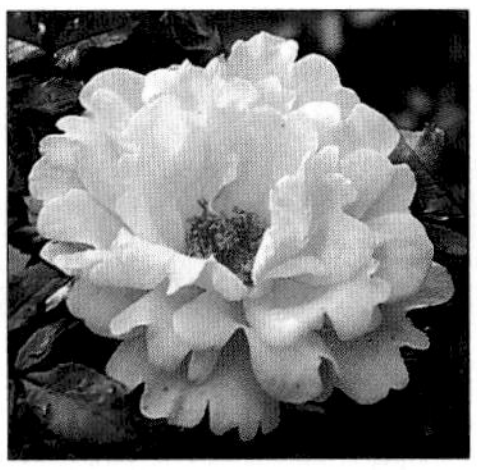
Rosa 'Valentine Heart'

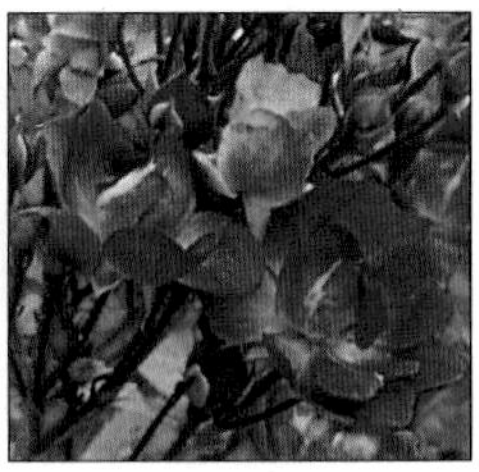
Rosa 'Veilchenblau'

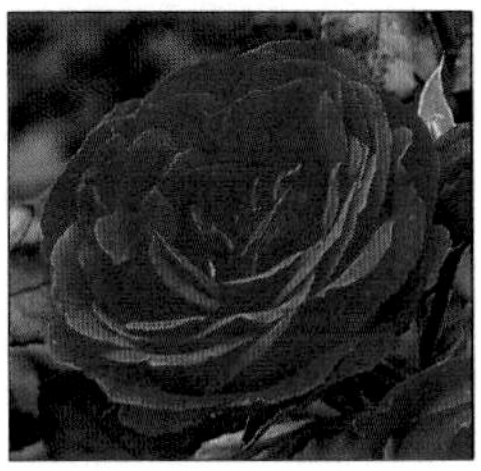
Rosa 'Warrior'

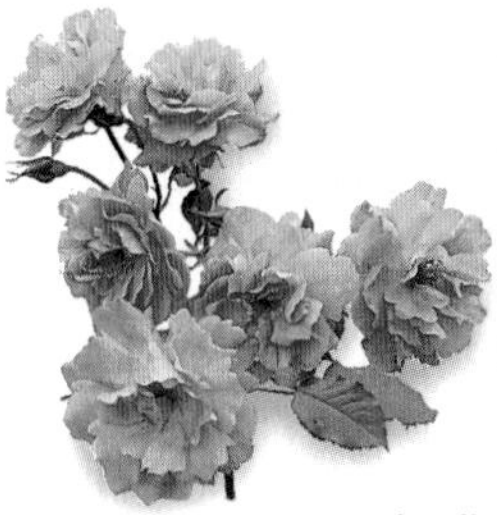
Rosa 'Westerland'

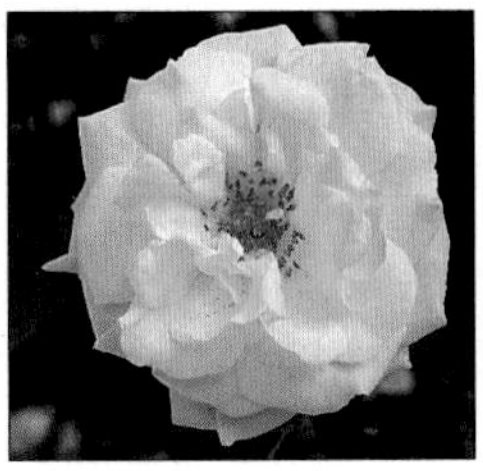
Rosa 'White Cockade'

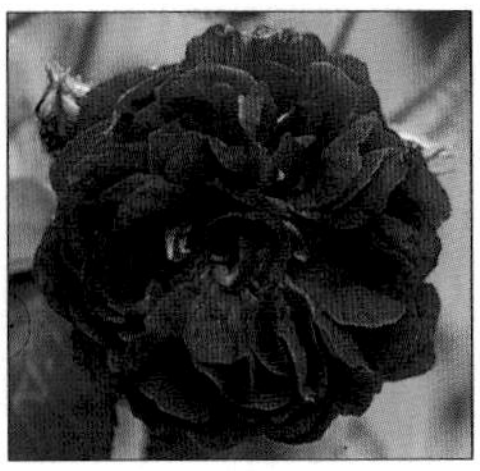
Rosa 'William Lobb'

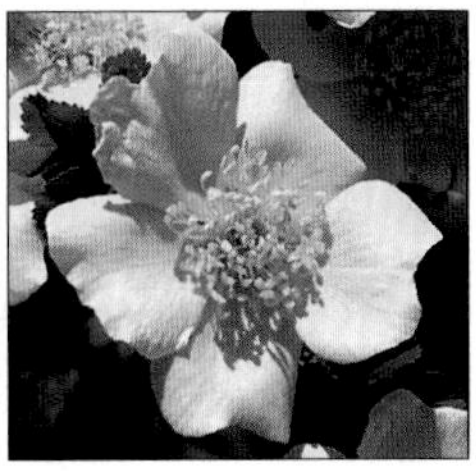
Rosa xanthina 'Canary Bird'

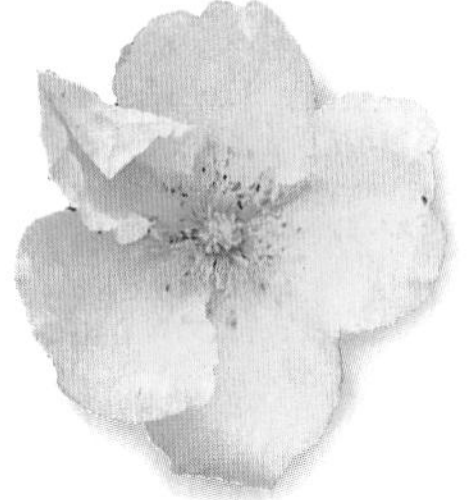
Rosa xanthina f. *hugonis*

with pale green leaves. Quartered-rosette, fully double, fragrant flowers, 8cm (3in) across, pale pink stippled with purple-crimson, are borne from summer to autumn. Prone to black spot. ↕ 2.2m (7ft), ↔ 1.5m (5ft). ✻✻✻

***R.* 'Veilchenblau'** ▣ ♀ syn. *R.* 'Blue Rambler', *R.* 'Violet Blue'. Vigorous rambler with light green leaves. In summer, bears large clusters of many cupped, double, fruit-scented violet flowers, 3cm (1¼in) across, streaked with white. ↕↔ 4m (12ft). ✻✻✻

***R.* 'Vent d'Eté'** see *R.* 'Surrey'.

***R.* 'Vick's Caprice'.** Upright, bushy Hybrid Perpetual rose with light green leaves. Pink buds open to cupped, fully double, fragrant, pale pink flowers, 10cm (4in) across, striped with pink and with irregular centres, from summer to autumn. Flowers may ball in rain. ↕ 1.2m (4ft), ↔ 1m (3ft). ✻✻✻

***R.* 'Ville de Chine'** see *R.* 'Chinatown'.

***R.* 'Violacea'**, syn. *R.* 'La Belle Sultane'. Tall, smooth-stemmed Gallica rose with sparse grey-green foliage. In summer, bears cupped to flat, single, fragrant, violet-purple flowers, 10cm (4in) across, with golden stamens. ↕ 2.2m (7ft), ↔ 1.5m (5ft). ✻✻✻

***R.* 'Violet Blue'** see *R.* 'Veilchenblau'.

R. virginiana ♀ syn. *R. lucida*. Species rose of erect, suckering habit, with shiny, light to mid-green leaves composed of 5–9 obovate to oblong-elliptic leaflets, 2.5–6cm (1–2½in) long, reddening in autumn. Cupped to flat, single, pale to bright pink flowers, 5–7cm (2–3in) across, are borne singly or in clusters of up to 8 blooms in summer; they are followed by spherical, ruby-red hips in autumn. ↕ 1.2m (4ft), ↔ 1.5m (5ft). E. North America. ✻✻✻

***R.* 'Viridiflora'** see *R.* x *odorata* 'Viridiflora'.

***R.* 'Warm Welcome'** ♀ syn. *R.* 'Chewizz'. Stiff, arching miniature climber with many dark green leaves. Small clusters of urn-shaped, semi-double, orange-red flowers, 4cm (1½in) across, are borne freely from summer to autumn. ↕↔ 2.2m (7ft). ✻✻✻

***R.* 'Warrior'** ▣ Low-growing cluster-flowered bush rose with light green foliage, purplish green when young. Cupped, crisp-petalled, double, blood-red flowers, 8cm (3in) across, are borne from summer to autumn. ↕ 40cm (16in), ↔ 45cm (18in). ✻✻✻

***R.* 'Wedding Day'.** Rampant rambler producing shiny, mid-green leaves with lance-shaped leaflets. Large clusters of flat, single, fruit-scented, creamy white flowers, 2.5cm (1in) across, ageing to pale pink, are borne in summer. ↕ to 8m (25ft), ↔ 4m (12ft). ✻✻✻

***R.* 'Wee Jock'**, syn. *R.* 'Cocabest'. Dense, compact dwarf cluster-flowered bush rose with abundant dark green leaves. From summer to autumn, high-centred buds open to rosette-shaped, fully double, deep crimson flowers, 4cm (1½in) across. ↕↔ 35cm (14in). ✻✻✻

***R.* 'Wendy Cussons'.** Strong-branching large-flowered bush rose with dark green leaves. Cherry-red buds open to high-centred, double, fragrant, cerise-pink flowers, 12cm (5in) across, from summer to autumn. ↕ 1m (3ft), ↔ 70cm (28in). ✻✻✻

***R.* 'Westerland'** ▣ ♀ syn. *R.* 'Korwest'. Vigorous, stiff-stemmed cluster-flowered shrub or climbing rose with bright green leaves. From summer to autumn, bears bold clusters of loosely formed, cupped, double, scented, apricot-orange flowers, 8cm (3in) across, suffused yellow. ↕ 2m (6ft), ↔ 1.2m (4ft) as a shrub; ↕ to 2.5m (8ft) as a climber. ✻✻✻

***R.* 'Whisky'** see *R.* 'Whisky Mac'.

***R.* 'Whisky Mac'**, syn. *R.* 'Tanky', *R.* 'Whisky'. Large-flowered bush rose with reddish green stems and glossy, dark green foliage. From summer to autumn, produces rounded, double, fragrant, light amber-yellow flowers, 10cm (4in) across. Prone to mildew. ↕ 75cm (30in), ↔ 60cm (24in). ✻✻

***R.* 'White American Beauty'** see *R.* 'Frau Karl Druschki'.

***R.* 'White Baby Rambler'** see *R.* 'Katharina Zeimet'.

***R.* 'White Cockade'** ▣ ♀ Upright, shrubby, large-flowered climber with dark green leaves. From summer to autumn, bears rounded, fully double, milk-white flowers, 9cm (3½in) across. ↕ 2.2m (7ft), ↔ 1.5m (5ft). ✻✻✻

***R.* 'White Cover'** see *R.* 'Kent'.

***R.* 'White Magic'** see *R.* 'Class Act'.

***R.* 'White Pet'** see *R.* 'Little White Pet'.

***R.* 'White Wings'.** Large-flowered bush rose with dark green leaves. Cupped to flat, single, scented white flowers, 8cm (3in) across, with chocolate-brown stamens, open from summer to autumn. ↕ 1m (3ft), ↔ 60cm (24in). ✻✻✻

R. wichuraiana see *R. wichurana.*

R. wichurana, syn. *R. wichuraiana* (Memorial rose). Vigorous, climbing, semi-evergreen species rose, mound-forming as ground cover, producing numerous small, shiny, dark green leaves comprised of 5–9 elliptic to broadly ovate leaflets, to 2.5cm (1in) long. Cupped to flat, single, clover-scented white flowers, 4.5cm (1¾in) across, with prominent golden yellow stamens, are borne in loose clusters of 6–10 in late summer. Ovoid to spherical hips are orange-red to dark red, and to 1.5cm (½in) long. ↕ 2m (6ft), ↔ 6m (20ft). E. China, Korea, Japan, Taiwan. ✻✻✻

***R.* 'William Allen Richardson'.** Noisette climbing rose with arching, branching growth and shiny, dark green leaves. From summer to autumn, urn-shaped buds open to quartered-rosette, double, scented, apricot-yellow flowers, 4.5cm (1¾in) across, paler towards the petal margins. ↕ 3m (10ft), ↔ 2.5m (8ft). ✻✻✻

***R.* 'William Lobb'** ▣ ♀ syn. *R.* 'Duchesse d'Istrie'. Vigorous Moss rose with arching, prickly stems, abundant mossy growth, and mid-green leaves. Cupped, fully double, scented, purple to lavender-grey flowers, 8cm (3in) across, are borne in summer. Best grown on a support. ↕↔ 2m (6ft). ✻✻✻

***R.* 'Williams' Double Yellow'** see *R.* x *harisonii* 'Williams' Double Yellow'.

***R.* 'William III'.** Suckering, spreading Scots rose with wiry stems and grey-green leaves. In early summer, bears cupped, semi-double, scented flowers,

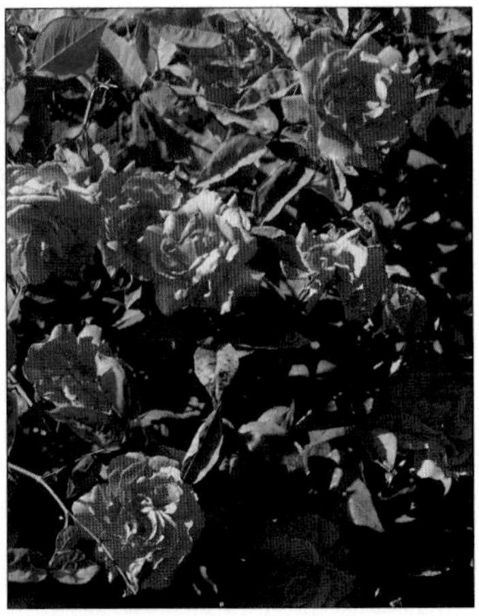

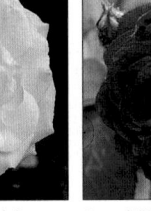
Rosa 'Zéphirine Drouhin'

4.5cm (1¾in) across, magenta-crimson shaded purplish red or lilac, followed by spherical, brownish red hips in autumn. ↕ 50cm (20in), ↔ 80cm (32in). ✻✻✻

R. xanthina*.** Species rose of shrubby, dense growth,with reddish green stems and fern-like, greyish green leaves, each with 7–13 broadly elliptic to obovate leaflets, 1–2cm (½–¾in) long. Loosely formed, cupped to flat, semi-double, scented yellow flowers, 5cm (2in) across, are borne, usually singly, along the stems in late spring. ↕↔ 2.5m (8ft). N. China, Korea. ✻✻✻. **'Canary Bird'** ▣ ♀ syn. *R.* 'Canary Bird', is arching in habit, with cupped, single, musk-scented yellow flowers borne in spring, sometimes sparsely later; ↕ 3m (10ft), ↔ to 4m (12ft). **f. *hugonis ▣ ♀ syn. *R. hugonis* (Father Hugo's rose, Golden rose of China) produces cupped, single, lightly scented, pale yellow flowers, 4.5cm (1¾in) across, in late spring; ↔ 2m (6ft); W. and C. China. **f. *normalis*** bears single flowers.

***R.* 'Yellow Cécile Brunner'** see *R.* 'Perle d'Or'.

***R.* 'Yesterday'** ♀ syn. *R.* 'Tapis d'Orient'. Polyantha bush rose of uneven growth, with shiny, mid-green leaves. Sprays of rosette-shaped, semi-double, scented, lilac-pink to rose-violet flowers, 2.5cm (1in) across, are borne very freely from summer to autumn. ↕↔ 1–1.5m (3–5ft). ✻✻✻

***R.* 'Young Mistress'** see *R.* 'Regensberg'.

***R.* 'Yvonne Rabier'** ♀ Compact Polyantha rose with abundant bright green leaves. From summer to autumn, bears rounded, fully double, lightly scented, creamy white flowers, 4.5cm (1¾in) across. ↕↔ 40cm (16in). ✻✻✻

***R.* 'Zéphirine Drouhin'** ▣ ♀ (Thornless rose). Bourbon rose with lax, open, thorn-free growth and mid-green leaves. From summer to autumn, freely bears loosely cupped, double, fragrant, deep pink flowers, 8cm (3in) across. Good as a climber or hedge. ↕ to 3m (10ft), ↔ 2m (6ft). ✻✻✻

***R.* 'Zigeunerknabe'** ♀ syn. *R.* 'Gipsy Boy'. Vigorous, lanky Bourbon rose with coarse, dark green leaves. Cupped to flat, double, scented, purplish crimson flowers, 8cm (3in) across, with prominent golden yellow stamens, are borne from summer to autumn. ↕ 2m (6ft), ↔ 1.2m (4ft). ✻✻✻

***R.* 'Zonta Rose'** see *R.* 'Princess Alice'.

ROSCOEA

ZINGIBERACEAE

Genus of about 18 species of tuberous perennials from meadows, slopes, and partially forested areas in the Himalayas and China. They are cultivated for their unusual, hooded, orchid-like flowers, which have prominent, entire or 2-lobed lips. The flowers are surrounded by overlapping bracts, and are produced on leafy stems from the leaf axils in summer or autumn. The arching leaves are stem-sheathing and linear, or lance-shaped to oblong-ovate. Roscoeas thrive in cool climates; grow in a peat bed, a woodland garden, or a damp, shady border.

• **HARDINESS** Fully hardy to frost hardy; will survive temperatures to -20°C (-4°F) if planted very deep.

• **CULTIVATION** Plant tubers 15cm (6in) deep in winter or early spring. Grow in moderately fertile, humus-rich, leafy, moist but well-drained soil, in a cool, sheltered site in partial shade. In frost-prone areas, apply a deep winter mulch.

• **PROPAGATION** Sow seed in containers in a cold frame as soon as ripe. Divide in spring.

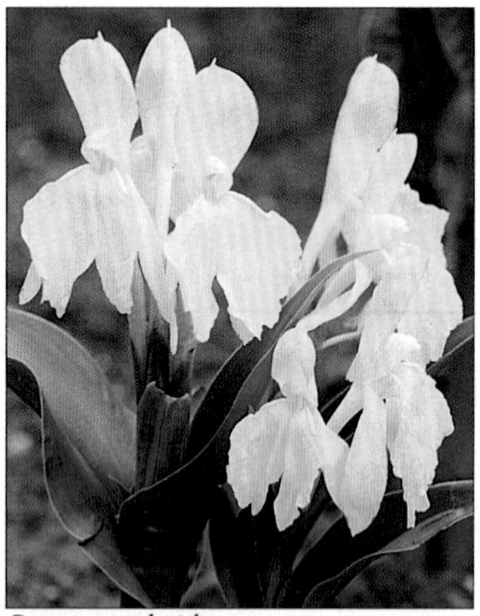

Roscoea cautleoides

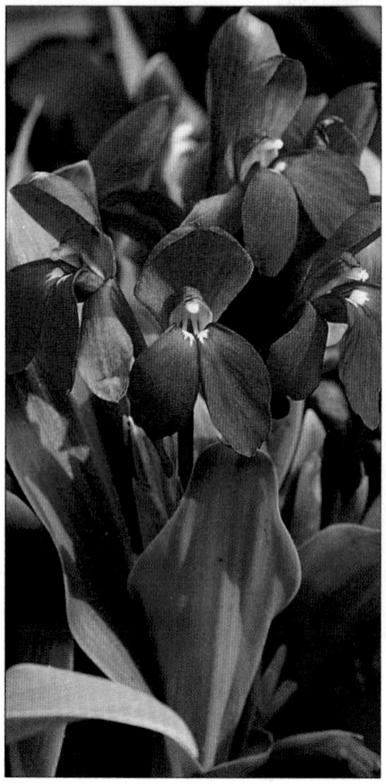

Roscoea humeana

• **PESTS AND DISEASES** Slugs and vine weevils may be a problem.

R. auriculata. Tuberous perennial with 3–10 linear to broadly lance-shaped, dark green leaves, to 25cm (10in) long. Rich purple flowers, 3.5cm (1½in) across, are produced from the upper leaf axils in late summer or autumn. ↕25–55cm (10–22in), ↔15cm (6in). Nepal, India (Sikkim). *** (borderline)

***R. capitata* of gardens** see *R. scillifolia.*

R. cautleoides ■ ♀ Tuberous perennial with 1–4 linear to lance-shaped, deep to mid-green leaves, 40cm (16in) long, usually to 15cm (6in) long at flowering. In midsummer, produces yellow, white, or purple flowers, 4cm (1½in) across, from the upper leaf axils. ↕ to 55cm (22in), ↔15cm (6in). China (Sichuan, Yunnan). *** (borderline)

R. humeana ■ ♀ Sturdy, tuberous perennial bearing a succession of up to 10 rich purple flowers, 4cm (1½in) across, from the upper leaf axils in early summer. The 1 or 2, rarely 3, oblong to ovate, deep green leaves, to 22cm (9in) long, are usually only partially developed at flowering time. ↕15–25cm (6–10in), ↔15cm (6in). China (Sichuan, Yunnan). *** (borderline)

R. procera see *R. purpurea.*

R. purpurea ■ syn. *R. procera, R. purpurea* var. *procera.* Tuberous perennial with 4–8 lance-shaped to oblong-ovate, deep green leaves, to 25cm (10in) long. Purple, occasionally white or bicoloured flowers, 6cm (2½in) across, are produced in succession from the upper leaf axils in early and mid-summer. ↕25–40cm (10–16in), ↔15cm (6in). Himalayas. *** (borderline).

var. *procera* see *R. purpurea.*

R. scillifolia, syn. *R. capitata* of gardens. Slender, tuberous perennial with 1–5 linear to linear-lance-shaped, mid-green leaves, 6–12cm (2½–5in) long. In summer, produces 2–4 blackish pink or purplish pink flowers, 2cm (¾in) across, on leafless stalks above the leaves. May seed freely. ↕35cm (14in), ↔8cm (3in). China (Yunnan). *** (borderline)

▷ **Rose** see *Rosa*
- **Apothecary's** see *Rosa gallica* var. *officinalis*
- **Austrian copper** see *Rosa foetida* 'Bicolor'
- **Austrian yellow** see *Rosa foetida*
- **Autumn damask** see *Rosa* x *damascena* var. *semperflorens*

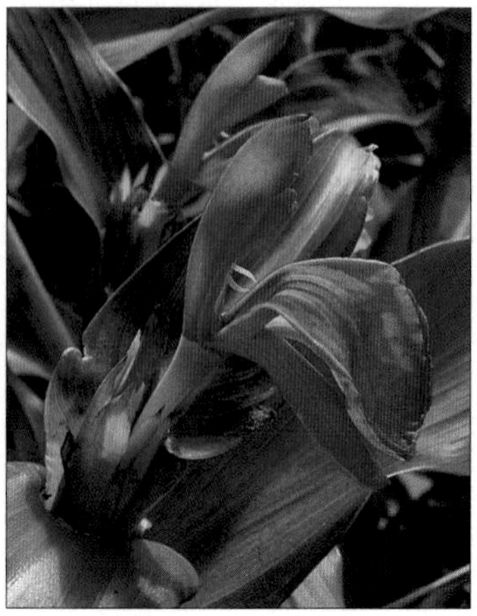

Roscoea purpurea

▷ **Rose cont.**
- **Burnet** see *Rosa pimpinellifolia*
- **Burr** see *Rosa roxburghii*
- **Camellia** see *Rosa laevigata*
- **Cherokee** see *Rosa laevigata*
- **Chestnut** see *Rosa roxburghii*
- **Chickasaw** see *Rosa bracteata*
- **Chinquapin** see *Rosa roxburghii*
- **Christmas** see *Helleborus niger*
- **Common moss** see *Rosa* x *centifolia* 'Muscosa'
- **Cotton** see *Hibiscus mutabilis*
- **Crested moss** see *Rosa* x *centifolia* 'Cristata'
- **Crimson damask** see *Rosa gallica* var. *officinalis*
- **Desert** see *Adenium*
- **Double velvet** see *Rosa* 'Tuscany Superb'
- **Double white banksian** see *Rosa banksiae*
- **Eglantine** see *Rosa eglanteria*
- **Father Hugo's** see *Rosa xanthina* f. *hugonis*
- **Fortune's double yellow** see *Rosa* x *odorata* 'Pseudindica'
- **Four seasons** see *Rosa* x *damascena* var. *semperflorens*
- **Great white** see *Rosa* 'Alba Maxima'
- **Green** see *Rosa* x *odorata* 'Viridiflora'
- **Guelder** see *Viburnum opulus*
- **Hedgehog** see *Rosa rugosa*
- **Incense** see *Rosa primula*
- **Jacobite** see *Rosa* 'Alba Maxima'
- **Japanese** see *Rosa rugosa*
- **Lenten** see *Helleborus orientalis*
- **Macartney** see *Rosa bracteata*
- **Memorial** see *Rosa wichurana*
- **Montpellier rock** see *Cistus monspeliensis*
- **Musk** see *Rosa moschata*
- **Myrrh-scented** see *Rosa* 'Splendens'
- **Nootka** see *Rosa nutkana*
- **Old black** see *Rosa* 'Nuits de Young'
- **Old blush China** see *Rosa* x *odorata* 'Pallida'
- **Old glory** see *Rosa* 'Gloire de Dijon'
- **Painted damask** see *Rosa* 'Leda'
- **Parsons' pink China** see *Rosa* x *odorata* 'Pallida'
- **Persian yellow** see *Rosa foetida* 'Persiana'
- **Pompon** see *Rosa* 'De Meaux'
- **Portland** see *Rosa* 'Portlandica'
- **Provins** see *Rosa gallica* var. *officinalis*
- **Ramanas** see *Rosa rugosa*
- **Red moss** see *Rosa* 'Henri Martin'
- **Rock** see *Cistus, Helianthemum*
- **Rosa mundi** see *Rosa gallica* var. *officinalis* 'Versicolor'
- **Sacramento** see *Rosa stellata* var. *mirifica*
- **Scotch** see *Rosa pimpinellifolia*
- **Scots** see *Rosa pimpinellifolia*
- **Single white banksian** see *Rosa banksiae* var. *normalis*
- **Slater's crimson China** see *Rosa* x *odorata* 'Semperflorens'
- **Snowbush** see *Rosa* 'Dupontii'
- **Summer damask** see *Rosa* x *damascena*
- **Sun** see *Cistus, Helianthemum*
- **Sydney rock** see *Boronia serrulata*
- **Thornless** see *Rosa* 'Zéphirine Drouhin'
- **Winged thorn** see *Rosa sericea* subsp. *omeiensis* f. *pteracantha*
- **Wood** see *Merremia tuberosa*
- **Yellow banksian** see *Rosa banksiae* 'Lutea'
- **York and Lancaster** see *Rosa* x *damascena* 'Versicolor'

▷ **Rose bay** see *Nerium oleander*

▷ **Rosebay, East Indian** see *Tabernaemontana divaricata*

▷ **Rose campion** see *Lychnis coronaria*

▷ **Rosemary** see *Rosmarinus, R. officinalis*
- **Australian** see *Westringia fruticosa*
- **Bog** see *Andromeda*
- **Common bog** see *Andromeda polifolia*
- **Wild** see *Dampiera rosmarinifolia*

▷ ***Roseocactus fissuratus*** see *Ariocarpus fissuratus*

▷ **Rose of Castille** see *Rosa* x *damascena* var. *semperflorens*

▷ **Rose of China** see *Hibiscus rosa-sinensis*
- **Golden** see *Rosa xanthina* f. *hugonis*

▷ **Rose of heaven** see *Silene coeli-rosa*

▷ **Rose of Jericho** see *Selaginella lepidophylla*

▷ **Rose of Lancaster, Red** see *Rosa gallica* var. *officinalis*

▷ **Rose of Sharon** see *Hypericum calycinum*

▷ **Rose of York, White** see *Rosa* 'Alba Maxima'

▷ **Roseroot** see *Rhodiola rosea*

▷ **Rosewood, Brazilian** see *Tipuana tipu*

▷ **Rosinweed** see *Grindelia, Silphium*

ROSMARINUS

Rosemary

LABIATAE/LAMIACEAE

Genus of 2 species of evergreen shrubs found in rocky sites, woodland, and scrub in the Mediterranean region, and cultivated for their aromatic foliage and flowers. The leaves are opposite and narrowly linear; the 2-lipped, tubular flowers are borne in short, few-flowered, axillary whorls. Grow rosemary in a shrub or mixed border, in a herb garden, against a sunny wall, or as a hedge. Low-growing cultivars, such as *R. officinalis* 'Prostratus', are ideal for a rock garden or the top of a dry wall. The leaves are commonly used as a culinary herb.

• **HARDINESS** Frost hardy; *R. officinalis* and most cultivars will withstand falls to -10°C (14°F) in well-drained soil.

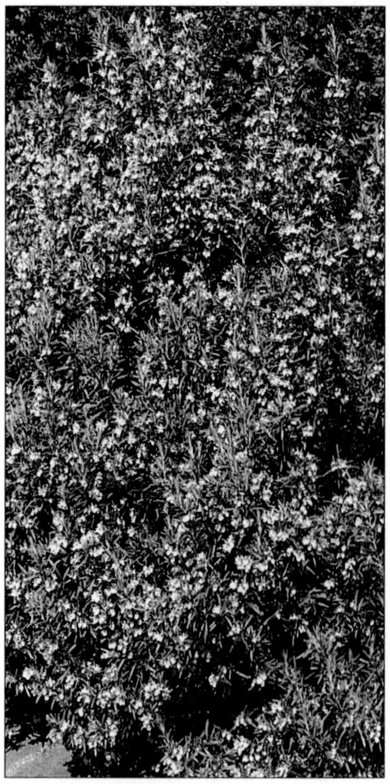

Rosmarinus officinalis

R

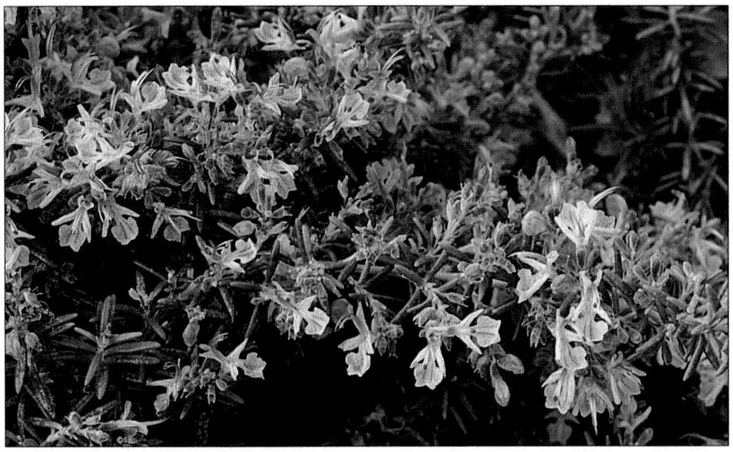

Rosmarinus officinalis 'Prostratus'

• **CULTIVATION** Grow in well-drained, poor to moderately fertile soil in full sun. Pruning group 9. Trim hedges after flowering.
• **PROPAGATION** Sow seed in containers in a cold frame in spring. Root semi-ripe cuttings in summer.
• **PESTS AND DISEASES** Honey fungus may be a problem.

***R. eriocalyx* of gardens** see *R. officinalis* 'Prostratus'.
***R. lavandulaceus* of gardens** see *R. officinalis* 'Prostratus'.
R. officinalis ■ (Rosemary). Upright to rounded, dense, bushy, aromatic, evergreen shrub with linear, leathery, dark green leaves, to 5cm (2in) long, white-felted beneath. Whorls of tubular, 2-lipped, purple-blue to white flowers, 1cm (½in) long, are produced from the upper leaf axils from mid-spring to early summer, and often again in autumn. ↕↔ 1.5m (5ft). Mediterranean. ✲✲. **'Aureovariegatus'** see 'Aureus'. **'Aureus'**, syn. 'Aureovariegatus', 'Gilded', produces yellow-marked leaves. **'Benenden Blue'**, syn. 'Collingwood Ingram', has narrow, dark green leaves and vivid blue flowers. **'Collingwood Ingram'** see 'Benenden Blue'. **'Fastigiatus'** see 'Miss Jessopp's Upright'. **'Gilded'** see 'Aureus'. **'Miss Jessopp's Upright'** ♕ syn. 'Fastigiatus', 'Pyramidalis', is vigorous and upright; ↕↔ 2m (6ft). **'Prostratus'** ■♕ syn. *R. eriocalyx* of gardens, *R. lavandulaceus* of gardens, is prostrate and the least hardy variant; ↕ 15cm (6in). **'Pyramidalis'** see 'Miss Jessopp's Upright'. **'Roseus'** has pink flowers. **'Severn Sea'** ♕ has a spreading habit, with arching branches and bright blue flowers; ↕ 1m (3ft). **'Tuscan Blue'** is upright, bearing dark blue flowers.

ROSSIOGLOSSUM

ORCHIDACEAE

Genus of 6 species of epiphytic, evergreen orchids from rainforest, up to altitudes of 2,700m (9,000ft), in Central America. At its apex, each conical to ovoid, dark grey-green pseudobulb produces 1–3 broadly oval, dark green to grey- or bluish green leaves, marked brown at the bases. Erect or arching, few-flowered racemes of showy, yellow and brown flowers are produced from the base of new growth from autumn to winter. Use as houseplants.
• **HARDINESS** Frost tender.
• **CULTIVATION** Cool-growing orchids. Grow in epiphytic orchid compost, with added leaf mould and sphagnum, in bright filtered light. In summer, provide good ventilation and, as new growth begins, water freely, applying a balanced liquid fertilizer monthly; keep just moist in winter. See also p.46.
• **PROPAGATION** Divide when the plant fills the pot and "flows" over the sides.
• **PESTS AND DISEASES** Prone to red spider mites, aphids, and mealybugs.

R. grande ♕ syn. *Odontoglossum grande* (Clown orchid, Tiger orchid). Epiphytic orchid with elliptic to lance-shaped, leathery, dark or bluish green leaves, 10–20cm (4–8in) long. From autumn to winter, bears erect racemes of 4–8 rich, glossy, chestnut-brown and yellow flowers, 12cm (5in) across, spotted red, brown, or yellow, with white lips. ↕ 35cm (14in), ↔ 20cm (8in). Mexico, Guatemala. ❀ (min. 10°C/50°F; max. 30°C/86°F)

ROTHMANNIA

RUBIACEAE

Genus of 25–30 species of evergreen shrubs and small trees from woodland and open savannah in tropical Africa, the Seychelles, Madagascar, and Asia. The leaves are simple and usually in opposite pairs, but sometimes in threes. They are cultivated for their bell- or funnel-shaped flowers, each with 5 spreading petal lobes, borne singly or in terminal and axillary clusters or cymes. Where temperatures fall below 7–10°C (45–50°F), grow in a cool or temperate greenhouse. In milder climates, grow at the base of a warm, sunny wall or in a shrub border.
• **HARDINESS** Frost tender.
• **CULTIVATION** Under glass, grow in loamless or loam-based potting compost (JI No.2) in full light, with shade from hot sun. When in growth, water freely with soft water and apply a balanced liquid fertilizer monthly; water sparingly in winter. Outdoors, grow in moist but well-drained, fertile, neutral to acid soil in full sun with some midday shade. Pruning group 1; plants under glass may need restrictive pruning.
• **PROPAGATION** Sow seed at 16°C (61°F) in spring. Root semi-ripe cuttings with bottom heat in summer.
• **PESTS AND DISEASES** Whiteflies, stem mealybugs, and root mealybugs may be a problem under glass.

R. capensis ⚲ syn. *Gardenia capensis, G. rothmannia* (Candlewood). Spreading tree with grey to brown bark. The broadly lance-shaped or elliptic to ovate leaves, 5–10cm (2–4in) long, are lustrous, deep green with conspicuous, sunken veins above, paler green beneath. Solitary, funnel-shaped, fragrant, white, cream, or yellow flowers, to 8cm (3in) long, are borne in summer. ↕ to 14m (46ft), ↔ to 7m (22ft). South Africa. ❀ (min. 7–10°C/45–50°F)
R. globosa ⚲ syn. *Gardenia globosa* (September bells). Spreading, large shrub or small tree with dark grey to brown bark. Inversely lance-shaped to lance-shaped or elliptic leaves, 6–12cm (2½–5in) long, are bright green with yellow, pink, or maroon veins, more obvious beneath than above. Narrowly bell-shaped, fragrant, ivory to white, occasionally pink-tinged flowers, to 4cm (1½in) long, with arching to reflexed petal lobes, are produced singly or in small clusters in the leaf axils in summer. ↕ 3–7m (10–22ft), ↔ 2–3.5m (6–11ft). South Africa. ❀ (min. 7–10°C/45–50°F)

▷ **Rowan** see *Sorbus aucuparia*
Hubei see *S. hupehensis*
▷ **Royal palm** see *Roystonea*

ROYSTONEA

Royal palm

ARECACEAE/PALMAE

Genus of about 10 species of single-stemmed palms found in moist, rich soil on the Caribbean islands and adjacent coasts. The trunks may be columnar, or swollen in the middle or at the bases, each topped by a crownshaft and a tuft of pinnate, feather-shaped, bright mid-green leaves. The tiny, cup-shaped, 3-petalled flowers are borne in panicles just below the crownshaft. In frost-prone climates, grow young plants in a warm greenhouse. In tropical regions, use as lawn specimens or in an avenue.
• **HARDINESS** Frost tender.

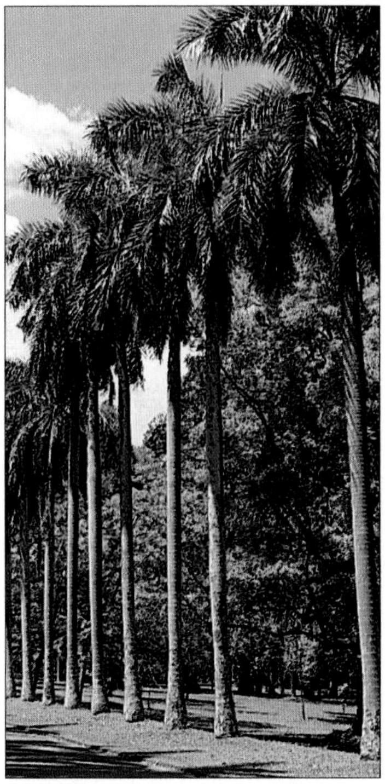

Roystonea regia

• **CULTIVATION** Under glass, grow in loamless potting compost in full light, shaded from hot sun. When in growth, water freely and apply a balanced liquid fertilizer monthly; water moderately in winter. Pot on or top-dress in spring. Outdoors, grow in moderately fertile, moist but well-drained soil in full sun.
• **PROPAGATION** Sow seed at 27°C (81°F) in spring.
• **PESTS AND DISEASES** Red spider mites, mealybugs, and scale insects may be a problem under glass.

R. borinquena ♈ syn. *R. caribaea.* Medium-sized palm with a spindle-shaped trunk ringed with old leaf scars. The arching leaves, up to 3m (10ft) long, have many narrow, linear, rich green leaflets in 2 double ranks. Cup-shaped cream flowers, with green-purple anthers, are borne in panicles, 1m (3ft) long, usually in summer. ↕ to 18m (60ft), ↔ to 6m (20ft). Puerto Rico (including Vieques), US Virgin Islands (St. Croix). ❀ (min. 15°C/59°F)
R. caribaea see *R. borinquena.*
R. regia ■♈ Tall palm with a sturdy trunk, usually thickened at the base and again in the middle, becoming thinner towards the crownshaft. Leaves 3–5m (10–15ft) long, have many linear, rich green leaflets arranged in several ranks. Cup-shaped white flowers are borne in panicles, to 1m (3ft) long, usually in summer. ↕ to 25m (80ft), ↔ to 10m (30ft). Cuba. ❀ (min. 15°C/59°F)

▷ **Rubber plant** see *Ficus elastica*

RUBUS

ROSACEAE

Genus of 250 or more species of often prickly or bristly, deciduous or evergreen shrubs and climbers, occasionally herbaceous perennials, found worldwide in a range of habitats from coastal sand dunes to thickets, woodland, forest, and mountain slopes. The leaves are alternate and entire, lobed, palmate, or pinnate, each with 3 to many, usually toothed leaflets. The saucer- to cup-shaped, 4- or 5-petalled flowers are borne in racemes or panicles, sometimes singly or in few-flowered clusters, and are pink, white, red, or purple.

Blackberries or brambles (*R. fruticosus*), raspberries (*R. idaeus*), and hybrids between these and other species are grown for their edible fruits. Ornamental species are grown for their flowers, their foliage, and sometimes their attractive winter shoots, and are suitable for a shrub border. Prostrate species provide good ground cover in sun or shade. Vigorous species are best grown in a wild or woodland garden.
• **HARDINESS** Fully hardy to frost hardy.
• **CULTIVATION** Grow in well-drained, moderately fertile soil. Grow deciduous species cultivated for their winter shoots in full sun; grow evergreen or semi-evergreen species in sun or partial shade. Pruning group 7 for *R. biflorus, R. cockburnianus, R. thibetanus*; group 2 for other deciduous species and cultivars; group 11 for *R. henryi*, after flowering, although pruning is seldom needed.
• **PROPAGATION** Divide *R. odoratus* in autumn. Root greenwood cuttings of deciduous species and cultivars in summer, or hardwood cuttings in early

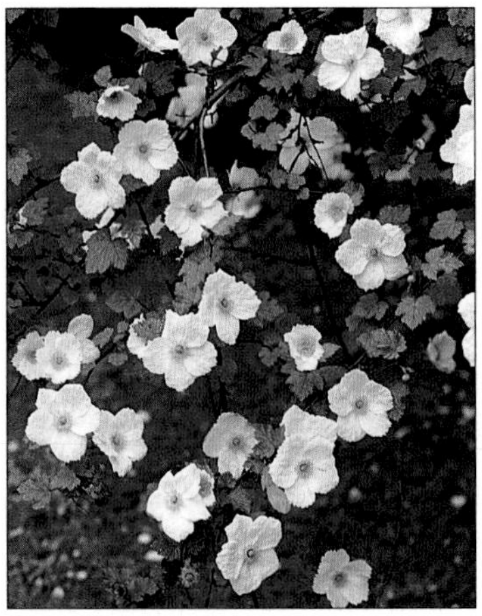

Rubus 'Benenden'

winter. Root semi-ripe cuttings of evergreens in summer. Detach rooted pieces of prostrate evergreens between autumn and spring.

• **PESTS AND DISEASES** Grey mould (*Botrytis*) may be a problem.

***R.* 'Benenden'** ■ 🏆 Spreading, deciduous shrub with arching, thornless branches, peeling bark, and broadly ovate, shallowly 3- to 5-lobed, dark green leaves, 6–8m (2½–3in) long. Solitary, rose-like, saucer-shaped, pure white flowers, to 7cm (3in) across, are borne profusely in late spring and early summer. ↕↔ 3m (10ft). ❄❄❄
***R.* 'Betty Ashburner'.** Prostrate, evergreen shrub with erect then arching shoots, densely covered in red bristles. Heart-shaped, shallowly 5-lobed, wavy-margined, glossy, mid-green leaves, 6cm (2½in) long, are deeply veined above, glaucous beneath. In summer, produces racemes of saucer-shaped white flowers, 2cm (¾in) across, from the leaf axils. ↕ 30cm (12in), ↔ indefinite. ❄❄❄
R. biflorus ■ Erect, prickly, deciduous shrub with chalky-white-bloomed young shoots, particularly conspicuous in winter. Ovate, pinnate leaves, to 25cm

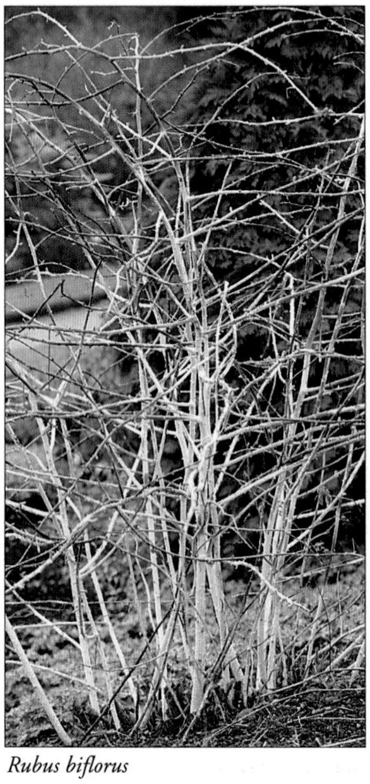

Rubus biflorus

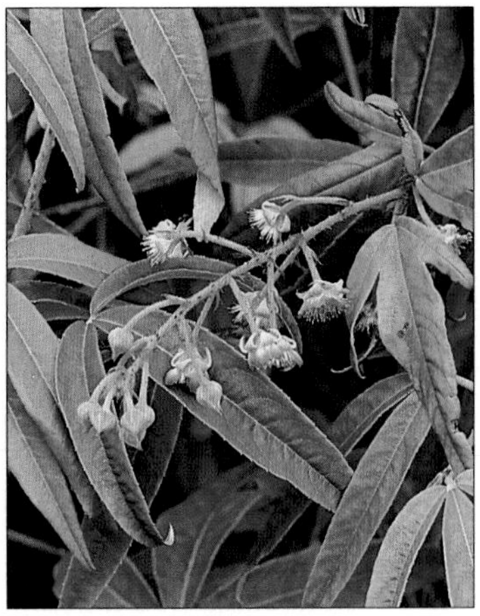

Rubus henryi var. *bambusarum*

(10in) long, each have 3, sometimes 5, ovate to elliptic, dark green leaflets, white-felted beneath. In summer, produces saucer-shaped white flowers, 2cm (¾in) across, singly or in clusters of 2 or 3 from the leaf axils, followed by edible, spherical yellow fruit, to 2cm (¾in) across. ↕↔ 3m (10ft). Himalayas, China. ❄❄❄. **var. *quinqueflorus***, the most commonly grown variant, has intensely white stems and bears clusters of 5 or more flowers.
R. calycinoides see *R. pentalobus.*
R. cockburnianus 🏆 Thicket-forming, deciduous shrub producing arching, prickly shoots with a brilliant white bloom in winter. Ovate, pinnate leaves, to 20cm (8in) long, with 5–7, sometimes 9, diamond-shaped or ovate-lance-shaped leaflets, are dark green above and white-hairy beneath, appearing greenish white overall. In summer, bears terminal racemes of saucer-shaped purple flowers, 1cm (½in) across, followed by spherical black, unpalatable fruit, to 1.5cm (½in) across. ↕↔ 2.5m (8ft). China. ❄❄❄
***R. fockeanus* of gardens** see *R. pentalobus.*
R. henryi* var. *bambusarum ■ Scrambling, evergreen climber with slender, spiny, white-hairy shoots and lance-shaped, deeply 3-lobed, glossy, dark green leaves, to 12cm (5in) long, white-felted beneath. Long racemes of cup-shaped pink flowers, 2cm (¾in) across, are borne in summer, followed by spherical, glossy black fruit, 1.5cm (½in) across. ↕ 6m (20ft). W. and C. China. ❄❄❄
R. odoratus (Flowering raspberry). Fast-growing, thicket-forming, deciduous

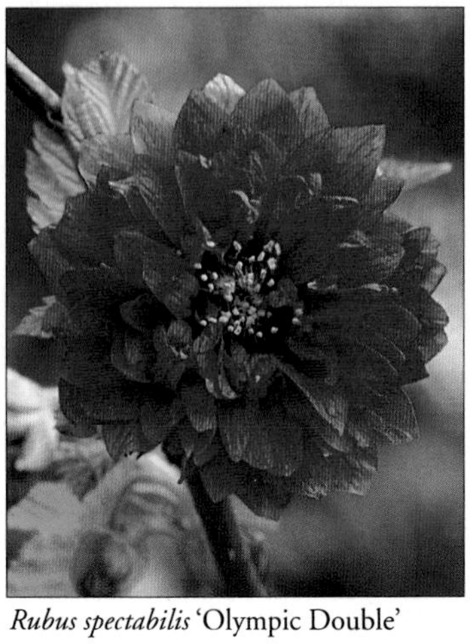

Rubus spectabilis 'Olympic Double'

shrub with spineless shoots and large, broadly ovate, 5-lobed, velvety, dark green leaves, to 24cm (10in) long. From early summer to early autumn, bears panicles of shallowly cup-shaped, fragrant, purple-pink flowers, to 5cm (2in) across; they are followed by tasteless, flattened hemispherical red fruit, to 2cm (¾in) across. ↕↔ 2.5m (8ft) or more. E. North America. ❄❄❄
R. pentalobus, syn. *R. calycinoides, R. fockeanus* of gardens. Prostrate, evergreen shrub with sparsely prickly shoots that root as they creep along the ground. The rounded, shallowly 3- to 5-lobed, glossy, dark green leaves, to 5cm (2in) long, are heart-shaped at the bases, with deeply impressed veins and wrinkled margins. In summer, bears solitary, saucer-shaped white flowers, 2cm (¾in) across, sometimes followed by spherical red fruit, to 10mm (½in) across. ↕ 10cm (4in), ↔ indefinite. Taiwan. ❄❄❄
***R. spectabilis* 'Flore Pleno'** see *R. spectabilis* 'Olympic Double'.
***R. spectabilis* 'Olympic Double'** ■ syn. *R. spectabilis* 'Flore Pleno'. Thicket-forming, deciduous shrub with upright, slightly prickly shoots and 3-palmate leaves, to 15cm (6in) long, composed of ovate, glossy, mid-green leaflets. Usually solitary, very showy, double, bright purple-pink flowers, 5cm (2in) across, open in mid-spring. ↕↔ 2m (6ft). ❄❄❄
R. thibetanus 🏆 Erect, thicket-forming, deciduous shrub with arching, prickly shoots, conspicuously white-bloomed in winter. Triangular, pinnate, dark green leaves, to 22cm (9in) long, have 7–13 lance-shaped to ovate leaflets, densely grey-hairy above, densely white-hairy beneath. In summer, saucer-shaped, red-purple flowers, 1cm (½in) across, are borne singly from the upper leaf axils or in few-flowered terminal racemes, followed by spherical black fruit, to 1.5cm (½in) across, with a whitish bloom. ↕↔ 2.5m (8ft). W. China. ❄❄❄
R. tricolor. Prostrate, evergreen shrub with both creeping and arching shoots, covered in conspicuous red bristles. Ovate, entire or very shallowly 3- to 5-lobed, glossy, dark green leaves, to 10cm (4in) long, are heart-shaped at the bases and white-hairy beneath. Saucer-shaped white flowers, 2.5cm (1in) across, open singly or in few-flowered terminal racemes in summer, followed by edible, raspberry-like red fruit, to 2.5cm (1in) across. ↕ 60cm (24in), ↔ indefinite. China (Sichuan, Yunnan). ❄❄❄
***R. ulmifolius* 'Bellidiflorus'.** Fast-growing, deciduous or semi-evergreen shrub of open habit, with long, arching, thorny shoots and 3- to 5-palmate leaves, to 12cm (5in) long, composed of ovate, dark green leaflets. Large panicles of hemispherical, double pink flowers, to 1.5cm (½in) across, are produced in mid- and late summer. ↕ 2.5m (8ft), ↔ 4m (12ft). ❄❄❄

RUDBECKIA

Coneflower

ASTERACEAE/COMPOSITAE

Genus of about 20 species of annuals, biennials, and perennials (some of which may be grown as annuals), with short rhizomes, from moist meadows and light woodland in North America. They have branched or unbranched stems, and most have alternate, simple to

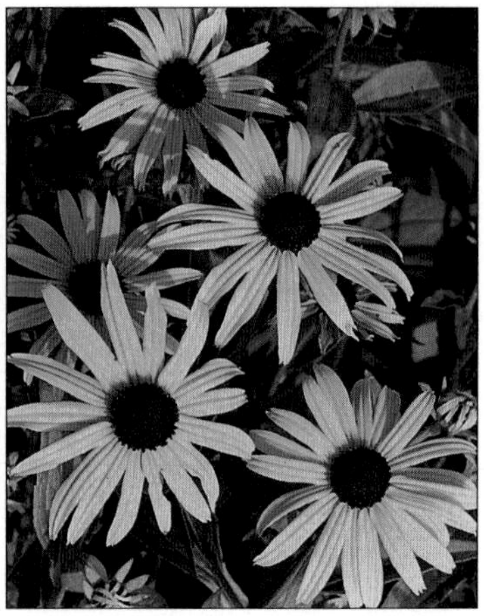

Rudbeckia fulgida var. *sullivantii* 'Goldsturm'

pinnatifid, occasionally pinnate, prominently veined leaves, toothed towards the tips. Usually solitary, daisy-like flowerheads, often with reflexed yellow ray-florets and conical centres consisting of black, brown, or green disc-florets, are borne on long stems over a long period from summer to autumn. Most are good for cut flowers. Grow in a border or naturalize in a meadow or woodland garden. Most cultivars of *R. hirta* are grown as annuals, and are good for bedding or for infilling in borders.

• **HARDINESS** Fully hardy to half hardy.

• **CULTIVATION** Grow in moderately fertile, preferably heavy but well-drained soil that does not dry out, in full sun or partial shade. *R. fulgida* var. *deamii* is more drought-tolerant than other species. On fertile soils, *R. laciniata* 'Golden Glow' may become invasive.

• **PROPAGATION** Sow seed of perennials in containers in a cold frame in early spring, or divide in autumn or spring. Sow seed of annuals and biennials at 16–18°C (61–64°F) in spring.

• **PESTS AND DISEASES** Slugs may damage young growth. *R. laciniata* 'Golden Glow' is susceptible to aphids.

***R.* 'Autumn Sun'** see *R.* 'Herbstsonne'.
R. columnifera see *Ratibida columnifera.*
R. deamii see *R. fulgida* var. *deamii.*
R. fulgida (Black-eyed Susan). Rhizomatous perennial with branched stems, long-stalked, oblong to lance-shaped, entire basal leaves, to 12cm (5in) long, and lance-shaped, toothed stem leaves; both are mid-green and slightly hairy with prominent veins. Daisy-like flowerheads, to 7cm (3in) across, with orange-yellow ray-florets and conical, blackish brown disc-florets, are borne from late summer to mid-autumn. ↕ to 90cm (36in), ↔ 45cm (18in). E. USA. ❄❄❄. **var. *deamii*** 🏆 syn. *R. deamii*, is free-flowering, and has very hairy stems with long-pointed, ovate or oval-ovate, toothed, rough basal and stem leaves; ↕ to 60cm (24in). USA (Indiana). **var. *speciosa***, syn. *R. newmanii, R. speciosa*, has elliptic to lance-shaped, almost sickle-shaped basal leaves and coarsely toothed stem leaves; USA (New Jersey to Alabama and Georgia). **var. *sullivantii***, syn. *R. sullivantii*, has broadly ovate to narrowly ovate-lance-shaped, less hairy, coarsely toothed, dark green basal leaves and

R

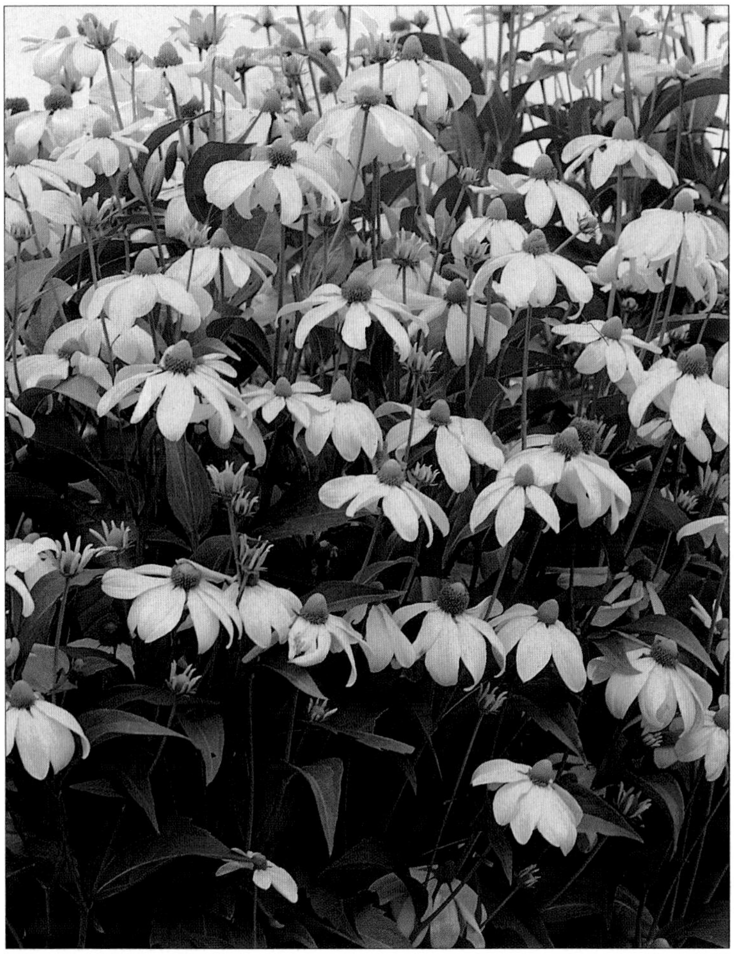

Rudbeckia 'Herbstsonne'

stem leaves, which become progressively smaller up the stems. The flowerheads are 8–9cm (3–3½in) across. USA (Michigan to Missouri, Connecticut to W. Virginia). **var. *sullivantii* 'Goldsturm'** ▣ ♀ has large, golden yellow flowerheads, 9–12cm (3½–5in) across, on shorter stems than the species; ↕ to 60cm (24in).
R. gloriosa see *R. hirta.*
***R.* 'Herbstsonne'** ▣ syn. *R.* 'Autumn Sun'. Upright, rhizomatous, clump-forming perennial with oval, toothed or slightly lobed, prominently veined, glossy, mid-green leaves, to 15cm (6in) long. From midsummer to early autumn, branching stems bear daisy-like flowerheads, 10–12cm (4–5in) across, with bright yellow ray-florets and high, conical centres of green disc-florets, becoming yellowish brown with age. ↕ to 2m (6ft), ↔ 90cm (36in). ❄❄❄
R. hirta, syn. *R. gloriosa* (Black-eyed Susan). Erect, stout-stemmed, branching, bristly biennial or short-lived perennial, often grown as an annual, with mid-green leaves. The basal leaves are ovate to diamond-shaped, sometimes slightly toothed, strongly 3-veined, and to 10cm (4in) long; stem leaves are usually narrower and ovate to lance-shaped. Daisy-like flowerheads, to 7cm (3in) across, with pale to golden yellow ray-florets and prominent, conical centres of deep brown-purple disc-florets, are borne from summer to early autumn. ↕ 30–90cm (12–36in), ↔ 30–45cm (12–18in). C. USA. ❄❄❄.
'Bambi' has flowerheads with bronze-brown, chestnut-brown, and golden

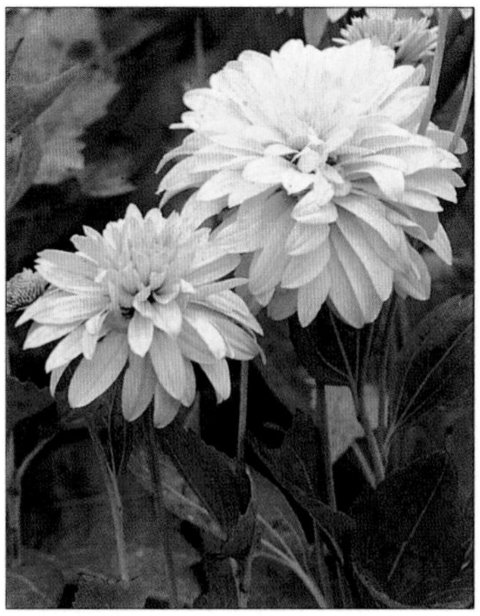

Rudbeckia laciniata 'Goldquelle'

yellow ray-florets; ↕ to 30cm (12in).
'Becky Mixed' ▣ is very dwarf, and has flowerheads with ray-florets in shades of lemon-yellow, golden yellow, and dark red or reddish brown; ↕ to 25cm (10in). **'Goldilocks'** has double and semi-double flowerheads with golden-orange ray-florets; ↕ to 60cm (24in). **'Green Eyes'** see 'Irish Eyes'. **'Irish Eyes'**, syn. 'Green Eyes', has flowerheads with bright yellow ray-florets and green disc-florets; ↕ 60–75cm (24–30in).
'Kelvedon Star' has flowerheads with deep golden yellow ray-florets, zoned in brownish red. **'Marmalade'** is bushy and compact, with large flowerheads, sometimes to 13cm (5in) across, with deep golden orange ray-florets; ↕ to 45cm (18in). **'Rustic Dwarfs'** ▣ has flowerheads with golden yellow, brownish red, or bronze-orange ray-florets, with some bicolours; ↕ to 60cm (24in). **'Sonora'** is compact, bearing flowerheads with bright yellow ray-florets; ↕ to 40cm (16in).
R. laciniata. Rhizomatous, hairless, glaucous perennial, forming loose clumps of tall, wiry stems, branched towards their tips. Basal leaves, to 10cm (4in) long, are pinnate or pinnatisect, each with deeply 3- to 5-lobed, toothed leaflets and prominent veins; stem leaves become less deeply lobed up the stems. Daisy-like flowerheads, 7–15cm (3–6in) across, with reflexed, pale yellow ray-florets and hemispherical to conical centres of greenish yellow disc-florets, are borne from midsummer to mid-autumn. ↕ 1.5m–3m (5–10ft), ↔ 1m (3ft). C. and E. North America. ❄❄❄.
'Golden Fountain' see 'Goldquelle'.
'Golden Glow' is very vigorous, bearing fully double flowerheads with yellow ray-florets; ↕ to 1.8m (6ft), ↔ 2–2.5m (6–8ft). **'Goldquelle'** ▣ ♀ syn. 'Golden Fountain', is compact, bearing double flowerheads with lemon-yellow ray-florets and green disc-florets that turn yellow as the flowerheads open; ↕ to 90cm (36in), ↔ 45cm (18in). **var. *hortensia*** is the name applied to all variants with double flowerheads.
R. newmanii see *R. fulgida* var. *speciosa.*
R. purpurea see *Echinacea purpurea.*
R. speciosa see *R. fulgida* var. *speciosa.*
R. sullivantii see *R. fulgida* var. *sullivantii.*

▷ **Rue** see *Ruta*
Common see *Ruta graveolens*
Fringed see *Ruta chalepensis*
Goat's see *Galega*

RUELLIA

syn. DIPTERACANTHUS

ACANTHACEAE

Diverse genus of about 150 species of evergreen perennials and soft-stemmed or woody shrubs and subshrubs, widely distributed in tropical America, warm parts of North America, and Africa and Asia, where they are found in meadows and at woodland margins. The leaves are opposite and entire, and may be stalked or stalkless. Funnel-shaped flowers are produced singly, in clusters from the leaf axils, or in terminal panicles. The tropical species, in particular, are cultivated for their attractive foliage and flowers, and are suitable for informal borders or plantings. In frost-prone climates, grow tender species in a warm greenhouse.

- **HARDINESS** Fully hardy to frost tender.
- **CULTIVATION** Under glass, grow in loamless potting compost in bright filtered light with high humidity. In the growing season, water freely and apply a balanced liquid fertilizer monthly; water moderately in winter. Pinch out the young shoots to encourage branching. Pruning group 10, after flowering. Outdoors, grow in any fertile, humus-rich, moist soil in a site in full sun or partial shade.
- **PROPAGATION** Sow seed at 19–24°C (66–75°F) in spring. Root softwood cuttings in spring or early summer.
- **PESTS AND DISEASES** Trouble free.

R. amoena see *R. graecizans.*
R. devosiana ▣ Hairy shrub with soft, purple-flushed stems and broadly lance-shaped, pale-veined, dark green leaves, to 8cm (3in) long, purple beneath. Funnel-shaped, lavender-blue-flushed white flowers, 4–5cm (1½–2in) long, with slender tubes and notched, spreading, purple-veined lobes, are produced singly from the leaf axils from spring to summer. ↕ 45cm (18in), ↔ 30cm (12in). Brazil. ❀ (min. 12°C/54°F)
R. graecizans, syn. *R. amoena.* Bushy shrub with soft, spreading stems and ovate to oblong, hairless, mid-green leaves, to 18cm (7in) long. Funnel-shaped scarlet flowers, 2.5cm (1in) long, each with one enlarged sepal, are borne in axillary clusters on long stalks from spring to summer. ↕ 60cm (24in), ↔ 45cm (18in). South America. ❀ (min. 12°C/54°F)

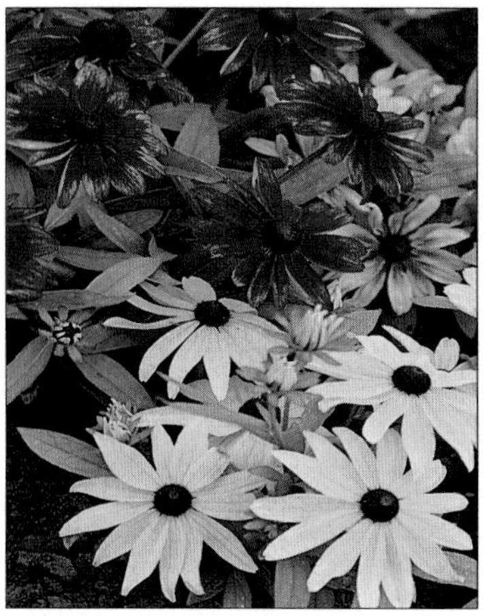

Rudbeckia hirta 'Becky Mixed'

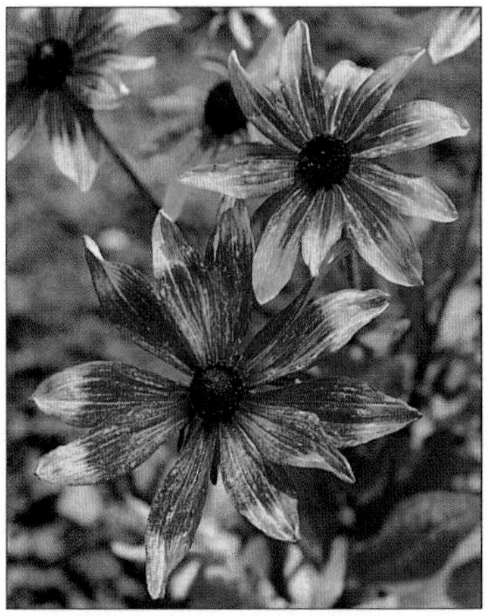

Rudbeckia hirta 'Rustic Dwarfs'

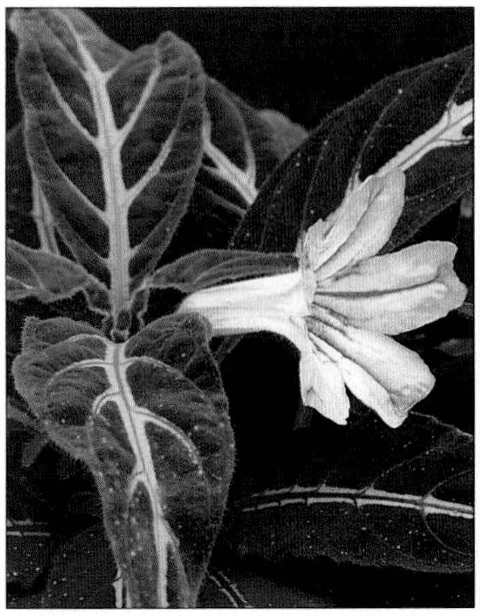

Ruellia devosiana

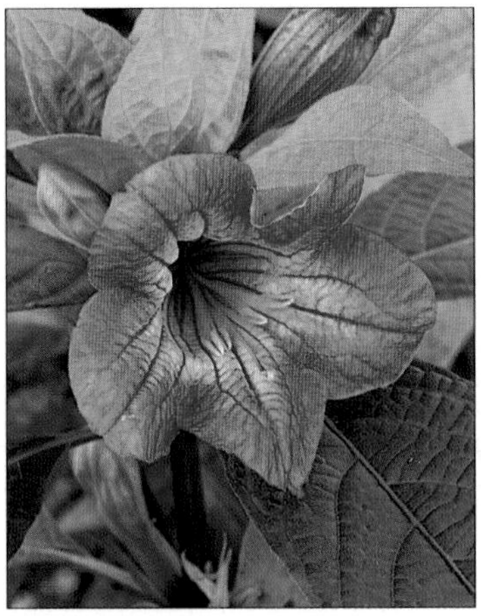

Ruellia macrantha

R. macrantha ■ (Christmas pride). Erect, soft-stemmed subshrub with lance-shaped, hairy, dull, dark green leaves, to 15cm (6in) long. From autumn to winter, funnel-shaped but slightly curved, rich purplish pink flowers, to 8cm (3in) long, with darker veins, are produced singly from the leaf axils. ↕ to 2m (6ft), ↔ 45cm (18in). Brazil. ❁ (min. 12°C/54°F)
R. makoyana ♀ (Monkey plant, Trailing velvet plant). Slender- and soft-stemmed, spreading, hairy perennial with ovate, silver-veined purple leaves, to 8cm (3in) long, dark purple beneath. In summer, produces funnel-shaped, carmine-pink flowers, 5cm (2in) long, singly from the leaf axils. ↕ to 60cm (24in), ↔ 45cm (18in). Brazil. ❁ (min. 12°C/54°F)

RUMEX

Dock

POLYGONACEAE

Genus of about 200 species of annuals, biennials, and usually tap-rooted, sometimes rhizomatous perennials from a range of habitats including mountains, wasteland, cultivated ground, and streamsides in N. temperate regions. Docks have simple, variably shaped, mainly basal leaves, which occasionally have wavy margins. In summer, the tiny, star-shaped, bisexual or unisexual flowers are borne in whorls in usually erect, dense, terminal panicles or racemes. They are followed by small, triangular, brown to red-brown fruit. Some species are invasive weeds; a few are grown for their decorative foliage or as herbs. Grow in a herbaceous or mixed border. All parts of docks may cause mild stomach upset if ingested; contact with the foliage may irritate skin.
- **HARDINESS** Fully hardy to half hardy.
- **CULTIVATION** Grow in moderately fertile, well-drained soil in full sun.
- **PROPAGATION** Sow seed *in situ* in spring. Docks also self-seed freely.
- **PESTS AND DISEASES** Susceptible to slug damage and aphids.

R. sanguineus ■ (Bloody dock, Red-veined dock). Tap-rooted, rosette-forming perennial with oblong-lance-shaped, mid- to dark green leaves, 5–15cm (2–6in) long, conspicuously veined blood-red or purple. In early and midsummer, erect, red-tinted flower stems bear panicles of tiny, star-shaped, green then red-brown flowers, 4mm (⅛in) across, followed by dark brown fruit. ↕ to 90cm (36in), ↔ 30cm (12in). Europe, N. Africa, S.W. Asia. ❄❄❄

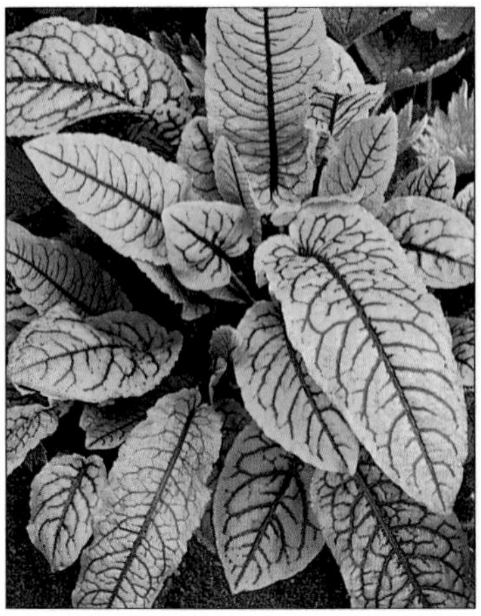

Rumex sanguineus

RUMOHRA

DRYOPTERIDACEAE

Genus of 50 species of epiphytic or terrestrial, rock-dwelling, evergreen ferns occurring in cool woodland or scrub in tropical regions of the S. hemisphere. They have scaly, creeping rhizomes covered in golden brown scales, and triangular, pinnate or 2- or 3-pinnate, leathery fronds. Spores are formed in conspicuous, large, circular spots, each covered with a centrally attached indusium. In frost-prone climates, grow in a warm greenhouse; in warmer areas, grow epiphytically or in a damp, shady border. The fronds are popular for flower arrangements.
- **HARDINESS** Frost tender.
- **CULTIVATION** Under glass, grow epiphytically on bark, or in shallow pots or hanging baskets in a mix of 1 part each of loam, medium-grade bark, and charcoal, 2 parts sharp sand, and 3 parts coarse leaf mould. Provide bright filtered light and moderate humidity. In growth, mist regularly, water freely, and apply a half-strength balanced liquid fertilizer monthly; water sparingly in winter. Outdoors, grow epiphytically or in moist, leafy, open, humus-rich soil in partial or light dappled shade.
- **PROPAGATION** Sow spores at 21°C (70°F) as soon as ripe, or separate rooted sections of rhizomes in early summer. See also p.51.
- **PESTS AND DISEASES** Trouble free.

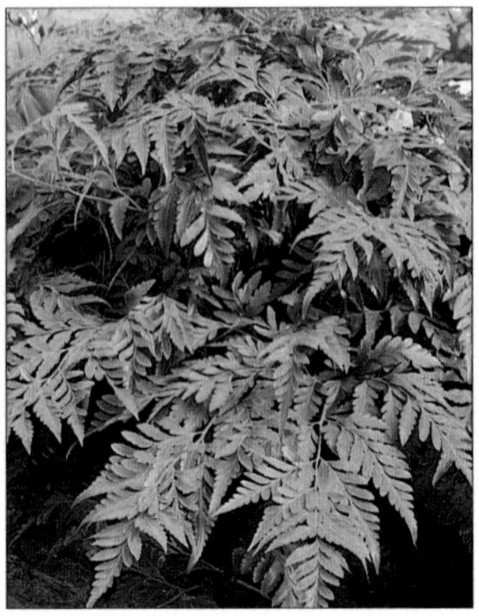

Rumohra adiantiformis

R. adiantiformis ■ ♀ (Leather fern). Evergreen, terrestrial or epiphytic fern, very variable in size, producing ovate or triangular, 2- or 3-pinnate, leathery, dark green fronds, to 90cm (36in) or more long; the fronds have narrowly diamond-shaped to oblong pinnae. ↕ 0.5–1.5m (20–60in), ↔ to 1m (3ft). Tropical and subtropical areas of S. hemisphere. ❁ (min. 10–13°C/50–55°F)

▷ **Running postman** see *Kennedia prostrata*

RUPICAPNOS

PAPAVERACEAE

Genus of about 30 species of almost stemless, evergreen perennials found on sunny mountain slopes or cliff faces in Spain and N. Africa. They have pinnate, finely dissected leaves with pinnatisect leaflets, and bear corymb-like racemes of tubular, 4-petalled, spurred flowers in summer. The short-lived *R. africana* is the most commonly cultivated species, and can be successfully grown in a scree bed or alpine house.
- **HARDINESS** Frost hardy. Will survive temperatures to -10°C (14°F), but will not tolerate winter wet.
- **CULTIVATION** Under glass, grow in a mix of 1 part each of loam and leaf mould and 2 parts grit, with additional tufa chippings, in full light. Water moderately in the growing season; keep just moist in winter. Self-seed freely under glass. Outdoors, grow in gritty, sharply drained soil in a scree bed, in full sun with protection from excessive winter wet.
- **PROPAGATION** Collect seed when almost ripe but still green, and sow immediately in containers in a cold frame.
- **PESTS AND DISEASES** Trouble free.

R. africana ■ Short-lived perennial producing basal clumps of fern-like, pinnate, bright grey-blue leaves, 8–10cm (3–4in) long, finely divided into pinnatisect leaflets, which may be linear, ovate, or oblong. Delicate, corymb-like racemes of 4-petalled, spurred, pinkish-purple flowers, to 1.5cm (½in) long, with dark purple tips, are borne over a long period in summer. ↕ 15cm (6in), ↔ 20cm (8in). Morocco (Rif Mountains). ❄❄. **subsp. *decipiens*** bears yellow-marked white flowers; S.W. Spain.

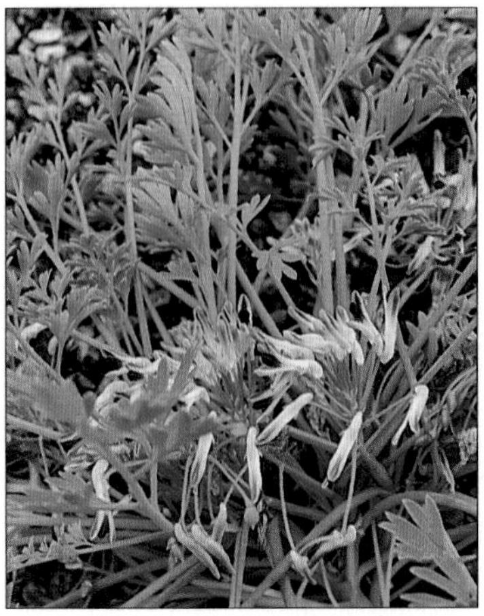

Rupicapnos africana

RUSCHIA

AIZOACEAE

Genus of about 350 species of shrubby or stemless, mat-forming, perennial succulents from semi-desert regions of Namibia and South Africa. Many species branch freely to form tufts or mats; others become shrubby, to 1m (3ft) tall. The leaves are arranged in pairs and are often boat-shaped. Daisy-like flowers open during the day in summer. In warm, dry climates, grow in a raised bed or desert garden. In frost-prone areas, grow prostrate species in a temperate greenhouse, or treat as frost-tender annuals and use for bedding, window-boxes, or hanging baskets.
- **HARDINESS** Frost tender.
- **CULTIVATION** Under glass, grow in standard cactus compost in full light with low humidity. Water moderately from spring to autumn, applying a dilute balanced liquid fertilizer once in late spring and once in late summer; keep dry in winter. Outdoors, grow in poor, gritty, sharply drained soil in full sun. See also pp.48–49.
- **PROPAGATION** Sow seed at 21°C (70°F) in early spring. Plant out seedlings to be grown as annuals when all danger of frost has passed. Root cuttings of stem sections from spring to summer.
- **PESTS AND DISEASES** Susceptible to mealybugs.

R. acuminata. Shrubby succulent with erect or almost prostrate, woody stems. Produces pairs of ovoid, bluntly keeled, sometimes toothed leaves, to 2.5cm (1in) long, with convex sides, narrowing towards the tips. They are roughly papillose, fleshy, and blue-green marked with dull green spots. In summer, bears solitary, terminal or axillary, daisy-like, white or pale pink flowers, 3cm (1¼in) across. ↕ 20cm (8in), ↔ 50cm (20in). South Africa (Eastern Cape). ❁ (min. 7°C/45°F)
R. derenbergiana see *Ebracteola derenbergiana.*
R. macowanii ■ Shrubby succulent with short, prostrate, woody stems and erect, fleshy branches. The fleshy, grey-green leaves, to 3.5cm (1½in) long, are boat-shaped to cylindrical, flat above and keeled beneath. In summer, bears solitary, terminal, daisy-like pink flowers, 2cm (¾in) across, with a darker pink stripe on each petal. ↕ 20cm (8in), ↔ 45cm (18in). South Africa (Western Cape, Northern Cape, Eastern Cape). ❁ (min. 7°C/45°F)
R. pusilla. Tufted, prostrate, almost stemless succulent with nearly spherical, fleshy, bright green leaves, 4mm (⅛in) long, keeled beneath. Solitary, terminal or axillary, daisy-like, pale pinkish white flowers, 1cm (½in) across, are produced in summer. ↕↔ 7cm (3in). South Africa (Western Cape, Northern Cape, Eastern Cape). ❁ (min. 7°C/45°F)
R. pygmaea. Mat-forming, prostrate succulent with very short, fleshy stems bearing 1 or 2 dissimilar pairs of ovoid or ellipsoid, fleshy, bright green leaves, to 5mm (¼in) long, keeled beneath, and more or less united almost to the tips. The leaf skins gradually shrivel to disclose a second pair of leaves, which are not united, and these become the

R

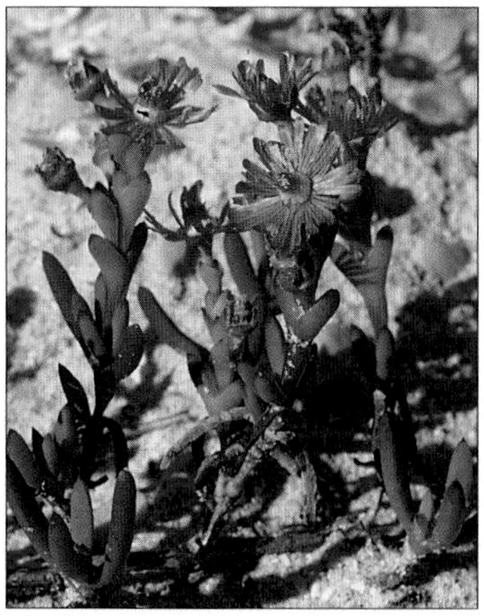

Ruschia macowanii

first pair of leaves of the following year's growth. Solitary, terminal or axillary, daisy-like, whitish pink flowers, to 2cm (¾in) across, are borne in summer. ↕↔ 8cm (3in). Namibia, South Africa (Western Cape, Northern Cape, Eastern Cape). ❁ (min. 7°C/45°F)

RUSCUS

Broom

LILIACEAE/RUSCACEAE

Genus of 6 species of rhizomatous, evergreen subshrubs from woodland in Madeira and the Azores, through Europe and N. Africa to Iran. The tiny, true leaves are replaced by flattened, leaf-like shoots (cladophylls) on which the flowers and showy red fruits are borne. The inconspicuous, star-shaped, green or greenish white flowers, to 2mm (1/16in) across, each have 6 tepals. *Ruscus* species are usually dioecious, and plants of both sexes are normally needed to obtain fruit; however, *R. aculeatus* sometimes bears hermaphrodite, self-fertile flowers. Grow in a dry, shady site. The stems may be dried in glycerine and used in floral arrangements. The berries of *R. aculeatus* may cause mild stomach upset if ingested.

- **HARDINESS** Fully hardy to frost hardy.
- **CULTIVATION** Grow in any but water-logged soil in sun or partial or full shade. Individual shoots are short-lived, but new ones are produced annually; cut out dead stems at the base in spring.
- **PROPAGATION** Sow seed in a seedbed, or in containers in a cold frame, as soon as ripe. Divide in spring.
- **PESTS AND DISEASES** Trouble free.

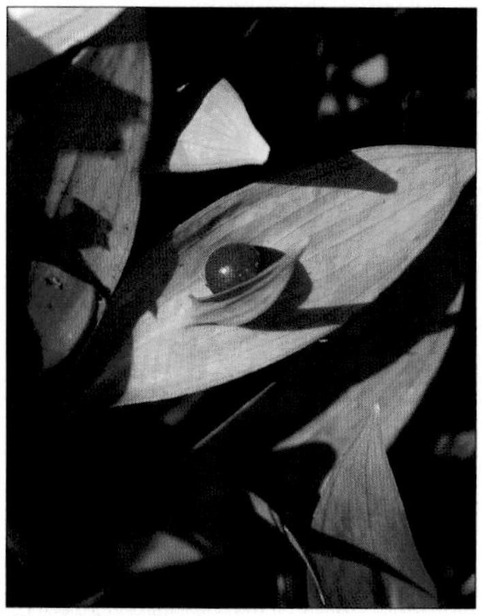

Ruscus hypoglossum

R. aculeatus (Butcher's broom). Clump-forming, rhizomatous subshrub with upright, branched shoots bearing ovate, spine-tipped, glossy, dark green cladophylls, to 2.5cm (1in) long. From late summer to winter, female plants produce spherical, bright red berries, 8mm (⅜in) across, on the upper sides of the cladophylls. ↕ 75cm (30in), ↔ 1m (3ft). Europe, N. Turkey, N. Africa, Azores. ❄❄❄

R. hypoglossum ▣ Clump-forming, rhizomatous subshrub producing arching, unbranched shoots and obovate to broadly ovate, glossy, mid-green cladophylls, to 10cm (4in) long. Female plants bear spherical red berries, 1cm (½in) across, on the upper sides of the cladophylls, from autumn to winter. ↕ 45cm (18in), ↔ 1m (3ft). Italy, Czech Republic to Turkey. ❄❄

R. hypophyllum. Rhizomatous, clump-forming subshrub with upright shoots and ovate, pointed, dark green cladophylls, to 10cm (4in) long. Female plants bear spherical red berries, 1cm (½in) across, on the upper or lower side of the cladophylls, from late summer to winter. Male and female flowers may be borne on the same plant. ↕ 60cm (24in), ↔ 1m (3ft). S.E. France, S. Spain, N. Africa, Sicily. ❄❄

▷ **Rush** see *Juncus*
  Corkscrew see *Juncus effusus* 'Spiralis'
  Dwarf Japanese see *Acorus gramineus* 'Pusillus'
  Egyptian paper see *Cyperus papyrus*
  Flowering see *Butomus*
  Japanese see *Acorus gramineus*
  Jointed see *Juncus articulatus*
  Mat see *Lomandra*
  Pale mat see *Lomandra glauca*
  Spiny-headed mat see *Lomandra longifolia*
  Variegated Japanese see *Acorus gramineus* 'Variegatus'
▷ **Rushes** see p.54

RUSSELIA

SCROPHULARIACEAE

Genus of about 50 species of evergreen or deciduous shrubs and subshrubs found at forest margins from Mexico and Cuba to Colombia. The pendent, rush-like stems bear opposite or whorled, often scale-like leaves. Showy, tubular, red, pink, or white flowers are borne in axillary cymes, or sometimes singly. *R. equisetiformis* is the only species commonly cultivated. In frost-prone areas, grow as houseplants, in a cool or temperate greenhouse, or in hanging baskets. In warmer climates, grow at the front of a shrub border, or allow to trail over the edges of a raised bed or wall.

- **HARDINESS** Frost tender.
- **CULTIVATION** Under glass, grow in loam-based potting compost (JI No.2) in full or bright filtered light. When in growth, water moderately and apply a balanced liquid fertilizer monthly; water sparingly in winter. Outdoors, grow in a sheltered site in well-drained, humus-rich, moderately fertile soil in full sun. Pruning group 9.
- **PROPAGATION** Divide rooted layers in spring; root softwood cuttings at any time of year.
- **PESTS AND DISEASES** Trouble free.

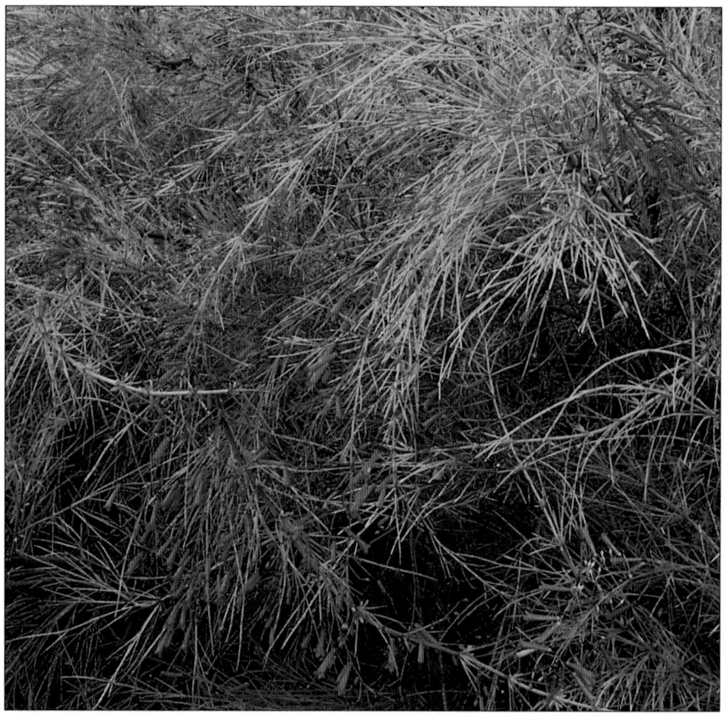

Russelia equisetiformis

R. equisetiformis ▣ 🏆 syn. *R. juncea* (Coral plant, Firecracker plant). Deciduous, branching subshrub with rush-like, erect and pendent, mid-green stems. The elliptic, scale-like, mid-green leaves, to 1.5cm (½in) long, fall early. Tubular scarlet flowers, to 3cm (1¼in) long, are borne in pendent cymes from spring to autumn. ↕ 1.5m (5ft), ↔ 2.5m (8ft). Mexico. ❁ (min. 10°C/50°F)

R. juncea see *R. equisetiformis.*

▷ **Russian vine** see *Fallopia baldschuanica*
▷ **Rusty leaf** see *Menziesia ferruginea*

RUTA

Rue

RUTACEAE

Genus of 8 species of deciduous or evergreen shrubs, subshrubs, and woody-based herbaceous perennials, occurring in dry, rocky habitats in the Canary Islands, the Mediterranean region, N.E. Africa, and S.W. Asia. They are cultivated for their aromatic foliage and flowers. The leaves are alternate, occasionally opposite, broadly ovate to rounded, and pinnatisect to pinnate. The unusual, 4- or 5-petalled, fringed or toothed yellow flowers are produced in terminal cymes. Rue is suitable for growing in a mixed or herbaceous border, or in a rock garden or herb garden. The foliage is sometimes used medicinally or very sparingly as a culinary flavouring. All parts of rue may cause severe discomfort if ingested; the foliage may cause photodermatitis on contact.

- **HARDINESS** Fully hardy to frost hardy.
- **CULTIVATION** Grow in moderately fertile, very well-drained soil in full sun or partial shade. Rue will thrive in a hot, dry site. Pruning group 10, in spring or after flowering.
- **PROPAGATION** Sow seed in containers in a cold frame in spring. Root semi-ripe cuttings in summer.
- **PESTS AND DISEASES** *Phytophthora* root rot may be a problem.

R. chalepensis (Fringed rue). Upright subshrub producing broadly ovate, 2- or 3-pinnatisect, aromatic, blue-green leaves, to 12cm (5in) long, with numerous oblong-lance-shaped or obovate lobes. Cup-shaped, dark yellow flowers, 2cm (¾in) across, each with 4 petals fringed with long hairs, are borne in open cymes in summer. ↕↔ 60cm (24in). S. Europe, N.E. Africa, S.W. Asia. ❄❄. **'Dimension Two'** is more spreading than the species, and almost prostrate.

R. graveolens (Common rue). Rounded to erect, evergreen shrub producing alternate, broadly ovate to rounded, 2-pinnatisect, aromatic, glaucous, blue-green leaves, to 15cm (6in) long, with numerous obovate lobes. Cymes of cup-shaped, 4-petalled, dull yellow flowers, 2cm (¾in) across, are borne in summer. ↕ 1m (3ft), ↔ 75cm (30in). S.E. Europe. ❄❄❄. **'Jackman's Blue'** ▣ 🏆 is more compact than the species, and has more intensely glaucous, blue-green foliage; ↕ 60cm (24in).

▷ **Rye,**
  Canadian wild see *Elymus canadensis*
  Wild see *Elymus*

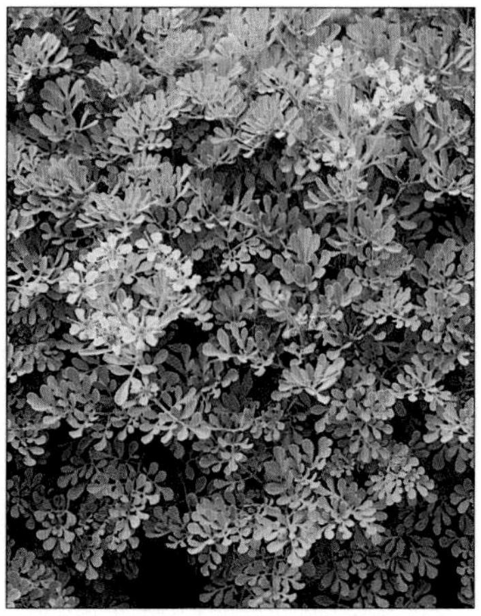

Ruta graveolens 'Jackman's Blue'

S

SABAL
Palmetto

ARECACEAE/PALMAE

Genus of 14 species of single-stemmed or stemless palms, chiefly from low-lying or swampy areas in tropical forest, from S. USA to N. South America, and from the West Indies. They have deeply divided, fan-shaped leaves, which often remain *in situ* when they die, forming a skirt-like bundle just below each crown. Panicles of 3-petalled flowers are borne between the leaves, usually in summer. In frost-prone areas, grow in a cool to warm greenhouse, a conservatory, or as houseplants. In warmer areas, plant the trees as lawn specimens and the stemless species in a shrub border.

• **HARDINESS** Frost tender.

• **CULTIVATION** Under glass, grow in well-drained, loam-based potting compost (JI No.2) in bright indirect light. During the growing season, water moderately and apply a balanced liquid fertilizer monthly. Pot on or top-dress in spring. Mist over lightly every day in summer. Keep just moist in winter. Outdoors, grow in moderately fertile, moist but well-drained soil in full sun with some midday shade.

• **PROPAGATION** Sow seed at 19–24°C (66–75°F) in spring.

• **PESTS AND DISEASES** Prone to red spider mites and scale insects under glass.

S. glabra see *S. minor.*
S. guatemalensis see *S. mexicana.*
S. mexicana ⚘ syn. *S. guatemalensis, S. texana* (Texas palmetto). Medium-sized palm with a columnar trunk that bears old leaf bases for several years. Fan-shaped, bright green, often yellowish green leaves, 1m (3ft) long, are divided up to halfway into many slender, pointed lobes. Bears cream flowers in panicles as long as or longer than the leaves, usually in summer. ↕ to 18m (60ft), ↔ to 4m (12ft). USA (Texas), Mexico, Guatemala. ❄ (min. 10–13°C/50–55°F)
S. minima see *S. minor.*
S. minor ▣ ✱ syn. *S. glabra, S. minima, S. pumila* (Dwarf palmetto, Scrub palmetto). Small palm with a short, buried stem (only the tip visible above the ground) and long-stalked, fan-shaped, blue-green leaves, 1–1.5m (3–5ft) long, divided at least to two-thirds into many slender lobes. Cream flowers are borne, usually in summer, in erect to arching panicles, to 2m (6ft) long. ↕ 1–2m (3–6ft), ↔ to 3m (10ft). S.E. USA. ❄ (min. 3–5°C/37–41°F)
S. palmetto ▣ ⚘ (Cabbage palmetto, Common blue palmetto). Large palm with a rough trunk, to 60cm (24in) in diameter. Bears compact, spherical heads of many fan-shaped, rich green leaves, to 2m (6ft) long, divided into numerous long, 2-lobed segments with thread-like filaments hanging between them. Cream flowers are borne in panicles just longer than the leaves, usually in summer. ↕ to 30m (100ft), ↔ 5–7m (15–22ft). USA (N. Carolina to Florida). ❄ (min. 5–7°C/41–45°F)
S. pumila see *S. minor.*
S. texana see *S. mexicana.*

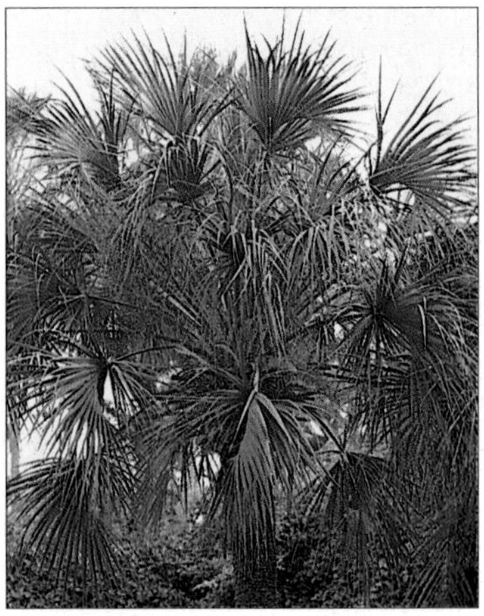

Sabal palmetto

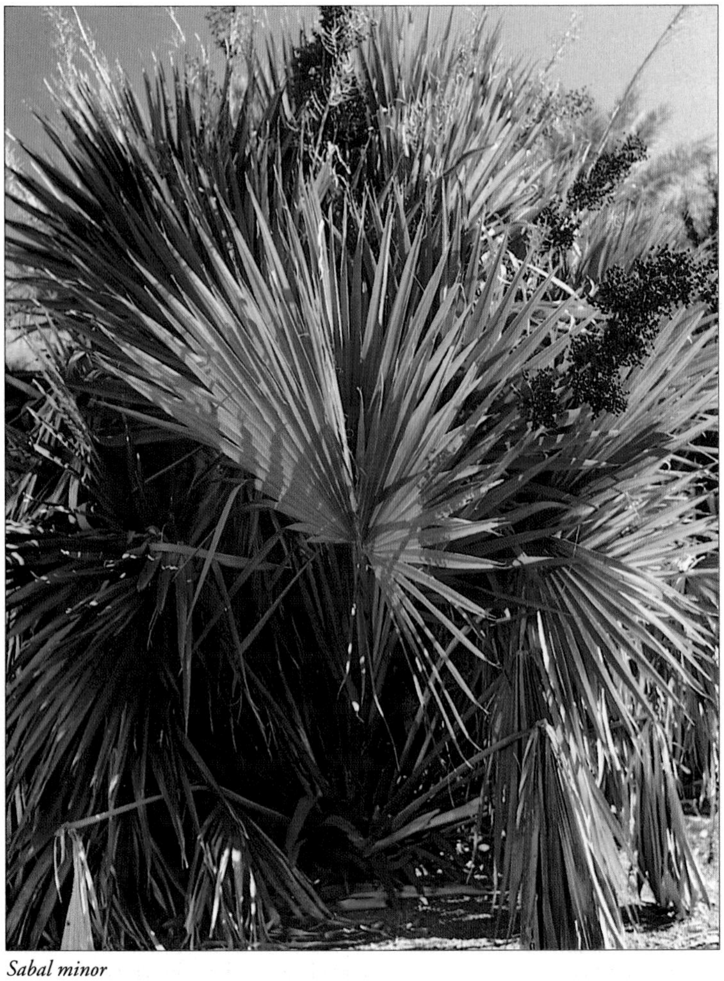

Sabal minor

▷ ***Sabina*** see *Juniperus*

SACCHARUM
syn. ERIANTHUS
Plume grass

GRAMINEAE/POACEAE

Genus of about 20 species of reed-like, tufted, clump-forming, or rhizomatous, perennial grasses found by riversides and in valley bottoms, widely distributed in warm-temperate and tropical regions. They are grown for their inflorescences and foliage. Leaves are narrowly lance-shaped to linear. Large, plume-like panicles of crowded flower spikes with silky-hairy spikelets are borne in pairs in summer and autumn. Effective at the back of a herbaceous or mixed border, against a warm, sunny wall, or as free-standing specimens. The cut panicles are useful in fresh and dried arrangements.

• **HARDINESS** Fully hardy to frost tender.

• **CULTIVATION** Grow in moderately fertile, well-drained soil in full sun, with shelter from cold, drying winds. Protect crowns from extreme cold with dry mulch or horticultural fleece. Remove any flowerheads left for winter effect by early spring. *S. ravennae* flowers most reliably after a long, hot summer.

• **PROPAGATION** Sow seed in containers under glass or in a cold frame in spring. Divide in mid-spring or early summer.

• **PESTS AND DISEASES** Trouble free.

S. ravennae. Robust, densely tufted, perennial grass with arching, linear leaves, 60–90cm (24–36in) long, that are grey-green with central white stripes, purple-tinted in autumn. In late summer and autumn, erect stems bear dense, upright panicles, to 60cm (24in) long, of softly hairy, silver-grey to purple flower spikes. ↕ 2–3m (6–10ft), ↔ 1.2m (4ft). Mediterranean to N. Africa. ✱✱ (hardy to about -8°C/18°F)

▷ **Sacred flower of the Incas** see *Cantua buxifolia*

SADLERIA

BLECHNACEAE

Genus of 7 species of evergreen, tree-like ferns from rainforest and exposed sites on lava flows in Hawaii. They each have a stout rhizome, crowned with large, divided fronds. The spores, unlike those of other tree ferns, such as *Cyathea* and *Dicksonia,* are borne in lines along the midribs of the frond segments. *S. cyatheoides* is the only species generally grown. In frost-prone areas, grow in a temperate greenhouse, a conservatory, or as houseplants. In warmer areas, grow in a shrub border, a woodland garden, or as a free-standing specimen.

• **HARDINESS** Frost tender.

• **CULTIVATION** Under glass, grow in equal parts medium-grade bark, perlite, and charcoal, in bright indirect to moderate light, and with moderate to high humidity. In growth, water moderately and apply a balanced liquid fertilizer monthly; keep just moist in winter. Outdoors, grow in moderately fertile, humus-rich, moist but well-drained, acid to neutral soil in partial to deep shade; shelter from cold, dry winds.

• **PROPAGATION** Sow spores at 21°C (70°F) as soon as ripe. See also p.51.

• **PESTS AND DISEASES** Trouble free.

S. cyatheoides. Tree-like fern with ovate, 2-pinnate, leathery fronds, 90cm (36in) long, dark green above, glaucous beneath; they have narrowly oblong pinnae, and numerous linear segments with the margins rolled under. ↕ 1.5m (5ft), ↔ 1.8m (6ft). USA (Hawaii). ❄ (min. 10°C/50°F)

▷ **Safflower** see *Carthamus, C. tinctorius*
▷ **Saffron,**
  False see *Carthamus tinctorius*
  Meadow see *Colchicum autumnale*
▷ **Saffron-spike** see *Aphelandra squarrosa*
▷ **Sage** see *Salvia*
  Autumn see *Salvia greggii*
  Blue see *Eranthemum pulchellum*
  Bog see *Salvia uliginosa*
  Common see *Salvia officinalis*
  Jerusalem see *Phlomis fruticosa, Pulmonaria saccharata*
  Jim see *Salvia clevelandii*
  Mealy see *Salvia farinacea*
  Pineapple see *Salvia elegans* 'Scarlet Pineapple'
  Purple see *Salvia officinalis* 'Purpurascens'
  Scarlet see *Salvia splendens*
▷ **Sagebrush** see *Artemisia, Seriphidium tridentatum*
▷ **Sage wood, South African** see *Buddleja salviifolia*

SAGINA
Pearlwort

CARYOPHYLLACEAE

Genus of about 20 species of compact, low-growing annuals and perennials found in a wide range of habitats, extensively distributed throughout the temperate regions of the N. hemisphere. They have linear to narrowly wedge-shaped leaves, arranged in pairs and joined at the bases around the stems. Minute, 4- or 5-petalled, rarely petalless white flowers are produced either singly or in few-flowered cymes. The majority of pearlworts are weeds; those described

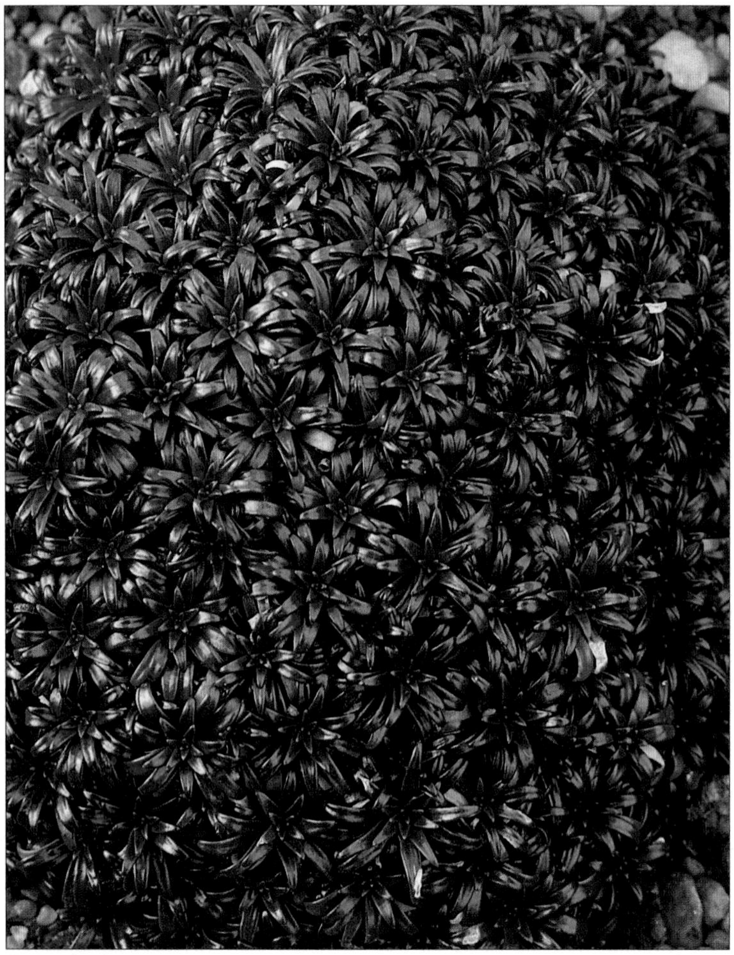

Sagina boydii

here are cultivated mainly for their dense mats or cushions of leaves, which provide effective ground cover. They are suitable for growing in a rock garden or paving crevice. Alternatively, grow in an alpine house.

• **HARDINESS** Fully hardy.

• **CULTIVATION** Grow in poor to moderately fertile, acid to neutral, moist but well-drained soil in full sun with some midday shade. *S. boydii* requires very sharply drained, poor soil, and tolerates partial shade. In an alpine house, grow in 3 parts grit or sharp sand and 1 part peat or leaf mould. Dislikes hot, dry conditions.

• **PROPAGATION** Sow seed in containers in a cold frame in autumn. Divide *S. subulata* in spring. Root individual rosettes of *S. boydii* as cuttings in early summer.

• **PESTS AND DISEASES** Prone to aphids or red spider mites under glass.

S. boydii ■ Very slow-growing, dense, cushion-forming perennial producing crowded rosettes of rigid, linear to narrowly wedge-shaped, recurved, glossy, dark green leaves, to 2cm (¾in) long. Bears tiny, solitary, normally petalless, mid-green flowers in summer. Best in an alpine house. ↕ 2.5cm (1in), ↔ 8cm (3in). Scotland. ✻✻✻

***S. glabra* 'Aurea'** see *S. subulata* 'Aurea'.

***S. subulata* 'Aurea'**, syn. *S. glabra* 'Aurea'. Mat-forming perennial with slender, rooting stems clothed in pointed, linear, yellow-green leaves, to 1cm (½in) long. In summer, bears solitary, 5-petalled white flowers, 4mm (⅛in) across, on stems to 4cm (1½in) long. Effective low ground cover in a rock garden or between paving stones. ↕ 1cm (½in), ↔ 20cm (8in) or more. W. and C. Europe. ✻✻✻

SAGITTARIA
Arrowhead

ALISMATACEAE

Genus of 20 species of marginal and submerged, herbaceous aquatic perennials and annuals, found mainly on muddy banks or in shallow water in temperate and tropical Europe, Asia, and North, Central, and South America. The often decorative leaves are aerial, floating, or submerged, and linear to elliptic, lance-shaped, ovate, or arrow-shaped. Panicles or racemes of whorled, 3-petalled, saucer-shaped white flowers are borne in summer. Most are excellent for the margins of a wildlife pool, where their tuberous rootstocks may spread; some (including *S. latifolia* and *S. sagittifolia*) produce walnut-sized tubers that attract waterfowl. Grow *S. subulata* in an aquarium for its attractive submerged leaves. In frost-prone areas, grow tender species in a pool in a cool or temperate greenhouse.

• **HARDINESS** Fully hardy to frost tender.

• **CULTIVATION** Outdoors, grow at the margins of a pool, in water no deeper than 22–30cm (9–12in), in full sun. Trim back spreading growth in late summer and remove faded flowers to prevent seeding. In an aquarium, grow in groups of 4 or 5 in a gravelly soil in bright indirect light, with a minimum temperature of 16°C (61°F). Under glass, grow in baskets at the margins of an indoor pool in bright filtered light, with a water temperature of 10°C (50°F). See also pp.52–53.

• **PROPAGATION** Sow seed as soon as ripe in containers standing in trays of shallow water. Remove runners, or collect and plant overwintering tubers, in spring.

• **PESTS AND DISEASES** Leaves may be damaged by water-lily aphid.

S. japonica see *S. sagittifolia* 'Flore Pleno'.

S. lancifolia. Stoloniferous, marginal aquatic perennial producing lance-shaped, leathery, pale green aerial leaves, 15–45cm (6–18in) long. In summer, bears several whorls of white flowers, 3–5cm (1¼–2in) across, on scapes to 2m (6ft) tall. ↕↔ 1.5m (5ft). Tropical and subtropical North, Central, and South America. ❁ (min. 10°C/50°F)

S. latifolia ■ (Duck potato, Wapato). Marginal aquatic perennial with large tubers and variable, mainly arrow-shaped aerial leaves, 10–30cm (4–12in) long. In summer, racemes of whorled white flowers, 3–4cm (1¼–1½in) across, are produced on the triangular flower stems, to 1.2m (4ft) tall. ↕ 45–90cm (18–36in), ↔ 90cm (36in). USA. ✻✻✻

S. sagittifolia (Japanese arrowhead). Marginal aquatic perennial bearing arrow-shaped aerial leaves, 25cm (10in) long, with 2 long, acute, basal lobes. In deep water, produces ribbon-like floating leaves, to 80cm (32in) long. In summer, scapes to 1m (3ft) tall bear racemes of white flowers, to 2.5cm (1in) across, with a purple spot at the base of each petal. ↕ 90cm (36in), ↔ indefinite. Eurasia. ✻✻✻. **'Flore Pleno'**, syn. *S. japonica*, is double-flowered.

S. subulata. Stoloniferous aquatic perennial bearing variable, usually linear, frequently bent or crooked submerged leaves, to 1m (3ft) long (depending on the depth of the water), with long, sharp-pointed or rounded tips. In shallow water, produces elliptic floating leaves, 5cm (2in) long. White flowers, 1.5–2cm (½–¾in) across, are borne in floating whorls of 1–3, in summer. ↕ to 60cm (24in), ↔ indefinite. E. USA. ✻

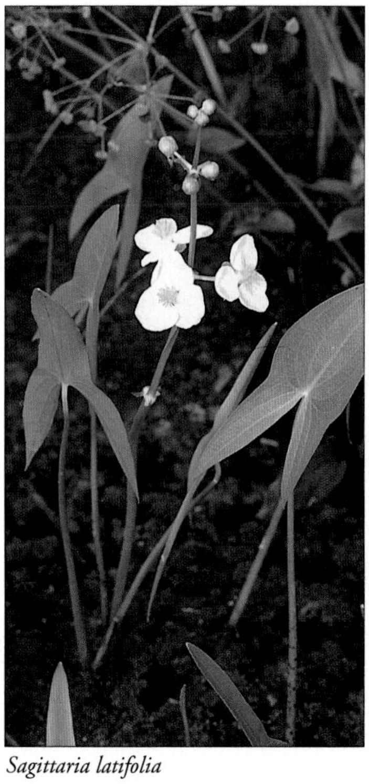

Sagittaria latifolia

▷**Sago, False** see *Cycas circinalis*
▷**Sago fern** see *Cyathea medullaris*
▷**Sago palm** see *Cycas, C. circinalis*
Japanese see *C. revoluta*
▷**Sailor caps** see *Dodecatheon hendersonii*
▷**St. Barbara's herb** see *Barbarea*
▷**St. Catherine's lace** see *Eriogonum, E. giganteum*
▷**St. Dabeoc's heath** see *Daboecia cantabrica*
▷**St. John's wort** see *Hypericum*
Perforate see *H. perforatum*

SAINTPAULIA
African violet

GESNERIACEAE

Genus of 20 species of low-growing, evergreen perennials found on banks, streamsides, on or among rocks, or as epiphytes on trees in a very small area of tropical E. Africa. Most are virtually stemless or have very short stems, and form rosettes of rounded to elliptic, somewhat succulent, usually hairy leaves. Trailing African violets produce the rosettes on extended stems, with the leaf-stalks usually longer than the leaf-blades. Flowers normally have 2 smaller petals at the top and 3 larger ones below, and are borne singly or in cymes.

There are over 2,000 cultivars, mainly derived from *S. ionantha*, with white, pink, red, blue, violet, bi- or multi-coloured flowers, 1–6cm (½–2½in) across, borne throughout the year. They may be single (5-petalled), semi-double (with small crests or lobes in the middle of the 5 petals), or fully double (with two or more layers of petals). The flowers are star-shaped, with all 5 petals of the same shape and size, or bell-shaped. Petal edges may be ruffled, rounded, frilled, or fringed. The leaves are usually mid- or dark green, and may be subtly feathered or flecked, or strongly variegated white, pink, or cream; most are broadly ovate to oval, and 4–20cm (1½–8in) long, including the stalks. Grow African violets as houseplants; most greenhouses or conservatories are too hot in summer and too cold in winter.

African violet cultivars are classified by rosette size into 5 groups (see below). The measurement given is the diameter of the rosette; the spread of each cultivar is the same as this.

MICRO-MINIATURE	less than 8cm (3in)
MINIATURE	8–16cm (3–6in)
SEMI-MINIATURE	16–21cm (6–8in)
STANDARD	21–40cm (8–16in)
LARGE	over 40cm (16in)

• **HARDINESS** Frost tender. Ideal temperature is 18–24°C (64–75°F).

• **CULTIVATION** Under glass, grow in well-drained loamless potting compost in bright filtered light and moderate to high humidity. At least 12 hours of light per day is needed for long-term flowering. Avoid direct summer sun, but position in the brightest light in winter; artificial light is useful. From early to

S

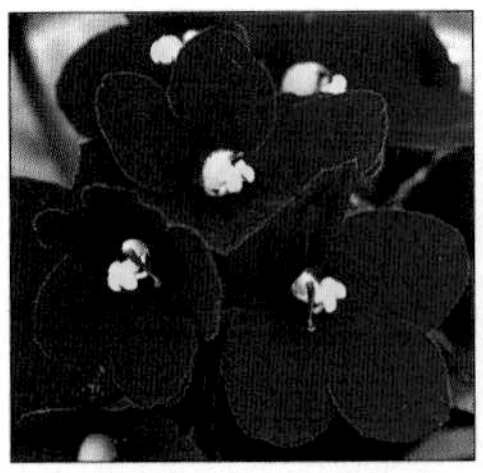
Saintpaulia 'Bright Eyes'

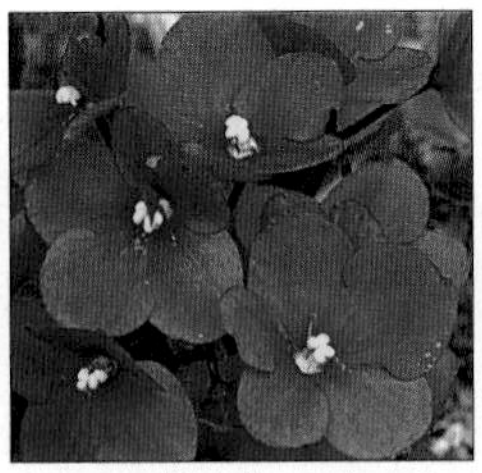
Saintpaulia 'Chantabent'

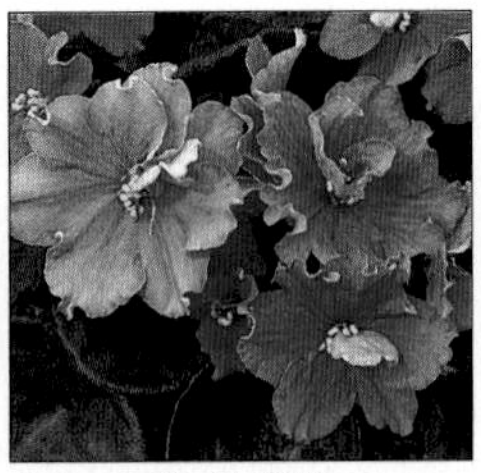
Saintpaulia 'Delft'

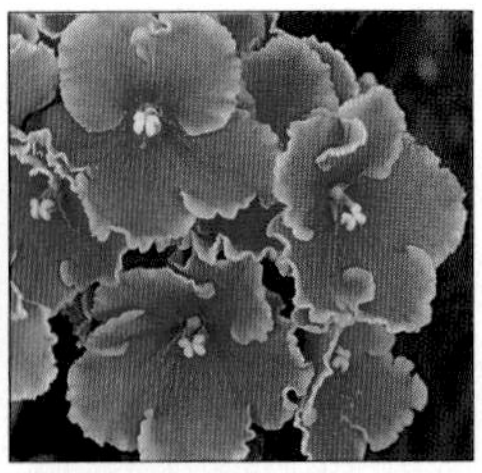
Saintpaulia 'Dorothy'

Saintpaulia 'Fancy Pants'

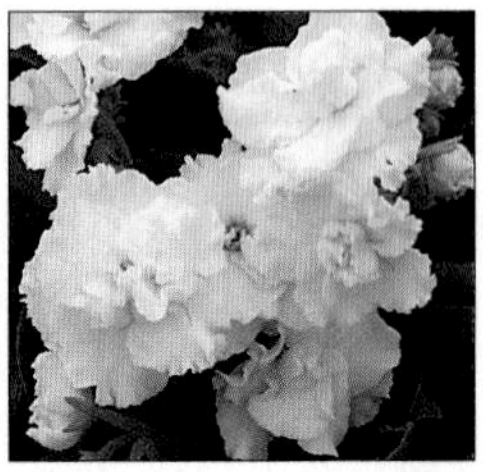
Saintpaulia 'Garden News'

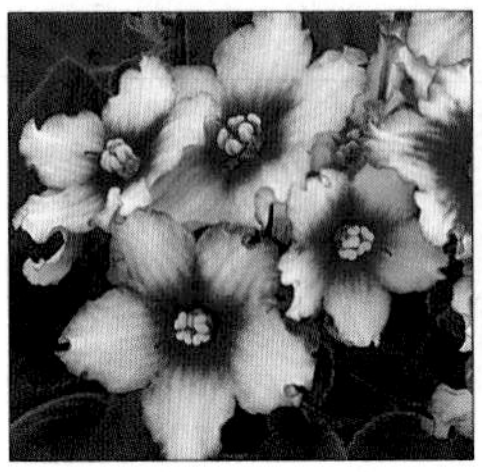

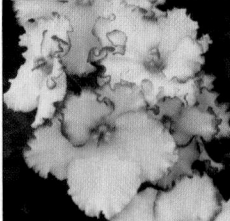
Saintpaulia 'Ice Maiden'

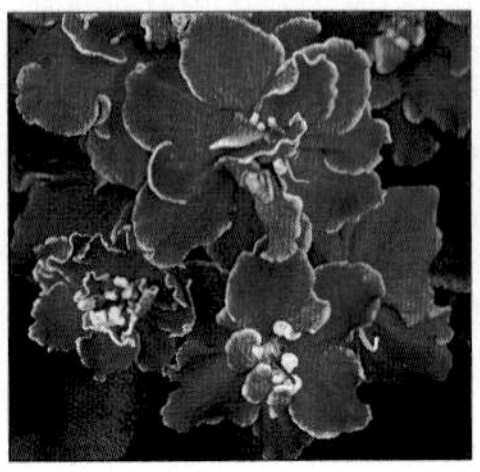
Saintpaulia 'Kristi Marie'

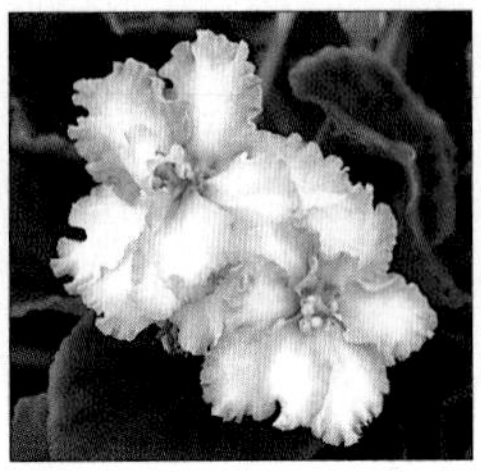
Saintpaulia 'Ms. Pretty'

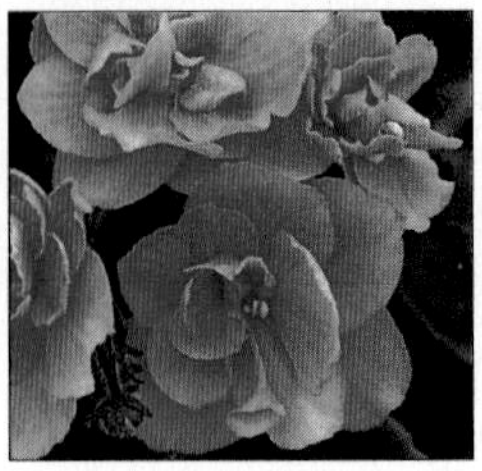
Saintpaulia 'Rococo Anna'

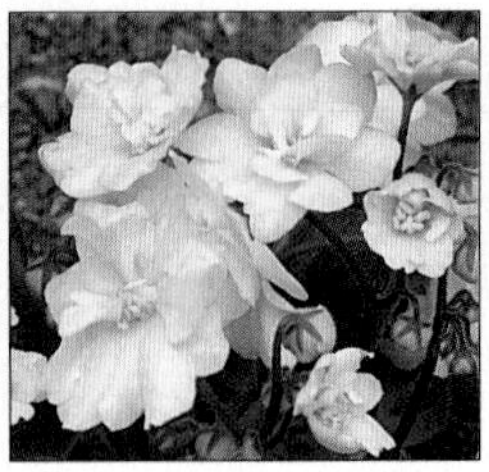
Saintpaulia 'Starry Trail'

Saintpaulia 'Zoja'

late summer, water moderately and apply a high potash and phosphate liquid fertilizer every 2 weeks, or add a quarter-strength fertilizer at every watering. Repot at least once a year, keeping to virtually the same container size; do not overpot.
• **PROPAGATION** Sow seed at 19–24°C (66–75°F) as soon as ripe or in early spring. Root leaf cuttings or suckers of cultivars at 24–27°C (75–81°F) in summer. Chimaeras (graft hybrids) will not come true from leaf cuttings.
• **PESTS AND DISEASES** Prone to aphids, mealybugs, thrips, tarsonemid mites, vine weevil larvae, grey mould (*Botrytis*), crown rot, and powdery mildew.

***S.* 'Bright Eyes'** ▣ ♀ (Standard group) Rosetted perennial with dark green leaves and single, deep blue flowers with prominent yellow pollen sacs. ↕ to 15cm (6in). ❄ (min. 15°C/59°F)
***S.* 'Chantabent'** ▣ (Semi-miniature group) Rosetted perennial bearing dark green leaves with deep red undersides. Produces large, single, violet-blue flowers. ↕ 10–15cm (4–6in). ❄ (min. 15°C/59°F)
***S.* 'Chantiana'.** (Miniature group) Rosetted perennial with light green leaves and fully double, light coral-pink flowers. ↕ 8–10cm (3–4in). ❄ (min. 15°C/59°F)
***S.* 'Chantora'.** (Miniature group) Rosetted perennial bearing pointed, dark green leaves with dark red undersides, and single, deep red flowers. ↕ 8–10cm (3–4in). ❄ (min. 15°C/59°F)
***S.* 'Colorado'** ▣ ♀ syn. *S.* 'Optimara Colorado'. (Standard group) Rosetted perennial with mid-green leaves. The single red flowers have frilled margins and bold yellow pollen sacs. ↕ 15–20cm (6–8in). ❄ (min. 15°C/59°F)
***S.* 'Dancin' Trail'.** (Semi-miniature group) Trailing, rosetted perennial with pointed, shiny, dark green leaves, red beneath, and fully double, magenta-red flowers. ↕ 10–15cm (4–6in). ❄ (min. 15°C/59°F)
***S.* 'Delft'** ▣ ♀ (Standard group) Strong-growing, rosetted perennial bearing mid-green leaves and large, semi-double, cornflower-blue flowers. ↕ 15cm (6in). ❄ (min. 15°C/59°F)
***S.* 'Dina Mo'.** (Standard group) Rosetted perennial bearing mid-green leaves and fully double, fuchsia-red flowers with narrow white margins. ↕ 15cm (6in). ❄ (min. 15°C/59°F)
***S.* 'Dorothy'** ▣ (Standard group) Rosetted perennial bearing long-stalked, light green leaves and large, single, rich pink flowers with frilled white margins. ↕ 15cm (6in). ❄ (min. 15°C/59°F)
***S.* 'Dyn-O-Mite'.** (Standard group) Rosetted perennial producing mid-green leaves with red undersides, and semi-double red flowers. ↕ 15cm (6in). ❄ (min. 15°C/59°F)
***S.* 'Fancy Pants'** ▣ (Standard group) Rosetted perennial bearing mid-green leaves and single white flowers with frilled red margins. ↕ 15–20cm (6–8in). ❄ (min. 15°C/59°F)
***S.* 'Fancy Trail'** ♀ (Standard group) Compact, rosetted, trailing perennial with shiny, variegated green and white leaves and fully double pink flowers. ↕ 15cm (6in). ❄ (min. 15°C/59°F)
***S.* 'Garden News'** ▣ ♀ (Standard group) Rosetted perennial bearing light green leaves and producing fully double white flowers, sometimes tinged pale lilac. ↕ 15cm (6in). ❄ (min. 15°C/59°F)
***S.* 'Granger's Wonderland'** see *S.* 'Wonderland'.
S. grotei. Trailing, branching perennial with stems to 40cm (16in) long, rooting at the nodes. The rounded leaves, 8cm (3in) long, have prominent veins and coarsely scalloped margins, and are produced on leaf-stalks to 25cm (10in) long. Cymes of 2 or 3 pale mauve flowers, 3cm (1¼in) across, with violet throats, are borne intermittently throughout the year. A parent of the trailing hybrids. ↕ 15–20cm (6–8in), ↔ 30–50cm (12–20in). Tanzania. ❄ (min. 15°C/59°F)
***S.* 'Ice Maiden'** ▣ ♀ (Standard group) Rosetted perennial bearing mid-green leaves and single white flowers with purple-blue markings. ↕ 15cm (6in). ❄ (min. 15°C/59°F)
S. ionantha. Stemless, rosette-forming perennial bearing ovate to oblong-ovate, scalloped, mid-green leaves, to 5cm (2in) long, paler beneath, on leaf-stalks 6cm (2½in) long. Cymes of 8–10 light to dark blue flowers, 2.5cm (1in) across, are produced intermittently throughout the year. ↕ to 10cm (4in), ↔ 15cm (6in). Tanzania. ❄ (min. 15°C/59°F)
***S.* 'King's Treasure'** ♀ (Standard group) Rosetted perennial bearing mid-green leaves and fully double, dark lavender-blue flowers, margined purple, each with a fine white, often green-tinged line at the extreme edges. ↕ 15cm (6in). ❄ (min. 15°C/59°F)
***S.* 'Kiwi Dazzler'.** (Standard group) Rosetted perennial with mid-green leaves. Bears fringed, single, bright red flowers, each with a central white stripe. A chimaera (graft hybrid), so propagate from suckers. ↕ 15cm (6in). ❄ (min. 15°C/59°F)
***S.* 'Kristi Marie'** ▣ (Standard group) Rosetted perennial bearing dark green leaves and producing fully double, dusky-red flowers, with white margins. ↕ 15–20cm (6–8in). ❄ (min. 15°C/59°F)
***S.* 'Lila'.** (Standard group) Rosetted perennial producing dark green leaves with red undersides and single, white-margined, lavender-blue flowers. ↕ 15cm (6in). ❄ (min. 15°C/59°F)

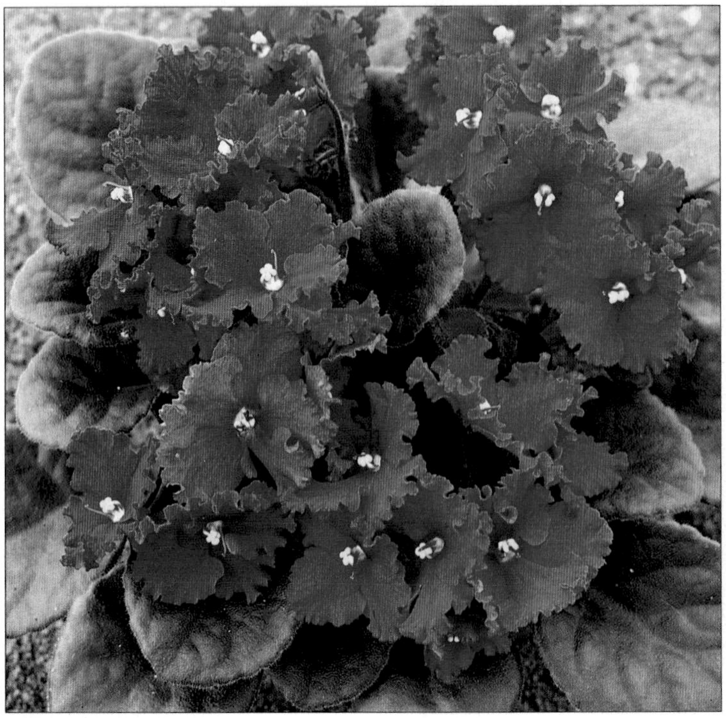
Saintpaulia 'Colorado'

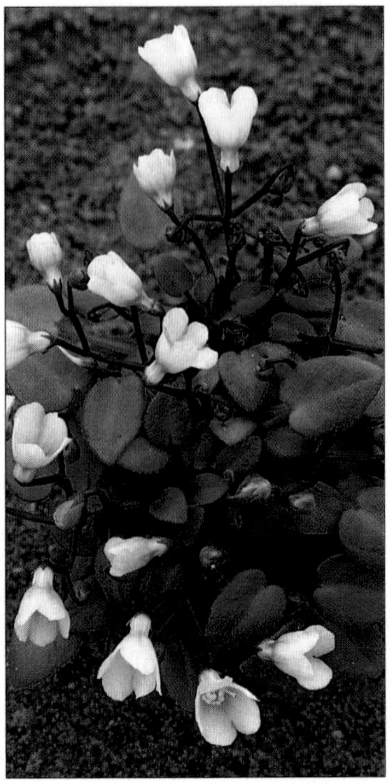

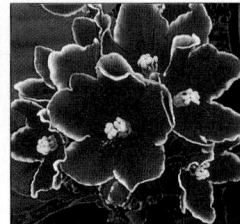
Saintpaulia 'Pip Squeek'

***S.* 'Maria'** 𝕐 (Standard group) Rosetted perennial bearing dark green leaves and large, single, clear pink flowers with frilled margins. ↕15cm (6in). ✿ (min. 15°C/59°F)
***S.* 'Midget Valentine'** 𝕐 (Miniature group) Rosetted perennial bearing shiny leaves, variegated green and white, and single, fuchsia-red flowers. ↕8–10cm (3–4in). ✿ (min. 15°C/59°F)
***S.* 'Moon Kissed'** 𝕐 (Semi-miniature group) Rosetted perennial bearing dark green leaves and fully double white flowers with fuchsia-pink markings. ↕8–13cm (3–5in). ✿ (min. 15°C/59°F)
***S.* 'Ms. Pretty'** ▣ (Standard group) Rosetted perennial bearing dark green leaves and single white flowers with fringed, pink margins. ↕15cm (6in). ✿ (min. 15°C/59°F)
***S.* 'Nortex's Snowkist Haven'.** (Standard group) Rosetted perennial producing pointed, quilted, mid-green leaves and bearing fringed, single white flowers. ↕15cm (6in). ✿ (min. 15°C/59°F)
***S.* 'Optimara Colorado'** see *S.* 'Colorado'.
***S.* 'Pip Squeek'** ▣ (Micro-miniature group) Rosetted, semi-trailing perennial producing tiny, pointed, dark green leaves and bearing single, light pink flowers. ↕8–10cm (3–4in). ✿ (min. 15°C/59°F)
***S.* 'Rococo Anna'** ▣𝕐 syn. *S.* 'Rococo Pink'. (Standard group) Rosetted perennial bearing mid-green leaves with very light green bases and pale undersides, and fully double, deep pink flowers. ↕15cm (6in). ✿ (min. 15°C/59°F)
***S.* 'Rococo Pink'** see *S.* 'Rococo Anna'.
S. shumensis. Compact, rosette-forming perennial with very short stems. Bears ovate to almost round, toothed leaves, 3.5cm (1½in) long, often with red-tinged veins beneath. Bears cymes of up to 5 pale mauve, almost white flowers, 2.5cm (1in) across, with deep purple eyes, intermittently throughout the year. ↕6–8cm (2½–3in), ↔ 8–12cm (3–5in). Tanzania. ✿ (min. 15°C/59°F)
***S.* 'Snuggles'.** (Miniature group) Rosetted perennial with dark green leaves, feathered and margined white, and large, semi-double pink flowers. ↕8–10cm (3–4in). ✿ (min. 15°C/59°F)
***S.* 'Starry Trail'** ▣𝕐 (Standard group) Rosetted, trailing perennial with dark green leaves. Bears narrow-petalled, semi-double to fully double white flowers, sometimes flushed pale pink. ↕15cm (6in). ✿ (min. 15°C/59°F)
***S.* 'Tomahawk'** 𝕐 (Standard group) Rosetted perennial producing dark green leaves and semi-double to fully double, dark red flowers, with fluted petals. ↕15–20cm (6–8in). ✿ (min. 15°C/59°F)
***S.* 'Wonderland'** 𝕐 syn. *S.* 'Granger's Wonderland'. (Large group) Rosetted perennial with wavy-margined, olive-green leaves and ruffled, semi-double, light blue flowers. ↕15cm (6in). ✿ (min. 10°C/50°F)
***S.* 'Zoja'** ▣ (Standard group) Rosetted perennial with mid-green leaves and large, single to semi-double, purple-blue flowers with a bold white line at the margin of each petal. ↕15cm (6in). ✿ (min. 10°C/50°F)

▷**Salal** see *Gaultheria shallon*

SALIX

Willow

SALICACEAE

Genus of approximately 300 species of normally dioecious, deciduous trees and shrubs found in habitats ranging from lowland meadows and riverbanks to sand dunes and mountain screes worldwide, except in Australia. They have simple, entire or toothed, usually alternate leaves, and bear very small flowers in usually erect catkins, before or with the foliage. Of diverse form, willows are cultivated for their habit (particularly the weeping willows), catkins (of which the males are usually the most striking), foliage, and sometimes coloured winter shoots. The largest willows are suitable only for a garden of large proportions; those with a weeping habit are especially effective by water. Grow smaller willows as specimen trees in a small garden, shrubby willows in a shrub border, and dwarf willows in a rock garden or trough.

• **HARDINESS** Fully hardy.

• **CULTIVATION** Grow in any deep, moist but well-drained soil in full sun; willows dislike shallow chalk soil. *S.* 'Erythroflexuosa' needs well-drained soil; the dwarf and alpine species need gritty, sharply drained soil. Pruning group 1 for most; group 7, every 1–3 years, for those grown for coloured winter shoots, and to rejuvenate old plants.

• **PROPAGATION** Root greenwood cuttings in early summer, or hardwood cuttings in winter.

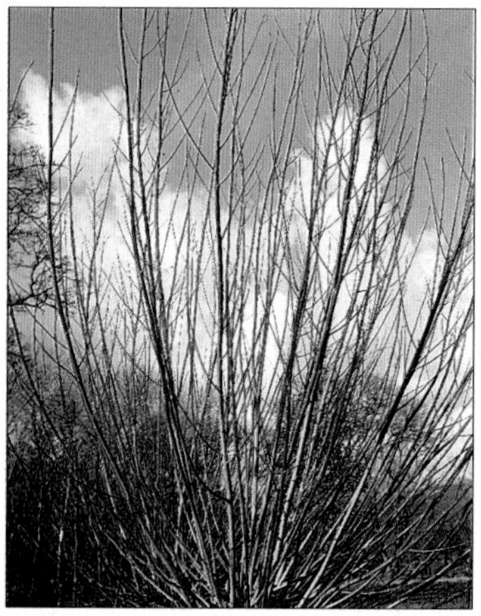

Salix alba var. *vitellina* 'Britzensis'

• **PESTS AND DISEASES** Aphids, caterpillars, leaf beetles, sawflies, willow scale, anthracnose, honey fungus, and rust may be a problem.

S. acutifolia ♀ Spreading tree with slender, arching, deep purple, white-bloomed shoots and narrowly lance-shaped, tapered, dark green leaves, to 10cm (4in) long. Silvery male catkins, 5cm (2in) long, with golden anthers, or pale green female catkins, 2–3cm (¾–1¼) long, are produced in early spring, before the leaves. ↕10m (30ft), ↔ 12m (40ft). Russia to E. Asia. ❄❄❄. **'Blue Streak'** 𝕐 is a male clone, and has blue-black shoots with a vivid blue-white bloom.
S. aegyptiaca ♀ syn. *S. medemii* (Musk willow). Strong-growing, bushy shrub or

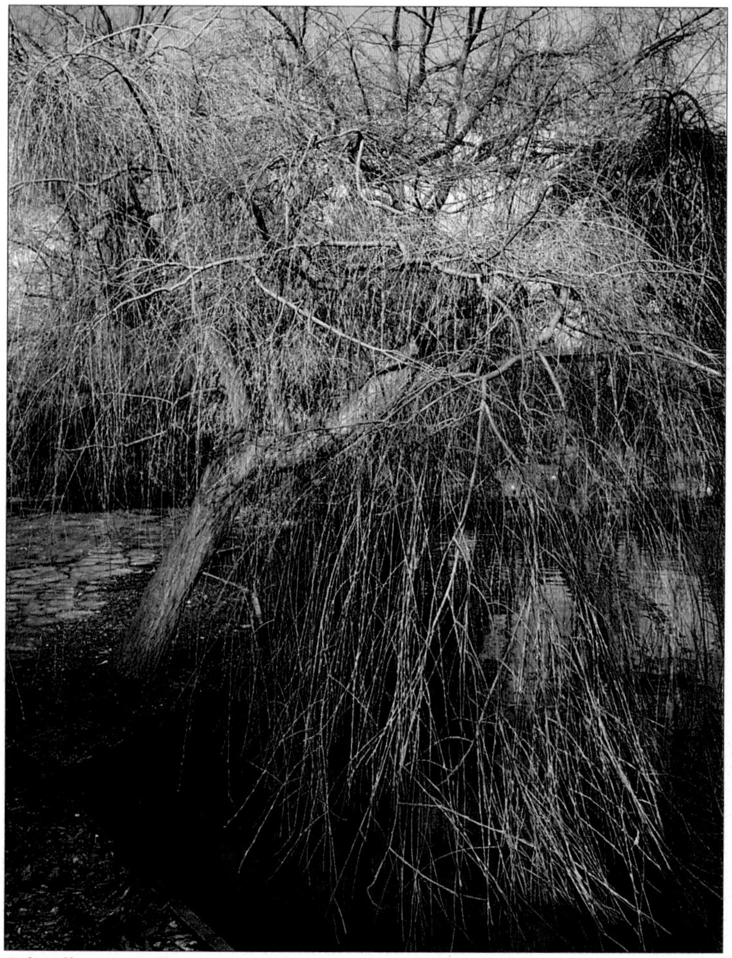

Salix alba var. *vitellina*

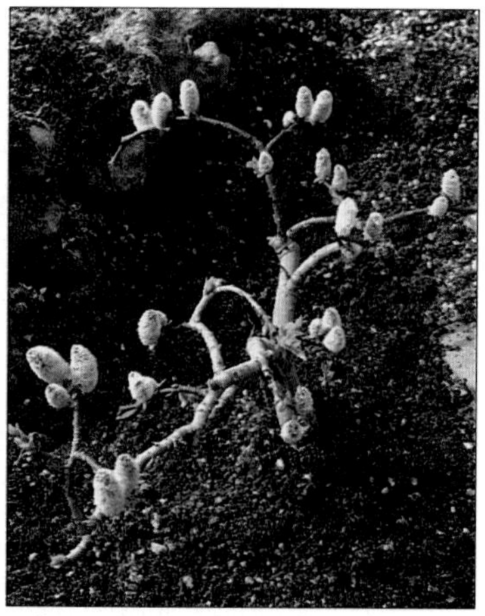

Salix apoda

tree with stout, red-purple shoots and oblong, toothed, dark green leaves, to 15cm (6in) long, with glaucous, hairy undersides. Fragrant grey catkins are produced in early spring, before the leaves: males are up to 4cm (1½in) long, with yellow anthers; females are up to 8cm (3in) long. ↕4m (12ft), ↔ 5m (15ft). Turkey, Armenia, Iraq, Iran, Afghanistan. ❄❄❄
S. alba ♀ (White willow). Very fast-growing, spreading tree with grey-pink to brown shoots and lance-shaped, saw-toothed, slender-pointed, dull green leaves, to 10cm (4in) long, silky-hairy when young, blue-green beneath. Yellow male catkins, to 5cm (2in) long, or stalkless, yellow-green female catkins, 3cm (1¼in) long, are produced in spring, with the leaves. ↕25m (80ft), ↔ 10m (30ft). Europe, N. Africa, C. Asia. ❄❄❄. **f. *argentea*** see var. *sericea*. **var. *caerulea*** (Cricket-bat willow) has upright branches and blue-green leaves. **var. *sericea*** 𝕐 syn. f. *argentea*, 'Sericea', 'Splendens' (Silver willow) has silvery grey leaves; ↕15m (50ft), ↔ 8m (25ft). **'Splendens'** see var. *sericea*. **'Tristis'** ♀ syn. *S. vitellina* 'Pendula', has a more weeping habit, and only produces female catkins. **'Tristis' of gardens** see *S.* x *sepulcralis* 'Chrysocoma'. **var. *vitellina*** ▣ (Golden willow) produces bright yellow to orange winter shoots. **var. *vitellina* 'Britzensis'** ▣𝕐 is a male clone, with bright orange-red winter shoots. **var. *vitellina* 'Chermesina'** is a male clone, with carmine-red young winter shoots.
S. apoda ▣ Prostrate shrub with obovate, leathery, dark green leaves, 2–8cm (¾–3in) long, hairy when young. Silky, silvery grey male catkins, 3cm (1¼in) long, which become pink-orange with maturity, are borne in early spring, before the leaves. Female clones are rarely cultivated. Suitable for large rock gardens. ↕20cm (8in), ↔ to 60cm (24in). E. Europe, Caucasus. ❄❄❄
S. arenaria see *S. repens* var. *argentea*.
S. babylonica ♀ (Weeping willow). Rounded, weeping tree with slender, pendent, green to brown shoots. Lance-shaped, saw-toothed, tapered, mid-green leaves, to 10cm (4in) long, are grey-green beneath. Slender, silvery green catkins are produced in spring, with the leaves: the males to 5cm (2in) long with yellow anthers, the females to 2.5cm (1in) long. Largely replaced in gardens by *S.* x *sepulcralis* 'Chrysocoma'. ↕↔ 12m (40ft). N. China. ❄❄❄. **'Annularis'** see

S

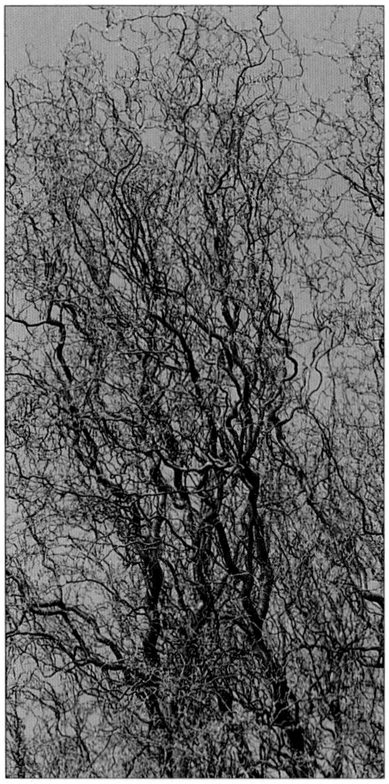

Salix babylonica var. *pekinensis* 'Tortuosa'

'Crispa'. **'Crispa'** ♀ syn. 'Annularis', is slow-growing and upright, and has curiously twisted leaves. **var. *pekinensis* 'Tortuosa'** ▣🏆♀ syn. *S. matsudana* 'Tortuosa', is fast-growing and upright. It has curiously twisted shoots that are particularly striking in winter, bright green, twisted leaves, and yellow-green catkins; ↕15m (50ft), ↔ 8m (25ft).

***S.* 'Blanda'** ♀ syn. *S.* x *pendulina* var. *blanda.* Spreading tree with weeping shoots and lance-shaped, tapered, glossy, dark green leaves, to 15cm (6in) long. Slender, silvery green, usually female catkins, to 3cm (1¼in) long, are produced in spring, with the leaves. ↕↔ 12m (40ft). ❄❄❄

S. bockii. Bushy shrub with slender, upright, grey-hairy shoots and oblong, glossy, bright green leaves, to 1.5cm (½in) long, with silky-hairy undersides. Usually female in cultivation; bears green catkins, 4cm (1½in) long, in early and mid-autumn. ↕↔ 2.5m (8ft). W. China. ❄❄❄

***S.* 'Boydii'** see *S.* x *boydii.*

S.* x *boydii ▣🏆 (*S. lapponum* x *S. reticulata*) syn. *S.* 'Boydii'. Very slow-growing, upright shrub with gnarled branches bearing almost rounded, rough-textured, prominently veined, grey-green leaves, 1–2cm (½–¾in) long. Occasionally produces insignificant female catkins on bare branches in early spring. Suitable for a rock garden or trough. ↕30cm (12in), ↔ 20cm (8in). Scotland (Angus Mountains). ❄❄❄

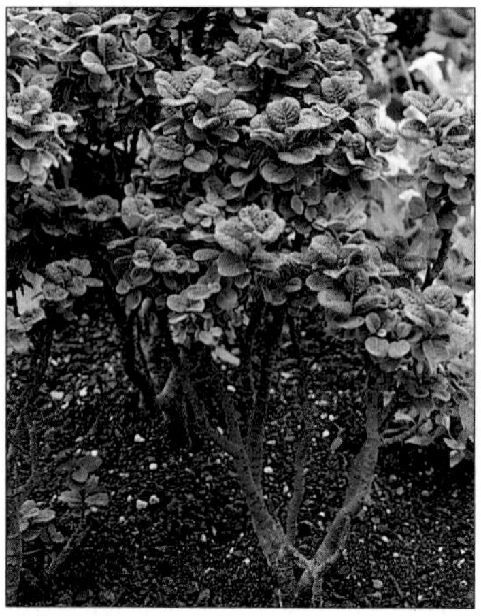

Salix x *boydii*

***S. caprea* 'Kilmarnock'** ▣🏆♀ syn. *S. caprea* 'Pendula' (Kilmarnock willow). Weeping tree with a dense head of stout, yellow-brown shoots and broadly elliptic, toothed leaves, to 10cm (4in) long, dark green above, grey-green beneath. Grey male catkins, 3cm (1¼in) long, studded with yellow anthers, are produced on the bare shoots in mid- and late spring. ↕1.5–2m (5–6ft), depending on grafting height, ↔ 2m (6ft). ❄❄❄

***S. caprea* 'Pendula'** see *S. caprea* 'Kilmarnock'.

S.* x *chrysocoma see *S.* x *sepulcralis* 'Chrysocoma'.

S. daphnoides ♀ (Violet willow). Initially upright, later spreading tree with purple young shoots, which are white-bloomed in winter, and narrowly oblong, saw-toothed, clearly stalked, dark green leaves, to 12cm (5in) long. Silky grey catkins, to 4cm (1½in) long, are produced in late winter and early spring, before the leaves; male catkins have yellow anthers. ↕8m (25ft), ↔ 6m (20ft). Europe to C. Asia. ❄❄❄. **'Aglaia'** ▣🏆 has glossy red shoots.

S. elaeagnos 🏆 syn. *S. incana* (Hoary willow). Dense, upright shrub with slender, grey-velvety, later red-yellow to almost brown shoots. The linear, entire, dark green leaves, to 20cm (8in) long, are grey when young, white-hairy beneath, and turn yellow in autumn. Produces slender green catkins, 3–6cm (1¼–2½in) long, in spring, as the leaves emerge; male catkins have yellow anthers. ↕3m (10ft), ↔ 5m (15ft). C. and S. Europe, S.W. Asia. ❄❄❄

***S.* 'Erythroflexuosa'** ♀ syn. *S.* 'Golden Curls', *S. matsudana* 'Tortuosa Aureopendula'. Spreading tree with arching branches and spirally twisted, orange-yellow young shoots. The twisted, lance-shaped, glossy, mid-green leaves, to 8cm (3in) long, are glaucous beneath. Produces slender, pale yellow catkins, 3–4cm (1¼–1½in) long, in spring, with the leaves. ↕↔ 5m (15ft). ❄❄❄

S. exigua ▣ (Coyote willow). Upright, thicket-forming, suckering shrub bearing slender shoots. Produces narrowly lance-shaped, tapered, grey-green leaves, to 10cm (4in) long, covered in silky, silvery grey hairs when young. Grey-yellow catkins, the males to 5cm (2in) long, the females to 6cm (2½in) long, are borne in spring, with the leaves. Grows well on sandy soils. ↕4m (12ft), ↔ 5m (15ft) or more. W. North America. ❄❄❄

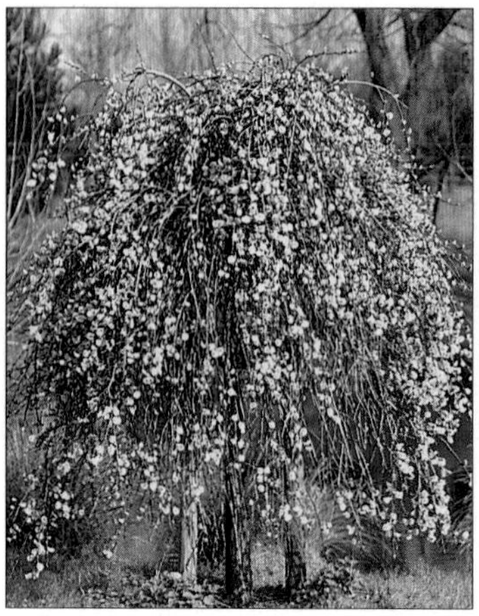

Salix caprea 'Kilmarnock'

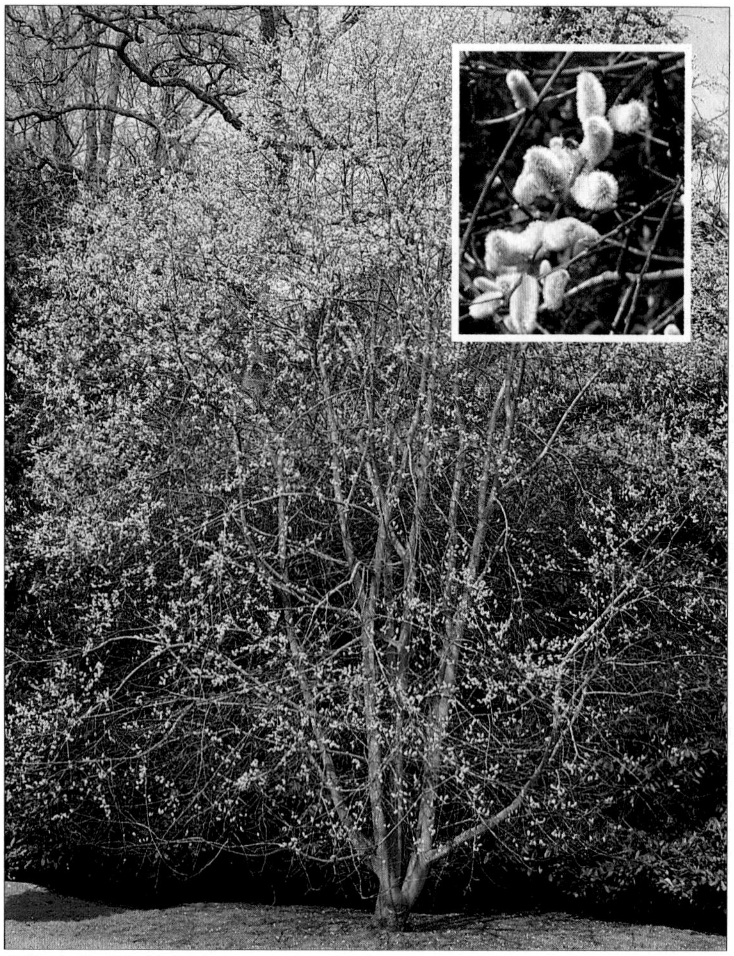

Salix daphnoides 'Aglaia' (inset: male catkins)

S. fargesii ▣ syn. *S. moupinensis* of gardens. Open, upright, stoutly branched shrub with glossy green young shoots that turn red-brown, and red winter buds. Produces oblong, finely saw-toothed, glossy, dark green leaves, to 18cm (7in) long, silky beneath. Slender green catkins, the males to 12cm (5in) long, the females to 18cm (7in) long, are borne in spring, with the leaves. ↕↔ 3m (10ft). C. China. ❄❄❄

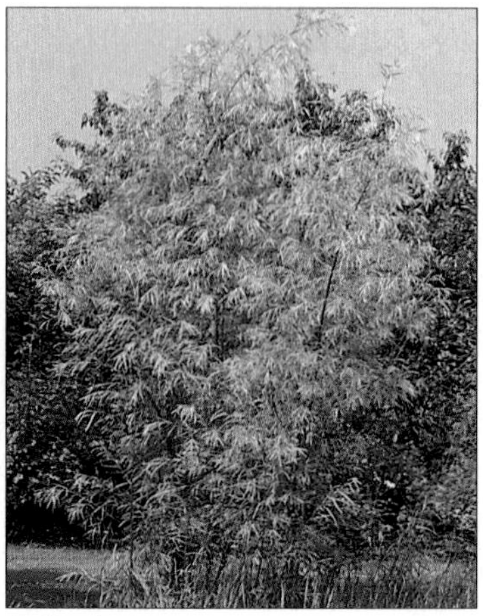

Salix exigua

S. fragilis ♀ (Crack willow). Spreading tree with brittle, olive-brown shoots. Bears lance-shaped, finely toothed, glossy, dark green leaves, to 15cm (6in) long, blue-green beneath. Bears slender, pendent green catkins, to 7cm (3in) long, in early spring, as the leaves emerge; male catkins have yellow anthers. ↕↔ 15m (50ft). Europe, N. Turkey, Russia (W. Siberia). ❄❄❄

***S.* 'Golden Curls'** see *S.* 'Erythroflexuosa'.

S. gracilistyla. Spreading, bushy shrub with arching shoots, silky-hairy when young, and oval, entire to finely toothed, silky-hairy, grey-green leaves, to 10cm (4in) long, turning glossy green. Silky grey catkins, to 4cm (1½in) long, are produced in early and mid-spring, before the leaves; male catkins have red anthers that turn bright yellow. ↕3m (10ft), ↔ 4m (12ft). E. Asia. ❄❄❄. **'Melanostachys'** ▣🏆 syn. var. *melanostachys*, *S. melanostachys*, is an upright male variant that bears black catkins with brick-red anthers.

***S. hastata* 'Wehrhahnii'** ▣🏆 Slow-growing, upright shrub with dark purple-brown shoots and oval, entire to finely toothed, bright green leaves, to 6cm (2½in) long. In early spring, bears conspicuous, silvery grey male catkins, to 7cm (3in) long, before the leaves. ↕↔ 1m (3ft). ❄❄❄

S. helvetica ▣🏆 (Swiss willow). Upright, many-branched shrub with oblong to ovate-lance-shaped, grey-green leaves, 1–3.5cm (½–1½in) long, smooth above, silver-downy beneath. In early spring, silver-grey catkins, to 5cm (2in) long, open from small golden

S

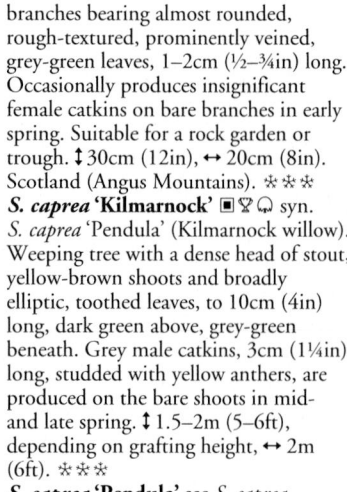

buds, before the leaves. ↕ 60cm (24in), ↔ 40cm (16in). Alps. ❄❄❄
S. hylematica of gardens see *S. lindleyana.*
S. incana see *S. elaeagnos.*
S. irrorata. Upright shrub producing slender purple shoots, which are white-bloomed in winter, and narrowly oblong, entire to sparsely toothed, short-stalked, bright green leaves, to 10cm (4in) long, glaucous beneath. Grey catkins, to 2.5cm (1in) long, are borne in early or mid-spring, before the leaves; male catkins have red anthers that turn yellow. ↕ 3m (10ft), ↔ 5m (15ft). S.W. USA. ❄❄❄
S. lanata ■ ♀ (Woolly willow). Compact, rounded, bushy shrub bearing stout shoots, white-woolly when young. The leaves are broadly rounded, wavy-margined, dull, dark green, to 6cm (2½in) long, and covered with silvery grey wool. Golden yellow male catkins, to 5cm (2in) long, or grey-yellow female catkins, to 8cm (3in) long, are produced in late spring, with the leaves. ↕ 1m (3ft), ↔ 1.5m (5ft). N. Europe. ❄❄❄. **'Stuartii'** see *S.* 'Stuartii'.
S. lindleyana, syn. *S. hylematica* of gardens, *S. nepalensis.* Dwarf, procumbent shrub with ovate-spoon-shaped, very glossy, pale green leaves, to 1cm (½in) long, densely set on short branchlets. Bears pinkish brown male catkins, to 1cm (½in) long, or short female catkins, 5mm (¼in) long, in spring, with the leaves. Spreads widely in moist, fertile soils, in partial shade. Much confused with *S. fruticulosa.* ↕ 4cm (1½in), ↔ 60cm (24in) or more. Himalayas. ❄❄❄
S. magnifica ♀ Q Broadly upright shrub or tree bearing stout, red-purple shoots and broadly oval, blue-green leaves, to 20cm (8in) long. Slender green catkins, the males to 18cm (7in) long, the females to 25cm (10in) long, are produced in late spring, after the leaves. ↕ 5m (15ft), ↔ 3m (10ft). W. China. ❄❄❄
S. 'Mark Postill'. Spreading shrub with stout green shoots, turning brown-purple, and broadly elliptic to rounded, glossy, dark green leaves, to 7cm (3in) long. Stout, initially silvery white, later green female catkins, to 5cm (2in) long, are produced over a long period in spring, before and with the leaves. ↕ 1m (3ft), ↔ 2m (6ft). ❄❄❄

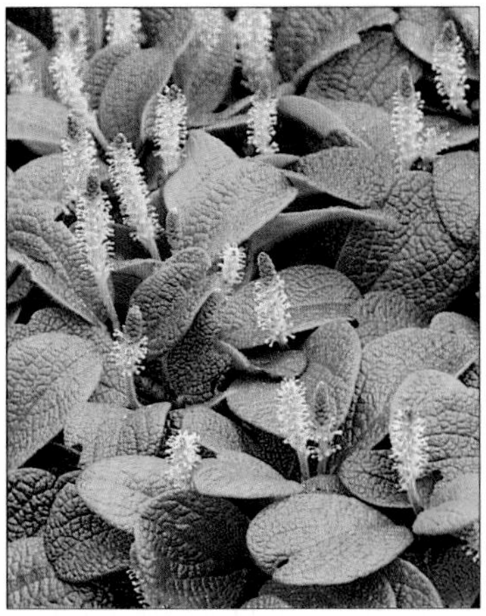
Salix reticulata

S. matsudana 'Tortuosa' see *S. babylonica* var. *pekinensis* 'Tortuosa'.
S. matsudana 'Tortuosa Aureopendula' see *S.* 'Erythroflexuosa'.
S. medemii see *S. aegyptiaca.*
S. melanostachys see *S. gracilistyla* 'Melanostachys'.
S. moupinensis of gardens see *S. fargesii.*
S. nepalensis see *S. lindleyana.*
S. x pendulina var. blanda see *S.* 'Blanda'.
S. pentandra Q (Bay willow). Spreading, bushy-headed tree with brown-green shoots and oval, finely glandular-toothed leaves, to 12cm (5in) long, glossy, dark green above, pale green beneath. Catkins, 5cm (2in) long, are produced in early summer, after the leaves: male catkins are yellow and very showy, with yellow anthers; female catkins are green. ↕↔ 10m (30ft). Eurasia. ❄❄❄
S. purpurea Q (Purple osier). Spreading shrub to upright tree with arching, frequently red-tinged shoots and often opposite, oblong, almost entire, dark green to blue-green leaves, to 8cm (3in) long. Slender, silvery green catkins, to 3cm (1¼in) long, are produced in early and mid-spring, before the leaves; male catkins have purple anthers that turn yellow. ↕↔ 5m (15ft). Europe, N. Africa, C. Asia. ❄❄❄. **'Nana'**, syn. 'Gracilis', is compact, bearing slender shoots and small, grey-green leaves, to 3.5cm (1½in) long. Suitable for growing as a low hedge; ↕ 1m (3ft), ↔ 1.5m (5ft).

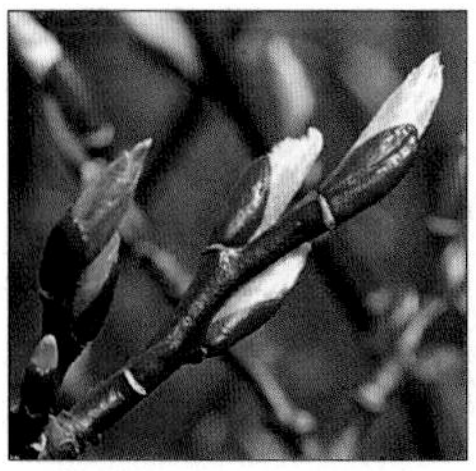
Salix fargesii

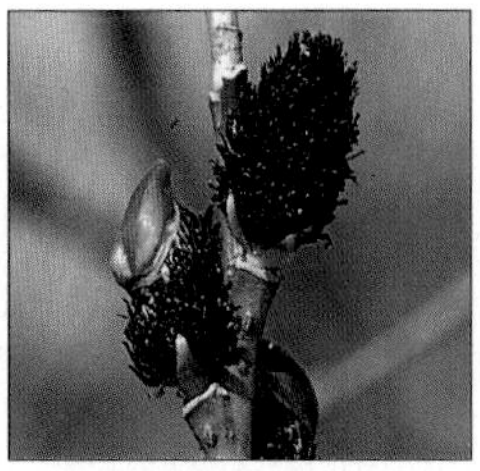
Salix gracilistyla 'Melanostachys'

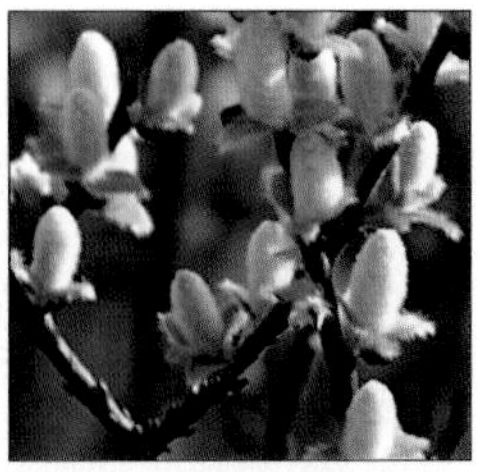
Salix hastata 'Wehrhahnii'

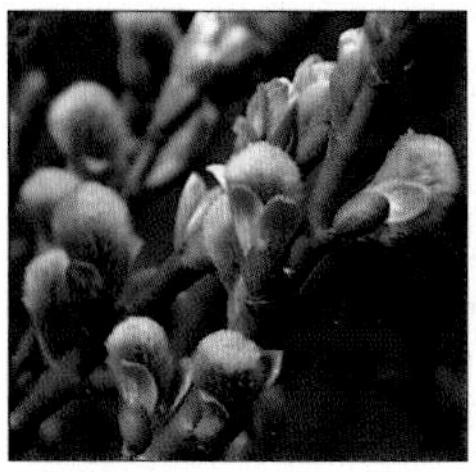
Salix helvetica

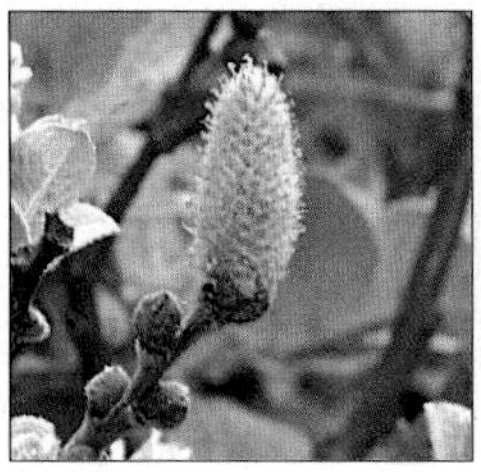
Salix lanata

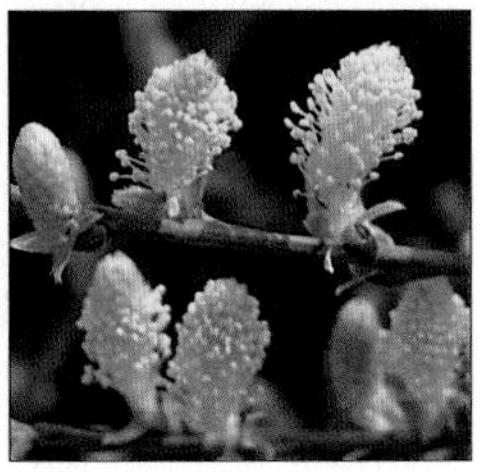
Salix repens

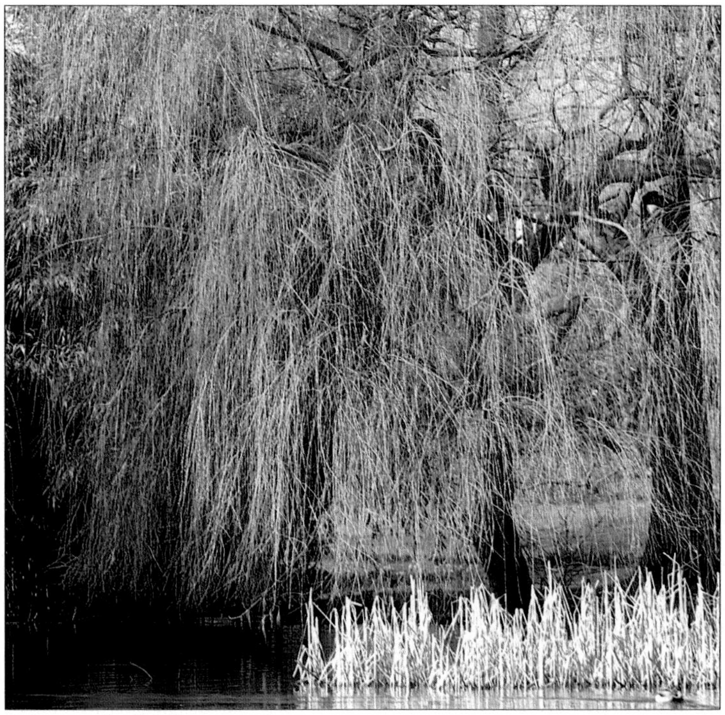
Salix x *sepulcralis* 'Chrysocoma'

S. repens ■ (Creeping willow). Prostrate shrub with slender shoots and oblong to oval, grey-green to bright green leaves, to 3.5cm (1½in) long, silvery beneath. Grey male catkins, to 2cm (¾in) long, with golden yellow anthers, are produced in mid- and late spring, before the leaves. ↕ to 60cm (24in), ↔ 1.5m (5ft) or more. Europe. ❄❄❄. **var. argentea**, syn. *S. arenaria,* is spreading, with creeping, initially upright, later arching shoots, and obovate, silky grey leaves, to 4cm (1½in) long. Catkins appear in mid-spring; ↕ 1m (3ft), ↔ 2m (6ft); N.W. Europe.
S. reticulata ■ ♀ Dwarf, prostrate shrub with rooting stems bearing rounded-ovate, glossy, dark green leaves, 1–4cm (½–1½in) long, conspicuously veined above, white-hairy beneath. In spring, bears slender yellow catkins, 2.5cm (1in) long, with pink tips. ↕ 8cm (3in), ↔ 30cm (12in). N. Europe, N. Asia, North America. ❄❄❄
S. retusa. Prostrate, carpeting shrub with rooting stems and ovate-oblong, notched, glossy, mid-green leaves, 1–3cm (½–1¼in) long, mostly clustered towards the twig tips. Bears upright grey catkins, to 2cm (¾in) long, in spring, as the leaves emerge. ↕ 10cm (4in), ↔ to 40cm (16in). Mountains of C. Europe. ❄❄❄
S. sachalinensis 'Sekka'. Vigorous, spreading shrub, forming large, dense thickets, with lance-shaped, shallowly scalloped, bright green leaves, to 12cm (5in) long. In early spring, bears showy, silvery grey male catkins, to 4cm (1½in) long, with golden anthers, on often curiously flattened, twisted red shoots. ↕ 5m (15ft), ↔ 10m (30ft). ❄❄❄
S. x sepulcralis 'Chrysocoma' ■ ♀ Q syn. *S. alba* 'Tristis' of gardens, *S.* x *chrysocoma, S.* x *sepulcralis* var. *chrysocoma* (Golden weeping willow). Fast-growing, wide-spreading tree with slender, golden yellow shoots, pendent to the ground, and narrowly lance-shaped, tapered, bright green leaves, to 12cm (5in) long. Slender catkins, to 5cm (2in) long, both yellow males and green females often present on the same plant, are produced with the leaves, in spring. ↕↔ 15m (50ft). ❄❄❄
S. x sepulcralis var. chrysocoma see *S.* x *sepulcralis* 'Chrysocoma'.
S. serpyllifolia (Thyme-leaved willow). Prostrate, carpeting shrub with rooting stems and obovate, glossy, mid-green leaves, 1cm (½in) long, that overlap and are pressed closely to the soil. Silvery green catkins, to 5mm (¼in) long, are borne with the leaves, in spring. Very similar to *S. retusa.* ↕ 2.5cm (1in), ↔ 30cm (12in). Alps. ❄❄❄
S. 'Stuartii', syn. *S. lanata* 'Stuartii'. Dwarf, slow-growing, bushy shrub with yellow-green winter shoots. Bears oblong, dark green leaves, to 5cm (2in) long, woolly when young, densely white-hairy beneath. Yellow-green, initially silky female catkins, to 5cm (2in) long, are borne from orange buds in early and mid-spring. ↕ 1m (3ft), ↔ 2m (6ft). ❄❄❄
S. viminalis Q (Common osier). Fast-growing, upright shrub or tree with glossy, yellow-green shoots and slender, linear, tapered, dark green leaves, to 15cm (6in) or more long, silver-hairy beneath. Dense, crowded green catkins, to 3.5cm (1½in) long, are produced in late winter and early spring, before the leaves; male catkins have yellow anthers. ↕ 6m (20ft), ↔ 5m (15ft). Eurasia. ❄❄❄
S. vitellina 'Pendula' see *S. alba* 'Tristis'.

▷**Sallee, White** see *Eucalyptus pauciflora*

SALPIGLOSSIS

SOLANACEAE

Genus of 2 erect to spreading, bushy, sticky-hairy annuals or short-lived perennials found on disturbed ground, in dry canyons, and on rocky slopes in the southern Andes. They have entire to wavy-margined or lobed, oval to lance-shaped, bright mid-green leaves, and

S

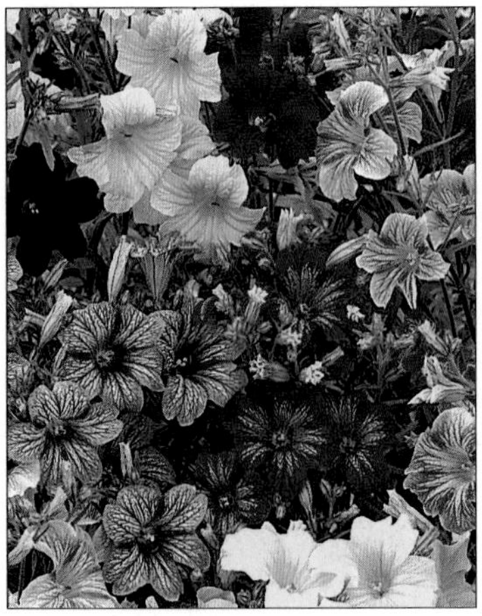

Salpiglossis sinuata Casino Series

produce funnel-shaped, richly coloured, red, yellow, bronze, violet-blue, or purple flowers from summer to autumn. Suitable for an annual, herbaceous, or mixed border where summers are warm, sunny, and reasonably dry. In cool-temperate regions, they are effective long-flowering container plants in a warm greenhouse or conservatory, and may be bedded out in summer. They provide moderately long-lasting cut flowers.

• **HARDINESS** Half hardy.

• **CULTIVATION** Under glass, grow in loamless or loam-based potting compost (JI No.2) in full light with shade from hot sun. During the growing season, maintain low to moderate humidity, water moderately, and apply a balanced liquid fertilizer every 2 weeks. Keep just moist in winter. Overwinter at 16–18°C (61–64°F). Outdoors, grow in moderately fertile, humus-rich, moist but well-drained soil in full sun; shelter from cold, drying winds. Dead-head to prolong flowering and maintain flower size. Provide brushwood support if grown in a slightly exposed site.

• **PROPAGATION** Sow seed at 18–24°C (64–75°F) in mid-spring, or in autumn or late winter for winter- or early spring-flowering container plants. In very mild areas, sow *in situ* in mid-spring.

• **PESTS AND DISEASES** Aphids, grey mould (*Botrytis*), and foot and root rots may be troublesome.

S

S. sinuata. Erect annual with slender, branching stems bearing alternate, long-stalked, narrowly to broadly lance-shaped, wavy-margined leaves, to 10cm (4in) long. From summer to autumn, broadly funnel-shaped, 5-lobed flowers, to 5cm (2in) across, in a wide variety of colours, and heavily veined in deeper or contrasting colours, are produced singly in the leaf axils of flowering stems. ↕ to 60cm (24in), ↔ to 30cm (12in). Peru, Argentina. ❄. **Bolero Hybrids** are less floriferous and more straggling than the other cultivars listed, and flower in shades of blue, orange, purple, red, or yellow. Cultivars of **Casino Series** ▣ 🏆 have good weather tolerance, and are compact, branching freely from the bases. Flowers are blue, purple, red, yellow, or orange, often heavily veined. **'Kew Blue'** has clear purple-blue flowers, conspicuously veined.

▷ **Salt tree** see *Halimodendron halodendron*

SALVIA

Sage

LABIATAE/LAMIACEAE

Genus of about 900 species of annuals, biennials, herbaceous and evergreen perennials, and shrubs, some rhizomatous or tuberous. Distributed worldwide in temperate and tropical regions (except in very hot, humid areas), they usually grow in sunny sites, including dry meadows, rocky slopes, scrub, light woodland, and moist grassland. They are frequently aromatic and often hairy; some species are very woolly, and others silver in appearance. The usually square stems bear opposite pairs of simple to pinnate, entire, toothed, notched, or scalloped leaves; basal leaves sometimes differ from stem leaves. Flowers are 2-lipped, the upper lips erect and hooded, the lower ones 2-toothed and more spreading. The calyces are sometimes colourful, and tubular to bell- or funnel-shaped; the often leaf-like, colourful bracts are ovate to diamond-shaped. The flowers are borne in panicles, or in axillary whorls on erect stems, forming more or less interrupted terminal spikes or racemes. Sages are effective in a sunny border, light woodland, or wildflower meadow. Annuals, and perennials grown as annuals, provide brilliant colour for bedding, infilling, or containers; less hardy sages may be grown in a cool or temperate greenhouse, either in a border or in large containers. *S. caespitosa* is suitable for a scree bed or alpine house. Many species attract bees; some have culinary or medicinal uses.

• **HARDINESS** Fully hardy to frost tender.

• **CULTIVATION** Under glass, grow in well-drained, loamless or loam-based potting compost (JI No.2 or 3) in full light with shade from hot sun. While in growth, water freely and apply a balanced liquid fertilizer monthly; water very sparingly in winter, except *S. canariensis*, *S. elegans* and its cultivars, and *S. leucantha*, which should be watered moderately. Maintain low to moderate humidity. Outdoors, grow in light, moderately fertile, humus-rich, moist but well-drained soil in full sun to light dappled shade. Small species with densely hairy or woolly leaves need sharp drainage and full sun. Protect these and frost-hardy species from excessive winter wet, and shelter from cold, drying winds. Pruning group 9, in spring.

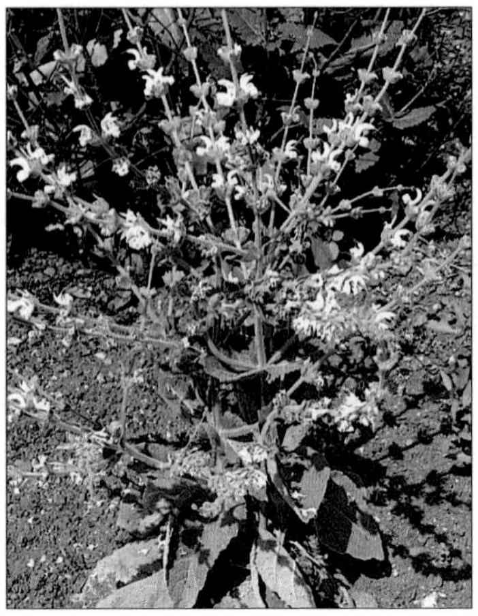

Salvia argentea

• **PROPAGATION** Sow seed as follows: annuals at 16–18°C (61–64°F) in mid-spring, biennials in containers in a cold frame in summer, and perennials in containers in a cold frame in spring; annuals and biennials may be sown *in situ* after all danger of frost has passed. Divide perennials in spring. For perennials and subshrubs, root basal or softwood cuttings in spring or early summer, or semi-ripe cuttings in late summer or autumn, with bottom heat.

• **PESTS AND DISEASES** Slugs and snails will attack young growth, as well as the fleshy rhizomes of *S. uliginosa*. Under glass, aphids, red spider mites, whiteflies, and foot and root rots may be troublesome.

S. aethiopis. Rosette-forming, monocarpic perennial or biennial with broadly ovate or elliptic to oblong, deeply toothed, white-woolly leaves, to 20cm (8in) long, clasping the erect upper stems. White, sometimes yellow-lipped flowers, 1.5cm (¾in) long, with persistent, broad, spiny bracts, are borne in branching, flat-topped, terminal panicles in mid- and late summer. ↕↔ 60cm (24in). C. and S. Europe to W. Asia. ❄❄❄

S. africana-lutea, syn. *S. aurea* (Sandsalie). Erect to spreading, rounded, evergreen shrub with sparsely to densely downy stems and rounded to narrowly obovate, densely white-woolly leaves, 1–4cm (½–1½in) long, sometimes minutely scalloped, and dotted with glands. From summer to late autumn, bears dense, terminal racemes of golden brown to red-brown or mauve flowers, 3–5cm (1¼–2in) long, with bell-shaped, purple-tinted calyces. ↕↔ to 1m (3ft). Sandy places in South Africa (Northern Cape, Eastern Cape, Western Cape). ❄

S. ambigens see *S. guaranitica* 'Blue Enigma'.

S. angustifolia see *S. azurea.*

S. argentea ▣ 🏆 Rosette-forming biennial or short-lived perennial producing ovate to oblong, toothed, silver-woolly leaves, to 20cm (8in) long. In mid- and late summer, bears many-branched, terminal panicles of white or pinkish-white flowers, to 3cm (1¼in) long, with grey calyces. ↕ 90cm (36in), ↔ 60cm (24in). S. Europe, N. Africa. ❄❄❄

S. aurea see *S. africana-lutea.*

S. azurea, syn. *S. angustifolia.* Erect, woody-based perennial with several to many simple or sparsely branched stems

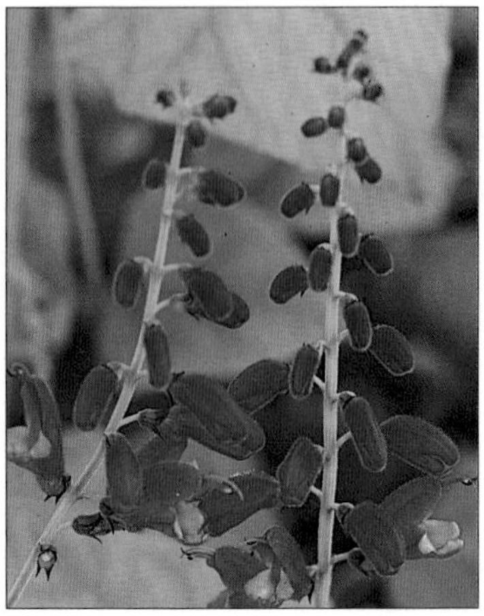

Salvia cacaliifolia

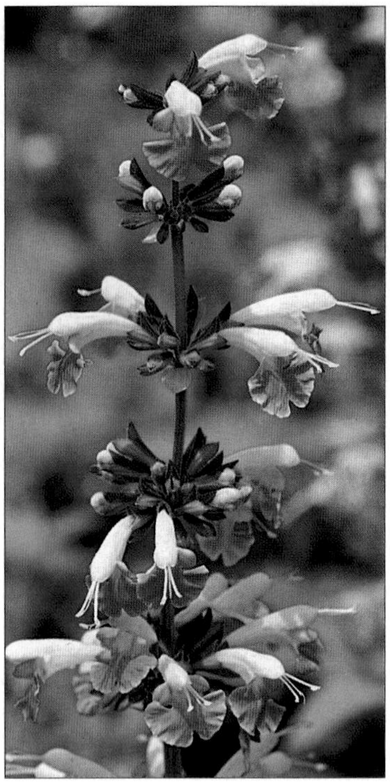

Salvia coccinea 'Coral Nymph'

bearing linear, elliptic, or lance-shaped, hairless or softly hairy, sometimes toothed, mid- to deep green leaves, 5–10cm (2–4in) long. From late summer to autumn, pure blue or white flowers, 1.5–2cm (½–¾in) long, are produced in dense, terminal racemes. ↕ to 1.5m (5ft), ↔ 60–90cm (24–36in). S.E. USA. ❄❄. **subsp. *pitcheri*** has very hairy stems; flowers are to 2.5cm (1in) long; S. USA.

***S. bacheriana* of gardens** see *S. buchananii.*

S. blepharophylla. Spreading, sub-shrubby, rhizomatous perennial bearing ovate to triangular, irregularly toothed, finely hairy, dark green leaves, 5cm (2in) long. From early summer to early autumn, branched stems bear loose, terminal racemes of bright scarlet flowers, to 2cm (¾in) long, with large lower lips and maroon calyces. ↕ 40cm (16in), ↔ 45cm (18in). Mexico. ❄

S. buchananii 🏆 syn. *S. bacheriana* of gardens. Woody-based perennial, spreading by runners, with erect, branching stems bearing spoon-shaped to ovate-lance-shaped, finely toothed, leathery, dark green leaves, to 7cm (3in) long. Velvet-hairy, magenta-red flowers, to 5cm (2in) long, with dark purplish brown calyces, are borne in loose, terminal racemes from midsummer to mid-autumn. ↕ 60cm (24in), ↔ 30cm (12in). Mexico. ❄

S. bulleyana, syn. *S. flava* var. *megalantha.* Clump-forming perennial with ovate or triangular-ovate, scalloped, prominently veined, sparsely hairy, wrinkled, mostly basal, mid-green leaves, to 12cm (5in) long. In mid- and late summer, bears terminal racemes of paired yellow flowers, to 3cm (1¼in) long, with purple-brown lower lips and bright green calyces. ↕ 40–90cm (16–36in), ↔ 60cm (24in). W. China. ❄❄❄

S. cacaliifolia ▣ 🏆 Erect, hairy perennial with more or less triangular, entire, mid-green leaves, to 10cm (4in) long. In early summer, branched stems

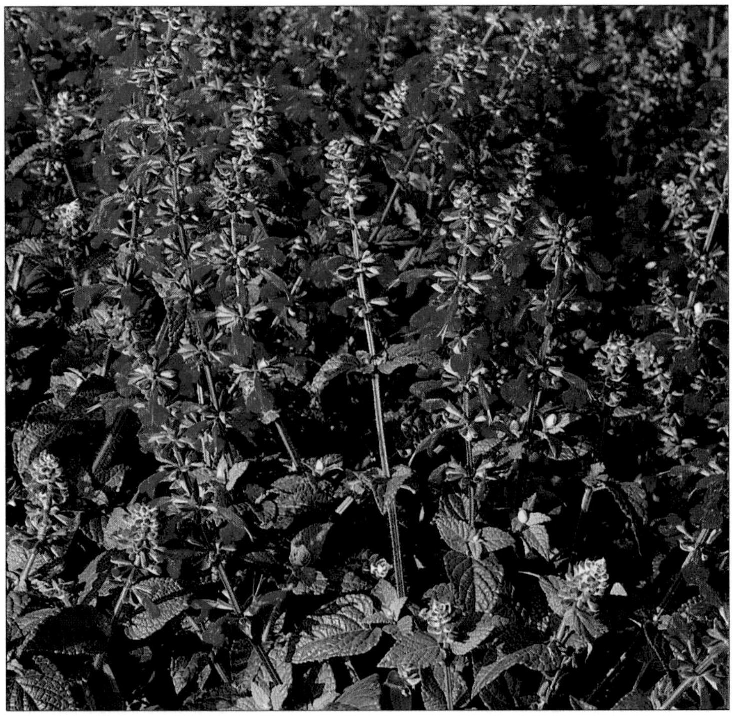
Salvia coccinea 'Lady in Red'

bear terminal panicles of paired, slightly hairy, deep blue flowers, to 2cm (¾in) long, with much shorter, bell-shaped calyces. ↕ 90cm (36in), ↔ 30cm (12in). Mexico, Guatemala. ❄
***S. caerulea* of gardens** see *S. guaranitica* 'Black and Blue'.
S. caespitosa. Woody-based, mat-forming perennial producing obovate, pinnatisect, silver-hairy leaves, 5cm (2in) long, each with a lance-shaped terminal segment. In summer, bears dense, terminal racemes of wide-tubed, lilac-pink flowers, to 3cm (1¼in) long, with broad lower lips. Resents winter wet. Suitable for an alpine house; can be grown in a scree bed if overhead protection provided in winter. ↕ 15cm (6in), ↔ 30cm (12in). Turkey (Anatolia). ❄❄
S. campanulata. Upright, robust-stemmed perennial with opposite, broadly ovate, mid-green leaves, to 12cm (5in) long, softly hairy on both surfaces and heart-shaped at the bases. In summer, whorls of yellow, rarely blue or purple flowers, 2.5cm (1in) long, each with a bell-shaped calyx, are borne in pairs on spreading panicles. ↕ to 1m (3ft), ↔ to 60cm (24in). Himalayas. ❄❄
S. canariensis. Erect, open, evergreen shrub with sparsely branched, white-downy stems. Lance-shaped to triangular, entire or notched, mid-green leaves, 6–15cm (2½–6in) long, each have 2 spreading lobes at the bases; they are covered with dense white down, at least beneath. From winter to spring, bears small, white to violet or purple flowers, to 2cm (¾in) long, in terminal panicles or racemes. ↕ 1–2m (3–6ft), ↔ 0.6–1.2m (2–4ft). Canary Islands. ⊛ (min. 7°C/45°F)
S. cardinalis see *S. fulgens.*
S. chamaedryoides. Low-growing, woody-based perennial with branching stems. Elliptic, finely scalloped, mid- to grey-green leaves, to 2cm (¾in) long, are covered in fine hairs, giving them a sage-green appearance. Deep blue flowers, 2.5cm (1in) long, with widely spreading lips, are borne in terminal racemes in late summer. ↕ 30cm (12in), ↔ 60cm (24in). USA (Texas), Mexico. ❄❄
S. clevelandii (Jim sage). Dwarf, rounded, evergreen shrub, branching mainly from the base, with usually downy stems, and ovate or oblong to elliptic or lance-shaped, wrinkled, toothed, mid-green leaves, to 2.5cm (1in) long. In summer, white, blue, or violet flowers, 1.5cm (½in) long, are borne in terminal whorls or short, simple to branched spikes. ↕ 40–60cm (16–24in), ↔ 30–60cm (12–24in). USA (California). ❄❄
S. coccinea. Erect, bushy annual or perennial with oval to heart-shaped, toothed, hairy, dark green leaves, to 6cm (2½in) long. From summer to autumn, soft cherry-red flowers, to 2cm (¾in) long, are borne in slender, open, terminal spikes. ↕ 60–75cm (24–30in), ↔ to 30cm (12in). Tropical South America. ❄. **'Coral Nymph'** ■ has coral-pink flowers; ↕ 40cm (16in). **'Lady in Red'** ■♀ produces red flowers; ↕ 40cm (16in). **'Snow Nymph'**, syn. 'White Lady', bears white flowers. **'Starry Eyed'** bears white, red, or coral-pink flowers. **'White Lady'** see 'Snow Nymph'.
***S. concolor* of gardens** see *S. guaranitica.*
S. confertiflora ■ Woody-based perennial with ovate, scalloped, yellow-green leaves, to 20cm (8in) long, that are densely woolly, especially beneath, and unpleasantly scented if crushed. From late summer to mid-autumn, the unbranched stems bear terminal spikes of orange-red flowers, 1cm (½in) long, with hairy, deep red calyces. ↕ to 1.2m (4ft), ↔ 60cm (24in). Brazil. ❄
S. deserta see *S.* x *sylvestris.*
S. discolor ■♀ Erect perennial with densely white-woolly, branched stems. Oblong-ovate, entire, mid-green leaves, to 6cm (2½in) long, are densely white-woolly beneath, less hairy above. In late summer and early autumn, bears long, terminal racemes of deep indigo-black flowers, to 2.5cm (1in) long, with finely white-hairy calyces. ↕ 45cm (18in), ↔ 30cm (12in). Peru. ❄
S. elegans. Soft-stemmed herbaceous perennial or subshrub with branching stems and ovate or almost triangular, hairless or softly hairy, toothed, mildly pineapple-scented, mid-green leaves, to 10cm (4in) long. Loose, terminal panicles of bright scarlet flowers, 2.5cm (1in) long, softly hairy inside, are produced from winter to spring. ↕ 2m (6ft), ↔ 1m (3ft). Mexico, Guatemala. ⊛ (min. 5°C/41°F). **'Scarlet Pineapple'** ■ syn. *S. rutilans* (Pineapple sage), has leaves that smell strongly of pineapple when crushed, and more densely hairy stems; it bears larger flowers, to 3.5cm (1½in) long; ↕ 90cm (36in), ↔ 60cm (24in).

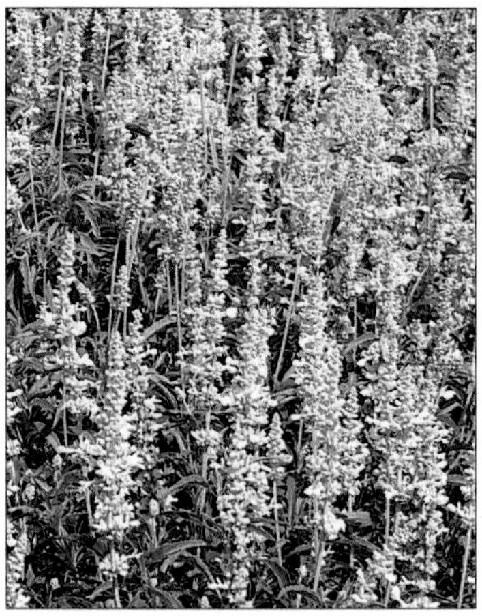
Salvia farinacea f. *alba*

S. farinacea (Mealy sage). Erect, bushy perennial, usually grown as an annual, with white-mealy stems bearing pointed, narrowly to broadly lance-shaped, wavy-margined, glossy, mid-green leaves, to 8cm (3in) long, white-hairy beneath. From summer to autumn, produces deep lavender-blue flowers, to 2cm (¾in) long, in tall, slender, dense, purple-stemmed, terminal or axillary spikes. It may be overwintered in moist peat, if kept frost-free. ↕ to 60cm (24in), ↔ to 30cm (12in), as an annual. USA (Texas), Mexico. ❄. **f. *alba*** ■ bears white flowers. **'Rhea'** is compact and early flowering, with intense dark blue flowers; ↕ to 35cm (14in). **'Strata'** has blue and white flowers. **'Victoria'** ■♀ has deep blue flowers and dense basal branching. **'White Porcelain'** has white flowers.
S. flava* var. *megalantha see *S. bulleyana.*
S. forskaohlei see *S. forsskaolii.*
S. forsskaolii, syn. *S. forskaohlei.* Clump-forming perennial producing ovate or deeply lobed, toothed, softly bristly, mostly basal, mid-green leaves, 5–30cm (2–12in) long, with heart-shaped bases. Stems are sometimes branched and, from early summer to early autumn, bear long, terminal or axillary spikes of white-tubed flowers, to 3cm (1¼in) long, with wide-spreading violet lips, the lower lips marked yellowish white. ↕ to 90cm (36in), ↔ 50cm (20in). Bulgaria, Turkey (Black Sea coast). ❄❄❄
S. fruticosa, syn. *S. triloba.* Bushy, evergreen shrub or subshrub with white-hairy, branched stems bearing simple or

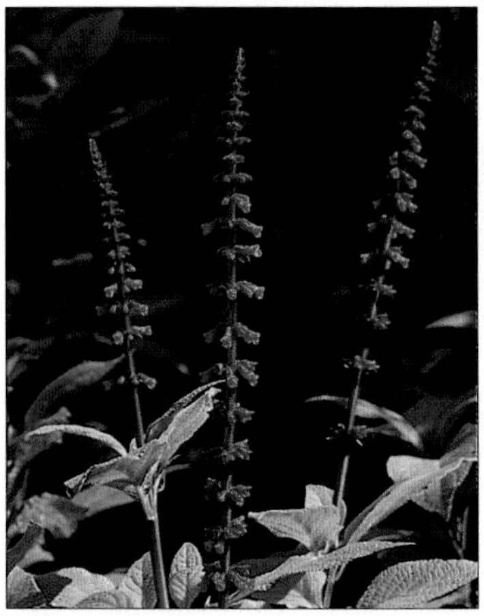
Salvia confertiflora

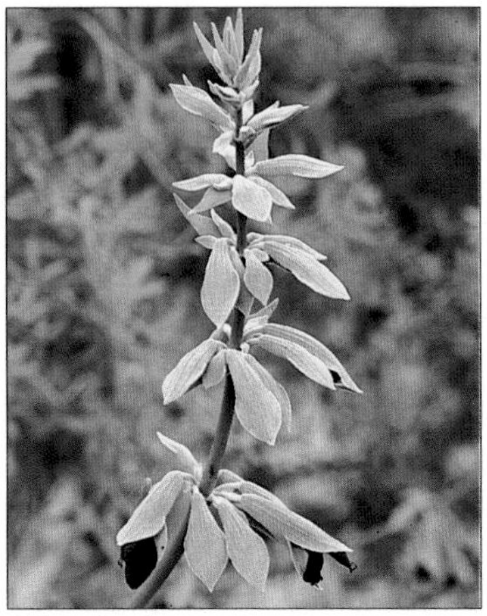
Salvia discolor

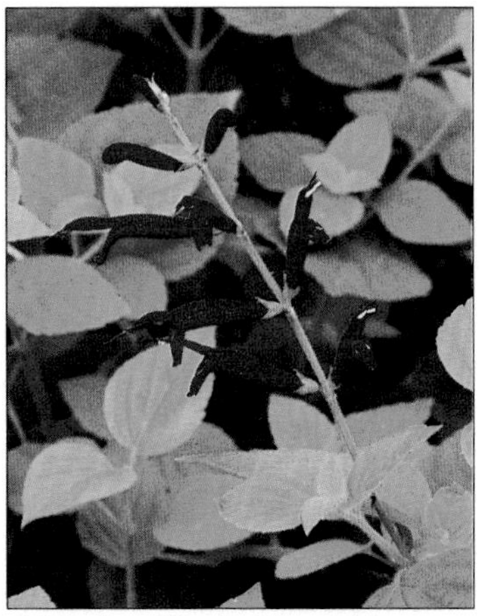
Salvia elegans 'Scarlet Pineapple'

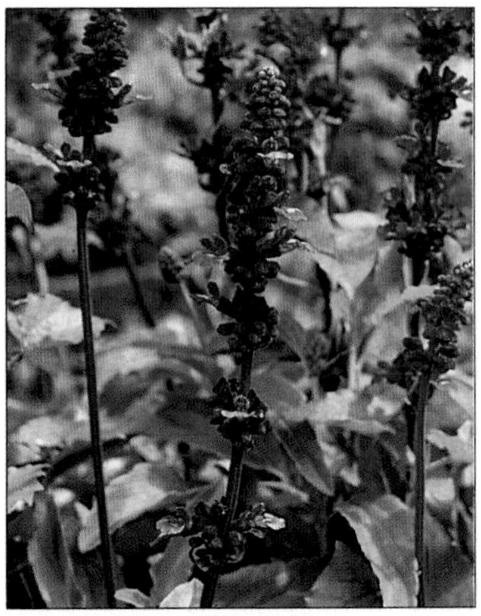
Salvia farinacea 'Victoria'

SALVIA

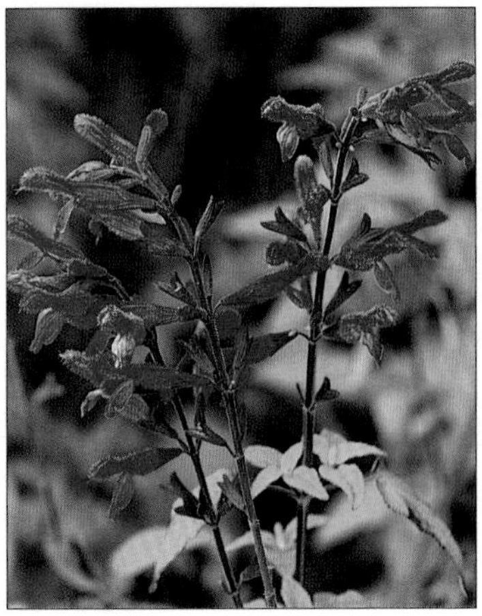

Salvia fulgens

pinnate, mid-green leaves, to 5cm (2in) long; the pinnate leaves each have 3 or 5 oblong-elliptic leaflets. In summer, bears purple, lilac-pink, or pink, rarely white flowers, to 2.5cm (1in) long, in terminal or axillary racemes. ↕ to 1.2m (4ft), ↔ to 80cm (32in). C. and E. Mediterranean. ✻✻

S. fulgens ■ ♀ syn. *S. cardinalis.* Woody-based perennial or evergreen subshrub, branching mainly from the base, with ovate to narrowly triangular, toothed or notched leaves, 6–12cm (2½–5in) long, rich green above, densely white-woolly beneath. Terminal or axillary spikes or racemes of red flowers, to 3cm (1¼in) long, with densely downy lower lips, are produced in summer. ↕ 50–100cm (20–39in), ↔ 40–90cm (16–36in). Mexico. ✻

S. gesneriiflora. Subshrubby perennial bearing ovate, scalloped, hairy, mid-green leaves, to 10cm (4in) long, with heart-shaped bases. From early spring to mid-autumn, many-branched stems bear terminal racemes of numerous softly hairy red flowers, 5cm (2in) long, with flattened upper lips. ↕ 60cm (24in), ↔ 20cm (8in). Mexico, Colombia. ✻

S. glutinosa (Jupiter's distaff). Clump-forming, sticky-hairy perennial with branched or unbranched stems and heart-shaped, toothed, mid-green leaves, to 20cm (8in) long. From midsummer to mid-autumn, bears loose, terminal racemes of softly hairy, pale yellow flowers, to 4cm (1½in) long, heavily spotted maroon and with reddish brown markings on the brighter yellow lower lips. ↕↔ 90cm (36in). C. and S. Europe to W. Asia. ✻✻✻

S

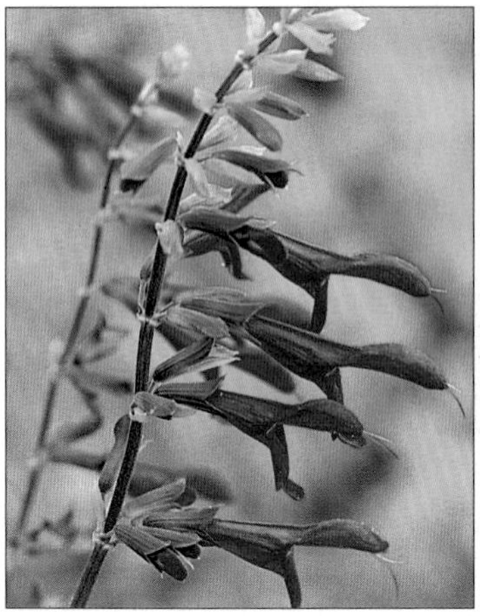

Salvia guaranitica 'Blue Enigma'

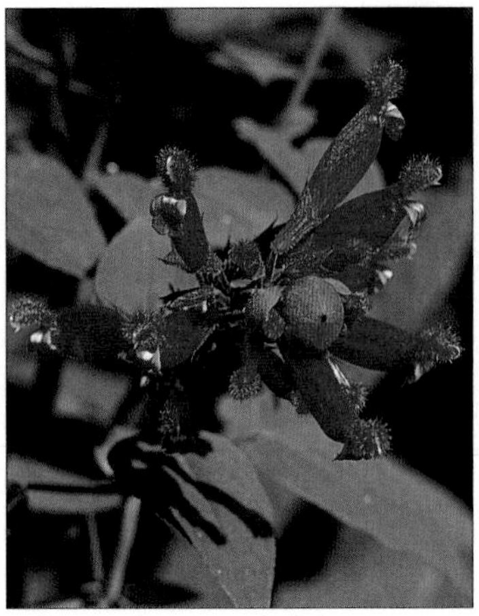

Salvia involucrata 'Bethellii'

S. grahamii see *S. microphylla.*

S. greggii (Autumn sage). Dwarf, evergreen shrub or sometimes erect, woody-based perennial, branching mainly from the base, with glandular-hairy stems. Ovate or elliptic to oblong or linear, leathery, entire, mid- to deep green leaves, 2–3cm (¾–1¼in) long, are hairless to softly hairy and dotted with glands. Paired, red to purple, pink, yellow, or violet flowers, 2cm (¾in) long, are borne in terminal racemes from late summer to autumn. ↕↔ 30–50cm (12–20in). USA (Texas), Mexico. ✻✻. **'Raspberry Royal'** has bright raspberry-red flowers; ↕ to 60cm (24in), ↔ 30cm (12in).

S. guaranitica ♀ syn. *S. concolor* of gardens. Subshrubby perennial with branched, dark green stems and ovate, pointed, slightly toothed, hairy, wrinkled, mid-green leaves, to 13cm (5in) long. Deep blue flowers, to 5cm (2in) long, with purplish blue calyces, are borne in terminal or axillary spikes from late summer to late autumn. ↕ 1.5m (5ft), ↔ 60cm (24in). Brazil, Uruguay, Argentina. ✻. **'Black and Blue'**, syn. *S. caerulea* of gardens, bears rich blue flowers with very dark purple-blue calyces; ↕ to 2.5m (8ft), ↔ 90cm (36in). **'Blue Enigma'** ■ syn. *S. ambigens,* bears fragrant, deep blue flowers with bright green calyces; ↔ 90cm (36in). **'Purple Splendour'** bears hairless leaves and purple flowers; ↔ 90cm (36in).

S. haematodes see *S. pratensis* Haematodes Group.

S. hians. Erect, sticky-hairy, pleasantly scented, somewhat short-lived perennial

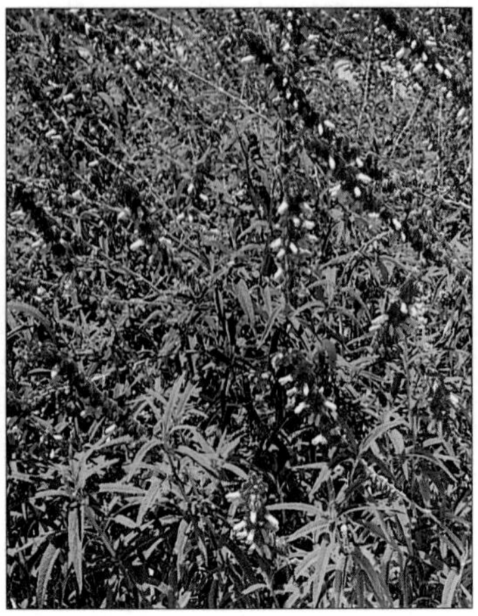

Salvia leucantha

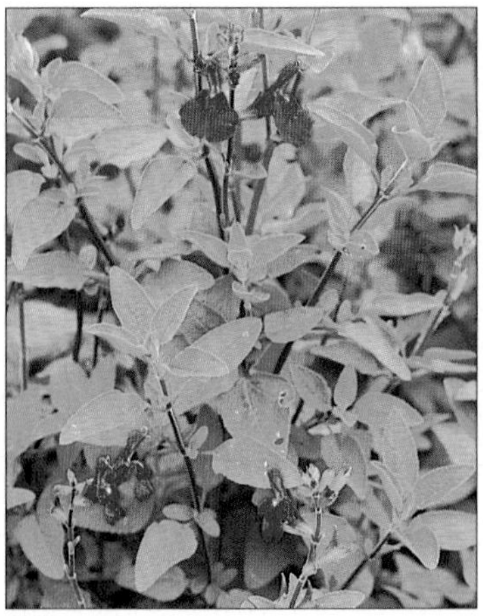

Salvia microphylla

with ovate, toothed, prominently veined, wrinkled, dark green leaves, to 15cm (6in) long. Branched stems bear terminal spikes of purplish blue flowers, to 3.5cm (1½in) long, with spreading lips, the lower lips white-marked, from early to late summer. ↕↔ 60cm (24in). Himalayas (mainly Kashmir). ✻✻✻

S. hispanica see *S. lavandulifolia.*

S. horminum see *S. viridis.*

S. involucrata ♀ Subshrubby perennial with sparsely branched stems and ovate, tapering, entire or notched, softly hairy, rich green leaves, to 12cm (5in) long. From late summer to mid-autumn, bears dense, terminal racemes of purplish red flowers, to 5cm (2in) long, with pink bracts that fall as the flowers open. ↕ 1.5m (5ft), ↔ 1m (3ft). Mexico. ✻✻. **'Bethellii'** ■ has slightly larger, more velvety leaves, and bright purplish crimson flowers. **'Deschampsiana'** has leaves that are narrowly acute at the tips, and more ovoid racemes of rose-pink flowers with bright red bracts and calyces; ↕ 90cm (36in).

S. x jamensis (*S. greggii* x *S. microphylla*). Bushy shrub with opposite, ovate to elliptic, toothed, mid-green leaves, 2–3.5cm (¾–1½in) long. In summer and autumn, red, rose-pink, salmon-pink, orange, or rarely creamy yellow flowers, 1–2.5cm (½–1in) long, are borne in opposite pairs in terminal racemes. ↕ 0.5–1m (20–39in), ↔ 50cm (20in). Mexico. ✻. **'Fuego'** bears bright, flame-red flowers. **'James Compton'** has leaves to 2cm (¾in) long, and bears racemes of deep crimson flowers, 2.5cm (1in) long; ↕ to 1m (3ft), ↔ 75cm (30in); ❀ (min. 5°C/41°F). **'La Luna'** bears creamy yellow flowers, the upper lips covered in buff-coloured hairs. **'Pat Vlasto'** has ovate-elliptic, entire leaves, 2cm (¾in) long, and pink-suffused orange flowers, 2–2.5cm (¾–1in) long; ↕ 1m (3ft), ↔ 75cm (30in); ❀ (min. 5°C/41°F)

S. jurisicii. Low-growing, hairy perennial with basal rosettes of ovate, scalloped, mid-green leaves, 10cm (4in) long, and many-branched stems producing pinnate leaves, 10cm (4in) long, each divided into 4–6 pairs of linear leaflets. From early to late summer, bears a profusion of terminal racemes of apparently upside-down, violet-blue flowers, to 1cm (½in) long, the upper lips covered with long, violet-blue hairs. ↕ to 60cm (24in), ↔ 45cm (18in). Yugoslavia (Serbia), Macedonia. ✻✻✻

S. lavandulifolia, syn. *S. hispanica.* Woody-based perennial with mostly basal, long-stalked, narrowly oblong, entire, grey- to white-woolly leaves, to 2.5cm (1in) long. In midsummer, blue-violet flowers, to 2.5cm (1in) long, are produced in terminal and axillary racemes. ↕ to 50cm (20in), ↔ 60cm (24in). Spain. ✻✻✻ (borderline)

S. lemmonii see *S. microphylla var. wislizenii.*

S. leucantha ■ ♀ (Mexican bush). Bushy, evergreen subshrub with white-downy stems when young, and ovate or lance-shaped to oblong or linear, toothed or scalloped, mid-green leaves, to 15cm (6in) long, wrinkled above, white-downy beneath. From winter to spring, produces terminal racemes of white flowers, to 1.5–2cm (½–¾in) long, with bell-shaped, downy, purple to lavender-blue calyces. ↕ 60–100cm (24–39in), ↔ 40–90cm (16–36in). Mexico, tropical Central America. ✻

S. microphylla ■ syn. *S. grahamii.* Moderately bushy, evergreen shrub or shrubby perennial bearing triangular-ovate to elliptic, softly hairy or hairless, mid- to deep green leaves, 1.5–4cm (½–1½in) long, with rounded teeth. From late summer to autumn, paired or whorled, deep crimson or, less commonly, magenta, pink, or purple flowers, 2.5cm (1in) long, are produced in terminal racemes. ↕ 90–120cm (3–4ft), ↔ 60–100cm (24–39in). USA (Arizona, New Mexico), Mexico. ✻✻. **var. *neurepia*** has pale green leaves, 3.5–5cm (1¼–2in) long, and produces cherry-red flowers, to 3cm (1¼in) long, mainly in autumn. **'Oxford'** bears deep rose-crimson flowers. **'Ruth Stungo'** has white-splashed leaves. **var. *wislizenii,*** syn. *S. lemmonii,* is more compact, with triangular leaves, to 3cm (1¼in) long, and dense spikes of vermilion or magenta flowers; ↕↔ 1m (3ft).

S. nemorosa. Erect, many-branched perennial with ovate or lance-shaped to oblong, notched, wrinkled, mid-green leaves, to 10cm (4in) long. From summer to autumn, bears violet to purple, or white to pink flowers, to 1cm (½in) long, with violet to purple bracts, in dense, terminal racemes. ↕ to 1m (3ft), ↔ 60cm (24in). Europe to C. Asia. ✻✻✻. **'East Friesland'** see 'Ostfriesland'. **'Lubecca'**, syn. *S.* x *superba* 'Lubecca', is dwarf and clump-forming, with greyish green leaves. From midsummer to early autumn, bears violet flowers with reddish purple

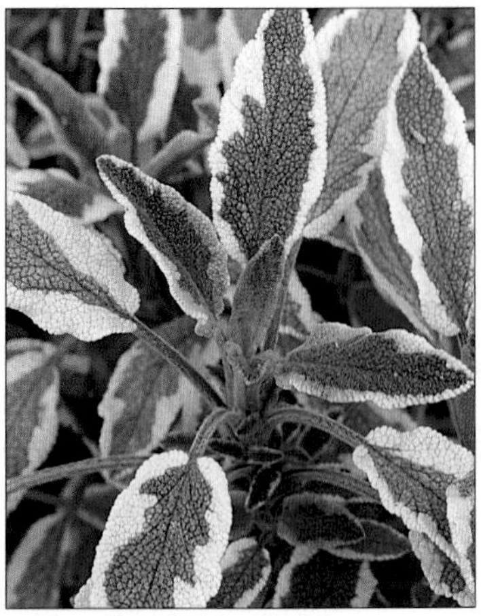

Salvia officinalis 'Tricolor'

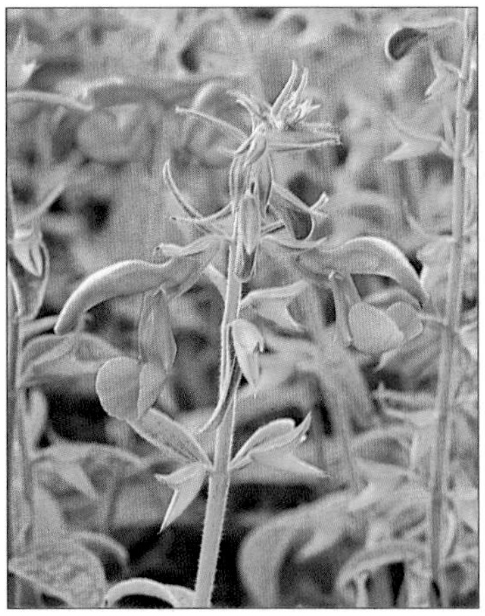

Salvia patens 'Cambridge Blue'

bracts that persist long after the flowers fall; ↕↔ 45cm (18in). **'Ostfriesland'**, syn. 'East Friesland', produces deep blue-violet flowers; ↕ 45cm (18in).
S. officinalis (Common sage). Subshrubby, erect, hairy, evergreen perennial with oblong-ovate, entire, grey-green-woolly, aromatic leaves, to 8cm (3in) long. Branched stems bear terminal or axillary racemes of lilac-blue flowers, 1.5cm (½in) long, in early and midsummer. A popular culinary herb. ↕ to 80cm (32in), ↔ 1m (3ft). Mediterranean, N. Africa. ❄❄❄. **'Aurea'** has a more compact habit, with oblong yellow leaves, and produces small spikes of purplish blue flowers in early summer; ↕ 30cm (12in), ↔ 45cm (18in). **'Icterina'** 🏆 has variegated yellow and green leaves. **'Kew Gold'** produces golden yellow leaves, sometimes flecked with green, and bears mauve flowers; ↕ 20–30cm (8–12in), ↔ 30cm (12in). **'Purpurascens'** 🏆 (Purple sage) has red-purple young leaves. **'Tricolor'** ◼ bears grey-green leaves, zoned cream and pink to purple; ❄❄
S. patens 🏆 Tuberous perennial with erect, branched stems bearing ovate, broadly ovate to triangular, or pentagonal, toothed, hairy, mid-green leaves, to 20cm (8in) long, with spear-shaped bases. From midsummer to mid-autumn, produces few-flowered, loose, sometimes branched, terminal racemes of paired, deep blue flowers, 5cm (2in) long, with wide open mouths. ↕ 45–60cm (18–24in), ↔ 45cm (18in). Mexico. ❄❄. **'Cambridge Blue'** ◼🏆 produces pale blue flowers.

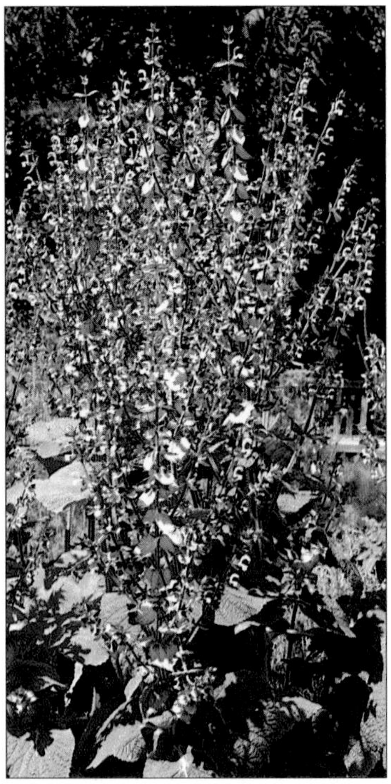

Salvia sclarea var. *turkestanica*

S. pratensis (Meadow clary). Clump-forming, woody-based perennial with ovate, blunt-tipped, toothed, wrinkled, mid-green basal leaves, to 15cm (6in) long, and few smaller stem leaves. In early and midsummer, erect, branched or unbranched, slightly sticky-hairy stems bear terminal spikes of violet, rarely pink or white flowers, 2–3cm (¾–1¼in) long. ↕ to 90cm (36in), ↔ 30cm (12in). Europe, Morocco. ❄❄❄. Cultivars of **Haematodes Group** ◼🏆 syn. *S. haematodes*, are short-lived plants with basal rosettes of large, broadly ovate, wavy-margined, dark green leaves, to 20cm (8in) long. Branched, reddish brown stems bear loose, spreading panicles of bluish violet flowers, with hairy upper lips and paler throats; Greece. **'Mittsommer'** produces loose spikes of sky-blue flowers with long, arched upper lips and darker blue calyces and bracts, throughout summer.
S. rutilans see *S. elegans* 'Scarlet Pineapple'.
S. sclarea (Biennial clary). Erect, many-branched, glandular-hairy perennial or biennial with ovate to oblong, notched to irregularly toothed, wrinkled, mid-green leaves, to 23cm (9in) long, with

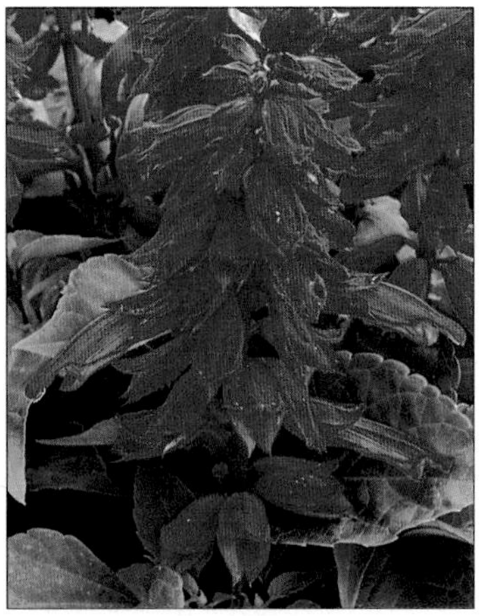

Salvia splendens 'Scarlet King'

heart-shaped or perfoliate bases. From spring to summer, bears many-flowered, terminal panicles or racemes of cream and lilac to pink or blue flowers, to 3cm (1¼in) long, with prominent lilac bracts. ↕ to 1m (3ft), ↔ 30cm (12in). Europe to C. Asia. ❄❄❄. **var. *turkestanica*** ◼ has pink stems bearing spikes of pink-flecked white flowers.
S. splendens (Scarlet sage). Erect, bushy perennial, usually grown as an annual, with oval, pointed, toothed, slightly hairy, pale to dark green leaves, to 7cm (3in) long. Long-tubed, bright red flowers, 1.5–5cm (½–2in) long, enclosed in red bracts, are borne in dense, terminal spikes from summer to autumn. ↕ to 40cm (16in), ↔ 23–35cm (9–14in). Brazil. ❄. The best of modern seed selections are compact, with very erect flower spikes. Grow red cultivars in full sun; pastel shades need shade from the hottest sun. **'Blaze of Fire'**, syn. 'Fireball', has pale green leaves and red flowers; ↕ 30–40cm (12–16in). Cultivars of **Cleopatra Series** ◼ produce flowers in red, salmon-pink, purple, or white; ↕ 30–40cm (12–16in). **'Fireball'** see 'Blaze of Fire'. **Phoenix Series** cultivars produce flowers in dark salmon-pink, pale salmon-pink, purple, white, red, or lilac; ↕ 26–30cm (10–12in). **'Rambo'** is very tall-growing, vigorous, and bushy, with dark green leaves and scarlet flowers; ↕ to 60cm (24in). **'Red Arrow'** has very dark green leaves, and produces scarlet flowers; ↕ to 30cm (12in). **'Red Riches'** 🏆 syn. 'Ryco', bears dark green leaves and scarlet flowers; ↕ 30–40cm (12–16in). **'Ryco'** see 'Red Riches'. **'Scarlet King'** ◼🏆 is compact and long-flowering, with dark green leaves and scarlet flowers; ↕ to 25cm (10in). **'Scarlet Queen'** bears bright scarlet flowers in early summer; ↕ 25cm (10in). **Sizzler Series** ◼ cultivars have flowers in bright shades of cerise-red, lavender-blue, salmon-pink, purple, scarlet, or white. They are early flowering, and available as single colours; ↕ 25–30cm (10–12in).
S. x superba 🏆 (*S. nemorosa* x *S.* x *sylvestris*). Clump-forming, erect, branched perennial with lance-shaped to oblong, scalloped, mid-green leaves, to 10cm (4in) long, slightly hairy beneath; the basal leaves are stalked, the stem leaves stalkless and sometimes stem-clasping. From midsummer to early autumn, bears slender, terminal racemes of bright violet or purple flowers, to 1.5cm (½in) long. ↕ 60–90m (26–36in), ↔ 45–60cm (18–24in). Garden origin. ❄❄❄. **'Lubecca'** see *S. nemorosa* 'Lubecca'.
S. x sylvestris (*S. nemorosa* x *S. pratensis*) syn. *S. deserta*. Clump-forming, erect, branched perennial bearing oblong-lance-shaped, scalloped, wrinkled, softly hairy, mid-green leaves, to 7cm (3in) long. Pinkish violet flowers, 1cm (½in) long, are produced in dense, terminal racemes in early and midsummer. ↕ 80cm (32in), ↔ 30cm (12in). Garden origin. ❄❄❄. **'Blauhügel'**, syn. 'Blue Mound', produces pure blue flowers; ↕ 50cm (20in), ↔ 45cm (18in). **'Blaukönigin'**, syn. 'Blue Queen', bears rich blue-violet flowers; ↕ 70cm (28in), ↔ 45cm (18in). **'Blue Mound'** see 'Blauhügel'. **'Blue Queen'** see

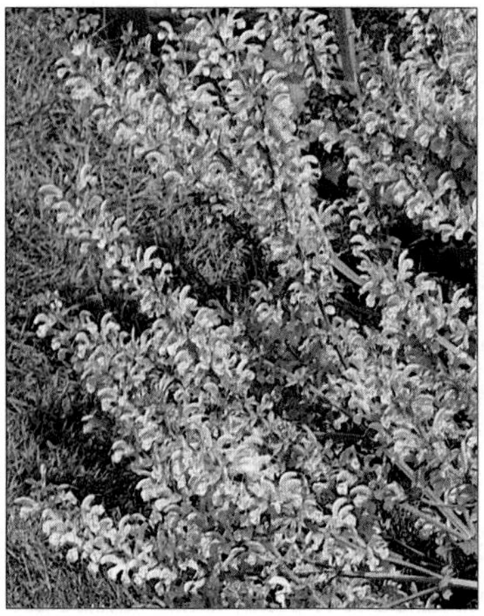

Salvia pratensis Haematodes Group

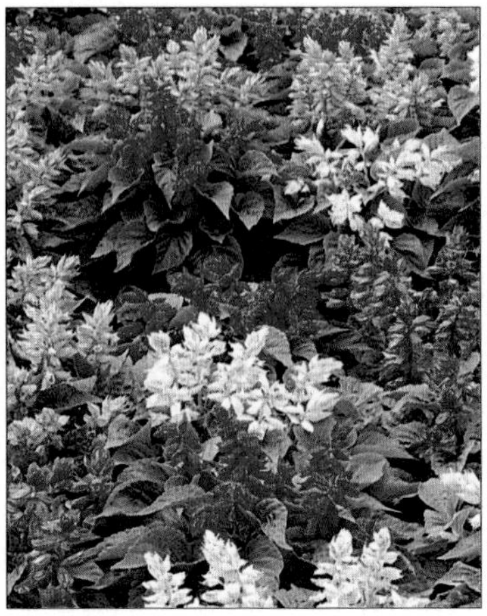

Salvia splendens Cleopatra Series

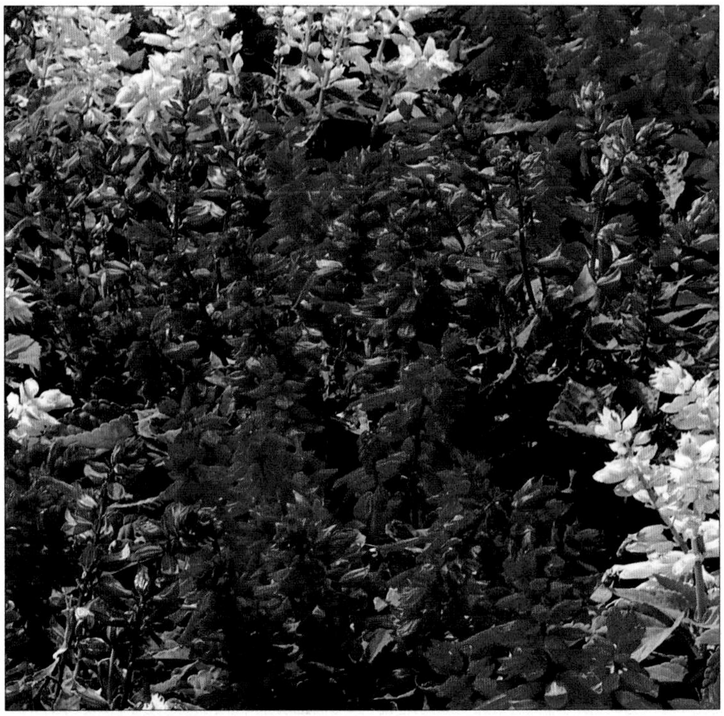

Salvia splendens Sizzler Series

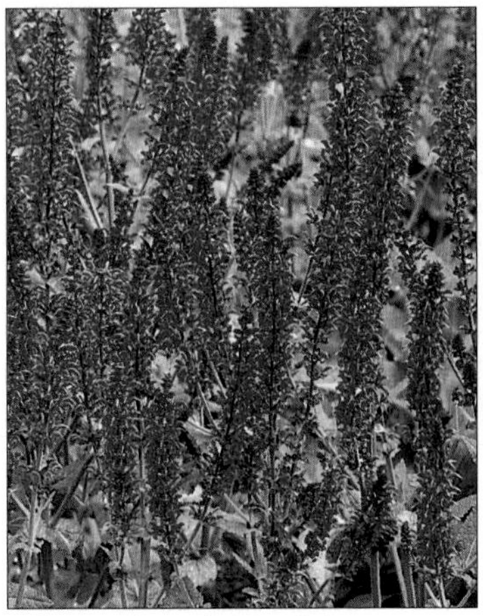
Salvia x *sylvestris* 'Mainacht'

'Blaukönigin'. **'Mainacht'** ■ syn. 'May Night', bears large, indigo-blue flowers, 2cm (¾in) long; ↕70cm (28in), ↔45cm (18in). **'May Night'** see 'Mainacht'. **'Rose Queen'** has rose-pink flowers and grey-tinted leaves; ↕75cm (30in).
S. triloba see *S. fruticosa.*
S. uliginosa ■🏆 (Bog sage). Clump-forming, moisture-loving, rhizomatous perennial with oblong-lance-shaped, deeply toothed, mid-green leaves, to 7cm (3in) long; they are well spaced out and become progressively smaller up the slender, branching stems. From late summer to mid-autumn, bears short, terminal racemes of clear blue flowers, 2cm (¾in) long. Needs moist soil and full sun. ↕ to 2m (6ft), ↔ 90cm (36in). Brazil, Uruguay, Argentina. ❄❄
S. verticillata. Erect herbaceous perennial with opposite, ovate or elliptic to oblong, softly glandular-hairy, mid-green leaves, to 13cm (5in) long, pinnatifid with a larger terminal lobe. In summer, produces branched racemes of violet to lilac-blue, rarely white flowers, 8mm (⅜in) long, in whorls of 20–40 blooms. ↕ to 90cm (36in), ↔ to 45cm (18in). Europe to W. Asia. ❄❄❄
S. viridis, syn. *S. horminum* (Annual clary). Erect, bushy annual with ovate to oblong, notched, hairy, mid-green leaves, 5cm (2in) long. In summer, bears terminal spikes of insignificant, whorled, pink to pale purple flowers, 8–15mm (⅜–½in) long, each whorl enclosed in 2 showy, pink, purple, or white bracts, to 4cm (1½in) long, with darker veins. Grow as a cut flower for the very long-lasting bracts. May also be dried. ↕45–50cm (18–20in), ↔ 23cm (9in).

S

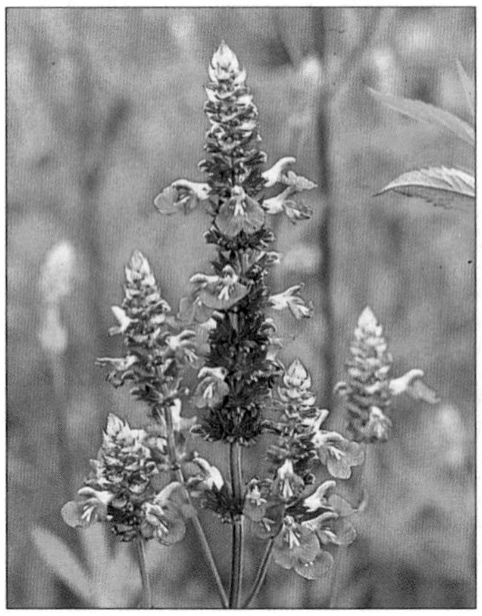
Salvia uliginosa

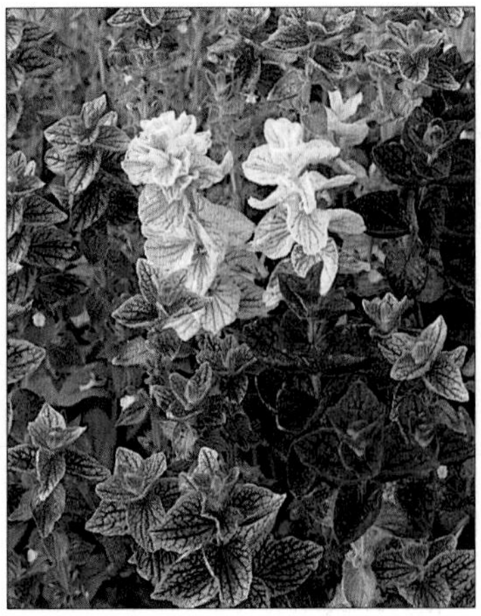
Salvia viridis 'Claryssa'

Mediterranean. ❄❄❄. **'Bouquet'**, syn. 'Monarch Bouquet', has blue, rose-pink, white, deep carmine-pink, or purple bracts; also available as single colours. **'Claryssa'** ■ is compact and very well-branched, with bracts in rose-pink, blue, purple, or white; also available as single colours; ↕ to 40cm (16in). **'Monarch Bouquet'** see 'Bouquet'. **'Oxford Blue'** has violet-blue bracts; ↕30cm (12in). **'Pink Sundae'** has bright carmine-pink bracts. **'White Swan'** has white bracts with green veins; ↕30cm (12in).

SALVINIA

SALVINIACEAE

Genus of 10 species of aquatic annual ferns found in stagnant or slow-moving water, with a wide tropical and sub-tropical distribution, especially in tropical Africa and Central and South America; they are also naturalized in some warm-temperate areas. Floating, rootless plants, they have very slender, irregularly branched stems, and bear mostly rounded to ovate leaves in pairs, with a third, finely dissected, root-like, submerged leaf. They are useful for an aquarium, where fish fry can hide in the submerged leaves. In tropical areas, grow in an outdoor pool. In frost-prone areas, grow in an outdoor pool during summer, then lift and store in winter.
• **HARDINESS** Frost tender.
• **CULTIVATION** In an aquarium, grow in nutrient-rich water at 18–24°C (64–75°F) in full light. Tilt the aquarium cover to prevent condensation forming on the leaves, as this may cause scorch in artificial light. Very invasive, so thin regularly. Outdoors, float on the surface of a still-water pool in full sun. In frost-prone areas, lift before the first frosts and store in shallow trays of sandy loam covered with 2.5–5cm (1–2in) of water, in a cool or temperate green-house. See also pp.52–53.
• **PROPAGATION** Separate stems in spring or summer.
• **PESTS AND DISEASES** Trouble free.

S. auriculata. Floating aquatic fern with whorls of 3 leaves, each consisting of an opposite pair of oval to ovate floating leaves, 3–4cm (1¼–1½in) long, covered with fine hairs, and one root-like submerged leaf adapted to a root function. ↔ indefinite. Central and South America. ❁ (min. 10°C/50°F)
S. natans ■ Floating aquatic fern bearing paired, elliptic, pale green leaves,

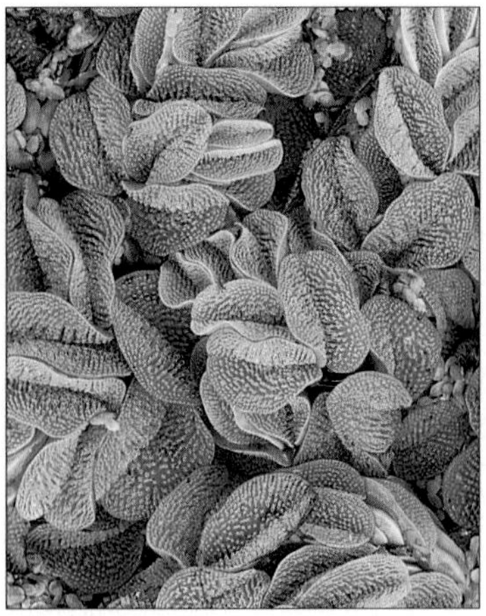
Salvinia natans

to 1.5cm (½in) long, with shiny brown hairs beneath, and a submerged, root-like frond, 2–7cm (¾–3in) long. ↔ indefinite. S. Europe, N. Africa, Asia. ❁ (min. 10°C/50°F)

SAMBUCUS

Elder

CAPRIFOLIACEAE

Genus of about 25 species of herbaceous perennials and deciduous shrubs and trees from woodland and thickets in temperate and subtropical regions of Eurasia, N. and tropical E. Africa, Australia, and North and South America. They are cultivated for their foliage, flowers, and fruits. They bear opposite, pinnate leaves and dense, flat-topped umbels or panicles of small, white to ivory flowers, followed by red, black, or white fruits. Elders are suitable for a mixed or shrub border, or a wild garden. Those with coloured leaves are effective as free-standing specimens. All parts may cause severe discomfort if ingested, although fruits are safe when cooked; contact with the leaves may irritate skin.
• **HARDINESS** Fully hardy.
• **CULTIVATION** Grow in moderately fertile, humus rich, moist but well-drained soil in full sun or partial shade; those with coloured leaves colour well in sun, but retain colour best in dappled shade. Pruning group 7, for those grown for their coloured or cut leaves; group 1 for the rest. Elders tolerate hard pruning as necessary to restrict size.
• **PROPAGATION** Sow seed in containers in an open frame in autumn. Take hardwood cuttings in winter, or green-wood cuttings in early summer.
• **PESTS AND DISEASES** Black fly infest the young shoots and foliage, and *Verticillium* wilt may be a problem.

S. canadensis (American elder). Upright shrub with stout shoots and pinnate leaves, to 30cm (12in) long, each composed of 9 or more elliptic to lance-shaped, toothed, light green leaflets. In midsummer, bears small white flowers in flattened panicles, to 20cm (8in) across, followed by spherical, purple-black fruit, to 5mm (¼in) across. ↕↔ 4m (12ft). North America. ❄❄❄. **'Aurea'** has golden yellow foliage and red fruit.
S. nigra (Black elder, Bourtree, Common elder, Elderberry, European elder). Upright, bushy shrub with stout shoots. Pinnate leaves, to 25cm (10in) long, each have 5 ovate, toothed, mid-green leaflets. Bears musk-scented white flowers in flattened panicles, to 20cm (8in) across, in early summer, followed by spherical, glossy black fruit, to 8mm (⅜in) across. ↕↔ 6m (20ft). Europe, N. Africa, S.W. Asia. ❄❄❄. **'Aurea'** 🏆 has golden yellow leaves borne on pink-flushed leaf-stalks. **'Aureomarginata'** bears yellow-margined, dark green leaves. **'Guincho Purple'** ■🏆 has dark green leaves, turning blackish purple then red in autumn, and pink-tinged flowers with purple stalks. **'Laciniata'** 🏆 syn. f. *laciniata*, has irregularly and finely cut leaflets.
S. racemosa (Red-berried elder). Bushy shrub with arching shoots and pinnate

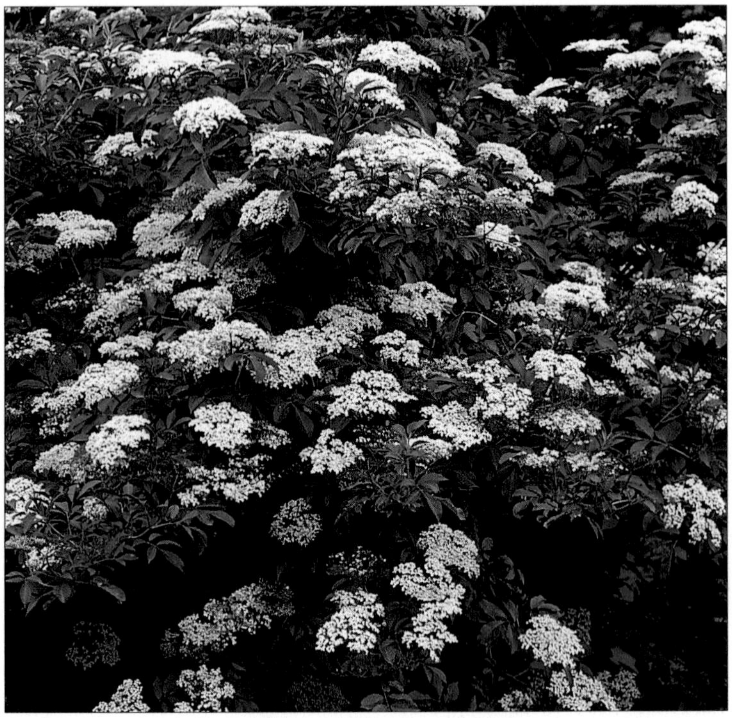
Sambucus nigra 'Guincho Purple'

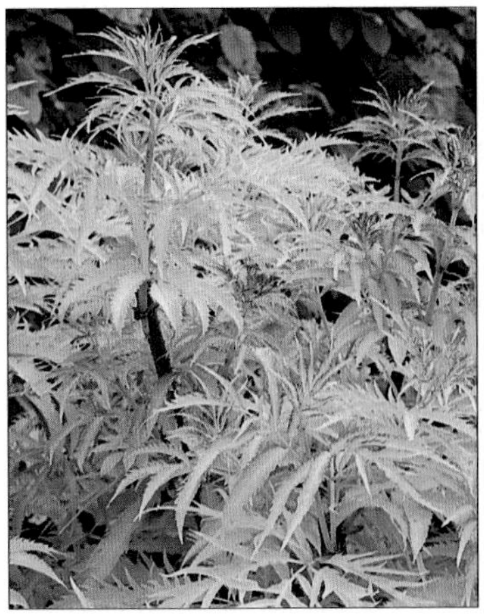
Sambucus racemosa 'Plumosa Aurea'

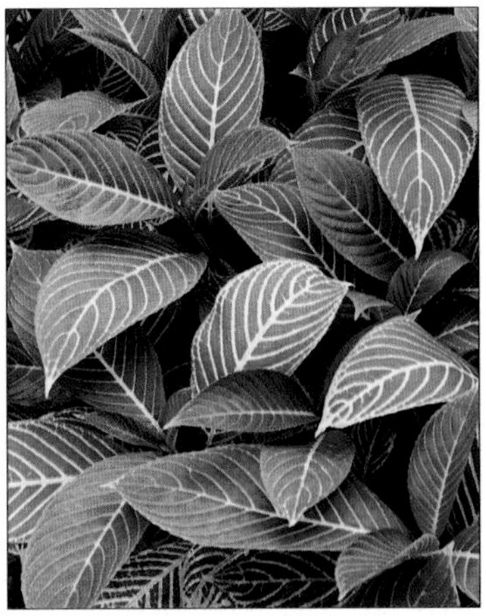
Sanchezia speciosa

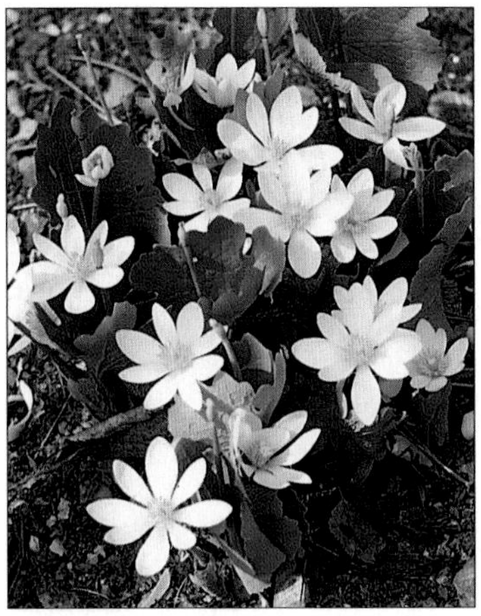
Sanguinaria canadensis

leaves, to 22cm (9in) long, each with usually 5 oval or ovate, toothed, dark green leaflets. In mid-spring, bears small, creamy yellow flowers in conical panicles, 8cm (3in) long, followed in summer by spherical, glossy red fruit, 4mm (⅛in) across. ↕↔ 3m (10ft). Europe, Russia (W. Siberia). ❄❄❄. **'Plumosa'** has purple new growth and finely cut leaflets. **'Plumosa Aurea'** ◼ has finely cut leaflets, bronze when young, turning golden yellow. Foliage may burn in hot sun. **'Sutherland Gold'** ♀ is similar to 'Plumosa Aurea', but less susceptible to sun scorch. **'Tenuifolia'** ♀ is mound-forming, with leaflets very finely cut into long, slender lobes; ↕ 1m (3ft), ↔ 2m (6ft).

SANCHEZIA

ACANTHACEAE

Genus of about 20 species of soft-stemmed evergreen shrubs and shrubby perennials from tropical rainforest in Central and South America. They have opposite pairs of simple, often entire leaves, and bear terminal or axillary spikes or panicles of tubular, showy, yellow, orange, red, or purple flowers, each with 5 small, rounded lobes, often with coloured bracts. Where temperatures drop below 15°C (59°F), grow in a warm greenhouse or conservatory, or as houseplants. In tropical areas, grow at the base of a warm, sunny wall, or in a shrub border.

- **HARDINESS** Frost tender.
- **CULTIVATION** Under glass, grow in loam-based potting compost (JI No.2) in bright filtered or full light, with shade from hot sun. In growth, water freely and apply a balanced liquid fertilizer every 2 or 3 weeks; water sparingly in winter. Outdoors, grow in moderately fertile, humus rich, moist but well-drained soil, in full sun with some midday shade, or in light dappled shade. Pruning group 8; plants under glass may need restrictive pruning in late winter.
- **PROPAGATION** Root softwood cuttings in spring or semi-ripe cuttings in summer, both with gentle bottom heat.
- **PESTS AND DISEASES** Red spider mites and scale insects may be a problem under glass.

S. glaucophylla see *S. speciosa.*
S. nobilis see *S. speciosa.*
S. speciosa ◼ syn. *S. glaucophylla, S. nobilis, S. spectabilis.* Moderately bushy shrub with sparsely branched, sturdy, sometimes obscurely angled, smooth, bright green stems and ovate-elliptic to oblong-lance-shaped, glossy, dark green leaves, 15–30cm (6–12in) long, with yellow-, ivory-, or white-banded midribs and main veins. In summer, bears terminal spikes of 6–10 yellow flowers, 4–5cm (1½–2in) long, with red bracts. ↕ 1.2–2.2m (4–7ft), ↔ 90–150cm (3–5ft). Ecuador, Peru. ❁ (min. 13–15°C/55–59°F)
S. spectabilis see *S. speciosa.*

SANDERSONIA

COLCHICACEAE/LILIACEAE

Genus of one species of tuberous, perennial climber from rocky areas and light woodland in South Africa. Related to *Gloriosa* and *Littonia*, it has alternate leaves, often tipped with tendrils, and solitary flowers. In frost-prone areas, grow in a temperate greenhouse or a conservatory. In frost-free areas, grow in a herbaceous border or among low shrubs.

- **HARDINESS** Half hardy.
- **CULTIVATION** Under glass, plant tubers 7–10cm (3–4in) deep in late winter or early spring, in 4 parts loam-based potting compost (JI No.2) and 1 part grit, in full light with some midday shade. In growth, water freely and apply a balanced liquid fertilizer every 4 weeks; dry off as leaves fade and keep dry while dormant. Stems need support. Outdoors, grow in moderately fertile to humus-rich, well-drained soil in full sun. Protect from excessive winter wet. In frost-prone areas, lift tubers in autumn and store in dry, frost-free conditions.
- **PROPAGATION** Sow seed at 18–24°C (64–75°F) as soon as ripe. Divide in autumn or winter.
- **PESTS AND DISEASES** Trouble free.

S. aurantiaca. Perennial climber with slender stems bearing scattered, lance-shaped, mid-green leaves, to 10cm (4in) long, some of which are tipped with tendrils. In summer, pendent, urn-shaped, bright orange flowers, 2.5cm (1in) long, are borne on downcurved stalks, 2–3cm (¾–1¼in) long, from the upper leaf axils. ↕ to 75cm (30in), ↔ 10cm (4in). South Africa. ❄

▷**Sandsalie** see *Salvia africana-lutea*
▷**Sandwort** see *Arenaria*
Corsican see *A. balearica*
Pink see *A. purpurascens*

SANGUINARIA

Bloodroot, Red puccoon

PAPAVERACEAE

Genus of one species of rhizomatous perennial occurring in moist woodland in E. North America. It is cultivated for its cup-shaped, white or pink-tinted flowers, which emerge from between the vertically folded leaves as they unfurl, in spring. *S. canadensis* is excellent for growing in a damp, shaded site in a rock garden, wild or woodland garden, or peat bed. The rhizomes exude red sap when cut, giving rise to the common name, bloodroot.

- **HARDINESS** Fully hardy.
- **CULTIVATION** Grow in moderately fertile, humus rich, moist but well-drained soil in deep or partial shade. Thrives in part-day sun where soils remain reliably moist.
- **PROPAGATION** Sow seed in containers in a cold frame in autumn, or divide rhizomes immediately after flowering.
- **PESTS AND DISEASES** Trouble free.

S. canadensis ◼ Rhizomatous perennial producing variably lobed, heart- to kidney-shaped, scalloped, bluish grey-green leaves, 15–30cm (6–12in) across when fully expanded. Solitary, cup-shaped, white, occasionally pink-tinted flowers, to 8cm (3in) across, emerge in spring as the leaves unfold. ↕ 15cm (6in), ↔ 30cm (12in) or more. E. North America. ❄❄❄. **'Plena'** ♀ produces many-petalled, double white flowers, which are longer-lasting than those of the species.

SANGUISORBA

Burnet

ROSACEAE

Genus of approximately 18 species of rhizomatous perennials, most occurring in damp meadows, with a few from dry, grassy or rocky sites, in temperate and cooler regions of the N. hemisphere. They produce alternate, pinnate leaves, with mostly oblong to elliptic, toothed, neatly veined leaflets, which in some species are glaucous. The leafy, wiry stems bear dense or loose, bottlebrush-like, terminal spikes of small, fluffy flowers, with red, pink, white, or greenish white sepals and prominent stamens, but no petals. Burnets are suitable for growing in a herbaceous or mixed border, and for naturalizing in a damp meadow garden or by water. Many species provide unusual flowers and foliage for cutting.

- **HARDINESS** Fully hardy.
- **CULTIVATION** Grow in any moderately fertile, moist but well-drained soil that does not dry out, in full sun or partial shade. Taller species usually require support. May become invasive.
- **PROPAGATION** Sow seed in containers in a cold frame in spring or autumn. Divide in spring or autumn.
- **PESTS AND DISEASES** Slugs may damage young leaves.

S. canadensis ◼ (Canadian burnet). Spreading, clump-forming, rhizomatous perennial with upright, simple or branched stems and pinnate, hairy leaves, to 25cm (10in) long, each composed of 7–17 oblong-lance-shaped to ovate leaflets. From midsummer to mid-autumn, long "cones" of green buds open from the bottom up, to form bottlebrush-like spikes, to 20cm (8in) long, of small, fluffy white flowers. ↕ to 2m (6ft), ↔ 1m (3ft). N.E. North America. ❄❄❄
S. obtusa. Rhizomatous perennial with upright stems, branched near the ends, bearing numerous pinnate, greyish green leaves, to 40cm (16in) long, each with 13–17 crowded, oblong-elliptic, almost stalkless leaflets. From mid- or late summer to early autumn, bears small, fluffy, rich pink flowers in short, nodding, bottlebrush-like spikes, 7cm (3in) long. ↕↔ to 60cm (24in). Japan. ❄❄❄
S. officinalis (Greater burnet). Clump-forming, rhizomatous perennial producing pinnate basal leaves, 50cm (20in) long, each with 7–25 oblong-elliptic leaflets; leaves on the erect, branching, often red stems are smaller. The small, red-brown to maroon flowers are borne in erect, very short, dense, ovoid spikes, 1.5–3cm (¾–1¼in) long, from early summer to mid-autumn. ↕ to 1.2m (4ft), ↔ 60cm (24in). Europe, N. and W. Asia, North America. ❄❄❄

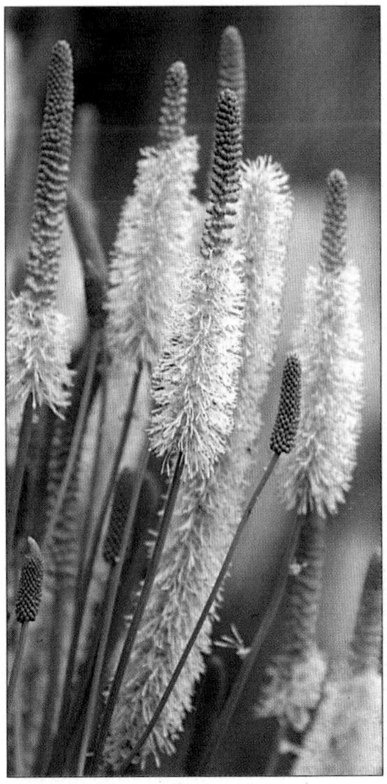
Sanguisorba canadensis

SANSEVIERIA

Bowstring hemp

AGAVACEAE/DRACAENACEAE

Genus of about 60 species of usually stemless, xerophytic, rhizomatous, evergreen perennials from dry, rocky habitats in tropical and subtropical Africa, Madagascar, India, and Indonesia. They are grown for their stiff, fleshy, linear to broadly ovate, upright or more or less spreading leaves, which may be flat, concave, or cylindrical; these are produced in clumps or squat rosettes from spreading, underground or partially exposed rhizomes. Mature plants infrequently bear low racemes or panicles of fragrant, nectar-rich, tubular, 6-lobed flowers in spring. In frost-prone areas, grow in a warm greenhouse or conservatory, or use as houseplants. In warmer areas, grow in a desert garden, in containers on a patio, or in a small courtyard garden. Tolerant of neglect.

- **HARDINESS** Frost tender.
- **CULTIVATION** Under glass, grow in 2 parts loam-based potting compost (JI No.2) and 1 part coarse grit, in bright filtered light or indirect light. In growth, water moderately and apply a half-strength balanced liquid fertilizer monthly; water sparingly in winter. Pot on only when pot-bound; leaf growth may stop if leaf-tips are damaged. Outdoors, grow in poor to moderately fertile, neutral to slightly alkaline, gritty soil in full sun. Protect from excessive winter wet.
- **PROPAGATION** Remove suckers, or divide, in spring. Root leaf sections with bottom heat from spring to autumn. Offspring from variegated cultivars will lack variegation if raised from leaf cuttings.
- **PESTS AND DISEASES** Vine weevil grubs may be a problem.

S. cylindrica. Very slow-growing, woody, rhizomatous perennial with 2-ranked, erect, cylindrical, fleshy, dark green leaves, to 1m (3ft) or more long, with lighter crossbands. Intermittently bears spike-like racemes, 35–75cm (14–30in) long, of tubular, pink or white flowers, 1.5–2.5cm (½–1in) long, the lobes with margins rolled outwards. ↕ to 1.5m (5ft), ↔ 60cm (24in). Angola. ❁ (min. 13°C/55°F)

S

S. trifasciata (Mother-in-law's tongue). Erect, rhizomatous perennial with pointed, lance-shaped, fleshy leaves, to

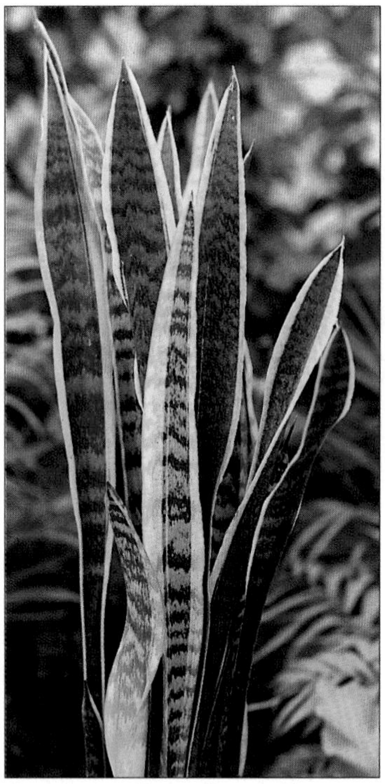

Sansevieria trifasciata 'Laurentii'

1.2m (4ft) or more long, horizontally marbled and banded dark and light green. Racemes, 30–75cm (12–30in) long, of tubular, green or greenish white flowers, 6–10mm (¼–½in) long, are produced intermittently. Dwarf cultivars are suitable for growing in bowls and pans. ↕ 1.2m (4ft), ↔ 50cm (20in). W. tropical Africa. ❁ (min. 13°C/55°F). **'Bantel's Sensation'** 🏆 has variable, slender, slightly spiralled, dark green leaves, to 60cm (24in) long, with intermittent, vertical cream stripes. **'Golden Hahnii'** ▣🏆 forms dwarf rosettes of broad leaves, to 20cm (8in) long, with bold, golden yellow, vertical stripes, particularly at the margins; rarely flowers; ↕↔ 12cm (5in). **'Hahnii'** 🏆 (Bird's nest) is dwarf, with rosettes of broad, mid-green leaves, 25cm (10in) long, crossbanded with darker green; rarely flowers; ↕ to 15cm (6in), ↔ 18cm (7in). **'Laurentii'** ▣🏆 has upright leaves, 45cm (18in) long, horizontally marbled mid- and dark green, with broad yellow margins; ↕ 1–1.2m (3–4ft). **'Silver Hahnii'** ▣ is dwarf, with rosettes of broad, dark green leaves, to 25cm (10in) long, banded silver; flowers are rarely borne; ↕↔ 12cm (5in).

SANTOLINA

ASTERACEAE/COMPOSITAE

Genus of 18 species of evergreen shrubs occurring in dry, rocky habitats in the Mediterranean. They have alternate, entire, pinnatisect, or pinnate, aromatic leaves, and tiny flowers borne in long-stemmed, dense, button-like heads, surrounded by several rows of involucral bracts. Each individual floret is tubular, usually hermaphrodite, and yellow or white; there are no ray-florets. They are grown mainly for their ornamental and aromatic foliage, and are suitable for a mixed or shrub border or a rock garden; they may also be used for ground cover, edging, or as low hedges.

- **HARDINESS** Frost hardy.
- **CULTIVATION** Grow in poor to moderately fertile, well-drained soil in full sun. Pruning group 10, in spring.
- **PROPAGATION** Sow seed in containers in a cold frame in autumn or spring. Root semi-ripe cuttings with bottom heat in late summer.
- **PESTS AND DISEASES** Trouble free.

S. chamaecyparissus 🏆 syn. *S. incana* (Cotton lavender). Compact, rounded shrub producing white-woolly young shoots, densely covered with slender, narrowly oblong, toothed to pinnatisect, grey-white leaves, to 4cm (1½in) long, with very fine, toothed divisions. Bright yellow flowerheads, to 1cm (½in) across, are borne on slender stems in mid- and late summer. ↕ 50cm (20in), ↔ 1m (3ft). W. and C. Mediterranean. ❄❄. **'Lambrook Silver'** has silver-grey leaves.

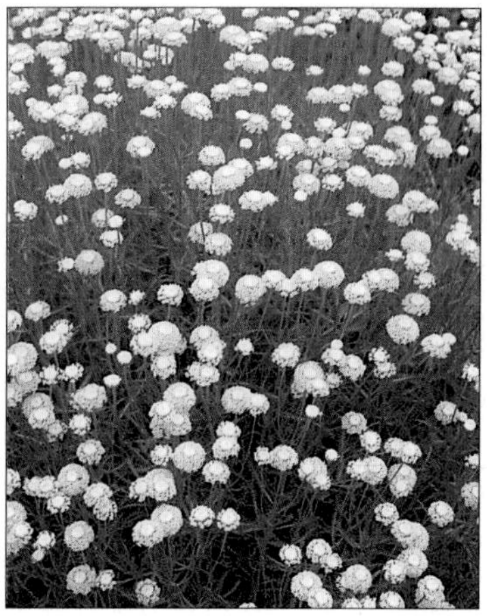

Santolina pinnata subsp. *neapolitana* 'Sulphurea'

'Lemon Queen' ▣ is compact, with lemon-yellow flowerheads; ↕↔ 60cm (24in). **'Pretty Carol'** is compact, with soft grey foliage; ↕↔ 40cm (16in). **'Small-Ness'** is dwarf; ↕↔ 20cm (8in). **subsp. *tomentosa*** see *S. pinnata*. **'Weston'** is very dwarf, with very silvery foliage; ↕ 15cm (6in), ↔ 20cm (8in).
S. incana see *S. chamaecyparissus*.
S. neapolitana see *S. pinnata* subsp. *neapolitana*.
S. pinnata, syn. *S. chamaecyparissus* subsp. *tomentosa*. Rounded, bushy shrub with slender, pinnate, hairless, slightly aromatic, mid-green leaves, to 4cm (1½in) long, with many cylindrical leaflets. Creamy white flowerheads, 2cm (¾in) across, are borne in midsummer. ↕ 75cm (30in), ↔ 1m (3ft). Italy. ❄❄.

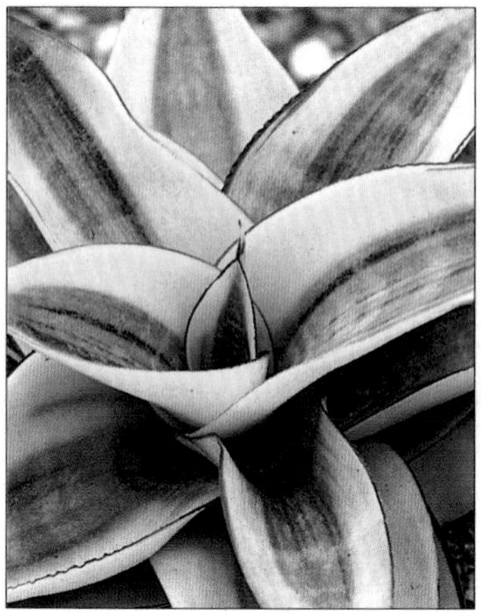

Sansevieria trifasciata 'Golden Hahnii'

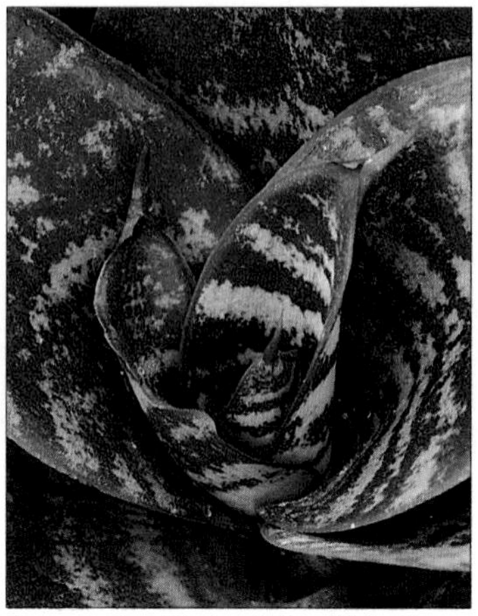

Sansevieria trifasciata 'Silver Hahnii'

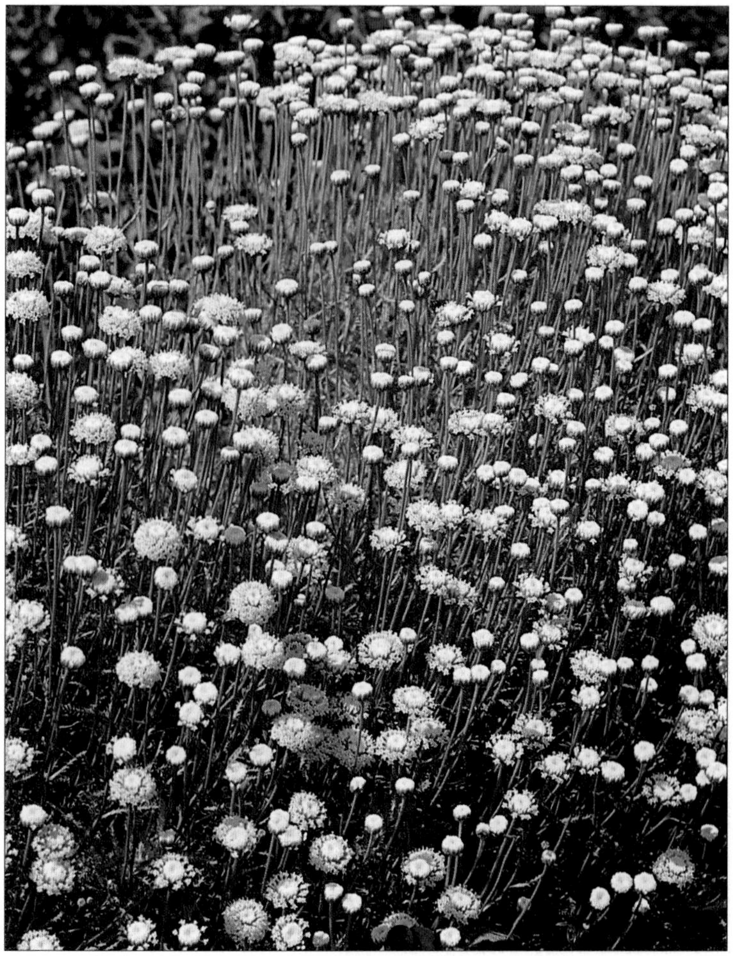

Santolina chamaecyparissus 'Lemon Queen'

Mainly represented in gardens by the following subspecies and its forms. **subsp. *neapolitana*** 🏆 syn. *S. neapolitana*, *S. tomentosa*, has aromatic, grey-green foliage and bright yellow flowerheads. **subsp. *neapolitana* 'Edward Bowles'** has grey-green foliage and creamy white flowerheads. **subsp. *neapolitana* 'Sulphurea'** ▣ has grey-green foliage and primrose-yellow flowerheads.
S. rosmarinifolia, syn. *S. virens*, *S. viridis*. Dense, rounded, bushy shrub with slender, finely cut, aromatic, bright green leaves, to 5cm (2in) long. Bright yellow flowerheads, 2cm (¾in) across, are produced at the end of slender shoots in midsummer. ↕60cm (24in), ↔ 1m (3ft). S.W. Europe. ❄❄.
'Primrose Gem' 🏆 has pale yellow flowerheads.
S. tomentosa see *S. pinnata* subsp. *neapolitana*.
S. virens see *S. rosmarinifolia*.
S. viridis see *S. rosmarinifolia*.

SANVITALIA
Creeping zinnia
ASTERACEAE/COMPOSITAE

Genus of 7 species of creeping and spreading annuals and perennials from rocky slopes and dry river washes in S.W. USA and Mexico. They have opposite, simple, oval leaves, and bear daisy-like, bright yellow, orange, or white flowerheads. Creeping zinnias provide colourful ground cover in an annual or herbaceous border, raised bed, or rock garden, or at the edge of a path. They are also suitable for a trough, or for containers on a patio. Modern cultivars are good for hanging baskets.
• **HARDINESS** Fully hardy.
• **CULTIVATION** Grow in moderately fertile, humus-rich, well-drained soil in full sun.
• **PROPAGATION** Sow seed *in situ* in autumn or spring. Delay thinning autumn-sown seedlings until spring.
• **PESTS AND DISEASES** Trouble free.

S. procumbens ▣ (Creeping zinnia). Prostrate, mat-forming annual with pointed, oval, mid-green leaves, to 6cm (2½in) long. Bears single, black-centred, bright yellow flowerheads, to 2cm (¾in) across, over a long period from early summer to early autumn. ↕to 20cm (8in), ↔ to 45cm (18in). Mexico. ❄❄❄. **'Gold Braid'** is compact, producing golden yellow flowerheads; ↕5–10cm

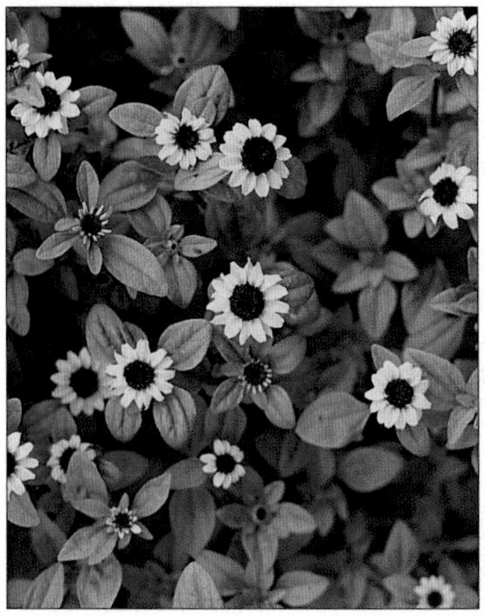
Sanvitalia procumbens

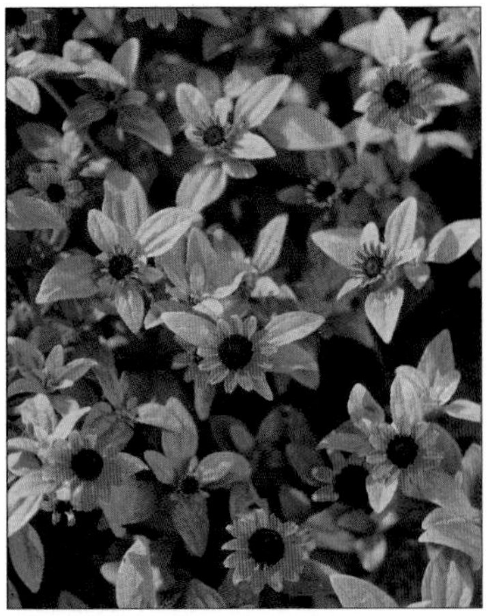
Sanvitalia procumbens 'Mandarin Orange'

(2–4in), ↔ 35cm (14in). **'Golden Carpet'** is dwarf, producing very dark green leaves and small, lemon-yellow flowerheads; ↕ to 10cm (4in). **'Mandarin Orange'** ▣ is compact, with semi-double orange flowerheads; ↕ to 10cm (4in), ↔ 35cm (14in).

SAPINDUS
SAPINDACEAE

Genus of 13 species of deciduous or evergreen trees, shrubs, and climbers, widely distributed in woodland and on riverbanks in warm-temperate, sub-tropical, and tropical regions. They are cultivated for their alternate, simple or pinnate leaves, axillary or terminal racemes or panicles of small, 4- or 5-petalled flowers, and fleshy, spherical fruits. They grow best in a continental climate, with long, hot summers, where they are effective shade trees. Useful for gardens with poor, dry soil.
• **HARDINESS** Fully hardy to frost tender.
• **CULTIVATION** Grow in poor to moderately fertile, well-drained soil in full sun, sheltered from cold winds. Pruning group 1.
• **PROPAGATION** Sow seed of hardy species in containers in a cold frame in spring, after cold stratification for 8 weeks. Sow seed of tender species at 16–18°C (61–64°F) in spring.
• **PESTS AND DISEASES** Trouble free.

S. drummondii ♀ (Western soapberry). Spreading, deciduous tree producing pinnate leaves, to 40cm (16in) long, with up to 18 lance-shaped, glossy, mid-green leaflets, turning golden yellow in autumn. Small, creamy white flowers are borne in conical, terminal panicles, to 25cm (10in) long, in late spring and early summer; they are followed by spherical, orange-yellow fruit, 1cm (½in) across. ↕15m (50ft), ↔ 10m (30ft). S. USA, N. Mexico. ❄❄❄ (borderline)

SAPONARIA
Soapwort
CARYOPHYLLACEAE

Genus of about 20 species of annuals and perennials, some with a woody rootstock, mostly from meadows or rocky areas in the mountains of Europe and S.W. Asia. Closely related to *Lychnis* and *Silene*, they differ in having flowers with 2 styles rather than 3 or 5.

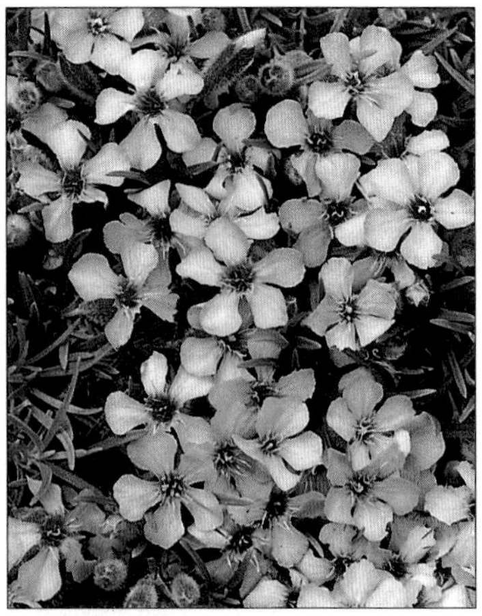
Saponaria caespitosa

They have opposite, entire, variably shaped, narrow leaves and abundant flat, 5-petalled, clawed flowers, usually in shades of pink, borne in loose or dense heads, panicles, or cymes. The genus includes compact plants, suitable for a rock garden, trough, or raised bed, and taller, spreading plants, useful for a herbaceous or mixed border.
• **HARDINESS** Fully hardy.
• **CULTIVATION** Grow border perennials in moderately fertile, well-drained, neutral to slightly alkaline soil in full sun. More compact species, such as *S. caespitosa*, require gritty, sharply drained soil. Cut *S. ocymoides* back hard after flowering, to maintain a compact habit.
• **PROPAGATION** Sow seed in containers in an open frame in autumn or spring. Divide border perennials in autumn or spring. Root softwood cuttings in early summer.
• **PESTS AND DISEASES** May be damaged by slugs and snails.

***S.* 'Bressingham'** 🏆 syn. *S.* 'Bressingham Hybrid'. Loose, mat-forming perennial with hairy, narrowly ovate-lance-shaped, mid-green leaves, to 1.5cm (½in) long. Bears many short-stemmed, panicle-like cymes of brilliant deep pink flowers, to 1cm (½in) across, in summer. Ideal for a trough or rock garden. ↕8cm (3in), ↔ 30cm (12in). ❄❄❄
***S.* 'Bressingham Hybrid'** see *S.* 'Bressingham'.
S. caespitosa ▣ Compact, densely tufted, mat-forming perennial with a woody rootstock and narrowly lance-

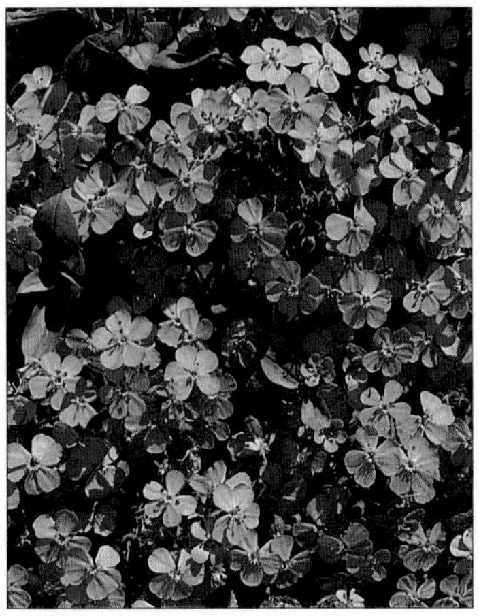
Saponaria ocymoides

shaped, mid-green leaves, 5mm (¼in) long. Few-flowered heads of pink to purple flowers, 1cm (½in) across, are borne just above the leaves in summer. ↕↔ 15cm (6in). Pyrenees. ❄❄❄
S. ocymoides ▣🏆 (Tumbling Ted). Spreading, mat-forming perennial with ovate-lance-shaped, hairy, bright green leaves, to 1cm (½in) long. A profusion of pink flowers, 1cm (½in) across, opens in loose, panicle-like cymes, in summer. May swamp smaller plants. ↕8cm (3in), ↔ 45cm (18in) or more. Mountainous areas from Spain to Yugoslavia. ❄❄❄. **'Alba'** is less vigorous, with white flowers. **'Rubra Compacta'** 🏆 has a neat, dense habit, and dark red flowers.
S. officinalis (Bouncing Bet, Soapwort). Upright perennial, spreading rapidly by rhizomes, with narrowly ovate, rough, prominently veined, mid-green leaves, 4–7cm (1½–3in) long. From summer to autumn, bears panicle-like cymes of pink, red, or white flowers, to 2cm (¾in) across. ↕60cm (24in), ↔ 50cm (20in). Europe. ❄❄❄. **'Alba Plena'** bears abundant double white flowers, pink in bud. **'Dazzler'**, syn. 'Taff's Dazzler', 'Variegata', has single pink flowers, and leaves heavily variegated cream. Less invasive than the species. **'Rubra Plena'** tends to spread, and has double red flowers that fade to pink. **'Taff's Dazzler'** see 'Dazzler'. **'Variegata'** see 'Dazzler'.
S. x olivana ▣🏆 (*S. pumilio* x *S. ocymoides*). Cushion-forming perennial with narrowly lance-shaped, mid-green leaves, 7mm (¼in) long. Produces branching stems around the edges of the cushion, each bearing heads of several pale pink flowers, 1.5cm (½in) across, in summer. ↕5cm (2in), ↔ 15cm (6in). Garden origin. ❄❄❄

▷ **Sapphire berry** see *Symplocos paniculata*
▷ **Sapphire flower** see *Browallia speciosa*
▷ **Sarana, Black** see *Fritillaria camschatcensis*

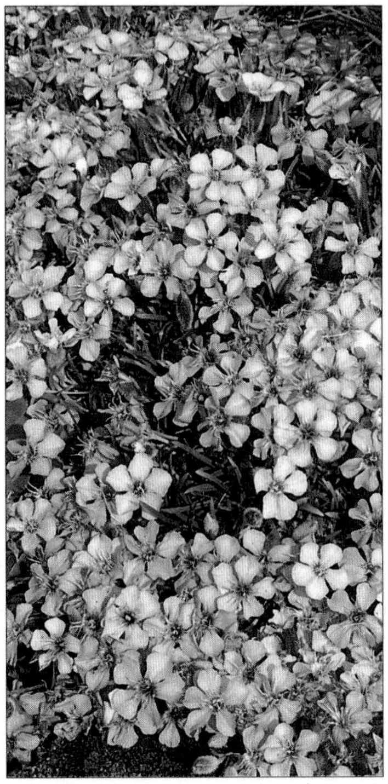
Saponaria x *olivana*

S

SARCOCAPNOS

PAPAVERACEAE

Genus of 3 or 4 species of dwarf, tufted annuals or perennials from cliff crevices in mountains throughout S.W. Europe and N. Africa. They are grown for their fleshy, simple or 2- or 3-ternate, finely divided leaves, to 15cm (6in) long, and for their terminal racemes of spurred flowers, similar to those of *Corydalis*, which are borne in spring and summer. Grow in a scree bed, raised bed, or in tufa; they are also delicate, short-lived plants for an alpine house.

• **HARDINESS** Frost hardy.

• **CULTIVATION** Grow in moderately fertile, sharply drained, alkaline soil, in full sun with some midday shade; protect from excessive winter wet. In an alpine house, grow in a mix of 2 parts grit and 1 part each loam and leaf mould, with additional tufa chippings.

• **PROPAGATION** Sow seed in containers in a cold frame as soon as ripe. Plants grown under glass often self-seed.

• **PESTS AND DISEASES** Aphids and red spider mites may be a problem under glass.

S. enneaphylla. Tuft-forming annual or short-lived perennial with brittle, branching stems bearing fern-like, 2- or 3-ternate, blue-green leaves, to 10cm (4in) long, consisting of ovate to elliptic leaflets with heart-shaped bases. In spring, produces racemes of 5–15 white or pink flowers, to 2cm (¾in) long, with short spurs. ↕↔ 15cm (6in). S. Spain, Morocco. ✻✻

SARCOCAULON

GERANIACEAE

Genus of about 15 species of freely branching, deciduous, succulent perennials and subshrubs from very dry areas of Angola, Namibia, and South Africa. Stem branches are armed with usually small thorns and have hard, resinous bark. The opposite leaves are of 2 types: primary, with long stalks that become spines, and secondary, with shorter stalks that may persist as blunt stumps in the axils of the primary leaves. Solitary, trumpet-shaped flowers are borne mostly from winter to summer. Where temperatures fall below 10°C (50°F), grow in a temperate or warm greenhouse or conservatory; in warmer climates, use in a desert garden.

• **HARDINESS** Frost tender.

• **CULTIVATION** Under glass, grow in standard cactus compost in full light with low humidity. In growth, water moderately, and apply a half-strength balanced liquid fertilizer monthly; water sparingly in winter, but mist lightly on warmer days. Outdoors, grow in poor to moderately fertile, sharply drained soil in full sun. Protect from excessive winter wet. See also pp.48–49.

• **PROPAGATION** Sow seed at 24°C (75°F) as soon as ripe.

• **PESTS AND DISEASES** Susceptible to mealybugs.

S. herrei. Shrubby, succulent perennial with spreading branches marked with leaf scars, and bearing thorns to 2.5cm (1in) long. Triangular to rounded, fleshy, 2- or 3-pinnatisect leaves, 1.5–2cm (½–¾in) long, are yellowish green with silky hairs. White and yellow flowers, 2cm (¾in) across, are borne in winter. ↕↔ to 30cm (12in). South Africa (Western Cape). ❀ (min. 10°C/50°F)

SARCOCOCCA

Christmas box, Sweet box

BUXACEAE

Genus of about 14 species of monoecious, evergreen, sometimes rhizomatous shrubs found in moist, shady places, forest, and thickets from China to the Himalayas and S.E. Asia. They are grown for their foliage, usually fragrant flowers, and berry-like fruits. The leaves are mainly alternate, rarely opposite, entire, and narrowly lance-shaped to broadly ovate or elliptic. Tiny, fragrant, petalless, white or whitish green male and female flowers, 5mm (¼in) long, are borne in small clusters or spikes in the leaf axils. The male flowers have conspicuous anthers; the females are produced below the males in the inflorescence. Grow as ground cover in a woodland garden, or use as a low, informal hedge. Tolerant of atmospheric pollution, dry shade, and neglect.

• **HARDINESS** Fully hardy to frost hardy.

• **CULTIVATION** Grow in moderately fertile, humus-rich, moist but well-drained soil in deep or partial shade. Full sun is tolerated if the soil remains moist. Shelter from cold, drying winds. Pruning group 8.

• **PROPAGATION** Sow seed in containers outdoors in autumn or spring. Take semi-ripe cuttings in late summer. Remove suckers in late winter.

• **PESTS AND DISEASES** Trouble free.

S. confusa ▣ 🏆 Dense, rounded, bushy shrub with elliptic, tapered, glossy, dark green leaves, to 6cm (2½in) long. Clusters of about 5 very fragrant white flowers are borne in winter, followed by spherical, glossy black fruit, 5mm (¼in) across. ↕ 2m (6ft), ↔ 1m (3ft). Probably W. China. ✻✻✻

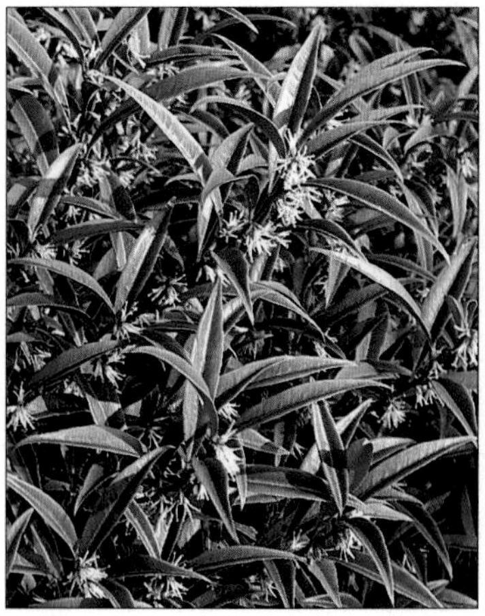

Sarcococca hookeriana var. *digyna* 'Purple Stem'

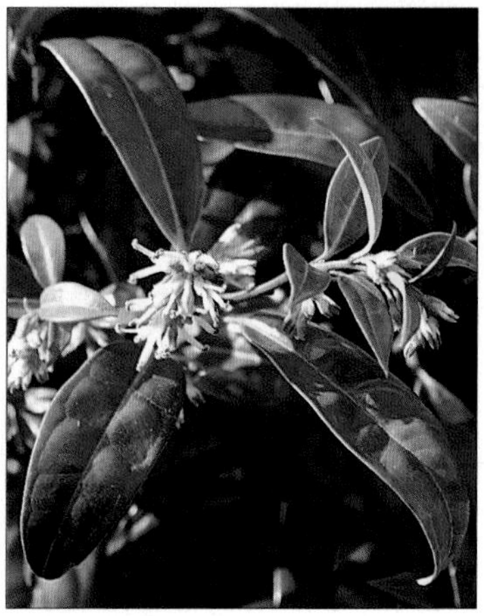

Sarcococca humilis

S. hookeriana 🏆 Rhizomatous, thicket-forming, suckering, compact shrub with lance-shaped to oblong, mid- to dark green leaves, to 9cm (3½in) long. Clusters of fragrant white flowers are borne in winter, followed by spherical, black or blue-black fruit, 5mm (¼in) across. ↕ 1.5m (5ft), ↔ 2m (6ft). W. China. ✻✻✻. **var. *digyna*** 🏆 has slender, tapered leaves, and male flowers with cream anthers. **var. *digyna* 'Purple Stem'** ▣ has young shoots flushed dark purple-pink, and pink-tinged flowers. **var. *humilis*** see *S. humilis*.

S. humilis ▣ syn. *S. hookeriana* var. *humilis*. Dwarf, clump-forming shrub, spreading by suckers, with erect shoots and oblong, glossy, dark green leaves, to 8cm (3in) long. In winter, bears clusters of fragrant, pink-tinged white flowers, the males with pink anthers, followed by spherical, dark blue-black fruit, 5mm (¼in) across. ↕ 60cm (24in), ↔ 1m (3ft). W. China. ✻✻✻

S. ruscifolia. Dense, bushy shrub with arching shoots and ovate, tapered, glossy, dark green leaves, to 6cm (2½in) long. Clusters of fragrant, creamy white flowers are produced in winter, and are followed by spherical, dark red fruit, 5mm (¼in) across. ↕↔ 1m (3ft). W. and C. China. ✻✻. **var. *chinensis*** 🏆 has narrowly ovate to lance-shaped leaves.

S. saligna. Thicket-forming shrub with erect shoots and narrowly lance-shaped, finely tapered leaves, to 14cm (5½in) long, dark green above, pale green beneath. In winter and early spring, bears spikes, to 1.5cm (½in) long, of unscented, greenish white flowers, followed by ovoid purple fruit, to 1cm (½in) long. ↕ 1m (3ft), ↔ 2m (6ft). Afghanistan to Nepal (Himalayas). ✻✻

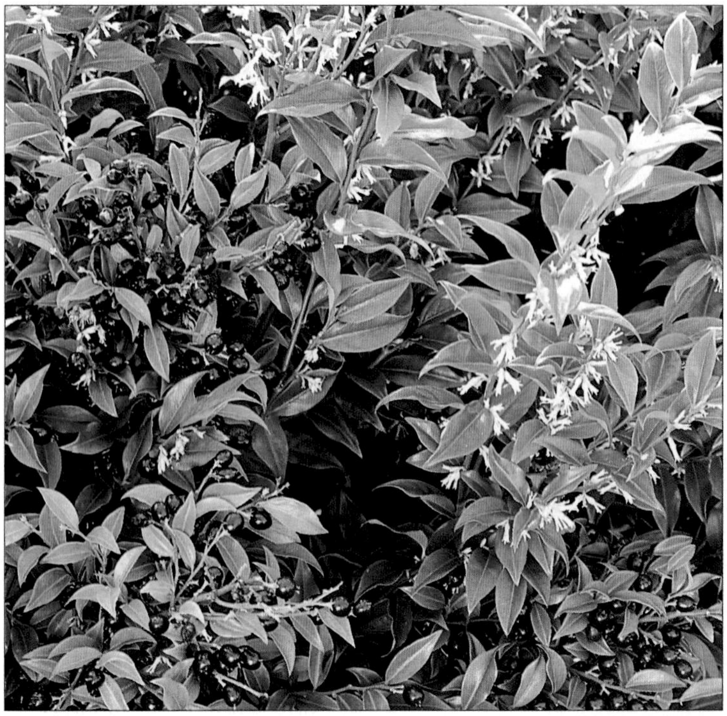

Sarcococca confusa

SARITAEA

BIGNONIACEAE

Genus of a single species of woody-stemmed, evergreen tendril climber from woodland in N. South America. It produces opposite pairs of leaves and cyme-like panicles of tubular-bell-shaped flowers, with 5 spreading petal lobes. Where temperatures fall below 10°C (50°F), grow in a temperate or warm greenhouse. In warmer regions, grow over a pergola or arch, or through the branches of a tree.

• **HARDINESS** Frost tender.

• **CULTIVATION** Under glass, grow in loam-based potting compost (JI No.2) in bright filtered light. When in growth, water freely and apply a balanced liquid fertilizer monthly; maintain moderate to high humidity. Water sparingly in winter. Outdoors, grow in moderately fertile, humus-rich, moist but well-drained soil, in full sun with some midday shade, or in partial shade. Pruning group 11, in early spring.

• **PROPAGATION** Sow seed at about 16°C (61°F) in spring. Root semi-ripe cuttings with bottom heat in late summer. Layer in early spring.

• **PESTS AND DISEASES** Red spider mites may be a problem under glass.

S. magnifica, syn. *Arrabidaea magnifica*. Vigorous, erect climber with leaves composed of 2 obovate, rich green leaflets, to 10cm (4in) long, those on the main climbing stems having hook-tipped tendrils. Cyme-like panicles of tubular-bell-shaped, pale purple to rose-pink flowers, 7–9cm (3–3½in) across, with light yellow to white, V-shaped markings inside, are borne in several flushes throughout the year. ↕ to 10m (30ft) or more. Colombia, Ecuador. ❀ (min. 10°C/50°F)

S

SARMIENTA

GESNERIACEAE

Genus of one species of small, shrubby, creeping, evergreen perennial growing epiphytically on trees in cool rainforest in temperate Chile. It has simple leaves in opposite pairs, and 5-lobed, tubular, axillary flowers. Where temperatures fall below 5°C (41°F), grow in a cool or temperate greenhouse, or conservatory. In milder areas, grow over mossy rocks, or epiphytically on a tree.

- **HARDINESS** Frost tender, but may survive short spells down to 0°C (32°F).
- **CULTIVATION** Under glass, grow in 2 parts loamless potting compost and 1 part each fine-grade granulated bark and leaf mould, or grow epiphytically. Provide bright indirect light. In growth, water freely, applying a balanced liquid fertilizer monthly. Mist daily in summer. Water sparingly in winter. Outdoors, grow in fertile, humus-rich soil, ideally mixed with sphagnum moss, in light dappled shade or partial shade.
- **PROPAGATION** Sow seed at 16–21°C (61–70°F) in spring. Root stem-tip cuttings in late summer, with bottom heat. Separate rooted stems in spring.
- **PESTS AND DISEASES** Red spider mites may infest plants grown under glass.

S. repens 🏆 syn. *S. scandens.* Creeping or low-climbing perennial with semi-woody, rooting stems and obovate to elliptic, minutely glandular, light to mid-green leaves, to 2.5cm (1in) long, with 3–5 shallow to deep teeth at the tips. In summer, bears solitary, pendent, tubular scarlet flowers, 2–2.5cm (¾–1in) long. ↕ prostrate, ↔ to 30cm (12in) or more. S. Chile. ⌂ (min. 5°C/41°F)
S. scandens see *S. repens.*

SARRACENIA

Pitcher plant

SARRACENIACEAE

Genus of 8 species of evergreen or deciduous, carnivorous perennials found in acid and nutrient-deficient bogs from the Canadian Arctic to Florida, USA. Short, stout rhizomes bear sparse, wiry roots and rosettes of phyllodes, some or all of which are modified into nectar-secreting, insect-catching pitchers. The mostly vertical, sometimes horizontal, attractively marked pitchers, 5–90cm (2–36in) long, have lateral wings and hooded lids. Mainly in spring, solitary, nodding or pendent, more or less cup-shaped flowers, with 4 or 5 sepals and 5 petals, are borne above the pitchers. Where temperatures fall below -5°C (23°F), grow in a cold or cool greenhouse or on a sunny window-sill. In warmer areas, grow on a damp, shaded peat terrace.

- **HARDINESS** Fully hardy to frost hardy.
- **CULTIVATION** Under glass, grow in half pots of 3 parts sphagnum moss and 1 part each leaf mould and lime-free coarse sand or grit, in full light with shade from hot sun. In growth, apply a balanced liquid fertilizer monthly. In summer, stand containers in trays of lime-free water. In winter, keep just moist, cool, and well ventilated. Outdoors, grow in humus-rich, moist but sharply drained, acid soil in full sun. Irrigate with lime-free water.
- **PROPAGATION** Sow seed of species at 16–21°C (61–70°F) in spring, after cold stratification for 2 weeks; place the pot in a tray of lime-free water. Prick out seedlings when 3 tiny pitchers appear. Divide in spring.
- **PESTS AND DISEASES** Prone to scale insects, mealybugs, aphids, and tortrix moth caterpillars.

S. drummondii see *S. leucophylla.*
S. flava ▣ 🏆 (Yellow trumpet). Very variable perennial bearing erect, yellow-green pitchers, 30–90cm (12–36in) long, with round mouths and raised lids, often veined red. Phyllodes that do not produce pitchers are linear, and persist throughout the winter. In spring, bears yellow flowers, to 10cm (4in) across. ↕ 50–100cm (20–39in), ↔ to 1m (3ft). USA (Virginia to Alabama, Florida). ❄❄. **'Burgundy'** has pitchers plum-coloured outside. **'Maxima'** has pitchers 90cm (36in) long, with purple-veined lids and stems.
S. leucophylla 🏆 syn. *S. drummondii* (White trumpet). Semi-evergreen perennial bearing erect, slender pitchers, 25–100cm (10–39in) long, with narrow wings and erect lids with wavy margins. The lids and tops are typically white, often with light or heavy purple-red netting, gradually merging into green bases. In spring, bears purple flowers, to 7cm (3in) across. ↕ 50–90cm (20–39in), ↔ to 1m (3ft). USA (Missouri to Florida). ❄❄
S. purpurea (Huntsman's cup). Very variable perennial bearing horizontal, purple-veined, purple or green pitchers, 5–50cm (2–20in) long, with upcurved ends, broad wings, and erect, entire, smooth, often glossy, broad lids. Dark purple-red and pink to dark red flowers, occasionally yellow, to 5cm (2in) across, are produced in spring. ↕ 10–15cm (4–6in), ↔ 1m (3ft). Canadian Arctic to USA (New Jersey). ❄❄❄. **subsp. *venosa*** has more inflated, rough, green to purple pitchers, with broader, wavy lids that extend beyond the mouths; flowers are purple or rose-pink; USA (New Jersey to Louisiana), naturalized in Ireland; ❄❄

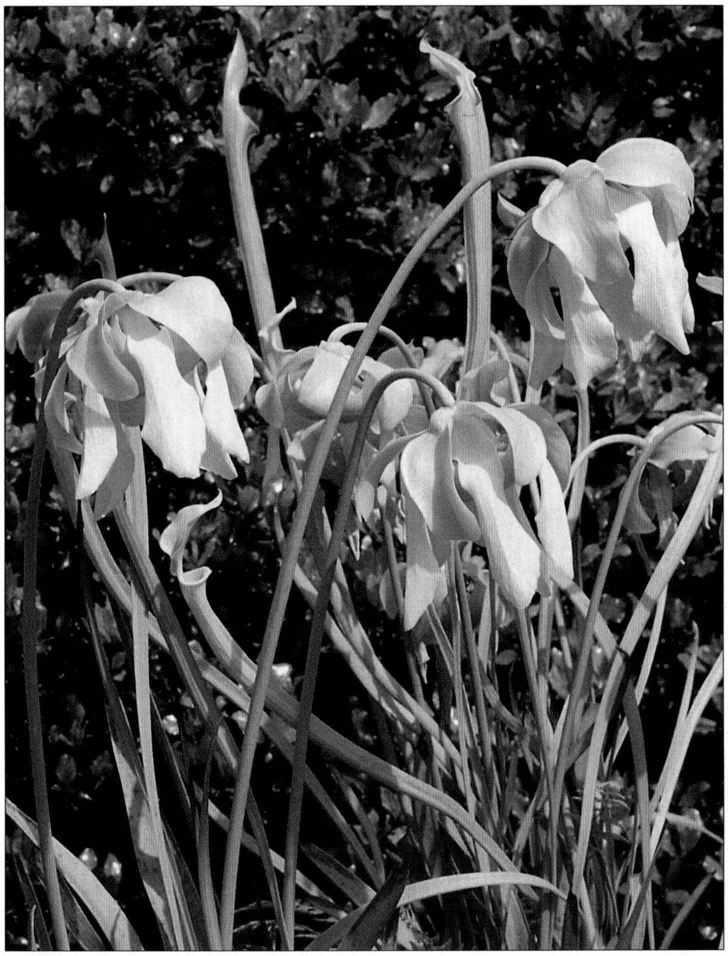

Sarracenia flava

SASA

GRAMINEAE/POACEAE

Genus of 40–50 species of small to medium-sized bamboos, with running rhizomes, closely related to *Sasaella,* to which several species of *Sasa* have now been transferred. They are found in damp hollows and woodland in Japan, Korea, and China. The ascending canes are smooth and cylindrical, with persistent, bristly sheaths and a white-waxy bloom beneath the nodes. The large, usually broad, thick, toothed, and tessellated leaves often wither at the margins in winter, giving a variegated effect. Use as ground cover under trees, or as a hedge; sasas tolerate deep shade.

- **HARDINESS** Fully hardy.
- **CULTIVATION** Grow in fertile, humus-rich, moist but well-drained soil in full sun to deep shade; tolerant of most soils, but avoid dry soils when planting in full sun. To restrict spread, plant in containers and plunge into the soil.
- **PROPAGATION** Divide or cut sections of the youngest rhizomes in spring.

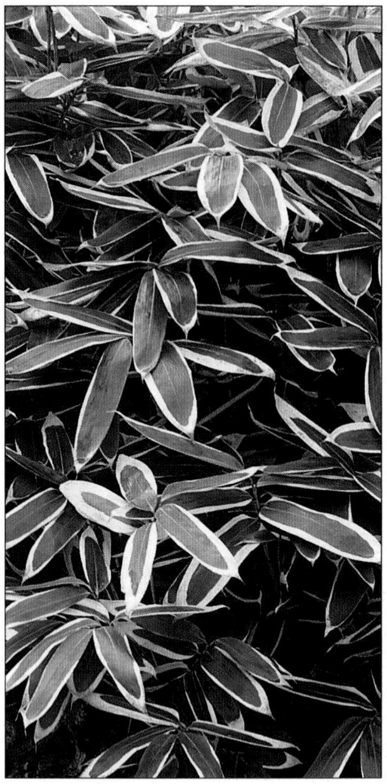

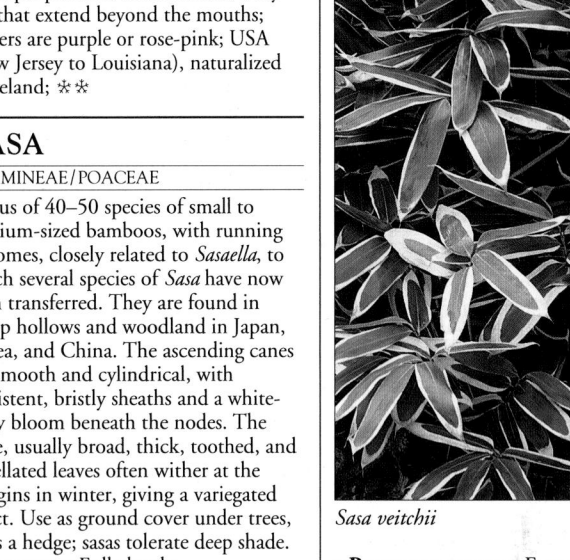

Sasa veitchii

- **PESTS AND DISEASES** Emergent shoots may be eaten by slugs.

S. albomarginata see *S. veitchii.*
S. humilis see *Pleioblastus humilis.*
***S. masumuneana* 'Albostriata'**, syn. *Sasaella masumuneana* f. *albostriata.* Low-growing, moderately spreading bamboo with very slender, green or brown canes, producing a single branch at each node. The narrowly elliptic, mid-green leaves, 10–19cm (4–7in) long, are conspicuously white-striped when young, becoming yellow as they mature in autumn, and fading in winter. ↕ to 1.5m (5ft), ↔ indefinite. ❄❄❄
S. palmata* f. *nebulosa. Vigorous bamboo with wide-spreading rhizomes and stout, upward-curved, usually purple-streaked canes that produce a single branch at each node. The broadly elliptic, tapered, smooth, glossy, bright green leaves, 35–40cm (14–16in) long, are paler green beneath, and have yellow midribs. The leaves generally wither at the margins and tips in winter. ↕ to 2m (6ft), ↔ indefinite. Japan. ❄❄❄
S. ramosa, syn. *Arundinaria vagans, Sasaella ramosa.* Extremely vigorous, low-growing bamboo with slender, glossy, bright green canes producing a single branch at each node. Elliptic, mid-green leaves, to 20cm (8in) long, have yellow midribs, and wither at the margins and tips in winter. ↕ 0.6–1.5m (2–5ft), ↔ indefinite. Japan. ❄❄❄
S. ruscifolia see *Shibataea kumasasa.*
S. veitchii ▣ syn. *S. albomarginata.* Moderately spreading bamboo with slender, glaucous, usually purple canes, producing a single branch at each node. The broadly lance-shaped-ovate, ribbed leaves are glossy, dark green, to 25cm (10in) long, and wither at the margins from late autumn. ↕ to 2m (6ft), usually 1–1.2m (3–4ft), ↔ indefinite. Japan. ❄❄❄

▷ ***Sasaella masumuneana* f. *albostriata*** see *Sasa masumuneana* 'Albostriata'
▷ ***Sasaella ramosa*** see *Sasa ramosa*

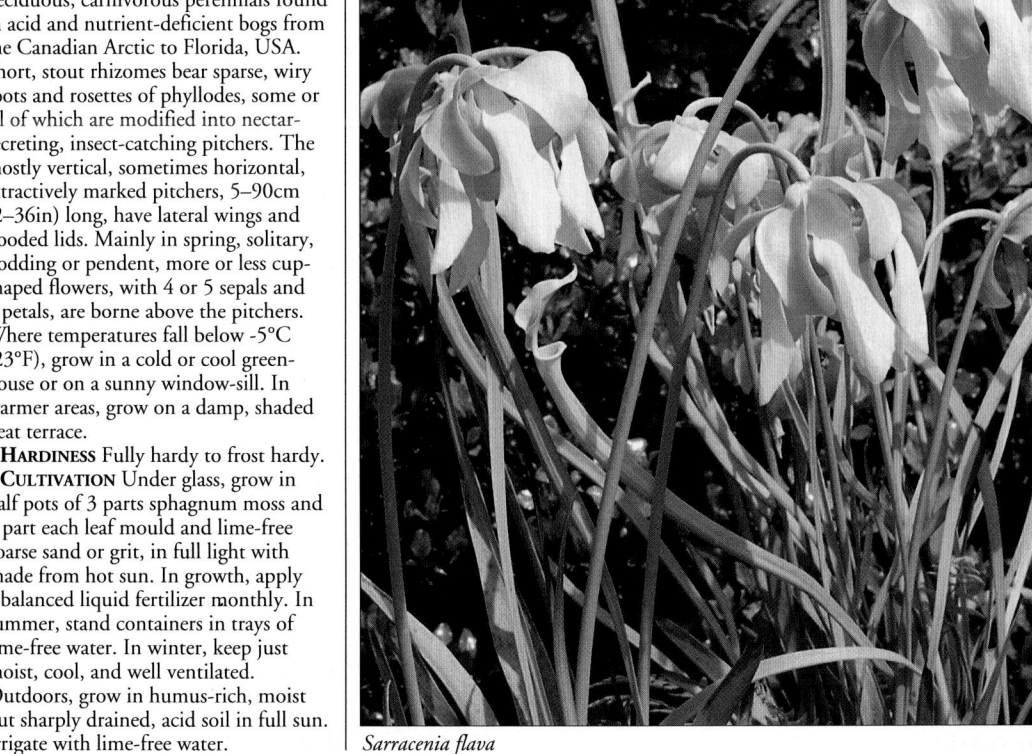

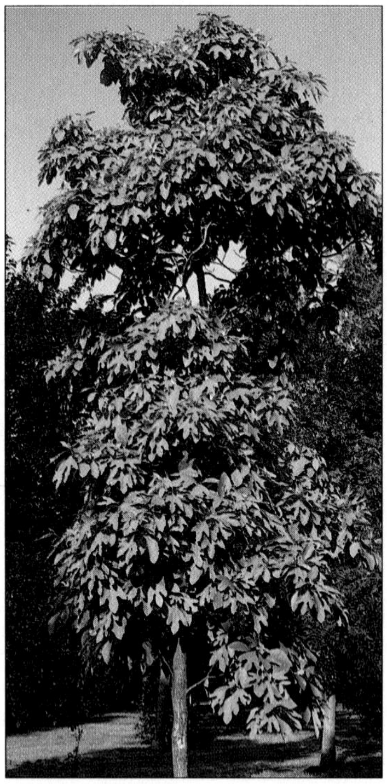

Sassafras albidum

SASSAFRAS

LAURACEAE

Genus of 3 species of generally dioecious, deciduous trees from woodland and thickets in China, Taiwan, and North America. They are cultivated for their stately habit and glossy, aromatic foliage, which colours attractively in autumn. They have deeply fissured bark, and produce alternate, often 1- to 3-lobed, elliptic, oval, ovate, or obovate leaves. Clustered racemes of small, yellow-green flowers are borne in spring, either before or as the leaves emerge. Where plants of both sexes are grown together, the flowers on female plants are followed by ovoid fruits. Grow as specimen trees in a woodland garden or at woodland margins.

- **HARDINESS** Fully hardy.
- **CULTIVATION** Grow in moist but well-drained, moderately fertile, humus-rich, preferably acid, deep soil in full sun or partial shade. Cut out suckers as they arise. Pruning group 1.
- **PROPAGATION** Sow seed in containers in a cold frame as soon as ripe. Take root cuttings in winter.
- **PESTS AND DISEASES** Trouble free.

S

S. albidum ▣ ◊ Broadly columnar to upright tree, spreading by suckers. The elliptic to ovate, entire or shallowly to deeply 3-lobed, aromatic, dark green leaves, to 15cm (6in) long, turn yellow to orange or purple in autumn. Tiny yellow flowers are produced in racemes to 5cm (2in) across, in spring, as the leaves emerge. If pollinated, the flowers on female plants are followed by red-stalked, ovoid, dark blue fruit, 1cm (½in) long. ↕ 25m (80ft), ↔ 15m (50ft). E. North America. ✲✲✲

▷ **Sassafras, Australian** see *Atherosperma moschatum*
▷ **Satin flower** see *Clarkia amoena, Lunaria, L. annua*
▷ **Satinwood** see *Phebalium squameum*

SATUREJA

Savory

LABIATAE/LAMIACEAE

Genus of approximately 30 species of annuals, perennials, and subshrubs, widely distributed throughout the N. hemisphere, occurring in dry, sunny sites and often found on cliffs. They are cultivated for their aromatic leaves, which are opposite, linear to lance-shaped, or oblong-obovate to spoon-shaped, and for their cyme-like or spike-like inflorescences; these consist of whorls of stalkless, tubular, 2-lipped flowers, borne in summer, which are attractive to bees and other insects. Suitable for growing in a mixed border or rock garden. *S. hortensis* and *S. montana* are used as culinary herbs.

- **HARDINESS** Fully hardy to frost hardy.
- **CULTIVATION** Grow in moderately fertile, well-drained, neutral to slightly alkaline soil in full sun. Protect from excessive winter wet. Cut back old shoots of subshrubs in early spring.
- **PROPAGATION** Sow seed at 13–16°C (55–61°F) in late winter or early spring; seed of *S. hortensis* may be sown *in situ* in spring or, in mild climates, in autumn. Take greenwood cuttings of subshrubs in summer.
- **PESTS AND DISEASES** Trouble free.

S. hortensis (Summer savory). Bushy, aromatic annual with linear to narrowly lance-shaped, fresh green leaves, to 3cm (1¼in) long. In summer, bears crowded or lax, whorl-like spikes of 2–5 white or pink flowers, to 7mm (¼in) long. ↕ 25cm (10in), ↔ to 30cm (12in). S.E. Europe. ✲✲
S. montana ▣ (Winter savory). Dwarf subshrub producing stalkless, linear to inversely lance-shaped, leathery, smooth or sparsely hairy, dark greyish green leaves, 0.5–3cm (¼–1¼in) long. For long periods throughout summer, bears whorls of up to 14 lavender-pink to purple flowers, to 8mm (⅜in) long, in dense, upright spikes. ↕ 40cm (16in), ↔ 20cm (8in). S. Europe. ✲✲✲.
'Prostrate White' ▣ is more compact, with erect white flower spikes; ↕↔ to 15cm (6in).
S. repanda see *S. spicigera.*
S. reptans see *S. spicigera.*
S. spicigera, syn. *S. repanda, S. reptans.* Creeping, aromatic subshrub with procumbent stems and linear to lance-shaped, mid-green leaves, to 2.5cm (1in)

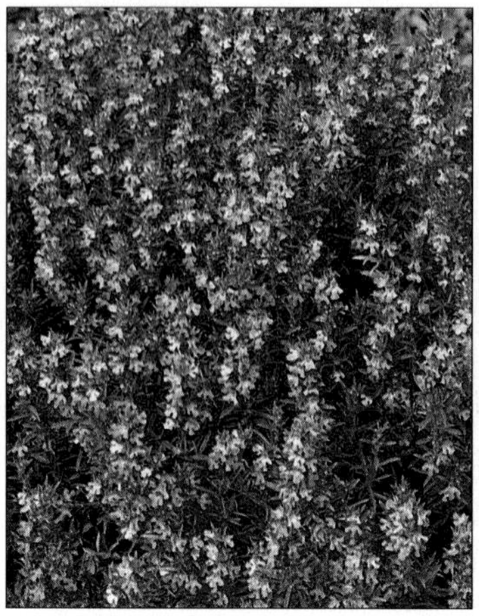

Satureja montana

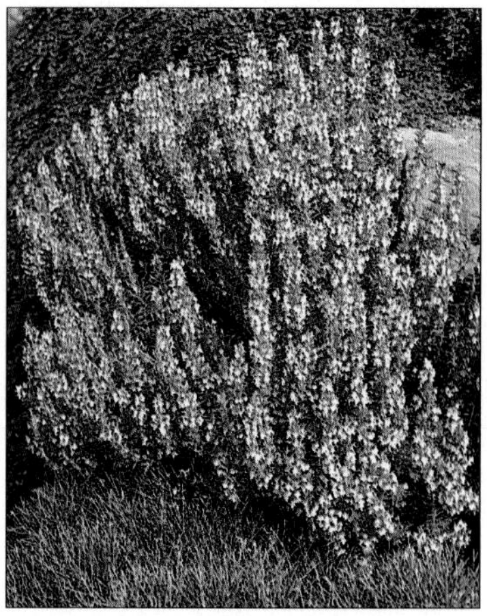

Satureja montana 'Prostrate White'

long. In summer, bears lax cymes of white flowers, 1cm (½in) long, in whorls of up to 16. ↕ 15cm (6in), ↔ 30cm (12in). Turkey, Iran, Caucasus. ✲✲✲

SAUROMATUM

ARACEAE

Genus of 2 species of tuberous perennials from woodland and shady cliffs in the Himalayas and E. and W. Africa, cultivated for their large spathes borne in spring or early summer, followed by single, pedate, long-stalked leaves. In frost-prone areas, grow in a cool greenhouse, or outdoors in summer; elsewhere, grow in a woodland garden.

- **HARDINESS** Frost tender.
- **CULTIVATION** Plant tubers 15cm (6in) deep in late winter. Under glass, grow in loam-based potting compost in bright filtered or indirect light. In growth, water moderately; keep completely dry in winter. Tubers will flower on a saucer without soil or water. Outdoors, grow in well-drained, fertile, humus-rich, neutral to slightly acid soil in partial shade.
- **PROPAGATION** Remove offsets when dormant in winter.
- **PESTS AND DISEASES** Trouble free.

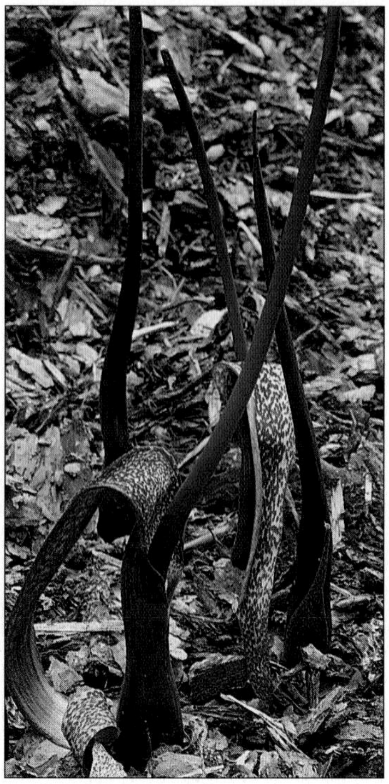

Sauromatum venosum

S. guttatum see *S. venosum.*
S. venosum ▣ syn. *S. guttatum* (Monarch of the East, Voodoo lily). Tuberous perennial with an oblong-lance-shaped, yellowish or greenish white spathe, 30–70cm (12–28in) long, heavily spotted purple, with a foul-smelling, greenish purple spadix, to 35cm (14in) long, produced in late spring and early summer. The spathe is followed by a single, rounded leaf, to 35cm (14in) long, with many oblong-lance-shaped segments. ↕ 30–45cm (12–18in), ↔ 15cm (6in). Himalayas. ❀ (min. 5°C/41°F)

▷ **Sausage tree** see *Kigelia*
▷ **Savin** see *Juniperus sabina*
▷ **Savory** see *Satureja*
Summer see *S. hortensis*
Winter see *S. montana*
▷ **Saw palm** see *Acoelorraphe*
Silver see *A. wrightii*

SAXEGOTHAEA

PODOCARPACEAE

Genus of one species of monoecious, evergreen, coniferous tree or shrub from dense forest in Chile and Argentina. It has whorled branches with irregularly set, yew-like foliage, and bears fleshy, spherical green female cones and tiny male cones. Grow in a woodland garden among other conifers or as a free-standing specimen.

- **HARDINESS** Fully hardy.
- **CULTIVATION** Grow in moderately fertile, well-drained, neutral to slightly acid soil, in full sun with some midday shade, or in partial shade. Shelter from cold, drying winds.
- **PROPAGATION** Take semi-ripe cuttings in late summer or early autumn.
- **PESTS AND DISEASES** Trouble free.

S. conspicua ▣ ◊ (Prince Albert's yew). Slender, conical, coniferous tree or shrub, bushy in cold areas, with smooth, purple-brown bark and whorled branches bearing green shoots. Linear to linear-lance-shaped, dark green leaves, to 3cm (1¼in) long, each have 2 silver crossbands beneath, and persist for 5 or 6 years. Fleshy, spherical, prickly, glaucous-green female cones, 1.5cm (½in) across, contain about 6 seeds, and develop from terminal clusters of scales in autumn. Male cones are cylindrical, dark purple, and borne at the bases of the shoots. ↕ to 20m (70ft), ↔ 5–8m (15–25ft). S. Chile to Argentina. ✲✲✲

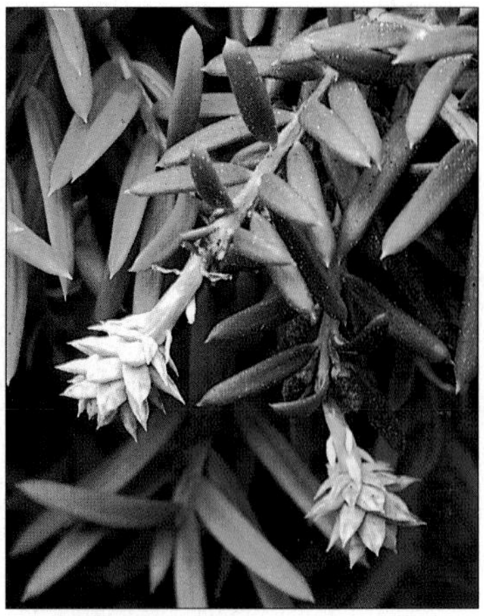

Saxegothaea conspicua

SAXIFRAGA

Saxifrage

SAXIFRAGACEAE

Genus of about 440 species of mostly mat- or cushion-forming, evergreen, semi-evergreen, or deciduous perennials, biennials, and a few annuals, mostly from mountains in the N. hemisphere. Those described are evergreen and perennial unless stated. Varying greatly in habit and leaf form, they produce flat, star-shaped, or shallowly cup-shaped flowers, either singly or in cymes, racemes, or panicles. The rosettes of monocarpic saxifrages die after flowering and are replaced by daughter rosettes. Saxifrages are suitable for rock gardens, mixed borders, and woodland gardens.

Saxifrages are classified botanically into sections, subsections, and series. Those of most horticultural value are as follows.

Section Gymnopera (Robertsonia) Saxifrages with evergreen, rosetted leaves, and flowers in panicles on leafless flower stems. Contains London pride (*S.* x *urbium*) and similar shade-lovers.
Section Irregulares (Diptera) Woodland plants with rosettes of basal, usually deciduous leaves (often evergreen under glass); flower panicles, on leafless stems, appear in summer and autumn.
Section Ligulatae (Euaizoonia) The silver or encrusted saxifrages, which have evergreen, monocarpic rosettes with a conspicuous calcareous (lime) encrustation. Cushion- or mat-forming; flower panicles are borne on leafy stems.
Section Porphyrion (Porophyllum) Cushion- or mat-forming, evergreen perennials with rosettes or leafy shoots, usually with lime-encrusted leaves. The section includes the following horticulturally important subsections. ***Engleria*** – saxifrages with rosettes of leaves alternately arranged, the margins translucent. Flower stems are leafy and distinct, with coloured bracts, and flowers have erect sepals largely hiding the pink, purple, white, or yellow petals, which have basal fringes of hairs; they are borne singly or in small cymes or racemes. ***Kabschia*** – saxifrages with leafy shoots, and alternate leaves with translucent margins. The leafy flowering stems are short or distinct (with up to 15 flowers), and bear white, pink, purple, or yellow flowers, singly or in small cymes or racemes. ***Oppositifoliae*** – saxifrages with opposite leaves, usually without translucent margins. Purple, pink, or white flowers are borne in short cymes of up to 3. Flowering stems are short and leafy or absent.
Section Saxifraga (Dactyloides) Perennial, rarely annual or biennial, usually evergreen saxifrages, sometimes summer-dormant; they produce bulbils. Of varied habit, their often leafy shoots form cushions or mats, with soft, lobed or scalloped leaves, lacking chalk glands. Bears cymes of white, rarely red, pink, or yellow flowers on usually leafy stems. Includes the mossy saxifrages.
Section Xanthizoon are mat- or cushion-forming, evergreen perennials with fleshy, narrow, stalkless leaves, with or without functional chalk glands. Yellow or orange flowers are borne in loose cymes on leafy stems.

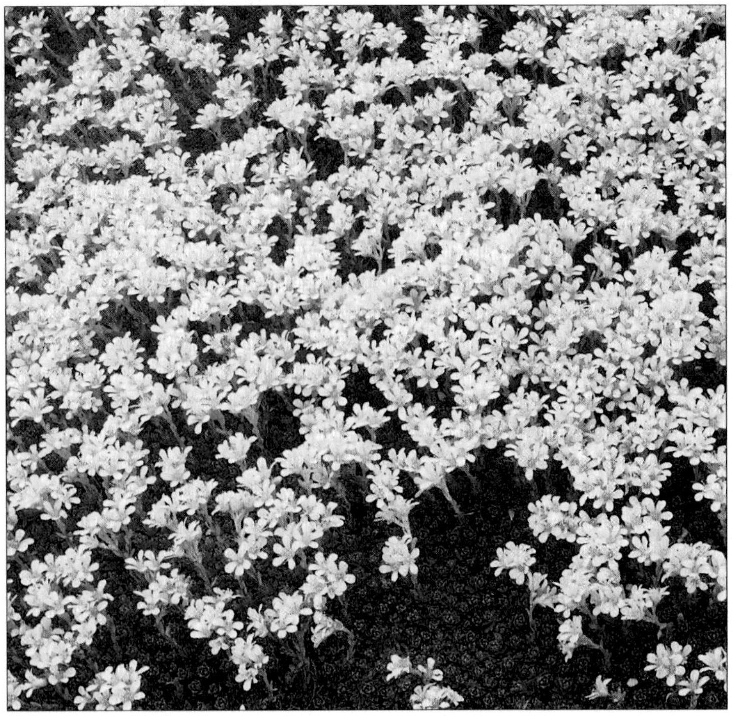

Saxifraga x *apiculata*

• **HARDINESS** Fully hardy; *S. stolonifera* and its cultivars are frost hardy.
• **CULTIVATION** Requirements fall broadly into 4 groups.
1. Grow in moist but well-drained, humus-rich soil in deep or partial shade. Suitable for a border or rock garden.
2. Grow in humus-rich, moist but very sharply drained, neutral to alkaline soil in light shade. Suitable for a rock crevice, scree bed, or alpine house.
3. Grow in moderately fertile, very well-drained, neutral to alkaline soil; keep roots moist. Tolerant of full sun in cool areas, but protect from hot sun in warm areas to prevent leaf scorch. Suitable for a rock garden or trough.
4. Grow in moderately fertile, very sharply drained, alkaline soil or scree in full sun. Suitable for a rock garden, trough, alpine house, or tufa. Some are intolerant of winter wet. In an alpine house, grow in shallow pans in 2 parts loam-based compost (JI No.1) and 1 part limestone chippings.
• **PROPAGATION** Sow seed in autumn in containers in an open frame. Divide herbaceous perennials in spring. Detach individual rosettes and root as cuttings in late spring or early summer.

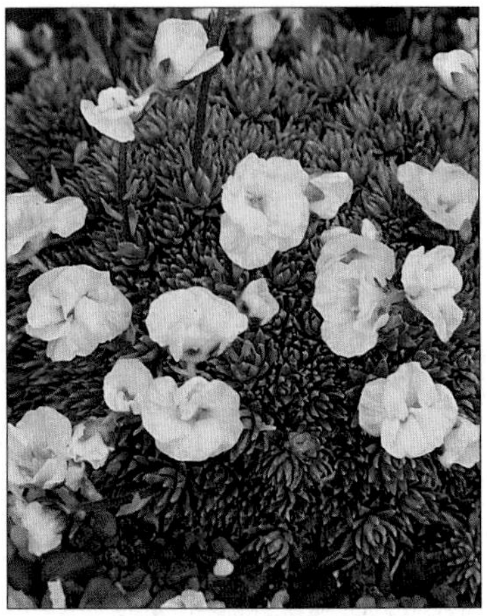

Saxifraga x *boydii* 'Hindhead Seedling'

• **PESTS AND DISEASES** Aphids, slugs, vine weevil grubs, and red spider mites may be a problem.

S. aizoides (Yellow mountain saxifrage). Mat-forming Xanthizoon saxifrage with branching stems bearing tight rosettes of linear to oblong, fleshy, glossy, mid- to dark green leaves, 0.4–2cm (⅛–¾in) long, with 2 short teeth near the tips, and bristly margins. In summer and early autumn, erect, hairy stems bear star-shaped, red-spotted, deep orange flowers, 8mm (⅜in) across, in few-flowered cymes. Cultivation group 2. ↕15cm (6in), ↔20cm (8in). Arctic, alpine areas of Europe, Asia, North America. ❄❄❄
S. aizoon see *S. paniculata.*
S.* x *anglica (*S. aretioides* x *S. lilacina* x *S. media*). Dense, mat- or rosette-forming Kabschia saxifrage with linear-oblong to spoon-shaped, dark green or grey-green to silver, encrusted leaves, 0.3–1.5cm (⅛–½in) long. Cup-shaped, pink to pink-purple flowers, to 2cm (¾in) across, are borne singly or in 2- or 3-flowered cymes in early and mid-spring. Cultivation group 3 or 4. ↕2–6cm (¾–2½in), ↔5–30cm (2–12in). Garden origin. ❄❄❄. **'Cranbourne'** 🏆 has linear, grey-green leaves and, in early summer, bears solitary, almost stemless, deep rose-pink flowers; ↕2.5cm (1in), ↔20cm (8in). **'Myra'**, syn. *S.* 'Myra', is very compact and slow-growing, with narrowly lance-shaped leaves, to 1cm (½in) long. Bears deep red-purple flowers, 1cm (½in) across, in early spring; ↕5cm (2in), ↔10cm (4in).
S.* x *apiculata ▣ (*S. marginata* x *S. sancta*). Cushion-forming Kabschia saxifrage with tight rosettes of linear-lance-shaped, slightly lime-encrusted, deep green leaves, 1cm (½in) long. Produces cymes of 4–12 cup-shaped yellow flowers, 8mm (⅜in) across, in early spring. Cultivation group 3. ↕10cm (4in) ↔30cm (12in). Garden origin. ❄❄❄. **'Gregor Mendel'** 🏆 has glossy, pale green leaves and pale yellow flowers. Good for a rock garden or wall.
S. aretioides. Compact Kabschia saxifrage bearing rosettes of pointed, oblong-lance-shaped, blue-green leaves, 5mm (¼in) long. Produces flat-topped cymes of up to 5 open cup-shaped yellow flowers, 8–10mm (⅜–½in) across, in early spring. Cultivation group 3. ↕8cm (3in), ↔15cm (6in). N.W. Spain, Pyrenees. ❄❄❄
***S.* 'Bob Hawkins'.** Mossy, mat-forming Saxifraga saxifrage with large, soft rosettes of deeply divided, linear, white-variegated, mid-green leaves, to 2cm (¾in) long. In summer, bears cymes of 5–12 upturned, cup-shaped, greenish white flowers, to 2cm (¾in) across, on upright stems. Cultivation group 2. ↕15cm (6in), ↔30cm (12in). ❄❄❄
S.* x *boydii (*S. aretioides* x *S. burseriana*). Dense, rosette-forming Kabschia saxifrage with linear to lance-shaped, often pointed, grey-green to silver-green leaves, 3–10mm (⅛–½in) long. In spring, cup-shaped yellow flowers, to 1.5cm (½in) across, are borne singly or in 2- or 3-flowered cymes. Cultivation group 3 or 4. ↕3–8cm (1¼–3in), ↔15cm (6in). Garden origin. ❄❄❄. **'Faldonside'** 🏆 is vigorous, with irregular cymes of star-shaped, bright yellow flowers, to 2.5cm (1in) across; ↕5cm (2in). **'Hindhead Seedling'** ▣ syn. *S.* 'Hindhead Seedling', has spiny, blue-green leaves, 5–10mm (¼–½in) long, and mostly solitary, yellow-centred, creamy white flowers, to 2.5cm (1in) across; ↕5cm (2in).
S. burseriana ▣ Kabschia saxifrage with firm rosettes of pointed, narrowly lance-shaped, lime-encrusted, grey-green leaves, to 1cm (½in) long. Solitary, cup-shaped white flowers, 1cm (½in) across, open on short red stems in early spring. Cultivation group 3 or 4. ↕to 5cm (2in), ↔15cm (6in). E. Alps. ❄❄❄. **'Gloria'** 🏆 has larger flowers, 3cm (1¼in) across, with yellow centres, on bright red stems.
S. callosa 🏆 syn. *S. lingulata.* Rosette-forming Ligulatae saxifrage with linear, lime-encrusted silver leaves, to 8cm (3in) long. In early summer, arching stems bear narrow panicles, 5–20cm (2–8in) long, of 3–7 star-shaped white flowers, 1cm (½in) across. Cultivation group 4. ↕25cm (10in), ↔20cm (8in). N.E. Spain, S.W. Alps, Apennines to S. Italy, Sicily, Sardinia. ❄❄❄
S. cochlearis. Dense, cushion-forming Ligulatae saxifrage with compact rosettes of spoon-shaped, mid-green leaves, 4cm

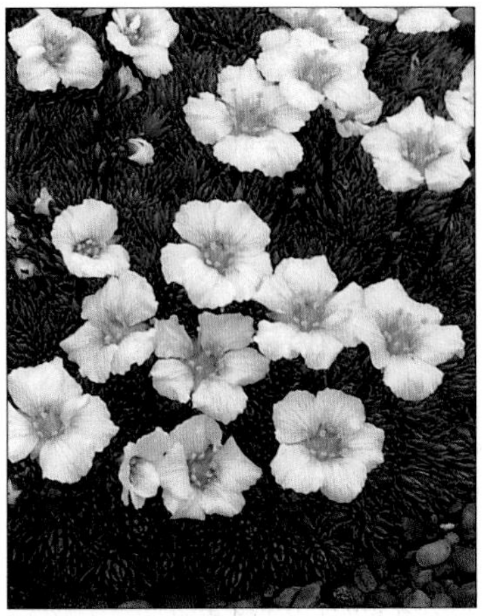

Saxifraga burseriana

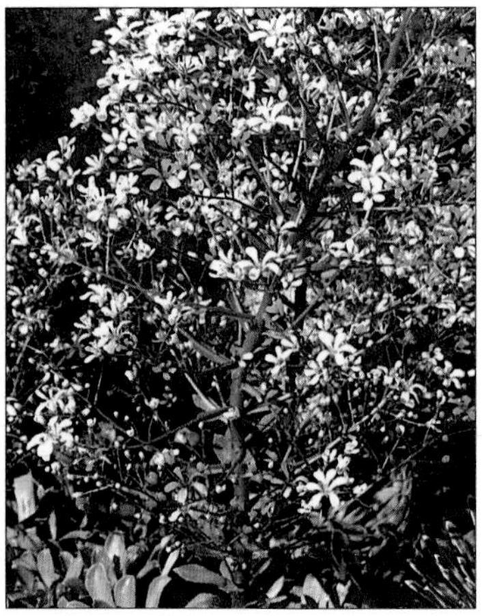

Saxifraga cotyledon

(1½in) long, with lime-encrusted margins. In early summer, bears densely hairy panicles, 6–10cm (2½–4in) long, of 15–25 (occasionally up to 60) rounded, sometimes red-spotted white flowers, 1cm (½in) or more across. Cultivation group 3 or 4. ↕ 20cm (8in), ↔ 15cm (6in). France (Maritime Alps). ❄❄❄. **'Minor'** is lower-growing, and has smaller rosettes; ↕ 10cm (4in).
S. cortusifolia. Deciduous or evergreen Irregulares saxifrage with loose rosettes of kidney-shaped to rounded, 5- or 7-lobed, fleshy, glossy, mid-green leaves, 5–8cm (2–3in) long, with scalloped margins. In late summer, produces pyramidal panicles, to 20cm (8in) long, of cup-shaped white flowers, to 3.5cm (1½in) across, spotted yellow or red.

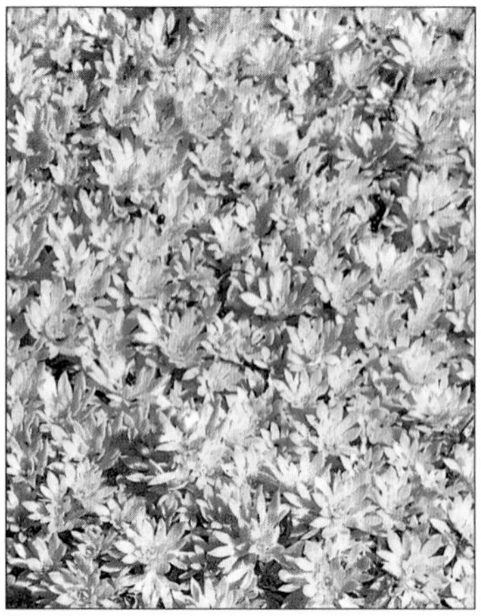

Saxifraga exarata subsp. *moschata* 'Cloth of Gold'

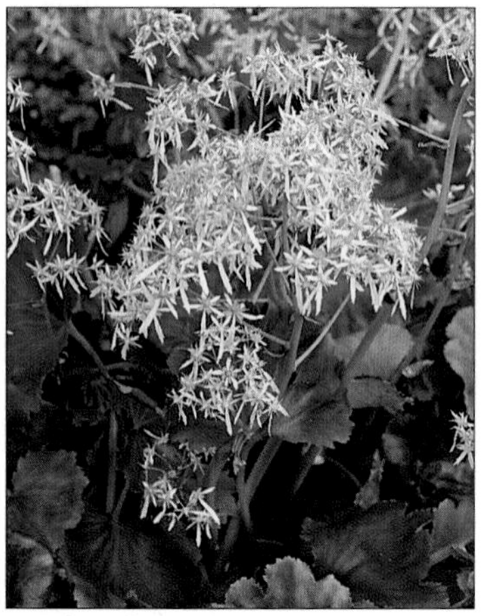

Saxifraga fortunei

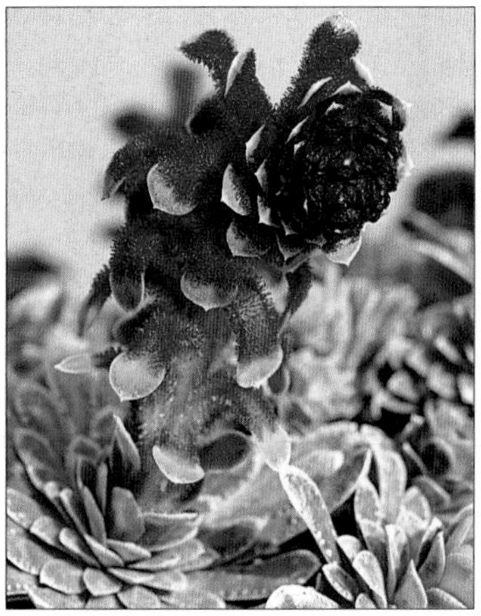

Saxifraga frederici-augusti subsp. *grisebachii* 'Wisley Variety'

Each flower has 3 or 4 upper petals and 1 or 2 much longer lower petals. Cultivation group 1. ↕ 15cm (6in), ↔ 20cm (8in). Japan. ❄❄❄. **var. *fortunei*** see *S. fortunei.*
S. cotyledon ■ Rosette-forming Ligulatae saxifrage with oblong to inversely lance-shaped, pale green leaves, to 8cm (3in) long, with lime-encrusted teeth. In late spring and early summer, bears loose, pyramidal panicles, to 70cm (28in) long, of cup-shaped white flowers, to 1cm (½in) across, often marked red. Cultivation group 3 or 4. ↕ 30–70cm (12–28in), ↔ 20cm (8in). Iceland, Scandinavia, Alps, Pyrenees. ❄❄❄
S. cuneifolia. Mat-forming Gymnopera saxifrage bearing rosettes of stalked, usually wedge-shaped, occasionally ovate to rounded, leathery, fresh green leaves, to 2.5cm (1in) long, purple beneath. In spring and early summer, produces loose panicles, 5–18cm (2–7in) long, of 3–12 (rarely up to 30) star-shaped white flowers, 7mm (¼in) across, frequently spotted yellow, sometimes red, on red-tinted stems. Cultivation group 1. ↕ 20cm (8in), ↔ 30cm (12in). Europe (Carpathians to Pyrenees). ❄❄❄
***S. exarata* subsp. *moschata*,** syn. *S. moschata.* Mossy, mat- or cushion-forming Saxifraga saxifrage with rosettes of variably shaped, entire or 3-lobed, pale green leaves, 0.4–2cm (⅛–¾in) long. From late spring to early autumn, bears flat-topped cymes of 1–7 star-shaped, cream or yellow, occasionally pink-tinted flowers, to 8mm (⅜in) across. Cultivation group 2. ↕ 10cm (4in), ↔ 30cm (12in). C. and S. Europe. ❄❄❄. **'Cloth of Gold'** ■ has golden foliage; best grown in shade.
S. ferdinandi-coburgi 🏆 Dense, irregular cushion-forming Kabschia saxifrage with rosettes of oblong-lance-shaped, chalk-grey, lime-encrusted leaves, to 8mm (⅜in) long, incurved at the tips. In early spring, produces cymes of 7–12 open cup-shaped, rich yellow flowers, 1cm (½in) across, on red-tinged stems. Cultivation group 3. ↕ 10cm (4in), ↔ 15cm (6in). Macedonia, N. Greece, E. Bulgaria. ❄❄❄
S. fortunei ■🏆 syn. *S. cortusifolia* var. *fortunei.* Deciduous or semi-evergreen, clump-forming Irregulares saxifrage with kidney-shaped to rounded, 7-lobed, mid-green leaves, 6–10cm (2½–4in) across, often red-purple beneath or purple-tinged with age; they have deeply heart-shaped bases and scalloped margins. In late summer or autumn, bears loose, pendent, red-stemmed panicles, to 50cm (20in) long, of white flowers, 1cm (½in) across, with 3 upper petals and 1 or 2 longer lower petals. Cultivation group 1. ↕↔ 30cm (12in). Japan. ❄❄❄. **'Rubrifolia'** is compact, with strongly red-suffused leaves and deep red stems; ↕↔ 20cm (8in).
S. frederici-augusti. Cushion-forming Engleria saxifrage with flat rosettes of obovate to spoon-shaped, grey-green, usually lime-encrusted leaves, 1–3.5cm (½–1½in) long. The red stems, which bear several leaves, and flower-stalks are partially covered in long, bright cherry-red to dark purple, glandular hairs. In late spring, produces slender racemes, 3–10cm (1¼–4in) long, of 15–25 cup-shaped, purplish pink flowers, 6mm (¼in) across. Cultivation group 4. ↕ 7–20cm (3–8in), ↔ to 15cm (6in). Macedonia, Albania, Greece, Bulgaria. ❄❄❄. **subsp. *grisebachii* 'Wisley Variety'** ■🏆 has spoon-shaped, silver-grey leaves, arching stems clothed in green-tipped, red-purple bracts, and red-purple flowers; ↕ 10cm (4in).
S. x geum ■ (*S. hirsuta* x *S. umbrosa*). Mat-forming Gymnopera saxifrage with rosettes of long-stalked, sparsely hairy, spoon-shaped, scalloped, mid-green leaves, to 8cm (3in) long. In summer, bears loose panicles, 6–20cm (2½–8in) long, of 2–12 star-shaped white flowers, 7–8mm (¼–⅜in) across, spotted with red. Cultivation group 1. ↕↔ 20cm (8in). Pyrenees. ❄❄❄
S. granulata ■ (Fair maids of France, Meadow saxifrage). Clump-forming, summer-dormant Saxifraga saxifrage with stem and root bulbils, and loose rosettes of kidney-shaped, toothed or scalloped, pale to mid-green leaves, to 3cm (1¼in) long. In late spring, bears panicles, 8–20cm (3–8in) long, of 10–20 rounded white flowers, to 1.5cm (½in) across, on sticky, erect stems. May be naturalized in grass. Cultivation group 2; tolerates full sun in moist soil. ↕ 20–35cm (8–14in), ↔ 30cm (12in). Europe (mostly W.), N. Africa. ❄❄❄. **'Plena'** has double flowers.
***S.* 'Hindhead Seedling'** see *S.* x *boydii* 'Hindhead Seedling'.
***S. x irvingii* 'Jenkinsiae'** ■🏆 syn. *S.* x *jenkinsiae.* Dense, mound-forming, slow-growing Kabschia saxifrage with tight rosettes of wedge-shaped, lime-encrusted, grey-green leaves, 7mm (¼in) long. In early spring, bears abundant solitary, open cup-shaped, dark-centred,

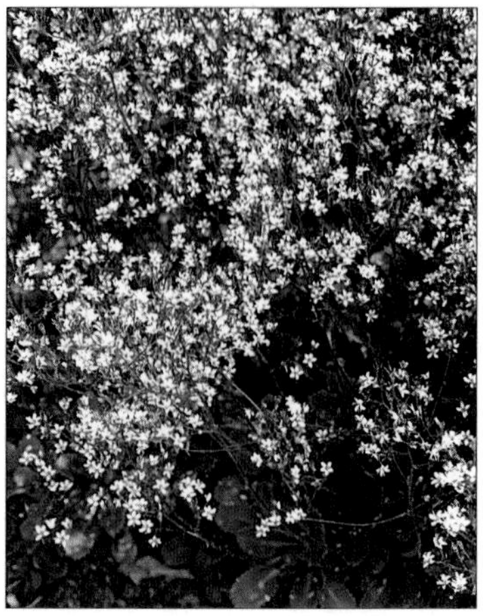

Saxifraga x *geum*

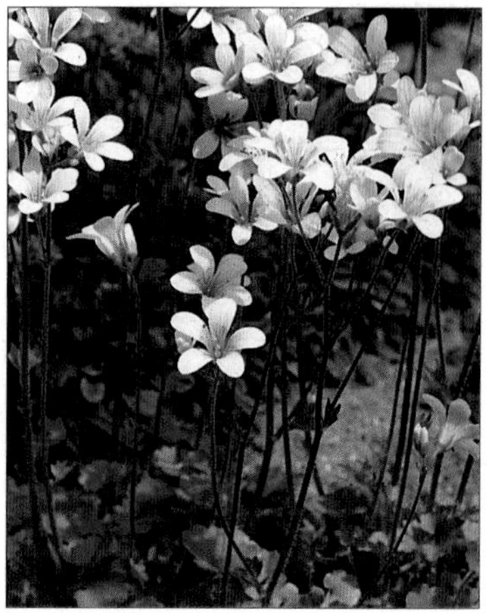

Saxifraga granulata

pale pink flowers, to 2cm (¾in) across, on short red stems. Cultivation group 3. ↕ 5cm (2in), ↔ 20cm (8in). ❄❄❄
S. x jenkinsiae see *S.* x *irvingii* 'Jenkinsiae'.
S. juniperifolia* subsp. *sancta see *S. sancta.*
***S.* 'Kathleen Pinsent'** ■🏆 Rosette-forming Ligulatae saxifrage with narrowly spoon-shaped, silvery leaves, 2–7cm (¾–3in) long, recurved at the tips. In late spring and early summer, bears arching panicles, to 20cm (8in) long, of open cup-shaped, rose-pink flowers, to 2cm (¾in) across. Cultivation group 3 or 4. ↕↔ to 20cm (8in). ❄❄❄
S. lingulata see *S. callosa.*
S. longifolia ■ (Pyrenean saxifrage). Ligulatae saxifrage with a single rosette of linear, lime-encrusted silver leaves, 6–11cm (2½–4½in) long, silver-grey beneath. After 3 or 4 years, produces a huge pyramidal panicle, to 70cm (28in) long, of up to 80 rounded, 5-petalled, open cup-shaped white flowers, 1cm (½in) across, in summer. Cultivation group 4. May only be propagated from seed. ↕ 60cm (24in), ↔ 20cm (8in). Pyrenees. ❄❄❄. **'Tumbling Waters'** see *S.* 'Tumbling Waters'.
S. marginata. Vigorous, cushion- to mat-forming Kabschia saxifrage with rosettes of narrowly elliptic to obovate, lime-encrusted, silver-grey leaves, to 1.5cm (½in) long. Compact panicles, 1–5cm (½–2in) long, of 5–9 open cup-shaped, white, sometimes pink-flushed flowers, to 2cm (¾in) across, are borne in early spring. Cultivation group 3. ↕ 8cm (3in), ↔ 30cm (12in). S. Italy, Balkans, Romania. ❄❄❄

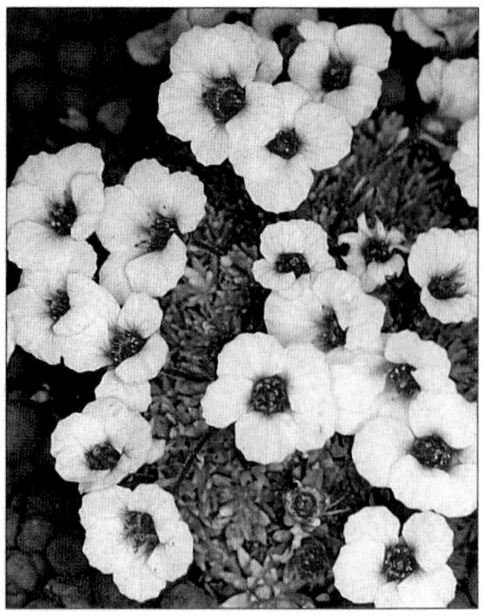

Saxifraga x *irvingii* 'Jenkinsiae'

S

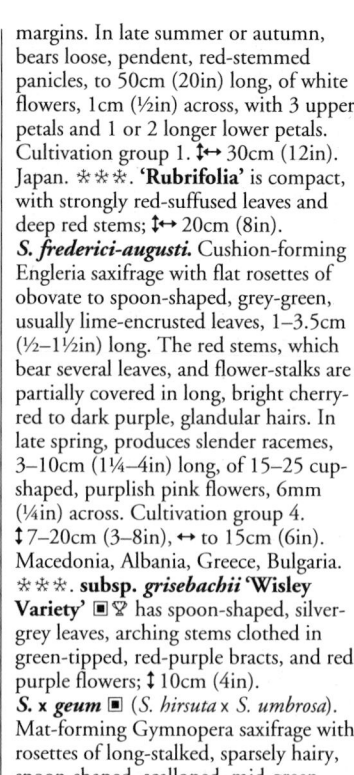

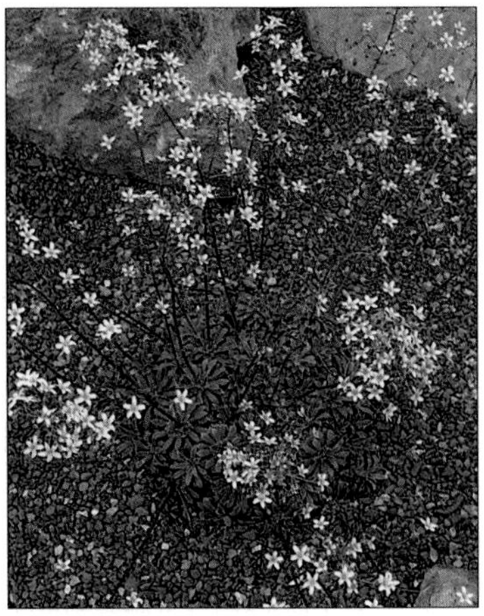

Saxifraga 'Kathleen Pinsent'

S. moschata see *S. exarata* subsp. *moschata.*
S. 'Myra' see *S.* x *anglica* 'Myra'.
S. oppositifolia ▣ (Purple saxifrage). Flat mat-forming Oppositifoliae saxifrage with rosettes of stiff, oblong or elliptic, dark green leaves, to 5mm (¼in) long, on branching stems. In early summer, bears solitary, almost stemless, cup-shaped, deep red-purple to pale pink or white flowers, to 2cm (¾in) across. Cultivation group 2. ↕ 2.5cm (1in), ↔ 20cm (8in) or more. Arctic, mountains of Europe, W. Asia, North America. ✲✲✲. **'Ruth Draper'** has large, bright rose-pink flowers, to 3cm (1¼in) across.
S. paniculata, syn. *S. aizoon.* Variable, mat-forming Ligulatae saxifrage bearing rosettes of incurved, broadly linear or narrowly obovate, grey-green leaves, 0.5–6cm (¼–2½in) long, with lime-encrusted margins. In early summer, numerous cup-shaped flowers open in narrow, flat panicles, 3–20cm (1¼–8in) long. The primary branches each have 1–3, rarely 4, rounded, creamy white, rarely pink flowers, to 1cm (½in) across. Cultivation group 4. ↕ 15cm (6in), ↔ 25cm (10in). Norway, C. and S.

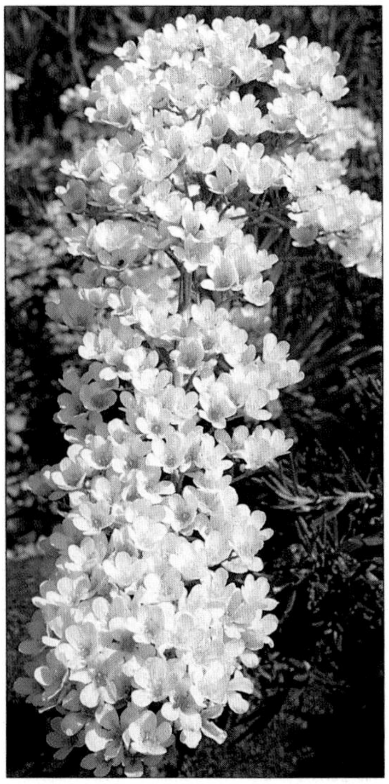

Saxifraga longifolia

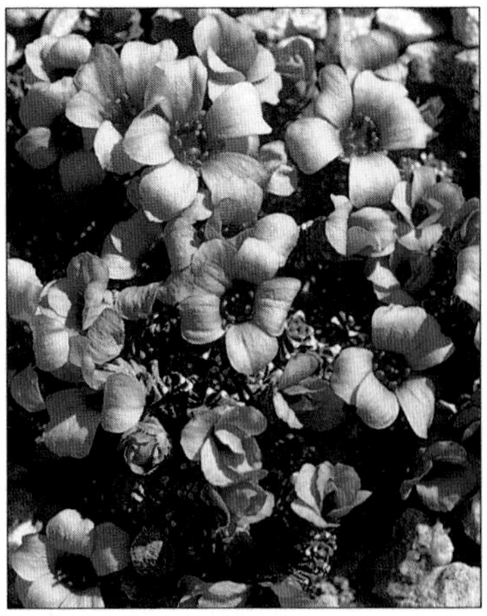

Saxifraga oppositifolia

Europe, Caucasus, Canada, Greenland, Iceland. ✲✲✲. **var. *baldensis*,** syn. 'Baldensis', 'Minutifolia', produces much smaller rosettes and red-tinged flower stems; ↕ 10cm (4in), ↔ 15cm (6in). **'Baldensis'** see var. *baldensis.*
'Minutifolia' see var. *baldensis.*
S. porophylla* var. *thessalica see *S. sempervivum.*
S. 'Primulaize' see *S.* x *primulaize.*
S.* x *primulaize (*S. aizoides* x *S.* x *urbium* or *S. umbrosa*), syn. *S.* 'Primulaize'. Loose, rosette-forming saxifrage, a hybrid of Section Xanthizoon and Section Gymnopera, resembling a miniature *S.* x *urbium.* Fleshy, narrowly ovate, glossy, mid-green leaves are 2–6cm (¾–2½in) long. In summer, bears loose panicles, 15cm (6in) long, of star-shaped, crimson- or salmon-pink flowers, to 1.5cm (½in) across. Cultivation group 1. ↕ 8cm (3in), ↔ 15cm (6in). Garden origin. ✲✲✲
S. primuloides see *S. umbrosa* var. *primuloides.*
S. sancta ▣ syn. *S. juniperifolia* subsp. *sancta.* Cushion-forming Kabschia saxifrage with rosettes of narrowly lance-shaped, lime-encrusted, bright green leaves, to 1cm (½in) long. Cymes of 3–7 upward-facing, open cup-shaped, deep yellow flowers, 7–9mm (¼–⅜in) across, with prominent anthers, are borne in spring. Cultivation group 3. ↕ 5cm (2in), ↔ 20cm (8in). N.E. Greece. ✲✲✲
***S. sarmentosa* 'Tricolor'** see *S. stolonifera* 'Tricolor'.
S. scardica. Dense, cushion-forming, slow-growing Kabschia saxifrage with firm rosettes of fleshy, oblong, lime-encrusted, blue-green leaves, to 1.5cm

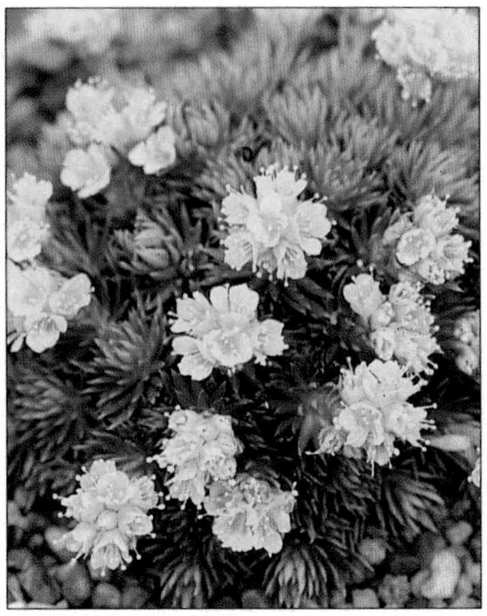

Saxifraga sancta

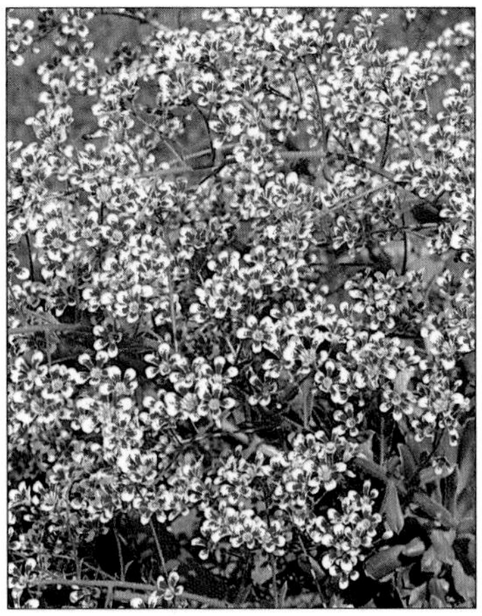

Saxifraga 'Southside Seedling'

(½in) long. In spring, bears cymes of 4–13 upward-facing, cup-shaped white flowers, to 1.5cm (½in) across, on red-tinted stems. Prefers light dappled shade. Cultivation group 3. ↕ 8cm (3in), ↔ 15cm (6in). Balkans. ✲✲✲
S. sempervivum, syn. *S. porophylla* var. *thessalica.* Loose, cushion-forming Engleria saxifrage with rosettes of linear, lime-encrusted, silvery green leaves, to 2cm (¾in) long. In spring, crozier-like, silver-hairy stems bear racemes, 2–8cm (¾–3in) long, of 7–20 pendent, open cup-shaped, deep reddish purple flowers, to 6mm (¼in) across. Cultivation group 4. ↕ 10cm (4in), ↔ 20cm (8in). Balkans, N.W. Turkey. ✲✲✲
S. 'Southside Seedling' ▣ 🏆 Mat-forming Ligulatae saxifrage similar to, and possibly a cultivar of, *S. cotyledon,* with rosettes of oblong to spoon-shaped, pale green leaves, to 12cm (5in) long. Arching panicles, 30cm (12in) long, of open cup-shaped white flowers, 1cm (½in) across, heavily spotted red, are borne in late spring and early summer. Cultivation group 3 or 4. ↕ 30cm (12in), ↔ 20cm (8in). ✲✲✲
S. spruneri. Cushion-forming, slow-growing Kabschia saxifrage. Hairy, oblong or spoon-shaped, lime-encrusted, mid-green leaves, to 7mm (¼in) long, are in small rosettes. In late spring, bears flat-topped cymes of 6–10 star-shaped, yellowish white flowers, to 1cm (½in) across. Cultivation group 3. ↕ 8cm (3in), ↔ 10cm (4in). Balkans. ✲✲✲
***S. stolonifera* 'Magic Carpet'** see *S. stolonifera* 'Tricolor'.
***S. stolonifera* 'Tricolor'** ▣ 🏆 syn. *S. sarmentosa* 'Tricolor', *S. stolonifera*

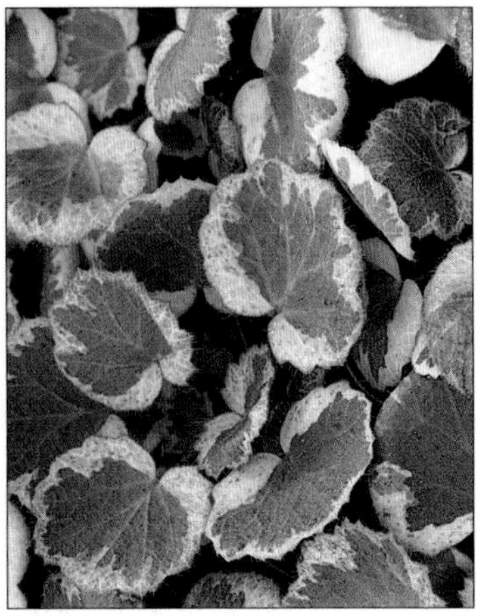

Saxifraga stolonifera 'Tricolor'

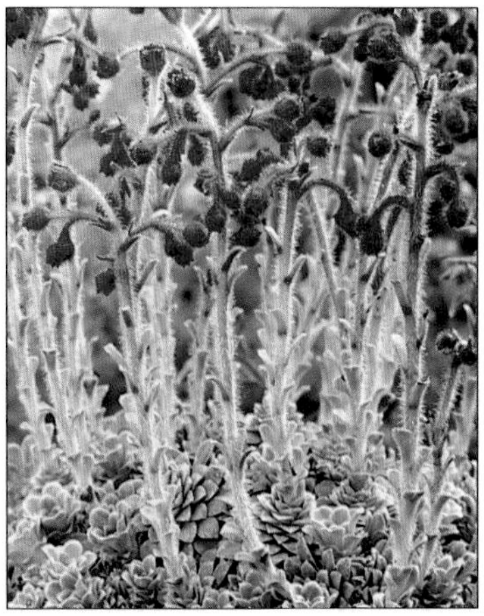

Saxifraga stribrnyi

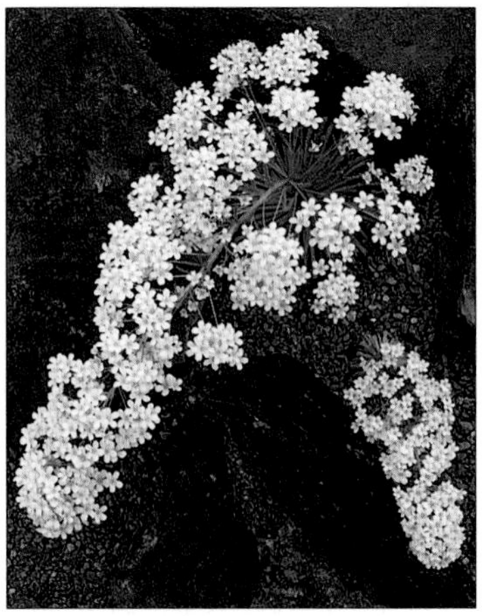

Saxifraga 'Tumbling Waters'

'Magic Carpet' (Mother of thousands). Stoloniferous, rosette- or tuft-forming Irregulares saxifrage with kidney-shaped to rounded, deeply cut, mid- to dark green leaves, 4–9cm (1½–3½in) long, strongly patterned in red and white. In summer, bears loose panicles, 20–40cm (8–16in) long, of tiny white flowers, to 8mm (⅜in) across, spotted yellow or red, with 3 or 4 upper petals and 1 or 2 longer lower petals, on slender, upright stems. Cultivation group 1. ↕↔ to 30cm (12in). ✲✲
S. stribrnyi ▣ Mound-forming Engleria saxifrage with tight rosettes of pointed, inversely lance-shaped to spoon-shaped, lime-encrusted, blue-green leaves, 1–2.5cm (½–1in) long. Bears branched, arching, crozier-like stems with racemes, 2–5cm (¾–2in) long, of 10–30 open cup-shaped, deep violet-purple flowers, to 1cm (½in) across, in late spring and early summer. Cultivation group 4. ↕ 10cm (4in), ↔ 20cm (8in). Balkans. ✲✲✲
S. 'Tumbling Waters' ▣ 🏆 syn. *S. longifolia* 'Tumbling Waters'. Slow-growing Ligulatae perennial with large, clustered rosettes of narrow, linear, lime-encrusted, silvery green leaves, to 15cm (6in) long. Bears dense, arching, conical panicles, 30–70cm (12–28in) long, of small, open cup-shaped white flowers, to 1cm (½in) across, in spring, after several years. Cultivation group 4. ↕ 45cm (18in), ↔ 30cm (12in). ✲✲✲
***S. umbrosa* var. *primuloides*,** syn. *S. primuloides.* Gymnopera saxifrage with neat, compact rosettes of ovate to spoon-shaped, crinkled, regularly scalloped leaves, to 8cm (3in) long, mid-

S

green above, reddish green beneath. Bears loose panicles, to 25cm (10in) long, of star-shaped, red-spotted white flowers, 6–8mm (¼–⅜in) across, in summer. Cultivation group 1. ↕↔ 30cm (12in). Pyrenees. ✻✻✻. **'Clarence Elliott'** see 'Elliott's Variety'. **'Elliott's Variety'**, syn. *S. primuloides* 'Clarence Elliott', *S. primuloides* 'Elliott's Variety', *S. umbrosa* var. *primuloides* 'Clarence Elliott', is more compact, with leaves to 6cm (2½in) long, and red-stemmed, rose-pink flowers, 8–10mm (⅜–½in) across; ↕↔ 15cm (6in).

S. x urbium 🏆 (*S. spathularis* x *S. umbrosa*) (London pride). Vigorous, spreading Gymnopera saxifrage with large rosettes of spoon-shaped, toothed, leathery, mid-green leaves, 2–4cm (¾–1½in) across. Upright, branching stems bear loose panicles, to 30cm (12in) long, of tiny, star-shaped, pink-flushed white flowers, to 8mm (⅜in) across, in summer. Good ground cover, even in poor soil. Cultivation group 1. ↕ 30cm (12in), ↔ indefinite. Garden origin. ✻✻✻

▷ **Saxifrage** see *Saxifraga*
Elephant-eared see *Bergenia*
Golden see *Chrysosplenium*
Meadow see *Saxifraga granulata*
Purple see *Saxifraga oppositifolia*
Pyrenean see *Saxifraga longifolia*
Yellow mountain see *Saxifraga aizoides*

SCABIOSA

Pincushion flower, Scabious

DIPSACACEAE

Genus of about 80 species of annuals, biennials, and perennials from sunny sites, dry meadows, and rocky slopes, mostly in the Mediterranean region, but also in the rest of Europe, the Caucasus, Africa, Asia, and Japan. They have mainly basal leaves, which are simple and entire or lobed, pinnatifid, or pinnatisect, and produce compound or solitary, blue, white, yellow, or pink flowerheads with domed, pincushion-like central florets and larger marginal florets. The smaller perennial species are ideal for a rock garden, while the taller ones are suitable for a sunny herbaceous or mixed border, or a wild garden; the annuals are excellent in borders. Long-flowering species and cultivars are ideal for window-boxes or containers on a patio. Many are also good for cutting. All are attractive to bees and butterflies.

S

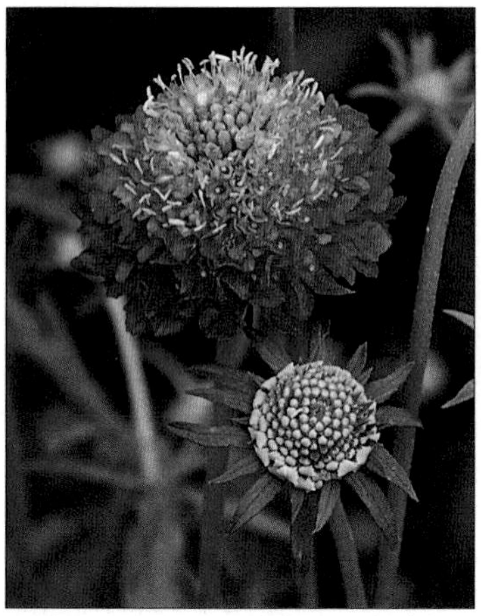

Scabiosa atropurpurea 'Blue Cockade'

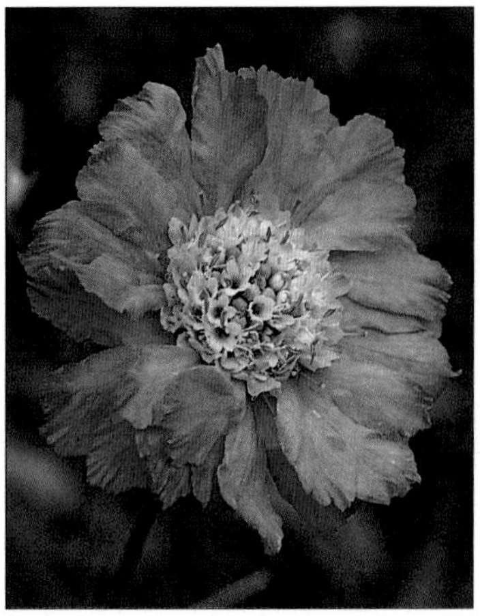

Scabiosa caucasica 'Clive Greaves'

• **HARDINESS** Fully hardy to frost hardy.
• **CULTIVATION** Grow in moderately fertile, well-drained, neutral to slightly alkaline soil in full sun. Protect from excessive winter wet. Dead-head to prolong flowering. Divide and replant perennials in fresh or replenished soil every 3 years.
• **PROPAGATION** Sow seed of annuals and biennials at 6–12°C (43–54°F) in early spring, or *in situ* in mid-spring; sow seed of perennials in containers in a cold frame as soon as ripe or in spring. Divide, or take basal cuttings of perennials, in spring.
• **PESTS AND DISEASES** Trouble free.

S. alpina see *Cephalaria alpina.*
S. arvensis see *Knautia arvensis.*
S. atropurpurea (Pincushion flower, Sweet scabious). Erect, branching, wiry-stemmed biennial or short-lived perennial with mid-green leaves, 3–12cm (1¼–5in) long: the basal leaves are oblong-spoon-shaped and entire or coarsely toothed; the stem leaves are pinnatifid, composed of entire or toothed segments. Solitary, fragrant, dark purple to lilac flowerheads, to 5cm (2in) across, are borne in summer. ↕ to

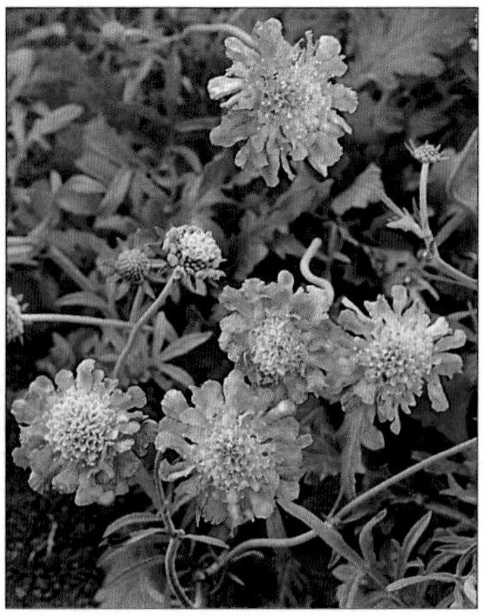

Scabiosa columbaria 'Butterfly Blue'

90cm (36in), ↔ to 23cm (9in). S. Europe. ✻✻✻. **'Blue Cockade'** ▣ has lavender-blue to purple-blue flowerheads, sometimes over 5cm (2in) across. **'Double'** is a mixture with fully double, white, dark purple, blue, or pink flowerheads, which need support. **'Dwarf Double'** is a mixture with fully double flowerheads in white, dark purple, blue, or pink; ↕ to 45cm (18in).
***S.* 'Butterfly Blue'** see *S. columbaria* 'Butterfly Blue'.
***S.* 'Butterfly Pink'** see *S. columbaria* 'Pink Mist'.
S. caucasica. Clump-forming perennial with lance-shaped, entire, grey-green basal leaves, to 15cm (6in) long, with partly winged stalks, and usually unbranched stems bearing pinnatifid leaves. Solitary, pale blue or lavender-blue flowerheads, to 8cm (3in) across, are borne in mid- and late summer. ↕↔ 60cm (24in). Caucasus, N.E. Turkey, N. Iran. ✻✻✻. **'Bressingham White'** has white flowerheads. **'Clive Greaves'** ▣ 🏆 produces lavender-blue flowerheads. **'Floral Queen'** has pale blue flowerheads; ↕ to 75cm (30in). **'Miss Willmott'** ▣ 🏆 has white flowerheads; ↕ to 90cm (36in).

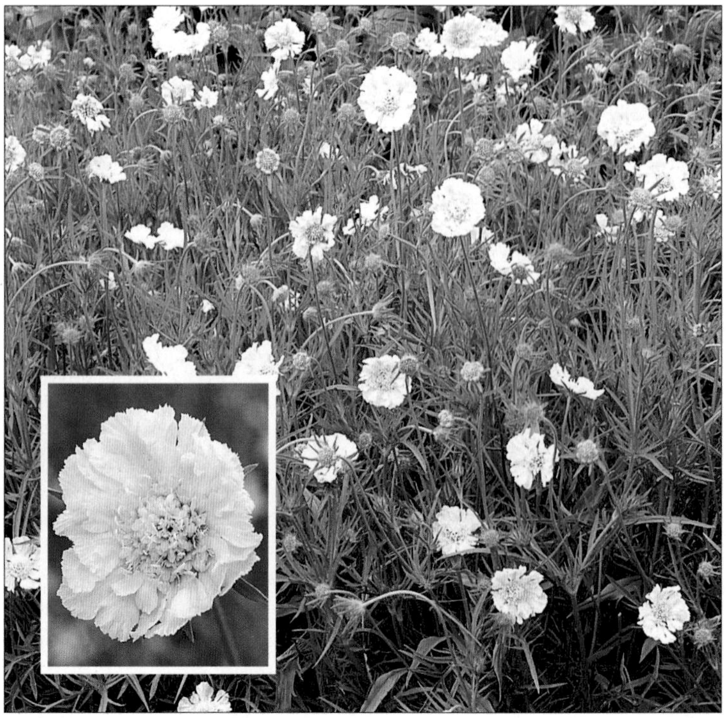

Scabiosa caucasica 'Miss Willmott' (inset: flower detail)

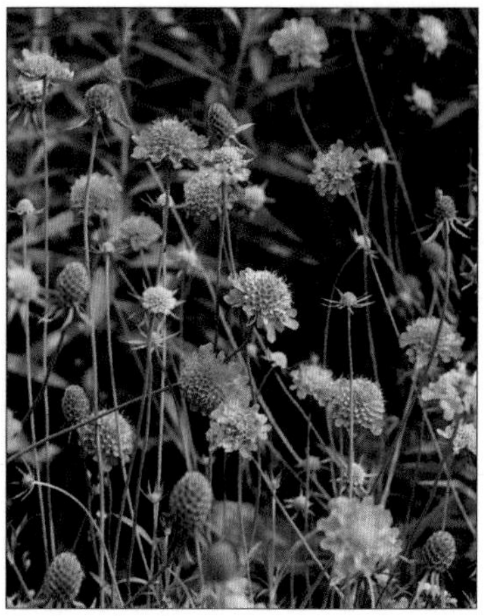

Scabiosa lucida

S. columbaria (Small scabious). Branched, hairy perennial with long-stalked, ovate to lance-shaped, simple or pinnatifid basal leaves, 5–15cm (2–6in) long, and pinnatifid, 2-pinnatifid, or pinnatisect stem leaves, the uppermost very finely divided; all are light, mid-, or greyish green. From summer to early autumn, bears solitary, bluish lilac flowerheads, to 4cm (1½in) across. ↕ 50–70cm (20–28in), ↔ to 1m (3ft) or more. Europe, W. Asia. ✻✻✻. The following cultivars are probably hybrids of *S. columbaria*. **'Butterfly Blue'** ▣ syn. *S.* 'Butterfly Blue', has grey-green leaves, and produces lavender-blue flowerheads in mid- and late summer; ↕↔ to 40cm (16in). **'Pink Mist'**, syn. *S.* 'Butterfly Pink', *S.* 'Pink Mist', is similar to 'Butterfly Blue', with grey-green leaves and deep pink flowerheads, paler in the centres, borne over long periods in summer; ↕↔ to 40cm (16in).
S. gigantea see *Cephalaria gigantea.*
S. graminifolia. Evergreen, clump-forming perennial with tufts of silver-hairy, entire, linear-lance-shaped, mid-green leaves, to 15cm (6in) long. In summer, solitary, spherical, lilac to violet flowerheads, to 4cm (1½in) across, are borne on stiff, slender stems. ↕ 25cm (10in), ↔ 30cm (12in). S. Europe. ✻✻✻. **'Pinkushion'** is mat-forming, with rose-pink flowerheads.
S. lucida ▣ Clump-forming, occasionally branched perennial producing tufts of ovate-lance-shaped, toothed basal leaves and pinnatifid stem leaves; both are silvery green and to 12cm (5in) long. In summer, solitary, pale lilac flowerheads, to 4cm (1½in)

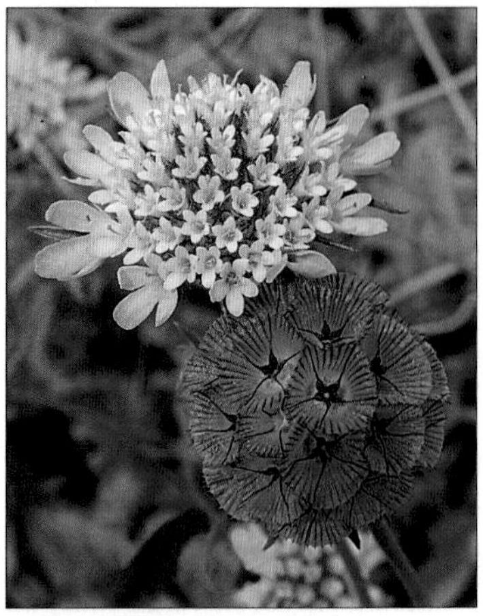

Scabiosa stellata 'Paper Moon'

across, are borne on slender, erect stems. ↕ 20cm (8in), ↔ 30cm (12in). C. Europe. ❄❄❄
***S.* 'Pink Mist'** see *S. columbaria* 'Pink Mist'.
S. rumelica see *Knautia macedonica.*
S. stellata. Erect, branching, wiry-stemmed, hairy annual with lance-shaped to ovate, pinnatifid, mid-green leaves, 18cm (7in) long. Solitary, spherical, pale blue flowerheads, to 3cm (1¼in) across, are borne in summer. They are followed by silvery cream seed heads, to 8cm (3in) across, formed by clustered, cup-shaped, green- or maroon-centred bracts, enlarged after flowering. The seed heads are excellent for dried flower arrangements. ↕ to 45cm (18in), ↔ 23cm (9in). S. Europe. ❄❄❄. **'Drum Stick'** ♀ has light blue flowerheads, turning bronze; ↕ to 30cm (12in). **'Paper Moon'** ▣ produces pale, watery blue seed heads. **'Ping Pong'** bears small white seed heads.
S. succisa see *Succisa pratensis.*
S. tatarica see *Cephalaria gigantea.*

▷**Scabious** see *Scabiosa*
Devil's bit see *Succisa pratensis*
Field see *Knautia arvensis*
Giant see *Cephalaria gigantea*
Sheep's bit see *Jasione laevis*
Shepherd's see *Jasione laevis*
Small see *Scabiosa columbaria*
Sweet see *Scabiosa atropurpurea*
Yellow see *Cephalaria gigantea*

SCADOXUS

Blood lily

AMARYLLIDACEAE

Genus of 9 species of bulbous and rhizomatous perennials from rocky cliffs and woodland in tropical regions of Africa and the Arabian Peninsula. They are closely related to *Haemanthus*, but are distinguished by the spiral arrangement of their leaves, and by their rhizomatous bulbs. They are cultivated for their spectacular, crowded, conical to spherical flowerheads of cylindrical red flowers, with 6 spreading or erect tepals, borne on leafless stems from spring to summer, and followed by spherical, yellow, orange, or red berries. In frost-prone areas, grow blood lilies in a temperate or warm greenhouse or conservatory; elsewhere, use in a border, or at the base of a warm, sunny wall.
• **HARDINESS** Frost tender.
• **CULTIVATION** Plant bulbs in autumn or winter with the necks at soil level.

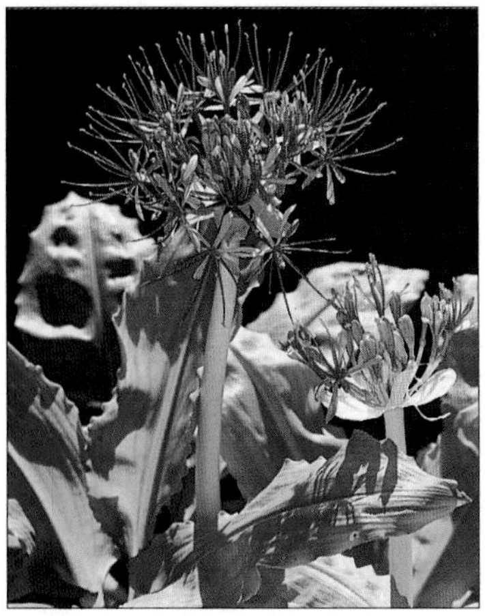

Scadoxus multiflorus subsp. *katherinae*

Under glass, grow in loam-based potting compost (JI No.2) in full light with shade from hot sun. Move into partial shade as buds open. When in active growth, water freely and apply a half-strength balanced liquid fertilizer monthly. Dry off completely as leaves fade. Pot on in spring if necessary. Outdoors, grow in moderately fertile, humus-rich, moist but well-drained soil in full sun or light dappled shade.
• **PROPAGATION** Sow seed at 19–24°C (66–75°F) as soon as ripe. Separate offsets in spring.
• **PESTS AND DISEASES** Trouble free.

S. multiflorus, syn. *Haemanthus multiflorus.* Bulbous perennial with semi-erect, broad, lance-shaped to ovate, basal leaves, to 30cm (12in) long. In summer, produces spherical heads, 10–15cm (4–6in) across, of up to 200 narrow-tepalled red flowers, with conspicuous stamens, followed by small orange berries, 5–10mm (¼–½in) across. ↕ to 60cm (24in), ↔ 15cm (6in). Tropical Africa, South Africa, Yemen. ❄ (min. 10–15°C/50–59°F). **subsp. *katherinae*** ▣ ♀ syn. *Haemanthus katherinae*, has wavy-margined leaves; ↕ to 1.2m (4ft); E. southern Africa.
S. puniceus, syn. *Haemanthus magnificus, H. natalensis, H. puniceus.* Bulbous perennial with semi-erect, elliptic, wavy-margined, basal leaves, to 30cm (12in) long, that form a "stem", to 50cm (20in) long, of sheathed leaf-stalks. From spring to summer, bears conical heads, 10cm (4in) across, of up to 100 tiny, yellowish green to pink or scarlet flowers, surrounded by conspicuous red bracts; they are followed by yellow berries, 1cm (½in) across. ↕ 50cm (20in), ↔ 15cm (6in). E. and southern Africa. ❄ (min. 10–15°C/50–59°F)

SCAEVOLA

GOODENIACEAE

Genus of about 96 species of mostly short-lived, mainly evergreen perennials, but also scrambling climbers, shrubs and small trees, occurring in habitats ranging from coastal dunes to damp, subalpine regions in Australia and Polynesia. They have alternate, rarely opposite, rounded to linear, entire or toothed leaves, and produce solitary or few-flowered cymes or racemes of distinctive, fan-shaped flowers. In frost-prone areas, grow in a cool greenhouse or conservatory, or grow outdoors in containers or hanging baskets during summer. In warmer climates, grow in a border.
• **HARDINESS** Frost tender, but may tolerate falls in temperature to around -3°C (27°F), or perhaps lower, if soil is very sharply drained.
• **CULTIVATION** Under glass, grow in loam-based potting compost (JI No.2) in bright indirect light. During the growing season, water freely and apply a balanced liquid fertilizer monthly. Keep just moist in winter. Outdoors, grow in moderately fertile, humus-rich, moist but well-drained soil in full sun or light dappled shade.
• **PROPAGATION** Sow seed at 19–24°C (66–75°F) in spring. Root softwood cuttings in late spring or summer, with bottom heat.
• **PESTS AND DISEASES** Trouble free.

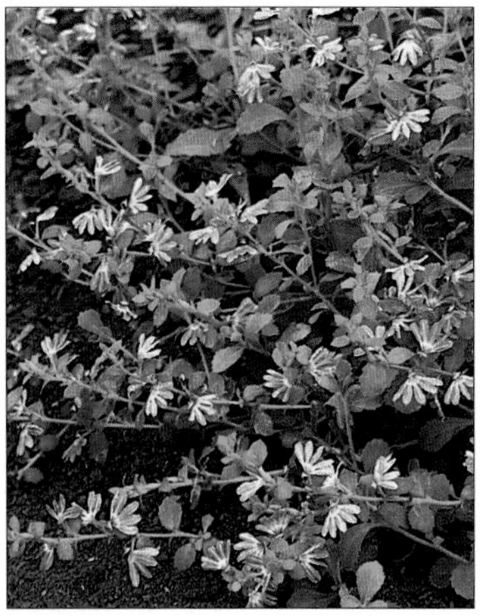

Scaevola aemula

S. aemula ▣ (Fairy fan-flower). Variable, tufted, evergreen perennial with spoon-shaped, toothed basal leaves, to 9cm (3½in) long, and smaller stem leaves, borne on erect or sometimes procumbent stems, with yellow or brown hairs. Leafy racemes of purple-blue or blue flowers, to 2.5cm (1in) across, are borne during summer. ↕↔ to 50cm (20in). S. and E. Australia. ❄ (min. 5°C/41°F). **'Blue Wonder'**, syn. *S.* 'Blue Wonder', is shrubby, with vigorous, trailing stems and inversely lance-shaped leaves, 1cm (½in) long. Lilac-blue flowers, 1cm (½in) across, are borne almost continuously and in great profusion from spring to autumn; ↕ to 15cm (6in), ↔ to 1.5m (5ft).
***S.* 'Blue Wonder'** see *S. aemula* 'Blue Wonder'.
***S.* 'Mauve Clusters'.** Vigorous, shrubby, evergreen perennial with a trailing habit and inversely lance-shaped leaves, 1cm (½in) long. Leafy racemes of lilac-mauve flowers, 1cm (½in) across, are borne freely for much of the year, but particularly in summer. ↕ 10–15cm (4–6in), ↔ to 1.5m (5ft). Australia. ❄ (min. 5°C/41°F)

▷**Scarlet runner** see *Kennedia prostrata*

SCHEFFLERA *syn.* BRASSAIA

ARALIACEAE

Genus of at least 900 species of mostly evergreen shrubs, trees, and climbers (some epiphytic when juvenile) from warm-temperate and tropical areas of S.E. Asia to the Pacific islands and Central and South America. They are grown mainly for their spiralled, fine, long-stalked, usually rounded, fully divided leaves, each with 3–30 stalked leaflets. In summer, autumn, or winter, mature trees bear compound umbels, panicles, racemes, or spikes of usually tiny flowers with 4 or 5 yellow-green to greenish red petals. The flowers are followed by mostly spherical or ovoid, black or purple fruits. In frost-prone areas, grow in a warm greenhouse or as houseplants. In warmer areas, grow at the back of a shrub border or as an informal hedge or windbreak.
• **HARDINESS** Half hardy to frost tender.
• **CULTIVATION** Under glass, grow in loam-based potting compost (JI No.2) in bright filtered or indirect light. In growth, water moderately and apply a balanced liquid fertilizer monthly; keep just moist in winter. Pot on in spring.

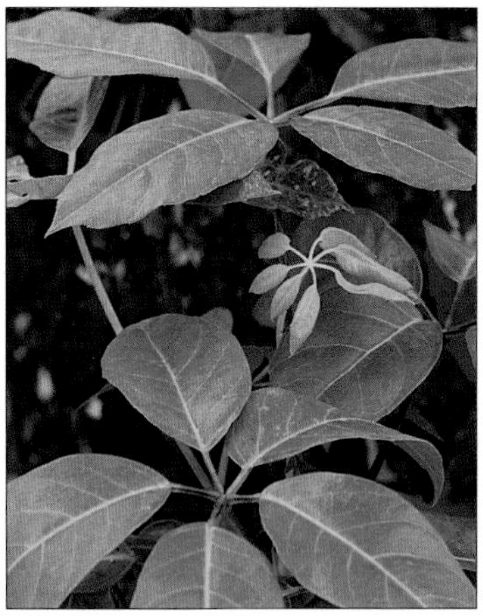

Schefflera actinophylla

Outdoors, grow in fertile, humus-rich, moist but well-drained soil in partial to deep shade. Shelter from cold, drying winds. Pruning group 1; clip hedges in late summer.
• **PROPAGATION** Sow seed at 19–24°C (66–75°F) in spring. Root semi-ripe cuttings with bottom heat in summer. Air layer in spring.
• **PESTS AND DISEASES** Scale insects, thrips, and mealybugs may be a problem under glass.

S. actinophylla ▣ ♀ ♀ syn. *Brassaia actinophylla* (Australian ivy palm, Octopus tree, Queensland umbrella tree). Erect, large shrub or small tree with stiff, thick, sparsely branched stems. Large leaves, 10–30cm (4–12in) long, divided into 7–16 ovate-oblong, leathery, glossy, deep bright green leaflets, to 30cm (12in) long, are borne in terminal rosettes on the branches. Leaves of juvenile plants have fewer, smaller leaflets than adult plants. Bears upright, terminal, compound panicles, to 80cm (32in) long, of tiny, brownish pink to red flowers in summer, followed by spherical black fruit. Often grown as juvenile plants. ↕ to 12m (40ft), ↔ to 6m (20ft). N. and N.E. Australia, S. and S.E. New Guinea. ❄ (min. 13°C/55°F)
S. elegantissima ▣ ♀ ♀ syn. *Aralia elegantissima, Dizygotheca elegantissima* (False aralia). Erect, sparsely branched, large shrub or small tree with leaves, 8–40cm (3–16in) long, composed of 7–11 linear, deeply toothed leaflets, 15–23cm (6–9in) long; when young, they are glossy, dark green above, dark brown-green beneath, with white

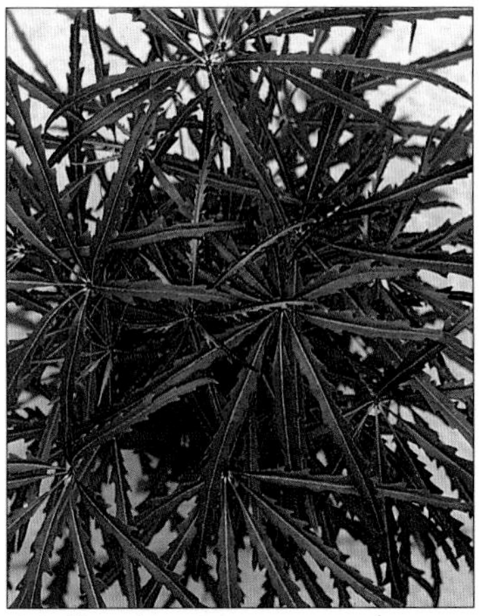

Schefflera elegantissima

S

midribs; adult plants have broader, stiffer, less glossy leaflets. In autumn and winter, bears yellowish green flowers in terminal umbels, to 30cm (12in) long, followed by spherical black fruit. ↕ 8–15m (25–50ft), ↔ 2–3m (6–10ft). New Caledonia. ❀ (min. 13–15°C/55–59°F)

S. heptaphylla ♀ syn. *S. octophylla* (Fukanoki, Ivy tree). Dense, spreading, evergreen or semi-evergreen tree with loose rosettes of leaves, to 13cm (5in) long, each composed of 6–8 elliptic to oblong-elliptic, glossy, deep green leaflets, 10–20cm (4–8in) long, often white beneath. From autumn to early winter, produces yellowish green flowers in terminal panicles, to 30cm (12in) long, followed by spherical, blue-black fruit. ↕ 12–25m (40–80ft), ↔ 5–10m (15–30ft). E. Asia, Philippines. ❀ (min. 13–15°C/55–59°F)

S. octophylla see *S. heptaphylla.*

SCHIMA

THEACEAE

Genus of one very variable species of evergreen tree or shrub extensively distributed in forest from S.W. China and the E. Himalayas to S.E. Asia. It is grown for the attractive spiral arrangement of its simple, glossy leaves, and for its fragrant, camellia-like flowers, usually solitary, sometimes in raceme-like inflorescences. In frost-prone areas, grow in a cool greenhouse; elsewhere, use as a specimen tree in a woodland garden.

• **HARDINESS** Half hardy.

• **CULTIVATION** Under glass, grow in lime-free (ericaceous) potting compost in bright filtered light or indirect light; provide moderate humidity. During the growing season, water freely and apply a balanced liquid fertilizer monthly; keep just moist in winter. Outdoors, grow in humus-rich, leafy, moist but well-drained, neutral to acid soil in full sun with some midday shade, or in partial shade. Shelter from cold, drying winds. Pruning group 1.

• **PROPAGATION** Sow seed at 6–12°C (43–54°F) in autumn. Root semi-ripe cuttings with bottom heat in late summer.

• **PESTS AND DISEASES** Trouble free.

S. argentea see *S. wallichii.*

S. khasiana see *S. wallichii.*

S. wallichii ♀ syn. *S. argentea, S. khasiana.* Broadly conical tree or shrub. The oblong, lance-shaped, ovate, or obovate, tapered leaves are entire, shallowly scalloped, or toothed, 7–24cm (3–10in) long, papery or leathery in texture, and glossy, dark green, with red veins, often reddish beneath. From late summer to autumn, red-tinged buds open to solitary, cup-shaped, fragrant white flowers, to 7cm (3in) across, with 5 or 6 rounded petals. ↕ 10m (30ft), ↔ 6m (20ft). Himalayas to S.E. Asia. ❄

SCHINUS

ANACARDIACEAE

Genus of about 30 species of usually dioecious, evergreen shrubs and trees occurring in woodland from Mexico to Uruguay. They are grown mainly for their alternate leaves, which may be simple or pinnate, entire or toothed. Tiny, 4- or 5-petalled flowers are borne in terminal or axillary panicles. When plants of both sexes are grown together, the flowers are followed on female plants by small, red to purple fruits (drupes). In frost-prone areas, grow in a temperate greenhouse or conservatory; elsewhere, use smaller species in a shrub border and larger ones as specimen trees.

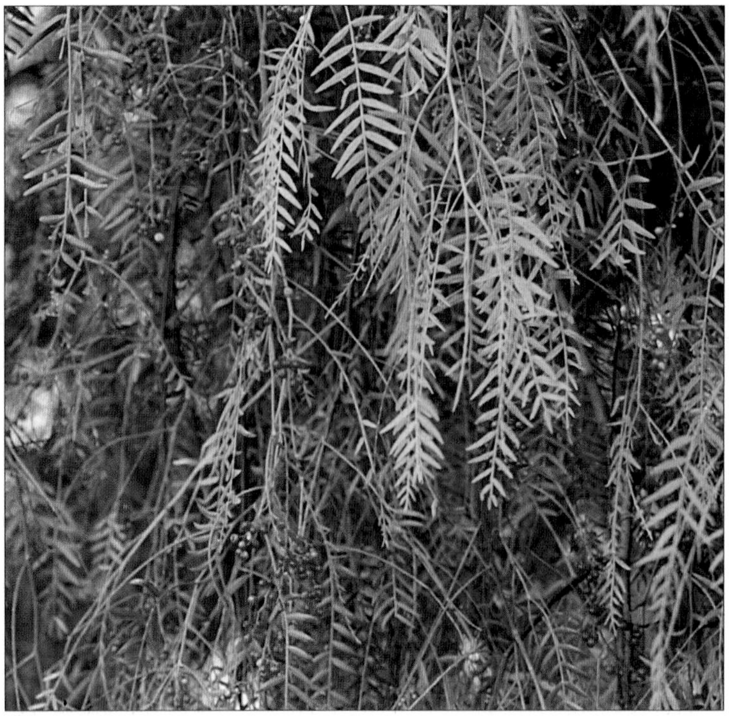

Schinus molle

• **HARDINESS** Half hardy to frost tender.

• **CULTIVATION** Under glass, grow in loam-based potting compost (JI No.2) in full light with shade from hot sun. When in active growth, water freely and apply a balanced liquid fertilizer monthly; water sparingly in winter. Outdoors, grow in moderately fertile, humus-rich, moist but well-drained soil in full sun, or with some midday shade. Pruning group 1.

• **PROPAGATION** Sow seed at 19–21°C (66–70°F) in spring. Root semi-ripe cuttings with bottom heat during late summer. Air layer in spring.

• **PESTS AND DISEASES** Scale insects and red spider mites may be troublesome under glass.

S. molle ▣ ♀ (Pepper tree, Peruvian mastic tree). Usually broad-headed tree with slender, pendent branches. The arching or semi-pendent, pinnate leaves, 10–30cm (4–12in) long, are composed of 19–41 narrow, lance-shaped, toothed, glossy, mid- to deep green leaflets. Pendent panicles, 8–20cm (3–8in) long, of tiny, whitish yellow flowers are borne from late winter to summer, followed by rose-pink fruit. ↕ 10–25m (30–80ft), ↔ 3–5m (10–15ft). Mexico, Brazil, Bolivia, Chile, N. Argentina, Paraguay, Uruguay. ❀ (min. 10°C/50°F)

S. terebinthifolius ♀ (Brazilian pepper tree, Christmas berry tree). Moderately bushy, large shrub or small tree with erect to spreading stems bearing pinnate leaves, 10–17cm (4–7in) long, with winged midribs and 3–13 (normally 7) oblong, deep green leaflets, which are paler beneath. From summer to autumn, produces panicles, to 15cm (6in) long, of tiny white flowers, followed by red fruit. Contact with the seeds may irritate skin and cause respiratory problems. ↕ 5–7m (15–22ft), ↔ 3–5m (10–15ft). Venezuela to Argentina, S. Brazil. ❀ (min. 7°C/45°F)

SCHISANDRA

SCHISANDRACEAE

Genus of about 25 species of twining, woody, monoecious or dioecious, deciduous or evergreen climbers found in woodland in E. Asia, with one species from S.E. USA. They are grown for their cup-shaped, red, pink, yellow, or white flowers, borne singly or in clusters or short spikes in the leaf axils, and for their spikes of spherical, brightly coloured fruits. Leaves are alternate, entire or toothed, and usually lance-shaped or ovate to elliptic. Both male and female plants of dioecious species must be grown to obtain fruit. Grow in woodland, or train on a wall or pergola.

• **HARDINESS** Fully hardy.

• **CULTIVATION** Grow in fertile, moist but well-drained soil in full sun or partial shade. Tie in shoots of young plants until established. Pruning group 12, in early spring.

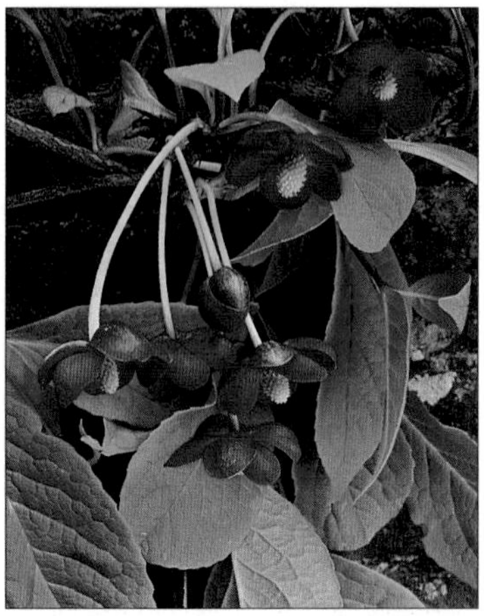

Schisandra rubriflora

• **PROPAGATION** Sow seed in containers in a cold frame as soon as ripe. Take greenwood cuttings in early or mid-summer; root semi-ripe cuttings in summer.

• **PESTS AND DISEASES** Trouble free.

S. chinensis. Twining, woody, deciduous climber with red shoots and producing elliptic to obovate, minutely toothed, glossy, dark green leaves, to 14cm (5½in) long. From late spring to summer, bears small clusters of cream to pale pink flowers, to 2cm (¾in) across; these are followed, on female plants, by pendent spikes, to 15cm (6in) long, of fleshy, red or pink fruit. ↕ 10m (30ft). E. Asia. ❄❄❄

S. henryi. Twining, woody, deciduous climber with angled shoots, winged when young, and oval, finely toothed, leathery, glossy, mid-green leaves, to 10cm (4in) long. In spring, bears small clusters of white flowers, 1cm (½in) across; these are followed, on female plants, by pendent spikes, to 7cm (3in) long, of fleshy red fruit. ↕ 3–4m (10–12ft). W. China. ❄❄❄

S. rubriflora ▣ Twining, woody, deciduous climber with slender red shoots and lance-shaped to narrowly elliptic or inversely lance-shaped, slightly toothed to entire, dark green leaves, to 12cm (5in) long, yellow in autumn. Produces solitary, dark crimson flowers, to 2.5cm (1in) across, from late spring to summer, followed, on female plants, by pendent spikes, to 15cm (6in) long, of fleshy red fruit. ↕ 10m (30ft). India, W. China, Burma. ❄❄❄

SCHIZACHYRIUM

GRAMINEAE/POACEAE

Genus of about 100 species of deciduous, perennial grasses native to grasslands worldwide. Closely related to *Andropogon*, they are distinguished by their solitary, terminal, obliquely branched racemes of stalked spikelets. Suitable for a herbaceous or mixed border. The flowerheads may be dried.

• **HARDINESS** Fully hardy.

• **CULTIVATION** Grow in moderately fertile, sharply drained soil in full sun. Cut down old stems in early winter.

• **PROPAGATION** Sow seed at 13–15°C (55–59°F), or divide, in spring.

• **PESTS AND DISEASES** Trouble free.

S. scoparium, syn. *Andropogon scoparius* (Little bluestem). Densely tufted, perennial grass, spreading slowly to form clumps of upright stems with linear, mid-green to grey-green leaves, to 45cm (18in) long, that turn purple to orange-red in autumn. From late summer to mid-autumn, bears narrow racemes, to 15cm (6in) long, of wispy, long-awned spikelets. ↕ to 1m (3ft), ↔ 30cm (12in). North America. ❄❄❄

SCHIZANTHUS

Butterfly flower, Poor man's orchid

SOLANACEAE

Genus of 12–15 erect to spreading, bushy, soft-stemmed, downy annuals, and some biennials, from dry, rocky slopes and canyons in Chile. They have alternate, pinnatisect to 3-pinnatisect or deeply lobed leaves. They are cultivated for their terminal cymes of showy, 2-

S

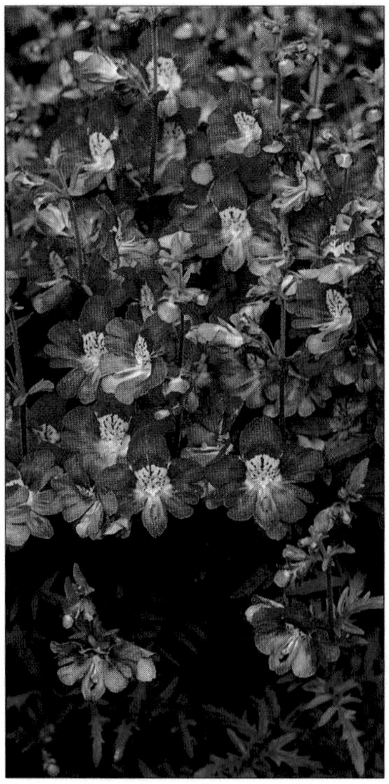

Schizanthus pinnatus 'Hit Parade'

lipped, orchid-like flowers of various colours, which are borne from spring to winter. In cool-temperate regions, grow either in a conservatory or cool greenhouse, as half-hardy annuals in a sheltered annual border, or in containers on a patio or in a courtyard garden. In warmer climates, grow in a border. They provide long-lasting cut flowers.

- **HARDINESS** Frost tender.
- **CULTIVATION** Under glass, grow in loam-based potting compost (JI No.2) in full light with shade from hot sun, or in bright filtered light. In growth, water moderately, and apply a high-potash liquid fertilizer every 2 weeks. Support flowering stems. Excessive heat produces elongated plants. Outdoors, grow in fertile, moist but well-drained soil in full sun. Pinch back young growth to promote bushiness.
- **PROPAGATION** Sow seed at 16°C (61°F) in mid-spring for summer- to autumn-flowering plants. Sow in late summer at 16°C (61°F) for winter-flowering container plants.
- **PESTS AND DISEASES** Aphids may be a problem under glass.

S. pinnatus (Poor man's orchid). Erect annual with almost fern-like, lance-shaped to inversely lance-shaped, pinnatisect to 3-pinnatisect, light green leaves, to 12cm (5in) long. From spring to autumn, bears terminal, open cymes of tubular, then flared, 2-lipped, white, yellow, pink, purple, or red flowers, to 8cm (3in) across; they often have yellow throats with violet markings, further streaked and spotted in contrasting colours. ↕ 20–50cm (8–20in), ↔ 23–30cm (9–12in). Chile. ⌂ (min. 5°C/41°F). **'Hit Parade'** ▣ has flowers with clear, contrasting markings; ↕ 23–30cm (9–12in). **'Star Parade'** is compact, with a distinctive pyramidal habit; ↕ 20–25cm (8–10in).

S. x wisetonensis (*S. grahamii* x *S. pinnatus*). Erect annual with lance-shaped to inversely lance-shaped, pinnatisect to 3-pinnatisect, light green leaves, to 12cm (5in) long. From spring to summer, bears terminal, open cymes of tubular, then flared, 2-lipped, white, pale blue, pink, or red-brown flowers, to 8cm (3in) across, often flushed yellow on the central lobe of the upper lips. ↕ to 45cm (18in), ↔ 23–30cm (9–12in). Garden origin. ⌂ (min. 5°C/41°F)

▷ ***Schizocodon*** see *Shortia*

SCHIZOPETALON

BRASSICACEAE/CRUCIFERAE

Genus of about 8 species of erect, slender-stemmed, hairy annuals from rocky slopes and disturbed ground in Chile. They have alternate, wavy-margined, toothed, simple or pinnatifid, linear to ovate leaves. From late spring to early autumn, they bear leafy racemes of star-shaped, white or purple flowers, each with 4 fringed petals. Grow at the edge of a border, in a rock garden or raised bed, or in containers. They are particularly effective grown near a patio or paved area where the evening scent of the blooms may be best appreciated.

- **HARDINESS** Frost hardy.
- **CULTIVATION** Grow in moderately fertile, well-drained soil in full sun.
- **PROPAGATION** Sow seed at 19–21°C (66–70°F) in mid-spring.
- **PESTS AND DISEASES** Trouble free.

S. walkeri. Upright, slightly branching annual producing deeply pinnatifid, linear to lance-shaped leaves, to 14cm (5½in) long. Terminal racemes of almond-scented, spreading, deeply cut, star-shaped, pure white flowers, to 4cm (1½in) across, are borne from summer to early autumn. ↕ 15–35cm (6–14in), ↔ 20cm (8in). Chile. ✻✻

SCHIZOPHRAGMA

HYDRANGEACEAE

Genus of 2 species of woody, deciduous root climbers from woodland and cliffs in China, Korea, and Japan. They bear opposite pairs of simple, long-stalked, entire or toothed, ovate, dark green leaves. Schizophragmas are cultivated for their showy flowerheads, similar to those of "lacecap" hydrangeas, but with large, conspicuous, bract-like, sterile, outer flowers. Best grown against a wall, fence, or large tree, to which the plant will attach itself by aerial roots.

- **HARDINESS** Fully hardy to frost hardy.
- **CULTIVATION** Grow in moderately fertile, humus-rich, moist but well-drained soil, in full sun or partial shade. Plant at least 60cm (24in) away from a host plant or support. Tie in to a support and train until established. Pruning group 11, in spring.
- **PROPAGATION** Take greenwood cuttings in early or midsummer; take semi-ripe cuttings in late summer.
- **PESTS AND DISEASES** Trouble free.

S. hydrangeoides. Woody root climber with long-stalked, broadly ovate, sharply toothed, dark green leaves, to 15cm (6in) long. In midsummer, small, slightly fragrant, creamy white flowers are borne in broad, flattened, terminal cymes, to 25cm (10in) across, with conspicuous, ovate, creamy, marginal bracts, to 6cm (2½in) long. ↕ 12m (40ft). Korea, Japan. ✻✻✻. **'Roseum'** has pink bracts.

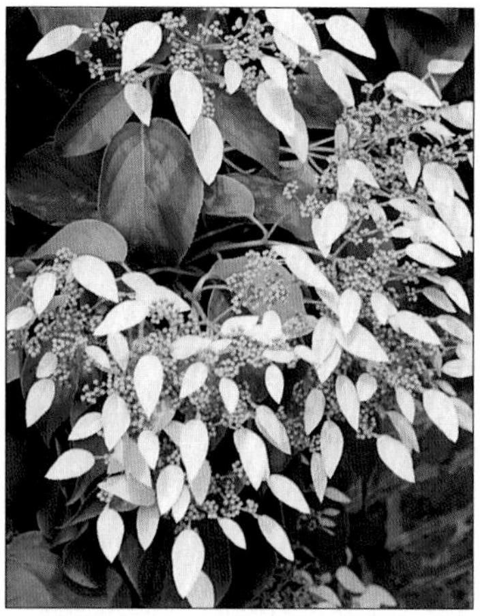

Schizophragma integrifolium

S. integrifolium ▣ 🏆 Woody root climber with long-stalked, ovate, entire or finely toothed, dark green leaves, to 18cm (7in) long. In midsummer, small, slightly fragrant, creamy white flowers are borne in broad, flattened, terminal cymes, to 30cm (12in) across, with conspicuous, ovate, creamy, marginal bracts, to 9cm (3½in) long. ↕ 12m (40ft). C. and W. China. ✻✻

S. viburnoides see *Pileostegia viburnoides.*

SCHIZOSTYLIS

Kaffir lily

IRIDACEAE

Genus of a single species of virtually evergreen, rhizomatous perennial from damp water-meadows and streambanks in southern Africa. Kaffir lilies are cultivated for their showy, gladiolus-like spikes of open cup-shaped flowers, which are produced from late summer to early winter. They are suitable for growing at the front of a herbaceous or mixed border, at the base of a warm, sunny wall, or in a small courtyard garden. *S. coccinea* and its cultivars are also effective grown *en masse* in large

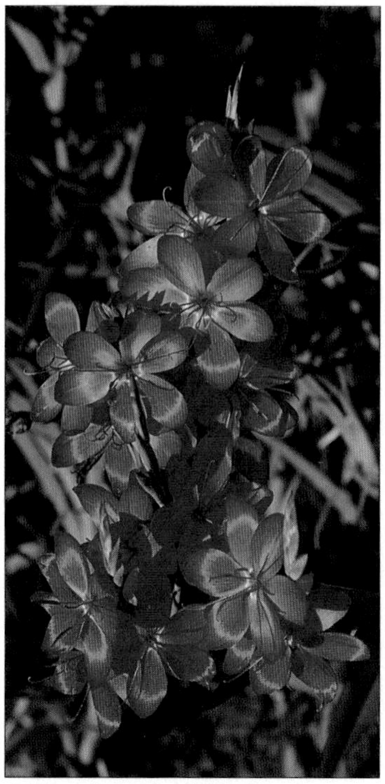

Schizostylis coccinea 'Major'

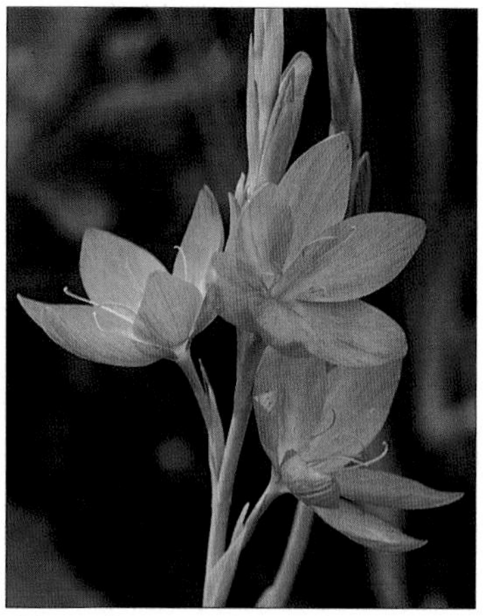

Schizostylis coccinea 'Sunrise'

containers in a cool greenhouse, where they will flower for long periods during the winter months. Excellent for cut flowers.

- **HARDINESS** Hardy to -10°C (14°F), although flower spikes will be damaged by frost.
- **CULTIVATION** Grow in moderately fertile, moist but well-drained soil in full sun. Keep the roots moist. Shelter from cold, drying winds. Provide an organic mulch in winter.
- **PROPAGATION** Sow seed at 13–16°C (55–61°F) in spring. Divide species and cultivars in spring.
- **PESTS AND DISEASES** Trouble free.

S. coccinea. Vigorous, clump-forming, rhizomatous perennial with erect, keeled, narrow, sword-shaped leaves, to 40cm (16in) long, with distinct midribs. Spikes of 4–14 open cup-shaped scarlet flowers, 2cm (¾in) across, are produced in autumn. ↕ to 60cm (24in), ↔ 30cm (12in). South Africa, Lesotho, Swaziland. ✻✻. **var. *alba*** bears white flowers. **'Grandiflora'** see 'Major'. **'Jennifer'** 🏆 is robust, bearing large, mid-pink flowers, 5–6cm (2–2½in) across, in late summer. **'Major'** ▣ 🏆 syn. 'Grandiflora', is robust, producing large red flowers, 5–6cm (2–2½in) across, on stiff stems in late summer. **'Sunrise'** ▣ 🏆 syn. 'Sunset', produces large, salmon-pink flowers, 5–6cm (2–2½in) across, in autumn. **'Sunset'** see 'Sunrise'. **'Viscountess Byng'** ▣ bears pale pink flowers, 3cm (1¼in) across, with narrow petals, in late autumn; its flowers are particularly vulnerable to damage by frost.

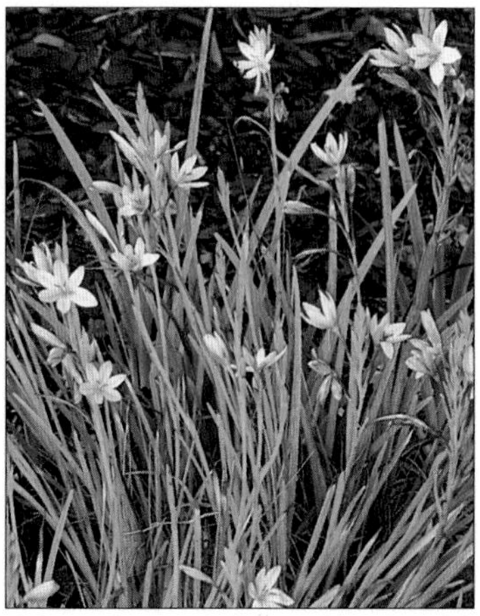

Schizostylis coccinea 'Viscountess Byng'

S

SCHLUMBERGERA

Christmas cactus

CACTACEAE

Genus of about 6 species of bushy, epiphytic or rock-dwelling, perennial cacti from tropical rainforest in S.E. Brazil, cultivated for their attractive flowers. Erect then pendent, fleshy stems are divided into flattened, oblong or obovate, normally truncate, leaf-like segments, usually with marginal, often prominent notches, almost tooth-like in some species. The areoles often have a few fine bristles; those near the tips of the upper segments bear open trumpet-shaped, narrow-petalled flowers, most in late winter and early spring, others in summer or autumn. Where temperatures fall below 10°C (50°F), grow Christmas cacti as houseplants, or in a temperate or warm greenhouse. In warmer areas, they are suitable for growing in a raised bed in a courtyard garden.

- **HARDINESS** Frost tender.
- **CULTIVATION** Under glass, grow in epiphytic cactus compost in bright indirect light. Water moderately and maintain moderate humidity. Apply a high-potash liquid fertilizer every 4 weeks when in growth; keep just moist after flowering. Repot every 3 or 4 years in spring. Outdoors, grow in humus-rich, acid to neutral, moist but well-drained soil, with added leaf mould and grit, in light dappled to partial shade. Protect from excessive rain; shelter from strong winds. Buds may drop in dry conditions. See also pp.48–49.
- **PROPAGATION** Sow seed at 19–21°C (66–70°F) in spring, or take cuttings of stem sections in spring or early summer.
- **PESTS AND DISEASES** Susceptible to mealybugs.

S. bridgesii see *S.* x *buckleyi*.

***S.* 'Bristol Beauty'.** Epiphytic cactus with oblong, bright green stem segments, 2.5cm (1in) long, with 4–6 marginal notches. In late winter and early spring, produces reddish purple flowers, 7cm (3in) long, with silvery white tubes. ↕ to 35cm (14in), ↔ 30cm (12in). ❄ (min. 10°C/50°F)

S.* x *buckleyi 🏆 (*S. russelliana* x *S. truncata*) syn. *S. bridgesii* (Christmas cactus). Epiphytic cactus with oblong or obovate, truncate, scalloped, mid-green stem segments, 2–5cm (¾–2in) long. Produces bright red flowers, to 7cm (3in) long, in late winter. ↕ to 35cm (14in), ↔ 1m (3ft). Garden origin. ❄ (min. 10°C/50°F)

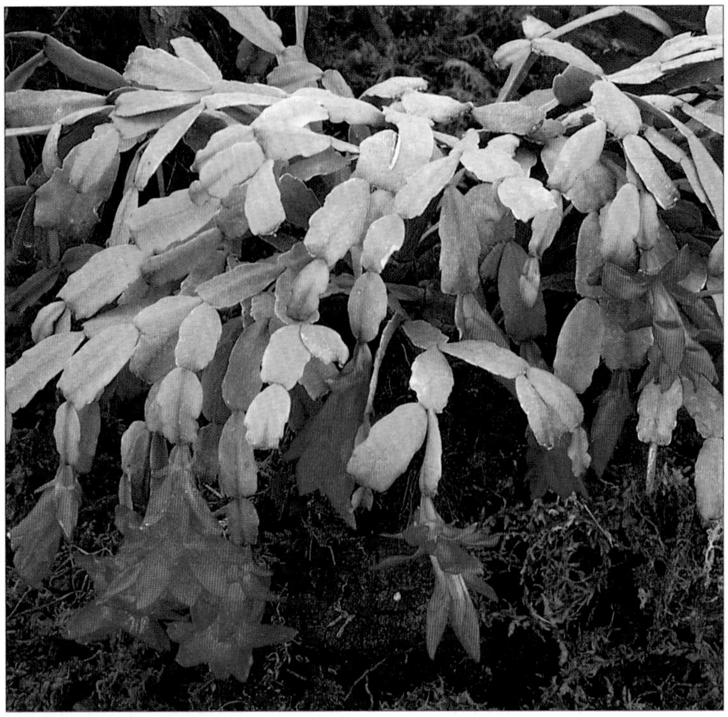

Schlumbergera 'Spectabile Coccineum'

***S.* 'Gold Charm'** ▣ Epiphytic cactus with oblong, mid-green stem segments, 3–5cm (1¼–2in) long, with 6–8 prominent, tooth-like marginal notches. Flowers, 6cm (2½in) long, are yellow in autumn but may turn pinkish if kept below 14°C (57°F). ↕ to 30cm (12in), ↔ 30cm (12in). ❄ (min. 10°C/50°F)

S. opuntioides, syn. *Epiphyllanthus obovatus*. Epiphytic or rock-dwelling cactus with thick, obovate to oblong, deep green stem segments, 5–7cm (2–3in) long, often tinged red, bearing white areoles, with minute spines, on both surfaces and margins. Deep pink flowers, 6cm (2½in) long, are borne in spring. Allow houseplants a brief, dry period after flowering. ↕ to 40cm (16in), ↔ 22cm (9in). S.E. Brazil. ❄ (min. 10°C/50°F)

***S. orssichiana*.** Epiphytic cactus with oblong, dark green stem segments, to 5cm (2in) long, with 4–6 prominent, tooth-like marginal notches, with areoles set in the angles. White flowers, to 9cm (3½in) long, purplish pink towards the petal tips, are borne from late summer to winter. ↕ to 30cm (12in), ↔ to 35cm (14in). S.E. Brazil. ❄ (min. 10°C/50°F)

***S.* 'Spectabile Coccineum'** ▣ Epiphytic cactus with oblong, dark green stem segments, to 2.5cm (1in) long, with 3–5 tooth-like marginal notches. Bears bright red flowers, to 8cm (3in) long, in late winter and early spring. ↕ to 28cm (11in), ↔ 25cm (10in) or more. ❄ (min. 10°C/50°F)

S. truncata ▣ syn. *Zygocactus truncatus* (Crab cactus). Epiphytic cactus with oblong, bright green stem segments, 4–6cm (1½–2½in) long, with 4–8 prominent, tooth-like marginal notches. Deep pink, red, orange, or white flowers, to 8cm (3in) long, are borne from late autumn to winter. ↕ to 30cm (12in), ↔ 30cm (12in). S.E. Brazil. ❄ (min. 10°C/50°F)

***S.* 'Wintermärchen'.** Epiphytic cactus bearing oblong, glossy, mid-green stem segments, 4cm (1½in) long, with 4–6 tooth-like marginal notches. Delicate pale pink, almost white flowers, 6–7cm (2½–3in) long, are produced in late autumn, and turn pinkish white in winter. ↕ to 35cm (14in), ↔ 30cm (12in). ❄ (min. 10°C/50°F)

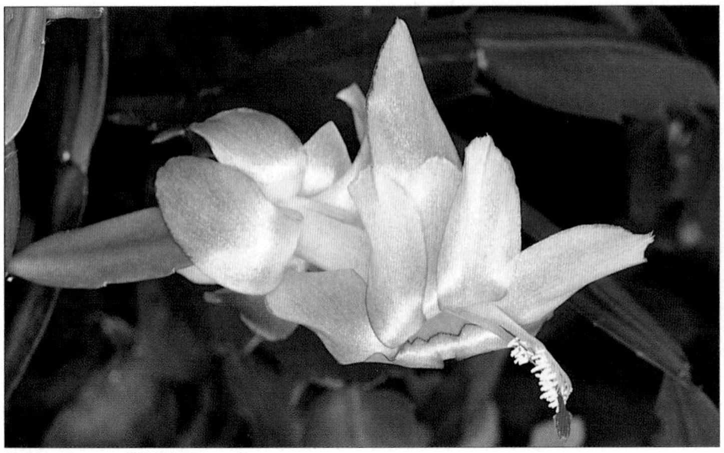

Schlumbergera 'Gold Charm'

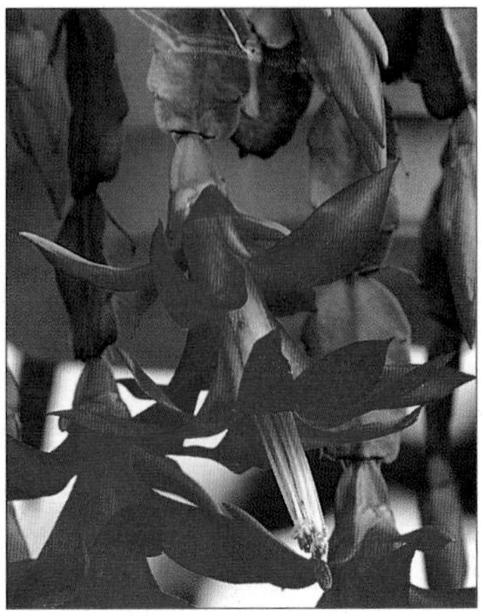

Schlumbergera truncata

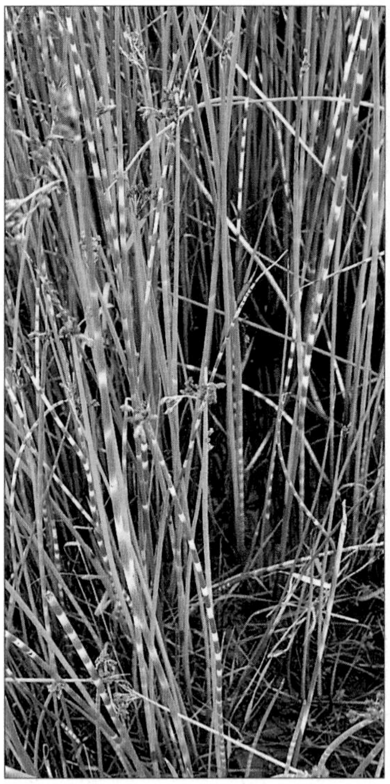

Schoenoplectus lacustris subsp. *tabernaemontani* 'Zebrinus'

SCHOENOPLECTUS

CYPERACEAE

Genus, formerly included in *Scirpus*, of 80 species of evergreen, rhizomatous, marginal aquatic perennials and annuals usually found on the banks of lakes and slow-running streams, almost world-wide. Leaves are grass-like and are often borne under water. Insignificant flowers are borne in inflorescences on cylindrical or 3-angled stems, in summer. The plant described is grown for its striped stems, and is suitable for cultivation in a bog garden, or as a marginal aquatic plant in still or slow-moving water.

- **HARDINESS** Fully hardy.
- **CULTIVATION** Grow in fertile, wet soil, or in water up to 30cm (12in) deep, in full sun. In small pools, restrict growth by cutting back the rhizomes annually. See also pp.52–53.
- **PROPAGATION** Root sections of rhizome from mid-spring to mid-summer.
- **PESTS AND DISEASES** Trouble free.

***S. lacustris* subsp. *tabernaemontani* 'Zebrinus'** ▣ (Club-rush). Rhizomatous perennial with virtually leafless, grey-green stems banded creamy white, arising at intervals along the rhizome. Bears branched clusters, 5–10mm (¼–½in) across, of brown spikelets from early to late summer. Cut reverting stems back to the rhizomes. ↕ 1m (3ft), ↔ 60cm (24in) or more. ***

SCHOMBURGKIA

ORCHIDACEAE

Genus, closely related to *Laelia*, of about 12–15 species of large, evergreen, epiphytic or lithophytic orchids from rainforest and moist cliffs or rocks, at low to medium altitudes in the West Indies and tropical America. They have stout, elongated, spindle-shaped to cylindrical, sometimes hollow pseudo-

S

bulbs, each with 1–3 leathery, semi-rigid, ovate to oblong leaves. Racemes or panicles of showy flowers are produced from the tips of the pseudobulbs, and may be extremely long.
• **HARDINESS** Frost tender.
• **CULTIVATION** Intermediate-growing orchids. Grow in epiphytic orchid compost in containers or slatted baskets. In the growing season, water freely and apply a half-strength balanced liquid fertilizer every 4 weeks; provide high humidity and bright indirect light. Water sparingly and provide full light in winter. See also p.46.
• **PROPAGATION** Divide when the plant "overflows" the sides of the container. Remove backbulbs and pot them up separately.
• **PESTS AND DISEASES** Scale insects, red spider mites, aphids, whiteflies, and mealybugs may be troublesome.

S. tibicinis, syn. *Myrmecophila tibicinis.* Epiphytic orchid with stoutly cylindrical, hollow pseudobulbs and 2 or 3 elliptic to oblong leaves, 45cm (18in) long. Variable, fragrant, brown to rich purple flowers, 6cm (2½in) across, with yellow, white, and purple lips, are produced in extended racemes, 1.5m (5ft) or more long, in summer. ↕↔ 60cm (24in). Mexico to Panama. ❀ (min. 13°C/55°F; max. 30°C/86°F)

SCHOTIA

CAESALPINIACEAE/LEGUMINOSAE

Genus of 4 or 5 species of deciduous or semi-evergreen shrubs and trees from open deciduous woodland, dry woodland, and scrub in southern Africa. They are cultivated for their pinnate leaves, and for their 5-petalled, red or pink flowers, which are borne in summer in axillary or terminal panicles, often on bare stems and sometimes directly from older wood. Where temperatures regularly fall below 0°C (32°F), grow in a cool or temperate greenhouse. In milder climates, use in a shrub border or as specimen plants.
• **HARDINESS** Half hardy to frost tender, but may withstand temperatures down to -5°C (23°F) if the wood has been well ripened in summer.
• **CULTIVATION** Under glass, grow in loam-based potting compost (JI No.2) in full light. During the growing season, water moderately and apply a balanced liquid fertilizer monthly; water sparingly in winter. Outdoors, grow in moderately fertile, well-drained soil in full sun with shelter from cold, drying winds. Pruning group 1.
• **PROPAGATION** Sow seed at 13–16°C (55–61°F) in spring. Root semi-ripe cuttings with bottom heat in summer.
• **PESTS AND DISEASES** Whiteflies and red spider mites may be troublesome under glass.

S. brachypetala ♀ (African walnut, Tree fuchsia, Weeping boerboon). Spreading to arching, semi-evergreen, large shrub or small tree with red-brown bark and grey twigs. The pinnate leaves, to 18cm (7in) long, each have 8–15 oblong or oval leaflets, which emerge rose-red and mature through copper to bright green. From summer to late autumn, bears fragrant flowers in nodding to pendent, usually crowded panicles, to 13cm (5in) across, on leafless or almost leafless twigs; each flower has 5 minute petals and 4 spreading crimson sepals, to 1cm (½in) long. Bean-like pods, 5–17cm (2–7in) long, contain large seeds that are edible when roasted. ↕ 10–15m (30–50ft), ↔ 5–10m (15–30ft). Zimbabwe, Mozambique, South Africa (Northern Transvaal, KwaZulu/Natal), Swaziland. ✲ (borderline)

SCHWANTESIA

AIZOACEAE

Genus of 10 species of dwarf, compact, cushion-forming, perennial succulents from hillsides and lowlands of Namibia and S. South Africa. They have unequal pairs of fleshy, keeled, bluish green leaves, and bear daisy-like, bright yellow flowers, which open during the day, in summer. Where temperatures fall below 10°C (50°F), grow in a temperate or warm greenhouse; in warmer climates, schwantesias are suitable for cultivation in a desert garden.
• **HARDINESS** Frost tender.
• **CULTIVATION** Under glass, grow in standard cactus compost in full light with shade from hot sun; provide low humidity. During the growing season, water moderately and apply a balanced liquid fertilizer monthly; keep just moist in winter. Outdoors, grow in poor to moderately fertile, humus-rich, sharply drained soil in full sun. Protect from excessive rain in summer and winter. See also pp.48–49.
• **PROPAGATION** Sow seed at 19–21°C (66–70°F) in spring. Divide offsets from spring to early summer.
• **PESTS AND DISEASES** Prone to aphids while flowering.

S. herrei. Cushion-forming, succulent perennial with 2 or 3 pairs of 3-angled, keeled, fleshy, pale blue-green leaves, 2.5–3.5cm (1–1½in) long, sometimes with a few terminal teeth. Bright yellow flowers, 4cm (1½in) across, are borne in summer. ↕↔ 14cm (5½in). Namibia, South Africa (Northern Cape, Western Cape). ❀ (min. 10°C/50°F)
S. ruedebuschii ▣ Clump-forming, succulent perennial producing slightly angular, very fleshy, white-mottled, greyish green leaves, 3–5cm (1¼–2in) long, the upper surfaces slightly convex, the lower ones more rounded, and the tips widening and bearing 3–7 thick blue teeth, to 4mm (⅛in) long. Bright pale yellow flowers, to 4cm (1½in) across, are borne in summer. ↕ 10cm (4in), ↔ 15cm (6in). Namibia, South Africa (Northern Cape, Western Cape). ❀ (min. 10°C/50°F).

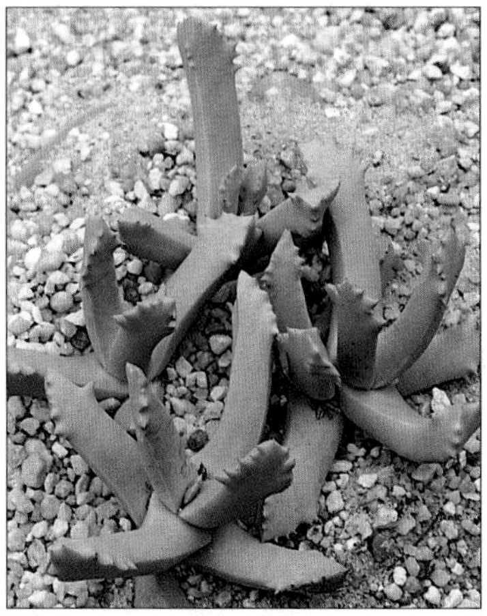
Schwantesia ruedebuschii

SCIADOPITYS

SCIADOPITYACEAE/TAXODIACEAE

Genus of one species of monoecious, evergreen, coniferous tree from forest in Japan. It has peeling, red-brown bark, and the glossy, linear leaves, sometimes in fused pairs, are borne in whorls at the shoot-tips, like the spokes of an umbrella. Use as a specimen tree.
• **HARDINESS** Fully hardy.
• **CULTIVATION** Grow in moderately fertile, moist but well-drained, neutral to slightly acid soil, in full sun with some midday shade, or in partial shade. May need several years training to maintain a central leader.
• **PROPAGATION** Sow seed in containers in a cold frame in spring, or take semi-ripe cuttings in late summer.
• **PESTS AND DISEASES** Trouble free.

S. verticillata ▣ ♀ ◊ (Japanese umbrella pine). Conical or columnar-conical tree with red-brown bark, peeling in ribbons, and brown shoots. Linear, grooved, glossy, dark green leaves, 5–12cm (2–5in) long, olive-green beneath, are borne in terminal whorls of 15–25, and persist for 3 or 4 years. Single, ovoid female cones, 5–8cm (2–3in) long, ripen in the second year. Spherical male cones, 3–8mm (⅛–⅜in) across, are borne in clusters. ↕ 10–20m (30–70ft), ↔ to 6–8m (20–25ft). S. Japan. ✲✲✲

SCILLA

HYACINTHACEAE/LILIACEAE

Genus of about 90 species of bulbous perennials found in a range of habitats including subalpine meadows, rocky slopes, woodland, and sea shores in Europe, southern Africa, and Asia. They are grown for their terminal racemes or corymbs of small, usually blue but also pink, purple, or white, bell-shaped to flat, or star-shaped flowers, borne in spring, summer, and autumn. Most have semi-erect, linear to elliptic, sometimes channelled, basal leaves. Naturalize under trees and shrubs or in grass; small species are suitable for an alpine house.
• **HARDINESS** Fully hardy to half hardy.
• **CULTIVATION** Plant bulbs 8–10cm (3–4in) deep in late summer or early autumn. Under glass, grow in 2 parts loam-based potting compost (JI No.2) and 1 part each leaf mould and grit. Provide full light. When in growth, water freely; keep dry during summer dormancy. *S. peruviana* does not have a dormant period. Outdoors, grow in moderately fertile, humus-rich, well-drained soil in full sun or partial shade.
• **PROPAGATION** Sow seed in containers in a cold frame as soon as ripe. Divide and pot up offsets when dormant.
• **PESTS AND DISEASES** Prone to viruses.

S. adlamii see *Ledebouria cooperi.*
S. amethystina see *S. litardierei.*
S. amoena. Small, bulbous perennial with 3–5 flaccid, linear, basal leaves, 15–22cm (6–9in) long, emerging before the small, compact racemes of 3–6 star-

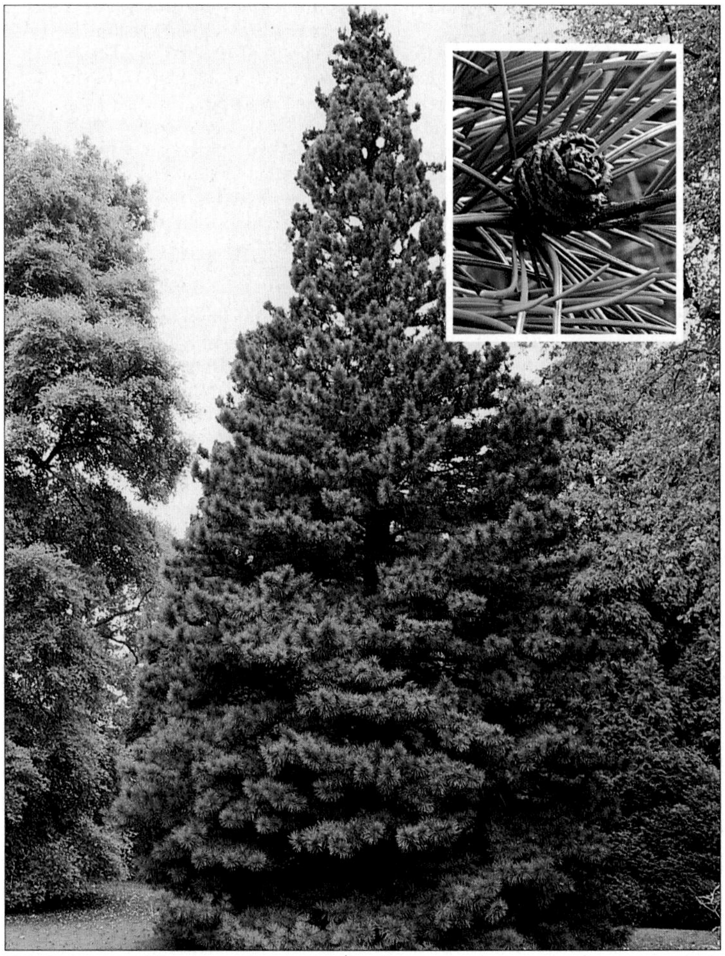
Sciadopitys verticillata (inset: female cone detail)

S

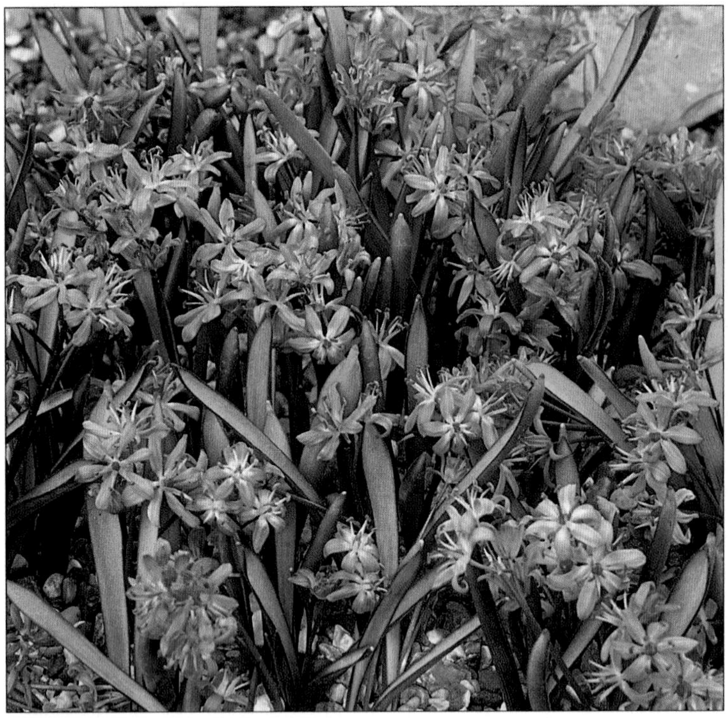
Scilla bifolia

shaped blue flowers, 1.5–2cm (½–¾in) across, in spring. Similar to *S. bithynica* but lacks bracts. Good for naturalizing. ↕15–20cm (6–8in), ↔5cm (2in). Probably S.E. Europe. ✻✻✻

S. bifolia ■🏆 Small, bulbous perennial with 2 semi-erect, broadly linear, basal leaves, 5–20cm (2–8in) long, borne in early spring, at the same time as slightly one-sided racemes of up to 10 star-shaped, blue to purple-blue flowers, 2.5–4cm (1–1½in) across. Excellent for naturalizing. ↕8–15cm (3–6in), ↔5cm (2in). C. and S. Europe, Turkey. ✻✻✻

S. bithynica. Small, bulbous perennial with 3–5 flaccid, linear, basal leaves, to 20cm (8in) long, borne in spring, at the same time as compact, conical racemes of 6–12 star-shaped blue flowers, to 2cm (¾in) across. Excellent for naturalizing. ↕10–15cm (4–6in), ↔8cm (3in). Bulgaria, Turkey. ✻✻✻

S. campanulata see *Hyacinthoides hispanica.*

S. chinensis see *S. scilloides.*

S. cilicica. Bulbous perennial, sometimes confused with *S. hohenackeri*, producing 3 or 4 erect, broadly linear, basal leaves, 15–25cm (6–10in) long, in autumn. In spring, bears loose racemes of 5–15 star-shaped, pale or lavender-blue flowers, 2–3cm (¾–1¼in) across, with reflexed segments. Easily grown in a bulb frame or alpine house. ↕15–35cm (6–14in), ↔8cm (3in). Turkey. ✻✻

S. cooperi see *Ledebouria cooperi.*

S. hispanica see *Hyacinthoides hispanica.*

S. hohenackeri. Bulbous perennial, similar to *S. cilicica*, with 3–5 flaccid, linear, basal leaves, 10–25cm (4–10in) long, produced in spring before loose racemes of 4–12 star-shaped, pale blue flowers, 1.5cm (½in) across, with reflexed segments. Easily grown in partial shade. ↕10–20cm (4–8in), ↔5cm (2in). Azerbaijan, Iran. ✻✻✻

S. japonica see *S. scilloides.*

S. liliohyacinthus. Small, clump-forming, bulbous perennial with relatively large, lily-like bulbs, with yellow scales. In late spring, produces a basal cluster of 6–10 erect, inversely lance-shaped, glossy leaves, 15–30cm (6–12in) long, and dense, conical racemes of 5–20 star-shaped, bright lilac-blue to purplish blue, rarely white flowers, 1.5cm (½in) across. Prefers a cool site. ↕15–25cm (6–10in), ↔7cm (3in). S.W. France, Spain. ✻✻✻

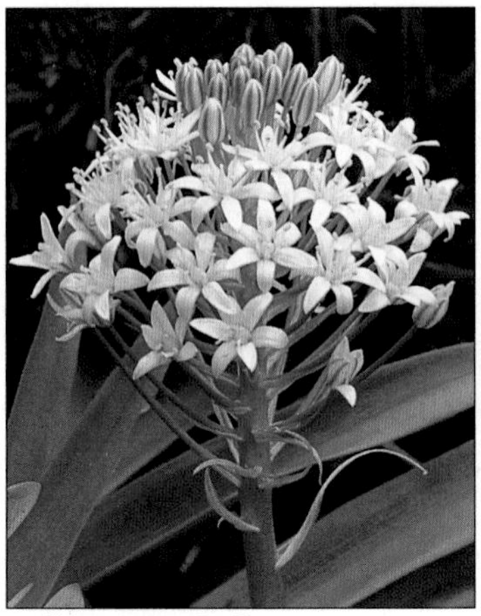
Scilla peruviana f. *alba*

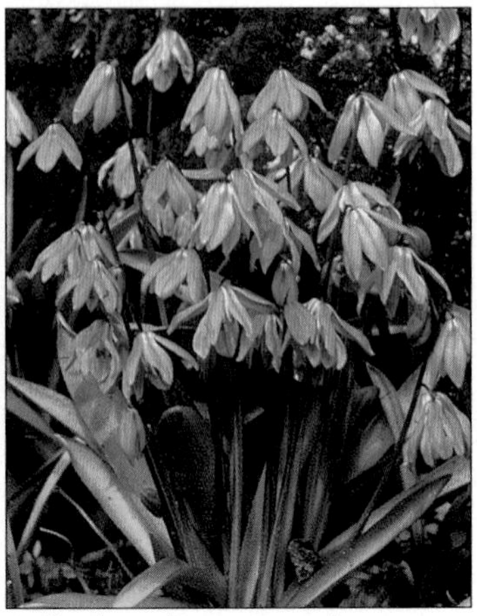
Scilla siberica 'Spring Beauty'

S. litardierei, syn. *S. amethystina, S. pratensis.* Clump-forming, bulbous perennial with a basal cluster of 3–6 semi-erect, linear leaves, 15–30cm (6–12in) long, borne in early summer, at the same time as dense racemes of 15–35 star-shaped, pale bluish violet flowers, 6mm (¼in) across. ↕10–20cm (4–8in), ↔5cm (2in). Coast of former Yugoslavia. ✻✻✻

S. mischtschenkoana, syn. *S. tubergeniana.* Dwarf, bulbous perennial with 3–5 semi-erect, linear to inversely lance-shaped, basal leaves, 4–10cm (1½–4in) long, borne in late winter or early spring. At the same time, racemes of 2–6 star-shaped, silvery blue flowers, 2cm (¾in) across, with darker stripes, open just above the ground. Stems and racemes gradually elongate. ↕10–15cm (4–6in), ↔5cm (2in). Georgia, Armenia, Azerbaijan, Iran. ✻✻✻

S. natalensis. Bulbous perennial with 4–8 semi-erect, lance-shaped, basal leaves, to 20cm (8in) long when they emerge at flowering time, later growing to 30–60cm (12–24in). Tall racemes of up to 100 flattish, light violet-blue, pink, or white flowers, 1.5cm (½in) across, are produced in summer. The flowering stems gradually elongate. ↕30–120cm (12–48in), ↔8cm (3in). South Africa, Lesotho. ✻

S. non-scripta see *Hyacinthoides non-scripta.*

S. nutans see *Hyacinthoides non-scripta.*

S. peruviana. Virtually evergreen, clump-forming, bulbous perennial with a basal cluster of 5–15 semi-erect, lance-shaped leaves, 40–60cm (16–24in) long, developing in autumn as older leaves fade. In early summer, produces tall, conical racemes of 50–100 star-shaped, deep purplish blue or white flowers, 1.5cm (½in) across. ↕15–30cm (6–12in), ↔10cm (4in). Portugal, Spain, Italy, N. Africa. ✻✻. **f. *alba*** ■ has large heads of white flowers.

S. pratensis see *S. litardierei.*

S. scilloides, syn. *S. chinensis, S. japonica.* Slender, bulbous perennial with 2–7 semi-erect, flaccid, linear, basal leaves, 15–25cm (6–10in) long, borne in late summer and early autumn, with slender racemes of 40–80 star-shaped, mauve-pink flowers, 4mm (⅛in) across. Easily grown in full sun or in an alpine house. ↕15–20cm (6–8in), ↔5cm (2in). China, Korea, Taiwan, Japan (including Ryukyu Islands). ✻✻✻

S. siberica 🏆 (Siberian squill). Bulbous perennial with 2–4 semi-erect, broadly linear, basal leaves, 10–15cm (4–6in) long, produced in spring, at the same time as loose racemes of up to 4 or 5 pendent, bowl-shaped, bright blue flowers, 1.5cm (½in) across. Stems gradually elongate. ↕10–20cm (4–8in), ↔5cm (2in). Ukraine, Russia, Georgia, Azerbaijan, N. Iran. ✻✻✻. **'Alba'** has white flowers. **'Atrocoerulea'** see 'Spring Beauty'. **'Spring Beauty'** ■ syn. 'Atrocoerulea', has deep blue flowers; ↕to 20cm (8in).

S. socialis see *Ledebouria socialis.*

S. tubergeniana see *S. mischtschenkoana.*

S. violacea see *Ledebouria socialis.*

▷ ***Scindapsus aureus*** see *Epipremnum aureum*

▷ ***Scindapsus pictus* 'Argyraeus'** see *Epipremnum pictum* 'Argyraeum'

SCIRPOIDES

CYPERACEAE

Genus, formerly included in *Scirpus*, of one species of deciduous or semi-evergreen, fleshy-rooted, rhizomatous, perennial sedge found in damp, sandy, coastal areas and damp or wet meadows inland, from Europe to S.W. Asia. *S. holoschoenus* has almost leafless stems, and produces long-stalked, spherical flowerheads from midsummer to early autumn. Suitable for a wild garden. Grow *S. holoschoenus* 'Variegatus' at the margins of a pool or in a bog garden.

- **HARDINESS** Fully hardy.
- **CULTIVATION** Grow in moderately fertile, constantly moist soil in full sun. Submerge in water to 23cm (9in) deep if grown as a marginal aquatic plant. Cut back stems left for winter effect by early spring. See also pp.52–53.
- **PROPAGATION** Sow seed at 6–12°C (43–54°F) in spring, in permanently moist seed compost. Divide between mid-spring and early summer.
- **PESTS AND DISEASES** Trouble free.

S. holoschoenus, syn. *Scirpus holoschoenus* (Round-headed club-rush). Tufted perennial with upright, smooth, rounded, mid-green stems, to 1m (3ft) long, turning orange-brown in autumn; they occasionally bear linear, round-tipped, rough-margined, mid-green, basal leaves. From midsummer to early autumn, produces lax, terminal umbels of dense, long-stalked, spherical heads, 1cm (½in) long, consisting of ovoid, pale brown spikelets. ↕1m (3ft), ↔45cm (18in). Europe, S.W. Asia. ✻✻✻. **'Variegatus'** has leaves and stems ringed yellow.

▷ ***Scirpus holoschoenus*** see *Scirpoides holoschoenus*

▷ ***Scirpus lacustris* 'Spiralis'** see *Juncus effusus* 'Spiralis'

SCLEROCACTUS

syn. ANCISTROCACTUS

CACTACEAE

Genus, closely allied to and sometimes merged with *Pediocactus*, of 3 or 4 species of depressed-spherical to club-shaped or cylindrical, perennial cacti from relatively arid areas of the USA and Mexico. They have a long, fleshy tap root and deeply notched or warty ribs. The areoles are nectar-secreting and bear

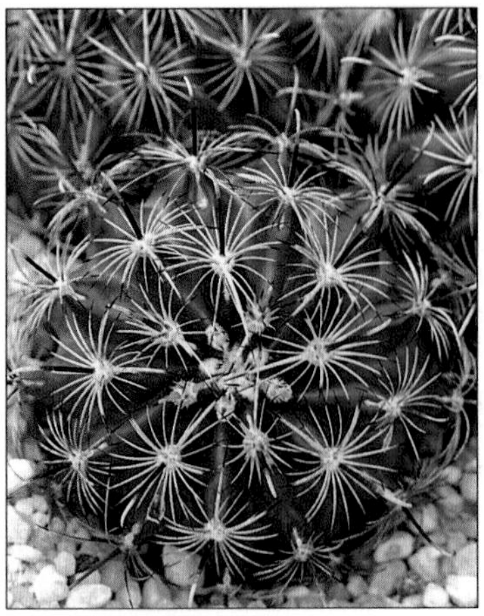
Sclerocactus scheeri

S

prominent spines, the centrals often slightly hooked; flowering areoles extend in a furrow. Diurnal, trumpet-shaped flowers are borne in summer, followed by juicy, ovoid to cylindrical or club- or barrel-shaped, mid-green fruits, scaly on the upper part, smooth below. Where temperatures fall below 7–10°C (45–50°F), grow in a temperate greenhouse; elsewhere, use in a desert garden.
• **HARDINESS** Frost tender.
• **CULTIVATION** Under glass, grow in standard cactus compost in full light with shade from hot sun. When in growth, water moderately and apply a half-strength balanced liquid fertilizer monthly; keep completely dry in winter. Outdoors, grow in poor to moderately fertile, sharply drained, neutral to slightly alkaline soil in full sun with some midday shade. See also pp.48–49.
• **PROPAGATION** Sow seed at 16–21°C (61–70°F) in spring. Graft on to a sturdy rootstock of *Cereus peruvianus* or *Hylocereus undatus* in early summer.
• **PESTS AND DISEASES** Prone to mealybugs.

S. scheeri ■ syn. *Ancistrocactus megarhizus, A. scheeri, Echinocactus scheeri.* Spherical to narrowly club-shaped, dark green, perennial cactus bearing about 13 ribs with warts that have areoles at the tips, and yellow spines (12–20 radials to 1cm (½in) long and 1–4 centrals to 5cm (2in) long, the lowest hooked). Bears greenish yellow flowers, 3cm (1¼in) across, in summer. ↕12cm (5in), ↔ 8cm (3in). USA (Texas), Mexico. ⊛ (min. 7–10°C/45–50°F)
S. uncinatus, syn. *Ancistrocactus uncinatus, Echinocactus uncinatus, Glandulicactus uncinatus, Hamatocactus uncinatus.* Depressed-spherical to short-cylindrical, bluish green, perennial cactus with 13 ribs. Hairy areoles bear prominently hooked, reddish brown spines (7–11 radials to 5cm (2in) long; 1–4 centrals, the upper 3, where present, nearly straight or incurved, and to 2.5cm (1in) long, the lowest one strongly hooked, ascending, and to 9cm (3½in) long). In summer, bears deep pinkish red to brownish red flowers, 2.5cm (1in) across. ↕ 20cm (8in), ↔ 10cm (4in). USA (Texas), N. to C. Mexico. ⊛ (min. 7–10°C/45–50°F).
var. *crassihamatus*, syn. *Ancistrocactus crassihamatus, Ferocactus crassihamatus, Glandulicactus crassihamatus, Hamatocactus crassihamatus*, has large areoles with red spines (7 or 8 radials to 3cm (1¼in) long and 1–4 centrals to 5cm (2in) long, the lowest spine hooked). Flowers, 2cm (¾in) across, have white-margined purple tepals; ↕ to 10cm (4in), ↔ to 15cm (6in); Mexico.

SCOLIOPUS

LILIACEAE/TRILLIACEAE

Genus, allied to *Trillium*, of 2 species of herbaceous perennials found in woodland in the W. USA. They have short, underground stems and usually paired, ovate or oblong to elliptic, boldly veined, basal leaves, sometimes with brown-purple markings. In spring, stalkless umbels of flowers, each with 3 narrow, upright inner tepals and 3 spreading outer tepals, arise directly from buds on the rootstock. Grow for their unusual but malodorous flowers

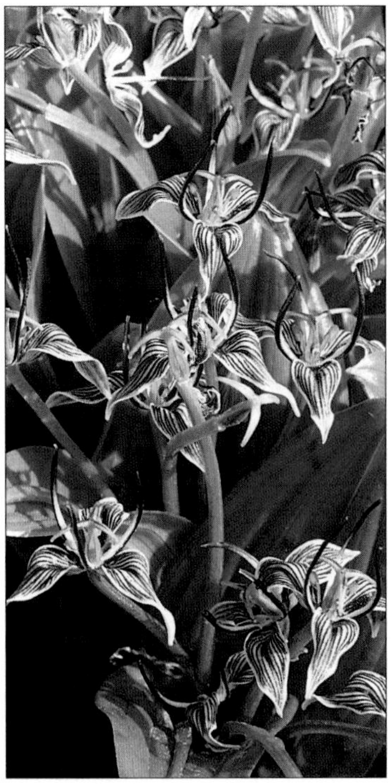

Scoliopus bigelovii

and attractive foliage in a rock garden, peat bed, or alpine house.
• **HARDINESS** Hardy to -10°C (14°F).
• **CULTIVATION** Grow in humus-rich, leafy, moist but well-drained, acid to neutral soil in deep to partial shade. Provide a dry winter mulch. In an alpine house, grow in loamless potting compost with added leaf mould in filtered light.
• **PROPAGATION** Sow seed in containers in a cold frame as soon as ripe.
• **PESTS AND DISEASES** Young foliage may be damaged by slugs and snails.

S. bigelovii ■ syn. *S. bigelowii* (Footed adder's tongue, Stink pod). Compact herbaceous perennial producing pairs of broadly oblong to elliptic, boldly veined, purple-mottled, dull dark green leaves, 10–20cm (4–8in) long. In early spring, bears umbels of 3–12 trillium-like flowers, to 5cm (2in) across, with narrow, erect, deep purple inner tepals, and greenish white outer tepals, striped brown-purple. ↕ 10cm (4in), ↔ 15cm (6in). USA (California). **
S. bigelowii see *S. bigelovii.*

▷ ***Scolopendrium vulgare*** see *Asplenium scolopendrium*

SCOPOLIA

SOLANACEAE

Genus of 5 species of rhizomatous, creeping perennials from woodland in C. and S. Europe, and Siberia (Russia) to the Himalayas, China, and Japan. Scopolias have alternate, simple, entire, boldly veined leaves. They die back after producing solitary, pendent, bell-shaped flowers in spring. Grow in woodland. All parts are highly toxic if ingested.
• **HARDINESS** Fully hardy.
• **CULTIVATION** Grow in humus-rich, leafy, moist but well-drained, neutral to slightly alkaline soil in partial shade.
• **PROPAGATION** Sow seed in containers in a cold frame in autumn, or *in situ* in autumn or spring. Divide in spring.
• **PESTS AND DISEASES** Trouble free.

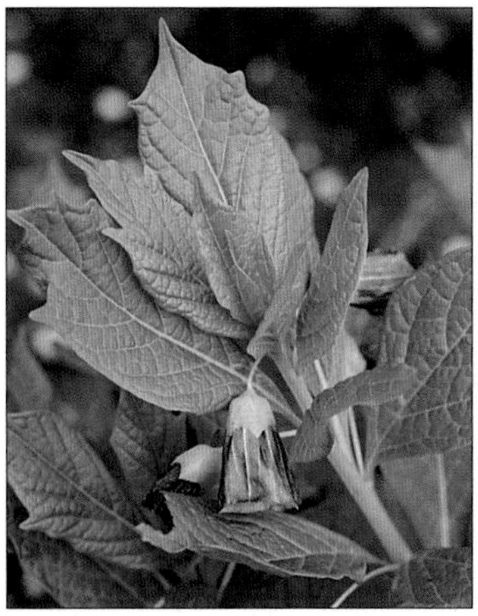

Scopolia carniolica

S. carniolica ■ Creeping, rhizomatous perennial with ovate or ovate-oblong, pointed, veined, wrinkled leaves, to 20cm (8in) long. Solitary, 5-pointed, bell-shaped, brownish purple to red flowers, 2.5cm (1in) long, yellow-green inside, are borne from the leaf axils in mid- and late spring. ↕↔ to 60cm (24in). C. and S.E. Europe, Caucasus. ***.
subsp. *hladnikiana* has brighter, buff-yellow flowers, greenish yellow inside.

▷**Scorpion weed** see *Phacelia*
▷**Scots heather** see *Calluna vulgaris*
▷**Scots pine** see *Pinus sylvestris*

SCROPHULARIA

Figwort

SCROPHULARIACEAE

Genus of about 200 species of subshrubs and herbaceous perennials, mainly found in marshes, moist meadows, woodland, scrub, and drier wasteland in N. temperate regions, with a few species occurring in tropical North and Central America. Often coarse and unpleasantly scented, they have erect, square stems, opposite, simple, entire or toothed, scalloped or lobed leaves, and small,

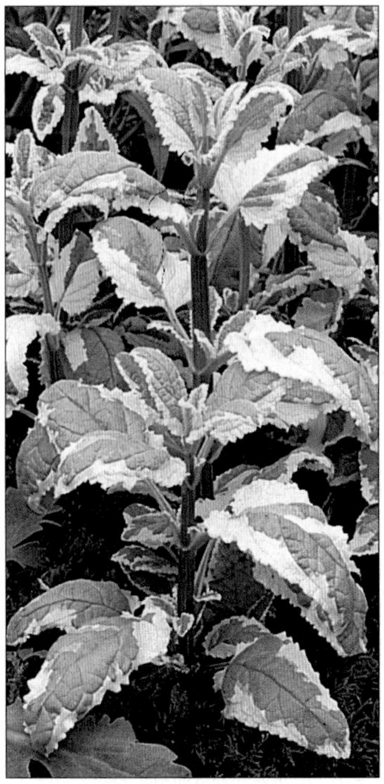

Scrophularia auriculata 'Variegata'

2-lipped, foxglove-like, greenish yellow, purple, or red flowers, borne in terminal, panicle-like cymes. Suitable for a wild or woodland garden. *S. auriculata* may also be grown as a marginal aquatic plant.
• **HARDINESS** Fully hardy to half hardy.
• **CULTIVATION** Grow in humus-rich, moist but well-drained soil in dappled to partial shade. If *S. auriculata* and its cultivars are grown as marginal aquatic plants, submerge to about 15cm (6in) deep. See also pp.52–53. To maintain *S. auriculata* 'Variegata' as a foliage plant, remove flowering stems as they form.
• **PROPAGATION** Sow seed of perennials *in situ* in autumn or spring. *S. auriculata* 'Variegata' will not come true from seed. Divide in spring. Root basal cuttings in a cold frame in spring, or root softwood cuttings in summer.
• **PESTS AND DISEASES** Prone to damage from slugs, caterpillars, and figwort weevils.

S. aquatica see *S. auriculata.*
S. auriculata, syn. *S. aquatica* (Water betony, Water figwort). Marginal aquatic perennial, or moisture-loving herbaceous perennial. Erect, square, winged stems produce ovate, wrinkled, toothed, dark green leaves, 5–25cm (2–10in) long. Panicle-like cymes of 2-lipped, yellowish green flowers, to 1cm (½in) long, each with a brown upper lip, are borne above the leaves from early summer to early autumn. ↕↔ 90cm (36in). W. Europe. ***.
'Variegata' ■ bears leaves boldly marked cream.

SCUTELLARIA

Helmet flower, Skullcap

LABIATAE/LAMIACEAE

Genus of about 300 species of erect or spreading annuals, rhizomatous and clump-forming herbaceous perennials, and, more rarely, subshrubs, widespread in temperate regions and on mountains in tropical areas. Leaves are opposite and entire, rarely pinnatifid or toothed. The tubular, 2-lipped, blue, violet, yellow, or white flowers, often with coloured bracts, are borne singly or in pairs from the leaf axils, or in terminal spikes or racemes. Grow smaller species in a rock garden or alpine house; use taller species at the front of a herbaceous border.
• **HARDINESS** Fully hardy to frost hardy.
• **CULTIVATION** Grow in moderately fertile, light, gravelly, well-drained, neutral to alkaline soil in full sun or light dappled shade. In very cold areas, apply a deep winter mulch. In an alpine house, grow in equal parts loam, leaf mould, and grit.
• **PROPAGATION** Sow seed in containers in a cold frame in autumn. Divide in autumn or spring. Take basal and softwood cuttings in late spring or early summer.
• **PESTS AND DISEASES** Prone to aphids and red spider mites under glass.

S. alpina. Spreading, tuft-forming perennial with ovate, toothed, hairy, grey-green leaves, to 2.5cm (1in) long. In summer, bears erect purple flowers, 2.5cm (1in) long, with yellow-white lower lips, in dense, 4-angled racemes. ↕ 15cm (6in), ↔ 30cm (12in). S. Europe to Russia (Siberia). ***

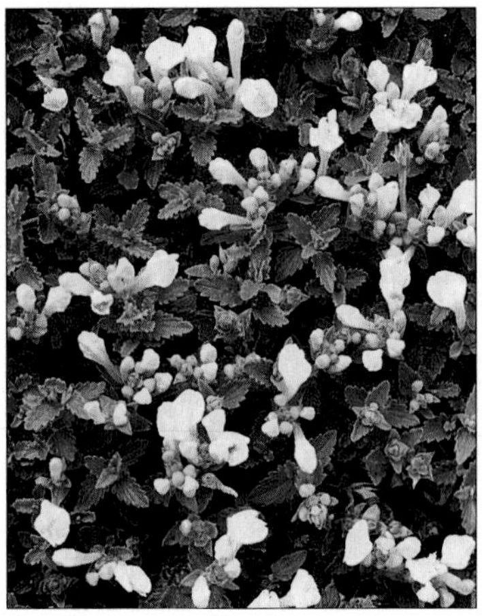

Scutellaria orientalis

S. baicalensis. Bushy perennial with angular, decumbent then erect, purple-tinged stems, and short-stalked, lance-shaped, hairy-margined, mid-green leaves, to 4cm (1½in) long. From early summer to early autumn, produces dense, one-sided racemes of hairy flowers, to 2.5cm (1in) long, upper lips dark blue, lower lips paler. ‡↔ 20–30cm (8–12in). Mongolia, China, Japan. ✻✻✻

S. indica. Slender, upright, rhizomatous perennial with white-hairy, shallowly toothed, broadly ovate to heart-shaped, mid-green leaves, to 2.5cm (1in) long. Bears dense, 4-angled racemes of long-tubed, grey-blue or rarely white flowers, to 2cm (¾in) long, in summer. ‡↔ to 20cm (8in). Mountains of China, Korea, Japan. ✻✻✻. **var. *parvifolia*,** syn. var. *japonica*, has lilac-blue flowers; ‡25cm (10in), ↔30cm (12in).

S. orientalis ■ Woody-based, rhizomatous perennial with grey-hairy, rooting stems, and ovate-oblong to broadly ovate, deeply toothed to pinnatisect, dark green leaves, 1.5cm (½in) long, grey-woolly beneath. In summer, bears dense, erect, 4-angled racemes of bright yellow flowers, 1.5–3cm (½–1¼in) long, marked red on the lower lips, and with yellow-green or purple-tinted bracts. ‡25cm (10cm), ↔ 30cm (12in). S.E. Europe. ✻✻✻

▷**Sea buckthorn** see *Hippophae rhamnoides*
▷***Seaforthia elegans*** see *Ptychosperma elegans*
▷**Sea kale** see *Crambe maritima*
▷**Sea lavender** see *Limonium, L. latifolium*
▷**Sea onion** see *Urginea maritima*
False see *Ornithogalum longibracteatum*
▷**Sea pink** see *Armeria*
▷**Sedge** see *Carex*
Bowles' golden see *Carex elata* 'Aurea'
Drooping see *Carex pendula*
Hook see *Uncinia*
Leatherleaf see *Carex buchananii*
Mace see *Carex grayi*
Palm branch see *Carex muskingumensis*
Pendulous see *Carex pendula*
Variegated russet see *Carex saxatilis* 'Ski Run'
Weeping see *Carex pendula*
▷**Sedges** see p.54
▷***Sedirea japonica*** see *Aerides japonica*

SEDUM syn. HYLOTELEPHIUM

Stonecrop

CRASSULACEAE

Genus of about 400 species of usually succulent annuals and evergreen, semi-evergreen, or deciduous biennials, perennials, subshrubs, and shrubs, a few of which are sometimes included in the genus *Hylotelephium*. They are widely distributed, most found in mountains of the N. hemisphere, but some in arid areas of South America. Stonecrops are very variable, with alternate, opposite, or whorled, fleshy, cylindrical or flattened leaves and usually terminal, often compound, cymes, panicles, or corymbs of generally star-shaped and 5-petalled flowers, borne mostly in summer and autumn. Grow hardy species in a rock garden or at the front of a herbaceous or mixed border. In frost-prone climates, grow tender species as houseplants, or in a temperate greenhouse or conservatory. All parts of the plants may cause mild stomach upset if ingested; contact with the sap may irritate skin.

• **HARDINESS** Fully hardy to frost tender.

• **CULTIVATION** Under glass, grow tender species in a mix of 3 parts loam-based potting compost (JI No.2), 2 parts grit, and 1 part leaf mould, in full light with good ventilation. In growth, water moderately and apply a half-strength balanced liquid fertilizer every month; water sparingly in winter. Outdoors, grow in moderately fertile, well-drained, neutral to slightly alkaline soil in full sun. Vigorous species tolerate light shade. Cut back spreading species after flowering, to maintain shape. Divide larger, herbaceous species every 3 or 4 years to improve flowering.

• **PROPAGATION** Sow seed of hardy species in containers in a cold frame in autumn. Sow seed of annuals and biennials at 13–16°C (55–61°F) in early spring, or *in situ* in mid-spring. Sow tender species at 15–18°C (59–64°F) in early spring. Divide in spring. For perennials, subshrubs, and shrubs, take softwood cuttings of non-flowering shoots in early summer.

• **PESTS AND DISEASES** Outdoors, prone to slugs and snails; may be affected by fungal and bacterial crown and root rots. Under glass, prone to aphids, and may be infested by scale insects, mealy-bugs, and vine weevil grubs.

S. acre ■ (Biting stonecrop, Common stonecrop, Wallpepper). Mat-forming, evergreen perennial with erect or trailing stems densely clothed in overlapping, triangular, pale green leaves, to 6mm (¼in) long. Flat-topped cymes, 2.5–4cm (1–1½in) across, of star-shaped, yellow-green flowers, 1.5cm (½in) across, are produced in abundance over long periods in summer. ‡5cm (2in), ↔ 60cm (24in) or more. Europe, Turkey, N. Africa. ✻✻✻. **'Aureum'** ■ bears bright yellow leaves.

S. aizoon, syn. *S. maximowiczii*. Rhizomatous, deciduous perennial with a stout rootstock and upright, unbranched, hairless stems bearing alternate, stalkless, ovate-lance-shaped, coarsely toothed, light green leaves, to 8cm (3in) long. In summer, produces star-shaped yellow flowers, 1.5cm (½in) across, with conspicuous stamens, in terminal, flattened, cyme-like clusters, to 4cm (1½in) across. ‡↔ 45cm (18in). Russia (Siberia), China, Japan. ✻✻✻. **'Aurantiacum'** ■ has dark red stems, dark green leaves, and red-tinted buds opening to yellow-orange flowers, followed by spherical to ovoid red fruit. **'Euphorbioides'** is more compact, and has deeper yellow flowers; ‡35cm (14in), ↔ 30cm (12in).

S. alboroseum see *S. erythrostictum*.

***S.* 'Autumn Joy'** see *S.* 'Herbstfreude'.

S. caeruleum. Branching, spreading annual with alternate, spoon-shaped, ovate to oblong-ovate, pale green leaves, 1–2cm (½–¾in) long. In summer, bears star-shaped, 7-petalled, pale blue flowers, 6mm (¼in) across, in cymes to 2.5cm (1in) across. Leaves and stems gradually flush red during flowering. Self-seeds freely. ‡10–15cm (4–6in), ↔ to 15cm (6in). France (Corsica), Italy (Sardinia, Sicily), coastal Tunisia and Algeria. ✻✻✻

S. cauticola 🏆 Trailing, stoloniferous, sometimes woody-based, deciduous perennial with purple-tinged stems bearing opposite, bluntly toothed, rounded to spoon-shaped or obovate, grey-green leaves, to 2.5cm (1in) long. In early autumn, branching stems bear terminal, slightly rounded, panicle-like cymes, to 10cm (4in) across, of star-shaped, pink-purple flowers, to 9mm (⅜in) across, ageing to carmine-red. ‡8cm (3in), ↔ 30cm (12in). Japan. ✻✻✻

S. crassipes see *Rhodiola wallichiana*.

S. erythrostictum, syn. *Hylotelephium roseum, S. alboroseum*. Clump-forming, deciduous perennial, similar to *S. spectabile*, with unbranched, spreading, woody stems bearing usually opposite, ovate, sometimes toothed, glaucous, grey-green leaves, to 8cm (3in) long. In late summer, bears terminal, corymb-like clusters, to 15cm (6in) across, of star-shaped, greenish white flowers, 1cm (½in) across, with pink carpels. ‡30cm (12in), ↔ 60cm (24in). E. Asia. ✻✻✻. **'Mediovariegatum'** produces larger flower clusters, and leaves with central, creamy white splashes, which are especially striking in spring. Grow in partial shade and cut out reverting green shoots; ↔ 45cm (18in).

S. ewersii. Low-branching, deciduous perennial with opposite, stalkless, rounded to broadly ovate, entire or slightly toothed, grey-blue leaves, to 2cm (¾in) long, heart-shaped at the bases. In summer, produces dense, rounded cymes, to 10cm (4in) across, of star-shaped, pinkish red flowers, to 8mm (⅜in) across. Similar to, but often later flowering than *S. cauticola*. ‡8cm (3in), ↔ 30cm (12in). C. Asia, Himalayas, Mongolia, China. ✻✻✻

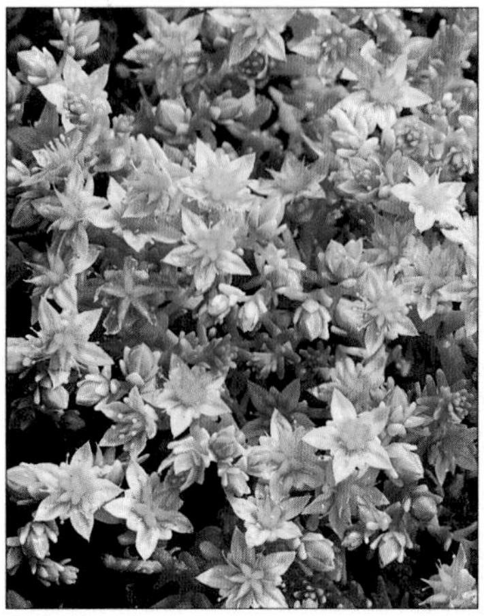

Sedum acre

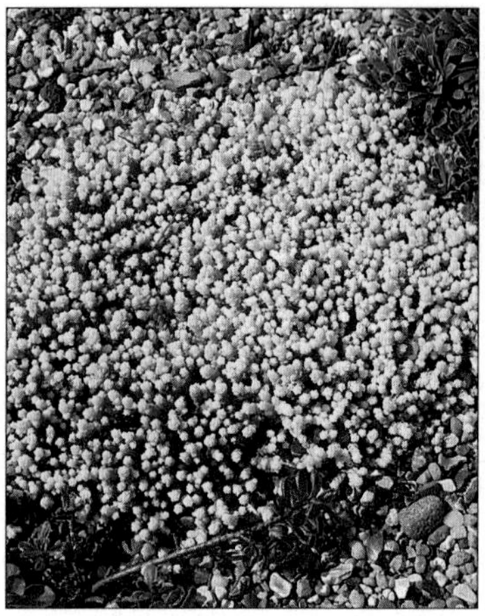

Sedum acre 'Aureum'

S. frutescens. Shrubby, semi-evergreen perennial bearing woody, branching stems, to 1cm (½in) thick, clothed in papery, peeling bark. Alternate, pointed, linear-elliptic, bright green leaves, 2–6cm (¾–2½in) long, are usually produced in terminal clusters. In summer, star-shaped white flowers, to 1.5cm (½in) across, are produced in few-flowered, terminal cymes. ‡ to 1m (3ft), ↔ 40cm (16in). Mexico. ❄ (min. 5–7°C/41–45°F)

***S.* 'Herbstfreude'** 🏆 syn. *S.* 'Autumn Joy'. Clump-forming, bushy deciduous perennial with unbranched, glaucous, mid-green stems bearing alternate, oblong to obovate, toothed, glaucous, dark green leaves, to 12cm (5in) long. In early autumn, produces flat corymbs, to 20cm (8in) across, of star-shaped flowers, 5mm (¼in) across, deep pink at first, then turning through pinkish bronze to copper-red. ‡↔ to 60cm (24in). ✻✻✻

S. heterodontum see *Rhodiola heterodonta*.

S. humifusum ■ Mat-forming, evergreen perennial with creeping, branching stems bearing tight rosettes of overlapping, blunt, obovate, mid-green leaves, 4mm (⅛in) long, ageing to red. Solitary, terminal, bright yellow flowers, 9mm (⅜in) across, are borne in early summer. ‡1cm (½in), ↔ 10cm (4in). Mexico. ✻✻

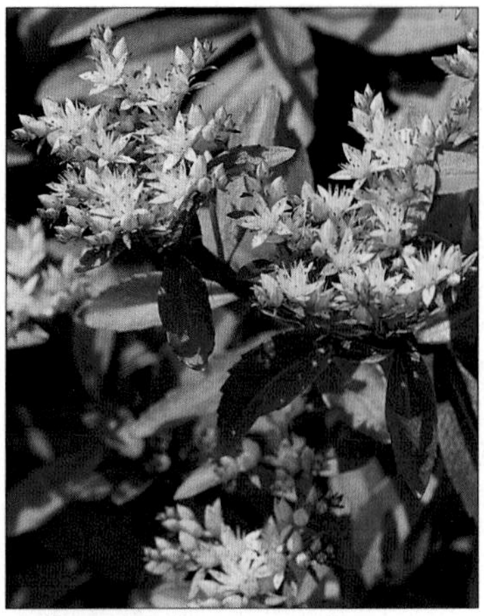

Sedum aizoon 'Aurantiacum'

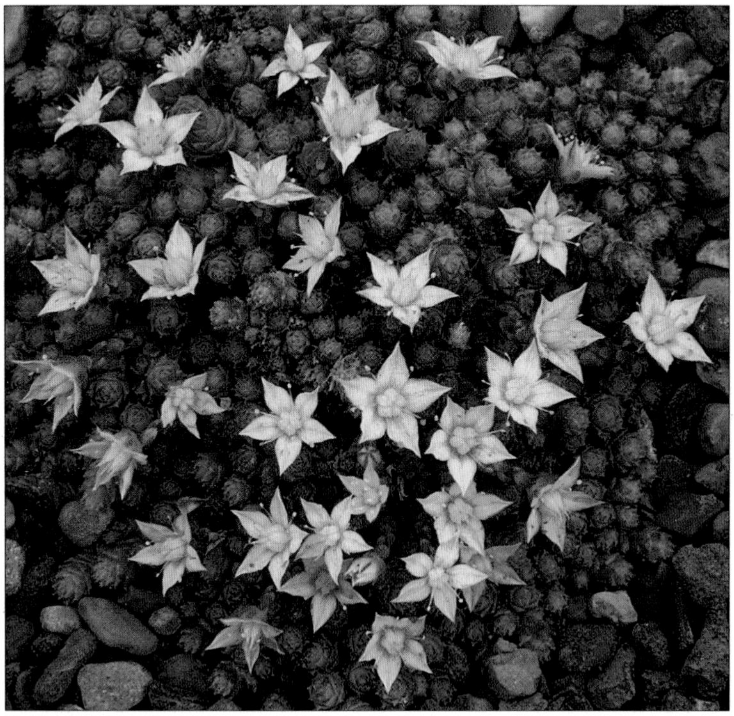

Sedum humifusum

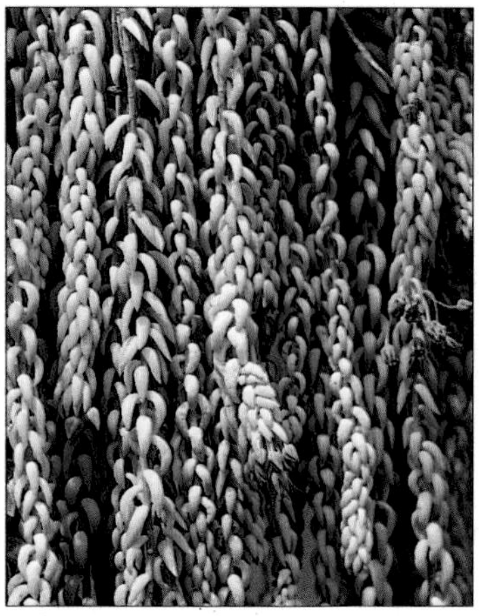

Sedum morganianum

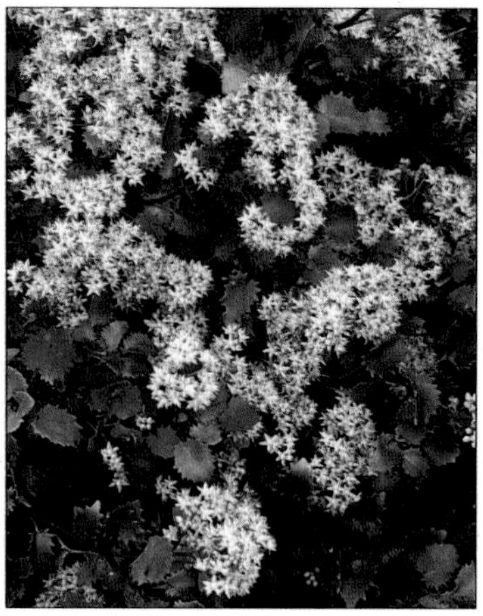

Sedum populifolium

S. kamtschaticum ♀ Clump-forming, semi-evergreen perennial with stout rhizomes and alternate, inversely lance-shaped to spoon-shaped, glossy, deep green leaves, to 4cm (1½in) long, coarsely toothed towards the tips. In late summer, bears short-stemmed, flat cymes, to 5cm (2in) across, of star-shaped, deep golden yellow flowers, 1.5cm (½in) across, opening from pink buds. ↕ 10cm (4in), ↔ 25cm (10in). Russia (Siberia, Kamchatka), N. and C. China, Japan. ❄❄❄. **'Variegatum'** ■ ♀ has pink-tinted, mid-green leaves with cream margins, and yellow flowers, ageing to crimson. Tolerant of partial shade.
S. lydium ■ Stem-rooting, mat-forming, evergreen perennial with tight rosettes of cylindrical, red-tipped, bright to mid-green leaves, to 6mm (¼in) long. In summer, bears flat-topped, terminal corymbs, 2.5cm (1in) across, of star-shaped white flowers, 6mm (¼in) across. ↕ 5cm (2in), ↔ 20cm (8in). W. and C. Turkey. ❄❄❄
S. maximowiczii see *S. aizoon.*
S. morganianum ■ ♀ Pendent, evergreen perennial (prostrate in the wild) with fleshy, woody-based stems and bearing alternate, oblong-lance-shaped, fleshy, glaucous, greenish blue leaves, to 2cm (¾in) long. In spring and summer, star-shaped, pale pink to deep scarlet-purple flowers, 1cm (½in) across, are produced in cymes to 2.5cm (1in) across. ↕↔ 30cm (12in). Mexico. ❁ (min. 5–7°C/41–45°F)
S. obtusatum ■ syn. *S. rubroglaucum.* Evergreen perennial with terminal rosettes of spoon-shaped, blunt-tipped, glaucous, mid-green leaves, 0.5–2.5cm (¼–1in) long, flushed crimson in autumn. In summer, bears star-shaped, bright yellow flowers, to 1cm (½in) across, in flat, panicle-like cymes, to 10cm (4in) across. ↕ 5cm (2in), ↔ 20cm (8in). USA (California). ❄❄❄
S. oxypetalum. Many-branched, semi-evergreen perennial with fleshy, woody stems, clothed in papery, peeling bark. The alternate, inversely lance-shaped to obovate, minutely papillose, greyish green leaves are 5cm (2in) long. Diurnal, star-shaped, fragrant, pink or dull red flowers, to 1.5cm (½in) across, usually with pink-marked petals, open in cymes 4cm (1½in) across, in summer. ↕ 50–90cm (20–36in), ↔ 45cm (18in). Mexico. ❁ (min. 5–7°C/41–45°F)
S. pilosum. Densely grey-hairy, rosette-forming, evergreen biennial. Incurved, oblong to narrowly spoon-shaped, dark green leaves are to 2cm (¾in) long. Bears dense, flat corymbs, 5cm (2in) across, of many short-stemmed, bell-shaped, rose-red flowers, 9mm (⅜in) across, in summer. ↕ 8cm (3in), ↔ 15cm (6in). W. Asia (Turkey to Iran). ❄❄
S. populifolium ■ Slowly spreading, deciduous subshrub with slightly decumbent, branched, dark brown stems bearing alternate, ovate, toothed, light green leaves, to 4cm (1½in) long, heart-shaped at the bases. Corymb-like cymes, 5cm (2in) across, of star-shaped, fragrant white flowers, 1cm (½in) across, pink-tinged on the reverse, are borne in late summer and early autumn. ↕ 20–30cm (8–12in), ↔ 45cm (18in). Russia (Siberia). ❄❄❄
S. reflexum see *S. rupestre.*
S. rhodiola see *Rhodiola rosea.*
S. rosea see *Rhodiola rosea.*
S. rosea* var. *heterodontum see *Rhodiola heterodonta.*
S. rubroglaucum see *S. obtusatum.*
S. rubrotinctum. Evergreen subshrub with numerous arching, rooting, branching stems bearing alternate, blunt, cylindrical, mid-green leaves, 1.5cm (½in) long, often flushed red. Loose, many-flowered cymes, 4cm (1½in) across, of star-shaped, pale yellow flowers, 1cm (½in) across, are borne in winter. ↕ 24cm (10in), ↔ 20cm (8in). Mexico. ❄❄ (borderline)
***S.* 'Ruby Glow'** ■ ♀ Low-growing deciduous perennial with spreading, unbranched red stems bearing opposite, elliptic, toothed, green-purple leaves, 5cm (2in) long. Numerous loose cymes, 6cm (2½in) across, of star-shaped, ruby-red flowers, 1cm (½in) across, are produced from midsummer to early autumn. ↕ 25cm (10in), ↔ 45cm (18in). ❄❄❄
S. rupestre ■ syn. *S. reflexum* (Stone orpine). Vigorous, mat-forming, evergreen perennial with alternate, pointed, cylindrical, grey-green leaves, to 1–2cm (½–¾in) long. Upright, leafy, woody stems bear terminal, umbel-like cymes, 6cm (2½in) across, of star-shaped yellow flowers, 1.5cm (½in) across, pendent in bud, but erect as they open in summer. Spreads freely; best in a large rock garden. ↕ 10cm (4in), ↔ 60cm (24in) or more. Mountains of C. and W. Europe. ❄❄❄
S. sarcocaule see *Crassula sarcocaulis.*

Sedum 'Ruby Glow'

S

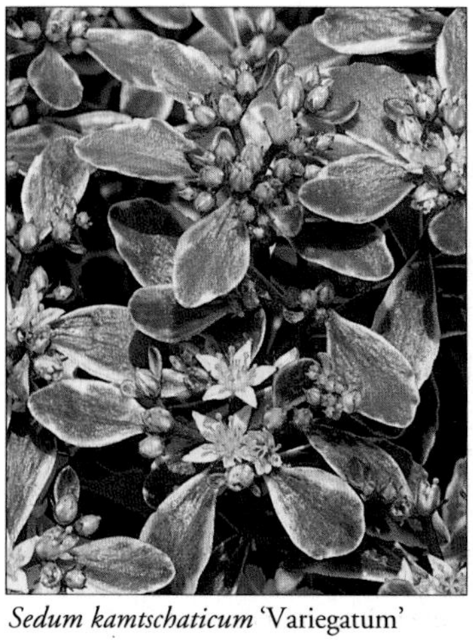

Sedum kamtschaticum 'Variegatum'

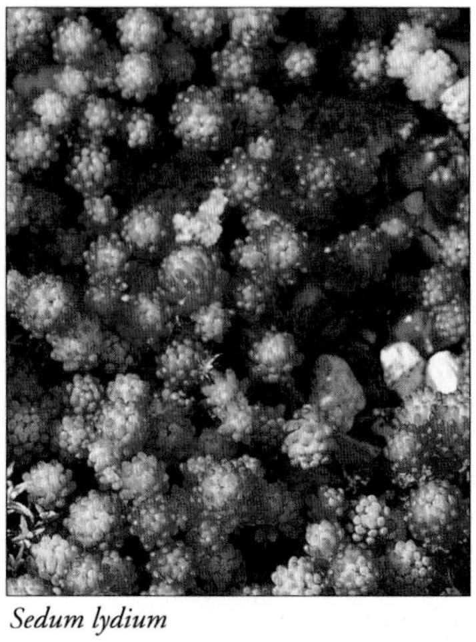

Sedum lydium

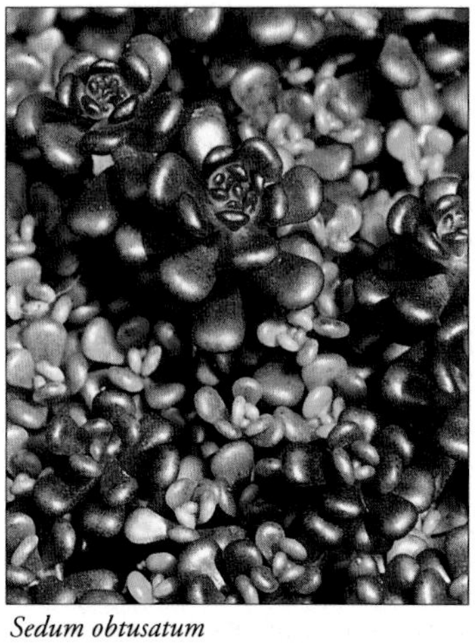

Sedum obtusatum

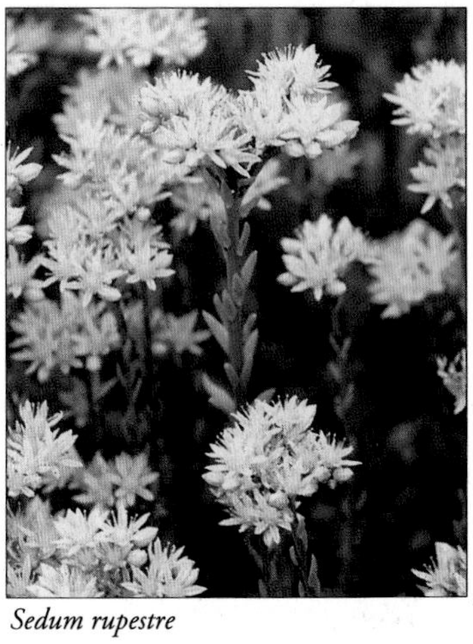

Sedum rupestre

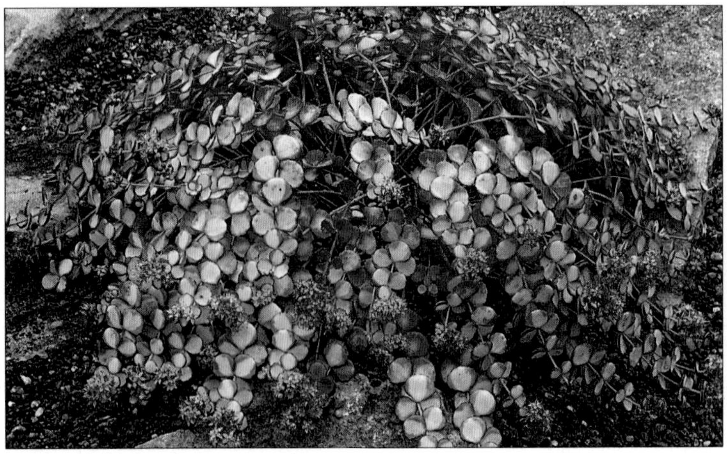

Sedum sieboldii 'Mediovariegatum'

S. sempervivoides. Rosette-forming, evergreen biennial producing pointed, ovate to diamond-shaped, hairy, blue-green leaves, to 3cm (1¼in) long, flushed red-purple at the bases. In summer, bears domed, corymb-like panicles, 4–5cm (1½–2in) across, of many star-shaped, carmine-red flowers, 1.5cm (½in) across. Dislikes winter wet; best in an alpine house. ↕ 10cm (4in), ↔ 15cm (6in). Caucasus, Georgia, N. Iran, S.W. Asia. ❄❄

S. sieboldii. Spreading, tuberous, tufted, deciduous perennial with whorls of 3 rounded, glaucous, blue-green, occasionally purple-tinted leaves, to 2cm (¾in) long, some irregularly toothed and red-margined towards the tips. Star-shaped pink flowers, to 1.5cm (½in) across, are borne in flat-topped cymes,

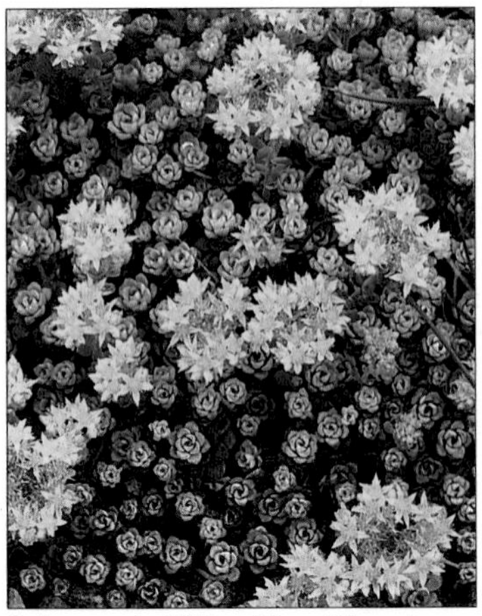

Sedum spathulifolium 'Cape Blanco'

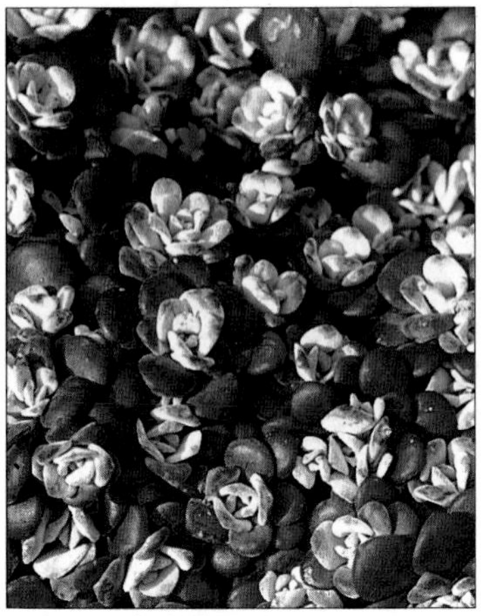

Sedum spathulifolium 'Purpureum'

6cm (2½in) across, in late summer. Use as a houseplant, or in an alpine house. ↕ 10cm (4in), ↔ 20cm (8in). Japan. ❄❄. **'Mediovariegatum'** ▣ ♀ syn. 'Foliis Mediovariegatis', 'Foliis Variegatis', 'Variegatum', has glaucous-blue leaves, marbled cream and occasionally with red margins.

S. spathulifolium. Vigorous, mat-forming, evergreen perennial with branching, fleshy stems bearing terminal rosettes of brittle, spoon-shaped, silvery or mid-green leaves, to 2cm (¾in) long, usually tinted bronze-purple. Short-stemmed, star-shaped, bright yellow flowers, 1.5cm (½in) across, are borne in flat cymes, 2.5cm (1in) across, in summer. Tolerates light shade. ↕ 10cm (4in), ↔ 60cm (24in). W. North America. ❄❄❄. **'Cape Blanco'** ▣ ♀ syn. 'Cappa Blanca', has the innermost leaves of its rosettes heavily powdered with white bloom. **'Purpureum'** ▣ ♀ produces leaves richly suffused reddish purple.

S. spectabile ♀ (Ice plant). Clump-forming, deciduous perennial. Upright, unbranched green stems bear opposite or whorled, ovate to elliptic or obovate, slightly scalloped, toothed, grey-green leaves, to 8cm (3in) long. In late summer, star-shaped pink flowers, to 1cm (½in) across, with prominent stamens, are borne in dense, flat cymes, to 15cm (6in) across, often causing the stems to bend. Attractive to bees. ↕↔ 45cm (18in). China, Korea. ❄❄❄. **'Brilliant'** ▣ ♀ bears flowers with bright pink petals and darker pink carpels and anthers. **'Carmen'** is a slightly darker mauve-pink. **'Iceberg'** has paler green leaves than the species, and pure white flowers; ↕ 30–45cm (12–18in), ↔ 35cm (14in). **'Septemberglut'**, syn. 'September Glow', has glowing, rich pink flowers; ↕ to 50cm (20in).

S. spurium. Vigorous, mat-forming, evergreen perennial with branching red stems bearing opposite, obovate, toothed, mid-green leaves, to 2.5cm (1in) long. Star-shaped, pinkish purple or white flowers, 2cm (¾in) across, are produced in rounded corymbs, 4cm (1½in) across, in late summer. ↕ 10cm (4in), ↔ 60cm (24in) or more. Caucasus, Armenia, N. Iran. ❄❄❄. **'Dragon's Blood'** see 'Schorbuser Blut'. **'Purple Carpet'** see 'Purpurteppich'. **'Purpurteppich'**, syn. 'Purple Carpet', is compact, with deep plum-purple leaves and dark purplish red flowers. **'Schorbuser Blut'** ▣ ♀ syn. 'Dragon's

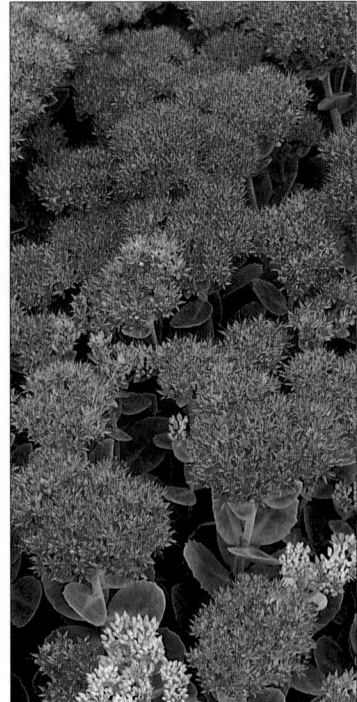

Sedum spectabile 'Brilliant'

Blood', has green leaves, purple-tinted when mature, and deep pink flowers.

S. telephium (Orpine). Clump-forming, rhizomatous, deciduous perennial. Erect, unbranched, pale green stems bear alternate, oblong to oblong-ovate, toothed, glaucous, grey-green leaves, to 8cm (3in) long. Dense, axillary and terminal cymes, to 12cm (5in) across, of star-shaped, purplish pink flowers, to 1cm (½in) across, are borne in late summer and early autumn. ↕ to 60cm (24in), ↔ 30cm (12in). Europe, Russia (Siberia), China, Japan. ❄❄❄. **subsp. *maximum* 'Atropurpureum'** ▣ ♀ has glaucous, very dark purple stems and leaves, and smaller cymes of pink flowers with orange-red centres, appearing buff-white; ↕ 45–60cm (18–24in). **'Munstead Dark Red'** has purple-tinted, dark green leaves and dark purplish red flowers, becoming even darker with age; ↕ to 60cm (24in).

***S.* 'Vera Jameson'** ♀ Deciduous perennial with spreading purple stems and opposite, ovate, toothed, glaucous, purple-pink leaves, to 10cm (4in) long, appearing almost pink at flowering time. In late summer and early autumn, bears

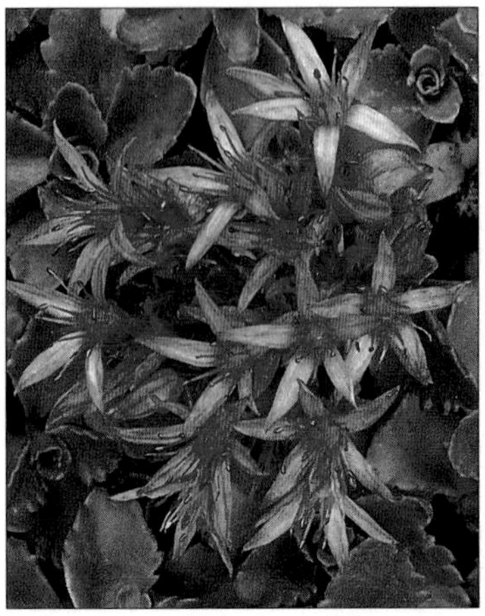

Sedum spurium 'Schorbuser Blut'

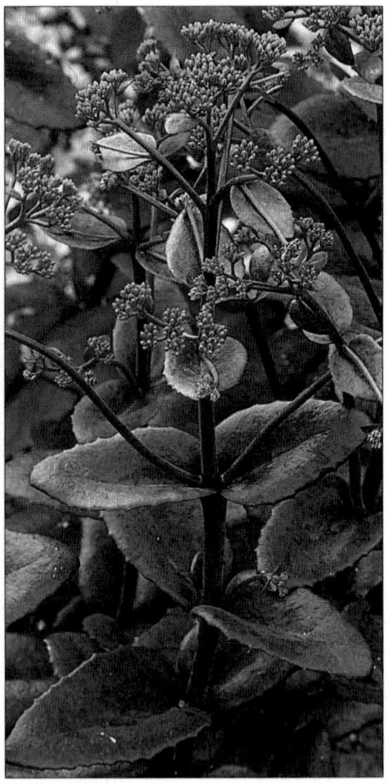

Sedum telephium subsp. *maximum* 'Atropurpureum'

rounded cymes, 6cm (2½in) across, of star-shaped, soft rose-pink flowers, 6–10mm (¼–½in) across. ↕ 20–30cm (8–12in), ↔ 45cm (18in). ❄❄❄

S. wallichianum see *Rhodiola wallichiana.*

S. weinbergii see *Graptopetalum paraguayense.*

▷ ***Seemannia gymnostoma*** see *Gloxinia gymnostoma*

SELAGINELLA

SELAGINELLACEAE

Genus of approximately 700 species of evergreen, rhizomatous perennials found in a range of habitats, from semi-desert to rainforest, mostly in tropical regions, with some species in temperate and alpine zones. Grown for their foliage, they vary from small, moss-like tufts to tall, scrambling plants. They have long, creeping, branched stems, often rooting along their length, which are clothed in scale-like leaves, to 3mm (⅛in) long. Spores form in small, leafy, terminal spikes. Use as ground cover or in hanging baskets. In frost-prone areas,

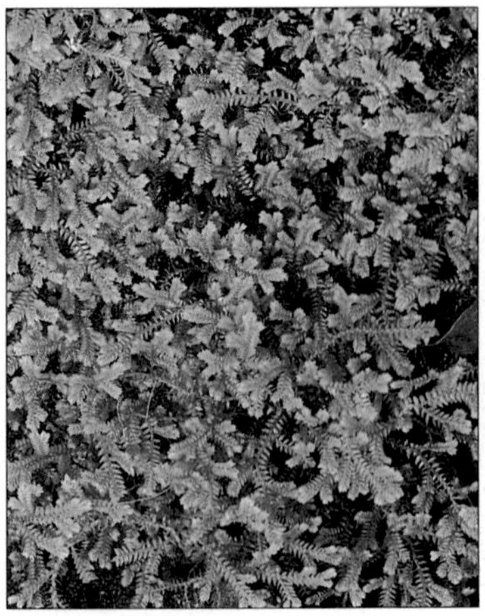

Selaginella kraussiana

S

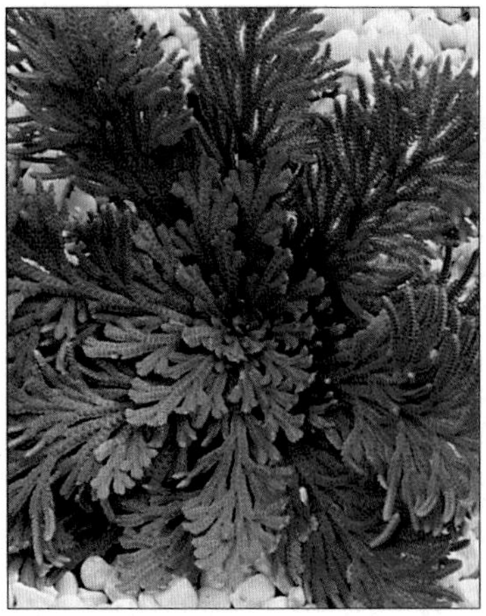

Selaginella lepidophylla

grow in a cool, temperate, or warm greenhouse, or as houseplants.
• **HARDINESS** Frost tender.
• **CULTIVATION** Under glass, grow in a mix of 2 parts loam-based potting compost (JI No.2) and 1 part leaf mould, in bright filtered or indirect light; *S. uncinata* and *S. willdenovii* are best in bright filtered light. In growth, water freely and apply a balanced liquid fertilizer monthly. Maintain high humidity. Keep just moist in winter. Outdoors, grow in moderately fertile, humus-rich, moist but well-drained, neutral to slightly acid soil in partial shade. *S. lepidophylla* tolerates drier conditions and prefers alkaline soil. Shelter from cold, drying winds.
• **PROPAGATION** Sow spores at 21°C (70°F) as soon as ripe. Divide rhizomes or rooted stems in spring.
• **PESTS AND DISEASES** Trouble free.

S. emmeliana see *S. pallescens*.
S. kraussiana ■ 🏆 (Krauss's spikemoss). Mat-forming perennial producing trailing stems clothed in pinnatisect, bright green foliage. ↕ 2.5cm (1in), ↔ indefinite. Tropical and southern Africa, Azores. ❄ (min. 5–7°C/ 41–45°F). **'Aurea'** has yellow-green foliage. **'Brownii'** 🏆 forms small cushions; ↕ 5cm (2in), ↔ 15cm (6in). **'Variegata'** 🏆 produces cream-splashed foliage.
S. lepidophylla ■ (Resurrection plant, Rose of Jericho). Small, spreading perennial with dense tufts of dark green leaves. When dry, curls into a ball that opens into a flat rosette when soaked with water. Dry plants are often sold

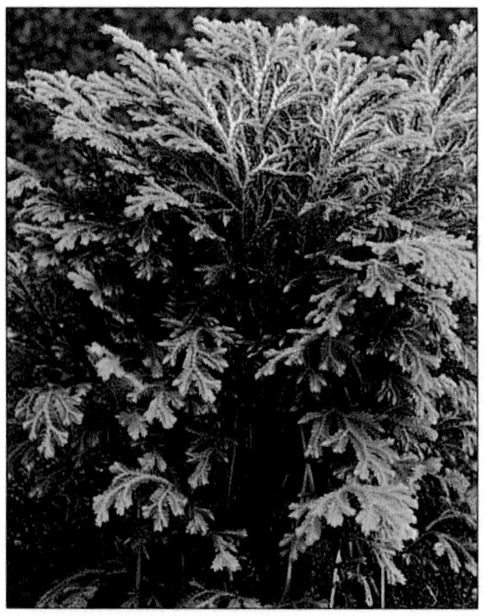

Selaginella martensii

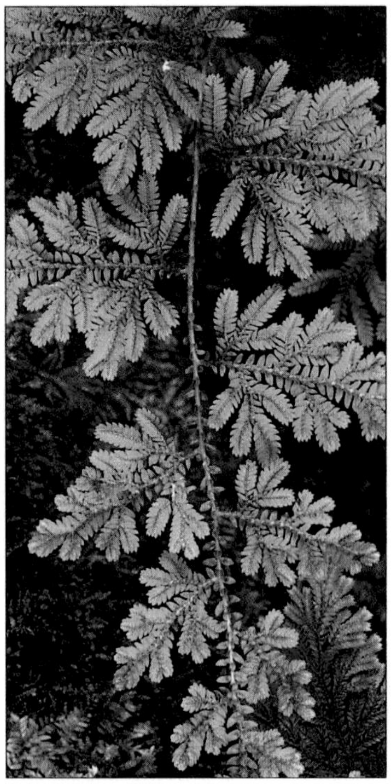

Selaginella willdenovii

as curiosities. ↕ to 8cm (3in), ↔ 15cm (6in). USA (Arizona, Texas) to Peru. ❄ (min. 5–7°C/41–45°F)
S. martensii ■ 🏆 Trailing perennial with many-branched stems bearing frond-like, glossy, bright green foliage. ↕ to 15cm (6in), ↔ 20cm (8in). Central America. ❄ (min. 5–7°C/41–45°F). **'Variegata'** has white-flecked foliage.
S. pallescens, syn. *S. emmeliana*. Perennial with a densely tufted stem, branching from the base, with short, much-divided branches. Leaves are light yellow-green, white beneath. ↕ to 15cm (6in), ↔ 30cm (12in). North America to N. Colombia and Venezuela. ❄ (min. 10–15°C/50–59°F)
S. umbrosa. Perennial with erect, regularly branched, red-tinged stems, and triangular, 3-pinnate branches with light green leaves. ↕ to 40cm (16in), ↔ indefinite. Central and South America. ❄ (min. 10–15°C/50–59°F)
S. uncinata 🏆 Perennial with slender, trailing, rooting stems bearing alternate, short, pinnate branches and leaves with a distinct metallic blue sheen. ↕ 2.5–5cm (1–2in), ↔ indefinite. China. ❄ (min. 5–7°C/41–45°F)
S. willdenovii ■ Perennial climber with a nearly leafless stem bearing densely branched, leafy sideshoots. Leaves are mid-green, ageing to pinkish yellow or plum, with a metallic blue sheen. ↕ 3–6m (10–20ft) or more. Himalayas to S. China and Indonesia. ❄ (min. 10–15°C/50–59°F)

SELAGO

SCROPHULARIACEAE

Genus of about 150 species of evergreen shrubs, subshrubs, and annuals from grassland, rocky places, moist sites, and forest margins in tropical Africa and South Africa. Their simple, often very narrow leaves are usually clustered or solitary, and borne at alternate nodes or occasionally in opposite pairs. Selagos are grown mainly for their heads, spikes, corymbs, or panicles of usually small, tubular flowers, each with 5 spreading petal lobes. In frost-prone climates, grow in a temperate greenhouse. In milder areas, grow at the front of a shrub border, in a raised bed, or at the base of a warm, sunny wall. *S. serrata* is also effective grown in a container in a courtyard garden.
• **HARDINESS** Frost tender, although some may survive temperatures near 0°C (32°F).
• **CULTIVATION** Under glass, grow in loam-based potting compost (JI No.2) in full light with shade from hot sun, or in bright filtered light. In growth, water freely, and apply a balanced liquid fertilizer monthly; maintain low to moderate humidity. Keep just moist in winter. Outdoors, grow in moderately fertile, humus-rich, moist but well-drained soil in full sun. Dead-head regularly. Pruning group 9.
• **PROPAGATION** Sow seed at 13–15°C (55–59°F) in spring. Root softwood cuttings in spring or early summer, with bottom heat. Layer or air layer in spring or early summer.
• **PESTS AND DISEASES** Red spider mites may be a problem under glass.

S. serrata. Initially erect, then spreading to decumbent, evergreen shrub with crowded, stalkless, obovate or oblong, boldly toothed, firm, deep green leaves, to 2.5cm (1in) long. Fragrant purple to pale blue flowers are borne in compact corymbs, to 5cm (2in) across, in summer. ↕↔ 30–90cm (12–36in). South Africa. ❄ (min. 5°C/41°F)

SELENICEREUS

CACTACEAE

Genus of approximately 20 species of mostly scandent or semi-pendent, epiphytic or rock-dwelling, perennial cacti from forest and woody areas of Texas (USA), Mexico, Central America, Colombia, and the West Indies. They produce short-hairy, generally spiny areoles, and most have aerial roots. Stems are slender, ribbed, or, more rarely, angled or flattened. The large, trumpet-shaped, mainly nocturnal flowers are usually borne in summer. In areas where temperatures fall below 15°C (59°F), grow in a warm greenhouse, in hanging baskets or in containers with support for climbing stems. In warmer climates, grow in containers in a courtyard garden, or at the base of a warm, sunny wall.
• **HARDINESS** Frost tender.
• **CULTIVATION** Under glass, grow in epiphytic cactus compost in bright indirect to moderate light. In the growing season, water freely and apply a half-strength balanced liquid fertilizer monthly; keep just moist in winter. Maintain moderate to high humidity. Outdoors, grow in moderately fertile, humus-rich, moist but sharply drained, neutral to slightly alkaline soil, with additional grit and leaf mould, in light dappled to partial shade. See also pp.48–49.
• **PROPAGATION** Sow seed at 16–19°C (61–66°F) as soon as ripe or in spring. Root cuttings of stem segments in a closed, slightly shaded propagating case in spring or summer.
• **PESTS AND DISEASES** Scale insects and mealybugs may be a problem.

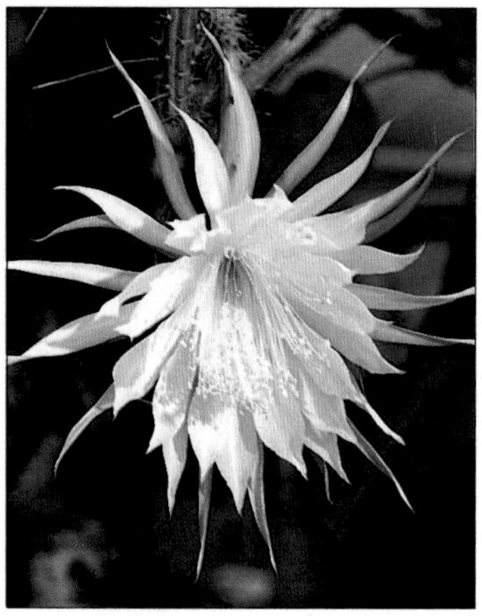

Selenicereus grandiflorus

S. anthonyanus, syn. *Cryptocereus anthonyanus*. Semi-pendent, scandent, epiphytic cactus with flattened, leaf-like, bright green stems, 7–15cm (3–6in) across, with prominent marginal notches, 4.5cm (1¾in) deep, forming lobes. The areoles bear 2–4 short, pale brown spines. In summer, produces nocturnal, fragrant, yellowish or creamy white flowers, 12cm (5in) long, with maroon-red outer segments. ↕ to 75cm (30in), ↔ indefinite. S.E. Mexico. ❄ (min. 15°C/59°F)
S. chrysocardium see *Epiphyllum chrysocardium*.
S. grandiflorus ■ (Queen of the night). Scandent, epiphytic cactus producing 5- to 8-ribbed, mid-green stems, 1–2.5cm (½–1in) thick, with areoles bearing 6–18 yellow spines that turn grey. The nocturnal, fragrant white flowers, 30cm (12in) long, with spreading, pale yellowish brown outer segments, are borne in summer. ↕ 5m (15ft). Mexico, West Indies. ❄ (min. 15°C/59°F)
S. hamatus. Scandent, epiphytic cactus with 3- or 4-angled, dark green stems, 1.5cm (½in) thick, bearing hooked warts. The areoles have 5–9 white or brown spines. The nocturnal, scented white flowers are 20–35cm (8–14in) long, with yellow and red outer segments, and produced during summer. ↕ 4m (12ft). Mexico, West Indies. ❄ (min. 15°C/59°F)
S. innesii. Scandent or trailing, epiphytic cactus with 4- or 5-ribbed, mid-green stems, 1cm (½in) thick, and woolly areoles bearing 1 or 2 thick, pale yellow spines and 3–7 slender ones. In summer, produces diurnal white flowers, 4–5cm (1½–2in) long, with extended petals, to 6cm (2½in) across, the outer petals tinged magenta-pink; some plants produce only male flowers, others produce only female. ↕ to 2m (6ft). West Indies (St. Vincent). ❄ (min. 15°C/59°F)
S. pteranthus. Scandent, epiphytic cactus with 4- to 6-angled, purplish green stems, 2.5–5cm (1–2in) thick, and white-woolly areoles bearing 6–12 thick, yellowish grey spines. Nocturnal, white or pale cream flowers, 30cm (12in) long, with long, slender, recurved, pale purple outer segments, are produced in summer. ↕ 4m (12ft). Mexico. ❄ (min. 15°C/59°F)
S. wercklei. Semi-pendent, freely branching, epiphytic cactus with mid-green stems, 1cm (½in) thick, each with

up to 12 shallow ribs. Areoles are mostly spineless, but a few brown spines form on the flower tubes. Nocturnal white flowers, 15cm (6in) long, with red outer segments, are produced in summer. ↕75cm (30in), ↔ indefinite. Costa Rica. ❀ (min. 15°C/59°F)

▷**Self-heal** see *Prunella*
Large see *P. grandiflora*

SELINUM

APIACEAE/UMBELLIFERAE

Genus of 6 species of tap-rooted perennials from rocky slopes, mountain meadows, and scrub in temperate areas of Europe and the Himalayas. The tall stems bear finely cut leaves and large, flattish umbels of small, star-shaped white flowers, rarely purple-tinged. Few species are grown, but *S. wallichianum* is suitable for an informal mixed or shrub border or a woodland garden, and is effective grown as a specimen to display the tiered effect of its floral umbels.

- **HARDINESS** Fully hardy.
- **CULTIVATION** Grow in moderately fertile, moist but well-drained soil in full sun or partial shade. Tolerant of a wide range of conditions.
- **PROPAGATION** Sow seed in containers in a cold frame as soon as ripe; prick out into deep containers as soon as possible to avoid tap-root damage. Divide carefully in early spring; selinums resent disturbance.
- **PESTS AND DISEASES** Overwintering buds are especially prone to slug and snail damage. Powdery mildew may be a problem in dry conditions.

S. tenuifolium see *S. wallichianum*.
S. wallichianum ■ syn. *S. tenuifolium*. Clump-forming perennial with erect, branched stems, usually shaded or lined reddish purple, as are the leaf-stalks, which are 20–30cm (8–12in) long. Triangular leaf-blades, to 50cm (20in) long, are 2- or 3-pinnate, the final segments elliptic and toothed. Tiny, star-shaped white flowers are borne in terminal umbels, to 20cm (8in) across, from midsummer to early autumn. ↕ to 1.8m (6ft), ↔ 60cm (24in). W. Pakistan, Himalayas, India. ❄❄❄

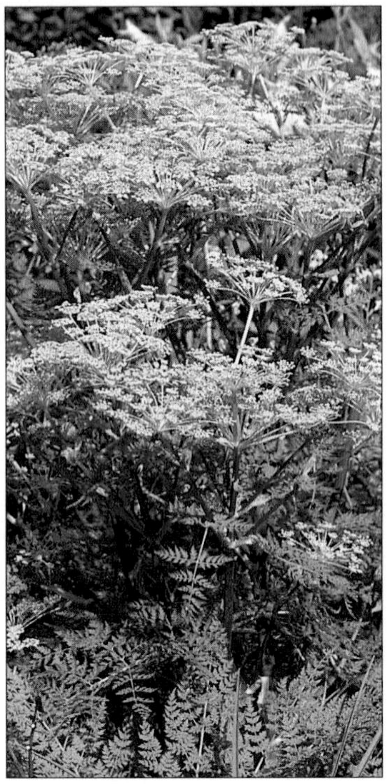
Selinum wallichianum

SEMELE

Climbing butcher's broom

LILIACEAE/RUSCACEAE

Genus of one species of evergreen, woody climber from laurel forest in S. Spain, S.E. France, Sicily, N. Africa, and the Canary Islands. The true leaves are scale-like, their function taken over by leaf-like stems, on which clusters of tiny, star-shaped, 6-tepalled flowers are borne in late spring and early summer. These are sometimes followed by single-seeded, orange-red berries. In frost-prone areas, grow as a foliage plant in a cool greenhouse. In warmer climates, use to provide handsome foliage cover on a warm, sunny wall.

- **HARDINESS** Half hardy.
- **CULTIVATION** Under glass, grow in loam-based potting compost (JI No.2) in full light with shade from hot sun, or in bright filtered light. In growth, water moderately and apply a balanced liquid fertilizer monthly; water sparingly in winter. Maintain low to moderate humidity. Outdoors, grow in moderately fertile, well-drained soil in full sun. Provide the stems with support. Pruning group 11, in late winter or early spring.
- **PROPAGATION** Sow seed at 16–19°C (61–66°F) in spring. Divide in spring.
- **PESTS AND DISEASES** Trouble free.

S. androgyna (Liana). Moderately bushy, twining climber, with the main stems arising at ground level, bearing lance-shaped to ovate, sometimes shallowly lobed, glossy, mid-green, leaf-like stems, to 2.5cm (1in) long. Clusters of 2–6 tiny, star-shaped cream flowers are produced in late spring and early summer; the females are 6mm (¼in) across, the males 9mm (⅜in) across. ↕5–7m (15–22ft). S. Spain, S.E. France (Hyères Isles), Sicily, N. Africa, Canary Islands. ❄

SEMIAQUILEGIA

RANUNCULACEAE

Genus of 7 species of small, sometimes short-lived perennials from mountain habitats in E. Asia. They resemble columbines (*Aquilegia*), but have spurless flowers, swollen or pouched at the bases, borne in corymb-like panicles in spring or summer. Leaves are ternate or 2-ternate, and often further divided. They are most effective when grown in a rock garden.

- **HARDINESS** Fully hardy.
- **CULTIVATION** Grow in moderately fertile, humus-rich, moist but well-drained, neutral to slightly acid soil in full sun with some midday shade, or in partial shade. Provide shelter from cold, drying winds.
- **PROPAGATION** Sow seed in containers in a cold frame as soon as ripe.
- **PESTS AND DISEASES** Susceptible to damage by slugs and snails.

S. ecalcarata ■ Short-lived, erect perennial with long-stalked, 2-ternate, mid-green leaves, to 8cm (3in) long, the leaflets purple beneath. In early summer,

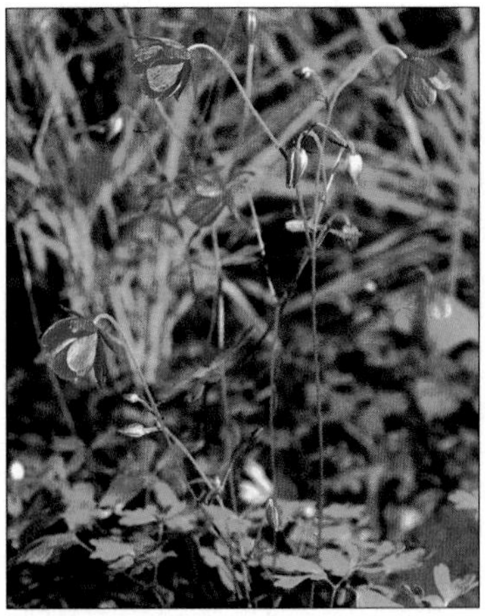
Semiaquilegia ecalcarata

produces loose, corymb-like panicles of pendent, open bell-shaped, dusky pink to deep purple-red flowers, 1.5cm (½in) long. ↕30cm (12in), ↔ 20cm (8in). W. China. ❄❄❄

SEMIARUNDINARIA

GRAMINEAE/POACEAE

Genus of 10–20 species of tall, upright bamboos from deciduous woodland, upland slopes, and ravines in China and Japan. They generally have running rhizomes, but form dense clumps in cool climates. Smooth, cylindrical canes, with short-lived cane-sheaths, some with upper internodes grooved or flattened, produce 3–7 branches at each node, with tessellated, narrowly lance-shaped leaves. Grow in a woodland garden, as a specimen plant, or as an informal hedge.

- **HARDINESS** Fully hardy to frost hardy.
- **CULTIVATION** Grow in moderately fertile, humus-rich, moist but well-drained soil in full sun or light dappled shade.
- **PROPAGATION** Divide, or cut up sections of youngest rhizomes, in spring.
- **PESTS AND DISEASES** Young shoots may be damaged by slugs.

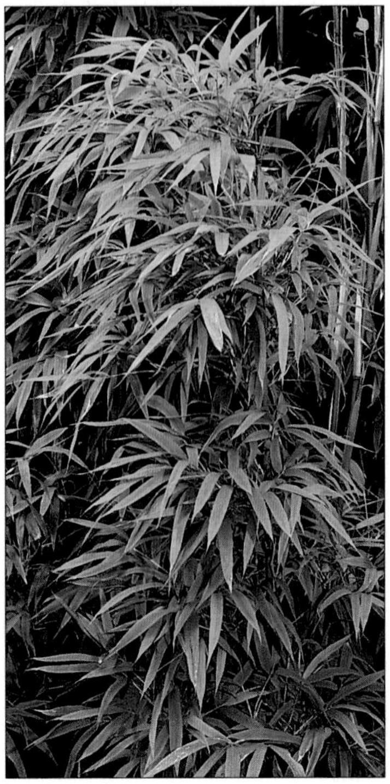
Semiarundinaria fastuosa

S. fastuosa ■ 🏆 syn. *Arundinaria fastuosa* (Narihira bamboo). Tall, erect, tree-like bamboo, either with spreading rhizomes or forming dense clumps. The shining, mid-green canes are striped purple-brown, markedly so when young; cane-sheaths open to reveal polished, deep red-purple interiors. Bears lance-shaped, glossy, mid-green leaves, 12–15cm (5–6in) long, mainly on the upper part of the plant. ↕ to 7m (22ft), ↔ 2m (6ft) or more. Japan. ❄❄❄

▷**Seminole bread** see *Zamia pumila*

SEMPERVIVUM

Houseleek

CRASSULACEAE

Genus of about 40 species of dense, mat-forming, evergreen succulent perennials, mainly from the mountains of Europe and Asia. They bear rosettes of thick, pointed leaves, often with bristle-fringed margins, and sometimes covered with a web of white hairs. Flat, branching, terminal, panicle-like cymes of star-shaped, white, yellow, red, or purple flowers are borne on upright stems in summer. The rosettes die after flowering, but are replaced by new, offset rosettes, borne on lateral runners. Numerous cultivars of hybrid origin are available. Grow in a rock garden, scree bed, wall crevice, or trough, or in containers in an alpine house.

- **HARDINESS** Fully hardy.
- **CULTIVATION** Grow in poor to moderately fertile, sharply drained soil, with added grit, in full sun. Some, particularly softly hairy species, resent winter wet, and are best grown in an alpine house in areas with wet winters. In an alpine house, grow in a mix of equal parts loam-based potting compost (JI No.2) and grit. See also pp.48–49.
- **PROPAGATION** Sow seed in containers in a cold frame in spring. Root offsets in spring or early summer.
- **PESTS AND DISEASES** May be affected by *Endophyllum sempervivi* (rust).

S. arachnoideum ■ 🏆 (Cobweb houseleek). Mat-forming, rosetted succulent with fleshy, obovate, mid-green to red leaves, to 1cm (½in) long. The rosettes, 1–2.5cm (½–1in) across, are cobwebbed with white hairs. In summer, bears flat cymes, to 2.5cm (1in) across, of reddish pink flowers on leafy stems. ↕8cm (3in), ↔ 30cm (12in). Europe (Alps, Apennines, Carpathians). ❄❄❄

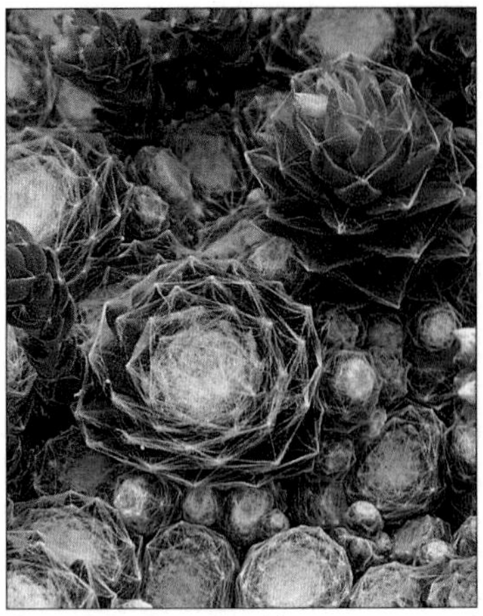
Sempervivum arachnoideum

S

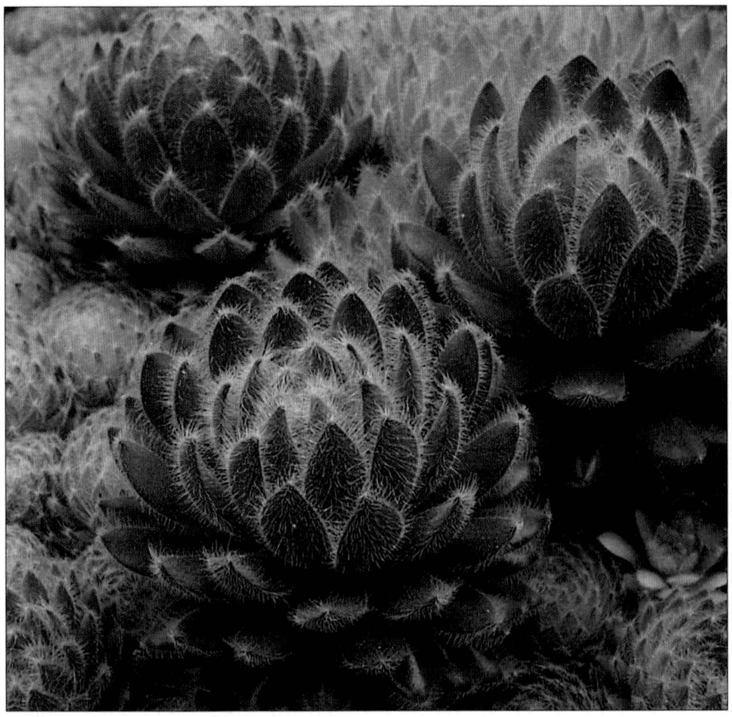
Sempervivum ciliosum

S. arboreum see *Aeonium arboreum.*
S. balsamiferum see *Aeonium balsamiferum.*
S. ciliosum ■ ♀ Mat-forming succulent with very hairy rosettes, to 5cm (2in) across, of incurved, inversely lance-shaped, grey-green leaves, 2.5cm (1in) long, convex on both surfaces. Bears flat, compact cymes, 2.5cm (1in) across, of greenish yellow flowers in summer. Best in an alpine house. ↕ 8cm (3in), ↔ 30cm (12in). Former Yugoslavia, Bulgaria, N.W. Greece. ✻✻✻
S. 'Commander Hay' ♀ Succulent, similar to *S. tectorum*, bearing rosettes, to 10cm (4in) across, of inversely lance-shaped, glossy, deep red-purple leaves, to 4cm (1½in) long, with mid-green tips. In summer, produces cymes, 5–10cm (2–4in) across, of greenish red flowers. ↕ 10cm (4in), ↔ 30cm (12in). ✻✻✻
S. complanatum see *Aeonium tabuliforme.*
S. giuseppii ■ Vigorous, mat-forming succulent with rosettes, 2.5–3.5cm (1–1½in) across, of ovate, pea-green leaves, 1.5cm (½in) long, hairy when young, and dark-spotted at the tips. Red flowers are produced in cymes, 3.5cm (1½in) across, in summer. ↕ 8cm (3in), ↔ 30cm (12in). Spain. ✻✻✻
S. grandiflorum. Variable, mat-forming succulent bearing rosettes, 5–10cm (2–4in) across, of sharp-pointed, oblong-triangular, very hairy, dark green leaves, 2.5–5cm (1–2in) long, which are often tipped with brown. In summer, yellow flowers, stained purple at the bases, are produced in cymes 10cm (4in) across. Prefers acid soil. ↕ 10cm (4in), ↔ 30cm (12in). Europe (W. and C. Alps). ✻✻✻
S. haworthii see *Aeonium haworthii.*
S. helveticum see *S. montanum.*
S. hirtum see *Jovibarba hirta.*
S. masferreri see *Aeonium sedifolium.*
S. montanum ■ syn. *S. helveticum.* Vigorous, mat-forming succulent with clustered, open rosettes, 2–8cm (¾–3in) across, of sharp-pointed, inversely lance-shaped, finely hairy, fleshy, dull, dark green leaves, to 1cm (½in) long. Red-purple flowers are borne in loose cymes, to 6cm (2½in) across, in summer. Hybridizes freely. ↕ 10cm (4in), ↔ 30cm (12in) or more. C. Europe. ✻✻✻
S. nobile see *Aeonium nobile.*
S. patens see *Jovibarba heuffelii.*
S. soboliferum see *Jovibarba sobolifera.*

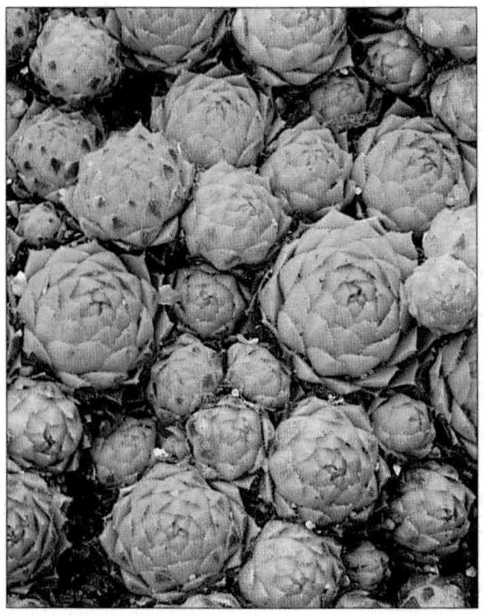
Sempervivum giuseppii

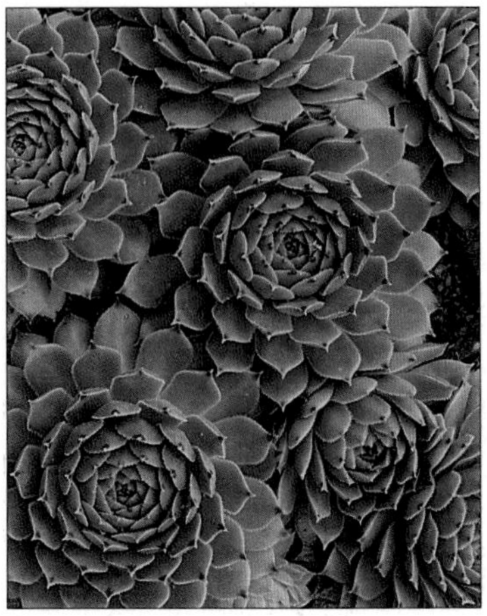
Sempervivum montanum

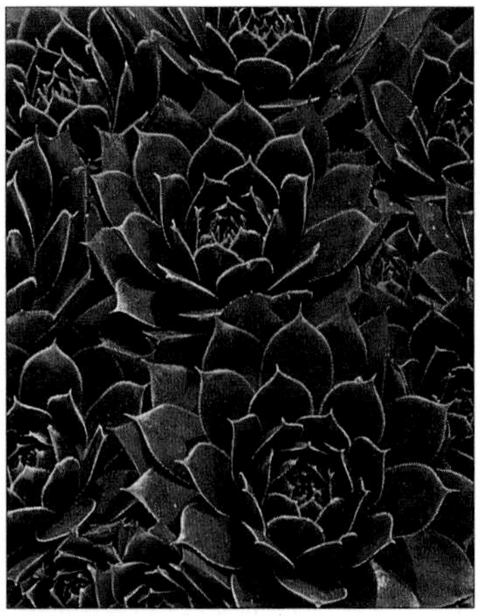
Sempervivum tectorum

S. tectorum ■ ♀ (Common houseleek). Mat-forming succulent with open rosettes, to 10cm (4in) across, of thick, obovate to narrowly oblong, bristle-tipped, blue-green leaves, to 4cm (1½in) long, often suffused red-purple. In summer, bears cymes, 5–10cm (2–4in) across, of red-purple flowers on upright, hairy stems. ↕ 15cm (6in), ↔ 50cm (20in). Mountains of S. Europe. ✻✻✻

▷**Seneca** see *Polygala*

SENECIO

ASTERACEAE/COMPOSITAE

Large genus of more than 1,000 species of annuals, biennials, herbaceous perennials, climbers, shrubs, and small trees, some of them succulent. They are found worldwide in habitats ranging from mountains to sea shores, and in dry to moist soils. Basal leaves are entire or variably lobed, sometimes white or silver; stem leaves, if present, are smaller and alternate. The flowerheads, either solitary or borne in corymbs, are usually terminal and daisy-like (some species lack ray-florets), and yellow, white, red, blue, or purple, sometimes orange; they mainly have yellow, sometimes purple disc-florets. Use annuals for bedding, or in containers; grow small perennials in a scree bed or rock garden, and tall ones in a border or wild garden. In frost-prone areas, grow tender species in a cool or temperate greenhouse. All parts may cause severe discomfort if ingested.

• **HARDINESS** Fully hardy to frost tender.

• **CULTIVATION** For ease of reference, cultivation has been grouped as follows:
1. Grow in poor, gritty, sharply drained soil in full sun.
2. Grow in moderately fertile, well-drained soil in full sun.
3. Grow in moderately fertile, moist to boggy soil (such as in a bog garden) in full sun or partial shade.
4. Under glass, grow in a mix of 2 parts loam-based potting compost (JI No.1) and 1 part each leaf mould and grit in full light with good ventilation. When in growth, water moderately and apply a balanced liquid fertilizer monthly. Maintain moderate humidity. Keep just moist in winter. Outdoors, in frost-free areas, grow as for group 2.
5. Under glass, grow in a mix of 2 parts loam-based potting compost (JI No.1) and 1 part each leaf mould and grit in full light with good ventilation. When in growth, water moderately, maintain low humidity, and apply a half-strength balanced liquid fertilizer monthly. Keep just moist in winter at a minimum of 7–10°C (45–50°F). Outdoors, in frost-free areas, grow as for group 1, in neutral to slightly alkaline soil.

Pruning group 8 or 9 for shrubs; group 11, after flowering, for climbers.

• **PROPAGATION** Sow seed in spring: for cultivation groups 2, 4, and 5 at 19–24°C (66–75°F); for groups 1 and 3 in containers in a cold frame. Divide groups 1 and 3 and *S. doronicum* in spring; take basal cuttings in early spring. Divide groups 4 and 5 as growth begins; take softwood cuttings in early summer or semi-ripe cuttings in mid- or late summer. Take semi-ripe cuttings of silver and white forms of group 2 in mid- or late summer.

• **PESTS AND DISEASES** Prone to rust, particularly *S. cineraria* and its cultivars. Whiteflies, aphids, and red spider mites may be a problem under glass.

S. abrotanifolius. Evergreen subshrub with spreading or erect, hairless or downy stems, and 2- or 3-pinnatisect, glossy, dark green leaves, to 8cm (3in) long, the upper leaves less divided. From midsummer to early autumn, bears yellow to orange-scarlet flowerheads, to 4cm (1½in) across, singly or in few-flowered corymbs. Cultivation group 1. ↕ 15–45cm (6–18in), ↔ 30cm (12in). Mountains of C. and E. Europe. ✻✻✻
S. articulatus (Candle plant). Erect, perennial succulent with cylindrical, jointed, fleshy, grey-veined, silvery blue stems, each segment to 15cm (6in) long. Bears ovate, 3- to 5-lobed, stalked, blue-green leaves, to 5cm (2in) long. Yellow flowerheads, 1cm (½in) across, are borne in small corymbs from spring to autumn. Cultivation group 5. ↕ to 60cm (24in), ↔ indefinite. South Africa. ❀ (min. 7°C/45°F). **'Variegatus'** ■ has bold, pink or cream marks and shading on the leaves and flowerheads.
S. bicolor* subsp. *cineraria see *S. cineraria.*

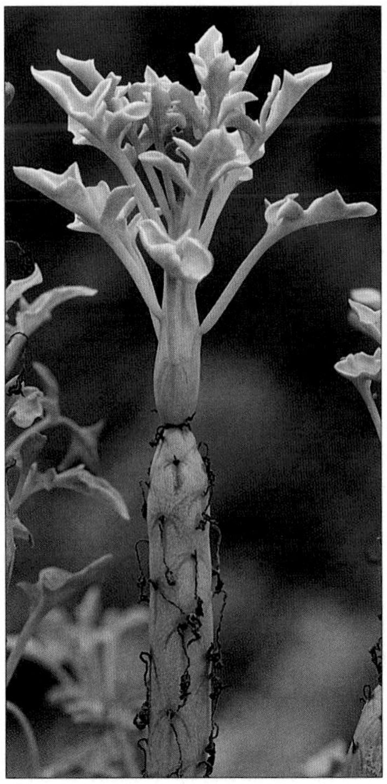
Senecio articulatus 'Variegatus'

S

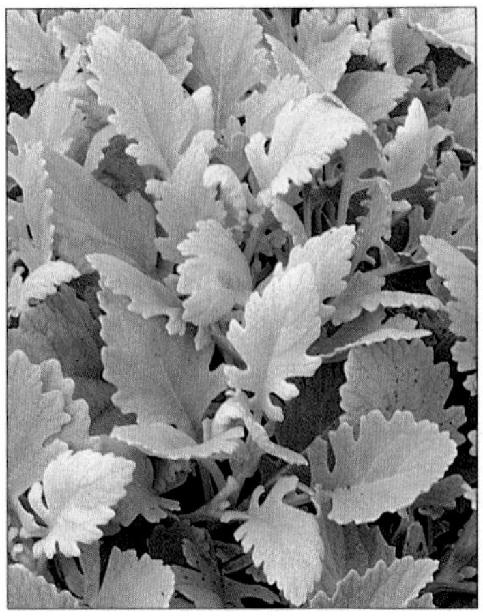
Senecio cineraria 'Cirrus'

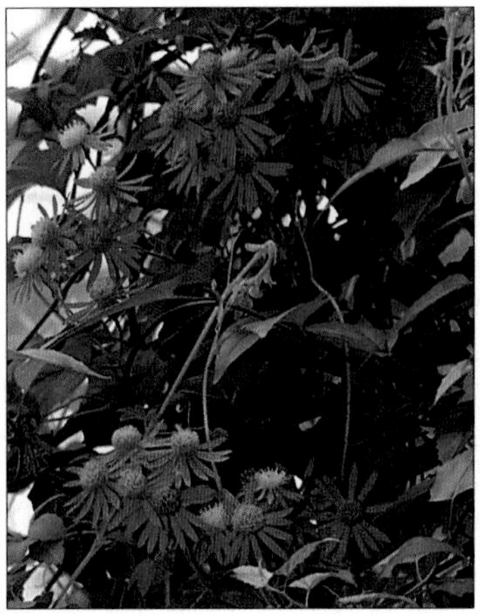
Senecio confusus

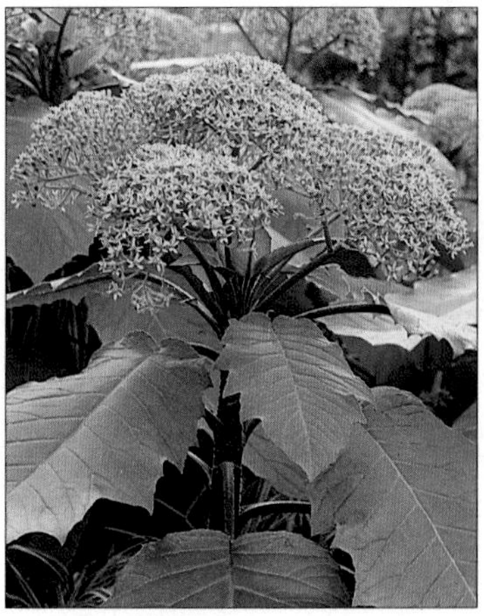
Senecio grandifolius

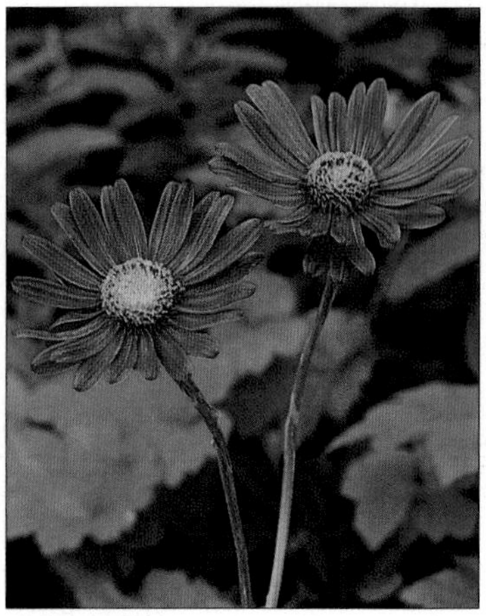
Senecio pulcher

S. bidwillii see *Brachyglottis bidwillii.*
S. candicans see *S. cineraria.*
S. cineraria, syn. *Cineraria maritima, S. bicolor* subsp. *cineraria, S. candicans, S. maritimus.* Mound-forming, evergreen subshrub or shrub, usually grown as an annual, with ovate to lance-shaped or elliptic, shallowly to deeply pinnatisect or pinnate, felted, silvery grey leaves, to 15cm (6in) long. Loose corymbs of mustard-yellow flowerheads, to 2.5cm (1in) across, are borne in midsummer, in the second year after sowing. Cultivation group 2. Dead-head regularly. ↕↔ to 60cm (24in). W. and C. Mediterranean. ❄❄. Dwarf cultivars, with a range of foliage characteristics, are popular. **'Alice'** has deeply cut, silver-stained white leaves; ↕↔ 30cm (12in). **'Cirrus'** ■ produces elliptic, finely toothed or lobed, silvery green to white leaves; ↕↔ 30cm (12in). **'Silver Dust'** ■♀ has deeply pinnatisect, lacy, almost white leaves; ↕↔ 30cm (12in). **'White Diamond'** ♀ has deeply divided, almost oak-like, grey-white leaves; usually grown as a perennial; ↕30–40cm (12–16in), ↔ 30cm (12in).
S. clivorum see *Ligularia dentata.*
S. compactus see *Brachyglottis compacta.*
S. confusus ■ syn. *Pseudogynoxys chenopodioides.* Moderately bushy, evergreen, twining climber with lance-shaped to narrowly ovate, thick, toothed, mid-green leaves, to 8cm (3in) long. Fragrant flowerheads, 5cm (2in) across, are bright orange fading to red, and are profusely borne in small, axillary and terminal corymbs, mainly in summer. Cultivation group 4. ↕ to 6m (20ft) or more. Mexico to Honduras. ❀ (min. 7–10°C/45–50°F)
S. cruentus see *Pericallis* x *hybrida.*
S. doronicum (Leopard's bane ragwort). Clump-forming, deciduous perennial with upright, sometimes branched stems and ovate to lance-shaped or elliptic, toothed, dark green leaves, to 25cm (10in) long, cobweb-hairy beneath. Bright orange-yellow to rich yellow flowerheads, to 6cm (2½in) across, are borne singly or in loose corymbs in early and midsummer. Cultivation group 2. ↕15–40cm (6–16in), ↔ 30cm (12in). Mountainous regions of C. and S. Europe. ❄❄❄
***S.* Dunedin Hybrids** see *Brachyglottis* Dunedin Hybrids.
S. elaeagnifolius see *Brachyglottis elaeagnifolia.*
S. elegans. Erect annual with branched stems and oblong-ovate, pinnately lobed or coarsely toothed, deep green leaves, to 8cm (3in) long. In summer, bears corymbs of flowerheads, 2.5cm (1in) across, with yellow disc-florets and purple, reddish purple, or occasionally white ray-florets. Cultivation group 2. ↕ to 60cm (24in), ↔ to 35cm (14in). South Africa. ❄❄
S. grandifolius ■ syn. *Telanthophora grandifolia.* Evergreen shrub, rounded when young, but becoming erect, with very thick, sparsely branched, purple-downy stems bearing ovate to elliptic, usually wavy-lobed, sometimes toothed, semi-lustrous, mid- to deep green leaves, 20–45cm (8–18in) long, downy, rust-brown beneath. Small, 5-rayed, bright yellow flowerheads, to 1cm (½in) across, are borne in dense, widely domed corymbs, to 30cm (12in) across, mainly in winter. Cultivation group 4. ↕↔ 2–3m (6–10ft), sometimes more. Mexico. ❀ (min. 7–10°C/45–50°F)
S. greyi see *Brachyglottis greyi.*
***S. greyi* of gardens** see *Brachyglottis* Dunedin Hybrids.
S. hectoris see *Brachyglottis hectoris.*
S. huntii see *Brachyglottis huntii.*
S.* x *hybridus see *Pericallis* x *hybrida.*
S. laxifolius see *Brachyglottis laxifolia.*
***S. laxifolius* of gardens** see *Brachyglottis* Dunedin Hybrids.
S. leucostachys see *S. viravira.*
S. macroglossus (Cape ivy, Natal ivy). Evergreen, twining climber with semi-succulent growth at first, then eventually woody stems, which branch moderately. Triangular to spear-shaped, mid-green leaves, to 8cm (3in) long, have 3–5 pointed lobes. Flowerheads, 5–6cm (2–2½in) across, with white to pale yellow ray-florets, are usually borne singly, sometimes in twos or threes, in summer and winter. Cultivation group 4, with shade from midday sun. ↕ to 3m (10ft), sometimes more. Zimbabwe to Mozambique, E. South Africa. ❀ (min. 5–7°C/41–45°F). **'Variegatus'** ■♀ has foliage with irregular, cream to light yellow margins.
S. maritimus see *S. cineraria.*
S. mikanioides, syn. *Delairea odorata* (German ivy, Parlour ivy). Evergreen, twining climber with succulent young stems, woody when mature. Fleshy, bright green leaves, 8–10cm (3–4in) across, are triangular to triangular-ovate, with 5–7 broad, pointed lobes. Small, groundsel-like yellow flowerheads, 8mm (⅜in) across, without ray-florets, are borne in dense, axillary and terminal corymbs, 8cm (3in) across, from autumn to early winter. Cultivation group 4. ↕ to 6m (20ft). South Africa. ❀ (min. 3–5°C/37–41°F)
***S.* 'Moira Read'** see *Brachyglottis* Dunedin Hybrids 'Moira Read'.
S. monroi see *Brachyglottis monroi.*
S. przewalskii see *Ligularia przewalskii.*

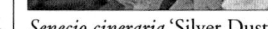

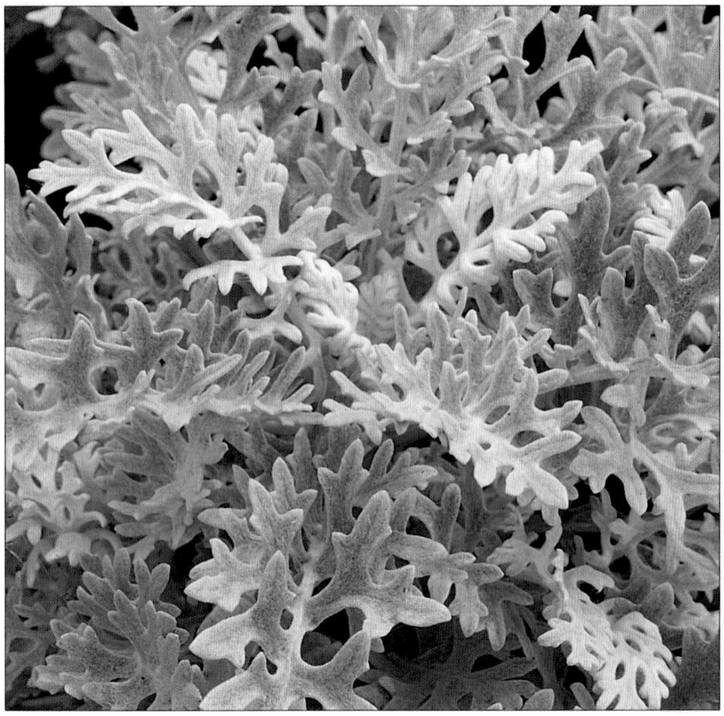
Senecio cineraria 'Silver Dust'

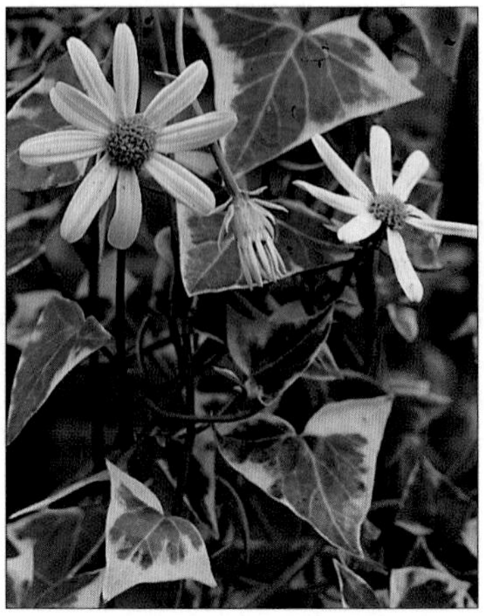
Senecio macroglossus 'Variegatus'

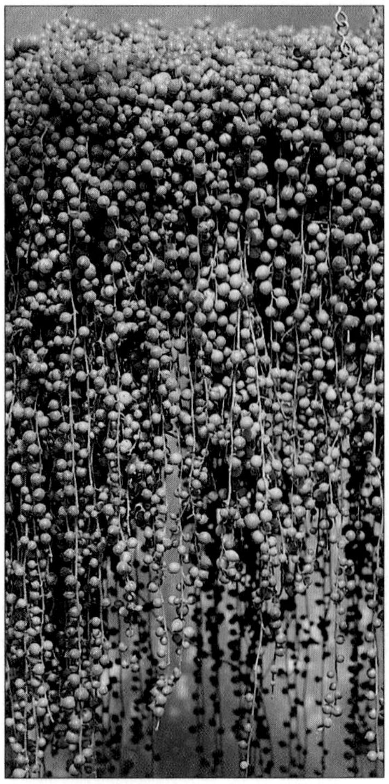
Senecio rowleyanus

S

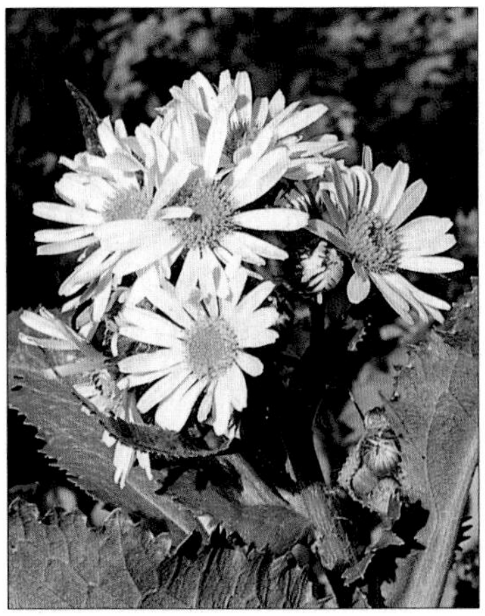

Senecio smithii

S. pulcher ■ Erect, deciduous or semi-evergreen perennial, woolly in early growth, becoming hairless, with leathery, mid-green leaves, to 20cm (8in) long. Basal leaves are elliptic with scalloped margins; stem leaves are lance-shaped with toothed margins. In mid- and late autumn, bears solitary corymbs of carmine-purple flowerheads, 5–8cm (2–3in) across. Cultivation group 4; may survive outdoors in a sheltered, sunny site, in cool, deep, fertile soil; severe weather harms leaves and flowers. ↕45–60cm (18–24in), ↔ 50cm (20in). S. Brazil, Uruguay, Argentina. ❄❄

S. radicans. Mat-forming, perennial succulent with prostrate, rooting stems and cylindrical, straight or slightly curved, fleshy, glaucous, mid-green leaves, to 2.5cm (1in) long, each with a darker stripe down the middle. Solitary or paired white flowerheads, 3–5mm (1/8–1/4in) across, are borne sporadically during the year. Cultivation group 5. ↕8–10cm (3–4in), ↔ 15–30cm (6–12in). South Africa. ❄❄

S. reinholdii see *Brachyglottis rotundifolia.*

S. reniformis see *Cremanthodium reniforme.*

S. rotundifolius see *Brachyglottis rotundifolia.*

S. rowleyanus ■ syn. *Kleinia rowleyana* (String of beads). Pendent or creeping, perennial succulent with adventitious roots on the stems and spherical, slightly pointed, mid-green leaves, to 1cm (1/2in) long. Bears solitary, funnel-shaped, cinnamon-scented white flowerheads, to 1cm (1/2in) long, with protruding brown stamens, in summer. Cultivation group 5. ↕60cm (24in) or more, ↔ indefinite. S.W. Africa. ❅ (min. 7–10°C/45–50°F)

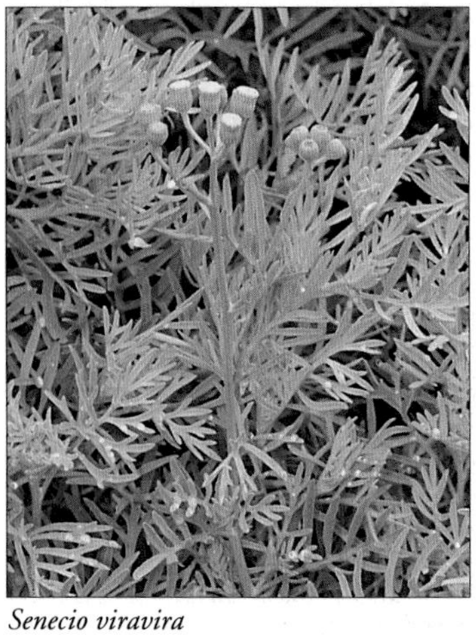

Senecio viravira

S. scandens. Evergreen, twining climber, woody-based and usually bushy when mature, with ovate or narrowly triangular, almost entire to sharply toothed or lobed, bright green leaves, to 10cm (4in) long. From autumn to winter, bears yellow flowerheads, 1.5cm (1/2in) across, in panicle-like corymbs, 13cm (5in) across. Cultivation group 4. ↕2.5–5m (8–15ft). E. Asia. ❅ (min. 7°C/45°F)

S. serpens, syn. *Kleinia repens.* Shrubby, perennial succulent with semi-erect, fleshy, blue-frosted shoots, 7mm (1/4in) thick. Cylindrical, fleshy, waxy, bluish grey leaves, to 3cm (1 1/4in) long, grooved on the upper surfaces, are crowded at the stem and branch tips. In summer, bears whitish yellow flowerheads, 1cm (1/2in) long, lacking ray-florets. Cultivation group 5. ↕↔ 30cm (12in). South Africa. ❅ (min. 7°C/45°F)

S. smithii ■ Vigorous, deciduous, clump-forming, woolly perennial with oblong-ovate, toothed, leathery, glossy, dark grey-green basal and stem leaves, to 30cm (12in) long. From early to late summer, stout, upright, unbranched stems bear large corymbs, 10–15cm (4–6in) across, of numerous yellow-centred white flowerheads, to 5cm (2in) across. Cultivation group 3, but best in moist soil. ↕ to 1.2m (4ft), ↔ 60cm (24in). S. Chile, W. Argentina, Falkland Islands. ❄❄❄

S. stapeliiformis see *Kleinia stapeliiformis.*

***S.* 'Sunshine'** see *Brachyglottis* Dunedin Hybrids 'Sunshine'.

S. tanguticus, syn. *Ligularia tangutica, Sinacalia tangutica* (Chinese groundsel). Clump-forming, deciduous perennial with upright, unbranched black stems and ovate, deeply pinnatisect, jagged, dark green leaves, to 18cm (7in) long. In early and mid-autumn, bears pyramidal panicles or loose corymbs of bright yellow flowerheads, 2mm (1/16in) across. Cultivation group 3; invasive, so best in a large, wild garden, near water. ↕ to 1.2m (4ft) or more, ↔ 1.1m (3 1/2ft). N.W. China. ❄❄❄

S. viravira ■ 🏆 syn. *S. leucostachys.* Open, spreading, evergreen subshrub with densely white-hairy shoots and deeply pinnatisect, silvery white leaves, to 8cm (3in) long, with 5–9 linear lobes that are usually further divided. Loose corymbs of small, pale yellow flowerheads, 5mm (1/4in) across, without ray-florets, are produced from summer to autumn. Cultivation group 2. ↕60cm (24in), ↔ 1m (3ft). Argentina. ❄❄

SENNA

CAESALPINIACEAE/LEGUMINOSAE

Genus, often included in *Cassia,* of about 260 species of evergreen and deciduous trees, shrubs, and perennials from semi-desert, scrub, and savannah in dry, tropical and warm-temperate regions. Leaves are alternate and pinnate, with linear to nearly rounded leaflets. Sennas are cultivated for their yellow or rarely white, pea-like flowers, borne in terminal or axillary racemes, corymbs, or panicles. In frost-prone climates, grow in a temperate or warm greenhouse. In frost-free areas, grow in a shrub border.

• **HARDINESS** Frost tender.

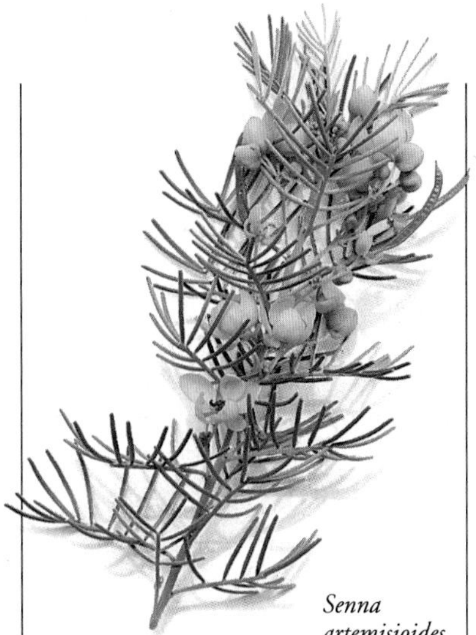

Senna artemisioides

• **CULTIVATION** Under glass, grow in loam-based potting compost (JI No.2) in full light and moderate humidity. In growth, water moderately and apply a balanced liquid fertilizer monthly; water sparingly in winter. Outdoors, grow in moist but well-drained, moderately fertile soil in full sun. Pruning group 1; may need restrictive pruning under glass.

• **PROPAGATION** Sow seed at 18–24°C (64–75°F) in spring. Divide perennials in spring. Root semi-ripe cuttings with bottom heat in summer.

• **PESTS AND DISEASES** Trouble free.

S. alata ♀ syn. *Cassia alata* (Empress candle plant). Erect to spreading, evergreen shrub or small tree. Broadly oblong to obovate, pinnate leaves, 20–75cm (8–30in) long, have 14–28 oblong, bright green leaflets. Bears numerous bright yellow flowers, to 2.5cm (1in) across, in tall, erect, axillary racemes, 15–60cm (6–24in) long, mainly from late summer to autumn; flowers are protected by broad, yellowish green bracts when in bud. ↕2–10m (6–30ft), ↔ 2–5m (6–15ft). Africa to S.E. Asia, Pacific islands, tropical America. ❅ (min. 5–7°C/41–45°F)

S. artemisioides ■ 🏆 syn. *Cassia artemisioides* (Silver cassia). Erect to spreading, evergreen shrub with pinnate leaves, 3–6cm (1 1/4–2 1/2in) long, composed of 6–8 short, narrowly linear, thickly downy, grey-green leaflets. Stems are covered in ash-white hairs. Bears axillary racemes, to 8cm (3in) long, of 4–12 fragrant, pale to rich yellow flowers, to 1cm (1/2in) across, intermittently throughout the year. ↕1–2m (3–6ft), ↔ 1m (3ft). Australia (Northern Territory, South Australia, New South Wales). ❅ (min. 10–13°C/50–55°F)

S. corymbosa ■ ♀ syn. *Cassia corymbosa.* Erect to spreading, evergreen shrub or small tree producing pinnate, yellowish-green leaves, 40–90cm (16–36in) long, with 6–8 oblong-lance-shaped leaflets. Axillary corymbs, 10cm (4in) across, of up to 20 golden yellow flowers, to 2cm (3/4in) across, are borne in late summer. ↕2–4m (6–12ft), ↔ 1.5–3m (5–10ft). Argentina, Uruguay. ❅ (min. 5–7°C/41–45°F)

S. didymobotrya ♀ syn. *Cassia didymobotrya.* Erect to spreading, evergreen shrub or small tree with pinnate, mid-green leaves, 10–50cm (4–20in) long, composed of 16–32 elliptic-obovate leaflets. Numerous golden yellow flowers, to 3cm (1 1/4in) across, with blackish brown bracts covering the buds, are borne in tall, erect, terminal or axillary racemes, 15–60cm (6–24in) long, mainly from late summer to autumn. ↕2.5m (8ft), ↔ 1.5–3m (5–10ft). Tropical Africa; naturalized in India, Malaysia. ❅ (min. 13°C/55°F)

S. x floribunda (*S. multiglandulosa* x *S. septentrionalis*) syn. *Cassia corymbosa* var. *plurijuga, C. x floribunda.* Many-branched, evergreen or deciduous shrub with pinnate, mid-green leaves, 6–8cm (2 1/2–3in) long, comprising 12 oblong-elliptic leaflets. From summer to winter, often-branched, axillary racemes, 10cm (4in) long, produce up to 20 rich yellow flowers, to 2cm (3/4in) across. ↕1–3m (3–10ft), ↔ 1–2.5m (3–8ft). Garden origin. ❅ (min. 7°C/45°F)

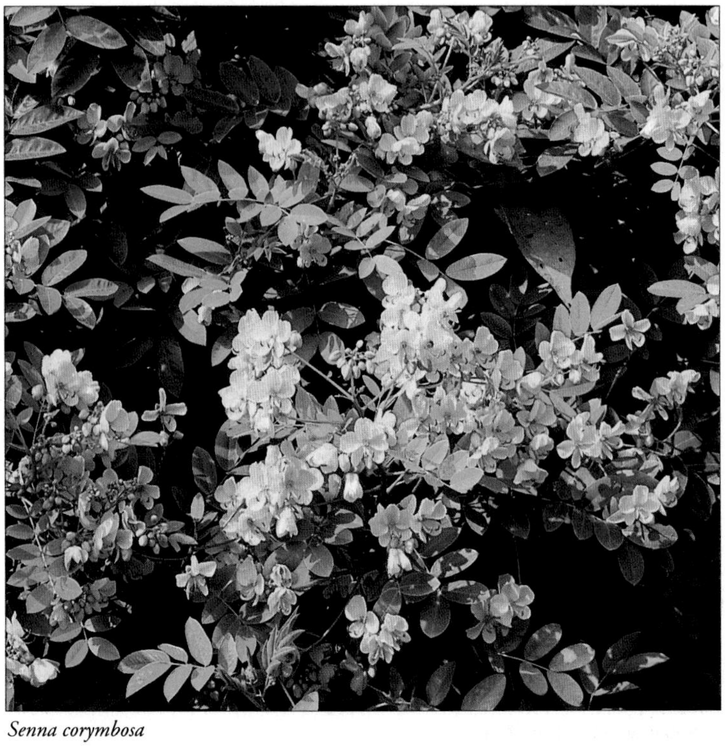

Senna corymbosa

S

S. siamea ⚲ syn. *Cassia siamea* (Kassod tree). Open, fast-growing, evergreen tree with hairless young stems. Pinnate, deep yellow-green leaves, 10–35cm (4–14in) long, each have 14–24 narrowly elliptic to oblong leaflets. Dense, erect, terminal, corymb-like panicles, 15–35cm (6–14in) long, of 10–60 yellow flowers, to 2cm (¾in) across, are borne from spring to summer. ↕10m (30ft), ↔7m (22ft). Indonesia, Malay Peninsula. ❀ (min. 16–18°C/61–64°F)

S. sturtii. Spreading or rounded, evergreen shrub. Pinnate, mid-green leaves, 4–5cm (1½–2in) long, have 4–16 linear to elliptic leaflets. In early summer, bears short, axillary racemes, to 10cm (4in) across, of 4 or 5 yellow flowers, 1cm (½in) across. ↕1–2m (3–6ft), ↔1–1.5m (3–5ft). Australia. ❀ (min. 10°C/50°F)

▷**Senna,**
Bladder see *Colutea, C. arborescens*
Scorpion see *Coronilla emerus*
▷**Sensitive plant** see *Mimosa pudica*
▷**September bells** see *Rothmannia globosa*

SEQUOIA

TAXODIACEAE

Genus of one species of very tall, fast-growing, monoecious, evergreen, coniferous tree from coastal forest in California and Oregon, USA. It has thick, soft bark, whorled branches when young, and yew-like foliage. Useful where a tall, evergreen tree is needed quickly; it thrives in climates with cool, damp summers, and is tolerant of pollution and wind. It is one of the few conifers that will coppice, or make new shoots from the base if cut down. The genus contains the tallest tree and also some of the oldest trees in the world.

- **HARDINESS** Fully hardy.
- **CULTIVATION** Grow in moderately fertile, moist but well-drained soil in full sun to light dappled shade.
- **PROPAGATION** Sow seed in containers in a cold frame in spring. Root softwood cuttings in summer, or semi-ripe cuttings in late summer or autumn.
- **PESTS AND DISEASES** Trouble free.

S. sempervirens ◼♀◊ (Coastal redwood). Columnar-conical tree with horizontal or downcurved branches, thick, fissured, soft, red-brown bark, and mid-green, later red-brown shoots with decurrent leaf bases. The hard, linear, sharp-pointed, deep green leaves, 2cm (¾in) long, silvery white beneath, are 2-ranked. On very strong shoots, the leaves are scale-like. Cones are spherical-cylindrical: the terminal, mid-green female cones, 3cm (1¼in) long, ripen in their first autumn; the tiny, terminal and axillary, brownish green male cones are to 4mm (⅛in) long. ↕to 112m (365ft), but mainly 20–30m (70–100ft), ↔6–9m (20–28ft). USA (coastal California and Oregon). ❄❄❄. **'Adpressa'** has short, broad leaves, to 1cm (½in) long, creamy white when young and lying flat along the shoots; ↕6–9m (20–28ft), ↔4–6m (12–20ft). **'Pendula'** produces arching branches with pendent branchlets. **'Prostrata'** is dwarf, with spreading branches and broader, glaucous, dark green leaves; ↕to 1.5m (5ft), ↔2–3m (6–10ft).

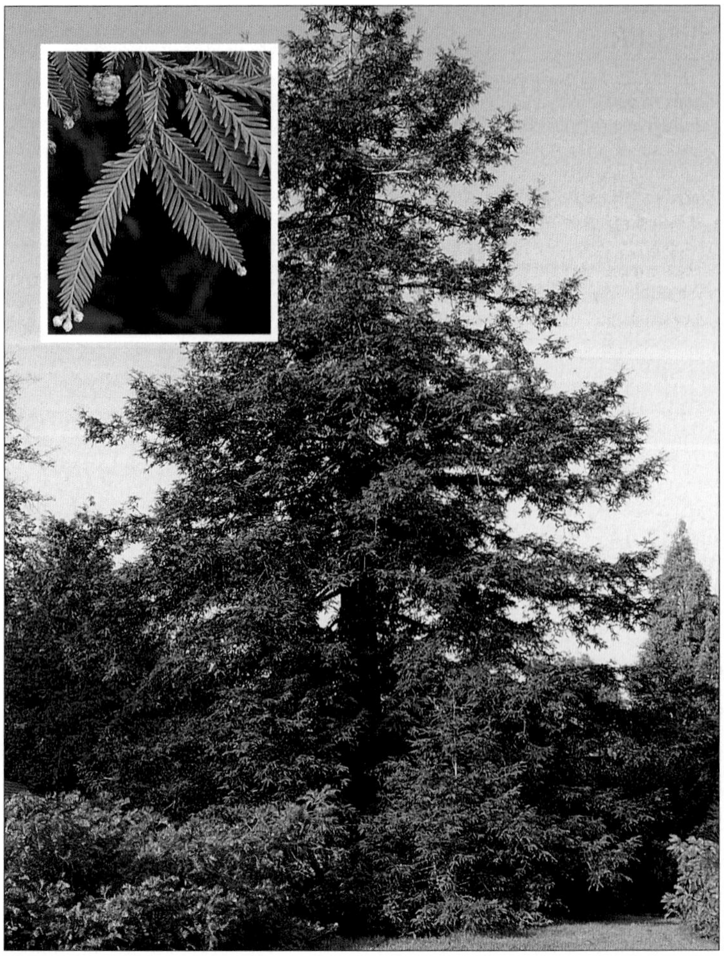

Sequoia sempervirens (inset: leaf and cone detail)

SEQUOIADENDRON

TAXODIACEAE

Genus of one species of monoecious, evergreen, coniferous tree from forest in the mountains of California, USA. It is related to *Sequoia* but has narrowly wedge-shaped leaves and thicker, harder bark, and cones that ripen in the second year rather than the first; it thrives in a cooler, drier atmosphere than *Sequoia*. An excellent, but very tall specimen tree.

- **HARDINESS** Fully hardy.
- **CULTIVATION** Grow in moderately fertile, well-drained soil in full sun or light dappled shade.
- **PROPAGATION** Sow seed in containers in a cold frame in spring. Root softwood cuttings in summer, or semi-ripe cuttings in late summer.
- **PESTS AND DISEASES** Susceptible to honey fungus.

S. giganteum ◼♀◊ (Big tree, Giant redwood, Sierra redwood, Wellingtonia). Conical tree, becoming columnar, with downcurved branches, very thick, fissured, red-brown bark, and mid-green, later red-brown shoots. Awl-shaped, grey-green leaves, to 7mm (¼in) long, are arranged radially and point forwards on the shoots. Bears ovoid, mid-green female cones, 4.5cm (1¾in) long, ripening brown and persisting for several years. ↕25–80m (80–260ft), ↔7–10m (22–30ft). USA (Sierra Nevada, California). ❄❄❄. **'Pendulum'** has pendent side branches, giving a curtain-like effect, although the main shoot grows rather erratically.

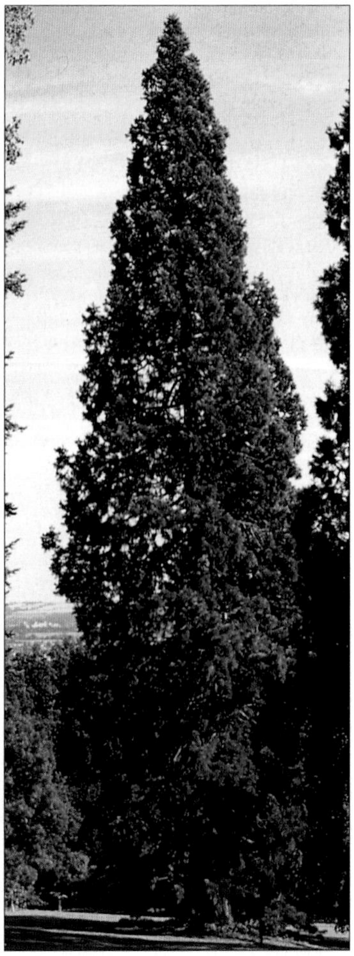

Sequoiadendron giganteum

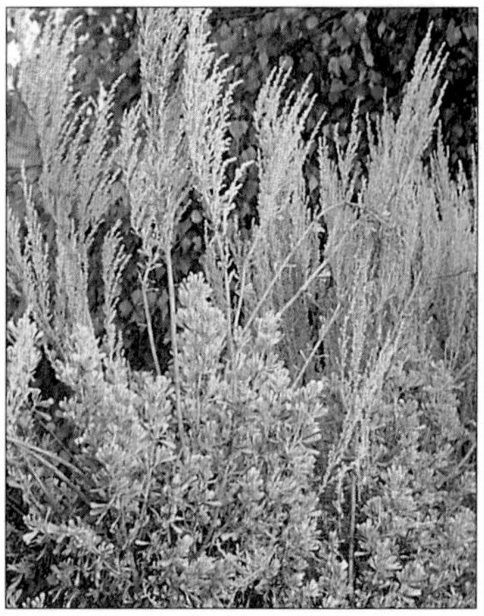

Seriphidium tridentatum

SERIPHIDIUM

ASTERACEAE/COMPOSITAE

Genus of 60–130 species of annuals, herbaceous or evergreen perennials, and mainly evergreen subshrubs from dry steppes, chaparral, and rocky or stony ground in Europe, N. Africa, temperate Asia, and North America. They are grown for their silver or grey, alternate, simple, pinnatisect, often aromatic leaves. Yellow to purple flowerheads, consisting only of disc-florets, are borne in terminal or axillary spikes, panicles, or racemes in summer or autumn. Grow in a shrub border. Tolerant of neglect.

- **HARDINESS** Fully hardy to half hardy.
- **CULTIVATION** Grow in poor to moderately fertile, dry, sharply drained soil in full sun. Pruning group 9.
- **PROPAGATION** Sow seed in containers in a cold frame in spring. Root semi-ripe cuttings in late summer, with bottom heat.
- **PESTS AND DISEASES** Trouble free.

S. nutans, syn. *Artemisia nutans.* Woody-based, evergreen perennial producing 2- or 3-pinnatisect, aromatic, silvery grey leaves, 5–10cm (2–4in) long, with small, linear lobes. In late summer and early autumn, bears pale yellow flowerheads, 6mm (¼in) across, in dense, leafy, pyramidal panicles, to 12cm (5in) long. ↕to 1m (3ft), ↔60cm (24in). S.E. Russia. ❄❄❄

S. tridentatum ◼ syn. *Artemisia tridentata* (Sagebrush). Woody-based, evergreen perennial or spreading sub-shrub with a short trunk or few stems, white-woolly at first, becoming pale brown as bark forms. Densely clustered, wedge-shaped, aromatic, silvery grey-downy leaves, 1–4cm (½–1½in) long, often have 3-toothed tips. In mid-autumn, bears feathery, greyish white or yellow flowerheads, to 4mm (⅛in) across, in slender panicles, to 45cm (18in) long. ↕↔to 2.5m (8ft). USA (S. California). ❄❄❄ (borderline)

SERISSA

RUBIACEAE

Genus of one species of small, evergreen shrub from moist, open woodland in S.E. Asia. Its leaves are simple, borne in opposite pairs, and foetid when crushed. Small, funnel-shaped flowers, with tubular calyces and 4–6 spreading petal lobes, are borne singly or in clusters in

summer. Where temperatures fall below 7°C (45°F), grow in a temperate greenhouse, mainly as a foliage plant. In warmer areas, grow at the base of a house wall, in a shrub border, or as a low hedge.
• **HARDINESS** Frost tender.
• **CULTIVATION** Under glass, grow in loam-based potting compost (JI No.2) in full light with shade from hot sun. When in growth, water moderately and apply a balanced liquid fertilizer monthly; water sparingly in winter. Outdoors, grow in moderately fertile, moist but well-drained soil in full sun. Shelter from cold, drying winds. Pruning group 9. Trim hedges after flowering or in late winter.
• **PROPAGATION** Root softwood cuttings in spring or early summer, or semi-ripe cuttings in late summer, both with bottom heat. Layer in spring.
• **PESTS AND DISEASES** Scale insects may be a problem under glass.

S. foetida, syn. *S. japonica.* Wiry-stemmed, eventually domed, bushy shrub producing crowded, tiny, ovate, leathery, deep green leaves, to 2cm (¾in) long. In summer, pink buds open to star-shaped white flowers, to 1.5cm (½in) across. ↕ 30–60cm (12–24in), ↔ 30–75cm (12–30in). S.E. Asia. ❀ (min. 7°C/45°F). **'Flore Pleno'** is smaller, with double flowers; ↕ to 45cm (18in), ↔ 30cm (12in). **'Variegata'** has leaves with cream margins. **'Variegated Pink'** has cream-margined foliage and bears a profusion of pink flowers.
S. japonica see *S. foetida.*

SERRURIA
PROTEACEAE

Genus, related to *Protea*, of about 55 species of evergreen shrubs from dry heathland scrub in South Africa. They have alternate, usually finely divided leaves, and bear dense heads of small, 4-petalled flowers from early spring to autumn, surrounded in *S. florida* by showy, petal-like bracts. In frost-prone areas, grow in a temperate greenhouse. In warmer areas, grow in a shrub border or at the base of a warm, sunny wall.
• **HARDINESS** Frost tender, but may survive short spells at about 0°C (32°F).
• **CULTIVATION** Under glass, grow in 1 part loam-based potting compost (JI No.1) and 3 parts 50/50 mix of perlite and peat (or coir) in full light, with good ventilation. During the growing season, water moderately; after the first year, apply a half-strength phosphate-free liquid fertilizer monthly. Water sparingly in winter. Outdoors, grow in poor to moderately fertile, well-drained, neutral to slightly acid soil in full sun. May become chlorotic if deficient in magnesium. Pruning group 1; may need restrictive pruning under glass.
• **PROPAGATION** Sow seed singly in pots at 16–21°C (61–70°F) as soon as ripe or in spring. Root semi-ripe cuttings in late summer, with bottom heat.
• **PESTS AND DISEASES** Trouble free.

S. florida ■ (Blushing bride). Airy shrub with erect, purple-tinged branches bearing pinnate or 2-pinnate, greyish green leaves, 4–6cm (1½–2½in) long, with numerous almost cylindrical, sharp-pointed leaflets. From spring

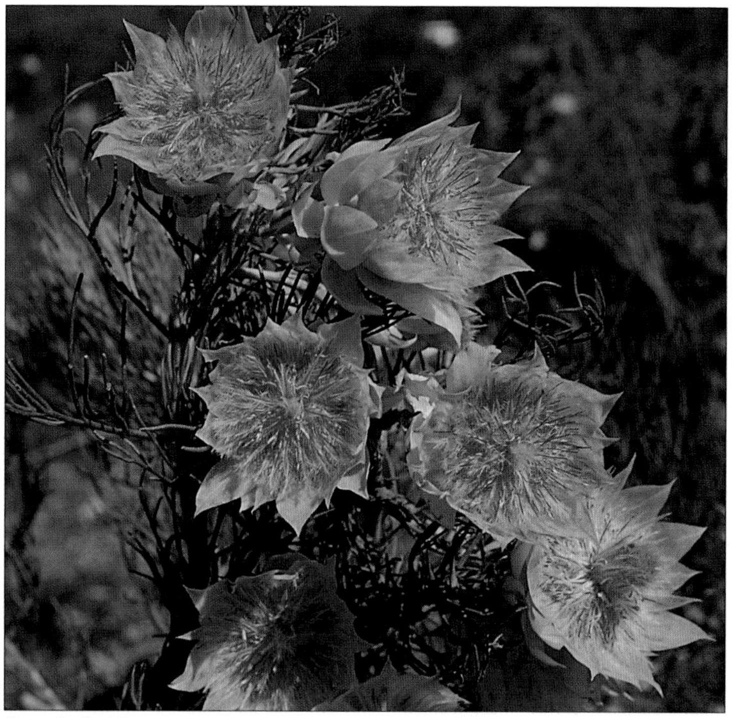
Serruria florida

to autumn, produces salmon-pink flowerheads, 2–2.5cm (¾–1in) across, each with a cup-shaped ring of pink-tinted white bracts. ↕ 1.5–2m (5–6ft), ↔ 1–1.5m (3–5ft). South Africa (Western Cape, Eastern Cape). ❀ (min. 7–10°C/45–50°F)

▷**Serviceberry, Allegheny** see *Amelanchier laevis*
▷**Service tree** see *Sorbus domestica*
▷**Service tree of Fontainebleau** see *Sorbus latifolia*

SESBANIA syn. DAUBENTONIA
LEGUMINOSAE/PAPILIONACEAE

Genus of about 50 species of short-lived, evergreen perennials, shrubs, and small trees found on streambanks and on moist soils in tropical and subtropical regions worldwide. Sesbanias are cultivated for their showy, pea-like flowers, borne in loose racemes from the leaf axils in summer. The leaves are alternate and pinnate, with many leaflets, each leaf terminating in a short extension of the axis. In frost-prone areas, grow in a cool to warm greenhouse, or in a conservatory. In warmer areas, grow in a shrub border, or at the base of a warm, sunny wall.
• **HARDINESS** Frost tender, but a few species, including *S. punicea*, may survive temperatures around 0°C (32°F), if wood has been well ripened in summer.
• **CULTIVATION** Under glass, grow in loam-based potting compost (JI No.2) in full light. In growth, water freely and apply a balanced liquid fertilizer monthly. Water sparingly in winter. Outdoors, grow in moderately fertile, moist but well-drained soil in full sun. Pruning group 9.
• **PROPAGATION** Sow seed at 15–19°C (59–66°F) in spring. Root semi-ripe cuttings in late summer, with bottom heat.
• **PESTS AND DISEASES** Prone to red spider mites and whiteflies under glass.

S. punicea ♀ syn. *Daubentonia punicea.* Erect to spreading, large shrub or small tree. Pinnate leaves, 20–30cm (8–12in) long, have 6–20 pairs of oblong, mid- to deep green leaflets. In summer, bears pea-like, red-purple flowers, 2cm (¾in) across, in racemes to 10cm (4in) long. ↕ 2–4m (6–12ft), ↔ 1.5–2.5m (5–8ft). S. Brazil, N.E. Argentina, Uruguay. ❀ (min. 5°C/41°F)

SESLERIA
GRAMINEAE/POACEAE

Genus of 33 species of tufted or clump-forming, evergreen, perennial grasses found mainly in damp or dry grasslands in the hills and mountains of Europe. They bear narrow, usually linear leaves and dense, spherical to cylindrical, spike-like panicles of flowers. Cultivated mainly for their colourful foliage, they are suitable for the front of a herbaceous or mixed border, in a rock garden, or in a wildflower meadow.
• **HARDINESS** Fully hardy.
• **CULTIVATION** Grow in moderately fertile, well-drained, neutral to slightly alkaline soil in full sun or light dappled shade.

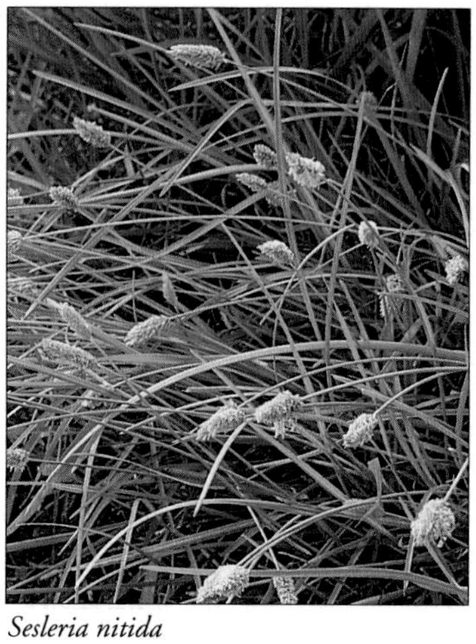
Sesleria nitida

• **PROPAGATION** Sow seed in containers in a cold frame in spring or autumn. Divide in spring.
• **PESTS AND DISEASES** Trouble free.

S. albicans, syn. *S. caerulea* subsp. *calcarea* (Blue moor grass). Vigorous, densely tufted, mound-forming, evergreen perennial with round-tipped, flat or channelled, linear, pale blue-grey leaves, to 30cm (12in) long, glossy, dark green beneath. Bears bluish purple, rarely greenish white spikelets, in dense, ovoid panicles, to 1–3cm (½–1¼in) long, just above the foliage from mid-spring to early summer. ↕ to 30cm (12in), ↔ 25cm (10in). Europe. ***
S. caerulea* subsp. *calcarea see *S. albicans.*
S. heufleriana (Balkan moor grass). Densely tufted, mound-forming, evergreen perennial with linear, bright green leaves, to 45cm (18in) long, greyish green beneath, and initially glaucous. White spikelets, ageing to deep purple, are borne in panicles 1–3cm (½–1¼in) long, from late spring to late summer. ↕ to 60cm (24in), ↔ 45cm (18in). S.E. Europe. ***
S. nitida ■ (Nest moor grass). Densely tufted, mound-forming, evergreen perennial with smooth, linear, sharp-pointed, pale grey-green to grey-blue leaves, to 45cm (18in) long. In late spring and early summer, long stems bear panicles, 2–3cm (¾–1¼in) long, of whitish green spikelets. ↕ to 60cm (24in), ↔ 40cm (16in). C. and S. Italy. ***

▷***Setcreasea purpurea*** see *Tradescantia pallida* 'Purpurea'
▷***Setcreasea striata*** see *Callisia elegans*
▷**Sevenbark** see *Hydrangea arborescens*
▷**Seville orange** see *Citrus aurantium*
▷**Shadbush** see *Amelanchier, A. canadensis*
▷**Shallon** see *Gaultheria shallon*
▷**Shamrock** see *Oxalis, Trifolium repens*
▷**Shamrock pea** see *Parochetus africana*
▷**Shasta daisy** see *Leucanthemum x superbum*
▷**Shaving brush plant** see *Haemanthus albiflos*
▷**Sheepberry** see *Viburnum lentago*
▷**Sheep's bit** see *Jasione*
▷**Shell flower** see *Moluccella laevis, Pistia, P. stratiotes*

SHEPHERDIA
ELAEAGNACEAE

Genus of 3 species of dioecious, evergreen or deciduous shrubs or small trees found in rocky and sandy habitats, and on streambanks, in North America. They have opposite, simple, ovate or oblong leaves and, in spring, before the leaves appear, bear short spikes or racemes of tiny, tubular, petalless flowers, each with a 4-lobed calyx. On female plants, the flowers are followed by spherical or ovoid, red or yellowish red fruits. Valued for their ornamental fruit and foliage, shepherdias are suitable for the back of a mixed or shrub border; they are particularly useful on poor, dry soils, and excellent for sites in exposed coastal regions. Male and female plants must be grown together to obtain fruit.
• **HARDINESS** Fully hardy.
• **CULTIVATION** Grow in moderately fertile, well-drained, neutral to slightly alkaline soil in full sun. Pruning group 1.

• **PROPAGATION** Sow seed in containers in a cold frame in autumn. Root greenwood cuttings in early summer, with gentle bottom heat.
• **PESTS AND DISEASES** Trouble free.

S. argentea (Buffalo berry). Upright, bushy, deciduous shrub, often tree-like, with oblong leaves, to 5cm (2in) long, covered in silvery scales. In spring, produces insignificant, yellow-green flowers, followed on female plants by ovoid, sour-tasting, bright red fruit, 5mm (¼in) long. ↕↔ 4m (12ft). North America. ❄❄❄

SHIBATAEA

GRAMINEAE/POACEAE

Genus of about 5 species of low-growing, clump-forming, evergreen bamboos from deciduous woodland and valley slopes in China and Japan. They have slowly spreading rhizomes and slender canes, slightly flattened on one side and slightly bent at the nodes, creating a zigzag effect. Each node bears 2–5 short branches with narrowly ovate to elliptic, tessellated leaves. Grow for their foliage in a mixed border, a gravel planting, or a container on a patio, or, if densely planted, as ground cover.
• **HARDINESS** Fully hardy.
• **CULTIVATION** Grow in moderately fertile, moist but well-drained or damp soil in partial shade, or in full sun where soil stays damp in spring and summer.
• **PROPAGATION** Divide or transplant sections of young rhizomes in spring.
• **PESTS AND DISEASES** Young shoots may be damaged by slugs.

S. kumasasa ■ syn. *Sasa ruscifolia.* Evergreen, clump-forming bamboo with short-jointed, greenish brown canes and abundant long-stalked, broadly lance-shaped, taper-pointed, rich dark green leaves, 5–11cm (2–4½in) long. New shoots appear very early in spring. ↕ 0.6–1.5m (2–5ft), ↔ 60cm (24in). Japan. ❄❄❄

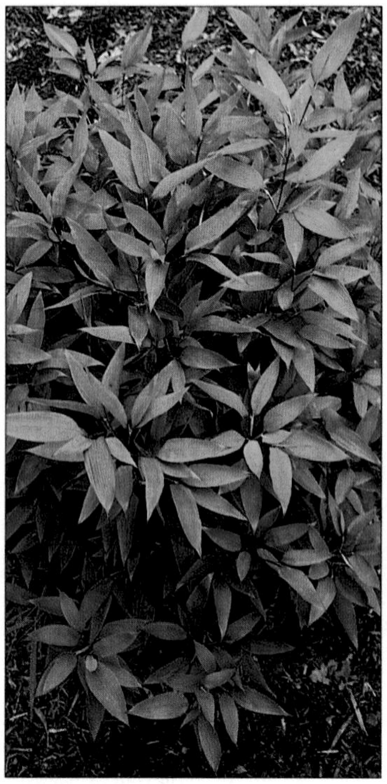

Shibataea kumasasa

▷**Shield, Carolina water** see *Cabomba caroliniana*
▷**Shield fern** see *Polystichum*
Hard see *P. aculeatum*
Prickly see *P. aculeatum*
Soft see *P. setiferum*
▷**Shingle plant** see *Rhaphidophora celatocaulis*
▷**Shinleaf** see *Pyrola*
▷**Shoo-fly** see *Nicandra, N. physalodes*
▷**Shooting star** see *Dodecatheon, D. meadia, Thymophylla tenuiloba*

SHORTIA syn. SCHIZOCODON

DIAPENSIACEAE

Genus of 6 species of evergreen perennials, spreading by runners, from woodland in E. Asia, with one species from North America. The rounded, heart-shaped, or elliptic, toothed, leathery, glossy, usually dark green leaves often turn red in autumn and winter. Bell-, trumpet-, or funnel-shaped, white or deep pink flowers, with toothed or deeply fringed petals, are borne either singly or in terminal racemes, in spring. These attractive, shade-loving plants are suitable for cultivation in a rock garden, peat bed, open glade in a woodland garden, or an alpine house. They grow best in areas with cool, damp summers.
• **HARDINESS** Fully hardy; without snow cover, buds may be damaged by frost.
• **CULTIVATION** Grow in humus-rich, leafy, moist but well-drained, acid soil in deep to partial shade. Difficult to grow in dry climates, even with frequent watering. Under glass, grow in lime-free (ericaceous) potting compost, and keep cool and well ventilated, with moderate to high humidity.
• **PROPAGATION** Sow seed in containers in a cold frame as soon as ripe; keep moist at all times. Remove small, rooted runners carefully in spring; shortias dislike root disturbance. Take basal cuttings in early summer.
• **PESTS AND DISEASES** Prone to slugs and snails outdoors; may be infested with aphids under glass.

S. galacifolia (Oconee bells). Clump-forming perennial with rounded, blunt-toothed, glossy, dark green leaves, 2–7cm (¾–3in) long, with wavy margins, turning bronze-red in autumn. In late spring, bears solitary, funnel-shaped white flowers, to 2.5cm (1in) across, often flushed pink, with toothed petals and pink calyces. ↕ 15cm (6in), ↔ 25cm (10in). E. USA. ❄❄❄

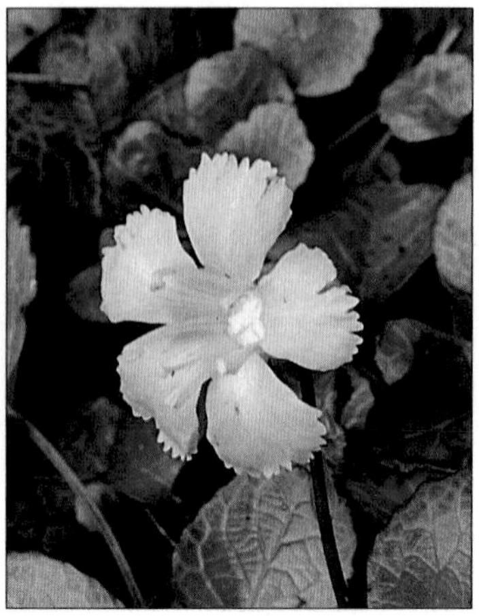

Shortia uniflora 'Grandiflora'

S. soldanelloides. Mat-forming perennial producing ovate to rounded, coarsely toothed, glossy, dark green leaves, 5cm (2in) long, rounded or heart-shaped at the bases. In late spring, bears narrowly trumpet-shaped, deep pink flowers, to 2.5cm (1in) across, with deeply fringed petals, usually in one-sided racemes. ↕ 10–30cm (4–12in), ↔ 25cm (10in). Japan. ❄❄❄. **var. *ilicifolia*** has smaller leaves with triangular teeth, and white or rarely pink flowers.
***S. uniflora* 'Grandiflora'** ■ Vigorous, mat-forming perennial with rounded, toothed, glossy, mid-green leaves, 2–7cm (¾–3in) long, heart-shaped at the bases and with wavy margins. In spring, bears a profusion of solitary, widely bell-shaped, shell-pink flowers, 5cm (2in) across, with toothed petals. ↕ 15cm (6in), ↔ 25cm (10in). Japan. ❄❄❄

▷**Shot plant, Indian** see *Canna*
▷**Shower tree, Golden** see *Cassia fistula*
▷**Shrimp bush** see *Justicia brandegeeana*
▷**Shrimp plant** see *Justicia brandegeeana*
▷**Shrubs** see pp.34–35

SIBIRAEA

ROSACEAE

Genus, closely related to *Spiraea*, of one species of deciduous shrub found on cliffs and in rocky places in E. Europe, Russia (Siberia), and China. The leaves are alternate (occasionally appearing whorled on short, lateral shoots), entire, linear-oblong to narrowly obovate, and mid- or blue-green. Racemes of tiny, cup-shaped, white or yellowish green flowers are produced in summer; the flowers are usually either male or female. Grow *S. laevigata* for its foliage and flowers in a mixed or shrub border.
• **HARDINESS** Fully hardy.
• **CULTIVATION** Grow in moderately fertile, well-drained, neutral to slightly alkaline soil in full sun. Pruning group 2 or 4.
• **PROPAGATION** Sow seed in containers in a cold frame in autumn or spring. Root softwood cuttings in spring or summer, with gentle bottom heat.
• **PESTS AND DISEASES** Trouble free.

S. altaiensis see *S. laevigata.*
S. laevigata, syn. *S. altaiensis.* Spreading, sparsely branched shrub with stout, purple-brown shoots and linear-oblong to narrowly obovate, mid- or blue-green leaves, to 10cm (4in) long. Tiny, cup-shaped, white or yellowish green flowers are borne in terminal racemes, to 12cm (5in) long, in early summer. ↕ 1m (3ft), ↔ 1.5m (5ft). Russia (Siberia), Balkans, W. China. ❄❄❄

SIDALCEA

False mallow, Prairie mallow

MALVACEAE

Genus of approximately 20–25 species of annuals and perennials, some rhizomatous, occurring in grassland, woodland glades, and on mountain streamsides in W. and C. North America. They form clumps of rounded to kidney-shaped, palmately lobed or toothed, mid-green basal leaves, from

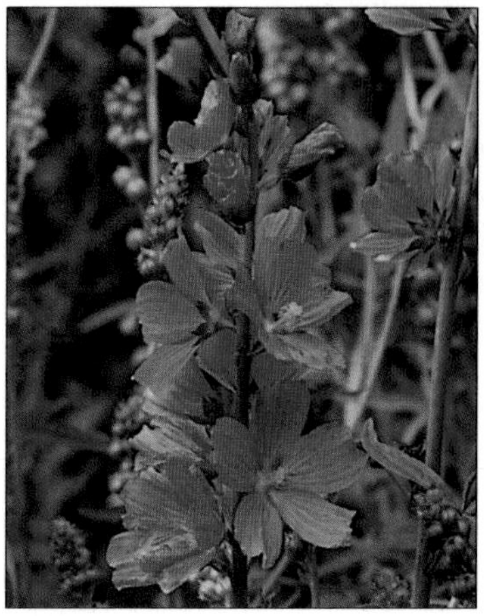

Sidalcea malviflora 'Elsie Heugh'

which arise erect, sometimes branched, stiff, flowering stems. The flowering stems produce palmately lobed, mid-green stem leaves and long-lasting, hollyhock-like, white, pink, or purple-pink flowers in dense, upright, terminal racemes. Each flower has 5 spreading, sometimes fringed, silky petals and numerous prominent stamens. Sidalceas are suitable for growing in a mixed or herbaceous border, and provide good cut flowers.
• **HARDINESS** Fully hardy.
• **CULTIVATION** Grow in moderately fertile, humus-rich, moist but well-drained, light, sandy, neutral to slightly acid soil in full sun. Sidalceas will tolerate a wide range of soil conditions, but resent waterlogging. Provide a dry winter mulch of bracken or straw during prolonged frosty periods without protective snow cover. Cut stems back hard after flowering, to prevent seed formation and to encourage a further flush of blooms.
• **PROPAGATION** Sow seed in containers in a cold frame in autumn or spring. Divide cultivars in autumn or spring.
• **PESTS AND DISEASES** Prone to slug damage and susceptible to rust.

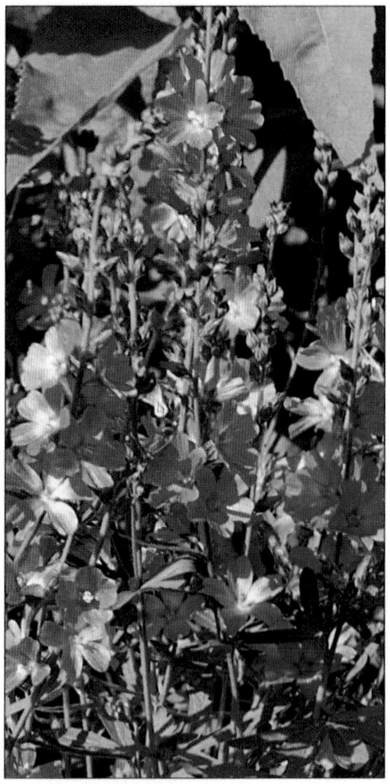

Sidalcea malviflora 'Oberon'

S

S. candida. Rhizomatous perennial with rounded, 7-lobed basal leaves, to 20cm (8in) long, and smaller, rounded leaves on the erect, unbranched stems. Dense racemes of open funnel-shaped, white or cream flowers, to 2.5cm (1in) across, are produced in mid- and late summer. ↕30–80cm (12–32in), ↔45cm (18in). USA (Wyoming, Nevada, Utah, Colorado, New Mexico). ❄❄❄

S. malviflora (Checkerbloom). Erect to slightly decumbent perennial producing rounded to kidney-shaped, shallowly lobed basal leaves, 4–8cm (1½–3in) long, and more deeply lobed stem leaves. In early and midsummer, bears racemes of funnel-shaped, pink or lilac-pink flowers, 5cm (2in) across. ↕ to 1.2m (4ft), ↔45cm (18in). USA (Oregon, California), Mexico (Baja California). ❄❄❄. Most of the cultivars described are hybrids between *S. candida* and *S. malviflora*. **'Croftway Red'** has rich reddish pink flowers; ↕90cm (36in). **'Elsie Heugh'** ■ has large, satin-textured, purple-pink flowers, the petals fringed; ↕90cm (36in). **'Loveliness'** is compact, with pale pink flowers; ↕75cm (30in). **'Oberon** ■ has clear rose-pink flowers. **'Puck'** is compact and upright, bearing deep pink flowers in midsummer; ↕ to 40cm (16in). **'Reverend Page Roberts'** has silvery, pale rose-pink flowers. **'Sussex Beauty'** has satin-textured, clear pink flowers. **'William Smith'** 🏆 has deep rose-pink flowers, tinted salmon-pink; ↕90cm (36in).

SIDERITIS

LABIATAE/LAMIACEAE

Genus of about 100 species of annuals, perennials, and evergreen shrubs and subshrubs from coastal plains to forest or laurel-covered clifftops in the Mediterranean and Atlantic islands. They are grown mainly for their simple, often softly hairy or white-woolly leaves, arranged in opposite pairs. Tubular to bell-shaped, 2-lipped flowers are borne in whorled spikes in summer. They need long, hot summers to thrive. In warm, dry climates, grow at the front of a mixed or shrub border, in a rock garden, or in a small courtyard garden. Where winters are cold and damp, grow as foliage plants in a cool greenhouse.

• **HARDINESS** Half hardy to frost tender.

• **CULTIVATION** Under glass, grow in loam-based potting compost (JI No.1) in full light. When in growth, water moderately and apply a balanced liquid fertilizer monthly; water sparingly in winter. Outdoors, grow in moderately fertile, sharply drained, neutral to slightly alkaline soil in full sun. Provide a dry winter mulch. Pruning group 9.

• **PROPAGATION** Sow seed of tender species at 13–16°C (55–61°F) in spring; sow seed of hardier species in containers in a cold frame in spring. Divide perennials in early spring. Root softwood cuttings of shrubs in late spring, with bottom heat; take semi-ripe cuttings in late summer.

• **PESTS AND DISEASES** Trouble free.

S. candicans. Erect to spreading, many-branched shrub with ovate to heart-shaped, densely white-woolly, scalloped leaves, 5–10cm (2–4in) long. In summer, bears erect, terminal spikes, 15–28cm (6–11in) long, of 20–30 small, light yellow flowers, 8mm (⅜in) long, tipped orange and red-brown. ↕60–90cm (24–36in), ↔45–80cm (18–32in). Canary Islands (Tenerife). ❄

▷ ***Sieversia reptans*** see *Geum reptans*
▷ ***Sigmatostalix radicans*** see *Ornithophora radicans*

SILENE

Campion, Catchfly

CARYOPHYLLACEAE

Genus of about 500 species of annuals, biennials, and deciduous or evergreen perennials, some subshrubby, widely distributed in habitats ranging from open woodland to meadows and mountain screes in the N. hemisphere; most occur around the Mediterranean, but some are found in the mountains of tropical Africa and in South America. The variable leaves are opposite, linear to ovate or obovate, and entire. The flowers have 5 often notched or split, clawed petals and a tubular, often conspicuously inflated calyx; they are borne singly or in sprays, clusters, broad or narrow panicle-like cymes, or corymb-like panicles. Most silenes are easily grown, and often self-seed freely. Smaller perennials are excellent for a rock garden, and taller ones for the front of a herbaceous border, or for a wild garden. Use annuals as bedding in mixed or annual borders. Some silenes resent winter wet and are best grown in a scree bed or alpine house.

• **HARDINESS** Fully hardy to half hardy.

• **CULTIVATION** Grow in moderately fertile, well-drained, neutral to slightly alkaline soil in full sun or light dappled shade. *S. hookeri* needs acid soil. *S. dioica* 'Rosea Plena' needs moist but well-drained soil in light dappled shade. Grow smaller alpine species in sharply drained, gritty soil in a scree bed, or in a mix of equal parts loam-based potting compost (JI No.2) and sharp grit, in containers in an alpine house.

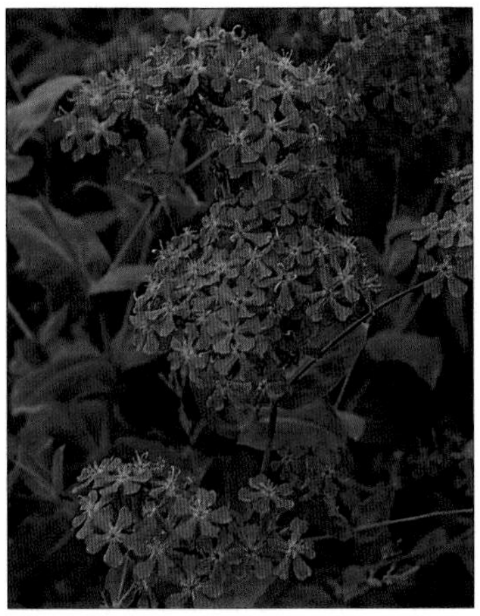

Silene armeria 'Electra'

• **PROPAGATION** Sow seed of perennials in containers in a cold frame in autumn. Sow seed of hardy annuals *in situ* in autumn or spring; sow half-hardy annuals at 16–19°C (61–66°F) in spring and harden off before planting out after last frosts. Divide rooted offshoots of *S. dioica* 'Rosea Plena' from midsummer to autumn. Root basal cuttings of perennials in spring.

• **PESTS AND DISEASES** Outdoors, susceptible to slug and snail damage; under glass, often infested by aphids, whiteflies, and red spider mites. *S. dioica* 'Rosea Plena' is prone to smut fungus and, in dry conditions, to powdery mildew.

S. acaulis (Moss campion). Very dwarf, evergreen perennial forming moss-like cushions of tiny, linear, bright green leaves, 6–10mm (¼–½in) long. In summer, produces solitary, almost stemless, deep pink, sometimes white flowers, to 1cm (½in) across, with entire or notched petals. Suitable for a scree bed, but rarely bears abundant flowers in cultivation. ↕5cm (2in), ↔20cm (8in). Arctic, mountains of Eurasia, North America. ❄❄❄

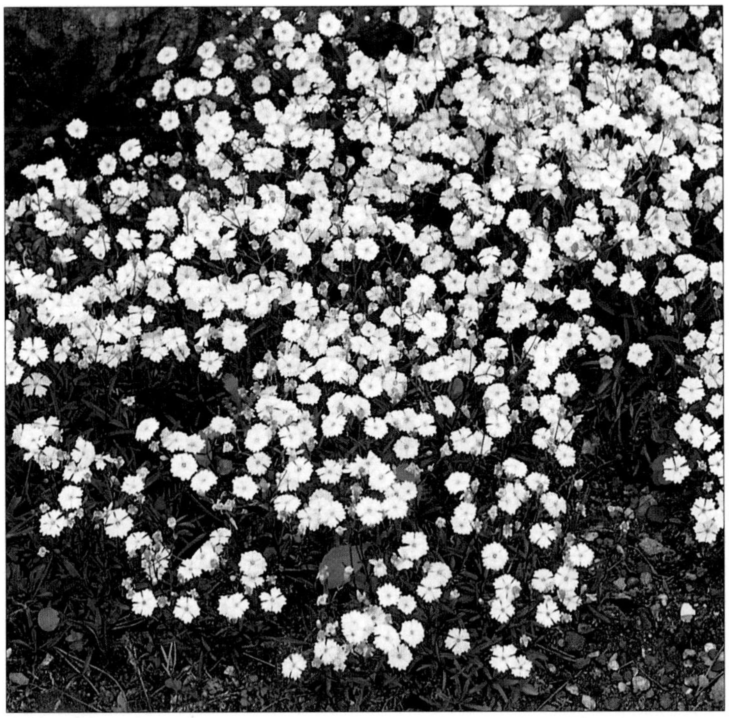

Silene alpestris

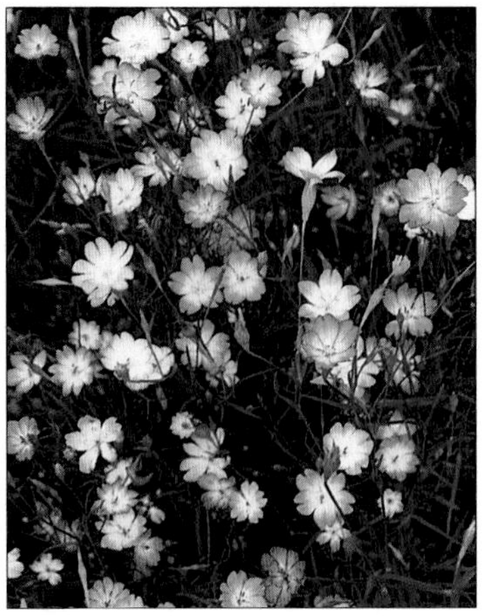

Silene coeli-rosa

S. alpestris ■ syn. *Heliosperma alpestris.* Loosely tufted, branching, evergreen perennial with linear-lance-shaped, mid-green leaves, to 3cm (1¼in) long. In early summer, bears open sprays of rounded, white, sometimes pink-flushed flowers, 1cm (½in) across, with fringed petals. ↕15cm (6in), ↔20cm (8in). Europe (E. Alps). ❄❄❄

S. armeria. Sticky-hairy annual or biennial with upright stems. Produces grey-green leaves, 1–4cm (½–1½in) long, the basal leaves spoon-shaped, the stem leaves lance-shaped. In late summer, bears broad, dense, rounded, corymb-like panicles of deep carmine-pink flowers, to 1.5cm (½in) across, with shallowly notched petals. Treat as an annual. ↕30cm (12in), ↔15cm (6in). C. and S. Europe. ❄❄❄. **'Electra'** ■ is very free-flowering.

S. coeli-rosa ■ syn. *Agrostemma coeli-rosa, Lychnis coeli-rosa, Viscaria elegans* (Rose of heaven). Erect, slender, hairless annual with oblong to lance-shaped, grey-green leaves, 1–5cm (½–2in) long. In summer, bears loose, long-stalked clusters of spreading, white-centred, rose-pink flowers, to 2.5cm (1in) across, with deeply notched petals and prominently toothed calyces. Good for cut flowers. ↕ to 50cm (20in), ↔ to 15cm (6in). Mediterranean. ❄❄❄. **Angel Series** cultivars flower in 2 separate, soft, clear colours; ↕25–30cm (10–12in). **'Blue Angel'** has lavender-blue flowers. **'Rose Angel'** ■ has deep pink-magenta flowers.

***S. conica* 'Balletje Balletje'.** Erect, slender, sticky-stemmed annual with narrowly lance-shaped, grey-green

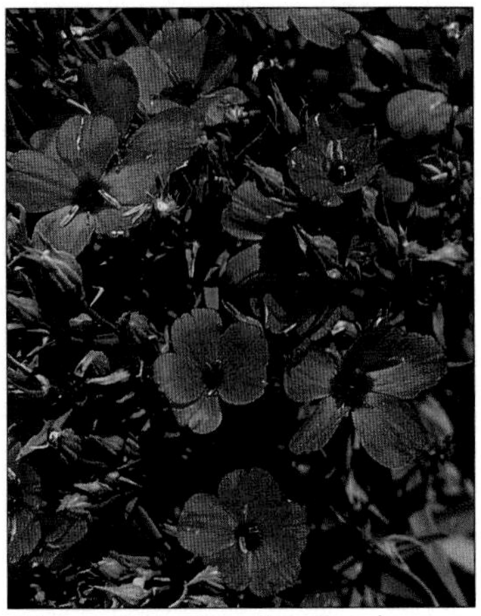

Silene coeli-rosa 'Rose Angel'

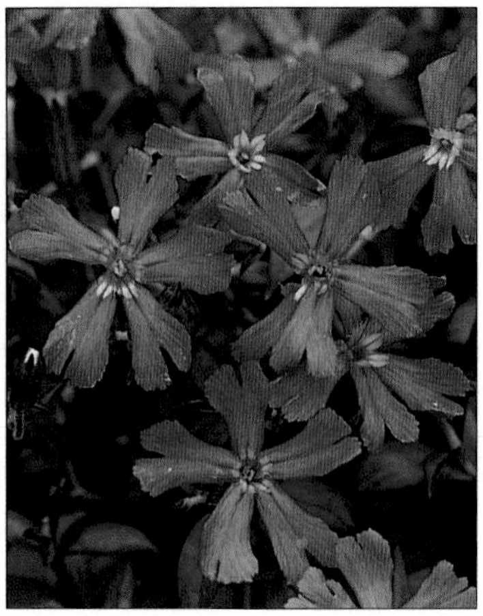
Silene keiskei var. *minor*

leaves, 1–4cm (½–1½in) long. In summer, produces cymes of 5–30 rose-pink flowers, to 5mm (¼in) across, but is grown for its oval, sticky-hairy, grey-green calyces, with bright green ribs, which enlarge in fruit and are good for flower arrangements. ↕ 15–50cm (6–20in), ↔ to 15cm (6in). ✽✽✽

***S. dioica* 'Rosea Plena'.** Clump-forming, semi-evergreen perennial with erect, branched flowering stems. Bears dark green leaves, most to 9cm (3½in) long, the basal leaves obovate, the stem leaves oblong-obovate, becoming smaller and almost stalkless towards the stem tips. From late spring to midsummer, bears loosely branched, panicle-like cymes of large, rounded, double flowers, 4cm (1½in) across, with notched, dusky-pink petals, white at the bases. ↕ to 80cm (32in), ↔ 45cm (18in). ✽✽✽

***S. elisabethae*,** syn. *Melandrium elisabethae*. Tufted, semi-evergreen perennial with loose rosettes of lance-shaped, glossy, mid-green leaves, 6cm (2½in) long. In early summer, spreading stems bear usually solitary, large, deep red-purple flowers, 5cm (2in) across, with 2-lobed petals. Resents winter wet. ↕ to 25cm (10in), ↔ 15cm (6in). Limestone screes in the Italian Alps. ✽✽✽

***S. hookeri*.** Tufted, prostrate, deciduous perennial with lance-shaped, grey-hairy, mid-green leaves, 5–7cm (2–3in) long. In late summer, bears solitary, clear pale pink to salmon-pink flowers, to 6cm (2½in) across, with very deeply lobed white petals. Resents winter wet; needs acid soil. ↕ to 5cm (2in), ↔ to 15cm (6in). USA (California). ✽✽✽

S

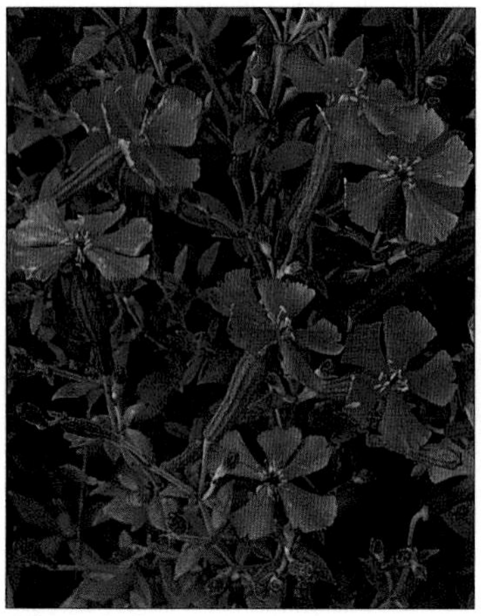
Silene schafta

S. keiskei* var. *minor ■ Tufted, evergreen perennial, similar to *S. elisabethae*, with hairy, narrowly lance-shaped, dark green leaves, to 3cm (1¼in) long, on slender stems. Bears loosely branching sprays of deep rose-pink flowers, 2–3cm (¾–1¼in) across, with shallowly notched petals, in late summer. ↕ 10cm (4in), ↔ 20cm (8in). Japan. ✽✽✽

***S. maritima* 'Flore Pleno'** see *S. uniflora* 'Flore Pleno'.

S. pendula (Nodding catchfly). Erect to spreading, glandular-hairy, bushy annual with ovate to lance-shaped, hairy, mid-green leaves, to 6cm (2½in) long. In summer, bears loose clusters of slightly pendent, single or double, pale pink flowers, to 1.5cm (½in) across, with prominently toothed calyces. Good for edging or for hanging baskets. ↕↔ 15–23cm (6–9in). Mediterranean. ✽✽✽. **'Peach Blossom'** has double flowers, opening deep rose-pink and maturing through pale pink to white, showing a range of colours at the same time on a single plant; ↕ 15cm (6in). **'Snowball'** has double white flowers. **'Triumph'** has double, deep pinkish red flowers.

S. schafta ■ ♀ Clump-forming, slender-stemmed, semi-evergreen perennial with lance-shaped, bright green leaves, 1–2cm (½–¾in) long. Profusely bears sprays of long-tubed, deep magenta flowers, 2cm (¾in) across, with notched petals, from late summer to autumn. Suitable for a rock garden. ↕ 25cm (10in), ↔ 30cm (12in). W. Asia. ✽✽✽. **'Shell Pink'**, syn. 'Ralph Haywood', has clear pale pink flowers.

***S. uniflora* 'Flore Pleno'**, syn. *S. maritima* 'Flore Pleno', *S. vulgaris* subsp. *maritima* 'Flore Pleno' (Double sea campion). Lax, prostrate, deeply rooting, semi-evergreen perennial with fleshy, lance-shaped, grey-green leaves, to 2cm (¾in) long, fringed with fine hairs. In summer, erect, branching stems produce double white flowers, to 2.5cm (1in) across, with deeply cut petals, either singly or in few-flowered clusters. ↕ 15cm (6in), ↔ 20cm (8in). ✽✽✽

***S. vulgaris* subsp. *maritima* 'Flore Pleno'** see *S. uniflora* 'Flore Pleno'.

▷ **Silk cotton tree** see *Bombax, Ceiba*
Red see *Bombax ceiba*
White see *Ceiba pentandra*
▷ **Silk-tassel bush** see *Garrya elliptica*
▷ **Silk tree** see *Albizia julibrissin*
Floss see *Chorisia speciosa*
▷ **Silk vine** see *Periploca graeca*
▷ **Silkweed** see *Asclepias*

SILPHIUM

Prairie dock, Rosinweed

ASTERACEAE/COMPOSITAE

Genus of about 20 species of tall herbaceous perennials from fields, prairies, and open woodland and scrub (some in moister areas) in Canada and C. and E. USA. Their erect, sparsely branched stems exude resinous sap with a strong turpentine-like scent. The opposite or alternate, coarse leaves, sometimes all basal, are lance-shaped to ovate or triangular, some toothed or pinnatifid. Sunflower-like yellow flowerheads are borne in branching corymbs. Excellent for naturalizing in a wild or woodland garden.

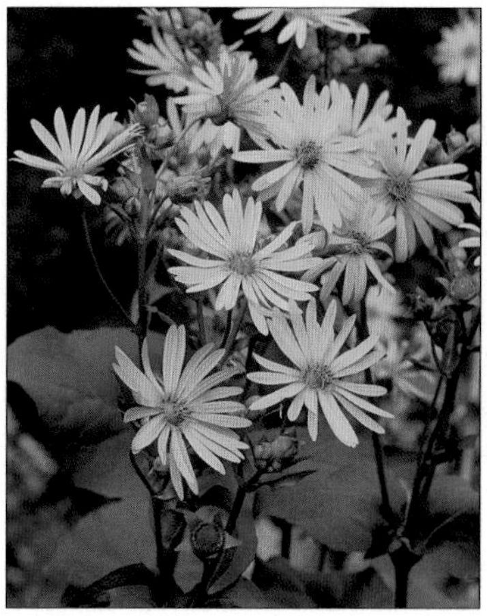
Silphium perfoliatum

• **HARDINESS** Fully hardy.
• **CULTIVATION** Grow in moderately fertile, moist, deep, neutral to slightly alkaline soil in full sun or partial shade; best in heavy soil. *S. perfoliatum* prefers damper soil.
• **PROPAGATION** Sow seed in containers in a cold frame as soon as ripe. Divide in spring.
• **PESTS AND DISEASES** Trouble free.

S. laciniatum (Compass plant, Pilot plant, Polar plant). Upright, clump-forming perennial with stiffly hairy stems bearing alternate, erect, pinnatifid or 2-pinnatifid, fern-like, hairy leaves, to 50cm (20in) long, becoming smaller up the stems; the flat sides face east and west, hence the plant's common names. In late summer and early autumn, bears terminal, narrow, raceme-like corymbs of nodding yellow, eastward-facing flowerheads, to 12cm (5in) across, with darker disc-florets. ↕ to 3m (10ft), ↔ 60cm (24in). E. and C. USA. ✽✽✽

S. perfoliatum ■ (Cup plant). Erect, hairless or nearly hairless, clump-forming perennial producing opposite, triangular-ovate, coarsely toothed, bristly leaves, to 35cm (14in) long, with winged stalks. The upper leaves are perfoliate. From midsummer to early autumn, bears terminal, open-branched, corymb-like inflorescences of yellow flowerheads, to 8cm (3in) across, with darker disc-florets. ↕ to 2.5m (8ft), ↔ 1m (3ft). North America (Ontario to Oklahoma and Georgia). ✽✽✽

▷ **Silver bell** see *Halesia*
▷ **Silver berry** see *Elaeagnus commutata*
▷ **Silver fir** see *Abies, A. alba*
European see *A. alba*
▷ **Silver net leaf** see *Fittonia verschaffeltii* var. *argyroneura*
▷ **Silver thatch** see *Coccothrinax fragrans*
▷ **Silver torch** see *Cleistocactus strausii*
▷ **Silver tree** see *Leucadendron argenteum*
▷ **Silver vine** see *Actinidia polygama*

SILYBUM

ASTERACEAE/COMPOSITAE

Genus of 2 species of erect, rosette-forming, thistle-like annuals or biennials from the mountains of E. Africa and from stony slopes, steppes, and thickets in W. Africa, the Mediterranean, and Europe to C. Asia. They have broad, shallowly to deeply lobed, obovate to inversely lance-shaped, spiny, light to dark green leaves, and bear spherical,

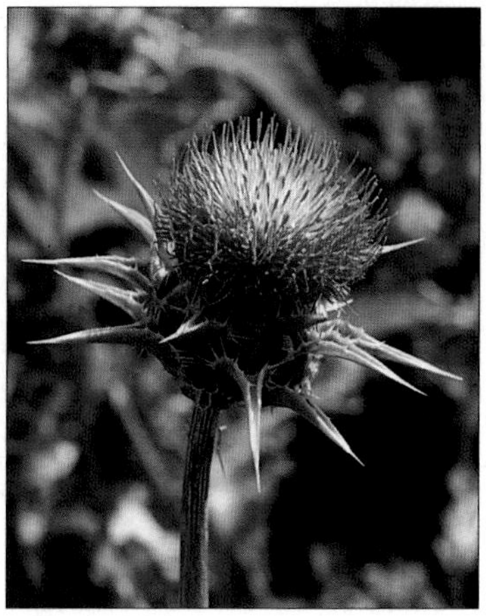
Silybum marianum

single, purple-pink flowerheads, enclosed in spiny bracts. Cultivated for their foliage and flowers, silybums are suitable for growing in a mixed or herbaceous border or a gravel garden.
• **HARDINESS** Fully hardy.
• **CULTIVATION** Grow in poor to moderately fertile, well-drained, neutral to slightly alkaline soil in full sun. Protect from excessive winter wet. Remove flowering stems as they form, to retain foliage effect.
• **PROPAGATION** Sow seed *in situ* in late spring or early summer and thin seedlings to 60cm (24in) apart. To grow for foliage effect alone, sow in a cold greenhouse in late winter or very early spring; prick out into 9cm (3½in) containers and grow on to plant out in late spring.
• **PESTS AND DISEASES** Prone to slug and snail damage.

S. marianum ■ (Blessed Mary's thistle). Rosette-forming biennial with a flat, basal rosette of deeply lobed, obovate, spiny, heavily white-veined and marbled, glossy, dark green leaves, to 50cm (20in) long. In the second year after sowing, bears thistle-like, slightly scented, purple-pink flowerheads, to 5cm (2in) across, from summer to autumn. ↕ to 1.5m (5ft), ↔ 60–90cm (24–36in). S.W. Europe to Afghanistan, N. Africa. ✽✽✽

▷ ***Sinacalia tangutica*** see *Senecio tanguticus*
▷ ***Sinarundinaria jaunsarensis*** see *Yushania anceps*
▷ ***Sinarundinaria murieliae*** see *Fargesia murieliae*
▷ ***Sinarundinaria nitida*** see *Fargesia nitida*

SINNINGIA

GESNERIACEAE

Genus, including species formerly classified under *Gloxinia* and *Rechsteineria*, of about 40 species of tuberous perennials and deciduous or evergreen, low-growing shrubs from tropical forest in Central and South America. They have usually ovate to elliptic, fleshy leaves, in opposite pairs or in whorls of 6 or more, often crowded at the stem bases. They are grown for their showy, solitary or clustered, tubular, trumpet-shaped, or bell-shaped flowers, generally borne in summer. In frost-prone areas or in areas with high winter rainfall, grow as

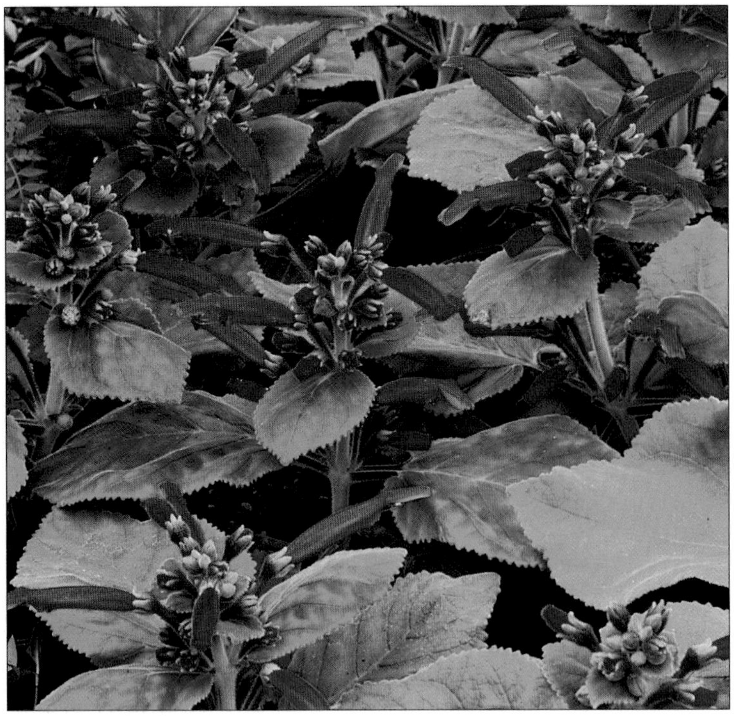

Sinningia cardinalis

houseplants or in a warm greenhouse or conservatory. In frost-free areas, they are suitable for a trough, raised bed, peat bed, terrace, or woodland garden.
• **HARDINESS** Frost tender.
• **CULTIVATION** Under glass, grow in loamless potting compost in bright filtered or indirect light. Most are best maintained with high humidity at 18–24°C (64–75°F); grow *S. cardinalis* and *S. pusilla* at 19°C (66°F) or more. In the growing season, water moderately and apply a half-strength high-potash fertilizer every 2 weeks. Dry off tubers in autumn and keep completely dry in winter. Start into growth in early spring in shallow trays of peat; pot up individually into 9–10cm (3½–4in) containers when young shoots are 5–7cm (2–3in) long. Outdoors, grow in moist but well-drained, humus-rich, acid to neutral soil in light dappled or partial shade.
• **PROPAGATION** Surface-sow seed at 15–21°C (59–70°F) in spring. Divide tubers in spring. Take stem-tip cuttings of miniature species and cultivars in late spring or early summer. Root leaf cuttings in spring or summer, with bottom heat.

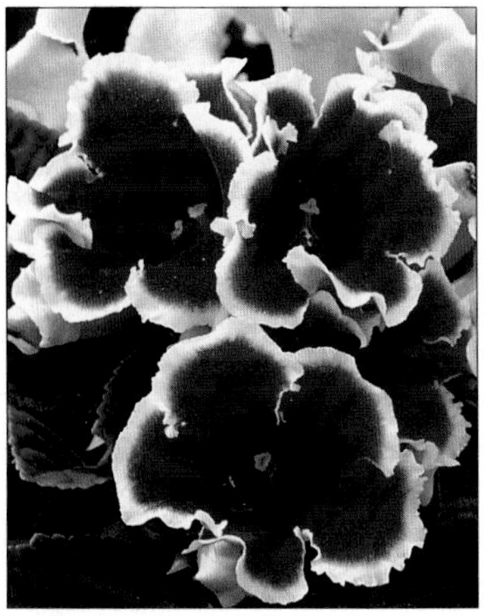

Sinningia 'Switzerland'

• **PESTS AND DISEASES** Leafhoppers and western flower thrips may be a problem.

S. canescens ♀ syn. *Rechsteineria leucotricha*, *S. leucotricha* (Brazilian edelweiss). Upright, densely woolly, tuberous perennial. Whorls of obovate, sage-green leaves, to 15cm (6in) long, are covered with silvery white hairs. In summer, short-lived, nodding, narrowly tubular, pinkish orange-red to rose-pink flowers, 2.5cm (1in) long, are borne in clusters of 3–5. ↕ 30cm (12in), ↔ 35cm (14in). Brazil. ❀ (min. 15°C/59°F)
S. cardinalis ■ (Cardinal flower, Helmet flower). Tuberous perennial with short white hairs covering both the stems and the pairs of ovate, scalloped, mid-green leaves, 7–15cm (3–6in) long. Clustered, upwardly angled, hooded, tubular, blood-red flowers, 5cm (2in) long, open in succession for up to 3 months from late summer to autumn. ↕↔ to 30cm (12in). Brazil. ❀ (min. 15°C/59°F)
S. leucotricha see *S. canescens.*
***S.* 'Mont Blanc'.** Rosette-forming, tuberous perennial with ovate, velvety, mid-green leaves, 20–24cm (8–10in) long. In summer, bears solitary, erect, trumpet-shaped, pure white flowers, 4cm (1½in) long. ↕ to 30cm (12in), ↔ 45cm (18in). ❀ (min. 15°C/59°F)
***S. pusilla*.** Prostrate, miniature perennial with pea-sized tubers, bearing pairs of ovate, hairy, dark olive-green leaves, to 1cm (½in) long, red-veined beneath. Solitary, nodding, tubular lilac flowers, 2cm (¾in) long, with white throats, are produced on hairy stalks, 1cm (½in) long, in summer. Blooms almost continuously in a terrarium. ↕↔ 2.5–5cm (1–2in). Brazil. ❀ (min. 15°C/59°F). **'White Sprite'** bears white flowers.
S. regina (Cinderella slippers). Tuberous perennial with pairs of ovate to elliptic, finely scalloped, dark green leaves, 10–20cm (4–8in) long, velvety above and pale green in the vein areas. Clusters of 4–6 nodding, trumpet-shaped, rich purple flowers, 5cm (2in) long, each with a pale yellow band, are produced in summer. ↕ 20cm (8in), ↔ 35cm (14in). Brazil. ❀ (min. 15°C/59°F)
***S. speciosa*,** syn. *Gloxinia speciosa* (Florists' gloxinia). Tuberous perennial with rosettes of ovate to oblong, scalloped, dark green leaves, 20–30cm (8–12in) long, covered with velvety hairs, and red-flushed beneath. Produces solitary or clustered, nodding, tubular-bell-shaped, red, violet-blue, or white flowers, 3.5cm (1½in) long, in summer. ↕↔ 30cm (12in). Brazil. ❀ (min. 15°C/59°F)
***S.* 'Switzerland'** ■ Tuberous perennial with rosettes of ovate, velvety, mid-green leaves, 20–24cm (8–10in) long. In summer, produces solitary, upright, trumpet-shaped, bright scarlet flowers, 4cm (1½in) long, with wavy white margins. ↕ to 30cm (12in), ↔ 45cm (18in). ❀ (min. 15°C/59°F)
***S.* 'Waterloo'.** Rosette-forming, tuberous perennial with ovate, velvety, mid-green leaves, 20–24cm (8–10in) long. In summer, bears solitary, upright, trumpet-shaped, bright scarlet flowers, 4cm (1½in) long. ↕ to 30cm (12in), ↔ 45cm (18in). ❀ (min. 15°C/59°F)

▷ ***Sinocalamus giganteus*** see *Dendrocalamus giganteus*

SINOCALYCANTHUS

CALYCANTHACEAE

Genus of one species of deciduous shrub, related to *Calycanthus*, occurring in woodland in China. It produces simple, opposite leaves and is grown for its showy, single white flowers, borne in early summer. Use in a shrub border or wild garden.
• **HARDINESS** Fully hardy.
• **CULTIVATION** Grow in moderately fertile, humus-rich, moist but well-drained soil in full sun, or with some midday shade. Shelter from cold, drying winds. Pruning group 1.
• **PROPAGATION** Sow seed in containers in a cold frame in autumn. Root softwood cuttings in late spring or early summer, with bottom heat.
• **PESTS AND DISEASES** Trouble free.

***S. chinensis*,** syn. *Calycanthus chinensis.* Spreading shrub with broadly oval, short-tapered, glossy, mid-green leaves, to 15cm (6in) long. Cup-shaped, slightly pink-flushed white flowers, 7cm (3in) across, marked white and maroon inside, are produced singly, close to the shoot-tips, in early summer. ↕ 3m (10ft), ↔ 4m (12ft). E. China. ***

SINOFRANCHETIA

LARDIZABALACEAE

Genus of one species of twining, woody, dioecious, deciduous climber occurring in woodland in China. It has alternate, 3-palmate leaves, and produces pendent racemes of tiny white flowers; on female plants, these are followed by grape-like berries. Cultivated for its attractive foliage and fruit, it may be grown through a tree, over a large shrub, or against a wall. Female plants can bear fruit without a male.
• **HARDINESS** Fully hardy.
• **CULTIVATION** Grow in moderately fertile, humus-rich, moist but well-drained soil in full sun or partial shade. Pruning group 11, in spring.
• **PROPAGATION** Sow seed in containers in a cold frame in autumn. Root softwood cuttings in late spring or early summer.
• **PESTS AND DISEASES** Trouble free.

S. chinensis. Twining, woody climber with glaucous, purple-spotted stems and long-stalked leaves, to 15cm (6in) long, composed of 3 ovate, dark green leaflets, glaucous beneath. In late spring, bears tiny white flowers in pendent racemes, to 10cm (4in) long. In summer, female plants produce spherical, grape-like purple berries, to 2cm (¾in) long. ↕ 12m (40ft). W. and C. China. ***

SINOJACKIA

STYRACACEAE

Genus of 2 species of deciduous shrubs or small trees from woodland in China. They are valued for their small racemes of white flowers, which are borne close to the tips of short, leafy shoots in late spring and early summer. The leaves are simple and alternate. Grow sinojackias in a woodland garden among other trees and shrubs.
• **HARDINESS** Fully hardy.
• **CULTIVATION** Grow in moderately fertile, humus-rich, moist but well-drained, acid soil in full sun with some midday shade, or in partial shade. Avoid very exposed sites. Pruning group 1.
• **PROPAGATION** Sow seed in containers in a cold frame in autumn. Root greenwood cuttings in early summer, with bottom heat.
• **PESTS AND DISEASES** Trouble free.

S. rehderiana ■ ◯ Bushy shrub, or sometimes spreading tree, with elliptic to elliptic-obovate, glossy, dark green leaves, to 9cm (3½in) long. In late spring and early summer, produces pendent, star-shaped white flowers, 2cm (¾in) across, with yellow stamens. ↕↔ to 5m (15ft). E. China. ***
S. xylocarpa ◯ Bushy shrub, or sometimes spreading tree, with obovate, glossy, dark green leaves, to 8cm (3in) long, wedge-shaped at the bases and with pointed tips. Star-shaped white flowers, 2.5cm (1in) across, with yellow stamens, are borne in late spring and early summer. ↕↔ to 6m (20ft). E. China. ***

S

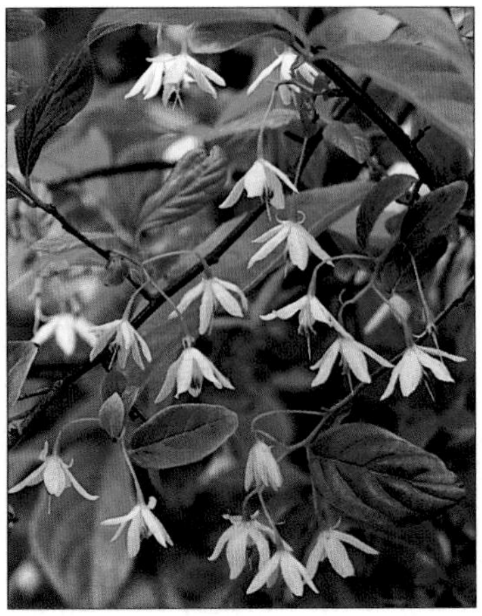

Sinojackia rehderiana

SINOWILSONIA

HAMAMELIDACEAE

Genus of one species of monoecious, deciduous shrub or small tree, related to witch hazels (*Hamamelis*), found on streambanks in the mountains of China. It has simple, alternate leaves, and is mainly cultivated for its catkin-like racemes of small flowers, borne in late spring before the leaves. Grow in a shrub border or woodland garden.

- **HARDINESS** Fully hardy.
- **CULTIVATION** Grow in moist but well-drained, moderately fertile, humus-rich, acid soil, in full sun with some midday shade, or in partial shade. Shelter from cold, drying winds. Pruning group 1.
- **PROPAGATION** Sow seed in containers in a cold frame in autumn. Root green-wood cuttings with bottom heat in early summer.
- **PESTS AND DISEASES** Trouble free.

S. henryi Spreading shrub or small tree with broadly oval to elliptic, tapered, bristle-toothed leaves, to 18cm (7in) long. In late spring, bears catkin-like racemes of small green flowers: males are 6cm (2½in) long, females are to 3cm (1¼in) long, and elongate to 15cm (6in) in fruit. The fruit are woody, 2-valved capsules, 2cm (¾in) across. ↕ 8m (25ft), ↔ 5m (15ft). C. and W. China. ❄❄❄

▷ ***Siphonosmanthus delavayi*** see *Osmanthus delavayi*

SISYRINCHIUM

IRIDACEAE

Genus of about 90 species of annuals and rhizomatous perennials, some of which are semi-evergreen. Native to North and South America (although some are widely naturalized elsewhere), they thrive in habitats ranging from mountainous areas to meadows and coastal sands. They produce clumps of linear to sword-shaped, mostly basal leaves, often forming fans. In spring and summer, upright, often winged stems bear star-, cup-, or shallowly trumpet-shaped, blue, yellow, mauve, white, or rarely pink flowers, either singly or in umbel-like clusters of 2–8; each cluster is enclosed in a pair of spathe bracts. Grow smaller species in a rock garden or gravel planting, taller species in a herbaceous border. In frost-prone areas, grow half-hardy plants in a cool green-

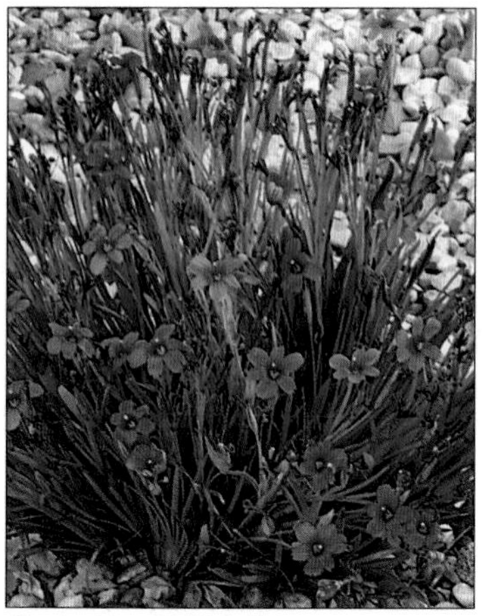

Sisyrinchium 'E.K. Balls'

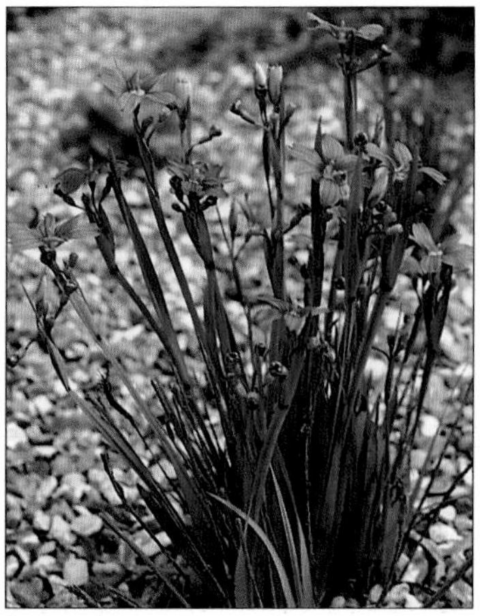

Sisyrinchium graminoides

house or alpine house. Some species self-seed freely. A few species, especially the larger perennials, are shallow rooted, and may die suddenly after several years.

- **HARDINESS** Fully hardy to half hardy.
- **CULTIVATION** Grow in poor to moderately fertile, well-drained, neutral to slightly alkaline soil in full sun. Protect from excessive winter wet.
- **PROPAGATION** Sow seed in containers in a cold frame in autumn or early spring. Divide in spring.
- **PESTS AND DISEASES** May be affected by root rot outdoors, and infested by aphids and red spider mites under glass.

S. angustifolium see *S. graminoides*.
***S.* 'Ball's Mauve'** see *S.* 'E.K. Balls'.
***S. bellum* of gardens** see *S. idahoense*.
S. bermudiana see *S. graminoides*.
***S. birameum* of gardens** see *S. graminoides*.
***S.* 'Biscutella'.** Clump-forming, semi-evergreen perennial with linear leaves, to 18cm (7in) long. In summer, upright stems bear a succession of individually short-lived, shallowly trumpet-shaped, dull yellow flowers, 2cm (¾in) across, heavily veined and suffused brownish purple. ↕ 30cm (12in), ↔ 15cm (6in). ❄❄❄
S. boreale see *S. californicum*.
S. brachypus see *S. californicum*.
S. californicum, syn. *S. boreale*, *S. brachypus*. Short-lived, semi-evergreen perennial with sword-shaped, grey-green leaves, to 15cm (6in) long. In summer, broadly winged stems bear a succession of star-shaped, dark-veined, bright yellow flowers, 1–2cm (½–¾in) across. Self-seeds freely. ↕ 60cm (24in), ↔ to 15cm (6in). W. North America (Vancouver to California). ❄❄
S. douglasii see *Olsynium douglasii*.
***S.* 'E.K. Balls'** ▣ syn. *S.* 'Ball's Mauve'. Clump-forming, semi-evergreen perennial with fans of narrow, sword-shaped leaves, to 25cm (10in) long. Erect stems bear individually short-lived, star-shaped mauve flowers, 2cm (¾in) across, in summer. ↕ 25cm (10in), ↔ 15cm (6in). ❄❄❄
S. graminoides ▣ syn. *S. angustifolium*, *S. bermudiana*, *S. birameum* of gardens (Blue-eyed grass). Clump-forming, semi-evergreen perennial with linear leaves, to 50cm (20in) long. In summer, erect stems bear a long succession of individually short-lived, iris-like, deep blue, yellow-throated flowers, 2cm (¾in) across. Self-seeds freely. ↕ 50cm (20in), ↔ 15cm (6in). North America. ❄❄❄

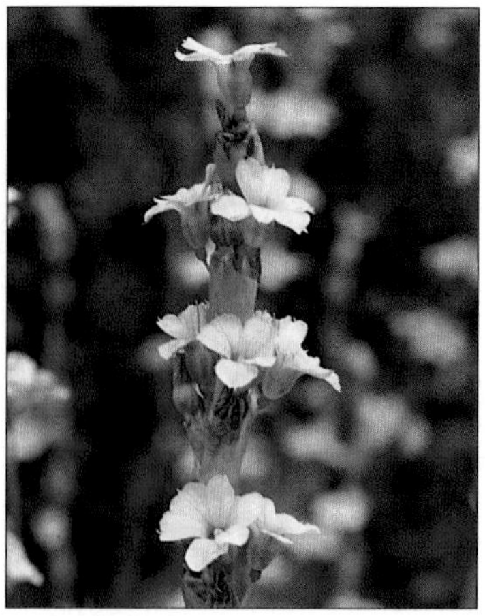

Sisyrinchium striatum

S. grandiflorum see *Olsynium douglasii*.
S. idahoense, syn. *S. bellum* of gardens, *S. macounii*. Clump-forming, semi-evergreen perennial with narrowly linear leaves, 7–30cm (3–12in) long. Upright stems bear star-shaped, deep violet-blue flowers, 2.5cm (1in) across, with yellow throats, during summer. Self-seeds freely. ↕ 12cm (5in), ↔ 15cm (6in). USA (Washington and Idaho to California). ❄❄❄. **'Album'**, syn. *S.* 'May Snow', has white flowers with yellow throats.
S. macounii see *S. idahoense*.
***S.* 'May Snow'** see *S. idahoense* 'Album'.
***S.* 'North Star'** see *S.* 'Pole Star'.
S. odoratissimum see *Olsynium biflorum*.
***S.* 'Pole Star'**, syn. *S.* 'North Star'. Clump-forming, semi-evergreen perennial with linear leaves, to 40cm (16in) long. In summer, erect stems bear a succession of star-shaped white flowers, to 3cm (1¼in) across. ↕↔ to 15cm (6in). ❄❄❄
S. striatum ▣ syn. *Phaiophleps nigricans*. Clump-forming, evergreen perennial with linear to lance-shaped, iris-like but 2-ranked, stiff, greyish green leaves, to 40cm (16in) long. In early and midsummer, unbranched stems bear stalkless clusters of open cup-shaped, pale yellow flowers, 2.5cm (1in) across, with tepal backs striped purple-brown. ↕ to 90cm (36in), ↔ 25cm (10in). Chile, Argentina. ❄❄❄. **'Aunt May'** ▣ syn. 'Variegatum', is less vigorous, with leaves striped creamy yellow; ↕ to 50cm (20in). **'Variegatum'** see 'Aunt May'.

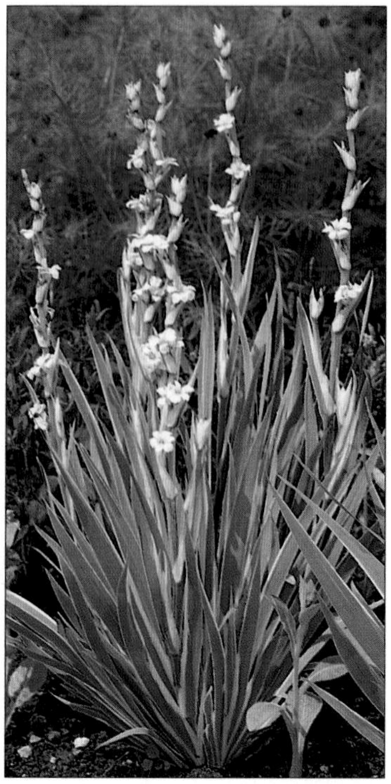

Sisyrinchium striatum 'Aunt May'

▷ **Sitka spruce** see *Picea sitchensis*

SKIMMIA

RUTACEAE

Genus of 4 species of monoecious or dioecious, occasionally hermaphrodite, evergreen shrubs and trees found in woodland from the Himalayas to S.E. Asia, China, and Japan. They are grown for their attractive leaves, flowers, and fruits. Leaves are alternate, simple, aromatic, obovate to inversely lance-shaped or elliptic, and mainly borne in terminal clusters. In spring, they bear terminal panicles of star-shaped flowers, strongly scented in some species, followed, on female and hermaphrodite plants, by fleshy, spherical, red or black fruits. Skimmias are suitable for a shrub border or woodland garden. With dioecious species, both male and female plants are needed to obtain fruit. Skimmias tolerate shade, atmospheric pollution, and neglect. The fruits may cause mild stomach upset if ingested.

- **HARDINESS** Fully hardy.
- **CULTIVATION** Grow in moderately fertile, humus-rich, moist but well-drained soil in light dappled shade to deep shade; *S.* x *confusa* 'Kew Green' tolerates full sun. May become chlorotic

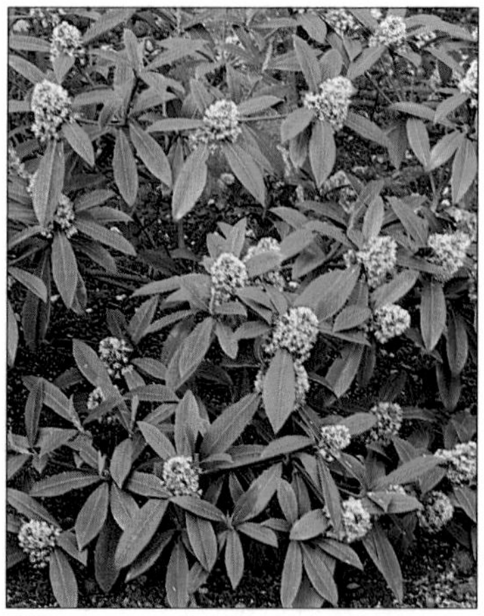

Skimmia x *confusa* 'Kew Green'

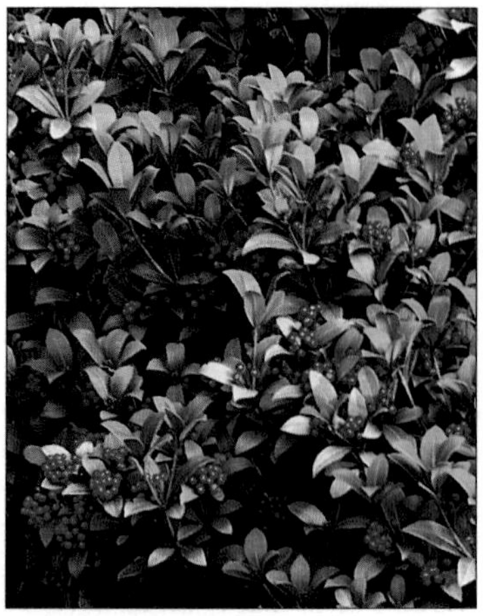

Skimmia japonica

S

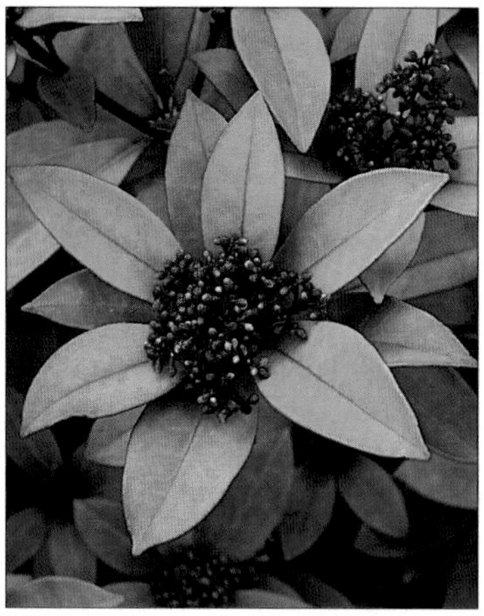

Skimmia japonica 'Bronze Knight'

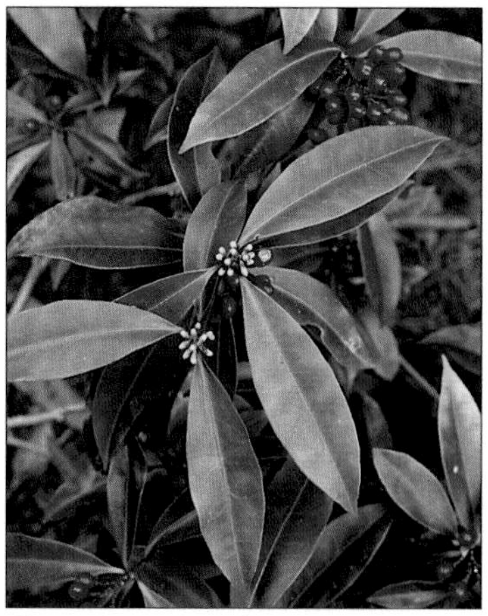

Skimmia japonica subsp. *reevesiana*

on poor, dry soil or if over-exposed to sun. Pruning group 8, if necessary.
• **PROPAGATION** Sow seed in containers in a cold frame in autumn. Root semi-ripe cuttings with bottom heat in late summer.
• **PESTS AND DISEASES** Prone to scale insects.

S. anquetilia. Creeping or erect, dome-shaped shrub producing inversely lance-shaped to oblong-elliptic, leathery, strongly aromatic, dark or yellowish green leaves, to 18cm (7in) long. In mid- and late spring, bears small, yellow-green flowers, 4mm (⅛in) across, in compact, nearly spherical panicles, 5cm (2in) across, followed on female plants by scarlet fruit, 1cm (½in) across. ↕↔ 2m (6ft). W. Himalayas. ❄❄❄
***S. x confusa* 'Kew Green'** ■ 🏆 Compact, dome-shaped shrub with inversely lance-shaped to elliptic, pointed, aromatic, mid-green leaves, to 11cm (4½in) long. Fragrant, creamy white male flowers, 3–5mm (⅛–¼in) across, open in dense, conical panicles, to 15cm (6in) long, in spring. ↕ 0.5–3m (1½–10ft), ↔ 1.5m (5ft). ❄❄❄
***S. x foremanii* of gardens** see *S. japonica* 'Veitchii'.
S. japonica ■ Dome-shaped to erect or creeping shrub with oval to obovate or inversely lance-shaped, slightly aromatic, dark green leaves, to 10cm (4in) long. Fragrant white flowers, 6mm (¼in) across, sometimes tinged pink or red, often opening from red buds, are borne in dense panicles, to 8cm (3in) long, in mid- and late spring; they are followed on female plants by red fruit, 8mm (⅜in) across. ↕↔ to 6m (20ft). China, Japan, S.E. Asia. ❄❄❄. **'Bowles' Dwarf'** is compact, with leaves to 4cm (1½in) long, and red winter flower buds; both male and female clones are available; ↕ 15cm (6in), ↔ 45cm (18in). **'Bronze Knight'** ■ is a male clone of open habit, with dark red winter buds. **'Cecilia Brown'** has large fruit clusters. **'Foremanii'** see 'Veitchii'. **'Fragrans'** 🏆 syn. *S. laureola* 'Fragrant Cloud', is an erect, compact, free-flowering male clone, with narrowly oval leaves; ↕↔ 1m (3ft). **'Fructu Albo'** ■ has green flower buds and white fruit; ↕ 60cm (24in), ↔ 1m (3ft). **'Nymans'** 🏆 is a spreading female clone, with inversely lance-shaped leaves; ↕ 1m (3ft), ↔ 2m (6ft). **subsp. *reevesiana*** ■ syn. *S. reevesiana*, is hermaphrodite, with narrowly elliptic, tapered leaves and ovoid fruit; ↕ to 7m (22ft), ↔ 90cm (36in); China, Taiwan. **subsp. *reevesiana* 'Robert Fortune'** 🏆 is hermaphrodite, with pale green leaves margined dark green. **'Rogersii'** is a dense female clone, with thick, twisted leaves and abundant fruit; ↕↔ 75cm (30in). **'Rubella'** ■ 🏆 is a compact male clone, with red-margined leaves, and dark red flower buds in autumn and winter. **'Veitchii'**, syn. *S.* x *foremanii* of gardens, 'Foremanii', is a vigorous, upright female clone. **'Wakehurst White'** has white fruit.
***S. laureola* 'Fragrant Cloud'** see *S. japonica* 'Fragrans'.
S. reevesiana see *S. japonica* subsp. *reevesiana.*

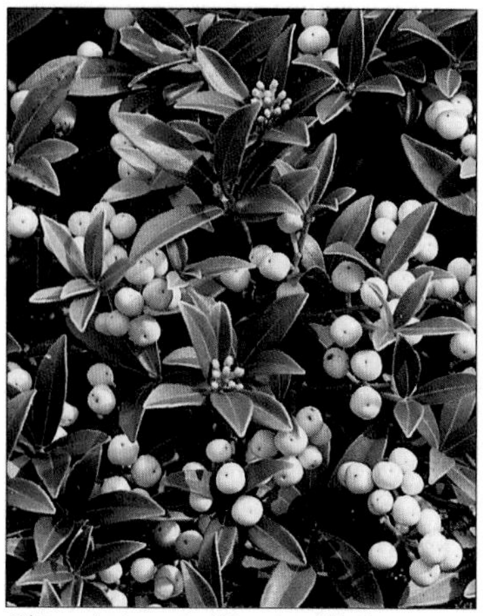

Skimmia japonica 'Fructu Albo'

▷**Skull cap** see *Scutellaria*
▷**Skunk cabbage** see *Lysichiton*
White see *L. camtschatcensis*
Yellow see *L. americanus*
▷**Sky flower** see *Duranta erecta*
▷**Slipper flower** see *Calceolaria*
▷**Slipperwort** see *Calceolaria*
▷**Sloe** see *Prunus spinosa*
▷**Smallweed** see *Calamagrostis*

SMILACINA

False Solomon's seal

CONVALLARIACEAE/LILIACEAE

Genus of 25 species of mainly rhizomatous perennials from woodland in Asia and North and Central America. Similar to Solomon's seal (*Polygonatum*), they have unbranched, often arching stems with alternate, ovate-lance-shaped, stalkless or short-stalked leaves, and bear terminal racemes or panicles of star-shaped, short-stalked, scented, creamy white flowers, followed by green berries, usually ripening to red. Excellent in a woodland garden or shaded border.
• **HARDINESS** Fully hardy.
• **CULTIVATION** Grow in moderately fertile, humus-rich, lime-free, moist but well-drained soil in light dappled shade or deep shade. Shelter from cold winds.
• **PROPAGATION** Sow seed in containers in a cold frame in autumn. Divide rhizomes in spring.
• **PESTS AND DISEASES** Trouble free.

S. racemosa ■ 🏆 syn. *Maianthemum racemosum* (False spikenard). Clump-forming, rhizomatous perennial with narrowly ovate or elliptic, pointed, prominently veined, mid-green leaves, to 15cm (6in) long, downy beneath and yellow in autumn. Terminal panicles of many white to creamy white, sometimes green-tinged flowers, 6mm (¼in) across, are produced in mid- and late spring, occasionally followed by green, later red berries. ↕ to 90cm (36in), ↔ 60cm (24in). North America, Mexico. ❄❄❄

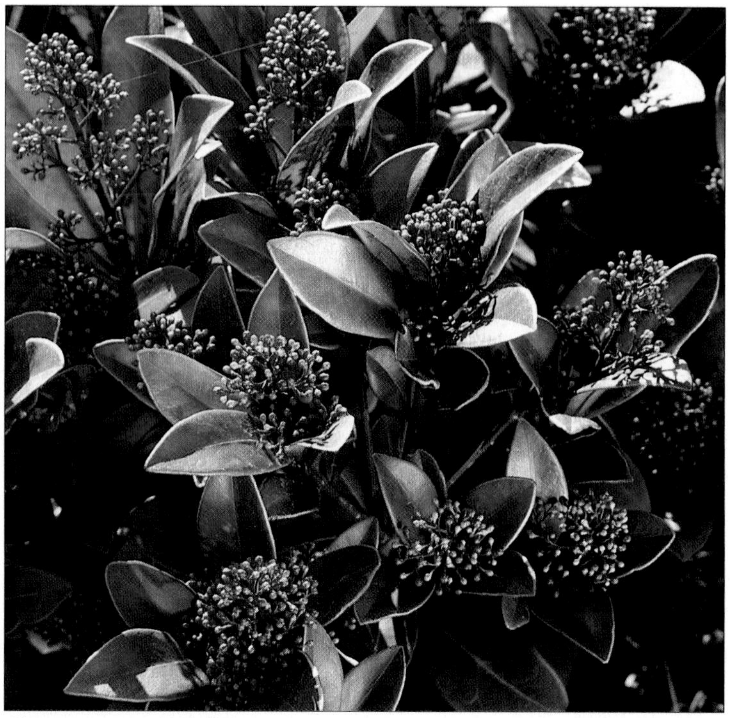

Skimmia japonica 'Rubella'

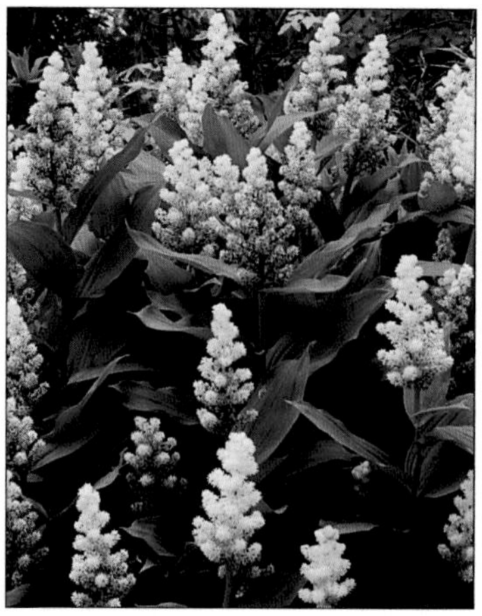

Smilacina racemosa

SMILAX

LILIACEAE/SMILACACEAE

Genus of about 200 species of usually dioecious, woody, deciduous or evergreen climbers, and herbaceous perennials, grown for their foliage and fruits. They are widespread in tropical and temperate regions, in woodland and thickets. The alternate, simple, sometimes shallowly lobed leaves are lance-shaped to elliptic, or broadly ovate to rounded, some truncate or heart-shaped at the bases; they have curled tendrils, and are often borne on prickly stems. The small, star-shaped flowers are green, greenish white, yellow, or brown, and are followed by spherical, black or red berries. Train into a tree, on to a pillar, or against a warm, sunny wall. In frost-prone areas, grow tender species in a temperate or warm greenhouse.
• **HARDINESS** Frost hardy to frost tender.
• **CULTIVATION** Grow against a support in moderately fertile, well-drained soil in full sun or partial shade. Pruning group 11, after flowering.
• **PROPAGATION** Sow seed in containers in a cold frame in autumn. Divide in autumn or spring.
• **PESTS AND DISEASES** Trouble free.

S. china. Scrambling, woody, deciduous climber with sparsely prickly shoots and broadly ovate to rounded, tapered, dark green leaves, to 8cm (3in) long. Small umbels of tiny, yellow-green flowers, 2–3mm (1/16–⅛in) across, are borne in spring, followed on female plants by spherical, bright red berries, 8mm (⅜in) across, in autumn. ↕ 5m (15ft). China, Korea, Japan. ❄❄

SMITHIANTHA

Temple bells

GESNERIACEAE

Genus of 4 species of rhizomatous perennials from moist, tropical woodland and rocks in Mexico, grown for their flowers and foliage. They have opposite, heart-shaped, fleshy leaves, with a velvet sheen of fine, red or purple hairs. Terminal racemes of nodding,

S

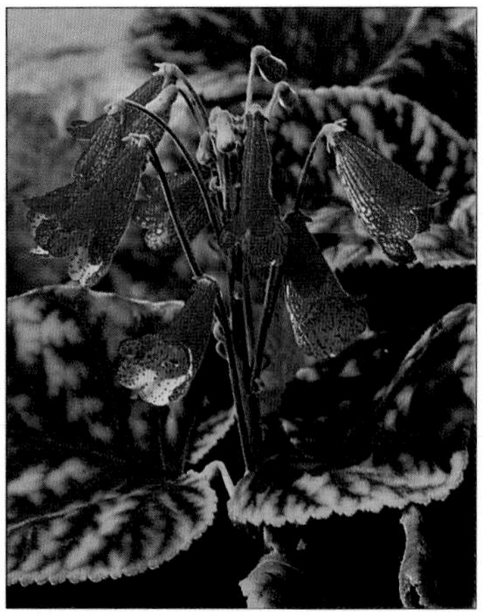

Smithiantha 'Orange King'

tubular to tubular-bell-shaped, red, orange, or yellow flowers are borne in summer and autumn. In frost-prone climates, grow in a temperate or warm greenhouse, in a conservatory, or as houseplants. In frost-free areas grow in a border or lightly shaded raised bed; they grow best in areas with dry winters.

• **HARDINESS** Frost tender.

• **CULTIVATION** Under glass, grow in half pots of well-drained, loamless potting compost. Provide high humidity and bright filtered to indirect light. In growth, water moderately and apply a quarter-strength high-potash liquid fertilizer at each watering; maintain at 19°C (66°F). Keep completely dry when dormant in winter. Pot on each spring, and water sparingly until in full growth. Do not overwater. Outdoors, grow in moderately fertile, humus-rich, moist but well-drained, neutral to slightly acid soil, in full sun with some midday shade, or in light dappled shade. Protect from winter wet.

• **PROPAGATION** Sow seed at 15–18°C (59–64°F), or divide rhizomes, in spring.

• **PESTS AND DISEASES** Prone to aphids.

S. cinnabarina, syn. *Naegelia cinnabarina.* Rhizomatous perennial with stem-sheathing, heart-shaped, densely red-hairy, deep green leaves, 15cm (6in) long, marked purple along the veins. From summer to autumn, bears brick-red flowers, 3.5cm (1½in) long, paler or white-spotted in the throats. ↕ to 45cm (18in), ↔ 30cm (12in). Mexico. ❄ (min. 10°C/50°F)

S

***S.* 'Orange King'** ▣ Rhizomatous perennial with heart-shaped, scalloped, densely red-purple-hairy, rich mid-green leaves, 15cm (6in) long, marked dark red along the veins. From summer to autumn, bears orange flowers, 3–4cm (1¼–1½in) long, with red-spotted throats and yellow lips. ↕↔ 60cm (24in). ❄ (min. 10°C/50°F)

S. zebrina, syn. *Gesneria zebrina, Naegelia zebrina.* Rhizomatous perennial producing heart-shaped, deep green leaves, 18cm (7in) long, marked darker green and purple-brown along the veins. Scarlet and yellow flowers, 3.5cm (1½in) long, with red-spotted yellow throats, are borne in summer. ↕ to 75cm (30in), ↔ 35cm (14in). Mexico. ❄ (min. 10°C/50°F)

▷**Smoke bush** see *Cotinus, C. coggygria*
▷**Smoke tree, American** see *Cotinus obovatus*

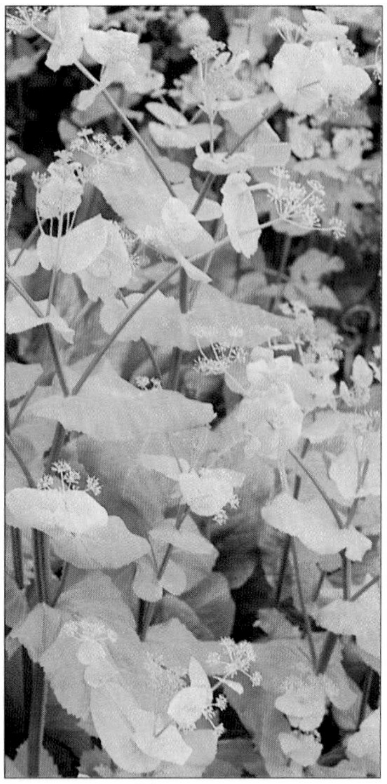

Smyrnium perfoliatum

SMYRNIUM

APIACEAE/UMBELLIFERAE

Genus of approximately 8 erect, branching biennials or short-lived, monocarpic perennials found in rocky places, scrub, fields, and at woodland margins in Europe, Africa, and W. Asia. They produce broadly oblong, divided basal leaves and rounded, usually entire upper leaves. In late spring and early summer, they bear branched, terminal umbels of numerous tiny, greenish yellow flowers. Ideal for naturalizing in a large border or in a wild or woodland garden. They also provide unusual cut flowers.

• **HARDINESS** Fully hardy.

• **CULTIVATION** Grow in moderately fertile, moist but well-drained soil in full sun to partial shade. Will also naturalize well in grass.

• **PROPAGATION** Sow seed *in situ* in autumn or late spring, or in containers in a cold frame in spring. Germination is often erratic.

• **PESTS AND DISEASES** Trouble free.

S. perfoliatum ▣ (Perfoliate Alexanders). Upright biennial with stout, ribbed stems, pinnate or 2-pinnate basal leaves, 5–20cm (2–8in) long, and perfoliate, simple, rounded, bract-like, bright yellow-green upper leaves, 3–10cm (1¼–4in) long, borne on the flowering stems. Many tiny flowers are produced in dome-shaped, 7- to 12-rayed umbels, to 10cm (4in) across, in spring of the second year after germination. ↕ 0.6–1.5m (2–5ft), ↔ 60cm (24in). N. Czech Republic, Slovakia, S. Europe, N. Africa, S.W. Asia. ❄❄❄

▷**Snail bean** see *Vigna caracalla*
▷**Snail flower** see *Vigna caracalla*
▷**Snakeroot** see *Polygala*
White see *Eupatorium rugosum*
▷**Snake root, Black** see *Cimicifuga racemosa*
▷**Snapdragon** see *Antirrhinum*
Dwarf see *Chaenorhinum*
Violet twining see *Maurandella antirrhiniflora*
▷**Sneezeweed** see *Helenium autumnale*
▷**Sneezewort** see *Achillea ptarmica*
▷**Snowball bush** see *Viburnum macrocephalum*
Japanese see *Viburnum plicatum*
▷**Snowball tree** see *Viburnum opulus* 'Roseum'
▷**Snowbell** see *Soldanella*
Alpine see *Soldanella alpina*
American see *Styrax americanus*
Fragrant see *Styrax obassia*
Japanese see *Styrax japonicus*
Least see *Soldanella minima*
▷**Snowberry** see *Symphoricarpos, S. albus* var. *laevigatus*
▷**Snow bush** see *Breynia disticha*
▷**Snowdrop** see *Galanthus*
Common see *G. nivalis*
▷**Snowdrop tree** see *Halesia*
▷**Snowflake** see *Leucojum*
Spring see *Leucojum vernum*
Summer see *Leucojum aestivum*
Water see *Nymphoides indica*
▷**Snow in summer** see *Cerastium tomentosum, Ozothamnus thyrsoideus*
▷**Snow in the jungle** see *Porana paniculata*
▷**Snow on the mountain** see *Euphorbia marginata*
▷**Soapberry, Western** see *Sapindus drummondii*
▷**Soapwort** see *Saponaria, S. officinalis*

SOBRALIA

ORCHIDACEAE

Genus of about 50 species of mostly large, evergreen, terrestrial, occasionally epiphytic orchids from Central America and tropical South America, occurring at altitudes of up to 3,400m (11,300ft), sometimes on rocks by streams. They have slender, cane-like stems, with foliage borne along almost all the stem length. The leathery, mid-green leaves are oblong to broadly oval or lance-shaped, and often folded. Short-lived, cattleya-like blooms, with a delicate, papery texture, are borne in succession every 3–4 days, at the stem tips.

• **HARDINESS** Frost tender.

• **CULTIVATION** Cool-growing orchids. Grow in containers of terrestrial orchid compost in bright filtered light, and maintain moderate to high humidity. When in active growth, water freely, mist the foliage daily, and apply a quarter-strength balanced liquid fertilizer monthly. Water sparingly in winter. Pot on when the plant fills the container and "flows" over the sides. See also p.46.

• **PROPAGATION** Divide after flowering. Offshoots may be rooted successfully in spring.

• **PESTS AND DISEASES** Red spider mites, aphids, whiteflies, and mealybugs may be troublesome.

S. macrantha. Terrestrial or epiphytic orchid producing lance-shaped leaves, 15–30cm (6–12in) long. Delicate, papery, white to pink-purple flowers, 15–18cm (6–7in) across, with yellow on the lips, are borne from spring to summer. ↕ 2m (6ft), ↔ 1.2m (4ft). Mexico to Costa Rica. ❄ (min. 11–13°C/52–55°F; max. 30°C/86°F)

SOLANDRA

Chalice vine

SOLANACEAE

Genus of 8 species of woody-stemmed, evergreen, scrambling climbers found in tropical forest in Mexico, the West Indies, and South America. They are grown for their large, solitary, funnel- or trumpet-shaped, night-scented flowers, each with 5 reflexed lobes. The lustrous, rich green leaves are alternate, simple, ovate to obovate, and usually leathery. Where temperatures fall below 7–10°C (45–50°F), grow chalice vines in a temperate greenhouse. In warmer climates, use to clothe a pergola, arch, or wall.

• **HARDINESS** Frost tender.

• **CULTIVATION** Under glass, grow in loam-based potting compost (JI No.2) in full light with shade from hot sun. During the growing season, water moderately and apply a balanced liquid fertilizer every 4 weeks. Water more sparingly in winter. Outdoors, grow in moderately fertile, humus-rich, moist but well-drained soil in full sun. Provide support for the climbing stems. Pruning group 11, in late winter or early spring, if necessary to restrict size.

• **PROPAGATION** Sow seed at 16–18°C (61–64°F) in spring. Root semi-ripe cuttings with bottom heat in summer. Air layer in spring.

• **PESTS AND DISEASES** Red spider mites and scale insects may be troublesome under glass.

S. grandiflora. Vigorous, semi-scandent climber with robust, sparsely branched stems clothed in elliptic to obovate leaves, to 13cm (5in) long. In spring, produces funnel-shaped, violet-tinged white flowers, 15–24cm (6–10in) long, which become tawny yellow with age. ↕ to 12m (40ft) or more. Jamaica. ❄ (min. 7–10°C/45–50°F)

S. hartwegii see *S. maxima.*

S. maxima ▣ syn. *S. hartwegii, S. nitida* (Cup of gold). Scandent, moderately dense climber producing branching stems clothed in elliptic leaves, to 15cm (6in) long. Trumpet-shaped yellow flowers, 15–20cm (6–8in) long, with purple veins, are produced in summer; the inside of each flower is marked with purple ridges. ↕ to 12m (40ft). Mexico to Colombia and Venezuela. ❄ (min. 7–10°C/45–50°F)

S. nitida see *S. maxima.*

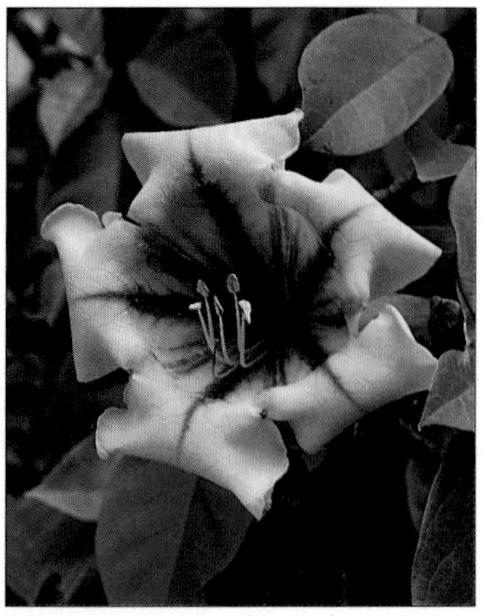

Solandra maxima

SOLANUM syn. LYCIANTHES

SOLANACEAE

Genus of about 1,400 species of annuals, biennials, herbaceous perennials, and evergreen, semi-evergreen, and deciduous shrubs, trees, and twining climbers from a range of habitats worldwide. The genus includes a number of vegetables, such as potato (*S. tuberosum*) and aubergine (*S. melongena*), and also ornamental plants, described below, which are cultivated for their flowers and decorative fruits. The leaves are alternate, and entire, lobed, or pinnately divided. The small, 5-petalled, bell- or shallowly trumpet-shaped, sometimes star-shaped, blue, purple, or white, yellow-anthered flowers are borne singly or in cymes, cyme-like umbels, corymbs, or panicles, from spring to autumn, later followed by fruits. Train climbers on a warm, sunny wall. Shrubs are suitable for a sheltered border. In frost-prone regions, grow tender species in a cool or temperate greenhouse. All parts of most species, especially the fruits of *S. capsicastrum* and *S. pseudocapsicum*, can cause severe discomfort if ingested.

• **HARDINESS** Frost hardy to frost tender.

• **CULTIVATION** Under glass, grow in loam-based potting compost (JI No.2) in full light with shade from hot sun, or in bright indirect light. In growth, water freely, apply a balanced liquid fertilizer monthly, mist daily, and maintain moderate humidity. Apply a high-potash liquid fertilizer every 2 or 3 weeks to *S. capsicastrum* and *S. pseudocapsicum* until fruit ripens. Water sparingly when dormant. Outdoors, grow in moderately fertile, moist but well-drained, neutral to slightly alkaline soil in full sun. Support plants and tie in young shoots regularly. Pruning group 9 for shrubs; group 12 for climbers, after flowering.

• **PROPAGATION** Sow seed at 18–20°C (64–68°F) in spring. Root semi-ripe cuttings of shrubs and climbers with gentle bottom heat from summer to early autumn.

• **PESTS AND DISEASES** Prone to aphids, red spider mites, tomato spotted wilt, and grey mould (*Botrytis*), under glass.

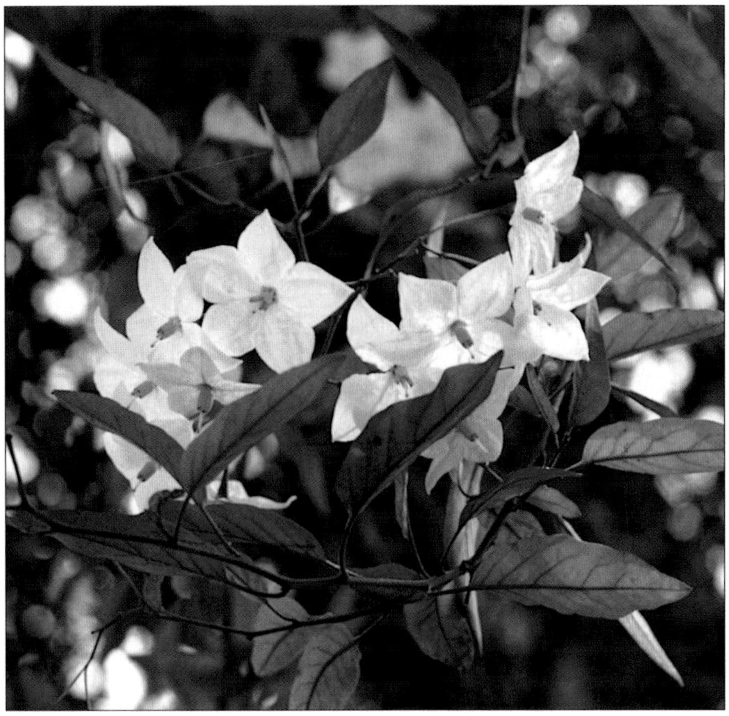

Solanum jasminoides 'Album'

S. aviculare (Kangaroo apple). Erect to spreading, open, evergreen, hairless shrub with narrowly lance-shaped, simple to irregularly pinnatifid, deep green leaves, 12–20cm (5–8in) long. In spring and summer, bears axillary cymes, 5–13cm (2–5in) across, of 3–8 shallowly lobed, blue-purple or white flowers, 3–4cm (1¼–1½in) across, followed by ovoid green fruit, 1.5cm (½in) long, ripening yellow. ↕ 1.8–3.5m (6–11ft), ↔ 1.5–2.5m (5–8ft). Australia (Queensland to Tasmania), New Zealand. ✲

S. capsicastrum (False Jerusalem cherry, Winter cherry). Erect, bushy, evergreen, downy-stemmed shrub, often grown as a winter-fruiting annual. Oblong to lance-shaped, wavy-margined leaves, 5–7cm (2–3in) long, are downy, dark green. In summer, bears axillary cymes, 5cm (2in) long, of star-shaped white flowers, to 1.5cm (½in) across, followed by oblong-ellipsoid to ovoid, pointed, red or orange-red fruit, 2cm (¾in) or more long. ↕↔ 30–60cm (12–24in), in containers. Brazil. ❄ (min. 5°C/41°F)

S. crispum (Chilean potato tree). Fast-growing, scrambling, evergreen or semi-evergreen climber with ovate, dark green leaves, to 12cm (5in) long. In summer, bears fragrant, lilac- to purple-blue flowers, 2.5cm (1in) across, in terminal corymbs, to 15cm (6in) across; they are followed by yellowish white fruit, 6–9mm (¼–⅜in) across. ↕ 6m (20ft). Peru, Chile. ✲✲. **'Glasnevin'** ■♀ syn. 'Autumnale', bears deep purple-blue flowers from summer to autumn.

S. jasminoides (Potato vine). Scrambling, evergreen or semi-evergreen climber with narrowly ovate to lance-shaped, glossy, dark green leaves, to 5cm (2in) long, sometimes 3- to 5-lobed or with separate ovate leaflets at the bases. In summer and autumn, bears fragrant, blue-white flowers, 2.5cm (1in) across, with yellow anthers, in terminal and axillary clusters, 5–7cm (2–3in) across, followed by ovoid black fruit, 9mm (⅜in) across. ↕ 6m (20ft). Brazil. ✲. **'Album'** ■♀ has white flowers.

S. laciniatum (Kangaroo apple). Vigorous, erect, evergreen shrub with purple-tinged shoots and lance-shaped to deeply pinnatisect, mid-green leaves, to 20cm (8in) long. In summer and autumn, bears dark blue flowers, 5cm (2in) across, in axillary cymes, to 15cm (6in) long, followed by ovoid, bright orange fruit, 2cm (¾in) long. ↕ 2m (6ft), ↔ 1.5m (5ft). Australia, New Zealand. ✲

S. pseudocapsicum (Christmas cherry, Jerusalem cherry, Winter cherry). Erect, bushy, evergreen shrub, often grown as a winter-fruiting annual. Wavy-margined, elliptic leaves, to 8cm (3in) long, are glossy, dark green. In summer, bears axillary cymes, 5cm (2in) across, of up to 3 star-shaped white flowers, to 1.5cm (½in) across, followed by long-lasting, spherical, red, yellow, or orange-red fruit, 1.5–2cm (½–¾in) across. ↕↔ 30–45cm (12–18in), in containers. E. South America. ❄ (min. 5°C/41°F). **'Cherry Jubilee'** has white, yellow, or orange fruit. **'Fancy'** is compact, with bright scarlet fruit; ↕ to 30cm (12in). **'Joker'** is dwarf, with yellow fruit turning orange and red; ↕↔ 20cm (8in). **'Jubilee'** is dwarf, with pale lime-green fruit, ripening deep orange; ↕↔ 15cm (6in). **'Red Giant'** ■ has large, orange-red fruit, to 2.5cm (1in) across.

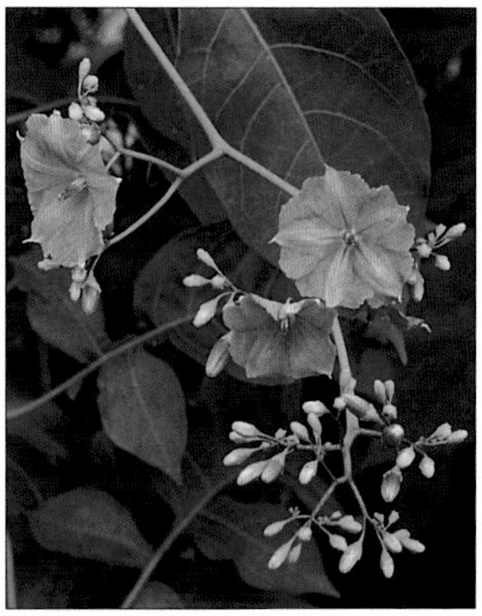

Solanum wendlandii

S. rantonnetii, syn. *Lycianthes rantonnetii* (Blue potato bush). Lax, evergreen shrub, usually many-branched when mature, producing ovate to lance-shaped, often wavy-margined, smooth, mid- to deep green leaves, 6–10cm (2½–4in) long. In summer and autumn, bears axillary clusters, to 6cm (2½in) across, of 2–5 shallowly trumpet-shaped, dark blue to violet-blue or pale blue flowers, 1–2.5cm (½–1in) across, with paler blue or yellow-tinged centres, followed by ovoid red fruit, 2.5cm (1in) long. ↕↔ 1–2m (3–6ft). Paraguay, Argentina. ❄ (min. 7°C/45°F). **'Royal Robe'** ■ has fragrant, deep violet-blue flowers with yellow centres.

S. seaforthianum (Italian jasmine, St. Vincent lilac). Spreading, evergreen, hairless, scandent climber with broadly elliptic, rich green leaves, 10–20cm (4–8in) long, either entire or pinnatifid with 3–9 lobes. In summer, bears blue, purple, pink, or white flowers, to 2cm (¾in) across, in pendent panicles, to 15cm (6in) across, followed by ovoid red fruit, 6–10mm (¼–½in) across. ↕ to 6m (20ft). Tropical South America. ❄ (min. 7–10°C/45–50°F)

S. wendlandii ■ (Paradise flower, Potato vine). Spreading, evergreen or semi-evergreen, scrambling climber with hooked barbs on the stems and foliage. Bright green leaves, 10–25cm (4–10in) long, are pinnate (with 8–13 leaflets), oblong with heart-shaped bases, or 3-palmate. In summer, bears shallowly trumpet-shaped, lilac-blue flowers, 4–6cm (1½–2½in) across, in terminal, pendent, cyme-like panicles, to 15cm (6in) long, followed by spherical to ovoid orange fruit, 8–10cm (3–4in) across. ↕ 5m (15ft) or more. Costa Rica. ❄ (min. 7–10°C/45–50°F). **'Albescens'** has off-white flowers.

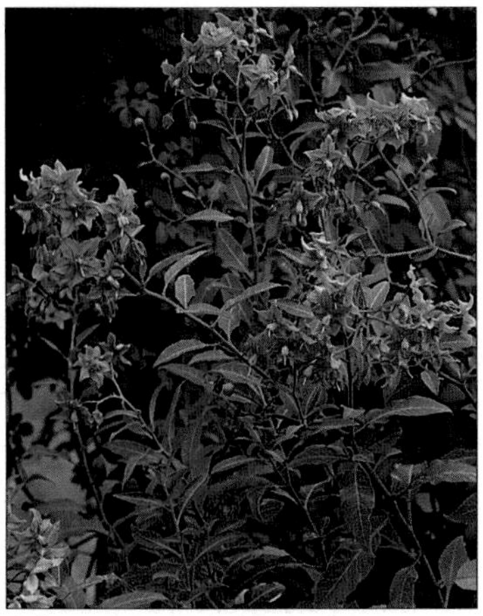

Solanum crispum 'Glasnevin'

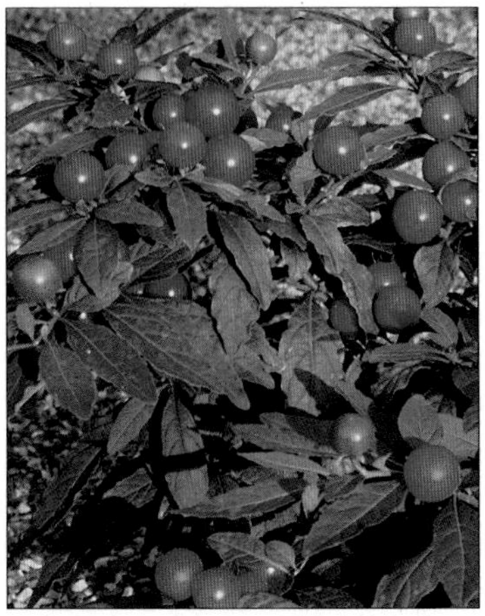

Solanum pseudocapsicum 'Red Giant'

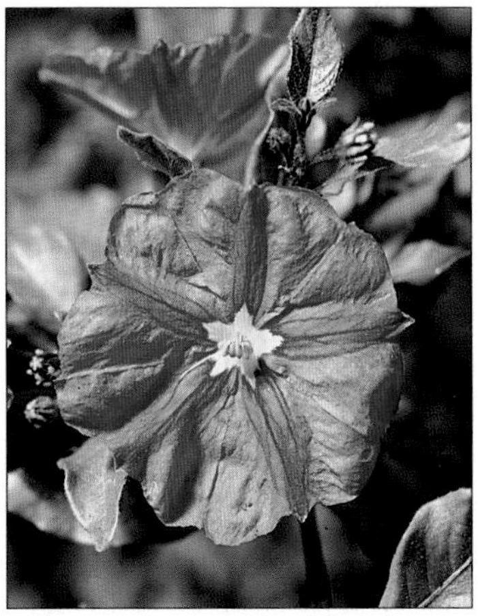

Solanum rantonnetii 'Royal Robe'

S

SOLDANELLA

Snowbell

PRIMULACEAE

Genus of about 10 species of small, spring-flowering, evergreen perennials from the mountains of Europe, usually found in alpine turf or among rocks, often flowering through the melting snow. They have basal rosettes of long-stalked, rounded or kidney-shaped, leathery leaves. The nodding to pendent, funnel- or bell-shaped, purple to white flowers have fringed petals and are borne in umbels, rarely singly. Grow in a rock garden, alpine house, or peat bed.

- **HARDINESS** Fully hardy.
- **CULTIVATION** Grow in humus-rich, moist, sharply drained soil in full sun with some midday shade, or in partial shade in warm areas. Top-dress with sharp grit, and protect from excessive winter wet. Under glass, grow in shallow pans of equal parts lime-free (ericaceous) potting compost, leaf mould, and grit.
- **PROPAGATION** Sow seed as soon as ripe in containers in a cold frame. Divide in early spring.
- **PESTS AND DISEASES** Young growth is prone to slug and snail damage.

S. alpina ■ (Alpine snowbell). Clump-forming perennial with thick, rounded to kidney-shaped, dark green leaves, 4cm (1½in) long. In early spring, each erect scape bears 2–5 nodding, funnel-shaped, bluish violet flowers, to 1.5cm (½in) long, with fringed petals cut to half their lengths and marked red inside. ↕↔ 12cm (5in). C. and S. Europe. ❄❄❄

S. carpatica ♀ Clump-forming perennial with rounded, dark green leaves, 5cm (2in) long, violet-purple beneath. In early spring, each scape bears 2–5 funnel-shaped, violet-blue flowers, to 1.5cm (½in) across, resembling those of *S. alpina*, but more freely borne, with fringed petals cut to two-thirds of their lengths. ↕↔ 15cm (6in). E. Europe (W. Carpathians). ❄❄❄

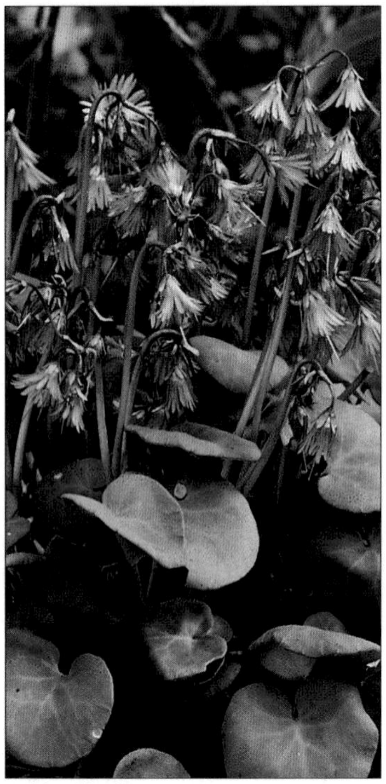

Soldanella alpina

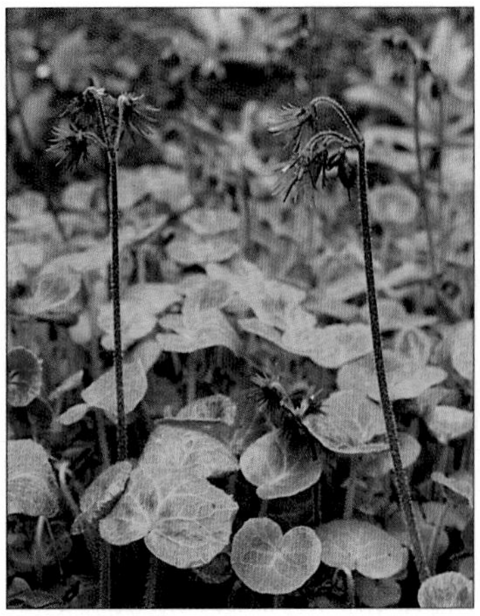

Soldanella villosa

S. minima (Least snowbell). Dwarf, clump-forming perennial with rounded, glossy, mid-green leaves, 1cm (½in) long. In early spring, scapes bear usually solitary, narrowly bell-shaped, white or pale blue flowers, to 1.5cm (½in) long, with darker streaks, the fringed petals cut to a quarter of their lengths. ↕ 10cm (4in), ↔ 20cm (8in). S. central Europe (E. Alps, C. Apennines). ❄❄❄

S. montana. Mound-forming perennial producing shallowly toothed, rounded or kidney-shaped, bright green leaves, 2–7cm (¾–3in) long, violet-tinted beneath. In early spring, each scape bears 3–10 pendent, bell-shaped, lavender-blue flowers, to 2cm (¾in) long, with fringed petals cut to three-quarters of their lengths. ↕ 30cm (12in), ↔ 20cm (8in). S. central Europe (N. Alps, Carpathians, Balkan peninsula). ❄❄❄

S. villosa ■ Vigorous, clump-forming perennial with rounded, hairy-stalked, mid-green leaves, 7cm (3in) long, paler green beneath. In early spring, each scape bears 3 or 4 nodding, bell-shaped violet flowers, 1.5cm (½in) long, with fringed petals cut to three-quarters of their lengths. Relatively easy to grow. ↕ 30cm (12in), ↔ 20cm (8in). S.W. Europe (W. Pyrenees). ❄❄❄

▷**Soldiers and sailors** see *Pulmonaria officinalis*

SOLEIROLIA syn. HELXINE

URTICACEAE

Genus of one species of vigorous, dwarf, monoecious, evergreen perennial from moist, shaded sites in W. Mediterranean islands. It is cultivated for its fresh green foliage, and tolerates a wide range of conditions. Where temperatures fall below -5°C (23°F), grow as a houseplant, in a terrarium, or in a cool to warm greenhouse or conservatory. In warmer areas, it provides ground cover in difficult sites outdoors, but is often invasive; it is difficult to eradicate.

- **HARDINESS** Fully hardy (borderline); becomes deciduous below 0°C (32°F).
- **CULTIVATION** Under glass, grow in loam-based potting compost (JI No.1) with added grit, in full light with shade from hot sun, or in partial shade. When in growth, water freely; water sparingly in winter. Outdoors, grow in any soil in sun or shade. May be damaged by frost, but quickly recovers in spring.
- **PROPAGATION** Divide in late spring.
- **PESTS AND DISEASES** Trouble free.

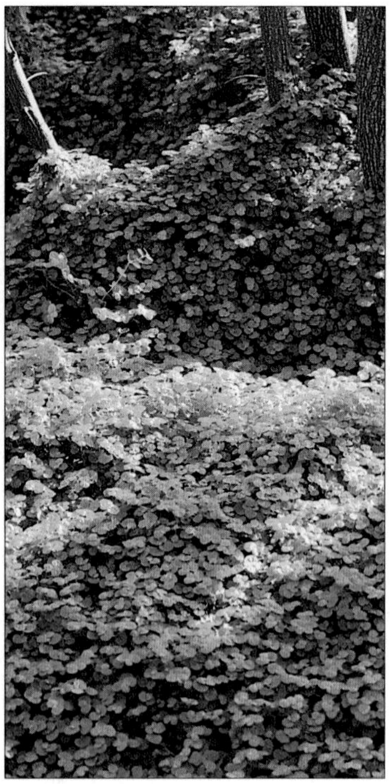

Soleirolia soleirolii

S. soleirolii ■ syn. *Helxine soleirolii* (Baby's tears, Mind your own business, Mother of thousands). Slender, mat-forming perennial with branched, translucent, pale green, sometimes pink-tinted stems and alternate, rounded, minutely hairy, short-stalked leaves, 2–6mm (1/16–¼in) long. Produces tiny, solitary, tubular, 4-lobed, pink-tinged white flowers from the leaf axils in summer. ↕ 5cm (2in), ↔ indefinite. W. Mediterranean islands. ❄❄❄ (borderline). **'Aurea'**, syn. 'Golden Queen', has gold-green leaves. **'Golden Queen'** see 'Aurea'. **'Silver Queen'** see 'Variegata'. **'Variegata'**, syn. 'Silver Queen', has variegated silver leaves.

SOLENOPSIS syn. ISOTOMA

CAMPANULACEAE

Genus of about 25 species of annuals and perennials from dry, exposed sites in Australia as well as Central and South America. They have alternate, lobed to pinnatisect, linear to ovate or oblong leaves, and bear solitary, terminal or axillary, long-tubed, salverform flowers, each with 5 usually narrow, star-like petal lobes. In frost-prone areas, grow in a temperate or warm greenhouse, in containers, or use for summer bedding. In warmer climates, grow as accent plants in a border or for bedding. Contact with the sap may irritate skin.

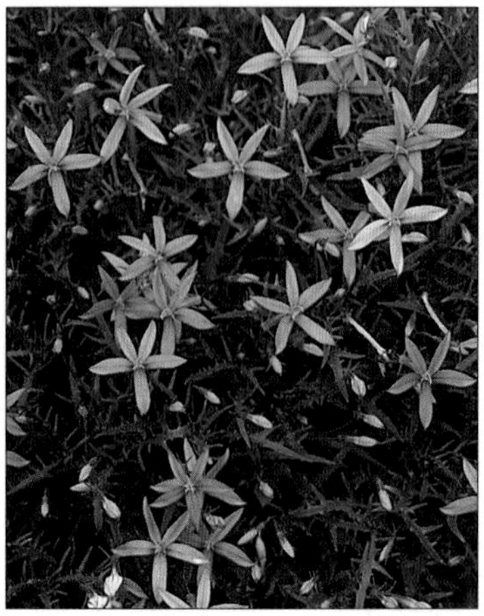

Solenopsis axillaris

- **HARDINESS** Frost tender.
- **CULTIVATION** Under glass, grow in loam-based potting compost (JI No.2) in full light. When in growth, water moderately and apply a balanced liquid fertilizer every 4 weeks; maintain low humidity. Water sparingly in winter. Outdoors, grow in moderately fertile, well-drained soil in full sun. In frost-prone areas, plant out after last frosts. Dead-head regularly.
- **PROPAGATION** Sow seed at 16–18°C (61–64°F) in spring. Root softwood cuttings in summer.
- **PESTS AND DISEASES** Aphids may be a problem in hot, dry conditions.

S. axillaris ■ syn. *Isotoma axillaris, Laurentia axillaris.* Woody-based perennial with erect, branched stems bearing ovate, pinnatisect leaves, 3–12cm (1¼–5in) long, with very narrow lobes. Star-shaped, pale to deep blue flowers, to 4cm (1½in) across, are borne in great abundance from spring to late autumn. ↕↔ 30cm (12in). Australia. ❀ (min. 7°C/45°F)

SOLENOSTEMON

Coleus, Flame nettle, Painted nettle

LABIATAE/LAMIACEAE

Genus of about 60 species of evergreen, bushy, erect to spreading, subshrubby perennials from forest in tropical Africa and Asia. They are mainly cultivated for their opposite, coarsely toothed, often hairy, mostly ovate, colourful leaves. Throughout the year, they bear raceme-like whorls of tiny, tubular, 2-lipped, blue, white, or purple flowers. In frost-prone climates, grow in a temperate greenhouse or as houseplants, or use outdoors as summer bedding. In warmer areas, coleus are good bedding plants for shady positions.

- **HARDINESS** Frost tender.
- **CULTIVATION** Under glass, grow in loam-based potting compost (JI No.3) in bright filtered to moderate light. In growth, water freely and apply a high-nitrogen fertilizer every 2 weeks. Keep just moist in winter. Pot on annually in spring. Outdoors, grow in humus-rich, moist but well-drained soil, enriched with well-rotted organic matter. Provide a sheltered position in full sun or partial shade. Water freely in dry weather. Pinch out young shoots to promote bushiness.
- **PROPAGATION** Surface-sow seed at 22–24°C (72–75°F) in early spring. Root softwood cuttings with bottom heat in spring or summer.
- **PESTS AND DISEASES** Mealybugs, scale insects, and whiteflies may be a problem under glass.

S. scutellarioides, syn. *Coleus blumei* var. *verschaffeltii* (Flame nettle, Painted nettle). Finely hairy, evergreen perennial, usually grown as an annual or short-lived perennial for its foliage. Semi-succulent, 4-angled stems bear broadly to narrowly ovate, toothed, sometimes frilly-margined, multi-coloured leaves, to 15cm (6in) long, often heart-shaped at the bases and hairy beneath.

S

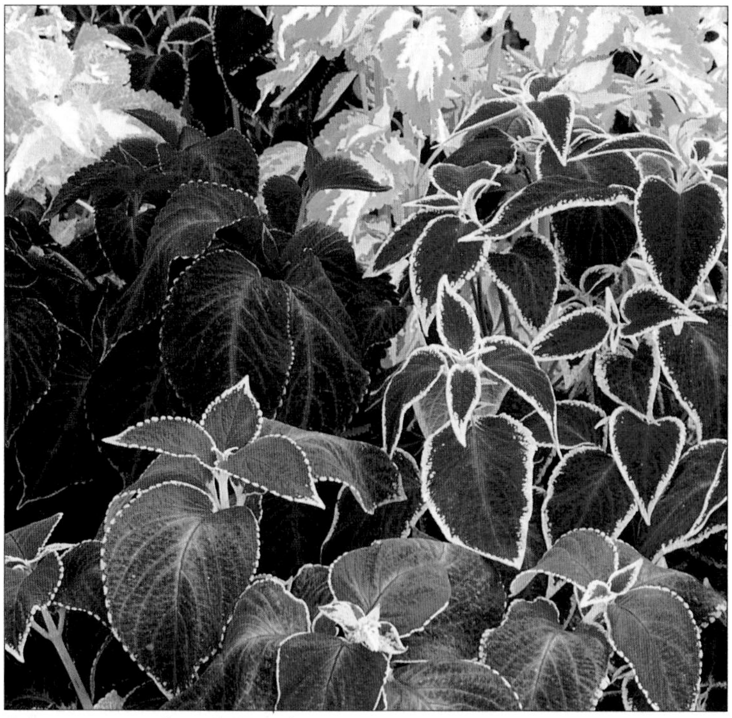

Solenostemon scutellarioides Wizard Series

Terminal, whorled racemes, to 15cm (6in) long, of tiny, blue or white flowers, 1.5cm (½in) long, are borne at any time of year. Dead-head to maintain foliage colour. ↕↔ to 60cm (24in), in containers. S.E. Asia (including Malaysia). ❀ (min. 4°C/39°F). Seed selections and named cultivars are usually highly patterned, the light to dark green leaves veined and freckled pink, red, yellow, purple, brown, or creamy white. **'Pineapple Beauty'** is vigorous, with yellow-green leaves that turn gold, and with brown-purple markings at the bases and on the stems; excellent for training into pyramids or standards; ↕↔ 50–100cm (20–39in). **Rainbow Series** cultivars are vigorous and good for summer bedding; ↕ to 40cm (16in). **'Royal Scot'** is bushy, with long-pointed, triangular leaves, bright red with green-brown centres and deeply lobed yellow margins. Cultivars of **Wizard Series** ▣ are compact, and branched from the base; ↕ to 20cm (8in).

SOLIDAGO

Aaron's rod, Golden rod

ASTERACEAE/COMPOSITAE

Genus of about 100 species of woody-based perennials occurring on roadsides, prairies, and riverbanks; most are found in North America, a few in South America and Eurasia. They are valued for their small, elongated flowerheads, borne in one-sided, upward-facing racemes or spike-like panicles. Stiff, branched stems bear alternate, narrowly elliptic to lance-shaped, entire or toothed, prominently veined, usually mid-green leaves, 10–30cm (4–12in) or more long. Most species are coarse and invasive, and are best grown in a wild garden, although *S. virgaurea* subsp. *minuta* is suitable for a rock garden. Named hybrids are robust, less invasive, and more colourful, with slightly larger flowerheads. They are ideal for a late-summer border or wild garden, and provide good cut flowers.

• **HARDINESS** Fully hardy.
• **CULTIVATION** Grow in poor to moderately fertile, preferably sandy, well-drained soil in full sun. Remove flowered stems to prevent seeding.
• **PROPAGATION** Divide in autumn or spring.
• **PESTS AND DISEASES** Powdery mildew may be a problem.

***S.* 'Crown of Rays'**, syn. *S.* 'Strahlenkrone'. Erect, clump-forming perennial with mid-green leaves. Bears golden yellow flowerheads in flattened, radiating, corymb-like panicles, to 25cm (10in) long, in mid- and late summer. ↕ 60cm (24in), ↔ 45cm (18in). ❄❄❄
***S.* 'Goldenmosa'** ▣♀ Compact, bushy perennial with wrinkled, mid-green

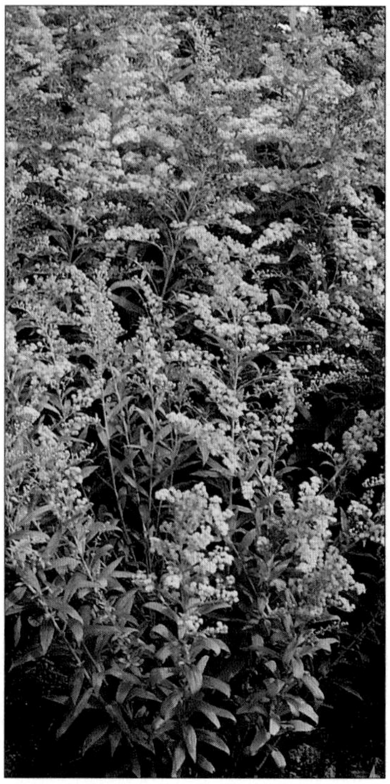

Solidago 'Goldenmosa'

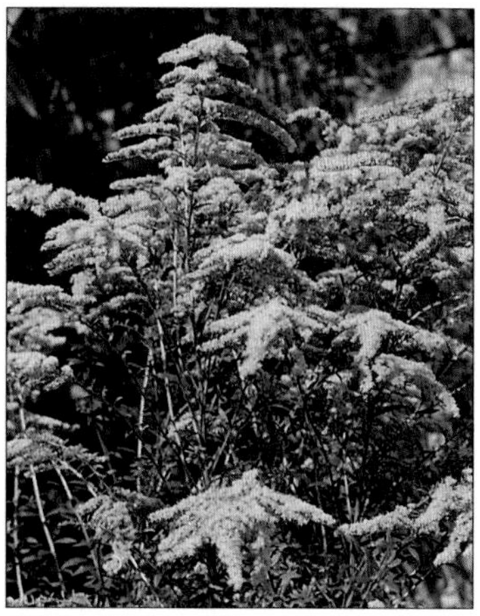

Solidago 'Golden Wings'

leaves. In late summer and early autumn, bears yellow-stalked, bright yellow flowerheads in conical panicles, to 30cm (12in) long. ↕ to 75cm (30in), ↔ 45cm (18in). ❄❄❄
***S.* 'Golden Wings'** ▣ Erect perennial with mid-green leaves, and spreading, corymb-like panicles, to 25cm (10in) long, of golden yellow flowerheads borne in late summer and early autumn. Thrives in poor soil. ↕ to 1.8m (6ft), ↔ 90cm (36in). ❄❄❄
***S.* 'Lemore'** see x *Solidaster luteus* 'Lemore'.
***S.* 'Loddon Gold'.** Erect perennial with mid-green leaves. In late summer and early autumn, bears deep yellow flowerheads in conical panicles, to 20cm (8in) long. ↕ to 90cm (36in), ↔ 45cm (18in). ❄❄❄
***S.* 'Strahlenkrone'** see *S.* 'Crown of Rays'.
S. virgaurea* subsp. *alpestris see *S. virgaurea* subsp. *minuta*.
S. virgaurea* subsp. *minuta, syn. *S. virgaurea* subsp. *alpestris*. Mound-forming perennial with leathery, lance-shaped, toothed, mid-green leaves, 2–10cm (¾–4in) long. From late summer to autumn, bears compact, erect, spike-like racemes, 3cm (1¼in) long, of deep yellow flowerheads, 6–8mm (¼–⅜in) across. Good for a rock garden, in moist soil. ↕ 5–20cm (2–8in), ↔ 20cm (8in). N., C., and E. Europe. ❄❄❄

x SOLIDASTER

ASTERACEAE/COMPOSITAE

Hybrid genus of one clump-forming perennial, possibly the result of a cross between *Solidago canadensis* and *Aster ptarmicoides*. It is valued for its daisy-like yellow flowerheads, profusely borne from midsummer to early autumn. The leaves are alternate, and lance-shaped to linear-elliptic or narrowly inversely lance-shaped. Suitable for a mixed or herbaceous border; the flowers are good for cutting.

• **HARDINESS** Fully hardy.
• **CULTIVATION** Grow in moderately fertile, well-drained soil in full sun.
• **PROPAGATION** Divide, or take basal cuttings, in spring.
• **PESTS AND DISEASES** Prone to powdery mildew in dry summers.

x *S. hybridus* see x *S. luteus*.
x *S. luteus* ▣ syn. x *S. hybridus*. Clump-forming perennial with erect, branched

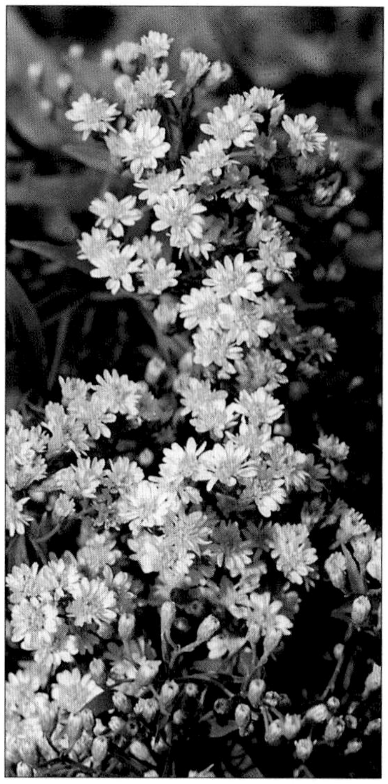

x *Solidaster luteus*

stems bearing leaves to 15cm (6in) long, toothed at the tips. From midsummer to early autumn, bears branched, corymb-like panicles of daisy-like flowerheads, to 1cm (½in) across, with pale yellow ray-florets and golden yellow disc-florets. ↕ to 90cm (36in), ↔ 30cm (12in). Garden origin. ❄❄❄. **'Lemore'** ♀ syn. *Solidago* 'Lemore', has pale lemon ray-florets; ↕↔ to 80cm (32in).

SOLLYA

PITTOSPORACEAE

Genus, related to *Billardiera*, of 3 species of evergreen, twining climbers or scandent shrubs or subshrubs found in light woodland in Australia. They are cultivated for their 5-petalled, bell-shaped, usually blue flowers, which are terminally borne, either singly or in pendent cymes, from summer to autumn. Stalkless, narrow, entire or slightly wavy-margined, oblong to ovate or obovate leaves are arranged alternately or in spirals. Where temperatures fall below 5°C (41°F), grow in a cool or temperate greenhouse. In warmer areas, train over an arch, pergola, or shrub.

• **HARDINESS** Frost tender, but may survive temperatures near to 0°C (32°F).
• **CULTIVATION** Under glass, grow in loam-based potting compost (JI No.2) in full light with shade from hot sun, or in bright filtered light. During the growing season, water moderately and apply a balanced liquid fertilizer monthly; maintain low to moderate humidity. Water sparingly in winter. Outdoors, grow in moderately fertile, humus-rich, moist but well-drained soil in full sun with some midday shade, or in light dappled shade. Apply a dry winter mulch. Support the climbing stems. Pruning group 12, in late winter or early spring.
• **PROPAGATION** Sow seed at 10–16°C (50–61°F) in spring. Root softwood cuttings in late spring or early summer.
• **PESTS AND DISEASES** Red spider mites may be troublesome under glass.

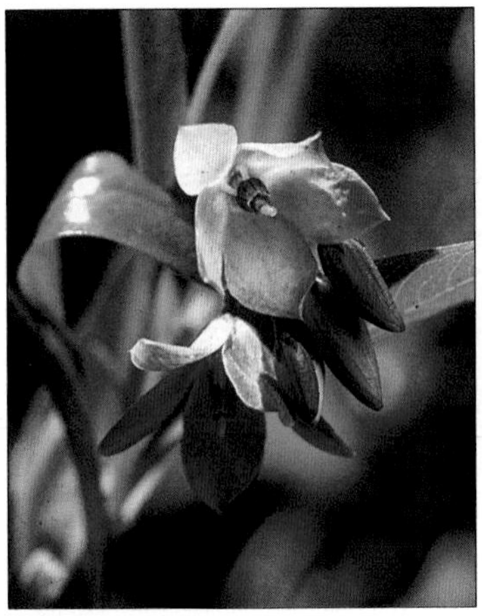

Sollya heterophylla

S. fusiformis see *S. heterophylla.*
S. heterophylla ▣ ♀ syn. *S. fusiformis* (Bluebell creeper). Weak-stemmed, eventually bushy, twining climber with ovate to narrowly oblong or obovate, mid- to deep green leaves, 2.5–5cm (1–2in) long, paler beneath. Bell-shaped blue flowers, 1.5cm (½in) across, are borne singly or in cymes of 4–8 or more, from early summer to autumn; they are followed by edible, cylindrical blue berries, to 2.5cm (1in) long. ↕1.5–2m (5–6ft). Australia (Western Australia). ✻ (borderline)

▷**Solomon's seal** see *Polygonatum*
Common see *Polygonatum* x *hybridum*
False see *Smilacina*
Whorled see *Polygonatum verticillatum*

SONERILA

MELASTOMATACEAE

Genus of about 175 species of evergreen perennials and small shrubs from tropical woodland in Asia, cultivated for their foliage and flowers. The leaves are opposite, whorled, or in basal rosettes, and mainly oval to elliptic, with bold veins. Flowers are star-, saucer-, or cup-shaped, and are borne in curved, spike-like racemes or corymbs. In frost-prone regions, grow in a warm greenhouse or conservatory, as houseplants, or in a terrarium. In warmer climates, use as ground cover among shrubs.
• **HARDINESS** Frost tender.
• **CULTIVATION** Under glass, grow in half pots or shallow pans of loamless potting compost with added fine-grade, granulated bark, in bright filtered light. Maintain steady temperatures and high humidity to prevent leaf drop. When in growth, water moderately and apply a half-strength balanced liquid fertilizer monthly. Keep just moist in winter. Pot on in spring; trim regularly to maintain dense growth. Outdoors, grow in humus-rich, moist but well-drained, acid to neutral soil with added leaf mould and grit, in light dappled to partial shade. Shelter from cold, drying winds.
• **PROPAGATION** Root softwood cuttings with bottom heat in spring or summer.
• **PEST AND DISEASES** Trouble free.

S. margaritacea ♀ Evergreen perennial with weak, 4-angled red stems bearing opposite, ovate to lance-shaped, glossy, dark green leaves, 10cm (4in) long, with numerous oval, pearl-white spots above, purple veins beneath, and purple-red leaf-stalks. Racemes of 8–10 star-shaped, 3-petalled, reddish pink flowers, 1cm (½in) long, are borne from summer to autumn. ↕↔ 25cm (10in). Burma to Indonesia (Java). ❀ (min. 19°C/66°F). **'Argentea'** (Pearly sonerila) has claret-red leaves, densely spotted silver. **'Hendersonii'** ▣ has dark olive-green leaves, covered with white spots above, and purple-red beneath.

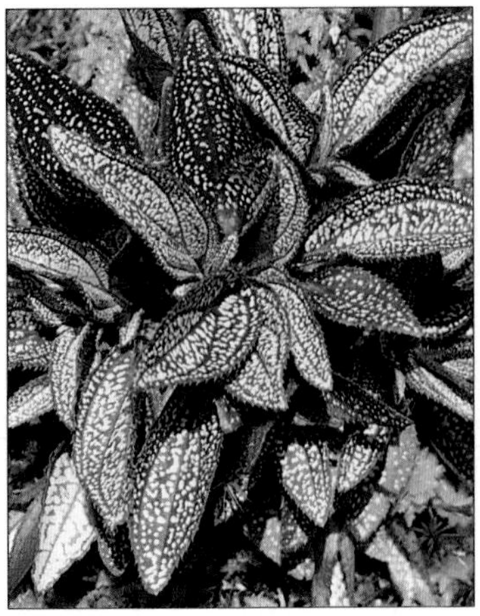

Sonerila margaritacea 'Hendersonii'

▷**Sonerila, Pearly** see *Sonerila margaritacea* 'Argentea'

SOPHORA

LEGUMINOSAE/PAPILIONACEAE

Genus of about 50 species of herbaceous perennials and deciduous and evergreen trees and shrubs, widely distributed in tropical and temperate regions, found mostly in dry valleys and woodland, and on rocky slopes of hills and mountains. They are cultivated for their elegant, alternate, pinnate leaves and racemes or panicles of pea-like flowers, with upright standards or with all petals forward-pointing. Grow in a shrub border, or as specimen plants. In frost-prone areas, grow tender sophoras at the base of a warm, sunny wall, or in a temperate or warm greenhouse. They need long, hot summers to flower well.
• **HARDINESS** Fully hardy to frost tender.
• **CULTIVATION** Grow in moderately fertile, well-drained soil in full sun. Pruning group 1.
• **PROPAGATION** Sow seed in containers in a cold frame as soon as ripe. Root semi-ripe cuttings of evergreen species with bottom heat in summer or autumn. Graft *S. japonica* cultivars in late winter.
• **PESTS AND DISEASES** Trouble free.

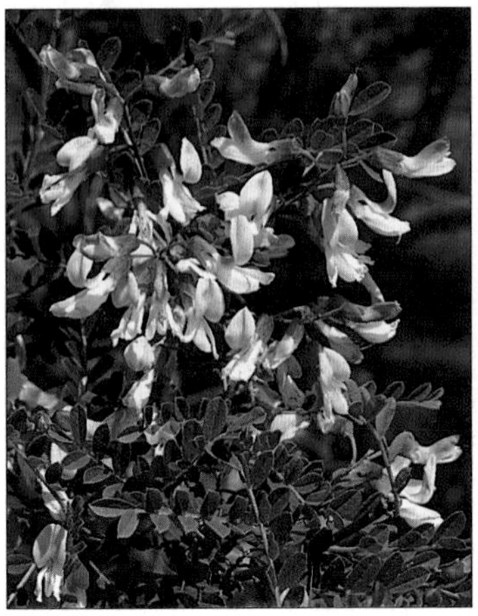

Sophora davidii

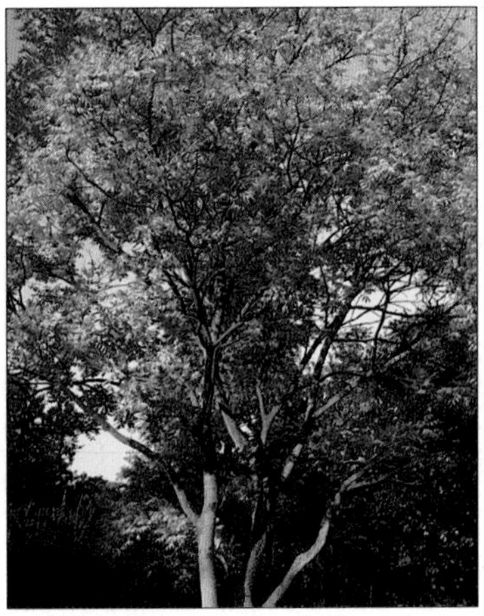

Sophora japonica 'Violacea'

S. davidii ▣ syn. *S. viciifolia.* Bushy or spreading, deciduous shrub with pinnate leaves, to 9cm (3½in) long, each composed of up to 17 oval or obovate, grey-green leaflets. In late spring and early summer, produces terminal racemes, to 15cm (6in) long, of small, pea-like, purple-blue and white flowers, to 2cm (¾in) long. ↕2.5m (8ft), ↔ 3m (10ft). China. ✻✻✻
S. japonica ♀ Q (Japanese pagoda tree). Spreading, deciduous tree with pinnate leaves, to 25cm (10in) long, composed of up to 17 ovate to lance-shaped, glossy, dark green leaflets that turn yellow in autumn. In late summer and early autumn, mature trees bear small, fragrant, pea-like white flowers, 1.5cm (½in) long, in terminal panicles to 30cm (12in) long. ↕ to 30m (100ft), ↔ 20m (70ft). China, Korea. ✻✻✻. **'Pendula'** Q has long, pendent branches, and rarely flowers; ↕↔ 3m (10ft). **'Violacea'** ▣ has white flowers tinged lilac-pink.
S. microphylla Q syn. *Edwardsia microphylla.* Spreading, evergreen, small tree or shrub producing pinnate leaves, to 15cm (6in) long, each with up to 40 pairs of ovate or elliptic-oblong, dark green leaflets, borne on silky shoots. In spring, bears small, axillary, pendent racemes, to 5cm (2in) long, of pea-like, dark yellow flowers, 5cm (2in) long, with all petals pointing forwards. ↕↔ 8m (25ft). New Zealand, Chile. ✻✻. **'Sun King'** ▣ is bushy, and bears long-lasting flowers in late winter and early spring; ↕↔ 3m (10ft); ✻✻✻
S. tetraptera ♀ Q (Kowhai). Spreading, evergreen tree or shrub with pinnate leaves, to 17cm (7in) long, each composed of up to 20 pairs of ovate or elliptic-oblong, dark green leaflets. In late spring, produces racemes, to 6cm (2½in) long, of 4–10 golden yellow flowers, to 5cm (2in) long, with all the petals pointing forwards. ↕10m (30ft), ↔ 5m (15ft). New Zealand. ✻✻
S. viciifolia see *S. davidii.*

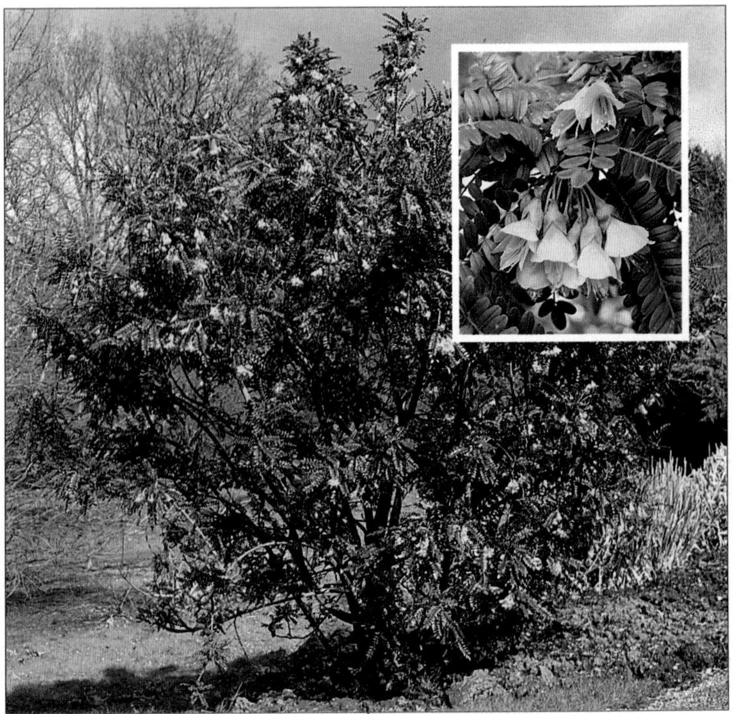

Sophora microphylla 'Sun King' (inset: flower detail)

x SOPHROLAELIO-CATTLEYA

ORCHIDACEAE

Trigeneric hybrid genus of evergreen orchids derived from crosses between *Sophronitis, Laelia,* and *Cattleya.* They are vegetatively similar to laeliocattleyas and brassolaeliocattleyas, and all are loosely referred to as cattleyas. The spindle-shaped or elongated pseudobulbs support 1 or 2 semi-rigid, elliptic leaves, to 15cm (6in) long. Flowers 10cm (4in) across, in a range of rich colours from vibrant reds to fiery oranges and yellows, are borne singly or in racemes of up to 6 blooms; they are produced from the bases of the pseudobulbs at any time of year.
• **HARDINESS** Frost tender.
• **CULTIVATION** Intermediate-growing orchids. Grow in containers of terrestrial orchid compost. During the growing season, provide bright indirect light, and water freely; apply a half-strength

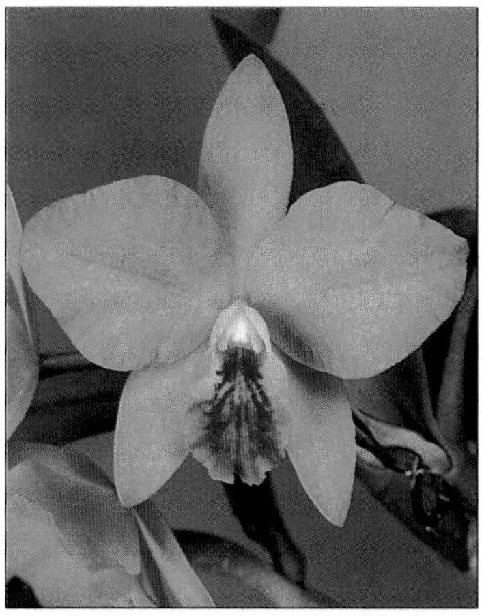

x *Sophrolaeliocattleya* Hazel Boyd 'Apricot Glow'

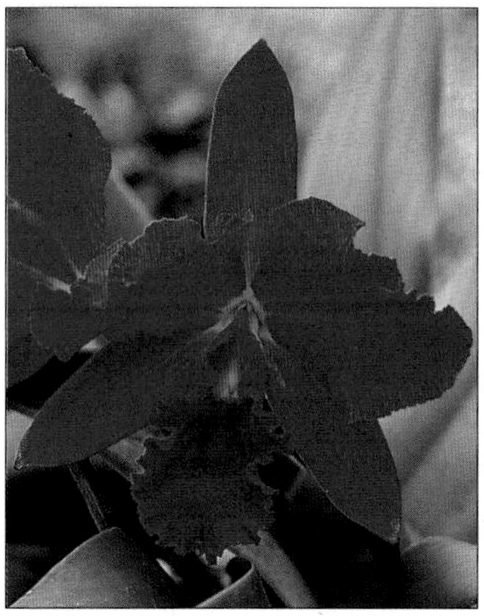

x *Sophrolaeliocattleya* Trizac 'Purple Emperor'

balanced liquid fertilizer monthly; mist daily and maintain high humidity. In winter, provide full light and water sparingly. See also p.46.
• **Propagation** Divide when the plant "overflows" the container. Remove backbulbs and pot them up separately.
• **Pests and diseases** Scale insects, red spider mites, aphids, and mealybugs may be troublesome.

x *S.* Hazel Boyd 'Apricot Glow' ▣ Evergreen orchid with spindle-shaped pseudobulbs and elliptic leaves, 10cm (4in) long. Bears racemes of rich orange-red flowers, marked red on the lips, at any time of year. ↕ 20cm (8in), ↔ 30cm (12in). ❁ (min. 13°C/55°F; max. 30°C/86°F)
x *S.* Jewel Box 'Dark Waters'. Evergreen orchid with spindle-shaped pseudobulbs and elliptic-ovate leaves, 10cm (4in) long. Produces racemes of deep vibrant red flowers at any time of year. ↕↔ 30cm (12in). ❁ (min. 13°C/55°F; max. 30°C/86°F)
x *S.* Tangerine Jewel. Evergreen orchid with elongated pseudobulbs and elliptic leaves, 10cm (4in) long. Orange-yellow flowers, 10cm (4in) across, are borne in racemes at any time of year. ↕↔ 30cm (12in). ❁ (min. 13°C/55°F; max. 30°C/86°F)
x *S.* Trizac 'Purple Emperor' ▣ Evergreen orchid with spindle-shaped pseudobulbs and elliptic leaves, 10cm (4in) long. Bears racemes of deep purple flowers at any time of year. ↕↔ 30cm (12in). ❁ (min. 13°C/55°F; max. 30°C/86°F)

Sophronitis

ORCHIDACEAE

Genus of about 8 species of small, evergreen, epiphytic or lithophytic orchids from E. Brazil and Paraguay, found at medium altitudes in humid, shady cloud forest. They have small, elongated to oval, often clustered pseudobulbs, each with a single leathery, ovate to elliptic or oblong, purple-tinted, dark green leaf. Richly coloured flowers are borne singly, or in short-stemmed racemes of up to 5 flowers, at any time of year. The plants resemble miniature cattleyas, and will interbreed with them and other related genera to produce brilliantly coloured hybrids, such as the sophrolaeliocattleyas.
• **Hardiness** Frost tender.
• **Cultivation** Cool-growing orchids. Grow in epiphytic orchid compost in small containers or wooden slatted baskets, or epiphytically on bark. In growth, provide bright indirect light, water moderately, and maintain high humidity; apply a half-strength balanced liquid fertilizer monthly. In winter, admit full light and water more sparingly. See also p.46.
• **Propagation** Divide when the plant "overflows" the sides of the container.
• **Pests and diseases** Prone to red spider mites, aphids, and mealybugs.

S. coccinea ♡ syn. *S. grandiflora.* Epiphytic orchid with small, oval or spindle-shaped pseudobulbs and elliptic to ovate, purple-tinted, sometimes glaucous, dark green leaves, 3–6cm (1¼–2½in) long. Bears yellow to red or pinkish red flowers, 6–7cm (2½–3in) across, at any time of year. ↕ 5cm (2in), ↔ 10cm (4in). E. Brazil. ❁ (min. 11–13°C/52–55°F; max. 30°C/86°F)
S. grandiflora see *S. coccinea.*

Sorbaria

ROSACEAE

Genus of 10 species of suckering, deciduous shrubs, often with star-shaped hairs, mainly occurring on riverbanks from the Himalayas to E. Asia. They are cultivated for their elegant foliage and flowers. The leaves are alternate and pinnate; the 5-petalled, star-like white flowers are borne in large, conical, terminal panicles in mid- and late summer. Sorbarias are good for a large shrub border, a wild or woodland garden, where they may form thickets, or for a waterside planting.
• **Hardiness** Fully hardy.
• **Cultivation** Grow in moderately fertile, moist but well-drained, neutral to slightly alkaline soil in full sun to partial shade. Remove excess suckers to restrict spread. Pruning group 2 or 6.
• **Propagation** Sow seed in containers in a cold frame in autumn. Take semi-ripe cuttings in midsummer. Transplant rooted suckers in autumn or winter.
• **Pests and diseases** Trouble free.

S. aitchisonii see *S. tomentosa* var. *angustifolia.*
S. arborea see *S. kirilowii.*
S. kirilowii ▣ syn. *S. arborea, Spiraea arborea.* Vigorous, spreading shrub with arching shoots and pinnate leaves, to 30cm (12in) long, each composed of 13–17 (rarely 9) lance-shaped, tapered,

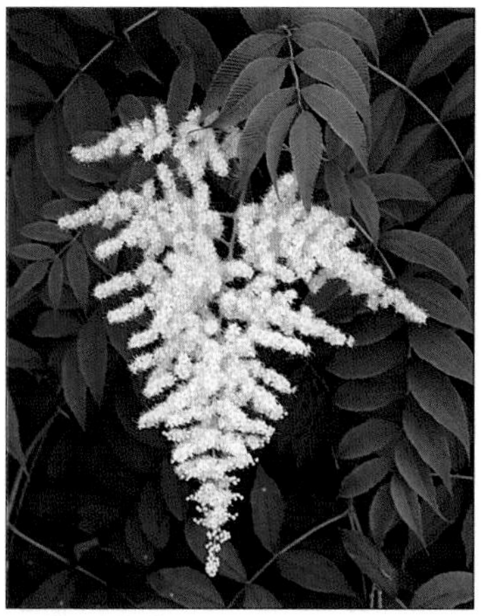

Sorbaria kirilowii

dark green leaflets. In mid- and late summer, bears white flowers, to 6mm (¼in) across, in terminal, arching, conical panicles, to 40cm (16in) long. ↕↔ 1.3–8m (4½–25ft). W. China, S.E. Tibet. ❄❄❄
S. lindleyana see *S. tomentosa.*
S. sorbifolia ▣ syn. *Spiraea sorbifolia.* Upright, thicket-forming shrub with erect branches and pinnate leaves, to 25cm (10in) long, each with up to 25 lance-shaped or oblong, tapered, dark green leaflets. In mid- and late summer, produces small white flowers, to 8mm (⅜in) across, in erect, terminal, conical panicles, to 25cm (10in) long. ↕ 2m (6ft), ↔ 3m (10ft). N. Asia, Japan. ❄❄❄
S. tomentosa, syn. *S. lindleyana.* Strong-growing, spreading shrub with pinnate leaves, to 45cm (18in) long, composed of up to 23 lance-shaped, tapered, dark green leaflets. In mid- and late summer, bears small, creamy white flowers, 6mm (¼in) across, in terminal, conical panicles, to 40cm (16in) long. ↕↔ 6m (20ft). Himalayas. ❄❄❄. **var. *angustifolia***, syn *S. aitchisonii, Spiraea aitchisonii*, is shorter, with red shoots and slender leaflets; ↕↔ 3m (10ft); Afghanistan to W. Nepal.

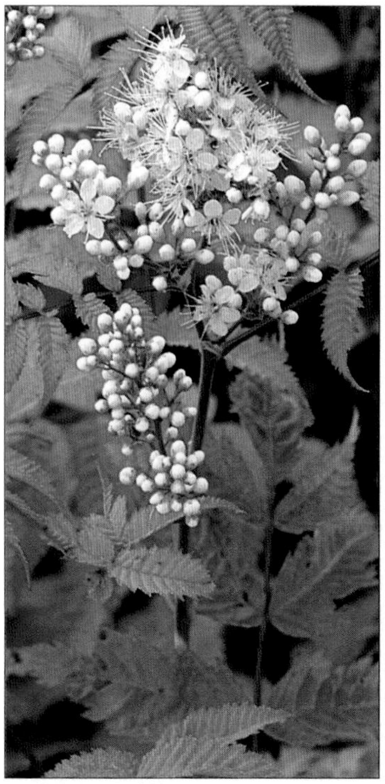

Sorbaria sorbifolia

Sorbus

ROSACEAE

Genus of about 100 species of deciduous trees and shrubs, widely distributed in N. temperate regions, found in woodland, on hills and mountains, and on scree. *Sorbus* species and cultivars are valued for their ornamental leaves, which are alternate, variable, and either simple and toothed to lobed, or pinnate; they often colour well in autumn. They are also grown for their terminal, sometimes panicle-like corymbs of small, white, rarely pink flowers, 0.8–2cm (⅜–¾in) across, borne in spring or early summer, and for their mostly spherical, white, yellow, orange, red, or brown fruits (berries). Tolerant of atmospheric pollution, they are ideal as specimen trees in a small garden, or wild or woodland garden. The raw fruit may cause mild stomach upset if ingested.
• **Hardiness** Fully hardy to frost hardy.
• **Cultivation** Grow in moderately fertile, humus-rich, well-drained soil in full sun or light dappled shade. *Sorbus* species and cultivars with pinnate leaves grow best in moist but well-drained, acid to neutral soil. *S. aria* will thrive on dry, chalky soil as well as on acid soil. Pruning group 1, if necessary.
• **Propagation** Sow seed in containers in a cold frame in autumn. Take greenwood cuttings in early summer; not all will root readily. Bud in summer. Graft in winter.
• **Pests and diseases** Prone to aphids, blister beetles, red spider mites, scale insects, sawfly larvae, canker, silver leaf, honey fungus, and fireblight.

S. alnifolia △ (Korean mountain ash). Broadly conical tree with simple, ovate to lance-shaped, toothed, dark green leaves, to 10cm (4in) long, turning yellow to orange or red in autumn. In mid-spring, bears dense corymbs, 8cm (3in) across, of small white flowers, followed in autumn by spherical, deep pink to red berries, 1cm (½in) across. ↕ 20m (70ft), ↔ 8m (25ft). E. Asia. ❄❄❄
S. americana ▣ ♤ (American mountain ash). Rounded tree or shrub producing pinnate leaves, to 25cm (10in) long, each with up to 15 oblong to lance-shaped, toothed, light green leaflets, turning yellow or red in autumn. In late spring and early summer, bears dense corymbs, 14cm

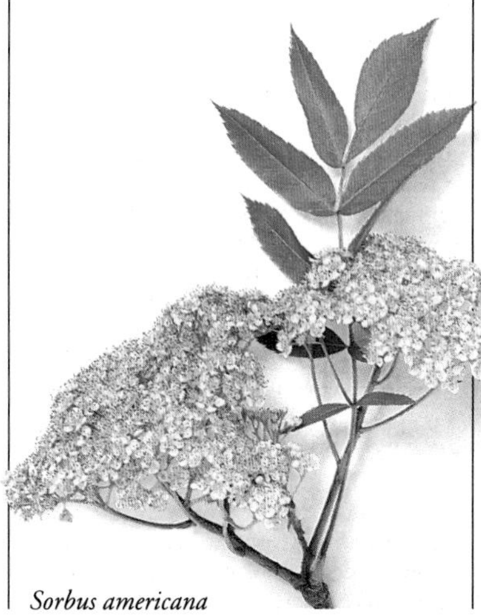

Sorbus americana

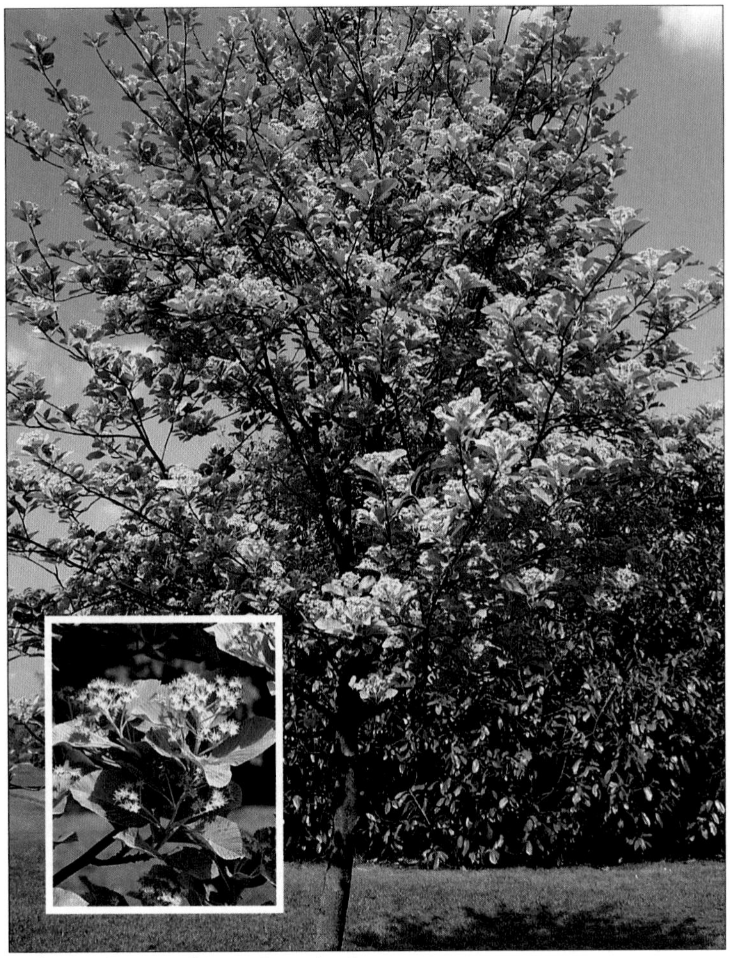

Sorbus aria 'Lutescens' (inset: flower detail)

(5½in) across, of white flowers, followed by spherical, orange-red berries, 8mm (⅜in) across. ↕ 10m (30ft), ↔ 7m (22ft). E. North America. ❄❄❄
S. aria ◯ (Whitebeam). Broadly columnar tree producing simple, elliptic to broadly ovate or obovate, toothed, glossy, dark green leaves, to 12cm (5in) long, white-hairy beneath. White flowers are borne in corymbs 8cm (3in) across, in late spring; they are followed by ovoid to spherical, brown-speckled, dark red berries, 1cm (½in) across. ↕ 10–25m (30–80ft), ↔ 10m (30ft). Europe. ❄❄❄. **'Chrysophylla'** has golden yellow juvenile leaves; ↕ 10m (30ft), ↔ 7m (22ft). **'Decaisneana'** see 'Majestica'. **'Lutescens'** ▣ 𝕐 is compact in habit, with silvery grey, later grey-green foliage; ↕ 10m (30ft), ↔ 8m (25ft). **'Magnifica'** has large, very glossy leaves, to 12cm (5in) long. **'Majestica'** 𝕐 syn. 'Decaisneana', has leaves to 15cm (6in) or more long.
S. aucuparia ▣ ◯–◯ (Mountain ash, Rowan). Broadly conical to rounded tree with mid- to dark green leaves, turning red or yellow in autumn. Leaves are oblong-lance-shaped to elliptic, to 20cm (8in) long, with 1 or 2 pairs of separate leaflets at the bases, or pinnate, with up to 12 oblong-lance-shaped, sharply toothed leaflets. In late spring, bears white flowers in corymbs to 12cm (5in) across, followed by spherical, orange-red berries, 8mm (⅜in) across. ↕ 15m (50ft), ↔ 7m (22ft). Europe, Asia. ❄❄❄. **'Aspleniifolia'** has leaflets pinnately divided at the bases. **'Beissneri'** ◯ syn. *S. moravica* 'Laciniata', is upright, with coppery bark, and red shoots and leaf-stalks; yellow-green leaves turn yellow in autumn; ↕ 10m (30ft), ↔ 5m (15ft). **'Cardinal Royal'** ◯ is upright and vigorous, and fruits profusely. **'Fastigiata'** ◯ syn. *S. decora* var. *nana*, *S. scopulina* of gardens, is dense in habit, with upright branches, conical when mature; it bears dark red berries, 1cm (½in) across; ↕ 8m (25ft), ↔ 5m (15ft). **'Fructu Luteo'** 𝕐 ◯ syn. 'Xanthocarpa', is spreading, with orange-yellow berries; ↕↔ 8m (25ft). **var. *pluripinnata*** see *S. scalaris*. **'Sheerwater Seedling'** 𝕐 ◯ is narrowly upright; ↕ 10m (30ft), ↔ 5m (15ft). **'Xanthocarpa'** see 'Fructu Luteo'.
S. cashmiriana ▣ 𝕐 ◯ Spreading tree or shrub with pinnate leaves, to 20cm (8in) long, composed of 17–21 lance-shaped, dark green leaflets. In late spring, bears pink or white flowers in corymbs 12cm (5in) across, followed by spherical white berries, to 1.5cm (½in) across, pink-tinged at first. ↕ 8m (25ft), ↔ 7m (22ft). W. Himalayas. ❄❄❄
S. 'Chinese Lace' ◯ Upright tree with pinnate leaves, to 20cm (8in) long, composed of numerous deeply cut, elliptic to oblong, dark green leaflets. Small white flowers, in corymbs to 15cm (6in) across, are produced in late spring, followed by spherical, orange-red berries, 1cm (½in) across. ↕ 6m (20ft), ↔ 5m (15ft). ❄❄❄
S. commixta ▣ ◯ syn. *S. discolor* of gardens, *S. reflexipetala*. Compact, broadly conical tree or shrub with erect branches and pinnate leaves, to 25cm (10in) long, each with up to 17 elliptic to lance-shaped, tapered, dark green

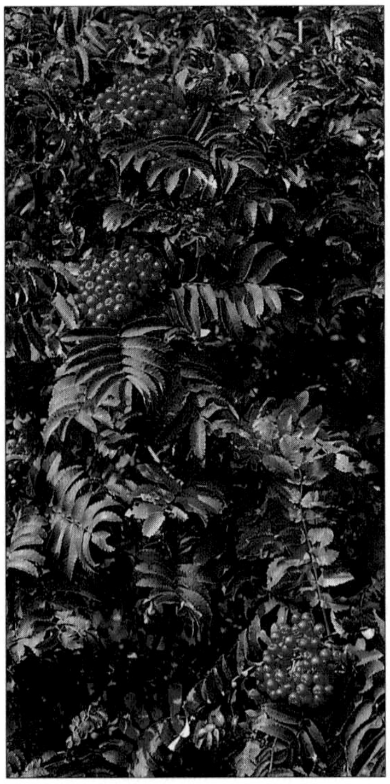

Sorbus aucuparia

leaflets, turning yellow to red or purple in autumn. In late spring, bears white flowers in corymbs 15cm (6in) across, followed by spherical, orange-red or red berries, 8mm (⅜in) across. ↕ 10m (30ft), ↔ 7m (22ft). Korea, Japan. ❄❄❄. **'Embley'** 𝕐 has bright red leaves in late autumn, and fruits profusely.
S. conradinae see *S. esserteauana*.
S. conradinae of gardens see *S. pohuashanensis*.
S. cuspidata see *S. vestita*.
S. decora ▣ ◯ Upright tree or shrub with pinnate leaves, to 15cm (6in) long, composed of up to 15 elliptic to oval-lance-shaped, dark blue-green leaflets, turning orange-red in autumn. In late spring, bears white flowers in corymbs to 10cm (4in) across, followed by spherical, bright red berries, 1cm (½in) across. ↕ 8m (25ft), ↔ 5m (15ft). Canada (Newfoundland), Greenland, N.E. USA. ❄❄❄. **var. *nana*** see *S. aucuparia* 'Fastigiata'.
S. discolor of gardens see *S. commixta*.
S. domestica ◯ (Service tree). Broadly columnar tree with pinnate leaves, to 20cm (8in) long, composed of up to 21 narrowly oblong, dark green leaflets, turning yellow or red in autumn. In late spring, bears white flowers in conical corymbs, 10cm (4in) across; they are followed by spherical or pear-shaped, yellow-green, red-flushed berries, to 3cm (1¼in) across. ↕ 20m (70ft), ↔ 12m (40ft). C. and S. Europe, N. Africa, Turkey, Caucasus, Ukraine (Crimea), Moldavia. ❄❄❄. **'Maliformis'** see f. *pomifera*. **f. *pomifera***, syn. 'Maliformis', bears spherical berries. **f. *pyriformis*** ▣ syn. var. *pyrifera*, 'Pyriformis', produces pear-shaped berries.
S. esserteauana ◯ syn. *S. conradinae*. Spreading tree with large, pinnate leaves, to 25cm (10in) long, composed of up to 15 oblong-lance-shaped, tapered, dark green leaflets, white-felted beneath, turning red in autumn. In late spring, bears white flowers in corymbs 12cm (5in) across, followed by spherical, dark red berries, 8mm (⅜in) across. ↕↔ 10m (30ft). China (W. Sichuan). ❄❄❄. **'Flava'** has orange-yellow berries.
S. folgneri 'Lemon Drop' ◯ Arching tree with slightly pendent branches and simple, narrowly ovate, dark green leaves, to 10cm (4in) long, white beneath. In late spring, produces white flowers, in corymbs 10cm (4in) across, followed by ovoid, bright yellow berries, 1cm (½in) across. ↕↔ 8m (25ft). ❄❄❄
S. forrestii ◯ Spreading tree with pinnate leaves, to 20cm (8in) long, composed of up to 19 elliptic-oblong, dark blue-green leaflets. In late spring, bears white flowers in corymbs 10cm (4in) across, followed by spherical white berries, 1cm (½in) across, tinged dark pink at the tips. ↕↔ 6m (20ft). China (N.W. Yunnan). ❄❄❄
S. glabrescens see *S. hupehensis*.
S. hupehensis 𝕐 ◯ syn. *S. glabrescens* (Hubei rowan). Broadly columnar tree with pinnate leaves, to 15cm (6in) long, each with up to 15 ovate, blue-green leaflets, turning red in autumn. In late spring, bears pyramidal, panicle-like corymbs, to 12cm (5in) long, of white flowers, followed by spherical white berries, 8mm (⅜in) across, slightly flushed pink. ↕↔ to 8m (25ft). China (Hubei). ❄❄❄. **var. *obtusa*** ▣ syn. 'Rosea', has berries ripening dark pink.
S. x hybrida of gardens see *S.* x *thuringiaca*.
S. intermedia ◯ (Swedish whitebeam). Compact, rounded tree with elliptic to oblong-elliptic, toothed, dark green leaves, to 12cm (5in) long, lobed near the bases. In late spring, bears dense corymbs, 12cm (5in) across, of white flowers, followed by ovoid-oblong,

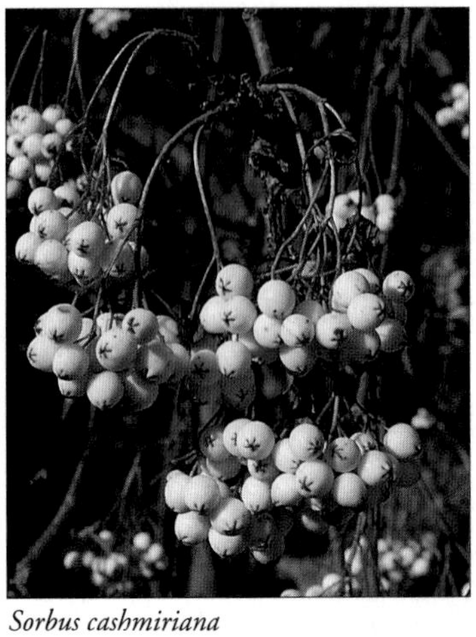

Sorbus cashmiriana

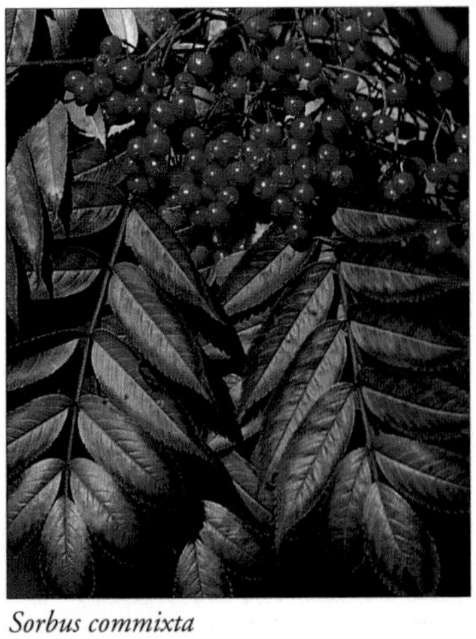

Sorbus commixta

S

SORBUS

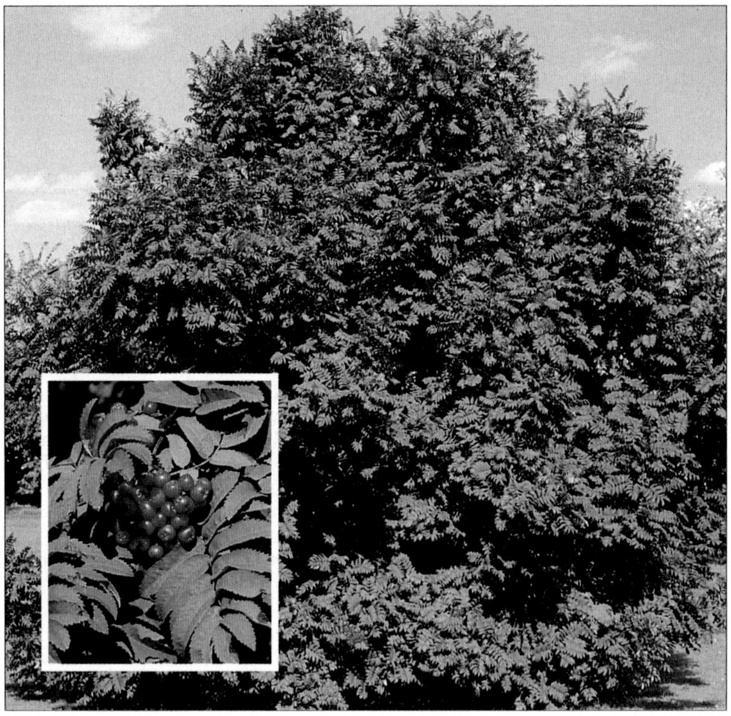

Sorbus decora (inset: fruit detail)

bright red berries, 1.5cm (½in) long. ↕↔ 12m (40ft). N.W. Europe. ❄❄❄

***S.* 'Joseph Rock'** ▣ ♀ ○ Broadly upright tree with pinnate leaves, to 15cm (6in) long, composed of up to 21 narrowly oblong, sharply toothed, bright green leaflets, turning orange, red, and purple in autumn. In late spring, bears white flowers, in corymbs 10cm (4in) across, followed by spherical, pale yellow, later orange-yellow berries, 1cm (½in) across. Prone to fireblight. ↕ 10m (30ft), ↔ 7m (22ft). ❄❄❄

S.* x *kewensis ♀ ○ (*S. pohuashanensis* x *S. aucuparia*) syn. *S. pohuashanensis* of gardens. Slow-growing, rounded, shrubby tree with pinnate leaves, to 30cm (12in) long, composed of 4–9 pairs of oblong-elliptic or oblong-lance-shaped, coarsely toothed, mid-green leaflets. In late spring, bears white flowers in corymbs 13cm (5in) across, followed by ovoid, bright red berries, 8mm (⅜in) across. ↕ 2.5m (8ft), ↔ 2m (6ft). Garden origin. ❄❄❄

S. koehneana ♀ ○ Spreading, small tree or shrub with pinnate leaves, to 15cm (6in) long, composed of up to 25 or more oblong to ovate, sharply toothed, dark green leaflets. In late spring, produces small corymbs, 8cm (3in) across, of white flowers, followed by small, spherical, mid-green berries, 6mm (¼in) across, ripening to white, on red stalks. Often confused with *S. fruticosa*, which is very similar but only grows to 2m (6ft) in height. ↕ 5m (15ft), ↔ 6m (20ft). China. ❄❄❄

***S. lanata* of gardens** see *S. vestita*.

S. latifolia ○ (Service tree of Fontainebleau). Broadly columnar tree with broadly elliptic, sharply toothed, glossy, dark green leaves, to 10cm (4in) long, lobed towards the bases. In late spring, bears white flowers in corymbs 8cm (3in) across, followed by spherical, yellow-brown berries, 1cm (½in) across. ↕ 10–20m (30–70ft), ↔ 5–8m (15–25ft). W. Europe. ❄❄❄

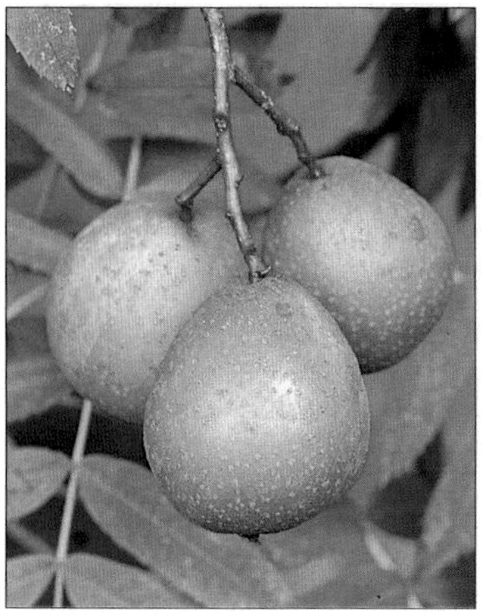

Sorbus domestica f. *pyriformis*

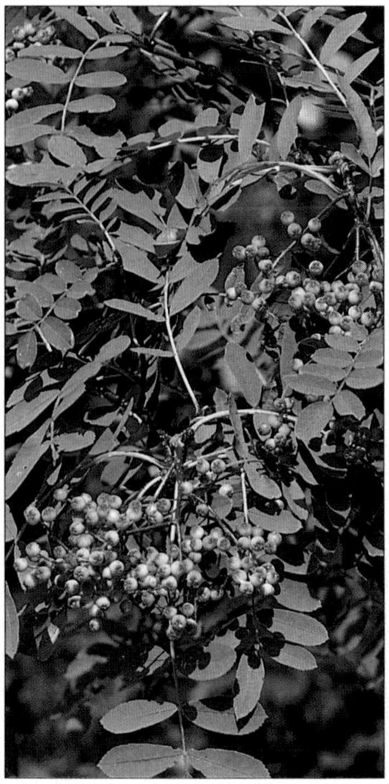

Sorbus hupehensis var. *obtusa*

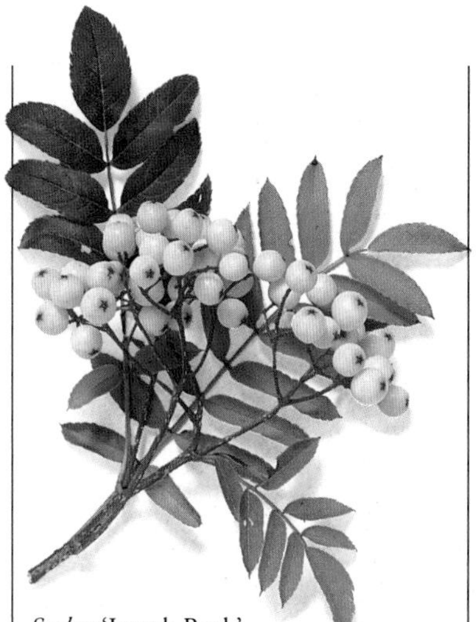

Sorbus 'Joseph Rock'

S. megalocarpa ○ Spreading tree or shrub with arching branches and oval, finely toothed, dark green leaves, to 25cm (10in) long, red when young and in autumn. In early spring, bears pungent, creamy white flowers in dense corymbs, to 15cm (6in) across, before or with the young leaves, followed by ovoid, russet-brown berries, 3cm (1¼in) long. ↕ 8m (25ft), ↔ 10m (30ft). C. to S. China. ❄❄❄

S. microphylla ○ Elegant, spreading tree or shrub with pinnate leaves, to 17cm (7in) long, each with up to 33 oblong, sharply toothed, dark green leaflets, red in autumn. In late spring, bears small corymbs, to 8cm (3in) across, of pale pink to almost crimson flowers, followed by spherical, white or pink berries, 8mm (⅜in) across. ↕↔ 6m (20ft). W. China, E. Himalayas. ❄❄❄

***S.* 'Mitchellii'** see *S. thibetica* 'John Mitchell'.

***S. moravica* 'Laciniata'** see *S. aucuparia* 'Beissneri'.

***S.* 'Pearly King'** ○ Spreading tree with slender shoots and pinnate leaves, to 15cm (6in) long, each comprising up to 17 elliptic, glossy, dark green leaflets, turning yellow or red in autumn. In late spring, bears white flowers in corymbs 10cm (4in) across, followed by spherical pink, later white-flushed berries, 1.5cm (½in) across. ↕↔ 6m (20ft). ❄❄❄

S. pohuashanensis ○ syn. *S. conradinae* of gardens. Spreading tree with pinnate leaves, to 18cm (7in) long, composed of up to 15 elliptic to oblong-lance-shaped, dark green leaflets. In late spring, produces dense corymbs, to 12cm (5in) across, of white flowers, followed by

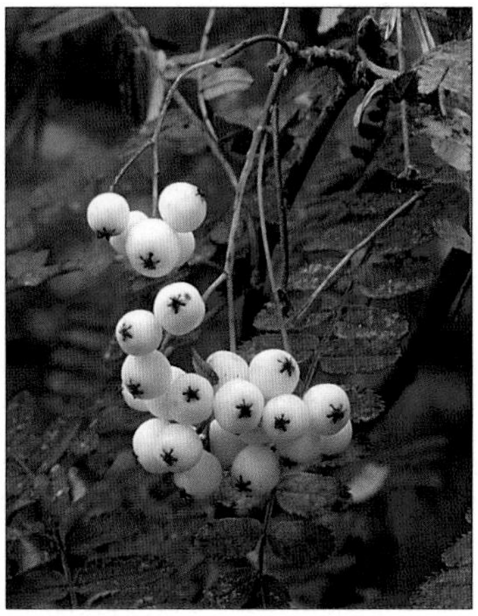

Sorbus prattii

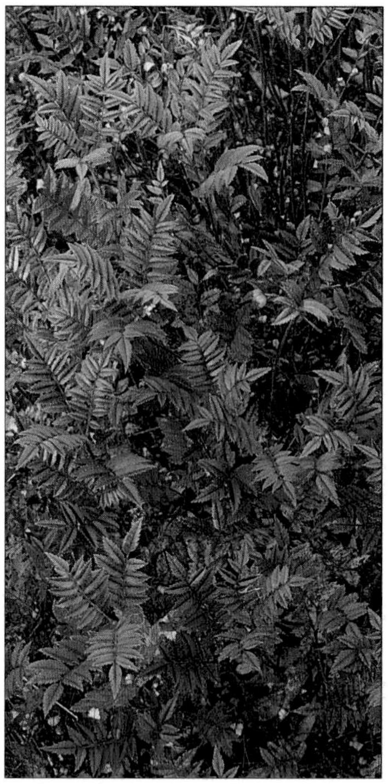

Sorbus reducta

spherical red berries, 8mm (⅜in) across. ↕ to 20m (70ft), ↔ 8m (25ft). Probably N. China. ❄❄❄

***S. pohuashanensis* of gardens** see *S.* x *kewensis*.

S. prattii ▣ ○ Spreading tree with pinnate leaves, to 15cm (6in) long, composed of up to 31 oblong, sharply toothed, dark green leaflets. In late spring, bears small corymbs, 8cm (3in) across, of white flowers, followed by spherical green berries, 8mm (⅜in) across, ripening to white. ↕↔ 6m (20ft). China (Sichuan). ❄❄❄

S. reducta ▣ ♀ Thicket-forming, usually suckering shrub with upright shoots. Pinnate leaves, to 10cm (4in) long, composed of up to 15 ovate, glossy, dark green leaflets, turn red and purple in autumn. In late spring, bears white flowers in small, open corymbs, to 8cm (3in) across, followed by spherical, crimson then white berries, 1cm (½in) across. ↕ 1–1.5m (3–5ft), ↔ 2m (6ft) or more. W. China. ❄❄❄

S. reflexipetala see *S. commixta*.

S. sargentiana ▣ ♀ ○ Broadly upright, slow-growing tree with stout shoots and large, sticky red winter buds. Large, pinnate leaves, to 35cm (14in) long,

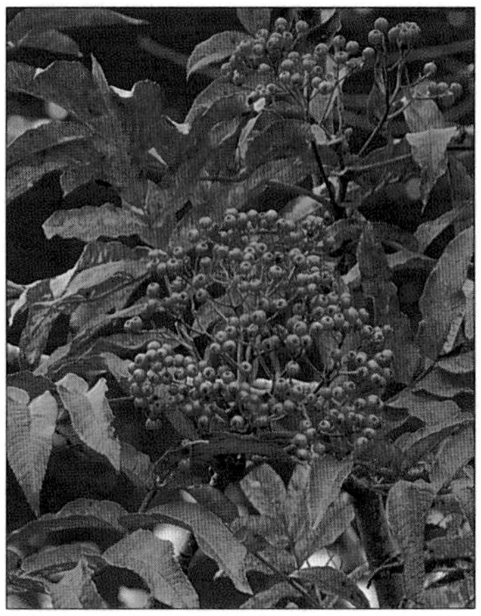

Sorbus sargentiana

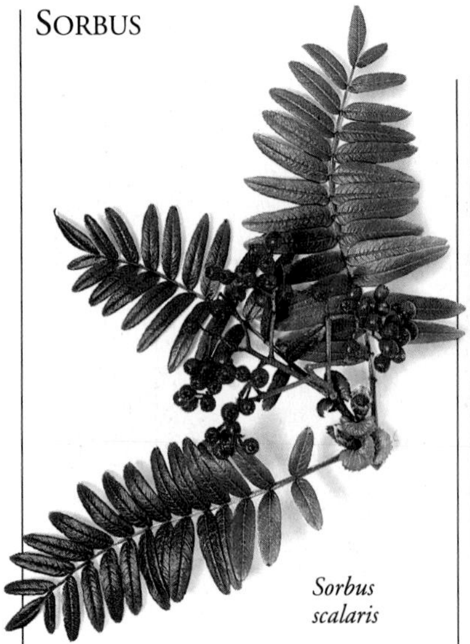

Sorbus scalaris

each with up to 13 oblong-lance-shaped, dark green leaflets, turn orange and red in autumn. In early summer, bears white flowers in broad corymbs, 20cm (8in) across, followed by spherical red berries, 8mm (3/8in) across. ↕↔ 10m (30ft). W. China. ❄❄❄

S. scalaris ▣ ♀ ♤ syn. *S. aucuparia* var. *pluripinnata*. Spreading tree with pinnate leaves, to 20cm (8in) long, composed of up to 33 narrowly oblong, glossy, dark green leaflets, turning red and purple in late autumn. In late spring and early summer, bears flattened corymbs, 15cm (6in) across, of white flowers, followed by spherical red berries, 6mm (1/4in) across. ↕↔ 10m (30ft). China (W. Sichuan). ❄❄❄

S. scopulina. Erect shrub with pinnate leaves, 3–6cm (1¾–2½in) long, each composed of up to 15 oblong-lance-shaped, dark green leaflets. In late spring and early summer, bears white flowers in corymbs to 10cm (4in) across, followed by spherical, glossy red berries, 1cm (½in) across. ↕ to 2m (6ft), ↔ 1.5m (5ft). North America (British Columbia to New Mexico). ❄❄❄

***S. scopulina* of gardens** see *S. aucuparia* 'Fastigiata'.

S. thibetica ♤ Broadly conical tree with elliptic to rounded, sharply toothed, dark green leaves, to 13cm (5in) long, densely white-hairy when young, remaining white-hairy beneath when mature. In late spring and early summer, bears white flowers in corymbs to 6cm (2½in) across, followed by spherical to pear-shaped green berries, 1.5cm (½in) across, ripening orange or yellow. ↕ 20m (70ft), ↔ 15m (50ft). S.W. China,

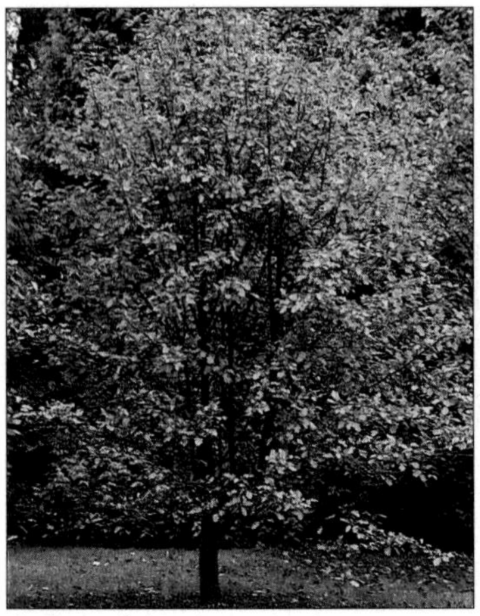

Sorbus x *thuringiaca*

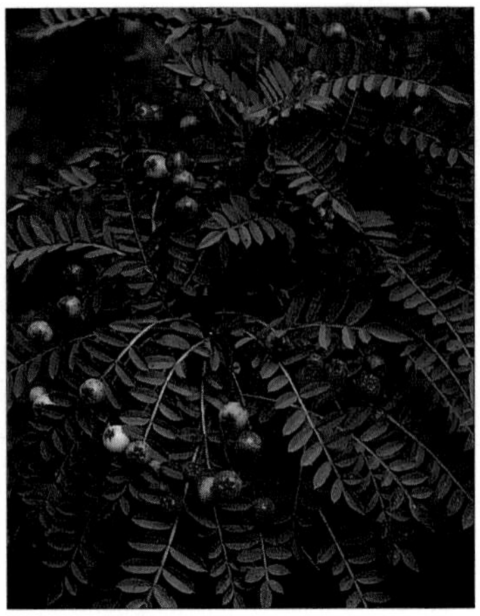

Sorbus vilmorinii

Himalayas. ❄❄❄. **'John Mitchell'** ♀ syn. *S.* 'Mitchellii', produces broadly rounded leaves.

S.* x *thuringiaca ▣ ♤ (*S. aria* x *S. aucuparia*) syn. *S.* x *hybrida* of gardens. Compact, broadly conical tree with ovate to elliptic, deeply lobed, glossy, dark green leaves, warm yellow-brown in autumn, to 15cm (6in) long, often with separate leaflets at the bases. In late spring, bears white flowers in corymbs to 12cm (5in) across, followed by spherical to ellipsoid, bright red berries, 1cm (½in) across. ↕ to 15m (50ft), ↔ 8m (25ft). Europe. ❄❄❄. **'Fastigiata'** ♢–♤ is very compact and narrowly upright, becoming broadly conical with age.

S. vestita ♤ syn. *S. cuspidata*, *S. lanata* of gardens. Broadly conical tree with simple, elliptic, sharply toothed, sometimes shallowly lobed leaves, to 20cm (8in) long. Leaves are white-hairy when young; mature leaves are glossy, dark green above, white-hairy beneath. In late spring, bears white-woolly corymbs, to 8cm (3in) across, of white flowers, followed by spherical, brown-speckled, yellow-green berries, 2cm (¾in) across. ↕ to 25m (80ft), ↔ 10m (30ft). Himalayas, N. Burma. ❄❄❄

S. vilmorinii ▣ ♀ ♤ Spreading shrub or tree with arching branches and pinnate leaves, to 15cm (6in) long, composed of up to 29 glossy, dark green leaflets. In late spring and early summer, bears white flowers in corymbs 10cm (4in) across, followed by spherical, dark red berries, 1cm (½in) across, ageing pink then white. ↕↔ 5m (15ft). S.W. China. ❄❄❄

***S.* 'Wilfrid Fox'** ♢–♤ Upright tree, broadly conical when mature, with elliptic, glossy, dark green leaves, to 12cm (5in) long, densely white-hairy beneath. White flowers are produced in corymbs 10cm (4in) across, in late spring, followed by spherical, yellow-brown, red-flushed berries, to 1.5cm (½in) across. ↕ 15m (50ft), ↔ 10m (30ft). ❄❄❄

SORGHASTRUM

GRAMINEAE/POACEAE

Genus of about 16 species of clump-forming, annual and perennial grasses from prairies and savannah in Africa and tropical and temperate North, Central, and South America. They are cultivated for their open or narrow, terminal panicles of late-summer flowerheads (which may be dried and dyed), and for their linear, flat or rolled leaves. Suitable for a mixed or herbaceous border.

- **HARDINESS** Fully hardy to frost tender.
- **CULTIVATION** Grow in moderately fertile, well-drained soil in full sun. Protect from excessive winter wet.
- **PROPAGATION** Sow seed in containers in a cold frame in spring. Divide in mid-spring or early summer.
- **PESTS AND DISEASES** Trouble free.

S. avenaceum see *S. nutans.*

S. nutans, syn. *S. avenaceum* (Indian grass, Wood grass). Slowly spreading, perennial grass forming loose clumps of erect stems with arching, broadly linear, bluish green leaves, to 60cm (24in) long. From summer to autumn, produces narrow, terminal panicles, to 35cm (14in) long, of golden brown spikelets. ↕ 1.2m (4ft), ↔ 60cm (24in). E. and C. USA. ❄❄❄. **'Sioux Blue'** is strongly erect, with metallic blue-green leaves, turning purple in autumn, and glossy, red-brown spikelets with yellow anthers.

▷**Sorrel** see *Oxalis*
▷**Sorrel tree** see *Oxydendrum arboreum*
▷**Sourwood** see *Oxydendrum arboreum*
▷**Southernwood** see *Artemisia abrotanum*
▷**Sowbread** see *Cyclamen*
▷**Spanish bayonet** see *Yucca aloifolia*
▷**Spanish chestnut** see *Castanea sativa*
▷**Spanish dagger** see *Yucca gloriosa*
▷**Spanish shawl** see *Heterocentron elegans*

SPARAXIS

Harlequin flower

IRIDACEAE

Genus of 6 species of cormous perennials from moist, rocky sites in South Africa. They are grown for their loose spikes of up to 5 widely funnel-shaped, brightly coloured flowers, borne in spring or summer. The sword-, sickle-, or lance-shaped, ribbed leaves, are often produced in an erect, basal fan. In frost-prone regions, grow in a cool greenhouse, or outdoors at the base of a warm, sunny wall in summer. In warmer areas, use in a raised bed or at the front of a border.

- **HARDINESS** Half hardy.
- **CULTIVATION** Plant corms 10cm (4in) deep. Under glass, plant in early to late autumn in loam-based potting compost (JI No.2), with added sand and leaf mould, in full light with shade from hot sun. Water sparingly when in growth, and keep cool; dry off as flowers fade. Keep completely dry when dormant. Outdoors, plant in late autumn in moderately fertile, well-drained soil in full sun. Shelter from cold, drying winds. Provide a dry winter mulch.
- **PROPAGATION** Sow seed in containers in a cold frame as soon as ripe. Remove offsets when corms are dormant.
- **PESTS AND DISEASES** Trouble free.

S. elegans, syn. *Streptanthera cuprea*, *Streptanthera elegans.* Cormous perennial with basal fans of sword-shaped leaves, 8–25cm (3–10in) long. In spring and summer, bears up to 5 stems, each with a spike of up to 5 widely funnel-shaped, orange or red, rarely white flowers, 4cm (1½in) long, fading to pink, and marked with yellow and violet. ↕ 10–30cm (4–12in), ↔ 8cm (3in). South Africa (Western Cape). ❄

S. fragrans. Cormous perennial with basal fans of lance- or sickle-shaped leaves, to 30cm (12in) long. In spring and summer, bears spikes of up to 6 flattish, widely funnel-shaped flowers, 5–6cm (2–2½in) long, with cream, yellow, red-purple, or violet-purple lobes, sometimes with darker markings, and yellow, purple, or black tubes. ↕ 8–45cm (3–18in), ↔ 8cm (3in). South Africa (Western Cape). ❄. **subsp. *grandiflora***, syn. *S. grandiflora*, is less vigorous, bearing reddish purple flowers with yellow tubes.

S. grandiflora see *S. fragrans* subsp. *grandiflora.*

S. pillansii. Cormous perennial with basal fans of 8 or 10 narrowly sword-

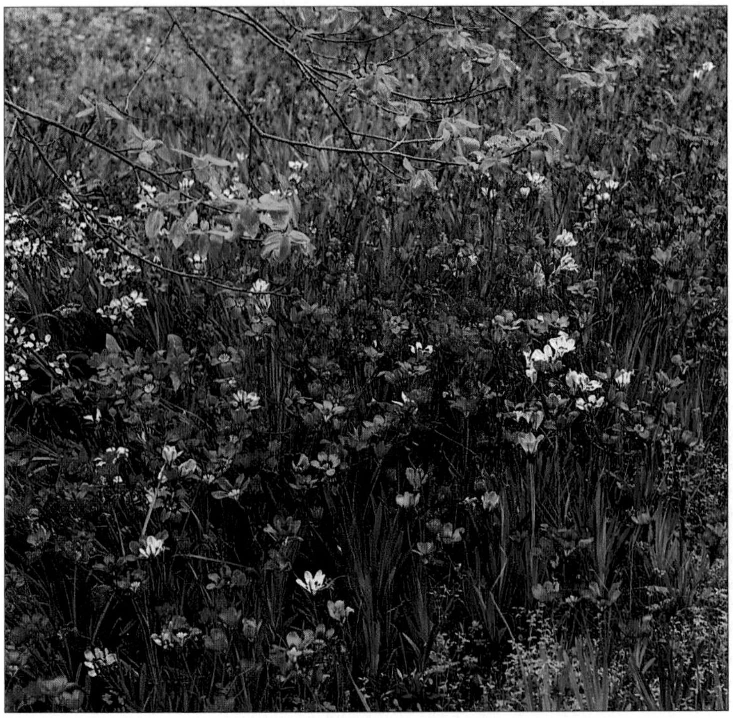

Sparaxis tricolor

S

shaped leaves, to 35cm (14in) long. In spring, bears 2–4 stems, each with spikes of 4–9 flattish, widely funnel-shaped flowers, to 6cm (2½in) across, with rose-pink lobes, marked yellow and purple-edged at the bases, and yellow tubes. ↕ to 60cm (24in), ↔ 8cm (3in). South Africa (Western Cape, Northern Cape). ❄

S. tricolor ▣ Cormous perennial with basal fans of erect, lance-shaped leaves, to 30cm (12in) long. From spring to early summer, produces 1–5 stems that bear 2–5 widely funnel-shaped, orange, red, or purple flowers, 5–8cm (2–3in) across, each with a black or dark red central mark. ↕ 10–40cm (4–16in), ↔ 8cm (3in). South Africa (Western Cape). ❄

SPARGANIUM

Burr reed

SPARGANIACEAE/TYPHACEAE

Genus of 21 species of deciduous or semi-evergreen, rhizomatous, marginal aquatic perennials, widely distributed in temperate regions worldwide, where they form vigorous stands of lush growth at the edges of lakes and rivers. Strong rhizomes support erect, linear, deep green, sometimes brown-green leaves, and produce spikes or racemes of inconspicuous, spherical, male and female flowerheads, followed by fleshy, burr-like fruits. Best grown in the shallows of a large wildlife pool.

- **HARDINESS** Fully hardy.
- **CULTIVATION** Grow in large drifts in a shallow pool margin, to 45cm (18in) deep, in full sun or partial shade. In winter, leave the foliage to provide shelter for wildlife. Remove dead foliage in spring. See also pp.52–53.
- **PROPAGATION** Sow seed at 15°C (59°F) as soon as ripe. Divide in spring.
- **PESTS AND DISEASES** Trouble free.

S. emersum. Vigorous, submerged, floating, or erect, semi-evergreen, marginal aquatic perennial with erect, boldly keeled, linear leaves, 20–50cm (8–20in) long, longer and wider on sterile plants. In summer, erect, unbranched flower spikes, 20–80cm (8–32in) long, bear densely packed, spherical, white to yellow-green flowerheads, to 2.5cm (1in) across, followed by ellipsoid, spiky brown fruit, 4–6mm (⅛–¼in) across. ↕ 20–70cm (10–28in), ↔ indefinite. Eurasia, North America. ❄❄❄

S. erectum, syn. *S. ramosum.* Vigorous, erect, rarely floating or submerged, semi-evergreen, marginal aquatic perennial with keeled, linear leaves, 1.5m (5ft) long. In summer, branched flower spikes, 20–100cm (8–39in) long, bear spherical, greenish brown flowerheads, 1–2cm (½–¾in) across, followed by ellipsoid to conical, prickly brown fruit, 6–9mm (¼–⅜in) across. ↕ 1.5m (5ft), ↔ indefinite. Eurasia. ❄❄❄

S. minimum see *S. natans.*

S. natans, syn. *S. minimum.* Slender, floating, deciduous or semi-evergreen, marginal aquatic perennial with thin, flat, translucent, dark green, submerged, sometimes floating leaves, 6–40cm (2½–16in) long. In summer, floating stems, 8–40cm (3–16in) long, bear unbranched spikes, 50–150cm (20–60in) or more long, of spherical, brownish green flowerheads, 1–2cm (½–¾in) across, followed by ovoid, spiky, green or brown fruit, 6–10mm (¼–½in) across. ↔ indefinite. Arctic, Eurasia, North America. ❄❄❄

S. ramosum see *S. erectum.*

▷ ***Sparmannia*** see *Sparrmannia*

SPARRMANNIA

syn. SPARMANNIA

TILIACEAE

Genus of 3–7 species of evergreen shrubs and small trees found in open woodland in tropical Africa, South Africa, and Madagascar. They are grown for their 4-petalled, white or pink to purple flowers, each with a showy boss of stamens, produced in long-stalked umbels from the upper leaf axils. Leaves are alternate, simple or palmately 3- to 7-lobed, toothed, narrow to broadly ovate, and often heart-shaped at the bases. In frost-prone climates, grow in a cool or temperate greenhouse. In warmer areas, grow sparrmannias in a shrub border.

- **HARDINESS** Frost tender.
- **CULTIVATION** Under glass, grow in loam-based potting compost (JI No.3) in full light. When in growth, water freely and apply a balanced liquid fertilizer monthly. Water sparingly in winter. Outdoors, grow in fertile, moist but well-drained soil in full sun. Pruning group 9, in late winter. Needs restrictive pruning under glass.
- **PROPAGATION** Sow seed at 15–18°C (59–64°F) in spring. Root semi-ripe cuttings with bottom heat in summer. Air layer in spring.
- **PESTS AND DISEASES** Whiteflies and red spider mites may be troublesome under glass.

S. africana ▣ ♀ ♢ (African hemp). Large shrub or small, upright tree with vigorous, many-branched, hairy stems and long-stalked, ovate to broadly ovate or rounded, shallowly palmately lobed, hairy, light green leaves, to 21cm (8in) long. In late spring and early summer, bears umbels of up to 20 cup-shaped white flowers, 3–4cm (1¼–1½in) across, with long, yellow and red-purple stamens. ↕ 3–6m (10–20ft), ↔ 2–4m (6–12ft). South Africa. ❁ (min. 7°C/45°F). **'Flore Pleno'**, syn. 'Plena', produces double flowers. **'Plena'** see 'Flore Pleno'. **'Variegata'** has leaves marked with white.

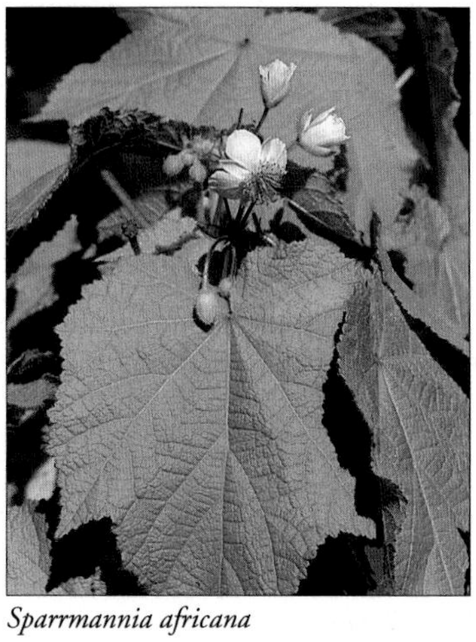

Sparrmannia africana

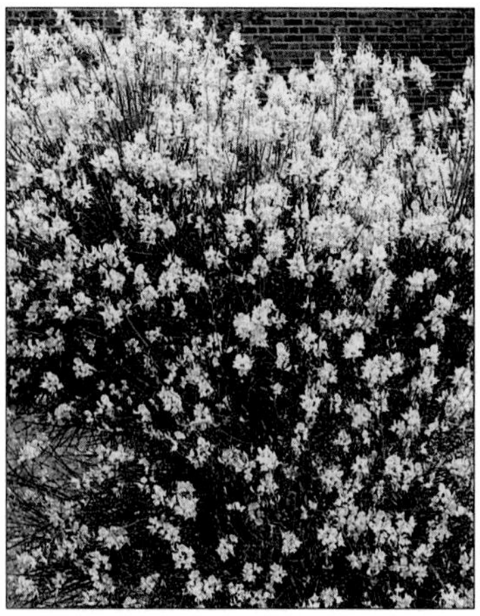

Spartium junceum

SPARTIUM

Broom, Spanish broom

LEGUMINOSAE/PAPILIONACEAE

Genus of a single species of deciduous shrub occurring in dry places, open woodland, and on roadsides mainly in the Mediterranean region, including Portugal. *S. junceum* is cultivated for its terminal racemes of fragrant, pea-like yellow flowers and rich dark green, broom-like stems. The leaves are sparse, alternate, simple, and dark green. It is suitable for a shrub border or for growing against a warm, sunny wall.

- **HARDINESS** Frost hardy.
- **CULTIVATION** Grow in moderately fertile, well-drained soil in full sun. Thrives in coastal situations and on chalky soils. Pruning group 9. To renovate older specimens, cut back to the ground in spring.
- **PROPAGATION** Sow seed in containers in a cold frame in autumn or spring. May self-seed.
- **PESTS AND DISEASES** Young plants may be damaged by rabbits.

S. junceum ▣ ♀ Upright shrub with slender, dark green shoots and few linear-oblong to narrowly lance-shaped, dark green leaves, to 3cm (1¼in) long, silky-hairy beneath. A profusion of fragrant, pea-like, golden yellow flowers, 2.5cm (1in) long, is borne in terminal racemes, to 45cm (18in) long, from early summer to early autumn; flowers are followed by flattened, dark brown seed pods, to 8cm (3in) long. ↕↔ 3m (10ft). S. Europe, Ukraine (Crimea), Turkey, Syria, N. Africa. ❄❄

SPATHIPHYLLUM

ARACEAE

Genus of 36 species of rhizomatous, evergreen perennials occurring in damp tropical forest in Indonesia, the Philippines, and tropical North, Central, and South America. They are cultivated for their stately, long-stemmed, white or cream-coloured spathes, set against dark green, lance-shaped, inversely lance-shaped, or oblong-ovate leaves with prominent midribs. In frost-prone climates, grow in a warm greenhouse or in a conservatory. In warmer regions, they are suitable for a humid, shady border. Some *Spathiphyllum* species can be grown as houseplants. All parts of the plants may cause mild stomach upset if

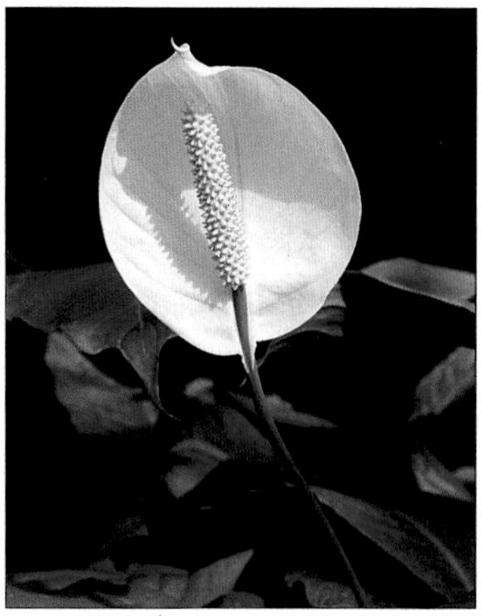

Spathiphyllum 'Mauna Loa'

ingested, and contact with the sap may irritate skin.

- **HARDINESS** Frost tender.
- **CULTIVATION** Under glass, grow in well-drained, loamless compost or loam-based potting compost (JI No.2). Water freely in growth, applying a balanced liquid fertilizer monthly; maintain high humidity. Provide bright indirect light throughout the year. Pot on when root growth has overfilled the container. Outdoors, grow in moist but well-drained, humus-rich soil in deep shade.
- **PROPAGATION** Sow seed at 23–27°C (73–81°F) as soon as ripe, or in spring on sphagnum moss. Divide in winter or immediately after flowering.
- **PESTS AND DISEASES** Trouble free.

S. 'Mauna Loa' ▣ ♀ Vigorous but compact, rhizomatous perennial with inversely lance-shaped, glossy, dark green leaves, to 30cm (12in) long. Oval, fragrant, pure white spathes, to 20cm (8in) long, surrounding green and white spadices, to 8cm (3in) long, are produced in spring and summer. ↕ 1m (3ft), ↔ 60cm (24in). ❁ (min. 15°C/59°F)

S. wallisii ▣ Rhizomatous perennial with lance-shaped-elliptic to oblong-elliptic, wavy-margined, dark green leaves, to 35cm (14in) long. Ovate to oblong-elliptic, fragrant white spathes, to 17cm (7in) long, ageing to green, and surrounding green and white spadices, to 10cm (4in) long, are borne above the foliage in spring and summer. ↕ 65cm (26in), ↔ 50cm (20in). Costa Rica, Panama, Colombia, Venezuela. ❁ (min. 10°C/50°F)

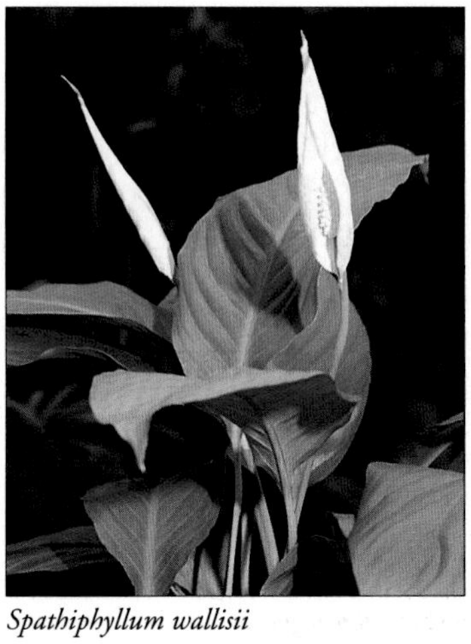

Spathiphyllum wallisii

SPATHODEA

African tulip tree

BIGNONIACEAE

Genus of one species of usually evergreen tree from forest margins and gorges in tropical Africa. It is grown for its showy, bell-shaped flowers and large, pinnate leaves. Where temperatures fall below 13°C (55°F), grow *S. campanulata* in a warm greenhouse; it seldom blooms in containers. In tropical climates, use as a specimen tree.

- **HARDINESS** Frost tender.
- **CULTIVATION** Under glass, grow in large containers or in a greenhouse border, in loam-based potting compost (JI No.3) in full light. When in growth, water freely and apply a balanced liquid fertilizer monthly; water sparingly in winter. Outdoors, grow in fertile, moist soil in full sun. Pruning group 1; needs restrictive pruning under glass, in late winter or after flowering.
- **PROPAGATION** Sow seed at 18–24°C (64–75°F) in spring. Root semi-ripe cuttings with bottom heat in summer. Air layer in spring.
- **PESTS AND DISEASES** Red spider mites may be troublesome under glass.

S. campanulata ■ ♀ Moderately branched, open, leafy tree with opposite, pinnate leaves, to 45cm (18in) long, each comprising 9–19 oblong to ovate, leathery, deep green leaflets. Terminal racemes or panicles of asymmetrical, bell-shaped, yellow-rimmed, scarlet to blood-red flowers, 5–10cm (2–4in) long, yellowish green inside, are borne mainly in spring and summer; they have a crêpe-like texture, fox-like scent, and abundant nectar. Large, woody, canoe-shaped seed pods release papery-winged seeds. ↕ 18–25m (60–80ft), ↔ 10–18m (30–60ft). Tropical Africa. ❀ (min. 13–15°C/55–59°F)

▷ **Spatterdock** see *Nuphar*
  American see *N. advena*
▷ **Speargrass** see *Aciphylla, A. colensoi*
▷ **Spearmint** see *Mentha spicata*
▷ **Spearwort,**
  Greater see *Ranunculus lingua*
  Lesser see *Ranunculus flammula*
▷ ***Specularia speculum-veneris*** see *Legousia speculum-veneris*
▷ **Speedwell** see *Veronica*
  Digger's see *Parahebe perfoliata*
  Germander see *Veronica chamaedrys*
  Prostrate see *Veronica prostrata*
  Rock see *Veronica fruticans*
  Silver see *Veronica spicata* subsp. *incana*

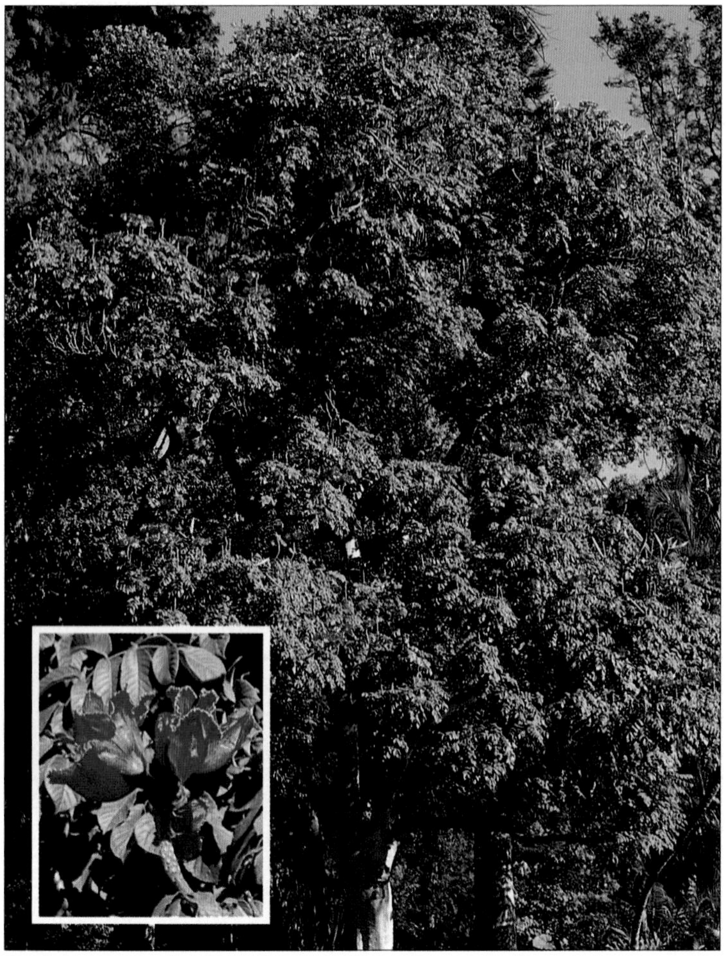

Spathodea campanulata (inset: flower detail)

SPHAERALCEA

syn. ILIAMNA

False mallow, Globe mallow

MALVACEAE

Genus of about 60 species of downy annuals, perennials, and deciduous or evergreen subshrubs and shrubs found in well-drained sites (many on mountain slopes, in wasteland, or in scrub) in warmer regions of North America, with a few in South America and southern Africa. The upright or decumbent stems bear spirally arranged, linear-lance-shaped to rounded, simple or lobed to palmate, toothed leaves. Saucer- or cup-shaped, mallow-like flowers, the stamens joined into a column around the styles, are produced singly or in racemes or panicles from summer to autumn. Suitable for a gravel garden, raised bed, or stony bank, with protection from excessive winter wet; may also be grown in a cold greenhouse.

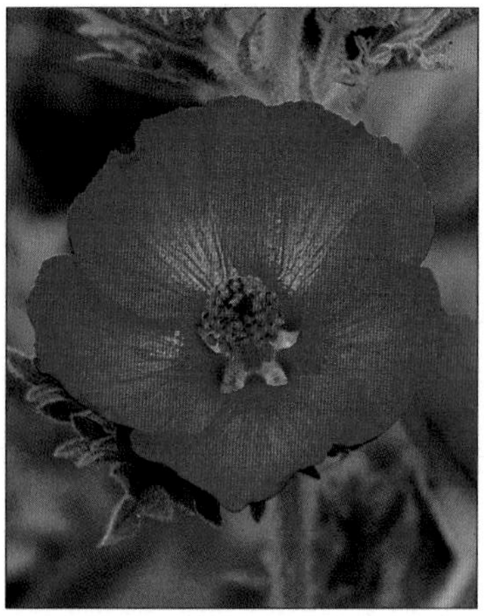

Sphaeralcea munroana

- **HARDINESS** Fully hardy to half hardy.
- **CULTIVATION** Outdoors, grow in moderately fertile, sharply drained, gravelly soil in full sun; in colder areas, plant in a warm, dry, sheltered position, and protect from winter wet. Under glass, grow in loam-based potting compost (JI No.2) with added grit, in full light. When in growth, water moderately and apply a balanced liquid fertilizer monthly. Water sparingly in winter. Repot annually in early spring.
- **PROPAGATION** Sow seed at 13°C (55°F) in spring. Divide perennials as growth begins in spring. Root basal or softwood cuttings with bottom heat in spring or early summer.
- **PESTS AND DISEASES** Hollyhock rust may be a problem.

S. coccinea, syn. *Malvastrum coccineum* (Prairie mallow). Spreading, grey- or white-hairy perennial with rounded, deeply 3- to 5-lobed, mid-green leaves, to 4cm (1½in) long, each lobe further divided. Decumbent, branching stems bear short, terminal racemes of cup-shaped, orange to red flowers, to 4cm (1½in) across, throughout summer. ↕ to 60cm (24in), ↔ 35cm (14in). S. Canada, C. and S.W. USA. ❄❄❄

S. fendleri. Hairy, subshrubby perennial with upright, branching stems and ovate to oblong, 3-lobed, toothed leaves, to 6cm (2½in) long, mid-green above, paler and often densely white-hairy beneath. From early summer to mid-autumn, saucer-shaped, reddish orange to pinkish violet flowers, to 2.5cm (1in) across, are borne in tight, axillary panicles, forming long, interrupted spikes. ↕ 1.2m (4ft), ↔ 45cm (18in). S.W. USA. ❄❄

S. munroana ■ Grey-hairy perennial with upright, unbranched stems and ovate to almost diamond-shaped, shallowly 3- to 5-lobed or scalloped, mid-green leaves, to 6cm (2½in) long. From midsummer to early autumn, bears saucer-shaped, reddish orange flowers, 2.5cm (1in) across, in many-flowered, axillary and terminal panicles. ↕ to 80cm (32in), ↔ 45cm (18in). W. North America. ❄❄❄

▷ **Spicebush** see *Calycanthus*
▷ **Spice bush** see *Lindera benzoin*
▷ **Spider flower** see *Cleome*
  Brazilian see *Tibouchina urvilleana*
▷ **Spider lily,**
  Golden see *Lycoris aurea*
  Red see *Lycoris radiata*
▷ **Spider orchid** see *Brassia lawrenceana*
▷ **Spider plant** see *Chlorophytum comosum, Cleome hassleriana*
▷ **Spignel** see *Meum athamanticum*
▷ **Spikemoss, Krauss's** see *Selaginella kraussiana*
▷ **Spikenard, False** see *Smilacina racemosa*
▷ ***Spiloxene capensis*** see *Hypoxis capensis*
▷ **Spinach,**
  Chinese see *Amaranthus tricolor*
  Red mountain see *Atriplex hortensis*
▷ **Spindle,**
  Japanese see *Euonymus japonicus*
  Winged see *Euonymus alatus*
▷ **Spindle tree** see *Euonymus*

SPIRAEA

ROSACEAE

Genus of about 80 species of deciduous or semi-evergreen shrubs found in rocky places, thickets, woodland, at woodland margins, and on riverbanks, widely distributed in N. temperate regions of Europe, Asia, and North America, including Mexico. The alternate leaves are entire, toothed, or lobed, and are decorative in some species. Spiraeas are cultivated mainly for their terminal, umbel-like racemes, panicles, cymes, or corymbs of small, mostly saucer-, cup-, or bowl-shaped, white, yellow, pink, or purple flowers; these are 0.5–1cm (¼–½in) across, or sometimes slightly larger, and profusely borne in spring or summer. Grow in a mixed or shrub border. Compact spiraeas are ideal for a rock garden; use low-growing variants of *S. japonica* as ground cover; use taller spiraeas as informal hedging.

- **HARDINESS** Fully hardy, although new growth on early-flowering species and cultivars may be damaged by late frosts.
- **CULTIVATION** Grow in fertile, moist but well-drained soil in full sun. Pruning group 2 for spiraeas flowering on previous year's wood; group 6 for those flowering on current season's wood (*S.* x *billiardii* and *S. douglasii*).
- **PROPAGATION** Take greenwood cuttings in summer. Divide suckering species, such as *S.* x *billiardii* and *S. douglasii*, in late autumn or early spring.
- **PESTS AND DISEASES** Trouble free.

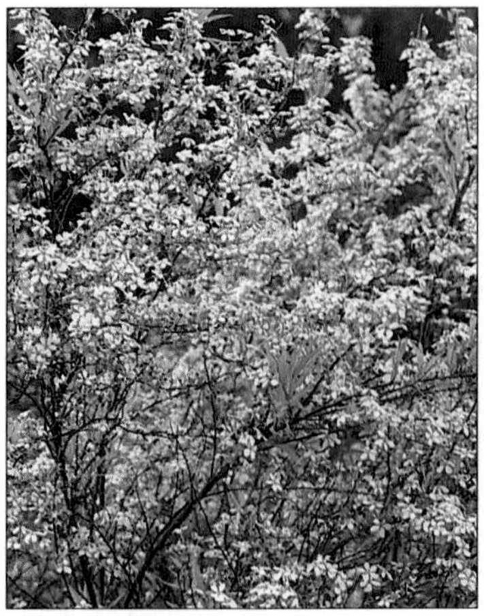

Spiraea 'Arguta'

S

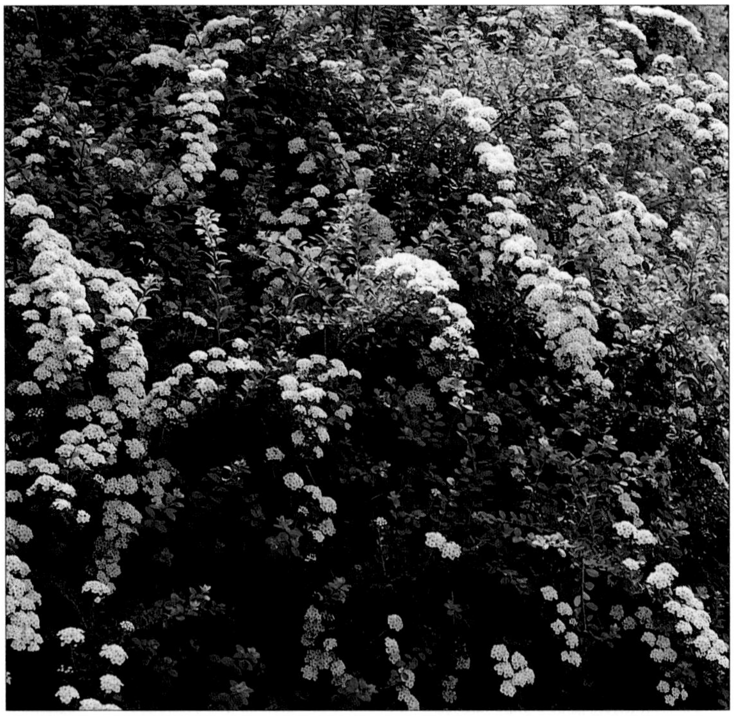
Spiraea canescens

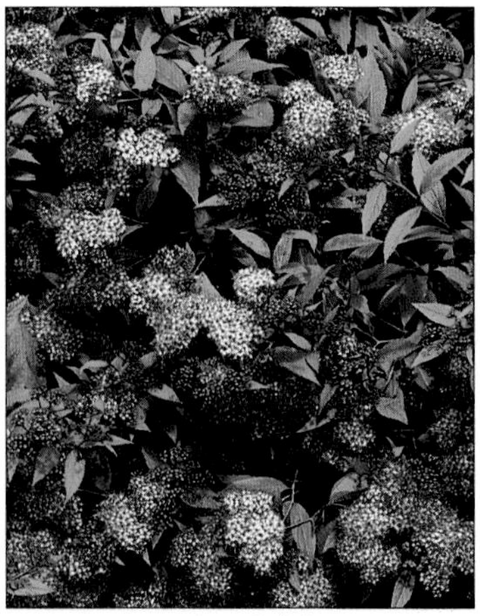
Spiraea japonica 'Froebelii'

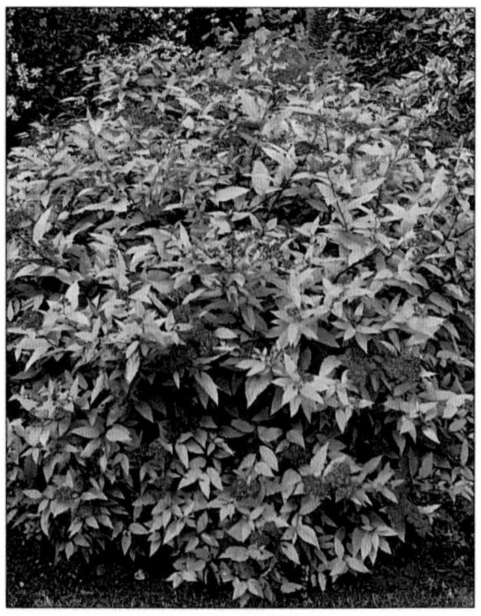
Spiraea japonica 'Goldflame'

S. aitchisonii see *Sorbaria tomentosa* var. *angustifolia.*
S. albiflora see *S. japonica* var. *albiflora.*
S. arborea see *Sorbaria kirilowii.*
***S.* 'Arguta'** ■ (Bridal wreath, Foam of May). Dense, rounded, deciduous shrub with slender, arching shoots and lance-shaped to narrowly oblong, toothed, bright green leaves, to 4cm (1½in) long. In spring, produces saucer-shaped white flowers in terminal corymbs, to 6cm (2½in) across, on short, leafy, lateral branches of the previous season's growth. ↕↔ 2.5m (8ft). ❄❄❄
S. aruncus see *Aruncus dioicus.*
S.* x *billiardii (*S. douglasii* x *S. salicifolia*). Upright, thicket-forming, suckering, deciduous shrub with oval to narrowly oblong, toothed, mid- or dark green leaves, to 10cm (4in) long. Cup-shaped, purple-pink flowers are borne in dense, terminal panicles, to 20cm (8in) long, in mid- and late summer. ↕ 1–2m (3–6ft), ↔ to 2m (6ft). Garden origin. ❄❄❄. **'Triumphans'** has dark green leaves, 6cm (2½in) long; ↕↔ 2.5m (8ft).
S.* x *bumalda see *S. japonica* 'Bumalda'.
S. canescens ■ Upright, deciduous shrub with arching shoots and elliptic to obovate, grey-green leaves, to 2.5cm (1in) long, toothed at the tips. Bowl-shaped, creamy white flowers, in corymbs to 5cm (2in) across, are borne at the tips of short, lateral shoots in mid- and late summer. ↕ 3m (10ft), ↔ 2m (6ft). Himalayas. ❄❄❄
S. cantoniensis ■ Spreading, deciduous or semi-evergreen shrub with arching shoots and lance-shaped, toothed, blue-green leaves, to 6cm (2½in) long. In early summer, short, lateral shoots bear corymbs, to 5cm (2in) across, of bowl-shaped white flowers. ↕ 2m (6ft), ↔ 3m (10ft). ❄❄❄. **'Flore Pleno'**, syn. 'Lanceata', has double white flowers. **'Lanceata'** see 'Flore Pleno'.
S. crispifolia see *S. japonica* 'Bullata'.
S. douglasii. Vigorous, suckering, erect, thicket-forming, deciduous shrub with narrowly oblong, dark green leaves, to 10cm (4in) long, toothed at the tips and densely grey-felted beneath. In early and midsummer, bears bowl-shaped, purple-pink flowers in dense, terminal panicles, to 20cm (8in) long. ↕ 2.5m (8ft), ↔ 1.5m (5ft). W. North America. ❄❄❄. **subsp. *menziesii***, syn. *S. menziesii*, has pink flowers, and leaves without felt beneath.
S. japonica. Clump-forming, deciduous shrub with erect shoots. Ovate to lance-shaped, sharply toothed, dark green leaves, to 12cm (5in) long, are grey-green beneath. In mid- and late summer, bears bowl-shaped, pink or white flowers in terminal corymbs, to 20cm (8in) across. ↕ 2m (6ft), ↔ 1.5m (5ft). China, Japan. ❄❄❄. **'Alba'** see var. *albiflora.* **var. *albiflora***, syn. 'Alba', *S. albiflora*, has pale green leaves, and white flowers in corymbs 10cm (4in) across; ↕ 60cm (24in), ↔ 90cm (36in). **'Allgold'** has golden yellow leaves and pink flowers; ↕ 45cm (18in), ↔ 60cm (24in). **'Anthony Waterer'** ■ 🏆 has dark pink flowers, and leaves often margined creamy white, bronze-red when young; ↕ to 1.5m (5ft). **'Bullata'**, syn. *S. crispifolia*, is slow-growing and compact, with small, very dark green leaves, to 2.5cm (1in) long, and deep pink flowers in corymbs 8cm (3in) across; ↕ to 40cm (16in), ↔ to 50cm (20in). **'Bumalda'**, syn. *S.* x *bumalda*, has bronze young leaves and dark pink flowers; ↕↔ 1m (3ft). **'Froebelii'** ■ has bronze-red young leaves and large corymbs of deep pink flowers. **'Golden Princess'** ■ has bronze-red, later bright yellow leaves, red in autumn, and bright purplish pink flowers. **'Goldflame'** ■ 🏆 has bronze-red young leaves, turning bright yellow then mid-green, and dark pink flowers; ↕↔ 75cm (30in). **'Little Princess'** ■ forms a dense mound, with small leaves, 2.5cm (1in) long, and rose-pink flowers in corymbs 4cm (1½in) across; ↕ 50cm (20in), ↔ 1m (3ft). **'Nana'** 🏆 syn. 'Nyewoods', forms a dwarf mound, with small leaves, to 1cm (½in) long, and dark pink flowers in corymbs 2.5cm (1in) across; ↕ 45cm (18in), ↔ 60cm (24in). **'Nyewoods'** see 'Nana'. **'Shiburi'** see 'Shirobana'. **'Shirobana'** 🏆 syn. 'Shiburi', has both dark pink and white flowers on each plant; ↕↔ 60cm (24in).
S. menziesii see *S. douglasii* subsp. *menziesii.*
S. nipponica. Upright to spreading, deciduous shrub with arching branches and ovate to rounded, dark green leaves, 1.5–3cm (½–1¼in) long, entire or with a few teeth at the tips, bluish green beneath. In midsummer, bowl-shaped white flowers open in terminal corymbs, 2.5–4cm (1–1½in) across. ↕↔ 1.2–2.5m (4–8ft). Japan. ❄❄❄. **'Halward's Silver'** is erect but compact, and flowers freely; ↕↔ 1m (3ft). **'Snowmound'** ■ 🏆 syn. var. *tosaensis* of gardens, is fast-growing and spreading. **var. *tosaensis* of gardens** see 'Snowmound'.

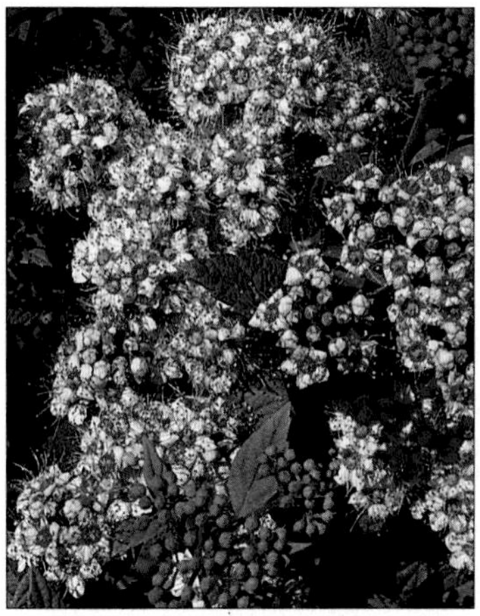
Spiraea japonica 'Little Princess'

S

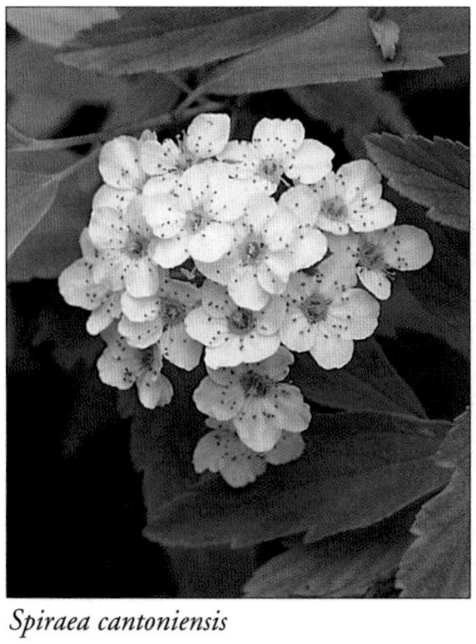
Spiraea cantoniensis

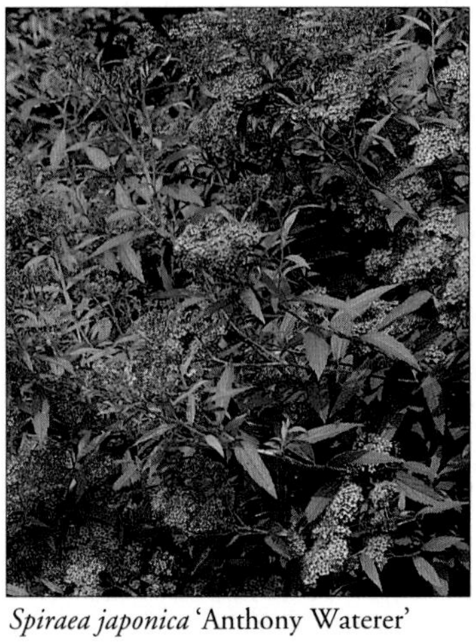
Spiraea japonica 'Anthony Waterer'

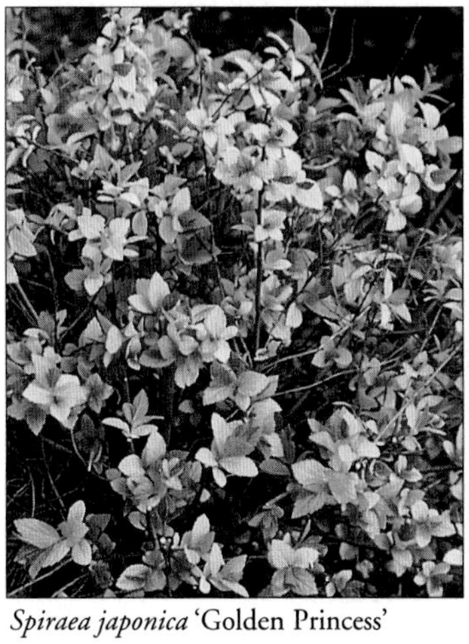
Spiraea japonica 'Golden Princess'

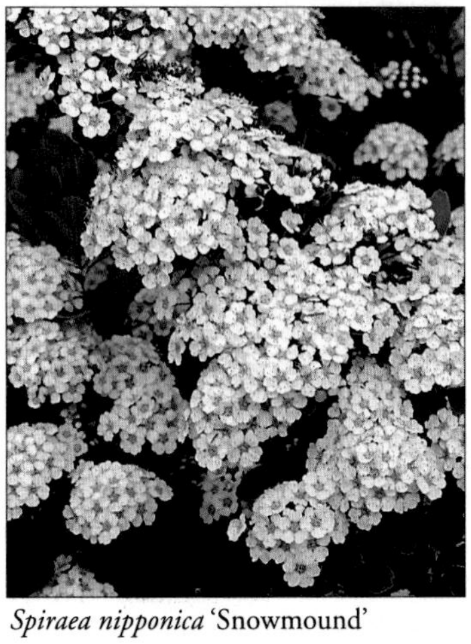
Spiraea nipponica 'Snowmound'

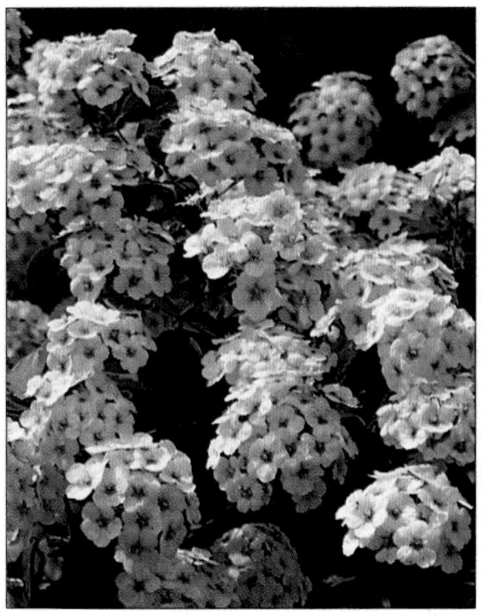

Spiraea x *vanhouttei*

S. opulifolius see *Physocarpus opulifolius.*
S. palmata see *Filipendula palmata.*
S. prunifolia, syn. *S. prunifolia* 'Plena'. Arching, deciduous shrub with ovate, finely toothed leaves, to 4.5cm (1¾in) long, glossy, bright green above, grey-downy beneath, turning bronze-yellow to red in autumn. Double white flowers are produced in stalkless corymbs, to 6cm (2½in) across, on short laterals along the shoots, in mid- and late spring. ↕↔ 2m (6ft). China, Taiwan, Japan. ❄❄❄. **'Plena'** see *S. prunifolia.*
***S.* 'Snow White'**, syn. *S. trichocarpa* 'Snow White'. Bushy, deciduous shrub with arching shoots and ovate, bright mid-green leaves, to 5cm (2in) long, with a few teeth at the tips. Small, cup-shaped white flowers are borne in dense corymbs, to 5cm (2in) across, on short laterals, in late spring and early summer. ↕↔ 2m (6ft). ❄❄❄
S. sorbifolia see *Sorbaria sorbifolia.*
S. thunbergii ♀ Dense, bushy, deciduous or semi-evergreen shrub with arching branches and slender, lance-shaped, sparsely toothed, light green leaves, to 4cm (1½in) long. In spring and early summer, bears bowl- or saucer-shaped white flowers in stalkless corymbs, to 5cm (2in) across, on short laterals along the shoots. ↕ 1.5m (5ft), ↔ 2m (6ft). China, Japan. ❄❄❄
***S. trichocarpa* 'Snow White'** see *S.* 'Snow White'.
S. ulmaria see *Filipendula ulmaria.*
S.* x *vanhouttei ▣ ♀ (*S. cantoniensis* x *S. trilobata*). Compact, bushy, deciduous shrub with slender, arching shoots. The diamond-shaped to obovate leaves, to 4.5cm (1¾in) long, are scalloped or coarsely toothed, occasionally 3- to 5-lobed at the tips, and dark green above, blue-green beneath. Bowl-shaped white flowers are borne in dense corymbs, to 5cm (2in) across, on short laterals along the shoots, in early summer. ↕ 2m (6ft), ↔ 1.5m (5ft). Garden origin. ❄❄❄. **'Pink Ice'** is slow-growing, with white-flecked leaves.
S. veitchii. Upright, deciduous shrub with long, arching shoots, red when young, and elliptic to oblong, entire, mid-green leaves, to 5cm (2in) long, glaucous beneath. In early and mid-summer, bears bowl-shaped white flowers in dense corymbs, 6cm (2½in) across, on short laterals along the shoots. ↕ 4m (12ft), ↔ 3m (10ft). W. and C. China. ❄❄❄

▷ **Spiraea, Rock** see *Petrophytum*

Spiranthes

ORCHIDACEAE

Genus of about 50 species of usually small, evergreen or deciduous, terrestrial or rarely epiphytic orchids from grassland or woodland habitats, often close to water, in temperate and tropical regions, mainly in North America, with a few in Europe and Asia. They have tuberous roots and basal rosettes of papery or fleshy, lance-shaped or ovate to almost rounded leaves. Tiny white flowers are borne in spiral racemes along erect stems. May form large colonies outdoors.
• **Hardiness** Fully hardy to frost tender.
• **Cultivation** Cool-growing orchids. Under glass, grow in terrestrial orchid compost in bright filtered light. In growth, water freely and apply fertilizer at every third watering. Keep almost dry and frost-free when dormant. Outdoors, plant hardy species, when dormant, in moist but well-drained, fertile, humus-rich, leafy soil in a sheltered site in partial shade. Provide a deep, dry winter mulch in frost-prone areas. See also p.46.
• **Propagation** Divide tubers when dormant.
• **Pests and diseases** Susceptible to red spider mites and aphids under glass.

S. cernua ▣ (Nodding ladies' tresses). Deciduous, terrestrial orchid producing broadly linear, acute leaves, 5–24cm (2–10in) long. Bears racemes of almost translucent white flowers, 5mm (¼in) long, with yellow centres, in autumn. ↕ 60cm (24in), ↔ 8cm (3in). E. Canada, USA. ⊛ (min. 2°C/36°F) in containers.

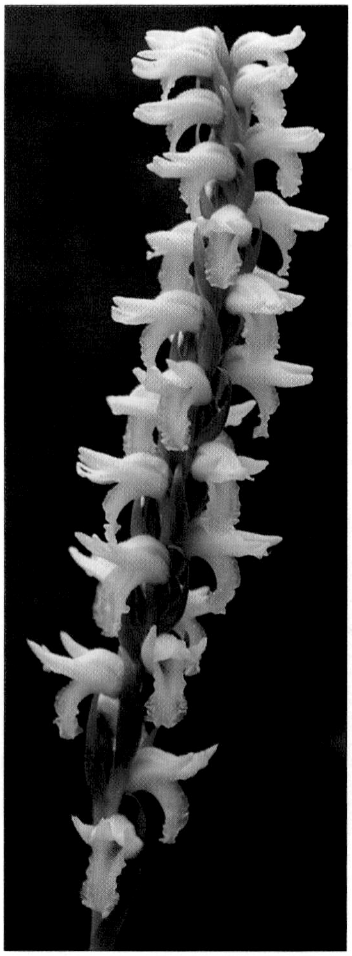

Spiranthes cernua

▷ ***Spironema fragrans*** see *Callisia fragrans*
▷ **Spleenwort** see *Asplenium*
Maidenhair see *A. trichomanes*
Mother see *A. bulbiferum*
Shining see *A. oblongifolium*
▷ **Spotted dog** see *Pulmonaria officinalis*
▷ **Spotted orchid** see *Dactylorhiza*
Heath see *D. maculata*

Sprekelia

AMARYLLIDACEAE

Genus of a single species of bulbous perennial occurring on rocky slopes in Mexico and Guatemala. It has semi-erect, strap-shaped, basal leaves, and is grown for its large, showy, 6-tepalled red flowers, sometimes marked or striped yellow, borne in spring. In frost-prone areas, grow in a temperate greenhouse or conservatory; in warmer areas, grow in a sunny border.
• **Hardiness** Frost tender.
• **Cultivation** Plant in autumn with the neck and shoulders of the bulb above soil level. Under glass, grow in loam-based potting compost (JI No.3) in full light. When in growth, water moderately and apply a half-strength balanced liquid fertilizer every 2 weeks after flowering. Reduce water as foliage fades; keep almost dry when dormant. Repot every 2–3 years. Outdoors, grow in well-drained, moderately fertile soil in full sun. Roots resent disturbance.
• **Propagation** Separate offsets when dormant in early autumn.
• **Pests and diseases** Trouble free.

S. formosissima ▣ ♀ (Aztec lily, Jacobean lily). Bulbous perennial with strap-shaped, mid-green leaves, to 50cm (20in) long. In spring, produces solitary, bright scarlet to deep crimson flowers, 12cm (5in) across, each with a broad, erect upper tepal, 2 narrower, horizontal tepals, and 3 narrow, pendent tepals. ↕ 15–35cm (6–14in), ↔ 15cm (6in). Mexico, Guatemala. ⊛ (min. 7–10°C/45–50°F)

▷ **Spring beauty** see *Claytonia*
▷ **Spruce** see *Picea*
Black see *P. mariana*
Brewer see *P. breweriana*
Caucasian see *P. orientalis*
Colorado see *P. pungens*
Dragon see *P. asperata*
Engelmann see *P. engelmannii*
Hondo see *P. jezoensis* subsp. *hondoensis*

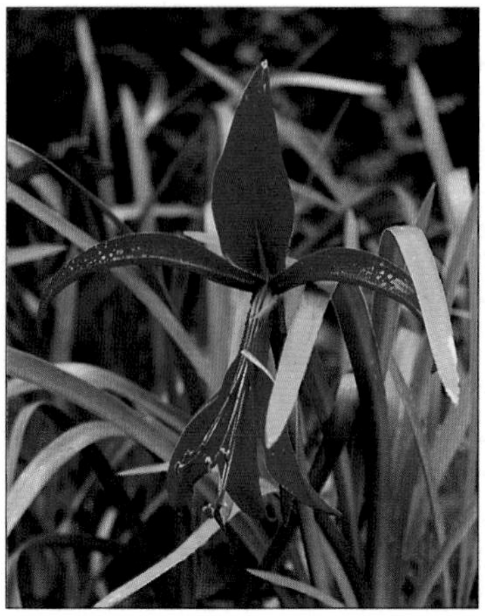

Sprekelia formosissima

▷ **Spruce cont.**
Lijiang see *P. likiangensis*
Morinda see *P. smithiana*
Norway see *P. abies*
Oriental see *P. orientalis*
Purple-cone see *P. purpurea*
Sargent see *P. brachytyla*
Serbian see *P. omorika*
Sitka see *P. sitchensis*
Taiwan see *P. morrisonicola*
White see *P. glauca*
▷ **Spurge** see *Euphorbia*
Caper see *E. lathyris*
Cypress see *E. cyparissias*
Hairy see *E. pilosa*
Honey see *E. mellifera*
Portland see *E. portlandica*
Wood see *E. amygdaloides*
▷ **Squill,**
Sea see *Urginea maritima*
Siberian see *Scilla siberica*

Stachys syn. Betonica

Betony, Hedge nettle, Woundwort

LABIATAE/LAMIACEAE

Genus of about 300 species of annuals, mostly rhizomatous and stoloniferous perennials, and a few evergreen shrubs, widely distributed in a range of habitats, including mountains, dry, rocky hills, scrub, wasteland, meadows, forest clearings, and streamsides, especially in N. temperate regions. The leaves on the square stems are short-stalked or stalkless, opposite, and become progressively smaller up the stems; basal leaves are lance-shaped or elliptic to ovate, entire to scalloped or toothed, wrinkled, prominently veined, hairy and stalked. Many species are aromatic, occasionally unpleasantly so. The tubular, 2-lipped, often hooded, usually white, yellow, pink, red, or purple flowers are borne in racemes or spikes of axillary whorls. Most are attractive to bees and butterflies. Grow taller perennials in a mixed or herbaceous border. *S. byzantina* is ideal as edging or as ground cover. Low-growing, hairy-leaved species, such as *S. candida, S. citrina,* and *S. lavandulifolia,* are suitable for a dry bank, gravel garden, raised bed, or rock garden, but need protection from excessive winter wet; they are best grown in an alpine house. Grow *S. sylvatica* in a wild garden.
• **Hardiness** Fully hardy to frost hardy.
• **Cultivation** Outdoors, grow in well-drained, moderately fertile soil in full sun; *S. macrantha, S. officinalis,* and *S. sylvatica* tolerate partial shade. Grow

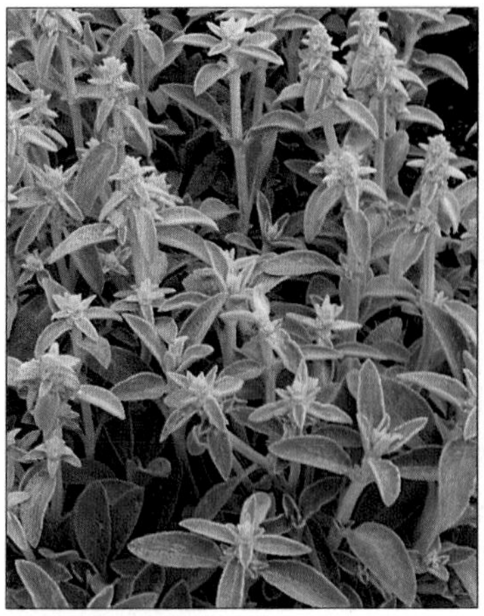

Stachys byzantina

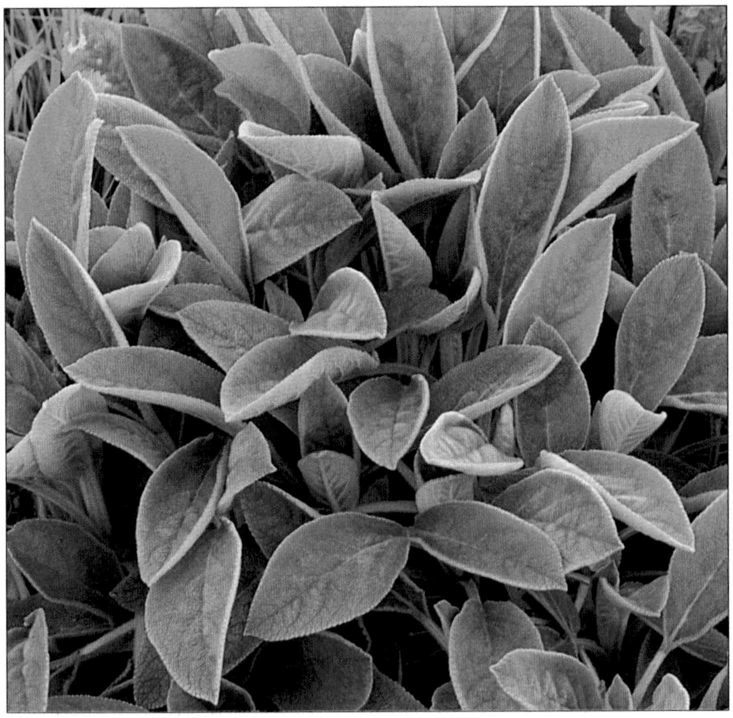

Stachys byzantina 'Big Ears'

rock garden species in sharply drained, gritty soil in a sunny site; protect from excessive winter wet. In an alpine house, grow in loam-based potting compost (JI No.2) with added grit, in full light.
• **PROPAGATION** Sow seed in containers in a cold frame in autumn or spring. Divide or remove rooted sections of perennials in spring as growth begins. Take greenwood cuttings of shrubs and subshrubs in early summer.
• **PESTS AND DISEASES** Slugs may be a problem. *S. byzantina*, in particular, is susceptible to powdery mildew.

S. betonica see *S. officinalis.*
S. byzantina ◼ syn. *S. lanata, S. olympica* (Lambs' ears, Lambs' lugs, Lambs' tails, Lambs' tongues). Mat-forming, densely white-woolly perennial with rosettes of entire, oblong-elliptic to lance-shaped, thick, wrinkled, veined, grey-green leaves, to 10cm (4in) long. Erect stems bear interrupted spikes of woolly, pink-purple flowers, 1.5cm (½in) long, from early summer to early autumn. ↕45cm (18in), ↔60cm (24in). Caucasus to Iran. ❄❄❄. **'Big Ears'** ◼ has large, greyish white-felted, mid-green leaves, 25cm (10in) long, and purple flowers. **'Cotton Boll'**, syn. 'Sheila McQueen', has leaves 11cm (4½in) long, and clusters of modified flowers forming cotton-wool-like balls along the stems. **'Primrose Heron'** ◼ syn. *S.* 'Primrose Heron', has yellowish grey leaves. **'Sheila McQueen'** see 'Cotton Boll'. **'Silver Carpet'** ◼ syn. *S.* 'Silver Carpet', is non-flowering, and has intensely silvered, greyish white leaves.
S. candida ◼ Spreading subshrub producing rounded, white-felted, grey-green leaves, to 2.5cm (1in) long. In summer, bears leafy spikes of hooded white flowers, 1cm (½in) or more long, streaked and spotted purple. ↕15cm (6in), ↔30cm (12in). S. Greece. ❄❄❄
S. citrina. Spreading, woody-based perennial producing elliptic to ovate-oblong, minutely round-toothed, grey-hairy, soft, lime-green leaves, to 5cm (2in) long. Short, dense, sometimes interrupted spikes of sulphur-yellow flowers, 2–2.5cm (¾–1in) long, are borne in summer. ↕20cm (8in), ↔30cm (12in). Turkey. ❄❄❄
S. coccinea. Spreading, softly hairy perennial with entire, ovate-lance-shaped or oblong-triangular, wrinkled, veined, mid-green leaves, to 7cm (3in) long. Upright stems bear slender spikes of narrow scarlet flowers, to 2cm (¾in) long, from mid-spring to mid-autumn. ↕60cm (24in), ↔45cm (18in). USA (Arizona, Texas) to Mexico. ❄❄
S. grandiflora see *S. macrantha.*
S. lanata see *S. byzantina.*
S. lavandulifolia. Spreading, woody-based perennial with oblong-lance-shaped, toothed, grey-hairy, grey-green leaves, 2–6cm (¾–2½in) long. Upright spikes of purplish pink flowers, to 1.5cm (½in) long, are produced in summer. ↕↔30cm (12in). Turkey, Iraq. ❄❄❄
S. macrantha, syn. *S. grandiflora, S. spicata.* Erect, hairy perennial with rosettes of broadly ovate, scalloped, wrinkled, veined, dark green leaves, to 7cm (3in) long, heart-shaped at the bases. Dense spikes of hooded, pinkish purple flowers, 3cm (1¼in) long, are produced on erect stems from early summer to early autumn. ↕60cm (24in), ↔30cm (12in). Caucasus, N.E. Turkey, N.W. Iran. ❄❄❄. **'Superba'** ◼ has slightly deeper pinkish purple flowers.
S. officinalis ◼ syn. *Betonica officinalis, S. betonica* (Bishop's wort, Wood betony). Erect, almost hairless to densely hairy perennial with rosettes of ovate-oblong to oblong, scalloped, wrinkled, veined, mid-green leaves, to 12cm (5in) long, heart-shaped at the bases. Upright stems bear dense, oblong spikes of reddish purple, pink, or white flowers, to 1.5cm (½in) long, from early summer to early autumn. ↕60cm (24in), ↔30cm (12in). Europe. ❄❄❄. **'Rosea Superba'** has rose-pink flowers and slightly paler green leaves.
S. olympica see *S. byzantina.*
S. 'Primrose Heron' see *S. byzantina* 'Primrose Heron'.
S. 'Silver Carpet' see *S. byzantina* 'Silver Carpet'.
S. spicata see *S. macrantha.*
S. sylvatica (Hedge woundwort). Unpleasant smelling, creeping, glandular-hairy perennial producing heart- to lance-shaped, toothed, mid-green leaves, 4–14cm (1½–5½in) long. Spikes of usually white-marked, dull reddish purple, occasionally pink or white flowers, to 1.5cm (½in) long, are borne from summer to autumn. ↕to 1m (3ft), ↔40–120cm (16–48in). Europe, W. Asia. ❄❄❄

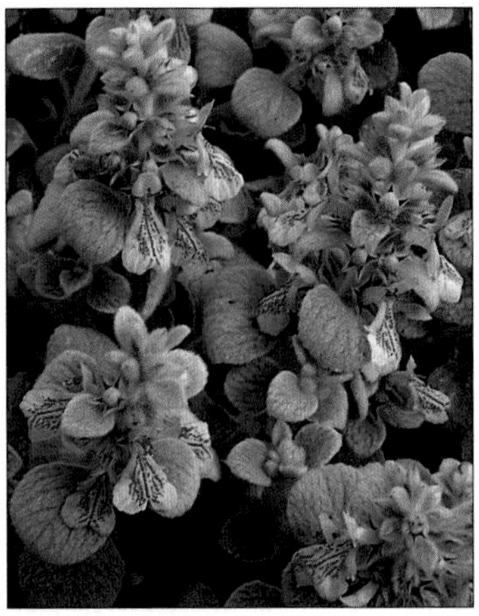

Stachys candida

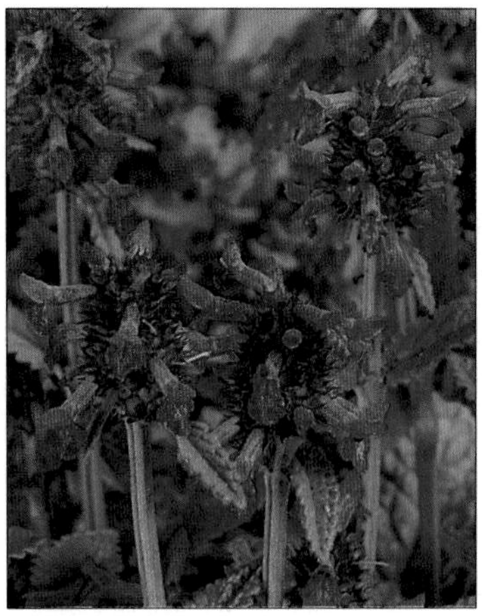

Stachys officinalis

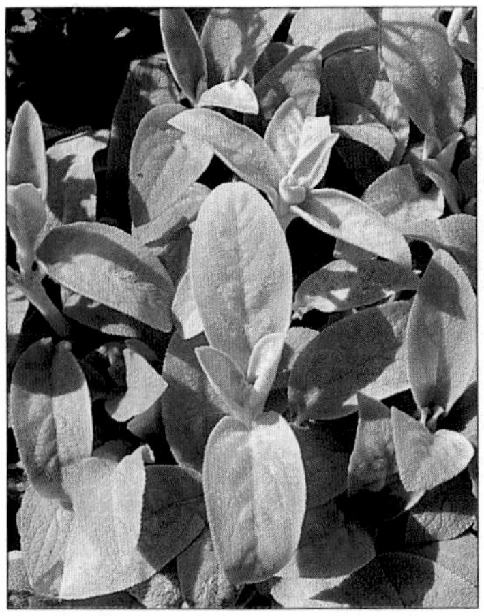

Stachys byzantina 'Primrose Heron'

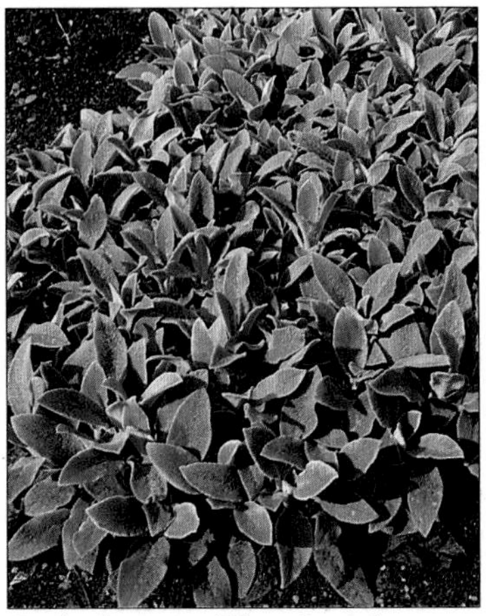

Stachys byzantina 'Silver Carpet'

Stachys macrantha 'Superba'

STACHYURUS

STACHYURACEAE

Genus of about 6 species of deciduous or semi-evergreen shrubs, occasionally small trees, found in woodland and thickets in the Himalayas and E. Asia. They are cultivated for their pendent racemes of small, 4-petalled flowers, produced from the leaf axils on bare shoots, before the leaves emerge. The alternate, simple, usually lance-shaped-oblong to broadly ovate, toothed leaves are borne on slender, glossy, red-brown shoots. Suitable for a shrub border, or for growing in a woodland garden or against a wall.
• **HARDINESS** Fully hardy.
• **CULTIVATION** Grow in light, moist but well-drained, humus-rich, fertile, acid soil in full sun or partial shade, with shelter from cold, drying winds. Pruning group 1; cut out flowered shoots to the base on mature plants, after flowering. S
• **PROPAGATION** Sow seed in containers in a cold frame in autumn. Take heeled, semi-ripe cuttings in summer.
• **PESTS AND DISEASES** Trouble free.

S. chinensis. Spreading, deciduous shrub with arching shoots and ovate, abruptly pointed, dark green leaves, to 12cm (5in) long. Bell-shaped, pale yellow flowers, 8mm (⅜in) across, are borne in racemes, to 13cm (5in) long, in late winter and early spring. ↕2m (6ft), ↔4m (12ft). China. ❄❄❄
S. praecox 🏆 Open, spreading, deciduous shrub with arching, red-purple shoots and ovate, tapered, mid-green leaves, to 18cm (7in) long. Bell-shaped, pale yellow-green flowers, 8mm (⅜in) across, are borne in racemes, to 10cm (4in) long, in late winter and early spring, ↕1–4m (3–12ft), ↔3m (10ft).

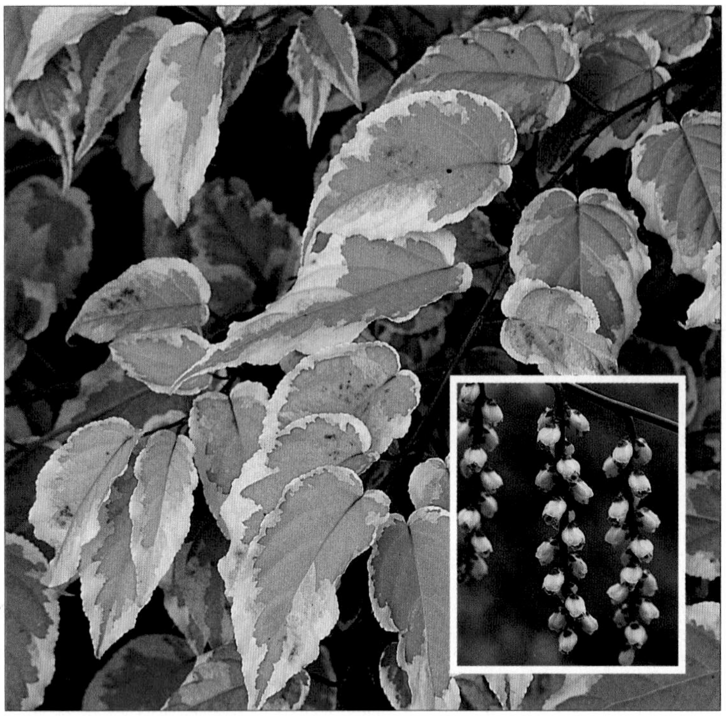

Stachyurus praecox 'Magpie' (inset: flower detail)

Japan. ❄❄❄. **'Magpie'** ■ is less vigorous than the species, with broad, creamy white margins to the leaves; ↕1.5m (5ft), ↔ 2m (6ft).

▷**Staff tree** see *Celastrus scandens*
▷**Stagger-bush** see *Lyonia mariana*
▷**Staghorn, South American** see *Platycerium alicorne*
▷**Staghorn fern** see *Platycerium*
Common see *P. bifurcatum*

STANGERIA

STANGERIACEAE

Genus of one species of fern-like cycad found in dry, open woodland and scrub in South Africa. It has a swollen, woody, largely underground stem, from the tip of which it produces rosettes of oval to oblong, pinnate leaves, which lack the leathery texture typical of cycads. Separate male and female, cone-like spikes ("cones") of flowers are borne from the centres of the rosettes, usually in summer. In frost-prone regions, grow *S. eriopus* in a warm greenhouse or as a houseplant. In warmer climates, grow in a border, or as a specimen plant.
• **HARDINESS** Frost tender.
• **CULTIVATION** Under glass, grow in a mix of equal parts loam, grit, coarse bark, and leaf mould, in bright filtered light with high humidity. In growth, water freely and apply a foliar fertilizer monthly. Water sparingly in winter. Pot on or top-dress in spring. Outdoors, grow in fertile, humus-rich, moist but well-drained soil in dappled shade.
• **PROPAGATION** Surface-sow seed on damp sand at 24–30°C (75–86°F) in spring. Pot up as soon as the tap root begins to form.
• **PESTS AND DISEASES** Susceptible to mealybugs and scale insects under glass.

S. eriopus ■ Fern-like cycad with a cylindrical to turnip-shaped stem or trunk, to 10cm (4in) across, with only the tip above ground. Bears one to several rosettes of long-stalked, pinnate leaves, 0.25–2m (¾–6ft) long, each with 10–40 lance-shaped to oblong, wavy, often papery, olive- to deep green leaflets, with entire or toothed margins. Cylindrical, felted, grey to yellow-brown flowering cones, to 18cm (7in) long, are produced mainly in summer. ↕ to 1m (3ft) or more, ↔ 1–2m (3–6ft). South Africa (Eastern Cape, KwaZulu/Natal). ❁ (min. 15°C/59°F)

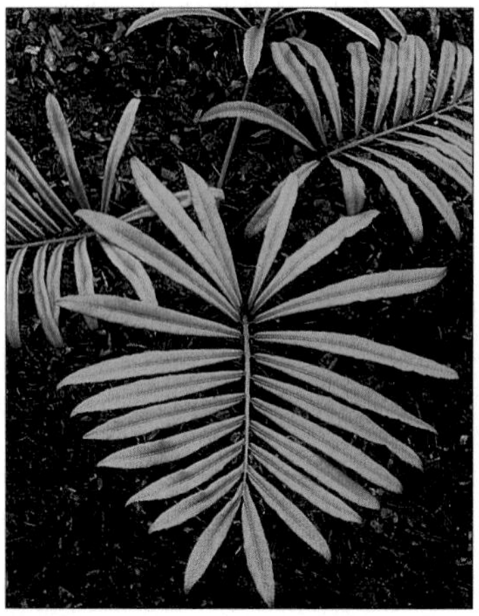

Stangeria eriopus

STANHOPEA

ORCHIDACEAE

Genus of about 30 species of evergreen, epiphytic orchids from moist forest, 1,000–2,000m (3,250–7,000ft) high, in Mexico and Central and South America. The conical, ribbed pseudobulbs each bear a single, large, semi-rigid, folded, elliptic to oblong-lance-shaped leaf. Pendent racemes of 2–10 very fragrant, short-lived flowers arise from the bases of the pseudobulbs over a long period.
• **HARDINESS** Frost tender.
• **CULTIVATION** Cool- to intermediate-growing orchids. Grow epiphytically on bark, or in epiphytic orchid compost in moss-lined, slatted baskets, to allow the pendent racemes to spread freely downwards. Provide high humidity and bright filtered light in summer, and full light in winter. In full growth, water and mist freely, and apply a half-strength balanced liquid fertilizer monthly. Water sparingly when inactive, which may be in early summer. See also p.46.
• **PROPAGATION** Divide when the plants "overflow" their containers, or remove backbulbs and pot up separately.
• **PESTS AND DISEASES** Susceptible to red spider mites, aphids, and mealybugs.

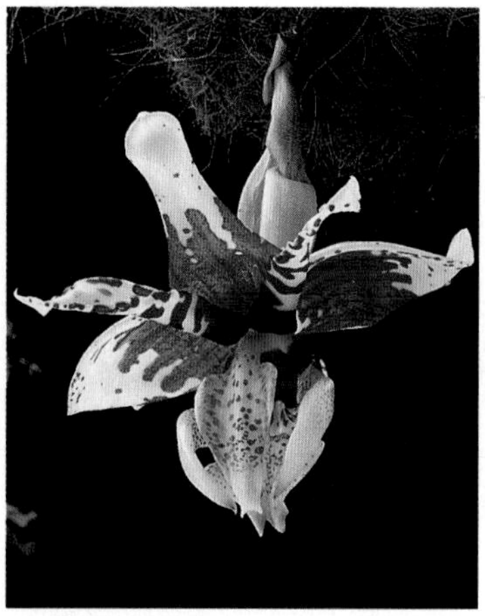

Stanhopea tigrina

S. oculata. Epiphytic orchid with one broadly elliptic or broadly lance-shaped leaf, 45cm (18in) long. Pendent racemes of waxy, maroon-spotted, light yellow, orange, or white flowers, 12cm (5in) across, are borne in summer or autumn. ↕45cm (18in), ↔ 60cm (24in). S. Mexico to Venezuela, N. Peru. ❁ (min. 11–13°C/52–55°F; max. 30°C/86°F)
S. tigrina ■♀ Epiphytic orchid with one broad, oblong leaf, 40cm (16in) long. Pendent racemes of fleshy yellow flowers, 15cm (6in) across, with dark red markings, are borne from summer to autumn. ↕45cm (18in), ↔ 60cm (24in). Mexico. ❁ (min. 11–13°C/52–55°F; max. 30°C/86°F)
S. wardii. Epiphytic orchid with one elliptic leaf, 30–45cm (12–18in) long. Pendent racemes of yellow-orange flowers, 12cm (5in) across, lightly spotted purple, are borne in summer. ↕45cm (18in), ↔ 60cm (24in). S. Mexico to Venezuela, N. Peru. ❁ (min. 11–13°C/52–55°F; max. 30°C/86°F)

STAPELIA

Carrion flower

ASCLEPIADACEAE

Genus of about 45 species of perennial succulents from low, hilly, often rocky terrain, mainly in tropical and southern Africa. They have generally erect, angular, coarsely toothed, fleshy stems, which branch from the bases to form large clumps. The rudimentary, fleshy leaves are borne at the tips of the stem teeth. Diurnal, star-shaped, often foul-smelling, solitary or clustered flowers, pollinated by blowflies and bluebottles, are produced in summer, usually from the stem bases. Where temperatures fall below 11°C (52°F), grow in a temperate or warm greenhouse. In warm, dry areas, grow in a raised bed or desert garden. Many species originally included in *Stapelia* are now classified as *Orbea*, *Orbeopsis*, *Huernia*, and other genera.

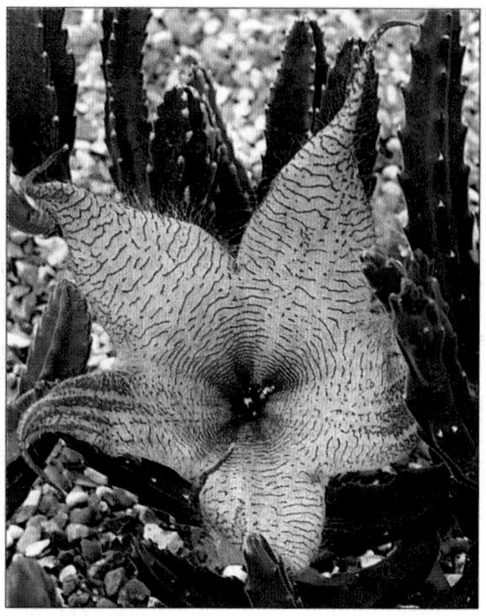

Stapelia gigantea

• **HARDINESS** Frost tender.
• **CULTIVATION** Under glass, grow in a mix of equal parts loam-based potting compost (JI No.2) and grit; top-dress with grit. Provide full light with shade from hot sun, and low humidity. When in growth, water moderately and apply a low-nitrogen fertilizer monthly. Water very sparingly at other times. Outdoors, grow in moderately fertile, gritty, sharply drained soil, in full sun with some midday shade. See also pp.48–49.
• **PROPAGATION** Sow seed at 18–21°C (64–70°F) in spring. Separate rooted sections, or take cuttings of stem sections, from spring to summer.
• **PESTS AND DISEASES** Susceptible to mealybugs, root mealybugs, and black root rot.

S. europaea see *Caralluma europaea.*
S. flavirostris see *S. grandiflora.*
S. gigantea ■♀ syn. *S. nobilis.* Very variable, clump-forming succulent with erect, 4-angled, velvety, light green stems, 3cm (1¼in) thick, with small teeth. In summer, produces malodorous, pale ochre-yellow and dark red flowers, 25–35cm (10–14in) across, with silky red hairs, numerous minute, transverse red wrinkles, and petals with white-hairy margins. ↕ to 20cm (8in), ↔ indefinite. E. southern Africa. ❁ (min. 11°C/52°F)
S. grandiflora ■ syn. *S. flavirostris.* Clump-forming succulent with erect, toothed, mid-green stems, 2–3cm (¾–1¼in) thick, with slightly winged angles, and covered with minute, velvety hairs. In summer, bears dull, purplish red flowers, to 22cm (9in) across, with hairy margins and wrinkled lobes, lined

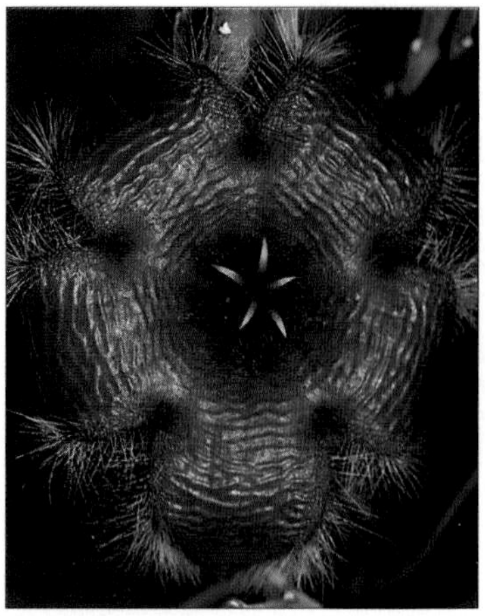

Stapelia grandiflora

S

with purple and yellow, becoming rich dull purple at the tips. ↕ to 30cm (12in), ↔ indefinite. South Africa (Western Cape, Eastern Cape), Lesotho. ❅ (min. 11°C/52°F)
S. nobilis see *S. gigantea.*
S. variegata see *Orbea variegata.*

STAPELIANTHUS

ASCLEPIADACEAE

Genus, closely related to *Huernia,* of about 8 species of perennial succulents from hilly lowlands in S. and S.W. Madagascar. They have often prostrate, 4- to 8-angled, fleshy, branching stems, which root down as the plant spreads; the stems sometimes have rudimentary leaves. Diurnal flowers are borne singly or in clusters from leaf axils at the bases of the stems in summer; each flower has a corona forming an erect, 5-lobed head above the staminal column. Where temperatures fall below 10°C (50°F), grow in a temperate or warm greenhouse. In warm, dry climates, use in a desert garden.
- **HARDINESS** Frost tender.
- **CULTIVATION** Under glass, grow in shallow pans in a mix of equal parts loam-based potting compost (JI No.2) and grit; top-dress with grit. Provide bright filtered light and low humidity. In growth, water moderately and apply a low-nitrogen fertilizer monthly. Water sparingly at other times. Outdoors, grow in gritty, sharply drained, moderately fertile soil in full sun with some midday shade. See also pp.48–49.
- **PROPAGATION** Sow seed at 18–21°C (64–70°F) in spring. Take cuttings of stem sections in spring and summer.
- **PESTS AND DISEASES** Trouble free.

S. hardyi. Mat-forming succulent with prostrate, 4- to 6-angled, greyish green stems, 8mm (3/8in) thick, producing small, rudimentary leaves at the tips. Bell-shaped, fleshy, yellowish pink and purplish brown flowers, 1.5cm (1/2in) across, with triangular, pointed lobes, densely covered in soft, purplish brown hairs, are borne in summer. ↕ 8cm (3in), ↔ 15cm (6in). Madagascar. ❅ (min. 10°C/50°F)
S. madagascariensis. Semi-erect or creeping succulent with 6- to 8-angled, red-spotted, grey-green stems, to 8mm (3/8in) thick, with tubercles bearing small, thin, linear, scale-like leaves. In summer, produces bell-shaped, pale yellow, red-marked flowers, to 2cm (3/4in) across; they have triangular, broadly spreading lobes with red papillae on the upper surfaces. ↕ to 5cm (2in), ↔ 12cm (5in). Madagascar. ❅ (min. 10°C/50°F)

STAPELIOPSIS

ASCLEPIADACEAE

Genus of 5 or 6 species of perennial succulents from hilly lowlands of Namibia and South Africa. They have 4-angled, fleshy, minutely hairy, usually toothed, purple-spotted, mid-green stems; in some species these bear tiny leaves. Diurnal, stalked, urn-shaped flowers develop from the bases of new shoots in summer. Where temperatures fall below 10°C (50°F), grow in a temperate or warm greenhouse. In warm, dry areas, use in a desert garden.
- **HARDINESS** Frost tender.
- **CULTIVATION** Under glass, grow in shallow pans in a mix of equal parts loam-based potting compost (JI No.2) and grit; top-dress with grit. Provide bright filtered light and low humidity. In the growing season, water moderately and apply a low-nitrogen fertilizer monthly. Water sparingly at other times. Outdoors, grow in moderately fertile, gritty, sharply drained soil in full sun, with midday shade. See also pp.48–49.
- **PROPAGATION** Sow seed at 18–21°C (64–70°F) in spring. Take cuttings of stem sections in spring and summer.
- **PESTS AND DISEASES** Trouble free.

S. pillansii, syn. *Pectinaria pillansii.* Clustering succulent with usually prostrate, 4-angled, dark green stems, 1cm (1/2in) thick, with prominent brown teeth. Red flowers, 7mm (1/4in) across, pale red inside, with watery papillae, are produced at ground level in summer. ↕ 8cm (3in), ↔ 18cm (7in). South Africa (Eastern Cape). ❅ (min. 10°C/50°F)
S. urniflora. Clump-forming succulent with prostrate, brown-marked, rounded, 4-angled, minutely papillose, greyish green, partially subterranean stems, 2cm (3/4in) thick. The stems have laterally compressed teeth, and tiny, scale-like, deciduous leaves, to 2mm (1/16in) long. Red flowers, 1.5cm (1/2in) across, hairless outside, densely hairy and papillose inside, are borne in summer. ↕↔ to 8cm (3in). Namibia. ❅ (min. 10°C/50°F)

STAPHYLEA

Bladdernut

STAPHYLEACEAE

Genus of about 11 species of deciduous shrubs or small trees found in woodland and thickets in N. temperate regions. They are grown for their bell- or cup-shaped, white, cream, or pink flowers, borne in terminal panicles, and for their curious, bladder-like, 2- or 3-lobed fruits. The opposite leaves are pinnate or 3- to 5-palmate. Suitable for a shrub border or woodland garden.

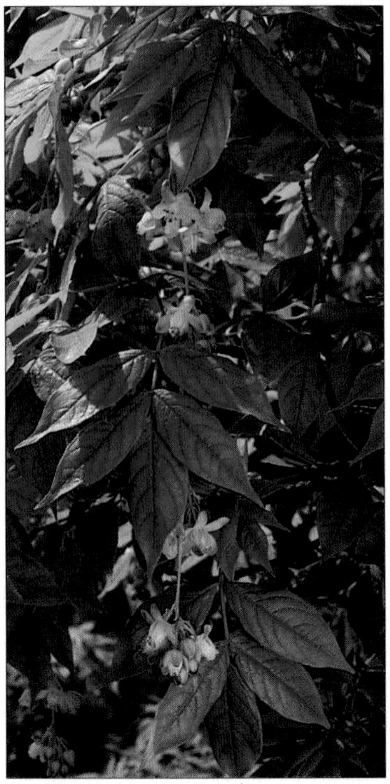
Staphylea pinnata

- **HARDINESS** Fully hardy.
- **CULTIVATION** Grow in any moist but well-drained soil in full sun or partial shade. Pruning group 1 or 2.
- **PROPAGATION** Sow seed in containers in a cold frame in autumn. Root greenwood cuttings in early summer, or semi-ripe cuttings in midsummer, both with bottom heat.
- **PESTS AND DISEASES** Trouble free.

S. colchica ♀ Upright shrub with stout shoots and pinnate, glossy, mid-green leaves, each with 3–5 ovate-oblong leaflets, 4–9cm (1½–3½in) long. In late spring, bears bell-shaped, fragrant white flowers, to 2cm (3/4in) long, in panicles to 12cm (5in) long; they are followed by greenish white fruit, to 10cm (4in) long. ↕↔ 3.5m (11ft). Caucasus. ❄❄❄
S. holocarpa ♀ Upright shrub or spreading, small tree bearing 3-palmate, blue-green leaves with oblong to lance-shaped leaflets, 3–10cm (1¼–4in) long. Bell-shaped, white to pink flowers, to 1.5cm (1/2in) long, are borne in nodding panicles, to 10cm (4in) long, in mid- and late spring, before the leaves; they are followed by greenish white fruit, to 5cm (2in) long. ↕ 10m (30ft), ↔ 6m (20ft). China. ❄❄❄. **'Rosea'** ♀ has bronze young leaves and pink flowers.
S. pinnata ■ (Bladdernut). Upright shrub with stout shoots and pinnate leaves, each comprised of 5–7 ovate-oblong leaflets, 5–10cm (2–4in) long, dark green above, slightly glaucous beneath. In late spring and early summer, bears bell-shaped, fragrant, pink-tinged white flowers, 1cm (1/2in) long, in pendent panicles, to 10cm (4in) long; they are followed by greenish white fruit, to 4cm (1½in) long. ↕↔ 5m (15ft). Europe, Turkey, Caucasus. ❄❄❄

▷**Star cluster** see *Pentas lanceolata*
Egyptian see *P. lanceolata*
▷**Starfish plant** see *Cryptanthus*
▷**Starflower** see *Calytrix, Hypoxis, Mentzelia*
▷**Starfruit** see *Damasonium*
▷**Star glory** see *Ipomoea quamoclit*
▷**Star-of-Bethlehem** see *Campanula isophylla, Ornithogalum, O. umbellatum*
▷**Star of the veldt** see *Dimorphotheca sinuata*
▷**Starwort,**
Autumn see *Callitriche hermaphroditica*
Water see *Callitriche*
▷**Statice** see *Limonium, L. sinuatum, Psylliostachys*
Tatarian see *Goniolimon tataricum*
▷***Statice bellidifolia*** see *Limonium bellidifolium*
▷***Statice minuta*** see *Limonium minutum*
▷***Statice spicata*** see *Psylliostachys spicata*
▷***Statice suworowii*** see *Psylliostachys suworowii*

STAUNTONIA

LARDIZABALACEAE

Genus of up to 16 species of twining, woody, mostly dioecious, evergreen climbers occurring in woodland from Burma to Taiwan and Japan. They are cultivated for their handsome, alternate, palmate leaves, for their bell-shaped flowers, borne in few-flowered, axillary racemes, and for their ellipsoid, edible

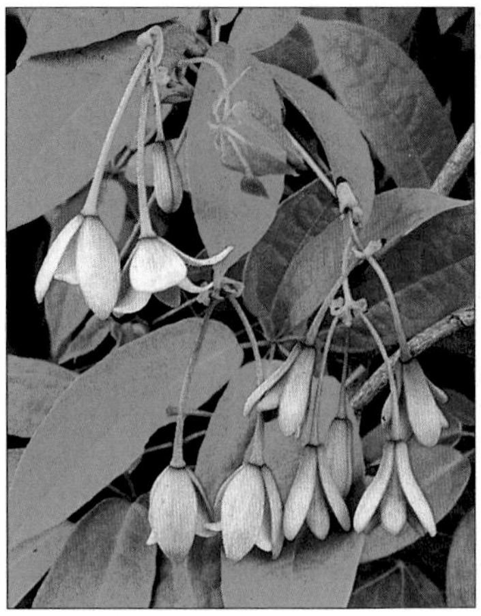
Stauntonia hexaphylla

fruits. Grow over a large shrub or through a tree, or train on wires against a wall. In areas of severe frost, grow stauntonias in a cool greenhouse.
- **HARDINESS** Frost hardy to frost tender.
- **CULTIVATION** Under glass, grow in loam-based potting compost (JI No.3) in full light, with shade from hot sun. When in full growth, water freely and apply a balanced liquid fertilizer every 4 weeks. Water sparingly in winter. Outdoors, grow in fertile, well-drained soil, in a warm, sheltered site in full sun or partial shade, with suitable support. Pruning group 11, in early spring.
- **PROPAGATION** Sow seed at 13–16°C (55–61°F) in spring. Take semi-ripe cuttings in summer.
- **PESTS AND DISEASES** Trouble free.

S. hexaphylla ■ Fast-growing, dioecious, evergreen climber producing 3- to 7-palmate, mid- to dark green leaves, to 15cm (6in) long, with oval to elliptic, leathery leaflets. Racemes of cup-shaped, fragrant, violet-tinged white flowers, 2cm (3/4in) across, are borne in spring. If pollinated, females produce ellipsoid, edible purple fruit, 5cm (2in) long. ↕ 10m (30ft) or more. S. Korea, Japan. ❄❄

▷***Steironema ciliata*** see *Lysimachia ciliata*

STENANTHIUM

LILIACEAE/MELANTHIACEAE

Genus of about 5 species of bulbous perennials from moist slopes in grassland or open woodland on Sakhalin Island (Russia), and in North America, including Mexico. They have arching, grass-like, mostly basal leaves and erect, slender stems bearing terminal racemes or panicles of small, bell- or star-shaped flowers. Grow in a border, peat bed, or in woodland.
- **HARDINESS** Fully hardy to frost hardy.
- **CULTIVATION** Plant bulbs 10cm (4in) deep in autumn, in moist but well-drained, moderately fertile, humus-rich, neutral to acid soil, in a sheltered site in partial shade. They dislike hot, dry conditions.
- **PROPAGATION** Sow seed in containers in a cold frame as soon as ripe.
- **PESTS AND DISEASES** Trouble free.

S. angustifolium see *S. gramineum.*
S. gramineum, syn. *S. angustifolium.* Bulbous perennial with 4 erect, linear,

keeled, channelled, bright green, basal leaves, 30–40cm (12–16in) long. In summer, bears star-shaped, fragrant, white or greenish white to purple flowers, to 2cm (¾in) across, in dense, often arching panicles, to 60cm (24in) long. ↕ 1–2m (3–6ft), ↔ 30cm (12in). S.E. USA. ❄❄. **var. *robustum*,** syn. *S. robustum*, has broader leaves and white or green flowers; ↕ to 1.8m (6ft)

S. robustum see *S. gramineum* var. *robustum*.

STENOCACTUS

syn. ECHINOFOSSULOCACTUS

CACTACEAE

Genus of about 10 species of variable, simple, rarely clustering, spherical, perennial cacti from shaded lowlands in Mexico. The stems have numerous, frequently undulating ribs, often with tubercles, and well-spaced areoles bearing variable spines, which are curved or straight, sometimes flat and dagger-like. Bell- or funnel-shaped, sometimes striped flowers develop from the crowns in spring, often in clusters. In frost-prone areas, grow as houseplants or in a temperate greenhouse. In warm, dry climates, use in a desert garden.

- **HARDINESS** Frost tender.
- **CULTIVATION** Under glass, grow in standard cactus compost in full light with low humidity. When in growth, water moderately and apply a low-nitrogen liquid fertilizer at every third or fourth watering. Keep completely dry at other times. Outdoors, grow in poor, humus-rich, gritty, sharply drained soil in full sun, with some midday shade. See also pp.48–49.
- **PROPAGATION** Sow seed at 21°C (70°F) in early spring.
- **PESTS AND DISEASES** Susceptible to aphids while flowering.

S. coptonogonus ▣ syn. *Echinofossulocactus coptonogonus*. Simple cactus producing a depressed-spherical to spherical, grey to blue-green stem with 10–14 deeply scalloped, acute ribs. White areoles bear 3–5 flat, upward-curving, pale brownish red spines, fading to very pale brown, the upper spines to 3cm (1¼in) long, the lower ones to 1.5cm (½in). In spring, bears clusters of funnel-shaped, white to purple flowers, 3cm (1¼in) long, with a pink-purple or violet mid-stripe on each petal. ↕ to 10cm (4in), ↔ 16cm (6in). C. Mexico. ❀ (min. 7°C/45°F)

S

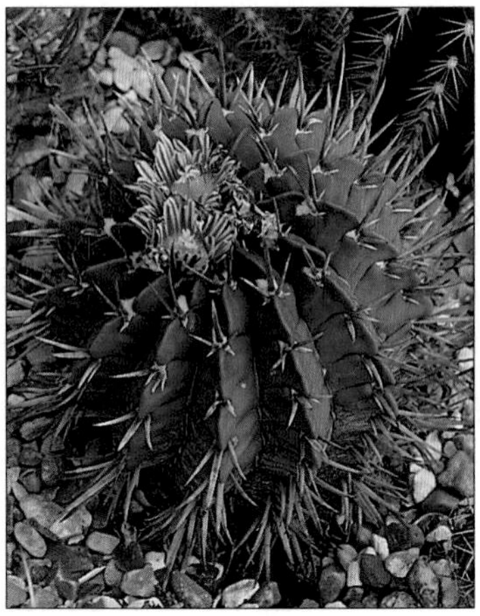

Stenocactus coptonogonus

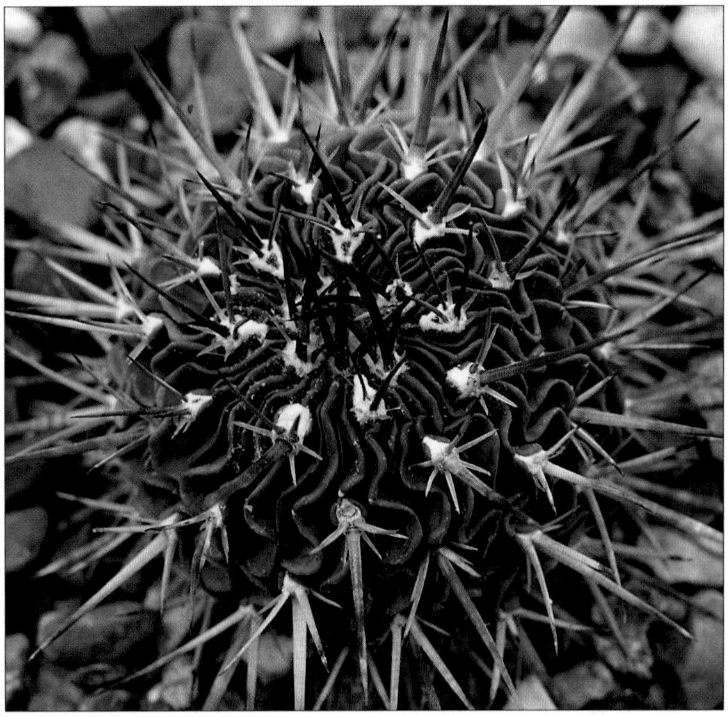

Stenocactus obvallatus

S. crispatus, syn. *Echinofossulocactus lamellosus*. Simple or clustering cactus with spherical, dark green to blue-green stems, each with 26–60 wavy ribs. White-woolly areoles bear brown-tipped white spines: 6–10 flat, straight radials, to 2cm (1¾in) long; 3 or 4 flattened, slightly curved centrals, 3.5cm (1½in) long. Solitary, funnel-shaped, carmine-red flowers, 4cm (1½in) long, are borne in spring. ↕ 10cm (4in), ↔ 8cm (3in). C. to S. Mexico. ❀ (min. 7°C/45°F)

S. multicostatus, syn. *Echinofossulocactus multicostatus*. Simple or clustering cactus producing flattened-spherical to spherical, pale green stems with 100 or more wavy ribs; each rib bears about 2 white-woolly areoles with 6–18 flat, straight or curved, yellow or grey spines, the upper ones to 8cm (3in) long, the lower to 1.5cm (½in). In spring, bears clusters of funnel-shaped flowers, 2.5cm (1in) long, pinkish purple or white with a purplish violet or faint pink stripe on each petal. ↕↔ 10cm (4in). N.E. Mexico. ❀ (min. 7°C/45°F)

S. obvallatus ▣ syn. *Echinofossulocactus pentacanthus, E. violaciflorus*. Simple cactus producing a spherical, greyish blue-green stem with 20–50 wavy-margined ribs. White areoles bear 5–12 flat, straight or curved, greyish brown spines, the upper and lateral ones to 5cm (2in) long, the lower to 1cm (½in). In spring, bears solitary, funnel-shaped, pale yellow or pale pink flowers, 2cm (¾in) long, with a purplish red stripe on each petal. ↕↔ 8cm (3in). N. and E. central Mexico. ❀ (min. 7°C/45°F)

STENOCARPUS

PROTEACEAE

Genus of up to 22 species of evergreen shrubs and trees from Malaysia, New Caledonia, and Australia. The trees usually grow in rainforest; the shrubs are found in open scrub, often along water-courses. They have alternate, simple to pinnatifid leaves and, in summer, bear axillary umbels of tubular, cream to red flowers, each with a knob-shaped stigma protruding through a split on the lower side of the tube. In frost-prone areas, use in a temperate greenhouse as foliage plants (flowering is rare in containers). In warmer areas, use as specimen plants.

- **HARDINESS** Frost tender, but some species may survive brief falls in temperature to around 0°C (32°F).
- **CULTIVATION** Under glass, grow in loam-based potting compost (JI No.3) in full light, shaded from hot sun. When in growth, water moderately and apply a balanced liquid fertilizer every month. Water sparingly in winter. Outdoors, grow in fertile, humus-rich, moist but well drained soil in full sun, with some midday shade; shelter from cold, drying winds. Pruning group 1; may need restrictive pruning under glass.
- **PROPAGATION** Sow seed at 15–20°C (59–68°F) as soon as ripe or in spring (seedlings take about 7 years to flower). Root semi-ripe cuttings with bottom heat in summer.
- **PESTS AND DISEASES** Trouble free.

S. sinuatus ▣ ◊ (Firewheel tree). Slow-growing, columnar tree with erect branches and branchlets. The leathery, wavy-margined, glossy, deep green leaves, 60cm (24in) long, are sometimes red beneath, and may be oblong-lance-shaped or deeply lobed, with up to 8 lance-shaped lobes, to 10cm (4in) long. Plants over 3m (10ft) tall bear wheel-like umbels of 12–20 scarlet flowers, to 2.5cm (1in) long, in summer. ↕ 20–30m (70–100ft), ↔ 5–15m (15–50ft). Australia (Queensland, New South Wales). ❀ (min. 7–10°C/45–50°F)

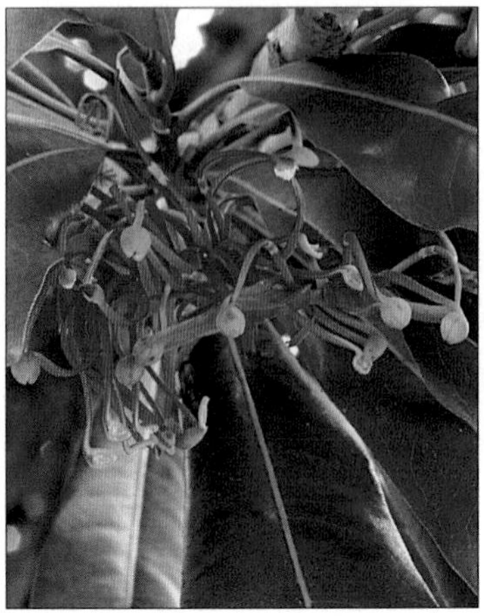

Stenocarpus sinuatus

STENOCEREUS

CACTACEAE

Genus of about 25 species of tree-like or shrubby, sometimes clump-forming, perennial cacti found on low hillsides in the USA (Arizona), Mexico, Central America, Colombia, Venezuela, and the West Indies. The prominently ribbed stems are often densely spined. The funnel- or bell-shaped, usually nocturnal flowers, borne in spring or summer, are followed by ovoid, fleshy, spiny fruits. Where temperatures fall below 13°C (55°F), grow in a warm greenhouse. In warmer climates, use in a desert garden.

- **HARDINESS** Frost tender.
- **CULTIVATION** Under glass, grow in a mix of 3 parts standard cactus compost and 1 part leaf mould, in full light with low humidity. From mid-spring to early autumn, water moderately and apply a low-nitrogen liquid fertilizer monthly. Keep completely dry at other times. Outdoors, grow in poor to moderately fertile, humus-rich, sharply drained, gritty soil in full sun. See also pp.48–49.
- **PROPAGATION** Sow seed at 21°C (70°F) in spring. Take cuttings of stem sections in summer.
- **PESTS AND DISEASES** Prone to scale insects and aphids while flowering.

S. eruca ▣ syn. *Machaerocereus eruca* (Creeping devil). Bushy, creeping cactus that roots all along its prostrate, 10- to 12-ribbed, mid-green stems, 4–10cm (1½–4in) thick, with only the stem tips erect. Brown areoles bear pale yellow to white spines (about 20 radials, 1 flattened, dagger-like central). In spring, produces nocturnal, funnel-shaped, white or pale yellow, sometimes pink-tinged flowers, 10–14cm (4–5½in) long. ↕ to 30cm (12in), ↔ indefinite. N.W. Mexico. ❀ (min. 13°C/55°F)

S. marginatus, syn. *Marginatocereus marginatus*. Tree-like cactus with erect, freely branching, 5- to 7-ribbed, dark greyish green stems, to 30cm (12in)

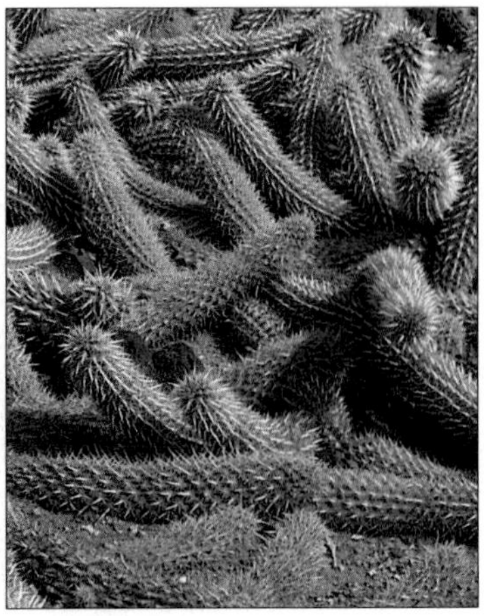

Stenocereus eruca

thick. Brown-woolly areoles bear brown spines (7–9 radials, 1 or 2 centrals), which fall as the plant matures. Diurnal, bell-shaped white flowers, red outside, 4–5cm (1½–2in) long, are produced at the stem tips in summer. ↕↔ 6m (20ft). C. and S. Mexico. ❀ (min. 13°C/55°F)
S. thurberi, syn. *Lemaireocereus thurberi*. Columnar cactus, branching from the base to form clumps, with erect, greyish green stems, 10–20cm (4–8in) thick, with 12–19 prominent ribs. Brown areoles bear almost black or brown spines (7–10 radials, 1–3 longer centrals). Mainly nocturnal, funnel-shaped, purple or pink flowers, 6–8cm (2½–3in) long, with red sepals, are borne in summer. ↕ 3–7m (10–22ft), ↔ 1m (3ft). USA (Arizona), Mexico (Baja California). ❀ (min. 13°C/55°F)

▷ ***Stenolobium stans*** see *Tecoma stans*

STENOMESSON
syn. URCEOLINA
AMARYLLIDACEAE

Genus of about 20 species of bulbous perennials from rocky, upland slopes and meadows in the Andes, South America. They are grown for their umbels of pendent, tubular, brightly coloured flowers, borne on solid, sometimes 4-angled stems mainly from spring to summer. The semi-erect, linear to lance-shaped, occasionally channelled or keeled, basal leaves often elongate after flowering. In frost-prone areas, grow in a temperate greenhouse or conservatory. In warmer areas, grow in a border.
• **HARDINESS** Half hardy to frost tender.
• **CULTIVATION** Plant in autumn with the neck and shoulders of the bulb above soil level. Under glass, grow in loam-based potting compost (JI No.2) in full light, shaded from hot sun. Water sparingly until in active growth, then water moderately and apply a balanced liquid fertilizer every 2 weeks. Reduce water as leaves wither, and keep barely moist when dormant. Pot on every 3 years. Outdoors, grow in well-drained, moderately fertile soil in a sheltered site in full sun; protect with a mulch in winter. Roots resent disturbance.
• **PROPAGATION** Sow seed at 16–18°C (61–64°F) in spring. Divide in autumn.
• **PESTS AND DISEASES** Trouble free.

S. coccineum. Bulbous perennial with narrow, strap-shaped leaves, to 30cm (12in) long, which appear as the flowers open, and then elongate. Umbels of 4–8 nodding, tubular, bright crimson flowers, 4cm (1½in) long, are produced from spring to summer. ↕ 30cm (12in), ↔ 15cm (6in). Peru. ❀ (min. 7–10°C/45–50°F)

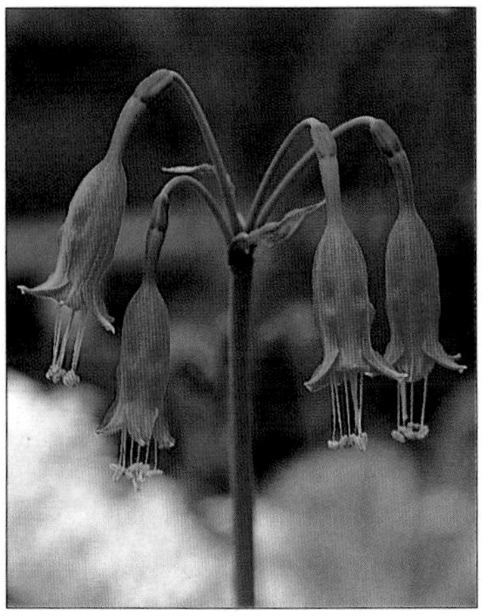

Stenomesson miniatum

S. incarnatum see *S. variegatum*.
S. miniatum ■ syn. *Urceolina pendula*, *U. peruviana*. Bulbous perennial bearing umbels of 3–6 pendent, tubular, bright red or orange flowers, 3–3.5cm (1¼–1½in) long, with protruding stamens, from spring to summer. Narrow, strap-shaped leaves, to 40cm (16in) long, develop after the flowers. ↕ 30cm (12in), ↔ 15cm (6in). Peru, Bolivia. ❀ (min. 7–10°C/45–50°F)
S. variegatum, syn. *S. incarnatum*. Bulbous perennial with strap-shaped leaves elongating to 60–75cm (24–30in) long after flowering. In spring, usually 4-angled stems bear umbels of up to 6 pendent, tubular, white, yellow, pink, or scarlet flowers, to 13cm (5in) long, sometimes with bands of another colour, all with a green mark on each tepal. ↕ 40–60cm (16–24in), ↔ 24cm (10in). Ecuador, Peru, Bolivia. ❀ (min. 7–10°C/45–50°F)

STENOTAPHRUM
GRAMINEAE/POACEAE

Genus of about 6 species of annual and perennial grasses, widespread in tropical and subtropical regions worldwide, on seashores or near the coast, occasionally inland. The creeping or ascending stems root at the nodes, and bear linear to lance-shaped, flat or folded, upright leaves, sheathing at the bases. Greenish brown spikelets are borne in axillary and terminal racemes. *S. secundatum* and *S. secundatum* 'Variegatum' are the most commonly grown, and are valued for their foliage. In frost-prone climates, treat perennials as annuals, or grow in a cool greenhouse as ground cover or in hanging baskets. Use as lawn grasses in tropical and subtropical climates; *S. secundatum* 'Variegatum' is also suitable for a border.
• **HARDINESS** Frost tender.
• **CULTIVATION** Under glass, grow in loam-based potting compost (JI No.2) in full light. When in growth, water freely and apply a balanced liquid fertilizer every 2 weeks. Water sparingly in winter. Container-grown plants thrive and continue to look attractive if given a winter minimum temperature of 12°C (54°F). Outdoors, grow in moist but well-drained, fertile soil in full sun. In frost-prone areas, plant out only when danger of frost has passed.
• **PROPAGATION** Divide in spring. Take nodal cuttings in late spring or during summer.
• **PESTS AND DISEASES** Trouble free.

S. secundatum (Buffalo grass, St. Augustine grass). Stoloniferous, prostrate, evergreen, perennial grass. Almost rigid, flattened, branching stems bear linear-oblong, flat to folded, bluish green leaves, to 15cm (6in) long. In late summer and early autumn, produces greenish brown, flattened, spike-like racemes, to 10cm (4in) long. ↕ 15cm (6in), ↔ indefinite. Central America, tropical South America. ❀ (min. 5°C/41°F). **'Variegatum'** ♀ has pale green leaves with ivory-white stripes.

STENOTUS
ASTERACEAE/COMPOSITAE

Genus of 18 species of tufted, evergreen subshrubs found in dry, rocky places in W. North America. They produce mainly basal, alternate, leathery, simple, entire leaves and solitary, daisy-like flowerheads. Grow in a rock garden.
• **HARDINESS** Fully hardy to frost hardy.
• **CULTIVATION** Grow in gritty, poor to moderately fertile, sharply drained soil in full sun.
• **PROPAGATION** Sow seed in containers in a cold frame in spring.
• **PESTS AND DISEASES** Trouble free.

S. acaulis, syn. *Haplopappus acaulis*. Mat-forming subshrub producing erect, slender stems and inversely lance-shaped, tapered, dark green leaves, to 6cm (2½in) long. Solitary, daisy-like yellow flowerheads, to 2.5cm (1in) across, are borne in summer. ↕ 15cm (6in), ↔ 45cm (18in). W. USA. ✻✻✻

STEPHANANDRA
ROSACEAE

Genus, related to *Spiraea*, of 4 species of suckering, deciduous shrubs occurring in thickets and at woodland margins in E. Asia. They have attractive leaves, which are alternate, narrowly ovate to ovate, lobed, and sharply toothed, and have good autumn colour. The tiny, star-shaped, greenish white or yellow-green flowers are produced in terminal, corymb-like panicles during summer. Suitable for a shrub border.
• **HARDINESS** Fully hardy.
• **CULTIVATION** Grow in moist but well-drained, fertile soil in full sun or partial shade. Pruning group 2.
• **PROPAGATION** Separate rooted suckers from autumn to early spring. Take greenwood cuttings in early summer, semi-ripe cuttings in summer, or hardwood cuttings in late autumn.
• **PESTS AND DISEASES** Trouble free.

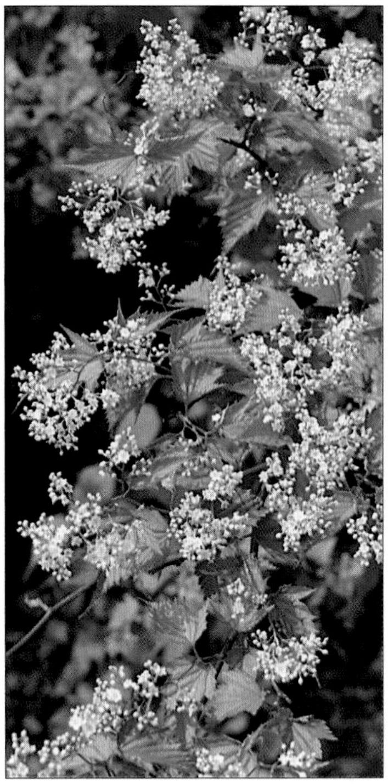

Stephanandra tanakae

S. incisa. Thicket-forming shrub with arching shoots, rich brown in winter, and ovate, sharply lobed, toothed, mid-green leaves, to 8cm (3in) long, turning orange-yellow in autumn. Greenish white flowers are produced in panicles, to 8cm (3in) long, in early summer. ↕ to 2m (6ft), ↔ 3m (10ft). Korea, Japan, Taiwan. ✻✻✻. **'Crispa'** ■ has deeply lobed, wavy-margined leaves; ↕ 60cm (24in).
S. tanakae ■ Thicket-forming shrub with arching, orange-brown shoots and broadly ovate, 3- to 5-lobed, sharply toothed, mid-green leaves, to 12cm (5in) long, turning orange and yellow in autumn. In early and midsummer, bears yellow-green flowers in panicles to 10cm (4in) long. ↕↔ 3m (10ft). Japan. ✻✻✻

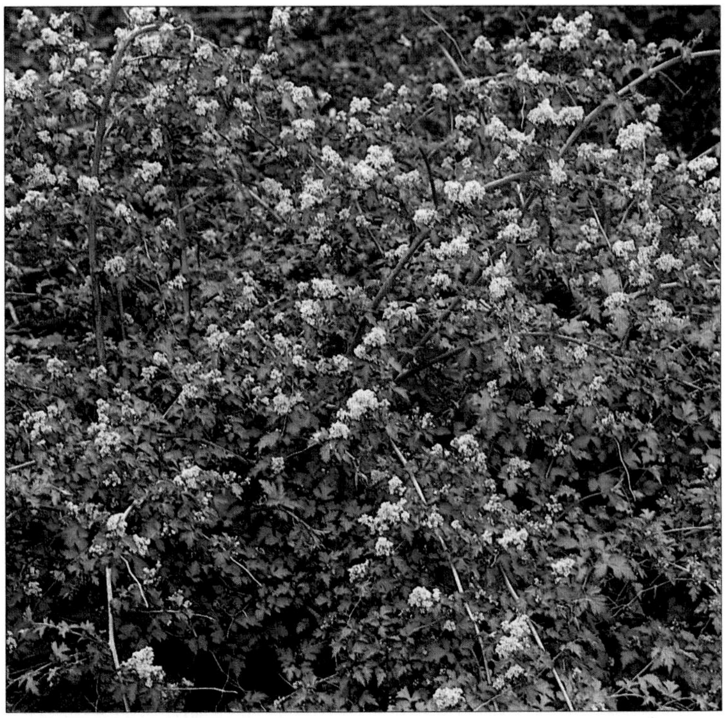

Stephanandra incisa 'Crispa'

S

STEPHANOCEREUS

CACTACEAE

Genus of one species of columnar, rarely branching, ribbed, perennial cactus from stony, rocky sites in E. Brazil. The stems, with rings of bristles at the joints, eventually develop woolly cephaliums at the tips; during summer, the tips bear tubular, nocturnal flowers, followed by ovoid, mid-green fruit, 5cm (2in) long, which take many weeks to ripen. Where temperatures fall below 13°C (55°F), grow *S. leucostele* in a warm greenhouse. In warmer areas, use in a desert garden.

• **HARDINESS** Frost tender.

• **CULTIVATION** Under glass, grow in standard cactus compost with added limestone chips, in full light with low humidity. In spring and summer, water moderately and apply a low-nitrogen liquid fertilizer every 4–5 weeks. Water sparingly at other times. Outdoors, grow in sharply drained, gritty, poor, humus-rich, neutral to alkaline soil in full sun. See also pp.48–49.

• **PROPAGATION** Sow seed at 24°C (75°F) in spring.

• **PESTS AND DISEASES** Trouble free.

S. leucostele. Erect, columnar cactus with 12- to 18-ribbed, blue-green stems, to 10cm (4in) thick. Close-set, white-hairy areoles each bear about 22 spines (20 white to yellow radials, 1 or 2 longer yellow centrals). In summer, the densely woolly cephalium produces white flowers, to 7cm (3in) long, with scaly yellow tubes. ↕ to 3m (10ft), ↔ 45cm (18in). E. Brazil. ✿ (min. 13°C/55°F)

STEPHANOTIS

ASCLEPIADACEAE

Genus of 5–15 species of evergreen, woody-stemmed climbers from tropical woodland in Africa, Madagascar, and Asia. They are grown for their strongly perfumed, waxy, tubular, usually white flowers, each with 5 spreading lobes, borne in short-stalked, axillary cymes. Leaves are opposite, ovate to elliptic, and leathery. Where temperatures fall below 15°C (59°F), grow in a warm greenhouse or as houseplants. In warmer areas, train over a pergola or on a wall.

• **HARDINESS** Frost tender.

• **CULTIVATION** Under glass, grow in loamless or loam-based potting compost (JI No.3) in full light, with shade from hot sun. In the growing season, water and mist freely, and apply a balanced liquid fertilizer every 2 or 3 weeks. Water sparingly in winter. Outdoors, grow in moderately fertile, humus-rich, moist but well-drained soil in full sun, with some midday shade. Support climbing stems. Pruning group 11, in late winter or early spring.

• **PROPAGATION** Sow seed at 18–21°C (64–70°C) in spring. Root semi-ripe cuttings with bottom heat in summer.

• **PESTS AND DISEASES** Under glass, may be infested by red spider mites, scale insects, mealybugs, and root mealybugs.

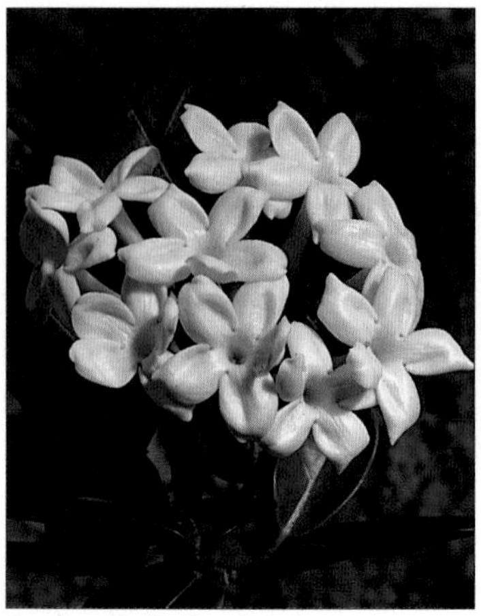

Stephanotis floribunda

S. floribunda ■ ♀ syn. *S. jasminoides* (Bridal wreath, Floradora, Madagascar jasmine). Sparsely branched, twining climber with oval to broadly elliptic, thick, glossy, mid- to deep green leaves, to 10cm (4in) or more long. From spring to autumn, bears cymes of 3–6 fragrant, waxy white flowers, 4–6cm (1½–2½in) long. ↕ 3–6m (10–20ft) or more. Madagascar. ✿ (min. 15°C/59°F)

S. jasminoides see *S. floribunda.*

▷ ***Sterculia acerifolia*** see *Brachychiton acerifolius*

▷ ***Sterculia diversifolia*** see *Brachychiton populneus*

▷ ***Sterculia platanifolia*** see *Firmiana simplex*

STERNBERGIA

Autumn daffodil

AMARYLLIDACEAE

Genus of about 8 species of bulbous perennials found on stony hillsides, in fields, and in sparse scrub or pine woodland from S. Europe and Turkey to C. Asia. They are cultivated for their crocus-like, mainly solitary, funnel- or goblet-shaped, occasionally narrow-tepalled and star-like, usually bright yellow flowers, borne on leafless stems. The erect, basal leaves are linear or strap-shaped to narrowly lance-shaped. Grow in a sunny rock garden. In frost-prone areas, grow all species except *S. lutea* and *S. sicula* in an alpine house or bulb frame; they are intolerant of winter wet.

• **HARDINESS** Frost hardy.

• **CULTIVATION** Plant bulbs 15cm (6in) deep in late summer; plant *S. candida* and *S. fischeriana* 20cm (8in) deep. Under glass, grow in equal parts loam, leaf mould, and sharp sand, in full light. Water sparingly in growth, reduce water as leaves wither, and keep completely dry when dormant. Outdoors, grow in sharply drained, moderately fertile soil in full sun. Allow large clumps to form; divide only if flowering is impaired.

• **PROPAGATION** Sow seed at 13–16°C (55–61°F) as soon as ripe. Separate offsets when dormant.

• **PESTS AND DISEASES** Prone to narcissus viruses. May be infested with large and small narcissus bulb flies and eelworms.

S. candida ■ Bulbous perennial with lance- to strap-shaped, grey-green leaves, 15cm (6in) long, followed in late winter and early spring by cup-, goblet-, or funnel-shaped, fragrant white flowers, 5cm (2in) across. ↕ 10–20cm (4–8in), ↔ 10cm (4in). S.W. Turkey. ❄❄

S. clusiana, syn. *S. macrantha.* Bulbous perennial producing funnel-shaped yellow flowers, 7cm (3in) across, in

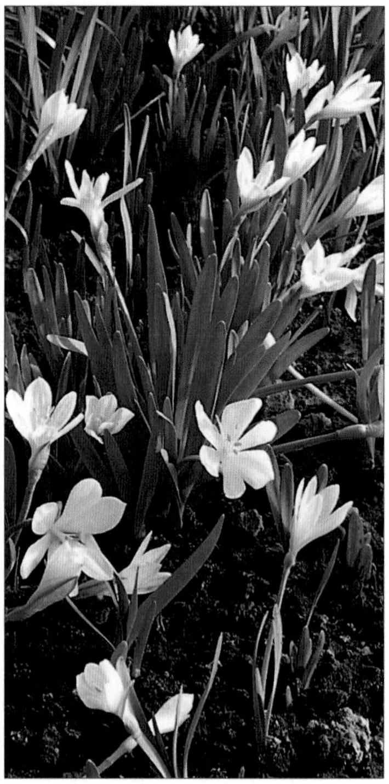

Sternbergia candida

autumn, before the strap-shaped, grey-green leaves, to 30cm (12in) long, develop. ↕ 10cm (4in), ↔ 8cm (3in). Turkey, Israel, Jordan, Iran. ❄❄

S. fischeriana. Bulbous perennial with goblet-shaped, pale yellow flowers, 3.5cm (1½in) across, borne in winter, after the strap-shaped, glossy, dark grey-green leaves, to 35cm (14in) long. Tends to divide into small, non-flowering bulbs. ↕ 8–15cm (3–6in), ↔ 8cm (3in). Caucasus to India (Kashmir). ❄❄

S. lutea ■ Very free-flowering, bulbous perennial producing goblet-shaped, deep yellow flowers, 4cm (1½in) across, in autumn, at the same time as narrowly lance-shaped, deep green leaves, to 30cm (12in) long. ↕ 15cm (6in), ↔ 8cm (3in). Spain to Afghanistan. ❄❄

S. macrantha see *S. clusiana.*

S. sicula. Variable, bulbous perennial with very narrow, strap-shaped, dark green leaves, 25cm (10in) long, with central grey stripes; these emerge before or with the star-shaped, deep yellow flowers, 1.5–3.5cm (½–1½in) across, with rounded or pointed segments, in autumn. ↕ 7cm (3in), ↔ 5cm (2in). Italy (including Sicily), Greece (including Aegean Islands, Crete), W. Turkey. ❄❄

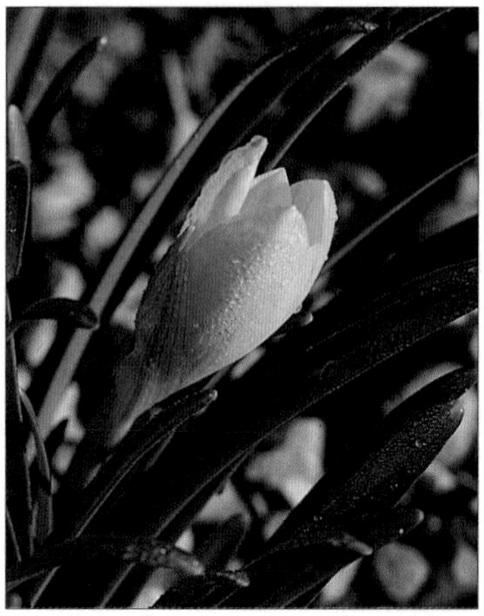

Sternbergia lutea

STEWARTIA syn. STUARTIA

THEACEAE

Genus, related to *Camellia,* of 15–20 species of deciduous or evergreen trees and shrubs from woodland in E. Asia and S.E. USA. They are grown for their often peeling bark, their simple, usually toothed leaves, which colour well in autumn, and their cup-shaped white flowers with bold stamens, borne in the leaf axils. Use as specimens in woodland.

• **HARDINESS** Fully hardy to frost hardy.

• **CULTIVATION** Grow in moist but well-drained, moderately fertile, humus-rich, neutral to acid soil in full sun or light dappled shade, with shelter from strong winds. They resent transplanting. Pruning group 1.

• **PROPAGATION** Sow seed in containers in a cold frame in autumn. Take green-wood cuttings in early summer, or semi-ripe cuttings in mid- to late summer. Layer in autumn.

• **PESTS AND DISEASES** Trouble free.

S. koreana see *S. pseudocamellia* Koreana Group.

S. malacodendron ☼ Broadly columnar, deciduous tree or upright, bushy shrub with ovate, finely toothed, dark green leaves, to 10cm (4in) long, downy beneath. Rose-like white flowers, 10cm (4in) across, cup-shaped at first, with purple stamens and often purple streaks on the petals, are borne singly along the shoots in midsummer. ↕ 7m (22ft), ↔ 3m (10ft). S.E. USA. ❄❄

S. monadelpha ■ ☼–◐ Broadly columnar to conical, deciduous tree or shrub with peeling, grey and red-brown bark. Ovate, elliptic, or lance-shaped, toothed, glossy, dark green leaves, to 10cm (4in) long, turn orange and red in autumn. In midsummer, cup-shaped white flowers, 4cm (1½in) across, with creamy filaments and violet anthers, are borne singly or in pairs along the shoots. ↕ to 25m (80ft), ↔ 8m (25ft). Korea, S. Japan. ❄❄❄

S. ovata. Broadly upright, bushy, deciduous shrub bearing ovate to lance-shaped, toothed or entire, dark green leaves, to 15cm (6in) long, red-tinged when young, downy beneath, turning orange and red in autumn. Rose-like, cup-shaped white flowers, to 10cm (4in) across, with creamy yellow or rose-pink stamens, are produced singly along the shoots in mid- and late summer. ↕ 6m (20ft), ↔ 4m (12ft). S.E. USA. ❄❄❄

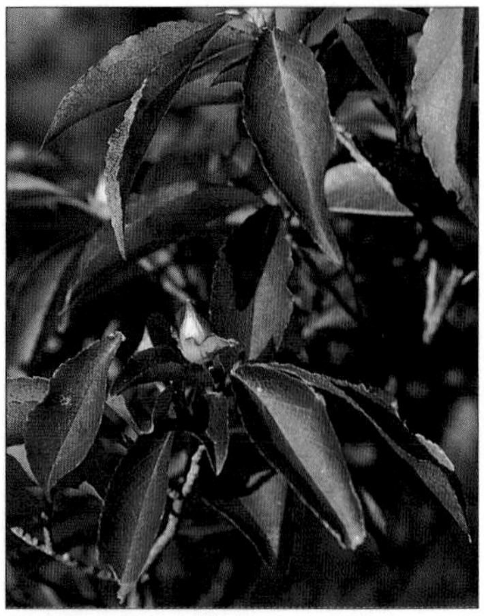

Stewartia monadelpha

S

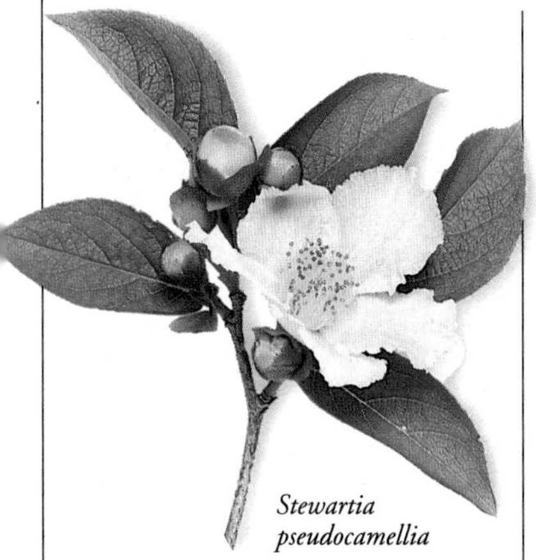

Stewartia pseudocamellia

S. pseudocamellia ▣🏆◊ Broadly columnar, deciduous tree with peeling, pink to red-brown and grey bark. Ovate to elliptic, finely toothed, dark green leaves, to 10cm (4in) long, turn yellow to orange and red in autumn. Rose-like, cup-shaped white flowers, 6cm (2½in) across, with creamy yellow stamens, are borne singly or in pairs along the shoots in midsummer. ↕20m (70ft), ↔8m (25ft). Japan. ❄❄❄. **Koreana Group** 🏆 syn. S. *koreana, S. pseudocamellia* var. *koreana*, has flowers that open more widely, to 7cm (3in) across; Korea.
S. sinensis 🏆△ Broadly conical, deciduous tree with peeling, red-brown bark and ovate or elliptic, toothed, dark green leaves, to 10cm (4in) long, turning brilliant red in autumn. Rose-like, cup-shaped, fragrant white flowers, 5cm (2in) across, are borne singly along the shoots in midsummer. ↕20m (70ft), ↔7m (22ft). C. and E. China. ❄❄❄

STIGMAPHYLLON

MALPIGHIACEAE

Genus of about 110 species of evergreen, woody-stemmed climbers, shrubs and perennials occurring in tropical woodland in Central and South America and the Caribbean, with one species from West Africa. They have simple or lobed, sometimes toothed leaves, borne in opposite pairs or nearly alternately. From spring to autumn, wide open, 5-petalled flowers are produced in short, dense, corymb-like racemes. In frost-prone areas, grow in a temperate greenhouse. In warmer climates, grow over a pergola or arch, or allow to cascade from a tree.
• **HARDINESS** Frost tender.
• **CULTIVATION** Under glass, grow in loamless or loam-based potting compost (JI No.3) in full light, shaded from hot sun. In growth, water freely and apply a balanced liquid fertilizer every 4 weeks. Water sparingly in winter. Outdoors, grow in fertile, moist soil in full sun with some shade. Support climbing stems. Pruning group 11, in late winter.
• **PROPAGATION** Root semi-ripe cuttings with bottom heat in summer. Layer in autumn or spring.
• **PESTS AND DISEASES** Trouble free.

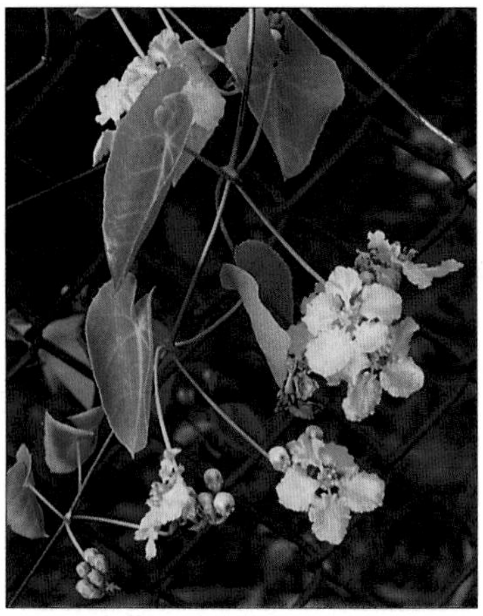

Stigmaphyllon ciliatum

S. ciliatum ▣ Twining, evergreen climber with slender, branched stems and broadly ovate, hairy-margined, light green leaves, 4–10cm (1½–4in) long, each with 2 ear-shaped lobes at the bases. Axillary, corymb-like racemes of 3–7 saucer-shaped, rich bright yellow flowers, 3–4cm (1¼–1½in) across, are produced in autumn; each flower has 1 small and 4 large, rounded, clawed, fringed petals. ↕5–8m (15–25ft). Belize to Uruguay. ❁ (min. 7–10°C/45–50°F)

▷**Stinking Benjamin** see *Trillium erectum*
▷**Stinking gladwyn** see *Iris foetidissima*
▷**Stinking madder** see *Putoria calabrica*
▷**Stinking nightshade** see *Hyoscyamus niger*
▷**Stink pod** see *Scoliopus bigelovii*
▷**Stinkwort** see *Helleborus foetidus*

STIPA syn. ACHNATHERUM

Feather grass, Needle grass, Spear grass

GRAMINEAE/POACEAE

Genus of about 300 species of bristly, tufted, evergreen or deciduous, perennial (rarely annual) grasses from open woodland and stony slopes in temperate and warm-temperate regions worldwide. They have linear, pleated, inrolled, occasionally flat leaves, and bear narrow panicles of flattened spikelets, often with long, feathery or bristly awns, from early summer to autumn. They are grown for their habit, and also for their attractive

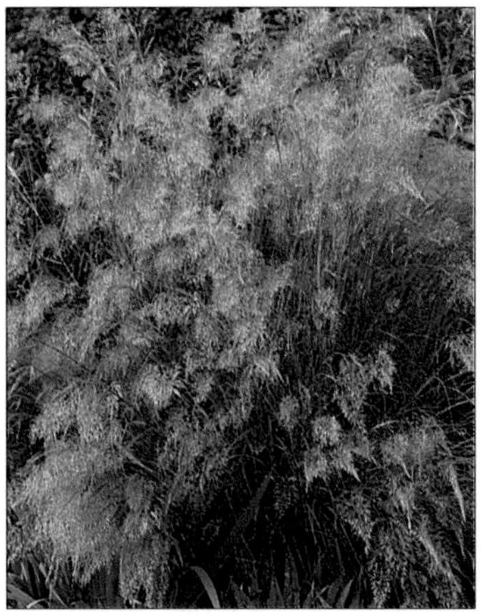

Stipa calamagrostis

inflorescences, which may be dried and dyed for use in flower arrangements. Use in a mixed or shrub border. *S. gigantea* is effective set against a dark backdrop of shrubs or conifers.
• **HARDINESS** Fully hardy to frost hardy; *S. arundinacea* will withstand short periods around -10°C (14°F).
• **CULTIVATION** Grow in moderately fertile, medium to light, well-drained soil in full sun; *S. arundinacea* tolerates heavier soils and partial shade. Cut back deciduous species in early winter; remove dead leaves on evergreens in early spring.
• **PROPAGATION** Sow seed in containers in a cold frame in spring. Divide from mid-spring to early summer.
• **PESTS AND DISEASES** Trouble free.

S. arundinacea ▣ (Pheasant's tail grass). Loosely tufted, rhizomatous, evergreen perennial producing arching, linear, flat or inrolled, leathery, dark green leaves, to 30cm (12in) long, streaked orange-brown in summer, and turning orange-brown all over in winter. From mid-summer to early autumn, bears pendent panicles, to 75cm (30in) long, of purplish green spikelets. ↕1m (3ft), ↔1.2m (4ft). New Zealand. ❄❄

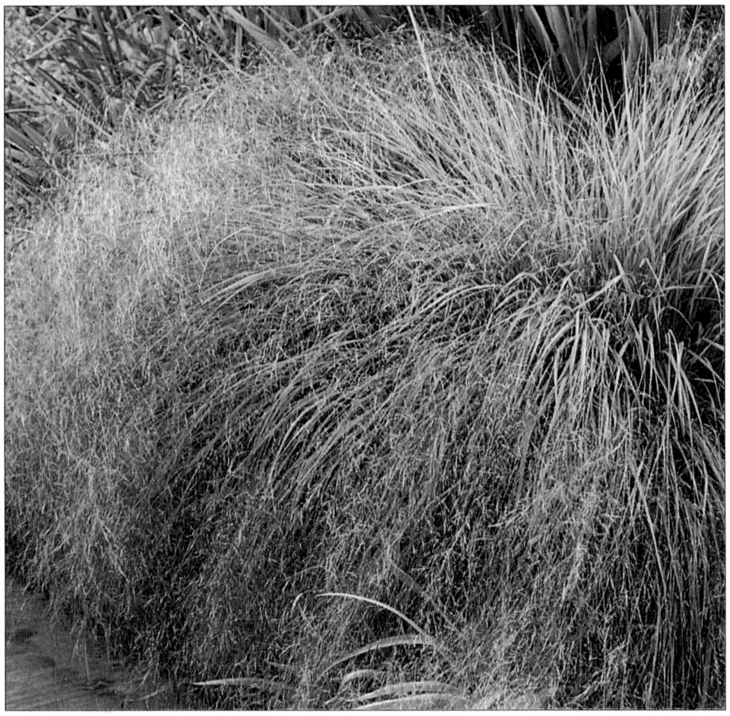

Stipa arundinacea

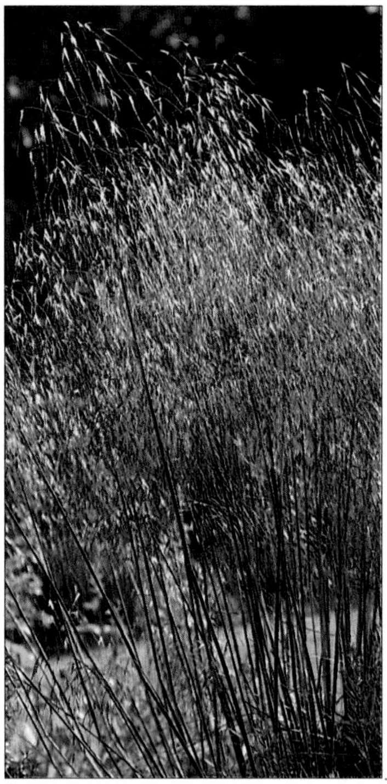

Stipa gigantea

S. calamagrostis ▣ syn. *S. lasiogrostis.* Densely tufted, deciduous perennial with mounds of arching, linear, inrolled, blue-green leaves, to 30cm (12in) long. In summer, bears silvery, purple-tinted to buff spikelets in nodding, feathery, lax panicles, to 80cm (32in) long. ↕1m (3ft), ↔1.2m (4ft). S. Europe. ❄❄❄
S. gigantea ▣🏆 (Giant feather grass, Golden oats). Densely tufted, evergreen or semi-evergreen perennial forming lax clumps of linear, inrolled, mid-green leaves, to 70cm (28in) long. Bristled, silvery, purplish green spikelets, turning gold when ripe, are borne in long-stemmed, oat-like panicles, to 50cm (20in) long, in summer. ↕to 2.5m (8ft), ↔1.2m (4ft). Spain, Portugal. ❄❄❄
S. lasiogrostis see *S. calamagrostis.*
S. splendens. Densely tufted, deciduous perennial forming large mounds of arching, linear, pleated, dark green leaves, to 50cm (20in) long. Purple-tinted white spikelets, in large, loose panicles, to 50cm (20in) long, are borne above the foliage in early and mid-summer. ↕to 2.5m (8ft), ↔1.2m (4ft). C. Asia, Russia (Siberia), Chile. ❄❄❄
S. tenuissima ▣ Densely tufted, deciduous perennial with erect, narrowly

S

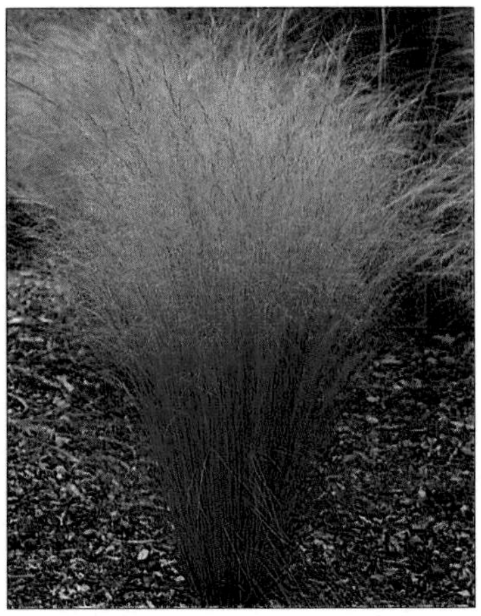

Stipa tenuissima

linear to filament-like, tightly inrolled, bright green leaves, 30cm (12in) or more long. Throughout summer, bears a profusion of narrow, nodding, softly feathery panicles, to 30cm (12in) long, greenish white at first, becoming buff. The whole plant billows in the slightest breeze. ↕ 60cm (24in), ↔ 30cm (12in). USA (Texas, New Mexico), Mexico, Argentina. ❄❄❄

▷ **Stock** see *Matthiola, M. incana*
Night-scented see *Matthiola longipetala* subsp. *bicornis*
Virginia see *Malcolmia maritima*

STOKESIA
Stokes' aster

ASTERACEAE/COMPOSITAE

Genus of one species of erect perennial from conifer woods on moist, acid soil in S.E. USA. The evergreen, simple, smooth leaves are entire, sometimes with spines towards the bases, and are borne in basal rosettes. The long-lasting, colourful, terminal, cornflower-like flowerheads are solitary or produced in few- to many-flowered corymbs; they are good for cutting. Grow in a warm position in a herbaceous border.

• **HARDINESS** Fully hardy.

• **CULTIVATION** Grow in light, fertile, moist but well-drained, acid soil in full sun. Liable to rot in damp, heavy soils. Provide twiggy support. Dead-head to prolong flowering. Provide a deep, dry mulch in areas with severe winters.

• **PROPAGATION** Sow seed in containers in a cold frame in autumn. Divide in spring, or take root cuttings in late winter.

• **PESTS AND DISEASES** Trouble free.

S. laevis ■ Rosette-forming, evergreen perennial with elliptic to lance-shaped, mid-green basal leaves, to 20cm (8in) long, slightly spiny near the bases, and with conspicuous, pale greenish white midribs. From midsummer to early autumn, upright stems, with smaller, stalkless leaves, bear solitary, terminal, cornflower-like flowerheads, to 10cm (4in) across; these have spreading, fringed ray-florets in purplish blue, pink, or white, and disc-florets in paler or darker shades of the same colours. ↕ to 60cm (24in), ↔ 45cm (18in). S.E. USA. ❄❄❄. **'Blue Star'** has large, light blue flowerheads with whitish blue disc-florets. **'Silver Moon'** has silvery white flowerheads.

S

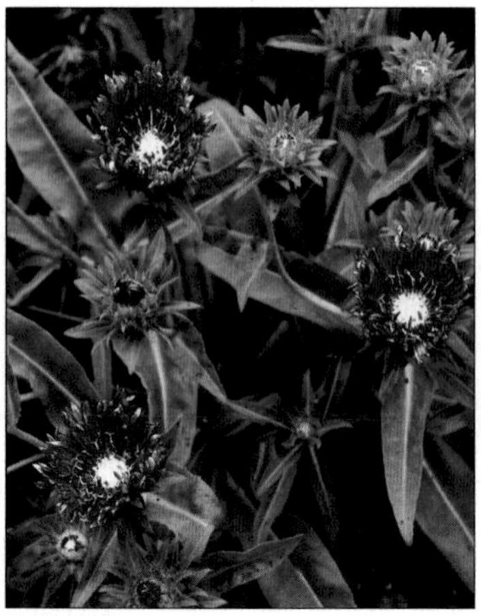

Stokesia laevis

STOMATIUM

AIZOACEAE

Genus of about 40 species of mainly mat-forming, perennial succulents from semi-desert areas of Botswana and South Africa. They have very short stems and unequal pairs of angular or rounded, often keeled, rough, fleshy leaves, sometimes with marginal teeth and white or transparent dots. Solitary, daisy-like, scented flowers are borne in the middle of the stems in summer; they often open in late afternoon and stay open all night. In frost-prone areas, grow in a temperate greenhouse. In warm, dry areas, use in a desert garden or raised bed.

• **HARDINESS** Frost tender.

• **CULTIVATION** Under glass, grow in standard cactus compost in full light. From spring to summer, apply a low-nitrogen fertilizer monthly and water moderately. Water very sparingly at other times. Outdoors, grow in sandy, poor, humus-rich, sharply drained soil in full sun. See also pp.48–49.

• **PROPAGATION** Sow seed at 19–24°C (66–75°F), or take cuttings of stem sections, from spring to summer.

• **PESTS AND DISEASES** Susceptible to aphids while flowering.

S. agninum. Clustering succulent with pairs of 3-angled to semi-cylindrical, oblong, obtuse, very convex and keeled, dull grey-green leaves, 4–5cm (1½–2in) long, roughened by green papillae, and sometimes with 3–5 short, marginal teeth. Pale yellow flowers, 2–2.5cm (¾–1in) across, open in late afternoon or early evening in summer. ↕ 5cm (2in), ↔ 45cm (18in). South Africa (Western Cape). ❀ (min. 7°C/45°F). **var. *integrifolium*** ■ has smooth leaves.
S. patulum. Clustering succulent with crowded pairs of 3-angled to semi-cylindrical, pale greyish green leaves, 2cm (¾in) long, with rough white dots, and with 2–9 pointed tubercles on the upper surfaces. Pale yellow flowers, 2cm (¾in) across, open in the evening in summer. ↕ 3cm (1¼in), ↔ 45cm (18in). South Africa. ❀ (min. 7°C/45°F)

▷ **Stone cress** see *Aethionema*
▷ **Stonecrop** see *Sedum*
Biting see *S. acre*
Common see *S. acre*
▷ **Stone orpine** see *Sedum rupestre*
▷ **Stone pine** see *Pinus pinea*
▷ **Stone plant** see *Lithops*

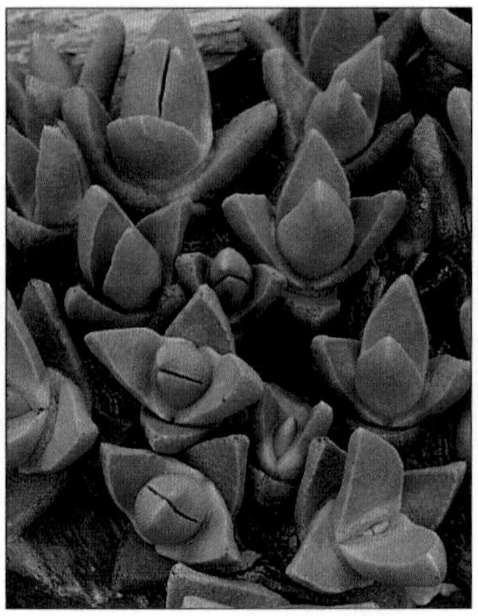

Stomatium agninum var. *integrifolium*

▷ **Storax** see *Styrax officinalis*
▷ **Stork's bill** see *Erodium*
▷ ***Strangweja spicata*** see *Bellevalia hyacinthoides*
▷ ***Stranvaesia*** see *Photinia*
S. davidiana see *P. davidiana*
S. nussia see *P. nussia*

STRATIOTES

HYDROCHARITACEAE

Genus of one species of vigorous, dioecious, submerged aquatic perennial found in still and slow-moving water in Eurasia. It has rosettes of narrow, prickly, saw-toothed, submerged leaves, which rise to the surface at flowering time. An attractive foliage plant for a sunny pool, it acts to some extent as a filter and oxygenator, but must be kept in check.

• **HARDINESS** Fully hardy.

• **CULTIVATION** In summer, scatter new plants into a pool of slightly alkaline water over 30cm (12in) deep. Remove runners as necessary to control spread.

• **PROPAGATION** Detach winter buds or young plantlets in spring.

• **PESTS AND DISEASES** Trouble free.

S. aloides (Water soldier). Aquatic perennial with short runners producing stalkless rosettes of linear to lance-shaped, sharp-pointed, toothed, deep olive-green leaves, to 50cm (20in) long. In midsummer, bears cup-shaped, white, sometimes pink-tinged flowers, 3cm (1¼in) across, from 2-leaved bracts: the males in pairs or threes, the females solitary. ↔ indefinite. Eurasia. ❄❄❄

▷ **Strawberry** see *Fragaria*
Indian see *Duchesnea indica*
Mock see *Duchesnea indica*
▷ **Strawberry bush** see *Calycanthus floridus*
▷ **Strawberry tree** see *Arbutus, A. unedo*
Grecian see *A. andrachne*
▷ **Strawflower** see *Bracteantha bracteata, Rhodanthe*

STRELITZIA
Bird of paradise

STRELITZIACEAE

Genus of about 5 species of clump-forming, evergreen perennials found in habitats ranging from riverbanks to open glades in the bush of South Africa. They have large, long-stalked, mostly oblong to lance-shaped leaves with woody bases forming a "trunk" that may reach 10m (30ft) tall. Their exotic inflorescences, produced intermittently from the leaf axils, consist of usually horizontal, waxy, stiff, boat-shaped spathes, from the top of which crest-like flowers arise sequentially, often in contrasting colours; they are very long-lasting when cut. In frost-prone areas, grow in a warm greenhouse; move outdoors in summer. In warmer areas, grow as specimen plants.

• **HARDINESS** Frost tender.

• **CULTIVATION** Under glass, grow in large containers or in a greenhouse border in loam-based potting compost (JI No.3). Provide full light with shade from hot sun, and ventilate freely when temperatures exceed 20°C (68°F). In the growing season, water freely and apply a balanced liquid fertilizer monthly. Water sparingly in winter. Top-dress annually and repot every second year.

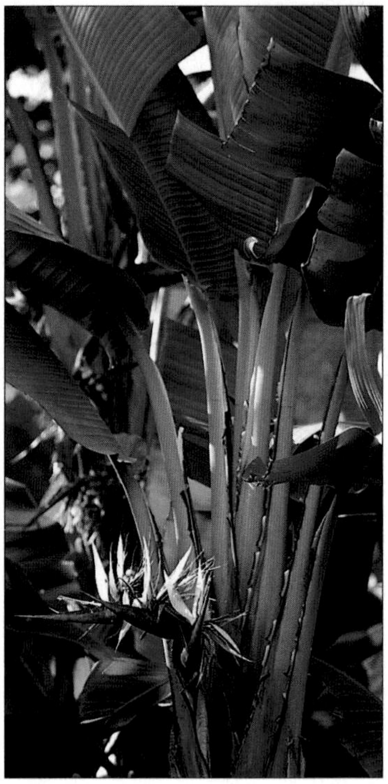

Strelitzia nicolai

Outdoors, grow in fertile, moist but well-drained soil in full sun or partial shade, with shelter from strong winds.

• **PROPAGATION** Sow seed at 18–21°C (64–70°F), or divide rooted suckers, in spring. Seed-raised plants may take 3 or more years to flower.

• **PESTS AND DISEASES** Susceptible to scale insects.

S. alba. Clump-forming perennial with oblong to lance-shaped leaf-blades, 2m (6ft) long, on leaf-stalks 1m (3ft) long. Bears purple-glaucous spathes, 25–30cm (10–12in) long, with white flowers, 20cm (8in) long, usually in spring. ↕ to 10m (30ft), ↔ to 3m (10ft). South Africa (Western Cape, Northern Cape, Eastern Cape). ❀ (min. 10°C/50°F)
S. juncea, syn. *S. reginae* var. *juncea.* Clump-forming perennial with rush-like leaves, 50cm (20in) long, without leaf-blades. From winter to spring, produces green spathes, 12cm (5in) long, and flowers, 3–4cm (1¼–1½in) long, with orange calyces and blue corollas. ↕ to 1.5m (5ft), ↔ 1m (3ft). South Africa (Eastern Cape). ❀ (min. 10°C/50°F)
S. nicolai ■ Clump-forming perennial with oblong leaf-blades, 1.5m (5ft) long,

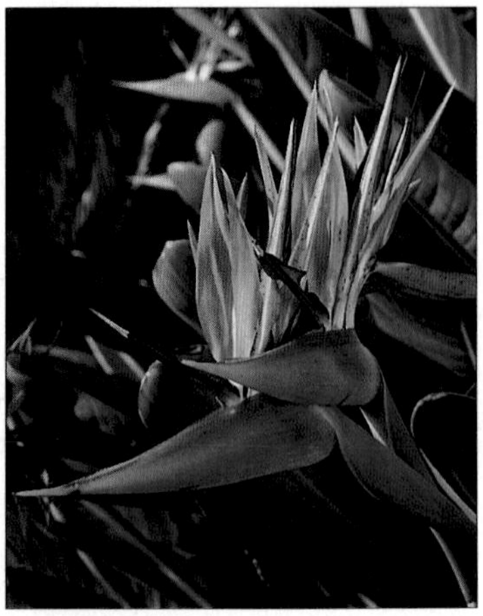

Strelitzia reginae

rounded or heart-shaped at the bases, on leaf-stalks 2m (6ft) long. In spring, bears 3–5 brownish red spathes, 40–45cm (16–18in) long, and white flowers, 20cm (8in) long, with light purplish blue corollas. Needs ample space. ↕ to 10m (30ft), ↔ to 5m (15ft). South Africa (Northern Cape, Eastern Cape, KwaZulu/Natal). ❅ (min. 10°C/50°F)

S. reginae ■ 🏆 (Crane flower). Clump-forming perennial with oblong-lance-shaped leaf-blades, to 50cm (20in) long, with round or tapered bases, on stalks to 1m (3ft) long. From winter to spring, bears purple- and orange-flushed green spathes, 12cm (5in) long, and flowers 10cm (4in) long, with orange or yellow calyces and blue corollas. ↕ to 2m (6ft), ↔ to 1m (3ft). South Africa. ❅ (min. 10°C/50°F). **'Humilis'**, syn. 'Pygmaea', is dwarf, forming dense clumps, and has ovate-oblong leaves; it grows well in containers; ↕ 80cm (32in). **'Pygmaea'** see 'Humilis'. **var. *juncea*** see *S. juncea*.

▷ ***Streptanthera cuprea*** see *Sparaxis elegans*

▷ ***Streptanthera elegans*** see *Sparaxis elegans*

STREPTOCARPUS

Cape primrose

GESNERIACEAE

Genus of about 130 species of annuals and perennials, some monocarpic, or rarely subshrubs, often found in rain-forest, sometimes as epiphytes, and on damp banks and rocks or in grassland. They occur from tropical to southern Africa, in Madagascar, and in China, with 4 species from S.E. Asia. Linear to rounded, hairy, often mid-green, veined, wrinkled leaves are borne singly or in opposite pairs on erect, fleshy stems, or in stemless rosettes. Cymes of tubular, often 2-lipped flowers, with 5 spreading lobes, are axillary or borne from the leaf rosettes. In frost-prone areas, grow in a temperate or warm greenhouse. Use in a humid, shady border in warmer areas.

• **HARDINESS** Frost tender.

• **CULTIVATION** Under glass, grow in loamless potting compost in bright filtered light, with shade from hot sun. When in growth, water freely, allowing compost to dry out between waterings (overwatering results in basal rot); apply a high-potash fertilizer every 2 weeks. Reduce humidity and keep just moist in winter. Repot annually in spring. Remove faded flowers and stalks to discourage seeding. Outdoors, grow in fertile, leafy, humus-rich, moist but well-drained soil in partial shade.

• **PROPAGATION** Surface-sow seed in late winter or spring, at 18°C (64°F). Divide, or take leaf cuttings, in spring or early summer. Root stem-tip cuttings, 5–8cm (2–3in) long, of bushy and trailing plants in spring, with bottom heat.

• **PESTS AND DISEASES** Leafhoppers, mealybugs, thrips, tarsonemid mites, and vine weevil larvae may be a problem.

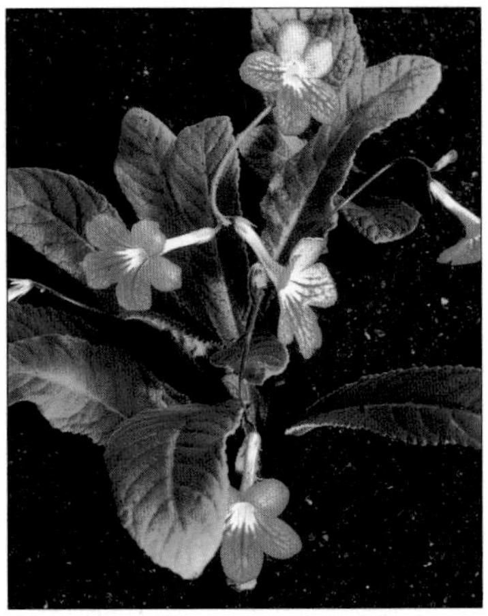

Streptocarpus 'Constant Nymph'

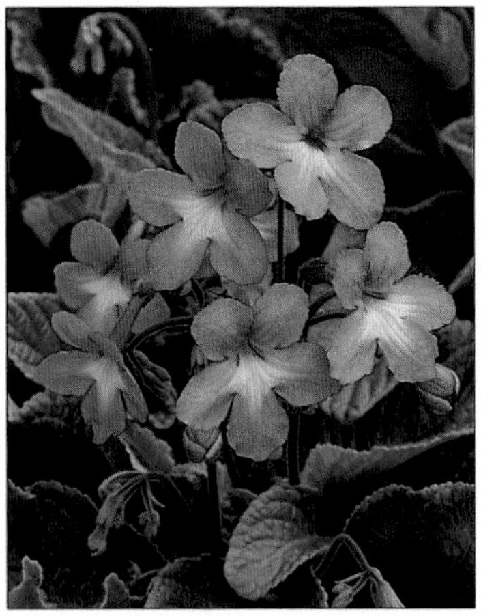

Streptocarpus 'Lisa'

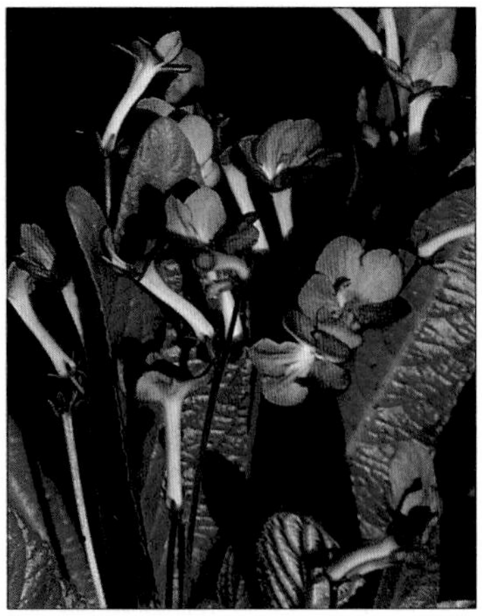

Streptocarpus 'Nicola'

***S.* 'Albatross'** 🏆 Robust, rhizomatous perennial with rosettes of broad, strap-shaped, finely hairy leaves, 25cm (10in) long. Cymes of up to 5 yellow-throated white flowers, 6cm (2½in) across, open from spring to autumn. ↕ 30cm (12in), ↔ 55cm (22in). ❅ (min. 10°C/ 50°F)

S. caulescens ■ Erect perennial with fleshy, deep brown stems and opposite, elliptic to ovate, softly hairy leaves, 6cm (2½in) long. Cymes of 6–12 violet or white flowers, 1.5–2cm (½–¾in) across, with purple throats, are borne through-out the year. ↕↔ to 60cm (24in). Kenya, Tanzania. ❅ (min. 10°C/50°F)

***S.* 'Concord Blue'.** Erect, bushy perennial producing fleshy stems and opposite, rounded, softly hairy leaves, 2.5cm (1in) long. Cymes of many mid-blue flowers, 2cm (¾in) across, open from spring to autumn. ↕ 30cm (12in), ↔ 50cm (20in). ❅ (min. 10°C/50°F)

***S.* 'Constant Nymph'** ■ Stemless, rhizomatous perennial with rosettes of lance-shaped, finely hairy leaves, to 30cm (12in) long. From spring to autumn, bears cymes of up to 5 blue flowers, 6cm (2½in) across, with pale yellow throats and deep violet veins on the 3 lower lobes. ↕ 30cm (12in), ↔ 60cm (24in). ❅ (min. 10°C/50°F)

***S.* 'Heidi'** 🏆 Rhizomatous perennial with rosettes of strap-shaped, finely hairy leaves, to 22cm (9in) long. From spring to autumn, bears cymes of up to 5 clear blue flowers, 6cm (2½in) across, with purple markings on the lower 3 lobes. ↕ 24cm (10in), ↔ 45cm (18in). ❅ (min. 10°C/50°F)

***S.* 'Joanna'.** Vigorous, rhizomatous perennial with rosettes of strap-shaped, finely hairy leaves, 35cm (14in) long. From spring to autumn, bears cymes of up to 5 frilled, deep velvet-red flowers, 8cm (3in) across, with darker markings. ↕ 30cm (12in), ↔ 75cm (30in). ❅ (min. 10°C/50°F)

***S.* 'Kim'** ■ 🏆 Rhizomatous perennial with rosettes of strap-shaped, finely hairy leaves, 15cm (6in) long. From spring to summer, bears cymes of many dark purple flowers, 3.5cm (1½in) across, with white throats. ↕ 20cm (8in), ↔ 35cm (14in). ❅ (min. 10°C/50°F)

***S.* 'Lisa'** ■ 🏆 Rhizomatous perennial with rosettes of strap-shaped, finely hairy leaves, 30cm (12in) long. Many cymes of up to 5 white-throated, shell-pink flowers, 6cm (2½in) across, open from spring to autumn. ↕ 35cm (14in), ↔ 65cm (26in). ❅ (min. 10°C/50°F)

***S.* 'Nicola'** ■ Rhizomatous perennial with erect rosettes of strap-shaped, finely hairy leaves, 20cm (8in) long. From spring to autumn, bears many cymes of up to 5 semi-double, deep pink flowers, 3cm (1¼in) across. ↕ 35cm (14in), ↔ 45cm (18in). ❅ (min. 10°C/50°F)

S. rexii. Rhizomatous perennial with rosettes of strap-shaped, blunt-tipped, finely hairy leaves, to 30cm (12in) long. Violet-tinged white, or violet flowers, 3.5–4.5cm (1½–1¾in) across, with violet lines on the lower lobes, are borne usually singly or in pairs, or in cymes of up to 6, from spring to autumn. ↕ to 25cm (10in), ↔ to 50cm (20in). South Africa (Western Cape, Eastern Cape, S. KwaZulu/Natal). ❅ (min. 10°C/50°F)

S. saxorum ■ 🏆 Prostrate, sparsely branched, woody-based perennial with opposite, elliptic to ovate, finely hairy, thick, grey-green leaves, 2.5cm (1in) long. Axillary, pale lilac, white-throated flowers, 3cm (1¼in) across, are borne singly or in pairs, in spring and early summer. ↕ 15cm (6in), ↔ 60cm (24in). E. Africa. ❅ (min. 10°C/50°F)

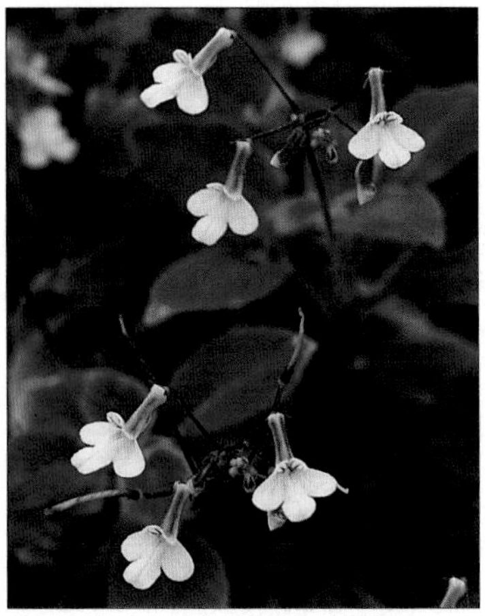

Streptocarpus caulescens

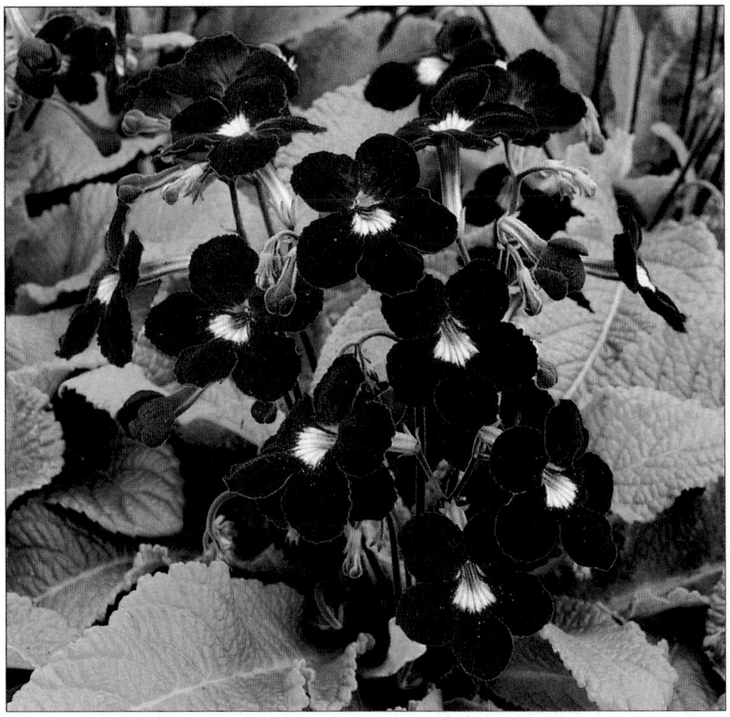

Streptocarpus 'Kim'

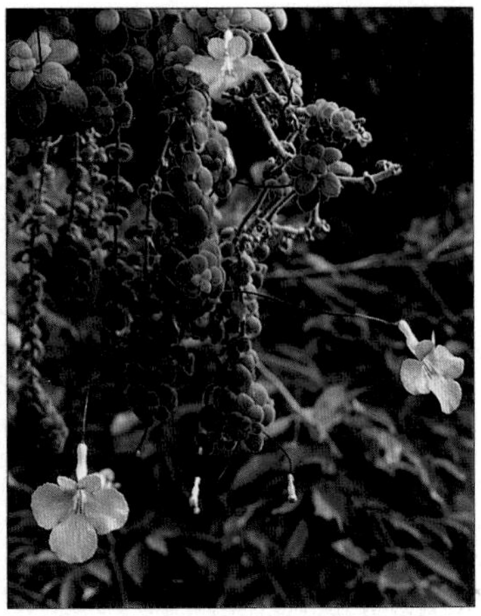

Streptocarpus saxorum

STREPTOSOLEN

SOLANACEAE

Genus of one species of evergreen shrub found in open woodland from Colombia to Peru and Ecuador, grown for its clusters of colourful, salverform flowers. It is loosely scrambling, with alternate, simple leaves. Below 7°C (45°F), grow in a cool or temperate greenhouse. In warmer areas, grow against a wall or among other shrubs.

• **HARDINESS** Frost tender; may survive temperatures near to 0°C (32°F).

• **CULTIVATION** Under glass, grow in loam-based potting compost (JI No.3) in full light with shade from hot sun. When in growth, water freely and apply a balanced liquid fertilizer monthly. Water sparingly in winter. Outdoors, grow in fertile, moist but well-drained soil in full sun. Pruning group 8 or 9, in late winter or early spring; group 13 if wall-trained; may need restrictive pruning under glass.

• **PROPAGATION** Root softwood cuttings in early summer, or semi-ripe cuttings in mid- to late summer, both with bottom heat. Layer in late summer.

• **PESTS AND DISEASES** Whiteflies, red spider mites, and aphids may be troublesome under glass.

S. jamesonii ▣ ♡ (Marmalade bush). Tall, slender-stemmed shrub, semi-scandent unless annually pruned, with ovate to elliptic, finely wrinkled, mid- to deep green leaves, 2.5–5cm (1–2in) long. From late spring to late summer, produces yellow to orange-yellow flowers, 3–4cm (1¼–1½in) long, with slender, twisted tubes and spreading petal lobes, in large, terminal corymbs, to 15cm (6in) across. ↕ 2–3m (6–10ft), ↔ 1–2.5m (3–8ft). Colombia, Ecuador, Peru. ❀ (min. 7°C/45°F)

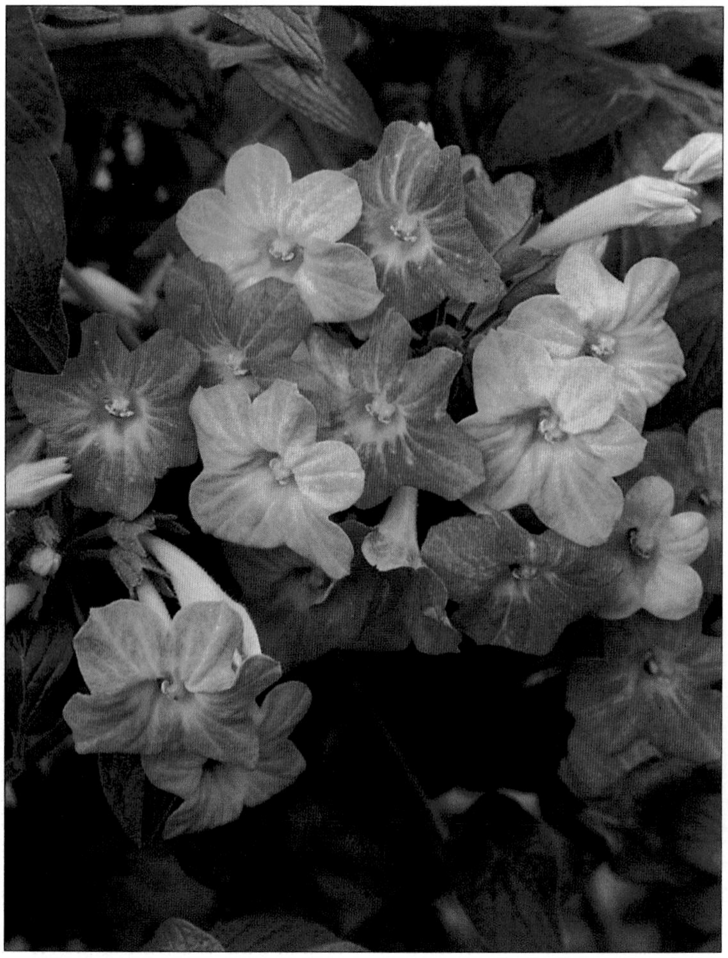

Streptosolen jamesonii

▷**String of beads** see *Senecio rowleyanus*

STROBILANTHES

ACANTHACEAE

Genus of 250 species of evergreen or deciduous perennials or soft-stemmed shrubs from woodland margins in Asia and Madagascar. They are grown for their tubular to funnel-shaped, 2-lipped, often hooded, 5-lobed, blue to purple, white, or rarely yellow flowers, borne in terminal or axillary, usually cone-shaped inflorescences, sometimes loose panicles or spikes. The leaves are opposite, ovate to lance-shaped or elliptic, entire or toothed, often in unequal pairs. In frost-prone areas, grow hardy species in a herbaceous border; grow tender species as summer bedding or in a warm greenhouse. In warmer areas, use in a border.

• **HARDINESS** Mostly frost tender; *S. atropurpureus* is fully hardy.

• **CULTIVATION** Under glass, grow in loam-based potting compost (JI No.2) in full light with shade from hot sun. In growth, water freely; apply a balanced liquid fertilizer every 4 weeks. Water moderately in winter. Outdoors, grow in light, fertile, free-draining soil in full sun or partial shade. Pinch out young growth to induce bushiness. In frost-prone climates, protect *S. atropurpureus* with a dry winter mulch. Pruning group 9 for shrubby species; they may need restrictive pruning under glass.

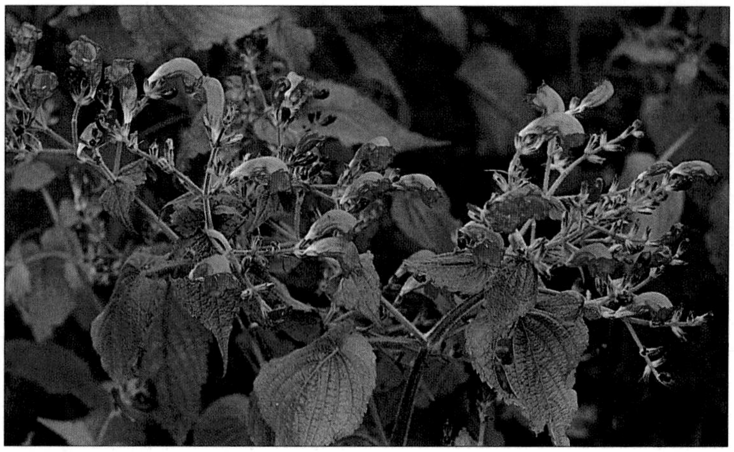

Strobilanthes atropurpureus

• **PROPAGATION** Sow seed at 13–18°C (55–64°F) in spring. Root basal or softwood cuttings in spring or early summer, with bottom heat.

• **PESTS AND DISEASES** Red spider mites may be troublesome.

S. anisophyllus. Small subshrub with unequal pairs of lance-shaped, toothed, dark green leaves, 9cm (3½in) long. Tubular, lavender-blue flowers, 2.5cm (1in) long, with curved corolla tubes, are borne in cone-shaped inflorescences in spring and winter. ↕ 1–2m (3–6ft), ↔ 75cm (30in). Himalayas. ❀ (min. 12°C/54°F)

S. atropurpureus ▣ Erect, branching perennial with long-stalked, ovate, toothed, dark green leaves, 10cm (4in) long. Dense spikes of tubular, indigo or purple flowers, 4cm (1½in) long, are produced in summer. ↕ 1.2m (4ft), ↔ 1m (3ft). N. India. ❄❄❄

S. dyerianus ♡ (Persian shield). Soft-stemmed shrub with unequal pairs of elliptic, toothed, dark green leaves, to 15cm (6in) long, flushed purple with a silver overlay above, dark purple beneath. Bears short spikes of funnel-shaped, pale blue flowers, 3cm (1¼in) long, in autumn. ↕ 1.2m (4ft), ↔ 1m (3ft). Burma. ❀ (min. 12°C/54°F)

STROMANTHE

MARANTACEAE

Genus of 13 species of evergreen, rhizomatous herbaceous perennials from forest floors and clearings in Central and South America. They are grown for their foliage and showy flower bracts. Obovate, ovate, elliptic, or lance-shaped to linear-lance-shaped leaves are borne basally and on the slender, often many-branched stems. Cup-shaped, yellow, red, or white flowers, with colourful bracts, are borne in racemes or panicles, often several on a stem, in winter, spring, and summer. In frost-prone areas, grow in a warm greenhouse. In warmer areas, use in a damp, humid border.

• **HARDINESS** Frost tender.

• **CULTIVATION** Under glass, grow in a greenhouse border in loamless or loam-based potting compost (JI No.3) in bright filtered light, allowing a free root run. In growth, water freely, maintain high humidity, and apply a low-nitrogen liquid fertilizer every 2 or 3 weeks. Water moderately in winter. Outdoors, grow in moist, fertile soil in full sun or dappled shade.

• **PROPAGATION** Sow seed at 18°C (64°F) in early spring. Divide when dormant or after flowering, minimizing root damage.

• **PESTS AND DISEASES** Red spider mites may be troublesome in dry conditions.

S. jacquinii, syn. *S. lutea.* Rhizomatous perennial with branching stems and oblong-ovate to elliptic, mid-green leaves, 35cm (14in) long. In winter and spring, bears pale yellow flowers, 9mm (⅜in) long, with bright yellow bracts, in panicles 5–8cm (2–3in) across. ↕ 3m (10ft), ↔ 1m (3ft). Panama, Colombia, Venezuela. ❀ (min. 10°C/50°F)

S. lutea see *S. jacquinii.*

S. sanguinea. Erect, rhizomatous perennial. Branching stems bear lance-shaped to linear-lance-shaped, dark olive-green leaves, 50cm (20in) long, red beneath and 2-ranked at the bases. Bears white-petalled flowers, to 1cm (½in) long, with orange-red sepals, among red bracts, in panicles 5–8cm (2–3in) across, in winter and spring. ↕ to 1.5m (5ft), ↔ 1m (3ft). Brazil. ❀ (min. 10°C/50°F)

STROMBOCACTUS

CACTACEAE

Genus of one species of perennial cactus from rocky fissures in C. Mexico. It has a mainly flattened-spherical stem, with ribs divided into prominent tubercles, spirally arranged; the areoles produce a few bristles, which fall as the plant matures. It produces solitary, funnel-shaped flowers from the crown in summer, followed by thin-walled, dry fruit containing minute seeds. Where temperatures drop below 10°C (50°F), grow in a warm greenhouse; in warmer climates, use in a desert garden.

• **HARDINESS** Frost tender.

• **CULTIVATION** Under glass, grow in standard cactus compost, with added limestone chips, in full light and low humidity. Water moderately in spring and summer, applying a balanced liquid fertilizer every 3 or 4 weeks. Keep completely dry at other times. Outdoors, grow in gritty, sharply drained, poor, humus-rich, preferably neutral to slightly alkaline soil in full sun. See also pp.48–49.

• **PROPAGATION** Sow seed at 21°C (70°F) in spring; seedlings may be difficult to establish.

• **PESTS AND DISEASES** Trouble free.

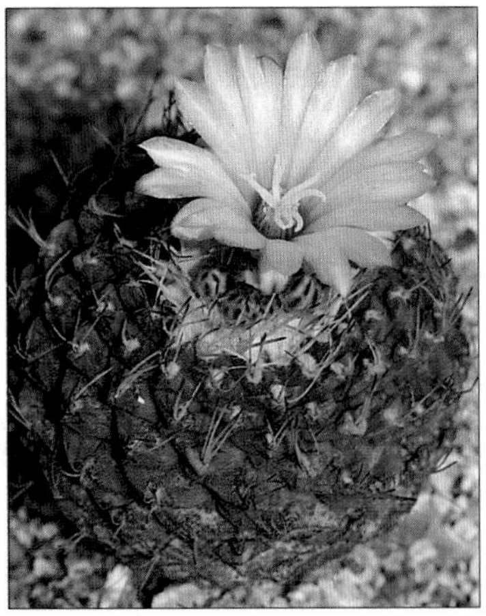

Strombocactus disciformis

S. disciformis ■ Simple, occasionally offsetting, flattened-spherical, greyish green cactus, bearing a few persistent, off-white, dark-tipped spines at the crown and 12–18 ribs closely set with diamond-shaped tubercles. Each tubercle has a central white areole bearing 1–5 bristly white radial spines (there are no centrals). Produces funnel-shaped, white or yellow flowers, with red throats, 3cm (1¼in) across, by day in summer. ↕↔ to 12cm (5in). C. Mexico. ❁ (min. 10°C/50°F)

STRONGYLODON

LEGUMINOSAE/PAPILIONACEAE

Genus of about 20 species of evergreen shrubs or woody-stemmed, twining climbers from tropical woodland in S.E. Asia and the Pacific islands. Alternate, 3-palmate leaves have lance-shaped to rounded leaflets, the terminal one largest. From winter to summer, they bear pendent racemes of pea-like, red, orange, blue, or bluish green flowers with pointed, upturned keel petals. Below 15°C (59°F), grow in a warm greenhouse. In warmer areas, train over an arch or pergola.

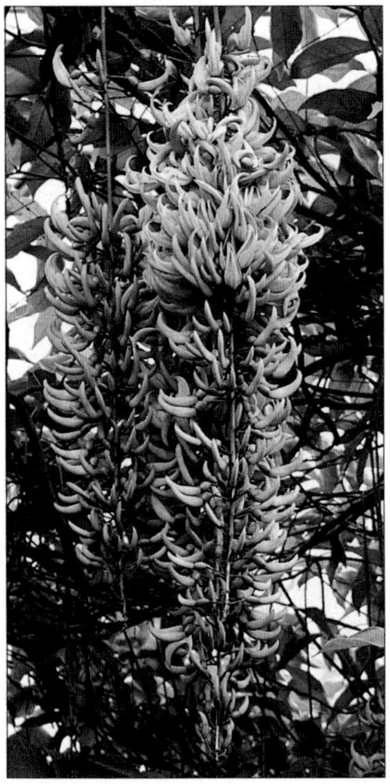

Strongylodon macrobotrys

• **HARDINESS** Frost tender.
• **CULTIVATION** Under glass, grow in loam-based potting compost (JI No.3) in full light with shade from hot sun. In growth, water freely; apply a balanced liquid fertilizer every 2 or 3 weeks. Water moderately to sparingly in winter. Outdoors, grow in fertile, humus-rich, neutral to acid soil in full sun or partial shade. Support climbing stems. Pruning group 11; or 12, after flowering.
• **PROPAGATION** Sow seed at 27–30°C (81–86°F) as soon as ripe. Root semi-ripe stem sections in summer, with bottom heat. Air layer in spring.
• **PESTS AND DISEASES** Scale insects may be troublesome under glass.

S. macrobotrys ■ (Emerald creeper, Jade vine). Strong-growing, evergreen, twining climber. Leaves, to 15cm (6in) long, with 3 oblong to elliptic leaflets, are pinkish bronze, turning glossy, rich green. From winter to spring, rarely in summer, bears pea-like, luminous, blue-green flowers, 8cm (3in) long, in dense racemes, 40–90cm (16–36in) long. ↕ to 20m (70ft). Philippines. ❁ (min. 15°C/59°F)

▷ ***Stuartia*** see *Stewartia*

STYLIDIUM

STYLIDIACEAE

Genus of about 150 species of annuals, herbaceous perennials, and subshrubs from dry scrub in Australia (one species from New Zealand). They are grown for their glossy, grass-like foliage and their flowers. The usually very narrow leaves, to 50cm (20in) long, are alternate or in basal rosettes. Pink, white, yellow, or purple flowers are borne in racemes, panicles, or corymbs in summer. The flowers are asymmetrical: each has 5 petals, one very small, with a central column combining stamens and style. A trigger action in the stamens aids insect pollination. In frost-prone areas, grow in a cool to temperate greenhouse. In warmer areas, use in a sunny border.
• **HARDINESS** Frost tender.
• **CULTIVATION** Under glass, grow in loamless or loam-based potting compost (JI No.2) in full light. When in full growth, water sparingly and apply a balanced liquid fertilizer monthly. Keep almost dry in winter. Outdoors, grow in well-drained, fertile soil in full sun.
• **PROPAGATION** Sow seed at 13–18°C (55–64°F), or divide, in spring.
• **PESTS AND DISEASES** Trouble free.

S. graminifolium (Trigger plant). Tufted perennial with basal rosettes of stiffly erect to arching, linear leaves, to 24cm (10in) long. Produces tiny, pink to magenta flowers in terminal, erect, narrow racemes, to 30cm (12in) long, in summer. ↕ 30cm (12in), ↔ 45cm (18in). Australia. ❁ (min. 7°C/45°F)

STYLOPHORUM

PAPAVERACEAE

Genus of 3 species of herbaceous perennials from woodland in E. Asia and E. North America. The pinnatisect leaves have long stalks in the basal rosettes, and are stalkless on the upright, branching, ridged stems. The flowers are saucer-shaped, poppy-like, and yellow or

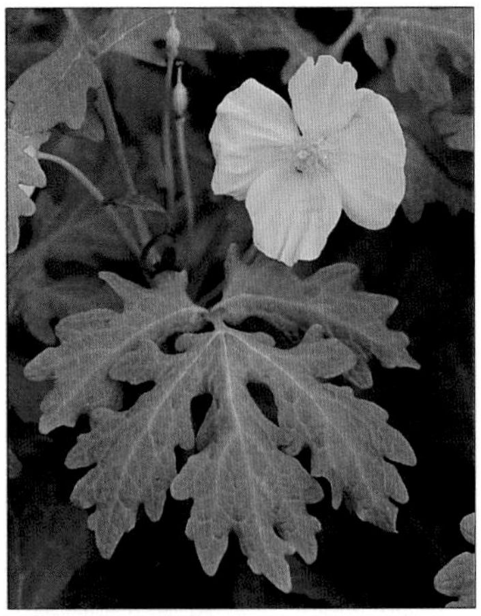

Stylophorum diphyllum

orange, borne in terminal umbels in spring and summer. Stylophorums are attractive plants for a woodland garden, a shady border among shrubs, or a large rock garden. They may self-seed.
• **HARDINESS** Fully hardy.
• **CULTIVATION** Grow in moist, moderately fertile, humus-rich soil in deep or partial shade.
• **PROPAGATION** Sow seed in containers in a cold frame in autumn. Divide in spring; may be slow to re-establish.
• **PESTS AND DISEASES** May be attacked by slugs and snails.

S. diphyllum ■ (Celandine poppy). Downy, rosette-forming perennial with deeply incised, hairy, mid-green leaves, 20–30cm (8–12in) long, each with 5–7 oblong-obovate, irregularly scalloped and toothed lobes. Bright golden yellow flowers, to 2.5cm (1in) across, are borne in summer. ↕↔ to 30cm (12in). E. USA. ❄❄❄

STYPHELIA

EPACRIDACEAE

Genus of 12 species of wiry-stemmed, evergreen shrubs from dry forest and woodland; they occur in Australia, except for one species found in New Guinea. They have small, simple, aromatic, rigidly leathery leaves, arranged alternately or in spirals. Long, slender, tubular flowers, each with 5 reflexed or rolled-back lobes, are borne singly or in small groups from the upper leaf axils in summer. In frost-prone areas, grow in a cool greenhouse. In milder climates, grow in a shrub border.
• **HARDINESS** Half hardy to frost tender.
• **CULTIVATION** Under glass, grow in lime-free (ericaceous) potting compost in full light with good ventilation. In the growing season, water moderately and apply a balanced liquid fertilizer monthly. Water sparingly in winter. Outdoors, grow in fertile, humus-rich, neutral to acid soil in full sun. Pruning group 10, after flowering.
• **PROPAGATION** Sow seed at 6–12°C (43–54°F) as soon as ripe or in spring. Root semi-ripe cuttings in summer, with bottom heat. Layer in spring.
• **PESTS AND DISEASES** Trouble free.

S. colensoi see *Cyathodes colensoi.*
S. triflora (Pink fivecorner). Erect, moderately dense shrub bearing elliptic to oblong-elliptic leaves, 1.5–3cm (½–1¼in) long, with sharp points. In summer, tubular, 5-angled, usually pink to red, occasionally cream or pale yellow-green flowers, 2cm (¾in) long, with strongly rolled-back lobes, are produced singly or in twos or threes. ↕ 0.4–2m (16–72in), ↔ 60–90cm (24–36in). S.W. Australia. ❄

STYRAX

STYRACACEAE

Genus of approximately 100 species of deciduous or evergreen shrubs and small trees found in woodland and thickets in Europe, Asia, and North America, including Mexico. Of graceful habit, they have alternate, short-stalked, variably shaped, entire or toothed leaves. The dainty, nodding, bell-shaped or cup-shaped, fragrant white flowers may be solitary, borne in pendent, terminal or axillary racemes or panicles, or produced in clusters on short branchlets; they appear on the previous year's wood in spring or summer. Grow in a woodland garden.
• **HARDINESS** Fully hardy to frost hardy.
• **CULTIVATION** Grow in moist but well-drained, fertile, humus-rich, neutral to acid soil in full sun or partial shade, with shelter from cold, drying winds. Pruning group 1.
• **PROPAGATION** Sow seed as soon as ripe; keep at 15°C (59°F) for 3 months, then at 0–5°C (32–41°F) for 3 months; keep seedlings frost-free until they are established. Take greenwood cuttings in summer.
• **PESTS AND DISEASES** Trouble free.

S. americanus (American snowbell). Rounded, deciduous shrub with elliptic to oblong, entire or toothed, dark green leaves, to 8cm (3in) long. Nodding, bell-shaped white flowers, 2cm (¾in) long, with narrow, backward-curving petals, are produced singly or in small clusters of up to 4 from the leaf axils, in early and midsummer. ↕ 3m (10ft), ↔ 2.5m (8ft). S.E. USA. ❄❄❄
S. hemsleyanus ♀ Broadly columnar, deciduous tree with oval to obovate, toothed, dark green leaves, to 12cm (5in) long. Bell-shaped white flowers, 1.5cm (½in) long, are borne in terminal racemes or few-branched panicles, to 15cm (6in) long, in early summer. ↕ 8m (25ft), ↔ 5m (15ft). C. China. ❄❄❄
S. japonicus ■ ♀ (Japanese snowbell). Graceful, spreading, deciduous tree bearing elliptic-oblong, minutely toothed, glossy, mid- to dark

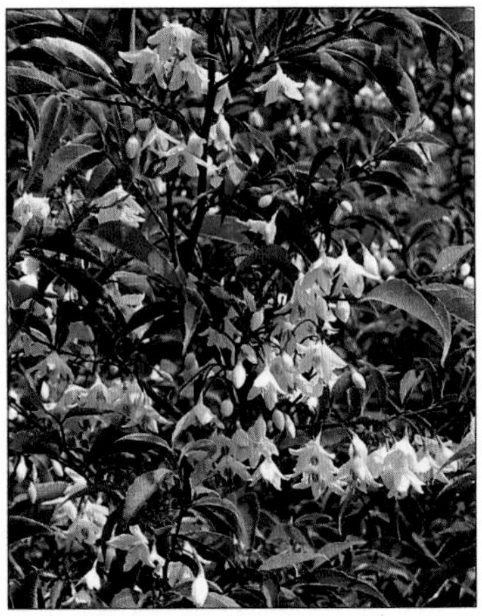

Styrax japonicus

S

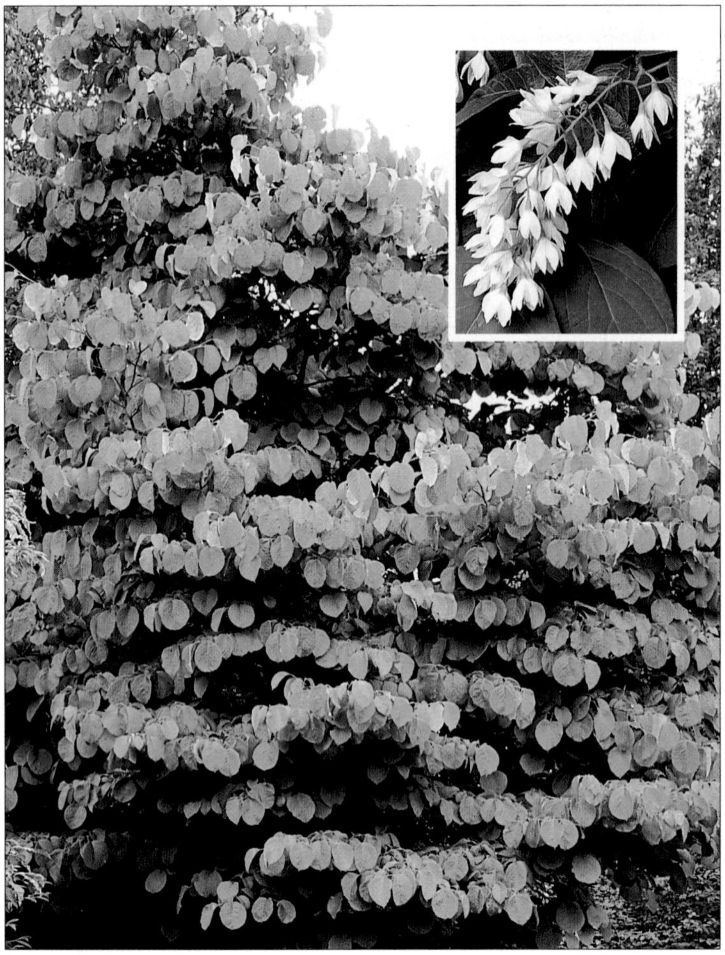

Styrax obassia (inset: flower detail)

green leaves, to 10cm (4in) long, turning yellow or red in autumn. Bell-shaped, white, sometimes pink-tinged flowers, 1.5cm (½in) long, are produced singly or in clusters of 3–6 along the undersides of the branches, in early and midsummer. ↕ 10m (30ft), ↔ 8m (25ft). China, Korea, Japan. ❄❄❄. **'Pink Chimes'** bears a profusion of pink flowers.

S. obassia ▣♀♡ (Fragrant snowbell). Broadly columnar, deciduous tree bearing elliptic to rounded, dark green leaves, 7–15cm (3–6in) long, distinctly toothed except towards their bases, and blue-grey beneath, turning yellow in autumn. Bell-shaped white flowers, 2.5cm (1in) long, are produced in spreading, terminal racemes, to 20cm (8in) long, in early and midsummer. ↕ 12m (40ft), ↔ 7m (22ft). N. China, Korea, Japan. ❄❄❄

S. officinalis ▣♡ (Storax). Spreading, deciduous shrub or tree with ovate, entire, dark green leaves, grey-white beneath, to 8cm (3in) long. Bell-shaped white flowers, 2.5cm (1in) long, are produced in pendent clusters of 3–8 near the shoot tips, in early summer. ↕ 6m (20ft), ↔ 5m (15ft). S. Europe, S.W. Asia. ❄❄

S. wilsonii. Rounded, bushy, deciduous shrub with slender shoots and oval to diamond-shaped, dark green leaves, to 2.5cm (1in) long, with a few teeth near the tips. Broadly bell-shaped white flowers, 1.5cm (½in) across, are borne singly or in clusters of up to 4 along the shoots, in early summer. ↕↔ 2.5m (8ft). W. China. ❄❄❄

S

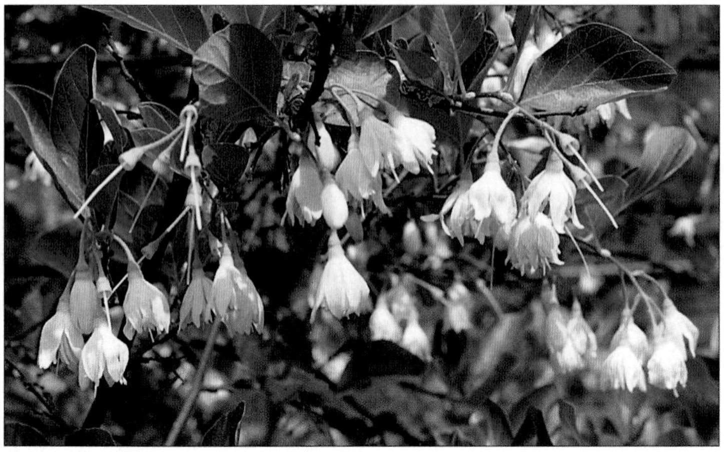

Styrax officinalis

SUCCISA

DIPSACACEAE

Genus of one species of perennial found in boggy meadows and moorland from Europe to W. Siberia, and in N.W. Africa. Minutely hairy, it bears rosettes of obovate to elliptic basal leaves and erect or decumbent stems with smaller, narrower leaves. Its pincushion-like flowerheads, late- and long-flowering, are similar to those of *Scabiosa*. Grow in a damp wild garden or meadow.

• **HARDINESS** Fully hardy.

• **CULTIVATION** Grow in poor to moderately fertile, peaty soil that is moist at least through the growing season, in full sun or partial shade.

• **PROPAGATION** Sow seed in containers in a cold frame in autumn or spring. Root basal cuttings in spring.

• **PESTS AND DISEASES** Trouble free.

S. pratensis, syn. *Scabiosa succisa* (Blue buttons, Devil's bit scabious). Rosette-forming, rhizomatous perennial with thin, branched, softly hairy stems and obovate to elliptic, usually entire, mainly basal leaves, to 30cm (12in) long. From midsummer to late autumn, bears solitary, pincushion-like, violet, rarely white or pink flowerheads, to 2.5cm (1in) across. ↕ 15–60cm (6–24in), ↔ to 60cm (24in). Europe, N.W. Africa, Caucasus, Russia (W. Siberia). ❄❄❄

▷**Succulents** see pp.48–49
▷**Sugar-almond plant** see *Pachyphytum oviferum*
▷**Sugarberry** see *Celtis occidentalis, C. reticulata*
▷**Sugarbush** see *Protea repens*
▷***Sulcorebutia*** see *Rebutia*
S. rauschii see *R. rauschii*
▷**Sulphur flower** see *Eriogonum gracilipes, E. umbellatum*
▷**Sumach** see *Rhus*
Dwarf see *Rhus copallina*
Fragrant see *Rhus aromatica*
Scarlet see *Rhus glabra*
Shining see *Rhus copallina*
Smooth see *Rhus glabra*
Stag's horn see *Rhus typhina*
Velvet see *Rhus typhina*
Venetian see *Cotinus coggygria*
▷**Summer-sweet** see *Clethra*
▷**Sundew** see *Drosera*
Cape see *D. capensis*
▷**Sundrops** see *Oenothera, O. fruticosa, O. perennis*
Ozark see *O. macrocarpa*
▷**Sunflower** see *Helianthus, H. annuus*
Dark-eye see *Helianthus atrorubens*
Mexican see *Tithonia, T. rotundifolia*
Thin-leaved see *Helianthus decapetalus*
Willow-leaved see *Helianthus salicifolius*
Woolly see *Eriophyllum*
▷**Sun plant** see *Portulaca grandiflora*
▷**Supple Jack** see *Berchemia scandens*

SUTERA

SCROPHULARIACEAE

Genus of 130 species of annuals, soft-stemmed perennials, and small, woody, evergreen shrubs, mostly from woodland margins in South Africa. They have opposite, toothed, scalloped, or lobed leaves. From summer to autumn, white, pale mauve, or blue, salverform flowers, with tubular corollas and 5 spreading lobes, are produced singly from the leaf axils or in axillary or terminal cymes, racemes, spikes, or panicles. In frost-prone areas, use as summer bedding or grow in a temperate greenhouse. In warmer areas, grow as border edging.

• **HARDINESS** Frost tender.

• **CULTIVATION** Under glass, grow in loam-based potting compost (JI No.2) in full light. In the growing season, water freely and apply a balanced liquid fertilizer every 4 weeks. Water sparingly in winter. Outdoors, grow in well-drained, fertile soil in full sun.

• **PROPAGATION** Sow seed at 13–18°C (55–64°F), or divide, in spring. Root stem-tip cuttings in spring or summer, with bottom heat.

• **PESTS AND DISEASES** Prone to aphids.

S. grandiflora (Purple glory plant). Many-branched perennial, woody at the base, with elliptic, deeply scalloped leaves, 2.5cm (1in) long. From summer to autumn, produces racemes, 30cm (12in) long, of salverform, lavender-blue, white-throated flowers, 2–3cm (¾–1¼in) long. ↕ 1m (3ft), ↔ 60cm (24in). South Africa. ✾ (min. 5°C/41°F)

SUTHERLANDIA

LEGUMINOSAE/PAPILIONACEAE

Genus of 5 species of evergreen shrubs found on dry slopes and grassland in southern Africa. They are grown for their showy, pea-like, red to purple flowers, borne in slender, axillary racemes from late spring to summer, and for their bladder-like fruits. Leaves are alternate and pinnate. In frost-prone climates, grow in a cool greenhouse; in milder areas, plant at the base of a sunny wall.

• **HARDINESS** Frost tender; may survive short periods close to 0°C (32°F).

• **CULTIVATION** Under glass, grow in loam-based potting compost (JI No.2), with added sharp sand, in full light. During growth, water moderately and apply a balanced liquid fertilizer monthly. Water sparingly in winter. Outdoors, grow in well-drained, poor to moderately fertile soil in full sun; dry soils are tolerated. Pruning group 8; may need restrictive pruning under glass, in late winter.

• **PROPAGATION** Sow seed at 15°C (59°F) in spring. Root semi-ripe cuttings in summer, with bottom heat.

• **PESTS AND DISEASES** Earwigs and red spider mites may be a problem.

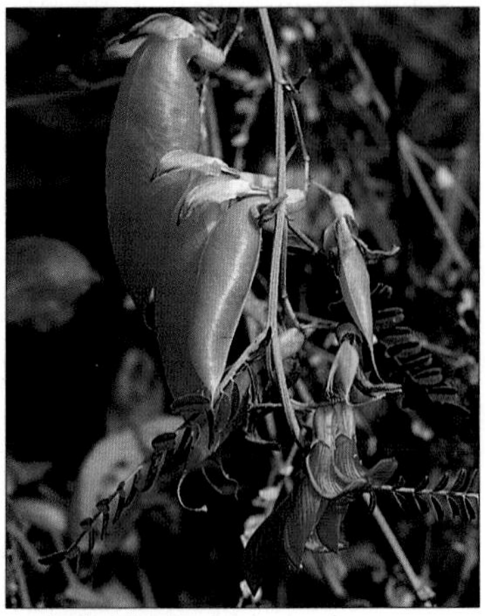

Sutherlandia frutescens

S. frutescens ▣ (Balloon pea, Duck plant). Evergreen shrub with slender, erect, twiggy, white-downy stems and pinnate, hairy, grey-green leaves, 6–10cm (2½–4in) long, each composed of 13–21 small, oblong to linear-elliptic leaflets on densely white-downy midribs. From late spring to summer, bears racemes, to 8cm (3in) long, of pea-like, bright red flowers, 2.5–5cm (1–2in) long, followed by inflated, broadly ellipsoid to almost spherical, greenish yellow, occasionally red-flushed seed pods, to 5cm (2in) long. ↕0.6–2m (2–6ft), ↔ 1–1.5m (3–5ft). Southern Africa. ❀ (min. 5°C/41°F)

SWAINSONA
syn. SWAINSONIA

LEGUMINOSAE/PAPILIONACEAE

Genus of 50 species of annuals, perennials, and subshrubs occurring on stony slopes and grassland and in open woodland in Australia (one species in New Zealand). They have alternate, pinnate leaves and pea-like, usually purple, sometimes white, pink, yellow, orange, or red flowers, with very broad standard petals, borne in erect, axillary racemes from spring to summer. In frost-prone areas, grow in a cool greenhouse. Elsewhere, use in a border.

- **HARDINESS** Frost tender.
- **CULTIVATION** Under glass, grow in loam-based potting compost (JI No.2), with added sharp sand, in full light. In growth, water moderately and apply a low-phosphate fertilizer monthly. Water sparingly in winter. Outdoors, grow in sharply drained, moderately fertile soil in full sun. Pruning group 10, after flowering (or late winter, if under glass).
- **PROPAGATION** Sow pre-soaked seed at 15°C (59°F) in spring. Root semi-ripe cuttings in summer, with bottom heat.
- **PESTS AND DISEASES** Red spider mites may be a problem under glass.

S. galegifolia ▣ Loose, evergreen subshrub with spreading to semi-scandent stems. Pinnate leaves, 5–8cm (2–3in) long, have 11–21 small, oblong, grey- to deep green leaflets. From spring to summer, bears racemes, 8–15cm (3–6in) long, of red, pink, purple, or blue flowers, 1.5cm (½in) long. ↕↔ 1–2m (3–6ft). Australia (Queensland, New South Wales). ❀ (min. 5–7°C/41–45°F). **'Albiflora'** has pure white flowers and light green leaves. **'Violacea'** bears rose-red to purple flowers.

▷***Swainsonia*** see *Swainsona*
▷**Swallow-wort** see *Asclepias curassavica*
▷**Swan plant** see *Gomphocarpus physocarpus*
▷**Sweet basil** see *Ocimum basilicum*
▷**Sweetbells** see *Leucothoe racemosa*
▷**Sweet briar** see *Rosa eglanteria*
▷**Sweet Cicely** see *Myrrhis, M. odorata*
▷**Sweetcorn** see *Zea mays*
▷**Sweet gale** see *Myrica gale*
▷**Sweet gum** see *Liquidambar styraciflua*
  Oriental see *L. orientalis*
▷**Sweetheart plant** see *Philodendron scandens*
▷**Sweetheart vine** see *Ceropegia linearis* subsp. *woodii*
▷**Sweet pea** see *Lathyrus odoratus*
▷**Sweet pepper bush** see *Clethra, C. alnifolia*
▷**Sweetshrub, Common** see *Calycanthus floridus*
▷**Sweetspire** see *Itea virginica*
▷**Sweet sultan** see *Amberboa, A. moschata*
▷**Sweet William** see *Dianthus barbatus*
  Wild see *Phlox divaricata*
▷**Sweetwood** see *Glycyrrhiza glabra*
▷***Swida alba*** see *Cornus alba*
▷***Swida alternifolia*** see *Cornus alternifolia*
▷***Swida amomum*** see *Cornus amomum*
▷***Swida controversa*** see *Cornus controversa*
▷**Swiss chard** see *Beta vulgaris* subsp. *cicla*
▷**Swiss cheese plant** see *Monstera deliciosa*
▷**Switch grass** see *Panicum virgatum*
▷**Switch ivy** see *Leucothoe fontanesiana*

SYAGRUS syn. ARECASTRUM

ARECACEAE/PALMAE

Genus of 32 species of often low-growing, single- or cluster-stemmed, sometimes stemless palms, from habitats including shrubby vegetation to woodland, often on rocky ridges, in South America. Leaves are pinnate, arranged in spiralling, terminal tufts; the ovoid, 3-petalled flowers appear in spikes or panicles between them. In frost-prone climates, grow in a temperate or warm greenhouse, or as houseplants. In warmer areas, use tall species as lawn specimens, and smaller ones in a shrub border.

- **HARDINESS** Frost tender.
- **CULTIVATION** Under glass, grow in loam-based potting compost (JI No.3) in bright filtered light. In growth, water freely; apply a balanced liquid fertilizer monthly. Water sparingly in winter. Pot on or top-dress in spring. Outdoors, grow in fertile, moist but well-drained soil in full sun or partial shade.
- **PROPAGATION** Sow seed at 27°C (81°F) in spring.
- **PESTS AND DISEASES** Red spider mites may be troublesome under glass.

S. flexuosa ▣✱ (Palmito do campo). Small palm with slender, single or clustered stems bearing pinnate leaves, 1–2m (3–6ft) long, composed of many linear, mid- to deep green leaflets each side. Green flowers appear in panicles, to 45cm (18in) or more long, usually in summer. ↕2–5m (6–15ft), ↔ 2–4m (6–12ft). Brazil. ❀ (min. 13°C/55°F)
S. petraea ✱ Usually stemless palm with pinnate leaves, to 1m (3ft) long, composed of many linear, rich green leaflets in 2 flat ranks. Green flowers are borne in simple or branched spikes, to 30cm (12in) long, usually in summer. ↕ to 1m (3ft), ↔ 2m (6ft) or more. Bolivia, Brazil. ❀ (min. 13°C/55°F)
S. romanzoffiana ✱ syn. *Arecastrum romanzoffianum* (Queen palm). Small to medium-sized palm with a sturdy trunk, sometimes swollen around the middle. Pinnate leaves are 3–5m (10–15ft) long, each with many linear, mid-green leaflets borne singly or in clusters of 2–5. Orange-glanded green flowers are borne in panicles, to 1m (3ft) long, usually in summer. ↕ to 20m (70ft), ↔ 6–10m (20–30ft). Brazil. ❀ (min. 13°C/55°F)
S. weddelliana see *Lytocaryum weddellianum.*

▷**Sycamore** see *Acer pseudoplatanus*
  American see *Platanus occidentalis*
  California see *Platanus racemosa*

x SYCOPARROTIA

HAMAMELIDACEAE

Hybrid genus of one species of semi-evergreen shrub with alternate, simple, glossy, dark green leaves and dense clusters of flowers. Grow in a shrub border, as a specimen plant on a lawn, or in light woodland.

- **HARDINESS** Fully hardy.
- **CULTIVATION** Grow in moderately fertile, moist but well-drained, neutral to acid soil in full sun or partial shade. Pruning group 1.
- **PROPAGATION** Take semi-ripe cuttings in summer.
- **PESTS AND DISEASES** Trouble free.

x *S. semidecidua* (*Parrotia persica* x *Sycopsis sinensis*). Spreading shrub with oblong-elliptic, glossy, dark green leaves, to 8cm (3in) long; some turn yellow in autumn. In spring, brown-woolly flower buds reveal dense clusters, 2.5cm (1in) across, of bright red anthers surrounded by small brown bracts. ↕4m (12ft), ↔ 6m (20ft). Garden origin. ❄❄❄

SYCOPSIS

HAMAMELIDACEAE

Genus of 7 species of evergreen shrubs and trees from woodland in China, the Himalayas, and S.E. Asia. They bear alternate, simple, ovate to oblong, entire or finely toothed leaves and, in spring, racemes or heads of small, petalless, male or bisexual flowers. Only *S. sinensis* is

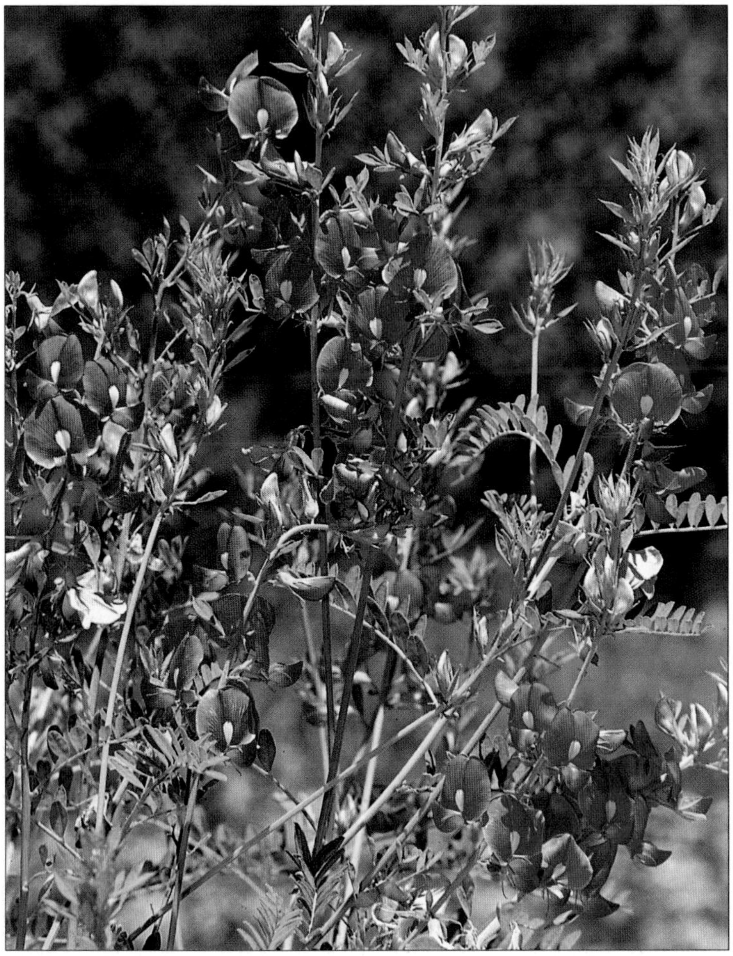

Swainsona galegifolia

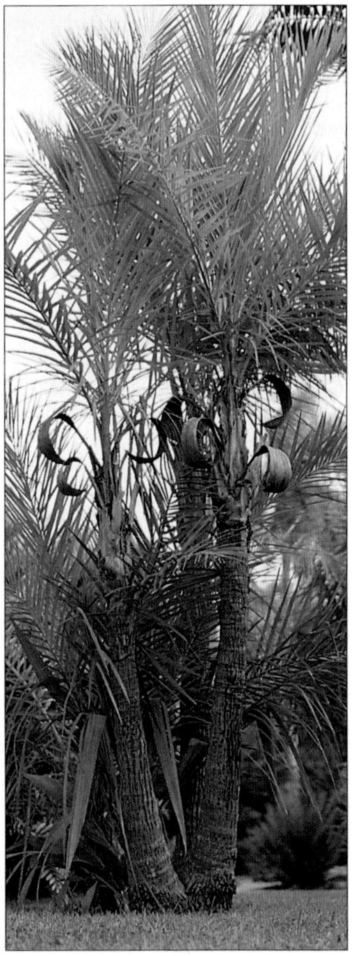

Syagrus flexuosa

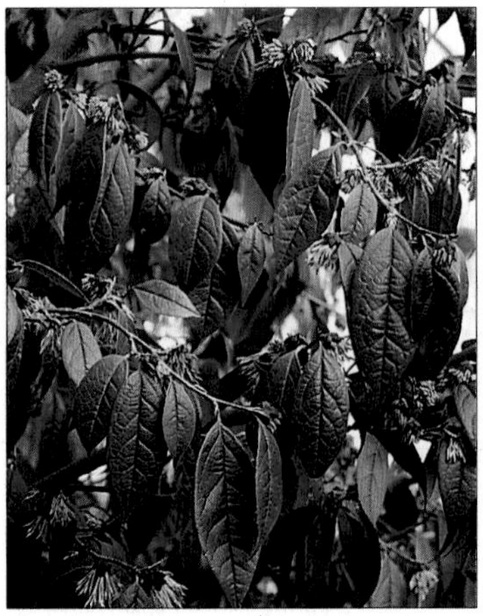

Sycopsis sinensis

generally cultivated, for its flowers; use in a shrub border or woodland garden.
• **HARDINESS** Frost hardy to frost tender.
• **CULTIVATION** Grow in moist but well-drained, moderately fertile, humus-rich, neutral to acid soil in full sun or partial shade, sheltered from strong, and cold, drying winds. Pruning group 1.
• **PROPAGATION** Sow seed as soon as ripe, in lime-free (ericaceous) seed compost in containers in a cold frame. Take semi-ripe cuttings in summer.
• **PESTS AND DISEASES** Trouble free.

S. sinensis ◼ Conical shrub with upright branches and oblong, leathery, dark green leaves, to 10cm (4in) long, pale green beneath. In spring, short, dense clusters, 2.5cm (1in) across, of brown-felted buds open to reveal petalless flowers with red anthers and yellow filaments. ↕ 6m (20ft), ↔ 4m (12ft). C. China. ❄❄

SYMPHORICARPOS

Snowberry

CAPRIFOLIACEAE

Genus of about 17 species of deciduous shrubs found in woodland and thickets and on prairies and plains in W. China and North and Central America. They are grown for their spherical or ovoid, fleshy, white to pink, or dark blue or purple fruits, which last well into winter, and their tiny, bell- or funnel-shaped, nectar-rich, white to pink flowers, which attract bees. The flowers are borne singly or in terminal or axillary clusters, spikes, or dense racemes. The leaves are simple

S

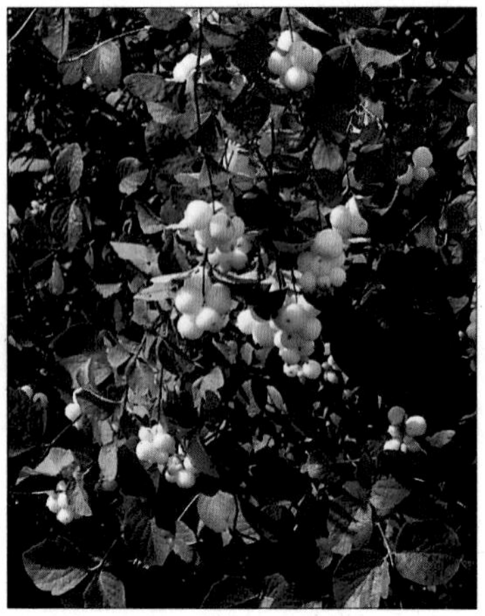

Symphoricarpos albus var. *laevigatus*

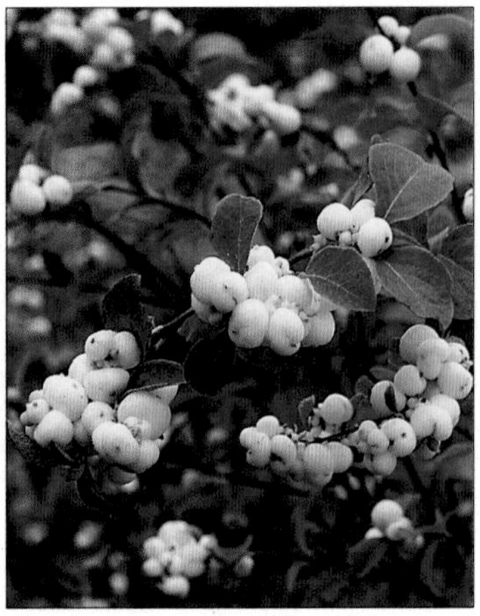

Symphoricarpos x *doorenbosii* 'White Hedge'

and opposite. Very hardy, and tolerant of poor soil, pollution, and exposed sites. Good for a shrub border, screen, or informal hedge. Use *S.* x *chenaultii* 'Hancock' as ground cover. Fruits may cause mild stomach upset if ingested; contact with them may irritate skin.
• **HARDINESS** Fully hardy.
• **CULTIVATION** Grow in any fertile, reasonably well-drained soil in full sun or partial shade. Pruning group 1 or 2.
• **PROPAGATION** Divide in autumn if suckering. Take greenwood cuttings in summer, or hardwood cuttings in autumn.
• **PESTS AND DISEASES** Trouble free.

S. albus* var. *laevigatus ◼ syn. *S. rivularis* (Snowberry). Thicket-forming shrub with upright, arching shoots and oval to oval-oblong, rarely lobed, dark green leaves, to 5cm (2in) long. Tiny, bell-shaped pink flowers are produced in pairs on spike-like racemes in summer, followed by spherical, pure white fruit, 1cm (½in) across. ↕↔ 2m (6ft). W. North America. ❄❄❄
S.* x *chenaultii (*S. microphyllus* x *S. orbiculatus*). Upright, many-branched shrub with ovate, dark green leaves, to 2.5cm (1in) long, glaucous and densely hairy beneath. In late summer, bears short spikes of small, open bell-shaped, greenish white flowers, followed by spherical, red-stippled white fruit, 6mm (¼in) across. ↕ 2m (6ft), ↔ 1.2m (4ft). Garden origin. ❄❄❄. **'Hancock'** is low and spreading, self-layering to form a broad mound; bears white flowers and sparse, dark pink fruit; ↕↔ 3m (10ft).
S.* x *doorenbosii (*S. albus* var. *laevigatus* x *S.* x *chenaultii*). Thicket-forming shrub with elliptic to broadly ovate, dark green leaves, 2–4cm (¾–1½in) long, lighter beneath. In mid- and late summer, bears short racemes of small, bell-shaped, greenish white flowers, followed by dense clusters of spherical white fruit, to 1.5cm (½in) across, with a pink blush. ↕ 2m (6ft), ↔ indefinite. Garden origin. ❄❄❄. **'Mother of Pearl'** has arching shoots bearing dense crops of fruit. **'White Hedge'** ◼ is compact and upright, with white fruit; ↕ 1.5m (5ft).
S. microphyllus. Upright shrub with ovate, blue-green leaves, to 6cm (2½in) long, with pointed tips, softly hairy beneath. In late summer, bears small, cup-shaped white flowers, which are solitary, in axillary pairs, or in short, terminal spikes, followed by spherical,

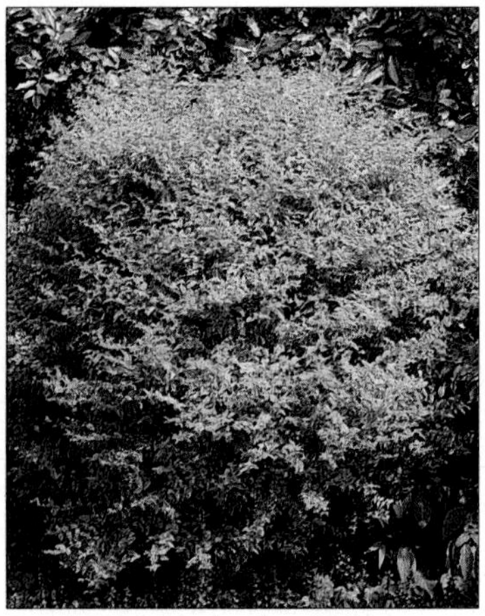

Symphoricarpos orbiculatus 'Foliis Variegatis'

semi-translucent, pink or white fruit, 8mm (⅜in) across. ↕ 1–2m (3–6ft), ↔ 0.6–1.2m (2–4ft). Mexico. ❄❄❄
S. orbiculatus (Coralberry, Indian currant). Dense, bushy shrub with broadly elliptic to ovate, dark green leaves, to 3cm (1¼in) long. In late summer and early autumn, bears dense clusters of tiny, bell-shaped, white, sometimes pink-tinged flowers, followed by ovoid-spherical, dark purple-red fruit, 6mm (¼in) across. Fruits most freely after a hot summer. ↕↔ 2m (6ft). E. USA, Mexico. ❄❄❄. **'Foliis Variegatis'** ◼ syn. 'Variegatus', has irregularly yellow-margined leaves.
S. rivularis see *S. albus* var. *laevigatus.*

SYMPHYANDRA

CAMPANULACEAE

Genus of about 12 species of often monocarpic, sometimes rhizomatous perennials from mountains in the E. Mediterranean and the Caucasus to C. Asia and Korea. They are grown for their tubular-bell-shaped or bell-shaped flowers, borne on branched stems in racemes, corymbs, or panicles over long periods in summer. Leaves are long-stalked, often heart-shaped, toothed, hairy, and mainly basal. Grow in a herbaceous or mixed border, or rock garden. They are very free-flowering, but usually short-lived. May self-seed.
• **HARDINESS** Fully hardy.
• **CULTIVATION** Grow in light, fertile, well-drained soil in full sun or light dappled shade. Often die after flowering; collect seed and propagate regularly.

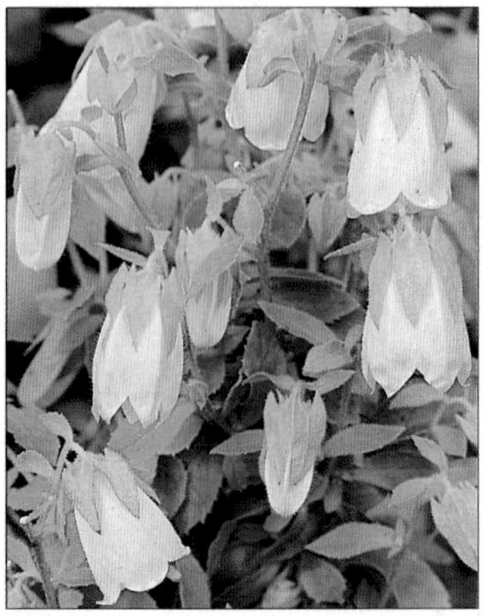

Symphyandra hofmannii

• **PROPAGATION** Sow seed at 13°C (55°F) in winter or early spring, or in containers in a cold frame when ripe.
• **PESTS AND DISEASES** Susceptible to slugs and snails, especially new growth.

S. armena. Upright or spreading, densely hairy, rhizomatous perennial with long-stalked, pointed, heart-shaped, velvety-hairy, irregularly lobed and toothed leaves, to 25cm (10in) long. During summer, produces pendent, bell-shaped, velvet-textured, white or pale blue flowers, to 2cm (¾in) long, usually in terminal corymbs, sometimes solitary. ↕ to 50cm (20in), ↔ to 30cm (12in). Caucasus, Turkey, Iran. ❄❄❄
S. hofmannii ◼ Rosette-forming, usually short-lived, often monocarpic perennial with ovate to lance-shaped, toothed basal leaves, 15cm (6in) long, with winged stalks. Erect stems produce a few alternate, shorter-stalked leaves, and, from early to late summer, they bear terminal racemes of long-lasting, pendent, tubular-bell-shaped, hairy, white to cream flowers, to 3cm (1¼in) long. ↕ 30–60cm (12–24in), ↔ 30cm (12in). Bosnia & Herzegovina. ❄❄❄
S. pendula, syn. *Campanula ossetica.* Arching, spreading, often woody-based perennial with broadly ovate, hairy, pale green leaves, to 15cm (6in) long, heart-shaped at the bases, and with round-toothed margins. In summer, bears short panicles of bell-shaped, velvet-textured, creamy white flowers, to 5cm (2in) long. ↕ to 50cm (20in), ↔ to 30cm (12in). Caucasus. ❄❄❄
S. wanneri ◼ syn. *Campanula wanneri.* Upright, downy, monocarpic perennial with rosettes of lance-shaped, roughly hairy, irregularly toothed leaves, to 10cm (4in) long, stalkless or with winged stalks. Bears pendent, narrowly bell-shaped, deep violet-blue flowers, to 3.5cm (1½in) long, in pyramidal, terminal or axillary panicles, over long periods in summer. ↕↔ to 30cm (12in). Mountains of Romania, Bulgaria, Serbia, Montenegro, Macedonia. ❄❄❄

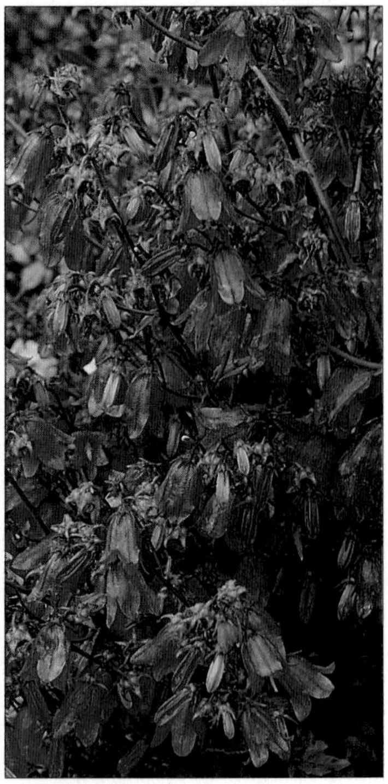

Symphyandra wanneri

SYMPHYTUM

Comfrey

BORAGINACEAE

Genus of 25–35 species of coarse, sometimes invasive, bristly or hairy, rhizomatous perennials from damp, often shady habitats, including woodland, scrub, wasteland, streamsides, and roadsides, in Europe, N. Africa, and W. Asia. Some are used medicinally or for liquid plant food or green manure. They have fleshy roots and long-stalked, oblong- to ovate-lance-shaped or elliptic, wrinkled, prominently veined, mostly basal leaves. Erect, usually branched stems often become decumbent; they bear smaller, more or less stalkless leaves and terminal cymes of pendent, tubular flowers in blue, purple, pink, yellowish white, or white. Excellent ground-cover plants for a shady border or woodland garden, but they can be rampant. Roots and leaves may cause severe discomfort if ingested; contact with foliage may irritate skin.

- **HARDINESS** Fully hardy.
- **CULTIVATION** Grow in moist, moderately fertile soil in full sun or partial shade. Site carefully as all but variegated cultivars may be very invasive; even small pieces of detached root will form new plants. Remove flower stems of variegated cultivars as they form, to keep the foliage attractive. For plant food, grow *S. officinale* and *S.* x *uplandicum* in a permanent, sunny site in a vegetable garden; mulch with well-rotted manure in spring; compost the leaves, or steep in water until decayed, in summer; then use the liquid obtained diluted 1:20.
- **PROPAGATION** Sow seed in containers in a cold frame in autumn or spring. Divide in spring. Take root cuttings in early winter.
- **PESTS AND DISEASES** Trouble free.

S. caucasicum ■ Clump-forming, hairy, rhizomatous perennial with rosettes of oblong-lance-shaped to ovate-lance-shaped, mid-green leaves, to 25cm (10in) long. Bears cymes of bright blue flowers, to 1.5cm (½in) long, on erect then decumbent stems from early to late summer. ↕↔ 60cm (24in), later spreading widely. Caucasus, Iran. ❄❄❄

***S.* 'Goldsmith'** ■ syn. *S. ibericum* 'Jubilee', *S. ibericum* 'Variegatum', *S.* 'Jubilee'. Spreading, hairy, rhizomatous perennial with ovate-lance-shaped, dark green leaves, to 25cm (10in) long, with gold and cream markings. Bears cymes of pale blue, cream, or pink flowers, to 1.5cm (½in) long, in mid- and late spring. ↕↔ 30cm (12in). ❄❄❄

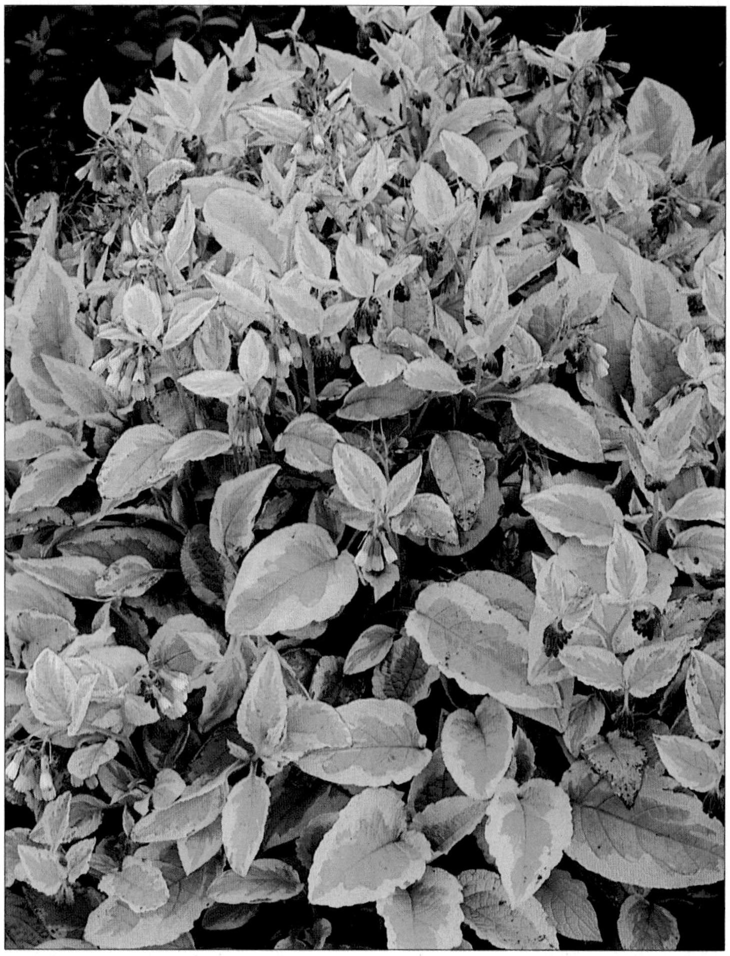

Symphytum 'Goldsmith'

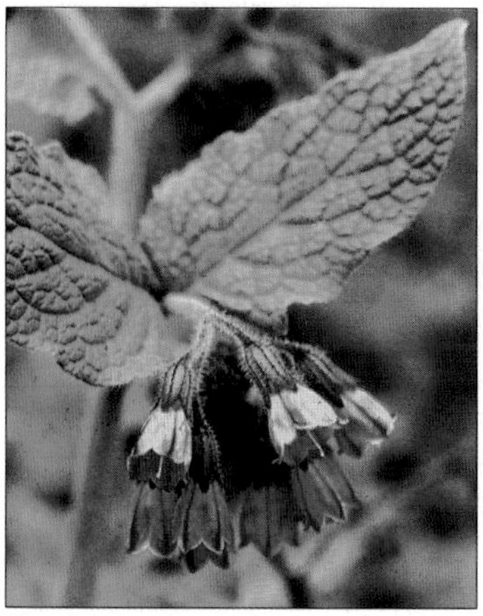

Symphytum caucasicum

***S. grandiflorum* of gardens** see *S. ibericum*.

***S.* 'Hidcote Blue'.** Erect then decumbent, hairy, rhizomatous perennial with ovate to elliptic, mid-green leaves, to 25cm (10in) long. In mid- and late spring, cymes of red buds open to pale blue flowers, to 1.5cm (½in) long, fading with age. ↕↔ 45cm (18in). ❄❄❄

***S.* 'Hidcote Pink'**, syn. *S.* 'Roseum'. Erect then decumbent, hairy, rhizomatous perennial with ovate to elliptic, mid-green leaves, to 25cm (10in) long. Cymes of pale pink and white flowers, to 1.5cm (½in) long, fading with age, are produced in mid- and late spring. ↕↔ 45cm (18in). ❄❄❄

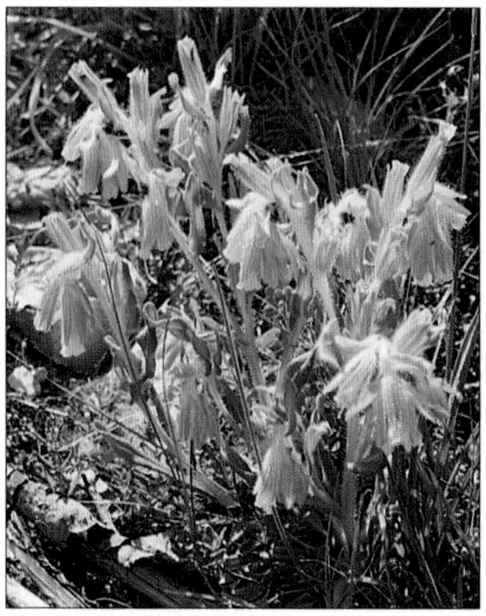

Symphytum tuberosum

S. ibericum, syn. *S. grandiflorum* of gardens. Erect then decumbent, hairy, rhizomatous perennial. Ovate to elliptic or ovate-lance-shaped, mid-green leaves, are to 25cm (10in) long. In late spring and early summer, cymes of red-tipped buds open to pale yellow flowers, to 1.5cm (½in) long. ↕ 40cm (16in), ↔ 60cm (24in), later more. Turkey (N.E. Anatolia), Georgia. ❄❄❄. **'Jubilee'** see *S.* 'Goldsmith'. **'Variegatum'** see *S.* 'Goldsmith'.

***S.* 'Jubilee'** see *S.* 'Goldsmith'.

S. officinale (Common comfrey). Vigorous, clump-forming perennial with winged, upright stems and coarse, hairy, ovate to lance-shaped, dark green leaves, 25cm (10in) long, with winged stalks. From late spring to summer, bears forked cymes of purple-violet, pink, or creamy yellow flowers, to 2cm (¾in) long. ↕ to 1.5m (5ft), ↔ to 2m (6ft) or more. Europe, W. Asia. ❄❄❄. Non-invasive, sterile clones, such as **'Bocking'**, are available.

***S. peregrinum* of gardens** see *S.* x *uplandicum*.

***S.* 'Roseum'** see *S.* 'Hidcote Pink'.

S. tuberosum ■ (Tuberous comfrey). Coarse, creeping perennial producing tuberous rhizomes. Upright, hairy stems bear ovate to lance-shaped, dark green leaves, to 25cm (10in) long, and in early summer produce spiralled cymes of pale yellow flowers, 1.5–2cm (½–¾in) long. ↕ 40–60cm (16–24in), ↔ to 1m (3ft). Europe (Pyrenees to Balkans), N.W. Turkey. ❄❄❄

S.* x *uplandicum (*S. asperum* x *S. officinale*), syn. *S. peregrinum* of gardens. Erect, bristly perennial bearing oblong to elliptic-lance-shaped, mid-green, basal leaves, to 35cm (14in) long, decurrent at the bases. From late spring to late summer, many-branched stems bear cymes of pinkish blue buds, opening to blue-purple flowers, to 2cm (¾in) long. ↕ 2m (6ft), ↔ 1.2m (4ft) or more. Garden origin (naturalized in N. Europe). ❄❄❄. **'Variegatum'** ■ 🏆 has greyish green leaves with broad and irregular cream margins, and pale lilac-pink flowers. Liable to revert, especially if roots are damaged or in poor soil; ↕ 90cm (36in), ↔ 60cm (24in).

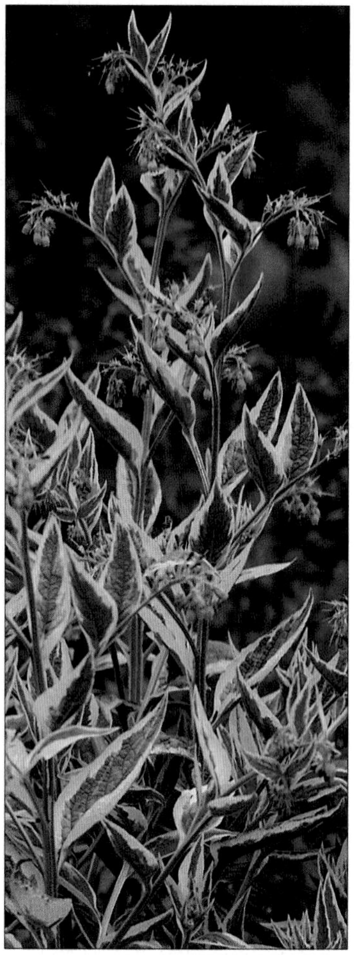

Symphytum x *uplandicum* 'Variegatum'

SYMPLOCOS

SYMPLOCACEAE

Genus of about 250 species of evergreen or deciduous trees and shrubs widely distributed, mainly in woodland, from E. Asia to Australasia and in North and South America. Leaves are alternate and simple. Star-shaped, 5-petalled, usually yellow or white flowers are produced singly or in racemes, panicles, or spikes, followed by blue, black, purple, or white ovoid fruits. Only *S. paniculata* is generally cultivated, for its flowers and fruit; grow in a shrub border. It fruits best when several seedlings are planted together, and in hot summers.

- **HARDINESS** Fully hardy to frost tender.
- **CULTIVATION** Grow in fertile, moist but well-drained, neutral to acid soil in full sun, avoiding very exposed positions. Pruning group 1.
- **PROPAGATION** Sow seed in containers in a cold frame in autumn. Take greenwood cuttings in summer.
- **PESTS AND DISEASES** Trouble free.

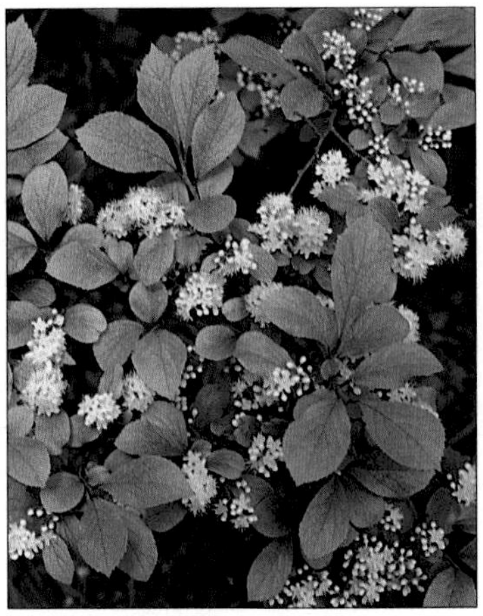

Symplocos paniculata

S. paniculata ▣ ♀ (Sapphire berry). Deciduous, upright, bushy shrub or spreading tree with elliptic to oblong-obovate, finely toothed, sparsely hairy, dark green leaves, to 8cm (3in) long. In late spring and early summer, small, star-shaped, fragrant white flowers, with many prominent stamens, are borne in terminal panicles to 8cm (3in) long, before ovoid, metallic blue fruit, 8mm (⅜in) across. ↕↔ 5m (15ft), rarely to 12m (40ft). Himalayas, E. Asia. ✻✻✻

SYNADENIUM

EUPHORBIACEAE

Genus of about 20 species of evergreen shrubs and small trees from dry slopes and banks in tropical Africa to the Mascarene Islands. Their smooth, fleshy stems contain a milky sap. Leaves are alternate, simple, obovate or lance-shaped, and fleshy; insignificant, petal-less flowers are borne from the upper leaf axils. *S. compactum* var. *rubrum* is most often grown, for its foliage. Where temperatures fall below 10°C (50°F), grow in a temperate or warm greenhouse, or as a houseplant. In warmer, dry areas, grow in a shrub border. All parts of *Synadenium* species are highly toxic if ingested; sap may irritate skin.

- **HARDINESS** Frost tender.
- **CULTIVATION** Under glass, grow in loam-based potting compost (JI No.2), with added sharp sand, in full light. In growth, water moderately and apply a balanced liquid fertilizer monthly. Water sparingly in winter. Outdoors, grow in moderately fertile, well-drained soil in full sun. Pruning group 9; may need restrictive pruning under glass.
- **PROPAGATION** Sow seed at 15–20°C (59–68°F) in spring. Root semi-ripe cuttings in summer, with bottom heat.
- **PESTS AND DISEASES** Root mealybugs may be a problem under glass.

S. compactum* var. *rubrum, syn. *S grantii* 'Rubrum', *S. grantii* var. *rubrum*. Erect, succulent shrub, eventually moderately bushy, with obovate, finely toothed red leaves, 8–18cm (3–7in) long, red-purple beneath. Throughout the year, bears cup-shaped, yellow-green floral bracts with red glands, in cymes 10–15cm (4–6in) long. ↕ to 3m (10ft), ↔ to 2m (6ft). ❀ (min. 10°C/50°F)
***S. grantii* 'Rubrum'** see *S. compactum* var. *rubrum*.
S. grantii* var. *rubrum see *S. compactum* var. *rubrum*.

SYNGONIUM

ARACEAE

Genus of 33 species of evergreen, root climbers from woodland in tropical Central and South America. The alternate leaves are initially simple and ovate to triangular, becoming larger, long-stalked, arrow-shaped, then 3- to 5-lobed or pedate as the plants mature. Tiny, petalless flowers are borne on spadices surrounded by pale green and cream to purplish green spathes, which often become bright red at fruiting time. They rarely flower in cultivation, and are grown for foliage. Where temperatures fall below 15°C (59°F), grow in a warm greenhouse or as houseplants. In warmer climates, use as ground cover, or to clothe a wall. All parts may cause mild stomach upset if ingested; contact with the sap may irritate skin.

- **HARDINESS** Half hardy to frost tender.
- **CULTIVATION** Under glass, grow in loamless potting compost, in bright indirect light for green-leaved species, or in bright filtered light for variegated ones. Provide moderate humidity. When in growth, water freely and apply a balanced liquid fertilizer every 3 or 4 weeks. Water moderately in winter. Support with a moss pole. Outdoors, grow in fertile, moist soil in light dappled or partial shade. Pruning group 11, in late winter or early spring.
- **PROPAGATION** Root stem-tip cuttings or leaf-bud cuttings in summer, with bottom heat.
- **PESTS AND DISEASES** Mealybugs and red spider mites may be a problem under glass.

S. auritum, syn. *Philodendron auritum* of gardens, *P. trifoliatum* (Five fingers). Sparsely branched trailer or climber. Juvenile leaves are ovate to triangular, often arrow-shaped, glossy, mid- to deep green, and to 15cm (6in) long; mature leaves are pedate, each with usually 3 or 5 elliptic, deep green leaflets, the central

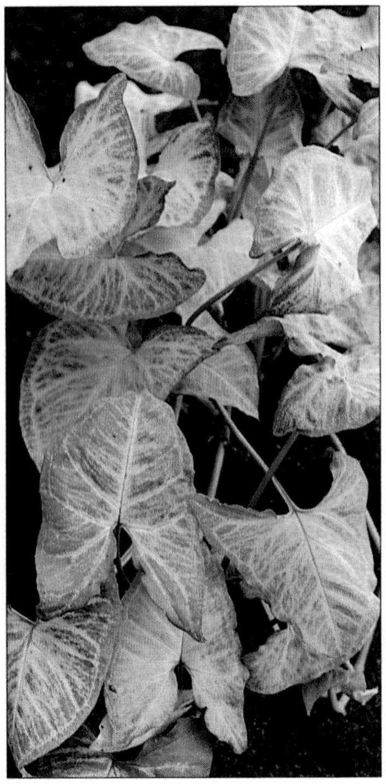

Syngonium podophyllum

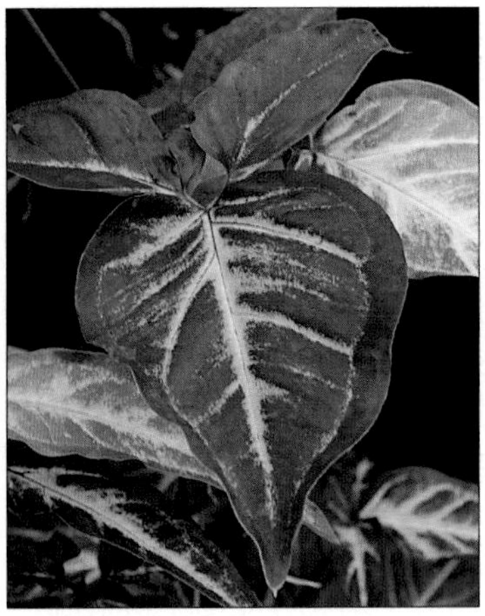

Syngonium podophyllum 'Trileaf Wonder'

one broadly elliptic and 10–30cm (4–12in) long, the others much smaller. In summer, green and cream spathes, to 9cm (3½in) long, are borne in groups from the leaf axils. ↕ to 3m (10ft) or more. Cuba, Jamaica, Haiti, Dominican Republic. ❀ (min. 15°C/59°F).
'Fantasy' has white-mottled leaves.
S. erythrophyllum. Sparsely branched climber with ovate juvenile leaves, heart-shaped at the bases, to 10cm (4in) long; adult leaves are each composed of 3 elliptic leaflets, the central one largest, 10–22cm (4–9in) long, pale at first, then very dark green above and purple-flushed beneath. Green and white spathes, 8–11cm (3–4½in) long, with longer spadices, are produced from the leaf axils in summer. ↕ 2–3m (6–10ft) or more. Panama. ❀ (min. 15°C/59°F)
S. podophyllum ▣ ♀ syn. *Nephthytis triphylla* of gardens (Goosefoot). Sparsely branched climber, compact or trailing when young. Juvenile leaves, 7–14cm (3–5½in) long, are ovate with heart-shaped bases; when mature they are arrow-shaped, later pedate, each with 5–11 elliptic leaflets, the largest leaflet 16–40cm (6–16in) long; all are dark green above, sometimes with grey-green markings, paler beneath. In summer, green and greenish white to cream or, more rarely, yellow spathes, 11cm (4½in) long, are borne in groups of 4–11 from the leaf axils. ↕ 1–2m (3–6ft) or more. Mexico to Brazil. ❀ (min. 15°C/59°F). **'Trileaf Wonder'** ▣ produces leaves with silvery grey veins. **'Variegatum'** has arrow-shaped leaves splashed creamy white.

SYNNOTIA

IRIDACEAE

Genus, sometimes included in *Sparaxis*, of 5 species of small, spring-flowering, cormous perennials from low-altitude grassland and scrub in South Africa. They have basal fans of 2-ranked, linear or oblong to lance-shaped leaves. Branched or unbranched stems bear short spikes of funnel-shaped, cream, yellow, lilac, or mauve flowers, hooded like gladioli. In frost-prone areas, grow in a cool greenhouse or bulb frame. In warmer areas, grow in a sunny border.

- **HARDINESS** Half hardy.
- **CULTIVATION** Plant corms in autumn, 10cm (4in) deep. Under glass, grow in loam-based potting compost (JI No.2), with added sand and leaf mould, in full light. Keep cool and only slightly moist until roots are well developed. Water sparingly when in growth, and dry off as the leaves wither; keep dry and frost-free when dormant in summer. Outdoors, grow in a warm, sheltered site in moderately fertile, well-drained soil in full sun. Provide a dry winter mulch, and keep dry in summer.
- **PROPAGATION** Sow seed at 16°C (61°F) as soon as ripe, or in spring. Remove offsets when dormant.
- **PESTS AND DISEASES** Trouble free.

S. variegata. Cormous perennial with a fan of oblong, basal leaves, each to 15cm (6in) long. In spring, an unbranched or 1- to 3-branched stem produces up to 7 hooded flowers, 3cm (1¼in) across, evenly coloured yellow and violet, or lavender-blue to deep purple with yellow stripes on the lower lips and in the throats. ↕ 15–40cm (6–16in), ↔ 8cm (3in). South Africa (Western Cape). ✻. **var. *metelerkampiae*** has a branched stem, each branch bearing a sparse spike of violet flowers, marked orange on each of the lower 3 petals.

SYNTHYRIS

SCROPHULARIACEAE

Genus of about 14 species of tufted, low-growing, usually rhizomatous perennials, mainly from woodland in W. and C. North America. They have radical, heart-shaped, kidney-shaped, or pinnatifid leaves. Unbranched, leafy, upright stems produce narrow, upright, spike-like racemes of small, tubular to bell-shaped, violet to blue, or rarely pink or white flowers, mainly in spring. Grow in a woodland or rock garden, or at the front of a shady, herbaceous border. Grow *S. pinnatifida* var. *lanuginosa* in a scree bed or alpine house; it is hard to grow and flower buds often abort.

- **HARDINESS** Fully hardy, but intolerant of winter wet.
- **CULTIVATION** Grow in fertile, moist but well-drained, humus-rich soil in partial or deep shade. For *S. pinnatifida* var. *lanuginosa*: in a scree bed, grow in gritty, poor to moderately fertile, humus-rich soil in full sun with some midday shade; in an alpine house, use a mix of equal parts loam, leaf mould, and grit, water moderately when in growth, and keep just moist in winter.
- **PROPAGATION** Sow seed in containers in an open frame in autumn. Divide in early spring as growth begins.

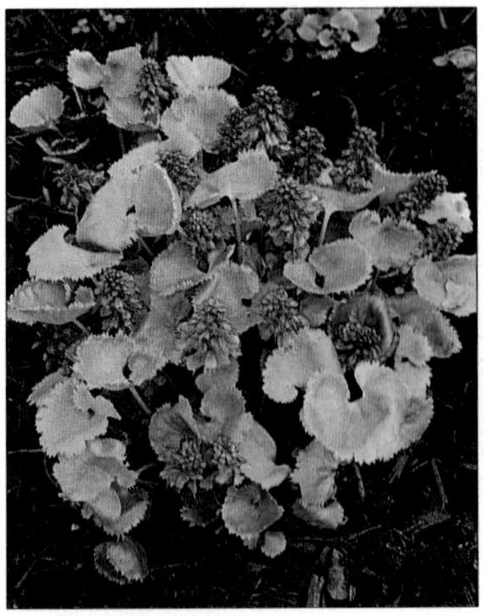

Synthyris missurica

S

• **PESTS AND DISEASES** Prone to attack by slugs and snails. Aphids and red spider mites may damage *S. pinnatifida* var. *lanuginosa* under glass.

S. missurica ■ Clump-forming herbaceous perennial with rounded-heart-shaped to kidney-shaped, shallowly lobed, bluntly toothed, leathery, dark green leaves, to 5cm (2in) across. Over long periods in spring, bears tubular-bell-shaped, deep lavender-blue flowers, to 2cm (¾in) long, with prominent styles and anthers, in abundant dense, upright, spike-like racemes, 5–10cm (2–4in) long. ↕ to 25cm (10in), ↔ to 30cm (12in). Arctic Canada to N. and C. USA. ❄❄❄
S. pinnatifida. Clump-forming herbaceous perennial bearing ovate, pinnate, mid-green leaves, to 10cm (4in) long, with linear, toothed segments. In late spring, produces racemes 10–15cm (4–6in) long, of tubular, lavender-blue flowers, to 5cm (2in) long, with silver calyces. ↕↔ to 15cm (6in). USA (Washington). ❄❄❄. **var. *lanuginosa*** forms a low mound, with silvery grey leaves, and bears deep blue flowers, to 2cm (¾in) long, in racemes 3–6cm (1¼–2½in) long; ↕ to 10cm (4in).
S. reniformis. Clump-forming, evergreen perennial with shallowly round-lobed, rounded-heart-shaped, dark green leaves, to 5cm (2in) long, paler beneath. In spring, bears bell-shaped, blue, pink, or white flowers, to 9mm (⅜in) long, in short racemes, to 3cm (1¼in) long. ↕ to 15cm (6in), ↔ to 25cm (10in). USA (Washington, Oregon). ❄❄❄
S. stellata ■ Clump-forming herbaceous perennial with rounded-heart-shaped, hairy, dark green leaves, to 5cm (2in) across, deeply and doubly toothed. From spring to early summer, bears dense, spike-like racemes, 8–15cm (3–6in) long, of bell-shaped, violet-blue flowers, to 6mm (¼in) long, with conspicuous, sharply toothed bracts. ↕ to 15cm (6in), ↔ to 25cm (10in). USA (Washington, Oregon). ❄❄❄

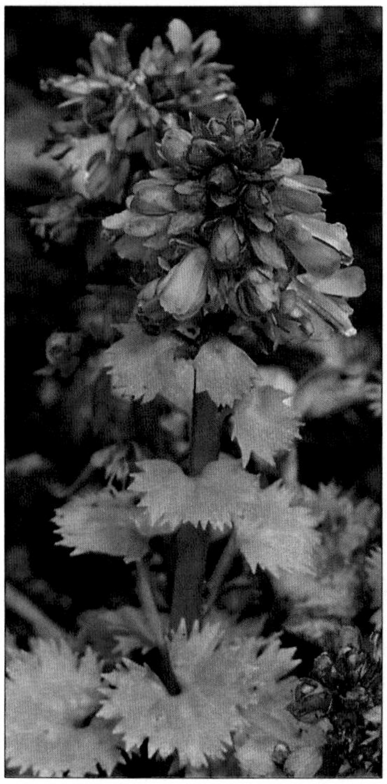

Synthyris stellata

SYRINGA

Lilac

OLEACEAE

Genus of about 20 species of deciduous shrubs and trees found in woodland and scrub from S.E. Europe to E. Asia. They are grown for their often pyramidal or conical panicles of small, tubular, usually very fragrant flowers, which may be white, pink, almost red to magenta, lilac (light purplish pink), or blue. They have opposite, entire, lance-shaped to rounded, usually ovate, rarely pinnate leaves. Most garden cultivars are grouped under *S. vulgaris*. Grow lilacs in a shrub border or as specimen trees.
• **HARDINESS** Fully hardy, but late frosts may damage new growth.
• **CULTIVATION** Grow in fertile, humus-rich, well-drained, neutral to alkaline soil in full sun. Mulch regularly. Dead-head newly planted lilacs before fruits form. Pruning group 1 or 2, but prune only lightly; group 1 for *S. reticulata*, *S. vulgaris*, and cultivars; *S. vulgaris* tolerates hard renovation pruning.
• **PROPAGATION** Sow seed in containers in a cold frame as soon as ripe or in spring. Take greenwood cuttings, or layer, in early summer. Graft in winter or bud in midsummer.
• **PESTS AND DISEASES** May be affected by lilac blight, honey fungus, leaf miners, thrips, and willow scale.

S. afghanica see *S. protolaciniata*.
S. x chinensis (*S.* x *persica* x *S. vulgaris*) (Rouen lilac). Bushy shrub with arching branches and oval leaves, to 8cm (3in) long. In late spring, produces fragrant, lilac-purple flowers in large, nodding panicles, to 15cm (6in) long. ↕↔ 4m (12ft). Garden origin. ❄❄❄. **'Alba'** ■ bears white flowers. **'Saugeana'** has lilac-red flowers.
S. emodi (Himalayan lilac). Vigorous, upright shrub with stout shoots and elliptic-oblong leaves, to 15cm (6in) long. Unpleasantly scented, pale lilac flowers are produced in large, upright panicles, to 15cm (6in) long, in early summer. ↕ 5m (15ft), ↔ 4m (12ft). Afghanistan, Himalayas. ❄❄❄
S. 'Fountain'. Upright shrub with ovate, tapered leaves, 5–15cm (2–6in) long, mid-green above, blue-green and softly hairy beneath. In early summer, bears single, pale pink flowers in narrow, conical, nodding panicles, to 15cm (6in) long. ↕ 3–4m (10–12ft), ↔ 2–3m (6–10ft). ❄❄❄
S. x hyacinthiflora (*S. oblata* x *S. vulgaris*). Spreading shrub, upright when young, with broadly heart-shaped leaves, bronze when young, often purple in autumn. In mid- and late spring, bears fragrant, single or double, variably coloured flowers, in large panicles, to 12cm (5in) long. ↕↔ 5m (15ft). Garden origin. ❄❄❄. **'Alice Eastwood'** bears double, claret-purple flowers in slender panicles. **'Blue Hyacinth'** ■ has single, lilac to blue flowers. **'Clarke's Giant'** ■ has large, single flowers, purple in bud, opening lilac, in panicles to 30cm (12in) long. **'Cora Brandt'** ■ has double white flowers in large, open panicles, 20–23cm (8–9in) long. **'Esther Staley'** ■🏆 is vigorous, with profuse single, lilac-pink flowers opening from mauve-red buds.
S. 'Isabella' see *S.* x *prestoniae* 'Isabella'.

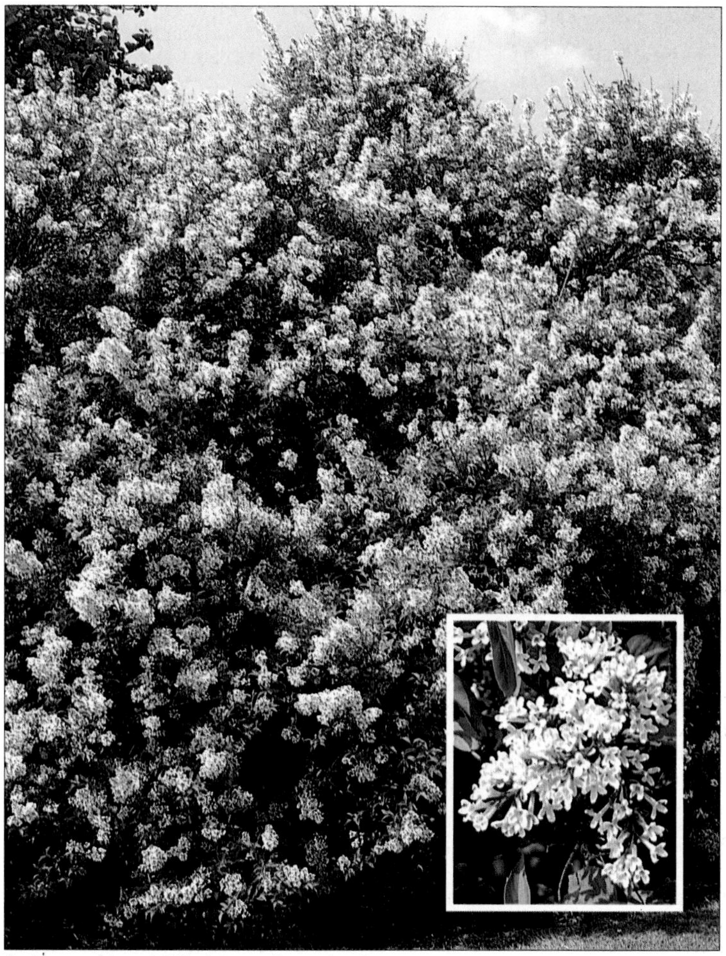

Syringa x *chinensis* 'Alba' (inset: flower detail)

S. x josiflexa (*S. josikaea* x *S. komarowii* subsp. *reflexa*). Upright shrub with ovate to oblong-lance-shaped, mid-green leaves, 8–15cm (3–6in) long, white-hairy beneath. In early summer, bears fragrant, lavender-pink flowers in conical to cylindrical panicles, 10–20cm (4–8in) long. ↕ 3m (10ft), ↔ 2m (6ft). Garden origin. ❄❄❄. **'Bellicent'** 🏆 has tapered, dark green leaves, and bears clear pink flowers in late spring and early summer; ↕ 4m (12ft), ↔ 5m (15ft).
S. x laciniata ■ (*S. protolaciniata* x *S. vulgaris*). Spreading shrub with lance-shaped to pinnate leaves, to 8cm (3in) long, composed of up to 9 narrowly elliptic, dark green leaflets. Fragrant lilac flowers, in panicles to 10cm (4in) long, are produced in late spring. ↕ 2m (6ft), ↔ 3m (10ft). Garden origin. ❄❄❄
S. meyeri. Compact, rounded shrub with oval leaves, 1–3cm (½–1¼in) long. Bears fragrant, bluish pink or lavender-pink flowers in small panicles, 3–8cm (1¼–3in) long, in late spring and early summer. ↕ 1.5–2m (5–6ft), ↔ 1.2m (4ft). ❄❄❄. **'Palibin'** ■🏆 syn. *S. palibiniana* of gardens, *S. patula* of gardens, *S. velutina* of gardens, is slow-growing, with lavender-pink flowers in dense panicles, to 10cm (4in) long; ↔ 1.5m (5ft).

S

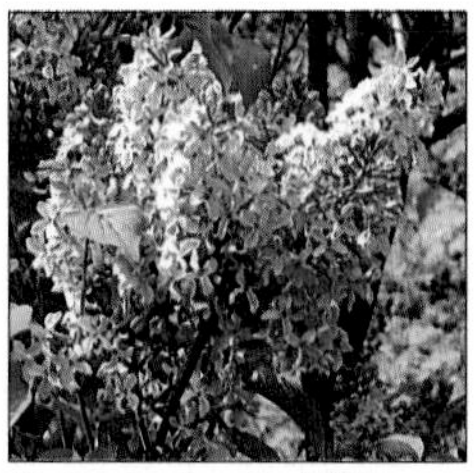

Syringa x *hyacinthiflora* 'Blue Hyacinth'

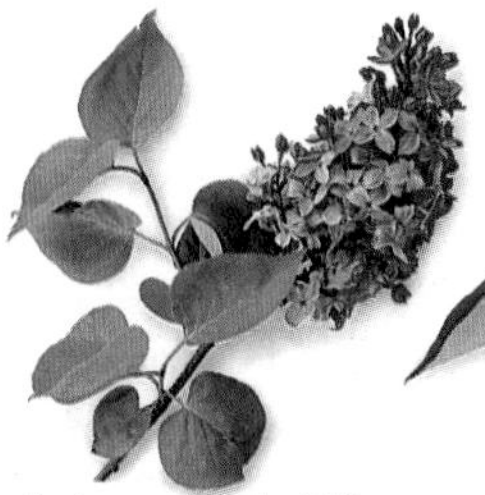

Syringa x *hyacinthiflora* 'Clarke's Giant'

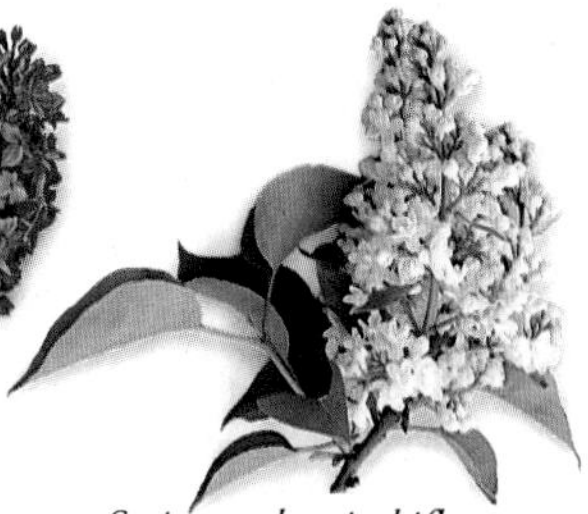

Syringa x *hyacinthiflora* 'Cora Brandt'

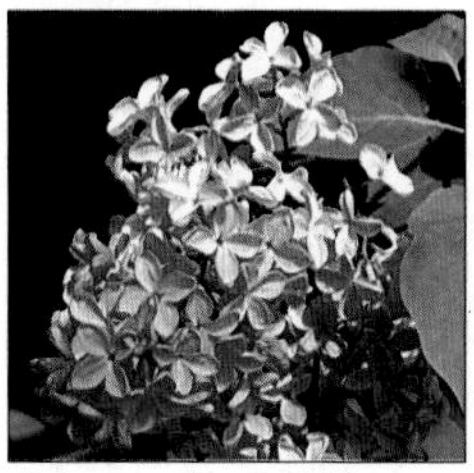

Syringa x *hyacinthiflora* 'Esther Staley'

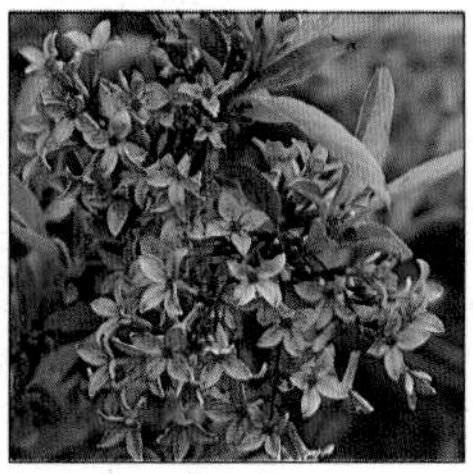

Syringa x *laciniata*

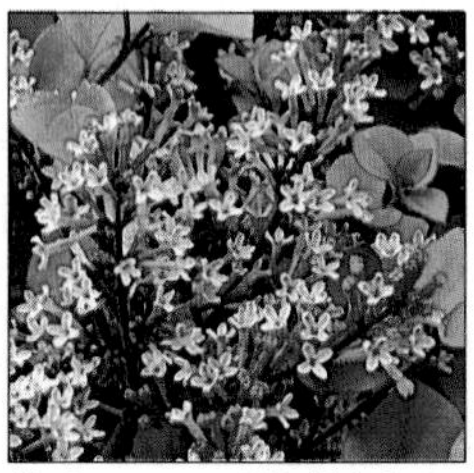

Syringa meyeri 'Palibin'

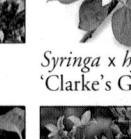

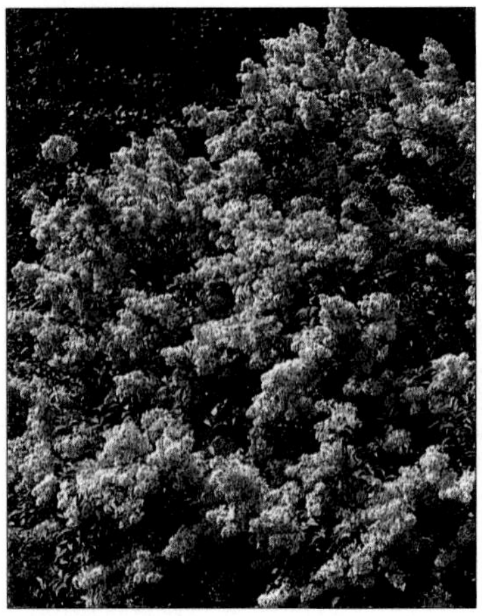

Syringa x *persica*

S. microphylla see *S. pubescens* subsp. *microphylla*.
S. oblata* var. *dilatata 🗨 Vigorous, upright, later spreading shrub or small tree with broadly heart-shaped, tapered leaves, to 8cm (3in) long, bronze when young, then glossy, mid-green, turning purple in autumn. Fragrant, pale lilac flowers, in broad panicles, to 12cm (5in) long, are produced in mid-spring. ↕↔ 5m (15ft). Korea. ✻✻✻
***S. palibiniana* of gardens** see *S. meyeri* 'Palibin'.
S. patula see *S. pubescens* subsp. *patula*.
***S. patula* of gardens** see *S. meyeri* 'Palibin'.
S. pekinensis see *S. reticulata* subsp. *pekinensis*.
S. x persica ▣🏆 (*S. afghanica* x *S. laciniata*) (Persian lilac). Compact, bushy shrub with lance-shaped, rarely 3-lobed, dark green leaves, to 6cm (2½in) long. In late spring, profusely bears fragrant purple flowers in small, dense panicles, to 5cm (2in) long. ↕↔ 2m (6ft). Garden origin. ✻✻✻. **'Alba'** 🏆 has white flowers.
S. pinnatifolia. Open, upright shrub with peeling bark on older branches. Each pinnate leaf, to 6cm (2½in) long, has up to 11 ovate to lance-shaped, dark green leaflets. In late spring, bears fragrant, lilac-flushed white flowers, in panicles to 7cm (3in) long. ↕ to 4m (12ft), ↔ 2.5m (8ft). W. China. ✻✻✻
S. x prestoniae ◊ (*S. reflexa* x *S. villosa*). Vigorous, upright shrub or small tree with oval, dark green leaves, to 15cm (6in) long. In early summer, bears fragrant, white, pink, lavender-pink, lavender-blue, violet, magenta, or deep purple flowers in large, erect to nodding panicles, 10–16cm (4–6in) long. ↕↔ 4m (12ft). Garden origin. ✻✻✻. **'Audrey'** has dark pink flowers. **'Coral'** bears pale pink flowers, fading to nearly white. **'Elinor'** 🏆 bears pale lavender-blue flowers from purple buds. **'Isabella'**, syn. *S.* 'Isabella', flowers purple-pink.
S. protolaciniata, syn. *S. afghanica*. Graceful, open, spreading shrub with slender, purplish brown shoots and pinnate leaves, to 7cm (3in) long, each with 3–9 narrowly elliptic to lance-shaped, dark green leaflets. In late spring, bears fragrant lilac flowers, in panicles to 7cm (3in) long. ↕ 3m (10ft), ↔ 1.5m (5ft). W. China. ✻✻✻
S. pubescens. Erect, spreading, often bushy shrub with slender branches, red-green when young, and lance-shaped to ovate or elliptic, glossy, dark green leaves, to 9cm (3½in) long, densely grey-white-hairy beneath. In spring and early summer, bears strongly scented, white-throated, purplish lilac flowers, in panicles to 12cm (5in) long. ↕ to 6m (20ft), ↔ 6m (20ft). N. central China. ✻✻✻. **subsp. *microphylla***, syn. *S. microphylla*, is conical and spreading or upright. Lilac-pink flowers are borne in small panicles, to 7cm (3in) long, in early summer, often again in autumn; W. China. **subsp. *microphylla* 'Superba'** ▣🏆 has rose-pink flowers. After initial flowering, it blooms irregularly until autumn. **subsp. *patula***, syn. *S. patula*, has dull green leaves, 5–11cm (2–4½in) long, with purple young shoots. Purplish lilac flowers, in nodding panicles, open from lilac buds; ↕ 4m (12ft), ↔ 2m (6ft); N. China, Korea. **subsp. *patula* 'Miss Kim'** 🏆 is similar to subsp. *patula*, but mound-forming; leaves may turn purple in autumn; ↕ 2m (6ft), ↔ 1.5m (5ft).
S. reflexa 🏆 Vigorous, upright shrub with stout shoots and oval, dark green leaves, to 15cm (6in) long. Bears rich purple-pink flowers in slender, nodding panicles, to 16cm (6in) long, in late spring and early summer. ↕↔ 4m (12ft). C. China. ✻✻✻
S. reticulata ◊ Upright shrub or broadly conical tree with an oval crown

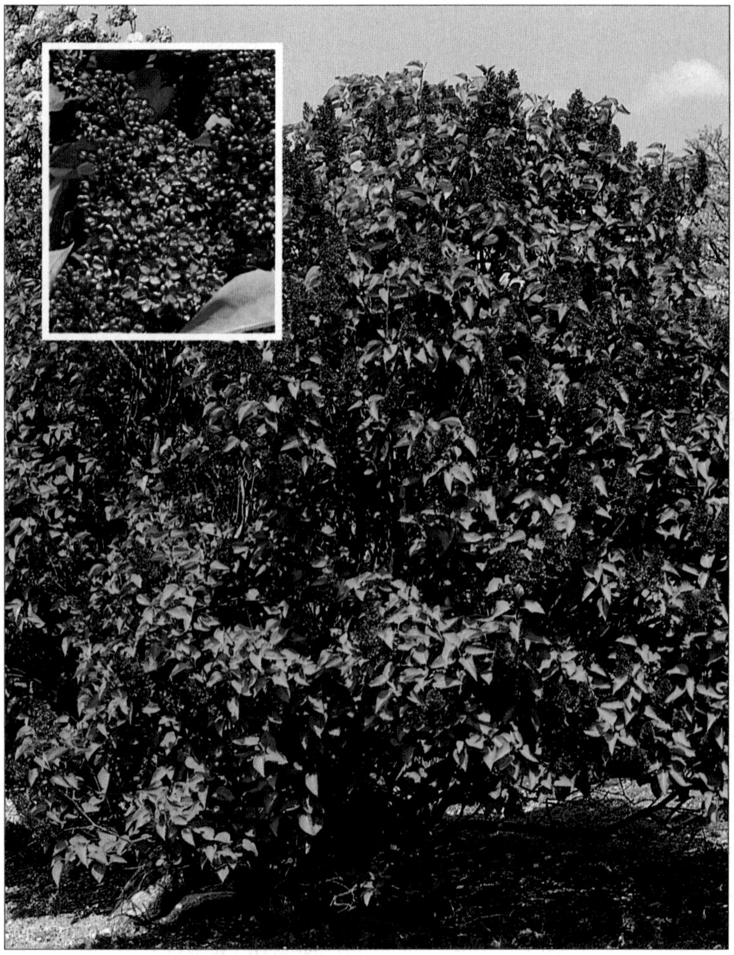

Syringa vulgaris 'Monge' (inset: flower detail)

and reddish brown, shining bark when young. Leaves are lance-shaped to ovate, sharp-pointed, and to 15cm (6in) long. Bears fragrant, creamy white flowers, in large, showy panicles, to 20cm (8in) long, in early and midsummer. ↕ 10m (30ft), ↔ 6m (20ft). Japan. ✻✻✻. **'Ivory Silk'** is compact, and flowers profusely, even when young; ↕ 3–4m (10–12ft), ↔ 2m (6ft). **subsp. *pekinensis*** 🗨 syn. *S. pekinensis*, is spreading, with arching branches and dark green leaves, to 8cm (3in) long; ↕↔ 5m (15ft); Mongolia, N. China.
S. x swegiflexa (*S. reflexa* x *S. sweginzowii*). Upright shrub with purple-grey young stems and oblong-lance-shaped to oval leaves, 5–12cm (2–5in) long. Fragrant pink flowers, opening from deep red buds, are produced in nearly cylindrical, nodding panicles, 10–20cm (4–8in) long, in late spring and early summer. ↕ 4m (12ft), ↔ 2.5m (8ft). Garden origin. ✻✻✻
S. sweginzowii ▣ Upright shrub with red-purple shoots and elliptic-oblong to lance-shaped leaves, to 10cm (4in) long. Fragrant, pale pink to lilac-pink or white flowers, in upright panicles, to 20cm (8in) long, are produced in late spring and early summer. ↕ 4m (12ft), ↔ 2.5m (8ft). S.W. China. ✻✻✻

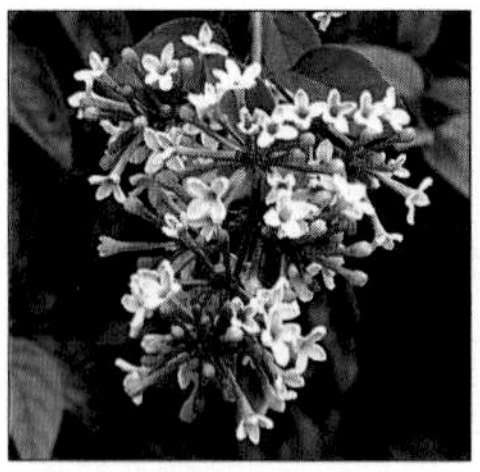

Syringa pubescens subsp. *microphylla* 'Superba'

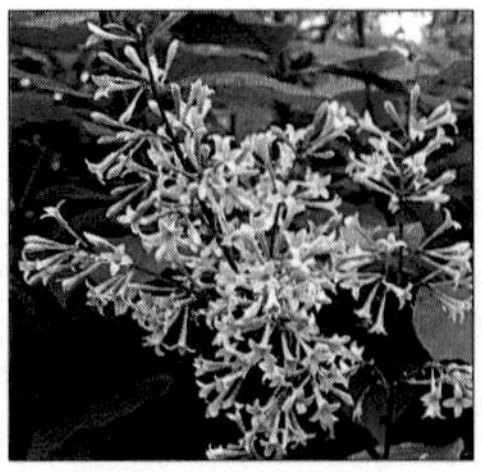

Syringa sweginzowii

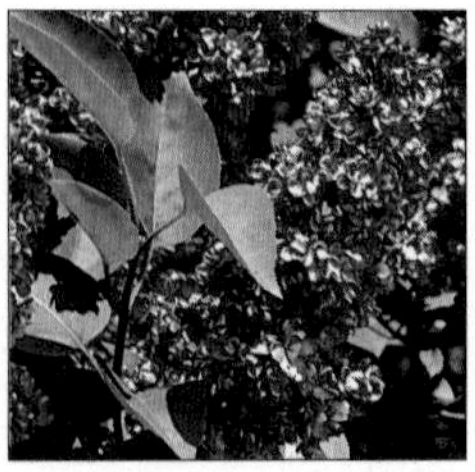

Syringa vulgaris 'Charles Joly'

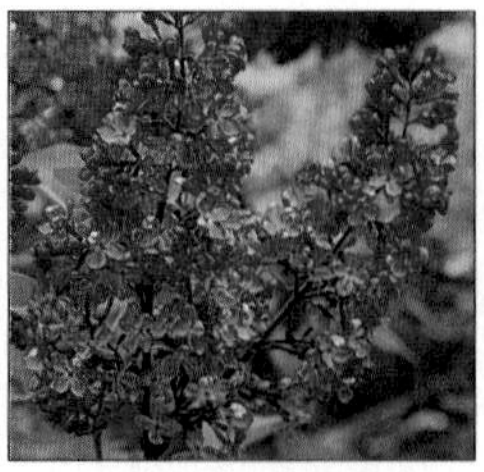

Syringa vulgaris 'Charles X'

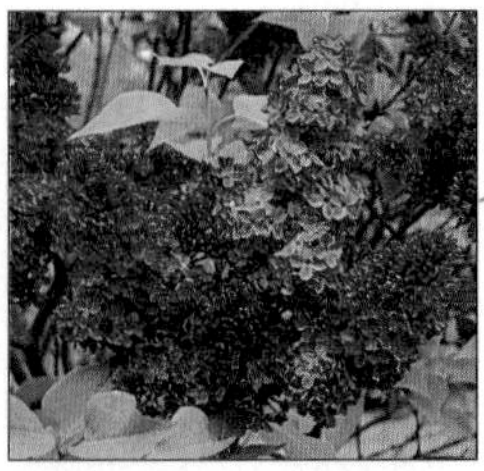

Syringa vulgaris 'Congo'

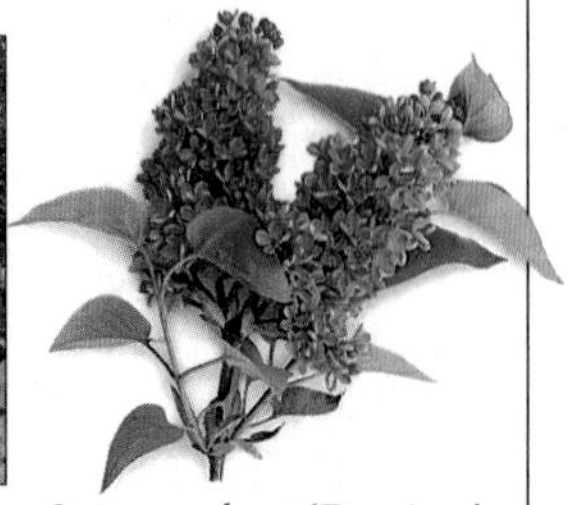

Syringa vulgaris 'Decaisne'

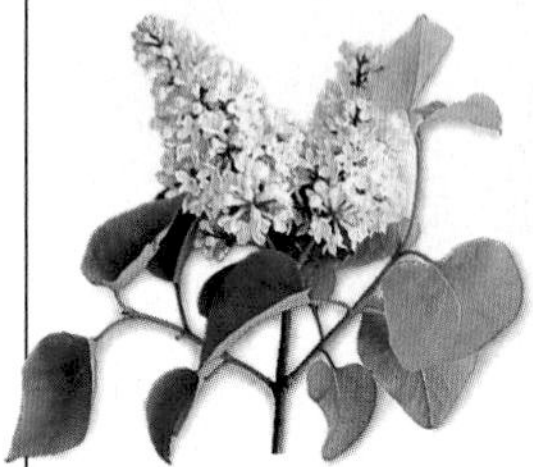

Syringa vulgaris 'Jan van Tol'

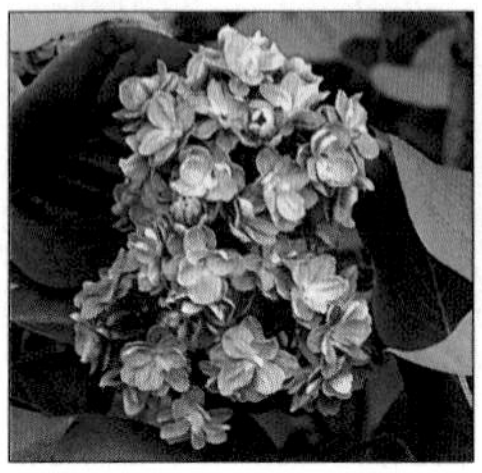

Syringa vulgaris 'Katherine Havemeyer'

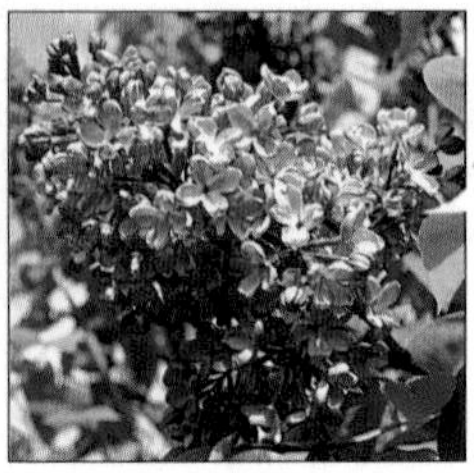

Syringa vulgaris 'Maréchal Foch'

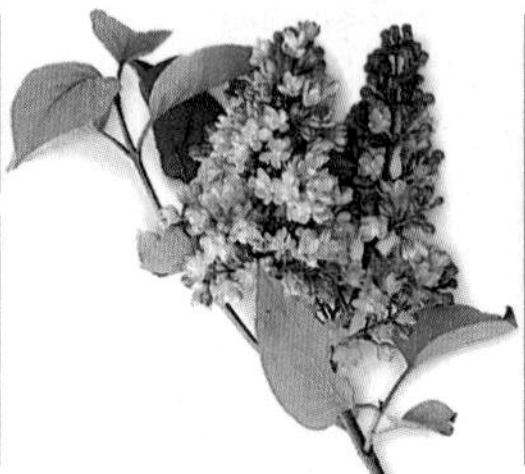

Syringa vulgaris 'Michel Buchner'

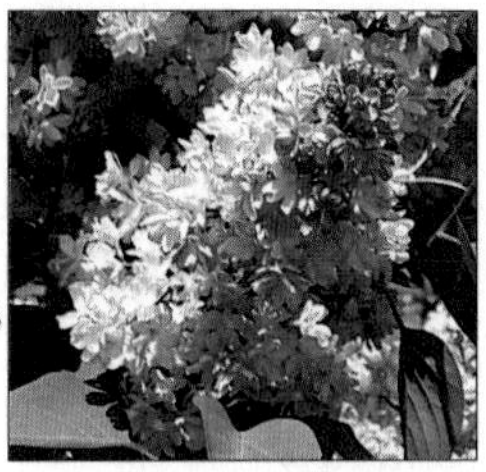

Syringa vulgaris 'Mme Antoine Buchner'

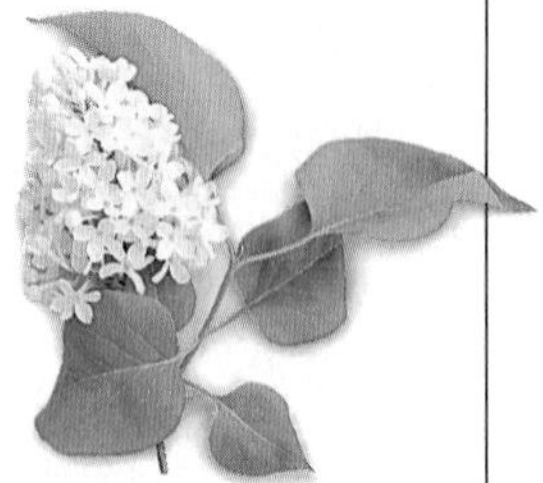

Syringa vulgaris 'Mme Florent Stepman'

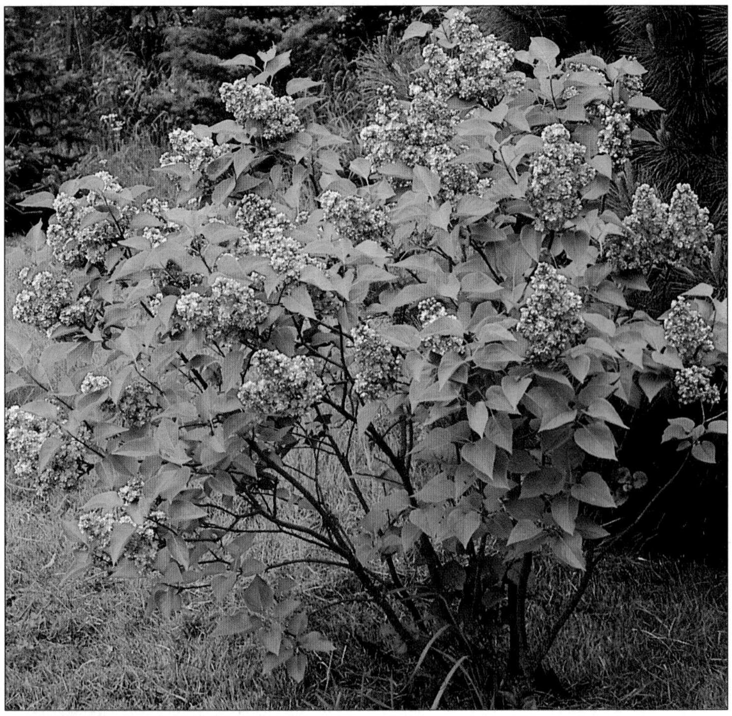

Syringa vulgaris 'Président Grévy'

***S. velutina* of gardens** see *S. meyeri* 'Palibin'.
S. villosa. Compact, rounded shrub with upright shoots and ovate to oblong leaves, to 20cm (8in) long. Fragrant pink flowers, in large, conical panicles, to 20cm (8in) long, are produced in late spring and early summer. ↕↔ 4m (12ft). N. China. ❄❄❄
S. vulgaris ♀ (Common lilac). Spreading shrub or small tree, upright when young, with heart-shaped to ovate leaves, to 10cm (4in) long. Very fragrant, single or double lilac flowers are produced in dense, conical panicles, to 10–20cm (4–8in) long, in late spring and early summer. ↕↔ 7m (22ft). E. Europe. ❄❄❄. **'Alphonse Lavallée'** bears double, lilac-blue flowers, from purple buds. **'Ami Schott'** bears double, cobalt-blue flowers. **'Andenken an Ludwig Späth'** ♀ syn. 'Souvenir de Louis Spaeth', produces slender panicles, to 30cm (12in) long, of single, dark purple-red flowers. **'Belle de Nancy'** produces large panicles of double, mauve-pink flowers, from purple buds. **'Cavour'** bears upright panicles of single, violet-blue flowers. **'Charles Joly'** ■ ♀ bears double, dark purple flowers. **'Charles X'** ■ produces single, purple-red flowers. **'Christophe Colomb'**, syn. 'Christopher Columbus', bears single, deep lilac-pink flowers. **'Congo'** ■ bears large, single, dark lilac-purple flowers, from purple-red buds. **'Decaisne'** ■ is compact, with many single, light purplish blue flowers; ↕ to 2.5m (8ft), ↔ 1.5m (5ft). **'Edith Cavell'** bears panicles, to 30cm (12in) long, of large, double, creamy white flowers. **'Firmament'** ♀ produces single, light blue flowers. **'Glory of Horstenstein'** see 'Ruhm von Horstenstein'. **'Jan van Tol'** ■ bears panicles, to 35cm (14in) long, of single, pure white flowers. The vigorous **'Katherine Havemeyer'** ■ ♀ bears double, lavender-blue flowers, from purple buds. **'Lucie Baltet'** bears single, pale pink flowers, from purple-pink buds. **'Maréchal Foch'** ■ bears single, carmine-pink flowers. **'Maréchal Lannes'** bears double, pale violet flowers. **'Masséna'** bears loose panicles of large, single, dark purple flowers. **'Maud Notcutt'** produces single, pure white flowers. **'Michel Buchner'** ■ bears large panicles, to 30cm (12in) long, of double, rose-lilac, white-centred flowers. **'Mme Antoine Buchner'** ■ ♀ bears slender panicles of double, pale mauve-pink flowers, from dark purple-red buds. **'Mme Florent Stepman'** ■ bears large panicles, to 25cm (10in) long, of single white flowers. **'Mme F. Morel'** ■ produces large panicles of single, dark mauve-pink flowers. **'Mme Lemoine'** ■ ♀ bears compact panicles of large, double white flowers, from creamy buds. **'Monge'** ■ bears a profusion of very large, single, dark purple-red flowers. **'Montaigne'** bears double, pale pink flowers, from purple-pink buds. **'Mont Blanc'** produces large panicles, to 35cm (14in) long, of single white flowers. **'Mrs. Edward Harding'** ■ ♀ bears large panicles, to 25cm (10in) long, of double, purple-red flowers. **'Night'** bears single, dark purple flowers. **'Olivier de Serres'** bears large panicles, to 35cm (14in) long, of large, double, lavender-blue flowers, from purple-blue buds. **'Paul Hariot'** bears slender panicles of large, double, dark violet-red flowers. **'Paul Thirion'** ■ produces double, lilac-pink flowers, from dark purple-red buds. **'Président Grévy'** ■ bears very large panicles, to 25cm (10in) long, of double, lilac-blue flowers, from red-violet buds. **'Primrose'** ■ bears small panicles of fragrant, single, pale creamy yellow flowers. **'Ruhm von Horstenstein'**, syn. 'Glory of Horstenstein', is vigorous, with compact panicles of single, dark lilac-red flowers. **'Souvenir de Louis Spaeth'** see 'Andenken an Ludwig Späth'. **'Vestale'** ♀ bears many single, pure white flowers. **'Victor Lemoine'** bears slender panicles of double, pale lavender-pink to lilac-blue flowers. **'Violetta'** bears long, slim panicles of double, dark violet flowers.
S. yunnanensis ■ Upright shrub with elliptic-oblong leaves, to 10cm (4in) long. Fragrant, pale pink to nearly white flowers, in large, upright or semi-pendent panicles, to 15cm (6in) long, are produced in early summer. ↕ 3m (10ft), ↔ 2.5m (8ft). W. China. ❄❄❄

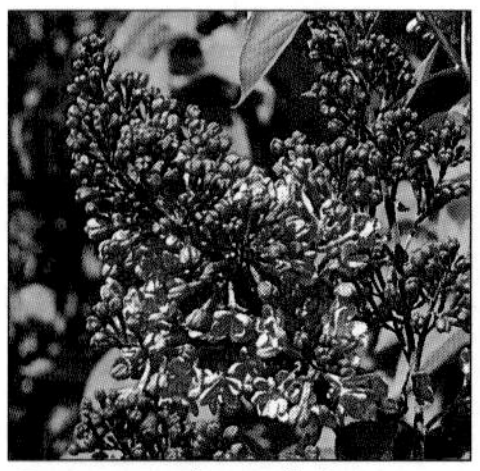

Syringa vulgaris 'Mme F. Morel'

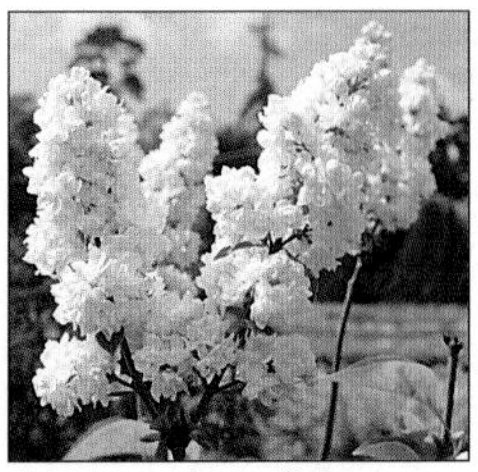

Syringa vulgaris 'Mme Lemoine'

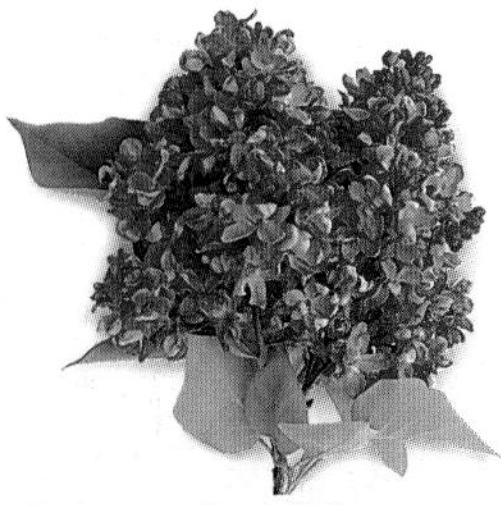

Syringa vulgaris 'Mrs. Edward Harding'

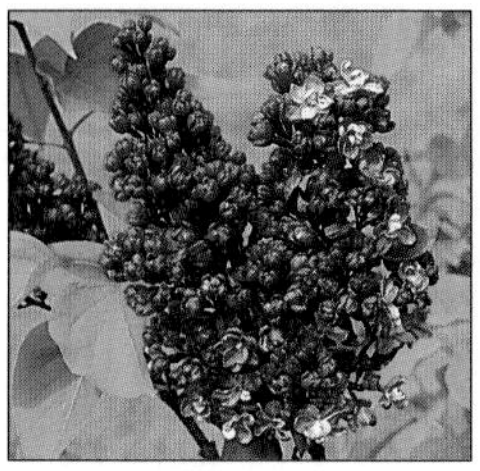

Syringa vulgaris 'Paul Thirion'

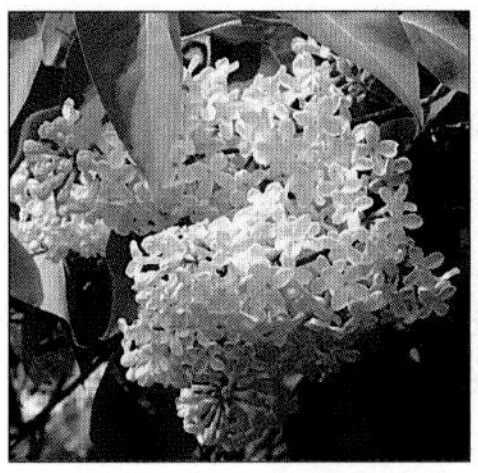

Syringa vulgaris 'Primrose'

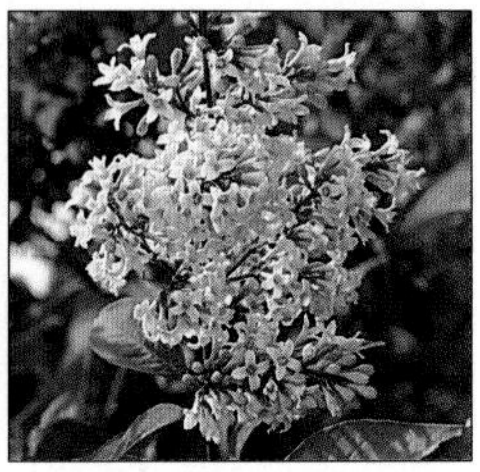

Syringa yunnanensis

SYZYGIUM

MYRTACEAE

Genus of 400–500 species of aromatic, evergreen shrubs and trees, mostly from woodland and rainforest throughout tropical regions. They have opposite, leathery leaves and terminal or axillary cymes or panicles of saucer-shaped, 4- or 5-petalled flowers, each with a prominent boss of stamens. These are followed by fleshy, spherical to pear-shaped or oblong, red, purple, or white berries. The dried flower buds of *S. aromaticum* are the cloves of commerce. In frost-prone areas, grow in a temperate or warm greenhouse. In warmer climates, grow in a shrub border.
• **HARDINESS** Half hardy to frost tender.
• **CULTIVATION** Under glass, grow in loam-based potting compost (JI No.3) in full or bright indirect light. In spring and summer, water moderately; apply a balanced liquid fertilizer monthly.

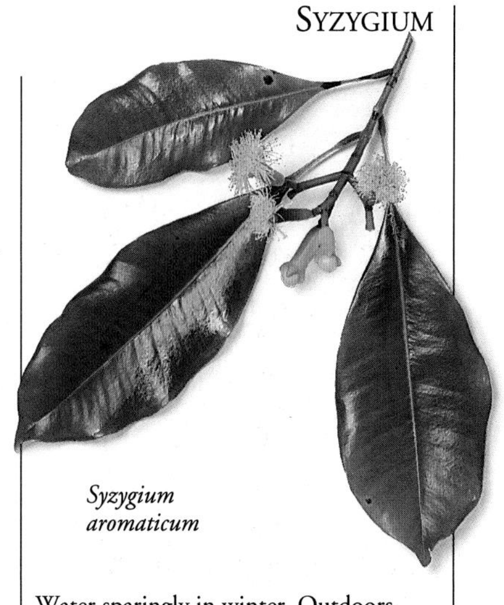

Syzygium aromaticum

Water sparingly in winter. Outdoors, grow in deep, fertile, moist, but well-drained soil in full sun or partial shade. Pruning group 1.
• **PROPAGATION** Sow seed at 15–18°C (59–64°F), or 27°C (81°F) for *S. aromaticum*, in spring. Root greenwood cuttings in early summer, or semi-ripe cuttings in mid- to late summer, both with bottom heat. Air layer in spring.
• **PESTS AND DISEASES** Trouble free.

S. aromaticum ■ ♀ syn. *Eugenia aromatica* (Clove). Small, bushy, roughly conical to columnar tree, with oval-lance-shaped, clove-scented leaves, 8–13cm (3–5in) long, pink-flushed when young, then lustrous, deep green above. In late summer, bears terminal panicles of 3–20 flowers, 1.5–2cm (½–¾in) long, with tiny, pink-tinted petals, which fall on opening, and a small brush of slender yellow stamens; flowers are followed by ellipsoid purple fruit, 8mm (⅜in) long. ↕ to 15m (50ft), ↔ 3–5m (10–15ft). Indonesia (Moluccas). ⌂ (min. 22–25°C/72–77°F)
S. paniculatum ■ ♀ syn. *Eugenia australis* of gardens, *E. paniculata* (Brush cherry). Erect to spreading, bushy, large shrub or small tree with flaky, patterned, cream, pink, and light brown bark. Obovate to elliptic or lance-shaped leaves, 5–9cm (2–3½in) long, reddish bronze when young, become shiny, deep green. In summer, bears a few small white flowers, 1–2.5cm (½–1in) long, with many yellow stamens, in terminal and axillary panicles, followed by ovoid, pink, red, purple, or white fruit, to 2cm (¾in) long. ↕ to 10m (30ft) or more, ↔ 3–10m (10–30ft). Australia (Queensland). ⌂ (min. 7°C/45°F)

S

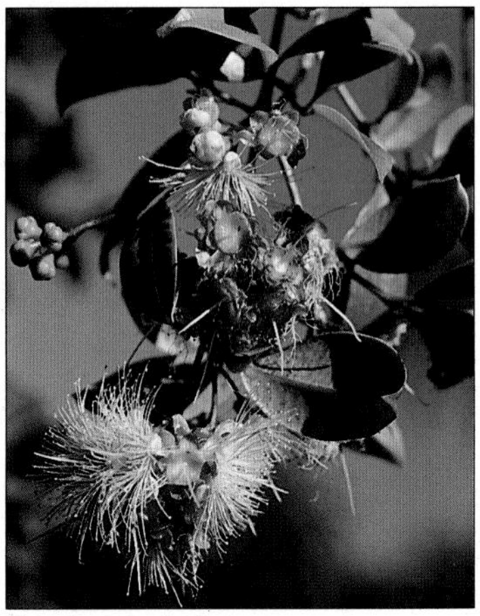

Syzygium paniculatum

T

TABEBUIA

BIGNONIACEAE

Genus of about 100 species of evergreen or deciduous trees and shrubs found in a variety of habitats, from swamp margins to thickets and rainforest, in Central and South America, and the West Indies. They are grown mainly for their foliage, although flowers may form once plants reach about 3m (10ft) tall. They have mostly opposite, long-stalked, simple or fully divided, 3- to 7-palmate leaves, with the central leaflet longer than the others. The 3- to 5-lobed, tubular to bell-shaped flowers are produced in showy, terminal panicles, usually in spring. Where temperatures fall below 8–15°C (46–59°F), grow in a temperate or warm greenhouse. In warmer areas, grow the larger species as specimens, the shrubby ones in a border.

• **HARDINESS** Frost tender.

• **CULTIVATION** Under glass, grow in loam-based potting compost (JI No.3), in full light with shade from hot sun. In the growing season, water freely and apply a balanced liquid fertilizer monthly; water sparingly in winter. Outdoors, grow in fertile, moist soil in full sun. Pruning group 1; may need restrictive pruning under glass.

• **PROPAGATION** Sow seed at 16°C (61°F) as soon as ripe or in spring. Insert semi-ripe cuttings with bottom heat in summer. Air layer in spring.

• **PESTS AND DISEASES** Red spider mites may be a problem under glass.

T. chrysantha ■ ♀ Rounded to spreading, deciduous tree bearing 5-palmate leaves, consisting of lance-shaped to obovate, entire or toothed leaflets, the central ones to 18cm (7in) long; the leaflets are mid-green, with a light covering of star-shaped hairs on the upper surfaces, more densely hairy beneath. Trumpet-shaped, sweetly scented, golden yellow flowers, 2.5–8cm

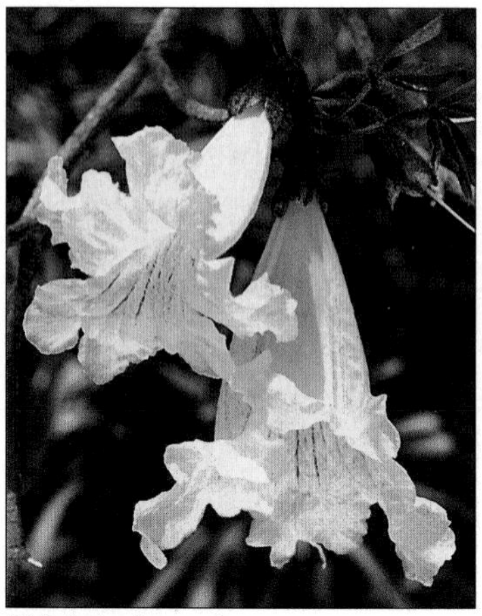

Tabebuia chrysantha

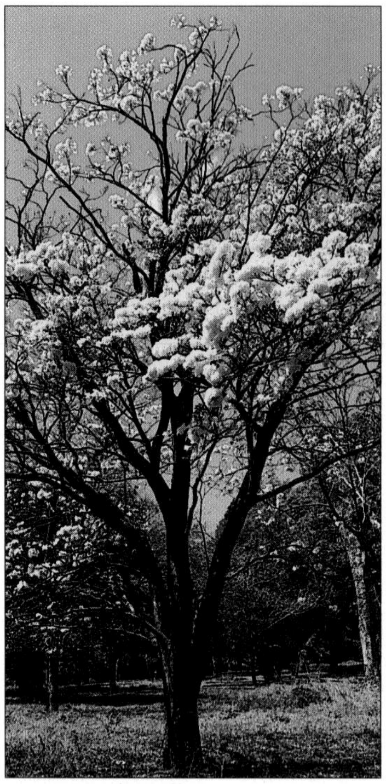

Tabebuia serratifolia

(1–3in) long, are produced in panicles in spring. ↕25m (80ft), ↔ 18m (60ft). Mexico to Colombia, Venezuela. ❄ (min. 8°C/46°F)

T. donnell-smithii see *Cybistax donnell-smithii.*

***T. pentaphylla* of gardens** see *T. rosea.*

T. rosea ♀ syn. *T. pentaphylla* of gardens (Pink poui, Pink tecoma, Rosy trumpet tree). Broadly upright, evergreen or deciduous tree with a long, smooth trunk, branching near the top. The 5-palmate leaves have oblong to ovate-elliptic, leathery, scaly, mid- to dark green leaflets, the central ones to 30cm (12in) long. Funnel-shaped, white, pink, or lilac flowers, 5–10cm (2–4in) long, with yellow eyes fading to white, are produced in pairs in dense panicles, in spring. ↕20–25m (70–80ft), ↔ 10–15m (30–50ft). Mexico to Colombia, Venezuela. ❄ (min. 10–15°C/50–59°F)

T. serratifolia ■ ♀ (Guayacan polvillo, Yellow poui). Ascending to spreading, deciduous shrub or medium-sized tree bearing 3- to 5-palmate leaves with oblong-lance-shaped, mid-green leaflets, to 17cm (7in) long, with rounded teeth. From winter to spring, produces dense panicles of funnel-shaped yellow flowers, 5–6cm (2–2½in) long, each with 5 crimped lobes. ↕ to 12m (40ft) (but slow-growing), ↔ to 20m (70ft). Trinidad, Colombia, Venezuela. ❄ (min. 10–15°C/50–59°F)

TABERNAEMONTANA

APOCYNACEAE

Genus of at least 100 species of rounded to upright, evergreen trees and shrubs found in tropical areas worldwide, in a variety of habitats, from rocky coppices to forests. They have opposite, simple, usually oblong to elliptic leaves, and are grown for their salverform flowers, each with 5 wide-spreading lobes, produced in sparsely branched, terminal cymes over a long period in summer. In areas where temperatures fall below 10–13°C (50–55°F), grow in a temperate or warm greenhouse. Elsewhere, grow in a shrub border or small courtyard garden.

• **HARDINESS** Frost tender.

• **CULTIVATION** Under glass, grow in loam-based potting compost (JI No.3) in full light. In the growing season, water moderately and apply a balanced liquid fertilizer monthly; water sparingly in winter. Outdoors, grow in moist, fertile soil in full sun. Pruning group 9, in early spring.

• **PROPAGATION** Sow seed at 16–20°C (61–68°F) in spring. Insert semi-ripe cuttings in summer, with bottom heat in cool areas. Layer or air layer in spring.

• **PESTS AND DISEASES** Scale insects and aphids may be a problem under glass.

T. coronaria see *T. divaricata.*

T. divaricata, syn. *Ervatamia coronaria, T. coronaria* (Crepe jasmine, East Indian rosebay, Paper gardenia). Spreading, bushy, many-branched shrub with elliptic-oblong, wavy-margined, thin, glossy, mid- to dark green leaves, 7–15cm (3–6in) long, paler beneath. In summer, bears cymes of 4–6 salverform, waxy, pure white flowers, 5cm (2in) across, fragrant at dusk and after dark. ↕2–3m (6–10ft) or more, ↔ 1.5–2.5m (5–8ft). India to China (Yunnan), Thailand. ❄ (min. 10–13°C/50–55°F). **'Flore Pleno'** has double flowers.

▷ **Tacamahac** see *Populus balsamifera*

TACCA

TACCACEAE

Genus of 10 species of stemless perennials, with solid tubers or upright, scarred rhizomes, from semi-evergreen, monsoon forest in West Africa and S.E. Asia, grown for their handsome foliage and unusual flowers. Lance-shaped to elliptic or obovate, entire or palmately or pinnately lobed leaves, often with purplish green leaf-stalks, are widely spaced or crowded on the rootstock. Nodding, bell-shaped flowers are borne in umbels, each umbel surrounded by 4 leaf-like floral bracts. Each flower also has a distinctive, narrow, thread-like appendage, to 25cm (10in) long. In frost-prone areas, grow in a warm greenhouse; in humid tropical climates, grow in a shady border.

• **HARDINESS** Frost tender.

• **CULTIVATION** Under glass, grow in a mix of equal parts leaf mould and coarse bark, with added slow-release fertilizer, in bright filtered light. Water freely all

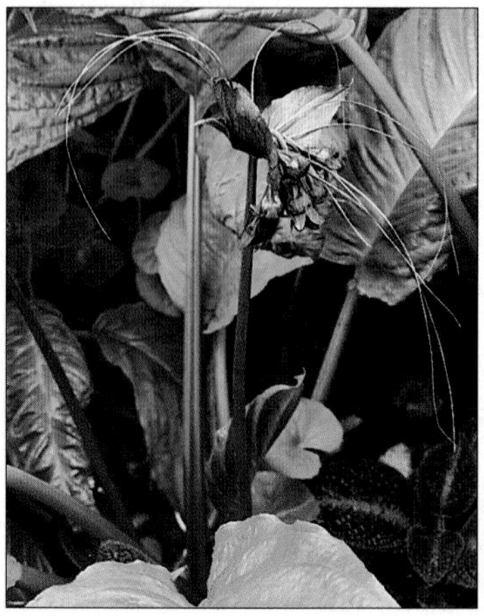

Tacca chantrierei

year; in summer, mist regularly and apply a half-strength foliar fertilizer monthly. Pot on every 2 or 3 years, removing old, decaying rhizomes. Outdoors, grow in fertile, moist but well-drained, leafy, acid soil in partial shade.

• **PROPAGATION** Surface-sow seed at 22–27°C (72–81°F) in spring. Divide, or take transverse sections of rhizomes with at least one bud, in spring. Dust cut surfaces with fungicide.

• **PESTS AND DISEASES** Red spider mites, tarsonemid mites, and grey mould (*Botrytis*) may be a problem.

T. chantrierei ■ (Bat flower, Cat's whiskers, Devil flower). Erect, rhizomatous perennial with oblong or lance-shaped leaves, 17–55cm (7–22in) long, dark green above and paler beneath. In summer, umbels of 5-petalled green flowers, each with 2 pairs of green, brown, or black floral bracts and dark green, maroon, or black, thread-like appendages, 25cm (10in) long, are borne on scapes to 65cm (26in) long. ↕↔ 1m (3ft). N.E. India, S.E. Asia. ❄ (min. 13°C/55°F)

T. integrifolia (Bat flower). Erect, rhizomatous perennial with oblong or lance-shaped leaves, 7–65cm (3–26in) long, dark green above and mid-green beneath. In summer, umbels of purple-red or brown flowers, surrounded by 4 green or deep purple floral bracts, are borne on scapes to 1m (3ft) long; the inner 2 flowers are white, green, or purple, with pale green, thread-like appendages, 20cm (8in) long, suffused violet and darkening with age. ↕ to 1.2m (4ft), ↔ 75cm (30in). E. India to S. China, Thailand, Malaysia, Indonesia (Sumatra, Java), Borneo. ❄ (min. 13°C/55°F)

▷ ***Tacitus bellus*** see *Graptopetalum bellum*

▷ ***Tacsonia* x *exoniensis*** see *Passiflora* x *exoniensis*

▷ ***Tacsonia mollissima*** see *Passiflora mollissima*

▷ ***Tacsonia van-volxemii*** see *Passiflora antioquiensis*

TAGETES

ASTERACEAE/COMPOSITAE

Genus of about 50 species of erect, bushy, strongly aromatic annuals and herbaceous perennials. They are found on hot, dry slopes and in valley bottoms from New Mexico, USA, to Argentina; one species occurs in Africa. The many hybrids and cultivars are derived mainly from *T. erecta, T. patula,* and *T. tenuifolia.* The almost fern-like leaves are usually opposite, pinnatifid to pinnate, with conspicuous glands, and mid- to dark green. Daisy-like or double, carnation-like flowerheads are produced singly or in cyme-like clusters from late spring to autumn. Germination from the large, easily handled seeds is rapid, and blooms appear within a few weeks of sowing. The African marigolds are excellent for formal bedding, whereas the French, Afro-French, and Signet marigolds are more suitable for the edge of a mixed border. All are good in containers and provide long-lasting cut flowers. Contact with the foliage may aggravate skin allergies. Four main hybrid groups are in cultivation:

African marigolds (African Group) Compact annuals, derived from *T. erecta*, with angular, hairless stems and pinnate, sparsely glandular leaves, 5–10cm (2–4in) long, each with 11–17 narrowly lance-shaped, pointed, sharply toothed leaflets, to 5cm (2in) long. Large, densely double, pompon-like, terminal flowerheads, usually to 12cm (5in) across, each with 5–8 or more ray-florets and numerous orange to yellow disc-florets, are produced from late spring to autumn. ↔ to 45cm (18in).
French marigolds (French Group) Compact annuals, derived from *T. patula*, with hairless, purple-tinged stems and pinnate leaves, to 10cm (4in) long, with lance-shaped to narrowly lance-shaped, toothed leaflets, to 3cm (1¼in) long. Solitary, usually double flowerheads, typically to 5cm (2in) across, with few to many red-brown, yellow, orange, or parti-coloured ray-florets and usually several disc-florets in a wide range of colours, are borne singly or in cyme-like inflorescences from late spring to autumn. ↔ to 30cm (12in).
Afro-French marigolds (Afro-French Group) Bushy annuals, derived from crosses of *T. erecta* and *T. patula*, with angular to rounded stems, branched and sometimes stained purple, and pinnate leaves, 5–13cm (2–5in) long, with lance-shaped leaflets, to 5cm (2in) long. Numerous small, single or double, yellow or orange flowerheads, usually 2.5–6cm (1–2½in) across, often marked red brown, are borne singly or in cyme-like inflorescences from late spring to autumn. ↔ 30–40cm (12–16in).
Signet marigolds (Signet Group) Upright annuals, derived from *T. tenuifolia*, with cylindrical, simple or many-branched stems and pinnate leaves, 5–13cm (2–5in) long, with narrowly lance-shaped, toothed leaflets, to 2cm (¾in) long. Many single flowerheads, usually to 2.5cm (1in) across, with yellow or orange florets (few ray-florets and several disc-florets), are borne in cyme-like inflorescences from late spring to autumn. ↔ to 40cm (16in).

• **HARDINESS** Half hardy.
• **CULTIVATION** Grow in moderately fertile, well-drained soil in full sun. Dead-head to prolong flowering and water freely during dry seasons. The densely double flowerheads of the African marigolds tend to rot in wet seasons. In containers, use a loam-based potting compost (JI No.2); during the growing season, water freely and apply a balanced liquid fertilizer weekly.
• **PROPAGATION** Sow seed *in situ* in late spring, or at 21°C (70°F) in early spring.
• **PESTS AND DISEASES** Red spider mites, whiteflies, slugs, snails, foot rot, and grey mould (*Botrytis*) may cause problems under glass.

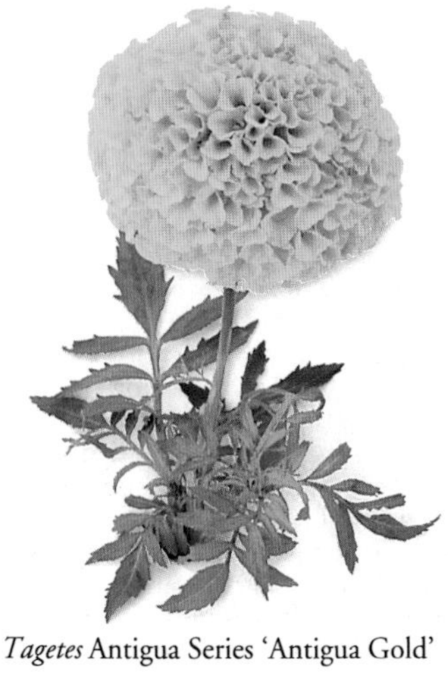
Tagetes Antigua Series 'Antigua Gold'

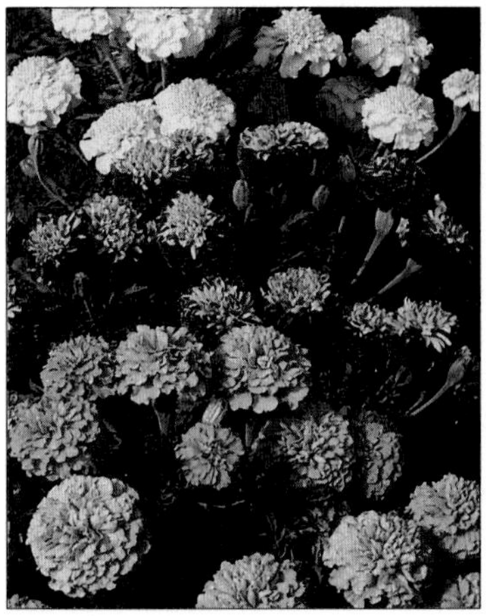
Tagetes Boy Series

***T.* Antigua Series.** African marigolds producing orange, lemon-yellow, golden yellow, or primrose-yellow flowerheads, from late spring to early autumn. ↕ to 30cm (12in). ✻. **'Antigua Gold'** ▣ has rich golden yellow flowerheads.
***T.* Aurora Series.** French marigolds bearing densely double, broad-petalled, light to golden yellow, orange, or mahogany-red flowerheads, with some unusual bicolours, from late spring to early autumn. ↕ 20–25cm (8–10in). ✻
***T.* Beaux Series.** Afro-French marigolds bearing double flowerheads in shades of rich golden yellow, orange with a red splash, or copper-red, from late spring to early autumn. ↕ 35cm (14in). ✻
***T.* Bonanza Series.** French marigolds that produce double flowerheads in deep orange-mahogany with gold margins, golden orange-mahogany, or orange-yellow-mahogany, in summer. ↕ 30cm (12in). ✻
***T.* Boy Series** ▣ Compact French marigolds that produce double, crested flowerheads in a range of colours, including shades of golden yellow, yellow, orange, or reddish brown, with deep orange or yellow crests, in late spring and early summer. ↕ to 15cm (6in). ✻. **'Boy O'Boy'** is available as a mixture. **'Golden Boy'** has deep red flowerheads with orange crests. **'Spry Boy'** has deep mahogany flowerheads with bright yellow crests.
***T.* Disco Series.** French marigolds that produce single, weather-resistant flowerheads in a range of colours, including yellow, golden yellow with mahogany markings, golden red, and red-orange, from late spring to early autumn. ↕ 20–25cm (8–10in). ✻
***T.* Excel Series.** African marigolds bearing primrose-yellow, yellow, golden yellow, or orange flowerheads, from late spring to early autumn. ↕ to 30cm (12in). ✻
***T.* Gem Series.** Signet marigolds that bear flowerheads in lemon-yellow, deep orange, or bright orange with darker markings, from late spring to early autumn. ↕ to 23cm (9in). ✻. **'Lemon Gem'** ▣ has lemon-yellow flowerheads. **'Tangerine Gem'** ▣ has deep orange flowerheads.

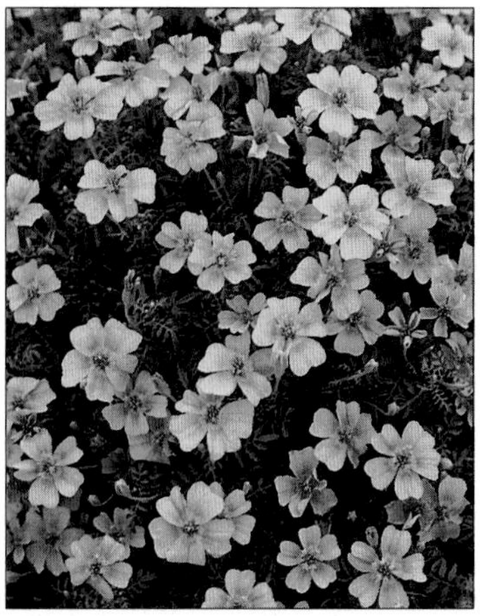
Tagetes Gem Series 'Tangerine Gem'

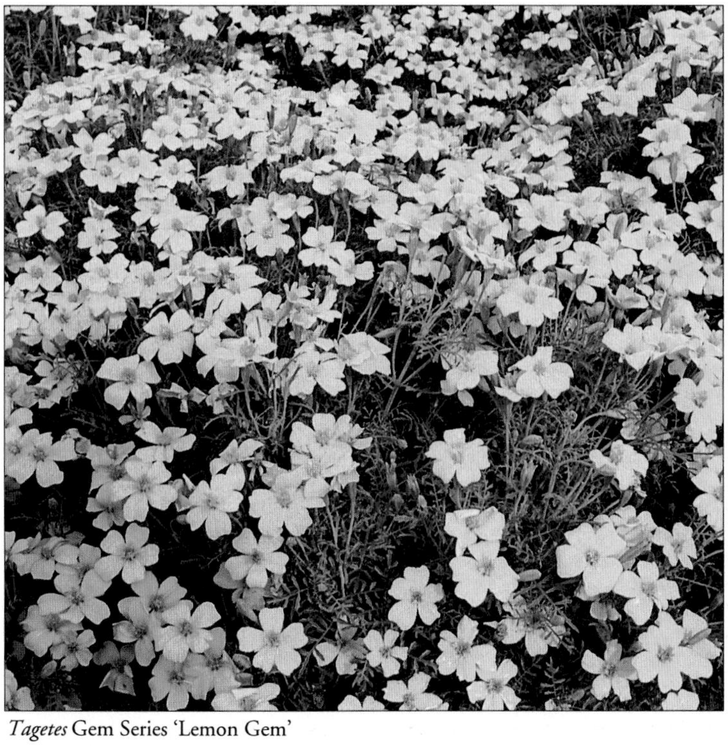
Tagetes Gem Series 'Lemon Gem'

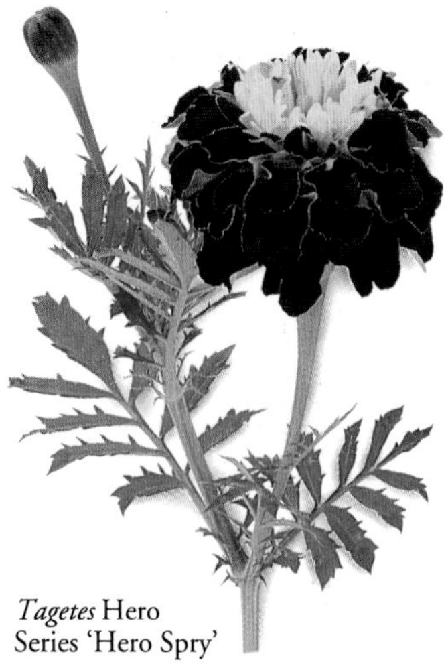
Tagetes Hero Series 'Hero Spry'

***T.* Hero Series.** French marigolds that bear large, double flowerheads, to 6cm (2½in) across, in yellow, golden yellow, orange, red, or mahogany, with crested yellow centres, from late spring to early autumn. ↕ 20–25cm (8–10in). ✻. **'Hero Spry'** ▣ produces flowerheads with mahogany outer petals and crested yellow centres.
***T.* Lady Series.** African marigolds bearing orange, primrose-yellow, yellow, or golden yellow flowerheads, from late spring to early autumn. ↕ 40–45cm (16–18in). ✻
***T.* Marvel Series.** Compact African marigolds bearing densely double flowerheads in gold, orange, yellow, lemon-yellow, or in a formula mixture of colours, from late spring to early autumn. ↕ 45cm (18in). ✻
***T.* Mischief Series.** French marigolds bearing single flowerheads in mahogany-red, yellow, or golden yellow, with some bicolours, from late spring to early autumn. ↕ to 30cm (12in) or more. ✻
***T.* 'Naughty Marietta'** ▣ French marigold producing single, deep yellow flowerheads, with maroon-red markings at the petal centres, from late spring to early autumn. ↕ 30–40cm (12–16in). ✻
***T.* Safari Series.** French marigolds bearing double, broad-petalled flowerheads in a range of colours, including golden yellow with mahogany-red splashes, soft pale yellow, tangerine-orange, and scarlet, from late spring to early autumn. ↕ 20–25cm (8–10in). ✻.

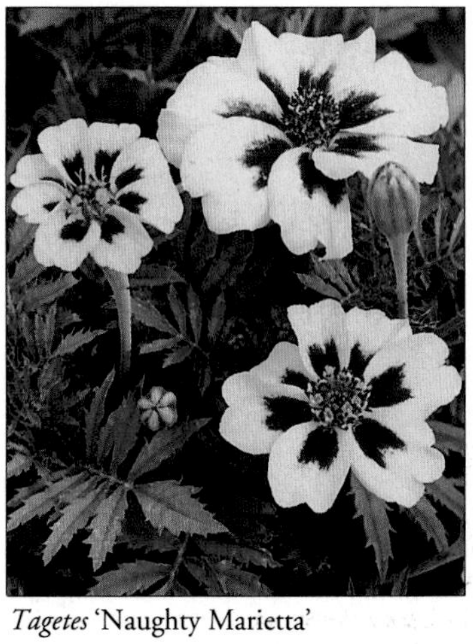
Tagetes 'Naughty Marietta'

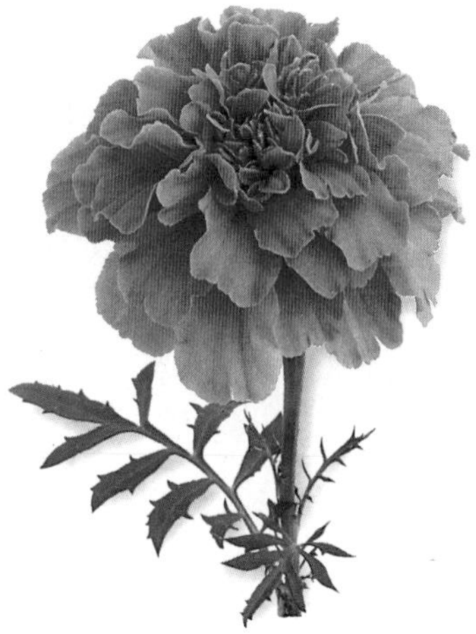

Tagetes Safari Series 'Safari Tangerine'

'Safari Tangerine' ■ produces rich tangerine-orange flowerheads.
***T.* Solar Series** ■ Afro-French marigolds bearing large, densely double flowerheads, to 8cm (3in) across, in colours including orange with red flecking, sulphur-yellow, and golden yellow, some with crested centres, from late spring to early autumn. ‡35cm (14in). ✻. **'Solar Gold'** has abundant non-crested, golden yellow flowerheads.
***T.* 'Starfire'.** Signet marigold producing flowerheads in a range of colours that includes yellow, golden yellow, and red, with some bicolours, in late spring and early summer. ‡15–20cm (6–8in). ✻
***T.* 'Vanilla'** ■ African marigold producing creamy white flowerheads, from late spring to early autumn. ‡to 35cm (14in). ✻

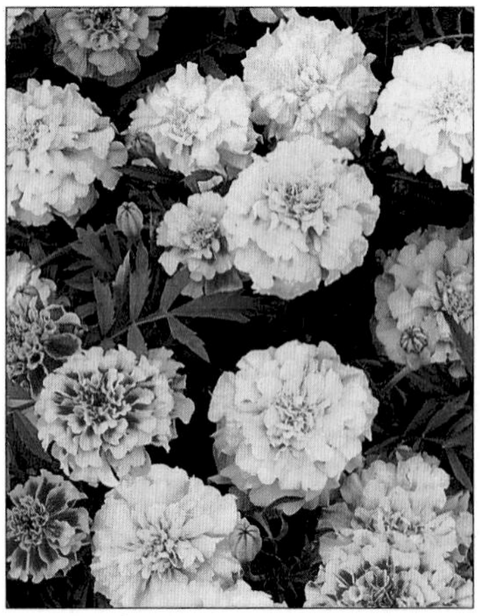

Tagetes Solar Series

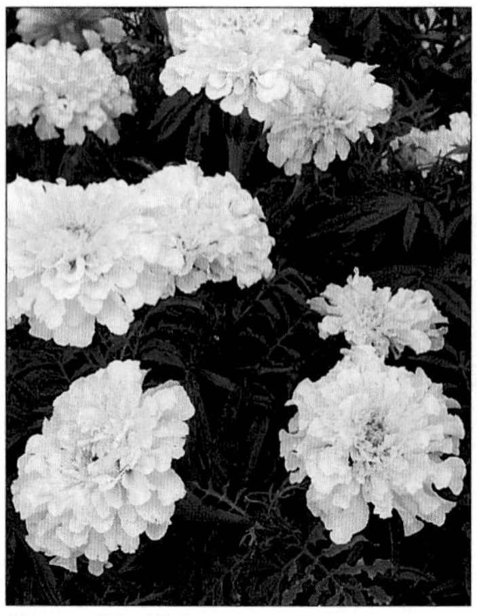

Tagetes 'Vanilla'

***T.* Voyager Series.** Compact African marigolds producing large, yellow or orange flowerheads, to 10cm (4in) across, from late spring to early autumn. ‡30–35cm (12–14in). ✻
***T.* Zenith Series.** Afro-French marigolds producing flowerheads in yellow, golden yellow, lemon-yellow, red, or orange, from late spring to early autumn. ‡30cm (12in). ✻

▷**Tail flower** see *Anthurium*
▷***Talbotia elegans*** see *Vellozia elegans*

TALINUM
Fameflower
PORTULACACEAE

Genus of 50 species of annuals, biennials, and often succulent and woody-based perennials, found in dry grassland and scrub in tropical and subtropical regions of Africa and North and Central America. The smooth, often succulent, usually deciduous but sometimes semi-evergreen leaves are arranged in attractive rosettes or in opposite pairs on short or elongated stems arising from a tuberous or fleshy rootstock. Showy, cup- to saucer-shaped flowers are borne singly or in cymes or panicles; although short-lived, they may be produced over a long period in summer. Grow in a rock garden. In cool areas, grow tender species in a temperate or warm greenhouse, or on a sunny window-sill.
• **HARDINESS** Fully hardy to frost tender.
• **CULTIVATION** Under glass, grow in standard cactus compost in full light and with good ventilation. In the growing season, water moderately, applying a balanced liquid fertilizer once or twice; keep just moist at other times. Outdoors, grow in well-drained, poor to moderately fertile soil in full sun.
• **PROPAGATION** Sow seed at 15–18°C (59–64°F) in spring or as soon as ripe. Divide mat- or rosette-forming species in spring.
• **PESTS AND DISEASES** Susceptible to greenfly.

T. caffrum. Succulent, deciduous perennial, sometimes biennial, with a thickened, tuberous, caudex-like rootstock, short, erect or prostrate stems, and inversely lance-shaped, linear, or oval, fleshy, mid-green leaves, 2.5–13cm (1–5in) long. Solitary, cup-shaped, pale lemon-yellow flowers, 1–2cm (½–¾in) across, open during daytime in summer. ‡↔15cm (6in). Namibia and Angola to Kenya. ❀ (min. 10°C/50°F)
T. okanoganense ■ Prostrate, mat- or cushion-forming, semi-evergreen perennial with succulent stems bearing cylindrical, fleshy, grey-green leaves, to 1cm (½in) long. The basal portions of the leaf midribs are retained as bristles in winter. Solitary, short-stemmed, saucer-shaped white flowers, to 2cm (¾in) across, tinged pink or yellow and with yellow stamens, are borne over several weeks in summer. Grow in an alpine house or trough. ‡to 5cm (2in), ↔ to 20cm (8in). W. North America. ✻✻✻
T. paniculatum (Jewels of Opar). Tuberous-rooted, deciduous perennial with erect, usually unbranched stems, becoming somewhat woody with age, and elliptic or obovate, mid-green leaves, to 10cm (4in) long. Many-flowered, terminal panicles of bowl-shaped, red or yellow flowers, to 2.5cm (1in) across, are produced in summer. ‡1m (3ft), ↔60cm (24in). S. USA to Central America. ❀ (min. 15°C/59°F)
T. spinescens. Dense, cushion-forming, semi-evergreen perennial with succulent stems, clothed in spines and thickening with age, and cylindrical, fleshy, grey-green leaves, 1–3cm (½–1¼in) long. The basal portions of the leaf midribs are usually retained as bristles in winter. Produces loose, cyme-like panicles of 1–5 short-stemmed, saucer-shaped, dark magenta flowers, to 1.5cm (½in) across, in summer. ‡to 10cm (4in), ↔ to 15cm (6in). W. North America. ✻✻✻

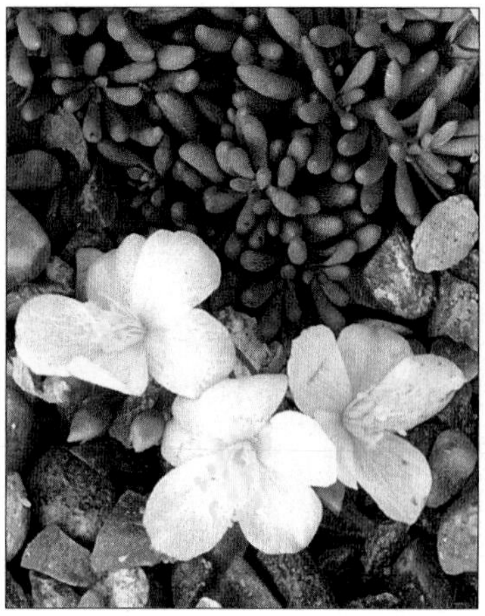

Talinum okanoganense

▷**Tamarisk** see *Tamarix*

TAMARIX
Tamarisk
TAMARICACEAE

Genus of 54 species of deciduous shrubs and small trees from coastal sites and dry or marshy, often salt-rich areas inland, from W. Europe and the Mediterranean to E. Asia and India. They are grown for their attractive, feathery foliage, consisting of small, scale- or needle-like leaves, and their plume-like, often leafy racemes of small flowers. They are useful for a shrub border in an inland garden, but may also be used as a windbreak or hedge in an exposed coastal area, and for growing on light, sandy soils.
• **HARDINESS** Fully hardy.
• **CULTIVATION** Grow in full sun, in well-drained soil in coastal areas, or in moister soil inland. Shelter from cold, drying winds in inland gardens; in coastal areas, they are resistant to strong winds. Prune regularly, or they may become top-heavy and unstable. Cut back young plants almost to ground level after planting. Pruning group 2 for spring-flowering species; group 6 for those flowering in late summer.
• **PROPAGATION** Sow seed as soon as ripe in containers in a cold frame. Take hardwood cuttings in winter or semi-ripe cuttings in summer.
• **PESTS AND DISEASES** Trouble free.

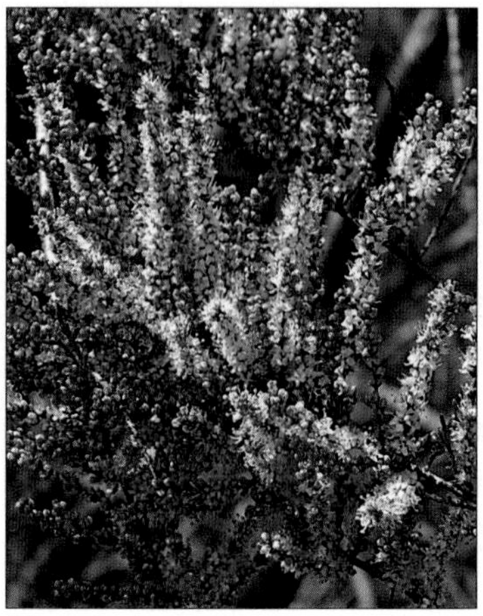

Tamarix ramosissima

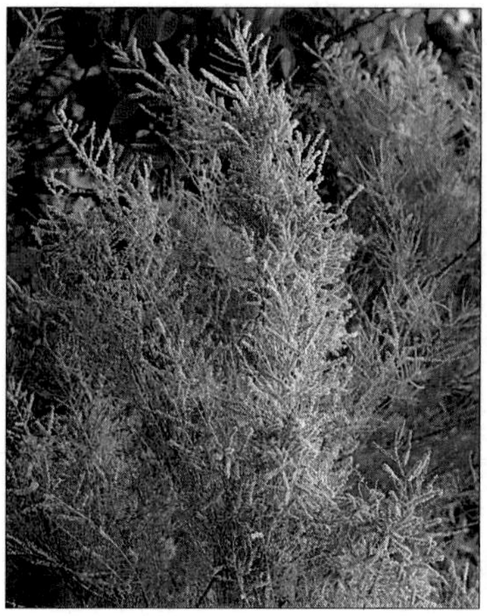

Tamarix ramosissima 'Pink Cascade'

T. parviflora. Spreading shrub with arching purple shoots and pointed leaves, 3mm (⅛in) long. In late spring, 4-petalled, pale pink flowers are borne in dense, lateral racemes, to 5cm (2in) long, on the old shoots. ‡5m (15ft), ↔6m (20ft). S.E. Europe. ✻✻✻
T. pentandra see *T. ramosissima.*
T. ramosissima ■ 🏆 syn. *T. pentandra.* Graceful shrub or small tree with arching, red-brown shoots and pointed leaves, to 4mm (⅛in) long. In late summer and early autumn, 5-petalled pink flowers are produced in dense racemes, to 7cm (3in) long, on the new shoots. ‡↔5m (15ft). S.E. Europe to Asia. ✻✻✻. **'Pink Cascade'** ■ has rich pink flowers.
T. tetrandra 🏆 Shrub or small tree with arching, purple-brown shoots and needle- or scale-like leaves, to 4mm (⅛in) long. Bears 4-petalled, light pink flowers in lateral racemes, to 5cm (2in) long, on the old shoots, in mid- and late spring. ‡↔3m (10ft). E. Balkans, W. Asia, S. former USSR. ✻✻✻

▷**Tampala** see *Amaranthus tricolor*

TANACETUM
syn. BALSAMITA, PYRETHRUM
ASTERACEAE/COMPOSITAE

Genus of about 70 species of annuals and evergreen and herbaceous perennials and subshrubs from mountains, cliffs, meadows, and dry slopes in N. temperate regions. They have simple or pinnate to 3-pinnate, entire, toothed, or scalloped, mostly aromatic, mainly basal leaves that are sparsely to densely hairy and sometimes silver. Stem leaves, where present, are spirally arranged, usually smaller and less divided, and may be stalkless. Terminal, daisy- or button-like flowerheads, borne singly or in corymbs, have yellow disc-florets and sometimes barely discernible, white, red, or yellow ray-florets. This diverse genus includes

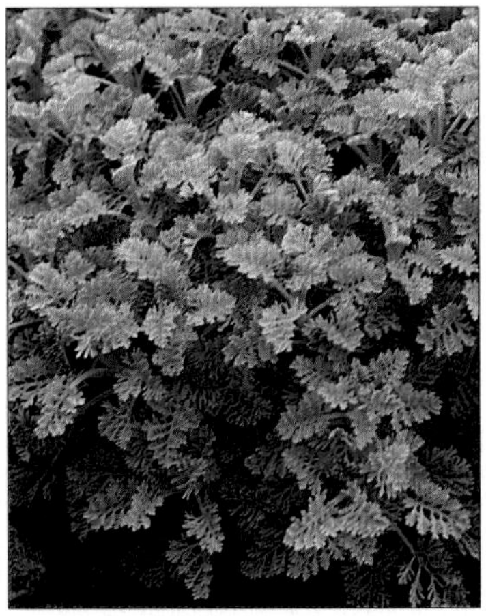
Tanacetum argenteum

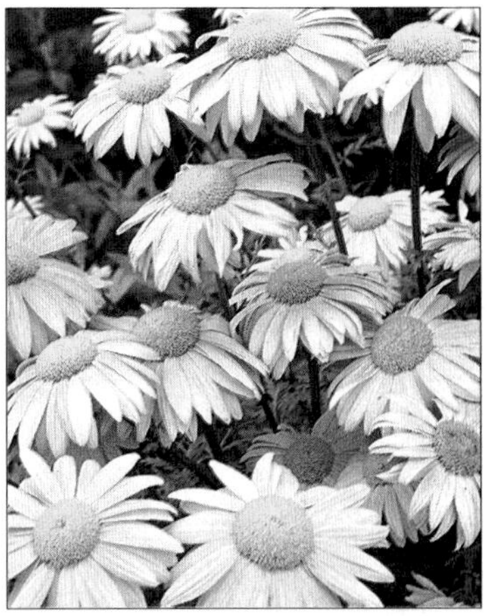
Tanacetum coccineum 'Eileen May Robinson'

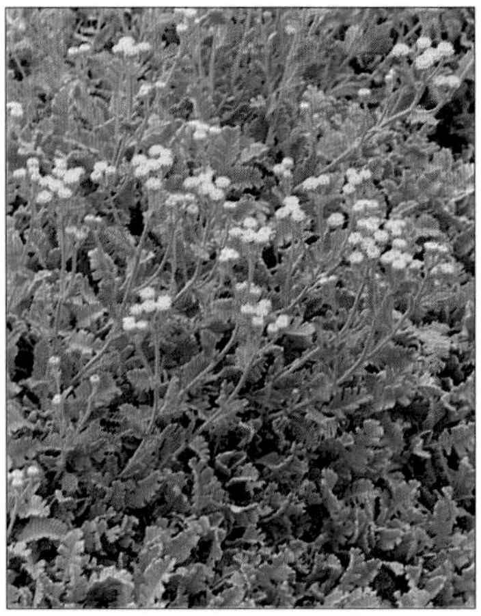
Tanacetum densum subsp. *amani*

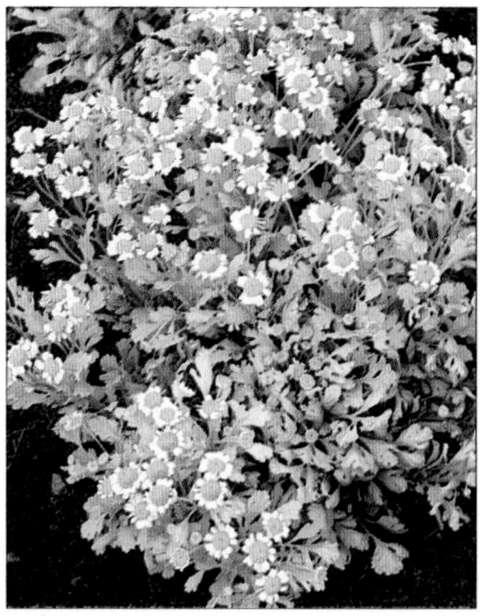
Tanacetum parthenium 'Golden Moss'

species suitable for a rock garden, a herb garden, or border edging. *T. coccineum* and its cultivars are suitable for a border and produce good cut flowers. Some have aromatic foliage, which may be dried for use in pot-pourri; several have medicinal qualities. Contact with the foliage may aggravate skin allergies.

• **HARDINESS** Fully hardy to half hardy.

• **CULTIVATION** Grow in well-drained, preferably sandy soil in full sun, although most will tolerate any soil that is not wet and heavy. *T. balsamita* produces leafier growth in partial shade. Grow mound-forming, dwarf, white- or silver-leaved species in sharply drained, poor to moderately fertile soil. Cut back *T. coccineum* and its cultivars as the flowers fade, in order to encourage a second flowering. *T. parthenium* and its cultivars self-seed prolifically.

• **PROPAGATION** Sow seed at 10–13°C (50–55°F) in late winter or early spring. Divide perennials, or root basal cuttings, in spring. Insert softwood cuttings of *T. parthenium* and *T. ptarmiciflorum* in early summer; in winter, young plants of *T. ptarmiciflorum* are best kept in a cool greenhouse .

• **PESTS AND DISEASES** Aphids, chrysanthemum eelworm, and leaf miners may be a problem.

T. argenteum ▣ syn. *Achillea argentea.* Mat-forming, usually evergreen, woody-based perennial with branching, densely white-woolly stems. Ovate, 2-pinnate, bright silvery white leaves, 2–7cm (¾–3in) long, have 5–9 pairs of divided to narrowly lance-shaped leaflets. In summer, daisy-like white flowerheads, 4mm (⅛in) across, are borne singly or in corymbs. Suitable for a rock garden or border edging. ↕ to 20cm (8in), ↔ to 30cm (12in). Mediterranean. ✻✻✻

T. balsamita, syn. *Balsamita major, Chrysanthemum balsamita* (Alecost, Costmary). Mat-forming, woody-based, rhizomatous perennial with oblong to elliptic, scalloped, softly silver-hairy basal leaves, to 30cm (12in) long, and smaller, stalkless leaves on erect stems. Numerous flowerheads, to 1.5cm (½in) across, with tiny white ray-florets and yellow disc-florets, are borne in corymbs in late summer and early autumn. Grown for its balsam-scented foliage (used in pot-pourri), and suitable for a herb garden. ↕ to 90cm (36in), ↔ 45cm (18in). Europe to C. Asia. ✻✻✻

T. coccineum, syn. *Chrysanthemum coccineum, Pyrethrum coccineum, P. roseum* (Painted daisy, Pyrethrum). Bushy, hairless, herbaceous perennial with erect stems and elliptic-oblong, pinnatisect or 2-pinnatisect, dark green, mainly basal leaves, to 12cm (5in) long, consisting of 10–14 narrowly lance-shaped, toothed segments. Daisy-like flowerheads to 7cm (3in) across, with white, pink, or red ray-florets and yellow disc-florets are produced in early summer. ↕ 45–75cm (18–30in), ↔ 45cm (18in). Caucasus, S.W. Asia. ✻✻✻. **'Brenda'** ▣🏆 bears deep cerise-pink flowerheads; ↕ 70–80cm (28–32in). **'Eileen May Robinson'** ▣🏆 has pale, rich pink flowerheads; ↕ 70–80cm (28–32in). **'James Kelway'** 🏆 produces brilliant deep crimson-pink flowerheads; ↕ 60cm (24in). **'Snow Cloud'** has white flowerheads; ↕ 60cm (24in).

T. densum* subsp. *amani ▣ syn. *Chrysanthemum densum.* Mound-forming, usually evergreen, woody-based perennial with white-downy stems and ovate to broadly elliptic, 2-pinnatisect, downy, grey-white leaves, 2–5cm (¾–2in) long, finely cut into 10–25 inversely lance-shaped segments. In summer, bears flat corymbs of 3–7 daisy-like yellow flowerheads, 5–10mm (¼–½in) across, each with 12–15 yellow ray-florets, to 4mm (⅛in) long. *T. densum* is similar to *T. haradjanii*, but female ray-florets are absent on the latter. Grow in a rock garden. ↕ to 25cm (10in), ↔ to 20cm (8in). Turkey. ✻✻✻

T. haradjanii, syn. *Chrysanthemum haradjanii.* Mat-forming, woody-based, evergreen perennial with silver-white, downy stems. Oblong-elliptic to ovate, 2- or 3-pinnatisect, silvery grey leaves, to 5cm (2in) long, are composed of 4 or 5 pairs of narrowly lance-shaped, entire or further divided segments. Daisy-like yellow flowerheads, 2–4mm (¹⁄₁₆–⅛in) across, are borne in loose corymbs in late summer. Suitable for a rock garden. ↕ to 15cm (6in), ↔ to 20cm (8in). Syria, Turkey. ✻✻✻

T. parthenium ▣ syn. *Chrysanthemum parthenium, Pyrethrum parthenium* (Feverfew). Short-lived, bushy, aromatic, woody-based perennial with ovate, pinnatisect or 2-pinnatisect, softly hairy basal leaves, to 8cm (3in) long, with 3–5 paired, scalloped or entire segments; smaller, less divided, shorter-stalked leaves are produced on the erect stems. Daisy-like flowerheads, to 2.5cm (1in) across, with yellow disc-florets and white ray-florets, are borne in dense corymbs in summer. Suitable for border edging. ↕ 45–60cm (18–24in), ↔ 30cm (12in). Europe, Caucasus. ✻✻✻. **'Aureum'** has golden yellow leaves, and produces single, yellow-tinted white flowerheads. **'Ball's Double White'** has double white flowerheads. **'Butterball'** bears double yellow flowerheads. **'Golden Moss'** ▣ is dwarf and carpet-forming, with moss-like yellow leaves; ↕ to 10cm (4in). **'Plenum'** ▣ has fully double white flowerheads; ↕ 35cm (14in). **'Santana'** is dwarf, producing double flowerheads, and will flower at any time of year when grown in

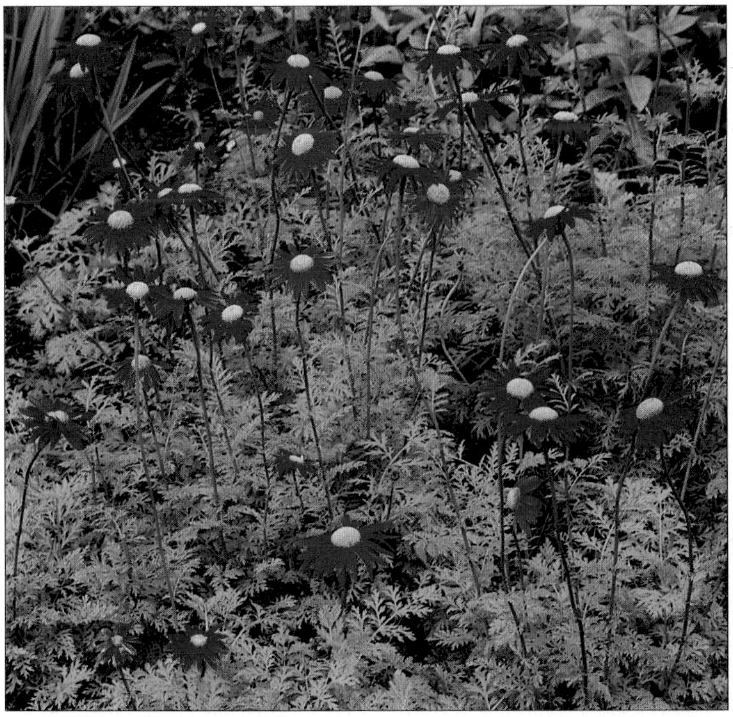
Tanacetum coccineum 'Brenda'

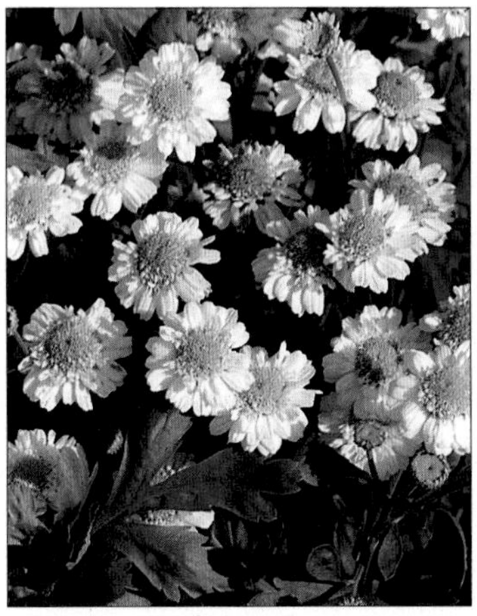
Tanacetum parthenium

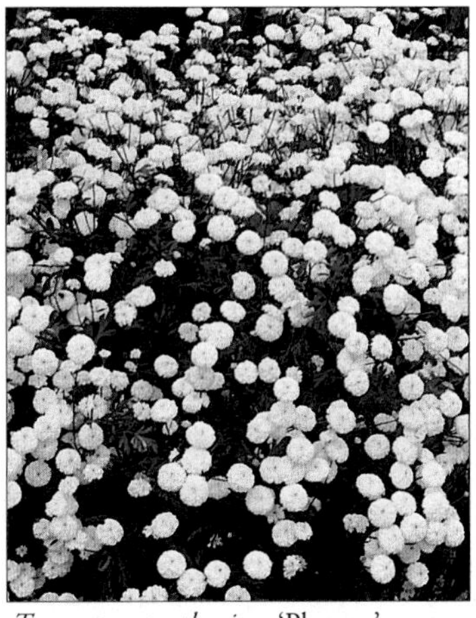
Tanacetum parthenium 'Plenum'

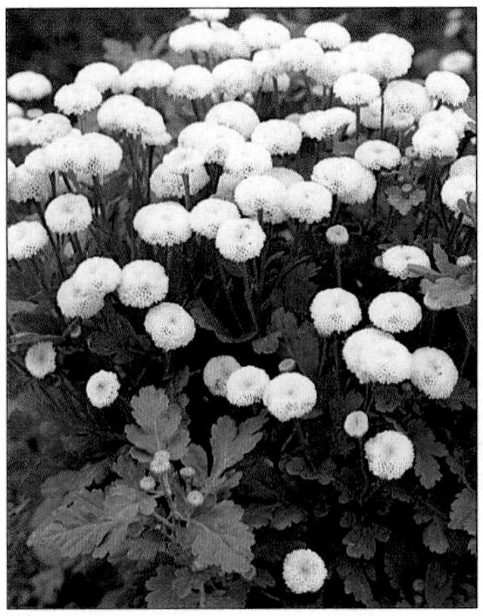
Tanacetum parthenium 'Snowball'

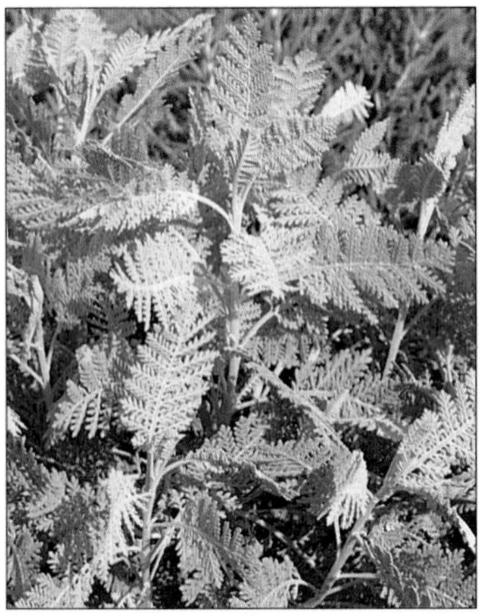
Tanacetum ptarmiciflorum

containers; ↕ 20cm (8in), ↔ 15cm (6in). **'Snowball'** ▣ has pompon-like, fully double, ivory-white flowerheads; ↕ 30cm (12in), ↔ 15cm (6in).
T. ptarmiciflorum ▣ syn. *Pyrethrum ptarmiciflorum.* Woody-based perennial, often grown as an annual, with erect stems. Elliptic to oblong-ovate, 2- or 3-pinnatisect, silver-hairy basal and stem leaves, to 10cm (4in) long, have 8–22 linear-elliptic, scalloped segments. Daisy-like white flowerheads, to 2.5cm (1in) across, with yellow disc-florets, are borne in dense corymbs in late summer. Suitable for border edging. ↕ 60cm (24in), ↔ 40cm (16in). Canary Islands (Gran Canaria). ❄
T. vulgare, syn. *Chrysanthemum vulgare* (Common tansy). Vigorous, erect, deciduous perennial with alternate, oblong, pinnate leaves, to 10cm (4in) long, comprising up to 12 oblong or lance-shaped, pinnately lobed or toothed leaflets. Bears button-shaped, bright yellow flowerheads, to 1cm (½in) across, in flat-topped corymbs, 14cm (5½in) across, in summer. Suitable for a herb garden. ↕ 60–90cm (24–36in), ↔ 45cm (18in). Europe. ❄❄❄

T

TANAKAEA syn. TANAKEA
Japanese foam flower

SAXIFRAGACEAE

Genus of one species of dioecious, rhizomatous, evergreen perennial from wet, rocky, shaded sites in Japan. *T. radicans* is an attractive creeping plant, with basal leaf rosettes and upright, leafless stems bearing dense panicles of minute white flowers in late spring and early summer. Grow in a moist, shaded site in a woodland or rock garden.

• **HARDINESS** Fully hardy.
• **CULTIVATION** Grow in moist, humus-rich, peaty soil in full or partial shade.
• **PROPAGATION** Separate rooted portions of rhizome in spring.
• **PESTS AND DISEASES** Trouble free.

T. radicans. Dense, spreading perennial with basal rosettes of ovate to broadly lance-shaped or oblong, leathery leaves, 2–8cm (¾–3in) long, rounded or heart-shaped at the bases, dark green above, paler beneath. In late spring and early summer, mainly unisexual, star-shaped white flowers, to 3mm (⅛in) across, with prominent anthers, are borne in dense panicles, 5–15cm (2–6in) long. ↕ to 10cm (4in), ↔ to 30cm (12in). Japan (Shikoku, Kyushu). ❄❄❄

▷ ***Tanakea*** see *Tanakaea*
▷ **Tanekaha** see *Phyllocladus trichomanoides*
▷ **Tangerine** see *Citrus reticulata*
▷ **Tanguru** see *Olearia albida*
▷ **Tansy, Common** see *Tanacetum vulgare*

TAPEINOCHILUS

COSTACEAE/ZINGIBERACEAE

Genus of about 15 species of evergreen, rhizomatous perennials from tropical forest in Malaysia, Indonesia, New Guinea, and N.E. Australia. They are cultivated mainly for their spectacular inflorescences of red bracts. The obovate leaves, to 15cm (6in) long, are spirally arranged on bamboo-like stems. In frost-prone areas, grow in a warm greenhouse; in humid tropical climates, grow in a shady border.

• **HARDINESS** Frost tender.
• **CULTIVATION** Under glass, grow in loam-based potting compost (JI No.3), with added leaf mould, in bright indirect light or deep shade, with high humidity. In spring and summer, water freely and apply a balanced liquid fertilizer monthly; water moderately in winter. Outdoors, grow in fertile, leafy, humus-rich soil in deep shade.
• **PROPAGATION** Sow seed at 20°C (68°F) in early spring. Divide in spring.
• **PESTS AND DISEASES** Trouble free.

T. ananassae. Clump-forming perennial with long, narrowly obovate, sharply pointed leaves, 15cm (6in) long. In summer, leafless stems, 45–120cm (18–48in) long, bear cone-like inflorescences of many recurved, overlapping, vivid red bracts, 10cm (4in) across, resembling red pineapples; they often cover the small yellow flowers. ↕ to 2m (6ft), ↔ 1m (3ft). Indonesia (Moluccas). ⌂ (min. 20°C/68°F)

▷ **Tarata** see *Pittosporum eugenioides*
▷ **Taro** see *Colocasia, C. esculenta*
  Blue see *Xanthosoma violaceum*
  Giant see *Alocasia macrorrhiza*
  Imperial see *Colocasia esculenta* 'Illustris'
▷ **Tarragon** see *Artemisia dracunculus*
▷ **Tarweed** see *Grindelia*
▷ ***Tasmannia*** see *Drimys*
  T. aromatica see *D. lanceolata*
▷ **Tassel flower** see *Amaranthus caudatus, Emilia*
▷ **Tassel-white** see *Itea virginica*

TAXODIUM
Swamp cypress

TAXODIACEAE

Genus of 2 species of upright, conical, monoecious, deciduous or semi-evergreen, coniferous trees found in swampy forest or by river margins from S.E. USA to Guatemala. The shoots are of 2 types: deciduous (without buds), which fall in autumn, and persistent (with buds), from which only the leaves fall. The narrowly lance-shaped or linear leaves are arranged alternately, radially, or in 2 ranks. Male cones occur in groups; female cones are scattered. They are late to come into leaf and to assume the spectacular autumn colours for which they are renowned. Grow as specimen trees; they are especially suited to very wet sites, where they produce aerial roots (known as pneumatophores or "knees") at water level.

• **HARDINESS** Fully hardy.
• **CULTIVATION** Grow in any moist or wet, preferably acid soil in full or partial shade.
• **PROPAGATION** Sow seed in containers in a cold frame in spring. Graft cultivars in late winter.
• **PESTS AND DISEASES** Trouble free.

T. ascendens see *T. distichum* var. *imbricarium.*
T. distichum ▣ 🏆 💧 (Swamp cypress). Conical tree, becoming columnar and often ragged with age, due to its brittle branches and pale brown, shallowly fissured bark. The alternate (almost opposite), narrowly lance-shaped, pale green leaves, 2cm (¾in) long, turning rust-brown in autumn, are 2-ranked on deciduous shoots. On persistent shoots, leaves are small and scale-like. Spherical green female cones, 3cm (1¼in) across, ripen to brown in autumn; pendent red male cones expand in winter. ↕ 20–40m (70–130ft), ↔ 6–9m (20–28ft). S.E. USA. ❄❄❄. **var. *imbricarium***, syn. *T. ascendens*, var. *imbricatum* (Pond cypress) is narrowly conical, with dull brown bark and radial leaves, 5–10mm (¼–½in) long, lying flat on erect shoots; ↕ 10–20m (30–70ft), ↔ to 6m (20ft). **var. *imbricarium* 'Nutans'** ▣ 🏆 has erect foliage shoots, becoming pendent when mature. **var. *imbricatum*** see var. *imbricarium.*

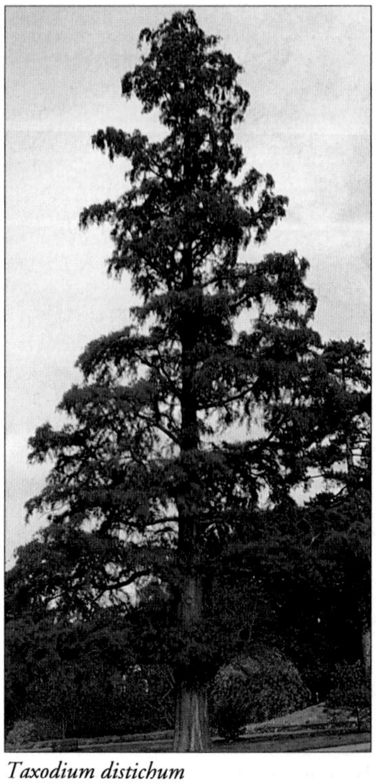
Taxodium distichum

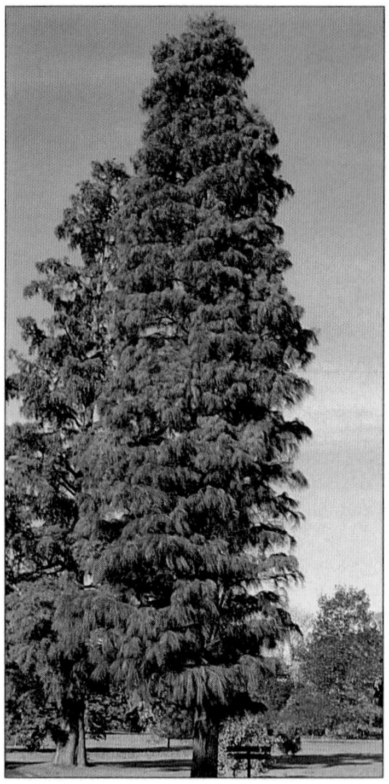
Taxodium distichum var. *imbricarium* 'Nutans'

TAXUS
Yew

TAXACEAE

Genus of 5–10 species of broadly rounded to upright, dioecious, evergreen, coniferous, large shrubs or small trees found in forest extending from N. temperate areas to the Philippines and Central America. Yews are grown for their reddish-brown, frequently peeling bark, and their linear, dark green leaves, often paler beneath; these are spirally arranged but often appear 2-ranked. On the female plants, single-seeded, oblong-ovoid fruits are produced in open, fleshy arils. Grow as specimen plants or use for hedging and topiary; the prostrate forms make good ground cover, even in dense, dry shade. Most tolerate exposure, dry soils, and urban pollution. All parts (but not the arils) are highly toxic if ingested.

• **HARDINESS** Fully hardy.
• **CULTIVATION** Grow in any well-drained, fertile soil, including chalky or acid soils, in sun or deep shade. Trim hedging in summer and early autumn. Can withstand renovation pruning.
• **PROPAGATION** Sow seed as soon as ripe in containers in a cold frame, or in a seedbed; seed may take 2 or more years to germinate. Insert semi-ripe cuttings in late summer or early autumn; take cuttings from strongly upright shoots (except for prostrate cultivars), otherwise they may not form a strong leading shoot. Graft cultivars in early autumn.
• **PESTS AND DISEASES** Resistant to most diseases, except *Phytophthora* root rot. May be damaged by tortrix moth caterpillars, vine weevil, and yew scale.

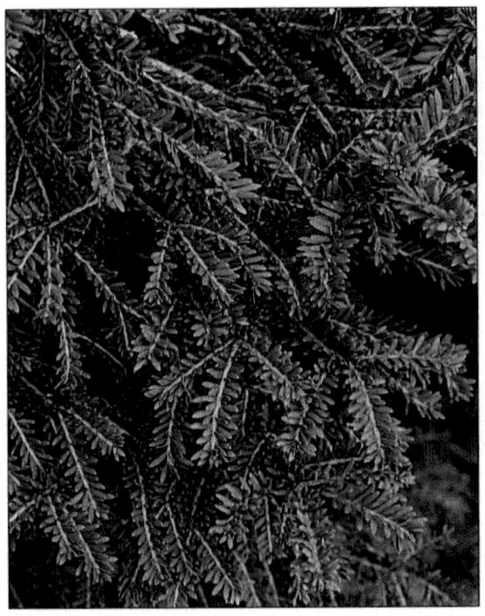
Taxus baccata 'Adpressa'

T. baccata 🏆 ◯ (Yew). Broadly conical tree with spreading, horizontal branches, scaly, purple-brown bark, and shoots that remain green for several years. Linear, glossy or matt, dark green leaves, 2–3cm (¾–1¼in) long, paler beneath, are 2-ranked and parted either side of the shoots. Yellow male cones are borne in spring. Fruit consist of single green seeds with juicy, sweet, usually red arils, 1cm (½in) across. ↕ 10–20m (30–70ft), ↔ 8–10m (25–30ft). Europe, N. Africa to Iran. ❄❄❄. **'Adpressa'** ▣ ◯ is a dense, spreading, female shrub, with short, wide, abruptly pointed leaves, to 1.5cm (½in) long; ↕ 6m (20ft), ↔ 4m (12ft). **'Dovastonii Aurea'** ▣ 🏆 ◯ is a small, female tree, with spreading branches, pendent branchlets, and yellow-margined leaves borne on golden yellow shoots; ↕ 3–5m (10–15ft), ↔ 2m (6ft). **'Fastigiata'** ▣ 🏆 ◯ (Florence Court yew, Irish yew) is columnar and female, with radially set leaves; ↕ to 10m (30ft), ↔ 6m (20ft). **'Fastigiata Aurea'** ◯ is female, similar to 'Fastigiata', but has variegated leaves with gold patches; ↕ 6m (20ft), ↔ 3m (10ft). **'Fastigiata Aureomarginata'** 🏆 ◯ is female, similar to 'Fastigiata', but with leaves margined bright yellow; ↕ 3–5m (10–15ft), ↔ 1–2.5m (3–8ft). **'Repandens'** 🏆 is a female shrub, and does not form leaders but spreads over the ground, forming a mound; ↕ to 60cm (24in), ↔ 5m (15ft). **'Repens Aurea'** 🏆 is a female shrub that is similar to, and may even be the same as 'Dovastonii Aurea', but is propagated from sideshoots and thus forms only spreading ground cover; ↕↔ 1–1.5m (3–5ft). **'Standishii'** 🏆 ◯ is narrow and

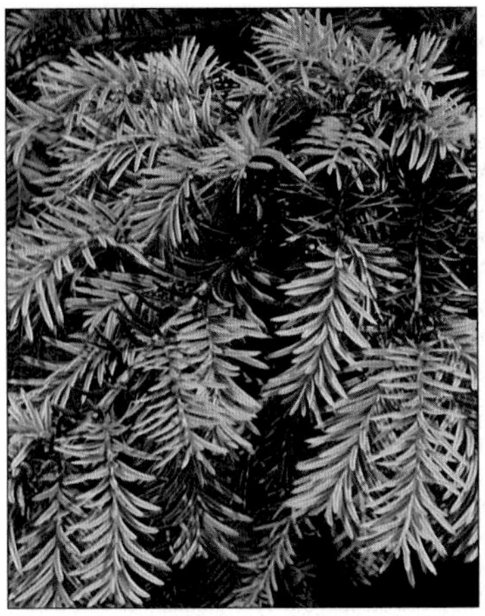
Taxus baccata 'Dovastonii Aurea'

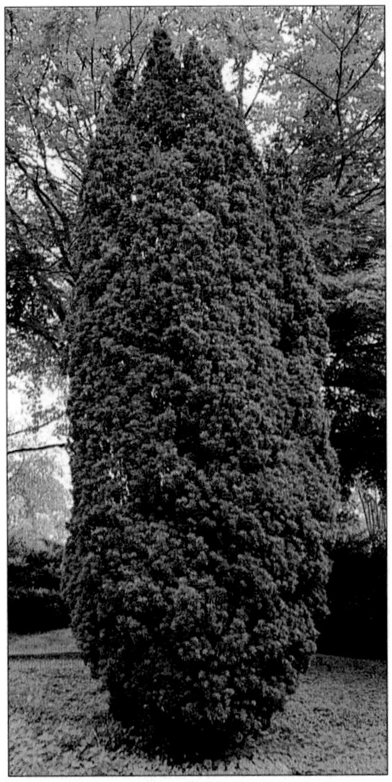
Taxus baccata 'Fastigiata'

columnar, a miniature female selection of 'Fastigiata', and produces golden yellow leaves; ↕ 1.5m (5ft), ↔ 60cm (24in).

T. cuspidata ▣ ◯ (Japanese yew). Broadly columnar shrub or small tree with linear, spiny-tipped, dark green leaves, 1.5–2.5cm (½–1in) long, tawny or yellow-green beneath, turning red-green over winter, and narrowly parted either side of the shoots. Scarlet arils are 0.5–1cm (¼–½in) across. Much hardier in cold areas than *T. baccata.* ↕ 10–15m (30–50ft), ↔ 6–8m (20–25ft). N.E. China, Japan. ❄❄❄. **f. *nana*** is a spreading shrub, with erect shoots and radial leaves, and is mainly male in cultivation; ↕ 2–4m (6–12ft); Japan (Honshu). **f. *nana* 'Densa'** is a low-growing, broad, flattened, female shrub; ↕ 1.2m (4ft), ↔ to 6m (20ft).

T. x media ◯–◯ (*T. baccata* x *T. cuspidata*). Rounded to upright tree combining the vigour of *T. baccata* with the hardiness of *T. cuspidata.* The distinctly 2-ranked, oblong to needle-like, pointed, flat, olive- to dark green leaves, 1.5–3cm (½–1¼in) long, have prominent white midribs and are slightly red-flushed in winter. Scarlet

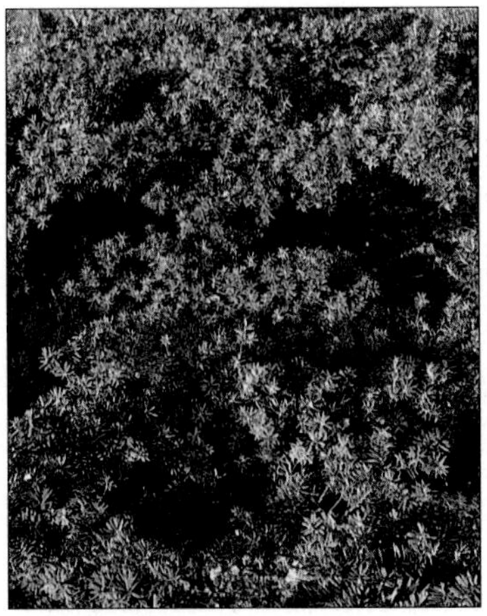
Taxus cuspidata

arils are 5–10mm (¼–½in) across. ↕↔ to 6–8m (20–25ft). Garden origin. ❄❄❄. **'Brownii'** ◯ is female, dense and spherical, with short, parted, widely-spaced, dark green leaves, 1.5–2cm (½–¾in) long; ↕ to 2.5m (8ft), ↔ to 3.5m (11ft). **'Hicksii'** 🏆 ◯ is probably male, and columnar in habit, similar to *T. baccata* 'Fastigiata' but more open, with more radially set, dark green leaves; ↕ 6–8m (20–25ft), ↔ 2–3m (6–10ft), later to 6m (20ft).

▷**Tea,**
Labrador see *Ledum groenlandicum*
Oswego see *Monarda didyma*
Sweet see *Osmanthus fragrans*
▷**Teasel** see *Dipsacus*
▷**Tea tree** see *Leptospermum*
Duke of Argyll's see *Lycium barbarum*
New Zealand see *Leptospermum scoparium*
Woolly see *Leptospermum lanigerum*

TECOMA *syn.* TECOMARIA

BIGNONIACEAE

Genus of about 12 species of evergreen climbers, scrambling shrubs, and upright trees, found on rocky slopes and in valleys in southern Africa and from S. USA to Argentina. The opposite leaves are pinnate or sometimes 3-pinnate, with ovate-oblong to rounded leaflets. Narrowly bell- to funnel-shaped, 5-lobed, yellow, orange, or red flowers are produced in dense, terminal racemes or panicles between winter and summer. In frost-prone areas, grow in a cool or temperate greenhouse or conservatory. In warmer climates, grow as specimen plants; the scrambling species may be trained over an arch.

• **HARDINESS** Frost tender; *T. capensis* may survive brief spells near 0°C (32°F).

• **CULTIVATION** Under glass, plant directly into a border or grow in large tubs of loam-based potting compost (JI No.3) in full light. During the growing season, water freely and apply a half-strength balanced liquid fertilizer monthly; water sparingly in winter. Outdoors, grow in moist but well-drained, fertile soil in full sun. Pruning group 8 for early-flowering species; group 9 for late-flowering species, in early spring. Plants under glass need restrictive pruning and benefit from thinning of overcrowded stems.

• **PROPAGATION** Sow seed at 18–21°C (64–70°F) in spring. Insert semi-ripe

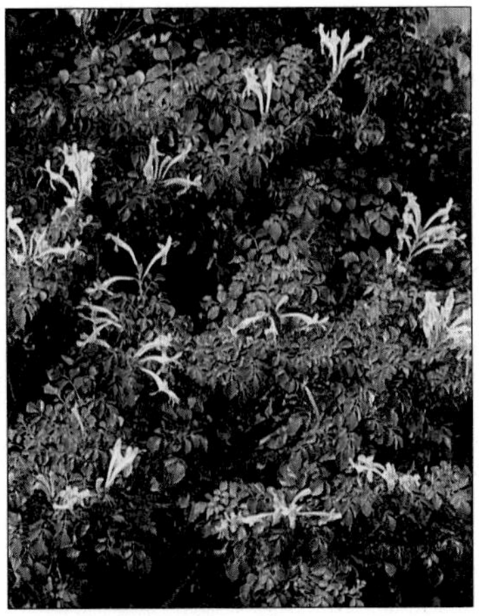
Tecoma capensis 'Aurea'

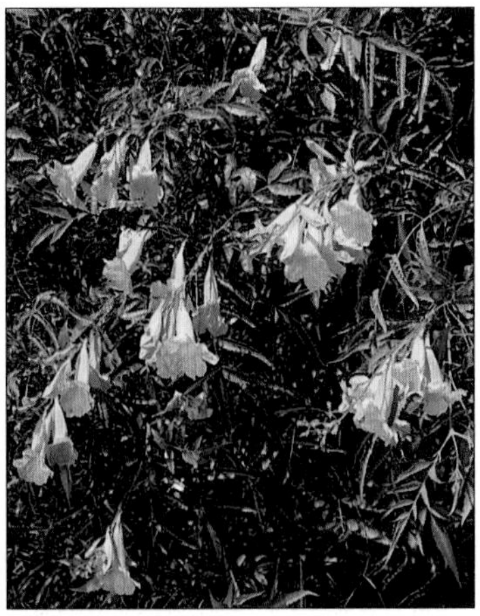
Tecoma stans

cuttings with bottom heat in summer. Layer *T. capensis* in spring or autumn.

• **PESTS AND DISEASES** Red spider mites and whiteflies may be troublesome under glass.

T. australis see *Pandorea pandorana.*

T. capensis 🏆 syn. *Bignonia capensis, Tecomaria capensis, T. petersii* (Cape honeysuckle). Erect, scrambling, evergreen shrub with slender stems and pinnate, lustrous, mid- to dark green leaves, to 15cm (6in) long, each with 5–7 elliptic-ovate to roughly diamond-shaped, toothed leaflets. Racemes, to 15cm (6in) long, of slender, tubular, orange to scarlet flowers, 6–7cm (2½–3in) long, are produced mainly in summer. ↕ 2–7m (6–22ft), ↔ 1–3m (3–10ft). Southern Africa. ❅ (min. 5°C/41°F). **'Apricot'** is compact, with vivid apricot-orange flowers; ↕ to 1.5m (5ft), ↔ 1m (3ft). **'Aurea'** ▣ bears yellow flowers, to 5cm (2in) long; ↕ 4m (12ft), ↔ 2m (6ft). **'Lutea'** is slow-growing, with dark yellow flowers; ↕ 2m (6ft), ↔ 1m (3ft).

T. grandiflora see *Campsis grandiflora.*

T. radicans see *Campsis radicans.*

T. ricasoliana see *Podranea ricasoliana.*

T. stans ▣ ◯ syn. *Bignonia stans, Stenolobium stans* (Trumpet bush, Yellow bells, Yellow elder). Open, ascending, large shrub or small tree, often with several slim trunks if grown as a tree. Pinnate leaves, to 35cm (14in) long, each have 5–13 oblong-ovate to lance-shaped, toothed, bright green leaflets. Funnel-shaped, bright yellow flowers, 5cm (2in) long, are produced in terminal racemes or panicles, to 15cm (6in) long, from late winter to summer. ↕ 5–9m (15–28ft), ↔ 3–5m (10–15ft). S. USA to Guatemala, Argentina. ❅ (min. 7–10°C/45–50°F)

▷**Tecoma, Pink** see *Tabebuia rosea*

TECOMANTHE

BIGNONIACEAE

Genus of 5 species of woody-stemmed, evergreen, twining climbers from tropical woodland in Indonesia, New Guinea, the Solomon Islands, and Australasia. They are grown for their funnel-shaped, 5-lobed flowers, borne in pendent racemes from the bare branches, below the leafy stems. The opposite leaves are pinnate or sometimes 3-palmate. Where temperatures fall below 15°C (59°F), grow in a warm

greenhouse. In tropical areas, train over an arch or pergola, or grow against a warm wall.
• **HARDINESS** Frost tender.
• **CULTIVATION** Under glass, grow in loam-based potting compost (JI No.3) in full light with shade from hot sun. Provide strong support. In the growing season, water freely, applying a balanced liquid fertilizer monthly; water sparingly in winter. Outdoors, grow in fertile, moist but well-drained soil, in full sun with some midday shade. Pruning group 11, in spring.
• **PROPAGATION** Sow seed at 18–21°C (64–70°F) in spring. Insert semi-ripe cuttings with bottom heat in summer. Layer in spring.
• **PESTS AND DISEASES** Red spider mites and mealybugs may be troublesome under glass.

T. dendrophila. Evergreen, twining climber with sparsely branched stems, particularly when young, and pinnate leaves, 7cm (3in) long, each consisting of 3–5 ovate or oblong-lance-shaped, rich green leaflets. In summer, produces racemes of 1–12 flowers, 7–11cm (3–4½in) long, with deep pink to rose-purple tubes, becoming yellow at the top, and yellow lobes, suffused and veined pink or purple. ↕ to 15m (50ft) or more. Indonesia (Moluccas), New Guinea, Solomon Islands. ❀ (min. 13–15°C/55–59°F)
T. speciosa. Evergreen, twining climber with sparsely branched stems when young, and pinnate leaves, to 6cm (2½in) long, each with 5 broadly obovate, thick, lustrous, deep green leaflets. In autumn, bears light, almost luminous, yellow-green flowers, 6–8cm (2½–3in) long, with downy lobes, in dense racemes of 1–10. ↕ 10m (30ft) or more. New Zealand (Three Kings Islands). ❀ (min. 13–15°C/55–59°F)

▷ ***Tecomaria*** see *Tecoma*
T. capensis see *T. capensis*
T. petersii see *T. capensis*

TECOPHILAEA
LILIACEAE/TECOPHILAEACEAE

Genus of 2 species of cormous perennials, originally from subalpine grassland in South America but probably now extinct in the wild. They have narrowly lance-shaped, basal leaves, and bear crocus-like, brilliantly coloured flowers on leafless stems in spring. They are suitable for a rock garden or raised bed, but, in all except completely frost-free areas, should be grown in a bulb frame, cold greenhouse, or alpine house to protect the early growth from frost.
• **HARDINESS** Frost hardy, but early leaves are liable to frost damage.
• **CULTIVATION** Under glass, plant 5cm (2in) deep, in a mix of equal parts loam-based potting compost (JI No.2) and sharp sand in full light. In the growing season, water moderately; reduce water gradually as the leaves die down to keep corms warm and dry during summer dormancy. Outdoors, grow in well-drained, sandy soil in full sun.
• **PROPAGATION** Sow seed in containers in a frost-free frame, in autumn or as soon as ripe. Remove offsets in late summer.
• **PESTS AND DISEASES** Trouble free.

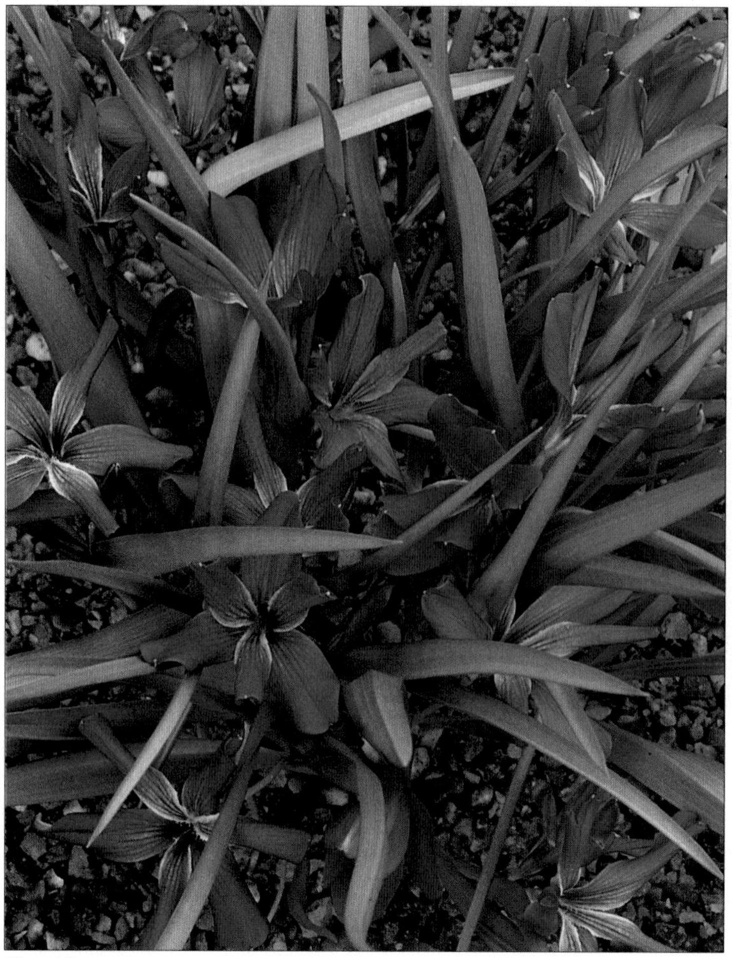
Tecophilaea cyanocrocus

T. cyanocrocus ■ ♀ (Chilean blue crocus). Small, cormous perennial with semi-erect, narrowly lance-shaped, basal leaves, to 13cm (5in) long. In spring, bears 1 or 2 open funnel-shaped, intense gentian-blue flowers, 4–5cm (1½–2in) long, with white throats and faint white veins. ↕ 8–10cm (3–4in), ↔ 5cm (2in). Chile. ✲✲. **var. *leichtlinii*** ♀ has pale blue flowers with large white centres. **var. *violacea*** has deep violet flowers.

▷ **Teddy bear plant** see *Cyanotis kewensis*
▷ ***Telanthophora grandifolia*** see *Senecio grandifolius*

TELEKIA
ASTERACEAE/COMPOSITAE

Genus of 2 species of imposing, erect, herbaceous perennials found in moist woodland and beside streams in scrub, from C. and S. Europe to the Caucasus, Turkey, Ukraine, Belorussia, and Russia. The basal leaves are long-stalked, ovate and coarsely toothed; the alternate stem leaves have shorter stalks. Solitary flowerheads, with long, narrow yellow ray-florets, tubular yellow disc-florets, ageing to brown, and 3 or 4 rows of overlapping involucral bracts, are produced in branching sprays from early summer to early autumn. *Telekia* species make effective specimen plants for a damp woodland or wild garden, or beside water.
• **HARDINESS** Fully hardy.
• **CULTIVATION** Grow in moist, not too fertile soil, in partial shade with shelter from strong winds. They may self-seed.
• **PROPAGATION** Sow seed in containers as soon as ripe. Divide in spring.
• **PESTS AND DISEASES** Young leaves may be damaged by slugs.

T. speciosa, syn. *Buphthalmum speciosum.* Spreading, rhizomatous perennial with ovate, coarsely scalloped to toothed, aromatic, somewhat limp leaves, 30cm (12in) or more long, heart-shaped at the bases, on stalks to 20cm (8in) long. The coarse, upright stems have smaller, almost clasping leaves. In late summer and early autumn, loose, branching sprays of solitary, daisy-like yellow flowerheads, 6–9cm (2½–3½in) across, are produced on long peduncles. ↕ to 2m (6ft), ↔ 1m (3ft). S.E. Europe, Caucasus, Ukraine, Belorussia, Russia. ✲✲✲

▷ ***Telesonix jamesii*** see *Boykinia jamesii*

TELLIMA
Fringe cups
SAXIFRAGACEAE

Genus of one species of rosette-forming, hairy herbaceous perennial from cool, moist woodland in W. North America. The mainly basal leaves are heart-shaped or triangular to kidney-shaped, scalloped or toothed, and 5- to 7-lobed. Small, bell-shaped flowers, with 5 tiny petals, fringed into linear segments, relatively large calyces, and 10 stamens, are borne in terminal racemes in late spring and midsummer. Fringe cups are drought-tolerant and suitable for ground cover in a shrub border or woodland garden.
• **HARDINESS** Fully hardy.

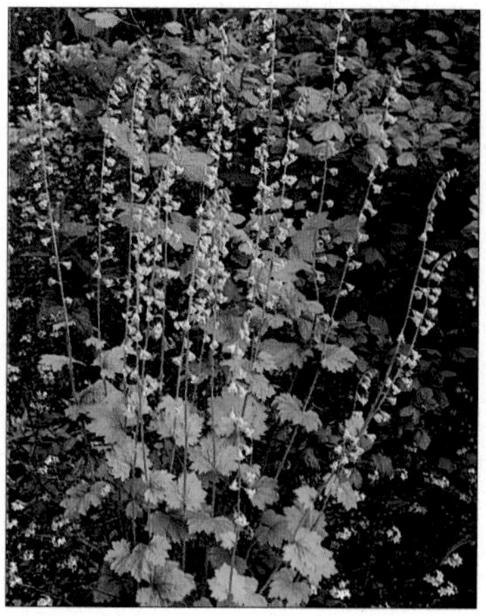
Tellima grandiflora

• **CULTIVATION** Grow in moist, humus-rich soil in partial shade, although will tolerate dry soil and full sun. Self-seeds freely.
• **PROPAGATION** Sow seed in containers in a cold frame as soon as ripe or in spring. Divide in spring.
• **PESTS AND DISEASES** Leaves may be attacked by slugs.

T. grandiflora ■ Rosette-forming perennial with hairy, heart-shaped or triangular to kidney-shaped, 5- to 7-lobed, scalloped leaves, 5–10cm (2–4in) long. From late spring to midsummer, erect, hairy stems bear terminal racemes, to 30cm (12in) long, of 15–30 white to greenish white flowers, to 8mm (⅜in) long, with greenish white calyces. ↕ to 80cm (32in), ↔ 30cm (12in). North America (Alaska to California). ✲✲✲. **'Perky'** has smaller leaves, and bears red flowers; ↕ to 40cm (16in), ↔ 25cm (10in). **'Purpurteppich'** has leaves tinged purplish red in summer, dark purple leaf-stalks, and pink-fringed green flowers; ↕ to 60cm (24in).

TELOPEA
Waratah
PROTEACEAE

Genus of 4 species of evergreen shrubs or small trees occurring in drought-prone woodland in Australia. The alternate leaves are simple, leathery, and sometimes toothed or lobed. *Telopea* species are cultivated mainly for their paired, tubular flowers, 2–2.5cm (¾–1in) long, which are split on the lower sides. Each flower has 4 short lobes, with the margins rolled under, and a prominent stigma. The flowers are surrounded by overlapping, coloured bracts and are produced in dense, terminal, umbel-like heads in spring or summer; they are followed by boat-shaped, woody seed pods. In frost-prone climates, grow in a cool greenhouse. In warmer areas, they are suitable for a shrub border.
• **HARDINESS** Half hardy to frost tender.
• **CULTIVATION** Under glass, grow in loam-based potting compost (JI No.2), with additional sharp sand, in full light or bright filtered light. During the growing season, water freely and apply a low-nitrate, low-phosphate fertilizer monthly; water sparingly in winter. Outdoors, grow in moist but well-drained, sandy, slightly acid soil in full sun or partial shade. Pruning group 8.

• **PROPAGATION** Sow seed in containers in a cold frame as soon as ripe. Insert semi-ripe or leaf-bud cuttings with bottom heat in summer.
• **PESTS AND DISEASES** Trouble free.

T. mongaensis ▣ (Braidwood waratah, Monga waratah). Erect, bushy shrub producing inversely lance-shaped, round-tipped, matt, dark green leaves, 10–15cm (4–6in) long. From late spring to summer, produces flowerheads 8–10cm (3–4in) across, each consisting of a ring of pale green to pale pink bracts and abundant tubular red flowers. ↕ 2–3m (6–10ft) or more, ↔ 1.5–2.5m (5–8ft). Australia (New South Wales). ✲
T. oreades ▣◐ (Gippsland waratah, Victorian waratah). Large, moderately bushy shrub or sometimes small, broadly upright tree with inversely lance-shaped to obovate, matt, dark green leaves, 15–20cm (6–8in) long, with pointed tips. In late spring and summer, bears flowerheads 9cm (3½in) across, each consisting of a ring of light green or pink bracts and tubular red flowers. ↕ to 3m (10ft) as a shrub, to 10m (30ft) as a tree, ↔ 1.5–3m (5–10ft) or more. Australia (Victoria). ✲
T. speciosissima (Common waratah, Sydney waratah). Large shrub, bushy when young, often becoming untidy with age, with narrowly obovate, round-tipped, mid-green leaves, to 25cm (10in) long, usually toothed above the middle. Flowerheads, 10–15cm (4–6in) across, each consisting of a ring of red bracts and many tubular red flowers, the outer flowers maturing first, are borne in spring. ↕ 3m (10ft), ↔ 1.5–2m (5–6ft). Australia (New South Wales). ✲
T. truncata ◐ (Tasmanian waratah). Many-branched shrub or, rarely, small tree with lance-shaped to obovate, usually entire leaves with recurved margins, to 10cm (4in) long, dull green and hairless above, silver-hairy beneath. In early summer, produces flowerheads 5–8cm (2–3in) across, each consisting of

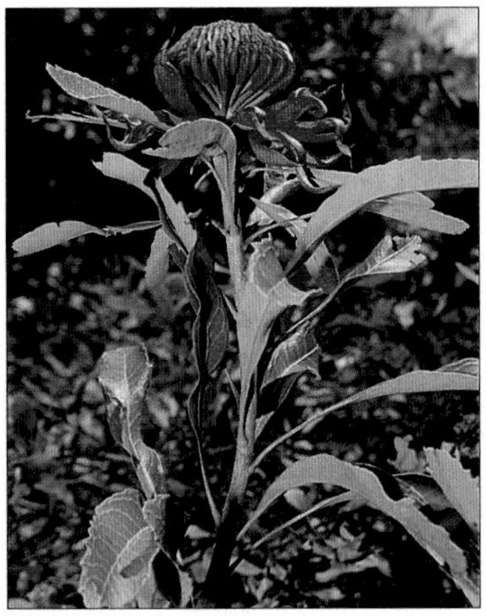

Telopea oreades

a ring of inconspicuous, hairy, rust-red bracts and 10–20 tubular red, rarely yellow flowers, all maturing at the same time. ↕ to 8m (25ft), ↔ 1.5–3m (5–10ft). Australia (Tasmania). ✲

▷ **Temple bells** see *Smithiantha*

TEMPLETONIA

LEGUMINOSAE / PAPILIONACEAE

Genus of 11 species of upright to rounded, evergreen shrubs and sub-shrubs found in dry, open scrub and drought-prone woodland in Australia. Angular or grooved, sometimes spiny branches bear alternate, simple, obovate to oblong leaves. They are grown for their pea-like flowers, borne singly or in clusters from the leaf axils, between autumn and spring. Where temperatures fall below 5–7°C (41–45°F), grow in a cool or temperate greenhouse. Elsewhere, grow in a shrub border.
• **HARDINESS** Frost tender.
• **CULTIVATION** Under glass, grow in loam-based potting compost (JI No.2) in full light. In the growing season, water freely, applying a balanced liquid fertilizer monthly; water sparingly in

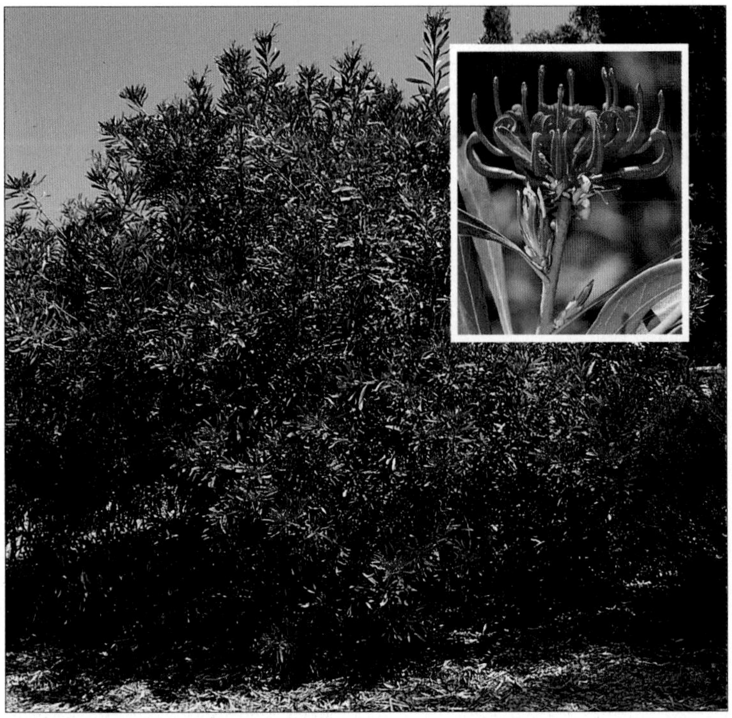

Telopea mongaensis (inset: flowerhead detail)

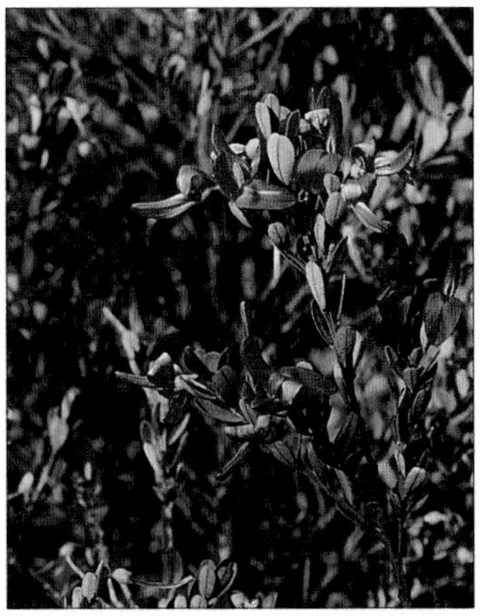

Templetonia retusa

winter. Outdoors, grow in moist but well-drained, fertile soil in full sun. Pruning group 8; plants under glass may need restrictive pruning.
• **PROPAGATION** Sow pre-soaked seed at 16°C (61°F) in spring. Insert semi-ripe cuttings with bottom heat in summer. Layer in spring.
• **PESTS AND DISEASES** Red spider mites may be troublesome under glass.

T. retusa ▣ (Cockies' tongues, Coral bush, Flame bush). Evergreen shrub, bushy when young, with alternate, obovate to oblong, leathery, glaucous, deep green leaves, 1.5–4cm (½–1½in) long. Crimson, sometimes pink or yellow-white flowers, 3–5cm (1¼–2in) long, are borne singly from the leaf axils from winter to spring. ↕ 1–3m (3–10ft), ↔ 1–2m (3–6ft). S. and W. Australia. ❀ (min. 5–7°C/41–45°F)

▷ **Terebinth** see *Pistacia terebinthus*

TERMINALIA

COMBRETACEAE

Genus of 200 species of deciduous and evergreen trees, frequently buttressed, found in tropical woodland worldwide. The attractive, simple, entire, broadly obovate to oblong or elliptic leaves are either transparent or minutely pitted with transparent spots, and arranged alternately, in spirals, or in nearly opposite pairs. Insignificant, petalless, tubular flowers are borne in axillary or terminal spikes or panicles, followed by one-seeded fruits. Where temperatures fall below 13°C (55°F), grow in a temperate or warm greenhouse. In tropical climates, grow as specimen or shade trees, hedges, or windbreaks.
• **HARDINESS** Frost tender.
• **CULTIVATION** Under glass, grow in loam-based potting compost (JI No.2), with additional sharp sand, in full light. During the growing season, water moderately and apply a balanced liquid fertilizer monthly; water sparingly in winter. Outdoors, grow in moderately fertile, sandy soil in full sun. Pruning group 1; plants grown under glass need restrictive pruning.
• **PROPAGATION** Sow seed at 18–24°C (64–75°F) in spring. Layer in spring.
• **PESTS AND DISEASES** Trouble free.

T. catappa ◐ (Indian almond). Dense, spreading, deciduous tree, the branches of young specimens forming horizontal whorls. Broadly obovate to obovate, lustrous, dark green leaves, to 25cm (10in) long, borne in rosette-like clusters at the branch tips, turn red before falling. Petalless flowers have white calyces, with tubes to 1cm (½in) long, and are borne in axillary spikes, to 16cm (6in) long, in summer; they are followed by narrowly winged, ellipsoid, red, yellow, or green fruit, 5–7cm (2–3in) long, with edible seeds. ↕ 20–35m (70–120ft), ↔ 15–20m (50–70ft). Tropical Asia, Malaysia, N. Australia, Polynesia. ❀ (min. 13–15°C/55–59°F)

TERNSTROEMIA

THEACEAE

Genus of 85 species of evergreen trees and shrubs occurring in woodland in mainly tropical regions of Asia, Africa, and North and South America. They are cultivated for their handsome, usually entire, leathery leaves, their many-stamened flowers, produced singly or sometimes in small clusters, and their usually pendent, spherical, fleshy, greenish yellow then bright red fruit. *T. gymnanthera* is the most commonly cultivated species. Grow as a specimen plant, in a shrub border, or against a shady wall, or use for hedging. In frost-prone climates, grow tender species in a conservatory or cool greenhouse.
• **HARDINESS** Frost hardy to frost tender.
• **CULTIVATION** Under glass, grow in lime-free (ericaceous) compost in bright filtered light. In the growing season, water freely, applying a balanced liquid fertilizer monthly; water sparingly in winter. Outdoors, grow in moist but well-drained, humus-rich, acid soil in partial shade. Pruning group 8; plants grown under glass may need restrictive pruning. Trim hedges after flowering.
• **PROPAGATION** Sow seed as soon as ripe in containers in a cold frame. Insert semi-ripe cuttings with bottom heat in late summer.
• **PESTS AND DISEASES** Trouble free.

T. gymnanthera, syn. *T. japonica*. Rounded, evergreen shrub. Elliptic to inversely lance-shaped, leathery, glossy, very dark green leaves, to 10cm (4in) long, turning bronze in cold weather, are usually clustered at the shoot tips. White flowers, 1cm (½in) across, are produced singly or in small clusters from the leaf axils, in late spring and early summer; they are followed by spherical, greenish yellow berries, 2.5cm (1in) long, ripening to red. ↕↔ 3m (10ft). China, Taiwan, Japan. ✲✲ (borderline). **'Variegata'** has leaves margined with creamy white, and tinged pink in winter; ✲
T. japonica see *T. gymnanthera*.

▷ ***Testudinaria elephantipes*** see *Dioscorea elephantipes*

TETRACENTRON

TETRACENTRACEAE

Genus of one species of deciduous tree found in mountain woodland in S.W. and C. China, the Himalayas, and N. Burma, cultivated for its attractive foliage and flower spikes. The alternate, simple leaves have stipule-like flanges on the stalks. Small, petalless, bisexual yellow flowers are produced in pendent

T

spikes in summer. *T. sinense* is suitable for a woodland garden.
- **HARDINESS** Fully hardy, but young growth may be damaged by late frosts.
- **CULTIVATION** Grow in well-drained soil in sun or partial shade. Shelter from cold, drying winds. Pruning group 1.
- **PROPAGATION** Sow seed in a seedbed in autumn. Insert semi-ripe cuttings with bottom heat in summer.
- **PESTS AND DISEASES** Trouble free.

T. sinense ♀ Graceful, spreading, deciduous tree with ovate or heart-shaped, tapered, scalloped, dark green leaves, to 12cm (5in) long, turning red in autumn. Tiny yellow flowers are borne in slender, pendent spikes, to 15cm (6in) long, from the shoot tips in summer. ↕ 17–30m (56–100ft), ↔ 10m (30ft). Himalayas, S.W. and C. China, N. Burma. ❄❄❄

TETRADIUM
syn. EUODIA, EVODIA
RUTACEAE

Genus of 9 species of upright to rounded, deciduous or evergreen trees and shrubs found in woodland from the Himalayas to E. and S.E. Asia, and cultivated for their attractive foliage, flowers, and dense clusters of fruit. They have opposite, usually pinnate leaves. Cup-shaped flowers, each with 4 or 5 usually hooded petals, are borne in terminal or axillary corymbs or panicles. Oval to pear-shaped or spherical green fruits, with 1–5 follicles, each 1- or 2-seeded, are produced in late summer or autumn. Tetradiums make handsome specimen trees for a lawn or woodland garden. In frost-prone areas, grow tender species in a cool or temperate greenhouse.
- **HARDINESS** Fully hardy to frost tender.
- **CULTIVATION** Grow in well-drained soil in full sun or partial shade. Pruning group 1.
- **PROPAGATION** Sow seed in a seedbed in autumn. Insert root cuttings in midwinter.
- **PESTS AND DISEASES** Trouble free.

T. daniellii ▣ ♀ syn. *Euodia daniellii, E. hupehensis.* Spreading, deciduous tree bearing pinnate leaves, to 40cm (16in) or more long, each with up to 11 elliptic, ovate, or lance-shaped, glossy, dark green leaflets, turning yellow in autumn. Small, aromatic white flowers, with yellow anthers, are produced in domed, terminal corymbs, to 15cm (6in) across, in late summer and early autumn; they are followed by dense clusters of spherical, red-brown to black fruit, 8mm (3/8in) across. ↕↔ 15m (50ft). S.W. China, Korea. ❄❄❄

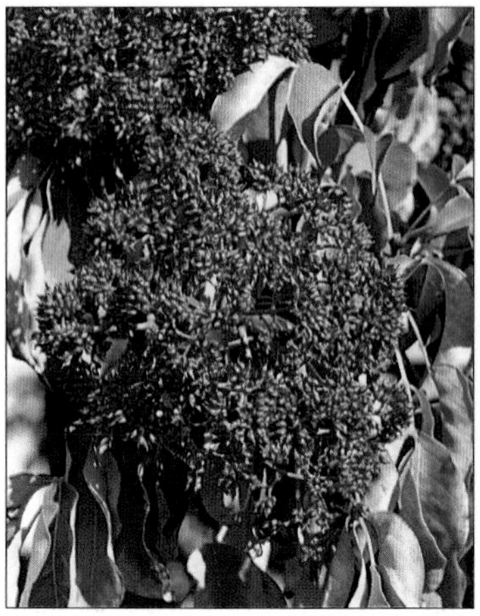
Tetradium daniellii

TETRANEMA
SCROPHULARIACEAE

Genus of 2 species of shrubby, evergreen perennials from moist, shady situations at altitudes up to 1,200m (4,000ft) in Mexico and Guatemala. They are cultivated for their decorative flowers, produced over a long period in summer. The many flower stems bear terminal clusters of trumpet-shaped, 2-lipped, violet, lilac, or mauve flowers, the upper lips 2-lobed, the lower ones 3-lobed; the stems arise from neat rosettes of obovate or oblong, scalloped, leathery leaves. In frost-prone areas, grow in a warm greenhouse or as houseplants. In warmer areas, grow in a shady border.
- **HARDINESS** Frost tender.
- **CULTIVATION** Under glass, grow in loam-based potting compost (JI No.2) in bright filtered light with moderate to high humidity. In summer, water freely and apply a balanced liquid fertilizer monthly; water moderately at other times. Pot on in spring. Outdoors, grow in well-drained soil in partial shade.
- **PROPAGATION** Sow seed at 18–21°C (64–70°F) as soon as ripe or in spring. Divide established clumps in spring.
- **PESTS AND DISEASES** Aphids may be a problem.

T. mexicanum see *T. roseum.*
T. roseum ▣ ♀ syn. *T. mexicanum* (Mexican foxglove, Mexican violet). Evergreen perennial with obovate, dark green leaves, to 12cm (5in) long. In summer, trumpet-shaped, 2-lipped, lilac or mauve flowers, 1.5cm (1/2in) across, with darker markings, are produced on stems to 20cm (8in) long. ↕ 20cm (8in), ↔ 15cm (6in). Mexico. ❀ (min. 13°C/55°F)

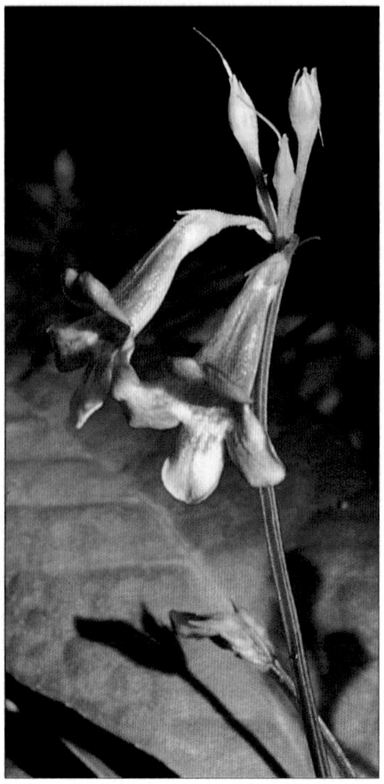
Tetranema roseum

TETRANEURIS
ASTERACEAE/COMPOSITAE

Genus of about 35 species of aromatic annuals and short-lived herbaceous perennials from plains, prairies, and mountain screes in W. and C. USA. They are grown for their aromatic foliage and flowers. Alternate, narrowly linear to lance-shaped or inversely lance-shaped, occasionally lobed, very hairy leaves are usually arranged in basal rosettes, but are occasionally distributed along the stems. The mostly solitary, daisy-like yellow flowerheads are borne in early summer. Grow in a sunny scree bed or alpine house.
- **HARDINESS** Fully hardy.
- **CULTIVATION** Outdoors, grow in sharply drained, gritty soil in full sun, protected from excessive winter wet. In an alpine house, use a mix of 2 parts grit and 1 part each loam and leaf mould. Water moderately when in growth, avoiding the foliage, and sparingly in winter.
- **PROPAGATION** Sow seed as soon as ripe in an open frame.
- **PESTS AND DISEASES** Aphids and red spider mites may prove troublesome under glass.

T. acaulis, syn. *Hymenoxys acaulis.* Tap-rooted perennial with crowded, basal rosettes of narrowly inversely lance-shaped, very hairy, grey-green leaves, 2–8cm (1/4–3in) long. Usually solitary yellow flowerheads, to 5cm (2in) across, are borne on upright, hairy stems in early summer. ↕↔ to 15cm (6in). USA (Idaho to N. Dakota, Texas, and New Mexico). ❄❄❄

TETRAPANAX
ARALIACEAE

Genus of one species of suckering, evergreen shrub or small tree occurring in woodland in S. China and Taiwan. It is grown for its large, alternate, palmately lobed leaves, its umbels of flowers, borne in panicle-like, woolly inflorescences with conspicuous bracts, and its clusters of black fruit. In frost-prone areas, grow against a warm wall, in a container moved under cover in winter, or in a cool greenhouse. In warmer climates, grow in a sheltered border. The flowers are particularly attractive to bees.
- **HARDINESS** Frost hardy (borderline).
- **CULTIVATION** Under glass, grow in loam-based potting compost (JI No.2), in full light with shade from hot sun. During the growing season, water freely and apply a balanced liquid fertilizer monthly; water sparingly in winter. Outdoors, grow in any well-drained soil in full sun, sheltered from strong winds. In order to restrict the spread of established clumps, remove suckers at the extremities. Where top-growth is killed by frost, *T. papyrifer* may be almost herbaceous, growing again from below ground. Pruning group 1 or 7.
- **PROPAGATION** Sow seed in containers in a cold frame in autumn. Remove suckers in spring or summer.
- **PESTS AND DISEASES** Trouble free.

T. papyrifer ♀ ♀ syn. *Aralia papyrifer, Fatsia papyrifera, T. papyriferus* (Rice-paper plant). Thicket-forming, sparsely branched, evergreen shrub or small tree with stout shoots. The 5- to 11-lobed leaves, to 50cm (20in) or more across, scaly, mid-green above and felted pale green beneath, are clustered at the shoot tips. In autumn, produces umbels, 1cm (1/2in) across, of white flowers in panicle-like inflorescences, to 50cm (20in) long, followed by spherical fruit, to 3mm (1/8in) across. ↕↔ 5m (15ft) or more. S. China, Taiwan. ❄❄ (borderline)
T. papyriferus see *T. papyrifer.*

TETRASTIGMA
VITACEAE

Genus of about 90 species of evergreen and deciduous tendril climbers found in tropical woodland from Indonesia and Malaysia to N. Australia. They are grown mainly for their alternate, mostly fully divided, sometimes lobed, palmate to pedate leaves. Tiny, 4-petalled flowers are borne in cyme-like, axillary umbels or clusters in summer, followed by grape-like black berries. In areas where temperatures fall below 15°C (59°F), grow in a warm greenhouse or as houseplants. In tropical climates, train over a wall or a tree stump.
- **HARDINESS** Frost tender.
- **CULTIVATION** Under glass, grow in loam-based potting compost (JI No.3), with additional leaf mould, in bright filtered or bright indirect light, with moderate to high humidity. In the growing season, water freely, applying a balanced liquid fertilizer monthly; water moderately in winter. The climbing stems need support. Outdoors, grow in moist, fertile soil in partial or dappled shade. Pruning group 11, in spring.
- **PROPAGATION** Insert semi-ripe cuttings with bottom heat in summer. Layer in spring.
- **PESTS AND DISEASES** Red spider mites may be a problem under glass.

T. voinierianum ▣ ♀ syn. *Cissus voinieriana, Vitis voinieriana* (Chestnut vine, Lizard plant). Strong-growing,

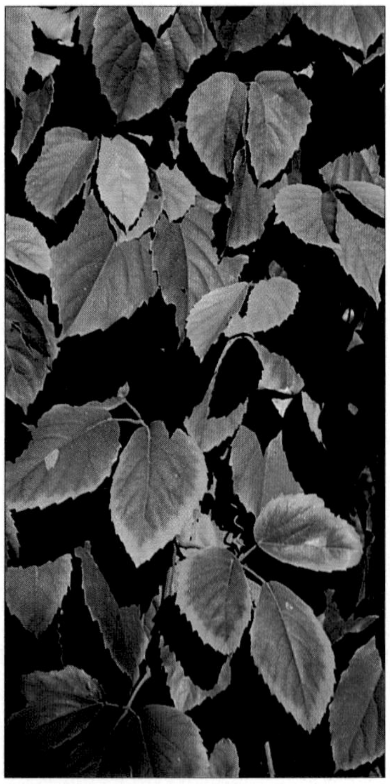
Tetrastigma voinierianum

evergreen climber with sturdy, hairy, densely red-brown stems. Leaves are 3- to 5-palmate, 15–40cm (6–16in) long, with broadly diamond-shaped to obovate, coarsely toothed leaflets, to 25cm (10in) long, lustrous, dark green above and brownish yellow-hairy beneath. Yellowish green flowers are borne in dense, axillary umbels or clusters, 5cm (2in) across, on mature plants in summer; they are followed by small, acidic berries. ↕ to 15m (50ft) or more. Laos. ❀ (min. 15°C/59°F)

TETRATHECA

TREMANDRACEAE

Genus of at least 20 species of small, evergreen shrubs from heathland and drought-prone forest in Australia, grown for their flowers and attractive, heather-like habit. The tiny, linear to rounded leaves are arranged alternately, in whorls, or in opposite pairs. Solitary, nodding, cross-, star-, or cup-shaped, 4- or 5-petalled flowers are borne from the upper leaf axils in spring and summer. In frost-prone regions, grow in a cool greenhouse. In milder areas, grow in a shrub border.

• **HARDINESS** Half hardy; *T. ciliare* may survive brief spells at a few degrees below 0°C (32°F).

• **CULTIVATION** Under glass, grow in lime-free (ericaceous) potting compost in full light, with shade from hot sun, and with good ventilation. In growth, water freely and apply a half-strength balanced liquid fertilizer monthly; water sparingly in winter. Outdoors, grow in humus-rich, neutral to acid soil in full sun with some midday shade. Pruning group 10, after flowering.

• **PROPAGATION** Surface-sow seed at 13–16°C (55–61°F) in spring. Insert semi-ripe cuttings with bottom heat in summer. Air layer in spring.

• **PESTS AND DISEASES** Trouble free.

T. ciliare. Twiggy, tufted shrub with wiry, densely hairy stems and whorls of 3 broadly ovate, mid- to dark green leaves, 5mm (¼in) long, fringed with hairs. From spring to summer, cup-shaped, rose-pink flowers, 1–2cm (½–¾in) across, with 4 oblong petals, are produced from the upper leaf axils. ↕↔ 40–50cm (16–20in). S. Australia. ❄

TEUCRIUM

LABIATAE/LAMIACEAE

Genus of approximately 300 species of herbaceous perennials and evergreen and deciduous shrubs and subshrubs, found mainly in thickets, woodland, dry, rocky places, and mountainous areas worldwide, especially in the Mediterranean region. Teucriums are grown for their attractive habit, aromatic foliage, and whorled clusters or racemes of 2–6 tubular to bell-shaped, sometimes 2-lipped flowers. The leaves, arranged in opposite pairs, are simple or lobed, and entire or toothed. Teucriums have a variety of garden uses: the small species, to 30cm (12in) tall, are suitable for a rock garden, raised bed, or trough; grow the shrubs, such as *T. fruticans,* in a sheltered border or against a warm, sunny wall, or use for hedging in mild climates.

• **HARDINESS** Fully hardy to frost hardy.

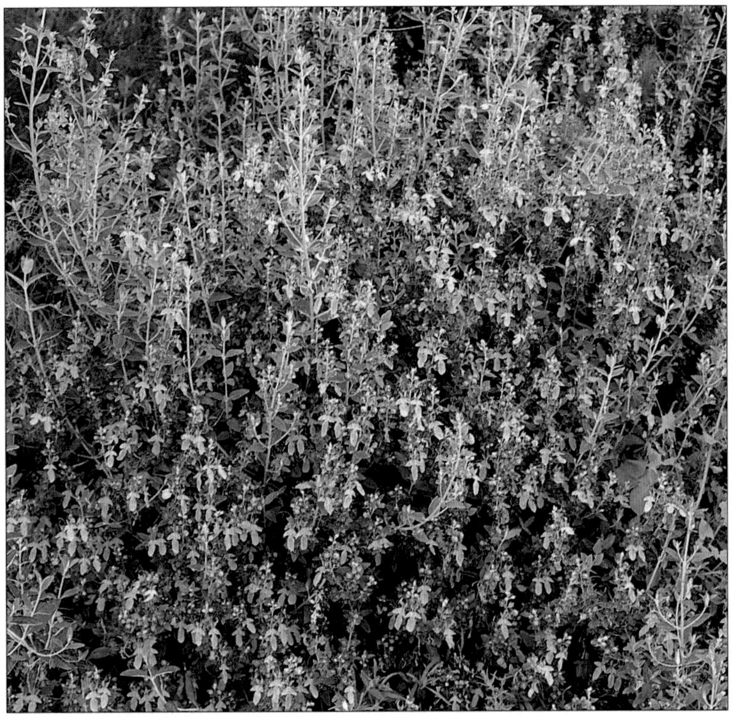

Teucrium fruticans

• **CULTIVATION** Grow in well-drained, preferably neutral to alkaline soil in full sun; the smallest species retain their compact habit better on poor, gritty soil. Pruning group 7 for *T. fruticans.*

• **PROPAGATION** Sow seed in containers in a cold frame as soon as ripe. Insert softwood cuttings in early summer, or semi-ripe cuttings in midsummer, both with bottom heat. Overwinter young plants of frost-hardy species in a cool greenhouse.

• **PESTS AND DISEASES** Trouble free.

T. aroanium, syn. *T. aroanum.* Low-growing, evergreen subshrub producing branching, stoloniferous, densely hairy stems and ovate or elliptic to oblong, aromatic, silver-hairy leaves, to 2cm (¾in) long. In summer, 2-lipped purple flowers, to 2cm (¾in) long, are borne in short-stemmed, axillary clusters. ↕ to 8cm (3in), ↔ to 20cm (8in). S. Greece. ❄❄❄

T. aroanum see *T. aroanium.*

T. fruticans ▣ (Shrubby germander, Tree germander). Bushy, evergreen shrub with arching, white-woolly shoots and aromatic, ovate to lance-shaped, grey-green leaves, to 2cm (¾in) long, white-woolly beneath. In summer, whorls of pale blue flowers, 2.5cm (1in) long, with prominent stamens, are borne in terminal racemes, to 10cm (4in) long. ↕ 60–100cm (24–39in), ↔ 4m (12ft). W. Mediterranean. ❄❄. **'Azureum'** 🏆 has dark blue flowers.

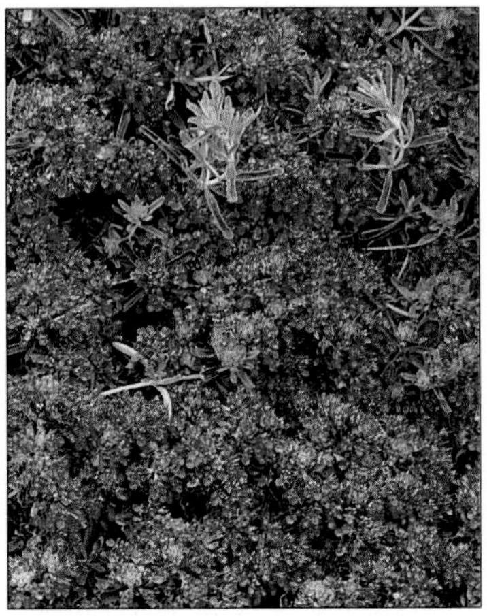

Teucrium polium

T. polium ▣ Mound-forming, deciduous subshrub with decumbent to erect, white- to tawny-woolly stems. Bears stemless, linear or oblong to lance-shaped, wrinkled, white-woolly, grey-green leaves, to 3.5cm (1½in) long. In summer, 2-lipped, purple or yellow flowers, to 1cm (½in) long, are borne in abundant dense, flat-topped, terminal clusters. ↕↔ 30cm (12in). Mediterranean to W. Asia. ❄❄❄

T. subspinosum. Shrubby perennial with ascending, twisted, branching, white-woolly stems, with short spines on the branchlets, and diamond-shaped to lance-shaped or linear, grey-green leaves, to 7mm (¼in) long, often densely white-woolly beneath. In summer, 2-lipped pink flowers, to 8mm (⅜in) long, are produced in loose, terminal racemes, to 5cm (2in) long. ↕↔ 20cm (8in). Balearic Islands (Majorca). ❄❄❄

THALIA

MARANTACEAE

Genus of 12 species of evergreen or herbaceous, marginal aquatic perennials found at the swampy margins of lakes and ponds from S.E. USA to Argentina, including the West Indies, with one species in tropical Africa. They have handsome, long-stalked, ovate-lance-shaped leaves, and bear unusual violet flowers, with enlarged staminodes, in 2 ranks in long-stalked, branched panicles. In frost-prone areas, grow in a pool in a cool greenhouse. In warmer areas, grow as specimen plants in and around a tropical pool or bog garden.

• **HARDINESS** Half hardy to frost tender; if well below water level, *T. dealbata* survives occasional temperatures to -5°C (23°F) but then becomes deciduous.

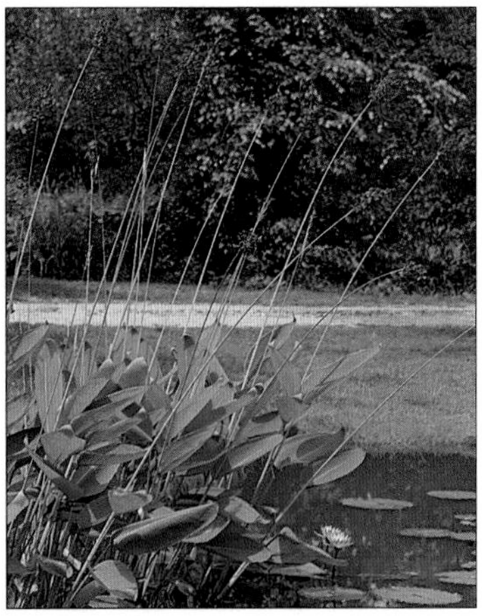

Thalia dealbata

• **CULTIVATION** Grow in a large aquatic planting basket of fertile, loamy soil, or in deep, humus-rich mud in water up to 15cm (6in) deep, at the edge of a sunny pool. In summer, apply a proprietary aquatic plant fertilizer monthly. Remove old leaves and flowers regularly. Under glass, grow in baskets of loam-based potting compost (JI No.3) in full light, with a minimum temperature of 10°C (50°F). See also pp.52–53.

• **PROPAGATION** Sow seed at 16–21°C (61–70°F) in moist propagating compost, as soon as ripe or in spring. Divide in spring.

• **PESTS AND DISEASES** Trouble free.

T. dealbata ▣ Evergreen, marginal aquatic perennial producing ovate to lance-shaped, white-floury, grey-green leaves, 50cm (20in) long, on leaf-stalks 30–60cm (12–24in) long. In summer, violet flowers, 1.5–2cm (½–¾in) across, are borne in slender panicles, to 20cm (8in) long. ↕ 2–3m (6–10ft), ↔ 2m (6ft). S. USA, Mexico. ❄ (borderline)

T. geniculata. Evergreen, marginal aquatic perennial bearing ovate to lance-shaped, grey-green leaves, to 60cm (24in) long, on leaf-stalks to 1.8m (6ft) long. In summer, bears violet flowers, 1.5–2cm (½–¾in) across, in lax, pendent panicles, to 20cm (8in) long. ↕↔ 2m (6ft). Tropical Africa, USA (Florida) to Argentina, West Indies. ❄ (borderline)

THALICTRUM

Meadow rue

RANUNCULACEAE

Genus of about 130 species of rhizomatous or tuberous perennials found by streams, in meadows, and in moist, shady, often mountainous areas worldwide (except Australasia), mainly in N. temperate regions. The usually erect stems bear alternate, ternate to 4-ternate or 2- to 4-pinnate, sometimes glaucous leaves with lobed or toothed leaflets, the end leaflet longer than the others. The many tiny, petalless flowers are borne in axillary or terminal corymbs, racemes, or panicles; they have petal-like sepals and often numerous showy stamens and pistils in white, yellow, pink, lilac-pink, or violet, giving a fluffy effect. Grown for their attractive foliage and flowers, the taller species are excellent background plants for a border, or a wild or woodland garden; the smaller species are suitable for a

shady rock garden, peat bed, or alpine house. Except for *T. aquilegiifolium* and *T. flavum*, most grow best in areas with cool, damp summers. In frost-prone climates, grow tender species in a cool greenhouse.
• **HARDINESS** Fully hardy to frost tender.
• **CULTIVATION** Grow in moist, humus-rich soil in partial shade; *T. flavum* subsp. *glaucum* tolerates drier soil and more sun. Grow smaller, alpine species in moist, humus-rich, acid soil in cool partial shade. Tall species and cultivars need staking. Divide and replant *T. delavayi* 'Hewitt's Double' every 2 or 3 years to maintain vigour. All start into growth in mid- or late spring, so take care to avoid damage to dormant plants when cultivating earlier in the year.
• **PROPAGATION** Sow seed in containers in a cold frame as soon as ripe or in early spring. Divide as new growth begins in spring; divisions may be slow to re-establish. *T. delavayi* 'Hewitt's Double' is sterile, and may be increased only by division.
• **PESTS AND DISEASES** Susceptible to powdery mildew in dry conditions. Slugs may be a problem.

T. aquilegiifolium ■ Erect, clump-forming, rhizomatous perennial with 2- or 3-pinnate, hairless leaves, to 30cm (12in) long, composed of obovate, wavy-margined leaflets. Clustered, fluffy flowers, 8–10mm (3/8–1/2in) long, with greenish white sepals, falling to reveal numerous bright purple-pink or white stamens, are produced in spreading, flat-topped, terminal panicles on glaucous stems in early summer. ↕ to 1m (3ft), ↔ 45cm (18in). Europe to temperate Asia. ✲✲✲. **'Purple Cloud'** see 'Thundercloud'. **'Thundercloud'** 🏆 syn. 'Purple Cloud', has dark purple stamens. **'White Cloud'** has yellow-tipped white stamens.
T. chelidonii. Erect, clump-forming, rhizomatous perennial bearing 2- or 3-pinnate or ternate, hairless leaves, to 45cm (18in) long, with ovate to almost rounded, many-toothed leaflets. During late summer and early autumn, fluffy flowers, to 2.5cm (1in) across, with conspicuous mauve sepals and shorter, pendent yellow stamens, are produced in terminal and axillary panicles. ↕ 0.3–2.5m (1–8ft), ↔ 60cm (24in). C. and E. Himalayas. ✲✲✲
T. delavayi 🏆 syn. *T. dipterocarpum* of gardens. Erect, hairless, clump-forming, rhizomatous perennial with slender

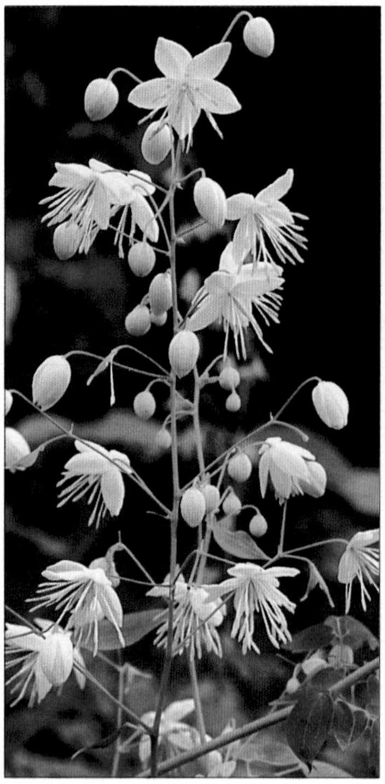
Thalictrum delavayi 'Album'

stems, shaded dark purple, and usually 2- or 3-pinnate or ternate leaves, to 35cm (14in) long, with entire or 3-lobed leaflets. From midsummer to early autumn, numerous long-stalked, fluffy flowers, to 2.5cm (1in) across, with large, lilac to white sepals, 1.5cm (1/2in) long, and clusters of yellowish white stamens, are borne in widely branching, pyramidal, terminal and axillary panicles. ↕ 1.2m (4ft) or more, ↔ 60cm (24in). E. Tibet to W. China. ✲✲✲. **'Album'** ■ has flowers with white sepals. **'Hewitt's Double'** ■ 🏆 lacks stamens but has more numerous rich mauve sepals, forming long-lasting, rounded, pompon-like flowers.
T. diffusiflorum. Erect, clump-forming, rhizomatous perennial, similar to *T. chelidonii*, bearing 2- or 3-pinnate or ternate, greyish green, basal leaves, to 20cm (8in) long, with rounded, almost circular, slightly toothed, finely hairy leaflets. In summer, bears fluffy flowers, 2.5cm (1¼in) across, with light pinkish mauve sepals and much shorter, pendent yellow stamens, in loose, few- to many-flowered, axillary and terminal panicles. ↕ 90cm (36in) or more, ↔ 30cm (12in). S.E. Tibet. ✲✲✲

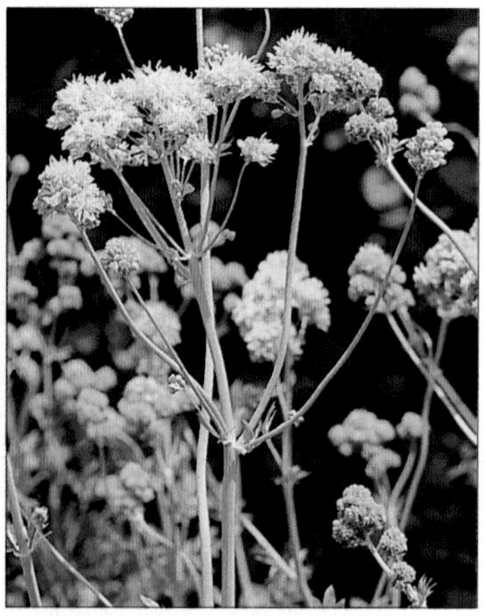
Thalictrum flavum subsp. *glaucum*

***T. dipterocarpum* of gardens** see *T. delavayi.*
T. flavum (Yellow meadow rue). Clump-forming, rhizomatous perennial producing 2- or 3-pinnate, hairless leaves, to 40cm (16in) long, composed of obovate, 3- or 4-lobed leaflets. In summer, numerous fragrant flowers, 5mm (1/4in) long, with small yellow sepals and longer, erect, bright yellow stamens, are produced in erect, compact, narrowly ovoid, axillary and terminal panicles on stout, furrowed stems. ↕ to 1m (3ft), ↔ 45cm (18in). Europe to Caucasus, Russia (Siberia). ✲✲✲. **subsp. *glaucum*** ■ 🏆 syn. *T. speciosissimum*, has glaucous stems and foliage, the leaflets with prominent veins beneath, and larger panicles of paler, sulphur-yellow flowers; ↔ 60cm (24in); Portugal, Spain, N.W. Africa. **'Illuminator'** has bright green leaves, emerging yellow-green, and lemon-yellow flowers; ↕ 1.2m (4ft).
T. kiusianum ■ Mat-forming perennial with short rhizomes and fern-like, ternate or 2-ternate, dark blue-green leaves, to 12cm (5in) long, with ovate, 3- to 5-lobed leaflets. Pale pinkish mauve flowers, to 1cm (1/2in) across, with conspicuous stamens, are borne in few-flowered, short-stemmed corymbs in early summer. Grow in a damp, shady peat bed, trough, rock garden, or alpine house. Prefers peaty soil. ↕ to 10cm (4in), ↔ to 30cm (12in). Japan. ✲✲✲
T. orientale. Slow-growing, clump-forming, rhizomatous perennial with fern-like, 2-ternate, blue-green leaves, to 12cm (5in) long, with rounded, 3-lobed leaflets. Deep pinkish blue flowers, 1.5cm (1/2in) long, are produced in few-flowered, wiry-stemmed corymbs in late spring and early summer. Difficult to propagate. ↕↔ to 30cm (12in). Greece to Caucasus. ✲✲✲
T. rochebruneanum. Upright, hairless, clump-forming, rhizomatous perennial with 3- or 4-ternate leaves, to 45cm (18in) long, composed of obovate to elliptic, entire or lobed leaflets. White or lavender-pink flowers, 1.5cm (1/2in) long, with pendent stamens, are produced in loose panicles in summer. ↕ 90cm (36in), ↔ 30cm (12in). Japan. ✲✲✲
T. speciosissimum see *T. flavum* subsp. *glaucum.*

▷ ***Thamnocalamus falconeri*** see *Himalayacalamus falconeri*
▷ ***Thamnocalamus spathaceus* of gardens** see *Fargesia murieliae*
▷ **Thatch,**
Brittle see *Thrinax morrisii*
Buffalo see *Thrinax morrisii*
Silver see *Coccothrinax fragrans*
▷ **Thatch palm** see *Thrinax, T. parviflora*

THELOCACTUS

CACTACEAE

Genus of about 11 species of spherical to short-cylindrical, ribbed or warty, perennial cacti occurring in arid regions of S.W. USA and C., E., and N. Mexico. In summer, large, funnel- to bell-shaped, diurnal flowers are borne on or near the slightly depressed crowns. In areas where temperatures fall below 7°C (45°F), grow *Thelocactus* species as houseplants, or in a cool or temperate greenhouse. In warm, dry climates, they are suitable for a border with other cacti, or for a desert garden.
• **HARDINESS** Frost tender.
• **CULTIVATION** Under glass, grow in standard cactus compost in full light, with low humidity. From mid-spring to early autumn, water moderately, applying fertilizer 2 or 3 times; keep completely dry at other times of year. Outdoors, grow in poor to moderately fertile, gritty, sharply drained soil in full sun. See also pp.48–49.
• **PROPAGATION** Sow seed at 21°C (70°F) in spring. Detach offsets in spring or early summer.
• **PESTS AND DISEASES** Mealybugs may be a problem.

T. bicolor ■ 🏆 syn. *Ferocactus bicolor.* Simple, rarely clustering cactus bearing spherical, often slightly elongated, bluish green stems. Each rib has 8–13 straight or spirally arranged, warty ribs. Areoles, which have nectar-secreting glands, produce red, yellow, or white spines (8–18 radials and 4 slightly longer centrals, the uppermost of which is flat). Funnel-shaped, red-throated, dark purple-pink flowers, 4–8cm (1½–3in) across, are produced in summer. ↕ 15–20cm (6–8in), ↔ 10cm (4in). USA (Texas), N. and E. Mexico. ❀ (min. 7°C/45°F)
T. leucacanthus. Often offsetting cactus producing spherical to cylindrical, pale green stems, each bearing 7–14 straight or slightly spiralling, conical, warty ribs. Areoles with nectar-secreting glands produce yellow, red, grey, or black

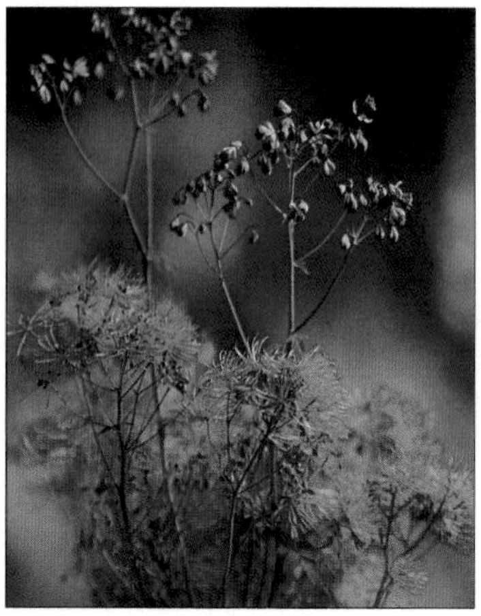
Thalictrum aquilegiifolium

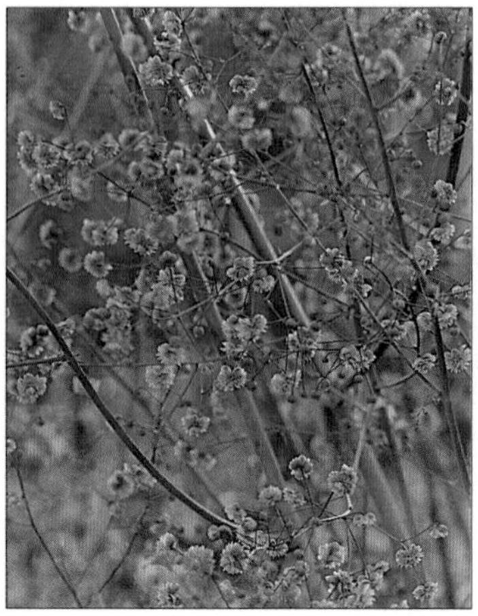
Thalictrum delavayi 'Hewitt's Double'

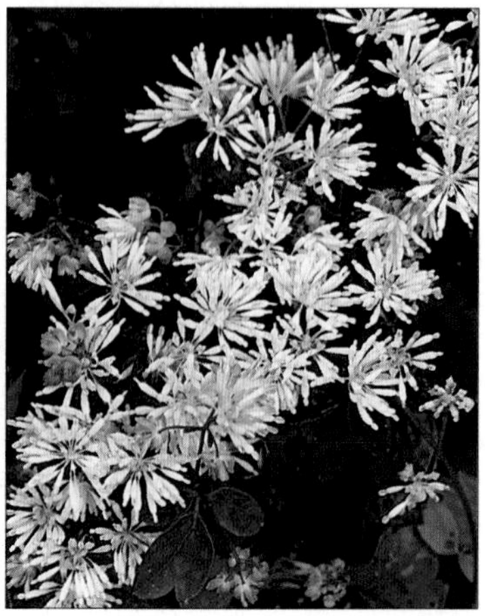
Thalictrum kiusianum

T

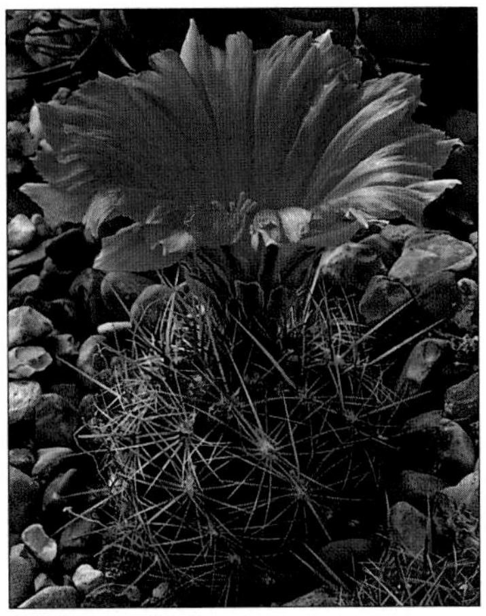

Thelocactus bicolor

spines (6–20 yellow, sometimes red-tinged radials and 1–3 yellow, red, or black centrals). Short-tubed, funnel-shaped, pale to deep yellow to magenta flowers, 4–5cm (1½–2in) across, are produced in summer. ↕ to 15cm (6in), ↔ to 20cm (8in). C. Mexico. ❀ (min. 7°C/45°F)

T. macdowellii, syn. *Echinocactus macdowellii.* Sometimes clustering cactus producing spherical to club-shaped, pale green stems, each bearing 20–25 conical, warty ribs. The white-felted areoles are densely arranged, and produce glassy, transparent, white or pale yellow spines (15–20 radials and 3 or 4 yellowish white centrals, the centrals longer than the radials). Funnel-shaped magenta flowers, 5cm (2in) or more across, are produced in summer. ↕ to 15cm (6in), ↔ 10cm (4in). N.E. Mexico. ❀ (min. 7°C/45°F)

T. setispinus, syn. *Ferocactus setispinus, Hamatocactus setispinus.* Solitary cactus, later offsetting, producing spherical to short-cylindrical, dark green stems. Each stem has 12–15 notched, often wavy ribs. Rounded to elliptic, straw-coloured areoles produce white or brown spines (9–17 white or red-tinged radials and 1 pale yellow, sometimes red-tinged, hooked central). Funnel-shaped, red-throated yellow flowers, to 5cm (2in) across, are produced from summer to autumn. ↕ 20cm (8in), ↔ 12cm (5in). USA (Texas), N.E. Mexico. ❀ (min. 7°C/45°F)

▷ ***Thelycrania*** see *Cornus*
T. alba see *C. alba*

THELYPTERIS

THELYPTERIDACEAE

Genus of 2 species of deciduous, terrestrial ferns found in swamps and bogs in temperate regions throughout the world. The lance-shaped, pinnate fronds, comprising deeply lobed pinnae, arise from creeping rhizomes. Sori, which have no protective indusia, form on the undersides of the fronds. Grow in a moist border, or plant at the edge of a pond; *T. palustris* may be invasive.

• **HARDINESS** Fully hardy.
• **CULTIVATION** Grow in any moist, moderately fertile soil in full sun or partial shade.
• **PROPAGATION** Sow spores at 15°C (59°F) as soon as ripe. Divide in spring or summer. See also p.51.
• **PESTS AND DISEASES** Trouble free.

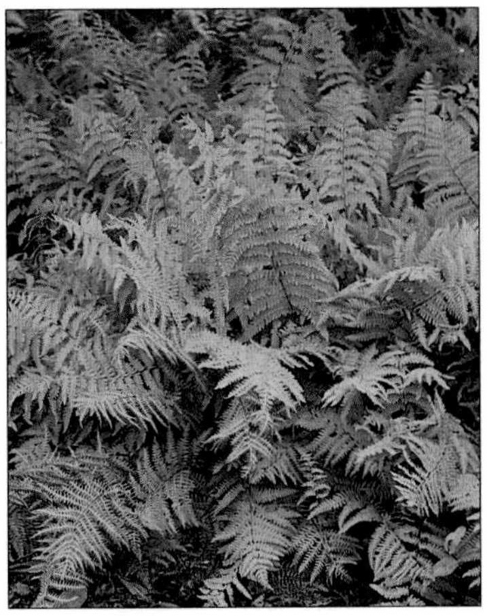

Thelypteris palustris

T. hexagonoptera see *Phegopteris hexagonoptera.*

T. palustris ■ (Marsh fern). Deciduous fern producing long, creeping rhizomes and long-stalked, erect, lance-shaped, pinnate, pale green sterile fronds, to 40cm (16in) long, each consisting of up to 25 pairs of narrowly lance-shaped, deeply lobed pinnae. Fertile fronds, 90cm (36in) long, which are produced only in good light, have pinnae with narrower lobes. The abundant sori may produce a brown haze over the colony in late summer. ↕ 60cm (24in), ↔ to 1m (3ft). Europe, Asia. ❄❄❄

T. phegopteris see *Phegopteris connectilis.*

THERMOPSIS

LEGUMINOSAE/PAPILIONACEAE

Genus of approximately 20 species of rhizomatous perennials from grassy mountainsides, light woodland, and streamsides in Siberia (Russia), N. India, E. Asia, and North America. They are cultivated for their attractive foliage and lupin-like flowers. Erect stems bear alternate, stalked, 3-palmate leaves, some silver-hairy, with persistent, leafy stipules; the similar basal leaves are produced in smaller numbers. Pea-like, yellow or purple flowers, with rounded standard petals and roughly equal-sized keel and wing petals, are borne in terminal or axillary racemes. Suitable for a mixed or herbaceous border, or a wild-flower garden; *T. rhombifolia* is invasive and best grown in a wild garden. The flowers are attractive to bees.

• **HARDINESS** Fully hardy.
• **CULTIVATION** Grow in light, well-drained, fertile, loamy soil in full sun or partial shade, although they will tolerate a range of conditions. Usually long-lived, they have tough roots that resent disturbance.
• **PROPAGATION** Sow seed at 10–13°C (50–55°F) in spring, transplanting seedlings to their final position as soon as possible. Division is difficult, and divisions are very slow to re-establish.
• **PESTS AND DISEASES** Slugs and aphids may be a problem.

T. caroliniana see *T. villosa.*
T. montana see *T. rhombifolia.*
T. rhombifolia ■ syn. *T. montana.* Rhizomatous perennial producing unbranched stems and 3-palmate leaves, to 11cm (4½in) long, with broadly ovate leaflets. The stems and lower leaf surfaces are softly silver-hairy. In early summer, yellow flowers, 2.5cm (1in) long, are produced in erect, terminal racemes. ↕ 90cm (36in), ↔ 60cm (24in). USA (Rocky Mountains to New Mexico). ❄❄❄

T. villosa, syn. *T. caroliniana* (Carolina lupin). Rhizomatous perennial with stout, few-branched or branchless, hairless stems. The 3-palmate leaves, to 10cm (4in) long, have elliptic, obovate, or lance-shaped leaflets, hairless above, glaucous and silky-hairy beneath. In late spring and early summer, downy yellow flowers, to 2cm (¾in) long, are produced in erect, compact, terminal racemes. ↕ 1–1.5m (3–5ft), ↔ 60cm (24in). USA (North Carolina to Georgia). ❄❄❄

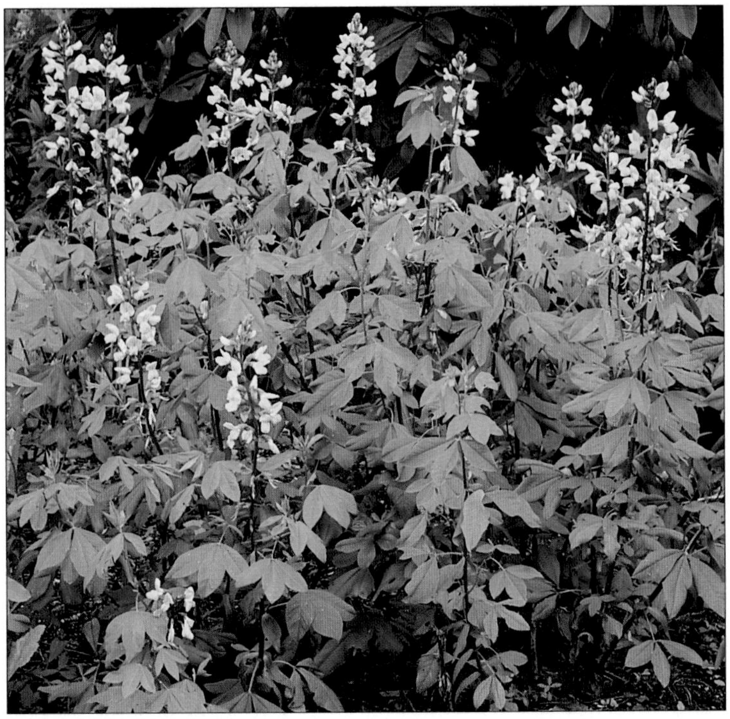

Thermopsis rhombifolia

THESPESIA

MALVACEAE

Genus of 17 species of mainly evergreen shrubs and trees, closely allied to *Hibiscus*, occurring throughout the world in a wide range of habitats, often in coastal areas of tropical regions. They are grown for their cup-shaped flowers, each with 5 spreading petals, produced singly or in clusters from the leaf axils. The leaves are alternate, simple, mainly lance-shaped to broadly ovate, or palmately 5- to 9-lobed. In areas where temperatures fall below 13–15°C (55–59°F), grow in a warm greenhouse. In tropical climates, grow as specimen plants, screens, or windbreaks, especially in coastal areas.

• **HARDINESS** Frost tender.
• **CULTIVATION** Under glass, grow in loam-based potting compost (JI No.3) in full light. In growth, water freely, applying a balanced liquid fertilizer monthly; water sparingly in winter. Outdoors, grow in moist but well-drained, fertile soil in full sun. Pruning group 1; plants under glass may need restrictive pruning.
• **PROPAGATION** Sow seed at 16°C (61°F) in spring. Insert semi-ripe cuttings with bottom heat in summer. Air layer in spring or summer.
• **PESTS AND DISEASES** Susceptible to red spider mites and whiteflies under glass.

T. populnea ♀ (Portia tree). Erect to spreading, bushy, evergreen tree bearing long-stalked, heart-shaped to ovate, light to mid-green leaves, 6–12cm (2½–5in) long, with nectar-bearing zones at the bases of the midribs. Solitary yellow flowers, 5–8cm (2–3in) across, with maroon-marked centres, open in sequence throughout the year in warm areas; they fade to dull purple. ↕ 10–15m (30–50ft), ↔ 5–8m (15–25ft). Coastal tropics. (min. 13–15°C/55–59°F)

THEVETIA

APOCYNACEAE

Genus of 8 species of evergreen shrubs and small trees from woodland, often near coastal areas, in tropical North and South America and the West Indies. They are cultivated for their showy, funnel-shaped flowers, with 5 overlapping petals, produced singly or in cymes from spring to autumn. They have alternate, simple, mostly linear to ovate leaves. Where temperatures fall below 13–15°C (55–59°F), grow in a temperate or warm greenhouse. In warmer climates, grow in a shrub border. The seeds are highly toxic if ingested.

• **HARDINESS** Frost tender.
• **CULTIVATION** Under glass, grow in loam-based potting compost (JI No.2) in full light and with good ventilation. During the growing season, water freely and apply a balanced liquid fertilizer monthly; water sparingly in winter. Outdoors, grow in moist but well-drained, fertile soil in full sun. Pruning group 1; plants under glass need restrictive pruning.
• **PROPAGATION** Sow seed at 18–21°C (64–70°F) in spring. Insert semi-ripe cuttings with bottom heat in summer.
• **PESTS AND DISEASES** Trouble free.

T

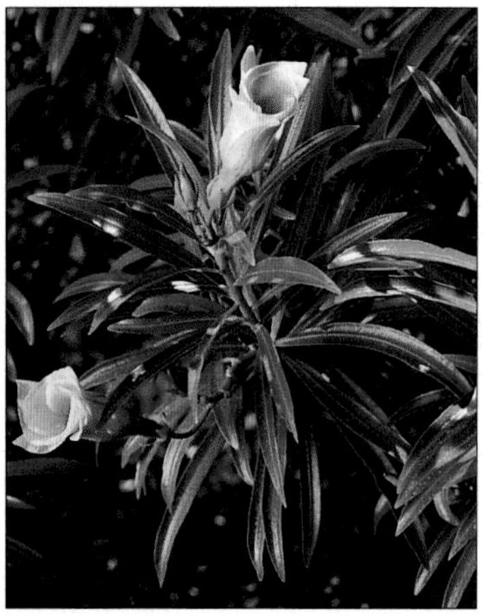

Thevetia peruviana

T. neriifolia see *T. peruviana.*
T. peruviana ◼♀ syn. *T. neriifolia.* Erect, open shrub or small tree bearing narrowly lance-shaped, lustrous, mid- to dark green leaves, 8–15cm (3–6in) long. Fragrant, apricot-yellow flowers, to 7cm (3in) long, are produced in few-flowered cymes near the shoot-tips from spring to autumn; they are followed by triangular-ovoid, semi-fleshy, red, later black seed pods, each of which contains 1 or 2 nut-like seeds. ↕ 2–8m (6–25ft), ↔ 1–3m (3–10ft). Tropical America. ⊛ (min. 13–15°C/55–59°F). **'Alba'** has white flowers.

▷**Thistle,**
Blessed Mary's see *Silybum marianum*
Carline see *Carlina*
Cotton see *Onopordum*
Globe see *Echinops*
Mountain see *Acanthus montanus*
Mountain sow see *Cicerbita alpina*
Scotch see *Onopordum*
Stemless Carline see *Carlina acaulis*

THLASPI

BRASSICACEAE/CRUCIFERAE

Genus of about 60 species of annuals, biennials, and short-lived perennials found in alpine pasture, in mountain woodland, or among rocks and screes in N. temperate regions. They produce oblong or spoon-shaped to broadly ovate or rounded, entire or toothed leaves, usually in rosettes, and are grown for their racemes of 4-petalled, cross-shaped flowers, borne from spring to early summer. Suitable for growing in a sunny rock garden, scree bed, or alpine house.
• **HARDINESS** Fully hardy.
• **CULTIVATION** Grow in gritty, humus-rich, sharply drained soil in full sun with some midday shade. In an alpine house, use a mix of equal parts loam, leaf mould, and sharp grit.
• **PROPAGATION** Sow seed as soon as ripe in containers in an open frame. May self-seed.
• **PESTS AND DISEASES** Slugs and snails may be a problem.

T. bulbosum. Tufted, tuberous-rooted perennial with rosettes of ovate to ovate-oblong or rounded, entire or toothed, glaucous, dark green leaves, to 2.5cm (1in) long. Deep purple-violet flowers, 6–8mm (¼–⅜in) across, with spoon-shaped petals, are produced in loose, spike-like racemes in spring. ↕ to 10cm (4in), ↔ to 20cm (8in). C. Greece, Aegean Islands. ❄❄❄
T. cepaeifolium* subsp. *rotundifolium. Short-lived, tufted perennial bearing broadly ovate to almost rounded, deep green leaves, to 1.5cm (½in) long. From spring to early summer, fragrant, deep violet-blue flowers, 1cm (½in) long, are produced in short-stemmed, congested, head-like racemes. ↕↔ to 10cm (4in). Europe (Alps, Apennines). ❄❄❄
T. macrophyllum see *Pachyphragma macrophyllum.*

▷**Thorn,**
Chinese box see *Lycium barbarum*
Christ's see *Euphorbia milii* var. *splendens, Paliurus spina-christi*
Cockspur see *Crataegus crus-galli*
Glastonbury see *Crataegus monogyna* 'Biflora'
Jerusalem see *Paliurus spina-christi, Parkinsonia aculeata*
Kangaroo see *Acacia paradoxa*
Tansy-leaved see *Crataegus tanacetifolia*
Washington see *Crataegus phaenopyrum*
▷**Thorns, Crown of** see *Euphorbia milii*
▷**Thorow-wax** see *Bupleurum*
▷**Thousand mothers** see *Tolmiea menziesii*
▷**Three-men-in-a-boat** see *Tradescantia spathacea*
▷**Thrift** see *Armeria*
Sea see *A. maritima*

THRINAX

Thatch palm

ARECACEAE/PALMAE

Genus of 7 species of single-stemmed palms, found in forested areas on well-drained, often limestone soils, from sea-level to 1,200m (4,000ft), in the USA (Florida), Mexico, Belize, and the Caribbean islands. The long-stalked, fan-shaped, palmately lobed leaves are borne in a terminal, almost spherical head. Small, cup-shaped flowers, each composed of a fused, 3-lobed calyx and a 3-lobed corolla, are borne in panicles between the leaves. In frost-prone areas, grow in a warm greenhouse or as house-plants. In tropical regions, grow in a shrub border or as specimen plants on a lawn.

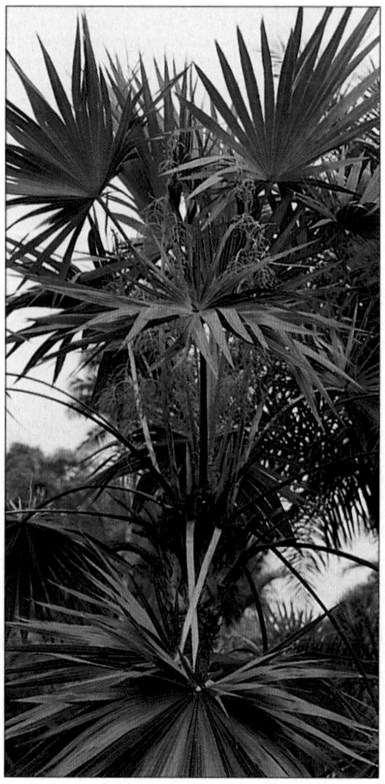

Thrinax morrisii

• **HARDINESS** Frost tender.
• **CULTIVATION** Under glass, grow in loam-based potting compost (JI No.3) in full light or bright filtered light. During growth, water freely and apply a balanced liquid fertilizer monthly; water sparingly in winter. Pot on or top-dress in spring. Outdoors, grow in moist but well-drained, fertile soil in full sun.
• **PROPAGATION** Sow seed at 27°C (81°F) in spring.
• **PESTS AND DISEASES** Red spider mites may be a problem under glass.

T. bahamensis see *T. morrisii.*
T. microcarpa see *T. morrisii.*
T. morrisii ◼🌴 syn. *T. bahamensis, T. microcarpa, T. ponceana* (Brittle thatch, Buffalo thatch, Key palm). Small palm with a slim, erect stem. Leaves, 75cm (30in) long, are divided to halfway into 33–58 narrow lobes, densely white- to tan-scaly beneath when young, then glabrous blue-green above; they have fibrous-based leaf-stalks, to 80cm (32in) long. White to yellow or orange flowers are borne in loose, arching panicles, to 1.5m (5ft) long, usually in summer. ↕ 5–10m (15–30ft), ↔ 2–3.5m (6–11ft). USA (Florida), Cuba, West Indies. ⊛ (min. 16°C/61°F)
T. parviflora 🌴 (Broom palm, Thatch palm). Small to medium-sized palm with a slim stem. Leaves, to 1m (3ft) long, are divided to halfway into 35–60 narrow lobes, sparsely scaly beneath, rich green above; they have leaf-stalks 40–130cm (16–54in) long. Fragrant, cream to yellow flowers are produced in panicles, 0.5–1.7m (20–66in) long, usually in summer. ↕ 6–13m (20–43ft), ↔ 1.5–3.5m (5–11ft). Jamaica. ⊛ (min. 16°C/61°F)
T. ponceana see *T. morrisii.*

▷**Throatwort** see *Campanula trachelium*
Blue see *Trachelium caeruleum*

THRYPTOMENE

Heath myrtle

MYRTACEAE

Genus of 25 species of upright to spreading, evergreen shrubs, found on rocky slopes and heathland in Australia, and grown for their flowers and foliage. The wiry stems bear small, simple, oblong or obovate to inversely lance-shaped leaves in opposite pairs, and produce an abundance of saucer-shaped flowers, each with 5 petals and 5 tepals, from winter to summer. In frost-prone areas, grow in a cool greenhouse. In milder climates, grow heath myrtles in a shrub border.
• **HARDINESS** Frost tender.
• **CULTIVATION** Under glass, grow in lime-free (ericaceous) potting compost in full light with good ventilation. During the growing season, water moderately and apply a half-strength, balanced liquid fertilizer monthly; water sparingly in winter. Outdoors, grow in light, well-drained, moderately fertile, neutral to acid soil in full sun. Pruning group 10, after flowering.
• **PROPAGATION** Surface-sow seed at 13°C (55°F) in spring. Insert semi-ripe cuttings with bottom heat in summer.
• **PESTS AND DISEASES** Trouble free.

T. calycina. Spreading, bushy shrub with crowded, tiny, oblong to inversely lance-shaped, aromatic, dark green leaves, 0.8–1.5cm (⅜–½in) long. From winter to spring, axillary, white, pink, or pink and white flowers, 6mm (¼in) across, with yellow centres that age to red, are borne singly or in clusters of 2 or 3. ↕↔ 1.5–2.5m (5–8ft). Australia (Victoria). ⊛ (min. 4–5°C/39–41°F)

THUJA *syn.* PLATYCLADUS

Arborvitae

CUPRESSACEAE

Genus of 6 species of narrowly to broadly conical, sometimes columnar, monoecious, evergreen, coniferous trees found in forests in E. Asia and North America. Scale-like, narrowly wedge- to diamond-shaped leaves, borne in 2 ranks of opposite pairs, are usually aromatic when bruised. The small, erect, variably shaped female cones have scales that hinge from the base; male cones are small and ovoid. Grow as specimen trees; most are suitable for hedging. The dwarf cultivars may be grown in a rock garden. Contact with the foliage may aggravate skin allergies.
• **HARDINESS** Fully hardy.
• **CULTIVATION** Grow in deep, moist but well-drained soil in full sun. Shelter from cold, drying winds, especially when young. Trim hedging in spring and late summer.

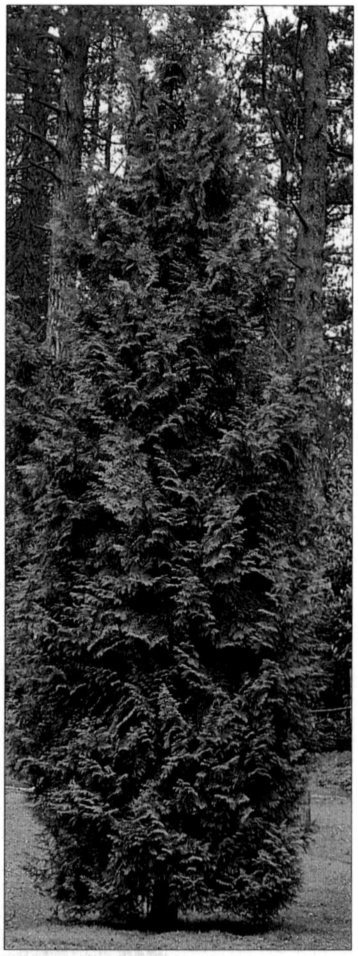

Thuja koraiensis

T

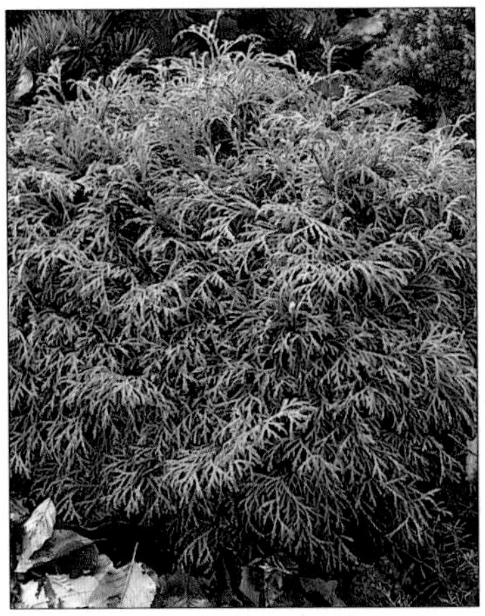

Thuja occidentalis 'Caespitosa'

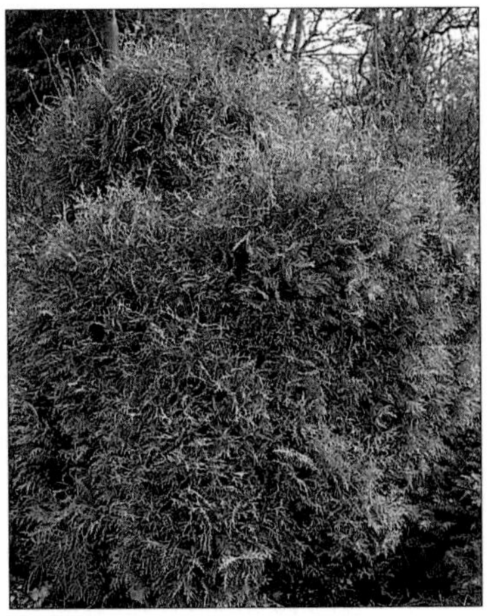

Thuja occidentalis 'Rheingold'

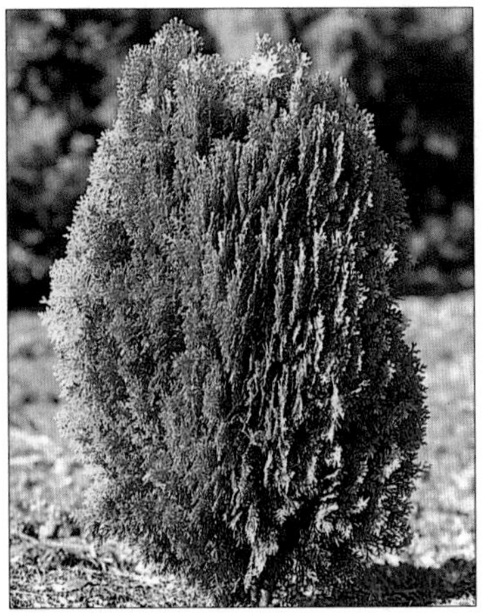

Thuja orientalis 'Semperaurea'

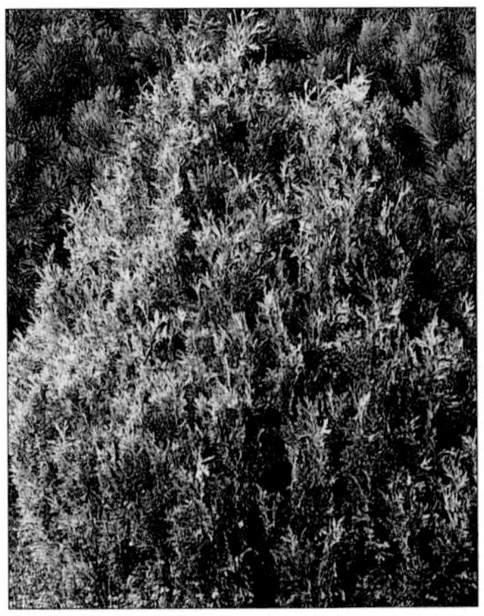

Thuja plicata 'Stoneham Gold'

• **PROPAGATION** Sow seed in late winter in containers in a cold frame. Insert semi-ripe cuttings in late summer.
• **PESTS AND DISEASES** Prone to scale insects, *Coryneum* canker, and aphids. Leaves are susceptible to *Keithia* disease, which may be fatal in young seedlings.

T. koraiensis ■◊–△ Small, conical tree with often trailing branchlets and flattened shoots. Scale-like leaves are triangular on the main shoots and diamond-shaped on the young shoots, bright mid-green above and vivid silver beneath. Ellipsoid brown female cones, 0.8–1.5cm (3/8–1/2in) long, each have 4 pairs of scales. ↕ to 10m (30ft), ↔ to 5m (15ft). N.E. China, Korea. ❄❄❄
T. occidentalis ◊ (White cedar). Small, rounded, conical tree with billowing branches and shredding, orange-brown bark. Scale-like, ovate, yellowish green leaves, pale or greyish green beneath, each with a prominent, raised dorsal gland, are apple-scented. Ovoid female cones, 1cm (1/2in) long, each have 8–10 pairs of smooth scales. ↕ 10–20m (30–70ft), ↔ 3–5m (10–15ft). E. North America. ❄❄❄. **'Caespitosa'** ■ is a very slow-growing, cushion- or bun-shaped shrub; ↕ to 30cm (12in), ↔ to 40cm (16in). **'Filiformis'** is mound-forming, with pendent, whip-like shoots; ↕ to 8m (25ft). **'Golden Globe'** is a dwarf, spherical shrub, with bright golden yellow leaves; ↕↔ 1m (3ft). **'Hetz Midget'** ■ is a slow-growing, spherical, dwarf bush; ↕↔ 80cm (32in). **'Holmstrup'** 🏆 is a dense, conical bush, with vertical sprays of mid-green leaves; ↕ to 4m (12ft). **'Little Champion'** is a spherical shrub, with bright green leaves; ↕↔ 1m (3ft). **'Rheingold'** ■🏆 is a conical bush, with golden yellow leaves, pink-tinted when young; ↕ 1–2m (3–6ft). **'Smaragd'** 🏆 is a dwarf, conical, compact shrub, with bright green leaves; ↕ 1m (3ft), ↔ 80cm (32in). **'Wansdyke Silver'** is dwarf and conical, with variegated, silver-white leaves; ↕ 1.5m (5ft), ↔ 60cm (24in).
T. orientalis ◊–♢ syn. *Biota orientalis, Platycladus orientalis*. Conical or irregularly crowned tree with fibrous, red-brown bark and flat, vertical, irregularly arranged sprays of scale-like, blunt, triangular, unscented, mid-green or yellow-green leaves, which often turn bronze in winter. Upright, flask-shaped, grey-bloomed female cones, 2cm (3/4in) long, have 3 or 4 pairs of scales, each with 2 prominent, dorsal, reflexed hooks. ↕ to 15m (50ft), ↔ to 6m (20ft). China, Iran. ❄❄❄. **'Aurea Nana'** 🏆 is dwarf, with yellow-green leaves, fading to bronze in winter; ↕ to 60cm (24in). **'Elegantissima'** 🏆 is a conical bush, with golden yellow leaves that slowly age to yellow-green and turn bronze over winter; ↕ to 5m (15ft). **'Semperaurea'** ■ is an ovoid bush, with golden yellow new growth; ↕ to 3m (10ft).
T. plicata ■◊–♢ (Western red cedar). Tall, columnar-conical tree, developing billowing lower branches with fissured, red-brown bark and flat, horizontal or hanging sprays of foliage. Scale-like, ovate, mid- to dark green leaves, whitish green beneath, have small dorsal glands. Oblong-ellipsoid female cones, to 1.5cm (1/2in) long, have 4 or 5 pairs of scales, with a small, terminal hook on each scale. ↕ 20–35m (70–120ft), ↔ 6–9m (20–30ft). W. North America. ❄❄❄. All of the following, except 'Zebrina', are shrubs. **'Atrovirens'** 🏆 is good for hedging, and has very dark green leaves. **'Aurea'** 🏆 has golden yellow leaves. **'Hillieri'** is dwarf, with blue-green leaves; ↕↔ 2–3m (6–10ft). **'Stoneham Gold'** ■🏆 is conical, with bright gold new leaves, ageing to dark green; ↕↔ to 2m (6ft). **'Zebrina'** △ is a broadly conical tree, with yellow-striped leaves; ↕ 12–15m (40–50ft), ↔ 4m (12ft).

THUJOPSIS

CUPRESSACEAE

Genus of one species of monoecious, slow-growing, evergreen, coniferous tree, related to *Thuja*, found in forest in Japan. *T. dolabrata* has shredding bark, 4-ranked, scale-like leaves, and a large, prominent, central prickle on each cone scale. A fine specimen tree in woodland.
• **HARDINESS** Fully hardy.
• **CULTIVATION** Grow in moist but well-drained, fertile, humus-rich soil in full sun with shelter from cold, dry winds.
• **PROPAGATION** Sow seed in containers in a cold frame in late winter or early spring. Insert semi-ripe cuttings in late summer.
• **PESTS AND DISEASES** Trouble free.

T. dolabrata 🏆◊–♢ (Hiba). Conical to cylindrical tree with brown bark, shredding in grey strips, and 4-ranked, thick, scale-like, shiny-margined, glossy, dark green leaves, silvery white beneath; spreading side leaves are hatchet- or boat-shaped. Spherical, blue-grey female cones, 1cm (1/2in) across, with leathery scales, ripen to brown; cylindrical male cones are dark violet. ↕ to 20m (70ft), ↔ 6–9m (20–30ft). Japan. ❄❄❄. **'Nana'** is dwarf, with lighter leaves; ↕ 1m (3ft), ↔ 80cm (32in). **'Variegata'** ■ has mid-green foliage with white patches; ↕ 10m (30ft), ↔ 4m (12ft).

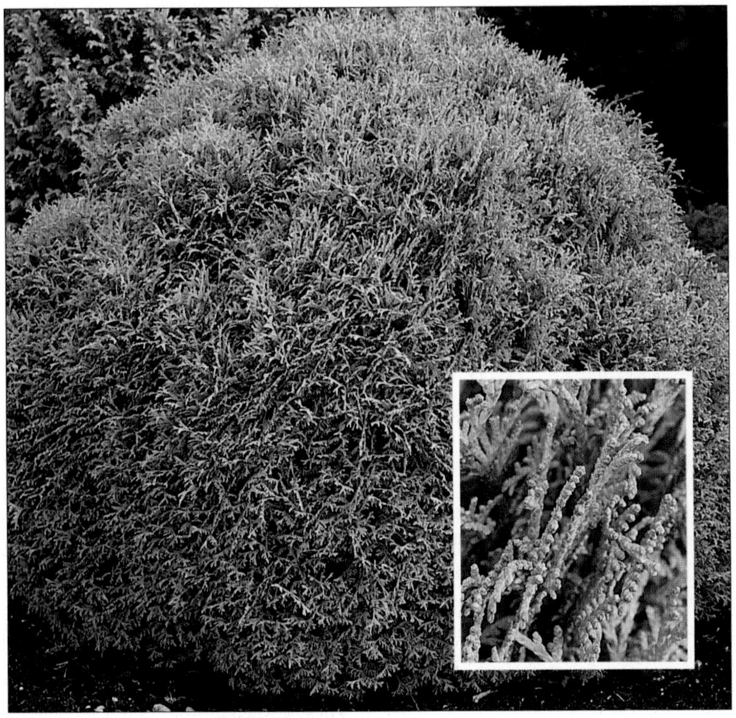

Thuja occidentalis 'Hetz Midget' (inset: leaf detail)

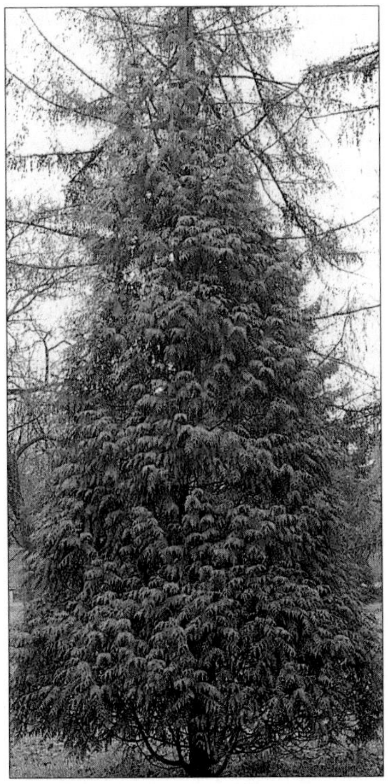

Thuja plicata

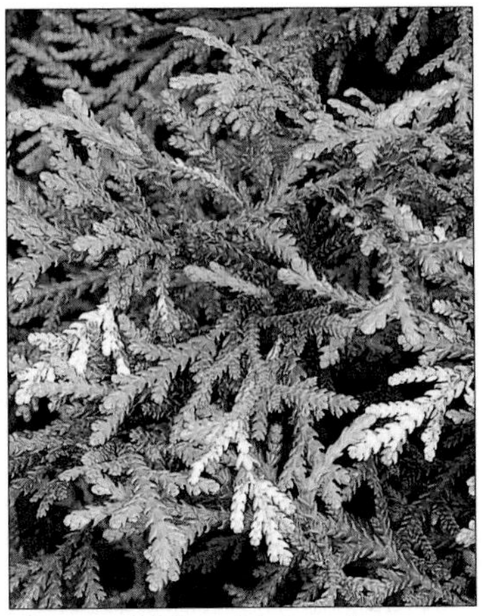

Thujopsis dolabrata 'Variegata'

THUNBERGIA

ACANTHACEAE

Genus of about 100 species of annuals, evergreen perennials, including many twining climbers, and some shrubs, from tropical and southern Africa, Madagascar, and warm to tropical Asia. They occur on forest floors or in rocky areas, or climb through forest trees or shrubs. They are grown for their often showy, salverform to trumpet-shaped, blue, yellow, orange, red, or white flowers, each with 5 usually spreading lobes, borne singly from the leaf axils or in terminal racemes, mainly in summer. The opposite, elliptic or ovate to almost rounded leaves are sometimes lobed or toothed. In frost-prone areas, grow in a temperate or warm greenhouse; *T. alata*, *T. gregorii*, and their cultivars may be grown outdoors as annuals in a sheltered site. In warmer areas, grow shrubs and perennials in a border; the climbers are suitable for training over an arch, pergola, or tree.

- **HARDINESS** Half hardy to frost tender.
- **CULTIVATION** Under glass, grow in loam-based potting compost (JI No.3) in full light with shade from hot sun. Support the climbing stems. In growth, water freely, applying a balanced liquid fertilizer monthly; water sparingly in winter. Outdoors, grow in moist but well-drained, fertile soil in full sun. Tropical climbers require partial shade. Pruning group 11 for climbers, in early spring; group 9 for shrubs. All may need restrictive pruning under glass.
- **PROPAGATION** Sow seed at 16–18°C (61–64°F) in spring. Insert greenwood cuttings in early summer, or semi-ripe cuttings in mid- or late summer, both with bottom heat. Layer in spring.
- **PESTS AND DISEASES** Red spider mites, whiteflies, and scale insects may be a problem under glass.

T. alata ▣ (Black-eyed Susan). Evergreen, perennial, twining climber, often grown as an annual, with ovate-triangular, toothed, mid-green leaves, to 8cm (3in) long, usually with angular basal lobes and narrowly winged stalks. Produces numerous axillary, solitary, salverform flowers, 3–4cm (1¼–1½in) across, usually bright orange or yellow, sometimes creamy white, either with or without chocolate-purple centres from summer to autumn. ↕ to 2.5m (8ft) as a perennial, 1.5–2m (5–8ft) as an annual.

T

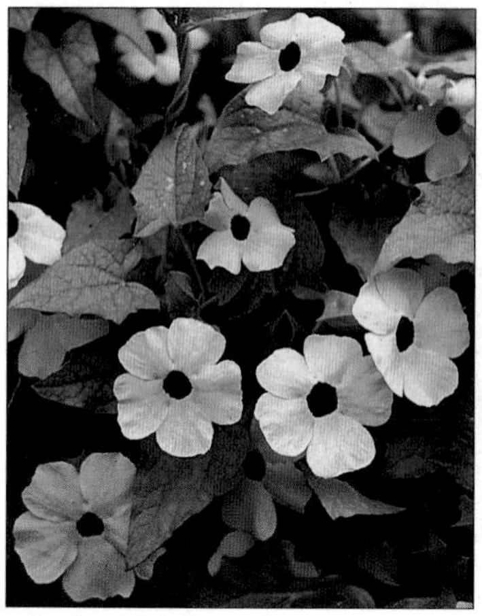

Thunbergia alata

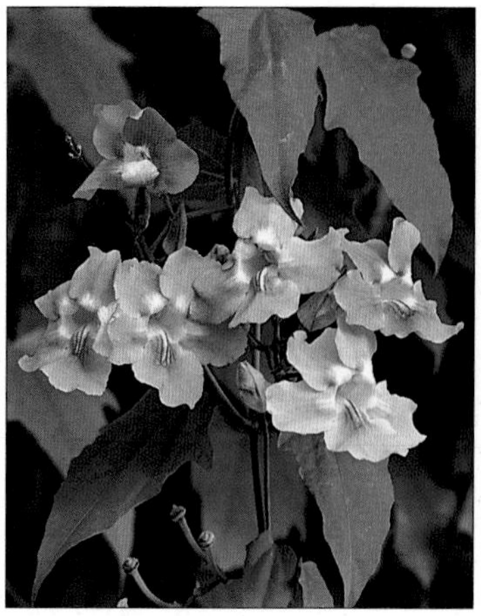

Thunbergia grandiflora

Tropical Africa. ❄ (min. 7–10°C/45–50°F). **Suzie Hybrids** have dark-centred, orange-yellow or white flowers.

T. coccinea. Moderately to sparsely branched, evergreen, perennial, twining climber with narrowly elliptic-ovate, toothed, dark green leaves, to 20cm (8in) long. Tubular, orange-red flowers, 2.5cm (1in) long, with reflexed lobes, are produced in loose, pendent racemes, 15–45cm (6–18in) long, from winter to spring. ↕ 3–8m (10–25ft). India, Burma. ❄ (min. 10–13°C/50–55°F)

T. erecta (Bush clock vine, King's mantle). Often creeping or mat-forming, evergreen perennial or bushy, spreading shrub, with ovate to oblong, semi-lustrous, dark green leaves, 3–8cm (1¼–3in) long, sometimes with a few broad teeth. Solitary, trumpet-shaped, creamy yellow flowers, to 7cm (3in) long, with deep blue-purple lobes, are produced from the leaf axils in summer. ↕↔ to 2m (6ft). Tropical W. Africa to South Africa. ❄ (min. 7°C/45°F)

T. gibsonii see *T. gregorii.*

T. grandiflora ▣ 🏆 (Bengal clock vine, Blue trumpet vine). Vigorous, woody-stemmed, evergreen, perennial, twining climber. Ovate-elliptic to heart-shaped, toothed or lobed, dark green leaves, 10–20cm (4–8in) long, are softly hairy. Trumpet-shaped, lavender-blue to violet-blue, occasionally white flowers, 8cm (3in) long, with yellow throats, are borne singly or in pendent racemes, to 10cm (4in) long, in summer. ↕ 5–10m (15–30ft). N. India. ❄ (min. 10–13°C/50–55°F)

T. gregorii ▣ syn. *T. gibsonii.* Woody-based, evergreen, perennial, twining

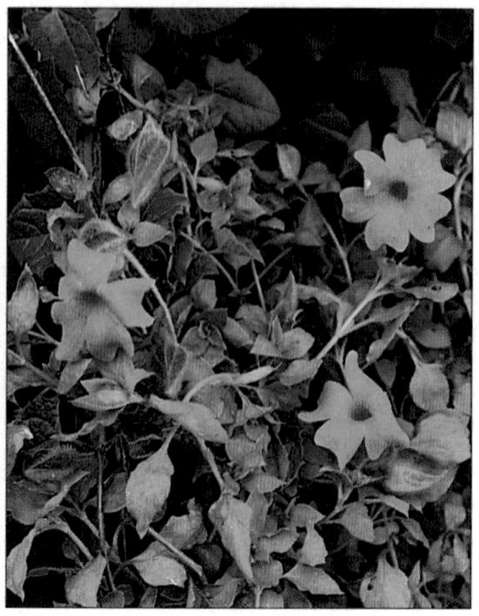

Thunbergia gregorii

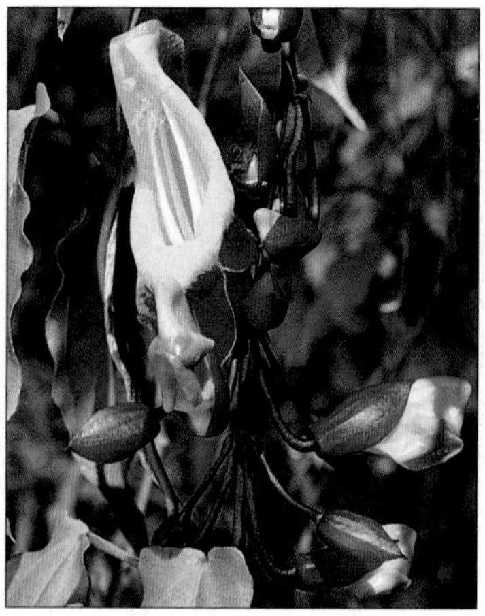

Thunbergia mysorensis

climber, often grown as an annual, with slender, bristly-hairy stems and ovate-triangular, softly hairy, mid-green leaves, to 8cm (3in) long. In summer, bears solitary, salverform, clear orange flowers, 4.5cm (1¾in) across. ↕ to 4m (12ft) or more as a perennial, to 2.2m (7ft) as an annual. Tropical Africa. ❄ (min. 10–13°C/50–55°F)

T. mysorensis ▣ 🏆 Vigorous, woody-stemmed, evergreen, perennial, twining climber with slender, sparsely branched shoots, at least when young. Narrowly elliptic, slender-pointed, toothed, dark green leaves, 10–15cm (4–6in) long, are prominently veined. In spring, hooded, 2-lipped yellow flowers, 5cm (2in) long, with brownish red to purple tubes, and almost erect, arching, tongue-like upper lips, are produced in pendent racemes, to 18cm (7in) long. ↕ to 6m (20ft) or more. India (Nilgiri Hills). ❄ (min. 13–15°C/55–59°F)

▷ **Thyme** see *Thymus*
Basil see *Acinos arvensis*
Caraway see *Thymus herba-barona*
Curly water see *Lagarosiphon*
Garden see *Thymus vulgaris*
Lemon-scented see *Thymus x citriodorus*
Mother of see *Acinos arvensis*

THYMOPHYLLA

ASTERACEAE/COMPOSITAE

Genus of 10–12 species of erect to spreading, bushy, strongly aromatic annuals, biennials, perennials, and sub-shrubs from dry slopes and prairies in the USA, Mexico, and Central America. Alternate or opposite leaves are entire to pinnatisect. The abundant small, daisy-like, bright yellow or orange flowerheads are borne from spring to summer. Use *T. tenuiloba*, the most commonly grown species, for summer bedding, or grow in a container or hanging basket.

- **HARDINESS** Frost hardy.
- **CULTIVATION** Grow in well-drained, moderately fertile soil in full sun.
- **PROPAGATION** Sow seed at 10–13°C (50–55°F) in mid-spring, and plant out after last frosts. Alternatively, sow seed *in situ* in mid- to late spring.
- **PESTS AND DISEASES** Trouble free.

T. tenuiloba ▣ (Dahlberg daisy, Golden fleece, Shooting star). Branching annual, rarely a short-lived perennial, with almost fern-like, pinnatisect, pungent leaves, 0.8–2.5cm (⅜–1in)

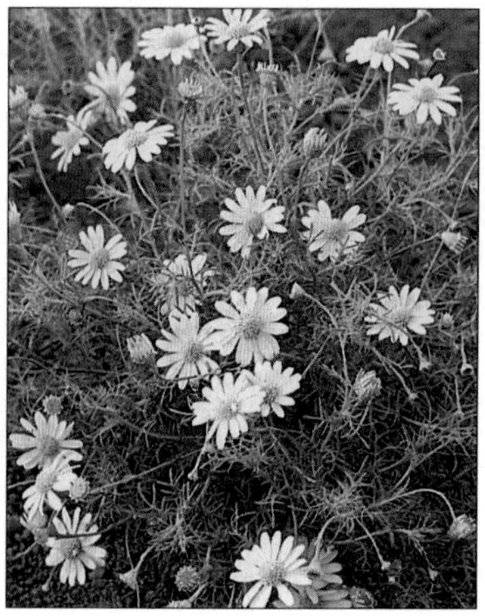

Thymophylla tenuiloba

long, with 7–15 long, linear lobes. From spring to summer, produces upturned, star-shaped, bright yellow flowerheads, to 1.5cm (½in) across. ↕↔ to 30cm (12in). USA (Texas), Mexico. ✲✲

THYMUS

Thyme

LABIATAE/LAMIACEAE

Genus of approximately 350 species of woody-based, aromatic, evergreen perennials, shrubs, and subshrubs, found mainly on calcareous soils and in dry grassland throughout Eurasia. They produce small, opposite, oval to linear leaves. In summer, they produce usually terminal, whorled racemes, heads, or clusters of tubular, 2-lipped, usually pink, purple, or white flowers, mostly 4–8mm (⅛–⅜in) long, often with conspicuous bracts. Some thymes, such as *T. x citriodorus*, *T. herba-barona*, and *T. vulgaris*, have culinary uses, and are usually grown in herb gardens. Most are ideal low shrubs or mat-forming plants for a sunny border or rock garden. The prostrate species, such as *T. polytrichus* or *T. serpyllum*, are suitable for planting in paving crevices, where they release their fragrance when trodden on. Some, such as *T. cilicicus*, need protection from winter wet and are best grown in an alpine house. All are attractive to bees. Many cultivars described here under *T. serpyllum* are probably of hybrid origin, and their status is botanically uncertain.

- **HARDINESS** Fully hardy to frost hardy.
- **CULTIVATION** Grow in well-drained, neutral to alkaline soil in full sun. After flowering, cut vigorous thymes back hard to retain compactness. In an alpine house, use a mix of equal parts loam, leaf mould, and grit. Pruning group 10, in spring, for upright, shrubby species.
- **PROPAGATION** Sow seed in containers in a cold frame in spring. Divide in spring. Insert semi-ripe cuttings in mid- or late summer, or softwood cuttings in early summer. Separate rooted stem sections in spring or summer, and pot on until re-established.
- **PESTS AND DISEASES** Trouble free.

T. azoricus see *T. caespititius.*

T. caespititius, syn. *T. azoricus*, *T. micans.* Dense, mat- or mound-forming subshrub with branching, woody stems and hairy, narrowly spoon-shaped, dark green leaves, to 1cm (½in) long. In late spring and early summer, bears whorled heads of pale rose-pink, lilac, or white flowers, pressed against the foliage. ↕ to 5cm (2in), ↔ to 30cm (12in). Spain, Portugal. ✻✻✻

T. cilicicus ▣ Compact, cushion- to tussock-forming subshrub with upright, minutely hairy shoots bearing stalkless, linear, prominently veined, dark green leaves, to 1cm (½in) long, finely hairy beneath and at the margins. In early summer, bears lilac or mauve flowers in dense, hemispherical heads. ↕ to 15cm (6in), ↔ to 20cm (8in). Turkey. ✻✻

T. x citriodorus (*T. pulegioides* x *T. vulgaris*) (Lemon-scented thyme). Bushy, rounded shrub with branching stems and narrow, oval-diamond-shaped to lance-shaped, more or less hairless, mid-green leaves, to 1cm (½in) long. In summer, pale lavender-pink flowers, with leaf-like bracts, are borne in irregular, oblong heads. ↕ to 30cm (12in), ↔ to 25cm (10in). Garden origin. ✻✻✻. **'Anderson's Gold'** see 'Bertram Anderson'. **'Archer's Gold'** has mid-green leaves with narrow, golden yellow margins. **'Aureus'** ▣🏆 has gold-dappled leaves. **'Bertram Anderson'** ▣🏆 syn. 'Anderson's Gold', has grey-green leaves, strongly suffused yellow. **'Golden King'** is upright, with gold-margined leaves; ↕ 25cm (10in), ↔ to 45cm (18in). **'Silver Queen'** 🏆 has cream-variegated leaves.

T. doerfleri. Compact, spreading subshrub with prostrate, hairy stems and linear, fragrant, mid- to dark green, hairy leaves, 0.8–1.5cm (⅜–½in) long. Purplish pink flowers are produced in whorled racemes in summer. ↕ 15cm (6in), ↔ 45cm (18in). Albania. ✻✻✻. **'Bressingham'** ▣ is prostrate and mat-forming, with grey-green leaves and clear pink flowers; ↕ 10cm (4in), ↔ 35cm (14in).

T. 'Doone Valley' ▣ Mat-forming subshrub with lance-shaped, dark olive-green leaves, to 1cm (½in) long, with yellow spots. Lavender-pink flowers, opening from crimson-red buds, are borne in rounded heads in summer. ↕ 12cm (5in), ↔ 35cm (14in). ✻✻✻

T. herba-barona (Caraway thyme). Dwarf, loosely mat-forming, wiry-branched subshrub bearing ovate to lance-shaped, caraway-scented, dark green leaves, to 7mm (¼in) long. Pale pink flowers are produced in loose, irregular, oblong to hemispherical heads

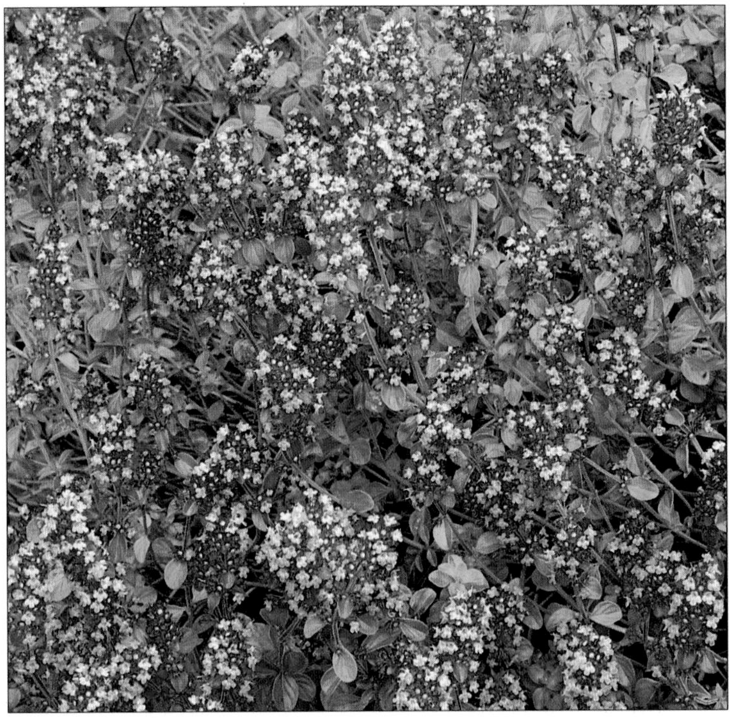

Thymus pulegioides

in midsummer. ↕ to 10cm (4in), ↔ to 20cm (8in). Corsica, Sardinia. ✻✻✻

T. leucotrichus ▣ Dwarf, creeping subshrub with narrowly lance-shaped, hairy, grey-green leaves, 4–9mm (⅛–⅜in) long. Whorled clusters of pale purplish pink flowers are produced in late spring. ↕ to 15cm (6in), ↔ to 20cm (8in). Greece, Turkey. ✻✻✻

T. longiflorus ▣ Densely branched subshrub with ascending, hairy shoots bearing hairy, narrowly elliptic to linear, greyish green leaves, to 1cm (½in) long, with the margins rolled under. Pink flowers with ovate, leathery, greenish purple bracts are borne in spike-like whorls in summer. ↕ to 30cm (12in), ↔ to 25cm (10in). S. Spain. ✻✻

T. mastichina. Vigorous, erect subshrub with upright, hairy shoots and ovate to elliptic-lance-shaped, often shallowly scalloped, mid-green leaves, 1.5cm (½in) long. In summer, bears spherical heads of abundant white flowers. ↕ to 30cm (12in), ↔ to 40cm (16in). Spain, Portugal. ✻✻✻

T. membranaceus. Spreading, rounded shrub with ascending shoots and linear, grey-green leaves, to 1.5cm (½in) long. In summer, bears ovoid heads of long-tubed white flowers, to 1cm (½in) long, with conspicuous, greenish white bracts. Grow in an alpine house or a warm garden. ↕↔ to 20cm (8in). S. Spain. ✻✻

T. micans see *T. caespititius.*

T. polytrichus, syn. *T. praecox.* Creeping, mat-forming subshrub with woody, prostrate, branching stems and narrowly obovate, dark green leaves, 8mm (⅜in) long, fringed with minute hairs. Pale to deep purple, occasionally off-white flowers are borne in terminal heads in summer. ↕ to 5cm (2in), ↔ to 60cm (24in) or more. S. Europe. ✻✻✻. **subsp. *britannicus* var. *albus*,** syn. *T. praecox* subsp. *arcticus* var. *albus*, has softly hairy stems, obovate leaves, and white flowers.

T. praecox see *T. polytrichus.*

T. praecox* subsp. *arcticus* var. *albus see *T. polytrichus* subsp. *britannicus* var. *albus.*

***T. praecox* 'Coccineus'** see *T. serpyllum* var. *coccineus.*

T. pulegioides ▣ Spreading subshrub with semi-erect, 4-angled stems and oblong-lance-shaped, strongly aromatic, mid-green leaves, 0.6–2cm (¼–¾in) long. In late spring and early summer, bears short, irregular, whorled racemes of pink to purple flowers. ↕ 5–25cm (2–10in), ↔ 30cm (12in). Europe. ✻✻✻

T. richardii. Spreading to loosely mat-forming subshrub with ovate, aromatic, mid-green leaves, 0.9–1.5cm (⅜–½in) long. Whorled racemes of purple flowers are produced in late spring. ↕ 12cm (5in), ↔ 30cm (12in). Spain (Balearic Islands), Italy (Sicily), Croatia. ✻✻✻. **subsp. *nitidus*** has narrowly ovate leaves, to 1cm (½in) long; Italy (Sicily). **subsp. *nitidus* 'Peter Davis'** ▣ is bushy, with grey-green leaves, to 8mm (⅜in) long, and numerous pink flowers; ↕ 15cm (6in), ↔ 5cm (2in).

T. serpyllum. Mat-forming subshrub with finely hairy, trailing stems and linear to elliptic or elliptic-ovate, mid-green leaves, 4–8mm (⅛–⅜in) long. Purple flowers are borne in congested whorls in summer. ↕ 25cm (10in), ↔ 45cm (18in). Europe. ✻✻✻. **'Annie Hall'** ▣ has pale purple-pink flowers. **var. *coccineus*** ▣🏆 syn. *T. praecox* 'Coccineus', has crimson-pink flowers. **'Elfin'** ▣ forms dense mounds of foliage, and seldom flowers freely; ↕ to 8cm (3in), ↔ to 10cm (4in). **'Minimus'** is compact, producing lance-shaped leaves, to 4mm (⅛in) long, and pink flowers; ↕ 5cm (2in), ↔ 10cm (4in). **'Minor'** is compact, with lance-shaped leaves, to 5mm (¼in) long, and pink flowers; ↕ 12cm (5in). **'Pink Chintz'** 🏆 has grey-green leaves and flesh-pink flowers. **'Snowdrift'** bears clear white flowers.

T. vulgaris (Garden thyme). Bushy, cushion-forming, spreading subshrub with linear to elliptic, finely hairy, aromatic, grey-green leaves, 0.6–1.5cm (¼–½in) long. In late spring and early summer, bright purple to white flowers are produced in whorled racemes. ↕ 15–30cm (6–12in), ↔ 40cm (16in). W. Mediterranean to S. Italy. ✻✻✻. **'Aureus'** has leaves suffused yellow. **'Silver Posie'** ▣ has white-margined leaves.

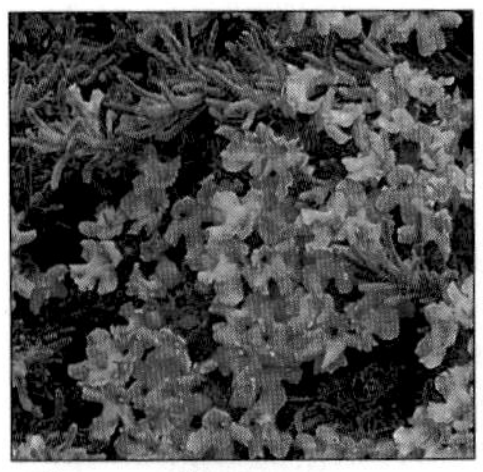

Thymus cilicicus

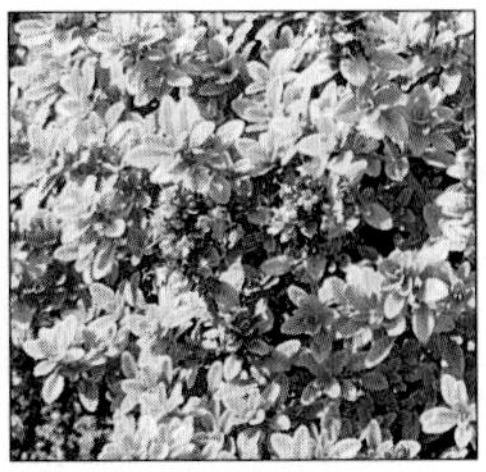

Thymus x *citriodorus* 'Aureus'

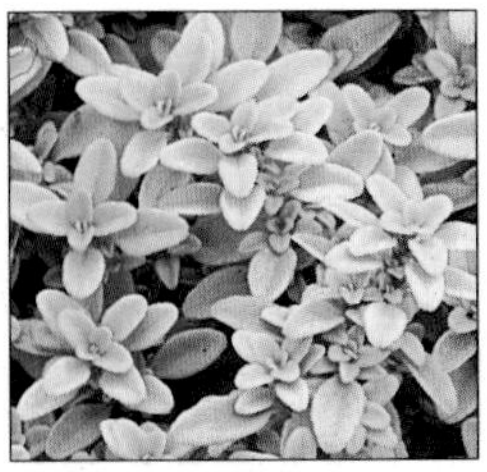

Thymus x *citriodorus* 'Bertram Anderson'

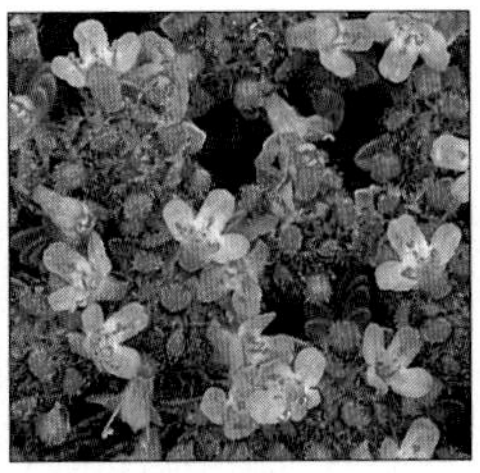

Thymus doerfleri 'Bressingham'

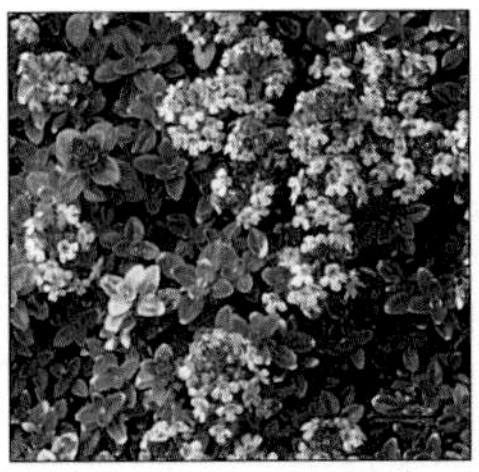

Thymus 'Doone Valley'

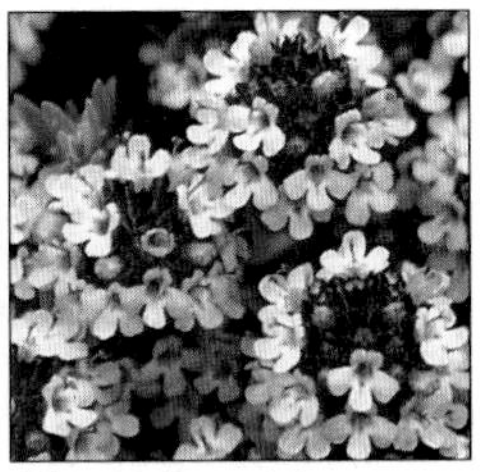

Thymus leucotrichus

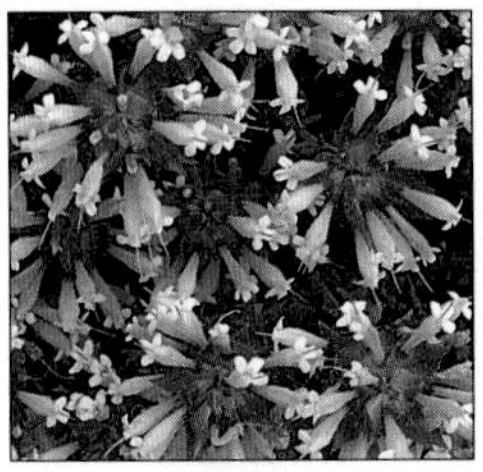

Thymus longiflorus

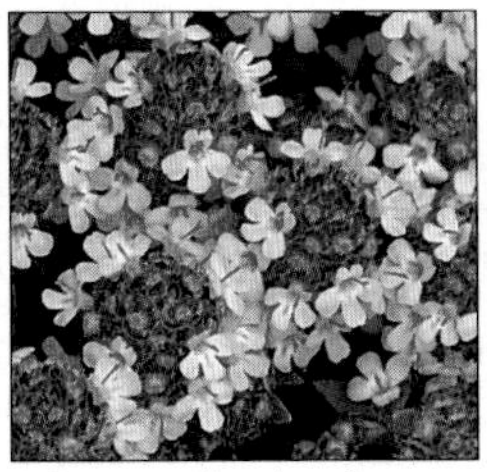

Thymus richardii subsp. *nitidus* 'Peter Davis'

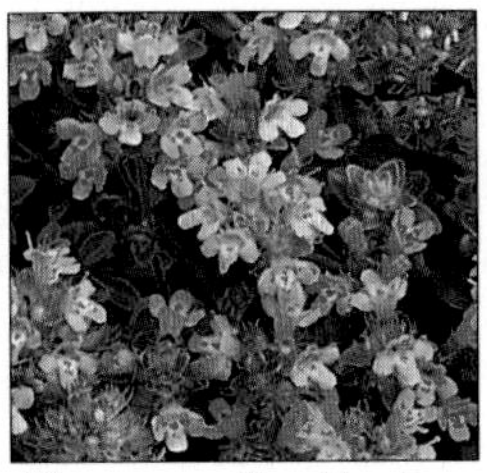

Thymus serpyllum 'Annie Hall'

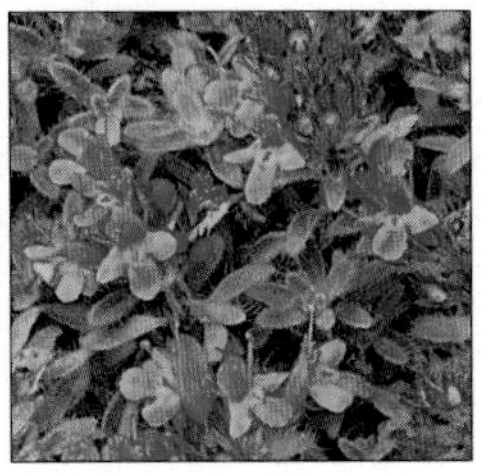

Thymus serpyllum var. *coccineus*

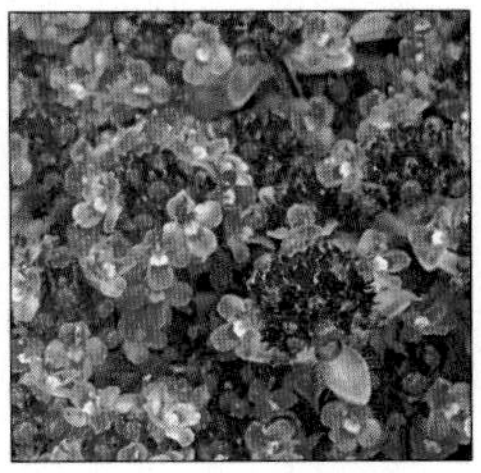

Thymus serpyllum 'Elfin'

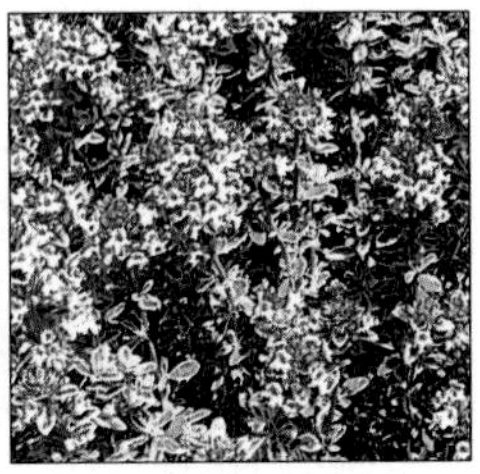

Thymus vulgaris 'Silver Posie'

T

TIARELLA

Foam flower

SAXIFRAGACEAE

Genus of about 7 species of rhizomatous herbaceous perennials from woodland and streambanks in E. Asia and North America. The mainly basal, ovate to heart-shaped or rounded, toothed, sometimes long-stalked leaves are simple or palmately 3- to 5-lobed, occasionally 7-lobed, or 3-palmate; they are pale to mid-green, often turning shades of reddish copper in autumn and winter, and have conspicuous veins and sparse, bristly hairs. The tiny, star-shaped, fluffy, white or pinkish white flowers, 5–10mm (¼–½in) across, are borne in terminal panicles or racemes over a long period from spring to summer. Grow as ground cover in a woodland garden or shady border; *T. cordifolia* spreads freely.

• **HARDINESS** Fully hardy.

• **CULTIVATION** Grow ideally in cool, moist, humus-rich soil, although they tolerate a wide range of soil conditions. Provide deep or partial shade. Protect from excessive winter wet.

• **PROPAGATION** Sow seed in containers in a cold frame in spring or as soon as ripe. Divide in spring.

• **PESTS AND DISEASES** Leaves may be damaged by slugs.

T. cordifolia ■ 🏆 (Foam flower). Vigorous, rhizomatous perennial, spreading by stolons, with hairy, 3- to 5-lobed, ovate, pale green leaves, to 10cm (4in) long, heart-shaped at the bases, tinted bronze-red in autumn. Creamy white flowers are borne in a profusion of upright, spike-like racemes, 10–30cm (4–12in) long, in summer. ↕ 10–30cm (4–12in), ↔ to 30cm (12in) or more. North America. ✻✻✻. **var. *collina*** see *T. wherryi*.

***T.* 'Maple Leaf'.** Clump-forming, herbaceous or semi-evergreen perennial, without stolons, producing rosettes of broadly ovate, 5-lobed, mid-green, red-flushed leaves, 5–12cm (2–5in) long. From late spring to midsummer, bears white, pink-flushed flowers in racemes, 15–30cm (6–12in) long. ↕↔ to 30cm (12in). ✻✻✻

T. trifoliata ■ Clump-forming, rhizomatous perennial, without stolons, producing 3-palmate basal leaves, to 8cm (3in) long, with 3-lobed, hairy, mid-green leaflets, veined dark green; the 2 or 3 stem leaves have short stalks.

T

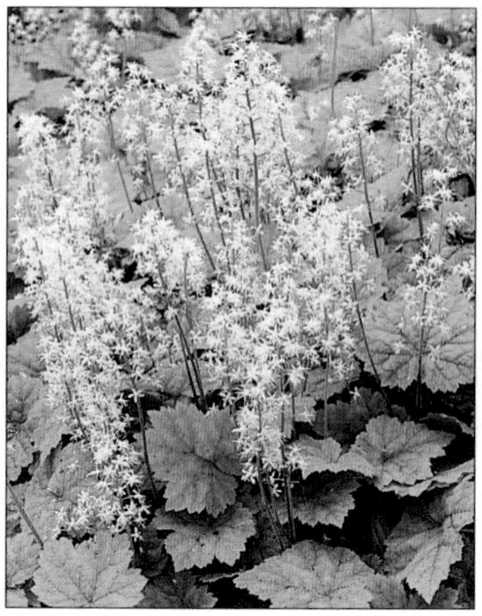

Tiarella cordifolia

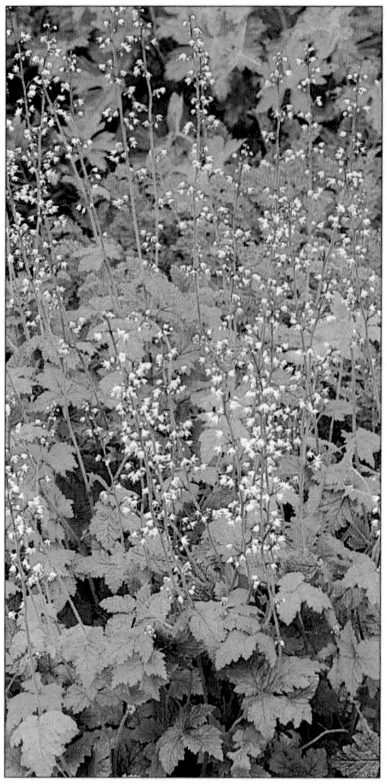

Tiarella trifoliata

Pendent white flowers are produced in loose panicles, 15–50cm (6–20in) long, opening from pinkish white buds from late spring to midsummer. ↕ to 50cm (20in), ↔ 30cm (12in). North America (Alaska to Oregon). ✻✻✻

T. wherryi 🏆 syn. *T. cordifolia* var. *collina*. Compact, slow-growing, clump-forming perennial, without stolons, producing hairy, ovate, sharply 3-lobed, maroon-tinted, pale green leaves, to 14cm (5½in) long, heart-shaped at the bases. White, sometimes pink-tinged flowers are borne in brown-stemmed, slender, spike-like racemes, 15–35cm (6–14in) long, in late spring and early summer. Prefers moist shade. ↕ to 20cm (8in), ↔ to 15cm (6in). USA (Appalachians). ✻✻✻. **'Bronze Beauty'** has dark red-bronze foliage and light pinkish white flowers.

TIBOUCHINA

MELASTOMATACEAE

Genus of about 350 species of evergreen shrubs and subshrubs or herbaceous perennials, some of them climbing, found in rainforest in Mexico, the West Indies, and from tropical South America to N. Argentina (mainly Brazil). Large, elliptic, ovate, or lance-shaped, leathery leaves, usually with 1–3 pairs of prominent, primary veins, are borne in opposite pairs. Saucer- to cup-shaped, mostly 5-petalled flowers are produced singly, in threes, or in long panicles. Where temperatures fall below 7°C (45°F), grow in a cool or temperate greenhouse. In warmer areas, grow in a shrub border.

• **HARDINESS** Frost tender.

• **CULTIVATION** Under glass, grow in loam-based potting compost (JI No.3) in full light with shade from hot sun. During growth, water freely and apply a balanced liquid fertilizer monthly; water sparingly in winter. Outdoors, grow in moist, fertile soil in full sun. Pruning group 9; plants grown under glass need restrictive pruning in late winter.

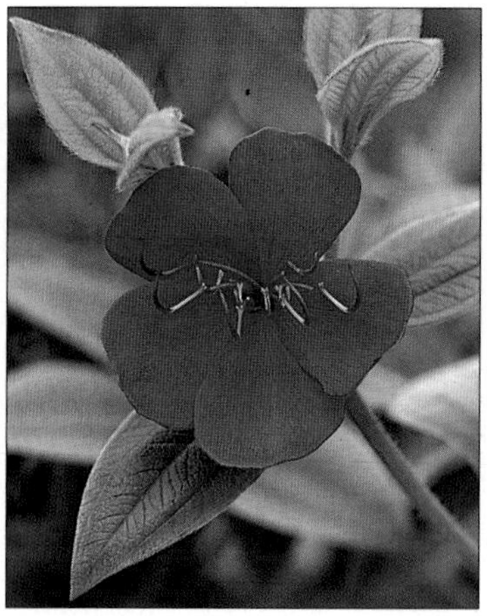

Tibouchina urvilleana

• **PROPAGATION** Sow seed at 16°C (61°F) in spring. Root softwood cuttings in late spring or semi-ripe cuttings in summer, both with bottom heat.

• **PESTS AND DISEASES** Prone to oedema, red spider mites, and aphids under glass.

T. organensis, syn. *T. semidecandra* subsp. *floribunda* of gardens (Glory bush). Open, erect shrub with 4-angled, hairy stems and ovate-oblong, velvety-hairy, greyish green leaves, to 15cm (6in) long, sometimes maturing to bright scarlet. From summer to autumn, produces open, leafy panicles of satin-textured, saucer-shaped, bluish purple flowers, 10cm (4in) or more across. ↕ 3–6m (10–20ft), ↔ 2–3m (6–10ft). S.E. Brazil. ✿ (min. 5–7°C/41–45°F)

***T. semidecandra* of gardens** see *T. urvilleana*.

***T. semidecandra* subsp. *floribunda* of gardens** see *T. organensis*.

T. urvilleana ■ 🏆 syn. *Pleroma macrantha*, *T. semidecandra* of gardens (Brazilian spider flower, Glory bush). Erect to spreading shrub with 4-angled, red-hairy stems and oblong-ovate to ovate or elliptic, velvety-hairy, mid- to dark green leaves, 5–7cm (2–3in) long. From summer to autumn, bears leafy panicles of satin-textured, saucer-shaped, reddish purple flowers, 7–10cm (3–4in) across, with dark, hooked stamens. ↕ 3–6m (10–20ft), ↔ 2–3m (6–10ft). Brazil. ✿ (min. 3–5°C/39–41°F)

▷**Tickseed** see *Coreopsis*
▷**Tidy tips** see *Layia platyglossa*
▷**Tiger flower** see *Tigridia*, *T. pavonia*
▷**Tiger jaws** see *Faucaria*

TIGRIDIA

Peacock flower, Tiger flower

IRIDACEAE

Genus of 23 species of bulbous perennials from seasonally dry sands and grassland, occasionally among rocks, in Mexico and Guatemala. They have mostly basal, narrowly lance-shaped to sword-shaped leaves. The attractive, short-lived, brightly coloured summer flowers, either upright and iris-like or pendent and bell-shaped, have 3 large, spreading outer segments and 3 shorter inner ones. In frost-free climates, grow in a border; in frost-prone areas, grow outdoors and lift in autumn, or grow permanently as container plants in a cool greenhouse or conservatory.

• **HARDINESS** Frost tender.

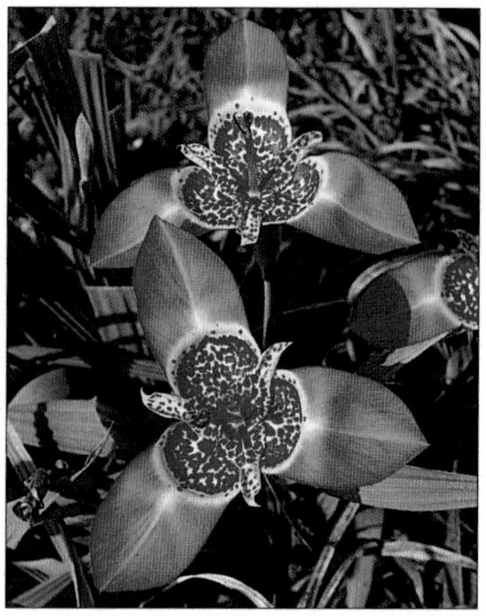

Tigridia pavonia

• **CULTIVATION** Plant 10cm (4in) deep. Outdoors, grow in well-drained, preferably sandy, fertile soil in full sun. In cold areas, lift bulbs after flowering and overwinter in dry sand at about 10°C (50°F). Under glass, grow in loam-based potting compost (JI No.2), with added sharp sand. Water freely when in growth and keep dry when dormant; repot annually in spring.

• **PROPAGATION** Sow seed at 13–18°C (55–64°F) in spring. Separate offsets when dormant (taking care to avoid plants affected by viruses).

• **PESTS AND DISEASES** Prone to viruses.

T. meleagris. Bulbous perennial with branched stems bearing 1 or 2 lance-shaped leaves, 20–30cm (8–12in) long; basal leaves are only rarely produced. In summer, bears 2–6 pendent, widely bell-shaped, pale pink to maroon flowers, 3cm (1¼in) across, with darker spots. ↕ 25–60cm (10–24in), ↔ 10cm (4in). Mexico. ✿ (min. 8–12°C/46–54°F)

T. pavonia ■ (Peacock flower, Tiger flower). Bulbous perennial with lance-shaped leaves, 20–50cm (8–20in) long, borne in a basal fan. In summer, bears occasionally branched stems, each with 1–3 stem leaves and a succession of iris-like, orange to pink, red, yellow, or white flowers, 10–15cm (4–6in) across, mostly with contrasting central marks. ↕ 1.5m (5ft), ↔ 10cm (4in). Mexico. ✿ (min. 8–12°C/46–54°F)

TILIA

Lime, Linden

TILIACEAE

Genus of 20–45 species of deciduous trees occurring in woodland in Europe, Asia, and North America. They are cultivated for their stately habit, their foliage and flowers, and, in some cases, for their colourful winter shoots. The ovate to rounded leaves, arranged alternately on slender stalks, are toothed or lobed, with tapered to pointed tips and heart-shaped bases. On old trees, the smooth, silver-grey bark becomes fissured. Small, cup-shaped, fragrant, creamy white to yellow flowers are borne in slender, axillary cymes with long stalks; the stalks are fused with the upper surfaces of large, narrowly elliptic or inversely lance-shaped, membranous bracts, usually pale yellow or green, to 15cm (6in) long. The flowers are followed by dry, nut-like fruits. Grow as free-standing specimens or avenue trees.

TILIA

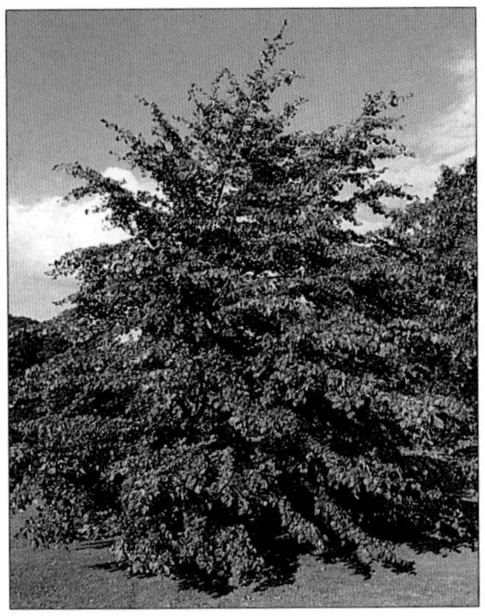

Tilia cordata 'Rancho'

The flowers attract bees, although the nectar of *T. tomentosa* and *T.* 'Petiolaris' may be toxic, especially to bumblebees.

- **HARDINESS** Fully hardy.
- **CULTIVATION** Grow in moist but well-drained soil in full sun or partial shade. Avoid very dry conditions and exposure to strong winds. Limes prefer alkaline or neutral soil, but they tolerate acid soil. *T.* x *europaea* often produces dense thickets of shoots from the base and from burrs on the trunk; remove these every few years by cutting back to the trunk in early spring. Pruning group 1.
- **PROPAGATION** Stratify seed for 3–5 months and sow in containers in a cold frame in spring, or sow as soon as ripe in a seed bed in autumn; garden-collected seed may yield hybrids of variable quality. Bud in late summer on to seedling understock of *T. platyphyllos* or *T. tomentosa*. Remove suckers in winter.
- **PESTS AND DISEASES** Susceptible to honey fungus, *Phytophthora* root rot, gall mites on the leaves, scale insects on the bark, and aphids that produce sticky honeydew.

T. americana (American lime, Basswood). Broadly columnar tree with broadly ovate to rounded, dark green leaves, matt above, glossy beneath, to 20cm (8in) long. Pendent cymes of 10–15 yellow flowers, 1.5cm (½in) across, are produced in midsummer. ↕25m (80ft), ↔15m (50ft). C. and E. North America. ❄❄❄. **'Fastigiata'** is conical, with upright branches; ↔8m (25ft). **'Redmond'** syn. *T.* x *euchlora* 'Redmond', is dense and broadly conical; ↕14m (46ft), ↔7m (22ft).

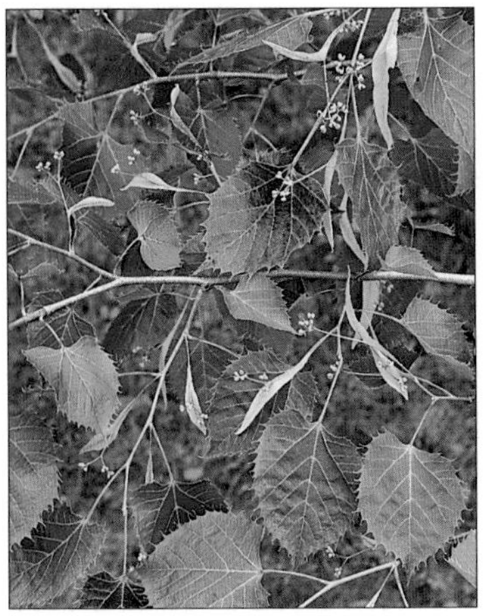

Tilia henryana

T. caroliniana (Carolina basswood). Dense, rounded tree with ovate, dark green leaves, to 9cm (3½in) long, paler and hairy beneath. In early summer, bears pale yellow flowers, 1.5cm (½in) across, in pendent cymes of 10–15. ↕10–12m (30–40ft), ↔8m (25ft). S.E. USA. ❄❄❄

T. cordata (Small-leaved lime). Broadly columnar tree with rounded, dark green leaves, to 8cm (3in) long, blue-green and smooth beneath except for tufts of brown hairs in the leaf axils; leaves turn yellow in autumn. Produces cymes of up to 10 pale yellow flowers, 2cm (¾in) across, in midsummer. ↕25m (90ft), ↔15m (50ft). Europe, Caucasus. ❄❄❄. **'Greenspire'** is vigorous and conical; ↕15m (50ft), ↔7m (22ft). **'Rancho'** is open in habit when young, becoming narrowly conical, with glossy leaves; ↕15m (50ft), ↔8m (25ft).

***T. dasystyla* of gardens** see *T.* x *euchlora.*

T.* x *euchlora syn. *T. dasystyla* of gardens. Rounded tree with branches that become slightly pendent with age. The rounded to broadly ovate, toothed leaves, 5–10cm (2–4in) long, are heart-shaped at the bases, glossy, dark green above and pale green with tufts of hairs in the axils of the veins beneath. Cymes of 3–7 yellowish white flowers, 1.5cm (½in) across, are borne in midsummer. Remains free of aphids, and therefore also of sticky honeydew. ↕20m (70ft), ↔15m (50ft). Garden origin. ❄❄❄.

'Redmond' see *T. americana* 'Redmond'.

T.* x *europaea (*T. cordata* x *T. platyphyllos*) syn. *T. intermedia*, *T.* x *vulgaris* (Common lime). Broadly columnar tree with broadly ovate to rounded, dark green leaves, to 10cm (4in) long, paler beneath. Cymes of up to 10 pale yellow flowers, 2cm (¾in) across, are borne in midsummer. ↕35m (120ft), ↔15m (50ft). Europe. ❄❄❄. **'Wratislaviensis'** has bright yellow young leaves, turning yellowish green; ↕20m (70ft), ↔12m (40ft).

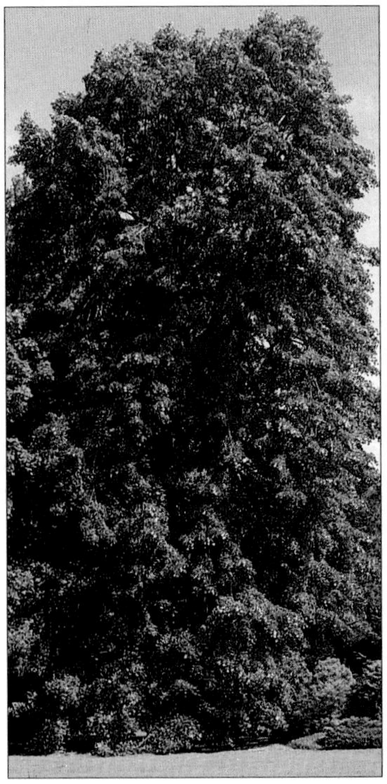

Tilia 'Petiolaris'

T. henryana Spreading tree with broadly ovate, glossy, bright green leaves, to 12cm (5in) long, brown-hairy and paler beneath, red-tinged when young, and with long, bristle-like teeth. In late summer and early autumn, bears cymes of up to 25 small, creamy white flowers, 1.5cm (½in) across. ↕↔ to 25m (80ft). C. China. ❄❄❄

T. intermedia see *T.* x *europaea.*

T. japonica (Japanese lime). Broadly columnar tree with rounded, dark green leaves, to 8cm (3in) long, blue-green beneath. Pendent cymes of 4–10 pale yellow flowers, 1.5cm (½in) across, are produced in midsummer. ↕20m (70ft), ↔6m (20ft). E. China, Japan. ❄❄❄

T. mongolica (Mongolian lime). Rounded tree or shrub with glossy, dark green leaves, to 4cm (1½in) long, blue-green beneath, and red when young; they are rounded to triangular, and deeply cut into 3 sharply toothed lobes, often with 2 lateral lobes. Pale yellow flowers, 2cm (¾in) across, are produced in pendent cymes of up to 30 in early summer. ↕18m (60ft), ↔12m (40ft). Mongolia, N. China. ❄❄❄

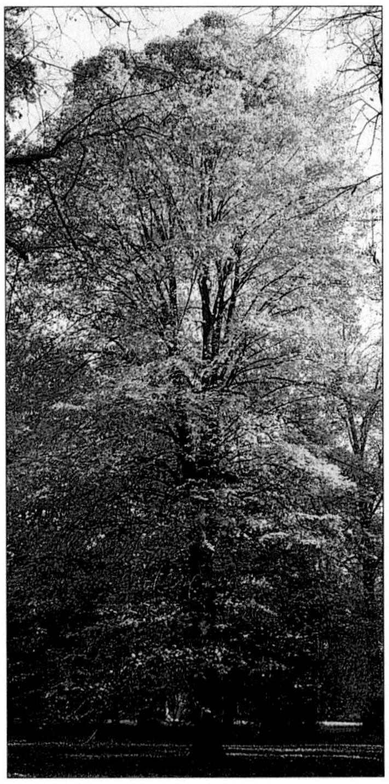

Tilia platyphyllos

T. oliveri Spreading tree with broadly ovate, dark green leaves, to 12cm (5in) long, tapering to sharp points at the tips, densely white-hairy beneath. Pendent cymes of 6–10 pale yellow flowers, 1cm (½in) across, are produced in midsummer. ↕15m (50ft), ↔10m (30ft). C. China. ❄❄❄

T. petiolaris see *T.* 'Petiolaris'.

***T.* 'Petiolaris'** syn. *T. petiolaris*, *T. tomentosa* 'Petiolaris' (Pendulous silver lime). Broadly columnar tree with weeping branches, pendent shoots, and long-stalked, rounded, dark green leaves, to 8cm (3in) long, densely white-hairy beneath. Produces pendent cymes of up to 10 fragrant, pale yellow flowers, to 1.5cm (½in) across, in late summer. ↕30m (100ft), ↔20m (70ft). ❄❄❄

T. platyphyllos (Large-leaved lime). Broadly columnar tree with rounded to broadly ovate, dark green leaves, 8–15cm (3–6in) long, paler and usually densely hairy beneath, turning yellow in autumn. Produces pendent cymes of 3–5 pale yellow flowers, 2cm (¾in) across, in midsummer. ↕30m (100ft), ↔20m (70ft). Europe. ❄❄❄. **'Princes Street'** is upright, with bright red winter shoots. **'Rubra'** (Red-twigged lime) has red winter shoots.

T. tomentosa (European white lime, Silver lime). Broadly columnar tree with rounded to broadly ovate, sometimes lobed, dark green leaves, to 10cm (4in) long, densely white-hairy beneath. In summer, bears cymes of up to 10 very fragrant white flowers, to 1.5cm (½in) across. ↕30m (100ft), ↔20m (70ft). S.E. Europe, S.W. Asia. ❄❄❄.

'Petiolaris' see *T.* 'Petiolaris'.

T.* x *vulgaris see *T.* x *europaea.*

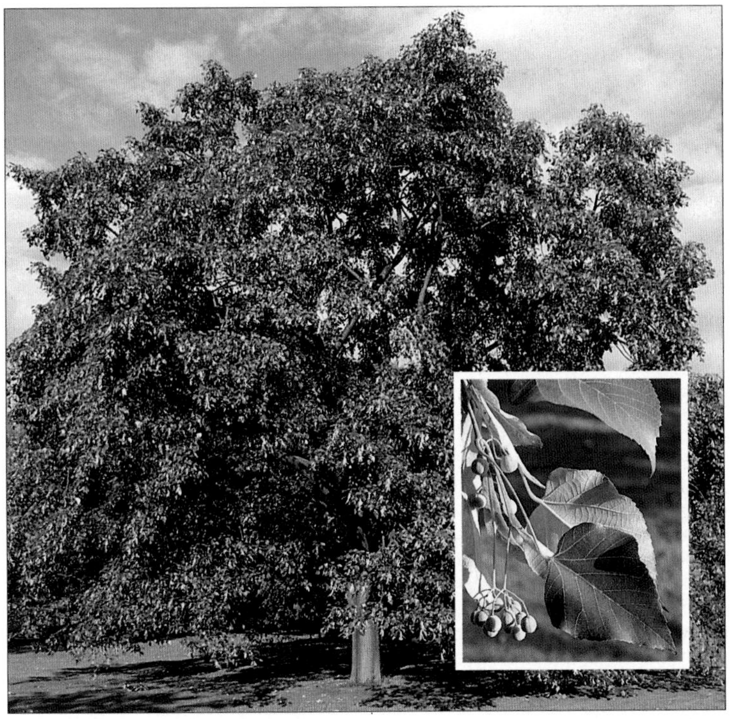

Tilia oliveri (inset: leaf and fruit detail)

T

TILLANDSIA

TILLANDSIA

Air plant

BROMELIACEAE

Genus of over 400 species of epiphytic, terrestrial, or rock-dwelling, evergreen perennials (bromeliads) from scrub and woodland in S. USA, the West Indies, and Central and South America. The entire, often scaly leaves are strap-shaped to narrowly triangular to linear, sometimes tapering to fine threads; they are mainly borne in rosettes, with a few along the slender stems, and sometimes have prominent sheaths. Most species have tubular to funnel-shaped flowers, each with 3 sepals and 3 petals, often with spreading terminal lobes; they are borne among usually colourful floral bracts, generally opening in daytime in spring or autumn. The flowers may be solitary but are usually in 2 or more opposite rows, forming small, dense racemes or spikes, which are sometimes grouped into compound inflorescences; the flowers are borne mainly at the ends of scapes that have sometimes dense or colourful bracts. Where temperatures fall below 7°C (45°F), grow in a temperate greenhouse or conservatory, or as houseplants. In warmer areas, grow the epiphytic species on a tree; the rock-dwelling and terrestrial species may also be grown in a rock garden, on bark or tree branches placed on the ground, or beneath trees or shrubs.

• **HARDINESS** Frost tender.

• **CULTIVATION** Under glass, grow epiphytically in bright indirect light, with moderate to high humidity; rock-dwelling species prefer full light with shade from hot sun, and will tolerate low humidity. From late spring to mid-autumn, mist daily with rainwater and apply a quarter-strength low-nitrogen liquid fertilizer monthly. In winter, mist once or twice a week. Grow terrestrial species, and *T. cyanea* and *T. lindenii*, in containers of terrestrial bromeliad compost, with the bases of the leaves at or just above the surface, in bright filtered light. In growth, water freely and apply a half-strength, low-nitrogen fertilizer monthly; keep just moist in winter. Outdoors, grow epiphytic species in a tree in moist partial shade. Grow terrestrial and rock-dwelling species in coarse, open, leafy soil in partial or dappled shade. See also p.47.

• **PROPAGATION** Sow seed at 27°C (81°F) in spring, on to bundles of conifer twigs and sphagnum moss; mist daily. Detach offsets in spring.

• **PESTS AND DISEASES** Vulnerable to aphids while flowering.

T

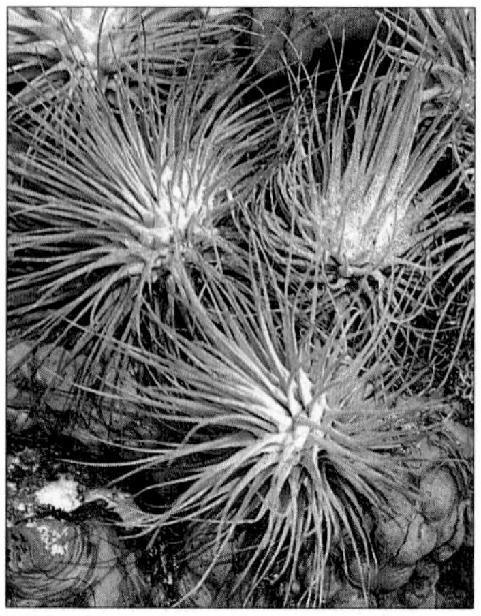

Tillandsia argentea

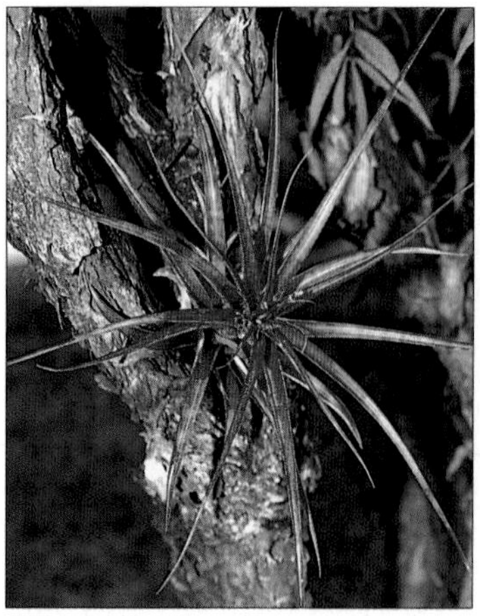

Tillandsia brachycaulos

T. aeranthos, syn. *T. dianthoidea.* Epiphytic, cushion-forming perennial with fine-scaly stems bearing narrowly lance-shaped, often keeled, rigid, densely grey-scaly, mid-green leaves, 10cm (4in) or more long. In spring, bears cylindrical spikes of 5–20 slender, funnel-shaped, dark blue flowers, 2.5cm (1in) long, with bright rose-pink floral bracts. ↕↔ to 30cm (12in). S. Brazil, N.E. Argentina, Paraguay, Uruguay. ❄ (min. 7°C/45°F)

T. argentea ■ Epiphytic perennial with a rhizomatous, curved, short, branched stem bearing dense rosettes of narrowly linear, silvery white-scaly, pale green leaves, 6–9cm (2½–3½in) long. Bears simple spikes of 6–8 tubular, bright red or blue flowers, 3cm (1¼in) long, with salmon-pink floral bracts, in spring. ↕↔ to 25cm (10in). Mexico, Guatemala, Cuba, Jamaica. ❄ (min. 7°C/45°F)

T. bergeri. Rock-dwelling perennial with rosettes of narrowly triangular, grey-scaly, mid-green leaves, 10cm (4in) long. In spring, produces simple spikes of 7–12 funnel-shaped, blue and white flowers, 3cm (1¼in) long, fading to rose-pink, with grey-green floral bracts. ↕ to 18cm (7in), ↔ 15cm (6in). Argentina. ❄ (min. 7°C/45°F)

T. brachycaulos ■ Stemless, epiphytic perennial with rosettes of slender, linear to lance-shaped, arching, densely green-scaly or silver-grey-scaly, dark green leaves, 12–26cm (5–10in) long, with thread-like tips and prominent sheaths, turning bright red when in flower. In spring, bears short spikes of 1 or 2 erect, tubular violet flowers, to 7cm (3in) long, with red floral bracts, clustered into a head. ↕↔ 25cm (10in). S. Mexico, Central America. ❄ (min. 7°C/45°F)

T. caput-medusae ■ Stemless, epiphytic perennial with rosettes of narrowly awl-shaped, tapered, recurved, pale green leaves, 15cm (6in) or more long; the leaf-blades are covered with spreading, coarse, silver-grey hairs, and have ovate sheaths inflated to form hollow pseudobulbs. Suberect or curved spikes of 6–12 slender, tubular blue flowers, 3–4cm (1¼–1½in) long, with red floral bracts, are produced in late spring. ↕ 15–40cm (6–16in), ↔ to 24cm (10in). Mexico, Central America. ❄ (min. 7°C/45°F)

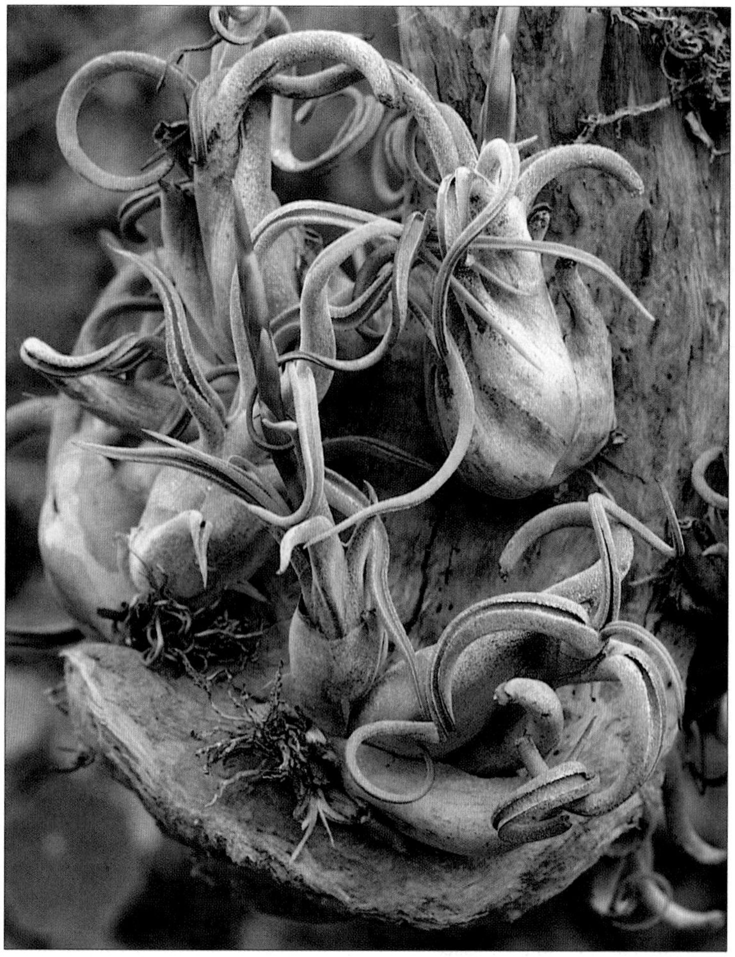

Tillandsia caput-medusae

T. crocata. Short-stemmed, untidy, sometimes branched, epiphytic or rock-dwelling perennial with 2 rows of linear, coarse, grey-hairy, mid-green leaves, 10–15cm (4–6in) long. In spring or autumn, produces simple spikes of 3 or 4 funnel-shaped, bright canary-yellow flowers, 2cm (¾in) long, with green, heavily grey-scaled floral bracts. ↕ to 20cm (8in), ↔ to 15cm (6in). Brazil, Argentina. ❄ (min. 7°C/45°F)

T. cyanea ■ Epiphytic perennial with stemless rosettes of linear-triangular, semi-erect then recurved, dark green leaves, to 35cm (14in) long, red-striped near the bases. Flattened, paddle-shaped, almost stalkless spikes of 20 funnel-shaped, rich violet flowers, to 3cm (1¼in) long, with spreading petals and rose-pink floral bracts, are produced in late spring or autumn. ↕ to 30cm (12in), ↔ to 40cm (16in). Ecuador. ❄ (min. 7°C/45°F)

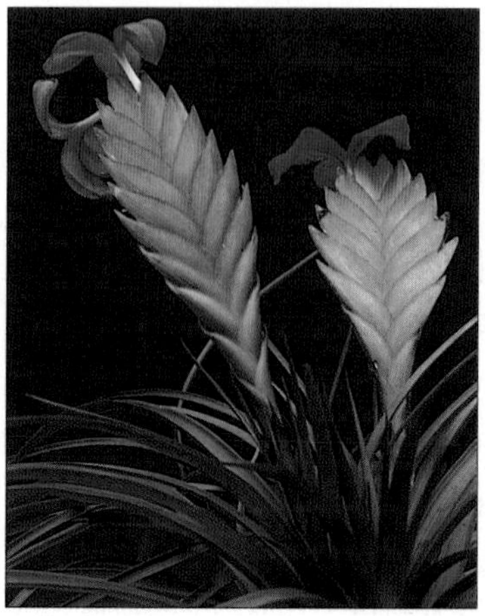

Tillandsia cyanea

T. dianthoidea see *T. aeranthos.*

T. fasciculata ■ Epiphytic perennial with stemless rosettes of narrowly triangular, spreading, sparsely hairy or silver-grey-hairy, brittle, pale grey-green leaves, to 30cm (12in) long, with brown sheaths. In late spring, spikes of red to yellow floral bracts and erect, tubular, white and purple flowers, to 6cm (2½in) long, usually 3 or 4 at a time, are borne in compound inflorescences. ↕↔ 30cm (12in) or more. S. USA, West Indies, Mexico to Colombia and Peru. ❄ (min. 7°C/45°F)

T. gardneri. Epiphytic or rock-dwelling perennial bearing dense rosettes of narrowly triangular, densely scaly, silver-

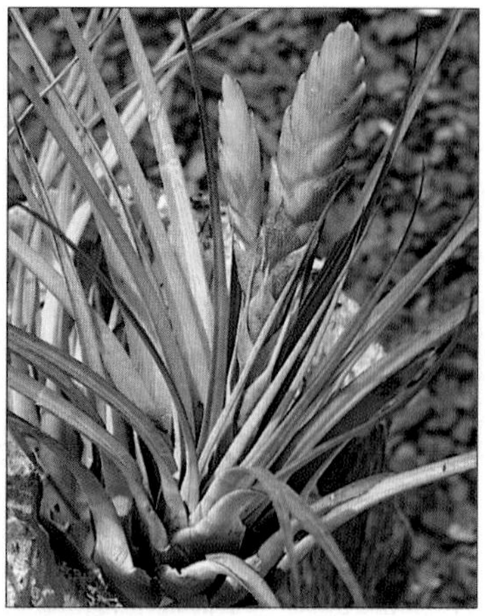

Tillandsia fasciculata

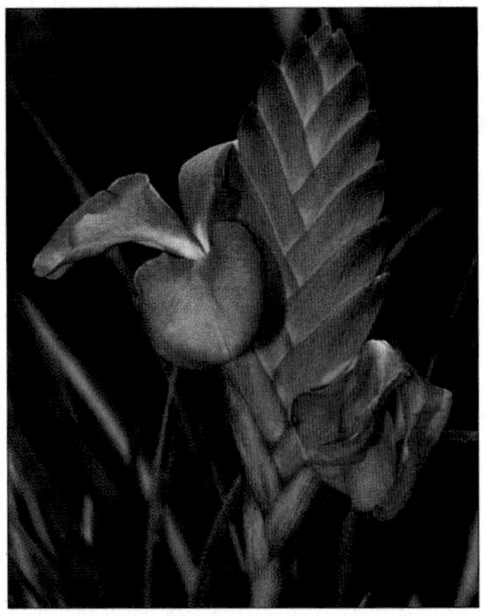

Tillandsia lindenii

grey leaves, 10–27cm (4–11in) long, the lower ones recurved. Compound inflorescences, each consisting of 4–12 spikes of 3–12 slender, funnel-shaped, rose-pink to pale lavender-pink flowers, to 2cm (¾in) long, with green to pink floral bracts, are produced in late spring. ↕↔ 25cm (10in). Colombia to E. Brazil, Trinidad. ❄ (min. 7°C/45°F)

T. imperialis. Stemless, epiphytic or rock-dwelling perennial producing dense rosettes of slender, lance-shaped, sparsely scaly, mid-green or slightly purple leaves, to 40cm (16in) long. In autumn, spikes of 3 or 4 erect, tubular violet flowers, to 6cm (2½in) long, with brilliant red floral bracts, are borne in compound, cone-shaped inflorescences. ↕↔ 50cm (20in). C. and S. Mexico. ❄ (min. 7°C/45°F)

T. ionantha. Freely clustering, epiphytic or terrestrial perennial with dense rosettes of linear, incurved or recurved, coarsely scaly, greyish green leaves, to 4cm (1½in) long, turning red in late spring. Solitary, tubular, violet-blue and white flowers, to 4.5cm (1¾in) long, with white floral bracts, are borne in simple spikes in spring. ↕ 12cm (5in), ↔ 10cm (4in) or more. Mexico, Central America. ❄ (min. 7°C/45°F)

T. leiboldiana. Stemless, epiphytic perennial with funnel-shaped rosettes of slender, lance-shaped, mid-green leaves, to 15cm (6in) long, with flat, brown-scaly sheaths. Branched spikes of 3–8 tubular violet flowers, 3cm (1¼in) long, with red or purple floral bracts, are produced in late spring. ↕↔ 30–60cm (12–24in). Mexico, Central America. ❄ (min. 7°C/45°F)

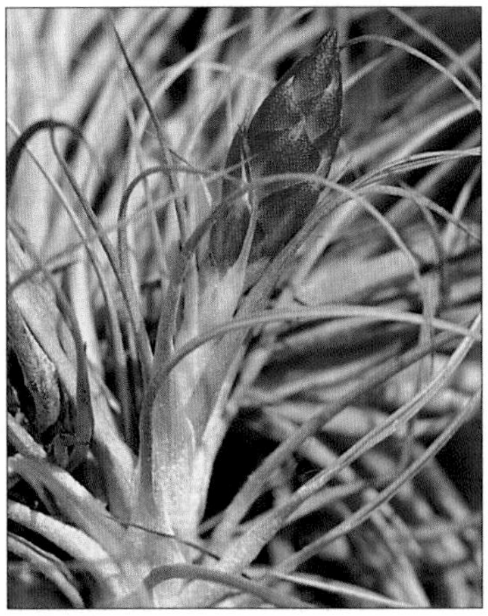

Tillandsia stricta

T. lindenii ■ 🏆 (Blue-flowered torch). Epiphytic perennial with funnel-shaped rosettes of linear-triangular, arching, dark green leaves, 40cm (16in) long, striped reddish purple. In late spring or autumn, green to purple-pink floral bracts and funnel-shaped, white-eyed, deep purple-blue flowers, 7cm (3in) long, with spreading petals, are borne in lance-shaped spikes, each with 2 ranks of up to 20 flowers. ↕ 40cm (16in), ↔ 60cm (24in). N.W. Peru. ❄ (min. 7°C/45°F)

T. multicaulis ■ Epiphytic perennial with dense, funnel-shaped rosettes of linear, pale brown-scaly, mid-green leaves, 30–40cm (12–16in) long. In late spring, simple, sword-shaped spikes of 9–12 tubular blue flowers, 7cm (3in) long, with greenish white sepals and red floral bracts, are produced from the leaf axils on scapes with green bracts. ↕↔ 40cm (16in). Mexico, Central America. ❄ (min. 7°C/45°F)

T. punctulata. Stemless, epiphytic perennial forming symmetrical rosettes of linear, bright green and purplish green leaves, to 45cm (18in) long, with almost black sheaths. In late spring, bears erect spikes of 4–6 tubular, white-tipped violet flowers, 3–5cm (1¼–2in) long, with green floral bracts, sometimes grouped into compound inflorescences; scapes have red bracts. ↕↔ 45cm (18in). Mexico to Panama. ❄ (min. 7°C/45°F)

T. recurvata. Epiphytic or terrestrial perennial with simple or branched stems bearing linear, recurved, grey-scaly, mid-green leaves, 3–17cm (1¼–7in) long, in 2 rows. In autumn, produces simple spikes of 1–5 slender, funnel-shaped,

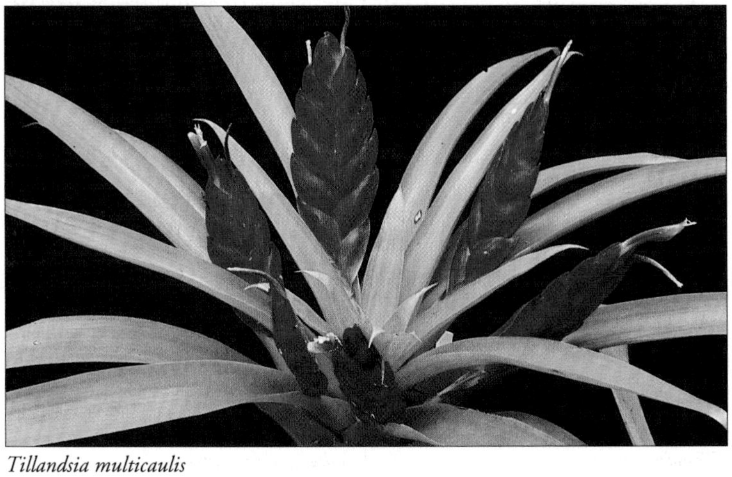

Tillandsia multicaulis

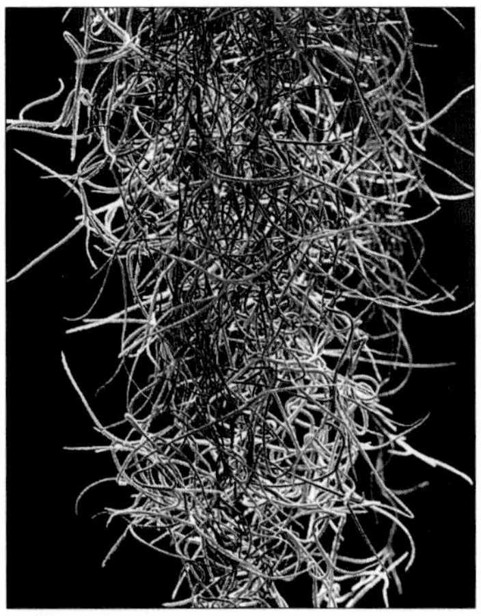

Tillandsia usneoides

erect, pale violet or white flowers, to 1.5cm (½in) long, with green sepals and green or silver, grey-scaly floral bracts. ↕↔ 10–20cm (4–8in). S. USA, Central and South America. ❄ (min. 7°C/45°F)

T. stricta ■ Clump-forming, short-stemmed, epiphytic perennial with dense rosettes of narrowly triangular, grey-scaly, pale green leaves, 6–18cm (2½–7in) long. In spring, bears slender, pendent, cone-shaped spikes of 40 or more slender, funnel-shaped, blue or purple flowers, 2cm (¾in) or more long, with yellowish white to rose-pink floral bracts. ↕↔ 10–20cm (4–8in). Venezuela and Trinidad to N. Argentina. ❄ (min. 7°C/45°F)

T. usneoides ■ (Spanish moss). Pendent, epiphytic perennial with branching, rootless, wiry stems, to 3mm (⅛in) thick, bearing cylindrical, densely grey-scaly, grey-green leaves, 2.5–5cm (1–2in) long. Solitary, tubular, fragrant, greenish yellow or pale blue flowers, to 1cm (½in) long, with green or silver, grey-scaly floral bracts, are produced in late spring or autumn. ↕ 8m (25ft), ↔ indefinite. S. USA, Central and South America, West Indies. ❄ (min. 7°C/45°F)

TIPUANA

Tipu tree

LEGUMINOSAE/PAPILIONACEAE

Genus of one species of semi-evergreen tree found in tropical forest in South America, and cultivated for its attractive habit and flowers. *T. tipu* has mainly alternate, pinnate leaves and arching to pendent, terminal or axillary racemes or panicles of pea-like flowers. Where temperatures fall below 10°C (50°F), grow in a cool or temperate greenhouse; flowers are seldom produced when grown in a container. In warmer areas, grow as a shade or avenue tree.

- **HARDINESS** Frost tender.
- **CULTIVATION** Under glass, grow in loam-based potting compost (JI No.2) in full light. From late spring to early autumn, water freely and apply a balanced liquid fertilizer monthly; water sparingly in winter. Outdoors, grow in moist but well-drained, fertile soil in full sun. Pruning group 1; plants grown under glass need restrictive pruning after flowering.
- **PROPAGATION** Sow seed at 15°C (59°F) in spring.
- **PESTS AND DISEASES** Red spider mites may be troublesome under glass.

T. speciosa see *T. tipu*.

T. tipu ♀ syn. *T. speciosa* (Brazilian rosewood, Pride of Bolivia, Tipu tree). Freely branching, rounded tree bearing pinnate leaves, to 45cm (18in) long, with 9–25 oblong to elliptic, mid- to bright green leaflets with notched tips, downy beneath. In spring, pea-like flowers, 2–2.5cm (¾–1in) across, with crimped, bright yellow to apricot petals, veined rust-red, are borne in racemes to 30cm (12in) long, followed by broadly winged, short, ovoid, woody seed pods. ↕ 10–30m (30–100ft), ↔ 8–15m (25–50ft). Bolivia, Brazil, Argentina. ❄ (min. 7–10°C/45–50°F)

▷**Tipu tree** see *Tipuana, T. tipu*

TITANOPSIS

AIZOACEAE

Genus of 5 or 6 species of short-stemmed, fleshy-rooted, succulent herbaceous perennials, readily forming dense mats or clumps, found in semi-desert areas of Namibia and South Africa. The erect, spoon-shaped to 3-angled, fleshy leaves, thickly crowded with tubercles at the tips, are arranged in attractive basal rosettes. Solitary, daisy-like, yellow or orange flowers are borne during daytime from late summer to early spring. In areas where temperatures fall below 10°C (50°F), grow in a bowl garden indoors or in a warm greenhouse. In warmer climates, grow in a desert garden.

- **HARDINESS** Frost tender.
- **CULTIVATION** Under glass, grow in deep containers in a mix of 3 parts standard cactus compost and 1 part limestone chippings; provide full light and low humidity. From spring to late summer, water moderately, applying a balanced liquid fertilizer 3 or 4 times; keep dry at other times. Outdoors, grow in sharply drained, gritty, alkaline soil in full sun. See also pp.48–49.
- **PROPAGATION** Sow seed at 21°C (70°F) in spring or early summer.
- **PESTS AND DISEASES** Vulnerable to greenfly while flowering.

T. calcarea ■ Clump-forming succulent with crowded, basal rosettes of spoon-shaped, bluish green, sometimes white-tinged leaves, 6–8cm (2½–3in) long, with reddish or greyish white tubercles. Produces bright golden yellow to orange flowers, 2cm (¾in) across, from late summer to autumn. ↕ 3cm

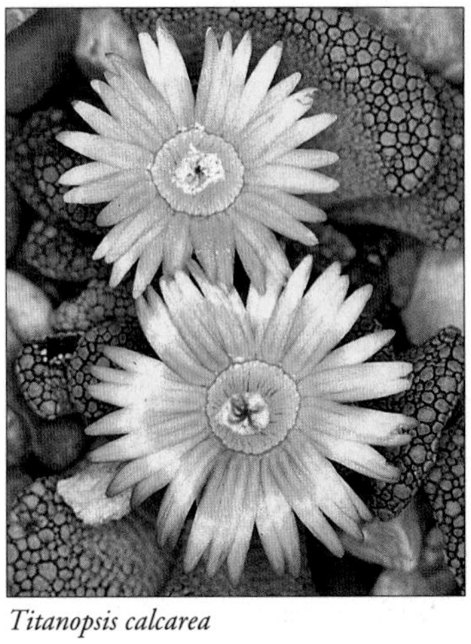

Titanopsis calcarea

T

(1¼in), ↔ 10cm (4in). South Africa (Western Cape). ❁ (min. 10°C/50°F)
T. schwantesii. Clump-forming succulent with basal rosettes of spoon-shaped, light grey-blue, sometimes red-tinged leaves, 3cm (1¼in) long, with rounded bases, 3-angled tips, and yellowish brown tubercles. Pale yellow flowers, to 2cm (¾in) across, are borne from autumn to early winter. ↕ 3cm (1¼in), ↔ 10cm (4in). Namibia. ❁ (min. 10°C/50°F)

TITHONIA

Mexican sunflower

ASTERACEAE/COMPOSITAE

Genus of 10 erect, bushy, stout-stemmed, sometimes woody-based, frequently hairy annuals, perennials, and shrubs, found in thickets and scrub in Mexico and Central America. Alternate, occasionally opposite, entire or lobed leaves each have 3 prominent veins. Large, long-stemmed, mostly solitary flowerheads are borne from late summer to autumn. *T. rotundifolia*, the most commonly grown species, lends height to a mixed or annual border, and provides long-lasting cut flowers.

• **HARDINESS** Half hardy.

• **CULTIVATION** Grow in well-drained, moderately fertile soil in full sun, with shelter from strong winds. Support tall cultivars, water in dry weather, and dead-head to prolong flowering. They grow poorly in cool, overcast weather.

• **PROPAGATION** Sow seed at 13–18°C (55–64°F) in mid- to late spring. Plant out when all danger of frost has passed. Alternatively, sow seed *in situ* in late spring. If seedlings are subjected to cold, leaves turn yellow.

• **PESTS AND DISEASES** Young foliage may be attacked by slugs and snails.

T. rotundifolia, syn. *T. speciosa* (Mexican sunflower). Robust, branching annual with long, triangular-ovate, entire or occasionally 3-lobed, toothed leaves, 8–30cm (3–12in) long, hairy beneath. Bright orange or orange-red flowerheads, to 8cm (3in) across, similar to those of single-flowered dahlias, are borne from late summer to autumn. ↕ to 2m (6ft), ↔ 30cm (12in). Mexico to Central America. ❄. **'Goldfinger'** is compact, with vivid, rich orange flower-heads; ↕ to 75cm (30in). **'Sundance'** has bright orange flowerheads. **'Torch'** ■ has vivid red or orange-red flowerheads.
T. speciosa see *T. rotundifolia.*

T

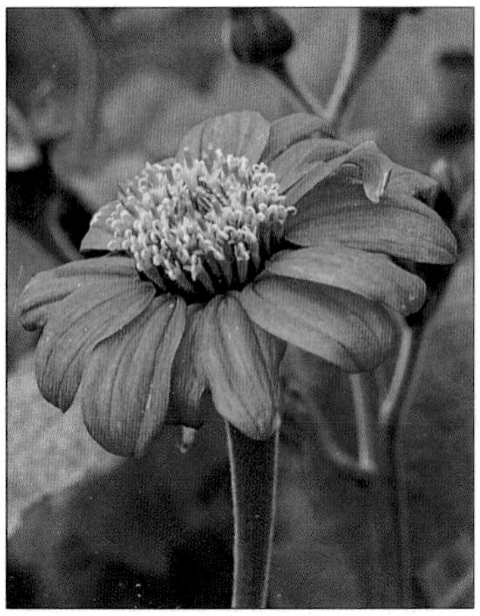

Tithonia rotundifolia 'Torch'

▷**Ti tree** see *Cordyline fruticosa*
▷**Toadflax** see *Linaria, L. vulgaris*
Alpine see *L. alpina*
Purple-net see *L. reticulata*
▷**Toad-shade** see *Trillium sessile*
▷**Tobacco plant** see *Nicotiana*

TODEA

OSMUNDACEAE

Genus of 2 species of large, terrestrial, evergreen ferns found in open places in tropical and warm-temperate rainforest in South Africa, Australia, New Guinea, and New Zealand. Massive, erect, hairy rhizomes bear crowns of upright 2-pinnate, leathery fronds, with spores along the veins. In frost-prone climates, grow *T. barbara* in a temperate or warm greenhouse. In warmer areas, grow as a specimen plant or in light woodland.

• **HARDINESS** Frost tender.

• **CULTIVATION** Under glass, grow in 1 part each of loam, medium-grade bark, and charcoal, 2 parts sharp sand, and 3 parts leaf mould, in bright filtered light, with moderate humidity. In growth, water freely and apply a balanced liquid fertilizer monthly; water moderately to sparingly in winter. Outdoors, grow in moist, fertile soil in partial shade.

• **PROPAGATION** Sow spores at 21°C (70°F) as soon as ripe. Divide in early summer, but only after several trunks have developed. See also p.51.

• **PESTS AND DISEASES** Susceptible to mealybugs under glass.

T. barbara 🏆 Tree-like fern with stout black rhizomes and short, thick trunks, to 80cm (32in) tall. Glossy, bright green fronds, to 2m (6ft) long, have lance-shaped, pinnatifid pinnae. ↕ to 2m (6ft), ↔ to 1.5m (5ft). South Africa, Australia, New Zealand. ❁ (min. 5°C/41°F)

▷**Toe toe** see *Cortaderia richardii*

TOLMIEA

Pick-a-back plant, Youth-on-age

SAXIFRAGACEAE

Genus of one species of fast-spreading, hairy herbaceous perennial occurring in coniferous woodland in W. North America. It is unusual in that young plants are produced on the leaves, where leaf-stalk and blade meet. Leafy stems bear erect racemes of small, cup-shaped, greenish purple flowers with 3 stamens. Grow as ground cover in a woodland garden or as a foliage houseplant.

• **HARDINESS** Fully hardy.

• **CULTIVATION** Grow in cool, moist, humus-rich soil in partial or deep shade. Sun will scorch the leaves, especially of *T. menziesii* 'Taff's Gold'. Under glass, grow in fertile, loam-based potting compost (JI No.2) in bright filtered or indirect light. In growth, water freely and apply a balanced liquid fertilizer monthly; water sparingly in winter.

• **PROPAGATION** Sow seed in containers in a cold frame in autumn. Divide in spring. Remove and pot up plantlets from the leaves in mid- to late summer, or peg leaves into potting compost and remove plantlets when rooted.

• **PESTS AND DISEASES** Trouble free.

T. menziesii 🏆 (Thousand mothers). Clump-forming, hairy perennial with creeping rhizomes and mainly basal,

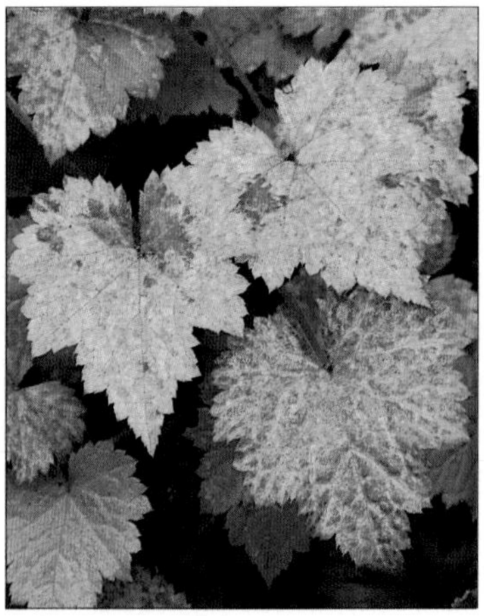

Tolmiea menziesii 'Taff's Gold'

long-stalked, kidney-shaped, shallowly lobed, toothed, conspicuously veined, pale to lime-green leaves, to 12cm (5in) long. In late spring and early summer, produces one-sided racemes of 20–50 slightly scented flowers, to 1cm (½in) long, with orange anthers; the sepals are pale green, heavily shaded and lined purple-brown, with thread-like, purple-brown petals recurved between them. ↕ 30–60cm (12–24in), ↔ 1–2m (3–6ft). W. North America. ❄❄❄. **'Maculata'** see 'Taff's Gold'. **'Taff's Gold'** ■🏆 syn. 'Maculata', has paler green leaves, spotted and mottled cream and pale yellow.

TOLPIS

ASTERACEAE/COMPOSITAE

Genus of 20 frequently mat-forming annuals and perennials from dry, sandy areas in the Azores and the Canary Islands, the Mediterranean region, N.E. Africa, and Ethiopia. The mainly ovate to lance-shaped, toothed or lobed, bright green basal leaves are usually arranged in rosettes, while the branching stems support pinnate or lobed leaves. Leaves and stems contain a milky latex. Daisy-like, bright yellow flowerheads emerge over a long period from spring to summer. Suitable for the front of a mixed or annual border.

• **HARDINESS** Fully hardy.

• **CULTIVATION** Grow in well-drained, light, moderately fertile soil in full sun. Dead-head to prolong flowering.

• **PROPAGATION** Sow seed *in situ* in mid-spring.

• **PESTS AND DISEASES** Trouble free.

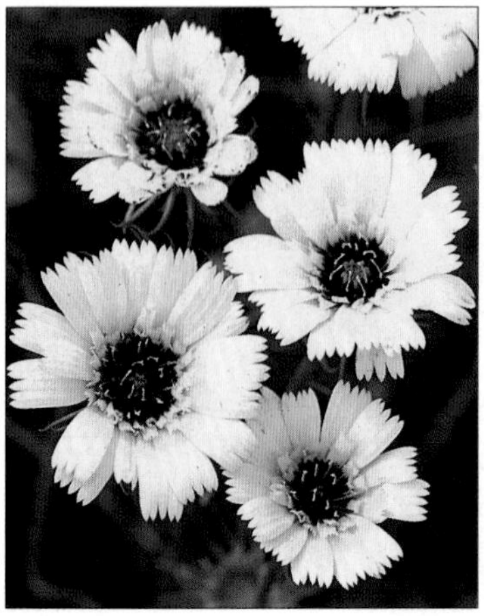

Tolpis barbata

T. barbata ■ Annual with mostly basal, lance-shaped to oblong, toothed, hairy, bright green leaves, 2–10cm (¾–4in) long. From spring to summer, solitary or clustered, bright yellow flowerheads, 1–3cm (½–1¼in) across, with fringed margins and dark maroon centres, are borne singly or in clusters, on sparsely leaved, branching stems. ↕ to 60cm (24in), usually less, ↔ 30cm (12in). Mediterranean. ❄❄❄

TOONA

MELIACEAE

Genus of about 6 species of deciduous or semi-evergreen trees found in woodland from E. Asia to Australasia. They are grown for their alternate, pinnate leaves and small, cup-shaped, fragrant, greenish white or white flowers, which are borne in large, terminal or axillary panicles. *T. sinensis*, the most common species in cultivation, is an effective specimen tree. It grows best in areas with hot summers, where it is a useful shade or street tree.

• **HARDINESS** Fully hardy.

• **CULTIVATION** Grow in fertile, well-drained soil in full sun. Pruning group 1.

• **PROPAGATION** Sow seed in containers in a cold frame in autumn. Insert root cuttings in late winter.

• **PESTS AND DISEASES** Trouble free.

T. sinensis ■🏆 syn. *Cedrela sinensis.* Broadly columnar, deciduous tree with peeling brown bark. Aromatic leaves, to 60cm (24in) long, have up to 26 ovate-lance-shaped to oblong, papery leaflets, bronze-red to pink when young, turning yellow in autumn. In midsummer, bears small, fragrant, white or greenish white flowers in pendent, terminal panicles, to 30cm (12in) long. ↕ 15m (50ft), ↔ 10m (30ft). China. ❄❄❄. **'Flamingo'** has vivid pink young leaves, turning creamy yellow then bright green.

▷**Toothwort, Purple** see *Lathraea clandestina*

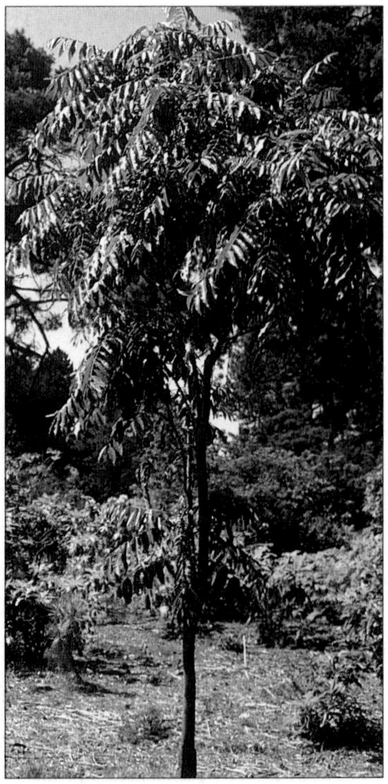

Toona sinensis

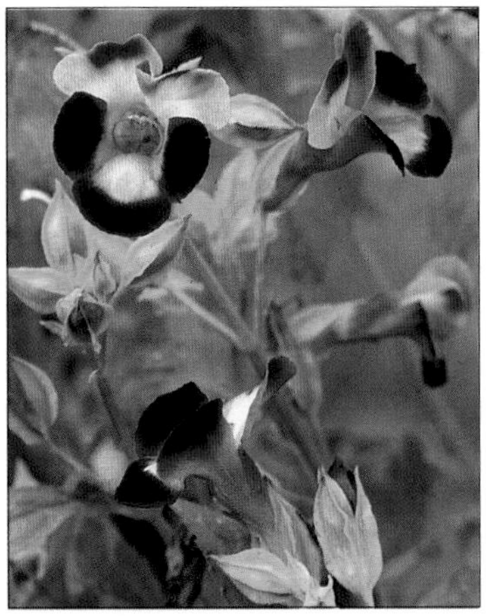

Torenia fournieri

TORENIA

Wishbone flower

SCROPHULARIACEAE

Genus of 40–50 erect to spreading, bushy, sometimes softly hairy annuals and perennials found in woodland, at altitudes up to 3,000m (10,000ft), in tropical Africa and Asia. They are grown for their short, showy, terminal or axillary racemes of tubular then flaring, 2-lipped flowers, the upper lips slightly 2-lobed, the lower ones markedly 3-lobed, produced in summer. The opposite leaves are mostly broadly to narrowly ovate or lance-shaped, and may be entire or toothed. *T. fournieri* is the most commonly cultivated species: use for summer bedding, or grow at the front of an annual or mixed border; it is also grown as a summer-flowering houseplant or cool-greenhouse plant.
• **HARDINESS** Frost tender.
• **CULTIVATION** Under glass, grow in loam-based potting compost (JI No.2) in bright filtered light, providing good ventilation. In the growing season, water freely and apply a high-potash liquid fertilizer every 2 or 3 weeks. Pinch out stem tips to promote bushiness. Outdoors, grow in fertile, moist but well-drained soil in partial shade.
• **PROPAGATION** Sow seed at 18°C (64°F) in mid-spring; harden off and plant out when all danger of frost has passed.
• **PESTS AND DISEASES** Trouble free.

T. fournieri ■ (Wishbone flower). Erect, smooth annual with long-stalked, pointed, ovate to narrowly ovate, toothed, pale green leaves, 4–5cm (1½–2in) long. In summer, produces abundant lilac-blue flowers, to 3.5cm (1½in) long, the lower lips deep purple and the throats marked yellow. ↕ 30cm (12in), ↔ 15–23cm (6–9in). Tropical Asia. ❀ (min. 5°C/41°F). Cultivars of **Clown Series** ■ are compact, and produce white, pink, deep purple, or lavender-blue flowers; ↕ 20–25cm (8–10in). **Panda Series** cultivars are more compact, producing white, pink, purple, or lavender-blue flowers; ↕ 10–20cm (4–8in).

▷**Tormentil** see *Potentilla erecta*

TORREYA

Nutmeg yew

TAXACEAE

Genus of 7 species of dioecious, evergreen, coniferous shrubs or trees found in woodland in Asia and North America. The flattened, lance-shaped, 2-ranked leaves are yew-like, but hard and spine-tipped. The common name refers to the single-seeded, ovoid or ovoid-ellipsoid female, cone-like structures ("cones"); they may take 2 years to ripen, maturing to olive- or plum-like fruits. The male "cones" are white and spherical. Nutmeg yews are vigorous, small to medium-sized specimen trees. *T. californica* thrives in areas with cool, damp summers, whereas other species grow best in areas with summers that are warm and humid.
• **HARDINESS** Fully hardy.

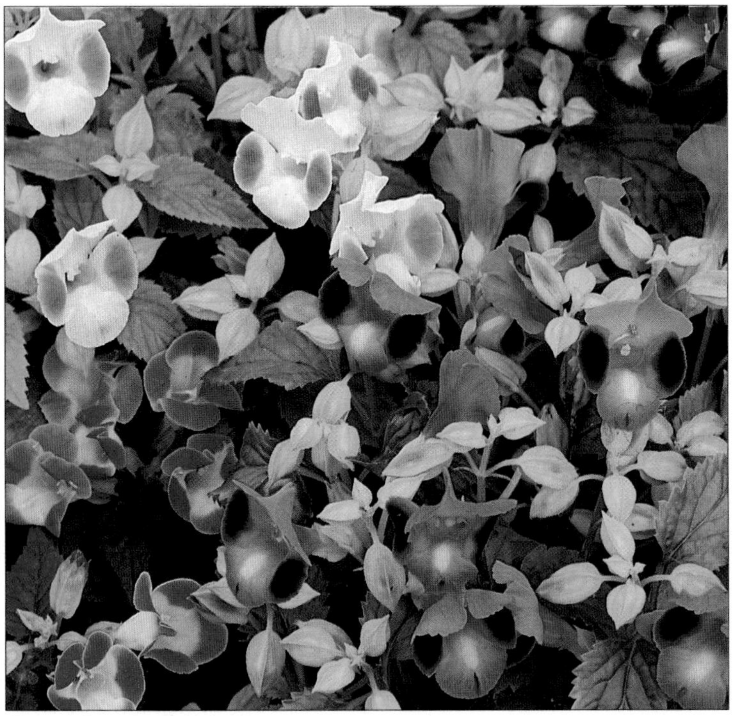

Torenia fournieri Clown Series

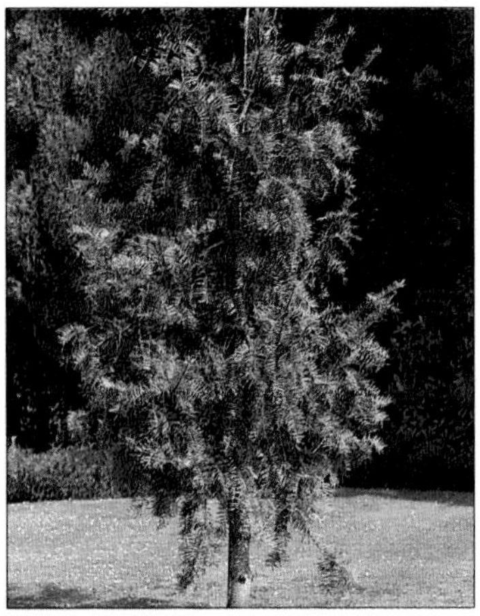

Torreya californica

• **CULTIVATION** Grow in fertile, moist but well-drained soil in full sun or light dappled shade. Provide shelter from cold, drying winds.
• **PROPAGATION** Sow seed in containers in a cold frame or in a seed bed, as soon as ripe; the seed may take 2 or more years to germinate. Insert semi-ripe cuttings in late summer; use cuttings from strongly upright growth to form leading shoots.
• **PESTS AND DISEASES** Trouble free.

T. californica ■ ◯ (California nutmeg tree). Broadly conical tree with whorled branches, red-brown or brown bark, becoming scaly, and green shoots with pointed buds. Produces spreading, 2-ranked, narrowly lance-shaped, tapered, yellowish green leaves, 3–5cm (1¼–2in) long, and ellipsoid or obovoid, purplish green female "cones", to 4cm (1½in) long. ↕ to 25m (80ft), ↔ to 8m (25ft). USA (C. California). ✻✻✻
T. nucifera ◯–◯ Upright to broadly conical tree with opposite branchlets and linear, glossy, dark green leaves, 2–3cm (¾–1¼in) long, in 2 opposite ranks, separated by a broad, V-shaped channel. Ellipsoid female "cones" are olive-green, 2.5cm (1in) long. ↕ to 15m (50ft), ↔ 8m (25ft). S. Japan. ✻✻✻

▷**Totara, Alpine** see *Podocarpus nivalis*
▷***Tovara*** see *Persicaria*
T. virginiana see *P. virginiana*

TOWNSENDIA

ASTERACEAE/COMPOSITAE

Genus of about 20 species of compact, occasionally stemless annuals and evergreen, often monocarpic perennials found in open, freely draining habitats in mountainous areas of W. North America. The alternate leaves are linear to spoon-shaped, entire, and smooth to densely hairy. Solitary, short-stemmed, aster-like flowerheads are produced in summer. Suitable for a rock garden, trough, or alpine house.
• **HARDINESS** Fully hardy.
• **CULTIVATION** Grow in gritty, sharply drained soil in full sun. Protect from excessive winter wet. In an alpine house, grow in a mix of equal parts loam, leaf mould, and sharp sand.
• **PROPAGATION** Sow seed as soon as ripe in containers in a cold frame. Propagate regularly as plants are often short-lived.
• **PESTS AND DISEASES** Susceptible to aphids and red spider mites under glass.

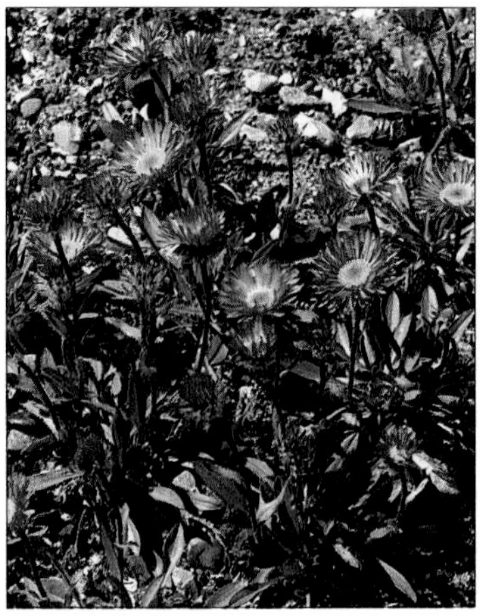

Townsendia formosa

T. formosa ■ Upright, clump-forming, rhizomatous perennial with spoon-shaped to inversely lance-shaped leaves, to 8cm (3in) long, with finely hairy midribs and margins. In summer, one to several solitary flowerheads, 3cm (1¼in) across, with pale violet ray-florets, mauve beneath, and yellow disc-florets, are produced on upright stems, 10cm (4in) long. ↕ to 60cm (24in), ↔ to 15cm (6in). S.W. USA. ✻✻✻
T. parryi. Clump-forming, short-lived perennial with spoon-shaped, slightly fleshy leaves, to 10cm (4in) long, smooth above and bristly-hairy beneath. One to several solitary flowerheads, to 3cm (1¼in) across, with violet-blue or lavender-blue ray-florets and yellow disc-florets, are borne on upright stems, 5–15cm (2–6in) long, in early summer. ↕ to 15cm (6in), ↔ to 10cm (4in). N.W. North America. ✻✻✻

▷***Toxicodendron*** see *Rhus*
T. succedaneum see *R. succedanea*
T. vernicifluum see *R. verniciflua*

TRACHELIUM

syn. DIOSPHAERA

CAMPANULACEAE

Genus of about 7 species of small, sometimes cushion-forming, often woody-based perennials, usually found in calcareous soils in the Mediterranean region. The tiny, narrowly lance-shaped to oblong or almost rounded leaves are alternate and simple. Tubular flowers, each with 5 spreading petal lobes, are solitary or, more usually, produced in corymbs. Grow *T. caeruleum* and other tall species and cultivars in an annual, mixed, or herbaceous border; their flowers are excellent for cutting. Dwarf tracheliums, such as *T. asperuloides*, are suitable for a rock garden, scree bed, trough, or alpine house.
• **HARDINESS** Fully hardy to half hardy.
• **CULTIVATION** Grow in well-drained soil in full sun with some midday shade. *T. asperuloides* prefers more sharply drained, alkaline soil, and needs protection from excessive winter wet. In an alpine house, grow in deep containers in a mix of equal parts loam, leaf mould, and sharp sand.
• **PROPAGATION** Sow seed of half-hardy species at 13–16°C (55–61°F) in early spring, or *in situ* in late spring. Sow seed of fully hardy species as soon as ripe in containers in a cold frame. Insert softwood cuttings in early summer.

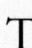

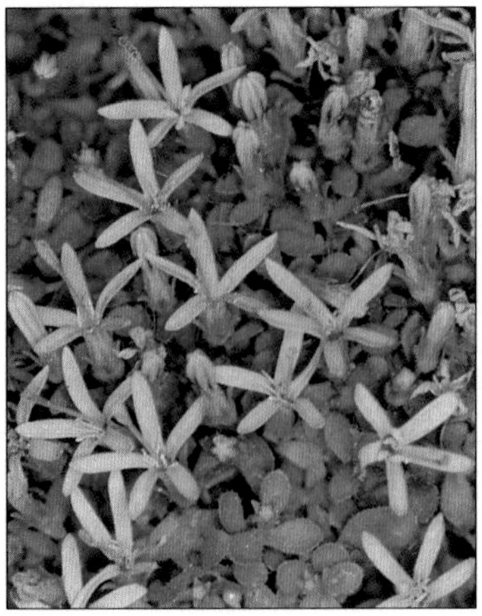

Trachelium asperuloides

• **PESTS AND DISEASES** Aphids and red spider mites may prove troublesome under glass.

T. asperuloides ■ syn. *Diosphaera asperuloides.* Dense, cushion-forming perennial with thread-like stems bearing minute, overlapping, ovate-rounded, glossy, mid-green leaves, 6mm (¼in) long. In late summer, bears abundant, tubular, lavender-blue or white flowers, 6mm (¼in) across, singly or in corymbs of up to 5, on very short flower-stalks in the upper leaf axils. ↕ to 5cm (2in), ↔ to 15cm (6in). S. Greece. ❄❄❄

T. caeruleum ♀ (Blue throatwort). Erect perennial, grown as an annual in frost-prone climates, with pointed, oval to lance-shaped, toothed, mid-green leaves, 8cm (3in) long. In summer, bears lightly scented, deep violet-blue or white flowers, to 7mm (¼in) across, in dense, dome-shaped, terminal corymbs on long, branching, red-flushed stalks. ↕ 1–1.2m (3–4ft), ↔ 30cm (12in). W. and C. Mediterranean. ❄. **'Purple Umbrella'** has deep purple flowers. **'White Veil'** has white flowers.

TRACHELOSPERMUM

APOCYNACEAE

Genus of about 20 species of woody, evergreen, twining climbers found in woodland from India to Japan. They are grown for their attractive foliage and fragrant flowers. Opposite, lance-shaped to broadly ovate leaves are borne on stems that contain a milky latex. Small, salverform flowers, with cylindrical tubes and 5 spreading, slightly twisted lobes, are produced in terminal or axillary cymes, followed by pendent, pod-like fruits (seldom borne in areas with cool summers). Grow against a warm, sunny wall; in areas prone to severe frosts, grow in a cool greenhouse.

• **HARDINESS** Frost hardy.

• **CULTIVATION** Outdoors, grow in fertile, well-drained soil in full sun or partial shade; provide shelter from cold, drying winds. Under glass, grow in loam-based potting compost (JI No.3) in full light with shade from hot sun. During the growing season, water freely and apply a balanced liquid fertilizer monthly. Water sparingly in winter. Pruning group 11, in early spring.

• **PROPAGATION** Insert semi-ripe cuttings with bottom heat in summer. Layer in autumn.

• **PESTS AND DISEASES** Trouble free.

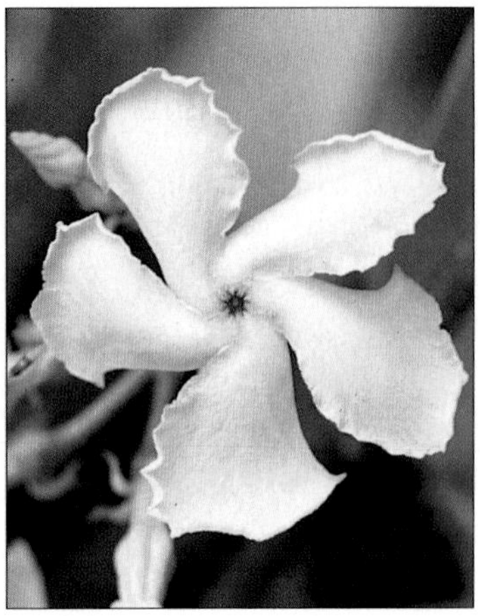

Trachelospermum jasminoides

T. asiaticum ♀ Woody, evergreen, twining climber bearing oval, glossy, dark green leaves, to 5cm (2in) long. Fragrant, creamy white flowers, 2cm (¾in) across, which age to yellow, are produced in terminal cymes in mid- and late summer. ↕ 6m (20ft). Korea, Japan. ❄❄

T. jasminoides ■ ♀ (Confederate jasmine, Star jasmine). Woody, evergreen, twining climber with oval, glossy, dark green leaves, to 10cm (4in) long, turning bronze-red in winter. In mid- and late summer, pure white flowers, 2.5cm (1in) across, are produced in terminal and axillary cymes. ↕ 9m (28ft). China, Korea, Japan. ❄❄

TRACHYCARPUS

ARECACEAE/PALMAE

Genus of 6 species of usually single-stemmed, sometimes clustering, dioecious, evergreen palms occurring in temperate and mountain forest in subtropical Asia. They are cultivated for their attractive habit, their terminal, fan-shaped leaves, palmately lobed to half their length or more, and their cup-shaped flowers, surrounded by bowl-shaped, white or brown bracts. The flowers are followed by spherical or kidney-shaped fruits. Fan palms are small enough to be grown in a restricted area, such as a courtyard; they are also effective specimen trees.

• **HARDINESS** Frost hardy.

• **CULTIVATION** Grow in well-drained, fertile soil in full sun or light dappled shade, sheltered from strong or cold, drying winds.

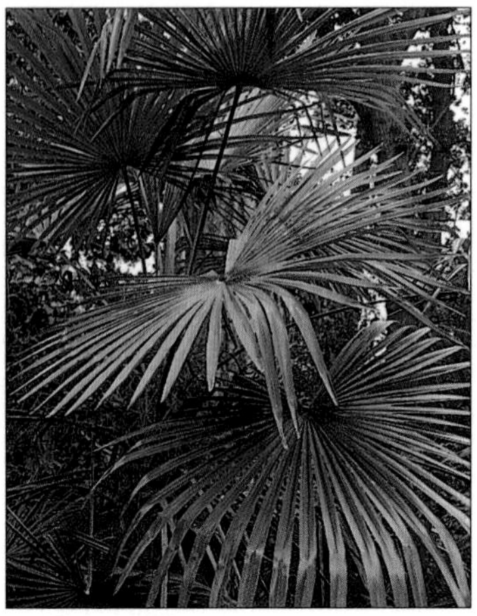

Trachycarpus fortunei

• **PROPAGATION** Sow seed in spring or autumn at 24°C (75°F).

• **PESTS AND DISEASES** Trouble free.

T. fortunei ■ ♀ ♣ (Chusan palm). Unbranched, single-stemmed, evergreen palm with a head of fan-shaped, dark green leaves, 45–75cm (18–30in) long, with numerous pointed segments variously lobed to half their length or more. Small yellow flowers are borne in large, pendent panicles, 60cm (24in) or more long; they emerge from close to the leaf bases in early summer. Female plants bear spherical, blue-black fruit, 1cm (½in) across. ↕ to 20m (70ft), ↔ 2.5m (8ft). Origin unknown. ❄❄. **'Nanus'** has a short or almost non-existent trunk and stiffer leaf-blades, to 30cm (12in) long.

TRACHYMENE

syn. DIDISCUS

APIACEAE/UMBELLIFERAE

Genus of 12 or more species of erect, branching annuals, biennials, and perennials from moist woodland and swamps to dry sandhills and subalpine areas in Australia and the W. Pacific. The lacy leaves are ternate or 2-ternate, usually with linear leaflets, or rarely with 2 leaflets or palmately divided. Dainty, terminal umbels of tiny, star-shaped, white, pink, or blue flowers are borne in summer. Grow *T. coerulea*, the species most commonly cultivated, at the front of an annual or mixed border, or in a cool greenhouse. It provides long-lasting cut flowers.

• **HARDINESS** Half hardy.

• **CULTIVATION** Under glass, grow in loam-based potting compost (JI No.2) in full light with shade from hot sun. In summer, water moderately and apply a high-potash liquid fertilizer every 2 or 3 weeks. Outdoors, grow in light, well-drained, moderately fertile soil in a sheltered site in full sun. Provide twiggy support.

• **PROPAGATION** Sow seed at 15°C (59°F) in mid-spring, or sow *in situ* in late spring. Germination is slow.

• **PESTS AND DISEASES** Trouble free.

T. coerulea, syn. *Didiscus coeruleus* (Blue lace flower). Stiff-stemmed annual or biennial with pale green leaves, to 10cm (4in) long, divided into 2 or 3 narrow, 3-lobed leaflets. Lightly scented, lavender-blue flowers are produced in long-stemmed, rounded umbels, to 5cm (2in) across, in summer. ↕ to 60cm (24in), ↔ 23cm (9in). W. Australia. ❄

TRADESCANTIA

COMMELINACEAE

Genus of about 65 species of creeping, trailing, or tuft-forming, fibrous- or tuberous-rooted, evergreen perennials from woodland, scrub, or disturbed ground in North, Central, and South America. The leaves are alternate, usually fleshy, lance-shaped to ovate, often purple-flushed or variegated, and hairy or hairless. Short-lived, spreading, usually saucer-shaped flowers, each with 3 petals and 3 sepals, are produced in terminal or axillary cymes, which are fused in pairs, with paired, boat-shaped bracts. Hardy tradescantias are suitable for a mixed or herbaceous border. In

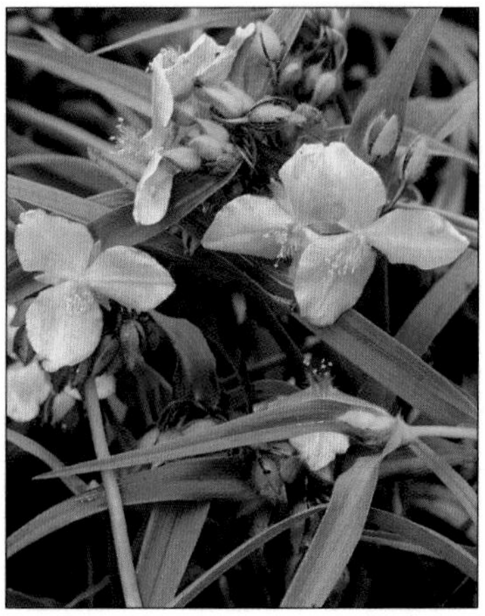

Tradescantia Andersoniana Group 'J.C. Weguelin'

warm regions, grow the tender species beneath shrubs or for ground cover; in frost-prone areas, grow in a temperate or cool greenhouse, as houseplants, or in a conservatory; they are especially effective in hanging baskets. Contact with the foliage may irritate skin.

• **HARDINESS** Fully hardy to frost tender.

• **CULTIVATION** Under glass, grow in loamless or loam-based potting compost (JI No.2) in bright filtered light. When in active growth, water moderately and apply a balanced liquid fertilizer every 4 weeks; water sparingly in winter. Pinch growing tips to encourage bushiness, and remove plain green foliage from variegated cultivars. Pot on each spring. Outdoors, grow in moist, fertile soil in full sun or partial shade. After flowering, cut back flowered stems to prevent seeding and to encourage further flowers.

• **PROPAGATION** Insert stem-tip cuttings, 5–8cm (2–3in) long, of the tender tradescantias at any time; root in cutting compost or water, then pot up into soil-based compost (JI No.1). Divide hardy species and cultivars in autumn or spring.

• **PESTS AND DISEASES** Susceptible to aphids, grubs, and vine weevil.

***T. albiflora* 'Albovittata'** see *T. fluminensis* 'Albovittata'.

***T. albiflora* 'Variegata'** see *T. fluminensis* 'Variegata'.

T. x andersoniana see *T.* Andersoniana Group.

***T.* Andersoniana Group**, syn. *T.* x *andersoniana.* Tufted, clump-forming perennials with erect, branching stems and arching, narrowly lance-shaped, pointed, hairless, slightly fleshy, mid-green, often purple-tinted leaves, to 35cm (14in) long. Blue, purple, rose-pink to rose-red, or white flowers, 2.5–4cm (1–1½in) across, each have 3 wide-open, triangular petals and fluffy-hairy stamen filaments; they are borne in succession in paired, terminal cymes from early summer to early autumn. ↕ 40–60cm (16–24in), ↔ 45–60cm (18–24in). ❄❄❄. **'Carmine Glow'** see 'Karminglut'. **'Iris Prichard'** has white flowers, shaded pale blue. **'Isis'** ♀ produces large, dark blue flowers. **'J.C. Weguelin'** ■ ♀ has large, pale blue flowers. **'Karminglut'**, syn. 'Carmine Glow', has carmine-red flowers. **'Osprey'** ■ ♀ has large white flowers with blue stamen filaments. **'Purewell**

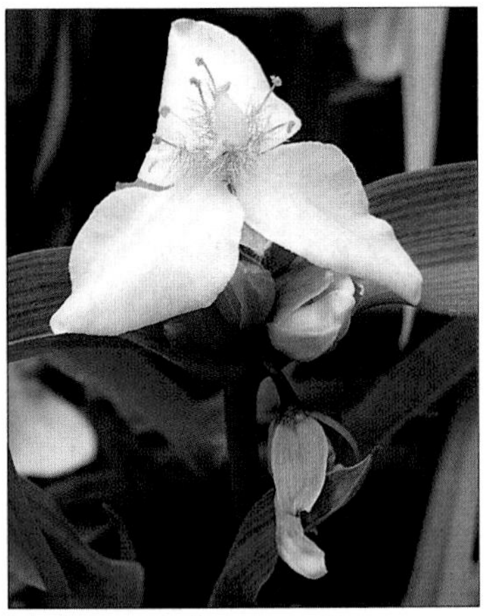
Tradescantia Andersoniana Group 'Osprey'

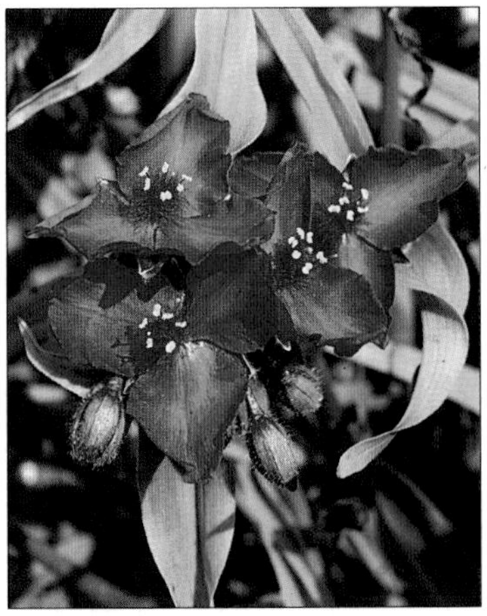
Tradescantia Andersoniana Group 'Purple Dome'

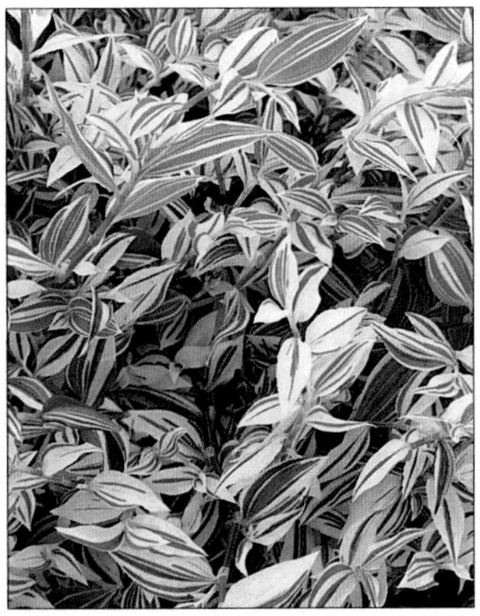
Tradescantia fluminensis 'Albovittata'

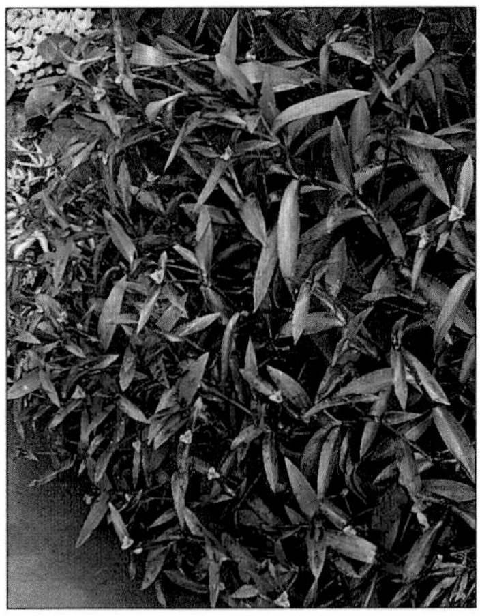
Tradescantia pallida 'Purpurea'

Giant' ■ produces large, purple to rose-red flowers; ↕↔ 45cm (18in). **'Purple Dome'** ■ produces large, rich purple flowers. **'Red Cloud'** has cerise-red flowers; ↕↔ 45cm (18in). **'Zwanenburg Blue'** has large, dark blue flowers.
T. blossfeldiana see *T. cerinthoides.*
T. cerinthoides, syn. *T. blossfeldiana.* Vigorous, creeping or ascending perennial with stout, branching stems and elliptic-oblong to narrowly ovate, very fleshy, deep green leaves, 15cm (6in) long, hairless above, and deep purple and densely hairy beneath. Paired, terminal or axillary cymes of pink and white flowers are produced intermittently throughout the year. ↕ 90cm (36in), ↔ 45cm (18in). Brazil. ❄ (min. 10–16°C/50–61°F).

'Variegata' 🏆 has leaves with bold buff stripes, light pink above.
T. fluminensis (Wandering Jew). Trailing perennial with thin, pointed, ovate to ovate-oblong, usually hairless, light green leaves, 2–10cm (¾–4in) long, often stained purple beneath. White flowers are produced in paired, terminal or axillary cymes intermittently throughout the year. ↕ 15cm (6in), ↔ 20cm (8in). Brazil to N. Argentina. ❄ (min. 10–16°C/50–61°F). **'Albovittata'** ■ syn. *T. albiflora* 'Albovittata', has light green leaves with white longitudinal stripes, and purple undersides that partially show through the almost transparent upper surfaces. **'Aurea'** 🏆 has yellow-striped leaves. **'Variegata'** ■ syn. *T. albiflora* 'Variegata', has leaves variably striped green, white, purple, or cream.
T. navicularis see *Callisia navicularis.*
***T. pallida* 'Purple Heart'** see *T. pallida* 'Purpurea'.
***T. pallida* 'Purpurea'** ■ 🏆 syn. *Setcreasea purpurea, T. pallida* 'Purple Heart'. Trailing perennial producing ascending purple stems. Large, pointed, narrowly oblong leaves, 8–15cm (3–6in) long, are V-shaped in section, and fleshy, hairless, rich violet-purple. In summer, bears bright pink flowers in paired, terminal cymes. Leaves colour best in bright sunlight and when the root zone is slightly dry and cramped. ↕ 20cm (8in), ↔ to 40cm (16in). E. Mexico. ❄ (min. 10–16°C/50–61°F)
T. pexata see *T. sillamontana.*
T. purpusii see *T. zebrina* 'Purpusii'.
T. sillamontana ■ 🏆 syn. *T. pexata, T. velutina* (White velvet). Trailing perennial with upright, later spreading, silky-hairy stems and ovate, fleshy, silky-hairy, grey-green leaves, 4–6cm (1½–2½in) long. Magenta-pink flowers are borne in paired, terminal cymes in summer. ↕ 30cm (12in), ↔ to 45cm (18in). N. Mexico. ❄ (min. 10–16°C/50–61°F)
T. spathacea ■ syn. *Rhoeo discolor, R. spathacea* (Moses-in-the-cradle, Three-men-in-a-boat). Clump-forming perennial with rosettes of semi-erect, linear-lance-shaped, fleshy, hairless leaves, 20–35cm (8–14in) long, dark green above and deep purple beneath. White flowers are produced in paired, axillary cymes, which are surrounded by prominent, long-lasting purple bracts, throughout the year. ↕↔ 30cm (12in). Central America. ❄ (min. 10–16°C/50–61°F). **'Vittata'** 🏆 has leaves with numerous longitudinal, pale yellow stripes.
T. velutina see *T. sillamontana.*
T. zanonia, syn. *Campelia zanonia.* Clump-forming perennial with erect or decumbent stems and broadly elliptic to inversely lance-shaped, hairless, membranous, dark green leaves, 24cm (10in) long. White flowers are borne in paired, axillary cymes, surrounded by 2 leafy bracts, from summer to winter. ↕ 2.2m (7ft), ↔ 1m (3ft). Mexico to Brazil, West Indies. ❄ (min. 10–16°C/50–61°F). **'Mexican Flag'** has leaves with longitudinal white stripes and red margins, sometimes silvery beneath.

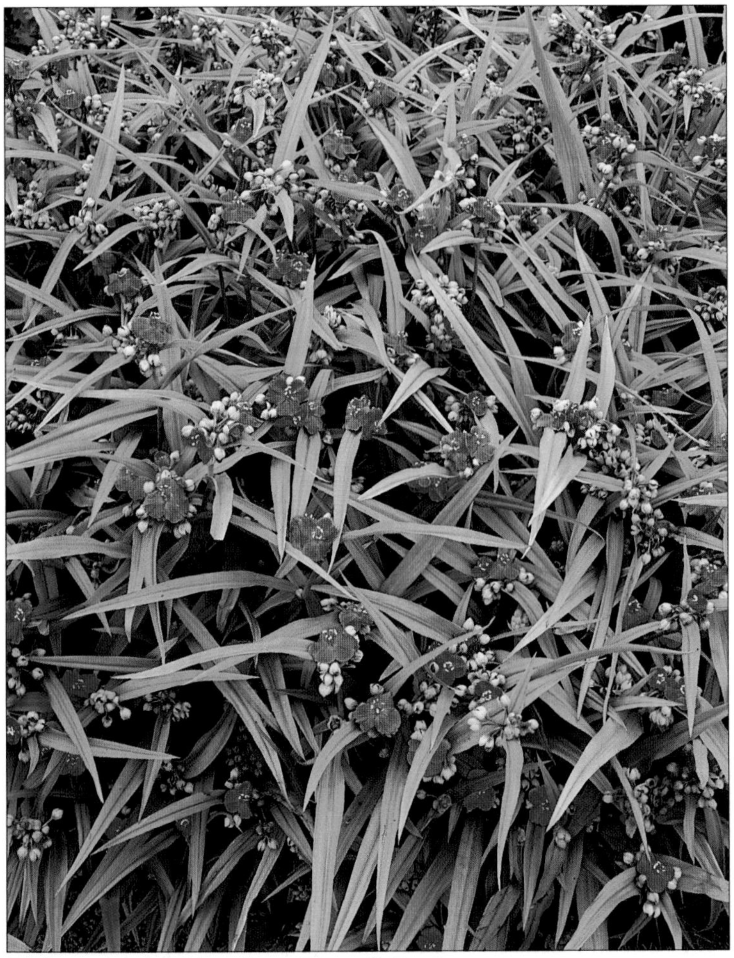
Tradescantia Andersoniana Group 'Purewell Giant'

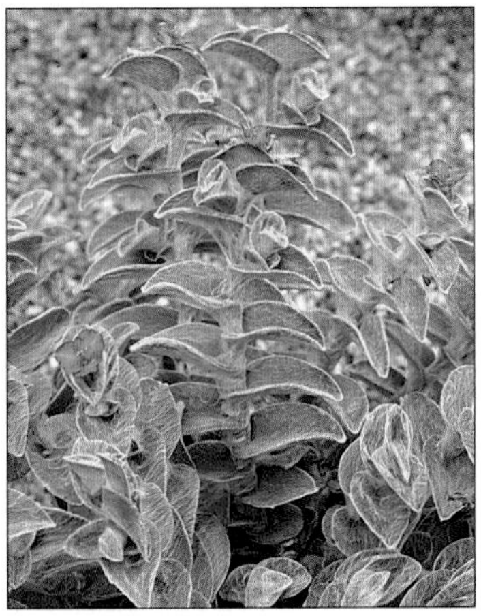
Tradescantia sillamontana

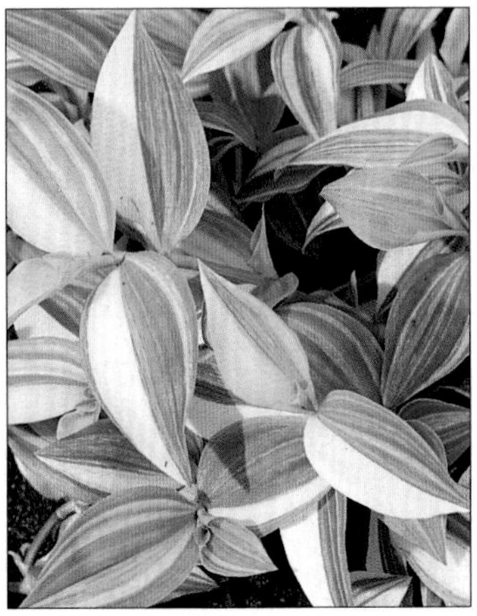
Tradescantia fluminensis 'Variegata'

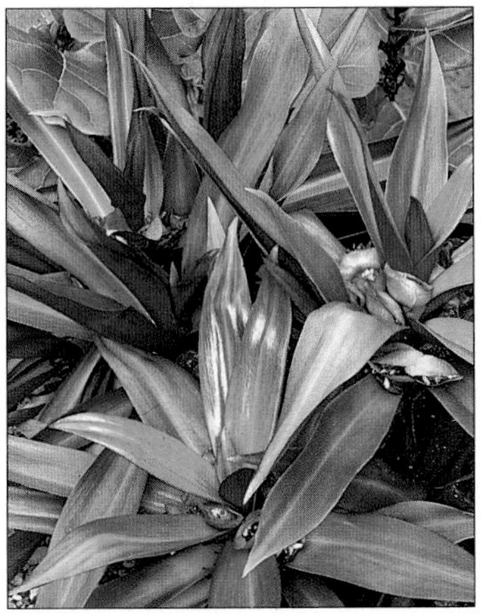
Tradescantia spathacea

T

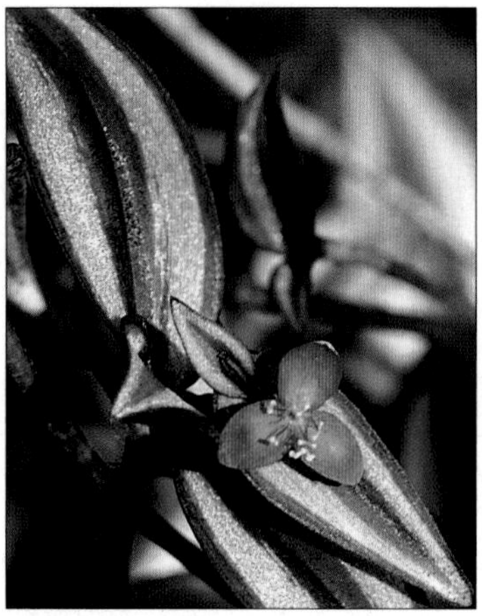

Tradescantia zebrina

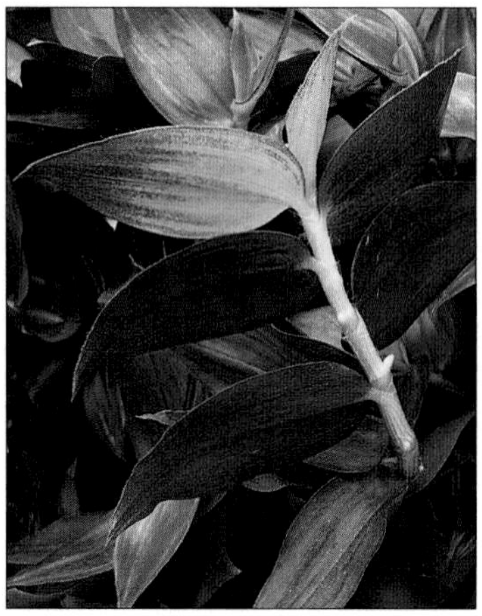

Tradescantia zebrina 'Purpusii'

T. zebrina ▣♀ syn. *Zebrina pendula* (Wandering Jew). Trailing perennial with ovate-oblong to broadly ovate, fleshy, hairless, bluish green leaves, to 10cm (4in) long; 2 longitudinal stripes, silver-green above and rich purple beneath, mark each leaf. Purple-pink to purple-blue flowers are produced in paired, terminal cymes intermittently throughout the year. ↕15cm (6in), ↔ 20cm (8in). S. Mexico. ❀ (min. 10–16°C/50–61°F). **'Purpusii'** ▣♀ syn. *T. purpusii, Zebrina purpusii*, has rich bronze-purple leaves and pink flowers. **'Quadricolor'** ♀ has leaves striped green, cream, pink, and silver.

TRAPA

Water chestnut

TRAPACEAE

Genus of about 30 species of submerged aquatic annuals from still or slow-moving water in C. Europe, E. Asia, and Africa. The creeping, floating stems bear linear submerged leaves and rosettes of ovate or almost triangular to diamond-shaped, toothed, mottled floating leaves, hairy beneath, with spongy, swollen leaf-stalks. Small, solitary, tubular, white or lilac flowers are followed by inflated, spiny fruits. In frost-prone areas, grow in baskets in a cold-greenhouse pool, or float rosettes on the surface of an outdoor pool after last frosts. In warmer climates, grow in an outdoor pool.

• **HARDINESS** Half hardy to frost tender.
• **CULTIVATION** Plant in baskets of loam-based potting compost (JI No.3) in full light, at no less than 10°C (50°F); or, in frost-prone areas, float rosettes on

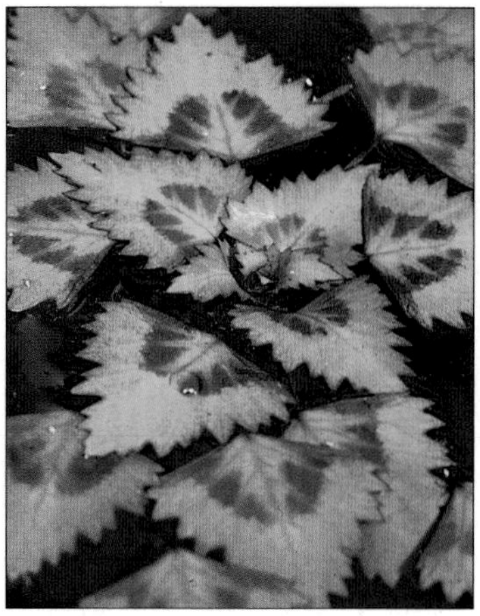

Trapa natans

still, shallow, nutrient-rich, acid water in full sun. See also pp.52–53.
• **PROPAGATION** Collect seed in autumn. Store frost-free in water or wet moss over winter; sow in spring, at 13–18°C (55–64°F), in wet compost.
• **PESTS AND DISEASES** Trouble free.

T. natans ▣ (Jesuit's nut, Water caltrops, Water chestnut). Clump-forming, aquatic annual. Roughly diamond-shaped, floating leaves, 2.5cm (1in) across, have red-tinged leaf-stalks, 5–8cm (2–3in) long. White flowers are borne from the leaf axils in summer, followed by 4-angled, spiny, hard black fruit, to 5cm (2in) across. ↔ indefinite. Eurasia, Africa. ✲ (borderline)

▷ **Traveller's joy** see *Clematis*
▷ **Traveller's tree** see *Ravenala*
▷ **Tree fern** see *Cyathea*
  Black see *Cyathea medullaris*
  Hawaiian see *Cibotium glaucum*
  Soft see *Dicksonia antarctica*
  Woolly see *Dicksonia antarctica*
▷ **Tree heath** see *Erica arborea*
▷ **Tree-ivy** see x *Fatshedera lizei*
▷ **Tree of heaven** see *Ailanthus altissima*
▷ **Trees** see pp.32–33
▷ **Tree tomato** see *Cyphomandra*
▷ **Trefoil,**
  Double bird's foot see *Lotus corniculatus* 'Plenus'
  Moon see *Medicago arborea*
▷ ***Trichinium manglesii*** see *Ptilotus manglesii*
▷ ***Trichocereus bridgesii*** see *Echinopsis lageniformis*
▷ ***Trichocereus candicans*** see *Echinopsis candicans*
▷ ***Trichocereus grandiflorus*** see *Echinopsis huascha*
▷ ***Trichocereus huascha*** see *Echinopsis huascha*
▷ ***Trichocereus shaferi*** see *Echinopsis schickendantzii*
▷ ***Trichocereus spachianus*** see *Echinopsis spachiana*

TRICHODIADEMA

AIZOACEAE

Genus of about 30 species of mainly small, tuberous, fibrous, or woody-based, shrubby, succulent perennials found in dry, hilly areas in Namibia, South Africa, and Ethiopia. The long-lasting, solitary, short-stalked, daisy-like, terminal flowers are borne on long or short stems in daytime, from spring to autumn. Semi-cylindrical to cylindrical

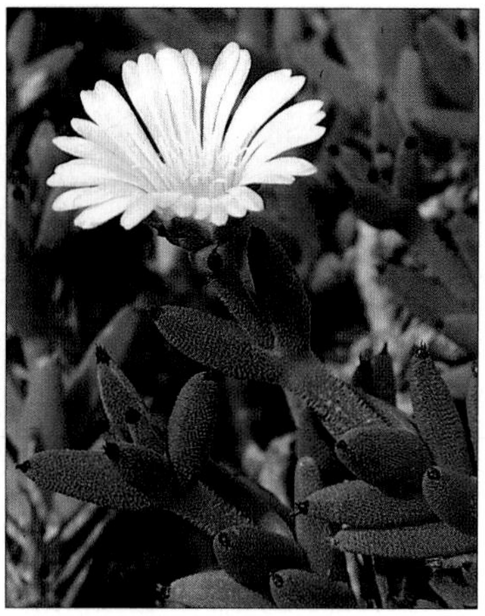

Trichodiadema mirabile

leaves are sparsely covered with minute papillae, producing a glistening effect, and the leaf tips bear clusters of stiff, spreading or erect, shiny bristles. Below 7°C (45°F), grow in a temperate greenhouse. In warm, dry areas, grow in a border with other succulents.

• **HARDINESS** Frost tender.
• **CULTIVATION** Under glass, grow in standard cactus compost in full light, with low humidity. In growth, water moderately and apply a low-nitrogen fertilizer every 3 or 4 weeks; keep dry at other times. Outdoors, grow in gritty, sharply drained, poor to moderately fertile soil in full sun. See also pp.48–49.
• **PROPAGATION** Sow seed at 19–24°C (66–75°F), or insert cuttings of stem sections, in spring or summer.
• **PESTS AND DISEASES** Susceptible to mealybugs early in the season.

T. bulbosum ♀ Semi-erect, short- to long-stemmed succulent with an almost caudex-like, tuberous rootstock and semi-cylindrical, grey-papillose leaves, to 8mm (3/8in) long, with white bristles. Deep red flowers, 2cm (3/4in) across, are borne from spring to autumn. ↕20cm (8in), ↔ 30cm (12in). South Africa (Eastern Cape). ❀ (min. 7°C/45°F)

T. mirabile ▣ Short-stemmed, often prostrate succulent with a fibrous rootstock, and stems covered with bristly white hairs. Semi-cylindrical, finger-like leaves, to 2.5cm (1in) long, are flat above, and have blunt tips with stiff, dark brown bristles. White flowers, 4cm (1½in) across, are produced in summer. ↕10cm (4in), ↔ 12cm (5in) or more. South Africa (Eastern Cape, Karoo). ❀ (min. 7°C/45°F)

TRICHOSANTHES

CUCURBITACEAE

Genus of 15 species of monoecious or dioecious, annual and perennial tendril climbers found in woodland and scrub from Indonesia and Malaysia to the Pacific islands. They are grown mainly for their colourful, ornamental, mostly ovoid or spherical gourd fruits, which are edible when young. The alternate leaves are ovate to rounded, and simple or palmately 3- to 9-lobed. Parasol-like, fringed, 5-lobed flowers are produced from the upper leaf axils in summer, the females singly, the males in racemes or, rarely, singly. In frost-prone areas, grow in a warm greenhouse; elsewhere, train over a pergola, arch, or tree stump.

• **HARDINESS** Frost tender.
• **CULTIVATION** Under glass, grow in loam-based potting compost (JI No.3) in full light with shade from hot sun, with high humidity. During growth, water freely and apply a balanced liquid fertilizer every 2 weeks. Water sparingly in winter. For good fruit production, pollinate by hand. Outdoors, grow in moist but well-drained, fertile soil in full sun. Provide support for climbing stems.
• **PROPAGATION** Sow seed at 20°C (68°F) in spring. Insert softwood cuttings with bottom heat in summer.
• **PESTS AND DISEASES** Susceptible to red spider mites and whiteflies under glass.

T. anguina see *T. cucumerina* var. *anguina*.

T. cucumerina. Dioecious, annual climber with slender, 5-angled stems and rounded-kidney-shaped to broadly ovate, 5- to 7-lobed, toothed, rich green leaves, 6–13cm (2½–5in) long. Bears pure white flowers, 5cm (2in) across, in summer. Ovoid to conical fruit, 6cm (2½in) long, are yellowish green with red seeds. ↕3–5m (10–15ft) or more. India to Malaysia and N. Australia. ❀ (min. 15°C/59°F). **var. *anguina***, syn. *T. anguina* (Serpent cucumber, Snake gourd), has shallowly to deeply 3- to 7-lobed leaves, to 15cm (6in) long, and slender, twisted, pointed fruit, 0.3–2m (1–6ft) long, white-striped when young, orange when ripe; Pakistan to India.

▷ ***Trichosma suavis*** see *Eria coronaria*
▷ ***Tricuspidaria lanceolata*** see *Crinodendron hookerianum*

TRICYRTIS

Toad lily

CONVALLARIACEAE/LILIACEAE

Genus of about 16 species of rhizomatous or stoloniferous herbaceous perennials occurring in moist woodland and on mountains and cliffs from the E. Himalayas to the Philippines. Erect or arching, usually hairy stems bear alternate, sometimes 2-ranked, oblong to lance-shaped, pointed, pale to dark green, usually stem-clasping leaves; they are often glossy, sometimes spotted darker green, and have prominent veins. The flowers are star-shaped, open bell-shaped, or funnel-shaped with the tips opened out. They each have 6 tepals, the outer 3 with basal bulges, and are borne singly or in clusters from the leaf axils, or in terminal or axillary cymes. Toad

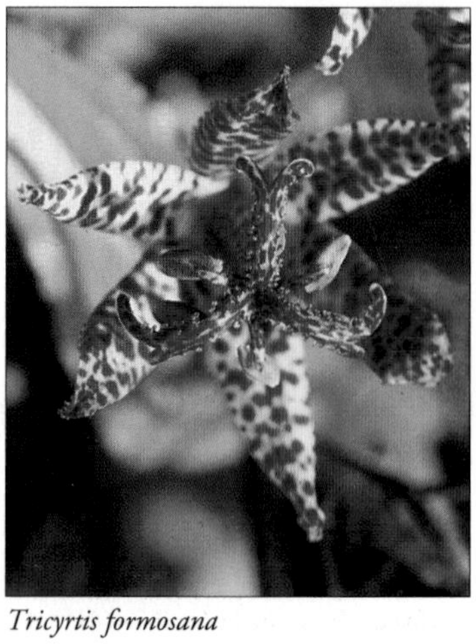

Tricyrtis formosana

T

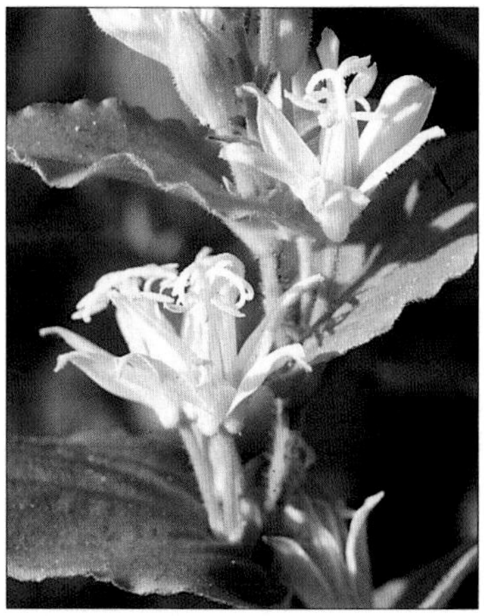

Tricyrtis hirta var. *alba*

lilies are suitable for a woodland garden, a shady border, or a peat bank.

• **HARDINESS** Fully hardy.

• **CULTIVATION** Grow in moist but well-drained, humus-rich soil in deep or partial shade. *T. latifolia* tolerates drier conditions and may spread widely. *T. macrantha* and *T. macrantha* subsp. *macranthopsis* prefer deep shade and very moist soil. In colder areas, grow the late-blooming species in a sheltered, warm but not sunny position to encourage flowering before frosts. Provide a deep winter mulch in areas where prolonged cold is not accompanied by snow cover.

• **PROPAGATION** Sow seed as soon as ripe in containers in a cold frame; where frost is severe, overwinter young plants in a cold greenhouse for the first winter. Divide in early spring, when dormant.

• **PESTS AND DISEASES** Slugs and snails may attack young spring growth.

T. bakeri see *T. latifolia.*

T. flava. Clump-forming perennial with short rhizomes, erect, softly hairy stems, and broadly ovate, veined, mid-green leaves, to 14cm (5½in) long, often with dark purplish green spots. In early autumn, upward-facing, star-shaped yellow flowers, to 2.5cm (1in) across, spotted brownish-purple, are borne singly or in clusters from the upper leaf axils. ↕ 30–50cm (12–20in), ↔ 30cm (12in). Japan. ❄❄❄. **subsp. *ohsumiensis*** see *T. ohsumiensis.*

T. formosana ■ ♀ syn. *T. stolonifera.* Rhizomatous perennial, spreading by stolons, with erect, somewhat zig-zagging, softly hairy stems, and inversely lance-shaped to ovate, veined, glossy, dark green leaves, to 12cm (5in) long, spotted darker purplish green. In early autumn, produces branched, terminal cymes of upward-facing, star-shaped, white to pinkish white or pinkish purple flowers, 2.5–3cm (1–1¼in) across; they are spotted reddish purple inside, with yellow tepal bases and heavily red-spotted white stigmas. ↕ to 80cm (32in), ↔ 45cm (18in). Taiwan. ❄❄❄

T. hirta, syn. *T. japonica.* Clump-forming, rhizomatous perennial with densely hairy stems and lance-shaped, veined, hairy, pale green leaves, to 15cm (6in) long, heart-shaped at the bases. From late summer to mid-autumn, erect, funnel-shaped, purple-spotted white flowers, to 3cm (1¼in) long, with purple stigmas and spreading then recurved tepals, are produced singly or in clusters from the leaf axils, or in

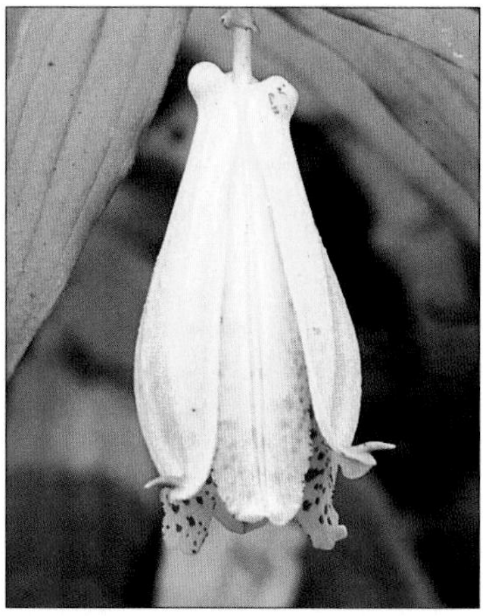

Tricyrtis macrantha subsp. *macranthopsis*

terminal or axillary cymes. ↕ to 80cm (32in), ↔ 60cm (24in). Japan. ❄❄❄. **var. *alba*** ■ has green-flushed white flowers with pink-tinged anthers. **'Miyazaki'** bears white flowers, spotted lilac-purple, in the leaf axils all along the stems; ↕ to 90cm (36in), ↔ 45cm (18in). **'White Towers'** has erect stems, and bears upward-facing white flowers, with pink-tinged stamens, in most of the leaf axils; ↕ to 60cm (24in), ↔ 30cm (12in).

T. japonica see *T. hirta.*

T. latifolia, syn. *T. bakeri.* Spreading, clump-forming perennial with short rhizomes, erect to arching, hairy stems, and broadly ovate-oblong, veined, glossy, mid-green leaves, to 15cm (6in) long, with heart-shaped bases, spotted darker green when young. In early and midsummer, produces upward-facing, trumpet- then star-shaped flowers, to 2.5cm (1in) across, with spreading, brown-spotted tepals, yellow inside and greenish yellow outside, in branched, terminal cymes. ↕ to 80cm (32in), ↔ 90cm (36in). China, Japan. ❄❄❄

T. macrantha. Tufted perennial with short rhizomes, arching or decumbent, brown-hairy stems, and ovate to lance-shaped, veined, glossy, dark green leaves, 10–15cm (4–6in) long, heart-shaped at the bases. In early and mid-autumn, bears pendent, bell-shaped, deep yellow flowers, 3–4cm (1¼–1½in) long, with thick, fleshy tepals, spotted red-brown inside, in few-flowered cymes from the upper leaf axils. ↕ 40–80cm (16–32in), ↔ 30cm (12in). Japan. ❄❄❄. **subsp. *macranthopsis*** ■ syn. *T. macranthopsis,* has hairless stems, with leaves to 17cm (7in) long, and bears axillary or terminal cymes in mid- and late autumn.

T. macranthopsis see *T. macrantha* subsp. *macranthopsis.*

T. ohsumiensis ■ syn. *T. flava* subsp. *ohsumiensis.* Clump-forming perennial with short rhizomes, erect to arching, hairy stems, and oblong-lance-shaped, veined, pale green leaves, 5–20cm (2–8in) long, marked darker green, the lower ones larger and elliptic-oblong. In early autumn, upward-facing, broadly bell-shaped yellow flowers, 2.5–3cm (1–1¼in) long, faintly brown-spotted inside, especially the stigmas, are borne singly or in axillary clusters. ↕ to 50cm (20in), ↔ 23cm (9in). Japan. ❄❄❄

T. perfoliata. Spreading, rhizomatous perennial with almost decumbent, zig-zagging, hairless stems. Perfoliate, broadly lance-shaped, veined, leathery, glossy, mid-green leaves, 7–18cm (3–7in) long, have long, tapered tips. Upward-facing, funnel-shaped yellow flowers, to 3cm (1¼in) long, sparsely spotted brownish red, are borne singly from the upper leaf axils in late spring. ↕ to 70cm (28in), ↔ 25cm (10in). Japan. ❄❄❄

T. stolonifera see *T. formosana.*

TRIFOLIUM

Clover

LEGUMINOSAE/PAPILIONACEAE

Genus of about 240 species of erect or creeping annuals, biennials, and herbaceous perennials, usually found on scree or in grassy meadows or scrub worldwide, except in Australasia, and mainly in the N. hemisphere. The 3-

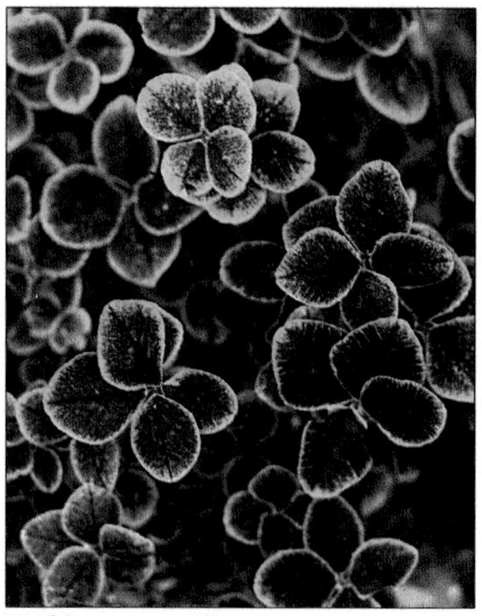

Trifolium repens 'Purpurascens Quadrifolium'

palmate leaves, rarely up to 7-palmate, have entire or toothed leaflets, usually with stipules. Small, pea-like flowers are produced in heads or in short, terminal or axillary spike-like racemes (or, rarely, singly), in spring or summer, and are attractive to bees. Many clovers are invasive weeds. The others are suitable for a border or a wildflower garden.

• **HARDINESS** Fully hardy.

• **CULTIVATION** Grow in moist but well-drained, neutral soil in full sun.

• **PROPAGATION** Sow seed in containers in a cold frame in spring. Divide, or detach and replant rooted stems, in spring.

• **PESTS AND DISEASES** Trouble free.

T. incarnatum (Crimson clover, Italian clover). Erect, bushy, downy-stemmed annual with 3-palmate leaves, to 3cm (1¼in) long, with obovate-wedge-shaped leaflets, finely toothed towards the tips. In spring and summer, bears oblong, spike-like racemes, to 1.5cm (½in) across, of 5–8 deep red to creamy yellow flowers. ↕↔ 20–50cm (8–20in). S. and W. Europe. ❄❄❄

***T. pratense* 'Dolly North'** see *T. pratense* 'Susan Smith'.

***T. pratense* 'Goldnet'** see *T. pratense* 'Susan Smith'.

***T. pratense* 'Susan Smith',** syn. *T. pratense* 'Dolly North', *T. pratense* 'Goldnet'. Mat-forming perennial with 3-palmate leaves, to 3.5cm (1½in) long, with obovate to broadly elliptic, entire leaflets, usually notched at the tips, with vein-like gold markings, hairy beneath. In early and midsummer, bears dense, spherical to ovoid, axillary, spike-like racemes, to 2cm (¾in) across, of 5–9 pink flowers. ↕ 15cm (6in), ↔ 45cm (18in). ❄❄❄

T. repens (Dutch clover, Shamrock, White clover). The species is very invasive, and a weed of lawns. **'Purpurascens Quadrifolium'** ■ is a vigorous, rhizomatous, stem-rooting perennial with 4-palmate leaves, 2–3cm (¾–1¼in) long, divided into inversely heart-shaped leaflets with deep purple maroon centres and narrow, mid-green margins. Small, pea-like white flowers are produced in dense, umbel-like racemes, 1.5–2cm (½–¾in) across, in summer. ↕ to 10cm (4in), ↔ indefinite. Europe. ❄❄❄.

▷**Trigger plant** see *Stylidium graminifolium*

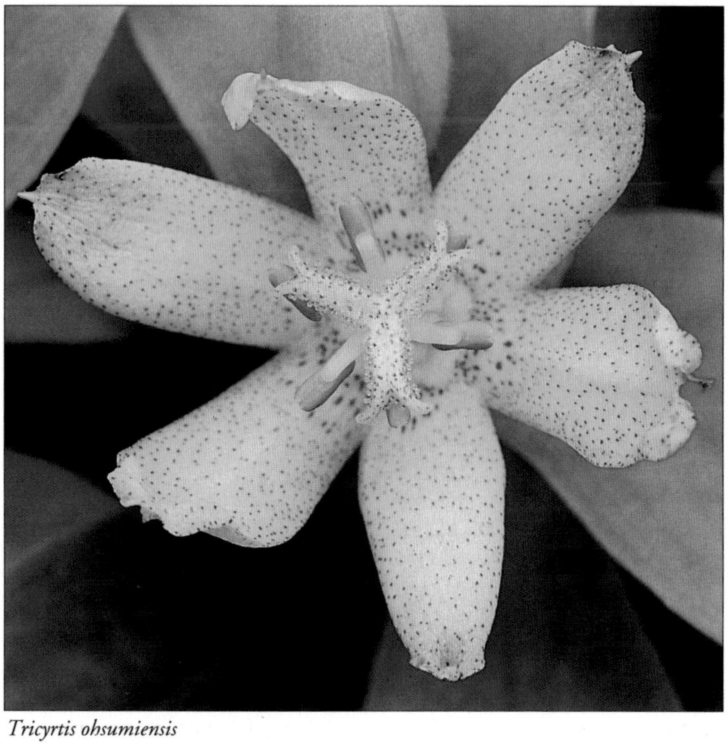

Tricyrtis ohsumiensis

TRILLIUM

Trinity flower, Wake robin, Wood lily

LILIACEAE/TRILLIACEAE

Genus of about 30 species of rhizomatous, deciduous perennials, occurring mainly in woodland and scrub in North America, with a few species in the W. Himalayas and N.E. Asia. Erect, rarely procumbent, short stems each bear an apical whorl of 3 lance-shaped or elliptic to ovate or diamond-shaped, net-veined, often silver- or purple-marbled leaves. Upright or nodding, terminal, solitary, funnel- or cup-shaped flowers, with whorls of 3 leaf-like, often reflexed outer sepals, and 3 inner petals, are either stalkless supported by the leaves, or stalked and borne above or below the leaves. Suitable for a moist, shady border or woodland garden. Grow the smallest species, *T. nivale* and *T. rivale*, on a peat bank, where they will not be overwhelmed by other plants.

- **HARDINESS** Fully hardy.
- **CULTIVATION** Grow in moist but well-drained, deep, humus-rich, preferably acid to neutral soil, although some will grow in moderately alkaline soils, in deep or partial shade. Mulch annually in autumn with leaf mould.
- **PROPAGATION** Sow seed as soon as ripe in containers in a shaded cold frame; leaves will not usually appear until the second spring, and plants take 5–7 years to reach flowering size. Divide rhizomes after flowering, ensuring that each section has at least one growing point; divisions may be slow to re-establish. Alternatively, cut out the growing point from the rhizome after flowering, which stimulates formation of offsets.
- **PESTS AND DISEASES** Young leaves may be damaged by slugs and snails.

T. catesbaei, syn. *T. catesbyi*, *T. nervosum*, *T. stylosum*. Slender, clump-forming perennial with red-pink-tinted stems and almost stalkless, elliptic to ovate, deeply veined leaves, to 7cm (3in)

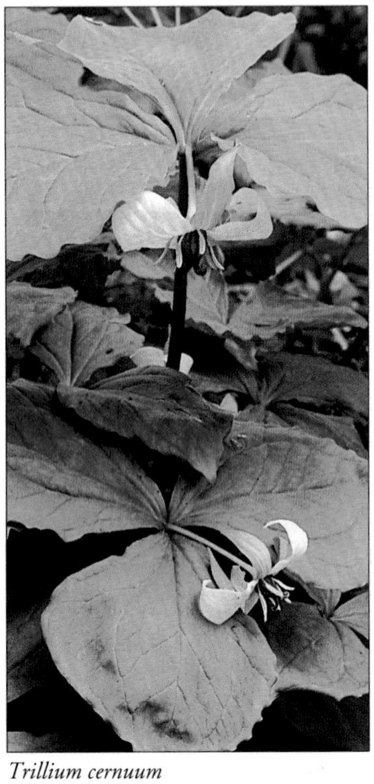

Trillium cernuum

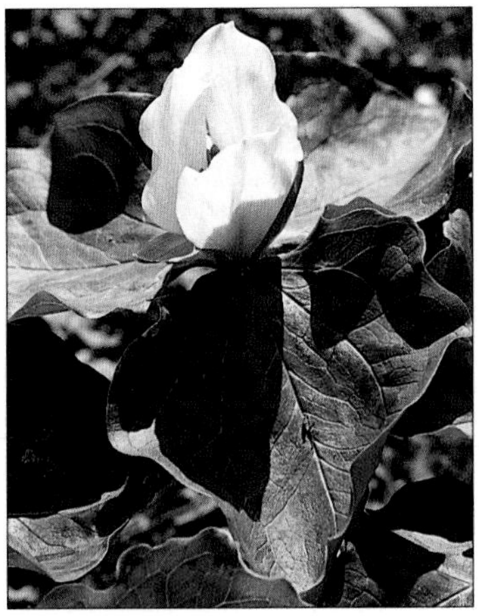

Trillium chloropetalum

long. Stalked, nodding, pale to deep pink flowers, with ovate to heart-shaped petals, to 5cm (2in) long, reflexed, mid-green sepals, and pale green ovaries, are borne beneath or among the leaves in spring and summer. ↕ to 50cm (20in), ↔ to 15cm (6in). S.E. USA. ***

T. catesbyi see *T. catesbaei*.

T. cernuum ■ Clump-forming perennial with short-stalked, broadly diamond-shaped, abruptly pointed, mid-green leaves, 5–15cm (2–6in) long, with moderately conspicuous veining. Pale pink, sometimes reddish brown, occasionally white flowers, with recurved, wavy petals, to 2cm (¾in) long, prominent purple stamens, and dark red ovaries, are borne on reflexed, pendent stalks, beneath or among the leaves, in spring. ↕ to 60cm (24in), ↔ to 25cm (10in). E. North America. ***. **f. *album*** has white flowers.

T. chloropetalum ■ ♀ Robust, clump-forming perennial with thick, hairless, red-green stems. Stalkless, broadly ovate to diamond-shaped, dark green leaves, 10–20cm (4–8in) long, are variably marbled greyish cream or maroon. Upright, stalkless, fragrant flowers, with obovate, greenish white, yellow, or brownish purple petals, 5–10cm (2–4in) long, and spreading, lance-shaped sepals, are borne above or among the leaves, in spring. ↕ to 40cm (16in), ↔ to 20cm (8in). USA (California). ***

T. cuneatum, syn. *T. sessile* of gardens. Robust, upright, clump-forming perennial with stalkless, broadly ovate-rounded, often pointed, mid-green leaves, to 20cm (8in) long, marked pale or silver-green. In spring, upright, stalkless, musk-scented, dark maroon flowers, with wedge-shaped petals, 5cm (2in) or more long, and purple-tipped, olive-green sepals, are borne above the leaves. Similar to *T. sessile*; often sold under that name. ↕ 30–60cm (12–24in), ↔ to 30cm (12in). S.E. USA. ***

T. erectum ■ ♀ (Birth root, Stinking Benjamin). Vigorous, upright perennial with stalkless, broadly ovate, mid-green leaves, to 20cm (8in) long. In spring, stalked, upright or outward-facing flowers, with pointed, elliptic, spreading or incurved petals, to 8cm (3in) long, are borne above the leaves; flowers are deep red-purple, occasionally white or yellow, with purple-tinted green sepals and purple ovaries. ↕ to 50cm (20in), ↔ to 30cm (12in). E. North America. ***. **f. *albiflorum*** has white or pale pink petals with dark purple ovaries.

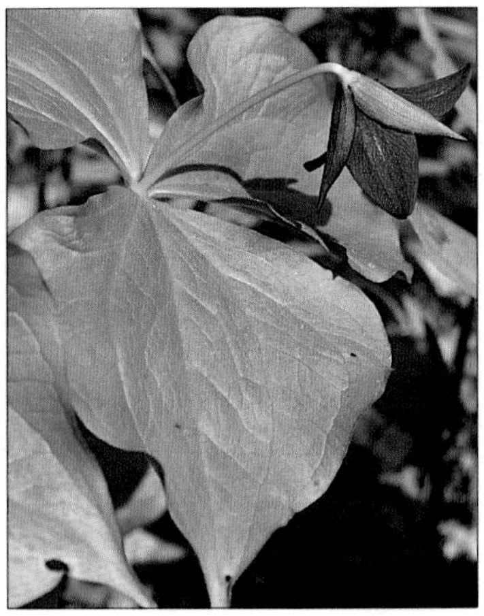

Trillium erectum

T. grandiflorum ■ ♀ (Wake robin). Vigorous, clump-forming perennial with almost stalkless, ovate to rounded, dark green leaves, to 30cm (12in) long. In spring and summer, pure white flowers, often fading to pink, with green sepals, are produced above the leaves; they are stalked, erect or outward-facing, cupped at first, then opening widely, with broadly ovate, slightly wavy petals, to 8cm (3in) long, reflexing near the tips. ↕ to 40cm (16in), ↔ 30cm (12in) or more. E. North America. ***. **'Flore Pleno'** ♀ is slower-growing, with very attractive, formal double flowers. Several variants with slightly differing double flowers are grown under this name.

T. kamtschaticum. Upright perennial with stalkless, ovate to diamond-shaped, abruptly pointed, dark green leaves, to

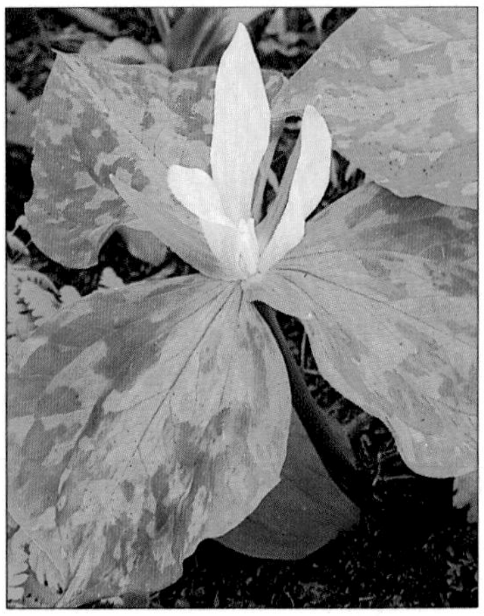

Trillium luteum

15cm (6in) long. Stalked, upright flowers, with ovate white petals, to 4.5cm (1¾in) long, sometimes purple-flushed with age, and dark green sepals, are produced above the leaves in late spring and early summer. ↕ to 25cm (10in), ↔ to 20cm (8in). E. Asia. ***

T. luteum ■ ♀ Upright, clump-forming perennial with stalkless, elliptic to broadly ovate, abruptly pointed, mid-green leaves, to 15cm (6in) long, heavily marked paler green. Stalkless, upright, sweet-scented, golden- or bronze-green flowers, with inversely lance-shaped to obovate or narrowly elliptic petals, to 9cm (3½in) long, and lance-shaped, mid-green sepals, are produced above the leaves in spring. ↕ to 40cm (16in), ↔ to 30cm (12in). S.E. USA. ***

T. nervosum see *T. catesbaei*.

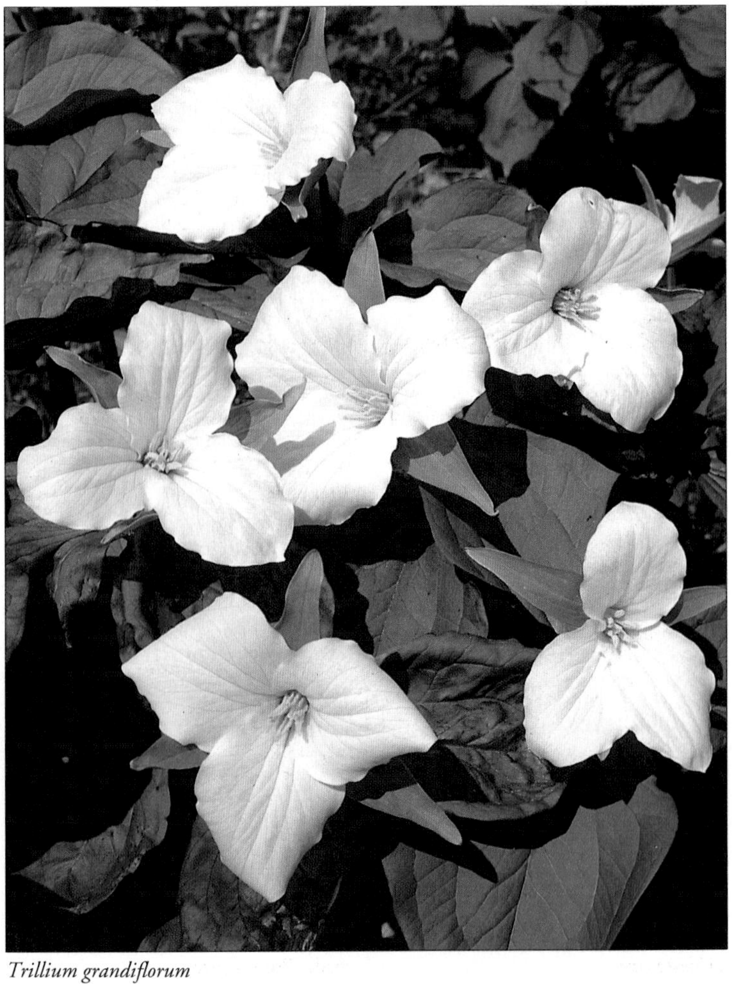

Trillium grandiflorum

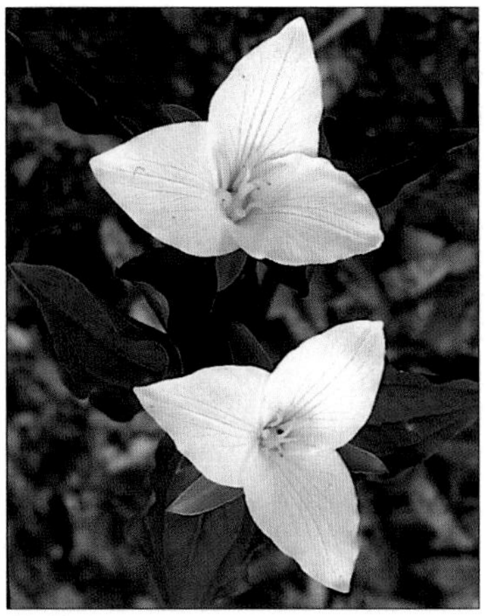

Trillium ovatum

T. nivale (Dwarf white wood lily, Snow trillium). Compact, clump-forming perennial with stalked, ovate, dark bluish green leaves, to 3.5cm (1½in) long. Bears short-stalked, upright, pure white flowers, with oblong petals, to 4cm (1½in) long, and green sepals and ovaries, above the leaves in early spring. Not easy to grow. ↕ to 12cm (5in), ↔ to 10cm (4in). S.E. USA. ❄❄❄
T. ovatum ■ Clump-forming perennial with red-green stems and stalkless, diamond-shaped, pointed, dark green leaves, to 15cm (6in) long, each with 5 conspicuous sunken veins. In spring, stalked, upright, musk-scented, pure white flowers, fading to pink or red, with spreading, ovate petals, 2.5–7cm (1–3in) long, and green sepals, are borne above the leaves. ↕ to 50cm (20in), ↔ to 20cm (8in). W. North America. ❄❄❄
T. recurvatum. Upright, clump-forming perennial with lance-shaped to elliptic, mottled, mid-green leaves, to 8cm (3in) long, tapering to short stalks. In spring, upright, stalkless, deep maroon, occasionally white or yellow flowers are produced above the leaves; they have lance-shaped to ovate petals, to 5cm (2in) long, clawed at the bases, and strongly recurving green sepals. ↕ to 40cm (16in), ↔ to 30cm (12in). E. USA. ❄❄❄
T. rivale ■ ♀ Dwarf, upright perennial with stalked, ovate, pointed, mid-green leaves, to 3cm (1¼in) long. In spring, stalked, upright, white or pale pink flowers, spotted purple at the bases, with diamond-shaped to ovate petals, to 2.5cm (1in) long, and green sepals, are produced above the leaves. Similar to

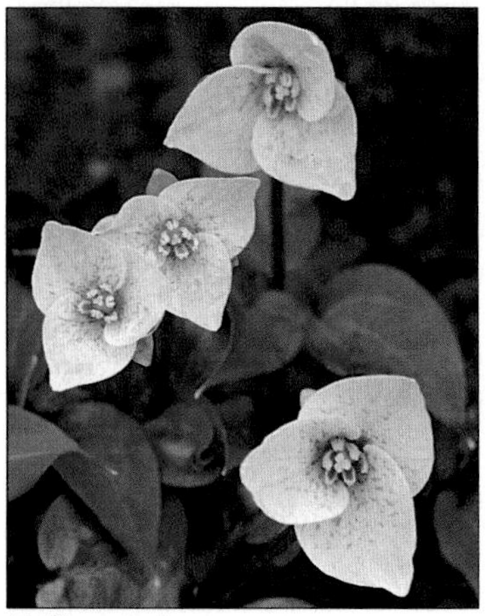

Trillium rivale

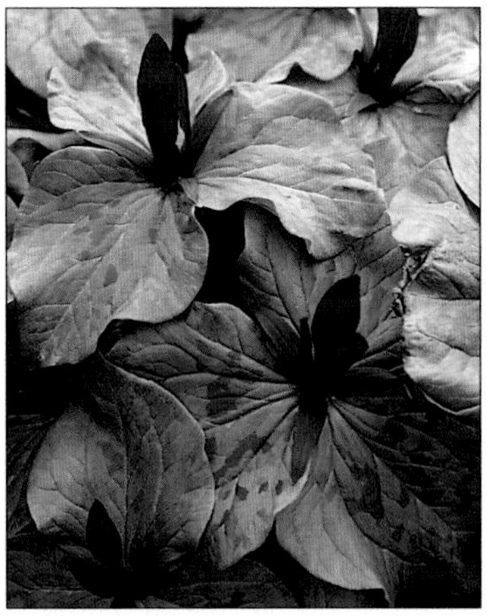

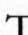

Trillium sessile

T. nivale, but easier to grow. ↕ to 12cm (5in), ↔ to 15cm (6in). W. USA. ❄❄❄
T. sessile ■ (Toad-shade, Wake robin). Upright, clump-forming perennial with stalkless, broadly elliptic to rounded, deep green leaves, to 12cm (5in) long, marbled pale green, grey-white, and bronze-maroon. Stalkless, upright, red-maroon, rarely greenish yellow flowers, with lance-shaped petals, to 4.5cm (1¾in) long, and spreading, maroon-flushed green sepals, are borne above the leaves in late spring. ↕ to 30cm (12in), ↔ to 20cm (8in). N.E. USA. ❄❄❄
***T. sessile* of gardens** see *T. cuneatum.*
T. stylosum see *T. catesbaei.*
T. undulatum (Painted trillium, Painted wood lily). Graceful, clump-forming perennial with erect, pale green stems, flushed pink at the bases, and stalked, narrowly ovate, tapered, dark blue-green leaves, to 15cm (6in) long. In late spring, stalked, upright, white or very pale pink flowers, with wavy petals, to 3cm (1¼in) long, with dark red, V-shaped marks at the bases and maroon-margined, dark green sepals, are borne above the leaves. Not easy to grow; needs moist, acid soil. ↕ to 30cm (12in), ↔ to 15cm (6in). E. USA. ❄❄❄
T. viride. Upright perennial with sometimes downy stems, and stalkless, lance-shaped to elliptic, mid-green leaves, 8–15cm (3–6in) long, spotted white above. Stalkless, upright, malodorous, yellow-green flowers, sometimes maroon at the bases, occasionally completely maroon, with narrowly lance-shaped petals, to 7cm (3in) long, and green sepals, are borne above the leaves in spring. ↕ to 40cm (16in), ↔ to 20cm (8in). USA (Illinois, Missouri). ❄❄❄

▷**Trillium,**
Painted see *Trillium undulatum*
Snow see *Trillium nivale*
▷**Trinity flower** see *Trillium*

TRIPETALEIA
syn. ELLIOTTIA
ERICACEAE

Genus of 2 species of deciduous shrubs found in mountain woodland in Japan. They are cultivated for their terminal panicles of attractive, 3-petalled, sometimes 4- or 5-petalled flowers. Grow in a peat, rock, or woodland garden.
• **HARDINESS** Fully hardy.
• **CULTIVATION** Grow in moist but well-drained, humus-rich, acid soil in partial shade. Pruning group 1.
• **PROPAGATION** Sow seed in containers in a cold frame in autumn. Insert softwood cuttings in summer.
• **PESTS AND DISEASES** Trouble free.

T. paniculata, syn. *Elliottia paniculata.* Upright, deciduous shrub with alternate, obovate to narrowly ovate-elliptic, dark green leaves, to 6cm (2½in) long. From midsummer to early autumn, pink-tinged white flowers, 2cm (¾in) across, with 3 or 5 narrow, twisted petals, are borne in upright, terminal panicles, to 15cm (6in) long. ↕↔ 1.5m (5ft). Japan. ❄❄❄

TRIPTERYGIUM
CELASTRACEAE

Genus of 2 or 3 species of deciduous, scrambling to twining climbers from deciduous woodland in E. Asia. They have large, alternate, ovate or broadly ovate to elliptic leaves. Abundant tiny, 5-petalled, saucer-shaped flowers are borne in terminal panicles, followed by prominently winged fruits. *T. regelii*, the most commonly cultivated species, is suitable for training on a house wall or over a pergola, tree, or tall tree stump. In frost-prone areas, grow half-hardy species in a cool greenhouse.
• **HARDINESS** Frost hardy to half hardy.
• **CULTIVATION** Grow in moist but well-drained, fertile soil in full sun. Pruning group 11, in spring.
• **PROPAGATION** Sow seed in containers in a cold frame as soon as ripe. Root semi-ripe cuttings in summer with bottom heat. Layer in early spring.
• **PESTS AND DISEASES** Trouble free.

T. regelii. Bushy, twining climber, often loosely shrubby when young, producing slightly angled, warty stems and long-stalked, ovate or broadly ovate to elliptic, slender-pointed, toothed, bright green leaves, 8–13cm (3–5in) long. In summer, small, saucer-shaped, green-tinted white flowers are borne in leafy panicles, to 25cm (10in) long, followed by 3-winged, pale green to light brown fruit, 1.5–2cm (½–¾in) long. ↕ to 10m (30ft). China, Korea, Japan. ❄❄

▷ ***Tristagma* 'Rolf Fiedler'** see *Ipheion* 'Rolf Fiedler'
▷ ***Tristagma uniflorum*** see *Ipheion uniflorum*
▷ ***Tristania conferta*** see *Lophostemon confertus*

TRITELEIA
ALLIACEAE/LILIACEAE

Genus of about 15 species of cormous perennials, closely related to *Brodiaea*, mainly found in grassland, chaparral, and pine woodland in W. USA. They are cultivated for their umbels of funnel-shaped flowers, borne on leafless stems. The semi-erect, narrowly linear, basal leaves usually die away by flowering time. Suitable for a warm, sunny, mixed or herbaceous border. In areas prone to severe frosts, grow in a cold greenhouse or alpine house.
• **HARDINESS** Frost hardy.
• **CULTIVATION** Plant corms 8cm (3in) deep in autumn. Outdoors, grow in light, sandy, fertile soil in full sun. Under glass, grow in loam-based potting compost (JI No.2), with added sharp

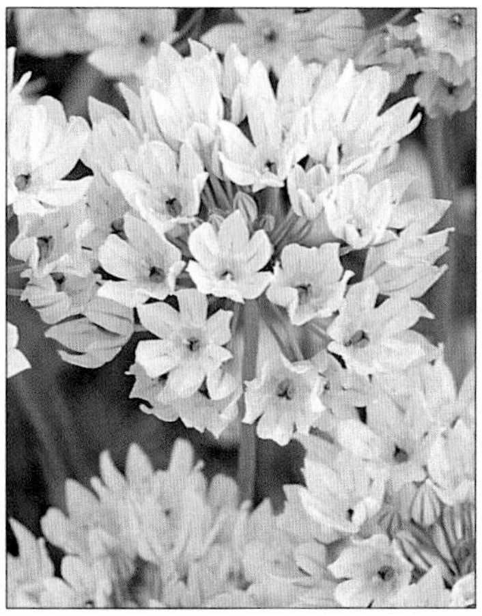

Triteleia hyacinthina

sand, in full light. After planting, water sparingly until leaves appear. In growth, water freely and apply a half-strength balanced liquid fertilizer monthly. Reduce water gradually after flowering; keep warm and dry when dormant.
• **PROPAGATION** Sow seed at 13–16°C (55–61°F) as soon as ripe or in early spring; seed-grown plants take 3–5 years to reach maturity. Separate corms when dormant.
• **PESTS AND DISEASES** Trouble free.

T. hyacinthina ■ syn. *Brodiaea hyacinthina, B. lactea.* Cormous perennial with linear, basal leaves, 10–40cm (4–16in) long. Flat umbels, 10cm (4in) across, of up to 20 or more white or pale blue flowers, 1.5cm (½in) long, are produced in late spring and early summer. ↕ to 70cm (28in), ↔ 5cm (2in). W. USA. ❄❄
T. ixioides, syn. *Brodiaea ixioides, B. lutea.* Cormous perennial with linear, basal leaves, 10–40cm (4–16in) long. Open umbels, 12cm (5in) across, of up to 25 yellow flowers, 1–2.5cm (½–1in) long, with purple midribs, are produced in early summer. ↕ to 60cm (24in), ↔ 8cm (3in). W. USA. ❄❄
T. laxa ■ syn. *Brodiaea laxa.* Showy, cormous perennial with linear, basal leaves, 20–40cm (8–16in) long. In early summer, produces loose umbels, 16cm (6in) across, of up to 25 pale to deep purple-blue flowers, 2–5cm (¾–2in) long, rarely white or shading to white at the bases. ↕ to 70cm (28in), ↔ 5cm (2in). W. USA. ❄❄. **'Koningin Fabiola'**, syn. 'Queen Fabiola', has purple-blue flowers, 5cm (2in) long.

T

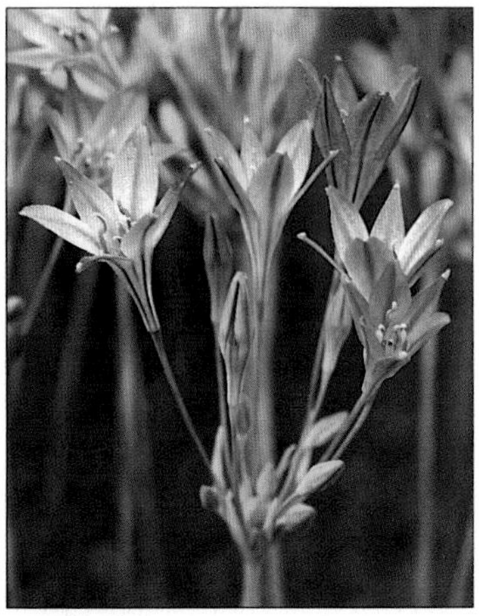

Triteleia laxa

T. peduncularis, syn. *Brodiaea peduncularis.* Cormous perennial with linear, basal leaves, 20–40cm (8–16in) long. In summer, produces lax umbels, 35cm (14in) across, of up to 20 white or pale blue flowers, 3cm (1¼in) long. ↕ to 40cm (16in), ↔ 8cm (3in). USA (California). ❄❄

TRITONIA

IRIDACEAE

Genus of 28 species of cormous perennials, closely related to *Crocosmia*, found mainly on grassy or stony hillsides in South Africa and Swaziland. They are grown for their slender spikes of funnel- or cup-shaped, colourful flowers. The 2-ranked leaves are usually linear to lance-shaped. Grow in a warm, sunny, mixed or herbaceous border. In frost-prone areas, grow half-hardy species in a cool greenhouse or conservatory.

- **HARDINESS** Frost hardy to half hardy.
- **CULTIVATION** Plant 10cm (4in) deep. Under glass, grow in loam-based potting compost (JI No.2), with added sharp sand, in full light. After flowering, water sparingly, until leaves appear; in full growth, water freely. As leaves wither after flowering, reduce water gradually to ensure a warm, dry dormancy. Repot annually. Outdoors, grow in light, well-drained, preferably sandy soil, in a sheltered site in full sun. Provide a deep, dry winter mulch. Avoid excessive moisture, especially when dormant.
- **PROPAGATION** Sow seed at 13–16°C (55–61°F) as soon as ripe. Remove offsets when dormant
- **PESTS AND DISEASES** Trouble free.

T. crocata, syn. *T. fenestrata, T. hyalina.* Cormous perennial with erect, lance-shaped, basal leaves, 5–30cm (2–12in) long. Spikes of up to 10 cup-shaped, orange to pinkish red flowers, 1.5cm (½in) long, are produced on arching, wiry stems in spring. ↕ 20–50cm (8–20in), ↔ 8cm (3in). South Africa (Western Cape, Eastern Cape). ❄. **'Princess Beatrix'** ■ bears brilliant orange-red flowers. **'White Glory'** has amber-tinged white flowers.

T. disticha, syn. *Crocosmia rosea.* Cormous perennial with erect, linear or lance- or sword-shaped, basal leaves, 25–70cm (10–28in) long. In mid- and late summer, irregular, funnel-shaped, orange-red, red, or pink flowers, 2cm (¾in) long, are borne in many-flowered spikes, on arching, branched stems.

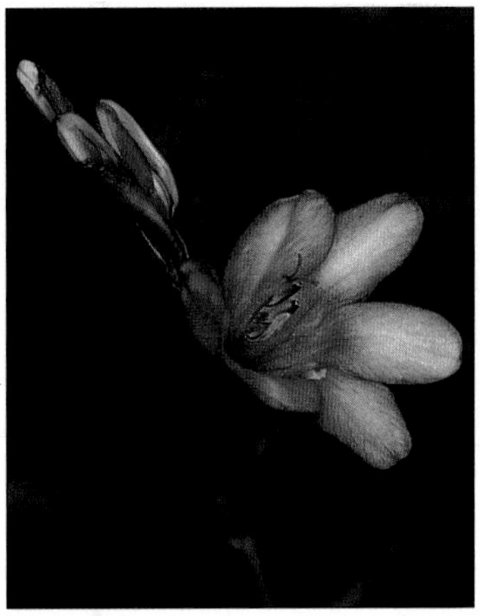
Tritonia disticha subsp. *rubrolucens*

↕ 50–100cm (20–39in), ↔ 5cm (2in). South Africa (Western Cape, Eastern Cape, Kwazulu/Natal). ❄❄. **subsp. *rubrolucens*** ■ syn. *T. rosea, T. rubrolucens*, bears a succession of open funnel-shaped pink flowers, 2.5–3.5cm (1–1½in) across, in one-sided spikes on wiry stems; South Africa (Eastern Cape, Orange Free State, Kwazulu/Natal, Eastern Transvaal), Swaziland.

T. fenestrata see *T. crocata.*

T. hyalina see *T. crocata.*

T. longiflora see *Ixia paniculata.*

T. rosea see *T. disticha* subsp. *rubrolucens.*

T. rubrolucens see *T. disticha* subsp. *rubrolucens.*

TROCHODENDRON

TROCHODENDRACEAE

Genus of one species of evergreen tree or large shrub from forest in Japan, Korea, and Taiwan. *T. aralioides* is grown for its handsome, spirally arranged leaves and its racemes of unusual, vivid green flowers. Grow in a woodland garden among other trees and shrubs.

- **HARDINESS** Frost hardy.
- **CULTIVATION** Grow in moist but well-drained, neutral to slightly acid soil in full sun or dappled shade. Shelter from cold, drying winds. Pruning group 1.
- **PROPAGATION** Sow seed in containers in a cold frame in autumn. Insert semi-ripe cuttings in summer.
- **PESTS AND DISEASES** Trouble free.

T. aralioides ■ ♀ Broadly columnar tree or large, rounded shrub with broadly ovate to elliptic, tapered, glossy, dark green leaves, to 12cm (5in) long. Racemes, to 12cm (5in) long, of 10–20 or more flowers are borne at the shoot-tips in late spring and early summer; the petalless, bright green flowers, 2cm (¾in) across, each consist of numerous stamens radiating from a central green disc. ↕ 10m (30ft), ↔ 8m (25ft). Japan (including Ryukyu Islands), Korea, Taiwan. ❄❄

TROLLIUS

Globeflower

RANUNCULACEAE

Genus of about 24 species of buttercup-like, hairless, clump-forming herbaceous perennials from moist or wet meadows in cool-temperate areas of Europe, Asia, and North America. They produce numerous fibrous roots, and basal rosettes of stalked, palmately lobed leaves, the lobes further divided or toothed. Erect stems usually bear a few mainly stalkless leaves. Both the basal and stem leaves are usually mid-green, sometimes glossy. Terminal, solitary, spherical to bowl-shaped flowers, with reduced or linear, petal-like sepals, nectary-bearing petals, and numerous stamens, are borne in spring or summer. Grow in a moist border or bog garden, or beside a pond or stream, or naturalize in a damp meadow garden.

- **HARDINESS** Fully hardy.
- **CULTIVATION** Grow in moist, deep, fertile, preferably heavy soil, which does not dry out, in full sun or partial shade. Cut stems back hard after first flush of flowers; apply a balanced liquid fertilizer to encourage further blooming. Earlier-flowering species and cultivars may be forced gently in a temperate greenhouse, to produce early flowers for cutting.
- **PROPAGATION** Sow seed in containers in a cold frame as soon as ripe or in spring; seed may take 2 years to germinate. Divide as new growth begins or immediately after flowering.
- **PESTS AND DISEASES** Powdery mildew may be a problem.

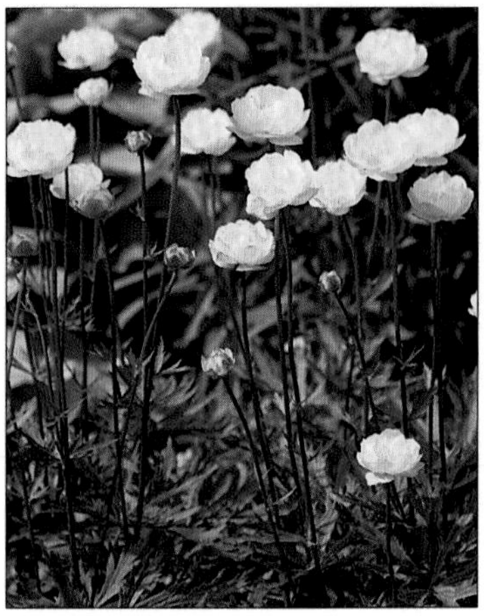
Trollius x *cultorum* 'Alabaster'

T. chinensis ■ syn. *T. ledebourii* of gardens. Clump-forming perennial bearing 5-lobed basal leaves, to 12cm (5in) long, with broadly lance-shaped, lobes divided into sharply toothed segments; the stem leaves are smaller. In midsummer, shallowly bowl-shaped, light orange-yellow flowers, 5cm (2in) across, with long petals, are produced on stout, furrowed stems. ↕ to 90cm (36in), ↔ 45cm (18in). N.E. China. ❄❄❄

***T. x cultorum* cultivars.** Clump-forming perennials with 5-lobed, toothed, glossy basal leaves, 18cm (7in) long, with lance-shaped lobes divided into toothed segments; stem leaves are smaller and more finely divided. Bowl-shaped flowers, 2.5–6cm (1–2½in) across, are borne from mid-spring to midsummer. ↕ to 90cm (36in), ↔ 45cm (18in). ❄❄❄. **'Alabaster'** ■ is less vigorous than most cultivars, and bears pale primrose-yellow flowers in mid- and late spring; ↕ to 60cm (24in), ↔ to 40cm (16in). **'Earliest of All'** ■ bears clear yellow flowers, 7cm (3in) across, in mid-spring; ↕ 50cm (20in), ↔ 40cm (16in). **'Feuertroll'**, syn. 'Fireglobe', produces rich orange-yellow flowers, with deeper orange stamens, in late

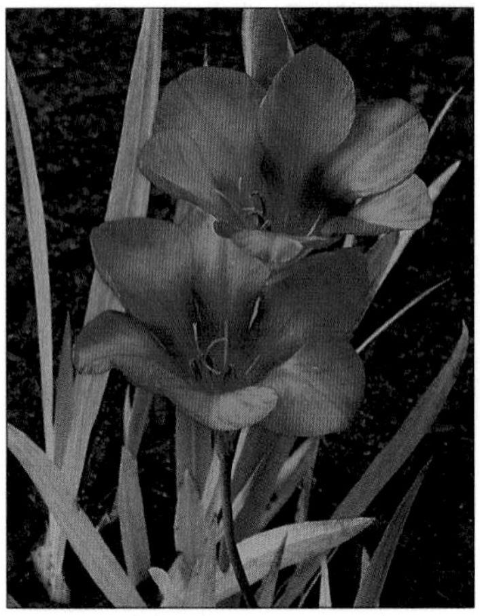
Tritonia crocata 'Princess Beatrix'

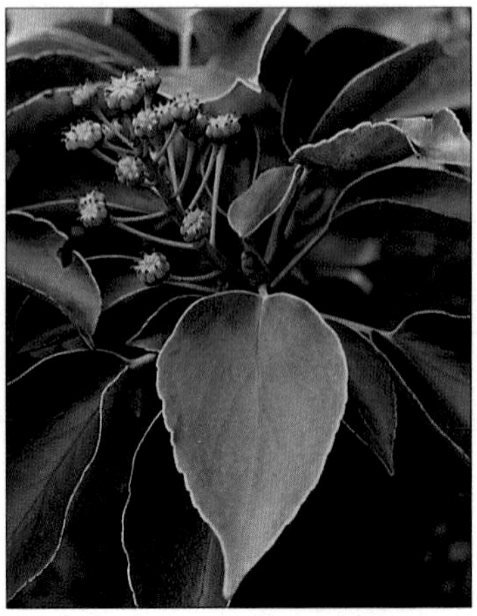
Trochodendron aralioides

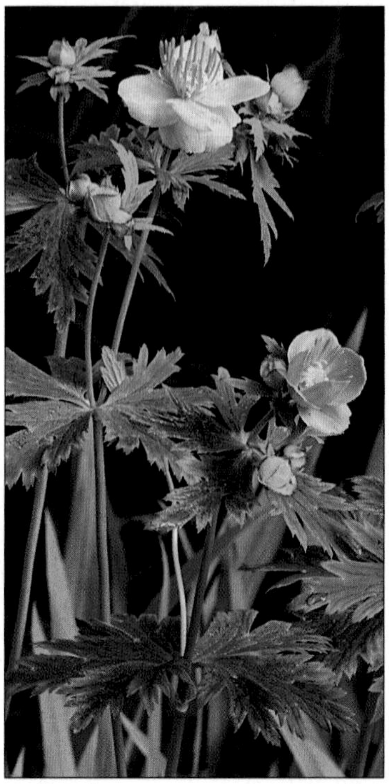
Trollius chinensis

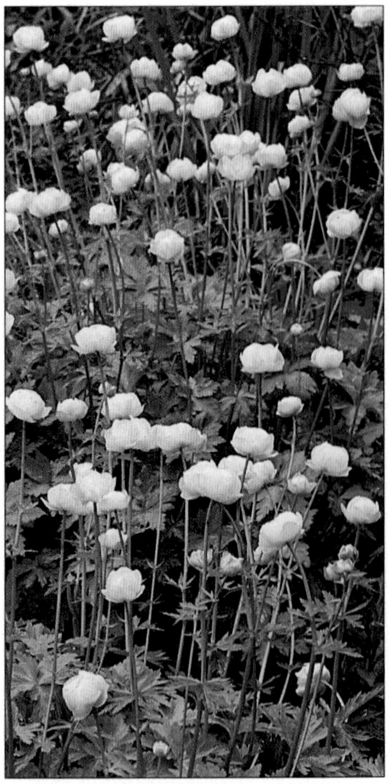
Trollius x *cultorum* 'Earliest of All'

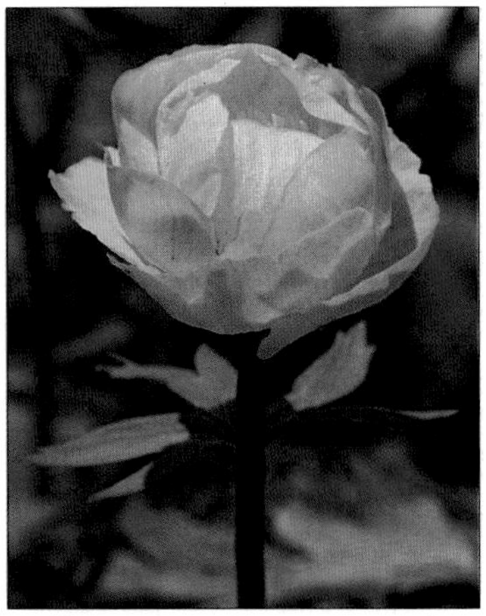

Trollius x *cultorum* 'Orange Princess'

spring; ↕ to 65cm (26in), ↔ 40cm (16in). **'Fireglobe'** see 'Feuertroll'. **'Gold Fountain'** see 'Goldquelle'. **'Goldquelle'** 🏆 syn. 'Gold Fountain', bears yellow flowers, 7cm (3in) across, in early and midsummer; ↕ to 70cm (28in). **'Lemon Queen'** bears pale yellow flowers, 7cm (3in) across, in late spring and early summer; ↕ 60cm (24in). **'Orange Princess'** ▣ 🏆 bears orange-gold flowers in late spring and early summer.

T. europaeus (Common European globeflower). Clump-forming, very variable perennial bearing 5-lobed basal leaves, to 12cm (5in) long, with wedge-shaped, deeply divided and toothed lobes. Erect, rarely branched stems produce smaller leaves and spherical, lemon-yellow flowers, 5cm (2in) across, in early and midsummer. ↕ 80cm (32in), ↔ 45cm (18in). Europe, Caucasus, North America. ✲✲✲. **'Canary Bird'** bears pale lemon-yellow flowers over a long period.

***T. ledebourii* of gardens** see *T. chinensis.*

T. pumilus ▣ Clump-forming, tufted perennial bearing 5-lobed, glossy basal leaves, 2–7cm (¾–3in) long, with oblong to lance-shaped, toothed lobes. In late spring and early summer, bears cup-shaped, deep golden yellow flowers, 2–3.5cm (¾–1½in) across, often red or purple-crimson on the outside. ↕ to 30cm (12in), ↔ to 20cm (8in). Himalayas, E. Tibet, China. ✲✲✲

T. yunnanensis. Clump-forming, tufted perennial bearing 3- to 5-lobed, glossy basal leaves, 5–12cm (2–5in) long, with ovate, toothed lobes; the stem leaves are similar but smaller. In late spring and early summer, produces cup-shaped, golden yellow flowers, 2–6cm (¾–2½in) across. ↕ to 70cm (28in), ↔ to 30cm (12in). S.W. China. ✲✲✲

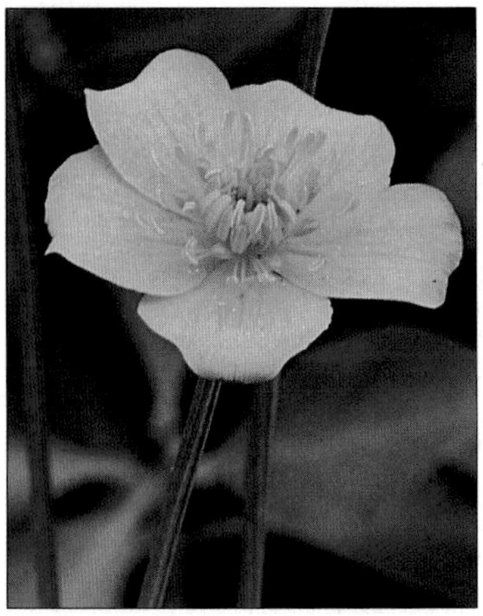

Trollius pumilus

▷**Trompetilla, Scarlet** see *Bouvardia ternifolia*

TROPAEOLUM

TROPAEOLACEAE

Genus of 80–90 species of hairless, climbing, trailing, or bushy annuals and herbaceous perennials, many with tuberous roots, found mainly in cool, mountainous areas in Central and South America. The alternate, rounded, peltate leaves are entire or palmately lobed to palmate with 5–7 lobes or leaflets; they have long leaf-stalks, which are used as the method of attachment in climbing species. Roughly funnel-shaped flowers, with 5 showy, clawed petals, often with prominent spurs, and 5 inconspicuous, pointed sepals, are borne singly from the leaf axils. Grow climbing tropaeolums over a fence, trellis, pergola, or non-flowering shrub, or allow to trail on a bank or dry wall. *T. polyphyllum* is suitable for a raised or scree bed, or a large rock garden. The dwarf, bushy *T. majus* hybrids and cultivars are effective in an annual bed or border; the trailing or semi-trailing variants are excellent for hanging baskets or other containers. In frost-prone areas, grow tender perennials in a cool greenhouse or conservatory. The leaves and flowers of annual tropaeolums are edible, and the young fruits of *T. majus* can be pickled.

• **HARDINESS** Frost hardy to frost tender.

• **CULTIVATION** Grow in moist but well-drained, moderately fertile soil, in full sun. *T. majus* and its hybrids and cultivars flower best in poorer soils; *T. speciosum* prefers moist, humus-rich, neutral to acid soil in full sun or partial shade, but with roots and lower stems in cool shade. Support the climbing stems. In frost-prone areas, lift the tubers of *T. tuberosum* and store in a frost-free place until the following spring. Under glass, grow in loam-based potting compost (JI No.2), with added fine grit, in full light with shade from hot sun. Plant those with running rootstocks directly into a border; tuberous tropaeolums need deep containers. During growth, water freely and apply a balanced liquid fertilizer monthly; reduce water as leaves wither and keep barely moist when dormant. *T. azureum* and *T. tricolorum* are both dormant in summer; start into growth in early autumn, and water sparingly in autumn and winter.

• **PROPAGATION** Sow seed of annuals at 13–16°C (55–61°F) in early spring or *in situ* in mid-spring. Sow seed of perennials in containers in a cold frame as soon as ripe; germination is often erratic. Separate tubers in autumn, when dormant. Divide *T. speciosum* carefully in early spring. Insert stem-tip cuttings in late summer with bottom heat. Root basal or stem-tip cuttings of selected cultivars, such as *T. majus* 'Hermine Grasshoff', in spring or early summer.

• **PESTS AND DISEASES** Caterpillars of cabbage white butterflies, flea beetles, black fly, and slugs may be troublesome. *T. majus* and its hybrids and cultivars are susceptible to whiteflies and viruses.

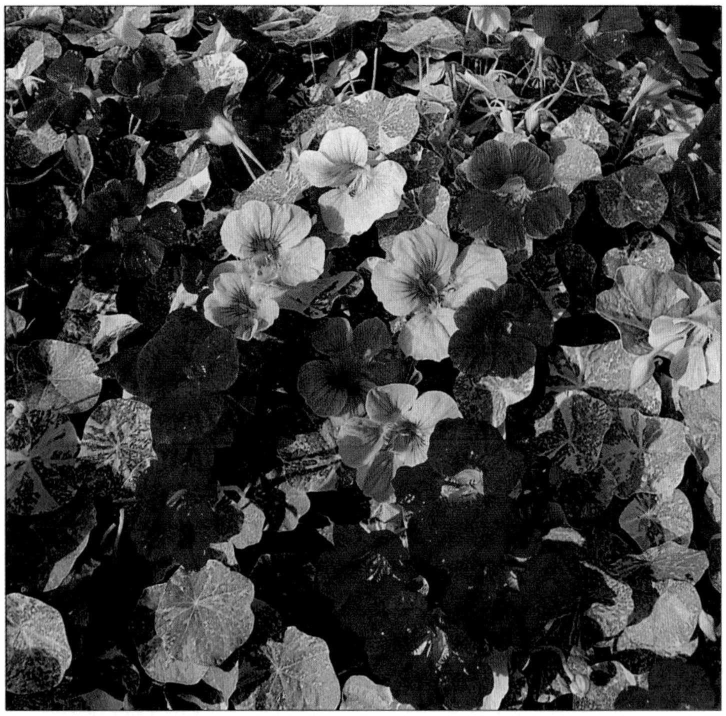

Tropaeolum Alaska Series

T. aduncum see *T. peregrinum.*

***T.* Alaska Series** ▣ 🏆 Dwarf, bushy annuals, derived from *T. majus*, with light green leaves, speckled and marked creamy white. Single flowers, in shades of yellow, orange, mahogany, or cream, are borne from summer to autumn. ↕ to 30cm (12in), ↔ to 45cm (18in). ✲

T. azureum. Perennial climber with an ovoid tuber and 5- to 9-palmate or palmately lobed, pale or mid-green leaves, 2cm (¾in) across, with lance-shaped leaflets or lobes. Short-spurred, sky-blue flowers, 1.5–2cm (½–¾in) across, with whitish cream or yellow centres, are borne in late spring. ↕ 60–100cm (24–39in). Chile. ✲

T. canariense see *T. peregrinum.*

***T.* 'Empress of India'.** Dwarf, bushy annual, derived from *T. majus*, with purple-green leaves. From summer to autumn, produces semi-double, velvety, rich scarlet flowers. ↕ to 30cm (12in), ↔ to 45cm (18in). ✲

***T.* Gleam Series.** Vigorous, semi-trailing annuals, derived from *T. majus*, bearing semi-double flowers in scarlet, orange, yellow, or pastel shades from summer to autumn. ↕ to 40cm (16in), ↔ to 60cm (24in). ✲

***T.* Jewel Series** ▣ Dwarf, bushy annuals, derived from *T. majus*, bearing semi-double and double, yellow, pink-orange, scarlet, or crimson flowers from early summer to autumn; flowers are sometimes covered by the foliage. ↕ to 30cm (12in), ↔ to 45cm (18in). ✲

T. majus (Indian cress, Nasturtium). Strong-growing, annual climber, sometimes scrambling, with rounded to kidney-shaped, wavy-margined, light green leaves, 2.5–6cm (1–2½in) long. From summer to autumn, bears long-spurred, red, orange, or yellow flowers, 5–6cm (2–2½in) across. Many cultivars often attributed to *T. majus*, and with similar characteristics to the species, are of hybrid origin, and are described in this account under their cultivar names. ↕ 1–3m (3–10ft), ↔ 1.5–5m (5–15ft). Bolivia to Colombia. ❀ (min. 3°C/37°F). **'Hermine Grasshof'** has double, bright red flowers, and may only be propagated by stem-tip cuttings.

***T.* 'Peach Melba'** ▣ Dwarf, bushy annual, derived from *T. majus*, bearing semi-double, creamy yellow flowers with orange-red centres, from summer to autumn. Best in a container. ↕ 23–30cm (9–12in), ↔ to 45cm (18in). ✲

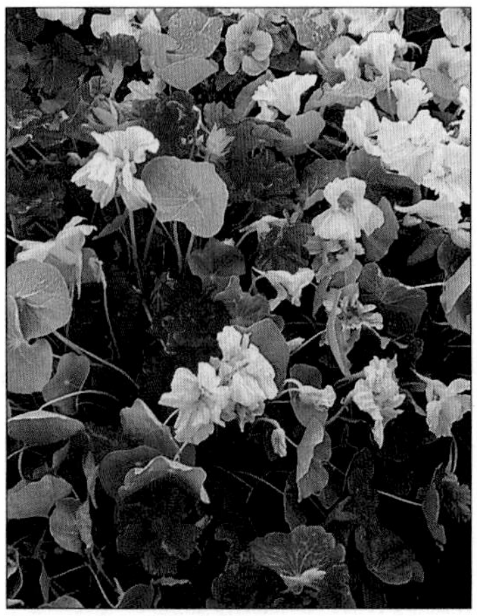

Tropaeolum Jewel Series

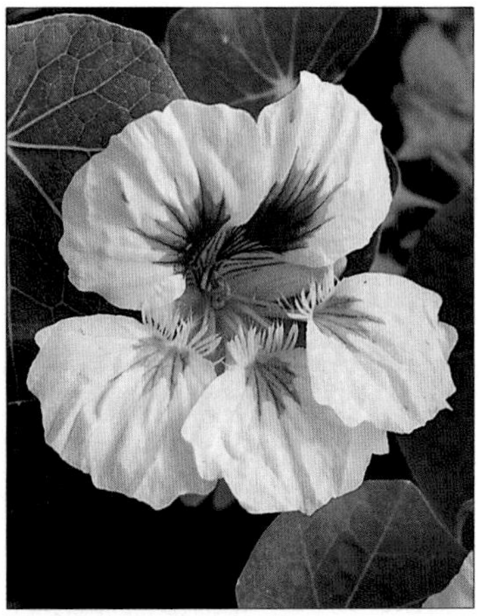

Tropaeolum 'Peach Melba'

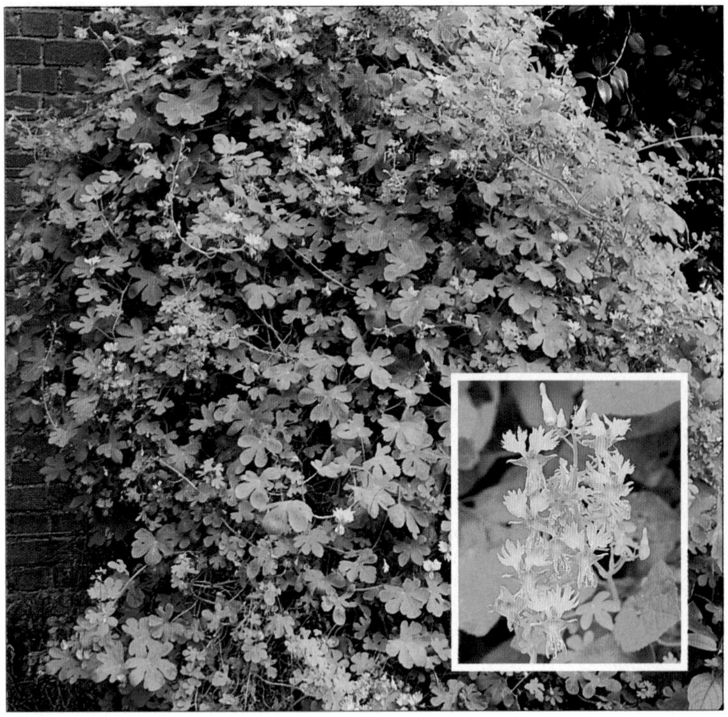

Tropaeolum peregrinum (inset: flower detail)

T. peregrinum ■ syn. *T. aduncum*, *T. canariense* (Canary creeper). Strong-growing, annual climber with 5-lobed, light to greyish green leaves, 2.5–5cm (1–2in) long. From summer to autumn, produces hook-spurred, bright yellow flowers, 2.5cm (1in) across; they have 3 tiny lower petals and 2 large, erect upper ones, which are toothed and fringed like tiny birds' wings. ↕2.5–4m (8–12ft). Ecuador, Peru. ❀ (min. 3°C/37°F)
T. polyphyllum ■ Trailing herbaceous perennial with an elongated, rhizome-like tuber and deeply 5- to 9-lobed, glaucous, blue-green leaves, to 8cm (3in) long. Long-spurred, rich yellow to orange flowers, 4cm (1½in) across, are produced among long, trailing masses of foliage over a long period in summer. ↕5–8cm (2–3in), ↔ to 1m (3ft). Chile, Argentina. ❄❄
T. speciosum ■ 🏆 (Flame creeper, Flame nasturtium). Slender, perennial climber with deep-rooting, long, thin, fleshy white rhizomes. The 5- to 7-palmate, mid- to dark green leaves, 4cm (1½in) long, are composed of obovate to wedge-shaped leaflets. From summer to autumn, bears long-spurred, bright vermilion flowers, 2cm (¾in) across, with long-clawed petals, the lower 3 of which are larger than the others; flowers are followed by spherical blue fruit with persistent red calyces. ↕to 3m (10ft) or more. Chile. ❄❄
***T.* Tom Thumb Series.** Dwarf, bushy annuals, derived from *T. majus*, bearing single, yellow, orange, red, salmon-pink, or rose-pink flowers from summer to autumn; flowers are sometimes covered by the foliage. ↕to 24cm (10in), ↔ to 35cm (14in). ❄
T. tricolor see *T. tricolorum.*
T. tricolorum 🏆 syn. *T. tricolor.* Tuberous-rooted, perennial climber with ovoid, often irregular tubers. Very slender stems bear rounded, 5- to 7-palmate, light green leaves, to 4cm (1½in) long, with narrowly elliptic to narrowly obovate, 5- to 7-lobed leaflets. From winter to early summer, bears flowers, 3cm (1¼in) long, with lantern-shaped, maroon-tipped, orange-scarlet calyces, short, orange to yellow petals, and long, upturned, red to yellow or purple spurs. ↕1–2m (3–6ft). Chile. ❄
T. tuberosum. Perennial climber with large, purple-marbled yellow tubers and 3- to 6-lobed, greyish green leaves, 5cm (2in) long. Long-spurred, cup-shaped

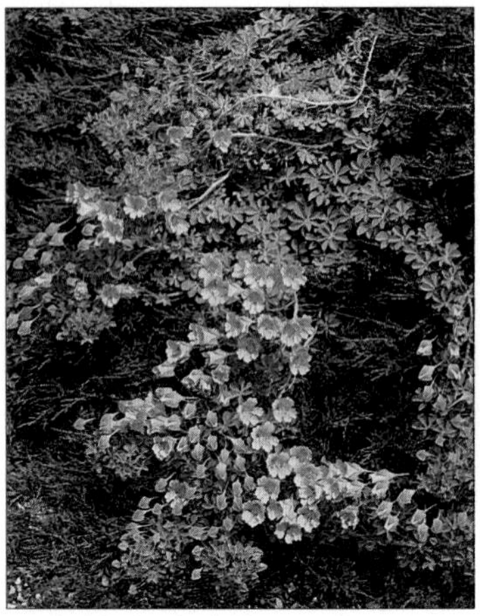

Tropaeolum polyphyllum

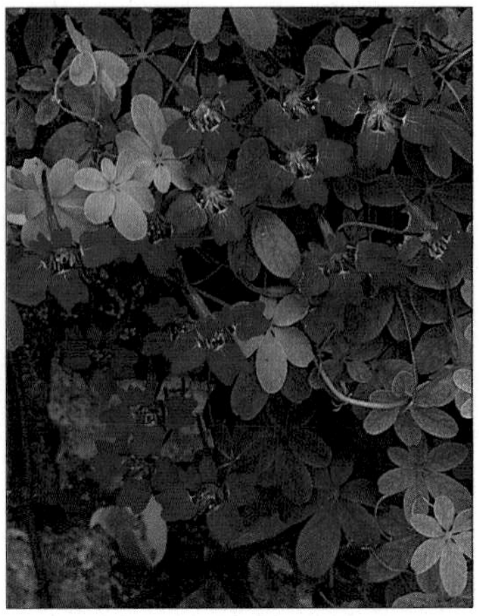

Tropaeolum speciosum

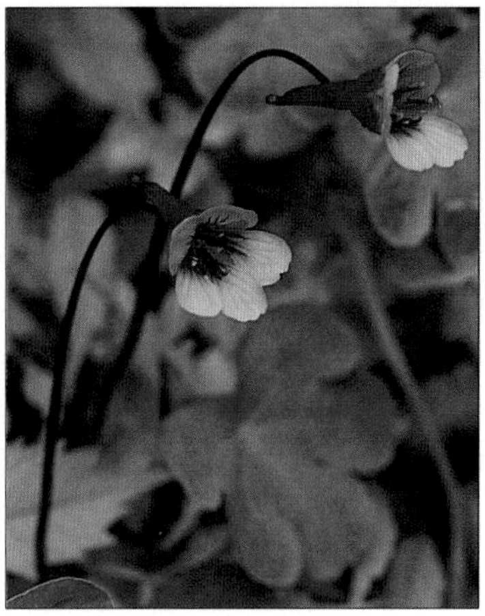

Tropaeolum tuberosum var. *lineamaculatum* 'Ken Aslet'

flowers, 3–4cm (1¼–1½in) long, with orange-red sepals and deep yellow to orange-yellow petals, with brown veins inside, are produced from midsummer to autumn. ↕2–4m (6–12ft). Colombia, Ecuador, Peru, Bolivia. ❄. **var. *lineamaculatum* 'Ken Aslet'** ■ 🏆 is the most common cultivar, and has orange flowers. **var. *piliferum* 'Sidney'** has more slender, rhizome-like tubers and orange flowers, 2–3cm (¾–1¼in) long.
***T.* Whirlybird Series** 🏆 Dwarf, bushy annuals, derived from *T. majus.* Non-spurred, single to semi-double flowers, in colours including reds, pinks, yellows, and oranges, are produced well above the foliage, from summer to autumn. ↕to 24cm (10in), ↔ to 35cm (14in). ❄. **'Whirlybird Cream'** has creamy yellow flowers; ❀ (min. 3–5°C/37–41°F)

▷**Trumpet,**
Evening see *Gelsemium sempervirens*
Golden see *Allamanda cathartica*
Herald's see *Beaumontia grandiflora*
Water see *Cryptocoryne*
White see *Sarracenia leucophylla*
Yellow see *Sarracenia flava*
▷**Trumpet bush** see *Tecoma stans*
▷**Trumpet creeper** see *Campsis*
Chinese see *C. grandiflora*
Common see *C. radicans*
▷**Trumpet tree, Rosy** see *Tabebuia rosea*
▷**Trumpet vine** see *Campsis*
Blue see *Thunbergia grandiflora*
Chinese see *Campsis grandiflora*
Pink see *Podranea ricasoliana*

TSUGA
Hemlock

PINACEAE

Genus of 10 or 11 species of evergreen, monoecious, coniferous trees found in forest from the Himalayas to N. Burma, W. Vietnam, China, Taiwan, and Japan, and in North America. Flattened, usually linear leaves, with silvery white bands beneath, are radially arranged or 2-ranked, and vary in length along the shoots. The small, ovoid-oblong to almost spherical, terminal, pale to mid-brown female cones become pendent, similar to those of *Picea*, but with few scales; male cones are almost spherical, 3–5mm (⅛–¼in) across, and borne at the tips of lateral shoots. The leading shoot is pendent. Tsugas are excellent specimen trees and very shade-tolerant, especially when young. *T. heterophylla* is suitable for hedging. The dwarf cultivars are all suitable for bonsai work.
• **HARDINESS** Fully hardy.
• **CULTIVATION** Grow in humus-rich, moist but well-drained, acid to slightly alkaline soil in full sun or partial shade, providing shelter from cold, drying winds. Trim hedges from early to late summer.
• **PROPAGATION** Sow seed in containers in a cold frame in spring. Root semi-ripe cuttings in late summer or early autumn.
• **PESTS AND DISEASES** Susceptible to butt rot fungus.

T. canadensis ■ △ (Eastern hemlock). Broadly conical tree, often having several stems, with deeply furrowed, purplish grey bark and small-budded, slender, grey-hairy shoots. Linear, finely toothed, mid-green leaves, to 2cm (¾in) long, taper from the bases and are 2-ranked with a wide parting below; a few very short leaves lie flat along the shoots with their silver undersides uppermost. Oblong-conical female cones are 2cm (¾in) long. ↕to 25m (80ft), ↔ to 10m (30ft). E. North America. ❄❄❄. **'Aurea'** is compact and slow-growing, with golden yellow young foliage, turning greener with age; ↕8m (25ft), ↔ 4m (12ft). **'Bennett'** is dwarf and vase-shaped, forming a central "nest", with short, light green leaves; ↕1.5m (5ft), ↔ 2m (6ft). **'Cole's Prostrate'**, syn. 'Coles', is low-growing and suitable for ground cover; ↕30cm (12in), ↔ 1m (3ft). **'Gracilis'** is a slow-growing, dwarf shrub with pendent branch tips; ↕↔ 1m (3ft). **'Jeddeloh'** ■ 🏆 is hemispherical, and similar to 'Bennett', with bright green leaves; ↕1.5m (5ft), ↔ 2m (6ft). **'Pendula'** 🏆 syn. f. *pendula*, is a slow-growing, spreading, mound-forming shrub, with pendent branches, and is very effective hanging over a bank or wall; ↕to 4m (12ft), ↔ to 8m (25ft).
T. caroliniana △ (Carolina hemlock). Conical or ovoid, twiggy tree with shallowly fissured, red-brown bark and shiny, red-brown shoots with short hairs in the grooves. Round-tipped, entire, dark green leaves, 1–2cm (½–¾in) long, are 2-ranked, widely parted above, and somewhat irregular and sparse. Ovoid to ellipsoid female cones are 2.5–3.5cm (1–1½in) long. ↕15–20m (50–70ft), ↔ to 8m (25ft). USA (Appalachians from Virginia to Georgia). ❄❄❄
T. diversifolia △ (Northern Japanese hemlock). Broadly conical, later domed tree, usually having several stems, with

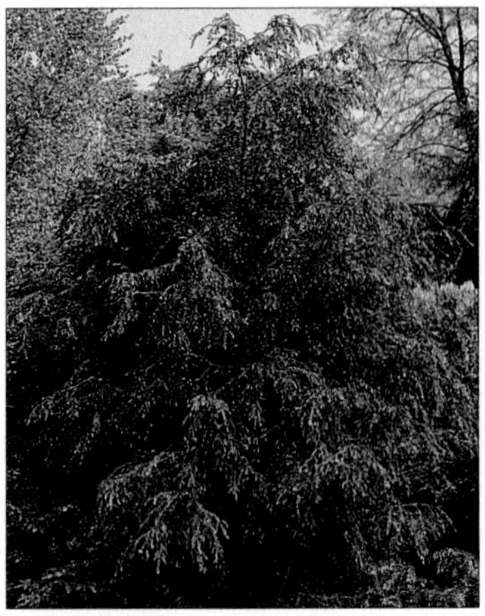

Tsuga canadensis

T

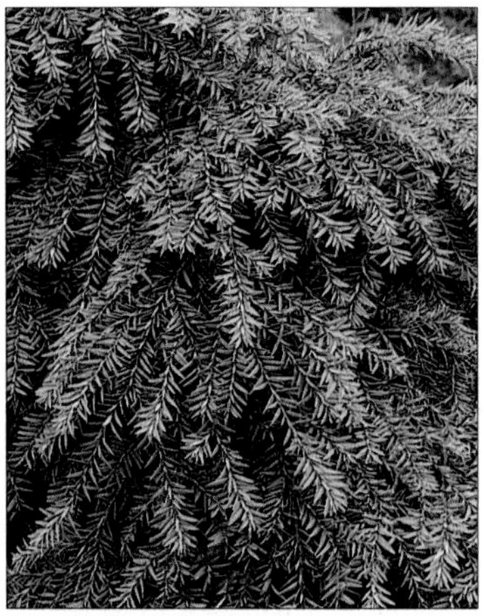

Tsuga canadensis 'Jeddeloh'

orange-brown bark and orange shoots with short, fine hairs. Linear leaves are very glossy, dark green, 0.5–1.5cm (¼–½in) long, and 2-ranked with a wide parting above, broader and more densely packed towards the rounded, notched shoot-tips. Ovoid female cones are up to 2cm (¾in) long. ↕ to 15m (50ft), ↔ to 8m (25ft). N. Japan. ❄❄❄
T. heterophylla 🏆◊ (Western hemlock). Narrowly conical tree with cracked, purple-brown bark, horizontal branches with pendent tips, and brownish grey shoots with long brown hairs. Blunt, round-tipped, narrowly elliptic-oblong, finely toothed, very glossy, dark green leaves, 0.5–2cm (¼–¾in) long, are 2-ranked with a wide parting beneath. Ovoid female cones are 2cm (¾in) long. Very shade-tolerant but requires shelter from wind. ↕ 20–40m (70–130ft), ↔ 6–10m (20–30ft). W. North America (Alaska to California). ❄❄❄
T. mertensiana ◊ (Mountain hemlock). Columnar-conical tree with scaly, purple to red-brown bark and hairy, red-brown shoots. Thick, blunt-tipped, linear, entire, glaucous blue or grey-green leaves, 1.5–2.5cm (½–1in) long, are convex on both sides, and radially arranged. Female cones are oblong-cylindrical, 4–8cm (1½–3in) long, and have reflexed scales when fully open. ↕ 15m (50ft), ↔ 6m (20ft). W. North America (Alaska to California). ❄❄❄. **'Glauca'** ▣◊–△ is slow-growing and dwarf, with glaucous, silver-grey foliage; ↕ 3m (10ft), ↔ 2m (6ft).
T. sieboldii △ (Southern Japanese hemlock). Broadly conical tree having several stems with smooth, dark grey bark, later cracked, and stiff, shiny, buff shoots. Linear, entire leaves, 0.7–2cm (¼–¾in) long, with notched tips, glossy, dark green above and pale green or dull white beneath, are variable in length and arrangement. Ovoid female cones are 2.5cm (1in) long. ↕ 15m (50ft), ↔ to 8m (25ft). S. Japan. ❄❄❄

TSUSIOPHYLLUM

ERICACEAE

Genus of one species of dwarf, semi-evergreen shrub found in woodland in Japan. It is cultivated for its umbel-like clusters of small, tubular-bell-shaped white flowers, borne in early summer, and is an attractive addition to a peat bed or woodland garden.
• **HARDINESS** Frost hardy.
• **CULTIVATION** Grow in moist, humus-rich, acid soil in partial shade. Provide shelter from cold, drying winds. Pruning group 8.
• **PROPAGATION** Sow seed as soon as ripe in containers in a cold frame. Insert semi-ripe cuttings in summer.
• **PESTS AND DISEASES** Trouble free.

T. tanakae. Prostrate, spreading shrub with short, hairy branches and alternate, ovate to lance-shaped or inversely lance-shaped, very hairy, dark green leaves, 1–3cm (½–1¼in) or more long. Dense clusters of 2–6 silky-hairy white flowers, 7–10mm (¼–½in) long, each with 4 or 5 spreading petal lobes, are produced at the shoot-tips in early summer. ↕ to 50cm (20in), ↔ to 20cm (8in). Japan (Honshu). ❄❄

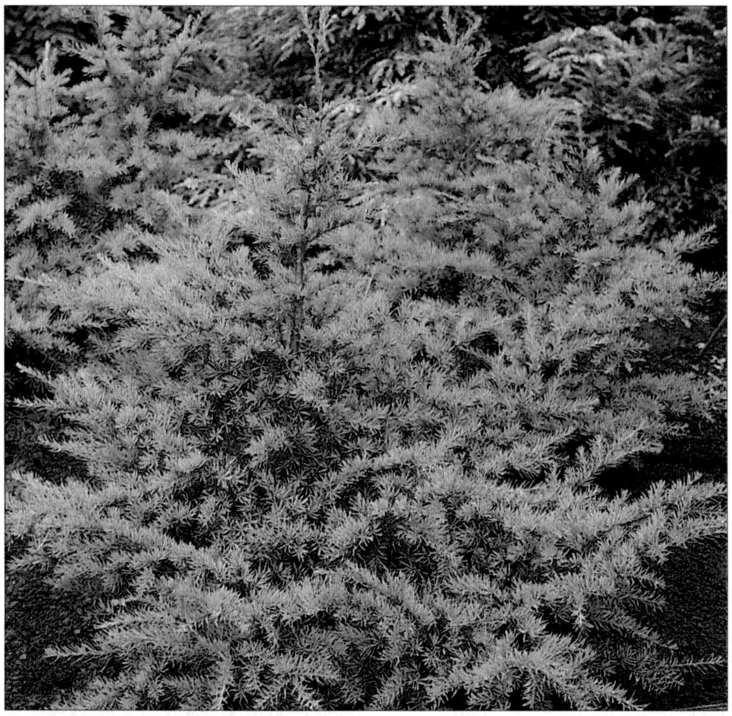

Tsuga mertensiana 'Glauca'

TUBERARIA

CISTACEAE

Genus of about 12 species of annuals and perennials from scrub, heath, and woodland in C. and S. Europe. The simple, lance-shaped to almost rounded leaves are borne in basal rosettes, and occasionally on the upright flowering stems. Terminal cymes of shallowly cup-shaped yellow flowers, sometimes with purple or red spots, are borne in late spring and summer. Grow annuals in a mixed or annual border, and perennials in a sunny border or warm rock garden.
• **HARDINESS** Fully hardy to frost hardy.
• **CULTIVATION** Grow in any well-drained soil in full sun.
• **PROPAGATION** Sow seed at 13–16°C (55–61°F) in early spring. Seed of annuals may also be sown *in situ* in mid- to late spring. Separate rooted rosettes, or take rosettes as cuttings, in spring.
• **PESTS AND DISEASES** Leaves may be damaged by slugs and snails.

T. guttata, syn. *Helianthemum guttatum.* Erect, rosette-forming, hairy annual with wavy-margined, mid-green, prominently 3-veined leaves, 2.5–8cm (1–3in) long; the basal leaves are elliptic or obovate, the stem leaves linear-oblong or linear-lance-shaped. In summer, bears terminal cymes of short-lived, long-stalked, cup-shaped yellow flowers, to 3cm (1¼in) across, each petal spotted maroon-red at the base. ↕↔ to 30cm (12in). C. and S. Europe. ❄❄❄
T. lignosa, syn. *Helianthemum tuberaria.* Spreading, rosette-forming, woody-based perennial with hairy, obovate to lance-shaped or elliptic, dark green leaves, to 6cm (2½in) long. Loose, terminal cymes of bright yellow flowers, 2.5–3cm (1–1¼in) across, without spots, are produced from early to late summer. ↕ to 40cm (16in), ↔ 40cm (16in). W. Mediterranean. ❄❄

▷**Tuberose** see *Polianthes tuberosa*

TULBAGHIA

ALLIACEAE/LILIACEAE

Genus of about 24 species of clump-forming, mainly deciduous, sometimes semi-evergreen, rhizomatous or bulbous perennials found in various habitats, some mountainous, in tropical and temperate southern Africa. Basal, strap-shaped to linear, hairless, sometimes grey-green leaves have a smell similar to that of onions or garlic. Umbels of dainty, usually purple or white flowers, sometimes fragrant, especially at night, are borne over a long period between late spring and autumn. The flowers are tubular, each with 6 spreading tepals and a small, trumpet-like corona. Grow in a sunny border or rock garden. In frost-prone areas, grow in a cool greenhouse or conservatory, particularly *T. alliacea*, which has overwintering leaves.
• **HARDINESS** Frost hardy to frost tender; most frost-hardy species tolerate short periods at temperatures to -10°C (14°F).
• **CULTIVATION** Under glass, grow in well-drained, loam-based potting compost (JI No.2) in full light. Water freely when in growth; reduce water when in flower, and again as the leaves wither; keep almost dry when dormant.

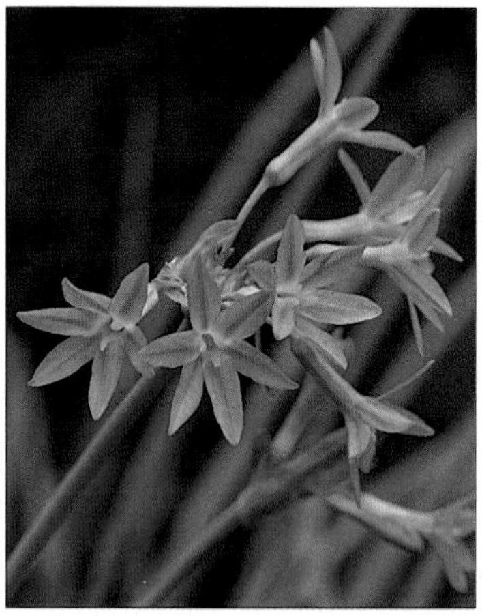

Tulbaghia simmleri

Outdoors, grow in well-drained, moderately fertile, humus-rich, loamy soil in full sun. In frost-prone areas, provide a dry winter mulch.
• **PROPAGATION** Sow seed in containers in a cold frame as soon as ripe, or in spring. Seed germinates easily, and the seedlings quickly reach flowering size. Divide most species in spring; divide *T. alliacea* in late summer.
• **PESTS AND DISEASES** Susceptible to aphids and whiteflies under glass.

T. alliacea. Semi-evergreen, rhizomatous perennial bearing clusters of narrowly linear leaves, to 20cm (8in) long. In late spring and early summer, produces terminal umbels of fragrant, purple-tinged, greenish white flowers, 1cm (½in) long; the flowers have brownish red coronas. ↕ to 45cm (18in), ↔ 20cm (8in). Zimbabwe, South Africa (Northern Cape, Eastern Cape, Western Cape). ❄❄
T. capensis. Rhizomatous perennial with clusters of narrowly linear leaves, to 30cm (12in) long. Terminal umbels of greenish purple flowers, to 1.5cm (½in) long, with purplish brown coronas, are produced in early and midsummer. ↕ to 60cm (24in), ↔ 25cm (10in). South Africa (Namaqualand to Western Cape). ❄❄
T. fragrans see *T. simmleri.*
T. pulchella see *T. simmleri.*
T. simmleri ▣ syn. *T. fragrans, T. pulchella.* Bulbous perennial with clusters of linear leaves, 30–60cm (12–24in) long (wider than in most species). Large, terminal umbels of fragrant, light to deep purple flowers, to 2cm (¾in) long, are produced in early and midsummer. ↕ to 60cm (24in), ↔ 25cm (10in). South Africa (Eastern Transvaal). ❄❄
T. violacea. Vigorous, clump-forming perennial with corm-like rhizomes and narrowly linear, greyish green leaves, to 30cm (12in) long. Large, terminal umbels of fragrant lilac flowers, 2cm (¾in) long, are produced from mid-summer to early autumn. ↕ 45–60cm (18–24in), ↔ 25cm (10in). South Africa (Eastern Cape, KwaZulu/Natal, Eastern Transvaal). ❄❄. **'Silver Lace'**, syn. 'Variegata', has cream-striped leaves and larger flowers, 2–4cm (¾–1½in) long.

▷**Tulip** see *Tulipa*
Cape see *Haemanthus coccineus*
Lady see *Tulipa clusiana*
Mariposa see *Calochortus*
Water-lily see *Tulipa kaufmanniana*

TULIPA syn. AMANA

Tulip

LILIACEAE

Genus of about 100 species of bulbous perennials found in usually hot, dry situations, from sea level and steppes to alpine areas, in temperate Europe, Asia and the Middle East, although they are at their most diverse in C. Asia. Tulips have linear to broadly ovate, hairy or hairless, sometimes channelled or wavy-margined, mostly mid- or grey-green leaves; they are generally borne at the base, although in some species and cultivars they are arranged alternately on the usually hairless, sometimes hairy or downy flower stems, and decrease in size up the stem. The upright, terminal flowers, each with 6 tepals (often referred to as petals), are borne singly or in clusters of up to 12. Tulip cultivars have single or double flowers, mainly ovoid or goblet- to bowl-shaped or lily-like, sometimes fringed (see panel below), and are available in a wide range of single, mixed, or variegated colours. Variegation (i.e. breaks in colour) may be caused by a virus, although healthy tulips may also be variegated.

Tulips are valued in beds and borders for their brilliant colours. Some smaller species, such as *T. kaufmanniana* and *T. tarda*, are suitable for a rock garden. If ingested, all parts may cause mild stomach upset, and contact with any part may aggravate skin allergies.

For horticultural purposes, tulips are divided into the following groups, which are chiefly defined by their flower characteristics. This replaces the older divisions (given in brackets below).

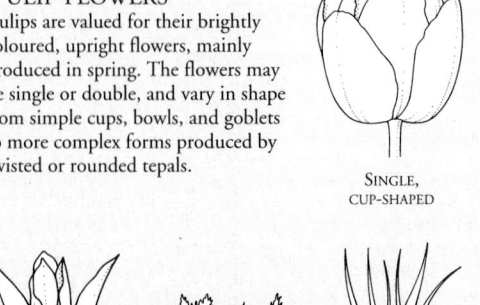

Single Early Group (Division 1)
Cup-shaped flowers, to 7cm (3in) across, are white to dark purple, often margined, "flamed", or flecked with a contrasting colour. Early and mid-spring-flowering. Leaves are 10–35cm (4–14in) long. Suitable for bedding or a mixed border; use low-growing cultivars in containers. ↕15–45cm (6–18in).
Double Early Group (Division 2)
Fully double, bowl-shaped flowers, to 8cm (3in) across, are dark red to yellow or white, often margined or flecked with another colour. Mid-spring-flowering. Leaves are 10–35cm (4–14in) long. Suitable for bedding and containers. ↕30–40cm (12–16in).
Triumph Group (Division 3)
Single, cup-shaped flowers, to 6cm (2½in) across, are produced in a wide range of colours, including dark purple to red, pink, yellow, or white, often margined or flecked with a contrasting colour. Mid- or late spring-flowering. Leaves are 10–35cm (4–14in) long. Suitable for bedding, and good for cut flowers. ↕35–60cm (14–24in).
Darwin Hybrid Group (Division 4)
Single, ovoid flowers, to 7cm (3in) across, are often very brightly coloured in shades of yellow, pink, orange, or red, usually flushed, "flamed", or margined with a different colour, and often with contrasting bases. Mid- or late spring-flowering. Leaves are upright, 10–35cm (4–14in) long. Not to be confused with the old Darwin tulips (see Single Late Group). Suitable for bedding, and good for cut flowers. ↕50–70cm (20–28in).
Single Late Group (Division 5)
Cup- or goblet-shaped flowers, to 7cm (3in) across, sometimes several to a stem, are white to yellow, pink, red, or almost black, often with contrasting margins. Late spring-flowering. Leaves are 10–35cm (4–14in) long. Includes the old Darwin and cottage tulips. Suitable for bedding, and good for cut flowers. ↕45–75cm (18–30in).
Lily-flowered Group (Division 6)
Elegant, single, goblet-shaped flowers, to 8cm (3in) across, with reflexed, pointed tips to the tepals, are white to yellow, or pink to shades of red and magenta, sometimes margined, "flamed", or flushed with a contrasting colour. Late spring-flowering. Leaves are 10–40cm (4–16in) long. Excellent for formal bedding. ↕45–65cm (18–26in).
Fringed Group (Division 7)
Single, cup-shaped flowers, to 8cm (3in) across, are white, yellow, pink, red, or violet, with fringed margins, usually in a different colour. Late spring-flowering. Leaves are 10–40cm (4–16in) long. Suitable for a border, and good for cut flowers. ↕35–65cm (14–26in).
Viridiflora Group (Division 8)
Single, cup- or almost closed bowl-shaped flowers, to 8cm (3in) across, are sometimes entirely green, margined with another colour, or white to yellow, red, or purple, "flamed" or striped green, with contrasting centres. Late spring-flowering. Leaves are 10–40cm (4–16in) long. Ideal for a mixed border, and good for cut flowers. ↕40–55cm (16–22in).
Rembrandt Group (Division 9)
Single, cup-shaped flowers, to 8cm (3in) across, are white, yellow, or red, with black, brown, bronze, purple, red, or pink stripes or "feathers", caused by a virus. Often termed "broken" tulips. Late spring-flowering. Leaves are 10–35cm (4–14in) long. Suitable for a mixed border, and good for cut flowers. ↕45–65cm (18–26in)
Parrot Group (Division 10)
Single, cup-shaped flowers, to 10cm (4in) across, are white to pink or violet-blue, often unevenly striped with different colours, including green. The tepals are finely and irregularly cut. Late spring-flowering. Leaves are 10–35cm (4–14in) long. Ideal for a border; good for cut flowers. ↕35–65cm (14–26in).
Double Late Group (peony-flowered) (Division 11)
Fully double, bowl-shaped flowers, to 12cm (5in) across, are white to purple, sometimes margined or "flamed" in a different colour. Late spring-flowering. Leaves are 10–40cm (4–16in) long. Suitable for bedding or a border. ↕35–60cm (14–24in).
Kaufmanniana Group (Division 12)
T. kaufmanniana and hybrids mainly derived from it. Single, bowl-shaped flowers, 8–10cm (3–4in) across, are frequently multicoloured, usually with distinctively coloured bases. Early or mid-spring-flowering. Leaves, 8–25cm (3–10in) long, are sometimes marked bronze, red, or purple. Ideal for a rock garden or border. ↕15–30cm (6–12in).
Fosteriana Group (Division 13)
T. fosteriana and hybrids mainly derived from it. Single, bowl-shaped flowers, to 12cm (5in) across, are white to yellow or dark red, sometimes margined or "flamed" in another colour, and with contrasting bases. Mid-spring-flowering.

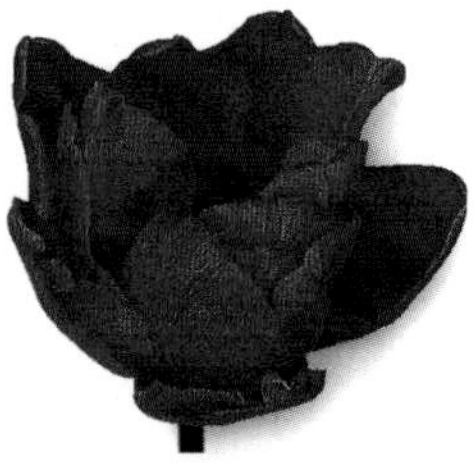

Tulipa 'Abba'

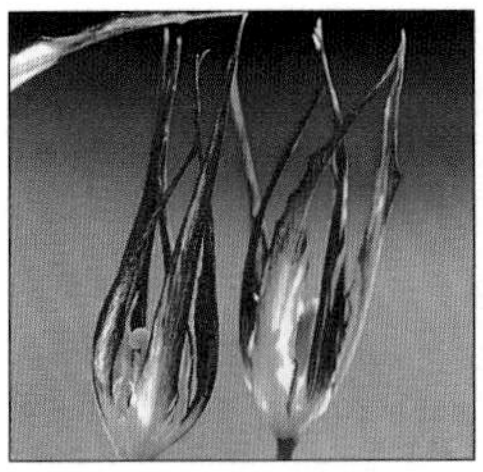

Tulipa acuminata

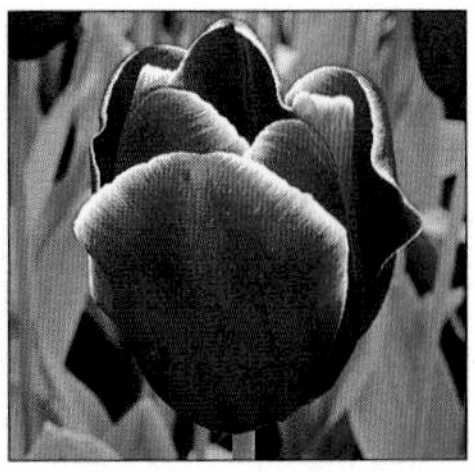

Tulipa 'African Queen'

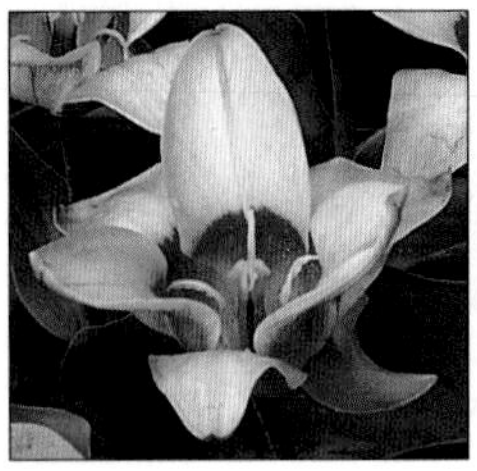

Tulipa 'Ancilla'

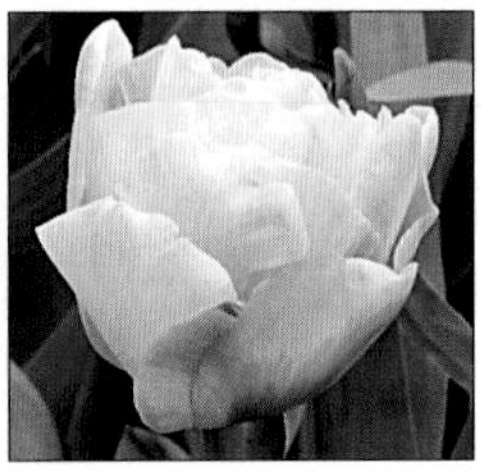

Tulipa 'Angélique'

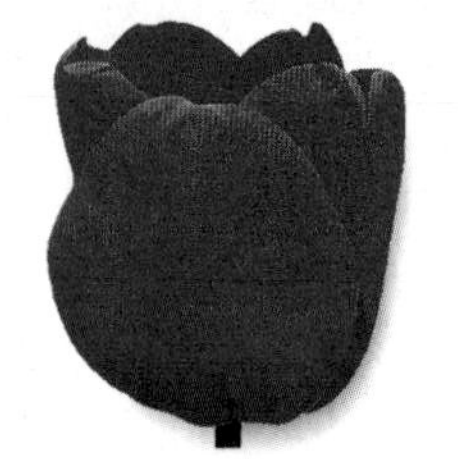

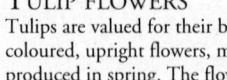

Tulipa 'Apeldoorn'

Leaves, 5–30cm (2–12in) long, are usually light bright green to dark green, sometimes marked red-purple. Suitable for a border. ↕20–65cm (8–26in).
Greigii Group (Division 14)
T. greigii and hybrids mainly derived from it. Single, bowl-shaped flowers, to 10cm (4in) across, are yellow to red, sometimes "flamed" or margined in a different colour, and with contrasting bases. Usually early or mid-spring-flowering. Broad, spreading, usually wavy-margined, blue-grey leaves, 5–18cm (2–7in) long, have dark bluish maroon markings. Grow in a rock garden or border. ↕15–30cm (6–12in).
Miscellaneous Group (Division 15)
All species and hybrids not included in other divisions. There are two informal sections: low-growing, 10–20cm (4–8in) tall, with star-shaped flowers, 5–8cm (2–3in) across, with pointed tepals; and taller-growing, 20–35cm (8–14in) or more tall, with mainly bowl-shaped flowers, 6–15cm (2½–6in) across, mostly with rounded bases and tepals. Late winter- to late spring-flowering. Grow in a rock garden. Keep dry in summer. The smallest ones may also be grown in a bulb frame or alpine house. *T. sprengeri* and *T. sylvestris* are suitable for naturalizing in fine grass.

- **HARDINESS** Fully hardy.
- **CULTIVATION** Grow in fertile, well-drained soil in full sun, sheltered from strong winds: *T. sprengeri* and *T. tarda* prefer humus-rich, peaty soil; rock garden species and cultivars prefer more sharply drained soil. All dislike excessive wet. Plant at a depth of 10–15cm (4–6in) in late summer or autumn; allow for a spread of 8–13cm (3–5in) for most tulips, and 13–15cm (5–6in) for Greigii and Kaufmanniana Group tulips, which have spreading leaves. Dead-head and remove any fallen tepals after flowering. The species, and many Greigii and Kaufmanniana Group tulips, may be left in the ground for several years. For those belonging to other groups, lift bulbs annually, once the leaves have died down, and ripen in a cold greenhouse. Replant the largest bulbs, and grow on smaller ones in a nursery bed for a year. Smaller tulips may be grown in containers in a bulb frame or alpine house, in a mix of equal parts loam, leaf mould, and sharp sand. In growth, water moderately, applying a balanced liquid fertilizer weekly for 3 or 4 weeks after flowering; keep dry in summer, and repot annually. Early-flowering and Triumph Group tulips are sometimes prepared for forcing, in a

TULIP FLOWERS

Tulips are valued for their brightly coloured, upright flowers, mainly produced in spring. The flowers may be single or double, and vary in shape from simple cups, bowls, and goblets to more complex forms produced by twisted or rounded tepals.

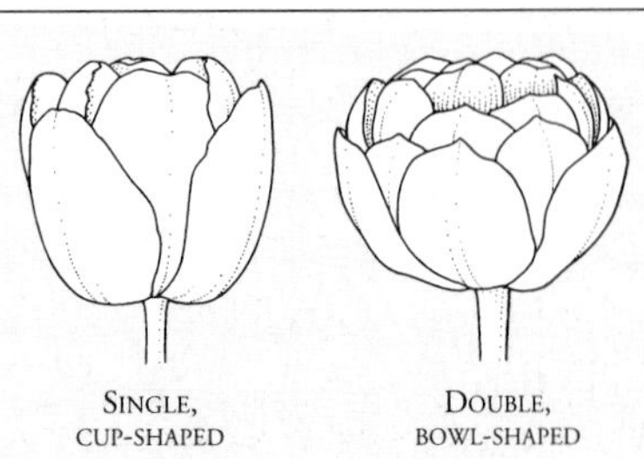

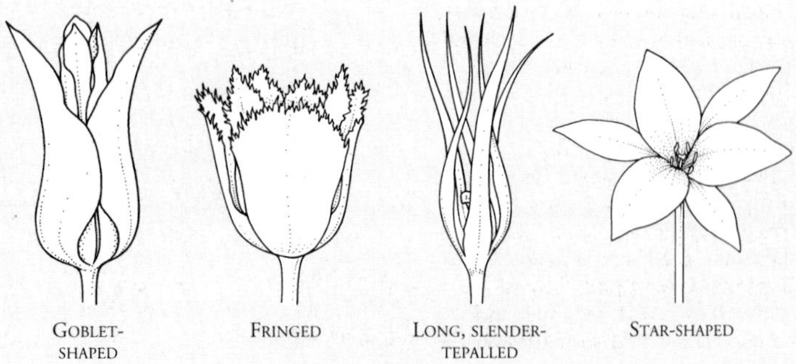

T

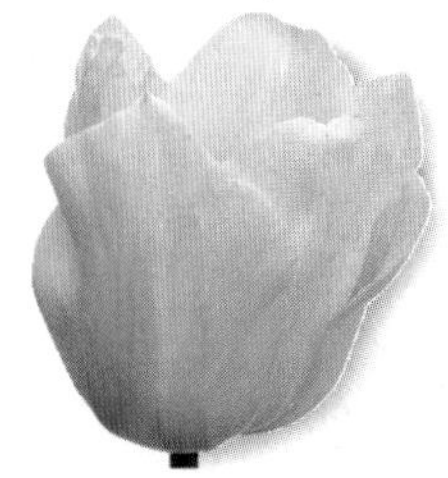
Tulipa 'Apricot Beauty'

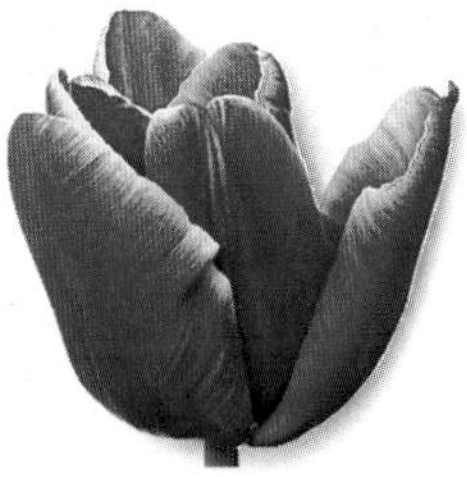
Tulipa 'Arabian Mystery'

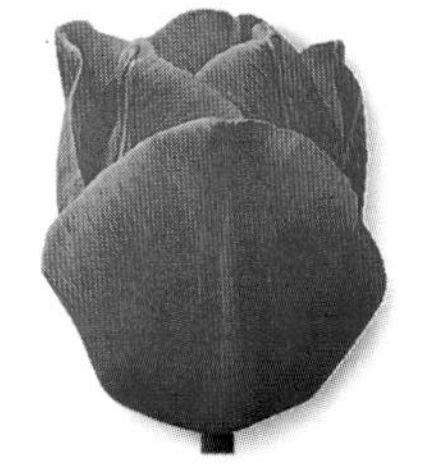
Tulipa 'Attila'

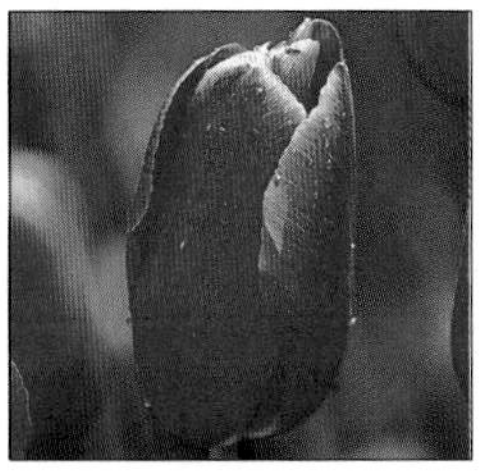
Tulipa 'Balalaika'

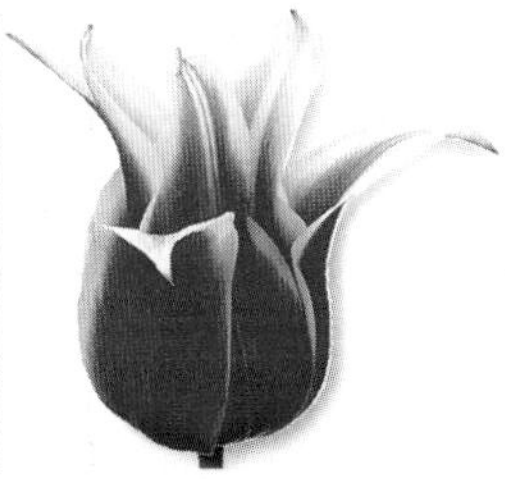
Tulipa 'Ballade'

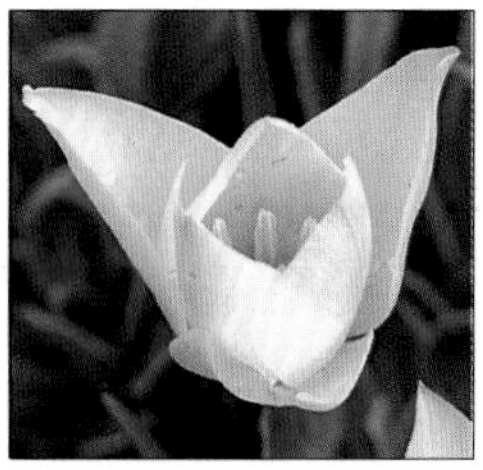
Tulipa batalinii

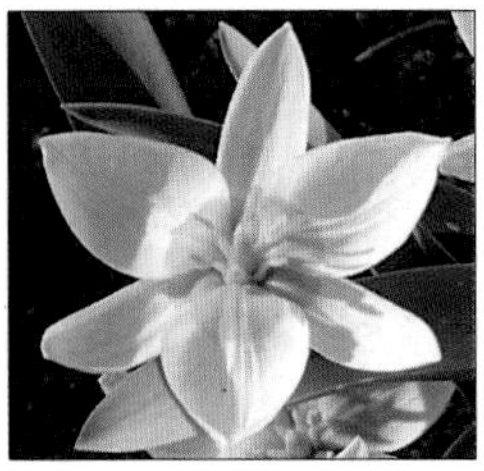
Tulipa biflora

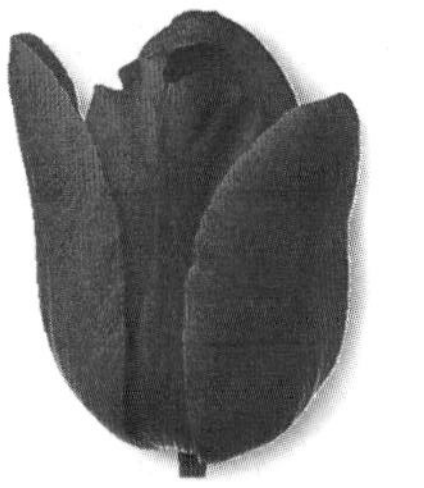
Tulipa 'Bing Crosby'

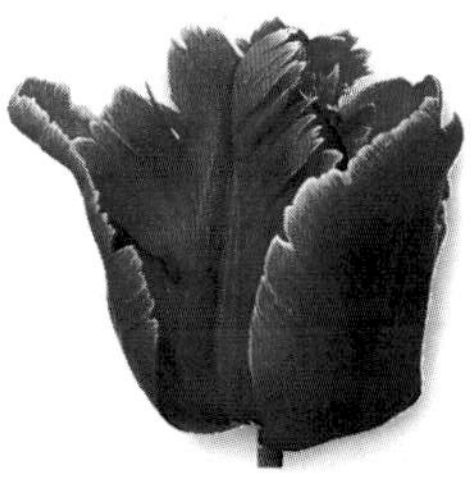
Tulipa 'Bird of Paradise'

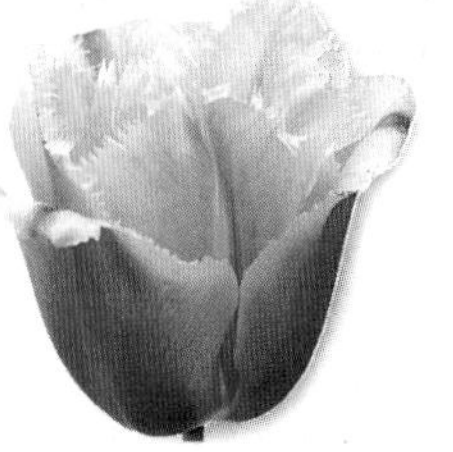
Tulipa 'Blue Heron'

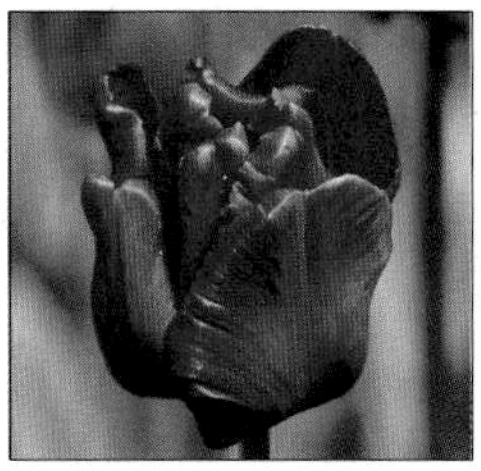
Tulipa 'Blue Parrot'

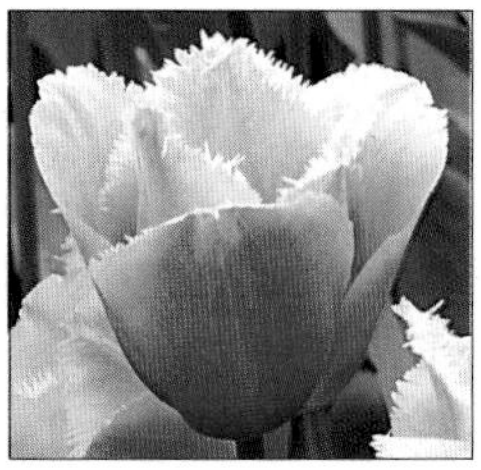
Tulipa 'Burns'

similar manner to hyacinths (see *Hyacinthus*), except that tulip bulbs should be kept in a cool, dark place until leaf-tips show, then brought indoors or into a greenhouse at 10°C (50°F). Raise the temperature gradually to no more than 18°C (64°F) when leaves reach 10cm (4in) long.

• **PROPAGATION** Sow seed of species in containers in a cold greenhouse or frame in autumn; it may take 4–7 years for flowers to be produced. Separate offsets of species and cultivars after lifting in summer, replant, and grow on.

• **PESTS AND DISEASES** Bulb rots may affect tulips in poorly drained soil. Aphids spread tulip-breaking virus from Rembrandt Group tulips to other tulips. Also prone to tulip fire, slugs, and stem and bulb eelworms.

***T.* 'Abba'** ■ Double Early Group tulip producing glowing tomato-red flowers, flushed dull cardinal-red and sometimes irregularly feathered yellow. Mid-spring-flowering. ↕30cm (12in). ***

***T.* 'Abra'.** Triumph Group tulip bearing yellow-margined, reddish brown flowers in mid-spring. ↕40cm (16in). ***

T. acuminata ■ Miscellaneous Group tulip with 2–7 linear to lance-shaped, sometimes wavy-margined, hairless, glaucous, grey-green leaves, to 30cm (12in) long. Solitary flowers, 10cm (4in) long, with long, pointed tepals and rounded bases, are produced on hairless or finely downy stems in early and mid-spring. Flowers are pale red or yellow, usually tinged red or green. Stamens have reddish brown anthers and yellow or white filaments. ↕50cm (20in). Garden origin. ***

***T.* 'African Queen'** ■ Triumph Group tulip bearing dark purplish red flowers, fading at the margins, with purple-margined, primrose-yellow basal marks. Insides are dark ruby-red with yellowish white or white margins and purple anthers. Mid-spring-flowering. ↕40cm (16in). ***

T. aitchisonii see *T. clusiana*.

***T.* 'Aladdin'.** Lily-flowered Group tulip bearing yellow-margined scarlet flowers in late spring. ↕45cm (18in). ***

***T.* 'Ancilla'** ■♀ Kaufmanniana Group tulip producing soft pink flowers, flushed rose-red, with red inner and outer basal rings. Mid-spring-flowering. ↕15cm (6in). ***

***T.* 'Angélique'** ■ Double Late Group tulip with pale pink flowers, flushed with paler and darker shades of pink, with lighter margins and, occasionally, green or yellow bases. Mid-spring-flowering. ↕30cm (12in). ***

***T.* 'Apeldoorn'** ■ Darwin Hybrid Group tulip bearing cherry-red flowers with signal-red margins. Insides are signal-red with yellow-bordered black marks and black anthers. Mid-spring-flowering. ↕60cm (24in). ***

***T.* 'Apeldoorn's Elite'** ♀ Darwin Hybrid Group tulip with red-feathered, buttercup-yellow flowers, flushed yellowish green at the bases outside, with black anthers and black basal marks inside. Mid-spring-flowering. ↕60cm (24in). ***

***T.* 'Apricot Beauty'** ■ Single Early Group tulip producing soft salmon-pink flowers, later with orange margins, in mid-spring. Good for forcing. ↕35cm (14in). ***

***T.* 'Apricot Jewel'.** Miscellaneous Group tulip bearing apricot flowers, flushed orange at the bases, in early and mid-spring. ↕35cm (14in). ***

***T.* 'Arabian Mystery'** ■ Triumph Group tulip bearing dark purple flowers, with white margins, in mid-spring. ↕45cm (18in). ***

***T.* 'Aristocrat'** ♀ Single Late Group tulip producing white-margined, soft purplish violet flowers in late spring. ↕60cm (24in). ***

***T.* 'Artist'** ■ Viridiflora Group tulip bearing purple and salmon-pink flowers, green-flushed salmon-pink inside, in late spring. ↕45cm (18in). ***

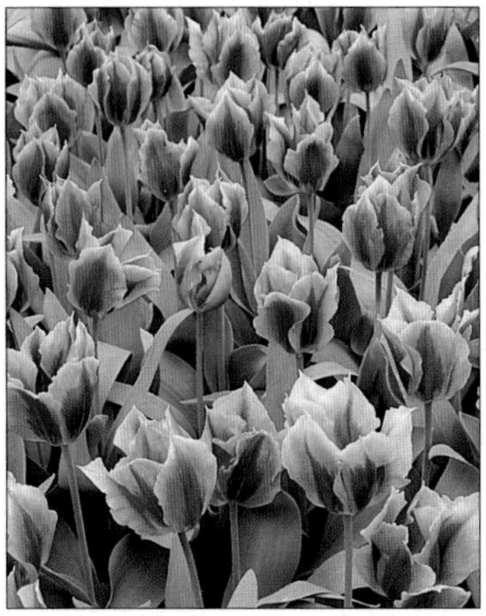
Tulipa 'Artist'

***T.* 'Attila'** ■ Triumph Group tulip bearing light purplish violet flowers in mid-spring. Good for forcing. ↕40cm (16in). ***

T. aucheriana ♀ Miscellaneous Group tulip with 2–5 linear, channelled, hairless, glaucous, mid-green leaves, to 15cm (6in) long. In mid-spring, bears star-shaped pink flowers, to 7cm (3in) across, with yellow centres and stamens, singly or, occasionally, in twos or threes. ↕10–25cm (4–10in). Iran. ***

T. australis see *T. sylvestris*.

***T.* 'Avignon'.** Single Late Group tulip with red flowers, fire-red towards the margins and flushed yellowish white at the bases. Insides are tomato-red with yellow basal marks, greenish red at the margins, and with yellow anthers. Late spring-flowering. ↕50cm (20in). ***

T. bakeri see *T. saxatilis*.

***T.* 'Balalaika'** ■ Single Late Group tulip bearing glowing bright red flowers with yellow basal marks inside and black anthers. Late spring-flowering. ↕55cm (22in). ***

***T.* 'Ballade'** ■♀ Lily-flowered Group tulip bearing white-margined, reddish magenta flowers with white-margined yellow basal marks inside. Late spring-flowering. ↕50cm (20in). ***

***T.* 'Ballerina'.** Lily-flowered Group tulip producing lemon-yellow flowers with blood-red flames, orange-yellow veins at the margins, and star-shaped yellow bases. Insides are capsicum-red, feathered marigold-orange, with pale golden yellow anthers. Late spring-flowering. ↕60cm (24in). ***

***T.* 'Baronesse'.** Single Late Group tulip producing rose-red flowers with broad white margins and bluish white bases. Insides are white with red feathers, pale blue and yellow basal marks, and dark brown anthers. Late spring-flowering. ↕45cm (18in). ***

T. batalinii ■♀ Miscellaneous Group tulip with 3–9 linear, sickle-shaped, hairless, grey-green leaves, to 15cm (6in) long, with wavy red margins. In early and mid-spring, produces solitary, bowl-shaped, pale yellow flowers, to 8cm (3in) across, with rounded bases and dark yellow or bronze marks inside. Stamens have yellow anthers and black or yellow filaments. ↕35cm (14in). Uzbekistan. ***

***T.* 'Bellona'.** Triumph Group tulip bearing scented, golden yellow flowers in mid-spring. ↕40cm (16in). ***

***T.* 'Bestseller'.** Single Early Group tulip producing bright copper-orange flowers in mid-spring. ↕35cm (14in). ***

***T.* 'Bienvenue'.** Darwin Hybrid Group tulip bearing canary-yellow flowers with dark yellowish pink flames and yellow-green bases. Insides are bright golden yellow, flamed capsicum-red, with black basal marks. Mid-spring-flowering. ↕60cm (24in). ***

T. biflora ■ syn. *T. polychroma*. Miscellaneous Group tulip with 1 or 2 linear, hairless, grey-green leaves, to 18cm (7in) long. Star-shaped, fragrant, red-margined white flowers, to 4cm (1½in) across, have yellow bases, and are flushed greenish grey or greenish pink outside. Stamens have yellow anthers, often tipped dark purple or black, and yellow filaments. Flowers are borne singly or in twos or threes, on upright stems from late winter to spring. ↕10cm (4in). Kazakhstan, E. Turkey, Iran, Afghanistan, Tajikistan. ***

***T.* 'Bing Crosby'** ■ Triumph Group tulip producing glowing scarlet flowers in mid-spring. ↕40cm (16in). ***

***T.* 'Bird of Paradise'** ■ Parrot Group tulip with orange-margined, cardinal-red flowers. Insides are scarlet, feathered dark red, with bright yellow bases and purple anthers. Late spring-flowering. ↕55cm (22in). ***

***T.* 'Blue Heron'** ■ Fringed Group tulip producing purple-fringed, violet-purple flowers. Insides are cobalt-violet with white stripes and bases, and black anthers. Late spring-flowering. ↕60cm (24in). ***

***T.* 'Blue Parrot'** ■ Parrot Group tulip with bright violet-blue flowers, bronze-purple inside. Late spring-flowering. ↕60cm (24in). ***

***T.* 'Bright Gem'.** Miscellaneous Group tulip bearing orange-flushed, sulphur-yellow flowers with bronze-orange basal marks. Early and mid-spring-flowering. ↕35cm (14in). ***

***T.* 'Brilliant Star'.** Single Early Group tulip bearing bright vermilion flowers in mid-spring. ↕20cm (8in). ***

***T.* 'Burgundy Lace'.** Fringed Group tulip bearing fringed, wine-red flowers in late spring. ↕60cm (24in). ***

***T.* 'Burns'** ■ Fringed Group tulip bearing bright light pink flowers, with

TULIPA

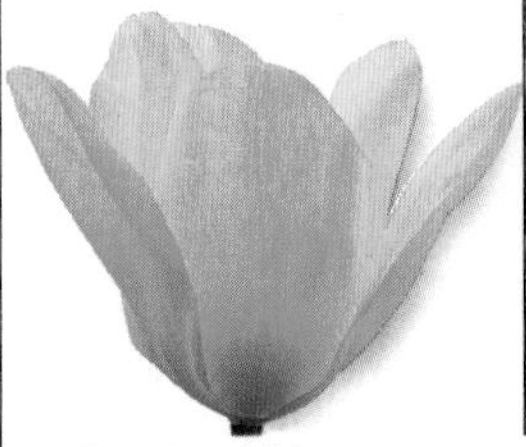
Tulipa 'Candela'

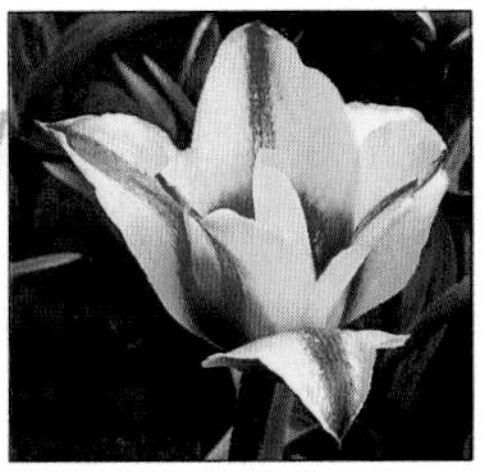
Tulipa 'Cape Cod'

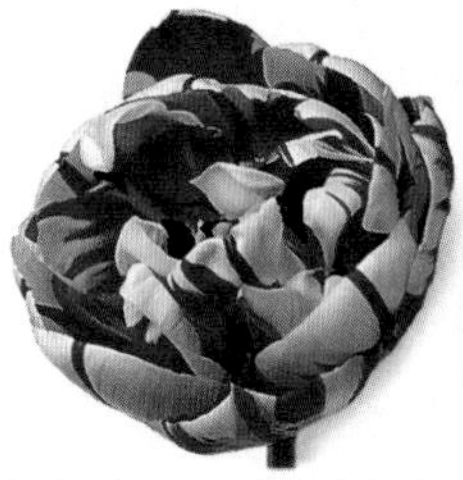
Tulipa 'Carnaval de Nice'

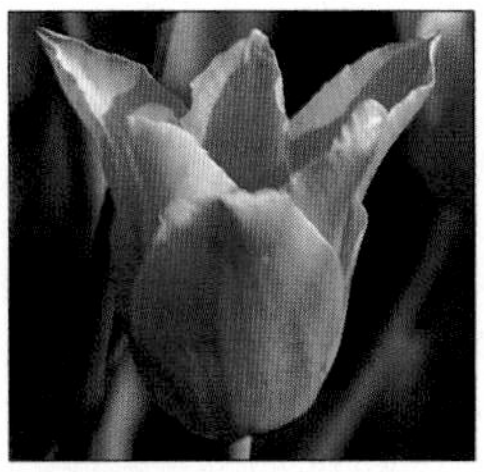
Tulipa 'China Pink'

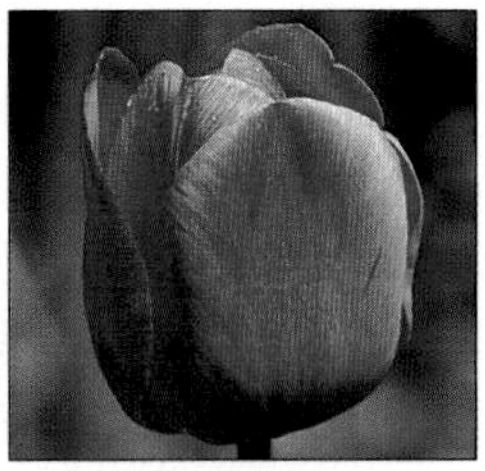
Tulipa 'Clara Butt'

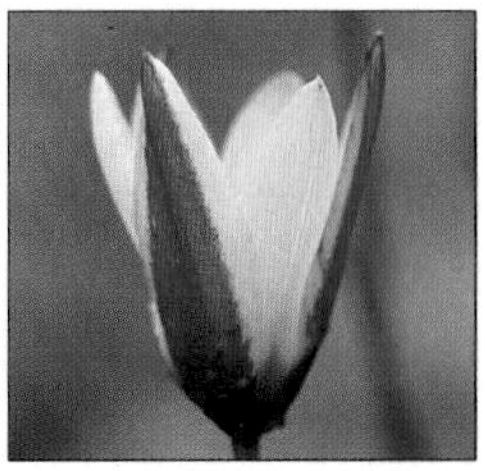
Tulipa clusiana

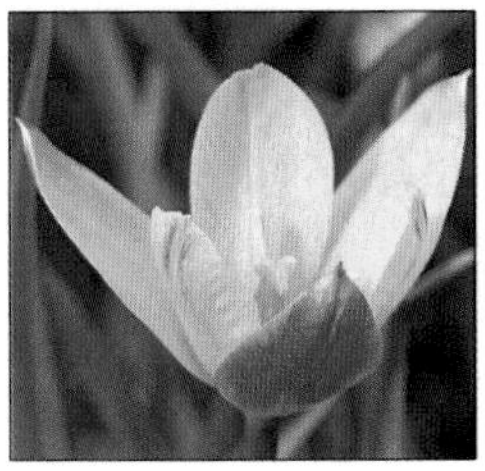
Tulipa clusiana var. *chrysantha*

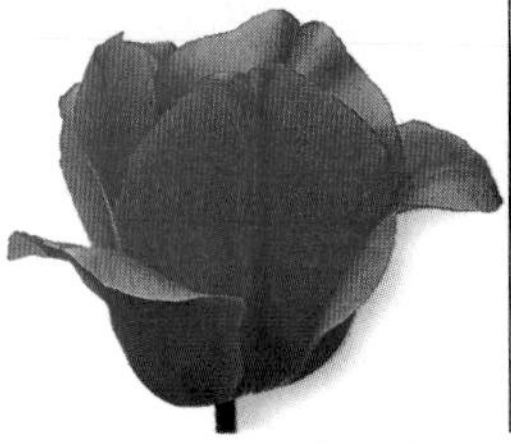
Tulipa 'Don Quichotte'

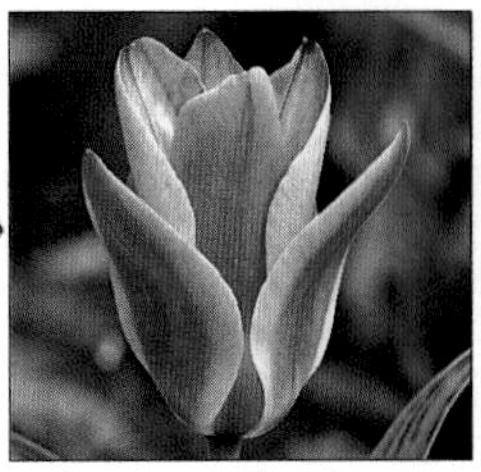
Tulipa 'Dreamboat'

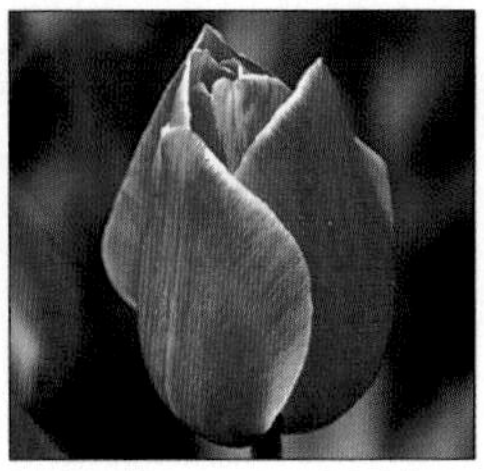
Tulipa 'Dreaming Maid'

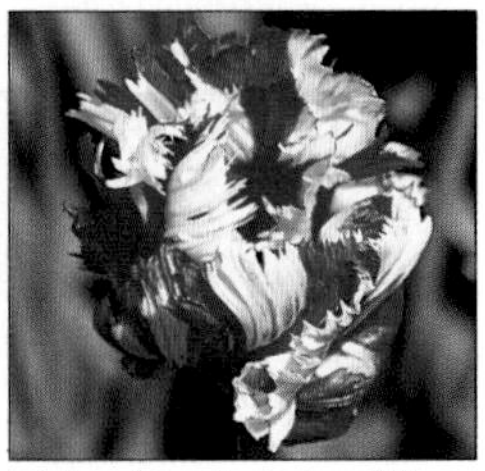
Tulipa 'Estella Rijnveld'

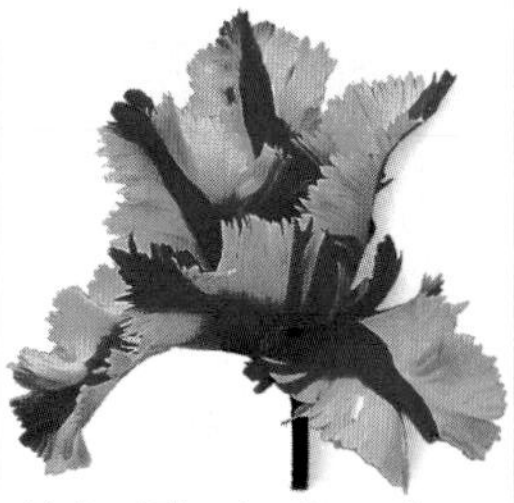
Tulipa 'Flaming Parrot'

greyish white bases outside, in late spring. Insides are pinkish red with ivory-white bases, violet margins, and yellow anthers. ↕50cm (20in). ❄❄❄
T. 'Buttercup'. Greigii Group tulip bearing yellow-margined, carmine-red flowers, dark golden yellow inside, with red-marked yellow bases. Mid-spring-flowering. Leaves are marked dark bluish maroon. ↕25cm (10in). ❄❄❄
T. 'Candela' ■ Fosteriana Group tulip producing large, pure yellow flowers, with black anthers, in mid-spring. ↕35cm (14in). ❄❄❄
T. 'Cape Cod' ■ Greigii Group tulip bearing apricot-yellow flowers, with red central stripes on the tepals, in mid-spring. Leaves are marked dark bluish maroon. ↕20cm (8in). ❄❄❄
T. 'Carnaval de Nice' ■ Double Late Group tulip bearing white flowers, with dark red feathers and markings, in late spring. ↕40cm (16in). ❄❄❄
T. 'China Pink' ■ Lily-flowered Group tulip bearing pink flowers, with white bases inside, in late spring. ↕50cm (20in). ❄❄❄
T. *chrysantha* see *T. clusiana* var. *chrysantha*.
T. 'Clara Butt' ■ Single Late Group tulip bearing deep salmon-pink flowers in late spring. ↕60cm (24in). ❄❄❄

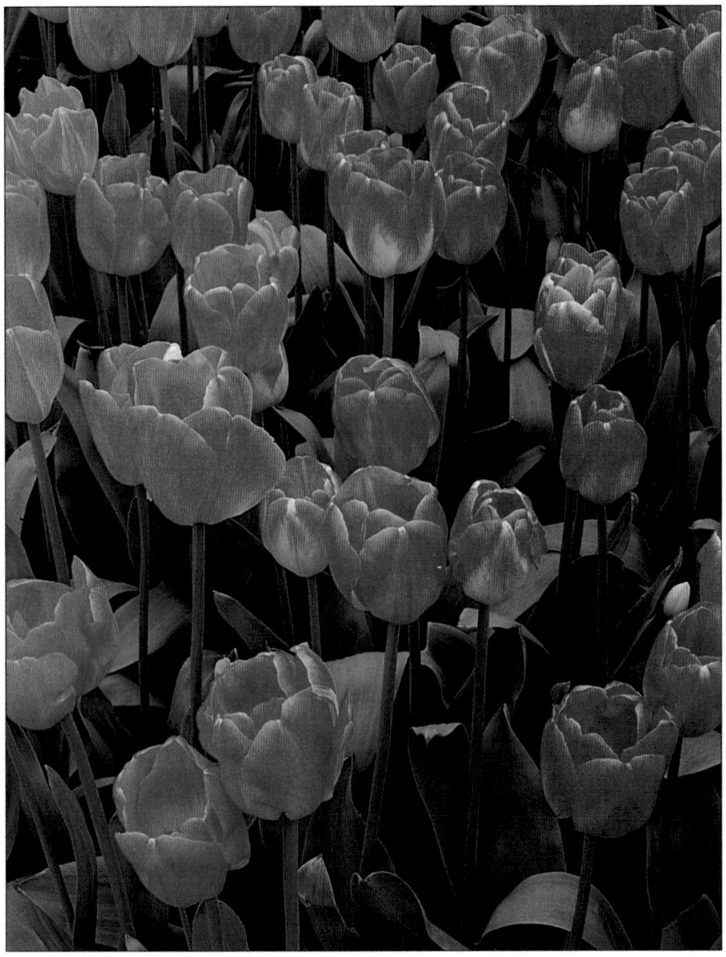
Tulipa 'Dreamland'

T. *clusiana* ■ syn. *T. aitchisonii* (Lady tulip). Miscellaneous Group tulip with 2–5 linear, hairless, glaucous, grey-green leaves, to 15cm (6in) long, sometimes wavy-margined. Bowl-shaped, later star-shaped flowers, to 10cm (4in) across, with rounded bases, are produced singly or in pairs in early and mid-spring. Flowers are white, striped dark pink outside, with purple or crimson basal marks and purple stamens. ↕30cm (12in). Iran to Himalayas. ❄❄❄. **var. *chrysantha*** ■♀ syn. *T. chrysantha*, *T. stellata* var. *chrysantha*, has up to 3 yellow flowers, tinged red or brownish purple outside, with yellow anthers. **var. *stellata***, syn. *T. stellata*, has star-shaped flowers with yellow basal marks.
T. 'Cordell Hull'. Single Late Group tulip bearing white-flamed red flowers in late spring. ↕60cm (24in). ❄❄❄
T. 'Corona'. Kaufmanniana Group tulip bearing red flowers, pale yellow inside, in mid-spring. Leaves are marked purple. ↕25cm (10in). ❄❄❄
T. 'Corsage' ♀ Greigii Group tulip bearing rose-pink flowers, with yellow margins and bronze bases, in mid-spring. Insides are rose-red with golden yellow feathers. Leaves are marked dark bluish maroon. ↕25cm (10in). ❄❄❄
T. 'Couleur Cardinal'. Triumph Group tulip producing plum-purple flowers, dark crimson-scarlet inside, in mid-spring. ↕35cm (14in). ❄❄❄
T. *dasystemon* of gardens see *T. tarda*.
T. 'Dawnglow'. Darwin Hybrid Group tulip bearing pale apricot flowers, flushed carmine-pink, with greenish yellow bases. Insides are yellow-orange with purple anthers. Mid-spring-flowering. ↕60cm (24in). ❄❄❄
T. 'Destiny'. Parrot Group tulip producing carmine-pink flowers, with creamy white bases and bronze anthers, in late spring. ↕45cm (18in). ❄❄❄
T. 'Diana'. Single Early Group tulip producing white flowers in mid-spring. ↕35cm (14in). ❄❄❄
T. 'Don Quichotte' ■ Triumph Group tulip producing cherry-pink flowers in late spring. ↕40cm (16in). ❄❄❄
T. 'Dreamboat' ■ Greigii Group tulip producing red-tinged, amber-yellow flowers with red-marked, green-bronze bases. Mid-spring-flowering. Leaves are marked dark bluish maroon. ↕20cm (8in). ❄❄❄
T. 'Dreaming Maid' ■ Triumph Group tulip producing white-margined violet flowers in mid-spring. ↕50cm (20in). ❄❄❄
T. 'Dreamland' ■ Single Late Group tulip producing cream-flamed red flowers. Insides are pinkish red with white bases and yellow anthers. Late spring-flowering. ↕60cm (24in). ❄❄❄
T. 'Early Harvest' ♀ Kaufmanniana Group tulip bearing dark pinkish red flowers with yellow margins and bases, and bronze-green basal marks. Insides are yellow with vivid, reddish orange markings and pale yellow anthers. Mid-spring-flowering. Leaves are marked purple. ↕25cm (10in). ❄❄❄
T. *edulis*, syn. *Amana edulis*. Miscellaneous Group tulip with 6 linear, hairless, mid-green leaves, 15–25cm (6–10in) long. In late winter and early spring, star-shaped white flowers, 6cm (2½in) across, veined reddish brown or purple outside, with yellow-margined, dark purple basal marks and yellow anthers, are borne singly or in pairs. The 2 or 3 linear bracts below each flower distinguish it from other species. ↕20cm (8in). N.E. China, Korea, Japan. ❄❄❄
T. 'Elizabeth Arden'. Darwin Hybrid Group tulip producing violet-flushed, dark salmon-pink flowers with yellow and white bases. Mid-spring-flowering. ↕55cm (22in). ❄❄❄
T. 'Engadin' ♀ Greigii Group tulip bearing yellow-margined, blood-red flowers, dark golden yellow with blood-red stripes inside. Mid-spring-flowering. Leaves are marked dark bluish maroon. ↕20cm (8in). ❄❄❄
T. 'Esperanto'. Viridiflora Group tulip bearing pinkish red flowers with green-flamed midveins, which fade to reddish brown, greenish brown bases, and greenish yellow anthers. Late spring-flowering. Leaves are margined white. ↕50cm (20in). ❄❄❄
T. 'Estella Rijnveld' ■ syn. *T.* 'Gay Presto'. Parrot Group tulip producing fringed, white-flamed red flowers in late spring. ↕55cm (22in). ❄❄❄
T. 'Fancy Frills'. Fringed Group tulip producing deep rose-red flowers with whitish pink fringes, ivory-white bases, and pale yellow anthers. Late spring-flowering. ↕45cm (18in). ❄❄❄
T. 'Flaming Parrot' ■ Parrot Group tulip with deep yellow flowers, flamed

T

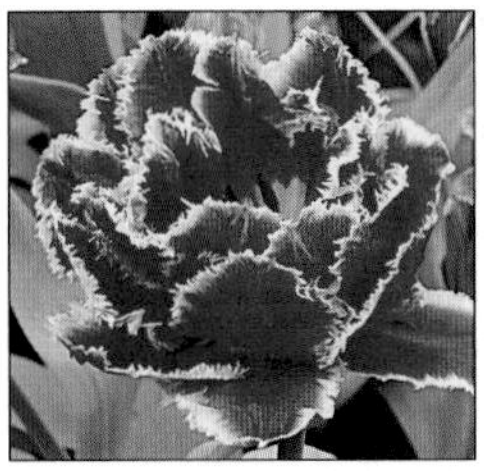
Tulipa 'Fringed Beauty'

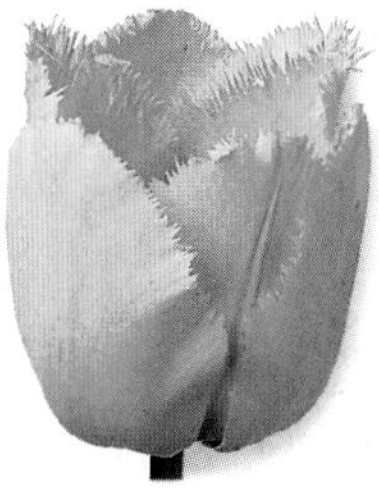
Tulipa 'Fringed Elegance'

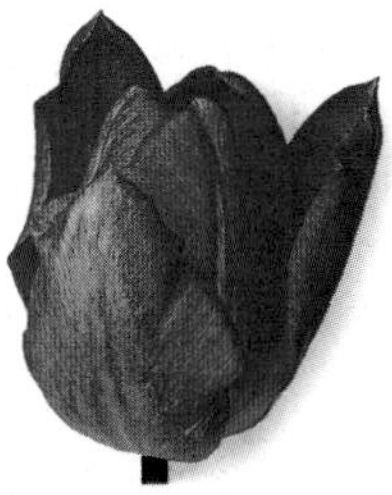
Tulipa 'Generaal De Wet'

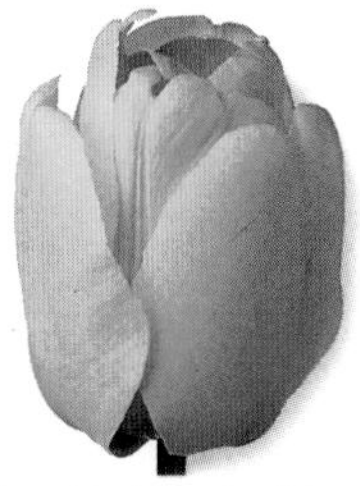
Tulipa 'Golden Apeldoorn'

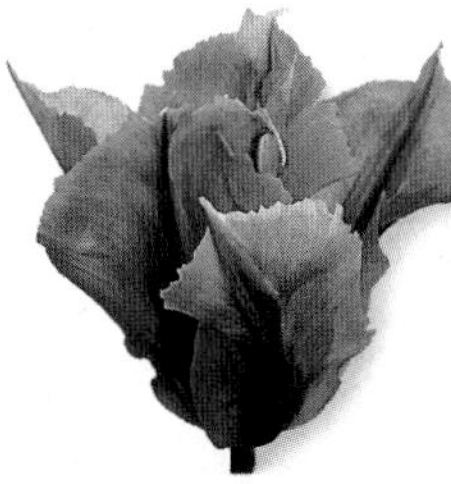
Tulipa 'Golden Artist'

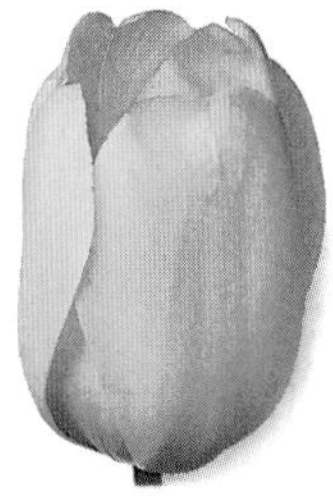
Tulipa 'Golden Oxford'

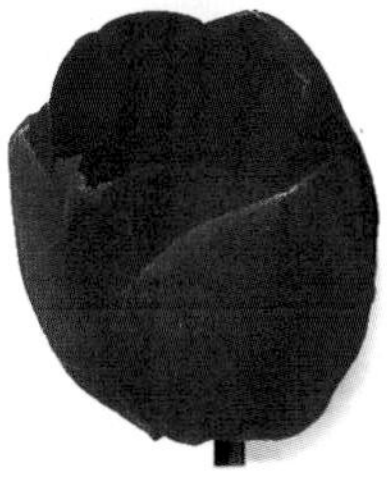
Tulipa 'Gordon Cooper'

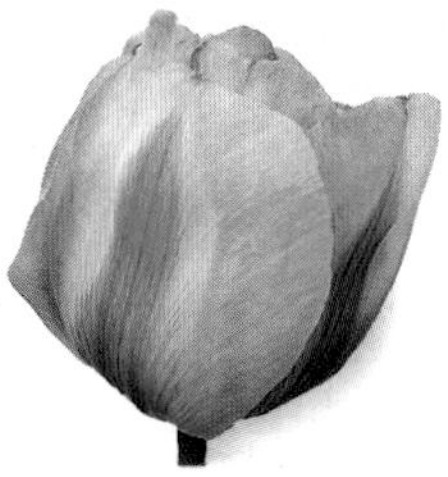
Tulipa 'Groenland'

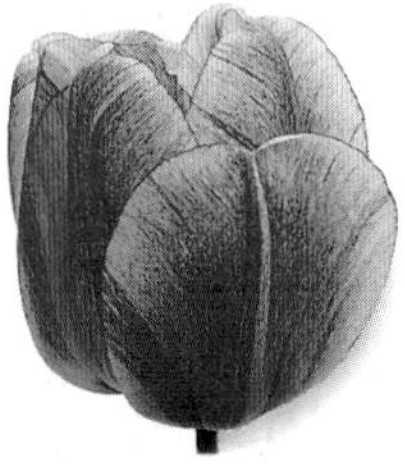
Tulipa 'Gudoshnik'

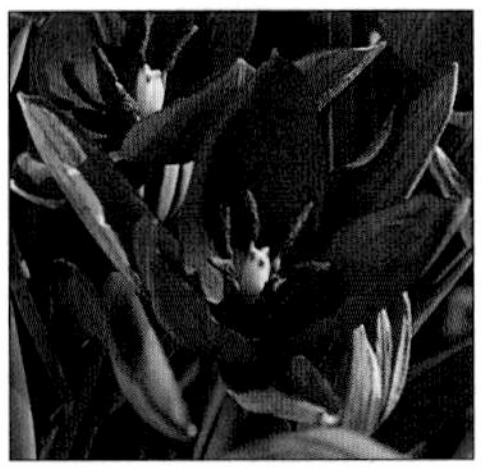
Tulipa hageri 'Splendens'

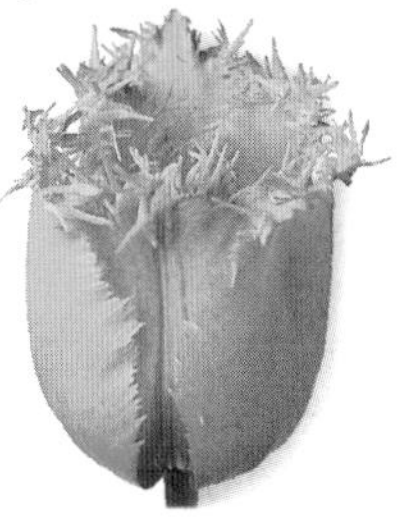
Tulipa 'Hamilton'

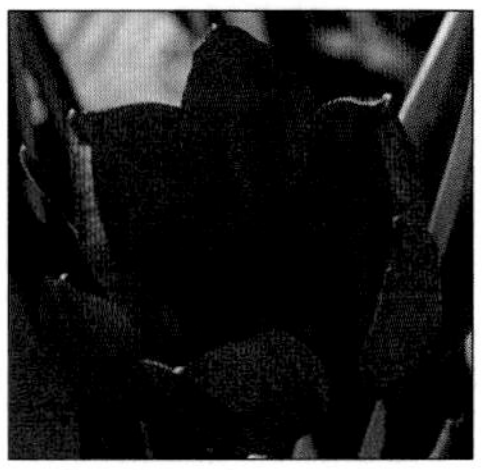
Tulipa humilis

dark red, and with primrose-yellow bases. Insides are primrose-yellow with glowing blood-red flames, and purple-black anthers. Late spring-flowering. ↕55cm (22in). ❄❄❄

T. fosteriana. Fosteriana Group tulip with 3–6 oblong to broadly ovate, light grey-green leaves, to 30cm (12in) long, downy above. Bowl-shaped, slightly fragrant flowers, to 20cm (8in) across, with rounded bases, are borne singly on slightly downy stems in early and mid-spring. Flowers are bright red with yellow-margined, purplish black basal marks. Stamens have purplish black anthers and black or yellow filaments. ↕45cm (18in). Kazakhstan, Uzbekistan, Tajikistan. ❄❄❄. **'Princeps'** has orange-scarlet flowers, scarlet inside, with greenish bronze basal marks.

***T.* 'Fringed Beauty'** ■ Fringed Group tulip producing vermilion flowers, with golden yellow fringes, in late spring. ↕35cm (14in). ❄❄❄

***T.* 'Fringed Elegance'** ■ Fringed Group tulip bearing primrose-yellow flowers, with paler fringes, and sometimes with pink markings, in late spring. Insides are brilliant greenish yellow with bronze-green basal marks and purple anthers. ↕35cm (14in). ❄❄❄

***T.* 'Garden Party'.** Triumph Group tulip bearing white flowers, carmine-red at the margins. Insides are feathered carmine-red with white bases. Mid-spring-flowering. ↕45cm (18in). ❄❄❄

***T.* 'Gay Presto'** see *T.* 'Estella Rijnveld'.

***T.* 'Generaal de Wet'** ■ syn. *T.* 'General de Wet'. Single Early Group tulip bearing fragrant, golden orange flowers, with dark orange shading, in mid-spring. ↕40cm (16in). ❄❄❄

***T.* 'General de Wet'** see *T.* 'Generaal de Wet'.

***T.* 'Georgette'.** Single Late Group tulip producing red-margined yellow flowers, several per stem, in late spring. ↕45cm (18in). ❄❄❄

***T.* 'Gerbrand Kieft'.** Double Late Group tulip bearing glowing purple-red flowers, with pure white margins, in late spring. ↕45cm (18in). ❄❄❄

T. gesneriana. Miscellaneous Group tulip with 2–7 lance-shaped to ovate-lance-shaped, hairless or finely downy, mid-green leaves, to 30cm (12in) long. Solitary flowers, to 12cm (5in) across, cup-shaped at first, opening to star-shaped, with rounded bases, are borne on hairless or finely downy stems in early to late spring. Flowers are red, orange, yellow, or purplish red, sometimes marked yellow or black at the bases, with purple or yellow stamens. The original parent of many garden cultivars. ↕45cm (18in). Probably garden origin; naturalized in parts of the Mediterranean. ❄❄❄

***T.* 'Giuseppe Verdi'** ■ Kaufmanniana Group tulip bearing yellow-margined, carmine-red flowers, golden yellow with small red marks inside, in mid-spring. Leaves are marked purple. ↕20cm (8in). ❄❄❄

***T.* 'Golden Apeldoorn'** ■ Darwin Hybrid Group tulip producing golden yellow flowers, with black anthers, in mid-spring. Inside, star-shaped black bases have bronze-green borders. ↕60cm (24in). ❄❄❄

***T.* 'Golden Artist'** ■ Viridiflora Group tulip producing golden orange flowers, with green stripes on the tepals, in late spring. ↕45cm (18in). ❄❄❄

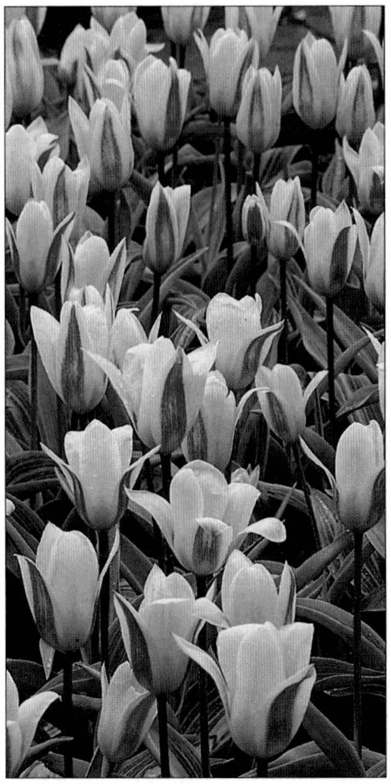
Tulipa 'Giuseppe Verdi'

***T.* 'Golden Mirjoran'.** Triumph Group tulip producing dark rose-red flowers, with light yellow margins, in mid-spring. Insides are sulphur-yellow with broad, cherry-red margins and purple-brown anthers. ↕45cm (18in). ❄❄❄

***T.* 'Golden Oxford'** ■ syn. *T.* 'Topic'. Darwin Hybrid Group tulip producing pure yellow flowers, sometimes narrowly margined red, with black anthers, in mid-spring. ↕60cm (24in). ❄❄❄

***T.* 'Gordon Cooper'** ■ Darwin Hybrid Group tulip with red flowers, maturing to pink, with signal-red margins and bluish black and yellow basal marks. Insides are glowing signal-red with black anthers. Mid-spring-flowering. ↕60cm (24in). ❄❄❄

***T.* 'Grand Duc'** see *T.* 'Keizerskroon'.

***T.* 'Greenland'** see *T.* 'Groenland'.

T. greigii. Greigii Group tulip with 2–7 oblong-lance-shaped to lance-shaped, sometimes wavy-margined, glaucous, grey-green leaves, to 25cm (10in) long, streaked or marked reddish or dark purple, and often downy above. In early spring, densely downy, pink- or brown-tinged stems bear solitary, bowl-shaped, red or yellow flowers, to 14cm (5½in) across; they are often orange-stained outside, with yellow-rimmed, blackish purple basal marks and black stamens. ↕50cm (20in). Tajikistan. ❄❄❄

***T.* 'Greuze'.** Single Late Group tulip producing violet-purple flowers in late spring. ↕55cm (22in). ❄❄❄

***T.* 'Groenland'** ■ syn. *T.* 'Greenland'. Viridiflora Group tulip producing green flowers, with rose-pink margins, in late spring. ↕45cm (18in). ❄❄❄

***T.* 'Gudoshnik'** ■ Darwin Hybrid Group tulip bearing yellow flowers with red spots, rose-pink flames, bluish black basal marks, and black anthers. Mid-spring-flowering. ↕60cm (24in). ❄❄❄

T. hageri. Miscellaneous Group tulip with 2–7 lance-shaped, hairless, light green leaves, to 20cm (8in) long, often margined reddish purple. In early and mid-spring, bears star-shaped flowers, 6–9cm (2½–3½in) across, singly or in clusters of up to 4, on hairless stems. The buff flowers are mostly green-tinged outside. Inside, they are dull red with black, sometimes yellow-margined basal marks, dark green or brown anthers, and green filaments, sometimes tinged purple. ↕35cm (14in). Bulgaria, Greece, W. Turkey. ❄❄❄. **var. *nitens*** has orange-scarlet flowers and glaucous leaves. **'Splendens'** ■ has crimson-scarlet flowers, brownish red inside.

***T.* 'Hamilton'** ■ Fringed Group tulip producing buttercup-yellow flowers, with darker yellow fringes and anthers, in late spring. ↕50cm (20in). ❄❄❄

***T.* 'Hans Mayer'.** Darwin Hybrid Group tulip bearing buttercup-yellow flowers, flamed translucent vermilion, with light green bases. Insides are golden yellow with vermilion flames and dark brown bases. Brown anthers have a violet glow. Mid-spring-flowering. ↕60cm (24in). ❄❄❄

***T.* 'Heart's Delight'.** Kaufmanniana Group tulip bearing dark rose-red flowers with pale rose-pink margins and red-marked, golden yellow bases. Insides are ivory-white. Early spring-flowering. Leaves are marked purple. ↕20cm (8in). ❄❄❄

***T.* 'Hollywood'.** Viridiflora Group tulip producing green-tinged red flowers, with yellow basal marks, in late spring. ↕50cm (20in). ❄❄❄

T. humilis ■ Miscellaneous Group tulip with 2–5 linear, channelled, hairless, glaucous, grey-green leaves, to 15cm (6in) long. In early and mid-spring, star-shaped flowers, to 7cm (3in) across, are produced singly, or sometimes in twos or threes. Flowers are pale pink to purplish pink or magenta, often tinged greyish green outside, with yellow, olive-green, or blue-black basal marks, and frequently margined yellow or white. Stamens have yellow, brown, purple, or black anthers and yellow filaments. ↕to 25cm (10in). S. and E. Turkey, N. Iraq, N. and W. Iran, Azerbaijan. ❄❄❄

***T.* 'Ile de France'.** Triumph Group tulip producing cardinal-red flowers with dark bronze-green basal marks and narrow, yellowish brown margins. Insides are blood-red. Mid- and late spring-flowering. ↕60cm (24in). ❄❄❄

***T.* 'Inzell'.** Triumph Group tulip producing ivory-white flowers, with yellow anthers, in mid-spring. ↕45cm (18in). ❄❄❄

***T.* 'Jewel of Spring'** 🏆 Darwin Hybrid Group tulip producing red-margined, sulphur-yellow flowers, with greenish black bases and black anthers, in mid-spring. ↕60cm (24in). ❄❄❄

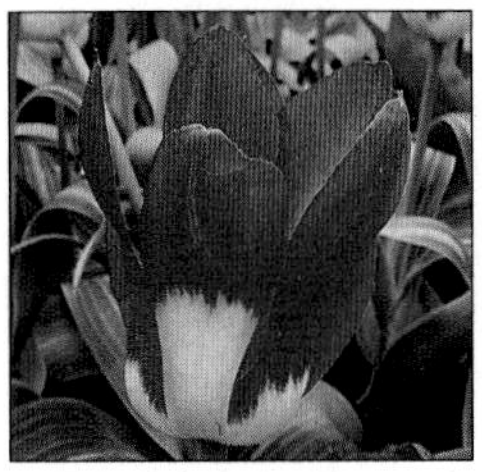
Tulipa 'Juan'

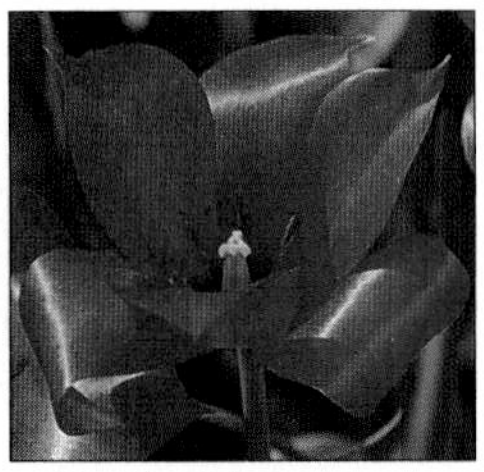
Tulipa linifolia

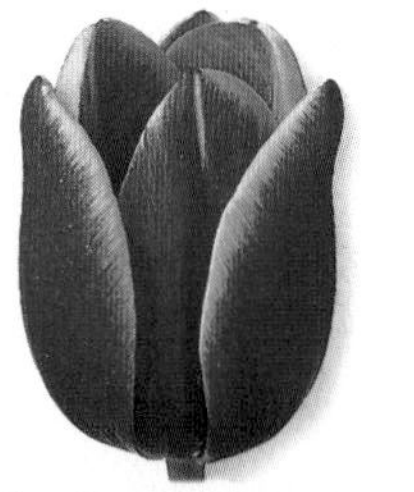
Tulipa 'Lustige Witwe'

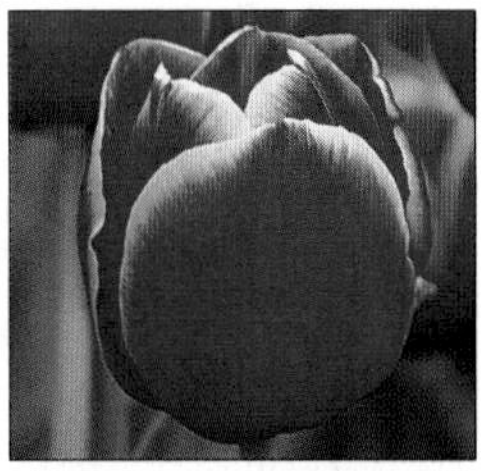
Tulipa 'Margot Fonteyn'

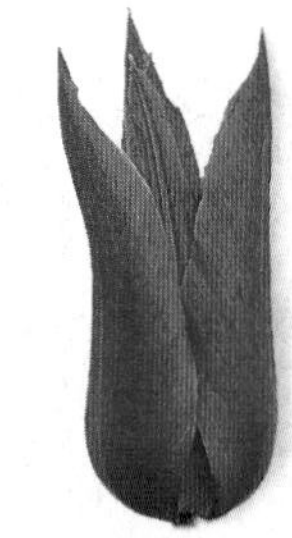
Tulipa 'Mariette'

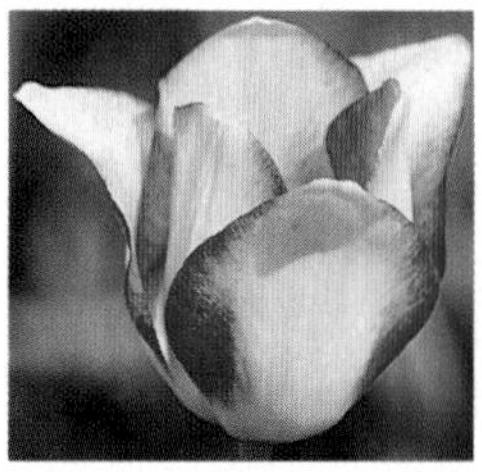
Tulipa marjolletii

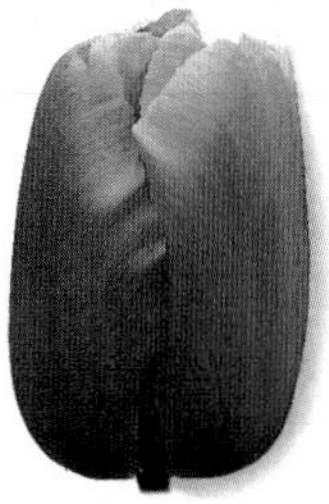
Tulipa 'Menton'

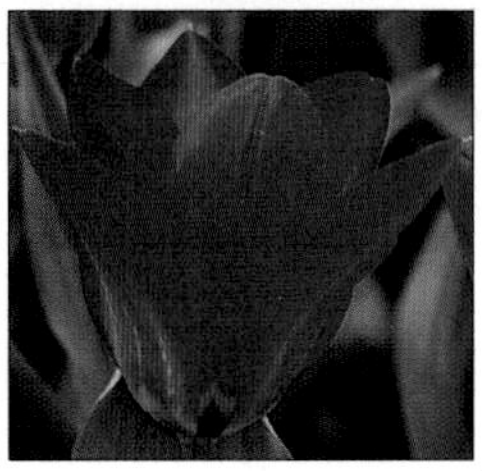
Tulipa 'Mme Lefeber'

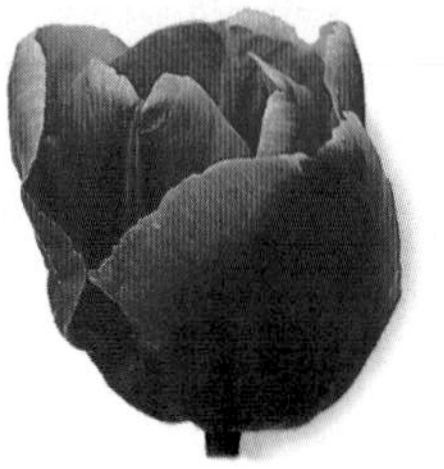
Tulipa 'Orange Monarch'

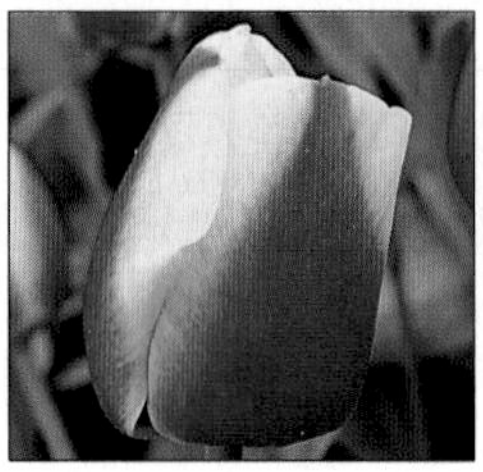
Tulipa 'Oriental Splendour'

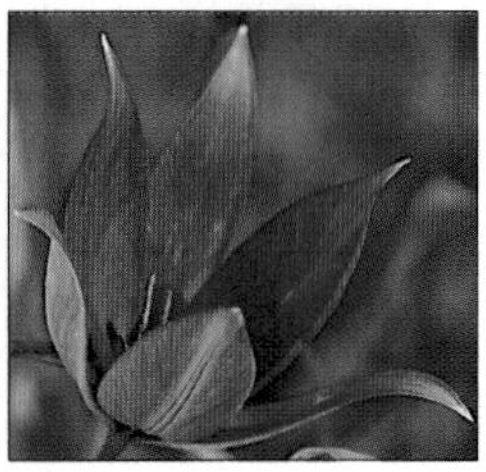
Tulipa orphanidea

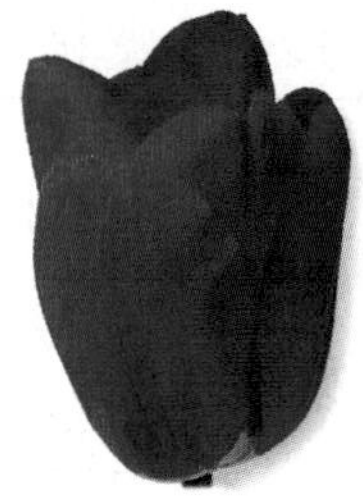
Tulipa 'Oxford'

***T.* 'Joffre'.** Single Early Group tulip producing yellow flowers, with subtle, light to dark red shades, in early spring. ↕30cm (12in). ❄❄❄

***T.* 'Johann Strauss'.** Kaufmanniana Group tulip bearing currant-red flowers, margined sulphur-yellow, with golden yellow bases. Insides are ivory-white. Early spring-flowering. Leaves are marked purple. ↕20cm (8in). ❄❄❄

***T.* 'Juan'** ■ Fosteriana Group tulip producing pink-tinged, dark orange flowers, with yellow bases and anthers, in mid-spring. Leaves are marked reddish brown. ↕25cm (10in). ❄❄❄

T. kaufmanniana (Water-lily tulip). Kaufmanniana Group tulip with 3–5 lance-shaped to inversely lance-shaped, slightly wavy-margined, hairless, grey-green leaves, to 25cm (10in) long. Bowl-shaped flowers, 3–12cm (1¼–5in) across, are borne singly or in clusters of up to 5, on slightly downy, often red-tinged stems in early and mid-spring. Flowers are cream or yellow, flushed pink or greyish green outside, or pink, orange, or red, often with contrasting basal marks. Stamens are yellow with twisted anthers. ↕to 25cm (10in). Kazakhstan, Uzbekistan, Tajikistan, Kyrgyzstan. ❄❄❄

***T.* 'Kees Nelis'.** Triumph Group tulip bearing blood-red flowers, with orange-yellow margins, in mid-spring. ↕40cm (16in). ❄❄❄

***T.* 'Keizerskroon'** ■♀ syn. *T.* 'Grand Duc'. Single Early Group tulip bearing broadly yellow-margined scarlet flowers in mid-spring. ↕30cm (12in). ❄❄❄

***T.* 'Kingsblood'** ♀ Single Late Group tulip bearing cherry-red flowers, with scarlet margins, in late spring. ↕60cm (24in). ❄❄❄

T. kolpakowskiana ♀ Miscellaneous Group tulip with 2–4 erect, linear, deeply channelled, hairless, wavy-margined, grey-green leaves, to 20cm (8in) long. In early and mid-spring, bowl-shaped yellow flowers, 3.5–7cm (1½–3in) across, marked crimson, orange, or olive-green outside, with yellow stamens, are produced singly or in clusters of up to 4. ↕20cm (8in). Uzbekistan, Afghanistan. ❄❄❄

T. linifolia ■♀ Miscellaneous Group tulip with 3–9 linear-sickle-shaped, hairless, grey-green leaves, to 8cm (3in) long, with wavy red margins. Bowl-shaped red flowers, to 8cm (3in) across, are produced in early and mid-spring. The rounded flower bases have blackish purple, often yellow-margined marks; stamens have dark purple or yellow anthers and black or yellow filaments. ↕20cm (8in). Uzbekistan, N. Iran, Afghanistan. ❄❄❄

***T.* 'Longfellow'.** Greigii Group tulip bearing black-based vermilion flowers, striped lighter red, and signal-red inside, in mid-spring. Leaves are marked dark bluish purple. ↕30cm (12in). ❄❄❄

***T.* 'Lustige Witwe'** ■ syn. *T.* 'Merry Widow'. Triumph Group tulip bearing glowing dark red flowers, margined pure white, in mid-spring. ↕40cm (16in). ❄❄❄

***T.* 'Magician'** see *T.* 'Magier'.

***T.* 'Magier'**, syn. *T.* 'Magician'. Single Late Group tulip bearing white flowers, with violet-blue margins, in late spring. ↕55cm (22in). ❄❄❄

***T.* 'Maja'.** Fringed Group tulip bearing fringed, pale mimosa-yellow flowers, brilliant greenish yellow inside, with bronze-yellow bases and yellow anthers, in late spring. ↕50cm (20in). ❄❄❄

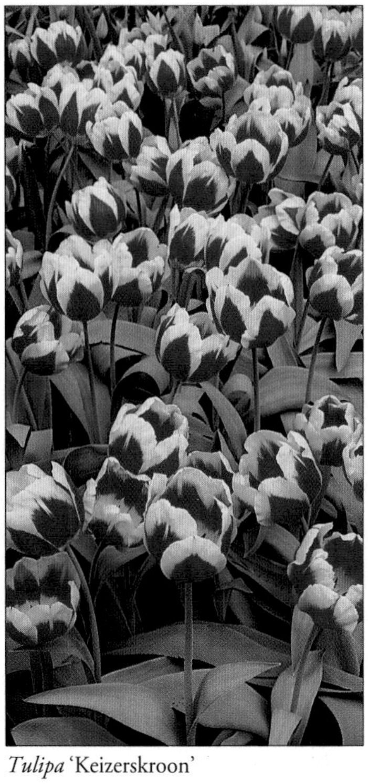
Tulipa 'Keizerskroon'

***T.* 'Margot Fonteyn'** ■ Triumph Group tulip bearing yellow-margined, cardinal-red flowers with yellow bases. Insides are bright red with lighter margins and black anthers. Mid-spring-flowering. ↕40cm (16in). ❄❄❄

***T.* 'Mariette'** ■ Lily-flowered Group tulip bearing satin-textured, dark rose-pink flowers, with white bases inside, in late spring. ↕50cm (20in). ❄❄❄

T. marjolettii see *T. marjolletii*.

T. marjolletii ■ syn. *T. marjolettii*. Miscellaneous Group tulip with 2–7 lance-shaped to ovate-lance-shaped, hairless, grey-green leaves, to 30cm (12in) long. In early and mid-spring, hairless stems bear solitary, bowl-shaped, creamy white flowers, to 12cm (5in) across, with rounded bases, margined dark pink and flushed purple on the outside. Stamens have yellow anthers and blue-black filaments. ↕45cm (18in). Probably garden origin; naturalized in S.W. Europe. ❄❄❄

***T.* 'Martine Bijl'.** Triumph Group tulip bearing glowing blood-red flowers, with yellow bases and bluish black anthers, in mid-spring. ↕45cm (18in). ❄❄❄

***T.* 'Maytime'.** Lily-flowered Group tulip bearing reddish violet flowers, with narrowly white-margined yellow bases, in late spring. ↕50cm (20in). ❄❄❄

***T.* 'Maywonder'.** Double Late Group tulip bearing rose-pink flowers in late spring. ↕45cm (18in). ❄❄❄

***T.* 'Menton'** ■ Single Late Group tulip bearing pinkish red flowers with pale orange stripes at the margins, and green-marked, yellow and white bases. Insides are poppy-red with white veins and yellow anthers. Late spring-flowering. ↕60cm (24in). ❄❄❄

***T.* 'Merry Widow'** see *T.* 'Lustige Witwe'.

***T.* 'Miss Holland'.** Triumph Group tulip bearing blood-red flowers with signal-red flames and buttercup-yellow bases with greenish yellow margins. Insides are signal-red with dark brown anthers. Mid-spring-flowering. ↕45cm (18in). ❄❄❄

***T.* 'Mme Lefeber'** ■ syn. *T.* 'Red Emperor'. Fosteriana Group tulip bearing fire-red flowers in early spring. ↕35cm (14in). ❄❄❄

***T.* 'Monsella'.** Double Early Group tulip bearing canary-yellow flowers with blood-red flames, sulphur-yellow inside, in mid-spring. ↕30cm (12in). ❄❄❄

T. montana, syn. *T. wilsoniana*. Miscellaneous Group tulip with 3–6 narrowly lance-shaped, wavy-margined, channelled, hairless, grey-green leaves, to 15cm (6in) long. In early and mid-spring, produces solitary, bowl-shaped red flowers, to 8cm (3in) across, with rounded bases, sometimes with a small, dark green central mark on each flower. Stamens have yellow anthers and red filaments. ↕25cm (10in). Turkmenistan, N. Iran. ❄❄❄

***T.* 'Monte Carlo'.** Double Early Group tulip producing sulphur-yellow flowers, with small red feathers, in mid-spring. ↕30cm (12in). ❄❄❄

***T.* 'Mount Tacoma'.** Double Late Group tulip producing pure white flowers in late spring. ↕40cm (16in). ❄❄❄

***T.* 'New Design'.** Triumph Group tulip bearing light yellow flowers, the outsides fading to pinkish white and having pale fuchsia-red margins. Insides have apricot flames, buttercup-yellow bases, and dark brown anthers. Mid-spring-flowering. Leaves have pinkish white margins. ↕45cm (18in). ❄❄❄

***T.* 'Noranda'.** Fringed Group tulip bearing dark blood-red flowers with fringed, orange-tinted margins, green-yellow bases, and black anthers. Late spring-flowering. ↕50cm (20in). ❄❄❄

***T.* 'Orange Favourite'.** Parrot Group tulip producing fragrant, green-marked orange flowers, with yellow bases, in late spring. ↕55cm (22in). ❄❄❄

***T.* 'Orange Monarch'** ■ Triumph Group tulip bearing orange flowers, tinged red-pink, with orange-yellow bases. Insides are apricot-orange with purple anthers. Mid-spring-flowering. ↕40cm (16in). ❄❄❄

***T.* 'Oranje Nassau'.** Double Early Group tulip bearing blood-red flowers, flushed fire-red, in mid-spring. ↕30cm (12in). ❄❄❄

***T.* 'Oratorio'.** Greigii Group tulip bearing rose-pink flowers, with black bases, in early spring. Insides are apricot-pink. Leaves are marked dark bluish purple. ↕20cm (8in). ❄❄❄

***T.* 'Oriental Splendour'** ■ Greigii Group tulip with carmine-red flowers, lemon-yellow at the margins and inside, and with green and red basal markings. Early spring-flowering. Leaves are marked dark bluish purple. ↕30cm (12in). ❄❄❄

T

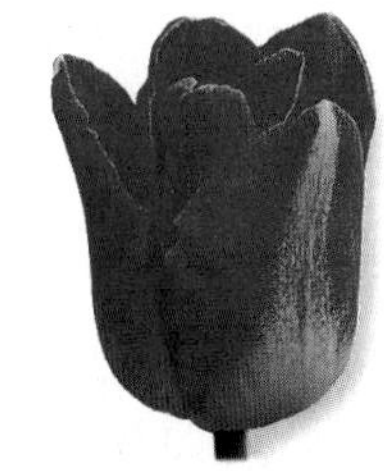
Tulipa 'Page Polka'

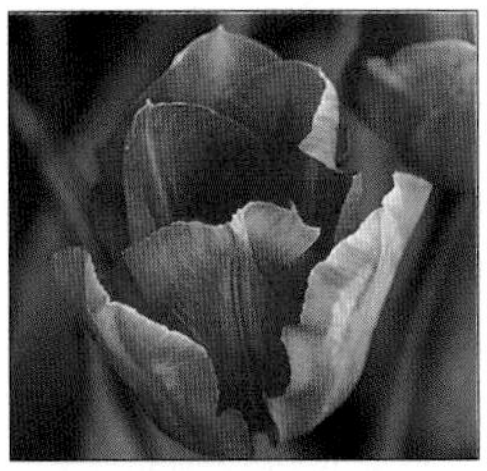
Tulipa 'Palestrina'

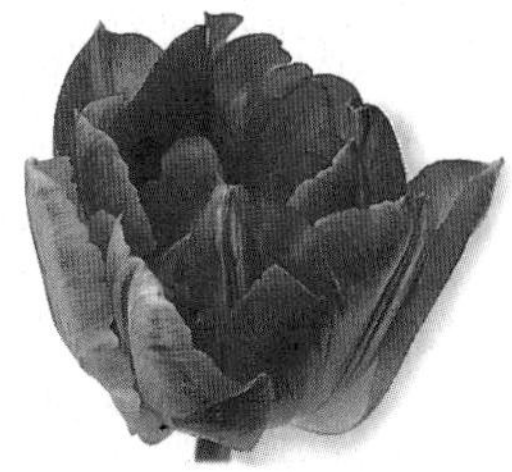
Tulipa 'Peach Blossom'

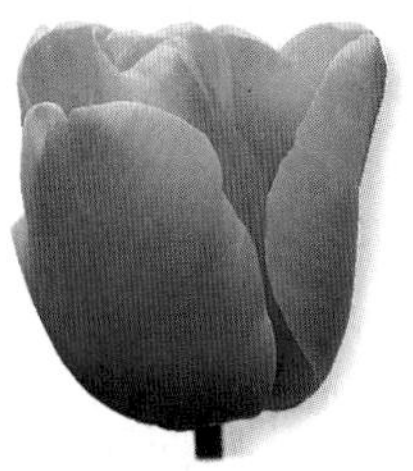
Tulipa 'Pink Diamond'

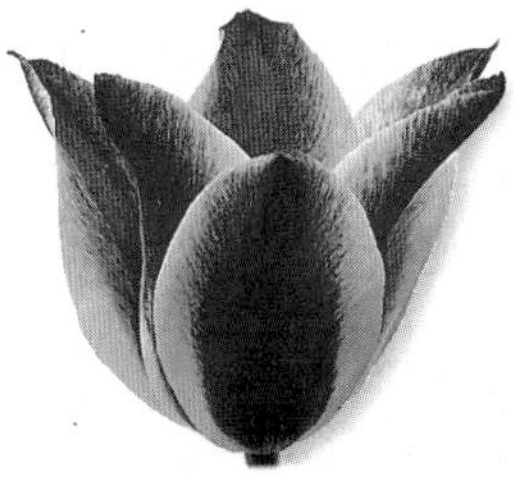
Tulipa 'Plaisir'

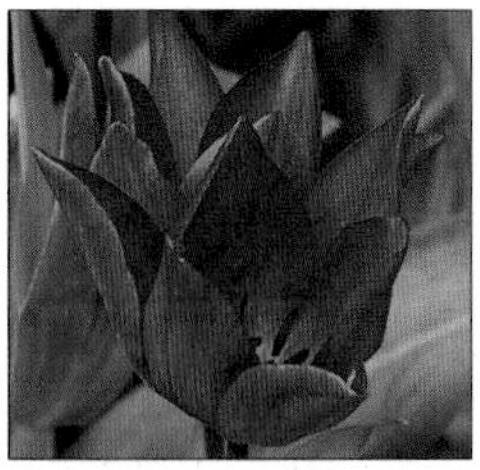
Tulipa praestans 'Van Tubergen's Variety'

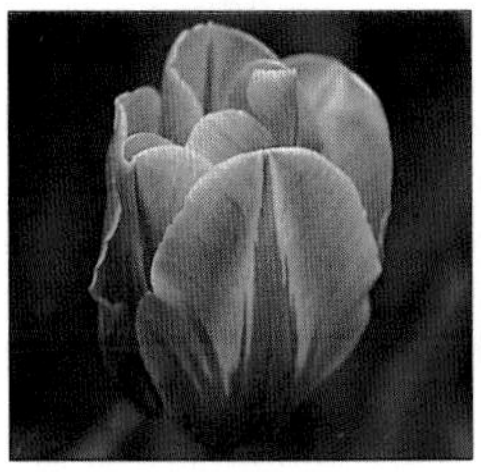
Tulipa 'Prinses Irene'

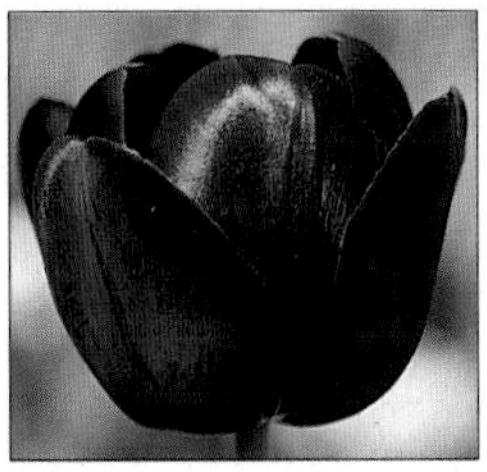
Tulipa 'Queen of Night'

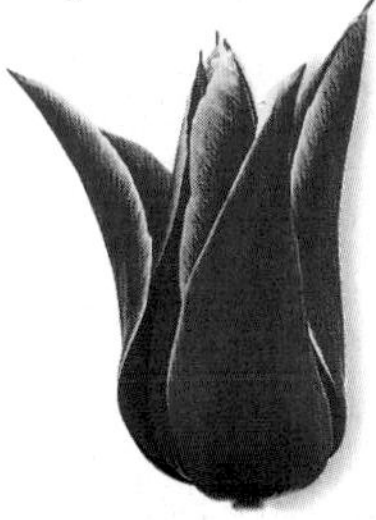
Tulipa 'Queen of Sheba'

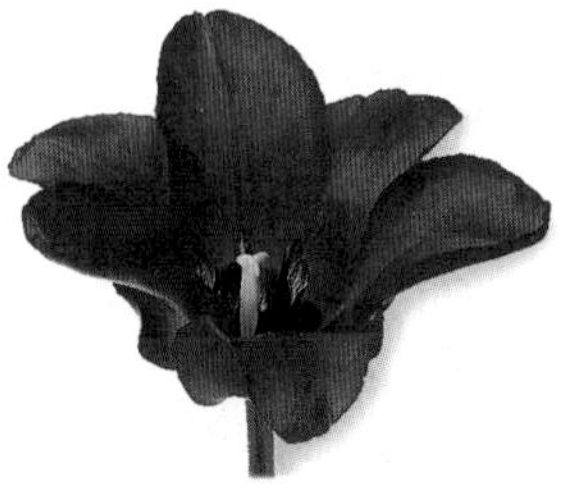
Tulipa 'Red Riding Hood'

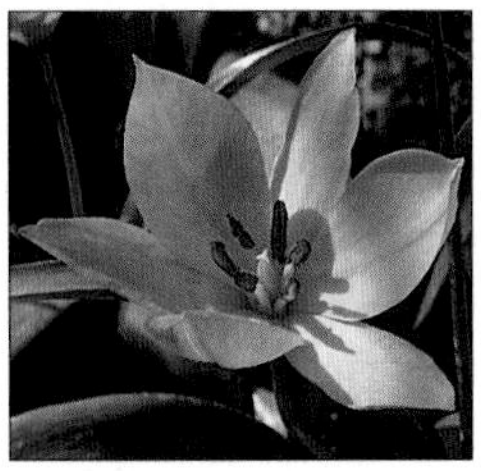
Tulipa saxatilis

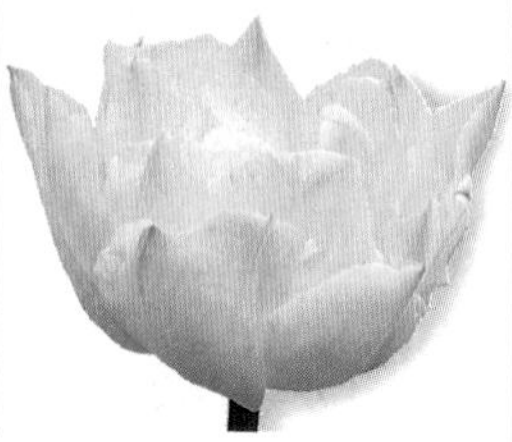
Tulipa 'Schoonoord'

T. orphanidea ■ Miscellaneous Group tulip with 2–7 lance-shaped, hairless, mid-green leaves, to 20cm (8in) long, often margined reddish purple. Star-shaped flowers, 3–6cm (1¼–2½in) across, are borne singly or in twos or threes, on hairless or downy stems in mid- and late spring. Flowers are buff, usually green-tinged outside; insides are pale to bright orange or brownish red, flushed red or rarely yellow, with black or dark green basal markings. Stamens have dark green or brown anthers and green, sometimes purple-tinged filaments. ↕35cm (14in). Bulgaria, Greece, W. Turkey. ❄❄❄
***T.* 'Oxford'** ■ 🏆 Darwin Hybrid Group tulip producing scarlet flowers, flushed purple-red, with sulphur-yellow bases. Insides are capsicum-red. Mid-spring-flowering. ↕60cm (24in). ❄❄❄
***T.* 'Page Polka'** ■ Triumph Group tulip producing dark red flowers, striped white outside, with white basal marks and yellow anthers. Mid-spring-flowering. ↕40cm (16in). ❄❄❄
***T.* 'Palestrina'** ■ Triumph Group tulip bearing salmon-pink flowers, green-tinged outside, in late spring. ↕50cm (20in). ❄❄❄
***T.* 'Passionale'.** Triumph Group tulip producing lilac-purple flowers, with dark purplish red flames, in mid-spring. Insides are beetroot-purple with purple-margined, tawny-yellow bases and light yellow anthers. ↕45cm (18in). ❄❄❄
***T.* 'Peach Blossom'** ■ Double Early Group tulip producing dark rose-pink flowers in mid-spring. Young flowers often have greenish white bases. ↕30cm (12in). ❄❄❄

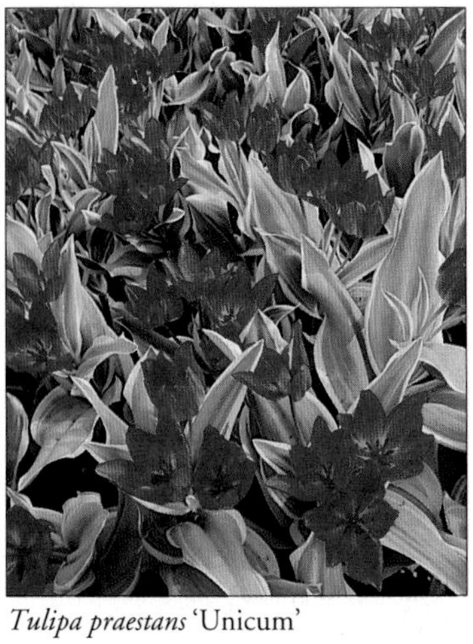
Tulipa praestans 'Unicum'

***T.* 'Peer Gynt'.** Triumph Group tulip bearing purple-margined, bright rose-pink flowers with yellow-spotted white bases. Insides are pink with purple-grey anthers. Mid-spring-flowering. ↕45cm (18in). ❄❄❄
***T.* 'Pink Diamond'** ■ Single Late Group tulip producing pink-purple flowers with paler margins. Insides are bright mid-pink with grey-yellow bases and yellow-green anthers. Late spring-flowering. ↕60cm (24in). ❄❄❄
***T.* 'Plaisir'** ■ 🏆 Greigii Group tulip bearing carmine-red flowers with sulphur-yellow margins and black and yellow bases. Insides are vermilion with sulphur-yellow margins. Early spring-flowering. Leaves are marked dark bluish maroon. ↕15cm (6in). ❄❄❄
T. polychroma see *T. biflora.*
T. praestans. Miscellaneous Group tulip with 3–6 erect, oblong or lance-shaped, keeled, downy, grey-green leaves, to 20cm (8in) long. In early and mid-spring, bowl-shaped, scarlet-orange flowers, 10–12cm (4–5in) across, are produced singly or in clusters of up to 5 on each of the minutely downy stems; stamens have yellow or purplish red anthers, and red filaments shading to yellow at the bases. Easily grown. ↕30cm (12in). Kazakhstan (Pamir Altai), Tajikistan. ❄❄❄. **'Fusilier'** 🏆 produces several very bright red flowers. **'Unicum'** ■ has variegated leaves with creamy white margins, and bears up to 5 capsicum-red flowers with small, light yellow bases and blue-black anthers. **'Van Tubergen's Variety'** ■ has up to 3 larger, bright orange-scarlet flowers, flushed yellow at the bases, with reddish brown anthers. ↕50cm (20in).
***T.* 'Prinses Irene'** ■ 🏆 Triumph Group tulip bearing unusual, orange and purple flowers in mid-spring. ↕35cm (14in). ❄❄❄
T. pulchella. Miscellaneous Group tulip with 2–5 linear, hairless, glaucous, grey-green leaves, to 15cm (6in) long. In early and mid-spring, star-shaped, light crimson or purple flowers, to 7cm (3in) across, with blue-black basal marks, are produced singly or sometimes in twos or threes. Stamens have purple anthers and blue filaments. ↕35cm (14in). Turkey, N. Iran, Turkmenistan, Uzbekistan, Afghanistan. ❄❄❄. **'Odalisque'** bears pale purple flowers with yellow basal marks. **'Persian Pearl'** produces rose-red flowers with yellow basal marks.
***T.* 'Purissima'** ■ syn. *T.* 'White Emperor'. Fosteriana Group tulip that produces pure white flowers in mid-spring. ↕35cm (14in). ❄❄❄
***T.* 'Queen of Night'** ■ Single Late Group tulip producing velvety, dark maroon flowers in late spring. ↕60cm (24in). ❄❄❄
***T.* 'Queen of Sheba'** ■ Lily-flowered Group tulip that produces glowing brownish red flowers, with orange margins, in late spring. ↕60cm (24in). ❄❄❄
***T.* 'Red Emperor'** see *T.* 'Mme Lefeber'.
***T.* 'Red Parrot'.** Parrot Group tulip producing raspberry-red flowers in late spring. ↕55cm (22in). ❄❄❄
***T.* 'Red Riding Hood'** ■ 🏆 Greigii Group tulip producing carmine-red flowers, scarlet inside, with black bases, in early spring. Leaves are marked dark bluish maroon. ↕20cm (8in). ❄❄❄

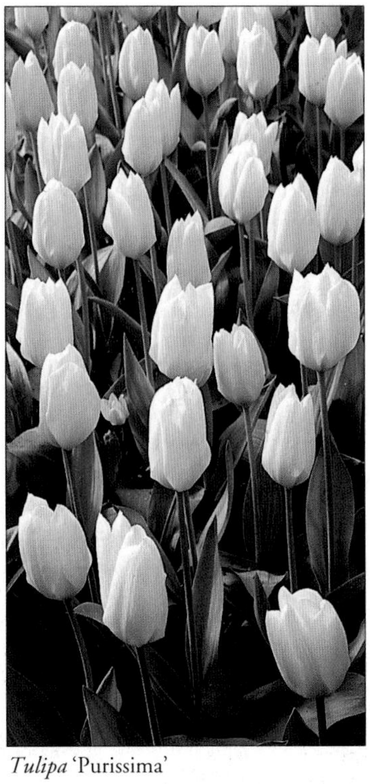
Tulipa 'Purissima'

***T.* 'Reginald Dixon'.** Fosteriana Group tulip with yellow-margined scarlet flowers. Insides are lemon-yellow with red-marked black bases. Mid-spring-flowering. ↕30cm (12in). ❄❄❄
***T.* 'Renown'.** Single Late Group tulip producing light carmine-red flowers with paler margins and blue-margined yellow bases. Late spring-flowering. ↕50cm (20in). ❄❄❄
***T.* 'Rococo'.** Parrot Group tulip bearing carmine-red flowers, margined fire-red, in late spring. ↕35cm (14in). ❄❄❄
***T.* 'Rondo'.** Fosteriana Group tulip producing yellow-margined vermilion flowers, golden yellow inside, with red-marked yellow bases. Mid-spring-flowering. ↕30cm (12in). ❄❄❄
***T.* 'Rosario'.** Triumph Group tulip producing dark pink flowers with large white bases. Insides are rose-pink with smaller, ivory-white bases. Mid-spring-flowering. ↕45cm (18in). ❄❄❄
T. saxatilis ■ syn. *T. bakeri.* Miscellaneous Group tulip, spreading by runners, with 2–4 linear, hairless, shiny, mid-green leaves, to 30cm (12in) long. In mid- and late spring, star-shaped, fragrant flowers, 6–8cm (2½–3in) across, are borne singly or in clusters of up to 4. Flowers are pink to lilac-purple with white-margined yellow marks. Stamens have yellow, purple, or brown anthers and yellow filaments. Tulips grown as *T. bakeri* are darker pink. ↕35cm (14in). Crete, W. Turkey. ❄❄❄
***T.* 'Schoonoord'** ■ Double Early Group tulip bearing pure white flowers in mid-spring. ↕30cm (12in). ❄❄❄
***T.* 'Shakespeare'.** Kaufmanniana Group tulip bearing carmine-red flowers, with salmon-pink margins and golden yellow bases, in mid-spring. Insides are scarlet-flushed salmon-pink. ↕25cm (10in). ❄❄❄
***T.* 'Shirley'.** Triumph Group tulip bearing ivory-white flowers, with narrow purple margins, white bases spotted pale purple, and brownish violet anthers, in late spring. ↕60cm (24in). ❄❄❄
***T.* 'Solva'.** Fosteriana Group tulip bearing pale vermilion flowers, yellow at the bases, in mid-spring. ↕35cm (14in). ❄❄❄
***T.* 'Sorbet'** 🏆 Single Late Group tulip bearing pinkish white flowers, creamy white at the bases, in late spring. Insides are white with carmine-red flames and yellow anthers. ↕60cm (24in). ❄❄❄

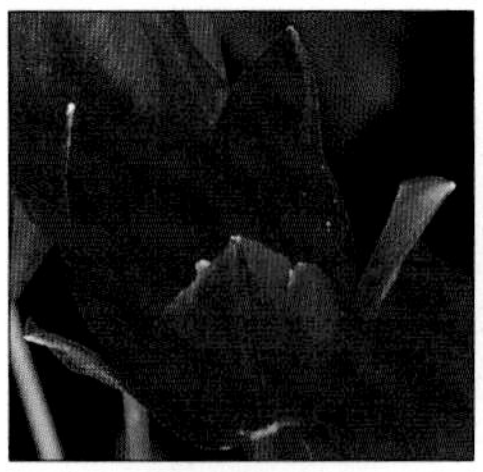
Tulipa sprengeri

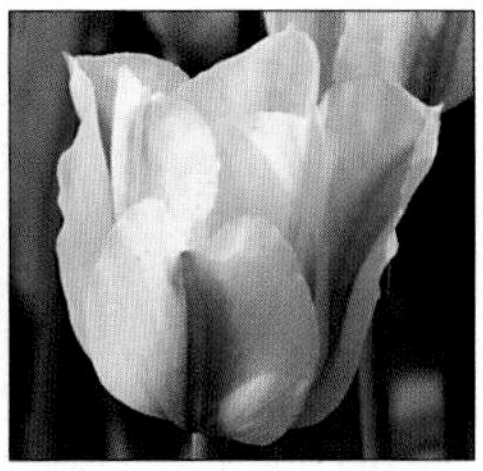
Tulipa 'Spring Green'

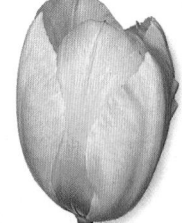

Tulipa 'Sweetheart'

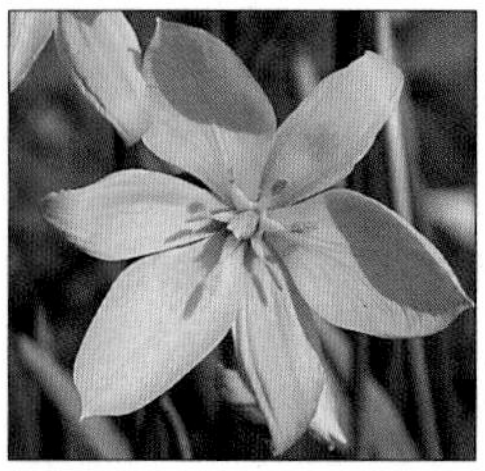
Tulipa sylvestris

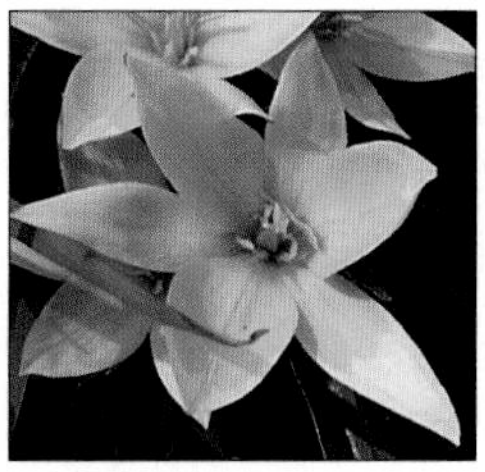
Tulipa tarda

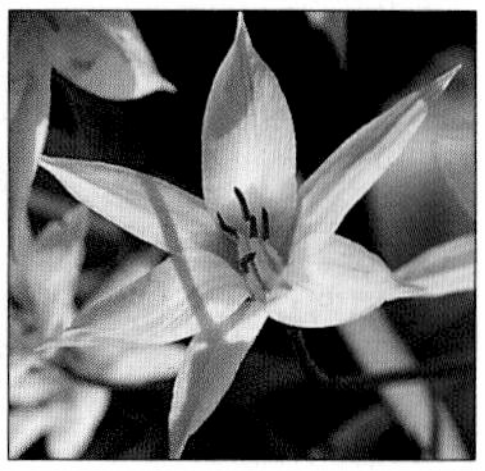
Tulipa turkestanica

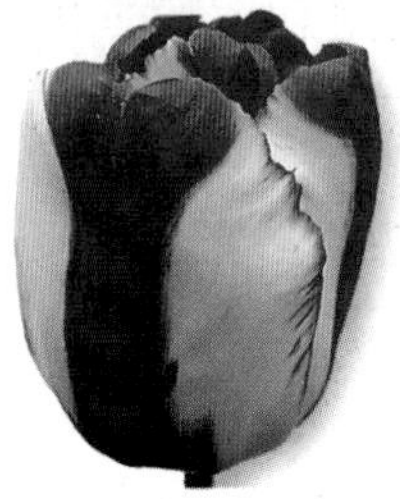
Tulipa 'Union Jack'

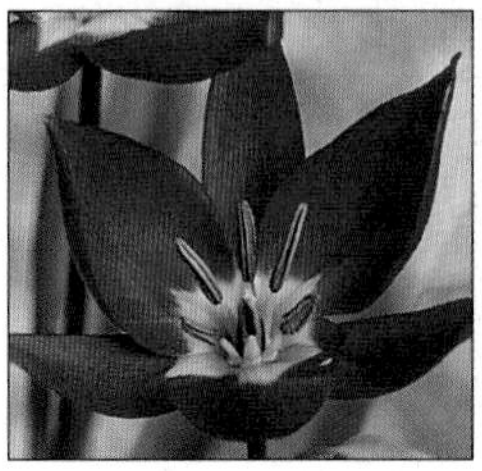
Tulipa violacea

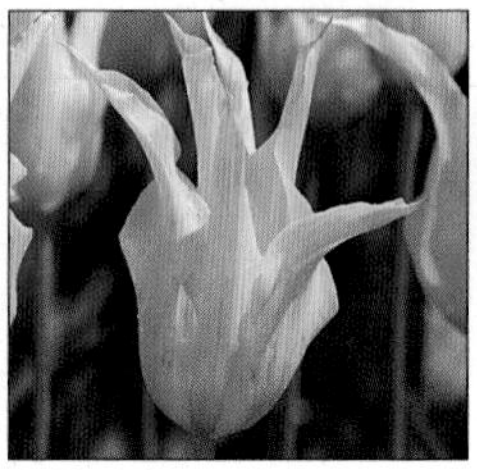
Tulipa 'West Point'

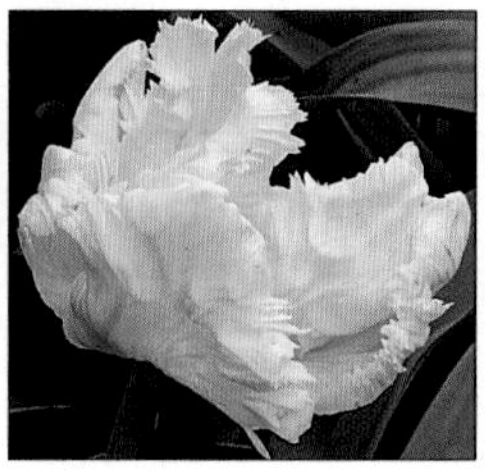
Tulipa 'White Parrot'

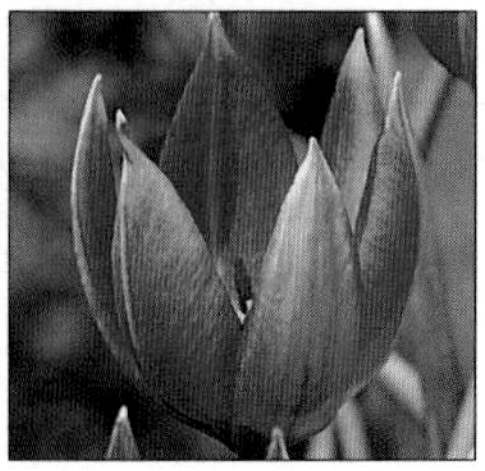
Tulipa whittallii

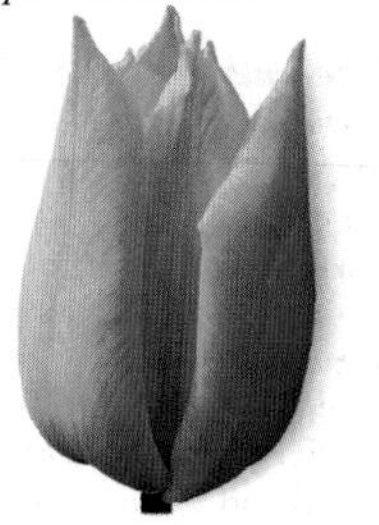
Tulipa 'Yokohama'

T. sprengeri ■ 🏆 Miscellaneous Group tulip with 5 or 6 linear, hairless, shiny, erect, mid-green leaves, to 25cm (10in) long. In early summer, solitary, goblet-shaped, red to orange-red flowers, 4.5–6cm (1¾–2½in) long, with yellow-buff bases, yellow anthers, and red filaments, are borne on smooth stems. One of the latest tulips to flower. Will self-seed and naturalize in sun or light woodland. ↕50cm (20in). Turkey (but no longer known in the wild). ✽✽✽
***T.* 'Spring Green'** ■ 🏆 Viridiflora Group tulip bearing green-feathered, ivory-white flowers, with light green anthers, in late spring. ↕40cm (16in). ✽✽✽
T. stellata see *T. clusiana* var. *stellata.*
T. stellata* var. *chrysantha see *T. clusiana* var. *chrysantha.*
***T.* 'Sweetheart'** ■ Fosteriana Group tulip bearing ivory-white flowers with lemon-yellow flames, broad, ivory-white margins, and yellow bases. Insides are deep yellow with ivory-white margins and yellow anthers. Mid-spring-flowering. ↕30cm (12in). ✽✽✽
***T.* 'Sweet Lady'.** Greigii Group tulip bearing peach-pink flowers with yellow-tinged, bronze-green bases and yellow anthers. Mid-spring-flowering. Leaves are marked dark bluish maroon. ↕20cm (8in). ✽✽✽
T. sylvestris ■ syn. *T. australis.* Miscellaneous Group tulip with 2–4 linear, channelled, glaucous, light green leaves, to 20cm (8in) long. In mid- and late spring, star-shaped, fragrant flowers, 6–8cm (2½–3in) across, pendent in bud then erect, are borne singly or in pairs. Flowers are yellow, occasionally cream, with green-flushed bases outside and yellow anthers. Easily grown. ↕45cm (18in). Origin unknown; naturalized in Europe and from N. Africa to the Middle East and Russia (Siberia). ✽✽✽
T. tarda ■ 🏆 syn. *T. dasystemon* of gardens. Miscellaneous Group tulip with 3–7 lance-shaped, recurved, often finely fringed, shiny, bright green leaves, to 12cm (5in) long. Produces 4–6 star-shaped flowers, to 6cm (2½in) across, in early and mid-spring. Flowers are white with a green tinge, sometimes red-tinged outside and yellow on the lower half inside. Stamens are yellow. ↕15cm (6in). C. Asia (Tien Shan). ✽✽✽
***T.* 'Texas Gold'.** Parrot Group tulip producing red-margined, bright golden yellow flowers. Late spring-flowering. ↕55cm (22in). ✽✽✽
***T.* 'Topic'** see *T.* 'Golden Oxford'.
***T.* 'Toronto'** 🏆 Greigii Group tulip bearing vermilion-tinged, pinkish red flowers, several to a stem, in mid-spring; insides are tangerine-red with buttercup-yellow bases, tinged bronze-green, and bronze anthers. Leaves are marked dark bluish maroon. ↕20cm (8in). ✽✽✽
T. turkestanica ■ 🏆 Miscellaneous Group tulip with 2–4 linear, grey-green leaves, to 15cm (6in) long. In early and mid-spring, up to 12 star-shaped, malodorous white flowers, 3–5cm (1¼–2in) across, flushed greenish grey or greenish pink outside, yellow or orange at the centres, are borne on hairy stems. Stamens have purple, brown, or purple-tipped yellow anthers, and yellow filaments. ↕30cm (12in). Kazakhstan, Tajikistan, N.W. China. ✽✽✽
***T.* 'Union Jack'** ■ Single Late Group tulip bearing ivory-white flowers, with raspberry-red flames and blue-margined white bases, in late spring. ↕60cm (24in). ✽✽✽
T. urumiensis 🏆 Miscellaneous Group tulip with 2–4 linear, sometimes slightly glaucous, mid-green leaves, to 12cm (5in) long. Star-shaped yellow flowers, 5–7cm (2–3in) across, flushed lilac or reddish brown outside, with yellow stamens, are produced singly or in pairs in early spring. ↕15cm (6in). N.W. Iran. ✽✽✽
***T.* 'Viking'.** Double Early Group tulip bearing scarlet-flamed, greenish red flowers. Insides are signal-red with slight yellow feathering, canary-yellow bases, and purple anthers. Mid-spring-flowering. ↕30cm (12in). ✽✽✽
T. violacea ■ Miscellaneous Group tulip with 2–5 linear, channelled, hairless, glaucous, grey-green leaves, to 15cm (6in) long. Produces star-shaped violet-purple flowers, 7cm (3in) across, with yellow or blue-black basal marks and purple stamens, singly or sometimes in clusters of 3, in early and mid-spring. ↕25cm (10in). S. and E. Turkey, N. Iraq, N. and W. Iran, Azerbaijan. ✽✽✽
T. vvedenskyi. Miscellaneous Group tulip with 4 or 5 lance-shaped, reflexed, often very finely downy, glaucous, grey-green, crimped leaves, to 30cm (12in) long. Solitary, bowl-shaped flowers, to 20cm (8in) across, with rounded bases, are produced on bristly, sometimes purple-tinged stems in early and mid-spring. Flowers are red with black or yellow basal marks, violet or yellow anthers, and brown or yellow filaments. ↕50cm (20in). Kazakhstan, C. Asia (Tien Shan). ✽✽✽. **'Tangerine Beauty'** has bright red flowers, orange inside, with pale yellow basal marks; stamens have purple anthers and yellow filaments.
***T.* 'West Point'** ■ Lily-flowered Group tulip producing primrose-yellow flowers in late spring. ↕50cm (20in). ✽✽✽
***T.* 'White Emperor'** see *T.* 'Purissima'.
***T.* 'White Parrot'** ■ Parrot Group tulip producing pure white flowers in late spring. ↕55cm (22in). ✽✽✽
T. whittallii ■ Miscellaneous Group tulip with 2–7 lance-shaped, hairless, mid-green leaves, to 20cm (8in) long, often with reddish purple margins. In early and mid-spring, bears star-shaped flowers, 3–6cm (1¼–2½in) across, singly or in clusters of up to 4 on hairless stems. Flowers are bright bronze-orange, usually green-tinged outside, with black, sometimes yellow-margined basal marks inside. Stamens have dark green or brown anthers, and purple or green filaments. ↕35cm (14in). Bulgaria, Greece, W. Turkey. ✽✽✽
***T.* 'Willemsoord'.** Double Early Group tulip bearing carmine-red and white flowers in mid-spring. ↕30cm (12in). ✽✽✽
T. wilsoniana see *T. montana.*
***T.* 'Wirosa'.** Double Late Group tulip with cream-margined, wine-red flowers in late spring. ↕40cm (16in). ✽✽✽
***T.* 'Yellow Purissima'.** Fosteriana Group tulip with canary-yellow flowers, broadly flamed deep yellow. Insides are bright golden yellow with greenish yellow anthers. Mid-spring-flowering. ↕35cm (14in). ✽✽✽
***T.* 'Yokohama'** ■ Single Early Group tulip producing tapered yellow flowers, with yellow anthers, in mid-spring. ↕30cm (12in). ✽✽✽
***T.* 'Zampa'** 🏆 Greigii Group tulip producing primrose-yellow flowers, with bronze and green bases, in mid-spring. Leaves are marked dark bluish maroon. ↕25cm (10in). ✽✽✽

▷**Tulip tree** see *Liriodendron, L. tulipifera*
African see *Spathodea*
Chinese see *Liriodendron chinense*
▷**Tumbling Ted** see *Saponaria ocymoides*
▷***Tunica saxifraga*** see *Petrorhagia saxifraga*
▷**Tunic flower** see *Petrorhagia saxifraga*
▷**Tupelo** see *Nyssa, N. sylvatica*
Chinese see *N. sinensis*
▷***Turbinicarpus schmiedickeanus*** see *Neolloydia schmiedickeana*
▷**Turkscap lily,**
American see *Lilium superbum*
Common see *Lilium martagon*
Scarlet see *Lilium chalcedonicum*
▷**Turpentine tree** see *Pistacia terebinthus*
▷**Turtlehead** see *Chelone, C. glabra*
▷**Tussock grass** see *Cortaderia, Deschampsia cespitosa*
Plumed see *Chionochloa conspicua*
▷**Tutsan** see *Hypericum androsaemum*

TWEEDIA syn. OXYPETALUM

ASCLEPIADACEAE

Genus of one species of evergreen, twining, scrambling subshrub from scrub and rocky areas in S. Brazil and Uruguay. It has simple, opposite leaves and produces stalked, axillary and terminal cymes of short, tubular, 5-petalled, salverform flowers. In frost-prone areas, grow as an annual or in a cool greenhouse. In warmer climates, grow in a border or among other small shrubs.
• **HARDINESS** Frost tender.
• **CULTIVATION** Under glass, grow in loam-based potting compost (JI No.2)

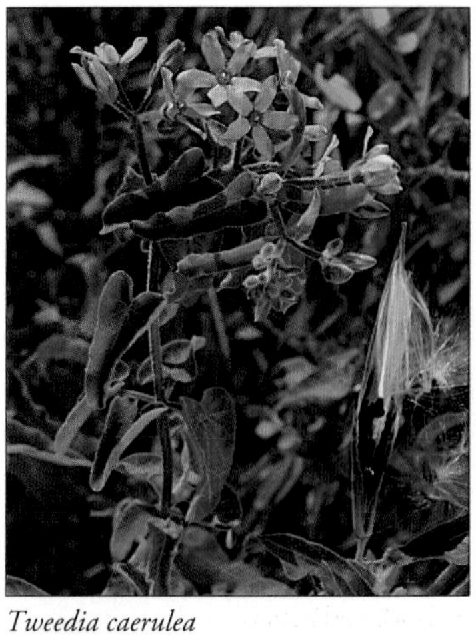
Tweedia caerulea

T

in full light. In the growing season, water freely and apply a balanced liquid fertilizer monthly; water sparingly in winter. Outdoors, grow in moist but well-drained, fertile soil in full sun. Support the climbing stems. Pruning group 13, in early spring.
• **PROPAGATION** Sow seed at 15°C (59°F) in spring. Insert softwood cuttings with bottom heat in summer.
• **PESTS AND DISEASES** Trouble free.

T. caerulea ■ 🏆 syn. *Amblyopetalum caeruleum, Oxypetalum caeruleum.* Erect, evergreen subshrub with twining, white-hairy stems and oblong-lance-shaped, downy, light green leaves, 5–10cm (2–4in) long, usually heart-shaped at the bases. From summer to early autumn, oblong-petalled, sky-blue flowers, 2–2.5cm (¾–1in) across, pink-flushed in bud and ageing to purple, are borne in small, 3- or 4-flowered cymes. ↕60–100cm (24–39in). S. Brazil to Uruguay. ❁ (min. 3–5°C/39–41°F)

▷**Twinberry** see *Lonicera involucrata*
▷**Twin-flower** see *Linnaea*
▷**Twin leaf** see *Jeffersonia*

TYLECODON

CRASSULACEAE

Genus of 20–30 species of bushy, succulent, deciduous shrubs, similar to *Cotyledon* and at one time included in that genus. They are found in deserts and partially shaded areas of Namibia and South Africa. The linear to ovate, spoon-shaped, or almost cylindrical leaves are alternate or borne in crowded spirals. Mainly bell-shaped, upright to pendent flowers have calyces with club-shaped hairs, and are borne in complex, many-branched, panicle-like cymes. In warm, dry, winter-rainfall areas, they are summer-dormant, suitable for a border with other succulents. In areas where temperatures fall below 7°C (45°F), grow in a temperate greenhouse. The leaves of *T. papillaris* subsp. *wallichii* are highly toxic if ingested.
• **HARDINESS** Frost tender.
• **CULTIVATION** Under glass, grow in standard cactus compost in full light, with low humidity. In growth, water moderately and apply a half-strength, low-nitrogen liquid fertilizer every 4–6 weeks; keep dry when leafless, and water moderately as growth resumes. Pot on as or just before new growth begins. Outdoors, grow in sharply drained, humus-rich, sandy or gritty soil in full sun. Pruning group 1. See also pp.48–49.
• **PROPAGATION** Sow seed at 19–24°C (66–75°F), or insert cuttings of stem sections, in late spring or summer.
• **PESTS AND DISEASES** Prey to mealybugs.

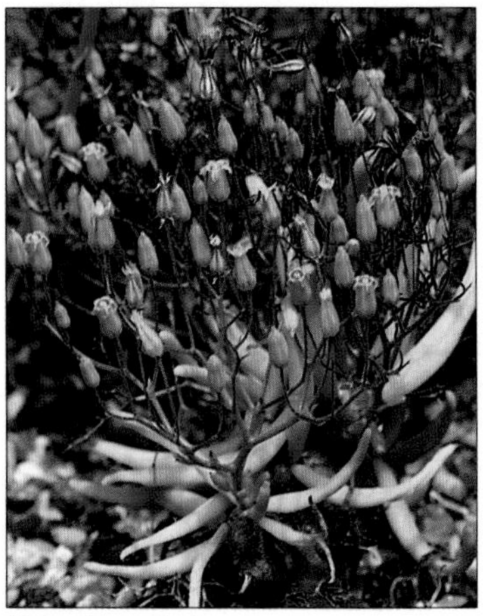
Tylecodon reticulatus

T. paniculatus, syn. *Cotyledon paniculata* (Butter tree). Succulent shrub producing soft, swollen, fleshy stems and short, thick, fleshy, warty branches, all covered with papery yellow bark. Obovate-spoon-shaped, fleshy, bright green leaves, to 11cm (4½in) long, are initially hairy with smooth margins, becoming completely hairless before falling. In spring, nodding, yellow-striped, dark reddish brown flowers, 1.5cm (½in) long, are borne in panicle-like cymes, 60cm (24in) long. ↕to 2m (6ft), ↔ 1m (3ft). Namibia, South Africa (Northern Cape, Western Cape, Eastern Cape). ❁ (min. 7°C/45°F)
T. papillaris* subsp. *wallichii, syn. *Cotyledon wallichii, T. wallichii.* Succulent shrub with fleshy stems and branches, covered with prominent, persistent leaf bases. Short-lived, linear-cylindrical, grey-green leaves, 5–12cm (2–5in) long, grooved above, die back from the branch tips. Pendent, tubular, pale greenish yellow flowers, 2cm (¾in) long, are borne in panicle-like cymes, to 70cm (28in) long, in autumn and winter. ↕↔ 30cm (12in). South Africa (Western Cape, Karoo). ❁ (min. 7°C/45°F)
T. reticulatus ■ syn. *Cotyledon reticulata* (Barbed-wire plant). Stumpy, succulent shrub with short, thick, fleshy stems, covered with peeling grey-brown bark, and soft, spongy branches covered in leaf scars. Linear to almost cylindrical, downy, soft, brown-tipped, yellowish green leaves, 1.5–5cm (½–2in) long, are compressed or grooved above. In winter, bears erect, yellowish green flowers, 1cm (½in) long, in panicle-like cymes, to 30cm (12in) long. Dead inflorescences persist, forming a tangle of weak, silvery thorns that envelops the plant. ↕↔ 30cm (12in). Namibia, South Africa (Western Cape, Karoo). ❁ (min. 7°C/45°F)
T. wallichii see *T. papillaris* subsp. *wallichii*

TYPHA

Bulrush, Cat's tail, Reedmace

TYPHACEAE

Genus of 10–15 species of monoecious, marginal aquatic herbaceous perennials from temperate and tropical regions worldwide. They form dense, robust stands of vegetation around lakes and large ponds. Thick rhizomes spread in shallow water, producing long, linear, mostly basal leaves and poker-like brown flower spikes, borne among the foliage but overtopped by the leaf tips. Clusters of male and female flowers are produced on the same spike. Bulrushes are usually only suitable for planting around a large wildlife pool, where deep water prevents their spread; *T. minima* is the only species suitable for a small pool or tub. The flower spikes are used in dried flower arrangements.
• **HARDINESS** Fully hardy.
• **CULTIVATION** Grow in water to 30–40cm (12–16in) deep, with ample space and depth of mud for the root system. Flexible liners may be punctured by the rhizome tips of the larger species. Pick flowerheads for drying early in the season, and seal them with lacquer.
• **PROPAGATION** Divide rootstock in spring.
• **PESTS AND DISEASES** Trouble free.

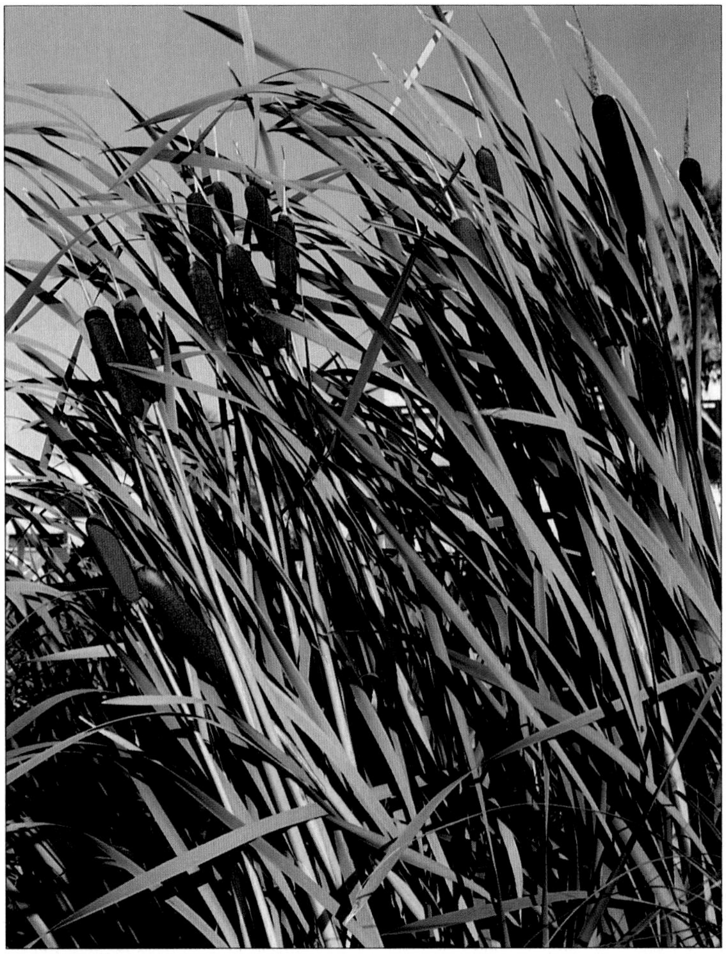
Typha latifolia

T. angustifolia (Lesser bulrush, Narrow-leaved reedmace, Soft flag). Aquatic perennial with linear leaves, to 1.5m (5ft) long, sheathed at the bases. Brown flower spikes, 8–20cm (3–8in) long, are borne in midsummer; male and female flowers are 3–8cm (1¼–3in) apart, the females with dark reddish brown scales. ↕1.5m (5ft), ↔ indefinite. Europe, N. and C. Asia, N. Africa, North to South America. ***
T. latifolia ■ (Bulrush, Cat's tail). Aquatic perennial with strap-shaped leaves, to 2m (6ft) or more long, with open-sheathed bases. Dark brown flower spikes, 15–22cm (6–9in) long, are borne in summer; male and female flowers are close together, no more than 2.5cm (1in) apart, the females becoming white-mottled with age. ↕2m (6ft) or more, ↔ indefinite. Europe, Asia, N. Africa, North America. ***. **'Variegata'** ■ is much less vigorous, and has leaves with longitudinal cream stripes; ↕0.9–1.2m (3–4ft).
T. minima ■ Slender, aquatic perennial with narrowly linear leaves, 20–75cm (8–30in) long. Dark brown flowers are produced in cylindrical spikes, 1.5–5cm (½–2in) long, the female flowers borne immediately above the males, in mid- and late summer. ↕to 75cm (30in), ↔ 30–45cm (12–18in). Eurasia. ***

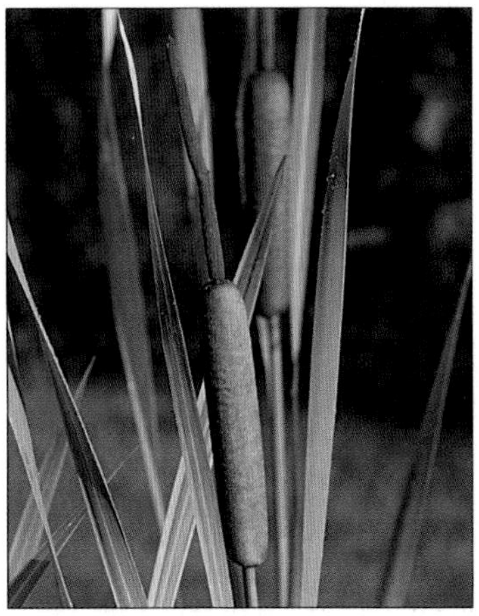
Typha latifolia 'Variegata'

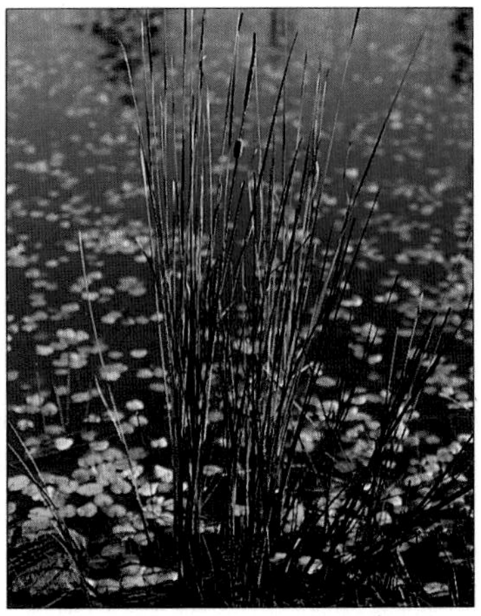
Typha minima

U

UEBELMANNIA

CACTACEAE

Genus of 3–5 species of simple, perennial cacti found in humid, moist areas in the mountains of E. Brazil. The mostly spherical to cylindrical stems have smooth or finely warty, sometimes scaly ribs, and spiny areoles. Diurnal, solitary, funnel-shaped yellow flowers are produced near the crown in summer. In areas where temperatures drop below 15°C (59°F), grow in a warm greenhouse; in warmer climates, they are useful in a border.

- **HARDINESS** Frost tender.
- **CULTIVATION** Under glass, grow in acid standard cactus compost in full light. From mid-spring to early autumn, water moderately and apply a low-nitrogen liquid fertilizer every 6–8 weeks. Mist daily in summer. In winter, keep completely dry, but mist frequently on warm days. Outdoors, grow in gritty, moderately fertile, sharply drained, acid soil in full sun. See also pp.48–49.
- **PROPAGATION** Sow seed at 24°C (75°F) in spring. Often difficult to grow unless grafted.
- **PESTS AND DISEASES** Trouble free.

U. buiningii. Cactus with spherical, sometimes slightly elongated, greenish red-brown to deep chocolate stems, each with about 18 ribs, totally covered with minute, waxy scales. Close-set areoles each bear 6–8 semi-erect (some slightly curved), black-tipped, yellow-brown spines. Funnel-shaped, bright yellow flowers, 2cm (¾in) across, are borne in summer. ↕ 10–12cm (4–5in), ↔ 8cm (3in). E. Brazil. ❀ (min. 15°C/59°F)
U. pectinifera ▣ Cactus with spherical to cylindrical, reddish green to reddish brown stems, later elongating, each with 15–20 prominently margined, smooth ribs and minute, off-white scales (sometimes absent in cultivation). Close-set areoles each bear 3–6 comb-like, light grey to nearly black spines. Funnel-shaped yellow flowers, to 1cm (½in) across, are borne in summer. ↕ 50–80cm (20–32in), ↔ 15cm (6in). E. Brazil. ❀ (min. 15°C/59°F)

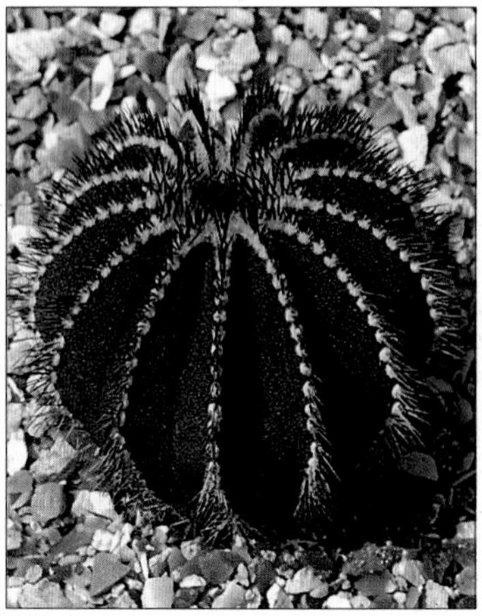
Uebelmannia pectinifera

UGNI

MYRTACEAE

Genus of 5–15 species of densely leafy, evergreen shrubs or trees found in forest and scrub in South America. They have opposite, small, elliptic to ovate, simple, leathery leaves, and produce solitary, cup- or bowl-shaped flowers from the leaf axils of young shoots, followed by edible, spherical berries. *U. molinae*, the only species usually cultivated, is valued for its foliage, flowers, and fruit. Grow in a sheltered border or use as hedging. In frost-prone areas, grow tender species in a cool greenhouse.

- **HARDINESS** Frost hardy to frost tender.
- **CULTIVATION** Grow in any moist but well-drained soil in full sun or partial shade. In frost-prone climates, shelter from cold, dry winds. Pruning group 1.
- **PROPAGATION** Root semi-ripe cuttings in late summer, with bottom heat.
- **PESTS AND DISEASES** Trouble free.

U. molinae ♀ syn. *Eugenia ugni, Myrtus ugni* (Chilean guava). Upright shrub or tree with elliptic to ovate, glossy, dark green leaves, to 3.5cm (1½in) long. Nodding, bowl-shaped, fragrant, pink-tinged white flowers, 1cm (½in) across, are produced singly from the leaf axils in late spring, followed by spherical, aromatic, dark red berries, 1cm (½in) across, in autumn. ↕ 1.5m (5ft), ↔ 1m (3ft). Chile, W. Argentina. ❄❄

ULEX

Furze, Gorse

LEGUMINOSAE/PAPILIONACEAE

Genus of about 20 species of spiny, evergreen shrubs from heaths and hillsides, woodland margins, and rocky sites in W. and C. Europe and N. Africa. As young seedlings, they have alternate leaves, which are quickly replaced by long-lasting green spines. They are grown for their axillary, pea-like yellow flowers, borne singly, in clusters, or in racemes, virtually all year round in mild climates. Suitable for a shrub border and as a low hedge. The seeds may cause mild stomach upset if ingested.

- **HARDINESS** Fully hardy.
- **CULTIVATION** Grow in poor, sandy, acid to neutral, well-drained soil in full sun. May become very leggy on rich soil. Pruning group 10, after flowering, every 2 or 3 years.
- **PROPAGATION** Sow seed in containers in a cold frame in autumn or spring. Take semi-ripe cuttings in summer.
- **PESTS AND DISEASES** Trouble free.

U. europaeus ▣ (Furze, Gorse, Whin). Upright to rounded, densely bushy shrub with spine-tipped green shoots and rigid leaves reduced to deeply grooved spines, to 2.5cm (1in) long. Solitary, axillary, pea-like, coconut-scented, bright yellow flowers, 2cm (¾in) long, are produced intermittently throughout the year but mainly over a long period in spring. Dark brown seed pods, to 2cm (¾in) long, are borne in summer. ↕ to 2.5m (8ft), ↔ 2m (6ft).

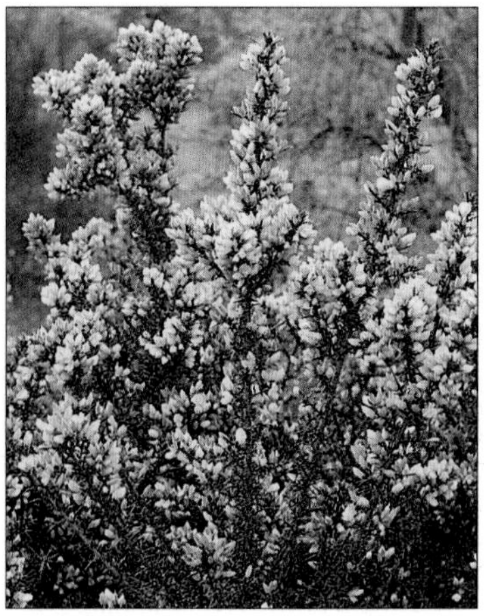
Ulex europaeus

W. and C. Europe. ❄❄❄. **'Flore Pleno'** 🏆 has double flowers and no fruit. **'Strictus'** (Irish gorse) is less spiny, with upright shoots.
U. gallii (Dwarf gorse). Spreading shrub with spine-tipped green shoots and rigid leaves reduced to slightly grooved spines, to 2.5cm (1in) long. From late summer to autumn, bears solitary, axillary, pea-like, bright yellow flowers, 1.5cm (½in) long; dark brown seed pods, to 1.5cm (½in) long, are produced in spring. ↕ 1.5–2m (5–6ft), ↔ 1.5m (5ft). W. Europe. ❄❄❄

▷ **Ulmo** see *Eucryphia cordifolia*

ULMUS

Elm

ULMACEAE

Genus of about 45 species of deciduous, rarely semi-evergreen trees and, very rarely, shrubs, occurring in woodland, thickets, and hedgerows in N. temperate regions. They have alternate, ovate to elliptic, obovate, or rounded, toothed leaves, usually with very unequally sized bases, and often attractively coloured in autumn. Clusters of tiny, bell-shaped flowers, each with 4–9 segments joined at the bases, are usually produced from axillary buds in spring, but sometimes from leafy buds in autumn; the flowers are very quickly followed by fruits, each consisting of a seed surrounded by a green to brown, rounded to elliptic, membranous wing. Cultivated for their habit and foliage, elms are mainly grown as specimen trees. *U.* x *hollandica* 'Jacqueline Hillier' is suitable for a shrub border and for hedging.

- **HARDINESS** Fully hardy.
- **CULTIVATION** Grow in any well-drained soil in full sun or partial shade. Pruning group 1.
- **PROPAGATION** Sow seed in containers outdoors in autumn or spring. Take greenwood cuttings in summer, or remove rooted suckers in autumn. Bud weeping trees in summer, or graft in winter.
- **PESTS AND DISEASES** Dutch elm disease is usually fatal; *U.* x *hollandica* 'Jacqueline Hillier', *U. parvifolia* and its cultivars, *U. pumila*, and *U.* 'Sapporo Autumn Gold' are partially resistant. A number of Asiatic species are, at present, the most disease-resistant. Elms may also be affected by honey fungus. Aphids, leafhoppers, and gall mites may be a problem.

U. americana ♀ (American white elm). Graceful, rounded, deciduous tree with pendent branch tips and ovate to elliptic, toothed, dark green leaves, to 15cm (6in) long, turning bright yellow in autumn. Tiny red flowers are produced in early spring, followed in mid- and late spring by winged green fruit, 1cm (½in) across. ↕↔ 30m (100ft). E. North America (E. of the Rocky Mountains). ❄❄❄
U. angustifolia see *U. minor* subsp. *angustifolia*.
U. angustifolia* var. *cornubiensis see *U. minor* 'Cornubiensis'.
***U.* 'Camperdownii'** see *U. glabra* 'Camperdownii'.
U. carpinifolia see *U. minor*.

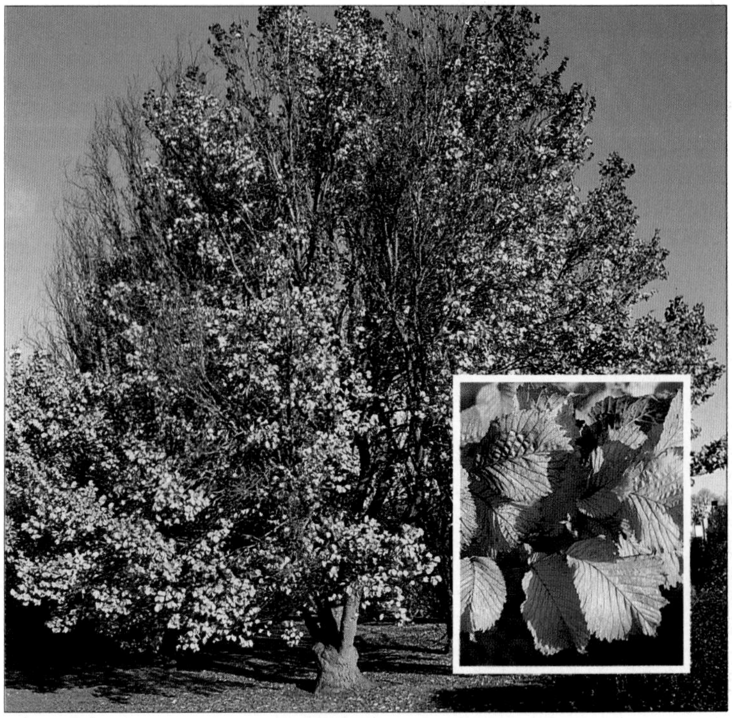
Ulmus glabra 'Exoniensis' (inset: leaf detail)

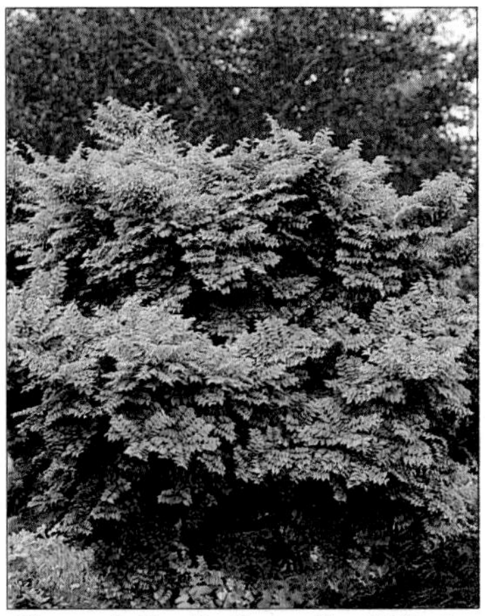

Ulmus x *hollandica* 'Jacqueline Hillier'

U. carpinifolia* var. *cornubiensis see *U. minor* 'Cornubiensis'.
U. carpinifolia* var. *sarniensis see *U. minor* 'Sarniensis'.
***U.* 'Commelin'** see *U.* x *hollandica* 'Commelin'.
***U.* 'Dicksonii'** see *U. minor* 'Dicksonii'.
***U.* x *elegantissima* 'Jacqueline Hillier'** see *U.* x *hollandica* 'Jacqueline Hillier'.
U. glabra (Wych elm). Rounded, deciduous tree with broadly obovate, double-toothed, dark green leaves, to 15cm (6in) long, lobed at the tips, and rough above, downy beneath, turning yellow in autumn. Tiny red flowers are produced in early spring, followed by clustered, winged green fruit, 2.5cm (1in) across, in late spring. ↕ 35–40m (120–130ft), ↔ 25m (80ft). Europe, S.W. Asia. ❄❄❄. **'Camperdownii'** syn. *U.* 'Camperdownii' (Camperdown elm) is weeping, with twisted branches and toothed to double-toothed, dark matt green leaves, to 20cm (8in) long; ↕↔ 8m (25ft). **'Exoniensis'** (Exeter elm) is narrowly columnar when young, broadening with age, and has upright branches bearing clustered, twisted, and folded leaves; ↕ 15m (50ft), ↔ 8m (25ft).
U.* x *hollandica (probably *U. glabra* x *U. minor*) (Dutch elm). Broadly columnar, deciduous tree with a short trunk and wide-spreading to often arching or pendent branches. Broadly elliptic, pointed, double-toothed, dark green leaves, 7–12cm (3–5in) long, initially rough above, becoming glossy, turn yellow in autumn. Tiny red flowers are produced in early spring, followed by winged green fruit, 2cm (¾in) across, in late spring. ↕ 35m (120ft), ↔ 25m (80ft). Europe. ❄❄❄. **'Commelin'** syn. *U.* 'Commelin', is narrower in habit, with more upright branches and oval, toothed, bright green leaves, to 10cm (4in) long, smooth above, downy beneath, turning yellow in autumn. Flowers are produced in late spring, followed by fruit 1cm (½in) across, in late summer. ↕ 25m (80ft), ↔ 15m (50ft). **'Jacqueline Hillier'** syn. *U.* x *elegantissima* 'Jacqueline Hillier', is a slow-growing, rounded, bushy shrub with elliptic-lance-shaped, double-toothed leaves, to 3.5cm (1½in) long, rough above, densely arranged in 2 rows along the shoots, and lasting until early winter; flowers are not usually produced. ↕↔ 2.5m (8ft). **'Vegeta'** syn. *U.* 'Vegeta' (Huntingdon elm) is fast-growing and broadly upright, with erect branches, pendent outer shoots, and broadly elliptic, ovate, or obovate, toothed, slightly rough leaves that turn yellow in autumn. ↕ 35m (120ft).
U. minor syn. *U. carpinifolia* (European field elm, Smooth-leaved elm). Broadly columnar, deciduous tree with arching branches and pendent shoots. Bears ovate, glossy, mid-green leaves, to 10cm (4in) long, smooth above, downy along the veins beneath and in the vein axils, and with double-toothed margins; they turn yellow in autumn. Very small red flowers are produced in early and mid-spring, followed by winged green fruit, 1cm (½in) across, in late spring. ↕ 30m (100ft), ↔ 20m (70ft). Europe, N. Africa, S.W. Asia. ❄❄❄. **subsp. *angustifolia*** syn. *U. angustifolia* (Goodyer's elm) has a rounded canopy and elliptic or obovate to inversely lance-shaped, double-toothed, glossy, mid- to deep green leaves, 5–13cm (2–5in) long, paler beneath. Flowers are produced in early spring, followed by fruit to 1.5cm (½in) across, in summer. S. Europe, N. Africa, S.W. Asia. **'Cornubiensis'** syn. *U. angustifolia* var. *cornubiensis*, *U. carpinifolia* var. *cornubiensis* (Cornish elm) is conical when young, becoming columnar and round-topped when mature, with upright branches. S.W. England. ↔ 15m (50ft). **'Dicksonii'** syn. 'Sarniensis Aurea', *U.* 'Dicksonii', *U.* 'Wheatleyi Aurea' (Cornish golden elm, Dickson's golden elm) is slow-growing, compact, and broadly conical, with broadly oval, toothed, glossy, bright golden yellow leaves, to 6cm (2½in) long; flowers are produced in spring, but only rarely. ↕ 10m (30ft), ↔ 6m (20ft). **'Sarniensis'** syn. *U. carpinifolia* var. *sarniensis* (Jersey elm, Wheatley elm) is compact and conical, with upright branches and broadly elliptic to obovate, toothed, smooth, glossy, mid-green leaves, to 7cm (3in) long; flowers are produced in early spring. ↔ 10m (30ft). **'Sarniensis Aurea'** see 'Dicksonii'.
U. parvifolia (Chinese elm). Spreading, deciduous or semi-evergreen tree with pendent shoots and flaking bark marked orange and brown. Elliptic, toothed, leathery, glossy, dark green leaves, to 6cm (2½in) long, with bases of almost equal size with matted hair beneath, may turn yellow or red in late autumn or early winter. Tiny red flowers are produced from late summer to autumn; they are followed by winged green fruit, 8mm (⅜in) across, in late autumn. ↕ 18m (60ft), ↔ 8–12m (25–40ft). China, Korea, Japan. ❄❄❄. **'Frosty'** is slow-growing and shrubby, with small, white-margined leaves, less than 2.5cm (1in) long; ↕↔ 2.5m (8ft). **'Hokkaido'**, syn. var. *pygmaea*, is slow-growing, with small leaves, to 4cm (1½in) long, and corky bark. **var. *pygmaea*** see 'Hokkaido'.
U. procera (English elm). Broadly upright, deciduous tree with a dense crown, broadest at the top. Broadly ovate to obovate, dark green leaves, to 10cm (4in) long, are rough above, paler and thinly hairy beneath, with coarsely double-toothed margins; they turn yellow in late autumn. Tiny red flowers are produced in early spring, followed by winged green fruit, to 1.5cm (½in) across, in late spring. ↕ 40m (130ft), ↔ 15m (50ft). UK. ❄❄❄
U. pumila (Siberian elm). Broadly upright, deciduous tree with narrowly elliptic to lance-shaped or ovate, tapered, toothed, dark green leaves, 3–10cm (1¼–4in) long, smooth above, hairy beneath, especially when young. Tiny red flowers are produced in early spring, followed by winged green fruit, 1cm (½in) across, in late spring. ↕ 20–30m (70–100ft), ↔ 12m (40ft). Russia (E. Siberia), S. Kazakhstan, N. China. ❄❄❄
***U.* 'Sapporo Autumn Gold'** Fast-growing, broadly conical, deciduous tree with upright branches. Oval, toothed, smooth, glossy, dark green leaves, to 8cm (3in) long, red-tinged when young, turn yellow-green in autumn. Flowers are not usually produced. ↕ 18m (60ft), ↔ 12m (40ft). ❄❄❄
***U.* 'Vegeta'** see *U.* x *hollandica* 'Vegeta'.
***U.* 'Wheatleyi Aurea'** see *U. minor* 'Dicksonii'.

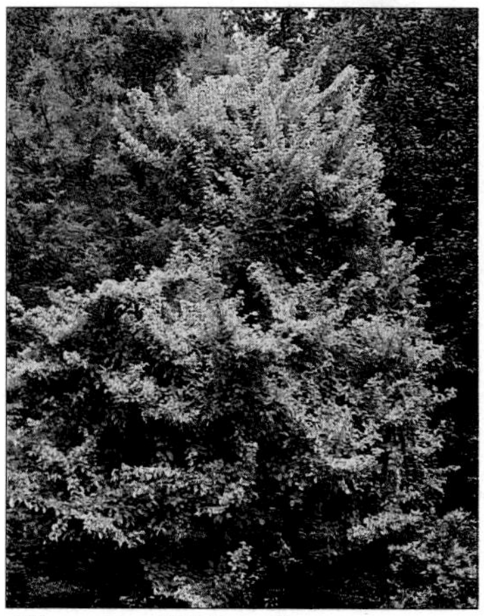

Ulmus minor 'Dicksonii'

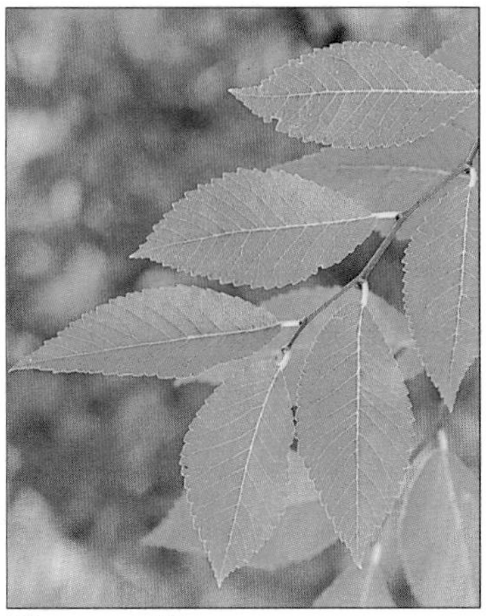

Ulmus parvifolia

UMBELLULARIA

LAURACEAE

Genus of one species of evergreen tree, with alternate, entire leaves, from coniferous forest in W. USA. It is grown for its aromatic foliage, although the scent of the crushed leaves may induce headaches and nausea in some people. Grow as a specimen tree in a woodland garden or other sheltered site.

- **HARDINESS** Frost hardy.
- **CULTIVATION** Grow in any well-drained soil in full sun. In frost-prone climates, shelter from cold, drying winds. Pruning group 1.

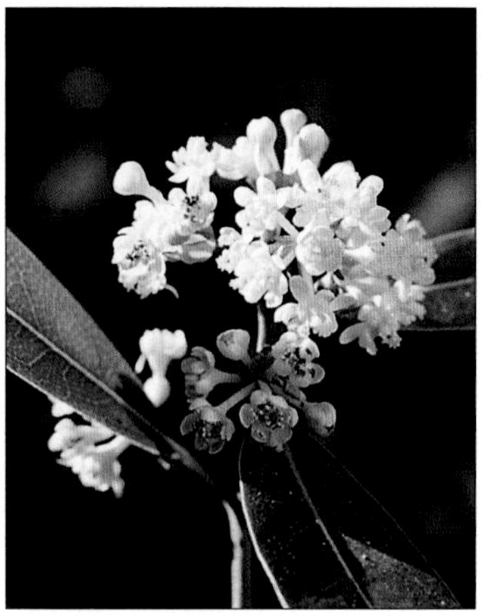

Umbellularia californica

- **PROPAGATION** Sow seed in containers in a cold frame in autumn. Insert semi-ripe cuttings in summer.
- **PESTS AND DISEASES** Trouble free.

U. californica (California laurel, Headache tree). Rounded, evergreen tree with elliptic to oblong, leathery, very aromatic, bright green leaves, to 10cm (4in) long. Umbels of up to 10 small, salverform, yellow-green flowers, 1cm (½in) across, are produced from the leaf axils in late winter and spring, followed by ovoid purple berries, 2.5cm (1in) long. ↕ 18m (60ft), ↔ 12m (40ft). USA (S. Oregon, N. California). ❄❄❄ (borderline)

▷ **Umbrella leaf** see *Diphylleia cymosa*
▷ **Umbrella pine** see *Pinus pinea*
Japanese see *Sciadopitys verticillata*
▷ **Umbrella plant** see *Cyperus alternifolius*
▷ **Umbrella tree** see *Magnolia macrophylla*, *M. tripetala*
Queensland see *Schefflera actinophylla*

UNCINIA

Hook sedge

CYPERACEAE

Genus of about 35–45 species of tufted, evergreen, monoecious perennials, some rhizomatous, occurring in damp, tussocky grassland, moist woodland, or swamps throughout S. temperate zones, except southern Africa. They have smooth, 3-angled to cylindrical stems and flat or shallowly channelled, grass-like leaves. The flowering stems bear spikes, with the male flowers at the top of the spike and the females beneath. The female flowers give rise to hooked, nut-like fruits. Several species are grown for their colourful leaves; they are suitable for the front of a border, or gravel plantings. In frost-prone climates, grow frost-tender species in a cool greenhouse.

- **HARDINESS** Frost hardy to frost tender; those described here will tolerate temperatures to about -10°C (14°F) for short periods.
- **CULTIVATION** Grow in moderately fertile, humus-rich, moist but well-drained soil in full sun or light dappled shade.
- **PROPAGATION** Sow seed at 13°C (55°F) in spring. Divide between late spring and midsummer.
- **PESTS AND DISEASES** Trouble free.

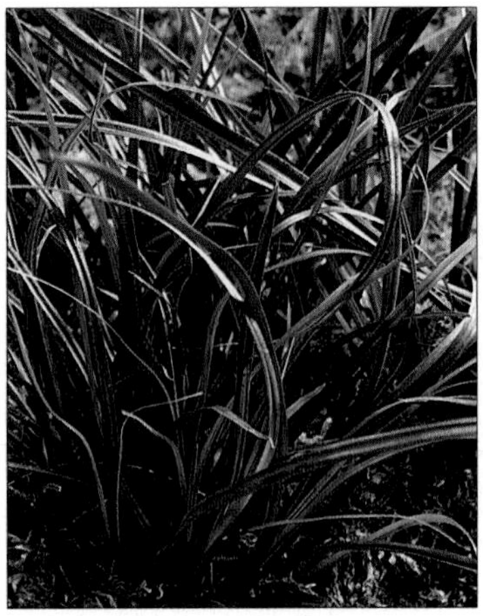

Uncinia rubra

U. rubra ■ Evergreen perennial, loosely tufted or with short rhizomes. Rigid, upright, 3-angled stems bear flat or inrolled, abruptly pointed, shiny leaves, to 35cm (14in) long; both stems and leaves are greenish red to rich reddish brown. Dark brown to black flowers are produced in narrow spikes, to 6cm (2½in) long, in mid- and late summer. ↕30cm (12in), ↔35cm (14in). New Zealand. ✲✲

U. uncinata. Densely tufted, evergreen perennial, similar to *U. rubra* but smaller, with rigid, upright stems and flat, rough-margined, pale brown to red-brown leaves, 5–10cm (2–4in) long. Bears dark brown flowers in narrow spikes, 15cm (6in) long, in mid- and late summer. ↕25cm (10in), ↔30cm (12in). New Zealand. ✲✲

▷ **Unicorn plant** see *Proboscidea*
Common see *P. louisianica*
▷ ***Uniola latifolia*** see *Chasmanthium latifolium*
▷ ***Urceolina*** see *Stenomesson*
U. pendula see *S. miniatum*
U. peruviana see *S. miniatum*

URGINEA

HYACINTHACEAE/LILIACEAE

Genus of about 100 species of bulbous perennials found on dry, rocky hillsides, on sandy soils near coasts, or on plains or savannah, mostly in tropical Africa, with a few in the Mediterranean. They have narrowly linear, basal leaves, and are grown for their star- or saucer-shaped flowers, produced in long, erect, dense racemes on leafless stems in summer and autumn. Grow in a sunny border. In frost-prone areas, grow half-hardy and frost-tender species in a cool greenhouse.

• **HARDINESS** Frost hardy to frost tender.
• **CULTIVATION** Under glass, grow in loam-based potting compost (JI No.2), with added sharp sand, in full light. Water freely when in growth. Keep just moist when dormant. Outdoors, grow in sandy or stony, poor to moderately fertile, sharply drained soil in full sun. Protect from winter wet.
• **PROPAGATION** Sow seed at 13–18°C (55–64°F) when ripe. Remove offsets in summer.
• **PESTS AND DISEASES** Trouble free.

U. maritima (Sea onion, Sea squill). Bulbous perennial producing dense racemes, 30cm (12in) or more long, of many tiny, star-shaped white flowers, 6mm (¼in) across, with green or purple midveins, in late summer and early autumn. Erect, narrow, basal leaves, 30–100cm (12–39in) long, appear in autumn, after the flowers. ↕1.5m (5ft), ↔30cm (12in). Mediterranean. ✲

URSINIA

ASTERACEAE/COMPOSITAE

Genus of about 40 species of annuals and evergreen perennials and subshrubs from dry savannah in South Africa, Namibia, Botswana, and Ethiopia. They are cultivated mainly for their flowers; a few species are grown for their foliage. The alternate leaves may occasionally be simple, but are usually pinnatifid, pinnatisect, or pinnate, often hairy or downy, and frequently aromatic. Daisy-like, yellow, orange, or red flowerheads, usually solitary, sometimes in corymbs, are borne on long stalks well above the foliage. Grow annual species at the front of a border or at the base of a house wall. Where winter temperatures fall below 0°C (32°F), grow perennials and subshrubs in a cool greenhouse or treat as annuals. Alternatively, lift before the first frosts and overwinter in frost-free conditions. In milder areas, grow in a border or small courtyard garden.

• **HARDINESS** Half hardy to frost tender.
• **CULTIVATION** Under glass, grow in loam-based potting compost (JI No.1) in full light. In growth, water freely and apply a balanced liquid fertilizer every 4 weeks. Water sparingly in winter. Outdoors, grow in sandy, fertile, well-drained soil in full sun.
• **PROPAGATION** Sow seed at 13–18°C (55–64°F) in spring. Take softwood cuttings in summer.
• **PESTS AND DISEASES** Trouble free.

U. anethoides. Bushy, evergreen perennial, usually grown as an annual, with crowded, pinnatisect, thinly hairy or hairless leaves, 2.5–4cm (1–1½in) long, with linear, almost cylindrical lobes. In summer, bears solitary, golden yellow flowerheads, 2.5cm (1in) across, with purple disc-florets. ↕45cm (18in), ↔35cm (14in). South Africa. ✲

U. anthemoides ■ Erect, bushy annual with pinnatisect, slightly hairy, scented, light green leaves, 2–6cm (¾–1½in) long, with slender, flat or thread-like lobes. In summer, bears solitary, purple-centred, yellow-orange flowerheads, to 6cm (2½in) across, each ray-floret zoned in maroon-red or copper-purple on the underside. ↕to 40cm (16in), ↔to 30cm (12in). South Africa (Northern Cape, Western Cape, Eastern Cape). ✲

U. chrysanthemoides. Erect, spreading, woody-based, evergreen, short-lived perennial, sometimes grown as an annual, with rooting stems. Bears softly hairy or hairless, scented, silvery grey-green leaves, 5cm (2in) long, which may be pinnate, 2-pinnate, or occasionally entire, all on the same plant. Produces solitary flowerheads, 3–6cm (1¼–2½in) across, with yellow or occasionally red or white ray-florets, sometimes copper-tinted beneath, mainly in summer. ↕30–45cm (12–18in), ↔60–75cm (24–30in). South Africa (Northern Cape, Western Cape, Eastern Cape). ❁ (min. 5–7°C/41–45°F). **var. *geyeri***, syn. 'Geyeri', *U. geyeri*, has dull green leaves, very white-woolly at first. Rich crimson-red flowerheads, 2.5–6cm (1–2½in) across, with red-black disc-florets, are produced in summer. ↕to 90cm (36in), ↔to 30cm (12in)

U. geyeri see *U. chrysanthemoides* var. *geyeri.*

U. sericea. Bushy, evergreen subshrub with pinnate or pinnatisect, silver-silky-hairy leaves, to 8cm (3in) long. In summer, produces solitary yellow flowerheads, to 3cm (1¼in) across, on very long stalks. ↕↔to 70cm (30in). South Africa (Northern Cape, Western Cape, Eastern Cape). ❁ (min. 5–7°C/41–45°F)

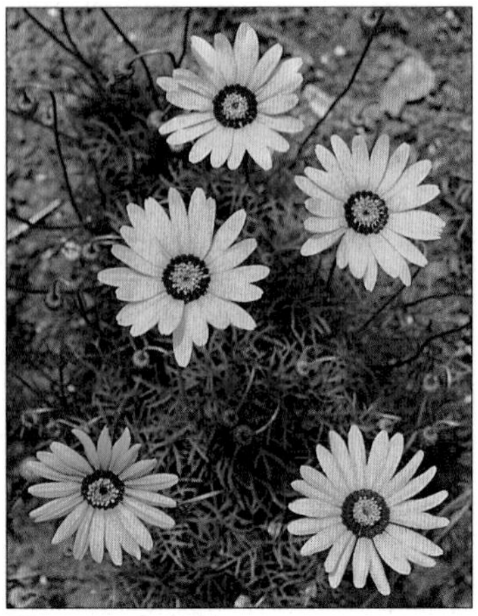

Ursinia anthemoides

UTRICULARIA

Bladderwort

LENTIBULARIACEAE

Genus of approximately 180 species of terrestrial, epiphytic, or free-floating aquatic annuals and perennials found worldwide in stagnant, shallow water, or growing on rainforest trees. They are insectivorous, and thrive in water that attracts mosquito larvae. Generally rootless, they have mainly submerged stems, either loosely anchored or free-floating, and thread-like or linear to rounded leaves with traps (bladders) adapted to catch and absorb insects. The flowers, solitary or in racemes, are usually borne on leafless stems above the water, and are supported by a whorl of spongy, floating leaves. Grow in an outdoor pool. In frost-prone areas, grow tender species in a warm aquarium. The hardy species may also be grown in a cold-water aquarium.

• **HARDINESS** Fully hardy to frost tender.
• **CULTIVATION** Outdoors, grow in acid water that warms up quickly in spring, in full sun. In an aquarium, grow in full light in soft, algae-free water; frost-tender species need a water temperature of 19°C (66°F), hardy species 12–15°C (54–59°F). See also pp.52–53.
• **PROPAGATION** Collect buds that sink to the bottom of the pool or aquarium after flowering and replant. Divide mats of floating foliage in summer.
• **PESTS AND DISEASES** Trouble free.

U. exoleta see *U. gibba.*

U. gibba, syn. *U. exoleta.* Floating aquatic annual or perennial with mat-forming stolons. Slender stems produce feathery, bladder-bearing leaves, to 8cm (3in) long. In midsummer, pouched, red-veined yellow flowers, to 6mm (¼in) long, are borne above the water, either singly or in a 2- to 5-flowered raceme, 20cm (8in) long. ↔20cm (8in). Spain, Portugal, Israel, southern Africa, China, Japan, Australia, New Zealand, North America, Argentina. ❁ (min. 7°C/45°F)

UVULARIA

Merrybells

CONVALLARIACEAE/LILIACEAE

Genus of 5 species of rhizomatous perennials from woodland in E. North America. They have erect, simple or branched stems, the upper parts bearing alternate, stalkless or perfoliate, ovate to lance-shaped, hairless or downy leaves. Pendent, tubular-bell-shaped, 6-tepalled yellow flowers are produced on long, slender stalks, and are usually solitary (occasionally in pairs) and terminal. Excellent for a peat bed, shady border, or woodland garden.

• **HARDINESS** Fully hardy.
• **CULTIVATION** Grow in fertile, humus-rich, moist but well-drained soil in deep or partial shade.
• **PROPAGATION** Sow seed in containers in a cold frame as soon as ripe. Divide in early spring.
• **PESTS AND DISEASES** Very susceptible to slugs and snails, especially in spring.

U. grandiflora ■ ♀ (Large merrybells). Slowly spreading, rhizomatous perennial with sometimes 2-branched stems bearing ovate-lance-shaped, downward-pointing, perfoliate, mid-green leaves, to 13cm (5in) long, softly hairy beneath. Solitary or paired, pendent, tubular-bell-shaped, sometimes green-tinted, yellow flowers, 5cm (2in) long, with free, slightly twisted tepals, and stamens longer than styles, are borne in mid- and late spring. ↕to 75cm (30in), ↔30cm (12in). E. North America. ✲✲✲. **var. *pallida*** has paler yellow flowers.

U. perfoliata. Slowly spreading, creeping, rhizomatous perennial with sometimes 2-branched stems bearing downward-pointing, ovate-lance-shaped, perfoliate, mid-green, hairless leaves, to 10cm (4in) long. A few solitary or paired, pendent, tubular-bell-shaped, pale yellow flowers, to 3.5cm (1½in) long, with free, slightly twisted tepals, the tips spreading, and stamens shorter than styles, are borne in late spring and early summer. ↕to 60cm (24in), ↔30cm (12in). E. North America. ✲✲✲

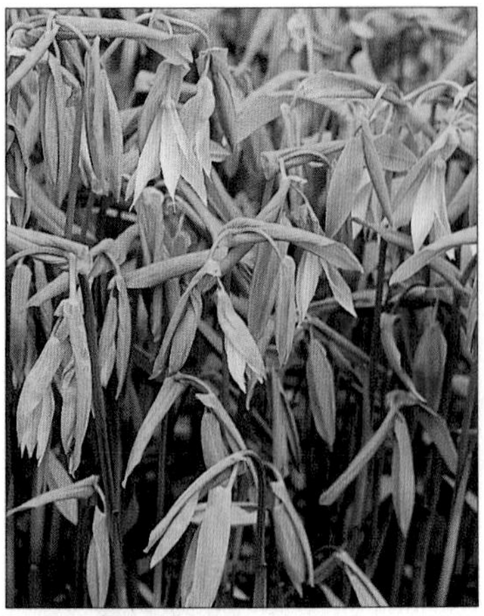

Uvularia grandiflora

U

V

VACCINIUM
Bilberry, Blueberry, Cranberry, Whortleberry

ERICACEAE

Genus of about 450 species of evergreen, semi-evergreen, or deciduous shrubs and trees, widely distributed throughout arctic and tropical regions, occurring in a variety of habitats from heath and moorland to bogs and woodland. They are valued for their ornamental foliage, flowers, and berries. The leathery leaves are alternate, and may be lance-shaped to elliptic, ovate, or rounded, with entire or toothed margins; in some of the deciduous species, the leaves provide brilliant autumn colour. The small, urn- or bell-shaped to cylindrical flowers are white, green, pink, or red, and are produced either singly in the leaf axils or in terminal or axillary racemes in spring and summer. The flowers are followed by edible, usually spherical berries; some species, including *V. angustifolium* var. *laevifolium*, *V. corymbosum*, and *V. macrocarpon*, are grown primarily for their fruits (blueberries and cranberries). Vacciniums are best suited to a woodland garden.

• **HARDINESS** Fully hardy to frost hardy.

• **CULTIVATION** Grow in acid, peaty or sandy, moist but well-drained soil in full sun or partial shade. Pruning group 1 for deciduous species; group 8 for evergreens.

• **PROPAGATION** Sow seed in containers in a cold frame in autumn. Take greenwood cuttings of deciduous species in early summer, and semi-ripe cuttings of evergreens in mid- to late summer. Layer in late summer.

• **PESTS AND DISEASES** May be affected by *Phytophthora* crown and root rot.

V. angustifolium* var. *laevifolium ■ (Lowbush blueberry). Spreading, densely branched, deciduous shrub with lance-shaped, minutely toothed, glossy, dark green leaves, to 4cm (1½in) long, turning red in autumn. Bell-shaped, white, sometimes pink-tinged flowers, 1cm (½in) long, are borne in pendent, axillary and terminal racemes, to 5cm (2in) long, in mid- and late spring; they are followed by edible, sweet, spherical, blue-black berries, to 1.5cm (½in) across. ↕↔ 10–60cm (4–24in). E. North America. ❄❄❄

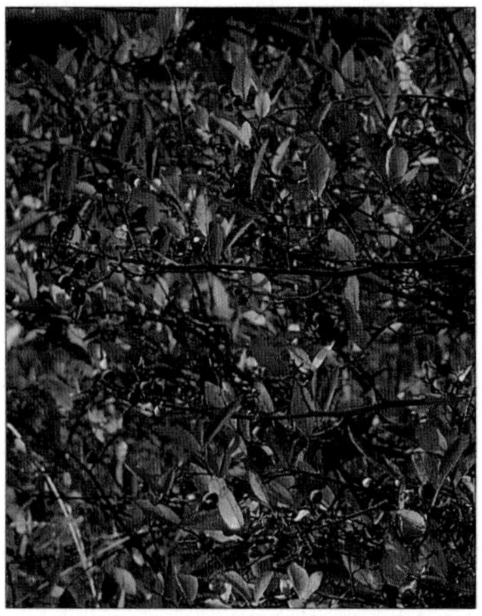
Vaccinium angustifolium var. *laevifolium*

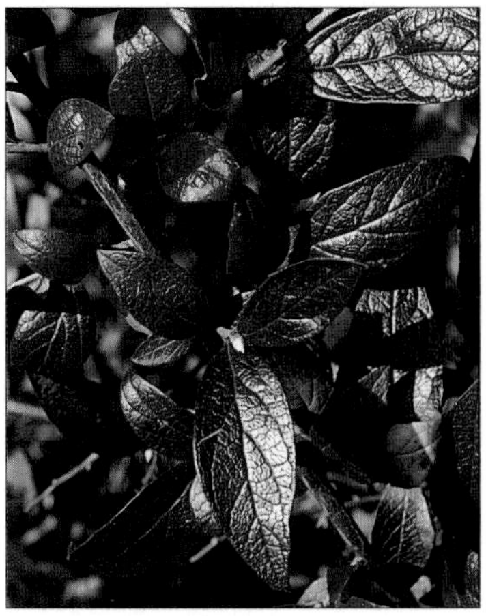
Vaccinium arctostaphylos

V. arctostaphylos ■ (Caucasian whortleberry). Erect, densely branched, deciduous shrub with red-brown young shoots and elliptic, entire, dark green leaves, to 10cm (4in) long, coloured red and purple in autumn. Bell-shaped, pink-tinged white flowers, 8mm (⅜in) long, are produced in pendent, axillary racemes, to 5cm (2in) long, in early summer; they are followed by edible, spherical, purple-black berries, 8mm (⅜in) across. ↕ 3m (10ft), ↔ 2m (6ft). Bulgaria, Turkey, Caucasus. ❄❄❄

V. caespitosum (Dwarf bilberry). Low-growing, rapidly spreading, densely branched, deciduous shrub with elliptic to obovate, entire or toothed, dark green leaves, 1.5–3.5cm (½–1½in) long. In late spring and early summer, produces pendent, urn-shaped, white to pink flowers, 5mm (¼in) long, singly from the leaf axils; flowers are followed by edible, spherical, blue-black fruit, 6mm (¼in) across. ↕ to 15cm (6in), ↔ 60cm (24in), or more. N. and W. North America. ❄❄❄

V. corymbosum ■ 🏆 (Highbush blueberry, Swamp blueberry). Upright, dense, many-branched, deciduous shrub with arching shoots and lance-shaped to elliptic, entire or toothed, mid-green

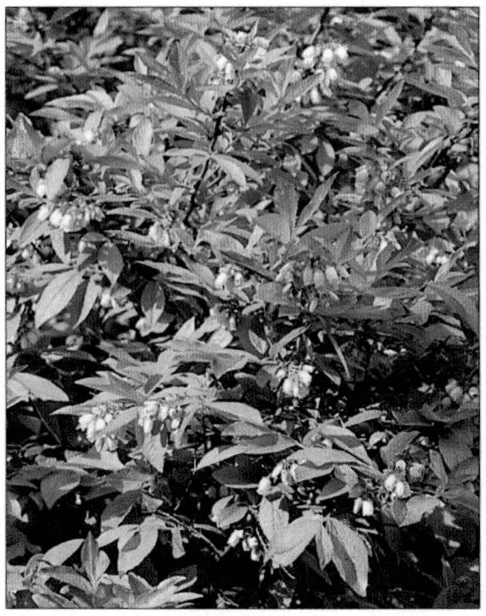
Vaccinium corymbosum

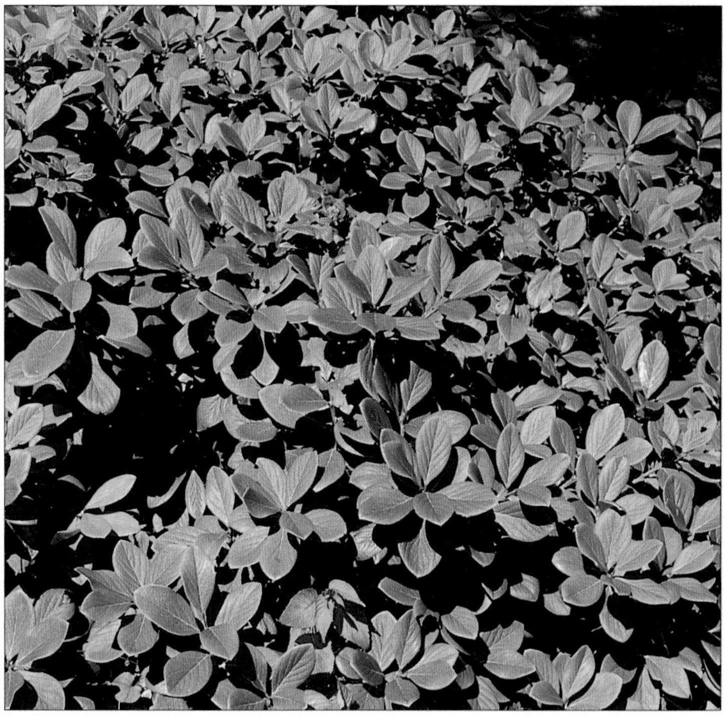
Vaccinium glaucoalbum

leaves, to 9cm (3½in) long, turning yellow or red in autumn. In late spring and early summer, produces pendent, terminal racemes, to 5cm (2in) long, of cylindrical, white, sometimes pink-tinged flowers, 1cm (½in) long; they are followed by edible, sweet, spherical, blue-black berries, to 1cm (½in) across. ↕↔ 1.5m (5ft). E. North America. ❄❄❄

V. crassifolium (Creeping blueberry). Vigorous, procumbent, mat-forming, evergreen shrub with oval-elliptic to rounded, finely toothed, thick, leathery, dark green leaves, 0.8–1.5cm (⅜–½in) long, paler beneath. In late spring and early summer, bears pendent, urn-shaped, white to pink or rose-red flowers, 4mm (⅛in) long, in loose, terminal and axillary racemes, to 5cm (2in) long; they are followed by edible, spherical, purple-black fruit, to 1cm (½in) across. ↕ to 45cm (18in), ↔ 1m (3ft). S.E USA. ❄❄❄ (borderline). **'Well's Delight'** has a looser, broader habit, and prefers partial shade; ↕ to 20cm (8in), ↔ 60cm (24in) or more.

V. cylindraceum 🏆 Upright, semi-evergreen shrub with lance-shaped, finely toothed, glossy, dark green leaves, to 6cm (2½in) long, retained until shortly before new growth begins in spring. In late summer and early autumn, bears cylindrical, red-tinged green flowers, 9–15mm (⅜–½in) long, in pendent, dense, axillary racemes, 5cm (2in) long; they are followed by edible, spherical, blue-black berries, 1cm (½in) long. ↕ 2.5m (8ft), ↔ 2m (6ft). Azores. ❄❄

V. delavayi. Compact, spreading, evergreen shrub with densely arranged, obovate to elliptic, entire, leathery, dark green leaves, to 1.5cm (½in) long, red-tinged when young. Tiny, pendent, urn-shaped, pink-flushed, creamy white flowers, 6mm (¼in) long, are produced singly or in clusters of 2–4 from the leaf axils in early summer; they are followed by edible, spherical, deep red berries, 5mm (¼in) across. ↕ 60cm (24in), ↔ 90cm (36in). S.W. China. ❄❄

V. floribundum, syn. *V. mortinia* (Mortiña). Spreading, evergreen shrub bearing arching shoots densely covered with ovate, glandular-toothed, dark green leaves, to 1cm (½in) long, red when young. In early summer, produces dense, pendent, axillary racemes, to 5cm (2in) long, of cylindrical pink flowers, 6mm (¼in) long; they are followed by edible, spherical red berries, 5mm (¼in) across. ↕ 1m (3ft), ↔ 2m (6ft). Ecuador, Peru. ❄❄

V. glaucoalbum ■ 🏆 Spreading, mound-forming, dense, evergreen shrub producing elliptic, dark green leaves, to 6cm (2½in) long, bright bluish white beneath, either entire or with bristle-like teeth. Cylindrical, pink-tinged white flowers, 6mm (¼in) long, are borne in pendent, axillary racemes, to 7cm (3in) long, in late spring and early summer; they are followed by edible, spherical, white-bloomed, blue-black berries, 8mm (⅜in) across. ↕ 50–120cm (20–48in), ↔ 1m (3ft). E. Himalayas to China, Tibet, N. Burma. ❄❄

V. macrocarpon (Cranberry). Prostrate, mat-forming, evergreen shrub with slender shoots and elliptic-oblong, entire, dark green leaves, to 2cm (¾in) long, bronze in winter. In summer, pendent, slender-stalked, bell-shaped pink flowers, 1cm (½in) across, with 4 slender, reflexed lobes, are produced singly from the leaf axils or in clusters of 2–10; they are followed by edible, spherical red berries, to 2cm (¾in) across. Best in cool, moist soil in sun. ↕ 15cm (6in), ↔ indefinite. E. North America. ❄❄❄

V. mortinia see *V. floribundum*.

V. moupinense. Compact, rounded, evergreen shrub with densely arranged, elliptic-oblong to obovate, entire, leathery, glossy, dark green leaves, to 1cm (½in) long. Tiny, urn-shaped, dark red-brown flowers, 5mm (¼in) long, are produced in pendent, axillary racemes, to 2.5cm (1in) long, in late spring and early summer; they are followed by edible, spherical, purple-black berries,

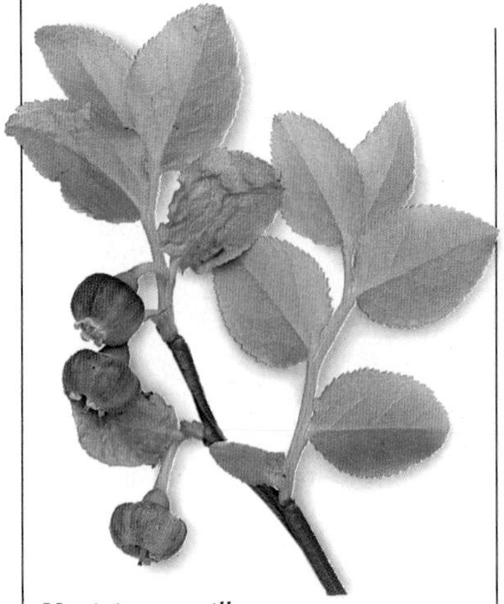
Vaccinium myrtillus

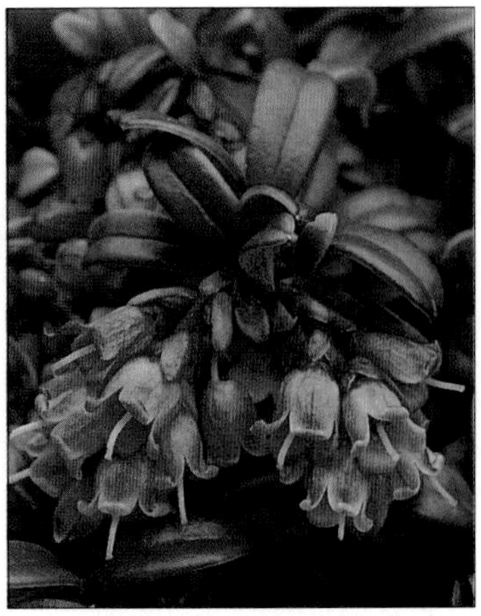
Vaccinium vitis-idaea subsp. *minus*

6mm (¼in) across. ↕ 60cm (24in), ↔ 90cm (36in). W. China. ✻✻✻
V. myrtillus ■ (Bilberry, Whinberry, Whortleberry). Vigorous, creeping, deciduous shrub with dense, upright stems and oval-elliptic, finely toothed, glossy, bright green leaves, 1–3cm (½–1¼in) long, often colouring red in autumn. In late spring and early summer, pendent, axillary, rounded, urn-shaped pink flowers, 6mm (¼in) long, are produced singly or in pairs. Flowers are followed by edible, spherical, blue-black berries, 6–10mm (¼–½in) across. May be invasive in fertile soils. ↕ to 30cm (12in), ↔ indefinite. Europe to N. Asia. ✻✻✻
V. nummularia. Spreading, low-growing, evergreen shrub with arching, brown-bristly stems. Rounded to elliptic, finely toothed, leathery, wrinkled, glossy, bright green leaves, 1–2.5cm (½–1in) long, are margined with red-brown bristles. In late spring, urn-shaped, red-tipped, pale pink flowers, 5mm (¼in) long, are produced in pendent racemes, to 5cm (2in) long, from leaf axils near the shoot tips; they are followed by edible, broadly ovoid black berries, 6mm (¼in) across. ↕ to 30cm (12in), ↔ to 60cm (24in). Himalayas (Sikkim, Bhutan). ✻✻✻ (borderline)
V. ovatum (Box blueberry). Upright, bushy, evergreen shrub with arching shoots and densely arranged, ovate, finely toothed, leathery, glossy, dark green leaves, to 3cm (1¼in) long, bronze when young. In late spring and early summer, produces cylindrical or urn-shaped, pink-flushed white flowers, 6mm (¼in) long, in dense, nodding, axillary racemes, 2.5cm (1in) long; flowers are followed by edible, spherical, glossy black berries, 6mm (¼in) across. ↕ 4m (12ft), ↔ 3m (10ft). W. North America (British Columbia to California). ✻✻
V. parvifolium (Red whortleberry). Upright, deciduous shrub with oblong, entire, blue-green leaves, to 3cm (1¼in) long, turning brilliant red in autumn. Small, rounded, urn-shaped, white, sometimes pink-tinged flowers, 4–6mm (⅛–¼in) long, are produced singly or in pairs from the leaf axils in late spring and early summer. Flowers are followed by edible, spherical, coral-red berries, 1cm (½in) across. ↕ 3m (10ft), ↔ 2m (6ft). W. North America (Alaska to California). ✻✻✻

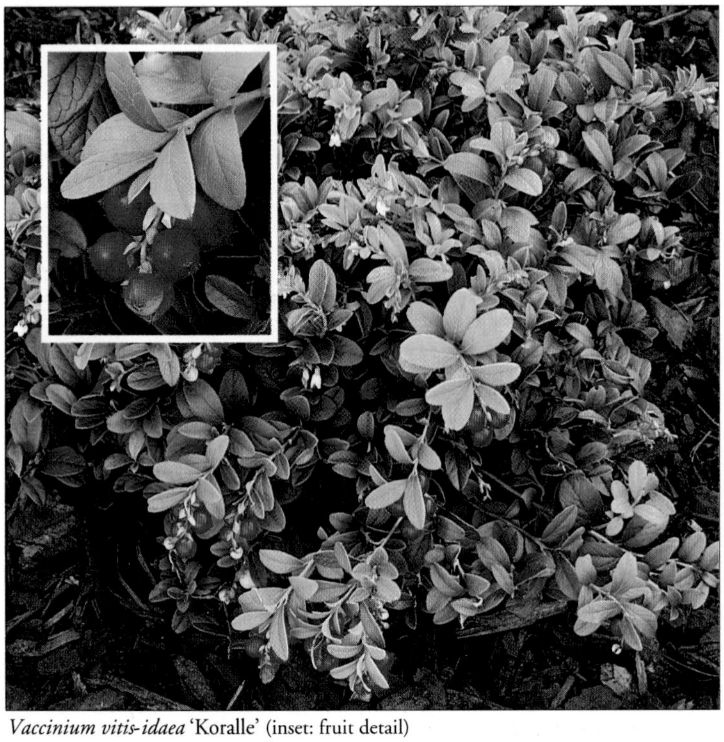
Vaccinium vitis-idaea 'Koralle' (inset: fruit detail)

V. praestans. Dwarf, deciduous shrub with sparse, creeping and ascending shoots. Broadly elliptic to obovate, indistinctly toothed, pale green leaves, 2.5–5cm (1–2in) long, are blunt or sharp-pointed at the tips and tapering at the bases, turning red in autumn. In early summer, produces bell-shaped, pink-flushed white flowers, 6mm (¼in) long, either singly or in few-flowered, pendent, axillary racemes, to 5cm (2in) long; they are followed by edible, spherical, bright red berries, 1cm (½in) across. ↕ to 10cm (4in), ↔ to 30cm (12in). N.E. Asia. ✻✻✻
V. vitis-idaea (Cowberry). Creeping, evergreen shrub, spreading by means of underground rhizomes, and bearing obovate, glossy, dark green leaves, to 2.5cm (1in) long, often shallowly notched at the tips. In late spring and early summer, produces bell-shaped, white to deep pink flowers, 6mm (¼in) long, in dense, nodding, terminal racemes, to 2.5cm (1in) long; they are followed by edible but acidic, spherical, bright red berries, 6mm (¼in) across. ↕ 25cm (10in), ↔ indefinite. Arctic and alpine regions of N. Eurasia, Japan, North America. ✻✻✻. **'Koralle'** ■ ♀ produces abundant fruit, to 9mm (⅜in) across. **subsp. *minus*** ■ is shorter, with smaller leaves, to 1.5cm (½in) long, and deep pink flowers; ↕ 20cm (8in); Arctic and alpine North America.

▷**Valerian** see *Centranthus, Valeriana*
Common see *Valeriana officinalis*
Greek see *Polemonium caeruleum*
Red see *Centranthus ruber*

VALERIANA

Valerian

VALERIANACEAE

Genus of 200 or more species of annuals, often rhizomatous or tap-rooted herbaceous perennials, semi-evergreen subshrubs, and usually evergreen shrubs. They are found throughout the world, except in Australasia, and occur in moist woodland, meadows, or at streamsides, often in mountainous regions; the alpine species grow in scree or rock crevices. The opposite leaves are often aromatic, but not always pleasantly so; they are generally simple, although the non-shrubby species often produce pinnate or pinnatifid stem leaves as well as basal rosettes of simple leaves. The small, unisexual or bisexual, salverform flowers are pink to lavender-pink, white, or yellow, and are borne in terminal, panicle- or corymb-like cymes in summer. The few species in cultivation are herbaceous perennials, grown for their attractive flowers. Valerians are suitable for growing in an informal, cottage-style garden, herbaceous border, or herb garden, or for naturalizing in a wild garden.

- **HARDINESS** Fully hardy.
- **CULTIVATION** Grow in any, preferably moist soil in full sun or dappled shade. Tall-stemmed species and cultivars may require support.
- **PROPAGATION** Sow seed in containers outdoors, or take basal cuttings, in spring. Divide in spring or autumn.
- **PESTS AND DISEASES** Trouble free.

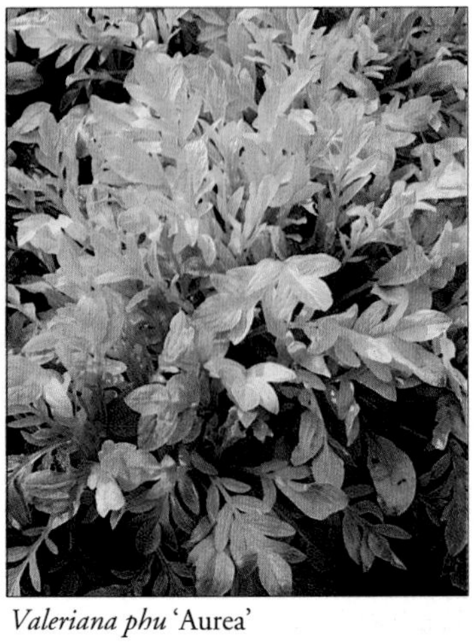
Valeriana phu 'Aurea'

V. officinalis (All heal, Common valerian). Upright, clump-forming perennial with short rhizomes producing fleshy, branching stems. The aromatic, bright green, basal and stem leaves are pinnate, to 20cm (8in) long, each with 7–10 pairs of lance-shaped, toothed leaflets. Branched, rounded, corymb-like cymes of salverform, bisexual, pink or white flowers, to 5mm (¼in) long, are borne throughout summer. ↕ 1.2–2m (4–6ft), ↔ 40–80cm (16–32in). W. Europe. ✻✻✻
***V. phu* 'Aurea'** ■ Clump-forming, rhizomatous perennial with simple or pinnatifid, elliptic to inversely lance-shaped, aromatic basal leaves, to 20cm (8in) long, and pinnatifid, pinnatisect, or pinnate stem leaves; pinnate leaves have 3 or 4 pairs of elliptic leaflets. All leaves are soft yellow in spring, turning lime- to mid-green by summer. In early summer, branching stems bear panicle-like corymbs of small, salverform, bisexual white flowers, 4mm (⅛in) long. ↕ to 1.5m (5ft), ↔ 60cm (24in). ✻✻✻

VALLEA

ELAEOCARPACEAE

Genus of one species of evergreen shrub or tree found in scrub in the Andes from Colombia to Bolivia. It has spirally arranged, simple or occasionally lobed leaves, and produces cup-shaped flowers, each with 5 sepals and 5 petals, in small, axillary and terminal cymes. Where temperatures fall below 0°C (32°F), grow in a cool greenhouse. In warmer areas, use in a courtyard garden or border, or plant against a warm, sunny wall.

- **HARDINESS** Frost hardy (borderline).
- **CULTIVATION** Under glass, grow in lime-free (ericaceous) potting compost in full or bright filtered light. When in growth, water moderately and apply a balanced liquid fertilizer monthly. Water sparingly in winter. Outdoors, grow in moderately fertile, neutral to acid, moist but well-drained soil in full sun or partial shade. Pruning group 9; may require restrictive pruning under glass.
- **PROPAGATION** Sow seed at 6–12°C (43–54°F), ideally as soon as ripe. Root semi-ripe cuttings with bottom heat in mid- or late summer.
- **PESTS AND DISEASES** Red spider mites may be a problem under glass.

V. stipularis ♀ Erect to spreading shrub or tree, freely branching, at least when mature. Almost fleshy, leathery, deep green leaves, 3–12cm (1¼–5in) long, are lance-shaped to broadly ovate,

V

rounded to heart-shaped at the bases, and sometimes lobed. Cymes of cup-shaped, crimson to dark rose-red flowers, 2–2.5cm (¾–1in) across, with darker veins, are produced from spring to summer. ↕ 3–5m (10–15ft), ↔ 2–4m (6–12ft). N. South America (Colombia to Bolivia). ✻✻ (borderline)

▷ ***Vallota speciosa*** see *Cyrtanthus elatus*

VANCOUVERIA

BERBERIDACEAE

Genus, closely allied to *Epimedium*, of about 3 species of creeping, rhizomatous perennials, some of them evergreen, from rocky hillside scrub or coniferous woodland in W. USA. They are grown for their ternate or 2-ternate, thick, sometimes leathery, basal leaves, and for their loose panicles of nodding flowers, each with 6 reflexed petals and 12 sepals, borne on wiry stems in late spring and summer. Suitable for ground cover in a large rock garden or woodland garden.

- **HARDINESS** Fully hardy to frost hardy.
- **CULTIVATION** Grow in moderately fertile, humus-rich, leafy, moist but well-drained soil in partial shade. Shelter from cold, drying winds.
- **PROPAGATION** Sow seed in containers in a cold frame as soon as ripe. Divide in spring.
- **PESTS AND DISEASES** Vine weevil may be a problem.

V. chrysantha. Creeping, evergreen, rhizomatous perennial with ternate or 2-ternate, thick, leathery, glossy, dark green, basal leaves, to 45cm (18in) long, glaucous and paler beneath, composed of usually 9, rarely 3 or 5, rounded, diamond-shaped leaflets, 4cm (1½in) long, with thickened, wavy margins. From late spring to summer, leafless stems bear loose panicles of 4–15 yellow flowers, to 1cm (½in) long. ↕ to 30cm (12in), ↔ to 60cm (24in) or more. USA (S.W. Oregon, N. California). ✻✻✻
V. hexandra ▣ Creeping, deciduous, rhizomatous perennial with 2-ternate, normally basal leaves, to 45cm (18in) long, each composed of 9 or more variable, ovate, smooth-textured, bright green leaflets, 7cm (3in) long, white-hairy when young. In late spring and early summer, leafless stems bear loose panicles of 6–45 white flowers, to 1.5cm (½in) long. Seldom spreads as widely as *V. chrysantha.* ↕↔ to 40cm (16in). USA (Washington to California). ✻✻✻

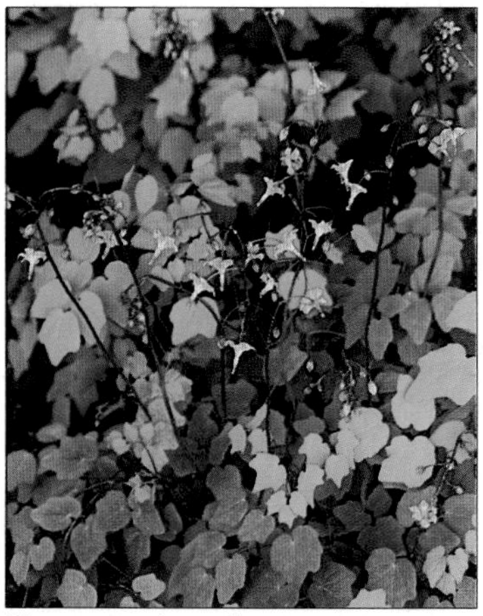

Vancouveria hexandra

VANDA

ORCHIDACEAE

Genus of 30–40 species of evergreen, epiphytic, monopodial orchids found in exposed sites in scrub forest at altitudes of 1,500m (5,000ft) from India to S.E. Asia and the Philippines, and south to Australia. They have stout, simple stems, the tips of which bear 2-ranked, strap-shaped to linear, leathery, semi-rigid, mid-green leaves, often lobed or toothed at the tips. Aerial roots form on the lower part of the stems. The flowers, borne in axillary, occasionally terminal racemes, are often large, showy, and intricately coloured on their sepals, with small lips. A range of richly coloured hybrids is available.

- **HARDINESS** Frost tender.
- **CULTIVATION** Intermediate-growing orchids. Grow in epiphytic orchid compost in slatted baskets in full light with shade from hot sun. In summer, water freely, apply fertilizer at every third watering, and mist plants twice daily. Water moderately in winter. See also p.46.
- **PROPAGATION** Remove offsets that arise at the base of the plants, or root cuttings of stem sections, in spring.
- **PESTS AND DISEASES** Susceptible to red spider mites, aphids, and mealybugs.

V. caerulea. Unbranched, epiphytic orchid producing curved, linear leaves, to 25cm (10in) long. In autumn and winter, bears long, pendent racemes of clear blue flowers, 5–10cm (2–4in) across, often chequered darker blue; the lips are dark violet-blue with whitish blue lateral lobes. ↕ 60cm (24in), ↔ 30cm (12in). India, Burma, Thailand. ❀ (min. 13–16°C/55–61°F; max. 30°C/86°F)
V. Kasem's Delight (*V.* Sun Tan x *V.* Thospol). Unbranched, epiphytic orchid with linear leaves, 15cm (6in) long. Flowers, 10cm (4in) across, in a combination of deep mauve and indigo, are borne in long, pendent racemes intermittently throughout the year. ↕ 60cm (24in), ↔ 30cm (12in). ❀ (min. 13–16°C/55–61°F; max. 30°C/86°F)
V. Rothschildiana ▣ 🏆 (*Euanthe sanderiana* x *V. caerulea*). Unbranched, epiphytic orchid with curved, linear leaves, 15cm (6in) long. Dark-veined, violet-blue flowers, 10cm (4in) across, are borne in long, pendent racemes intermittently throughout the year. ↕ 60cm (24in), ↔ 30cm (12in). ❀ (min. 13–16°C/55–61°F; max. 30°C/86°F)
V. sanderiana see *Euanthe sanderiana.*
V. tessellata. Unbranched, epiphytic orchid with curved, linear leaves, to 45cm (18in) long. In autumn, produces long, pendent racemes of variable flowers, 5cm (2in) across, yellow-green or very pale blue, chequered brown, with white-margined, violet to blue lips. ↕ 60cm (24in), ↔ 30cm (12in). India, Sri Lanka, Burma, Malaysia. ❀ (min. 13–16°C/55–61°F; max. 30°C/86°F)
V. tricolor. Unbranched, epiphytic orchid with curved, linear leaves, 45cm (18in) long. Fragrant flowers, 5–7cm (2–3in) across, are usually pale yellow, heavily patterned red-brown, with purple-striped, violet-red lips; they are borne in long, erect to spreading racemes in winter. ↕ 1m (3ft), ↔ 30cm (12in). Laos, Indonesia (Java). ❀ (min. 13–16°C/55–61°F; max. 30°C/86°F)

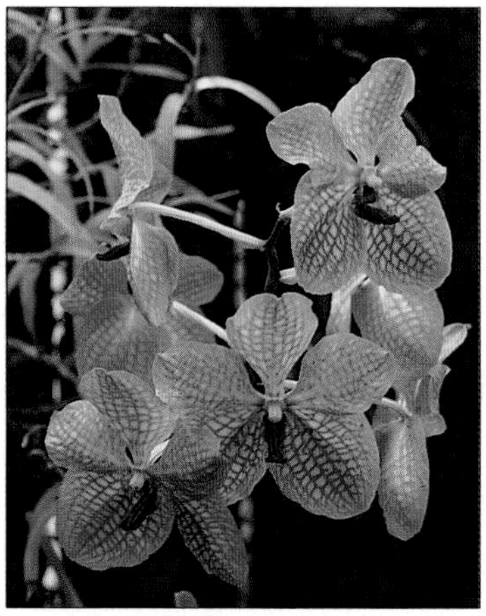

Vanda Rothschildiana

▷ **Varnish tree** see *Rhus verniciflua*
▷ **Vase plant** see *Aechmea fasciata*
▷ **Vegetable sheep** see *Haastia, H. pulvinaris, Raoulia eximia*

VEITCHIA

ARECACEAE/PALMAE

Genus of 18 species of single-stemmed palms found in tropical rainforest, from sea level to 650m (2,100ft), from the Philippines and New Caledonia to Fiji and the New Hebrides. Oblong, pinnate leaves are produced in terminal tufts above a distinctive crownshaft; bowl-shaped, 3-petalled flowers are borne in panicles just beneath the foliage, and are followed by showy, red to orange fruits. In frost-prone climates, grow in a warm greenhouse or as houseplants. In warmer areas, use small species in a courtyard or border, and grow tall species on a lawn.

- **HARDINESS** Frost tender.
- **CULTIVATION** Under glass, grow in loam-based potting compost (JI No.3) with added peat and sharp sand, in full light. Pot on or top-dress in spring. When in growth, water freely and apply a balanced liquid fertilizer monthly. Water sparingly in winter. Outdoors, grow in fertile, moist but well-drained soil in full sun.
- **PROPAGATION** Sow seed at 24°C (75°F) in spring.
- **PESTS AND DISEASES** Red spider mites may be troublesome under glass.

V. joannis Ŧ syn. *Kentia joannis.* Tall palm with a slender, columnar trunk, to 28cm (11in) across. Erect to arching, mid- to deep green leaves, to 3m (10ft) or more long, each have 70–80 narrowly linear, arching leaflets. Greenish yellow flowers, 1cm (½in) across, are produced in panicles to 1m (3ft) long, usually in summer; they are followed by ovoid, orange-red fruit, 5–6cm (2–2½in) long. ↕ to 30m (100ft), ↔ to 6m (20ft). Fiji. ❀ (min. 15°C/59°F)
V. merrillii ▣ Ŧ syn. *Adonidia merrillii* (Christmas palm, Manila palm). Small palm with a slender trunk, to 26cm (10in) across, which tapers towards the crownshaft. Strongly arching, matt, mid- to deep green leaves, 1–2m (3–6ft) long, each have 40–60 strap-shaped leaflets, pale green and scaly beneath. Green to yellow-green flowers, 2cm (¾in) across, are borne in panicles to 1m (3ft) long, usually in summer; they are followed by ovoid crimson fruit, to 3cm (1¼in) long, which are at their most colourful during winter. ↕ to 5–6m (15–20ft), ↔ 2–3.5m (6–11ft). Philippines (Palawan Islands). ❀ (min. 15°C/59°F)

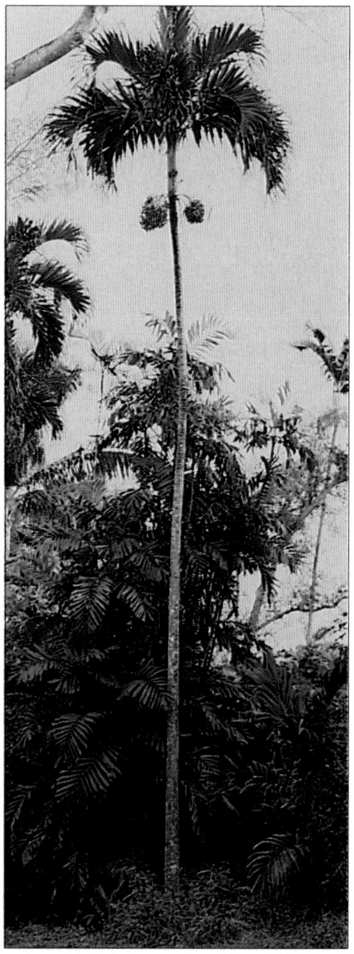

Veitchia merrillii

VELLOZIA

VELLOZIACEAE

Genus of 124 species of xerophytic, sometimes tree-like, evergreen perennials occurring on rocky, windswept cliffs or outcrops in scrub or woodland in tropical Africa, Madagascar, and tropical N., C., and S. America. They are grown for their fragrant, white, yellow, blue, purple, or violet flowers, which are bell-, funnel-, or star-shaped, and borne singly on long stalks. The narrowly elliptic to lance-shaped, toothed, rigid, often sharp-edged leaves are produced in tufts at the tops of woody stems, which can reach 4m (12ft) high. In frost-prone regions, grow in a warm greenhouse in containers or in hanging baskets. In dry, tropical areas, grow in a rock garden or desert garden. Vellozias often appear dead in drought conditions but quickly bear new leaves after watering or rainfall.

- **HARDINESS** Frost tender.
- **CULTIVATION** Under glass, grow in loam-based potting compost (JI No.2) with added peat and sharp sand, in full light. Water sparingly during the growing season; keep almost dry in winter. Outdoors, grow in moderately fertile, sharply drained soil in full sun.
- **PROPAGATION** Sow seed at 19–24°C (66–75°F), or divide, in spring.
- **PESTS AND DISEASES** Trouble free.

V. elegans, syn. *Barbacenia elegans, Talbotia elegans.* Evergreen perennial with firm, arching stems and narrow, lance-shaped, mid-green leaves, to 21cm (8in) long, with slender points. Pale lilac buds open to solitary, star-shaped, pure white flowers, 3cm (1¼in) across, in spring. ↕ 15–20cm (6–8in), ↔ 20cm (8in). South Africa (KwaZulu/Natal). ❄ (min. 16°C/61°F)

▷**Velour philodendron** see *Philodendron melanochrysum*

VELTHEIMIA

HYACINTHACEAE/LILIACEAE

Genus of 2 species of bulbous perennials from grassy and rocky hillsides in South Africa. They are grown for their rosettes of thick, wavy leaves, and for their terminal racemes of pendent, spring flowers, similar in form to those of red hot pokers (*Kniphofia*). In frost-prone areas, grow in a temperate greenhouse or as houseplants. In warmer areas, grow in a warm, sunny border.

- **HARDINESS** Frost tender.
- **CULTIVATION** Plant in autumn with the neck of each bulb just above the soil surface. Under glass, grow in loam-based potting compost (JI No.2) with added sharp sand, in full sun. In growth, water moderately and apply a low-nitrogen liquid fertilizer every 2 weeks. Reduce watering as the leaves fade, and keep just moist when dormant. Repot only when congested, to avoid root disturbance. Outdoors, grow in moderately fertile, well-drained soil in full sun.
- **PROPAGATION** Sow seed at 19–24°C (66–75°F) in autumn. Remove offsets in late summer.
- **PESTS AND DISEASES** Trouble free.

V. bracteata ▣ 🏆 syn. *V. capensis* of gardens, *V. undulata, V. viridifolia.* Robust, bulbous perennial with basal rosettes of broad, strap-shaped, thick, spreading, wavy, glossy, dark green leaves, to 35cm (14in) long and 10cm (4in) across. In spring, bears dense, terminal racemes of up to 60 pendent, tubular, yellow-spotted, pinkish purple flowers, 4cm (1½in) long, on stout, erect, yellow-spotted purple stems. ↕ 45cm (18in), ↔ 30cm (12in). South Africa. ❄ (min. 5–7°C/41–45°F). **'Rosalba'** has red-tinted yellow flowers.

V. capensis 🏆 syn. *V. glauca, V. roodeae, V. viridifolia* of gardens. Bulbous perennial producing basal rosettes of erect, narrowly lance-shaped, thick, glaucous, bluish green leaves, to 30cm (12in) long and 4cm (1½in) across, with wavy margins. In spring, stout green stems, flecked with purple, bear terminal racemes of pendent, tubular flowers, 2–3cm (¾–1¼in) long, varying from white with red spots to pink with green or red markings. Similar to *V. bracteata*, but more delicate and less easy to grow. ↕ 45cm (18in), ↔ 30cm (12in). South Africa (Western Cape). ❄ (min. 5–7°C/41–45°F)

***V. capensis* of gardens** see *V. bracteata.*
V. glauca see *V. capensis.*
V. roodeae see *V. capensis.*
V. undulata see *V. bracteata.*
V. viridifolia see *V. bracteata.*
***V. viridifolia* of gardens** see *V. capensis.*

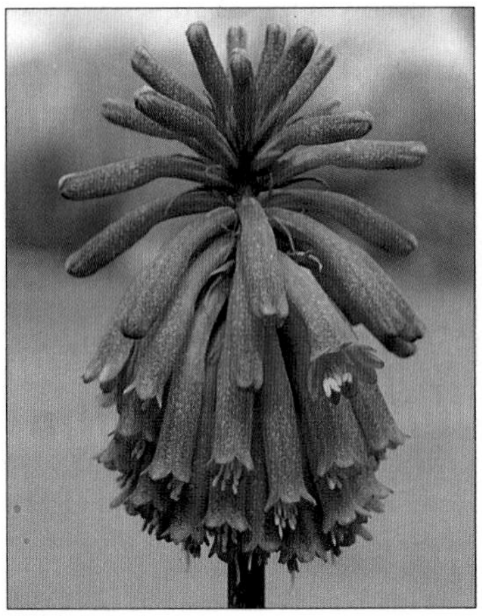
Veltheimia bracteata

▷**Velvet, White** see *Tradescantia sillamontana*
▷**Velvet bent** see *Agrostis canina*
▷**Velvet plant** see *Gynura aurantiaca*
Purple see *Gynura aurantiaca*
Royal see *Gynura aurantiaca*
Trailing see *Ruellia makoyana*
▷ **x *Venidioarctotis*** see *Arctotis, A.* Harlequin Hybrids
▷ ***Venidium*** see *Arctotis*
V. fastuosum see *A. fastuosa*
▷**Venus fly trap** see *Dionaea, D. muscipula*
▷**Venus's looking glass** see *Legousia speculum-veneris*

VERATRUM

LILIACEAE/MELANTHIACEAE

Genus of about 45 species of imposing, vigorous perennials, with poisonous black rhizomes, from damp meadows and open woodland throughout the N. hemisphere. The alternate, pleated, prominently veined, mid- to dark green leaves are broadly elliptic to ovate at the bases of the stout, erect stems, usually becoming smaller and more lance-shaped further up the stems. Numerous small, star-shaped, white, green, reddish brown, or almost black flowers are borne in summer, followed by spherical seed heads. The flowers are borne in large, terminal panicles, with unisexual (male) and bisexual flowers in the same inflorescence. Grow in a moist, shady site in a mixed or herbaceous border, a peat bed, or in a woodland or wild garden. All parts are highly toxic if ingested. Contact with the foliage may irritate the skin.

- **HARDINESS** Fully hardy.

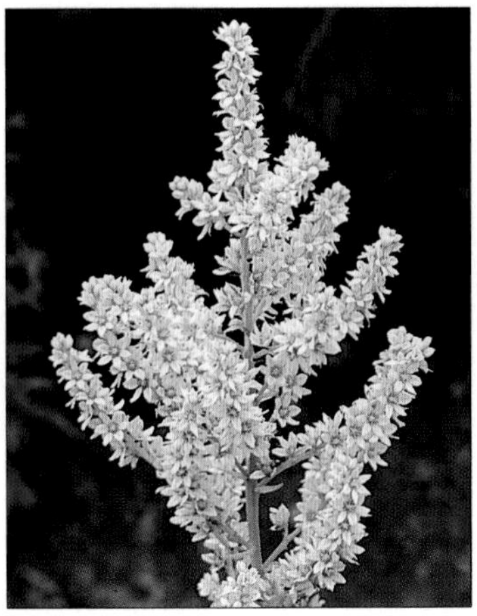
Veratrum album

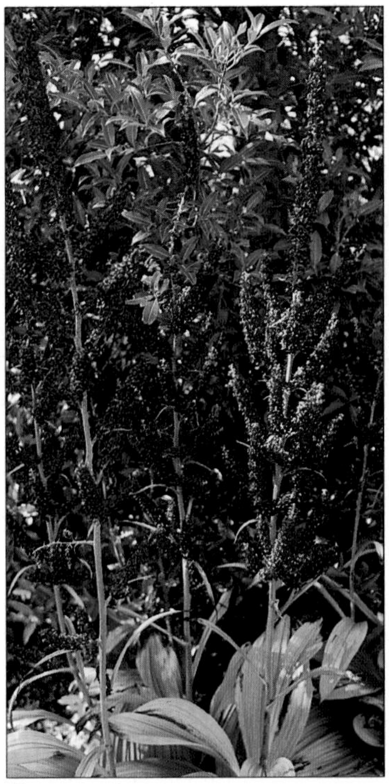
Veratrum nigrum

- **CULTIVATION** Grow in deep, fertile, moist but well-drained soil, with added well-rotted organic matter, in a site in partial shade, or in full sun where the soil does not dry out; *V. viride* tolerates wet soil. Provide shelter from cold, drying winds.
- **PROPAGATION** Sow seed in containers in a cold frame as soon as ripe. Divide in autumn or early spring.
- **PESTS AND DISEASES** Susceptible to slug and snail damage.

V. album ▣ (False hellebore, White hellebore). Rhizomatous perennial with ovate to broadly elliptic, pleated basal leaves, to 30cm (12in) long, and a few stem leaves. All leaves are hairless above, hairy-veined beneath. In early and mid-summer, bears numerous star-shaped, greenish white to white flowers, 1.5–2cm (½–¾in) across, in erect, terminal, freely branched panicles, to 60cm (24in) long. ↕ to 2m (6ft), ↔ 60cm (24in). Europe, N. Africa, N. Asia. ❄❄❄

V. nigrum ▣ 🏆 Rhizomatous perennial producing broadly elliptic, pleated basal leaves, to 35cm (14in) long, and a few stem leaves. All foliage is hairless. In mid- and late summer, numerous star-shaped, unpleasantly scented, reddish brown to almost black flowers, 1.5cm (½in) across, with green-striped backs, are borne in terminal panicles, 45cm (18in) long; the lower branches are often horizontal or slightly pendent. ↕ 60–120cm (24–48in), ↔ 60cm (24in). Europe to Russia (Siberia), China, Korea. ❄❄❄

V. viride (Indian poke). Rhizomatous perennial with ovate to broadly elliptic, pleated basal leaves, to 30cm (12in) long, and a few stem leaves. All leaves are hairless above and hairy beneath. In early and midsummer, numerous star-shaped, green to yellowish green flowers, to 2cm (¾in) across, are produced in terminal panicles, to 60cm (24in) long, with slightly pendent lower branches. ↕ to 2m (6ft), ↔ 60cm (24in). E. North America. ❄❄❄

VERBASCUM syn. CELSIA

Mullein

SCROPHULARIACEAE

Genus of 360 species, most of which are biennials, with a few annuals, perennials, and subshrubs, some semi-evergreen or evergreen. They are found mainly on dry, stony hillsides, wasteland, and in open woodland in Europe, N. Africa, and W. and C. Asia. Usually hairy, sometimes woolly plants, they have large, alternate, simple, entire, scalloped, lobed, or toothed, soft-textured basal leaves, which often form large rosettes, and smaller, often stalkless stem leaves. Most produce one or a few tall, erect stems bearing flowers in dense spikes or racemes, but some may have flowers clustered within the rosette centres. The generally short-stemmed or stemless, outward-facing, saucer-shaped flowers are usually yellow, occasionally purple, red, brownish red, or white; each has a short tube with 5 wide-spreading lobes, and sometimes coloured filament hairs. Individual flowers are short-lived, but they are very numerous and flowering takes place over a long period. Semi-evergreen species are grown as much for their overwintering rosettes of white-woolly leaves, built up during the first year, as for their flowers.

Most cultivated mulleins are hybrids. Rosette-forming and short-lived, they have ovate to oblong, mid- to greyish green leaves, and generally bear large, showy, saucer-shaped flowers, to 4cm (1½in) across, in more or less branched racemes, 30–100cm (12–39in) long.

Hybrids and larger species are good for growing in a large, mixed or herbaceous border or gravel bed, or for naturalizing in a wild or woodland garden. Smaller species, including *V. dumulosum, V. pestallozae,* and *V. spinosum,* are suitable for a rock garden or alpine house.

- **HARDINESS** Fully hardy to frost hardy.
- **CULTIVATION** Grow in alkaline, poor, well-drained soil in full sun. In fertile soil, they grow larger and need support. Protect alpines from winter wet. In an alpine house, use a mix of equal parts loam-based potting compost (JI No.2) and grit.
- **PROPAGATION** Sow seed of biennials and perennials in containers in a cold frame in late spring or early summer; biennials sown at 13–18°C (55–64°F) in early spring may flower and die in their first year. Divide perennials in spring, or take root cuttings in winter. Take semi-ripe cuttings of shrubby species in late summer.
- **PESTS AND DISEASES** Powdery mildew, some moth caterpillars, and figwort weevil may be a problem.

V. acaule, syn. *Celsia acaulis.* Rosette-forming, evergreen perennial producing ovate, rough, grey-green, basal leaves, to 5cm (2in) long, with coarsely toothed margins. In midsummer, bears saucer-shaped yellow flowers, 2cm (¾in) across, either singly or in clusters, from the centres of the rosettes. Best in a dry wall or alpine house. ↕ to 5cm (2in), ↔ to 15cm (6in). Mediterranean. ❄❄❄

V. arcturus, syn. *Celsia arcturus.* Rosette-forming, evergreen subshrub or semi-evergreen, woody-based perennial, usually grown as an annual or biennial.

V

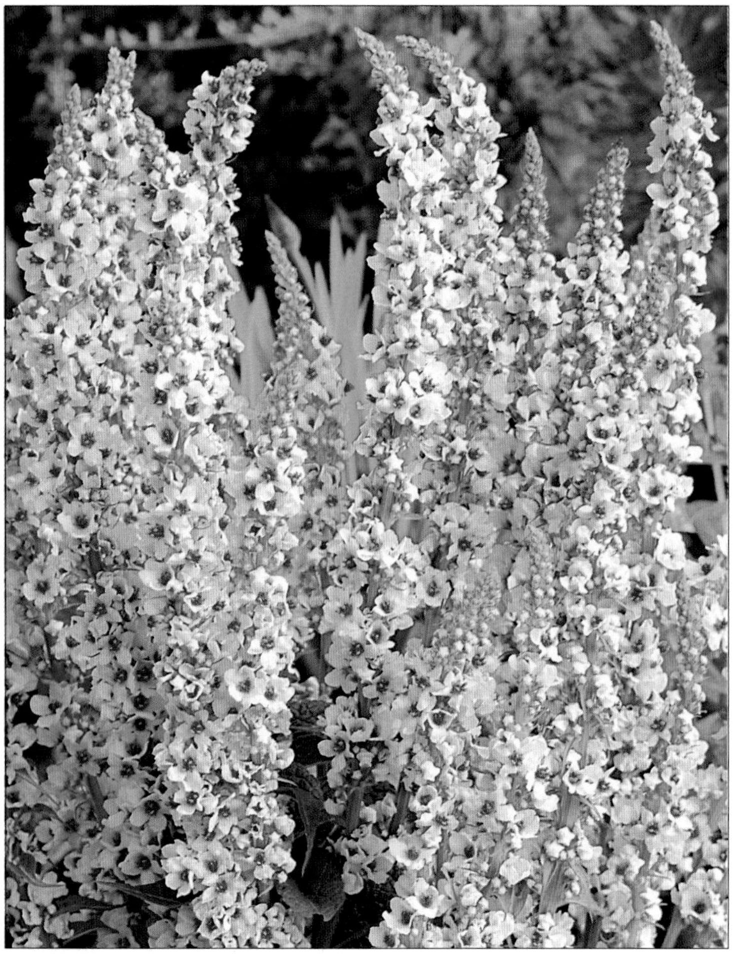

Verbascum chaixii f. *album*

Oblong to lance-shaped, pinnatifid, softly downy, grey-green, basal leaves, to 15cm (6in) long, each have a large terminal lobe, and lateral lobes that are progressively smaller towards the base. In summer of the second year, bears saucer-shaped yellow flowers, to 2.5cm (1in) across, in erect, loose racemes, to 20cm (8in) long. Protect against frost in winter. ↕ 30–60cm (12–24in), ↔ 30cm (12in). Greece (Crete). ❄❄

V. bombyciferum 🏆 syn. *V. broussa.* Rosette-forming biennial or short-lived, evergreen perennial covered with silky silver hairs. It has ovate-oblong, densely white-woolly, basal leaves, to 35cm (14in) long. Saucer-shaped, sulphur-yellow flowers, to 4cm (1½in) across, are borne in erect, dense, sparsely branched spikes, 60–120cm (24–48in) long, in summer. ↕ to 1.8m (8ft), ↔ to 60cm (24in). Turkey. ❄❄❄. **'Silver Lining'**, often cultivated as an annual, has silvery white, very silky-hairy foliage.

V. broussa see *V. bombyciferum.*

V. chaixii (Nettle-leaved mullein). Rosette-forming, semi-evergreen perennial producing long-stalked, ovate-oblong, grey-hairy, mid-green basal leaves, 5–25cm (2–10in) long, with scalloped margins, and sometimes lobed towards the bases. Densely white-woolly stems bear short-stalked leaves on the middle section of the stem, and more rounded, stalkless upper leaves. Saucer-shaped, pale yellow flowers, to 2.5cm (1in) across, with purple filament hairs, are borne in slender panicles, to 40cm (16in) long, from mid- to late summer. ↕ to 90cm (36in), ↔ 45cm (18in). C., E., and S. Europe. ❄❄❄.

f. *album* ■ produces white flowers with mauve centres.

***V.* 'C.L. Adams'.** Erect, semi-evergreen perennial with ovate to lance-shaped, wrinkled, mid-green leaves, to 20cm (8in) long. Saucer-shaped, deep yellow flowers, 3cm (1¼in) across, with reddish purple filament hairs, are borne in erect, branched spikes, 30–60cm (12–24in) long, from early to late summer. ↕ to 2m (6ft), ↔ 30cm (12in). ❄❄❄

***V.* 'Cotswold Queen'** ■ Erect, semi-evergreen perennial with ovate to lance-shaped, wrinkled, grey-green leaves, to 20cm (8in) long. From early to late summer, bears erect, unbranched spikes, 30–60cm (12–24in) long, of saucer-shaped yellow flowers, to 4cm (1½in) across, with purple filament hairs. ↕ 1.2m (4ft), ↔ 30cm (12in). ❄❄❄

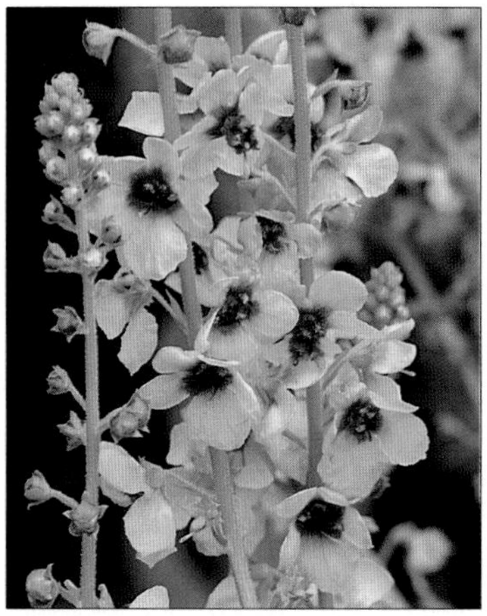

Verbascum 'Cotswold Queen'

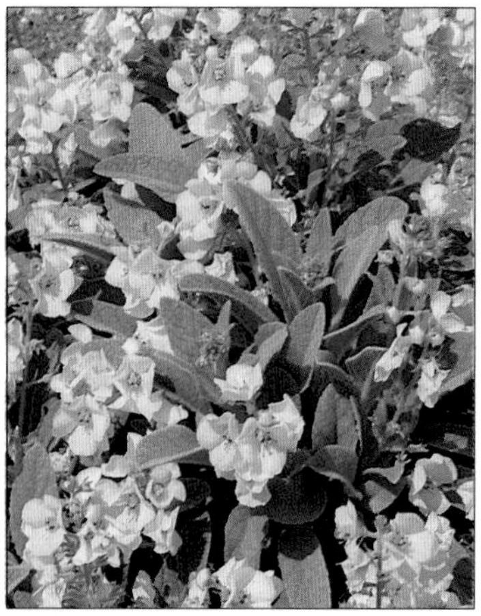

Verbascum dumulosum

V. densiflorum, syn. *V. thapsiforme.* Rosette-forming biennial or short-lived, semi-evergreen perennial with a dense covering of grey-yellow hairs and oblong to elliptic, wavy-margined, mid- to dark green, basal leaves, to 45cm (18in) long. In summer, produces erect, branching spikes, 60–90cm (24–36in) long, of closely set clusters of saucer-shaped, bright yellow, sometimes white flowers, to 5cm (2in) across. ↕ 1.2–1.5m (4–5ft), ↔ to 60cm (24in). Europe, Russia (Siberia). ❄❄❄

V. dumulosum ■ 🏆 Spreading, evergreen subshrub with white-downy stems and elliptic, entire to scalloped, felted-hairy, grey or grey-green leaves, 1.5–5cm (½–2in) long. In late spring and early summer, produces a succession of short racemes, to 15cm (6in) long, of saucer-shaped yellow flowers, to 1.5cm (½in) across, with small, red-purple eyes. Grow on its side in a wall crevice, or in a gravel or scree bed. ↕ to 25cm (10in), ↔ to 40cm (16in). S.W. Turkey. ❄❄❄

***V.* 'Gainsborough'** ■ 🏆 Rosette-forming, semi-evergreen perennial with ovate to elliptic, wrinkled, grey-green leaves, 25cm (10in) long. From early to late summer, bears pyramidal panicles, to 75cm (30in) long, of saucer-shaped, soft yellow flowers, 2.5cm (1in) across. ↕ to 1.2m (4ft), ↔ 30cm (12in). ❄❄❄

***V.* 'Helen Johnson'** 🏆 Rosette-forming, evergreen perennial producing ovate to lance-shaped, wrinkled, finely downy, grey-green leaves, 20cm (8in) long. From early to late summer, bears saucer-shaped, light pinkish brown flowers, 3cm (1¼in) across, with purple filament hairs, in erect, branched spikes

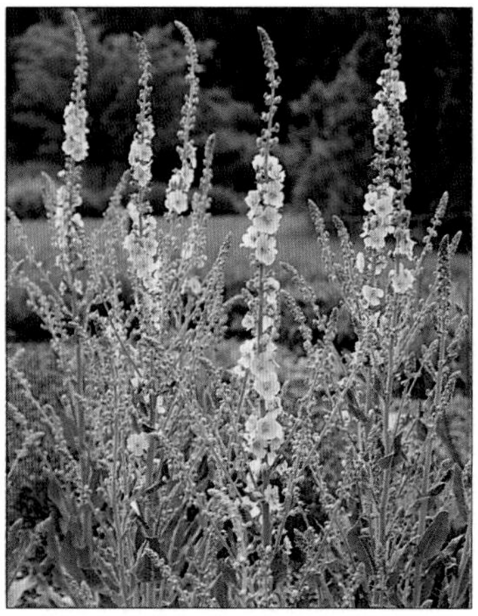

Verbascum 'Gainsborough'

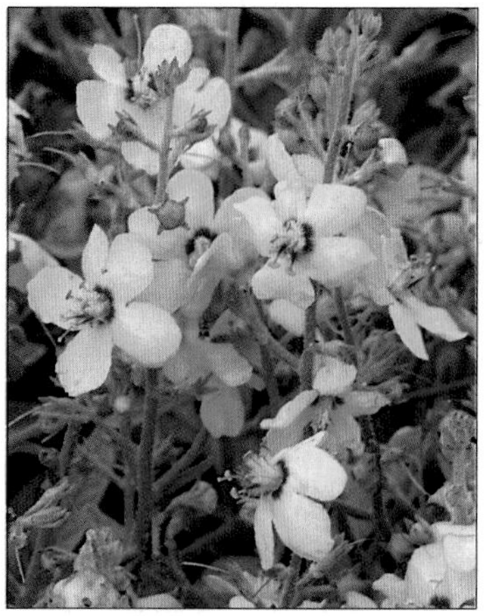

Verbascum 'Letitia'

to 45cm (18in) long. ↕ 90cm (36in), ↔ 30cm (12in) or more. ❄❄❄

***V.* 'Letitia'** ■ 🏆 Dense, rounded, evergreen subshrub with stiff, branching stems bearing oblong-lance-shaped, irregularly toothed or lobed, grey-green leaves, 3cm (1¼in) long. Produces an abundance of almost flat, clear yellow flowers, 1.5cm (½in) across, with reddish purple centres, in short racemes, 10cm (4in) long, over long periods in summer. Suitable for a raised bed, rock garden, or alpine house. Needs sharply drained soil. ↕ to 25cm (10in), ↔ to 30cm (12in). ❄❄❄

V. longifolium* var. *pannosum see *V. olympicum.*

***V.* 'Mont Blanc'.** Rosette-forming, semi-evergreen perennial producing ovate to lance-shaped, wrinkled, finely white-downy, pale grey-green, basal leaves, to 30cm (12in) long. Upright, unbranched, slender racemes, to 50cm (20in) long, of saucer-shaped, pure white flowers, to 3cm (1¼in) across, are borne from early to late summer. ↕ 90cm (36in), ↔ 30cm (12in). ❄❄❄

V. nigrum ■ (Dark mullein). Rosette-forming, deciduous or semi-evergreen perennial with ovate-oblong, scalloped,

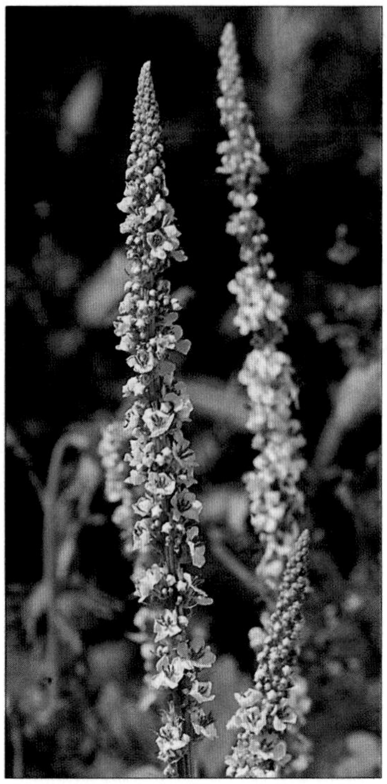

Verbascum nigrum

long-stalked, mid- to dark green basal leaves, 15–40cm (6–16in) long; the leaves become progressively shorter-stalked up the stems, then stalkless and more rounded; all leaves are heart-shaped at the bases, hairless above, and slightly grey-woolly beneath. From midsummer to early autumn, usually unbranched, ridged stems, with long hairs, bear slender racemes, 50cm (20in) long, of clustered, saucer-shaped, dark yellow flowers, to 2.5cm (1in) across, with violet filament hairs. ↕ 90cm (36in), ↔ 60cm (24in). Europe to Russia (Siberia). ❄❄❄

V. olympicum ▣ syn. *V. longifolium* var. *pannosum.* Rosette-forming, densely grey-white-woolly, often monocarpic perennial with broadly lance-shaped, entire, short-stalked, mid-green, mainly basal leaves, usually 15cm (6in) long, sometimes to 60cm (24in). Branching stems, which form a candelabra shape, bear stalkless leaves; from early to late summer of the second or third year, they bear panicles, to 75cm (30in) or more long, of clustered, saucer-shaped, golden yellow flowers, 3cm (1¼in) across, with yellowish white filament hairs. Often dies after flowering. ↕ to 2m (6ft), ↔ 60cm (24in). Greece. ❄❄❄

V. pestallozae. Dwarf, many-branched, evergreen subshrub with stems and mid-green leaves clothed in densely felted, white, yellow, or tawny-brown hairs. In summer, bears elliptic to lance-shaped, entire, basal leaves, 2.5–4cm (1–1½in) long, and short racemes, to 15cm (6in) long, of saucer-shaped yellow flowers, 2cm (¾in) across. ↕ to 25cm (10in), ↔ to 40cm (16in). Turkey. ❄❄❄

V. phoeniceum (Purple mullein). Rosette-forming biennial or short-lived, evergreen perennial with short-stalked, ovate, slightly scalloped, wrinkled, conspicuously veined, dark green basal leaves, to 15cm (6in) long, sparsely softly hairy or hairless, and a few stalkless stem leaves. In late spring and early summer, bears slender racemes, 75cm (30in) long, of saucer-shaped, white, pink, or violet to dark purple flowers, to 3cm (1¼in) across, with violet filament hairs. ↕ to 1.2m (4ft), ↔ 45cm (18in). S. Europe, N. Africa to C. Asia (Altai Mountains). ❄❄❄

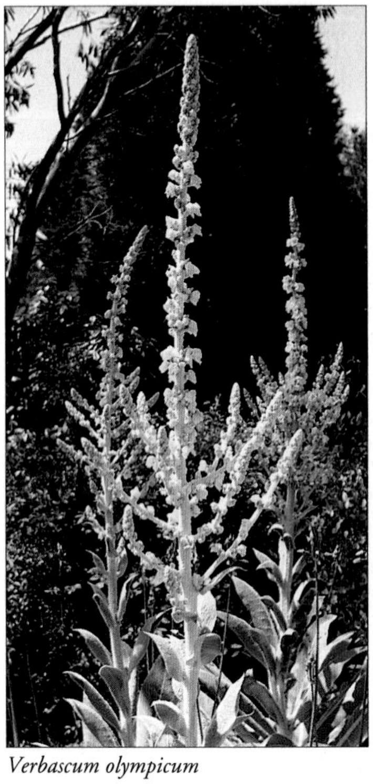

Verbascum olympicum

***V.* 'Pink Domino'** 🏆 Rosette-forming, semi-evergreen perennial with ovate to lance-shaped, wrinkled, dark purplish green leaves, 20cm (8in) long. From early to late summer, produces saucer-shaped, deep rose-pink flowers, 3cm (1¼in) long, with darker purple filament hairs, in erect, unbranched spikes, 70cm (28in) long. ↕ 1.2m (4ft), ↔ 30cm (12in). ❄❄❄

V. spinosum. Slow-growing, hummock-forming, intricately branched, semi-evergreen subshrub with woody grey shoots terminating in sharp spines. The oblong-lance-shaped, woolly, grey-white leaves, 1.5–5cm (½–2in) long, are irregularly toothed or lobed. In summer, bears twiggy panicles, to 5cm (2in) long, of saucer-shaped yellow flowers, to 2cm (¾in) across, with short lilac filament hairs. ↕ to 25cm (10in), ↔ to 40cm (16in) or more. Greece (Crete). ❄❄❄

V. thapsiforme see *V. densiflorum.*

V. thapsus (Aaron's rod, Great mullein). Robust, grey- or white-woolly, rosette-forming biennial with elliptic to oblong, entire or finely scalloped, mid-green, basal leaves, to 50cm (20in) long. In the summer of the second year, produces a stout, erect, usually unbranched, densely woolly stem, terminating in a spike-like raceme, to 75cm (30in) long, of saucer-shaped yellow flowers, to 3cm (1¼in) across. Suitable for a wildflower border. ↕ 1.2–2m (4–6ft), ↔ to 45cm (18in). Eurasia. ❄❄❄

VERBENA *syn.* GLANDULARIA

VERBENACEAE

Genus of about 250 species of annuals, perennials, and subshrubs, some of them tuberous or rhizomatous, occurring in usually open and sunny habitats, such as prairies, wasteland, and roadsides, and in open woodland (some species prefer dry sites, others moist). Almost all are from tropical and temperate regions of North, Central, and South America; a few are from S. Europe. The erect or procumbent, square stems have usually opposite, toothed, sometimes lobed to pinnatifid leaves, and bear small flowers in dense, terminal spikes, panicles, cymes, or corymbs, occasionally singly. The flowers, often brightly coloured, are salverform, each with a tubular corolla spreading at the mouth, and slightly 2-lipped, with 2 upper petals and 3 lower ones. Verbenas are long-flowering, but only a few species are fully hardy. There are numerous hybrids, which are ideal for an annual border, for edging, or for growing in containers, including hanging baskets; a few are suitable for a herbaceous border.

• **HARDINESS** Fully hardy to frost tender. Frost-hardy species often survive falls in temperature to -10°C (14°F).

• **CULTIVATION** In containers, grow in loam-based potting compost (JI No.2) with added sharp sand, in full sun. Water freely in growth, and apply a balanced liquid fertilizer monthly. Water more sparingly in winter. Outdoors, grow in moist but well-drained, moderately fertile soil in full sun. In frost-prone areas, protect with a dry winter mulch.

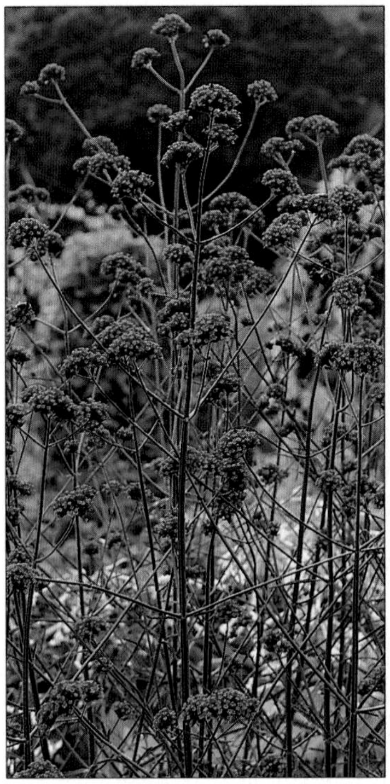

Verbena bonariensis

• **PROPAGATION** Sow seed at 18–21°C (64–70°F) in autumn or early spring. Divide perennials in spring. Take stem-tip cuttings in late summer.

• **PESTS AND DISEASES** Aphids, thrips, and leafhoppers may be a problem, especially in dry conditions. Vulnerable to slug damage. Most verbenas are very susceptible to powdery mildew.

***V. alpina* of gardens** see *V.* x *maonettii.*

V. bonariensis ▣ syn. *V. patagonica.* Stiff, upright, open clump-forming perennial with rough, branching stems bearing a few oblong-lance-shaped, wrinkled, clasping leaves, to 13cm (5in) long, with toothed margins and hairy beneath. Salverform, lilac-purple flowers, 6mm (¼in) across, are borne in panicle-like cymes, to 5cm (2in) across, from midsummer to early autumn. ↕ to 2m (6ft), ↔ 45cm (18in). South America (Brazil to Argentina). ❄❄

V. chamaedrifolia see *V. peruviana.*

V. chamaedrioides see *V. peruviana.*

V. corymbosa ▣ Spreading, rhizomatous perennial with erect, branched stems and stalkless, oblong or ovate, toothed, rough leaves, 2.5–6cm (1–2½in) long, often lobed at the bases. From early to late summer, bears salverform, red-purple flowers, 1cm (½in) across, in dense, corymb-like panicles, 5–8cm (2–3in) across. ↕ 1–2m (3–6ft), ↔ 60cm (24in). South America (S. Chile, Argentina). ❄❄

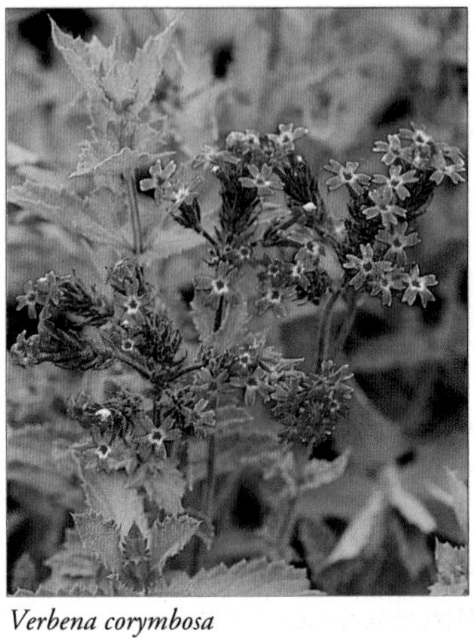

Verbena corymbosa

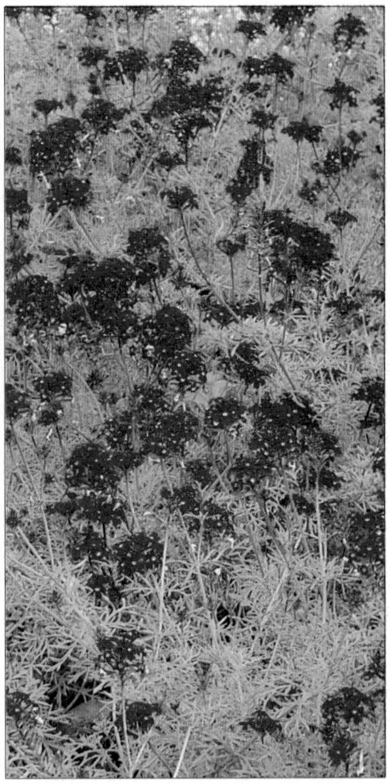

Verbena x *hybrida* 'Imagination'

V. hastata. Upright, clump-forming perennial with stems sometimes branched near the top. Bears stalked, mainly lance-shaped, pointed, toothed leaves, to 15cm (6in) long, the lowest ones spear-shaped. From early summer to early autumn, produces stiff panicles, 5–10cm (2–4in) across, of numerous salverform, violet-blue to pinkish purple, occasionally white flowers, 5mm (¼in) across. ↕ to 1.5m (5ft), ↔ 60cm (24in). E. North America. ❄❄❄

V.* x *hortensis see *V.* x *hybrida* cultivars.

***V.* x *hybrida* cultivars**, syn. *V.* x *hortensis.* Erect and bushy, or spreading and mat-forming, hairy perennials, usually grown as annuals, with ovate to oblong, toothed, rough, mid- to dark green leaves, 5–10cm (2–4in) long, either stalkless or with short stalks. In summer and autumn, they bear tight, corymb-like panicles, to 8cm (3in) or more across, of tiny, salverform, sometimes scented, white, pink, red, yellow,

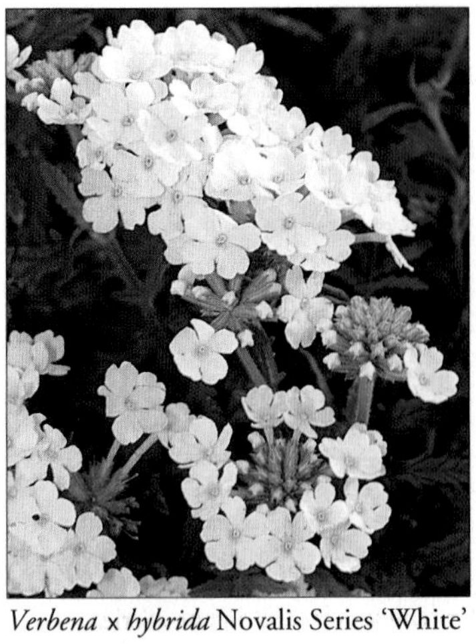

Verbena x *hybrida* Novalis Series 'White'

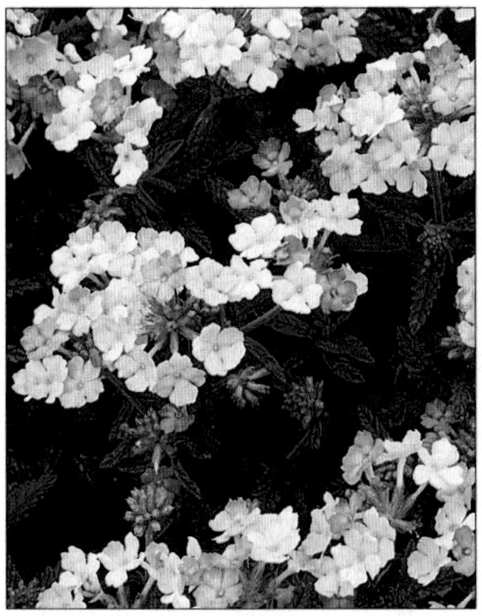

Verbena x *hybrida* 'Peaches and Cream'

or purple-blue flowers, 1–2.5cm (½–1in) across, each usually with a white eye. ↕ to 45cm (18in), ↔ 30–50cm (12–20in). ✻. Cultivars of **Derby Series** are erect and bushy, producing flowers in a full range of colours, biased slightly towards pink and red shades; ↕ to 25cm (10in). **'Imagination'** ▣ is spreading and mound-forming, with pinnatifid leaves and deep violet-blue flowers; good for hanging baskets. It is sometimes listed under *V. speciosa.* Cultivars of **Novalis Series** are erect and bushy, with almost spherical corymbs, 5–8cm (2–3in) across, of white-eyed flowers in rose-pink, deep blue, pinkish red, and scarlet, as well as single-colours in bright scarlet, white, or rose-pink; ↕ to 25cm (10in). **Novalis Series 'White'** ▣ has pure white flowers. **'Peaches and Cream'** ▣ is spreading and branching, with pastel orange-pink flowers, ageing to apricot-yellow, then creamy yellow. **Romance Series** ▣ cultivars are erect and bushy, producing white-eyed flowers in deep wine red, intense scarlet, carmine-rose-red, and blue-purple, as well as single colours of white, bright scarlet, dark rose, or lavender-pink; ↕ to 25cm (10in). **Sandy Series** ▣🏆 cultivars are compact and erect, with flowers in rose-pink, rose-pink with white eyes, magenta, scarlet, or white; colour mixtures are available. **'Showtime'** is bushy and fairly slow-growing, bearing flowers in a wide range of colours.

***V.* 'Lawrence Johnston'** 🏆 Spreading perennial with ovate to oblong, toothed leaves, to 10cm (4in) long. Salverform, cardinal-red flowers, 1cm (½in) across, are borne in large corymbs, 5cm (2in)

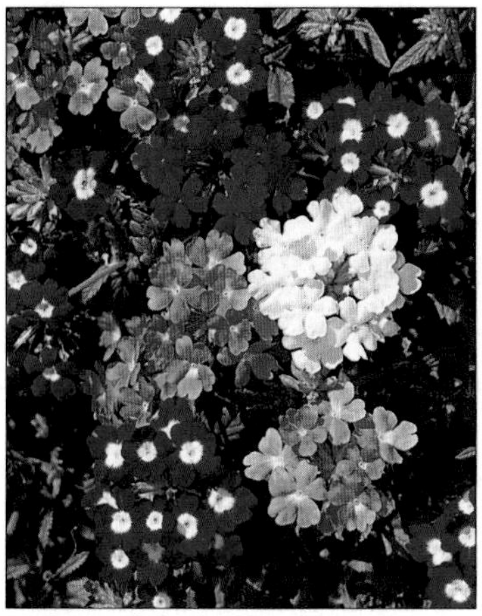

Verbena x *hybrida* Romance Series

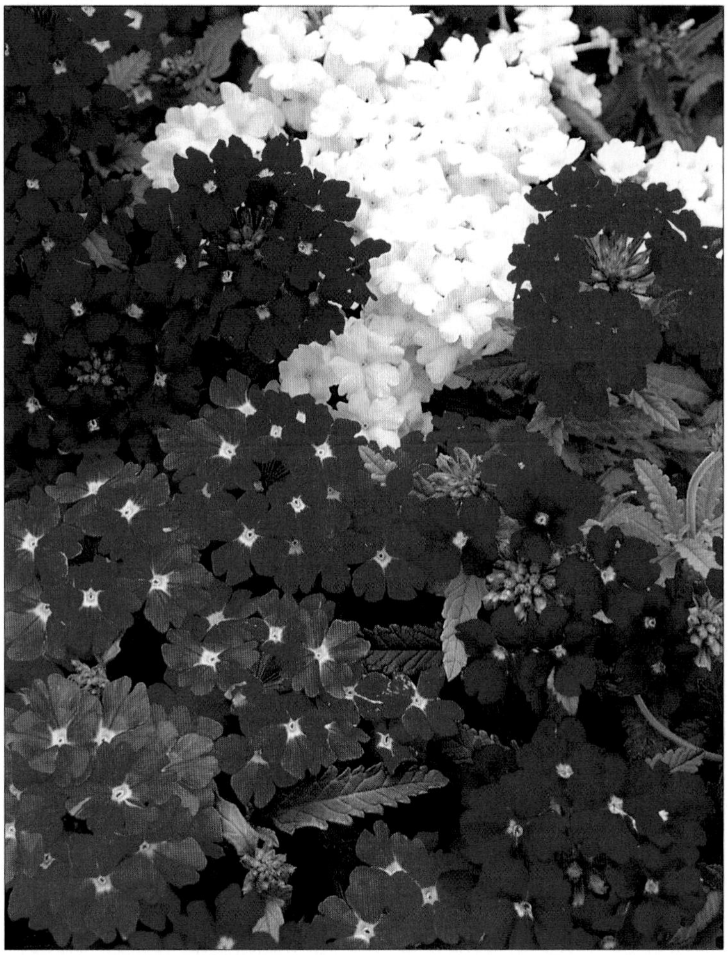

Verbena x *hybrida* Sandy Series

across, in summer and early autumn. ↕ 45cm (18in), ↔ 60cm (24in). ✻✻

***V.* 'Mahonettii'** see *V.* x *maonettii.*

***V.* x *maonettii*,** syn. *V. alpina* of gardens, *V.* 'Mahonetti' (Italian verbena). Spreading, prostrate perennial with finely cut, pinnatifid leaves, to 2.5cm (1in) long. Produces short spikes of red-violet flowers, to 1cm (½in) across, with white-margined lobes, in summer. ↕ to 5cm (2in), ↔ to 30cm (12in). ✻✻

V. patagonica see *V. bonariensis.*

***V. peruviana*,** syn. *V. chamaedrifolia, V. chamaedrioides.* Fast-growing, mat-forming, semi-evergreen perennial with slender, ascending stems clothed in closely set, oblong-lance-shaped, toothed leaves, 5cm (2in) long, with short stalks. From summer to autumn, bears salver-form, rich scarlet flowers, 1cm (½in)

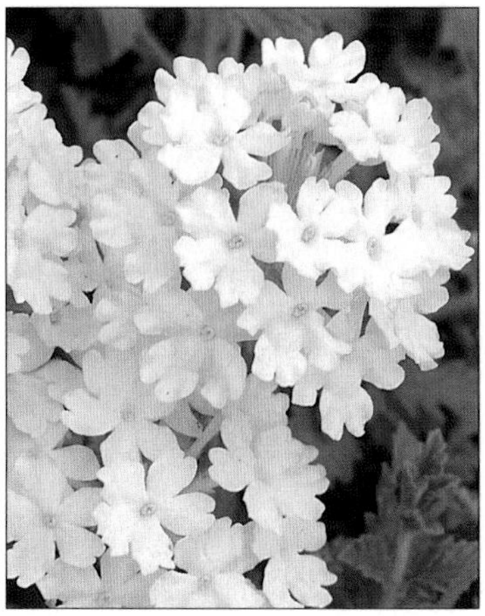

Verbena peruviana 'Alba'

across, in flat-topped, corymb-like spikes, 5cm (2in) across. ↕ to 7cm (3in), ↔ 1m (3ft). South America (S. Brazil to Argentina). ✻✻. **'Alba'** ▣ produces white flowers.

V. rigida 🏆 syn. *V. venosa.* Erect to spreading, hairy, tuberous perennial, grown as an annual, with stalkless, oblong, toothed, rough leaves, to 8cm (3in) long. In summer, bears salverform, fragrant, bright purple or magenta flowers, 5mm (¼in) across, in lax corymbs, to 5cm (2in) across, gradually lengthening and becoming spike-like with age. ↕ 45–60cm (18–24in), ↔ to 40cm (16in). South America (S. Brazil, Argentina). ✻✻. **'Lilacina'** has violet-blue flowers. **'Polaris'** forms dense clumps, and has rigid leaves to 7cm (3in) long; from early summer to early

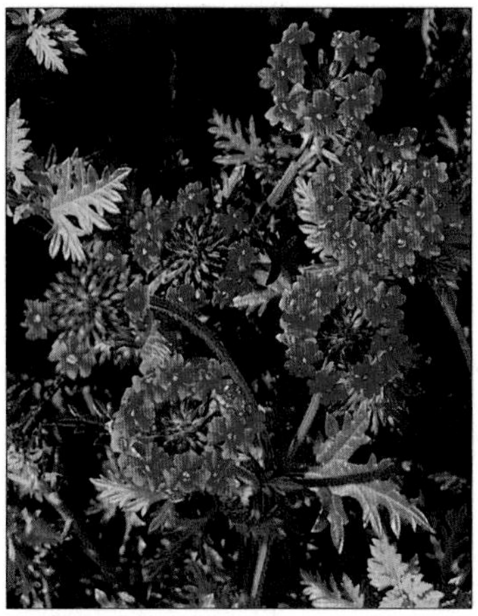

Verbena 'Sissinghurst'

autumn, bears silver-blue flowers, 8mm (⅜in) across, in corymbs 5cm (2in) across; ↕ to 60cm (24in), ↔ 30cm (12in).

***V.* 'Saint Paul'** see *V.* 'Sissinghurst'.

***V.* 'Silver Anne'** 🏆 Upright, spreading perennial with ovate-oblong, shallowly cut, rough, stalked leaves, 10cm (4in) long. Corymbs, 4cm (1½in) across, of salverform, sweetly scented flowers, 1cm (½in) across, bright pink at first and fading to silver-white with age, open in succession in summer and autumn, giving a multi-toned effect. ↕ to 30cm (12in), ↔ 60cm (24in). ✻✻

***V.* 'Sissinghurst'** ▣🏆 syn. *V.* 'Saint Paul'. Mat-forming perennial with ovate, pinnatifid, dark green leaves, to 3cm (1¼in) long. Salverform, magenta-pink flowers, 1cm (½in) across, are borne in corymbs, 2.5cm (1in) across, from late spring to autumn, but most prolifically in summer. ↕ to 20cm (8in), ↔ to 1m (3ft). ✻✻

V. tenuisecta. (Moss verbena). Usually prostrate to decumbent, sometimes erect, aromatic annual or perennial with 3-lobed leaves, to 3.5cm (1½in) long, the lobes pinnatifid, with linear, entire or toothed segments. Salverform, lilac, mauve, purple, white, or blue flowers are borne in corymb-like spikes, to 5cm (2in) across, from summer to autumn. ↕ to 50cm (20in), ↔ to 23cm (9in). S. South America. ✻✻✻

V. venosa see *V. rigida.*

▷**Verbena,**
Italian see *Verbena* x *maonettii*
Lemon see *Aloysia triphylla*
Moss see *Verbena tenuisecta*

VERNONIA

Ironweed

ASTERACEAE/COMPOSITAE

Genus of about 1,000 species of annuals, perennials, climbers, subshrubs, shrubs, and trees from mainly tropical and subtropical habitats, ranging from moist meadows to dry woodland. Most occur in South America, some in Africa, Asia, Australasia, and North America. Species from more northerly habitats are usually annuals or herbaceous perennials; those from the tropics are mainly woody. Only the perennials are cultivated. They have upright stems bearing alternate, simple, entire or toothed, stalkless leaves, and flat, corymb-like cymes of tubular, purple or reddish pink, rarely white flowerheads, becoming rust-coloured with age. Grow in a wild garden or mixed border.

- **HARDINESS** Fully hardy to frost tender.
- **CULTIVATION** Grow in any light, moderately fertile, moist soil in full sun or partial shade. Dead-head regularly.
- **PROPAGATION** Sow seed in containers in a cold frame in spring. Divide in spring or autumn.
- **PESTS AND DISEASES** Slugs may be a problem.

V. noveboracensis. Upright herbaceous perennial with branching stems bearing lance-shaped, entire to toothed leaves, to 20cm (8in) long. From late summer to mid-autumn, bears loose, flat, corymb-like cymes of tubular, red-purple or white florets, in fluffy heads, 1cm (½in) across. ↕ to 2m (6ft), ↔ 60cm (24in). USA (Massachusetts to Mississippi and Georgia). ✻✻✻

VERONICA

Speedwell

SCROPHULARIACEAE

Genus of about 250 species of annuals, perennials (including some marginal aquatics), and mostly deciduous subshrubs, some of them rhizomatous. They occur in swamps and moist meadows and grassland, or in open woodland to dry, sunny meadows, rocky hills, and scree, mainly in Europe. The linear to broadly lance-shaped, or oblong to rounded, entire or toothed, stalkless or short-stalked leaves are usually produced in opposite pairs, although those on the flowering stems can be alternate or whorled. Small, outward-facing flowers, 5–15mm (¼–½in) across, in purple, blue, pink, or white, are borne in long, axillary or terminal racemes or spikes, or singly from the leaf axils, from spring to autumn. The petals form a short tube, with 4 or 5 spreading, often unequally sized lobes; each flower has only 2 functional stamens. Good for a mixed or herbaceous border. Use cushion- or mat-forming veronicas in a rock garden; grow less vigorous species and cultivars in a trough or in an alpine house.

• **HARDINESS** Fully hardy to frost hardy.

• **CULTIVATION** Outdoors, grow alpines and rock garden veronicas in poor to moderately fertile, well-drained soil in full sun. Protect species with felted leaves from winter wet. In an alpine house, grow in a mix of equal parts loam, leaf mould, and grit. Grow border veronicas in loamy, moderately fertile, moist but well-drained soil in full sun or partial shade. Grow *V. beccabunga* in wet soil, or in water to 12cm (5in) deep, in full sun; see also pp.52–53.

• **PROPAGATION** Sow seed in containers in a cold frame in autumn. Divide perennials in autumn or spring; for *V. beccabunga*, divide, or take stem-tip cuttings, in summer. Take softwood cuttings of subshrubs in spring.

• **PESTS AND DISEASES** May suffer from downy mildew, powdery mildew, and leaf spot.

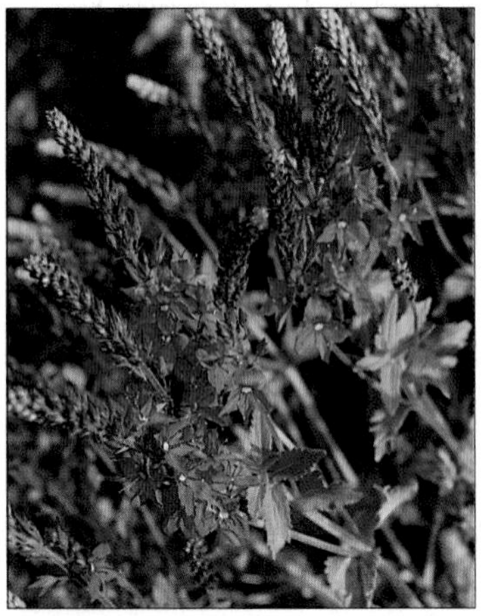

Veronica austriaca subsp. *teucrium* 'Kapitän'

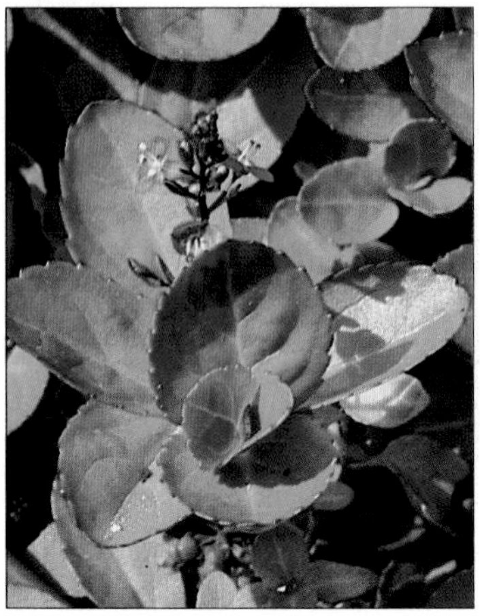

Veronica beccabunga

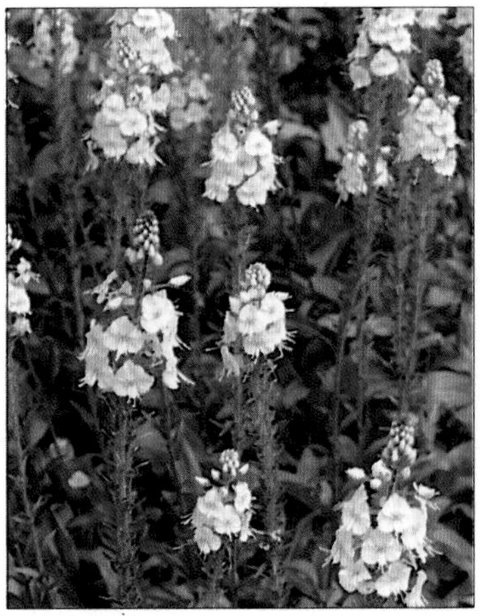

Veronica gentianoides

V. austriaca* subsp. *teucrium, syn. *V. teucrium.* Mat-forming perennial with ovate to oblong, scalloped or deeply toothed, hairy, greyish green leaves, to 7cm (3in) long. Upright stems bear abundant erect, terminal, spike-like racemes, 10–15cm (4–6in) long, of saucer-shaped, deep bright blue flowers over a long period in summer. ↕ to 90cm (36in), ↔ to 60cm (24in). N. temperate Europe. ✲✲✲. **'Kapitän'** ■ has gentian-blue flowers; ↕ to 30cm (12in), ↔ to 40cm (16in). **'Shirley Blue'** 🏆 bears erect racemes, 6–10cm (2½–4in) long, of vivid blue flowers from late spring to midsummer; ↕ to 25cm (10in), ↔ 30cm (12in).

V. beccabunga ■ (Brooklime). Usually evergreen, marginal aquatic perennial with creeping, branching, hollow, fleshy stems, rooting at the nodes, and ovate to rounded, entire or toothed, fleshy mid-green leaves, 1–4cm (½–1½in) long. Saucer-shaped, white-centred blue flowers are borne in loose, erect, axillary racemes, to 12cm (5in) long, from late spring to late summer. ↕ 10cm (4in), ↔ indefinite. Eurasia. ✲✲✲

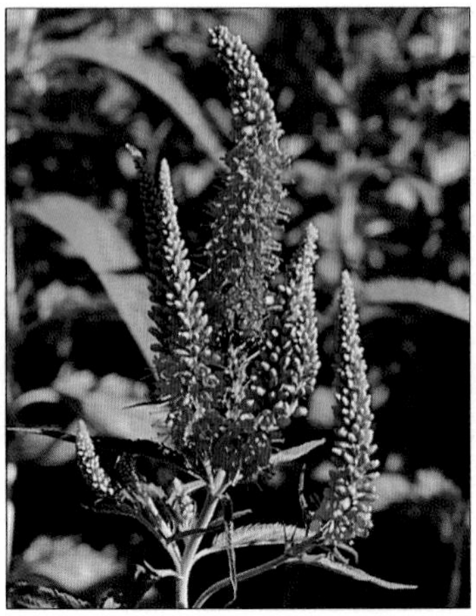

Veronica longifolia

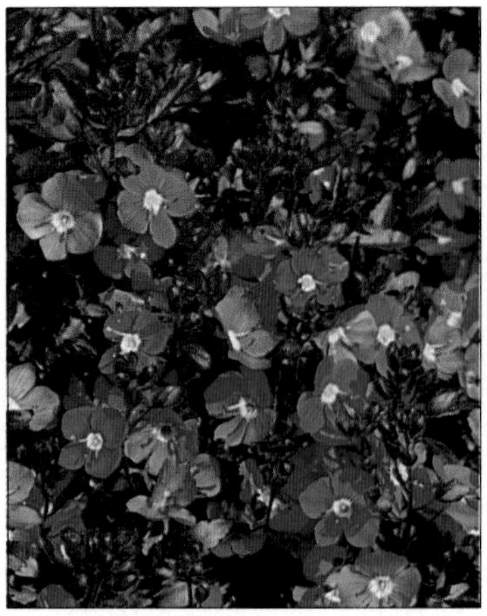

Veronica peduncularis

V. chamaedrys (Germander speedwell). Spreading, slender-stemmed, branching, rhizomatous perennial with stalkless, ovate to lance-shaped, toothed, bright green leaves, to 4cm (1½in) long. From summer to autumn, bears saucer-shaped, white-eyed, bright blue flowers in erect, slender, paired, axillary racemes, 8–15cm (3–6in) long. ↕ 30–50cm (12–20in), ↔ 50–80cm (20–32in). Europe, Caucasus, Russia (Siberia). ✲✲✲

V. cinerea 🏆 Woody-based, white-felted, subshrubby, evergreen perennial with prostrate, branching stems and linear, entire, mid-green, densely silvery white-woolly leaves, to 1.5cm (½in) long. In early summer, bears abundant terminal racemes, 2–3cm (¾–1¼in) long, of saucer-shaped, deep blue or blue-purple flowers. ↕ to15cm (6in), ↔ to 30cm (12in). E. Mediterranean, Turkey. ✲✲✲

V. fruticans, syn. *V. saxatilis* (Rock speedwell). Mat-forming, woody-based, branching perennial or subshrub with obovate to narrowly oblong, entire or slightly scalloped, mid-green leaves, to 2cm (¾in) long. In summer, bears erect, terminal racemes, to 5cm (2in) long, of saucer-shaped, deep blue flowers with dark red eyes. ↕ to 8cm (3in), ↔ to 20cm (8in). N.W. Europe, mountains of Spain to C. Europe, Balkans. ✲✲✲

V. gentianoides ■🏆 Mat-forming perennial with basal rosettes of broadly lance-shaped, entire or slightly scalloped, thick, dark green leaves, to 8cm (3in) long. In early summer, bears shallowly cup-shaped, pale blue, rarely darker blue or white flowers in erect, terminal racemes, 8–25cm (3–10in) long.

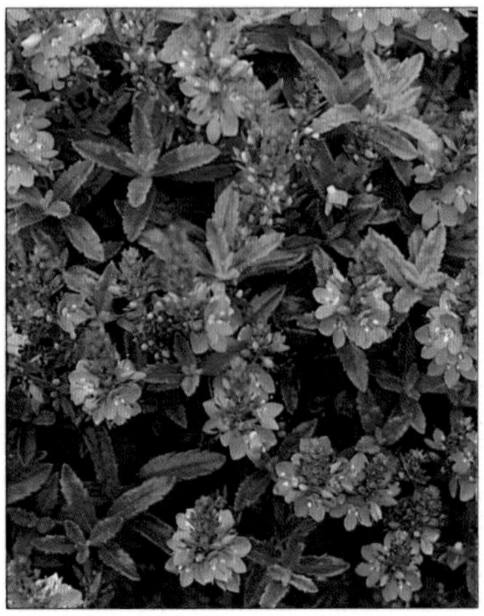

Veronica prostrata

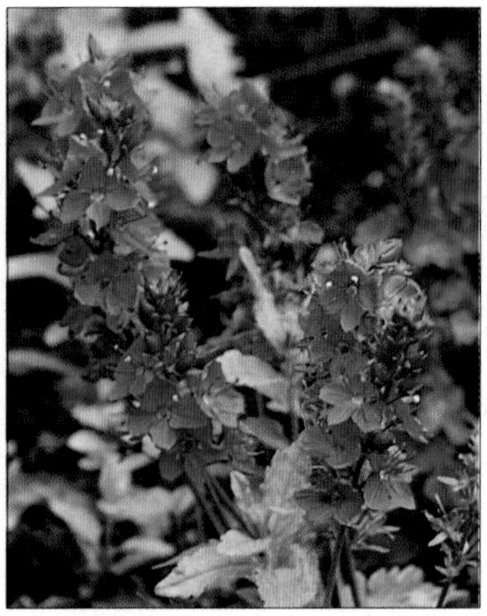

Veronica prostrata 'Trehane'

↕↔ 45cm (18in). Ukraine (Crimea), N. and C. Turkey, Caucasus. ✲✲✲. **'Variegata'** has white-variegated leaves and blue flowers.

V. incana see *V. spicata* subsp. *incana.*

V. kellereri see *V. spicata.*

V. longifolia ■ Variable, upright perennial with lance-shaped to linear, pointed, toothed, mid-green leaves, to 12cm (5in) long, either opposite or in whorls of 3, usually on unbranched stems. In late summer and early autumn, bears tubular, 5-lobed, lilac-blue flowers in dense, erect, terminal racemes, to 25cm (10in) long. ↕ to 1.2m (4ft), ↔ 30cm (12in). N. and C. Europe to Russia (Siberia), E. Asia. ✲✲✲. **'Blauriesin'**, syn. 'Foerster's Blue', is bushy, with bright, deep blue flowers; ↕ to 75cm (30in). **'Foerster's Blue'** see 'Blauriesin'.

V. pectinata. Dense, mat-forming, evergreen, subshrubby perennial with elliptic to oblong, deeply toothed, grey leaves, to 2.5cm (1in) long. Saucer-shaped, white-eyed, deep blue flowers are borne in short, erect, axillary racemes, 6–25cm (2½–10in) long, in summer. ↕ to 8cm (3in), ↔ to 20cm (8in). E. Balkans, Turkey. ✲✲✲. **'Rosea'** has pink flowers.

V. peduncularis ■ Mat-forming perennial with branching rhizomes and prostrate to ascending, freely branched stems bearing ovate to lance-shaped, toothed, glossy, purple-tinged, mid-green leaves, 0.5–2.5cm (¼–1in) long. Produces abundant erect, axillary racemes, 4–8cm (1½–3in) long, of saucer-shaped, deep blue flowers, with small white eyes, over a long period from early spring to summer. ↕ to 10cm

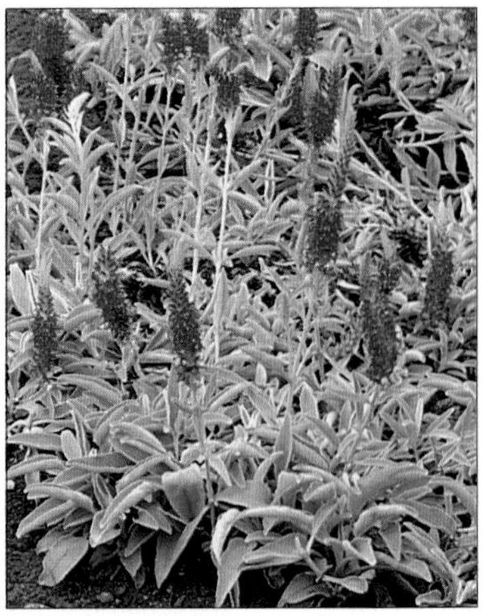

Veronica spicata subsp. *incana*

V

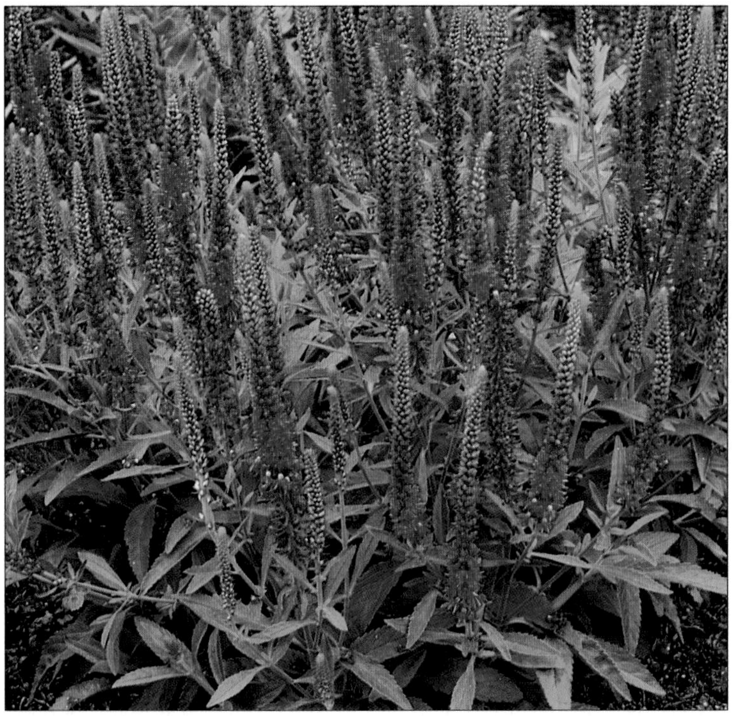

Veronica spicata 'Rotfuchs'

(4in), ↔ 60cm (24in) or more. Turkey, Caucasus, Ukraine. ✽✽✽. **'Georgia Blue'**, syn. 'Oxford Blue', is vigorous, very free-flowering, and easily grown. **'Oxford Blue'** see 'Georgia Blue'.
V. perfoliata see *Parahebe perfoliata.*
V. prostrata ■ 🏆 syn. *V. rupestris* (Prostrate speedwell). Mat-forming perennial with short, branched, decumbent stems bearing linear-oblong to ovate, toothed, bright to mid-green leaves, 0.8–2.5cm (3/8–1in) long. In early summer, produces erect, terminal, spike-like racemes, 2–4cm (3/4–1½in) long, of saucer-shaped, pale to deep blue flowers. ↕ to 15cm (6in), ↔ to 40cm (16in). Europe. ✽✽✽. **'Loddon Blue'** bears bright blue flowers; ↕ to 20cm (8in). **'Mrs. Holt'** produces pale pink flowers. **'Trehane'** ■ has yellow-green or golden leaves and deep blue flowers.
V. rupestris see *V. prostrata.*
V. saxatilis see *V. fruticans.*
V. spicata, syn. *V. kellereri.* Mat-forming perennial with decumbent, simple, rooting stems, and ascending to erect, flowering stems bearing oblong-lance-shaped to linear, toothed, hairy leaves, to 8cm (3in) long. Star-shaped, bright blue flowers, with long purple stamens, open in erect, dense, pyramidal, terminal racemes, to 30cm (12in) long, from early to late summer. ↕ 30–60cm (12–24in), ↔ 45cm (18in). Europe to Turkey, C. and E. Asia. ✽✽✽. **'Barcarolle'** freely bears pink flowers; ↕ 30cm (12in). **'Heidekind'** has silver-grey leaves and short spikes of raspberry-pink flowers; ↕ 30cm (12in). **'Icicle'**, syn. 'White Icicle', has white flowers; ↕ 60cm (24in). **subsp. *incana*** ■ syn. *V. incana* (Silver speedwell), is entirely silver-hairy, and has purple-blue flowers; ↕↔ 30cm (12in); Russia. **subsp. *incana* 'Saraband'**, syn. *V. incana* 'Saraband', has violet-blue flowers above densely hairy, silver-grey foliage. **subsp. *incana* 'Wendy'** 🏆 syn. *V. incana* 'Wendy', has a looser habit, with grey leaves and bright blue flowers; ↕ 45cm (18in). **'Red Fox'** see 'Rotfuchs'. **'Romiley Purple'** is bushy, with lateral racemes of dark violet flowers; ↕ 45cm (18in). **'Rotfuchs'** ■ syn. 'Red Fox', has very deep pink flowers; ↕↔ 30cm (12in). **'White Icicle'** see 'Icicle'.
V. teucrium see *V. austriaca* subsp. *teucrium.*
V. virginica see *Veronicastrum virginicum.*

VERONICASTRUM

SCROPHULARIACEAE

Genus of 2 species of erect perennials, one from Siberia, one from North America, occurring in open woodland, scrub, prairies, meadows, and grassy mountain sites. Imposing in stature, they have whorls of 3–7 more or less horizontal, simple, toothed leaves. They bear veronica-like racemes of salverform, white to pale pink or bluish purple flowers, terminally and from the upper leaf axils; each flower has a long, slender tube and 4 or 5 short lobes. Use to add height to a mixed summer border.
• **HARDINESS** Fully hardy.
• **CULTIVATION** Grow in moderately fertile, humus-rich, moist soil in full sun or partial shade.

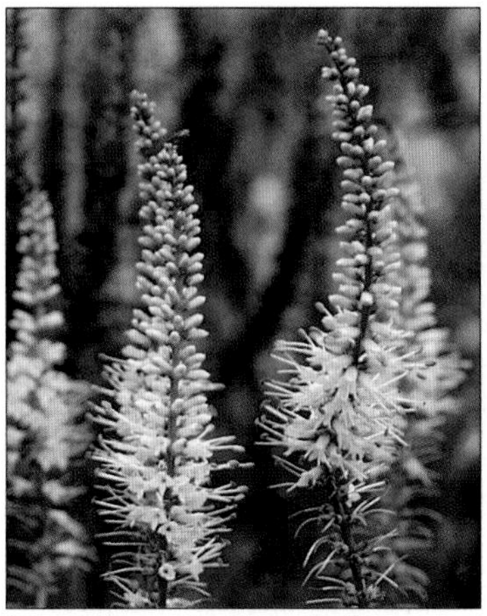

Veronicastrum virginicum f. *album*

• **PROPAGATION** Sow seed in containers in a cold frame in autumn. Divide in spring.
• **PESTS AND DISEASES** Prone to downy mildew, powdery mildew, and leaf spot.

V. virginicum, syn. *Veronica virginica* (Culver's root). Erect, usually hairless perennial with unbranched stems bearing lance-shaped to inversely lance-shaped, pointed, toothed, dark green leaves, to 15cm (6in) long, in whorls of 3–7. From midsummer to early autumn, bears tubular, white to pink or bluish purple flowers, 7mm (¼in) long, with protruding stamens, in slender, dense, terminal and axillary racemes. ↕ to 2m (6ft), ↔ 45cm (18in). North America (Ontario to Texas). ✽✽✽. **f. *album*** ■ has white flowers.

VERTICORDIA

MYRTACEAE

Genus of about 50 species of heath-like, evergreen shrubs from usually sandy or gravel heathland in Australia. They are grown for their leafy racemes or corymbs of showy flowers, produced terminally or from the upper leaf axils; each flower has 5 feathery, often coloured sepals and 5 entire or toothed petals. The leathery leaves are small, simple, and usually borne in opposite pairs. Where winter temperatures fall below 7°C (45°F), grow in a temperate greenhouse. In warmer, dry climates, use in a border.
• **HARDINESS** Frost tender.
• **CULTIVATION** Under glass, grow in lime-free (ericaceous) potting compost with added sharp sand, in full light. In growth, water moderately and apply a low-phosphate, low-nitrogen fertilizer monthly. Water sparingly in winter. Outdoors, grow in moderately fertile, neutral to acid, sharply drained soil in full sun. Pruning group 8 or 9; may need restrictive pruning under glass.
• **PROPAGATION** Sow seed at 13–18°C (55–64°F) in spring. Take semi-ripe cuttings in summer.
• **PESTS AND DISEASES** Red spider mites may be a problem under glass.

V. grandis (Scarlet featherflower). Usually erect, sparsely branched, open shrub with crowded, rounded, semi-glossy, greyish to deep green leaves, 0.8–1.5cm (3/8–½in) long. From spring to summer, bears deep bright scarlet to pink flowers, 2–2.5cm (3/4–1in) across, in dense corymbs, to 12cm (5in) across, either terminally or from the upper leaf axils. ↕↔ 1–2m (3–6ft). W. Australia. ❀ (min. 7°C/45°F)
V. plumosa ■ (Featherflower). Erect, bushy shrub with crowded, linear, cylindrical, grey-green leaves, 1cm (½in) long. Terminal corymbs, 3cm (1¼in) across, of many pink or white flowers, to 9mm (3/8in) wide, are borne from spring to autumn. ↕↔ to 90cm (36in). Granite outcrops in S.W. Australia. ❀ (min. 7°C/45°F)

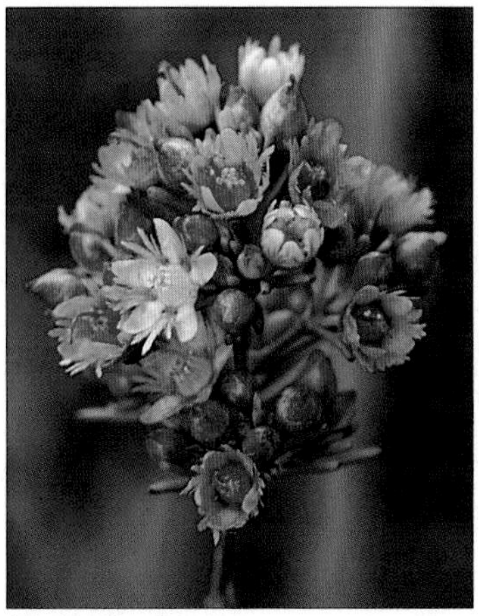

Verticordia plumosa

VESTIA

SOLANACEAE

Genus of one species of evergreen shrub found in woodland in Chile, cultivated for its attractive but malodorous foliage and flowers. The leaves are alternate, obovate to elliptic, and glossy, dark green. The pendent, pale yellow flowers are borne singly or in clusters. Best grown in a sheltered border or against a sunny wall in frost-prone areas. Where temperatures fall much below -5°C (23°F), grow in a cool greenhouse.
• **HARDINESS** Frost hardy.
• **CULTIVATION** Under glass, grow in loam-based potting compost (JI No.2) in full light, shaded from hot sun. In growth, water moderately and apply a balanced liquid fertilizer monthly. Water sparingly in winter. Outdoors, grow in any well-drained soil in full sun. In frost-prone areas, shelter from cold, drying winds in winter. Pruning group 8.
• **PROPAGATION** Sow seed in containers in a cold frame in autumn, or take semi-ripe cuttings in summer.
• **PESTS AND DISEASES** Trouble free.

V. foetida ■ 🏆 syn. *V. lycioides.* Erect, evergreen shrub with glossy, dark green leaves, to 5cm (2in) long, unpleasantly scented when crushed. Pendent, tubular, pale yellow flowers, to 3cm (1¼in) long, with protruding stamens, are produced singly or in clusters from the leaf axils from mid-spring to midsummer. ↕ 2m (6ft), ↔ 1.5m (5ft). Chile. ✽✽
V. lycioides see *V. foetida.*

▷**Vetch** see *Hippocrepis*
Bitter see *Lathyrus linifolius* var. *montanus*
Horseshoe see *Hippocrepis*
Kidney see *Anthyllis vulneraria*
▷**Vetchling,**
Common see *Lathyrus pratensis*
Meadow see *Lathyrus pratensis*
Spring see *Lathyrus vernus*

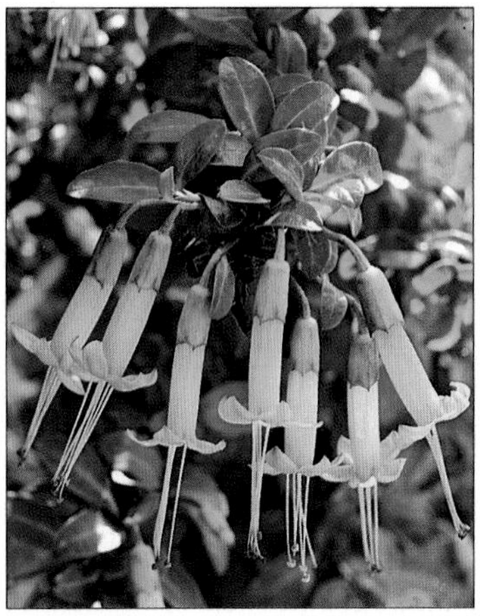

Vestia foetida

VIBURNUM

VIBURNUM

CAPRIFOLIACEAE

Genus of 150 or more species of evergreen, semi-evergreen, and deciduous shrubs, sometimes trees, from thickets and woodland, mainly in N. temperate regions, but extending to S.E. Asia and South America. They are cultivated for their foliage, flowers, and fruits. The mostly lance-shaped to rounded, entire or toothed, sometimes lobed leaves are arranged in opposite pairs, occasionally in whorls of 3; they are often rough and prominently veined, and, in most deciduous species, colour attractively in autumn. The sometimes fragrant, white or cream, pink-flushed, or wholly pink flowers are salverform to tubular, or tubular-trumpet-shaped, each with 5 usually spreading lobes. They are borne in terminal or axillary panicles, clusters, corymbs, or cymes, which are often spherical or domed. Some species have flowers in flattened heads, similar to those of "lacecap" hydrangeas, in which the small, fertile central flowers are surrounded by larger, flat or saucer-shaped, sterile ray-florets. The ornamental fruits are usually spherical or ovoid, and may be red, blue, or black.

Viburnums are suitable for a shrub border or woodland garden. Grow *V. macrocephalum* against a wall. Many show self-incompatibility; fruiting is often best if several seedlings of the same species are planted together so that cross-pollination can occur. The fruits of viburnums may cause mild stomach upset if ingested.

- **HARDINESS** Fully hardy to frost hardy.
- **CULTIVATION** Grow in any moderately fertile, moist but well-drained soil in full sun or partial shade. *V. lantanoides* needs lime-free soil. In frost-prone regions, shelter evergreen viburnums from cold, drying winds. Pruning group 1 for evergreens; group 8 for deciduous viburnums. *V. tinus* and most deciduous viburnums tolerate hard pruning.
- **PROPAGATION** Sow seed in containers in a cold frame, or in a seed bed, in autumn. Take greenwood cuttings of deciduous viburnums, and semi-ripe cuttings of evergreens, in summer.
- **PESTS AND DISEASES** Aphids and viburnum beetles may be a problem, particularly on *V. lantana*, *V. opulus*, and *V. tinus*. *V. tinus* is susceptible to whiteflies. All are prone to honey fungus and leaf spot.

V. acerifolium ▣ (Dockmackie, Possum-haw). Upright, deciduous shrub with maple-like, 3-lobed, dark green leaves, to 12cm (5in) long, turning orange, red, and purple in autumn. In early summer, bears small, tubular white flowers, 5mm (¼in) across, in long-stalked cymes, 8cm (3in) across, at the shoot-tips. Ovoid red fruit, 8mm (⅜in) long, ripen to purple-black. ↕ 1–2m (3–6ft), ↔ 1.2m (4ft). E. North America. ***

V. alnifolium see *V. lantanoides.*

V. betulifolium. Upright, deciduous shrub with arching branches and ovate, tapered, toothed, glossy, dark green leaves, to 10cm (4in) long. In early summer, bears small, salverform white flowers, 5mm (¼in) across, in domed terminal corymbs, to 10cm (4in) across; they are followed by pendent clusters of spherical, bright red fruit, 6mm (¼in) across. ↕↔ 3m (10ft). W. and C. China. ***

V. x bodnantense (*V. farreri* x *V. grandiflorum*). Upright, deciduous shrub with ovate to oblong, toothed, dark green leaves, to 10cm (4in) long, bronze when young. Heavily scented, tubular, rich rose-red to white-pink flowers, to 1cm (½in) across, are borne in dense, terminal and axillary clusters, to 7cm (3in) across, on bare wood, over a long period from late autumn to spring. Virtually sterile, producing a few small, spherical, blue-black or purple fruit, 3–6mm (⅛–¼in) across. ↕ 3m (10ft), ↔ 2m (6ft). Garden origin. ***. Mainly grown as the following cultivars. **'Charles Lamont'** ♀ bears bright pink flowers. **'Dawn'** ▣ ♀ has dark pink flowers, ageing to white, strongly flushed pink. **'Deben'** ♀ bears white flowers, faintly pink-flushed in winter.

V. x burkwoodii (*V. carlesii* x *V. utile*). Open, rounded, bushy, evergreen shrub producing ovate, sparsely toothed, glossy, dark green leaves, to 10cm (4in) long. Tubular, fragrant white flowers, 1cm (½in) across, in domed, terminal corymbs, to 9cm (3½in) across, open from pink buds in mid- and late spring; they are followed by flattened, ellipsoid red fruit, 1cm (½in) long, ripening to black in autumn. ↕↔ 2.5m (8ft). Garden origin. ***. **'Anne Russell'** ▣ ♀ is compact and deciduous, with fragrant flowers; ↕ 2m (6ft), ↔ 1.5m (5ft). **'Chenaultii'** is compact, with pale pink flowers and leaves that turn bronze in autumn; ↕↔ 1.5m (5ft). **'Fulbrook'** ♀ syn. *V.* 'Fulbrook', has very fragrant white flowers. **'Park Farm Hybrid'** ♀ produces dark pink flowers, fading to white, in broad corymbs, to 12cm (5in) across; some leaves turn orange and red in autumn.

V. x carlcephalum ▣ ♀ (*V. carlesii* x *V. macrocephalum*). Rounded, bushy, deciduous shrub with broadly heart-shaped, irregularly toothed, dark green leaves, 12cm (5in) long, turning red in autumn. Tubular-trumpet-shaped, fragrant white flowers, 1.5cm (½in) across, in domed, terminal corymbs, 15cm (6in) across, open from pink buds in late spring. ↕↔ 3m (10ft). Garden origin. ***

V. carlesii ▣ Dense, bushy, deciduous shrub with ovate, irregularly toothed, dark green leaves, to 10cm (4in) long, often turning red in autumn. In mid- and late spring, pink buds open to tubular, very fragrant, white or pink-flushed white flowers, 1cm (½in) across, produced in domed, terminal corymbs, to 8cm (3in) across; they are followed by ellipsoid red fruit, 6mm (¼in) long, ripening to black. ↕↔ 2m (6ft). Korea, Japan (Tsushima Island). ***. **'Aurora'** ♀ has red buds, opening to pink flowers. **'Diana'** has bronze young leaves, and red buds opening to purple-pink flowers that fade to white.

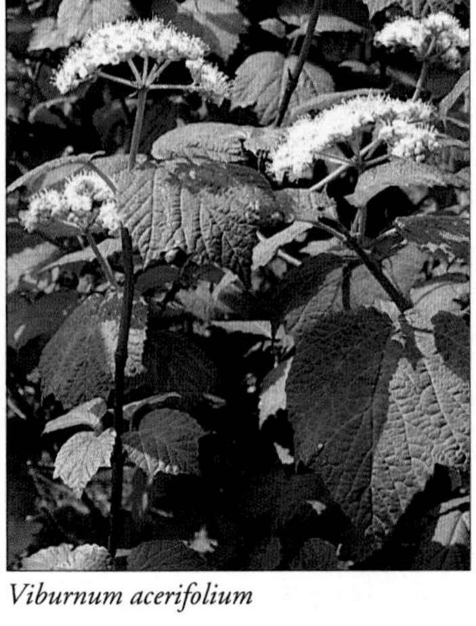

Viburnum acerifolium

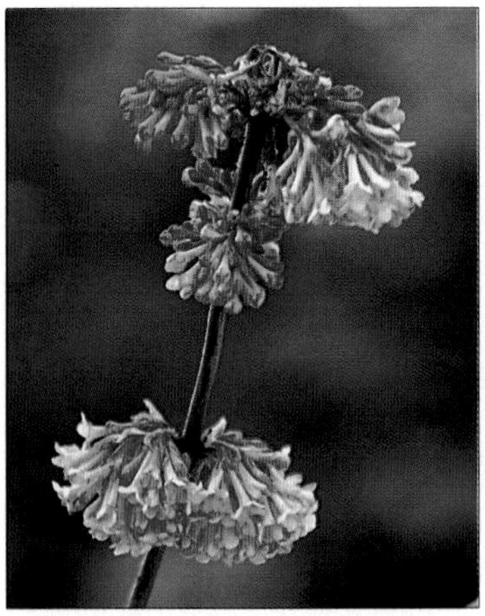

Viburnum x *bodnantense* 'Dawn'

V. 'Chesapeake' ▣ Compact, dense mound-forming, semi-evergreen shrub with ovate, slightly wavy-margined, leathery, glossy, dark green leaves, to 10cm (4in) long. Pink buds open to salverform, fragrant white flowers, 1cm (½in) across, borne in domed, terminal corymbs, 9cm (3½in) across, in mid- and late spring. It is virtually sterile, bearing no fruit. ↕ 2m (6ft), ↔ 3m (10ft). ***

V. cinnamomifolium ♀ ◐ Rounded, open, evergreen shrub, sometimes a small tree, with elliptic, tapered, sparsely toothed, conspicuously 3-veined, dark green leaves, dark green above, paler beneath, to 15cm (6in) long. In early summer, produces tiny, tubular white flowers, 4mm (⅛in) across, in loose, terminal cymes, 12–17cm (5–7in) across. Flowers are followed by ovoid, glossy, blue-black fruit, 4mm (⅛in) long. ↕↔ 5m (15ft), to 6m (20ft) high as a tree. W. China. **

V. davidii ▣ ♀ Dome-shaped, compact, evergreen shrub with oval, indistinctly toothed, 3-veined, dark green leaves, to 15cm (6in) long. Tiny, tubular white flowers, 4mm (⅛in) across, are borne in flattened, terminal cymes, 7cm (3in) across, in late spring; they are followed by ovoid, metallic-blue fruit, 6mm (¼in) long. Both male and female plants are needed to produce fruit. ↕↔ 1–1.5m (3–5ft). W. China. ***

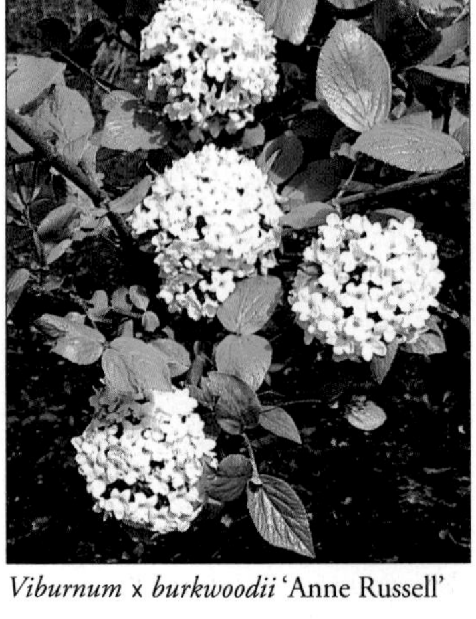

Viburnum x *burkwoodii* 'Anne Russell'

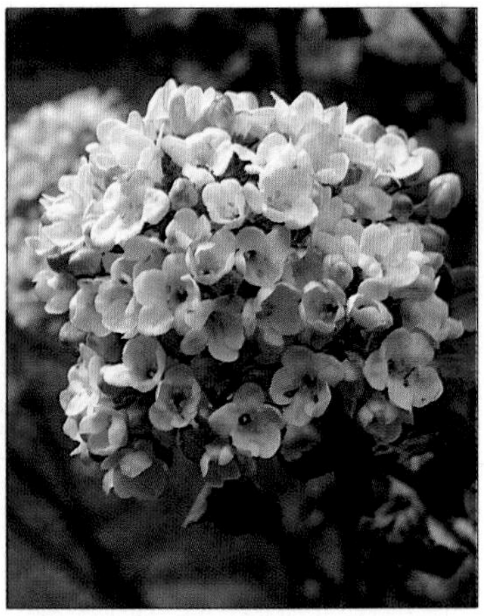

Viburnum x *carlcephalum*

V. dentatum ▣ (Southern arrow-wood). Upright, deciduous shrub with arching branches and ovate to rounded, coarsely toothed, dark green leaves, to 11cm (4½in) long, turning yellow or red in autumn. Tiny, tubular white flowers, 4mm (⅛in) across, are borne in flattened, terminal corymbs, 10cm (4in) across, in late spring and early summer; they are followed by ovoid, blue-black fruit, 8mm (⅜in) long. ↕↔ 3m (10ft). E. North America. ***

V. dilatatum. Upright, deciduous shrub producing broadly ovate to rounded or obovate, coarsely toothed, dark green leaves, to 12cm (5in) long, turning bronze to red in autumn. Small, salverform white flowers, 5mm (¼in) across, are borne in domed, terminal corymbs, to 12cm (5in) across, in late spring and early summer. The flowers are followed by ovoid, bright red fruit, 8mm (⅜in) long. ↕ 3m (10ft), ↔ 2m (6ft). China, Japan. ***. **'Catskill'** ▣ is compact, with leaves turning yellow, orange, and red in autumn, and bears dark red fruit; ↕ 1.5m (5ft), ↔ 2.5m (8ft). **'Erie'** is mound-forming, bearing large cymes, to 15cm (6in) across, and a profusion of fruit, turning pink in winter; ↕ 2m (6ft), ↔ 3m (10ft). **'Xanthocarpum'** bears yellow fruit.

V. 'Eskimo'. Mound-forming, compact, semi-evergreen shrub producing ovate, leathery, glossy, dark green leaves, to

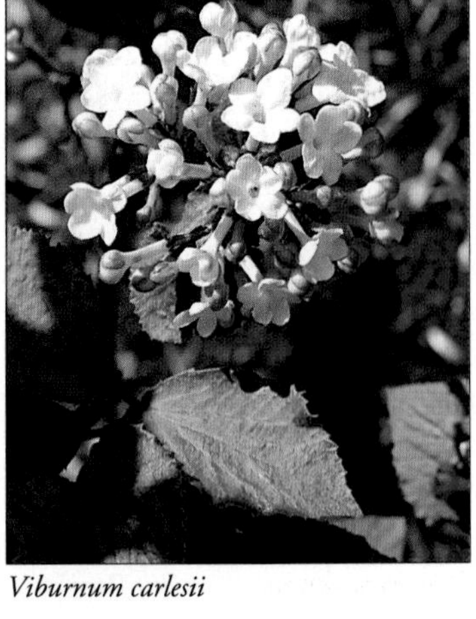

Viburnum carlesii

V

VIBURNUM

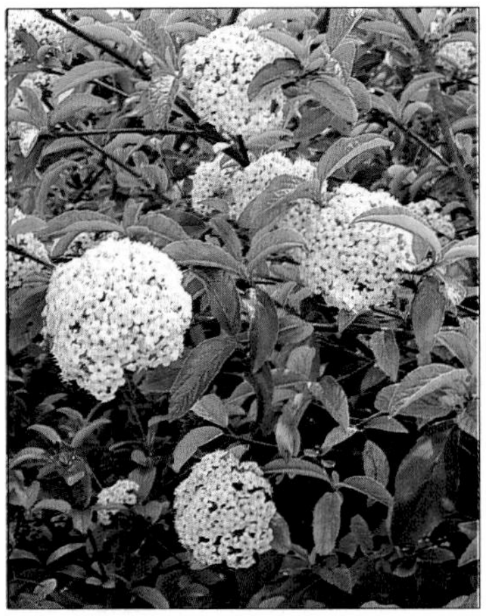

Viburnum 'Chesapeake'

10cm (4in) long. In mid- and late spring, pink-tinged cream buds open to tubular, pure white flowers, 1cm (½in) across, borne in dense, terminal, almost spherical corymbs, 10cm (4in) across. ↕↔ 1.5m (5ft). ❄❄❄

V. farreri ▣ 🏆 syn. *V. fragrans.* Erect, deciduous shrub with oval, toothed, dark green leaves, to 10cm (4in) long, bronze when young, turning red-purple in autumn. Tubular, fragrant, white or pink-tinged white flowers, 1cm (½in) long, are borne in dense, terminal and lateral clusters, to 5cm (2in) across, in late autumn and, in mild weather, in winter and early spring on bare stems; they are followed by spherical, bright red fruit, 5mm (¼in) long. ↕ 3m (10ft), ↔ 2.5m (8ft). N. China. ❄❄❄. **'Album'** see 'Candidissimum'. **'Candidissimum'**, syn. 'Album', has leaves that are pale green when young, and bears white flowers followed by pale yellow fruit. **'Nanum'** forms a dense mound, but is not free-flowering; ↕ 75cm (30in), ↔ 1m (3ft).

V. foetens. Upright, deciduous shrub with oblong, dark green leaves, to 10cm (4in) long. From late autumn to early spring, produces tubular, fragrant, white or pink-tinged white flowers, 5cm (2in) long, in flattened, terminal clusters, to 5cm (2in) across, on bare stems; they are followed by ovoid red fruit, to 1cm (½in) long, ripening to black. ↕↔ 2m (6ft). Himalayas. ❄❄❄

V. fragrans see *V. farreri.*

***V.* 'Fulbrook'** see *V.* x *burkwoodii* 'Fulbrook'.

***V.* x *globosum* 'Jermyns Globe'** ▣ Dense, rounded, evergreen shrub with

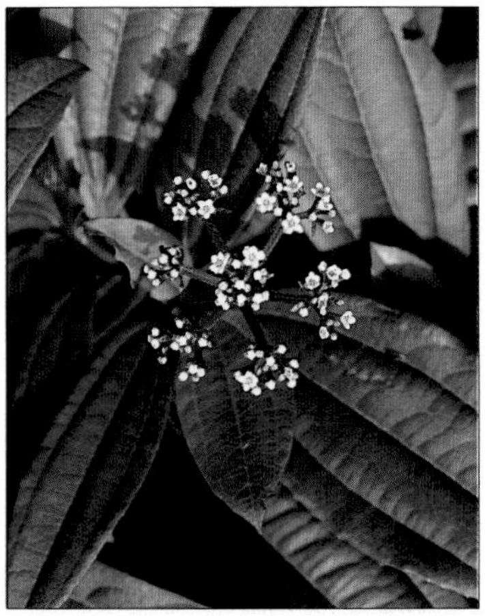

Viburnum davidii

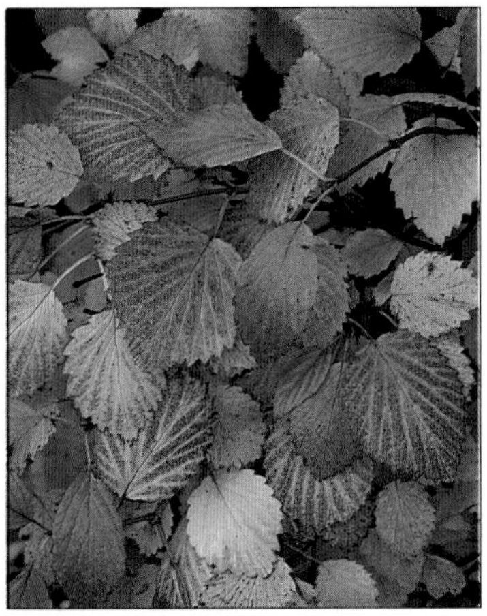

Viburnum dentatum

narrowly elliptic, tapered, dark green leaves, to 9cm (4½in) long, 3-veined at the bases. Masses of small, tubular white flowers, to 12mm (½in) across, are borne in flattened, terminal corymbs, 6cm (2½in) across, in late spring; they are followed by ovoid, metallic-blue fruit, 6mm (¼in) long. ↕ 2.5m (8ft), ↔ 3m (10ft). ❄❄❄

V. grandiflorum. Open, upright, deciduous shrub with stout shoots and elliptic, finely and irregularly toothed, dark green leaves, to 10cm (4in) long, turning dark purple in autumn. From winter to early spring, tubular, fragrant, pink-flushed white flowers, to 2cm (¾in) across, are produced on bare stems in flattened, terminal clusters, to 8cm (3in) across; they are followed by ovoid, black-purple fruit, to 2cm (¾in) long. ↕↔ 2m (6ft). Himalayas, W. China. ❄❄❄. **'Snow White'** has white flowers, flushed pink on the backs of the lobes, opening from dark pink buds.

V. harryanum. Upright, bushy, evergreen shrub with rounded, dark green leaves, to 2.5cm (1in) long, often in whorls of 3. Tiny, tubular white flowers, 3mm (⅛in) across, are produced in flattened, terminal, umbel-like cymes, 4cm (1½in) across, in late spring, followed by ovoid, glossy black fruit, 4mm (⅛in) long. ↕ 3m (10ft), ↔ 2.5m (8ft). W. China. ❄❄❄

V. japonicum. Rounded, evergreen shrub with stout shoots and ovate to rounded, leathery, sparsely toothed, glossy, dark green leaves, to 15cm (6in) long. Small, tubular, fragrant white flowers, 1cm (½in) across, in spherical cymes, to 10cm (4in) across, are borne

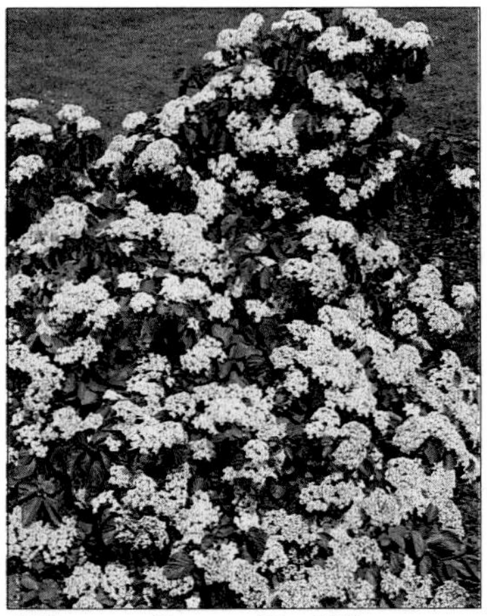

Viburnum dilatatum 'Catskill'

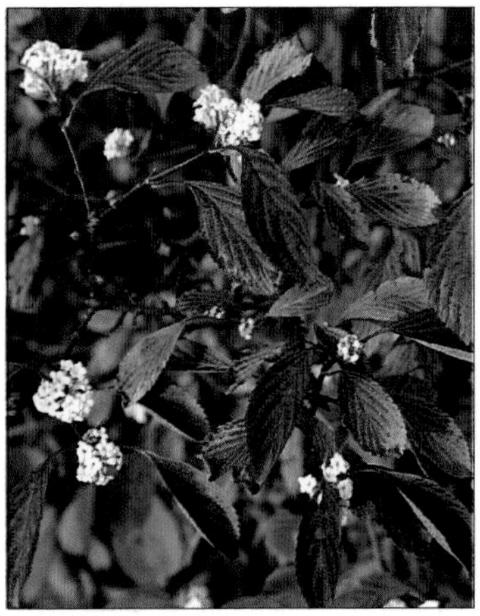

Viburnum farreri

in early summer, followed by ovoid, bright red fruit, 8mm (⅜in) long, which last into winter. ↕ 2m (6ft), ↔ 2.5m (8ft). Japan. ❄❄❄

V.* x *juddii ▣ 🏆 (*V. bitchiuense* x *V. carlesii*). Rounded, bushy, deciduous shrub with oval, dark green leaves, to 6cm (2½in) long, sometimes turning red in autumn. Small, salverform, fragrant, pink-tinged white flowers, 6mm (¼in) across, in almost spherical corymbs, to 9cm (3½in) across, open from pink buds in mid- and late spring. ↕ 1.2m (4ft), ↔ 1.5m (5ft). Garden origin. ❄❄❄

V. lantana (Wayfaring tree). Vigorous, upright, deciduous shrub with broadly ovate, finely toothed, grey-green leaves, to 12cm (5in) long, often turning red in autumn. Small, tubular white flowers,

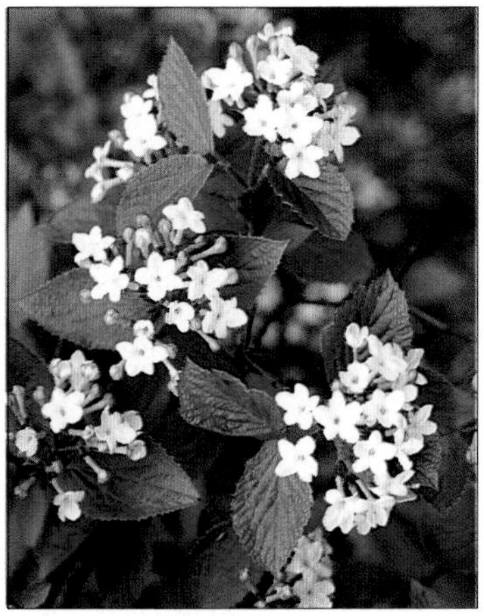

Viburnum x *juddii*

6mm (¼in) across, in loosely domed cymes, to 10cm (4in) across, are borne in late spring and early summer; they are followed by ovoid-oblong red fruit, 8mm (⅜in) long, ripening to black. ↕ 5m (15ft), ↔ 4m (12ft). Europe, N. Africa, S.W. Asia. ❄❄❄. **'Mohican'** is compact, with dark green foliage and orange-red fruit; ↕↔ 2.5m (8ft)

V. lantanoides, syn. *V. alnifolium* (Hobble bush). Spreading, deciduous shrub, the outer branches prostrate and rooting in the soil. Broadly ovate to rounded, irregularly toothed, dark green leaves, to 20cm (8in) long, turn yellow to red or purple in autumn. In late spring and early summer, bears lacecap-like, terminal cymes, to 12cm (5in) wide, of tubular, white, fertile central flowers, 3–4mm (⅛in) across, surrounded by

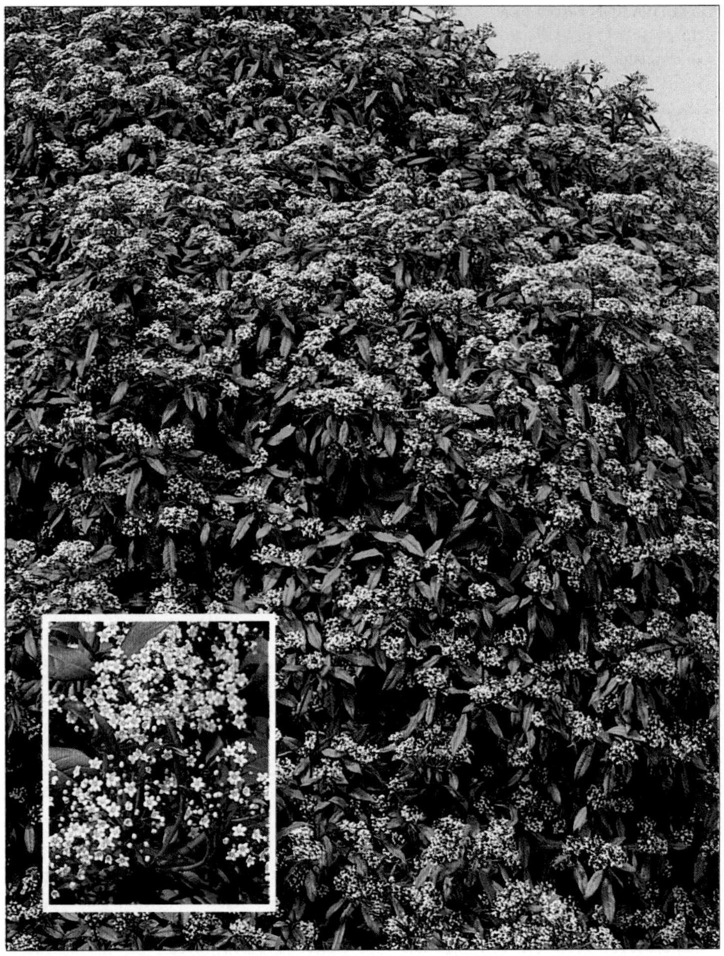

Viburnum x *globosum* 'Jermyns Globe' (inset: flower detail)

V

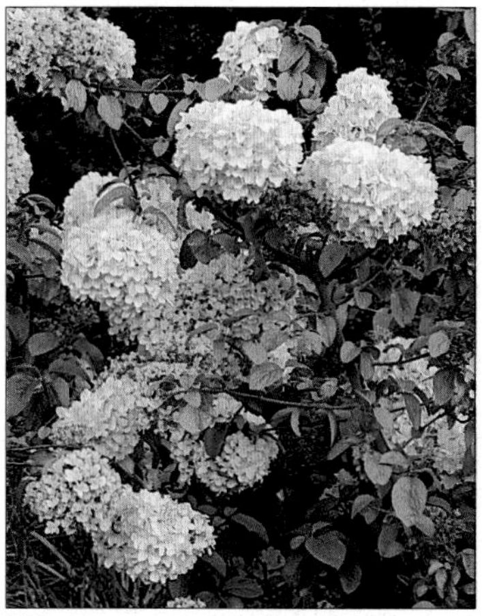

Viburnum macrocephalum

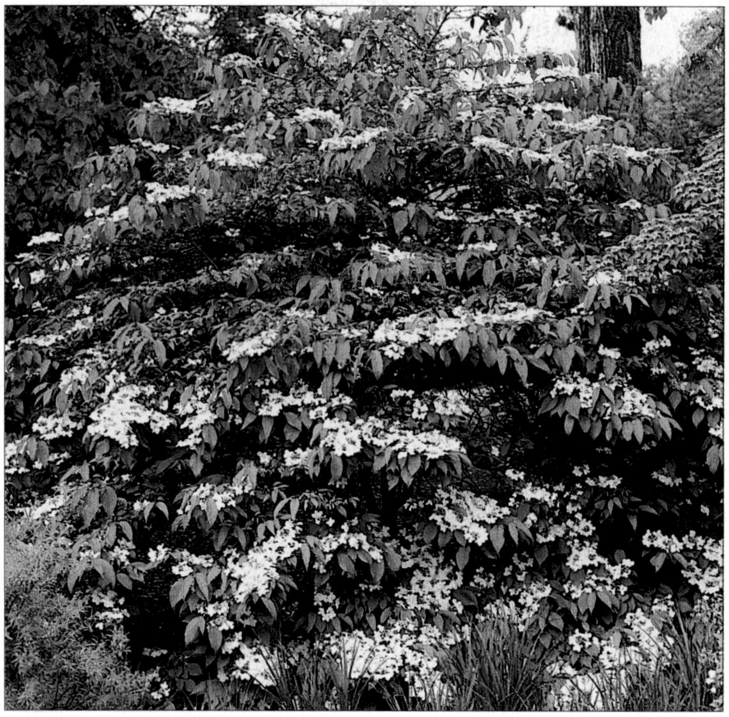

Viburnum plicatum 'Mariesii'

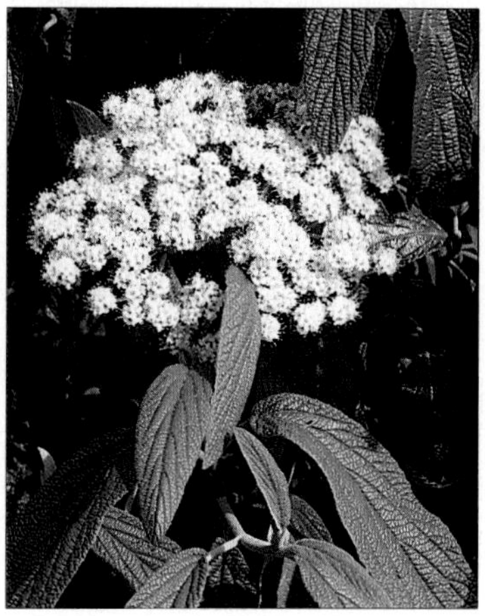

Viburnum rhytidophyllum

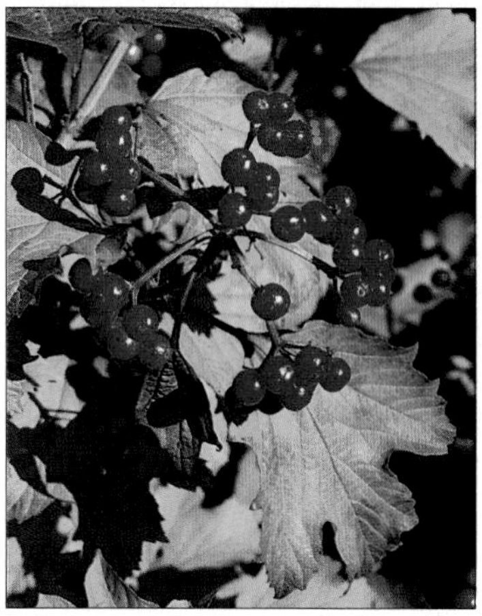

Viburnum opulus 'Compactum'

saucer-shaped, white, sterile ray-florets, to 2.5cm (1in) across; they are followed by ovoid red fruit, 8mm (3/8in) long, ripening to black-purple. Prefers partial shade. ↕ 2.5m (8ft), ↔ 4m (12ft). E. North America. ❄❄❄

V. lentago ◊ (Sheepberry). Vigorous, upright, deciduous shrub or small tree, producing oval, finely toothed, glossy, dark green leaves, to 10cm (4in) long, turning red and purple in autumn. Small, tubular, fragrant, creamy white flowers, to 5mm (1/4in) across, are borne in flattened, terminal cymes, to 11cm (4½in) across, in late spring and early summer, followed by ovoid, blue-black fruit, 1cm (½in) long. ↕ 4m (12ft), ↔ 3m (10ft). E. North America. ❄❄❄

V. macrocephalum ■ (Snowball bush). Rounded shrub, sometimes tree-like, semi-evergreen or evergreen in mild climates, deciduous where winters are severe, with ovate to elliptic, toothed, dark green leaves, to 10cm (4in) long. In late spring, salverform, sterile white flowers, 3cm (1¼in) across, are borne in dense, terminal cymes, to 15cm (6in) across. Does not bear fruit. ↕↔ 5m (15ft). Garden origin. ❄❄

V. mariesii see *V. plicatum* 'Mariesii'.

V. odoratissimum. Vigorous, bushy, evergreen shrub with oval, glossy, dark green leaves, to 20cm (8in) long. Small, tubular, fragrant white flowers, 6mm (1/4in) across, are produced in broadly conical panicles, 8–10cm (3–4in) long, in late spring, followed by ovoid red fruit, 1cm (½in) long, ripening to black. ↕↔ 5m (15ft). India, China, Burma, Philippines, Japan. ❄❄

V. opulus (Guelder rose). Vigorous, bushy, deciduous shrub with maple-like, usually 3-lobed, dark green leaves, to 10cm (4in) long, turning red in autumn. In late spring and early summer, bears flat, lacecap-like, terminal cymes, to 8cm (3in) across, composed of tubular, white, fertile central flowers, 2cm (3/4in) across, surrounded by showy, flat, white, sterile ray-florets, to 2cm (3/4in) across; they are followed by spherical, fleshy, bright red fruit, 8mm (3/8in) across. ↕ 5m (15ft), ↔ 4m (12ft). Europe, N. Africa, C. Asia. ❄❄❄. **var. *americanum*** see *V. trilobum*. **'Compactum'** ■🏆 is slow-growing and very dense; ↕↔ 1.5m (5ft). **'Roseum'** 🏆 syn. 'Sterile' (Snowball tree), has a rounded habit, with leaves that become purple-tinted in autumn; it bears large, white or green-tinted white, sterile flowers, 1cm (½in) long, sometimes turning pink, in spherical cymes, 5–6cm (2–2½in) across; ↕↔ to 4m (12ft). **'Sterile'** see 'Roseum'. **'Xanthocarpum'** ■🏆 produces bright yellow fruit.

V. plicatum (Japanese snowball bush). Spreading, bushy, deciduous shrub with heart-shaped, tapered, toothed, deeply veined, dark green leaves, to 10cm (4in) long, turning red-purple in autumn. In late spring, bears saucer-shaped, sterile white flowers, to 3cm (1¼in) across, in dense, spherical, terminal cymes, 8cm (3in) across. Does not produce fruit. ↕ 3m (10ft), ↔ 4m (12ft). Garden origin. ❄❄❄. **'Grandiflorum'** 🏆 has larger flowerheads, to 10cm (4in) across. The following cultivars have fertile central flowers and sterile outer florets; they are sometimes grouped under f. *tomentosum*. **'Lanarth'** has large, sterile florets, to 5cm (2in) or more across, and bears few fruit. **'Mariesii'** ■🏆 syn. *V. mariesii*, has distinctly layered, tiered branches, and produces few fruit. **'Nanum Semperflorens'**, syn. 'Nanum', 'Watanabei', *V. semperflorens, V. watanabei*, is low-growing and compact, blooming over a long period from late spring to autumn; ↕ 2m (6ft), ↔ 1.5m (5ft). **'Pink Beauty'** ■🏆 has white sterile florets maturing to pink. **'Rowallane'** 🏆 is compact, with leaves turning dark red-purple in autumn, and bears abundant red fruit; ↕↔ 2m (6ft). **f. *tomentosum***, syn. *V. tomentosum*, has flattened, lacecap-like cymes, to 10cm (4in) across, with tiny, fertile central flowers and larger, sterile outer florets, to 3cm (1¼in) across. Ovoid red fruit, 8mm (3/8in) long, ripen to black; China, Japan. **'Watanabei'** see 'Nanum Semperflorens'.

V. x pragense see *V.* 'Pragense'.

V. 'Pragense' ■🏆 syn. *V. x pragense*. Rounded, bushy, evergreen shrub with elliptic, deeply veined, wrinkled, wavy-margined, glossy, dark green leaves, to 10cm (4in) long. Tubular white flowers, 5–8mm (1/4–3/8in) across, opening from pink buds, are produced in domed, terminal, umbel-like cymes, to 10cm (4in) across, in late spring. ↕↔ 3m (10ft). ❄❄❄

V. propinquum. Compact, bushy, evergreen shrub with ovate-lance-shaped to elliptic, sparsely toothed, 3-veined, glossy, dark green leaves, to 9cm (3½in) long. Tiny, tubular, greenish white flowers, 4mm (1/8in) across, in flattened,

V

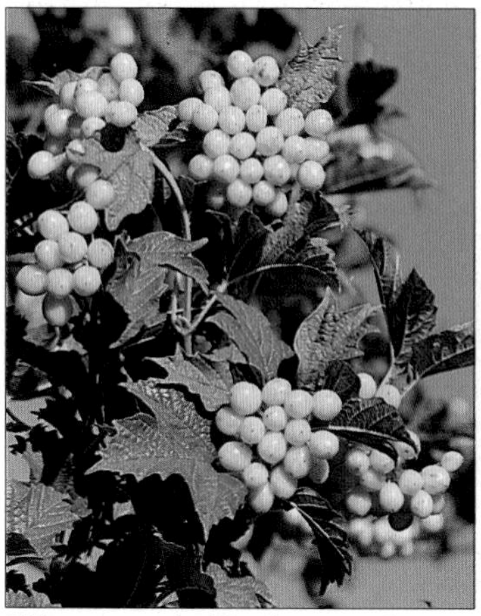

Viburnum opulus 'Xanthocarpum'

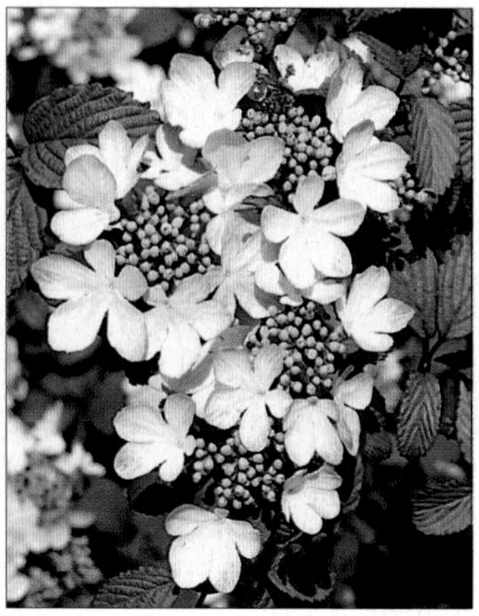

Viburnum plicatum 'Pink Beauty'

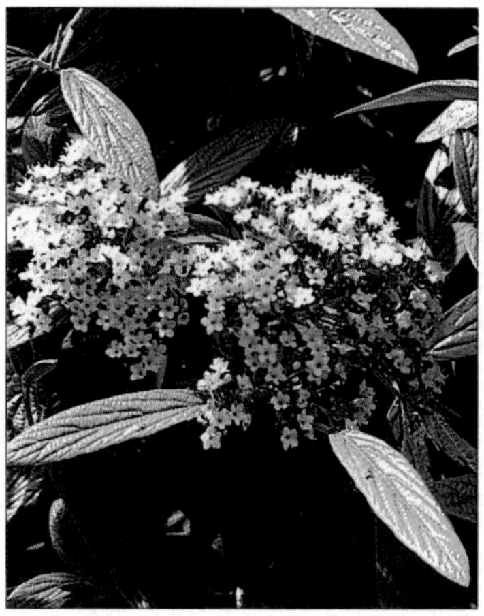

Viburnum 'Pragense'

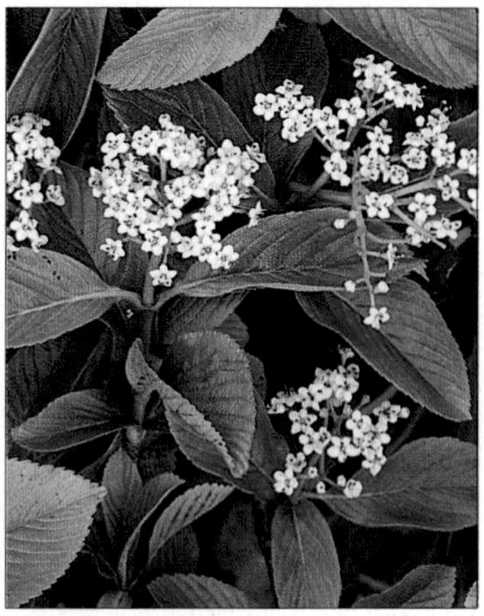

Viburnum sieboldii

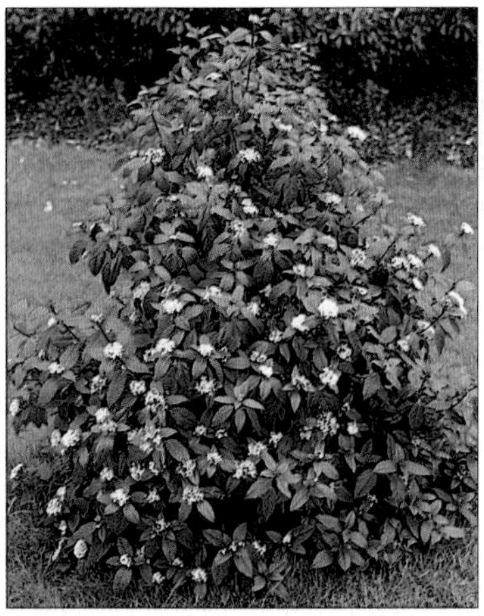

Viburnum tinus

terminal cymes, to 8cm (3in) across, are produced in late spring, sometimes followed by ovoid, blue-black fruit, 5mm (¼in) long. ↕3m (10ft), ↔2m (6ft). C. and W. China, Taiwan, Philippines. ❄❄

V.* x *rhytidophylloides (*V. lantana* x *V. rhytidophyllum*). Spreading, semi-evergreen shrub with arching shoots clothed in oblong, wavy-margined, dark green leaves, to 20cm (8in) long. In late spring, small, tubular, creamy white flowers, 5mm (¼in) across, are borne in flattened, terminal, umbel-like cymes, to 10cm (4in) across; they are followed by ovoid red fruit, 8mm (⅜in) long, which ripen to black. ↕3m (10ft), ↔4m (12ft). Garden origin. ❄❄❄. **'Willowwood'** has deeply veined, glossy leaves.

V. rhytidophyllum ■ Vigorous, erect, evergreen shrub with oblong to lance-shaped, wavy-margined, very deeply veined, glossy, dark green leaves, 20cm (8in) or more long. In late spring, bears small, tubular, creamy white flowers, 5mm (¼in) across, in dense, domed, terminal, umbel-like cymes, to 20cm (8in) across, followed by ovoid red fruit, 8mm (⅜in) long, ripening to glossy black. ↕5m (15ft), ↔4m (12ft). C. and W. China. ❄❄❄

V. sargentii. Bushy, deciduous shrub with maple-like, 3-lobed, toothed leaves, to 12cm (5in) long, bronze when young, often turning yellow or red in autumn. Flat, lacecap-like cymes, to 10cm (4in) across, with a central mass of tiny, tubular, white, fertile flowers surrounded by saucer-shaped, white, sterile ray-florets, 2cm (¾in) across, are borne in late spring. The flowers are followed by

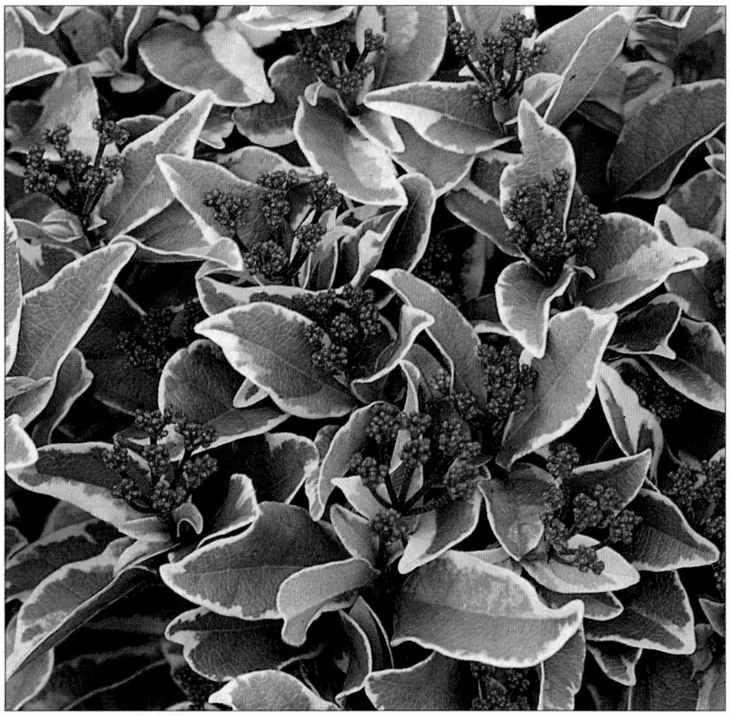

Viburnum tinus 'Variegatum'

spherical, bright red fruit, 1cm (½in) across. ↕↔3m (10ft). N.E. Asia. ❄❄❄.
'Flavum' produces yellow fruit.
'Onondaga' 🏆 has an upright habit, and produces dark bronze-purple foliage ageing to dark green, then turning red-purple in autumn. Fertile flowers are dark red in bud, opening pink-flushed white; ↔2m (6ft)

V. semperflorens see *V. plicatum* 'Nanum Semperflorens'.

V. sieboldii ■ Compact, spreading, large, deciduous shrub with arching shoots and elliptic to obovate, coarsely toothed, glossy, dark green leaves, to 12cm (5in) long. Small, tubular white flowers, 6mm (¼in) across, are borne in flattened, terminal cymes, to 10cm (4in) across, in late spring, and followed by ovoid pink fruit, 1cm (½in) long, which ripen to black. ↕4m (12ft), ↔6m (20ft). Japan. ❄❄❄

V. tinus ■ (Laurustinus). Compact, bushy, evergreen shrub with narrowly ovate to oblong, dark green leaves, to 10cm (4in) long. Bears small, salverform white flowers, 6mm (¼in) across, in flattened, terminal cymes, to 10cm (4in) across, over a long period in late winter and spring; they are followed by ovoid, dark blue-black fruit, 6mm (¼in) long. ↕↔3m (10ft). Mediterranean. ❄❄❄.
'Eve Price' ■🏆 is dense, with leaves to 8cm (3in) long, and pink flower buds.
'Gwenllian' 🏆 bears a profusion of pink-flushed white flowers opening from dark pink buds, and fruits freely.
'Lucidum' is vigorous, with very glossy leaves; each flower is 1cm (½in) across.
'Pink Prelude' has white flowers opening from pink buds and ageing to pink. **'Purpureum'** has young foliage tinged dark bronze-purple.
'Variegatum' ■ has leaves broadly margined with creamy yellow; needs more shelter than green-leaved forms.

V. tomentosum see *V. plicatum* f. *tomentosum.*

V. trilobum, syn. *V. opulus* var. *americanum.* Dense, rounded, deciduous shrub producing maple-like, 3-lobed, dark green leaves, to 12cm (5in) long, bronze when young, turning yellow to red in autumn. In late spring, bears flattened, lacecap-like, terminal cymes, to 10cm (4in) across, of tiny, tubular, white, fertile central flowers, 2cm (¾in) across, surrounded by showy, flat, white, sterile florets, to 2cm (¾in) across. The flowers are followed by edible, spherical red fruit, 8mm (⅜in) across. ↕5m (15ft), ↔4m (12ft). North America. ❄❄❄

V. watanabei see *V. plicatum* 'Nanum Semperflorens'.

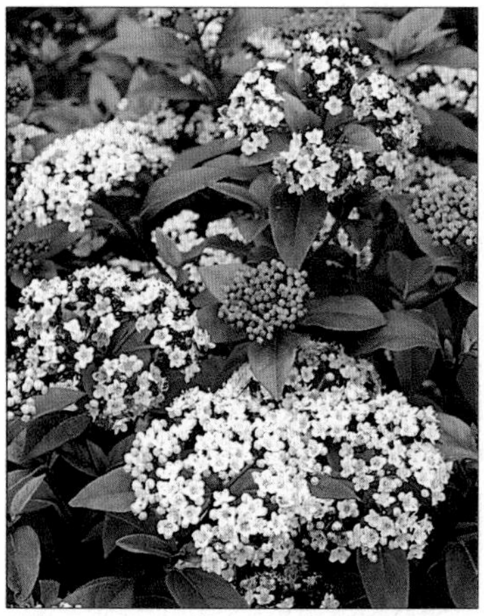

Viburnum tinus 'Eve Price'

VICTORIA

Giant water lily

NYMPHAEACEAE

Genus of 2 species of rhizomatous, submerged, deep-water aquatic annuals or perennials occurring in tropical South America, in the slow-moving backwaters of the Amazon. Their stout rhizomes support enormous, rounded, floating leaves, and bear night-blooming, water-lily-like flowers. In tropical gardens, grow in a large pool; elsewhere, grow as annuals in a heated pool in a warm greenhouse.

• **HARDINESS** Frost tender.

• **CULTIVATION** Outdoors, grow in a pool at least 1m (3ft) deep in full sun; grow in baskets, 1m (3ft) across and 60cm (24in) deep, of rich, loamy soil, with added well-rotted organic matter. Under glass, grow in baskets of loamy soil in an indoor pool with a water temperature of 21–24°C (70–75°F) in summer; provide full light. During the growing season, add pellets of slow-release fertilizer to the growing medium every 6 weeks. See also pp.52–53.

• **PROPAGATION** Collect the seeds when ripe and overwinter in distilled water. In early spring, sow at 29–32°C (84–90°F), covering seeds with 5–8cm (2–3in) of water.

• **PESTS AND DISEASES** Trouble free.

V. amazonica ■ (Amazon water lily, Royal water lily). Submerged, deep-water aquatic annual or perennial with stout rhizomes supporting rounded, mid-green, floating leaves, to 2m (6ft) long, reddish purple beneath; they have large prickles and vertical rims, to 10cm (4in), or occasionally 15cm (6in) high. In summer, bears many-petalled, water-lily-like white flowers, to 30cm (12in) across, ageing pink, with prickly sepals. ↔6m (20ft). South America (Amazon). ❅ (min. 25°C/77°F to remain perennial)

V. cruziana, syn. *V. trickeri* (Santa Cruz water lily). Submerged, deep-water aquatic annual or perennial with stout rhizomes supporting rounded, floating leaves, to 1.4m (4½ft) long, with vertical rims, to 20cm (8in) high. Leaves are mid-green above, densely softly hairy and reddish purple beneath, but the undersides are less highly coloured than those of *V. amazonica.* In summer, bears many-petalled, water-lily-like white flowers, to 10cm (4in) across, the sepals with basal prickles only. ↔6m (20ft). South America (Bolivia, Brazil, N. Argentina, Paraguay). ❅ (min. 22–25°C/72–77°F to remain perennial)

***V.* 'Longwood Hybrid'** (*V. amazonica* x *V. cruziana*). Submerged, deep-water aquatic annual or perennial with a stout rhizome supporting rounded, mid-green, floating leaves, to 2.5m (8ft) long, with reddish purple outer margins on the upturned rims. In summer, produces many-petalled, water-lily-like white flowers, to 30cm (12in) across, the sepals with basal prickles only. More free-flowering and hardier than its parents. ↔7m (22ft). Garden origin. ❅ (min. 22°C/72°F to remain perennial)

V. trickeri see *V. cruziana.*

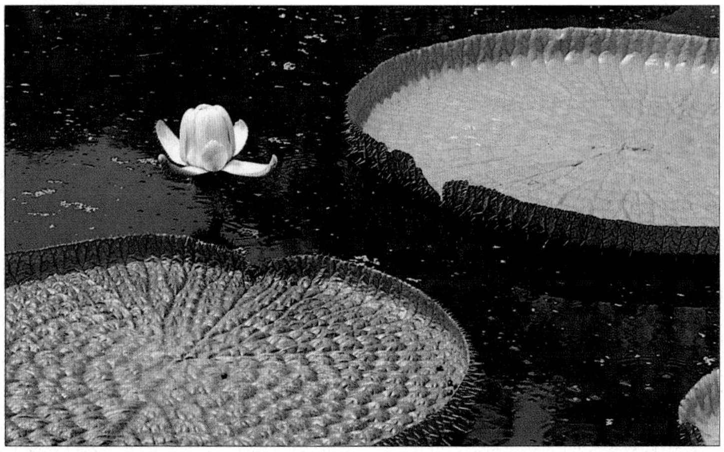

Victoria amazonica

VIGNA

LEGUMINOSAE/PAPILIONACEAE

Genus of about 150 species of erect and climbing or trailing annuals and evergreen perennials from woodland, scrub, and rocky areas in tropical regions of Africa, Asia, S. USA, and Central and South America. Most are cultivated as agricultural crops, for their edible pods and seeds (beans); the climbers are also grown as ornamentals, for their flowers, foliage, and seed pods. The alternate leaves are palmately lobed or 3-palmate with entire leaflets. Pea-like flowers with distinctive, coiled keel petals are borne in axillary clusters or racemes, often in alternate pairs, followed by linear, straight or curved pods. Where summer temperatures average less than 16°C (61°F), grow as annuals in a warm greenhouse. Elsewhere, grow over a pergola, arch, or tall tree stump.

• **HARDINESS** Frost tender.

• **CULTIVATION** Under glass, grow in loam-based potting compost (JI No.2) in full light. In the growing season, water freely and apply a balanced liquid fertilizer monthly; water sparingly in winter. Outdoors, grow in fertile, moist but well-drained soil in full sun. Support climbing stems. Pruning group 11, in early spring.

• **PROPAGATION** Sow seed at 13–18°C (55–64°F) in autumn or spring.

• **PESTS AND DISEASES** Susceptible to red spider mites and whiteflies under glass.

V. caracalla, syn. *Phaseolus caracalla* (Corkscrew flower, Snail bean, Snail flower). Fast-growing, evergreen, twining, perennial climber with sparsely branched stems and 3-palmate leaves, 15cm (6in) long, with ovate, downy, light to mid-green leaflets, 7–13cm (3–5in) long. From summer to autumn, and into winter if warm enough, bears erect, axillary racemes, to 30cm (12in) long, of pink, white, or yellow flowers 3–5cm (1¼–2in) across, with elongated and coiled keel and standard petals, the keels coiled like a snail's shell; flowers are followed by nearly cylindrical, green then brown fruit, 15–18cm (6–7in) long. ↕ 6–8m (20–25ft). Tropical South America. ❀ (min. 10–15°C/50–59°F)

▷ ***Villarsia nymphoides*** see *Nymphoides peltata*

VINCA

Periwinkle

APOCYNACEAE

Genus of 7 species of slender-stemmed, evergreen subshrubs and herbaceous perennials from woodland in Europe, N. Africa, and C. Asia. They are grown for their opposite, simple, lance-shaped to elliptic or ovate, often variegated leaves, and for their showy, long-stalked, star-like or salverform flowers, each with 5 petal lobes, borne singly in the leaf axils. Useful ground cover for a woodland garden, shrub border, or shady bank, but may be invasive. All parts may cause mild stomach upset if ingested.

• **HARDINESS** Fully hardy to frost hardy.

• **CULTIVATION** Grow in any but very dry soil, in full sun (for best flowering) or partial shade. To restrict growth, cut back hard in early spring.

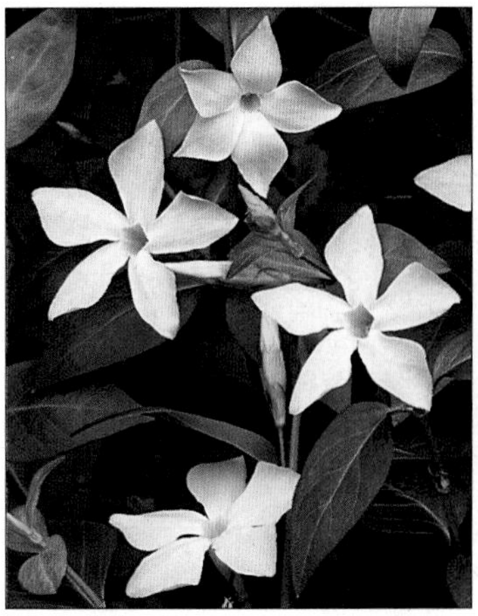

Vinca difformis

• **PROPAGATION** Divide from autumn to spring. Take semi-ripe cuttings in summer.

• **PESTS AND DISEASES** Prone to rust.

V. difformis ■ Prostrate, evergreen subshrub with usually narrowly lance-shaped, glossy, dark green leaves, to 7cm (3in) long. In late winter and early spring, upright shoots produce pale blue to nearly white flowers, to 4cm (1½in) across. ↕ 30cm (12in), ↔ indefinite. S.W. Europe, N. Africa. ❄❄

***V. herbacea* 'Hidcote Purple'** see *V. major* var. *oxyloba*.

***V. hirsuta* of gardens** see *V. major* var. *oxyloba*.

V. major (Greater periwinkle). Prostrate, evergreen shrub with arching shoots and ovate to lance-shaped, dark green leaves, to 9cm (3½in) long. Blue-violet or dark violet flowers, to 5cm (2in) across, are produced over a long period from mid-spring to autumn. ↕ 45cm (18in), ↔ indefinite. W. Mediterranean. ❄❄❄. **'Dartington Star'** see var. *oxyloba*. **'Elegantissima'** see 'Variegata'. **subsp. *hirsuta***, syn. var. *pubescens*, produces lance-shaped, distinctly hairy leaves; Georgia, Turkey. **'Maculata'** has leaves with yellow-green centres. **var. *oxyloba***, syn. 'Dartington Star', *V. herbacea* 'Hidcote Purple', *V. hirsuta* of gardens, produces dark violet-blue flowers with narrow, pointed lobes. **var. *pubescens*** see subsp. *hirsuta*. **'Reticulata'** has leaves conspicuously veined with yellow or cream when young, later dark green. **'Variegata'** ■ 🏆 syn. 'Elegantissima' has leaves margined creamy white.

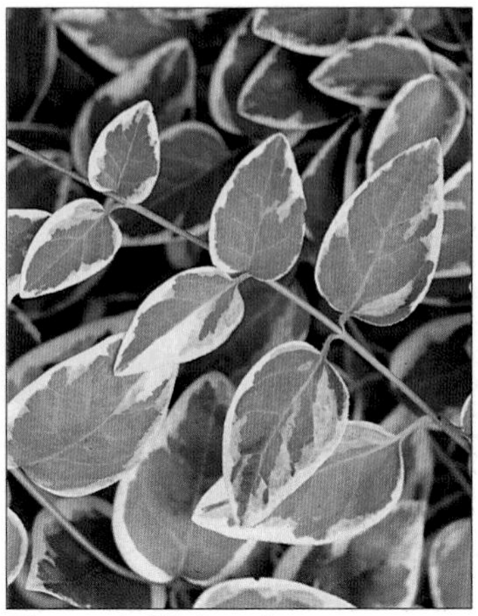

Vinca major 'Variegata'

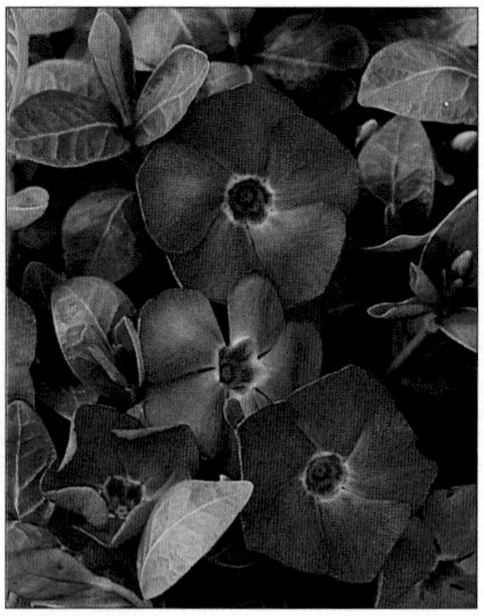

Vinca minor

V. minor ■ (Lesser periwinkle). Prostrate, mat-forming, evergreen shrub with long, trailing shoots and elliptic or lance-shaped, sometimes ovate, dark green leaves, to 5cm (2in) long. Over a long period from mid-spring to autumn, bears usually blue-violet, sometimes pale blue, reddish purple, or white flowers, 2.5–3cm (1–1¼in) across. ↕ 10–20cm (4–8in), ↔ indefinite. Europe, S. Russia, N. Caucasus. ❄❄❄. **f. *alba*** has white flowers. **'Alba Variegata'**, syn. 'Alba Aureavariegata', has leaves with pale yellow margins, and bears white flowers. **'Argenteovariegata'** 🏆 syn. 'Variegata', has leaves with creamy white margins, and produces light violet-blue flowers. **'Atropurpurea'** 🏆 syn. 'Purpurea', 'Rubra', has dark plum-purple flowers. **'Azurea Flore Pleno'** 🏆 syn. 'Caerulea Plena', has double, sky-blue flowers. **'Bowles' Blue'** see 'La Grave'. **'Bowles' Variety'** see 'La Grave'. **'Bowles' White'** bears white flowers, opening from pinkish white buds. **'Caerulea Plena'** see 'Azurea Flore Pleno'. **'Double Burgundy'** see 'Multiplex'. **'Gertrude Jekyll'** 🏆 is very compact, and profusely bears white flowers. **'La Grave'** 🏆 syn. 'Bowles' Blue', 'Bowles' Variety', bears lavender-blue flowers, 3cm (1¼in) across. **'Multiplex'**, syn. 'Double Burgundy', has double, plum-purple flowers. **'Purpurea'** see 'Atropurpurea'. **'Rubra'** see 'Atropurpurea'. **'Variegata'** see 'Argenteovariegata'.

V. rosea see *Catharanthus roseus.*

▷**Vine** see *Vitis*
- **Allegheny** see *Adlumia fungosa*
- **Balloon** see *Cardiospermum halicacabum*
- **Bengal clock** see *Thunbergia grandiflora*
- **Blue trumpet** see *Thunbergia grandiflora*
- **Bush clock** see *Thunbergia erecta*
- **Cat's claw** see *Macfadyena*
- **Chalice** see *Solandra*
- **Chestnut** see *Tetrastigma voinierianum*
- **Chinese trumpet** see *Campsis grandiflora*
- **Chocolate** see *Akebia*
- **Common cat's claw** see *Macfadyena unguis-cati*
- **Common coral** see *Kennedia coccinea*
- **Confederate** see *Antigonon leptopus*
- **Coral** see *Antigonon*
- **Cross** see *Bignonia*
- **Firecracker** see *Manettia cordifolia*

▷**Vine cont.**
- **Grape** see *Vitis*
- **Hemp** see *Mikania scandens*
- **Jade** see *Strongylodon macrobotrys*
- **Kangaroo** see *Cissus antarctica*
- **Kudzu** see *Pueraria lobata*
- **Lipstick** see *Aeschynanthus lobbianus*
- **Macquarie** see *Muehlenbeckia adpressa*
- **Madeira** see *Anredera cordifolia*
- **Mignonette** see *Anredera cordifolia*
- **Pink trumpet** see *Podranea ricasoliana*
- **Potato** see *Solanum jasminoides, S. wendlandii*
- **Rattan** see *Berchemia scandens*
- **Rosary** see *Ceropegia linearis* subsp. *woodii*
- **Russian** see *Fallopia baldschuanica*
- **Silk** see *Periploca graeca*
- **Silver** see *Actinidia polygama*
- **Staff** see *Celastrus, C. orbiculatus, C. scandens*
- **Sweetheart** see *Ceropegia linearis* subsp. *woodii*
- **Tara** see *Actinidia arguta*
- **Trumpet** see *Campsis*
- **Water** see *Cissus hypoglauca*
- **Wonga wonga** see *Pandorea pandorana*

VIOLA *syn.* ERPETION

Pansy, Violet

VIOLACEAE

Genus of about 500 species of annuals, biennials, evergreen, semi-evergreen, and deciduous perennials (some tufted or rhizomatous), and a few deciduous subshrubs, found in varied habitats in temperate regions worldwide. They have variable, entire to finely pinnatisect, mostly mid-green leaves with stipules. Some South American species are rosette-forming, and are very similar to sempervivums. The mostly unscented flowers, borne in the leaf axils, are usually solitary, rarely paired. Each has 5 petals: a spurred lower petal, 2 lateral petals, and 2 upward-facing upper petals. Most flower profusely over long periods in summer, and may self-seed freely.

Many cultivars within the genus are informally referred to as garden pansies, violas, or violettas; they are all derived from the complex hybridization of *V. tricolor*, *V. lutea*, *V. cornuta*, and other species. Garden pansies (*V.* x *wittrockiana* cultivars) are biennials or very short-lived perennials, with faintly scented or unscented, more or less rounded flowers with patterned "faces". They have a single-stemmed root system. Violas, often called "tufted pansies", are compact, tufted perennials with usually scented, more or less rounded, often patterned flowers with rays (lines in a deeper or contrasting colour), and a multi-stemmed root system. Violettas are similar to violas, but are even more compact, with small, sweetly fragrant, oval flowers, each with a central yellow mark and no rays.

The perennials and subshrubs are suitable for a rock garden, a scree bed, or the front of a border; a few are best in an alpine house. Treat garden pansies as annuals, biennials, or short-lived perennials: they are good for containers; some are suitable for summer bedding; plant winter- or spring-flowering types with spring-flowering bulbs.

• **HARDINESS** Fully hardy to half hardy.

V

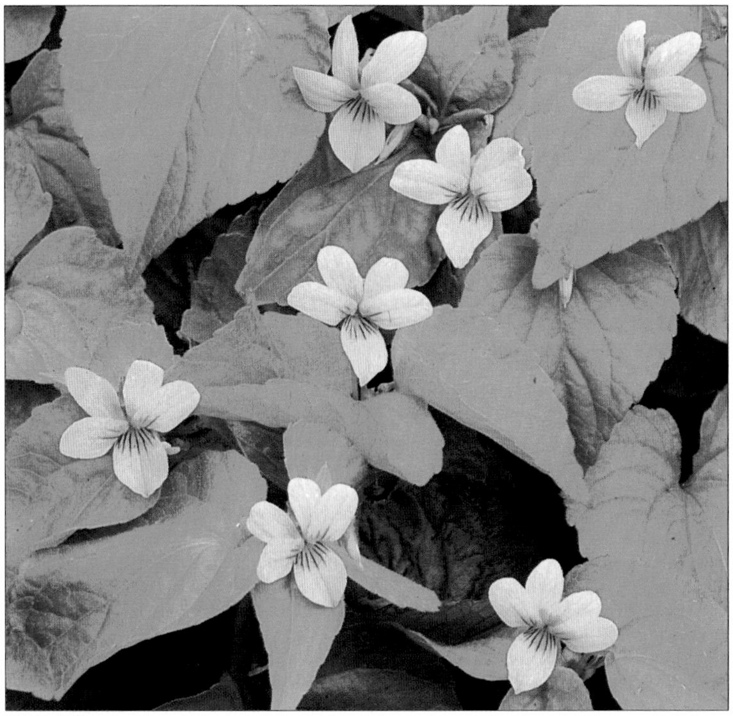

Viola biflora

• **CULTIVATION** Grow in fertile, humus-rich, moist but well-drained soil in full sun or partial shade. In a rock garden, grow in poor to moderately fertile, gritty, sharply drained soil in full sun or partial shade; protect from winter wet. In an alpine house, use a mix of equal parts loam, leaf mould, and grit or tufa chips. Dead-head to prolong flowering. After flowering, cut back vigorous plants, especially *V. cornuta*, to keep compact.
• **PROPAGATION** Sow seed in containers in a cold frame as soon as ripe or in spring; for garden pansies sow seed in late winter for early spring and summer flowering, or in summer for winter flowering. Divide *V. biflora*, *V. cornuta*, *V. elatior*, *V. glabella*, *V. hederacea*, *V. obliqua*, and *V. odorata* in spring or autumn. Take stem-tip cuttings of perennials and subshrubs in spring or late summer. Many viola species are short-lived, so propagate them regularly.
• **PESTS AND DISEASES** May be damaged by slugs, snails, aphids, red spider mites, and violet leaf midges. Susceptible to leaf spot; may also be affected by mosaic viruses, rust, and powdery mildew.

V. adunca (Hooked-spur violet, Western dog violet). Compact, tuft-forming, semi-evergreen perennial with procumbent stems bearing ovate to broadly ovate, finely toothed, smooth to slightly hairy leaves, to 4cm (1½in) long. In spring, bears scented, violet to lavender-blue flowers, 2cm (¾in) across, with white spurs, to 2cm (¾in) long, and white eyes. Suitable for a rock garden; self-seeds freely. ↕↔ to 8cm (3in). N. USA. ❄❄❄. **var. *minor*** see *V. labradorica*.
V. aetolica. Neat, clump-forming, short-lived, evergreen perennial with short, spreading stems and ovate to lance-shaped, scalloped leaves, to 2cm (¾in) long. In late spring and early summer, produces yellow flowers, to 2cm (¾in) across; the slightly darker lower petals have spurs to 6mm (¼in) long. ↕ to 8cm (3in), ↔ to 15cm (6in). E. Europe. ❄❄❄
V. beckwithii (Great Basin violet). Small, tufted, evergreen perennial with spreading stems and palmately 3-lobed, hairy, conspicuously veined leaves, 3cm (1¼in) long, each lobe pinnatifid with linear segments. In spring, bears solitary, slightly scented flowers, 2cm (¾in) across, with spurs to 2mm (1⁄16in) long; the 2 upper petals are deep reddish violet, the 3 lower ones pale lavender-blue with purple-veined yellow bases. Best in an alpine house; difficult to grow. ↕ 5–13cm (2–5in), ↔ to 10cm (4in). North America (Great Basin area). ❄❄❄
V. biflora ▣ (Twin-flowered violet). Dwarf, creeping herbaceous perennial with slender rhizomes and thin stems bearing kidney- to heart-shaped, toothed, pale green leaves, 3–4cm (1¼–1½in) long, with scalloped margins. In late spring and summer, bears solitary or paired, deep lemon flowers, 1.5cm (½in) across, veined dark purple-brown on the lower petals and with spurs to 3mm (⅛in) long. Prefers moist soil in partial shade. ↕ to 8cm (3in), ↔ to 20cm (8in). Europe to N. Asia, North America (Alaska, Rocky Mountains). ❄❄❄

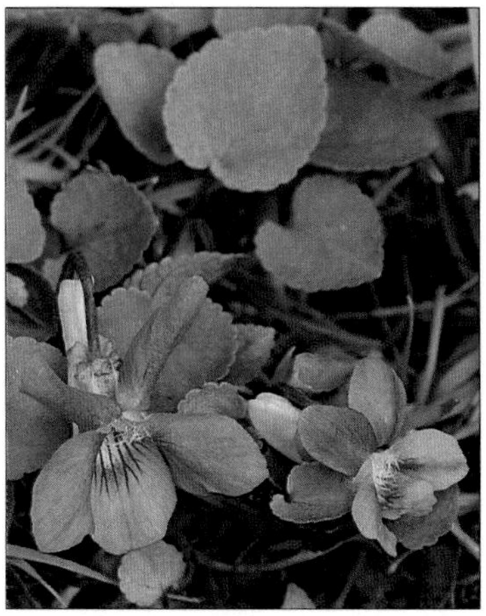

Viola canina

V. canina ▣ (Dog violet, Heath violet). Rhizomatous, semi-evergreen perennial with decumbent to erect stems and ovate to ovate-lance-shaped, entire leaves, 1–2cm (½–¾in) long, shallowly heart-shaped at the bases. In spring and early summer, bears solitary, bright blue or violet flowers, to 2.5cm (1in) across, each with a straight, pale yellowish green or white spur, 1cm (½in) long. ↕↔ 15–30cm (6–12in). Temperate Europe and W. Asia. ❄❄❄
V. cazorlensis ▣ Dwarf, woody-based, evergreen perennial with crowded, upright stems bearing very narrow, linear to inversely lance-shaped, entire leaves, to 1.5cm (½in) long. In late spring and early summer, produces narrow-petalled, pinkish purple flowers, 2cm (¾in) across, with notched lower petals, and slender spurs, to 3cm (1¼in) long. Difficult to grow; best in tufa or in an alpine house. ↕ to 8cm (3in), ↔ to 10cm (4in). S.E. Spain. ❄❄❄
V. cornuta ▣♀ (Horned violet, Viola). Spreading, rhizomatous, evergreen perennial with ascending stems and ovate, toothed leaves, 2–5cm (¾–2in) long, truncate at the bases. From spring to summer, produces abundant slightly scented flowers, to 3.5cm (1½in) across; they have widely separated, usually violet to lilac-blue petals, the lower ones with white markings, and slender spurs, to 1.5cm (½in) long. ↕ to 15cm (6in), ↔ to 40cm (16in) or more. Spain (Pyrenees). ❄❄❄. **var. *minor*** ♀ is smaller in all its parts, and produces white or lavender-blue flowers, 1.5–2cm (½–¾in) across; ↕ to 7cm (3in), ↔ to 20cm (8in).
V. cucullata see *V. obliqua*.
V. elatior, syn. *V. erecta*. Upright, sparsely branched, subshrubby perennial with deciduous, lance-shaped, toothed leaves, to 9cm (3½in) long, slightly heart-shaped at the bases. Bears scented, pale lavender-blue flowers, 2.5cm (1in) across, with spurs 2–4mm (1⁄16–⅛in) long, over long periods in late spring and early summer. Easily grown in moist soil. ↕ to 30cm (12in), ↔ to 15cm (6in). C., S., and E. Europe to W. Asia. ❄❄❄
V. erecta see *V. elatior*.
V. glabella (Stream violet). Vigorous, spreading, rhizomatous, deciduous or semi-evergreen perennial with upright or spreading stems and long-stalked, ovate or rounded, toothed, bright green leaves, 3–9cm (1¼–3½in) long, with heart-shaped bases. In late spring, bears deep yellow flowers, 2.5cm (1in) across, veined purple on the lower petals, and with short spurs, 2mm (1⁄16in) long. Prefers partial shade. ↕ to 20cm (8in), ↔ to 30cm (12in) or more. N.E. Asia, N.W. USA. ❄❄❄

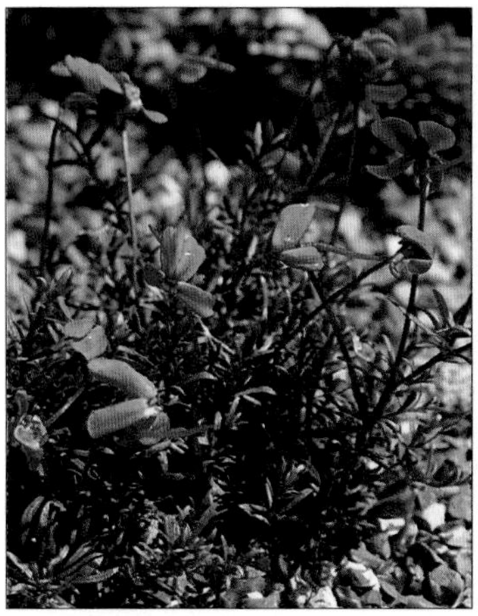

Viola cazorlensis

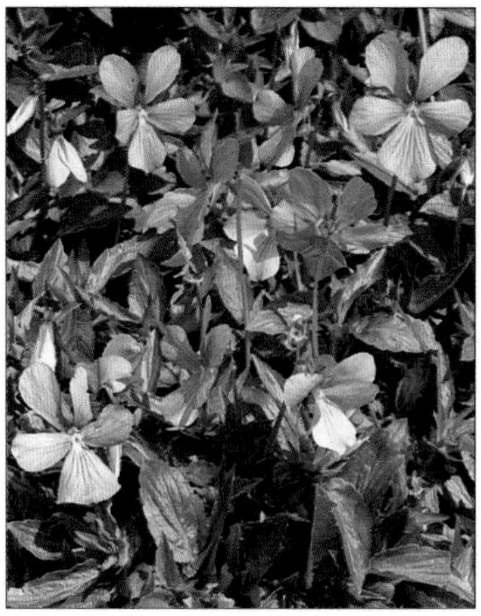

Viola cornuta

V. gracilis, syn. *V. velutina*. Mat-forming, evergreen perennial with erect or ascending stems and oblong to broadly ovate, variably toothed leaves, 2–3cm (¾–1¼in) long, with finely divided stipules. In summer, bears yellow-eyed, deep violet, occasionally yellow flowers, to 3cm (1¼in) across, with slender spurs, to 7mm (¼in) long. Needs full sun. ↕ to 10cm (4in), ↔ to 20cm (8in). Balkan Peninsula, Greece, Turkey. ❄❄❄
V. 'Haslemere' see *V.* 'Nellie Britton'.
V. hederacea, syn. *Erpetion hederaceum*, *E. reniforme*, *V. reniforme* (Australian violet, Ivy-leaved violet, Trailing violet). Mat-forming, evergreen perennial with slender stolons and short, erect, tufted stems bearing broadly ovate to kidney-shaped, entire or coarsely toothed, dark green leaves, to 3.5cm (1½in) long, with scalloped margins. In late summer, bears sometimes slightly scented flowers, to 2.5cm (1in) across, either spurless or with inconspicuous spurs, and with a rather flattened appearance; they may be white, cream, pale to dark violet, or sometimes white with violet patches. Best in an alpine house; prefers partial shade. Very vigorous; good ground cover in warm climates. ↕ to 10cm (4in), ↔ 20–30cm (8–12in). Australia. ❄❄
V. 'Huntercombe Purple' ▣♀ Spreading, clump-forming, evergreen

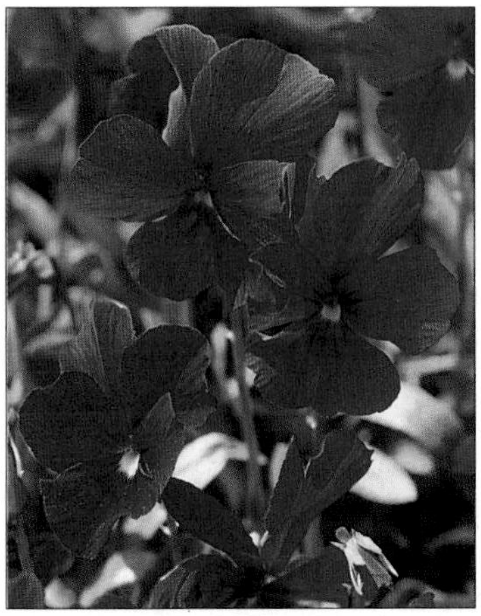

Viola 'Huntercombe Purple'

V

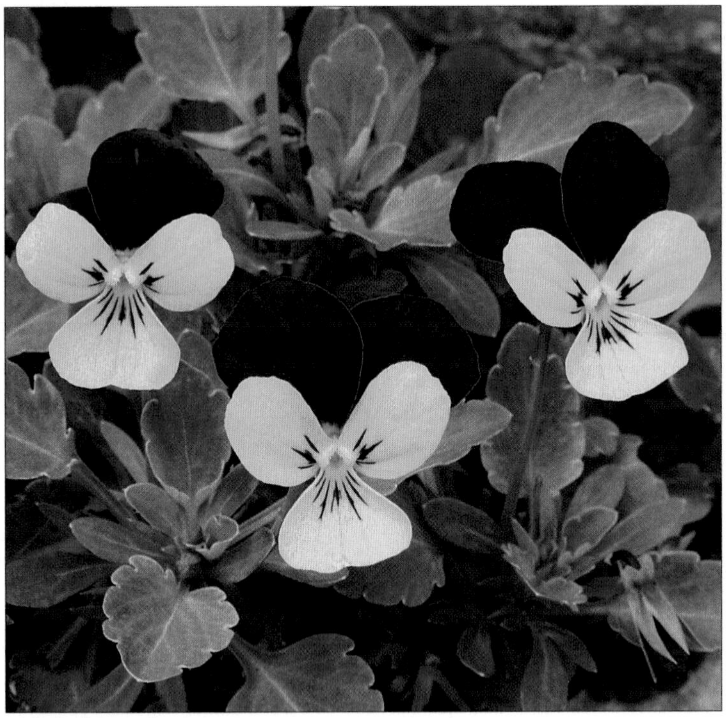

Viola 'Jackanapes'

perennial with upright stems and ovate, toothed leaves, to 2.5cm (1in) long. In spring and late summer, produces abundant deep violet-purple flowers, to 2.5cm (1in) across, with spurs 4–6mm (⅛–¼in) long. ↕ to 15cm (6in), ↔ to 30cm (12in). ❄❄❄

***V.* 'Irish Molly'.** Evergreen, usually short-lived perennial with spreading stems and broadly ovate, deeply cut leaves, to 3cm (1¼in) long. In summer, produces a long succession of dark gold flowers, to 3cm (1¼in) across, with brown centres, and spurs 4–6mm (⅛–¼in) long. Propagate regularly. ↕ to 15cm (6in), ↔ to 20cm (8in). ❄❄❄

***V.* 'Jackanapes'** ■ 🏆 Robust, clump-forming, evergreen perennial with spreading stems and ovate, toothed, bright green leaves, to 2.5cm (1in) long. In late spring and summer, bears flowers to 2cm (¾in) across, the upper petals deep violet-purple to almost brown, the lower ones golden yellow, streaked purple at the centres, and with spurs 1.5cm (½in) long. Propagate regularly. ↕ to 12cm (5in), ↔ to 30cm (12in). ❄❄❄

***V. labradorica*,** syn. *V. adunca* var. *minor* (Labrador violet). Spreading, clump-forming, semi-evergreen perennial with prostrate stems and heart- to kidney-shaped, finely toothed, dark green leaves, 2cm (¾in) long, flushed bronze-purple when young. Solitary, pale purple flowers, 1.5cm (½in) across, with short spurs, 6mm (¼in) long, are borne in spring and summer. ↕ to 8cm (3in), ↔ indefinite. Canada, N. USA, Greenland. ❄❄❄. **var. *purpurea* of gardens** see *V. riviniana* 'Purpurea'.

V. lutea*,** syn. *V. lutea* subsp. *elegans* (Mountain pansy). Slender, creeping, rhizomatous, evergreen perennial bearing ovate lower stem leaves and ovate to lance-shaped, shallowly scalloped or almost entire upper leaves, to 2cm (¾in) long. In late spring and early summer, bears flowers to 3cm (1¼in) across, in bright yellow, blue-violet, or red-violet, or all three colours combined, and with short spurs, 3–6mm (⅛–¼in) long. ↕↔ 7–15cm (3–6in). W. and C. Europe. ❄❄❄. **subsp. *elegans see *V. lutea*.

***V.* 'Nellie Britton'** ■ 🏆 syn. *V.* 'Haslemere'. Clump-forming, evergreen perennial with spreading stems bearing ovate to lance-shaped, toothed, glossy leaves, 3cm (1¼in) long. Pinkish mauve flowers, to 2.5cm (1in) across, with spurs 1cm (½in) long, are profusely borne over long periods in summer. ↕ to 15cm (6in), ↔ to 30cm (12in). ❄❄❄

***V. obliqua*,** syn. *V. cucullata* (Marsh blue violet). Spreading, stemless, rhizomatous, deciduous perennial with heart-shaped, toothed leaves, to 9cm (3½in) long. In late spring, solitary, blue-violet flowers, to 2cm (¾in) across, with short spurs to 2mm (¹⁄₁₆in) long, are borne above the leaves. Occasionally produces white flowers with blue eyes and blue veins. ↕ to 8cm (3in), ↔ to 25cm (10in). North America. ❄❄❄

V. odorata (English violet, Garden violet, Sweet violet). Rhizomatous, semi-evergreen perennial with slender stolons and short, erect stems that bear tufts of heart-shaped to rounded, toothed, bright green leaves, to 6cm (2½in) long. In late winter and early spring, produces sweetly scented, blue or white flowers, 2cm (¾in) or more across, with spurs to 5mm (¼in) long. Self-seeds freely; excellent for a wild or woodland garden. ↕ to 20cm (8in), ↔ 30cm (12in) or more. Probably W. and S. Europe; very widely naturalized elsewhere. ❄❄❄

V. papilionacea see *V. sororia*.

V. pedata ■ (Bird's-foot violet, Crow-foot violet). Stemless, clump-forming, semi-evergreen perennial with short, stout rhizomes and 3-lobed leaves, to 3cm (1¼in) long, the 2 lateral lobes themselves divided into 3–5 linear or spoon-shaped lobes. In late spring and early summer, bears yellow-centred, pale violet flowers, 3cm (1¼in) across, with widely spaced petals and short spurs, to 2mm (¹⁄₁₆in) long. Flowers are sometimes white or bicoloured, with deep purple upper petals and pale lavender-blue or white lower ones. Best in an alpine house. Needs well-drained, peaty, sandy soil. ↕ to 5cm (2in), ↔ to 10cm (4in). E. North America. ❄❄❄

V. pedatifida (Larkspur violet, Purple prairie violet). Small, clump-forming, semi-evergreen to deciduous perennial with 5- to 11-palmate leaves, to 3cm (1¼in) long, with very narrow leaflets. In spring and summer, bears deep violet-blue flowers, to 2cm (¾in) across, with bearded lower petals and short spurs, 4mm (⅛in) long. Self-seeds freely. ↕ to 12cm (5in), ↔ to 15cm (6in). C. North America. ❄❄❄

V. reniforme see *V. hederacea*.

V. riviniana (Common dog violet, Wood violet). Tufted, semi-evergreen perennial with basal tufts of ovate-rounded, toothed leaves, to 4cm (1½in) long, deeply heart-shaped at the bases. In late spring and early summer, bears pale violet-blue flowers, 1.5–2.5cm (½–1in) across, with notched, white or pale purple spurs, to 5mm (¼in) long. Suitable for a wild garden, in deep or partial shade. ↕ 10–20cm (4–8in), ↔ 20–40cm (8–16in). Europe, N. Africa. ❄❄❄. **'Purpurea'** ■ syn. *V. labradorica* var. *purpurea* of gardens, has dark purplish green leaves. Invasive, but excellent in a wild or woodland garden.

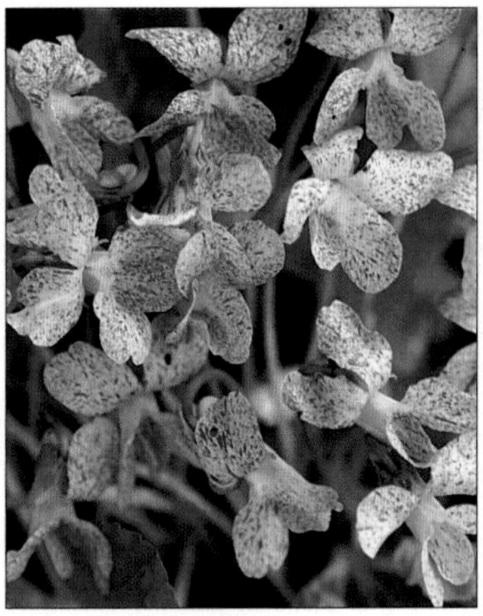

Viola sororia 'Freckles'

***V. sororia*,** syn. *V. papilionacea* (Sister violet, Woolly blue violet). Stemless, rhizomatous herbaceous perennial with ovate to rounded, sharp-pointed, scalloped leaves, to 10cm (4in) long, densely hairy beneath. In spring and summer, bears flowers to 2cm (¾in) across, with short spurs, to 3mm (⅛in) long. The flowers are sometimes deep violet-blue, but usually white, heavily speckled and streaked violet-blue around the centres. Self-seeds freely. ↕ to 10cm (4in), ↔ to 20cm (8in). E. North America. ❄❄❄. **'Freckles'** ■ bears white flowers, speckled violet-purple.

V. tricolor ■ (Heartsease, Love-in-idleness, Wild pansy). Tufted annual, biennial, or short-lived, evergreen perennial, sometimes rhizomatous, with spreading stems and ovate to heart-shaped, toothed leaves, to 3cm (1¼in) long. From spring to autumn, bears flowers, 2.5cm (1in) or more across, in shades of purple, lavender-blue, white, or yellow, with usually dark purple upper petals, lower petals often streaked dark purple, and spurs to 7mm (¼in)

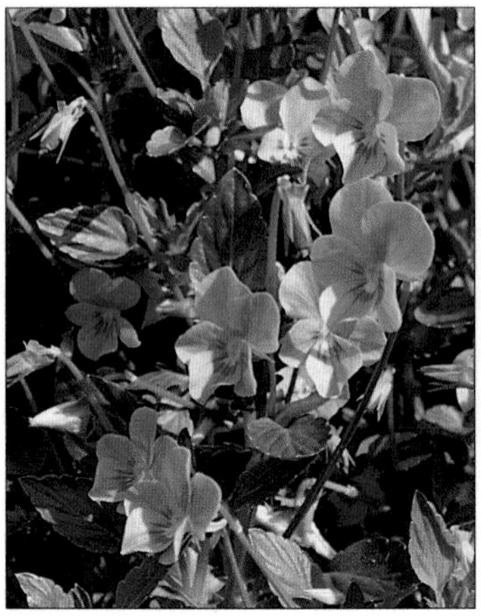

Viola 'Nellie Britton'

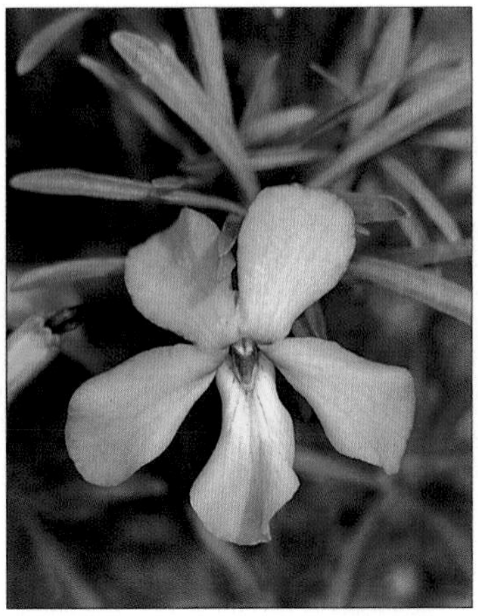

Viola pedata

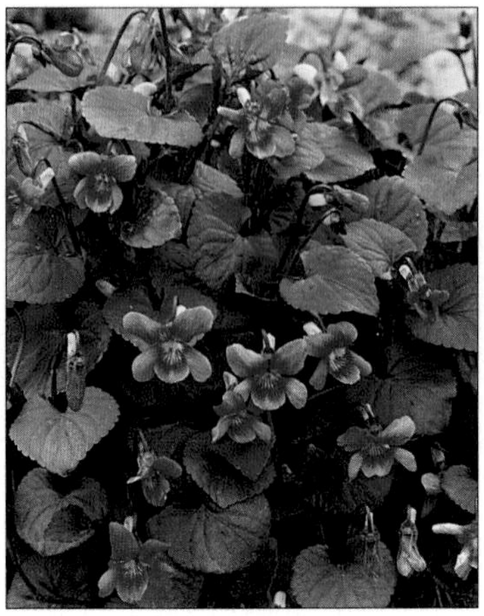

Viola riviniana 'Purpurea'

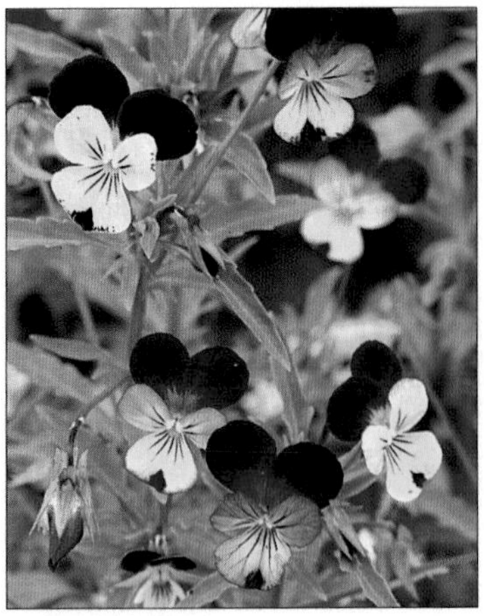

Viola tricolor

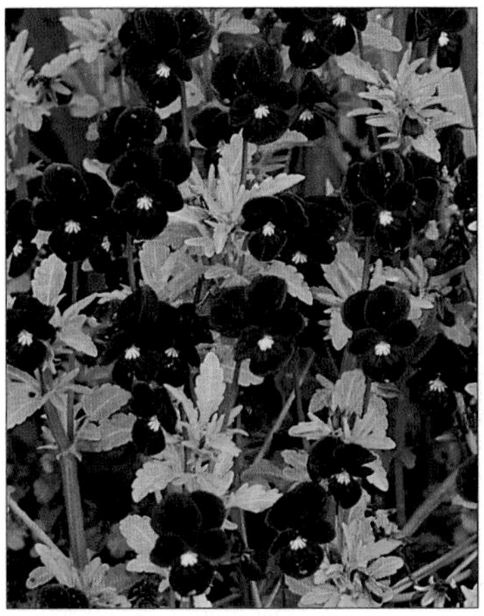
Viola tricolor 'Bowles' Black'

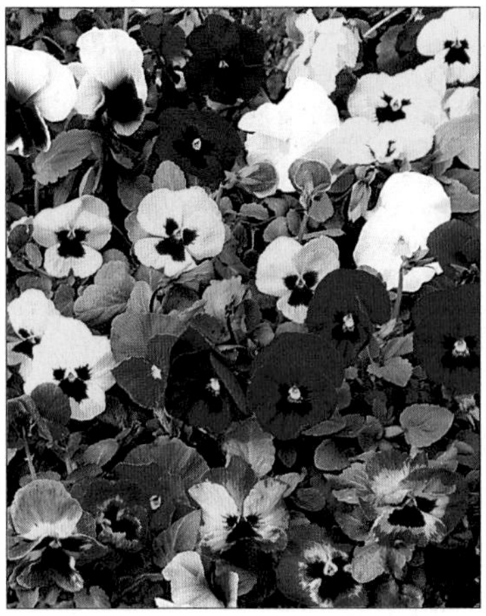
Viola x *wittrockiana* Forerunner Series

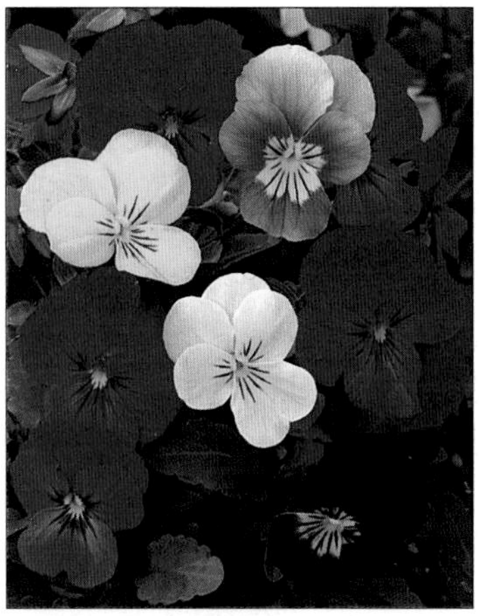
Viola x *wittrockiana* Princess Series

long. Very short-lived, but self-seeds prolifically. ↕ to 8–12cm (3–5in), ↔ to 10–15cm (4–6in). Europe, Asia. ✻✻✻. **'Bowles' Black'** ▣ has velvety, almost black flowers with small, golden yellow eyes. Seeds freely and comes almost true from seed; ↕ to 10cm (4in), ↔ to 20cm (8in). **'Prince Henry'** bears small, very dark purple flowers, 1.5–2cm (½–¾in) across, from spring to summer. **'Prince John'** bears small, bright yellow flowers, 1.5–2cm (½–¾in) across, from spring to summer.

V. velutina see *V. gracilis*.

***V.* x *wittrockiana* cultivars** (Pansy). Erect, bushy evergreen perennials, grown as annuals or biennials, derived from cross-breeding *V. altaica*, *V. cornuta*, *V. lutea*, and *V. tricolor*; they are usually larger and more robust than their parents. They have spreading stems and ovate to almost heart-shaped, shallowly lobed, shiny, mid- to deep green leaves, to 3.5cm (1½in) or more long. Flowers are 6–10cm (2½–4in) across, with the lateral petals overlapping the lower and upper petals, and with very short spurs. They may be either self-coloured, usually in blue, white, yellow, orange, pink, red, or purple; bicoloured; or the more traditional pansy type, bicoloured with central, face-like markings. Flowers are produced mainly from early spring to summer, some from autumn to winter. Other, usually smaller-flowered cultivars have been bred for winter and early spring flowering, and are excellent bedding plants during the coldest months. ↕ 16–23cm (6–9in), ↔ 23–30cm (9–12in). ✻✻✻. **Allegro Series** cultivars bear large flowers in a broad colour range, with or without markings, in winter and spring. **'Baby Lucia'** produces small, yellow-eyed, clear blue flowers in spring and summer. **'Bambini'** has small flowers, borne in spring and summer, in a wide colour range, most with contrasting white or yellow faces and "whiskered" central markings. **Bingo Series** cultivars flower in winter and spring, producing large blooms in a broad colour range, some with darker markings. **Clear Crystal Series** cultivars bear medium-sized flowers in summer, in a wide range of clear, single colours, without central markings. **'Cornetto'** produces small, very long-spurred, clear white flowers in spring and summer. **Crown Series** cultivars produce large flowers in a broad range of clear colours, in early spring and summer. **Crystal Bowl Series** cultivars are compact, and bear medium-sized, unmarked flowers in a wide range of clear colours, including white, in summer; ↕ 23cm (9in), ↔ 30cm (12in). **'Cuty'** bears small, yellow-eyed white flowers, with deep violet-purple upper petals, from spring to summer. **Delta Series** cultivars are compact and robust, bearing large flowers in a wide range of colours, some with darker markings, in early spring. **Fama Series** ▣ cultivars produce large flowers in winter and spring, in a wide range of single colours and in mixed colours. **Fanfare Series** cultivars are compact, producing medium-sized flowers in winter and spring, available in a broad range of single colours and bicolours; excellent for hanging baskets. Cultivars of **Forerunner Series** ▣ bloom in winter and spring, bearing medium-sized flowers in a range of bright single colours and bicolours. Cultivars of **Imperial Series** produce large flowers in a broad colour range, almost all with a deeper central mark, in winter and early spring; **'Imperial Frosty Rose'** is an unusual rose-pink with a deeper central mark; **'Imperial Gold Princess'** is bicoloured yellow and red. **Jewel Series** cultivars are compact and free-flowering, bearing small blooms in winter and spring, in yellow, blue, purple with pansy faces, and white with pansy faces. Cultivars of **Joker Series** 🏆 produce medium-sized, bi-coloured flowers in light blue, mahogany-gold, violet-gold, and mixed colours, with very strongly marked pansy faces, in summer; **'Jolly Joker'** ▣ blooms in spring and summer, and has medium-sized orange flowers, with deep purple upper petals and purple-margined lower petals. **'Pretty'** bears small yellow flowers, with rich mahogany-red upper petals, in spring and summer. **Princess Series** ▣ 🏆 cultivars are neat in habit, and produce small flowers in blue, cream, dark purple, bicoloured purple and white, or yellow, in spring and summer. **Rally Series** cultivars are free-flowering, producing medium-sized blooms in a broad range of colours, in winter and spring. Cultivars of **Regal Series** are compact, producing medium-sized flowers in a wide range of separate colours and a mixture of colours, all with darker markings, in winter and spring. **Super Chalon Giants** bears medium-sized to large, bicoloured flowers, with wavy, ruffled margins, in summer. **Ultima Series** 🏆 cultivars, blooming in winter and spring, have medium-sized flowers in a very broad range of colours, including bicolours. **Universal Series** ▣ 🏆 cultivars bear medium-sized flowers in winter and spring, in a broad range of colours, including bicolours, and sometimes with patterned faces. Cultivars of **Velours Series** have a neat habit, and bear small flowers in violet-blue, pale blue with deep blue markings, purple, and yellow, in spring and summer.

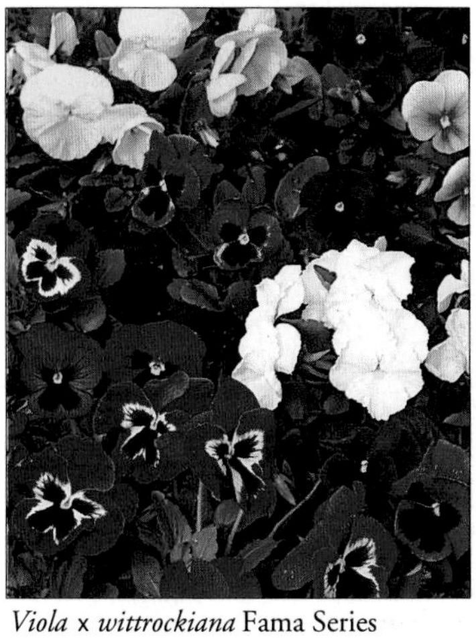
Viola x *wittrockiana* Fama Series

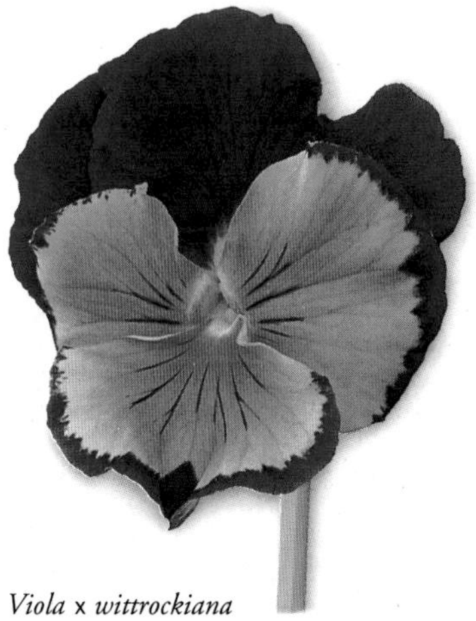
Viola x *wittrockiana*
Joker Series 'Jolly Joker'

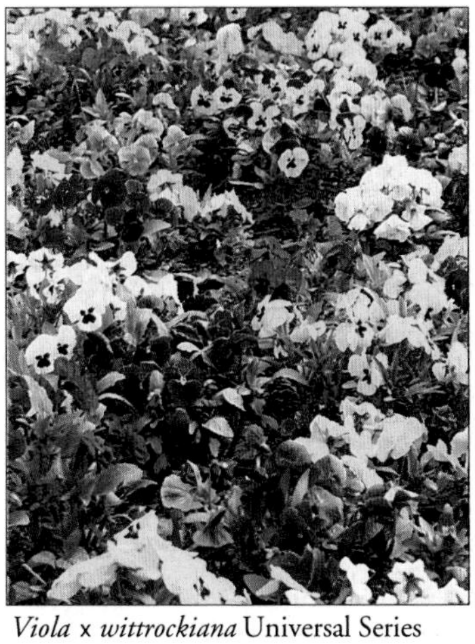
Viola x *wittrockiana* Universal Series

▷**Viola** see *Viola cornuta*
▷**Violet** see *Viola*
- **African** see *Saintpaulia*
- **Amethyst** see *Browallia*
- **Australian** see *Viola hederacea*
- **Bird's-foot** see *Viola pedata*
- **Bush** see *Browallia*
- **Common dog** see *Viola riviniana*
- **Crow-foot** see *Viola pedata*
- **Dame's** see *Hesperis matronalis*
- **Dog** see *Viola canina*
- **Dog's-tooth** see *Erythronium*
- **English** see *Viola odorata*
- **European dog's-tooth** see *Erythronium dens-canis*
- **Flame** see *Episcia*
- **Garden** see *Viola odorata*
- **Great Basin** see *Viola beckwithii*
- **Heath** see *Viola canina*
- **Hooked-spur** see *Viola adunca*
- **Horned** see *Viola cornuta*
- **Ivy-leaved** see *Viola hederacea*
- **Labrador** see *Viola labradorica*
- **Larkspur** see *Viola pedatifida*
- **Marsh blue** see *Viola obliqua*
- **Mexican** see *Tetranema roseum*
- **Persian** see *Exacum affine*
- **Philippine** see *Barleria cristata*
- **Purple prairie** see *Viola pedatifida*
- **Sister** see *Viola sororia*
- **Stream** see *Viola glabella*
- **Sweet** see *Viola odorata*
- **Trailing** see *Viola hederacea*
- **Twin-flowered** see *Viola biflora*
- **Water** see *Hottonia palustris*
- **Western dog** see *Viola adunca*
- **Wood** see *Viola riviniana*
- **Woolly blue** see *Viola sororia*

▷**Viper's bugloss** see *Echium vulgare*

VIRGILIA

LEGUMINOSAE/PAPILIONACEAE

Genus of 2 species of small, evergreen trees from forest edges and river valleys in coastal areas of South Africa. They have alternate, pinnate leaves, and are grown for their abundant pea-like flowers, borne in axillary or terminal racemes, occasionally in panicles. Where winter temperatures fall below 5–7°C (41–45°F), grow in a cool greenhouse. In milder areas, use as specimen trees.

• **HARDINESS** Frost tender, but may survive temperatures down to 0°C (32°F) provided the wood has been well ripened in summer.

• **CULTIVATION** Under glass, grow in ericaceous potting compost with added sharp sand, in full light. In growth, water moderately and apply a balanced liquid fertilizer every month; water sparingly in winter. Outdoors, grow in neutral to acid, poor to moderately fertile, moist but well-drained soil in full sun. Pruning group 1; may need restrictive pruning under glass.

V

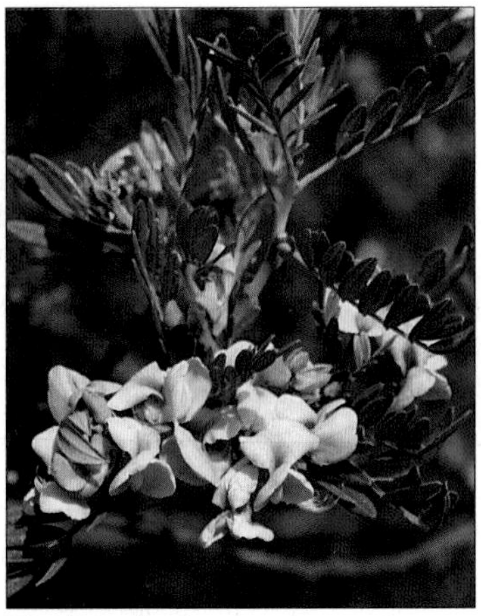

Virgilia oroboides

• **PROPAGATION** Sow seed at about 15°C (59°F) in spring, after soaking in hot water or after scarification.
• **PESTS AND DISEASES** Trouble free.

V. capensis see *V. oroboides*.
V. oroboides ■ ◇–◇ syn. *V. capensis*. Fast-growing shrub or small, rounded to broadly columnar tree, usually with several main stems, and with red-downy young growth. Pinnate leaves, 10–20cm (4–8in) long, each have 13–21 narrowly oblong, leathery, mid- to deep green leaflets, pale and densely woolly beneath, with thorn-like points. From spring to summer, bears racemes of up to 12 pea-like, fragrant, white, pink, purple, or crimson flowers, to 2cm (¾in) across. ↕ 5–9m (15–28ft), ↔ 3–5m (10–15ft). South Africa (Western Cape, Eastern Cape). ❄ (borderline)

▷ **Virginia creeper** see *Parthenocissus, P. quinquefolia*
Chinese see *P. henryana*
▷ **Virgin's bower** see *Clematis*
▷ ***Viscaria*** see *Lychnis*
V. elegans see *Silene coeli-rosa*
V. vulgaris see *Lychnis viscaria*

VITALIANA syn. DOUGLASIA

PRIMULACEAE

Genus of one species of tufted, mat- or cushion-forming, evergreen perennial, occurring in alpine and subalpine screes, rocks, and meadows in the mountains of C. and S. Europe. It has rosettes of small leaves, and is cultivated for its solitary flowers, produced in spring. Grow in a rock garden, scree bed, or alpine house.
• **HARDINESS** Fully hardy, but dislikes excessive winter wet.
• **CULTIVATION** Grow in leafy, moderately fertile, gritty, moist but sharply drained soil in full sun. Protect from winter wet. In an alpine house, grow in a mix of 1 part each loam and leaf mould, and 3 parts grit.
• **PROPAGATION** Sow seed in containers in an open frame as soon as ripe. Detach and root offsets in spring and early summer.
• **PESTS AND DISEASES** Susceptible to aphids and red spider mites under glass.

V. primuliflora ■ syn. *Androsace vitaliana, Douglasia vitaliana*. Tufted, mat- or cushion-forming, evergreen perennial with creeping stems and tight rosettes of linear to oblong-lance-shaped, pointed, usually hairy, pale green leaves, to 1cm (½in) long, with silver margins. In spring, bears solitary, almost stemless, tubular yellow flowers, to 2cm (¾in) across, with 5 spreading lobes. ↕ to 2.5cm (1in), ↔ to 25cm (10in). Mountains of S.W. and C. Europe, to S.E. Alps, and C. Apennines. ❄❄❄

VITEX

VERBENACEAE

Widespread genus of 250 species of deciduous or evergreen trees and shrubs, occurring mainly in tropical regions, often in woodland or dried-up river beds. They have opposite, fully divided, 3- to 7-palmate leaves, and produce terminal panicles, racemes, or cymes of tubular, 2-lipped flowers. *V. agnus-castus* and *V. negundo* are cultivated for their elegant foliage and late flowers, and may be grown in a shrub border or against a wall. In frost-prone areas, grow tender species in a warm greenhouse.
• **HARDINESS** Frost hardy to frost tender.
• **CULTIVATION** Grow in any well-drained soil in full sun. In frost-prone areas, shelter frost-hardy species from cold, drying winds. Pruning group 6.
• **PROPAGATION** Sow seed at 6–12°C (43–54°F) in autumn or spring. Take semi-ripe cuttings in summer.
• **PESTS AND DISEASES** Trouble free.

V. agnus-castus (Chaste tree). Open, spreading, deciduous shrub with 5- or 7-palmate leaves composed of slender, narrowly elliptic, pointed, entire or slightly toothed, aromatic, dark green leaflets, to 10cm (4in) or more long. Small, tubular, fragrant, lilac- to dark blue, sometimes white flowers are borne in slender upright, terminal panicles, to 13–18cm (5–7in) long, in early and mid-autumn. ↕↔ 2–8m (6–25ft). Mediterranean to C. Asia. ❄❄. **var. *latifolia*** ■ is more vigorous, with broader leaflets.
V. negundo. Bushy, deciduous shrub with 3- to 5-palmate, dark green leaves composed of lance-shaped, pointed, sharply toothed or entire leaflets, to 10cm (4in) long. In late summer and early autumn, bears small, tubular, pale violet-blue flowers in terminal panicles, to 22cm (9in) long. ↕↔ 3m (10ft). E. Africa, E. Asia. ❄❄

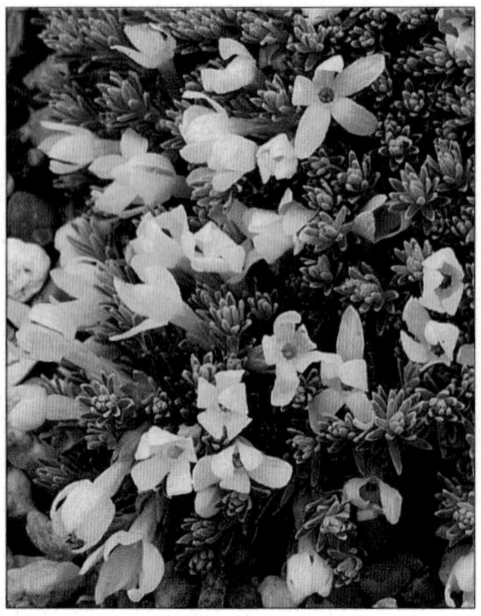

Vitaliana primuliflora

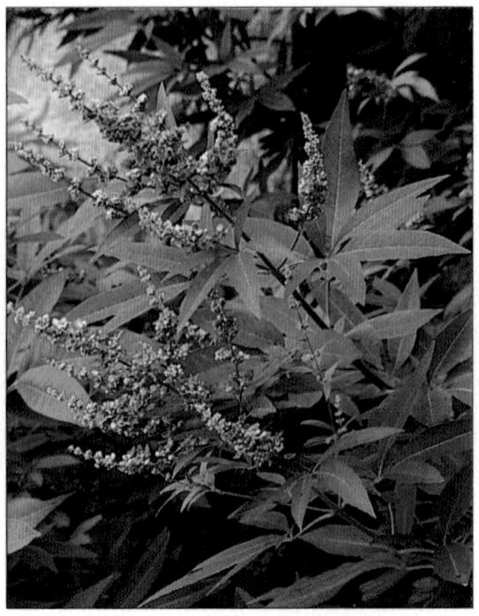

Vitex agnus-castus var. *latifolia*

VITIS

Grape vine, Vine

VITACEAE

Genus of about 65 species of woody, deciduous tendril climbers, occasionally shrubs, occurring in woodland, woodland margins, and thickets in N. temperate regions. They have flaking bark and alternate, simple to lobed, sometimes toothed leaves. Tiny green flowers are produced in panicles from the leaf axils in summer, and are followed by fruits (grapes), which in some species are edible or are used to make wine. The ornamental vines are cultivated for their foliage and fruits; grow over a trellis, pergola, or fence, or through a large shrub or tree, or train against a wall.
• **HARDINESS** Fully hardy.
• **CULTIVATION** Grow in well-drained, preferably neutral to alkaline, humus-rich soil in full sun or partial shade. Pruning group 11, in midwinter, and again in midsummer if necessary, to restrict growth; pruning group 12, if more formal training required.
• **PROPAGATION** Sow seed in containers in a cold frame in autumn or spring. Take hardwood cuttings in late winter, or root "vine eye" cuttings (with a single bud) in early spring. Layer in autumn.
• **PESTS AND DISEASES** May be affected by powdery mildew and honey fungus. Scale insects and mealybugs may be troublesome under glass.

V. aconitifolia see *Ampelopsis aconitifolia*.
V. amurensis (Amur grape). Vigorous, woody, deciduous climber, sometimes a shrub, with red-tinged young shoots and broadly ovate, often shallowly 3-lobed, sharply toothed, dark green leaves, to 30cm (12in) long, heart-shaped at the bases, and turning red and purple in autumn. Bears small, unpalatable, ovoid, white-bloomed black grapes, 1.5cm (½in) across, in late summer. ↕ 15m (50ft). China, Korea, Japan. ❄❄❄
***V.* 'Brant'** ♀ Vigorous, woody, deciduous climber with rounded, palmately 3- to 5-lobed, toothed, bright green leaves, to 22cm (9in) long, which turn bronze-red with green veins in autumn. In autumn, produces large bunches of edible, spherical, blue-black grapes, 1.5cm (½in) across. ↕ 7m (22ft) or more. ❄❄❄
V. capensis see *Rhoicissus capensis*.
V. coignetiae ■ ♀ Vigorous, woody, deciduous climber with large, heart-shaped, shallowly 3- to 5-lobed, shallowly to coarsely toothed, dark green

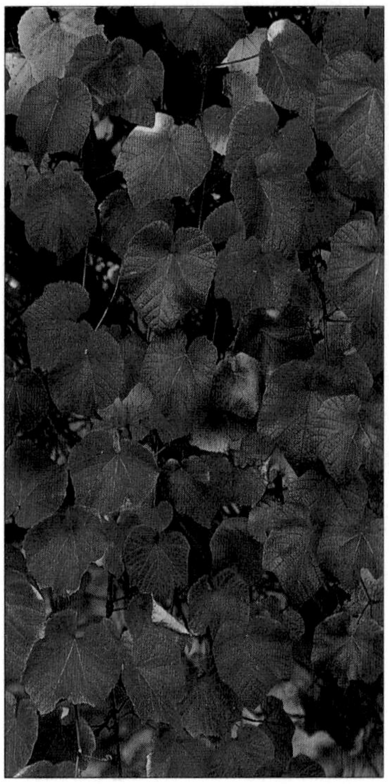

Vitis coignetiae

leaves, to 30cm (12in) long, with deeply impressed veins above and thickly brown-felted beneath; they turn bright red in autumn. Small, unpalatable, spherical, blue-black grapes, 1cm (½in) across, are produced in autumn. ↕ 15m (50ft). Korea, Japan. ❄❄❄
V. davidii. Woody, deciduous climber producing young shoots densely covered with short, rigid spines. Heart-shaped, shallowly lobed, toothed, glossy, dark green leaves, to 25cm (10in) long, blue-green or blue-grey beneath, turn scarlet in autumn. Produces edible, spherical black grapes, 1.5cm (½in) across, in autumn. ↕ 8m (25ft) or more. China. ❄❄❄
V. henryana see *Parthenocissus henryana*.
V. heterophylla see *Ampelopsis brevipedunculata* var. *maximowiczii*.
V. quinquefolia see *Parthenocissus quinquefolia*.
V. striata see *Cissus striata*.
V. thomsonii see *Parthenocissus thomsonii*.
***V. vinifera* 'Purpurea'** ■ ♀ Woody, deciduous climber with rounded, 3- to 5-lobed, toothed leaves, to 15cm (6in) long, grey-hairy at first, turning plum-

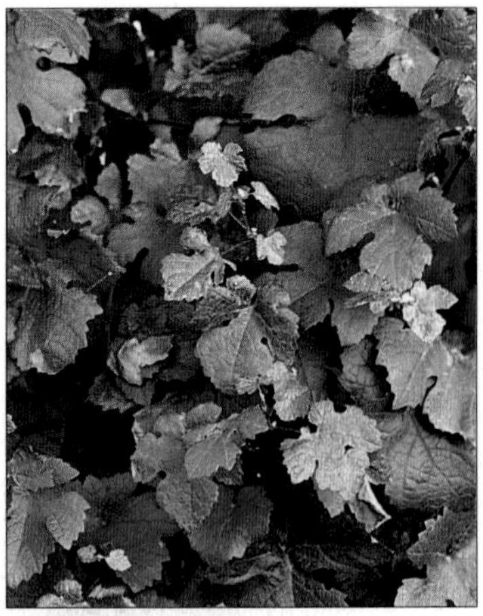

Vitis vinifera 'Purpurea'

purple, then dark purple in autumn. In autumn, produces small, unpalatable, spherical purple grapes, to 2cm (¾in) across. ↕7m (22ft). ❄❄❄
V. voinieriana see *Tetrastigma voinierianum.*

VRIESEA

BROMELIACEAE

Genus of about 250 species of rosette-forming, evergreen, mostly epiphytic perennials (bromeliads), closely related to *Tillandsia.* They occur in forested and rocky areas, to 2,500m (8,000ft) high, in Mexico, Central America, the West Indies, and South America. The mostly lance-shaped or linear leaves have smooth margins, are often finely scaly, and frequently have coloured cross-bands and other markings. Bract-like sheaths, sometimes colourful, are present at the leaf bases. The short-stalked flowers are variously shaped, with petals free or fused into a tube, often shorter than the sepals, each petal with 2 scales at the base on the inner surface; the flowers are usually borne in flattened, 2-ranked, spike-like racemes or panicles, with prominent floral bracts, produced on more or less erect scapes from the centres of the rosettes, in summer or autumn. Where temperatures drop below 15°C (59°F), grow in a warm greenhouse or as houseplants. In tropical gardens, grow epiphytically in a tree, or on mossy rocks.

- **HARDINESS** Frost tender.
- **CULTIVATION** Under glass, grow attached to pieces of bark or tree branches, or in containers of standard epiphytic bromeliad compost, in moderate light. During the growing season, keep the rosette centres filled with water, mist daily, and apply quarter-strength foliar fertilizer every 4–5 weeks. Keep just moist in winter. Outdoors, grow epiphytically in partial shade. See also p.47.
- **PROPAGATION** Sow seed at 19–24°C (66–75°F) when ripe. Remove offsets in spring.
- **PESTS AND DISEASES** Susceptible to scale insects.

V. carinata ■ (Lobster claw, Painted feather). Epiphytic bromeliad with funnel-shaped rosettes of arching, lance-shaped, pale green leaves, to 20cm (8in) long, broadly acute or rounded at the tips, and with broadly elliptic, red-tinged sheaths, 5–6cm (2–2½in) long.

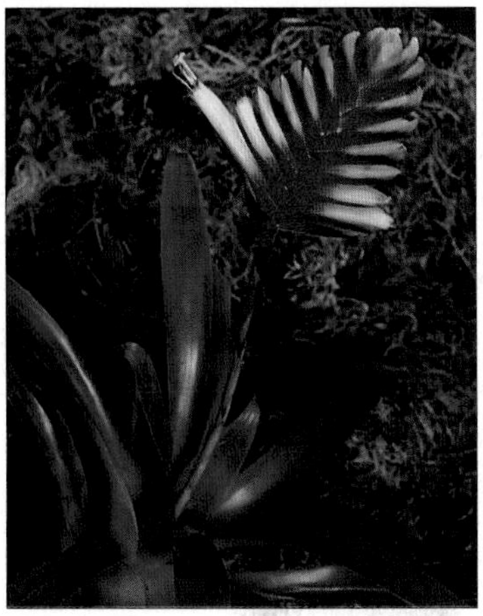

Vriesea carinata

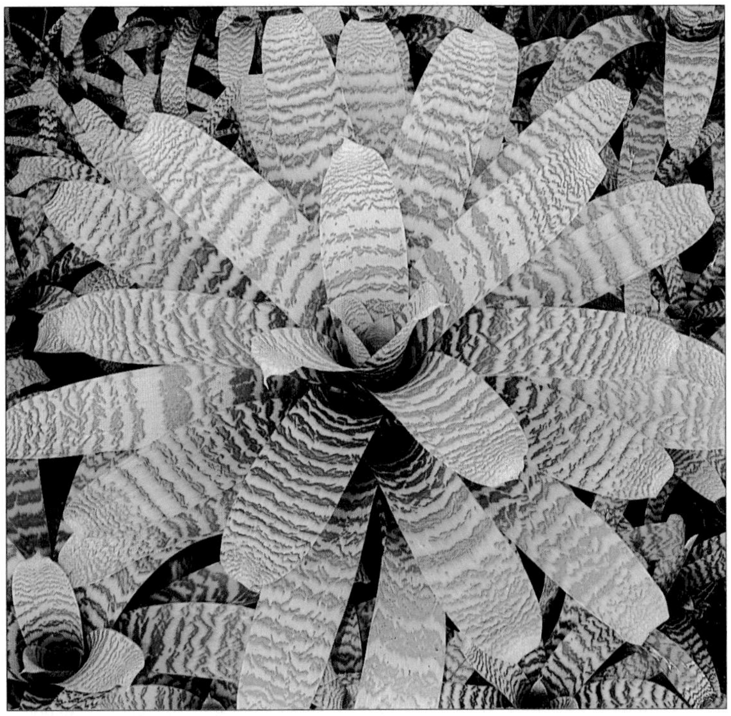

Vriesea hieroglyphica

In summer or autumn, scapes with green, purple, or red bracts bear spike-like racemes, 4–5cm (1½–2in) long, of tubular flowers, to 5cm (2in) long; the flowers have green-tipped yellow petals, keeled sepals, and red-based, yellow-green floral bracts. ↕ to 30cm (12in), ↔ 15–20cm (6–8in). Brazil. ❁ (min. 15°C/59°F)
V. fenestralis. Rock-dwelling or epiphytic bromeliad with funnel-shaped rosettes of recurved or arching, broadly linear, pale green leaves, to 40cm (16in) long, with rounded tips, each with a recurved thorn; the leaf-blades have dark green lines and purple circles beneath, and the broadly oval, yellowish green sheaths, 9–10cm (3½–4in) long, are spotted reddish brown. In summer, bears loose, spike-like racemes, to 30cm (12in) long, of green floral bracts and spreading, yellowish green or greenish white flowers, 6–7cm (2½–3in) long. ↕ to 1m (3ft), ↔ 35–50cm (14–20in). Brazil. ❁ (min. 15°C/59°F)
V. fosteriana 🏆 Epiphytic, probably also terrestrial bromeliad with stiff, dense, funnel-shaped rosettes of arching, broadly tongue-shaped, yellowish to deep green leaves, to 70cm (28in) long;

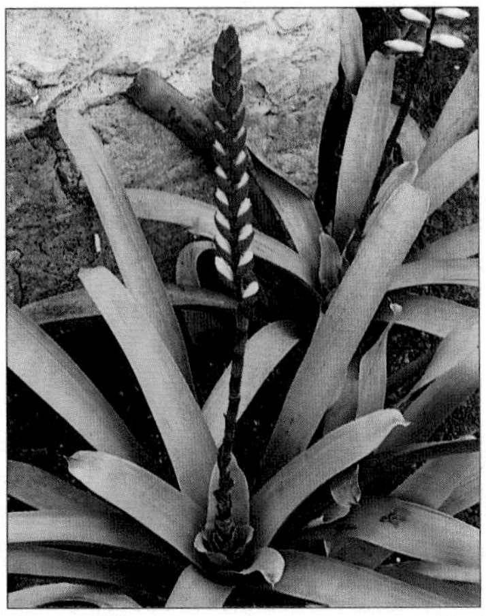

Vriesea platynema

they are cross-banded with purple or maroon, especially beneath, and have broadly oval, dark brown sheaths, 10–15cm (4–6in) long. In summer, bears loose, spike-like racemes, 40cm (16in) or more long, of yellow floral bracts and tubular flowers, 4.5cm (1¾in) long, with yellow petals and green sepals, all with reddish brown tips. ↕ to 1.5m (5ft), ↔ 1m (3ft). Brazil. ❁ (min. 15°C/59°F)
V. hieroglyphica ■ (King of bromeliads). Epiphytic bromeliad with dense, funnel-shaped rosettes of arching, strap-shaped, minutely scaly, yellowish green leaves, 50–80cm (20–32in) long, marked dark green above, purplish brown beneath; dark brown sheaths are 8–10cm (3–4in) long. In summer, produces branching, spike-like racemes or panicles, to 80cm (32in) long, of greenish yellow floral bracts and tubular-trumpet-shaped, sulphur-yellow flowers, to 6cm (2½in) long. ↕ to 1m (3ft), ↔ 80–100cm (32–39in). E. Brazil. ❁ (min. 15°C/59°F)
V. imperialis (Giant vriesea). Rock-dwelling bromeliad with funnel-shaped rosettes of flat or arching, lance-shaped, leathery, pale reddish green leaves, 1.5m (5ft) long, with broadly oval, green sheaths, to 20cm (8in) long. In summer, erect scapes bear glossy, maroon-red bracts and branching, pyramidal, spike-like racemes or panicles, 2m (6ft) or more long, with red floral bracts and tubular, yellow or white flowers, 10cm (4in) or more long. ↕ 3–5m (10–15ft), ↔ 1.5m (5ft) or more. E. Brazil. ❁ (min. 15°C/59°F)
V. platynema ■ Variable, epiphytic bromeliad with very dense, funnel-shaped rosettes of flaccid, strap-shaped, violet-tipped, dull green, often violet-striped leaves, 60cm (24in) long, often margined purple, and with broadly oval, dark brown sheaths, to 12cm (5in) long. In summer, bears loose, spike-like racemes, to 40cm (16in) long, of red or yellow floral bracts and tubular green flowers, to 4.5cm (1¾in) long, with yellow sepals. ↕ to 1m (3ft), ↔ 60cm (24in). West Indies, E. South America. ❁ (min. 15°C/59°F). **'Variegata'** has mid-green leaves, pale reddish purple beneath, with pale lines near the tips; E. Brazil.
V. psittacina 🏆 Variable, epiphytic bromeliad with broadly funnel-shaped rosettes of arching, strap-shaped, pale green leaves, 50cm (20in) long; the leaves have elliptic, green or pale brown sheaths, 7–9cm (3–3½in) long. In summer, produces slender, erect, spike-like racemes, to 30cm (12in) long, with yellow-tipped red, or entirely red or green, floral bracts, and spreading, sometimes green-tipped yellow flowers, 6cm (2½in) long. ↕ to 60cm (24in), ↔ 40–60cm (16–24in). Brazil, Paraguay. ❁ (min. 15°C/59°F)
V. saundersii 🏆 Rock-dwelling bromeliad with dense rosettes of arching, linear, thorn-tipped, grey-scaly, grey-green leaves, 30cm (12in) long; they have fine maroon spots beneath, and oval, yellowish brown sheaths, to 15cm (6in) long, with reddish brown spots. In summer, bears dense, spike-like racemes or panicles, 14cm (5½in) long, of pale or yellowish green floral bracts and tubular yellow flowers, 3.5cm (1½in) long, with pale or yellowish green sepals. ↕ 60–70cm (24–28in), ↔ 40cm (16in). E. Brazil. ❁ (min. 15°C/59°F)
V. splendens ■ 🏆 (Flaming sword). Variable, terrestrial or epiphytic bromeliad producing dense, funnel-shaped rosettes of arching, linear, bluish green leaves, to 80cm (32in) long, with broad, dark green, purple, or reddish brown cross-banding, and with indistinct sheaths. In summer, bears lance-shaped, spike-like racemes, to 55cm (22in) long, of thin, bright red floral bracts and tubular yellow flowers, 8cm (3in) long, with often red-tipped yellow sepals. ↕ to 1m (3ft), ↔ 30cm (12in). E. Venezuela to French Guiana. ❁ (min. 15°C/59°F)

▷**Vriesea, Giant** see *Vriesea imperialis*

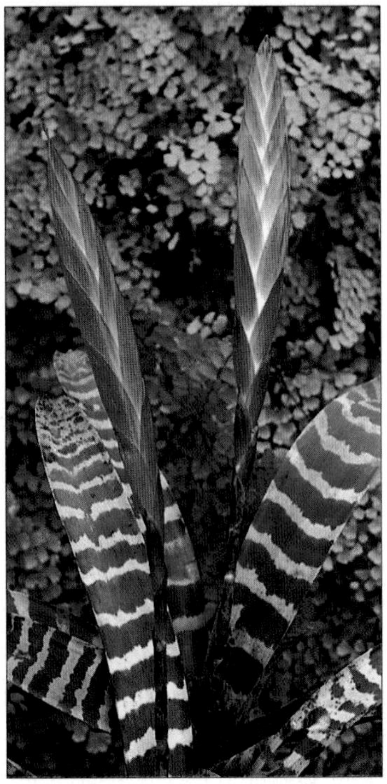

Vriesea splendens

V

W

WACHENDORFIA

HAEMODORACEAE

Genus of about 25 species of tuberous, evergreen perennials found on grassy slopes in South Africa. They have bright red tubers and large, broadly linear, pleated, parallel-veined, erect, basal leaves, sheathing one another at their bases and arranged in 2 opposite rows. They are grown for their large, terminal panicles of irregular, flat, star-shaped yellow flowers, with 6 tepals, borne on leafless stems. In frost-prone areas, grow in a cool greenhouse; for optimum flowering, plant directly into a greenhouse border. In frost-free areas, grow in a sheltered border.

• **HARDINESS** Half hardy.
• **CULTIVATION** Under glass, grow in loam-based potting compost (JI No.2), with additional sharp sand and peat or leaf mould, in full light. During the growing season, water freely and apply a balanced liquid fertilizer every month. Keep just moist when dormant. Outdoors, grow in fertile, reliably moist soil in full sun.
• **PROPAGATION** Sow seed at 13–18°C (55–64°F) in autumn or spring. Separate tubers in spring.
• **PESTS AND DISEASES** Susceptible to slug and snail damage.

W. thyrsiflora ■ Clump-forming, tuberous perennial with furry red roots and tubers. Arching, broadly linear, pleated, parallel-veined, basal leaves, to 1m (3ft) long, are hairless and fairly brittle. In early summer, produces dense panicles of star-shaped yellow flowers, to 3cm (1¼in) across. ↕ 1.5–2m (5–6ft), ↔ 45cm (18in). South Africa (Northern Cape, Western Cape, Eastern Cape). ❄

▷ **Waffle plant, Purple** see *Hemigraphis* 'Exotica'

WAHLENBERGIA

CAMPANULACEAE

Genus of about 150 species of mat-forming to upright annuals and perennials from mountains in Europe, South Africa, and Australasia. They have variable, usually alternate leaves, and are grown for their conspicuous, funnel-, bell-, saucer-, or star-shaped, usually violet, blue, or white flowers, borne singly or in cymes, in summer. Grow in a rock garden, peat bed, or alpine house.

• **HARDINESS** Fully hardy (borderline) to frost hardy.
• **CULTIVATION** Grow in well-drained, sandy, humus-rich soil in a sheltered site in partial shade. In an alpine house, grow in a mix of equal parts loam, leaf mould, and sharp sand.
• **PROPAGATION** Sow seed at 13–15°C (55–59°F) in early spring. Divide in spring. Propagate regularly.
• **PESTS AND DISEASES** May be damaged by slugs and snails.

W. albomarginata (New Zealand bluebell). Tufted, spreading, short-lived, rhizomatous perennial producing basal rosettes of elliptic to lance-shaped or ovate-spoon-shaped, hairy, leathery, mid-green leaves, to 2cm (¾in) long, with reddish brown margins, often purplish green beneath. Solitary, slender-stemmed, upward-facing, bell-shaped, blue, sometimes white flowers, 2.5cm (1in) across, usually with green veins, are produced in summer. ↕ 5–20cm (2–8in), ↔ to 20cm (8in). New Zealand. ❄❄❄ (borderline)
W. gloriosa ■ Tufted, rhizomatous perennial bearing lance-shaped, thick, dark green leaves, 2–3cm (¾–1¼in) long, with wavy, toothed margins. Solitary, upward-facing, widely bell-shaped, deep violet-blue flowers, 2cm (¾in) across, with darker veins, are produced in summer. ↕ to 5cm (2in), ↔ to 15cm (6in). Australia. ❄❄
W. pumilio see *Edraianthus pumilio.*
W. serpyllifolia see *Edraianthus serpyllifolius.*

▷ **Wake robin** see *Trillium, T. grandiflorum, T. sessile*

WALDSTEINIA

ROSACEAE

Genus of about 6 species of tufted, rhizomatous, herbaceous perennials found in woodland throughout N. temperate regions. They are grown mainly for their alternate, 3-palmate or palmately 3- to 7-lobed leaves, and for their saucer-shaped yellow flowers, borne singly or in cymes in late spring and early summer. They provide good ground cover in a woodland garden, on dry, shady banks, or at the front of a herbaceous border, but may be invasive.

• **HARDINESS** Fully hardy.
• **CULTIVATION** Grow in any moderately fertile soil in full or partial shade.
• **PROPAGATION** Sow seed in containers in a cold frame in autumn or spring. Divide in early spring.
• **PESTS AND DISEASES** Trouble free.

W. ternata ■ syn. *W. trifolia.* Vigorous, semi-evergreen perennial, spreading by rhizomes and stolons, with 3-palmate, shallowly lobed and toothed leaves, to 6cm (2½in) long, each composed of 2 almost diamond-shaped lateral leaflets and a rounded terminal leaflet. In late spring and early summer, bears loose cymes of 3–7 saucer-shaped, bright yellow flowers, 1.5cm (½in) across. ↕ to 10cm (4in), ↔ 60cm (24in) or more. C., E., and S. Europe, Russia (E. Siberia), China, Japan. ❄❄❄
W. trifolia see *W. ternata.*

▷ **Wallflower** see *Erysimum, E. cheiri*
Siberian see *E.* x *allionii*
Western see *E. asperum*
▷ **Wallpepper** see *Sedum acre*
▷ **Walnut** see *Juglans*
African see *Schotia brachypetala*
Black see *Juglans nigra*
Californian see *Juglans californica*
Common see *Juglans regia*
Japanese see *Juglans ailantifolia*
Manchurian see *Juglans mandshurica*
Texan see *Juglans microcarpa*
▷ **Wandering Jew** see *Tradescantia fluminensis, T. zebrina*
▷ **Wandflower** see *Dierama, Galax*
▷ **Wapato** see *Sagittaria latifolia*
▷ **Waratah** see *Telopea*
Braidwood see *T. mongaensis*
Common see *T. speciosissima*
Gippsland see *T. oreades*
Monga see *T. mongaensis*
Sydney see *T. speciosissima*
Tasmanian see *T. truncata*
Victorian see *T. oreades*

WASHINGTONIA

ARECACEAE/PALMAE

Genus of 2 species of single-stemmed palms from rocky, arid areas in S.W. USA and N. Mexico. Deeply lobed, fan-shaped leaves are borne in terminal heads that form a dense, shaggy thatch on the trunk as they die back. Because of the fire risk, this dead material is often removed in cultivation. Tubular, creamy white or creamy pink flowers, each with 3 petal lobes, are borne in slender, arching panicles between the leaves. In frost-prone climates, grow young plants as houseplants or in a temperate or warm greenhouse. In warmer areas, use as lawn specimens or as avenue trees.

• **HARDINESS** Frost tender.
• **CULTIVATION** Under glass, grow in loam-based potting compost (JI No.3), with added leaf mould and sharp sand, in full light. When in growth, water moderately and apply a balanced liquid fertilizer monthly; keep almost dry in winter. Outdoors, grow in fertile, well-drained soil in full sun.
• **PROPAGATION** Sow seed at 24°C (75°F) in spring.
• **PESTS AND DISEASES** Red spider mites and scale insects may be troublesome under glass.

W. filamentosa see *W. filifera.*
W. filifera ♕ ♆ syn. *W. filamentosa* (Desert fan palm, Northern washingtonia). Medium-sized to large palm with a robust, columnar trunk. Leaf-stalks are sharply toothed at the bases, and the fan-shaped, grey-green blades, 1.5–3m (5–10ft) long, are erect at first, then spreading and arching, with filaments hanging from the slender lobes. Dead foliage forms an even skirt that clothes the trunk from top to bottom. Bears tubular, creamy white flowers in panicles to 5m (15ft) long, usually in summer. ↕ 15–20m (50–70ft), ↔ 3–6m (10–20ft). USA (S. California, S. Arizona). ⌂ (min. 8–10°C/46–50°F)
W. robusta ■ ♆ (Thread palm). Tall, fast-growing palm with a slender trunk that gradually tapers from ground level to the crown. Leaf-stalks are sharply toothed throughout their length, and the fan-shaped, bright green blades, to

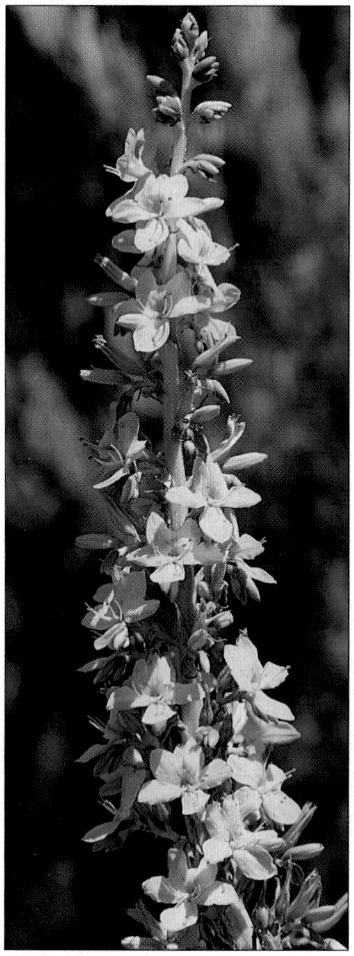

Wachendorfia thyrsiflora

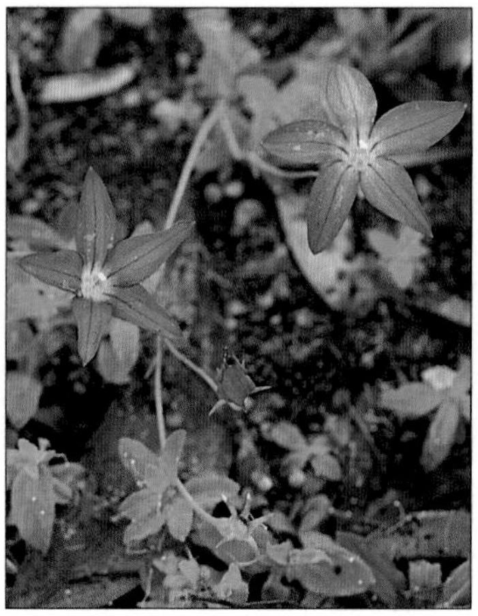

Wahlenbergia gloriosa

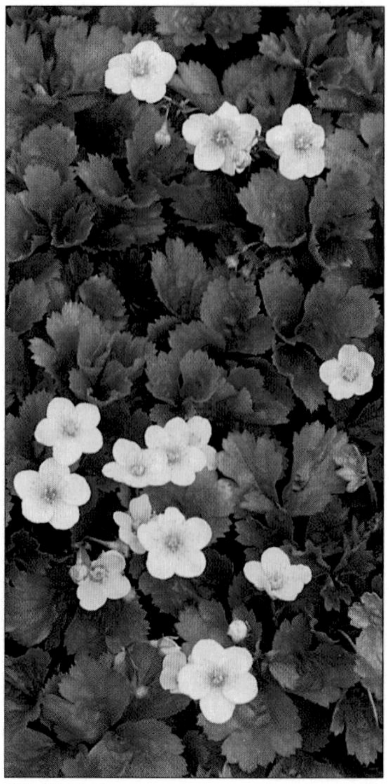

Waldsteinia ternata

W

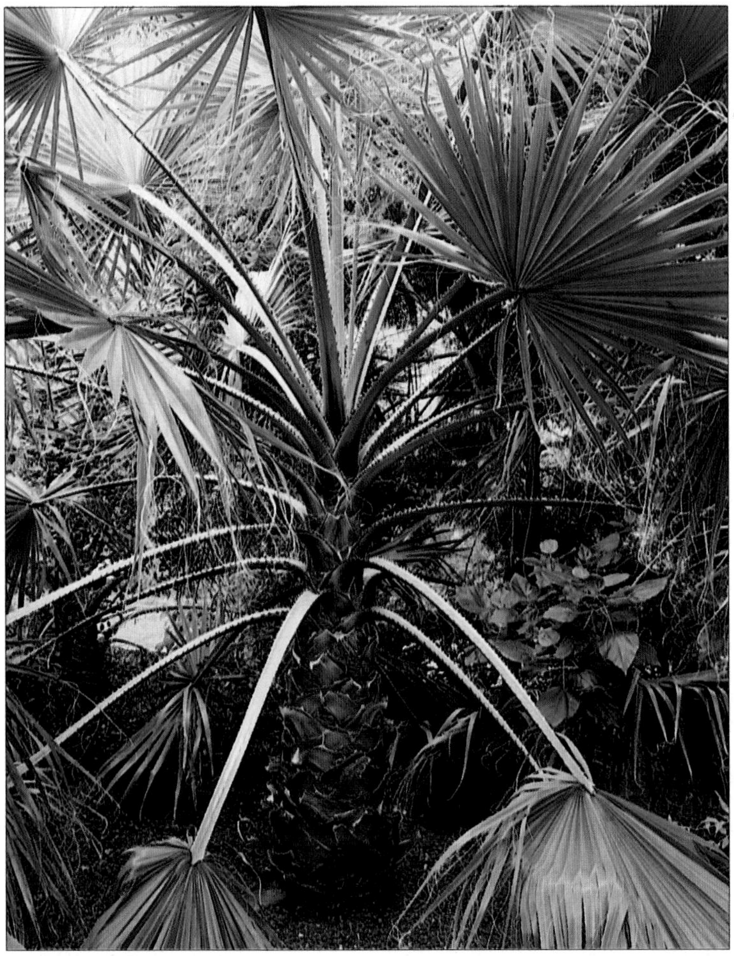

Washingtonia robusta

1m (3ft) long, have arching lobe tips, with inconspicuous or no filaments. Dead foliage forms a shaggy skirt that clothes the trunk. Tubular, creamy pink flowers are borne in panicles to 3m (10ft) long, usually in summer. Suitable for coastal gardens. ↕ to 25m (80ft), ↔ 2.5–5m (8–15ft). N. Mexico. ❀ (min. 8–10°C/46–50°F)

▷ **Washingtonia, Northern** see *Washingtonia filifera*
▷ **Water fringe** see *Nymphoides peltata*
▷ **Water lily** see *Nymphaea*
  Amazon see *Victoria amazonica*
  Australian see *Nymphaea gigantea*
  Cape blue see *Nymphaea capensis*
  Egyptian see *Nymphaea lotus*
  Giant see *Victoria*
  Royal see *Victoria amazonica*
  Santa Cruz see *Victoria cruziana*
  White see *Nymphaea alba*
  Yellow see *Nymphaea mexicana*
▷ **Watermint** see *Mentha aquatica*
▷ **Water shield, Carolina** see *Cabomba caroliniana*
▷ **Water soldier** see *Stratiotes aloides*

WATSONIA

IRIDACEAE

Genus of approximately 60 species of cormous perennials, usually found on rocky or grassy slopes and plateaux in South Africa and Madagascar. They have erect, usually sword-shaped, basal leaves, and are cultivated for their showy spikes of horizontal, tubular, red, orange, pink, or white flowers, with curved tubes and 6 tepal lobes; the flowers are borne on erect stems at various times of the year. They are only suitable for outdoor cultivation in regions where there is little or no frost. In frost-prone areas, grow in a cool greenhouse or conservatory; spring- and summer-growing species may be grown in a border outdoors, and lifted in autumn for storage in a dry, frost-free place.

• **HARDINESS** Half hardy.

• **CULTIVATION** Under glass, grow in loam-based potting compost (JI No.2), with added sharp sand and leaf mould, in full sun. In growth, water freely and apply a balanced liquid fertilizer every month. Keep just moist when dormant. Outdoors, grow in light, well-drained soil that does not dry out in summer. Where frost is likely, protect with a dry winter mulch.

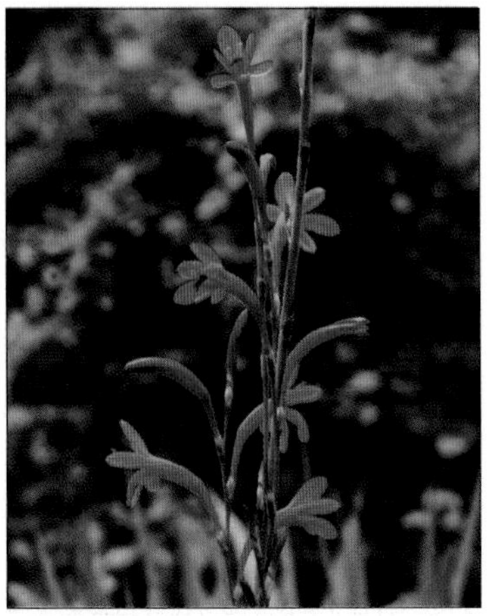

Watsonia pillansii

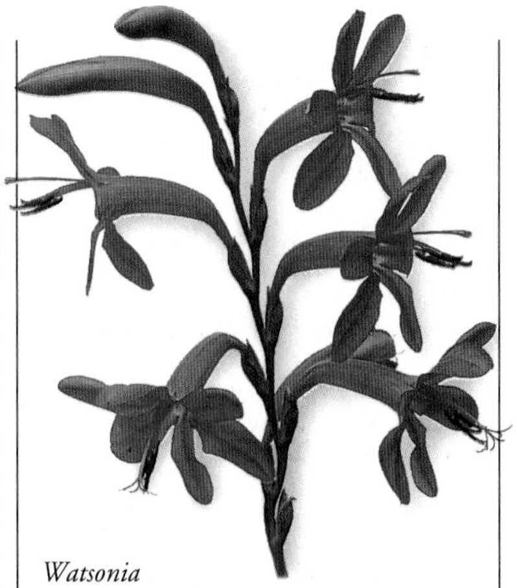

Watsonia 'Stanford Scarlet'

• **PROPAGATION** Sow seed at 13–18°C (55–64°F) in autumn. Divide in spring.

• **PESTS AND DISEASES** Trouble free.

W. aletroides. Clump-forming, cormous perennial with sword-shaped, glossy leaves, 20–40cm (8–16in) long, overtopped from late winter to spring by unbranched spikes of up to 12 tubular, orange-red flowers, 5cm (2in) long, the tepal lobes not spreading. ↕ 60cm (24in), ↔ 10cm (4in). South Africa (Western Cape). ✻

W. ardernei see *W. borbonica* subsp. *ardernei.*

W. beatricis see *W. pillansii.*

W. borbonica, syn. *W. pyramidata.* Clump-forming, cormous perennial with narrowly sword-shaped leaves, to 75cm (30in) long. In summer, bears branched spikes of up to 20 slightly irregular, bright pink flowers, 3cm (1¼in) long, with spreading tepal lobes and white lines at the base of each tepal. ↕ 1–1.5m (3–5ft), ↔ 10cm (4in). South Africa (Western Cape). ✻. **subsp. *ardernei***, syn. *W. ardernei*, has usually white, rarely pink flowers.

W. bulbillifera see *W. meriana* 'Bulbillifera'.

W. fourcadei. Robust, clump-forming, cormous perennial with sword-shaped leaves, 30–60cm (12–24in) long. Dense, branched spikes of 20–40 tubular, pink, orange, or red flowers, 6cm (2½in) long, are produced in spring and summer. ↕ 1.5m (5ft), ↔ 10cm (4in). South Africa (Western Cape). ✻

W. humilis. Slender, clump-forming, cormous perennial with lance-shaped leaves, to 30cm (12in) long. In spring or early summer, produces unbranched spikes of up to 12 tubular flowers, 3–4.5cm (1¼–1¾in) long, either white with pink outside, or pink with darker pink outside. ↕ 30cm (12in), ↔ 8cm (3in). South Africa (Western Cape). ✻

W. marginata. Clump-forming, cormous perennial with sword-shaped leaves, 75cm (30in) long. From spring to early summer, bears dense, branched spikes of few to many tubular, mauve-pink flowers, 2cm (¾in) long, with spreading tepal lobes and white and purple markings. ↕ to 2m (6ft), ↔ 15cm (6in). South Africa (Western Cape). ✻

W. meriana. Clump-forming, cormous perennial with sword-shaped leaves, 30–60cm (12–24in) long. In summer, produces branched spikes of up to 25 tubular flowers, 2–2.5cm (¾–1in) long, with spreading tepal lobes, in bright rose-red, rarely scarlet or white. ↕ 0.5–2m (1¾–6ft), ↔ 15cm (6in). South Africa. (Eastern Cape, Western Cape, KwaZulu/Natal). ✻. **'Bulbillifera'**, syn. *W. bulbillifera*, has flowers 3cm (1¼in) long, and produces bulbils among the flower spikes.

W. pillansii ■ syn. *W. beatricis.* Slender, clump-forming, cormous perennial producing sword-shaped leaves, 25–60cm (10–24in) long. From summer to autumn, bears branched spikes of 20–25 tubular, bright orange to orange-red flowers, to 5cm (2in) long, with spreading tepal lobes. ↕ 50–120cm (20–48in), ↔ 10cm (4in). South Africa (Western Cape, Eastern Cape, KwaZulu/Natal, Eastern Transvaal). ✻

W. pyramidata see *W. borbonica.*

***W.* 'Stanford Scarlet'** ■ Slender, clump-forming, cormous perennial with sword-shaped leaves, 40–100cm (16–39in) long. Bears unbranched spikes of 10–12 tubular, orange-scarlet flowers, 3cm (1¼in) long, with spreading tepal lobes, in late spring or summer. ↕ 0.8–1.4m (32–54in), ↔ 15cm (6in). ✻

▷ ***Wattakaka*** see *Dregea*
  W. sinensis see *D. sinensis*
▷ **Wattle** see *Acacia*
  Black see *Acacia mearnsii*
  Cape see *Albizia lophantha*
  Cootamundra see *Acacia baileyana*
  Drummond's see *Acacia drummondii*
  Early black see *Acacia decurrens*
  Green see *Acacia decurrens*
  Hedge see *Acacia paradoxa*
  Knife-leaf see *Acacia cultriformis*
  Ovens see *Acacia pravissima*
  Queensland silver see *Acacia podalyriifolia*
  Silver see *Acacia dealbata, A. retinodes*
  Swamp see *Acacia retinodes, Albizia lophantha*
  White sallow see *Acacia floribunda*
▷ **Wax flower** see *Eriostemon, Hoya, Jamesia americana*
  Long-leaf see *Eriostemon myoporoides*
  Philippine see *Etlingera elatior*
  Pink see *Eriostemon australasius*
▷ **Wax, Geraldton** see *Chamelaucium uncinatum*
▷ **Wax plant** see *Hoya carnosa*
▷ **Wax tree** see *Rhus succedanea*
▷ **Wayfaring tree** see *Viburnum lantana*
▷ **Weather prophet** see *Dimorphotheca pluvialis*

WEBEROCEREUS

CACTACEAE

Genus of about 5 species of climbing or pendent, epiphytic or rock-dwelling, perennial cacti from mostly rainforest habitats in Mexico, Guatemala, Nicaragua, Costa Rica, and Panama. They have aerial roots and spiny, fleshy stems that may be 3- or 4-angled, slender and cylindrical, or flat and leaf-like with scalloped margins. Nocturnal, cup- or funnel-shaped, pink or greenish or yellowish white flowers are produced in midsummer, followed by spherical to oblong, warty fruits with short, spiny or hairy areoles. Where temperatures drop below 15°C (59°F), grow in a warm greenhouse; in warmer climates, use outdoors in a courtyard garden or against a wall.

• **HARDINESS** Frost tender.

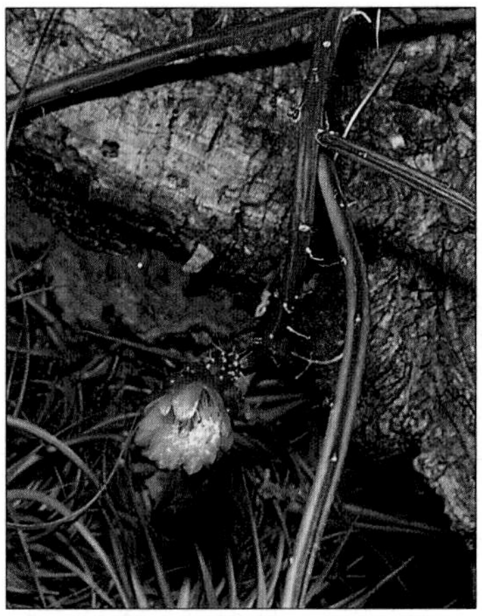

Weberocereus biolleyi

• **CULTIVATION** Under glass, grow in epiphytic cactus compost, with added leaf mould, in bright filtered light and high humidity. From spring to early autumn, water freely, apply a half-strength, balanced liquid fertilizer every 4 or 5 weeks, and mist daily with tepid water. Keep just moist at other times. Outdoors, grow in gritty, moderately fertile, sharply drained soil in partial shade. See also pp.48–49.
• **PROPAGATION** Sow seed at 19–24°C (66–75°F), or take cuttings of stem sections, both in spring or summer.
• **PESTS AND DISEASES** Scale insects may attack plants if left dry.

W. biolleyi ■ Mainly pendent cactus with cylindrical or irregularly 4-angled stems, 5mm (¼in) thick, sometimes branching. Small, white-woolly areoles occasionally bear 1–3 very short, fine yellow spines. Funnel-shaped, whitish pink flowers, 3–5cm (1¼–2in) long, with dark pink outer petals, are borne in midsummer. ↕ 80cm (32in), ↔ 30cm (12in). Costa Rica. ⊛ (min. 15°C/59°F)
W. bradei, syn. *Eccremocactus bradei.* Pendent cactus with flat, leaf-like, wavy-margined, jointed branches, to 10cm (4in) across; these produce small, pale brown-woolly areoles, each with one dark brown spine. Funnel-shaped white flowers, 6–7cm (2½–3in) long, with slightly expanding, fleshy petals, pale pink outside, are borne from the upper areoles from spring to autumn. ↕↔ 60cm (24in). Costa Rica. ⊛ (min. 15°C/59°F)
W. glaber, syn. *Werckleocereus glaber.* Climbing cactus with 3-angled, toothed, pale green stems, 2.5–4.5cm (1–1¾in) thick. Small, brown-woolly areoles bear 2–4 yellow or brown spines. Cup-shaped white flowers, 10–12cm (4–5in) long, with pale greenish brown outer petals, are borne in midsummer. ↕ 3m (10ft), ↔ 60cm (24in). Mexico, Guatemala, Costa Rica. ⊛ (min. 15°C/59°F)

WEDELIA

ASTERACEAE/COMPOSITAE

Genus of about 70 species of erect, prostrate, or climbing, hairy annuals, evergreen perennials and soft-stemmed or woody shrubs, found near coasts in tropical and subtropical regions. They have opposite, usually oblong to elliptic or obovate, toothed or lobed leaves, and are grown for their daisy-like yellow flowerheads, borne either singly or in few-headed clusters in summer. In frost-

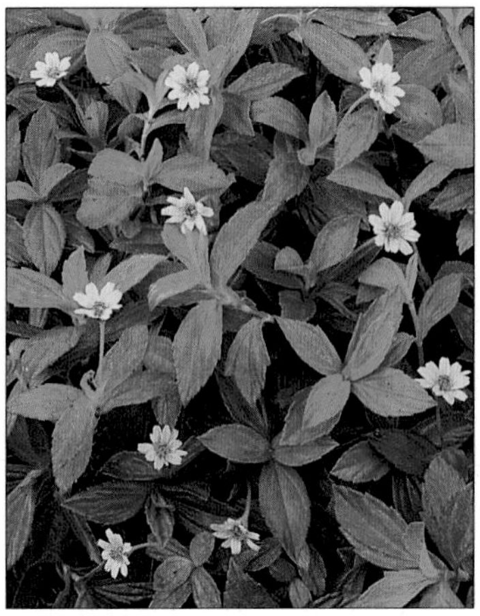

Wedelia trilobata

prone areas, grow as houseplants, or in a warm greenhouse, or use outdoors in summer in containers. In warmer areas, *W. trilobata* is a rampant ground-cover plant, and is also useful for growing in dry shade under trees.
• **HARDINESS** Frost tender.
• **CULTIVATION** Grow in any well-drained soil or potting compost.
• **PROPAGATION** Sow seed at 18°C (64°F), divide, or root stem-tip cuttings, at any time.
• **PESTS AND DISEASES** Trouble free.

W. trilobata ■ Creeping, evergreen perennial, rooting at the leaf nodes and spreading widely. The elliptic or obovate, mid- to dark green leaves, 12cm (5in) long, are usually 3-lobed, sometimes entire or barely lobed. Solitary, daisy-like yellow flowerheads, 2cm (¾in) across, are borne from late spring to autumn. ↕ 15–20cm (6–8in), ↔ 2m (6ft) or more. USA (Florida), West Indies, Central America, tropical South America. ⊛ (min. 13°C/55°F)

▷ **Weeping willow** see *Salix babylonica*
Golden see *Salix* x *sepulcralis* 'Chrysocoma'

WEIGELA

CAPRIFOLIACEAE

Genus of 12 species of mostly spreading to upright, deciduous shrubs found in scrub and woodland margins in E. Asia. They have opposite, oblong to ovate or elliptic, toothed leaves, usually up to 10cm (4in) long. Weigelas are cultivated for their showy, bell- to funnel-shaped, pink to red, sometimes white or yellow flowers; these are usually 4cm (1½in) long, and are borne singly or in corymbs or cymes of 3 or 4, usually on short lateral twigs on the previous year's branches. Suitable for a mixed or shrub border, or for open woodland.
• **HARDINESS** Fully hardy.
• **CULTIVATION** Grow in any fertile, well-drained soil in full sun or partial shade. Pruning group 2.
• **PROPAGATION** Sow seed in containers in a cold frame in autumn; weigelas hybridize readily, so seed may not come true. Root greenwood cuttings in early summer; semi-ripe cuttings with bottom heat in midsummer; hardwood cuttings from autumn to winter.
• **PESTS AND DISEASES** Leaves may be attacked by leaf and bud eelworm, and honey fungus.

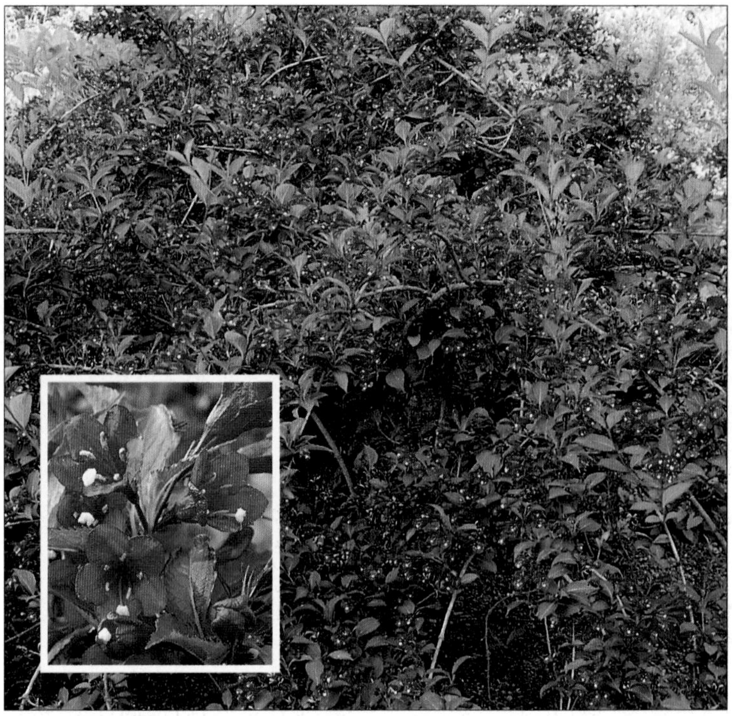

Weigela 'Eva Rathke' (inset: flower detail)

***W.* 'Abel Carrière'** ♀ Spreading shrub with oval, dark green leaves. Bell-shaped, dark pinkish red flowers, with yellow-spotted throats, open from purple-red buds in late spring and early summer. ↕↔ 2m (6ft). ❄❄❄
***W.* 'Briant Rubidor'**, syn. *W.* 'Olympiade'. Spreading shrub with oval, leaves, to 8cm (3in) long, yellow-green at first, turning bright yellow or sometimes becoming margined with yellow. In late spring and early summer, bears bell-shaped, dark ruby-red flowers, 3cm (1¼in) long. Best in partial shade. ↕↔ 2m (6ft). ❄❄❄
***W.* 'Bristol Ruby'.** Vigorous, upright shrub with oval, dark green leaves and usually bell-shaped, dark red flowers, opening from very dark red buds, in late spring and early summer. ↕ 2.5m (8ft), ↔ 2m (6ft). ❄❄❄
***W.* 'Bristol Snowflake'** see *W.* 'Snowflake'.
***W.* 'Candida'.** Spreading, bushy shrub with oval, bright green leaves and bell-shaped, pure white flowers, borne in late spring and early summer. ↕↔ 2.5m (8ft). ❄❄❄
***W.* 'Carnaval'.** Vigorous, upright shrub with oval, dark green leaves, to 10cm

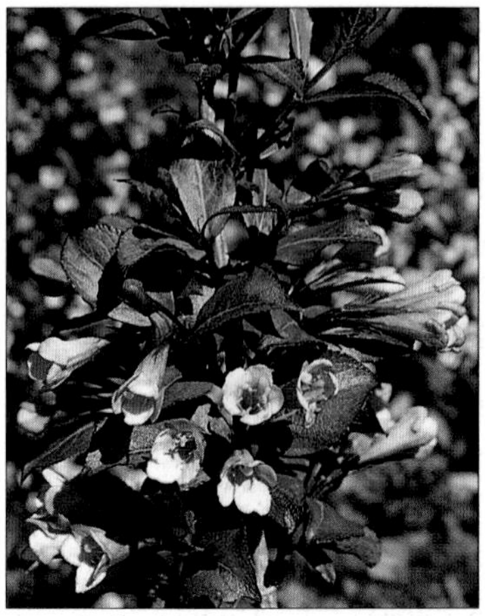

Weigela florida 'Foliis Purpureis'

(4in) or more long. Bell-shaped flowers, to 5cm (2in) long, in a combination of pale pink, white, and dark pink, are borne in late spring and early summer. ↕ 2.5m (8ft), ↔ 2m (6ft). ❄❄❄
***W.* 'Eva Rathke'** ■ Compact, upright shrub with oval, dark green leaves and broadly funnel-shaped, dark crimson flowers, opening from dark red buds in late spring and early summer. ↕↔ 1.5m (5ft). ❄❄❄
W. florida. Spreading shrub with arching shoots and oval, tapered, dark green leaves. Produces corymbs of funnel-shaped, dark pink flowers, 3cm (1¼in) long, pale pink to nearly white inside, in late spring and early summer. ↕↔ 2.5m (8ft). N. China, Korea. ❄❄❄.
'Foliis Purpureis' ■ ♀ has bronze-

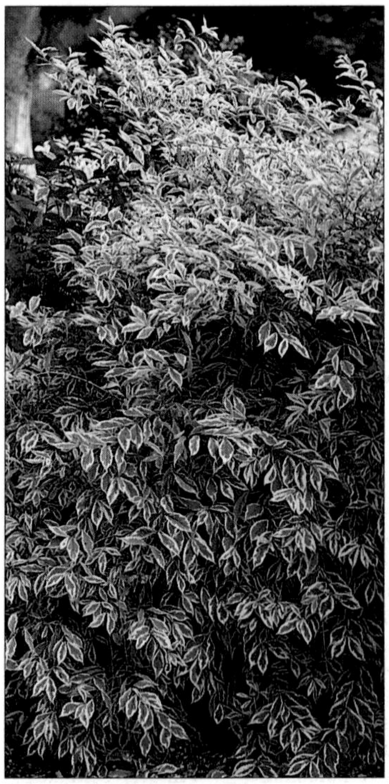

Weigela florida 'Variegata'

W

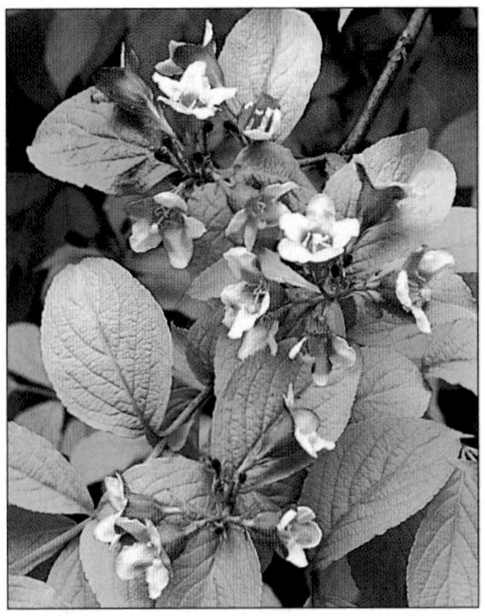

Weigela 'Looymansii Aurea'

green foliage; ↕ 1m (3ft), ↔ 1.5m (5ft).
'Variegata' ■ 🏆 is compact, with white-margined, grey-green leaves; ↕↔ 2–2.5m (6–9ft).
***W.* 'Looymansii Aurea'** ■ Slow-growing, spreading shrub with arching shoots and oval, golden yellow leaves, 8cm (3in) long, narrowly margined with red. Bears bell-shaped, pale pink flowers in late spring and early summer. Best in partial shade. ↕↔ 1.5m (5ft). ❄❄❄
W. middendorffiana. Upright shrub with oval, bright green leaves, to 8cm (3in) long. Bell-shaped, pale yellow flowers, often with conspicuous, orange or red throat markings, are borne in terminal cymes from mid-spring to midsummer. ↕↔ 1.5m (5ft). N.E. Russia, N. China, Korea, Japan. ❄❄❄
***W.* 'Minuet'.** Compact, spreading shrub with oval, bronze-green leaves, to 8cm (3in) long. Bears bell-shaped, slightly fragrant, dark pink flowers, with yellow throats, in late spring and early summer. ↕ 75cm (30in), ↔ 1.2m (4ft). ❄❄❄
***W.* 'Olympiade'** see *W.* 'Briant Rubidor'.
W. praecox. Upright shrub with oval, dark green leaves, hairy beneath. In late spring and early summer, bears corymbs of funnel-shaped, fragrant pink flowers with yellow throats. ↕ 2.5m (8ft), ↔ 2m (6ft). N.E. Russia, Korea, Japan. ❄❄❄.
'Variegata' 🏆 has leaves with creamy yellow margins that turn white with age.
***W.* 'Snowflake'**, syn. *W.* 'Bristol Snowflake'. Spreading shrub with ovate, dark green leaves and bell-shaped, pure white flowers, borne profusely in late spring and early summer. ↕ 1.2m (4ft), ↔ 1.5m (5ft). ❄❄❄

▷ ***Weingartia*** see *Rebutia*
W. neocumingii see *R. neocumingii*

WELDENIA

COMMELINACEAE

Genus of one species of tuberous perennial occurring in the mountains of Mexico and Guatemala. *W. candida* is grown for its rosettes of large, simple leaves and its stalkless cymes of cup-shaped white flowers. Grow in a raised bed; in regions with cool, damp winters, it is best grown in an alpine house.
• **HARDINESS** Frost hardy.
• **CULTIVATION** Grow in gritty, moderately fertile, sharply drained soil in full sun. Protect from winter wet. In an alpine house, grow in deep containers in a mix of equal parts loam, leaf mould,

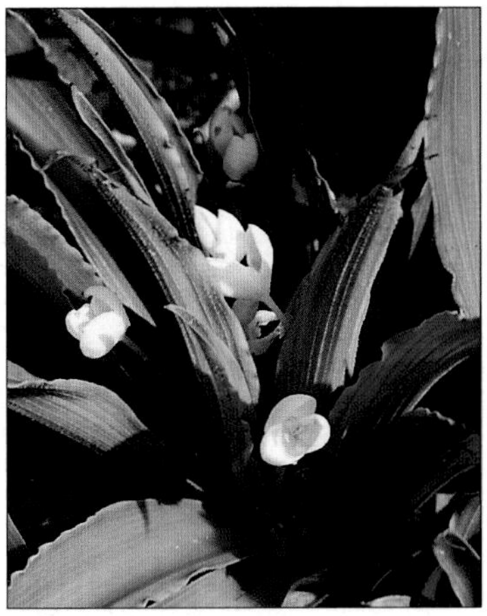

Weldenia candida

and grit. Water freely in growth; reduce water as leaves wither, and keep barely moist when dormant in winter. Repot annually in autumn.
• **PROPAGATION** Sow seed as soon as ripe in containers in a cold frame. Divide in spring. Take root cuttings in winter.
• **PESTS AND DISEASES** Aphids and whiteflies may be a problem under glass.

W. candida ■ Tuberous perennial with rosettes of lance-shaped, pointed, wavy-margined, slightly leathery leaves, 5–20cm (2–8in) long. In late spring and early summer, bears a long succession of upright, cup-shaped, pure white flowers, to 3cm (1¼in) across. ↕↔ to 15cm (6in). Mexico, Guatemala. ❄❄

▷ **Wellingtonia** see *Sequoiadendron giganteum*

WELWITSCHIA

WELWITSCHIACEAE

Genus of one species of prostrate, dioecious, evergreen perennial from deserts, mainly coastal, in Angola and Namibia. It has a large but relatively shallow tap root with many lateral roots just below ground level. The fleshy, leathery, mid- or grey-green leaves are strap-shaped, and the inflorescences are cone-like. In their natural habitat, male plants produce masses of pollen, which is carried on the wind to female plants. In summer, females can produce up to 100 conical to spherical floral cones, but there is no record of welwitschias blooming in cultivation, except in botanic gardens. Where temperatures

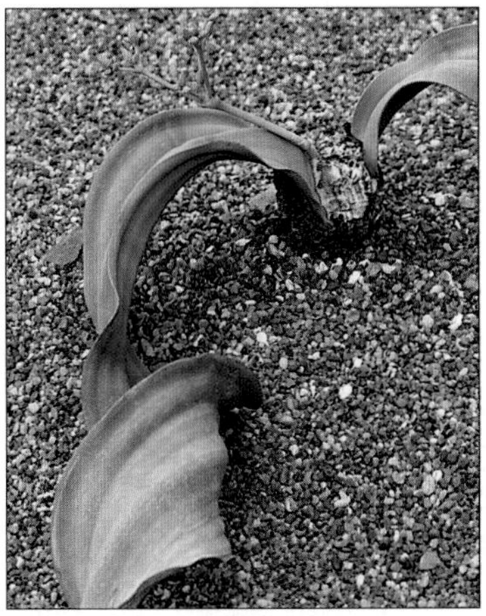

Welwitschia mirabilis

drop below 19°C (66°F), grow in a warm greenhouse; in warmer climates, use in a desert garden. Its adaptation to the extreme conditions of its natural habitat means it is difficult to cultivate.
• **HARDINESS** Frost tender.
• **CULTIVATION** Under glass, grow in a mixture of 2 parts sharp, granitic sand and 1 part each loam-based potting compost (JI No.2), peat, and leaf mould. Provide full light and low humidity. Grow in deep containers, or in a clay drainpipe, and top-dress with crushed limestone. From spring to autumn, water moderately and apply a balanced liquid fertilizer every 6–8 weeks. Keep completely dry in winter. Outdoors, grow in gritty, poor, sharply drained soil, with added leaf mould, in full sun. See also pp.48–49.
• **PROPAGATION** Sow seed at 19–24°C (66–75°F) as soon as ripe; sow in tall, narrow containers that allow for the growth of the tap root.
• **PESTS AND DISEASES** Trouble free.

W. bainesii see *W. mirabilis.*
W. mirabilis ■ syn. *W. bainesii.* Prostrate, dioecious, evergreen perennial with a short, conical caudex becoming swollen with age, often 1m (3ft) across in very old plants, and divided in half by a groove. The 2 strap-shaped, often curling, leathery, fleshy, mid- or grey-green leaves, 2m (6ft) or more long, grow from marginal grooves on the crown. Cones are produced in axillary cymes from the top of the caudex in summer: female cones, 5cm (2in) long, are brownish green; male cones, 3cm (1¼in) long, are reddish brown. ↕ 45cm (18in) or more, ↔ 4m (12ft). Angola, Namibia. ❀ (min. 19°C/66°F)

▷ ***Werckleocereus glaber*** see *Weberocereus glaber*

WESTRINGIA

LABIATAE/LAMIACEAE

Genus of about 25 species of rounded to erect, evergreen shrubs from dry coastal heathland, scrub, sands, and dry forest in Australia. They are cultivated for their flowers and foliage. The crowded, narrowly linear to ovate, rosemary-like leaves are produced in whorls of 3–5. The tubular, white to pale blue or mauve flowers are 2-lipped, the upper lip longer, erect and 2-lobed, the lower lip divided into 3 spreading lobes; the flowers are borne singly in the uppermost leaf axils or in terminal clusters. In frost-prone areas, grow in a cool greenhouse. In milder regions, use in a border, or as a hedge or screen.
• **HARDINESS** Frost tender, although some species (including *W. fruticosa*) may survive short spells just below 0°C (32°F).
• **CULTIVATION** Under glass, grow in loam-based potting compost (JI No.2), with added leaf mould and sharp sand, in full light. When in growth, water moderately and apply a balanced liquid fertilizer monthly. Water sparingly in winter. Outdoors, grow in moderately fertile, moist but well-drained soil in full sun. Pruning group 9; trim hedges in late spring and late summer. May need restrictive pruning under glass.
• **PROPAGATION** Sow seed at 13–18°C (55–64°F) in spring. Root greenwood

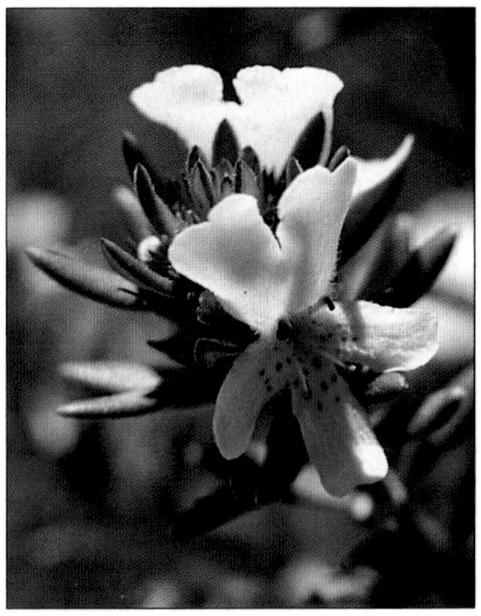

Westringia fruticosa

cuttings in early summer, or semi-ripe cuttings with bottom heat in midsummer.
• **PESTS AND DISEASES** Trouble free.

W. fruticosa ■ 🏆 syn. *W. rosmariniformis* (Australian rosemary). Erect, bushy, rounded shrub, at least when young, becoming more open as it matures, with linear to narrowly lance-shaped leaves, 1.5–2.5cm (½–1in) long, mid- to deep green above, white-felted beneath. Solitary, tubular, white to very pale blue flowers, 1.5cm (½in) across, with darker freckling in the throats, are borne in axillary cymes from late spring to early autumn. ↕↔ 1–1.5m (3–5ft). Australia (coastal New South Wales). ❀ (min. 5°C/41°F)
W. rosmariniformis see *W. fruticosa.*

▷ **Whauwhaupaku** see *Pseudopanax arboreus*
▷ **Wheat, Puffed** see *Briza maxima*
▷ **Wheatgrass, Intermediate** see *Elymus hispidus*
▷ **Whin** see *Ulex europaeus*
▷ **Whinberry** see *Vaccinium myrtillus*
▷ **Whitebeam** see *Sorbus aria*
Swedish see *S. intermedia*
▷ **White cup** see *Nierembergia repens*
▷ **White paint brush** see *Haemanthus albiflos*
▷ **White pine,**
Eastern see *Pinus strobus*
Japanese see *Pinus parviflora*
Mexican see *Pinus ayacahuite*
Western see *Pinus monticola*
▷ **Whitethorn, Coast** see *Ceanothus incanus*
▷ **White trumpet** see *Sarracenia leucophylla*
▷ **Whitey wood** see *Acradenia frankliniae*
▷ **Whitlow-wort** see *Paronychia*
▷ **Whorlflower** see *Morina longifolia*
▷ **Whortleberry** see *Vaccinium, V. myrtillus*
Caucasian see *V. arctostaphylos*
Red see *V. parvifolium*
▷ **Widow's tears** see *Commelina*

WIGANDIA

HYDROPHYLLACEAE

Genus of 5 species of evergreen, upright to spreading perennials, subshrubs, shrubs, and small trees occurring in woodland and roadsides in tropical USA, Central America, and South America. They are cultivated for their flowers and foliage. The large, alternate,

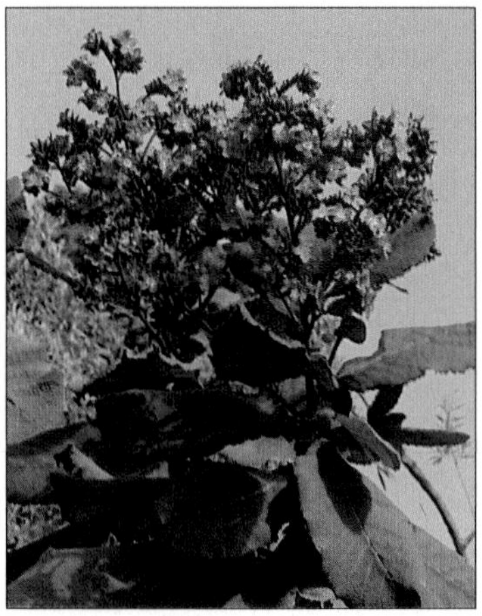

Wigandia caracasana

simple, oblong to broadly ovate, toothed leaves are covered in stinging hairs. Tubular-based, bell-shaped, usually lilac to violet flowers, with 5 broad, wide-spreading lobes, are borne in terminal panicles. Where temperatures fall below 5–7°C (41–45°F) in winter, grow in a cool or temperate greenhouse or use as annuals for summer bedding. In milder regions, grow as specimen plants. Contact with foliage may aggravate skin allergies.
• **HARDINESS** Frost tender.
• **CULTIVATION** Under glass, grow in loam-based potting compost (JI No.2) in full light. During the growing season, water moderately and apply a balanced liquid fertilizer monthly. Water sparingly in winter. Outdoors, grow in fertile, moist but well-drained soil in full sun. Pruning group 1; may need restrictive pruning under glass.
• **PROPAGATION** Sow seed at 13–18°C (55–64°F) in spring. Take greenwood cuttings in early summer.
• **PESTS AND DISEASES** Red spider mites may be troublesome under glass.

W. caracasana ▣ syn. *W. macrophylla.* Open, soft-stemmed, evergreen sub-shrub with robust, sparsely branched, yellow- to white-woolly stems. Long-stalked, ovate, coarsely toothed leaves, 30–60cm (12–24in) long, heart-shaped at the bases, are mid- to deep green above, hoary beneath. Bears bell-shaped, white-tubed, light violet flowers, 2cm (¾in) across, in large, terminal panicles, to 30cm (12in) or more long, mainly in summer. ↕ 3–4m (10–12ft), ↔ 2–3.5m (6–11ft). Mexico to Colombia. ❀ (min. 7°C/45°F)
W. macrophylla see *W. caracasana.*

▷ ***Wigginsia*** see *Parodia*
W. erinacea see *P. erinacea*
W. vorwerkiana see *P. erinacea*

WIKSTROEMIA

THYMELAEACEAE

Genus of approximately 70 species of deciduous or evergreen, spreading to upright shrubs and trees, closely related to *Daphne.* They are usually found in habitats ranging from dry slopes to wet woodland in mountainous areas from the Himalayas to E. Asia, Sri Lanka, Australia, and the Pacific islands. The alternate or opposite leaves are oblong-lance-shaped to broadly ovate. Tubular or salverform, usually yellow flowers are produced in terminal spikes, racemes, cymes, or, occasionally, panicles. They are seldom cultivated, but *W. canescens,* valued for its flowers, will grow in a sheltered position in a woodland garden. In frost-prone areas, grow the tender species in a cool or temperate greenhouse.
• **HARDINESS** Fully hardy to frost tender.
• **CULTIVATION** Grow in any well-drained soil in full sun to partial shade. In frost-prone areas, shelter from cold, drying winds. Pruning group 1.
• **PROPAGATION** Sow seed in containers in a cold frame in autumn.
• **PESTS AND DISEASES** Trouble free.

W. canescens. Upright, deciduous shrub with slender, arching shoots. Alternate to nearly opposite, elliptic leaves are up to 8cm (3in) long. In late summer and early autumn, purple flower buds open to tubular, yellow to greenish yellow flowers, 1.5cm (½in) long, each with a slender, slightly curved tube and 4 short lobes, in terminal cymes. ↕ 1.8m (6ft), ↔ 1.5m (5ft). Sri Lanka, Himalayas, China. ✲✲

▷ ***Wilcoxia albiflora*** see *Echinocereus leucanthus*
▷ ***Wilcoxia schmollii*** see *Echinocereus schmollii*
▷ **Wild flowers** see p.43
▷ **Wild Irishman** see *Discaria toumatou*
▷ **Wild Spaniard** see *Aciphylla colensoi*
▷ **Willow** see *Salix*
Bay see *Salix pentandra*
Coyote see *Salix exigua*
Crack see *Salix fragilis*
Creeping see *Salix repens*
Cricket-bat see *Salix alba* var. *caerulea*
Desert see *Pittosporum phillyreoides*
Golden see *Salix alba* var. *vitellina*
Golden weeping see *Salix* x *sepulcralis* 'Chrysocoma'
Hoary see *Salix elaeagnos*
Kilmarnock see *Salix caprea* 'Kilmarnock'
Musk see *Salix aegyptiaca*
Silver see *Salix alba* var. *sericea*
Swiss see *Salix helvetica*
Thyme-leaved see *Salix serpyllifolia*
Violet see *Salix daphnoides*
Weeping see *Salix babylonica*
White see *Salix alba*
Woolly see *Salix lanata*
▷ **Willow-bell** see *Campanula persicifolia* var. *planiflora*
▷ **Willow herb** see *Epilobium*

x WILSONARA

ORCHIDACEAE

Hybrid genus of evergreen orchids, derived from crosses between *Cochlioda, Odontoglossum,* and *Oncidium.* Conical, flattened pseudobulbs grow from a rhizome, each pseudobulb producing 1 or 2 soft, linear to lance-shaped leaves at its apex. The inflorescences, either tall panicles with 100 or more flowers, or shorter panicles of larger flowers, are produced from the bases of the pseudobulbs. The rounded, sometimes star-shaped flowers are very variably coloured, often having conspicuous markings.
• **HARDINESS** Frost tender.
• **CULTIVATION** Cool-growing orchids. Grow in epiphytic orchid compost in

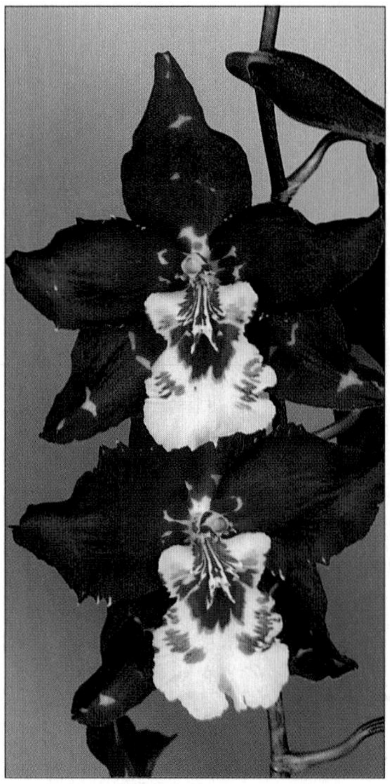

x *Wilsonara* Hambühren Stern 'Cheam'

containers that restrict the roots. In summer, provide bright filtered light and high humidity, water freely, applying a fertilizer at every third watering, and mist twice daily. In winter, admit full light, water sparingly, provide moderate humidity, and mist daily. See also p.46.
• **PROPAGATION** Divide when plants fill their containers and "flow" over the sides.
• **PESTS AND DISEASES** Aphids, red spider mites, and mealybugs may be a problem.

x *W.* Hambühren Stern 'Cheam' ▣ (*Oncidium tigrinum* x x *Odontioda* Lippestern). Evergreen orchid with 1 or 2 linear leaves, 23cm (9in) long. Almost circular flowers, 6cm (2½in) across, are rich brown and yellow, and are borne in long panicles at any time of year. ↕ 60cm (24in), ↔ 30cm (12in). ❀ (min. 10°C/50°F; max. 30°C/86°F)

▷ **Windflower** see *Anemone, A. nemorosa, Zephyranthes*
▷ **Winecups** see *Geissorhiza radians*
▷ **Wing nut** see *Pterocarya*
Caucasian see *P. fraxinifolia*
Chinese see *P. stenoptera*
Japanese see *P. rhoifolia*
▷ ***Wintera aromatica*** see *Drimys winteri*
▷ **Winter aconite** see *Eranthis, E. hyemalis*
▷ **Winterberry** see *Ilex verticillata*
Japanese see *Ilex serrata*
▷ **Wintergreen** see *Gaultheria procumbens, Pyrola*
Round-leaved see *Pyrola rotundifolia*
▷ **Winter heath** see *Erica carnea*
▷ **Winter's bark** see *Drimys winteri*
▷ **Wintersweet** see *Acokanthera oblongifolia, Chimonanthus, C. praecox*
▷ **Wire-netting bush** see *Corokia cotoneaster*
▷ **Wishbone flower** see *Torenia, T. fournieri*
▷ **Wistaria** see *Wisteria*

WISTERIA

Wistaria

LEGUMINOSAE/PAPILIONACEAE

Genus of about 10 species of twining, woody, deciduous climbers found in moist woodland and on streambanks in China, Korea, Japan, and C. and S. USA. They have alternate, pinnate, dark green leaves, to 35cm (14in) or more long, with ovate to lance-shaped or elliptic leaflets. They are cultivated for their showy, pea-like, fragrant flowers, borne in usually pendent racemes in spring or summer, followed by pendent, bean-like green seed pods. Train against a wall, into a tree, over an arch or pergola, or as a free-standing half-standard. The stems twine anticlockwise around the support. All parts may cause severe discomfort if ingested.
• **HARDINESS** Fully hardy, but flower buds may be damaged by late frosts.
• **CULTIVATION** Grow in fertile, moist but well-drained soil in full sun or partial shade. Wisterias growing into trees need no training. To train formally, after planting, prune back the leading shoot to 75–90cm (30–36in) above ground level. During the first growing season, tie in lateral shoots to the framework and cut back sublaterals to 2 or 3 buds. In the first winter, cut back laterals by one-third of their length, and sublaterals to 2 or 3 buds; cut back the leading shoot again, to 75–90cm (30–36in) above the point from which the topmost laterals branch. In subsequent years, repeat the pruning of the leader and selection of lateral shoots until the framework has been completed. Once established, in late summer cut back all shoots not needed to extend the framework, to within 15cm (6in) of the main branches; leave 4–6 leaves on each shoot. In midwinter, reduce these spurs further to 8–10cm (3–4in), leaving only 2 or 3 buds.
• **PROPAGATION** Take basal cuttings from sideshoots in early to midsummer and root with bottom heat. Layer in autumn, or graft in winter.
• **PESTS AND DISEASES** May be attacked by leaf spot, aphids, honey fungus, and brown scale.

W. brachybotrys (Silky wisteria). Twining climber with pinnate, softly hairy leaves, to 35cm (14in) long, each composed of 9–13 ovate to lance-shaped leaflets. Pea-like, fragrant, yellow-

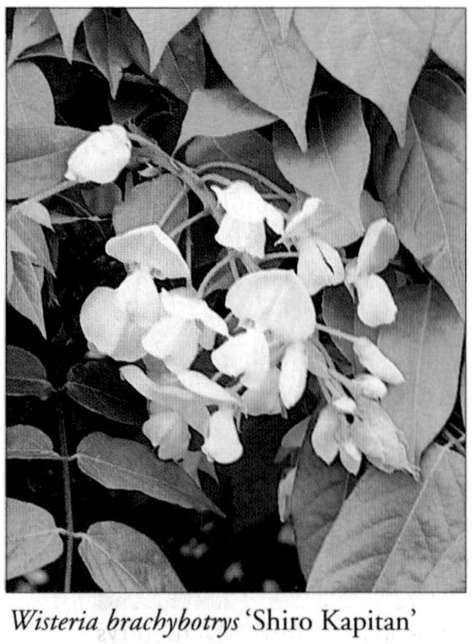

Wisteria brachybotrys 'Shiro Kapitan'

W

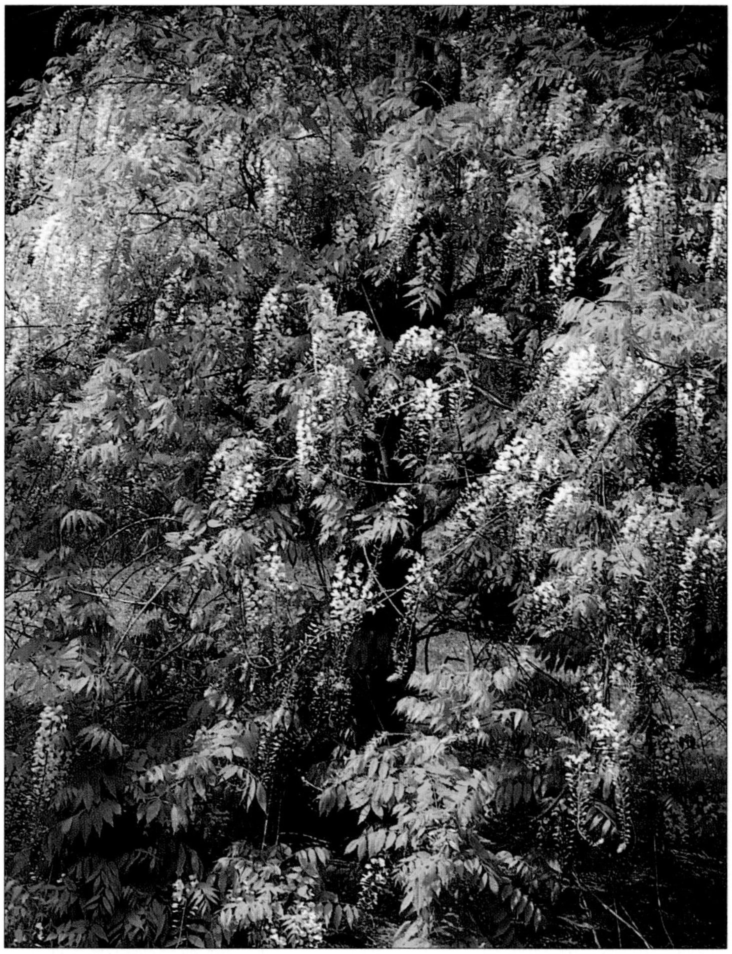

Wisteria floribunda 'Alba'

marked, violet to white flowers are produced in racemes, to 15cm (6in) long, in early summer; they are followed by bean-like, velvety green seed pods, to 20cm (8in) long. ↕ 9m (28ft) or more. Garden origin. ❄❄❄. **'Alba'** see 'Shiro Kapitan'. **f. *alba*** see 'Shiro Kapitan'. **'Alba Plena'** see 'Shiro Kapitan'. **'Murasaki Kapitan'**, syn. *W. venusta* 'Violacea', *W. venusta* f. *violacea*, has deep blue-violet flowers with prominent white, slightly yellow-tinged markings on the standards. **f. *plena*** see 'Shiro Kapitan'. **'Shiro Kapitan'** ▣ syn. 'Alba', f. *alba*, 'Alba Plena', f. *plena*, *W. venusta*, *W. venusta* 'Alba', *W. venusta* f. *alba*, *W. venusta* 'Alba Plena', produces white flowers with a yellow stain at the base of each standard. Double flowers are occasionally produced.

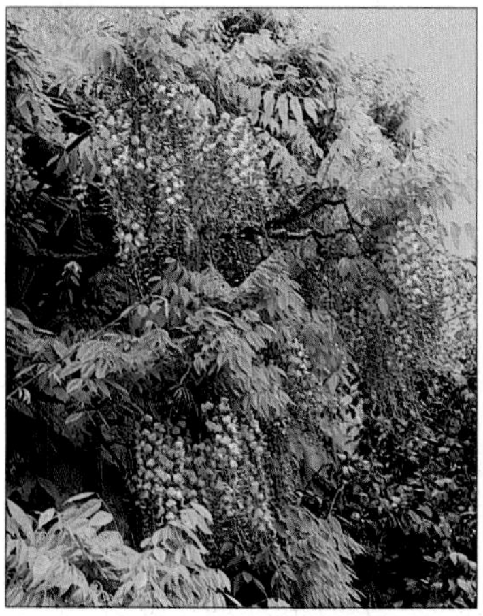

Wisteria floribunda 'Macrobotrys'

W. chinensis see *W. sinensis*.
W. floribunda (Japanese wisteria). Vigorous, twining climber with pinnate leaves, each composed of 11–19 ovate to lance-shaped leaflets. In early summer, pea-like, fragrant, blue to violet, pink, or white flowers, the standards marked with white and yellow, are produced in pendent racemes, to 30cm (12in) or more long, the flowers opening gradually from the bases to the tips; they are often followed by bean-like, velvety green seed pods, to 15cm (6in) long. ↕ 9m (28ft) or more. Japan. ❄❄❄. **'Alba'** ▣🏆 syn. 'Shiro Noda', bears white flowers in racemes to 60cm (24in) long. **'Black Dragon'** see 'Royal Purple'. **'Double Black Dragon'** see 'Violacea Plena'. **'Honbeni'** 🏆 syn. 'Honko', f. *rosea*, 'Rosea', has pink

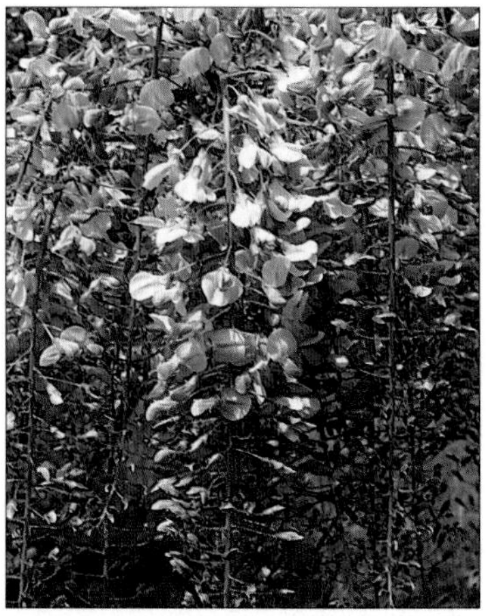

Wisteria x *formosa*

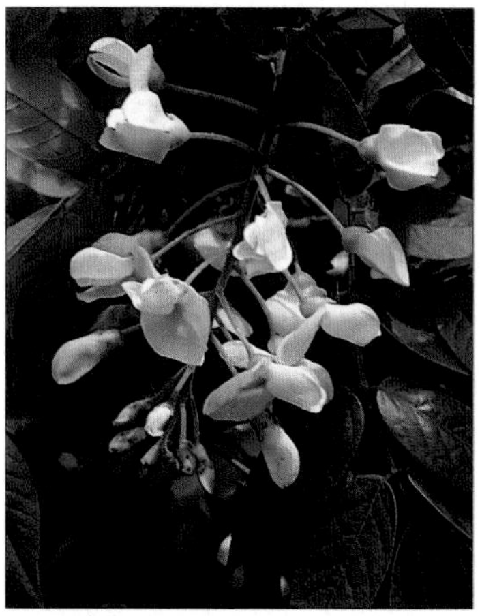

Wisteria sinensis 'Alba'

flowers in racemes to 45cm (18in) long. **'Honko'** see 'Honbeni'. **'Kokuryu'** see 'Royal Purple'. **'Kyushaku'** see 'Macrobotrys'. **'Macrobotrys'** ▣🏆 syn. 'Kyushaku', 'Multijuga', 'Naga Noda', has lilac-blue flowers in racemes 0.9–1.2m (3–4ft) long. **'Multijuga'** see 'Macrobotrys'. **'Naga Noda'** see 'Macrobotrys'. **'Rosea'** see 'Honbeni'. **f. *rosea*** see 'Honbeni'. **'Royal Purple'**, syn. 'Black Dragon', 'Kokuryu', has racemes, 30–50cm (12–20in) long, with purple-violet flowers. **'Shiro Noda'** see 'Alba'. **'Violacea Plena'**, syn. 'Double Black Dragon', 'Yae Kokyuryu', has double, violet-blue flowers. **'Yae Kokyuryu'** see 'Violacea Plena'.
W.* x *formosa ▣ (*W. floribunda* x *W. sinensis*). Vigorous, twining climber with pinnate leaves, each composed of 9–15, broadly ovate to elliptic leaflets. Pea-like, fragrant, violet-blue flowers, with white and yellow markings, are borne in pendent racemes, to 25cm (10in) long, in late spring and early summer, often followed by bean-like, velvety green seed pods, to 15cm (6in) long. ↕ 9m (28ft) or more. Garden origin. ❄❄❄
W. sinensis 🏆 syn. *W. chinensis* (Chinese wisteria). Vigorous, twining climber with pinnate leaves, each composed of 7–13 elliptic or ovate leaflets. Pea-like, fragrant, lilac-blue to white flowers, in dense, pendent racemes to 30cm (12in) long, are borne in late spring and early summer; they are often followed by bean-like, velvety green seed pods, to 15cm (6in) long. ↕ 9m (28ft) or more. China. ❄❄❄. **'Alba'** ▣🏆 has white flowers. **'Prolific'** bears many lilac-blue to pale violet-blue flowers. **'Sierra Madre'** has very fragrant, lavender-violet flowers with white-flushed standards.
W. venusta see *W. brachybotrys* 'Shiro Kapitan'.
***W. venusta* 'Alba'** see *W. brachybotrys* 'Shiro Kapitan'.
W. venusta* f. *alba see *W. brachybotrys* 'Shiro Kapitan'.
***W. venusta* 'Alba Plena'** see *W. brachybotrys* 'Shiro Kapitan'.
***W. venusta* 'Violacea'** see *W. brachybotrys* 'Murasaki Kapitan'.
***W. venusta* f. violacea** see *W. brachybotrys* 'Murasaki Kapitan'.

▷**Wisteria,**
Chinese see *Wisteria sinensis*
Japanese see *Wisteria floribunda*
Silky see *Wisteria brachybotrys*
South African see *Bolusanthus*
Water see *Hygrophila difformis*

▷**Witch hazel** see *Hamamelis*
Chinese see *H. mollis*
Japanese see *H. japonica*
Ozark see *H. vernalis*
Virginian see *H. virginiana*
▷ ***Wittia amazonica*** see *Disocactus amazonicus*
▷ ***Wittiocactus amazonicus*** see *Disocactus amazonicus*

WITTROCKIA

BROMELIACEAE

Genus, closely related to *Nidularium*, of 7 species of rosetted, stemless, evergreen, terrestrial, epiphytic, or rock-dwelling perennials (bromeliads) from mountain areas, to 900m (3,000ft) high, in Brazil. The linear, spiny-margined, scaly leaves, smooth near the tips, are often wide and colourful. In summer, spikes of tubular, usually blue flowers, with 3 separate sepals and 3 petals joined only at their tips, are produced among clusters of leaf-like bracts within the leaf rosettes. In areas where temperatures drop below 18°C (64°F), grow as houseplants or in a warm greenhouse; in warmer climates, use in a humid, moist border.
• **HARDINESS** Frost tender.
• **CULTIVATION** Under glass, grow in standard epiphytic or terrestrial bromeliad compost in bright filtered light. From late spring to early autumn, mist daily with tepid water to maintain moderate humidity, and apply a low-nitrogen liquid fertilizer every 3 or 4 weeks. Outdoors, grow in peaty, leafy, moderately fertile, moist but well-drained soil in a site in partial shade. See also p.47.
• **PROPAGATION** Sow seed at 19–24°C (66–75°F) in spring. Detach offsets in spring or summer.
• **PESTS AND DISEASES** Susceptible to mealybugs.

W. superba ▣ Terrestrial, epiphytic, or rock-dwelling, evergreen bromeliad producing linear, pointed, mid-green leaves, to 1m (3ft) long, narrower at the bases, and with brown scales, red tips, and spiny, red or green teeth. Compact, sunken inflorescences, 12cm (5in) wide, consisting of cone-shaped spikes of tubular blue flowers with pointed petals, surrounded by red bracts, are produced on very short scapes in summer. ↕↔ 1m (3ft) or more. E. Brazil. ❀ (min. 18°C/64°F)

▷**Woad** see *Isatis tinctoria*

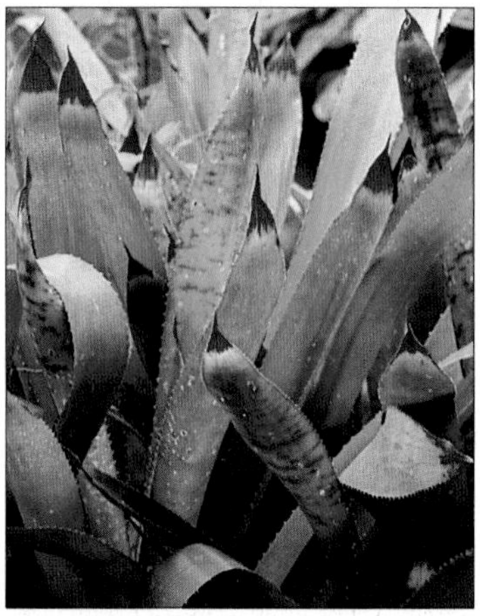

Wittrockia superba

W

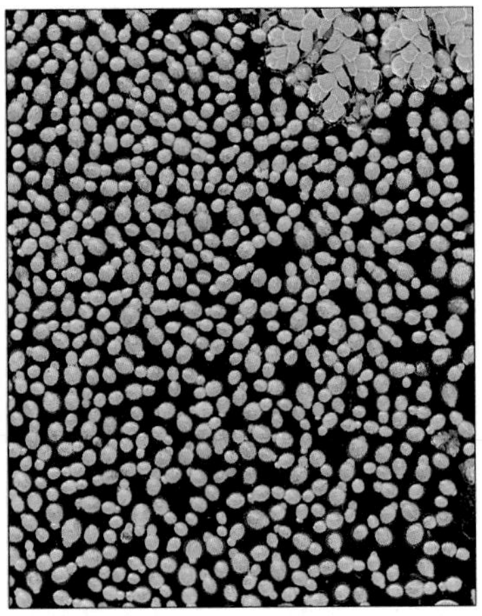
Wolffia arrhiza

WOLFFIA

LEMNACEAE

Genus of 8 species of semi-evergreen, floating aquatic perennials, similar to duckweeds (*Lemna*) but much smaller and lacking a root, with a wide distribution in Europe, Africa, W. Asia, India, Australia, North America, and E. Brazil. They are the smallest known flowering plants, grown mainly for their curiosity value. In frost-prone areas, grow in an aquarium. In warmer climates, grow in an outdoor pool.
- **HARDINESS** Half hardy to frost tender.
- **CULTIVATION** In an outdoor pool, grow in full sun. In an aquarium, grow at 15–28°C (59–82°F) in full light. See also pp.52–53.
- **PROPAGATION** Detach plantlets as they form.
- **PESTS AND DISEASES** Trouble free.

W. arrhiza ▣ Semi-evergreen, floating aquatic perennial with rootless, rounded, bright green fronds, 1mm (1/16in) across. Insignificant, green-tinged white flowers are produced in summer. ↔ indefinite. Europe, Africa, W. Asia, Australia. ❄

▷**Wolf's bane** see *Aconitum lycoctonum*
▷**Wombat berry** see *Eustrephus*
▷**Wonga wonga vine** see *Pandorea pandorana*
▷**Wood anemone** see *Anemone nemorosa*
▷**Woodbine** see *Lonicera periclymenum*
▷**Wood fern, Wallich's** see *Dryopteris wallichiana*
▷**Woodland star** see *Lithophragma*
▷**Wood lily** see *Trillium*
Dwarf white see *T. nivale*
Painted see *T. undulatum*
▷**Wood rose** see *Merremia tuberosa*
▷**Woodruff** see *Asperula*
Sweet see *Galium odoratum*
▷**Woodrush** see *Luzula*
Greater see *L. sylvatica*
Snowy see *L. nivea*

WOODSIA

DRYOPTERIDACEAE

Genus of approximately 25 species of small, tufted, deciduous, terrestrial or rock-dwelling ferns occurring in upland and mountainous regions, mainly in the N. hemisphere. They have erect, short rhizomes, and pinnate to 2-pinnate fronds with the pinnae sometimes pinnatifid. Sporangia are in cup-shaped

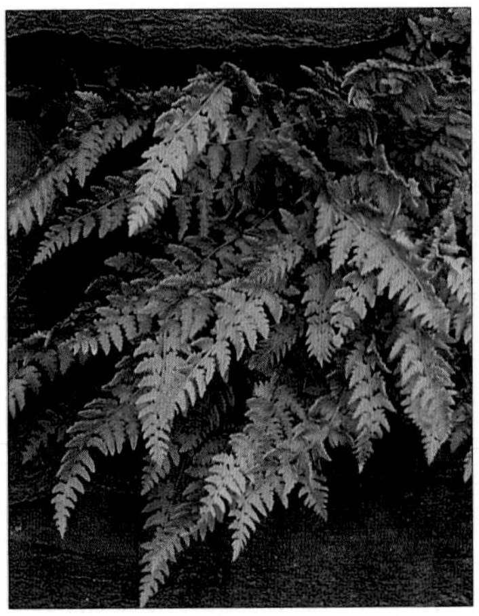
Woodsia polystichoides

indusia, which have often deeply cut fringes. Suitable for a rock garden.
- **HARDINESS** Fully hardy to frost hardy.
- **CULTIVATION** Grow in sharply drained but moist, fertile soil in partial shade. Position crowns above soil level and surround with small stones. *W. ilvensis* prefers acid soil.
- **PROPAGATION** Sow spores at 15–16°C (59–61°F) as soon as ripe. Divide when dormant. See also p.51.
- **PESTS AND DISEASES** Trouble free.

W. ilvensis (Rusty woodsia). Dwarf, tufted, terrestrial or rock-dwelling fern. In early spring, produces lance-shaped to oblong, pinnate, dull green fronds, to 15cm (6in) long, each composed of 7–25 pairs of ovate to lance-shaped, lobed pinnae, clothed with reddish brown hairs and scales. ↕ 15cm (6in), ↔ 10cm (4in). Arctic, Europe, North America. ❄❄❄
W. polystichoides ▣ (Holly-fern woodsia). Tufted, terrestrial or rock-dwelling fern. In early spring, produces lance-shaped, pinnate, pale green fronds, to 35cm (14in) long, softly hairy on both surfaces and scaly beneath; each is composed of 15–30 pairs of narrowly sickle-shaped or oblong pinnae, with slightly toothed margins. May be damaged by late frosts. ↕ 10–30cm (4–12in), ↔ 20–40cm (8–16in). E. Asia. ❄❄❄

▷**Woodsia,**
Holly-fern see *Woodsia polystichoides*
Rusty see *Woodsia ilvensis*

WOODWARDIA

Chain fern

BLECHNACEAE

Genus of approximately 10 species of evergreen or deciduous, terrestrial ferns found in damp, sheltered places in warm-temperate regions of Eurasia and North America. Some are creeping plants, found in acid bogs. Most are large, often with spreading and arching, usually pinnate fronds with pinnatifid pinnae, unfurling in spring; bulbils may be produced towards the tips of the fronds or on their upper surfaces. The chain-like arrangement of the sori on the undersides of the pinnae gives rise to the common name. Use to clothe a moist, shady bank, ideally near water.
- **HARDINESS** Fully hardy to frost hardy.
- **CULTIVATION** Grow in neutral, moderately fertile, damp soil in partial

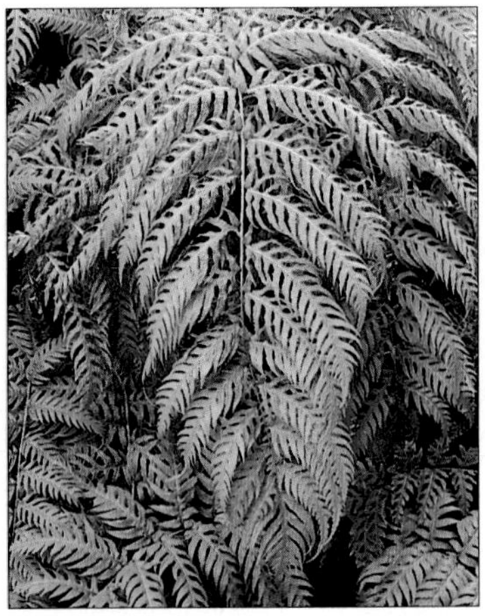
Woodwardia radicans

shade. In frost-prone climates, shelter from cold, drying winds and protect in winter with a dry mulch.
- **PROPAGATION** Sow spores at 16°C (61°F) in late summer or early autumn. Remove bulbils in autumn. Divide in spring. See also p.51.
- **PESTS AND DISEASES** Trouble free.

W. radicans ▣ ♀ (European chain fern). Evergreen fern with arching, broadly lance-shaped, pinnate, dark green fronds, to 2m (6ft) tall, producing bulbils near the tips; the pinnatifid pinnae, to 30cm (12in) long, are ovate-lance-shaped, with curved, lance-shaped, finely toothed segments. ↕ 1.8m (6ft), ↔ 3m (10ft). Atlantic islands, S.W. Europe. ❄❄
W. unigemmata (Asian chain fern). Evergreen fern very similar to *W. radicans*. New foliage emerges brilliant red and fades to brown then green. ↕ 1m (3ft), ↔ 3m (10ft). Himalayas, E. Asia. ❄❄❄ (borderline)

▷**Wormwood** see *Artemisia, A. absinthium*

WORSLEYA

Blue amaryllis

AMARYLLIDACEAE

Genus of one species of bulbous, evergreen perennial from moist mountain forests in Brazil. It has strap-shaped leaves, and is grown for its large umbels of funnel-shaped flowers, borne on leafless stems in winter. In frost-prone climates, it is suitable for a warm greenhouse or conservatory, although it does not easily flower. In warmer climates, grow in a warm, sunny border.
- **HARDINESS** Frost tender.
- **CULTIVATION** Plant bulbs with the necks just above soil level. Under glass, grow in loam-based potting compost (JI No.2), with added leaf mould and bark chips or sharp sand, in full light. In growth, water freely and apply a balanced liquid fertilizer monthly. Keep barely moist in winter, but do not allow the compost to dry out. Outdoors, grow in fertile, reliably moist but sharply drained soil in full sun.
- **PROPAGATION** Sow seed at 19–24°C (66–75°F) in spring.
- **PESTS AND DISEASES** Trouble free.

W. procera see *W. rayneri*.
W. rayneri, syn. *Hippeastrum procerum, W. procera*. Robust, bulbous, evergreen perennial with arching, strap-shaped leaves, to 1m (3ft) long. In winter, bears umbels of up to 14 funnel-shaped flowers, lilac-blue to white at the bases, 4cm (1½in) across, speckled mauve within; the tubes are 2cm (¾in) long, the curving lobes to 15cm (6in) long. ↕ 1–1.2m (3–4ft), ↔ 30cm (12in). Brazil. ❀ (min. 15°C/59°F)

▷**Woundwort** see *Stachys*
Hedge see *S. sylvatica*
▷**Wreath,**
Bridal see *Francoa, Spiraea* 'Arguta', *Stephanotis floribunda*
Purple see *Petrea volubilis*
Queen's see *Antigonon, Petrea volubilis*

WULFENIA

SCROPHULARIACEAE

Genus of about 6 species of rosette-forming, evergreen perennials from alpine meadows in C. and S.E. Europe, W. Asia, and the Himalayas. They are grown mainly for their spike-like racemes of tubular, 2-lipped, blue to pinkish purple or occasionally white flowers borne in summer. Leaves are inversely lance-shaped to broadly ovate or oblong. Suitable for a rock garden or wall crevice.
- **HARDINESS** Fully hardy.
- **CULTIVATION** Grow in gritty, humus-rich, moist but well-drained soil in full sun. Protect from winter wet.
- **PROPAGATION** Sow seed in containers in a cold frame in spring or autumn. Divide in spring.
- **PESTS AND DISEASES** Trouble free.

W. amherstiana ▣ Evergreen perennial with rosettes of obovate-oblong, coarsely scalloped, conspicuously veined, dark green leaves, 5–15cm (2–6in) long, sparsely hairy beneath. In summer, produces erect stems bearing lax, one-sided racemes, 4–20cm (1½–8in) long, of many small, narrowly tubular, pinkish purple flowers. ↕↔ to 20cm (8in). Afghanistan, W. Himalayas. ❄❄❄
W. carinthiaca. Evergreen perennial with rosettes of scalloped, inversely lance-shaped to obovate, shiny, dark green leaves, to 20cm (8in) long. In summer, bears dense, one-sided racemes, 6–10cm (2½–4in) long, of small, narrowly tubular, deep violet-blue flowers on erect stems. ↕↔ 25cm (10in) or more. S.E. Alps, Albania. ❄❄❄

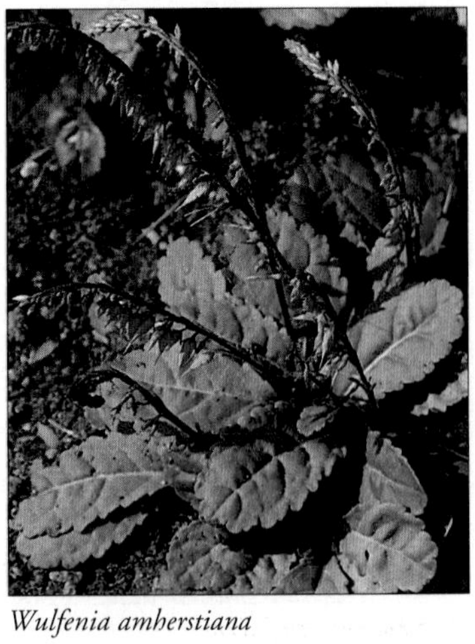
Wulfenia amherstiana

X

XANTHOCERAS

SAPINDACEAE

Genus of one species of erect, deciduous shrub found in scrub and at woodland margins in N. China. An unusual plant and rare in gardens, *X. sorbifolium* is cultivated for its alternate, pinnate leaves and attractive star-shaped, 5-petalled white flowers, borne in late spring. Suitable for a shrub border, for training against a wall, or for a sunny position in a woodland garden.

• **HARDINESS** Fully hardy.

• **CULTIVATION** Grow in fertile, well-drained soil in full sun; grows best in areas with very hot summers. In frost-prone climates, provide shelter from cold, drying winds in winter. Pruning group 1.

• **PROPAGATION** Sow seed in containers outdoors in autumn. Take root cuttings, or remove rooted suckers, in winter.

• **PESTS AND DISEASES** May be affected by coral spot.

X. sorbifolium ■ 🏆 Upright, deciduous shrub with stout shoots and pinnate leaves, to 30cm (12in) long, composed of up to 17 narrowly elliptic to lance-shaped, toothed, glossy, dark green leaflets. As the young leaves emerge in late spring, star-shaped white flowers, 3cm (1¼in) across, are terminally borne in upright panicles, 15–20cm (6–8in) long; yellow-green marks at the petal bases mature to brown. ↕ 4m (12ft), ↔ 3m (10ft). N. China. ❄❄❄

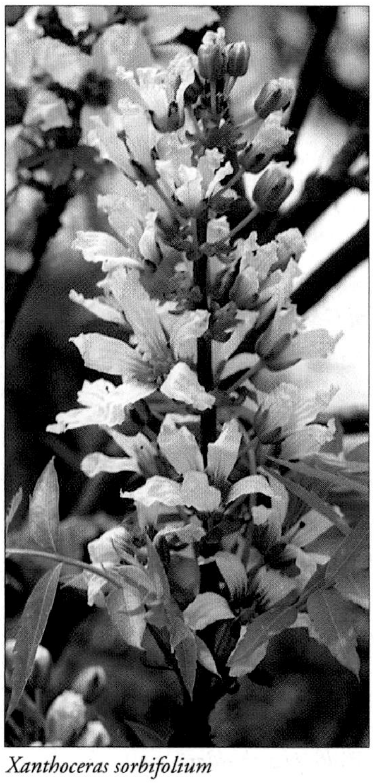

Xanthoceras sorbifolium

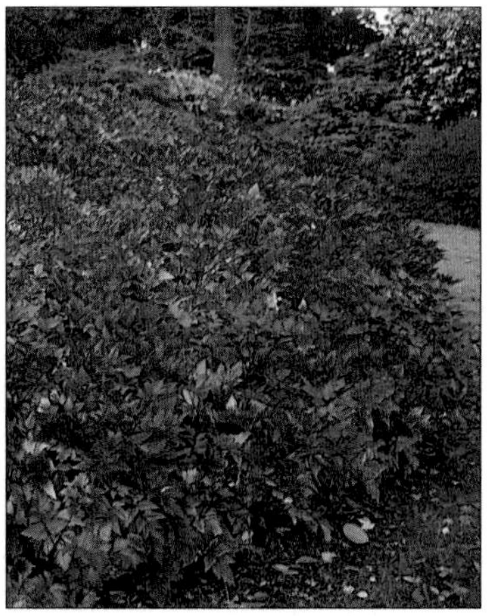

Xanthorhiza simplicissima

XANTHORHIZA

RANUNCULACEAE

Genus of one species of suckering, deciduous shrub found in moist woodland and on streambanks in E. USA. It is cultivated for its alternate, pinnate leaves, clustered at the shoot tips. Tiny, star-shaped, brown-purple flowers are produced in spring. Use *X. simplicissima* for ground cover in a shady position.

• **HARDINESS** Fully hardy.

• **CULTIVATION** Grow in moist but not waterlogged soil in full or partial shade. Pruning group 1 or 3.

• **PROPAGATION** Sow seed in containers outdoors in autumn. Divide in spring or autumn.

• **PESTS AND DISEASES** Trouble free.

X. apiifolia see *X. simplicissima.*

X. simplicissima ■ syn. *X. apiifolia* (Yellowroot). Thicket-forming shrub with erect shoots and bright green leaves to 30cm (12in) long, bronze at first, often red-purple in autumn, each with 3–5 ovate, deeply lobed, irregularly toothed leaflets. In spring, bears flowers in pendent racemes, to 10cm (4in) long, as the leaves emerge. ↕ 60cm (24in), ↔ 1.5m (5ft) or more. E. USA. ❄❄❄

XANTHOSOMA

Yautia

ARACEAE

Genus of up to 50 species of tuberous or thick-stemmed perennials from forest clearings in tropical USA and in Central and South America. They are grown for their edible, fleshy, long-stalked leaves, which may be arrow- to spear-shaped or pedately divided into 3–18 segments. Their cylindrical or spherical tubers or corms, which are white, orange, pink, or purple inside, are also edible, as are some of the stems. Inflorescences consist of a spadix within a taller spathe, and are borne intermittently throughout the year. In frost-prone areas, grow in a warm greenhouse or conservatory. In warmer areas, grow in a shady border.

• **HARDINESS** Frost tender.

• **CULTIVATION** Under glass, grow in containers that allow a free root run, in loam-based potting compost (JI No.2), with added leaf mould, in moderate light. In growth, water freely and apply a balanced liquid fertilizer every 2–3 weeks. Water moderately in winter. Outdoors, grow in slightly acid, leafy,

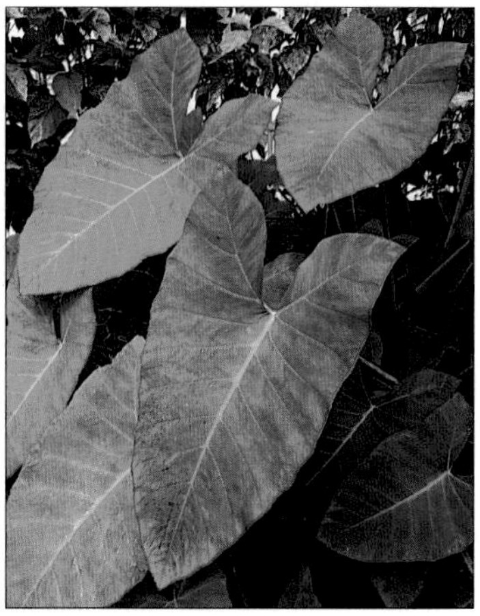

Xanthosoma violaceum

humus-rich, fertile, well-drained soil in partial shade. Avoid waterlogging.

• **PROPAGATION** Separate tubers at any time of year. Take soft-tip cuttings from young plants from spring to autumn.

• **PESTS AND DISEASES** Trouble free.

X. sagittifolium. Thick-stemmed, non-tuberous perennial with arrow-shaped, often white-spotted leaves, to 70cm (28in) long, with broad basal lobes, and leaf-stalks 1m (3ft) long. Greenish white spathes, 22cm (9in) long, surrounding white spadices, are borne intermittently. Stems are edible. ↕↔ 1m (3ft). Tropical USA, Central America, South America. ❀ (min. 13°C/55°F)

X. violaceum ■ (Blue taro). Tuberous perennial, stemless above ground. Arrow-shaped leaves, 70cm (28in) long, with almost triangular lobes, and dark purple leaf-stalks, 30–85cm (12–34in) long, have creamy white veins above, purple veins beneath and at the margins. Intermittently bears pale yellow spathes, 30cm (12in) long, around violet, dark red, or white spadices. Edible tubers are pink inside. ↕ 2.5m (8ft), ↔ 2m (6ft). Widely naturalized. ❀ (min. 13°C/55°F)

XERANTHEMUM

ASTERACEAE/COMPOSITAE

Genus of 6 species of erect, white-woolly, branching annuals from steppes and stony banks in the Mediterranean to S.W. Asia. They have linear to linear-elliptic, entire leaves, and are cultivated for their alternate, daisy-like, crimson-red, pink, white, lilac-blue, or mauve-blue flowerheads, enclosed within

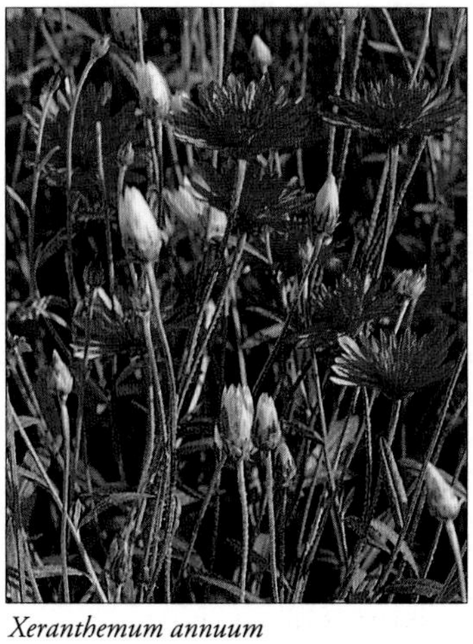

Xeranthemum annuum

papery bracts, borne in summer and autumn. Xeranthemums are suitable for an annual border, and provide long-lasting cut flowers for both fresh and dried arrangements.

• **HARDINESS** Half hardy.

• **CULTIVATION** Grow in moderately fertile, well-drained soil in full sun. Provide light support in exposed sites. Cut flowers for drying before they have fully opened and hang upside down in a cool, dark, well-ventilated area.

• **PROPAGATION** Sow seed at 16°C (61°F) in spring.

• **PESTS AND DISEASES** Trouble free.

X. annuum ■ Slender, upright annual, branched at the bases of the wiry stems, bearing linear-elliptic, entire, woolly, silver-green leaves, 2–6cm (¾–2½in) long. Branched heads of delicate, daisy-like, single to double, white, bright pink, crimson-red, or deep purple flowerheads, to 5cm (2in) across, are produced from summer to autumn. ↕ 25–75cm (10–30in), ↔ 45cm (18in). S.E. Europe to Caucasus, Iran. ❄. **'Snow Lady'** produces single white flowerheads.

XEROPHYLLUM

LILIACEAE/MELANTHIACEAE

Genus of 2 or 3 species of upright, rhizomatous, clump-forming perennials from dry slopes and open woodland in hilly and mountainous areas of North America. They are cultivated for their flowers and bold, architectural foliage. Woody, stem-like rhizomes produce numerous densely tufted, linear, finely tapered leaves, mid-green above and glaucous, blue-green beneath, with hard, rough or finely toothed margins. The leaves become progressively smaller towards the tips of the unbranched stems, each of which bears a dense, terminal raceme of small, funnel-shaped, white or yellowish white flowers in summer. They are suitable for growing in a sunny herbaceous border or in a Mediterranean garden.

• **HARDINESS** Fully hardy.

• **CULTIVATION** Grow in moderately fertile, moist but well-drained soil in full sun. In frost-prone areas, protect crowns with a dry winter mulch.

• **PROPAGATION** Sow seed in containers in a cold frame in autumn or spring. Divide crowns just before growth commences in spring.

• **PESTS AND DISEASES** Trouble free.

X. asphodeloides. Upright perennial with linear leaves, to 45cm (18in) long, mid-green above, glaucous, blue-green beneath, with rough margins. During summer, produces funnel-shaped, fragrant, yellow-white flowers, 1cm (½in) across, in dense, broad, rounded racemes, to 30cm (12in) long. ↕ to 1.5m (5ft), ↔ to 60cm (24in). E. Canada to USA (New Jersey to Tennessee, Georgia). ❄❄❄

X. tenax. Upright perennial with tufted, linear, stiff leaves, to 90cm (36in) long, mid-green above, glaucous, blue-green beneath, with rough margins. Produces funnel-shaped, white to cream flowers, 5mm (¼in) across, in dense racemes, to 60cm (24in) long, in summer. ↕↔ 75cm (30in). W. North America. ❄❄❄

Y

▷**Yam, Ornamental** see *Dioscorea discolor*
▷**Yanquapin** see *Nelumbo lutea*
▷**Yarrow** see *Achillea*
Golden see *Eriophyllum*
▷**Yautia** see *Xanthosoma*
▷**Yellow archangel** see *Lamium galeobdolon*
▷**Yellow bells** see *Tecoma stans*
▷**Yellowroot** see *Xanthorhiza simplicissima*
▷**Yellow trumpet** see *Sarracenia flava*
▷**Yellow wood** see *Cladrastis lutea*
▷**Yesterday, today, and tomorrow** see *Brunfelsia pauciflora*
▷**Yew** see *Taxus, T. baccata*
Florence Court see *Taxus baccata* 'Fastigiata'
Fortune plum see *Cephalotaxus fortunei*
Irish see *Taxus baccata* 'Fastigiata'
Japanese see *Taxus cuspidata*
Nutmeg see *Torreya*
Plum see *Cephalotaxus, C. harringtoniana*
Prince Albert's see *Saxegothaea conspicua*
▷**Ylang-ylang** see *Cananga odorata*
▷**Youth-on-age** see *Tolmiea*

YUCCA syn. HESPEROYUCCA

AGAVACEAE

Genus of about 40 species of rosette-forming or woody-based perennials (some species monocarpic), evergreen shrubs, and erect, eventually spreading, evergreen trees from hot, dry places, such as deserts, sand dunes, and plains, in North and Central America and the West Indies. They are cultivated for their bold, linear to lance-shaped or inversely lance-shaped, neatly or loosely rosetted leaves, and for their erect or rarely pendent panicles of bell-shaped to hemispherical, usually white flowers. Use as architectural specimens in a border or courtyard. In frost-prone areas, grow tender yuccas in a cool or temperate greenhouse, or conservatory.

- **HARDINESS** Fully hardy to frost tender.
- **CULTIVATION** Under glass, grow in loam-based potting compost (JI No.2) in full light. When in growth, water moderately and apply a balanced liquid fertilizer monthly. Water sparingly in winter. Outdoors, grow in any well-drained soil in full sun. Flowers may require hand-pollination to set seed. Remove spent flowering stems.
- **PROPAGATION** Sow seed in spring, at 13–18°C (55–64°F) for hardy yuccas, or at 19–24°C (66–75°F) for tender ones. Remove rooted suckers in spring. Take root cuttings in winter.
- **PESTS AND DISEASES** Susceptible to leaf spot; aphids may infest flowers.

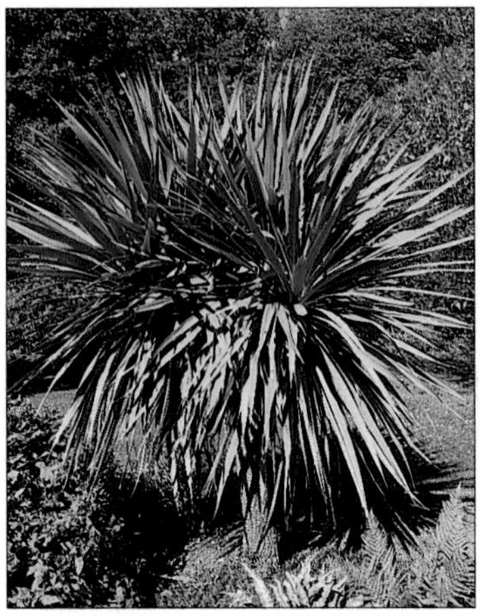

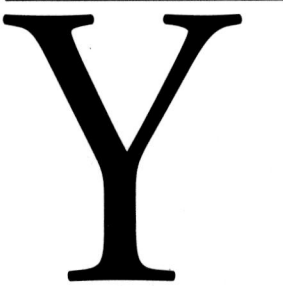

Yucca aloifolia

Y. aloifolia ▣ ◌ (Spanish bayonet). Slow-growing, rounded shrub or small tree with a simple or branched stem and densely arranged, linear to narrowly lance-shaped, toothed, dark green leaves, to 50cm (20in) long, each ending in a sharp, stiff point. From summer to autumn, bears stout, erect panicles, to 45cm (18in) long, of pendent, bell-shaped, white, sometimes purple-tinged flowers, 3cm (1¼in) long, held above the foliage. ↕ 8m (25ft), ↔ 4–5m (12–15ft). S.E. USA, Mexico, West Indies. ❅ (min. 7°C/45°F)

Y. elephantipes ♀ ◌ syn. *Y. guatemalensis* (Giant yucca, Spineless yucca). Large, upright shrub or usually small tree with several to many sparsely branched trunks arising near ground level. Narrowly lance-shaped, light to mid-green leaves, 60–100cm (24–39in) long, are stiffly leathery, with toothed margins. On mature plants, pendent, hemispherical, white to cream flowers, 3–4cm (1¼–1½in) long, are borne in dense, erect panicles, to 1m (3ft) long, from summer to autumn. ↕ to 10m (30ft), ↔ 5–8m (15–25ft). Mexico. ❅ (min. 10°C/50°F). **'Variegata'** ▣ produces leaves that are creamy white at the margins.

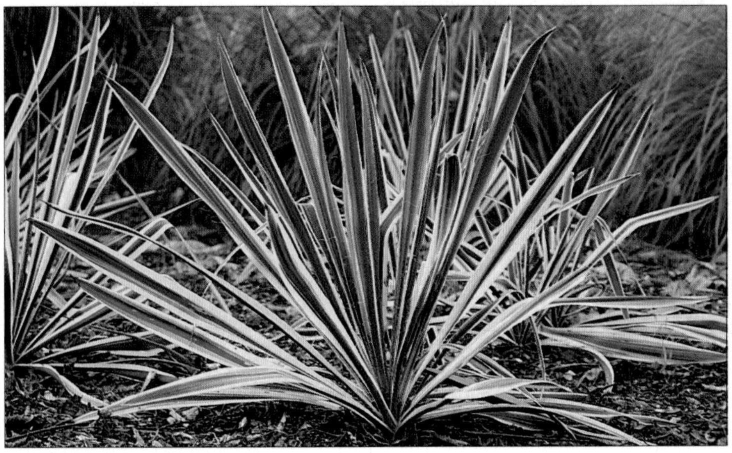

Yucca filamentosa 'Bright Edge'

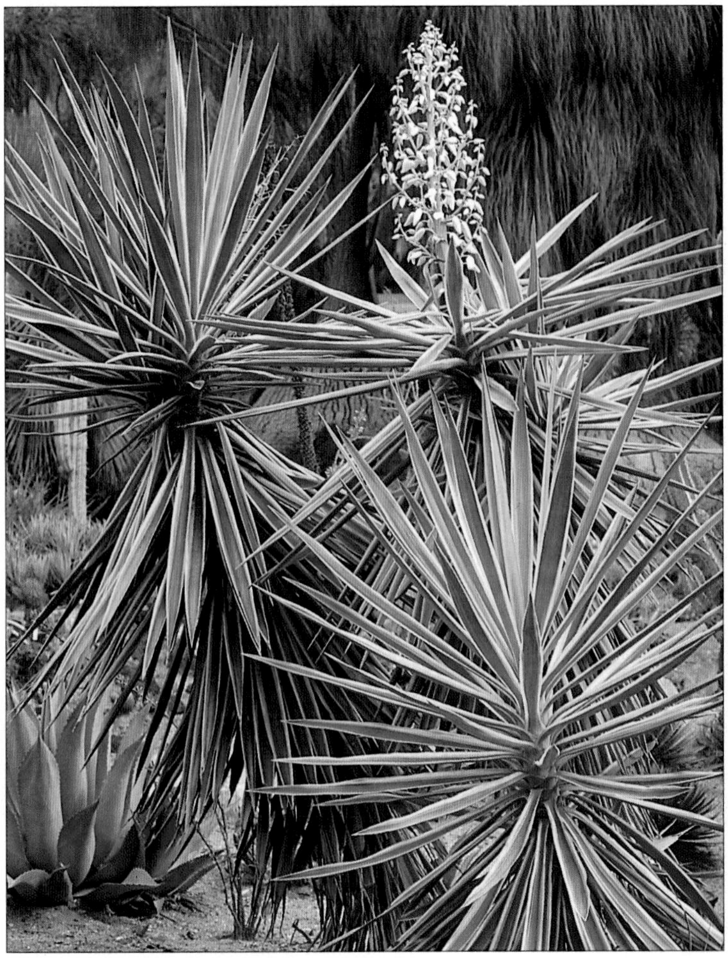

Yucca elephantipes 'Variegata'

Y. filamentosa ♀ (Adam's needle). Clump-forming shrub, stemless or almost so, with basal rosettes of inversely lance-shaped, rigid, dark green leaves, to 75cm (30in) long, margined with curly white threads. Nodding, bell-shaped white flowers, 5cm (2in) long, tinged green or cream, are borne in upright panicles, to 2m (6ft) or more long, in mid- and late summer. ↕ 75cm (30in), ↔ 1.5m (5ft). USA (New Jersey to Florida). ❄❄❄. **'Bright Edge'** ▣ ♀ has leaves with broad yellow margins. **'Variegata'** ♀ has white-margined, blue-green leaves, tinged pink in winter.

Y. flaccida. Clump-forming, almost stemless shrub bearing basal rosettes of lance-shaped, dark blue-green leaves, to 55cm (22in) long, fringed with curly or straight threads. Bears nodding, bell-shaped white flowers, 5cm (2in) long, in upright panicles, to 1.5m (5ft) or more long, in mid- and late summer. ↕ 55cm (22in), ↔ 1.5m (5ft). USA (N. Carolina to Alabama). ❄❄❄. **'Golden Sword'** ♀ has yellow-margined leaves. **'Ivory'** ♀ bears a profusion of spreading, green-tinged, creamy white flowers.

Y. gloriosa ▣ ♀ (Spanish dagger). Erect shrub with a stout stem, simple at first, later sparsely branched, bearing terminal tufts of narrowly lance-shaped, stiffly pointed, arching, leaves, to 60cm (24in) long, blue-green maturing to dark green, with entire to few-toothed margins. From late summer to autumn, produces pendent, bell-shaped, sometimes purple-tinged, white flowers, 5cm (2in) long, in upright panicles, to 2.5m (8ft) long. ↕↔ 2m (6ft). USA (N. Carolina to Florida). ❄❄. **'Nobilis'** has flowers with red petal backs, and blue-green leaves, the outer ones arched. **'Variegata'** ♀ has yellow-margined leaves.

Y. guatemalensis see *Y. elephantipes.*

Y. parviflora see *Hesperaloe parviflora.*

Y. recurvifolia ♀ Robust, tree-like shrub, sometimes with several trunk-like stems, sparsely branched with age. Bears lance-shaped, arching to strongly recurved, stiffly leathery, mid- to deep

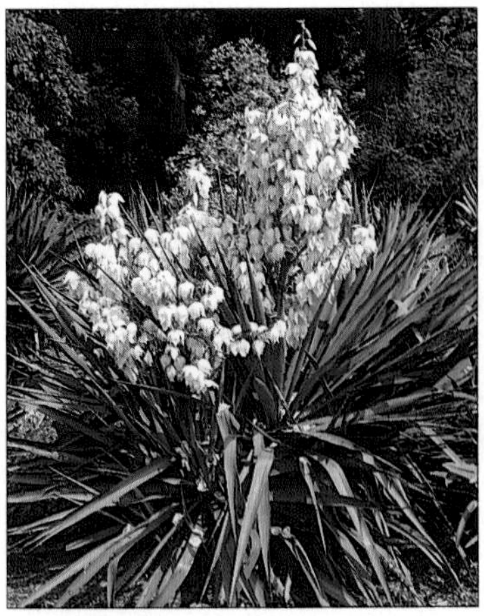

Yucca gloriosa

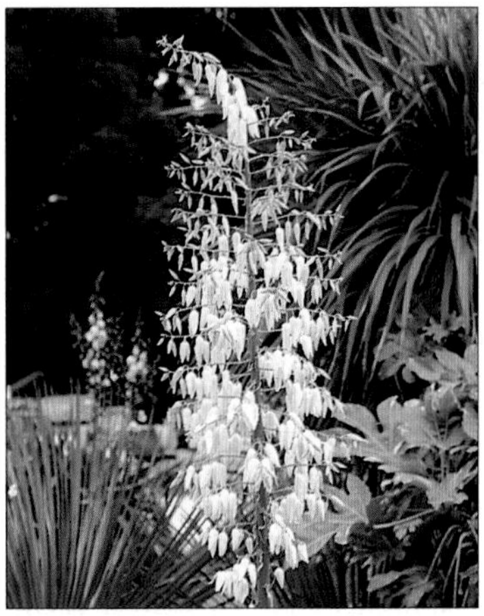

Yucca whipplei

green leaves, to 90cm (36in) long, blue-green when young, with entire to slightly toothed margins. Pendent, bell-shaped cream flowers, 6–8cm (2½–3in) long, open in upright panicles, to 2m (6ft) long, from late summer to autumn. ↕ 1.5–2.5m (5–8ft), ↔ 1.2–2m (4–6ft). USA (Georgia to Missouri). ❄❄❄

Y. whipplei ■ (Our Lord's candle). Clump-forming, stemless, monocarpic shrub with dense tufts of slender, linear, finely toothed, rigid, grey-green leaves, to 90cm (36in) long. Pendent, bell-shaped or hemispherical, fragrant, creamy white, sometimes purple-tinged flowers, 3.5cm (1½in) long, are borne in summer in upright panicles, to 2m (6ft) or more long. Propagate by seed; it may take many years to flower. ↕ 1m (3ft), ↔ 1.2m (4ft). USA (S. California, Arizona), N.W. Mexico. ❄❄

▷**Yucca,**
Giant see *Yucca elephantipes*
Spineless see *Yucca elephantipes*
▷**Yulan** see *Magnolia denudata*

YUSHANIA

Anceps bamboo

GRAMINEAE/POACEAE

Genus of 2 species of tall, evergreen, clump-forming bamboos found at high altitudes in the N.W. and C. Himalayas, Taiwan, and the Philippines. Cultivated for their lance-shaped to linear leaves, yushanias are suitable for use as hedging or screening, or as specimens, but they can be invasive.

• **HARDINESS** Fully hardy, although foliage may be damaged in extreme cold.
• **CULTIVATION** Grow in fertile, humus-rich, moist but well-drained soil in full sun or partial shade. In frost-prone areas, shelter from cold winds. Plant in large tubs plunged into soil to restrict spread.
• **PROPAGATION** Divide in spring.
• **PESTS AND DISEASES** Young shoots may be damaged by slugs.

Y. anceps 🏆 syn. *Arundinaria anceps, Arundinaria jaunsarensis, Sinarundinaria jaunsarensis* (Anceps bamboo). Tall, evergreen, rhizomatous bamboo forming dense, scattered clumps of shiny, dark green canes, straight and erect at first, arching with age. Pendent branchlets bear narrowly lance-shaped, mid-green leaves, 6–14cm (2½–5½in) long, rounded at the bases, with purple-tinted stalks. ↕ 4m (12ft) or more, ↔ indefinite. N.W. and C. Himalayas. ❄❄❄

Z

ZALUZIANSKYA

SCROPHULARIACEAE

Genus of about 35 species of sticky, low-growing annuals and evergreen perennials or subshrubs from grassland and rocky slopes in South Africa. They are grown for their terminal spikes of tubular, salverform, heavily scented flowers, with 5 spreading petal lobes; the flowers are usually deep red in bud, opening to white with red petal backs. The variably shaped leaves are entire or toothed, the lower ones opposite, the upper ones alternate. Suitable for a sunny rock garden or alpine house.

• **HARDINESS** Frost hardy.
• **CULTIVATION** Grow in moist but sharply drained, humus-rich soil in full sun. Cut back hard after flowering. In an alpine house, grow in a mix of equal parts loam, leaf mould, and grit. Water freely when in growth. Keep barely moist in winter.
• **PROPAGATION** Propagate regularly as plants are short-lived. Take stem-tip cuttings in summer, overwinter in frost-free conditions, and plant out in spring. Seed is not regularly produced in gardens; if available, sow at 10–13°C (50–55°F) as soon as ripe or in spring.
• **PESTS AND DISEASES** Aphids and red spider mites may be troublesome under glass.

Z. ovata ■ Clump-forming, evergreen perennial with branching, brittle stems bearing ovate, toothed, sticky, grey-green leaves, 4cm (1½in) long. Produces terminal spikes of salverform, crimson-backed white flowers, 2–2.5cm (¾–1in) across, each with 5 petal lobes, cleft into 2 further lobes; they open in sunshine, and are produced over a long period in summer. ↕ to 25cm (10in), ↔ to 60cm (24in). South Africa (Western Cape, Northern Cape, Eastern Cape, KwaZulu/Natal, Orange Free State), Lesotho. ❄❄

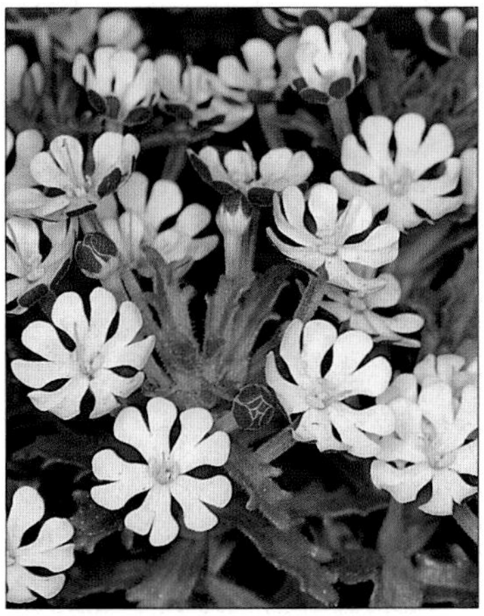

Zaluzianskya ovata

ZAMIA

ZAMIACEAE

Genus of about 30 species of mainly small, dioecious cycads found in scrub and pine woodland, and on dry slopes from North to South America. Most have short, swollen stems, some similar to palms; others, with tuberous, underground stems, resemble ferns. Zamias are grown for their habit and pinnate leaves, borne in terminal whorls or rosettes and often composed of many narrow, oblong or linear to ovate leaflets. They produce usually felted, single-sexed, cone-like flower spikes ("cones"), with male and female flowers borne on separate plants; the insignificant male cones are cylindrical, the females ovoid. In frost-prone areas, grow in a warm greenhouse or as houseplants. In tropical areas, site large species on a lawn and small ones in a shrub border.

• **HARDINESS** Frost tender.
• **CULTIVATION** Under glass, grow in loam-based potting compost (JI No.3), with added leaf mould and sharp sand, in full light with shade from hot sun. During the growing season, water freely and apply a balanced liquid fertilizer monthly. Water sparingly in winter. Outdoors, grow in fertile, moist but well-drained soil in full sun with some midday shade, or in partial shade.
• **PROPAGATION** Sow seed at 24°C (75°F) in spring.
• **PESTS AND DISEASES** Susceptible to scale insects and mealybugs under glass.

Z. floridana see *Z. pumila.*

Z. furfuracea (Cardboard palm). Small cycad with a partly underground, simple or rarely branched, cylindrical trunk. Bears terminal whorls of semi-erect to spreading, pinnate leaves, to 1m (3ft) long, each with up to 24 oblong or inversely lance-shaped to obovate, stiff, pale green leaflets, later olive-green, with red-brown hairs. Produces felted, red-brown female flower cones, 10–13cm (4–5in) long, usually in summer. ↕ to 1m (3ft), ↔ to 2m (6ft). Coast of E. Mexico. ❀ (min. 15°C/59°F)

Z. integrifolia see *Z. pumila.*

Z. loddigesii. Small cycad with a largely underground, sometimes branching trunk. Bears terminal whorls of semi-erect to spreading, pinnate leaves, to 1m (3ft) long, each with up to 54 narrowly lance-shaped, lustrous, bright green leaflets, toothed on their upper halves. Brownish green female flower cones, 5cm (2in) or more long, are generally produced in summer. ↕ 1.5m (5ft), ↔ to 1.7m (5½ft). Mexico, Guatemala. ❀ (min. 15°C/ 59°F). **var. *latifolia*** has lance-shaped to obovate leaflets.

Z. pumila ■ syn. *Z. floridana, Z. integrifolia* (Florida arrowroot, Guayiga, Seminole bread). Small cycad with a mainly underground, unbranched or branched trunk. Bears terminal rosettes of ascending to spreading, pinnate leaves, 60–120cm (24–48in) long, each with up to 60 linear to inversely lance-shaped, leathery, deep green leaflets, frequently toothed on their upper halves. Large, russet-green female flower cones, to 15cm (6in) long, are usually produced in summer. ↕ to 1.2m (4ft), ↔ 1.2–2m (4–6ft). USA (Florida), Cuba, West Indies. ❀ (min. 15°C/59°F)

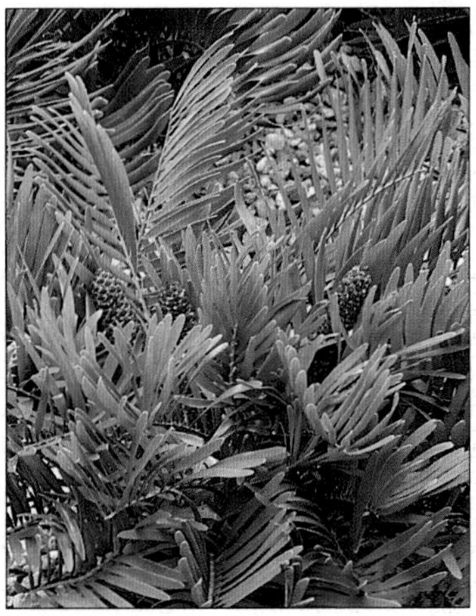

Zamia pumila

ZANTEDESCHIA

Arum lily

ARACEAE

Genus of 6 species of perennials, with tuberous rhizomes, found in moist soils, swamps, or lake margins in southern and E. Africa. They are grown for their unusual, white or brightly coloured spathes, borne in spring and summer. Most bear lance-shaped or narrowly to broadly arrow- or heart-shaped leaves. A number of hybrids have been developed. **Elliottiana hybrids** have broadly heart-shaped, usually mid- to dark green leaves, most covered with translucent white dots, and usually yellow spathes, 15cm (6in) long, surrounding golden yellow spadices. **Rehmannii hybrids** have lance-shaped, rarely spotted, mid- to dark green leaves, and white to pink or dark purple spathes, 12cm (5in) long, surrounding yellow spadices.

Z. aethiopica may be cultivated as a marginal aquatic. Where temperatures fall below 10°C (50°F), grow less hardy arum lilies in a warm greenhouse or as houseplants, or plant out in summer. All parts may cause mild stomach upset if ingested, and contact with the sap may irritate the skin.

• **HARDINESS** Fully hardy to frost tender.
• **CULTIVATION** Under glass, grow in loam-based potting compost (JI No.2) in full light. In growth, water freely and apply a balanced liquid fertilizer every 2 weeks until the flowers have faded. Keep just moist in winter. Outdoors, grow in humus-rich, moist soil in full sun. In frost-prone areas, protect *Z. aethiopica* with a deep winter mulch. As a marginal aquatic, grow *Z. aethiopica* in a planting basket 25–30cm (10–12in) across, filled with heavy loam soil, in water up to 30cm (12in) deep; see also pp.52–53.
• **PROPAGATION** Sow seed at 21–27°C (70–81°F) when ripe. Divide in spring.
• **PESTS AND DISEASES** Susceptible to various fungi and prone to aphids.

Z. aethiopica 🏆 (Arum lily). Clump-forming, rhizomatous perennial, evergreen in mild areas, with semi-erect, arrow-shaped, glossy, bright green leaves, to 40cm (16in) long. From late spring to midsummer, bears a succession of large, pure white spathes, to 25cm (10in) long, with creamy yellow spadices. ↕ 90cm (36in), ↔ 60cm (24in). South Africa, Lesotho. ❄❄. **'Apple Court Babe'** is much shorter; ↕ 60cm

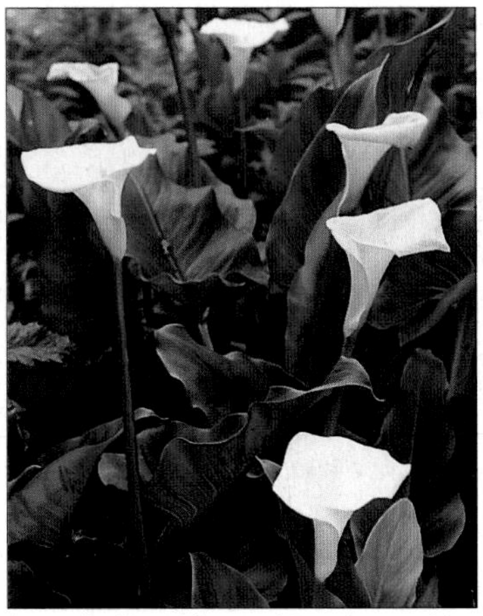

Zantedeschia aethiopica 'Crowborough'

(24in). **'Crowborough'** ▣ has spathes 10–15cm (4–6in) long; ❄❄❄ (borderline). **'Green Goddess'** ▣♀ has dull green leaves and white-centred, bright green spathes, 15–20cm (6–8in) long. **'Little Gem'** is dwarf and floriferous; ↕45cm (18in). **'White Sails'** has open white spathes, 10cm (4in) long.

Z. albomaculata, syn. *Z. melanoleuca.* Rhizomatous perennial with semi-erect, arrow-shaped, mid-green, basal leaves, to 45cm (18in) long, with translucent white spots. In summer, bears white to cream, pale yellow, or pale pink spathes, to 12cm (5in) long, each with a purple mark inside at the base, surrounding yellow spadices. ↕30–40cm (12–16in), ↔20cm (8in). Tropical Africa, South Africa, E. Africa. ❀ (min. 10°C/50°F)

Z. angustiloba see *Z. pentlandii.*

***Z.* 'Aztec Gold'.** Elliottiana hybrid with unspotted leaves. Golden yellow spathes are borne in summer, maturing to burnt orange. ↕55cm (22in), ↔20cm (8in). ❀ (min. 10°C/50°F)

***Z.* 'Black-eyed Beauty'.** Elliottiana hybrid with heavily white-spotted leaves. In summer, produces cream spathes, each with a black central mark in the throat. ↕30–40cm (12–16in), ↔15cm (6in). ❀ (min. 10°C/50°F)

***Z.* 'Black Magic'.** Elliottiana hybrid with heavily white-mottled leaves. Bears yellow spathes, with black throats, in summer. ↕75cm (30in), ↔20cm (8in). ❀ (min. 10°C/50°F)

***Z.* 'Dusty Pink'.** Rehmannii hybrid bearing rounded, mauve-pink spathes, with darker throats, in summer. ↕70cm (28in), ↔20cm (8in). ❀ (min. 10°C/50°F)

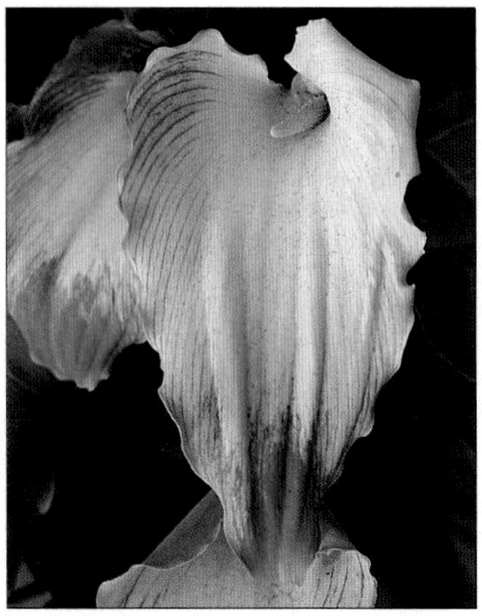

Zantedeschia aethiopica 'Green Goddess'

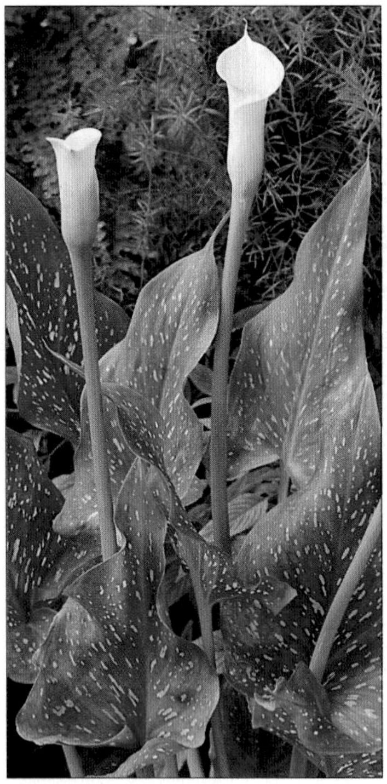

Zantedeschia elliottiana

Z. elliottiana ▣♀ (Golden arum). Rhizomatous perennial with erect, heart-shaped, dark green, basal leaves, to 45cm (18in) long, covered with translucent white spots. In summer, bears golden yellow spathes, 15cm (6in) long, with golden yellow spadices. ↕60–90cm (24–36in), ↔20cm (8in). Origin unknown. ❀ (min. 10°C/50°F)

***Z.* 'Golden Affair'.** Elliottiana hybrid with unspotted leaves. In summer, bears bright yellow spathes. ↕60cm (24in), ↔20cm (8in). ❀ (min. 10°C/50°F)

***Z.* 'Majestic Red'.** Elliottiana hybrid with unspotted leaves, and pointed, crimson spathes, borne in summer. ↕65cm (26in), ↔20cm (8in). ❀ (min. 10°C/50°F)

Z. melanoleuca see *Z. albomaculata.*

Z. pentlandii, syn. *Z. angustiloba.* Upright, rhizomatous perennial with erect, oblong-elliptic to oblong-lance-shaped, mid- to dark green, rarely spotted leaves, to 30cm (12in) long, arrow- or heart-shaped at the bases. In summer, bears bright golden to lemon-yellow spathes, to 12cm (5in) long, each marked dark purple inside at the base, and golden yellow spadices. ↕60–90cm (24–36in), ↔20cm (8in). ❄❄❄

Z. rehmannii ♀ (Pink arum). Rhizomatous perennial with semi-erect, lance-shaped, dark green, basal leaves. In summer, bears slender, white to pink or dark purple spathes, 12cm (5in) long, with yellow spadices. ↕40cm (16in), ↔28cm (11in). South Africa (Northern Transvaal, Eastern Transvaal), Swaziland. ❀ (min. 10°C/50°F)

ZANTHOXYLUM

RUTACEAE

Genus of about 250 species of broadly rounded to upright, spiny, deciduous or evergreen trees and shrubs, mainly from forest in Asia, Australia, North to South America, and Africa, usually in warmer regions. They have aromatic bark, and are grown for their alternate, usually pinnate leaves, dotted with minute glands, and for their fruits, which split to reveal seeds attached by short threads. They bear cymes or panicles of small, cup-shaped, green or yellowish green flowers from spring to summer; individual plants may be dioecious, or produce both unisexual and bisexual flowers. Suitable for use in a shrub border or as specimen trees. In frost-prone areas, grow tender species in a cool greenhouse.

- **HARDINESS** Fully hardy to frost tender.
- **CULTIVATION** Grow in fertile, well-drained soil in full sun or light dappled shade. Pruning group 1.
- **PROPAGATION** Sow seed in containers in a cold frame in autumn. Root semi-ripe cuttings in midsummer, with bottom heat. Take root cuttings in late winter.
- **PESTS AND DISEASES** Trouble free.

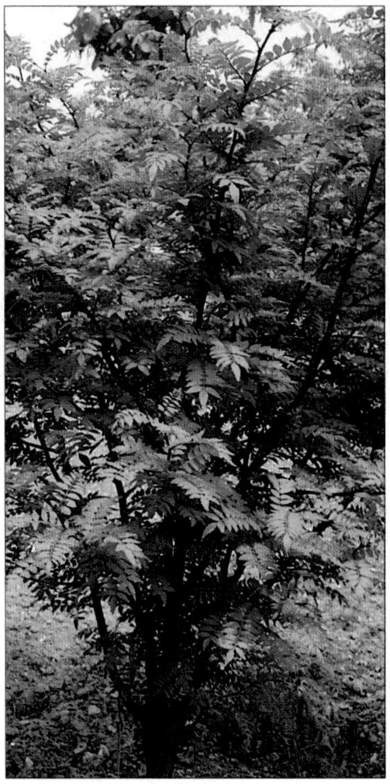

Zanthoxylum piperitum

Z. piperitum ▣ (Japan pepper). Bushy, spiny, deciduous shrub with pinnate, aromatic, glossy, dark green leaves, to 15cm (6in) long, each with 11–23 ovate, toothed leaflets, turning yellow in autumn. In early summer, bears panicles, 5cm (2in) long, of small, cup-shaped, yellow-green flowers from the leaf axils; they are followed by tiny, spherical, berry-like red fruit, which split to reveal black seeds. ↕↔2.5m (8ft). China, Korea, Japan, Taiwan. ❄❄❄

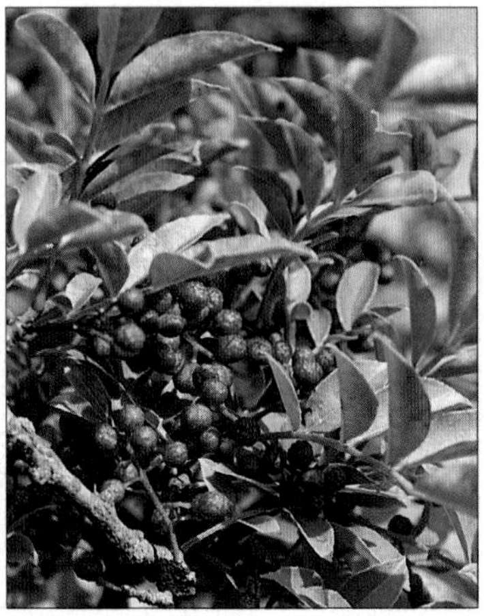

Zanthoxylum simulans

Z. simulans ▣⌒ Spreading, deciduous shrub or small tree with broad spines, sometimes with pendent shoots. Pinnate leaves, to 20cm (8in) long, each with up to 11 ovate-oblong, saw-toothed, glossy, dark green leaflets, become yellow to reddish yellow in autumn. In early summer, bears tiny, cup-shaped green flowers in cymes 5cm (2in) across, followed by spherical, warty red fruit, 5mm (¼in) across, which split to reveal glossy black seeds. ↕6m (20ft), ↔5m (15ft). China, Japan, Taiwan. ❄❄❄

ZAUSCHNERIA

Californian fuchsia

ONAGRACEAE

Genus of 4 species of subshrubby, evergreen or deciduous perennials, sometimes included in *Epilobium*, from dry slopes and chaparral or coastal sage brush in W. North America. The small, opposite or alternate, linear-lance-shaped to broadly ovate leaves are stalkless or virtually so. Californian fuchsias are grown for their profusion of tubular to funnel-shaped, usually scarlet flowers, borne in terminal racemes in late summer and autumn. Providing spectacular colour late in the season, they are suitable for a rock garden or dry-stone wall, or for a mixed or herbaceous border.

- **HARDINESS** Fully hardy to frost hardy.
- **CULTIVATION** Grow in moderately fertile, well-drained soil in full sun, with shelter from cold, dry winds.
- **PROPAGATION** Sow seed in containers in a cold frame in spring. Root basal cuttings in spring, with bottom heat.
- **PESTS AND DISEASES** Young growth may be damaged by slugs.

Z. californica, syn. *Epilobium californicum* ♀ Clump-forming, woody-based, evergreen or semi-evergreen, rhizomatous perennial producing lance-shaped to linear-lance-shaped, hairy, grey-green leaves, 1–4cm (½–1½in) long. Racemes of tubular, brilliant scarlet flowers, 2.5–4cm (1–1½in) long, are terminally borne over long periods in late summer and early autumn. ↕to 30cm (12in), ↔to 50cm (20in). USA (California). ❄❄❄ (borderline). **subsp. *angustifolia*** has linear, densely woolly leaves, and slightly shorter flowers; ↕to 50cm (20in). **subsp. *cana***, syn. *Epilobium canum, Z. cana*, is deciduous, with linear to oblong, grey-woolly to white silky-hairy leaves, and funnel-shaped, vermilion to scarlet flowers; ↕to 60cm (24in), ↔45cm (18in). **subsp. *cana* 'Dublin'** ▣♀ is deciduous, with bright red flowers; ↕to 25cm (10in), ↔to 30cm (12in). **subsp. *latifolia*** is spreading, with a non-woody base, and produces ovate to lance-shaped-ovate, finely hairy, mid-green to greyish green leaves. **'Solidarity Pink'** is less vigorous, and produces pale pink flowers; ↔to 30cm (12in).

Z. cana see *Z. californica* subsp. *cana.*

Z. septentrionalis, syn. *Epilobium septentrionale.* Mat-forming, non-woody, deciduous perennial with oval or lance-shaped to ovate, hairy, grey to grey-green leaves, 1–2.5cm (½–1in) long.

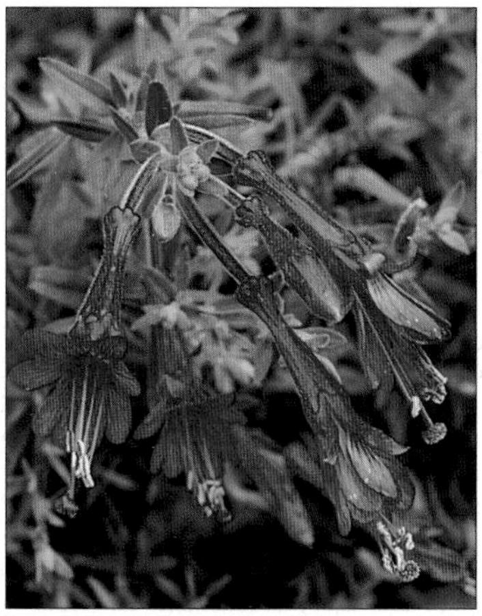

Zauschneria californica subsp. *cana* 'Dublin'

In late summer, bears racemes with a great profusion of short-stalked, tubular scarlet flowers, to 3cm (1¼in) long. ↕ 10–20cm (4–8in), ↔ to 20cm (8in). ✻✻✻

ZEA

GRAMINEAE/POACEAE

Genus of 4 species of annual, rarely perennial grasses found along field margins and on disturbed ground in Central America. The sturdy stems bear lance-shaped leaves in 2 ranks. They produce terminal, spike-like male panicles, each one with a solitary, stemless spikelet or "ear" on the inter-nodes; axillary female inflorescences consist of numerous spikelets arranged in longitudinal rows on a thickened axis. The female flowers, each with a long, silky style, are enclosed within a spathe bract or "husk", and are followed by a "cob" of fleshy kernels. *Z. mays* (maize) is an important cereal crop in tropical and temperate regions. A number of ornamental cultivars are valued for their brightly variegated leaves and for their multi-coloured cobs. Grow in a sheltered mixed border or as dot plants in summer bedding schemes.

• **HARDINESS** Half hardy.
• **CULTIVATION** Grow in a warm, sheltered site in fertile, moist but well-drained soil in full sun.
• **PROPAGATION** Sow seed at 18°C (64°F) in late winter or early spring, or *in situ* in late spring.
• **PESTS AND DISEASES** Occasionally attacked by aphids and sweetcorn smut.

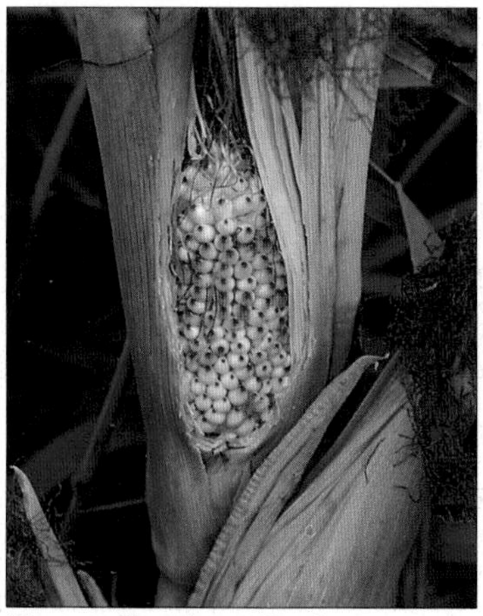

Zea mays 'Strawberry Corn'

Z. mays 𝕐 (Maize, Sweetcorn). Robust, erect, annual grass with pointed, lance-shaped, arching, wavy leaves, to 90cm (36in) long. In midsummer, produces a terminal panicle of spike-like male racemes, to 20cm (8in) long, and female inflorescences, also to 20cm (8in) long, enclosed within spathe bracts. The female flowers are followed in late summer and early autumn by cobs with flattened, usually yellow, sweet-tasting, edible grains, to 1cm (½in) long. ↕ to 4m (12ft), ↔ 60cm (24in) or more. Mexico. ✻. **'Harlequin'** has foliage striped green, red, and white, and cobs with deep red grains; ↕ 1.2m (4ft). **'Strawberry Corn'** ■ produces cobs with small, yellow to burgundy-red grains enclosed within yellow-green spathe bracts; ↕ 1.2m (4ft). **'Variegata'** has leaves boldly striped with creamy white; ↕ 90cm (36in).

▷ **Zebra plant** see *Aphelandra squarrosa, Calathea zebrina, Cryptanthus zonatus*
▷ ***Zebrina pendula*** see *Tradescantia zebrina*
▷ ***Zebrina purpusii*** see *Tradescantia zebrina* 'Purpusii'

ZELKOVA

ULMACEAE

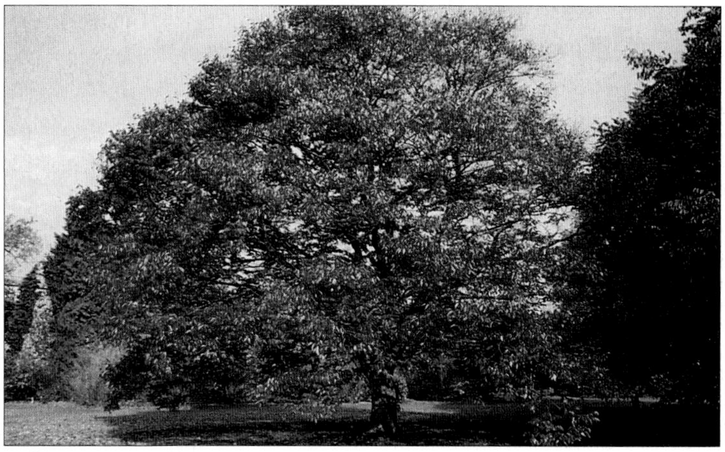

Zelkova serrata

Genus of about 6 species of deciduous, monoecious or hermaphrodite trees, occasionally shrubby, occurring in scrub and woodland in Sicily (Italy), Crete (Greece), N.E. Turkey, the Caucasus, N. Iran, and E. Asia. They are grown for their attractive habit and alternate, oval-oblong to ovate or elliptic, toothed, dark green leaves, which change colour to yellow, then orange-brown or red, in autumn. *Zelkova* species are closely related to, and often confused with elms (*Ulmus*), differing in their unwinged fruits and in their leaves, which are not oblique at the bases. The very small, inconspicuous, male or hermaphrodite green flowers are borne singly or in small clusters in spring, the males from the lower axils of the shoots, the hermaphrodites higher up; the flowers are followed by small, spherical green fruits. *Zelkova* species and cultivars are imposing specimen and avenue trees, most of them suitable for open parkland and larger gardens; *Z. abelicea* and dwarf cultivars of *Z. serrata* are better suited for use in smaller gardens.

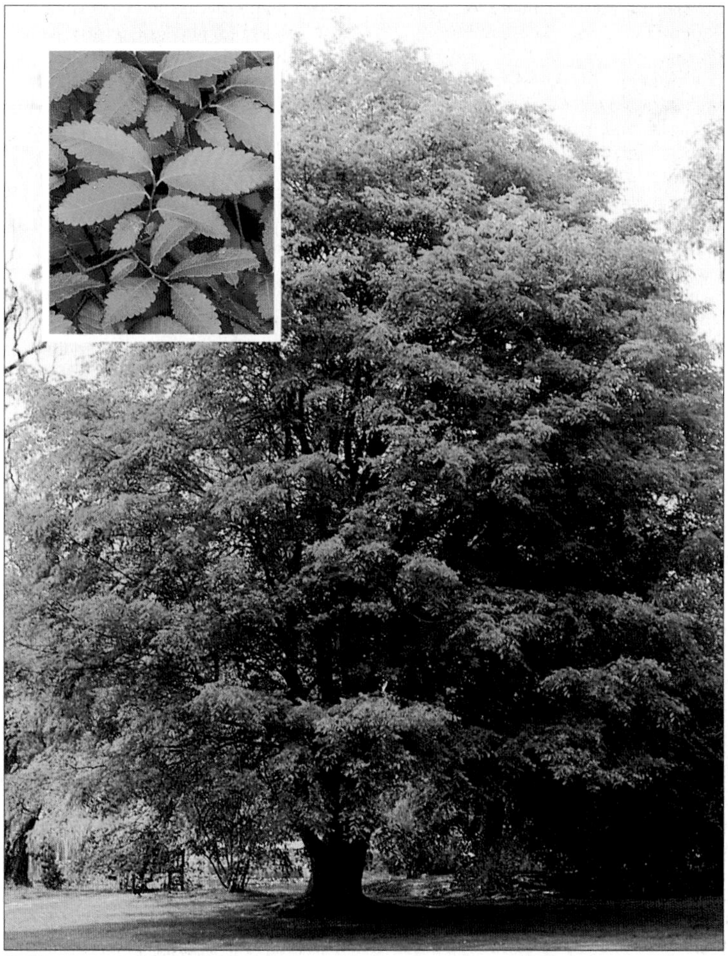

Zelkova carpinifolia (inset: leaf detail)

• **HARDINESS** Fully hardy.
• **CULTIVATION** Grow in deep, fertile, moist but well-drained soil in sun or partial shade. In frost-prone areas, protect from cold, drying winds. Pruning group 1.
• **PROPAGATION** Sow seed in containers outdoors in autumn. Take greenwood cuttings in summer (preferably from young plants). Graft in winter. Remove rooted suckers in winter.
• **PESTS AND DISEASES** Prone to bacterial canker, Dutch elm disease, and horse-chestnut scale.

Z. abelicea ⚲ syn. *Z. cretica*. Spreading, bushy-headed tree with white-hairy young shoots and ovate, thick-textured, glossy, dark green leaves, to 2.5cm (1in) long, each with up to 6 or 7 teeth on either side. ↕ 5m (15ft), ↔ 7m (22ft). Greece (Crete). ✻✻✻
Z. carpinifolia ■⚲ (Caucasian elm). Broadly upright tree, normally with a short, stout trunk from which arise many erect branches. Ovate, dark green leaves, slightly rough above, to 10cm (4in) long, each with about 10 broad teeth on either side, are orange-brown in autumn. ↕ 30m (100ft), ↔ 25m (80ft). Caucasus, N.E. Turkey, N. Iran. ✻✻✻
Z. cretica see *Z. abelicea.*
Z. keaki see *Z. serrata.*
Z. serrata ■𝕐⚲ syn. *Z. keaki* (Japanese zelkova). Spreading tree with smooth grey bark, peeling to reveal orange patches. Thin, narrowly ovate, tapered leaves, to 12cm (5in) long, each with up to 16 teeth on either side, are dark green, becoming yellow, orange, or red in autumn. ↕ to 30m (100ft), ↔ 18m (60ft). S. Korea, Japan, Taiwan. ✻✻✻. **'Goblin'** is dwarf and slow-growing, forming a dense, bushy shrub; ↕↔ 1m (3ft). **'Green Vase'** is vase-shaped, fast-growing, and graceful, with upright, arching branches, and leaves that turn orange-brown to bronze-red in autumn. **'Village Green'** is fast-growing, with red autumn coloration; it is resistant to Dutch elm disease.
Z. sinica ⚲ Broadly upright tree with a short trunk, numerous ascending branches, and peeling bark marked grey, orange, and brown. Ovate, thin, dark green leaves, to 9cm (4½in) long, each with up to 10 teeth on either side and entire at the tapered base, turn yellow or orange in autumn. ↕ 18m (60ft), ↔ 15m (50ft). C. and E. China. ✻✻✻

▷ **Zelkova, Japanese** see *Zelkova serrata.*

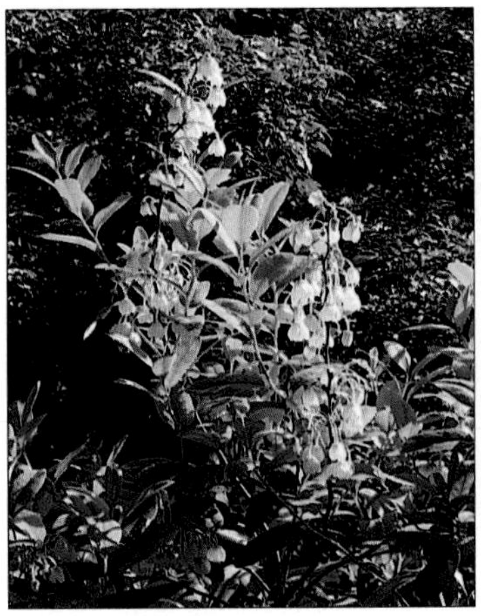

Zenobia pulverulenta

ZENOBIA

ERICACEAE

Genus of one species of spreading, deciduous or semi-evergreen shrub occurring in moist, sandy places and bogs in S.E. USA. It has oblong-ovate, toothed leaves, and is grown for its bell-shaped, fragrant white flowers. Suitable for a woodland garden.

• **HARDINESS** Fully hardy.

• **CULTIVATION** Grow in a sheltered site, in acid, humus-rich, moist soil in sun or partial shade. Plant in shade in areas where the soil dries out in summer. Pruning group 2 or 5, in midsummer.

• **PROPAGATION** Sow seed in containers outdoors in late winter. Take semi-ripe cuttings in summer.

• **PESTS AND DISEASES** Trouble free.

Z. pulverulenta ■ Spreading shrub with slender, arching shoots producing alternate, oblong-ovate, glaucous, blue-green to glossy, dark green leaves, to 8cm (3in) long, with toothed margins. Pendent, bell-shaped, scented white flowers, 1.2cm (½in) long, are borne in erect racemes, to 20cm (8in) long, in early and midsummer. ↕2m (6ft), ↔1.5m (5ft). USA (Virginia to South Carolina). ✻✻✻

ZEPHYRANTHES

syn. COOPERIA

Rain flower, Windflower

AMARYLLIDACEAE

Genus of about 71 species of bulbous perennials, some evergreen, found in grassland from North to South America. Closely related to *Habranthus*, they are grown for their erect, funnel-shaped to tubular, often crocus-like, white, yellow, pink, or red flowers, borne from spring to autumn, usually when the linear leaves emerge. In frost-prone areas, grow in an alpine house or cool greenhouse; *Z. candida* will thrive outside in a rock garden. Elsewhere, use in a rock garden or at the front of a sunny border.

• **HARDINESS** Frost hardy to frost tender.

• **CULTIVATION** Under glass, grow 10cm (4in) deep in loam-based potting compost (JI No.2), with added sharp sand, in full light. When in growth, water freely and apply a balanced liquid fertilizer every 4 weeks. Keep just moist in winter. Outdoors, grow in moist but well-drained soil in full sun. Protect from winter wet.

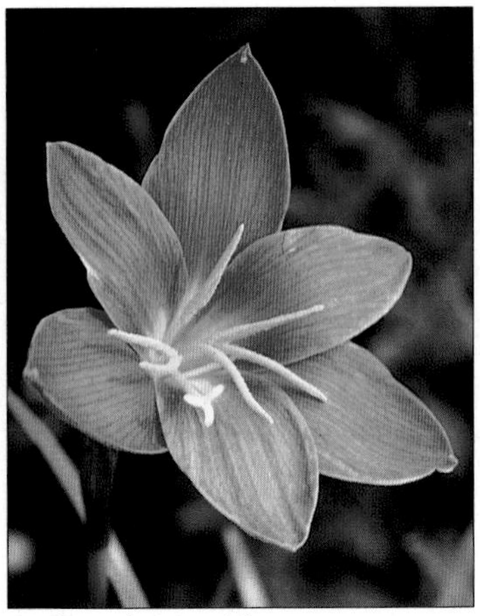

Zephyranthes grandiflora

• **PROPAGATION** Sow seed at 13–18°C (55–64°F) as soon as ripe. Separate offsets in spring.

• **PESTS AND DISEASES** Trouble free.

Z. andersonii see *Habranthus tubispathus.*

Z. atamasco (Atamasco lily). Deciduous, bulbous perennial with semi-erect, strap-shaped, basal leaves, to 40cm (16in) long. In spring or summer, bears funnel-shaped white flowers, 7cm (3in) long, the petals sometimes flushed with purple. ↕20–30cm (8–12in), ↔5cm (2in). S.E. USA. ✻

Z. candida. Deciduous, bulbous perennial with upright, narrowly linear, basal leaves, to 40cm (16in) long. Bears a succession of crocus-like, pure white flowers, 3cm (1¼in) long, occasionally tinted with red on the petal backs, from summer to early autumn. ↕10–20cm (4–8in), ↔8cm (3in). Argentina, Uruguay. ✻✻

Z. carinata see *Z. grandiflora.*

Z. citrina. Deciduous, bulbous perennial producing crocus-like, bright yellow flowers, 5cm (2in) long, above the erect, rush-like, basal leaves, to 30cm (12in) long, in autumn. ↕10–15cm (4–6in), ↔5cm (2in). Tropical South America. ✻

Z. grandiflora ■ syn. *Z. carinata, Z. rosea* of gardens. Deciduous, bulbous perennial with semi-erect, slender, linear, glossy, basal leaves, to 30cm (12in) long. In late summer and early autumn, bears funnel-shaped, bright pink flowers, 7cm (3in) long. An attractive greenhouse container plant. ↕20–30cm (8–12in), ↔5cm (2in). Central America. ✻

Z. robusta see *Habranthus robustus.*

Z. rosea. Deciduous, bulbous perennial with semi-erect, narrowly linear, basal leaves, to 20cm (8in) long. Short-tubed, funnel-shaped pink flowers, to 3cm (1¼in) long, are borne in autumn. ↕15–20cm (6–8in), ↔8–10cm (3–4in). Cuba, West Indies, Guatemala. ✻

***Z. rosea* of gardens** see *Z. grandiflora.*

ZIGADENUS

LILIACEAE/MELANTHIACEAE

Genus of 18 species of bulbous or rhizomatous, deciduous perennials from grassland and open woodland in North America, Mexico, and N.E. Asia. They are cultivated for their upright, terminal racemes or panicles of small, star-shaped, 6-tepalled, greenish white or yellowish

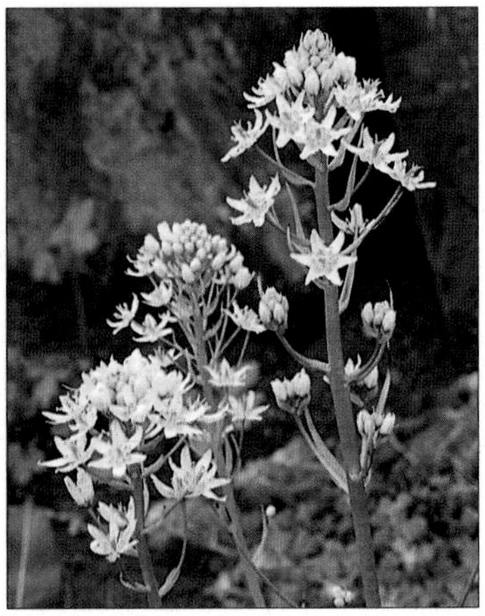

Zigadenus fremontii

white flowers, produced in summer. The leaves are mainly basal and linear, and often folded or keeled. Good for a shady border or woodland garden; grow *Z. fremontii* in a bulb frame. All parts are highly toxic if ingested.

• **HARDINESS** Frost hardy.

• **CULTIVATION** Grow in deep, fertile, moist but well-drained soil in full sun or partial shade; *Z. fremontii* prefers full sun. In a bulb frame, grow 15–20cm (6–8in) deep in equal parts loam-based potting compost (JI No.2) and grit.

• **PROPAGATION** Sow seed at 13–18°C (55–64°F) when ripe or in spring. Divide in spring or autumn.

• **PESTS AND DISEASES** Trouble free.

Z. elegans. Bulbous perennial with semi-erect, narrowly linear, grey-green, basal leaves, to 30cm (12in) long. Bears spikes of many star-shaped, greenish white flowers, 8mm (⅜in) across, with prominent, yellowish green nectaries, in mid- and late summer. ↕70cm (28in), ↔8cm (3in). North America (Alaska, Minnesota to Arizona). ✻✻

Z. fremontii ■ Robust, bulbous perennial with semi-erect, narrowly linear, greyish green, basal leaves, to 60cm (24in) long. Racemes or panicles of many star-shaped, creamy white flowers, 1.5cm (½in) across, are borne in early summer. Requires dry summer dormancy; best in a bulb frame. ↕70cm (28in), ↔8cm (3in). USA (S. Oregon) to Mexico (N. Baja California). ✻✻

Z. glaucus. Bulbous perennial with semi-erect, narrowly linear, greyish green, basal leaves, to 30cm (12in) long. In summer, bears racemes or panicles of many star-shaped, creamy white flowers, to 1cm (½in) across, suffused brown or purple. ↕to 60cm (24in), ↔to 8cm (3in). E. Canada, N.E. USA. ✻✻

Z. nuttallii. Slender, bulbous perennial with semi-erect, narrowly linear, mid- to dark green, basal leaves, to 45cm (18in) long. In summer, bears dense racemes of numerous tiny, star-shaped, creamy yellow flowers, 6–8mm (¼–⅜in) across. ↕30–60cm (12–24in), ↔8cm (3in). W. North America. ✻✻

Z. venenosus (Death camas). Bulbous perennial with semi-erect, narrowly linear, mid- to dark green, basal leaves, to 30cm (12in) long. In summer, produces slender racemes of numerous small, star-shaped, off-white flowers, 3–6mm (⅛–¼in) across. ↕70cm (28in), ↔8cm (3in). North America (W. Canada to Utah, New Mexico). ✻✻

ZINNIA

ASTERACEAE/COMPOSITAE

Genus of 20 species of spreading to erect annuals, perennials, and subshrubs from scrub and desert grassland, mainly in Mexico, but also in S.W. USA, and Central and South America. They have branching, angled or rounded stems and opposite, stalkless or almost stalkless, linear to ovate or elliptic, pale to mid-green leaves. Zinnias are cultivated for their solitary, long-stemmed, daisy-like, terminal flowerheads in a wide range of colours, including white, yellow, orange, red, purple, and lilac, some with white eyes. Use in an annual or mixed border, and for cutting. Smaller cultivars are suitable for edging, and for window-boxes or other containers.

• **HARDINESS** Frost tender.

• **CULTIVATION** Grow in fertile, humus-rich, well-drained soil in full sun. Dead-head to prolong flowering.

• **PROPAGATION** Sow seed at 13–18°C (55–64°F) in early spring, or *in situ* in late spring. Sow in succession for a longer flowering display.

• **PESTS AND DISEASES** Trouble free if grown in an open position to minimize attack by mildew.

***Z. angustifolia* of gardens** see *Z. haageana.*

***Z. angustifolia* 'Orange Star'** see *Z. haageana* 'Orange Star'.

***Z. angustifolia* 'Persian Carpet'** see *Z. haageana* 'Persian Carpet'.

Z. elegans. Upright, bushy annual bearing lightly hairy, ovate to lance-

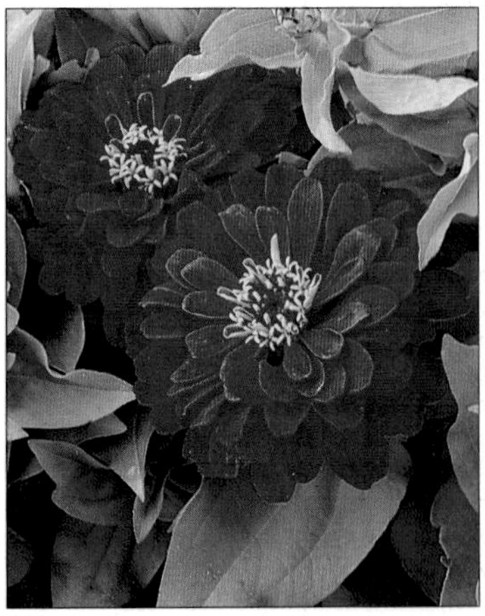

Zinnia elegans Dreamland Series 'Dreamland Scarlet'

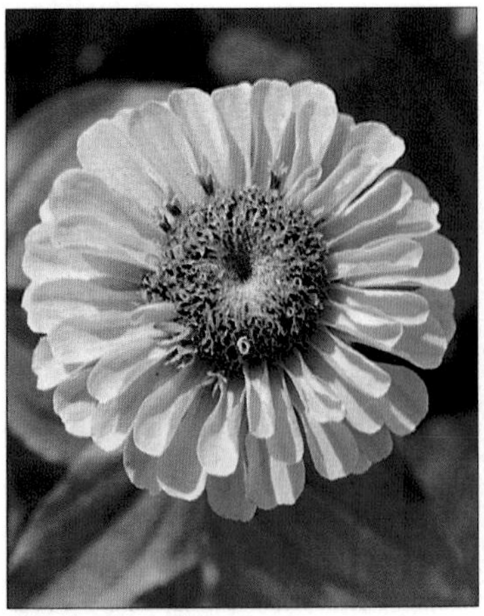

Zinnia elegans 'Envy'

Z

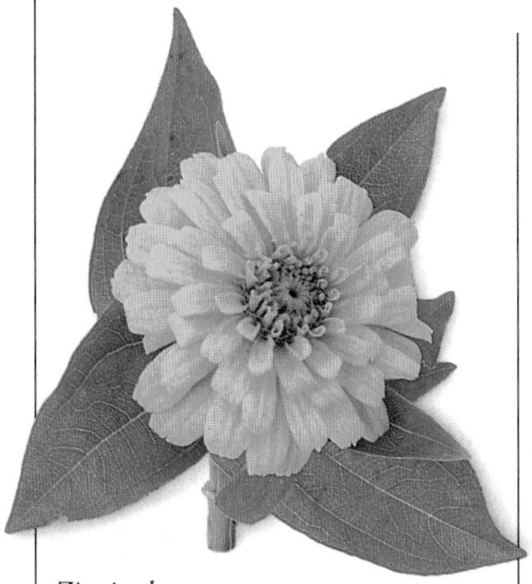

Zinnia elegans
Peter Pan Series 'Peter Pan Gold'

shaped leaves, to 8cm (3in) long. Daisy-like, broad-petalled purple flowerheads, to 4.5cm (1¾in) across, are produced in summer. ↕ 60–75cm (24–30in), ↔ 30cm (12in). Mexico. ❄ (min. 10°C/50°F). **'Belvedere'** is dwarf, with double, weather-resistant flowerheads in a broad colour range; ↕ to 30cm (12in). **Cactus-flowered Group** cultivars are tall-growing, with large, semi-double flowerheads, to 12cm (5in) across, like those of cactus dahlias, with long, narrow, quilled petals in a broad colour range; ↕ 60–90cm (24–36in). **Dreamland Series 'Dreamland Scarlet'** ■ is dwarf and compact, produces scarlet-orange blooms, and is ideal for containers or bedding; ↕ 20–25cm (8–10in). **'Envy'** ■ has semi-double, chartreuse-green flowerheads, and tolerates shade; ↕ to 75cm (30in). **Hobgoblin Series** cultivars are dwarf, sturdy, and bushy, with small, single, weather-resistant flowerheads in a broad colour range; good for bedding; ↕ to 45cm (18in). **Peter Pan Series** cultivars are extremely dwarf and compact; early-flowering with large flowers, to 10cm (4in) across; use in containers or as bedding plants; **'Peter Pan Gold'** ■ has golden yellow flowers. **'Ruffles'** has ruffled, fully double flowerheads, like those of pompon dahlias, in a wide colour range; good for cut flowers; ↕ to 60cm (24in). **Short Stuff Series** cultivars are dwarf and compact, with double flowerheads, to 6cm (2½in) across, in a broad colour range; ↕ to 25cm (10in). **Small World Series** cultivars are dwarf, with double flowerheads in a wide colour range,

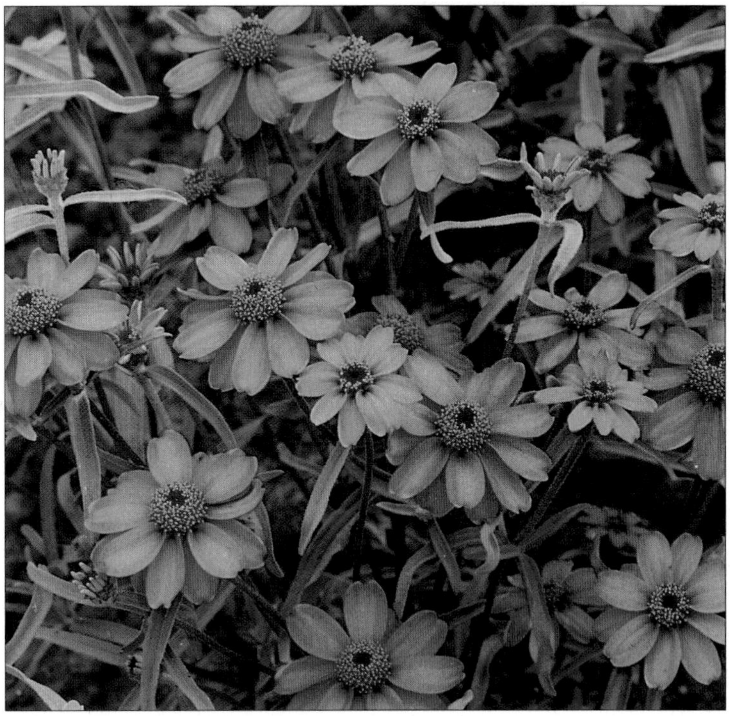

Zinnia haageana 'Orange Star'

including pale pink; ↕ to 45cm (18in). **'State Fair'** is tall-growing and very vigorous, with large, double, lavender, rose-pink, orange, purple, or scarlet flowerheads, to 8cm (3in) across; ↕ to 75cm (30in). **Thumbelina Series** ■ cultivars are very dwarf and spreading, with single or semi-double, weather-resistant, yellow, red, magenta, or pale pink flowerheads; ↕ to 15cm (6in).
Z. haageana, syn. *Z. angustifolia* of gardens, *Z. mexicana* (Mexican zinnia). Erect, bushy annual with oblong to linear or linear-lance-shaped leaves, to 7cm (3in) long, lightly covered in bristly hairs. Daisy-like, broad-petalled, bright orange flowerheads, to 3.5cm (1½in) across, are produced in summer. ↕ to 60cm (24in), ↔ to 30cm (12in). S.E. USA, Mexico. ✻. **'Classic'** see 'Orange Star'. **'Orange Star'** ■ syn. 'Classic', *Z. angustifolia* 'Orange Star', is dwarf and bushy in habit, and produces orange flowerheads; mildew-resistant and good for ground cover; ↕ to 25cm (10in). **'Persian Carpet'** ■ syn. *Z. angustifolia* 'Persian Carpet', is dwarf, compact, and spreading; produces small, semi-double and double, weather-resistant flowerheads, to 4cm (1½in) across, in a range of bicolours and tricolours; excellent for summer bedding; ↕ to 40cm (16in). **'Star White'** has white flowerheads with golden yellow centres.
Z. mexicana see *Z. haageana.*

▷ **Zinnia,**
Creeping see *Sanvitalia, S. procumbens*
Mexican see *Zinnia haageana*

ZIZANIA

Water oats, Wild rice

GRAMINEAE/POACEAE

Genus of 3 species of annual or perennial, marginal aquatic grasses from marshland and lake margins in E. Asia and North America. They are cultivated for their flat, linear leaves, produced on tall, reedy stems. Conical or pyramidal, feathery panicles of spikelets are borne from summer to autumn, followed by edible, rice-like seeds. Suitable for a large pond or wildlife pool. In frost-prone areas, grow tender species in a warm greenhouse.
• **HARDINESS** Fully hardy to frost tender.
• **CULTIVATION** Outdoors, grow at the edges of a large pool in full sun, in water to 23cm (9in) deep. See also pp.52–53.
• **PROPAGATION** Overwinter seed in trays of damp loam, and sow at 18°C (64°F) in early spring. As the seedlings emerge, cover with 5cm (2in) of water and maintain at the same temperature.
• **PESTS AND DISEASES** Trouble free.

Z. aquatica (Annual wild rice, Canadian wild rice, Water rice). Marginal aquatic annual with grass-like, linear, deep green leaves, to 1.2m (4ft) long. Pale green flowers are borne in pyramidal panicles, to 75cm (30in) long, in summer, followed by edible, rice-like seeds. ↕ 3m (10ft), ↔ 45cm (18in). North America. ✻✻✻

▷ ***Zygocactus truncatus*** see *Schlumbergera truncata*

ZYGOPETALUM

ORCHIDACEAE

Genus of about 20 species of evergreen, epiphytic or terrestrial orchids native to South America, occurring in warm, moist rainforest, sometimes on rocky outcrops or in leaf litter. They have conical to ovoid pseudobulbs, from the tops of which are produced 2 or more narrowly elongated, lance-shaped, leathery or fleshy leaves. Racemes of delicate, highly fragrant flowers, most of which are richly coloured with an attractive combination of green-brown and indigo-blue, arise from the bases of the pseudobulbs from autumn to spring.
• **HARDINESS** Frost tender.
• **CULTIVATION** Cool- to intermediate-growing orchids. Grow in standard epiphytic orchid compost in containers that will easily accommodate the root system, or in slatted baskets. During the growing season, provide high humidity and bright filtered light; water freely, and apply a quarter- to half-strength balanced liquid fertilizer at every third watering. In winter, admit full light and water sparingly. See also p.46.
• **PROPAGATION** Divide when the roots of the plant fill the container and "flow" over the sides. Alternatively, remove backbulbs and pot them up separately.
• **PESTS AND DISEASES** May be attacked by red spider mites, aphids, and mealybugs.

Z. mackaii ■ syn. *Z. mackayi.* Epiphytic orchid with fleshy, ovoid pseudobulbs and 2 or 3 pendent, lance-shaped, leathery, apical leaves, 30–50cm (12–20in) long. Upright racemes of 5–7 green flowers, to 8cm (3in) across, each one strongly barred in brown and with a heavily veined indigo-blue lip, are produced from autumn to winter. ↕ 30cm (12in), ↔ 45cm (18in). Brazil. ❄ (min. 11–13°C/52–55°F; max. 30°C/86°F)
Z. mackayi see *Z. mackaii.*
***Z.* Perrenoudii** (*Z. intermedium* x *Z. maxillare*). Epiphytic orchid with fleshy, ovoid pseudobulbs and 2 pendent, lance-shaped, leathery, apical leaves, 30cm (12in) long. Upright racemes of 5–12 green flowers, 5–7cm (2–3in) across, each one lightly barred in brown and with a heavily veined indigo lip, are produced from autumn to spring. ↕↔ 30cm (12in). ❄ (min. 11–13°C/ 52–55°F; max. 30°C/86°F)

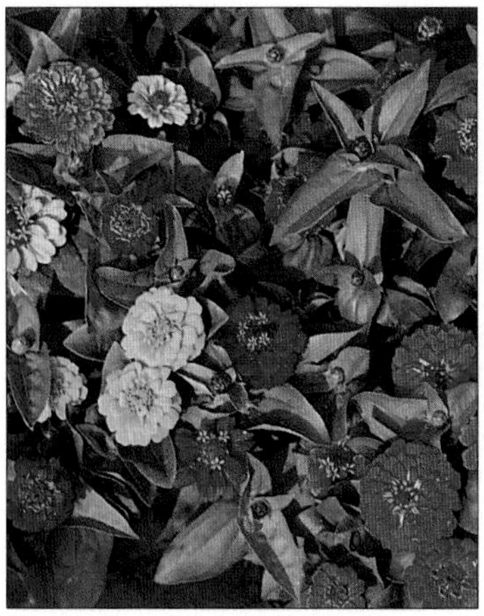

Zinnia elegans Thumbelina Series

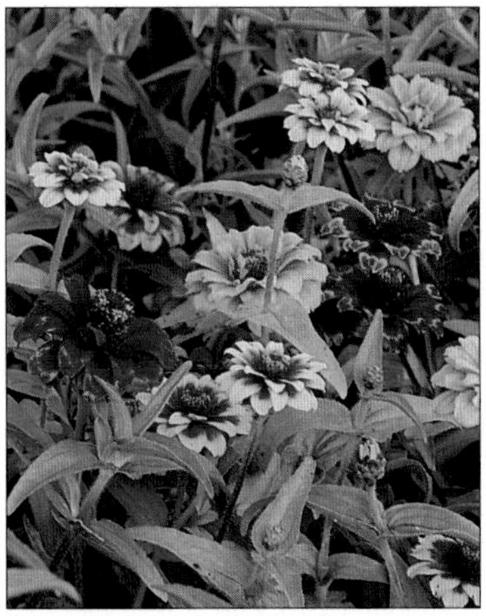

Zinnia haageana 'Persian Carpet'

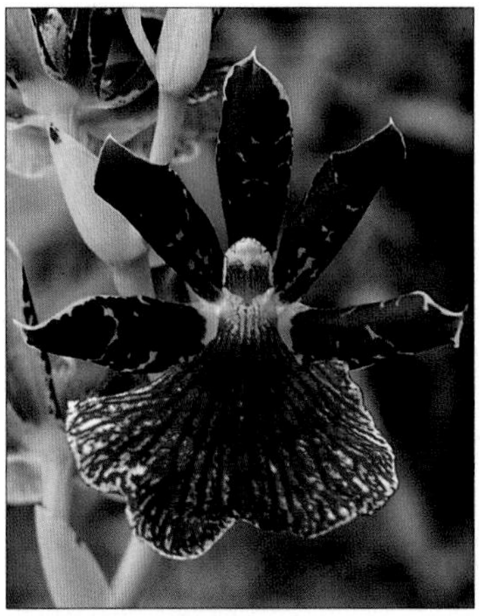

Zygopetalum mackaii

GLOSSARY OF TERMS

This glossary provides concise definitions of terms used throughout the encyclopedia, as well as a number of others commonly found in horticulture. For the sake of clarity, many of the terms are narrowly defined here, but may be interpreted differently in non-horticultural contexts. For an illustrated account of plant botany, cultivation, and ornamental plant groups, see the introductory pages (pp.10–54); an index for these appears on p.1080. Pests and diseases are defined on pp.30–31.

A

Accent plant Plant used in a formal bed or border to emphasize contrasts of height, colour, and/or texture.
Acicular *see* Linear, Needle.
Acid With a pH value below 7.
Acuminate With a long, tapering point.
Acute Ending in a short, sharp point.
Adpressed Pressed flat to the axis to which it is attached.
Adventitious Refers to a plant organ that occurs in an unusual location.
Aeration Loosening of the soil structure to allow free circulation of air.
Aerial root Root that emerges from the stem above ground level.
Air-layering Method of propagation whereby a cut in an aerial stem is covered with moist sphagnum moss and sealed in a plastic sleeve in order to induce rooting. *See also p.28.*
Alkaline With a pH value above 7.
Alpine 1. High-altitude plant from above the tree-line and usually snow-covered in winter. 2. Loosely, any plant suitable for a rock garden. *See also pp.40–41.*
Alpine house Unheated, well-ventilated greenhouse used to grow alpines and other perennial plants.
Alternate Describes organs, usually leaves, borne singly at each node, in 2 vertical rows, on either side of an axis.
Angiosperm Flowering plant that bears ovules, later seeds, enclosed in ovaries (as opposed to a gymnosperm that bears naked ovules, then seeds, in cones). *See also p.10.*
Annual Plant that completes its life-cycle in one growing season. *See also pp.42–43.*
Annulus 1. Corona or rim of the corolla in the plants of the Asclepiadaceae family. 2. In ferns, the part of the sporangium involved in spore dispersal.
Anther Part of the stamen that releases pollen; usually borne on a filament.
Apex (*pl.* apexes; *adj.* apical) Tip or growing point of an organ.
Apomixis (*adj.* apomictic) Asexual production of ripe seed. Offspring are clones – genetically identical to the parent.
Aquatic plant Plant that lives in water; free-floating, submerged, or rooted on the bottom with the leaves and flowers above water. *See also pp.52–53.*
Areole 1. Depressed or raised area bearing spines, branches, or flowers in cacti. 2. Small space outlined on a surface, such as an area of leaf between veins.
Aril Coat covering some seeds, often fleshy and brightly coloured.
Aroid Member of the Araceae family, characterized by an inflorescence composed of a spadix and spathe.
Arrow-shaped (sagittate) With a narrow, blunt or pointed tip, and widening at the base into 2 acute, downward-pointing lobes.
Asexual reproduction Process of producing new individuals by apomixis or vegetative propagation. *See also* Reproduction.
Auricle (*adj.* auricular) Ear-like lobe, often in pairs at the base of an organ.
Awn Stiff, bristle-like projection often found on grass seeds and spikelets.
Axil Upper angle between a part of a plant and the stem that bears it.
Axillary Borne in an axil. *See also* Terminal.
Axis (*pl.* axes) Rachis, stalk, or stem on which organs such as flowers, leaves, or leaflets are arranged.

B

Backbulb Dormant pseudobulb unique to orchids.
Bamboo Woody-caned plant belonging to the Gramineae family. *See also p.54.*
Bark Outermost layers of a woody stem, including all the living and non-living tissues outside the cambium.
Basal At the base of an organ or structure.
Basal leaf Leaf that grows from the lowest part of the stem.
Basal stem cutting Cutting taken from the base of a plant, usually herbaceous, in spring.
Beard 1. Awn. 2. Tuft or zone of hair.
Bed Area of ground, often set into a lawn, in which plants are grown.
Bedding plant Annual, biennial, or perennial planted to provide a temporary display of foliage and/or flowers.
Bell-shaped (campanulate) Describes a flower with a broad tube terminating in flared lobes.
Berry Fruit with soft flesh surrounding one or more seeds.
Bicoloured With 2 distinct colours.
Biennial Plant that completes its life-cycle in 2 years, growing in the first year, and flowering and fruiting in the second. *See also pp.10, 42–43.*
Bigeneric hybrid Offspring derived from crossing 2 different genera.
Binomial Two-part name derived from Latin or Greek, consisting of a genus name and a species, cultivar, group, series, or hybrid epithet, denoting an individual within a genus. *See also p.11.*
Bipinnate *see* Pinnate.
Bisexual (hermaphrodite) Refers to a flower that bears both male and female reproductive organs.
Bleed To weep sap.
Blind 1. Refers to a plant in which the growing point has been damaged. 2. Refers to plants, particularly bulbs, that do not flower.
Bloom 1. Flower or blossom. 2. Fine, waxy, whitish or bluish white coating. *See also* Glaucous, White-frosted.
Bog garden Waterlogged area used to grow plants found in bogs, marshes, wet pasture, and at water margins.
Bolt To produce flowers and seed prematurely.
Bonsai Production of dwarf trees or shrubs by pruning and root restriction.
Bottom heat Warmth radiated from below, usually via electrical cables, used in propagating cases to assist the rooting of cuttings and the germination of seed.
Bowl-shaped Describes a flower that is hemispherical with the sides straight or very slightly spreading at the tips.
Bract Modified leaf at the base of a flower or flowerhead. May be small and scale-like, or large, brightly coloured, and petal-like, or resemble normal foliage.
Bracteole Secondary bract sheathing a flower in an inflorescence, itself enclosed within a primary bract.
Branch Division of a stem, a trunk, or the axis of an inflorescence.
Branched-head standard Standard tree with a clear stem of 1.8m (6ft); the leader is cut back to develop an open crown. *See also p.33,* Central-leader standard.
Break To produce new growth as a result of pinching out.
Broad-leaved Describes trees and shrubs that have broad, flat, usually deciduous leaves – in contrast to the narrow, linear, usually evergreen needles of conifers.
Broken Type of marking in which the ground colour is striped with one or more contrasting colours, usually caused by viral infection; particularly applied to tulips.
Bromeliad Member of the Bromeliaceae family, characterized by showy inflorescences, frequently with brightly coloured bracts, and rosettes of often colourful leaves. *See also p.47.*
Bud Immature organ or shoot enclosing an embryonic branch, leaf, inflorescence, or flower.
Budding Method of propagation in which a vegetative bud of one plant is grafted on to another plant.
Bulb Modified, subterranean bud, with a short, thick stem and fleshy, scale leaves or leaf bases.
Bulb frame Glass or plastic frame used to provide a dry environment for bulbs during dormancy.
Bulbil Small, bulb-like organ borne in the axil of a leaf, bract, or occasionally flowerhead.
Bulblet Small bulb produced at the base of a parent bulb, often inside the tunic.
Bulbous 1. Describes a stem that is swollen at the base, usually underground. 2. Describes a plant with bulbs. 3. Loosely, refers to a plant with an underground storage organ such as a bulb, corm, tuber, or rhizome. *See also pp.44–45.*
Burr 1. Prickly, spiny, or hooked fruit, seed head, or flowerhead. 2. Woody outgrowth on the trunk of some trees.
Buttress root Fluted or swollen tree trunk that aids stability in shallow rooting conditions. *See also* Stilt root.

C

Cactus (*pl.* cacti) Stem succulent, member of the Cactaceae family. *See also pp.48–49.*
Calcareous Refers to soil with a high content of calcium carbonate (chalk) or magnesium carbonate. *See also* Lime.
Callus Thickened tissue that is formed by the cambium layer to aid healing around a wound.
Calyx (*pl.* calyces) Collective name for sepals, joined or separate, which form the outer whorl of the perianth.
Cambium Growth tissue directly below the bark of woody plants; its increase adds to the girth of roots and stems.
Campanulate *see* Bell-shaped.
Cane Hollow, slender, jointed stem, particularly characteristic of bamboos.
Capitulum *see* Flowerhead.
Capsule Dry fruit that splits open to disperse ripe seed.
Carnivorous (insectivorous) Applied to a plant that obtains nutrients by trapping and ingesting insects or other small creatures.
Carpel Female part of a flower consisting of a style, a stigma, and an ovary. *See also* Pistil.
Catkin Form of inflorescence, often pendent, consisting of scale-like bracts and tiny, unisexual, usually petalless flowers arranged in a spike.
Caudex (*pl.* caudices; *adj.* caudiciform) Swollen stem base of a woody-based plant such as a palm, a cycad, or some succulents.
Caudiciform Resembling or possessing a caudex.
Central Spine of a cactus, growing from the centre of an areole.
Central-leader standard Standard tree with a clear stem of 1.8m (6ft) or more, and lateral branches that taper from an erect central leader. *See also p.33,* Branched-head standard.
Central vein *see* Midrib.
Cephalium Woody, flower-bearing, densely spined area at the stem apex of some cacti. *See also* Pseudocephalium.
Chalky *see* Calcareous.
Channelled Lined with one or more longitudinal grooves.
Chimaera Plant composed of 2 or more genetically different tissues; the result of a mutation or of a graft hybrid.
Chipping *see* Scarify.
Chlorophyll Green pigment that absorbs energy from sunlight. *See also* Photosynthesis.
Chlorosis Loss of chlorophyll, and consequently the loss of green leaf coloration, caused by mineral deficiency, poor light levels, or disease.

Cladode *see* Phylloclade.
Cladophyll *see* Phylloclade.
Clay Very fertile, heavy, moisture-retentive soil, prone to compaction and surface capping.
Clay granules Moisture-retentive pellets of expanded clay. In hot, dry weather, the evaporation of water poured on to these granules increases humidity around houseplants.
Cleft Divided almost halfway to the centre. *See also* Sinus.
Climber Plant that climbs or clings by means of modified stems, roots, leaves, or leaf-stalks, using other plants or objects as support. *See also pp.36–37,* Scandent, Tendril.
Cloche Structure of glass or plastic panes or plastic sheeting, mainly used for cold-weather protection or for forcing early crops in open ground.
Clone A genetically identical group of plants derived from one individual by vegetative propagation or apomixis.
Cluster (fascicle) Arrangement of several inflorescences, leaves, stems, roots, or flowers that arise from a single point, or appear to do so.
Cold frame Unheated frame used for growing on fully hardy, frost-hardy, and half-hardy plants, usually situated outdoors.
Cold greenhouse Unheated but frost-free greenhouse. *See also p.24.*
Column Flower organ, mainly found in orchids, consisting of fused male and female reproductive parts.
Compaction Compression of soil, particularly saturated clay and silt soils, resulting in poor aeration. *See also* Surface-capping.
Compost *see* Cutting compost, Garden compost, JI No.1/2/3, Loam, Potting compost, Seed compost.
Compound Consisting of several parts, but still identifiable as single unit, such as a leaf divided into 2 or more leaflets.
Cone Woody, seed-bearing structure in gymnosperms, generally composed of an axis with many lateral scales.
Conifer (*adj.* coniferous) Mostly evergreen trees or shrubs, usually with needle-like, linear leaves, and seeds borne naked on the scales of cones. Often from cool-temperate zones.
Conservatory Glazed, heated or unheated structure attached to a house; often has poorer ventilation than a greenhouse. *See also p.24.*
Continental climate Weather conditions in the centre of a landmass, distant from coastal areas; the seasons are well defined, with hot summers and cold winters. *See also pp.18–19.*
Contractile Describes a root that is able to draw a bulb, corm, rhizome, or seedling deeper into the soil or closer to the surface.
Cool greenhouse Greenhouse with a minimum temperature of 2°C (35°F). *See also p.24.*
Cool-temperate Refers to a temperate climate with cold winters and warm summers.
Coppice (stool) To prune trees or shrubs close to ground level annually to promote strong growth.
Cordate *see* Heart-shaped.
Cordon Trained plant (usually a fruit tree) generally restricted to one main stem, occasionally 2–4 stems, by a careful system of training and pruning.
Corm (*adj.* cormous) Subterranean storage organ consisting of a solid stem or stem base, often enclosed in a tunic. Corms are replaced annually.
Cormlet Small corm that arises at or near the base of a mature one.
Corolla 1. Collective name for petals. 2. Inner whorl of perianth segments in some monocotyledons.
Corona A crown- or cup-like growth on a flower, between the corolla and the stamens, formed either by fused stamen filaments or from the perianth segments.
Corymb Broad, flat-topped or domed inflorescence of stalked flowers or flower-heads arising at different levels on alternate sides of an axis.
Cotyledon *see* Seed-leaf.
Crenate *see* Scalloped.
Crest 1. Tuft of hairs or soft bristles. 2. Raised ridge on a surface. *See also* Beard.
Cristate 1. Crested, or with a terminal tuft of hairs or other tissue. 2. Describes ferns with ruffled, usually forked fronds.
Crocks Broken pieces of clay pot, used to cover drainage holes in containers in order to provide free drainage and improve air circulation to the roots.
Cross To interbreed. *See also* Hybrid.
Cross-pollination When the stigma of a flower on one plant is dusted with the pollen from a different plant.
Cross-shaped (cruciform) Describes a flower with 4 petals, usually set at right-angles to each other in the form of a cross when viewed from above.
Crown 1. Growing point of a plant from which new shoots arise, at or just below the soil surface, at the junction with the roots. 2. Uppermost part of a tree or shrub. 3. Corona of a flower.
Crown bud Central flower bud growing at the tip of a shoot among other, usually smaller buds.
Crownshaft Upper section of a palm or cycad trunk, bearing leaves and inflorescences.
Crozier Coiled juvenile frond of a fern, similar in form to a bishop's crozier.
Cruciform *see* Cross-shaped.
Culm Jointed flowering stem of a grass.
Cultivar (*abbrev.* cv., contraction of "cultivated variety") Plant raised or selected in cultivation that retains distinct, uniform characteristics when propagated by appropriate means. *See also p.11, 42.*
Cuneate *see* Wedge-shaped.
Cup Corona of *Narcissus*, but only when shorter than the surrounding tepals.
Cup-shaped Describes a flower that is hemispherical with the sides straight or very slightly spreading at the tips; slightly narrower than bowl-shaped.
Cupule Cup-shaped whorl of hard, fused bracts surrounding the base of a fruit, as in beech nuts (*Fagus*).
Cutting Section of leaf, stem, or root separated from a plant and used for propagation. *See also p.29,* Basal stem cutting, Greenwood cutting, Hardwood cutting, Heel cutting, Leaf-bud cutting, Leaf cutting, Root cutting, Semi-ripe cutting, Softwood cutting, Stem-tip cutting.
Cutting compost Free-draining, low-nutrient compost that is used to root cuttings; usually based on fine-grade granulated bark, soil, peat (or peat substitute), perlite, or sand.
Cyathium (*pl.* cyathia) Inflorescence of *Euphorbia*, in which a cup-like involucre surrounds a single pistil and several male flowers, each with a single stamen; flowers are sometimes bisexual.
Cycad Member of the Cycadaceae family, mainly with stiff, palm-like leaves borne terminally from a short, stout trunk. *See also p.50.*
Cyme Flat or round-topped, branched inflorescence with each axis ending in a flower, the oldest at the centre, and the youngest arising in succession from the axils of bracteoles.

D

Damp down To wet the floor and staging in a greenhouse in order to raise humidity and lower the temperature. *See also* Mist.
Damping off Collapse of seedlings and young plants caused by fungi, which rot the bases of stems and roots.
Dead-head To remove spent flowerheads in order to prolong flowering and prevent self-seeding.
Deciduous 1. Shedding leaves annually at the end of the growing season. 2. Falling away when no longer functional, as with the petals of many flowers.
Decumbent Growing close to the ground but usually with upward-growing tips.
Decurrent Extending downwards from the point of attachment; often used to describe the attachment of a leaf to a stem.
Decussate *see* Rank.
Deep-water aquatic Plant that roots in water 30–90cm (12–36in) deep, and produces foliage and flowers at or above surface level.
Deltoid *see* Triangular.
Dentate *see* Toothed.
Depressed Describes a flattened, solid form.
Diamond-shaped (rhomboidal) Roughly oval but with acute angles at the base and tip, and obtuse angles midway down both sides.
Dicotyledon Angiosperm with 2 seed-leaves, net-veined leaves, a cambium layer (in many species), and floral parts usually in fours or fives. *See also* Monocotyledon.
Die-back Death of a shoot, beginning at the tip, due to damage or disease.
Digitate *see* Palmate.
Dioecious Bearing male and female flowers on separate plants, so that both male and female plants must be grown if fruit is required.
Disbud To remove surplus buds so that better quality flowers or fruit are borne.
Disc-floret Tiny, usually tubular flower, one of many that normally comprise the centre of a (composite) flowerhead.
Dissected *see* Divided.
Distichous *see* Rank.
Diurnal With activity taking place only in daylight, e.g. a flower that opens only during the day.
Divide To propagate a plant by splitting it into 2 or more parts, each with its own section of root system and one or more shoots or dormant buds.
Divided (dissected) Deeply cut into segments or lobes.
Dormancy (*adj.* dormant) Suspension of active growth in unfavourable conditions.
Dot plant Usually tall-growing plant, used singly in the design of a formal bed or border to accentuate contrasts of height, colour, and/or texture.
Double Describes a flower with more petals than in the normal wild state, and with few, if any, stamens.
Drainage 1. Movement of excess water through the soil or compost. 2. System designed to remove excess water rapidly from the soil.
Drill Narrow, straight furrow in the soil, in which seeds are sown.
Drupe Fruit consisting of one or several hard seeds (stones) surrounded by a fleshy outer covering.
Dwarf Small or slow-growing variant of a species resulting from hybridization, mutation, or specific cultivation methods. *See also* Bonsai.

E

Earth up To draw soil up around a plant to exclude light, promote the formation of roots from the stem, or provide winter protection.
Ellipsoid Describes a solid form, broadest at the centre, tapering towards each end; length is 2 times the width. It is wider than a spindle-shaped form, with the sides more curved.
Elliptic Describes a flat structure, broadest at the centre, tapering towards each end; length is 2 times the width.
Embryo Part of a seed from which a new plant develops.
Ensiform *see* Strap-shaped.
Entire Describes a continuous, untoothed, and unlobed margin, usually of a leaf.
Epicalyx (*pl.* epicalyces) 1. Whorl of bracts surrounding the calyx. 2. False calyx.
Epicormic Refers to strong shoots that develop from latent or adventitious buds under the bark of a tree or shrub, usually close to pruning cuts or wounds.
Epiphyte (*adj.* epiphytic) Plant that grows on another plant without obtaining food from it.
Erect Upright; perpendicular to the ground or to the point of attachment.
Ericaceous 1. Belonging to the Ericaceae family. 2. Heath-like or allied to the genus *Erica.* 3. Describes potting compost with a pH of 6.5 or less, suitable for growing acid-loving plants.
Espalier Fruit tree with pairs of branches trained horizontally from the central stem, in a single plane.
Etiolated Describes a plant that has abnormally elongated, often bleached shoots as a result of poor light levels.
Evergreen 1. Retaining leaves for more than one growing season. 2. Plant with the above characteristic.
Eye Centre of a flower, usually contrasting with the ground colour.

F

F1 hybrid Vigorous and uniform, first-generation offspring, derived from crossing 2 distinct, pure-bred lines. F2 hybrids result from self-pollination within a population of F1 hybrids; they do not come true.
Falcate *see* Sickle-shaped.

Fall Semi-pendent or spreading tepal of *Iris* flower.
Family Primary category in plant classification, between order and genus, encompassing genera that have natural characteristics that group them together. *See also p.11.*
Fancy Describes a flower that is flaked, flecked, or striped in contrast to the ground colour.
Fan palm Palm with fan-like, palmate rather than pinnate leaves.
Fan-shaped (flabellate) Wedge-shaped or semi-circular, with a pleated or boldly veined surface.
Farina (*adj.* farinaceous, farinose) *see* White-mealy.
Fascicle *see* Cluster.
Feathered 1. Describes a standard tree with a stem or trunk that is branched to the base with lateral "feathers". *See also p.33,* Central-leader standard. 2. Describes a flower with feather-like markings contrasting with the ground colour, particularly of some tulips.
Fern Non-flowering, vascular plant, often with feather-like fronds. *See also p.51.*
Fertile 1. Refers to organs that produce functional pollen, spores, or viable seed. 2. Describes soil with a high content of nutrients essential to plant growth.
Fertilization Sexual fusion of male and female elements, initiating seed development. *See also* Reproduction.
Fertilizer Nutrients added to soil or potting compost to promote the vigour of a plant. Nitrogen (N), phosphorus (P), and potassium (K) are the chief elements used in inorganic fertilizers. Organic fertilizers are based on decomposed plant or animal matter.
Filament 1. Stalk of the stamen attached to the anther. 2. Thread-like extension or hair.
Filiform *see* Linear.
Flabellate *see* Fan-shaped.
Flaked Describes a flower in which another colour overlies the ground colour in large splashes; particularly applied to some carnations (*Dianthus*) and tulips.
Floret Tiny, individual flower within a dense inflorescence, such as a grass flower in a spikelet, or a disc- or ray-floret in a (composite) flowerhead.
Flower Reproductive structure of angiosperms, usually consisting of an ovary or stamens, or both, most frequently encircled by a perianth of differentiated petals and sepals or undifferentiated tepals, and usually borne on a flower-stalk. *See also pp.16–17.*
Flowerhead (capitulum) Inflorescence consisting of a central group of tiny disc-florets, usually ringed by ray-florets, borne on a compressed axis or stem. Also referred to as a composite flowerhead.
Flowering plant *see* Angiosperm.
Flower-stalk (pedicel) Stalk supporting an individual flower or fruit singly or in an inflorescence.
Fluted With long, rounded, vertical grooves.
Foliar feed Dilute solution of fertilizer applied to leaves.
Follicle Dry fruit, formed from a single carpel, that splits along one side to release one or more seeds.
Force To induce unseasonal growth, flowering, or fruiting of a plant, usually under glass; achieved by manipulating the plant's environment.
Forma (*abbrev.* f.) Variant of a species, ranked below *varietas* (var.) in the nomenclatural hierarchy, distinguished by minor characteristics such as habit or the colour of the leaves, flowers, or fruits. *See also p.11.*
Formative pruning Training of young trees or shrubs to produce a framework of strong, evenly spaced stems or branches. *See also p.25.*
Frame Structure with a glass or plastic cover used for forcing, hardening off, propagation, or winter protection. *See also* Bulb frame, Cold frame, Propagating frame.
Free-tipped Refers to a conifer needle that is pressed flat to an axis with the tip extending beyond it.
Frond 1. Leaf of a fern. 2. Loosely, a large, compound leaf, such as a palm leaf.
Frost hardy Able to withstand temperatures down to -5°C (23°F).
Frost tender May be damaged by temperatures below 5°C (41°F).
Fruit Ripened ovary and any attached structures that ripen with it.
Fully hardy Able to withstand temperatures down to -15°C (5°F).
Fungus (*pl.* fungi; *adj.* fungal) Non-vascular, non-photosynthetic organism, such as a mould or mushroom, that obtains nutrients by absorbing organic compounds from its surroundings.
Funnel-shaped Describes a flower in which the perianth widens gradually from the base into a spreading, often lobed mouth, like a funnel.
Fusiform *see* Spindle-shaped.

G

Garden compost Humus-rich material formed by the decay of organic matter. Used as a mulch or to improve soil structure and nutrition.
Garden origin Applied to a plant that has been artificially bred or selected, rather than occurring in the wild.
Garigue Exposed Mediterranean habitat covered with scrub vegetation.
Genus (*pl.* genera; *adj.* generic) Primary category in plant classification, ranked between family and species. Encompasses species that share a wide range of characteristics. *See also p.11,* Binomial.
Germination Physical and chemical changes that occur as a seed begins to develop into a young plant.
Gesneriad Member of the Gesneriaceae family, including perennials, climbers, subshrubs, and small trees, many of which are epiphytic. *See also p.40.*
Glabrous Smooth and hairless.
Gland Cell, organ, or pore that secretes oils or other substances.
Glandular-hairy With gland-tipped hairs.
Glaucous With a blue-green, blue-grey, grey, or white bloom; usually refers to stems and leaves.
Globose *see* Spherical.
Globular *see* Spherical.
Glochid Small, barbed bristle or hair borne on the areole of a cactus.
Glume Thin, dry, membrane-like bract in the inflorescence of a grass or sedge, usually arranged in 2 ranks; may be a perianth segment, or support a spikelet or flower, depending on the species.
Graft hybrid Plant resulting from the combination of tissues from both scion and rootstock after grafting. *See also* Chimaera.
Grafting Method of propagation by which the scion of one plant and rootstock of another are artificially united so that they eventually function as one plant.
Granulated bark Bark ground to fine, medium, or coarse grade, often used in potting compost.
Grass Member of the Gramineae family, with round, hollow, or solid stems that have usually regularly spaced, solid nodes. The basic inflorescence is a spikelet, grouped into a panicle, raceme, or spike. *See also p.54.*
Greenhouse Structure glazed with glass or plastic, providing a controlled environment for the cultivation of plants. *See also p.24,* Cold greenhouse, Cool greenhouse, Temperate greenhouse, Warm greenhouse.
Green manure Practice of sowing quick-growing crops, e.g. clover (*Trifolium*), and digging them into the soil to rot and improve the humus content.
Greenwood cutting Cutting taken from the shoot-tip of a plant once the initial flush of spring growth has slowed; stems are slightly harder than those used for softwood cuttings.
Grex A collective term applied to all the progeny of an artificial cross from known parents of different taxa. Mainly applied to orchids. *See also p.11.*
Ground cover Applied to (usually) low-growing plants that quickly spread over the soil surface, helping to suppress weeds.
Ground frost Climatic effect when the temperature at or just beneath the surface of the soil falls to 0°C (32°F) or below.
Group Category of cultivated plants that denotes a collection of similar, named cultivars. *See also p.11,* Series.
Growing point (shoot-tip) Tip of a shoot from which new extension growth develops.
Growing season Part of the year when a plant is in active growth.
Grow on To grow young plants to a stage where they are ready to plant out or flower.
Growth habit *see* Habit.
Gymnosperm Tree or shrub, generally evergreen, that bears naked seeds in cones rather than enclosed in ovaries, e.g. conifers, cycads. *See also p.10.*

H

Habit Characteristic form, appearance, or mode of growth of a mature plant.
Habitat Natural environment in which a plant occurs in the wild.
Haft Narrow or constricted base of an organ, particularly the fall and standard petals of *Iris* flowers.
Half hardy Able to withstand temperatures down to 0°C (32°F).
Half-pot Container that is half the depth of a standard plant pot.
Half-standard Standard tree or shrub with a clear stem of 1–1.5m (3–5ft) from ground level to the lowest lateral branches.
Harden off To acclimatize young plants reared in a protective environment to cooler conditions outdoors by gradually introducing them to a cooler environment.
Hardiness Capacity of a cultivated plant to withstand adverse conditions; in general usage, its tolerance of low temperatures. *See pp.18–19.*
Hardwood Mature wood used for cuttings.
Hardwood cutting Cutting taken from mature wood from early autumn (after leaf fall) to early winter.
Hastate *see* Spear-shaped.
Heart-shaped (cordate) 1. Roughly ovate, pointed at the tip, and with a deep cleft at the centre of a rounded base. 2. Describes a base that is rounded with a deep cleft at the centre, which in leaves is where the leaf-stalk attaches.
Heel cutting Cutting consisting of vigorous sideshoot from a stem of the current season's growth, with a small piece of bark or older wood at the base.
Herb 1. Plant with practical properties, such as for culinary or medicinal use. 2. Botanically, any herbaceous plant.
Herbaceous border Area of land set aside for the cultivation of herbaceous plants.
Herbaceous plant Non-woody plant that dies back (loses top-growth and becomes dormant) at the end of the growing season, usually in autumn, overwintering by means of underground rootstocks. Some may develop a woody base. Growth resumes in spring.
Herbicide Chemical treatment used to control or eradicate weeds.
Hermaphrodite *see* Bisexual.
Hip Fleshy fruit of a rose.
Hose-in-hose Describes a double flower in which the corolla or calyx is duplicated, with one inserted in the throat of the other.
Houseplant Any plant grown for long periods indoors, often frost-tender species that would not survive outside in cold climates.
Humidity Measure of the air's moisture content as a percentage of saturated air (relative humidity/RH). In this encyclopedia, low humidity is below 50% RH; moderate humidity is 51–60% RH; high humidity is 61% RH and above. *See also p.24.*
Humus Slowly decomposed organic material found in soil; may also refer to rotted garden compost or leaf mould. Where lacking or deficient, it may be dug into soil to increase bacterial activity and improve structure.
Hybrid (cross) Naturally or artificially produced offspring of genetically distinct parents of different taxa. Hybrids show new characteristics and are often vigorous in growth. *See also* F1 hybrid, Graft hybrid, Intergeneric hybrid, Interspecific hybrid, Multigeneric hybrid, Trigeneric hybrid.

I

Incised Deeply, irregularly, and sharply toothed or lobed.
Incurved Bending inwards.
Indumentum Covering of hair or, more rarely, scales.
Indusium (*pl.* indusia) Tissue covering a sorus on a fern frond.
Infertile 1. Refers to a soil that is very low

in nutrients. 2. More loosely, applied to plants that do not flower or fruit for various reasons, but may do so if the conditions are right. *See also* Sterile.
Inflorescence Arrangement of flowers on a single axis. *See also* Catkin, Cluster, Corymb, Cyme, Flowerhead, Panicle, Raceme, Spadix, Spike, Umbel.
Insecticide Chemical treatment used to control or eradicate insect pests.
Insectivorous *see* Carnivorous.
Insert To place cuttings in a growing medium.
Intergeneric hybrid Result of crossing plants of 2 distinct, usually closely related genera.
Internode Section of stem between 2 nodes.
Interrupted Refers to a structure, usually an inflorescence, that is not continuous, such as the inflorescences of *Salvia* species.
Interspecific hybrid Result of crossing 2 species within the same genus.
Invasive Describes a vigorous plant that rapidly overwhelms more delicate neighbours, unless restricted in spread.
Inversely heart-shaped (obcordate) Inversely ovate, with a deep cleft at the centre of a rounded tip, and pointed at the base.
Inversely lance-shaped (oblanceolate) Broadest above the centre, tapering to a narrow basal point; length is 3–6 times the width.
Involucre (*adj.* involucral) Ring of crowded bracts (sometimes only one), sometimes conspicuous and often overlapping, around the base of a flowerhead or umbel.

JK

JI No. 1/2/3 (John Innes composts) Series of standardized potting composts containing 7 parts sterilized loam, 3 parts peat (or substitute), and 2 parts sand, to which is added varying amounts of ground limestone, hoof and horn, superphosphate, and potassium sulphate. *See also p.24.*
Keel 1. Prominent longitudinal ridge, usually on the underside of an organ such as a leaf, similar to the keel of a boat. 2. Two lower, fused petals of a pea-like flower.
Kidney-shaped (reniform) Roughly quarter-moon-shaped with blunt ends (on a leaf, the stalk is attached at the notched centre of the concave margin).

L

Labellum Lip, particularly applied to prominent third petal of *Iris* or orchid flowers. *See also* Lip.
Laced Describes a flower in which the colour of the petal margins and centre contrast with the ground colour.
Laciniate Describes a margin that is finely and irregularly cut.
Lamina *see* Leaf-blade.
Lanceolate *see* Lance-shaped.
Lance-shaped (lanceolate) Broadest below the centre, tapering to a narrow tip; length is 3–6 times the width.
Lateral 1. Located on or to the side of an axis or organ, such as lateral veins that arise from the midrib on a leaf surface. 2. Side-shoot from the stem of a plant.
Latex Milky-white sap or fluid that bleeds from some plants when the stem is cut or damaged; may be irritant.
Lath house Structure composed of light planks (laths) or trellis work used to protect plants from sun, wind, and rain and to acclimatize young, usually woody, plants before planting out in the garden.
Lax Loose, not compact.
Layering Method of propagation whereby a stem is pegged to the soil while still attached to the parent plant, to induce rooting. *See also* Air-layering, Mound-layering.
Leaching Removal of soluble nutrients from soil by the passage of water.
Leader 1. Main, usually central stem of a plant. *See also* Central-leader standard. 2. Terminal shoot of a main branch.
Leaf Plant organ, usually flattened and green, borne on a stem or branch, that fulfils the functions of photosynthesis, respiration, and transpiration. *See also pp.14–15.*
Leaf axil Angle formed between a leaf or leaf-stalk and the stem of a plant.
Leaf-blade (lamina) Thin, usually flat part of a leaf, excluding the leaf-stalk.
Leaf-bud cutting Cutting taken from a stem section, including a leaf-bud and leaf-stalk.
Leaf cutting Cutting taken from a leaf or section of a leaf.
Leaflet Single division of a compound leaf. Botanically, a pinna.
Leaf mould Fibrous, flaky, organic material composed of decayed leaves. Often found in woodland, and used as a peat substitute. *See also* Humus, Leaf-rich.
Leaf node Point at which a leaf arises from a stem.
Leaf-rich Describes soil that contains a high proportion of humus or leaf mould.
Leaf scar Raised area on a tree trunk, branch, or twig, where a leaf once grew.
Leaf-stalk (petiole) Part of a leaf, attached to the base or centre of the leaf-blade, that connects it to a stem or branch.
Legume *see* Pod.
Lenticel Raised pore on the surface of bark or some fruits, which provides access for air to the inner tissues.
Ligulate *see* Strap-shaped.
Limb 1. Broadened, flattened, and expanded part of a plant organ, usually a leaf or flower, extending from a narrower base. 2. Larger branch of a tree.
Lime Loosely, refers to compounds of calcium. Calcium content is used to measure soil pH. *See also* Calcareous.
Lime-free Refers to acidic soil. *See also* Peat.
Lime-tolerant Capable of growing in calcareous soil.
Linear (acicular, filiform) Long and narrow, with parallel margins, or almost so; length is 12 or more times the width.
Lingulate *see* Strap-shaped.
Lip Prominent lower lobe on a flower, formed by one or more fused petals or sepals. *See also* Labellum.
Liquid feed Water-diluted solution of fertilizers, often used for houseplants.
Lithophytic (saxicolous) Growing on or among rocks or stones.
Loam Highly fertile, well-drained but moisture-retentive soil, usually fibre- and humus-rich, and containing more or less equal parts of clay, sand, and silt.
Lobe Usually rounded segment, separated from adjacent segments by clefts extending halfway or less to the centre of an organ, such as a leaf. *See also* Palmately lobed.
Lorate *see* Strap-shaped.

M

Maquis Habitat consisting of dense shrub thickets, particular to Corsican and other Mediterranean coastlines.
Marginal aquatic Plant that requires permanently moist conditions, from pure mud to water 30–45cm (12–18in) deep.
Maritime climate Weather conditions experienced in coastal areas. Proximity to the sea or ocean brings exposure to strong winds, but usually moderates seasonal temperatures; rainfall occurs regularly throughout the year. *See also pp.18–19.*
Meristem Tip of a shoot or root in which cell division takes place. Undifferentiated cells are formed or differentiated into tissues that eventually become leaves, flowers, stems, or even whole plants.
Midrib (midvein) Primary, usually central vein running from the stalk to the tip of a leaf or leaflet.
Midvein *see* Midrib.
Mist To increase humidity under glass in summer by spraying very fine droplets of water into the air. *See also* Damp down.
Mixed border Area of ground in which herbaceous plants, annuals, bulbs, and shrubs are grown.
Monocarpic Refers to plants that flower and fruit once and then die. Monocarpic perennials may grow for several or many years before flowering.
Monocotyledon Angiosperm with a single seed-leaf, parallel-veined leaves, no cambium layer, and floral parts usually in threes. *See also* Dicotyledon.
Monoecious With separate male and female flowers borne on the same plant.
Monopodial Refers to a stem or rhizome growing indefinitely from an apical or terminal bud, not usually producing secondary branches.
Monotypic Having only one component, e.g. a genus containing a single species.
Mound-layering Method of propagation whereby the basal section of a stem is earthed-up to induce rooting.
Mulch Layer of material spread on the top of the soil around plants. Loose mulches, such as leaf-mould and garden compost, retain moisture, insulate roots, and can improve soil structure and add nutrients. Sheet mulches, such as black polythene, suppress weeds and also conserve moisture. *See also p.21.*
Multigeneric hybrid Result of crossing 3 or more genera, often over more than one generation.
Mutation *see* Sport.
Mycorrhizal Refers to a mutually beneficial association between a fungus and the roots of a plant.

N

Native Species that naturally grows wild in a particular area.
Naturalized Describes a species that apparently grows wild in a particular area, but is introduced and not native.
Nectar Sugary, liquid secretion that attracts some pollinators.
Nectary Gland, often a modified sepal, petal, or stamen, that secretes nectar.
Needle Stiff, linear leaf of a conifer.
Neutral With pH7, neither acid nor alkaline.
Node Point on a stem, sometimes swollen, at which leaves, leaf buds, and shoots arise.
Nodule Small, rounded swelling.
Nomenclature Standard system of naming plants and providing for the formation and use of the names. Cultivated plants are named in accordance with the International Code of Nomenclature for Cultivated Plants and the International Code for Botanical Nomenclature. *See also p.11.*
Non-vascular Describes plants that lack conductive tissue for the circulation of water and nutrients, for example fungi and mosses. *See also p.10.*
Non-woody *see* Soft-stemmed.
Nut Dry, non-splitting fruit with a hard or leathery shell surrounding a single seed (kernel).
Nutrients Minerals necessary for healthy metabolism and growth.

O

Obcordate *see* Inversely heart-shaped.
Oblanceolate *see* Inversely lance-shaped.
Oblong With 2 parallel sides of roughly equal length; length is 2–4 times the width.
Oblong-ovate Roughly oblong, rounded at both ends, and broader at one end than the other.
Obovate Refers to a flat form, egg-shaped in outline and broadest above the middle; length is 1½–2 times the width.
Obovoid Refers to a solid form, egg-shaped and broadest above the middle; length is 1½ times the width.
Offset Small plant that arises naturally by vegetative increase, as with many bulbous plants and succulents.
Of gardens Term used after the Latin name of a plant to denote that the name is commonly but incorrectly used.
Opposite Describes organs, usually leaves, borne in pairs at each node, in the same plane but on opposite sides of an axis.
Orbicular *see* Rounded.
Orchid Member of the Orchidaceae family, which contains 835 genera of perennials, more than half epiphytic, the rest terrestrial; they are characterized by their unique flower structure. *See also p.46.*
Organic 1. Carbon-based matter of plant or animal origin. 2. Gardening practices using only natural materials.
Osmunda fibre Chopped, dried roots of the fern genus *Osmunda*, used in orchid cultivation.
Oval Broadly elliptic, rounded at both ends, with slightly parallel sides in the middle; length is 1½–2 times the width.
Ovary Female organ of a flower, containing ovules.
Ovate Refers to a flat form, egg-shaped in outline and broadest below the middle; length is 1½ times the width.
Ovoid Refers to a solid form, egg-shaped, and broadest below the middle.
Ovule Part of the ovary from which seed develops after fertilization.
Oxygenator Fully submerged aquatic plant that releases oxygen into the water.

PQ

Palm Member of the Palmae or Arecaceae family. Usually solitary, sometimes multi-stemmed trees or shrubs with characteristic terminal rosettes of palmate or pinnate leaves. *See also p.50*, Fan palm.
Palmate Describes a compound leaf that is fully divided into leaflets arising from a single basal point; it is often also used loosely to mean lobed in a hand-like form. 3-palmate leaves are divided into 3 leaflets, and are often also referred to as trifoliolate, ternate, or, incorrectly, trifoliate. 5-palmate leaves are divided into 5 leaflets, and may also be described as digitate. *See also* Trifoliate.
Palmately lobed Describes a leaf that is deeply divided into 3–7, sometimes more, lobes. It is distinct from a palmate leaf in that the divisions do not extend to the basal point, so remain lobes rather than leaflets.
Pan Shallow dish used for growing alpine plants and sowing seed; often set into a raised bed.
Panicle Branched raceme. Loosely applied to freely branched, corymb-like or cyme-like inflorescences.
Papilla (*pl.* papillae, *adj.* papillose) Small, soft, wart-like projection.
Parasite Organism that derives nutrients directly from a host species, often to the detriment of the latter.
Pea-like Describes a flower structure found in many genera of the Leguminosae and Papilionaceae family, with an erect standard petal, 2 large, usually lateral wing petals, and 2 lower, keeled petals that may be fused at the base or on the lower side, enclosing the stamens and pistil.
Peat Moisture-retentive, humus-rich, acid, partially decayed organic matter, with a pH up to 6.5. Used mainly for potting compost and as a mulch. Derived from sedges (sedge peat) or sphagnum moss (sphagnum peat) and occurring in boggy, waterlogged conditions. Peat substitutes can be used where appropriate; they include animal wastes, coconut fibre (coir), garden compost, mushroom compost, worm-worked compost, granulated bark, and leaf mould.
Peat bed Area edged with peat blocks and filled with moist, peaty soil, for growing acid-loving plants.
Pectinate Arrangement of plant organs, usually leaves, in regular, comb-like rows, either in a single row or 2-ranked.
Pedate Describes a palmate or palmately divided leaf in which the basal lobes or leaflets are themselves lobed.
Pedicel *see* Flower-stalk.
Peduncle Stalk of an inflorescence.
Peltate Attached to the stalk at the centre or other point on the underside of a structure, such as a leaf, rather than at the margin.
Pendent Hanging downwards. Used synonymously with pendulous.
Perennial Plant that lives for more than 2 growing seasons; in horticulure, usually only applied to non-woody plants. *See also pp.10, 38–39.*
Perfoliate Describes stalkless leaves, arranged singly or in opposite pairs, with the bases united around the stem.
Perianth Collective term for the corolla and calyx, whether these are distinct from each other or undifferentiated.
Perianth segment Undifferentiated petal or sepal.
Perlite Light granules of volcanic minerals added to soil or to potting and seed compost to improve aeration.
Permeability Ease with which water passes through soil.
Perpetual-flowering Describes a plant that bears flowers more or less continuously throughout the year.
Persistent Remaining attached to the plant.
Pesticide Chemical treatment used to control or eradicate pests, diseases, or weeds.
Pests Loosely, vermin that feed on plants, and often transmit disease. *See also pp.30–31.*
Petal Modified leaf that makes up the corolla of a flower; generally brightly coloured. *See also* Perianth segment, Tepal.
Petaloid Similar to a petal in colour shape, and texture. *See also* Perianth segment, Tepal.
Petiole *see* Leaf-stalk.
pH Measure of acidity or alkalinity. Many garden plants prefer neutral to slightly acid soil with pH5.5–7.5. *See also* Acid, Alkaline, Neutral.
Photosynthesis Complex series of chemical reactions in green plants and some bacteria, in which energy from sunlight is absorbed by chlorophyll, and carbon dioxide and water are converted into sugars and oxygen.
Phylloclade (cladode, cladophyll) Stem that looks like and takes on the functions of a leaf.
Phyllode Expanded leaf-stalk that takes on the functions of a leaf.
Picotee Describes a flower with narrow petal margins contrasting with the ground colour.
Pinch out (stop) To remove soft growing points to encourage the bushy growth of sideshoots.
Pinna (*pl.* pinnae) Leaflet of a pinnate leaf or of a fern frond. *See also* Pinnate.
Pinnate Describes a compound leaf with leaflets (pinnae) arranged alternately or in opposite pairs on a central axis, with or without a terminal leaflet. 2-pinnate (bipinnate) leaves have pinnately divided leaflets. 3-pinnate (tripinnate) leaves have pinnately divided leaflets that are themselves pinnately divided.
Pinnatifid Describes a simple leaf with usually opposite pairs of lobes cut no deeper than half way to the midrib.
Pinnatisect Describes a simple leaf with usually opposite pairs of deep lobes cut almost to the midrib.
Pinnule *see* Segment.
Pistil Female reproductive organ of a flower, composed of one or several fused or separate carpels.
Plantlet 1. Older seedling. 2. Young, small plant that develops on a mature plant. *See also* Offset, Viviparous.
Pleach To intertwine the branches of a tree or shrub to form a hedge or screen.
Plumose 1. Feather-like, with long, fine, often branched hairs. 2. Applied to plume-like, finely branched inflorescences.
Plunge To sink a container to its rim in ashes, peat, sand, or soil to insulate the roots and prevent the plant drying out.
Pod (legume) 1. One-celled fruit of the Leguminosae family that splits along 2 sides to disperse ripe seed. 2. Loosely, any dry fruit that splits to disperse seed.
Pollard To cut branches back hard to the main trunk of a tree in order to restrict growth.
Pollen Grains released from anthers containing the male element necessary for fertilization.
Pollination Transfer of pollen from the anthers to the stigma of the same or a different flower. Can be performed by animals, insects, wind, or water, and, in the garden, by hand.
Pompon Describes a roughly spherical flower with tightly packed florets that are often curved inwards.
Pot on To remove a plant (usually a cutting or seedling) from an outgrown container, and place it with fresh compost in a larger container, with room for further growth.
Potting compost Well-drained but moisture-retentive growing medium used mainly for container-grown plants. Loam-based potting compost is based on loam mixed with peat (or substitute), and perlite, vermiculite, or sharp sand. Loamless potting composts are based on peat (or substitute), mixed with sphagnum moss and perlite or vermiculite. *See also p.24*, Ericaceous, JI No.1/2/3.
Pot up To insert a seedling or rooted cutting in potting compost in a container.
Pre-chill *see* Stratify.
Pre-soak To soak seed in recently boiled water for between 10 minutes and 72 hours, depending on the species, to soften the seedcoat prior to sowing.
Prick out To transfer seedlings or small cuttings from where they have been propagated into appropriate containers and compost, where they have room to grow.
Procumbent *see* Prostrate.
Propagate To increase plants by seed or by vegetative means. *See also pp.28–29*, Vegetative propagation.
Propagating case (propagator) Small, closed case with a transparent lid, used to provide a humid atmosphere under glass, usually with bottom heat, for rooting cuttings, germinating seed, or raising other plants.
Propagating frame Large case, normally unheated, used outdoors to root cuttings, germinate seed, or raise other plants.
Propagator *see* Propagating case.
Prostrate (procumbent) Describes a plant with spreading or trailing stems lying flat on the ground.
Pruinose *see* White-frosted.
Prune To remove twigs or branches from woody plants in order to maintain health, control size, train to a desired shape, or stimulate growth or the production of flowers or fruit. *See also pp.25–27*, Formative pruning, Renovation pruning, Restrictive pruning.
Pseudobulb Swollen, bulb-like stem, sometimes jointed, that acts as a storage organ for some sympodial orchids. *See also* Backbulb.
Pseudocephalium Woody, flower-bearing, densely spined area near the apex of some cacti. *See also* Cephalium.
Quilled Describes a flowerhead consistingof narrow, tubular ray-florets.

R

Raceme Inflorescence of stalked flowers radiating from a single, unbranched axis, the youngest flowers near the tip.
Rachis Main axis of a compound leaf or inflorescence.
Radial Spine at the perimeter of an areole on a cactus.
Radical Refers to basal leaves that grow from or near ground level. *See also* Rosette.
Rank Refers to a linear arrangement of leaves. 2-ranked (distichous) leaves are arranged in opposite pairs along a stem. 4-ranked (decussate) leaves are arranged in opposite pairs, each pair at right angles to the pair next to it.
Ray-floret Tiny, usually strap-shaped, tubular-based, outer flower of a (composite) flowerhead.
Receptacle Enlarged or elongated tip of the stem from which all parts of a simple flower arise.
Recurved Arched backwards.
Reflexed Arched or bent sharply back upon itself.
Remontant Refers to a plant that flowers more than once within a growing season, at distinct times.
Renewal pruning *see* Renovation pruning.
Reniform *see* Kidney-shaped.
Renovation pruning (renewal pruning) Hard pruning to rejuvenate an old or overgrown shrub. *See also p.25.*
Repot To remove a plant (usually mature) from an outgrown container, and re-establish it in a larger container.
Reproduction Process of producing new individuals by either sexual or asexual (vegetative) methods.
Respiration Absorption of oxygen and breakdown of carbohydrates within cells, releasing carbon dioxide and water and providing energy for metabolism.
Resting period *see* Dormancy.
Restrictive pruning Annual pruning to limit growth. *See also p.25.*
Reversion Genetic change within a sport or chimaera in which a plant or part of a plant reverts to its original character.
Rhizome (*adj.* rhizomatous) Horizontal, usually branching and fleshy stem, growing underground or, less often, at ground level.
Rhomboidal *see* Diamond-shaped.
Rib 1. Ridge, normally vertical, formed on the stem of a cactus. 2. Refers to the primary vein on a leaf.
Ripening 1. Maturing of fruit. 2. Maturing of young shoots (wood) on trees and shrubs, or of bulbs.
Ripewood cutting Cutting of a mature shoot taken from an evergreen plant, from late summer to early winter.
Rock-dwelling *see* Lithophytic.
Rock garden Area for growing alpines and rock plants among rocks, ideally set out naturally as rock outcrops.
Rock plant Any small plant grown in association with alpines, and with similar cultivation requirements. *See also pp.40–41.*
Root 1. Part of a plant, usually underground, that anchors it and absorbs water and nutrients from the soil. 2. To insert cuttings in a compost where they will produce roots. *See also pp.12–13*, Aerial root, Buttress root, Stilt root, Tap root.

Root ball Mass of roots and soil or compost attached to them, formed by a plant in a container or in the ground.
Root cutting Cutting taken from vigorous, young roots during winter.
Rootstock 1. Underground part of a plant. 2. Loosely, the crown and root system of any herbaceous perennial, from which new plants arise. 3. Plant upon which a scion is grafted.
Rosette 1. Dense whorl of leaves arising from the central point or crown of a plant, usually at or near ground level. 2. Whorled arrangement of petals or tepals.
Rounded (orbicular) Roughly or fully circular in outline.
Runner 1. Trailing stem, growing above ground and rooting at the nodes, where plantlets are produced. 2. Underground, spreading shoot producing upright shoots that form new plants at intervals.

S

Sac Space or chamber inside an ovary, anther, or fruit.
Sagittate *see* Arrow-shaped.
Salverform Describes a flower with a long, slim, tubular corolla that spreads out into more or less horizontal, flat lobes.
Sandy Describes dry, light, free-draining soil, low in nutrients, derived from quartz or sandstone.
Sap Juice that flows through conductive tissue of vascular plants.
Sapling Young tree.
Saprophyte Plant, usually lacking in chlorophyll, that absorbs nutrients from dead or decaying organic matter.
Saucer-shaped Describes a flat flower with the corolla lobes slightly upturned at the tips.
Savannah Flat, dry grassland habitat covered with low shrubs and dotted with small trees.
Saxicolous *see* Lithophytic.
Scale 1. Flat, membranous structure. 2. Dry leaf or bract, usually pressed flat to the axis to which it is attached.
Scalloped (crenate) Refers to a margin, generally of a leaf, with shallow, rounded teeth.
Scandent Describes a plant that climbs by means of flexible stems that grow over or through supports, attaching themselves loosely, if at all. *See also pp.36–37,* Climber.
Scape Leafless stem of a solitary flower or inflorescence.
Scarify 1. To treate chemically or abrade the hard outer casing of a seed before sowing, to increase rate of water uptake and thus rate of germination. 2. To remove moss and old grass from a lawn by raking. *See also p.28.*
Scion Shoot or part of a shoot that is bonded to the rootstock of a second plant by grafting.
Scree 1. Slope of unstable, rocky fragments, retaining little moisture, at the bottom of a cliff. 2. In gardens, a deep layer of stone chippings with a small proportion of loam, providing very sharp drainage for alpines and rock plants.
Scrub Habitat with poor or dry soil, covered with bushes and small trees.
Seed Ripened, fertilized ovule containing a dormant embryo capable of developing into an adult plant.
Seedbed Area of ground that has been dug over, raked, and firmed in preparation for sowing seed.
Seedcoat Outer casing of seed. *See also* Aril.
Seed compost Fine-textured, low-nutrient, moisture-retentive compost, formulated for the healthy germination and development of seeds and seedlings; also used for rooting cuttings.
Seed head Loosely refers to dry fruits. *See also* Capsule.
Seed-leaf (cotyledon) First leaf, pair of leaves, or occasionally group of leaves produced by a seed during germination.
Seedling Young plant raised from seed.
Segment 1. Subdivision of pinna on a pinnate leaf or frond; botanically known as a pinnule. 2. Any division of an organ, such as the lobe of a leaf or flower.
Self *see* Self-coloured.
Self-coloured (self) Describes a flower with a uniform colour.
Self-fertile (self-setting) Describes a plant that does not need pollen from a second individual in order to fertilize and set fruit. *See also* Self-pollinate.
Self-pollinate Process whereby pollen from the anthers of one flower reaches the stigma of a second flower on the same plant. *See also* Self-fertile.
Self-seed To regenerate from seed that is dispersed in the garden without human intervention.
Self-setting *see* Self-fertile.
Self-sterile Describes a plant that requires pollen from a second individual of the species, but not the same clone, to fertilize its flowers.
Semi-deciduous *see* Semi-evergreen.
Semi-double Describes a flower with 2 or 3 times the number of petals of a single flower, usually arranged in 2 or 3 rows.
Semi-evergreen Describes a plant that retains most or some of its foliage throughout the year.
Semi-ripe cutting Cutting taken from semi-mature wood in mid- or late summer, occasionally in early autumn.
Semi-ripe wood Refers to stems or shoots that have slowed down in growth and become semi-woody.
Sepal One part of the calyx, when it is composed of separate parts. Usually green and smaller than petals, but sometimes colourful and petal-like.
Series Name applied to a group of cultivars of annuals that share most of the same characteristics but differ from one another by one character (rarely more), usually colour. *See also pp.11, 42.*
Serrate Describes a finely toothed margin, usually of a leaf, with the teeth slightly curved as in a saw blade.
Sessile Refers to a stalkless or almost stalkless plant organ.
Set Refers to fertilized flowers that have developed fruit.
Sharp drainage Very free movement of excess water through the soil.
Sheath Tubular structure around a part of plant, such as a leaf base around a stem.
Shoot 1. First, erect growth of a seedling, before it becomes a stem. 2. Loosely applied to side-growths, twigs, or branches. *See also* Branch, Sideshoot, Stem.
Shoot-tip *see* Growing point.
Shrub Deciduous or evergreen perennial with multiple woody stems or branches, generally bearing branches from or near its base. *See also pp.34–35.*
Shrub border Area of ground set aside for the cultivation of shrubs.
Shrublet *see* Subshrub.
Shy-flowering 1. Reluctant to come into flower. 2. Bearing few blooms.
Sickle-shaped (falcate) Curving sideways in the manner of a scythe or sickle.
Sideshoot Lateral shoot that develops from the side of a main shoot.
Silt Moderately fertile, moisture-retentive soil, prone to compaction and surface-capping. Has finer soil particles than clay.
Simple Not divided into secondary units; for example, a leaf with a continuous surface, not cut into leaflets.
Single Describes a flower with the normal number of petals or tepals for the species, arranged in a single whorl. Also applied to (composite) flowerheads that have a single row of outer ray-florets with the centre filled with disc-florets.
Sinus Deep cleft between 2 lobes.
Slipper-shaped Describes a flower in which the corolla has a pouch-like form.
Soft-stemmed With a non-woody stem.
Soft-tip cutting *see* Stem-tip cutting.
Softwood Young, soft, unripened shoots of woody plants.
Softwood cutting Cutting taken from young, non-woody growth, from spring to early summer.
Soilless medium Growing medium based on substances other than soil. *See also* Clay granules, Perlite, Vermiculite.
Solitary Flower borne singly rather than in an inflorescence.
Sorus (*pl.* sori) Cluster of sporangia usually on the underside of a fern frond, almost always surrounded or covered by an indusium.
Spadix (*pl.* spadices) Fleshy axis of a spike or spike-like inflorescence, embedded with tiny sessile flowers, usually borne within a spathe.
Spathe Often prominent, fleshy, hood-like bract, surrounding a spadix.
Spathulate *see* Spoon-shaped.
Spear-shaped (hastate) Triangular, with 2 equal, roughly triangular, outward-pointing, basal lobes.
Species Basic category in plant classification, ranked below genus and consisting of similar individual plants that breed true in the wild. Characterized by a binomial. *See also p.11.*
Specimen plant Ornamental plant, normally a tree or shrub, grown usually in a prominent position, where it may be viewed from different angles.
Speculum Glossy raised area, varying from square- to diamond- or horseshoe-shaped, on the lip of some orchid flowers.
Sphagnum Genus of mosses which, when decomposed in bog conditions, is called sphagnum (or moss) peat. In fresh form, it is used to line hanging baskets, or is finely chopped and added to orchid compost.
Spherical (globose, globular) Applied to a round or almost round solid form.
Spike Inflorescence in which stalkless flowers are arranged on an unbranched axis.
Spikelet Small spike forming part of a compound inflorescence, particularly in grasses and bromeliads.
Spindle-shaped (fusiform) Applied to a solid form, broadest at the centre, tapering towards each end (narrower and with straighter sides than ellipsoid forms).
Spine Stiff, sharp-tipped, modified leaf or stem.
Spiny (spinose) Bearing stiff, sharp-tipped spines.
Spoon-shaped (spathulate) Narrow at the base, gradually broadening into a blunt, rounded tip.
Sporangium (*pl.* sporangia) Spore-producing organ on the underside of the fronds of all ferns (and other members of the order Pteridophyta). *See also p.51.*
Spore Basic unit of reproduction in many non-flowering plants, such as ferns, fungi, and mosses. *See also p.51.*
Sporeling Young plant raised from a spore.
Sport (mutation) Natural or induced genetic change, often exhibited as a variegated shoot or flower from the parent plant. Sports may be vegetatively propagated to give rise to new cultivars. *See also p.11.*
Spray Cluster of flowers or flowerheads arranged on a single, branched stem.
Spread Measure of an individual plant's horizontal growth. Spreads given in this encyclopedia correspond to the diameter of a mature plant (in perennials, after 3 years' growth) in an appropriate garden site.
Spur 1. Modified petal with a hollow, basal projection, often containing nectar. 2. Short branches or branchlets along the main branches, on which flowers and fruit are produced.
Stalk Stem-like organ joining a leaf, flower, flowerhead, or inflorescence to the stem of a plant. *See also* Flower-stalk, Leaf-stalk, Peduncle, Sessile.
Stamen Male part of a flower, composed of an anther, normally borne on a filament.
Staminode Sterile, modified stamen, either inconspicuous or resembling a narrow petal.
Standard 1. Tree or shrub trained to form a rounded head of branches at the top of a clear stem. *See also* Branched-head standard, Central-leader standard, Half-standard. 2. Uppermost petal of a pea-like flower, often large and brightly coloured. 3. Erect inner tepal of an *Iris* flower.
Star-shaped (stellate) Refers to a flower with widely spaced, narrow petals or tepals that radiate from a common central point.
Stellate *see* Star-shaped.
Stem Main axis of a plant, usually above ground, that supports structures such as branches, leaves, flowers, and fruit.
Stem-tip cutting (soft-tip cutting) Cutting taken from the soft tip of a non-flowering stem, usually from spring to autumn.
Sterile 1. Refers to any flower that is incapable of producing seeds. 2. Applied to trees in which the flowers may be self-sterile. 3. Refers to soils that have been deliberately treated with a chemical to kill weed seeds, pests, and diseases.
Stigma Tip of pistil, which receives pollen to fertilize the ovules.
Stilt root Stabilizing, obliquely angled, adventitious root produced from the trunks of trees adapted to shallow or waterlogged soil. *See also* Buttress root.

Stipule Leaf-like or bract-like structure borne, usually in pairs, at the point where a leaf-stalk arises from a stem.
Stolon (*adj.* stoloniferous) Arching, horizontal or trailing stem producing roots and new shoot at its tips.
Stomata Microscopic pores in the surface of the aerial parts of plants, allowing gaseous exchange. *See also* Transpiration.
Stool *see* Coppice.
Stop *see* Pinch out.
Strap-shaped (ensiform, ligulate, lorate) Narrow, with straight or curving sides; length is 6 (or more) times the width.
Stratify (pre-chill) To expose seed to cold in order to break dormancy, either by refrigeration before sowing, or by sowing outdoors in autumn or winter.
Strobilus (*pl.* strobili) Reproductive organ of a conifer. Male strobili resemble catkins; female ones resemble mature cones in miniature.
Style Part of the carpel or pistil connecting the ovary and the stigma.
Subalpine Applied to mountain areas between the foothills and the alpine slopes.
Submerged aquatic Plant that remains totally submerged below water.
Subshrub (shrublet) 1. Woody-based plant with soft-wooded stems. 2. Low-growing, woody-stemmed plant.
Subsoil Layer of soil below the topsoil, usually less fertile and of poor structure.
Subspecies (*abbrev.* subsp.) Category of plant classification, below species but higher in rank than *varietas* or *forma*. *See also p.11.*
Subtropical Refers to the high-temperature zone located between tropical and temperate regions. Rainfall occurs mainly as heavy downpours during the monsoon season.
Succulent Plant with fleshy leaves, roots, or stems (not bulbs, corms, rhizomes, or tubers) that are adapted for water storage; often native to arid areas. *See also pp.48–49.*
Sucker 1. Adventitious shoot arising below soil level, usually from the roots rather than from the stem or crown of the plant. 2. Shoot that arises from the stock of a grafted or budded plant.
Surface-capping When the soil surface bakes dry in summer, especially on clay and silt soils, resulting in poor aeration. *See also* Compaction.
Swamp Spongy, waterlogged habitat.
Synonym Name or epithet that is not the accepted one for the plant. *See also p.11.*
Sympodial Form of growth in which the terminal bud dies or ends in an inflorescence, and growth continues from lateral buds.

T

Tap root 1. Primary, sometimes swollen, downward-growing root of a plant from which the root system extends. 2. Loosely, any strongly downward-growing root.
Taxon (*pl.* taxa) Named group of organisms that is defined by a set of shared characters. Taxonomy is the science of classification, nomenclature, and identification of organisms. *See also p.10–11.*
Temperate Refers to zones located between the subtropics and the polar circles, which experience distinct seasons, without temperature extremes. Rainfall occurs throughout the year. *See also* Cool-temperate, Warm-temperate.
Temperate greenhouse Greenhouse with a minimum temperature of 7°C (45°F). *See also p.24.*
Tender Applied to plants that may be damaged by temperatures below 5°C (41°F). *See also* Frost tender.
Tendril Coiling, thread-like, modified leaf, leaflet, inflorescence, or shoot used by a climbing plant to attach itself to an adjacent support.
Tepal Petal or sepal of a flower, where the calyx and corolla are not clearly distinguished. *See also* Perianth segment, Petaloid.
Terminal Located at the end of a stem, shoot, or other organ. *See also* Axillary.
Ternate Arranged in groups of 3 around a common axis. *See also* Palmate.
Terrarium An enclosed, glass or plastic container in which plants are grown.
Terrestrial Describes a land plant that grows in soil, rather than epiphytically, as a parasite, or in water.
Tessellated With a bold, chequered pattern that contrasts with the ground colour; usually describes corolla markings.
Thin To remove a number of buds, flowers, seedlings, or shoots to improve the growth and quality of remaining ones.
Throat Opening of the tubular part of a flower, from where the petals or tepals spread.
Toothed (dentate) Describes a margin, usually of a leaf, with tooth-like, triangular indentations. Double-toothed margins have alternate large and small teeth.
Top-dress 1. To apply fertilizers or mulches to the soil surface around plants. 2. To apply organic and inorganic dressing to lawns to feed and improve the texture of the grass. 3. To apply material such as stone or grit, usually decorative, to the surface of the soil or potting compost around a plant, in order to improve drainage and reduce moisture loss. 4. To renew the upper layers of potting compost in a container instead of potting on the plant.
Topiary Clipping and training of shrubs or trees into free, geometric, or representational forms.
Topsoil Uppermost layer of the soil, usually the most fertile.
Trademark name Name licensed for commercial use, and distinct from a registered cultivar name. In this encyclopedia, the true cultivar name is usually given as a synonym if appropriate.
Trailing *see* Climber.
Train To prune and shape the growth of any plant.
Transpiration Evaporation of water from the leaves and stems of plants (mostly through stomata).
Tree Woody perennial with a crown of branches developing from the top of a usually single stem or trunk. *See also pp.32–33.*
Tree fern Large fern that develops a tree-like trunk in maturity. *See also p.51.*
Triangular (deltoid) With 3 sides of equal length. A triangular leaf is attached to the stem at a point midway along one side.
Trifoliate Arrangement of leaves that arise in groups of 3 from a single point.
Trifoliolate *see* Palmate.
Trigeneric hybrid Offspring of 3 genera, crossed over 2 generations.
Tripartite Divided almost to the base into 3 lobes or segments.
Tripinnate (3-pinnate) *see* Pinnate.
Tropical Refers to the zone between the Tropics of Cancer and Capricorn, with a hot, steamy climate that encourages lush plant growth. Rainfall may occur throughout the year or mainly during a monsoon season. *See also* Subtropical.
True (true-breeding) Term applied to plants that, when raised from seed, virtually reproduce the characteristics of the parents.
Trumpet-shaped Refers to a flower with a long, narrow tube, flaring at the throat into corolla lobes, which are usually arched backwards.
Truncate Ending abruptly as though cut off at a right-angle.
Trunk Rigid, woody, bark-covered stem of a tree.
Truss Compact cluster of flowers or fruit, particularly of rhododendrons.
Tuber (*adj.* tuberous) Swollen root or underground stem with storage tissue.
Tubercle (*adj.* tuberculate) Small, wart-like projection.
Tubular Refers to a plant organ, usually a flower, with perianth segments fully or partially fused to form a hollow tube.
Tufa Porous, moisture-retentive limestone rock, used for the cultivation of alkaline-loving, rock-dwelling alpines.
Tunic Membrane covering bulbs and corms, often papery but sometimes thick and leathery.
Turion Detached, often fleshy bud of an aquatic plant that overwinters at the bottom of a pond, regenerating in spring.
Turkscap Refers to a flower resembling a traditional Turkish cap with petals strongly reflexed.
Twining *see* Climber.

UV

Umbel Flat- or round-topped inflorescence in which numerous stalked flowers are terminally borne from a single point.
Unisexual Applied to a flower that is either male or female only, requiring pollination from a flower of the other sex.
Upright *see* Erect.
Urceolate *see* Urn-shaped.
Urn-shaped (urceolate) Describes a spherical to cylindrical or tubular flower contracted at or just below the mouth.
Variant Plant form that varies to some degree from the norm. Often loosely applied to any naturally occurring or artificially selected form of species.
Variegation Irregular arrangement of pigments, usually as result of mutation or sometimes disease.
Varietas (variety; *abbrev.* var.) Naturally occurring variant of a species, ranked taxonomically between subspecies and *forma*. *See also p.11.*
Variety *see* Varietas.
Vascular Containing conductive tissue, enabling sap to pass around the plant. *See also p.10,* Non-vascular.
Vegetative propagation Asexual techniques for increasing plants, by cuttings, division, grafting, or layering.
Vein Fibrous strand of vascular tissue that conducts sap through the plant.
Venation Pattern of leaf veins.
Ventilation Control of air movement under glass to avoid atmospheric stagnation and regulate temperature.
Vermiculite Light, mica-like mineral added to potting compost to improve aeration and moisture retention.
Viable Applied to seed capable of germination.
Viviparous Describes plant that forms plantlets on leaves, inflorescences, or stems. Also applied loosely to plants that produce bulbils or bulblets on these organs.

WX

Warm greenhouse Greenhouse with a minimum temperature of 13°C (55°F). *See also p.24.*
Warm-temperate Refers to a temperate climate with mild winters and hot summers.
Wasteland Weed-infested, desolate habitat.
Waterlogged Refers to soil that is saturated as a result of excessive rainfall, over-watering, or proximity to a water source, and which often drains very slowly.
Water plant *see* Aquatic plant.
Wedge-shaped (cuneate) Inversely triangular, or with straight sides tapering to the base.
Weed 1. Vigorous, invasive, or self-seeding plant competing with desired garden plants for moisture and nutrients. 2. Any plant growing where it is not wanted.
Weeping Describes a tree or shrub that is pendent in habit.
White-frosted (pruinose) With a whitish bloom. *See also* Glaucous.
White-mealy (farinaceous, farinose) With a white or yellow, floury or starchy texture.
Whorl Circular arrangement of 3 or more flowers, parts of a flower, leaves, or shoots, arising from a single point.
Wildflower garden Informal garden used to grow mainly indigenous plants.
Wild garden Informal area intended to resemble a natural habitat, such as a woodland or alpine meadow. *See also* Woodland garden.
Wing 1. Thin, flat or membranous extension of an organ. 2. Lateral petal in many orchids and members of the Leguminosae family. *See also* Pea-like.
Woodland garden Woodland in which non-indigenous trees and shrubs are grown with underplantings of shade-loving herbaceous plants and bulbs, and often with artificially created open glades.
Woody Describes the fibrous stems of certain perennials, such as trees and shrubs, that persist above ground throughout the year.
Woody-based perennial Perennial with a woody base but herbaceous stems.
Xerophytic Describes a plant adapted to survive in arid conditions, either by the reduction of stems and leaves to minimize water loss, or by having water-storage tissue, as in cacti and other succulents.

ACKNOWLEDGMENTS

Dorling Kindersley would like to thank the following:

Additional editorial assistance
Louise Abbott, Jane Aspden, Cathy Buchanan, Rebecca Davies, Claire Folkard, Robert Graham, Lindsay Harber, Lesley Malkin, Andrew Mikolajski, Gillian Emerson Roberts, Ray Rogers, Lyn Saville, Sue Spielberg.

Additional design assistance
Stephen Josland, Geoff Manders, Alistair Wardle.

Additional administrative assistance
Esther Beaton, David Bruce, Caroline Fanshawe, Melissa Gould, Angela-Marie Graham, Ros Searle, Meryl Silbert, Roma Sinclair.

Additional consultants
Darrell Apps, Nicola Brown, Tony Clements, Philip Eden, Martin F. Gardner, Mark Griffiths, Andrew Halstead, A.P. Hamilton, Ronald Hedge, P. Francis Hunt, Frances Hutchison, Sally Kington, Alan Leslie, Suzanne Maxwell, Susanne Mitchell, Diana Percy, James E. Richardson, Dr Johan van Scheepen, Nicola J. Sinclair, Philip Thomas, Peter Valder.

Additional photographers
Peter Anderson, Bill Balham, Paul Barker, Peter Chadwick, Roger Foley, Paul Goff, Steve Gorton, David Harding, Dr Alan Hemsley, Julian Holland, Neil Holmes, David Karonides, Jonathan Metcalf, Les Saucier, Roger Scruton, Steven Still, Darryl Sweetland, Alex Watson.

Colour correction
Pelican Graphics, London EC2.

Dorling Kindersley would also like to thank the following private individuals and staff at the locations and organisations listed below for their help with the photography for this encyclopedia. Unless otherwise stated, all are located in the UK.

Ingrid Adler, Canberra, A.C.T., Australia; African Violet Centre, Terrington St. Clement, Norfolk; Albert's Garden, Pialligo, A.C.T., Australia; I. Allen, Wraxall, Bristol, Avon; The Alpine Garden Society Centre, Pershore, Hereford & Worcs; Jacques Amand Ltd., Stanmore, Middx; Anglo Aquarium Plants, Enfield, Middx; Apple Court, Lymington, Hants; Arcadia Lily Ponds, Arcadia, N.S.W., Australia; Architectural Plants, Horsham, W. Sussex; David Austin Roses Ltd., Wolverhampton, W. Midlands; Australian National Botanic Gardens, Canberra, A.C.T., Australia; Aylett Nurseries Ltd., St. Albans, Herts; Steven Bailey Ltd., Lymington, Hants; Bill Baker, Tidmarsh, Reading, Berks; Bankstown Native Gardens, Picnic Point, N.S.W., Australia; Batsford Arboretum, Moreton-in-Marsh, Glos; Les & Nancy Beard, Warriewood, N.S.W., Australia; Bedgebury Pinetum, Bedgebury, Kent; Birch Farm Nursery, Gravetye, W. Sussex; Birmingham Botanic Gardens, Birmingham, W. Midlands; Joy Bishop, Lightwater, Surrey; Blackthorn Nurseries, (Sue & Robin White), Alresford, Hants; Bloomsbury Nursery and Garden, (Susan & Michael Oakley), Padworth Common, Reading, Berks; Bourne Brook Nurseries, (B. & H.M. Baker), Halstead, Essex; Rupert Bowlby, Reigate, Surrey; Bressingham Gardens, Diss, Norfolk; Bridgemere Nurseries, Nantwich, Cheshire; Brighton Town Council, Brighton, E. Sussex; British Gladiolus Society; British Orchid Growers' Association; Broadleigh Gardens, Taunton, Somerset; Brockings Exotics, North Petherwin, Cornwall; Bromeliad Society of N.S.W., (Bob Christoffel, Alice Williams), Australia; Brooklyn Botanic Garden, New York, USA; Mrs. Ruth Buckley, Clunton, Shropshire; Burncoose Nursery, Gwennap, Cornwall; Burnham Nurseries, Newton Abbott, Devon; Bushyfield Nursery, Herne, Kent; Buskers End, Bowral, N.S.W., Australia; Calwell Garden Connection, Calwell, A.C.T., Australia; Cambridge Alpines, Cottenham, Cambs; Cambridge Bulbs, Newton, Cambs; Cambridge Garden Plants, Horningsea, Cambs; Carnon Downs Garden Centre, Truro, Cornwall; Coby Causer, Sydney, N.S.W., Australia; Colin Chapman, Wyverstone, Suffolk; Beth Chatto Gardens, Elmstead Market, Colchester, Essex; Claylane Nursery, South Nutfield, Redhill, Surrey; Cloudhill Nursery, Olinda, VIC, Australia; Colegrave Seeds, Hallam, VIC, Australia; Colegraves Seeds Ltd., Banbury, Oxon; Colonial Cottage Nursery, Dural, N.S.W., Australia; Conifer Gardens Nursery, Ferny Creek, VIC, Australia; Coolwyn Conifers, Monbulk, VIC, Australia; Cottage Garden Roses, (John Scarman), Stretton, Staffs; Dr & Mrs. A.J. Cox, Marcliff, Warks; C.S.I.R.O. Forestry, (Nathan Caesar, David Spencer), Yarralumla, A.C.T., Australia; Derby City Council Leisure Services, Derby; Dibley's Nurseries, Llanelidan, Ruthin, Clwyd; Diggers Seeds, Dromana, VIC, Australia; Dingle Plants & Gardens, Pilsgate, Stamford, Lincs; Drummond Castle, Crieff, Perthshire; Drysdale Nursery, Fordingbridge, Hants; Drywood Nursery, (Ian Kirby), Holton, Northants; Duchy College, Camborne, Cornwall; Mr. & Mrs. E.W. Dyer, Welford-on-Avon, Warks; Eastgrove Cottage Garden Nursery, (Carol & Malcolm Skinner), Sankyns Green, Hereford & Worcs; E.C.C. International, St. Austell, Cornwall; Alan Edwards, Dorking, Surrey; Mrs. Sally Edwards, Horningsea, Cambs; Exbury Gardens, (Nicholas de Rothschild), Exbury, Hants; Fairchild Tropical Garden, (Mary E. Collins), Miami, Florida, USA; A.T. Farmer, Hanslope, Bucks; Fibrex Nurseries, Pebworth, Stratford-on-Avon, Warks; Field House Nurseries, Gotham, Nottingham; Floranova Ltd., Foxley, Dereham, Norfolk; Fortescue Garden Trust, Buckland, Monachorum, Devon; Four Seasons, Forncett St. Mary, Norwich, Norfolk; Derek Fox, Hockley, Essex; Jeremy Francis, Olinda, VIC, Australia; Fulbrooke Nursery, Westley Waterless, Newmarket, Suffolk; The Garden, Mawson, A.C.T., Australia; *Gardening Which?*, Capel Manor, Enfield, Middx; Garden of St. Erth, Blackwood, VIC, Australia; Garden World, Keysborough, VIC, Australia; Douglas Gardiner, Wimbledon, London; Glasgow Botanic Garden, Glasgow; Glebe Cottage Nursery, (Carol Klein), Warleigh, Devon; David Glen, Ascot, VIC, Australia; Glenedd Violets, Sutton Bridge, Lincs; Goldbrook Plants, Hoxne, Suffolk; Goscote Nurseries, Cossington, Leics; Pam Gossage, Oakenlea, Yeoville, Somerset; Hadspen Gardens, (Norrie & Sandra Pope), Castle Cary, Somerset; Hall Farm Nursery, Kinnerley, Shropshire; Johan Harder, Arcadia, N.S.W., Australia; Hardy Exotics Nursery, Whitecross, Cornwall; Hardy's Cottage Garden Plants, Whitchurch, Hants; Harvey & Son, Little Shelford, Cambs; Martin Harwood, Chobham, Surrey; Hayward's Carnations, Waterlooville, Hants; The Hon. Mrs. Peter Healing, Kemerton, Hereford & Worcs; Hibiscus Park Nursery, Warriewood, N.S.W., Australia; Sir Harold Hillier Gardens & Arboretum, Ampfield, Romsey, Hants; Malcolm Hillier, London; Hilltop Cottage, Guildford, VIC, Australia; Hinton Nurseries, Christchurch, Dorset; Judith Hitchings, Swalcliffe, Oxon; Mr. & Mrs. D. Hodges, Alkerton, Oxon; Holkam Gardens, Holkam, Norfolk; Holly Gate Nurseries, Ashington, W. Sussex; Honeysome Aquatic Nursery, Sutton, Cambs; Hopleys Plants Ltd., Much Hadham, Herts; The Hon. & Mrs. Simon Howard, Castle Howard, N. Yorks; Howard & Kooij's Nurseries, Wortham, Diss, Norfolk; J. Huish, Wraxall, Bristol; V.H. Humphrey, (Pauline Brown), Dorking, Surrey; Annie Huntington, Sudborough, Northants; Huntington Botanical Gardens, San Marino, CA., USA; Essie Huxley, Longley, TAS, Australia; Ian Huxley, Guildford, VIC, Australia; Brenda Hyatt, Chatham, Kent; Idon Croft Herbs, Staplehurst, Kent; W.E.Th. Ingwersen Ltd., East Grinstead, W. Sussex; Susan Irvine, Gisborne, VIC, Australia; Russell & Sue Jenner, Gould Farm Nurseries, Cranbrook, Kent; Barbara Jennings, Sandy Bay, TAS, Australia; Sally Johannsohn, Neika, TAS, Australia; Mr. & Mrs. Roy Joseph, Welshpool, Powys; Karoo Botanic Gardens, Cape Town, South Africa; Mr. S. Keeble, Wickhambrook, Suffolk; Kelways Nurseries, Langport, Somerset; Lisse Keukenhof, Holland; Kiftsgate Court Gardens, (Mr. & Mrs. J. Chambers), Chipping Campden, Glos; Kirstenboch Gardens, Worcester, South Africa; Lakeland Horticultural Society, Windermere, Cumbria; Lambley Nursery, Ascot, VIC, Australia; Langthorns Plantery, Little Canfield, Dunmow, Essex; Wendy Lauderdale, Kilmington, Wiltshire; Ledora Water Gardens, (Mr. Kuring-Gai), N.S.W., Australia; Leonardslee Gardens, Lower Beeding, W. Sussex; Pam & Peter Lewis, Buckland Newton, Dorset; Littlebrook Fuschias, (Carol Gubler), Aldershot, Hants; Little Treasures Nursery, Horsedowns, Cornwall; London Aquatic Company, Enfield, Middx; Longacres Nursery & Florist, Bagshot, Surrey; Lower Kennegy Nursery, Germoe Crossroads, Cornwall; Rob Magnus, Woodbridge, TAS, Australia; Mansell & Hatcher Ltd., Rawdon, Leeds; Marwood Hill Gardens, Marwood, Devon; Colin Mason, Kenilworth, Warks; Mattocks Roses, Courtney, Oxford; Dr Ronald McKenzie, Shilton, Burford, Oxon; Moidart Wholesale Nursery, Burradoo, N.S.W., Australia; Moles Seeds, Colchester, Essex; Monksilver Nursery, Cottenham, Cambs; National Chrysanthemum Society, Tamworth, Staffs; National Herb Garden, (Janet Walker), Washington, D.C., USA; The National Trust, Powis Castle, Welshpool, Powys; The National Trust, Tintinhull House, Yeovil, Somerset; Ness Gardens, Neston, South Wirral, Cheshire; The New York Botanical Garden (Michael Ruggiero, Gregory Piotrowski, Mobee Weinstein), New York, USA; Nielsen Plants, Hellingly, E. Sussex; Norgate's Plant Farm, (Dennis Norgate), Trentham, VIC, Australia; Northern Horticultural Society, Harrogate, N. Yorks; The Nurseries, (Ian Roger), Pickering, N. Yorks; Odiham Waterlily Collection, Basingstoke, Hants; Margaret Farquhar Ogilvie, The House of Pitmuies, by Forfar, Tayside; Old Court Nurseries, (Mr. & Mrs. P. Picton), Colwall, Malvern, Hereford & Worcs; Mr. M. Oviatt-Ham, Willingham, Cambs; Mr. & Mrs. R. Paice, Bourton-on-the-Hill, Glos; Pan-American Seeds, Abington, Cambs; Paradise Centre, Lamarsh, Bures, Suffolk; Paradise Park, Hayle, Cornwall; Park Green Nurseries, (Richard Ford), Stowmarket, Suffolk; *Passiflora* National Collection, Clevedon, Avon; Wendy & Michael Perry, Truro, Cornwall; Perryhill Nurseries, (Peter Chapman), Hartfield, E. Sussex; Pine Lodge Gardens, Cuddra, Cornwall; Pirianda Garden, Olinda, VIC, Australia; Michael Pitkin, Arcadia, N.S.W., Australia; Roger Platts, Mavesfield, E. Sussex; Potash Nursery, (R.J. Blythe), Stowmarket, Suffolk; Suz Price, Daylesford, VIC, Australia; Probus Gardens, Probus, Cornwall; Mr. & Mrs. T. Ratcliff, Little Thakeham, Storrington, W. Sussex; Reads Nursery, Loddon, Norfolk; Rhodes & Rockliffe Nursery, Nazeing, Essex; Mr. & Mrs. E.J. Rice, Saxlingham, Norfolk; Rickards Hardy Ferns, Tenbury Wells, Hereford & Worcs; Noel Riley, Arcadia, N.S.W., Australia; Dr M. Rogers, Ramsden, Oxon; Romantic Cottage Garden, Dromana, VIC, Australia; Royal Botanic Garden, Edinburgh; Royal Botanic Gardens, (Sue Wells), Hobart, TAS, Australia; Royal Botanic Gardens, (Jenny Evans), Kew, Surrey; Royal Botanic Gardens, Melbourne, VIC, Australia; Royal Botanic Gardens, Peradeniya, Sri Lanka; Royal Botanic Gardens, Sydney, N.S.W., Australia; Royal Canberra Golf Club, Yarralumla, A.C.T., Australia; Royal Horticultural Society, Vincent Square, London; Royal Horticultural Society, Hyde Hall Garden, Chelmsford, Essex; Royal Horticultural Society, Rosemoor Garden, Great Torrington, Devon; Royal Horticultural Society's Gardens, Wisley, Surrey; Royal National Rose Society, St. Albans, Herts; The Savill Garden & Valley Gardens, (John Bond), Windsor Great Park, Berks; Lord Saye & Sele, Broughton Castle, Banbury, Oxon; R.A. Scamp, Falmouth, Cornwall; Scarletts Nursery, West Bergholt, Suffolk; Scotts Nurseries Ltd., Merriott, Somerset; Rob & Dawn Senior, Marazion, Cornwall; Peter Simmons, North Chailey, E. Sussex; Singapore Botanic Gardens, Singapore; Springfield Gardens, (Andrew Boynton), Spalding, Lincs; Ashley Stephenson, Sydney, N.S.W., Australia; Stonecrop Gardens, (Caroline Burgess), Cold Spring, New York, USA; Stonehurst Nursery, Ardingly, W. Sussex; Stony Range Flora Reserve, Dee Why, N.S.W., Australia; Strybing Arboretum & Botanical Gardens, San Francisco, CA., USA; Sudeley Castle Gardens, (Lady Ashcombe), Winchcombe, Glos; Suttons Seeds Ltd., Torquay, Devon; Mr. & Mrs. R.J. Taylor, Dolton, Devon; Sue Templeton, Albury, N.S.W., Australia; Andrew Thompson, Cheltenham, VIC, Australia; David Trehane, Probus, Truro, Cornwall; Trehane Camellia Nursery, Wimborne, Dorset; Trewhella House, Daylesford, VIC, Australia; Trinidad Botanic Gardens, Trinidad; Tropical Botanic Gardens & Research Institute, Palode, Kerala, India; University Botanic Garden, Cambridge; University Botanic Gardens, Oxford; University of California Arboretum, Santa Cruz, CA., USA; University Parks, Oxford; University of Reading Botanic Garden, Reading, Berks; Unlimited Perennials, Albury, N.S.W., Australia; Unwins Seeds Ltd., Histon, Cambs; Rosemary Verey, Barnsley, Glos; Viburnum Gardens, Arcadia, N.S.W., Australia; Wakehurst Place, (Royal Botanic Gardens, Kew), Ardingly, W. Sussex; Walnut Tree Gardens, (Mrs. M. Oldaker), Little Chart, Kent; Graham Warwick, Burradoo, N.S.W., Australia; Peter Waster, Invergowrie, Perthshire; Waterperry Gardens, Wheatley, Oxon; Theresa Watts, Canberra, A.C.T., Australia; Mr. A. West, Hailey, Oxon; Westonbirt Arboretum (Hugh Angus), Westonbirt, Glos; Whitehouse Ivies, Fardham, Colchester, Essex; Garry Wood, Baxter, VIC, Australia; Ray Wood, Castle Howard, N. Yorks; Woodbank Nursery, (Ken & Lesley Gillanders), Longley, TAS, Australia; Wylde Court Rainforest, Newbury, Berks; Arthur Yates & Co., Milperra, N.S.W., Australia.

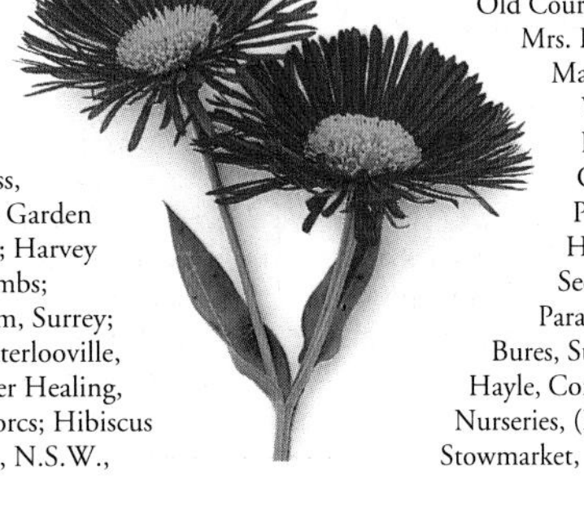

PHOTOGRAPHY CREDITS

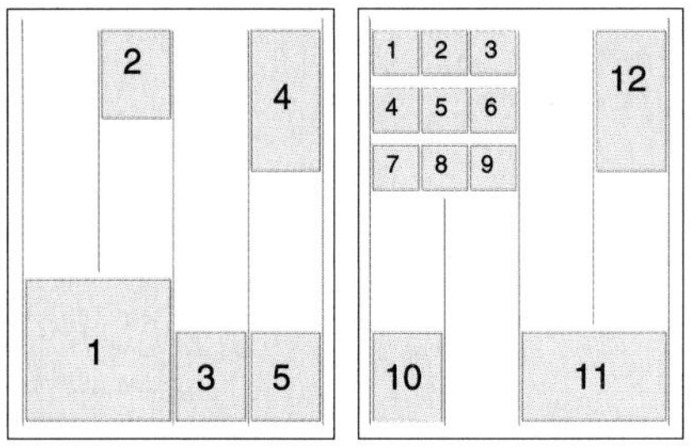

How to use the photography grid (above)
Photographs are numbered from top to bottom within each column of text, then left to right across the page. In the feature panels, photographs are numbered from left to right across each row, working from the top row to the bottom row (see panel on right-hand page above).

With the exception of those listed below, all photographs in the encyclopedia were taken by the photographers listed on p.6. Dorling Kindersley is grateful to the following agencies and photographers for their kind permission to reproduce images in the encyclopedia. To locate the photographs credited below, use the reference numbers given. The first in each pair of numbers is the page number on which the photograph appears; the second is its position number, determined by the order of photographs on each page (see left).

The Alpine Garden Society
533/10 • 569/1 • 721/1

Gillian Beckett
104/6 • 256/2 • 348/3 • 381/1 • 399/1 • 489/1 517/3 • 543/3 • 968/2

Biofotos
10/5 • 18/1 • 40/3 • 56/1 • 61/1 • 73/5 • 109/2 296/2 • 535/4 • 686/3 • 919/1

Christopher Brickell
87/2 • 174/6 • 175/3 • 220/4 • 259/2 • 299/2 355/1 • 362/3 • 384/1 • 931/3 • 970/4

Pat Brindley
359/4 • 436/4 • 618/1

Eric Catterall
168/7

Bruce Coleman Limited
18/2

Jack Elliott
142/1 • 281/5 • 415/4 • 460/6 • 560/9 • 672/1 735/2 • 1053/3

Nigel Farr
266/7

John Fielding
103/4 • 156/7 • 352/7

Fleurmerc B.V.
83/3 • 296/1 • 547/1 • 586/3 • 646/9 • 676/4

John Galbally
359/8 • 359/9 • 360/1 • 360/14 • 361/5

Garden Matters
560/5

Garden Picture Library
35/2 • 40/2 • 42/2 • 43/1 • 46/2 • 48/2 • 51/3 52/2 • 92/1 • 138/2 • 196/3 • 220/6 • 293/4 343/1 • 433/2 • 464/1 • 617/2 • 663/3 • 678/3 710/3 • 767/5 • 830/9 • 972/4 • 978/4 • 981/1

John Glover
44/2 • 127/1 • 307/2 • 322/2 • 556/1

Derek Gould
172/3 • 313/2 • 371/2 • 376/1 • 378/1 • 507/2 556/2 • 567/1 • 569/2 • 571/4 • 583/7 • 663/2 924/3 • 999/7 • 1065/2

Peter Harkness
890/1 • 890/5 • 890/13 • 893/10 • 896/3 • 897/8 900/5 • 902/6 • 903/3 • 903/4 • 903/5 • 903/6 905/9 • 907/4 • 907/12 • 908/6 • 908/11 • 909/11 911/13 • 913/1

Jerry Harpur
36/2 • 38/1 (designer: Beth Chatto) • 43/2 • 54/6

Derek Hewlett
339/7 • 339/11 • 341/13 • 342/2 • 342/12

Neil Holmes
648/5

Clive Innes
58/6 • 188/3 • 188/4 • 273/4 • 383/2 • 387/1 391/1 • 427/2 • 428/1 • 485/3 • 492/2 • 527/2 536/2 • 536/3 • 536/4 • 591/3 • 708/5 • 714/1 714/2 • 752/1 • 850/2 • 980/4 • 1015/2

International Flower Bulb Centre
471/9 • 472/4 • 473/4

Andrew Lawson
44/3 • 124/1 • 128/4 • 192/3 • 224/1 • 243/5 255/2 • 273/1 • 274/1 • 386/1 • 413/2 • 417/2 616/8 • 621/2 • 744/3 • 745/1 • 864/2 • 883/1 1067/2

Brian Mathew
121/2

Peter Maynard
558/2 • 562/4 • 562/8

Clive Nichols
34/2 • 53/1 (designer: Roger Platts) • 54/7 • 224/3 349/2

Vincent Page
896/8 • 904/12 • 907/1 • 913/3

Photos Horticultural
75/3 • 76/3 • 78/1 • 83/1 • 86/3 • 106/2 • 107/3 139/4 • 140/1 • 141/7 • 213/2 • 230/3 • 272/2 288/2 • 292/5 • 293/2 • 297/2 • 336/1 • 361/10 368/3 • 375/1 • 384/2 • 386/2 • 390/1 • 398/1 411/1 • 420/2 • 432/2 • 436/2 • 438/2 • 440/3 495/6 • 496/3 • 516/8 • 520/1 • 524/1 • 527/1 535/1 • 535/3 • 551/2 • 552/3 • 553/4 • 555/2 562/18 • 564/6 • 574/1 • 579/5 • 605/2 • 645/8 661/2 • 664/1 • 670/3 • 681/1 • 686/1 • 772/3 856/4 • 871/6 • 925/1 • 930/3 • 936/2 • 939/2 1000/1 • 1003/4 • 1004/1 • 1005/1 • 1011/3 1011/12 • 1017/4 • 1027/2 • 1062/1

Planet Earth Pictures
47/2 • 50/2

Plant Portraits Worldwide
61/5 • 73/1 • 74/3 • 77/2 • 91/2 • 102/2 • 109/1 113/4 • 118/1 • 121/1 • 138/1 • 138/3 • 138/4 157/3 • 158/2 • 161/3 • 176/1 • 190/1 • 193/1 206/3 • 222/3 • 259/4 • 268/3 • 273/2 • 288/3 311/2 • 319/2 • 325/1 • 348/1 • 350/1 • 350/2 368/4 • 376/2 • 377/1 • 379/3 • 382/2 • 420/7 461/1 • 474/10 • 485/4 • 506/4 • 524/3 • 541/2 542/2 • 609/1 • 639/2 • 649/3 • 685/4 • 697/2 704/6 • 731/2 • 747/2 • 750/1 • 751/1 • 791/2 805/3 • 815/3 • 1054/5

Martin Rickard
817/4

Sakata Seeds
432/1

Christine Skelmersdale
317/12 • 887/3 • 982/2

Harry Smith Collection
63/1 • 72/6 • 73/2 • 77/4 • 122/3 • 124/4 • 125/4 128/2 • 134/4 • 137/2 • 161/1 • 178/4 • 183/2 187/3 • 191/3 • 203/4 • 204/4 • 227/4 • 243/1 283/2 • 288/1 • 343/11 • 366/6 • 371/4 • 373/1 375/2 • 408/9 • 413/3 • 436/3 • 463/11 • 464/2 468/5 • 474/11 • 507/4 • 521/4 • 560/17 • 573/3 598/1 • 616/4 • 616/19 • 627/4 • 663/4 • 701/2 742/14 • 742/17 • 768/2 • 778/1 • 893/3 • 929/4 936/3 • 957/1 • 961/2 • 965/3 • 999/3 • 1031/12 1055/6 • 1071/2

Van Staaveren Aalsmeer B.V.
446/1 • 446/2

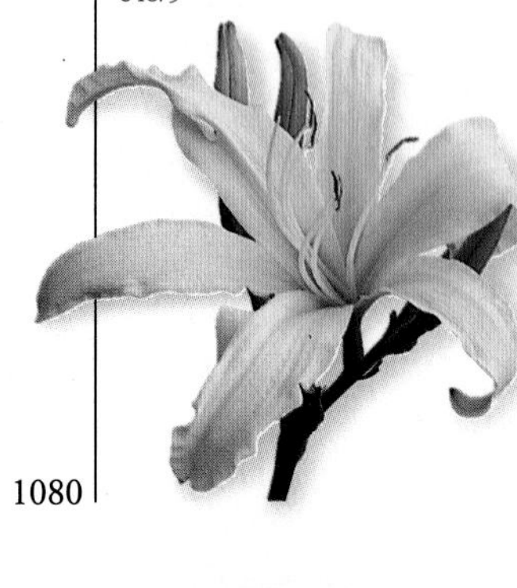

GENERAL INDEX

This index provides quick access to the general horticultural topics featured in the main introduction to the encyclopedia (pp.10–54). Plant names are not listed here, as these are presented in alphabetical sequence throughout the plant directory, together with cross-references to all synonyms and common names.

Visual glossary: Pruning groups

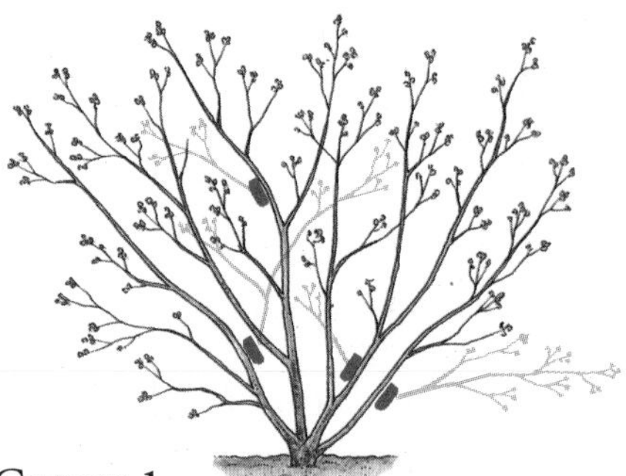

Group 1

Action In late winter or early spring, when dormant, remove misplaced or crossing shoots to maintain permanent, healthy framework.

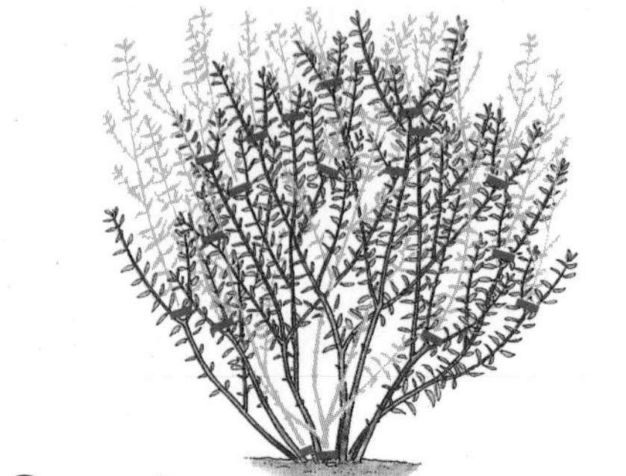

Group 2

Action After flowering, cut back flowered shoots to strong buds or young lower growth; on mature plants, also cut back a quarter to a fifth of old shoots to base.

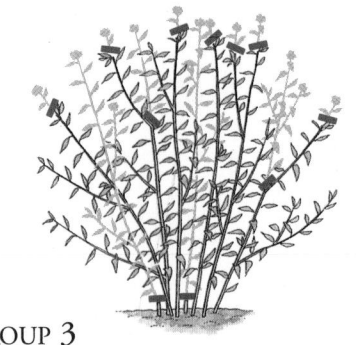

Group 3

Action After flowering, cut back flowered shoots to young sideshoots or to strong buds low down on branch framework.

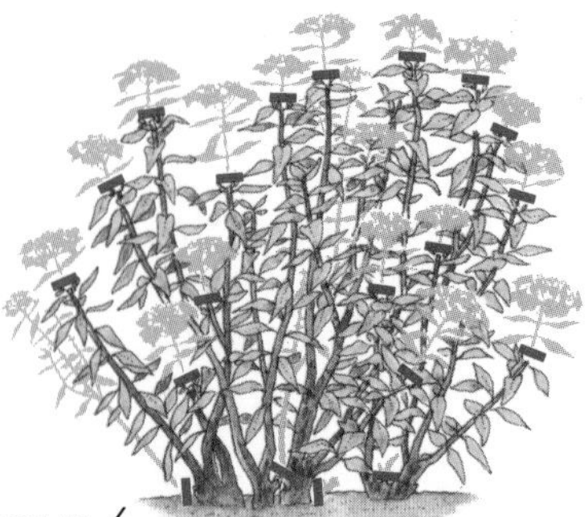

Group 4

Action Cut back to first bud or pair of buds below each flowerhead. Once established, cut back a third to a quarter of old shoots to base in early or mid-spring.

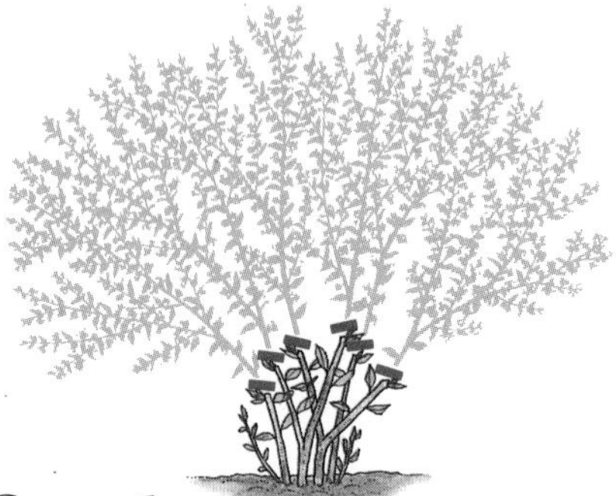

Group 5

Action After flowering, cut back all stems to strong buds, or to developing shoots close to base.

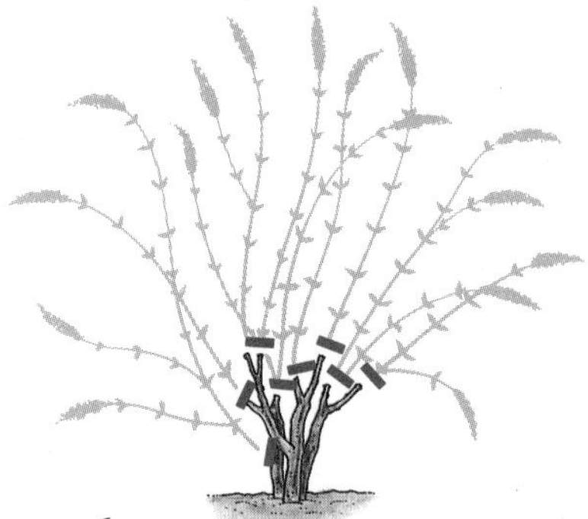

Group 6

Action In early spring, cut back to permanent framework or, for subshrubs and for drastic renovation, cut back flowered stems close to base.

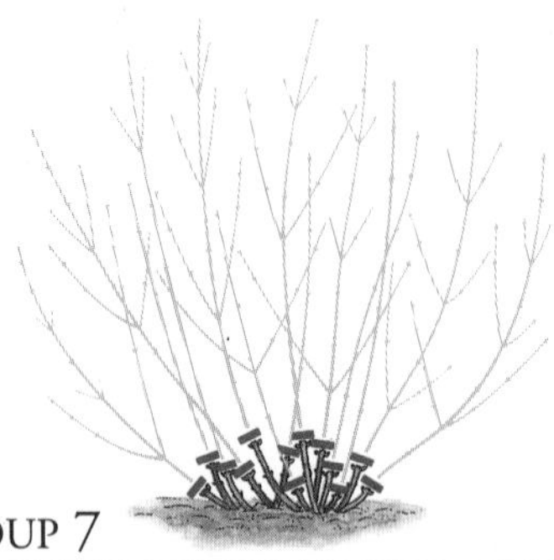

Group 7

Action In early spring, cut back stems to within 2 or 3 buds of base (suckering species close to base), or to permanent framework.

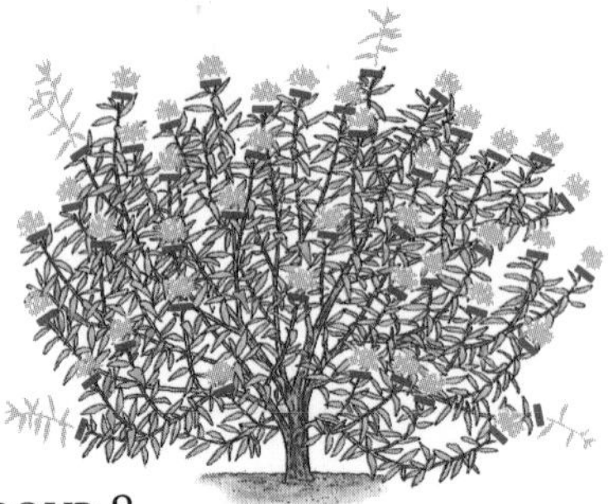

Group 8

Action After flowering, lightly trim or prune back shoots that spoil symmetry. Dead-head regularly if practical (unless fruit required).

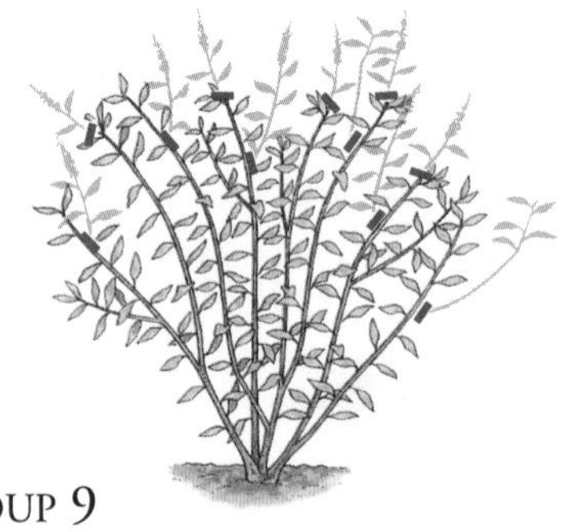

Group 9

Action In mid- or late spring, lightly trim or prune back shoots that spoil symmetry. Dead-head regularly if practical (unless fruit required).

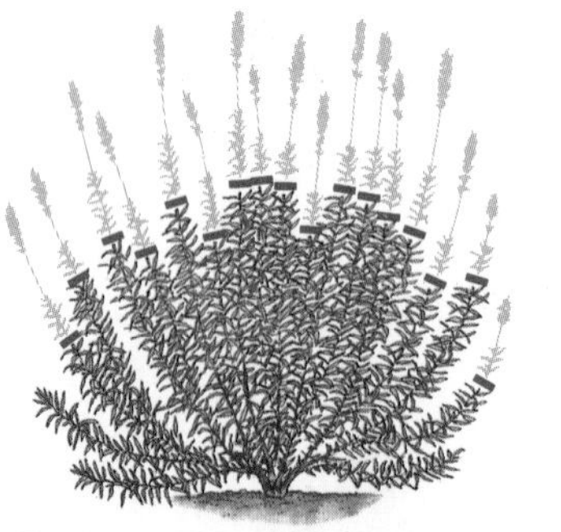

Group 10

Action After flowering, or in early or mid-spring, cut back flowered shoots to within 2.5cm (1in) of old growth.

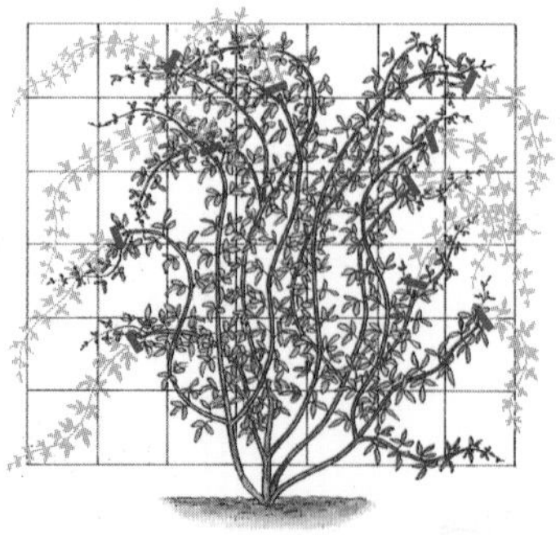

Group 11

Action After flowering, or in late winter or early spring, trim to fit available space; carry out renovation pruning as needed.

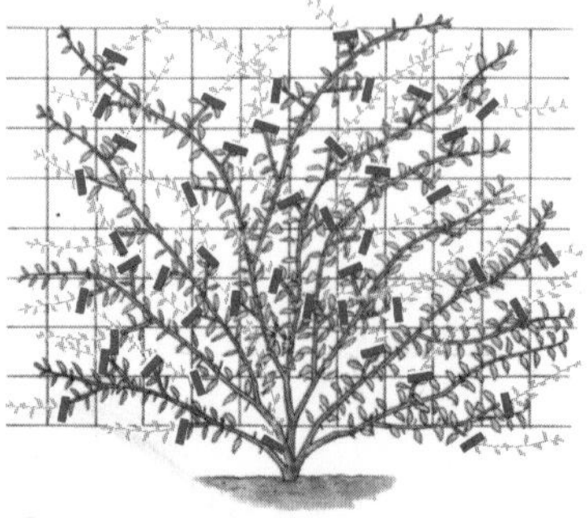

Group 12

Action After flowering, or in late winter or early spring, "spur prune" sideshoots to within 3 or 4 buds of permanent framework.

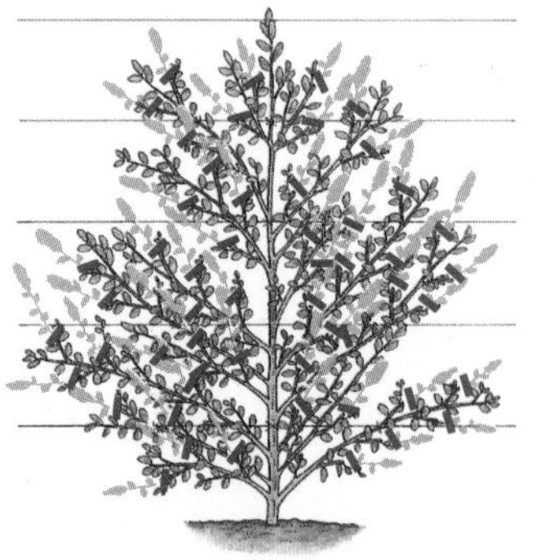

Group 13

Action After flowering, or in late winter or early spring, cut back flowered shoots to within 2–4 buds of permanent framework.